Maxcy-Rosenau-Last

PUBLIC HEALTH & PREVENTIVE MEDICINE

Maxcy-Rosenau-Last

PUBLIC HEALTH & PREVENTIVE MEDICINE

Sixteenth edition

Editor

MATTHEW L. BOULTON, MD, MPH

Senior Associate Dean
Pearl L. Kendrick Collegiate Professor of Global Health
Professor of Epidemiology and Preventive Medicine
University of Michigan School of Public Health
Ann Arbor, Michigan

Associate Editor

Robert B. Wallace, MD, MSc

Irene Ensminger Stecher Emeritus Professor of Epidemiology and Internal Medicine
University of Iowa College of Public Health
Iowa City, Iowa

Section Editors

Jared Baeten, MD, PhD • Grant Baldwin, PhD, MPH • Ana V. Diez Roux, MD, PhD, MPH • Sandro Galea, MD, DrPH, MPH • Karen Glanz, PhD, MPH • Paul Halverson, DrPH, MHSA • Timothy Jones, MD • Ruth Lynfield, MD • James Mercy, PhD • Maria C. Mora Pinzon, MD, MS • Ana Navas-Acien, MD, PhD, MPH • Karen Peterson, DSc • Patrick Remington, MD, MPH • Jonathan Samet, MD, MS • Judith Wasserheit, MD, MPH

Editorial Administration

Jillian B. Morgan, MPH

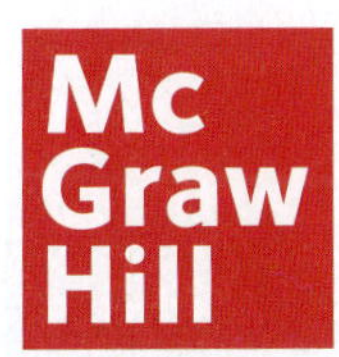

New York / Chicago / San Francisco / Athens / London / Madrid / Mexico City / New Delhi / Milan / Singapore / Sydney / Toronto

Maxcy-Rosenau-Last Public Health & Preventive Medicine, 16th Edition

1 2 3 4 5 6 7 8 9 LWI 26 25 24 23 22 21

ISBN 978-1-259-64451-1
MHID 1-259-64451-0

This book was set in Minion Pro by MPS Limited.
The editors were Susan Oldenburg, Michael Weitz, and Kim J. Davis.
The production supervisor was Richard Ruzycka.
Project management was provided by Jyoti Shaw, MPS Limited.
The designer was Mary McKeon.
The cover designer was W2 Design.

This book is printed on acid-free paper.

Library of Congress Cataloging-in-Publication Data

Names: Boulton, Matthew L., 1957- editor. | Wallace, Robert B., 1942- editor.
Title: Maxcy-Rosenau-Last public health & preventive medicine / editors, Matthew L. Boulton, Robert B. Wallace.
Other titles: Wallace/Maxcy-Rosenau-Last public health & preventive medicine | Maxcy-Rosenau-Last public health and preventive medicine
Description: Sixteenth edition. | New York: McGraw Hill, [2021] | Includes bibliographical references and index. | Summary: "The leading post-graduate reference-text spanning the fields of public health and preventive medicine"—Provided by publisher.
Identifiers: LCCN 2021008662 (print) | LCCN 2021008663 (ebook) | ISBN 9781259644511 (hardcover) (alk. paper) | ISBN 9781259644528 (ebook)
Subjects: MESH: Public Health | Preventive Medicine
Classification: LCC RA425 (print) | LCC RA425 (ebook) | NLM WA 100 | DDC 362.1—dc23
LC record available at https://lccn.loc.gov/2021008662
LC ebook record available at https://lccn.loc.gov/2021008663

To my parents,
The late Kenneth and Barbara Boulton

To my four remarkable children,
Kathryn, Sarah, Ravinath, and Nikhil

And to my wife, Chitra,
Whose steady counsel and loving support made my involvement in this project possible

Contents

Contributors

Francis Aboagye-Nyame
Pharmaceuticals & Health Technologies (PHT) Group
Management Sciences for Health
Arlington, Virginia
21. Global Health Systems: What Will It Take to Deliver on the Promise of Health for All?

Amit Acharya, BDS, MS, PhD
Advocate Aurora Health
Downers Grove, Illinois
60. Oral Health

Anna M. Acosta, MD
Division of Bacterial Diseases
National Center for Immunization and Respiratory Diseases
Centers for Disease Control and Prevention
Atlanta, Georgia
95. Diphtheria
97. Pertussis

Maria Acosta, MPH
College of Health & Social Sciences
Department of Health Education
San Francisco State University
San Francisco, California
185. Food and Physical Activity Environments: Influences on Diet and Physical Activity

Kesetebirhan Admasu, MD, MPH
RBM Partnership to End Malaria
Geneva, Switzerland
19. Evaluating Progress in Global Health: Global Health Measures That Build Capacity

Yazan A. Al-Ajlouni
New York University (NYU) School of Medicine
Department of Population Health
NYU Spatial Epidemiology Lab
New York, New York
31. Connecting Neighborhoods and Health: Methodological Approaches and Substantive Evidence

Sandra S. Albrecht, PhD, MPH
Department of Epidemiology
Columbia University Mailman School of Public Health
New York, New York
30. Race and Ethnic Health Disparities

Bereket Alemayehu, MD, MS, MSc
ICAP at Columbia University
Mailman School of Public Health
Columbia University
New York, New York
21. Global Health Systems: What Will It Take to Deliver on the Promise of Health for All?

Ibne K. Ali, PhD
Biologist
Waterborne Disease Prevention Branch
Division of Foodborne, Waterborne, and Environmental Diseases
National Center for Emerging and Zoonotic Infectious Diseases
Centers for Disease Control and Prevention
Atlanta, Georgia
117. Amebiasis
118. Amebic Meningoencephalitis

Mohsin Ali
Waterborne Disease Prevention Branch
Division of Foodborne, Waterborne, and Environmental Diseases
National Center for Emerging and Zoonotic Infectious Diseases
Centers for Disease Control and Prevention
Atlanta, Georgia
116. Giardiasis

Abdulsalam Alsulami, MD
University of Alabama at Birmingham
Birmingham, Alabama
123. Herpes Simplex Virus

Ala Alwan, MD, FRCP, FFPH
Professor of Practice of Global Health
London School of Hygiene and Tropical Medicine
Clinical Professor, Global Health, University of Washington
Director Emeritus
World Health Organization Eastern Mediterranean Region
Seattle, Washington
24. Addressing the Growing Burden of Chronic Noncommunicable Diseases

Sarah Amin, PhD, MPH
Assistant Professor and Director of Community Nutrition Education (SNAP-Ed & EFNEP)
Department of Nutrition and Food Sciences
University of Rhode Island
Kingston, Rhode Island
184. Strategies to Address Physical Activity in Schools

Olivia S. Anderson, PhD, RD
Clinical Assistant Professor
Department of Nutritional Sciences
School of Public Health
University of Michigan
Ann Arbor, Michigan
180. The Principles of Nutritional Sciences: Nutrients, Nutrition Recommendations, and Dietary Guidelines

Ting Fang Ang, MD, MPH
Department of Epidemiology
Boston University School of Public Health
Boston, Massachusetts
The Framingham Heart Study
Framingham, Massachusetts
161. Neurocognitive Disorder and Cognitive Decline

Grace D. Appiah, MD, MS
CDR, U.S. Public Health Service
Medical Epidemiologist
Division of Global Migration and Quarantine
National Center for Emerging and Zoonotic Infectious Diseases
U.S. Centers for Disease Control and Prevention
Atlanta, Georgia
110. Diseases Spread by Food and Water
114. Shigellosis

Tomás J. Aragón, MD, DrPH
Director and State Public Health Officer
California Department of Public Health
Assistant Adjunct Professor
University of California, Berkeley School of Public Health
Berkeley, California
82. Epidemiology and Control of Infectious Diseases

Christopher R. Armstrong, MD, MPH, MAEd, FACPM, FAsMA
Chief Medical Officer
U.S. Department of Labor, Office of Workers' Compensation Programs
Washington, DC
12. Aerospace Medicine

Katherine A. Artis, MD, MPH
Assistant Professor of Medicine
Oregon Health and Science University
VA Portland Health Care System
Portland, Oregon
56. Respiratory Diseases

Rhoda Au, PhD
The Framingham Heart Study
Framingham, Massachusetts
Department of Epidemiology
Boston University School of Public Health
Departments of Anatomy & Neurobiology and Neurology
Boston University School of Medicine
Boston, Massachusetts
161. Neurocognitive Disorder and Cognitive Decline

Rachael D. Aubert, PhD
Enteric Diseases Laboratory Branch
Division of Foodborne, Waterborne, and Environmental Diseases
National Center for Emerging and Zoonotic Infectious Diseases
Centers for Disease Control and Prevention
Atlanta, Georgia
110. Diseases Spread by Food and Water

Jared Baeten, MD, PhD
Professor of Global Health, Medicine, and Epidemiology
University of Washington
Seattle, Washington
Section Editor

Grant T. Baldwin, PhD, MPH
Director, Division of Overdose Prevention
National Center for Injury Prevention and Control
Centers for Disease Control and Prevention
Atlanta, Georgia
Section Editor

Casey P. Balio
Richard M. Fairbanks School of Public Health
Indiana University
Indianapolis, Indiana
48. Understanding Revenue and Delivery Models in the United States Healthcare System

Michael F. Ballesteros, PhD
Division of Analysis, Research and Practice Integration
National Center for Injury Prevention and Control
Centers for Disease Control & Prevention
Atlanta, Georgia
172. Fire and Burns

Solange Baptiste
International Treatment Preparedness Coalition
Gaborone, Botswana
21. Global Health Systems: What Will It Take to Deliver on the Promise of Health for All?

Barbara Baquero, PhD, MPH
Assistant Professor
Department of Community and Behavioral Health
University of Iowa College of Public Health
Iowa City, Iowa
42. Community Engaged Research

Natalie Bareis, PhD
Department of Psychiatry
Columbia University
New York, New York
163. Mood Disorders

Ruanne V. Barnbas, MD, DPhil
Associate Professor
Departments of Global Health, Allergy and Infectious Disease, and Pediatrics
University of Washington
Seattle, Washington
23. Control and Prevention of Infection Diseases of Global Significance

Christie M. Bartels, MD, MS
Assistant Professor
Division of Rheumatology
School of Medicine and Public Health
University of Wisconsin
Madison, Wisconsin
57. Musculoskeletal Disorders

Bradford Bartholow, PhD
Research and Evaluation Branch, Division of Violence Prevention
National Center for Injury Control and Prevention
Centers for Disease Control and Prevention
Atlanta, Georgia
177. Prevention of Youth Violence

Maneesh Batra, MD, MPH
Associate Professor, Departments of Pediatrics and Global Health
Associate Director, Pediatric Residency Program
Co-Director, UW Global WACh
University of Washington
Seattle, Washington
22. Reproductive Health and Child and Adolescent Health and Development

Amanda Beaudoin, DVM, PhD
Director of One Health Antibiotic Stewardship
Minnesota Department of Health
Saint Paul, Minnesota
153. Antibiotic Resistance and Stewardship

Angela J. Beck, PhD, MPH
Clinical Assistant Professor
Department of Health Behavior and Health Education
University of Michigan School of Public Health
Ann Arbor, Michigan
9. Public Health Practice in the United States

Leslie M. Beitsch, MD, JD
Chair, Dept. of Behavioral Sciences and Social Medicine
Center for Medicine and Public Health
Florida State University College of Medicine
Tallahassee, Florida
47. Health Policy Development

Mesfin A. Bekalu, PhD
Harvard T.H. Chan School of Public Health
The Dana-Farber-Cancer Institute
Dana-Farber Cancer Institute
Boston, Massachusetts
36. Health Communications

Beth P. Bell, MD, MPH
Clinical Professor
Department of Global Health
University of Washington School of Public Health
Seattle, Washington
26. Global Health Security and Response to Humanitarian Emergencies

Katharine M. Benedict, DVM, PhD
Waterborne Disease Prevention Branch
Division of Foodborne, Waterborne, and Environmental Diseases
National Center for Emerging and Zoonotic Infectious Diseases
Centers for Disease Control and Prevention
Atlanta, Georgia
116. Giardiasis

Rachel S. Bergmans, PhD
Department of Psychiatry
University of Michigan Medical School
Ann Arbor, Michigan
163. Mood Disorders

Micah L. Berman, JD
Associate Professor of Public Health and Law
The Ohio State University
Columbus, Ohio
13. Public Health Law

Naomi Beyeler, MPH, MCP
Global Health Policy Analyst
Institute for Global Health Sciences
University of California, San Francisco
San Francisco, California
18. Global Health Financing: Mechanisms, Trends, and Opportunities

Ipchita Bharali, MS
Policy Associate, Center for Policy Impact in Global Health
Duke Global Health Institute
Duke University
Durham, North Carolina
18. Global Health Financing: Mechanisms, Trends, and Opportunities

Zulfiqar A. Bhutta, PhD, MBBS, FRCPCH, FAAP
Centre for Global Child Health
The Hospital for Sick Children
Toronto, Ontario, Canada
23. Control and Prevention of Infection Diseases of Global Significance

Carina G. M. Blackmore, DVM, PhD, Dipl, ACVPM
Director, Division of Disease Control and Health Protection
State Epidemiologist
Florida Department of Health
141. Dengue, Chikungunya, and Zika Virus

Amy E. Blain, MPH
Meningitis and Vaccine Preventable Diseases Branch
National Center for Immunization and Respiratory Diseases
Centers for Disease Control and Prevention
Atlanta, Georgia
96. Tetanus

Steven N. Blair, PED
Department of Exercise Science
Arnold School of Public Health
University of South Carolina
Columbia, South Carolina
183. Physical Activity Epidemiology in Health and Disease

Drew Blakeman
Independent Consultant
New York
28. A Trained and Prepared Global Health Workforce Is Required to Achieve Impact

Jesse D. Blanton, DrPH
Epidemiologist
Division of Viral and Rickettsial Diseases
National Center for Zoonotic, Vectorborne, and Enteric Diseases
Centers for Disease Control and Prevention
Atlanta, Georgia
140. Viral Zoonoses—Rabies

Drew Blasco
School of Global Public Health
New York University
New York, New York
162. A Public Health Approach to Severe Mental Illness

Gail Bolan, MD
Director
Division of Sexually Transmitted Disease Prevention
Center for HIV, Hepatitis, STD and TB Prevention
Centers for Disease Control and Prevention
Atlanta, Georgia
120. Syphilis

Jessica L. Bonumwezi
Department of Psychology
Montclair State University
Montclair, New Jersey
165. Trauma- and Stressor-Related Disorders

Matthew L. Boulton, MD, MPH
Senior Associate Dean
Pearl L. Kendrick Collegiate Professor of Global Health
Professor of Epidemiology and Preventive Medicine
Professor of Health Management and Policy
University of Michigan School of Public Health
Professor of Internal Medicine
Infectious Diseases Division
Michigan Medicine
Ann Arbor, Michigan
92. Measles
106. Pneumococcal Infections

Richard S. Bradbury, PhD, FFSc RCPA, FASM, FACTM
Division of Parasitic Diseases and Malaria
Centers for Disease Control and Prevention
Atlanta, Georgia
124. Vector-borne Filariases
125. Hookworm Infection: Necatoriasis and Ancylostomiasis
126. Intestinal Nematode Infections
127. Tissue Nematodes

128. Schistosomiasis
129. Foodborne Trematode Infections
130. Taeniasis and Cysticercosis
131. Zoonotic Cestodes

Paula Braveman, MD, MPH
Professor of Family and Community Medicine
Founding Director, Center for Health Equity
University of California, San Francisco
San Francisco, California
29. The Social Determinants of Health

Simon J. Brooker, PhD, MSc
The Bill & Melinda Gates Foundation
Seattle, Washington
23. Control and Prevention of Infection Diseases of Global Significance

M. Alison Brooks, MD, MPH
Department of Medicine
Rheumatology Division
University of Wisconsin School of Medicine and Public Health
Madison, Wisconsin
57. Musculoskeletal Disorders

Andrew F. Brouwer, PhD, MS, MA
University of Michigan
Department of Epidemiology
Ann Arbor, Michigan
159. Introduction to Infectious Disease Modeling

Heidi E. Brown, PhD, MPH
Epidemiology and Biostatistics Department
Mel & Enid Zuckerman College of Public Health
University of Arizona
Tucson, Arizona
51. Cancer

Beau B. Bruce, MD, PhD
Enteric Diseases Epidemiology Branch
Division of Foodborne, Waterborne, and Environmental Diseases
National Center for Zoonotic and Emerging Infectious Diseases
Centers for Disease Control and Prevention
Atlanta, Georgia
111. Salmonella Infections (Nontyphoidal)

Elizabeth Bukusi, MBChB, MMed, MPH, PhD, PGD
Chief Research Officer, Kenya Medical Research Institute (KEMRI)
Research Professor, Departments of Obstetrics/Gynecology and Global Health
University of Washington
Seattle, Washington
Clinical Professor, University of California San Francisco
San Francisco, California
Honorary Lecturer, Aga Khan University
Nairobi, Kenya
22. Reproductive Health and Child and Adolescent Health and Development

Thomas A. Burke, PhD
Bloomberg School of Public Health
Johns Hopkins University
Baltimore, Maryland
78. Managing Environmental and Occupational Risks

Matthew J. Burton, MBBCh, PhD, MRCP, FRCOphth
London School of Hygiene and Tropical Medicine
London, United Kingdom
137. Trachoma

Elizabeth Cahoon, PhD
Division of Cancer Epidemiology and Genetics
Radiation Epidemiology Branch
National Cancer Institutes
Rockville, Maryland
68. Ionizing Radiation
69. Nonionizing Radiation

Stefanie Campbell, DVM, MS
Division of Vector-Borne Diseases
Centers for Disease Control and Prevention
Fort Collins, Colorado
143. Lyme Disease and Other Borrelia Infections

Paul Cantey, MD, MPH
Division of Parasitic Diseases and Malaria
Centers for Disease Control and Prevention
Atlanta, Georgia
124. Vector-borne Filariases

Jennifer Carns, PhD
Department of Bioengineering
Rice University
Houston, Texas
27. Emerging Technology Innovations in Global Health

Maribel Casas, PhD
ISGlobal
Barcelona, Catalonia, Spain
74. Early Life Environmental Exposures and Children's Health

Magdalena Cerdá, DrPH
Department of Population Health
New York University School of Medicine
New York, New York
165. Trauma- and Stressor-Related Disorders

Steven B. Cersovsky, MD, MPH, FACPM
Colonel (Retired), Medical Corps, U.S. Army
10. Military Preventive Medicine and Public Health

Basile Chaix, PhD
INSERM, Sorbonne Université
Institut Pierre Louis d'Epidémiologie et de Santé Publique IPLESP
Paris, France
31. Connecting Neighborhoods and Health: Methodological Approaches and Substantive Evidence

Kevin Chatham-Stephens, MD, MPH, FAAP
Centers for Disease Control and Prevention
National Center on Birth Defects and Developmental Disabilities
Division of Human Development and Disability
Atlanta, Georgia
110. Diseases Spread by Food and Water

William Checkley, MD, PhD
Division of Pulmonary and Critical Care
Johns Hopkins University School of Medicine
Baltimore, Maryland
71. Household Air Pollution in Low- and Middle-Income Countries

Cara Cherry, DVM
Centers for Disease Control and Prevention
Atlanta, Georgia
145. Q Fever

Peter Cherutich, MBChB, MPH, PhD
Ministry of Health
Nairobi, Kenya
20. Implementation Science: A New Research Paradigm to Accelerate Global Health Impact at Scale

Mary J. Choi, MD, MPH
Viral Special Pathogens Branch
Centers for Disease Control and Prevention
Atlanta, Georgia
139. Ebola and Other Viral Hemorrhagic Fevers

Stephen L. Cochi, MD, MPH
Senior Advisor
Global Immunization Division
Centers for Disease Control and Prevention
Atlanta, Georgia
98. Poliomyelitis

Pamela Collins, MD, MPH
Professor of Global Health
Professor of Psychiatry and Behavioral Science
University of Washington
Seattle, Washington
24. Addressing the Growing Burden of Chronic Noncommunicable Diseases

Lisa Conti, DVM, MPH
Deputy Commissioner and Chief Science Officer
Florida Department of Agriculture and Consumer Services
Tallahassee, Florida
84. One Health: A New Paradigm for Disease Prevention and Control

Jennifer R. Cope, MD, MPH
Medical Epidemiologist
Waterborne Disease Prevention Branch
Division of Foodborne, Waterborne, and Environmental Diseases
National Center for Emerging and Zoonotic Infectious Diseases
Centers for Disease Control and Prevention
Atlanta, Georgia
117. Amebiasis
118. Amebic Meningoencephalitis

Pierre-Olivier Cote, MPH
Centers for Disease Control and Prevention
National Center for Injury Prevention and Control
Atlanta, Georgia
174. Poisoning Prevention

Caitlin Cotter, DVM, MPH
Division of Vector-Borne Diseases
Centers for Disease Control and Prevention
Atlanta, Georgia
144. Rickettsial Infections

David B. Coultas, MD
Professor of Medicine
Oregon Health and Science University
Associate Chief of Staff-Education
VA Portland Health Care System
Portland, Oregon
56. Respiratory Diseases

Jean M. Cox-Ganser, PhD
National Institute for Occupational Safety and Health
Respiratory Health Division
Morgantown, West Virginia
76. Work-Related Asthma

Kathryn A. Crawford, MS, PhD
Environmental Studies Program
Middlebury College
Middlebury, Vermont
75. Environmental Endocrine-Disrupting Chemicals: Common Sources and Health Effects

Richard K. Crawford, MD
School of Medicine and Public Health
University of Wisconsin—Madison
Madison, Wisconsin
58. Diseases of the Nervous System

Amihan F. Crisostomo, MPH
College of Health & Social Sciences, Department of Health Education
San Francisco State University
San Francisco, California
185. Food and Physical Activity Environments: Influences on Diet and Physical Activity

Alex E. Crosby, MD, MPH
Division of Violence Prevention
National Center for Injury Prevention and Control
Centers for Disease Control and Prevention
Atlanta, Georgia
175. The Epidemiology and Prevention of Self-Directed Violence

Elizabeth Crouch, PhD
Rural and Minority Health Research Center
Arnold School of Public Health
University of South Carolina
Columbia, South Carolina
33. Rural America: Public Health Challenges and Opportunities

Pham Viet Cuong, PhD
Center for Injury Policy and Prevention Research
Hanoi University of Public Health
Hanoi, Viet Nam
25. Injury Prevention and Trauma Care: Global Perspectives

James W. Curran, MD, MPH
Dean, Rollins School of Public Health
Adjunct Professor
Emory University School of Medicine and Nell Hodgson Woodruff School of Nursing
Co-Director and Principal Investigator
Co-Director for Prevention Science
Atlanta, Georgia
87. The Epidemiology and Prevention of HIV and AIDS

Leila Cuttle, PhD, BSc
Queensland University of Technology
School of Biomedical Sciences
South Brisbane, Australia
172. Fire and Burns

Ashley Schappell D'Inverno, PhD
Division of Violence Prevention
National Center for Injury Prevention and Control
Centers for Disease Control and Prevention
Atlanta, Georgia
178. Intimate Partner Violence Prevention

James Damsere-Derry, PhD
Building and Roads Research Institute
Kumasi, Ghana
25. Injury Prevention and Trauma Care: Global Perspectives

Jason D. Daniel-Ulloa, PhD, MPH
Assistant Clinical Professor
Department of Community and Behavioral Health
University of Iowa College of Public Health
Iowa City, Iowa
42. Community Engaged Research

Andrew L. Dannenberg, MD, MPH
Affiliate Professor
Department of Environmental and Occupational Health Sciences
University of Washington School of Public Health
Seattle, Washington
44. Health Impact Assessment: A Tool for Promoting Healthier Communities

Michael Z. David, MD, PhD
Assistant Professor
Division of Infectious Diseases
Department of Medicine
University of Pennsylvania
Philadelphia, Pennsylvania
154. Staphylococcus aureus

Meghan F. Davis, DVM, MPH, PhD
Department of Environmental Health & Engineering
Bloomberg School of Public Health
Johns Hopkins University
Baltimore, Maryland
77. Infectious Diseases: Industrial Animal Operations

William Davis, DrPH
Centers for Disease Control and Prevention
Atlanta, Georgia
112. Cholera

Jesús de la Osa
Environment and Sustainability Agency
Zaragoza City Council
Zaragoza, Spain
67. Diseases Due to Physical Factors: Noise

Helen de Pinho, MBBCh, FCCH, MBA
Heilbrunn Department of Population and Family Health
Mailman School of Public Health
Columbia University
New York, New York
21. Global Health Systems: What Will It Take to Deliver on the Promise of Health for All?

Kevin M. De Cock, MD
CDC Kenya
Nairobi, Kenya
15. The History and Emergence of Global Health

Sarah DeGue, PhD
Senior Health Scientist
Division of Violence Prevention
Centers for Disease Control and Prevention
Atlanta, Georgia
179. Sexual Violence

Ann M. Dellinger, MPH, PhD
Division of Injury Prevention
National Center for Injury Prevention and Control
Centers for Disease Control and Prevention
Atlanta, Georgia
170. Road Safety and Injury Prevention

Cristine D. Delnevo, PhD, MPH, FAAHB
Professor
Director, Center for Tobacco Studies
Co-Leader of the Cancer Prevention and Control Program
Rutgers Cancer Institute of New Jersey
Department of Health Behavior, Society and Policy
Rutgers University School of Public Health
New Brunswick, New Jersey
166. Tobacco Use and Tobacco Use Disorder

Alfred DeMaria, Jr., MD
Bureau of Infectious Disease and Laboratory Sciences
Massachusetts Department of Public Health
Jamaica Plain, Massachusetts
158. Hepatitis C

Leslie K. Dennis, PhD, MS
Professor
Epidemiology and Biostatistics Department
Mel and Enid Zuckerman College of Public Health
University of Arizona
Tucson, Arizona
51. Cancer

Donna Denno, MD, MPH
Professor, Departments of Pediatrics and Global Health
University of Washington
Seattle, Washington
22. Reproductive Health and Child and Adolescent Health and Development

Kebede Deribe, MPH, PhD
Brighton and Sussex Centre for Global Health Research
Department of Global Health and Infection
Brighton and Sussex Medical School
University of Sussex, Brighton, United Kingdom
School of Public Health
College of Health Sciences
Addis Ababa University
Addis Ababa, Ethiopia
23. Control and Prevention of Infection Diseases of Global Significance

Julio Díaz, PhD
National School of Public Health
Carlos III Institute of Health
Madrid, Spain
67. Diseases Due to Physical Factors: Noise

Shane Diekman, PhD, MPH
Division of Global HIV & TB
Center for Global Health
Centers for Disease Control & Prevention
Atlanta, Georgia
172. Fire and Burns

Ana Diez Roux, MD, PhD, MPH
Dana and David Dornsife Dean and Distinguished University Professor of Epidemiology
Dornsife School of Public Health
Drexel University
Philadelphia, Pennsylvania
Section Editor

Jenny Dills, MPH
Division of Violence Prevention
National Center for Injury Prevention and Control
Centers for Disease Control and Prevention
Atlanta, Georgia
178. Intimate Partner Violence Prevention

Liming Dong, PhD
Department of Epidemiology
University of Michigan School of Public Health
Ann Arbor, Michigan
163. Mood Disorders

Ogobara K. Doumbo, MD, MsC, PhD
Faculty of Medicine
Department of Epidemiology of Parasitic Diseases
University of Bamako
Bamako, Mali
23. Control and Prevention of Infection Diseases of Global Significance

Alison Drake, MPH, PhD
Assistant Professor
Department of Global Health
University of Washington (UW)
Co-Director, Family Planning Decision-Support Scientific Priority Area
UW Center for Global Integrated Health of Women, Adolescents, and Children (Global WACh)
Seattle, Washington
22. Reproductive Health and Child and Adolescent Health and Development

Dimitri Drekonja, MD, MS
Chief, Infectious Disease Section
Minneapolis VA Health Care System
Associate Professor of Medicine
University of Minnesota
Minneapolis, Minnesota
157. Clostridioides difficile Infection

Christine DuBray, MD
Division of Parasitic Diseases and Malaria
Centers for Disease Control and Prevention
Atlanta, Georgia
124. Vector-borne Filariases

Dustin T. Duncan, ScD
New York University (NYU) School of Medicine
Department of Population Health
NYU Spatial Epidemiology Lab
New York, New York
31. Connecting Neighborhoods and Health: Methodological Approaches and Substantive Evidence

John R. Dunn, DVM, PhD
Tennessee Department of Health
Nashville, Tennessee
150. Leptospirosis

Alexis M. Eastman, MD
Department of Medicine
Division of Geriatrics
University of Wisconsin—Madison
Madison, Wisconsin
61. Health Promotion and Disability Prevention in Older Persons

David L. Eaton, PhD
University of Washington
Seattle, Washington
University of Arizona
Tucson, Arizona
64. Basic Toxicology and Mode of Action of Toxic Substances

William W. Eaton, PhD
Bloomberg School of Public Health
Department of Mental Health
Johns Hopkins University
Baltimore, Maryland
164. Anxiety Disorders

Jan M. Eberth, PhD
Rural and Minority Health Research Center
Arnold School of Public Health
University of South Carolina
Columbia, South Carolina
33. Rural America: Public Health Challenges and Opportunities

Marisa C. Eisenberg, PhD
Associate Professor of Epidemiology and Complex Systems
School of Public Health
University of Michigan, Ann Arbor
159. Introduction to Infectious Disease Modeling

Chris Elias, MD, MPH
Bill & Melinda Gates Foundation
Seattle, Washington
19. Evaluating Progress in Global Health: Global Health Measures That Build Capacity

Nikki Eller, MPH
Department of Global Health
University of Washington
Seattle, Washington
19. Evaluating Progress in Global Health: Global Health Measures That Build Capacity

Erin M. Ellis, PhD, MPH
Behavioral Research Program
National Cancer Institute
Bethesda, Maryland
38. Effective and Impactful Risk Communication

Wafaa M. El-Sadr
ICAP at Columbia University
Mailman School of Public Health
Columbia University
New York, New York
21. Global Health Systems: What Will It Take to Deliver on the Promise of Health for All?

W. Douglas Evans, PhD
Professor
Milken Institute School of Public Health
The George Washington University
Washington, DC
37. Social Marketing: Theory, Practice, and Research

Magdalena Fandiño-Del-Rio, MS
Division of Pulmonary and Critical Care
Johns Hopkins University School of Medicine
Department of Environmental Health & Engineering
Bloomberg School of Public Health
Johns Hopkins University
Baltimore, Maryland
71. Household Air Pollution in Low- and Middle-Income Countries

Mark D. Faries, PhD
Associate Professor and Extension Health Specialist
Texas A&M AgriLife Extension Service
Adjunct Associate Professor
Texas A&M School of Public Health
College Station, Texas
11. Lifestyle Medicine

Monica M. Farley, MD
Jonas A. Shulman Professor of Medicine/Infectious Diseases
Director, Division on Infectious Diseases
Emory University School of Medicine
Atlanta, Georgia
156. Streptococcus agalactiae (Group B Streptococcal) Disease

Kristen Fedak, MEM
Department of Environmental and Radiological Health Sciences
Colorado School of Public Health
Colorado State University
Fort Collins, Colorado
71. Household Air Pollution in Low- and Middle-Income Countries

Vincent L. Fenimore, PhD
School of Public Health
University of Nevada, Las Vegas
Las Vegas, Nevada
83. Principles of Disease Elimination and Eradication

Sara Fewer, MPP, MPH
Global Health Policy Analyst
Institute for Global Health Sciences
University of California, San Francisco
San Francisco, California
18. Global Health Financing: Mechanisms, Trends, and Opportunities

Mary-Margaret Fill, MD
Tennessee Department of Health
Nashville, Tennessee
150. Leptospirosis

Marc Fischer, MD, MPH
Arboviral Diseases Branch
Division of Vector-Borne Diseases
US Centers for Disease Control and Prevention
Fort Collins, Colorado
142. Diseases Transmitted Primarily by Arthropod Vectors: Viral Infections

W. Oscar Fleming, DrPH, MSPH
Clinical Assistant Professor, Department of Maternal and Child Health
Research Scientist, National Implementation Research Network
Frank Porter Graham Child Development Institute
University of North Carolina, Chapel Hill
Chapel Hill, North Carolina
49. Implementing Public Health Programs

Maria Foraster, PhD
ISGlobal
Barcelona, Catalonia, Spain
74. Early Life Environmental Exposures and Children's Health

Beverly L. Fortson, PhD
Senior Behavioral Scientist
Division of Violence Prevention
National Center for Injury Prevention and Control
Centers for Disease Control and Prevention
Atlanta, Georgia
176. Child Abuse and Neglect

Beth Frates, MD, FACLM, DipABLM
Clinical Assistant Professor
Harvard Medical School
Director of Wellness Programming
Stroke Institute for Research and Recovery
Spaulding Rehabilitation Hospital
Charlestown, Massachusetts
11. Lifestyle Medicine

Jeff French, PhD
CEO Strategic Social Marketing
Professor Brighton Business School
Brighton, United Kingdom
37. Social Marketing: Theory, Practice, and Research

Cindy R. Friedman, MD
Chief, Travelers' Health Branch
Division of Global Migration and Quarantine
National Center for Emerging Zoonotic and Infectious Diseases
Centers for Disease Control and Prevention
Atlanta, Georgia
119. Yersiniosis

Howard Frumkin, DrPH, MPH, MD
Head, Our Planet, Our Health Program
Wellcome Trust
Gibbs Building
London, United Kingdom
17. Global Environmental Changes Reshaping Health in the 21st Century

Katie Fullerton, MPH
Division of Foodborne, Waterborne, and Environmental Diseases
National Center for Emerging and Zoonotic Infectious Diseases
Centers for Disease Control and Prevention
Atlanta, Georgia
114. Shigellosis

Sandro Galea, MD, DrPH, MPH
Dean and Robert A. Knox Professor
School of Public Health
Boston University
Boston, Massachusetts
Section Editor

Deborah A. Galuska, PhD, MPH
Division of Nutrition, Physical Activity, and Obesity
Centers for Disease Control and Prevention
Atlanta, Georgia
181. Obesity Prevention and Control: A Public Health Perspective

Patricia J. Garcia, MD, MPH, PhD
Universidad Peruana Cayetano Heredia
Facultad de Salud Pública
Lima, Perú
19. Evaluating Progress in Global Health: Global Health Measures That Build Capacity

Renata Garcia, MD
Retina Department
Instituto Mexicano de Oftalmologia
Santiago De Queretaro
Queretaro, Mexixo
59. Visual Disorders

Robin L. García, MPH, RD
Nutrition Consultant
Department of Nutritional Sciences
School of Public Health
University of Michigan
Ann Arbor, Michigan
180. The Principles of Nutritional Sciences: Nutrients, Nutrition Recommendations, and Dietary Guidelines
185. Food and Physical Activity Environments: Influences on Diet and Physical Activity

Julia W. Gargano, PhD
Division of Viral Diseases
National Center for Immunization and Respiratory Diseases
Centers for Disease Control and Prevention
Atlanta, Georgia
100. Human Papillomavirus

Veronica Eva Helms Garrison, MPH
Office of Policy Development and Research
US Department of Housing and Urban Development
Washington, DC
32. Housing and Health

Paul A. Gilbert, PhD, ScM
Assistant Professor
Department of Community and Behavioral Health
University of Iowa College of Public Health
Iowa City, Iowa
42. Community Engaged Research

Julie Gilchrist, MD
Medical Epidemiologist
Division of Unintentional Injury Prevention
National Center for Injury Prevention and Control
Centers for Disease Control and Prevention
Atlanta, Georgia
173. The Epidemiology and Prevention of Drowning

Daniel Giovenco, PhD, MPH
Assistant Professor
Department of Sociomedical Sciences
Mailman School of Public Health
Columbia University
New York, New York
166. Tobacco Use and Tobacco Use Disorder

Karen Glanz, PhD, MPH
Perelman School of Medicine and School of Nursing
University of Pennsylvania
Philadelphia, Pennsylvania
35. Health Behavior Theories
Section Editor

Ingrid Glurich, PhD
Marshfield Clinic Research Institute
Marshfield, Wisconsin
60. Oral Health

William C. Goedel, BA
New York University (NYU) School of Medicine
Department of Population Health
NYU Spatial Epidemiology Lab
New York, New York
31. Connecting Neighborhoods and Health: Methodological Approaches and Substantive Evidence

Samantha Goldfarb, DrPH, MPH
Cross Appointment in Family & Child Sciences
Assistant Professor, College of Medicine
Florida State University
Tallahassee, Florida
47. Health Policy Development

Renee D. Goodwin, PhD, MPH
Department of Epidemiology and Biostatistics
Graduate School of Public Health and Health Policy
The City University of New York
Department of Epidemiology
Mailman School of Public Health
Columbia University
New York, New York
166. Tobacco Use and Tobacco Use Disorder

Stephen M. Graham, MB BS, FRACP, DTCH, PhD
University of Melbourne
Department of Paediatrics
Murdoch Children's Research Institute
Royal Children's Hospital
International Union Against Tuberculosis and Lung Disease
The Burnet Institute
Melbourne, Australia
23. Control and Prevention of Infection Diseases of Global Significance

James Graziano, MPH
Viral Special Pathogens Branch
Centers for Disease Control and Prevention
Atlanta, Georgia
139. Ebola and Other Viral Hemorrhagic Fevers

Patricia M. Griffin, MD
Enteric Diseases Epidemiology Branch
Division of Foodborne, Waterborne, and Environmental Diseases
Centers for Disease Control and Prevention
Atlanta, Georgia
113. Escherichia coli, Diarrheagenic

Oana R. Groene, PhD, MA
Project Manager Patient Activation and Health Competence
Gesundheir fur Billstedt/Horn UG [haftungsbeschrankt]
Hamburg, Germany
39. Health Literacy: An Update

Sarah Anne J. Guagliardo, PhD
Division of Parasitic Diseases and Malaria
Centers for Disease Control and Prevention
Atlanta, Georgia
129. Foodborne Trematode Infections

Danny Haddad, MD
Director, Global Vision Initiative
Assistant Professor of Opthalmology and Global Health
Emory University School of Medicine
Atlanta, Georgia
59. Visual Disorders

Tamara M. Haegerich, PhD
Centers for Disease Control and Prevention
National Center for Injury Prevention and Control
Atlanta, Georgia
174. Poisoning Prevention

Paul Halverson, DrPH, MHSA
Richard M. Fairbanks School of Public Health
Indiana University
Indianapolis, Indiana
Section Editor

Sarah A. Hamer, MS, PhD, DVM, DACVPM (Epidemiology)
Department of Veterinary Integrative Biosciences
Texas A&M University
College Station, Texas
132. Chagas Disease (American Trypanosomiasis)

Saima Hamid, PhD, MPH, MBBS
Health Services Academy
Islamabad, Pakistan
19. Evaluating Progress in Global Health: Global Health Measures That Build Capacity

Erin Hammer, MD
Departments of Family Medicine and Community Health and Orthopedics and Rehabilitation
Division of Sports Medicine
University of Wisconsin—Madison School of Medicine and Public Health
Madison, Wisconsin
57. Musculoskeletal Disorders

Sukwan Handali, MD
Division of Parasitic Diseases and Malaria
Centers for Disease Control and Prevention
Atlanta, Georgia
130. Taeniasis and Cysticercosis

Lori Kestenbaum Handy, MD, MSCE
Associate Medical Director, Infection Prevention & Control
Division of Infectious Diseases
Children's Hospital of Philadelphia
Philadelphia, Pennsylvania
90. Vaccine Innovation and Development

Eric Hanson, MD
Moran Eye Center
University of Utah Health
Salt Lake City, Utah
59. Visual Disorders

Luxme Hariharan, MD, MPH
Pediatric Ophthalmologist
Division of Pediatric Ophthalmology
Nicklaus Children's Hospital
Miami, Florida
59. Visual Disorders

Katherine Harripersaud
ICAP at Columbia University
Mailman School of Public Health
Columbia University
New York, New York
21. Global Health Systems: What Will It Take to Deliver on the Promise of Health for All?

Aaron M. Harris, MD, MPH, FACP
Team Lead, Prevention Branch
Division of Viral Hepatitis
National Center for HIV/AIDS, Viral Hepatitis, STD, and TB Prevention
Centers for Disease Control and Prevention
Atlanta, Georgia
101. Hepatitis B

Deborah S. Hasin, PhD
Columbia University
New York, New York
168. Marijuana Use in the U.S.: Trends, Consequences, Changing Laws

Barton F. Haynes, MD
Director, Duke Human Vaccine Institute
Frederic M. Hanes Professor of Medicine and Immunology
Duke University Medical Center
Durham, North Carolina
90. Vaccine Innovation and Development

Jessica M. Healy, PhD
Enteric Diseases Epidemiology Branch
Division of Foodborne, Waterborne, and Environmental Diseases
National Center for Emerging Zoonotic Infectious Diseases
Centers for Disease Control and Prevention
Atlanta, Georgia
111. Salmonella Infections (Nontyphoidal)

Christopher D. Heaney, PhD, MS
Department of Environmental Health and Engineering
Department of Epidemiology
Department of International Health
Johns Hopkins Bloomberg School of Public Health
Baltimore, Maryland
66. Participatory Research for Environmental Justice: Advancements in Community Science and Innovation

James R. Hebert, MSPH, ScD
Health Sciences Distinguished Professor
Department of Epidemiology and Biostatistics
Arnold School of Public Health, University of South Carolina
Director, Statewide Cancer Prevention & Control Program
Columbia, South Carolina
182. Nutritional Epidemiology

Craig W. Hedberg, PhD
Division of Environmental Health Sciences
School of Public Health
University of Minnesota
Minneapolis, Minnesota
109. Campylobacter

Katherine A. Hendricks, MD, MPH&TM
Bacterial Special Pathogens Branch
Division of High-Consequence Pathogens and Pathology
National Center for Emerging and Zoonotic Infectious Diseases
Centers for Disease Control and Prevention
Atlanta, Georgia
148. Anthrax

Paul K. Henneberger, MPH, ScD
National Institute for Occupational Safety and Health
Respiratory Health Division
Morgantown, West Virginia
76. Work-Related Asthma

Jeffrey H. Herbst, PhD
Research and Evaluation Branch, Division of Violence Prevention
National Center for Injury Control and Prevention
Centers for Disease Control and Prevention
Atlanta, Georgia
177. Prevention of Youth Violence

Martha Hijar, PhD
Professor, El Colegio de Morelos
Cuernavaca, Morelos, México
25. Injury Prevention and Trauma Care: Global Perspectives

Alison Hinckley, PhD
Division of Vector-Borne Diseases
Centers for Disease Control and Prevention
Fort Collins, Colorado
143. Lyme Disease and Other Borrelia Infections

Tracy N. Hipp, PhD
Assistant Professor
Department of Psychology
University of Memphis
Memphis, Tennessee
179. Sexual Violence

Katherine Hirono, MPH
President, Society of Practitioners of Health Impact Assessment
PhD Candidate
Global Public Health Unit, School of Social and Political Science
University of Edinburgh
Chrystal Macmillan Building
Edinburgh, Scotland, United Kingdom
44. Health Impact Assessment: A Tool for Promoting Healthier Communities

Megan G. Hofmeister, MD, MS, MPH
Division of Viral Hepatitis
Centers for Disease Control and Prevention
Atlanta, Georgia
102. Hepatitis A

Kristin M. Holland, PhD, MPH
Division of Violence Prevention
National Center for Injury Prevention and Control
Centers for Disease Control and Prevention
Atlanta, Georgia
175. The Epidemiology and Prevention of Self-Directed Violence

King K. Holmes, MD, PHD
Distinguished Professor Emeritus, Department of Global Health
Professor Emeritus, School of Public Health
Professor Emeritus, School of Medicine
Director Emeritus, Fred Hutch Center for AIDS Research (CFAR)
Co-Director Emeritus, Center for AIDS and STD
University of Washington
Seattle, Washington
15. The History and Emergence of Global Health

Stacy Holzbauer, DVM, MPH
Minnesota Department of Health
Career Epidemiology Field Officer
Centers for Disease Control and Prevention
Minneapolis, Minnesota
157. Clostridioides difficile Infection

Douglas B. Hornick, MD
Professor, UI Carver College of Medicine
Director of the TB Chest Clinic and Clinical Services
Division of Pulmonary, Critical Care, and Occupational Medicine
Iowa City, Iowa
88. Tuberculosis

Peter J. Hotez, MD, PhD
National School of Tropical Medicine
Baylor College of Medicine
Houston, Texas
126. Intestinal Nematode Infections

Debra Houry, MD, MPH
Centers for Disease Control and Prevention
National Center for Injury Prevention and Control
Atlanta, Georgia
174. Poisoning Prevention

Joel D. Howell, MD, PhD
Elizabeth Farrand Professor of the History of Medicine
Departments of Internal Medicine, History, and Health Services Management and Policy
University of Michigan
Ann Arbor, Michigan
1. History of Preventive Medicine, Public Health, and a Century After Milton J. Rosenau's Preventive Medicine and Hygiene

Victor H. Hu, MBBCh, PhD, FRCOphth
London School of Hygiene and Tropical Medicine
London, United Kingdom
137. Trachoma

James M. Hughes, MD
Professor Emeritus of Medicine
Emory University School of Medicine
Atlanta, Georgia
85. Emerging Microbial Threats to Health

Jennifer C. Hunter, DrPH, MPH
Centers for Disease Control and Prevention
Atlanta, Georgia
113. Escherichia coli, Diarrheagenic

Noreen A. Hynes, MD, MPH
Associate Professor
Division of Infectious Diseases
Department of Medicine
School of Medicine
Departments of International Health; Environmental Health and Engineering; and Population, Family, & Reproductive Health
Bloomberg School of Public Health
Johns Hopkins University
Associate Medical Director
Biocontainment Unit
Johns Hopkins Hospital
Baltimore, Maryland
81. Agents of Infection and Principles of Transmission

Chikwe Ihekweazu, MBBS, MPH
Director General
Nigeria Centre for Disease Control
Abuja, Nigeria
26. Global Health Security and Response to Humanitarian Emergencies

Kari Irvin, MS
Commander
United States Public Health Service
College Park, Maryland
107. Introduction to Food Safety

Dean Jamison, PhD
Emeritus Professor
Institute for Global Health Sciences
University of California, San Francisco
San Francisco, California
18. Global Health Financing: Mechanisms, Trends, and Opportunities

Yahya Jan, MD
Division of Nephrology and Hypertension
Indiana University School of Medicine
Indianapolis, Indiana
54. Genitourinary Disorders

Ilesh Jani, MD, PhD
Instituto Nacional de Saúde
Vila de Marracuene, Mozambique
21. Global Health Systems: What Will It Take to Deliver on the Promise of Health for All?

Robert Johnson, MD, MPH, MBA, FACPM, FAsMA
Clinical Associate Professor of Preventive Medicine
Department of Preventive Medicine and Community Health
University of Texas Medical Branch
Galveston, Texas
Senior Medical Director, Humana Government Business
San Antonio, Texas
12. Aerospace Medicine

Paul D. R. Johnson, MBBS, PhD, FRACP
Department of Infectious Diseases
Austin Health and Department of Medicine
University of Melbourne
Heidelberg, Victoria, Australia
WHO Collaborating Centre for Mycobacterium Ulcerans

Victorian Infectious Diseases Reference Laboratory
Peter Doherty Institute for Infection and Immunity
Melbourne, Victoria, Australia
136. Buruli Ulcer

Grace John-Stewart, MD, MPH, PhD
Professor, Departments of Global Health, Medicine, Epidemiology, and Pediatrics
Director, UW Global WACh
University of Washington
Seattle, Washington
22. Reproductive Health and Child and Adolescent Health and Development

Jeb Jones, PhD, MPH, MS
Department of Epidemiology
Emory University
Atlanta, Georgia
87. The Epidemiology and Prevention of HIV and AIDS

Timothy Jones, MD
Chief Medical Officer
Nashville, Tennessee
Section Editor

S. Patrick Kachur, MD, MPH, FACPM, FASTMH
Professor of Population and Family Health
Columbia University Mailman School of Public Health
New York, New York
89. Malaria

Lily Kamalyan, MA
Department of Psychiatry
HIV Neurobehavioral Research Program
University of California San Diego
Joint Doctoral Program in Clinical Psychology
San Diego State University/University of California San Diego
San Diego, California
162. A Public Health Approach to Severe Mental Illness

Mary Kamb, MD, MPH
Division of Parasitic Diseases and Malaria
Centers for Disease Control and Prevention
Atlanta, Georgia
126. Intestinal Nematode Infections

Thomas Kannampallil, PhD
Assistant Professor, Department of Anesthesiology & Institute for Informatics
Assoc. Chief Research Information Officer, School of Medicine
Washington University in St. Louis
St. Louis, Missouri
3. Precision Medicine

Edward L. Kaplan, MD
Professor Emeritus
Department of Pediatrics
University of Minnesota Medical School
Minneapolis, Minnesota
155. The Group A Streptococcus

Sharon L. R. Kardia, PhD
Millicent W. Higgins Collegiate Professor of Epidemiology
Department of Epidemiology
University of Michigan School of Public Health
Ann Arbor, Michigan
8. Genomic Determinants of Health and Applications in Public Health and Preventive Medicine

Beth E. Karp, DVM, MPH, DACVPM
Senior Veterinary Epidemiologist
Enteric Diseases Epidemiology Branch
Division of Foodborne, Waterborne, and Environmental Diseases
Centers for Disease Control and Prevention
Atlanta, Georgia
114. Shigellosis

David L. Katz, MD, MPH
Past President, American College of Lifestyle Medicine
Director, Prevention Research Center
Yale University/Griffin Hospital
Griffin Hospital, Second Floor
Derby, Connecticut
11. Lifestyle Medicine

Mark A. Katz, MD
Clalit Research Institute
Clalit Health Services
Ramat Gan, Israel
Ben Gurion University of the Negev
Beersheba, Israel
University of Michigan School of Public Health
Ann Arbor, Michigan
105. Influenza

Megan C. Kearns, PhD
Division of Violence Prevention
National Center for Injury Prevention and Control
Centers for Disease Control and Prevention
Atlanta, Georgia
178. Intimate Partner Violence Prevention

Colleen Kelley, MD, MPH
Associate Professor
Department of Medicine
Emory University
Atlanta, Georgia
87. The Epidemiology and Prevention of HIV and AIDS

Eileen Kennedy, ScD
Professor
Friedman School of Nutrition Science and Policy
Tufts University
Boston, Massachusetts
186. Nutrition and Global Food Systems

Gilbert J. Kersh, PhD
Division of Vector-Borne Diseases
Centers for Disease Control and Prevention
Atlanta, Georgia
144. Rickettsial Infections
145. Q Fever

Kiarri N. Kershaw, PhD, MPH
Department of Preventive Medicine
Northwestern University Feinberg School of Medicine
Chicago, Illinois
30. Race and Ethnic Health Disparities

Amira M. Khan, MBBS, DCH, MPH
Centre for Global Child Health
The Hospital for Sick Children
Toronto, Ontario, Canada
23. Control and Prevention of Infection Diseases of Global Significance

Ramni Khattar, MD
Department of Internal Medicine
University of New Mexico School of Medicine
Albuquerque, New Mexico
E1. Pneumoconiosis

Lonnie J. King, DVM, MS, MPA
Academy Professor and Dean Emeritus
College of Veterinary Medicine
Ohio State University
Columbus, Ohio
84. One Health: A New Paradigm for Disease Prevention and Control

Martyn Kirk, BAppSci (WIAE), MAppEpid (ANU), PhD (ANU)
Professor, National Centre for Epidemiology and Population Health
Research School of Population Health
The Australian National University
Acton, Australia
108. Acute Diarrheal Illness—An Overview

Robert D. Kirkcaldy, MD, MPH
Division of STD Prevention
National Center for HIV/AIDS, Viral Hepatitis, STD and TB Prevention
Centers for Disease Control and Prevention
Atlanta, Georgia
121. Gonorrhea

William M. P. Klein, PhD
Behavioral Research Program
National Cancer Institute
Bethesda, Maryland
38. Effective and Impactful Risk Communication

Terri Kleutsch, BA
Dental Division Administrator (Retired)
Family Health Center of Marshfield, Inc.
Winter, Wisconsin
60. Oral Health

Jennifer K. Knapp, PhD, MPH
Epidemiologist
WPRO Measles Rubella Focal Point
Global Immunization Division
US Centers for Disease Control and Prevention
Atlanta, Georgia
94. Rubella

Kirsten Koehler, PhD
Associate Professor
Bloomberg School of Public Health
Johns Hopkins University
Baltimore, Maryland
63. Exposures and Their Assessment, Including General and Occupational Environments
71. Household Air Pollution in Low- and Middle-Income Countries

Aaron D. Kofman, MD
Viral Special Pathogens Branch
Centers for Disease Control and Prevention
Atlanta, Georgia
139. Ebola and other Viral Hemorrhagic Fevers

Karen L. Kotloff, MD
Department of Pediatrics
University of Maryland School of Medicine
23. Control and Prevention of Infection Diseases of Global Significance

Jessica Kraus, MPP
Consultant, SEEK Development
Berlin, Germany
18. Global Health Financing: Mechanisms, Trends, and Opportunities

Kiersten J. Kugeler, PhD, MPH
Epidemiologist
Division of Vector-Borne Diseases
Centers for Disease Control and Prevention
Fort Collins, Colorado
147. Plague

Phoebe K. G. Kulik, MPH
Director of Workforce Development
Department of Health Behavior and Health Education
University of Michigan School of Public Health
Ann Arbor, Michigan
9. Public Health Practice in the United States

Kathryn Kundrod, PhD
Department of Bioengineering
Rice University
Houston, Texas
27. Emerging Technology Innovations in Global Health

Godwin Kwakye-Nuako, PhD
Department of Biomedical Sciences
College of Health and Allied Sciences
University of Cape Coast
Cape Coast, Ghana
134. Leishmaniasis

Maria Lahuerta, PhD, MPH
ICAP at Columbia University
Mailman School of Public Health
Columbia University
New York, New York
21. Global Health Systems: What Will It Take to Deliver on the Promise of Health for All?

Van Charles Lansingh, MD, PhD
Help Me See
Instituto Mexicano de Oftalmología I.A.P.
HelpMeSee Inc
New York, New York
Santiago De Querétaro
Querétaro, México
59. Visual Disorders

Paula M. Lantz, PhD
Associate Dean for Academic Affairs
Professor of Public Policy
Ford School of Public Policy
Professor of Health Management and Policy
School of Public Health
University of Michigan
Ann Arbor, Michigan
2. Population Health: Definitions, Tensions, and New Directions

Stephanie Lashway, MPH
Department of Epidemiology and Biostatistics
Mel and Enid Zuckerman College of Public Health
University of Arizona
Tucson, Arizona
51. Cancer

Anna R. Last, MBChB, PhD, MRCP
London School of Hygiene and Tropical Medicine
London, United Kingdom
137. Trachoma

A.C. Lauer, PhD
Microbiologist in the National Salmonella Reference Laboratory
Senior Assistant Scientist, United States Public Health Service
Centers for Disease Control and Prevention
Atlanta, Georgia
110. Diseases Spread by Food and Water

Christina M. Laukaitis, MD, PhD, FACP, FACMG
Associate Professor
University of Illinois
Urbana, Illinois
51. Cancer

Suzanne R. Lavoie, MD
Professor of Pediatrics and Internal Medicine
Children's Hospital of Richmond at VCU
Virginia Commonwealth University
Richmond, Virginia
122. Chlamydia and Other Sexually Transmitted Infections

Robin Lee, PhD, MPH
Centers for Disease Control and Prevention
National Center for Injury Prevention and Control
Atlanta, Georgia
171. Fall Burden and Prevention Across the Lifespan

Maija Leff, MPH
Project Director, Carolina Collaborative for Research on Work and Health
UNC Gillings School of Global Public Health
Chapel Hill, North Carolina
43. A Comprehensive Approach to Planning Public Health Programs and Policies

Fernanda C. Lessa, MD, MPH
Respiratory Diseases Branch
Centers for Disease Control and Prevention
Atlanta, Georgia
103. Haemophilus influenzae Infections

Gillian A. Levine, PhD, MPH
Departments of Global Health and Epidemiology
University of Washington
Seattle, Washington
23. Control and Prevention of Infection Diseases of Global Significance

Barry S. Levy, MD, MPH
Adjunct Professor of Public Health
Department of Public Health and Community Medicine
Tufts University School of Medicine
Boston, Massachusetts
14. Armed Conflict and Public Health

Megan A. Lewis, PhD
Director, Patient and Family Engagement Research Program
Center for Communication Science
RTI International
Seattle, Washington
3. Precision Medicine

Yuan L. Li, PhD
Respiratory Diseases Branch
National Center for Immunization and Respiratory Diseases
Centers for Disease Control and Prevention
Atlanta, Georgia
155. The Group A Streptococcus

Cristina Linares, PhD
National School of Public Health
Carlos III Institute of Health
Madrid, Spain
67. Diseases Due to Physical Factors: Noise

Laura Linnan, ScD
Senior Associate Dean, Academic and Student Affairs
Professor, Department of Health Behavior
Gillings School of Global Public Health
University of North Carolina
Chapel Hill, North Carolina
43. A Comprehensive Approach to Planning Public Health Programs and Policies

James A. Litch, MD, DTMH
Executive Director and Chief Research Officer
Global Alliance to Prevent Prematurity and Stillbirth
Lynnwood, Washington
23. Control and Prevention of Infection Diseases of Global Significance

Kailey Love, MBA, MS
Research Project Manager
College of Health Solutions
Arizona State University
Phoenix, Arizona
45. Structure and Function of the Public Health System in the United States

Sarah R. Lowe, PhD
Department of Social and Behavioral Sciences
Yale School of Public Health
165. Trauma- and Stressor-Related Disorders

Stephen P. Luby, MD
Infectious Diseases and Geographic Medicine
Stanford University
Stanford, California
23. Control and Prevention of Infection Diseases of Global Significance

Claressa E. Lucas, PhD
Respiratory Diseases Branch
Centers for Disease Control and Prevention
Atlanta, Georgia
115. A Multidisciplinary Approach for the Control and Prevention of Legionellosis

Russell V. Luepker, MD, MS
Mayo Professor
Division of Epidemiology and Community Health
School of Public Health
University of Minnesota
Minneapolis, Minnesota
52. Cardiovascular Disease

Nan Lv, PhD
Research Scientist
Center for Health Behavior Research
Institute for Health Research and Policy
University of Illinois at Chicago
Chicago, Illinois
3. Precision Medicine

Charles F. Lynch, MD, PhD
Department of Epidemiology
College of Public Health
Department of Pathology
College of Medicine
University of Iowa
Iowa City, Iowa
51. Cancer

Ruth Lynfield, MD
State Epidemiologist and Medical Director
Minnesota Department of Health
North St Paul, Minnesota
84. One Health: A New Paradigm for Disease Prevention and Control
Section Editor

Jun Ma, MD, PhD
Professor of Academic Internal Medicine and Geriatrics
Associate Head for Research, Department of Medicine
Director, Center for Health Behavior Research
Institute for Health Research and Policy
University of Illinois at Chicago
Chicago, Illinois
3. Precision Medicine

David C. Mabey, DM, FRCP, FMedSci
London School of Hygiene and Tropical Medicine
London, United Kingdom
137. Trachoma

Karin A. Mack, PhD
Division of Analysis, Research and Practice Integration
National Center for Injury Prevention and Control
Centers for Disease Control & Prevention
Atlanta, Georgia
172. Fire and Burns

Suman S Majumdar, FRACP
Burnet Institute
Melbourne, Australia
23. Control and Prevention of Infection Diseases of Global Significance

Ryan E. Malosh, PhD, MPH
Assistant Research Scientist, Epidemiology
School of Public Health
University of Michigan
Ann Arbor, Michigan
86. SARS CoV-2 and the COVID-19 Pandemic

Mona Marin, MD
National Center for Immunization and Respiratory Diseases
Centers for Disease Control and Prevention
Atlanta, Georgia
99. Varicella

Lauri E. Markowitz, MD
Division of Viral Diseases
National Center for Immunization and Respiratory Diseases
Centers for Disease Control and Prevention
Atlanta, Georgia
100. Human Papillomavirus

Michael Marks, MRCP, DTM&H, PhD
Clinical Research Department
Faculty of Infectious and Tropical Diseases
London School of Hygiene & Tropical Medicine
Hospital for Tropical Diseases
London, United Kingdom
138. Yaws

Mariel A. Marlow, PhD, MPH
Epidemiologist
Mumps, Varicella, and Zoster (MuVZ) Epidemiology Team
Viral Vaccine Preventable Diseases Branch/Division of Viral Diseases
National Center for Immunization and Respiratory Diseases
US Centers for Disease Control and Prevention
Atlanta, Georgia
93. Mumps

Khiya J. Marshall, DrPH
Research and Evaluation Branch, Division of Violence Prevention
National Center for Injury Control and Prevention
Centers for Disease Control and Prevention
Atlanta, Georgia
177. Prevention of Youth Violence

Rebecca M. Martin, PhD
Centers for Disease Control and Prevention
Atlanta, Georgia
28. A Trained and Prepared Global Health Workforce Is Required to Achieve Impact

Jennifer L. Matjasko, PhD, MPP
Research and Evaluation Branch, Division of Violence Prevention
National Center for Injury Control and Prevention
Centers for Disease Control and Prevention
Atlanta, Georgia
177. Prevention of Youth Violence

Sarah Mbaeyi, MD, MPH
Meningitis and Vaccine Preventable Diseases Branch
National Center for Immunization and Respiratory Diseases
Atlanta, Georgia
104. Meningococcal Disease

Sandra I. McCoy, PhD, MPH
Associate Professor, Division of Epidemiology
School of Public Health
University of California, Berkeley
Berkeley, California
82. Epidemiology and Control of Infectious Diseases

Paul S. Mead, MD, MPH
Chief, Bacterial Diseases Branch
Division of Vector-Borne Diseases
National Center for Emerging and Zoonotic Diseases
Centers for Disease Control and Prevention
Fort Collins, Colorado
146. Diseases Transmitted Primarily from Animals to Humans (Zoonoses): Tularemia

Arianna Rubin Means, PhD, MPH
Department of Global Health
University of Washington
Seattle, Washington
20. Implementation Science: A New Research Paradigm to Accelerate Global Health Impact at Scale

Felicita Medalla, MD, MS
Division of Foodborne, Waterborne, and Environmental Diseases
Centers for Disease Control and Prevention
Atlanta, Georgia
110. Diseases Spread by Food and Water

Zaal Meher-Homji, MBBS, DTMH
Department of Infectious Diseases
Austin Health and Department of Medicine
University of Melbourne
Heidelberg, Victoria, Australia
136. Buruli Ulcer

Nir Menachemi, PhD, MPH
Indiana University Richard M. Fairbanks School of Public Health
Indianapolis, Indiana
48. Understanding Revenue and Delivery Models in the United States Healthcare System

Shawna L. Mercer, MSc, PhD
Lead, National Neurological Conditions Surveillance System
Senior Scientific Advisor for Public Health Initiatives and Partnerships
Office of the Director
Center for Surveillance, Epidemiology, and Laboratory Services
Centers for Disease Control and Prevention
Atlanta, Georgia
41. Evidence-Based Community Interventions

James A. Mercy, PhD
Director, Division of Violence Prevention
National Center for Injury Control and Prevention
Centers for Disease Control and Prevention
Atlanta, Georgia
Section Editor

Diane Meyer, RN, MPH
Research Associate
Johns Hopkins Center for Health Security
Department of Environmental Health and Engineering
Bloomberg School of Public Health
Johns Hopkins University
Baltimore, Maryland
81. Agents of Infection and Principles of Transmission

Rafael Meza, PhD
Associate Chair and Associate Professor, Epidemiology
Associate Professor of Global Public Health
Co-Leader, Cancer Epidemiology and Prevention Program
Rogel Cancer Center
University of Michigan
Ann Arbor, Michigan
159. Introduction to Infectious Disease Modeling

Briana Mezuk, PhD
Department of Epidemiology
University of Michigan School of Public Health
Ann Arbor, Michigan
163. Mood Disorders

Olachi J. Mezu-Ndubuisi, MD, OD
Assistant Professor
Department of Pediatrics
Department of Ophthalmology and Visual Sciences
School of Medicine and Public Health
University of Wisconsin
Madison, Wisconsin
59. Visual Disorders

Rachel G. Miller, PhD
Research Assistant Professor
Department of Epidemiology
Graduate School of Public Health
University of Pittsburgh
Pittsburgh, Pennsylvania
53. Diabetes and Other Metabolic Disorders

Beyon Miloyan, PhD
Faculty of Health, School of Psychology and Health Sciences
Federation University
Ballarat, Victoria, Australia
164. Anxiety Disorders

Eric Mintz, MD, MPH
Team Lead, Global WASH Epidemiology
Waterborne Disease Prevention Branch
The Division of Foodborne, Waterborne, and Environmental Diseases (DFWED)
The National Center for Emerging and Zoonotic Infectious Diseases (*NCEZID*)
Centers for Disease Control and Prevention
Atlanta, Georgia
112. Cholera

Charles Mock, MD, PhD
Department of Global Health
The Harborview Injury Prevention and Research Center
University of Washington
Seattle, Washington
25. Injury Prevention and Trauma Care: Global Perspectives

Stephen M. Modell, MD, MS
Research and Dissemination Activities Director,
Center for Public Health and Community Genomics
University of Michigan School of Public Health
Ann Arbor, Michigan
8. Genomic Determinants of Health and Applications in Public Health and Preventive Medicine

Martha P. Montgomery, MD, MHS
Physician
Division of Viral Hepatitis
Centers for Disease Control and Prevention
Atlanta, Georgia
102. Hepatitis A

Arnold S. Monto, MD
Professor, Epidemiology
Professor, Global Public Health
Thomas Francis, Jr. Collegiate Professor of Public Health
University of Michigan
Acting Chair of the FDA's Vaccines and Related Biological Products Advisory Committee
Ann Arbor, Michigan
86. SARS CoV-2 and the COVID-19 Pandemic

Latetia V. Moore, PhD, MSPH
Division of Nutrition, Physical Activity, and Obesity
Centers for Disease Control and Prevention
Atlanta, Georgia
181. Obesity Prevention and Control: A Public Health Perspective

Maria C. Mora Pinzon, MD, MS
Assistant Scientist, Wisconsin Alzheimer's Institute
Research Fellow, Department of Family Medicine and Community Health
School of Medicine and Public Health
University of Wisconsin—Madison
Madison, Wisconsin
54. Genitourinary Disorders
Section Editor

Briana Moreland, MPH
Centers for Disease Control and Prevention
National Center for Injury Prevention and Control
Atlanta, Georgia
171. Fall Burden and Prevention Across the Lifespan

Oliver W. Morgan, PhD, MSc
Department of Health Emergency Information and Risk Assessment
Health Emergencies Programme
World Health Organization
26. Global Health Security & Response to Humanitarian Emergencies

Priya Morjaria, BSc, MCOptom, MPH, PhD
Faculty of Infectious and Tropical Diseases
Department of Clinical Research
London School of Hygiene & Tropical Medicine
London, United Kingdom
59. Visual Disorders

Wame Mosime
International Treatment Preparedness Coalition
Gaborone, Botswana
21. Global Health Systems: What Will It Take to Deliver on the Promise of Health for All?

Emily Mosites, PhD, MPH
Arctic Investigations Program
Division of Preparedness and Emerging Infections
National Center for Emerging and Zoonotic Infectious Diseases
Centers for Disease Control and Prevention
Anchorage, Alaska
155. The Group A Streptococcus

Melissa Mugambi, MD, PhD
Department of Global Health
University of Washington
Seattle, Washington
20. Implementation Science: A New Research Paradigm to Accelerate Global Health Impact at Scale

Nelly Mugo, MBChB, MMed, MPH
Department of Global Health
University of Washington
Seattle, Washington
Center for Clinical Research
Kenya Medical Research Institute
Thika, Kenya
23. Control and Prevention of Infection Diseases of Global Significance

Christopher J. L. Murray, MD, DPhil
Chair and Professor, Health Metrics Sciences
Institute Director, Institute for Health Metrics and Evaluation
University of Washington
Seattle, Washington
16. Transitions in Global Disease Burden

Immaculate Mutisya
CDC Kenya
Nairobi, Kenya
15. The History and Emergence of Global Health

Julie Mwabe
CDC Kenya
Nairobi, Kenya
15. The History and Emergence of Global Health

Rupa Narra, MD
Assistant Professor, Departments of Emergency Medicine and Pediatrics
New York University School of Medicine
New York, New York
112. Cholera

D. Maria Navarro, MD, MSc, MPH, PhD
Director of Patient Experience
Hospital Sant Joan de Deu
Barcelona, Spain
39. Health Literacy: An Update

Ana Navas-Acien, MD, PhD
Professor
Mailman School of Public Health
Columbia University
New York, New York
62. Environmental and Occupational Exposures: Sources, Characteristics, Consequences, and Control
65. Research Approaches in Environmental and Occupational Health
73. Metals and Health: Science and Practice
Section Editor

María E. Negrón Sureda, DVM, PhD, MS
Centers for Disease Control and Prevention
Atlanta, Georgia
149. Brucellosis

Kenrad E. Nelson, MD
Professor of Epidemiology and International Health
Bloomberg School of Public Health
Johns Hopkins University
Baltimore, Maryland
135. Leprosy

Paul E. Nevin, MPH
Department of Global Health
University of Washington
Seattle, Washington
25. Injury Prevention and Trauma Care: Global Perspectives

Phyllis Holditch Niolon, PhD
Division of Violence Prevention
National Center for Injury Prevention and Control
Centers for Disease Control and Prevention
Atlanta, Georgia
178. Intimate Partner Violence Prevention

Josie Noah, MPA, MPL
Senior Director
Advocacy, Prevention and Clinical Programs
SightLife
Seattle, Washington
59. Visual Disorders

Margaret Nolan, MD, MS
Department of Population Health Sciences
School of Medicine and Public Health
University of Wisconsin—Madison
Madison, Wisconsin
52. Cardiovascular Disease

Laura E. Norton, MD, MS
Assistant Professor of Pediatrics
Department of Pediatrics
Division of Infectious Diseases and Immunology
University of Minnesota Medical School
Minneapolis, Minnesota
153. Antibiotic Resistance and Stewardship

Francois Nosten, MD, PhD
Department of Medicine
University of Oxford
23. Control and Prevention of Infection Diseases of Global Significance

Greg Nycz
Director
Family Health Center of Marshfield, Inc.
Marshfield, Wisconsin
60. Oral Health

Sara E. Oliver, MD, MSPH
Epidemic Intelligence Service Officer
Division of Viral Diseases
Centers for Disease Control and Prevention
Atlanta, Georgia
103. Haemophilus influenzae Infections

Danielle C. Ompad, PhD
Associate Professor
New York University College of Global Public Health
Deputy Director
Center for Drug Use and HIV Research at the NYU Rory Meyers College of Nursing
New York University
College of Global Public Health
New York, New York
169. Prescription Drug Use and Misuse

Emily Oot, PhD
Boston University School of Medicine
Boston, Massachusetts
167. Alcohol and Health

Walter A. Orenstein, MD
Emory Vaccine Center and School of Medicine
Emory University
Atlanta, Georgia
83. Principles of Disease Elimination and Eradication

Robert R. Orford, MD, FAsMA
Medical Consultant, Mayo Clinic
Assistant Professor, Mayo Graduate School of Medicine
Scottsdale, Arizona
Associate Professor, University of Texas Medical Branch
Galveston, Texas
12. Aerospace Medicine

Stephen M. Ostroff, MD
Deputy Commissioner for Foods and Veterinary Medicine (Retired)
U.S. Food and Drug Administration
Silver Spring, Maryland
85. Emerging Microbial Threats to Health

Belinda Ostrowsky, MD, MPH, FIDSA, FSHEA
Prevention and Response Branch
Division of Healthcare Quality Promotion
Centers for Disease Control and Prevention
Atlanta, Georgia
152. Control of Infections in Institutions: Healthcare-Associated Infections

Ariel Pablos-Mendez, MD, MPH
Department of Medicine
Vagelos College of Physicians and Surgeons
Columbia University
New York, New York
21. Global Health Systems: What Will It Take to Deliver on the Promise of Health for All?

Nigel Paneth, MD, MPH
University Distinguished Professor
Departments of Epidemiology & Biostatistics and Pediatrics & Human Development
Michigan State University
College of Human Medicine
East Lansing, Michigan
160 Developmental Disabilities

Aloksagar Panny, BDS, MS
Research Specialist
Center for Oral and Systemic Health
Marshfield Clinic Research Institute
Marshfield Clinic Health System
Marshfield, Wisconsin
60. Oral Health

Edith A. Parker, DrPH, MPH
Dean
Professor, Department of Community and Behavioral Health
University of Iowa College of Public Health
Iowa City, Iowa
42. Community Engaged Research

Erin Parker, PhD
Centers for Disease Control and Prevention
National Center for Injury Prevention and Control
Atlanta, Georgia
174. Poisoning Prevention

Sai Paul
Department of Bioengineering
Rice University
Houston, Texas
27. Emerging Technology Innovations in Global Health

Lucia C. Pawloski, PhD
Division of Bacterial Diseases
National Center for Immunization and Respiratory Diseases
Centers for Disease Control and Prevention
Atlanta, Georgia
97. Pertussis

Veronica A. Pear, MPH
Violence Prevention Research Program
University of California, Davis
165. Trauma- and Stressor-Related Disorders

Jennifer Peel, PhD
Department of Environmental and Radiological Health Sciences
Colorado School of Public Health
Colorado State University
Fort Collins, Colorado
71. Household Air Pollution in Low- and Middle-Income Countries

Jason A. Penniecook, MD, MSc
Instituto de la Vision, Universidad de Montemorelos
Centro Mexicano de Salud Visual Preventiva
Collaborative Network for Quality in Eye Research (CONQUER)
Montemorelos, Mexico
59. Visual Disorders

Joseph F. Perz, DrPH, MA
Deputy Branch Chief, Public Health Programs
Prevention and Response Branch
Division of Healthcare Quality Promotion
Centers for Disease Control and Prevention
Atlanta, Georgia
152. Control of Infections in Institutions: Healthcare-Associated Infections

Amy Peterson, DVM, PhD
Division of Vector-Borne Diseases
Centers for Disease Control and Prevention
Atlanta, Georgia
144. Rickettsial Infections

Karen E. Peterson, DSc
Stanley M. Garn Collegiate Professor of Nutritional Sciences
Chair, Department of Nutritional Sciences
Professor, Department of Global Public Health
University of Michigan
Ann Arbor, Michigan
Section Editor

Jeff Pettey, MD
Moran Eye Center
University of Utah
Salt Lake City, Utah
59. Visual Disorders

Emily G. Pieracci, DVM, MPH, DACVPM
Veterinary Epidemiologist
Centers for Disease Control and Prevention
Atlanta, Georgia
140. Viral Zoonoses—Rabies

Ryan J. Piers, MA
Department of Psychological and Brain Sciences
Boston University
Boston, Massachusetts
161. Neurocognitive Disorder and Cognitive Decline

Yogan Pillay, PhD
National Department of Health
Republic of South Africa
Pretoria, South Africa
21. Global Health Systems: What Will It Take to Deliver on the Promise of Health for All?

Leah C. Pinckney, MPH
Department of Epidemiology
School of Public Health
University of Michigan
Ann Arbor, Michigan
91. Vaccine Decision-making and Vaccine Hesitancy

Jillian Pintye, RN, MPH, PhD
Department of Epidemiology
University of Washington
Seattle, Washington
23. Control and Prevention of Infection Diseases of Global Significance

Jonathan M. Platt, PhD, MPH
Department of Epidemiology
Mailman School of Public Health
Columbia University
New York, New York
166. Tobacco Use and Tobacco Use Disorder

Stanley A. Plotkin, MD
Emeritus Professor of Pediatrics
University of Pennsylvania
Vaxconsult
Doylestown, Pennsylvania
90. Vaccine Innovation and Development

Craig Evan Pollack, MD
Associate Professor
Bloomberg School of Public Health
Johns Hopkins University
Baltimore, Maryland
32. Housing and Health

Katie A. Ports, PhD
Behavioral Scientist
Division of Violence Prevention
National Center for Injury Prevention and Control
Centers for Disease Control and Prevention
Atlanta, Georgia
176. Child Abuse and Neglect

Ann M. Powers, PhD
Arboviral Diseases Branch
Division of Vector-Borne Diseases
US Centers for Disease Control and Prevention
Fort Collins, Colorado
142. Diseases Transmitted Primarily by Arthropod Vectors: Viral Infections

Joanna M. Prasher, PhD, MPH
Senior Advisor for Medical Countermeasures
Center for Preparedness and Response
Centers for Disease Control and Prevention
Atlanta, Georgia
6. Preparing for and Responding to Public Health Emergencies

Janice C. Probst, PhD
Rural and Minority Health Research Center
Arnold School of Public Health
University of South Carolina
Columbia, South Carolina
33. Rural America: Public Health Challenges and Opportunities

Wendy M. Purcell, PhD, FRSA
Harvard T.H. Chan School of Public Health
Boston, Massachusetts
80. Looking to the Future: Sustainability and Other Issues

Michael A. Purdy, PhD
Division of Viral Hepatitis
National Center for HIV/AIDS, Viral Hepatitis, STD and TB Prevention
Centers for Disease Control and Prevention
Atlanta, Georgia
102. Hepatitis A

Shamim A. Qazi, MBBS, MSc, MD
Consultant
Department of Maternal, Newborn, Child and Adolescent Health
World Health Organization
Geneva, Switzerland
23. Control and Prevention of Infection Diseases of Global Significance

Thomas Quade, MA, MPH, CPH, HFRSPH
Health Commissioner, Geauga County, Ohio
Past President, American Public Health Association
Chardon, Ohio
45. Structure and Function of the Public Health System in the United States

Linda Quan, MD
Seattle Children's Hospital
Seattle, Washington
173. The Epidemiology and Prevention of Drowning

Lesliam Quirós-Alcalá, PhD, MS
Johns Hopkins Bloomberg School of Public Health
Department of Environmental Health and Engineering
Baltimore, Maryland
63. Exposures and Their Assessment, Including General and Occupational Environments

Ingrid Rabe, MBChB, MMed
Arboviral Diseases Branch
Division of Vector-Borne Diseases
US Centers for Disease Control and Prevention
Fort Collins, Colorado
142. Diseases Transmitted Primarily by Arthropod Vectors: Viral Infections

Miriam Rabkin, MD, MPH
Associate Professor of Medicine & Epidemiology
Mailman School of Public Health
Columbia University
New York, New York
21. Global Health Systems: What Will It Take to Deliver on the Promise of Health for All?

Rohit Ramaswamy, PhD, MPH
Professor and Associate Director
Public Health Leadership Program
Professor, Department of Maternal and Child Health
Faculty Director, Online Global Health Certificate
Director, Center for Global Learning
University of North Carolina at Chapel Hill
Chapel Hill, North Carolina
49. Implementing Public Health Programs

Brian H. Raphael, PhD
Respiratory Diseases Branch
Centers for Disease Control and Prevention
Atlanta, Georgia
115. A Multidisciplinary Approach for the Control and Prevention of Legionellosis

Stephen C. Redd, MD
RADM, United States Public Health Service
Deputy Director for Public Health Service and Implementation Science
Centers for Disease Control and Prevention
Atlanta, Georgia
6. Preparing for and Responding to Public Health Emergencies

Susan E. Reef, MD
Global Immunization Division
Center for Global Health
Centers for Disease Control and Prevention
Atlanta, Georgia
94. Rubella

Susan Reid, LLB, MA
Director, Health Literacy New Zealand
Auckland, New Zealand
39. Health Literacy: An Update

Arthur Reingold, MD
Professor of Epidemiology
Chair, Division of Epidemiology
School of Public Health
University of California, Berkeley
Berkeley, California
82. Epidemiology and Control of Infectious Diseases

Patrick Remington, MD, MPH
Professor Emeritus
Director, Preventive Medicine Residency Program
Department of Population Health Sciences
School of Medicine and Public Health
University of Wisconsin—Madison

Kim D. Reynolds, PhD
Professor of School of Community and Global Health
Claremont Graduate University
Claremont, California
40. Health Promotion Interventions and Research

Rebecca Richards-Kortum, PhD
Department of Bioengineering
Rice University
Houston, Texas
27. Emerging Technology Innovations in Global Health

William Riley, PhD
Professor, Program for the Science of Health Care Delivery
Director, National Safety Net Advancement Center
College of Health Solutions
Arizona State University
Phoenix, Arizona
45. Structure and Function of the Public Health System in the United States

Barbara K. Rimer, DrPH
UNC Gillings School of Global Public Health
University of North Carolina at Chapel Hill
Chapel Hill, North Carolina
35. Health Behavior Theories

Charlene M.C. Rodrigues, MBChB (Hons), MRCPCH
Pediatrician Specialising in Infectious Diseases
University of Oxford
Department of Zoology
Oxford, United Kingdom
90. Vaccine Innovation and Development

Megan E. Romano, MPH, PhD
Department of Epidemiology
Geisel School of Medicine at Dartmouth
Lebanon, New Hampshire
75. Environmental Endocrine-Disrupting Chemicals: Common Sources and Health Effects

Corina R. Ronneberg, MS
Senior Research Specialist
Center for Health Behavior Research
Institute for Health Research and Policy
University of Illinois at Chicago
Chicago, Illinois
3. Precision Medicine

David A. Ross, BMBCh, MA, MSc, PhD
Consultant to the Partnership for Maternal, Newborn & Child Health
Geneva, Switzerland
22. Reproductive Health and Child and Adolescent Health and Development

Rima E. Rudd, ScD, MSPH
Senior Lecturer on Health Literacy, Education, and Policy
Department of Social and Behavioral Sciences
Harvard T.H. Chan School of Public Health
Boston, Massachusetts
39. Health Literacy: An Update

Ana M. Rule, PhD, MHS
Johns Hopkins Bloomberg School of Public Health
Department of Environmental Health and Engineering
Baltimore, Maryland
63. Exposures and Their Assessment, Including General and Occupational Environments

Jennifer Sacheck, PhD
Professor and Chair, Department of Exercise and Nutrition Sciences
Milken Institute School of Public Health
George Washington University
Washington, DC
184. Strategies to Address Physical Activity in Schools

Adnan Said, MD, MS
Department of Medicine, Gastroenterology and Hepatology, University of Wisconsin School of Medicine and Public Health and Wm S Middleton VAMC
Madison, Wisconsin
55. Gastrointestinal and Liver Disorders

Richard Saitz, MD
Boston University Schools of Public Health and Medicine
Boston Medical Center
Boston, Massachusetts
167. Alcohol and Health

Jonathan M. Samet, MD, MS
Dean and Professor
Departments of Epidemiology and Environmental and Occupational Health
Colorado School of Public Health
Aurora, Colorado
56. Respiratory Diseases
62. Environmental and Occupational Exposures: Sources, Characteristics, Consequences, and Control
65. Research Approaches in Environmental and Occupational Health
70. Air Pollution
78. Managing Environmental and Occupational Risks
Section Editor

Hillary Samples, PhD
Columbia University
New York, New York
168. Marijuana Use in the U.S.: Trends, Consequences, Changing Laws

Brisa N. Sánchez, PhD
Dornsife School of Public Health
Department of Epidemiology and Biostatistics
Drexel University
Philadelphia, Pennsylvania
185. Food and Physical Activity Environments: Influences on Diet and Physical Activity

Emma V. Sanchez-Vaznaugh, ScD, MPH
College of Health & Social Sciences, Department of Health Education
San Francisco State University
Center for Health Equity
University of California, San Francisco
San Francisco, California
185. Food and Physical Activity Environments: Influences on Diet and Physical Activity

Simon Sandh, MPH
Doctoral Student
New York University College of Global Public Health
New York University
College of Global Public Health
New York, New York
169. Prescription Drug Use and Misuse

Rengaswamy Sankaranarayanan, MD
Senior Research Fellow, International Agency on Research on Cancer
World Health Organization
24. Addressing the Growing Burden of Chronic Noncommunicable Diseases

Sarah G. H. Sapp, PhD
Division of Parasitic Diseases and Malaria
Centers for Disease Control and Prevention
Atlanta, Georgia
Oak Ridge Associated Universities
Oak Ridge, Tennessee
126. Intestinal Nematode Infections
127. Tissue Nematodes
129. Foodborne Trematode Infections
131. Zoonotic Cestodes

Shekar Saxena, MD, FRCPsych
Visiting Professor
Harvard T.H. Chan School of Public Health
Boston, Massachusetts
24. Addressing the Growing Burden of Chronic Noncommunicable Diseases

Marco Schäferhoff, PhD
Managing Director, Open Consultants
Berlin, Germany
18. Global Health Financing: Mechanisms, Trends, and Opportunities

Lauren Schwartz, PhD Student
Department of Epidemiology
University of Washington
Seattle, Washington
23. Control and Prevention of Infection Diseases of Global Significance

David M. Scollard, MD, PhD
Director (Retired)
National Hansen's Disease Programs
Baton Rouge, Louisiana
135. Leprosy

W. Evan Secor, PhD
Division of Parasitic Diseases and Malaria
Centers for Disease Control and Prevention
Atlanta, Georgia
128. Schistosomiasis

Hannah E. Segaloff, PhD, MPH
Department of Epidemiology
School of Public Health
University of Michigan
Ann Arbor Michigan
86. SARS CoV-2 and the COVID-19 Pandemic
105. Influenza

Randall Sell, ScD
Professor
Dornsife School of Public Health
Drexel University
Philadelphia, Pennsylvania
34. Considering Sexual Orientation, Gender Identity and Expression, and Sex Characteristics in Public Health

Rachel M. Shaffer, MPH, PhD
University of Washington
Seattle, Washington
64. Basic Toxicology and Mode of Action of Toxic Substances

Christine E. Sheffer, PhD
Professor of Oncology, Department of Health Behavior
Roswell Park Comprehensive Cancer Center
Buffalo, New York
166. Tobacco Use and Tobacco Use Disorder

Jessica R. Shoaff, MPH, PhD
Channing Division of Network Medicine
Brigham and Women's Hospital
Harvard Medical School
Department of Epidemiology
Harvard T.H. Chan School of Public Health
Boston, Massachusetts
75. Environmental Endocrine-Disrupting Chemicals: Common Sources and Health Effects

Robin P. Shook, PhD
Department of Pediatrics
Center for Children's Healthy Lifestyles
Children's Mercy Kansas City
Kansas City, Missouri
183. Physical Activity Epidemiology in Health and Disease

Paul A. Simon, MD, MPH
Los Angeles County Department of Public Health
Los Angeles, California
7. Public Health Surveillance

Tami H. Skoff, MS
Division of Bacterial Diseases
National Center for Immunization and Respiratory Diseases
Centers for Disease Control and Prevention
Atlanta, Georgia
97. Pertussis

Elaine M. Smith, PhD
Professor
Department of Epidemiology
University of Iowa
Iowa City, Iowa
51. Cancer

Akshay Sood, MD, MPH
Department of Internal Medicine
University of New Mexico School of Medicine
Albuquerque, New Mexico
E1. Pneumoconiosis

Agnes Soucat, MD, MPH, PhD
Director, Health Systems Governance and Financing Department
World Health Organization
Geneva, Switzerland
18. Global Health Financing: Mechanisms, Trends, and Opportunities

John D. Spengler, PhD, MS
Harvard T.H. Chan School of Public Health
Boston, Massachusetts
80. Looking to the Future: Sustainability and Other Issues

Emily A. Spieler, JD
Northeastern University School of Law
Boston, Massachusetts
79. Protecting Workers' Health, Safety, and Wellbeing

Donna Spruijt-Metz, PhD
Director, USC mHealth Collaboratory
Center for Economic and Social Research
Los Angeles, California
40. Health Promotion Interventions and Research

Ellery Lopez Starr, MD, MBA
Medical Director
Mexican Institute of Ophthalmology
Queretaro, Mexico
59. Visual Disorders

Saige Stortz, MA
The Graduate Center, CUNY
New York, New York
162. A Public Health Approach to Severe Mental Illness

Anne Straily, DVM, MPH, DACVPM
Veterinary Medical Officer
Center for Global Health, Parasitic Diseases Branch
Centers for Disease Control and Prevention
Atlanta, Georgia
151. Toxoplasmosis

Joanna M. Streck, PhD
Tobacco Research and Treatment Center
Division of General Internal Medicine
Department of Medicine
Department of Psychiatry
Harvard Medical School
Massachusetts General Hospital
Boston, Massachusetts
166. Tobacco Use and Tobacco Use Disorder

Nancy A. Strockbine, PhD
Chief, Escherichia Shigella Unit
Deputy Lead, PulseNet, Reference, Outbreak and Surveillance Team
Enteric Diseases Laboratory Branch
Division of Foodborne, Waterborne, and Environmental Diseases
National Center for Emerging, Zoonotic and Infectious Diseases
Centers for Disease Control and Prevention
Atlanta, Georgia
113. Escherichia coli, Diarrheagenic
114. Shigellosis

Patrick S. Sullivan, MD, FACS, FASCRS
Associate Professor of Surgery
Division of Surgical Oncology & Division of Colorectal Surgery
Department of Surgery
Chief Quality Officer
Division of Surgical Oncology
Department of Surgery
Emory University School of Medicine
Atlanta, Georgia
87. The Epidemiology and Prevention of HIV and AIDS

Jordi Sunyer, MD, PhD
ISGlobal
Barcelona, Catalonia, Spain
74. Early Life Environmental Exposures and Children's Health

Roland W. Sutter, MD, MPH&TM
Consultant
Centers for Disease Control and Prevention (Retired)
World Health Organization (Retired)
Geneva, Switzerland
98. Poliomyelitis

Diego Tamez, MD, MPH
School of Medicine and Public Health
University of Wisconsin—Madison
Madison, Wisconsin
53. Diabetes and Other Metabolic Disorders

Melody Tan, PhD, MSE
Department of Bioengineering
Rice University
Houston, Texas
27. Emerging Technology Innovations in Global Health

Jordan W. Tappero, MD, MPH
Global Health
Bill and Melinda Gates Foundation
26. Global Health Security and Response to Humanitarian Emergencies

Trisa Taro
International Treatment Preparedness Coalition
Gaborone, Botswana
21. Global Health Systems: What Will It Take to Deliver on the Promise of Health for All?

Robert V. Tauxe, MD, MPH
Director, Division of Foodborne, Waterborne, and Environmental Diseases
Deputy Director for Infectious Diseases
National Center for Emerging and Zoonotic Infectious Diseases
Centers for Disease Control and Prevention
Atlanta, Georgia
111. Salmonella Infections (Nontyphoidal)

Maria Tellez-Plaza, MD, PhD
National Center for Epidemiology
Institute of Health Carlos III
Madrid, Spain
73. Metals and Health: Science and Practice

Awoke Misganaw Temesgen, PhD
Clinical Assistant Professor
Institute of Health Metrics and Evaluation
University of Washington
Seattle, Washington
16. Transitions in Global Disease Burden

Steven M. Teutsch, MD, MPH
Center for Health Advancement
Fielding School of Public Health
University of California, Los Angeles
Los Angeles, California
7. Public Health Surveillance

Kirkby D. Tickell, MPH
Departments of Global Health and Epidemiology
University of Washington
Seattle, Washington
23. Control and Prevention of Infection Diseases of Global Significance

Tejpratap S.P. Tiwari, MD
Meningitis and Vaccine Preventable Disease Branch
Division of Bacterial Diseases
National Center for Immunization and Respiratory Diseases
Centers for Disease Control and Prevention
Atlanta, Georgia
95. Diphtheria
96. Tetanus

Stephanie M. Topp, PhD, MPH, MPhil (Oxon)
College of Public Health, Medical & Veterinary Sciences
James Cook University
Townsville, Queensland, Australia
21. Global Health Systems: What Will It Take to Deliver on the Promise of Health for All?

James C. Torner, PhD, MS
Professor and Head
Department of Epidemiology
College of Public Health
University of Iowa
Iowa City, Iowa
58. Diseases of the Nervous System

Maryann Turnsek, BS
Division of Foodborne, Waterborne, and Environmental Diseases
Enteric Diseases Laboratory Branch
Centers for Disease Control and Prevention
Atlanta, Georgia
112. Cholera

Jennifer B. Unger, PhD
Professor of Preventive Medicine
University of Southern California
Los Angeles, California
40. Health Promotion Interventions and Research

Diogo G. Valadares, PhD
Departments of Internal Medicine and Microbiology & Immunology
University of Iowa
Veterans' Affairs Medical Center
Iowa City, Iowa
CNPq
Brazil
134. Leishmaniasis

Chris A. Van Beneden, MD, MPH
Respiratory Diseases Branch
National Center for Immunization and Respiratory Diseases
Centers for Disease Control and Prevention
Atlanta, Georgia
155. The Group A Streptococcus

Jan Van Den Abbeele, PhD
Professor, Veterinary Protozoology Unit
Department of Biomedical Sciences
Institute of Tropical Medicine
Antwerp, Belgium
133. Human African Trypanosomiasis

Camila V. Ventura, MD, PhD
Department of Ophthalmology
Altino Ventura Foundation
HOPE Eye Hospital
Recife, Brazil
59. Visual Disorders

Antonio Vieira, DVM, MPH, PhD
Bacterial Special Pathogens Branch
Division of High-Consequence Pathogens and Pathology
National Center for Emerging and Zoonotic Infectious Diseases
Centers for Disease Control and Prevention
Atlanta, Georgia
148. Anthrax

K. Viswanath, PhD
Harvard T.H. Chan School of Public Health
The Dana-Farber-Cancer Institute
Dana-Farber Cancer Institute
Boston, Massachusetts
36. Health Communications

Kevin Vlahovich, MD, MS
Department of Internal Medicine
University of New Mexico School of Medicine
Albuquerque, New Mexico
E1. Pneumoconiosis

Caroline Voyles, MPH
Dornsife School of Public Health
Drexel University
Philadelphia, Pennsylvania
34. Considering Sexual Orientation, Gender Identity and Expression, and Sex Characteristics in Public Health

Martine Vrijheid, PhD
ISGlobal
Barcelona, Catalonia, Spain
74. Early Life Environmental Exposures and Children's Health

Timothy J. Wade, PhD, MPH
US EPA Office of Research and Development
National Health and Environmental Effects Research Laboratory
Epidemiology Branch
Research Triangle Park, North Carolina
72. Water Pollution

Abram L. Wagner, PhD, MPH
Department of Epidemiology
School of Public Health
University of Michigan
Ann Arbor, Michigan
91. Vaccine Decision-making and Vaccine Hesitancy
92. Measles
106. Pneumococcal Infections

Gregory R. Wagner, MD
Department of Environmental Health
Harvard T.H. Chan School of Public Health
Boston, Massachusetts
79. Protecting Workers' Health, Safety, and Wellbeing

Sana Waheed, MD
Assistant Professor
Department of Medicine
University of Wisconsin—Madison
Madison, Wisconsin
54. Genitourinary Disorders

Arnold Wald, MD
Department of Medicine, Gastroenterology and Hepatology
University of Wisconsin School of Medicine and Public Health and Wm S Middleton VAMC
Madison, Wisconsin
55. Gastrointestinal and Liver Disorders

Robert B. Wallace, MD, MSc
Irene Ensminger Stecher Emeritus Professor of Epidemiology and Internal Medicine
University of Iowa College of Public Health
Iowa City, Iowa
4. Epidemiology and Public Health
50. Screening for Early and Asymptomatic Conditions

Judd L. Walson, MD, MPH
Professor, Departments of Global Health, Pediatrics, Medicine (Division of Allergy and Infectious Disease) and Epidemiology
University of Washington
Seattle, Washington
23. Control and Prevention of Infection Diseases of Global Significance

Judith N. Wasserheit, MD, MPH
Department of Global Health
University of Washington
Seattle, Washington
19. Evaluating Progress in Global Health: Global Health Measures That Build Capacity
Section Editor

Louise K. Francois Watkins, MD, MPH
Division of Foodborne, Waterborne, and Environmental Diseases
National Center for Emerging and Zoonotic Infectious Diseases
Centers for Disease Control and Prevention
Atlanta, Georgia
119. Yersiniosis

Bryan J. Weiner, PhD
Department of Global Health
University of Washington
Seattle, Washington
20. Implementation Science: A New Research Paradigm to Accelerate Global Health Impact at Scale

David N. Weissman
National Institute for Occupational Safety and Health
Respiratory Health Division
Morgantown, West Virginia
76. Work-Related Asthma

Mark Weng, MD, MSc
National Center for HIV/AIDS, Viral Hepatitis, STD, and TB Prevention
Centers for Disease Control and Prevention
Atlanta, Georgia
102. Hepatitis A

Richard J. Whitley, MD
University of Alabama at Birmingham
Birmingham, Alabama
123. Herpes Simplex Virus

Cynthia G. Whitney, MD, MPH
Respiratory Diseases Branch
Centers for Disease Control and Prevention
Atlanta, Georgia
115. A Multidisciplinary Approach for the Control and Prevention of Legionellosis

Mary E. Wilson, MD
Departments of Internal Medicine and Microbiology & Immunology
University of Iowa
Veterans' Affairs Medical Center
Iowa City, Iowa
134. Leishmaniasis

Sacoby M. Wilson, PhD, MS
Maryland Institute for Applied Environmental Health
University of Maryland
College Park, Maryland
66. Participatory Research for Environmental Justice: Advancements in Community Science and Innovation

Alison Winstead, MD
National Center for Emerging and Zoonotic Infectious Diseases (NCEZID)
Division of Foodborne, Waterborne, and Environmental Diseases (DFWED)
Centers for Disease Control and Prevention
Atlanta, Georgia
113. Escherichia coli, Diarrheagenic

Kevin L. Winthrop, MD, MPH
Professor of Infectious Diseases, Public Health, and Ophthalmology
Oregon Health and Sciences University
Portland, Oregon
59. Visual Disorders

Michael D. Wirth, PhD
Department of Epidemiology and Biostatistics and Cancer Prevention and Control Program
Arnold School of Public Heath
University of South Carolina
Columbia, South Carolina
183. Physical Activity Epidemiology in Health and Disease

Kimberly Won, PhD, MPH
Health Scientist
Center for Global Health
Division of Parasitic Diseases and Malaria
Centers for Disease Control and Prevention
Atlanta, Georgia
124. Vector-borne Filariases

Yue Wu, PhD, MS, RD
Nutrition Research Associate
Department of Nutritional Sciences
School of Public Health
University of Michigan
Ann Arbor, Michigan
180. The Principles of Nutritional Sciences: Nutrients, Nutrition Recommendations, and Dietary Guidelines

Dong Roman Xu, PhD, MPP
Sun Yat-sen Global Health Institute (SGHI)
School of Public Health & Institute of National Governance
Sun Yat-sen University
Guangzhou, China
19. Evaluating Progress in Global Health: Global Health Measures That Build Capacity

Lingshu Xue, MS
Department of Epidemiology
Graduate School of Public Health
University of Pittsburgh
Pittsburgh, Pennsylvania
53. Diabetes and Other Metabolic Disorders

Gavin Yamey, MD, MPH, MA
Professor of Global Health and Public Policy
Director of the Center for Policy Impact in Global Health
Duke Global Health Institute
Duke University
Durham, North Carolina
18. Global Health Financing: Mechanisms, Trends, and Opportunities

Lawrence Yang, PhD
Vice Chair and Associate Professor
Social and Behavioral Sciences
New York University
Adjunct Associate Professor
Department of Epidemiology
Columbia University
New York, New York
162. A Public Health Approach to Severe Mental Illness

Abdo Yazbeck, PhD
Lead Economist
Health Systems Governance and Financing Department
World Health Organization
Geneva, Switzerland
18. Global Health Financing: Mechanisms, Trends, and Opportunities

Valerie A. Yeager, DrPH, MPhil
Associate Professor
Indiana University Richard M. Fairbanks School of Public Health
Department of Health Policy & Management
Indianapolis, Indiana
46. The Public Health Workforce

Merissa A. Yellman, MPH
Division of Injury Prevention
National Center for Injury Prevention and Control
Centers for Disease Control and Prevention
Atlanta, Georgia
170. Road Safety and Injury Prevention

Jonathan S. Yoder, MSW, MPH
Waterborne Disease Prevention Branch
Division of Foodborne, Waterborne, and Environmental Diseases
National Center for Emerging and Zoonotic Infectious Diseases
Centers for Disease Control and Prevention
Atlanta, Georgia
116. Giardiasis

Italo B. Zecca, MPH, PhD
Department of Veterinary Integrative Biosciences
Texas A&M University
College Station, Texas
132. Chagas Disease (American Trypanosomiasis)

Jon Zelner, PhD
Assistant Professor
Department of Epidemiology
Center for Social Epidemiology and Public Health (CSEPH)
University of Michigan School of Public Health
Ann Arbor, Michigan
159. Introduction to Infectious Disease Modeling

Janice C. Zgibor, RPh, PhD, CPH, FACE
Associate Professor of Epidemiology and Pharmacy
Director of Doctoral Program in Epidemiology
Director of COPH Doctor of Public Health Program
Department of Epidemiology and Biostatistics
College of Public Health
University of South Florida
Tampa, Florida
53. Diabetes and Other Metabolic Disorders

Jim Zhang, PhD
Duke University Nicholas School of the Environment
Durham, North Carolina
70. Air Pollution

Junying Zhao, PhD, MPH, MSc, MBBS
Institute for Mathematical Behavioral Sciences
University of California, Irvine
Irvine, California
5. Public Health Informatics

Kai Zheng, PhD, FACMI
Department of Informatics
University of California, Irvine
Irvine, California
5. Public Health Informatics

Brian J. Zikmund-Fisher, PhD
Professor, Health Behavior & Health Education
School of Public Health
Research Associate Professor, Internal Medicine
Medical School
University of Michigan
Ann Arbor, Michigan
91. Vaccine Decision-making and Vaccine Hesitancy

Kara Zivin, PhD
Department of Psychiatry
University of Michigan Medical School
Ann Arbor, Michigan
163. Mood Disorders

Foreword

The first edition of Milton Rosenau's textbook of *Preventive Medicine and Hygiene* was published in 1913. This book appears just over 100 years later. It is identified as the 16th edition, which is justifiable despite the change in the title, the publisher, the increased number of editors, contributors, and the changes in emphasis on concepts, themes, and topics.

Early in the twentieth century, Milton Rosenau was the pre-eminent scholar of the science, art, and practice of public health. Rosenau and Kenneth Maxcy, his successor as editor, identified pathogenic microbes as the most dangerous threats to population health. By the time Philip Sartwell took over from Kenneth Maxcy, the importance of epidemiology as the basic science of public health was recognized. Evidence-based public health practice was taking over from practice based on the observations and opinions of respected elders. Sartwell contributed a comprehensive summary of the science of epidemiology, and I enlarged on this during my time as editor. I also introduced chapters on the epidemiology of cancer, heart disease, and other "noncommunicable" conditions. More important, social and behavioral determinants of susceptibility to infectious pathogens such as ignorance and overcrowding were made explicit and discussed in chapters by experts in these domains. As knowledge and understanding expanded in the middle decades of the twentieth century, we became aware of the complex interconnections among causal factors that were often synergistic. The multifactoral causes of diseases of public health importance were recognized, and policies, strategies, and tactics to control and, if possible, to prevent such diseases were spelt out. The need for such comprehensive thinking and planning is well illustrated by the newly emergent public health problem of road traffic injury and death. Mitigation required road design that separated vehicles traveling in different directions at different speeds, limiting risks of collision at road junctions, etc., car design that protected drivers and passengers, and measures to ensure that drivers were well educated about safe operation of their cars, were fit to drive and their judgment was not impaired by use of alcohol, drugs, or prescribed medication.

Another set of scientific disciplines and technologies of increasing importance is environmental health. This examines threats to health caused by exposure to toxic chemicals, dusts, etc., often in workplaces and sometimes in dwellings adjacent to refineries, factories, etc., where these toxins are produced.

The editors and chapter authors of this most recent edition of *Public Health & Preventive Medicine* have reintroduced in modern guise, enlightened by current concepts of genetic determinants of disease, pertinent ideas derived from these concepts. The old debate about the relative importance of nature versus nurture in disease causation remains alive, enlightened now by technical advances and greatly increased knowledge and understanding. In truth, nature and nurture are equally important, a theme that is woven into the fabric of this exciting new edition.

John M. Last (September 22, 1926–September 11, 2019)
Editor, 11th, 12th, and 13th editions
November 2018

Preface

The first edition of Milton Rosenau's *Preventive Medicine and Hygiene*, the forbearer of the current text, was published over a century ago. Rosenau would go on to edit five more editions before he was followed by John Maxcy who served as editor for the 7th edition in 1952 after Rosenau's death. Maxcy was eventually succeeded in turn by John Last who was editor for the 11th, 12th, and 13th editions, thus establishing the Maxcy-Rosenau-Last moniker that remains with the text to this day. I was fortunate to communicate with John Last as I began my work on this project, and he was delighted to learn that a new edition was underway. He agreed to write a brief foreword, providing a direct link to the storied past of this book. Sadly, John passed away in October 2019 just shy of his 93rd birthday. However, the connection with the text's century-long lineage continues with Robert Wallace who coedited the 13th edition with John Last, served as editor for the 14th and 15th editions, and now Associate Editor for this, the 16th edition. I first met Bob several years ago when I became the Editor-in-Chief of the *American Journal of Preventive Medicine.* He was already an editor for the journal and graciously agreed to stay on with the new team. It was Bob who first approached me about serving as lead editor for this edition and for that I will always be grateful.

The *Maxcy-Rosenau-Last Public Health & Preventive Medicine* text has been with me the entirety of my professional life, and it would be hard to overstate the influence this book has had on me as a physician, public health practitioner, and academician. I purchased my first copy, the 11th edition, as a medical student almost 40 years ago. Although I had originally planned to be an evolutionary biologist, it was an encounter with public health through a reading of sociologist Paul Starr's Pulitzer Prize-winning 1982 book, *The Social Transformation of Medicine in America,* which irrevocably altered my career plans. Many years later, a chance meeting with Paul on an airport shuttle bus gave me an opportunity to share how important his book had been to my decision to enter medicine. The discovery of public health was a revelation for me, and I was seized with the idea of public health as my calling. I was further encouraged when I realized public health and preventive medicine were a recognized specialty in the field of medicine, which prompted my initial purchase of *Maxcy-Rosenau-Last Public Health & Preventive Medicine.* Although I eventually entered a Family Medicine residency at University of Michigan, it was the residency program in General Preventive Medicine and Public Health that originally drew me there, and I ended up serving as Director of the University of Michigan's Preventive Medicine Residency for 20 years. Following residency, I spent almost two decades in public health practice, initially at the Detroit-Wayne County Health Departments and years later culminating in my appointment as the Governor's Chief Medical Executive and State Epidemiologist before moving on to an academic career at the University of Michigan. Multiple editions of *Maxcy-Rosenau-Last* accompanied me throughout, and it would not be possible for me to recount the many times I have recommended the text to my students, preventive medicine residents, physician colleagues, and fellow faculty over the years.

It's been about 13 years since the last edition of this text was published, calling for a much-needed update to the rapidly expanding fields of preventive medicine and public health. Appearing for the first time in this edition are four new sections that will hopefully become indispensable to all future versions of the text including sections on Global Health (Section II); Health Disparities and Vulnerable Populations (Section III); Mental Health and Substance Use (Section IX); and Nutrition and Physical Activity (Section XI). These new sections are accompanied by major expansions of existing sections on Injury and Violence (Section X); Communicable Diseases (Section VIII); Noncommunicable and Chronic Conditions (Section VI); and Health Education, Health Behavior, and Health Communications (Section IV) along with a complete revision of the structure and content of Environmental and Occupational Health (Section VII). The addition of new sections and expansion of existing ones has resulted in a near doubling of chapters relative to prior editions and reflects the evolving and continually growing disciplines of public health and preventive medicine. I am especially pleased at the inclusion of an opening chapter on the history of this textbook set against the larger backdrop of preventive medicine's development including the origins of the American College of Preventive Medicine (ACPM) and the Association for Prevention Teaching and Research (APTR), the latter serving as the societal sponsor of this text for many years.

The public health and preventive medicine communities are currently confronting the COVID-19 pandemic, an unprecedented global health crisis that has affected every country worldwide. According to the WHO, as of March 2, 2021, there have been almost 15 million cases and over 2.5 million deaths from SARS-CoV-2, resulting in incalculable costs and profound disruption to the lives of people, societies, and countries everywhere. The pandemic has also underscored, perhaps in a way otherwise not possible, the vital role of public health and preventive medicine in addressing a global disaster of unimagined scale and, ultimately, in bringing it to an end. I remain confident we will prevail and hope that the information contained herein contributes to this and future efforts to promote health and prevent disease around the world in keeping with *Maxcy-Rosenau-Last Public Health & Preventive Medicine's* remarkable century of tradition.

Matthew L. Boulton
Ann Arbor, Michigan
March 2021

Acknowledgments

I would like to thank a number of colleagues whose assistance and support throughout this project made the publication of this text possible:

Kim J. Davis, Michael Weitz, and Rachel Norton of McGraw Hill Professional, Jyoti Shaw of MPS Limited, and Susan Oldenburg of McGraw Hill Professional, who collectively facilitated the overall production of this book. Their professionalism in all interactions made it a pleasure to work with them.

Jillian Morgan, who I have worked with for many years in her role as the outstanding Managing Editor of the *American Journal of Preventive Medicine* and applied those same invaluable skills in overseeing the administration of this textbook.

Robert B. Wallace, who served as Associate Editor for this text and first approached me about serving as Editor for this edition, which I deeply appreciate. As a widely respected and highly regarded scholar of preventive medicine and public health, Bob provided indispensable guidance and sage counsel throughout the entire process.

The section editors and chapter contributors who graciously donated their time and expertise as thought leaders in preventive medicine and public health.

And, finally, to John M. Last, who as an iconic figure in preventive medicine, public health, and epidemiology, served as lead editor of the 11th, 12th, and 13th editions and editor emeritus of the 14th and 15th editions of this text. John wrote the foreword for the 16th edition before his passing in fall 2019, building upon a legacy with this text perhaps matched only by Milton Rosenau as befits the title, *Maxcy-Rosenau-Last Public Health & Preventive Medicine*.

Section I

Section Editor
Matthew L. Boulton

Foundational Topics in Public Health and Preventive Medicine

CHAPTER

1 History of Preventive Medicine, Public Health, and a Century after Milton J. Rosenau's *Preventive Medicine and Hygiene*

Joel D. Howell

The first edition of this book was published in 1913 as Milton J. Rosenau's *Preventive Medicine and Hygiene*.[1] It has now persisted (and thrived) for well over a century. The editors that followed Rosenau included Kenneth Maxcy, John Last, and the current co-editors, Matthew L. Boulton and Bob Wallace. Rosenau's 1913 first edition was a path-breaking accomplishment when it first appeared, and its successors continue to be field-defining books well into the twenty-first century. This chapter will set the stage by discussing Rosenau's life and career, as well as by considering the state of public health and the tensions that existed in and around the writing of the first edition of book, especially regarding the relationship between public health and medicine. It will then shift to consider how and when the field of "preventive medicine" was created.

MILTON JOSEPH ROSENAU

Milton Joseph Rosenau was well-suited to write this book. Born in 1869, Rosenau had a career that witnessed some of most dramatic changes in ideas about disease and disease causation that the world has ever seen. Not only a witness to these events, he was associated with (and helped to shape) some of the most important institutions for the worlds of medicine and public health.[2,3]

Rosenau attended the oldest medical school in the country, the University of Pennsylvania. He graduated in 1889, only 7 years after the start of the microbiological revolution. The signal event in that epochal revolution came when the German scientist Robert Koch took advantage of new technological developments, such as improved microscopes, solid culture media, and dyes that could enable objects to be seen more clearly under the microscope, to fundamentally transform the way we think about disease through the first clear explication of what is now known as the "germ theory of disease." He not only identified the cause of tuberculosis—itself a massively significant finding, given that one out of every seven human beings was then dying of the disease—but also, and of much more importance, established a precise way of defining diseases that were caused by specific pathogenic organisms. Previously the actual cause of many diseases was a topic of heated debate. Was the disease caused by foul odors in the air? Or was it a consequence of rapid temperature change, or a family propensity to that disease? If people with a disease were found to harbor microorganisms within their body, were these microorganisms the cause of the disease, or a result of the disease? "Koch's postulates" provided answers to these questions. His postulates included specific, systematic steps that were necessary to establish a specific microorganism as the cause of a specific disease. As such, they offered a roadmap for scientists to study disease causation and opened the floodgates of scientific discovery. The discovery of *Mycobacterium tuberculosis* or the tubercle bacillus as the agent responsible for tuberculosis was soon followed by the discoveries of similarly specific agents for a wide range of diseases. It is truly difficult to overstate the incredible excitement the microbiological revolution created among physicians around the world.

Studying at one of the top medical schools in the United States, Rosenau doubtless shared in the excitement of these new scientific discoveries. However, these findings were coming from overseas. The United States did not at that time have scientific laboratories of any great sophistication. So, like so many others of his era who were to become leading lights in American healthcare and public health, Rosenau went abroad to study with the leaders of this new revolution in Berlin, Paris, and Vienna.[4]

Having become acquainted with the very latest research in the rapidly growing field of infectious diseases, Rosenau returned to the United States with a new set of skills and ideas. From 1890 to 1909, he worked in the United States Public Health Service including the last 10 years as the second Director of the U.S. Hygienic Laboratory. The Hygienic Laboratory had recently moved to a small building on the corner of 25th and E streets, NW, in Washington, DC. It was eventually to become the National Institutes of Health (NIH) in Bethesda, Maryland, the center of healthcare research in the country. Rosenau worked in the Hygienic Laboratory on direct therapeutic implications of the germ theory, including tetanus and diphtheria antitoxin. He helped establish standards for vaccine potency, which led to an increased role for the government in the supervision of vaccine production. This work had clear implications for preventive medicine. It was also part of a widespread move toward increasing centralization and standardization of therapeutic agents. In 1906, passage of the Pure Food and Drug Act marked another step toward consumer protection, one that led to creation of the Food and Drug Administration.

From the Hygienic Laboratory, Rosenau moved into a new phase of his career, working as an author and educator to create the next generation of public health practitioners. From 1909 to 1935, he held at Harvard the first chair of Preventive Medicine and Hygiene in an American medical school. He authored a book, *The Milk Question,* in 1912, addressing a crucial topic for public health and preventive medicine, as will be discussed below. In 1913 came his *magnum opus*, the first edition of this classic textbook, which has helped to train countless people for over 100 years. In 1936, Rosenau moved to the University of North Carolina as Professor of Epidemiology. There he built a new school of public health (1940), and continued in the mission of educating the next generation of public health practitioners, serving as dean until his death in 1946. His distinguished career included terms as president of the Society of American Bacteriologists (1934) and the American Public Health Association (APHA) (1944).

THE STATE OF PUBLIC HEALTH

When Rosenau wrote his book, the general topic of public health and preventive medicine had been around in various forms for some time. The subject was located under a variety of terms such as public health, public hygiene, sanitary science, sanitation, and others.[5] In the middle of the nineteenth century, few medical schools explicitly taught such subjects. One exception was the women's medical colleges, which paid more attention to teaching hygiene than the other, all-male schools.[6] One example was the Women's Medical College of Pennsylvania, founded in 1850 to train women physicians, in which preventive medicine and personal and public hygiene long played a central role in the curriculum. Another exception was the University of Maryland, which established a chair in Materia Medica, Therapeutics, Hygiene, and Medical Jurisprudence in 1833.[7] From 1861 to 1865, the U.S. Civil War forced medical schools to pay more attention to hygiene. Wounded troops required attention in field hospitals, which had to be kept clean. Most wartime deaths were not due to enemy fire but due to widespread epidemic diseases. Even before the advent of germ theory, sanitary scientists knew that powerful chemicals such as iodides, as well as disinfectants like lime and carbolic acid, were effective in not only reducing the morbid odors but also reducing the spread of diseases such as cholera.[5] U.S. medical schools responded to military needs for instruction in hygiene by creating new courses. By the end of the war, about a third of U.S. medical schools offered instruction in the subject.

Issues of public health were of great practical importance for other reasons. Epidemics, in which clusters of people came down with a disease, had been recognized for some time. One way of controlling (or at least mitigating) the spread of epidemic diseases was by quarantining people with the disease, or those who had been exposed to the disease. Smallpox and yellow fever were most common diseases quarantined in the early days of the country. If a ship arrived on which passengers or crew were suspected of having a contagious disease, it would be prevented from docking and sent to an isolated place until the incubation period had passed. By the eighteenth century, most U.S. cities on the Atlantic coast had passed quarantine laws and many had built pesthouses to hold potentially infectious immigrants. This was an effective, albeit harsh method of prevention. It was also one with significant economic consequences.

As industries became more effective and improved methods of transportation made increased trading possible, there was increasing profit to be made. In that setting, the idea of quarantine increased tension between those who wanted to see disease as being contagious and those who did not. The contagious advocates saw the cause of disease as being carried in individuals. For them, quarantine was an obvious intervention. The anticontagionist advocates saw the cause as more likely coming from the environment, such as rotting organic material. Rather than quarantine they advocated clean water, sewage disposal, and garbage disposal. While prior to 1882 neither side was able to clearly articulate microorganisms as the cause of disease, both advocated interventions that clearly "worked" in the sense of preventing disease. Rosenau had himself worked as a quarantine officer, and was personally familiar with the difficult decisions that had to be made.

By the 1880s, public health and preventive medicine were seen as important and scientific. Their practitioners organized to promote the public's health, forming the APHA in 1872. At the first conference, the association leadership opened with remarks that emphasized the importance of preventive medicine and made no distinction between public health and preventive medicine: "If … the medical profession was as much devoted to the practice of the art of preventing as it is in curing disease, there can be no doubt that many diseases which now decimate communities would disappear altogether."[8] The APHA was initially dominated by physicians, who made up some 80% of the early membership. Public health advocates and physicians often worked closely together, sharing similar outlooks and seeking similar goals.[9] Medical schools responded to this interest by devoting significant amounts of curricular time to related topics. At the University of Michigan in the 1890s, the medical school course in hygiene lasted about 80 hours. The intent was not to make all medical students sanitarians. Rather, the belief was that such material was essential to becoming a skilled physician.[6] Advocates saw the increasing importance of public health as obvious and likely to continue.

Meanwhile, large cities such as Boston and New York City started to create public health departments. These departments could coordinate inoculation campaigns, supply diagnostic laboratory testing, isolate patients with communicable diseases, and lead campaigns for clean water and pure milk. Public health movements were slower to reach into the more rural parts of the country. Even so, some public health innovations could have effects on the entire population, such as the decision to have salt manufacturers add a small amount of iodine to the salt that they sold. This simple intervention led to a dramatic decrease in the incidence of thyroid diseases.[10] Ideas about domestic application of preventive medicine incorporated older ideas of dirt and ideas with the new germ theory.[11]

So, when Rosenau sat down to write his *magnum opus* he did so in a world that saw clearly the value of public health and preventive medicine. It was a world that had been transformed by the discovery of the germ theory only a few decades earlier. Public health and preventive medicine seemed to have much to offer the population. But there was no definitive source to consult for information across the breadth of the field. Rosenau set out to create one.

THE BOOK

At 1034 pages (not including a 40-page index), *Preventive Medicine and Hygiene* certainly made a serious attempt to cover the waterfront of what was then preventive medicine. Although he thanked a number of people for help, Rosenau wrote all but a very few of the 1034 pages by himself. He was well-equipped to do so, having acquired a breadth of experience through his 23 years in public health, which he acknowledged in his preface. He noted that he had worked in several different places, both in the United States and abroad, including the tropics, which gave him a broad background from which to consider the field.

The book was divided into two major parts. The first dealt with individuals—what Rosenau termed the subject of "hygiene," and included chapters on communicable diseases, heredity, eugenics, and other subjects. The second part dealt with the environment, what he termed "sanitation," and included chapters on food, water, air, soil, vital statistics, and quarantine. He was careful to note that economics and social context played a central role in preventive medicine.

Perhaps not surprisingly, Rosenau started Chapter 1 with smallpox, a classic disease for anyone interested in public health. Smallpox was characterized by its tendency to lead to scars or blindness. It was known to spread explosively among populations where there was no immunity, as had happened when Europeans first came to North America. Prevention had long rested on the observation that survivors of the disease seemed to be immune to further illness. Based on that finding, families would intentionally expose their children to a mild case, hoping to prevent a more serious case later on. Sometimes this worked; sometimes the intentionally produced case turned out to be quite severe. In the late eighteenth century, the English physician and naturalist William Jenner had learned about intentional infection with cowpox. Cowpox was thought to produce a milder form of the disease, and still prevent the more serious smallpox. Jenner tried an experiment, injecting an 8-year-old boy, James Phipps, first with cowpox, and then with an active case of smallpox. Young Phipps did not come down with smallpox. In 1798 Jenner published the results. Smallpox vaccination quickly became widely established thereafter and was widely used in North America. Note that this example of preventive medicine was possible without any knowledge of the causative organism.

Moreover, Rosenau had personal experience with the disease. In 1895, he had been tasked with controlling a smallpox epidemic among about a thousand African Americans attempting to return across the border back to the United States from Mexico, in Eagle Pass, Texas. They were living in a camp, which Rosenau renamed "Camp Jenner," after the pioneering innovator. Rosenau attempted to control the outbreak using a new vaccines; some historians have suggested that the new vaccine may have had mixed and somewhat deleterious effects.[12] So not only was smallpox an important and well-known disease, it was one that Rosenau had himself tried to control in the community.

In his textbook, Rosenau described the disease in depth, including detailed instructions on how to vaccinate to prevent infections. It is worth noting that he explicitly discussed the problems caused by people who refused to be vaccinated. He carefully considered the science and the existing laws, and compared the results of compulsory vaccination laws in Germany with the existence of a "conscience clause" in England, which had led to many people remaining unvaccinated, to the detriment of the public health. Rosenau concluded that compulsory vaccination is the preferable public policy in order to prevent spread of the disease.

Rosenau discussed tuberculosis, which he dubbed the most frequent and widespread of all the major diseases, responsible for 9% of all deaths in the United States. What made the impact of tuberculosis even more striking was that those deaths were disproportionately found among the most productive members of society—30% of all deaths of people between ages of 15 and 60. Moreover, the disease was far more common among the poor than the well-to-do. Prevention was based on avoiding contact with infection and increasing personal resistance through improved hygiene. The disease, Rosenau averred, had become not just a medical, but also a sociological problem. He felt that adequate health insurance could be a major adjunct to medical treatment—and here again Rosenau looked to Germany to demonstrate the value of such insurance.

Cholera had been linked with contaminated drinking water long before Koch identified the organism that causes the disease in 1884. In 1854, the English physician John Snow carefully tracked cases of cholera and identified the source as a pump in the London Area of Soho, on Broad Street. Rosenau offered a detailed description of John Snow's exploits in his textbook, both in the section on infectious diseases and later in the section under diseases due to water. Rosenau saw quarantine as an effective means of prevention, albeit a method of control that often treated immigrants badly. Rosenau had personally witnessed the Hamburg epidemic of 1892 and traced the cause as recent immigrants from either Russia or France. On the whole, he saw cholera as a "signal" success story for public health. In the textbook he devoted considerable space to a detailed discussion of the theory of quarantines and to the procedures necessary for their implementation. He then went on to discuss a wide range of other diseases seen as communicable, including influenza, insect-borne diseases, and the common cold.

The book's Section II covered topics such as immunity, heredity, and eugenics. Rosenau saw immunity as the very foundation of preventive medicine. The field of immunology was a new and fruitful area of study, although Rosenau was well aware that people remained generally ignorant of the mechanism by which immunity was manifest. Gregor Mendel's laws of heredity had only recently been rediscovered, and the science of heredity was of enormous interest to numerous physicians. Like many others of the period, Rosenau saw what he called "the breeding of the fit and elimination of the unfit"—or, eugenics—as of particular importance for preventive medicine. One way of implementing this policy could be through sterilization of people thought to be carrying unwanted genes. Here Rosenau was a bit more hesitant than some of his contemporaries, opining that implementing eugenics through such a method "contains great possibilities for abuse and injustice."

In the next section, Section III, Rosenau turned his attention to what was termed sanitation. Here he included foods, both animal and plant. He took up questions about how much food people ought to eat and the problems that could come from ingesting adulterated food. He devoted considerable space to a discussion of milk. Adulterated milk was then a major public health concern, being responsible for more sickness and death than all other foods combined. Rosenau pointed out a number of factors that made milk a liquid especially prone to becoming adulterated with bacterial infection. Milk is a good culture medium for bacteria. It is hard to transport in a satisfactory condition, and it was routinely consumed when raw. Fortunately, there existed an effective way to effectively prevent milk-borne diseases. The noted French wine chemist Louis Pasteur had discovered that heating milk would make it safe to drink, in a process that now bears his name, "Pasteurization." In his book Rosenau notes that, "Next to water purification, Pasteurization is the most important single preventive measure in the field of sanitation." Indeed, Rosenau had already made a significant contribution to the process of Pasteurization. The high temperatures initially used for Pasteurization gave the milk an unpleasant "cooked milk" taste. Rosenau demonstrated that slower pasteurization at a lower temperature could make the milk safe without ruining the taste. But many Americans continued to consume their milk raw.

Sections IV, V, and VI dealt with air, soil, and water. Rosenau addressed how each of these environmental factors could play a role in creating disease. He gave special attention to the role of the public health professional and how best to effectively use the laboratory to assess the quality of the environment.

The remainder of the book, Sections VII–XII, dealt with the disposal of sewage and refuse, vital statistics, what we would today call "occupational diseases," schools, and disinfection. This section covered everything from the usual meaning of "sanitary" science to a detailed discussion of what makes a proper student desk.

MEDICINE AND PUBLIC HEALTH

If preventive medicine was, in fact, valuable, where should it be taught? And to whom? At the turn of the twentieth century, many healthcare professionals had the idea that preventive medicine should, and would, become central to the education of future physicians and be based within medical schools. And those advocates had allies with deep pockets. Founded by the oil magnate John D. Rockefeller in 1913, the Rockefeller Foundation had quickly become the most influential funder of health-related research and education in the world, and the Foundation saw prevention as absolutely central to medical care. In a 1920 report, the president of the Rockefeller Foundation offers insight into his ideas about preventive medicine. Writing this commentary as the United States was energized by an industrial boom in which railroads, factories, and automobiles were seen as key to the nation's progress, he said:

> "A railroad spends more money on train and track inspection than on wreck crews. The average automobile owner is on the watch for signs of motor trouble and does not wait until there is a breakdown. The factory manager looks solicitously after his machines and does all he can to guard against interruptions in production. The human body, which is vastly more complex than any machine, is in need of vigilant care and frequent examination. Yet for the most part it is neglected until pain and disability sound an unmistakable alarm. Then the doctor is called in and too often is expected to do the impossible."[13]

In other words, according to the president of the Rockefeller Foundation, preventive medicine ought to be the physician's central mission.

He wrote these words shortly after the end of World War 1 (WW1), a war that had offered a remarkable demonstration of the value of preventive medicine. Its value had been demonstrated by the success in almost completely eliminating the epidemics that previously had been characteristic of wars. Indeed, preventive medicine had "almost unlimited potentials and possibilities." Great Britain was considering establishment of a ministry of health, and observers thought that perhaps the United States should follow their lead and create a national department of health.[14]

But that sort of thinking was already starting to loose traction early in the twentieth century, as the essence of what was to be seen as "modern medicine" began to change. Germ theory and microscopes became increasingly associated not so much with the health of populations, but with new and exciting science and technology focused on individual people. Tools such as the newly invented X-ray machine and the electrocardiograph machine attracted excitement both within and outside of medicine. Animal experimentation led to the discovery of insulin and a treatment for diabetes—a development seen as truly miraculous, and one that offered hope to patients with other chronic, noninfectious diseases. Urbanization, improved transportation, and new diagnostic technology all contributed to the increasing importance of hospital care and the movement of medical education away from the community and into a hospital ward. Students no longer got to know patients in their home and community, but first met them on a hospital ward. All of this tended to make medicine look inward, to look at a person with a disease not in relationship to their environment, but rather to see in a sick person a set of bodily organs infected by a specially identified microorganism, or a set of physiological functions gone awry.

Medical education was in flux, moving from apprentice-based training and proprietary schools to laboratory experimentation and university-based education. But the considerable efforts of reformers, many supported by the Rockefeller Foundation, generally failed to do little to dissuade the medical schools from being increasingly focused on disease detection and treatment. As the amount of experimental science put into the curriculum went up, the amount of preventive medicine went down. The end result was physicians going into practice with insufficient understand of the basic principles of public health. A 1931 review of medical education concluded that teaching of preventive medicine was in general "desultory, uninteresting, and poorly … organized."[15]

The problem extended beyond simply the care of individual patients by a physician. The lack of education about preventive medicine and public health too-often meant that physicians did not understand the functioning of the local public health officers and how best to work with them. "Because of the advances of medical knowledge, the medical school curriculum has become so crowded that the social importance of preventive medicine and public health is seldom emphasized. This creates a blind spot which often persists throughout professional life and results at times in misunderstandings between the practicing physicians and the constituted health authorities of the community."[16]

Physicians had ample reasons to question public health. They debated whether they ought to be concerned only with the treatment of individual patients, or whether their concerns extended to the treatment of diseases through social measures, what was referred to as "sanitation."[5,9] As physicians became more powerful in their therapeutic interventions and more comfortable in their social standing, they sometimes perceived public health initiatives as encroaching on the importance of the individual doctor-patient relationship, or even their social standing, as some perceived a status difference between physicians in practice and public health physicians. Some physicians even saw public health programs as posing a threat to their newfound economic security, fearing that the free care provided by the clinic, along with the effectiveness of new prevention methods, would mean less work for them. While the visions of medicine and public health were not always in opposition, the increasing dominance of medicine's inward-looking vision combined with the increasing prevalence of hospital care meant that preventive medicine had a harder and harder time finding space in the medical schools.

But the field of public health was not static. It was growing and coming to include a wide range of sophisticated topics (as a glance at the 1913 edition of this textbook will make clear). And the new tools and techniques were having a positive effect on community health in general. For all of these reasons, Rosenau thought public health ought to be taught not as part of medical school training for physicians, but in an independent school. Early on he had helped to create a new training model for public health by combining courses at the Massachusetts Institute of Technology and Harvard to create the School for Health Officers. He noted that in 1915 hygiene was included as a major subject in only three medical schools (Harvard, the University of Michigan, and the University of Pennsylvania). Rosenau thought that despite the pedagogical advantages of having medical students conduct a sanitary survey, what was really needed was separate educational facilities to teach preventive medicine, and went on to make the case for separate schools of public health devoted to the topic:

> "The teaching of hygiene is becoming increasingly difficult, on account of the widening scope of the subject, including preventive medicine, sanitary engineering, vital statistics, epidemiology, industrial hygiene and public health activities generally. It has become necessary to establish special schools with graded courses to meet the demand of training men to become public health officers. It is slowly being recognized that the training received for the M.D. degree, even in our best medical schools, does not properly fit a man to enter public health work. Sanitation and hygiene has become a separate profession."[17]

Also published in 1915 was the Welch-Rose report. Authored by the founding dean of the Johns Hopkins School of Medicine and Wycliffe Rose of the Rockefeller Foundation, the report guided the Foundation's investments over the next few decades, starting with the opening of the Johns Hopkins School of Hygiene and Public Health the very next year. By 1947 a total of 10 university-based schools of public had been founded, thus helping to institutionalize a model of public health education as separate from medical education.[9]

Rosenau fought for a separate school of public health at Harvard, often more vigorously than his superiors. In 1914, he wrote to the Rockefeller Foundation and asked them to fund the public health school as a separate entity. But he failed to gain the support of his superiors before doing so. Harvard's president, Abbott Lawrence Lowell, made it very clear that Rosenau's appeal was that of a single voice, and did not have the support of the university as a whole. Perhaps as a result of Lawrence's opposition, the request was unsuccessful. Rosenau did live (barely) long enough to see the Harvard School of Public Health separate from the medical school in 1946.

ORGANIZATIONS AND PUBLICATIONS

It is one thing to have ideas about prevention, and it is another to put them into the curriculum of a professional school. It is quite another undertaking to create a specialty of preventive medicine, and it is to that process that we now turn. As this textbook went through subsequent editions after 1913, the field of preventive medicine made its way toward becoming a specialty, a specialty marked (as are most specialties) by special organizations, journals, and certifications. The move to specialization in preventive medicine did not take place in isolation, but took place within the context of a much broader move to specialization in general, especially in health-related areas.

During much of the nineteenth century, anyone who wanted to practice medicine was free to do so, whether or not they had ever received any training in the field. There were no licensure laws, no formal certification of skills necessary to set up practice as a physician. Generalism was the highest level of practice; specialists were often seen as incompetent quacks. This attitude began to change around the turn of the twentieth century. One of the main drivers toward specialization was the invention of new tools that required specific expertise to use, such as the ophthalmoscope or the X-ray machine. Another driver was the acquisition of specific skills, such as the ability to do surgery.

But how to identify someone as a specialist?[18] Around the turn of the twentieth century, states began to pass laws requiring that physicians obtain a license in order to legally practice. Being a specialist could have taken a similar path, and specialists could have been defined by state or federal licensure. Or, specialists could have come to be defined by a university degree, or by membership in a specialty society, or simply by having completed a training program. Instead, the choice was made to identify specialists as those who were certified by a specialty board. The first specialty board to be established was the American Board of Ophthalmology in 1917, soon followed by boards in Otolaryngology, Obstetrics and Gynecology, and Dermatology. In 1933–34 the Advisory Board for Medical Specialties (ABMS) was formed (later, in 1970, the American Board of Medical Specialties), in order to coordinate and approve medical specialization.

Still, before World War 2 (WW2) few physicians opted to become specialists. But WW2 served as a major stimulus for growth in specialization. Physicians went to war by the thousands. Once in the military they entered a medical department that at its peak was *three times* the size of the *entire* army in 1939. Decisions had to be made quickly about who was to be in charge, who was to be awarded a higher rank and more pay; those decisions were based on specialty certification. During the war, physicians saw the value of the latest scientific discoveries, in the form of advances such as penicillin and blood banking. When physicians returned home they found an expanded repertoire of opportunities for specialty training, including positions in an expanding VA system, as well as additional support in the form of the Serviceman's Readjustment Act of 1944, the GI Bill of Rights. Extramural support for research from the NIH was rapidly increasing, helping to create an environment conducive to specialization. WW2 thus increased the perceived relevance of board certification and offered additional training opportunities. And physicians responded; the numbers (and percentage) of board-certified physicians started to grow exponentially. It did not hurt that at mid-century the possibilities for improving the health of the nation seemed almost boundless.[19]

It was in this immediate postwar context that discussions about board certification in preventive medicine started in September 1946.[20] Two months after the initial conversation the Committee on Professional Education of the APHA considered a recommendation that "A specialty board for public health physicians would further stimulate more adequate preparation of health officers for their responsibilities."[20] The recommendation went on to propose just what that adequate training might consist of: an internship, an MPH, 5 years of training approved by Council on Medical Education and Hospitals of the American Medical Association (AMA), and the public health physician's specialty board examination. Military service could also be used to fulfill some of the requirements.

As with other medical specialties, certification was to be limited to physicians. In order to make this point clear, especially to the AMA, the original board, named in 1947, was called the "American Board of Physicians in Preventive Medicine and Public Health" (ABPPMPH). The next year the word "physicians" was dropped and it became the "American Board of Preventive Medicine and Public Health" (ABPMPH). At the same time the military services agreed that specialists in preventive medicine ought to receive special recognition. Congress followed suit by awarding substantial pay increases to all military physicians who became board certified. On June 29, 1948 the ABPMPH was officially incorporated. Approval of the board by the ABMS followed in 1949, thus establishing preventive medicine board certification as the 18th core board certification available for physicians.

While board certification was to be restricted to physicians, the ABPMPH recognized the importance of all types of practitioners to the field. Thus, an important early step was to set the annual meetings of the corporation to coincide with the annual meeting of the entire APHA. This made clear the close relationship between the two organizations.

One issue that commonly arises when new specialty groups are formed is what to do about people who have already been working in the field. Who would be able to examine the people who had created the organization itself and who be themselves writing the original examinations? To solve the problem, the bylaws provided that a "Founders Group" would be exempt from examination; they were "grandfathered" in. These were to be people who had attained "unquestioned eminence in the field," or those with at least 10 years of distinguished service. An early estimate was that 25–400 people would meet these criteria. However, in the end at least 637 were admitted as members of the Public Health Founders Group.

This new field of preventive medicine was to prove a dynamic one. Healthcare needs and organization always reflect larger societal changes. In addition to the aforementioned early-twentieth-century innovations in medical technology, the invention of the airplane was to have an especially broad impact. Following the Wright brothers' successful 1913 flight at Kitty Hawk, North Carolina, aviation had come to play an ever-more central role in the nation's activities. And with air travel came a new set of healthcare issues. Airplanes played a crucial role during both WW1 and WW2. The special issues that confronted pilots and others associated with aviation drew the attention of a dedicated group of medical practitioners. Following in the footsteps of other specialties, a group of physicians gathered to try to establish specialty status for people working in aviation medicine. An Interim Board of Aviation Medicine was appointed in 1949. In 1951 that group applied to the ABMS to become an officially designated specialty board.

However, the ABMS turned them down. The ABMS was concerned that there were only two training programs, both in military facilities. In response, additional training programs were established. But on the reapplication, the ABMS suggested that instead of trying to become a primary specialty, the aviation physicians approach the ABPMPH and attempt to become a subspecialty. There was ample precedent for the model of an overarching larger specialty with subspecialty boards. One such example was Internal Medicine. Founded in 1936, by 1940 the American Board of Internal Medicine had established subspecialty certification in four fields: cardiology, gastroenterology, tuberculosis, and allergy. The aviation medicine group approached Internal Medicine and other boards to learn from their experience. In 1953, the aviation medicine program was approved as a subspecialty of preventive medicine. As was the case with earlier boards, there were 193 physicians admitted as members of a Founders Group. Aviation gradually came to include space travel; in 1963 the name of the board was changed from "aviation medicine" to "aerospace medicine."

Another group of physicians shared interests and expertise in occupational medicine. Early pioneers in occupational medicine include Alice Hamilton, who early in the twentieth-century pioneered awareness of health problems in the lead and munitions industries, as well as being Harvard's first female faculty member. (Hamilton came to Harvard in 1919 and remained until she retired in 1935. Rosenau played a key role in her recruitment.) Occupational medicine became an increasingly important topic as the United States started to become a more industrial society. A subspeciality board in industrial health and occupational medicine was initially proposed in 1949. After some discussion, applicants began to be approved in 1955, including 129 members of a Founders Group. The first written examinations were given in 1957. A certification in general preventive medicine was approved in 1961. Subsequently, subspecialties were added in undersea medicine (1989, changed to undersea and hyperbaric medicine in 1999), medical toxicology (1992), clinical informatics (2010), and addiction medicine (2016).

Like many boards, the ABPM has moved toward mechanisms for time-limited certification and established recertification processes. Much more about the history of the AABPM can be found in the extremely thorough review by Alice Ring, on which much of this section is based.[20]

Another marker of specialty formation is the existence of specialty societies. In 1954, some 30 or so preventive medicine physicians gathered for an organizational meeting in St. Petersburg, Florida, to form the American College of Preventive Medicine (ACPM).[21] The interrelationships of this group with existing organizations can be inferred by the fact that the meeting was announced in the newsletter of the American Board of Preventive Medicine, and the meeting was held together with annual meeting of the Southern Branch of the APHA. While a national organization may have been innovative, public health physicians in several states had already taken the lead in forming academies of preventive medicine, including those in North Carolina, Illinois, New York, and Florida. A resolution to form a national ACPM was adopted. It quickly grew. After 2 years, the academy had members from almost all states in the United States, as well as Canada and Europe. One of the charter members of the Academy was Jonas Salk of the University of Pittsburg, whose work on the polio vaccine has saved countless children from contacting this once common disease.

The various professional groups associated with preventive medicine worked closely together. From the early 1960s, the ACPM worked to evaluate and accredit residency programs at the request of the Joint Residency Review Committee, the AMA Council on Medical Education and Hospitals, and the ABPM, including evaluations of programs at universities, on military bases, and in public health departments and industrial plants.

Another major achievement was the creation of a new journal for preventive medicine, the *American Journal of Preventive Medicine.* This journal grew out of a collaboration between ACPM and another organization, the Association of Teachers of Preventive Medicine (ATPM). The ATPM was founded in 1942. Starting in 1975, ATPM sponsored the *Journal of Community Health*, a journal conceived out of frustration that the right questions about healthcare delivery were not being asked. It was intended to highlight "practice, teaching, and research in community health." The journal saw itself as tightly linked with its official sponsor, the ATPM, and intended to offer extensive analyses of teaching programs.[22]

The next few years saw a serious effort to bring ATPM and ACPM closer together. This took the form of joint sponsorship of scientific meetings, and, perhaps most important, joint sponsorship of the *American Journal of Preventive Medicine*, which was first published in 1985.[23] The ATPM withdrew its sponsorship of the *Journal of Community Health* in 1984, which broadened its scope in 1985 to become "The Publication of Health Promotion and Disease Prevention."

In its inaugural issue of 1985, the *American Journal of Preventive Medicine* published an article laying out the importance of preventive medicine for the needs of the healthcare system. Other articles addressed causes of mortality, ways that public health could interact with clinical delivery, and questions about water purity—the latter a topic that would also have seemed central for preventive medicine practitioners a century earlier.

Having worked together to create a journal, and sharing much in the way of a leadership and common vision, one might have thought that ACPM and ATPM could join forces to better accomplish their goals. From 1989 to 1990, a joint affiliation task force considered the possibility of a merger of the two groups. Several meetings led to the creation of a draft constitution and bylaws for a merged organization. However, the merger did not take place, largely because of concerns each group of members had about the membership characteristics of the proposed new organization. The ACPM membership consisted exclusively of physicians, and some members were concerned about admitting nonphysicians as full members of the ACPM. The ATPM members were unhappy that under the proposed merger the president of the new organization would have to be a physician, a criteria that would leave out some of their members. The two organizations thus moved forward with many shared goals (not to mention a shared journal), but as two distinct entities.

In 2006, ATPM changed its name to the Association for Prevention Teaching and Research (APTR). It is now the national professional membership association for medical and health professions institutions and their faculty teaching and researching prevention and preventive medicine. It develops curricular resources, collaborates with federal agencies, organizes an annual meeting, and continues to co-sponsor AJPM. ACPM is made up of preventive medicine and public health physicians. Its goal is to represent and support its members as public health and health systems leaders and serves as the other co-sponsor of AJPM.

CONCLUSION

Public health and preventive medicine have changed quite a bit since this textbook was first published in 1913. New ideas and new tools have shaped what it means to practice preventive medicine. Certification, specialization, journals, and societies have been created. While impossible to know for certain, it seems likely that most of the people involved in these changes were familiar with, had read, or had been significantly influenced by one of the editions of this textbook that have been published since 1913.

Looking back at the original edition from the perspective of the present, it is not surprising that many things have changed. On the other hand, in some respects Rosenau seems to have nicely anticipated current issues and debates.

Smallpox is gone. After a worldwide effort to reach all naturally occurring cases of the disease, in 1979 the WHO formally declared that smallpox had been eradicated. On the other hand, over a century later Rosenau's discussion of vaccination seems eerily prescient. Albeit for different diseases, many contemporary events—such as the recent measles epidemic—raise many of the same arguments that Rosenau pointed out vis-à-vis smallpox inoculation.

While much less common, tuberculosis is still with us. Although Rosenau could not have even imagined antibiotic treatment as we know it today, almost everything else he recommended would still make complete sense. The disease, Rosenau averred in 1913, had become not just a medical, but also a sociological problem. Adequate health insurance was a major adjunct to medical treatment—and here Rosenau looked to Germany as an example of the value of such insurance. Today, we would tend to agree, and to make the points about healthcare coverage for many other diseases. Rosenau referred to Germany as an example of a system worth emulating. After WW1, he (and many other health reformers of the era) may have been slower to look to Germany as an example worthy of imitation. Today, as we grapple with questions about how best to organize healthcare delivery and financing, people continue to debate how (or if) we ought to turn to other countries for edification.

Quarantines are no longer as central a part of public health practice as they were in 1913. But they have not gone away, and continue to raise issues both ethical and operational, as recent experience with Ebola has demonstrated.

While Rosenau saw immunity as critically important, current ideas about the process are far different than he could have imagined.

And eugenics is no longer seen as acceptable, though we should note Rosenau's concerns about potential abuse using mandatory sterilization to carry out eugenic goals.

Preventive medicine is still the goal. Just how to get there is always a contested area. The hope is that early diagnosis will prevent more serious disease and prolong life. This led to the idea of annual examination, which dates back to the turn of the twentieth century.[24] Whether these examinations or screening tests achieve their goals of improving health remains, in many cases, a topic of active debate.

The chapter topics and content of this book have changed dramatically from the original 1913 edition. As has the authorship—Rosenau wrote much of the book himself, while today's version follows the usual twenty-first-century model of a multiauthor work. It is also being published (and read) electronically, a far different world than anyone in 1913 could have imagined. But in a broader (and perhaps more important) sense there are important continuities. The goals of preventive medicine remain essentially the same. The content of public health, as Rosenau emphasizes throughout, is inextricably embedded in the specific social context.[25,26] And the book serves as an introduction into a field of practice that was and continues to be essential for the health and well-being of all human beings.

References

1. Rosenau MJ. *Preventive Medicine and Hygiene*. New York: D. Appleton and Company; 1913. Available at https://babel.hathitrust.org/cgi/pt?id=mdp.39015009484430&view=image&seq=9.
2. Rosenau MJ. *AJPH*. 1946;35(5):530–1.
3. Rosenau MJ. *MMWR Weekly*. 1999;(40):907.
4. Bonner TN. *American Doctors and German Universities: A Chapter in International Intellectual Relations, 1870–1914*. Lincoln, NE: University of Nebraska Press; 1963.
5. Burnham JC. *Health Care in America: A History*. Baltimore, MD: Johns Hopkins University Press; 2015.
6. Leavitt JW. Public health and preventive medicine. In: Numbers RL, ed. *The Education of American Physicians*. Berkeley, CA: University of California Press; 1980, pp. 250–72.
7. Hannaway C, Dunglison R. In: Bynum WF, Bynum H, eds. *Dictionary of Medical Biography*. Westport, CT: Greenwood Press; 2007, pp. 440–1.
8. Terris M. Evolution of public health and preventive medicine in the United States. *AJPH*. 1975;65(2):161–9.
9. Brandt AM, Gardner M. Antagonism and accommodation: Interpreting the relationship between Public Health and Medicine in the United States during the 20th century. *AJPH*. 2000;90(5):707–15.
10. Semba RD. The impact of improved nutrition on disease prevention. In: Ward JW, Warren C, eds. *Silent Victories: The History and Progress of Public Health in Twentieth-Century America*. Oxford: Oxford University Press; 2007, pp. 170–2.
11. Tomes N. *The Gospel of Germs: Men, Women and the Microbe in American Life*. Cambridge, MA: Harvard University Press; 1999.
12. Mckiernan-Gonzalez J. *Fevered Measures: Public Health and Race at the Texas-Mexico Border 1848–1942*. Durham, NC: Duke University Press; 2012.
13. Vincent GE. *The Rockefeller Foundation: A Review for 1920, the Program for 1921*. New York: Rockefeller Foundation; 1921.
14. The progress of preventive medicine. *JAMA*. 1918;71(24):1999–2000.
15. Fee E. *Disease & Discovery: A History of the Johns Hopkins School of Hygiene and Public Health 1916–1939*. Baltimore, MD: Johns Hopkins University Press; 1987.
16. Miller JA, Baehr G, Corwin EHL. *Preventive Medicine in Modern Practice*. New York: PR Hoeber; 1942.
17. Rosenau MJ. The value of a sanitary service in the teaching of hygiene. *JAMA*. 1915;65:321–2.
18. Howell JD. The invention and development of American Internal Medicine. *J Gen Intern Med*. 1989;4:127–33.
19. Anderson OW, Rosen G. *An Examination of the Concept of Preventive Medicine*. New York: Health Information Foundation Research Series (12); 1960.
20. Ring AR. History of the American Board of Preventive Medicine. *Am J Prev Med*. 2002;22(4):296–319.
21. American College of Preventive Medicine. *50 Years of Leadership, Improving Health Yesterday, Today, and Tomorrow*. Washington, DC: ACPM; 2004.
22. Kane RL. By way of introduction. *J Community Health*. 1975;1(1):1–2.
23. Scutchfield FD. The Madeleine and the journal. *Am J Prev Med*. 2018;55(6):759–61.
24. Bullough B, Rosen G. *Preventive Medicine in the United States 1900–1990: Trends and Interpretations*. Canton, MA: Science History Publications, Watson Publishing; 1992.
25. Perdiguero E, Bernabeu J, Huertas R, et al. History of health: A valuable tool in public health. *J Epidemiol Community Health*. 2001;55:667–73.
26. Martin SC, Howell JD. One hundred years of clinical preventive medicine in America. *Prim Care*. 1989;16 (1):3–8.

CHAPTER

2

Population Health: Definitions, Tensions, and New Directions

Paula M. Lantz

Population health has long been a topic of great interest to population-based fields such as epidemiology, social demography, geography, and public health. It is both a set of social indicators and a field of scientific interest and professional practice. Historically, for at least two centuries, population health has primarily been focused on the distributions and patterns of health outcomes and their causes in populations—typically based on geography and/or governmental authority—and sociodemographic subgroups within populations. The overarching objective of population health is to elucidate how social, economic, environmental, and ecological factors and changes within societies manifest—in both positive and negative ways—in health outcomes at the population level.[1]

The general foci of population health has historically included: (a) systematically measuring rates of health, morbidity, injury, and mortality in populations; (b) elucidating the determinants of health at both individual and population level; (c) identifying and addressing risks to population health; and (d) identifying and evaluating interventions aimed at improving population health and reducing distributional disparities.[2,3]

The key methods and metrics used in population health research and policy (listed in Box 2-1) are defined in a plethora of books and articles.[1–6] Population health data typically come from vital registration systems, censuses, public health reporting systems, numerous public and private administrative databases, and surveys, all with strong attention to capturing data from the entire "denominator" or population base from the which the data are gathered and should validly represent.[5] Population-level indicators such as life expectancy, mortality rates across the life course, unintentional injury incidence, risk behavior levels, preventable hospitalization rates, etc., represent both exposures and investments at the micro, mezzo, and macro levels, and are important signals regarding the physical, mental, and social health of populations. Surveillance and research using these metrics is a powerful tool for making absolute and relative comparisons within and across countries and their subpopulations in the cross-section and over time.

Although there is broad agreement on the general set of metrics for measuring health outcomes within and across populations, there is significant variation in the definition, use, and application of the term "population health" in science, practice, and policy. More recently, over the past two decades, there has been an increase in the number of both complementary and contradictory definitions and uses of the term "population health" and related concepts. As such, this chapter covers key aspects of population health, primarily in the context of the United States, in the following sections:

- Brief history of the broad concept of population health
- Frameworks for understanding the social determinants of health in populations
- Population health and the related fields of public health and preventive medicine, and the emergence of population medicine and population health management
- Tensions between competing definitions of and approaches to population health
- Opportunities and challenges for the field of population health
- Conclusions

BRIEF HISTORY OF POPULATION HEALTH

There is ample historical evidence across societies of a long-standing understanding of both the individual and social causes of the devastating impact of disease, injury, and death in communities. Early public health efforts recognized the importance of living conditions or "public hygiene" in the areas of water, air, food, housing, and work environments for health, and also that the poor were much more likely to suffer from disease, injury, and early death than those in elite or wealthy social classes. For example, German physician Johan Peter Frank, in the late 1700s, wrote and spoke about how poverty or "the people's misery is the mother of diseases."[1,7]

In his research on the history of population health, Szreter documented that in the 18th century period of progressive Enlightenment thought, "the dual revolutions of Republican liberty and expanding commerce in Europe and the Americas introduced a new rationalist and democratic agenda."[1] In the midst of significant concerns about potential health and social risks associated with the explosive economic and urban growth fueled by the Industrial Revolution, the revelation that improved health and well-being were indeed possible created new social and political agendas.[1]

Similarly, Kunitz has posited that two revolutions have shaped the primary ways in which health within populations is currently understood.[6] The first was the Industrial Revolution in western Europe, which brought into stark focus the unequal distribution of the significant benefits and costs of industrialization in terms of social welfare and public health across socioeconomic strata. The second revolution was that of germ theory and bacteriology in the late 19th century, which greatly elucidated the role of biology and pathogenesis in disease incidence and progression. While the latter is foundational for modern medicine, it is the understanding of the social structural, economic, and political factors related to health and disease that are foundational for the field of population health. As Kunitz argues, it is essential to understand how the social context of populations—their history, culture, economy, and political institutions—produces and shapes health distributions within populations for both scientific and intervention purposes.[6]

Public health movements in Europe and the United States in the late 19th and early 20th centuries directed interventions toward the strong link between poverty and disease, including through mechanisms related to "hygiene" and infectious disease exposure.[8,9] Early efforts focused strongly on the risks for infectious disease in the physical environment and their patterning by socioeconomic status. However, with the "epidemiologic transition," or the shift from higher

BOX 2-1. Key Population Health Indicators and Measures

Population-Level Health Indicators
Life expectancy
Healthy life expectancy or health-adjusted life expectancy
Disability-free life expectancy
Years of healthy life
Quality-adjusted life years (QALYs)
Disability-adjusted life years (DALYs)
Compression of morbidity
Total fertility rate

Measures of Mortality
Overall crude mortality rate
Overall age-standardized mortality rate
Cause-specific mortality rate
Age-specific mortality
Perinatal mortality rate
Infant mortality rate
Child mortality rate
Maternal mortality rate
Premature mortality (before age 65)
Years of life lost to premature mortality

Measures of Disease and Injury Frequency
Period incidence
Cumulative incidence
Incidence density
Point prevalence
Period prevalence

Measures of Physical and Mental Health Status
Self-reported overall health status
Disease/condition incidence and prevalence
Depressive symptoms scales
Depression scales
GAD-7 scale
CAGE alcohol screening tests
K6 scale
SF-36 (36-Item Short Form Survey)
Quality of Well-Being Scale
Sickness Impact Profile
Adverse Childhood Experiences scale

Measures of Functioning and Disability
Disability rates
Physical functioning scales
Activities of daily living
Instrumental activities of daily living
Cognitive impairment

Measures of Health Risk
Tobacco use
Alcohol use
Body mass index
Physical activity
Sedentary life style
Sleep quantity and quality
Substance abuse/addiction
Sexual risk taking
Seat belt use
Helmet use
Occupational injury risk

Measures of Healthcare Access and Utilization
Health insurance coverage
Usual source of primary healthcare
Healthcare utilization
Compliance with healthcare recommendations including prescriptions
Reported foregoing healthcare because of concerns about costs
Clinical preventive service use (immunizations, screening tests, teeth cleaning, etc.)

Measures of Socioeconomic Indicators Important for Population Health
Poverty rate
Unemployment rate
Average household income
Bankruptcy and foreclosure rates
Percentage of household on public assistance
Percentage of single-parent households
Percentage of children receiving free or reduce-price lunch
Concentrated disadvantage scales
Concentrated affluence scales
Percent of adults 25+ with less than high school education
Percent of adults 18+ with less than eighth-grade education
High school graduation and dropout rates
Percentage of third-grade and tenth-grade students reading at grade level
Percentage of tenth-grade students at grade level in math
Density of voluntary organizations
Voter registration and turnout rates

Measures of Health and Social Inequity
Odd ratios (with proper controls)
Relative versus absolute difference comparisons
Life-expectancy stratified by gender, race, ethnicity, education, geography
Mapping techniques to reveal geographic variation in age-adjusted rates of morbidity/mortality
Inequality in morbidity/mortality rates: Gini Index, Index of Dissimilarity, Lorenz Curve
Measures of income inequality: Gini Index; Palma Ratio; Hoover Index
Racial residential segregation measures: Index of Dissimilarity; Entropy Index

morbidity and mortality from infectious disease to longer life expectancy with a significant increase in chronic disease, it was increasingly recognized that the poor and others with relatively lower social standing were seemingly at risk for *all* types of injury, morbidity, and mortality.[10]

In the mid-20th century, the field of social epidemiology emerged with a strong and articulated focus on unequal distributions of social, economic, and political exposures and resources as the primary drivers—through physical, biological, and psychosocial pathways—of social inequalities in the distribution of health outcomes within societies.[11] Central to the social epidemiologic perspective on population health is the understanding that, while the main causes of illnesses and their risk factors within societies change over time, the patterning of most measures of health by individuals' position within the socioeconomic structure of the population persists.

Key Population Health Constructs

Although populations comprise individuals and health is expressed in individual bodies, the field of population health is primarily interested in understanding and intervening upon the myriad factors and processes that work at levels above the individual. Many of risks and processes of interest to population health are group and population-level rather than individual-level phenomena (Box 2-1). For example, life expectancy is a population-level synthetic or simulated statistic that estimates the average life expectancy of a cohort of people born into a population if they—as an aggregate—were to go through life experiencing current age-specific mortality rates.[12]

In addition, population health scientists focus on critically important population-level processes such as herd immunity and tipping points in different types of disease outbreaks or epidemics. Many social demographers are interested in the interconnected patterns of migration, fertility, and mortality within populations and subpopulations. Social epidemiologists, for example, consider such questions as how economic recessions influence mortality rates in a population, and how both absolute and relative income inequality within populations influence its health patterns.[13,14] Of additional interest to population health scientists are the effects of organizational, neighborhood, community, and other mezzo-level phenomenon on individual health, including the influence of societal processes such as segregation on health disparities.[15,16]

Population Health and Risk Distributions

Rose articulated the important insight that an individual's risk of illness cannot be separated from the *risk distribution* within the population to which she/he belongs.[17] Key to this simple yet core insight is the recognition that there is a difference between *sick individuals* and *sick populations*. In the latter case, a disease or health condition becomes more prevalent in a society primarily because there has been an increase in the number of people at *some* rather than high risk. This way of thinking has important implications for prevention. If the strategy is to identify only those individuals at "high risk" for injury or disease, the incidence and prevalence of the condition will not be changed as much as if prevention efforts attempt to shift the distribution of all risk within the population.

For example, attempts to decrease the current high rates of diabetes mellitus in many countries are primarily focused on identifying people at high risk based on their body mass index or hemoglobin A1c levels. Identifying individuals who are at high risk and targeting them with diabetes prevention interventions can indeed reduce the rates at which those people at high risk end up with a diagnosis of Type II diabetes.[18] However, this type of strategy is quite inefficient if the overall goal is to reduce the incidence and prevalence of diabetes within the population. Population-level strategies that attempt to intervene on the environmental, social, and behavioral factors that lead to increased weight and sedentary lifestyles will shift the risk distribution of the *entire* population, and thus be more efficient and effective in terms of the overall health of the population.

Additional examples abound, including not only for the risk of chronic or infectious disease but also for the risk of mental illness, injury, and violence. For example, invoking Durkheim's classic insights about how the rate of suicide in a society is a result of social structures and processes, Berkman and Kiwachi observed that there "are myriad reasons why any individual commits suicide, yet such individuals come and go while the *social* rate of suicide remains predictable."[11]

Summary

Population health is focused on the distribution and social patterning of all health risks (biological, chemical, physical, social, behavioral, and psychological) and their outcomes within populations, which are more than the sum of the individuals within them.[19] The distributions of risk, illness, and health within populations are the core focus of research and intervention design. As such, population health focuses on the question of *why does a particular population or subpopulation have a specific distribution of risk* rather than why do some individual people get sick/injured when others do not? [17]

The result is that the greatest improvements in population health status and health equity within populations will result from attempting to answer the first question and figuring out how to shift or positively change the distribution of risk.[17,20] And the most effective way to impact population risk distributions is to intervene at levels about the individual (i.e., at the institutional, community, policy, and system levels). Simulation models and empirical analyses have demonstrated that low-cost population level interventions often have better benefit-cost ratios than interventions tailored to individuals at highest risk.[21]

FRAMEWORKS FOR UNDERSTANDING THE SOCIAL DETERMINANTS OF HEALTH

Social Ecological Model of Health

A key component of population health is the understanding of the myriad societal or social determinants of health and how these factors play out at multiple levels within society. The *social ecological model* of population health includes five levels at which social processes and factors produce both health and health disparities[22]:

1. **Intrapersonal level**: Factors within individuals such as knowledge, attitudes, and behaviors, along with genetic predispositions.
2. **Interpersonal level**: Factors that occur in relationships between individuals, such as peer influences, psychosocial support, family dynamics.
3. **Institutional level**: Factors and processes that occur within institutions in which individuals spend time, such as schools, churches, worksites, local organizations and agencies, etc.
4. **Community level:** Factors and process that occur in the neighborhoods and communities in which people live, work, and play, such as environmental exposures in air, water, and the housing stock, rates of crime and other safety issues, rates of poverty, unemployment and food security, community cohesion and social capital, community-level resources related to health and social services, etc.
5. **Systems level:** Macro-level factors such as large systems of institutions and the political economy; this includes macroeconomic factors like recession, inflation, and jobs creations; healthcare and health insurance systems, and public policies in myriad areas include taxation, employment, public education, housing, transportation, social welfare, crime and policing, environment, segregation, migration, civil rights, etc.

All levels in the model are embedded within and influenced by higher levels in the model; and all levels play a role in creating specific types of health distributions and disparities. In addition, all levels in the model provide opportunities for intervention, although it is the more "upstream" or mezzo (organizational or community) and macro (system) levels where interventions have the greatest impact for preventing, alleviating, or shifting the negative distributions of the fundamental causes of health risks within populations.

WORLD HEALTH ORGANIZATION CONCEPTUAL FRAMEWORK OF SOCIAL DETERMINANTS OF HEALTH

In 2010, the World Health Organization (WHO) introduced a detailed and multilevel conceptual framework of the social determinants of health and health inequities.[23] The WHO framework (Fig. 2-1) posits that health and well-being are determined by *social structural factors* at the macro level such as socioeconomic, political, and public policy contexts, with a strong focus on how these macro factors influence individuals' socioeconomic position (education, income, and occupation) within the social structures. In turn, these social structural factors and individuals' socioeconomic positions influence a broad set of intermediary social determinants at the mezzo and micro levels, including the material conditions or circumstances of living (housing, food, safety, etc.), health-related behaviors, biological factors, psychosocial processes, and personal healthcare services.

A robust finding from population health research in developed countries is that medical care (or individual healthcare services) is not a key factor in explaining levels of population health or social disparities in health outcomes within populations.[24,25] As such, in the WHO model, access to and use of healthcare services are considered as downstream determinants of health, primarily used after the onset of illness or disease.

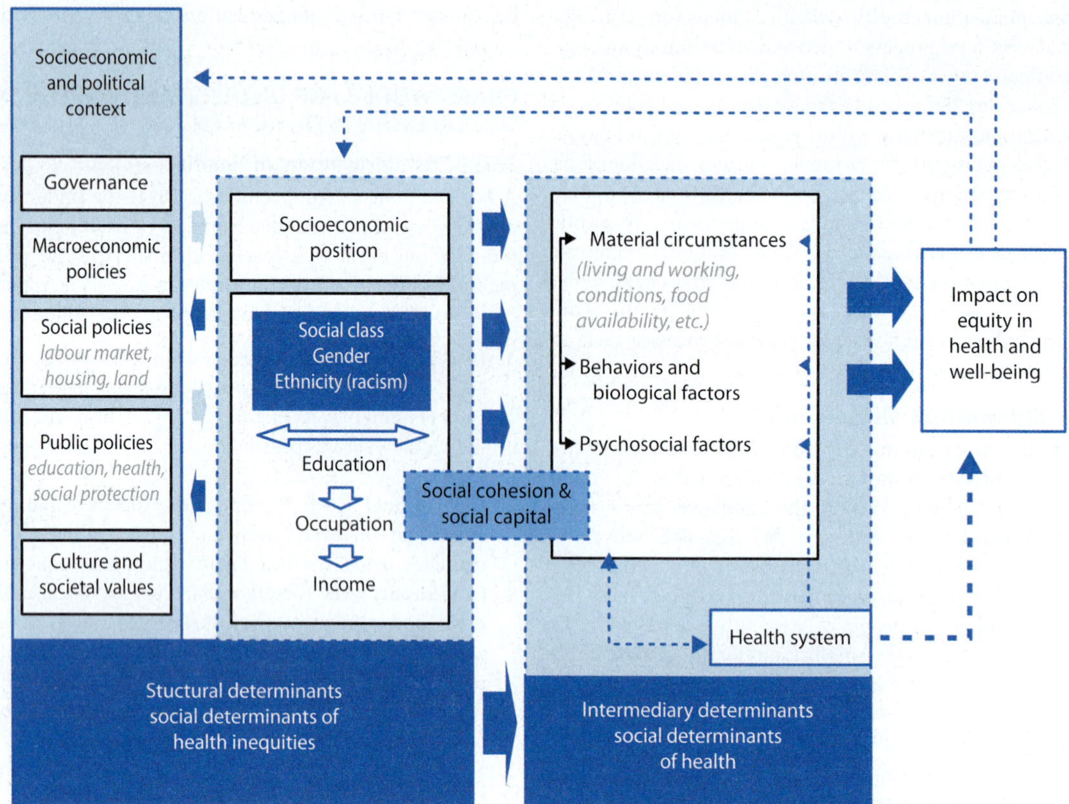

FIGURE 2-1. Word Health Organization Framework of the social determinants of health. Used with permission from Solar O, Irwin A. *A Conceptual Framework for Action on the Social Determinants of Health. Social Determinants of Health Discussion Paper 2 (policy and practice)*. Geneva, Switzerland: World Health Organization, 2010.

All of the factors in the WHO model work in multiple and often bidirectional ways to influence the expression of health at the micro, individual level. They also determine the social patterning of health and health inequities at the population level. The upstream factors—social structures/systems and public policy—are the driving force behind the strong patterns and disparities in health that are observed across socioeconomic, racial, ethnic, and other social factors. As Williams has articulated, "(s)ocial structure refers to enduring patterns of social life that shape an individual's attitudes and beliefs; behaviors and actions; and material and psychological resources."[26]

Key social structures that have been shown to be strongly related to socioeconomic and racial disparities in health include economic inequality, racism, discrimination, and segregation.[27] These macro-level social structures have a powerful impact on individuals' socioeconomic position and standing within society, which in turn fundamentally drives the material conditions of health (e.g., housing, food, safety, environmental quality, etc.) and access to healthcare.

Fundamental Causes Theory

To elucidate this critically important phenomenon in population health, Link and Phelan articulated the "fundamental causes" theory, which posits that the "enduring association" between socioeconomic status and health persists across time and societies because "SES embodies an array of resources, such as money, knowledge, prestige, power, and beneficial social connections that protect health no matter what mechanisms are relevant at any given time."[28] The fundamental cause perspective explains why the leading causes of morbidity and mortality are always patterned by socioeconomic position within societies, even though the actual causes change dramatically over time.

Public Policy in All Sectors Is Key to Population Health Improvement

All models of the social determinants of population health emphasize the importance of upstream social structural factors—including public policy—for both shaping health outcome distributions and also as a point of intervention. Public policy is a critically important lever for improving risk distributions within communities and the broader society. For example, a number of public policies and regulations related to education have had a positive impact on metrics of educational attainment and quality, including a reduction in racial disparities in key education metrics.[29] Tobacco control policies, including taxation, age of purchase laws, clean indoor air laws and public education campaigns, have all contributed to a sharp decline in smoking rates in the United States over the past several decades.[30]

CityHealth, a joint project of Kaiser Permanente and the de Beaumont Foundation, is promoting a package of evidence-based policy solutions that will shift population distribution risks and thus improve the health of communities and individuals living within them. The nine policies being promoted by this project are: (1) paid sick leave; (2) universal, high-quality pre-kindergarten; (3) affordable housing and inclusionary zoning; (4) complete streets (safe and accessible transportation); (5) alcohol sales control; (6) raising the legal age of retail tobacco sales to 21; (7) clean indoor air; (8) publically available food safety and restaurant inspection ratings; (9) healthy food procurement.[31]

While public policy can have a positive impact on individual health risks and risk distributions within communities and societies, it also can be a structural factor that contributes to or produces social inequalities that have a negative impact on health. That is, public policy is often the *cause* of the structural or macro-level forces that create health inequities within society. For example, the significant racial disparities in wealth in the United States stem in large part from social structures and public policies, including red-lining, that systematically hindered African Americans from access to mortgages and thus home ownership.[32] As another example of how public policy can fuel social and health disparities, land use planning and zoning policies have exacerbated the concentration of environmental hazards in lower income and racial minority neighborhoods, contributing to environmental racism and its impact on health.[33]

RELATED FIELDS OF PUBLIC HEALTH AND PREVENTIVE MEDICINE

Public Health

Although the field of population health has a long history of both science and practice, it also is a confusing endeavor to understand, given its overlap and conflation with a number of other health-oriented fields. Many people use the terms "population health" and "public health" interchangeably; and there is clearly a great deal of overlap in the focus and aims of these two fields of inquiry and practice. Both public health and population health are concerned with understanding and intervening upon the distributions of factors that both promote health and produce risks for health within populations, broadly defined.

Public health and population health are quite similar if the population in question is the total population in a geographic or geopolitically defined area such as a city, county, state, province, region, or country. If, however, the population in question is more narrowly defined, such as that of a healthcare provider or nursing home or Medicaid managed care plan, there are some key differences in the approaches. This more narrow definition of a population for research and intervention can better be defined as "population health management" (discussed in detail below). However, from the longer-standing historic perspective of population health described above, there is significant overlap between public health and population health.

Public health has been defined as "the science and art of preventing disease, prolonging life, and promoting health through the organized efforts and informed choices of society, organizations, public and private communities, and individuals."[34] In the U.S. context, public health is defined broadly as what "we as a society do collectively to assure the conditions in which people can be healthy."[35] Public health is primarily concerned with health *protection* (primarily in regard to protecting people from water, air, food, occupational, and other risks or hazards), health *promotion* and disease/injury *prevention* in populations, which can be defined in terms of geopolitical areas (cities, counties, states, countries, etc.), and/or in terms of social identities such as race, ethnicity, socioeconomic position, or LGBTQ status.

A central concept in all public health activities is prevention at three levels. *Primary prevention* involves interventions and efforts that attempt to prevent the actual incidence of illness or injury (e.g., immunizations; smoking prevention; speed limits). *Secondary prevention* entails interventions or measures that attempt to identify or diagnose a disease or health condition at an early stage so that the morbidity and mortality risk can be reduced (e.g., cancer screening for early detection; diet and exercise programs for people who are overweight). *Tertiary prevention* involves the treatment or rehabilitation of those who already have a disease or health condition in order to promote recovery or to prevent further decline in health status (e.g., diabetes management interventions; occupational therapy after a stroke).

While many different types of organizations and groups are engaged in public health activities, the building of a *public health system* is also considered to be a public or governmental responsibility. This public health system is comprised of public health agencies at the local, state, and federal level; public safety agencies; human service and charity organizations; healthcare providers; education and youth development organization; recreation and arts-related organization; economic and philanthropic organizations; and environmental agencies and organization. In turn, this public health system is responsible for providing ten essential services required for the health protection, promotion, and prevention goals of the public's health[35]:

1. Monitor health status to identify and solve community health problems.
2. Diagnose and investigate health problems and health hazards in the community.
3. Inform, educate, and empower people about health issues.
4. Mobilize community partnerships and action to identify and solve health problems.
5. Develop policies and plans that support individual and community health efforts.
6. Enforce laws and regulations that protect health and ensure safety.
7. Link people to needed personal health services and assure the provision of healthcare when otherwise unavailable.
8. Assure competent public and personal healthcare workforce.
9. Evaluate effectiveness, accessibility, and quality of personal and population-based health services.
10. Research for new insights and innovative solutions to health problems.

Given that "public health" is considered to be a practice- or action-based endeavor and given its broad range of essential services, public health action is informed by what is often referred to as the "public health sciences" including population sciences (epidemiology, demography, geography), biological sciences (e.g., pathophysiology, epigenetics), behavioral sciences (e.g., social psychology, addiction science), environmental science (e.g., toxicology, water chemistry), and social sciences (e.g., economics, political science, sociology, and anthropology).

Preventive Medicine

Preventive medicine is a specialty of medicine practiced by licensed physicians who are devoted to health promotion and disease prevention, and are primarily engaged in preventing rather than curing disease. What constitutes preventive medicine varies within and across countries.[36] In the U.S. context, preventive medicine is an area of medical practice recognized by the American Board of Medical Specialties with three main specialty areas: aerospace medicine, occupational medicine, and public health and general preventive medicine. Preventive medicine physicians can be board-certified in one or more of these specialty areas, with public health and general preventive medicine being the most common.

Preventive medicine training integrates clinical and public health skills, with a strong focus on primary, secondary, and tertiary prevention. As such, preventive medicine practitioners engaged in prevention-oriented work aimed at individuals, institutions, and communities in a wide variety of settings. Preventive medicine training involves the understanding of population health as the distribution of health risks and outcomes within and across populations and understanding the social determinants of health at multiple levels. Even so, preventive medicine practice is primarily at the micro and mezzo levels.

EMERGENCE OF POPULATION MEDICINE AND POPULATION HEALTH MANAGEMENT

Population Health in the Context of Healthcare Improvement

In 2003, Kindig and Stoddart attempted to clarify and expand the concept of population health by defining it as "the health outcomes of a group of individuals, including the distribution of such outcomes within the group…These groups are often geographic populations such as nations or communities, but can also be other groups such as employees, ethnic groups, disabled persons, prisoners, or any other defined group."[37] In an attempt to clarify the distinction between efforts to understand health risk and outcome distributions within populations at different levels, Kindig and Stoddard used the term "total population health" to refer to the health of *everyone* within a defined geopolitical unit such as a state, province, or nation.[37]

A strong and consistent finding from "total population health" research is that the United States spends a much greater percentage of its GDP on medical care than any other developed country, yet ranks in the bottom on most broad population-level indicators of health status (including overall life expectancy, infant mortality, obesity, injury, suicide, etc.).[24] The United States also experiences significant social disparities in most population health metrics, including by race, ethnicity, income, education, and place.[19,26,28]

A key response to this complex set of issues and problems was the Institute for Healthcare Improvement's 2007 introduction of the **Triple Aim Framework** to optimize healthcare system performance while addressing disparities in health outcomes: reduce *costs*, improve *quality*, and improve *population health*.[38] Building on the Kindig and Stoddard perspective regarding population health, IHI successfully developed and disseminated an important agenda for healthcare improvement that used the term "population health" to refer to the health of the groups of people for which healthcare delivery organizations/systems and health insurance plans were responsible.

This important trifecta of goals for healthcare improvement was woven into some key components of the Patient Protection and Affordable Care Act (ACA), reinforcing the central importance of "population health" within the context of health insurance reform.[38] Efforts to contain healthcare costs and improve quality should not come at the expense of the distribution of health-related risks and outcomes within the populations being impacted by public policy and healthcare system changes. As key actors in the healthcare industry worked to respond to the stark disconnect between healthcare investments and population health outcomes in the United States, they also started looking at the distribution of health outcomes in the patient and beneficiary populations for which they were responsible. In the context of the Triple Aim, "population health" embodies the recognition of the limits of medical care and the importance of the social determinants of health in the broad context of efforts to improve the quality and value of healthcare expenditures and health insurance design.

Because of this constrained definition of a "population," however, the Triple Aim movement promoted and popularized the term "population health" in a way that actually narrowed—rather than expanded—its historic meaning and focus. The ACA and other subsequent healthcare policy efforts and movements reinforced this perspective. This recent explicit focus on population health within the context of healthcare improvement has fueled significant growth in what is generally referred to as "population medicine" and "population health management."[39,40]

Population Medicine

The term "population medicine" has its origin in veterinary science as an evidence-based and multifaceted approach to promoting the health, productivity, and welfare of herds or other aggregates of food and fiber producing animals. Adapted for human health, population medicine is generally centered on the following five activities: (1) conducting epidemiologic research on host-agent-environmental interactions populations; (2) understanding spatial patterns of health and disease; (3) assessing policy and management systems on the production of health; (4) developing and monitoring surveillance systems; and (5) seeking cost-effective means of solving problems.[41]

Population medicine is a field of inquiry and practice that seeks to identify the optimal access to, delivery of, and use of medical care services in a human population, community, or group to achieve population health goals. With an explicit focus on efficiency, the primary focus of population medicine is to craft policy, management, and resource allocation decisions that optimize the role of services and interventions in producing prioritized health outcomes at the community or population level. Population medicine explicitly recognizes policy and management decisions as critically important intervention mechanisms along with individual healthcare services and treatments.

More recently, population medicine has been used to capture the planned activities of a healthcare delivery system that promote community health beyond the goals of those being individually treated or cared for within the system, often in collaboration with community-based partners.[41] A population medicine approach focuses on how medical care interacts with both the biological and social determinants of health, seeking to identify when and how to invest in medical care services versus when and how best to invest in other types of services and interventions, primarily at the micro and mezzo levels. Some examples of health system activities that embrace population medicine principles include patient case management models that involve assessing patients' social needs and circumstances and connecting them to key services and resources in the community.

Kindig views population medicine as being primarily focused on the impact of clinical/healthcare services on health yet recognizing the key role of the services provided by other sectors (such as business, education, social services, and public health) on health as well.[42] As such, the role of *multisector partnerships* is critically important in efforts to improve and address inequities in the health of a population. As Kindig wrote, "we should use the term *population medicine* to describe and promote efforts by leading clinical organizations to use their professional and financial base to actively participate and partner in improving total population health through a multisectoral approach to address broad health outcomes and disparity reductions."[42]

Similarly, IHI defines population medicine as "the design, delivery, coordination and payment of high-quality healthcare services to manage the Triple Aim for a population using the resources we have available to us within the healthcare system."[42] This includes such efforts as patient registries that gather data that can be used in risk stratification models, patient-centered medical home models, Accountable Care Organizations, and case-management approaches to proactively managing chronic disease.

Population Health Management

Motivated by the Triple Aim for healthcare improvement (reduce costs, increase quality, and improve population health), the burgeoning field of "population health management" is quite similar to population medicine. The Institute for Healthcare Improvement views population health management as a shift from a primary focus on the medical care provided to individual patients to an improved alignment between public policies, payment structures, and provider incentives for managing and paying for the healthcare services of a clearly defined or discrete population of patients. The view of IHI on this overlapping set of concepts is that the term "population management should be clearly distinguished from population health (which focuses on the broader determinants of health). From what we have seen through our work at IHI, population management as presently practiced is best conceptualized as *population medicine*."[43]

Sharfstein reported that the use of the term "population health" in the titles of scientific journal article almost doubled between 2010 and 2014 alone.[39] He also noted that "as originally conceived, the term encompassed the impact of income inequality, educational differences and unjust disparities. Since then, population health has come to mean many different things to many different people."[39] There is currently no consensus or consistency regarding the definition or use of the term "population health management." The terms "population health" and "population health management" and—to a lesser degree—"population medicine" are used interchangeably by the leaders of hospitals, healthcare delivery systems, health insurance plans, and myriad companies selling business analytic products and services to help organize and take advantage of patient clinical, financial, and social data.

Over the past two decades, there also has been tremendous growth in the number of schools, departments, and degree programs whose names include the words "population health" or "population health management." By the end of 2018, more than 60 universities and medical schools in the United States had a college, division, department, and/or degree program in either population health, population medicine, or population health management. The majority of these research and training programs emerged after 2010, and the number continues to grow. However, the definition of what "population health" actually means in the context of mission and activities of these endeavors continues to vary greatly.[40]

For example, Marc Gourevitch (professor and chair of the Department of Population Health at New York University Langone Medical Center) views population health as primarily concerned with "measuring and optimizing of the health of groups, and in doing so embraces the full range of determinants of health, including healthcare delivery" whereas public health is more generally focused on the factors that influence health and the levers for improvement that primarily exist outside of the personal healthcare delivery system.[43] Population health, from this perspective, is embedded within the healthcare delivery systems; and it is an approach that emphasizes preventive care and incorporates models of healthcare that are patient-centered, promote self-management, and recognize patient nonmedical determinants of health.[44] The six divisions of the NYU Department of Population Health are engaged in a wide variety of basic and intervention research projects, including the "Health and Behavior" division which includes a strong focus on healthful behavior change, early childhood health and development, health equity, and community service.

David Nash, founding dean of Jefferson College of Population Health, uses the terms "population health" and "population health management" interchangeably in much of his writing and speaking. As a leader in the field of population health management, Nash has articulated "four pillars" of population health: chronic care management; the quality and safety of patient care; healthcare policy and regulation; and a two-way relationship with the public health system.[45] The "population health mandate," according to Nash, fundamentally "seeks to create conditions that promote health, prevent adverse events, and improve outcomes."[44] From this perspective, population health management is an intentional expansion of the delivery of healthcare services to include recognition of patients' social circumstances through prevention and lifestyle change, improved care coordination with public health and social services, reducing or eliminating waste and error in healthcare delivery, eradicating healthcare disparities, and improving transparency and accountability within the system.[45]

Along with the growth in research and training programs in "population health" at institutions of higher learning, there has also been a simultaneous explosion of new business-oriented tools, products, and consulting services designed to improve the management of the healthcare use, costs, and outcomes of the populations for which healthcare systems and payers are financially responsible.[40] This "commodification" of population health management has further fueled its growth as part of the big business of healthcare management and analytics in the 21st century.

For example, ZeOmega—a company that provides healthcare management and software products to payers, providers, and value-based care organizations—states on its website: "If you ask ten healthcare professionals to define population health management (PHM), you're likely to get ten different responses; from risk identification and stratification to patient outreach, care coordination, dashboards and registries, and more."[46] ZeOmega claims that their approach to population health is broad, comprehensive, and incorporates Triple Aim thinking, with a different set of "key pillars" than those promoted by Nash: (1) program design and governance; (2) data integration and aggregation; (3) actionable intelligence; (4) holistic patient-centered care; and (5) stakeholder engagement.[46]

Despite all of the variation in the use and application of the concept of "population health management," the "population" of focus in the vast majority of efforts is comprised of the patients who make their way onto a health insurance plan and/or into healthcare delivery system's clinical and financial databases. In these efforts, the term "population" typically refers to individuals or patients who are covered by a health insurance plan or receive their care from a specific healthcare delivery organization or system.

TENSIONS BETWEEN COMPETING DEFINITIONS OF AND APPROACHES TO POPULATION HEALTH

Sharfstein describes the "strange journal of population health" as historically focusing on broadly defined populations and emphasizing policy approaches to the underlying causes of illness.[39] More recently, however, "population health" has become equated with "population health management" in healthcare delivery and policy circles, focused primarily on the health of groups covered by insurance plans or other types of patient aggregates, "limited to the group of people (health services providers) know, see, and track."[39] Although population health in this context does recognize the social determinants of health and focuses on partnerships between the healthcare system and public health agencies and community-based services, it remains a patient-centered and primarily biomedical approach to health at the individual rather than social level.

Medicalization

Despite the long history of "population health" from a public health and social policy perspective, the relatively new attention from the healthcare system has changed the focus, practice, and impact of population health improvement efforts. The shift from population health to population health management that began in the 1990s can be understood as the result of a strong and long-standing force within the modern biomedical system, what sociologist Peter Conrad refers to as the "engines of medicalization."[47]

Medicalization is a process by which social and behavioral issues are increasingly viewed through a biomedical lens, and come to be defined primarily as individual pathological or biological problems. The process of medicalization: (1) includes a strong focus on individual sickness/pathology; (2) gives medical and clinical experts the primary authority to "diagnose and treat" social problems within the boundaries of medical expertise and practice; (3) often creates new clinical services, treatments, and business services/products so that the "problem" or issue can be addressed medically; and (4) focuses attention and interventions downstream to the individual, intrapersonal level.[47]

There are myriad examples of medicalization. Between 1952 and 1973, homosexuality was medicalized as various types of personality and mental disorders in the *Diagnostic and Statistical Manual* of the American Psychiatric Association. A medicalized approach to the steep rise in the rate of people in the United States who are obese includes defining obesity as a disease, which in turn emphasizes individual treatment rather than community-based or public policy prevention approaches. Medicalization also includes the labeling of being at high risk for a chronic illness as a disease state in and of itself (e.g., diagnosing patients as having "pre-hypertension" or "pre-diabetes"), with such diagnoses needing a clinical treatment response, usually through prescription drugs.

Rates of attention deficit/hyperactivity disorder (ADHD) vary greatly across school districts in the United States, with higher rates in urban schools with a more diverse student body.[48] A medicalized approach to this problem defines social disparities in childhood behavioral problems such as ADHD primarily as differences in the incidence of brain disorders without acknowledging social disparities in children's home environments and racial differences in how teachers' react to students who are disruptive in the classroom. To further underscore this point, research has demonstrated that school districts with school-entry birthdate policies of September 1 have significantly higher rates of children with ADHD diagnoses than those with later birthday cut-offs, controlling for other observable factors. This is ostensibly because having a higher proportion of younger children in a classroom leads to more behavioral disruptions, which in turn is medicalized as individual pathology and treated with prescription drugs.

Concerns about the Medicalization of Population Health

Medicalization is not always a negative process. Medicalization can bring important attention and resources to population health problems. For example, the medicalization of smoking as "nicotine addiction syndrome" accelerated the research, development, and dissemination of effective nicotine replacement therapies for smoking cessation. However, the medicalization and commodification of population health as "population health management" has produced a strong downstream shift in the focus and approach of the field, which in turn raises a number of concerns about its potential to actually have an impact on the broad and important historic metrics of population health.

The first of these concerns can be described as "denominator shrinkage" or the move from focusing on populations based on broad sociopolitical criteria to small groups of people who temporarily share the same set of healthcare providers or insurance plan. This shift in the definition and focus of what constitutes "population health" severely narrows the focus of the field, including the number and types of people of interest for research, service, and policy attention.[40]

Second, population health management is primarily concerned with individual patients or insurance beneficiaries and thus tends to frame all of the population "problems" and their potential solutions at the micro, individual, and downstream level. Of course, population health management efforts emphasize the important role of partnerships, especially partnerships with community-based social service and public health agencies and organizations. However, the primary approach of population health management is to connect individuals with needed medical and social services and resources, primarily after a health condition or disease is already present. This ignores the mezzo and macro factors that are the root causes of the unequal distributions of health resources, risks, and outcomes across the life course in the total population.[49]

Recalling Nash's four pillars of population health, the focus is clearly at the individual patient level. The "policy" pillar is focused on health*care* policy and regulation related to personal healthcare services. The community is primarily viewed as a place where patients get their medications, their care is better coordinated, and they connect with needed social services. In the "public health" pillar, Nash recognizes the important primary prevention efforts of public health agencies yet also states that "local, state and national public health efforts must support and complement the work being done in the local healthcare institutions."[44]

Third, a medicalized view of population health that is focused at the individual or micro level fundamentally ignores or is timid about the macro-level factors (including social policy) that create and reinforce population health problems and inequities.[40,49]

Prior to the emergence of population health management, the field of population health was primarily focused on the social structural, systemic, and sociopolitical forces that create health disparities by place, socioeconomic position, race, ethnicity, gender, immigration status, and other social factors. However, with few exceptions, current population health management training, research, and practice are silent about the upstream institutional, systemic, and public policy drivers of population health problems and distributional disparities. This historic upstream/macro-level focus of the field is shrugged off by most population health management efforts as being outside of its scope because it involves political and social factors and that are fairly far removed from the healthcare coverage and delivery systems and their usual partners.[40]

A fourth and serious problem with the strong emergence of the population health management movement is the rampant conflation of terms, which reinforces all of the concerns discussed above. Given the strength of biomedical model, the concepts of "population health management" and "population medicine" have become significantly conflated with "population health." This is not surprising, given the existing and long-standing confusion between or conflation of "health" and "healthcare" and of "health disparities" with "healthcare disparities."[49] Ultimately, medicalization leads to a melding of the distinct concepts of health and healthcare, and thus gives further strength and credence to the fallacy that societal problems having to do with health primarily need to be solved with healthcare services and solutions.[40,47,49]

OPPORTUNITIES AND CHALLENGES FOR THE FIELD OF POPULATION HEALTH

Opportunities

Despite the numerous concerns outlined above, the emergence and growth of the population health management movement is providing significant opportunities for the general field of population of health. Without question, the increased attention to population health has been fueled by an increased understanding and appreciation of the nonmedical, social determinants of health within the healthcare system. This has led to a number of varied and important new types of programs and interventions that attempt to better assess patient social circumstances, identify patient social needs, and connect them with needed social and material resources such as food, housing, transportation, and behavioral health interventions. In addition, the growth in cross-sector collaborations and partnerships between healthcare system and public health agencies, community-based organizations and private sector businesses is important and encouraging.[39]

For example, with a number of community partners, Boston Medical Center is investing over $6 million dollars in housing affordability and stability programs in low-income areas of Boston, including investments in supportive housing for the homeless, a housing stabilization program for patients with complex medical needs, resources to assist families in fighting evictions, and a neighborhood food market.[50] In addition, significant attention is currently being given to ways in which Medicaid funding can be used or leveraged in terms of addressing upstream, nonmedical determinants of health.[51,52]

As another example, *Medical-Legal Partnership* projects have now been implemented in over 300 health systems, hospitals, community health centers, and Veterans Affairs facilities in 46 different states.[53] These partnerships are premised on the recognition that low-income patients often face, in addition to myriad health challenges, complex social problems regarding housing, employment, public benefits, and the criminal justice system that require legal expertise and assistance.[54] When embedded within healthcare environments, "lawyers can directly resolve specific problems for individual patients, while also helping clinical and non-clinical staff navigate system and policy barriers and transform institutional practice. Using legal expertise and services, the healthcare system can disrupt the cycle of returning people to the unhealthy conditions that would otherwise bring them right back to the clinic or hospital."[51]

In addition, as described above, there has been a significant growth in the number of degree programs and academic units that are devoted to research, training, and practice in the field of population health; and many of these efforts have embraced an approach to population health that extends upstream beyond the healthcare delivery system and micro-level or individual interventions and approaches. For example, William Tierney has documented the strategic process by which the mission, scope, and activities of a new Department of Population Health were developed at the Dell Medical School at the University of Texas, including consensus development through focus groups with stakeholders from the university, city/county government, community nonprofit organizations, and selected national academic leaders.[55] Although Tierney incorrectly asserts that "(p)opulation health is a relatively new concept," this Department of Population Health was designed to not only engage in efforts that would better "manage" patients but also push upstream to promote health and prevent disease. This new department includes a division dedicated to community engagement and health equity—a historically recognized cornerstone of population health—and a medical education division that will attempt to incorporate basic population health principles like social determinants of health and social epidemiology into the curriculum.[55]

There are myriad additional examples of innovative and promising approaches to population health improvement that are resulting from the increased attention that healthcare institutions, health insurance plans, and universities/academic medical centers are giving to population health. Among the large and growing array of population health management efforts underway in the United States, there are some exciting and positive activities that are indeed important and necessary. The primary goal of these efforts is to understand patients and their health issues in the context of their social, economic, and community circumstances, and in doing so recognizes the importance of partnerships with public health and other community-based organizations and also the importance of other fields of science including social epidemiology, health behavior change, health informatics, community psychology, among others.[1]

Challenges

Although one can certainly appreciate the relatively new and innovative activities that the healthcare industry is undertaking in the name of population health improvement, this progress should also be viewed in the context of what has been the historical focus and approach of the field of population health. From this broad and historical perspective comes the revelation that most of the current efforts in population health management are fundamentally limited in their intentions, foci, and approaches. While grounded in a social determinants of health framework, the training, research, and practice-based activities of the population health management movement are focused downstream, primarily at the intersection of the healthcare system and a limited range of observable social circumstances of patients who make their way to the system.

Population health management can be described as a collection of downstream efforts diligently working to identify and address both the biomedical and immediate social circumstances that affect patient healthcare and health status outcomes. Many people with longstanding commitments to population health and health equity are greatly encouraged that the healthcare system—with its vast resources and control of most of the country's investments in health—is building these efforts and has embraced an understanding of the social determinants of health.[40] From any perspective, this shift within the healthcare system is essential and necessary, even if the primary populations of interest are those of health plans or patient systems.

Nonetheless, if the fundamental goal of population health efforts is to improve health outcomes and health equity at the societal level, the current efforts regarding population health management and population medicine are quite insufficient. We must recognize the fundamental difference between macro- and system-level changes necessary to improve population health and the micro-level interventions and services being implemented under the guise of population health management. We must recognize the significant differences between:

- Upstream policy and community financing efforts aimed at increasing affordable housing within gentrifying urban neighborhoods versus downstream efforts that provide supportive housing to chronically homeless individuals
- Policy, financing, and access reforms for family planning services to ensure that all women are able to control the timing and spacing of their pregnancies versus home visiting programs for high-risk pregnant mothers
- Policy and community investments in the primary prevention of child abuse/neglect versus screening child patients for adverse childhood experiences
- Investments in public education system reform versus patient-centered interventions focused on health literacy
- Investments in affordable and efficient public transportation systems versus assisting patients with transportation to and from their medical appointments
- Income security and poverty prevention policies versus screening patients for trouble paying for prescriptions or keeping up with their utility bills

The labors of population health management that are building a bigger and stronger array of efforts to rescue individual people from downstream waters of poor health are important and necessary. However, these efforts are not sufficient for total population health and must not divert research, resources, and policy attention from the upstream forces that are pushing groups of people and their communities into the rivers of health inequity in the first place.[40]

SUMMARY AND CONCLUSIONS

For over two centuries, the development of "population health" as both a science and a field of practice has been centered upon the root understanding of the fundamental social determinants of health and health inequities within societies, the limits of personal healthcare services in addressing social factors and circumstances related to health, and the need for an upstream or macro-level focus on social structures, systems, and policies. In an effort to promote an expanded view of the social determinants of health and the limits of medical care, a so-called "population health" perspective became a corner stone of efforts to reframe and refocus healthcare and improvement and health insurance reform in the United States in the early 21st century.

Ironically, however, these efforts to enhance healthcare improvement by considering the socioeconomic situations, social and cultural backgrounds, and psychosocial behaviors of people within defined patient populations have actually served to *narrow* and medicalize "population health" as population medicine or population health management. And along with the co-opting of term "population health," there have been significant resource investments in education, research, information systems, data analytics, and policy actions that appear ignorant of the historic focus of population health and are focused downstream on narrowly defined groups of people who are "populations" only because they share fragmented and tenuous links to healthcare providers and payers. This is diverting attention and resources away from rather than closer to the well-researched and understood macro- and mezzo-level fundamental drivers of poor population health and social disparities in health.[10,19,28]

At this time, there is serious conflation between population health and population health management, just as there has long been a dangerous conflation between health and healthcare. This conflation or fuzziness is not going to go away with calls for more detailed or precise definitions and or with clearer lines of distinction for what should be within and outside of the scope of practice of healthcare professionals and the healthcare delivery system. A key point of this chapter, however, is that all healthcare practitioners—especially those engaged in preventive medicine and population medicine—need to understand the important distinctions between *population health* as an upstream scientific and policy-based approach for reaching broad societal health goals and *population health management* as a downstream approach to reaching for the Triple Aim of controlling costs, improving quality, and improving health outcomes in groups of people tied together by healthcare and/or health insurance providers.

In sum, the medicalization of population health as population health management is indeed bringing new attention and resources to the important role of social factors and socioeconomic conditions in the creation and persistent of health inequities. However, a view of population health that is grounded in the healthcare delivery system and focused on patients—even in the context of community-based partnerships—is extremely limited in fundamental ways.

The long-standing and historic perspective on total population health—with a strong focus on the physical, mental, and social well-being of an entire population—is only possible with significant resource investments and macro-level changes required to ensure that everyone enjoys a childhood without poverty or other adverse events, a high-quality education, access to jobs and economic security, safe and affordable housing, food security, efficient and affordable transportation, thriving neighborhoods and communities with safe water and air, and lives free from individual and systemic discrimination. This would enable the provision of high-quality healthcare for the "fine-tuning" of health problems, as opposed to using healthcare as the primary way to address the vulnerabilities and inequities that derive from complex social environments and extend far beyond the healthcare delivery system.[49]

Galea recently asked an important rhetorical question: *Is ignoring the causes and potential solutions to America's health indicators tacit complicity with a status quo that should be far from acceptable?*[56] If the primary training, research, and intervention activities of the field of population health do not return to the historical focus on the macro- and mezzo-level fundamental social determinants of health and health inequities, the field is indeed "complicit," as Galea suggests, in a status quo in which almost every type of health outcome across the life course varies significantly by socioeconomic status, race, ethnicity, and other social factors, in which the United States spends far more per capita on healthcare than any other country in the world yet continues to rank poorly on every metric that measures the actual health status of the population, and in which average life expectancy is actually decreasing.[20,57]

The relatively new and burgeoning field of population health management is in need of some critical re-evaluation and redirection. Amid the loud and revving engines of the medicalization of population health, there needs to be increased and steadfast action on policy reforms and other interventions that will influence and impact the key institutions, social systems, and public policies that drive population health outcomes and disparities in the first place. Otherwise, as Sharfstein laments, "we may find ourselves awash in population health efforts, without meaningful progress in the health of our population."[39]

References

1. Szreter S. The population health approach in historical perspective. *Am J Public Health*. 2003;93(3):421-31.
2. Young TK. *Population Health: Concepts and Methods*. New York, NY: Oxford University Press; 1998.
3. Parrish RG. Measuring population health outcomes. *Prevent Chronic Dis*. 2010;7(4):A71.
4. Lantz PM, Pritchard A. Socioeconomic indicators that matter for population health. *Prevent Chronic Dis*. 2010;7(4):A74.
5. Etches V, Frank J, DiRuggiero E, Manuel D. Measuring population health: a review of indicators. *Annu Rev Public Health*. 2006;27:29-55.
6. Kunitz SJ. *The Health of Populations: General Theories and Particular Realities*. New York, NY: Oxford University Press; 2007.
7. Anderson M. "The people's misery: mother of diseases": Johan Peter Frank (1790). *The Social Medicine Portal*. September 3, 2008. Available at https://www.socialmedicine.org/2008/09/03/history-of-social-medicine/the-peoples-misery-mother-of-diseases-johann-peter-frank-1790/. Accessed January 2, 2019.
8. Rosen G. *A History of Public Health: Revised and Expanded Edition*. Baltimore, MD: Johns Hopkins University Press; 2015.
9. Duffy J. *The Sanitarians: A History of American Public Health*. Urbana, IL: University of Illinois Press; 1990.
10. Omran AR. The epidemiologic transition. *Milbank Mem Fund Q*. 1971;49:509-38.
11. Berkman L, Kawachi I. *Social Epidemiology*. New York, NY: Oxford University Press; 2000.
12. Ho JY, Hendi AS. Recent trends in life expectancy across high income countries: retrospective observational study. *BMJ*. 2018;362:k2562.
13. Tapia Granados JA, Ionides EL. Population health and the economy: mortality and the great recession in Europe. *Health Eco*. 2017;26(12):e219-35.
14. Lynch JW, Davey Smith G, Kaplan GA, House JS. Income inequality and mortality importance to health of individual incomes, psychosocial environment, or material conditions. *BMJ*. 2000;320:1200-04.
15. Diez Roux AV, Mair C. Neighborhoods and health. *Ann NY Acad Sci*. 2010;1186:125-45.
16. Arcaya M, Tucker-Seeley R, Kim R, Schnake-Mahl A, So M, Subramanian SV. Research on neighborhood effects on health in the United States: a systematic review of study characteristics. *Soc Sci Med*. 2016;168:16-29.
17. Rose G. Sick individuals and sick populations. *Int J Epidemiol*. 1985;14:32-38.
18. Aziz Z, Absetz P, Oldroyd J, Pronk NP, Oldenburg B. A systematic review of real-world diabetes prevention programs: learning from the last 15 years. *Implement Sci*. 2015;10:172.
19. Evans R, Barer M, Marmor T. *Why Are Some People Healthy and Others Not? The Determinants of Health of Populations*. New York, NY: Aldine de Gruyter; 1994.
20. Keyes KM, Galea S. *Population Health Science*. Oxford: Oxford University Press; 2016.
21. Ahern J, Jones MR, Bakshis E, Galea S. Revisiting Rose: comparing the benefits and costs of population-wide and targeted interventions. *Milbank Q*. 2008;86(4):581-600.
22. Stokols D. Translating social ecological theory into guidelines for community health promotion. *Am J Health Promot*. 1996;10:282-98.
23. Solar O, Irwin A. *A Conceptual Framework for Action on the Social Determinants of Health. Social Determinants of Health Discussion Paper 2 (Policy and Practice)*. Geneva, Switzerland: World Health Organization; 2010.
24. Shroeder SA. We can do better—improving the health of the American people. *N Engl J Med*. 2007;357:1221-28.
25. McGinnis JM, Williams-Russo P, Knickman JP. The case for more active policy attention to health promotion. *Health Aff*. 2002;78-93.
26. Williams DR, Sternthal M. Understanding racial-ethnic disparities in health: sociological contributions. *J Health Soc Behav*. 2010;51(S):S15-S27.
27. Phelan JC, Link BG. Is racism a fundamental cause of inequalities in health? *Ann Rev Soc*. 2015;41:311-30.
28. Link BG, Phelan JC. McKeown and the idea that social conditions are fundamental causes of disease. *Am J Pub Health*. 2002;92(5):730-32.
29. Curry-Stevens A, Lopezrevorido A, Peters D. *Policies to Eliminate Racial Disparities in Education: A Literature Review*. Portland, OR: Center to Advance Racial Equity, Portland State University; 2013.
30. Levy DT, Tam J, Cuo C, Fong GT, Chaloupka F. The impact of implementing tobacco control policies: the 2017 Tobacco Control Scorecard. *J Pub Health Manage Practice*. 2018;24(5):448-57.
31. De Beaumont Foundation. CityHealth—A Project of the de Beaumont Foundation and Kaiser Permanente. Available at http://www.debeaumont.org/cityhealth/. Accessed January 4, 2019.
32. Shapiro TM. Race, homeownership and wealth. *Washington Univ J Law Policy*. 2006;20(4):53-74.
33. Salkin PE. Environmental justice and land use planning and zoning. *Touro Law*. 2003. Available at https://digitalcommons.tourolaw.edu/cgi/viewcontent.cgi?referer=https://www.google.com/&httpsredir=1&article=1570&context=scholarlyworks. Accessed January 4, 2019.
34. Banta HD, de Wit GA. Public health services and cost-effectiveness analysis. *Ann Rev Pub Health*. 2008;29:383-97.
35. Institute of Medicine. *The Future of the Public's Health in the 21st Century*. Washington, DC: The National Academies Press; 2003.

36. Peik SM, Mohan KM, Baba T, Donadel M, Labruto A, Loh LC. Comparison of public health and preventive medicine physician specialty training in six countries: identifying challenges and opportunities. *Med Teach.* 2016;38(11):1146-51.
37. Kindig D, Stoddart G. What is population health? *Am J Pub Health.* 2003;93:380-83.
38. Whittington JW, Nolan K, Lewis N, Torres T. Pursuing the Triple Aim: the first 7 years. *Milbank Q.* 2015;93(2):263-300.
39. Sharfstein JM. The strange journey of population health. *Milbank Q.* 2014;92(4):640-43.
40. Lantz PM. The medicalization of population health: who will stay upstream? *Milbank Q.* 2018. Available at https://www.milbank.org/quarterly/articles/the-medicalization-of-population-health-who-will-stay-upstream/.
41. Lewis N. Populations, population health, and the evolution of population management: making sense of terminology in US health care today. *Institute for Healthcare Improvement* blog post. March 19, 2014. Available at http://www.ihi.org/communities/blogs/population-health-population-management-terminology-in-us-health-care. Accessed January 4, 2019.
42. Kindig D. What are we talking about when we talk about population health? *Health Affairs* blog. April 6, 2015. Available at https://www.healthaffairs.org/do/10.1377/hblog20150406.046151/full/. Accessed January 4, 2019.
43. Gourevitch MN. Population health and the academic medical center: the time is right. *Acad Med.* 2014:89(4):544-49.
44. Nash DB, Fabius RJ, Skoufalos A, Clarke JL, Horowitz MR. *Population Health: Creating a Culture of Wellness.* Burlington, MA: Jones & Bartlett Learning; 2016.
45. Nash DB. *The Population Health Mandate: A Broader Approach to Patient Care Delivery.* San Diego, CA: The BoardRoom Press, 2012. Available at http://populationhealthcolloquium.com/readings/Pop_Health_Mandate_NASH_2012.pdf. Accessed January 4, 2019.
46. ZeOmega: What we do. Available at http://www.zeomega.com/population-health-management-five-pillars/. Accessed January 4, 2019.
47. Conrad P. The shifting engines of medicalization. *J Health Social Behav.* 46(1):3-14.
48. Layton TJ, Barnett ML, Hicks TR, Jena AB. Attention deficit-hyperactivity disorder and month of school enrollment. *N Engl J Med.* 2018;379:2122-30.
49. Lantz PM, Lichtenstein RL, Pollack HA. Health policy approaches to population health: the limits of medicalization. *Health Affairs.* 2007;26(5):1253-57.
50. Boston Medical Center website. "Boston Medical Center to invest $6.5 million in affordable housing to improve community health and patient outcomes, reduce medical costs." Available at https://www.bmc.org/news/press-releases/2017/12/07/boston-medical-center-invest-65-million-affordable-housing-improve. Accessed January 4, 2019.
51. Machledt D. *Addressing the Social Determinants of Health Through Medicaid Managed Care.* The Commonwealth Fund, Issue Brief, November, 2017. Available at http://www.commonwealthfund.org/publications/issue-briefs/2017/nov/social-determinants-health-medicaid-managed-care#/utm_source=social-determinants-health-medicaid-managed-care&utm_medium=Twitter&utm_campaign=Medicaid. Accessed January 4, 2019.
52. Goldberg SH, Lantz PM, Iovan S. Addressing social determinants of health through Medicaid: Expanding upstream interventions with federal matching funds and social impact investments under the 2016 Medicaid Managed Care Final Rule. Federal Reserve Bank of San Francisco. *Open Source Solutions*, No. 2, October 31, 2018.
53. National Center for Medical Legal Partnership website. The Need. Available at https://medical-legalpartnership.org/need/. Accessed January 4, 2019.
54. Tietlebaum J, Lawton E. The roots and branches of the medical-legal partnership approach to health: from collegiality to civil rights to health equity. *Yale J Health Policy Law Ethics.* 2017;17(2):Article 5.
55. Tierney WM. Use of stakeholder focus groups to define the mission and scope of a new department of population health. *J Gen Int Med.* 2018;33(7):1069-76.
56. Galea S. The complicity of the population health scientist. *Milbank Q.* 2018;96(2):227-30.
57. Murphey SL, Xu J, Kochanek KD, Arias E. Mortality in the United States, 2017. NCHS Data Brief, No. 328, November, 2018.

CHAPTER

3

Precision Medicine

Jun Ma • Corina R. Ronneberg • Nan Lv • Megan A. Lewis • Thomas Kannampallil

The goal of this chapter is to discuss the role and promise of precision medicine in public health and preventive medicine. This chapter is organized as follows: First, we define precision medicine and review its history and evolution. Second, we present an overview of comprehensive theoretical frameworks that can inform the conception and implementation of precision medicine to optimize its impact on individual and population health. Third, a brief discussion follows that highlights state-of-the-art technologies, data pipelines, and computational tools across multiple levels and contexts in accordance to theory and, importantly, how these can be leveraged to advance precision medicine in public health research and practice. Fourth, specific examples of precision medicine in action in both national and global contexts are presented. Finally, we discuss the future of precision medicine from the perspective of public health and preventive medicine in terms of achieving a vision for precision health.

EVOLUTION OF PRECISION MEDICINE

Definitions

Precision medicine is defined as "an emerging approach for disease treatment and prevention that takes into account individual variability in genes, environment, and lifestyle for each person."[1] Historically, the term "personalized medicine" has been used interchangeably with precision medicine, as both terms are interrelated and draw heavily from genomics; however, the two concepts have notable differences (see Table 3-1). The importance of a distinction in terminology arose from the concern that personalized medicine can be interpreted as treatment and prevention strategies that are "developed uniquely for an individual," whereas precision medicine's aims to explore "how treatment or prevention approaches can be developed based on the combination of genetic, environmental, and social factors which could be targeted to individuals or populations."[1,2] In other words, precision medicine is not limited to an individual, but holds great potential for developing population-wide interventions with targeted precision. Another reason for distinction is related to the commonly shared notion among physicians that medicine is already personalized since treatments are individualized based on a patient's clinical context and care trajectory.[3] However, such a definition of personalized medicine misses additional elements that precision medicine carries, specifically the focus on new and precise approaches to diagnostics and therapeutics.

Another important term to define is "precision public health" (see Table 3-1) which is an application of the precision medicine approach at the population level. This emphasizes the need for precision to broaden from its narrow focus on an individual to that of populations. However, the evolution of precision medicine is still ongoing; and there is likely a larger picture that we are moving toward. We offer a vision of the precision medicine approach that is to attain precision health, which we define in Table 3-1 and expand on in the *Future Direction: Precision Health* section of this chapter.

Need for Precision Medicine

The need for precision medicine arose from a combination of factors: a shift in disease pattern prevalence,[4] evolution of medical models reflecting recent advances in science and technology, and patient inputs and preferences. The past half century has witnessed an evolution and shift in disease patterns and resultant causes of mortality: the prevalence of infectious diseases has decreased, at a particularly accelerated rate in developed countries, while noncommunicable disease (NCD)

TABLE 3-1	KEY DEFINITIONS[a]
Precision medicine	An emerging approach for disease treatment and prevention that takes into account individual variability in genes, environment, and lifestyle for each person (U.S. National Library of Medicine)[1]
Personalized medicine	Tailoring of medical treatment to the individual characteristics of each patient. It does not literally mean the creation of drugs or medical devices that are unique to a patient, but rather the ability to classify individuals into subpopulations that differ in their susceptibility to a particular disease or their response to a specific treatment. Preventive or therapeutic interventions can then be concentrated on those who will benefit, sparing expense, and side effects for those who will not (President's Council of Advisors on Science and Technology)[4]
Precision public health	Improving the ability to prevent disease, promote health, and reduce health disparities in populations by: (1) applying emerging methods and technologies for measuring disease, pathogens, exposures, behaviors, and susceptibility in populations; and (2) developing policies and targeted public health programs to improve health (Centers for Disease Control and Prevention)[5]
Precision health	The attainment of a state of complete physical, mental, and social well-being at individual and population levels through enhanced abilities to optimally predict, prevent, and treat disease by accounting for variability in genes, environment, and lifestyle (current chapter authors)

[a]Although different definitions exist for each of these concepts, we have included the definitions from key literature on this topic.

prevalence has continued to rise, commonly referred to as the epidemiologic transition.[5,6] It is projected that over 75% of deaths globally in 2030 will be attributable to NCD.[5,6] Therefore, it is critical to identify environmental and lifestyle factors and their interplay with genetics responsible for the etiology, spread, and sustained burden of NCDs. Precision medicine offers immense promise for studying these factors, and also has the ability to provide tailored and targeted interventions aimed at health promotion and disease prevention.

Further, models of medicine (classified from P0 to P6) have evolved reflecting advances in science, technology, and patient preferences. The overarching goal of these models has been to characterize approaches for the practice of medicine across different domains. The original P0 model was strictly physician-centered; but it gradually evolved in to the P4 medicine model, which aimed to make medicine participatory, personalized, predictive, and preventive. This shift is what ultimately led to the development and application of precision medicine approaches. For instance, via integrative personal panomics profile analysis that combines information from genomic, transcriptomic, proteomic, metabolomic, and autoantibody profiles from an individual,[7,8] it is now possible to discover biological pathways and diagnostic or prognostic markers that are otherwise not readily apparent. It is, in turn, possible to develop new disease prediction models and novel targeted therapeutics accounting for granular interindividual variation. Of the omics,[9] genomics was the first to appear, and has received the greatest attention. The availability and knowledge of genomic information can be directly attributed to advances in genome sequencing. The first genome was sequenced in 2000 and the Human Genome Project (an international research effort aiming to sequence and map all human genes)[10] was completed in 2003 when the final sequence mapping of the human genome was published. Since then, we have seen increased speed and drastically lowered cost of genome sequencing.[11] It now takes as little as 1 hour to sequence a genome (as opposed to the 13 years it took to sequence the first one) and costs have plummeted from $95 million to $1000 per genome.[12] The Human Genome Project along with work being done as part of the Human Microbiome Project (which studies "microbial communities that live in and on our bodies and the roles they play in human health and disease")[13] and the Human Metabolome Database (a web-enabled metabolomic database that is now considered the standard metabolomic resource for human metabolic studies)[14] are some examples that hold great potential for revolutionizing our understanding of health and disease in the precision medicine paradigm. Precision medicine approaches have been intensely applied in a number of disease areas, with most of the work being done currently taking place in cancer research, as exemplified by the $1.8 billion Cancer Moonshot initiative. One of the objectives of this initiative is to leverage genomic data "to make more therapies available to more patients, whiwle also improving our ability to prevent cancer and detect it at an early stage."[15]

While immensely beneficial, the P0–P4 models excluded a critical aspect related to health and well-being: psychological health.[16] The P5 model was therefore developed and builds in psychocognitive variables [concordant with the World Health Organization (WHO) definition of health[17]], which may affect health and health behaviors (e.g., treatment compliance and adherence). By further integrating a person's "environmental factors and psychological profile,"[16] a physician can conceivably personalize prevention, and can inform patients on how to prevent certain diseases. In fact, P5 model emphasizes patient education and health promotion.

More recently, medicine has evolved yet again, to the P6 model, which adds a "public" element to the P5 model. The novelty of this addition is that it accounts for the ability of patients to not only access health information via the internet, but also actively utilize the "Health Web Science" (a combination of e-health, e-medicine, and telemedicine) to support optimal personalized health.[16] The ability of individuals to measure, store, and share their personal health data has reached new heights with the ballooning popularity of health sensor technologies in the last 20 years. The clinical, ethical, and legal implications are complex and controversial—and should not be overlooked. These factors notwithstanding, the more open, public form of medicine as reflected in the P6 model highlights unprecedented opportunities for precision medicine applications, such as continuous, passive health monitoring as well as just-in-time adaptive intervention development and delivery, where preventive care or treatment could be tailored and delivered through novel, accessible means—and precisely targeted in the right moment of *time* to the right *person* at the right *place*.

Precision Medicine Initiative

Precision medicine developed into a national priority in 2011 after a National Research Council (NRC) Committee was convened and tasked by the Director of the National Institutes of Health (NIH) to explore the "feasibility and need for a new taxonomy of human disease based on molecular biology," given the surge in genomic and molecular information available. The NRC concluded that a new taxonomy will lead to better healthcare, that the time for doing so is optimal, and that a new taxonomy should therefore be developed.[12] In order to create such a taxonomy, the NRC recommended that a system must first be developed for "acquiring and analyzing information relating to the molecular profiles and health histories of large numbers of individuals," and that the resulting data are made available to researchers. More specifically, the NRC recommended a pilot study for sequencing the genomes of ≥1 million individuals in order to build an Information Commons and Knowledge Network of Disease.[12] Shortly thereafter, in 2015, President Barack Obama announced the $215 million launch of the Precision Medicine Initiative intended to "accelerate biomedical discoveries and provide clinicians with new tools, knowledge, and therapies to select which treatments will work best for which patients."[18] Taken together, the NRC report along with the heavily funded Precision Medicine Initiative is the defining initiative that led to the recognition of precision medicine as a national paradigm and priority in health and healthcare.

The Precision Medicine Initiative is a long-term research endeavor[19] with two primary goals[1]: in the short term, to gain a better understanding of cancer and finding ways to "anticipate, prevent, diagnose, and treat" cancers, and[2] in the longer term, to generate knowledge around disease risk, underlying disease mechanisms, and prediction of optimal treatment, that can be extended to many diseases.[20] To meet these goals, several institutes of the NIH received considerable funding to develop a national voluntary research cohort of 1+ million individuals, to identify genomic drivers in cancer, to focus on database development, and to establish secure and private data exchanges.

The national research cohort, called "All of Us,"[21] has the mission to "accelerate health research and medical breakthroughs, enabling individualized prevention, treatment, and care for all of us." The program is currently underway, and with expected completion of enrollment by 2022. Despite all of the recent progress, challenges abound, including practical issues of data collection and integration for the future healthcare of patients enrolled in the All of Us initiative and, perhaps more far-reaching, philosophical concerns such as those highlighted below.

Challenges of Precision Medicine

Although precision medicine has had widespread support, it is not without its share of critics. The biggest concerns have been around the narrow focus and conceptualization in its application, its utility, and its cost-effectiveness for patient care. First, focusing on the Precision Medicine Initiative and its vision to explore variability in genes, environment, and lifestyle, it is important to point out the way it is currently being implemented is incongruent with its mission. The focus has disproportionately concentrated on biological mechanisms while important social, behavioral, and environmental mechanisms,[22] which have been proven to affect disease etiology and progression, have been largely ignored.[23] These multilevel determinants of health[24–26] are of paramount importance as they influence the risk, causation, and the ongoing burden of NCDs, a major global concern.[27] Additionally, to date, precision medicine has narrowly focused on individuals by relying on genetic and other molecular biological information for providing treatment and prevention for individuals. This focus on individual rather than population health[28] raises an important question around the scale of intended impact in disease prevention and treatment. Relatedly, it elicits a fear that federal funding would be diverted away from exploring important group differences in morbidity and mortality, and as a result, certain groups (e.g., low income, minority populations) would be adversely affected and experience exacerbated health disparities.[29] Critics of precision medicine therefore urge us to recognize that health is affected by much more than clinical care and genetics, and if we are to improve population health while also reducing health inequities, two major goals of the Healthy People 2020 initiative,[30] proper attention must be situated on the social-structural and behavioral factors that shape individual and population health.

A related, second criticism calls into question the utility and cost-effectiveness of precision medicine for public health.[29] Although precision medicine has had success in several areas of importance to public health (e.g., genomic screening for breast and ovarian cancers), scholars and practitioners alike have argued that most of precision medicine potentially helps only a small fragment of the population and does so at a steep cost, perhaps best exemplified by the development of the Ivacaftor drug, which is useful among only 5% of cystic fibrosis patients, took decades to develop, and costs $300,000/year/patient.[31] The "prevention paradox," a term coined by epidemiologist Geoffrey Rose,[23,32] posits that greater reductions in morbidity and mortality and improved public health benefits can be observed given a focus on people with average and low risk versus on those with the highest risk. In addition, other critics have opined that traditional medicine approaches including behavioral interventions are just as, if not more efficacious (as well as cost-effective) than precision medicine approaches, among the majority of the population, while individually tailored treatments may be most useful for detecting and treating rare conditions.[31,33] Lastly, despite the increased attention to identifying genetic variants and determinants of a disease, treatment solutions lag; in addition, there are many conditions with no treatment options, raising the question around the utility of narrowly focused precision medicine approaches.[33]

Opportunities for Precision Medicine in Public Health and Preventative Medicine

In spite of these concerns, there is considerable consensus that precision medicine holds great promise for advancing and revolutionizing healthcare and public health. However, to reach its full potential, it must be expanded both in how it is conceptualized and applied. This reconceptualization must go beyond the unidimensional focus on omics, and evolve to being multidimensional and dynamic, accounting for social, behavioral, and environmental determinants of health.[22] Therefore, theoretical frameworks are critical in this reconceptualization (discussed in the following section).

Fundamental to precision medicine is also advances in technology and data science with new data storage and management technologies, computational infrastructures, and robust analytic methods[2,22] that can leverage the derived knowledge of person, place, and time with precision to develop potent and targeted treatment and prevention approaches and deliver them at scale. Finally, the applicability of precision medicine should be expanded to focus beyond the individual, on populations, taking a precision public health approach (defined in Table 3-1). The latter part of this chapter will discuss how precision medicine has been applied to date in prevention and public health contexts, highlighting significant gaps that remain to be addressed, and end with a discussion around precision medicine's untapped potential as well as future directions in its quest to ultimately achieve precision health.

THEORETICAL FRAMEWORKS AND PRECISION HEALTH

The conceptions of precision medicine are undergoing expansion to extend beyond the initial focus on biology and individuals to encompass the multidimensional, complex, and dynamic influences on health and well-being. This expanded view of precision in health requires an acknowledgment of the influences of multiple levels on health, including biological, intra- and interpersonal, social, and environmental influences. In addition, precision entails that both science and practice be exact and accurate in the prediction of risk and protective factors, as well as accounting for the variability in health outcomes due to interventions or treatments. To be accurate, researchers and clinicians must be able to explain how a large array of factors lead to health outcomes, because the determinants of health and well-being are multifactorial. The potential breadth and complexity of the factors that need to be considered requires a theoretical perspective that can accommodate a holistic approach. This can aid in understanding how biology, person factors, and social and environmental factors interact to produce health. A systems perspective, hence, is a theoretical approach that can account for such complexities, and can be applied for understanding health problems, and potential interventions that can alleviate them.

Systems theory is an inter- and multidisciplinary study of systems that either occur naturally or are developed by human endeavor.[34,35] The boundaries of a system are typically defined by time, space, biological, social, and cultural dimensions. Now with the widespread use of computing, systems can be virtual.[36,37] How we define the boundaries of a system also impact how we describe and study a health problem, and the interventions that could improve the problem. This can be challenging as the definition of the components of a system can change by disciplinary perspectives, but it is helpful to take a systems perspective as it allows researchers and clinicians to understand problems holistically rather than piecemeal, thereby potentially increasing precision. Inherent in this approach is the examination of context when understanding health, and how these contextual dimensions are interdependent in creating or alleviating health risks. It may seem counterintuitive that understanding context would aid precision. However, to understand how interventions and treatments can be tailored to individuals and targeted to groups and populations, knowledge of contextual factors is critical. Reductionist approaches that focus on only one dimension of health, and ignore context, may not account for the variability that is needed for precision.

There have been many frameworks, theories, and conceptual models that draw on the ideas of a systems perspective (see Table 3-2), and that have evolved over time to account for more complex conceptions of health and illness. Some of these theories and models were developed as reactions to the biomedical model of health. The biomedical model of health primarily focuses on the physical or biological aspects of disease and illness as a way of understanding health, which from this perspective is usually defined as the absence of disease.[38] Over time, theory, research, and practice clearly have implicated many other domains as influential on and consequential to health. The biopsychosocial model, credited to George Engel, was proposed in reaction to the biomedical model's reductionistic and dualistic conception of illness,[39] and as a way to account for a broader set of factors that contribute to health and well-being, particularly psychological and social phenomenon.

Around the same time, in other disciplines, researchers were also conceptualizing how broader contextual factors influenced health and individual development over time. Bronfenbrenner's ecological systems theory[40] posited that multiple levels of interdependent influences impacted human development. This notion of multiple levels, and interdependence, ultimately became a central organizing framework for

TABLE 3-2 COMMON MODELS THAT DRAW ON A SYSTEMS APPROACH

Theoretical Models	Core Perspective	Major Proponents
Biopsychosocial model	In reaction to the traditional biomedical model, this model proposes that health is produced by the complex interaction between biological processes, psychological, and social factors.	Engel
Ecological systems theory	Proposed to account for the complex interaction of environmental factors in human development. First proposed to focus on the importance of the environment in a child's development.	Bronfenbrenner
Bioecological model	This model extends ecological systems thinking to include a stronger focus on the role of individual factors, including genetic and biological factors.	Bronfenbrenner and Ceci
Social ecological framework	Builds on and encompasses other models and emphasizes the interactions between people and environments and their interdependent nature. Also includes a greater focus on macro processes in producing health.	Stokols

social ecology[41] and models that stem from that tradition[37] put forth by Stokols and colleagues. Over time, Bronfenbrenner's model also incorporated more biological influences, including genetic influences on health and illness,[42] whereas the social ecology framework originally,[41,43,44] and continues to, emphasize individual experience in the context of more macroinfluences on health.[45–47] As these models started to encompass more areas of influence, over time, even the biopsychosocial model, which primarily focused on the clinical context,[48] started to view health and well-being from a more systems and dynamic perspective.[49]

Conceptually connected with these systems models, epigenetics has direct implications for understanding contextual factors in health, and implications for precision medicine. Epigenetics is the study of heritable changes in gene expression (phenotype) rather than changes in genetic code itself (genotype). Epigenetics involves chemical processes that are the mechanisms by which DNA gives instructions for gene expression. Epigenetic change occurs regularly and naturally, is reversible, and may be influenced by a host of behavioral, social, and environmental factors.[50] The connection with the models previously discussed is that environmental exposures, broadly defined, are thought to initiate these chemical processes, and potentially, alter gene expression. Epigenetic chemical processes can help explain how environmental exposures impact health across a person's lifetime. That is, environmental exposures can build up over time and affect genetic expression.[51] Originally, the environmental exposures thought to be important were physical in nature, such as exposure to toxic chemicals. However, the conceptualization has broadened over time and now behavioral, psychological, and social factors are considered important aspects of environmental exposure as well. This broader conceptualization of environmental exposure is sometimes referred to as the "exposome."[52,53] Research on the interaction of genomics and the exposome examines how various behavioral, psychological, and social factors produce health benefits or health risk in conjunction with cellular and molecular processes, which could lead to targeted interventions addressing multilevel factors in order to reduce risk and promote health.[54]

Despite stemming from different traditions, the systems models all acknowledge health as determined by a more complex interplay of biological, person, social, and environmental factors than initially conceived by the biomedical model. They have several common elements, principles, and concepts. Some of the key principles or concepts from these models can aid in fruitful expansion of the Precision Medicine Initiative by providing clearer ideas about who is at risk for developing disease or who is likely to benefit from a treatment or prevention strategy, when in the life course and in what context. These common elements are described below.

Multiple Levels of Analysis

Systems perspectives identify determinants of health at multiple levels of analysis.[37,40] Figure 3-1 shows a common depiction of a multilevel approach that considers both person and environmental factors proposed by Bronfenbrenner. Individuals and their biological, cognitive, or psychological characteristics are at the core of these models. Other levels depict environmental influences that surround the individual and vary in how direct or indirect their influence is thought to be. Microlevels reflect factors in the immediate environment such as interpersonal interactions, including those with family members, friends, or co-workers, which might be most proximal to the individual in space and time. The mesosystem reflects factors that might be linked to an individual via microlevel interactions and connections but are slightly more distal in time and space. These could be organizational and community connections, settings, or contexts, such as churches, community groups, and healthcare settings. The exosystem reflects environmental contexts that are more distal to an individual and might exert a more indirect influence. These factors could entail the broader community or geographical influences such as the composition of industry, neighborhoods, organizations, and services provided. The macrosystem reflects even broader social and cultural influences that may affect individuals as well as political and economic systems. While these factors are conceptualized to be more distal, they can have direct effects on individuals via policies, laws, and societal norms that sanction behavior. Finally, the chronosystem was added in later iterations of this model because of the inherent importance of time in determining the health and well-being of individuals as they move through the life course.

System Characteristics and Processes

Important processes that govern systems also relate to health and precision because they can help researchers and practitioners understand environments (i.e., levels) and individual reactions to environmental change over time.

Interdependence

Microlevels are nested within more macrolevels as shown in Fig. 3-1. Nesting implies potential interdependence between factors at different levels as reflected by the bidirectional arrows both between and within levels. Interdependence is an important factor to consider because it has the potential to aid in precision. For example, if researchers and practitioners can identify the points of leverage, defined as interdependent factors or conditions that exert a disproportionate influence on an individual's health, these points can aid in more precisely targeted interventions or treatments.

Mutual Influence

Interactions between people and environments are dynamic and governed by mutual influence. People react to the conditions in their social and physical environments, and act in ways to change

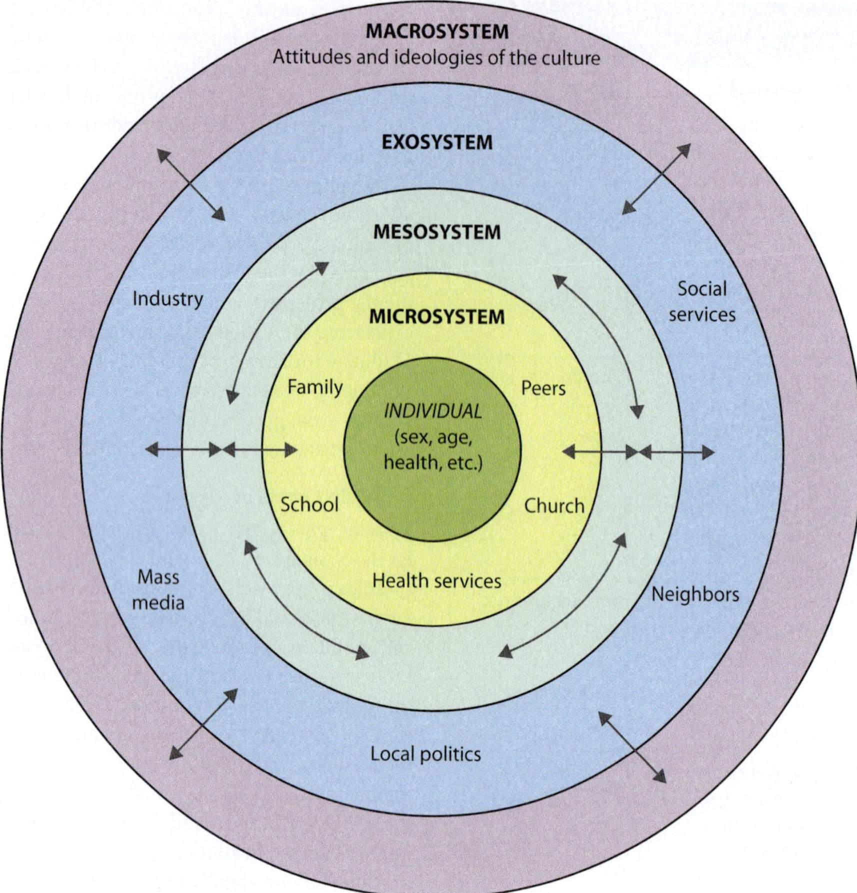

FIGURE 3-1. Bronfenbrenner's ecological systems model.

these conditions to better suit their needs or desires. Many times, this mutual influence is also reflected in repetitive cycles over time. Understanding and identifying cycles of behavior within particular environmental contexts, and how people seek to maintain the environment that either enhances health or risk, can provide a lens for identifying factors at both individual and environmental levels that need intervention or treatment.

Equifinality

In complex systems there is rarely one solution to a problem. The principle of equifinality suggests that there are multiple pathways to achieve outcomes, including health and well-being. This is an important principle for precision. Equifinality acknowledges variability in genetic, lifestyle, and environmental experiences among individuals and populations that needs to be considered and used in the promotion of health and treatment for a person or population. It encompasses the essence of a tailored versus one-size-fits all approach to health promotion.

Person and Environment Fit

Environments can be characterized by both objective and subjective dimensions that exert an influence on an individual's capability to enact behavior in health promoting ways (see Fig. 3-2).[40] In addition, individuals vary in their biological or psychological capacity to deal with and manage environments. For example, when environmental factors create stress and individual capacity is low then the potential for healthy outcomes is diminished. As shown in Fig. 3-2 when environments are too weak or strong in relationship to individual capacity, health outcomes vary. This concept can aid in precision by helping researchers and practitioners identify how person and environmental interactions can be combined to promote optimal health depending on characteristics of each dimension.[55]

To know if these models, principles, and concepts contribute to making the promotion of health and treatment of disease more precise, additional research is required. However, the field continues to move in the direction of conceiving of health and the environmental inputs that contribute to risk and protection more broadly,[56,57] with the promise that doing so will make the ideals of precision medicine a reality. To understand the complex interplay of genomics, behavior, and the social and physical environment, new developments in data sciences, refined measurement strategies that capture spatial and temporal influences, and the integration of multiple, large data streams need to be realized. Some of the theories and concepts presented here can provide a roadmap for making sense of these large data structures that are needed to operationalize precision medicine.

DATA AND PRECISION HEALTH

The emergence of big data has been simultaneously supported by the growth of tools and technologies that have increased our ability to organize, store, and manage data. Advances in database and computing technologies have sustained the development of multiple data-centered disciplines such as bioinformatics (using biologic/genetic data), clinical informatics (using patient data from electronic records), consumer health informatics (using naturalistic data on human behavior and health), and public health informatics (using informatics tools for addressing population health problems). Although these disciplines have emerged with independent research paradigms, the growth of the precision medicine paradigm has

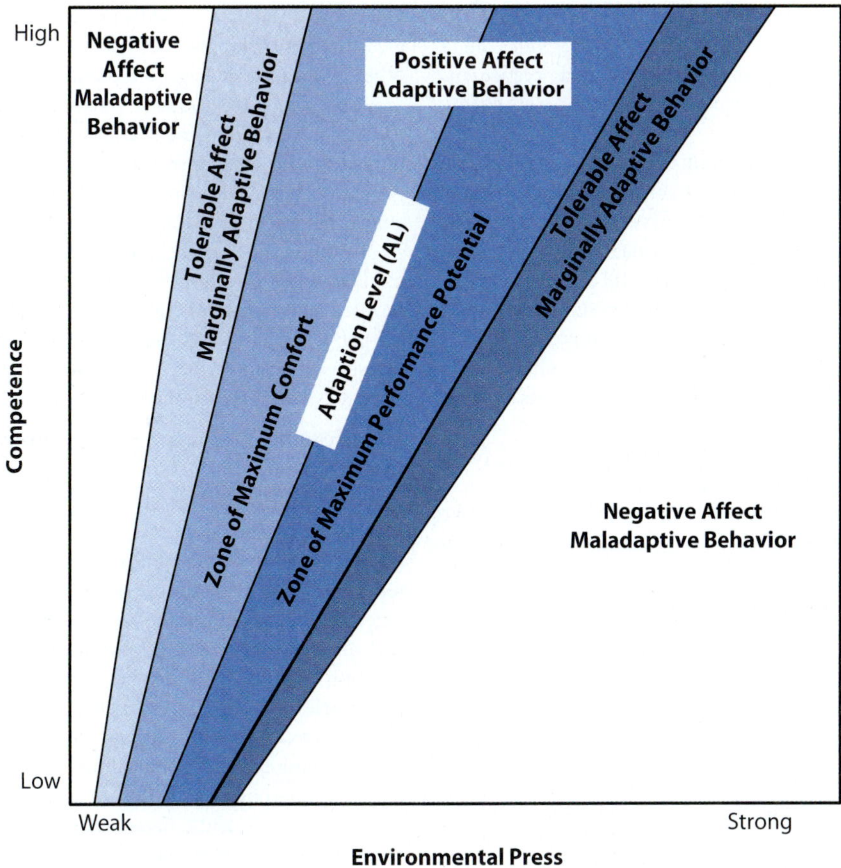

FIGURE 3-2. Person-environment fit model.

changed the ways in which research is conceived across these disciplines. Primarily, there has been an effort toward organizing and aligning siloed data across these disciplines to develop meaningful insights regarding overall human health.

Within the public health domain, a host of pragmatic and systems-oriented theories and strategies have been developed to guide the design and implementation of research, practice, and preventive practices. These efforts are situated in reconciling the goals of precision medicine, which begins with individuals, and that of public health, which begins with populations.[58] The bridge between the two has been data—more specifically, "big data"—a term generally applied to describe large quantities of data with complex dependencies and relationships.[59] An in-depth discussion of health informatics and big data analytics can be found in the corresponding chapter of this book. Here we briefly present the relevance of big data and analytic tools to precision public health.

The progress made in machine learning (ML) approaches in creating reliable insights regarding multiscaled data has been promising. ML, as opposed to conventional statistical approaches, relies on learning patterns and rules from the data.[60] In other words, ML techniques use a large number of predictor variables from the data, learning relationships that exist between them, and utilizing these learned relationships to predict outcomes. For example, for predicting hospital readmissions for patients, an ML algorithm can consider a host of variables including clinical conditions, severity of the clinical conditions, prior history of hospitalizations, medications, genomic data (when available), and other relevant sociodemographic variables from a patient's record. ML algorithms then utilize thousands of such patient records to "learn" patterns within variables that potentially predict readmissions. The self-learning aspect of ML algorithms makes it particularly attractive when dealing with millions of multifactorial data points such as the clinical situations of patients over time.

Within public health, the use of big data and associated data science approaches is fairly new. Examples of the application of predictive approaches include creation of precision maps for identifying growth deficiencies in children,[61] predicting poverty,[62] syndromic surveillance,[63] and monitoring infectious diseases.[64] For additional information and examples, please refer to the next section, *Applications of Precision Medicine in Public Health and Prevention*. In spite of the advantages, ML techniques have several disadvantages including requirement of large data sets, potential overfitting of data, and susceptibility to biases.[65] However, they are seen as indispensable for addressing complex challenges posed by big data.

Newer approaches such as deep learning[65,66] have dramatically improved the predictive capabilities of computational algorithms. Deep learning algorithms consist of multiple processing layers where representations are automatically learned for detection of patterns. Although there are limited examples of the use of deep learning for specific public health problems, they have been used in a variety of application. The applications have ranged from genomic analysis to clinical informatics and consumer health informatics. For example, Rajkomar et al.[66] used data from multiple hospitals to create a risk prediction model of medical events—in-hospital mortality, 30-day readmissions, and length of stay—that performed better than traditional models. The application of deep learning techniques has been more prominent in predicting consumer (patient)-centered applications for prediction of emotional states and sentiment analysis using patient-reported, unobtrusively captured activities or social media data via a variety of smartphone applications. For example,

Cao et al.[67] used a deep learning algorithm to predict changes in human mood based on changes in psychomotor activities on a mobile keyboard. Similar efforts of mood detection using deep learning tools have relied on participant responses at various points during the day.[68]

Deep learning algorithms show promise in integrating multiple structured and unstructured data sources from cohort studies, claims data, electronic health record (EHR) data, surveys, wearable devices, and sensors on mobile phones (i.e., naturalistic data on human behavior and health). However, significant challenges still exist for integrating multiscaled information—from genetic to environmental—in a meaningful manner that can translate data to knowledge.[69] This challenge primarily arises from the need to address the inherent data complexities—where the data "whole is not a sum of its parts"[70]—that affect its appropriate use for public health research and practice. One of the reasons for the lack of considerable progress is the lack of an integrated and coherent data and analytical infrastructure.

Tenenbaum et al.[69] provide a two-step process that should drive the infrastructure development: ability to translate data to knowledge and then translate knowledge into action. Within this framework, translation of data to knowledge would involve development of data standards that ensure data privacy, security and integrity, supporting data exchange.

Translating the available data to knowledge relies on developing clinical decision support that utilizes the data (and associated algorithms) for providing actionable information. The latter can include information at the point-of-care for decision support to information that can help in providing adequate surveillance of a community or population.[71] This would involve pragmatic and translational applications requiring development of sharable knowledge bases and the use of multiple delivery mechanisms for disease identification and management.[72] It must, however, be stated that the translation from data to point-of-care (or for surveillance) is still an emerging area of research.

APPLICATIONS OF PRECISION MEDICINE IN PUBLIC HEALTH AND PREVENTION

Early efforts on the development of translational work integrating systems perspectives and new data techniques have been undertaken in several domains in precision public health (see definition in Table 3-1). The goal of precision public health is to apply the precision medicine concept at the population level in order to improve public health. Whereas precision medicine aims to deliver the right health intervention to the right *person* at the right *place* and *time*, precision public health seeks to deliver the right health intervention to the right *population* at the right *place* and *time*.[73–75] It does so by building on the systems theory and providing tailored preventive interventions or treatments for targeted segments of the population. With advances in data pipelines and computational tools, applications of precision medicine in public health are rapidly expanding. The areas where most research has been carried out include cancer screening, prevention and survival, prevention and control of infectious and chronic diseases, population vulnerability and equity, and targeted public health policy.[76] In the following sections, we present several specific applications that utilize different streams of data and knowledge to enhance precision across levels according to the systems theory, thereby to better illustrate the concept of precision public health in action.

Individual-Level Applications

Advances in genomic research, focused on individuals' biological characteristics, paved the way for early applications of precision medicine. One example is the utilization of genomic screening for breast and ovarian cancers. About 2–7% of breast cancer and 10–15% of ovarian cancer patients carry mutations in *BRCA1* and *BRCA2*[77] and approximately 1 in 500 women have a BRCA mutation, which gives them a strikingly high risk for developing breast, ovarian, and other cancers. In 2005, genomic study evidence led to U.S. Preventive Services Task Force (USPSTF) recommendations, specifically that of *BRCA1* and *BRCA2* genetic counseling and testing for women who have a family history of breast and/or ovarian cancers. Similarly, genomics studies have provided evidence about Lynch syndrome and colorectal cancer, and as a result, in 2009 the Evaluation of Genomic Applications in Practice and Prevention Working Group recommended genetic testing for Lynch syndrome among patients with newly diagnosed colorectal cancer in order to reduce morbidity and mortality in their family members.[78] Both of these recommendations are also reflected in the two Healthy People 2020 objectives in the genomics area aimed at increasing genetic counseling and testing.

Microsystem-, Mesosystem-, and Chronosystem-Level Applications

Microsystem focuses on factors in the immediate environment such as interpersonal interactions (e.g., those with family members, friends, or co-workers), while meso- and chronosystems focus on the relationship between an individual's microsystems over time. Taken together, they highlight the need for considering behavioral, social, and environmental data across spatial and temporal contexts, in addition to individual biological data, which has inspired new lines of inquiries in multidimensional applications of precision medicine. One such example with promise is the EHR, which is in the process of developing beyond a clinical tool as currently implemented to be a robust, interoperable platform capable of linking genetic, clinical, social/behavioral, and different levels of environmental data in order to ultimately benefit population health management. Linking these contextual data, EHRs could help stratify a patient population into groups with different levels of disease risk, both inside and outside of the healthcare delivery system. It is important to underscore, however, that much work is still ahead to reach the end goal of efficient and effective population health management. Within the care delivery system, emerging research has shed light on the potential of utilizing EHR data to stratify patient populations with different degrees of control for common chronic diseases such as diabetes and hypertension and provide tailored treatment and follow-up to these patient groups.[79,80] These ongoing efforts support the Institute for Healthcare Improvement (IHI) Triple Aim framework for optimization of health system performance by simultaneously addressing patient experience of care, population health, and per capita cost of healthcare.[81] EHR data have also demonstrated utility to aid tailored disease management strategies outside of the care delivery system. For example, because NCDs are often found to cluster among geographic neighborhoods, centrally aggregated EHR data provided by clinics in nearby neighborhoods offer a new way to identify and target neighborhoods with the least effective control of diabetes.[82] Consequently, appropriate community-based diabetes management interventions can be designed and implemented based on the unique disease and risk factor profiles of high-risk neighborhoods.

Another example is the area of smoking cessation for the prevention of lung diseases. In order to maximize the efficiency of smoking cessation treatments,[83] researchers have not only identified genetic variants that may predict nicotine dependence, smoking cessation, and response to cessation pharmacotherapy, but also have included psychobehavioral, social, and environmental factors in public health efforts for smoking cessation. As a result, multilevel smoking cessation interventions have been designed and delivered based on the unique problems experienced by specific neighborhoods and have targeted intrapersonal (e.g., self-efficacy), interpersonal (e.g., social support from family, friends, and neighborhood), and environmental factors.[84] The latter have included neighborhood activities such as antitobacco campaign messages and pamphlets/posters on risks of passive smoke exposure to children, along with policy-related activities such as smoking guidelines or bans at community settings and events. The combined efforts addressing personal, interpersonal, to micro- as well as macrolevel factors have reduced smoking prevalence from 43% to 18% in the U.S. adults over the past half century.[85]

A further exemplary application of precision medicine in public health is the rapidly developing area of wearable technology for health and clinical research (referred to as *mhealth*) for unobtrusive sensing and monitoring of human activity across space and time.[86] Such mhealth interventions have been used to track physical activity,[87] mental health,[88] cardiovascular health,[89] and pain,[90] to name a few. While early research in this field was situated around merely providing descriptive frequencies of events (e.g., steps walked or calories burned), more recent efforts have shifted to focus on predicting potential clinical or health events based on tracked data and then delivering just-in-time, tailored interventions to curb the risk.[91] For example, in the smoking cessation example, psychobehavioral, social, and environmental factors can be measured during smoking cessation interventions using ecological momentary assessment (EMA) methods via smartphones and other portable devices. Risk for smoking relapse can then be predicted in real time using a weighted lapse risk estimator containing personal psychobehavioral data (e.g., smoke urge, stress, recent alcohol consumption, motivation to quit), social factors (e.g., interaction with people smoking), and microenvironmental factors (e.g., cigarette availability). In response to level of risk, just-in-time, tailored intervention messages could be delivered.[92] Furthermore, the related and emerging domain of spatial energetics which combines spatiotemporal location data (e.g., GPS) with time-matched energetics data (e.g., from the accelerometer of a smart phone) provides insights into contextual aspects of individual activities (e.g., where does a person walk?) and holds great potential for developing personalized, context-specific, and moment-in-time interventions to address major public health problems such as inactivity and obesity.[93]

Exosystem- and Macrosystem-Level Applications

The exo- and macrosystems are increasingly distal levels but nonetheless can have direct and indirect influences on individual and population health (e.g., through neighborhood characteristics, cultural values, social norms, economic systems, health policies). Research in precision public health around these systems has been underway, mainly in the area of precise disease surveillance, both nationally and globally.

One example is the development and use of "precision maps" to identify diseases and their prevalence so as to support community-based public health initiatives. The use of maps in identifying public health issues and challenges have been a staple strategy remaining at the forefront of public health research.[94] Beginning with John Snow's famous cholera maps in London in the nineteenth century, these efforts have focused on source, spread, and causal underpinnings of the prevalence of diseases or public health concerns. While much of the early research relied on coarse data (e.g., at a country level), more recent efforts have focused on generating "precision maps" regarding areas of interest.[94] An example that illustrates the use of layered data strategies and precision mapping, in asthma research, shows that asthma-related emergency department visits and hospitalizations among children are significantly associated with the density of housing code violations (e.g., the presence of mold or cockroaches),[95] asthma-related medication adherence, socioeconomic status, crime, and traffic in the neighborhood, among other individual, social, and environmental factors.[96] Following a precision maps approach, geomarkers of risk factors can be obtained from various sources, mapped at a granular scale, and new computational approaches can be employed, thus generating localized predictions. For instance, housing code violation density can be obtained from a city's Building, Health, and Property Maintenance database and asthma-related medication adherence from pharmacy chain data. Then metrics estimating asthma risk factors can be calculated using appropriate statistical methods. As noted above, coupled with the advances in EHRs, such contextual information could also be integrated into a patient's chart, providing clinicians with important, rich personal and environmental data. Precision maps therefore provide a sustainable approach for developing localized design interventions that can produce maximum impact on a local, state, national and, as described below, even international scale.

Developed countries, such as the United States and some European countries, are more mature in implementing precise disease surveillance. Unlike developed countries, developing countries have not yet been fully able to take advantage of the developments in precision public health, primarily because of the general lack of good-quality surveillance data and reliable laboratory testing that informs surveillance in many developing countries. Progress to precise disease surveillance is challenging without adequate funding devoted to this public health priority in the developing countries that confront a large burden of diseases.

The Bill & Melinda Gates Foundation, the largest philanthropic private foundation in the United States, is committed to this type of work, specifically to enhance global health and alleviate population health inequities.[97] For example, a Gates Foundation project found evidence of group B streptococci in the tissues of stillbirths in South Africa. The researchers found that Group B streptococcus infection is the reason why so many women in South Africa are losing their babies, and that women who have experienced such losses also have a sevenfold higher risk of subsequent losses in later pregnancies. This discovery was key in identifying an effectively targeted and economical preventive treatment. Antibiotics (e.g., penicillin) can effectively prevent group B streptococcal infections in newborns and, as a result, related death. It is also inexpensive to prescribe antibiotics to women at risk of losing their babies due to Group B streptococcus infection.[98]

Another example of precision medicine applied in global health also relates to disease surveillance, specifically using precision maps that identify the geographical distribution of disease worldwide. For example, during the outbreak of Zika virus in 2016, two at-risk neighborhoods of just 2.6 and 3.9 square kilometers in Miami were identified, leading to targeted travel advisories and mosquito control efforts focused on these areas.[98] A related example has to do with the finding that mosquitoes do not transmit certain viruses (including Zika) if they carry the Wolbachia virus. Therefore, Wolbachia-carrying mosquitoes can be distributed to displace wild-type mosquitoes and reduce Zika transmission. However, such programs on a global scale are expensive. Fortunately, precise disease surveillance data, combined with geospatial modeling, have identified an area of only 7 million (vs. originally nearly 50 million) square kilometers with 90% of the predicted disease burden, significantly reducing the area in need of intervention, making Wolbachia-based mosquito control possible and affordable for many countries including Colombia and Brazil.[98] Another application of precision mapping is witnessed in the effort to prevent child growth failure (i.e., stunting, wasting, and underweight for children under 5 years old) in Africa. By combining information on local climate and geography with geo-located information on growth failure in children gathered from surveys (over a 15-year period) and using Bayesian prediction approaches, researchers could determine growth failure patterns, locations with improvements, and predict the likelihood of future potential improvements.[61]

In addition, researchers have learned valuable lessons from the massive disaster caused by the 2014 Ebola outbreak in multiple countries of West Africa, particularly around the shortcomings in surveillance data availability and quality. This deadly epidemic highlighted the need for accurate surveillance data at the individual level (e.g., to identify who was infected or had contact with an infected person), at the interpersonal level (e.g., to identify where/how cases may have

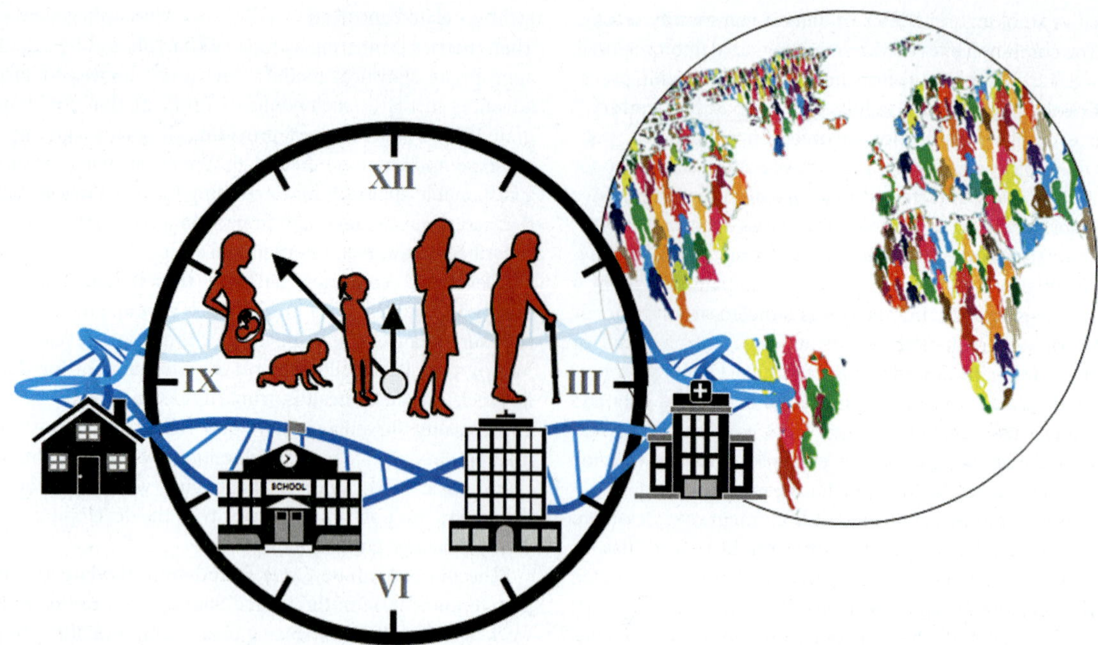

FIGURE 3-3. Precision health. It is defined as the attainment of a state of complete physical, mental, and social well-being at individual and population levels through enhanced abilities to optimally predict, prevent, and treat disease by accounting for variability in genes, environment, and lifestyle.

been infected), and at the population level (e.g., to identify the size and demographics of populations affected).[99] In response, recent research has focused on using mobile phone data as a new source of "real time" information that can identify individuals' mobility patterns, and consequently, be more effective in preventing future outbreaks.[100] Although global public health efforts are underway, in order for them to be more successful, there is a pressing need for investments in core infrastructure, disease surveillance, laboratory methods, and workforce training, particularly so in developing countries.

FUTURE DIRECTION: PRECISION HEALTH

In this chapter, we reviewed the evolution of precision medicine, described system theories as well as advances in technology and data science for the conception and implementation of precision medicine research, and presented exemplary applications of precision medicine in public health and prevention. We focused on underscoring the challenges and opportunities that lie ahead and, more importantly, for focusing on a vision for precision health. Precision health is a term that has been increasingly used in the literature but, to date, poorly defined. Building on the WHO definition of health that it is "a state of complete physical, mental, and social well-being and not merely the absence of disease or infirmity,"[101] we define precision health as the attainment of a state of complete physical, mental, and social well-being at individual and population levels through enhanced abilities to optimally predict, prevent, and treat disease by accounting for variability in genes, environment, and lifestyle.

In the pursuit of precision health many challenges abound, and we highlight a few that we consider fundamental. First, a better integrated, comprehensive framework that guides research and knowledge transfer must be developed and employed by those engaged in precision medicine research and practice. Although important work is underway in this constantly evolving field, it is fragmented without a unifying framework that would help in characterizing the ongoing research and directions for future research.

Second, new tools, technologies, and methods in this field must be critically evaluated as they are developed and implemented, and the field needs to be cautious with interpreting results derived from big data in order to prevent overestimation of findings. For example, during the 2013 influenza outbreak in the United States, Google Flu Trends dramatically overestimated peak influenza levels by analyzing influenza-related internet searches, compared to public health surveillance.[102] This is problematic because inaccurate surveillance data could lead to ineffective public health responses.

Third, more efforts are needed to obtain proper informed consents and ensure adequate protections for collecting, storing, and sharing health information. This is particularly important when biological, behavioral, social, and environmental data are being collected and shared among different stakeholders. It is critical to ensure ethical privacy and confidentiality so that, for instance, personal health data are not breached during storage, and genomic data are not used against an individual's employment and health insurance status.

Fourth, precision public health requires substantial infrastructure development and access to large-scale multilevel data. A precision health infrastructure (e.g., including health professionals, community engagement, laboratories, policies, logistics, etc.) would provide opportunities for integrating data from different sources and for efficiently utilizing multilevel population data to provide the right interventions to right populations. Appropriate infrastructure can also provide communities, states, and countries alike, the capacity to quickly respond to acute infectious outbreaks, monitor chronic disease patterns, effectively deliver interventions to target populations, and optimize the allocation of resources in space and time in order to improve the public's health and reduce health disparities.

In summary, precision medicine seeks to incorporate state-of-the-art technology and data science into medicine and healthcare so as to more precisely identify, prevent, and treat an individual's disease. The ultimate impact of the precision medicine movement on population health will depend on a foresighted integration with the public health approach. The latter relies on a systematic and iterative process of defining and monitoring the public's health problem, identifying risk and protective factors, developing and testing prevention strategies, and assuring widespread adoption. It is also important to acknowledge several realities that are central to the health of any population. These include that disease risk is a continuum rather than a dichotomy, that most often the majority of people in a population fall in the middle of the risk distribution with a small percentage at the extremes of high or low risk, and that an individual's risk of illness needs to be considered in relation to the disease risk for the population to which he or she belongs.[103] The precision medicine movement reflects advances in medicine and technology that have sharpened our abilities to attain greater precision in risk prediction, prevention, and treatment than ever previously possible. To realize the full potential of these advances—and many more on their way—for population health, requires an unwavering appreciation of the realities that shape population health as well as the efforts to achieve it. The ultimate goal of the precision medicine approach is to achieve precision health as defined above. The rapid scientific and technological advances inspire us to envision a future when we can harness data on important biological, behavioral, social, and environmental determinants of health, measure them by moment in time across life stages and social contexts, and robustly examine the intricate interactions of person, place, and time—among individuals and populations. We illustrate this vision in Fig. 3-3. Importantly, the vision of precision health shall be rooted in a resolute commitment to health for all.

References

1. US National Library of Medicine. What is precision medicine? 2018; https://ghr.nlm.nih.gov/primer/precisionmedicine/definition. Accessed October 5, 2018.
2. Khoury MJ. The shift from personalized medicine to precision medicine and precision public health: Words matter! 2016; https://blogs.cdc.gov/genomics/2016/04/21/shift/. Accessed October 5, 2018.
3. Jameson JL, Longo DL. Precision medicine—personalized, problematic, and promising. *N Engl J Med*. 2015;372(23):2229–34.
4. Mascie-Taylor CG, Karim E. The burden of chronic disease. *Science*. 2003;302(5652):1921–2.
5. World Health Organization. Noncommunicable diseases now biggest killers. 2008; http://www.who.int/mediacentre/news/releases/2008/pr14/en/.
6. World Health Organization. World health statistics. 2008.
7. Sandhu C, Qureshi A, Emili A. Panomics for precision medicine. *Trends Mol Med*. 2018;24(1):85–101.
8. Chen R, Snyder M. Promise of personalized omics to precision medicine. *Wiley Interdiscip Rev Syst Biol Med*. 2013;5(1):73–82.
9. Hasin Y, Seldin M, Lusis A. Multi-omics approaches to disease. *Genome Biol*. 2017;18:83.
10. National Human Genome Research Institute. All about the human genome project (hgp). 2015; https://www.genome.gov/10001772/all-about-the--human-genome-project-hgp/. Accessed October 15, 2018.
11. Feero W, Wicklund CA, Veenstra D. Precision medicine, genome sequencing, and improved population health. *JAMA*. 2018;319(19):1979–80.
12. National Research Council Committee. *Toward Precision Medicine: Building a Knowledge Network for Biomedical Research and a New Taxonomy of Disease*. Washington, DC: National Academies Press; 2011.
13. National Institutes of Health. Human microbiome project. 2018; https://commonfund.nih.gov/hmp. Accessed October 15, 2018.
14. Wishart DS, Feunang YD, Marcu A, et al. Hmdb 4.0: The human metabolome database for 2018. *Nucleic Acids Res*. 2018;46(D1):D608–17.
15. National Cancer Institute. Cancer moonshot. https://www.cancer.gov/research/key-initiatives/moonshot-cancer-initiative. Accessed October 5, 2018.
16. Bragazzi NL. From p0 to p6 medicine, a model of highly participatory, narrative, interactive, and "augmented" medicine: Some considerations on Salvatore Iaconesi's clinical story. *Patient Prefer Adherence*. 2013;7:353–9.
17. World Health Organization. About WHO. 2018. https://www.who.int/ Accessed October 15, 2018.
18. The White House. Fact sheet: President Obama's precision medicine initiative. 2015; https://obamawhitehouse.archives.gov/the-press-office/2015/01/30/fact-sheet-president-obama-s-precision-medicine-initiative. Accessed October 5, 2018.
19. US National Library of Medicine. What is the precision medicine initiative? 2018; https://ghr.nlm.nih.gov/primer/precisionmedicine/initiative. Accessed October 5, 2018.
20. Collins FS, Varmus H. A new initiative on precision medicine. *N Engl J Med*. 2015;372(9):793–5.
21. National Institutes of Health. The future of health begins with you. 2018; https://allofus.nih.gov. Accessed October 5, 2018.
22. Khoury MJ, Galea S. Precision medicine and population health: Dealing with the elephant in the room. 2016; https://blogs.cdc.gov/genomics/2016/08/17/precision-medicine-3/. Accessed October 5, 2018.
23. Chowkwanyun M, Bayer R, Galea S. "Precision" public health—Between novelty and hype. *N Engl J Med*. 2018;379(15):1398–1400.
24. World Health Organization. Social determinants of health. 2018; https://www.who.int/social_determinants/sdh_definition/en/. Accessed October 15, 2018.
25. Centers for Disease Control and Prevention. Social determinants of health: Know what affects health. 2018; https://www.cdc.gov/socialdeterminants/. Accessed October 15, 2018.
26. Agency for Healthcare Research and Quality. Population health: Behavioral and social science insights: A role for social and behavioral research. 2015; http://www.ahrq.gov/professionals/education/curriculum-tools/population-health/baldwin.html. Accessed October 5, 2018.
27. Arena R, Guazzi M, Lianov L, et al. Healthy lifestyle interventions to combat noncommunicable disease—A novel nonhierarchical connectivity model for key stakeholders: A policy statement from the American Heart Association, European Society of Cardiology, European Association for Cardiovascular Prevention and Rehabilitation, and American College of Preventive Medicine. *Eur Heart J*. 2015;36(31):2097–109.
28. Galea S, Bayer R. The precision medicine chimera. 2016; https://www.project-syndicate.org/commentary/precision-medicine-public-health-by-sandro-galea-and-ronald-bayer-2016-01?barrier=accesspaylog. Accessed October 5, 2018.
29. Bayer R, Galea S. Public health in the precision-medicine era. *N Engl J Med*. 2015;373(6):499–501.
30. Office of Disease Prevention and Health Promotion. About healthy people. 2018; https://www.healthypeople.gov/2020/About-Healthy-People. Accessed October 8, 2018.
31. Interlandi J. The paradox of precision medicine. 2016; https://www.scientificamerican.com/article/the-paradox-of-precision-medicine/. Accessed October 5, 2018.
32. Rose G. Strategy of prevention: Lessons from cardiovascular disease. *Br Med J*. 1981;282(6279):1847–51. PMC1506445.
33. Ramaswami R, Bayer R, Galea S. Precision medicine from a public health perspective. *Annu Rev Public Health*. 2018;39:153–68.
34. Miller JG. *Living Systems*. New York: McGraw-Hill; 1978.
35. von Bertanlaffy L. *Perspectives on General System Theory*. New York: George Braziller, Inc.; 1975.
36. Stokols D. *Social Ecology in the Digital Age*. San Diego, CA: Academic Press, Elsevier; 2018.
37. Stokols D. Establishing and maintaining healthy environments. Toward a social ecology of health promotion. *Am Psychol*. 1992;47(1):6–22.
38. National Research Council. *Biomedical Models and Resources: Current Needs and Future Opportunities*. Washington, DC: The National Academies Press; 1998.
39. Engel GL. The need for a new medical model: A challenge for biomedicine. *Science*. 1977;196(4286):129–36.
40. Bronfenbrenner U. Ecological systems theory. In: Kazdin AE, ed. *Encyclopedia of Psychology*. Vol. 3. Washington, DC: American Psychological Association; 2000.
41. Binder A, Stokols D, Catalano R. Social ecology: An emerging multidiscipline. *J Environ Educ*. 1975;7(2):32–43.
42. Bronfenbrenner U, Ceci SJ. Nature-nurture reconceptualized in developmental perspective: A bioecological model. *Psychol Rev*. 1994;101(4):568–86.
43. Emery F, Trist E. *Towards a Social Ecology: Contextual Appreciation of the Future in the Present*. London: Plenum Press; 1972.
44. Catalano R. *Health, Behavior and the Community: An Ecological Perspective*. New York: Pergamon Press; 1979.
45. Golden SD, McLeroy KR, Green LW, Earp JA, Lieberman LD. Upending the social ecological model to guide health promotion efforts toward policy and environmental change. *Health Educ Behav*. 2015;42(1 Suppl):8s–14s.
46. Misra S, Stokols D. A typology of people–environment relationships in the digital age. *Technol Soc*. 2012;34(4):311–25.
47. Stokols D, Lejano RP, Hipp J. Enhancing the resilience of human-environment systems: A social ecological perspective. *Ecol Soc*. 2013;18(1):7.
48. Borrell-Carrió F, Suchman AL, Epstein RM. The biopsychosocial model 25 years later: Principles, practice, and scientific inquiry. *Ann Family Med*. 2004;2(6):576–82.

49. Lehman BJ, David DM, Gruber JA. Rethinking the biopsychosocial model of health: Understanding health as a dynamic system. *Soc Personal Psychol Compass.* 2017;11(8):e12328.
50. Weinhold B. Epigenetics: The science of change. *Environ Health Perspect.* 2006;114(3):A160–7.
51. Sierra MI, Fernandez AF, Fraga MF. Epigenetics of aging. *Curr Genomics.* 2015;16(6):435–40.
52. Wild CP. Complementing the genome with an "exposome": The outstanding challenge of environmental exposure measurement in molecular epidemiology. *Cancer Epidemiol Biomarkers Prev.* 2005;14(8):1847–50.
53. Juarez PD, Matthews-Juarez P, Hood DB, et al. The public health exposome: A population-based, exposure science approach to health disparities research. *Int J Environ Res Public Health.* 2014;11(12):12866–95.
54. McBride CM, Koehly LM. Imagining roles for epigenetics in health promotion research. *J Behav Med.* 2017;40(2):229–38.
55. Lawton M, Nahemow L. Ecology and the aging process. In: Eisdorfer C, Lawton M, eds. *The Psychology of Adult Development and Aging.* Washington, DC: American Psychological Association; 1973.
56. Roth TL. Epigenetic mechanisms in the development of behavior: Advances, challenges, and future promises of a new field. *Dev Psychopathol.* 2013;25(4 Pt 2):1279–91.
57. Loi M, Del Savio L, Stupka E. Social epigenetics and equality of opportunity. *Public Health Ethics.* 2013;6(2):142–53.
58. Chowkwanyun M, Bayer R, Galea S. "Precision" public health—Between novelty and hype. *N Engl J Med.* 2018;379(15):1398–1400.
59. Mayer-Schönberger V, Cukier K. *Big Data: A Revolution That Will Transform How We Live, Work, and Think.* Boston, MA: Houghton Mifflin Harcourt; 2013.
60. Obermeyer Z, Emanuel EJ. Predicting the future—Big data, machine learning, and clinical medicine. *N Engl J Med.* 2016;375(13):1216.
61. Osgood-Zimmerman A, Millear AI, Stubbs RW, et al. Mapping child growth failure in Africa between 2000 and 2015. *Nature.* 2018;555(7694):41–45.
62. Jean N, Burke M, Xie M, et al. Combining satellite imagery and machine learning to predict poverty. *Science.* 2016;353(6301):790–4.
63. Paul MJ, Dredze M. *You are What you Tweet: Analyzing Twitter for Public Health.* Baltimore, MD:ICWSM; 2011.
64. Brownstein JS, Freifeld CC, Reis BY, Mandl KD. Surveillance Sans Frontieres: Internet-based emerging infectious disease intelligence and the healthmap project. *PLoS Med.* 2008;5(7):e151.
65. LeCun Y, Bengio Y, Hinton G. Deep learning. *Nature.* 2015;521(7553): 436–40.
66. Rajkomar A, Oren E, Chen K, et al. Scalable and accurate deep learning with electronic health records. *NPJ Digital Med.* 2018;1(1):18–27.
67. Cao B, Zheng L, Zhang C, et al. Deepmood: Modeling mobile phone typing dynamics for mood detection. *Proceedings of the 23rd ACM SIGKDD International Conference on Knowledge Discovery and Data Mining*; 2017.
68. Suhara Y, Xu Y, Pentland AS. Deepmood: Forecasting depressed mood based on self-reported histories via recurrent neural networks. *Proceedings of the 26th International Conference on World Wide Web*; 2017.
69. Tenenbaum JD, Avillach P, Benham-Hutchins M, et al. An informatics research agenda to support precision medicine: Seven key areas. *J Am Med Inform Assoc.* 2016;23(4):791–5.
70. Simon HA. *The Sciences of the Artificial.* Cambridge MA: MIT Press; 1996.
71. Ehrenstein V, Nielsen H, Pedersen AB, Johnsen SP, Pedersen L. Clinical epidemiology in the era of big data: New opportunities, familiar challenges. *Clin Epidemiol.* 2017;9:245–8.
72. Masys DR, Jarvik GP, Abernethy NF, et al. Technical desiderata for the integration of genomic data into electronic health records. *J Biomed Inform.* 2012;45(3):419–22.
73. Khoury MJ, Bowen MS, Clyne M, et al. From public health genomics to precision public health: A 20-year journey. *Genet Med.* 2018;20(6): 574–82.
74. Arnett DK, Claas SA. Precision medicine, genomics, and public health. *Diabetes Care.* 2016;39(11):1870–3.
75. Khoury MJ, Iademarco MF, Riley WT. Precision public health for the era of precision medicine. *Am J Prev Med.* 2016;50(3):398–401.
76. Weeramanthri TS, Dawkins HJS, Baynam G, et al. Editorial: Precision public health. *Front Public Health.* 2018;6:121.
77. Bellcross CA, Kolor K, Goddard KA, et al. Awareness and utilization of brca1/2 testing among U.S. primary care physicians. *Am J Prev Med.* 2011;40(1):61–6.
78. Evaluation of Genomic Applications in Practice and Prevention (EGAPP) Working Group. Recommendations from the EGAPP working group: Genetic testing strategies in newly diagnosed individuals with colorectal cancer aimed at reducing morbidity and mortality from Lynch syndrome in relatives. *Genet Med.* 2009;11(1):35–41.
79. Lv N, Xiao L, Simmons ML, et al. Personalized hypertension management using patient-generated health data integrated with electronic health records (empower-h): Six-month pre-post study. *J Med Internet Res.* 2017;19(9):e311.
80. Eggleston EM, Klompas M. Rational use of electronic health records for diabetes population management. *Curr Diab Rep.* 2014;14(4):479.
81. Berwick DM, Nolan TW, Whittington J. The triple aim: Care, health, and cost. *Health Aff (Millwood).* 2008;27(3):759–69.
82. Gabert R, Thomson B, Gakidou E, Roth G. Identifying high-risk neighborhoods using electronic medical records: A population-based approach for targeting diabetes prevention and treatment interventions. *PLoS One.* 2016;11(7):e0159227.
83. Chen LS, Horton A, Bierut L. Pathways to precision medicine in smoking cessation treatments. *Neurosci Lett.* 2018;669:83–92.
84. Andrews JO, Tingen MS, Jarriel SC, et al. Application of a CBPR framework to inform a multi-level tobacco cessation intervention in public housing neighborhoods. *Am J Community Psychol.* 2012;50(1-2):129–40.
85. U.S. Department of Health and Human Services. The health consequences of smoking—50 years of progress: A report of the surgeon general. Atlanta, GA: U.S. Department of Health and Human Services, Centers for Disease Control and Prevention, National Center for Chronic Disease Prevention and Health Promotion, Office on Smoking and Health; 2014.
86. Klasnja P, Pratt W. Managing health with mobile technology. *Interactions.* 2014;21(1):66–9.
87. Hurvitz PM, Moudon AV, Kang B, Saelens BE, Duncan GE. Emerging technologies for assessing physical activity behaviors in space and time. *Front Public Health.* 2014;2:2.
88. Donker T, Petrie K, Proudfoot J, et al. Smartphones for smarter delivery of mental health programs: A systematic review. *J Med Internet Res.* 2013;15(11):e247.
89. Chow CK, Redfern J, Hillis GS, et al. Effect of lifestyle-focused text messaging on risk factor modification in patients with coronary heart disease: A randomized clinical trial. *JAMA.* 2015;314(12):1255–63.
90. Parker SJ, Jessel S, Richardson JE, Reid MC. Older adults are mobile too! Identifying the barriers and facilitators to older adults' use of mHealth for pain management. *BMC Geriatr.* 2013;13(1):43.
91. Mohr DC, Zhang M, Schueller SM. Personal sensing: Understanding mental health using ubiquitous sensors and machine learning. *Annu Rev Clin Psychol.* 2017;13(1):23–47.
92. Hebert ET, Stevens EM, Frank SG, et al. An ecological momentary intervention for smoking cessation: The associations of just-in-time, tailored messages with lapse risk factors. *Addict Behav.* 2018;78:30–35.
93. James KL, Randall NP, Haddaway NR. A methodology for systematic mapping in environmental sciences. *Environ Evidence.* 2016;5(1):7.
94. Reich B, Haran M. Precision maps for public health. *Nature.* 2018; 555:32–33.
95. Beck AF, Huang B, Chundur R, Kahn RS. Housing code violation density associated with emergency department and hospital use by children with asthma. *Health Aff (Millwood).* 2014;33(11):1993–2002.
96. Beck AF, Sandel MT, Ryan PH, Kahn RS. Mapping neighborhood health geomarkers to clinical care decisions to promote equity in child health. *Health Aff (Millwood).* 2017;36(6):999–1005.
97. Bill & Melinda Gates Foundation. https://www.gatesfoundation.org/Who-We-Are. Accessed October 19, 2018.
98. Dowell S, Blazes D, Desmond-Hellmann S. Four steps to precision public health. *Nature.* 2006;540:189–91.
99. Cori A, Donnelly CA, Dorigatti I, et al. Key data for outbreak evaluation: Building on the Ebola experience. *Philos Trans R Soc Lond B Biol Sci.* 2017;372(1721).
100. Sacks JA, Zehe E, Redick C, et al. Introduction of mobile health tools to support Ebola surveillance and contact tracing in guinea. *Glob Health Sci Pract.* 2015;3(4):646–59.
101. World Health Organization. Constitution of WHO: Principles. https://www.who.int/about/mission/en/. Accessed November 12, 2018.
102. Butler D. When google got flu wrong. 2013; http://www.nature.com/news/when-google-got-flu-wrong-1.12413. Accessed December 13, 2018.
103. Institute of Medicine (US) Committee on Assuring the Health of the Public in the 21st Century. *The Future of the Public's Health in the 21st Century.* Washington, DC: National Academies Press; 2002.

CHAPTER

4

Epidemiology and Public Health

Robert B. Wallace

Epidemiology is the basic science and most fundamental practice of public health and preventive medicine. We can study health and disease by observing their effects on individuals, by laboratory investigation of experimental animals, and by measuring their distribution in the population. The epidemiologist uses each of these approached to investigate health and disease in populations. Epidemiology is therefore the scientific foundation for the practice of public health.

The word "epidemiology" comes from epidemic, which translated literally from the Greek means "upon the people." Historically, the earliest concern of the epidemiologist was to investigate, control, and prevent epidemics. This chapter deals with the scientific principles that are the foundation of epidemiology. It first addresses the sources and characteristics of information used to assess the health of populations. Next, some essential elements of the practice of epidemiology will be discussed, as well as challenges to that practice. Finally, the evolution and newer techniques for epidemiology in controlling and preventing health problems will be presented.

A BRIEF HISTORY OF EPIDEMIOLOGY

Epidemiology has roots in the Bible and in the writings of Hippocrates, as does much of Western medicine. The *Aphorisms of Hippocrates* (fourth to fifth century BC) contain many generalizations based on prolonged and careful observation of large numbers of cases. The introductory paragraph of *Airs, Waters, Places* offers timeless advice on good environmental epidemiology:

> Whoever would study medicine aright must learn of the following subjects. First he must consider the effect of each season of the year and the differences between them. Secondly he must study the warm and the cold winds, both those that are common to every country and those peculiar to a particular locality. Lastly, the effect of water on the health must not be forgotten. When, therefore, a physician comes to a district previously unknown to him, he should consider both its situation and its aspect to the winds. Similarly, the nature of the water supply must be considered. Then think of the soil, whether it be bare and waterless or thickly covered with vegetation and well-watered, whether in a hollow and stifling, or exposed and cold. Lastly consider the life of the inhabitants themselves, are they heavy drinkers and eaters and consequently unable to stand fatigue or, being fond of work and exercise, eat wisely but drink sparely?[1]

Epidemics of infection were serious concerns for physicians in ancient times, although often they could do little more than observe the victims and record mortality. Their limited knowledge rarely permitted effective intervention. Until the Renaissance in the fourteenth through sixteenth centuries, physicians based their approach more on impressions than real numbers. John Graunt is often regarded as the founder of vital statistics. He first published his numerical methods for examining health problems in *Natural and Political Observations on the Bills of Mortality* in 1662. He was the first to attempt this approach.

Epidemiology was first applied to the control of communicable diseases and public health through quarantine and isolation, even though ideas about disease transmission and microbiology and epidemiology were rudimentary. Johann Peter Frank, a physician who became "director-general of public health" (in modern terminology) to the Hapsburg Empire, systematized and codified many rules for personal and communal behavior in the eighteenth century. His work contributed to public health and is published in *System einer vollstandigen medicinischen Polizey* (1779).

Careful clinical observation, precise counts of well-defined cases, and demonstration of relationships between cases and the populations in which they occur all combine in the method upon which epidemiology depends. This method was first developed in the nineteenth century. Modern epidemiologists hold John Snow[2] in high esteem. He painstakingly collected the facts about sources of drinking water that he related to mortality rates from cholera in London. This proved a classic demonstration of the mode of transmission about 30 years before Koch isolated and identified the cholera *Vibrio*. Snow's great contemporary, William Farr,[3] defined and clarified many basic ideas of vital statistics and epidemiology. Among his most important contributions were the following: (a) the scope of epidemiology, (b) the concept of person-years, (c) the relationship between mortality rate and probability of dying, (d) standardized mortality ratios, (e) dose-response relationships, (f) herd immunity, (g) the relationship between incidence and prevalence, and (h) the concepts of retrospective and prospective study. He also developed the first effective classification of disease, the direct ancestor of the nosology that we still use today. *Vital Statistics* (1885), an edited volume of excerpts from Farr's annual reports to the registrar-general, is perhaps the most impressive textbook of epidemiology ever written, graced by beautiful writing and well-chosen tables to illustrate the text.

Methods of epidemiological investigation have evolved since the mid-nineteenth century. The case-control study reentered medicine from the social sciences in the third decade of the twentieth century. The cohort study came into use after World War II, as a means of identifying risks associated with heart disease, lung cancer, and other emerging public health problems. Epidemiological "experiments" as now conducted in randomized trials are essentially modern innovations. Statistical methods and electronic computation have greatly improved epidemiological analysis. Present indications suggest expanding potential and an exciting future for epidemiology. Population-based medicine makes community assessment and diagnosis important for determining the need for health services. An increasingly broad interface between clinical medicine and epidemiology is referred to as clinical epidemiology. Molecular epidemiology has allowed epidemiologists to link genetic and many other biomarkers to health conditions and physiological functions, thereby creating new potential approaches to interventions. New and enhanced study designs are rapidly adding to our understanding of cause-effect relationships in many chronic and disabling disorders, as well as acute conditions. Epidemiological methods continue to be used in many areas of science and practice.

What does this brief history of epidemiology tell us? First, the community and environment influence the health of humans, as do our own inherited characteristics. Second, knowing how a disease is transmitted permits us to control and prevent it, even though we may not know the causal agent. Third, even the simplest information about vital events, illnesses, and populations can detect and analyze epidemiological problems. Finally, epidemiology can help identify, investigate, analyze, control, and prevent a wide range of health problems.

DEFINITION OF EPIDEMIOLOGY

Epidemiology is both the basic science of public health and its most fundamental practice. Therefore, we need to examine both aspects of its meaning.

Science

Epidemiology was originally defined as the scientific study of epidemics. An epidemic is the occurrence in excess of normal for an illness, health event, or health-related behavior that occurs in a specific place or among a group. Reports of cholera by John Snow and childbed fever by Holmes are among the classic examples. In recent years, excessive use of tobacco, called by some "the brown plague," and the acquired immunodeficiency syndrome (AIDS) are examples of modern epidemics.

Because the word "epidemic" may lead to chaotic or emotional, unreasoned responses to health problems, journalists use the term more often than epidemiologists. Other words, such as outbreak and cluster, are employed by practicing public health professionals to perhaps avoid stoking unnecessary anxiety and fear among the public.

In current use, however, the definition of epidemiology is broader and recognizes the application of this basic science of public health to the control and prevention of health problems. The following definition, recently agreed upon by an international panel, is widely accepted:

> Epidemiology is the study of the distribution and determinants of health-related states and events in specified populations and the application of this study to the control of health problems.[4]

Some terms in this definition require discussion. *Distribution* relates to time, place, and person. The relevant population characteristics include location, age, sex, and race; occupation and other social characteristics; living places; susceptibility; and exposure to specific agents. In addition, the distribution of the exposed cases needs to examine time as a factor. Relationships in time reveal information about trends, cyclic or secular patterns, clusters, and intervals from exposure to inciting factors to the onset of disease.

Determinants include both causes and factors that influence the risk of disease. Many diseases have a single necessary cause. When the agent of disease causes a single, specific condition, as occurs with the tubercle bacillus and tuberculosis, we know the necessary cause. However, there are usually many other determinants. They fall into two broad groups: (a) host factors that determine the susceptibility of the individual and (b) environmental factors that determine the host's exposure to the specific agent. Human "host factors" include age, sex, race, genetic or constitutional makeup, physiologic state, nutritional condition, and previous exposure experiences. Environmental factors include all conditions of living. Among these factors are family size and composition; crowding; hygienic conditions; occupation; and geographic, climatic, and seasonal circumstances. Thus, the "environment" includes broad physical, biological, and social factors. Behavioral features of individuals or populations, often identified by the term "lifestyle," may include such factors as use of tobacco, alcohol, and automobiles. Past and present environment—including the period of intrauterine life—may influence both exposure and susceptibility to disease.

Practice

The practice of a science is best defined by what the scientist does. Langmuir pointed out that, "the basic operation of the epidemiologist is to count cases and measure the population in which they arise."[5] The practice of epidemiology, therefore, is the scientific process that detects, investigates, and analyzes health problems, followed by applying this information to the control and prevention of these problems. This practice requires health problems to be the subject of public health surveillance, epidemiological investigation, and analysis. The findings of this analysis linked to health policy can lead to the control and prevention programs intended to resolve health problems. Implementation and evaluation of control and prevention are also the responsibilities of the practicing epidemiologist as is the clear and persuasive communication of the scientific findings to the public, policy makers, and program staff.

Uses of Epidemiology

The most important use for epidemiology is to improve our understanding of health and disease—a goal shared by all the disciplines and branches of the biomedical sciences. Morris[6] defined seven uses of epidemiology: historical study, community assessment, working of health services, individual risks and chances, completing the clinical picture, identification of syndromes, and the search for causes (Table 4-1). Each deserves brief comment.

Trajectories of Epidemiology over Time

The classic question "Is health improving?" can be answered only by comparing experience (rates) over time; this is one essential routine activity in all health services. Sometimes when the data are closely examined, unexpected trends appear. For example, there have been substantial changes in disease states in communities over the years, such as decreases in lung cancer and heart attack, and increases in substance use. Again, these are critical in directing clinical and community control programs.

Community Assessment

What are the health problems? This question can be answered in many ways. For example, what proportion of school children have

TABLE 4-1 USES OF EPIDEMIOLOGY
Historical study: Is community health getting better or worse?
Community assessment: What actual and potential health problems are there?
Working of health services
Efficacy
Effectiveness
Efficiency
Individual risk and chances
Actuarial risks
Health hazard appraisal
Completing the clinical picture: different presentations of a disease
Identification of syndromes: "lumping and splitting"
Search for causes: case-control and cohort studies
Evaluation of presenting symptoms and signs
Clinical decision analysis

become regular cigarette smokers by various stages of their progress through school? Or what proportion of people always or never use seat belts when driving or riding in cars? Answers to such questions have prognostic and also diagnostic value, as well as impact on the organization and funding of clinical care and public health programs. Community assessment makes it possible to predict the impact of future health problems by known effects of many risk factors.

The Search for Causes of Illnesses and Conditions

This is the most obvious use for epidemiology. Most hypothesis-testing studies (discussed later) have the primary aim of identifying causal factors, or at least of risk factors for disease. This chapter cites many examples of such studies.

Presence and Types of Health Services

Are all needed services available, accessible, and used appropriately? Are children receiving necessary immunizations? Can pregnant women begin prenatal care at the appropriate time? Do known contacts of persons with sexually transmitted infections receive follow-up and treatment? Information on these and many other questions is often gathered routinely or by special surveys. Health service administrators should not just focus on these simple routine questions, but should also be alert to less obvious potential gaps in coverage. For example, the census and other studies assess the numbers of elderly persons who live alone. Are all or only a small portion of these sources known to relevant clinical and public health organization who provide healthcare and surveillance for these individuals?

Individual Risks and Chances

What is the risk that a person will die before the next birthday? Actuaries who evaluate the risks for persons seeking life insurance or other applications have calculated answers based on probabilities derived from experience. This has become a prominent activity of epidemiologists who work on risk assessment and has led to many new insights, for example, about occupational and environmental risks and the hazards associated with immunizations.[7]

Completing the Clinical Picture

In assessing the taxonomy and nomenclature of diseases and conditions, epidemiologists may be referred to as "lumpers or splitters" because epidemiological investigations sometimes make it possible to group together several differing manifestations of a condition or to separate seemingly identical diseases into more than one category. The latter are more common than the former; examples include the differentiation of hepatitis A from other infections and the distinction between several types of childhood leukemia. Examples of "lumping" include the identification of many manifestations of tuberculosis. At one time, each group of tubercular symptoms and signs had an earlier, now updated name, such as phthisis, consumption, or pleurisy. Addiction to tobacco is the underlying cause of a variety of outcomes. Among them are respiratory cancers, chronic obstructive pulmonary disease, and a portion of the risk of coronary heart disease. One of Morris' original illustrations of this use for epidemiology was the demonstration that myocardial infarction occurs commonly in women as well as in men. An important difference is that this condition occurs in women at older ages and may have varied clinical presentations. Last used the technique of "completing the clinical picture" to construct a model[8] of what might occur in the average general primary-care population. In the course of a year, facts known and seen by the physician may be amplified by epidemiological study even though they might be unidentified, undiagnosed, or in a single practitioner's experience and only constitute the submerged part of the "disease" iceberg. This can lead to more effective clinical decision making.[9]

Clinical epidemiologists have defined other uses for epidemiology. One important use is the evaluation of presenting symptoms and signs of disease. Analyzing the data in hospital charts and relating symptoms and complaints to final diagnoses makes it possible for an epidemiologist to study clinical outcomes, including assessing the adverse effects of therapy. A related use is clinical decision analysis.[9] This technique is a rigorous quantitative method used to decide the best method of managing patients with particular diseases. This procedure involves the use of algorithms and other analytical methods, in which the probability of an outcome for each different decision is predicted based on prior clinical studies.

An Overview of the Epidemiological Method

Epidemiologists use a wide range of scientific information, including clinical findings, laboratory data, and field observations. In the end, it is the reasoning of the epidemiologist that ties these facts together. This reasoning is the logic behind disease control and prevention measures.

Epidemiological reasoning is fundamental and straightforward. First, we define events or clinical cases using careful, specific, and objective observations. Next, we count these events or cases and orient them to time, place, and person. Then we determine the population at risk and calculate rates of occurrences for the events or clinical cases. We put the events or cases in the numerator according to their relevant characteristics. The next step involves using a denominator of the portion of the population at risk and characterizing this group in the same way as those in the numerator are characterized. At this point, we calculate rates of occurrence in the group of cases. These rates are then compared with the rates of occurrence in other population groups. Finally, using this information, we draw inferences about the events that define the health problem and the agent or agents that cause it. These rates also provide information about the host and the environmental factors that influence the risk of occurrence and the transmission of the health problem. Using this information and collaborating with other health professionals, we propose control measures and then continue the observations required to assess the control program.

In identifying a health problem or case, many kinds of clinical examination may be employed. The patient's history may reveal information about exposure to risk, incubation period, susceptibility, occupation, residence, course of disease, or other factors. Physical examination can classify individuals not only about whether they have the condition under study, but as to type, stage, and duration of disease. Laboratory tests are valuable for a similar purpose. In addition, they are essential in revealing clinically inapparent cases, and they often shed light on the pathogenesis of the condition. Field observations are the sine qua non of the epidemiological method.

Viral hepatitis is an example of the ways that clinical, laboratory, and field studies can interlock. "Epidemic jaundice," mentioned by Hippocrates, has occurred in wars from ancient times to the present. Medical investigators used needle biopsies, a technique developed in the 1940s, to show generalized parenchymal inflammation of the liver accompanied the acute disease. Epidemiological studies soon distinguished hepatitis A ("infectious hepatitis") from hepatitis B ("syringe jaundice"). Both were shown to be due to viruses. However, hepatitis A had the epidemiological features of a fecal-oral transmission. Hepatitis B, on the other hand, was clearly blood borne and transmitted by inadequately sterilized hypodermic needles or other medical equipment. No cross-immunity protected people with one form of hepatitis from the other. Subsequent studies showed further differences. Hepatitis A had a shorter incubation period, was more contagious, and had a briefer period of abnormal serum transaminase activity than did hepatitis B.[10] Later epidemiological studies revealed the pattern of sexual transmission of hepatitis B among

gay men. Later still, Blumberg and colleagues detected an antigen in the serum of patients who had multiple transfusions, which was clearly associated with hepatitis B.[11] A few years later, the virus was identified,[12] and in 1971, the particles were further confirmed as being the antigen that[13] was the hepatitis B surface antigen (HBsAg). HBsAg was extremely valuable in screening carriers for hepatitis B and in developing a vaccine. Vaccines developed independently in France and in the United States. After rigorous testing in laboratory and field trials, the vaccine's efficacy and safety were proven to prevent hepatitis B in susceptible individuals. Among their users are health professionals, patients in renal dialysis units, infants born to mothers carrying hepatitis B, and men who have sex with men. The virus of hepatitis A was soon after identified, paving the way for serological tests for hepatitis A antibody. Detection of this antibody, found in some 70% of adult urban Americans, suggested a high prevalence of subclinical cases. Vaccine preparation was made possible by such advances.

The epidemiological features of hepatitis B among men having sex with men (MSM) have been a useful model to follow in the investigation of AIDS. Both conditions have the same pattern of distribution in this subset of the population. Case-control studies have shown that many persons who contract AIDS, like hepatitis B, are MSM who engage in anal receptive intercourse and have multiple sexual partners.[14]

The tools employed in this illustration of the epidemiological method are clinical, immunological, microbiological, pathological, demographic, sociological, and statistical. None of these approaches is uniquely epidemiological; it is their employment in particular ways with particular objectives that is the epidemiological method.

In epidemiology, unlike in clinical medicine, the concern is not with individual cases but with all the cases in a defined population. Furthermore, the entire range of manifestations of the condition must be considered in relation to the population from which the cases arise.

Epidemiological Sequence

An orderly sequence characterizes epidemiology: observing, counting cases, relating cases to the population at risk, making comparisons, making scientific inferences, developing the hypothesis, testing the hypothesis, experimenting and intervening, and evaluating. This sequence describes the actions we take whenever a "new" condition occurs. The relationship between cigarette smoking and lung cancer illustrates the stages in this epidemiological sequence, and process of identifying of scientific progress:

1. *Observing.* Scientific observations on smoking and cancer appeared in the *Journal of the American Medical Association*[15] in 1920 and in the *New England Journal of Medicine*[16] in 1928. In the following decade, *Science* documented that smokers had a shorter life expectancy than did nonsmokers.[17]
2. *Counting cases or events.* Vital statistics trends showed an increase in deaths caused by lung cancer in the United States beginning in the 1930s.
3. *Relating cases or events to the population at risk.* Increased death rates from lung cancer reported in national vital statistics attracted the attention of health department officials. Registrars of vital statistics in countries where smoking was an established lifestyle characteristic reported a similar trend.
4. *Making comparisons.* Studies of British physicians reported by Doll and Hill[18] and of contacts of American Cancer Society volunteers reported by Hammond and Horn[19] in the 1950s provided definitive comparisons between smoking and lung cancer. In addition to identifying the threat to the health of the public, the studies of Doll and Hill established the contemporary criteria for establishing epidemiological associations and potential causation.[20]
5. *Developing the hypothesis.* Since cigarette smoke contains more than 2500 chemical components, some of which are carcinogenic in animals,[21] only a small logical step was required to go from inference to hypothesis.
6. *Testing the hypothesis.* The hypothesis that smoking caused lung cancer lent itself to testing by means of a case-control study. A small case-control study done in Germany during 1938–39 was overlooked in the turmoil of World War II. Epidemiological studies designed to test the hypothesis were conducted in postwar Britain by Doll and Hill[18] and in the United States by Hammond and Horn.[19] Both studies showed consistent relationships between the present occurrence of lung cancer and a history of cigarette smoking, with a dose-response relationship. Subsequent case-control studies produced similar results. Reports of cohort studies soon followed. Both kinds of investigations confirmed the association and demonstrated other adverse effects from smoking.[22]
7. *Making scientific inferences.* Several observations led to valid scientific inferences about the association of tobacco smoking and lung cancer. Among them were (a) clinical observations, (b) national trends in mortality from several countries associated with the increased prevalence of cigarette smoking, (c) epidemiological comparisons made in large groups representing different segments of national populations in more than one country, and (d) the biological effects of tobacco smoke. All of these observations led to the inference that smoking increased the risk of dying from this disease.
8. *Conducting experimental studies.* Laboratory animal studies with beagles showed that exposure to tobacco smoke produces the precancerous lesions followed by squamous cell carcinoma in both animals and humans.
9. *Intervening and evaluating.* Action by public health and voluntary health agencies reduced cigarette-smoking rates. A decline in mortality trends in smoking-related causes in the United States and other countries followed this reduction. One of the most important steps in this process was the issuance in 1964 of the first Surgeon General's *Report on Smoking and Health,* continuing in 2006, when a subsequent report on the harms of second-hand smoke was issued. Today, adult smoking rates in the United States and other countries are at their lowest levels since the 1950s.

FOUNDATIONS OF EPIDEMIOLOGICAL PRACTICE

Putting the epidemiological method into practice requires skill in a unique set of tasks, and these tasks are increasing in breadth and depth. Some of them have expanded to become disciplines of their own. Several of these, for example, public health law and ethics, genetics, and informatics, are covered in more detail elsewhere in this section of the textbook. Some of the basic elements are as follows.

Surveillance

Surveillance as an element of epidemiological practice is "the ongoing systematic collection, analysis, and interpretation of health data essential to the planning, implementation, and evaluation of public health practice, closely integrated with the timely dissemination of these data to those who need to know. The final link in the surveillance chain is the application of these data to prevention and control." This definition is part of the plan for the national coordination of disease surveillance of the U.S. national Centers for Disease Control and Prevention (CDC),[23] based on earlier work there. The surveillance of public health problems is a critical task for the practicing epidemiologist, and is described in more detail in a separate chapter in this book.

Investigation

Surveillance information can trigger epidemiological investigations by public health surveillance reports. Epidemiological investigations may begin because of any of a number of other initiating events, such as news articles, communications from parts of the healthcare system or other health departments or colleagues with similar responsibilities, as well as alternative surveillance systems. The investigation of an epidemiological problem, whether it is an epidemic of acute infection or a long-term condition such as cancer, begins with careful observation and a detailed description. The basic steps of an epidemiological investigation are discussed below.

Analysis

The analysis of epidemiological data goes through a series of orderly steps, beginning with a careful and detailed description of cases or events. The description ought to include direct observations of persons influenced by the health event. In addition, the environment in which they live and work, the risk factors related to the event, and information about the agents that might have caused the health problem require careful description. Additionally, the observations need to be quantified. The analysis can then progress to comparison groups. The epidemiologist then compares occurrence rates among groups according to specific characteristics of the groups, that is, looking for a dose-response relationship, and may ultimately reach the point of complex and sophisticated quantitative analysis.

Evaluation

Evaluation addresses well-defined problems, such as the effectiveness of a drug, vaccine, or control program. It involves the assessment of a problem-solving action. Consequently, the first essential step is a detailed description of the problem and the actions intended to solve it. Evaluation may include the assessment of the effectiveness of any specific control interventions, such as assessment of contraceptive effectiveness, vaccine application or disease eradication programs, removal of contaminated foods from stores and restaurants, or the effectiveness of screening for a particular cancer.

Other Essential Tasks in Epidemiological Practice

Communication, information systems, management, including team building and human relations, and consultation are essential but not unique to the practice of epidemiology.

Communication

Communicating epidemiological information clearly and persuasively is essential to effective practice. Just as a clinician must clearly explain to a patient the need for a medication or other treatment, an epidemiologist must persuade professional colleagues, government officials, and the public that epidemiological findings warrant action to control and prevent a health problem.

Information Systems

Please see the chapter 5 on public health informatics in this section.

Management and Teamwork

Epidemiologists also need to develop management skills because they rarely work alone. Even in the investigation of a small outbreak, the assistance of other public health staff or department or agencies/organizations may be essential. Subsequent analytic work often requires collaboration with statistical and data management personnel. In these circumstances, epidemiologists need to understand the basic concepts of management, beginning with planning and including organizing, team building, directing, and evaluating management.

Human relations are a key part of every management process. Epidemiologists cannot ignore these relationships. Practice and observation are the best ways to learn these skills. Many health professionals deal with human relations in a clinical, patient-to-professional situation. Epidemiological practice requires working in teams, although essential team members may not be professionals. Nonetheless, their skills are indispensable to conducting epidemiological work, and they deserve respect.

Consultation

Consultation with colleagues in epidemiology, other fields of public health, clinical medicine, or public groups is part of the professional practice. Consultation requires a special kind of communication skill; it is difficult to offer scientifically sound advice in a persuasive yet dispassionate manner. In many important epidemiological situations, identifying and assuring representation of all important stakeholders is essential.

Presentation Skills

The ability to present epidemiological information to professional and public groups is as much a part of epidemiology as doing a case count or computing a relative risk. This skill differs from that of consultation because a presentation is most often a single event in which an epidemiologist discusses the investigation, often presenting complex information orally and visually to a large group. Consultation, on the other hand, is a process that requires information gathering, often involves interviewing, and may conclude with a presentation. Distinguishing between these two is important because of the emphasis of skill in presentation. Without this skill, important epidemiological work may have little health or scientific impact.

Relationship to Other Public Health Professions

The unique discipline of epidemiology interacts with a host of other professions.

Biostatistics and Statistics

Statistics is closely allied to epidemiology. Epidemiologists need to know enough statistics to utilize various modeling and software applications, and to perform basic statistical tests. Statisticians support epidemiological studies in many ways; for example, helping determine sample size, choosing samples, ensuring data quality, selecting the correct approach to complex analysis, and interpreting findings.

Laboratory Science

Laboratory science is often the key to correctly identifying a disease agent and an environmental exposure. Microbiologists, immunologists, toxicologists, biochemists, demographers, and behavioral and survey research scientists all contribute to epidemiological investigations. Laboratory determinations help characterize host susceptibility and assess carrier and preclinical disease states, as well as applying and interpreting various biomarkers of exposures, agents, and diseases. Importantly, laboratory services often provide the greatest predictive capability possible in arriving at a case definition.

Health Policy

Epidemiologists optimize their contribution to public health when the problems they address influence health policy. Policy decisions often seem remote from the practice of epidemiology because epidemiologists may equate policy with politics. However, epidemiologists influence policy to some degree almost every time they issue a report.

Health Service and Program Management

Epidemiology often provides health service programs with information that in selected areas set the standards of care. Epidemiological evaluation of effectiveness may determine the product used in nationwide programs and the schedule for administering preventive agents, such as vaccines, or conducting screening examinations, such as cervical cancer screening with cytology.

INVESTIGATION

Investigation is one of the most fundamental elements of epidemiological practice, and will be further elaborated. An investigation is an examination for the purpose of finding out about something. It differs from surveillance because when doing an investigation one assumes that a problem already exists. Moreover, an investigation may use information from an established data-collection system, but it goes farther and gathers new information. Analysis, on the other hand, involves the study of a problem by breaking it down into its constituent parts. In carrying out an investigation, therefore, an epidemiologist must have some idea as to what analysis will ultimately be necessary.

Exactly what must be found out depends in part on what is already known. The classic epidemiological triad of host, agent, and environment first mentioned in the discussion of *determinants*, is a useful framework for thinking about epidemics. The epidemiologist often knows about the host as to signs and symptoms of an illness, or health event, and the number of people in the epidemic. This holds true for epidemics of infection, acute noninfectious problems, such as unexplained deaths in a hospital, and chronic disease problems, as illustrated by the occurrence of endometrial cancer and estrogen use.

When the investigation is complete, however, we must know about the host and have information on a wide range of risk factors for the health problem. In addition, we need detailed information about the agent to which the host is exposed and the environment of the exposure. Ultimately, we require effective control measures. This entails the epidemiologist knowing how the agent is transmitted and, if possible, its portal of entry.

Epidemiological investigations meet both public service and scientific needs. If, for example, a community faces a health problem that is likely to continue to spread and about which the approach to control is uncertain, then the epidemiologist has an important role. Epidemics of viral infections that occur in presumably immunized young people, as has been the case of measles epidemics on college campuses, illustrate this problem. Moreover, public concern may also require the epidemiologist to provide assurance that no epidemic exists and none is threatening. Concern about transmission of AIDS by exposure to medical waste in public places is one such example, even though this environmental problem is not a legitimate risk hazard for transmitting disease.

Scientific need is a second important reason for an epidemiologist to do a detailed field investigation. This kind of investigation led to the discovery of Ebola and Zika viruses and the agent causing Legionnaires' disease. Field investigation also identified the causal association between vinyl chloride exposure and angiosarcoma of the liver, as it was for oral contraceptive (OC) use and hepatocellular adenoma, and a wide range of other exposures and health conditions.

Preparing for an Investigation

Preparation for an epidemiological field investigation has three general elements: (a) notification of essential people and organizations, (b) identification of materials needed for the investigation, and (c) travel planning. The notification process will have begun before the epidemiologist departs for the field. However, initial reports require confirmation. In addition, the date and place of investigation, and its purpose, need the concurrence of supervisors, health officials, where the investigation is being done, and other officials whose regions may include that area. Failure to notify these individuals can bring the investigation to a halt, limit access to people who have essential information, or lead to a withdrawal of support personnel needed to complete the investigation. Before going to the field, materials must be assembled to help with the investigation. Depending on the nature of the problem, the epidemiologist may want rapid and rigorous scientific review of what is known about a given topic. In addition, other items may be useful. Among them are access to: (a) relevant, validated questionnaires, (b) digital data-collection tools and communications connections, (c) immediate and longer term data analysis capacity, and (d) a suite of tools for collecting environmental and human biomarkers and even tissues for further analysis, if healthcare and laboratory services are not immediately available.

Basic Steps of an Investigation

It is useful to present the basic process of conducting an investigation first. This will be followed by additional guidance and detail on specific elements of this process. There are two essential steps to be considered in every epidemiological investigation:

1. *Ensure the existence of an epidemic.* The first important decision is to determine if an epidemic exists. A preliminary count of people with similar symptoms is often the first criterion for this decision. Laboratory confirmation may be absent. It may even be inappropriate because of the urgent need to begin an investigation.
2. *Confirm the diagnosis.* The epidemiologist needs to know the diagnosis of the health problem being addressed, if at all possible. The number of cases is sometimes too great to do a history and physical examination on every person. Collection of laboratory specimens must then follow quickly, although decisions about epidemic control are often made before laboratory confirmation is available. Using this preliminary information, the epidemiologist must formulate a working or tentative case definition of the health problem, regardless of the medical sources available. The symptoms for the case definition are written down, as are the essential physical signs. Measurements of levels of severity of the health problem, or disease, must be determined. Confirming each reported case may not be possible, and laboratory specimens may be obtained on only 15–20% of the cases. In some large epidemics, a sample of cases gave the essential information about the agent, the host, the method of transmission, the portal of entry, and the environment of the disease. For example, this may happen during large food borne outbreaks.[24] Epidemiologists set up control measures more quickly using this approach than by an exhaustive detection of every ill individual.
3. *Estimate the number of cases.* Case finding often begins with a single report or a small cluster of cases. Initially, the epidemiologist casts a wide net, using a preliminary case definition that is sensitive and excludes as few true cases as possible. After making a preliminary estimate, the epidemiologist must make a key judgment. Should all cases be studied or is the epidemic so large that investigating a sample will lead to a decision more quickly? If only a sample is selected, then only the most severe cases should be studied because they are the ones of most value. Outlying observations deserve special attention because explaining their relationship to the epidemic is often the key to understanding its mode of spread. Given a workable definition, the epidemiologist must count the cases and collect data about them. Once the ill persons are identified, the characteristics of the illness from beginning to the present and the demographic characteristics of each individual need to be determined. Next, data on the places where the ill people live, work, and have traveled to, and the possible exposures that might lead to health impairment all must be documented. Among the questions the epidemiologist may want to answer are the following: What signs and symptoms are the most important? Are any of them pathognomonic? What is the laboratory test most likely to confirm the diagnosis? Can both the exposure to the presumed source and the severity of the illness be characterized at different levels? What must be done to identify the people with these problems? Should long-term follow-up be necessary? Are there any inapparent or subclinical cases? What role do they play in determining the future size of this epidemic or the susceptibility of the people in this community?
4. *Orient the data as to time, place, and person.* Data on each case must include the date of onset of the illness, the place where the person lives and/or became ill, and the characteristics of each individual, including age, sex, and occupation. A simple histogram, often called "the epidemic curve," shows the relationship between the occurrence of cases and their times of onset. The spatial relationships of cases are often shown best on a spot map. Maps, for instance, help show that the cases occurred in proximity to a body of water, a sewage treatment plant, or its outflow. Characterizing individuals by age, sex, and other relevant attributes permits the epidemiologist to estimate rates of occurrence and compare them with other appropriate community groups.
5. *Determine who is at risk of having the health problem.* The epidemiologist will calculate rates at which a health problem, or disease, occurs using the number of the population at risk as the denominator, while the number of those individuals with the problem form the numerator. If the original reports of an

illness come from a state surveillance system, then the first estimations of rates may be based on a state's population. However, if the epidemic occurs only in school-age children from a particular school, the population at risk may be only the children who attend that school. Those not ill must be characterized by the same attributes as those who are ill, that is, age, sex, grade in school, or classroom.

6. *Develop an explanatory hypothesis.* During a field investigation, comparing the rates of occurrence among those at greatest risk with other groups helps the epidemiologist develop hypotheses to explain the cause and transmission of a health problem. Besides examining rates, other approaches to developing hypotheses of cause include further, more detailed interviews with ill individuals or with local health officials and residents, careful examination of outlying cases, or describing the epidemic in more detail. Depending on the extent of the epidemiologist's field library, reference to current and historical literature can stimulate new hypotheses.
7. *Compare the hypothesis with the established facts.* The hypothesis that explains the epidemic must be consistent with all the facts the epidemiologist knows. If the hypothesis does not do so, then it must be reexamined. It should do more than just strengthen speculation, explaining the cases at the peak of the epidemic. The epidemiologist may need to repeat the interview of case subjects, reassess medical records, gather additional laboratory specimens, and repeat calculations.
8. *Plan a more systematic study.* When the initial field investigations and preliminary calculations are complete, the investigator may need to conduct one or more case-control studies. The data for such studies may be in hand, but more often additional information will be needed. It may be collected by either interviewing subjects in more detail or surveying the population. Sometimes, a serological survey or extensive sampling of the environment for chemical or biological agents will generate new facts. Sometimes a visual record helps, requiring extensive photography or video taping of a work process. If there is a food borne infection, a detailed food history is necessary. If a water borne infection is suspected, a food and liquid intake history stimulates additional causal associations. For example, a water borne epidemic may be discovered by knowing the number of glasses of water drunk by each person, thereby permitting the epidemiologist to estimate a dose-response relationship. An occupational illness might be determined by a jobsite exposure and the time and extent of exposure by those workers.
9. *Prepare a written report.* Preparing a written document is an essential step in any epidemiological investigation. An epidemic report need not be a publishable paper. However, it should be a benchmark in the conduct of an investigation, just as a hospital discharge summary is for patient care or a thesis is for the advancement of a scholar. The epidemic report is an essential public health document. It may be the basis for action by health officials, who may close a restaurant or face a major industry's attorneys in court. For the public, it may provide information for those concerned about the epidemic, its spread, and the likelihood that others will be involved. A report may have scientific epidemiological importance in documenting the discovery of a new agent, a new route of transmission, or a new and imaginative approach to epidemiological investigation. Moreover, many investigative reports are useful in teaching, but it is important to always be cognizant of need for protection of the identifying information of those involved in an in investigation—patients, professionals, and others.
10. *Propose measures for control and prevention.* The ultimate purpose of an epidemiological investigation is to control a health problem in a community. The epidemiologist is part of the team that develops the approach to control and prevention.

Selecting Study Methods for Investigations

Epidemiological investigations often start with case reports, evolve to become a series of cases, and then go on to include ecological studies, cross-sectional studies, or surveys that describe the problem and perhaps suggest causal hypotheses. Working with descriptive information from case reports or a series of cases is often the first step in a field or community investigation. For an epidemiologist concerned with the clinical details of an illness, the causal agent, the environmental facilitators, and other risk factors, additional information will be needed, as well as demographic, social, and other behavioral characteristics and possible exposures to biological, physical, or chemical agents are also essential.

Designing an investigation will depend on a large number of contingencies, including the social and physical environment in which it takes place; the extent of the problem at issue; available resources to conduct the activities, data-collection elements, and the hypothesized causal agents and mechanisms. The analysis of the investigation will mainly depend on these elements, as well as the scientific and study design elements that were used to construct the study. These would include the broad and increasing range of analytical designs available in the epidemiological toolbox. These will not be presented here, but will likely include both descriptive and analytical observational analytical designs and models, such as ecological, case-control, and cohort studies as well as more modern designs. It is not outside of the range of investigations to utilize experimental and quasiexperimental designs as circumstances allow, in order help substantiate or prove causal processes related to the epidemiological situation. Having biostatistical assistance in study design and analysis is always important and sometimes critical to achieving the best answers possible.

Gathering Information

Data gathering is an essential part of "finding out about something." Investigations most often involve interviewing and record review. Anytime an interview is required, a friendly, persuasive introduction should precede questioning. Training of interviewers, therefore, should include practicing both the introduction and the questions.

The form in which the information is gathered may differ from one investigation to another. In field investigations of epidemics or in surveys, such as childhood immunization surveys, a line listing of respondents and related elements may suffice. More complex investigations may require a more detailed data-collection process, such as using visual aids for improving response accuracy, which may include pictures of medication packages or various foods, or clinical physical signs such as a skin rash.

Identifying the respondent and recording respondent information for follow-up or record retrieval are among the first items gathered. If follow-up or verification of information is needed, then information about family, friends, and neighbors via further contact may also be important.

Responses to questions, both from interview and record abstraction, should be simple and in a form that is easy to code. Initial data collection of items, such as age, should be gathered in terms of individual years; grouping of these items is better done at the time of tabulation and analysis. Avoiding certain open-ended questions as much as possible may reduce the difficulties in tabulating and analyzing the resulting information, but sometimes at the risk of missing important and insightful observations. Pretesting the data gathering form or interview is essential. Simulating an interview with a respondent or abstracting a chart that represents a typical case should be followed by simulating some of the unlikely circumstances.[25]

Case-finding, that is, searching for and gathering information from subjects for the case and comparison groups, is essential to an investigation. Initially, a study should include a wide range of those at risk of the health problem. Being sure that the entire population at risk is being considered at the beginning of the investigation is generally easier than it is to make a second trip to the community.

The establishment of a surveillance system for study of the population at risk is an important element in ensuring the effectiveness of the control program that may be later invoked. This is often an essential element of an epidemiologist's responsibility in fulfilling a public need and carrying out a scientific study.

If members of the comparison group are matched to specific individuals in the case group, then the forms for both case and comparison individuals must be able to be linked for analysis. Choosing comparison groups can be challenging. The epidemiologist must think carefully before selecting the easiest way. If the cases, for example, are all hospitalized, the question of using control subjects from the hospital or from the neighborhoods where the cases normally lived deserves careful study because both groups should come from the environment where exposure occurred.

It is important to point out that one useful technique for collecting information in an epidemiological investigation and many other research situations is to employ formal qualitative methods. Much of the information acquired may be carried out through open-ended or semistructured interviews. These interviews can often be recorded and analyzed in various ways, including sophisticated programs that summarize prominent themes and other important elements.[26]

Using Judgment in Field Investigations

The judgment of experienced epidemiologists regarding field investigations rests on a series of questions. The first is: When do you do a field investigation? Public need and scientific importance are the most frequent determinants of this answer. A community faced with a health problem of uncertain cause that cannot be controlled or that has created public alarm can be a public health emergency. The community's urgent need may be satisfied only by an immediate, competent epidemiological investigation. Scientific importance, while rarely isolated from public need, is more often determined by the nature of the problem. For example, this was the case in Legionnaires' disease,[27] the initial studies on penicillinase-producing *Neisseria gonorrhoeae* infection,[28] and the more recent epidemic of Brazilian purpuric fever. A form of *Haemophilus aegypticus* with a new plasmid type caused this new condition.[29] In each of these instances, the etiologic agent required that an epidemiological investigation be done in the field with intensive and highly technical laboratory support.

Once in the field, when does an epidemiologist ask for help? Since a single health professional rarely carries out an epidemic investigation, key questions must be asked before the field work begins. Among the foremost are: Will there be enough people available to ensure a successful investigation? Will these people have the necessary skills? What are the technical support requirements, in terms of data collection and analysis, specimen gathering, computer science, and laboratory science? Since the answers to these questions will change as the investigation evolves, the epidemiologist must reexamine each of them repeatedly.

How detailed should an investigation be? This question is best answered by considering the reasons for undertaking the investigation. Responding to public need is the principal determinant. This needs to include recommendations for control measures and addressing public information requirements, even if the epidemiologist is not communicating with the media personally. After fulfilling this obligation, the epidemiologist needs to assess the value of the investigation regarding changes in health policy for a larger population. Finally, the epidemiologist must evaluate the overall scientific importance of the fieldwork.

Before leaving the site of a field investigation, the epidemiologist should have affirmative answers to four questions:

1. Is it possible to do a quantitative (or, alternatively, a qualitative) analysis of the data?
2. Is the analysis sufficient to permit the epidemiologist to make preliminary recommendations about control measures to local health and other officials?
3. Is it possible to give responsible officials a report that would permit them to initiate control measures and provide a credible explanation of the occurrence of the health problem to the public?
4. Will the person responsible for supervising the investigation from its institutional base find the report of the investigation acceptable?

If the epidemiologist cannot answer these questions satisfactorily, the investigation must continue. Epidemiologists who do field investigations should always be prepared to *go back for the facts*, but it is best to get all of the facts in the first place.

Communicating the investigative findings clearly is essential, particularly when the epidemiologist completes the fieldwork. Who needs to know these findings? As a rule, the epidemiologist informs those who reported the first cases in the epidemic first. They are the practitioners who will know if the facts are correct and the public health actions are sensible. If the official and professional personnel responsible for control of the health problem are not part of this group, then they, too, must receive a report. This report describes both the field investigation and the scientific rationale control and prevention. Then, those who permitted, enabled, or facilitated the field work should be told of the findings and proposed actions. This group deserves the courtesy of hearing from the investigator where possible, rather than only through public media. This promotes transparency, and paves the way for better community acceptance the next time an investigation occurs. Finally, the public and the media must be informed. The control and prevention actions are the responsibility of public officials in that community because these measures will occur in their community. Therefore, it is those officials rather than the investigating epidemiologist who should discuss the problem, the investigative findings, and the approach to control and prevention to the community and the media. The number of involved public health professionals may increase exponentially if the investigation has regional, national, or international implications.

General Interpretation of Investigative Data

Interpreting epidemiological data requires that causal associations between exposure and outcome be correctly identified as best as possible using specific objective criteria. Although interpreting epidemiological findings focuses on factors such issues as the appropriateness of analytical methods and models and measures of association, the identification of bias and statistical power and related issues, and these criteria include, but go beyond, measurement and chance. While the evolving processes for improving causal inference are of great import, it is beyond the scope of this chapter, but selected references are offered.[30–32] Readers may wish to consult modern textbooks of epidemiology and related quantitative fields. Often, the search for causal inference in research and data analysis has underlying principles and tools but also may have contingent methods that depend on the specific research theme at hand; some research treatises on causation that appear in journals dedicated to focused research topics or disciplines may be helpful.

Some Basic Criteria for Causal Interpretation

The initial criteria used to distinguish direct causal associations from indirect and artifactual ones have both historical and current practical values. Early causal criteria were applied to a study of epidemic infections by Koch[33] and can be stated as follows:

1. The causative agent must be recovered from all individuals with the disease.
2. The agent must be recovered from those with the disease and grown in pure culture.
3. The organism grown in pure culture must replicate the disease when introduced into susceptible animals.

Such rigorous criteria ensure that studies adhering to them are very likely to identify causal associations correctly. Nonetheless, they are restrictive, and, had they been adhered to inflexibly, some important epidemiological associations would not have been found. The association of smoking and lung cancer is one.

In the mid-1960s, criteria more suited to contemporary health problems became the topic of heated scientific debate. Austin Bradford Hill[20] in his first presidential address to the section of Occupational Medicine of the Royal Society of Medicine in England proposed a set of criteria more suited to contemporary health problems. Serious objections to the work of Hill and Sir Richard Doll were raised by many respected scientists, including Ronald Fisher. Contemporaneously, in the United States, the Surgeon General of the U.S. Public Health Service convened an Advisory Committee on Smoking and Health. This committee promoted use of criteria similar to those proposed by Hill. These criteria can be summarized as follows[34]:

1. *Chronological relationship:* Exposure to the causative factor must occur before the onset of the disease.
2. *Strength of association:* If all those with a health problem have been exposed to the agent believed to be associated with this problem and only a few in the comparison have been so exposed, the association is a strong one. In quantitative terms, the larger the relative risk, the more likely the association is causal.
3. *Intensity or duration of exposure:* If those with the most intense or longest exposure have the greatest frequency or severity of illness while those with less exposure are not as ill, then the association is likely to be causal. This can be measured by showing a biological gradient or a dose-response relationship.
4. *Specificity of association:* If an agent, or risk factor, can be isolated from others and shown to produce changes in the frequency of occurrence, or severity of the disease, the likelihood of a causal association is increased.
5. *Consistency of findings:* An association is consistent if it is confirmed by different investigators, in different populations, or by using different methods of study.
6. *Coherent and plausible findings:* This criterion is met when a plausible relationship between the biological and behavioral factors related to the association support a causal hypothesis. Evidence from experimental animals, analogous effects created by analogous agents, and information from other experimental systems and forms of observation are among the kinds of evidence to be considered.

Interpreting epidemiological data, therefore, requires two major steps. One, the criteria for a causal association must each be carefully evaluated. The second is an equally careful assessment to identify bias and evaluate the role of chance. Of interest, there has always been discussion and contention on the emphasis given to the role of chance. This led Bradford Hill to comment on tests of statistical significance: "such tests can, and should, remind us of the effects that the play of chance can create, and they will instruct us in the likely magnitude of those effects. Beyond that they contribute nothing to the 'proof' of our hypothesis."[20] This highlights the importance of using judgment in analysis.

The following points are important when applying judgment to epidemiological analysis. They are:

1. Start with data of good quality and know the strength and weakness of the data set in detail.
2. Make careful description of the first step.
3. Determine the population at risk as precisely as possible.
4. Selecting the comparison, or control, group is one of the most difficult judgments to make. As a rule, try to choose subjects for comparison who represent the case group and come from the place where the exposure under study is most likely to have occurred.
5. The strongest case for an epidemiological association is one that meets all of the causal criteria.
6. Carefully determine the role that bias, including confounding, may have played in distorting an association.
7. In assessing an association, do not rely solely on tests of statistical significance alone. With regard to this issue, Bradford Hill stated, "there are innumerable situations in which they [tests of statistical significance] are totally unnecessary—because the difference is grotesquely obvious, because it is negligible, or because, whether it be formally significant or not, it is too small to be of any practical importance."[20]

EVALUATION IN EPIDEMIOLOGY

Evaluation, for an epidemiologist, is the scientific process of determining the effectiveness and safety of a given measure intended to control or prevent a health problem. Evaluation can involve a clinical trial that tests effectiveness of a drug, vaccine, or medical device and the occurrence of adverse side effects. Evaluation also assesses intervention programs in communities, as was done with the fluoridation of water on the prevention of dental caries. Evaluation may also assess the effectiveness of measures to control an epidemic.

Those who work in evaluation make a distinction between the terms effectiveness, efficacy, and efficiency. The effectiveness of a therapeutic or preventive agent or an intervention procedure is determined during its use in a defined population. Efficacy, on the other hand, is evaluated in terms of the benefit that such an agent or procedure produces under the conditions of a carefully controlled trial. Efficiency evaluation assumes that therapeutic or preventive agents and intervention procedures are effective and safe. Efficiency, therefore, concerns the assessment of resources in terms of money, human effort, and time.

Characteristics of Epidemiological Evaluation

The epidemiological evaluation of a health problem has special characteristics. First, the health problem is usually well defined. This means that the epidemiologist does not need to be deeply concerned with questions such as "Is there an epidemic?" Second, because the problem definition is clearer, epidemiological evaluation customarily has specific and explicit objectives that can be quantified. Third, a case definition for the health problem has often been formulated in detail before the epidemiologist begins field work. Finally, careful planning of an evaluation study is often essential, so that a complex set of study design issues need to be carefully addressed.

Epidemiologists evaluate a wide range of issues. An epidemic of an infection, such as of COVID-19, may require a new evaluation of many "established" epidemiological methods. An unusual cluster of abnormal cytology reports may suggest either an unusual cluster of cancer cases or a problem with screening procedures for this condition. The epidemiologist may also evaluate therapeutic and preventive measures in carefully designed clinical trials in the community. Such measures may include an assessment of the effectiveness of social media interventions,[35] vaccine efficacy,[36] or promoting healthy workplace behaviors.[37] Epidemiologists may also evaluate programs intended to improve the health of entire communities, despite the specific method of intervention used, as is done in program evaluation. Worthwhile efforts like this have been made in controlling epidemics of infection and with programs to prevent unplanned pregnancy. In addition, carefully organized community trials have been used to evaluate the prevention of cardiovascular disease, nutritional deficiencies, and dental health conditions.

The need for carefully designed clinical and community trials to evaluate prevention programs and agents has led some writers to characterize this as "experimental epidemiology."[38]

The scientific desirability of carrying out randomized, blinded, and controlled clinical trial of a therapeutic or preventive intervention is undeniable. Nonetheless, epidemiologists may need to evaluate health problems in communities that exist, because a presumably effective form of intervention did not adequately prevent or treat a health problem. This arises in connection with vaccine efficacy during outbreaks, when a randomized trial is not feasible either in terms of resources or the urgency of the immediate problem.

Systematic Reviews and Meta-analysis

Systematic reviews and meta-analysis are critically important tools to combine and synthesize the results of different research studies. Meta-analysis uses statistical methods to obtain a numerical estimate of an overall effect of interest across studies. Its primary aim is to enhance the statistical power of research findings when numbers in the available studies are too small. It is more objective and quantitative than a narrative review. In public health and clinical medicine, meta-analysis is often applied by pooling results of small randomized controlled trials when no single trial has enough cases to show statistical significance, but there are many examples of meta-analyses of observational studies.

Although meta-analysis is an important tool for the epidemiologist, it has some pitfalls. First, the problems of bias take on greater importance. Publication bias results from the tendency of authors and editors to put studies into print that have positive findings in preference to those that show no association. In addition, authors tend to select or emphasize studies that confirm their own viewpoint by applying the criteria for inclusion in a meta-analysis that varies from one study to another, thereby supporting their own beliefs. There are many publications on the methods of systematic reviews and meta-analyses. For example, see Institute of Medicine[39] and Walker et al.[40]

EPIDEMIOLOGY APPROACHES THE FUTURE

Epidemiology, as the scientific basis for the practice of public health, has important applications to resolving high-priority contemporary health problems. This section highlights current, major applications, still very important, and some possible directions as epidemiological evolves and approaches its future.

Current Major Applications of Epidemiology

Epidemic Control

Epidemiology applied to the control of epidemics is still relevant to contemporary public health practice. While the AIDS pandemic is well recognized, epidemics of many other types also occur. A recent estimate, for example, indicated that several thousand epidemics occur in the United States each year, and major global diseases such influenza, tuberculosis, malaria, AIDS, and COVID-19 continue to be of great import.

Program Practices and Operations

Preventive and public health service programs that affect the health of large population groups and geographic areas are also importantly influenced by the work of epidemiologists. The package inserts for OC pills have information for women in their reproductive years that is taken directly from the findings of epidemiological studies. Safeguards against the risks of environmental and occupational exposures, such as those of radon, asbestos, vinyl chloride, and tobacco smoke, are based on epidemiological research. Immunization policy also rests on the scientific work of epidemiologists.

Policy Development

Epidemiology is essential to the development of scientifically responsible public health policy. Within the past decade and a half, the countries of North America have analyzed the health problems faced by their citizens and proposed important new approaches to policy development, focusing on nationwide health objectives. If these objectives are to be met, professionals throughout public health and preventive medicine will play essential parts. The role of epidemiology and its practicing professionals is, however, not always clearly recognized. Nonetheless, epidemiologists will be involved in carrying out every essential task of the profession. *Surveillance* will be required to provide a baseline description of the epidemiology of each health problem and the ways in which it changes and evolves. *Investigations* will be carried out in communities as unexpected clustering occurs of uncontrolled infections. In addition, emerging new infections, automotive and other vehicular injuries, suicides, homicides, workplace fatalities, disabling exposures to chemical and physical agents, and persisting problems of neoplasia and cardiovascular diseases continue to limit the quality of life. *Analysis* will uncover previously unknown risk factors and ineffective prevention measures. *Evaluation* will lead to the development of new community preventive services and improved clinical treatment. Effective communication will be increasingly important to epidemiology as complicated scientific studies influence the behavior of individuals and the laws and regulations that govern communities.

What evidence is there that epidemiology can have this kind of impact on the health of a population? The eradication of smallpox from our planet is one such bit of evidence. The role of epidemiology in this worldwide effort is now well documented. Health policy and planning tools for communities can show how they can use public health surveillance to define the baseline of the health problems they face; see: https://www.cdc.gov/healthyplaces/health_planning_tools.htm, for an important set of tools published by CDC through 2016. The provision of epidemic and epidemiological assistance by local, state, and national public health agencies illustrates the ways in which investigations influence public health. How the sum of all these actions influences health and the quality of living will be determined by the policies, programs, and practices through which they act. Epidemiology plays an important part in developing the scientific base for this kind of societal change. It seems fitting that epidemiologists also play a role in seeing that the outcome of these changes is a desired one.

Some Newer Directions for Epidemiological Research and Practice

More Interdisciplinary Relationships

With the general growth of science and its constituent disciplines, inevitably there will more interdisciplinary interactions as epidemiology approaches new, more complex public health challenges. Some disciplines include sustainability science, botany, agriculture, meteorology, bioinformatics, and a host of basic, molecular and genetic, and other "-omics" endeavors. This will necessitate new types of epidemiological training in research and practice. As suggested by Bedford et al.,[41] new interactions may be occurring in such areas as newer social science disciplines, emerging technologies, new forms of research and development, and the amalgamation of clinical disciplines that occur in "One Health."

Newer Approaches to Planning and Evaluation of the Organizational Aspects of Epidemiological Programs

New organizational structures in the management of epidemiological services and resources, and many administrative practices are changing. These programmatic directions are increasingly intersecting with "implementation science," to enhance the research-to-practice gap,[42] with a large dose of new methods of evaluation, which as noted above emphasize, for example, the differences between efficacy and effectiveness.

More Attention to the Economics of Public Health and Preventive Interventions

While there has been increasing economic analyses of the public health and preventive medicine enterprise, much more is needed. This includes areas where the effects of a degraded environment and ecology (due to natural or anthropogenic forces) must be evaluated with regard to combined macro- and microeconomic and health consequences, such as may occur with deforestation or the global wildlife trade.[43]

The Need for Quicker and More Effective Responses to Community Disasters

The plethora of natural and unnatural disasters have led to mandates to create more rapid and helpful responses to community preparedness during health emergencies, including pandemics such as the current COVID-19. Not only is the nature of the response critical, but so are the resulting longer term outcomes. These are important but intense challenges, regardless of the cause. Particularly with regard to the COVID-19 pandemic, Fineberg[44] has suggested a set of actions that need improvement, such as in establishing a unified community command structure, providing sufficient technical resources for health professionals, and greater ability to inspire and motivate the public. The needed for epidemiologist should acquire training in these areas and others.

The Importance of a Greater Understanding of the Health Effects of Psychological Stress

While the emphasis on physical diseases and their antecedent causes is important and understandable, much less is known about the nature, outcomes, and control of either individual or community-based stress responses. The biological base for human stress responses and their health manifestations is improving, and should be an expanded part of the epidemiologists approach to disease control, no matter the extent and severity of the underlying physical or mental conditions may be.[45]

Prediction Models and Life-Course Epidemiology

Because of the increasing amount of data on the health of communities, both in populations and in clinical settings, and increasing computing resources, there has been an increasing number of clinical prediction models being created, where health outcomes are predicted with increasing precision. These have many clinical themes, and they have become abundant. As with other prospective designs, however, problems emerge including redundant and nonstandardized approaches, varying ease of user access, lack of updating and contradictory outcomes, sometimes related to variation in the source populations. Some of these issues have been addressed[46] in a thoughtful way, and some modernization of these processes seems indicated.

For many years, there has been a similar approach, which has been called "life-course epidemiology." This has been a fruitful approach and as longer term cohort data become more available, it has become possible in some circumstances to, for example, apply prenatal or infant characteristics in both epidemiological and biological ways, to explore the natural history of exposures, diseases, and conditions to not only adult outcomes but also among older people.[47] This approach can expand knowledge in ways never before possible, and should be encouraged.

Promoting an "Epidemiology of Ecosystems" to Better Understand the Emergence of Diseases and Conditions

A number of disciplines, that while not new, have grown and further developed to help improve the understanding of why diseases occur, and how their manifestations and clinical outcomes differ from the way they used to be. These include broad topics such as ecology and ecosystems, plant and animal biology, biodiversity and evolution, and their genetic and other molecular tools. Through study of how species interact and evolve with each other, through processes such as parasitism, commensalism, pollination, and infection, it is possible to understand the persistence and evolution of ecosystems, and their impact on humans.[48] In fact, not surprisingly, there is good evidence that species that can make humans ill persist in ecosystems that have been changed by human habitation.[49] While the pathways of evolution of species and their conditions have been thought to be long-term, it is that shorter term changes, such as due to the industrial revolution, have led to shifts in important human physiological functions and predispositions to important chronic illnesses, even including natural selection.[50] All of this suggests the importance of epidemiological study and participation in understanding the contributions of ecology and evolution to human health change.

The Growth of Computational Modeling in Epidemiology

While modeling of epidemics and other population phenomena have been available for many years, and have made important contributions to understanding and forecasting health, social and behavioral complex events in many disciplines, applications after the start of the COVID-19 pandemic have caused increasing interest in their utility and methodology.[51] Such applications have been applied robustly for forecasting trends in the U.S. prevalence of smoking[52] and in assessing the effectiveness of face masks in managing the COVID-19 pandemic.[53] As such, as modeling assumes more important place in the epidemiologist's toolbox, it will provide more interactions with the statistical sciences.[54] Cross-disciplinary applications with such modeling activities as agent-based modeling,[55] network modeling, and geo-spatial modeling are also assuming a greater role in the field.

References

1. Lloyd GER, ed. *Hippocratic Writings*. Harmondsworth, England: Penguin; 1978.
2. Snow J. *On the Mode of Transmission of Cholera*. 2nd ed. London: Churchill; 1855 (reprinted New York: Commonwealth Fund; 1936).
3. Farr W. In: Humphreys NA, ed. *Vital Statistics*. London: *The Sanitary Institute*; 1885 (reprinted New York: New York Academy of Medicine; 1975).
4. Last JM, ed. *A Dictionary of Epidemiology*. 3rd ed. New York: Oxford University Press; 1995.
5. Langmuir AD. The territory of epidemiology: Pentimento. *J Infect Dis*. 1987;155:3.
6. Morris JN. *Uses of Epidemiology*. 3rd ed. Edinburgh, London: Churchill-Livingstone; 1975.
7. Task Force on Health Risk Assessment. *Determining Risks to Health: Federal Policy and Practice*. Dover, MA: Auburn; 1986.
8. Last JM. The iceberg completing the clinical picture in general practice. *Lancet*. 1963;2:28–31.
9. Felix HM, Simon LV. Conceptual frameworks in medical simulation. In: *StatPearls [internet]*. Treasure Island, FL: Stat Pearls Publishing; 2020 Aug 16.
10. Krugman S, Giles JP, Hammon J. Infectious hepatitis: Evidence for two distinctive clinical and immunological types of infection. *JAMA*. 1967;200:365–73.
11. Blumberg BS, Gerstley BJ, Hungerford , DA, et al. A serum antigen (Australia antigen) in Down's syndrome, leukemia and hepatitis. *Ann Intern Med*. 1967;66:924–31.
12. Dane DS, Cameron CH, Briggs M. Virus-like particles in serum of patients with Australia-antigen-associated hepatitis. *Lancet*. 1970;1:695–8.
13. Almeida JD, Rubenstein D, Stott EJ. New antigen-antibody system in Australia-antigen-positive hepatitis. *Lancet*. 1971;2:1225–6.
14. Jaffe HW, Choi K, Thomas PA, et al. National case-control study of Kaposi's sarcoma and *Pneumocystis carinii* pneumonia in homosexual men. Part I. Epidemiologic results. *Ann Intern Med*. 1983;99:145–51.
15. Broders AC. Squamous-cell epithelioma of the lip: A study of five hundred and thirty-seven cases. *JAMA*. 1920;74:10.
16. Lombard HL, Doering CR. Cancer studies in Massachusetts. 2. Habits, characteristics and environment of individuals with and without cancer. *N Engl J Med*. 1928;198:10.
17. Pearl R. Tobacco smoking and longevity. *Science*. 1938;87:2253.
18. Doll R, Hill AB. The mortality of doctors in relation to their smoking habits: A preliminary report. *Br Med J*. 1954;1:1451–5.
19. Hammond EC, Horn D. Smoking and death rates: Report on forty-four months of follow-up of 187,783 men. II. Death rates by cause. *JAMA*. 1958;166(1159–72):1294–1308.
20. Hill AB. The environment and disease: Association or causation? *Proc R Soc Med*. 1965;58:295–300.
21. U.S. Department of Health, Education, and Welfare. *Smoking and Health: A Report of the Surgeon General*. Washington, DC: U.S. Department of Health, Education, and Welfare, Public Health Service, U.S. Government Printing Office; 1979.
22. U.S. Department of Health and Human Services. *Reducing the Health Consequences of Smoking: 25 Years of Progress: A Report of Surgeon General*. DHHS Publication, No. (CDC) 89-8411; 1989.

23. For additional information on surveillance methodology and disease-specific surveillance, consult the Centers for Disease Control and Prevention website at www.cdc.gov, as well as the chapter on surveillance in this book.
24. Shaw KA, Wright K, Holloman K, et al. Salmonella outbreak after a large-scale food event in Virginia, 2017. *Public Health Rep.* 2020;135: 668–75.
25. Hilton CH. The importance of pretesting questionnaires: A field research example of cognitive pretesting the Exercise referral Quality of Life Scale. *Int J Soc Res Methodol.* 2017;20(1):1-14.
26. Chesebro JW, Borisoff DJ. What makes qualitative research qualitative? Qual Res Rep Commun. 2007;8(1):3–4.
27. Fraser DW, McDade JE. Legionellosis. *Sci Am.* 1979;241:4.
28. Centers for Disease Control. Penicillinase-producing *Neisseria gonorrhoeae*—United States, Worldwide. *MMWR.* 1979;28:8.
29. Fleming DW, Berkeley SF, Harrison LH, the Brazilian Purpuric Fever Group. Epidemic purpura fulminans associated with antecedent purulent conjunctivitis and *Haemophilus aegypticus* bacteremia in Brazilian purpuric fever. *Lancet.* 1987;2:757–63.
30. Aiello A, Green LW. Introduction to the Symposium: Causal inference and public health. *Annu Rev Public Health.* 2019;40:1–5.
31. Gershman B, Guo DP, Dahabreh IJ. Using observational data for personalized medicine when clinical trial evidence is limited. *Fertil Steril.* 2018;109(6):946–51.
32. Pingault J-B, O'Reilly PF, Schoeler T, et al. Using genetic data to strengthen causal inference in observational research. *Nat Rev Genet.* 2018;19(9):566–80.
33. Koch R. Uber bacteriologische Forschung. *Verh Ten Internat Med Cong Berlin.* 1891;1:35.
34. U.S. Department of Health, Education and Welfare. *Smoking and Health: A Report of the Surgeon General.* Washington, DC: U.S. Government Printing Office; 1964.
35. Zhang Y, Cao B, Wang Y, et al. When public health research meets social media: Knowledge mapping from 2000 to 2018. *J Med Internet Res.* 2020;22(8):e17582.
36. Levine MH, Abdullah S, Arabi YM, et al. Viewpoint of a WHO advisory group tasked to consider a closely-monitored challenge model of COVID-19 in healthy volunteers. *Clin Infect Dis.* 2020, ciaa1290, https://doi.org/10.1093/cid/icaa1290.
37. El Dib RP, Verbeek J, Atallah AN, et al. Interventions to promote the wearing of hearing protection. *Cochrane Database Syst Rev.* 2006;(2):CD005234.
38. Lilienfeld DE, Stolley PD. *Foundations of Epidemiology.* 3rd ed. New York: Oxford University Press; 1994.
39. Institute of Medicine. *Finding What Works in Health Care: Standards for Systematic Reviews.* Washington, DC: The National Academies Press; 2011.
40. Walker E, Hernandez AV, Kattan MW. Meta-analysis: Its strengths and limitations. *Cleve Clin J Med.* 2008;75(6):431–9.
41. Bedford J, Farrar J, Ihekweazu C, et al. A new twenty-first century science for effective for effective epidemic response. *Nature.* 2019;575(7781):130–6.
42. Bauer MS, Damschroder L, Hagedorn H, et al. An introduction to implementation science for the non-specialist. *BMC Psychol.* 2015;2:32.
43. Dobson AP, Pimm SL, Hannah L, et al. Ecology and economics for pandemic prevention. *Science.* 2020;369(6502):379–81.
44. Fineberg HV. Ten weeks to crush the curve. *N Engl J Med.* 2020;382 (17):e37.
45. Costa-Mattioli M, Walter P. The integrated stress response: From mechanism to disease. *Science.* 2020;368:eaat5314.
46. Adibi A, Sadatsfavi M, Ioannidis J. Validation and utility testing of clinical prediction models: Time to change the approach. *JAMA.* 2020;324:235–6.
47. Kuh D, Cooper R, Richards M, et al. A life course approach to healthy ageing: The HALCyon programme. *Public Health.* 2012;126:193–5.
48. Hecht LBB, Thompson PC, Rosenthal BM. Assessing the evolutionary persistence of ecological relationships: A review and preview. 2020. *Infect Genet Evol.* 2020;84:104441.
49. Ostfeld RS, Kessing F. Species that can make us ill thrive in human habitats. *Nature* 2020;584:346–7.
50. Corbett S, Courtiol A, Lummaa V, et al. The transition to modernity and chronic disease: Mismatch and natural selection. *Nat Rev Genet.* 2018;19:419–30.
51. Metcalf CJE, Morris DH, Park SW. Mathematical modeling to guide pandemic response. *Science.* 2020;369:368–70.
52. Mendez D, Warner KE, Courant PN. Has smoking cessation ceased? Expected trends in the prevalence of smoking in the United States. *Am J Epidemiol.* 1998;148:249–58.
53. Stutt ROJH, Retkute R, Bradley M, et al. A modeling framework to assess the likely effectiveness of facemasks in combination with 'lock-down' in managing the COVID-19 pandemic. *Proc Math Phys Eng Sci.* 2020;476(2238):20200376.
54. Tolles J, Luong BH. Modeling epidemics with compartmental models. *JAMA.* 2020;323(24):2515–6.
55. Tracy M, Cerda M, Keyes KM. Agent-based modeling in public health: Current applications and future directions. *Annu Rev Public Health.* 2018;39:77–94.

CHAPTER 5

Public Health Informatics

Kai Zheng • Junying Zhao

INTRODUCTION

The ability to collect, process, and act upon data is central to the mission of public health. In the past several decades, the advancement in informatics, particularly in the areas of electronic data exchange and advanced data analytics, has afforded public health workers and academicians an unprecedented set of tools to assemble and make sense of large volumes of data from diverse settings. This capability is further extended thanks to the now nearly ubiquitous adoption of electronic health records (EHRs) in U.S. hospitals and clinics,[1,2] higher performance computing and faster computer networks, and increased citizen participation in public health activities on social media. In this digital era, informatics has undoubtedly become a core competency for leaders and practitioners in public and population health.

The term "informatics" is an amalgamation of "information" and "automatic." It was first coined in 1957 by the German computer scientist Karl Steinbuch to describe automatic processing of information—usually through computing systems.[3] Today, it is used to broadly describe the study, design, and development of information technology for the good of people, organizations, and society.[4] In the last 15 years, biomedical and health informatics has been the fastest growing subdomain of informatics. Biomedical and health informatics is a scientific discipline that applies informatics principles to the advancement of life sciences research, health professions education, public health, and patient care.[5]

Public health informatics is, in turn, a subspecialty of biomedical and health informatics dedicated to serving the needs of public health practice, research, and learning.[6] Public health informatics concerns a broad range of activities relevant to the health of populations, rather than the medical care of individual patients. It also has strong links to government agencies such as the health departments at local, state, and national levels. Public health informatics applications thus have a predominant focus on surveillance, prevention, and routine collection of population-level data from communities (e.g., socioeconomic determinants of health) to inform health policy making and disaster planning. As defined by the American Medical Informatics Association,[7] public health informatics is:

> The application of informatics in areas of public health, including surveillance, prevention, preparedness, and health promotion. Public health informatics and the related population informatics, work on information and technology issues from the perspective of groups of individuals. Public health is extremely broad and can even touch on the environment, work and living places and more.

The field of public health informatics has developed substantially in the past decade. Its rise has revolutionized many public health processes, and contributed to the improved health of millions of lives. Public health informatics is a multidisciplinary field in nature, which is built upon many component sciences such as computer and information sciences, engineering, operation research, and cognitive and social sciences. According to Savel and Foldy,[8] the work of public health informatics comprises three major categories[1]: study and description of complex systems (e.g., models of disease transmission or public health nursing work flow)[2]; identification of opportunities to improve the efficiency and effectiveness of public health systems through innovative data collection or use of information; and[3] implementation and maintenance of processes and systems to achieve such improvements.

In the United States, the Centers for Disease Control and Prevention (CDC) has been a champion in promoting the concept of public health informatics and supporting the development of key public health informatics infrastructures, tools, and educational programs. Over a decade ago, the CDC started to construct the Public Health Information Network (PHIN), a nationwide fabric comprising interoperable public health information systems for facilitating transmission of health data (e.g., infectious disease incidents) from hospitals, physician offices, laboratories, and pharmacies to local and state health agencies, then to the CDC. Launched in 1996, the CDC's Public Health Informatics Fellowship Program is a flagship training program for professionals to acquire and apply expertise in public health informatics to solve complex public health challenges. Many colleges and universities in the United States, such as the University of Utah and Emory University, now offer public health informatics graduate degree programs or an MPH with a concentration in public health informatics.

In the following sections of this chapter, we first present a brief history of public health informatics as a scientific discipline, followed by a description of core technologies underlying modern public health information systems. Then, we describe several significant public health informatics infrastructures and applications that have led to paradigm shift in public and population health practices in areas such as monitoring and surveillance and control of the opioid epidemic, followed by a description of recent efforts on advancing public health informatics training and workforce development. We conclude the chapter with a discussion of emerging trends in public health informatics.

HISTORY OF PUBLIC HEALTH INFORMATICS

The need to monitor and control infectious diseases dated back to 10,000 BC when early smallpox appeared in Africa.[8] It spread from Egypt to Asia and Europe and claimed 3.5–7 million lives from 165 to 180 AD.[9,10] Europeans then spread the disease to the New World and caused a drastic decline of the Native American population.[11,12] Another significant disease, Black Death due to bacterium *Yersinia pestis*, struck Eurasia from 1347 to 1351 and ended with the Great

Plague of London in 1665. It was estimated to have killed 75–200 million people.[13] During the colonial times from 1500s to 1800s, American laws required the reporting of several contagious diseases such as cholera.[8] The British Civil Registration Act of 1836 also mandated registration of births and deaths.[14]

These events highlight the necessity of collecting public health information at the population scale and systematic methods at doing so began to emerge. In 1850 and 1854, William Farr and John Snow analyzed the cholera outbreak in London. They used mathematical and statistical methods to trace the cause, found that cholera was a waterborne disease, and advised successful interventions.[15] Statistical and graphical methods were also applied by Florence Nightingale to explain the causes of deaths in the British army during the 1850s Crimean War.[16] Similar methods were employed by Charles Joseph Minard in 1869 to study French army casualties during the war with Russia.[17] During the 1890s, the United States passed the immigration law that required health inspections of all immigrants to exclude "persons likely to become public charges, persons suffering from a loathsome or dangerous contagious disease."[18]

In the eighteenth and nineteenth centuries, medical breakthroughs such as immunization and antibiotics were made to effectively combat diseases threatening public health. Smallpox vaccine was first successfully developed by Edward Jenner in 1796 and produced for public vaccination required by the 1898 Vaccination Act and 1899 English Government Vaccine Establishment.[19] Alexander Fleming discovered penicillin in 1928.[20] Moreover, the antibacterial compound tyrothricin was first derived by Rene Dubos in 1939.[21] Both antibiotics effectively treated infections and significantly reduced bacteria-caused deaths during World Wars I and II.

However, more virulent and mutative viruses continue to cause pandemics. The 1918 Spanish flu, caused by the H1N1 subtype of the influenza A virus, was estimated to have infected one-third of the world population and resulted in 20–40 million deaths.[22] The 1968–69 Hong Kong flu, caused by the H3N2 subtype, led to deaths ranging from 750,000 to 2 million.[23] Human immunodeficiency virus infection and acquired immune deficiency syndrome (HIV/AIDS) was first clinically reported in 1981,[24] and has killed an estimated 35 million people worldwide as of 2017.[25] Severe acute respiratory syndrome (SARS) caused by a coronavirus, while infecting a smaller population (estimated at 8000), spread much faster via air travel across continents and led to a global outbreak within months in 2003.[26] Expected pandemic deaths exceed 700,000 per year worldwide with expected income and mortality costs of $80 and $490 billion.[27]

To better record, disseminate, and monitor epidemics, technologies have advanced from pencil and paper to telegraphs, tabulators, and computers. The invention of telegraph and standardization of the Morse code in the 1860s greatly facilitated communication and surveillance of critical health conditions such as the progress of 1918 Spanish Flu.[28] The first electronic tabulating system was invented by Herman Hollerith in 1889 to process the 1890 U.S. Census data.[29] IBM continued to develop faster tabulating machines since the 1930s until the early digital computers—Atanasoff-Berry Computer (ABC) and the Electronic Numerical Integrator and Computer (ENIAC)—were invented in England in 1943 and the United States in 1945, respectively.[30] IBM further produced mainframe computers starting in the 1950s and dominated business, research, and education sectors during the 1960s–70s. Leveraging the power of these capable computing systems, the National Library of Medicine and the then newly established CDC undertook a new digital method for collecting and visualizing public health data. The subsequent availability of microcomputers, together with the first internet ARPANET created in 1969, fostered the establishment of interconnected computer networks during the 1980s. It was the Illinois Department of Public Health that first developed a computer network for public health surveillance purposes during the 1985 salmonellosis outbreak. The resulting PHIN enhanced information sharing and communication between state and local health departments and the CDC.

The emerging professions specializing in applying information science and computing technologies to health spurred the development of many professional organizations. Founded in 1928, the American Health Information Management Association (AHIMA) is the premier association of health information management, a field devoted to effective management of health data.[31] With the advent and advancement of computers, the American Medical Informatics Association (AMIA) formed in 1988 from the merger of three organizations: the American Association for Medical Systems and Informatics; the American College of Medical Informatics; and the Symposium on Computer Applications in Medical Care. Further specialized, the Public Health Informatics Institute was established in 1992 with the support from the Robert Wood Foundation, devoted to nurturing the emerging field of public health informatics.[32]

Meanwhile, the abundant data and tools allowed governments at various levels to better prevent and control diseases and injuries to protect public health and safety. The CDC was established for this purpose in 1946. It started collection of digital data using mainframe computers during the 1960s, such as the National Health Interview Survey (NHIS) for general health[33] and the National Health and Nutrition Examination Survey (NHANES) for nutrition.[34] The CDC updated its computing and data capabilities over the next two decades for more efficient data collection and disease registration, including the Behavioral Risk Factor Surveillance System (BRFSS) for health behaviors[35] and the Surveillance, Epidemiology, and End Results (SEER) Program for cancer registries.[36] In 1960, the National Office of Vital Statistics and the National Health Survey merged to form the National Center for Health Statistics (NCHS) which has been part of the CDC since 1987.[37]

The 1995–2001 era of the World Wide Web was characterized by a recognized need to integrate data across disparate systems. The CDC reported that integrated information and surveillance systems "can join fragments of information by combining or linking the data systems that hold such information. What holds these systems together are uniform data standards, communications networks, and policy-level agreements regarding confidentiality, data access, sharing, and reduction of the burden of collecting data."[38] In 1998, the CDC planned to develop a syndromic surveillance system for early detection of outbreaks. It aimed to create a nationwide network by increasing links among surveillance sites and translating data into public health action.[39] In 1999, the Department of Defense also built a system to monitor health data for early detection of epidemics, called Electronic Surveillance System for the Early Notification of Community-based Epidemics (ESSENCE[40]). Since the 2001 anthrax and the September 11 attacks, strict security and (bio-)terrorism surveillance based on interconnected information systems has been implemented. The CDC's Early Aberration Reporting System (EARS) was modified into a standard surveillance tool for the health departments in New York City and the Washington, DC area.[41] Additional early detection capabilities and medical countermeasures to biological, chemical, radiological, and nuclear agents were also developed. Major programs included BioSense by the CDC,[42] Bioshield by the Department of Health and Human Services,[43] and BioWatch by the Department of Homeland Security.[44]

How to improve data interoperability while protecting patient and individual privacy has been a long-standing challenge in public health informatics. The Health Insurance Portability and Accountability Act of 1996 (HIPPA) protected individual health information maintained by the healthcare providers and payers. However, HIPPA also amended the Public Health Service Act, permitting disclosures without individual authorization when reporting information to public health agencies.[45] In 2004, the Office of the National Coordinator (ONC) for Health Information Technology began developing the

Nationwide Health Information Network, which was envisioned to be a set of standards and infrastructures for authorized users including public health entities to exchange health information in a real time and secure manner.[46] The Health Information Technology for Economic and Clinical Health Act of 2009 further provided financial incentives for providers to adopt and use EHRs in meaningful ways. This allowed providers to electronically report public health data, including laboratory test results and immunization records.[47]

Additionally, with the introduction of smartphones in 2002, mobile health (mHealth) technology has demonstrated great potential to collect and analyze personal health data for the purposes of public health, population health management, and reduction of health disparities.[48,49] As of 2017, more than 325,000 mHealth apps were available worldwide.[50] Moreover, "big data" oriented new data analytics techniques, such as deep learning, offer powerful artificial intelligence tools to the realm of public health. They have been applied and shown great promise in areas such as screening of breast and lung cancers,[51] detection of mental health conditions,[52] and diagnosis and care delivery in resource-poor global health settings.[53] However, currently, mHealth and healthcare AI have triggered many ethical and legal issues in terms of fairness, privacy, and cybersecurity beyond the scope of 1996 HIPPA. To ensure public safety, their quality and potential liability also need clear definitions, standardization, and regulation by government agencies such as the CDC, the Federal Communications Commission, and the Food and Drug Administration.

CORE TECHNOLOGIES

Electronic Data Exchange Standards

A key ingredient to the success of a public health infrastructure is the ability to exchange electronic health data between disparate clinical and public health information systems. This is particularly true for monitoring and surveillance programs that critically rely on[1] robust system interoperability using widely adopted data exchange protocols such as the standards developed by the Health Level 7 International (HL7), a not-for-profit, American National Standards Institute (ANSI)-accredited standards-developing organization devoted to facilitating exchange of electronic health information; and[2] accurate, complete, and timely data codified using formalized nomenclatures and taxonomies, such as the Logical Observation Identifiers Names and Codes (LOINC) for laboratory test names and the Systematized Nomenclature of Medicine (SNOMED) for test results.

Public health workers have in fact led the way in developing many data exchange standards in prevalent use today. These include the International Classification of Diseases (ICD) that was originally developed for the purpose of assembling mortality and morbidity statistics. Since 2009, as a result of the Health Information Technology for Economic and Clinical Health Act, significant efforts have been made to accelerate the adoption of EHRs and improve the interoperability between clinical information systems both within and across healthcare organizations. The results have greatly enhanced the capability of local, state, and nationwide public health informatics infrastructures to establish data interfaces with health system EHRs, laboratory information systems, and pharmacy information systems. More recently, the 21st Century Cures Act of 2016 further requires the Department of Health and Human Services and the Office of the National Coordinator for Health Information Technology to improve the interoperability of health information, in addition to including clauses that prohibit information blocking from healthcare to public health.

Currently, the effort to advance bidirectional electronic information flow between healthcare systems and public health agencies is spearheaded by the Digital Bridge initiative established in 2016 (digitalbridge.us). Governed by a body consisting of representatives from healthcare, public health, EHR vendors, and government agencies such as the CDC, the mission of the Digital Bridge is to "promote the use of national health IT infrastructure to alleviate the administrative burden and costs of outdated, siloed data exchange practices."[54] Since its inception, Digital Bridge has led several important efforts to engage multiple stakeholder communities to have constructive conversations in achieving common public health goals. Its most noteworthy project to date is the development of a standard-based, multijurisdictional approach to electronic case reporting that removes technical barriers for health system EHRs, regardless of their vendors and implementation context, to be able to automatically generate and transmit surveillance data to public health authorities.

Databases and Data Warehouses

The database is the foundation of most modern information systems. Relational databases, which organize data according to their inherent relations (e.g., a patient can have only one primary care physician at a time, and a physician can serve as the primary care physician for many patients), are the most widely used type of databases. In a typical relational design, data structures are "normalized" to ensure that the same piece of information is stored only once in order to improve data integrity and reduce redundancy.

The software platforms for managing relational databases are called relational database management systems (RDBMS). RDBMS most popularly used in public health informatics applications include Oracle, Microsoft SQL/Server, and open-source platforms such as MySQL and PostgreSQL. Relational databases are manipulated and queried using the Structured Query Language (SQL). A basic SQL query takes the form of *SELECT * FROM diagnosis, patient WHERE icd_10_code = 'E11.9' AND gender = 'F' AND diagnosis.patient_id = patient.patient_id*, which instructs the RDBMS to use the data stored across two data tables, *diagnosis* and *patient*, to retrieve all information about the patients who have been diagnosed with type 2 diabetes mellitus based on the ICD-10 code.

Relational databases are designed to record events and transactions in real time as they occur. As such, they are optimized to handle a large number of concurrent users, provide transaction control (to avoid conflicts when multiple users operate on the same data at the same time), and use normalized data structures to improve storage efficiency and writing and reading performance. To put the data in a form desirable for large-scale analytics, a data warehouse is often needed. Data warehouses integrate data from multiple relational or nonrelational databases and convert the data into aggregates optimized for analytics. During this "denormalized" process, data that are frequently queried together, such as patient sex and diagnosis information, can be stored in a single table rather spread across multiple tables. The result is less complex data structures that can be more easily understood by nontechnical users, as well as better performance for frequently executed data analytics tasks such as routine data reporting.

Geographic Information System

Geographic information systems (GIS) are software programs designed to store, manipulate, query, and analyze spatial or geographic data. They are particularly relevant to public health as many data sources of interest for public or population health purposes are geospatial in nature (e.g., contamination of water sources by state, county, or city). In 1854, John Snow mapped the cholera outbreak in London and traced the cause of infection to use of water from a specific pump.[55] This is the earliest known application of GIS in public health. Since then, the need to utilize geographic data to understand the pattern of incidence and spread of infectious diseases has led to the birth of new disciplines such as medical geography[56] and spatial epidemiology,[57] which use GIS tools to study how diseases and risk factors are associated with spatially distributed geographic or environmental features. Currently, the most widely used GIS platforms are ArcGIS developed by ESRI (Redlands, CA), and the open-source tool QGIS.

GIS uses data that contain geographic features and their attributes. Multiple sources of location-referenced data can be overlaid on top of one another in a GIS system to produce maps of interest (e.g., drug overdose deaths by state). Spatial analysis can be then applied to answer important public health questions, for example, how valley fever incidents correlate with the geographic distribution of coccidioides. The most commonly used spatial analysis in public health is spatial cluster analysis, which identifies nonrandom spatial distributions of disease cases, incidence, or prevalence.[58] Temporospatial analysis has also become increasingly popular, which allows public health workers to visualize and identify patterns related to the spatial spread of infectious diseases overtime. By analyzing common use of GIS, Fletcher-Lartey and Caprarelli identified three areas in public health in which GIS has been particularly successful[1]: understanding the sociocultural determinants of health,[2] disease surveillance and early warning systems, and[3] international collaboration on zoonotic parasitic diseases.[59]

Data Visualization and Visual Analytics

Data visualization, even in its most basic forms such as bar graphs and line charts, is an extremely powerful tool to help public health workers interpret complex data and convey important information effectively to policy makers and the general public. Visual analytics extends beyond static graphical presentations of data to offer an interactive approach to decision making that combines visualization, human factors, and data analysis.[60] As defined by Thomas and Cook, visual analytics is the "science of analytical reasoning facilitated by interactive visual interface."[61] It amplifies human cognition by increasing the memory and processing resources available to users, reducing the search for information, using visual representations to enhance the detection of patterns, enabling perceptual inference operations, and encoding information in a manipulable medium that allows for rapid exploration and sense making.[62]

In medicine, visual analytics is a valuable approach to helping clinicians visually inspect longitudinal patient records data to discern trends and abnormalities that are not otherwise apparent.[63,64] This has led to a proliferation of interactive visualization tools, such as LifeLines[65] and Timeline[66] designed to work with EHR or medical imaging data. In public health,[67] visual analytics has also been widely applied in areas such as exploring the relationships between demographics, behavior habits, and other health conditions and chronic diseases[68]; studying the pattern of outbreak of foodborne vibriosis[69]; and enhancing public health surveillance for injury prevention and control.[70]

D3 (d3js.org) is the most popularly used tool for creating web-based visual analytics applications, with a simplified version, dimple (dimplejs.org), for quicker development and deployment. D3, dimple, and D3-based extensions such as D3Plus (d3plus.org) provide powerful libraries to generate rich, interactive visualizations to allow real-time inspection and interpretation of complex data. They are the visualization engine underlying many web-based systems that offer visual analytics capability for public health. These include DataUSA (datausa.io), a comprehensive website that hosts a range of interactive visualizations of public U.S. government data including public health datasets (e.g., opioid-related deaths), and socioeconomic determinants of health (e.g., education and poverty rates). Another popularly used platform for visual analytics is Tableau (Tableau Software, Seattle, WA), an off-the-shelf commercial system for building data dashboards with interactive visual representations. Originally developed for business intelligence, Tableau has now been increasingly adopted by healthcare organizations for monitoring performance and outcomes,[71] and by public health agencies for analyzing population-level health indicators and program evaluation data.[72]

KEY PUBLIC HEALTH INFORMAITCS APPLICATIONS

Childhood Immunization Registry

Childhood immunization was first required by public schools in Boston to prevent the spread of smallpox in the 1850s.[73] Such requirements began at the local level and ultimately became statewide. However, state vaccination laws received significant resistance due to parents' religious beliefs or concerns about vaccine-related harms. In 1893 Chicago, less than 10% of the children were vaccinated a decade after the state law for mandatory vaccination was enacted.[74]

Social controversies sought legal resolutions. In 1922 *Zucht v. King*, the constitutionality of such a state law was challenged and heard by the U.S. Supreme Court. The Court upheld that the state vaccination law was constitutional. By 1963, 20 states had passed school vaccination laws.[74] Furthermore, in 1987 Maricopa County Health Department vs. Harmon, the Court of Appeals of Arizona held that the student's right to education can be overridden by the state vaccination law during outbreaks.[75] Despite these rulings, the measles outbreak in the United States during the period of 1989–91 with tens of thousands of infected cases and hundreds of deaths was found by the CDC to be caused by more than half of affected children being unvaccinated.[76] The lack of vaccination, believed to be a main contributing factor of the outbreak, highlighted the need for immunization registries.

However, a single nationwide immunization registry at the federal level was prohibited by the Congress. As an alternative, private foundations including the Robert Wood Johnson Foundation initiated the All Kids Count program in 1992, which provided financial support to assist states to develop state-level immunization registries. By 1997, all 50 states had successfully established their immunization registries.[77] Meanwhile, the Omnibus Budget Reconciliation Act for helping disadvantaged children receive vaccination for free was passed by the Congress in 1993 and implemented via the CDC's Vaccines for Children program.[78] Moreover, due to children's relocation, it required registries to be able to exchange information with each another. To achieve this goal, the CDC collaborated with HL7 to develop the standard for immunization record exchange and implemented it in 1999.[79]

As of 2017, more than 90% of children aged 19–35 months nationally have received vaccination for measles, mumps, rubella, polio, hepatitis B, and chickenpox.[80] As of 2019, 45 states as well as Washington DC grant exemptions due to religious reasons; and 15 states allow personal or philosophical objection to immunization.[81]

National Notifiable Diseases Surveillance System (NNDSS) and National Syndromic Surveillance Program (NSSP)

CDC's Division of Health Informatics and Surveillance operates several major public health informatics infrastructural programs. These include the National Notifiable Diseases Surveillance System (NNDSS) and the National Syndromic Surveillance Program (NSSP).

NNDSS is a large network of public health information systems. At the state and local level, health departments collect data from healthcare providers and laboratories. Health departments then notify the CDC of conditions deemed "notifiable" by the Council of State and Territorial Epidemiologists (CSTE) whose membership includes at least one representatives from each of the 50 states and DC. Through NNDSS, the CDC currently monitors approximately 120 conditions ranging from infectious diseases such as Zika, foodborne outbreaks such as *E. coli*, and noninfectious conditions such as lead poisoning. Each year, CSTE and CDC review and modify the notifiable condition list based on public health relevance as well as emerging priorities.

Instead of mandating a uniform system, NNDSS takes a standards-based approach to allow local and state health departments to develop or purchase their own systems as long as they conform to the National Electronic Disease Surveillance System architectural standards, such as using standardized HL7 messaging to send case notifications. This approach is crucial to the viability of NNDSS. It gives health departments the flexibility to adopt a system that is customized to the local needs and regulations, while maintaining the ability for the data to be readily shared across the network.

NSSP, on the other hand, is a cloud-based common platform operated by the CDC. Its mission is to promote timely collection of syndromic data from settings such as emergency departments, and urgent care for early detection and rapid assessment of bioterrorism-related events and disease outbreaks. NSSP was developed through a collaboration of the CDC, health departments at local, and state levels, and other federal agencies such as the Department of Defense and the Department of Veterans Affairs. The core component of NSSP is the BioSense Platform that provides public health workers standardized tools and procedures to collect, share, and analyze syndromic data. The BioSense Platform is the first CDC system fully operated in a cloud-based environment. It is also the only public health surveillance system in the United States that allows state and local health departments and the CDC to share health information across city, county, or state jurisdictions.

Prescription Drug Monitoring Program (PDMP)

The Prescription Drug Monitoring Program (PDMP) is a public health informatics infrastructure that has been implemented throughout the United States. PDMPs collect prescribing and dispensing data electronically submitted by pharmacies and dispensing practitioners. The data are then used by healthcare professionals, regulatory boards, and law enforcement agencies to support the effort in reducing prescription drug misuse and diversion. All 50 states, except Missouri, have had an operational PDMP by 2014.[82]

As of August 2018, all of these 49 states have passed state legislations mandating the use of PDMP, even though the exact definition of use and the enforcement mechanisms differ.[83] For example, the California PDMP, branded as the Controlled Substance Utilization Review and Evaluation System (CURES), is created and maintained by the California Department of Justice. Starting in October 2018, subject to certain exceptions, all prescribers are required to review the CURES database prior to prescribing a Schedule II, III, or IV controlled substance to a patient for the first time, and at least every 4 months thereafter if the substance remains part of the patient's treatment. Recent research has reported significantly reduction of opioid dosages dispensed, percentage of patients receiving opioids, and measures of high-risk prescribing in states with comprehensive mandatory use laws versus those without.[84]

PUBLIC HEALTH INFORMATICS TRAINING AND WORKFORCE DEVELOPMENT

Many public health informatics training and workforce development programs are now available, providing full- and part-time education ranging from graduate degree programs, fellowships, and certificates. For example, the University of Utah offers PhD and master-level programs in biomedical informatics with an application track in population and public health informatics.[85] The University of Texas offers dual degrees PhD/MPH and MS/MPH in biomedical informatics and public health.[86] Other universities such as Emory and the University of Illinois Chicago offer a master's program in public health informatics,[87,88] and the University of Chicago offers Masters in Biomedical Informatics with a concentration in population health Informatics.[89] CDC has been offering the Public Health Informatics Fellowship Program since 1996.[90] It provides 2-year onsite training for public health professionals to develop and apply skills in information and computer science and technology to public health issues. Between 2005 and 2010, the Robert Wood Johnson Foundation supported the National Library of Medicine in overseeing a Public Health Informatics Fellows Training Program.[91,92] Certificates in public health informatics are also offered by numerous universities, such as Johns Hopkins University,[93] University of Maryland,[94] University of North Carolina at Chapel Hill,[95] and City University of New York.[96] The certificate programs at the University of Pittsburgh and Loma Linda University specialize in biosurveillance and geoinformatics, respectively.[97,98]

Competency requirements for public health informatics have also been developed and continue to evolve. There is general recognition that competencies need to be tied to practice and that there are multiple pathways to achieving individual competency. In 1995, the CDC and the University of Washington (UW) collaborated on curriculum development to train public health workers for state immunization registries. Complementary to core public health competencies, three informatics-specific competencies were identified, including using information *per se* for public health practice; using information technology; and managing information technology projects.[99] In 2009, the CDC-UW coalition developed an expanded and tiered framework of public health informatics competencies. The resultant 13 competencies include setting strategies; knowledge management; using informatics standards; meeting user needs and requirements; supporting information systems development; IT project and program management; communication; evaluation; public health informatics research; development of interoperable systems; information security; and education and training.[100] Studies also surveyed and ranked the needs of majority public health practitioners in four domains: leadership and system thinking, financial planning and management, community dimensions of practice, and policy development and program planning.[101] There have been continued efforts to revise and update these public health informatics competencies and direct training resources accordingly.

EMERGING TRENDS

In the past 10 years, the most significant development in biomedical and health informatics was the passage of the 2009 Health Information Technology for Economic and Clinical Health Act (HITECT Act). The goal was to accelerate the adoption of certified EHRs across hospitals and physician-based offices in the United States by providing policy mandates and monetary incentives. As part of the HITECT Act, hospitals and eligible practitioners were required to adopt a certified EHR system by 2015 and demonstrated "meaningful use" of it.[102,103] The Meaningful Use Criteria cover a wide range of measures, from increasing the proportion of data entered in a structured, computer-processable manner to providing patients electronic access to their medical records. The Meaningful Use Criteria also emphasize interoperability of health IT, to make sure that health information can be readily exchanged across healthcare organizations as well as between healthcare organizations and government agencies such as the Centers for Medicare and Medicaid Services and the CDC.

A direct result of the HITECT Act is the now nearly ubiquitous adoption of certified EHRs in the United States. These systems have the potential to automatically prepare and submit public health data such as notifiable conditions, which could significantly reduce the burden of public health reporting by providers as well as improve timeliness and data quality. To realize this potential, the Digital Bridge initiative led in developing an electronic case reporting (eCR) framework to ensure consistent, standards-based implementation of eCR across all EHR systems and all healthcare organizations. These include standard triggering criteria for identifying potential cases that are reportable, and standard formats for data reporting. The Council of State and Territorial Epidemiologists (CSTE), the governance body that defines and updates the notifiable condition list, also oversaw the development of a Reportable Conditions Knowledge Management System (RCKMS) that can automatically determine if a suspected case is reportable based on the data submitted from EHRs. These efforts have made it possible to have fully automated electronic public health data reporting capabilities from nearly all healthcare providers across the United States.

Another significant development in the past decade is the rise of citizen science and the increasingly recognized value of utilizing user-generated content in social media for public health surveillance purposes. The Vaccine Adverse Event Reporting System (VAERS) is an exemplar of how citizens can be involved to participate in and contribute to public health activities. VAERS, jointly operated by the CDC and the Food and Drug Administration, is a postlicensure vaccine safety monitoring program. Any individual, including patients, parents, and family members, can report information to VAERS about adverse events that occurred after vaccination. The data provide public health officers early warning safety signals that may prompt subsequent studies and interventions. Despite limitations (e.g., issues due to underreporting and unverified reports), VAERS has proved to be a valuable tool for quickly uncovering recurring patterns of adverse events associated with vaccination and collecting information from patients and parents that may not be otherwise captured.[104]

Social media platforms, such as Facebook, Twitter, YouTube, and Instagram, have been a popular vehicle for individuals to share information and discuss contemporary issues, including those related to public and population health.[105,106] A majority of Americans across a wide range of the sociodemographic spectrum now use social media on a daily basis.[107] Many studies have shown preliminary success of monitoring social media postings to produce early warnings of disease outbreaks such as seasonal influenza,[108] predict emergency room visits related to conditions such as asthma and drug overdose,[109,110] and study mental health issues such as anxiety, depression, and suicidal ideation.[111,112] While not a method to replace conventional polling and population-based surveys, utilizing user-generated social media content has also proved to be a valuable supplemental source of information to understand public opinions regarding critical public health issues such as health policies (e.g., the Affordable Care Act),[113] sentiments toward vaccination,[114] and public reactions to public health crises such as the Zika outbreak.[115] The Department of Health and Human Services, through a challenge competition, created a website (nowtrending.hhs.gov) that uses Twitter data for health departments and other health entities to monitor trending health and build a baseline of trend data, both for a specified geographic area and at the national level.

Social media has also become a common platform for public health agencies to engage and communicate to the general public on important health topics.[116,117] For example, the CDC has established a strong presence on major social media platforms such as Facebook and Twitter in order to disseminate credible, science-based health information. The CDC also developed a guideline, "The Health Communicator's Social Media Toolkit," to provide guidance for designing effective social media-based communication strategies based on the agency's multiyear experience in leveraging social media in its health communication campaigns.[118] In addition, social media has been increasingly used as a venue to deliver health interventions, such as to influence parental vaccine behaviors[119]; prevent risks for eating disorders[120]; encourage HIV testing, linkage, adherence, and retention[121]; and improve the health outcomes of cancer survivors.[122] Despites concerns (e.g., on user privacy) and limitations (e.g., low online participation rate), there is optimism that social media can be a valuable approach to health communication and behavior modification by improving information sharing, social connectiveness, and peer support at relatively very low cost.

CONCLUSION

The field of public health informatics has grown substantially in the past few decades because of the rapid development in information and computer sciences and computing technologies. Public health informatics infrastructures and tools are now playing an indispensable role in enabling effective monitoring and surveillance, informed decision making, and improved population health. Today, it is difficult to imagine any public or population health programs would succeed without the support of public health informaticians. While challenges remain, it is reasonable to predict that public health will continue to benefit from further advancement in machine learning and artificial intelligence, better interoperability between clinical and public health information systems, and more widespread use of mHealth applications and social media. We believe that the recent revolution in public health as a result of the rise of public health informatics is just the beginning, and a brighter future awaits.

References

1. Office of the National Coordinator for Health Information Technology. Office-based Physician Electronic Health Record Adoption, Health IT Quick-Stat #50. https://dashboard.healthit.gov/quickstats/pages/physician-ehr-adoption-trends.php. Washington, DC, 2019.
2. Parasrampuria S, Henry J. *Hospitals' Use of Electronic Health Records Data, 2015–2017*. Washington DC: Office of the National Coordinator for Health Information Technology; 2019.
3. Steinbuch KW. *Informatik: Automatische Informationsverarbeitung (Informatics: Automatic Information Processing)*. Berlin: SEG-Nachrichten; 1957.
4. University of Washington Information School. What Is Informatics? https://ischool.uw.edu/programs/informatics/what-is-informatics. Seattle, WA, 2019.
5. American Medical Informatics Association. What is Informatics. https://www.amia.org/fact-sheets/what-informatics. Bethesda, MD, 2019.
6. Yasnoff WA, O'Carroll PW, Koo D, et al. Public health informatics: Improving and transforming public health in the information age. *J Public Health Manag Pract*. 2000;6(6):67–75.
7. American Medical Informatics Association. Public Health Informatics. https://www.amia.org/applications-informatics/public-health-informatics. Bethesda, MD, 2019.
8. Hinman AR. Surveillance of communicable diseases. Presented at the 100th Annual Meeting of the American Public Health Association, Atlantic City, NJ, November 15, 1972.
9. Zinsser H. *Rats, Lice and History*. Boston, MA: Little, Brown; 1935.
10. Littman RJ, Littman ML. Galen and the antonine plague. *Am J Philos*. 1973;94:243–55.
11. Duffy J. Smallpox and the Indians in the American colonies. *Bull Hist Med*. 1951;25:324–41.
12. Duffy J. *Epidemics in Colonial American*. Baton Rouge, LA: Louisiana State University Press; 1953.
13. Ziegler P. *The Black Death*. New York: John Day Company; 1969.
14. Cullen MJ. The making of the Civil Registration Act of 1836. *J Ecclesiast Hist*. 1974;25(1):39–59.
15. Eyler JM. The changing assessments of John Snow's and William Farr's cholera studies. *Soz Praventivmed*. 2001;46:225–32.
16. Cohen IB. Florence Nightingale. *Sci Am*. 1984;250(3):128–37.
17. Dursteler JC. The golden age of visualization. The digital magazine of InfoVis.net. https://www.infovis.net:5201/?num=111&%20lang=2. Accessed July 12, 2019.
18. Kondratas R. Images from the History of the Public Health Service. The National Library of Medicine. https://www.nlm.nih.gov/exhibition/phs_history/index.html. Accessed July 12, 2019.
19. Dixon CW. *Smallpox*. London: J. & A. Churchill; 1962.
20. Gould K. Antibiotics: From prehistory to the present day. *J Antimicrob Chemother*. 2016;71(3):572–5.
21. Van Epps HL. René Dubos: Unearthing antibiotics. *J Exp Med*. 2006;203(2):259.
22. Kilbourne ED. Influenza pandemics of the 20 century. *Emerg Infect Dis*. 2006;12(1):9–14.
23. Viboud C, Grais RF, Lafont BA, et al. Multinational impact of the 1968 Hong Kong influenza pandemic: Evidence for a smoldering pandemic. *J Infect Dis*. 2005;192(2):233–48.
24. Mandell GL, Bennett JE, Dolan R. *Principles and Practice of Infectious Diseases*. London: Churchill Livingstone; 2010.
25. Joint United Nations Programme on HIV and AIDS. Fact Sheet—Latest Global and Regional Statistics on the Status. https://www.unaids.org/en/resources/documents/2018/UNAIDS_FactSheet. Accessed July 12, 2019.

26. World Health Organization. Severe Acute Respiratory Syndrome. https://www.who.int/csr/sars/en/. Accessed July 12, 2019.
27. Fan VY, Jamison DT, Summers LH. The inclusive cost of pandemic influenza risk. National Bureau of Economic Research Working Paper No. 22137. Massachusetts, MA, March 2016.
28. Lombardo JS, Ross D. Disease surveillance, a public health priority. In: Lombardo JS, Buckeridge DL, eds. *Disease Surveillance: A Public Health Informatics Approach*. Hoboken, NJ: Wiley; 2007.
29. Hollerith H. The electric tabulating machine. *J R Stat Soc*. 1894;57(4):678–82.
30. Goldstine HH, Goldstine A. The electronic numerical integrator and computer (ENIAC). *Math. Tables Other Aids Comput*. 1946;2(15):97–110.
31. American Health Information Management Association. Who We Are. https://www.ahima.org/about/aboutahima. Accessed July 12, 2019.
32. Public Health Informatics Institute. https://www.phii.org/. Accessed July 12, 2019.
33. Center for Disease Control and Prevention. National Health Interview Survey. https://www.cdc.gov/nchs/nhis/index.htm. Accessed July 12, 2019.
34. Center for Disease Control and Prevention. National Health and Nutrition Examination Survey. https://www.cdc.gov/nchs/nhanes/about_nhanes.htm. Accessed July 12, 2019.
35. Center for Disease Control and Prevention. Behavioral Risk Factor Surveillance System. https://www.cdc.gov/brfss/. Accessed July 12, 2019.
36. National Cancer Institute. Surveillance, Epidemiology, and End Results Program. https://seer.cancer.gov/. Accessed July 12, 2019.
37. Hetzel AM. *History and Organization of the Vital Statistics System*. Hyattsville, MD: National Center for Health Statistics; 1997.
38. Centers for Disease Control and Prevention and Agency for Toxic Substances and Disease Registry Steering Committee on Public Health Information and Surveillance System Development. Integrating Public Health Information and Surveillance Systems: A Report and Recommendations. https://stacks.cdc.gov/view/cdc/7677/cdc_7677_DS1.pdf. Atlanta, GA, 1995.
39. Centers for Disease Control and Prevention. Preventing Emerging Infectious Diseases: A Strategy for the 21st Century. https://www.cdc.gov/mmwr/PDF/rr/rr4715.pdf. Atlanta, GA, 1998.
40. Lewis M, Pavlin J, Mansfield J, et al. Disease outbreak detection system using syndromic data in the greater Washington DC area. *Am J Prev Med*. 2002;23(3):180–6.
41. Hutwagner L, Thompson W, Seeman GM, et al. The bioterrorism preparedness and response Early Aberration Reporting System (EARS). *J Urban Health*. 2003;80:i89–96.
42. Centers for Disease Control and Prevention. BioSense—A National Initiative for Early Detection and Quantification of Public Health Emergencies. https://www.cdc.gov/MMWR/Preview/MMWRhtml/su5301a13.htm. Accessed July 12, 2019.
43. Russell PK. Project BioShield: What it is, why it is needed, and its accomplishments so far. *Clin Infect Dis*. 2007;45:68–72.
44. Institute of Medicine and National Research Council of the National Academies. *BioWatch and Public Health Surveillance: Evaluating Systems for the Early Detection of Biological Threats*. Washington, DC: National Academies Press; 2011.
45. Centers for Disease Control and Prevention. HIPAA Privacy Rule and Public Health: Guidance from CDC and the U.S. Department of Health and Human Services. https://www.cdc.gov/mmwr/preview/mmwrhtml/m2e411a1.htm. Accessed July 12, 2019.
46. Kass-Hout TA, Gray SK, Massoudi BL, et al. NHIN, RHIOs, and public health. *J Public Health Manag Pract*. 2007;13(1):31–4.
47. Goldstein MM, Pewen WF. The HIPAA Omnibus Rule: Implications for public health policy and practice. *Public Health Rep*. 2013;128(6):554–8.
48. Atienza AA, Patrick K. Mobile health: The killer App for cyberinfrastructure and consumer health. *Am J Prev Med*. 2011;40(5):S151–3.
49. Steinhubl SR, Muse ED, Topol EJ. The emerging field of mobile health. *Sci Transl Med*. 2015;7(283):283rv3.
50. Larson RS. A path to better-quality mHealth Apps. *JMIR Mhealth Uhealth*. 2018;6(7):e10414.
51. Neuman Y. Artificial intelligence in public health surveillance and research. In: Luxton DDLuxton DD, ed. *Artificial Intelligence in Behavioral and Mental Health Care*. San Diego, CA: Academic Press; 2016.
52. Benke K, Benke G. Artificial intelligence and big data in public health. *Int J Environ Res Public Health*. 2018;15(12):2796.
53. Wahl B, Cossy-Gantner A, Germann S, et al. Artificial intelligence (AI) and global health: How can AI contribute to health in resource-poor settings? *BMJ Global Health*. 2018;3:e000798.
54. Digital Bridge. What is Digital Bridge. https://digitalbridge.us/infoex/about/. Accessed July 12, 2019.
55. Snow J. On the mode of communication of cholera. *Edinb Med J*. 1856;1(7):668–70.
56. May JM. Medical geography: Its methods and objectives. *Soc Sci Med*. 1977;11(14–16):715–30.
57. Elliott P, Wakefield JC, Best NG, et al. Spatial *Epidemiology: Methods and Applications*. Oxford: Oxford University Press; 2000.
58. Auchincloss AH, Gebreab SY, Mair C, et al. A review of spatial methods in epidemiology, 2000–2010. *Annu Rev Public Health*. 2012; 33:107–22.
59. Fletcher-Lartey SM, Caprarelli G. Application of GIS technology in public health: Successes and challenges. *Parasitology*. 2016;143(4):401–15.
60. Keim D, Andrienko G, Fekete JD, et al. Visual analytics: Definition, process, and challenges. In: Kerren A, Stasko JT, Fekete JD, et al., eds. *Information Visualization*. Lecture Notes In Computer Science, Vol. 4950. Berlin, Heidelberg: Springer-Verlag; 2008, p. 154.
61. Thomas JJ, Cook KA. *Illuminating the Path*. Los Alamitos, CA: IEEE Computer Society Press; 2005.
62. Card SK, Mackinlay JD, Shneiderman B. *Readings in Information Visualization: Using Vision to Think*. San Francisco, CA: Morgan Kaufmann Publishers; 1999.
63. Caban JJ, Gotz D. Visual analytics in healthcare—Opportunities and research challenges. *J Am Med Inform Assoc*. 2015;22(2):260–2.
64. West VL, Borland D, Hammond WE. Innovative information visualization of electronic health record data: A systematic review. *J Am Med Inform Assoc*. 2015;22(2):330–9.
65. Plaisant C, Mushlin R, Snyder A, et al. LifeLines: Using visualization to enhance navigation and analysis of patient records. *Proc AMIA Symp*. 1998;76–80.
66. Bui AAT, Aberle DR, Kangarloo H. TimeLine: Visualizing integrated patient records. *IEEE Trans Inf Technol Biomed*. 2007;11:462–73.
67. Ola O, Sedig K. The challenge of big data in public health: An opportunity for visual analytics. *J Public Health Inform*. 2014;5(3):223.
68. Raghupathi W, Raghupathi V. An empirical study of chronic diseases in the United States: A visual analytics approach. *Int J Environ Res Public Health*. 2018;15(3):431.
69. Sims JN, Isokpehi RD, Cooper GA, et al. Visual analytics of surveillance data on foodborne vibriosis, United States, 1973–2010. *Environ Health Insights*. 2011;5:71–85.
70. Martinez R, Ordunez P, Soliz PN, et al. Data visualisation in surveillance for injury prevention and control: Conceptual bases and case studies. *Inj Prev*. 2016;22:i27–33.
71. Ko I, Chang H. Interactive visualization of healthcare data using Tableau. *Healthc Inform Res*. 2017;23(4):349–54.
72. Zakkar M, Sedig K. Interactive visualization of public health indicators to support policymaking: An exploratory study. *Online J Public Health Inform*. 2017;9(2):e190.
73. McAllister-Grum K. Pigments and vaccines: Evaluating the constitutionality of targeting melanin groups for mandatory vaccination. *J Leg Med*. 2017;37(1–2):217–47.
74. Hodge JG, Gostin LO. School vaccination requirements: Historical, social, and legal perspectives. *KY Law J*. 2001–2002;90(4):831–90.
75. Malone KM, Hinman AR. The public health imperative and individual rights. In: Goodman RA, Hoffman RE, Lopez W, et al. eds. *Law in Public Health Practice*. New York: Oxford University Press; 2003, p. 262.
76. Atkinson WL, Orenstein WA, Krugman S. The resurgence of measles in the United States, 1989–1990. *Annu Rev Med*. 1992;43:451–63.
77. Baker EL, Friede A, Moulton AD, et al. CDC's Information Network for Public Health Officials (INPHO): A framework for integrated public health information and practice. *J Public Health Manag Pract*. 1995;1(1):43–7.
78. Centers for Disease Control and Prevention. Vaccines for Children Program. https://www.cdc.gov/vaccines/programs/vfc/about/index.html. Accessed July 12, 2019.
79. Yasnoff WA, O'Carroll PW, Friede A. Public health informatics and the health information infrastructure. In: Shortliffe EH, Cimino JJ eds. *Biomedical Informatics: Computer Applications in Health Care and Biomedicine*. London: Springer; 2006.
80. Centers for Disease Control and Prevention. Immunization. https://www.cdc.gov/nchs/fastats/immunize.htm. Accessed July 12, 2019.

81. National Conference of State Legislatures. States with Religious and Philosophical Exemptions from School Immunization Requirements. http://www.ncsl.org/research/health/school-immunization-exemption-state-laws.aspx. Accessed July 12, 2019.
82. Prescription Drug Monitoring Program Training and Technical Assistance Center. Status of Prescription Drug Monitoring Programs. http://www.pdmpassist.org/pdf/PDMPProgramStatus2015.pdf. Accessed July 12, 2019.
83. Prescription Drug Monitoring Program Training and Technical Assistance Center. Mandatory PDMP Use. http://www.pdmpassist.org/pdf/Mandatory_Query_Conditions_20180801.pdf. Accessed July 12, 2019.
84. Haffajee RL, Mello MM, Zhang F, et al. Four states with robust prescription drug monitoring programs reduced opioid dosages. *Health Aff (Millwood)*. 2018;37(6):964–74.
85. University of Utah. Biomedical Informatics PhD & MS Application Track: Population & Public Health Informatics. https://medicine.utah.edu/dbmi/academics-education/phd-program/pphealth-informatics.php. Accessed July 12, 2019.
86. University of Texas. Dual Degree Programs in Public Health Informatics. https://sbmi.uth.edu/prospective-students/academics/dual-degree.htm. Accessed July 12, 2019.
87. Emory University. Applied Public Health Informatics. https://www.sph.emory.edu/departments/emph/tracks/applied-public-health-informatics/index.html. Accessed July 12, 2019.
88. University of Illinois at Chicago. MPH in Public Health Informatics. https://www.online.uillinois.edu/catalog/ProgramDetail.asp?ProgramID=319. Accessed July 12, 2019.
89. University of Chicago. Population Health Informatics. https://grahamschool.uchicago.edu/academic-programs/masters-degrees/biomedical-informatics/mscbmi-concentrations/population-health-informatics-concentration. Accessed July 12, 2019.
90. Centers for Disease Control and Prevention. Public Health Informatics Fellowship Program (PHIFP). https://www.cdc.gov/phifp/index.html Accessed July 12, 2019.
91. Robert Wood Johnson Foundation. Public Health Informatics Fellows Training Program. https://www.rwjf.org/en/library/research/2011/08/public-health-informatics-fellows-training-program.html. Accessed July 12, 2019.
92. U.S. National Library of Medicine. NLM's University-based Biomedical Informatics and Data Science Research Training Programs. https://www.nlm.nih.gov/ep/GrantTrainInstitute.html. Accessed July 12, 2019.
93. Johns Hopkins University. Certificate in Public Health Informatics. https://www.jhsph.edu/departments/health-policy-and-management/certificates/public-health-informatics/index.html. Accessed July 12, 2019.
94. University of Maryland. Public Health Informatics. https://academiccatalog.umd.edu/graduate/programs/public-health-informatics-z028/. Accessed July 12, 2019.
95. University of North Carolina at Chapel Hill. Public Health Informatics Certificate. https://chip.unc.edu/public-health-informatics-certificate/. Accessed July 12, 2019.
96. City University of New York. Population Health Informatics Certificate. https://sph.cuny.edu/academics/degrees-programs/certificate-programs/phi-certificate/. Accessed July 12, 2019.
97. University of Pittsburgh. Public Health Informatics and Biosurveillance. https://www.dbmi.pitt.edu/content/public-health-informatics-and-biosurveillance. Accessed July 12, 2019.
98. Loma Linda University. Health Geoinformatics—Certificate. http://llucatalog.llu.edu/public-health/health-geoinformatics-certificate/. Accessed July 12, 2019.
99. O'Carroll PW, Public Health Informatics Competency Working Group. Informatics competencies for public health professionals. August 2002. Seattle, WA.
100. Centers for Disease Control and Prevention, University of Washington School of Public Health and Community Medicine's Center for Public Health Informatics. Competencies for public health informaticians. Atlanta, GA, September 2009.
101. Hsu CE, Dunn K, Juo HH, et al. Understanding public health informatics competencies for mid-tier public health practitioners—A Web-based survey. *Health Informatics J*. 2012;18(1):66–76.
102. Blumenthal D. Stimulating the adoption of health information technology. *N Engl J Med*. 2009;360(15):1477–9.
103. Blumenthal D, Tavenner M. The "meaningful use" regulation for electronic health records. *N Engl J Med*. 2010;363(6):501–4.
104. Ren JJ, Sun T, He Y, et al. A statistical analysis of vaccine-adverse event data. *BMC Med Inform Decis Mak*. 2019;19(1):101.
105. Paul MJ, Dredze M. *Social Monitoring for Public Health*. San Rafael, CA: Morgan & Claypool Publishers; 2017.
106. Charles-Smith LE, Reynolds TL, Cameron MA, et al. Using social media for actionable disease surveillance and outbreak management: a systematic literature review. *PLoS One*. 2015;10(10):e0139701.
107. Pew Research Center. Use of Different Online Platforms by Demographic Groups. https://www.pewresearch.org/fact-tank/2019/04/10/share-of-u-s-adults-using-social-media-including-facebook-is-mostly-unchanged-since-2018/. Accessed July 12, 2019.
108. Alessa A, Faezipour M. A review of influenza detection and prediction through social networking sites. *Theor Biol Med Model*. 2018;15(1):2.
109. Ram S, Zhang W, Williams M, et al. Predicting asthma-related emergency department visits using big data. *IEEE J Biomed Health Inform*. 2015;19(4):1216–23.
110. Young SD, Zheng K, Chu LF, et al. Internet searches for opioids predict future emergency department heroin admissions. *Drug Alcohol Depend*. 2018;190:166–9.
111. De Choudhury M, Counts S, Horvitz E. Social media as a measurement tool of depression in populations. In: Proc. WebSci 2013: 5th ACM International Conference on Web Science, 47–56, 2013.
112. De Choudhury M, Kiciman E, Dredze M, et al. Discovering shifts to suicidal ideation from mental health content in social media. Proc SIGCHI Conf Hum Factor Comput Syst. 2016;2016:2098–110.
113. Davis MA, Zheng K, Liu Y, et al. Public response to Obamacare on Twitter. *J Med Internet Res*. 2017;19(5):e167.
114. Salathé M, Khandelwal S. Assessing vaccination sentiments with online social media: Implications for infectious disease dynamics and control. *PLoS Comput Biol*. 2011;7(10):e1002199.
115. Gui X, Wang Y, Kou Y, et al. Understanding the patterns of health information dissemination on social media during the Zika outbreak. *AMIA Annu Symp Proc*. 2017;820–9.
116. Gill HK, Gill N, Young SD. Online technologies for health information and education: A literature review. *J Consum Health Internet*. 2013;17(2):139–50.
117. Moorhead SA, Hazlett DE, Harrison L, et al. A new dimension of health care: Systematic review of the uses, benefits, and limitations of social media for health communication. *J Med Internet Res*. 2013;15(4):e85.
118. Center for Disease Control and Prevention. CDC Social Media Tools, Guidelines & Best Practices. https://www.cdc.gov/socialmedia/tools/guidelines/socialmediatoolkit.html. Accessed July 12, 2019.
119. Glanz JM, Wagner NM, Narwaney KJ. Web-based social media intervention to increase vaccine acceptance: A randomized controlled trial. *Pediatrics*. 2017;140(6). pii: e20171117.
120. McLean SA, Wertheim EH, Masters J, et al. A pilot evaluation of a social media literacy intervention to reduce risk factors for eating disorders. *Int J Eat Disord*. 2017;50(7):847–51.
121. Cao B, Gupta S, Wang J, et al. Social media interventions to promote HIV testing, linkage, adherence, and retention: Systematic review and meta-analysis. *J Med Internet Res*. 2017;19(11):e394.
122. Pope Z, Lee JE, Zeng N, et al. Feasibility of smartphone application and social media intervention on breast cancer survivors' health outcomes. *Transl Behav Med*. 2019;1;9(1):11–22.

CHAPTER

6

Preparing for and Responding to Public Health Emergencies

Joanna M. Prasher • Stephen C. Redd

INTRODUCTION

Protecting the public is a core function of the government. Usually, this function is thought of as a national security or military defense mission, but protecting the public from health threats is also a security function. Because large-scale health emergencies can cause loss of life and loss of confidence in government capacities, preparing for and responding to health emergencies is increasingly seen as an element of national security.[1,2]

Health emergencies have affected human society at least since the classical civilizations of Rome and Greece. For example, the Greek city-states of Athens and Sparta experienced a plague, of unknown cause, during the Peloponnesian War (431–404 BC). In 541 AD, the bacterium *Yersinia pestis* caused severe social disruption and widespread mortality in the Byzantine (Eastern Roman) Empire. During the fourteenth to eighteenth centuries, recurrent waves of the "Black Death" pandemics, caused by *Yersinia pestis*, occurred throughout Europe.[3] Events like the yellow fever outbreaks in Philadelphia in 1793 and in Memphis in 1878 similarly caused widespread death and destruction.[4] Large-scale natural disasters, such as droughts, earthquakes, volcanic eruptions, and floods have also led to the collapse of cities, and at times entire civilizations. For example, one leading theory is that a massive drought, potentially exacerbated by human deforestation, led to the collapse of the Mayan empire in Central America and Southern Mexico during the ninth-century AD.[5] All these events are more notable for the destruction they caused, and the sense of inevitability, than any semblance of an effective public health response. Today, advances in communication, organizational capacity, the logistical capacity to move resources at speed and scale, and scientific advances in diagnostics, vaccines, and therapeutics have created the capability to respond effectively to large-scale emergencies and mitigate their consequences in ways that in the past would have been unthinkable.

PUBLIC HEALTH EMERGENCY CATEGORIES

Public health emergencies can be defined as events that overwhelm the available capacity to respond. In the modern era, three types of public health emergencies, each requiring a distinct type of response, can be distinguished. These are natural disasters, which are predictable based on the historical record; manmade events (emergencies that are the result of human action, either intentional or accidental); and emerging threats caused by an unexpected or novel agent that leads to an unanticipated or unimagined severe epidemic or pandemic. Effective response to each of these requires systems that match the speed and scale of the response with the speed and scale of the emergency.

Natural disasters, such as hurricanes, earthquakes, tornadoes, flood, and tsunamis, typically cause destruction of physical infrastructure, and the severity of the event is directly related to the magnitude of this destruction. Government emergency response agencies (in the United States, e.g., the Federal Emergency Management Agency or FEMA) typically lead responses to these emergencies. These events can be considered "predictable" or anticipated events, as the season and location of their occurrence can be predicted, although the severity and exact timing cannot. For example, hurricanes occur in the summer months in southern U.S. states with shorelines on the Gulf of Mexico or the Atlantic Ocean. The number and magnitude of hurricanes anticipated to reach the United States in an individual year is estimated annually by the National Oceanic and Atmospheric Administration. Similarly, earthquakes and tornadoes occur in predictable geographies, but the timing of neither can be precisely anticipated.

The first response to such predictable, natural disaster emergencies includes search and rescue operations. Next, priority activities shift to the provision of food and shelter and restoration of services including power, water, sanitation, and communications. Reestablishing clinical services and public health capacities are then prioritized following the stabilization of these core services. Public health activities in these cases depend on the specific disaster, but often require health monitoring of populations living in shelters, ensuring access to preventive vaccination, and restoring public health surveillance and laboratory capacity to detect and address any increased transmission of diseases of public health significance. Given the frequency of natural disasters, these types of response capabilities are used regularly and, although every disaster has unique features, the systems used are familiar to the responder community. Logistical issues tend to dominate these responses—assuring that resources are delivered to populations in need at the time and scale needed.

The next type of public health emergency can be termed manmade events. These emergencies are those that are the result of human action, either intentional or accidental. In the United States, the World Trade Center and Pentagon attacks on September 11, 2001, and the anthrax attacks later that year, were events that changed the expectations for public health responses. The anthrax attack, in particular, revealed vulnerabilities in preparedness for an event for which there had been numerous warnings.[6] In autumn of that year several letters containing anthrax spores were mailed to government representatives and journalists. This led to significant public health and criminal investigations across multiple states and in the end, 22 people were infected and 5 died.[7] The public health system in the United States—which includes local and state health departments as well as federal entities—was not ready to respond at the speed and scale required. These events highlighted the need to develop detailed plans for such incidents, and to exercise these plans. Routine communication systems were inadequate to transmit essential information to critical decision makers at all levels, and to communicate rapidly changing information and guidance to the general public.

In the years after 2001, federal preparedness funding for these types of public health emergencies increased approximately 10-fold,[8–10] with a heavy initial emphasis on preparation for nonstate, terrorist attacks. Analysis of recent events has made clear that state actors are willing and able to use biologic, chemical, or radiological weapons, potentially at significantly greater scales than terrorist actors could employ, and this must also be considered in planning.[11–13]

While these increased resources and preparedness efforts prioritized readiness against intentional attacks, the public health community also realized that unintended accidents or chemical, biological, or radiological agent releases are also manmade events that require the same planning, exercising, and countermeasure availability as intentional attacks. The Federal Select Agent Program in the United States was developed, for example, to reduce the risks associated with laboratory work utilizing pathogens and toxins that could cause widespread illness in humans or animals, or that could have substantial adverse effects on agricultural interests, whether intentional or unintentional. The need for the program became apparent in 1995 when a U.S. citizen was able to obtain *Yersinia pestis*, a Category A agent, from the American Type Culture Collection (ATCC), a supplier of biological research materials, without having a demonstrated or appropriate need for the organism.[14,15] While there are multiple ways to categorize particular pathogens, U.S. Centers for Disease Control and Prevention (CDC) has categorized particular biological agents and toxins as Category A, B, or C, based on factors such as their transmission and mortality rates and their potential to cause social disruption (see Table 6-1 for the current lists and category descriptions). The individual placed an order using the state laboratory license number of the laboratory where he worked as a microbiologist. The ATCC only became suspicious when the individual called CDC because of a delay in arrival of the requested sample.[16] Following this incident, the U.S. Department of Health and Human Services (HHS) and the U.S. Department of Agriculture were charged with creating a system to track such microbial purchases. After the attacks of September 11, this program was expanded into a regulatory program including the following elements: creating a list of the most dangerous pathogens and toxins—called select agents and toxins; developing regulations to assure safe and secure handling of these select agents and toxins; and creating a system for registering laboratories using these pathogens. This system was to include: an inspection program to ensure compliance with regulations; a process for reporting theft, loss, or release of select agents; and enforcement mechanisms. With the rapid development of methods to manipulate bacterial and viral genomes, additional steps are being considered to assure safe and secure work with these new techniques.[17]

TABLE 6-1 BIOTERRORISM AGENTS[100]

Category/Definition	Agents/Diseases
Category A: High-priority agents include organisms that pose a risk to national security because they: • can be easily disseminated or transmitted from person to person; • result in high mortality rates and have the potential for major public health impact; • might cause public panic and social disruption; and • require special action for public health preparedness.	• Anthrax (*Bacillus anthracis*) • Botulism (*Clostridium botulinum* toxin) • Plague (*Yersinia pestis*) • Smallpox (variola major) • Tularemia (*Francisella tularensis*) • Viral hemorrhagic fevers, including Filoviruses (Ebola, Marburg) • Arenaviruses (Lassa, Machupo)
Category B: Second highest priority agents include those that: • are moderately easy to disseminate; • result in moderate morbidity rates and low mortality rates; and • require specific enhancements of CDC's diagnostic capacity and enhanced disease surveillance.	• Brucellosis (*Brucella* species) • Epsilon toxin of *Clostridium perfringens* • Food safety threats (*Salmonella* species, *Escherichia coli* O157:H7, *Shigella*) • Glanders (*Burkholderia mallei*) • Melioidosis (*Burkholderia pseudomallei*) • Psittacosis (*Chlamydia psittaci*) • Q fever (*Coxiella burnetii*) • Ricin toxin from *Ricinus communis* (castor beans) • Staphylococcal enterotoxin B • Typhus fever (*Rickettsia prowazekii*) • Viral encephalitis (alpha viruses, such as eastern equine encephalitis, Venezuelan equine encephalitis, and western equine encephalitis) • Water safety threats (*Vibrio cholerae*, *Cryptosporidium parvum*)
Category C: Third highest priority agents include emerging pathogens that could be engineered for mass dissemination in the future because of: • availability; • ease of production and dissemination; and • potential for high morbidity and mortality rates and major health impact.	• Emerging infectious diseases such as Nipah virus and hantavirus

The final category of public health emergency is those due to "emerging" threats. The West African Ebola epidemic of 2014–15 and the Zika epidemic in the Western Hemisphere of 2015–16 are examples of such unpredicted, emerging events. In each of these emergencies, the potential of the pathogen to create the kind of epidemic that emerged was unexpected and the nature of the epidemic was initially misunderstood. Ebola virus, first identified in 1976, had caused outbreaks of dozens to a few hundred cases in remote areas of Central and East Africa, but had not caused an outbreak in West Africa, where highly interconnected communities and poorly functioning healthcare and public health systems coexisted.[18] Even when the outbreak was initially recognized in March 2014, 4 months after the first case,[19] the general view was that it would be contained using the same measures that had been successful in controlling previous outbreaks. This failure of imagination delayed the mobilization of sufficient resources to control the outbreak for months.

The Zika virus, although identified in monkeys in 1947 and in humans in 1952,[20] was not suspected to cause birth defects until 2015, and was not confirmed as a cause of these defects until mid-2016.[21] This delay in recognition of the birth defect risk was at least partially because Zika was the first virus linked to birth defects since the rubella virus was identified as a cause of such in the early 1960s.[22] Furthermore, this was the first time that any member of this family of viruses (flaviviruses), which are predominantly transmitted by mosquito vectors, was definitively shown to cause birth defects.[21] New challenges for public health are emerging at the time of this writing as the world responds to the COVID-19 pandemic.

As these examples show, the defining characteristic of emerging public health threats is that they are unanticipated and often the initial perceptions around them turn out to be incomplete or inaccurate. Successful public health response to these events requires the capability to access and interpret new information in near real time. This type of response resiliency—interpreting and adapting response efforts to new information—is distinct from contingency planning in which anticipated or potential events are carefully considered and detailed alternative courses of action are developed during the response in preparation. In responses to emerging events, shorter feedback loops and continuous reassessment of major assumptions are essential.

Although each of these three types of emergencies has distinct features, some emergencies may compound features from more than one type or occur in contexts that present additional response challenges. For example, the 2011 Fukushima Daiichi nuclear disaster in Japan began as a magnitude 9.0–9.1 (moment magnitude scale) earthquake that led to a tsunami that washed over the protective wall. In this event, the earthquake and tsunami—a naturally occurring event—caused an estimated nearly 20,000 deaths and created a nuclear disaster through the destruction of the nuclear power plant (as a result of the placement of the reactor and loss of cooling capacity) and public communication failures.[23] This public health emergency therefore combined aspects of both a natural disaster and a manmade event; the public health response required had to address the needs generated by both types. In addition, the social and political context may affect the scope and scale of the emergency, and the challenge of providing an effective response. Increasingly, the need to respond in politically unstable areas of active civil strife hampers emergency response. For example, the 2018–19 Ebola response in the eastern Democratic Republic of Congo took place in an area marked by armed militias and criminal elements, which limited the ability to perform case identification and contact tracing.[24]

CONSIDERATIONS ON FOCUSING PREPAREDNESS EFFORTS

Given the range of possible emergencies, determining where to focus the limited resources and personnel available for pre-event preparations is a challenge for public health. In general, two approaches, each with its own strengths and drawbacks, have been taken: an approach that focuses on developing capabilities needed in any response (an all-hazards approach) or a scenario- or threat-based approach. Under the all-hazards approach, the focus is on building, exercising, and sustaining the public health capabilities that will be important for effective response to most if not all types of emergencies. These could include, for example, effective situational awareness tools or state-of-the-art laboratory capabilities. This approach does not require foreknowledge as to which emergency will be faced next and builds capacities within the public health infrastructure which also support routine public health efforts. Alternatively, under a scenario-based approach, the focus is on building and exercising those specific capabilities, assets, and plans that will be needed for effective response to one or more probable, high-consequence scenarios. This approach acknowledges that each type of emergency will be unique and allows for more detailed preparations. For example, large stockpiles of antibiotics will be required for postexposure prophylaxis of the population under a wide-area anthrax release scenario. Building and maintaining a stockpile of these antibiotics, and the other anthrax-specific medical countermeasures that will be needed (e.g., vaccine, antitoxins), will greatly enhance preparedness for this one particular threat. Such approaches however rely on calculating the risk posed by various agents or scenarios, and correctly choosing which to address. In practice, public health preparedness approaches often include aspects of both all-hazards and scenario-based planning. The decision as to how and to what degree each approach is resourced and maintained is ultimately a political and policy decision that may change over time.

EVOLUTION OF STRUCTURES TO MANAGE PUBLIC HEALTH EMERGENCIES

A series of real-world incidents, both naturally occurring and manmade, during the first decades of the twenty-first century demonstrated the importance of public health preparedness and response. In response to these events, both the United States and the global community have responded with an evolving body of legislation and governance structures to improve the ability for coordinated and effective public health response (summarized in Table 6-2).

The attacks on the World Trade Center and the Pentagon on September 11, 2001, and particularly the release, the following month, of anthrax-contaminated mail, led to an increased recognition within the United States of the critical role that public health must play in effective preparedness and response to such manmade emergencies. In addition to the conventional natural disaster response considerations, bioterrorism involves unique response issues such as the need for rapid characterization of the offending agent, mass decontamination, ready access to antidotes and medications, specialized medical training, and proper protective equipment for emergency responders. The recognition that the nation was not fully prepared to address such challenges led to the passage of a number of laws within the United States, including the Homeland Security Act of 2002 and the

TABLE 6-2 KEY PUBLIC HEALTH PREPAREDNESS AND RESPONSE GUIDANCE, LEGISLATION, AND STRUCTURES

Year	Guidance, Legislation, or Structure	Description
2002	U.S. Homeland Security Act	Established U.S. Department of Homeland Security
2002	U.S. Public Health Security and Bioterrorism Preparedness Act (Bioterrorism Act)	Called for increasing public health capabilities to prepare for and respond to bioterrorism and other public health emergencies
2004	U.S. Project BioShield Act	Supported and accelerated advanced research, development, procurement, and regulatory pathways for use of critical medical countermeasures
2005	Revision of the International Health Regulations	Expanded the International Health Regulations to cover all agents that could potentially cause public health emergencies of international concern (PHEIC), required the development and maintenance of core public health surveillance and response capacities in all signatories, and required rapid reporting to the World Health Organization (WHO) of all such events
2006	U.S. Pandemic and All-Hazards Preparedness Act (reauthorized in 2013)	Established the Assistant Secretary for Preparedness and Response within the U.S. Department of Health and Human Services and called for development of a National Health Security Strategy
2008	First U.S. National Response Framework	Laid out emergency response roles and responsibilities of the various Federal Departments and Agencies across 15 core capability areas and established central coordination across them.
2014	Global Health Security Agenda	Sought to increase global health security through multilateral and multisectoral approaches to combatting human and animal infectious disease threats
2015	Joint External Evaluation process adopted by WHO	A voluntary monitoring and evaluation framework to track implementation of the IHRs
2016	WHO establishment of the Health Emergencies Programme	Sought to improve WHO's capacity to lead and coordinate international health responses and contain disease outbreaks at their source

Public Health Security and Bioterrorism Preparedness and Response Act of 2002 (also known as the Bioterrorism Act). The Homeland Security Act, among other actions, created the new Cabinet-level Department of Homeland Security to prevent terrorism and protect the nation's borders.[25] The Bioterrorism Act called for building public health capabilities to prepare for and respond to bioterrorism and other public health emergencies.[26] As a first step, the Public Health Emergency Preparedness program (PHEP), building on a previous CDC Bioterrorism Preparedness and Response Program, was established by Congress and implemented by CDC.[27] Two years later, the Project BioShield Act of 2004 was passed to support and accelerate advanced research, development, procurement, and regulatory pathways for use of critical medical countermeasures that were lacking in the anthrax-attack response and could be needed to respond to future chemical, biological, radiological, or nuclear attacks.[28] Medical countermeasures include both pharmaceutical interventions (e.g., vaccines, antimicrobials, antidotes, and antitoxins) and nonpharmaceutical interventions (e.g., ventilators, diagnostics, personal protective equipment, and patient decontamination supplies) that are used to prevent, mitigate, or treat the adverse health effects of a deliberate, an unintentional, or a naturally occurring public health emergency.[29]

Internationally, the need for an effective global response to emergent public health threats was realized in the aftermath of the SARS outbreak of 2002–2003. During this outbreak, 8096 people worldwide became sick and 774 died,[30] and there was an estimated global decrease in gross domestic product of up to $15 billion (USD).[31] This experience was a wake-up call to the global community and accelerated the ongoing revision of the International Health Regulations (IHRs), which were completed in 2005.[32] The updated IHRs covered any agent or threat that could potentially cause public health emergencies of international concern (PHEIC), required the development and maintenance of core public health surveillance and response capacities in all signatories, and mandated rapid reporting to the World Health Organization (WHO) of all such events, to support an appropriate global response.[33]

In 2005 Hurricane Katrina made landfall in Louisiana as a Category 3 storm. Ultimately, this storm would be associated with nearly 1000 deaths[34] and cost $125 billion dollars in damages, making it the most costly hurricane in U.S. history to date.[35] A Congressional review of the response found that existing federal emergency management coordination efforts were ineffective.[36] In response to these findings, the Pandemic and All-Hazards Preparedness Act (PAHPA) of 2006 was enacted to improve and streamline national security and public health emergency response, in part by establishing a new Assistant Secretary for Preparedness and Response (ASPR) within the HHS.[2] The ASPR serves as the central focal point within HHS on all matters related to federal public health and medical preparedness and response for public health emergencies. PAHPA also called for development of a National Health Security Strategy to establish a strategic approach to enhance the security of the nation's health in times of crisis. The first Strategy was released by the ASPR in 2009 and these are updated every 4 years[1] and are roughly modeled on the Department of Defense Quadrennial Defense Review. In 2008, the National Response Framework (NRF), which also incorporated lessons learned from the Hurricane Katrina response, was promulgated, superseding the previous national response approach.[37] Under the NRF, federal emergency response efforts would be centrally coordinated by the National Security Council. It also laid out roles and responsibilities of the various Federal Departments and Agencies across 15 core capability areas called Emergency Support Functions (see Box 6-1).[37] Under this framework, federal public health and medical services (Emergency Support Function 8) would be coordinated by HHS and included a range of specific capabilities in this area.

While these policy changes were being implemented in the aftermath of the Hurricane Katrina response, decision makers turned their

BOX 6-1 Emergency Support Functions (ESF) and ESF Coordinators

ESF #1—Transportation

ESF Coordinator: Department of Transportation

Coordinates the support of management of transportation systems and infrastructure, the regulation of transportation, management of the Nation's airspace, and ensuring the safety and security of the national transportation system. Functions include but are not limited to:

- Transportation modes management and control
- Transportation safety
- Stabilization and reestablishment of transportation infrastructure
- Movement restrictions
- Damage and impact assessment

ESF #2—Communications

ESF Coordinator: DHS/Cybersecurity and Communications

Coordinates government and industry efforts for the reestablishment and provision of critical communications infrastructure, facilitates the stabilization of systems and applications from malicious cyber activity, and coordinates communications support to response efforts. Functions include but are not limited to:

- Coordination with telecommunications and information technology industries
- Coordination of the reestablishment and provision of critical communications infrastructure
- Protection, reestablishment, and sustainment of national cyber and information technology
- Resources
- Oversight of communications within the Federal response structures
- Facilitation of the stabilization of systems and applications from cyber events

ESF #3—Public Works and Engineering

ESF Coordinator: DOD/U.S. Army Corps of Engineers

Coordinates the capabilities and resources to facilitate the delivery of services, technical assistance, engineering expertise, construction management, and other support to prepare for, respond to, and/or recover from a disaster or an incident. Functions include but are not limited to:

- Infrastructure protection and emergency repair
- Critical infrastructure reestablishment
- Engineering services and construction management
- Emergency contracting support for life-saving and life-sustaining services

ESF #4—Firefighting

ESF Coordinator: USDA/U.S. Forest Service and HDS/FEMA/U.S. Fire Administration

Coordinates the support for the detection and suppression of fires. Functions include but are not limited to:
Support to wildland, rural, and urban firefighting operations

ESF #5—Information and Planning

ESF Coordinator: DHS/FEMA

Supports and facilitates multiagency planning and coordination for operations involving incidents requiring Federal coordination. Functions include but are not limited to:

- Incident action planning
- Information collection, analysis, and dissemination

ESF #6—Mass Care, Emergency Assistance, Temporary Housing, and Human Services

ESF Coordinator: DHS/FEMA
Coordinates the delivery of mass care and emergency assistance. Functions include but are not limited to:

- Mass care
- Emergency assistance
- Temporary housing
- Human services

ESF #7—Logistics

ESF Coordinator: General Services Administration and DHS/FEMA
Coordinates comprehensive incident resource planning, management, and sustainment capability to meet the needs of disaster survivors and responders. Functions include but are not limited to:

- Comprehensive, national incident logistics planning, management, and sustainment capability
- Resource support (e.g., facility space, office equipment and supplies, contracting services)

ESF #8—Public Health and Medical Services

ESF Coordinator: Department of Health and Human Services
Coordinates the mechanisms for assistance in response to an actual or potential public health and medical disaster or incident. Functions include but are not limited to:

- Public health
- Medical surge support including patient movement
- Behavioral health services
- Mass fatality management

ESF #9—Search and Rescue

ESF Coordinator: DHS/FEMA
Coordinates the rapid deployment of search and rescue resources to provide specialized life-saving assistance. Functions include but are not limited to:

- Structural collapse (urban) search and rescue
- Maritime/coastal/waterborne search and rescue
- Land search and rescue

ESF #10—Oil and Hazardous Materials Response

ESF Coordinator: Environmental Protection Agency
Coordinates support in response to an actual or potential discharge and/or release of oil or hazardous materials. Functions include but are not limited to:

- Environmental assessment of the nature and extent of oil and hazardous materials contamination
- Environmental decontamination and cleanup, including buildings/structures and management of contaminated waste

ESF #11—Agriculture and Natural Resources

ESF Coordinator: Department of Agriculture
Coordinates a variety of functions designed to protect the Nation's food supply, respond to plant and animal pest and disease outbreaks, and protect natural and cultural resources. Functions include but are not limited to:

- Nutrition assistance
- Animal and agricultural health issue response
- Technical expertise, coordination, and support of animal and agricultural emergency management
- Meat, poultry, and processed egg products safety and defense
- Natural and cultural resources and historic properties protection

ESF #12—Energy

ESF Coordinator: Department of Energy
Facilitates the reestablishment of damaged energy systems and components and provides technical expertise during an incident involving radiological/nuclear materials. Functions include but are not limited to:

- Energy infrastructure assessment, repair, and reestablishment
- Energy industry utilities coordination
- Energy forecast

ESF #13—Public Safety and Security

ESF Coordinator: Department of Justice/Bureau of Alcohol, Tobacco, Firearms, and Explosives
Coordinates the integration of public safety and security capabilities and resources to support the full range of incident management activities. Functions include but are not limited to:

- Facility and resource security
- Security planning and technical resource assistance
- Public safety and security support
- Support to access, traffic, and crowd control

ESF #14—Superseded by National Disaster Recovery Framework

ESF #15—External Affairs

ESF Coordinator: DHS
Coordinates the release of accurate, coordinated, timely, and accessible public information to affected audiences, including the government, media, NGOs, and the private sector. Works closely with state and local officials to ensure outreach to the whole community. Functions include, but are not limited to:

- Public affairs and the Joint Information Center
- Intergovernmental (local, state, tribal, and territorial) affairs
- Congressional affairs
- Private sector outreach
- All Hazards Emergency Response Operations Tribal

attention to the potential for an influenza pandemic. In 2005, a novel H5N1 avian influenza virus was identified in China in wild birds and poultry.[38] In rare instances, the virus caused human infection and had an approximately 60% mortality rate. The recognition of this threat, and closer examination of the historical influenza pandemics of the twentieth century—in 1918, 1957, and 1968—galvanized an intense worldwide effort to plan and prepare for an influenza pandemic. The United Nations established a global coordination office to oversee efforts to prepare for a pandemic, and to reduce the risk through better detection and response to avian outbreaks. In many countries, including the United States, the emergence of H5N1 led to a similar effort to shore up plans for pandemic response. In the United States, the White House released a strategy[39] and implementation plan[40] that called for hundreds of actions to be undertaken to improve national readiness for an influenza pandemic. Exercises of these capabilities also took place at all levels of government.

In April 2009, a novel influenza A strain (H1N1) was first detected in the United States in a 10-year-old patient in California.[41] The subsequent 2009 H1N1 pandemic differed in numerous ways from the severe pandemics that had been the basis for assumptions under the prior plans—the H1N1 pandemic was first recognized in the United States, it was most closely related to a swine influenza virus (not avian), and the case fatality rate, while varying widely across the globe, was far lower than the planning assumptions.[42] Even so, by the end of the outbreak, CDC estimated that 60.8 million people had been infected with this new influenza strain in the United States, and that 12,469 Americans had died.[43] Efforts to prepare for a severe influenza pandemic, in particular, improvements in surveillance systems, vaccine production, and public communication, supported a stronger H1N1 pandemic response than would have been the case otherwise. Federal investments made to build state and local public health response capacity for such incidents were also critical.[44] A national U.S. survey, conducted in January 2010 near the end of the pandemic response, found that 59% of the general public thought that the U.S. government had done a good or excellent job with the response.[45,46]

The 2014–16 Ebola epidemic in West Africa was the first and largest Ebola epidemic of its kind. It included widespread urban transmission and a massive death count of more than 11,300 people, predominantly in the African nations of Guinea, Liberia, and Sierra Leone.[47] As noted above, limited Ebola outbreaks had occurred sporadically in East and Central Africa since the initial identification of the virus in the Democratic Republic of Congo in 1976,[18] but the governments of West Africa were ill prepared to respond to this new, urbanized outbreak. There were also charges that the WHO and other international partners did not respond swiftly enough, or in a sustained enough manner, to avert the massive loss of life that ultimately resulted before the outbreak was controlled.[48] Within the United States, the arrival of medical personnel and travelers from the affected region at U.S. community hospitals led to a new recognition of challenges with management of even small numbers of Ebola patients despite the developed medical infrastructure available in the United States. In the aftermath of this experience, the HHS (in a collaboration between CDC and ASPR) funded development of the National Ebola Training and Education Center (NETEC).[49] This network of ten healthcare institutions from across the country sought to leverage their expertise and experience to increase national capacity to manage individuals infected with these types of pathogens.

In the aftermath of the 2014–16 Ebola outbreak, WHO amplified its operational capabilities to respond to future emergencies under the Health Emergencies Programme.[50] This new structure, established in August 2016, sought to improve WHO's capacity to lead and coordinate international health responses and contain disease outbreaks at their source. The Programme operates under a unified budget and is overseen by an independent oversight and advisory committee that reports its findings directly to the Executive Board of the WHO's World Health Assembly. The Programme supports countries in their preincident preparedness work, develops strategies to prevent and control high-threat infectious hazards, and leads WHO surveillance, risk assessment, and emergency response efforts. This reorganization led to the improved effectiveness of the WHO response during the 2018–19 Ebola outbreak in the Democratic Republic of the Congo (Equateur Province). WHO was able to quickly mobilize to address the outbreak and continue to assess the evolving epidemiological and security situation that impacted the global response.[51] In March 2019, WHO underwent a massive reorganization to modernize and strengthen its health leadership roles around the world, including its emergency response functions.[52] Under this structure, the Health Emergencies Programme is now housed under the new emergencies pillar, which is dedicated to global health security both before and during health crises.

At the same time the 2014–15 West Africa Ebola epidemic was unfolding, the United States joined WHO, 29 partner countries, and other international partners to launch the Global Health Security Agenda (GHSA) in 2014.[53] Eliciting political attention and calling for specific national actions across the prevention, detection, and response continuum, GHSA seeks to increase global health security through building each nation's capacity to prevent, detect, and respond to human and animal infectious disease threats. Many of the identified capabilities were those that could have been critical in stopping the 2014–16 Ebola outbreak.[54] A monitoring and evaluation framework to track implementation of the IHRs and achievement of the GHSA capabilities, the Joint External Evaluation (JEE) process, was adopted by WHO in 2015.[55] The JEEs are voluntary, external assessments of a country's capacity to prevent, detect, and respond to infectious diseases and other public health threats. The JEE process brings together experts from around the world to help a country assess its strengths and weaknesses in health security and identify priority actions to improve its health capacity. As of September 2019, 104 JEEs have been completed. Following a JEE, countries develop National Action Plans for Health Security (NAPHS) to identify the resources and actions needed to address the weaknesses. The NAPHS outlines a country's own priorities for improving health systems over the next 5 years to reduce the likelihood of disease outbreaks that could spread within their borders and to other countries. Many of these plans, including that developed by the United States following the U.S. JEE in 2016, are available online to promote transparency and the sharing of best practices across the world.[56] The GHSA partnership has grown over time and as of 2019 includes over 64 nations, international organizations, and nongovernmental stakeholders focused on building local capacity to enable countries to stop infectious diseases at their source and so reduce human suffering and global economic impact.[57]

MANAGEMENT OF PUBLIC HEALTH EMERGENCIES IN THE UNITED STATES

The medical and public health response to any disaster can be envisioned as occurring on multiple levels. There are the response needs on both the "micro" level (at the level of the individual, the family, or the medical practitioner, where most needs involve traditional medical practices such as the provision of patient care) and the "macro" level (the level of public and governmental entities such as local, state, and federal public health authorities). Traditional medical response and the management of individual patients have been extensively reviewed elsewhere and are beyond the scope of this chapter.[58,59] Here, we concentrate instead on the "macro" response of the public health community within the United States and the many governmental and nongovernmental institutions that might be called upon to respond to, and mitigate the health effects of natural disasters, manmade, or emerging emergencies.

Response to a public health emergency can constitute a complex undertaking requiring extensive cooperation among medical practitioners, civilian authorities, and officials at various levels of government. Depending on the emergency, healthcare providers will require a thorough understanding of the principles of disaster medicine, basic trauma management, humanitarian relief operations, infection control procedures, and principles of personal protection. Moreover, they will also need a working knowledge of the components of the U.S. local, state, and federal response systems in order to function optimally in the event of an event in their local area. Each practitioner and public health official should have a point of contact with such agencies and should be familiar with mechanisms for contacting them before a crisis arises. Conceptually, sharing resources across other jurisdictions or involving other sectors are ways to augment the available response capabilities. Disaster Risk Reduction, a strategy to involve multiple sectors in planning for disaster preparedness and response, is an example of how this idea can be considered as a strategy. In Disaster Risk Reduction planning, broad sectors of society are encouraged to participate in planning for preventive or response activities related to particular threats. This approach was codified in the *Sendai Protocol for Disaster Risk Reduction 2015–2030*.[60] Modern public health entities are called upon to marshal an increasing array of capabilities and to work with a complex web of interconnected partnerships to ensure they are prepared and ready to respond effectively, as dictated by the type and characteristics of the emergency.

Just as in emergency preparedness, the approach to public health emergency response in the United States has evolved over time, culminating in first the National Response Plan and then the National Response Framework (NRF), the most recent version of which was released in 2016.[37] The NRF is a guide to how the Nation responds to all types of disasters and emergencies. The NRF describes specific authorities and best practices for managing incidents that range from the serious but purely local to large-scale terrorist attacks or catastrophic natural disasters. It is built on scalable, flexible, and adaptable concepts identified in the National Incident Management System (NIMS), including use of the Incident Command System (ICS) to coordinate efforts and to align key roles and responsibilities across the Nation. The ICS was originally developed to better organize the response to a very particular type of emergency, wildfires in the United States in the 1970s.[61] It was then adopted by the National Fire Academy as the standard for all fire responses, by many states to manage various types of incident responses, and by the FEMA as the basis for their national emergency management capabilities for all types of hazards. Finally, Homeland Security Presidential Directive 5 (HSPD-5), released in 2003, directed the Department of Homeland Security to develop a NIMS, based on the ICS structure, which was to be adopted for incident response by all Federal departments and agencies, and all entities supported by them. As a result of its origins, ICS utilizes a hierarchical and unified command structure that was highly effective in firefighting and other similar environments. Public health agencies have adapted this approach to the traditionally more distributed decision processes practiced in the public health community.[62,63] CDC, for example, has developed a compatible incident management system (IMS) to manage the agency's response to public health emergencies.[64] The use of ICS to respond to public health emergencies is still a new field, and the optimal way to organize and ensure effectiveness in public health incidents continues to evolve. ICS, and the broader NRF, forms the basis for a planning and response effort, achievable in the United States and other developed nations. Efforts at disaster planning and response during complex emergencies and in developing nations can follow the core principles, despite inadequate infrastructure, severe resource constraints, the realities of often inadequate security, and all of the additional challenges inherent in such settings.[65]

The institutional response to any disaster, natural or manmade, begins at the local level, and it is here that preparation efforts are perhaps most critical.[66] In the past, public health and safety professionals and organizations concentrated their efforts primarily on emergency disaster relief. More recently, however, preincident preparedness, prevention, and mitigation have become increasingly expected and important public health activities. Within the United States, significant resources at all levels of government have been dedicated to improving the national capacity of the public health and medical systems to rapidly detect, confirm, prepare for, and respond to public health emergencies. Since 1999, CDC has provided financial support (through what became known as the PHEP) to assist state and local public health departments in improving their preparedness and response capabilities. This funding has helped health departments build and strengthen their abilities to effectively respond to a range of public health threats, including infectious diseases, natural disasters, and biological, chemical, nuclear, and radiological events. Preparedness activities funded by the PHEP cooperative agreement specifically target the development of emergency-ready public health departments that are flexible and adaptable. For example, while only 5% of public health departments had an ICS with preassigned roles in place before the anthrax attacks of 2001, now 100% of them do.[27,67] Before 2001, none of these entities had sufficient storage and distribution capacity for critical medicines and supplies that would be needed in a public health emergency; by 2016 100% had such capacity.[26,66] In 2011, CDC published the first national public health preparedness standards to provide capability benchmarks all state and local public health departments should be striving to achieve; these were later updated in 2018 (see Table 6-3).[68] The combination of these clear, nationwide standards and sustained financial support to state and local health departments over time has enabled significant improvements to be realized in national public health preparedness capabilities.[27]

Within the healthcare community, ASPR's Hospital Preparedness Program (HPP) prepares the healthcare system to save lives through providing funding and other assistance, through public health departments, to develop and support regional healthcare coalitions (HCCs). HCCs are groups of healthcare and response organizations that collaborate to prepare for and respond to medical surge events. HCCs incentivize diverse and often competitive healthcare organizations to work together and 85% of hospitals nationwide now belong to these groups.[99]

In 1999, in close partnership with the Federal Bureau of Investigation (FBI), and the Association of Public Health Laboratories (APHL), CDC developed a network of public and private laboratories, known as the "Laboratory Response Network," prepared to respond to potential biological and chemical threats and other public health emergencies.[69] These high-capability facilities exist within established local public health, military, veterinary, agricultural, food, environmental, and water-testing laboratories throughout the United States. Under this system, local hospital "Sentinel" (level A) laboratories would be capable of ruling out the presence of certain biological threat agents in clinical specimens. "Reference" (level B) laboratories in certain municipalities and regions would be capable of ruling in potential threat agents and performing susceptibility testing. On the biological side, approximately 120 domestic laboratories are members, representing all 50 states. On the chemical side, 53 laboratories are members, including 46 state and local public health laboratories that provide testing on clinical specimens to measure human exposure to toxic chemicals.[70]

Finally, CDC has built long-standing relationships and supports the development of public health surveillance capabilities at the federal and state, local, tribal, and territorial (SLTT) levels to ensure nationwide risk awareness and inform public health decision making. CDC's broader mission also supports development of biosurveillance capacity internationally to improve global health security.

TABLE 6-3 PUBLIC HEALTH EMERGENCY PREPAREDNESS AND RESPONSE CAPABILITIES

Domain	Capability
Community Resilience	Community Preparedness
	Community Recovery
Incident Management	Emergency Operations Coordination
Information Management	Emergency Public Information and Warning
	Information Sharing
Countermeasures and Mitigation	Medical Countermeasure Dispensing and Administration
	Medical Material Management and Distribution
	Nonpharmaceutical Interventions
	Responder Safety and Health
Surge Management	Fatality Management
	Mass Care
	Medical Surge
	Volunteer Management
Biosurveillance	Public Health Laboratory Testing
	Public Health Surveillance and Epidemiological Investigation

To support national emergency preparedness, the U.S. Congress passed legislation and appropriated funding to CDC to establish an integrated national public health surveillance system for early detection and rapid assessment of bioterrorism-related events. To meet this need, CDC launched BioSense in 2003.[71] The BioSense Platform has since evolved into a cloud-based, secure integrated electronic health information system with standardized analytic tools and processes.[72] CDC's National Syndromic Surveillance Program (NSSP) works with SLTT partners to expand national syndromic coverage and increase the number of healthcare facilities that transmit data to the system on a daily basis. As of 2019, 66% of the nation's emergency departments, representing 46 states and the District of Columbia, were submitting data to this system; data are available within 48 hours of Emergency Department visit.[73] By using a common platform, health officials can now analyze syndromic data to improve their common awareness of health threats over time and across regional boundaries.

Prompt and competent disaster response at the local level has always been critical to preserving life, providing for public safety, and safeguarding public health. When response requirements exceed local capabilities however, the local incident commander may request assistance from the state. The state can mobilize statewide resources, such as the National Guard and, as needed, their Weapons of Mass Destruction Civil Support Teams (WMD CST). WMD CSTs are positioned in every state and U.S. territory and in Washington, DC.[74] These specialized forces support civil authorities at a domestic chemical, biological, radiological, and nuclear or high-yield explosive incident site by identifying the agent or substances at work, assessing current or projected consequences, advising on response measures, and assisting with appropriate requests for additional follow-on state and federal military forces. States may also request assistance from neighboring jurisdictions through preexisting Emergency Management Assistance Compact (EMAC) that enable states to share resources during natural and manmade disasters, including terrorism.[75]

When response requirements exceed the capabilities available at the state or regional level, the state may request assistance from the federal government through a Stafford Act Declaration under the auspices of the NRF.[37] Under the NRF, federal consequence management is organized into 15 Emergency Support Functions (ESFs), with each ESF being the responsibility of a specific federal agency (Box 6-1). In addition, dozens of additional federal agencies can be tasked to provide assistance to these lead agencies. Federal disaster medical and public health support is provided for under ESF 8, and is primarily the responsibility of HHS, in coordination with 16 additional federal entities.

One of the assets HHS can bring to bear is the National Disaster Medical System (NDMS), managed by ASPR. The NDMS consists of specialized teams, comprising trained medical volunteers, who can arrive at a disaster site within hours.[76] These units include Disaster Medical Assistance Teams (DMATs), Trauma and Critical Care Teams (TCCTs), Disaster Mortuary Operational Response Teams (DMORTs), National Veterinary Response Teams (NVRTs), and Victim Information Center (VIC) Teams.[77] ASPR also maintains critical drugs and vaccines necessary to respond to a large-scale disaster. These pharmaceuticals are stockpiled at several locations throughout the country, available via the Strategic National Stockpile (SNS) program for rapid deployment to an affected area.

Expert epidemiological consultation is available from CDC often involving its Epidemic Intelligence Service (EIS). When disease outbreaks or other public health threats emerge, EIS officers investigate, identify the cause, rapidly implement control measures, and collect evidence to recommend preventive actions at the request of the jurisdiction. In the case of a potential bioterrorist attack, CDC, the United States Army Medical Research Institute of Infectious Diseases (USAMRIID), and the Department of Homeland Security's National Biodefense Analysis and Countermeasures Center (NBACC) provide state-of-the-art laboratories capable of sophisticated biological threat agent analysis. These laboratories, capable of banking specimens, probing for genetic manipulations, and operating at Biosafety Level 4, would provide backup to regional laboratories at the state and large local health departments.

In the event of a disaster, and especially in the event of a terrorist attack employing WMDs, the military could provide several unique forms of assistance. In addition to laboratory support, biological threat evaluation and medical consultation are available through USAMRIID. Analogous chemical response capabilities are available through the U.S. Army Medical Research Institute for Chemical Defense (USAMRICD), and radiological capabilities are available through the Armed Forces Radiobiology Research Institute (AFRRI). Moreover, the military can advise and support civilian authorities through the Chemical/Biological Rapid Response Team (CBRRT) and the Chemical/Biological Incident Response Force (CBIRF), a Marine Corps unit capable of reconnaissance, decontamination, and field treatment. Both the CBRRT and the CBIRF can be en route to a disaster site within hours of notification. Military support, when requested, would be subordinate to civilian authorities and would be tailored by the Joint Task Force for Civil Support, the component of the military's Northern Command (NORTHCOM) designated to provide command and control for all military assets involved in disaster response missions and contingencies within the United States.

UNITED NATIONS SYSTEM TO MANAGE EMERGENCIES

Similar to the U.S.-based approach, the first response to a public health emergency happening anywhere in the world will be locally managed and supported. If additional assistance is needed outside of internal country resources, assistance can be requested from WHO.[78] WHO supports emergency response worldwide in alignment with its Emergency Response Framework.[79] Under this framework, countries needing additional support to evaluate or respond to a public health emergency first work through one of the 150 country offices that WHO staffs and maintains around the world, and then through the six regional offices as needed. When a health emergency requires the engagement and resources of other sectors (e.g., refugee services, logistical support) WHO country offices can designate a "health cluster" coordinator that can marshal the expertise and resources of the nongovernmental organizations supporting health issues in the country on a routine basis to respond to the emergency. These country-level health clusters can also call upon the global health cluster leadership, based at WHO headquarters in Geneva, to access resources outside the country boundaries as needed.

If the emergency outstrips these local resources, WHO headquarters in Geneva previously worked through the Country Director to determine when and if to mobilize additional support. This system was shown to be insufficient during the 2014–16 Ebola outbreak in West Africa however, and was blamed for the "unjustifiable" delay in global response to this crisis.[80] Under the new Health Emergencies Programme, established in 2016 in response to these critiques, WHO headquarters may now rapidly deploy appropriate subject-matter experts and leadership staff to the field who have authority to lead the international response efforts on the ground, as well as more rapidly releasing funds from the WHO Contingency Fund as needed to support these efforts.[50] These leaders will continue to work with both the health cluster organizations, as well as other partners such as the Global Outbreak Alert and Response Network (GOARN),[81] to evaluate and support, for as long as needed, the public health emergency response.

Under the 2005 International Health Regulations, it is also WHO's responsibility to determine if an emergency represents a PHEIC. This designation is reserved for those emergencies that are determined to pose a public health risk to surrounding countries that may require additional and significant international action.[82] Designation of a PHEIC, which has occurred six times between 2009 and 2020, can lead to recommendations including surveillance measures, treatment guidelines, and travel and trade restrictions to contain the risk. Importantly, declaration of a PHEIC can also lead to increased global attention and critical resource contributions from member nations and other entities, to allow a truly global response to important public health threats.

TWENTY-FIRST-CENTURY THREATS

While much work has been done to prepare for the threats outlined in the preceding sections, public health must also develop strategies to deal with the threats of the future. We can anticipate six worldwide trends in the coming decades that will challenge public health emergency response. These trends include: (1) an increasing global population that is ever more concentrated in massive megacities; (2) continuing mass population movements and migration; (3) increasing speed and volume of international travel and globalization of trade; (4) climate change; (5) increasing exposure to zoonotic diseases; and (6) increasing digital communication and connections.

The world's population is growing rapidly, with a global population expected to reach 10 billion by 2060.[83] Of course, population growth is not occurring equally in every country. Poorer countries in Africa and Asia and some middle-income countries in Asia account for the bulk of growth. And, for the first time in history, population growth is occurring exclusively in urban areas.[84] By 2030 the world will have 43 megacities (those with more than 10 million inhabitants), most of which will be in these developing regions.[85] Population growth in urban areas, in particular in impoverished urban areas, has a number of consequences for health and for health emergencies. For one, poor hygiene and crowding create an increased risk for the spread of contagious diseases. The inequality of economic and health indicators also creates the potential for political instability, which can diminish the capability of governments to recognize and respond to health emergencies quickly and effectively.

Over the past 150 years, the speed of travel has increased dramatically, from horseback and horse drawn carriages to railroads, from railroads to propeller-driven aircraft, and finally to jet engine propelled aircraft. In the previous 50 years, speed of travel has plateaued with modern jet travel, but the number of travelers and trips has increased dramatically. Over 4 billion passengers were carried by the world's airlines in 2017.[86] And it is not only people that are increasingly moving across national borders. According to World Trade Organization data, worldwide there were more than $19 trillion (USD) in international exports in 2018.[87] It may be assumed that such increasing movement of people and products will lead to increased risks of communicable and infectious diseases traveling rapidly across the globe. A recent study of infectious disease spread across Europe within the last 10 years found that travel and trade, in combination with environmental factors, were key drivers of over 60% of all infectious disease events identified by the European Centre for Disease Prevention and Control.[89]

Global populations are also increasingly migrating or being forcibly displaced in large numbers. Toole and Waldman have described the insidious cycle of armed confrontation, famine, and population displacement.[88] In 1980 there were approximately 5 million refugees worldwide, but by 2018 this number had grown to 25.4 million, according to the United Nations High Commissioner for Refugees.[90] And this number does not include the 40 million internally displaced persons. In addition to those forcibly displaced by conflicts, experts estimate that by 2050 up to 1 billion people may be forced to migrate due to sudden or long-term environmental changes in their home countries including increasing droughts, desertification, and sea-level rise.[91] The public health problems of refugees and other displaced persons are often overwhelming, even in the absence of specific emergencies. Crude mortality rates among refugees and displaced populations frequently rise dramatically above baseline levels, principally due to nutritional shortages, environmental problems, and preventable infectious diseases. Public health emergency response in these settings must take these preexisting factors into consideration.

The changing global climate is likely to play an increasing role in driving future public health emergencies. The World Economic Forum recently reported that, climate change was linked to all of the top risks facing the world in 2019, except for the deliberate use of weapons of mass destruction and cyber/data security risks.[92] As noted above, such change is already driving population migration and this trend is expected to accelerate. Climate change is also resulting in changes in the geographic distribution of disease vectors (e.g., mosquitos) and is supporting the emergence of novel pathogens and pests that may threaten human health and food production.[93] Shifts of human and animal populations, in adapting to new environmental conditions, may lead to increased human-wildlife conflicts, including new opportunities for transmission of known or emerging zoonotic diseases.

As rapid as global travel is increasing, the flow of information is increasing even more rapidly. Based on a 2016 survey, a majority of U.S. adults get news from social media.[94] Among Canadians, 70% of internet users go online to look for health information.[95] In almost all instances, the ability to transmit information from one part of the world to another has changed the world for the better—supply chain management, global transmission of news, and the ability for person-to-person voice, and video communication were unthinkable before the 1990s. Public health will continue to develop new ways to leverage these new opportunities to provide useful information people need to protect their health and the health of their families, but such interconnectedness also can allow the swift propagation of inaccurate and harmful information. Violent ideologues can recruit remotely and catalyze attacks across the globe. Social media messages have the potential to augment rapidly without the possibility of validating or verifying the information being transmitted. As a result, false information can spread quickly. For example, in 2019 WHO highlighted vaccine hesitancy, the reluctance or refusal to vaccinate despite the availability of vaccines, as one of the 10 global health threats for that year. One key factor influencing the growth of such hesitancy in certain communities has been the spread and reinforcement of inaccurate safety and benefit data via social media and other online networks.[96] Public health will need to develop better tools and methodologies to address this rising concern in an ever-more interconnected age.

Additionally, healthcare and public health practice have become increasingly reliant on digital technologies and communication channels to treat patients, prevent disease, detect emerging threats, and respond quickly in emergencies. This reliance on technology however leads to a vulnerability to cyber-attacks, and, in fact, cyber threats are recognized as one of the greatest challenges facing the United States today.[97] Indeed, healthcare may present a particularly attractive target for cyber criminals, as a source of credit card data and employment and medical history information that can be used for fraud or identity theft. Beyond the economic risks however, lives may be at stake, as demonstrated with the 2017 "WannaCry" ransomware attack that crippled computer systems in 99 countries, including infecting at least 16 National Health Service hospitals in the United Kingdom.[98] While it is critical that public health continues to take advantage of the latest, cutting-edge technologies and platforms, increasing attention must be paid to ensuring these systems are safe and secure.

Of course, these trends do not exist independently of each other. With the increasingly tight connections of populations and information, events and communication from one location can affect another location in nearly instantaneously and unexpected ways.

PRIORITIES FOR THE FUTURE

To successfully combat both known and emerging threats within the dynamic context of the modern world, the response community needs to continue to innovate. Reviewing past responses and taking steps to improve where needed is critical, but insufficient to ensure future readiness. Looking ahead, public health can expect developments in two areas that will improve emergency responses.

First, data processing and communication technologies will continue to evolve rapidly. We need to be ready to explore these opportunities as they advance. For example, a system to understand community sentiment based on communication analyses, with privacy appropriately protected, could guide efforts to inform community members to take appropriate public health action. With faster and more specific disease surveillance efforts, the ability to rapidly gather and make comprehensible vast streams of data, and cutting-edge modeling efforts, public health can move from analyzing the past to making predictions about future emergencies and anticipating necessary interventions.

Second, advances in the life sciences will continue and accelerate. Advances in biology—from the ability to rapidly sequence whole genomes to *de novo* genome synthesis and real-time gene editing—will have revolutionary effects on medicine and the capability to respond to new threats. The development of production platforms that can be adapted within days to produce industrial-scale quantities of safe and effective vaccines against newly recognized pathogens is only one example of what the future may hold. However, these same technologies could potentially be used to create or modify existing pathogens to increase their pandemic potential. The response community needs to continue to work to make sure these technologies are safely harnessed to ensure the best response possible within available resources.

The public health consequences of emergencies are complex, multifactorial, wide ranging, and often long lasting. Knowledge and experience from many health disciplines, and the resiliency to identify and analyze evolving situations rapidly, will always be needed for effective emergency response.

References

1. Office of the Assistant Secretary for Preparedness and Response. National Health Security Strategy. https://www.phe.gov/Preparedness/planning/authority/nhss/Pages/default.aspx. Accessed August 28, 2019.
2. Pandemic and All-Hazards Preparedness Act, USC (2006).
3. Harper K. *The Fate of Rome*. Princeton, NJ: Princeton University Press; 2017.
4. Oldstone MBA. *Viruses, Plagues, & History*. New York, NY: Oxford University Press Inc.; 2010.
5. Turner BL, Sabloff JA. Classic Period collapse of the Central Maya Lowlands: Insights about human–environment relationships for sustainability. *Proc Natl Acad Sci U S A*. 2012; 109(35):13908–14.
6. Inglesby TV, Henderson DA, Bartlett JG, et al. Anthrax as a biological weapon: Medical and public health management. *JAMA*. 1999;281(18):1735–45.
7. Barras V, Greub G. History of biological warfare and bioterrorism. *Clin Microbiol Infect*. 2014;20:497–502.
8. Schuler A. Billions for Biodefense: Federal Agency Biodefense Funding, FY 2001–2005. *Biosecur Bioterror*. 2004;2(2).
9. Centers for Disease Control and Prevention. Public Health Preparedness: Strengthening the Nation's Emergency Response State by State. 2010.
10. Heinrich J. Bioterrorism: The Centers for Disease Control and Prevention's role in public health protection. 2002; https://www.gao.gov/assets/90/81756.html.
11. Warrick J. The message behind the murder: North Korea's assassination sheds light on chemical weapons arsenal. *The Washington Post*, July 6, 2017.
12. Morris S. Novichok poisonings: Were they linked and has source been found? *The Guardian*, July 11, 2018.
13. Barnard A, Gordon M. Worst chemical attack in years in Syria; U.S. blames Assad. *The New York Times*, April 4, 2017.
14. Miller J, Engelberg S, Broad W. *Germs: Biological Weapons and America's Secret War*. New York, NY: Simon & Schuster; 2002.
15. Centers for Disease Control and Prevention, US Department of Agriculture. Bioterrorism: A Brief History. 2017; https://www.selectagents.gov/history.html. Accessed September 20, 2019.
16. Stern JE. Larry Wayne Harris (1998). In: Tucker JB, ed. *Toxic Terror*. Cambridge, MA: MIT Press; 2000.
17. National Academies of Sciences, Engineering, and Medicine. *Biodefense in the Age of Synthetic Biology*. Washington, DC: The National Academies Press; 2018.
18. Centers for Disease Control and Prevention. Years of Ebola virus disease outbreaks. https://www.cdc.gov/vhf/ebola/history/chronology.html. Accessed August 28, 2019.
19. Baize S, Pannetier D, Oestereich L, et al. Emergence of Zaire Ebola virus disease in Guinea. *N Engl J Med*. 2014;371(15):1418–25.
20. World Health Organization. The history of Zika virus. https://www.who.int/emergencies/zika-virus/timeline/en/. Accessed August 27, 2019.
21. Rasmussen SA, Jamieson DJ, Honein MA, Petersen LR. Zika virus and birth defects—Reviewing the evidence for causality. *N Engl J Med*. 2016;374(20):1981–7.
22. Petersen LR, Jamieson DJ, Powers AM, Honein MA. Zika virus. *N Engl J Med*. 2016;374(16):1552–63.
23. International Atomic Energy Agency. The Fukushima Daiichi Accident: Report by the Director General and Technical Volumes. 2015.
24. Ilunga Kalenga O, Moeti M, Sparrow A, Nguyen V-K, Lucey D, Ghebreyesus TA. The ongoing Ebola epidemic in the Democratic Republic of Congo, 2018–2019. *N Engl J Med*. 2019;381(4):373–83.
25. Homeland Security Act of 2002, USC (2002).
26. Public Health Security and Bioterrorism Preparedness and Response Act of 2002, 594 (2002).
27. Murthy BP, Molinari NM, LeBlanc TT, Vagi SJ, Avchen RN. Progress in Public Health Emergency Preparedness—United States, 2001–2016. *Am J Public Health*. 2017;107(S2):S180–5.
28. Project BioShield Act of 2004, USC (2004).
29. US Department of Health and Human Services. 2017–2018 Public Health Emergency Medical Countermeasures Enterprise (PHEMCE) Strategy and Implementation Plan. December 2017; https://www.phe.gov/Preparedness/mcm/phemce/Documents/2017-phemce-sip.pdf. Accessed August 29, 2019.
30. World Health Organization. Summary of probable SARS cases with onset of illness from 1 November 2002 to 31 July 2003 2003; https://www.who.int/csr/sars/country/table2004_04_21/en/. Accessed August 28, 2019.
31. Keogh-Brown MR, Smith RD. The economic impact of SARS: How does the reality match the predictions? *Health Policy*. 2008;88(1):110–20.
32. Fidler D. Revision of the World Health Organization's International Health Regulations. 2004; https://www.asil.org/insights/volume/8/issue/8/revision-world-health-organizations-international-health-regulations. Accessed August 29, 2019.
33. World Health Organization. International Health Regulations (2005). 2016; Third Edition, https://www.who.int/ihr/publications/9789241580496/en/.
34. Brunkard J, Namulanda G, Ratard R. Hurricane Katrina deaths, Louisiana, 2005. *Disaster Med Public Health Prep*. 2005;2(4):215–23.
35. National Oceanic and Atmospheric Administration. Costliest U.S. tropical cyclones tables updated. 2018; https://www.nhc.noaa.gov/news/UpdatedCostliest.pdf.
36. Select Bipartisan Committee to Investigate the Preparation for and Response to Hurricane Katrina. A Failure of Initiative: Final Report of the Select Bipartisan Committee to Investigate the Preparation for and Response to Hurricane Katrina. February 15, 2006.
37. US Department of Homeland Security. National Response Framework. June 2016; Third Edition, https://www.fema.gov/media-library-data/1466014682982-9bcf8245ba4c60c120aa915abe74e15d/National_Response_Framework3rd.pdf.
38. World Health Organization. Weekly epidemiological record. 2005;80(47):409–16.
39. US Homeland Security Council. National Strategy for Pandemic Influenza. 2005.
40. US Homeland Security Council. National Strategy for Pandemic Influenza Implementation Plan. 2006.
41. Ginsberg M, Hopkins J, Maroufi A, et al. Swine influenza A (H1N1) infection in two children—Southern California, March–April 2009. *MMWR*. 2009;58(15):400–2.

42. Wong JY, Kelly H, Ip DK, Wu JT, Leung GM, Cowling BJ. Case fatality risk of influenza A (H1N1pdm09): A systematic review. *Epidemiology (Cambridge, Mass)*. 2013;24(6):830–41.
43. Shrestha SS, Swerdlow DL, Borse RH, et al. Estimating the burden of 2009 pandemic influenza A (H1N1) in the United States (April 2009–April 2010). *Clin Infect Dis*. 2011;52(Suppl 1):S75–82.
44. Redd SC, Frieden TR. CDC's evolving approach to emergency response. *Health Secur*. 2017;15(1):41–52.
45. SteelFisher GK, Blendon RJ, Bekheit MM, Lubell K. The public's response to the 2009 H1N1 influenza pandemic. *N Engl J Med*. 2010;362(22):e65.
46. Centers for Disease Control and Prevention. National Pandemic Influenza Plans. 2017; https://www.cdc.gov/flu/pandemic-resources/planning-preparedness/national-strategy-planning.html. Accessed August 28, 2019.
47. Centers for Disease Control and Prevention. 2014–2016 Ebola outbreak in West Africa. https://www.cdc.gov/vhf/ebola/history/2014-2016-outbreak/index.html. Accessed August 28, 2019.
48. Mackey TK. The Ebola outbreak: Catalyzing a "shift" in global health governance? *BMC Infect Dis*. 2016;16(1):699.
49. National Ebola Training and Education Center. Ready to Respond: Leading medical centers funded to train and prepare other U.S. health care facilities for Ebola and emerging threats. https://netec.org/. Accessed September 17, 2019.
50. World Health Organization. WHO's new Health Emergencies Programme. 2016; https://www.who.int/features/qa/health-emergencies-programme/en/. Accessed August 28, 2019.
51. World Health Organization. Ebola virus disease—Democratic Republic of the Congo 2019; https://www.who.int/csr/don/13-june-2019-ebola-drc/en/. Accessed August 28, 2019.
52. World Health Organization. WHO unveils sweeping reforms in drive towards "triple billion" targets. 2019; https://www.who.int/news-room/detail/06-03-2019-who-unveils-sweeping-reforms-in-drive-towards-triple-billion-targets. Accessed August 28, 2019.
53. Katz R, Sorrell EM, Kornblet SA, Fischer JE. Global health security agenda and the international health regulations: moving forward. *Biosecur Bioterror*. 2014;12(5):231–8.
54. Frieden TR, Damon I, Bell BP, Kenyon T, Nichol S. Ebola 2014—New challenges, new global response and responsibility. *N Engl J Med*. 2014;371(13):1177–80.
55. World Health Organization. IHR monitoring and evaluation framework. https://extranet.who.int/sph/ihrmef. Accessed August 29, 2018.
56. World Health Organization. National Action Plan for Health Security (NAPHS). https://extranet.who.int/sph/country-planning. Accessed August 29, 2019.
57. Global Health Security Agenda. https://www.ghsagenda.org/about. Accessed August 29, 2019.
58. Cieslak TJ, Christopher GW, Eitzen EM. Bioterrorism alert for health care workers. In: Fong IW, Alibek K, eds. *Bioterrorism and Infectious Agents: A New Dilemma for the 21st Century*. Boston, MA: Springer US; 2005, pp. 217–36.
59. Johannigman JA. Disaster preparedness: It's all about me. *Crit Care Med*. 2005;33(1)(Supplement):S22–8.
60. United Nations Office for Disaster Risk Reduction. Sendai Framework for Disaster Risk Reduction 2015–2030. 2015.
61. Bigley GA, Roberts KH. The Incident Command System: High-reliability organizing for complex and volatile task environments. *Acad Manag J*. 2001;44(6):1281–99.
62. Bochenek R, Grant M, Schwartz B. Enhancing the relevance of Incident Management Systems in Public Health Emergency Preparedness: A novel conceptual framework. *Disaster Med Public Health Prep*. 2015;9(4):415–22.
63. Jensen J, Waugh WL. The United States' experience with the Incident Command System: What we think we know and what we need to know more about. *J Contingencies Crisis Manag*. 2014;22(1):5–17.
64. Papagiotas SS, Frank M, Bruce S, Posid JM. From SARS to 2009 H1N1 influenza: The evolution of a Public Health Incident Management System at CDC. *Public Health Rep*. 2012;127(3):267–74.
65. Brooks J, Pinto M, Gill A, et al. Incident Management Systems and Building Emergency Management Capacity during the 2014–2016 Ebola epidemic—Liberia, Sierra Leone, and Guinea. *MMWR Suppl*. 2016;65:28–34.
66. Garrett L, Magruder C, Molgard C. Taking the terror out of bioterrorism: Planning for a bioterrorist event from a local perspective. *J Public Health Manag Pract*. 2000;6(4):1–7.
67. Khan AS. Public health preparedness and response in the USA since 9/11: A national health security imperative. *Lancet*. 2011;378(9794):953–6.
68. Centers for Disease Control and Prevention. Public Health Emergency Preparedness and Response Capabilities: National Standards for State, Local, Tribal, and Territorial Public Health. 2018.
69. Centers for Disease Control and Prevention. The Laboratory Response Network Partners in Preparedness. 2019; https://emergency.cdc.gov/lrn/index.asp. Accessed September 17, 2019.
70. Centers for Disease Control and Prevention. Frequently Asked Questions about the Laboratory Response Network (LRN). 2019; https://emergency.cdc.gov/lrn/faq.asp. Accessed September 17, 2019.
71. Centers for Disease Control and Prevention. National Syndromic Surveillance Program Overview. 2018; https://www.cdc.gov/nssp/overview.html. Accessed September 18, 2019.
72. Gould DW, Walker D, Yoon PW. The Evolution of BioSense: Lessons learned and future directions. *Public Health Rep*. 2017;132(1_suppl):7S–11S.
73. Centers for Disease Control and Prevention. National Syndromic Surveillance Program Participation. July 2019; https://www.cdc.gov/nssp/news.html#Participation. Accessed September 18, 2019.
74. United States National Guard. Weapons of Mass Destruction (WMD) Civil Support Team (CST). 2017.
75. Emergency Management Assistance Compact. What is EMAC? https://www.emacweb.org/index.php/learn-about-emac/what-is-emac. Accessed September 18, 2019.
76. Franco C, Toner E, Waldhorn R, Inglesby TV, O'Toole T. The National Disaster Medical System: Past, present, and suggestions for the future. *Biosecur Bioterror*. 2007;5(4):319–26.
77. Office of the Assistant Secretary for Preparedness and Response. NDMS Teams. https://www.phe.gov/Preparedness/responders/ndms/ndms-teams/Pages/default.aspx. Accessed September 3, 2019.
78. World Health Organization. About WHO. https://www.who.int/about. Accessed September 3, 2019.
79. World Health Organization. Emergency Response Framework. 2013.
80. Stocking B, Muyembe-Tamfun J-J, Shuaib F, Alberto-Banatin C, Frenk J, Kickbusch I. Report of the Ebola Interim Assessment Panel. 2015.
81. World Health Organization. Global Outbreak Alert and Response Network. https://extranet.who.int/goarn/. Accessed September 18, 2019.
82. World Health Organization. IHR Procedures concerning Public Health Emergencies of International Concern (PHEIC). 2005; https://www.who.int/ihr/procedures/pheic/en/. Accessed September 18, 2019.
83. United Nations Department of Economic and Social Affairs. World Population Prospects 2019: Highlights. 2019.
84. United Nations Department of Economic and Social Affairs. World Urbanization Prospects: The 2018 Revision: Final Report. 2019.
85. United Nations Department of Economic and Social Affairs. World Urbanization Prospects: The 2018 Revision: Key Facts. 2018.
86. Air Transport Action Group. Welcome to ATAG. https://www.atag.org/. Accessed September 20, 2019.
87. World Trade Organization. WTO Data Portal. https://data.wto.org/. Accessed September 20, 2019.
88. Toole MJ. The public health consequences of inaction: Lessons learned responding to sudden population displacement. In: Cahill KM, ed. *The Framework for Survival: Health, Human Rights, and Humanitarian Assistance in Conflicts and Disasters*. New York: Basic Books; 1993, pp. 144–58.
89. Semenza JC, Lindgren E, Balkanyi L, et al. Determinants and drivers of infectious disease threat events in Europe. *Emerg Infect Dis*. 2016;22(4):581–9.
90. United Nations High Commissioner for Refugees. Global trends: Forced displacement in 2017. June 25, 2018.
91. United Nations International Organization for Migration. Migration, environment and climate change: Assessing the evidence. 2009.
92. World Economic Forum. The Global Risks Report 2019: 14th Edition. 2019.
93. Scheffers BR, De Meester L, Bridge TCL, et al. The broad footprint of climate change from genes to biomes to people. *Science*. 2016;354(6313).
94. Gottfried J, Shearer E. News use across social media platforms 2016. 26 May 2016; https://www.journalism.org/2016/05/26/news-use-across-social-media-platforms-2016/. Accessed September 20, 2019.
95. Tonsaker T, Bartlett G, Trpkov C. Health information on the Internet: Gold mine or minefield? *Can Fam Physician*. 2014;60(5):407–8.

96. Dubé E, Laberge C, Guay M, Bramadat P, Roy R, Bettinger J. Vaccine hesitancy: An overview. *Hum Vaccin Immunother.* 2013;9(8):1763–73.

97. Coats DR. Worldwide threat assessment of the US Intelligence Community. January 29, 2019.

98. Lee BY. Friday's events showed how cyber attacks may hurt and kill people. *Forbes*, May 15, 2017.

99. Assistant Secretary for Preparedness and Response. Hospital Preparedness Program Factsheet. 2017; https://www.phe.gov/Preparedness/planning/hpp/Documents/hpp-intro-508.pdf. Accessed April 22, 2020.

100. Centers for Disease Control and Prevention. Bioterrorism Agents/Diseases, By Category. 2018; https://emergency.cdc.gov/agent/agentlist-category.asp. Accessed April 23, 2020.

CHAPTER 7

Public Health Surveillance

Paul A. Simon • Steven M. Teutsch

Public health surveillance is the cornerstone of public health practice, generating vital information for decision-making in nearly all aspects of public health work. Public health surveillance has been defined as "the ongoing systematic collection, analysis, and interpretation of health data essential to the planning, implementation, and evaluation of public health practice, closely integrated with the [timely] dissemination of these data to those who need to know and linked to prevention and control."[1] Important in this definition is the requirement that surveillance activities be closely aligned with public health actions to prevent and control disease, promote population health, and reduce health inequities.

Public health surveillance serves many purposes (Box 7-1). Surveillance is the primary means by which disease outbreaks are identified, characterized, and monitored to ensure effective control. Surveillance data are used to identify and address emerging health threats. Recent notable examples include the rapid spread of Zika virus in the South Pacific and the Americas beginning in 2007 and 2015, respectively,[2] the Ebola viral disease outbreak in West Africa in 2014,[3] and the rapid global spread of a novel new coronavirus (SARS-CoV-2) beginning in late 2019.[4] Surveillance is also important for detecting the resurgence of old threats, such as the steep increase in sexually transmitted infections in the United States beginning in 2013.[5] The importance of surveillance in protecting the public against acute health threats extends beyond communicable diseases to also include toxic environmental exposures, such as lead poisoning.[6]

BOX 7-1 Purposes of Surveillance

- Detecting and monitoring responses to disease outbreaks and epidemics
- Characterizing the natural history of disease
- Quantifying the magnitude of a health problem and monitoring trends over time
- Characterizing the geographic distribution of disease
- Identifying at-risk groups
- Monitoring patterns of antimicrobial resistance
- Detecting and monitoring responses to environmental hazards in community and workplace settings
- Identifying and characterizing health disparities
- Characterizing and tracking conditions in the environment that impact health, including the natural environment, built environment, and social environment
- Monitoring the safety of medical products
- Monitoring healthcare practices
- Supporting program planning, priority setting, and resource allocation decisions
- Informing policy development
- Evaluating impacts of public health programs and other interventions
- Generating causal hypotheses
- Supporting education and advocacy

Surveillance also supports health-promotion efforts, providing essential information on the incidence and prevalence of chronic health conditions, related health behaviors, unintentional injuries, and violence. In addition, surveillance is used to characterize and track the underlying conditions in community environments that impact health, including the social determinants of health.

Surveillance data provide important information for establishing public health priorities and determining how to best allocate resources. Surveillance information is used to inform program planning and policy development. Once programs and policies are implemented, surveillance data can be used to assess their impacts. Surveillance data are also often used to support advocacy efforts by helping to document the significance of a health issue in the population.

Surveillance data are generally descriptive in nature, documenting the magnitude and geographic distribution of disease over time within and across populations. Analyses focus on variables related to person, place, and time, thereby providing insights on potential at-risk groups, plausible modes of transmission, geographic clustering, and temporal trends. These analyses can be used to generate causal hypotheses and identify research needs but, unlike most research, are often limited in their ability to test causal hypotheses. However, surveillance databases can be an important resource for identifying and recruiting potential participants for research projects that can test for causal linkages.

HISTORICAL PERSPECTIVE

As early as the seventeenth century, events were taking place that laid the groundwork for modern surveillance systems. In Europe, medical science was becoming an established discipline and rudimentary healthcare systems were developing, creating an infrastructure for surveillance. New methods of classifying disease and illness were introduced by Thomas Sydenham, an English physician and leading diagnostician, creating a basic framework in which disease conditions could be defined for surveillance.[7]

During this period, advances were also made in the measurement of disease in populations. John Graunt, considered the founder of modern demography, published a book in 1662, entitled *Natural and Political Observations Made Upon the Bills of Mortality*, in which he reported his analyses of 50 years of weekly mortality statistics from London.[8] His work described patterns of mortality from bubonic plague and other diseases and led to the revelation that insights could be gained by examining patterns of disease in populations that were not apparent in examining disease in individuals. In the 1680s in Germany, Gottfried Wilhelm von Leibniz, a prominent mathematician and philosopher, advocated for health councils and analysis of mortality statistics to support health planning.[7] In nineteenth-century England and Wales, William Farr, considered one of the founders of modern surveillance, served as Superintendent of the Statistical Department in the General Register Office, where he created a more sophisticated system of disease classification and introduced more rigorous analysis of national and regional mortality statistics.[9] His work supported the efforts of John Snow in his landmark epidemiologic analyses of cholera outbreaks in London in the 1850s.

In the United States, similar efforts were underway, with a primary focus on control of infectious diseases.[7] The colony of Rhode Island passed a law in 1741 mandating tavern keepers report cases of communicable disease among their patrons, and more specifically in 1743 that they report cases of smallpox, yellow fever, and cholera. National reporting of vital statistics was established in 1850 and in 1893 Michigan became the first state to require reporting of designated infectious diseases. By 1901, all states had established mandatory reporting of tuberculosis, smallpox, and cholera.

While the states retained the legal authority to mandate reporting of disease to local and state government officials, an authority that persists to the present day, the federal government assumed the critical role of coordination and compilation of national statistics. In 1878, the forerunner of the Public Health Service (PHS) was established by Congress and in 1914 PHS epidemiologists were assigned to state health departments to assist in compiling and transmitting weekly disease reports via telegraph to PHS. By 1925, all states were participating in national morbidity reporting.

In the 1940s and 1950s, the prominence of surveillance in the public health enterprise greatly increased, in concert with the growth and influence of the Centers for Disease Control and Prevention (CDC), at that time referred to as the Communicable Disease Center. Led by CDC's chief epidemiologist, Alexander Langmuir, an outspoken champion for the use of surveillance to inform public health practice, the CDC established the Epidemic Intelligence Service (EIS) in 1951. EIS Officers, comprising physicians and other health professionals, were given basic training in field epidemiology and surveillance methods and then spent 2 years performing applied epidemiology and surveillance-related work across the United States and internationally. The EIS program has grown over time and similar field epidemiology training programs (FETP) have been established in many other countries over the past four decades.

Through the work of the staff at the CDC, the World Health Organization (WHO), and regional institutions, such as the European Centre for Disease Prevention and Control, awareness of the critical importance of surveillance in public health practice has grown considerably. Perhaps the best illustration is the central role that surveillance played in eradicating smallpox in the 1960s and 1970s, using a surveillance and containment strategy to rapidly identify and address pockets of smallpox activity with targeted vaccination in often hard to reach areas.[10] In addition, since the 1960s, application of surveillance methods has expanded far beyond infectious diseases to include chronic noninfectious diseases,[11] birth defects and developmental disabilities,[12] mental health conditions,[13] substance-use disorders,[14] intentional and unintentional injuries,[15,16] emergency preparedness and response,[17] environmental hazards in community and workplace settings,[18,19] health behaviors,[20] and healthcare quality.[21] Surveillance has also been used to detect adverse events associated with vaccines, other pharmaceuticals, and medical devices.[22] Surveillance has played a vital role in detecting and preventing the spread of healthcare-associated infections[23] and reducing medical errors in hospitals and medical practice more broadly.[21] Over the past decade, surveillance methods have also been used to track public health policies[24] and conditions in physical and social environments that impact health.[25]

In addition to the greatly broadened scope of surveillance applications, surveillance methodologies have also undergone tremendous change over the past 50 years. For example, advances in laboratory and other diagnostic methods have allowed for much greater precision in identifying and classifying disease. The advent of the computer and rapid growth in computational power have contributed to a plethora of new ways to process, analyze, and display surveillance data. The presence of the Internet and widespread connectivity have revolutionized the communication of surveillance information, including both the reporting and dissemination of surveillance data. The era of "big data" has created immense opportunities for collecting near real-time health information and yet poses significant challenges given the tremendous volume of available data and variability in data quality.

SURVEILLANCE SYSTEM PLANNING AND DESIGN

Determining the Need for Surveillance

An essential initial step in planning a surveillance system is to confirm the need for surveillance given the frequently scarce resources that will be required to establish and maintain the system. This determination should be made with input from key stakeholders, including representatives of impacted communities, those whose efforts will be needed to report surveillance information, those who will be responsible for managing the system, and potential users of the information to support public health interventions. Important factors to consider in determining the need for surveillance include[26]:

- the frequency of the condition being considered for surveillance (e.g., incidence or prevalence);
- the severity of the condition (e.g., case-fatality rate, crude or age-adjusted mortality, premature mortality, hospitalization rates, or disability-adjusted life years);
- the economic costs associated with the condition, including healthcare and lost productivity costs;
- the degree to which the condition is treatable or preventable;
- the level of communicability;
- the magnitude of disparities or inequities;
- evidence of a new or worsening public health threat; and
- priorities based on a consensus planning processes (e.g., Healthy People national health objectives, or a community process that prioritizes specific health conditions).

In some cases, widespread community concern or public interest may influence the decision on whether to implement surveillance. Political considerations may also come into play when, for example, one or more policymakers have strong concerns about a health issue and surveillance data are needed to address these concerns.

Defining Surveillance Objectives

Once the need for surveillance has been confirmed, it is imperative to clearly define the objectives of the planned surveillance system. Why is surveillance needed? How will the surveillance information be used? The answers to these questions will have important implications for the types of data that will be needed which, in turn, will influence how the surveillance system is designed and how costly it will be. For example, the primary objective of surveillance for many communicable diseases is to identify all cases in a given population as rapidly as possible to ensure that effective control measures are instituted swiftly for both cases and potential contacts to prevent secondary spread of disease. While desirable, this objective is usually only achieved for rare and particularly important conditions such as meningococcal disease and plague. Efforts to identify all or most cases in the population require the participation of an elaborate network of healthcare institutions and laboratories. In addition, it may require staff resources to actively search for cases and assist in collecting needed information, referred to as active surveillance. Active surveillance systems have been shown to have much greater sensitivity in identifying cases (also referred to as reporting completeness) relative to passive surveillance systems that do not include such outreach.[27] In some instances, passive systems may transition to active systems if circumstances change and higher quality data are required to address evolving surveillance objectives.

In contrast, surveillance objectives for some communicable diseases, such as influenza, can be met without identifying all cases, particularly when individual case follow-up is not needed. In addition, given the high incidence of influenza at its peak and the lack of a definitive diagnosis in many cases, ascertainment of all cases would not be feasible. In these instances, the primary surveillance objective may be to recognize at a population level when disease transmission is increasing and to identify high-risk groups that are most severely impacted so that public education and other community prevention measures can be effectively timed and targeted. This objective may be achievable with a sentinel surveillance system that engages a selected group of healthcare providers, hospitals, or laboratories for disease reporting.

Similarly, the primary objective of surveillance for some chronic noninfectious diseases, such as heart disease, diabetes, and asthma, may be to characterize population trends in prevalence over time and by demographic group and geographic area so that resources for treatment and prevention can be more effectively deployed. Given this objective, the design of this system may prioritize prevalence over incidence, exclude collection of personally identifying information since individual case follow-up is not needed, and not be as concerned with the timeliness of the data since trends in chronic disease prevalence are not likely to rapidly change.

Case Definitions

Well-crafted case definitions play a critical role in ensuring the success of surveillance systems. The criteria used to define a case must be as precisely and objectively measurable as possible to ensure that case counts can be accurately enumerated. Case definitions generally include elements of person, place, and time as well as specified diagnostic criteria that can include clinical signs and symptoms and/or laboratory test results. Cases definitions can further differentiate between confirmed, suspect, and probable cases based on the level of certainty of correct classification. For example, a case could be considered probable if the clinical criteria were satisfied but a confirmatory laboratory test had not yet been completed. Cases can also be classified as epidemiologically linked if an individual has had a clear exposure to another documented case but has not yet fulfilled the criteria needed for case confirmation. Epidemiologic linkage is sometimes established by molecular analysis of isolates from multiple cases.[28] This information is particularly helpful in outbreak investigations when determining the scope of the outbreak. The case definition for measles provides an example of the different elements that may be used to characterize a disease for the purposes of surveillance and outbreak investigations (Box 7-2).

Use of uniform criteria to define a case is essential for accurate comparison of case counts and rates across different populations. To ensure uniformity of case definitions for a core set of infectious and noninfectious diseases under surveillance across the United States, the Council of State and Territorial Epidemiologists (CSTE) has established a standard set of case definitions.[29] These definitions are used by state and local health departments across the United States to report cases to the CDC's National Electronic Disease Surveillance System (NEDSS). CSTE members meet annually in part to review and update these case definitions as needed as well as to propose new additions to the list of notifiable diseases under surveillance.

For some diseases, case definitions evolve over time to address changes in surveillance objectives or to accommodate advances in diagnostic tests or knowledge of the natural history of disease. For example, when the first cases of what would later become known as the Acquired Immunodeficiency Syndrome (AIDS) were reported in Los

BOX 7-2 Measles Case Definition, Council of State and Territorial Epidemiologists

Probable Case

In the absence of a more likely diagnosis, an illness that meets the clinical description with:

- No epidemiologic linkage to a laboratory-confirmed measles case; **and**
- Noncontributory or no measles laboratory testing.

Confirmed Case

An acute febrile rash illness[†] with:

- Isolation of measles virus[‡] from a clinical specimen; or
- Detection of measles-virus-specific nucleic acid from a clinical specimen using polymerase chain reaction; or
- IgG seroconversion or a significant rise in measles immunoglobulin G antibody using any evaluated and validated method; or
- A positive serologic test for measles immunoglobulin M antibody[§]; or
- Direct epidemiologic linkage to a case confirmed by one of the methods above.

(*Source:* Centers for Disease Control and Prevention; https://wwwn.cdc.gov/nndss/conditions/measles/case-definition/2013/.)

[†] Temperature does not need to reach $\geq$ 101°F/38.3°C and rash does not need to last $\geq$ 3 days.

[‡] Not explained by MMR vaccination during the previous 6–45 days.

[§] Not otherwise ruled out by other confirmatory testing or more specific measles testing in a public health laboratory.

Angeles, California in 1981, the etiologic agent was unknown and the clinical manifestations not well characterized. To increase the identification of possible cases, the initial case definition was constructed to maximize sensitivity, at the expense of specificity, by including a long list of opportunistic diseases without evidence of an alternative etiology. Over the next decade, the Human Immunodeficiency Virus (HIV) was identified as the causative agent, a diagnostic laboratory test was developed, and advances were made in the understanding of HIV disease manifestations. In response, the case definition was revised at least three times, with each successive iteration increasing the definition's sensitivity, specificity, and predictive value positive. This, in turn, resulted in more accurate surveillance statistics and also reduced workload by reducing the burden of investigating false positive cases.

Surveillance of conditions without a definitive laboratory or other diagnostic test can be challenging because the case definitions may rely on subjective clinical criteria that predispose to misclassification of cases. For example, surveillance of autism spectrum disorder (ASD) was established in the 1980s in response to concerns that the prevalence was increasing. Though surveillance data have confirmed this increase,[30] the interpretation of findings over time and across different surveillance systems has been challenging as the condition lacks a definitive biological marker and is defined by the presence of criteria that require considerable judgment in their application—"impaired reciprocal social interactions, delayed or unusual communication styles, and restricted or repetitive behavior."[31] Efforts to reduce misclassification have included provisions in the case definition that require that case status be determined based on an evaluation by a "qualified professional," that the information be abstracted from health and education records, and that the information be reviewed by an "ASD clinician reviewer." Descriptions of what constitute a qualified professional and a clinician reviewer are also included in the case definition.

Case definitions may also be limited by the need to collect information directly from individuals. For example, surveillance of some conditions, such as diabetes and asthma, may include the use of population-based surveys and reliance on an affirmative response to one or more survey questions (e.g., "Have you ever been told by a healthcare provider that you have diabetes?"). In these instances, it is important to use questions that have been validated in other surveys so that results are comparable across populations.

Case definitions used for surveillance of clinical syndromes, referred to as syndromic surveillance, may include abbreviated text fields that can be captured from a chief complaint or other brief description in a medical record, often in an emergency department. Syndromic surveillance can serve as an early warning system for detecting disease outbreaks, biologic or chemical terrorism events, or other acute public health threats. In addition, syndromic surveillance can be used to detect population-level health impacts associated with natural disasters.[32] For example, during extreme heat events, syndromic surveillance has been used to detect increases in heat-related illness,[33] and during wildfires to detect increases in respiratory illness.[34] These systems are often designed to detect "signals" of an emerging public health threat that may need to be confirmed with additional investigation.

Case definitions used for surveillance should be distinguished from diagnostic criteria used in the clinical setting. Clinical diagnosis may require a greater level of rigor than is needed or feasible in a case definition for surveillance. For example, with surveillance of a condition for which individual case follow-up is not needed and where the primary objective is to measure population-level trends, a case definition may have lower levels of sensitivity and specificity than would be required in a clinical setting, where accurate diagnosis is of paramount importance.

Data Sources for Surveillance

A large and growing number of data sources are used for surveillance and are generally selected either alone or in combination to best meet the objectives of the surveillance system. Many of these data sources are designed for purposes other than surveillance, such as to address administrative needs or support research. Hence it is important to select data sources that will best meet the needs of the surveillance system, taking into consideration cost, alignment with the population of interest, and quality of the data. Data quality can be considered across at least four dimensions—timeliness, completeness, accuracy, and representativeness. Their relative importance will vary based on the surveillance objectives.

Major data sources used for surveillance, along with their relative strengths and limitations, are described below.

Notifiable disease reports. A primary source of surveillance data on infectious diseases comes from notifiable disease reports. Healthcare providers, hospitals, laboratories, and others are mandated to report specified communicable diseases to public health authorities. In the United States, the legal requirement to report these diseases is delegated to the states, which carry out this authority through legislation, boards of health, or other administrative mechanisms. The CDC and CSTE collaborate to ensure that a core set of conditions are included for surveillance across all states.[35] However, there is variability among the states in the inclusion of additional conditions for surveillance as dictated by local and regional needs. The reporting requirement also generally specifies a time window in which a report must be made. For conditions that require urgent action, such as meningococcal infection, reporting is required immediately, while for conditions that require less time sensitive action, such as hepatitis B or C, the time window may be extended to a week.

Despite the importance of disease reporting for ensuring effective disease control intervention, compliance with reporting requirements is often suboptimal. In part, this reflects the burden of reporting procedures, including manual completion of case report forms and submission by mail or fax. However, gradual adoption of automated procedures and electronic submission of reports has reduced the burden and increased reporting completeness. In particular, the introduction of electronic reporting of laboratory results for specified reportable conditions has increased both the completeness and timeliness of reporting. However, additional clinical and non-clinical information often still needs to be collected from medical records to confirm the case and conduct needed follow-up as well as for describing population trends (e.g., information on location of residence and specified demographics such as race/ethnicity). The rapid growth in the use of electronic health records (EHRs) in medical clinics and hospitals over the past decade holds great promise for further improving the efficiency of data collection and reporting processes.[36]

Vital statistics. In most developed countries, nearly all births and deaths are recorded and registered with government offices. Birth certificates include vital information that can be used for surveillance of adverse birth outcomes, such as low birthweight births, premature births, and other birth complications. Birth data can also be used to populate other important public health data systems, such as immunization registries. In addition, birth certificate data can provide important information on maternal characteristics, such as age, race/ethnicity, and marital status, as well as place of residence to allow geographic analysis of trends. Death certificates include demographic information on the decedent and the underlying and contributing causes of death, classified using International Classification of Disease (ICD) codes. Death certificate data are the primary source of information for tracking the leading causes of death in the population, monitoring mortality trends, and identifying disparities in mortality across demographic groups and geographic areas. The data can also be used to assess trends in premature mortality (e.g., years of potential life lost) and life expectancy, and can be incorporated into calculations of disease burden as measured by disability-adjusted life years. Birth data can be linked with death data to track infant and maternal mortality and recorded causes of death.

An important strength of these databases is that there is nearly complete reporting of all births and deaths. However, the data may suffer from a lack of timeliness as there may be delays of months to several years before the official databases are available for analysis. In addition, information on birth and death certificates is relatively limited and may not provide the level of contextual information needed to inform public health efforts.

Hospital data. Data on the reasons for hospitalization are often captured in hospital discharge datasets. Though the data are collected largely for billing and other administrative purposes, the discharge diagnoses are ICD coded and, therefore, very useful for surveillance purposes. Hospital discharge datasets also often include ICD-coded discharge diagnoses for patients seen in emergency departments, allowing for a more comprehensive assessment of morbidity in the population. However, because most hospital discharge datasets do not include personally identifying information, they cannot be linked with other data sources to support surveillance efforts that require such linkage to provide a more complete assessment. In addition, there is often a 1- to 2-year delay in the availability of these datasets, making them less useful for surveillance systems that require more timely information.

Disease registries. Disease registries collect information on individuals with a particular disease or health condition. The most prominent of these are cancer registries, with an extensive network of registries having been established in many developed countries. Though these registries were developed primarily as a resource for research, they provide invaluable data for surveillance, allowing for tracking of cancer incidence and prevalence, and characterizing patterns across different populations. Cancer registries are generally well funded and have rigorous quality control measures, resulting in the collection of very high-quality data, as measured by the level of completeness and accuracy of the data. Completeness of reporting of cancer diagnoses is facilitated in many jurisdictions by a legal mandate to report this information and by trained staff who work with healthcare providers, hospitals, and pathology and other laboratories to ensure that all cases are reported and accurately classified. As with all surveillance data sources, however, these registries alone do not constitute a surveillance system, which, by definition, must also include a strong linkage with those responsible for cancer prevention and control efforts and related public health activities (e.g., tobacco control efforts).

Other registries that can support surveillance include birth defects registries and a variety of other registries that do not focus on a specific health condition but, rather, focus on the recruitment of a group of individuals with a common exposure or experience. For example, registries have been established for groups of employees who work in high-risk industries, and a registry was established in the aftermath of the September 11, 2001 World Trade Center attack to monitor potential health effects among first responders and others who were exposed to hazardous chemicals and debris.[37]

Health surveys. Both longitudinal and repeated cross-sectional health surveys generate a wealth of data that can be used for surveillance. Surveys are often used for surveillance of chronic noninfectious health conditions such as hypertension, diabetes, obesity, asthma, and arthritis, and for health behaviors such as tobacco use, alcohol and drug use, sexual-risk behavior, physical activity, and dietary practices. Examples include the Behavioral Risk Factor Surveillance System (BRFSS) and the Youth Risk Behavior Surveillance (YRBS) project, both directed by the CDC with implementation at the state level for BRFSS and in selected school districts for YRBS. Additional examples in the United States include the National Health Interview Survey and, at a state level, the California Health Interview Survey.

Most of these surveys are cross-sectional, providing prevalence estimates in defined populations, and are repeated at regular intervals to allow tracking of trends. The surveys collect detailed sociodemographic information that allows for examination of results across multiple subpopulations and stratification of results across variables not available in many other surveillance databases, such as household income and other measures of socioeconomic status. In addition, a wide range of topics are often covered in these surveys, providing opportunities to examine relationships between health behaviors, access to and utilization of healthcare and other services, and health outcomes.

Data from health surveys have important limitations. Because they are based on self-reported or proxy-reported information, the data are subject to response bias. An important exception is the National Health and Nutrition Examination Survey (NHANES), which collects data through structured interviews and through physical examinations and laboratory testing of blood and other biologic specimens.

In many surveys, response rates are low and so results may not be representative of the population of interest. To address this limitation, data weighting procedures are used to adjust for differential response across different subpopulations. However, unmeasured confounding may be introduced when large segments of the population are not well represented. In addition, sample frames may introduce bias. For example, few population-based surveys include those who are incarcerated, housed in other institutionalized settings, or are homeless. Telephone surveys are particularly challenged by low response rates and the rise in individuals and households that have dispensed with landlines, relying solely on cell phones. Given these challenges, the Internet has emerged as fertile ground for administering surveys, including Internet panels of cohorts that are recruited for multiple surveys. However, the degree to which these cohorts are representative of the general population is a concern, and their use for surveillance has not been well tested.

Surveys often do not have sufficiently large samples to generate results with the geographic precision needed to inform local public health planning efforts. In the United States, this is an important limitation of many federal and state surveys. To address this limitation, some local public health jurisdictions, including New York City,[38] Chicago,[39] and Los Angeles County,[40] have invested in their own population-based health surveys, with larger samples that allow for more granular demographic and geographic analysis. Given the importance of generating surveillance results at the community level to support public health actions, modeling techniques have been developed to generate indirect small area estimates when sample size is insufficient to produce reliable direct estimates.[41,42]

Census data. The census provides vitally important population estimates for calculating disease rates and for making valid comparisons across demographic subpopulations and geographic regions. In addition, accurate intercensal population estimates are essential for tracking temporal trends in rates. Census data are also an important source of information for surveillance of the social determinants of health. For example, U.S. census data can be used to track temporal trends and demographic and geographic variation in household income, education level, housing conditions or housing security, health insurance coverage, and other topics that are covered in special supplements to the census.[43]

However, it is also important to note the potential limitations of census data, including undercounting of persons who are homeless or members of stigmatized groups (e.g., certain immigrant groups). In addition, as with all self-reported data, there may be incomplete or inaccurate reporting of some information, particularly sensitive information such as household income or country of birth.

Data Collection

Data collection for surveillance generally operates under the principle of less is more. Given the need for the contributions of multiple stakeholders in the data collection process, there is a strong incentive to minimize response burden. Case report forms should be designed as efficiently and in as user-friendly a format as possible. Advances in technology over the past several decades have in many cases shifted data collection from manual completion of paper forms to use of laptop computers and tablets, including automated data collection and electronic submission of data.

Data elements should be selected carefully to address the objectives of the surveillance system and to confirm case status based on the criteria specified in the case definition. Additional information should be collected as needed for case follow-up and for analysis by person, place, and time. This includes, for example, information on demographic characteristics, date of diagnosis, date of case report, relevant historical information (e.g., recent travel history), relevant clinical and laboratory information, and vital status. If follow-up case investigation is anticipated, contact information for the case individual and the reporting entity will be required.

Surveillance systems may utilize a single data source or may require the use of multiple data sources for different purposes. For example, notifiable disease reports alone may be used to rapidly identify cases of infectious disease and intervene to prevent secondary transmission. Notifiable disease report data may be linked with mortality data to assess disease severity, as measured by case fatality rates. Analyses of notifiable disease data may be combined with analyses of hospital discharge data and mortality data to provide a more complete understanding of the burden of the disease in different populations to help focus community education and other prevention efforts.

Surveillance of diabetes provides a good example of how multiple data sources may be used to address different surveillance objectives and how decisions on which data sources to use may be influenced by their relative strengths and limitations, and by available resources. Developing strong systems of surveillance for diabetes has become a much higher priority over the past 30–40 years given its rising incidence and prevalence, associated medical complications, increased mortality, and substantial economic costs, including both healthcare and lost productivity costs. Most diabetes surveillance has utilized serial cross-sectional surveys to measure trends in diabetes prevalence. These population-based surveys are relatively costly and, therefore, challenging to implement at the community level. In addition, because of sample size limitations, results are generally only available at national and regional levels, limiting their utility for local community-level uses. To address this limitation, the CDC has used modeling techniques to generate indirect estimates of diabetes prevalence at county levels across the United States using data from the BRFSS.[44] Many local public health jurisdictions also utilize mortality data for diabetes surveillance. The survey and mortality data have been used primarily to track temporal trends and identify disproportionately impacted populations rather than for individual-level intervention.

However, the emergence of electronic reporting of laboratory and clinical information has created the opportunity for more timely reporting and potential follow-up at the individual patient and healthcare provider levels. For example, in 2005, New York City's Board of Health passed a regulation mandating electronic laboratory reporting of glycosylated hemoglobin (HbA1c) results.[45] Based on the communicable disease model of surveillance, the mandate included reporting of patient and provider names and contact information so that follow-up could be conducted with patients who have elevated Hb A1c levels, and with their physicians, to encourage interventions to achieve better glucose control.

Data Management

In designing a surveillance system, careful attention must be given to the data management infrastructure. This includes all steps involved in the collection, maintenance, analysis, and dissemination of the data. If data are received on paper forms, they are generally entered into an electronic database. Protocols must be developed to ensure accurate data entry, including measures such as random checks of the accuracy of entered data on a subset of cases and data ranges incorporated into the software to exclude implausible values. Increasingly, data are received electronically, necessitating a compatible and secure interface with the surveillance database. Given the growing complexity of electronic data systems and the need for connecting multiple systems, expertise in informatics has become an essential skillset to include on the surveillance team. This expertise is particularly important to assure that the surveillance database has the necessary security protections, including a secure storage environment, use of password protections, data encryption capacity as needed, redundant data storage, and routine back-ups of the data.

The surveillance database must be developed with a good understanding of the functions that will be required. For example, in some cases the surveillance database may be used solely for analysis and dissemination of aggregate results while other databases may need to maintain additional information to track the status of follow-up case investigations. In the former, access to the database may be limited to epidemiologists and other staff responsible for preparing datasets for analysis and completing the analyses, while the latter may require much broader access, including staff conducting field investigations.

Data may also need to be shared with other public health jurisdictions. For example, health departments may receive case reports on persons who are traveling or receiving medical care outside their areas of residence, necessitating a sharing of the reports with their local jurisdictions of residence. Data sharing also occurs across various levels of government. In most states in the United States, local health departments have the primary responsibility for collecting case reports and transmitting the data to the state health department. State health departments then report the data, without personal identifiers, to the CDC where national statistics are compiled. Globally, the updated International Health Regulations adopted in 2005 require countries that sign on to the agreement to report cases of selected health conditions of international concern to the WHO.[46]

Data analysis needs must be well defined prior to implementing surveillance and should be designed to address the surveillance objectives. For surveillance of rare conditions, such as human rabies, analyses may be limited to individual case descriptions. Diseases that are infrequent but spread rapidly, such as measles, will require time-sensitive analyses by person, place, and time to identify source cases and transmission pathways. This may require both temporal and spatial analyses, including use of geographic information systems (GIS) to generate maps. Analyses may also require consideration of contacts and social networks. Diseases that are seasonal, such as West Nile Virus, will require sensitive methods to detect temporal trends, such as weekly case counts. For influenza, analyses may include data from multiple sources, such as data on positive nasal swab isolates at sentinel provider sites, school absences, sales of antiviral medications, and patients presenting with respiratory illness at emergency departments.

Surveillance of chronic diseases and health behaviors may have very different analysis needs than those focused on communicable diseases that require immediate response. If data are obtained from surveys, analysis will require a knowledge of the sampling design and weighting factors. Descriptive analyses will likely be needed annually or at other regular intervals. Results will need to be stratified by predefined variables, including various demographic, social, and geographic variables. Depending on the level of granularity needed, having an adequate sample size may become a limiting factor. Confidence intervals will need to be calculated and criteria established for when to suppress a result because it is too unstable. Data tables and figures can be developed in advance to inform the analysis. GIS may also be needed to describe spatial patterns and associations. In addition, identifying "hot spots" may be important if EHR data are available and the surveillance objective is more rapid response with targeted community or health provider intervention.

Because case counts are strongly influenced by the size of the population under surveillance, analyses in which comparisons are being made across populations require calculation of rates. The validity of rate calculations is in part dependent on the accuracy of the population counts used in the calculation. Hence, the availability of high-quality population data is extremely important for surveillance analyses. Access to accurate intercensal population estimates are essential for assessing temporal trends in rates. Calculation of age-adjusted rates may be needed if the age distributions vary significantly across populations of interest.

Plans will also need to be established for disseminating the results of surveillance analyses. Essential in this process is defining the key stakeholders for dissemination. This group should be defined broadly and include all who may play a role in advancing the public's health. In some cases, these stakeholders will understand the important role they play and will actively seek the data. For example, many community organizations and other public health advocates frequently request surveillance data to support their advocacy efforts, funding requests, and planning activities. Healthcare systems may have an interest in the data for planning and priority setting. Those who assist health departments in responding to communicable disease and environmental health threats may actively seek the data to identify vulnerabilities and better prepare for emergencies. In other cases, key stakeholders may not be aware of the value of surveillance data in their work, or they may not know that it even exists. For example, one focus of public health efforts is to increase physical activity by encouraging land use and transportation planners to create environments that are more conducive to being physically active, including creating more infrastructure for walking and biking, and more compact development to reduce dependency on motor vehicles. However, many planners may not be aware of surveillance data, or their role in advancing these public health efforts. In these cases, surveillance staff have a responsibility to promote their data and ensure that it gets into the right hands.

There is a growing movement around increasing transparency of government activities, including providing the public more access to government data, with appropriate confidentiality protections in place. The provision of greater access to surveillance data can take different forms. For example, surveillance programs can make aggregate data available online as static tables and figures. Maps can also be made available and can be either static or interactive. Web-based data query systems have been developed that provide users the opportunity to run analyses tailored to their needs. Data dashboards are another frequent way in which data are presented online, highlighting change over time for a given surveillance indicator or variation across multiple indicators. An important limitation of these approaches is that users may not be well informed of the limitations of the data and may misinterpret findings.

Through all phases of data management, ensuring the confidentiality of the data is of critical importance. Government public health agencies are given much latitude to collect sensitive health information in the interests of protecting the public's health. For example, in the United States, access to and use of surveillance data by public health officials are specifically excluded from the rigorous restrictions on the sharing of protected health information, as defined in the federal Health Insurance Portability and Accountability Act (HIPAA). However, for surveillance systems that collect notifiable disease reports, the laws or administrative actions that mandate reporting also often include provisions on data confidentiality requirements and penalties for violation of these requirements. Other systems may not have these requirements in the law but, nonetheless, protocols for ensuring data confidentiality should be developed and all surveillance staff trained in their application.

COMMUNICATING SURVEILLANCE INFORMATION

Effective communication of surveillance information is essential for driving public health action and assuring that surveillance objectives are achieved. Communication can be distinguished from data dissemination in several important ways. Unlike data dissemination, which involves unidirectional sharing of data with outside parties, communication is a bidirectional process that includes both sharing surveillance findings and receiving feedback from key stakeholders. This feedback can help in the interpretation of the data, in determining what public health actions are needed based on the findings, and in identifying adjustments in the surveillance system that may be needed to increase its value. Implicit in the communication process is the need to translate the data into understandable and persuasive information that will engage target audiences. This should include clear explanations of the limitations of the data and the provision of contextual information that will aid in the interpretation of findings.

Effective communication requires that the target audiences be well defined. These may include public health colleagues, healthcare providers and systems, the general public, community organizations, employers, policymakers, the media, and any others who may have an interest or a role to play in advancing public health efforts. Public health colleagues may include those within a given government agency or in other agencies that may span various levels of government. Communication between city, county, state, and federal governments becomes very important when addressing a public health issue that crosses jurisdictional boundaries, as is often the case with disease outbreaks. In addition, communication and coordination across countries has become increasingly important with expansion of international travel and goods movement.

Products that will be used to communicate surveillance information should also be defined. For example, these may include surveillance reports, fact sheets, advisories, narrative reports, and press releases. Peer-reviewed journal articles are sometimes used to present surveillance results, but their value may be limited by the long time-period required for publication. However, some publications, such as the CDC's *Morbidity and Mortality Weekly Report* (MMWR) and WHO's *Weekly Epidemiological Record* are designed to provide more rapid communication of surveillance information on emerging health issues.

The objectives of the surveillance system often dictate the channels through which information is shared. For example, systems that prioritize detecting and responding to disease outbreaks will require direct communication via alerts and advisories distributed through email listservs. Direct communications by telephone, webinar, or private meetings may be needed to communicate time sensitive information and assure appropriate use of the surveillance information for disease control efforts. Public meetings may be needed to inform local residents, including the frequently challenging task of communicating risks and advising on precautionary measures without creating undue public alarm.

In situations where surveillance data suggest an acute health threat, designated staff must be prepared to respond to media inquiries. Proactive planning and development of a crisis communication plan is generally much more effective than reactive communications. In responding to media inquiries, designated spokespersons must have a strong understanding of the surveillance findings, associated risks, and planned response. This information is best organized into specified talking points, with a well-defined single overriding health communication objective determined prior to engaging in media interviews.[47]

Surveillance systems that focus on chronic conditions not subject to rapid change may prioritize a different set of communication products and channels. For example, annual surveillance reports may provide sufficient information for public health planning and priority-setting activities. Web-based data visualization products, such as interactive maps, may be used to more effectively engage various target audiences. Innovative ways of presenting and contextualizing data, such as the use of infographics, may be helpful in engaging important stakeholder groups. Meetings may be scheduled with elected officials and their staff to share surveillance data as a means of informing them on a priority issue. Advocacy organizations may use surveillance data in meetings with these officials to advocate for a policy intervention or lobby for a specific legislative proposal.

MONITORING AND EVALUATING SURVEILLANCE SYSTEMS

Surveillance often involves large and complex networks of individuals and institutions that provide and use the data as well as those responsible for operating the surveillance system. Given this complexity, it is important to establish a plan for monitoring the performance of the system to ensure that objectives are being met and the system is operating in an efficient and effective manner. When significant performance issues or questions arise, more formal evaluation of the system may be indicated. This is best done in a structured approach that includes a clear definition of the purpose of the evaluation and a determination of which internal and external stakeholders should be engaged to collect the needed information.[48]

Key attributes of the system that are important to consider for establishing performance metrics and for more formal evaluation include:

- *Simplicity.* Simplicity refers to both organizational structure and the ease in which the system functions. Systems should ideally be as simple as possible to meet the system's objectives. For example, does surveillance for a given condition require that all medical offices, hospitals, and laboratories participate or can adequate information be obtained from a more limited set of sentinel reporting sites? Are case report forms designed in user-friendly formats and are protocols for collecting and reporting the data straightforward? Are their clear lines of communication between those responsible for reporting the data and those receiving it?

- *Flexibility.* Flexibility refers to the degree to which the system can adapt to changing circumstances and needs. For example, case definitions may need to be modified as new diagnostic tests are introduced. Information collected in case reports may need to evolve as new treatment modalities and prevention strategies become available. Adjustments in methods of data transfer and storage may be required to address security threats and ensure the confidentiality of the data.
- *Data quality.* The quality of the data can be assessed both in relation to its accuracy and the completeness of reporting of data elements. While high-quality data are important, there may be acceptable trade-offs. For example, a certain level of error may be acceptable if operating costs are reduced and the ability of the system to achieve its objectives is not compromised. For example, population-based surveys are often used for surveillance of obesity in adults. These surveys rely on calculation of body mass index (BMI) based on self-reported height and weight, which has been documented to underestimate the true prevalence of obesity, particularly among older adults.[49] However, this approach may be sufficient to track trends over time and characterize disparities across subpopulations, while also saving considerable resources that would be needed to collect more accurate data by directly measuring height and weight.
- *Acceptability.* The success of surveillance is dependent on what is often a large number of external parties responsible for reporting data to the system. In addition, staff may face many challenges in operating the system. Hence, the acceptability of the system is a key attribute that can be assessed by tracking levels of participation in case reporting, conducting key informant interviews, and administering structured surveys, all of which can provide valuable information for improving the operation of the system.
- *Sensitivity.* Sensitivity is the proportion of cases in the population that are detected by the surveillance system, or the proportion of outbreaks detected by the system. Also referred to as reporting completeness, this is a particularly important metric for systems that are tracking health conditions that require action at the individual level, either in the management of the disease in a reported case or in preventing secondary spread. Low reporting completeness can also impede efforts to gain an accurate understanding of the magnitude and distribution of a disease in the population, resulting in inadequate information for planning services and allocating resources. Funding formulas, such as the distribution of federal funding for HIV prevention and treatment services to states and large local jurisdictions in the United States, are sometimes determined by case counts, creating an incentive for surveillance programs to maximize reporting completeness. Multiple data sources, such as hospitals, clinics, laboratories, and vital statistics, may be used to increase reporting completeness, though this must be counterbalanced with consideration of the yield versus the incremental cost of each added data source.
- *Predictive value positive.* Predictive value positive (PVP) is the proportion of cases reported to the system that are true cases. The lower the PVP, the higher the proportion of falsely reported cases. Challenges to achieving a high PVP most often occur with conditions that lack a definitive diagnostic test and include subjective elements in their case definition. Low PVP can also occur with surveillance of newly emerging diseases that have not yet been well characterized, leading to false diagnoses. For example, early in the HIV epidemic, some cases reported as AIDS were later determined to have been conditions associated with immunodeficiency that were unrelated to HIV infection. A low PVP can create additional costs and inefficiencies for a surveillance system as it results in unnecessary follow-up investigation of false positives (i.e., falsely reported cases). It can also lead to inaccurate aggregate surveillance statistics by inflating the number of cases and distorting their characteristics if the falsely reported cases differ from the true cases.
- *Representativeness.* Representativeness refers to the degree to which reported cases are an accurate representation of all cases in the population. As reporting completeness and PVP decline, representativeness becomes an issue of greater potential concern. In addition, representativeness is an important metric to consider with sentinel surveillance systems and systems that utilize surveys to collect information on a subset of the population using sampling methods.
- *Timeliness.* Timeliness refers to the time interval between when a case is diagnosed and when it is reported to the system. As with reporting completeness, timely reporting is particularly important for surveillance of acute and highly infectious conditions that require rapid follow-up. Timeliness may be of lesser importance for surveillance of chronic conditions that are not transmissible and do not undergo rapid shifts at the population level.
- *Usefulness.* An important consideration in all assessments of performance is the usefulness of the surveillance system. Is the system meeting its objectives? Are the surveillance findings reaching those who need the information and in what ways has the information been used so to support public health actions?

Performance monitoring and evaluation of surveillance systems need not address all of the attributes described above. These efforts should be tailored and focused on the specific attributes that most directly relate to the objectives of the surveillance system and should also be responsive to input provided by key stakeholders that participate in the system or rely on the surveillance findings. Ongoing monitoring and periodic evaluations using these criteria are essential so that systems can be modified or discontinued based on evolving needs.

ETHICAL CONSIDERATIONS IN SURVEILLANCE

Inherent in surveillance practice is the tension between the individual's right to privacy and autonomy and the public health imperative to protect and promote the public's health. Surveillance usually involves the collection of sensitive information, often linked to an individual's name or other identifying information and collected without informed consent. The information is sometimes used in ways that limit a person's freedom in the interests of the common good (e.g., isolation of patients with active tuberculosis or quarantine of unvaccinated persons exposed to measles). Surveillance activities are often exempted from the protections established by laws that regulate how personal health information in medical records may be used and shared. In addition, most surveillance activities are considered public health practice rather than research and, therefore, do not undergo review by institutional review boards (IRB).

However, the importance of ensuring that surveillance activities adhere to a well-defined set of ethical principles has become increasingly clear over the past 40 years, advanced to a large degree by the experience of the HIV epidemic. The early epidemic was characterized by great public fear of widespread transmission, associated with stigmatization and discrimination against groups disproportionately impacted by the epidemic. The gay and lesbian community organized in response and became very effective advocates for actions to address discrimination and accelerate efforts to identify effective treatments. Important among their concerns was the mandatory reporting of cases of AIDS and, later, reporting of HIV infection. Despite the need for high-quality surveillance data for quantifying the magnitude and evolution of the epidemic, there were well-justified concerns that the data might be used in some jurisdictions for nonpublic health purposes. There were further concerns that reporting by name would be a deterrent to HIV testing, driving at-risk groups underground and impeding HIV prevention efforts. This led to a period among some states in the United States in which code-based HIV reporting was implemented. This strategy was later discontinued when it was determined that it did not produce data of sufficient quality and did not allow for individual case follow-up, an activity of increasing importance as more effective HIV treatment options became available. Overall, the experience led to much greater communication between surveillance program staff and community advocates, a greater level of transparency of surveillance operations, and ultimately a greater level of public trust. In addition, the experience produced many best practices for protecting the confidentiality of surveillance data. Many laws and regulations that mandated HIV and AIDS reporting included strong confidentiality protections, including penalties for violation of these protections.

Despite this progress, some have called for more formalized ethical oversight of public health surveillance activities.[50] Others maintain that surveillance practice has a strong track record of adherence to ethical principles and that additional measures are not needed.[51] Recognizing that obtaining a person's consent to share their information is not feasible in many types of public health surveillance, Lee et al.[52] have defined the necessary conditions that provide an ethical justification for conducting surveillance without informed consent.[50] These include the requirement that surveillance activities only be used to support public health actions that improve population health, reduce health inequities, serve vulnerable populations, and prevent harm. In addition, efforts must be taken to ensure that data collected without informed consent be limited to the minimal essential data needed for effective public health action and that the data be maintained in a secure manner.

A 2017 the World Health Organization (WHO) report provides further delineation of the ethical issues that arise in surveillance practice, including guidelines on the ethical conduct of surveillance[53] (Box 7-3). Though these guidelines are framed around global health surveillance, they have relevance for surveillance at all levels, highlighting the importance of only using surveillance data for legitimate public health purposes, minimizing harm, and incorporating the concerns and perspectives of communities in planning and implementing surveillance and in the use of the data.

GLOBAL HEALTH SURVEILLANCE

While most surveillance systems operate within countries, the importance of global health surveillance and coordinating efforts across countries has become increasingly apparent over the past half century. The ability to travel virtually anywhere in world within a day and the expansion of human populations into previously remote areas has created opportunities for rapid spread of communicable disease, including novel and previously unrecognized pathogens. This is graphically illustrated by the most recent coronavirus-associated disease (COVID-19) pandemic, which over a period of several months spread to all major regions of the world.[4] Other examples include the emergence and rapid spread of an earlier coronavirus-associated illness, the Severe Acute Respiratory Syndrome (SARS) in 2003[54] and Zika virus in 2007.[2] In the case of SARS, caused by a previously unrecognized coronavirus distinct from the coronavirus associated with COVID-19, the illness was first reported in China but quickly spread to North America, South America, and Europe before it was contained. In contrast, human infection with Zika virus was first recognized in Nigeria in 1953 and was initially associated with a mild febrile illness. The virus was relatively quiescent over the next 50 years, until an outbreak was reported in Micronesia in 2007.[2] Over the next decade, rapid spread was documented in the South Pacific, South America, Central America, and the Caribbean, and was associated with more severe disease manifestations, including microcephaly and other manifestations of brain injury among infants born to mothers with infection.[55]

BOX 7-3 Ethical Guidelines for Public Health Surveillance, World Health Organization, 2017[51]

1. Countries have an obligation to develop appropriate, feasible, and sustainable public health surveillance systems. Surveillance systems should have a clear purpose and a plan for data collection, analysis, use, and dissemination based on relevant public health priorities.
2. Countries have an obligation to develop appropriate, effective mechanisms to ensure ethical surveillance.
3. Surveillance data should be collected only for a legitimate public health purpose.
4. Countries have an obligation to ensure that the data collected are of sufficient quality, including being timely, reliable, and valid, to achieve public health goals.
5. Planning for public health surveillance should be guided by transparent governmental priority setting.
6. The global community has an obligation to support countries that lack adequate resources to undertake surveillance.
7. The values and concerns of communities should be taken into account in planning, implementing, and using data from surveillance.
8. Those responsible for surveillance should identify, evaluate, minimize, and disclose risks for harm before surveillance is conducted. Monitoring for harm should be continuous, and, when any is identified, appropriate action should be taken to mitigate it.
9. Surveillance of individuals or groups who are particularly susceptible to disease, harm, or injustice is critical and demands careful scrutiny to avoid the imposition of unnecessary additional burdens.
10. Governments and others who hold surveillance data must ensure that identifiable data are appropriately secured.
11. Under certain circumstances, the collection of names or identifiable data is justified.
12. Individuals have an obligation to contribute to surveillance when reliable, valid, and complete data sets are required and relevant protection is in place. Under these circumstances, informed consent is not ethically required.
13. Results of surveillance must be effectively communicated to relevant target audiences.
14. With appropriate safeguards and justification, those responsible for public health surveillance have an obligation to share data with other national and international public health agencies.
15. During a public health emergency, it is imperative that all parties involved in surveillance share data in a timely fashion.
16. With appropriate justification and safeguards, public health agencies may use or share surveillance data for research purposes.
17. Personally identifiable surveillance data should not be shared with agencies that are likely to use them to take action against individuals or for uses unrelated to public health.

Used with Permission from WHO guidelines on ethical issues in public health surveillance. Geneva: World Health Organization; 2017.)

The significant morbidity and mortality associated with seasonal influenza and the ever-present threat of pandemic influenza are additional examples of the importance of a robust global surveillance infrastructure. A number of systems have been established to support global influenza surveillance, led by the WHO's Global Influenza Surveillance and Response System (GISRS).[56] Established in 1952, GISRS coordinates the collection and sharing of laboratory information on circulating influenza strains and influenza disease activity among participating countries, referred to as Member States. The system includes National Influenza Centers in regions across the world, national influenza reference laboratories, and FluNet, a web-based platform for influenza virological surveillance. The system supports influenza preparedness and response efforts at local, national, and international levels, providing vital information on circulating strains of the virus, including new and novel strains with potential for more severe disease and epidemic spread. The system also provides essential information for vaccine development in advance of each influenza season.

Global surveillance is also a priority for prevention and control of chronic noncommunicable diseases (NCDs) given that they account for the largest share of disease burden worldwide, including in resource poor countries.[57] The WHO leads and coordinates surveillance efforts across their Member States to track mortality, premature mortality, and prevalence of a broad array of NCDs, including mental health conditions. Surveillance also encompasses tracking the prevalence of behavioral health risks such as tobacco use, alcohol misuse, dietary practices, and physical activity. Surveillance of air pollution has been recently added given its importance as a risk factor for asthma and other chronic respiratory disease. WHO provides support in standardizing surveillance practices. For example, they have developed protocols and resource materials for surveillance of stroke, the second leading cause of death worldwide,[58,59] and for physical inactivity,[60] an important risk factor for cardiovascular disease, diabetes, and many types of cancer.

The establishment of effective global health surveillance systems can be challenging in several respects. First, there can be impediments to participation among countries with unstable governments and civil unrest. Second, coordination can be difficult across countries in conflict or with histories of conflict, either militarily or politically. Third, cooperation in reporting disease to international bodies may be suboptimal given the potential for disease control measures, such as travel advisories and restrictions, to have adverse economic and social impacts. Fourth, the necessary infrastructure for surveillance may be lacking in resource poor countries where organized health systems are not well developed, laboratory capacity is limited, and modern information and communication systems are lacking.

Despite these challenges, most countries in the world are engaged in global surveillance efforts. For example, the WHO recently published a NCD surveillance report with health profiles for 194 countries.[61] The report provides a standardized set of data that can be used by countries to establish national health objectives, plan, and gain support for disease control and prevention interventions, compare results with other countries, and identify opportunities for cross-national strategies to reduce the burden of NCDs. In addition, the report provides important baseline data for assessing progress over time.

FUTURE DIRECTIONS IN SURVEILLANCE

As public health practice continues to evolve, surveillance must adapt to meet the changing needs. Advances in information technology and the explosive increase in digital data available from a growing array of sources, including electronic health data systems and social media platforms, hold great promise for improving the quality and timeliness of surveillance data.

Several salient trends in public health practice have particularly important implications for the future of surveillance. First, over the past several decades, increasing attention has been given to the root causes of disease, including social, economic, and cultural factors (i.e., the social determinants of health) and attributes of the built and natural environments. The concept of "health-in-all" policies has been promoted, with greater attention to a health-equity focus in the policymaking process. Given public health's interest in prevention and the need to address these root causes, surveillance practice should continue to expand its focus beyond disease and behavioral-risk factors. For example, efforts to address conditions in the built environment as a means of increasing physical activity have been supported by active transportation surveillance systems that utilize transportation surveys to track pedestrian and bicycle activity.[62] Surveillance of the social determinants of health has become an additional area of focus.[25] Given the importance of policy as a lever for improving population health, policy surveillance has become a recognized public health practice.[24] Digital databases of laws and policies are expanding, allowing more systematic review of the policy landscape. Public health law practitioners are engaged in efforts to develop policy case definitions for more rigorous measurement and coding schemes that allow the various elements of policies to be better characterized.

Second, the growing movement toward greater integration of healthcare services and public health activities creates opportunities for strengthening surveillance, including enhanced coordination around disease reporting and increased communication and use of surveillance findings. Expansion of the use of EHRs over the past decade has provided great potential for more efficient, comprehensive, and timely disease reporting, supported in the United States by meaningful use requirements included in federal healthcare law.[63] EHR data are limited in that they only capture information on persons accessing healthcare services. However, among those receiving care, EHRs provide valuable clinical data that can supplement data collected through electronic laboratory reports. In addition, EHRs may provide a less costly alternative to health surveys in generating more timely prevalence estimates of chronic disease and behavioral-risk factors.[64]

Third, the need for near real-time information on patterns of communicable disease and potential bioterrorism and chemical terrorism threats has led to innovative analytic approaches and the use of social media to support surveillance. For example, automated spatial and temporal analyses of daily notifiable disease reports have allowed for more rapid detection of disease clusters and outbreaks.[65] Social media has been used to identity early indications of influenza activity,[66] enhance detection and response to disease outbreaks,[66] enhance detection and prediction of syphilis trends,[67] and identify cases of food-borne illness and potential links with unsafe restaurants.[68] The massive volume and variable quality of social media data create significant challenges for analysis and interpretation. However, advances in data analytics, including machine learning[69] and systems science methods,[70] are creating new opportunities to capitalize on these data.

In conclusion, the future effectiveness of public health surveillance will require adaptation to the evolving needs of public health practice and the ability to access, interconnect, and manage a rapidly expanding network of electronic data. New skillsets will be required of the surveillance workforce to analyze and interpret these data and to ensure that relevant and persuasive surveillance information reaches the right hands at the right time to inform public health actions and maximize population health impact.

References

1. Hall HI, Correa A, Yoon PW, Braden DR. Lexicon, definitions, and conceptual framework for public health surveillance. MMWR. 2012;61(Suppl; July 27, 2012):10–14.
2. Peterson LR, Jamieson DJ, Powers AM, Honein MA. Zika virus. *N Engl J Med.* 2016;374:1552–63.
3. Dixon MD, Schafer IJ. Ebola viral disease outbreak—West Africa, 2014. *MMWR.* 2014;63(25):548–51.
4. World Health Organization: Coronavirus 2019 (COVID-19) Situation Report—53. https://www.who.int/docs/default-source/coronaviruse/situation-reports/20200313-sitrep-53-covid-19.pdf?sfvrsn=adb3f72_2.

5. Centers for Disease Control and Prevention: New CDC analysis shows steep and sustained increases in STDs in recent years. https://www.cdc.gov/media/releases/2018/p0828-increases-in-stds.html.
6. Kennedy C, Yard E, Dignam T, et al. Blood lead levels among children aged <6 years—Flint, Michigan, 2013-2016. *MMWR.* 2016;65(25):650–4.
7. Thacker SB. Historical development. In: Lee LM, Teutsch SM, Thacker SB, St. Louise MELee LM, Teutsch SM, Thacker SB, St. Louise ME, eds. *Principles and Practice of Public Health Epidemiology.* New York: Oxford University Press; 2010, pp. 1–3.
8. Morabia A. Epidemiology's 350th anniversary: 1662–2012. *Epidemiology.* 2013;24:179–83.
9. Langmuir AD. William Farr: Founder of modern concepts of surveillance. *Internat J Epidem.* 1976;5(1):13–18.
10. Henderson DA. Surveillance of smallpox. *Internat J Epidem.* 1976;5(1):19–28.
11. Thacker SB, Stroup DF, Rothenberg RB. Public health surveillance for chronic conditions: A scientific basis for decisions. *Statist Med.* 1995;14: 629–41.
12. WHO/CDC/ICBDSR: Birth defects surveillance: A manual for programme managers. Geneva: World Health Organization; 2014.
13. Freeman EJ, Colpe LJ, Strine TW, et al. Public health surveillance for mental health. *Prev Chronic Dis.* 2010;7(1):1–7.
14. Substance Abuse and Mental Health Services Administration, Public health surveillance systems. https://www.samhsa.gov/capt/tools-capt-learning-resources/public-health-surveillance-systems.
15. Paulozzi LJ, Mercy J, Frazier L, Annest JL. CDC's National Violent Death Reporting System: Background and methodology. *Inj Prev.* 2004;10: 47–52.
16. Horan JM. Mallonee: Injury surveillance. *Epidemiol Rev.* 2003;25:24–42.
17. Sosin DM, Hopkins RS. Public health surveillance for preparedness and emergency response: Biosurveillance for human health. In: Lee LM, Teutsch SM, Thacker SB, St. Louise ME, eds.Lee LM, Teutsch SM, Thacker SB, St. Louise ME, eds. *Principles and Practice of Public Health Epidemiology.* New York: Oxford University Press; 2010, pp. 306–20.
18. National Institute for Occupational Health Surveillance, Centers for Disease Control and Prevention, Worker Health Surveillance. https://www.cdc.gov/niosh/topics/surveillance/default.html.
19. Macdonald SC, Pertowski CA, Jackson RJ. Environmental health surveillance. *J Public Health Manag Pract.* 1996;2(4):45–9.
20. Pickens CM, Pierannunzi C, Garvin W, Town M. Surveillance for certain health behaviors and conditions among states and selected local areas—Behavioral Risk Factor Surveillance System, United States, 2015. *MMWR.* 2018;67(9):1–90.
21. Murray JF, Richards C. Healthcare quality and safety: The monitoring of administrative information systems and the interface with public health surveillance. In: Lee LM, Teutsch SM, Thacker SB, St. Louise MELee LM, Teutsch SM, Thacker SB, St. Louise ME, eds. *Principles and Practice of Public Health Epidemiology.* New York: Oxford University Press; 2010, pp. 321–38.
22. Seligman PJ, Gross TP, Miles Braun M, Arrowsmith JB. PostMarket surveillance of medical products in the United States. In: Lee LM, Teutsch SM, Thacker SB, St. Louise MELee LM, Teutsch SM, Thacker SB, St. Louise ME, eds. *Principles and Practice of Public Health Epidemiology.* New York: Oxford University Press; 2010, pp. 339–56.
23. Centers for Disease Control and Prevention: Healthcare-Associated Infections: HAI Data. https://www.cdc.gov/hai/data/index.html.
24. Burris S, Hitchcock L, Ibrahim J, Penn M, Ramanathan T. Policy surveillance: A vital public health practice comes of age. *J Health Policy Law.* 2016;41(6):1151–73.
25. Parrish RG, McDonnell SM, Remington PL. Surveillance for the determinants of population health. In: Lee LM, Teutsch SM, Thacker SB, St. Louis MELee LM, Teutsch SM, Thacker SB, St. Louis ME, eds. *Principles and Practice of Public Health Surveillance.* New York: Oxford University Press; 2010, pp. 275–305.
26. Teutsch SM. Considerations in planning a surveillance system. In: Lee LM, Teutsch SM, Thacker SB, St. Louis MELee LM, Teutsch SM, Thacker SB, St. Louis ME, eds. *Principles and Practice of Public Health Surveillance.* New York: Oxford University Press; 2010, pp. 18–31.
27. Vogt RL, LaRue D, Klauke DN, Jillson DA. Comparison of an active and passive surveillance system of primary care providers for hepatitis, measles, rubella, and salmonellosis in Vermont. *Am J Public Health.* 1983;73:795–7.
28. Bender JB, Hedberg CW, Besser JM, Boxrud DJ, MacDonald KL, Osterholm MT. Surveillance for *Escherichia coli* O157:H7 infections in Minnesota by molecular subtyping. *N Engl J Med.* 1997;337:388–94.
29. Centers for Disease Control and Prevention: Surveillance Case Definitions for Current and Historical Conditions. https://wwwn.cdc.gov/nndss/conditions/.
30. Baio J, Wiggins L, Christensen DL, et al. Prevalence of Autism Spectrum Disorder among children aged 8 years—Autism and Developmental Disabilities Monitoring Network, 11 sites, United States, 2014. *MMWR.* 2018;67(6):1–23.
31. Centers for Disease Control and Prevention: Development Disabilities: Official MADDSP and MADDS Surveillance Case Definitions. https://www.cdc.gov/ncbddd/developmentaldisabilities/casedefinitions.html.
32. Buehler JW, Whitney EA, Smith D, Prietula MJ, Stanton SH, Isakov AP. Situational uses of syndromic surveillance. *Biosecur Bioterr Biodef Strat, Pract, Science.* 2009;7(2):165–77.
33. Mamou F, Henderson T. Analysis of heat illness using Michigan Emergency Department Syndromic Surveillance. *Online J Public Health Inform.* 2013;5(1):e139.
34. Johnson JM, Hicks L, McClean C, Ginsberg M. Leveraging syndromic surveillance during the San Diego Wildfires, 2003. In Syndromic Surveillance: Reports from a National Conference, 2004. *MMWR.* 2005;54(Suppl):190.
35. Centers for Disease Control and Prevention: 2020 National Notifiable Conditions. https://wwwn.cdc.gov/nndss/conditions/notifiable/2020/.
36. Birkhead GS, Klompas M, Shah N. Uses of electronic health records for public health surveillance to advance public health. *Health Affairs.* 2015;36:345–59.
37. NYC 9/11 Health, World Trade Center Registry. https://www1.nyc.gov/site/911health/about/wtc-health-registry.page.
38. NYC Health, Community Health Survey. https://www1.nyc.gov/site/doh/data/data-sets/community-health-survey.page.
39. Public Health: Healthy Chicago, Healthy Chicago 2.0. https://www.chicago.gov/city/en/depts/cdph/provdrs/healthychicago.html.
40. Simon PA, Wold CM, Cousineau MR, Fielding JE. Meeting the data needs of a local health department: The Los Angeles County Health Survey. *Am J Public Health.* 2001;91:1950–2.
41. Haomiao J, Muennig P, Borawski E. Comparison of small-area analysis of techniques for estimating county-level outcomes. *Am J Prev Med.* 2004;26(5):453–60.
42. Wang Y, Ponce NA, Wang P, Opsomer JD, Yu H. Generating health estimates by zip code: A semiparametric small area estimation approach using the California Health Interview Survey. *Am J Public Health.* 2015;105:2534–40.
43. United States Census Bureau: Current Population Survey (CPS). https://www.census.gov/programs-surveys/cps/about.html.
44. Centers for Disease Control and Prevention: Methods and References for County-Level Estimates and Ranks and State-Level Modeled Estimates. https://www.cdc.gov/diabetes/pdfs/data/calculating-methods-references-county-level-estimates-ranks.pdf.
45. Steinbrook R. Facing the diabetes epidemic—Mandatory reporting of glycosylated hemoglobin values in New York City. *N Engl J Med.* 2006;354(6):545–8.
46. Baker MG, Fidler DP. Global public health surveillance under New International Health Regulations. *Emerging Infect Dis.* 2006;12(7):1058–65.
47. Remington PL, Nelson DE. Communicating public health surveillance information for action. In: Lee LM, Teutsch SM, Thacker SB, St. Louis ME, eds. Lee LM, Teutsch SM, Thacker SB, St. Louis ME, eds. *Principles and Practice of Public Health Surveillance.* New York: Oxford University Press; 2010, pp. 146–65.
48. Centers for Disease Control and Prevention. Updated guidelines for evaluating public health surveillance systems: Recommendations from a guidelines working group. *MMWR.* 2001;50(No. RR-13):1–36.
49. Kuczmarski MF, Kuczmarski RJ, Najjar M. Effects of age on validity of self-reported height, weight, and body mass index: Findings from the Third National Health and Nutrition Examination Survey, 1988–1994. *J Am Diet Assoc.* 2001;101(1):28–34.
50. Fairchild A, Bayer R. Ethics and the conduct of public health surveillance. *Science.* 2004;303:631–2.
51. Middaugh, JP, Hodge JG, Cartter ML. The ethics of public health surveillance (letter). *Science.* 2004;304:681–2.
52. Lee LM, Heilig CM, White A. Ethical justification for conducting public health surveillance without patient consent. *Am J Public Health.* 2012;102: 38–44.
53. World Health Organization: WHO guidelines on ethical issues in public health surveillance, 2017. https://www.who.int/ethics/publications/public-health-surveillance/en/.

54. Hughes JM. The SARS response—Building and assessing an evidence-based approach to future global microbial threats. *N Engl J Med.* 2003;290(24):3251–43.

55. Honein MA, Jamieson DJ. Monitoring and preventing Congenital Zika syndrome. *N Engl J Med.* 2016;375(24):2393–4.

56. World Health Organization: Global Influenza Surveillance and Response System (GISRS). https://www.who.int/influenza/gisrs_laboratory/en/.

57. World Health Organization: Global Health Observatory Data: NCD Mortality and Morbidity. https://www.who.int/gho/ncd/mortality_morbidity/en/.

58. World Health Organization: STEPwise Approach to Stroke Surveillance. https://www.who.int/ncds/surveillance/steps/stroke/en/.

59. Truelsen T, Bonita R, Jamrozik K. Surveillance of stroke: A global perspective. *Int J Epidemiol.* 2001;30(Suppl 1):S11–16.

60. Hallal PC, Andersen LB, Bull FC, Guthold R, Haskell W, Ekelund U. Global physical activity levels: Surveillance progress, pitfalls, and prospects. *Lancet.* 2012;380:247–57.

61. World Health Organization: Noncommunicable diseases: Country Profiles, 2018. https://www.who.int/nmh/publications/ncd-profiles-2018/en/.

62. Whitfield GP, Paul P, Wendel AM. Active transportation surveillance—United States, 1999–2012. *MMWR.* 2015;64(7):1–17.

63. Centers for Disease Control and Prevention: Meaningful Use. https://www.cdc.gov/ehrmeaningfuluse/introduction.html.

64. Klompas M, Cocoros NM, Menchaca JT, et al. State and local chronic disease surveillance using electronic health records. *Am J Public Health.* 2017;107:1406–12.

65. Greene SK, Peterson ER, Kapell D, Fine AD, Kulldorff M. Daily reportable disease spatiotemporal cluster detection, New York City, New York, USA, 2014–2015. *Emerg Infect Dis.* 2016;22:1808–12.

66. Charles-Smith LE, Reynolds TL, Cameron MA, et al. Using social media for actionable disease surveillance and outbreak management: A systematic literature review. *PLoS One.* 2015;10(10):e0139701.

67. Young SD, Mercer N, Weiss RE, Torrone EA, Aral SO. Using social media as a tool to predict syphilis. *Prev Med.* 2018;109:58–61.

68. Sadilek A, Caty S. DiPrete L., et al. Machine-learned epidemiology: Real-time detection of foodborne illness at scale. *Digital Med.* 2018;1:36.

69. Mooney SJ, Pejaver J. Big data in public health: Terminology, machine learning, and privacy. *Annu Rev Public Health.* 2018;39:95–112.

70. Luke DA, Stamatakis KA. Systems science methods in public health: Dynamics, networks, and agents. *Ann Rev Public Health.* 2012;33: 357–76.

CHAPTER

8

Genomic Determinants of Health and Applications in Public Health and Preventive Medicine

Sharon L. R. Kardia • Stephen M. Modell

INTRODUCTION: TRANSITIONS IN PUBLIC HEALTH GENOMICS

Over the past 20 years, the field of genomics and public health genomics has changed rapidly. The sequencing of the first human genome, complete in 2003 and costing approximately ~$2 billion dollars, catalyzed monumental and wide-ranging shifts in research, technology, medicine, public health, business, and law. For example, technology and informatics have progressed to a level where sequencing of individual genomes is now becoming commonplace, costing only ~$1000 per person for high-quality sequence. With large amounts of new genomic information flowing into research across many disciplines, it is fundamentally changing our understanding of human variation and its relationship to disease globally.

We are at the very beginning of cataloging all the different genome variation being discovered along with annotating their molecular characteristics and distributions across populations and across an individual's genome. Moreover, the analysis and interpretation of the health consequences of the millions (soon to be billions) of DNA sequence variants discovered will remain a major challenge. National and international projects are sequencing 100,000s–1,000,000s of genomes and integrating them with clinical and epidemiological data to discover new genes for important health outcomes and to begin to assess clinical validity/utility. However, the translation of new genomic knowledge into improvements in health has been relatively slow for a variety of reasons, including the difficulty in estimating the clinical and population relevance of mutations and determining the appropriate use of this new genetic information within the economic and legal landscape of today's healthcare and public health sectors.

In this chapter, we cover key concepts used to talk about genetics in populations and provide an overview of key advances in genomics as they are applied clinically and in public health settings, using the lens of primary, secondary, and tertiary prevention. In particular, we will discuss examples of genetic testing and how they differ across the lifespan. We will also explore the use of genetics in common diseases—specifically, heart disease and cancer. Then, we will provide an overview of the CDC's Public Health Genomics program's tiered system for moving newly discovered variants into a process of evaluation of clinical validity and utility, and how it aligns with core public health functions. Major ethical, legal, and social issues underlying the integration of genetic knowledge into healthcare and public health practices will be described. Finally, we will discuss how shifts in population health infrastructure (e.g., health information exchanges) along with low-cost genomic information could give rise to a whole range of precision health advances from precision prevention to precision medicine to precision population health.

POPULATION—GENETICS PRINCIPLES

The "genome" may be considered as the set of genes carried by an individual. The human genome has evolved as an efficient mechanism for perpetuating the human species and maintaining human health since the earliest hominids arose in Africa 3.6–4 million years ago.[1] Conserved genetic sequences, maintained by natural selection, help to preserve essential biological functions from species to species. Environments can change, human beings may move to new locations, and disease agents can shift. For example, the hemoglobin S allele associated with sickle cell anemia has an adaptive advantage in malaria-ridden areas, but is disadvantageous where exposure to malarial parasites is less common.[2] Genetic variation acted upon by natural selection is the key to species preservation and survival, but also to individual vulnerability. Public health genetics applies advances in genetics and genomics toward health promotion and disease prevention in the population.[3] Genetics researchers in public health and medicine attempt to elucidate those components of genetic variation responsible for health and disease, and to develop preventive, diagnostic, and therapeutic measures to intervene.[4]

From a practical standpoint, physicians and public health practitioners today do not need to know most classic population genetic principles (e.g., Hardy-Weinberg equilibrium, genetic drift, etc.) but a few key concepts and terms—namely, gene pool, allele frequency, single nucleotide polymorphism, founder effects, bottlenecks, linkage disequilibrium, and admixture—will help when reading today's genomic literature and interpreting genetic information that is relevant to a community or population.

The Human Gene Pool

The increased ability to perform whole-genome sequencing is transforming our understanding of the human gene pool. It is much more diverse, personal, and larger than many geneticists expected. For example, the sequencing of ~58,000 individuals from diverse backgrounds in the United States as a part of a National Institutes of Health program entitled the TransOmic Precision Medicine (TOPMed) project[5] provides a window into the extent of human genetic variation that might be seen in a modern urban community (see Table 8-1).

First of all, the immense number of variations found (i.e., ~410 million) in a relatively small number of individuals (~58,000) highlights the genetic uniqueness of each person in a community. Over 46% of the variations detected were "singletons" (~189,000,000) meaning that only one person had the mutation. Following Mendelian genetic principles, 50% of their first-degree relatives might also carry that mutation, but the probability of another unrelated person carrying the mutation is likely well below 1/100,000. While only a small fraction of the variants fell into the category of potentially functional mutations (0.4%), the number of potentially functional mutations is

TABLE 8-1 VARIATION FOUND IN ~58,000 DIVERSE HUMAN GENOMES

	Total	Singletons (%)	Average per Individual
Total variants	~410M	~189M (46%)	3.78M
Single nucleotide variant	~381M	~175M (46%)	3.58M
Insertion/Deletion	~29M	~14M (47%)	197,000
Newly discovered	~323M	~178M (55%)	30,300
Single nucleotide variant	~298M	~165M (55%)	25,900
Insertion/Deletion	~25M	~13M (52%)	~4,350
Gene coding variation			
Nonsynonymous	~1.53M	~677K (43%)	~11,700
Stop/Splice site	~105K		~11,500
Synonymous	~1.53M		~480
Insertion/Deletion			
Frameshift	113K	67.9K	~130
Inframe	~55.8K	27.1K	~100

quite large (~1.5M nonsynonymous, ~105K stop/splice site, ~113K frameshift mutations) and will require very large studies to understand their influences on health outcomes. Moreover, most of the functional variants will have allele frequencies in the population less than 1%. Up until recently, it would have been impossible to conceptualize how to make inferences about the effects of very rare potentially deleterious mutations, but there are multiple avenues of research possible. Over the next decade, we can expect to see millions of people have their whole genomes sequenced and the total number of variants in the human gene pool will easily reach into the billions, since a large fraction of these mutations are likely to be "private'" mutations (i.e., singletons) only carried by a single individual or family.

Genotype Frequency and Allele Frequency

In order to estimate the prevalence of a particular DNA sequence mutation in a population, geneticists use a variety of statistics. *Genotype frequency* is the easiest to calculate because it is the most natural way to represent genetic information measured in individuals. Within an individual, the genome contained in each cell is determined by 46 chromosomes, 23 inherited from the mother and 23 from the father. Therefore, each person will have two possible forms (also known as alleles)—one maternal, one paternal—of any mutation found at a particular location on a chromosome known to vary in a population. For example, if a particular location on chromosome 1 is known to vary in a population such that most people have an adenine (A) nucleotide on one of their chromosomes and fewer people have a guanine (G) at that exact same location, then the "A" allele and "G" allele will be found in three genotype forms (AA, AG, and GG) in the community. The prevalence of the AA, AG, and GG genotypes are called the *genotype frequencies* in the population. Often, the *minor allele frequency* (MAF)—in this case for the "G" allele—is calculated using a simple algebraic derivation of the binomial formula ($p^2 + 2pq + q^2$) and is used to easily compare populations. For very rare mutations (e.g., found through newborn screening) it may not make sense to estimate the proportion of people who carry the mutation. Instead, the statistic of choice is *allele count* (AC). For example, if only three people have a mutation in population, then the allele count or AC = 3. On the other hand, if this *single nucleotide variant* (SNV) is present in the population at a frequency of 1% or greater, then it is considered a polymorphism and referred to as a *single nucleotide polymorphism* (SNP).

Founder Effect

All mutations found in the human gene pool first arose within a single individual, who then passed on that mutation to their children, and those individuals then passed it on to their children, and so on. In many instances throughout human history, small numbers of people migrated to new areas and through successive generations a particular deleterious mutation became prevalent in the population, so much so that specific medical and public health approaches are warranted. One notable example is a 10 kb deletion in the low-density lipoprotein receptor (*LDLR*) gene that was traced to the founder, one male within the five to seven families from France that settled in Quebec. This mutation is associated with familial hypercholesterolemia (FH) and found at a frequency of 57.5%, which is much greater than expected from random mating. Because of assortative mating, Quebec has the highest frequency of homozygous FH in the world requiring a different mindset toward preventing heart attacks in this specialized population.[6]

Bottleneck Effects

A closely related population genetic concept to the founder effect is the impact of a population bottleneck, whereby, only a modest fraction of people in a particular geographical region survived some major climactic event and the survivors' genetic variations are magnified in today's populations. One such example is the CCR5 mutation that was discovered to provide immunity from HIV infection.[7] This mutation is found in a pattern and frequency that has led geneticists to believe that it conferred a selective advantage during the bubonic plagues of the middle ages in Europe, which eliminated 30–60% of the population.[8]

Linkage Disequilibrium

As mentioned earlier, all mutations first arise in an individual and then are passed down through the generations. When a mutation occurs in an individual, it happens within the context of a chromosomal region that already has an array of historical variation. The array of variation in a chromosomal region on a single chromosome is called a *haplotype* and often the entire haplotype is passed through the generations since meiosis only involves a small number of recombinations between homologous chromosomes in gamete formation. The probability of observing one mutation in a particular genomic region thus becomes correlated with observing the other mutations contained in the haplotype. This phenomenon is known as *linkage disequilibrium* because mutations "linked" together in a particular chromosomal region are not found independently of each other (i.e., not at equilibrium). Linkage disequilibrium patterns differ across people from different ancestries because these correlations will decay with time as meiotic recombination breaks the frequency associations over many generations. For example, individuals with African ancestry have much less linkage disequilibrium than individuals of European ancestry.[9]

Admixture

People from different regions of the world have different mutational spectra, meaning that there are differences in both the mutations and their frequencies. These differences are also reflected in the haplotypes and their frequencies, often resulting in different linkage disequilibrium patterns. When people from different regions of the world migrate to new areas and these groups have children with individuals from those regions, the children's genomes represent both ancestries' haplotypes. Consequently, admixture is another source of correlation between mutations at different positions across the genome. The United States with its three centuries of migration has had a large amount of admixture of European, African, Asian, and Native American ancestries so allele frequencies and linkage disequilibrium patterns reflect a complex demographic and genetic history.

A single chapter on genomics in the context of preventive medicine does not provide adequate space to fully explore key concepts that anyone trying to utilize genomic information in a community should know. However, there are many additional texts that provide more in-depth molecular and population genetic background.[1,2,10,11]

GENETIC TESTING IN THE LIFE COURSE

Using Genetic Information to Prevent Disease

One broad way of looking at the range of public health genetic and genomic activities is through the lens of prevention. Different genetic relationships pertaining to the initiation, clinical manifestation, or progression of a disease map onto different levels of prevention. Primary prevention activities are geared toward intervening before health effects can occur—prior to disease manifestation.[12] Genetic carrier testing is one example of what people normally think of as primary prevention, as it entails taking steps to help a family avoid the disease from ever occurring. "Secondary prevention," which equates with many forms of screening, seeks to halt disease at the very earliest stages after it has begun to manifest. Newborn screening for inborn errors of metabolism is a classic example of secondary prevention. "Tertiary prevention" may be thought of as treatment, after a person has developed disease. Providers engage in tertiary prevention when they deliver treatments in an attempt to forestall or prevent advanced disease or further the complications of disease. The entire field of pharmacogenomics is focused upon improving tertiary prevention efforts, as well as reducing the deleterious effects of adverse drug reactions.

In this section, we provide an overview of key advances in genomics as they are applied clinically and in public health settings, using the lens of primary, secondary, and tertiary prevention. In particular, we discuss examples of genetic testing and how they differ across the lifespan. Public health programs are especially geared toward addressing or detecting disease at the earliest stages or before it can significantly manifest. In a review of nineteen state genetics plans, the three most common genetic programs covered birth defects, newborn screening, and childhood and adult genetic conditions such as sickle cell disease.[13] Genetic conditions with which a person may be born, such as cystic fibrosis (CF) and sickle cell disease, have been addressed by both the medical and public health communities. Public health is geared toward the entire life course, thus this review will begin with carrier or preconceptual genetic testing.

Carrier Testing

The Goals of Carrier Testing

Carrier testing is a type of genetic testing used to determine if a person is a carrier for a specific autosomal or X-linked recessive condition. It is often referred to as "carrier screening," especially when the means by which a person is identified for testing are indirect—for example, through the genetic status of another relative. If both members of a couple carry a recessive mutation, the possibility of a child being born with that condition is 1-in-4. In a sense, carrier identification and education represent a form of "genotypic prevention" by allowing couples to prevent the transmission of a specific genetic condition. Juengst recommends that the focus be on the couple's and family's welfare (a fetus has not yet been conceived), rather than the adoption of carrier testing to modify the spread of the condition in the population at large.[14]

Carrier testing often times takes place in the context of reproductive healthcare, allowing prospective parents to be informed of their options for family planning and subsequent prenatal diagnosis.[15] It is typically recommended on the basis of family history for a specific genetic condition, and for populations with a comparatively high incidence, such as Ashkenazic Jewish populations that display a comparatively high prevalence of hereditary breast and ovarian cancer (*BRCA1/2* mutations), Tay-Sachs disease, and Gaucher disease. Some authorities have recommended population-wide carrier testing or carrier screening in the case of CF and spinal muscular atrophy. Conditions that have been tested for at the preconceptual stage, either individually or as part of test panels, include CF, spinal muscular atrophy, Tay-Sachs disease, sickle cell anemia, and Fragile X syndrome. Early carrier testing programs for Tay-Sachs disease were a joint effort between medical and public health authorities. Because of the lethality of the condition and the decision to be made regarding fetal termination, efforts directed at this condition have progressed more on an individualized as opposed to population basis. Public health efforts have focused on CF and sickle cell disease carrier testing. CF carrier testing contains elements that involve both the at-risk couple and family, and will be described below. Sickle cell genetic testing will be detailed in the section to follow.

Cystic Fibrosis Carrier Testing

CF is a multisystem disease which presents the classic triad of obstructive pulmonary disease, pancreatic insufficiency, and elevated sweat chloride.[16,17] The basic pathophysiology involves abnormal thickening of respiratory and digestive secretions and tubular blockage, and decreased salt reabsorption. Symptoms typically appear early in childhood, before 2 years of age. In addition to persistent respiratory difficulties, infants may present with malabsorption, vitamin deficiency, and poor weight gain. CF is an autosomal recessive disorder, with carrier parents having a 1-in-4 chance of giving birth to an affected child with any pregnancy. Disease incidence and carrier frequency vary with the specific population. It is most common in Caucasians and Ashkenazic Jews, with disease incidences of 1/3200 and 1/3300, respectively. The condition is less frequent in other racial-ethnic groups: Latino (1/11,500); African American (1/17,000); and Asian American (1/25,500).[16] The Cystic Fibrosis Mutation Database lists more than 2070 genetic variants of the *CFTR* gene.[18] Homozygous F508del mutations are responsible for three-quarters of cases in the Caucasian population, but less than 50% of cases for the other groups.[16] Other common mutations associated with CF include G542X, R553X, W1282X, N1303K, 621 + 1 G-to-T, 1717-1 G-to-A, and R117H.[17]

In 2001, a three-organization steering committee [American College of Medical Genetics and Genomics (ACMG), American College of Obstetricians and Gynecologists (ACOG), National Institutes of Health (NIH)-National Human Genome Research Institute (NHGRI)] introduced a 25 mutation CF carrier screening panel based on an allele frequency of 0.1% or greater in the general U.S. population. A 2004 review by the ACMG, which evaluated mutation distribution amongst various ethnic groups, removed 1078delT and I148T from the list, narrowing the standard screening panel to 23 mutations. However, in a California study involving Latino CF patients, the detection rate was only 65% using this basic screening panel.[19] Farrell and Fost argue that the standard recommended panel is unnecessarily limited, especially given that commercial testing for 86 CF mutations has become routine, and that it should be expanded to cover mutations more prevalent in a variety of racial-ethnic groups.[20] Expanded testing (expanded mutation panels, gene sequencing) should also be considered in instances where a positive family history exists but genetic testing has yielded no identifiable mutation.[16] Consumer education is quite important here, as the existence of extended panels should be brought to the attention of couples requesting further literature.

The original NIH Consensus panel, attended by experts in medicine, genetics, economics, and public health, as well as healthcare consumer organizations and the lay public, recommended that all pregnant women and couples planning a pregnancy, regardless of ethnicity, should be offered CF carrier testing.[21] After a more narrow recommendation by ACOG in 2001 suggesting testing simply be made "available" to other ethnic groups, in 2005 ACOG reversed its decision and reaffirmed the original Consensus panel recommendation of testing for all ethnicities. Carrier testing is typically conducted early in prenatal care, but is ideally performed preconceptually, allowing parents to explore the full range of options. A number of testing approaches exist for the couple (concurrent testing of both partners, sequential or two-step testing of both members of a couple, couple-based testing separating simultaneous sampling from selective testing) and extended family (cascade screening).[21] For practical reasons, testing of the preconceptual or pregnant woman is the most widespread practice. If she is found to be at risk, the partner may then be tested. Standard risk assessment incorporates both the risk of transmitting a CF allele and population carrier frequencies. Bayesian analysis can be employed for more accurate risk determination in a variety of circumstances, including consideration of ethnic differences. Carrier testing has the goal of informing the couple for planning purposes, whether it be preparation for a child bearing a given genetic condition, or arranging for various reproductive options. A carrier screening program in Italy resulted in a significant reduction of CF birth incidence from about 4 per 10,000 newborns at program start in 1993, to about 1.5 per 10,000 by 2007.[16]

Cascade Screening

Once a proband (the person serving as the starting point for a genetic study of a family) comes to light, relatives have the opportunity to ascertain whether they themselves carry the responsible mutation. "Cascade screening" operates in snowball fashion, with the relatives of a patient first being tested, then their spouse if the relative is found to be positive, and onward to additional family members. Cascade carrier screening is a major prevention technique in that newly identified heterozygotes are found to have at least one CF allele they could transmit. The Centers for Disease Control and Prevention (CDC) have reported on the statistical success and cost-effectiveness of cascade screening applied to another condition that can begin with the young in at-risk families and that often lies undetected—FH.[22] Findings on uptake rates vary widely. An observational study from Victoria, Australia reported that 11.8% of informed relatives of children born from 2000 to 2004 and screened for CF subsequently engaged in testing.[23] CF testing uptake rates of 40.7% over a 25-year period were reported for informed relatives in a retrospective study out of western Brittany, France, an area where CF is relatively common.[24] Planning a pregnancy or expecting a child was a critical factor among many of the relatives who underwent testing. The authors note three public health impacts: (1) the ability to detect numerous carriers among relatives; (2) the detection of new at-risk couples; and (3) the reassurance granted the one quarter of relatives who were noncarriers of the familial mutation. In a prospective longitudinal study of the impact of CF newborn screening on families in Toronto, newborn carrier result communication to relatives was high, occurring in 92% of detected newborn carriers, yet only 35% of relatives expected the carrier results to influence their family planning.[25] These studies suggest two generalizable conclusions regarding carrier screening: (1) stage of life serves as a filter on whether a couple related to the proband wishes to undergo genetic testing; and (2) perceived seriousness (high prevalence; about to have children) is a critical factor in receptivity to genetic testing.

Prenatal Screening and Testing

Prenatal Screening Programs

Genetic screening is a strategy used in a population to check for the possibility of future disease (genetic risk) when no signs or symptoms of illness are apparent. Public health departments in several states (e.g., California, Iowa, and Maryland) have mounted programs to screen for prenatal risk as a conduit to subsequent genetic testing when indicated. The California Prenatal Screening Program offers three modalities: (1) sequential integrated screening (blood draws at two time points + nuchal translucency ultrasound); (2) serum integrated screening (blood draws at two time points); and (3) quad marker screening (one blood draw between 15 and 20 weeks).[26] The quad screen is a maternal blood screen that tests for four specific substances: alpha-fetoprotein, human chorionic gonadotropin, estriol, and inhibin-A. It replaces the former triple screen and earlier maternal serum alpha-fetoprotein screening. Levels of these four components vary with week of gestation; aberrant values suggest the possibility of a fetal developmental abnormality and the need for further work up. These levels serve as indicators of the potential existence of open neural tube defects (spina bifida, anencephaly), trisomy 21 or Down syndrome, trisomy 18, abdominal wall defects, and several other conditions, both congenital and noncongenital. The individual state programs address this shared set of conditions.

Program descriptions mention the risk of a prenatal blood test ("no greater than any other blood test") and that the results of the screen may cause anxiety. Controversy exists in that earlier brochures describing the program in California tended to interpret a negative result too positively, discounting the possibility of false negatives, and failed to mention that abortion might be recommended.[27] These shortcomings have been corrected in recent versions of the brochure, though the question of whether public health efforts should operate in an area where abortion is a possible recommendation is an issue of ongoing debate among public health authorities.[28] Information on these programs details that two primary options exist: (1) to plan for the birth of a baby with special care needs and (2) to choose to end the pregnancy if the couple so chooses. The programs also describe two other public health-related features: (1) research and (2) prevention. The proposed research takes two forms: (A) research for program evaluation, much like what takes place when states use residual newborn blood spots for program quality control and (B) research that will improve the health of mothers and their children, part of the California Biobank Program. The Connecticut Department of Public Health expanded upon this idea in 2007 when it proposed using funding from the PREEMIE Act of 2006 to link prenatal biobanks of public health departments to elucidate genetic susceptibilities leading to complex disease and adverse health events.[29] The legislation allocated $3 million annually to CDC to link population-based biobanks with medical records and health database systems.

Birth Defects Programs

The screening programs also offer an initial vantage point for providing prospective mothers and couples planning a pregnancy with information on preventing birth defects, principally through adequate intake of folic acid. Action taken to avoid birth defects constitutes primary prevention, while newborn screening and follow-up constitute secondary prevention (early in disease manifestation).[30] Birth defects affect 3% of babies born each year, cause short- and long-term morbidities, and are the leading cause of infant death in the United States.[31] Affected infants are more than twice as likely to be born preterm (<37 weeks gestation), account for at least 20% of infant deaths, and represent a leading cause of death in early childhood.[32] Birth defects are collectively more prevalent than infant mortality, very low birth weight (<1500 g), and early preterm birth (<32 weeks gestation). Surviving infants can experience chronic conditions with lifelong health and financial implications for self and family. From a public health perspective, the severity of birth defects and the needs they engender heighten the challenge to formulate a comprehensive population-based response. Prevalence and survival for many types of birth defects vary by race/ethnicity, posing additional challenges.

According to St. Louis et al., the estimated total number of live births with cardiovascular birth defects in the United States from 1999 to 2007 is 21,151; for central nervous system defects the estimate is 5613; and for ear defects the number is 2186.[31] Spina bifida without anencephaly represents 3915 of the CNS cases. Kirby reports the estimated annual number of spina bifida cases for 2004–06 is 1460, with a prevalence of 3.50 cases per 10,000 live births.[32] Consumption of the recommended amount of folic acid or vitamin B9 before and during early pregnancy can help prevent major birth defects such as anencephaly and spina bifida.[33] Preventive solutions are straightforward and not dependent on the condition's genetic complexity. The recommended amount, especially for women who desire pregnancy, is 400 micrograms (mcg) daily. Folic acid has been added to some foods, such as enriched breads, corn flour, pastas, rice, and cereal, and is a constituent of many multivitamins. Public health messages are often context dependent, so the recommended intake for expectant mothers may not be appropriate for adults over 50, for whom the recommendation is to rely on a balanced diet rather than depending on supplements containing extra folate.[34]

Sickle Cell Prenatal Testing and Associated Public Health Programs

While prenatal genetic testing is the next public health tool in the arsenal of addressing genetic conditions, public health departments have come to view it from the perspective of health across the lifespan. Prospective mothers who themselves harbor a recessive trait require attention to health as they plan to have a child and undergo pregnancy and delivery, which includes tending to the health of the newborn. Public health has devoted considerable attention to sickle cell disease since the passage of the National Sickle Cell Anemia Control Act of 1972. The population approach to sickle cell disease has evolved since that time, with prenatal testing being one prong of a multifaceted preventive health effort.

The presence of sickle hemoglobin (Hb S) in red blood cells is distinctive to sickle cell disease. The sickle cell mutation is autosomal recessive. Persons who are heterozygous are carriers and are referred to as having sickle cell trait (SCT). Individuals who are homozygous or compound homozygous for the mutation experience sickle cell disease (SCD). Sickle cell disease in the United States occupies four possible genotypes: (1) sickle cell anemia (Hb SS) and (2) sickle-hemoglobin C disease (Hb SC); and two types of beta-thalassemia (SB^{+}-thalassemia and SB^{0}-thalassemia).[35] Sickle cell disease is the most common; states reported 1800 births with this condition in 2006. Although frequencies differ, it is important to note that SCD affects people and families of varied background. It is more common in those with an ancestry from sub-Saharan Africa, Spanish-speaking regions (South America, Cuba, Central America), Saudi Arabia, India, and Mediterranean countries (Turkey, Sicily, Greece, and Italy).[36] The heterozygote state (AS) bears a selective advantage in malaria endemic areas, where it exists in population equilibrium.[2]

Hemoglobinopathy data collection and public/provider education are important constituents of core public health assessment and policy development functions. From 2010 to 2012, the CDC in collaboration with the NIH National Heart, Lung, and Blood Institute funded the Registry and Surveillance System for Hemoglobinopathies (RuSH) project to collect state-specific information on people with SCD and thalassemia.[37] The seven participating states created fact sheets describing these conditions and project results, and developed papers relaying what was learned about the health of youth and adults in their respective areas. Michigan identified the need to discuss with parents a "talk early/talk often" strategy to teach children and young adults the importance of ongoing health needs such as genetic counseling, oral health, maternal, and reproductive health.[36] Special attention by primary care providers and specialists who see patients outside the emergency department setting is needed between the ages of 18 and 30, when young adults are struggling with age-related transition in care as well as the possibility of pregnancy. In the follow-up PHRESH (Public Health Research, Epidemiology, and Surveillance for Hemoglobinopathies) project, three states (California, Mississippi, and Georgia) received CDC funding to expand and learn more about the information collected during the RuSH Project.[38] Activities to promote health and prevent disease complications focused on adequate vaccination to reduce risk of infection, early and continuous screening (especially transcranial Doppler screening for youth 0–18 years), and the provision of proper treatments.

A life course approach to support individuals with these genetic conditions must also incorporate the needs of prospective mothers. CDC-based education materials describe: (1) the causes of sickle cell disease and trait; (2) the role of the genetic counselor; (3) availability of parental testing through medical facilities, local public health departments, and SCD community-based organizations; (4) types of prenatal testing; and (5) steps to assure a healthy pregnancy.[39] Public health has prioritized the use of family history in risk assessment, not just as a responsibility of the genetic counselor, but as a way to make families aware of conditions requiring attention. Family health history tools such as the U.S. Surgeon General's "My Family Health Portrait" and Genetic Alliance's "Does it run in the family?" are available online.[40] If the mother has SCD, state and national resources advocate a balanced message conveying that a healthy pregnancy is possible, but that intensified monitoring is required to minimize risk of complications such as preterm delivery and low birth weight.

The public health approach to sickle cell disease and other recessive conditions calls for reducing morbidity and mortality to optimize the mother's health and allow planning for a baby with SCT, SCD, or another hemoglobinopathy, with the use of prenatal testing to aid in decisions about proceeding with the pregnancy.[35] Amniocentesis, performed around 14–19 weeks postconception, and chorionic villus sampling (CVS), performed around 9–13 weeks, remain the mainstay diagnostic approaches, though noninvasive prenatal testing (NIPT) has emerged on the market as an initial screening option. If NIPT is used, ACOG recommends that other prenatal tests be used beyond NIPT.[41] Amniocentesis and CVS are well-validated procedures, but have a recognizable miscarriage rate, about 1/400 and slightly greater than 1%, respectively, despite being the conventional diagnostic alternatives.

Utilization and outcomes of hemoglobinopathy carrier screening and prenatal testing programs vary by country. In Greece, where thalassemia constitutes the most frequent genetic disorder, the National Thalassaemia Prevention Programme has decreased the incidence of thalassemia major and sickle cell syndromes.[42] In Cyprus, surveys conducted by the Cyprus National Thalassaemia Screening Programme between 1986 and 2010 have registered a decrease in the frequency of beta-thalassemia carriers of about 1.89% over this period.[43] The cause of this overall decrease is subject to interpretation, however, since population selective pressure for thalassemia mutations has decreased since the eradication of malaria in that country in 1948. Despite one in every four individuals in Ontario, Canada belonging to an ethnic group with a high carrier frequency for alpha- and beta-thalassemia, the majority of at-risk pregnancies are missed by current approaches to carrier screening, genetic counseling, and prenatal diagnosis.[44] In a hospital-based study in New York City, 72% of mothers continued their pregnancies when hemoglobin SS disease was prenatally diagnosed after 20 weeks' gestation.[45] In a population-based study in Rochester, New York in which 53 pregnant women, most of whom were African American with known sickle cell trait, were offered free prenatal testing, 28 declined testing.[46] Of the remaining 25 women, 3 received a diagnosis of sickle cell disease in their child-to-be and continued their pregnancies. This observation underscores the value of public health educational efforts which can reach large numbers of people, such as "know your status" public awareness campaigns, and of making information on health risks and personal options available to couples who learn their risk.[35,36,47]

Newborn Screening

The Growth of Newborn Screening

For the most part, newborn screening has been aimed at detecting rare inborn errors of metabolism that are effectively prevented given early detection and dietary modification of the mother and newborn. Population screening for such conditions is based on a number of technical and ethical criteria which have been mapped out since Wilson and Jungner first developed a set of programmatic screening criteria 50 years ago.[48] Importance to the community—prevalence and seriousness of the consequences—is the first listed principle upon which decisions about screening should be made.

In practice, newborn screening began with a simple test for phenylketonuria (PKU) developed by Dr. Robert Guthrie in 1963.[49] The original test involved filter paper soaked with the infant's serum, but it quickly evolved into the now well-recognized procedure of drying a small amount of blood from the infant's heel, and punching out a small disc of the blood spot for testing. In subsequent years the test for PKU became mandatory in 37 states, and by the end of the 1960s and early 1970s, screening for many other severe metabolic conditions at the neonatal stage became the standard in hospitals throughout the United States, including congenital hypothyroidism, sickle cell disease, and maple syrup urine disease. Sickle cell disease and CF, both autosomal recessive conditions, were added to the newborn screening roster in 1973 [with Health Resources and Services Administration (HRSA) funding in 1988] and 1985, respectively.[50,51] Due to its frequency and the ability of providers to prevent and manage sickle cell disease, as of January 2006, all 50 states plus Puerto Rico and the Virgin Islands have implemented universal screening newborn screening for SCD.[35]

The number of core conditions suggested for screening enlarged to 25 with the development of updated guidelines in 2002 by ACMG, charged with this task by HSRA's Maternal and Child Health Bureau.[52] These conditions constituted the original Recommended Universal Screening Panel or RUSP. The adoption of tandem mass spectrometry (MS-MS) by many states, spurred by the availability of the technology and backing by commercial and advocacy groups, led half the states to screen for more than 22 disorders by 2005. A second body, the Secretary's Advisory Committee on Heritable Disorders in Newborns and Children (ACHDNC), worked closely with ACMG to get the RUSP adopted and establish a protocol for evaluating additional conditions for inclusion. By November of 2016, the RUSP contained 60 recommended conditions. The recommended conditions include disorders detectable through MS-MS, endocrine and hemoglobin disorders, CF, and other recent additions.[53] State panels have correspondingly expanded beyond the assessment of simply metabolic disorders. Preventability and treatability are criteria that have risen to the fore. In recommending the three most recent conditions for inclusion, Spinal Muscular Atrophy, Mucopolysaccharidosis Type I, and X-linked Adrenoleukodystrophy, the Advisory Committee acknowledged that state newborn screening programs would require 1–5 years to begin screening these conditions, and that funding would be required to obtain the necessary test platform and complete professional training on the appropriate protocols, both of which are ongoing efforts.[53]

Although the current RUSP has led to consensus on a common set of 35 core and 26 secondary conditions requiring screening, a great deal of variation remains between states.[54] As of 2016, eight states fell short of the number of core conditions recommended by the RUSP whereas seven states screened for almost all of the original 60 core conditions.[55] Forty-two state screening panels matched or exceeded the recommended set of newborn screens. A population-wide prevalence study of all neonates born between July 2005 and July 2010 also demonstrated considerable variation between racial-ethnic groups.[56] The above observations imply a deftness needed in addressing the analysis and interpretation of newborn screening findings, and the solutions—technical and social—that may be required. Despite the evolving complexity of newborn screening, it should be noted that success—prevention of morbidity and mortality—is achievable. The history of newborn screening shows that a significant reduction in SCD-related deaths was achieved in children after implementation of universal newborn screening and comprehensive follow-up care in Connecticut in 1990.[35,57] Ongoing public health research is required to assess clinical utility as further rare conditions are considered for addition to the current list.[58]

Whole-Genome Sequencing

It is conceivable that MS-MS could one day be replaced by newborn Whole-Genome Sequencing (WGS), which would further expand the list of critically assessed conditions, possibly by including susceptibility to cardiovascular disease, diabetes, or mental health disorders, and enable the construction of a "genetic report card" for every infant.[59–61] Such expansion requires close technical and ethical scrutiny, more so than did the move to MS-MS. Unique considerations posed by whole-genome or exome sequencing applied to newborn screening include: (1) shape of consent, which may require alternative scenarios such as opting-in and tiered consent[62]; (2) ability to distinguish pathogenic from benign variants and variants of unknown significance (a currently ongoing effort)[62,63]; (3) revamping of the public health and healthcare systems to handle the massive amounts of information generated[60]; (4) assurance of treatment and follow-up (requires consensus on individualized vs. population-wide approaches)[60]; and (5) equal availability and accessibility to infants born in different jurisdictions (calling for population-based coverage).[62] Randomized clinical trials of infants receiving genomic sequencing vs. conventional newborn screening are taking place as part of the BabySeq Project, funded by the U.S. National Institute of Child Health and Human Development (NICHD) and NHGRI.[64]

State-run Biobanks

Like their prenatal counterpart, newborn screening programs can also have a research-oriented arm. The California Biobank Program collects maternal blood samples in the first and second trimesters and stores for research newborn blood spots drawn 1–3 days after birth.[65] The Michigan Neonatal Biobank, part of the Michigan BioTrust for Health, stores blood spots, like California, separate from identifying information.[66] Uses to which the samples have been put include checking for methylation patterns in autism, ADHD, and coronary heart disease; gestational exposure to tobacco; and health outcomes of babies conceived by in-vitro fertilization. Such applications are not without controversy, and both biobanks have a community values advisory board to provide recommendations. Ethical issues that have been voiced include: (1) maintenance of samples over time vs. destruction after the immediate newborn period; (2) time at which parental consent is obtained; (3) opt-in/opt-out policy for samples collected prior to biobank initiation; (4) retention of identifiers; (5) inadvertent use by outside sources without parental authorization; and (6) means of storing enlarged genetic information should analysis be expanded through mRNA microarray analysis or whole-genome sequencing.[67,68]

From Genetic Association Studies to Genomic Applications to Improve Health

Evidentiary Approach to Genetics and Genomics

It is only a matter of time before germline genome sequencing beyond the newborn period becomes a routine procedure as a part of healthcare and preventive services. Estimates already indicate that the average person carries 20–30 clinically relevant mutations, based on today's standards.[69] Many more potentially functional mutations are likely to be elucidated. The vast majority have just been discovered, are rare, and have yet to be studied (see Table 8-1). Numerous questions arise as to how to best manage the evaluation of evidence and the promotion of work to catalog and convey the information accumulating about whether a particular genomic mutation is relevant (or not relevant) for use by practitioners. For simplicity, we provide a brief overview of the key evidence development process needed before broad introduction of new genetic testing or use of new genetic information in a healthcare setting or public health setting can be prudently suggested. In general, three levels of evidence must be gathered and verified—analytic validity, clinical validity, and clinical utility—before suitable evidence-based guidelines can be established.

Analytic Validity

In most initial genetic epidemiology or clinical studies, the main focus is on identifying which genomic variants are associated with a health outcome. Much time is spent on the design and execution of the study (e.g., case-control and cohort studies). Reliable and validated measures of health outcomes, genetic variants, biomarkers, anthropometric, and demographic factors often must be carefully collected in order to properly control for variation due to population characteristics when modeling the association between genotype and disease. Given the shift to genomic measures of variation (e.g., whole-genome sequencing) with extraordinary multiple testing issues, dozens of epidemiological studies must pool their results together to have adequate power to discover and replicate associations before a genomic association with disease is accepted.[70] Such pooling is especially prominent in multi-institutional genome wide association studies (GWAS) where the individual and cumulative effect of multiple SNPs is being assessed. In most cases, the main goal is to estimate in some fashion the probability of disease, response to treatment, recurrence, or survival if a person has a risk-conferring mutation, compared to if they do not. The *analytic validity* of these findings is directly related to whether the studies utilized proper epidemiological study designs, data collection principles, and statistical methods when estimating the genetic effects and making inferences about the relationship between the genomic variants and the health outcome(s) (see Teutsch et al.[71] for more details).

Clinical Validity

To demonstrate the *clinical validity* of a genetic test, it must be assessed within clinical populations or settings that reflect real-world implementation of the genetic test (e.g., diagnosis, therapeutic decision-making, newborn screening, prenatal screening, etc.). Here the key goal is to obtain real-world estimates of the probability of disease, response to treatment, recurrence, or survival if a person has a risk-conferring mutation, compared to if they do not, in the settings and situations in which the genetic test will be utilized. These estimates provide a basis from which to begin calculating important metrics such as positive/negative predictive value, number of lives saved, number of adverse drug reactions averted, or cost savings due to early detection, more precise treatment, and fewer disease sequelae for those carrying the deleterious mutations and/or for the community at large. Establishing the clinical validity of a genetic test also must estimate the added value of using the genetic or genomic information beyond the current standard of care.

Clinical Utility

Given the complexities of modern healthcare and public health, the incorporation of a genetic test into preventive services or clinical care takes much more forethought and planning than just obtaining estimates of key metrics of health benefit. The *clinical utility* of a genetic test, its usefulness and relevance, is evaluated through the offering of the genetic test in the actual practice setting and a thorough evaluation of all of the key delivery steps, as well as the impact on health outcomes. Evaluating the clinical utility of genetic test covers many more operational components of a genetic test, such as: (1) can the genetic mutation be detected reliably within a clinical laboratory setting (e.g., CLIA certified); (2) have physicians been trained to interpret the test correctly; (3) does adequate patient education exist; (4) have the laboratory results been appropriately integrated into automated clinical-decision support systems; (5) how/will the genetic test be covered by payers; and (6) are there any ethical, legal, or social issues that must be addressed for both patient and healthcare or public health practitioner to adequately use the genetic test? These are just a few of the many complexities involved in assessing the clinical utility in addition to the primary question of "Did the incorporation of the genetic test improve health outcomes within the practice setting?" Once clinical utility has been established, evidence-based guidelines for widespread implementation should be made available through professional associations.

Center for Disease Control and Prevention's Three-Tiered System

In response to the growing interest in incorporating genomic findings into practice, the CDC Office of Public Health Genomics created a three-tier system to help clarify when sufficient evidence has been accumulated to warrant implementation into healthcare and/or public health practice settings[72,73]:

- Tier 1: Genes and variants that have evidence-based guidelines established based on numerous studies of their clinical validity and clinical utility.
- Tier 2: Genes and variants that have well-established clinical validity, but not sufficient evidence of clinical utility.
- Tier 3: Genes and variants with established genetic associations but inadequate evidence of clinical validity or utility. Also, Tier 3 contains genetic variants with guidelines against their use.

Many of the classical and more heavily published genetic conditions have applications that fit under the CDC Tier 1 heading. For example, genetic testing for the CF F508del mutation, and newborn screening of 31 core conditions originally suggested by the Secretary's Advisory Committee on Heritable Disorders in Newborns and Children, have been extensively validated and are considered Tier 1 applications.[72] Three major forms of childhood and adult genetic testing are also classified as Tier 1 applications: (1) genetic counseling and *BRCA1*/*BRCA2* testing for hereditary breast and ovarian cancer; (2) diagnostic screening of colorectal cancer cases for Lynch syndrome and cascade screening of at-risk relatives; and (3) physiological plus DNA testing for FH individually and in relatives.[74] Certain forms of pharmacogenomic testing, such as *KRAS* testing for the use of cetuximab in metastatic colorectal cancer, are considered Tier 1, while others—*KRAS* testing for the administration of compounds in this drug category for nonsmall cell lung cancer—remain Tier 2. These strategies, since they are aimed at slowing disease progression, represent tertiary, more clinically oriented prevention. Direct-to-consumer (DTC) personal genetic testing for various common diseases often fits under Tier 3. With a few exceptions, attempts by companies to market disease-oriented testing have met with FDA calls to cease activity until the claim for a DTC test's medical benefit has been fully justified.

Adult and Childhood Genetic Testing

Categories of Genetic Testing

Given its preventive orientation, public health genomics is mostly concerned with detecting genetic mutations that will have an impact after birth, often later in life, both for a given individual and other at-risk family members. Diagnostic genetic testing is used to identify or rule-out the genetic basis of a clinical condition. Predictive genetic testing identifies mutations that increase a person's risk of developing a disorder, such as certain types of cancer.[75] Presymptomatic testing can be used to determine whether a person will develop a disorder in the future, such as FH, before signs and symptoms appear. All forms of genetic testing within a family can benefit from knowledge about the mutation identified in an original proband or index case. When specific genetic testing applications are likely to have a significant impact on public health based on available evidence-based guidelines and recommendations, they are considered "Tier 1" genetic or genomic applications. The CDC has prioritized three Tier 1 varieties of predictive and diagnostic genetic testing[74]:

- Hereditary breast and ovarian cancer (HBOC), which leads to an increased risk for breast, ovarian, tubal, peritoneal, and prostate cancers, and melanoma, due to mutations in *BRCA1* and *BRCA2* genes
- Hereditary nonpolyposis colorectal cancer or Lynch syndrome (LS), which leads to an increased risk for colorectal, endometrial, ovarian, and other cancers connected with mutations in mismatch-repair genes
- FH, posing an increased risk for heart disease or stroke due to mutations resulting in very high cholesterol levels from childhood onward

Heart disease and cancer are the first and second leading causes of mortality in the United States, though Survey of Epidemiology and End Results (SEER) findings suggest cancer may take the lead by 2020.[76] Nearly 2 million people in the United States are at an increased risk for adverse health outcomes due to genetic mutations in one of these three conditions spanning the two major disease categories.[74] Early detection and intervention can help reduce morbidity and mortality in at-risk individuals.

Hereditary Breast and Ovarian Cancer

Hereditary breast and ovarian cancer makes up 3–10% of all breast cancer, and 10–15% of all ovarian cancer cases.[77,78] The major mutations in HBOC are within two genes—*BRCA1* and *BRCA2*—that produce tumor suppressor proteins which help prevent cells from growing and dividing too rapidly or in an uncontrolled manner.[79] Transmission occurs in an autosomal dominant fashion. The lifetime cancer risks associated with having these mutations are 44–87% (breast cancer); 20–50% (ovarian cancer); and 7% (male breast and pancreatic cancer). The carrier frequency for deleterious *BRCA1* and *2* mutations is 1/800–1/300 in the general population, and 1/40 for individuals of Ashkenazi Jewish ancestry.[77,80] Specific allelic mutations have been associated with founder mutations and a population bottleneck in persons of Jewish ancestry. Other ethnic populations, such as the Norwegian, Dutch, and Icelandic peoples, show a higher prevalence of specific pathogenic variants associated with founder mutations and genetic drift.[79,81]

National Comprehensive Cancer Network (NCCN) Clinical Practice Guidelines indicate HBOC should be suspected in individuals with[78,82]:

- A personal or family history of breast cancer diagnosed at a young age (under 50 years)
- Multiple relatives having either breast or ovarian cancer
- A relative with primary cancers of both breasts
- Presence of ovarian or of male breast cancer
- Breast cancer diagnosed at any age in persons of Ashkenazi Jewish ancestry

The U.S. Preventive Services Task Force (USPSTF) recommends that primary care providers screen women who have family members with breast, ovarian, tubal, or peritoneal cancer to identify a family history that may be associated with an increased risk from carrying *BRCA1* or *2* mutations. Women with positive screening results should receive genetic counseling and, where indicated after counseling, BRCA genetic testing.[83] Healthy People 2020 has incorporated the USPSTF recommendations into its genomics objectives.[84] The National Cancer Institute has developed a Breast Cancer Risk Assessment Tool.[85] Family history resources are available from Genetic Alliance ("Does It Run in the Family?" Toolkit) and from states like the Michigan Department of Health and Human Services (hand-held "Cancer Family History Guide").[86,87]

State public health department approaches to HBOC, as outlined by the CDC, include: (1) enhancing cancer registry reporting, including "bidirectional" reporting between the state health department and the partner health system; (2) developing and tracking BRCA surveillance indicators to follow the implementation of Tier 1 recommendations, including the Healthy People 2020 BRCA objective; (3) instituting educational outreach to the public and health professional groups; and (4) informing evidence-based policy making among healthcare payers.[78,88] Additional activities include promoting and carrying out cascade screening among family members. Investigation of factors influencing communication between family members at risk for HBOC is ongoing.[89]

BRCA genetic testing has been found to be cost-effective in studies looking at genetic testing and mastectomy for women with breast cancer and their at-risk family members[90] and for women of Ashkenazi Jewish ancestry.[91] Decision analysis of *BRCA1/2* testing in American Ashkenazi Jewish women deduced $8300/QALY gained could be attained through such testing to avert ovarian cancer.[92] On a population level, *BRCA1/2* genetic testing represents a form of precision health in that it can be used with other biomarkers to stratify susceptibility and disease outcomes into subgroups reflecting underlying disease heterogeneity and response to interventions.[93,94] More than 1800 *BRCA1* pathogenic variants have been identified to date.[82] New challenges arise because of the low frequency of deleterious mutations identified in multigene germline panels and the possibility of identifying variants of uncertain significance for *BRCA1* and *BRCA2* when next-generation sequencing is employed.[95]

Lynch Syndrome

An estimated 150,000 new colorectal cancer (CRC) cases are diagnosed annually in the United States. About one third have a familial basis, and 3–5% are due to high penetrance cancer syndromes.[96] Lynch syndrome (LS) is the most commonly inherited CRC syndrome, accounting for about 4200 new cases of CRC in the United States per year.[97] The inheritance pattern is autosomal dominant. The most common LS mutations are in the germline mismatch repair (MMR) genes *MLH1*, *MSH2*, *MSH6*, and *PMS2*, and in *EPCAM* genes.[80,98] More than 250 different pathogenic variants in *MLH1* and 190 in *MSH2* have been reported.[99] These genes are directly and indirectly involved in the repair of errors occurring in DNA copying during cell division.[100] Estimates suggest that as many as 1 in 300 people may be a carrier for one of these mutations.[98] The most frequent cancer associated with LS is in the gastrointestinal tract—the colon, rectum, and stomach. Women have an increased risk of developing endometrial and ovarian cancer. SEER results show that CRC incidence is especially increased in young adults over age 30.[101,102] The lifetime cancer risks for LS in particular are 54–74% (males—colon); 30–52% (females—colon) (mean age of onset 27–46 years); 25–60% (endometrium); 6–13% (stomach); 4–12% (ovary); and 2–18% (hepatobiliary tract).[103,104] Colon polyps appear earlier but are less abundant and harder to detect than polyps for other colorectal cancers.[100]

Family history is very important in the diagnosis of Lynch syndrome and should be suspected if any of the following apply:

- The individual has a personal history of colorectal (CRC) or endometrial (EC) cancer before the age of 50.
- One or more first-degree relatives have been diagnosed with colorectal or endometrial cancer <50 years of age.
- The individual has a personal history of CRC or EC and another LS-related cancer.
- Three or more relatives have been diagnosed with LS-related cancers, regardless of age.[105,106]

Individuals suspecting the presence of a familial condition can start by using the U.S. Surgeon General's "My Family Health Portrait" and sharing the results with their personal physician.[107] Clinical prediction algorithms incorporating personal and family history exist, the most recent being the $PREMM_5$, which is user-friendly.[108] Tumor status is assessed through microsatellite instability (MSI), immunohistochemistry (IHC), and *BRAF* mutation testing. The CDC-supported Evaluation of Genomic Applications in Practice and Prevention (EGAPP) Working Group determined the analytical validity and clinical adequacy of these screens in decisions to proceed with MMR mutation testing in CRC cases, and offering of genetic testing to their relatives.[109] Based on this conclusion, Healthy People 2020 recommended that all those newly diagnosed with colorectal cancer should be offered Lynch syndrome testing, combined with informing relatives about their increased risk.[84] Testing with a multigene (*MLH1*, *MSH2*, etc.) panel is generally considered more cost-effective than serial single-gene testing.[104] While next-generation tumor sequencing of CRC as a whole has been productive in terms of yielding novel pathogenic variants,[110] the yield for LS has been quite low. Difficulty in interpreting functional significance and lack of supporting validation by other studies continue to be a challenge.[111]

A more basic shortcoming is that the vast majority of families with a history of CRC do not know they may have LS, or even that a genetic test is available.[108] State health departments have been active in promoting and implementing self-identification of at-risk individuals and families.[112] The Colorado Department of Public Health and Environment sent targeted information about hereditary CRC to 430 medical providers and 200 at-risk cases. Connecticut reported back 2471 cancer registry cases with two or more LS-related primary tumors to provider institutions. In a review by Grosse of LS cost-effectiveness studies published between 2010 and 2015, all but one of five looking at the universal offering of testing to adult CRC patients and two examining the testing of patients up to age 70 proved cost-effectiveness based on the threshold value of $100,000 per life-year or QALY gained.[113] Provider education is an important activity since so many LS cases are missed. Health department activities have included relaying information on LS, EGAPP guidelines, and listings of cancer genetic counselors to providers, as well as making available a telephone information line staffed by genetic counselors.[112] National resource and information sharing is being undertaken by Lynch Syndrome Screening Network member organizations.[114]

Familial Hypercholesterolemia

FH is the most common cardiovascular disease with Mendelian inheritance. With a prevalence of 1/500–1/200, it affects approximately 600,000 people in the United States.[115,116] FH is thought to account for 2–3% of myocardial infarctions in persons <60 years of age. The inheritance pattern is autosomal dominant.[117] An estimated 70–95% of FH results from heterozygous mutations in one of four genes—*LDLR* (low-density lipoprotein receptor) (85–90% of patients with the FH phenotype); *APOB* (1–12% of patients); *PCSK9* (2–4%); and *APOE* (~3%).[118,119] The University College of London *LDLR* Familial Hypercholesterolemia Database reports more than 1288 different variants.[120] The database also contains more than 45 *PCSK9* mutations.[121] Though many of the currently identified *PCSK9* SNPs remain investigational for FH, this family of genetic variants has already generated a new class of lipid-lowering drugs under trial—anti-*PCSK9* antibodies.[115,122] About 20% of definite FH is causally unaccounted for; it is believed that only a small proportion is due to as of yet undiscovered single gene mutations, as opposed to polygenic or multifactorial causes.[118,123] Like HBOC, the higher prevalence of FH mutations in specific populations (e.g., Amish, Christian Lebanese, South African Ashkenazi Jewish, and French Canadians) is thought to be due to founder effects.[115]

FH is characterized by severely elevated LDL cholesterol (LDL-C) levels leading to atherosclerosis in the coronary arteries and proximal aorta at an early age, coronary artery disease (CAD), and xanthomas of the eyelids and tendons.[115] Untreated men are at 50% risk for a fatal or nonfatal coronary event by age 50; untreated women at 30% risk by age 60. The considerably rarer homozygous form (HoFH) can be either strictly homozygous or compound homozygous, the latter arising when parents are unrelated. Individuals with HoFH experience severe CAD by their mid-1920s, and are likely to either receive coronary bypass surgery or stent insertion, or perish from related disease by their teenage years.

Threshold levels of LDL-C and total cholesterol have been established both for children and adults that warrant clinical suspicion, then establish a diagnosis of FH.[115] Four major sets of clinical criteria are in use: the (1) Dutch Lipid Clinic Network; (2) UK Simon Broome Familial Hypercholesterolemia Registry; (3) American Heart Association; and (4) US MedPed Program Diagnostic Criteria.[115,118,124] Personal or family history of premature cardiovascular disease and/or CAD are important components in these assessments. An actual diagnosis of FH in family members, high levels of LDL-C, early onset (<50 years) of CAD, and xanthomas suggest a positive family history. Serial single-gene testing and multigene panels are used to secure the diagnosis and identify the responsible pathogenic variant. It should be noted that certain health plans may not reimburse for the costs of genetic testing, and that some companies test for only a small number of mutations.[118]

A major public health goal is to provide information to policymakers allowing them to make evidence-based decisions about ascertainment (e.g., type of testing and testing in relatives) and treatment (e.g., age to start on medications) issues.[116] The Connecticut Department of Public Health added questions relating to FH to its Behavioral Risk Factor Surveillance System survey. The Michigan Sudden Cardiac Death of the Young Surveillance and Prevention Project charted 23 deaths over a 3-year period and notified 17 next-of-kin of the potential heritable cause.[125] Immediate causes of death included coronary atherosclerosis as well as heart arrhythmia, which also constitute a public health challenge in that in many instances it has a heritable basis.[126] Several primary and secondary prevention measures were recommended, from provider education to development of emergency response protocols for the extended family.

According to the U.S. National Institute for Health and Care Excellence (NICE), cascade screening using cholesterol testing with or without DNA analysis should be performed on relatives of probands to identify previously unknown FH cases and provide those family members with life-saving treatment.[116] The CDC, based on the NICE Guidelines, considers cascade screening of relatives of people diagnosed with FH as a Tier 1 application. FH is a condition that remains seriously underdiagnosed; testing relatives can bring many new cases to light.[116,127] Cascade screening in the Netherlands identified, on average, eight relatives with FH for each proband.[128] While the United States has created policies for universal cholesterol screening of adults (USPSTF) and children (National Heart, Lung, and Blood Institute; American Pediatric Association), implementation has been slow.[129] Promotion of testing in at-risk family members is an additional public health goal. The West Virginia Department of Health and Human Resources, for example, offers LDLR testing and a detailed family history to at-risk family members, and is working on a statewide registry of patients to help identify other family members.[116]

Familial Hypercholesterolemia and Precision Health

Investigators are currently assessing the use of polygenic risk scores (PRS) to identify those in the top risk stratum of the population. Family history, information about genetic variants such as SNPs ("G-scores") and lifestyle and environmental factors ("E-scores") combine to yield a single index or overall risk score for a given disease (e.g., subclinical coronary atherosclerosis, extreme high-density lipoprotein, colorectal cancer).[130–132] Phenotypic information is collected through various precision health means—electronic health records (EHRs), online patient or research participant follow-up, and mobile devices such as smartphone apps.[94,133] For FH, such scoring has shown relevance as a diagnostic factor in predicting disease severity at the individual level, but not in distinguishing likelihood of a mutation, as opposed to multifactorial causes, as the source of disease.[134] Khera and colleagues have shown that genetic risk scores can identify 2.5% of all individuals with a fourfold increased risk for coronary disease that is similar to monogenic disease risk. They also observed similar patterns with genetic risk scores for severe obesity and breast cancer.[135] The ongoing GeneRISK-study in Finland has found that about a third of patients who were told they have an elevated risk of developing cardiovascular disease, based on clinical factors and a high PRS, made weight- and smoking-related changes to their lifestyle.[136] Public health authorities have adopted a cautiously hopeful approach, which remains a Tier 3 genomic application at present despite DTC companies marketing such panels in advance of full investigation.[137]

SOCIETAL CONSIDERATIONS

The Affordable Care Act and Insurance Barriers

The Affordable Care Act (ACA) has had a wide-ranging impact on many facets of healthcare and population health, including making provision for the coverage of genetic screening. For example, it requires most states to cover the federal RUSP with no cost sharing.[138] The ACA coverage mandate does not include counseling, follow-up testing, medical foods (such as phenylalanine-free medical formula), and ongoing healthcare. These charges are usually included in negotiated newborn care reimbursement, but as newborn screening expands to include conditions with later onset, problems may arise with third-party coverage. Few state programs have budget items allowing adequate funding of all six recognized newborn screening components (the above plus education, tracking, diagnosis, and evaluation).[139] Ultimately, full attention to newborns is a question of distributive justice facing the members of society and their elected representatives.

Prior to the ACA, consumers and their insurers paid from $995 (DNA Traits) to $3100 (Myriad Genetics) for *BRCA1/2* testing, and healthcare plans used 56 criteria by which to set coverage criteria for genetic counseling and testing.[140] The ACA covers *BRCA1/2* counseling, and testing where indicated, at no cost. However, racial-ethnic minorities have only partially benefited from such coverage. A post-ACA University of South Florida/Florida Department of Public Health study of 1622 women with medical record-verified invasive breast cancer drawn from the Florida State Cancer Registry revealed African Americans were 16.6 times less likely than whites to have discussed the possibility of *BRCA1/2* genetic testing with a healthcare provider and 5.6 times less likely to have had genetic testing; and Spanish-speaking Latino Americans were two times less likely than whites to have discussed the possibility of genetic testing.[141] The investigators found lack of private insurance to be a significant contributing factor.

Genetic testing for familial cancer syndromes is gradually shifting from single-gene analysis to multigene panels. A multi-institutional review of payer coverage found that although 76% of payers had coverage policies for such panels, none of those reviewed covered the panels as a whole.[142] Seventy-seven percent considered the panels investigational, with the remainder limiting coverage to those panels on which all the genes were considered medically necessary. Genetic counselors wrestle with this issue by adjusting coverage requests to a portion of the panel, an unsatisfactory long-term solution. The current situation stands to impact racial-ethnic minorities more so than whites, since multigene panels are more likely to detect variants of uncertain significance in these groups.[143]

Technology Inequities

Screening colonoscopies are fully covered as part of the Medicare initial preventive physical examination, and by many private insurers under the ACA. More frequent use of colonoscopy for high-risk surveillance is outside the scope of the U.S. Preventive Services Task Force CRC recommendations since they have a preventive, rather than diagnostic, orientation. Consequently, both LS genetic testing and surveillance for LS adenomas are not included in the ACA provisions. An examination of Latino CRC patients with tumors displaying microsatellite instability in an inner-city Dallas County, TX hospital found that the majority were <50 years of age and uninsured.[144] Cost concerns with LS genetic testing and molecular screening may be a factor in underutilization of these procedures within Latino communities.

Colorectal cancer carries with it many private, so far unidentified, mutations which due to their rarity are only found in a single family or small population. PRS hold much promise for primary prevention of cancer and cardiovascular disease in the larger population. The concern is that PRS as it exists today is several times more accurate in individuals of European vs. other ancestries.[145] The disparity is a consequence of Eurocentric biases in genome- and phenome-wide association studies.[146] Greater diversity in patient sampling and more vigorous efforts in summary statistic dissemination could help close this gap.

Systematic investigation of the societal impact of whole-genome and exome sequencing is formative at this point. The National Human Genome Research Institute, NCI, and National Institute on Minority Health and Health Disparities (NIMHD) have funded a Clinical Sequencing Exploratory Research (CSER) consortium to investigate the effectiveness of integrating genomic sequencing into clinical care, taking into account population diversity and range of impacted healthcare settings.[147] The consortium supports five pediatric and one adult extramural clinical project, the latter focusing on hereditary cancer risk. Each project aims to enroll 60% of participants from non-European or underserved populations, or populations known to experience poorer medical outcomes. Participant perception of personal utility is a high-priority area.

Considering the different applications of such technologies, a distinction exists between genomic knowledge applied to individuals and groups, such as families, and genomic information applied to populations. Cascade screening is valuable for individuals and their families, but preventive medicine experts and public health authorities also have to balance that consideration against the need to prioritize actions realizing the greatest good for underserved geographic areas or populations, including the delivery of basic healthcare services and overcoming the health effects of racial residential segregation. Indeed, county of residence, supported by data from the National Center for Health Statistics and population counts from the Census Bureau, may in the end be the most telling indicator of mortality risk and practical instrument of precision health.[148]

Health Information Exchanges

Over the next several decades, the foundation of public health genomics is likely to drastically shift, not only because of the affordable nature of whole-genome sequencing, but as a result of advances in health information technology combined with public and private sector engagement to create Health Information Exchanges (HIEs). HIEs facilitate the electronic movement of health-related information (e.g., EHRs, personal health records, public health registry information) among organizations (e.g., hospitals, providers, departments of health, laboratories, pharmacies) according to nationally recognized standards. While the original impetus behind the development of HIEs was to facilitate patient care coordination through the sharing of electronic health information, the potential benefit to population health surveillance and research are enormous.

The overall goal is to improve efficiency, reduce costs, improve safety, and monitor quality of health systems. In doing so, HIEs also provide a solution to the many technical, legal, organizational, and funding challenges of performing high-quality research and surveillance at a population level. HIEs link data stored by multiple relevant stakeholders and in multiple systems while ensuring patient confidentiality and data security. HIEs provide real time access to health data for anyone within the public–private partnership's health information networks across a state and in the near future across the nation. The vast majority of individuals in the United States already have their health data shared through their state's HIE, and improved interoperability means this data is integrated with public health agency data including newborn blood spot screening, newborn hearing screening, Women, Infants, and Children (WIC) programs, blood lead level screening programs, genetic services and early intervention programs, as well as immunization, blood lead, birth defects, and cancer registries.[149]

For health systems that are piloting whole-genome sequencing of their patients, the ability to link their patient data with all other health data on those individuals creates an unparalleled clinical and epidemiological resource for estimating the analytic and clinical validity of the vast number of potentially functional mutations that are being discovered. It also lays the foundation for rapid advances in the emerging areas of precision medicine,[133,150] precision prevention,[151] and precision public health[94] in an inclusive manner.

Conclusion: The Future of Genomics in Healthcare and Public Health

The field of public health genomics has grown considerably since the first edition of this chapter by Patricia A. Baird and Charles R. Scriver was written in 1998 (the 14th edition of this volume). Population genetic principles remain integral to an understanding of the diseases under study in communities, but the array of conditions has expanded beyond its monogenic precursors to a myriad of allelic mutations, single nucleotide polymorphisms, and multifactorial chronic conditions. In exploring the importance of these alterations and the interventions that might be employed, preventive medicine and public health must continue to adopt an evidentiary, "show me" approach. A major translational challenge of the basic discoveries being made is to assess the added value of a test compared with or in addition to existing disease screening or intervention approaches based on age, family history, and interacting environmental risk factors.[152]

A number of Tier 1 conditions and genetic applications have passed the evidentiary test and are currently in widespread use. Networks continue to be formed to promote assessment of at-risk family members via cascade screening. Research to elucidate subtle genetic variants with a cumulative effect on individual and population health, to uncover the constitution of private mutations, and probe the meaning of variants of uncertain significance proceeds at a vigorous pace. This chapter has described correlated means of genetic assessment, such as large GWAS studies, whole-genome and exome sequencing, and the development of population-relevant risk scores. Each of these avenues deserves socioethical and scientific analysis and assessment, with room for public input.

The research system as a whole is also shifting to allow greater interoperability of patient information and research results. Until recently, it would have been impossible to conceptualize how to make inferences about the effects of very rare potentially deleterious mutations, but there are multiple avenues of research possible. National efforts to create secure and rapid mechanisms for health information exchange between healthcare providers within a state or nationally to help establish continuity between a patient's care across providers will have the added benefit of greatly accelerating the study of large numbers of individuals in communities. These pursuits will eventually lead to the linkage of genomic information with an individual's EHR.

Though thousands of genomic associations with diseases have been published, very few of these associations have moved into the Tier 1 or even Tier 2 category. The public's interest in genomics and the plethora of well-conducted association studies have been a major impetus for direct-to-consumer genetic testing companies to offer risk estimates and scores that satisfy the public's desire for information about their own genetic risks and ancestries. While recognizing the popular interest in genomic information, public health authorities caution that such information should be factored into the impact evaluation and outcomes review of ongoing studies as part of an evidentiary framework. Perhaps the simplest yet easiest to forget message is that basic tools like family health history and the use of national health statistics provide the most enabling means of directing health resources to where they are most needed. The paradox of preventive and public health genomics is that the majority of genomic discoveries are like grapes ripening on the vine, not yet ready for use. The growing volume of genomic and applicational discoveries is a source of great promise, yet we must continually assess the advantages and disadvantages of introducing them into communities and populations.

References

1. Cummings , M. *Human Heredity: Principles and Issues*. 5th ed. Pacific Grove, CA: Brooks/Cole; 2000.
2. Cavalli-Sforza LL, Bodmer W. *The Genetics of Human Populations*. Mineola, NY: Dover Publications; 2013.
3. Mikail CN. *Public Health Genomics: The Essentials*. San Francisco: Jossey-Bass; 2008.
4. Khoury MJ, Bedrosian SR, Gwinn M, et al. Human genome epidemiology: The road map revisited. In: Khoury MJ, Bedrosian SR, Gwinn M, Higgins JPT, Ioannidis JPA, Little JKhoury MJ, Bedrosian SR, Gwinn M, Higgins JPT, Ioannidis JPA, Little J, eds. *Human Genome Epidemiology*. 2nd ed. New York: Oxford University Press; 2010; pp. 3–12.
5. Gibbons GH. Charting our future together: Turning discovery science into cardiovascular health. *Circulation*. 2017;136(7):615–7.
6. Vohl M-C, Moorjan S, Roy M, et al. Geographic distribution of French-Canadian low-density lipoprotein receptor gene mutations in the Province of Quebec. *Clin Genet*. 1997;52(1):1–6.
7. Hill AV. The genomics and genetics of human infectious disease susceptibility. *Annu Rev Genomics Human Genet*. 2001;2:967–77.
8. Zajac V. Evolutionary view of the AIDS process. *J Int Med Res*. 2018;46(10):4032–8.
9. Rotimi CN, Bentley AR, Doumatey AP, et al. The genomic landscape of African populations in health and disease. *Hum Mol Genet*. 2017;26 (R2):R225–36.
10. Nielsen R, Slatkin M. *An Introduction to Population Genetics: Theory and Applications*. Sunderland, MA: Sinauer Associates; 2013.
11. Khoury MJ, Beaty TH, Cohen BH. *Fundamentals of Genetic Epidemiology*. New York: Oxford University Press; 1993.
12. Centers for Disease Control and Prevention. Picture of America—Prevention. https://www.cdc.gov/pictureofamerica/pdfs/picture_of_america_prevention.pdf. Atlanta, GA. 2019.
13. Wang G, Watts C. The role of genetics in the provision of essential public health services. *Am J Public Health*. 2007;97(4):620–5.
14. Juengst ET. "Prevention" and the goals of medicine. *Hum Gene Ther*. 1995;6(12):1595–605.
15. McGowan ML, Cho D, Sharp RR. The changing landscape of carrier screening: Expanding technology and options? *Health Matrix Clevel*. 2013;23:15–33.
16. Dungan JS. Carrier screening for cystic fibrosis. *Obstet Gynecol Clin North Am*. 2010;37(1):47–59.
17. Goetzinger KR, Cahill AG. An update on cystic fibrosis screening. *Clin Lab Med*. 2010;30(3):533–43.
18. Hospital for Sick Children: Cystic fibrosis mutation database. http://www.genet.sickkids.on.ca/StatisticsPage.html. Toronto, ON. 2011.
19. Alper OM, Wong L-J, Yong S, et al. Identification of novel and rare mutations in California Hispanics and African American cystic fibrosis patients. *Hum Mutat*. 2004;24(4):353.
20. Farrell PM, Fost N. Prenatal screening for cystic fibrosis: Where are we now? *J Pediatr*. 2002;141(6):758–63.
21. Langfelder-Schwind E, Kloza E, Sugarman E, et al. Cystic fibrosis prenatal screening in genetic counseling practice: Recommendations of the National Society of Genetic Counselors. *J Genet Couns*. 2005;14(1):1–15.
22. Knowles JW, Rader DJ, Khoury MJ. Cascade screening for familial hypercholesterolemia and the use of genetic testing. *JAMA*. 2017;318(4):381–2.
23. McClaren BJ, Metcalfe SA, Aitken M, et al. Uptake of carrier testing in families after cystic fibrosis diagnosis through newborn screening. *Eur J Hum Genet*. 2010;18(10):1084–9.
24. Dugueperoux I, L'Hostis C, Audrezet M-P, et al. Highlighting the impact of cascade carrier testing in cystic fibrosis families. *J Cyst Fibros*. 2016;15(4):452–9.
25. Bombard Y, Miller F, Berg CJ. A secondary benefit: The reproductive impact of carrier results from newborn screening for cystic fibrosis. *Genet Med*. 2017;19(4):403–11.
26. California Department of Public Health. California Prenatal Screening Program. https://www.cdph.ca.gov/Programs/CFH/DGDS/CDPH%20Document%20Library/PNS%20Documents/Patient%20Booklet%20Consent_ENG-ADA.pdf. Richmond, CA. 2017.
27. Faden RR, Chwalow AJ, Orel-Crosby E, et al. What participants understand about a maternal serum alpha-fetoprotein screening program. *Am J Public Health*. 1985;75(12):1381–4.
28. Khoury MJ. Relationship between medical genetics and public health: Changing the paradigm of disease prevention and the definition of a genetic disease. *Am J Med Genet*. 1997;71(3):289–91.

29. Kelley K, Stone C, Manning A, Swede H. Population-based biobanks and genetics research in Connecticut. https://portal.ct.gov/-/media/Departments-and-Agencies/DPH/dph/Genomics/BiobanksPolicyBriefpdf.pdf?la=en. Hartford, CT. 2007.
30. Khoury MJ. From genes to public health: The applications of genetic technology in disease prevention. Genetics Working Group. *Am J Public Health*. 1996;86(12):1717–22.
31. St. Louis AM, Kim K, Browne M, et al. Prevalence trends of selected major birth defects: A multi-state population-based retrospective study, United States, 1999 to 2007. *Birth Defects Res*. 2017;109(18):1442–50.
32. Kirby RS. The prevalence of selected major birth defects in the United States. *Semin Perinatol*. 2017;41(6):333–44.
33. Centers for Disease Control and Prevention. Folic acid helps prevent some birth defects. https://www.cdc.gov/features/folicacidbenefits/index.html. Atlanta, GA. 2019.
34. Sawaengsri H, Bergethon PR, Qui WQ, et al. Transcobalamin 776C->G polymorphism is associated with peripheral neuropathy in elderly individuals with high folate intake. *Am J Clin Nutr*. 2016;104(6):1665–70.
35. Yusuf HR, Lloyd-Puryear MA, Grant AM, et al. Sickle cell disease: The need for a public health agenda. *Am J Prev Med*. 2011;41(6S4):S376–383.
36. Michigan Department of Health and Human Services. A public health strategic plan to address sickle cell disease across the lifespan: 2015–2018. https://www.michigan.gov/documents/mdhhs/MDHHS_Final_SCD_Strategic_Plan_504325_7.pdf. Lansing, MI. 2015.
37. Centers for Disease Control and Prevention. Registry and Surveillance System for hemoglobinopathies (RuSH). https://www.cdc.gov/ncbddd/hemoglobinopathies/rush.html. Atlanta, GA. 2017.
38. Centers for Disease Control and Prevention. Public health research, epidemiology, and surveillance for hemoglobinopathies (PHRESH). https://www.cdc.gov/ncbddd/hemoglobinopathies/phresh.html. Atlanta, GA. 2017.
39. Centers for Disease Control and Prevention. Sickle cell disease and pregnancy. https://www.cdc.gov/ncbddd/sicklecell/pregnancy.html. Atlanta, GA. 2017.
40. Centers for Disease Control and Prevention. Family health history: Tools and resources. https://www.cdc.gov/genomics/famhistory/famhist_tools_resources.htm. Atlanta, GA. 2017.
41. American College of Obstetricians and Gynecologists. Screening for fetal aneuploidy. ACOG Practice bulletin no. 163. *Obstetr and Gynecol.* 2016;127:5:e123–37.
42. Theodoridou S, Alemayehou M, Prappas N, et al. Carrier screening and prenatal diagnosis of hemoglobinopathies. A study of indigenous and immigrant couples in northern Greece, over the last 5 years. *Hemoglobin*. 2008;32(5):434–9.
43. Kyrri AR, Kalogerou E, Loizidou D, et al. The changing epidemiology of beta-thalassemia in the Greek-Cypriot population. *Hemoglobin*. 2013;37(5):435–43.
44. Basran RK, Patterson M, Walker L, et al. Prenatal diagnosis of hemoglobinopathies in Ontario, Canada. *Ann N Y Acad Sci*. 2005;1054:507–10.
45. Wang X, Seaman C, Paik M, et al. Experience with 500 prenatal diagnoses of sickle cell diseases: The effect of gestational age on affected pregnancy outcome. *Prenat Diagn*. 1994;14(9):851–7.
46. Rowley PT. Prenatal screening for hemoglobinopathies. I. A prospective regional trial. *Am J Hum Genet*. 1991;48(3):439–46.
47. Dormandy E, Gulliford M, Bryan S, et al. Effectiveness of earlier antenatal screening for sickle cell disease and thalasaemia in primary care: Cluster randomized trial. *BMJ*. 2010;341:c5132.
48. Wilson JMG, Jungner G. Principles and practice of screening for disease. *Public Health Papers*. 34. Geneva: World Health Organization; 1968, pp. 1–163.
49. Gonzalez J, Willis MS. Robert Guthrie, MD, PhD: Clinical chemistry/microbiology. *Lab Med*. 2009;40(12): 748–9.
50. Benson JM, Therrell BL, Jr. History and current status of newborn screening for hemoglobinopathies. *Semin Perinatol*. 2010;34(2):134–44.
51. Farrell PM, Kosorok MR, Rock MJ, et al. Newborn screening for cystic fibrosis: A paradigm for public health genetics policy development. In: Khoury MJ, Burke W, Thomson EJKhoury MJ, Burke W, Thomson EJ, eds. *Genetics and Public Health in the 21st Century*. New York: Oxford University Press; 2000, pp. 405–29.
52. U.S. National Institute of Child Health and Human Development. Brief history of newborn screening. https://www.nichd.nih.gov/health/topics/newborn/conditioninfo/history. Rockville, MD. 2017.
53. U.S. Health Resources & Services Administration. Conditions added to the Recommended Uniform Screening Panel (RUSP) by the Secretary. https://www.hrsa.gov/advisory-committees/heritable-disorders/rusp/previous-nominations.html. Rockville, MD. 2019.
54. Baby's first test: Conditions screened by state. https://www.babysfirsttest.org/newborn-screening/states. Washington, DC. 2019.
55. Johnson T, Wile M. State newborn health screening policies. http://www.ncsl.org/research/health/state-newborn-health-screening-policies.aspx. Washington, DC. 2017.
56. Feuchtbaum L, Carter J, Dowray S, et al. Birth prevalence of disorders detectable through newborn screening by race/ethnicity. *Genet Med*. 2012;14(11):937–45.
57. Frempong T, Pearson HA. Newborn screening coupled with comprehensive follow-up reduced early mortality of sickle cell disease in Connecticut. *Conn Med*. 2007;71(1):9–12.
58. Grosse SD. Assessing the evidence for clinical utility in newborn screening. In: Khoury MJ, Bedrosian SR, Gwinn M, Higgins JPT, Ioannidis JPA, Little JKhoury MJ, Bedrosian SR, Gwinn M, Higgins JPT, Ioannidis JPA, Little J, eds. *Human Genome Epidemiology*. 2nd ed. New York: Oxford University Press; 2010, pp. 517–32.
59. Botkin JR, Rothwell E. Whole genome sequencing and newborn screening. *Curr Genet Med Rep*. 2016;4(1):1–6.
60. Knoppers BM, Senecal K, Borry P, Avard D. Whole-genome sequencing in newborn screening programs. *Sci Transl Med*. 2014;6(229):229cm2.
61. Tarini BA, Goldenberg AJ. Ethical issues with newborn screening in the genomics era. *Annu Rev Genomics Hum Genet*. 2012;13:381–93.
62. Friedman JM, Cornel MC, Goldenberg AJ, et al. Genomic newborn screening: Public health policy considerations and recommendations. *BMC Med Genomics*. 2017;10(9):9.
63. Bodian DL, Klein E, Iyer RK, et al. Utility of whole-genome sequencing for detection of newborn screening disorders in a population cohort of 1,696 neonates. *Genet Med*. 2016;18(3):221–30.
64. Genomes to People (G2P). The BabySeq Project. https://www.genomes2people.org/research/babyseq. Boston, MA. 2019.
65. California Department of Public Health. California Biobank Program (CBP). https://www.cdph.ca.gov/Programs/CFH/DGDS/Pages/cbp/Information-For-Researchers-and-Health-Care-Providers.aspx. Richmond, CA. 2019.
66. Michigan BioTrust for Health. Michigan Neonatal Biobank—Community. https://mnb.wayne.edu/community. Detroit, MI. 2017.
67. Modell SM, Citrin T, Platt JE, Kardia SLR. Distinctive features of public health ethics in the domain of expanded genetic screening and population biobanking. In: Pope JPope J, ed. *Patient Rights: Ethical Perspectives, Emerging Developments and Global Challenges*. Hauppauge, NY: Nova Science Publishers; 2015, pp. 1–27.
68. Haak PT, Busik JV, Kort EJ, et al. Archived unfrozen neonatal blood spots are amendable to quantitative gene expression analysis. *Neonatology*. 2009;95(3):210–6.
69. Bodian DL, McCutcheon JN, Kothiyal P, et al. Germline variation in cancer-susceptibility genes in a healthy, ancestrally diverse cohort: Implications for individual genome sequencing. *PLoS One*. 2014;9(4):e94554.
70. Manolio T. Case-control and cohort studies in the age of genome-wide associations. In: Khoury MJ, Bedrosian SR, Gwinn M, Higgins JPT, Ioannidis JPA, Little JKhoury MJ, Bedrosian SR, Gwinn M, Higgins JPT, Ioannidis JPA, Little J, eds. *Human Genome Epidemiology*. 2nd ed. New York: Oxford University Press; 2010, pp. 100–19.
71. Teutsch SM, Bradley LA, Palomaki GE, et al. The evaluation of genomic applications in Practice and Prevention (EGAPP) initiative: Methods of the EGAPP Working Group. In: Khoury MJ, Bedrosian SR, Gwinn M, Higgins JPT, Ioannidis JPA, Little JKhoury MJ, Bedrosian SR, Gwinn M, Higgins JPT, Ioannidis JPA, Little J, eds. *Human Genome Epidemiology*. 2nd ed. New York: Oxford University Press; 2010, pp. 458–81.
72. Centers for Disease Control and Prevention, Office of Public Health Genomics. Tier table database. https://phgkb.cdc.gov/PHGKB/topicStartPage.action. Atlanta, GA. 2018.
73. Dotson WD, Douglas MP, Kolor K. Prioritizing genomic applications for action by level of evidence: A horizon-scanning method. *Clin Pharmacol Ther*. 2014;95(4):394–402.
74. Centers for Disease Control and Prevention, Office of Public Health Genomics. Tier 1 genomics applications and their importance to public health. https://www.cdc.gov/genomics/implementation/toolkit/tier1.htm. Atlanta, GA. 2014.
75. U.S. National Library of Medicine, Genetics Home Reference. What are the types of genetic tests? https://ghr.nlm.nih.gov/primer/testing/uses. Rockville, MD. 2019.

76. Weir HK, Anderson RN, Coleman King SM, et al. Heart disease and cancer deaths—Trends and projections in the United States, 1969–2020. *Prev Chronic Dis*. 2016;13:E17.
77. Illinois Department of Public Health. BRCA1 & BRCA2. http://www.dph.illinois.gov/topics-services/life-stages-populations/genomics/brac1-2. Springfield, IL. 2019.
78. Centers for Disease Control and Prevention, Office of Public Health Genomics. More Detailed Information on Key Tier 1 Applications—Hereditary Breast and Ovarian Cancer (HBOC). https://www.cdc.gov/genomics/implementation/toolkit/hboc_1.htm. Atlanta, GA. 2014.
79. U.S. National Cancer Institute. BRCA Mutations: Cancer Risk and Genetic Testing. https://www.cancer.gov/about-cancer/causes-prevention/genetics/brca-fact-sheet. Bethesda, MD. 2018.
80. Coughlin SS, Burke W. Public health assessment of genetic predisposition to cancer. In: Khoury MJ, Burke W, Thomson EJKhoury MJ, Burke W, Thomson EJ, eds. *Genetics and Public Health in the 21st Century*. New York: Oxford University Press; 2000, pp. 151–71.
81. Fackenthal JD, Olopade OI. Breast cancer risk associated with BRCA1 and BRCA2 in diverse populations. *Nat Rev Cancer*. 2007;7(12):937–48.
82. Petrucelli N, Daly MB, Pal T. *BRCA1*- and *BRCA2*-associated hereditary breast and ovarian cancer. In: Adam MP, Ardinger HH, Pagon RA, et al., eds.Adam MP, Ardinger HH, Pagon RA, et al., eds. *GeneReviews*. Seattle: University of Washington; 2016, pp. 1–43.
83. U.S. Preventive Services Task Force. Final recommendation statement: BRCA-related cancer: Risk assessment, genetic counseling, and genetic testing. https://www.uspreventiveservicestaskforce.org/Page/Document/RecommendationStatementFinal/brca-related-cancer-risk-assessment-genetic-counseling-and-genetic-testing. Rockville, MD. 2013.
84. U.S. Department of Health and Human Services. Healthy People 2010: Genomics. https://www.healthypeople.gov/2020/topics-objectives/topic/genomics. Washington, DC. 2014.
85. U.S. National Cancer Institute. The Breast Cancer Risk Assessment Tool. https://bcrisktool.cancer.gov. Bethesda, MD. 2019.
86. Genetic Alliance. "Does it run in the family?" Toolkit. http://www.geneticalliance.org/publications/fhhtoolkit. Washington, DC. 2012.
87. Michigan Department of Health and Human Services. Family history and HBOC. https://www.michigan.gov/mdhhs/0,5885,7-339-73971_4911_4916_47257_68337-356290--,00.html. Lansing, MI. 2019.
88. Trivers K, Rodriguez JL, Cox SL, et al. The activities and impact of state programs to address hereditary breast and ovarian cancer, 2011–2014. *Healthcare (Basel)*. 2015; 3(4):948–63.
89. Lieberman S, Lahad A, Tomwer A, et al. Familial communication and cascade testing among relatives of *BRCA* population screening participants. *Genet Med*. 2018;20(11):1446–54.
90. Tuffaha HW, Mitchell A, Ward RL, et al. Cost-effectiveness analysis of germ-line BRCA testing in women with breast cancer and cascade testing in family members of mutation carriers. *Genet Med*. 2018;20(9):985–94.
91. Manchanda R, Patel S, Antoniou AC, et al. Cost-effectiveness of population based BRCA testing with varying Ashkenazi Jewish ancestry. *Am J Obstet Gynecol*. 2017;217(5):578.e1–12.
92. Rubinstein WS, Jiang H, Dellefave L, et al. Cost-effectiveness of population-based BRCA1/2 testing and ovarian cancer prevention for Ashkenazi Jews: A call for dialogue. *Genet Med*. 2009;11(9):629–39.
93. Ponte A, Greenberg S, Greendale K, Senier L. Moving the needle on action around evidence-based screening for hereditary conditions: Preparing state chronic disease directors to advance precision public health. *Public Health Rep*. 2019;134(3):228–33.
94. Khoury MJ, Bowen MS, Clyne M, et al. From public health to precision public health: A 20-year journey. *Genet Med*. 2018;20(6):574–82.
95. Afghahi A, Kurian AW. The changing landscape of genetic testing for inherited breast cancer predisposition. *Curr Treat Options Oncol*. 2017;18(5):27.
96. Grover S, Syngal S. Risk assessment, genetic testing, and management of Lynch Syndrome. *J Natl Compr Canc Netw*. 2010;8(1):98–105.
97. Centers for Disease Control and Prevention, Office of Public Health Genomics. More detailed information on key Tier 1 applications—Lynch syndrome. https://www.cdc.gov/genomics/implementation/toolkit/lynch_1.htm. Atlanta, GA. 2014.
98. American Society of Clinical Oncology, Cancer.Net. Lynch syndrome. https://www.cancer.net/cancer-types/lynch-syndrome. Alexandria, VA. 2018.
99. Campbell H, Hawken S, Theodoratou E, et al. Colorectal cancer. In: Khoury MJ, Bedrosian SR, Gwinn M, Higgins JPT, Ioannidis JPA, Little JKhoury MJ, Bedrosian SR, Gwinn M, Higgins JPT, Ioannidis JPA, Little J, eds. *Human Genome Epidemiology*. 2nd ed. New York: Oxford University Press; 2010, pp. 249–77.
100. U.S. National Library of Medicine, Genetics Home Reference. Lynch syndrome. https://ghr.nlm.nih.gov/condition/lynch-syndrome. Rockville, MD. 2019.
101. Bhandari A, Woodhouse M, Gupta S. Colorectal cancer is a leading cause of cancer incidence and mortality among adults younger than 50 years in the USA: A SEER-based analysis with comparison to other young-onset cancers. *J Invest Med*. 2017;65(2):311–15.
102. Ahnen DJ, Wade SW, Jones WF, et al. The increasing incidence of young-onset colorectal cancer: A call to action. *Mayo Clin Proc*. 2014;89(2):216–24.
103. Illinois Department of Public Health. Lynch Syndrome: For health care professionals. http://www.dph.illinois.gov/topics-services/life-stages-populations/genomics/lynch-syndrome-hcp. Springfield, IL. 2019.
104. Kohlmann W, Gruber SB. Lynch syndrome. In: Adam MP, Ardinger HH, Pagon RA, et al., eds. *GeneReviews*. Seattle: University of Washington; 2018, pp. 1–34.
105. Michigan Department of Health and Human Services. Lynch syndrome (LS). Available at https://www.michigan.gov/mdhhs/0,5885,7-339-73971_4911_4916_47257_68337-357147--,00.html. Lansing, MI. 2019.
106. Gupta S, Provenzale D, Regenbogen SE, et al. NCCN guidelines: Genetic/familial high-risk assessment: Colorectal, Version 3.2017. *J Natl Compr Canc Netw*. 2017;15(12):1465–75.
107. Centers for Disease Control and Prevention, Office of Public Health Genomics. My family health portrait. https://phgkb.cdc.gov/FHH/html/index.html. Atlanta, GA. 2018.
108. Kastrinos F, Uno H, Ukaegbu C, et al. Development and validation of the $PREMM_5$ model for comprehensive risk assessment of Lynch syndrome. *J Clin Oncol*. 2017;35(19):2165–72.
109. Evaluation of Genomic Applications in Practice and Prevention (EGAPP) Working Group. Recommendations from the EGAPP Working Group: Genetic testing strategies in newly diagnosed individuals with colorectal cancer aimed at reducing morbidity and mortality from Lynch syndrome in relatives. *Genet Med*. 2009;11(1):35–41.
110. Esteban-Jurado C, Vila-Casadesus M, Garre Pilar, et al. Whole-exome sequencing identifies rare pathogenic variants in new predisposition genes for familial colorectal cancer. *Genet Med*. 2015;17(2):131–42.
111. Valle L. Recent discoveries in the genetics of familial colorectal cancer and polyposis. *Clin Gastroenterol Hepatol*. 2017;15(6):809–19.
112. Centers for Disease Control and Prevention, Office of Public Health Genomics. Lynch syndrome phase 1. www.cdc.gov/genomics/implementation/toolkit/lynch_2.htm. Atlanta, GA. 2014.
113. Grosse SD. When is genomic testing cost-effective? Testing for Lynch syndrome in patients with newly-diagnosed colorectal cancer and their relatives. *Healthcare (Basel)*. 2015;3(4):860–78.
114. Mange S, Belcross C, Cragun D, et al. Creation of a network to promote universal screening for Lynch syndrome: The Lynch Syndrome Screening Network. *J Genet Counsel*. 2015;24(3):421–7.
115. Youngblom E, Parianai M, Knowles JW. Familial hypercholesterolemia. In: Adam MP, Ardinger HH, Pagon RA, et al., eds. *GeneReviews*. Seattle: University of Washington; 2016, pp. 1–31.
116. Centers for Disease Control and Prevention, Office of Public Health Genomics. More detailed information on key Tier 1 applications—Familial hypercholesterolemia. https://www.cdc.gov/genomics/implementation/toolkit/fh_1.htm. Atlanta, GA. 2014.
117. U.S. National Library of Medicine, Genetics Home Reference. Hypercholesterolemia. https://ghr.nlm.nih.gov/condition/hypercholesterolemia. Rockville, MD. 2019.
118. Rosenson RS, Durrington P. Familial hypercholesterolemia in adults: Overview, edited by Freeman MW, Saperia GM. https://www.uptodate.com/contents/familial-hypercholesterolemia-in-adults-overview. Waltham, MA. 2019.
119. Cenarro A, Etxabarria A, de Castro-Oros I, et al. The p.Leu167del mutation in APOE gene causes autosomal dominant hypercholesterolemia by down-regulation of LDL receptor expression in hepatocytes. *J Endocrinol Metab*. 2016;101(5):2113–21.
120. Usifo E, Leigh SE, Whittall RA, et al. Low-density lipoprotein receptor gene familial hypercholesterolemia variant database: Update and pathological assessment. *Ann Human Genet*. 2012;76(5):387–401.
121. Malo J, Parajuli A, Walker S. PCSK9: From molecular biology to clinical applications. *Ann Clin Biochem*. 2020;57(1):7–25.

122. El Khouri P, Elbitar S, Ghaleb Y, et al. PCSK9 mutations in familial hypercholesterolemia: From a groundbreaking discovery to anti-PCSK9 therapies. *Curr Atheroscler Rep*. 2017;19(12):49.

123. Williams RR, Hopkins PN, Wu LL, Hunt SC. Applying genetic strategies to prevent atherosclerosis. In: Khoury MJ, Burke W, Thomson EJKhoury MJ, Burke W, Thomson EJ, eds. *Genetics and Public Health in the 21st Century*. New York: Oxford University Press; 2000, pp. 463–85.

124. FH Foundation. Familial hypercholesterolemia. https://thefhfoundation.org/fh-diagnosis-management-and-family-screening. Pasadena, LA. 2015.

125. Mukerji S, Hanna B, Duquette D, et al. Sudden cardiac death of the young in Michigan: Development and implementation of a novel mortality review system. *J Community Health*. 2010;35(6):689–97.

126. Modell SM, Bradley DJ, Lehmann MH. Genetic testing for long QT syndrome and the category of cardiac ion channelopathies. *PLoS Curr*. 2012;4:e4f9995f69e6c7.

127. Centers for Disease Control and Prevention, Office of Public Health Genomics. Cascade screening for familial hypercholesterolemia in the United States: Public health impact and challenges. https://blogs.cdc.gov/genomics/2017/07/25/cascade_screening. Atlanta, GA. 2017.

128. Wonderling D, Umans-Eckenhausen MA, Marks D, et al. Cost-effectiveness analysis of the genetic screening program for familial hypercholesterolemia in The Netherlands. *Semin Vasc Med*. 2004;4(1):97–104.

129. Modell SM, Greendale K, Citrin T, Kardia SLR. Expert and advocacy group consensus findings on the horizon of public health genetic testing. *Healthcare (Basel)*. 2016;4(1):E14.

130. Natarajan P, Young R, Stitziel NO, et al. Polygenic risk score identifies subgroup with higher burden of atherosclerosis and greater relative benefit from statin therapy in the primary prevention setting. *Circulation*. 2017;135(22):2091–2101.

131. Dron JS, Wang J, Low-Kam C, et al. Polygenic determinants in extremes of high-density lipoprotein cholesterol. *J Lipid Res*. 2017;58(11):2162–70.

132. Hansen MF, Johansen J, Sylvander AE, et al. Use of multigene-panel identifies pathogenic variants in several CRC-predisposing genes in patients previously tested for Lynch Syndrome. *Clin Genet*. 2017;92(4):405–14.

133. Mamlin BW, Tierney WM. The promise of information and communication technology in healthcare: Extracting value from the chaos. *Am J Med Sci*. 2016;351(1):59–68.

134. Ghaleb Y, Elbitar S, El Khoury P, et al. Usefulness of the genetic risk score to identify phenocopies in families with familial hypercholesterolemia? *Eur J Hum Genet*. 2018;26(4):570–578.

135. Khera AV, Chaffin M, Aragam KG, et al. Genome-wide polygenic scores for common diseases identify individuals with risk equivalent to monogenic mutations. *Nat Genet*. 2018;50(9):1219–24.

136. Karow J. ASHG: High Polygenic Risk Score for heart disease motivates patients to make lifestyle changes. https://www.genomeweb.com/cardiovascular-disease/ashg-high-polygenic-risk-score-heart-disease-motivates-patients-make#.XVqB_-hKi70. 2018.

137. Khoury MJ, Mensah GA. Is it time to integrate Polygenic Risk Scores into clinical practice? Let's do the science first and follow the evidence wherever it takes us! https://blogs.cdc.gov/genomics/2019/06/03/is-it-time. 2019.

138. Costich JF, Durst AL. The impact of the Affordable Care Act on funding for newborn screening services. *Public Health Rep*. 2016;131(1):160–6.

139. Therrell BL, Williams D, Johnson K, et al. Financing newborn screening: Sources, issues, and future considerations. *J Public Health Manag Pract*. 2007;13(2):207–13.

140. Latchaw M, Ormond K, Smith M, et al. Health insurance coverage of genetic services in Illinois. *Genet Med*. 2010;12(8):525–31.

141. Cragun D, Weidner A, Lewis C, et al. Racial disparities in BRCA testing and cancer risk management across a population-based sample of young breast cancer survivors. *Cancer*. 2017;123(13):2497–2505.

142. Clain E, Trosman JR, Douglas MP, et al. Availability and payer coverage of BRCA1/2 tests and gene panels. *Nat Biotechnol*. 2015;33(9):900–2.

143. Ricker C, Culver JO, Lowstuter K, et al. Increased yield of actionable mutations using multi-gene panels to assess hereditary cancer susceptibility in an ethnically diverse clinical cohort. *Cancer Genet*. 2016;209(4):130–7.

144. Cruz-Correa M, Perez-Mayoral J, Dutil J, et al. Hereditary cancer syndromes in Latino populations: Genetic characterization and surveillance guidelines. *Hered Cancer Clin Pract*. 2017;15:3.

145. Martin AR, Kanai M, Kamatani Y, et al. Clinical use of current polygenic risk scores may exacerbate health disparities. *Nat Genet*. 2019;51(4):584–91.

146. Roberts MC, Khoury MJ, Mensah GA. Perspective: The clinical use of polygenic risk scores: Race, ethnicity, and health disparities. *Ethn Dis*. 2019;29(3):513–6.

147. Amendola LM, Berg JS, Horowitz CR, et al. The Clinical Sequencing Evidence-Generating Research Consortium: Integrating genomic sequencing in diverse and medically underserved populations. *Am J Hum Genet*. 2018;103(3):319–27.

148. Mokdad AH, Dwyer-Lindgren L, Fitzmaurice C, et al. Trends and patterns of disparities in cancer mortality among US counties, 1980-2014. *JAMA*. 2017;317(4):388–406.

149. Association of State and Territorial Health Officials. State options for enhancing health information exchange for MCH systems. http://www.astho.org/Maternal-and-Child-Health/Collaborations/MCH-and-Health-Information-Exchange-Issue-Brief. Arlington, VA. 2012.

150. Hulsen T, Jamuar SS, Moody AR, et al. From big data to precision medicine. *Front Med (Lausanne)*. 2019;6:34.

151. Barrett MA, Humblet O, Hiatt RA, Adler NE. Big data and disease prevention: From quantified self to quantified communities. *Big Data*. 2013;1(3):168–75.

152. Khoury MJ, Feero WG, Chambers DA, et al. A collaborative translational research framework for evaluating and implementing the appropriate use of human genome sequencing to improve health. *PLoS Med*. 2018;15(8):e1002631.

CHAPTER

9

Public Health Practice in the United States

Angela J. Beck • Phoebe K. G. Kulik

INTRODUCTION

Public health is the science of protecting and improving the health of populations, from small, local communities to entire countries and even regions of the world. It focuses on "what we, as a society, do collectively to assure the conditions in which people can be healthy."[1] Public health is charged with preventing epidemics and the spread of disease; protecting against environmental hazards; preventing injuries; promoting healthy behaviors; responding to disasters and assisting communities in recovery; and assuring the quality and accessibility of health services.[2] Core to public health's mission of health promotion and disease prevention is addressing the ***social determinants of health***—the conditions in the environments in which people live, work, and play that affect health outcomes and can disadvantage communities, often on the basis of characteristics including race, class, gender, wealth, and sexual orientation, among others.[3] Unequal distribution of resources and power contribute to avoidable and unjust health inequities in populations.[4] Public health works at multiple levels: through programs and policies that aim to address broader structural and systems factors that impact health; by implementing community interventions that focus on the social, behavioral, and environmental needs of specific populations; and through programs that help prompt individual behavior change that can improve health status. ***Public health practice*** refers to the implementation of programs and delivery of these services to improve the public's health. This chapter summarizes:

- The history of public health practice
- The core functions and essential services of public health
- The cross-sector partnerships critical for effective public health practice
- The importance of evidence-based decision making in public health
- The distinction between public health practice and public health research
- The alignment of academia and public health practice

HISTORY OF PUBLIC HEALTH PRACTICE

Public health practice in the late nineteenth to twentieth centuries is sometimes referred to as Public Health 1.0.[5] It was during this time that the health of a population came to also be seen as a public and societal concern, rather than solely the result of individual choices.[1] Increasing urban and industrial environments led to the rise of sanitation and hygienic issues, resulting in the creation of some of the key infrastructures of the public health system. In London, the 1842 *General Report on the Sanitary Conditions of the Labouring Population of Great Britain* by Edwin Chadwick and the Poor Law Commission influenced the Public Health Act of 1848 and the establishment of national and local boards of health in England and Wales.[1,6] In the United States, survey reports highlighting issues with poor sanitation similarly prompted the development of boards of health.[1] Two such influential reports were *The Sanitary Condition of the Labouring Population of New York* by John Griscom in 1848 and the 1850 *Report of the Massachusetts Sanitary Commission* by Lemuel Shattuck. Over the next 50 years, state and local health departments continued to form across the country, along with public health laboratories accompanied by new scientific advances in the investigation and control of disease.[1] In the early 1900s, health departments broadened their scope of services to incorporate clinical care and health education to address contagious disease and to promote health more generally. As the twentieth century got underway, an epidemiologic transition occurred in the United States as leading causes of death shifted from infectious etiologies to noncommunicable and chronic illnesses resulting in major changes in the burden of disease.[7,8]

Public Health 2.0 refers to public health practice in the second half of the twentieth century.[5] In alignment with political and social values of the times, governmental public health at the federal, state, and local levels expanded programs focused on supporting vulnerable populations.[1] These included new programmatic emphases on maternal and child health, mental health, and Medicaid/Medicare, among other priorities. Over time, key organizations worked to define parameters and standards for the field of public health during this era, as described later in this chapter.[1,5]

Public Health 3.0 denotes contemporary public health practice in the twenty-first century. This characterization represents an initiative of the U.S. Department of Health and Human Services that seeks to bolster a public health system that can address population health challenges and the social determinants of health through cross-sectoral collaboration.[5] Five recommendations form the foundation for this vision:

1. Public health leaders should serve in the role of **Chief Health Strategist** and act as a convener of partners within their communities.
2. Public health departments should establish structured **cross-sector partnerships** that lend toward shared resources and greater capacity for action.
3. National **accreditation** criteria should be updated to support Public Health 3.0 efforts.
4. High-quality, **actionable data** should be accessible at granular levels across the country, and clear metrics to evaluate public health practice especially as it relates to the social determinants of health and health equity should be developed.
5. **Funding models** should be enhanced and sustained to support Public Health 3.0-type practice.

Conceptualization of the purpose of and partners in the public health system continues to evolve to support advances in population health outcomes.

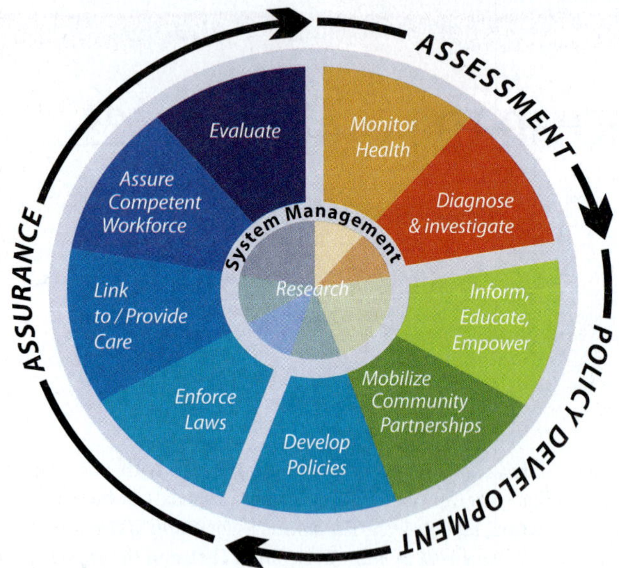

FIGURE 9-1. The ten Essential Public Health Services.

CORE FUNCTIONS AND ESSENTIAL SERVICES OF PUBLIC HEALTH

The ***public health system*** includes "all public, private, and voluntary entities that contribute to the delivery of essential public health services within a jurisdiction."[9] Central to the system are state, local, tribal, and territorial public health agencies, many of which have legal authority and responsibility for ensuring the health of the public through programs, services, and other means. Other entities comprising a component of the public health system include those that deliver primary care, behavioral health, or social services. Faith-based institutions, community centers, schools, various types of nonprofit organizations, and policy makers also contribute to the public health system.

In 1988, during the Public Health 2.0 period, a landmark Institute of Medicine (IOM)[1] report asserted that the public health system was in "disarray" and emphasized a need for the field to better define its purpose and contribution to population health.[1,5] Prompted by this report, a collection of key stakeholders representing national public health professional organizations and federal agencies that were engaged in public health work convened a committee that articulated the ten Essential Public Health Services that describe the public health activities all communities should undertake. The Essential Public Health Services align with the three core functions of public health designated by the IOM: assessment, policy development, and assurance (Fig. 9-1).[9] They include:

1. Monitor health status to identify and solve community health problems
2. Diagnose and investigate health problems and health hazards in the community
3. Inform, educate, and empower people about health issues
4. Mobilize community partnerships and action to identify and solve health problems
5. Develop policies and plans that support individual and community health efforts
6. Enforce laws and regulations that protect health and ensure safety
7. Link people to needed personal health services and assure the provision of healthcare when otherwise unavailable
8. Assure competent public and personal healthcare workforce
9. Evaluate effectiveness, accessibility, and quality of personal and population-based health services
10. Research for new insights and innovative solutions to health problems

The ten Essential Public Health Services form the foundation for public health practice activities.

CROSS-SECTOR PUBLIC HEALTH PRACTICE

As suggested in the vision for Public Health 3.0, public health practice and the implementation of the ten Essential Public Health Services is greatly enhanced by leveraging partnerships. While the Essential Public Health Services define the role of governmental public health agencies, the actual responsibility for carrying them out lies with the public health system as a whole.[10] Similarly, addressing the social determinants of health requires a systems-thinking approach. The Centers for Disease Control and Prevention (CDC), the nation's leading public health agency, provides examples of how public health agencies and partner institutions can incorporate the social determinants of health into delivery of the Essential Public Health Services (Table 9-1).[2,11]

Health equity, defined as everyone having "a fair and just opportunity to be as healthy as possible … requires removing obstacles to health such as poverty, discrimination, and their consequences."[4] Tackling major societal and social issues like these is beyond the scope of public health alone, of course, although doing so clearly has the potential for exerting a tremendous positive impact on population health. Rather, successfully addressing these challenges necessitates institutional and sociopolitical changes that involve working together with a range of stakeholders who have the capacity and authority to influence practice in their respective spheres.[10] Several major initiatives since the 1970s have shaped the discussion of partnerships within the field of public health by providing frameworks and strategies through which to pursue population health.

Collective Impact

The Public Health 3.0 framework emphasizes creativity in partner engagement, recognizing that professionals in other disciplines such as community organizing, business, and many others may bring different perspectives and approaches to problem solving.[5] Related to this is the idea of ***collective impact***, a framework for collaboration in which partnerships from different sectors come together around a common goal. These initiatives "involve a centralized infrastructure, a dedicated staff, and a structured process that leads to a common agenda, shared measurement, continuous communication, and mutually reinforcing activities among all participants."[12] These elements are common to a variety of approaches to partner-based work and collaboration.

Health in All Policies

Health in All Policies is an approach to cross-sectoral collaboration with global origins. The concept originated in Europe, building over time since the 1978 World Health Organization *Declaration of Alma-Ata* that emphasized the importance of aligning efforts between health services and other sectors for population health outcomes.[13,14] The 2013 *Helsinki Statement on Health in All Policies* defines it as "an approach to public policies across sectors that systematically takes into account the health implications of decisions, seeks synergies, and avoids harmful health impacts in order to improve population health and health equity."[14] That same year, the Public Health Institute and American Public Health Association released a guide for state and local governments in the United States that outlines five key elements of Health in All Policies initiatives:

[1] In 2015, the Institute of Medicine became the National Academy of Medicine. It is a member of the National Academies of Sciences, Engineering, and Medicine.

TABLE 9-1 ESSENTIAL PUBLIC HEALTH SERVICE ACTIVITIES AND SOCIAL DETERMINANTS OF HEALTH (SDOH)

Essential Public Health Service	Example Activities	Ways to Address SDOH
1. Monitor health status	Community health assessment; registries	Include SDOH measures in community health assessments; engage communities in assessment efforts
2. Diagnose and investigate	Investigate infections and water-, food-, and vector-borne disease outbreaks	Include community-level determinants of health in investigations (e.g., address deteriorating housing conditions to prevent lead poisoning and other health hazards)
3. Inform, educate, and empower	Health education and health promotion programming	Ensure education efforts address social and structural determinants of health inequities (e.g., structural racism). Ensure access to culturally and linguistically appropriate approaches to community health
4. Mobilize community partnerships	Partner with private sector, civic groups, nongovernmental organizations, faith community	Engage partners associated with SDOH (e.g., housing authorities, law enforcement, schools, and community organizations)
5. Develop policies	Strategic planning; community health improvement planning	Leverage evidence-based policies in nonhealth sectors that affect SDOH and health outcomes (e.g., safe and affordable housing policies). Develop community health improvement plans that address SDOH
6. Enforce laws	Review and enforce regulations and laws that affect public health	Develop strategies to ensure enforcement of existing regulations and laws that affect SDOH (e.g., housing and health codes, laws to prevent violence against women and children)
7. Link to/provide care	Establish links with primary care; engage in activities that ensure access to care	Educate community members about eligibility for and access to programs such as: Medicaid, Supplemental Nutrition Assistance Program. Ensure essential health benefits are provided equitably
8. Assure competent workforce	Public health workforce development and training; public health workforce research	Support staff training efforts that help workers incorporate SDOH into job responsibilities. Promote hiring of workforce that reflects population being served
9. Evaluate	Program evaluation and continuous quality improvement activities	Ensure evaluation and research designs include interventions that address SDOH inequity. Use performance management and quality improvement methods to explore and address root causes of health problems
10. Research	Identifying and sharing best practices; public health services and systems research	Expand research agendas to include SDOH and health outcomes. Use community-based participatory research designs. Apply evidence-based practices to address health inequity and demonstrate improved health outcomes

1. They **promote health, equity, and sustainability** through specific policies, programs, and processes, and by embedding these considerations into government decision-making processes.
2. They **support intersectoral collaboration** by connecting in an ongoing and authentic manner the entities whose work influences the social determinants of health.
3. They **benefit multiple partners** and take a win-win approach.
4. They **engage stakeholders** so that initiatives take into account community perspectives and result in meaningful impact on population health.
5. They **create structural or procedural change** so that the Health in All Policies lens becomes an institutionalized approach to decision making with the necessary infrastructure to support it.[13]

One tool for conducting Health in All Policies work is the ***health impact assessment*** (HIA), which can be used to determine the potential or expected health effects of a nonhealth-focused policy or decision.[15,16] These assessments often use mixed methods—quantitative/qualitative, primary/secondary data collection—in a specified five-step process that includes: screening to determine if an HIA is relevant to the policy at hand; scoping to identify possible stakeholders and relevant data; assessment of baseline conditions and projections of possible outcomes; recommendations to optimize the effect of the proposed policy; reporting to key stakeholders and decision makers; and monitoring and evaluation of the HIA process, its use, and the actual versus predicted health outcomes.[15,16]

In 2016, the Public Health—Seattle & King County local health department in the state of Washington conducted a rapid HIA regarding the South Park Community Center Open Space Design Plan.[17] In this case, Seattle Parks & Recreation aimed to address a community priority focused on improving the South Park Community Center by upgrading existing play areas as well as adding new areas. Although this was a positive effort, the community was concerned about the play area's proximity to a major highway. In response, the parks and recreation department partnered with the local health department, which implemented the HIA over 2 months to assess potential health impacts for design considerations. Data-collection methods included literature and secondary data reviews, air-quality sampling and noise testing, and qualitative input from subject-matter experts. Importantly, these experts represented nine different organizations and agencies, including a hospital, department of transportation, nonprofits, and local residents, among others. In the end, the health department found a number of negative and neutral possible impacts related to air quality, environmental noise, crime and safety, and social and mental health. They therefore anticipated that the design would be unlikely to substantially increase physical activity among the residents. The HIA concluded with seven recommendations for moving the improvement project forward but in a way that would benefit the community's health. The local health department also featured this HIA initiative in their larger, more comprehensive report around climate change and health.[18] In this plan, accounting for climate and health in policy and planning decisions is one of 15 key strategies that consider principles of health equity, community engagement, Health in All Policies, and systems thinking when working with myriad stakeholders and decision makers.

A state-based example is that of Vermont, where the Governor issued an executive order to form an interagency Health in All Policies Task Force in 2015.[19] This formal structure followed prior work of the Vermont Department of Health that focused on HIAs and collaborations with other (cross-sector) partners.[20] The Task Force included eight state agencies, which together have authority to implement broad-reaching initiatives. Activities of the Task Force have included, for example, inventorying best practices for Health in All Policies, conducting HIAs, creating a performance dashboard, and conducting a Total Health Expenditure Analysis to better understand investments in health across sectors. Some of the lessons learned across these initiatives as documented by the Vermont Department of Health are the importance of visible commitment from leadership, succession planning, having dedicated staff to implement projects, and framing activities to focus on mutual benefit.[19,20]

The Health in All Policies framework has also been implemented at the national level in countries around the world. A number of examples come from Central and South America. In Ecuador, the 2013–17 Plan Nacional Para el Buen Vivir (National Plan of Good Living) placed health within objectives related to the environment and workplace, and the plan as a whole addressed numerous social determinants of health.[21,22] In Guatemala, the 2012 Zero Hunger Plan involved numerous national and global partners including government, nonprofits, and other organizations to address malnutrition and food insecurity.[23] These are just two examples of many from across the globe, and they illustrate how Health in All Policies work may be a broad-facing approach or alternatively focus on a specific issue.

Interprofessional Education and Practice

Competencies that promote successful partnering across sectors are defined within the domains of interprofessional education (IPE) and practice. ***IPE*** is "when two or more professions learn about, from and with each other to enable effective collaboration and improve health outcomes."[24] Collaborative practice follows as professionals from different backgrounds work "with patients, their families, carers, and communities to deliver the highest quality of care across settings" by providing comprehensive services.[24] The Interprofessional Education Collaborative established a set of *Core Competencies for Interprofessional Collaborative Practice* in 2016 to guide IPE and practice efforts (Table 9-2).[25]

IPE and collaborative practice have been widely promoted by national associations, academic accrediting bodies, and formal legislation. The Patient Protection and Affordable Care Act of 2010 included provisions to promote interprofessional health teams for patient-centered medical homes, to include IPE within health professions graduate education, and to provide funding to rural physician training grants that include interprofessional partnerships.[26] IPE is a curricular focus area for students in public health, medicine, nursing, social work, and other health professions.[27] The literature suggests that interprofessional teams and training with other disciplines can be beneficial in a number of ways. For example, teamwork can enable resiliency to adjust to unforeseen changes, team members with different expertise can inform complex decisions, and effective team processes can promote effective communication.[28]

Though much discussion on IPE focuses on interaction between the health professions, it is not limited to those disciplines. Rather, the concept of IPE applies to a variety of public health partnerships such as those related to emergency preparedness and response activities.[24] In these situations, the range of stakeholders needed often goes beyond public health and healthcare to include law enforcement, other types of government workers, faith leaders, those working in food banks and other safety net nonprofits, etc. Moreover, the community itself is an important stakeholder in any population health activity. Factors that may help or hinder successful emergency preparedness and response efforts include trust between community and institutions, existing community engagement practices (e.g., meetings), cultural priorities, available resources, inclusion of vulnerable groups, and timelines, among others.[29] One can see how skills in working in teams, communicating effectively, understanding roles and lines of authority, and working with mutual respect would be necessary in an emergency situation beyond just the scope of the clinical healthcare team.

TABLE 9-2 CORE COMPETENCIES FOR INTERPROFESSIONAL COLLABORATIVE PRACTICE

Domain	Competency
Values/Ethics for Interprofessional Practice	Work with individuals of other professions to maintain a climate of mutual respect and shared values
Roles/ Responsibilities	Use the knowledge of one's own role and those of other professions to appropriately assess and address the healthcare needs of patients and to promote and advance the health of populations
Interprofessional Communication	Communicate with patients, families, communities, and professionals in health and other fields in a responsive and responsible manner that supports a team approach to the promotion and maintenance of health and the prevention and treatment of disease
Teams/Teamwork	Apply relationship-building values and the principles of team dynamics to perform effectively in different team roles to plan, deliver, and evaluate patient/population-centered care and population health programs and policies that are safe, timely, efficient, effective, and equitable

EVIDENCE-BASED DECISION MAKING IN PUBLIC HEALTH

While cross-sector and collaborative interprofessional practice are essential components for successful delivery of public health services, developing effective programs and policies are a primary goal for promoting and protecting the public's health. ***Evidence-based public health*** uses scientific findings to drive decisions about implementing public health programs or policies to improve population health outcomes.[30] This is important because the public health system has limited resources. Every dollar must be used wisely and this evidence can help ensure that interventions that work well are appropriately tailored and disseminated to communities that need them, and that ineffective interventions are modified before further implementation. An example of a national resource to support evidence-based public health is the Community Preventive Services Task Force, which was established by the U.S. Department of Health and Human Services to evaluate strengths and limitations of scientific studies about community-based health promotion programs and assess effectiveness.[31] Their findings are regularly published as *The Community Guide*.

Evidence-based public health is useful for public health practitioners developing programs and policies, for policy makers who make funding decisions about such initiatives, and for stakeholders who will be affected by the programs and policies. To adopt evidence-based public health, the following are needed:

- Accessible scientific information on the programs and policies most likely to be effective in promoting health
- The ability to translate that information on evidence-based practices and align it with the realities of the real world environment
- Dissemination of the information at state and local levels for adoption[30]

The type of data-driven evidence needed to inform public health programming decisions can take many forms. Epidemiologic data are generally quantitative in nature and provides descriptive statistics about health problems in a community, while qualitative data provides important additional context to the numbers and statistics. Stakeholder input, particularly from community members impacted by the proposed programs, helps identify potential barriers, unintended consequences, or facilitators that the quantitative data may not reveal. Results of policy or program evaluations are another important form of evidence that assess the efficiency and effectiveness of interventions in public health practice. This evidence is presented in the scientific literature, in public health surveillance data and community health needs assessment reports, and in reports and presentations documenting the findings of program evaluations. Summaries of town halls, focus groups, and other forums that engage community members and stakeholders are other forms of evidence used to inform public health decisions.

Decision making in public health practice is influenced in part by the best available research evidence, but also by the characteristics, needs, and values of the community being served; available resources to implement a program or policy; and the environment and organizational context of the community and its stakeholders.[30] Public health problems are always complex—considering all factors that determine whether an intervention may succeed or fail in a community is important. The scientific literature alone cannot do that. It is but one critical element to be considered as part of an evidence-based decision-making process.

Brownson and colleagues have proposed a seven-stage framework for adopting evidence-based public health.[30] The steps are nonlinear, and may have feedback loops and multiple iterations throughout each stage. To start the process, a community assessment determines the assets, resources, needs, and concerns of the community being served. This can happen through surveying a community and collecting qualitative data from community members. Next, the public health issue should be quantified—epidemiologic data are essential to this process. Third, public health practitioners should develop a concise statement of the public health issue. Following this, a scientific literature review determines what is known about the issue and what interventions have been effective in addressing the issue in similar communities. Fifth, program and policy options should be developed and prioritized. This information will need to be shared with the policy makers who control the necessary resources and with stakeholders who would be impacted by the program or policy, such as the community members. Next, an action plan is developed and the chosen intervention is implemented. The final step of the process is key—evaluating the policy or program. It is tempting to use all project resources on program implementation; however, if planners forgo program or policy evaluation, it is impossible to tell whether any improvement in population health outcomes is a result of the intervention or other factors. The results of the program evaluation then inform future community assessments (Fig. 9-2).[30,32]

By most accounts, the evidence-based public health framework is intuitive. It makes sense to implement this process to maximize the effectiveness of the public health interventions we pursue—so why is this strategy not always used? Several factors create challenges to adopting the evidence-based public health process. These may include lack of political will on the part of policy makers, deficits in relevant/timely research, lack of information systems to generate the necessary data to inform interventions, or lack of resources or leadership to support the process.[30] Facilitators to the process include effective dissemination of timely research, having advocates of the evidence empowered within organizations to help drive change and innovation, and having strong leadership within the institution. The organization's leadership influences

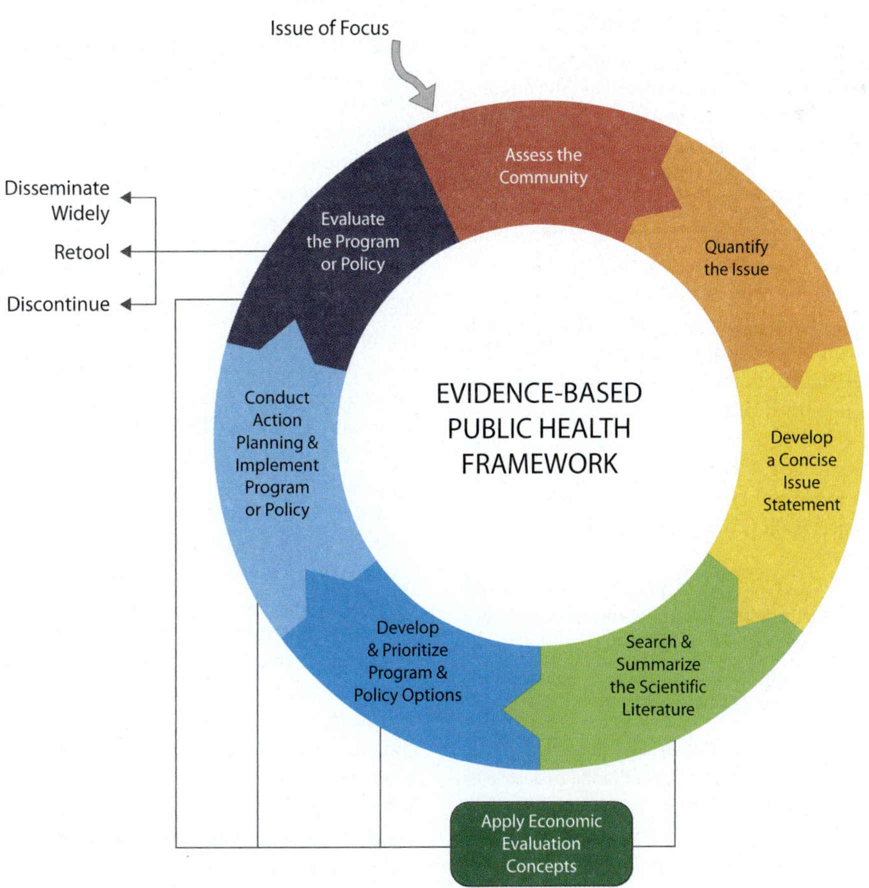

FIGURE 9-2. Evidence-based public health framework.

the organizational culture and the resource allocation toward evidence-based public health. Having sufficient funding and political backing to support evidence-based program and policy interventions is essential. Finally, training the workforce with the skills needed to adopt the seven stages of the evidence-based public health framework helps facilitate this process.[30]

In revisiting the cross-sector partnership approaches of Health in All Policies and IPE discussed earlier, these strategies illustrate the importance and possible complexities of evaluation and evidence-based practice. Health in All Policies initiatives vary in their implementation across settings—they might use numerous different tools like HIAs, and can range from formal to informal efforts, legislative or organizational policy, broad or issue-specific focus, and may or may not explicitly address health equity.[33,34] The latter may depend on the receptivity of political contexts to health equity concepts or it may be determined by the ways in which funding agencies such as foundations choose to focus their opportunities for support.[33] This versatility of Health in All Policies as an approach and set of principles means it is widely applicable but can also complicate evaluations. The length of time and amount of resources it may take to develop and implement Health in All Policies changes are challenges to evaluation, as is the difficulty in collecting data at a level to demonstrate a causal relationship with population health outcomes.[33,34] Similarly, IPE and collaborative practice are recommended by key national associations, but further evaluation of their impact on both learning and patient/population outcomes as well as clear evidence-based methods are needed.[35-39] It is possible that IPE has the potential to improve the elements of the Triple Aim of healthcare—quality of care, cost, and patience experience.[38,39] However, as with Health in All Policies, outcome evaluation is difficult due to the variations in which IPE and collaborative practice are implemented and the layers of variables outside of the learning experience or collaboration that may also impact results.[35-39]

Surveillance Data to Inform Public Health Practice

As noted earlier, one of the ten Essential Public Health Services is to monitor health. ***Public health surveillance*** is defined as "the ongoing, systematic collection, analysis, and interpretation of health data."[40] Surveillance is used to determine baseline rates of disease, detect epidemics and outbreaks, describe the extent of a problem, identify and describe populations at risk, monitor changes in a disease, assess interventions and control strategies, and aid in resource allocation.[40] Surveillance can provide valuable information about public health issues, but it can be resource intensive. To decide which diseases to surveil, public health professionals consider factors such as the public health importance of the problem; the ability to prevent, control, or treat the problem; and the capacity of the health system to implement control measures for an identified problem.[40] Once it is decided to conduct surveillance on a disease or condition of interest, an operational definition is needed. A ***case definition*** is a set of uniform epidemiologic, laboratory, and clinical criteria used to define a disease for public health surveillance. It allows for consistent and comparable reporting across jurisdictions.

A ***surveillance system*** is a collection of processes and components that enable public health practitioners to monitor a condition of interest. Surveillance systems have been described as the "informational nervous system" for public health practice.[40] The enabling components of surveillance systems can include:

- Laboratory diagnostics to detect or confirm health conditions;
- Information technologies to support the surveillance processes of data collection, analysis, and dissemination;
- Clinician consultation and reporting; education and training of clinicians, public health professionals, and laboratory workers; legislation, regulations, and policies that support the conduct of surveillance;
- Systems and directories for disseminating alerts, bulletins, clinical guidelines, and prevention recommendations; and
- Program administration and management, and human factors (e.g., multisector communications and relationships).[40]

The ultimate goal of public health surveillance systems is to increase the efficiency and effectiveness of the public health system, particularly the governmental public health system, in monitoring and controlling both familiar and new conditions and diseases of interest.

An example of a public health surveillance system is the National Notifiable Diseases Surveillance System, which is housed at the CDC.[41] This system helps to monitor, control, and prevent approximately 120 diseases, including Zika virus, foodborne outbreaks from *Escherichia coli*, and lead poisoning as examples. The Council of State and Territorial Epidemiologists, which has one voting member from each state, works closely with the CDC to determine which conditions reported to public health departments should be nationally notifiable. Public health departments across the country gather and use data on these diseases to inform programs and policies to keep their communities safe. Health departments are mandated to report this information to the CDC, which uses the data to monitor and address public health issues on regional and national levels.

How does a surveillance system work in practice? Consider the factors previously summarized that contribute to a well-functioning surveillance system. First, jurisdictional laws and regulations mandate the case reporting of certain infectious and noninfectious conditions to public health departments. When a notifiable condition is diagnosed in a clinician's office, for example, that clinician is required to report the case to the health department. This is important because without the legal mandate to report into the surveillance system with data and information, its utility would be greatly limited.

Once a notifiable condition is reported, the public health departments work with healthcare providers, laboratories, hospitals, clinics, and other partners to collect additional data about the health condition. Each health department has established its own structure and workforce for engaging in surveillance activities—these structures tend to vary depending on the size and resources of the health department and the population it serves. If the condition is considered nationally notifiable, the public health department voluntarily provides these data to the CDC. The compilation and analysis of these data benefit the state and local health departments and support regional and national disease monitoring. In addition to health information exchange and electronic health information systems, the CDC also provides support to health departments through funding, workforce training, and other tools. Finally, information dissemination needs to occur to appropriately inform public health policies and programs. Dissemination can refer to the sharing of information among CDC and public health departments as well as health departments sharing information with healthcare partners and the public.

This is one example of a public health surveillance system, but collectively they work to monitor incidence, patterns, and trends of infectious and noninfectious conditions and other health outcomes in populations. As surveillance systems can be resource-intensive and costly, it is important to evaluate the effectiveness and utility of the system regularly. Evaluations help determine whether the public health problem being monitored should remain under surveillance. In addition, evaluations can prompt reflection on characteristics and attributes of the system, such as how it operates, what case definitions are being used, whether it is cost effective, and whether it is simple, flexible, and acceptable to participants. A well-functioning system should have the necessary epidemiologic characteristics including a sufficiently high sensitivity, positive predictive value, and representativeness to accurately characterize the condition or disease.[40]

Community Health Assessments

Another type of evidence that informs public health decision making is data collected from ***community health assessments***. Community health assessments differ from data collected through surveillance in that they aim to involve community voice in data collection, analysis, and subsequent program planning and implementation. This means public health professionals need strong working relationships with community partners and the public. Community health assessment is a process that uses quantitative and qualitative methods to systematically collect and analyze health data within a specific community.[42,43] These health data include information on risk factors, quality of life, social determinants of health, determinants of inequity, morbidity, mortality, community assets, and information on how well the public health system provides essential services. Community health assessments should be part of ongoing broader community health improvement processes, which use assessment data to identify and prioritize issues, develop and implement strategies for action, and establish accountability to ensure measurable health improvement. These processes are often outlined in a community health improvement plan.

Incentives exist for health assessments to be conducted at the local level in communities. The Public Health Accreditation Board, which is a national voluntary accreditation program for local health departments, requires a community health assessment to be completed before health departments may apply for formal accreditation.[42] In addition, as a component of regulations within the Patient Protection and Affordable Care Act of 2010, the U.S. Internal Revenue Service instituted requirements for hospitals to conduct community health needs assessments if they are seeking to adopt or maintain a nonprofit status.[42] The assessment is intended to inform the community benefit practices of hospitals and health systems. The dual requirements of health departments and nonprofit hospitals yields an opportunity for the public health and healthcare systems to work collaboratively to engage and empower the communities they serve, and ensure their work is addressing population needs of highest priority.

Several tools, models, and frameworks exist to guide public health and healthcare professionals on how to conduct a community health assessment. The most widely used method of performing community health assessment and planning in public health is guided by the Mobilizing for Action through Planning and Partnerships (MAPP) framework, developed by the National Association of County and City Health Officials with support from the CDC. It involves all components of the local public health system—the health department, community organizations, and agencies that contribute to the mission of public health. The MAPP framework includes several steps and four separate assessments (Fig. 9-3).[44] MAPP begins with organizing the community—the organizations, agencies, and stakeholders—into a group to engage with and inform the remainder of the steps. A visioning process follows, which prompts the group to describe the desired health status of the community several years in the future. This step relies heavily on community engagement and deliberative forums with the public to identify values and prioritize strategic directions. Next, four separate assessments are conducted which focus on: community themes and strengths, the local public health system, community health status, and forces of change (which refers to the trends, factors, and events that are likely to influence community health and quality of life, or impact the work of the local public health system). The quantitative and qualitative data generated from these assessments permit community members to identify the most important health issues in the community and formulate goals and strategies to address them. This work leads to the action cycle, which includes planning, implementing, and evaluating policies and programs undertaken.[42–45]

In public health, an important tool for measuring population health outcomes that can inform community health assessments is

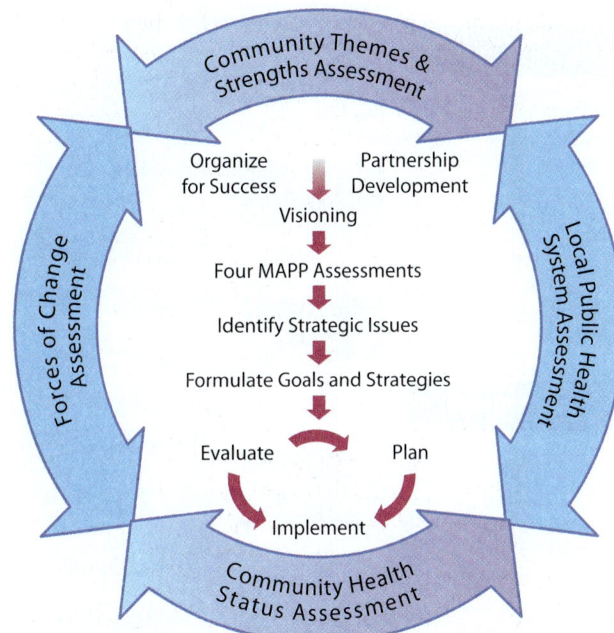

FIGURE 9-3. The mobilizing for action through planning and partnerships model.

the County Health Rankings Model. The University of Wisconsin Population Health Institute developed this model to rank the health of the more than 3000 counties in the United States since 2010 in what is described as a "population health checkup."[46] Rankings are compiled using county-level measures from a variety of national and state data sources. The measures are standardized and weighted to create scores. The County Health Rankings Model takes many factors influencing health into account (Fig. 9-4).[46] The rankings consider both ***health outcomes*** (e.g., morbidity and mortality) and ***health factors*** (e.g., health behaviors, access to clinical care, social and economic factors, and the physical environment). In doing so, this model attempts to quantify and account for some of the upstream factors, or the social determinants, that are so critical for understanding and influencing population health outcomes. The relative weighting of the health factors shows that those more likely to be addressed by public health interventions—health behaviors, social and economic factors, and the physical environment—collectively make up 80% of the ranking weight, while clinical care factors make up 20%.[46] The importance of public health's contribution to population health is clear in this model, which also permits intra- and interstate comparisons of the health status of counties.

Data from surveillance efforts, community health assessments, and initiatives such as the County Health Rankings, are examples of evidence that inform decision making in public health practice.

PUBLIC HEALTH PRACTICE AND RESEARCH

The functions and essential services of public health require practitioners to gather data—often from human subjects—analyze it, and use it to develop public health programs or policies. Does this make public health practice a form of research? The short answer to this is no, public health practice necessitates the use of research methods but is not, in itself, research. This distinction is based on the original purpose of the activity. Research generates or contributes to generalizable knowledge that benefits those beyond the participating community.[47] Practice, however, aims to prevent disease or injury and improve the health of the participating community. Surveillance, emergency response, and program evaluation are key components of public health practice that have been identified as having potential overlap with research.[47,48] The Council of State and Territorial

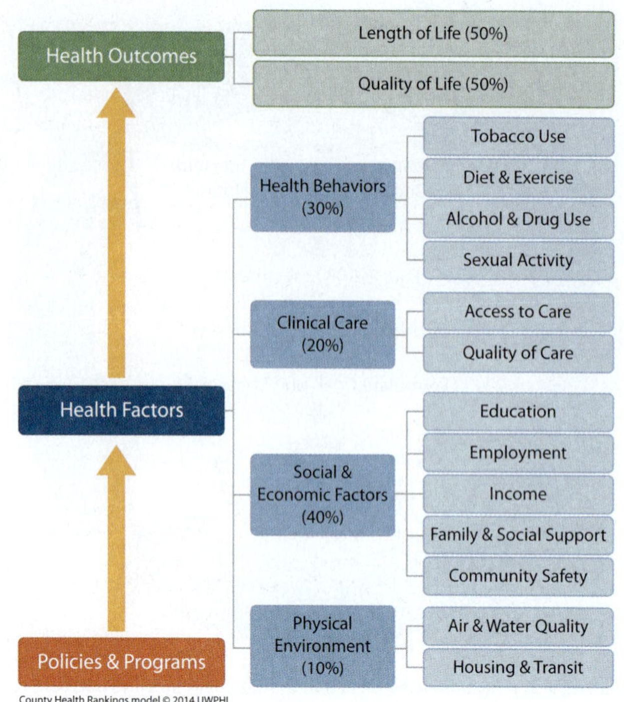

FIGURE 9-4. County health rankings model.

Epidemiologists has outlined essential characteristics of public health practice to include: "(1) specific legal authorization for conducting the activity; (2) governmental duty to perform the activity to protect the public's health; (3) direct performance or oversight of the activity by a governmental public health authority, or authorized partner, accountable to the public; (4) legitimacy of involving nonvolunteers; and (5) activities supported by ethical principles that focus on populations while respecting the dignity and rights of individuals."[47,48]

Despite the establishment of a priori purpose as a distinguishing factor to delineate practice from research, overlap remains. For example, activities intended to improve the health of a community that are not led by an authorized public health agency are likely to be considered research. This distinction is important because it determines whether activities require oversight by an Institutional Review Board to ensure ethical conduct of research. Activities involving human subjects for public benefit or service programs that are conducted or approved by a health department official, for example, would be exempt from Institutional Review Board review.[49] Ultimately, public health practice and research supplement and complement each other in the overall goal to improve population health. Using research to inform public health practice is equally as important as conducting practice-based research to ensure effective translation and adoption by public health practice.

Public Health Services and Systems Research

Public health services and systems research (PHSSR) is an area of study that aims to improve the effectiveness of public health practice. In this context, ***systems*** refers to the governmental public health agencies that provide the ten Essential Public Health Services along with the public and private sector institutions that have public health missions. ***Services*** broadly refers to "programs, direct services, policies, laws, and regulations designed to protect and promote the public's health and prevent disease and disability at the population level."[50] Much in the way health services research looks for relationships among organizational, structural, and financial factors and individual clinical service outcomes, PHSSR examines the organization, finance, and delivery of public health services in communities and the impact of these services on public health outcomes.[51] In 2012, a consortium of partners was convened to develop a national research agenda for PHSSR as a way of advancing efforts in the field through identifying and prioritizing the most pressing research questions that could positively impact public health practice. A total of 72 research questions were developed across three themes: public health workforce; public health system structure and performance; and public health financing and economics.[51] This call to action has raised visibility and funding investment in research that can improve the public health system infrastructure to better support public health practice.

ALIGNING ACADEMIA AND PUBLIC HEALTH PRACTICE

Reports released by the Institute of Medicine, now the National Academy of Medicine, have repeatedly recommended better alignment between schools and programs of public health and public health practice.[1,10] Recent public health workforce research findings indicate that improvement is still needed. The 2017 Public Health Workforce Interests and Needs Survey shows that 14% of the governmental public health workforce lacks a formal degree in public health,[52] despite the fact that the number of accredited schools and programs granting public health degrees has increased substantially over the past few decades. In 2000, a combined total of 7521 bachelor's, master's and doctoral public health degrees were conferred in the United States, compared to 26,306 in 2015, representing an increase of nearly 350% in public health-related degrees granted.[53] However, this growth in public health academic programs has not translated to a substantive influx of workers with public health degrees into public health practice.

Two key agencies have made an intentional effort to further bridge public health academia and practice—the Association of Schools and Programs of Public Health, which is the national membership organization for accredited public health degree-granting institutions, and the Council on Education for Public Health (CEPH), which accredits public health schools and programs. For example, CEPH engaged public health practice stakeholders to revise the curriculum requirements for Master of Public Health degrees to be more practice-focused. The updated requirements, released in 2016, aim to align the educational content and competencies taught by public health academic institutions with the skills needed of the public health workforce and emphasize applied practice experiences and exposure to interprofessional practice.

Academic institutions also play a role in public health workforce development by providing training to the broad range of public health professionals in practice. Federally funded Public Health Training Centers are administered by schools of public health and work with other academic and practice partners to deliver high-quality continuing education for the field. The training opportunities incorporate the Core Competencies for Public Health Professionals established by the Council on Linkages between Academia and Public Health Practice.[54] The core competencies are a set of skills for public health practice that align with the 10 Essential Public Health Services. Building on these core competencies, a set of eight strategic skills were identified by a consortium convened by the de Beaumont Foundation.[55] These are cross-cutting skills in which public health professionals of all disciplines should be competent, and include: systems thinking, change management, persuasive communication, data analytics, problem solving, diversity and inclusion, resource management, and policy engagement. Public Health Training Centers and other public health training entities focus their products around the core competencies and strategic skills. These opportunities are heavily subscribed to by state and local health department workers.

The past few decades have seen increased professionalization of public health. Although there is no unifying credential for public health workers, a National Board of Public Health Examiners was established in 2005 as an independent body whose purpose is to ensure that public health professionals have mastered foundational knowledge and skills needed to deliver Essential Public Health Services. The Certified in Public Health exam is a voluntary credential available to public health professionals who meet specific eligibility requirements. Similarly, a few disciplines within public health practice also have credentials such as Certified Health Education Specialists and Registered Environmental Health Specialists. Further, the Public Health Accreditation Board provides guidance around workforce development benchmarks for public health departments seeking voluntary accreditation. As public health curriculum requirements begin to better align with the skills and knowledge required for public health worker certification and the workforce needs of entities within the public health system, the ability of the collective workforce to deliver the Essential Public Health Services and improve population health outcomes should be strengthened.

References

1. Institute of Medicine. *The Future of Public Health*. Washington, DC: The National Academies Press; 1988.
2. Centers for Disease Control and Prevention. United States Public Health 101. https://www.cdc.gov/publichealthgateway/publichealthservices/pdf/usph101.pdf. Atlanta, GA. 2013.
3. Office of Disease Prevention and Health Promotion. Healthy People 2020: Social determinants of health. https://www.healthypeople.gov/2020/topics-objectives/topic/social-determinants-of-health. Washington, DC. 2014.
4. Braveman P, Arkin E, Orleans T, Proctor D, Plough A. What is health equity? And what difference does a definition make? https://www.rwjf.org/en/library/research/2017/05/what-is-health-equity-.html. Princeton, NJ, Robert Wood Johnson Foundation. 2017.
5. DeSalvo KB, Wang , YC, Harris A, Auerbach J, Koo D, O'Carroll P. Public health 3.0: A call to action for public health to meet the challenges of the 21st century. *Prev Chronic Dis*. 2017;14(E78):1–9.
6. Fee E, Brown TM. The public health act of 1848. *Bull World Health Organ*. 2005;83(11):866–7.
7. Gaziano JM. Fifth phase of the epidemiologic transition: The age of obesity and inactivity. *JAMA*. 2010;303(3):275–6.
8. Olshansky SJ, Ault AB. The fourth stage of the epidemiologic transition: The age of delayed degenerative diseases. *Milbank Q*. 1986;64(3):355–91.
9. Centers for Disease Control and Prevention. The Public Health System & 10 Essential Public Health Services. https://www.cdc.gov/publichealthgateway/publichealthservices/essentialhealthservices.html. Atlanta, GA. 2018.
10. Institute of Medicine. *The Future of the Public's Health in the 21st Century*. Washington, DC: The National Academies Press; 2003.
11. Centers for Disease Control and Prevention. Ten Essential Public Health Services and how they can include addressing the social determinants of health inequalities. https://www.cdc.gov/publichealthgateway/publichealthservices/pdf/Ten_Essential_Services_and_SDOH.pdf. Atlanta, GA. 2020.
12. Kania J, Kramer M. Collective impact. *Stanford Social Innovation Review*. 36–41, Winter 2011.
13. Rudolph L, Caplan J, Ben-Moshe K, Dillon, L. Health in all policies: A guide for state and local governments. https://www.phi.org/uploads/files/Health_in_All_Policies-A_Guide_for_State_and_Local_Governments.pdf. Washington, DC and Oakland, CA, American Public Health Association and Public Health Institute. 2013.
14. World Health Organization. Health in all policies: Helsinki statement: Framework for country action. https://www.who.int/healthpromotion/frameworkforcountryaction/en/. Geneva, Switzerland, WHO Press. 2014.
15. Gottlieb L, Egerter S, Braveman P. Health Impact Assessment: A tool for promoting health in all policies. Issue Brief 11. https://www.rwjf.org/en/library/research/2011/05/health-impact-assessment.html. Princeton, NJ, Robert Wood Johnson Foundation Commission to Build a Healthier America. 2011.
16. Wernham A, Teutsch SM. Health in All Policies for big cities. *J Public Health Manag Pract*. 2015;21(1 Suppl):S56–65.
17. Lee S, Shumann A. South Park Community Center Open Space Design Plan: Rapid Health Impact Assessment (HIA) findings & recommendations. https://www.kingcounty.gov/depts/health/environmental-health/healthy-communities/~/media/depts/health/environmental-health/documents/hia/south-park-commmunity-center-hia.ashx. Seattle, WA, The Healthy Community Planning Program, Public Health-Seattle & King County Environmental Health Services Division. 2016.
18. Climate and Health Action Team, Public Health-Seattle & King County. Blueprint for addressing climate change and health. https://www.kingcounty.gov/services/environment/climate/strategies/climate-change-health-blueprint.aspx. Seattle, WA, 2020.
19. Vermont Department of Health. Creating cross-sector action and accountability for health in Vermont: Guidance from a rural state. http://www.healthvermont.gov/sites/default/files/documents/pdf/ADM_CoH_Guide.pdf. Burlington, VT. 2018.
20. Association of State and Territorial Health Officials. Health in All Policies: Vermont's push for cross-sector collaboration among state agencies. http://www.astho.org/HiaP/VT-Push-for-Cross-Sector-Collaboration-Among-State-Agencies/. Arlington, VA. 2020.
21. World Health Organization. Health in All Policies (HiAP) framework for country action. https://www.who.int/cardiovascular_diseases/140120HPRHiAPFramework.pdf. Geneva, Switzerland. 2014.
22. Republic of Ecuador National Planning Council. National Plan for Good Living, 2013–2017, summarized version. http://www.planificacion.gob.ec/wp-content/uploads/downloads/2013/12/Buen-Vivir-ingles-web-final-completo.pdf. Quito, Ecuador, National Secretariat of Planning and Development. 2013.
23. Fortune K, Becerra F, Buss P, Solar O, Ribeiro P, Keahon GE. Health in All Policies: Perspectives from the region of the Americas. *Oxford Research Encyclopedia of Global Public Health*. Oxford, England: Oxford University Press; 2019.
24. Health Professions Network Nursing and Midwifery Office, Department of Human Resources for Health, World Health Organization. Framework for action on interprofessional education & collaborative practice. https://apps.who.int/iris/bitstream/handle/10665/70185/WHO_HRH_HPN_10.3_eng.pdf?sequence=1. Geneva, Switzerland, WHO Press. 2010.
25. Interprofessional Education Collaborative. Core competencies for interprofessional collaborative practice: 2016 update. https://hsc.unm.edu/ipe/resources/ipec-2016-core-competencies.pdf. Washington, DC, Interprofessional Education Collaborative. 2016.
26. Patient Protection and Affordable Care Act, Pub L No. 111-148, 2010.
27. Interprofessional Education Collaborative: IPEC members. https://www.ipecollaborative.org/membership.html. 2019.
28. Salas E, Zajac S, Marlow SL. Transforming health care one team at a time: Ten observations and the trail ahead. *Group Organ Manag*. 2018;43(3):357–81.
29. Ramsbottom A, O'Brien E, Ciotti L, Takacs J. Enablers and barriers to community engagement in public health emergency preparedness: A literature review. *J Community Health*. 2018;43:412–20.
30. Brownson RC, Fielding JE, Maylahn CM. Evidence-based public health: A fundamental concept for public health practice. *Annu Rev Public Health*. 2009;30:175–201.
31. U.S. Department of Health and Human Services: About the Community Preventive Services Task Force. https://www.thecommunityguide.org/task-force/about-community-preventive-services-task-force. 2019.
32. Allen P, O'Connor JC, Best LA, Lakshman M, Jacob RR, Brownson RC. Management practices to build evidence-based decision-making capacity for chronic disease prevention in Georgia: A case study. *Prev Chronic Dis*. 2018;15:170482.
33. Hall RL, Jacobson PD. Examining whether the Health-in-All-Policies approach promotes health equity. *Health Aff (Millwood)*. 2018;37(3):364–70.
34. Gase LN, Schooley T, Lee M, Rotakhina S, Vick J, Caplan J. A practice-grounded approach for evaluating Health in All Policies initiatives in the United States. *J Public Health Manag Pract*. 2017;23(4):339–47.
35. American Public Health Association. Promoting interprofessional education. Policy Number 20088. https://www.apha.org/policies-and-advocacy/public-health-policy-statements/policy-database/2014/07/23/09/20/promoting-interprofessional-education. 2008.
36. Institute of Medicine. *Measuring the Impact of Interprofessional Education on Collaborative Practice and Patient Outcomes*. Washington, DC: The National Academies Press; 2015.
37. Morano C, Domiani G. Interprofessional education at the Meso level: Taking the next step in IPE. *Gerontol Geriatr Educ*. 2019;40(1):43–54.
38. Brandt B, Nawal Lutfiyya M, King JA, Chioreso C. A scoping review of interprofessional collaborative practice and education using the lens of the triple aim. *J Interprof Care*. 2014;28(5):393–9.

39. Earnest M, Brandt B. Aligning practice redesign and interprofessional education to advance triple aim outcomes. *J Interprof Care.* 2014;28(6):497–500.
40. Groseclose SL, Buckeridge DL. Public Health Surveillance Systems: Recent advances in their use and evaluation. *Annu Rev Public Health.* 2017;38:57–79.
41. Centers for Disease Control and Prevention. National Notifiable Diseases Surveillance System. https://wwwn.cdc.gov/nndss/. Atlanta, GA. 2019.
42. Lamberth CD, Scutchfield FD. Community health assessment, planning, and implementation. In: Erwin PC, Brownson RCErwin PC, Brownson RC, eds. *Scutchfield and Keck: Principles of Public Health Practice.* 4th ed. Boston, MA: Cengage Learning; 2017.
43. National Association of County and City Health Officials. Community health assessment and improvement planning. https://www.naccho.org/programs/public-health-infrastructure/performance-improvement/community-health-assessment. Washington, DC. 2019.
44. National Association of County and City Health Officials. Achieving healthier communities through MAPP: A user's handbook. Washington, DC. 2015.
45. National Association of County and City Health Officials. Mobilizing for action through planning and partnerships. https://www.naccho.org/programs/public-health-infrastructure/performance-improvement/community-health-assessment/mapp. Washington, DC. 2019.
46. Remington PL, Catlin BB, Gennuso KP. The county health rankings: Rationale and methods. *Popul Health Metr.* 2015;13:11.
47. Otto JL, Holodniy M, DeFraites RF. Public health practice is not research. *Am J Public Health.* 2014;104(4):596–602.
48. Hodge JG, Gostin LO, CSTE Advisory Committee. Public health practice vs. research: A report for public health practitioners including cases and guidance for making distinctions. http://www.cste2.org/webpdfs/CSTEPHResRptHodgeFinal.5.24.04.pdf. 2004.
49. U.S. Department of Health and Human Services. Human subjects regulations decision charts. https://www.hhs.gov/ohrp/regulations-and-policy/decision-charts/index.html. Washington, DC. 2016.
50. Scutchfield FD, Perez DJ, Monroe JA, Howard AF. New Public Health Services and Systems Research agenda: Directions for the next decade. *AM J Prev Med.* 2012;42(5S1):S1–5.
51. Consortium from Altarum Institute, Centers for Disease Control and Prevention, the Robert Wood Johnson Foundation, and the National Coordinating Center for Public Health Services and Systems Research. A national research agenda for Public Health Services and Systems. *Am J Prev Med.* 2012;42(5S1):S72–8.
52. de Beaumont Foundation. Public health workforce interest and needs survey: 2017 National findings. https://www.debeaumont.org/phwins/. Bethesda, MD, de Beaumont Foundation. 2018.
53. Leider JP, Coronado F, Beck AJ, Harper E. Reconciling supply and demand for state and local public health staff in an era of retiring baby boomers. *Am J Prev Med.* 2018;54(3):334–40.
54. Council on Linkages Between Academia and Public Health Practice. Core competencies for public health professionals. http://www.phf.org/resourcestools/Documents/Core_Competencies_for_Public_Health_Professionals_2014June.pdf. 2014.
55. de Beaumont Foundation. Building skills for a more strategic public health workforce: A call to action. Bethesda, MD. 2017.

CHAPTER

10

Military Preventive Medicine and Public Health*

Steven B. Cersovsky

"The General has nothing more at heart, than the Health of the Troops."

– General George Washington[1]

"The prevention of disease is the highest object of medical science. . . . Medical officers . . . strengthen the hands of the Commanding General by keeping his army in the most vigorous health, thus rendering it, in the highest degree, efficient for enduring fatigue and privation, and for fighting."

– Major Jonathan Letterman, Medical Director, Army of the Potomac[2]

"Probably no activity pays in the military service such huge dividends as preventive medicine."

– Major General Merritte Ireland, Army Surgeon General[3]

INTRODUCTION AND PURPOSE

Military service is a hazardous occupation. Although the image that often jumps to mind is of service members—soldiers, sailors, airmen, and Marines—under fire in combat, the reality is that relatively few ever find themselves engaged in direct fighting with an adversary, and most separate from the military after one term of service (about 5 years). However, the process of becoming a service member (training), the military occupational specialties required in today's armed forces, and deployments to austere or less-developed areas of the world, expose the majority of military personnel to a wide range of potential health threats. This creates a challenge for preventive medicine physicians and other public health specialists, but one that makes for an exciting career and yields tremendous rewards.

The potential exposures of any one service member over his or her time in service, and the resulting health effects, are dependent on many factors, including predisposing characteristics (e.g., genetics, pre-existing conditions, fitness level), job-related activities (e.g., physical training, weapons training, use of equipment), and location (e.g., type of installation, deployment-related threats, climate). A service member's lifecycle is characterized by frequent displacement, usually every 2–3 years, periods of separation from family members for training or operational missions, and job-related tasks that are frequently associated with physical and psychological stressors and may expose the individual to a variety of known and unknown biological, chemical, and physical agents. Preventing illness and disability in service members is critical to any military's ability to effectively complete its mission, and it is preventive medicine and public health experts who develop and assist commanders in implementing the policies, programs, and countermeasures to maintain the health and readiness of the force.

Military operations take many forms, from traditional warfare to humanitarian assistance, disaster response, and other stability and support operations, collectively known as Operations Other Than War. In today's world, most military operations are joint, meaning more than one branch of service is engaged, and they are increasingly multinational. Although large conflicts are fairly infrequent and last for a few years at most—the ongoing operations since 9/11 being exceptions in modern history—the U.S. military is engaged continuously in missions around the globe and maintains a presence in most countries. The total number of military personnel stationed or deployed overseas has declined since the Vietnam War, a result of technological advances and changes in strategic priorities, global diplomacy, national politics, economic conditions, and military doctrine. With smaller numbers of personnel, the importance of any one service member in achieving mission success is increased, and that has altered the role of military preventive medicine from its historical focus on prevention to one that now includes human performance optimization.

The effectiveness of a military force is dependent on its ability to "fight tonight," commonly referred to as "readiness." The readiness of a military unit is determined by the status of both its personnel and materiel (i.e., equipment) and can be measured using a variety of indicators. Personal, or individual, readiness includes medical readiness (i.e., health) as well as being fully trained in tactics, techniques, and procedures (TTPs) and proficient in the use of all equipment required to successfully execute the mission requirements. Military preventive medicine and public health professionals are critical in ensuring optimal health and fitness so service members can achieve their maximum state of personal readiness. In recent years, the approach to health readiness has been codified in holistic frameworks such as Total Force Fitness (TFF, a program of the Chairman of the Joint Chiefs of Staff, Fig. 10-1), Holistic Health and Fitness [H2F, a program of the Army's Training and Doctrine Command (TRADOC)], and Preservation of the Force and Family [POTFF, a program of the Special Operations Command (SOCOM)]. Each addresses health in reference to component domains such as physical, psychological, social, and behavioral, and each provides support to family and community health as well, recognizing that individual service member readiness is only maximized in the context of healthy families and communities.

Despite its importance and vast scope, military preventive medicine and public health is only a small fraction of the overall Military Health System (MHS) and comprises approximately 3% of the Defense Health Program budget. As in the civilian sector, direct

*Disclaimer: The views expressed herein are those of the author and do not necessarily reflect those of the Department of Defense.

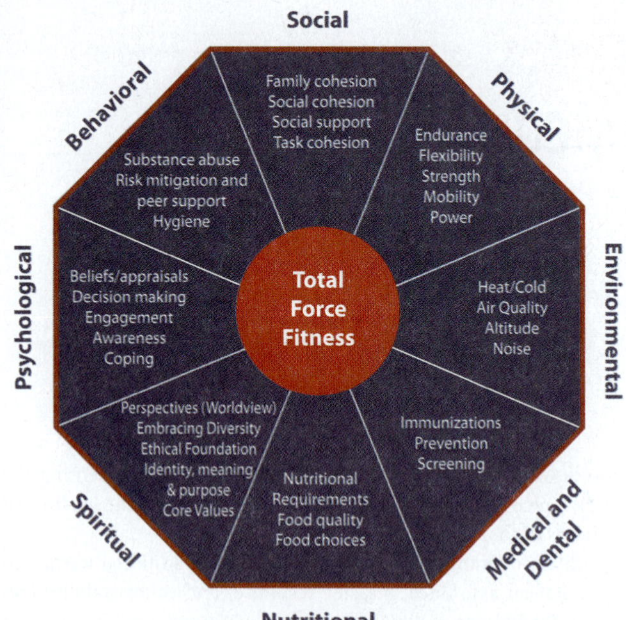

FIGURE 10-1. The domains of total force fitness. (*Source:* From Defense Suicide Prevention Office, Fiscal Year 2012 Annual Report.)

patient care consumes almost all of the healthcare resources, and attempts to shift from a healthcare system to a "system for health" have made little progress. Across the Department of Defense (DoD), preventive medicine and public health experts are engaged in the full spectrum of classic and military-specific public health activities, from health surveillance to risk characterization and communication, health promotion to injury prevention, industrial hygiene to entomology, environmental sciences, and engineering to toxicology. They are involved in research and development of new vaccines and other countermeasures; vector control; occupational and environmental medicine; hearing protection; vision conservation; chemical, biological, and nuclear surety; food protection; global health engagement; and so very much more. Given the breadth and depth of military preventive medicine, this chapter can only provide a basic understanding and appreciation of the subject.

To that end, the purpose of this chapter is to describe selected concepts, principles, and elements of preventive medicine and public health as organized and practiced in the military context. Although the fundamentals are similar to preventive medicine practice in the civilian world, there are unique aspects of the MHS, characteristics of the populations served, and occupational and environmental health threats associated with military service that deserve specific attention. Legters and Llewellyn, in a previous edition of this text, described military preventive medicine as "a unique brand of occupational medicine, one that deals with the prevention and treatment of diseases and injuries resulting from work in military occupations and operational environments."[1] This captures the primary focus of preventive medicine practitioners in the military—the majority of their work is appropriately centered on protecting the health of service members, especially those in an active duty status—but they also have responsibilities to those serving in a reserve status, military retirees, family members, and DoD civilian employees.

The chapter is organized to provide a broad overview of military preventive medicine, starting with a brief historical background, a summary of the MHS, and a short discussion of how preventive medicine is organized and operates in both garrison and deployed environments. Brief sections on specific health threats associated with military personnel and operations follows, and the chapter ends with some speculation on the future challenges in military preventive medicine practice. Additional resources for further reading are provided.

A BRIEF HISTORY OF MILITARY PREVENTIVE MEDICINE

The concepts and practices of what we know today to be preventive medicine have been critical to the success of military operations throughout history. Armed forces able to preserve the health of their personnel—the most critical component of their "fighting strength"—had an immense advantage over those whose personnel succumbed to disease and injury. From the earliest historical texts, it is clear that successful military commanders recognized the importance of personal hygiene, sanitation, and individual and collective countermeasures to prevent disease and injury in their formations. For example, the Old Testament books of Leviticus, Numbers, and Deuteronomy describe the preventive medicine functions of the Levites, Jewish priests Garrison called the "hygienic police" of the army of Israel.[2] They were responsible for regulating safe food and water, personal hygiene, communicable disease prevention, outbreak response, health education, and advising military leaders on camp sanitation and preserving the health of the soldiers, what we now call force health protection. These were distinct functions from those of physicians who treated disease and injury. The success of the Israelites in maintaining healthy military (and civilian) personnel is credited to the wisdom and leadership of Moses, who George Washington called "the wisest General that ever lived"[3] and who Percival Wood described as the equivalent of a modern Minister of Public Health.[4] The Mosaic sanitary code would be referenced by General Washington hundreds of times in his writings.

General Washington also relied on contemporary experts in preventive medicine and hygiene, including his own military physicians. The British surgeons general, Sir John Pringle and Dr. Richard Brocklesby, the former often referred to as the founder of modern military preventive medicine, directly influenced the medical officers in the Continental Army. Pringle, a close friend of Benjamin Franklin, established rules of hygiene for soldiers, including requirements for adequate ventilation of barracks and hospitals; wear of proper clothing; avoidance of overcrowding; mitigation of exposure to heat, cold, and dampness; management of fatigue; waste disposal; campsite selection; and methods to ensure safe sources of food and water.[5] His concept of military hospitals as sanctuaries for the sick and wounded that should be excluded as targets of enemy attacks was eventually codified in the Geneva Conventions and the establishment of the International Red Cross.[6] Brocklesby succeeded Pringle and expanded on concepts from infection control to the importance of good discipline and enforcement of hygiene orders by line commanders.[7] During this same period, James Lind of the Royal Navy ensconced hygiene in England's naval forces and published his famous treatise on the prevention of scurvy by inclusion of citrus fruits in the diets of sailors,[8] a practice adopted by American forces during the Revolution. Other important publications of the time that influenced Washington and his medical officers in the coming conflict were Gerard van Swieten's book on diseases of importance to armies, translated into English in 1762 and reprinted in 1776,[9] and an appendix on camp and military hospitals authored by John Jones, a professor of surgery at King's College in New York City, in 1775.[10]

The American Revolutionary War established several foundational practices in military preventive medicine. General Washington issued orders and made hundreds of references to protecting the health of his soldiers, tasking his subordinate commanders with the responsibility to enforce hygiene and sanitation practices to prevent disease and ensure the ability of the army to fully and successfully execute military operations. Benjamin Rush, who briefly served as a senior physician the Continental Army, elaborated on Pringle's principles in his "Directions for Preserving the Health of Soldiers"[11] and emphasized the importance of physicians as senior advisers to commanders as well as their enforcement of regulations on camp sanitation and individual hygienic practices. Baron von Steuben, the Prussian officer who joined George Washington at Valley Forge during the winter of 1778–9 and was put in charge of training the troops, produced in his "Regulations for the Order and Discipline of the Troops of the United States"[12] what would become the first Congressionally approved directive that contained instructions for disease prevention and health promotion in the American military.

However, arguably the most significant event in early military preventive medicine was Washington's decision to inoculate his troops against smallpox. In the first 2 years of the war, hundreds of soldiers in the Continental Army died from the disease, and it was a major factor in the failure of the Quebec campaign. Fear of contracting the disease even had a negative impact on recruiting new soldiers. Vaccination against smallpox using cowpox would not be discovered by Jenner for another two decades, and inoculation with the smallpox virus itself was not without consequences. At the time, however, the mortality from naturally acquired smallpox was about 16%, compared to 0.33% from inoculated smallpox,[6] and future success on the battlefield was in jeopardy if something was not done to mitigate the disease. In April 1776, John Morgan, Physician in Chief to the Army, recommended universal inoculation, and in January 1777 General Washington wrote to Morgan's successor, William Shippen, "Finding the small pox to be spreading much and fearing that precaution can prevent it from running thro' the whole of our Army, I have determined that the Troops shall be inoculated."[13] Later that year, inoculation of recruits became standard practice. The result was substantial; smallpox was no longer a threat to military operations, and the inoculation program was even described as the medical profession's "most important contribution to the winning of our national independence."[14]

Most modern principles of military preventive medicine were established by the end of the American Revolution (Box 10-1). Based on his experiences in the Continental Army, James Tilton published his "Economical Observations on Military Hospitals and the Prevention and Cure of Diseases Incident to an Army" in 1813. He was recalled from retirement to serve as Surgeon General of the Army during the War of 1812 following Congressional legislation and Presidential regulations adopted in 1813 that created a new Medical Department of the Army with more clearly defined responsibilities and authorities for the Surgeon General and other medical officers.[15] Tilton's design for military hospitals, which were adopted near the end of the Revolution to reduce transmission of infection, were expanded upon in practice by Joseph Lovell, demonstrating that infectious diseases could be controlled without the microbiological knowledge that would be discovered later. Lovell advanced the field of epidemiology by introducing the collection and reporting of vital statistics, he required the keeping of meteorological registers to investigate the association of disease with climate, and he established the Library of the Surgeon General's Office, which later became what is now the National Library of Medicine.[6]

The Crimean War (1854–6) was a reminder of the consequences of poor sanitation and failures in leadership. Dysentery, cholera, scurvy, and typhus fever caused mortality in as much as 20% of the British and French troops at various times.[16] The work of Florence Nightingale, arguably the first public health nurse, was noteworthy and impactful, but it was the public outcry that led the government to respond by creating the Royal Sanitary Commission. This organization consisted of leading civilian experts who were able to exert great influence on the British Army leaders and their medical officers, and they elevated the profession of Army medicine through a series of regulations and publications. The commission produced the first government report on sanitation practices and outcomes associated with warfare, and their work led to the establishment of the Royal Army Medical School in 1860. There, Edmund Parkes taught military preventive medicine, and his *Manual of Practical Hygiene* would become a standard text during the latter half of the nineteenth century in both England and the United States.[17] Lessons learned by the British as a result of their experience in Crimea would influence the approach to disease prevention employed by the Union Army during the American Civil War.

The first months of the Civil War saw an ineffective Army Medical Department's struggle to support a rapidly growing force of regular soldiers and volunteers. President Lincoln, in response to civilian experts who were aware of the Army's problems and familiar with the British experience, approved establishment of the United States Sanitary Commission in June 1861. Early on, the Commission was able to influence the reorganization of the Medical Department of the Army, including elevating the Surgeon General to general officer grade, enlarging his staff, and creating a cadre of medical inspectors to oversee matters of sanitation. As the Commission's authority and responsibilities grew, its medical officers became more active in the Army's preventive medicine activities, such as expanding the Camp Inspection Service and producing important documents on all matters of military hygiene and disease prevention that were used widely by military physicians and commanders in the field.[18] These publications provided guidance on the prevention and treatment of dysentery, typhus, measles, gangrene, venereal disease (VD), scurvy, pneumonia, and other military-relevant diseases; use of vaccination against smallpox; and the newly introduced practice of administering quinine as prophylaxis against malaria (which was endemic in the eastern and southern United States at the time). There was also a dedicated pamphlet outlining the 40 "Rules for Preserving the Health of the Soldier."[19] Importantly, the Commission was able to secure the appointment of William Alexander Hammond as Surgeon General in 1862, and convince General McClellan to appoint Jonathan Letterman as medical director of the Army of the Potomac. In addition to championing preventive medicine, Hammond established the Army Medical Museum, which would become the foundation for military preventive medicine education programs and home for

BOX 10-1 Principles of Military Preventive Medicine Established during the American Revolution

- Command responsibility for the preservation of the health of the troops
- Use of medical officers as advisers to line officers
- Discipline
- Personal hygiene; cleanliness
- Diet and nutrition
- Clothing and shoes
- Avoidance of exposure to extreme heat, cold, wetness, and fatigue
- Morale and recreation
- Health education
- Immunization
- Consideration of health factors in campsite selection
- Avoidance of crowding
- Camp sanitation
- Waste disposal
- Selection and protection of water supplies
- Isolation and quarantine
- Medical intelligence

Source: Adapted from Bayne-Jones S. *The Evolution of Preventive Medicine in the United States Army, 1607–1939.* Washington: Office of the Surgeon General, Department of the Army, 1968.[6]

future bacteriology and pathology laboratories; required medical officers to report monthly on medical and surgical data, including the relation of sanitation to diseases; and compiled a 600-page treatise on general and military hygiene.[20]

The period from the end of the Civil War to the Spanish-American War saw a decrease in the size of U.S. forces, but important advances in military preventive medicine and medical science in general. This was the era of discovery in microbiology, with the work of Pasteur, Koch, Lister, and others transforming the biological sciences. In the military, increased attention was paid to improving sanitation and hygiene at camps, posts, and stations, with new regulations, inspection regimes, and reporting requirements enacted.[6] Perhaps the most influential figure in the history of military preventive medicine, George Miller Sternberg became Army Surgeon General in 1893. An acclaimed bacteriologist in his own right, Sternberg established important Army laboratories to further work in the emerging scientific fields, and he founded the Army Medical School, located in the Army Medical Museum building in Washington, DC, to train medical officers on environmental sanitation, microbial causes of communicable diseases, and scientific approaches to disease prevention and control, becoming the first school of preventive medicine and public health in the United States. Sternberg chartered several important boards and commissions to investigate and advise on specific issues; Captain Walter Reed, one of the four original faculty members of the Army Medical School, would be chosen to lead such groups studying typhoid fever in Army camps during the Spanish-American War, and, later, yellow fever in troops sent to Cuba.[21]

The brief Spanish-American War (1898) pointed out several challenges for the military. Outbreaks of typhoid fever in camps of volunteers hastily assembled to increase the size of the Army pointed out continuing problems with sanitation and hygiene. Troops deployed to Cuba found new threats in the form of malaria, yellow fever, and various causes of diarrhea. Lessons in leadership and enforcement of hygienic practices by commanders had to be relearned, and it became clear that military physicians required additional training beyond that of civilian medical practice to be effective in preventing and treating health threats associated with military service, in particular tropical diseases.[6] The military's work in tropical medicine accelerated in the early twentieth century. Walter Reed confirmed Carlos Finlay's hypothesis that yellow fever was transmitted by a mosquito and proved that the disease was caused by a virus. Their work led to vector control practices and, ultimately, to a yellow fever vaccine. In Puerto Rico, Bailey Ashford discovered that the severe anemia in the local population was caused by hookworm infection, leading to the global campaign for control of hookworm disease by the Rockefeller Foundation. A series of Army Medical Research Boards in the Philippines conducted extensive work in human and animal parasitic diseases endemic to the region, and from their work came advances in the prevention and treatment of dengue, malaria, plague, and rinderpest. "The Golden Age of Tropical Medicine" had arrived, due in large part to the efforts of the Army, Navy, and USPHS.[22]

In Havana, Cuba, William Crawford Gorgas began applying the knowledge gained from Reed's work to free the city from malaria and yellow fever. His antimosquito brigades eliminated breeding sites, installed screening in patient treatment centers, and employed fumigation to eliminate adult mosquitoes.[23] Gorgas then turned his attention to eliminating the vectorborne disease threat in Panama, a critical accomplishment that made construction of the Panama Canal possible from 1904 to 1914.[24] During this same period, Frederick Russell introduced compulsory vaccination against typhoid fever in the U.S. Army (based on the British practice in the Boer War); Carl Darnall developed a system for chlorination of drinking water; William Lyster modified the process for use in the field; and Edward Munson formed the Army Shoe Board to improve military footwear, which would increase the mobility of the infantry in conflicts to come.[6,24]

When World War I started in Europe in 1914, the U.S. military was focused primarily in the Southern Department, the border region with Mexico, engaging in operations against Mexican General Francisco Villa. The Army gained experience in field sanitation practices, and in conjunction with important policy and organizational changes, found itself better prepared to enter WWI in 1917. However, the rapid mobilization of American forces was not without challenge. In about 18 months, the Army increased in size from 200,000 to over 3.7 million, resulting in hastily built and crowded training camps, where outbreaks of measles, mumps, and meningococcal meningitis were common.[25] Perhaps most attention, however, was directed toward the prevention and control of VD. Although not a new problem for military preventive medicine, social and cultural taboos had shifted such that sexually transmitted infections were now discussed openly in the context of improving the moral character of American society. Commissions and boards were formed, local- and national-level civilian health and service organizations joined the fight against VD, and even Congress got involved, authorizing the Secretary of War to take all steps necessary to combat the scourge. Zones around training camps were created in which alcohol sales were banned and prostitution was prohibited. Educational campaigns were launched and more leisure activities were provided within the camps to occupy the trainees during their idle time.[25]

The most serious epidemics in camps, and later on the battlefield, were those of pneumonia. Gorgas, now the Army Surgeon General, created a Pneumonia Board of civilian experts to assist military bacteriologists, pathologists, epidemiologists, and other specialists in combatting respiratory infections. (This group continued during World War II as the Army Epidemiological Board, became the Armed Forces Epidemiological Board in 1950, and still exists today as the Defense Health Board.) The Board would become invaluable in the military response to the influenza pandemic of 1918–19. Influenza had a tremendous impact on the American Expeditionary Force (AEF), with an estimated 25% becoming ill, almost 800,000 soldiers hospitalized in the United States and France, and mortality rates of 5–50%, depending on complications and coinfections, especially pneumonia. More than 57,000 soldiers died from influenza and secondary pneumonias, exceeding the total number of combat deaths during the war.[26]

Gorgas also expanded the preventive medicine staff in the Office of the Surgeon General and gave them additional authority and responsibility for sanitary inspections, operating laboratories, and training medical officers.[25] But on the battlefields of Europe, the medical assets of the AEF operated mostly independent of the Surgeon General. General Pershing placed his chief medical adviser, the AEF Surgeon, on his general staff and gave him the autonomy and authority to direct medical activities in the theater, providing an agility that was needed during combat operations and establishing a precedent for the command and control of overseas military operations that persists in today's combatant commands. Although preventive medicine officers in the AEF were constantly challenged with the poor sanitation of trench warfare, responding to outbreaks of influenza, diarrhea, and scabies,[25] the health of the force was considered to be generally good.[6]

The improvements made in the practice of field preventive medicine were the result of the coevolution of several scientific disciplines. Near the end of the war, the sanitary inspector for Second Army, AEF, was Hans Zinsser. A renowned bacteriologist, epidemiologist, and sanitarian, Zinsser may have been one of the first preventive medicine officers to link the disciplines of medical science, epidemiology, environmental engineering, laboratory science, and administration in what has become the standard for modern military preventive medicine. His publication on sanitation practices in a field army outlined the duties of "sanitary squads," today called field sanitation teams, established standards for disease prevention and control, and described the fundamentals of field epidemiology that became the foundation of current doctrine.[27]

WWI was also responsible for directing the attention of medical officers to two other problems associated with warfare: mental health disorders and the use of chemical weapons. While mental health disorders were not new to military forces, the sheer numbers of cases of "shell shock" in the British, Canadian, and French hospitals caught the attention of Gorgas, who put together a commission to study the problem in anticipation of the United States entering the war. Although the primary focus was on preparing to treat and/or evacuate those affected, the experts introduced the concept of screening for mental conditions to avoid sending those most susceptible into combat.[28] The medical department also had a role in gas warfare as it was the Surgeon General who was initially given the responsibility for developing and furnishing gas masks and other equipment to protect American forces from chemical attacks.[29] (This responsibility was transferred to a newly created Chemical Warfare Service in June 1918.) To achieve this, a dedicated manufacturing facility was constructed in Long Island City, New York, which employed just under 4700 civilians at its peak.[6] It was quickly realized that such a facility required some type of sanitary enforcement to protect the workers from hazards and exposures associated with the manufacturing and testing processes. The Office of the Surgeon General partnered with the Bureau of Mines to create the "Sanitary Supervision of Gas Factories," which provided oversight of worker safety and health in all government and contractor facilities working in the gas warfare industry.[30] This first foray into occupational health and industrial hygiene for civilian workers by military preventive medicine would expand greatly during World War II.

In the immediate aftermath of WWI, preventive medicine officers in Europe found themselves part of an occupying force that needed to reestablish sanitation and other public health activities in devastated areas. This new function was not something the U.S. military had prepared for, and civil affairs, as it would become known, required new policies and procedures. Fortunately, an experienced chief sanitary officer with the Third Army stationed in Trier, Walter Bensel, was able to work with and provide support to the German public health services to meet the needs of the civilian population. At the local level, military preventive medicine officers worked with their civilian public health counterparts to share information on cases of communicable disease and coordinate responses to outbreaks of typhoid fever, diphtheria, and influenza.[31]

In the period between the World Wars, medical science and public health would advance more rapidly than ever. Antibiotics were discovered, starting with penicillin in 1929, along with the protocols for both treatment of bacterial infections and use of these drugs for prophylaxis and to eliminate carrier states. Virology became a more prominent field of science, and new laboratory techniques such as serology were developed. A new antimalarial drug, atabrine, was introduced as a substitute for quinine.[6] In public health, epidemiology and sanitary engineering became more prominent disciplines, educational programs in preventive medicine expanded as more schools of public health were established, and work on noncommunicable disease control efforts, such as injury prevention, industrial exposures, psychiatric disorders, and nutritional deficiencies, started to gain more prominence, as did the burgeoning field of aviation medicine. In the military, budget pressures following the Great Depression and a series of reorganizations and personnel shortages lowered the prominence of preventive medicine until, in 1940, James Simmons was ordered to Washington, DC, to establish the Army's Preventive Medicine Service in preparation for the potential of the United States to enter World War II.[25]

As in the run-up to WWI, a rapid mobilization of American men to increase the size of the U.S. military forces, including the first use of a national draft, resulted in crowded conditions in training camps and the expected increase in cases of communicable disease. Clean water and waste disposal were challenges, as was the familiar problem of VD; the USPHS was once again called on to support prevention efforts in the communities around military camps. Over the course of the war, Simmons directed a preventive medicine staff in the Office of the Surgeon General that eventually swelled to 53 officers, one-sixth of the OTSG, and oversaw important advancements in public health. As the U.S. military moved into tropical areas, Simmons expanded education and training in tropical medicine for military officers, established yellow fever immunization requirements, and started a medical intelligence division to gather data on endemic diseases and other health threats across the globe. In the wake of Italy's surrender, he charted a typhus commission to investigate and deploy countermeasures, including the use of DDT to control lice during outbreaks in Naples, and prevent epidemics in POWs, civilian refugees, and concentration camp survivors.[32]

Civil affairs again gained prominence in occupied areas, as military sanitarians supported local public health personnel to protect the health of the civilian populations as they rebuilt societies devastated by war. Medical research was accelerated, with vaccines against Japanese encephalitis (1944) and influenza (1945) used to protect military personnel against these diseases for the first time. On the home front, Simmons helped establish the Armored Force Research Lab to evaluate the ergonomics and hazardous exposures associated with armored vehicles such as tanks. He also called upon Johns Hopkins University, which had previously supported the Army by providing public health education, to establish an Army Industrial Hygiene Laboratory to protect civilian munitions workers in the hundreds of production facilities across the country.[33] (This lab would relocate to Aberdeen Proving Ground, MD, where it grew over time and changed names several times, becoming what is now the Army Public Health Center.) As a result of Simmons' leadership and efforts of preventive medicine personnel throughout the military, deaths from disease would reach their lowest levels as a percentage of total deaths in U.S. military forces since the birth of the nation.[34]

Unfortunately, in what had become, and continues to be, a cycle of relearning old lessons, failures to prevent disease and injury highlighted the critical importance of command emphasis. General MacArthur quickly came to understand this after malaria incapacitated significant numbers of U.S. forces in the Pacific; he realized that medical advice and supplies were only as good as his commanders' willingness to prioritize them and take action, including ensuring the education and training of leaders and troops on disease and injury prevention as well as holding commanders accountable for enforcing good discipline and ensuring use of countermeasures.[35] A similar lesson would be (re)learned in Europe during the winter of 1944–5 when 90,000 cold weather injuries immobilized General Patton's infantry due to failure of commanders to provide the proper winter clothing in favor of ammunition and gasoline, a decision General Omar Bradley admitted to making after the war.[36]

In contrast, British Lieutenant General William Slim demonstrated what effective leadership can do to improve the health of a military force. Slim assumed command of the 14th Army during the China-Burma-India campaign in 1943. His initial assessment of his troops was grim: malaria, dysentery, hepatitis A, various skin diseases, and scrub typhus were out of control. On an annualized basis, 84% of his soldiers got malaria, and his overall disease and nonbattle injury (DNBI) evacuation rate was 12 per 1000 per day, 120 times greater than his evacuation rate for battle injuries.[37] Slim developed a medical plan that included a heavy emphasis on prevention and forward treatment, but its success relied on what the British called "medical discipline." He issued orders such as requiring antimalarial medication to be taken under supervision, and he relieved commanders who failed to enforce them, using regular medical surveillance and surprise blood testing of whole units to determine if the medication was being taken regularly.[38] The results of Slim's actions were dramatic, with DNBI rates plummeting, evacuations cut to 1 per

1000 per day, and the 14th Army successfully recapturing lands from the Japanese by 1945.[37]

Both infectious diseases and cold weather would challenge the U.S. military again in Korea. The primary infectious concern was malaria, and chloroquine prophylaxis was used during the transmission season, successfully reducing the impact of the disease on combat operations.[39] However, a new problem emerged as service members stopped their chemoprophylaxis while aboard ships heading home: they developed malaria. The temperate form of *Plasmodium vivax* was inadequately prevented or treated with chloroquine alone, and studies were quickly conducted to find a new drug that could eliminate the parasites from a patient's liver, where they were able to elude chloroquine. Primaquine was shown to be effective in this regard, and it was added to the chemoprophylaxis regimen, a practice still in use today.[40] Preparation for the effects of the harsh Korean winters, however, was inadequate. Education on prevention of cold weather injuries was deficient, and soldiers were not provided appropriate uniforms and protective footwear.[41] Better planning and command emphasis led to improvements the following winter, but once again important lessons in prevention and the need for "medical discipline" were learned the hard way.[42]

The Vietnam War brought new challenges. *Falciparum* malaria in southeast Asia was developing resistance to chloroquine, altering the chemoprophylaxis regimen from weekly dosing to daily, which required additional supervision and testing to ensure compliance.[43] Bacterial and fungal skin infections, along with immersion foot (tropical type), became the dominant medical conditions, in some units reducing combat strength by 50%.[44] Operations in the Mekong delta, where up to 90% of the land is covered in water, required soldiers to patrol for days submerged in flooded rice paddies. Knowledge concerning the prevention, diagnosis, and treatment of skin disease was limited, and the lack of DNBI reporting meant the problem went unnoticed at higher levels of command.[44] In response, teams of experts were mobilized to study the problem and make recommendations, including from the AFEB and the Walter Reed Army Institute of Research, resulting in significant changes to regulations and individual commanders' actions.[45] Units began tracking medical data and nonavailability of personnel, testing new types of footwear and skin ointments, and ultimately implemented guidance on duration of exposure (i.e., limiting patrol length in wet conditions) and requirements for recovery (a drying period). The results were dramatic: lost man-days from skin diseases dropped by two-thirds.[46]

U.S. Forces would not mobilize again in large numbers until the first Gulf War in 1990. During Operations Desert Shield and Desert Storm, DNBI rates were the lowest of any previous conflict, approximately half the rate seen during Vietnam, and less than one-quarter those of WWII or Korea.[47] Improvements in medical intelligence, well-established and understood preventive medicine policies and practices, enforcement of those by commanders, and time to prepare for the operation all contributed to the low rates. The Gulf War, however, cast a long shadow, as service members began complaining of multisymptom illnesses for which there were no clear etiologies. The low DNBI rates continued in the recent wars in Iraq and Afghanistan, and like the first Gulf War, most of the health conditions we now associate with the conflicts, and continue to study, became manifest in the affected service members months or years after they returned home. While musculoskeletal injuries (MSKI) were the most frequent cause of morbidity, in-theater hospitalization, and medical evacuation, mental health conditions have captured the most attention as suicide rates have risen along with diagnoses of depression and posttraumatic stress disorder, among others. Delayed-onset, chronic health impacts of environmental exposures also echo the aftermath of the first Gulf War, led by concern over respiratory effects from air pollution, including that caused by burn pits used by the military for waste disposal. More information on these topics is covered later in this chapter.

While most of what we know today as the basic principles of military preventive medicine were known at the time of the American Revolution, and despite the frequent lapses in remembering lessons learned from prior conflicts, steady progress in reducing the impact of disease and injury on military operations is readily apparent. Great leaders, visionary physicians, and innovative scientists, both military and civilian, armed with advances in knowledge and technological breakthroughs, contributed to changes in policy and doctrine; education and training; materiel; and the TTPs used by all service members to protect themselves and their units from medical threats. With improved health and readiness, military forces can achieve highly degrees of combat effectiveness. Perhaps as important, the prevention or mitigation of long-term disability resulting from medical threats during military operations allows veterans to live long, productive lives and continue to contribute to the country for which they sacrificed so much while in uniform. Society as a whole benefits from the continued productivity of veterans as they transition to become civilian workers and the reduced need for long-term healthcare spending. While much of the attention in military medicine is focused on battlefield trauma and the most effective ways to save the lives of service members injured in combat, a most critical capability to be sure, history has demonstrated repeatedly that preventive medicine is the greatest force multiplier.

THE MILITARY HEALTH SYSTEM

The modern U.S. armed forces, similar to most other major militaries in the modern world, are composed of branches or Services: Army, Navy, Air Force, Marine Corps. Each Service has an active component—Service members who are full-time employees of the Department of Defense—and a reserve component consisting of individuals who have civilian occupations but who maintain military roles and train regularly to be ready if called upon ("activated") to serve. In the United States, the reserve component is further divided into units under federal control (Reserves) and those under state control (National Guard). The President is the Commander in Chief of the federal armed forces, while the governors of the states and territories have jurisdiction over their National Guard forces (unless/until they are federalized). The United States has three other uniformed services, one of which, the U.S. Coast Guard (USCG), is also an armed force but is part of the Department of Homeland Security (DHS); the other two, the Commissioned Corps of the U.S. Public Health Service (PHS) and the National Oceanographic and Atmospheric Administration (NOAA), are not armed forces and are part of the Department of Health and Human Services (DHHS) and DHS, respectively.

The MHS serves approximately 9.4 million beneficiaries worldwide, including active duty personnel, reservists, retirees, and family members, with a budget of over $50 billion per year. In fiscal year 2017, there were over 106 million outpatient visits, over 1 million hospitalizations, over 110,000 births, and almost 120 million prescriptions filled in the MHS.[48] The MHS operates its own facilities, approximately 50 hospitals and over 600 medical and dental clinics, but also relies on civilian healthcare providers in its network, especially in remote locations and for specialized care. Active duty military personnel and their dependents have universal access to care that is centrally funded, i.e., there are no out-of-pocket costs, including referral care in the private sector. All healthcare providers in the MHS hospitals and medical and dental clinics are salaried military or civilian government employees or contracted civilian personnel. Options that increase provider choice, including use of private sector services without referral, and coverage for nonactive duty personnel and family members, are available with a combination of deductibles and copays. Separated Service members can obtain medical services from the Department of Veterans Affairs (VA) for service-connected conditions, and retired Service members have access to either DoD or VA treatment facilities.

In addition to healthcare delivery, the MHS provides medical education, medical research and development, and public health services. It is led by the Assistant Secretary of Defense for Health Affairs who reports to the Undersecretary of Defense for Personnel and Readiness. Historically, each branch of service (Army, Navy, and Air Force) has operated its own treatment facilities, medical research programs, and public health organizations. (The Marine Corps does not have organic medical assets; medical support is provided by the Navy.) Based on successes with joint medical operations on the battlefield, in 2011 the Deputy Secretary of Defense chartered a task force to provide recommendations for long-term governance of the MHS in an effort to improve outcomes related to access, quality, and safety as well as to achieve cost savings through more efficient, integrated medical services.[49] This led to the establishment of the Defense Health Agency (DHA) in 2013 to assume responsibility for a portfolio of shared medical services, activities, and facilities. Led by a three-star general officer, the DHA became fully operational in 2015, and in 2016 Congress further directed the consolidation of the management and administration of all military treatment facilities (MTFs) under the DHA with the passage of the National Defense Authorization Act (NDAA) for Fiscal Year 2017.[50] Two years later, in the NDAA for Fiscal Year 2019, Congress further directed the transfer of the Service-level public health centers—the Army Public Health Center, the Navy and Marine Corps Public Health Center, and parts of the United States Air Force School of Aerospace Medicine—to the DHA.[51] Installation-level preventive medicine and public health assets that are part of an MTF will transfer to DHA as a result of the NDAA for Fiscal Year 2017, but preventive medicine units organic to operational units will remain with their commands.

The DHA, in addition to managing the DoD's health benefit (known as TRICARE), including provision of care at all DoD-owned treatment facilities and the purchased care contracts, was created to serve as a combat support agency for the DoD's Combatant Commands. In this latter role, the DHA is responsible for medical readiness policies and procedures for all Service members as well as the education and training of military medical personnel. A DoD Directive issued in September 2013 formally directed the agency to "optimize readiness to deploy medically ready forces and ready medical forces" and to advise and assist the Chairman of the Joint Chiefs of Staff, combatant commanders, and other leaders on health readiness, including "public health matters."[52] The DHA includes a Public Health Division (PHD) that supports commanders and their medical staffs with advanced global health surveillance capabilities; standardized deployment health assessment tools; immunization policy guidance and clinical support; and oversight of veterinary services, including both military working animal care and ensuring safe food and water sources for service members worldwide.[53]

The central epidemiologic resource for U.S. military is the Armed Forces Health Surveillance Branch (AFHSB) of the DHA. The AFHSB operates the Defense Medical Surveillance System (DMSS), one of the most comprehensive longitudinal databases in existence, containing billions of records on service members from 1990 to the present. The system includes demographic data, outpatient visits, hospitalizations, immunization records, reportable medical events, health risk appraisals, history of assignments and deployments, deployment health assessments, and casualty data (Fig. 10-2). Data in the DMSS can be linked to the Department of Defense Serum Repository (DoDSR), also operated

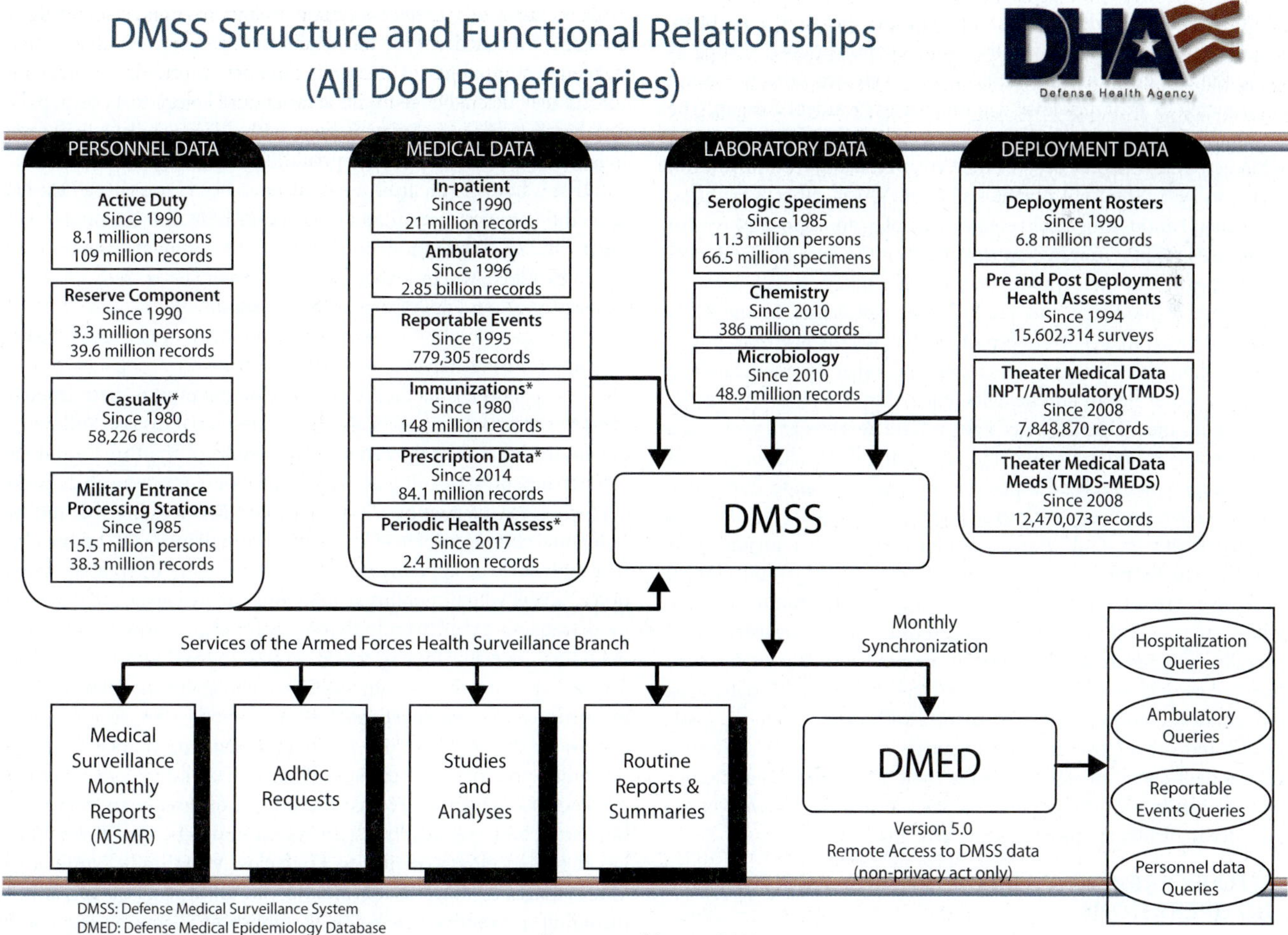

FIGURE 10-2. Defense Medical Surveillance System data structure. (*Source:* From Armed Forces Health Surveillance Branch, Public Health Division, Defense Health Agency.)

by the AFHSB, which houses over 62 million serial serum specimens obtained primarily from routine human immunodeficiency virus testing of more than 10 million service members starting in 1989.[54] While the DMSS and DoDSR are used predominantly by epidemiologists and researchers to study important, military-relevant questions, commanders, and medical personnel in the field, as well as senior defense leaders, also rely on the AFHSB to assess medical threats and provide evidence to inform decision-making. The AFHSB integrates data from partners such as the National Center for Medical Intelligence, open source reports, its own Global Emerging Infections Surveillance (GEIS), the Early Notification of Community-Based Epidemics (ESSENCE) system, and the DMSS to provide near real-time updates and assessments of global health events.[55] The AFHSB also publishes the *Medical Surveillance Monthly Report (MSMR)*, a monthly, peer-reviewed journal on health surveillance topics relevant to military service as well as intermittent reports of special interest, such as results of outbreak investigations in military populations.[56]

The Department of Veterans Affairs

U.S. Service members who have separated from the military may receive medical care for service-related health conditions in any of the 144 medical centers and over 1200 outpatient locations operated by the Department of Veterans Affairs (VA). Now a separate, cabinet-level department in the Executive Branch, the VA traces its history to the early days of the United States, when individual states and communities cared for their veterans. The Federal government established the first national care facility at the end of the Civil War, but the system grew significantly during World War I, and Congress established the Veterans Bureau in 1921. President Hoover, in an executive order signed in 1930, consolidated the Bureau with other government-operated programs for veterans into the Veterans Administration. World War II would drive the next expansion, including more healthcare facilities and expanded benefits, such as the GI Bill, but it was not until 1988 that the Veterans Administration was elevated to a cabinet-level department by President Reagan. The VA renamed its component departments, and the former Department of Medicine and Surgery became the Veterans Health Administration (VHA) in 1991. The VHA operates all of the VA's healthcare facilities, which also conduct medical research and play an important role in healthcare provider training (approximately 60% of medical residents spend a portion of their training in a VHA hospital).[57]

Preventive medicine and public health specialists in the DoD work closely with their counterparts in the VA on research, policy and program development, education, and other efforts related to service member health and benefits. Public health in the VA is organized under the VHA's Office of Patient Care Services and includes a strong focus on understanding and addressing the health impacts of known deployment-related exposures (e.g., Agent Orange, burn pits), illnesses or syndromes specific to an operation or region (e.g., illnesses associated with the Gulf War), conditions with higher incidence or prevalence in veterans (e.g., posttraumatic stress disorder), and clinical preventive care for veterans (e.g., tobacco cessation, immunizations). Long-term cohort studies of veterans, exposure-specific registries, and carefully designed research protocols are used to better understand potential associations between military service and health outcomes, both acute and chronic. The VA partners with major academic institutions and other governmental organizations, and often convenes independent panels of experts via the National Academies and other premier institutions to provide the best-available, evidence-based guidance to healthcare providers and veterans.[58]

MILITARY PREVENTIVE MEDICINE ORGANIZATION AND OPERATIONS

Unlike the civilian public health system in the United States, which operates mostly independent of healthcare delivery, military public health at the installation level is often aligned with or managed by the local medical treatment facility, especially in the Army and Navy. There are also preventive medicine assets that are organic to, or can be deployed with, operational military forces, such as the Army's preventive medicine detachments or the Navy's preventive medicine units. The Air Force's public health and aerospace medicine assets (e.g., flight surgeons) are mostly assigned to operational units (wings) and remain an organic medical asset of that unit whether at their home base or deployed. At higher echelons, there may be regional preventive medicine assets that operate in support of the installation-level resources, and each Service has a central public health organization to provide highly specialized functions and advanced expertise, similar to the role of the Centers for Disease Control and Prevention or a large state health department in its support of city and county public health resources.

In general, military preventive medicine and public health at the installation level includes the core functions of medical surveillance, epidemiology, health promotion, environmental health, occupational health, industrial hygiene, veterinary public health, and health physics (radiation safety and protection). The size and extent of specific services are dependent on the mission(s) of the units operating at a given installation. Preventive medicine and occupational and environmental medicine physicians are often the chiefs of installation-level public health resources and serve as the public health emergency officer for that installation, while also providing clinical services such as travel medicine, flight physicals, and other occupation-specific exams. At higher echelons, these physicians are often directing larger public health organizations, serving as advisors to senior military leaders, developing and evaluating service- or theater-level policies and programs, conducting medical research, and/or teaching in academic programs, such as one of the residency programs and/or the Uniformed Services University of the Health Sciences. Depending on the branch of service, type of installation/environment, and unique mission requirements of the units supported, preventive medicine officers may be challenged with a varied and complex set of population-based issues. An Army arsenal, with a large civilian workforce engaged in munitions work, is quite different from an Army installation that is home to an airborne division; a Navy submarine base has some different concerns than an Air Force base training pilots to fly supersonic jets. Operations in deployed environments present their own difficulties, whether they involve a Navy fleet at sea, a forward air base, or ground operations on foreign soil.

The responsibilities of preventive medicine and public health personnel during deployments begin well before troops leave their home installation. A medical threat assessment must be performed to identify the presence and magnitude of potential disease and injury threats in the area of operations. The nature of the threats and the countermeasures to mitigate them must be communicated to the deploying service members, especially countermeasures that rely on individual actions or behaviors, such as compliance with taking chemoprophylaxis or applying insect repellent. Early in combat operations, during which mobility is high and enemy engagement may be more frequent, reliance on individual countermeasures is high. Once the operation stabilizes and forces remain in fixed locations, such as forward operating bases, more sophisticated environmental countermeasures can be employed, such as area support for vector control and waste disposal. During the deployment, preventive medicine personnel conduct medical surveillance and respond to identified problems to prevent or reduce the impact of disease and injury on individual and unit readiness. In recent conflicts, the U.S. military has deployed alongside and worked closely with allied militaries. This requires significant coordination in all aspects of operations, including preventive medicine. Establishing common standards and procedures ahead of time, as is done among members of the North Atlantic Treaty Organization (NATO), helps ensure disease and injury prevention practices are supported and implemented by all service members and their leaders, regardless of nationality. In many cases, military preventive medicine personnel will also work with local national military and/or civilian public health authorities to assist them with improving the health of their own population, especially if forces remain in the region over time.

Upon redeployment, service members are assessed using standardized questionnaires to collect information on potential exposures and health conditions they experienced while deployed, once as they leave theater and return home, and again approximately 6 months later. This information is used both as a screening mechanism to identify individuals who may require further care or other interventions and as part of the each service member's longitudinal data set maintained as part of the DoD's health surveillance system. Military preventive medicine and public health professionals continue to monitor and support service members throughout the redeployment period as some health outcomes related to the deployment may not develop for months or years later.

SELECTED HEALTH THREATS TO MILITARY PERSONNEL

Military operations expose service members to unique health threats, from extreme environments on land, sea, and in the air, to physical and psychological stressors associated with prolonged deployments. From the first day of entry-level training, soldiers, sailors, airmen, and Marines are challenged with tasks and conditions that put their physical and mental health at risk. Many of these are well known and well characterized, and while some are prevented or mitigated through use of proven countermeasures, others persist as vexing problems for which solutions have yet to be developed or discovered. While it is impossible to cover all threats to service members' health in this chapter, those having the greatest adverse impact and/or highlighting unique aspects of military service will be reviewed.

Musculoskeletal Injuries

As one might expect in a population of highly active, predominantly young adults training and working in military occupations with high physical demands, MSKI are the most significant cause of morbidity and disability in service members. Their adverse impact on readiness is staggering, accounting for more than 3 million medical encounters annually and over 25 million limited duty days. About half of all service members experience one or more injuries per year, and the most commonly injured anatomic sites include the back and lower extremities, especially the knee.[59] The most common causes of MSKI are physical training and sports, led by running and road marching, followed by other training activities such as weightlifting and sports such as basketball.[60] Slips/trips/falls and motor vehicle injuries are other important causes of MSKI and contribute a greater proportion of injury-related hospitalizations. The impact and causes of MSKI are mostly consistent across operational and training environments, but with some variability in risk by occupation.[61] During deployments, military personnel experience injuries remarkably similar to those which occur in garrison. Despite exposure to the obvious dangers of combat, where injuries can be much more severe due to penetrating and nonpenetrating trauma, MSKI remain the most common reason for both in-theater medical treatment and for medical evacuation, and those MSKI are mostly the result of personal training and sports/athletics during off-duty hours. In the recent combat theaters of Iraq and Afghanistan, nonbattle injuries, mostly MSKIs, were responsible for 1.5- to 2-fold more air evacuations out of theater than combat-related injuries.[62]

MSKIs in the military are more commonly the result of cumulative micro-trauma than acute events, the former with a rate approximately fourfold higher than the latter[63] and accounting for 85% more limited duty days.[64] Historically, the military has used ICD-10 disease groups for conducting MSKI surveillance, but this has often obfuscated the true burden of MSKI as most of the diagnoses in the "musculoskeletal diseases" group are actually injuries from cumulative microtrauma, such as pain and inflammation of joints and tendons. (The "injuries and poisonings" group is also mostly MSKI.) Thus, the Army Public Health Center developed a more accurate taxonomy based on the energy transfer that is the cause of the injury to tissue.[65] Not only does this improve the accuracy of injury surveillance, it provides an effective means of communicating the injury burden to military commanders and better informs potential interventions. Initial application of the new taxonomy demonstrated that of all injuries in Army active duty personnel in 2017, 97% were due to mechanical energy transfer, 83% were MSKIs, and 76% were the result of cumulative micro-trauma; the lower back and knee were the sites of almost one-third of all mechanical injuries; almost one-half occurred to some part of the lower extremity.[66]

Risk factors for MSKI in the military can be grouped into intrinsic and extrinsic factors, most of which are modifiable (Table 10-1) and related to overtraining. There is an important paradox to understand here: while the best predictor of an increased risk of MSKI is poor aerobic fitness, which is improved by activities such as running, too much running is the greatest cause of MSKI. In other words, like many medications, what is protective at a low-to-moderate dose is harmful at high doses. Faster run times as measured during physical fitness testing have been shown to be associated with reduced risk of MSKI in military trainee populations[67–70] and operational forces.[61,71] When combined with sex and body composition, subpopulations of higher risk are evident, with poor aerobic fitness and either too low or too high body mass index (BMI) associated with increased risk of MSKI.[70] Low BMI is also specifically associated with increased risk of stress fractures in both male and female basic trainees.[72]

Recent studies have pointed out the problems with current military training regimens, especially in basic (initial) military training. High amounts of low-intensity endurance training (e.g., running) has negative effects on training adaptation and increases the risk of MSKI, especially in recruits entering the military with higher BMI and lower levels of general fitness.[73] On the other end of the spectrum, highly fit recruits require variation in the training stimulus to prevent a plateau in performance.[74] New approaches to individualize training, vary the training stimuli, and incorporate interval training, which can improve performance while decreasing exposure to MSKI risk, are being evaluated. One nonmodifiable risk factor, being female, is being re-examined with the recent integration of women into what were historically all-male combat roles, such as infantry. While studies have repeatedly shown military women to have approximately twice the risk of injury as men, this is primarily due to lower levels of aerobic fitness; studies that controlled for fitness demonstrated a similar MSKI injury rate among military women and men.[75]

Although not as significant as physical training and sports on overall MSKI burden in the military, there are unique injury risks related to specific subpopulations, tasks, activities, and environments. Parachuting; mounting/dismounting large vehicles and other land-, sea-, and aircraft; obstacle courses; and operating military equipment, such as some weapons systems, contribute to acute injuries in the form of strains/sprains and fractures from impact forces and slips/trips/falls. To take one example, military paratroopers engage in an inherently dangerous activity where injury risk is affected by multiple factors, including equipment used (e.g., parachute type, combat load), type of jump (e.g., static line, freefall), type of platform (e.g., plane, helicopter), weather conditions (e.g., temperature, wind speed), time of day, terrain of the drop zone, and operational setting (e.g., training, combat). Most injuries occur at ground impact, which occurs at 10–15 miles per hour or more, depending on many of the factors mentioned above.[76] Injury rates vary in studies of military paratroopers from as low as 1 injury per 1000 jumps in daylight from balloons to 29 per 1000 in a mass tactical assault exercise with full combat gear at night in inclement weather.[77] Attempts to reduce

TABLE 10-1 RISK FACTORS FOR MSKI IN MILITARY SERVICE MEMBERS

RF Category		RF Name	Effect on MSKI Risk
Intrinsic			
	Demographic	Female sex	Increases
		Older age	Increases
	Anatomic	High foot arches	Increases
		Knock knees	Increases
		High Q angles	Increases
	Physical fitness	Low aerobic fitness	Increases
		Low muscle endurance	Increases
		Muscle strength	No effect
		Low and high flexibility	Increases
		Low and high BMI (body composition)	Increases
	Health behaviors	Inactivity/sedentary lifestyle	Increases
		Tobacco use	Increases
		Prior injury	Increases
Extrinsic	Activities	Running (distance)	Increases
		Physical training other than running (amount)	Increases
		Acceleration of training (rapid increases)	Increases
		Obstacle courses	Increases
		Road marching/load carriage	Increases
		Job duties	Increases
	Interventions	Standardized training; reduced running	Decreases
		Ability groups for running	Decreases
		Cross-training to replace running	Decreases
		Back brace	No effect
		Running shoe type	No effect
		Boots vs. running shoes	No effect
		Insoles/orthotics	Inconclusive
		Training surface	Inconclusive
		Stretching before exercise	Inconclusive

Source: Adapted from Jones, Hauschild, and Canham-Chervak, Musculoskeletal training injury prevention in the U.S. Army: Evolution of the science and the public health approach. Journal of Science and Medicine in Sport. 21(2018), 1139-1146.

parachuting injuries, such as improving parachute design and use of ankle braces, have been mixed. Repeated studies in the 1990s showed the parachute ankle brace to be effective in reducing ankle injuries by 40–50%, but lack of acceptance by paratroopers, citing discomfort and impracticality of use during exercises and missions, prevented widespread adoption.[78]

Behavioral (Mental) Health Conditions

Behavioral (mental) health conditions are second to MSKI in number of outpatient medical encounters and lost duty days, and they are first in number of hospitalized bed-days. The most common mental health conditions responsible for outpatient medical encounters and number of individuals affected among active component service members are adjustment disorders, followed by anxiety disorders, mood disorders, and substance abuse disorders; the conditions responsible for the most hospitalized bed-days are mood disorders, followed by substance abuse disorders and adjustment disorders.[59] In Iraq and Afghanistan, behavioral health conditions were the third most common reason for air evacuation out of theater, accounting for 10–12% of the total, after MSKI at 31–34% and battle injuries at 16–20%.[62]

Pre-existing mental health disorders, like certain other physical ailments, are often disqualifying for military service if they are disclosed or otherwise detected during the medical screening process. Serving in the military can expose individuals to stressors and other risk factors that can lead to the development or exacerbation of various behavioral health conditions, most classically what is now called posttraumatic stress disorder (PTSD). Of great concern over the past decade or so has been the increase in suicides among current and former service members. Historically, suicide rates were lower in military populations than age- and sex-adjusted civilian populations, but rates in the military, most notably in the Army and Marine Corps, began increasing in 2004 and exceeded those of the comparable U.S. civilian population in 2008.[79] In response, the Army partnered with the National Institute of Mental Health, Harvard University, the Uniformed Services University, University of Michigan, the University of California-San Diego, and other leading academic and military organizations on an initial $60 million, 5-year program to comprehensively study the problem of suicide, suicide-related behavior and other mental/behavioral health issues.[80] The Army Study to Assess Risk and Resilience in Service members (Army STARRS), began in 2010 and was continued in 2015 for another 5 years as STARRS-Longitudinal Study (STARRS-LS). To date, these researchers have published almost 90 peer-reviewed journal articles.[81] In addition to providing important insights in risk and protective factors associated with behavioral health in the military, novel approaches using machine learning to develop predictive risk models allow for targeted preventive interventions in those individuals at risk for suicidal behavior, interpersonal violence, and various psychiatric disorders.[82–84] Unfortunately, despite this effort and many others funded by the DoD and VA, the challenge of preventing suicides in active duty service members and veterans persists, and rates continue to remain elevated. New approaches using predictive analytics, improved risk assessment tools, incorporation of novel theories such as the concept of moral injury,[85] and more effective means to destigmatize mental illness in the military culture are among the many ongoing efforts to seek effective solutions to this complex problem.

Although the term "mental health" is still used in some military reporting, the DoD favors the use of the term "behavioral health" to encompass clinically diagnosed mental health or psychological disorders. This was a change in the mid-2000s to help reduce the stigma associated with mental health conditions and encourage Service members and other beneficiaries to seek care. The Vice Chief of Staff of the Army (VCSA) at that time, General Peter Chiarelli, led efforts to address the suicide problem and its antecedent behavioral health conditions, issuing first the "Red Book," formally titled "Army Health Promotion, Risk Reduction, Suicide Prevention Report 2010,"[86] followed by the "Gold Book," officially titled "Army 2020: Generating Health & Discipline in the Force Ahead of the Strategic Reset Report 2012,"[87] both of which described a holistic approach to this major threat to force health and readiness. Chiarelli also advocated the American Psychiatric Association drop "disorder" from "posttraumatic stress disorder" in the *Diagnostic and Statistical Manual (DSM)* as a way to communicate to victims of PTSD that stress following trauma was not an illness or indication of mental frailty but rather a normal stress reaction or injury that could be managed with help from trained professionals.[88] Although posttraumatic stress has remained a "disorder" in *DSM-5*, the military continues to work to reduce the stigma associated with seeking help for behavioral health conditions, as well as to eliminate other potential barriers to care. For example, the Services moved some military behavioral health providers out of clinical facilities and embedded them in operational units where they could regularly engage with their fellow service members (build relationships), focus on prevention, intervene early, and treat in place (i.e., service members would not have to go to the clinic and risk feeling stigmatized). New behavioral health assessment tools were incorporated into the routine screenings and counseling sessions between service members and their leaders. Annual training requirements were expanded to include instruction in suicide prevention, mindfulness, and other methods of stress reduction, recognition of indicators of high-risk behavior, intervention techniques (e.g., Ask-Care-Escort), and ways to access help from medical and nonmedical experts.

The recent wars in Iraq and Afghanistan have been noteworthy for the injuries caused by blasts from improvised explosive devices (IEDs); traumatic brain injury (TBI), especially the most common form, mild TBI (mTBI) or concussion, has been called one of the "signature wounds" of these conflicts.[89] Understanding the association of mTBI with depression, PTSD and other mental health conditions have been a focus of much research. During the period 2000 through the first quarter of 2018, over 380,000 service members have been diagnosed with TBI, 82% of them mTBI,[90] and it is likely many more remain undiagnosed. TBI has been shown to increase the risk of mood disorders, anxiety disorders (including PTSD), substance abuse, sleep disorders, and psychosis.[91] The co-occurrence of TBI and PTSD can complicate diagnosis and lead to worse symptoms, many of which are common to both conditions, as well as to other psychiatric disorders, but the relative role of TBI in experiencing postconcussive symptoms or developing PTSD remains uncertain.[92,93] One of the biggest challenges in studying these problems in the context of military operations is the difficulty in controlling for the many confounders that exist (e.g., combat intensity, quality, and duration of sleep).[94] Abnormalities in sleep (quality, duration, etc.) have been of specific interest, both as a target of treatment for TBI and PTSD, but also as a risk factor for the development and severity of these conditions.[95]

Infectious Diseases

Infectious diseases have had significant adverse effects on military operations throughout history, and although their impact on the readiness of modern forces has been greatly reduced, challenges remain. Whether the current, relatively low threat environment will continue, given the emergence of antimicrobial resistance and changes in pathogenicity of various organisms, is impossible to predict. Importantly, most of the infectious disease threats faced today are known prior to the deployment of military forces into an endemic area, and most of these infections are preventable. The widespread use of individual preventive countermeasures, such as effective vaccines, chemoprophylaxis, insect repellents, and protective clothing, along with administrative and engineering controls, such as policies restricting contact with animals (administrative), use of food and water sanitation protocols (administrative and engineering), or area spraying to reduce insect vectors (engineering), minimize the risk of exposure to infectious organisms.

Disease and nonbattle injuries tend to be highest early in deployments when conditions are austere. Early in Iraq and Afghanistan, the most common infectious diseases affecting the United States and coalition partners were gastrointestinal illnesses, primarily diarrhea, and respiratory infections, both of which resolve relatively quickly but can decrease operational efficiency in affected units. In one study of over 15,000 service members deployed to Iraq or Afghanistan early in the conflicts (2003–04), 75% reported diarrhea, and 69% indicated a respiratory illness; of those with diarrhea, 46% reported decreased job performance for an average of 2 days.[96] While gastrointestinal and respiratory infections tend to be common in almost all military operations, infectious disease threats specific to a given geographic area can impact readiness. The classic example is malaria, and although the threat in Afghanistan was limited to *Plasmodium vivax*, which has low mortality but can still take a service member "out of the fight," and there was essentially no threat in Iraq, one Marine unit that left Iraq for a mission in Liberia (very high risk) failed to initiate or comply fully with chemoprophylaxis and use of insect repellents, resulting in up to 80 cases of *falciparum* malaria, several of whom required hospitalization in stateside ICUs.[97] One new threat early in Iraq demonstrates another failure to comply with preventive countermeasures, as well as lack of area-wide vector control measures: leishmaniasis. Transmitted by the bite of a sandfly, U.S. forces had not experienced this disease in large numbers since World War II, and by end of 2004 there were over 1300 cases.[98] Almost all the cutaneous form, which is not life-threatening, the infection can still interfere with activities and can be difficult to treat. Like other vectorborne diseases, leishmaniasis is preventable by employing personal protective measures, collectively referred to as the DoD Insect Repellent System, and consisting of the proper wearing of a permethrin-treated uniform, applying an approved insect repellent to exposed skin, and using permethrin-treated bed nets.[99]

Although a very different situation, the DoD's response to the Ebola outbreak in West Africa in 2014, Operation United Assistance, was largely an infectious disease success story. The deployment of almost 3000 U.S. military personnel to Liberia, the first ever deployment of the armed forces to control an infectious disease outbreak, was carefully planned and executed to prevent U.S. service members from becoming infected, despite other challenges.[100] The major threat, however, was not Ebola, as the U.S. military was not sent to treat patients, but rather the same *falciparum* malaria that affected the Marines in 2003. As with any large troop movement overseas, there were also concerns about the usual gastrointestinal and respiratory pathogens. Strict adherence to chemoprophylaxis and the DoD Insect Repellent System resulted in 32 cases of febrile illness over the 4-month deployment and no cases of malaria. The average prevalence of illness was 1.8%, of which most were gastrointestinal (33%), respiratory (22%), and dermatologic (20%).[101] The one preventive medicine failure, however, was in educating senior military and political leaders about the minimal Ebola risk to U.S. personnel and what appropriate screening and monitoring processes should be; instead, a policy of quarantine-like monitoring of all returning service members for 21 days in dedicated compounds was adopted despite being in opposition to the scientific evidence and in conflict with the procedures being used by other, nonmilitary medical organizations, including those in direct contact with Ebola patients.

The heightened concern about public perception or fear of a service member "bringing home" Ebola was unwarranted, but redeploying military personnel can certainly contribute to the spread of communicable diseases. The classic case of the influenza pandemic of 1918–19 is often cited as an example of this, and it is likely the mobilization and redeployment of troops to Europe played a significant role in transmission of the virus. Where initial exposure to the virus occurred, and to what strain(s), remains unclear as a fairly mild influenza-like illness affected service members in mobilization camps as well as those stationed in the trenches of France in the spring of 1918. Several experts believe, however, that the conditions in the trenches allowed for a more virulent strain to enter the U.S. personnel serving there, and it was they who brought it back stateside, arriving on ships in late August 1918 in Boston, and spreading the virus to nearby Camp Devens. Before any travel ban could be enforced, troops left Devens for Camp Upton, on Long Island, taking influenza there, and then further spread west and south eventually infected service members at camps throughout the country by late September.[26] Civilians working in and around the camps spread the virus into their local communities. The epidemic peaked in October, but in the end influenza and the associated secondary bacterial pneumonias would kill more U.S. service members during WWI than enemy fire.

Respiratory Infections in Basic Combat Training

Individuals joining the military as enlisted soldiers, sailors, airmen, or Marines enter basic training, a month's-long regimen to prepare them physically, mentally, socially, and culturally for service in the armed forces. The population dynamics of initial entry training—young adults from all geographic regions and socioeconomic backgrounds—along with the immunologic stress they experience from the physical and psychological exertion of training, crowding, and periodic deficiencies in personal hygiene and barracks sanitation, make these groups especially susceptible to respiratory infections. While some pathogens are common in other populations as well, there are at least two that are somewhat unique to basic trainees and have historically caused significant morbidity and loss of training time: adenovirus and Group A beta-hemolytic streptococcus (GABHS).

Data from the late 1950s and early 1960s indicated that adenoviruses caused hospitalization of approximately 10% of trainees, and during peak transmission in the winter months it was the cause of almost three-quarters of all respiratory disease. Infections occurred in the first 3 weeks of training, and serotypes 4 and 7 were responsible for the majority of cases.[102] Oral vaccines against these two serotypes were developed and routinely administered to trainees beginning in 1971; adenovirus infections dropped dramatically and remained low until the late 1990s, when the sole manufacturer ceased production (1996) and the last stocks were exhausted (1999).[103] Adenovirus quickly re-emerged as a predominant cause of respiratory disease in basic trainees, the majority of cases due to serotype 4,[104,105,106] and several notable outbreaks occurred until a new vaccine was licensed in 2011.[107] Following reintroduction of the vaccines, adenovirus disease declined 100-fold, as did all-cause acute respiratory disease in military trainee populations.[108] All new basic trainees continue to receive the two oral vaccines, and acute respiratory disease rates have remained at historically low levels.

A second infectious threat to basic trainees is GABHS. Periodic outbreaks in trainee populations after World War II led to studies in the 1950s to improve on the use of oral penicillin for prophylaxis, resulting in a regimen of injectable, high-dose benzathine penicillin G (BPG) that protects trainees from GABHS infection for several weeks.[109] Military training centers continued the practice of providing incoming trainees with a dose of BPG, known as tandem prophylaxis, until the mid-1970s to early 1980s when the centers began terminating the program due to a perceived decrease in the risk of severe streptococcal disease, such as acute rheumatic fever and pneumonia. Outbreaks at the Navy training center in San Diego (1986), Fort Leonard Wood (1988), and Lackland Air Force Base (1989) led to resumption of GABHS prophylaxis programs.[110] Fort Leonard Wood discontinued BPG use again in 1989 and 1993, only to see GABHS rates increase within months. Future interruptions in the supply of BPG would see the pattern repeated, further reinforcing the importance of prophylaxis in preventing severe GABHS disease.[111] Currently, all military basic training sites use some regimen of BPG prophylaxis, with penicillin-allergic trainees provided an alternative drug, such as a weekly dose of oral azithromycin for 4 weeks, except Fort Jackson, South Carolina. Variation in practice is based on the epidemiology at the specific location and decades of research, and for reasons still not understood today, the risk factors at each training are different. Fort Jackson has not had a GABHS outbreak despite never having a BPG prophylaxis program, while Navy and Marine Corps training centers administer an additional dose (or two) later in the training cycle, either year-round or only during high transmission season.[110]

Climate-related Illnesses and Injuries

Environmental extremes, particularly heat and cold, have been significant factors in military operations for millennia. In this century, morbidity and mortality from heat-related illnesses have far exceeded those of cold weather injuries, both in garrison and during deployments, due to a combination of geography, mission-related stressors, and advances in protective clothing (specifically cold weather gear). Most of the U.S. military's major training and force projection installations are in southern states, which continue to experience increasing average daily temperatures and longer periods of extreme heat days. Overseas deployments of personnel since 2001 have been primarily to the desert regions of southwest Asia and other hot climates. The exertional heat stress of military tasks performed in these environments can rapidly exceed the human body's physiological compensatory mechanisms, and without early recognition and intervention, can lead to severe organ damage and death. Despite awareness, education, and detailed doctrine on prevention of heat illness for military personnel and their leaders, these conditions have steadily increased over the past 5 years.

The DoD focuses on two types of heat illness: heat exhaustion and heat stroke.[112] The former, and less severe of the two, results from failure to maintain cardiac output due to physical exertion and environmental heat stress, resulting in an elevated core body temperature (38–40°C) and physical collapse, but no significant central nervous system (CNS) dysfunction. Heat stroke is characterized by severe hyperthermia (core body temperature of >40°C) and organ damage, including profound CNS dysfunction (e.g., delirium, seizures, coma).[113] In 2018, there were 578 incident cases of heat stroke (crude incidence rate = 0.45 per 1000 person-years) and 2214 (1.71 per 1000 p-yrs) of heat exhaustion among active component service members, but the risk is concentrated in young males (<20 years old) in the Army and Marine Corps in combat arms specialties (e.g., infantry, armor), and mostly in those still in initial entry training (12.55 per 1000 person-years).[114] This demographic is likely subjected to the greatest heat stress due to high metabolic heat production (strenuous physical activity over extended periods of time) and high environmental heat (training/operating in locations with high temperature and humidity), exacerbated by cumulative exposure and, in many cases, by the use of required protective clothing and equipment, dehydration, inadequate nutrition, and sleep deprivation. New recruits may arrive to basic training with additional risk factors, such as poor levels of fitness, elevated BMI, a minor illness, or taking certain medications; they may also be poorly acclimatized to heat, especially if they are coming from cooler climates. Genetic factors likely contribute to elevated risk in African Americans and Asian/Pacific Islanders. Fortunately, basic trainees are prohibited from using alcohol or taking dietary supplements, both of which can also contribute to risk of heat illness and are common in military personnel after completion of initial training. A final risk factor common in the military is overmotivation; a desire to avoid failure and to keep up with peers can cause individuals to ignore warning signs and/or reduce the likelihood of reporting symptoms to leaders or medical personnel.[115]

Two important and related conditions, exertional rhabdomyolysis and exertional hyponatremia, have the same risk factors and affect the same risk groups described above but may present without any elevation in core body temperature. Rhabdomyolysis is characterized by damage to skeletal muscle, often due to high-intensity, repetitive activity over time, especially in situations where the individual is unaccustomed to the type and degree of exertion. The accumulation of myoglobin from damaged muscle cells can cause renal failure, compartment syndrome, metabolic acidosis and lead to dysrhythmias and CNS dysfunction.[116] As with heat exhaustion and heat stroke, incident cases have increased in the Army and Marine Corps over the past 5 years.[117] Exertional hyponatremia (serum, plasma, or blood sodium below 135 milliequivalents per liter) in the military is often associated with overhydration in an attempt to prevent or treat suspected heat illness.[118] The signs and symptoms can often appear similar to heat stroke, which may be associated with dehydration, so obtaining a serum sodium level as quickly as possible is important to differentiate the two. Hyponatremia can rapidly lead to pulmonary and cerebral edema, the latter causing mental status changes, seizures, coma, and death. Nausea and emesis are common. Excessive sodium loss in sweat and earlier onset of sweating during exercise are associated with poor fitness levels, another reason this condition is frequently seen early in military training.

While elimination of heat-related medical outcomes is likely not possible given the nature of military operations, prevention of the worst outcomes is achievable with strict adherence to published guidance and recognition and treatment of early signs and symptoms. New trainees, cadre, and other leaders in high-risk environments must be trained on heat-related and exertional illnesses; high-risk service members must be closely monitored; strenuous activities should be preceded by graded preconditioning; and training events and other activities must be conducted according to established work/rest cycles and hydration protocols. When signs and symptoms occur, front-line medics must be fully trained and equipped to intervene early and appropriately. While there are no evidence-based standards for returning someone to full duty following a heat-related or exertional illness, medical providers should carefully evaluate individual risk and seek consultation with an appropriate expert as needed to minimize the likelihood of a future heat-related illness.

Other Deployment-related Environmental Exposures

The health effects of war are not always apparent during deployment or even soon after. Service members may develop delayed-onset, chronic illnesses that they attribute to potential environmental exposures during combat operations, even if no specific threats are identified or if exposures to known hazards occurred infrequently and/or at very low levels. Given the paucity of exposure data, passage of time, and the multifactorial nature of many illnesses, a definitive link to military-related exposures can rarely be determined. In the absence of scientific evidence, or sometimes despite data to the contrary, political decisions end up determining whether veterans receive compensation for medical care or disabilities after their period of active military service. In the past 50 years, several incidents of specific environmental exposures during military operations have highlighted the challenge for military preventive medicine and public health professionals, including Agent Orange in Vietnam; Kuwaiti oil well fires and a nerve agent release during the destruction of the Khamisiyah storage bunker in Operation Desert Storm; chromium and sulfur exposures during Operation Iraqi Freedom; and burn pit emissions in both Iraq and Afghanistan.

Agent Orange, one of many defoliants used in Vietnam to prevent enemy forces from using the forest canopy to hide their movements and positions, was contaminated with a type of dioxin associated to varying degrees of scientific confidence with specific adverse health outcomes.[119] To what extent individual service members were exposed, for how long, and whether the exposure led to a bioavailable dose that caused an illness is not knowable, so presumptions of exposure and associations with specific diseases are used to establish eligibility for compensatory benefits. Decades later, in the preparation leading up to the first Gulf War, the potential for exposure to oil well fires was predicted, and personnel were prepared to collect environmental sampling data to inform health risk assessments for specific geographical areas. But without individual location data, which was not collected during the conflict, estimated exposure to combustion products and the associated health risks had to be established using complex modeling based on retrospective analysis of where service members were likely to have been.[120] Concern about the oil well fires and other possible exposures, such as pesticides, chemical and biological warfare agents, various infectious diseases, and depleted uranium, independent of or interacting with various immunizations, chemoprophylaxis medications, and psychological stressors, became a significant focus of the DoD and VA when veterans of the Gulf War developed various health conditions years after their return to the United States. "Persian Gulf War Syndrome" or "Gulf War Illness" as it would become known resulted in numerous studies, investigations, and expert panels that, again, highlighted the challenges in establishing causative links between veterans' postwar illnesses and potential exposures during their deployment.[121]

Even in smaller, more circumscribed exposure incidents, the absence of individual-level exposure data precludes any definitive conclusions about health effects. As a group of U.S. troops were leaving Iraq in March 1991, they destroyed munitions bunkers in Khamisiyah, unintentionally releasing sarin nerve agent that was stored in one of the bunkers. Modeling by the CIA and DoD established the exposure area and probable levels at various distances from the site, which informed health outcome studies of the service members in the plume. While at least one study reported an association between exposure to the sarin plume and an increased risk of death from brain cancer,[122] the finding was questioned by other experts and found by the National Academies committee to be inadequate to establish an association.[121] Other studies based on self-reported questionnaire data indicate no association with the Khamisiyah event and subsequent morbidity.[123,124] Even today, the lack of data and resulting uncertainty of the science continue to pose a risk communication challenge for DoD and VA public health, and there will never be sufficient evidence to definitively support or refute health-related claims of harm from this battlefield exposure. In addition, despite important changes to deployment health surveillance, this problem will persist in future conflicts.

In large part as a result of the concern surrounding veterans' complaints of health problems resulting from their service during the first Gulf War, but also due to the relative success of the military in reducing acute illness and injury, the scope of military preventive medicine widened considerably to include a greater emphasis on low-level exposures and combinations of exposures that might lead to long-term health effects. In the wake of numerous governmental expert panels and publications in the 1990s, the Institute of Medicine's (IOM) 2000 report, Protecting Those Who Serve: Strategies to Protect the Health of Deployed U.S. Forces, set forth a series of recommendations that would improve force health protection, including documentation of medical encounters in theater, recording of service members' locations during deployment, more robust environmental exposure data and monitoring, an integrated health risk assessment paradigm, a comprehensive health surveillance system, and effective and timely communication of risks to inform rapid decision-making by commanders.[125] The military had already been working on implementing improvements, but activity increased significantly when it became clear on 11 September 2001 that another war was imminent.

The conflicts in Iraq and Afghanistan were the first to make use of in-theater electronic health records, web-based medical surveillance systems, daily location reporting, and increased environmental assessments of both troop locations and potential military targets. While these and other advances in force health protection contributed to low DNBI rates, the problem of linking exposures to health outcomes at the individual level remained unsolved, especially the long-term health effects of low-level exposures, whether intermittent or continuous. Despite increases in environmental sampling of base camps, the results were still representative of only the small area sampled and only at that one point in time. Individual location data were not continuous, and even with daily reporting, it was not possible to capture all locations visited by any one individual and for what duration of time, and, in the absence of an acute illness for which a service member seeks medical care, documentation of any concerns about potential exposures and adverse health effects are only systematically collected at the time of redeployment and again approximately 6 months later. While the self-reported information from these electronic assessments can be compared to a service member's predeployment questionnaire and annual periodic health assessments, all of which are required by DoD policy, the accuracy and completeness of the data are insufficient to determine causal links between exposures and outcomes.

Even in the case of known or predicted exposures, it can be difficult to determine what level of exposure should be considered safe. For many chemicals, there are published threshold values and exposure limits developed by government agencies and professional groups that are based on acute risk, and the military adopts them where applicable. In addition, the Army Public Health Center has developed additional guidance for lower-level continuous chemical exposures occurring over a 1-year period for deployed military personnel.[126] However, the experience with burn pits in Iraq and Afghanistan has demonstrated that science and medicine are still far from solving complex exposure scenarios, especially those where the exposure is mixed, intermittent, and occurs in the context of other hazards.

There are two ways to manage waste (trash) during a military operation: burn it or bury it. In most cases, operational considerations make the first option the better one, and in locations throughout Iraq and Afghanistan, waste was primarily disposed of in large, open burn pits. Although most are designed and located to minimize exposure of personnel to the smoke generated, winds shift and preventing any exposure is impossible. As service members developed illnesses in theater or even years later after returning home, many recalled the billowing black smoke and presumed a link between that potential exposure source and their health condition. Not as obvious, but arguably more significant, were the ubiquitous hazards of particulate matter (PM) from windblown dust, diesel exhaust, and other sources of local pollution. Air sampling over several years at the largest burn pit in Iraq, located at Joint Base Balad, documented periodic, low levels of volatile organic compounds, polycyclic aromatic hydrocarbons, and other chemicals, but very high levels of $PM_{2.5}$, the respirable constituent of PM, as much as twice the U.S. National Ambient Air Quality Standards.[127] A series of studies and reviews by experts, including the IOM, concluded that none of the individual chemicals from burn pits were likely to be associated with adverse health outcomes, but that PM levels were of more concern, and that deployment to Southwest Asia in general may be associated with respiratory conditions in susceptible individuals.[127]

Limitations in methodology, however, do not absolve any source of exposure as risk assessments do not look at mixtures of chemicals, nor are there standards from low-level and/or intermittent exposures over long periods of time. In the end, the IOM was unable to conclude whether burn pit emissions could be associated with long-term health outcomes.[128] Given the scientific limitations and ongoing concern among veterans about their exposures to burn pits, the fiscal year 2013 NDAA required the VA to establish a registry for these veterans, and the DoD expanded participation to currently serving service members.[129-132] Ongoing research studies continue to assess these and other potential exposures on the battlefield, but the continued inability to capture continuous, individual-level exposure data will preclude any definitive conclusions confirming or refuting links between specific exposures and health outcomes in individual service members. As with Agent Orange, in the end the decision to care for military personnel who claim their illnesses are the result of their service in Iraq and/or Afghanistan will largely be a political one.

THE FUTURE OF MILITARY PREVENTIVE MEDICINE

It is always difficult to predict the future, but that is precisely what senior military and political leaders spend a great deal of time doing. Using information from the best sources and experts available, they are charged with preparing to win the next war. In many ways, the future looks more challenging than ever. Despite the unprecedented levels of global peace and prosperity we experience today, the U.S. military must plan, train and equip for the worst-case scenario(s) should social, political, and/or economic forces cause changes that threaten the United States or its allies. The military dominance the United States has enjoyed for decades is unlikely to continue as other competitor nations close the technology gap and utilize tactics, such as cyberwarfare, that do not require large expenditures or industrial facilities to produce traditional weaponry and other material. Subjects once limited to science fiction novels have become topics of serious discussion: artificial intelligence; autonomous systems (e.g., vehicles, weapons); genetic engineering (as applied to both people and pathogens); space-based systems, both offensive and defensive; and many others. Most emerging technologies, while created to benefit society, can also be used to its detriment, so-called dual-use technology. As these technologies become cheaper and more accessible, even small groups of nonstate actors, such as terrorist organizations, will acquire the capabilities to do great harm. Where future conflicts take place is also likely to change. The rise of megacities and increased migration to these urban centers in the wake of climate change and other stressors increases the likelihood that future conflicts will take place in and around these large metropolitan areas.

So what does this mean for military medicine, and specifically military preventive medicine and public health? The core missions of disease and injury prevention and health promotion and optimization will remain, but the threats will change; existing threats may increase or decrease while new and emerging threats will require rapid identification, characterization, and development of countermeasures. New weapons systems, protective equipment, and other material being developed require health hazard assessments to ensure they do not expose the users (service members) to unintended harm, whether from noise, toxic byproducts, blast overpressure, vibration, heat, or many other potential hazards. New operating microenvironments introduce the potential for new health threats; for example, subterranean tunnels under large urban centers (e.g., subways, sewers) with limited airflow could concentrate airborne toxins, so troops operating in that setting may require specific personal protective equipment. Military units in the future are likely to be smaller, operate more autonomously, and be dispersed or isolated, which has significant implications for prevention and treatment of illnesses and injuries, as well as potential adverse effects on mental health. But the greatest driver of change in the practice of military preventive medicine, both as a destabilizing force that can increase the risk of armed conflict or require more frequent military support to provide humanitarian assistance and disaster response in affected populations, and as a source of new or increasing health threats, is climate change.

As climate change continues unabated, the most fragile of societies will find it increasingly difficult to obtain needed resources (e.g., food, water), large populations may be forced to migrate to areas with those resources, potentially leading to social conflict, insecurity, and instability. Economic hardship and social discontent create pressure on political leaders, which can trigger military actions to quell internal unrest or attempt to obtain needed resources from other countries through force. This increases the potential role for United States and other allied military personnel to respond as a stabilizing force. The increased frequency and severity of extreme weather events can also drive migration, but response to the devastation of the events themselves could increasingly result in calls for the United States and other militaries to provide humanitarian assistance in the aftermath of the disaster. In addition, as happened for the first time in 2014 with Ebola in West Africa, a large infectious disease outbreak could require a military response to expand treatment centers and provide resources to prevent further spread. Military preventive medicine plays a lead role in these types of missions.

The direct health effects of climate change will affect the readiness of military personnel, increasing the risk of heat-related illnesses, infectious diseases, and respiratory conditions. Mental health conditions are also associated with climate change, whether a direct effect of being victimized by a weather-related disaster or as a consequence of responding to assist in disaster recovery operations. Personnel living in and around military installations along the coasts will experience the effects of sea-level rise, potentially destroying property and forcing displacement, while those living on or near inland bases, which are mostly located in the southern half of the country, will be forced to live with increasing days of high heat and humidity, resulting in more days of poor air quality. In all locations, extreme weather events will likely increase, causing physical, mental, and economic challenges for those affected.

Global health surveillance, a key mission of military preventive medicine, is critical for detecting and monitoring new and emerging disease threats, especially infectious diseases, which are expected to increase as vectors of disease transmission, such as mosquitoes and ticks, expand their habitat; warmer oceans result in increases in toxic algal blooms; and weather-related events disrupt water and waste treatment infrastructure, leading to increased exposure to gastrointestinal pathogens. Military personnel operating in other countries will need accurate medical threat assessments to inform their use of preventive countermeasures, and new countermeasures, from vaccines and chemoprophylaxis drugs to uniforms and protective equipment, will need to be developed to address the range of new threats identified. Compounding the infectious disease threat is the increase in antimicrobial resistance among many pathogens and the lack of new antibiotics in development to combat this problem. As with the influenza pandemic in 1918, and more recently wounded service members returning from Iraq with multidrug-resistant *Acinetobacter baumannii* infections,[133] military personnel move globally and can play a role in the transmission of disease to civilian populations. Infection prevention and control on the battlefield is as important as in hospitals and other fixed medical treatment facilities outside of the combat theater.

Given the broad scope of current and future health threats to military personnel, and with the ever-present concern over resourcing and restructuring of preventive medicine and public health in the DoD, the challenges facing military preventive medicine physicians and their other public health colleagues are significant. However, with challenges come opportunities, and the historical successes of military and civilian preventive medicine professionals demonstrate clearly that the impact of effective preventive strategies and procedures can serve as a force multiplier on the battlefield. Keeping service members healthy and ready to fight and win the nation's wars is the ultimate charge of military preventive medicine, and the proud profession will continue to pursue this goal as long as militaries remain critical institutions in human society.[134-138]

ADDITIONAL RESOURCES

There is obviously much missing here. The preventive medicine and public health challenges facing the military are numerous and complex, and there are always new or re-emerging threats requiring attention. Detailed information on the topics touched on here, and much more, can be found in various volumes of the Textbooks of Military Medicine and other specialty texts published by the Borden Institute, an agency of the U.S. Army Medical Department Center and School. All publications are free of charge and can be found at https://www.cs.amedd.army.mil/borden/. The AFHSB's MSMR, repeatedly referenced herein, is a rich source of analyses of military medical surveillance data. It is published monthly at https://health.mil/Military-Health-Topics/Combat-Support/Armed-Forces-Health-Surveillance-Branch/Reports-and-Publications/Medical-Surveillance-Monthly-Report. The websites of the individual service public health centers, listed below, are excellent sources of information on past and current topics of interest in military preventive medicine. Finally, the Human Performance Resource Center (HPRC) of the Consortium for Health and Military Performance (CHAMP) at the Uniformed Services University of the Health Sciences (USUHS) maintains an excellent website at https://www.hprc-online.org, as well as the most excellent dietary supplement resource, Operation Supplement Safety, at https://www.opss.org.

U.S. Army Public Health Center: https://phc.amedd.army.mil/

Navy and Marine Corps Public Health Center: https://www.med.navy.mil/sites/nmcphc

U.S. Air Force School of Aerospace Medicine: https://www.wpafb.af.mil/afrl/711hpw/USAFSAM/

References

1. Washington G. *General Orders*. New York: s.n., August 5, 1776.
2. Letterman J. *Medical Recollections of the Army of the Potomac*. New York: D. Appleton and Company; 1866.
3. Ireland MW. The Medical Service in a Theater of Operations. *Military Surgeon*, Vol. 62. 1928, pp. 573–91.
4. Legters LJ, Llewellyn CH. Military medicine. In: JM Last, FB Wallace, eds. *Maxcy-Rosenau-Last Public Health and Preventive Medicine*, Vol. 71. 13th ed. Norwalk: Appleton & Lange; 1992, p. 1141.
5. Garrison FH. *Notes on the History of Military Medicine*. Washington, DC: Association of Military Surgeons; 1922. Reprinted from the Military Surgeon, 1921–22.
6. Washington G. Instructions for soldiers in the service of the United States concerning the means of preserving health: Of cleanliness. In: Baynes-Jones S. ed. *The Evolution of Preventive Medicine in the United States Army, 1607–1939*. Headquarters, Peeks-Kill: Office of Surgeon General; October 1777.
7. Wood P. *Moses: The Founder of Preventive Medicine*. New York: The Macmillan Company; 1920.
8. Pringle J. *Observations on the Diseases of the Army*. First American Edition (1810), Philadelphia, PA: Edward Earle (pub). London: A. Millar, D. Wilson, T. Payne; 1752.
9. Bayne-Jones S. *The Evolution of Preventive Medicine in the United States Army, 1607–1939*. Washington, DC: Office of the Surgeon General, Department of the Army; 1968.
10. Brocklesby R. *Oeconomical and Medical Observations, in Two Parts, from the Year 1758 to the Year 1763, inclusive: Tending to the Improvement of Military Hospitals, and to the Cure of Camp Diseases, incident to Soldiers*. London: T. Becket and P.A. De Hondt; 1764.
11. Lind J. *A Treatise on the Scurvy, in Three Parts, Containing An Inquiry into the Nature, Causes, and Cure, of that Disease*. London: A. Millar; 1757.
12. van Swieten G. *The Diseases Incident to Armies with the Method of Cure*. Philadelphia, PA: R. Bell; 1776.
13. Jones J. *Plain Concise Practical Remarks on the Treatment of Wounds and Fractures: Appendix on Camp and Military Hospitals*. New York: John Holt; 1775.
14. Rush B. *Directions for Preserving the Health of Soldiers*. Lancaster: John Dunlap; 1777.
15. Steuben FW. *Regulations for the Order and Discipline of the Troops of the United States: Part I*. Philadelphia, PA: Styner and Cist; 1779.
16. Washington G. Letter from George Washington to William Shippen, Jr. *Founders Online*. Headquarters, Morristown: National Archives; February 6, 1777.
17. Blake JB. Diseases and medical practice in Colonial America. *International Record of Medicine and General Practice Clinics*, Vol. 171. 1958, pp. 350–63.
18. Gillett MC. *The Army Medical Department, 1775–1818*. Washington, DC: U.S. Army Center of Military History; 2004.
19. Fielding H. The Statistical Lessons of the Crimean War. Garrison The Association of Military Surgeons of the United States. *The Military Surgeon*, Vol. 41. 1917, pp. 457–73.
20. Parkes EA. *A Manual of Practical Hygiene: Prepared Especially for Use in the Medical Service of the Army*. 3rd ed. London: John Churchill & Sons; 1869.
21. Stillé CJ. *History of the United States Sanitary Commission*. Philadelphia, PA: J.B. Lippincott & Co.; 1866.

22. Hammond WA, ed. *Military Medical and Surgical Essays Prepared for the United States Sanitary Commission*. Philadelphia, PA: J.B. Lippincott & Co.; 1864.

23. Hammond WA, ed. *A Treatise on Hygiene with Special Reference to Military Service*. Philadelphia, PA: J.B. Lippincott & Co.; 1863.

24. Craig SC. *In the Interest of Truth: The Life and Science of Surgeon General George Miller Sternberg*. Fort Sam Houston: Borden Institute, Office of the Surgeon General; 2013.

25. Meleney HE. Tropical medicine in United States military history. *Bull N Y Acad Med*. 1942;18:329–37.

26. Gorgas WC. *A Short Account of the Results of Mosquito Work in Havana, Cuba*, Vol. 12. In: Pilcher JE, ed. Carlisle: The Association of Military Surgeons, Journal of the Association of Military Surgeons. 1903, pp. 133–9.

27. Wintermute BA. *Public Health and the U.S. Military: A History of the Army Medical Department, 1818–1917*. New York: Routledge; 2011.

28. Gillett MC. *The Army Medical Department 1917–1941*. Washington, DC: U.S. Army Center of Military History; 2009.

29. Byerly CR. The U.S. military and the influenza pandemic of 1918–1919. *Public Health Rep*. 2010;125(Suppl 3):82–91.

30. Zinsser H, ed. The Sanitation of a Field Army. James Robb Church. Washington, DC: The Association of Military Surgeons of the United States, 1919, *The Military Surgeon*, Vol. 44, pp. 445–64, 571–81.

31. Army Medical Department. *Medical Department of the U.S. Army in the World War: Neuropsychiatry*. Washington, DC: Government Printing Office; 1929.

32. Army Medical Department. *Medical Department of the United States Army in the World War: Division of Gas Defense*, Vol. 1, Chapter 17. Washington, DC: Government Printing Office. 1923, pp. 504–11.

33. Army *Medical Department. Medical Department of the United States Army in the World War: Medical Aspects of Gas Warfare*, Vol. 14. Washington, DC: Government Printing Office; 1926.

34. Army Medical Department. *Medical Department of the United States Army in the World War: Administration: Department of Sanitation and Public Health, German Occupied Territory*, Vol. 2, Chapter 29. Washington, DC: Government Printing Office; 1927.

35. Marble S. Brigadier General James Stevens Simmons (1890–1954), Medical Corps, United States Army: A career in preventive medicine. *J Med Biog*. 2012; 3–10.

36. Cook WL. Occupational health and industrial medicine. In: Hoff EC ed. *Preventive Medicine in World War II*, Vol. IX. Washington, DC: Office of the Surgeon General, Department of the Army; 1969, pp. 101–202.

37. Reister FA. *Medical Statistics in World War II*. Washington, DC: Office of the Surgeon General, Department of the Army; 1975.

38. Hoff EC, ed. Communicable diseases: Malaria. *Preventive Medicine in World War II*, Vol. 6. Washington, DC: Office of the Surgeon General, Department of the Army; 1963.

39. Bradley ON. *A Soldier's Story*. New York: Henry Holland Co.; 1951.

40. Withers BG, Craig SC. The historical impact of preventive medicine at war. In: Kelley PW, ed. *Military Preventive Medicine: Mobilization and Deployment*, Vol. 1. Washington, DC: The Borden Institute, Office of the Surgeon General; 2003, p. 2.

41. Slim W. *Defeat Into Victory*. London: Cassell and Company; 1956.

42. Coggeshall LT. Treatment of malaria. *Am J Trop Med*. 1952; 124–31.

43. Archambeault CP. Mass antimalarial therapy in veterans returning from Korea. *J Am Med Assoc*. 1954;154:1411–15.

44. Cowdrey AE. The Medic's War. *United States Army in the Korean War*. Washington, DC: Center of Military History, US Army; 1987.

45. Orr KD, Fainer DC. *Cold Injuries in Korea During Winter of 1950–51*. Fort Knox, KY: Army Medical Research Laboratory; 1951.

46. Neel S. Medical support of the U.S. Army in Vietnam, 1965–1970. *Vietnam Studies*. Washington, DC: Center of Military History, Department of the Army; 1973.

47. Ewell JJ, Hunt IA. Sharpening the combat edge. *Vietnam Studies*. Washington, DC: Center of Military History, Department of the Army; 1974.

48. Allen AM, Taplin D, Lowy JA, Twigg L. Skin infections in Vietnam. *Mil Med*. 1972;137:295–301.

49. Allen AM. Skin diseases in Vietnam, 1965–72. In: Ognibene AJ, ed. *Internal Medicine in Vietnam*. Washington, DC: Center of Military History, Department of the Army; 1977.

50. Withers BG, Erickson RL, Petruccelli BP, Hanson RK, Kadlec RP. Preventing disease and non-battle injury in deployed units. *Mil Med*. 1994;159:39–43.

51. Defense Health Agency. *The Defense Health Agency 2017 Stakeholder Report*. Falls Church, VA: Defense Health Agency; 2018.

52. Department of Defense Task Force on Military Health System Governance. *Department of Defense Task Force on Military Health System Governance Final Report*. Department of Defense; 2011.

53. United States Congress. National Defense Authorization Act of 2017. Washington, DC, 2016.

54. United States Congress. National Defense Authorization Act of 2019. Washington, DC, 2018.

55. Deputy Secretary of Defense. Department of Defense Directive 5136.13. Washington, DC, September 30, 2013.

56. Military Health System. Combat Support. *Military Health System*. [Online] June 8, 2019. https://www.health.mil/Military-Health-Topics/Combat-Support.

57. Military Health System. Department of Defense Serum Repository. *health.mil*. [Online] August 8, 2019. https://www.health.mil/Military-Health-Topics/Combat-Support/Armed-Forces-Health-Surveillance-Branch/Data-Management-and-Technical-Support/Department-of-Defense-Serum-Repository.

58. Military Health System. Integrated Biosurveillance. *Health.mil*. [Online] August 8, 2019. https://www.health.mil/Military-Health-Topics/Combat-Support/Armed-Forces-Health-Surveillance-Branch/Integrated-Biosurveillance.

59. Military Health System. Medical Surveillance Monthly Report. *Health.mil*. [Online] August 15, 2019. https://health.mil/Military-Health-Topics/Combat-Support/Armed-Forces-Health-Surveillance-Branch/Reports-and-Publications/Medical-Surveillance-Monthly-Report.

60. U.S. Department of Veterans Affairs. About VA: History—VA History. [Online] August 8, 2019. https://www.va.gov/about_va/vahistory.asp.

61. U.S. Department of Veterans Affairs. Public Health. [Online] August 8, 2019. https://www.publichealth.va.gov.

62. Armed Forces Health Surveillance Branch. Absolute and Relative Morbidity Burdents Attributable to Various Illnesses and Injuries, Active Component, U.S. Armed Forces, 2018. *MSMR*. 2019;26:2–10.

63. Jones BH, Hauschild VD. Physical training, fitness, and injuries: Lessons learned from military studies. *J Strength Cond Res*. 2015;29:S57–64.

64. Anderson MK, Grier T, Canham-Chervak M, Bushman TT, Jones BH. Occupation and other risk factors for injury among enlisted U.S. Army soldiers. *Public Health*. 2015;129:531–8.

65. Hauret KG, Pacha L, Taylor BJ, Jones BH. Surveillance of disease and nonbattle injuries during US Army operations in Afghanistan and Iraq. *US Army Med Dep J*. 2016;15–23.

66. Armed Forces Health Surveillance Branch. *2018 Health of the DoD Force*. Armed Forces Health Surveillance Branch, 2019.

67. Schuh-Renner A, Canham-Chervak M, Grier TL, Hauschild VD, Jones BH. Expanding the injury definition: Evidence for the need to include musculoskeletal conditions. *Public Health*. 2019;169:69–75.

68. Army Public Health Center. *Public Health Information Paper 12-01-0717: A Taxonomy of Injuries for Public Health Monitoring and Reporting*. Aberdeen Proving Ground: Army Public Health Center; 2017.

69. Hauschild VD, Schuh-Renner A, Lee T, Richardson MD, Hauret K, Jones BH. Using causal energy categories to report the distribution of injuries in an active population: An approach used by the U.S. Army. *J Sci Med Sport*. 2019;22:997–1003.

70. Sharma J, Heagerty R, Dalal S, Banerjee B, Booker T. Risk factors associated with musculoskeletal injury: A prospective study of British Infantry recruits. *Curr Rheumatol Rev*. 2019;15:50–58.

71. Hall LJ. Relationship between 1.5-mile run time, injury risk and training outcome in British Army recruits. *J Roy Army Med Corps*. 2017;163:376–82.

72. Nye NS, Pawlak MT, Webber BJ, Tchandja JN, Milner MR. Description and rate of musculoskeletal injuries in Air Force Basic Military Trainees, 2012–2014. *J Athl Train*. 2016;51:858–65.

73. Jones BH, Hauret KG, Dye SK, et al. Impact of physical fitness and body composition on injury risk among active young adults: A study of army trainees. *J Sci Med Sport*. 2017;20 (Suppl 4):S17–22.

74. Rappole C, Grier T, Anderson MK, Hauschild V, Jones BH. Associations of age, aerobic fitness, and body mass index with injury in an operational army brigade. *J Sci Med Sport*. 2017;20 (Suppl 4):S45–50.

75. Knapik J, Montain SJ, McGraw S, Grier T, Ely M, Jones BH. Stress fracture risk factors in basic combat training. *Int J Sports Med*. 2012;33:940–6.

76. Kyrolainen H, Pihlainen K, Vaara JP, Ojanen T, Santtila M. Optimising training adaptations and performance in military environment. *J Sci Med Sport*. 2018;21:1131–8.

77. Burley SD, Drain JR, Sampson JA, Groeller H. Positive, limited and negative responders: The variability in physical fitness adaptation to basic military training. *J Sci Med Sport*. 2018;21:1168–72.

78. Bell NS, Mangione TW, Hemenway D, Amoroso PJ, Jones BH. High injury rates among female army trainees: A function of gender? *Am J Prev Med*. 2000;18(Suppl 1):141–6.

79. Knapik JJ, Craig SC, Hauret KG, Jones BH. Risk factors for injuries during military parachuting. *Aviat Space Environ Med*. 2003;74: 768–74.

80. U.S. Army Public Health Center. *Injuries Among Military Paratroopers: Current Evidence and Data Gaps*. Aberdeen Proving Ground: U.S. Army Public Health Center; 2019. Technical Information Paper.

81. Knapik JJ, Spiess A, Swedler DI, Grier TL, Darasjy SS, Jones BH. Systematic review of the parachute ankle brace injury risk reduction and cost effectiveness. *Am J Prev Med*. 2010;38(Suppl 1):S182–8.

82. Nock MK, Deming AC, Fullerton CS, et al. Suicide among soldiers: A review of psychosocial risk and protective factors. *Psychiatry*. 2013;76:97–125.

83. Ursano RJ, Colpe LJ, Heeringa SG, et al. The Army Study to Assess Risk and Resilience in Servicemembers (Army STARRS). *Psychiatry*. 2014;77:107–119.

84. Study to Assess Risk & Resilience in Service members-Longitudinal Study. Publications. *STARRS-LS*. [Online] August 9, 2019. https://starrs-ls.org/#/list/publications.

85. Kessler RC, Stein MB, Petukhova MV, et al. Predicting suicides after outpatient mental health visits in the Army Study to Assess Risk and Resilience in Servicemembers (Army STARRS). *Mol Psychiatry*. 2017;22:544–51.

86. Nock MK, Millner AJ, Joiner TE, et al. Risk factors for the transition from suicide ideation to suicide attempt: Results from the Army Study to Assess Risk and Resilience in Servicemembers (Army STARRS). *J Abnorm Psychol*. 2018;127:139–49.

87. Rosellini AJ, Stein MB, Benedek DM, et al. Predeployment predictors of psychiatric disorder symptoms and interpersonal violence during combat deployment. *Depress Anxiety*. 2018;35:1073–80.

88. Koenig, HG, Youssef, NA, Pearce, M. Assessment of moral injury in veterans and active duty military personnel with PTSD: A review. *Front Psychiatry*. 2019;10:1–15.

89. Department of the Army. *Army Health Promotion, Risk Reduction, Suicide Prevention Report 2010*. Department of the Army, 2010.

90. Department of the Army. *Army 2020: Generating Health & Discipline in the Force Ahead of the Strategic Reset Report 2012*. Department of the Army, 2012.

91. Sagalyn D. *Army General Calls for Changing Name of PTSD*. November 4, 2011. PBS Newshour.

92. Brundage JF, Taubman SB, Hunt DJ, Clark LL. Whither the "Signature Sounds of the War" after the war: Estimates of incidence rates and proportions of TBI and PTSD diagnoses attributable to background risk, enhanced ascertainment, and active war zone service, active component, U.S. Armed Forces. *MSMR*. 2015;22:2–11.

93. Defense and Veterans Brain Injury Center. *DoD Worldwide Numbers for TBI*. Defense and Veterans Brain Injury Center, 2018.

94. Bahraini NH, Breshears RE, Hernandez TD, Schneider AL, Forster JE, Brenner LA. Traumatic brain injury and posttraumatic stress disorder. *Psychiatr Clin North Am*. 2014;37:55–75.

95. Yurgil KA, Barkauskas DA, Vasterling, JJ, et al. Association between traumatic brain injury and risk of posttraumatic stress disorder in active-duty marines. *JAMA Psychiatry*. 2014;71:149–57.

96. Porter KE, Stein MB, Martis B, et al. Postconcussive symptoms (PCS) following combat-related traumatic brain injury (TBI) in veteran with posttraumatic stress disorder (PTSD): Influence of TBI, PTSD, and depression on symptoms measured by the Neurobehavioral Symptom Inventory (NSI). *J Psychiatr Res*. 2018;102:8–13.

97. Hoge CW, Castro CA. Treatment of generalized war-related health concerns: Placing TBI and PTSD in context. *JAMA*. 2014;312:1685–6.

98. Gilbert KS, Kark SM, Gehrman P, Bogdanova Y. Sleep disturbances, TBI and PTSD: Implications for treatment and recovery. *Clin Psychol Rev*. 2015;40:195–212.

99. Sanders JW, Putnam SD, Frankart C, et al. Impact of illness and non-combat injury during operations Iraqi freedom and enduring freedom (Afghanistan). *Am J Trop Med*. 2005;73:713–19.

100. Whitman TJ, Coyne PE, Magill AJ, et al. An outbreak of *Plasmodium falciparum* malaria in U.S. Marines deployed to Liberia. *Am J Trop Med Hyg*. 2010;83:258–65.

101. Stahlman S, Williams VF, Taubman SB. Incident diagnoses of leishmaniasis, active and reserve components, U.S. Armed Forces, 2001–2016. *MSMR*. 2017;24:2–7.

102. Army Public Health Center. DoD Insect Repellent System. *Army Public Health Center*. [Online] August 10, 2019. https://phc.amedd.army.mil/topics/envirohealth/epm/Pages/DoD-Insect-Repellent-System.aspx.

103. Joint and Coalition Operational Analysis. *Operation UNITED ASSISTANCE: The DOD Response to Ebola in West Africa*. Joint and Coalition Operational Analysis, Joint Staff J-7, 2016.

104. Cardile AP, Murray CK, Littell CT, et al. Monitoring exposure to ebola and health of U.S. military personnel deployed in support of ebola control efforts—Liberia, October 25, 2014–February 27, 2015. *MMWR*. 2015;64:690–4.

105. Gray GC, Callahan JD, Hawksworth AW, Fisher CA, Gaydos JC. Respiratory diseases among U.S. military personnel: Countering emerging threats. *Emerg Infect Dis*. 1999; 379–87.

106. Hoke CH, Hawksworth A, Snyder CE. Initial assessment of impact of adenovirus type 4 and type 7 vaccine on febrile respiratory illness and virus transmission in military basic trainees. *MSMR*. 2012; 2–5.

107. Barraza EM, Ludwig SL, Gaydos JC, Brundage JF. Reemergence of adenovirus type 4 acute respiratory disease in military trainees: Report of an outbreak during a lapse in vaccination. *J Infect Dis*. 1999;179:1531–3.

108. Kolavic-Gray SA, Binn LN, Sanchez JL, et al. Large epidemic of adenovirus type 4 infection among military trainees: Epidemiological, clinical and laboratory studies. *Clin Infect Dis*. 2002;35:808–18.

109. Russell KL, Hawksworth AW, Ryan MAK, et al. Vaccine-preventable adenoviral respiratory illness in US military recruits, 1999–2004. *Vaccine*. 2006;24:2835–42.

110. Sanchez JL, Cooper MJ, Myers CA, et al. Respiratory infections in the U.S. Military: Recent experience and control. *Clin Microbiol Rev*. 2015; 743–800.

111. Radin JM, Hawksworth AW, Blair PJ, et al. Dramatic decline of respiratory illness among US military recruits after the renewed use of adenovirus vaccines. *Clin Infect Dis*. 2014;59:962–8.

112. Schreier AJ, Hockett VE, Seal JR. Mass prophylaxis of epidemic Streptococcal infections with Benzathine Penicillin G: Experience at a Naval Training Center during the winter of 1955–56. *N Engl J Med*. 1958;258:1231–8.

113. Webber BJ, Kieffer JW, White BK, Hawksworth AW, Graf PCF, Yun HC Chemoprophylaxis against group A Streptococcus during military training. *Prev Med*. 2019;118:142–9.

114. Lee S, Eick A, Ciminera P. Respiratory disease in army recruits: Surveillance Program overview, 1995–2006. *Am J Prev Med*. 2008;24:389–95.

115. Armed Forces Health Surveillance Branch. *Armed Forces Reportable Medical Events: Guidelines and Case Definitions*. Defense Health Agency, 2017.

116. Atha WF. Heat-related illness. *Emerg Med Clin N Am*. 2013;31: 1097–108.

117. Armed Forces Health Surveillance Branch. Update: Heat illness, Active component, U.S. Armed Forces, 2018. *MSMR*. 2019;26:15–20.

118. Knapik JJ, Epstein Y. Exertional heat stroke: Pathophysiology, epidemiology, diagnosis, treatment, and prevention. *J Spec Oper Med*. 2019;19:108–16.

119. Knapik JJ, O'Connor FG. Exertional rhabdomyolysis: Epidemiology, diagnosis, treatment, and prevention. *J Spec Oper Med*. 2016;16:65–71.

120. Armed Forces Health Surveillance Branch. Update: Exertional rhabdomyolysis, active component, U.S. Armed Forces, 2014–2018. *MSMR*. 2019;26:21–25.

121. O'Brien KK, Montain SJ, Corr WP, Sawka MN, Knapik JJ, Craig SC. Hyponatremia associated with overhydration in U.S. Army trainees. *Mil Med*. 2001;166:405–10.

122. Committee to Review the Health Effects in Vietnam Veterans of Exposure to Herbicides (Tenth Biennial Update). *Veterans and Agent Orange: Update 2014*. Board on the Health of Select Populations, Institute of Medicine. Washington, DC: National Academies Press; 2016.

123. U.S. Army Environmental Hygiene Agency. *Kuwait Oil Fire Health Risk Assessment, Final Report, No. 39-26-L192-91*. Aberdeen Proving Ground, MD: U.S. Army Environmental Hygiene Agency; 1994.

124. National Academies of Sciences, Engineering, and Medicine. *Gulf War and Health: Volume 10: Update of Health Effects of Serving in the Gulf War, 2016*. Washington, DC: National Academies Press; 2016.

125. Bullman TA, Mahan CM, Kang HK, Page WF. Mortality in US Army Gulf War veterans exposed to 1991 Khamisiyah Chemical Munitions Destruction. *Am J Public Health.* 2005;95:1382–8.

126. Mahan CM, Page WF, Bullman TA, Kang HK. Health effects in Army Gulf War veterans possibly exposed to chemical munitions destruction at Khamisiyah, Iraq: Part I. Morbidity associated with potential exposure. *Mil Med.* 2005;170:935–44.

127. Page WF, Mahan CM, Kang HK, Bullman TA. Health effects in Army Gulf War veterans possibly exposed to Chemical Munitions Destruction at Khamisiyah, Iraq: Part II. Morbidity associated with notification of potential exposure. *Mil Med.* 2005;170:945–51.

128. Institute of Medicine. *Protecting Those Who Serve: Strategies to Protect the Health of Deployed U.S. Forces.* Washington, DC: National Academies Press; 2000.

129. U.S. Army Public Health Command. *Technical Guide 230: Environmental Health Risk Assessment and Chemical Exposure Guidelines for Deployed Military Personnel.* Aberdeen Proving Ground, MD: U.S. Army Public Health Command; 2013.

130. Baird CP, Harkins DK, edsBaird CP, Harkins DK, eds. *Airborne Hazards Related to Deployment.* Fort Sam Houston, TX: Borden Institute, Office of the Surgeon General; 2015.

131. Institute of Medicine. *Long-Term Health Consequences of Exposure to Burn Pits in Iraq and Afghanistan.* Washington, DC: National Academies Press; 2011.

132. U.S. Department of Veterans Affairs. VA's Airborne Hazards and Open Burn Pit Registry. *Public Health.* [Online] August 12, 2019. https://www.publichealth.va.gov/exposures/burnpits/registry.asp.

133. Scott P, Deye G, Srinivasan A, et al. An outbreak of multidrug-resistant *Acinetobacter baumannii-calcoaceticus* complex infection in the US Military Health Care System associated with military operations in Iraq. *Clin Infect Dis.* 2007;44:1577–84.

134. U.S. Congress. National Defense Authorization Act for Fiscal Year 2017. *Public Law 114-328.* Washington, DC: U.S. Government Publishing Office; December 2016.

135. Jones BH, Hauschild VD, Canham-Chervak M. Musculoskeletal training injury prevention in the U.S. Army: Evolution of the science and the public health approach. *J Sci Med Sport.* 2018;21:1139–46.

136. Cowan DN, Jones BH, Shaffer RA. Musculoskeletal injuries in the military training environment. In: Kelley P, ed. *Military Preventive Medicine: Mobilization and Deployment,* Vol. 1. Washington, DC: Borden Institute, Office of the Surgeon General; 2003, pp. 195–210.

137. Patel AA, Hauret KG, Taylor BJ, Jones BH. Non-battle injuries among U.S. Army soldiers deployed to Afghanistan and Iraq, 2001–2013. *J Saf Res.* 2017;60:29–34.

138. Chairman of the Joint Chiefs of Staff. Chairman of the Joint Chiefs of Staff Instruction 3405.01. *Chairman's Total Force Fitness Framework.* September 1, 2011.

CHAPTER 11

Lifestyle Medicine

Beth Frates • Mark D. Faries • David L. Katz

INTRODUCTION

Lifestyle Medicine focuses on empowering people to adopt and sustain healthful habits in order to reach their optimal level of health. The World Health Organization (WHO) defines health as, "a state of complete physical, mental, and social well-being and not merely the absence of disease or infirmity."[1,2] As defined by the Merriam Webster Dictionary, *lifestyle* means "the typical way of life of an individual, group, or culture," and *medicine* means "the science and art dealing with the maintenance of health and the prevention, alleviation, or cure of disease."[3] Together, the two words, *lifestyle medicine*, form a burgeoning domain in healthcare that seeks to not only add years to people's lives, but also life to their years.

The American College of Lifestyle Medicine (ACLM) states, "Lifestyle Medicine is the use of evidence-based lifestyle therapeutic approaches, such as a plant-predominant dietary lifestyle, regular physical activity, adequate sleep, stress management, avoidance of risky substance use, and other non-drug modalities to treat, often reverse, and prevent lifestyle-related, chronic disease."[4] By examining a person's daily activities; how they move, what they eat, when they sleep, how they manage stress, with whom they connect and spend time, and if they abstain from toxic substances (e.g., smoking), a healthcare practitioner is working with a patient's lifestyle to optimize their physical, mental, and social well-being.

Hippocrates expressed some of the main tenets of this field with his words, "Let food be thy medicine and medicine be thy food," "Walking is man's best medicine," and, "If we could give every individual the right amount of nourishment and exercise, not too little and not too much, we would have found the safest way to health."[5] Although the basic principles of lifestyle medicine have been discussed for centuries, their adaptation into a modern medical discipline is relatively new, as the ACLM was founded in 2004, and is actively evolving.

An Evidence-Based Practice

Research published in the past three decades demonstrates the impact that lifestyle practices can have on health with a focus on routine exercise, a healthful diet, not smoking, and maintaining a weight within a healthy BMI range.[6–9] In 1993, a landmark paper in JAMA posited that the "actual," or root causes of death were not the diseases cited on death certificates (e.g., heart disease, cancer, and stroke), but instead the underlying behaviors and exposures largely responsible for the development of these diseases, including smoking, poor diet, lack of physical activity, and excessive alcohol consumption. In fact, the authors estimated that approximately 80% of premature death in the United States was due to poor lifestyle.[6] In 2004, another JAMA review revealed similar results.[10]

The evidence that unhealthy lifestyles not only cause disease but that healthful lifestyles could, in fact, *prevent* disease was demonstrated in Germany, where researchers estimated that 80% of chronic disease could be avoided by (1) not smoking, (2) maintaining a body mass index (BMI) in the healthy range, (3) being physically active, and (4) adhering to a healthful diet consisting of high intake of fruits, vegetables, whole-grain bread, and low consumption of meat.[7] Over the years, research studies have revealed the importance of maintaining a weight within the healthy BMI range,[11] exercising regularly,[12] eating nutritious foods,[13,14] reducing stress,[15,16] not smoking,[17] and cultivating meaningful social connections.[18] It is on the basis of such evidence that healthful lifestyle practices have been equated to "medicine," and a modern medical discipline devoted to their application has developed.

The growing body of research behind lifestyle medicine spans from cell to culture. Understanding how diets influence endothelial cell function,[19] serotonin levels,[20] glucose control,[21] inflammation,[22] prostate cancer,[23] breast cancer,[24] multiple sclerosis,[25] and many other conditions informs how lifestyle medicine practitioners prescribe dietary patterns to patients. Research on exercise describes how it influences myocytes and insulin sensitivity.[21] In addition, research has helped to better understand sleep and its impact on the levels of appetite hormones, including ghrelin and leptin,[26] how caffeine competes with the same receptor as adenosine which is a natural chemical that helps promote sleep,[27] how blue wavelength light from devices like cell phones, computers, and tablets interrupts the release of melatonin from the pineal gland[28] that can delay the onset of sleep.[29]

Evidential support for lifestyle medicine at the cultural level have been exhibited by the work of the Blue Zones group examining different cultures around the globe that have the highest number of centenarians, such as Okinawa (Japan), Sardinia (Italy), Nicoya (Costa Rica), Icaria (Greece), and among the Seventh-day Adventists in Loma Linda, California,[30] and by migration and community-wide studies, such as the North Karelia Project[31] and Shape Up in Somerville, Massachusetts.[32]

Physician "core competencies" for prescribing lifestyle medicine were introduced in 2010 through a collaboration of ACLM and the American College of Preventive Medicine (ACPM).[33–36] These competencies revolved around five main domains of practice: leadership, knowledge, assessment skills, management skills, and the use of office and community support. These competencies help guide physicians in the capable practice of lifestyle medicine, including understanding the impact that healthful habits can have on the prevention, treatment, and reversal of disease, the importance of practicing these healthful habits themselves, and performing assessments to evaluate the lifestyle "vital signs," such as tobacco use, alcohol consumption, diet, physical activity, body mass index, stress level, sleep, and emotional well-being.

In October 2017, the first Board Examination created and administered by the American Board of Lifestyle Medicine was held to certify physicians and allied healthcare providers in lifestyle medicine. Physicians can be certified as lifestyle medicine physicians and those with PhDs, Masters Degrees, and other allied healthcare providers can be certified as lifestyle medicine specialists. Those who adhere to the tenets of lifestyle medicine and practice them with their patients are generally referred to as lifestyle medicine practitioners, but this does not imply certification in the field. The American Board of Medical Specialties (ABMS) does not offer general certificates or subspecialty certificates in lifestyle medicine,[35] but is a long-term goal for the field.

The interest in lifestyle medicine is international, and there is a Lifestyle Medicine Global Alliance (LMGA) in collaboration with the ACLM.[36] The clinical interest in lifestyle medicine is paralleled with an academic interest. A growing number of medical schools are incorporating lifestyle medicine into their education in a parallel format with lifestyle medicine interest groups (LMIG), elective courses on lifestyle medicine,[37] embedding the lifestyle medicine concepts into current core courses, and offering full core courses on the topic.[38]

Comparing Lifestyle Medicine to Conventional Medicine and Other Areas of Medicine

Lifestyle medicine is different from conventional medicine, in that its core principles and tenets are to use daily healthful habits to prevent, treat, and reverse disease. The field places a unique emphasis on the importance of a healthy lifestyle. Medication is sometimes used by some lifestyle medicine physicians, but the goal is to reduce the amount of medication whenever possible. Lifestyle medicine practitioners use exercise prescriptions, nutrition prescription, sleep prescriptions, stress resiliency prescriptions, and social connection prescriptions. Lifestyle medicine practitioners use exercise, diet, sleep, stress resiliency, social connection, and smoking cessation as methods not just to prevent pathology, but also to treat, and even reverse, diseases such as diabetes, heart disease, and stroke. The evidence of efficacy is discussed in section "Evidence of Efficacy for Lifestyle Medicine." They may also prescribe cessation or modification of substance use. Other nonconventional areas in medicine also use lifestyle as medicine, including integrative medicine, functional medicine, and preventive medicine. What sets lifestyle medicine apart is its devotion to lifestyle as medicine, and its sole focus on it as a specialty. Figure 11-1 demonstrates the differences between these areas.

Integrative medicine uses lifestyle counseling when working with patients. The National Institutes of Health (NIH) defines integrative healthcare as bringing "conventional and complementary approaches together in a coordinated way. It emphasizes a holistic, patient-focused approach to healthcare and wellness—often including mental, emotional, functional, spiritual, social, and community aspects—and treating the whole person rather than, for example, one organ system. It aims for well-coordinated care between different providers and institutions."[39] Therapies, not routinely utilized by conventional physicians but used by some integrative medicine practitioners, include acupuncture, Ayurveda, homeopathy, naturopathy, Chinese or Oriental medicine, massage, body movement therapies, Tai Chi, yoga, dietary supplements, herbal therapy, electromagnetic therapy, Reiki, Qigong, meditation, biofeedback, hypnosis, art therapy, dance therapy, music therapy, visualization, and guided imagery.[40]

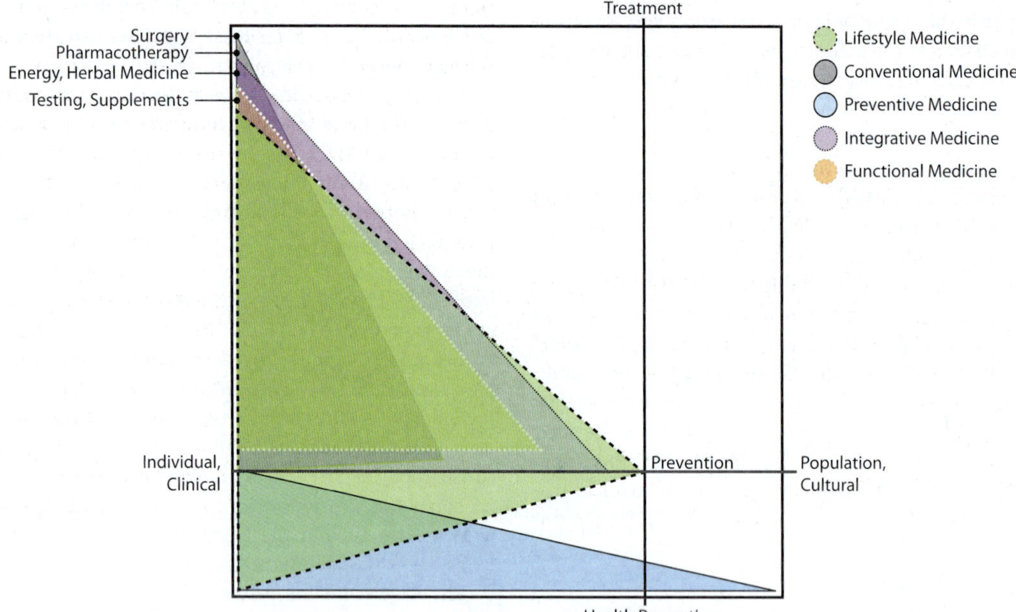

FIGURE 11-1. A Venn diagram showing the overlap and distinctions of lifestyle medicine, conventional medicine, preventive medicine, integrative medicine, and functional medicine. Disciplines are characterized by (1) the modalities they include, exclude, and emphasize; (2) their focus on treatment versus prevention and health promotion; and (3) their focus on individual clinical care versus population health.

Lifestyle medicine, represented in light green, is unique in its exclusive emphasis of nutrition, exercise, sleep, stress management, social connections, and substance use cessation or modification for clinical benefit. Lifestyle medicine encompasses both treatment and prevention, with a preferential emphasis on individual patient care rather than population health.

Conventional medicine, represented in gray, uses the modalities of lifestyle medicine, but relies preferentially on pharmacotherapy, technology, and surgery to treat patients. The emphasis is on treatment over prevention, and individuals over population health.

Preventive medicine, represented in light blue, uses the modalities of lifestyle medicine and conventional medicine to treat individual patients, but with a primary focus on prevention and health promotion. Preventive medicine is also the only discipline in this group with a major emphasis on population health.

Integrative medicine, represented in purple, uses the modalities of lifestyle and conventional medicine to treat individual patients, and extends to other modalities as well, including but not limited to supplements, herbs, and energy medicine. The discipline extends to prevention, but the primary focus is on treatment of the individual patient.

Functional medicine, represented in brown/orange, uses the modalities of lifestyle and conventional medicine. The preferential focus is on identifying biochemical imbalances through blood, stool, and skin testing and then correcting those imbalances with targeted supplements. The discipline is primarily devoted to treatment rather than prevention, and to individual patient care rather than population health.

Integrative medicine encompasses most of conventional medicine and adds to it. Surgery is the one area that does not play a large role in routine integrative medicine, although integrative medicine practitioners can be surgeons.

Functional medicine practitioners work with diet, exercise, sleep, stress reduction, and social connection. In addition, they have a focus on key common system pathways from health to disease (e.g., inflammation, oxidative stress); the role of diet, stress, and physical activity; the emerging sciences of genomics, proteomics, and metabolomics; and the effects of environmental toxins (in the air, water, soil, etc.) on health.[41] The use of blood, stool, and skin testing as well as treatment with prescriptive food plans, nutritional supplements, and herbs in addition to lifestyle changes is routine. The focus is on defining the biology and biochemistry of the problem and fixing any imbalance. The emphasis on genomics, proteomics, and metabolomics from preconception through pregnancy and the entire lifespan is a unique feature of functional medicine.

Preventive medicine is described as "focuses on the health of individuals, communities, and defined populations. Its goal is to protect, promote, and maintain health and well-being and to prevent disease, disability, and death."[34]

Preventive medicine has three main areas: aerospace medicine, occupational medicine, and public health and general preventive medicine. Preventive medicine practitioners "combine population-based public health skills with knowledge of primary, secondary, and tertiary prevention-oriented clinical practice in a wide variety of settings." Preventive medicine physicians use conventional medicines and interventions. However, the focus is on prevention, and lifestyle changes are used routinely as are conventional medicines. There is a greater focus on public health in the practice of preventive medicine than any other area of medicine. Lifestyle medicine also encompasses the area of public health but not to the same extent.

CORE COMPONENTS OF LIFESTYLE MEDICINE

The core components or "six pillars" of lifestyle medicine are typically catalogued as follows: (1) nutrition, (2) exercise, (3) stress, (4) sleep, (5) social connections, and (6) substance use cessation or modification (e.g., tobacco and alcohol). These appear under different but related names; in association with various mnemonics; and with the list slightly expanded through "splitting," or attenuated through "lumping"; the fundamental components, however, are subject to little dissent.

Nutrition

Diet is recognized as one of the leading contributors to chronic disease and premature death in the United States.[42] Poor diet is estimated to cause approximately 678,000 deaths every year, because of the significant role nutrition plays in heart disease, cancer, and type 2 diabetes.[43]

The most recent dietary guidelines for Americans focus on a healthy eating pattern that consists of a variety of nutrient dense whole foods including vegetables from all subgroups, legumes, fruits, whole grains, and a variety of protein foods.[44] In plate form (i.e., MyPlate), the recommendations emphasize 50% of the plate be vegetables and fruit, while 75–100% of the plate be whole, plant-based foods, depending on how healthy proteins are varied. Similarly, the Harvard Healthy Plate created by nutrition experts at the Harvard School of Health (Fig. 11-2) also emphasizes that plant-based choices make up at least three quarters of the plate.[45] The mechanisms of the healthful benefits of whole plants are likely diverse, and relate, in part, to the rich array of nutrient compounds native to plants, such as phytonutrients and antioxidants,[46–51] fiber content, volume, satiation, and the displacement of alternatives from the diet, including highly processed foods made from plants, and animal foods.

When the major diets (Table 11-1), including the low carb, low fat/vegetarian/vegan, low glycemic, Mediterranean, mixed/balanced diets, and Paleolithic, were compared, and the healthy components were identified and compared, more similarities among them than differences were found.[52] For example, they all limited refined starches, added sugars, processed foods, and certain fats including trans fats, while emphasizing whole, plant foods with or without lean meats, fish, poultry, or seafood. In addition, a diet rich in vegetables, fruit, and other whole, plant foods has been recommended for its potential environmental impacts.[53]

Lifestyle medicine practitioners seek to empower patients to adopt a whole foods plant-based diet. In many cases, they need to work with patients to transition them away from the Standard American Diet (SAD) of processed foods and limited whole foods,[54] to a prescription that has been summarized as, "Eat food [whole food], not too much, mostly plants."[55] Moving people closer to the dietary pattern that is best for health takes time and collaboration with the patient.[56] With some patients, the lifestyle medicine practitioner might refer the patient to a licensed nutrition professional for more in-depth analysis and counseling about dietary patterns.

Exercise

Physical activity has been shown to lower blood pressure, help control blood sugars, control weight, help prevent obesity, and help prevent bone loss.[57] In addition, there is evidence that it can improve sleep, reduce stress, and increase endurance, energy, and stamina.[58] Physical activity guidelines have been established for aerobic activity, strength training, flexibility, and balance training.

For aerobic activity, the United States Health and Human Services Department (USHHS) recommends accumulating at least 150 minutes of moderate-intensity physical activity per week, and/or at least 75 minutes of vigorous-intensity physical activity, with the goal of reaching 300 minutes of moderate-intensity or 150 minutes of vigorous-intensity physical activity per week.[59] Increased fitness levels in middle-age are associated with lower risk for morbidity and mortality.[60] At the cellular level, aerobic activity has been shown to promote a positive effect on oxidative stress, if performed at least three times a week for $\geq$2 months.[48] In terms of benefits to the brain, routine aerobic activity has been shown to increase the volume of the hippocampus, which is the area of the limbic system in the brain that is intricately involved with consolidating memory.[61]

The United States Health and Human Services Department recommends strength training twice a week on nonconsecutive days. Since adults begin to lose muscle mass at age 30, approximately 3–5% per decade, it is essential that patients work strength training into their routine as early as possible.[62] If they do not do so, then by age 50, some patients might lose 10% of their muscle mass.

Flexibility is critical for maintaining the full range of motion around the joints and for avoiding injury. Stretching is recommended to be performed when the muscles are warm, in a period of at least 5–10 minutes. Both *static* stretching, held for 30–60 seconds per stretch[63] and *dynamic* stretching can be a part of a healthy activity prescription.

Balance exercises are recommended to help people function optimally, avoid falls, and prevent injury, especially in the elderly. The recommendations are to perform balance training three times a week for 20- to 30-minute sessions.[64,65] Exercises that incorporate balance training include Tai Chi, yoga, or work with equipment that challenges stability such as a balance and stability board or Bosu ball.

Lifestyle medicine practitioners might write a specific physical activity plan or exercise prescription for the patient to achieve various health outcomes, or refer the patient to an exercise physiologist, disease- or disability-specific exercise specialist (e.g., cancer exercise specialist, adapted exercise specialist), physical therapist, or fitness professional for more detailed prescriptions and/or one-on-one training. Patients are encouraged to check with their primary care physician prior to engaging in any new physical activity or exercise routine.

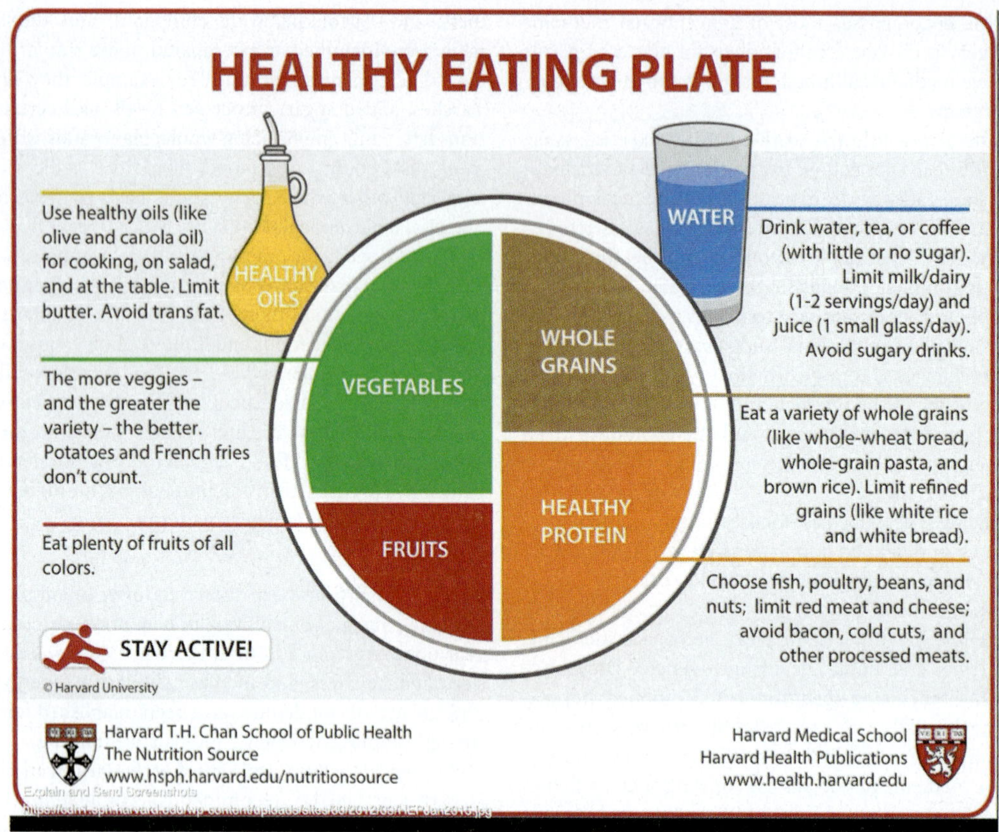

FIGURE 11-2. Harvard Healthy Eating Plate. (*Source*: Used with permission from Harvard University. Copyright © 2011 Harvard University. For more information about The Healthy Eating Plate, please see The Nutrition Source, Department of Nutrition, Harvard T.H. Chan School of Public Health, thenutritionsource.org, and Harvard Health Publications, health.harvard.edu.)

Stress

Lifestyle medicine practitioners work with patients to help them better manage stress. Too much stress leads to physical and emotional complaints. It is estimated that 60–80% of visits to medical doctors are stress related.[66] Excessive stress is associated with many different medical conditions, including obesity,[67] heart disease and elevated blood pressure,[68] depression and anxiety,[69] thyroid dysfunction and lower immune function,[70] decreased bone density,[71] disrupted sleep,[72] and impaired wound healing.[73] Research demonstrates that chronic stress can have a negative impact on the brain, specifically the hippocampus.[74]

Some stress that is manageable may increase productivity and create the state of flow, defined as "being completely involved in an activity for its own sake. The ego falls away. Time flies. Every action, movement, and thought follows inevitably from the previous one, like playing jazz. Your whole being is involved, and you're using your skills to the utmost."[75] To be in flow, a person's skill level must meet the challenge at hand. There is some stress leading to flow. Eustress may occur when there is a job to complete or a deadline to meet. When the challenge is too great for a person's skill level, they can experience anxiety and experience increased stress or even distress. If the challenge is too simple, they can experience boredom. Knowing how to match a task to a person's skill level will allow people to experience more flow. People who experience flow more often may have a greater sense of fulfillment and satisfaction.[76,77] Lifestyle medicine practitioners work with patients to help them achieve flow and avoid distress.

Stress resiliency techniques, including the relaxation response,[78] mindfulness-based stress reduction (MBSR)[79] meditation, and deep breathing, can all help to reduce the sympathetic response and increase the parasympathetic response, allowing for relaxation.[80] Also, other theoretical approaches can be employed, such as training in productive appraisals of stressors (e.g., cognitive flexibility, positive reframing), as well as improving both emotional and problem-focused forms of coping with stress.[81] Each patient requires a different approach depending on their situation. In some cases, the lifestyle medicine practitioner may recommend local classes for meditation, relaxation, MBSR, or yoga for patients to attend on their own, and in other cases they may refer the patient to a social worker, therapist, psychologist, or psychiatrist for individual work.

Sleep

The National Sleep Foundation recommends 7–9 hours of sleep per night for adults. It is estimated that one-third of the population gets less than the recommended amount of sleep.[82] A systematic review and meta-analysis of 16 prospective studies suggests that sleeping less than 6–8 hours a night is associated with approximately a 12% increase in their risk of premature death.[83] Lack of sleep is associated with depression, anxiety, heart disease, stroke, metabolic dysfunction, impaired immunity, substance use, decreased cognition, decreased performance and decreased memory, impaired decision making, fatigue, work-related accidents, suicide risk, and car accidents.[84] Behavioral determinants for poor sleep include shift work, travel to a new time zone, and simply skimping on sleep by going to bed too late. Different sleep disorders can include circadian rhythm disorders, sleep apnea, insomnia, and restless leg syndrome.

Routine practices that help people get sound sleep include going to bed and waking up at the same time each day, reserving the bedroom for sleep and sex only, keeping the temperature in the bedroom cool in the range of 60–70 degrees, and keeping the bedroom quiet and completely dark.[85,86] One of the signals for sleep is a drop in core body temperature. Thus, keeping the bedroom cool helps as does

TABLE 11-1 BASIC VARIETIES OF DIETARY PATTERNS, PROPOSED HEALTH BENEFITS, AND THEIR COMPATIBLE ELEMENTS

Diet	Description[a]	Health Benefits Relate to:
DASH[b]	Focus is on lowering blood pressure. Includes vegetables, fruits, whole grains, nuts/seeds, legumes, mostly nonfat dairy products, lean meats, poultry and fish, nontropical vegetable oils, and low-sodium foods.	Whole plant foods; low-sodium foods; low-fat dairy
Flexitarian	Focus is on allowing for a varied, "flexible" diet plan. Mostly a whole food, vegetarian diet that sometimes includes meat, fish, and/or poultry.	Whole plant foods
Low carb	Focus is on the restriction of total carbohydrate intake from all sources below some threshold (e.g., 45% of daily calories). Includes lean meats, poultry, seafood, eggs, mostly nonstarchy vegetables, whole fruits, nuts and seeds, variety of fats, with or without dairy/nondairy products. Limits grains, legumes, and added sugars.	Whole plant foods; avoids refined starches and added sugars
Low fat	Focus is on the restriction of total fat intake from all sources below some threshold (e.g., 20% of daily calories). Includes lean meats, poultry and fish, fruits and vegetables, grains, legumes, and low-fat dairy products. May include limited amounts of nuts, seeds, nut butters, olives, avocado, cooking oils, fatty fish, and eggs.	Whole plant foods; avoids harmful fats
Mediterranean	Focus is on mimicking the common themes of the traditional dietary pattern that prevails in Mediterranean countries. Includes vegetables, fruits, nuts and seeds, whole grains, legumes, low-fat dairy products, seafood and lean poultry. Emphasis on olive oil, herbs, spices, and red wine (in moderation).	Whole plant foods; emphasis on healthful fats (monounsaturates)
Ornish[c]	Focus is on a whole, plant-based, limited sugar, and low-fat approach derived from prior research with heart disease reversal. Includes vegetables, fruits, whole grains, legumes, nonfat dairy products, egg whites, and limited nuts and seeds.	Whole plant foods; avoids harmful fats
Paleo	Focus is on emulating the dietary pattern of our Stone Age ancestors. Includes a variety of meats (e.g., grass-fed, game), wild fish and seafood, free-range eggs, whole fruits and vegetables, nuts and seeds, with or without nondairy milk. Limits legumes, grains, dairy products, refined sugars, added salt, and processed foods.	Whole plant foods; minimizes processed foods; free range meats
Pescatarian	Focus is on healthy whole food diet that includes seafood (fin fish and shellfish), vegetables, fruits, grains, legumes, nuts, seeds, dairy products, and eggs. May include highly processed dairy and plant-based foods. Excludes all other animal products.	Whole plant foods; avoids harmful fats
Vegan	Focus is on 100% plant-based foods, and excluding all animal products. Includes vegetables, fruits, grains, legumes, nuts, and seeds.	Whole plant foods; avoids harmful fats
Vegetarian	Focus is on healthy whole food diet that includes vegetables, fruits, grains, legumes, nuts, seeds, dairy products, and eggs. Excludes all other animal products.	Whole plant foods; avoids harmful fats
Whole food Plant based	Focus is on consuming only whole foods, from nature. A subtype of a vegan diet that includes vegetables, fruits, intact whole grains, nuts, seeds, and legumes, with minimal processed foods. Excludes added oils, sugars, or concentrated fats.	Whole plant foods; avoids harmful fats; minimizes processed foods; avoids refined starches and added sugars
Compatible Elements		
Limited refined starches, added sugars, processed foods; limited intake of certain fats; emphasis on whole plant foods, with or without lean meats, fish, poultry, and seafood.		

[a]Descriptions emphasize a balanced, healthful version of each diet, and are not meant to accommodate all possible healthy or unhealthy variations of each diet.
[b]Dietary Approaches to Stop Hypertension.
[c]Ornish Plan for Reversing Heart Disease.
Sources: Katz & Meller, 2014; Diet ID, Inc (dietid.com).

wearing socks at bedtime, which will allow for peripheral vasodilation.[87–89] Another signal for sleep is the release of melatonin from the pineal gland in the brain. Blue wavelength light interferes with the release of melatonin,[90,91] and electronic devices emit this spectrum of light. Thus, it is recommended that patients turn off all screens including computer, tablet, phone, and television at least 1 hour prior to bedtime.[92] If people need to use an electrical device, there are apps that can diminish the emission of blue light. Other lifestyle tips for good sleep are to avoid alcohol before bed. Alcohol may aid in the initiation of sleep, but it can disrupt sleep and lead to poor-quality sleep.[93,94] Another chemical that disrupts sleep is caffeine. Coffee, tea, diet sodas, chocolate, and some medications have caffeine in them. Caffeine competes with the same receptor as adenosine. Adenosine builds up throughout the day, and high levels are a signal for sleep. This signal is transmitted when adenosine binds with its receptor. When caffeine binds to the same receptor, there is an opposite effect, because the adrenal glands receive the signal to release adrenaline to "rev up" the sympathetic system.[95] Since the half-life for caffeine is about 5 hours, the recommendations are to limit the intake of caffeine to the morning and avoid it after 12 o'clock pm.[95]

A lifestyle medicine practitioner assesses patients' sleep by asking them routine questions like time of sleep and time of awakening, requesting they fill out a sleep log that tracks the number of hours they sleep, how they feel when they wake up. Adjustments in lifestyle can often cure sleep problems. However, a sleep specialist can help identify the specific sleep condition a patient is experiencing, and help find successful strategies to address the problem. For example, restless leg syndrome may require a neurological workup (NIH, RLS) and snoring might be caused by sleep apnea, which is a risk factor for stroke and requires specific interventions like a continuous positive airway pressure (CPAP) machine.[96] The lifestyle medicine practitioner needs to have a deep understanding of sleep, be able to perform a routine sleep evaluation, and know when to send the patient elsewhere for further evaluation.

Social Connections

Social connections constitute the fifth pillar of lifestyle medicine. Maslow's Hierarchy of Needs reveals love and a sense of belongingness are key needs for humans to satisfy. Absence of a feeling of connection can lead to isolation and loneliness. *Loneliness* is a risk factor for increased morbidity and mortality, and an independent risk factor for heart disease.[97] It is defined as, "the discrepancy between a person's desired and actual social relationships."[98] In contrast to *isolation*, which is a measure of one's lack of social connections/interactions, loneliness is an emotional response to social isolation.[98]

One of the first studies to examine impact of social connections on rate of death was completed in 1979.[99] Researchers used the 1965 Human Population Laboratory survey of a random sample of 6928 adults in Alameda County, California and then examined mortality rates at a 9-year follow-up. They found that people with the highest number of connections were the least likely to die of any cause in the 9-year span of the study. Calculating mortality risk in a community and correlating it to level of social engagement in 10,720 subjects who were patients in 53 family practices in the United Kingdom revealed that mortality risk was greater in the medium and low social engagement groups than it was in those with the highest level of social engagement.[100] Low social connectivity is associated with development and progression of cardiovascular disease, recurrent heart attack, atherosclerosis, high blood pressure, cancer, delayed cancer recovery, and slower wound healing.[18] It is not just the number, but also the quality of these connections that matters. In a meta-analysis of 148 studies, including 308,849 participants, the results indicated that there was a 50% increased likelihood of survival for participants with stronger social relationships.[101]

High-quality connections are defined as relationships that are mutually supportive and have emotional carrying capacity, can handle the expression of both positive and negative emotions, and involve people who feel comfortable expressing themselves.[102] These types of relationships are resilient, and if there is a disagreement or problem they can learn and grow from them.

Lifestyle medicine practitioners work to identify those patients who are experiencing loneliness by asking open-ended questions and creating a strong sense of connection that allows for open communication between practitioner and patient. Also, they can help patients identify opportunities to make connections as well as identify ways to cultivate high-quality connections.

Substance Abuse

Substance use and the area of addictions is its own specialty in medicine; however, lifestyle medicine practitioners need to be familiar with the diagnosis and treatment of substance use disorders. Smoking and alcohol are the areas where the lifestyle medicine practitioner will most likely be involved with counseling, provided that alcohol consumption is part of diet and lifestyle, and smoking is a lifestyle practice, albeit an unhealthful one. Counseling patients in these areas relies heavily on motivational interviewing (MI) and behavior change techniques, which are discussed later in the chapter (see section "Lifestyle in Medicine Limitations").

Research on the Mediterranean diet indicates that some alcohol can be cardioprotective,[103] and The American Heart Association (AHA) recommends limiting alcohol to one serving a night for women and two for men.[104] One drink is considered 12 ounces of beer, 5 ounces of wine, and 1.5 ounces of distilled spirits.[105] Serving sizes are reviewed with patients for a basic understanding of the recommendations, since restaurants and bars do not often comply with these guidelines. The AHA and the Center for Disease Control both recommend, "If you don't drink, don't start,"[82,104] due to the risk of alcohol use disorder. If cancer prevention is the goal, then abstaining from alcohol is the recommendation.[106]

Lifestyle medicine practitioners routinely ask patients about smoking and alcohol use, and identifying difficulty with these substances is an important part of the practice. They counsel patients on smoking cessation, using alcohol in moderation or alcohol cessation. Some patients will require a referral to an addictions specialist, an alcohol rehabilitation center, or other organizations specializing in treatment of addictions like Alcoholics Anonymous. The holistic focus of lifestyle medicine is germane to the opioid crisis salient in the United States as this is being written,[107] as the dangers of opioid addiction warrant an urgent response that should not involve the neglect of pain.[108,109]

EVIDENCE OF EFFICACY FOR LIFESTYLE MEDICINE

This section highlights the evidence that provides a foundation for lifestyle *in* medicine (clinical models of care) and lifestyle *as* medicine (cultural models). More in-depth reviews of the evidence can be found elsewhere.[110]

Lifestyle *in* Medicine

Cardiovascular Disease

While the role of healthy lifestyles in the *prevention* of cardiovascular disease and mortality is promoted through current physical activity and dietary recommendations, public health and medical practitioners might be less aware of the role of lifestyle medicine in the *treatment* and possible *reversal* of cardiovascular disease. To highlight, the Lifestyle Heart Trial was an early catalyst for the heightened attention to the ability of comprehensive lifestyle changes (low-fat vegetarian diet, no smoking, stress management, moderate exercise) to promote the regression of severe coronary atherosclerosis (i.e., heart disease reversal) within 1 year, without the use of lipid-lowering drugs.[111]

Researchers utilizing a very low-fat, plant-based diet in combination with cholesterol-lowering drugs were able to clinically arrest or "reverse" coronary artery disease in patients with severe coronary artery disease.[112] The original cohort was followed for 12 years (1 woman, 23 men), being asked to maintain the plant-based diet and individualized cholesterol-lowering medication. By 1998, 6 nonadherent patients had sustained 13 new cardiac events, while 11 of the adherent patients experienced angiographic confirmation of disease arrest and regression, no coronary events or interventions.[113]

On a larger scale, the Lyon Diet Heart Study was a randomized controlled trial (RCT) that tested the effectiveness of a Mediterranean-type diet on composite measures of coronary recurrence rate after a first myocardial infarction in free-living participants.[114] After 46 months, those following the Mediterranean-style diet had a 50–70% lower risk of recurrent heart disease, including cardiac death and nonfatal heart attacks, angina, stroke, heart failure, and pulmonary embolism.

While current evidence supports the use of lifestyle in prevention, treatment, and possible reversal of cardiovascular disease, especially as Centers for Medicare and Medicaid Services now cover intensive lifestyle therapies as an alternative to coronary artery bypass grafting (CABG). The evidence also highlights the need for more research, including RCTs, on optimal intensity, duration, mode, and long-term follow-up, alongside innovations of measurement and intervention.[115–117]

Type 2 Diabetes

Lifestyle interventions have support for both the prevention and treatment of type 2 diabetes, including physical activity and various dietary patterns (e.g., Mediterranean-type, vegetarian, vegan).[118] The evidence is strong enough, at present, for promotion of lifestyle change as standard for medical care for diabetes.[119]

A landmark RCT from the Diabetes Prevention Program Research Group compared a lifestyle-modification intervention (healthy low-calorie, low-fat diet, moderate-intensity physical activity, behavior modification education) to a Metformin prescription group and placebo group in over 3000 nondiabetic persons from 1996 to 2001. The results suggest that the lifestyle intervention was more effective than Metformin in reducing the incidence of diabetes after 4 years.[120]

For treatment (beyond self-management), the evidence is weaker than that for prevention of type 2 diabetes. However, it is interesting to note that lifestyle, particularly dietary modification, was the primary therapy for diabetes before exogenous insulin became available. There is now evidence to suggest a possibility of type 2 diabetes remission. A 4-year RCT found an intensive lifestyle intervention to be associated with a partial remission of diabetes, compared to a control group who received diabetes support and education.[121] While more research is needed, it is an exciting possibility that the traditional concern of irreversibility of insulin-dependent diabetes mellitus could be challenged with intensive lifestyle interventions.

Stroke

Evidence from scientific reviews of multiple research designs have highlighted the association of lifestyle behaviors, including a healthy diet, not smoking, and an active lifestyle with the reduced risk of stroke, dementia, and cognitive decline.[122–124] In a prospective study, nearly 50% of all stroke cases and 54% of ischemic stroke cases were attributable to low-risk lifestyle, including not smoking, a healthy weight, modest alcohol consumption, achieving moderate physical activity, and a healthy diet score.[125] These same modifiable lifestyle predictors were compiled into quintiles of a "Healthy Heart Score," finding that poorer scores were related with a 2.9-fold higher risk of total mortality from cardiovascular disease, including a greater risk of death due to stroke.[126]

From a treatment perspective, prospective trials and RCTs have found an important role of lifestyle interventions on secondary stroke prevention, while also highlighting the need for emphasis on longer interventions that target multiple behavior change techniques.[115,127,128] Evidence also supports the use of physical activity, exercise, and nutrition for enhanced physical and cognitive benefits during stroke recovery, as well as unique challenges of adopting lifestyle changes.[129]

Cancer

Observable cancer risk cannot be sufficiently accounted for by accumulation of intrinsic processes, such as rates of endogenous mutation, being heavily influenced by extrinsic factors.[130] Over 40% of both the incidence of and deaths from cancer have been attributed to modifiable risk factors, including cigarette smoking, excess body weight, alcohol intake, consumption of red and processed meat, low consumption of fruits and vegetables, dietary fiber and dietary calcium, physical inactivity, ultraviolet radiation, and cancer-related infections.[131–133] As a result, the American Cancer Society (ACS) and the American Institute for Cancer Research (AICR) support lifestyle recommendations for cancer prevention.[134,135]

Modifiable lifestyle factors have also been implicated in the survivorship and treatment of cancer. For survivorship, the ACS provides lifestyle changes, highlighted by healthy nutrition and physical activity.[136] The efficacy of physical activity, especially aerobic exercise, is positive on the progression of cancer; however, considerable methodological heterogeneity precludes meaningful conclusions at this time.[137] Advantages of lifestyle modification following treatment have also been implicated across bladder,[138] breast,[139] colon,[140,141] and prostate cancers.[142,143] For possible cancer reversal, low-risk prostate cancer patients receiving comprehensive lifestyle changes have exhibited reduced PSA levels, cancer cell growth, and need for conventional cancer treatment, alongside increased relative telomere length within 5 years.[142–144] Like type 2 diabetes, the possibility of cancer reversal provides an exciting new frontier for future research, exhibited by advancements in epigenetics.[145]

LIFESTYLE *IN* MEDICINE LIMITATIONS

Despite the growing evidence, the best practices for clinical implementation strategies are unknown, which highlight methodological difficulties in lifestyle medicine research. There is the general concern that RCTs, the "gold standard," are incapable, ethically at least, to test how lifestyle behaviors influence morbidity and mortality.[146] While RCTs often can be applied to lifestyle medicine, they cannot be the source of information about lifetime effects on longevity and vitality. Lifestyle medicine calls for advances in evidence gathering. In response, at the writing of this chapter, a taskforce is underway to develop an easy, more effective tool for evaluating the evidence related to lifestyle medicine clinical questions, called Hierarchies of Evidence Applied to Lifestyle Medicine.[147]

As with any medication prescription, dose-response should also be considered. A strong dose-response effect has been found with physical activity, or perhaps more appropriately "physical fitness," where plateauing increases in activity volume and fitness produce increased reduction in mortality risk.[148–151] Any lifestyle intervention will presumably produce a similar dose-response effect. For example, can one conclude that three, individualized lifestyle counseling session of 15–45 minutes each, spread over the first 3 years of a 10-year study period is enough to produce a change in healthy lifestyles to the point of reducing risk and incidence of a chronic disease?[152] Studies of lifestyle interventions in clinical practice settings can lead to negative outcomes for doing too little. By way of analogy, a study of parachutes would prove them ineffective if the parachutes were too small to slow a free-fall, or deployed too late.[153] That would not disprove the utility of parachutes; it would only disprove the utility of inadequate parachutes.

Intensive therapeutic lifestyle change programs, such as the Lifestyle Heart Trial[154] and the Comprehensive Health Improvement Program,[155] can provide insight for clinical models, including dose-response and successful intervention qualities, alongside methodological difficulties that are applicable to all lifestyle intervention research. Dietary intake, for instance, is a well-known challenge, with measures of self-report serving as a convenient proxy for the costly inconvenience of metabolic ward studies. Physical activity levels and sleep are easier to measure objectively but still can contribute to substantial measurement error. Assessing the number and quality of social connections relies on the patient's opinion and self-reporting, which has its limitations as a research tool due to social desirability bias, misinterpretation of questions, recall bias, and limited responses, which can encourage participants to select an answer even if it might not accurately reflect their situation.[156]

Currently, the clinical setting is not optimally designed to support the multifactorial and synergistic practice of lifestyle medicine, as shared within a similar set of issues and concerns for lifestyle interventions in the workplace.[157] There are also concerns of practitioner competencies,[33,158] practice constraints (e.g., billing/reimbursement models, shared medical appointments, time to consult with patients, etc.), lack of patient referral options or practices, patient follow-up, and patient-provider interaction characteristics that influence patient adoption of lifestyle prescriptions (e.g., message framing, stigmatization, medical triggers, barriers to lifestyle prescriptions, practitioner's own health and lifestyle choices, etc.). These concerns must be elucidated to better understand the shortcomings of lifestyle medicine interventions in the clinical setting, and to establish models of best practice.

These challenges are greatly compounded by modern cultures that conspire directly against the lifestyle medicine guidance a clinician may provide. Counseling about physical activity is confronted by a world of labor-saving technologies right outside the clinic door. Counseling about diet is even more emphatically undermined by the ubiquity of fast-food outlets and the aggressive marketing of food all but engineered to undermine clinical goals.[159] Hectic schedules and stress conspire against recommendation for both stress management and sleep. The notion that clinical counseling might overcome direct confrontations with cultural defaults is at best an unconfirmed hypothesis, and at worst—not merely unproved, but also unlikely.

These difficulties should not preclude innovations and adaptations to clinical practice, however, as clinicians have an opportunity both to (a) compensate to the extent possible for toxic effects of cultural defaults and (b) to lead and champion efforts to change those defaults. Structures supportive of these roles include alternative fee and/or reimbursement models, new tools for assessing and prescribing lifestyle medicine, team-based approaches, and other tools to deliver lifestyle medicine digitally. The goal, in the end, is to make the clinical setting optimally effective at delivering lifestyle medicine, and thus maximize its contributions.

LIFESTYLE *AS* MEDICINE

Despite any advances in the clinical concept that lifestyle *is* medicine, there will be limitations of a clinical remedy for a cultural malady. The current progression of culture and society that encourages people to be sedentary and eat poorly provides an unreasonable task for clinical interventions, alone, to solve.

Thus, consideration can be made for the "lifestyle *as* medicine" approach, emphasizing the environmental accessibility and cultural influence on lifestyles that either increase or decrease the risk of disease, as illustrated by the Blue Zone Project,[160] North Karelia Project,[161] Stanford 5 City Project,[162,163] and Shape Up Somerville.[164] These efforts might be the most conducive for larger public health impact than clinical interventions alone. Such approaches will not be without challenges, encouraging people to navigate physical and social environments, tradition, public policy, industry, and media. However, these challenges provide an opportunity to inspire innovation for cooperative effort (e.g., True Health Initiative, One Health, Cooperative Extension), alongside future solutions for cultural influence and change.[165] Until or unless culture promotes health, there is a lot more work for clinicians to do. By guiding people to healthful choices, clinicians raise awareness and pave the way for culture-wide change. Over time, there could (and should) be a shift from a clinical emphasis that is directed at overcoming and changing cultural obstacles, to a cultural emphasis, where the defaults become health-promoting.

IMPLEMENTATION OF LIFESTYLE MEDICINE

Individual Care

The Patient

With any medication, there is the concern of adherence. This concern in lifestyle medicine is perhaps more pronounced, due to the complexities of adopting behaviors required to precipitate the prevention, treatment, and reversal of disease.[166,167] For example, the European Potsdam Study found achieving four healthy lifestyle factors (not smoking; BMI < 30 kg/m^2; ≥ 3.5 hours/week of physical activity; adherence to a diet high in fruits, vegetables, and whole grain, and low meat consumption) had nearly an 80% lower risk of developing a chronic disease.[168] However, only 9% of these participants achieved all four factors, while only 3% of Americans were estimated to achieve four similar factors.[169]

With the vast literature on factors that influence health behavior initiation and maintenance, the present review will focus on common settings for lifestyle medicine (e.g., primary care). More specifically, the patient, with consideration for any healthy lifestyle change, engages a "patient path" that is initiated with a triggering event (e.g., screening, diagnosis), followed by an individualized response or reaction, and then a level of engagement in a behavior change process to stay in line with a lifestyle medicine prescription.

The Trigger

Screenings and/or diagnoses in primary care, public health, and fitness settings are aimed at providing awareness and motivation for change in behavior. According to the Feedback-Processing Model of Self-Regulation, a desire to change is initiated with a perceived discrepancy about oneself in relation to a standard or goal.[170] For example, during a body weight screening, a patient finds she weighs more than an ideal body weight. The perceived discrepancy can act as "trigger" or spark for efforts to reduce the discrepancy. Much of the research in this area has focused on weight control, revealing that the response to the triggering experience is complex; able to enhance motivation for a myriad of reasons, from appearance to health risk (i.e., medical trigger),[171–174] or diminish motivation and inspire avoidance.[175–180] For example, being diagnosed as overweight, told to lose weight, or even being weighed is a self-reported reason for avoiding healthcare and other medical triggers, such as cancer screenings.[181–183]

The Response

Medical triggers are not benign in their impact on patient experience, suggesting that an emotional response from the patient provides a glimpse into a theorized level of effort to initiate change,[170] as well as behavioral choices to cope or "deal with" the experience.[180,184] The motivational response is similarly complex, so the inclination to dichotomize patients as motivated or not can mask a more comprehensive understanding. It is possible that certain types of motivation are more beneficial for sustainable lifestyle change, especially those that emphasize autonomy or *self*-determined sources of motivation versus *other*-determined sources (e.g., motivated due to pressure from the practitioner).[185–188]

Motivation, itself, is influenced by other factors. For example, a patient's attitude about a behavior, subjective norms of those most important to the patient, and perception of behavioral control can influence one's intention to change.[189] There is possibility that patients' progress or digress (i.e., relapse) through "stages of change," all of which vary in their presumption of motivation, as well as the tactics to influence movement through the stages (i.e., processes of change).[190] Such theoretical perspectives, which are foundational to public health, can be also utilized in lifestyle medicine contexts, or combined to create novel approaches to clinical care (e.g., The Pressure System Model).[191]

The Process

Patients must then enact the process of monitoring and changing their behavior to stay in line with a lifestyle medicine prescription (i.e., self-regulation). For example, a patient discovers he is diabetic, is frustrated, thus motivated to reduce blood sugar via a prescribed diet. However, he quickly realizes the complexities of monitoring and changing his dietary behavior, alongside the social and physical environments that tempt and test inadequacies in his self-regulatory abilities, such as awareness, self-control, self-confidence, goal shaping, cognitive flexibility, transcendence, and planning skills, leading to self-regulatory failure.[166,167,192–196] Early in the change process, living within an environment that works against health, as we experience today, mandates the patient garner and maintain self-regulatory proficiency, while the environment that encourages health allows the dependence on self-regulation to wane. Thus, efforts to improve the "patient path" for behavior change must align with systemic and cultural changes, alongside a team care approach to positively influence medication adherence, when lifestyle is the medicine.

The Practitioner

Lifestyle medicine practitioners can employ a number of approaches to help patients in their behavior change process. On one end of the spectrum, the practitioner can simply provide awareness and advice on lifestyle change. On the other end, the practitioner can engage in individualized prescriptions, counseling, and health and wellness coaching, aimed at "self-directed, lasting changes, aligned with their values, which promote health and wellness and, thereby, enhance well-being."[197] The practitioner can also function as a change agent at the community and cultural level, advocating for systemic modifications that enable the adoption of lifestyle as medicine.[198]

There are randomized controlled, prospective, retrospective, and qualitative research studies that demonstrate the value of health and wellness coaching for behavior change.[199,200] Common coaching strategies include helping the patient set goals, creating a mechanism for accountability, educating the patient in areas of importance and interest to the particular patient, and encouraging self-discovery.[201] When lifestyle medicine practitioners are using the coach approach, they are focused on sharing information that is appropriate for the patient, listening to more than the patient's words, including listening to body language, tone of voice, and facial expressions, asking open-ended questions which allow the patient to share important information as well as potentially uncover obstacles and motivators for change, and allowing the patient to find their own answers to problems that are getting in the way of their progress.[200]

Most lifestyle medicine practitioners who are physicians, nurses, and other allied healthcare providers are accustomed to being the experts, as they are trained to diagnose and treat medical problems. They are used to telling patients what to do, as they are the experts in medical diagnosis and treatment. With behavior change, the patient is the expert in his or her own life and lifestyle: knowing what has worked in the past, knowing the obstacles in the way, and understanding the motivations for change. In this way, the lifestyle medicine practitioner needs to be more like a coach and let the patient be the expert. In many cases, the practitioner learns important information by asking specific questions, which elucidate the patient's barriers to change, called impediment profiling. Patients may not immediately recognize their barriers but when asked relevant questions, their obstacles become more obvious.[202] After identifying the impediments, the practitioner can work with the patient on a tailored intervention.[203] Listening to the patient and using their prior experiences to help them be successful with a new attempt at lifestyle modification is an important part of behavior change counselling.[204] Spending 20 minutes asking the patients questions and holding a discussion about how to incorporate physical activity into the week is more effective for increasing minutes spent exercising than a routine visit where physical activity is not a focus, but spending 20 minutes telling the patients why they should exercise and that they should exercise does not increase minutes spent exercising compared to a routine visit.[205]

Motivational interviewing, defined as "a client-centered, directive method for enhancing intrinsic motivation to change by exploring and resolving ambivalence," can also be utilized in lifestyle medicine practice.[206] It is a style of interviewing that encourages the patient to do most of the talking, focused on the advantages of changing (i.e., "change talk").

There are four strategies that are commonly used in motivational interviewing, also called the OARS (Open-ended questions; Affirmations; Reflections; Summaries). Open-ended questions invite the patient to take time to reflect and craft an extensive answer to a question, whereas closed-ended questions invite the patient to answers with one word, usually yes or no. Affirmations are statements that acknowledge and appreciate any positive movement toward a healthy change. Reflections are statements that reflect the sentiments of the patient, often paraphrases of what the patient said. Summaries synthesize conversations, and state the main points in a clear concise manner.

One of the main goals in behavior change counseling is to make a solid connection with the patient, so that even if the patient is not ready for change, when they are ready, they will be open to discussing it with the practitioner. One simple way to make a connection with a patient is to express empathy. In a correlational study, primary care physicians scoring higher in self-reported empathy were more likely to have patients with good control of hemoglobin A1c and good LDL control.[207]

One of the core competencies in lifestyle medicine is to practice healthy lifestyle behaviors.[33] A correlational study revealed that physicians who exercised were more likely to counsel their patients on exercise. And, specifically physicians who strength trained counseled on strength training. Physicians who performed aerobic exercises counseled on aerobic exercise. However, if a physician did not perform strength training exercises, then they did not counsel on it.[208] One study in which subjects watched videos of physicians counseling patients demonstrated that physicians who disclosed information about their own healthy habits such as taking an apple to work for a snack or walking to work for exercise were rated as more motivating and believable than those who simply gave advice on exercise and diet.[209]

Team Care

A key feature of lifestyle medicine is the dedication to a team-approach in interdisciplinary healthcare.[33] The practitioner cannot do it all, and will likely minimize effectiveness in lifestyle adoption without assistance from team members who are internal and/or external to their practice. Commonly, the team care approach includes more traditional members, such as cooperating physicians of various specialties, nurses, physician assistants, and administrative support. Although less common in traditional medicine, lifestyle medicine practitioners find great benefit in exercise specialists, therapists, coaches and nutrition specialists, registered dieticians, and chefs (e.g., culinary medicine) who emphasize compatible lifestyle prescriptions.

Community Care

Lifestyle medicine practitioners extend the notion of team care beyond the clinical setting to the community. The physical and social aspects of communities that span the social ecological spectrum, including their social, governmental, educational, industrial, environmental, public health, and Cooperative Extension, provide a framework and strong influence on patients' access and abilities to adopt healthy lifestyle prescriptions. Physical environments can improve access, and help make health the "easy" choice, thus minimizing the need for strong self-regulatory abilities. The social environment, including a supportive culture of health and wellness, also provides a strong influence on lifestyle adoption and maintenance. Such an influence is exhibited by the Blue Zones, which represent the cultures throughout the world who have the highest percentage of centenarians, at ten times greater rates than the United States.[30] Of the nine common denominators of a healthy lifestyle, these populations belonged to faith-based communities, put families first, and had strong social circles and networks (i.e., the "right tribe").

In addition, when adequate education aimed at increasing knowledge, skills, and abilities to adopt a healthy lifestyle is unavailable within the clinical setting, the lifestyle medicine practitioner must depend on such offerings within the community across the prevention spectrum. For example, public health entities, such as state health services and local healthcare systems, can provide health screening opportunities and education in secondary prevention, such as diabetes self-management and classes. Also, the state's Cooperative Extension Service provides a network of local family and community health personnel and educational programs focused on the primary prevention of chronic disease by teaching people how to apply the results of scientific research.[210] Further, full prevention spectrum efforts might also include nonprofit organizations, faith-based organizations, local churches, and fitness centers to extend the possibilities for coordinated, community care.

THE FUTURE OF LIFESTYLE MEDICINE

Within the "lifestyle *is* medicine" approach, there are opportunities to develop new clinical models, reimbursement mechanisms, technologies, and digital platforms to support them. Innovations can also include team care approaches, not only in the clinical setting, but also within the community, leveraging existing resources such as Cooperative Extension and public health entities and services. With respect to the aforementioned "patient path," there is much to be learned and done to expand provider knowledge, confidence, and abilities in lifestyle prescription, including their patient interactions that maximize motivation and adherence to the prescriptions, as well as the processes that maximize patient involvement in clinical interventions or community-based programs found to be effective in healthy lifestyle adoption. Put another way, there is a bright future for innovations in medication adherence, with lifestyle as the medicine.

While the current limitations and potential future of lifestyle medicine encourage the clinical advancement of "lifestyle *is* medicine" approach, all evidence to date reinforces a strong emphasis on the "lifestyle *as* medicine" approach. Where healthy living prevails, it is because culture makes healthful choices the default choices—either by design (e.g., North Karelia Project) or by fortuitous, historical happenstance (e.g., the world's Blue Zone populations). The cultural malady of poor health highlights the limits to clinical solutions, while also emphasizing the spectrum of need from individual to family to community to public policy at local, state, and national levels to achieve a culture of health.

In addition, acknowledgment is made that a healthful lifestyle cannot occur absent of a healthy, thriving, and sustainable planet, which encourages multidisciplinary frameworks and systematic approaches to the conjoined challenge of public and planetary health. The One Health Initiative can serve as a guide to unite professionals from medicine, veterinary medicine, public health, environmental specialists, public policy experts, and others working to improve the health of the population and the sustainability of the planet.[211] However, with an original emphasis on infectious disease, there is no current model or consensus of a One Health approach to chronic disease prevention, although the dots are being connected. An unhealthy eating pattern is the leading risk factor for premature death in the United States; food systems accommodating the demand for such patterns are a main contributor to adverse environmental effects and changes as well.[212] The effect of eating patterns of the Dietary Guidelines for Americans (DGA) to environmental sustainability has been highlighted, including room for much improvement.[213] The EAT–*Lancet* Commission recently addressed the need to feed a growing global population through a universal healthy reference diet that also achieves environmentally sustainable food system while also defining sustainable food systems that will minimize damage to our planet.[214] Yet, dietary transitions to healthier lifestyle patterns also provide downstream challenges, such as enhanced production of healthier foods, increased availability, and impact on industry innovation, revenue, and jobs.

Advances and successes to date in lifestyle medicine have spurred current enthusiasm, rapid growth of the field, and the establishment of lifestyle medicine as a valued discipline with individual and public health implications. Lifestyle medicine positively impacts humans, animals, and the planet. This discipline sets itself apart by promoting prescriptions for six specific pillars: exercise, healthful eating, stress resiliency, sleep, social connection, smoking cessation, and alcohol moderation or elimination. These prescriptions place lifestyle medicine in a pivotal position to help transition the current state of healthcare in the United States. The future poses the challenges of addressing the planet as a marquee patient, and achieving health-promoting culture change at scale. The future is also bright with opportunity, as there is ever more innovation taking this best of medicine from research to practice, from cell to culture, from individual health to public health, and from disease care to healthcare.

References

1. World Health Organization. Constitution of the World Health Organization as adopted by the International Health Conference, New York, 19–22 June 1946; signed on 22 July 1946 by the representatives of 61 States (Official Records of the World Health Organization, no. 2, p. 100) and entered into force on 7 April 1948. In Grad, FP. The Preamble of the Constitution of the World Health Organization. *Bulletin of the World Health Organization*. 2002;80(12):982.
2. Used with permission from World Health Organization. Constitution of the World Health Organization --Basic Documents, Forty-fifth edition, Supplement, October 2006.
3. Used with permission from Merriam-Webster. Available at https://www.merriam-webster. com/dictionary/lifestyle+/Medicine+/distress+/eustress. Accessed November 2018.
4. American College of Lifestyle Medicine. Core Competencies. Available at http://www.lifestylemedicine.org/Core-Competencies. Accessed November 2018.
5. Hippocrates. *Hippocratic Writings*. Chicago, IL: Encyclopedia Britannica; 1955.
6. McGinnis JM, Foege WH. Actual causes of death in the United States. *JAMA*. 1993;270:2207–12.
7. Ford ES, Bergmann MM, Kroger J, Schienkiewitz A, Weikert C, Boeing H. Healthy living is the best revenge: Findings from the European Prospective Investigation into Cancer and Nutrition-Potsdam study. *Arch Intern Med*. 2009;169:1355–62.
8. Kvaavik E, Meyer HE, Tverdal A. Food habits, physical activity and body mass index in relation to smoking status in 40–42 year old Norwegian woman and men. *Prev Med*. 2004;38(1):1–5.
9. Bodai BI, Nakata TE, Wong WT, et al. Lifestyle medicine: A brief review of its dramatic impact on health and survival. *Perm J*. 2018;22:17–25.
10. Mokdad AH, Marks JS, Stroup DF, et al. Actual causes of death in the United States, 2000. *JAMA*. 2004;291(10):1238–45.
11. Pi-Sunyer X. The medical risks of obesity. *Postgrad Med*. 2009;121(6):21–33.
12. Warburton DE, Nicol CW, Bredin SS. Health benefits of physical activity: The evidence. *CMAJ*. 2006;174(6):801–9.
13. Lourida I, Soni M, Thompson-Coon J, et al. Mediterranean diet, cognitive function, and dementia: A systematic review. *Epidemiology*. 2013;24:479–89.
14. Skerrett PJ, Willett WC. Essentials of healthy eating: A guide. *J Midwifery Womens Health*. 2010; 55(6):492–501.
15. Rozanski A, Bairey CN, Krantz DS, et al. Mental stress and the induction of silent myocardial ischemia in patients with coronary artery disease. *N Engl J Med*. 1988;318:1005–12.
16. Schneiderman N, Ironson G, Siegel SD. Stress and health: Psychological, behavioral, and biological determinants. *Ann Rev Clin Psychol*. 2005;1:607–28.
17. Saha SP, Bhalla DK, Whayne TF, Gairola C. Cigarette smoke and adverse health effects: An overview of research trends and future needs. *Int J Angiol*. 2007;16(3):77–83.
18. Umberson D, Montez JK. Social relationships and health: A flashpoint for health policy. *J Health Soc Behav*. 2010;51(1), S54–66.
19. Tuso P, Stoll SR, Li WW. A plant-based diet, atherogenesis, and coronary artery disease prevention. *Perm J*. 2015;19(1):62–7.
20. Strasser B, Gostner JM, Fuchs D. Mood, food, and cognition: Role of tryptophan and serotonin. *Curr Opin Clin Nutr Metab Care*. 2016;19(1):55–61.
21. Ujvari D, Hulchiy M, Calaby A, Nybacka A, Bystrom B, Hirschberg AL. Lifestyle intervention up-regulates gene and protein levels of molecules involved in insulin signaling in the endometrium of overweight/obese women with polycystic ovary syndrome. *Hum Reprod*. 2014;29:1526–35.
22. Sears B. Anti-inflammatory diets. *J Am Coll Nutr*. 2015;34(Suppl 1):14–21.
23. Ornish D, Magbanua MJ, Weidner G, et al. Changes in prostate gene expression in men undergoing an intensive nutrition and lifestyle intervention. *Proc Natl Acad Sci U S A*. 2008;105:8369–74.
24. Barnard RJ, Hong Gonzalez J, Liva ME, Ngo TH. Effects of a low-fat, high-fiber diet and exercise program on breast cancer risk factors in vivo and tumor cell growth and apoptosis in vitro. *Nutr Cancer*. 2006;55:28–34.
25. Bagur MJ, Murcia MA, Jimenez-Monreal AM, et al. Influence of diet in multiple sclerosis: A systematic review. *Adv Nutr*. 2017;8(3):463–72.
26. Dashti HS, Scheer FA, Jacques PF, Lamon-Fava S, Ordovas JM. Short sleep duration anddietary intake: Epidemiologic evidence, mechanisms, and health implications. *Adv Nutr*. 2015;6(6):648–59.
27. Urry E, Landolt HP. Adenosine, caffeine, and performance: From cognitive neuroscience of sleep to sleep pharmacogenetics. *Curr Top Behav Neurosci*. 2015;25:331–66.
28. Touitou Y, Reinberg A, Touitou D. Association between light at night, melatonin secretion, sleep deprivation, and the internal clock: Health impacts and mechanisms of circadian disruption. *Life Sci*. 2017;173:94–106.

29. Moderie C, Van der Maren S, Dumont M. Circadian phase, dynamics of subjective sleepiness and sensitivity to blue light in young adults complaining of a delayed sleep schedule. *Sleep Med.* 2017;34:148–55.
30. Buettner D, Skemp S. Blue Zones: Lessons from the world's longest lived. *Am J Lifestyle Med.* 2016;10(5):318–21.
31. Vartiainen E. The north Karelia project: Cardiovascular disease prevention in Finland. *Glob Cardiol Sci Pract.* 2018;2018(2):13.
32. Coffield E, Nihiser AJ, Sherry B, et al. Shape up Somerville: Change in parent body mass indexes during a child-targeted, community-based environmental change intervention. *Am J Pub Health.* 2015;105(2):e83–9.
33. Lianov L, Johnson M. Physician competencies for prescribing lifestyle medicine. *J Am Med Assoc.* 2010;304(2):202–3.
34. American College of Preventive Medicine. Available at https://www.acpm.org/page/preventivemedicine.
35. American Board of Medical Specialties (ABMS). Available at https://www.abms.org/.
36. American College of Lifestyle Medicine. Available at https://lifestylemedicine.org/ACLM/About.
37. Pojednic R, Frates E. A parallel curriculum in lifestyle medicine. *Clin Teach.* 2017;14(1):27–31.
38. Pojednic RM, Trilk J, Phillips EM. Lifestyle medicine curricula: An initiative to include lifestyle medicine in our nation's medical schools. *Acad Med.* 2015;90(7):840–1.
39. National Institutes of Health, National Center for Complementary and Integrative Health. Available at https://nccih.nih.gov/health/integrative-health.
40. Johns Hopkins Medicine Health Library, Types of Complementary and Alternative Medicine. Available at https://www.hopkinsmedicine.org/healthlibrary/conditions/complementary_and_alternative_medicine/types_of_complementary_and_alternative_medicine_85,P00189.
41. The Institute for Functional Medicine. Reversing the Chronic Disease Trend: Six Steps to Better Wellness. Available at https://p.widencdn.net/xazlwe/Intro_Functional_Medicine.
42. The US Burden of Disease Collaborators. The State of US Health, 1990–2016: Burden of diseases, injuries, and risk factors among US states. *JAMA.* 2018;319(14):1444–72.
43. Available at https://cspinet.org/eating-healthy/why-good-nutrition-important.
44. United States Department of Agriculture. Available at https://www.cnpp.usda.gov/2015-2020-dietary-guidelines-americans.
45. Harvard TH. Chan School of Public Health. Healthy Eating Plate. Available at https://www.hsph.harvard.edu/nutritionsource/healthy-eating-plate/.
46. De Lorgeril M, Salen P, Martin JL, et al. Effect of a Mediterranean type of diet on the rate of cardiovascular complications in patients with coronary artery disease. Insights into the cardioprotective effect of certain nutriments. *J Am Coll Cardiol.* 1996;28(5):1103–8.
47. Sarker U, Oba S. Salinity stress enhances color parameters, bioactive leaf pigments, vitamins, polyphenols, flavonoids and antioxidant activity in selected Amaranthus leafy vegetables. *J Sci Food Agric.* 2019;99(5):2275–84.
48. Neves MF, Cunha MR, Paula R. Effects of nutrients and exercises to attenuate oxidative stress and prevent cardiovascular disease. *Curr Pharm Des.* 2018;24(40):4800–6.
49. Esteban R, Buezo J, Becerril JM, et al. Modified atmosphere packaging and dark/light refrigerated storage in green leafy vegetables have an impact on nutritional value. *Plant Foods Hum Nutr.* 2019;74(1):99–106.
50. Ko JH, Arfuso F, Sethi G, et al. Pharmacological utilization of bergamottin, derived from grapefruits, in cancer prevention and therapy. *Int J Mol Sci.* 2018;19(12):4048.
51. Paur I, Lilleby W, Bohn SK, et al. Tomato-based randomized controlled trial in prostate cancer patients: Effects on PSA. *Clin Nutr.* 2017;36(3):672–9.
52. Katz DL, Meller J. Can we say what diet is best for health. *Annu Rev Public Health.* 2014;35:83–103.
53. Willett W, Rockström J, Loken B, et al. Food in the Anthropocene: The EAT–Lancet Commission on healthy diets from sustainable food systems. *Lancet.* 2019;393(10170):447–92.
54. Grotto D, Zied E. The standard American diet and its relationship to the health status of Americans. *Nutr Clin Pract.* 2010;25(6):603–12.
55. Pollan M. *In Defense of Food: An Eater's Manifesto.* New York: Penguin Press; 2008.
56. Holli BB. Using behavior modification in nutrition counselling. *J Am Diet Assoc.* 1988;88(12):1530–6.
57. Hwang MY. Why you should exercise. *JAMA.* 1999;281(4):394.
58. Sharma A, Madaan V, Perry FD, et al. Exercise for mental health. *Prim Care Companion J Clin Psychiatry.* 2006;8(2):106.
59. Office of Disease Prevention and Health Promotion. Physical Activity Guidelines. Available at https://health.gov/paguidelines/.
60. Howden EJ, Sarma S, Lawley JS, et al. Reversing the cardiac effects of sedentary aging in middle age—A randomized controlled trial. *Circulation.* 2018;137:1549–60.
61. ten Brinke LF, Bolandzadeh N, Nagamatsu LS, et al. Aerobic exercise increases hippocampal volume in older women with probable mild cognitive impairment: A 6-month randomised controlled trial. *Br J Sports Med.* 2015;49(4):248–54.
62. Keller K, Engelhardt M. Strength and muscle mass loss with aging process: Age and strength loss. *Muscles Ligaments Tendons J.* 2013;3(4):346–50.
63. Behm DG, Blazevich AJ, Kay AD, McHugh M. Acute effects of muscle stretching on physical performance, range of motion, and injury incidence in healthy active individuals: A systematic review. *App Physiol Nutr Metabol.* 2016;41(1):1–11.
64. Brachman A, Kamieniarz A, Michalska J, Pawlowski M, Slomka KJ, Juras G. Balance training programs in athletes—A systematic review. *J Hum Kinet.* 2017;58:45–64.
65. Lesinski M, Hortobagyi T, Muehlbauer T, Gollhofer A, Granacher U. Effects of balance training on balance performance in healthy older adults: A systematic review and meta-analysis. *Sports Med.* 2015;45(12):1721–38.
66. Nerurkar A, Bitton A, Davis RB, Phillips RS, Yeh F. When physicians counsel about stress: Results of a national study. *JAMA Intern Med.* 2013;173(1):76–7.
67. Sinha R, Jastreboff AM. Stress as a common risk factor for obesity and addiction. *Biol Psychiatry.* 2013;73(9):827–35.
68. Chauvet-Gelinier JC, Bonin B. Stress, anxiety and depression in heart disease patients: A major challenge for cardiac rehabilitation. *Ann Phys Rehab Med.* 2017;60(1):6–12.
69. Cohen BE, Edmondson D, Kronish IM. State of the art review: Depression, stress, anxiety, and cardiovascular disease. *Am J Hypertens.* 2015;28(11):1295–302.
70. Zhang J, Huang J, Aximujiang K, Xu C, Ahemaiti A, Wu G, Zhong L, Yunusi K. Thyroid dysfunction, neurological disorder and immunosuppression as the consequences of long-term combined stress. *Sci Rep.* 2018;8(1):4552.
71. Furlan PM, Ten Have T, Cary M, et al. The role of stress-induced cortisol in the relationship between depression and decreased bone mineral density. *Biol Psychiatry.* 2005;57(8):911–7.
72. Eskildsen A, Fentz HN, Andersen LP, Pedersen AD, Kristensen SB, Andersen JH. Perceived stress, disturbed sleep, and cognitive impairments in patients with work-related stress complaints: A longitudinal study. *Stress.* 2017;20(4):371–8.
73. Cano Sanchez M, Lencel S, Boulanger E, Neviere R. Targeting oxidative stress and mitochondrial dysfunction in the treatment of impaired wound healing: A systematic review. *Antioxidants.* 2018;7(8):98.
74. Kim EJ, Pellman B, Kim JJ. Stress effects on the hippocampus: A critical review. *Learn Mem.* 2015;22(9):411–6.
75. Csikszentmihalyi M. *Flow: The Psychology of Optimal Experience.* New York: Harper & Row; 1990.
76. Asakawa, K. Flow experience, culture, and well-being: How do autotelic Japanese college students feel, behave, and think in their daily lives? *J Happiness Stud.* 2010;11(2):205–23.
77. Ullen F, de Manzano O, Almeida R, et al. Proneness for psychological flow in everyday life: Associations with personality and intelligence. *Pers Individ Differ.* 2012;52(2):167–72.
78. Bhasin MK, Denninger JW, Huffman JC, et al. Specific transcriptome changes associated with blood pressure reduction in hypertensive patients after relaxation response training. *J Altern Complement Med.* 2018;24(5):486–504.
79. Worthen M, Cash E. Stress Management. 2019 Jan 19. StatPearls [Internet]. Treasure Island (FL): StatPearls Publishing; 2018 Jan. Available at http://www.ncbi.nlm.nih.gov/books/NBK513300/PubMed. PMID: 30020672.
80. Park ER, Traeger L, Vranceanu AM, et al. The development of a patient-centered program based on the relaxation response: The relaxation response resiliency program (3RP). *Psychosomatics.* 2013;54(2):165–74.
81. Lazarus RS, Folkman S. Transactional theory and research on emotions and coping. *Eur J Pers.* 1987;1:141–69.
82. Centers for Disease Control and Prevention (CDC). Available at https://www.cdc.gov/sleep/index.html.

83. Cappuccio FP, Elia L, Strazzullo P, Miller MA. Sleep duration and all-cause mortality: A systematic review and meta-analysis of prospective studies. *Sleep*. 2010;33(5):585–92.

84. McEwen BS, Karatsoreos IN. Sleep deprivation and circadian disruption: Stress, allostasis, and allostatic load. *Sleep Med Clin*. 2015;10(1):1–10.

85. Irish LA, Kline CE, Gunn HE, Buysse DJ, Hall MH. The role of sleep hygiene in promoting public health: A review of empirical evidence. *Sleep Med Rev*. 2015;22:23–36.

86. Onen SH, Onen F, Bailly D, Parquet P. Prevention and treatment of sleep disorders through regulation of sleeping habits. *Presse Med*. 1994;23(10):485–9.

87. Buysse DJ, Reynolds CF III, Kupfer DJ. Effects of diagnosis on treatment recommendations in chronic insomnia—A report from the APAlNIMH DSM-IV field trial. *Sleep*. 1997;20(7):542–52.

88. Ko Y, Lee JY. Effects of feet warming using bed socks on sleep quality and thermoregulatory responses in a cool environment. *J Physiol Anthropol*. 2018;37(1):13.

89. Sleep.org. Available at https://www.sleep.org/articles/temperature-for-sleep/.

90. Tosini G, Ferguson I, Tsubota K. Effects of blue light on the circadian system and eye physiology. *Mol Vis*. 2016;22:61–72.

91. Zhao ZC, Zhou Y, Tan G, Li J. Research progress about the effect and prevention of blue light on eyes. *Int J Opthalmol*. 2018;11(12):1999–2003.

92. Gellis LA, Lichstein KL. Sleep hygiene practices of good and poor sleepers in the United States: An internet-based study. *Behav Ther*. 2009;40(1):1–9.

93. Chueh KH, Guilleminault C, Lin CM. Alcohol consumption as a moderator of anxiety and sleep quality. *J Nurs Res*. 2019;27(3):e23.

94. Colrain IM, Nicholas CL, Baker FC. Alcohol and the sleeping brain. *Handbook of Clinical Neurology*. Vol. 125. New York: Elsevier; 2014:415–31.

95. Woteki CE, et al. *Caffeine for the Sustainment of Mental Task Performance: Formulations for Military Operations. Institute of Medicine (US) Committee on Military Nutrition Research*. Washington, DC: National Academies Press; 2001.

96. Nair R, Radhakrishnan K, Chatterjee A, et al. Sleep apnea-predictor of functional outcome in acute ischemic stroke. *J Stroke Cerebrovasc Dis*. 2019;28(3):807–14.

97. Valtorta NK, Kanaan M, Gilbody S, Hanratty B. Loneliness, social isolation and risk of cardiovascular disease in the English longitudinal study of ageing. *Eur J Prev Cardiol*. 2018;25(13):1387–96.

98. House JS, Landis KR, Umberson D. Social relationships and health. *Science*. 1988;241:540–45.

99. Berkman L, Syme L. Social networks, host resistance, and mortality: A nine-year follow-up study of alameda county residents. *Am J Epidemiol*. 1979;109(2):186–204.

100. Sampson EL, Bulpitt CJ, Fletcher AE. Survival of community-dwelling older people: The effect of cognitive impairment and social engagement. *J Am Geriatr Soc*. 2009;57(6):985–91.

101. Holt-Lunstad J, Smith TB, Layton JB. Social relationships and mortality risk: A meta-analytic review. *PLoS Med*. 2010;7(7):e1000316.

102. Dutton JE, Heaphy ED. *"The Power of High Quality Connections," Positive Organizational Scholarship*. San Francisco, CA: Berrett-Koehler Publishers; 2003.

103. Georgousopoulou EN, Mellor DD, Naumovski N, et al. Mediterranean lifestyle and cardiovascular disease prevention. *Cardiovasc Diagn Ther*. 2017;7(Suppl 1):S39–47.

104. American Heart Association (AHA). Available at https://www.heart.org/.

105. National Institute on Alcohol Abuse and Alcoholism (NIAAA). What is a standard drink? Available at https://www.niaaa.nih.gov/alcohol-health/overview-alcohol-consumption/what-standard-drink.

106. Cao Y, Willett WC, Rimm EB, et al. Light to moderate intake of alcohol, drinking patterns, and risk of cancer: Results from two prospective US cohort studies. *BMJ*. 2015;351:h4238.

107. Leonhardt D. "Opioid Overreaction." Available at https://www.nytimes.com/2019/03/29/opinion/opioid-crisis-chronic-pain.html.

108. Rogers AH, Bakhshaie J, Orr MF, et al. Health literacy, opioid misuse, and pain experience among adults with chronic pain. *Pain Med*. 2020;21(4):670–6.

109. Arnold JF, Arshonsky JH, Bloch KA, et al. Opioid abuse prevention and treatment: Lessons from South Carolina. *J Public Health Manag Pract*. 2019;25(3):221–8.

110. Bodai BI, Nakata TE, Wong WT, et al. Lifestyle medicine: A brief review of its dramatic impact on health and survival. *Perm J*. 2018;22.

111. Ornish D, Brown SE, Billings JH, et al. Can lifestyle changes reverse coronary heart disease? The Lifestyle Heart Trial. *Lancet*. 1990;336(8708):129–33.

112. Esselstyn CB Jr, Ellis SG, Medendorp SV, Crowe TD. A strategy to arrest and reverse coronary artery disease: A 5-year longitudinal study of a single physician's practice. *J Fam Pract*. 1995;41(6):560–9.

113. Esselstyn CB. Updating a 12-year experience with arrest and reversal therapy for coronary heart disease (an overdue requiem for palliative cardiology). *Am J Cardiol*. 1999;84(3):339–41.

114. Kris-Etherton P, Eckel RH, Howard BV, Jeor SS, Bazzarre TL. Lyon diet heart study: Benefits of a Mediterranean-Style, National Cholesterol Education Program/American Heart Association Step I dietary pattern on cardiovascular disease. *Circulation*. 2001;103(13):1823–5.

115. Deijle IA, Van Schaik SM, Van Wegen EE, Weinstein HC, Kwakkel G, Van den Berg-Vos RM. Lifestyle interventions to prevent cardiovascular events after stroke and transient ischemic attack: Systematic review and meta-analysis. *Stroke*. 2017;48(1):174–9.

116. Doughty KN, Del Pilar NX, Audette A, Katz DL. Lifestyle medicine and the management of cardiovascular disease. *Curr Cardiol Rep*. 2017;19(11):116.

117. Williams MA, Kaminsky LA. Healthy lifestyle medicine in the traditional healthcare environment, primary care and cardiac rehabilitation. *Prog Cardiovasc Dis*. 2017;59(5):448–54.

118. Levesque C. Therapeutic lifestyle changes for diabetes mellitus. *Nurs Clin North Am*. 2017;52(4):679–92.

119. American Diabetes Association. Lifestyle management: Standards of medical care in diabetes—2018. *Diabetes Care*. 2018;41:S38–50.

120. Knowler WC, Barrett-Connor E, Fowler SE, et al. Reduction in the incidence of type 2 diabetes with lifestyle intervention or metformin. *N Engl J Med*. 2002;346(6):393–403.

121. Gregg EW, Chen H, Wagenknecht LE, et al. Association of an intensive lifestyle intervention with remission of type 2 diabetes. *JAMA*. 2012;308(23):2489–96.

122. Galimanis A, Mono ML, Arnold M, Nedeltchev K, Mattle HP. Lifestyle and stroke risk: A review. *Curr Opin Neurol*. 2009;22(1):60–8.

123. Lourida I, Soni M, Thompson-Coon J, et al. Mediterranean diet, cognitive function, and dementia: A systematic review. *Epidemiology*. 2013;24(4):479–89.

124. Shatenstein B, Barberger-Gateau P. Prevention of age-related cognitive decline: Which strategies, when, and for whom? *J Alzheimers Dis*. 2015;48(1):35–53.

125. Chiuve SE, Rexrode KM, Spiegelman D, Logroscino G, Manson JE, Rimm EB. Primary prevention of stroke by healthy lifestyle. *Circulation*. 2008;118(9):947–54.

126. Sotos-Prieto M, Mattei J, Cook NR, et al. Association between a 20-year cardiovascular disease risk score based on modifiable lifestyles and total and cause-specific mortality among US men and women. *J Am Heart Assoc*. 2018;7(21):e010052.

127. Jönsson AC, Delavaran H, Lövkvist H, et al. Secondary prevention and lifestyle indices after stroke in a long-term perspective. *Acta Neurol Scand*. 2018;138(3):227–34.

128. Kono Y, Yamada S, Yamaguchi J, et al. Secondary prevention of new vascular events with lifestyle intervention in patients with noncardioembolic mild ischemic stroke: A single-center randomized controlled trial. *Cerebrovasc Dis*. 2013;36(2):88–97.

129. Parappilly BP, Mortenson WB, Field TS. Exploring perceptions of stroke survivors and caregivers about secondary prevention: A longitudinal qualitative study. *Disabil Rehabil*. 2020;42(14):2020–6.

130. Wu S, Powers S, Zhu W, Hannun YA. Substantial contribution of extrinsic risk factors to cancer development. *Nature*. 2016;529(7584):43.

131. Calle EE. Obesity and cancer. *BMJ*. 2007;335(7630):1107.

132. Madigan M, Karhu E. The role of plant-based nutrition in cancer prevention. *J Unexplored Med Data*. 2018;3:9.

133. Islami F, Goding Sauer A, Miller KD, et al. Proportion and number of cancer cases and deaths attributable to potentially modifiable risk factors in the United States. *CA Cancer J Clin*. 2018;68(1):31–54.

134. American Cancer Society. Guidelines on nutrition and physical activity for cancer prevention. Available at https://www.cancer.org/healthy/eat-healthy-get-active/acs-guidelines-nutrition-physical-activity-cancer-prevention.html.

135. American Institute for Cancer Research. Available at http://www.aicr.org/reduce-your-cancer-risk/recommendations-for-cancer-prevention/.

136. American Cancer Society. Nutrition and physical activity guidelines for cancer survivors. Available at https://www.cancer.org/

health-care-professionals/american-cancer-society-prevention-early-detection-guidelines/nupa-guidelines-for-cancer-survivors.html.

137. Ashcraft KA, Peace RM, Betof AS, Dewhirst MW, Jones LW. Efficacy and mechanisms of aerobic exercise on cancer initiation, progression, and metastasis: A critical systematic review of in vivo preclinical data. *Cancer Res*. 2016;76(14):4032–50.

138. Kwan ML, Garren B, Nielsen ME, Tang L. Lifestyle and nutritional modifiable factors in the prevention and treatment of bladder cancer. *Urol Oncol*. 2019;37(6):380–6.

139. Falavigna M, Lima KM, Giacomazzi J, et al. Effects of lifestyle modification after breast cancer treatment: A systematic review protocol. *Syst Rev*. 2014;3(1):72.

140. Oberguggenberger A, Meraner V, Sztankay M, et al. Health behavior and quality of life outcome in breast cancer survivors: Prevalence rates and predictors. *Clin Breast Cancer*. 2018;18(1):38–44.

141. Satia JA, Campbell MK, Galanko JA, James A, Carr C, Sandler RS. Longitudinal changes in lifestyle behaviors and health status in colon cancer survivors. *Cancer Epidemiol Biomarkers Prev*. 2004;13(6):1022–31.

142. Ornish D, Weidner G, Fair WR, et al. Intensive lifestyle changes may affect the progression of prostate cancer. *J Urol*. 2005;174(3):1065–70.

143. Ornish D, Lin J, Chan JM, Epel E, et al. Effect of comprehensive lifestyle changes on telomerase activity and telomere length in men with biopsy-proven low-risk prostate cancer: 5-year follow-up of a descriptive pilot study. *Lancet Oncol*. 2013;14(11):1112–20.

144. Frattaroli J, Weidner G, Dnistrian AM, et al. Clinical events in prostate cancer lifestyle trial: Results from two years of follow-up. *Urology*. 2008;72(6):1319–23.

145. Ornish D, Magbanua MJ, Weidner G, et al. Changes in prostate gene expression in men undergoing an intensive nutrition and lifestyle intervention. *Proc Natl Acad Sci USA*. 2008;105(24):8369–74.

146. Guthrie GE. Uncovering the truth. *Am J Lifestyle Med*. 2017;12(1):49–50.

147. Katz DL, Karlsen MC, Chung M, et al. Hierarchies of Evidence Applied to Lifestyle Medicine (HEALM): Introduction of a strength-of-evidence approach based on a methodological systematic review. *BMC Med Res Methodol*. 2019;19(1):178.

148. Arem H, Moore SC, Patel A, et al. Leisure time physical activity and mortality: A detailed pooled analysis of the dose-response relationship. *Jama Intern Med*. 2015;175(6):959–67.

149. Blair SN, Kohl HW, Paffenbarger RS, et al. Physical fitness and all-cause mortality: A prospective study of healthy men and women. *JAMA*. 1989;262(17):2395–401.

150. Lee I, Skerrett PJ. Physical activity and all-cause mortality: What is the dose-response relation? *Med Sci Sports Exerc*. 2001;33(6 Suppl):S459–71.

151. Williams PT. Dose-response relationship of physical activity to premature and total call-cause and cardiovascular disease mortality in walkers. *PLoS One*. 2013;8(11):e78777.

152. Jørgensen T, Jacobsen RK, Toft U, Aadahl M, Glümer C, Pisinger C. Effect of screening and lifestyle counselling on incidence of ischaemic heart disease in general population: Inter99 randomised trial. *BMJ*. 2014;348:g3617.

153. Katz D. Lifestyle medicine and the parable of the tiny parachute. 2014. Available at https://www.huffpost.com/entry/diet-and-nutrition_b_5596931.

154. Ornish D, Scherwitz LW, Billings JH, et al. Intensive lifestyle changes for reversal of coronary heart disease. *JAMA*. 1998;280(23):2001–7.

155. Morton D, Rankin P, Kent L, Dysinger W. The Complete Health Improvement Program (CHIP) history, evaluation, and outcomes. *Am J Lifestyle Med*. 2016;10(1):64–73.

156. Choi BCK, Pak AWP. A catalog of biases in questionnaires. *Preventing Chronic Disease*. 2005;2(1):A13.

157. Wolfenden L, Goldman S, Stacey FG, et al. Strategies to improve the implementation of workplace-based policies or practices targeting tobacco, alcohol, diet, physical activity and obesity. *Cochrane Database Syst Rev*. 2018;11(11):CD012439. Available at https://www.cochranelibrary.com/cdsr/doi/10.1002/14651858.CD012439.pub2/abstract.

158. Dysinger WS. Lifestyle medicine competencies for primary care physicians. *Virtual Mentor*. 2013;15(4):306.

159. Moss M. The extraordinary science of addictive junk food. 2013. Available at https://www.nytimes.com/2013/02/24/magazine/the-extraordinary-science-of-junk-food.html.

160. Buettner D, Skemp S. Blue Zones: Lessons from the world's longest lived. *Am J Lifestyle Med*. 2016;10(5):318–21.

161. Puska P, Vartiainen E, Nissinen A, Laatikainen T, Jousilahti P. Background, principles, implementation, and general experiences of the North Karelia Project. *Global Heart*. 2016;11(2):173–8.

162. Farquhar JW, Fortmann SP, Flora JA, et al. Effects of communitywide education on cardiovascular disease risk factors: The Stanford Five-City Project. *JAMA*. 1990;264(3):359–65.

163. Fortmann SP, Flora JA, Winkleby MA, Schooler C, Taylor CB, Farquhar JW. Community intervention trials: Reflections on the Stanford Five-City Project experience. *Am J Epi*. 1995;142(6):576–86.

164. Economos CD, Hyatt RR, Goldberg JP, et al. A community intervention reduces BMI z-score in children: Shape Up Somerville first year results. *Obes*. 2007;15(5):1325–36.

165. Katz DL, Frates EP, Bonnet JP, Gupta SK, Vartiainen E, Carmona RH. Lifestyle as medicine: The case for a true health initiative. *Am J Health Promot*. 2018;32(6):1452–8.

166. Faries MD. Why we don't "just do it" understanding the intention-behavior gap in lifestyle medicine. *Am J Lifestyle Med*. 2016;10(5):322–9.

167. Faries MD, Abreu A. Medication adherence, when lifestyle is the medicine. *Am J Lifestyle Med*. 2017;11(5):397–403.

168. Ford ES, Bergmann MM, Kröger J, Schienkiewitz A, Weikert C, Boeing H. Healthy living is the best revenge: Findings from the European Prospective Investigation into Cancer and Nutrition—Potsdam study. *Arch Intern Med*. 2009;169(15):1355–62.

169. Reeves MJ, Rafferty AP. Healthy lifestyle characteristics among adults in the United States, 2000. *Arch Intern Med*. 2005;165(8):854–7.

170. Carver CS, Scheier MF. *On the Self-Regulation of Behavior*. Cambridge: Cambridge University Press; 2001.

171. Beeken RJ, Mahdi S, Johnson F, Meisel SF. Intentions to prevent weight gain in older and younger adults: The importance of perceived health and appearance consequences. *Obes Facts*. 2018;11(2):83–92.

172. Gorin AA, Phelan S, Hill JO, Wing RR. Medical triggers are associated with better short- and long-term weight loss outcomes. *Prev Med*. 2004;39(3):612–6.

173. LaRose JG, Leahey TM, Hill JO, Wing RR. Differences in motivations and weight loss behaviors in young adults and older adults in the National Weight Control Registry. *Obes*. 2013;21(3):449–53.

174. Wing RR, Phelan S. Long-term weight loss maintenance. *Am J Clin Nutr*. 2005;82:222–5.

175. Heatherton TF, Baumeister RF. Binge eating as escape from self-awareness. *Psychol Bull*. 1991;110(1):86–108.

176. Maphis LE, Martz DM, Bergman SS, Curtin LA, Webb RM. Body size dissatisfaction and avoidance behavior: How gender, age, ethnicity, and relative clothing size predict what some won't try. *Body Image*. 2013;10(3):361–8.

177. Millstein RA, Carlson SA, Fulton JE, et al. Relationships between body size satisfaction and weight control practices among US adults. *Medscape J Med*. 2008;10(5):119.

178. Neumark-Sztainer D, Wall M, Eisenberg ME, Story M, Hannan PJ. Overweight status and weight control behaviors in adolescents: Longitudinal and secular trends from 1999 to 2004. *Prev Med*. 2006;43(1):52–59.

179. Schwartz MB, Brownell KD. Obesity and body image. *Body Image*. 2004;1(1):43–56.

180. Faries MD, Bartholomew JB. Coping with weight-related discrepancies: Initial development of the WEIGHTCOPE. *Women Health Issues*. 2015;25(3):267–75.

181. Drury CA, Louis M. Exploring the association between body weight, stigma of obesity, and health care avoidance. *J Am Acad Nurse Pract*. 2002;14(12):554–61.

182. Beeken RJ, Wilson R, McDonald L, Wardle J. Body mass index and cancer screening: Findings from the English Longitudinal Study of Ageing. *J Med Screen*. 2014;21(2):76–81.

183. Wee CC, McCarthy EP, Davis RB, Phillips RS. Screening for cervical and breast cancer: Is obesity an unrecognized barrier to preventive care? *Ann Intern Med*. 2000;132(9):697–704.

184. Consedine NS, Magai C, Krivoshekova YS, Ryzewicz L, Neugut AI. Fear, anxiety, worry, and breast cancer screening behavior: A critical review. *Cancer Epidemiol Biomarkers Prev*. 2004;13(4):501–10.

185. Roesch SC, Weiner B. A meta-analytic review of coping with illness: Do causal attributions matter? *J Psychosom Res*. 2001;50(4):205–19.

186. Deci EL, Ryan RM. *Intrinsic Motivation and Self-determination in Human Behavior*. New York, NY: Springer Science & Business Media; 1985.

187. Ng JY, Ntoumanis N, Thøgersen-Ntoumani C, et al. Self-determination theory applied to health contexts: A meta-analysis. *Perspect Psychol Sci*. 2012;7(4):325–340.

188. Teixeira PJ, Carraça EV, Markland D, Silva MN, Ryan RM. Exercise, physical activity, and self-determination theory: A systematic review. *Int J Behav Nutr Phys Act*. 2012;9(1):78.

189. Ajzen I. The theory of planned behavior. *Organ Behav Hum Decis Process.* 1991;50:179–211.
190. Prochaska JO, Velicer WF. The transtheoretical model of health behavior change. *Am J Health Stud.* 1997;12(1):38–48.
191. Katz DL. Behavior modification in primary care: The pressure system model. *Prev Med.* 2001;32(1):66–72.
192. Baumeister RF, Heatherton TF. Self-regulation failure: An overview. *Psychol Inquiry.* 1996;7(1):1–5.
193. Carver CS, Scheier MF. Self-regulation and its failures. *Psychol Inquiry.* 1996;7(1):32–40.
194. Hall PA, Fong GT. Temporal self-regulation theory: A model for individual health behavior. *Health Psychol Rev.* 2007;1(1):6–52.
195. Karoly P. Mechanisms of self-regulation: A systems view. *Ann Rev Psychol.* 1993;44(1):23–52.
196. Rasmussen HN, Wrosch C, Scheier MF, Carver CS. Self-regulation processes and health: The importance of optimism and goal adjustment. *J Personal.* 2006;74(6):1721–4.
197. National Board for Health and Wellness Coaching. Available at https://nbhwc.org/.
198. Vine M, Hargreaves MB, Briefel RR, et al. Expanding the role of primary care in the prevention and treatment of childhood obesity: A review of clinic and community-based recommendations and interventions. *J Obes.* 2013;2013(11):172035.
199. Frates EP, Moore MA, Lopez CN, McMahon GT. Coaching for behavior change in physiatry. *Am J Phys Med Rehabil.* 2011;90(12):1074–82.
200. Frates EP, Bonnet J. Collaboration and negotiation: The key to therapeutic lifestyle change. *Am J Lifestyle Med.* 2016;10(5):302–12.
201. Wolever RQ, Simmons LA, Sforzo GA, et al. A systematic review of the literature on health and wellness coaching: Defining a key behavioral intervention in healthcare. *Global Adv Health Med.* 2013;2(4):38–57.
202. Katz DL, Boukhalil J, Lucan SC, et al. Impediment profiling for smoking cessation. Preliminary experience. *Behav Modif.* 2003;27(4):524–37.
203. O'Connell M, Lucan SC, Yeh MC, et al. Impediment profiling for smoking cessation: Results of a pilot study. *Am J Health Promot.* 2003;17(5):300–03.
204. Miller RW, Rollnick S. *Motivational Interviewing: Preparing People to Change Addictive Behavior.* 3rd ed. New York, NY: The Guilford Press; 2013.
205. Hollisdon M, Thorogood M, White I, Foster C. Advising people to take more exercise is ineffective: A randomized controlled trial of physical activity promotion in primary care. *Int J Epidemiol.* 2002;31:808–15.
206. Miller RW, Rollnick S. *Motivational Interviewing: Preparing People to Change Addictive Behavior.* 2nd ed. New York, NY: The Guilford Press; 2002.
207. Hojat M, Louis DZ, Markham FW, Wender R, Rabinowitz C, Gonnella JS. Physicians' empathy and clinical outcomes for diabetic patients. *Acad Med.* 2011;86:359–64.
208. Abramson S, Stein J, Schaufele M, et al. Personal exercise habits and counselling practices of primary care physicians: A national survey. *Clin J Sports Med.* 2000;10(1):40–8.
209. Frank E, Breyan J, Elon L. Physician disclosure of healthy personal behaviors improves credibility and ability to motivate. *Arch Fam Med.* 2000;9(3):287–90.
210. Rogers EM. The adoption process: Part I. *Journal of Extension.* 1963;1(1):16–22.
211. Barrett MA, Osofsky SA. *BioScience.* 2017;67(12):1026–8.
212. Tuomisto HL. Importance of considering environmental sustainability in dietary guidelines. *Lancet Planet Health.* 2018;2(8):e331–2.
213. Blackstone NT, El-Abbadi NH, McCabe MS, et al. Linking sustainability to the healthy eating patterns of the dietary guidelines for Americans: A modelling study. *Lancet Planet Health.* 2018;2(8):e344–52.
214. Willett W, Rockström J, Loken B, et al. Food in the Anthropocene: The EAT–Lancet Commission on healthy diets from sustainable food systems. *Lancet.* 2019;393(10170):447–92.

CHAPTER 12

Aerospace Medicine

Robert Johnson • Christopher R. Armstrong • Robert R. Orford

INTRODUCTION

Aerospace medicine is a preventive medicine specialty focusing on the health of crewmembers and passengers of air and space vehicles, and the people who support the operation of such vehicles. In contrast to most physicians who evaluate and care for persons with abnormal physiology (illness) in normal (terrestrial) environments, aerospace medicine specialists evaluate and assist healthy individuals and individuals with abnormal physiology to function optimally in abnormal (nonterrestrial), remote, isolated, extreme, or enclosed environments under conditions of physical and psychological stress. While aerospace medicine began with the balloon flights of the Montgolfier brothers in the late 1700s and the experiments of Paul Bert a century later, the field grew quickly after the demonstration of controlled powered flight by the Dayton, Ohio-based Wright brothers at Kittyhawk, North Carolina, in 1903. Thousands of civilian and military aircraft were built and flown before and during World War I, with rapid technological advances. Commercial aviation began in the 1920s, initially in unpressurized aircraft flying short distances at low altitudes. Pressurized aircraft in the 1930s allowed higher, further, and faster flights. During World War II, the need for air superiority dictated the development of breathing systems and pressure suits to allow pilots to fly even higher and faster, and with greater maneuverability.[1]

In April 1961, Soviet cosmonaut Yuri Gagarin was the first to orbit the earth, followed in February 1962 by American astronaut John Glenn. After a successful series of orbital, lunar, and space laboratory missions, the United States, Russia, and 14 other nations began construction on the International Space Station (ISS) in 1998. The ISS, a habitable artificial satellite in low earth orbit, has been continuously occupied since 2000. Manned missions to lunar orbit, Earth's moon, asteroids, and Mars are now in the planning stages.[2]

From the earliest days of flight, there have been thousands of aviation accidents resulting in injury and death—including 18 cosmonaut and astronaut fatalities during spaceflight. Nevertheless, aviation safety has greatly improved over time (Fig. 12-1).

THE SPECIALTY OF AEROSPACE MEDICINE

Shortly after World War II, the Aero Medical Association initiated activities, which led to the establishment of a training program for medical specialists in the field of Aviation Medicine. In 1953, the Advisory Board for Medical Specialties and the American Medical Association (AMA) Council on Medical Education and Hospitals authorized the American Board of Preventive Medicine (ABPM) to offer certification in Aviation Medicine. The ABPM certified the first group of specialists in Aviation Medicine that same year. In 2018, there were 1231 physicians holding active certificates of specialization in Aerospace Medicine issued by the ABPM.[3]

With the advent of space flight, both the Aero Medical Association and the specialty changed names to reflect activities in both air and space. The Aero Medical Association changed its name to the Aerospace Medical Association (AsMA) in 1959 and the ABPM changed the name of the specialty to Aerospace Medicine in 1963 (for more details, see https://www.theabpm.org/about-us/history-of-the-board/).

In 1989, the American Board of Medical Specialties and the AMA Council on Medical Education approved the ABPM's application to offer a subspecialty certificate in Undersea Medicine. (The name was changed to Undersea and Hyperbaric Medicine in 1999.) In addition to its other applications, Hyperbaric Medicine is used to treat altitude-induced decompression sickness in aviators due to flight in unpressurized aircraft, rapid decompression at altitude, and high-altitude reconnaissance missions.

TRAINING AND EDUCATION IN AEROSPACE MEDICINE

Few physicians have the opportunity to gain experience in Aerospace Medicine until their postgraduate years. Civilian physicians with an interest in aviation often turn to the Federal Aviation Administration (FAA) for orientation and training as an aviation medical examiner (AME) or to the International Civil Aviation Organization (ICAO) for training as a designated medical examiner. AMEs perform aeromedical physical examinations and issue medical certificates on behalf of the FAA. Military physicians with an interest in aviation often request training to become a flight surgeon. Flight surgeon training includes an introduction to altitude physiology, visual systems, night vision, toxicology, aviation protective equipment, stress and fatigue, gravitational forces, noise and vibration, spatial disorientation, and aircraft accident investigation. Flight surgeons provide occupational, preventive, and primary-care medical support to military aviators and aviation support personnel in garrison and while deployed. Historically, most physicians who have entered the field of Aerospace Medicine have done so during their military service.

Residency Programs

Aerospace Medicine is one of the smallest medical specialty training programs in the United States, both with regard to the number of training sites and number of residents. Its program is similar in structure to the training programs in Occupational Medicine and Preventive Medicine. The University of Texas, College of Medicine, Galveston, sponsors the only civilian residency program. It is affiliated with the National Aeronautics and Space Administration (NASA). The Department of Defense (DoD) sponsors three programs. The DoD programs include the Air Force program at the United States Air Force School of Aerospace Medicine, Wright-Patterson Air Force Base, Ohio; the Navy program at the Naval Aerospace Medical Institute, Pensacola, Florida; and the Army Program at the School of

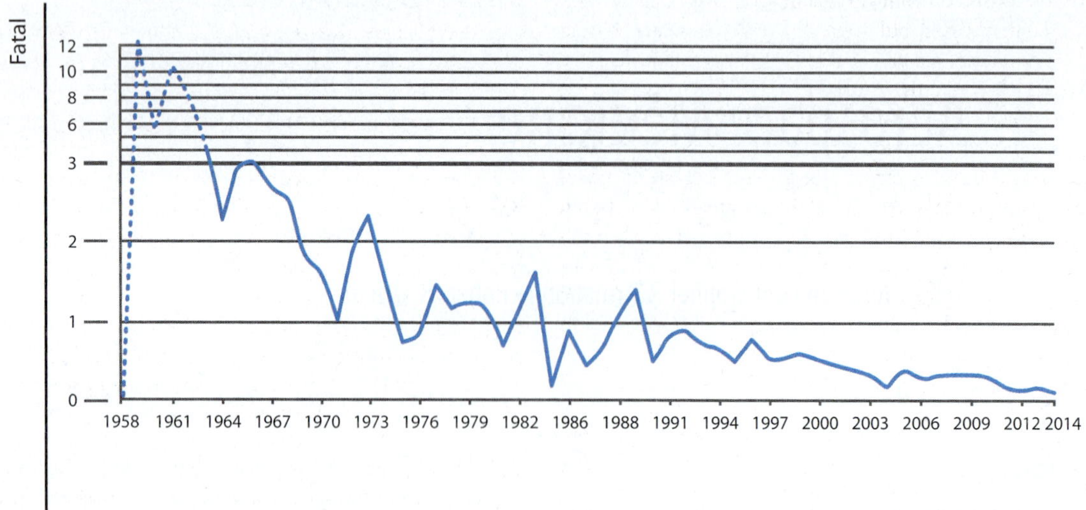

FIGURE 12-1. Yearly accident rate per million flights. Adapted with permission from Airbus (2017). A Statistical Analysis of Commercial Aviation Accidents 1958-2016. Retrieved from https://flightsafety.org/wp-content/uploads/2017/07/Airbus-Commercial-Aviation-Accidents-1958-2016-14Jun17-1.pdf.

Army Aviation Medicine, Fort Rucker, Alabama. Approximately 50 residents were in training in 2018.[4] An average of 29 candidates sat for the certifying examination each year from 2007 to 2017.[3]

THE AEROSPACE MEDICINE ENVIRONMENT

Aerospace Medicine is unique among medical specialties due to the physical characteristics of the environment in which flight takes place, the need to ensure that aircrew and passengers are fit to fly, and the need to optimize the health and safety of aircrew and passengers in the flight environment. Aerospace environmental stressors affecting humans include hypoxia, reduced atmospheric pressure, thermal extremes, brief and sustained acceleration, ionizing radiation, and microgravity. Aerospace medical practitioners apply preventive medicine principles in the selection, monitoring, and health maintenance of aircrew, and apply human factors knowledge to reduce the occurrence and effect of human error in aviation and space systems.

Atmosphere and Altitude

The earth's atmosphere is maintained through a balance between gravity (downward force) and air pressure (upward force) on atmospheric gases. The chemical and physical properties of the atmosphere are dynamic, varying with altitude, latitude, geographic location, time of day, and season. In addition, they are affected by the earth's rotation, incoming solar radiation, ozone, and greenhouse gases. For practical purposes, the component gasses and their relative percentages in the atmosphere remain more or less constant up to an altitude of approximately 90 km. The major constituents of the atmosphere are nitrogen (78%) and oxygen (21%). The remaining 1% of the atmosphere consists of argon, carbon dioxide, helium, krypton, xenon, hydrogen, methane, and other trace chemical compounds. The actual percentages of these constituents vary with the water content of the atmosphere, which is altitude dependent. As one ascends, the air becomes dryer. Regardless of the altitude within the aeronautical frame of reference, the percentage of oxygen remains relatively constant. The difference is that the partial pressure of oxygen is much reduced at altitude. Consequently, the physiological availability of oxygen is reduced. At sea level, the column of air creates an atmospheric pressure of 760 mm Hg, 760 torr, or 1013.2 millibars. As one ascends in altitude, there is less of a column of air and thus less air pressure. However, this relationship is not linear; the density of the air decreases exponentially. Consequently, at a height of 5.5 km the air density is one-half that found at sea level, and at 11 km the density is one-quarter. In practice, the actual heights are greater because of the effects of seasonal variations of temperature, which also varies air density since cooler air is denser than warmer air.

Unlike greenhouse gases, ozone is relevant to aviation. Ozone (O_3) is an oxidant gas produced in the upper atmosphere by the photodissociation of molecular oxygen. It is present in measurable concentrations from an altitude of 10 to 35 km, with maximum density at around 22 km. Ozone has significant, negative health effects—particularly on the upper airways and lungs—and is present at the cruising altitude of commercial aircraft. Since aircraft collect and concentrate air for use on board, it must be treated using a catalytic converter to remove the ozone and protect the health of crew and passengers.

Oxygen and Hypoxia

Hypoxia, or deficiency in the amount of oxygen reaching the tissues, has devastating effects on normal physiological function. While there are many causes of hypoxia, in aviation, oxygen deficiency at increased altitudes is due to the reduced oxygen partial pressure in inspired air. The alveolar partial pressure of oxygen is, therefore, reduced. Gas exchange in the alveoli at altitude is limited further by the presence of water vapor and carbon dioxide. Considering that water vapor pressure at normal body temperature is 47 mm Hg and the alveolar carbon dioxide pressure is 40 mm Hg, the ambient pressure must exceed 87 mm Hg for any air exchange to occur in the lungs. Even if the aviator is breathing 100% oxygen, if the ambient pressure of oxygen is less than 87 mm Hg, it is impossible to overcome the gas pressures already present in the alveoli in order to provide oxygen.

Hypoxia is particularly dangerous because its signs and symptoms produce little discomfort and no pain. Between an altitude of 2000 and 3000 m, the subtle symptoms may produce deficiencies in night vision and some drowsiness. Unfortunately, as the altitude increases and the partial pressures decrease, intellectual impairment can be an early manifestation of hypoxia—compromising the ability of an individual to behave rationally. Cognition is slowed, and mathematical calculations are difficult to perform. Both memory and judgment are diminished, and reaction time is delayed. Hypoxia can be treated rapidly at altitudes between 3000 and 10,000 m by administering oxygen. Successful treatment of hypoxia between 10,000 and 14,000 m requires positive pressure oxygen. Hypoxia must be prevented at altitudes greater than 14,000 m by enclosing the individual in a pressurized system with supplied oxygen.

At altitude, particularly in passenger-carrying aircraft, the body of the aircraft acts as a pressure vessel. To reduce the weight of the air on board, reduce the tension on the hull, and reduce the risk of rapid depressurization, cabin altitude for most commercial aircraft is set at approximately 2500 m at normally traveled altitudes, which is comfortable and well tolerated by most people. Although passengers will note some pressure changes in the ears or sinuses, the change is gradual and rarely causes pain or discomfort. Occasionally, passengers with a compromised pulmonary or cardiovascular system may require supplemental oxygen since their reserve is inadequate to compensate for these relatively small changes in oxygen partial pressure. In the absence of a pressurized cabin (as in military aircraft flying at high altitude), the aviator wears a self-contained pressure system and uses a pressurized oxygen mask. In the event of a passenger aircraft decompression at high altitude, supplemental oxygen systems are available for safety reasons. The most commonly used oxygen storage system on commercial airlines uses solid chemicals that, when activated, produce oxygen. Aircraft also carry a limited number of personal oxygen delivery devices on board for use in responding to unexpected medical events.

Acceleration and Biomechanical Forces

Acceleration occurs when the velocity of an object changes in direction or in magnitude. Changes in acceleration are conveyed using the term gravitational force or g-force, with 1 g being the gravitational acceleration at the earth's surface, which is 9.8 m/s^2. During World War I, fighter pilots were the first aviators to report visual changes when they engaged in a pullout or during aerial combat. Human centrifuge research later demonstrated the occurrence of blackout during sustained acceleration, which is achieved when the body has sufficient time to reach equilibrium with the effects of the acceleration. In this context, g can be used to estimate relative weight. For example, a pilot flying a maneuver in an aircraft in which he or she sustains 4 g would feel an increase in body weight from 175 to 700 pounds, and a flight helmet weighing 10 pounds would be experienced as weighing 40 pounds. Changes in mass also affect the body's hydrostatic blood column and cardiovascular function. In a normal terrestrial environment, the hydrostatic column from the heart to the eye is 30 cm; but in a 6 g acceleration environment, it becomes pressure gradient equivalent to 180 cm. The body's blood pressure is unable to overcome the hydrostatic pressure, and blood flow to the eyes is quickly lost, with unconsciousness from lack of blood to the brain following shortly thereafter. When tested on a centrifuge using a standard protocol, a typical aviator, relaxed, and without any protective devices, experiences visual blackout between 4 and 5.5 g. The same aviator, when allowed to strain to increase blood pressure, is able to increase his or her tolerance by an additional 0.5–1.5 g. The rate of onset of acceleration and its duration also affect tolerance.

Anti-g suits and other mechanical devices are used to protect the aviators from the effects of acceleration. Anti-g suits use g-modulated compressed air-filled bladders to compress the lower torso (abdomen, thighs, and calves). The bladders inflate when a sensor is stimulated by acceleration, increasing g tolerance by 2 g. Combined with a straining maneuver, tolerance may increase further to about 9 g. Other mechanisms used to enhance pilot g tolerance include orienting the long axis of the body more perpendicular to the acceleration vector, and positive pressure breathing to increase intrathoracic pressure. The need for protection from the effects of transitory acceleration has also influenced the development of restraint devices, such as lap belts and shoulder harnesses, the design of crew space to reduce the possibility of unwanted contact with the structural components of the airframe, improvements in seat structure to reduce mechanical failure, and changes to the design of airframes to increase their ability to absorb energy in the event of a mishap. Escape systems such as ejection seats and capsules have been designed to carry the occupant free of the aircraft or spacecraft during uncontrolled descent or other adverse conditions. These systems are specifically designed to remain within human tolerance.

Other biomechanical forces in aerospace systems include severe noise and vibration, which may adversely affect performance and health. Personal protection, prevention, and engineering mitigation are key to their management.

Spatial Disorientation

Our complex neurosensory system allows us to maintain balance and orientation on the surface of the earth, but it is inadequate for the three-dimensional dynamic aerospace environment. Vision is by far the most important sensory modality for maintaining our spatial orientation. Deprived of visual cues, the vestibular system becomes our major source of orientation in terrestrial environments. Proprioception (sense of body position) helps fine tune the visual-vestibular interface. However, an individual with a poorly functioning or nonfunctioning vestibular system can perform well as long as visual cues are adequate. In the flight environment, the aviator is exposed to far more complex motion inputs than our physiological system is designed to process. Visual cues may conflict with motion and velocity cues processed by the vestibular system. These conflicting cues may cause severe spatial disorientation or induce motion sickness. Visual illusions during flight may cause a pilot to perceive a position in free space that is inaccurate. Particularly at night or in conditions of poor visibility, a pilot may be misled by their vestibular system in the absence of visual cues. Vestibular illusions can result in aircraft mishaps that are often catastrophic and may be fatal.

Disorientation accidents account for 15% of military and civilian aviation mishaps. Ninety percent of the accidents ascribed to special disorientation include fatalities. Mitigation measures include modifying flight procedures to reduce the opportunity for disorientation; improving the ease of interpretation of information presented by flight instruments; increasing proficiency in instrument flying, which gives pilots the confidence to overcome false sensory input; and educating pilots regarding physiological frailty and the need for dependence on and acceptance of flight instrument information.

Space and Microgravity

The transition from the terrestrial to the space environment is not a well-demarcated line, but a continuum that varies with altitude depending upon the parameter discussed. The aircraft wings and other aerodynamic control surfaces including rudders and ailerons of conventional aircraft become ineffective at an altitude of 100 km because the atmosphere is insufficiently dense and cannot create the necessary force to provide lift. This altitude is known as the von Kármán line. It is often considered the boundary between our atmosphere and space—even though the earth's atmosphere is still detectable to 960 km. Typical orbital altitudes for human spaceflight are between 192 and 576 km. At these altitudes, the air density is so low that there is no practical method for compressing atmospheric gases to supply sufficient pressure and oxygen for the craft's inhabitants; a 100% contained and recirculating air supply is needed. Occupants must also be protected from the extreme cold of the ambient environment. While in orbital flight, astronauts experience a sensation of weightlessness even though g forces are not zero, just very small, so the term microgravity is used. This occurs when the gravitational force vector is counterbalanced by the centrifugal force imparted to the vehicle as it travels tangentially to the earth's surface. Long-term exposure to microgravity has been extensively studied during human habitation of the International Space Station. The effects of microgravity and other human risks of spaceflight are enumerated in Fig. 12-2.

The earth's atmosphere serves as an insulator to shield us from many of the potential dangers of space radiation. Once a person is in space, this protection is no longer available, and exposure to ionizing radiation becomes a concern. Three types of radiation present hazards: primary cosmic radiation, geomagnetically trapped radiation (also known as the Van Allen radiation belt), and radiation produced by solar flares. Solar flares are composed of x-rays, gamma rays, and may include protons, all of which are hazardous to exposed astronauts. However, the hull of a spacecraft provides more protection against these forms of radiation than against cosmic radiation, which has much higher energy levels.

Human Risks of Spaceflight

Grouped by Hazards – 30 Risks & 2 *Concerns*

Altered Gravity Level	Radiation	Hostile/Closed Environment–Spacecraft Design
• Vision alterations • Renal stone formation • Sensorimotor alterations • Bone fracture • Impaired performance • Reduced aerobic capacity • Adverse health effects • Urinary retention • Orthostatic intolerance • Back pain • Cardiac rhythm problems • *Effects of medication* • *Intervertebral disk damage*	• Exposure to space radiation **Distance from Earth** • Limited in-flight medical capabilities • Toxic medications **Isolation** • Adverse cognitive or behavioral conditions • Performance & behavioral health decrements	• CO_2 exposure • Inadequate food/nutrition • Inadequate human-system interaction design • Injury from dynamic loads • Injury during EVA • Celestial dust exposure • Altered immune response • Hypobaric hypoxia • Sleep loss & work overload • Decompression sickness • Toxic exposure • Hearing loss • Sunlight exposure

FIGURE 12-2. The effects of microgravity and other human risks of spaceflight. Grouped by hazards—30 risks and 2 concerns. (*Source:* From Clément G: Human Research Program Human Health Countermeasures Element Evidence Report: Artificial Gravity, Version 6.0, National Aeronautics and Space Administration, Houston, Texas 2015. Available online at https://humanresearchroadmap.nasa.gov/evidence/other/AG%20Evidence%20Report.pdf.)

OPERATIONAL AEROSPACE MEDICINE

Physicians practicing Aerospace Medicine as a clinical specialty must be astute clinicians familiar with both the flight environment and the unique physical and psychological challenges presented by the operational settings in which their patients work. Aircrew stressors vary with the type of flight vehicle—from a single-seat light aircraft to the multicrewmember International Space Station. For heuristic reasons, these operational settings are divided into civil aviation, military aviation, high-altitude terrain and polar environments, and space operations.

Civil Aviation

Civil aviation includes commercial and private aviation including recreational flying. Airlines represent an international industry, which transports over 3.5 billion passengers annually. After the deregulation of the airline industry in the United States in 1978, air commuter and air taxi operations grew to fill the vacuum left when the major airlines pulled out of smaller airports. Most large corporations in the United States either own or lease aircraft for business purposes. Other commercial activities include air ambulance service; flight training; aerial application of herbicides, insecticides, and fertilizers; air cargo; and commercial parcel delivery. In 2015, the most recent year for which data are available, more than 31% of commercial aircraft departures occurred in North America and four of the world's ten busiest airports were located in the United States.[5] There are approximately 575,000 active pilots in the United States. With the exception of balloon, glider, and Sport Pilots, all aviators certificated by the FAA are required to have an initial aeromedical physical examination prior to issuance of their certificate, and periodic assessments as long as they continue to fly. To examine these aviators, the FAA has designated 2735 physicians as AMEs. These physicians have undergone special training conducted under the auspices of the FAA and often have had experience as military flight surgeons, and are often private pilots. The physical examinations they perform adhere to rigorous protocols, and detailed physical standards have been promulgated.

The class of the certificate exercised by the aviator dictates, in part, the periodicity and sophistication of the physical examination. The airline captain must meet more stringent standards, more frequently, than the private pilot.[6] In all cases, the FAA's Civil Aeromedical Institute (CAMI) reviews the physical examination report. CAMI receives approximately 1400 physical examination reports each business day.

In addition, there are over 14,000 FAA air traffic controllers serving 20,000 airports located throughout the United States. Like pilots, air traffic controllers are required to meet detailed physical standards and undergo aeromedical physical examinations on a regular basis.

Finally, CAMI is responsible for conducting research on ways to protect the health and safety of commercial flight deck and cabin crewmembers, private pilots, and passengers. To this end, the Institute has conducted research on and recommended standards for emergency aircraft lighting, egress systems, restraint systems, breathing equipment, emergency breathing devices, and flotation systems.

Military Aviation

The U.S. Air Force has by far the widest range of aeronautical activities—mostly fixed-wing, with aeromedical evacuation (AE) being a major operational competency. Low and slow describes some Air Force missions, while other aircraft operate into the fringes of space. Large transport aircraft are capable of nearly endless flight with air-to-air refueling. With rest facilities and multiple crewmembers, these large aircraft can simply keep on flying. Current fighter aircraft are capable of readily exceeding the physiological tolerance of the pilot with rapid onset, high *g* forces. The response of fighter aircraft is so fast that controls are now electronic rather than hydraulic or mechanical. Since the 1950s, it has been predicted that aeronautical design would one day take aircraft performance beyond the performance capabilities of the pilot. That day has arrived.[7]

U.S. Army Aerospace Medicine specialists provide primary and specialty care while leading and conducting advanced aviation and occupational medicine programs across the full spectrum of operational environments, mostly for rotary-wing aircrew. They care for the most complicated, valuable, variable, and vulnerable component of modern military aviation—the human operator. Despite advances in technology, automation, and unmanned systems, human factors remain the major cause of aviation mishaps. The mission of Army Aviation Medicine specialists is made even more challenging by the need to prepare for the future military aviation operational environment, which will be more lethal, contested, dispersed, and complex—characterized by hybrid conventional and nonstate adversaries and operations in complex terrain, cyber threats, and space.

Aerospace Medicine specialists in the U.S. Navy are responsible for maintaining the health of carrier strike groups (CSGs), the primary operational formations of the United States Navy. The typical

CSG includes an aircraft carrier, at least one cruiser, as many as four destroyers, a fast combat support ship, and a carrier air wing (CVW). The CVW includes a mixture of 65–70 fixed-wing and rotary-wing aircraft organized into eight squadrons. Aerospace Medicine specialists are responsible, not only for the health maintenance of the flight crews, but also for maintaining the health of the entire CSG, including approximately 7500 sailors, Marines, and civilians. They are the Senior Medical Officers for this isolated community and oversee all aspects of clinical care (inpatient and outpatient), health maintenance, epidemiological surveillance, and medical disaster preparedness aboard ship. Neither fixed-wing AE nor rotary-wing medical evacuation (MEDEVAC) is core competency of the Navy. The Navy has neither aircraft nor personnel dedicated to these missions. When the needs of a critically ill or injured sailor, Marine, or civilian exceed the capabilities of the CSG, the Senior Medical Officer, using his or her knowledge of clinical medicine, the flight environment, and the unique challenges presented by the operational setting, must determine if and when to recommend how and to where patients are evacuated.

U.S. Marine Corps flight surgeons provide both rotary-wing and fixed-wing aircrew and aviation support personnel with the full range of occupational, preventive, and primary-care medical support both in garrison and while deployed. Their practice of Aerospace Medicine is characterized by frequent deployments to remote locations, high tempo operations, austere facilities, and harsh environments. Planning for deployment—gathering intelligence, identifying threats, developing threat mitigation strategies, and developing emergency plans—is the defining characteristic of their medical practice. Medical contingency response planning for manmade and natural disasters in the civilian community requires these same skills.

High-Altitude Terrain and Polar Environments

Aerospace Medicine specialists are uniquely qualified to provide medical support for scientific expeditions, high-adventure travel, and military operations in high-altitude terrain and polar environments. Temperature and altitude extremes in these environments result in exaggerated or atypical physiologic responses. They place significant stress on all personnel assigned. Symptoms of altitude illness typically occur above 8000 feet (2.44 km); with rapid ascent, they will be experienced by approximately 25% of personnel. Cold-induced deficits of the thyroid hormones, T3 and T4, may contribute to the fatigue, irritability, and depression suffered by approximately 50% of Antarctic residents who over-winter on the ice. Mission planning must include sufficient personnel to cover the decreased work capacity of personnel living in these harsh environments. Predeployment medical screening is essential; conditions such as diabetes, hypertension, and cardiac arrhythmias worsen with exposure to cold or altitude. Personal hygiene, food safety, communicable disease surveillance, and occupational safety programs cannot be neglected; unplanned loss of personnel due to illness or injury may delay or even prevent mission accomplishment. Evacuation of the ill and injured depends on the availability of transportation, the weather, and mission requirements. In polar environments, rapidly changing weather and visual illusions make flying much more challenging. Evacuation is nearly impossible during polar winters and weather delays are common even in the polar summer.[8]

Space Operations

As experience has accumulated with human-days in space and monitoring of increasing numbers of astronauts in the space environment, medical concerns have focused on the physiological effects of null gravity. Based on our experience during short duration flights, the biomedical challenges include space adaptation syndrome (space motion sickness), cardiovascular deconditioning, loss of red cell mass, and bone mineral loss. During the Space Transportation System (shuttle) operations, the first two challenges were of primary concern. Up to one-third of shuttle crewmembers experienced space adaptation syndrome. This syndrome occurs in the early segments of orbital flight and may adversely affect mission performance. Fluid shift and deconditioning effects occurred even during the relatively short duration of the shuttle orbital missions. Performance during orbit does not appear to be compromised, but with increasing g forces upon reentry, performance decrements are possible. As preparations proceed for a continuous habitat in space, loss of red cell mass and bone mineral loss have become more of a concern.

The International Space Station introduced additional challenges for maintaining astronauts on long duration missions. Environmental control systems were required to maintain potable water and uncontaminated air for long periods. Microbe overgrowth had to be prevented. Food and sanitation issues needed to be addressed, with resupply providing only one solution. Health maintenance surveillance, emergency medical treatment, crew work-rest cycles, and psychological considerations also presented new challenges.

In December 2017, the President signed Space Policy Directive-1, which directed NASA to work with international and commercial partners, and to refocus its efforts on returning to the moon for long-term exploration and utilization, followed by human missions to Mars and deeper into the solar system. Human spaceflight in low-Earth orbit will transition to commercial operations, which support NASA and the needs of an emerging private sector market. Long-duration U.S. human spaceflight operations will extend to lunar orbit. Long-term robotic exploration of the Moon will be followed by human exploration of the Moon in preparation for human missions to Mars and beyond.[9]

In December 2008, NASA awarded the privately held, American aerospace manufacturer and space transportation services company, Space Exploration Technologies Corporation (SpaceX), a (US) $1.6 billion contract to resupply the International Space Station (ISS). In July 2009, SpaceX's Falcon 1 became the first privately developed, liquid fuel rocket to deliver a commercial satellite to Earth orbit. SpaceX's Dragon spacecraft became the first private spacecraft to visit the ISS in May 2012. In September 2014, NASA awarded a (US) $2.6 billion contract to SpaceX to fly American astronauts, and February 2018 saw the first flight of SpaceX's Falcon Heavy rocket, capable of carrying large payloads to orbit and supporting missions as far as the Moon or Mars.[10]

In addition to transporting cargo and crewmembers to the ISS for the government, commercial space firms are developing new markets—including suborbital space tourism. In October 2004, SpaceShipOne became the first civilian venture to enter suborbital space flight. That same year, Congress directed the FAA to develop regulations establishing requirements for crew and space flight participants (passengers) involved in private space flight. The regulations require launch operators to inform passengers of the risks of space travel generally and the risks of space travel in the operator's vehicle in particular. The regulations also include training and general security requirements for space flight participants. In addition, they establish requirements for crew notification, medical qualifications and training, and requirements governing environmental control and life support systems.[11]

AEROSPACE MEDICAL PRACTICE

While it is not possible in this chapter to cover all of the duties and responsibilities of physicians practicing in the civil aviation, military aviation, and space sectors, there are some areas that are of particular interest to readers. These include planning for air travel with a medical condition, handling medical events that may occur on commercial aircraft, medical devices on aircraft, and AE. Circadian asynchronization, or jet lag, will also be discussed.

Routine Air Travel with Medical Conditions

Unexpected medical events occur on commercial aircraft at a rate of one medical event for every 30,000–40,000 passengers, or one for every 600 flight departures. These events may occur *de novo*, or air travel may trigger a medical situation in an already predisposed passenger. Such passengers include, among others, those suffering from a serious or unstable medical condition while travelling to seek medical attention elsewhere, returning to a home city with a terminal disease to die, traveling from another country where they have had surgery ("medical tourism"), and pregnant women whose labor starts prematurely.

The prevention of in-flight medical emergencies through planning and preparation before the flight is the responsibility of the passenger and their primary-care physician. Passengers should ensure that their basic and travel-related immunizations are current, carry (on their person or in carry-on luggage) sufficient medication for the duration of their trip (preferably with a few extra in case of a delay), and bring copies of their prescriptions (drug name, dose, and method of administration), in case a medication has to be refilled during the course of their trip.

Medical clearance may be required, particularly in the case of lung disease, heart disease, recent surgery, or pregnancy. Disqualifying conditions include a recent heart attack or stroke, active seizure disorder or recent head trauma, active TB, measles, mumps, chicken pox, meningitis, or infectious diseases of international health concern, term pregnancy, unstable diabetes, unstable psychosis, recent surgery (especially open heart or brain surgery), significant chronic obstructive pulmonary disease, and SCUBA diving within 24 hours prior to flight. Passengers with concerns about a pre-existing medical condition should check the airline website or contact either a reservations agent or the airline medical department for advice. The Aerospace Medical Association has published *Health Tips for Air Travel* for use by airline passengers.[12]

Airline gate agents and flight attendants are trained to identify passengers who are not fit to fly. When such a case is identified, they will utilize guidelines adopted by the airline or rely upon the advice of a medical person, typically an airport physician, an airline physician, or a third-party medical service. In some cases (e.g., when onboard oxygen is needed) it may not be possible to accommodate the passenger at the gate, so the earlier the notification of special medical needs or accommodations is made, the better. Preflight medical screening is particularly important in preventing the international spread of communicable diseases.

The concerned physician must exercise good clinical judgment, weighing the risks and benefits of air transportation for their patients, and considering the severity of the condition and time en route. The Aerospace Medical Association (AsMA) provides guidelines for use by physicians about medical conditions that may require special attention.[13] The International Air Transport Association (IATA) has also developed general guidelines for physicians to use when counselling patients about the risks of air travel. Many passengers have impairments that limit their activities. In the United States, the Americans with Disabilities Act Accessibility Guidelines apply to airports, and the Air Carrier Access Act applies to aircraft. Airlines are expected to make reasonable accommodations for passengers with disabilities, such as those in wheelchairs, on oxygen from a canister or portable oxygen concentrator, carrying CPAP devices or other essential medical equipment,[14] and those accompanied by service animals or emotional support animals.[15] Seriously ill or injured passengers may be carried by some commercial airlines (as an alternative to using an air ambulance service), but advance notice and approval are always required. Seats may be removed for installation of a stretcher or bed and ancillary equipment, which may be housed in its own compartment within a wide body aircraft. One or more attendants are required to accompany the seriously ill passenger.

Air Travel with Infants and Children

Infants and children can safely travel by air, but they often have poor Eustachian tube function, which makes them susceptible to ear pain on decent. Activities that facilitate swallowing help to maintain Eustachian tube patency. Nasal decongestants are helpful for the same reason.

While children younger than 2 years of age are permitted to sit in the lap of an adult while traveling on board a commercial airliner, the FAA, National Transportation Safety Board, and American Academy of Pediatrics do not recommend this practice. Children who weigh less than 40 pounds must be restrained in a child safety seat approved by the FAA for use on board aircraft. Many airlines have policies that require child safety seats to be placed in window seats to prevent them from blocking the escape path in an emergency. Airlines may require unapproved child safety seats to be checked as baggage. Children who weigh more than 40 pounds can use the aircraft seatbelt. More information is available online on the commercial airline websites or on FAA websites resources.

Airline Medical Events

Passenger safety is the primary responsibility of flight attendants. In addition to learning to handle emergency procedures such as emergency evacuation and extinguishing cabin fires, most flight attendants are trained in first aid and basic life support, including cardiopulmonary resuscitation (CPR) and the use of automated external defibrillators (AEDs).

In the event of an in-flight medical emergency that exceeds their skill level, cabin crews will ask for assistance from physicians or any other medical personnel on board. Ground-based medical support is usually available as well. Rarely, aircraft diversions may be required for a passenger to receive a higher level of care than is available onboard, and deaths—though extremely uncommon—do occur. Under United States and international law, the Captain, or pilot-in-command of an aircraft is responsible for, and the final authority as to, the operation of an aircraft. This includes responsibility for the safety of the passengers and crewmembers during flight.[16]

Although a medical professional may respond to an emergency on board, he or she is usually not trained to deal with serious situations outside a clinical setting, and may lack familiarity with the cabin environment and with the contents of the Emergency Medical Kit. They may also have questions concerning legal liability for the advice they provide or actions they take in the event of a medical emergency. In the United States, the Federal Aviation Medical Assistance Act of 1998 limits liability of medically qualified passengers who offer such assistance. In some other countries, there is a duty of care in the event of an emergency medical condition on board, although the likelihood of enforcement is low. With advances in radio communication, real-time communication with a ground-based medical service (GBMS) became possible, as an adjunct to or replacement for onboard medical assistance. Today, around 65% of world passenger traffic is covered by companies specializing in GBMS support for airlines, or by airline medical departments. Contact between an onboard medical volunteer and a GBMS before medical action is taken is optimal, particularly with respect to diversion decisions. Working with a GBMS relieves the onboard medical volunteer of much of the decision-making responsibility; essentially, they become the eyes and hands of the GBMS.

There is no clear-cut definition of what constitutes an in-flight medical event. From a GBMS perspective, a medical event occurs when the crewmember places a call to the telemedicine center, but such a call does not necessarily occur. This explains the wide variation of statistics found in the literature. Most medical events are benign in nature and can be handled effectively in-flight. Neurologic complaints are common on short-haul flights, whereas gastrointestinal complaints predominate on longer flights.

Syncope, most often vasovagal in origin, and often accompanied by urination or mild jerking of the limbs, is the single most frequent concerning event occurring in-flight.[17]

It is relatively easy to manage. A quick assessment for a more serious condition such as stroke, hypoglycemic episodes in diabetes, etc., is warranted for unconsciousness lasting more than a minute. An evolving stroke is serious, and most cases would benefit from diversion. In-flight seizures, resulting from medication disruption due to circadian rhythm changes, fatigue, hypoxia, or alcohol ingestion, occur rarely. An isolated seizure with prompt recovery is no reason to divert. However, prolonged or recurrent episodes, including "status epilepticus," may be life threatening and diversion for immediate care may be necessary to avoid anoxic brain damage. Injectable diltiazem may be available in the emergency medical kit for use by competent medical authority, particularly on international flights.

Chest pain requires rapid assessment of ischemic heart disease risk factors and a history of previous cardiac diagnoses by talking to the patient or an accompanying person. The usual approach is to provide a regular strength aspirin (or four baby aspirins), which may be chewed to accelerate absorption through the oral mucosa. Aspirin is available in the medical kit. Sublingual nitrates may be utilized on a case-by-case basis, particularly where they have been previously prescribed, except in the case of hypotension or in a patient who has recently (48–72 hours) used erectile dysfunction medications. GBMS is extremely helpful in such cases, by analyzing diversion options and activating EMS teams at the destination. In cases where an EKG or GBMS is not available, a typical chest pain lasting more than 30 minutes or a pain that does not resolve after adequate doses of nitrates is concerning enough for a diversion to be considered. For commercial aircraft, the Pilot in Command has the responsibility to make diversion decisions.

One in every 5–8 million passengers die in-flight, most from sudden cardiac arrest, often associated with underlying cardiac ischemic heart disease. Ventricular fibrillation is the usual mechanism of death. Flight attendants and most medical professionals are trained to perform CPR and to utilize an AED. Since 2004, in the United States, AEDs have been required on aircraft carrying 15 or more passengers and are the norm on most international airliners and in airports. In around 25% of cardiac arrests in-flight where a shock was administered, passengers survived to reach a hospital. In some cases, multiple shocks are needed. Recovery of spontaneous circulation after a shock delivered by an AED is an unequivocal indication for early landing. The AED should continue to be attached for the remainder of the flight until the patient is handed over to the medical team upon arrival. After 30 minutes of CPR with no shock recommended by the AED, a victim may be presumed dead and CPR efforts may be discontinued.[18]

Declaration of death is a legal matter and does not need to be made at the exact time the passenger dies. A formal declaration of death should wait until arrival at the destination to avoid jurisdictional problems regarding where the passenger was declared dead. Disposition of the decedent for the remainder of the flight is not a medical issue.

Allergic reactions are not common, but cases of anaphylaxis do occur in-flight, often associated with peanut or other food allergy. Passengers with a known allergic condition prone to anaphylaxis should carry their medication in their hand luggage; epinephrine and bronchodilator inhalers are provided in the onboard emergency medical kits carried by most airlines.[19]

Aircraft are required by the Federal Aviation Administration (FAA) to carry one or more first aid kits for minor emergencies not requiring medical assistance. First-Aid kits contain splints, scissors, and a variety of bandages. The FAA also mandates an Emergency Medical Kit. The required contents of the expanded kit are listed in Box 12-1. (EMK) for emergency use by a physician or other healthcare provider. In May 2004, the FAA mandated an expansion of the medical kit. Since 2005, the FAA has also required airlines to provide one or more AEDs aboard. The FAA Reauthorization Act of 2018 requires evaluation and revision of the FAA EMK by the FAA Administrator within 1 year. International and U.S. airlines may provide additional medications and equipment, including cardioactive drugs, benzodiazepines, narcotics, and telemetry equipment.

Trans-meridian Dyssynchronous or "Jet Lag"

Pilots, other aircrew, and passengers are affected by travel across time zones, which confuses the body's circadian rhythm (biological clock). This results in fatigue and insomnia, and may lead to other physical symptoms including disorientation, lightheadedness, headaches, appetite changes, bowel irregularity, mood changes, and performance problems. Adjustment takes on average one day per time zone crossed and for most people, jet lag is worse flying eastward than westward, but there is considerable individual variability. Traveling north to south within the same time zone produces no jet lag. Many measures are available to reduce jet lag, including adjusting sleep/wake time before departure by one hour per time zone to be crossed until the destination time zone is reached (most useful for domestic travel), changing meals to the new time, eating light meals, avoiding alcohol, and using exposure to bright light in the morning for west-to-east travel and at night for east-to-west travel prior to departure. Most travelers find that leaving during daylight

BOX 12-1 FAA Medical Kit Contents for Commercial Airliners

Sphygmomanometer (Blood pressure cuff)
Stethoscope
Airways, oropharyngeal (3 sizes): 1 pediatric, 1 small adult, and 1 large adult or equivalent
Self-inflating manual resuscitation device with 3 masks (1 pediatric, 1 small adult, and 1 large adult or equivalent) 1:3 masks
CPR mask (3 sizes), 1 pediatric, 1 small adult, and 1 large adult, or equivalent
IV Admin Set: Tubing w/2 Y connectors
2 Alcohol sponges
Adhesive tape, 1-inch standard roll adhesive
Tape scissors
Tourniquet
Saline solution, 500 cc
Protective nonpermeable gloves or equivalent
6 Needles (2–18 ga., 2–20 ga., 2–22 ga., or sizes necessary to administer required medications)
4 Syringes (1–5 cc, 2–10 cc, or sizes necessary to administer required medications)
4 Analgesic, non-narcotic, tablets, 325 mg
4 Antihistamine tablets, 25 mg
2 Antihistamine injectable, 50 mg, (single-dose ampule or equivalent)
2 Atropine, 0.5 mg, 5 cc (single-dose ampule or equivalent)
4 Aspirin tablets, 325 mg
Bronchodilator, inhaled (metered-dose inhaler or equivalent)
Dextrose, 50%/50 cc injectable, (single-dose ampule or equivalent)
2 Epinephrine 1:1000, 1 cc, injectable, (single-dose ampule or equivalent)
2 Epinephrine 1:10,000, 2 cc, injectable, (single-dose ampule or equivalent)
2 Lidocaine, 5 cc, 20 mg/ml, injectable (single-dose ampule or equivalent)
10 Nitroglycerin tablets, 0.4 mg
Basic instructions for use of the drugs in the kit

Source: FAA Reauthorization Act of 2018. Department of Transportation, Federal Aviation Administration. http://www.gpo.gov/fdsys/pkg/CFR-2013-title14-vol3/pdf/CFR-2013-title14-vol3-part121-appA.pdf.

hours minimizes subsequent jet lag symptoms. Caffeine may be used in moderation to maintain wakefulness. Hydration, exercise in flight and after arrival, and showering on arrival or at the destination may mitigate fatigue. Stimulants such as modafinil and armodafinil have been used, particularly by military pilots, but may be habit-forming. Similarly, hypnotics such as zolpidem or zaleplon can induce sleep at the proper time at the destination, but can cause short-term amnesia and may be habit-forming if taken frequently. Melatonin may help in some cases, but can make symptoms worse in others. The USAF does not recommend melatonin for use by pilots. Other supplements and aromatherapy have been tried, but are not well studied.

PATIENT MOVEMENT AND SAFETY IN THE AVIATION ENVIRONMENT

Air travel is demonstrably the safest mode of travel for the average, healthy passenger, but the physical stressors characteristic of the aviation environment can exacerbate many medical conditions. Noise, vibration, decreased humidity, and altitude-dependent changes in air pressure, the partial pressure of oxygen, and temperature can adversely affect both patients and passengers with medical conditions. There are few absolute contraindications to transporting patients by air. Patients who suffer from dysbarism, acute myocardial infarction, pneumothorax, or air embolism can be moved with relative safety, provided appropriate precautions are taken and preparations made. Assuming that maximum effort has been made to stabilize the patient, the question should be asked, "Are the benefits of air transportation real, and do they justify the clinical risks and financial costs of transport by air?"

Air Medical Transport

There are four generally recognized categories of air medical transport: AE, MEDEVAC, search and rescue (SAR), and casualty evacuation (CASEVAC). While there is overlap and there are exceptions, in most cases, AE involves the transportation of a patient between hospitals, over a relatively longer distance, via fixed-wing aircraft. MEDEVAC usually involves the transportation of a patient from the point of injury to a hospital, over a relatively shorter distance, via rotary-wing aircraft. SAR usually involves a government agency finding and removing a victim from an endangering environment using rotary-wing aircraft. CASEVAC is unique to the military; it involves the transportation of a patient using any available means, ground or air—sometimes under enemy fire.

Some aircraft, such as the C-130 *Hercules,* can be overpressurized to maintain the cabin below sea level pressure at operational altitudes. This capability makes the C-130 especially useful for transporting patients suffering from air embolism and decompression sickness, medical conditions that are likely to be exacerbated by the pressure changes routinely experienced in flight.

Not all medical equipment are safe and effective in the aviation environment. Medical equipment must be battery-powered or compatible with the aircraft power supply. It must be compact and unaffected by vibration and the variations in barometric pressure and temperature associated with changes in altitude. In addition, medical equipment must not interfere with or be affected by aircraft communication and navigation equipment; equipment approved for use on one type, model, or series aircraft may not be suitable for use on another. Automated and amplified equipment (e.g., cardiac rhythm monitors and Doppler stethoscopes) is preferred due to the vibration and increase in ambient noise after engine start.

There is no generally accepted staffing model for air medical transport flights. The number and qualifications of medical personnel on board will depend on the size of the aircraft and the mission. Medical personnel must have the medical skills necessary to complete the mission, be familiar with the aircraft, and understand the impact of the aviation environment on patient care. Fundamental skills include the ability to work in a restricted physical space, the ability to integrate into a team, knowledge of radio operations, flexibility, creativity, and sound judgment.

The DoD has the greatest experience with transporting seriously ill and injured patients. The military AE system employing large transport aircraft represents the nation's main resource for fixed-wing medical transport. Commercial air ambulance services are available in all large communities in the United States. Most visible is the medical center helicopter used to transfer critically ill and injured patients and neonates to tertiary medical facilities. Commercial airlines are frequently requested to carry ill or injured passengers. The airline and the airline's medical adviser should be contacted as early as possible in the planning process to assess if transfers of this type are available. Some airlines will accept stretcher-bound patients and at least one airline has a patient transport compartment module, which can be fitted into the cabin. At least one adequately qualified person must accompany the stretcher-bound patient.

AEROSPACE PUBLIC HEALTH

Cabin Air Quality

Commercial passenger aircraft cabins are pressurized to a cabin altitude of approximately 2400 m. Bleed air is taken from the engine by a compressor upstream of the combustor and passed through a heat exchanger to reduce the temperature. The air passes through a catalytic convertor to remove ozone, which could otherwise irritate the nose, throat, and respiratory system of passengers. Ventilation of the cockpit is independent of cabin ventilation. In the cabin, it is mixed with filtered air from the recirculation fans. As new air enters the cabin, an equivalent amount of air is exhausted.

Recirculated air passes through a high efficiency particulate arresting filter, which traps more than 99% of all bacteria and clustered viruses, into a mixing chamber. On most aircraft, the airflow is 50% outside air and 50% filtered air. The average air exchange rate is 20–30 times per hour on a commercial aircraft, which is comparable to the exchange rate in an operating theater or commercial kitchen and much higher than that in a typical office (five to ten times per hour). However, since a passenger aircraft is a crowded environment, the ventilation rate per person is lower. Aircraft air is dry, with a humidity of 10–25%, in contrast to 30–65% in most office and home environments.[20] Prior to takeoff, the fuselage transmits more heat from the sun to the interior than the forced air system (powered by the auxiliary power unit, or APU) can remove, while at altitude, the fuselage temperature is around −50°C, contributing to cabin air cooling. Studies have demonstrated that levels of chemical and biological contaminants in aircraft are less than levels in many offices and other workplaces, with no evidence of pollutants occurring in cabin air at levels exceeding available health and safety standards and guidelines.[21,22]

Disease Transmission and Vector Control

There is a large potential for the global spread of infectious diseases, particularly through air travel. This has been of concern to the World Health Organization (WHO), ICAO, other international agencies, the U.S. CDC and other nations for many years given the increasing interdependence of human societies, and increased efficiency of human transportation.[23] Viruses are more contagious than bacteria. Antigenic shift and antigenic drift occur regularly with influenza viruses, and the emergence of new infectious diseases such as Severe Acute Respiratory Syndrome (SARS), Middle East Respiratory Syndrome (MERS), and Coronavirus Disease 2019 (COVID-19), together with the emergence and dissemination of drug-resistant TB and other organisms have increased the level of concern.

Transmission may occur between passengers, crew, and others through direct contact with surfaces touched by infected persons or by coughing or sneezing (droplet and airborne transmission).

Because of the way air is circulated on passenger aircraft, infection usually occurs between passengers who are seated in the same row or in the row ahead and behind. Transmission of measles, influenza, and tuberculosis has been documented, though the risk is low.[24] Risk is increased when the aircraft ventilation system is inoperative on the ground and an APU is not in use. Travel information from international, national, and regional health authorities regarding outbreaks is the most cost-effective measure for preventing travel-related infectious diseases. It is inexpensive and does not burden travelers. Travel information allows travelers to cancel planned trips, avoid areas at greatest risk, or use personal protective equipment. Media coverage, which serves to disseminate this information can be helpful, but may sometimes be inaccurate or misleading. Handwashing and facemasks reduce transmission of infectious agents to others if used, but have limited value when used by uninfected passengers. To minimize the risk of spreading infections, travelers who are unwell, particularly if they have a fever, should delay travel until they have recovered. Airlines may deny boarding to passengers who appear to be infected with a communicable disease when symptoms or fever are present. Entry and exit screening is of limited value. Entry screening using thermal detection, declaration, medical examination, or laboratory tests is expensive and not very effective because of high false positive and false negative rates. Exit screening is cheaper (fewer airports), but the cost is borne by the host country which, as the source of the infectious agent, derives no direct benefit. Contact tracing may be of benefit particularly with respect to follow-up of exposed passengers, but it is expensive, passenger manifests may be incomplete, and exposed passengers may be difficult to locate several days after arrival at their destination.[25]

Global planning to contain the international spread of infectious agents is essential and is ongoing through the WHO, IATA, and the Centers for Disease Control and Prevention. Vector control may be performed in the host country airport, and air curtains may be used to prevent insects from entering open aircraft doors. Disinfection, or the use of pesticides sprayed inside aircraft in-flight after leaving an area with potential insect vectors is required by 21 countries. However, crew and passengers may complain about pesticide exposure. Control of animals, which are infectious disease reservoirs, and of fomites (baggage, cargo, clothing, etc.) is difficult. Inspections are often incomplete. Passengers may hide food products, or not admit to visiting farms or areas of epidemic outbreaks. Insects may be carried on or in luggage. Quarantine (isolating exposed travelers) is effective, but expensive for airlines and public health departments, takes time, and compliance is low and difficult to enforce. The delay between identification of a problem and making contact with those who may have been exposed to an infectious agent averages three days for returning passengers. Travel restriction is of limited effectiveness and politically controversial. Nevertheless, identifying a single case early in an epidemic and breaking the chain of transmission can be an effective public health strategy.

Environmental Impact

Noise

While susceptibility to noise-induced hearing loss is variable, prolonged exposure to sound louder than 85 dBA and brief exposure to extremely loud noise are potentially hazardous. The engines, other mechanical systems, and aerodynamics of powered aircraft and rotorcraft generate significant noise, which is particularly noticeable near airports. Supersonic flight generates shock waves (sonic booms) which can exceed 200 dB. The United States Aircraft Noise Abatement Act of 1968, Noise Pollution and Abatement Act of 1972, and Quiet Communities Act of 1978 require aircraft and airport noise control abatement procedures. Substantial efforts have been made by aircraft manufacturers to reduce noise at the source through changes in the design of engines. FAA regulations and the regulated airports minimize noise by controlling takeoff and landing patterns, including engine power adjustments.[24] Nearby communities often limit aircraft operations during the late night and early morning hours. Supersonic flight is not authorized by FAA regulation outside military operations areas. Internationally, ICAO has standards governing aircraft noise.

Air Pollution and Macroenvironmental Effects

Aircraft engine emissions are 70% carbon dioxide (CO_2), 29% water, and less than 1% NO_x, SO_x, and other gases and particulates. Carbon dioxide is a greenhouse gas, and CO_2 from aircraft represents 2.5% of all fossil fuel emissions. However, because they are released in the upper atmosphere, aircraft emissions are believed to contribute 3.5–4% of all radiative forcing (warming). Ground vehicles and APUs at airports produce additional emissions that contribute to air pollution. Air pollution is regulated in the United States by the Clean Air Act, and internationally by the ICAO through its CORSIA program (Carbon Offsetting and Reduction Scheme for International Aviation), which has the ambitious target of 80% reduction in global aviation emissions by 2035 relative to 2020. In addition to having a potential impact on global warming and climate change, aircraft emissions also affect the distribution of ozone in the atmosphere, contributing to the ozone thinning that forms at the poles each year. The effect is small, however, when compared with ground-based pollutant sources.[26]

The Future

Aerospace Medicine practitioners employ clinical medicine, physiology, toxicology, epidemiology, and the techniques of Public Health to maintain individual health and healthy populations. The field has grown dramatically since Dr. Louis Bauer published his seminal work on the subject in 1926. The focus of Aerospace Medicine has expanded from developing physical standards for aviators to the care of aviation support personnel, the AE of the ill and injured, the safety of passengers with chronic health conditions, the prevention of pandemics enabled by domestic and international air travel, the physiological challenges of space exploration, and the safety of civilians who will soon travel to the edge of outer space and beyond. As the technology of flight improves, so too will the medical support for those who find themselves in remote, isolated, extreme or enclosed environments under conditions of physical and psychological stress.

References

1. Engle E, Lott A. *Man in Flight*. Ann Arbor, MD: Leeward Publications; 1979.
2. International Space Exploration Coordination Group (ISECG). The Global Exploration Roadmap, 3rd edition. http://www.globalspaceexploration.org. The Netherlands. 2018.
3. Christopher J. Ondrula, JD, Executive Director, AmBoardPrevMed, email communication, July 25, 2018.
4. Accreditation Council for Graduate Medical Education. 2016–2017 Data Book. https://apps.acgme.org/ads/public/. Chicago, IL. 2017.
5. International Civil Aviation Organization. Appendix 1. Tables Relating to the World of Air Transport in 2015. https://www.icao.int/sustainability/Pages/FactsFigures.aspx.
6. Federal Aviation Administration, A: Guide for Aviation Medical Examiners. https://www.faa.gov/about/office_org/headquarters_offices/avs/offices/aam/ame/guide/. Washington, DC. 2018.
7. Clarke TF, DeHart RL, Erikson NS, et al. Aviation medicine in unique environments. In: Davis JR, Johnson R, Stepanek J, et al., eds. *Fundamentals of Aerospace Medicine*. 4th ed. Philadelphia, PA: Lippincott Williams & Wilkins; 2008, pp. 624–52.
8. Reed HL, Reedy, KR, Palinkas LA, et al. Impairment in cognitive and exercise performance during prolonged Antarctic residence: Effect of thyroxine supplementation in the polar triiodothyronine syndrome. *J Clin Endocrinol Metab*. 2001;86(1):110–6.
9. Presidential Memorandum on Reinvigorating America's Human Space Exploration Program, December 11, 2017. https://www.whitehouse.gov/presidential-actions/presidential-emorandum-reinvigorating-americas-human-space-exploration-program/. Washington, DC. 2017.

10. SpaceX: Company. https://www.spacex.com/about, 2018.
11. 14 Code of Federal Regulation (CFR) Parts 401, 415, 431, 435, 440 and 460.
12. Aerospace Medicine Association. https://www.asma.org/asma/media/asma/Travel-Publications/HEALTH-TIPS-FOR-AIRLINE-TRAVEL-Trifold-2013.pdf. Alexandria, VA. 2013.
13. Aerospace Medical Association. http://www.asma.org/asma/media/asma/travel-publications/medguid.pdf. Alexandria, VA. 2003.
14. International Air Transport Association. http://www.iata.org/publications/Pages/medical-manual.aspx.
15. Department of Transportation. http://airconsumer.ost.dot.gov/rules/382short.pdf. Federal Air Regulations (FAR) 91.3 (a) and FAR 121.535 (d).
16. Peterson DC, Martin-Gill C, Guyette FX, et al. Outcomes of medical emergencies on commercial airline flights. *N Engl J Med.* 2013;368:2075–83.
17. International Air Transport Association. https://www.iata.org/whatwedo/safety/health/Documents/death-on-board-guidelines.pdf.
18. Department of Transportation, Federal Aviation Administration. http://www.gpo.gov/fdsys/pkg/CFR-2013-title14-vol3/pdf/CFR-2013-title14-vol3-part121-appA.pdf. Washington, DC. 2013.
19. Giaconia C, Orilli A, Di Gang A. Air quality and relative humidity in commercial aircrafts: An experimental investigation on short-haul domestic flights. *Build Environ.* 2013;67:69–81.
20. Bagshaw M. Cabin air quality: A review of current aviation medical understanding, 2013. https://www.asma.org/asma/media/asma/Travel-Publications/Cabin-Air-Quality-A-review-of-current-aviation-medical-understanding-Jul13.pdf. Alexandria, VA. 2018.
21. European Aviation Safety Agency. www.easa.europa.eu/document-library/research-projects/facts-about-cabin-air-quality-board-large-transport-aircraft. Cologne, GE. 2018.
22. Mangili A, Gendreau M. Transmission of infectious diseases during commercial air travel. *Lancet.* 2005;365 (9463):12–18.
23. Moser MR, Bender TR, Margolis HS et al. An outbreak of influenza aboard a commercial airliner. *Am J Epidemiol.* 1979;110:1–6.
24. CDC. Guidelines for the investigation of contacts of persons with infectious tuberculosis. *MMWR.* 2005;54(RR15):1–37.
25. Airport Noise Compatibility Planning, Part 150 and Airport Noise and Access Restrictions, Part 161.
26. Federal Aviation Administration. Aviation & Emissions, A Primer. https://www.faa.gov/regulations_policies/policy_guidance/envir_policy/media/AEPRIMER.pdf. Washington, DC. 2005.

CHAPTER

13 Public Health Law

Micah L. Berman

INTRODUCTION

It is hard to overstate the law's importance to public health. Because law is one of the key mechanisms though which we order economic and social interactions, nearly every major advance in public health has been the result—at least in part—of changes in law.

Consider, for example, vaccinations. It was groundbreaking science that enabled the development of vaccines that can prevent a host of communicable diseases. However, it was the legal mandates (now in place in all 50 states) requiring vaccination as a condition of attendance in public and private schools that facilitated their near-universal uptake. Other legal interventions at the federal, state, and local level were then put to place to ensure that vaccines remain available and safe and that low-income families have access to free or reduced-cost vaccines. When new outbreaks of vaccine-preventable diseases occur (including outbreaks of previously well-contained diseases, like measles), states ideally revisit and update their laws as needed.[1]

Similar stories detailing the productive (and often complex) merger of public health science and law can be told about tobacco control, motor vehicle safety, occupational health, the decline in foodborne illnesses, and many other public health issues.[2] As the vaccination example illustrates, law typically does not provide a complete one-time fix for public health challenges; rather, attention must be paid to a law's impact, and laws much be updated, amended, or rescinded as conditions and social norms change.

As the practice of public health changes, public health law necessarily evolves alongside it. Public health departments in the United States were set up and organized with the mission of containing the infectious diseases that were at one time the leading causes of death. Today, with noncommunicable diseases and injuries as the leading causes of death and disability, new types of legal interventions are needed. In addition, because there are well-funded industries fueling many of today's greatest public health challenges (e.g., the tobacco, alcohol, sugar, and firearms industries), efforts to expand the reach of public health regulation is being increasingly countered by aggressive legal and political pushback. Thus, being able to build public and political support for effective public health action is increasingly a required skill set for public health professionals.

This chapter focuses on public health law in the United States. It surveys the legal authority of the various levels of government to pursue policies that promote health, the main constitutional protections relevant to public health, and the role of administrative agencies. It then discusses the practice of public health law, exploring key public health law skills, intersectoral collaboration, and the challenge posed by industries that may seek to block effective public health policies.

PUBLIC HEALTH LAW POWERS AND GOVERNMENT STRUCTURE

In the U.S. legal system, power is divided vertically (between the federal, state, and local levels of government) and horizontally (between the legislative, executive, and judicial branches of government at each level). Each lawmaking or regulatory body must act within the limits of its legal authority and must respect applicable constitutional constraints. An understanding of the authority of the various players in the U.S. legal system—and the relationships between them—is the starting point for considering how and by whom legal interventions could be developed to improve health. Otherwise, considerable effort could be wasted researching or advocating for interventions that are likely to be struck down in court.

LEGISLATIVE AUTHORITY

Federal Public Health Powers

At the federal level, legislative (i.e., lawmaking) authority is vested in the U.S. Congress. Congress can exercise only those powers specifically granted to it by the Constitution (referred to as "enumerated powers"). This limitation, though, still leaves it with tremendous authority to pass laws relating to public health. Congress can use its powers to regulate interstate commerce, to levy taxes, or to spend money "for the public welfare" to pursue nearly any public health objective.

Past court decisions interpreting Congress's constitutional power to regulate interstate commerce confirm that its reach is extensive. It has been used to uphold federal "civil rights laws, criminal laws, licensing requirements, laws regulating food and drugs, insurance regulations, and more."[3] This Commerce Clause power is not limitless, however. In a 1995 case, the Supreme Court ruled that a federal law prohibiting individuals from carrying a gun in a school zone could not be upheld under the Commerce Clause power because "[t]he possession of a gun in a school zone is in no sense an economic activity,"[4] and in 2012, the Court ruled that the Affordable Care Act's mandate for each individual to obtain health insurance coverage was not authorized by the Commerce Clause because it "compels individuals to become active in commerce," instead of regulating existing commercial relationships.[5]

With its power to tax, Congress can raise money to fund public health initiatives, and it can also discourage unhealthy behaviors and incentivize health-promoting actions. For example, the federal cigarette tax discourages smoking, while the Earned Income Tax Credit serves to reduce poverty and thereby improve health, particularly for single mothers and children.[6] In the same 2012 case that concluded that the "individual mandate" exceeded Congress's Commerce Clause authority, the Supreme Court held that the mandate—because it was enforced through a tax penalty—was a valid exercise of Congress's power to tax.[5]

Finally, Congress has the power to spend money "for the public welfare," and much of what the federal government does to promote public health is done by appropriating funds. Congress, for example, funds the Centers of Disease Control and Prevention (CDC), which conducts public health surveillance and research, assists in responding to public health emergencies, and provides financial support to state, local, and tribal public health entities. Funding can also be used as a lever to prompt policy change at the state level. In 1984, for instance, Congress passed a law withholding some transportation funding from states that did not raise their minimum drinking age to 21. All states eventually responded by raising the age. Even though Congress arguably lacked the authority to directly set a national drinking age, the Supreme Court upheld this indirect approach.[7] In 2012, however, the Supreme Court concluded that if the conditions placed on federal funding were so "coercive" as to deprive states of autonomy over their own decision-making, such an arrangement would exceed Congress's constitutional powers.[5]

State and Local Public Health Powers

Unlike Congress, the state legislatures that make the laws at the state level are not limited to enumerated powers. Instead, they possess inherent "police power" authority to regulate for the health, safety, and welfare of their citizens. (In this context the term "police" does not refer to police departments; it refers to the older meaning of the word "police"—to keep order.) In the foundational case of *Jacobson v. Massachusetts* (1905), the Supreme Court explained that the states can enact "health laws of every description" to "protect the public health and the public safety," so long as such laws have a reasonable public health justification and do not violate constitutional rights.[8] In the *Jacobson* case, the Supreme Court upheld a requirement for mandatory smallpox vaccinations in the face of smallpox outbreak.

Local governments are technically subdivision of the state in which they are located. Local governmental authority therefore depends on the specifics of each state's law. Some states grant broad "home rule" authority to each jurisdiction, essentially enabling them to exercise the full police power of the state (so long as local laws do not conflict with state law). Other states take the opposite approach and allow local governments to exercise only those powers that have been specifically delegated to them by the state.

Preemption

A major issue in public health law is the vertical distribution of power between different levels of government. Though federal, state, and local governmental entities ideally work collaboratively to tackle public health challenges, sometimes they have sharply conflicting policy approaches. Under the Supremacy Clause of the Constitution, federal law takes precedence over state and local laws in the event of a conflict. This is referred to as the doctrine of *preemption*. Indeed, not only do federal laws prevail in the event of a conflict, but Congress—so long as it is acting within the limits of its enumerated powers—can block (or "preempt") state and local lawmaking on a particular subject. This preemption can be direct, though a clear statement by Congress that it intends to block state- and local-level regulation ("express preemption"), or indirect, when a federal regulatory scheme is deemed to be so pervasive that it does not leave room for state and local regulation ("implied preemption").

Federal preemption can be problematic from a public health perspective because it prevents state and local governments from enacting laws that may be more protective of health than the national standard. For example, in 1965, Congress passed the Federal Cigarette Labeling and Advertising Act, requiring health warnings on cigarette packages. Though this law may have helped to inform the public about the dangers of smoking, it also included a provision that prevented state and local governments from mandating stronger warnings or regulating tobacco advertising and promotion.[9] In retrospect, it is likely that this trade-off was, on balance, bad for public health. In the absence of such preemption, the likely result would have been far stronger warnings and more forceful regulation of tobacco advertising (though there might have been substantial state-by-state variation in the strength of these measures).

A similar dynamic plays out at the state level. Because local governments are subdivisions of the state in which they are located, the state has the authority to limit the scope of their legislative power. Preemptive state laws are often pushed by industries or groups seeking to avoid local regulation. At the urging of the National Rifle Association, for instance, most states have enacted laws limiting the authority of local governments to pursue gun control measures.

REGULATORY AUTHORITY

In addition to the vertical distribution of power between the federal government, states, and localities, there is also the *horizontal* distribution of authority between the different branches of government. Much of the public health law is administrative law, meaning that it relates to the regulatory actions of federal, state, and local public health (and related) agencies. These regulatory agencies are part of the executive branch of government. As such, their job is to implement and enforce laws passed by the legislature. Depending on the scope of a legislative enactment, implementing a particular law may give regulators great authority to design creative public health interventions. At the same time, though, regulators must follow directives issued by the chief executive (the president at the federal level, and the governor at the state level), and their actions are subject to review by the courts.

At the federal level, an alphabet soup of regulatory agencies and cabinet departments—FDA, OSHA, EPA, etc.[10]—have the primary responsibility for ensuring that we have safe workplaces, healthy (or at least nontoxic) food, rigorously tested pharmaceuticals, and so forth. At the state and local levels, health departments do the day-to-day work of enforcing food and sanitation codes, conducting safety inspections, controlling infectious diseases, and, in many cases, providing preventive health services like tobacco cessation counseling and testing for sexually transmitted diseases.

If the legislature authorizes them to do so, agencies can issue their own rules, referred to as *regulations*. Regulations provide additional or more detailed requirements than those set forth in statutes. For example, a law passed by a state legislature may broadly authorize the commercial sale of marijuana but leave it to a state agency to issue regulations regarding who can become a licensed retailer, how licenses are issued and renewed, requirements for preventing sales to underage individuals, restrictions on advertising and promotion, penalties for violations, and more. Deferring such detailed questions to agencies rulemaking is common because agencies are considered to be the subject-matter experts with specialized knowledge and resources that the legislature (which much address many more topics) does not possess.

At the federal level (and broadly paralleled at the state level as well), the public is afforded an opportunity to comment on proposed regulations before they are finalized. The agency must consider and respond to the comments it receives. Comments are most often filed by the companies that would have to follow the regulation being proposed, but all members of the public can engage in this "notice and comment" process through the website Regualtions.Gov. Once a final regulation is issued, it has the force of law.

Traditionally public health agencies have been given very broad powers to do what they consider necessary to protect the public health. This reflects the recognition that public health decisions should be made by public health experts, as well as the desire for agencies to have sufficiently flexible authority to respond to new and unexpected health challenges. Regulations are easier and quicker to change than legislation and can be modified on an emergency basis. This is important when the health agency is dealing with problems such as emerging infectious diseases or changing standards of practice based on new scientific discoveries.

Even with broad delegations, there can be questions about when agencies are overstepping their bounds. This tends to come up when agencies try to respond to new public health challenges and use previously untested regulatory tools. For example, the lawsuit challenging New York City's attempt to regulate the portion size of sugar-sweetened beverages centered on the scope of the New York City Board of Health's authority. Was the Board's rule limiting the size of cups that could be used to serve beverages like Coke and Pepsi simply a new way to implement the Board's broad authority to "control … communicable and chronic diseases"? Or was the Board improperly setting "new policy, rather than carrying out preexisting legislative policy"?[11] By a narrow margin, New York State's highest court ruled that it was the latter and invalidated the rule not because it was bad policy, but because the Board, in its view, did not have the authority to issue it.

CONSTITUTIONAL LIMITATIONS

At all levels of government, laws and regulations must respect rights guaranteed by the Constitution or else they can be invalided through a court challenge. Thus, to be upheld, laws and regulations must be (1) within a legislative body or regulatory agency's authority, (2) not preempted by higher level of government, and (3) consistent with the Constitution. Importantly, the Constitution only provides limits on actions by governmental entities, not by private parties (though analogous protections against private action may be enacted through legislation). Though the Constitution's Bill of Rights was originally interpreted to limit only to the actions of the federal government, the Supreme Court later established that it generally applies to the actions of state and local governments as well. A few of the Constitution's protections that have specific relevance to public health are reviewed below. Notably, the U.S. Constitution—unlike the constitutions of many other countries—does not provide for positive rights like a "right to health." For the most part, the Constitution tells the government what it *cannot* do, not what it must do.

Freedom of Speech and Religion

Among other provisions, the First Amendment to the Constitution protects freedom of speech and the free exercise of religion. The protection for freedom speech takes some types of regulation that might protect public health off of the table. For instance, it prevents the government from regulating publications that contain inaccurate or even dangerous health information. Accordingly, the government cannot regulate internet sites that provide misleading or false information about vaccines unless the information is part of an advertisement for a product. Though this often poses a challenge to public health, it is the flip side of a First Amendment that broadly protects personal autonomy. Preventing the government from censoring individuals' expression also provides citizens with the ability to challenge the government when it is wrong. It is important to ensure that the government is *actually* protecting public health, not just claiming to do so. To provide a recent example, in Flint, Michigan, "some government officials disregarded the risk the water posed, denied the increasingly clear threat the public faced, … and rejected solutions that would have ended [the] crisis sooner"; it was public pressure that finally forced the government to acknowledge the high levels of bacteria and lead in the city's water and to take corrective action.[12]

Unlike individual expression, commercial advertising may be subject to regulation. Over the past several decades, however, the Supreme Court has expanded the scope of First Amendment protection provided to such "commercial speech," even when it is promoting harmful products. Commercial speech that is false or misleading can be prohibited, but beyond that, the Supreme Court has moved toward the view that the government cannot "prevent[] the dissemination of truthful commercial information in order to prevent members of the public from making bad decisions with the information."[13] Thus, it has become increasingly difficult for governments to use the regulation of advertisements (e.g., alcohol ads) as a public health tool. Instead, they must rely more on other tools like taxes or product regulation that do not raise First Amendment concerns. Concurrently, the courts have become more skeptical of compelled warnings—like black box warning labels on a product's packaging—that seek to inform consumers of a product's harms, concluding that such warnings can, in some cases, violate the First Amendment rights of the companies required to convey them.[14]

The First Amendment's Free Exercise Clause protects the right to practice one's religion free from governmental interference. There is occasionally tension between religious rights and public health, such as when adherents to a particular faith claim the right to be exempted from otherwise applicable public health laws, like vaccination requirements. In 1990, the Supreme Court ruled that the First Amendment did not protect Native Americans from being fired for the ceremonial use of the drug peyote.[15] Since that time, the Court has generally held to the rule that a "neutral law of general applicability" (one not designed to single out a particular religion or religious practice) need not contain an exemption for religious objectors. Governments can, however, pass laws that provide protections for religious practices that go beyond what is required by the Constitution.

Due Process of Law

The Fifth Amendment provides that "No person shall … be deprived of life, liberty, or property without due process of law," and the Fourteenth Amendment, enacted after the Civil War, specifies that this guarantee is also applicable to the states. Courts have interpreted the Due Process Clause to provide both substantive rights and procedural rights. Substantively, the Due Process Clause prohibits the government from taking away one's "fundamental rights" (e.g., the right to bodily integrity or the right to custody of one's children) without a "compelling state interest." The procedural protections embodied in the Due Process Clause ensure that a wider range of rights cannot be restricted unless the government provides for a fair process, including prior notice and a hearing conducted by a neutral decision-maker.

Both the courts and public health authorities, however, have not always been adequately protective of due process rights. In the troubling case of *Buck v. Bell* (1927), for example, the Supreme Court endorsed the use of forced sterilization as a method of promoting the now-discredited theory of eugenics,[16] a "belief that societies could improve public health and welfare through the systematic prevention of reproduction by genetically inferior humans."[3] Under the guise of public health, states involuntarily sterilized an estimated 65,000 women between the 1920s and the 1970s.

During the 2014 Ebola outbreak—and, more recently, during the novel coronavirus (COVID-19) pandemic—public health entities were required to consider what the Due Process Clause allowed in terms of *quarantine* (confinement of a person exposed to a disease) and *isolation* (confinement of a person with an infectious disease). Both quarantine and isolation are longstanding public health measures designed to prevent infectious diseases from spreading, but they also raise "in the starkest possible terms the fundamental ethical conflict of public health—the clash between individual and population rights and interests."[17] The response to COVID-19 also involved the extensive use of "social distancing" measures like prohibitions on mass gatherings (concerts, sports events, etc.) and the closure of schools and businesses. These measures, intended to slow the spread the virus in the absence of a vaccine or effective medical countermeasures, had not been used extensively in over 100 years. Accordingly, they raised a host of unanswered legal issues and provoked hundreds of lawsuits raising Due Process and other legal claims. As of this writing, "few courts have clearly identified the Fourteenth Amendment substantive due process rights implicated by coronavirus emergency measures, and even fewer have found community mitigation measures to run afoul of them."[18] Nonetheless, it is likely that the COVID-19 pandemic will lead some state governments to revise their current statutes to provide clearer authorization for (and, perhaps, limitations on) the issuance of social distancing measures in the future.

Equal Protection

The Equal Protection Clause, also found in both the Fifth and the Fourteenth Amendments, promises "equal protection of the law." Like "due process of law," this is another promise that has not always been respected by public health authorities. Prior to World War II, for instance, quarantines were "frequently applied disparately and invidiously against vulnerable populations."[18]

As interpreted by the Supreme Court, the Equal Protection Clause not does prohibit the government from making meaningful distinctions between different categories of people. For example, public health laws regularly prohibit individuals under a certain age (usually 18 or 21) from engaging in risky activities or using harmful products. Courts have never considered such laws to be a violation of the Equal Protection Clause. However, judicial review is heighted when laws make distinctions based on *suspect classes* or *semi-suspect classes*.

Laws that treat groups different on the basis of race or national origin involve suspect classes. Laws that make explicit distinctions between such groups are presumptively invalid and are almost never upheld. Things are more complicated, however, when a law does not make such distinctions on its face but instead impacts racial or ethics groups differently in practice. Such laws may contribute to health disparities (e.g., zoning decisions that concentrate toxic emissions in minority neighborhoods), but they can be more difficult to challenge on equal protection grounds. As a general rule, clear evidence that the law was designed to further a racially discriminatory purpose is necessary to invalidate such laws.[19]

Laws that make distinctions on the basis of gender provide an example of a semisuspect classification. This standard acknowledges that there may be valid reasons to treat men and women differently, but that gender-based distinctions may also be grounded in prejudice or outmoded stereotypes. In *Califano v. Westcott* (1979), for instance, the Supreme Court struck down a law that provided aid to families with an unemployed father, but not to families with an unemployed mother. The Court wrote that the law reflected the "baggage of sexual stereotypes," and that "[l]egislation that rests on such presumptions, without more, cannot survive scrutiny under the Due Process Clause[.]"[20] Courts are still divided on whether laws that make distinctions on the basis of sexual orientation similarly trigger a heightened standard of review.

If there is not suspect or semisuspect class involved, it is far less likely (though not impossible) that a law will be found to violate the Equal Protection Clause. Note, however, that "although categories such as age and disability do not receive heightened scrutiny under the [Supreme] Court's Equal Protection Clause jurisprudence, there are separate civil rights laws prohibiting discrimination on these bases."[3]

Other Constitutional Protections

Numerous other constitutional protections may arise in various public health contexts. For instance, the Second Amendment's "right … to keep and bear arms" has increasingly been used to challenge gun-related regulations[21]; the Fourth Amendment's protection against "unreasonable searches and seizures" limits the actions of public health agencies investigating potential health code violations[22]; and the Fifth Amendment's prohibition on taking property without just compensation may come into play in public health emergencies (if, e.g., the government needs to seize a hotel to use as a quarantine facility) and in other public health contexts as well.[23]

THE PRACTICE OF PUBLIC HEALTH LAW

The previous section outlined the basic legal framework in which policymakers issue health-related laws and regulations. However, it is important to remember that in practice, public health law is not solely (or even primarily) the province of lawyers. Lawyers bring specialized knowledge and training to the table, but the day-to-day work of advancing public health through law relies on many diverse "law-related activities—policy development, analysis, advocacy, enforcement, monitoring, and evaluation—that are performed by people without formal legal training, sometimes in collaboration with lawyers, and sometimes not."[3] *Anyone* interested in public health should realize that law is a critical determinant of health and that they have a role to play in advancing policies that can improve health and well-being.

This section discusses the skills needed to effectively engage in the practice of public health law. It then briefly highlights two central challenges likely to define the future of public health law: the need for intersectoral collaboration to tackle complex social determinants of health, and the role of corporate interests that actively oppose public health policies.

ESSENTIAL PUBLIC HEALTH LAW SKILLS

In 2016, a collaboration funded by the CDC and the Robert Wood Johnson Foundation developed a list of "five essential public health law services"—the key links in a chain necessary to advance sound public health policies.[24] Most of these key "services" require expertise beyond legal knowledge. These five services are:

1. **Access to evidence and expertise:** Public health policy should flow from public health evidence. Like the field of public health more generally, public health law's strength comes from its grounding in epidemiology and other public health sciences. Conducting high-quality research in a way that can inform policy requires building connections across disciplinary lines.
2. **Expertise in designing legal solutions:** In-depth knowledge of the legal system, as described above, is necessary to ensure that a policy idea can be translated into a technically sound proposal that will minimize loopholes, ensure compliance, and survive legal challenges.
3. **Building political will:** A proposal must be turned into a law or regulation to have an impact on health. Having the facts and evidence on your side is rarely sufficient to effectuate policy change—such information must be combined with effective advocacy campaigns that can sway decision makers and prompt them to act. This mobilization requires partnerships with advocacy organizations and affected communities.
4. **Implementing, enforcing, and defending legal solutions:** Getting a law passed is not the end of the process. Declaring victory after a law is passed and moving on to the next issue is a common mistake. Sustained vigilance is needed to ensure that implementation of a law is sufficiently resourced and effectively carried out. Laws (especially controversial ones) may also be challenged in court, and preparations for defending such lawsuits need to be initiated before the law is passed.
5. **Policy surveillance and evaluation:** The final key skill is the ability to evaluate whether or not a law is working as intended. Scientifically sound evaluations (in both the short-term and the long-term) are critical to building a knowledge base that can inform other communities that may be considering similar measures. Best practices for policy surveillance and evaluation have been developed over the past decade and continue to evolve.[25]

No individual person is expected to be equally competent at all of these skills, but anyone interested in public health policy should develop some familiarity with these five skills and consider how they can join (or build) a network that is proficient in all of them. Also critical to consider is how these skills can be used not just to advance health, but to address the significant health disparities that currently skew health outcomes by race, geography, educational attainment, and other factors.

HEALTH AND EQUITY IN ALL POLICIES

Historically, health departments have focused the majority of their efforts on food safety, sanitation, and the control of infectious disease. These functions remain important, but because of past successes in controlling infectious diseases, the leading causes of death today are noncommunicable diseases such as a heart disease, cancer, and stroke, as well as unintentional (e.g., car crashes) and intentional (e.g., gun violence) injuries. The laws that structure health agencies and give them their powers have, for the most part, not kept pace with these changes. Moreover, many key public health issues—infant mortality, gun violence, obesity, and others—impact particular communities in different ways, often as a result of past and ongoing patterns of discrimination. For example, "Native Americans and Alaskan Natives have an infant mortality rate that is 60% higher than the rate for their white counterparts," and "LGBT youth are more likely than their non-LGBT peers to be bullied, commit suicide, engage in sexual risk behaviors, and run away or be forced to leave home."[26]

Health agencies alone are not well suited to tackling the social determinants that are the key drivers of poor health and health disparities: concentrated poverty and residential segregation; limited educational and economic opportunities; exposure to crime and violence; and more. This recognition has prompted a turn toward a "Health and Equity in All Policies" (HEiAP) approach to policymaking, which recognizes that a spectrum of public agencies and resources must be enlisted to address widespread and complex public health problems that have multiple causes and multiple solutions.[27] States and communities around the country are gradually putting in place procedures that require health and equity to be considered, and affected communities to be consulted, when making a wide range of policy decisions.[28] Though the effect of these initiatives remains to be seen, it is clear that public health law's future success will depend on such cross-sector collaborations.

INDUSTRY INFLUENCE

Unlike the deadly and debilitating infectious diseases of the past—e.g., smallpox and polio—many of the major public health challenges of today—e.g., obesity, tobacco use, gun violence, and alcohol abuse—are fueled by powerful industries that have a profit motive to sell more and more of their products. All of these industries have powerful lobbying operations in Washington, DC and in state capitals around the country, and they can put pressure on legislators in numerous ways.[29] They can also afford to aggressively litigate legal challenges to public health laws that threaten their profitability.

Countering such industry influence is challenging, especially at the federal level. For instance, even though polls consistently showed that an overwhelming *90%* of Americans supported a bill that would have expanded background checks for gun purchases, the gun lobby's political muscle was widely credited with keeping the measure from passing through Congress.[30] Additionally, the phenomenon of "regulatory capture"—when government agencies become too closely aligned with the interests of the industry they are supposed to be regulating—can undermine the effectiveness of regulatory oversight. Those interested in public health policy must study these "corporate determinants of health" and strategies for addressing them.[31] Such responses may include a focus on local policymaking, where industry influence is generally less pronounced (though state-level preemption may pose a challenge), or efforts to exposure industry-driven narratives, such as the false narrative that obesity is due primarily to a lack of individual willpower.

CONCLUSION

For all of the key public health challenges of our time—COVID-19, opioid addiction, tobacco use, vaccine hesitancy, antimicrobial resistance, obesity, and more—law has been and will continue to be central to the nation's collective response. However, although law is a powerful tool available for advancing public's health, it can be a difficult one to wield, particularly in politically polarized times. Well-funded industries lobby against effective health policy interventions; legislators shy away from policies they view as too paternalistic or controversial; courts question whether public health is even a "substantial government interest"[14]: the barriers to effective public health legal interventions are often high, and new cross-sectoral and community partnerships are needed to overcome them. Despite the manifold challenges, the payoff is worth the effort. Millions upon millions of lives have been saved by vaccine mandates, tobacco control measures, occupational health standards, and other public health policy interventions—most of which were highly controversial when first proposed. The same remains true now: putting in place (and defending in court) the "controversial" public health measures that are needed today will save lives—not just one by one, but on a massive scale.

Acknowledgments

Rhianna Wardian assisted with the research for this chapter. Edward P. Richards, III and Katharine C. Rathbun authored the previous edition of this chapter, and some brief passages from the previous edition were retained.

References

1. Gostin LO, Ratzan SC, Bloom BR. Safe vaccinations for a healthy nation: increasing US vaccine coverage through law, science, and communication. *JAMA*. 2019;321:1969–70.
2. Centers for Disease Control and Prevention. Ten great public health achievements—United States, 1900–1999. *MMWR Morb Mortal Wkly Rep*. 1999;48:241–3.
3. Burris S, Berman ML, Penn M, Holiday TR. *The New Public Health Law: A Transdisciplinary Approach to Practice and Advocacy*. New York: Oxford University Press; 2018.
4. *United States v. Lopez*, 514 U.S. 549 (1995).
5. *Nat'l Fed'n of Indep. Bus. v. Sebelius*, 567 U.S. 519 (2012). Congress later eliminated the tax penalty for failing to comply with the individual mandate.
6. Evans WN, Garthwaite CL. Giving mom a break: The impact of higher EITC payments on maternal health. *Am Econ J Econ Policy*. 2014;6:258–90.
7. *South Dakota v. Dole*, 483 U.S. 203 (1987).
8. *Jacobson v. Massachusetts*, 197 U.S. 11 (1905).
9. Federal Cigarette Labeling and Advertising Act, Pub. L. No. 89-92 (1965). This law was later amended in 1969, 1984, and 2009. The 2009 amendments provided more flexibility to state and local governments to regulate tobacco advertising and promotion.
10. The FDA is the U.S. Food and Drug Administration, which is part of the Department of Health and Human Services. OSHA is the Occupational Safety and Health Administration, which is part of the Department of Labor. EPA is the Environmental Protection Agency, which is a cabinet-level department.
11. *New York Statewide Coal. of Hispanic Chambers of Commerce v. New York City Dep't of Health & Mental Hygiene*, 16 N.E.3d 538, 549 (N.Y. 2014).
12. *In re Flint Water Cases*, 329 F. Supp. 3d 369 (E.D. Mich. 2018).
13. *Thompson v. Western States Med. Ctr.*, 535 US 357 (2002).
14. *R.J. Reynolds Tobacco Co. v. U.S. Food & Drug Admin*, 696 F.3d 1205 (D.C. Cir. 2012).
15. *Employment Div., Dept. of Human Resources of Oregon v. Smith*, 494 U.S. 872 (1990).
16. *Buck v. Bell*, 274 U.S. 200 (2007).
17. Rothstein MA. From SARS to Ebola: Legal and ethical considerations for modern quarantine. *Ind Health L Rev.* 2015;12:227–80.
18. Wiley LF. Democratizing the law of social distancing. *Yale J Health Policy Law Ethics* (forthcoming 2020). Parmet WE. Quarantining the law of quarantine: Why quarantine law does not reflect contemporary constitutional law. *Wake Forest J L & Pol'y.* 2018;9:1–33.
19. *Washington v. Davis*, 426 U.S. 229 (1976).
20. *Califano v. Westcott*, 443 U.S. 76 (1979) (internal citations and quotation marks omitted).
21. *District of Columbia v. Heller*, 554 U.S. 570 (2008).
22. *Camara v. Municipal Court*, 387 U.S. 523 (1967).
23. *Philip Morris, Inc. v. Harshbarger*, 159 F.3d 670 (1st Cir. 1998).
24. Burris S, Ashe M, Blanke D, et al. Better health faster: The 5 essential public health law services. *Public Health Rep.* 2015;131:747–53.

25. Burris S, Wagenaar AC, Swanson J, Ibrahim JK, Wood J, Mello MM. Making the case for laws that improve health: A framework for public health law research. *Milbank Q.* 2010;88:169–210.

26. National Academies of Science, Engineering, and Medicine. *Communities in Action: Pathways to Health Equity*. Washington, DC: National Academies Press; 2017.

27. Gase LN, Pennotti R, Smith KD. "Health in All Policies": Taking stock of emerging practices to incorporate health in decision making in the United States. *J Public Health Manag Pract.* 2013;19:529–40.

28. Wernham A, Teutsch SM. Health in all policies for big cities. *J Public Health Manag Pract.* 2015;21(Suppl 1):S56–65.

29. Wiist WH. *The Bottom Line or Public Health: Tactics Corporations Use to Influence Health and Health Policy and What We Can Do to Counter Them*. New York: Oxford University Press; 2010.

30. Berman ML. Lethal but legal: Corporations, consumption, and protecting public health (book review). *J Legal Med.* 2014;35:601–8.

31. McKee M, Stuckler, D. Revisiting the corporate and commercial determinants of health. *Am J Public Health.* 2018;108:1167–70.

CHAPTER 14

Armed Conflict and Public Health

Barry S. Levy

INTRODUCTION

Armed conflict causes serious and widespread consequences for public health. It accounts for much injury, disease, disability, and premature death and damages the health-supporting infrastructure of society. It contaminates the air, water, and soil and harms the physical environment. It forcibly displaces people and violates human rights and international treaties. It diverts human and financial resources away from healthcare, public health, and social services; it often leads to more violence.[1]

Definitions

The Uppsala Conflict Data Program (UCDP), a data-collection program on organized violence that is based at Uppsala University in Sweden, divides organized violence into three categories: state-based conflict, nonstate conflict, and one-sided violence. It defines state-based armed conflict as: "A contested incompatibility between two parties—at least one of which is the government of a state—that concerns government or territory or both, where the use of armed force by the parties results in at least 25 battle-related deaths in a calendar year."[2] It defines *war* as "a state-based conflict that results in [at least] 1,000 battle-related deaths in a year."[2] The UCDP further divides state-based conflict into the following three categories:

- "Interstate conflicts are fought between two or more governments of states;
- Intrastate conflicts are fought between a government of a state and one or more rebel groups; and
- Internationalized intrastate conflicts are intrastate conflicts in which one or both sides receive troop support from an external state."[2]

Among these three categories, intrastate conflicts ("civil wars") are the most frequent, generally accounting for more than 80% of all conflicts globally, and interstate conflicts are the least frequent, although they lead to a very large number of deaths.[2]

According to the World Health Organization (WHO), there are three categories of violence: collective violence; self-directed violence, such as suicide; and interpersonal violence, such as intimate partner violence.[3] Collective violence includes armed conflict; state-sponsored violence, such as genocide and torture; and organized crime, such as gang warfare and banditry.[3] WHO defines armed conflict as "the instrumental use of violence by people who identify themselves as members of a group—whether this group is transitory or has a more permanent identity—against another group or set of individuals in order to achieve political, economic, ideological, or social objectives."[3]

Number of Armed Conflicts

During 2018, there were active armed conflicts in 27 countries: 11 in sub-Saharan Africa, 7 in the Middle East and North Africa, 7 in Asia and Oceania, 1 in Europe, and 1 in the Americas. Most of these conflicts were intrastate conflicts occurring within a country between one or more armed nonstate groups and government forces. One of the conflicts was between countries (between Pakistan and India). Two of the conflicts were waged between armed groups that aspired to statehood and government forces (conflicts between the Palestinian and Israel, and between the Kurds and Turkey). Three of the intrastate conflicts had more than 100,000 conflict-related deaths during 2018: the war in Afghanistan (with more than 43,000 reported deaths in 2018), the war in Yemen (with more than 30,000 reported deaths), and the war in Syria (with more than 30,000 reported deaths). In addition, armed conflicts in the following countries were associated with more than 1000 deaths in 2018: Iraq, Nigeria, Somalia, the Democratic Republic of the Congo, Turkey, the Philippines, Mali, Ethiopia, South Sudan, Cameroon, Egypt, the Central African Republic, and Libya.[4]

In recent decades, most intrastate armed conflicts have occurred in low- and middle-income countries (LMICs), often resulting in high mortality. For example, in the civil war in the Democratic Republic of the Congo, there were an estimated 5.4 million war-related deaths between August 1998 and April 2007—an estimated 2.1 million of which occurred *after* the formal conclusion of the war in 2002.[5] As another example, during the 30-year civil war in Ethiopia, approximately 1 million people died—about half of whom were noncombatant civilians.[6]

Causes of Armed Conflict

There are numerous underlying and precipitating causes of armed conflict. Underlying and contributory causes of war include disputes over territory, attempts at gaining or enhancing government power, enmity among ethnic groups, militarism, the international arms trade, social and economic inequities, and deterioration of public services.

It appears that there are increasing risks for armed conflict.[7] Reasons include the weakening of multinational alliances and international institutions,[8] proliferation of nuclear weapons,[9] climate change,[10] decreasing access to freshwater,[11] and forced displacement of people.[12]

Health and Environmental Consequences of Armed Conflict

Morbidity and Mortality

During the twentieth century, armed conflict, genocide, and mass murder accounted for the deaths of an estimated 191 million people, more than half of whom were noncombatant civilians.[13] During the current century, armed conflict continues to cause thousands of deaths among noncombatant civilians annually.[14,15]

Many civilians who have died during armed conflict were innocent bystanders. Many were specifically targeted. And many died of illness resulting from damage to the societal infrastructure—facilities and systems for healthcare, public health services, food and water supply, sanitation, transportation, communication, and electrical power.

Among noncombatant civilians, women and children represent especially vulnerable populations during armed conflict and its aftermath. Women—most notably those who are single and/or unaccompanied, displaced, partners of returned combatants, and survivors in postconflict zones—are at especially high risk of rape or other attacks, injuries, illnesses, and premature death.[16] Children are at increased risk of morbidity and mortality during armed conflict and its aftermath because of injuries or deaths from antipersonnel landmines and unexploded ordnance (UXO), acute and chronic malnutrition, mental health problems, displacement, and forced military service as child soldiers.[17] In addition, economic sanctions, which have often been imposed before, during, or after armed conflict, have led to shortages of food and essential medicines, especially impacting women and children.[18]

Over the course of the twentieth century, the percentage of wartime deaths among noncombatant civilians apparently increased; however, this statement is difficult to confirm because of the many obstacles to obtaining reliable data on civilian deaths during war.[19] Nevertheless, a major analysis of civilian casualties in modern warfare concluded that "it seems more than fair to conclude that since the turn of the twentieth century, civilian deaths have outnumbered military deaths in nearly all wars."[20]

Reasonably accurate estimates have been made of the number of civilian deaths during specific wars. For example, of the more than 15 million deaths during World War I,[21] an estimated 6.8 million (about 45%) were deaths of civilians.[22] Of the approximately 65.6 million deaths during World War II,[23] an estimated 45.9 million (about 70%) were deaths of civilians.[24] During the 1960s, an estimated 63% of wartime deaths were deaths of civilians; during the 1980s, an estimated 74% of war-time deaths were deaths of civilians.[25]

Recent studies performed on civilian deaths during armed conflict have utilized advanced epidemiologic methods. A review paper on the adverse consequences of the Iraq War concluded that the number of war-related deaths among Iraqi noncombatants was at least 116,903.[26] As of February 2020, an ongoing register indicated that there were between 184,868 and 207,759 documented civilian deaths from violence since the 2003 start of the Iraq War.[27] Reports from other major war zones have stated that, between October 2001 and October 2018, there were 38,480 direct deaths of civilians in Afghanistan and 23,372 direct deaths of civilians in Pakistan.[28]

The civil war in Syria has accounted for much morbidity and mortality among civilians. For example, a study found, between 2011 and 2016, 101,453 deaths due to war-related violence there among civilians, accounting for about 71% of all conflict-related violent deaths during this period. Of the 17,401 violent deaths among children during this period, about 42% were due to air bombardments, 38% to shelling, 11% to shooting, 5% to executions, 4% to ground-level explosives, and almost 1% to chemical weapons.[29] As of January 2020, there were 380,636 documented deaths in the civil war in Syria, including 115,490 civilians.[30]

Statistics are critical to understanding the nature and magnitude of injuries, illnesses, and deaths due to armed conflict. However, accurate data concerning armed conflict are difficult to obtain. In addition, statistics avoid the human dimension of the carnage of armed conflict. As my longtime colleague Victor Sidel often said, "Statistics are people with the tears washed away."

Survivors of wars are often physically and mentally scarred for the rest of their lives. Many are chronically disabled as a result of war-related injuries. Many are psychologically impaired due to physical or sexual assaults or having been forced to (a) serve in the military against their will, (b) witness the execution of family members, and/or (c) flee their homes and communities. Psychological trauma may lead to antisocial behavior, such as aggression toward others, and long-term anxiety, depression, and posttraumatic stress disorder (PTSD). During armed conflict, children may experience adverse childhood experiences, such as suffering from violence or abuse, witnessing conflict-related violence in their homes or communities, or having family members or friends injured or killed.

Results of specific studies illustrate the mental health impacts of armed conflict:

- A study of U.S. veterans of Iraq and Afghanistan wars found that the prevalence of reporting a mental health problem within 1 year after the end of deployment was 19% among military personnel returning from Iraq and 11% among those returning from Afghanistan.[31]
- Another study, which was performed on Iraq War veterans 1 year after returning from combat, found that 17% met screening criteria for PTSD.[32]

A meta-analysis, which was performed on U.S. veterans of the wars in Iraq and Afghanistan, based on 33 studies involving 4.9 million veterans, estimated that 23% had PTSD.[33] A systematic review, based on 16 articles, found that a history of PTSD is associated with (a) higher rates of morbidity and mortality and (b) an increased risk for suicidal behavior.[34] Long-term mental health problems have also been documented among child soldiers,[35] former prisoners of war,[36] and military peacekeepers.[37] Studies have also documented the long-term mental health impacts of armed conflict on noncombatant women and children, including the following:

- A cross-sectional study of psychiatric disorders among Cambodian refugees in the United States, which was performed more than 20 years after the end of the Cambodian civil war and refugee resettlement, found persistently high rates of trauma-associated psychiatric disorders, such as PTSD and major depression.[38]
- A study of exposure to violence and mental health of refugee children from the Middle East who were seeking asylum in Denmark found that 67% suffered from anxiety and 30% from sleep disturbance.[39]
- A study of civilian women in Herzegovina who had been exposed to traumatic war and postwar events had a significantly higher prevalence of PTSD (28%) than women who were not directly exposed (4.4%), and they manifested significantly more posttraumatic symptoms, such as anxiety and depression.[40]

A systematic review of the effects of war, terrorism, and armed conflict on young children, based on 35 studies that included 4365 young children, found that these effects include PTSD and posttraumatic stress symptoms, behavioral and emotional symptoms, sleep problems, disturbed play, and psychosomatic symptoms.[41]

Damage to the Health-supporting Infrastructure

Much of the morbidity and mortality during war and its aftermath is caused by damage to, or total destruction of, the health-supporting infrastructure of society. During the civil war in the Democratic Republic of the Congo, the vast majority of the more than 5 million deaths were due to damage to societal infrastructure, including facilities and systems for healthcare, public health services, and food and water supply.[42]

Environmental Consequences

Armed conflict and the preparation for armed conflict cause many adverse impacts on the physical environment. In urban environments, bombing and shelling destroy buildings, water and sanitation systems, and transportation networks. In rural environments, bombing and shelling destroy farm buildings, irrigation systems, roads, and other key components of the agriculture sector. Armed conflict causes unintended consequences; for example, bombs dropped during the Vietnam War produced craters that filled with water, which became breeding ponds for mosquitoes that transmitted malaria.

Military forces use substantial amounts of nonrenewable resources, such as timber and minerals as well as fossil fuels, the burning of which contributes to ambient air pollution and climate change. Many military activities, such as production, storage, and use of weapons, generate toxic and radioactive wastes that contaminate air, soil, surface water, and groundwater.

Military activities have destroyed ecosystems. For example, the U.S. military's use of chemical defoliants, such as Agent Orange during the Vietnam War, destroyed forests and their ecosystems. Military forces have deployed antipersonnel landmines, which have made large tracts of land uninhabitable and uncultivatable—sometimes for decades.[43]

Forced Displacement

Globally, as of February 2020, there were 25.9 million refugees, 41.3 million internally displaced people, and 3.5 million asylum seekers.[44] Many of them had been forced to flee their homes and communities during armed conflict to try to avoid injuries, illnesses, and death; protect their personal security; and meet their basic needs. Some sought refuge with friends or families elsewhere within their own countries. Others fled to other countries, where they received assistance from bilateral aid agencies and international organizations. Those internally displaced within their own countries often found it difficult to meet their basic needs and were vulnerable to malnutrition, infectious diseases, and injuries as well as physical and sexual trauma by criminals and military personnel.

Violation of Human Rights

Armed conflict often violates *political and civil rights,* which relate to democracy and freedom, as well as *social and economic rights,* which relate to social justice. These rights are embodied in international human rights, treaties, declarations, and laws, such as the Charter of the United Nations, the Universal Declaration of Human Rights, the International Covenant on Social and Political Rights, and the Convention on the Prevention and Punishment of the Crime of Genocide.

Armed conflict also violates *life integrity rights,* which transcend both political and civil rights and social and economic rights. Life integrity rights "include the right to life; the right to personal inviolability—not to be hurt; the right to be free of arbitrary seizure, detention, and punishment; the freedom to own one's body and labor; the right to free movement without discrimination; and the right to create and cohabit with family."[45]

Illustrative violations of international humanitarian and human rights law include the following:

- Direct assaults on civilians by conventional means;
- Ethnic cleansing and extrajudicial killings;
- Direct assaults on civilians caused by indiscriminate weapons;
- Indirect assaults on civilian populations; and
- Violations of medical neutrality.

International laws to protect human rights during war include humanitarian law and human rights law.

During the eighteenth century, the category of human rights law that addresses the obligations of combatants—since known as humanitarian law—was established. These combat-related obligations established rights of people and institutions to be protected during war. In 1782, a treaty between the United States and Prussia ensured that, if there were a war between these two countries, women and children, scholars, farmers, artisans, and others who were unarmed and were residing in unfortified places—and all people whose occupations were for "the common subsistence and benefit of mankind"—should not be "molested."[46] These treaties established the principle that noncombatant civilians are not legitimate targets during war[47]—a concept that was ultimately enshrined in The Hague Conventions of 1899 and 1907 and the Geneva Conventions of 1949.[48] The aforementioned international peace conferences in The Hague led to The Hague Conventions on the Laws and Customs of War. The Hague Convention of 1899, the first major treaty of international humanitarian law, addressed treatment of spies and prisoners of war; prohibition of weapons, arms, or material "of a nature to cause superfluous injury"; obligation to warn before bombardment; the duty to spare hospitals and buildings devoted to religion, arts, and charity; and the administration of occupied territory.[49] The Hague Convention of 1907 reaffirmed the 1899 convention and addressed compensation for belligerents when regulations were violated.

In 1920, the Covenant of the League of Nations helped to settle nonviolently some disputes that could have led to armed conflict.[50] Its first objective was "the acceptance of obligations not to resort to war." The Covenant stated that any war or threat of war would be a matter of concern to the entire League of Nations, and that the League was mandated to "take any action that may be deemed wise and effectual to safeguard the peace of nations."[50]

In 1928, the United States and 10 other countries signed A Treaty Providing for the Renunciation of War as an Instrument of National Policy—since known as the Kellogg-Briand Pact. Eventually, 66 nations acceded to the Pact, which still remains in force. It condemned recourse to war and renounced war as a national policy instrument. In short, it outlawed war. Parties agreed that any disputes among them should only be resolved by peaceful means. However, the Pact lacked an enforcement mechanism.[51]

Given the numerous wars that have occurred since 1928, one could mistakenly conclude that the Kellogg-Briand Pact was an utter failure. However, after the Pact entered into force, countries no longer had the legal right to wage war or to benefit from armed conflict by retaining territory—or people—afterward.[52] The Kellogg-Briand Pact not only changed the law, but it also changed behavior. Between 1816 and 1928, there had been about one territorial conquest globally every 10 months; since World War II, there has been only one every 4 years. In addition, the average annual amount of territory seized as a result of war has decreased from 114,088 square miles between 1816 and 1928 to 5772 square miles since World War II. Furthermore, from 1929 to 1948, much land that had been seized before 1948 *was returned to the countries that had previously held that land.*[52]

In 1938, the League of Nations adopted a resolution that further protected noncombatant civilians during armed conflict. The resolution stated that any aerial attack on military objectives "must be carried out in such a way that civilian populations in the neighborhood are not bombed through negligence."[53]

In June 1945, shortly after the end of World War II, the United Nations Charter was adopted in San Francisco. It stated, in part: "Armed force shall not be used, save in the common interest." It further stated: "All Members shall refrain in their international regulations from the threat or use of force against the territorial integrity or political independence of any state, or in any other manner inconsistent with the Purposes of the United Nations." The Charter described limited conditions under which the Security Council could authorize use of armed force and conditions in which UN member states could use armed force in self-defense.[54]

In 1949, representatives of 64 nations met in Geneva to adopt four conventions—now called the Geneva Conventions, which addressed the conditions of armed forces who were wounded or sick in the field and at sea, treatment of prisoners of war, and protection of civilians during war. The Conventions stated that individuals not actively

According to UNHCR: "Refugees are people fleeing conflict or persecution"; they "are defined and protected in international law, and must not be expelled or returned to situations where their life and freedom are at risk." "Internally displaced people stay within their own country and remain under the protection of the government, even if that government is the reason for their displacement." Asylum seekers are people "whose request for sanctuary has yet to be processed."

participating in hostilities should be protected against violence to life and person, cruel treatment, torture, humiliation, degrading treatment, and summary execution.[55] In 1977, added to the 1949 Geneva Conventions were two protocols related to protection of victims of international and noninternational conflict.[56]

In 1987, the Convention against Torture and Other Cruel, Inhuman, or Degrading Treatment or Punishment entered into force. The Convention defines torture as "any act by which severe pain or suffering, whether physical or mental, is intentionally inflicted on a person," by or with the acquiescence or approval of an agent of the state, for purposes such as the obtaining of a confession, punishment for an act committed or suspected of having been committed, intimidation or coercion, or discrimination. It stated: "Each State Party shall take effective legislative, administrative, judicial or other measures to prevent acts of torture in any territory under its jurisdiction." It further stated: "No exceptional circumstances whatsoever, whether a state of war or a threat of war, internal political instability or any other public emergency, may be invoked as a justification of torture."[57] Making countries and individuals accountable is central to preventing torture. Civil, criminal, or administrative laws and regulations can be used to implement this accountability. After the U.S. government chose not to prosecute two people who designed and implemented the Central Intelligence Agency's program of torture in the years following the 9/11 attacks, some victims filed civil suits against those responsible for torturing them; on the eve of the trial, the case was settled.[58]

Military Expenditures and the Diversion of Resources

Global military expenditures in 2018 were estimated at $1.822 billion—more than in any other year since the end of the Cold War in 1991.[59] These expenditures represented 2.1% of gross domestic product (GDP) globally—$239 per person.[59] The United States, with $649 billion (3.2% of its GDP) in military expenditures, accounted for more than one-third of the global total. U.S. military expenditures were 45% greater than that of next four countries combined: China ($250 billion), Saudi Arabia ($67.6 billion), India ($66.5 billion), and France ($63.8 billion).[59]

Military expenditures divert huge amounts of human and financial resources from health and human services and other societal needs. Illustrative of this diversion of resources, the United States ranks first among countries in both military expenditures and export of conventional weapons, but 43rd in infant mortality rate and 30th in life expectancy.[60,61] The ratio of health expenditures to military expenditures per capita varies among countries (Table 14-1).

President Dwight D. Eisenhower accurately described this diversion of resources in 1953 when he said: "Every gun that is made, every warship launched, every rocket fired signifies, in the final sense, a theft from those who hunger and are not fed, those who are cold and not clothed. This world in arms is not spending money alone. It is spending the sweat of its laborers, the genius of its scientists, the hopes of its children."[62]

Armed Conflict Leads to Further Violence

Armed conflict often creates a cycle of violence, including self-directed violence and interpersonal violence. Military veterans often return home while continuing to behave with a "battlefield mentality," sometimes leading to acts of violence against family members or others in their communities.

Armed conflict teaches people, including children, that violence is an acceptable—if not the preferred—method for resolving conflicts. It is therefore not surprising that the activity of teenage gangs is often similar to that of military forces.

Countries are sometimes plagued by ethnic violence that continues from one generation to the next. It has been said that, after years of "an-eye-for-an-eye" retaliation, everyone has become blind.

Types of Weapons

Conventional Weapons

Conventional weapons, which include small arms and light weapons, explosives, and incendiaries, account for most of the carnage in armed conflicts. Among conventional weapons, small arms (firearms) are the weapons of choice and sometimes the sole weapons used. Small arms—pistols, revolvers, rifles, shotguns, submachine guns, and assault rifles—all can be easily carried and used by individuals, and are generally inexpensive and easy to maintain. Heavy conventional weapons and weapon systems include battle tanks, armored combat vehicles, large-caliber artillery systems, combat aircraft, attack helicopters, warships, and missiles or missile systems.[63]

TABLE 14-1 COMPARISON OF HEALTH AND MILITARY EXPENDITURES, SELECTED COUNTRIES

Country	Population (in millions) (2018)[a]	Per-Capita Health Expenditures (2018 or latest available)[b]	Per-Capita Military Expenditures (2018)[c]	Ratio of Per-Capita Health Expenditures to Per-Capita Military Expenditures
Japan	126.5	$4,766	$368	12.95
Germany	82.9	$5,986	$597	10.03
Brazil	209.5	$1,282	$133	9.64
United Kingdom	66.5	$4,070	$752	5.41
United States	327.2	$10,586	$1,983	5.34
Turkey	82.3	$1,227	$231	5.31
France	67.0	$4,965	$952	5.22
India	1,352.6	$209	$49	4.27
China	1,392.7	$688	$180[d]	3.82[d]
South Korea	51.6	$3,192	$835	3.82
Russia	144.5	$1,514	$425	3.56

[a]The World Bank. Population, total. https://data.worldbank.org/indicator/SP.POP.TOTL. Accessed February 28, 2020.
[b]Organisation for Economic Co-operation and Development. Health spending. https://data.oecd.org/healthres/health-spending.htm. Accessed February 28, 2020.
[c]Derived from: Tian N, Fleurant A, Kuimova A, et al. I. Global developments in military expenditure. In: *Stockholm International Peace Research Institute. SIPRI Yearbook 2019: Armaments, Disarmament and International Security*. Oxford, UK: Oxford University Press; 2019, p. 194; and The World Bank. Population, total. https://data.worldbank.org/indicator/SP.POP.TOTL. Accessed February 28, 2020.
[d]Based on estimated military spending for 2018.

The international arms trade provides conventional weapons to armies, militias, insurgent groups, and individuals throughout the world. It increases availability of small arms, which enables people to resort to violence as a means of resolving disputes. It leads to domestic and community violence. It contributes to armed conflict and the threat of armed conflict. In addition, it diverts resources.

For 2018, the annual value of the international arms trade was estimated at approximately $60 billion—not including domestic sales of small arms. During the 2014–18 period, the volume of the international arms trade in major conventional weapons increased by 7.8% over the previous 5-year period, to reach its highest level since the end of the Cold War. In 2018, the five largest arms exporting countries were the United States ($10.5 billion), Russia ($6.4 billion), France ($1.7 billion), Germany ($1.3 billion), and China ($1.0 billion),[59] and the five largest recipients of major conventional weapons were Saudi Arabia ($3.8 billion), Australia ($1.6 billion), China ($1.6 billion), India ($1.5 billion), and Egypt ($1.5 billion).[59]

Explosive Remnants of War

Explosive remnants of war, which consist of antipersonnel landmines, UXO, and abandoned explosive ordnance, pose long-term threats of injury or death in many countries affected by armed conflict. Those injured or killed by explosive remnants of war are generally noncombatant civilians, primarily low-income adults and children living in rural areas of LMICs that are, or have previously been, in war zones. Because injuries resulting from explosive remnants of war tend to occur in remote areas, many victims die before they can receive medical care. Explosive remnants of war often remain in place for many years after armed conflict, posing long-term threats to nearby residents and internally displaced people—and making large areas uncultivatable and uninhabitable. At least 82 countries have been affected socioeconomically by explosive remnants of war.[64]

A systematic mixed-studies review of the effect of explosive remnants of war on global public health, based on 54 studies, yielded the following findings: More men than women were injured or killed by landmines or UXO. The mean age of casualties ranged from approximately 19 to 38 years in various studies. At the time of injury, victims were likely to be performing an activity of economic necessity. Across 12 of these studies, the proportion of casualties due to landmines or UXO among those younger than 18 years of age ranged from 22% to 55%. In these studies, among all landmine and UXO victims, 28–83% had one or more limbs amputated. Landmines and UXO adversely affected "internally displaced populations and returning refugees, physical security, economic productivity, child health and educational attainment, food security, and agriculture."[65]

The production and deployment of antipersonnel landmines has substantially decreased since the Convention on the Prohibition of the Use, Stockpiling, Production and Transfer of Anti-Personnel Mines and on Their Destruction (the Anti-Personnel Mine Ban Convention or the Mine Ban Treaty) entered into force in 1997. The four core aims of the Convention are ensuring universal adherence, destroying stockpiled mines, clearing mine areas, and assisting victims. As of February 2020, there were 164 countries (states parties) and one additional signatory (the Marshall Islands) to the Mine Ban Treaty. Thirty-two other countries had neither signed nor ratified it, including the United States, China, and Russia; most of these countries do not actually use or produce antipersonnel landmines.[66] In 2018, it was estimated that as many as 30 of the countries that had neither signed nor ratified the treaty were stocking antipersonnel landmines; the largest stockpilers and their estimated stockpiles were Russia (more than 26 million), Pakistan (6 million), India (4–5 million), China (less than 5 million), and the United States (3 million).[67]

Chemical Weapons

Chemical weapons are designed to kill or disable people by toxic mechanisms. They are relatively easy to produce and deploy, and their effects are often devastating. Chemical weapons have been deployed to target military personnel and noncombatant civilians. People are vulnerable because chemical weapons are silent and difficult to detect. Chemical agents, which can persist for long periods of time, can contaminate food, water, and the physical environment.

There are four major categories of traditional chemical agents:

- *Asphyxiants* include: (a) simple asphyxiants, such as carbon dioxide and nerve gases, which displace oxygen in confined or closed spaces, leading to oxygen deficiency; and (b) chemical asphyxiants, such as carbon monoxide and cyanides, which interfere with cellular respiration, oxygen transport, or both, thereby causing tissue hypoxia.
- *Cholinesterase inhibitors*, which include the nerve agents sarin and VX, inhibit the enzyme acetylcholinesterase leading to cholinergic overstimulation.
- *Respiratory tract irritants (choking agents)* include chlorine and lacrimogenic agents ("tear gas").
- *Vesicants and skin caustics (blister agents)* include sulfur mustard, arsenical vesicants (such as lewisite), and halogenated oximes.[68]

The toxicologically relevant features of chemical agents and their mechanisms of toxic action have been described in detail elsewhere.[69]

Chemical weapons have been used since about 1000 BCE, when China's military used arsenical smoke as a weapon. During the Peloponnesian War (460–445 BCE), Sparta used noxious smoke and flame against cities. During World War I (1914–18), France used ethyl bromoacetate grenades against Germany; Germany used xylyl bromide against Russia; Germany used chlorine gas against the Allies, which responded with chlorine gas; Germany used phosgene and diphosgene against France, which responded with hydrogen cyanide and cyanogen chloride; and Germany used mustard gas against France. During World War II (1939–45), chemical agents were used to kill millions of people in Nazi concentration camps.

Between 1919 and 1988, there were at least eight other armed conflicts—in Russia, Morocco, Abyssinia, Manchuria, Yemen, Vietnam, Iraq, and Iran—in which chemical weapons were used.[68] In addition, in 1994 and 1995, a Japanese cult, Aum Shinrikyo, released sarin, a highly toxic nerve agent, in a terrorist attack in subways in two Japanese cities, killing 19 people and injuring thousands. Since 2012, Syrian President Bashar al-Assad has used chemical weapons, likely sarin and chlorine gas, during the Syrian civil war at least 13 times, killing hundreds of noncombatant civilians.[70]

A total of 71,000 tons of chemical weapons have been declared. Russia, which has declared 40,000 tons, and the United States, which has declared 30,000 tons, represent the two countries with the vast majority of declared chemical weapons. Six other countries, including Albania, India, Iraq, South Korea, Libya, and Syria, have also declared chemical weapons.[71]

The Chemical Weapons Convention (CWC), which came into force in 1997, bans the development, production, acquisition, stockpiling, transfer, and use of chemical weapons. It requires each participating country to destroy its chemical weapons and facilities that produce these weapons as well as weapons it has abandoned in other participating countries. The CWC also places restrictions and obligations on civilian chemical industries regarding production, processing, and use of relevant chemicals. The Organisation for the Prohibition of Chemical Weapons was established in The Hague to ensure implementation of the provisions of the CWC. As of February 2020, 193 countries had signed the CWC; one country (Israel) had signed, but not yet ratified it; and three countries (Egypt, North Korea, and South Sudan) had neither signed nor ratified it.[72] The use of chemical weapons in Syria by Bashar al-Assad has been in clear violation of the CWC.

Development of chemical weapons based on traditional technologies may have reached its limit; however, further development of chemical weapons is occurring, based on modern scientific and technical disciplines.[71] A recently recognized concern is a category of highly dangerous organophosphorus chemical warfare agents known as Novichoks; these agents have not been included in formalized CWC schedules.[73]

Biological Weapons

Biological weapons are composed of bacteria, viruses, and other microorganisms and their toxins, which can cause illness in humans and can adversely affect agricultural resources and food supplies. Biological weapons evoke fear because they cannot be seen, can spread easily from person to person, and can cause horrific diseases.

Over the past 2600 years, there have been a number of reports of the use of biological weapons, but many of these have not been verified.[74] Exposure to biological agents has been confirmed in several instances, including the following:

- In the mid-1700s, during the French and Indian War, a British commander sent smallpox-infected blankets to Native Americans.
- During World War I, the German military implemented a global campaign to spread infectious diseases, such as anthrax and glanders, in animals.
- During World War II, Japan used biological agents that caused the deaths of thousands of Chinese civilians.
- In 1942, the British government contaminated Gruinard Island, which is off the coast of Scotland, with anthrax spores during a test of biological agents on sheep.
- In 1979 near Sverdlovsk, a Soviet military research facility accidentally released anthrax spores, which caused at least 76 fatal cases of anthrax.
- In 1984 in Oregon, more than 750 people developed *Salmonella* gastroenteritis after members of a religious commune deliberately contaminated restaurant food.
- In 2001, a person or persons who have never been identified disseminated anthrax spores through the United States Postal Service, causing 23 cases of anthrax, five of which were fatal.

A detailed history of the use of biological weapons has provided a critical review of the literature on the history of biological warfare and related activities.[74]

To promote preparedness for potential terrorist attacks, the Centers for Disease Control and Prevention (CDC) has identified three categories of biological agents:

- Category A consists of biologic agents that can be easily disseminated or transmitted from person to person, result in high mortality rates, have the potential for a major public health impact, might cause public panic and social disruption, and require special action for public health preparedness. Agents in this category include those that cause anthrax, botulism, plague, smallpox, tularemia, and viral hemorrhagic fevers, such as filoviruses (including the Ebola virus), the Marburg virus, and arenaviruses (including the Lassa virus).[75]
- Category B includes biological agents that are moderately easy to disseminate, result in moderate morbidity rates and low mortality rates, and require specific enhancements of CDC's diagnostic capacity and enhanced disease surveillance. Biologic agents include those that cause brucellosis, glanders, melioidosis, psittacosis, Q fever, typhus fever, viral encephalitis, water safety threats (such as *Vibrio cholera* and *Cryptosporidium parvum*), and food safety threats (such as *Salmonella* and *Shigella* species, and *Escherichia coli* O157:H7), as well as epsilon toxin of *Clostridium perfringens*, ricin toxin from castor beans, and staphylococcal enterotoxin B.[75]
- Category C agents include emerging pathogens that could be engineered for mass dissemination in the future because of availability, ease of production and dissemination, and potential for high morbidity and mortality rates as well as major health impact, such as Nipah virus and hantavirus.[75]

The Convention on the Prohibition of the Development, Production and Stockpiling of Bacteriological (Biological) and Toxin Weapons and on Their Destruction—often referred to as the Biological Weapons Convention (BWC)—was the first international treaty to ban an entire category of weapons of mass destruction. It entered into force in 1975. The BWC bans the development, production, transfer, or use of biological weapons.[76] As of February 2020, a total of 183 countries had signed and ratified the BWC; four countries had signed, but not ratified it; and 10 countries, including the United States, had not signed or ratified it.

Although the BWC states that use of biological weapons would be "repugnant to the conscience of mankind," implementation of this treaty has been less than satisfactory. At one of the recent BWC Review Conferences, state parties agreed only on a small number of issues, "which could put into question the role the BWC should play in countering biological threats in the future."[77] There is much evidence of a lack of political will or interest in the BWC among its states parties, as reflected in limited provision of reports by states parties and inadequate financial support of the Convention.[78]

Nuclear Weapons

Nuclear weapons, which release vast amounts of energy by fission and/or fusion, generate huge explosive forces, create extraordinarily high temperatures, and emit ionizing radiation. They have had profound global consequences for more than 70 years. The detonation by the United States Air Force of nuclear weapons over Hiroshima and Nagasaki, Japan, in August 1945 at the end of World War II, caused by the end of that year more than 200,000 deaths—due to heat, blast force, and ionizing radiation.

Atomic bomb survivors of Hiroshima and Nagasaki have been studied for 63 years by the Atomic Bomb Casualty Commission and its successor, the Radiation Effects Research Foundation. The primary component of this research, the Life Span Study, which gathered and analyzed information on mortality and cancer incidence of approximately 120,000 atomic bomb survivors and control subjects, found that the survivors experienced increased rates of various malignancies, including leukemia and cancers of the oral cavity, esophagus, stomach, colon, liver, lung, skin (nonmelanocytic), female breast, ovary, urinary bladder, brain/central nervous system, and thyroid. The highest excess relative risks were found for cancers of the bladder, female breast, and lung followed by cancers of the brain/central nervous system, ovary, thyroid, colon, and esophagus. The highest excess absolute risks were found for cancers of the female breast, stomach, colon, lung, liver, bladder, and thyroid.[79] The Adult Health Study, a clinical follow-up of a subset of about 20,000 subjects from the Life Span Study, found increased occurrence of noncancer effects among survivors, including cataracts, thyroid nodules, hyperparathyroidism, heart disease, and stroke.[79] Psychological and social effects, especially anxiety and somatization symptoms, among survivors have been documented.[80]

More than 2000 nuclear weapons tests, extensive research, and large-scale production of nuclear weapons has led to contamination of air, water, and soil, causing human disease and damage to ecosystems. Many people residing downwind of open-air nuclear tests received large doses of radiation; hundreds of thousands of them likely developed cancer.[81,82]

As of February 2020, nine countries—the United States, Russia, the United Kingdom, France, China, Israel, India, Pakistan, and North Korea—possessed almost 13,475 nuclear weapons; the United States and Russia had 91% of them.[83] Current concerns include the proliferation of nuclear weapons, an accidental launch of nuclear weapons,[84] a terrorist attack by nonstate actors, and the huge costs of maintaining and modernizing of nuclear weapons arsenals—which represent a major diversion of resources.

Even a limited nuclear war, such as between India and Pakistan, could cause a "nuclear winter" with widespread famine.[85] A more extensive nuclear war could kill millions of people and threaten the survival of the human species. As Daniel Ellsberg, an activist and former U.S. military analyst, stated in his 2017 book *The Doomsday Machine: Confessions of a Nuclear War Planner*: "The arsenals and plans of the two superpowers represent not only an insuperable obstacle to an effective global antiproliferation campaign: they are themselves a clear and present existential danger to the human species, and most others."[86]

Several international treaties pertain to the possession, proliferation, testing, and other aspects of nuclear weapons:

- *The Partial Test Ban Treaty (PTBT) of 1963*: This treaty prohibited tests of nuclear weapons in the atmosphere, under water, and in outer space.
- *The Comprehensive Nuclear-Test-Ban Treaty (CTBT)*: This treaty, considered to be an expansion of the PTBT, prohibits explosions of nuclear weapons, but does not prohibit computer simulations and subcritical tests. As of February 2020, the CTBT had been ratified by 168 countries and signed, but not ratified, by another 16. However, entry into force of the CTBT requires ratification by the 44 nuclear-capable countries; by February 2020, only 36 of these countries had ratified the CTBT and eight had not, including China, Egypt, India, Iran, Israel, North Korea, Pakistan, and the United States.
- *The Treaty on the Nonproliferation of Nuclear Weapons (the Nuclear Nonproliferation Treaty or NPT)*: This treaty restricts the transfer of certain technologies related to nuclear weapons. It commits countries possessing nuclear weapons to "good-faith negotiations" on nuclear disarmament. As of February 2020, a total of 191 countries had ratified the treaty, including all five of the nuclear-armed countries that it recognizes: China, France, Russia, the United Kingdom, and the United States.
- *The Treaty of the Prohibition of Nuclear Weapons (TPNW)*: This treaty, which is similar to the chemical and BWCs, bans nuclear weapons, including their possession. This treaty makes it illegal for its parties to develop, test, produce, acquire, possess, store, transfer, transport, plan to use (or threaten to use), or actually use nuclear weapons. The treaty also requires that nuclear-armed countries that become parties to the treaty destroy their nuclear weapons and terminate their nuclear-weapons programs. It also mandates that parties assist victims of nuclear weapons testing and use, and it also requires that areas contaminated by nuclear weapons be environmentally remediated.[87] As of February 2020, the treaty had been signed by 81 countries and ratified by 35; however, none of the nuclear-armed countries had either signed or ratified the treaty.

Armed Conflict Due to Climate Change and to Shortage of Freshwater

Climate change is causing major environmental consequences, including global warming, changes in precipitation, extreme weather events, and sea-level rise.[88,89] Since the mid-1800s, ambient temperature has risen about 1°C (1.8°F) and is likely to increase 1°C or substantially more by the year 2100.[90] In addition, heat waves are hotter, more frequent, and longer lasting.[91] Climate change is also contributing to extremes of precipitation, with increased rainfall and a higher risk of flooding in some areas, decreased rainfall with higher risk of drought in other areas, and, in many areas, a higher proportion of precipitation occurring in the form of downpours. Climate change is also causing, in some regions, more frequent hurricanes, cyclones, and other extreme weather events.[90] Extremes of precipitation and warmer temperatures are reducing crop yields and, in turn, reducing food security.[92]

Average sea level, which increased about 8 inches during the past 100 years (about the same amount as during the previous 2000 years),[93] will probably increase at least 12 more inches by 2100. Given recent reports of increases in the melting rates of the Greenland Ice Sheet and parts of Antarctica, sea-level rise by the end of this century may be substantially more.[94,95]

Climate change causes or contributes to the incidence of a variety of health consequences: heat-related disorders; respiratory and allergic disorders, such as exacerbations of asthma and allergic rhinitis; vectorborne, waterborne, and foodborne infectious diseases; injuries from extreme weather events; and mental health problems.[88] Higher ambient temperature also reduces worker productivity, especially in tropical areas, resulting in adverse economic consequences.[96]

The Intergovernmental Panel on Climate Change has projected that, in the absence of effective adaptation measures, climate change will adversely impact production of major crops in areas where temperature increases are 2°C or more above late-twentieth-century temperature.[97] By 2050, climate change could cause more than 25 million cases of malnutrition in children.[98]

Decreased food security and decreased availability of freshwater are forcibly displacing many people, increasing risks to their health and safety and the risks for socioeconomic and political instability and armed conflict. By 2050, climate change could displace 200 million people.[99]

Although climate change is rarely the only cause of armed conflict, it can contribute to the start or persistence of conflict.[100,101] Many studies in different time periods and in different geographical locations as well as two large meta-analyses have addressed the association between climate change and conflict.[102,103] One of these meta-analyses, which pooled data from 60 longitudinal studies, concluded that deviations from the normal range of precipitation and from mild ambient temperature significantly increased the risk of conflict, especially in poorer populations.[102] (Some experts have been critical of this meta-analysis, although the authors have appropriately responded to these critiques.[104,105]) The other meta-analysis, based on pooled data from 50 quantitative studies, led to a similar conclusion.[103] The following is an example of the sequence of conditions that can lead to armed conflict: Increased temperature and/or droughts or floods can (a) cause crop failures and damage to farmland, leading to (b) food shortages, loss of income, and distress migration by farmers and their families from rural to urban areas, leading to (c) socioeconomic and political instability, and (d) armed conflict.

In addition to climate change, population growth and other factors are contributing to water shortages, especially in Africa, the Middle East, and South Asia. Water scarcity affects at least 700 million people globally. In addition, another 1.6 million face economic water shortages, in which countries lack the infrastructure to optimally utilize water from rivers and aquifers.[106] In addition to causing health impacts, an inadequate supply of water can lead to shortages of food and energy and may restrict industrial development.

Water-related conflicts have been increasing, primarily during the past three decades (Table 14-2).[107] (The sharp increases in this century may represent, in part, an artifact of increased reporting.) Most of these conflicts have occurred in the context of violence, although water-related armed conflict has occurred relatively infrequently.[107]

Scarcity of water is infrequently the only cause of water-related conflicts. Underlying causes of these conflicts include dependency on only one major water source, high population growth and rapid urbanization, modernization, and industrialization, and a history of armed combat and poor relations between countries and among groups within countries.

Sharing of water between countries is common, with about 60% of water flowing into all rivers being shared by two or more countries. While this shared use of water represents a potential cause of conflict, cooperative agreements have been developed and implemented in many shared river basins.[108]

TABLE 14-2 WATER CONFLICTS, 1800–2019, BY YEAR BEGUN

Time Period	Number of Conflicts Begun	Average Number Per Year
1800–1899	14	0.14
1900–1999	177	1.77
2000–2009	220	22.00
2010–2019	466	46.60

Source: Adapted from Gleick PH. The water conflict chronology. 2019. http://worldwater.org/water-conflict/. Accessed February 28, 2020.

Genocide

Genocide (ethnic cleansing), which has occurred in the midst of armed conflict, is a crime under international law. As defined in the Convention on the Prevention and Punishment of the Crime of Genocide (1948), "Genocide means any of the following acts committed with intent to destroy, in whole or in part, a national, ethnical, racial or religious group, as such:

1. Killing members of the group;
2. Causing serious bodily or mental harm to members of the group;
3. Deliberately inflicting on the group conditions of life calculated to bring about its physical destruction in whole or in part;
4. Imposing measures intended to prevent births within the group; and
5. Forcibly transferring children of the group to another group."[109]

Examples of genocide have included the following: 1 million ethnic Armenians, Assyrians, and Greeks killed in the Ottoman Empire from 1915 to 1923; 6 million Jews and 5 million Slavs, Roma, people with disabilities, Jehovah's Witnesses, homosexuals, and political and religious dissidents killed in the Holocaust in Europe from 1933 to 1945; 800,000 Tutsis and moderate Hutus killed in the Rwandan genocide in 1994; and 300,000 people, mainly Muslims, killed in Darfur, Sudan, in 2004.[110] Genocide may begin with pogroms (violent riots intended to persecute, injure, or kill members of a specific ethnic or religious group), such as Kristallnacht (the Night of Broken Glass), a pogrom against Jews carried out by paramilitary forces and civilians throughout Nazi Germany in November 1938.

The United Nations has permitted intervention, including use of armed force, in some genocides. It authorized intervention in 1999 in Kosovo to prevent ethnic cleansing of Kosovar Albanians. However, it did not intervene in the Rwandan genocide in 1994. In this context, debate continues on both (a) how "genocide" is defined and documented and (b) the authority of the United Nations or individual countries to intervene in genocide.

There have been several other genocides in which the United States and other countries have not intervened. A detailed analysis has demonstrated how U.S. governmental officials and other U.S. citizens convinced themselves that refugees who had escaped from these genocides were exaggerating their reports, that intervention would have been of no use, and that these genocides were not as significant as those in the past.[111]

What Needs To Be Done

Preventing Armed Conflict and Its Adverse Health Consequences

The following two public health frameworks of prevention, among others, can be used to identify opportunities to prevent armed conflict and to minimize its health consequences.

1. *Primordial, primary, secondary, and tertiary prevention*: Primordial prevention examines root causes of (or risk factors for) armed conflicts, such as militarism, enmity among ethnic groups, and social and economic inequities. Primary prevention prevents war or other forms of armed conflict before they begin. Secondary prevention prevents or minimizes the consequences of armed conflict after it has begun. And tertiary prevention treats or improves the health and environmental consequences of war, including:
   - Restoring essential services and systems;
   - Rehabilitating and reintegrating people who have been severely injured or psychologically impaired due to armed conflict;
   - Repairing damage to the physical and sociocultural environments;
   - Advocating for prompt return and restoration of communities and livelihoods;
   - Opposing forced relocation or forced return of people to insecure environments;
   - Promoting and supporting programs for truth, justice, and reconciliation; and
   - Implementing additional measures to prevent more violence.

   Considering the above four types of prevention can help identify opportunities to break cycles of violence and help achieve peace.[112]
2. *The host-agent-environment framework*: Applying this framework, "host" represents people at risk, "agent" represents weapons and the military, and "environment" represents the conditions in which people live (Fig. 14-1). Strategies can be developed within this framework to prevent armed conflict and its health consequences, such as the following:
   - *Strategies aimed at people*, including promoting understanding and tolerance, social and economic interdependence among nations, nonviolent resolution of conflicts, and developing the popular and political will to prevent armed conflict and its consequences;
   - *Strategies aimed at weapons and the military*, including controlling the arms trade, reducing or eliminating weapons of mass destruction, reducing military expenditures, and intervening in conflicts to prevent their becoming violent; and
   - *Strategies to improve the conditions in which people live*, including protecting human rights and civil liberties, reducing poverty and economic disparities, improving education and employment opportunities, and ensuring personal security and legal protections.

Roles of Health Professionals

Health professionals can play important roles in preventing armed conflict and minimizing its health consequences.[113–115] These roles include the following:

- Educating other health professionals, policymakers, and the general public;
- Documenting the health consequences of armed conflict;
- Developing strategies to prevent armed conflict and its health consequences;
- Advocating for policies and actions to prevent armed conflict and minimize its adverse health consequences; and
- Treating the victims of armed conflict.

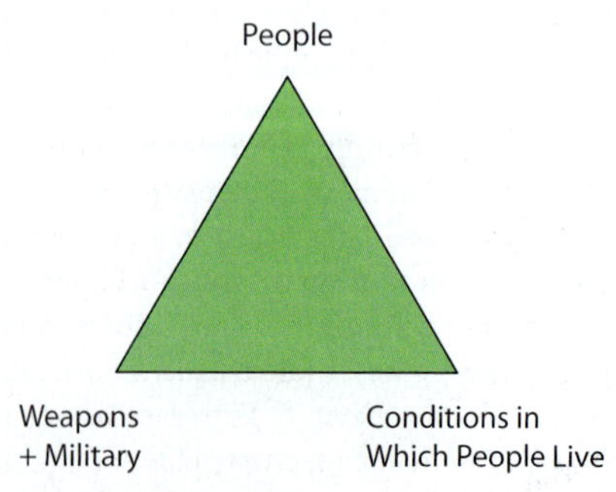

FIGURE 14-1. Armed Conflict and the host-agent-environment framework

Educating Other Health Professionals, Policymakers, and the General Public

Health professionals can actively participate in informing, educating, and communicating information to other health professionals, political leaders and policymakers, and the general public about the adverse health consequences of armed conflict. An especially important role is educating others about the hazards of nuclear weapons and ways to prevent nuclear war.[116]

Health professionals can also educate themselves and others about the causes of war, including militarism. Some observers propose that militarism be considered a psychosocial disease, one that masks the inherent irrationality of war.[117]

Peace and health are interrelated. Peace is necessary for nations and their citizens to achieve their full health potential. Armed conflict adversely affects both the health of individuals and the health of nations. Rights related to peace and health are enshrined in several international treaties and conventions.[118] The "Peace through Health" approach consists of health workers adopting a public health perspective concerning armed conflict, working to prevent or reduce violence as a cause of morbidity and mortality, and promoting peace as an important determinant of health for all people.[119]

Documenting the Health Consequences of Armed Conflict

Assessing and documenting the adverse health consequences of armed conflict can be done with public health surveillance, epidemiological studies, and rapid assessment activities. It is difficult to accurately document the adverse health consequences of armed conflict for a number of reasons, including inadequate or absent data systems, social breakdown, forced migration, reporting biases, difficulties in distinguishing between combatants and noncombatant civilians, inadequate attention to civilian mortality and morbidity, and the "fog of war."[120] Assessing and documenting the health consequences of armed conflict have been hampered by the lack of adequate resources, adequate coordination, and adequate mechanisms to prevent bias.

Assessing the health consequences of armed conflict is important not only in its aftermath, but also in the midst of armed conflict. It is important to gather and analyze data on the health consequences in order to adequately respond to the needs of civilian populations that are adversely affected—to ensure that prompt and appropriate care is provided to those who have been injured or are suffering other health consequences, such as malnutrition or infectious disease. It is also critically important for health professionals to be involved in the investigation and documentation of violations of human rights and of medical neutrality during armed conflict and its aftermath.[121]

An independent mechanism, established and maintained by a United Nations agency or a multilateral organization, is needed to investigate, document, and report on the health consequences of armed conflict.[120] In addition, programs need to be established to train individuals in methodologies for studying, documenting, and reporting on the adverse health effects of armed conflict on population health.

Developing Strategies to Prevent Armed Conflict and Its Health Consequences

Strategies need to be developed to prevent armed conflict and its health consequences. For example, a surveillance framework should be established to identify risk factors that indicate the likelihood of imminent armed conflict, the identification of which could lead to interventions to prevent violence. In addition, measures need to be implemented to better protect noncombatant civilians and to maintain medical neutrality to ensure access to medical care and public health services during armed conflict.[122,123]

Advocating for Policies and Actions to Prevent Armed Conflict and Minimize Its Health Consequences

Health professionals can play important advocacy roles. Advocacy is often most effective by working with professional associations, such as the American Public Health Association, the American Medical Association, the American Nursing Association, and the National Association of Social Workers, and with nongovernmental organizations, such as Physicians for Human Rights as well as Physicians for Social Responsibility and other national affiliates of the International Physicians for the Prevention of Nuclear War.

There are many relevant advocacy activities, such as:

- Promoting nonviolent conflict resolution;
- Decreasing military spending and the international trade in conventional weapons;
- Working for the abolition of nuclear weapons[124];
- Strengthening and promoting adherence to the CWC, the BWC, and the Mine Ban Treaty;
- Supporting peace-promoting and peacekeeping activities[125];
- Protecting noncombatant civilians and ensuring medical neutrality during armed conflict;
- Ensuring that human rights are respected, protected, and fulfilled; and
- Ensuring access to medical care for people who have been physically or mentally injured and/or displaced during armed conflict.

Treating the Victims of Armed Conflict

Health professionals have important roles in treating the victims of armed conflict, for both their physical and psychosocial disorders and impairments. Health professionals should always maintain medical neutrality, given their obligation to treat injured or ill noncombatant civilians and military personnel (including prisoners of war), regardless of their nationality or affiliation. Health professionals also have important roles in humanitarian emergencies related to armed conflict, such as providing clinical and public health services in camps for refugees and others displaced by armed conflict. They also have important roles to play in improving health in the aftermath of armed conflict, including restoring health facilities and health systems, training health workers, and addressing social determinants of health.

Ethical dilemmas may arise for physicians and other health professionals serving in the military. In battlefield and other situations, they may be faced with difficult problems of mixed agency, in which they have obligations to optimize the "fighting strength" of the military and to protect national security, while at the same time working in the best interests of individual soldiers. Physicians may also face ethical dilemmas concerning (a) participating in military research related to health and (b) obeying orders that conflict with their values and ethical assessments of situations.[126]

Although they may lack a local perspective or a keen understanding of factors related to the conflict, external health professionals (those who do not live in the zone of combat) may bring with them connections to international aid organizations as well as entities that may help bring an end to conflict or offer protection for noncombatant civilians and health workers. An important focus needs to be placed on psychosocial interventions for children affected by armed conflict—interventions that are vitally important for breaking cycles of violence.[127,128]

CONCLUSION

Health professionals have many vital roles to play in preventing or minimizing the health consequences of armed conflict. However, the only way to prevent all of the adverse health consequences of armed conflict is to totally eliminate armed conflict.[129]

ACKNOWLEDGMENT

The author acknowledges the excellent assistance of Heather McStowe, who assisted with literature review and prepared the manuscript.

References

1. Levy BS, Sidel VW, eds. *War and Public Health*. 2nd ed. New York: Oxford University Press; 2008.
2. Themnér L, Wallensteen P. Patterns of organized violence, 2002–11. In: *Stockholm International Peace Research Institute. SIPRI Yearbook 2013: Armaments, Disarmament and International Security*. Oxford, UK: Oxford University Press; 2013, pp. 41–2.
3. Krug EG, Dahlberg LL, Mercy JA, et al. Collective violence. In: *World Report on Violence and Health*. Geneva: World Health Organization; 2002, p. 215. http://www.who.int/violence_injury_prevention/violence/global_campaign/en/chap8.pdf?ua=1. Accessed April 16, 2019.
4. Stockholm International Peace Research Institute. *SIPRI Yearbook 2019: Armaments, Disarmament and International Security*. Oxford, UK: Oxford University Press; 2019, p. 33.
5. Coghlan B, Ngoy P, Mulumba F, et al. *Mortality in the Democratic Republic of Congo: An Ongoing Crisis*. International Rescue Committee. New York: International Rescue Committee; 2007, p. ii. https://www.rescue.org/sites/default/files/document/661/2006-7congomortalitysurvey.pdf. Accessed April 16, 2019.
6. Kloos H. Health impacts of war in Ethiopia. *Disasters*. 1992;16:347–54.
7. Levy BS. Increasing risks for armed conflict: Climate change, food and water insecurity, and forced displacement. *Int J Health Serv*. 2019;49:682–91.
8. Goodman PS. The post-World War II order is under assault from the powers that built it. *The New York Times*. March 26, 2018. https://www.nytimes.com/2018/03/26/business/nato-european-union.html. Accessed April 29, 2019.
9. Haberman C. 'This is not a drill': The threat of nuclear annihilation. *The New York Times*. May 13, 2018. https://www.nytimes.com/2018/05/13/us/nuclear-threat-retro-report.html. Accessed April 29, 2019.
10. Levy BS, Sidel VW. Collective violence caused by climate change and how it threatens health and human rights. *Health Hum Rights*. 2014;16:32–40.
11. Levy BS, Sidel VW. Editorial: Water rights and water fights: Preventing and resolving conflicts before they boil over. *Am J Public Health*. 2011;101(5):778–80.
12. Toole MJ. Forced migrants: Refugees and internally displaced persons. In: Levy BS, ed. *Social Injustice and Public Health*. 3rd ed. New York: Oxford University Press; 2019, pp. 213–28.
13. Rummel RJ. *Death by Government: Genocide and Mass Murder since 1900*. New Brunswick, NJ, and London: Transaction Publications; 1994.
14. Tirman T. *The Death of Others: The Fate of Civilians in America's Wars*. New York: Oxford University Press; 2011.
15. Slim H. *Killing Civilians: Method, Madness, and Morality in War*. New York: Columbia University Press; 2008.
16. Ashford M-W. The impact of war on women. In: Levy BS, Sidel VW, eds. *War and Public Health*. 2nd ed. New York: Oxford University Press; 2008, pp. 193–206.
17. Levy BS, Sidel VW. War, terrorism, and children's health. In: Landrigan PJ, Etzel RA, eds. *Textbook of Children's Environmental Health*. New York: Oxford University Press; 2014, pp. 537–45.
18. Ali MM, Blacker J, Jones G. Annual mortality rates and excess deaths of children under five in Iraq, 1991–98. *Popul Study (Camb)*. 2003;57:217–26.
19. Roberts A. Lives and statistics: Are 90% of war victims civilians? *Survival*. 2010;52:115–36.
20. Epps V. Civilian casualties in modern warfare: The death of the Collateral Damage Rule. Georgia Journal of International and Comparative Law. August 28, 2013. https://digitalcommons.law.uga.edu/cgi/viewcontent.cgi?article=1036&context=gjicl. Accessed April 23, 2019.
21. Hoschschild A. *To End All Wars: A Story of Loyalty and Rebellion, 1914–1918*. New York: Houghton Mifflin Harcourt Publishing Company; 2011.
22. White M. Source list and detailed death tolls for the primary megadeaths of the twentieth century. Necrometrics. http://necrometrics.com/20c5m.htm. Accessed April 23, 2019.
23. Ferguson N. *The War of the World: Twentieth-Century Conflict and the Descent of the West*. New York: Penguin Press; 2006.
24. White M. National death tolls for the Second World War. Necrometrics. http://necrometrics.com/ww2stats.htm#ww2chart. Accessed April 23, 2019.
25. Sivard RL. *World Military and Social Expenditures 1996 (16th ed.)*. 1996. http://www.ruthsivard.com/wmse96selections.html. Accessed April 23, 2019.
26. Levy BS, Sidel VW. Adverse health consequences of the Iraq War. *Lancet*. 2013;381:949–58.
27. Iraq Body Count. https://www.iraqbodycount.org/. Accessed February 29, 2020.
28. Crawford NC. *Human Cost of the Post-9/11 Wars: Lethality and the Need for Transparency*. Watson Institute for International and Public Affairs, Brown University, Providence, Rhode Island, November 2018. https://watson.brown.edu/costsofwar/files/cow/imce/papers/2018/Human%20Costs%2C%20Nov%208%202018%20CoW.pdf. Accessed April 23, 2019.
29. Guha-Sapir D, Schlüter B, Rodriguez-Llanes JM, et al. Patterns of civilian and child deaths due to war-related violence in Syria: A comparative analysis from the Violation Documentation Center dataset, 2011–16. *Lancet Glob Health*. 2018;6:103–10.
30. Syrian Observatory for Human Rights. http://www.syriahr.com/en/?p=152189. Accessed February 29, 2020.
31. Hoge CW, Auchterlonie JL, Milliken CS. Mental health problems, use of mental health services, and attrition from military service after returning from deployment to Iraq or Afghanistan. *JAMA*. 2006;295:1023–32.
32. Hoge CW, Terhakopian A, Castro CA, et al. Association of posttraumatic stress disorder with somatic symptoms, healthcare visits, and absenteeism among Iraq war veterans. *Am J Psychiatry*. 2007;164:150–3.
33. Fulton JJ, Calhoun PS, Wagner HR, et al. The prevalence of posttraumatic stress disorder in Operation Enduring Freedom/Operation Iraqi Freedom (OEF/OIF) veterans: A meta-analysis. *J Anxiety Disord*. 2015;31:98–107.
34. Pompili M, Sher L, Serfaini G, et al. Posttraumatic stress disorder and suicide risk among veterans. *J Nerv Ment Dis*. 2013;201:802–12.
35. Bayer CP, Klasen F, Adam H. Association of trauma and PTSD symptoms with openness to reconciliation and feelings of revenge among former Ugandan and Congolese child soldiers. *JAMA*. 2007;298:555–9.
36. O'Donnell C, Cook JM, Thompson R, et al. Verbal and physical aggression in World War II former prisoners of war: Role of posttraumatic stress disorder and depression. *J Trauma Stress*. 2006;19:859–66.
37. Gray MJ, Bolton EE, Litz BT. A longitudinal analysis of PTSD symptom course: Delayed-onset PTSD in Somalia peacekeepers. *J Consult Clin Psychol*. 2004;72:909–13.
38. Marshall GN, Shell TL, Elliott MN, et al. Mental health of Cambodian refugees 2 decades after resettlement in the United States. *JAMA*. 2005;294:571–9.
39. Montgomery E, Foldspang A. Seeking asylum in Denmark: Refugee children's mental health and exposure to violence. *Eur J Public Health*. 2005;15:233–7.
40. Pine DS, Castillo J, Masten A. Trauma, proximity, and developmental psychopathology: The effects of war and terrorism on children. *Neuropsychopharmacology*. 2005;30:1781–92.
41. Slone M, Mann S. Effects of war, terrorism and armed conflict on young children: A systematic review. *Child Psychiatry Hum Dev*. 2016;47:950–65.
42. Coghlan B, Brennan R, Ngoy P, et al. *Mortality in the Democratic Republic of Congo: Results from a Nationwide Survey*. New York: International Rescue Committee and Burnet Institute; 2004.
43. Westing AH. The impact of war on the environment. In: Levy BS, Sidel VW, eds. *War and Public Health*. 2nd ed. New York: Oxford University Press; 2008, pp. 69–84.
44. UNHCR: The UN Refugee Agency. Figures at a glance. https://www.unhcr.org/figures-at-a-glance.html. Accessed February 28, 2020.
45. Annas GJ, Geiger HJ. War and human rights. In: Levy BS, Sidel VW, eds. *War and Public Health*. 2nd ed. New York: Oxford University Press; 2008, p. 37.
46. Friedman I, ed. *The Law of War: A Documentary History*. New York: Random House; 1972, p. 150.
47. Gnaedinger A, Director-General of the International Committee of the Red Cross. *The Protection of Civilians in Armed Conflict*. Statement to the United Nations Security Council, December 10, 2002. https://unispal.un.org/DPA/DPR/unispal.nsf/0/4D0C7607540DEF7685256C8E0059A814. Accessed April 18, 2019.
48. International Committee of the Red Cross. Rule 1: The Principle of Distinction between Civilians and Combatants. http://www.icrc.org/customary-ihl/eng/docs/v1_rul_rule1. Accessed April 18, 2019.
49. Convention (II) with Respect to the Laws and Customs of War on Land and its annex: Regulations concerning the Laws and Customs of War on Land. The Hague, July 29, 1899. https://ihl-databases.icrc.org/ihl/INTRO/150?OpenDocument. Accessed April 18, 2019.

50. Covenant of the League of Nations. http://avalon.law.yale.edu/20th_century/leagcov.asp. Accessed April 18, 2019.
51. The Kellogg-Briand Pact. http://avalon.law.yale.edu/subject_menus/kbmenu.asp. Accessed April 18, 2019.
52. Hathaway OA, Shapiro SJ. Outlawing war? It actually worked. *The New York Times*, September 2, 2017. https://www.nytimes.com/2017/09/02/opinion/sunday/outlawing-war-kellogg-briand.html. Accessed April 18, 2019.
53. Schindler D, Toman J. *The Laws of Armed Conflict: A Collection of Conventions, Resolutions and Other Documents.* 4th ed. Dordrecht, The Netherlands: Martinus Nijhoff Publishers; 2004.
54. United Nations Charter. https://www.un.org/en/charter-united-nations/. Accessed April 18, 2019.
55. Convention (IV) relative to the Protection of Civilian Persons in Time of War. Geneva, August 12, 1949. https://ihl-databases.icrc.org/ihl/385ec082b509e76c41256739003e636d/6756482d86146898c125641e004aa3c5. Accessed April 18, 2019.
56. Protocol Additional to the Geneva Conventions of 12 August 1949, and relating to the Protection of Victims of International Armed Conflicts (Protocol I), June 8, 1977. https://ihl-databases.icrc.org/ihl/INTRO/470. Accessed April 18, 2019.
57. United Nations Human Rights Office of the High Commissioner. Convention against Torture and Other Cruel, Inhuman or Degrading Treatment or Punishment. https://www.ohchr.org/en/professionalinterest/pages/cat.aspx. Accessed April 18, 2019.
58. Rubenstein LS, Iacopino V. Preventing torture. In: Levy BS, ed. *Social Injustice and Public Health (Third Edition).* New York: Oxford University Press; 2019, p. 567.
59. Stockholm International Peace Research Institute. *SIPRI Yearbook 2019: Armaments, Disarmament and International Security.* Oxford, UK: Oxford University Press; 2019, p. 194.
60. Central Intelligence Agency. The World Factbook: Infant Mortality Rate. https://www.cia.gov/library/publications/resources/the-world-factbook/rankorder/2091rank.html. Accessed February 28, 2020.
61. Central Intelligence Agency. The World Factbook: Life Expectancy at Birth. https://www.cia.gov/library/publications/the-world-factbook/rankorder/2102rank.html. Accessed February 28, 2020.
62. Eisenhower DD. *The Chance for Peace.* Address delivered before the American Society of Newspaper Editors, Washington, DC, April 16, 1953. https://www.eisenhower.archives.gov/all_about_ike/speeches/chance_for_peace.pdf. Accessed April 3, 2019.
63. United Nations. General and complete disarmament: A Second Review Conference of the Parties to the Convention on the Prohibition of Military or Any Other Hostile Use of Environmental Modification Techniques, A/RES/46/36, December 6, 1991. http://www.un.org/documents/ga/res/46/a46r036.htm. Accessed April 8, 2019.
64. Borrie J. *Explosive Remnants of War: A Global Survey.* London: Landmine Action; 2003, p. 11.
65. Frost A, Boyle P, Autier P, et al. The effect of explosive remnants of war on global public health: A systematic mixed-studies review using narrative synthesis. *Lancet Public Health.* 2017;2:e286–96.
66. International Campaign to Ban Landmines. Treaty status: The Mine Ban Treaty. http://www.icbl.org/en-gb/the-treaty/treaty-status.aspx. Accessed February 29, 2020.
67. International Campaign to Ban Landmines—Cluster Munition Coalition. *Landmine Monitor 2018*:16. http://www.the-monitor.org/media/2918780/Landmine-Monitor-2018_final.pdf. Accessed February 29, 2020.
68. Lee EC, Bleek PC, Kales SN. Chemical weapons. In: Levy BS, Sidel VW, eds. *Terrorism and Public Health.* 2nd ed. New York: Oxford University Press; 2012, pp. 183–202.
69. Schwenk M. Chemical warfare agents: Classes and targets. *Toxicol Lett.* 2018;293:253–63.
70. Arms Control Association. Timeline of Syrian chemical weapons activity, 2012–2019. https://www.armscontrol.org/factsheets/Timeline-of-Syrian-Chemical-Weapons-Activity. Accessed February 29, 2020.
71. Pitschmann V. Overall view of chemical and biochemical weapons. *Toxins* 2014;6:1761–84.
72. Chemical Weapons Convention. https://www.opcw.org/chemical-weapons-convention. Accessed February 29, 2020.
73. Kloske M, Witkiewicz A. Novichoks: The A group of organophosphorus chemical warfare agents. *Chemosphere.* 2019;221:672–82.
74. Carus WS. The history of biological weapons use: What we know and what we don't. *Health Secur.* 2015;13:219–55.
75. Centers for Disease Control and Prevention. Emergency preparedness and response: Bioterrorism Agents/Diseases. https://emergency.cdc.gov/agent/agentlist-category.asp. Accessed April 3, 2019.
76. Convention on the Prohibition of the Development, Production and Stockpiling of Bacteriological (Biological) and Toxin Weapons and on Their Destruction. https://www.un.org/disarmament/wmd/bio/. Accessed April 18, 2019.
77. Feakes D. The Biological Weapons Convention. *Rev Sci Tech.* 2017;36:621–8.
78. Millett K. Financial woes spell trouble for the Biological Weapons Convention. *Health Secur.* 2017;15:320–2.
79. Douple EB, Mabuchi K, Cullings HM, et al. Long-term radiation-related health effects in a unique human population: Lessons learned from the atomic bomb survivors of Hiroshima and Nagasaki. *Disaster Med Public Health Prep.* 2011;5:S122–33.
80. Yamada M, Izumi S. Psychiatric sequelae in atomic bomb survivors in Hiroshima and Nagasaki two decades after the explosions. *Soc Psychiatry Psychiatr Epidemiol.* 2002;37:409–15.
81. International Physicians for the Prevention of Nuclear War, and Institute for Energy and Environmental Research. Radioactive Heaven and Earth: The Health and Environmental Effects of Nuclear Weapons Testing In, On and Above the Earth. New York: Apex Press; 1991.
82. Prăvălie R. Nuclear weapons test and environmental consequences: A global perspective. *AMBIO.* 2014;43:729–44.
83. Ploughshares Fund. World nuclear weapon stockpile. Updated January 13, 2020. https://www.ploughshares.org/world-nuclear-stockpile-report. Accessed February 29, 2020.
84. Forrow L, Blair BG, Helfand I, et al. Accidental nuclear war—A post-Cold War assessment. *N Engl J Med.* 1998;338:1326–31.
85. Baum S. The risk of nuclear winter. Federation of American Scientists, May 29, 2015. https://fas.org/pir-pubs/risk-nuclear-winter/. Accessed April 18, 2019.
86. Ellsberg D. *The Doomsday Machine: Confessions of a Nuclear War Planner.* New York: Bloomsbury USA; 2017, p. 20.
87. Egeland K, Hugo TG, Løvold M, Nystuen G. The nuclear weapons ban treaty and the non-proliferation regime. *Med Confl Surviv.* 2018; 34:74–94.
88. Levy BS, Patz JA, eds. *Climate Change and Public Health.* New York: Oxford University Press; 2015.
89. Luber G, Lemery J. *Global Climate Change and Human Health: From Science to Practice.* San Francisco, CA: Jossey-Bass; 2015.
90. Stocker TF, Qin D, Plattner G-K, et al., eds. Climate change 2013: The Physical Science Basis. Contribution of Working Group 1 to the Fifth Assessment of the Intergovernmental Panel on Climate Change; 2013. https://www.ipcc.ch/report/ar5/wg1/. Accessed April 19, 2019.
91. Basu R. Disorders related to heat waves. In: Levy BS, Patz JA, eds. *Climate Change and Public Health.* New York: Oxford University Press; 2015, pp. 87–103.
92. Myers SS, Smith MR, Guth S, et al. Climate change and global food systems: Potential impacts on food security and undernutrition. *Annu Rev Public Health* 2017;38:259–77.
93. Field CB, Barros VR, Dokken DJ, et al., eds. Climate Change 2014: Impacts, Adaptation, and Vulnerability. Contribution of Working Group II to the Fifth Assessment Report of the Intergovernmental Panel on Climate Change; 2014. https://www.ipcc.ch/report/ar5/wg2/. Accessed April 19, 2019.
94. Schwartz J. Greenland's melting ice nears a 'tipping point,' scientists say. *The New York Times.* January 21, 2019. https://www.nytimes.com/2019/01/21/climate/greenland-ice.html. Accessed April 19, 2019.
95. Pierre-Louis K. Antarctica is melting three times as fast as a decade ago. *The New York Times.* June 13, 2018. https://www.nytimes.com/2018/06/13/climate/antarctica-ice-melting-faster.html. Accessed April 19, 2019.
96. Kjellstrom T, Briggs D, Freyberg C, et al. Heat, human performance, and occupational health: A key issue for the assessment of global climate change impacts. *Annu Rev Public Health.* 2016;37:97–112.
97. Porter JR, Xie L, Challinor AJ, et al. Food security and food production systems. In: Field CB, Barros VR, Dokken DJ, et al., eds. *Climate Change 2014: Impacts, Adaptation, and Vulnerability. Part A: Global and Sectoral Aspects. Contribution of Working Group II to the Fifth Assessment Report of the Intergovernmental Panel on Climate Change.* Cambridge, UK and New York, NY: Cambridge University Press; 2014, pp. 485–533.

98. Phalkey RK, Aranda-Jan C, Marx S, et al. Systematic review of current efforts to quantify the impacts of climate change on undernutrition. *Proc Natl Acad Sci U S A.* 2015;112:E4522–9.
99. Swing WL. Foreword. In: IOM International Organization for Migration. *Migration, Environment and Climate Change: Assessing the Evidence.* Geneva, Switzerland: International Organization for Migration, 2009.
100. Levy BS, Sidel VW, Patz JA. Climate change and collective violence. *Annu Rev Public Health.* 2017;38:241–57.
101. Levy BS, Sidel VW. Collective violence caused by climate change and how it threatens health and human rights. *Health Hum Rights.* 2014;16:1–9.
102. Hsiang SM, Burke M, Miguel E. Quantifying the influence of climate on human conflict. *Science.* 2013;341(6151):1235367.
103. Hsiang SM, Burke M. Climate, conflict, and social stability: What does the evidence say? *Climatic Change.* 2014;123:39–55.
104. Bohannon J. Study links climate change and violence, battle ensues. *Science.* 2013;341:444–5.
105. Hsiang SM, Burke M, Miguel E. Supplementary materials for quantifying the influence of climate on human conflict. *Science.* 2013;341(6151). http://science.sciencemag.org/content/suppl/2013/07/31/science.1235367.dc1/hsiang.sm.pdf.
106. United Nations. Water scarcity. http://www.unwater.org/water-facts/scarcity/. Accessed April 19, 2019.
107. Gleick PH. The water conflict chronology. https://www.worldwater.org/water-conflict/. Accessed February 28, 2020.
108. Levy BS. Water and armed conflict. In: Selendy JMH, ed. *Water and Sanitation-Related Diseases and the Changing Environment: Challenges, Interventions, and Preventive Measures.* Hoboken, NJ: John Wiley & Sons, Inc; 2019, pp. 53–7.
109. United Nations General Assembly. Convention on the Prevention and Punishment of the Crime of Genocide, General Assembly Resolution 260 A (III), Article II. January 12, 1951. https://www.ohchr.org/en/professionalinterest/pages/crimeofgenocide.aspx. Accessed April 3, 2019.
110. Sidel VW, Levy BS. Genocide (text box). In: Levy BS, Sidel VW, eds. *Social Injustice and Public Health.* 2nd ed. New York: Oxford University Press; 2013, pp. 303–4.
111. Power S. *"A Problem From Hell": America and the Age of Genocide.* New York: Basic Books; 2002.
112. Arya N. Peace through Health I: Development and use of a working model. *Med Confl Surv.* 2004;20:242–57.
113. Buhmann C, Santa Barbara J, Arya N, Melf K. The roles of the health sector and health workers before, during and after violent conflict. *Med Confl Surv.* 2010;26:4–23.
114. Wiist WH, Baker K, Arya N, et al. The role of public health in the prevention of war: Rationale and competencies. *Am J Public Health.* 2014;104:e34–7.
115. Wiist WH, White SK. *Preventing War and Promoting Peace: A Guide for Health Professionals.* Cambridge, UK: Cambridge University Press; 2017.
116. Lown B. *Prescription for Survival: A Doctor's Journey to End Nuclear Madness.* San Francisco, CA: Berrett-Koehler Publishers, Inc.; 2008.
117. Coulter NA. Militarism: A psychosocial disease. *Med War.* 1992;8:7–17.
118. Arya N. Peace and health: Bridging the north-south divide (Editorial). *Med Confl Surv.* 2017;33:87–91.
119. Arya N, Santa Barbara J. *Peace through Health: How Health Professionals Can Work for a Less Violent World.* Sterling, VA: Kumarian Press; 2008.
120. Levy BS, Sidel VW. Documenting the effects of armed conflict on population health. *Annu Rev Public Health.* 2016;37:205–18.
121. Geiger HJ, Cook-Deegan RM. The role of physicians in conflicts and humanitarian crises: Case studies from the field missions of Physicians for Human Rights, 1988 to 1993. *JAMA.* 1993;270:616–20.
122. Mullan Z. Medical neutrality: Resetting the moral compass. *Lancet.* 2016;4:e215.
123. Benton A, Atshan S. "Even war has rules": On medical neutrality and legitimate non-violence. *Cult Med Psychiatry* 2015;40:151–8.
124. Helfand I, Sidel VW. Docs and nukes—Still a live issue. *N Engl J Med.* 2015;373:1901–3.
125. Johnson RJ 3rd. A literature review of medical aspects of post-cold war UN peacekeeping operations: Trends, lessons learnt, course of action and recommendations. *J R Army Med Corps.* 2016;162:250–5.
126. Sidel VW, Levy BS. Physician-soldier: A moral dilemma? In: Beam TE, Sparacino LR, specialty editors. *Military Medical Ethics: Volume 1 (Textbooks of Military Medicine).* Falls Church, VA: Office of the Surgeon General, United States Army; Washington, DC: Borden Institute, Walter Reed Army Medical Center; and Bethesda, MD: Uniformed Services University of the Health Sciences; 2003, pp. 293–312.
127. Peltonen K, Punamäki R-L. Preventive interventions among children exposed to trauma of armed conflict: A literature review. *Aggress Behav.* 2010;36:95–116.
128. Brown FL, de Graaff AM, Annan J, Betancourt TS. Annual research review: Breaking cycles of violence—A systematic review and common practice elements analysis of psychological interventions for children and youth affected by armed conflict. *J Child Psychol Psychiatry.* 2017;58:507–24.
129. Snyder BF, Ruyle LE. The abolition of war as a goal of environmental policy. *Sci Total Environ.* 2017;605–606:347–56.

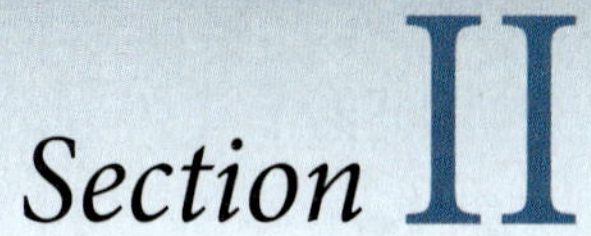

Section II

Section Editors
Judith N. Wasserheit and Jared Baeten

Global Health

CHAPTER 15

The History and Emergence of Global Health*

Kevin M. De Cock • Immaculate Mutisya • Julie Mwabe • King K. Holmes

WHAT IS GLOBAL HEALTH?

Global health is concerned with the health of all people on our planet, recognizing that the world is interconnected and that a health threat anywhere can become a threat everywhere. Hunter and Fineberg proposed a definition of global health as "public health for the world,"[1] demanding further interrogation of what is public health. In an oft-cited report, the U.S. Institute of Medicine regarded public health as what society "does collectively to assure the conditions for people to be healthy,"[2] a usefully comprehensive definition that can encompass clinical, preventive, and promotive as well as structural interventions to influence health in diverse contexts.

The philosophy of global health acknowledges the globalization of public health risks, not only the spread of infectious agents but also of other threats to public health such as tobacco use, consumption of sugar-laden drinks, unhealthy lifestyles promoting noncommunicable diseases (NCDs), unsafe or counterfeit medicines, and other factors undermining health.[3] Specific threats such as infectious agents may spread more quickly today than in earlier times because of the increased extent and speed of travel; it is now possible to traverse the world within the incubation period of most infectious diseases.

Noninfectious agents such as unhealthy foods and drinks, legal and illicit drugs, and other toxic substances are commonly distributed through increasingly globalized supply chains and marketing strategies.[4] Health is affected by the dissemination of ideas, behaviors, and cultural and recreational practices which reach and influence all corners of the world in an ever shorter time, spreading as effectively as infectious diseases. The Internet, social media, and other forms of modern communications have linked faraway places, just as air travel has bridged the physical distance that formerly kept them apart.

While global health is most definitively concerned with the well-being of our whole planet, it is also committed to health equity and concentrates much of its attention to more disadvantaged groups and areas. Encompassing priority populations, regions, and countries under a single term has proved problematic, not least because of dynamic socioeconomic development across the world. The term "Third World," often used synonymously with the "developing world," originated in the mid-twentieth century as a political concept describing countries not aligned with the First and Second Worlds, which referred, respectively, to nations affiliated to NATO or the communist Eastern Bloc. Recognition that poorer countries, described earlier as "underdeveloped and later as "developing," were mostly found in the world's southern hemisphere led to concepts of the "Global North" and "Global South" to indicate the rich and poor worlds.

All these terms have proved unsatisfactory and inconsistent over time with changes in the global landscape. The World Bank now usefully divides countries of the world into four categories based on Gross National Income per capita: high income; higher middle income; lower middle income; and low income. This categorization is reviewed annually, and countries can move up or down in the classification according to economic change. The current threshold to be defined a low-income country is a Gross National Income per capita of $1025 or less, equivalent to an income of less than $2.80 per day. While the terms "Third World" and "developing countries" remain part of the lexicon because of longstanding usage, global health science is best served by objective categorization of countries. Even the World Bank's classification suffers from deficiencies such as its obscuring of gross inequities within countries, potentially hiding priority areas or populations worthy of global health attention.

Historically, conquest of the New World brought an exchange of plants, animals, and pathogens. Indigenous people in the New World and Oceania had no immunity to smallpox, measles, or whooping cough. Cholera epidemics spread widely from South Asia, facilitated by maritime trade. The nineteenth century heralded the beginning of modern microbiology and infectious disease epidemiology, such as when John Snow famously traced the origin of an ongoing cholera epidemic to the Broad Street pump in London. The work of early microbiologists Pasteur, Lister, Koch, and Neisser soon followed, clarifying the role of microbial pathogens in causing pandemics. Sulfonamides, penicillin, waste disposal, sanitation, water chlorination, vaccines, and diagnostics were some of the advances that subsequently helped define the novel specialties of infectious diseases and public health. Today, we have emerging "super bugs," resistant to these and most other antimicrobials. Antimicrobial resistance (AMR) is very rapidly increasing in the microbes of humans and animals not only from widespread over use of antimicrobial agents but also by the geographic carriage and spread of the infectious agents. The 2016 report on Global Health from the National Academy of Medicine in the United States listed AMR as a very high priority (listed as the number two of fourteen priorities, just after "improving international emergency response coordination").[5]

In parallel with the socioeconomic changes that underlie our altered experience of health there have been natural and manmade changes to the environment, and to our very planet itself. The World Health Organization (WHO) has estimated an additional 250,000 deaths per year between 2030 and 2050 will be attributable to climate-associated increases in malnutrition, malaria, diarrhea, and heat stress, especially in elderly people.[6] Spillover effects on state and regional security are inevitable. The World Economic Forum has identified climate change as the single greatest threat to global stability[7] because of its considerable consequences on the health and development of low- and middle-income countries.

*The content of this chapter does not necessarily represent the views of the U.S. Department of Health and Human Services or the Centers for Disease Control and Prevention. The authors have no relevant financial affiliations or conflicts to disclose.

Public health has characterized challenges to populations in terms of outbreaks caused by infectious agents, toxic exposures, nutritional factors, or psychological conditions but there is now realization that the biggest threats to health may be environmental in nature. The immediate greatest uncertainty in global health may be the ultimate health impact of climate change. Broad shocks, such as climate change, make it more difficult to separate the exposed from the unexposed, a challenge to traditional epidemiology that compares health outcomes in relation to specific risk factors. The boundaries of global health have been suggested as inadequate in their lack of recognition of damage to the broader environment and the term "Planetary Health"[8] has been coined, referring to "the health of human civilization and the state of the natural systems on which it depends."

Public health and, necessarily, global health, are inherently political in nature since their practice involves the setting of priorities, the associated allocation of resources, and the effectiveness of prevention and service delivery systems. Global health is underpinned by diverse disciplines and science, especially epidemiology that usefully describes health inequities. Addressing health inequities is one of the prime aims of global health whose social basis includes commitment to social justice, defined as a fair distribution of the benefits and burdens of society.[9] This understanding of what global health is and does implies acceptance of the role and nature of the social determinants of health,[10] and of the so-called intersectoral policies for health, that fall into four broad categories: taxes and subsidies; regulation and related reinforcement mechanisms; built environments; and information. There are determinants that extend beyond individual behaviors or choices without minimizing the importance of the latter. Examples include taxation of tobacco; control of air pollution; access to healthcare; safe water supply; etc.[11] Global health, in short, strives to achieve the best health outcomes for every individual in the world.

THE ORIGINS AND EVOLUTION OF GLOBAL HEALTH

Global health's documentation in recent years has little or nothing to say about the medicinal experiences of indigenous peoples who lived in countries and continents for thousands of years before the arrival of explorers, armies, and adventurers of the European colonizing nations in the second half of the second millennium AD.

During the past 20 years, global health programs have grown dramatically. These programs have changed and diversified in focus, face new challenges and opportunities, and continue to evolve. Today, there are a wealth of useful online descriptions of who are the "Key Actors" or "Key Players" in global health, and what they are doing. There are also critiques of the "Global Health System." Modern understanding of global health has its origins in tropical medicine developed by colonizing European countries such as Great Britain, France, Belgium, Portugal, Germany, and the Netherlands in the nineteenth century and extending to the period of gaining independence from the colonial powers in the 1950s and 1960s. The legacy of this epoch extends to the present day, captured in the names and archives of institutes such as the London School of Hygiene and Tropical Medicine and the Liverpool School of Tropical Medicine in the United Kingdom, and the Institute of Tropical Medicine in Antwerp, Belgium. These institutes fulfilled the same responsibilities of academic medical institutions that pertain today: teaching, clinical work, research, and administrative and civic duties.

In addition to the military, the tropical regions of the world attracted civil servants, missionaries, traders, diverse travelers, and their dependents, all of whom required assistance to prevent or address the medical challenges associated with warm climates and unsanitary conditions. As many as one in three Europeans who ventured to West Africa in the late eighteenth and early nineteenth centuries failed to return, giving the region its fearsome reputation as "the White Man's Grave."[12] Malaria was a constant threat in tropical Africa and a leading cause of death, as were intermittent epidemics of yellow fever.[13] In Europe, with the work of giants such as Louis Pasteur, Joseph Lister, and Robert Koch, the science of microbiology advanced and the concept of microbial causes of disease became increasingly accepted. In parallel, major progress occurred in understanding of tropical diseases, their spread, and pathogenesis, through the contributions of scientists such as Sir Patrick Manson and Sir Ronald Ross. Manson, who while working in China demonstrated that filariasis was transmitted by a mosquito, is widely described as the father of tropical medicine.[14] Credit for proving that malaria was also a mosquito-transmitted disease went to Ross, a contribution for which he was awarded the Nobel Prize in Physiology or Medicine in 1902.[15]

Tropical medicine flourished and broadened as a discipline, dominated by the study of parasites, viruses, and vectors. The provision of medical care to colonial servants and travelers in the tropics or upon their return home, as well as the medical needs of military personnel deployed overseas, ensured that clinical medicine featured prominently in the evolving science. Interest and investment grew from beyond the European powers and in 1913, the Rockefeller Foundation was established in New York City, with the aim of "promoting the well-being of humanity throughout the world."[16] Although much broader in its portfolio today, the initial work of the Foundation concentrated on medical science, public health infrastructure and education, and tropical medicine. The Rockefeller Foundation committed resources to attacking specific diseases through research as well as public health interventions, targeting, for example, hookworm and yellow fever. The Foundation exemplified an early commitment to "vertical" approaches to disease intervention and also invested resources in the concept of disease eradication.

Tropical medicine in the minds of many became synonymous with clinical parasitology and diseases of poverty, and for a long time was distinct from the broader study and practice of infectious diseases. In the 1970s, the Rockefeller Foundation established its Great Neglected Diseases of Mankind program that set up a global network bridging basic science, clinical, and social sciences.[17] WHO launched its Tropical Diseases Research Programme in 1975, focusing on five parasitic and one bacterial disease: malaria, leishmaniasis, trypanosomiasis, schistosomiasis, filariasis, and leprosy.[18,19] These efforts were the precursors of today's concept of "neglected tropical diseases," characterized by WHO as a group of diverse conditions affecting the poorest in the world that had over time received inadequate attention.[19,20]

Terminology evolved in parallel with these developments, and "tropical medicine" became viewed as quaint and outdated.[21] "Geographic medicine" shed the colonial heritage that was associated with tropical medicine and in development circles, the term "international health" became increasingly used.[22,23] The late 1950s and the 1960s saw most former colonies obtain their independence; India had become independent in 1947. Postindependence, the world was divided into "developed" and "developing" countries, the latter mostly in the global south. The high-income countries of the north channeled funds into development assistance which invariably had a health component, often prioritizing maternal and child health through efforts focused on family planning, immunization, diarrheal disease control, and nutritional support. A north-south divide existed, with an emphasis on primary healthcare and preventive medicine in the resource-poor south that fostered tension between clinical services in hospitals and the needs of community medicine.[24]

Seminal documents in the evolution toward global health included the 1992 report from the U.S. Institute of Medicine on emerging infections[25]; the 1993 World Development Report ("Investing in Health")[26]; and the 2000 report of the Commission on Macroeconomics and Health.[27] Earlier outbreaks of viral hemorrhagic fevers, such as Marburg virus disease in Germany and Yugoslavia in 1967,[28] Lassa fever in Nigeria in 1969,[29] and Ebola virus disease in the Democratic Republic of Congo in 1976,[30] had drawn attention to northern vulnerability to exotic diseases of the south. Acquired immunodeficiency syndrome (AIDS), the end-stage manifestation of human immunodeficiency virus (HIV) infection, was first described from Los Angeles in 1981[31] but was quickly recognized to be widespread in sub-Saharan Africa.[32,33] The 1993 report[26] from the World Bank cogently argued that disease and death in Africa were disproportionately influenced by three conditions that were inadequately addressed, HIV/AIDS, malaria, and tuberculosis. The report highlighted the need for investment in clinical services, including surgical services, for the common conditions of ill-health, pregnancy, and injuries. The Commission on Macroeconomics and Health put forward the case that health was an essential driver of development and that the health sector should not be seen simply as a financial burden but a sound investment.

Perhaps the first time that the word "global" was used in the official lexicon was in the late 1980s when WHO's Special Programme on AIDS, the first world response to the pandemic, changed its name to the "Global Programme on AIDS" (widely referred to as GPA).[34] By the early 2000s, with the launch of the Millennium Development Goals (MDGs), creation of the Global Fund to Fight AIDS, Tuberculosis and Malaria,[35] establishment of the U.S. President's Emergency Plan for AIDS Relief (PEPFAR),[36] and the later initiation of the President's Malaria Initiative,[37] nomenclature had definitively shifted to global health.

In the 15th edition of this textbook, published 10 years ago, the chapter on International and Global Health gave an excellent overview of the rapidly developing field of global health, describing emerging globalization and interconnectedness of countries; selected health and development indicators of the burden of disease by region, and differential income levels for low- and middle-income countries; the role of Multilateral Agencies like WHO in the global eradication of smallpox, as well as the roles of UNICEF, UNDP, WORLD BANK, and UNAIDS in global health; the role of so-called bilateral agencies such as U.S. Agency for International Development (USAID) in country-to-country assistance; the work of international Non-Governmental Organizations (NGOs) such as the International Red Cross; the outstanding work of Médecins Sans Frontières (Doctors without Borders); and the work of philanthropic organizations, like the Bill and Melinda Gates Foundation, which has become a major player and contributor in global health.

In his recent memoir, William Foege, former Director of the U.S. Centers for Disease Control and Prevention (CDC), who played a key role in the eradication of smallpox, provided an important perspective in the implementation of global health programs. Dr. Foege related how, in the past, the CDC leader, David Sencer, had asked him to form a CDC committee to advise him on how CDC could best serve global health. Dr. Foege recalled that Sencer "...realized that what is good for the world is ultimately good for global health." When Dr. Foege became CDC Director, he felt that "Having the entire organization steeped in global health, rather than having a special program for global health, is best."[38]

EMERGENCE OF UNIVERSITY-BASED GLOBAL HEALTH PROGRAMS

The rapid emergence of academic programs into the global health field over the past decade is an important and relatively new phenomenon. There had been several very important examples of universities with academic programs that have long played an important role in International Health—for example—the London School of Hygiene and Tropical Medicine, Johns Hopkins University, the University of Liverpool School of Tropical Medicine, the University of Heidelberg International Health Program, the Institute of Tropical Medicine in Antwerp, and others.

However, U.K. universities now have a Global Health Research League Table, listing many U.K. global health programs. The Consortium of Universities for Global Health (CUGH), founded in the United States and Canada in 2008, now has 175 member academic institutions. Many have developed very large global health programs during the past 10 years. Interactive Global Maps show where each university now has a diversity of research, educational, or clinical health service programs (e.g., see University of Washington Department of Global Health Interactive World Map, with 699 projects in 134 countries; and the Johns Hopkins University Center for Global Health's Bloomberg School of Public Health Map of Global Health Projects throughout the world). An analysis of global health partnerships between North American and international institutions indicated that most believed these partnerships were constructive and useful.[39]

GLOBAL HEALTH GOVERNANCE

How a problem is defined strongly influences how society addresses it. Global health can usefully be analyzed through the lenses of development, security, and public health, each with its own motivations, modes of engagement and action, and supervision.[3] Richer countries invest in health interventions in faraway places for reasons that are both altruistic and self-centered; they aim to protect their own populations against disease threats, to promote economic development in poorer countries since healthy peoples and families are more likely to be productive and financially independent, to maintain political stability; and for humanitarian reasons. Protection of international travelers, of deployed military troops, civil servants and other workers, and of trading routes and practices are additional reasons to address health comprehensively and across the world.

In 2015 member states of the United Nations committed to the Sustainable Development Goals (SDGs), a broad and universal road map toward poverty elimination, protection of the planet, and promotion of human well-being. The 17 SDGs follow on from the MDGs, which covered the 15-year period from 2000. Although the SDGs and their 169 targets are interconnected, the ones most directly related to health are SDG1 (No Poverty); SDG2 (Zero Hunger); SDG3 (Good Health and Well-being); SDG5 (Gender Equality); SDG6 (Clean Water and Sanitation), and SDG17 (Partnerships). Along with funding trends, the call to action that the SDGs represent is among the strongest determinants of global health action.

A panoply of official and private actors now occupy the global health space which is much more complex than it was a few decades ago. Diverse agencies of the United Nations operate as multilateral agents in the health sector, most notably WHO, which is considered the specialized agency for health.[40] UNICEF focuses on the well-being of mothers, adolescents, and children,[41] the United Nations Population Fund on reproductive health,[42] the World Food Programme on food and nutrition,[43] the United Nations High Commissioner for Refugees on refugee issues,[44] among others. The World Bank is a major funder in global health.[45] The diversity of United Nations agencies, the need for coordination, and the potential for conflict and overlap is illustrated by the complexity of HIV/AIDS actions supported through the Joint United Nations Programme on HIV/AIDS (UNAIDS).[46]

In addition to the traditional bilateral donor agencies such as USAID, the United Kingdom's Department for International Development, and others from different high-income countries, NGOs, civil society groups, faith-based organizations, and private foundations are also active in global health. The best-financed foundation is the Bill and Melinda Gates Foundation, which in 2016 donated $1.2 billion to global health[47]; this approximates or is more than what WHO receives as "assessed contributions" from its 194 member states. Additional funding to WHO is provided as "voluntary contributions" from member states as well as other donors including the Bill and Melinda Gates Foundation, and these funds are often earmarked.

The governing body of WHO is the World Health Assembly, constituted by all member states, which comes together once annually. While this is historically the body with overall authority in global health and claims to represent essentially all countries and peoples of the world, its decision-making process is slow and cumbersome, and other actors in global health have moved to fill gaps in policies and practice. Nonetheless, WHO retains unique convening authority to bring people and countries together in a neutral way around specific health challenges, and its normative work such as provision of technical guidelines is widely respected. Although the luster of United Nations' agencies work in global health, and especially that of WHO, has faded, there remain important functions best delivered through the multilateral bodies, including coordination, presentation of global health data, tracking of financial needs and resources, advocacy, and provision of normative guidance.

A recent phenomenon is the active role in global health played by civil society groups and NGOs, which can often act more swiftly than traditional agents and are less constrained by political and other factors. Activists working in the HIV/AIDS field, for example, have exerted great pressure on formal agencies and governments to change policies and practice.[48] NGOs dealing with refugee health or specific infectious disease priorities can disproportionately influence what services are delivered where. Médecins Sans Frontières, set up in France in 1971, is active in emergency situations throughout the world, including in war zones, and has a well-justified reputation for expertise in hemorrhagic fevers, including Ebola.[49] All these groups actively contribute to the evolution of global health practice, highlighting the conservative nature and rigidity of some of the traditional institutions, but they operate with less accountability.

With the greatly increased bilateral funding for global health that was made available in the earlier part of this century, agencies of major donor countries, such as CDC[50] and USAID, have deployed hundreds of staff around the world. Amid the great changes that have occurred, a constant has been the role of faith-based and missionary organizations some of which have been working around the world since the early days of the colonial period. It has been estimated that as much as 40% of healthcare in sub-Saharan Africa is delivered through the faith-based sector, some of whose staff work in the most difficult and isolated areas for long periods of time.[51]

GLOBAL HEALTH FUNDING

Health spending worldwide remains very unequal: more than 80% of the world's population lives in low- and middle-income countries which account for only about 20% of global health expenditure.[52] In 2017, $37.4 billion of development assistance was provided to low- and middle-income countries to maintain or improve health.[53] The United States, the United Kingdom, and Germany provided $12.4, $3.3, and $2.0 billion, respectively, which represented 0.06%, 0.10%, and 0.05% of these countries' GDP. Other nations, though contributing smaller dollar figures, stood out as providing assistance from a substantial fraction of their GDP. The United Kingdom and Luxembourg devoted the highest fractions of their GDP to development assistance for health (DAH), dedicating 0.103% and 0.102%, respectively. By this metric, the United States was the sixth most generous contributor. Across health areas, maternal, newborn, and child health received the largest percentage of DAH funding in 2017 (31.0%) followed by HIV/AIDS (24.2%) and health systems strengthening and sector-wide approaches (11.3%).[53]

The health sector is an important source of real economic growth globally and particularly in low- and middle-income countries. While bilateral development agencies disburse a majority of DAH (34% between 1990 and 2017), substantial direct funding or at least investment in overall global health was provided by multilateral agencies such as The World Bank and WHO. Public–private partnerships such as the Global Fund to Fight AIDS, Tuberculosis, and Malaria (the Global Fund) and the Global Alliance for Vaccines and Immunization (GAVI) disbursed $4.6 and $1.5 billion, respectively. The public–private partnership UNITAID, which has focused especially on commodities and medicines, has pioneered an innovative financing mechanism based on a small tax on airline tickets levied by participating countries. Although some bodies have seen growth in their funding over the last decade, including the Global Fund, Gavi, NGOs, and private foundations, the period 2010–17 has witnessed a plateauing of DAH.

Despite this levelling off of direct health assistance, global health spending overall has continued to climb due to countries' own expenditures and investments. Total health spending for 2015 was estimated to be $9.7 trillion, up 4.7% from the prior year, and accounted for 10% of the world's total economy. It is estimated that this figure will reach $20.4 trillion in 2040. While this is a large increase over the $9.7 trillion spent in 2015, wide variations remain in resources available per person across and within income groups, geographic regions, and countries.[53,54]

Overall, the health sector has consistently grown faster than the general economy over the past 15 years. Between 2000 and 2015, the global health economy has grown in real terms at an average annual rate of 4.0%, compared with 2.8% for the global economy.[55] Investing in health not only leads to healthier lives, it also generates employment, fosters social and political stability, drives technological innovation, and contributes to higher productivity and economic output. Dramatic increases in total spending on HIV/AIDS since 2000 have mitigated a major global health crisis. However, the vulnerability of low-income and high-burden countries to reductions in direct health assistance is a critical issue. Tracking resources for HIV/AIDS and other specific diseases can illuminate the countries that are most vulnerable to future reductions in assistance for health and can be used to gauge progress toward goals such as the MDGs, now surpassed by the SDGs.[56]

With some sources of health spending growing and other types remaining steady, and with major variations in spending from country to country, it is important to understand the sources of health funding, how funds are spent, and how this spending aligns with health needs. This information is critical for planning and is a necessary catalyst for change as countries aim to close the gap on the unfinished agenda of the MDGs; move toward universal health coverage (UHC) in the SDGs era; contain the overwhelming impact of major diseases like HIV/AIDS, tuberculosis, and malaria; and strengthen preparedness and response capacity for unexpected shocks.

BURDEN OF DISEASE AND PRIORITY SETTING

Traditionally, WHO was the prime source of data on disease burden and trends, and its website remains an essential resource for health information and recommendations.[40] In recent time, the Institute for Health Metrics and Evaluation (IHME) at the University of Washington has taken central place with its "Global Burden of Disease" work, which is regularly published in the medical journal *The Lancet* and as individual reports.[57] With strong funding, including from the Bill and Melinda Gates Foundation, IHME is able to devote resources and staff to complex data collection and analyses in a way not possible at the less generously funded multilateral agencies. For data on HIV/AIDS, the most widely followed source of information is UNAIDS.[57,58] Nonetheless, regular reports from WHO on malaria,[59] tuberculosis,[60] neglected tropical diseases,[61] and other subjects remain important resources.

No single parameter fully describes the relative importance or impact of different diseases. Traditional measures to compare the health status of different countries have included infant and under-5 mortality rates (U5MRs), maternal mortality ratios (MMR), and life expectancy. In the typical low-income countries of the late twentieth century, close to half the population was under the age of 15 years and almost half of all deaths occurred in children under 5 years of age. Fertility rates, the average number of children per woman in the population, have tended to be high where child mortality rates were high.

As child mortality has declined through better infectious disease prevention and control, there has been a tendency for fertility rates to fall also and the relative proportion of deaths in adults versus in children has increased, a phenomenon referred to as the demographic transition. The epidemiologic transition refers to the shift from infectious to NCDs as the leading causes of death.

In 2016, there were an estimated 55 million deaths across the world.[61] Although total deaths increased slightly, age standardized mortality declined, and global life expectancy increased by a decade between 1990 and 2016, reaching 71.8 years.[61] The greatest impact on life expectancy, the average age of death for the whole population, results from reduction in child mortality. Advances in living standards and in preventive, promotive, and curative health interventions slowly increase adult longevity. With the demographic and health transitions occurring across the world, though at different rates and starting points in different settings, some infectious diseases have become less important and NCDs have emerged as major causes of mortality (Fig. 15-1 and Table 15-1). In low- and middle-income countries, the ongoing transitions mean a dual health burden with high rates of communicable and increasing rates of NCDs.

NCDs, often occurring in later life, increasingly predominate, and greater focus will be on preventable disease and premature death and how to measure the extent of loss of healthy life. There have been rare but striking shocks, which have caused precipitous increase in adult mortality and reduced life expectancy in different countries. These have included the AIDS epidemic before the advent of effective treatment; wars; genocides; breakdown of health systems, in addition to widespread alcohol abuse, in Russia after the political changes in Eastern Europe in the 1990s; and the current opioid epidemic in the United States.

For all these reasons, classic parameters such as child and maternal mortality are increasingly inadequate to describe the health status of populations. At the same time, simply charting causes of death in rank order ignores the burden of disease while people are alive, so it is important to assess the amount of years of healthy life that could have been saved or disease and death that could have been avoided. "Years of life lost" measure the amount of years at the population level between actual age of death and an arbitrarily defined life expectancy. "Disability-adjusted life years" assess the amount of fully active life lost due to a particular condition, thus combining both premature mortality and disability. Added to all these parameters should be measures of cost-effectiveness, what health can be gained for what monetary expenditure. Figure 15-1 shows leading causes of death and years of life lost, although tremendous heterogeneity exists across countries.

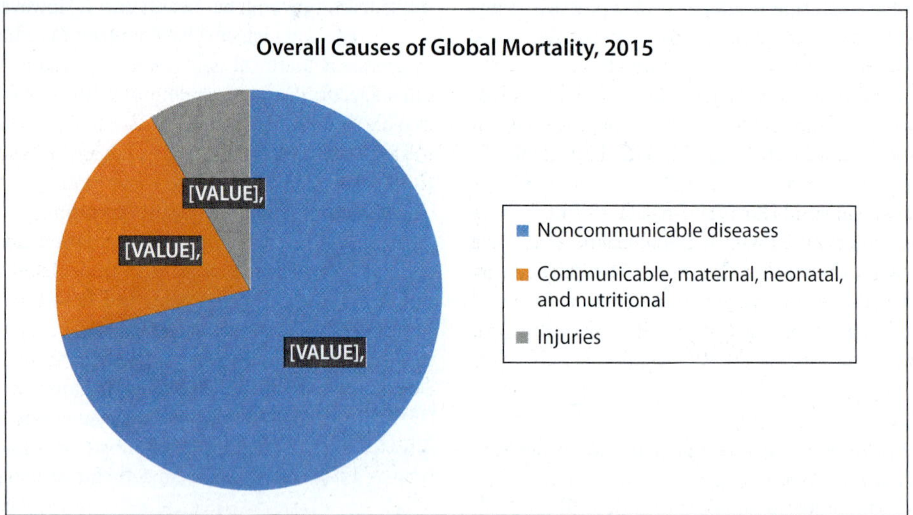

FIGURE 15-1. Overall causes of global mortality, 2015.
(*Source:* From GBD 2015 Morality and Causes of Death Collaborators. *Lancet.* 2016;388:1459–544.[57])

TABLE 15-1 LEADING GLOBAL CAUSES OF DEATH, NUMBER OF DEATHS, AND YEARS OF LIFE LOST, 2015

Cause of Death in Rank Order	Number of Deaths (Thousands)	Cause of Years of Life Lost, in Rank Order
Cardiovascular disease	17921.0	Ischemic heart disease
Neoplasms	8764.6	Cerebrovascular disease
Injuries	4725.1	Lower respiratory infections
Chronic respiratory disease	3795.5	Neonatal preterm causes
Diabetes	3409.3	Diarrheal diseases
Lower respiratory infections	2736.7	Neonatal encephalopathy
Neurologic diseases	2258.9	HIV/AIDS
Neonatal causes	2163.2	Road injuries
Diarrheal diseases	1312.1	Malaria
Chronic liver disease	1292.1	Chronic obstructive pulmonary disease
HIV/AIDS	1192.6	Congenital anomalies
Tuberculosis	1112.6	Tuberculosis
Malaria	730.5	Lung cancer

Source: GBD 2015 Mortality and Causes of Death Collaborators. *Lancet.* 2016;388:1459–544.[57]

One might expect that funding for global health would be aligned with agreed-upon priorities based on objective epidemiologic and financial measurements. Many other considerations, however, go into decisions concerning health financing including advocacy, political pressure, and historical factors. Emergencies, such as the West African epidemic of Ebola in 2014–16, can result in rapid mobilization of large sums of money; commitments to the PEPFAR and the Global Fund are longstanding earmarks; and the funding and efforts that go toward polio eradication exceed resources for other more common diseases. By contrast, financial allocations to NCDs, mental health, and injuries are disproportionately low compared to their global burden. Perhaps the most neglected of basic services is access to safe drinking water and sanitation. Although the separation of human feces from drinking water though provision of safe water and sewage systems formed the basis of the public health revolution in the nineteenth century, more than 40% of the world's population are affected by water scarcity, over 650 million people lack access to improved drinking water sources, and almost 900 million still resort to open defecation.

MATERNAL AND CHILD HEALTH

The health and well-being of mothers, neonates, infants, and children were identified as an important medical priority as early as the eighteenth century.[62] Maternal health refers to the health of mothers during pregnancy, childbirth and in the postpartum period, and child health to the health of children from birth through adolescence. Child health focuses on several periods with different challenges, neonatal health referring to the first 28 days of life, infant health from 0 to 12 months, and under-5 health dealing with children below 5 years.[63]

Attention to maternal and child health has expanded and become prioritized globally as evidenced by its specific inclusion under the MDGs (MDG 5: Improve maternal health)[35] and SDGs (SDG3.1: By 2030 reduce the global MMR to less than 70 per 100,000 live births).[64] Ending preventable deaths in neonates and in children under 5 and reducing global maternal mortality are key priorities in global health. Adverse pregnancy and neonatal outcomes, such as preterm delivery, stillbirth, and low birth weight, are often related to the health of the mother. Infant and child mortality in low- and middle-income settings are largely related to the lack of access to preventive services such as immunization while maternal mortality reflects more complex interactions across the health system including services for clinical care. The great majority of maternal and child deaths occur in low- and middle-income countries, with Africa having the greatest burden.[65]

In 2015, it was estimated that 300,000 women die during pregnancy and childbirth annually and nearly 1 million have severe complications during pregnancy, childbirth, or during the postpartum period.[66] Data on maternal deaths are captured by the MMR, the number of maternal deaths per 100,000 live births. Globally, the MMR has almost halved between 1990 and 2015 when it was estimated at 216 per 100,000 live births.[66] Some 19 countries, all in sub-Saharan Africa, have MMRs of 500/100,000 live births or greater. Sub-Saharan Africa accounts for two-thirds of all maternal deaths. In absolute numbers, because of their large populations, Nigeria and India contribute a third of maternal deaths. The lifetime risk of maternal mortality in high-income countries is of the order of 1:3300, while in the worst performing countries of West and Central Africa it is approximately 1:20.[66]

More than a quarter (27%) of all maternal deaths are due to severe bleeding, mostly after childbirth (postpartum hemorrhage). Sepsis (11%), unsafe abortion (8%), and hypertension during pregnancy (14%) are other major causes. Diseases that complicate pregnancy (indirect causes), including malaria, anemia, and HIV, account for about 28% of maternal deaths. Inadequate access to quality care during pregnancy, coupled with high fertility rates, due to unmet need for contraception and other family planning or reproductive health services, increase the lifetime risk of maternal death.

The decline in deaths in children under 5 from approximately 12.7 million in 1990 to 5.9 million in 2015 is one of the greatest achievements in global health; the U5MR over this period declined by 56%, from 91 to 43/100,000 live births.[67,68] Despite these advances, global disparities remain extreme: the risk of death in children under-5 in sub-Saharan Africa remains 1 in 13, compared with 1 in 189 in high-income countries. Overall, about 80% of under-5 deaths in 2016 occurred in South Asia and in sub-Saharan Africa; six countries accounted for half of all childhood deaths: India, Nigeria, Pakistan, the Democratic Republic of Congo, Ethiopia, and China. The highest risk of death remains in the first month of life, and trends in neonatal mortality rates have declined less than death rates in older age groups. These findings illustrate the interaction of high population numbers, adverse health indices,[67] and the urgent need for improved access to effective pediatric health services.

The global distribution of under-5 mortality, and especially that of neonatal mortality, broadly tracks that of maternal deaths. In terms of causes of neonatal deaths, complications due to premature births account for 35% of newborn deaths, followed by delivery-related complications (24%), sepsis (15%), congenital abnormalities (11%), pneumonia (6%), tetanus (1%), diarrhea (1%), and other causes of death (7%). Low birth weight is a major risk factor and indirect cause of newborn death. Newborn deaths account for just under half of child deaths (40%), followed by pneumonia (14%), diarrhea (10%), injuries (5%), malaria (7%), HIV/AIDS (2%), measles (1%), and other causes of death (18%).[67] Undernutrition significantly increases children's vulnerability to these conditions, as does the lack of access to clean water and sanitation.

Interventions that have contributed to improved child outcomes include growth monitoring, oral rehydration therapy for diarrheal disease, immunization, and promotion of breastfeeding.[67] In addition to continued emphasis on such basic and low-cost interventions, integration of disease-specific efforts such as prevention of mother-to-child transmission of HIV and use of insecticide-impregnated bed nets to prevent malaria are critically important. Neonatal welfare requires interventions to reduce maternal deaths, especially skilled care at birth and emergency obstetric care, keeping newborns warm and dry, and treating severe newborn infections. Other effective child health interventions include improved access to and use of clean water, sanitation, and hygiene practices like handwashing, improved nutrition, treatment of acute malnutrition, and the treatment of neglected tropical diseases. Strengthening health systems and increasing access to services, including through community-based clinics, are also important, and interventions have been found to be more effective when integrated within a comprehensive continuum of care.[68]

The welfare of children is profoundly affected by the general level of socioeconomic development, and MCH requirements have been given attention within the current SDGs that are broader than the MDGs that were operational over the period 2000–15. SDG2 aims to "end hunger, achieve food security and improved nutrition, and promote sustainable agriculture."[64] SDG3 aims to "ensure healthy lives and promote well-being for all at all ages," and has as specific targets reduction of the global MMR to less than 70 per 100,000 live births and an end to preventable deaths of newborns and under-5 children to at least as low as 12 per 1000 live births for neonatal mortality reduction, and for under-5 mortality, to at least as low as 25 per 1000 live births.[53] Support is required for global initiatives to assure adequate nutrition and food security to prevent growth retardation, stunting, and micronutrient deficiency.

Funding for MCH has remained among the top global health priorities, with financing from multiple sources including multilateral organizations, bilateral donor agencies, and philanthropists and foundations accounting for between one-quarter and one-third of DAH. Support for child health grew more rapidly than support for maternal health in the earlier years that global health funding was expanding.[69]

Health, including MCH, does not exist in a vacuum and for primary healthcare and public health interventions to succeed, there is need for leadership, good governance, and robust health systems that include adequate numbers of trained health workers. Political will and addressing sociocultural and religious barriers are key to success. Lastly, to track progress on the broader SDGs, there is need to improve measurement of vital statistics including registration of births and deaths; stronger disease-specific surveillance; understanding of causes of maternal and childhood deaths; and enhanced efforts to assure reliable Mother and Child Health and Nutrition indicators.

EMERGENCE OF GLOBAL COMMUNICABLE DISEASES

Microbes and humans have been constant companions, and an historic perspective of the continuing global emergence of the communicable diseases of humans was interpreted by the late Stanley Falkow. He described how the challenges of global diseases have only begun to be assessed and addressed, but in fact have been emerging and evolving over millennia. Understanding the origins and factors influencing the changing pandemics over the years could help us understand, predict, prevent, and cope with future global health threats, including the pandemic of NCDs.

All plagues have their origins in prior events, yet they always seem to catch societies by surprise. For most of human history, mankind lived in small, nomadic hunter-gatherer groups, largely isolated from neighbors. Development has been perpetual and continuous, leading a transition from agricultural to later industrial lifestyles, mixing and crowding of human populations, travel over distances, and contact with animals and new microbes, insects, rodents, and waste. Men and women evolved with their own microbiomes and microbes of other species; over half of emerging infectious diseases have a zoonotic origin. The world's most important current infection, HIV, crossed into humans from chimpanzees; falciparum malaria may have had its origin in gorillas; and microbial infections as diverse as measles, Hansen's disease (leprosy), and syphilis adapted themselves to man. As populations grew, human settlements and large cities arose, trade routes developed, plants and animals were domesticated, and plagues arose, such as the Black Death in the fourteenth century, likely due to *Yersinia pestis*.

THE BIG THREE

HIV/AIDS

Global health has been dominated in recent time by attention to three infectious diseases: HIV/AIDS, tuberculosis, and malaria. The advocacy, technical investment, and funding devoted to these three has had widespread ripple effects on health systems and other health threats.[70] Other major killers such as the hepatitis viruses have received much less attention.

In 2017, an estimated 36.9 million people were living with HIV, 940,000 persons became newly infected, and 1.3 million died.[71] AIDS mortality peaked around 2005, coinciding with the beginning of massive efforts to scale up access to antiretroviral therapy (ART).[57] Recognition that ART virtually eliminates infectiousness in persons whose viral load is suppressed[72,73] has made access to HIV testing and treatment of all infected persons a priority[74–76] leading UNAIDS to launch its 90:90:90 agenda: 90% of persons with HIV to be diagnosed, 90% of whom have access to ART, and 90% of whom have suppressed viral load.[77] By mid-2017 almost 22 million persons living with HIV were receiving ART globally.[71]

Sub-Saharan Africa, where HIV is transmitted predominantly by heterosexual sex, is the most heavily affected region. Rates of HIV infection in Central and West Africa are lower for reasons not fully understood although higher rates of male circumcision, which provides approximately 60% protection against HIV acquisition in men,[78] may be relevant. Despite the lesser severity of the epidemic in Central and West Africa, scale-up of ART should still be accelerated there.[79,80]

In most of the rest of the world HIV epidemics are described as concentrated rather than generalized, meaning they affect key populations at special risk such as men who have sex with men (MSM), people who inject drugs, and sex workers. The relative importance of each of these key populations varies internationally. For example, in Central and South America, MSM are most heavily affected. In Eastern Europe and Central Asia, which is seeing the steepest increases in HIV infection, the epidemic is driven by injected drug use. MSM seem at increased risk everywhere. While injected drug users can suffer explosive epidemics, harm reduction interventions have proved successful in containing HIV spread. Remarkable progress has been made worldwide in preventing HIV transmission through blood or blood products, and in eliminating, in some countries, or greatly reducing the transmission of HIV from mother to child. Despite the progress, HIV/AIDS remains the world's leading infectious disease challenge and the concerted response has had profound and wide-ranging influence on the conceptualization and implementation of global health activities.

Tuberculosis

In 2017, there were an estimated 10 million new cases of tuberculosis and 1.3 million deaths.[60] Twenty-five percent of cases were in the African region, and 62% in South East Asia or the Western Pacific. Five countries, three in southern Africa, had an annual incidence greater than 500/100,000 per year. According to WHO, tuberculosis is now causing more deaths than any other single infectious agent.

Tuberculosis is one infection but acts like three different diseases: classic tuberculosis, HIV-associated tuberculosis, and multidrug or extensively drug-resistant disease. HIV-associated tuberculosis accounts for 13% of world cases but for 22% of all deaths.[60] HIV infection greatly increases the risk of tuberculosis infection turning into tuberculosis disease; because southern Africa has high rates of both infections, it is this part of the world that has the highest rate of HIV-associated tuberculosis.[60] Close to half of all cases of HIV-positive cases of tuberculosis worldwide occur in southern Africa, and over three quarters in sub-Saharan Africa as a whole. There are approximately 600,000 cases annually of multidrug or extensively drug-resistant tuberculosis and a quarter of a million deaths, almost half of all those in India, China, and Russia.[60]

Tuberculosis has not had the political attention that HIV or malaria have received although this now may be changing. Scientific progress in terms of new drug development has been slow and the greatest recent advances have been in the area of diagnostics, especially with the introduction of molecular-based tests. Major challenges include incomplete detection of active cases of tuberculosis; inadequate diagnosis and treatment of drug-resistant disease; lack of use of preventive therapy; the persistent challenge of tuberculosis in persons living with HIV, despite access to ART; and prevention of tuberculosis transmission in congregate settings such as hospitals and prisons. Shortening treatment duration below 6 months with novel drugs and developing an efficacious vaccine are scientific priorities.

Malaria

WHO estimates that there were some 216 million cases of malaria in 2017, and 445,000 deaths[59] estimates from IHME (Table 15-1) were somewhat different. Between 2010 and 2016, malaria incidence rates are estimated to have declined by 18%; estimated mortality rates were heterogeneous but reduced by over one-third in Africa. Approximately 90% of cases and deaths were in WHO's Africa Region, with the rest in the South-East Asia and Eastern Mediterranean Regions. Because of the ecology of its vectors, malaria is geographically restricted to tropical regions and 80% of disease burden is concentrated in 15 countries. Almost all cases and deaths in Africa were due to *Plasmodium falciparum*, the most pathogenic of malaria parasites. The clinical impact of malaria in Africa is greatest in infants, children, and pregnant women with clinical presentations of cerebral malaria and severe anemia in the pediatric age range, and increased risk of preterm delivery and low birth weight as pregnancy outcomes. Malaria incidence and adverse outcomes are more frequent in HIV-infected pregnant women and children.

Approaches to malaria prevention and control include provision of insecticide-impregnated bed nets to populations in malaria-endemic regions; treatment with effective therapy, especially artemisinin-based combination therapy (ACT), based on parasitological diagnosis; indoor residual spraying with insecticide; intermittent therapy in pregnancy; and interventions to contain seasonal epidemics.

Although there has been substantial improvement in access to essential commodities, and the majority of patients treated in African public sector health facilities receive ACTs based on a malaria diagnostic test, less than half of households have one bed net for every two persons. Increasing emphasis globally is being placed on malaria elimination, meaning zero indigenous cases, and approximately 21 countries across the world, some in Africa, have been identified as potentially meeting this goal by 2020. By contrast, malaria remains a leading cause of child deaths in some other countries, especially in Central and West Africa. Major threats to continued progress toward malaria control and elimination include unpredictable financing, climate change affecting the ecology of the vector, conflict in malarious areas, resistance on the part of the vector to insecticides, and parasite resistance to drugs. A great concern is the resistance to artemisinin that is emerging in the Mekong Delta in South-East Asia.[81]

NEGLECTED TROPICAL DISEASES

Neglected tropical diseases are a group of conditions that include many encompassed in the old view of tropical medicine, although they may seem an assortment of diverse diseases not easily categorized elsewhere. As defined by WHO,[20] they include viral, bacterial, parasitic, fungal and chlamydial infections, as well as some noncommunicable conditions. Deep mycoses, scabies and other ectoparasites, and snakebite were added to the list in 2017.[61]

The term "neglected tropical diseases" gained prominence around 2005, after the MDGs had begun to be pursued, global health funding had greatly increased, and belated recognition occurred that the focus on HIV/AIDS, tuberculosis, and malaria left many important conditions behind.[19] WHO established a Neglected Tropical Diseases Department, and a specialist journal (*PLoS Neglected Tropical Diseases*) was established.[19]

A number of common themes link these various conditions, especially the fact that they affect over a billion of the most underprivileged people in the world, and that they occur most frequently, though not exclusively, in tropical, low-income countries. Many rarely kill but cause very longstanding infections or complications, and they have chronic and debilitating effects that interfere with daily activities such as farming and other work, blunt cognitive development, and impair school performance, may result in adverse pregnancy outcomes, and can cause disfiguring effects and blindness. These are not just medical conditions but causes of suffering, stigmatization, and exclusion, and an important impediment to socioeconomic development.

Box 15-1 shows the 20 conditions that WHO defines as neglected tropical diseases. Leishmaniasis, trypanosomiasis, schistosomiasis, filariasis, and onchocerciasis are classic tropical diseases that were included in earlier tropical medicine initiatives.[18,19] Buruli ulcer and Hansen's disease are chronic mycobacterial infections, yaws and trachoma being spirochetal and rickettsial infections, respectively.

BOX 15-1 Neglected Tropical Diseases as Defined by WHO

Chagas disease (South American trypanosomiasis),
Dengue and chikungunya
Dracunculiasis (guinea-worm disease)
Echinococcosis (hydatid disease)
Foodborne trematodiases
Human African trypanosomiasis (sleeping sickness)
Leishmaniasis (cutaneous and visceral, "kala azar")
Hansen's disease (Leprosy)
Lymphatic filariasis
Mycetoma, chromoblastomycosis, and other deep mycoses
Onchocerciasis (river blindness)
Rabies
Scabies and other ectoparasites
Schistosomiasis (bilharzia)
Soil-transmitted helminthiases
Snakebite envenoming
Taeniasis/Cysticercosis
Trachoma
Yaws (Endemic treponematoses)

Soil-transmitted helminthic infections such as ascariasis and hookworm are geographically widespread and not restricted to the tropics. Guinea worm disease has reduced vastly in incidence and prevalence thanks to efforts at eradicating the condition, the only disease currently slated for eradication other than polio.[83] Inclusion of viral diseases such as rabies, dengue, and chikungunya may seem arbitrary when other viral pathogens, especially other arboviruses, are excluded.[21]

WHO has categorized five groups of interventions to address neglected tropical diseases: preventive chemotherapy; innovative and intensified case management; vector ecology and management; use of veterinary public health services; and safe water, sanitation, and hygiene (WASH).[20] Examples of these different approaches include mass drug administration of drugs such as diethylcarbamazine and albendazole for elimination of filariasis, or ivermectin for onchocerciasis; praziquantel, sometimes delivered through school programs, is used for schistosomiasis. Case management through specific drug therapy is necessary for treatment of conditions such as human African trypanosomiasis (sleeping sickness), visceral leishmaniasis, and Hansen's disease. Vector ecology and management are relevant for diseases such as dengue and onchocerciasis. Veterinary public health services target conditions such as rabies. WASH interventions are required for guinea worm disease and trachoma.

NONCOMMUNICABLE DISEASES

NCDs are chronic conditions that result from interaction of host, environmental, and behavioral factors such as genetics, diet, physical activity, occupation, and tobacco, alcohol, and other drug use.[20] Although previously overshadowed by infectious diseases in low-income settings, NCDs have always existed throughout the world in varying proportions. NCDs are generally grouped into four categories—cardiovascular disease, chronic respiratory conditions, diabetes, and cancer—although this excludes some diseases such as the rheumatologic disorders or mental illness.

NCDs have always been present in low-income and tropical settings, where clinical medicine deals with three sets of conditions (i) the infectious diseases associated with poverty, such as sexually transmitted infections, diarrheal diseases, tuberculosis, and pneumonia; (ii) the classic tropical diseases such as malaria, which are ecologically restricted; and (iii) chronic diseases such as hypertension. Changes in lifestyle and unhealthy behaviors, such as smoking or excessive consumption of alcohol or sugar-laden drinks, affect the whole world, albeit at different rates, and the spectrum of disease worldwide has changed remarkably rapidly. Cardiovascular conditions such as rheumatic heart disease and diseases such as diabetes can be devastating conditions in poor societies with limited access to healthcare. Nonetheless, this category of conditions did not feature in earlier views of tropical medicine or international health, but very much concern modern approaches to global health.[3]

On a worldwide basis, NCDs are the most prevalent diseases in the world and the leading cause of death, responsible for about 70% of global mortality or approximately 40 million deaths annually.[84] Almost half of deaths from NCDs are from cardiovascular disease, and almost a quarter from cancers. Although rates of many NCDs may be higher in older age groups or in high-income countries, the absolute number is greater in low- and middle-income countries, and the global burden of NCDs continues to escalate. A particular feature in low-income settings is the emergence of a dual burden of disease, so that infectious and tropical diseases are still prevalent but NCDs, with their risk factors such as smoking, lack of exercise, unhealthy diet, and excess alcohol consumption, are increasing in frequency. A public health priority is addressing what must be considered premature mortality, deaths from NCDs before the "normal" life expectancy, representing between one-third and one-half of NCD deaths. Over three-quarters of such premature mortality occurs in low- and middle-income settings. Men suffer greater premature mortality than women, from NCDs as well as from other causes such as injuries, and this sex-specific inequity may be widening.

The majority of NCDs can be treated but not cured, and they tend to be lifelong. For this reason, prevention is especially important, both primary prevention (preventing the disease occurring in the first place), and secondary prevention (preventing progression or further complications). Political decision makers and others often think instinctively of tertiary medical care as the required response to NCDs, whereas policy initiatives, structural interventions, lifestyle changes, prevention of the *major* causes of NCDs (which actually include many of the infectious diseases, especially in low-income countries), and public health action can save more lives at less cost. The clinical approach to NCDs entails screening, detection, treatment, and palliative care.

WHO published the Global Action Plan for the Prevention and Control of NCDs 2013–20, and has provided guidance on enabling policy interventions and "best buys" for the four leading risk factors for NCDs, namely tobacco use, excessive alcohol use, unhealthy diet, and physical inactivity.[82,84] Critical policy actions include implementing or adopting the protocols of the WHO Framework Convention on Tobacco Control (WHO FTC); implementing WHO guidance on reducing alcohol use; and implementing global guidance on diet and physical activity. Some of the most important specific interventions include increasing taxes and prices for tobacco products and alcohol, restricting their advertising, reducing salt and sugar intake, and promoting physical exercise.

CONVERGENCE OF INFECTIOUS DISEASES AND NONCOMMUNICABLE DISEASES

As important as these specific policy interventions and best buys are for the prevention of NCDs, there is a growing awareness that infections really are, in fact, among the major causes of many of the so-called NCDs. For example, persistent infections account for an estimated attributable fraction of more than 50% of cancers in some regions in Sub-Saharan Africa.[85,86] Another important example is rheumatic heart disease caused by streptococcal infection. The World Health Federation found that, worldwide, in 2015, 33.4 million people had rheumatic heart disease, and at least 319,000 died from it.[87] Just a few examples of other "NCDs" that represent long-term complications of specific infectious diseases include cirrhosis and hepatocellular carcinoma (related to chronic hepatitis B and C virus infections); cervical cancers (human papillomavirus); peptic ulcer disease (*Helicobacter pylori*); blindness (onchoceriasis); epilepsy (cysticercosis) and brain damage; immune complex nephropathy (malaria); and stunted growth with impaired cognitive function in children (worm infestations).[88]

An article from Nigeria listed 59 infectious diseases that have played a role in the emergence of NCDs.[89] Recent reviews have further emphasized that dividing diseases into infectious diseases and NCDs is problematic.[85,86] Reddy and Hunter have asserted that even the term "noncommunicable diseases" is a misnomer—because it includes some diseases—such as cancers of the liver, stomach, and cervix noted above—that are caused by infections.[90,91]

Conversely, it is also clear that NCDs can increase susceptibility to major infections that can result in death or chronic morbidity, particularly in low- and middle-income countries, where prevalence of infection is high. Thus there is growing emphasis on the convergence of NCDs and infectious diseases in low- and middle-income countries,[90] and on the double burden of NCDs and infectious diseases in these countries.[88]

We should therefore be asking not only "what will be the global impact of AMR and of contaminated water and environments on increasing infectious disease morbidity and mortality?" but also "what will be the global impact of emerging AMR and contaminated waters and environment on the so-called "noncommunicable diseases"? Thus, coordination of programs for prevention, detection, treatment, and cure of infectious diseases should be designed to be synergistic with the important programs for detection, treatment, and cure of NCDs.

MENTAL HEALTH, INJURIES, AND SURGICAL CARE

Mental health and injuries are widespread causes of disease and death but receive little attention in global health discussion. As early as 1993, the World Development Report drew attention to the need for surgical services for injuries in low- and middle-income countries. The provision of medical and surgical care in conflict and war zones is a specialized area of work that some NGOs have prioritized, and the experience that military medical services have obtained in war settings has influenced the practice of trauma care for civilian populations.

MENTAL HEALTH

Mental health is defined by WHO as "a state of well-being in which every individual realizes his or her own potential, can cope with the normal stresses of life, can work productively and fruitfully, and is able to make a contribution to her or his community."[92] Mental disorders—in various forms and intensities—affect most of the population in their lifetime.[93] Despite the MDGs success in reducing the overall health gap between rich and poor countries, and considerable achievements for infectious diseases such as malaria or HIV/AIDS, this last generation of development goals did not include any reference to mental illness, despite the global impact of these conditions, and their cross-cutting impact on eight of the MDGs.[94] In September 2015, mental health was included in the SDGs.[95] In her Keynote address to the United Nations General Assembly, former WHO Director-General Dr. Margaret Chan noted that "The inclusion of NCDs under the health goal is a historical turning point. Finally these diseases are getting the attention they deserve."[95]

According to WHO, one in four people in the world will be affected by mental or neurological disorders at some point in their lives. Around 450 million people currently suffer from such conditions, placing mental disorders among the leading causes of ill health and disability worldwide.[95] Yet, in spite of the very considerable burden and their associated adverse human, economic, and social effects, global policy makers and funders have so far not prioritized treatment and care of people with mental illness. People with severe mental illness have up to 60% higher chances of dying prematurely from NCDs.[95] Different reasons have been proposed for the underestimation of the burden of mental illness: "(i) the overlap between psychiatric and neurological disorders; (ii) the grouping of suicide and behaviors associated with self-injury as a separate category outside the boundary of mental illness; (iii) the conflation of all chronic pain syndromes with musculoskeletal disorders; (iv) the exclusion of personality disorders in mental illness disease burden calculations; and (v) inadequate consideration of the contribution of severe mental illness to mortality from associated causes."

UHC, included under the SDGs,[55] offers opportunities for addressing this neglect of mental illnesses, which constitute, along with all cardiovascular plus circulatory disorders, the leading causes of global disease burden.[55] Achieving effective coverage will demand global commitment to increase funding for mental illness, better allocate resources, trained workforce for mental health, and improve integration of services for mental illness with other health services.

INJURIES AND SURGICAL CARE

Traditionally, surgical initiatives in global health were implemented as disease-specific, vertical interventions to meet targeted needs in resource-poor settings of the world.[55] More recent efforts to expand the breadth of such services include WHO's Emergency and Essential Surgical Care programme[96] and the World Bank's Disease Control Priorities project,[97] both of which promote the implementation of essential packages of interventions at first-level hospitals in low- and middle-income countries.

Remarkable gains have been made in global health in the past 25 years, but progress has not been uniform.[98] Mortality and morbidity from common conditions needing surgery have grown in the world's poorest regions, both in real terms and relative to other health gains. As low- and middle-income countries expand their economies and basic public health improves, NCDs and injuries comprise a growing proportion of the disease burden.[98,99] The failure to appreciate the role of surgery in addressing important public health problems is the main cause of disparities in surgical care worldwide.[99]

The lack of surgical care takes a serious human and economic toll and can lead to acute, preventable, life-threatening complications. In other instances, lack of access to care results in chronic disabilities that make productive employment impossible and impose a burden on family members and society.[97] The Lancet Commission on Global Surgery was launched in January 2014 to address the gaps in knowledge and policy around surgical services. The Commission brought together an international, multidisciplinary team of collaborators from more than 110 countries and 6 continents.[100] It was estimated that 5 billion people lack access to safe, affordable surgical and anesthesia care when needed and an additional 143 million operations are required to address emergency and essential conditions in low- and middle-income countries.[100] Additionally, of the 313 million procedures undertaken worldwide each year, only 6% occur in the poorest countries where over a third of the world's population lives. Unmet need is greatest in eastern, western, and central sub-Saharan Africa and South Asia.[100] Without urgent and accelerated investment in surgical scale up, low- and middle-income countries will continue to have losses in economic productivity, estimated cumulatively at U.S. $12.3 trillion between 2015 and 2030.[100]

Surgery should be considered an "indivisible, indispensable part of healthcare."[101] In 2015, the World Health Assembly passed a resolution strengthening emergency and essential surgical care and anesthesia as a component of UHC.[102] Although barriers such as accessibility, availability, affordability, and acceptability of surgical care as well as lack of a trained workforce hinder improvements in low- and middle-income countries, interventions to improve surgical care in these settings can be cost effective.[103] The misconception that surgical care is too costly[100] must be corrected, including by clear definition of its role in service provision and of what constitutes appropriate and minimum levels of surgical intervention.

UNIVERSAL HEALTH COVERAGE, HEALTH SECURITY, AND NATIONAL PUBLIC HEALTH INSTITUTES

Universal Health Coverage

UHC is about ensuring that people have access to the healthcare they need without suffering financial hardship or, worse, catastrophic impoverishment. UHC allows countries to make the most of their strongest asset: human capital. Health is a foundational investment in human capital and in economic growth—without good health, children are unable to go to school and adults are unable to go to work. In recent years, UHC has gained global momentum, with the World Health Assembly and the United Nations General Assembly calling on countries to "urgently and significantly scale up efforts to accelerate the transition toward universal access to affordable and quality healthcare services."[55] Along with the separate but allied subject of health security, UHC is perhaps the dominant theme in current global health discourse.[55]

In September 2015, it was agreed that health coverage should be universal. The UN General Assembly adopted UHC as part of the overall commitment to the SDGs. Included under SDG3 is a target to "achieve universal health coverage, including financial risk protection, access to quality essential healthcare services, and access to safe, effective, quality, and affordable essential medicines and vaccines for all."[64] SDG1, with the aim of ending poverty in all its forms everywhere, is also in peril without UHC, as hundreds of millions of people are impoverished by health expenses every year. UHC therefore cuts across SDGs that have health implications and brings hope of better health and protection for the world's poorest.

Achieving UHC is an ambitious goal and will require the commitment of countries to mobilize sustained resources. In particular, progress will depend on the capacity of societies to collectively mobilize resources for health and to redistribute them for better health, greater equity, and increased social cohesion. Multilateral institutions such as the World Bank, WHO, UNICEF, and others, along with bilateral development agencies, have rallied behind the concept of UHC. Leadership of WHO has made UHC the agency's highest and all-encompassing priority, with an emphasis on evidence and data as means to achieve it.[104] The collective aim is to galvanize the health sector, countries, development partners, civil society, and the private sector toward the common goal of UHC, including pandemic preparedness, and to highlight country success and breakthrough experiences to accelerate the progress of UHC. A philosophic basis underlying the concept of UHC is commitment to equity, the need to promote policies increasing equity, and avoiding those that would widen inequities. The "grand convergence" envisaged under the SDGs, of under-5 and infectious disease mortality attaining reduced and relatively similar levels across countries, would be the logical and aspired outcome of policies and strategies developed over many years aiming to deliver cost-effective interventions for the major health challenges of low- and middle-income countries.[26,105,106]

Even as countries themselves shoulder more of their own health expenditures, DAH will remain an important element in global health architecture.[53] External funds, predominantly from high-income countries and resources, will continue to support global public goods such as pandemic preparedness and response, funding for international organizations, health and biomedical research, and funding for transnational challenges such as AMR and climate change.

Financing will obviously be the Achilles heel of UHC, and the experience of high-income countries where demands on health services continually outstrip resources is salutary. Commitment to UHC will require finance ministries re-examining the priorities of the public sector as well as envisaging continuous search for health-promoting increases in revenue such as increased taxation on tobacco, alcohol, and unhealthy foods and beverages, and reducing subsidies on fossil fuels. Political decisions will be required concerning the extent of private sector involvement in UHC and optimal targeting of public sector resources, universal or to the most poor. Transparency into pooled health resources and efficiency of the health service delivery process will be critical. Collecting the most comprehensive, comparable, and accurate health financing data and forecasting will be imperative.

Despite the promises of UHC, the current challenges are daunting. Recent World Bank and WHO estimates from 2017 suggest that at least half the world's people do not have full coverage of essential services. More than 1 billion have uncontrolled hypertension, more than 200 million women have inadequate coverage for family planning, and over 20 million infants do not receive a third dose of the vaccine against diphtheria, tetanus, and pertussis. In addition, some 800 million people spend more than 10% of their annual budget on healthcare, and 100 million people are pushed into extreme poverty each year because of out-of-pocket health expenses.[107]

The allocation of health spending toward UHC needs to be balanced with spending on other critical health areas, including health emergency preparedness, health promotion, and capital investments such as hospitals. A country's physical infrastructure, education systems, governance, and leadership at the national and local levels all play into attainment of UHC: each in its own way has the potential to substantially accelerate or constrain a country's progress toward equitable health coverage for all.[52] The path to universal coverage involves important policy choices and inevitable trade-offs. The way that pooled funds—which can come from a variety of sources, such as general government budgets, compulsory insurance contributions (payroll taxes), and household and/or employer prepayments for voluntary health insurance—are organized, used, and allocated, influences greatly the direction and progress of reforms toward universal coverage.[52]

HEALTH SECURITY AND NATIONAL PUBLIC HEALTH INSTITUTES

Distinct from the concept of UHC, but relevant to the health of all, is the issue of global health security. During the 2014–16 Ebola epidemic that ravaged Guinea, Liberia, and Sierra Leone,[108,109] those countries' health systems broke down and delivery of routine services was disrupted.[110] Epidemics of measles resulted from interruption of vaccination programs, maternal health services ceased functioning, and interventions for malaria control stopped.[111,112] The results were that more people likely died from health systems failure than from Ebola itself. The West African Ebola epidemic, unprecedented in its severity and geographic extent, brutally exposed the underlying weakness of systems that allowed it to spread so rapidly and extensively.[113,114]

WHO has defined the building blocks that constitute a health system,[115] although physical infrastructure may require more emphasis. In low-income settings, weaknesses such as poor communications systems, irregular access to clean water and sanitation, unreliable electricity supplies, and lack of Internet access severely handicap aspirations of UHC and health security.

For public health and health security, priority requirements include strong surveillance and health information systems; workforce capacity, including in epidemiology and management; strong laboratory systems; supplies and commodity management and distribution; and the ability to use data including through implementation science and operational research.[116] There is increasing support for the concept of national public health institutes, the paradigm for which is the U.S. Centers for Disease Control and Prevention (CDC), playing a key role in assuring a country's preparedness and response capacity.[50,117–119] Specific requirements for this capability are captured under WHO's International Health Regulations,[120] revised in 2005 after the outbreak of Severe Acute Respiratory Syndrome (SARS) 2 years earlier.[121] The Global Health Security Agenda[122] is a multicountry initiative that was launched in 2014 to enhance countries' capacity to "prevent, detect, respond" to old or emerging health threats by focusing on 11 so-called "action packages" (Box 15-2). The African Union has established an Africa CDC to establish early warning and response surveillance systems, respond to emergencies, build capacity, and provide technical expertise to address health crises in a timely and effective manner. As an African-owned institution, the Africa CDC is uniquely positioned to join traditional partners in protecting the health of the continent. It will also join the international networks of public health institutions to share information and improve surveillance of public health threats.

BOX 15-2 Global Health Security Action Packages: "Prevent, Detect, Respond"

- "Prevent 1": Antimicrobial Resistance
- "Prevent 2": Zoonotic Disease
- "Prevent 3": Biosafety and Biosecurity
- "Prevent 4": Immunization
- "Detect 1": National Laboratory System
- "Detect 2 and 3": Real-Time Surveillance
- "Detect 4": Reporting
- "Detect 5": Workforce Development
- "Respond 1": Emergency Operations Centers
- "Respond 2": Linking Public Health with Law and Multisectoral Rapid Response
- "Respond 3": Medical Countermeasures and Personnel Deployment Action Package

Disease surveillance and outbreak response activities are the first and most evident responsibilities for a national public health agency. Useful infrastructure and management approaches may include development of an emergency operations center and an incident management system for dealing with complex emergencies.[123] With time, experience, and capacity, national public health institutes may take on additional responsibilities such as directing specific infectious disease programs such as for HIV/AIDS, tuberculosis, or malaria; overseeing public health programs for MCH, immunization, and environmental health; addressing population risk factors relevant to NCDs; issuing best practice guidelines; delivering health information and promotion; and providing essential national health statistics based on surveillance and vital registration data.[124]

Robust national public health institutes can assure transparency concerning the health of the nation. Although separate from usual perceptions of UHC, health security and the public health functions delivered by a national public health institute are vital elements for comprehensive and sustainable UHC.

GLOBAL DISEASE CONTROL PRIORITIES: A SYSTEMATIC APPROACH, GENERALIZABLE, CORRECT POLICIES, AND GUIDELINES

The third edition of "Disease Control Priorities in Developing Countries" (DCP3), with inputs from over 500 global health experts from around the world, defines five platforms from which interventions should be delivered: population-based; community level; health center; first-level hospital; and referral hospital.[106,125] Twenty-one essential packages were proposed (e.g., maternal and newborn health; child health; tuberculosis; cancer; etc.), which could be grouped under clusters (Age-Related; Infectious Diseases; NCD and Injury; Health Services). A total of 218 specific interventions were defined for essential universal healthcare, with a smaller subset of these designated as the highest priority packages that should be affordable in many low-income countries and would deliver the greatest health benefit for the resources invested.[125] All nine volumes of DCP3 analyses have been made freely available online by the World Bank.

DCP3's ninth volume presents a succinct overview and summary of the entire DCP3 series, with a focus on the main findings of DCP3—both the Intersectoral Policy Priorities and the Essential Universal Health Coverage platforms of logistically related channels for delivery of packages of conceptually related interventions, and their costs. This volume assesses how to achieve the "Biggest Bang for the Buck" in global disease control; and has developed intersectoral and fiscal policies, based upon good science, complemented by "informed judgement."

DCP3 emphasizes that in selections of potential packages, the key steps for a country, include (1) extending population coverage through insurance; (2) reducing out-of-pocket expenses through "financial risk tools"; and (3) prioritizing packages of essential services based upon affordability and cost-effectiveness, and supported by public finance and insurance programs. DCP3 focuses on the principal causes of morbidity and mortality, as discussed previously:

Of the mortality attributed to NCDs, 80% fell into four groups:

1. Cardiovascular disease (CVD) and strokes
2. Diabetes
3. Cancer
4. Chronic lung disease

These four groups all are attributable in large part to shared risk factors that include:

1. Tobacco
2. Unhealthy diet and obesity
3. Low physical activity
4. Alcohol consumption

Prevention Interventions recommended as "Best Buy" policies that address these risk factors include:

1. Tobacco control
2. Reduced air pollution (to reduce CVD, cancer, and chronic obstructive pulmonary disease)
3. Media campaigns
4. Physical exercise
5. Healthy diet

The Individual Healthcare Priorities for NCDs include treatment for diabetes and for hypertension.

For UHC, the "Best Buy" interventions proposed globally for NCDs in order of importance are:

1. Tobacco taxation
2. Decrease in alcohol consumption
3. Improving diets (e.g., decreasing fat, palm oil)

For injuries (responsible for 9–10% of all deaths per year), one-third are attributable to road traffic events, mostly involving young people. The Best Buys in public health to prevent these deaths due to traffic-related injuries include enforcement of speed limits and seat belt use, and enforcing helmet requirements.

For UHC, three actions are prioritized:

1. Expand population coverage to include the poor, marginalized, uninsured, and laborers (e.g., through governmental healthcare insurance)
2. Improve financial risk protection (e.g., through universal healthcare coverage)
3. Design packages to respond to health needs—for example, based on 218 priorities, with 108 listed as highest priorities for low-income countries

GLOBAL HEALTH AND THE FUTURE

Global health will continue to evolve in parallel with broader sociopolitical, scientific, and cultural developments. In terms of programmatic implementation, key drivers will be trends in DAH and domestic health spending, as well as the quest for the SDGs. UHC will remain a goal, though one difficult to achieve, and public health can play a useful role in setting appropriate expectations, re-orienting political attention to prevention and population-level interventions, and measuring and communicating health trends. Global health actors will continue to diversify and the centralization of authority in WHO or the World Health Assembly will likely continue to diminish as individual country capacity is enhanced.

Some of the greatest global health inequities remaining concern maternal mortality and child survival, justifying continued prioritization of maternal and child health services. Two diseases, polio and dracunculiasis (guinea worm), remain targeted for eradication[83]; complete extinction of a disease, thus far only achieved for smallpox, represents the ultimate in health equity. As eradication gets closer to being a reality, the remaining foci of transmission become more challenging to address and both efforts have seen unexpected setbacks. Endemic transmission of polio only persists in three countries, Afghanistan, Pakistan, and Nigeria. In all three countries, physical security related to conflict and terrorism is the biggest obstacle to success.

Numerous external factors will continue to influence global health including conflict and terrorism; population displacement, refugee crises, and migration; environmental and climate change; cultural pressures and their influence on lifestyles; and demographics. If climate change is the most unpredictable factor for the future of global health, perhaps the most neglected or underestimated is demographic change. From today's 7.6 billion, world population is expected to reach 8.6 billion by 2030, and, by the end of the century, 11.2 billion.[126] Despite encouraging reductions in fertility, Africa's population growth greatly exceeds that of the rest of the world and the proportion of the world's population that is African will likely reach 40% by 2100, from today's 17%. By the end of the century, the great majority of youth in the world will be African. The potential benefits from economic and market activity are considerable, as are the dangers from unemployment, crime, uncontrolled migration, and unmet health needs. By contrast, a large number of countries, many in Europe and including Japan, are experiencing aging and shrinking populations, with implications for increased demand on health and social services.

While there is concern about inadequate preparedness in case of terrorism, bioterrorism or war, the most likely and devastating challenge to health security would be an outbreak of infection with highly pathogenic airborne agent that could rapidly develop into a pandemic. Novel influenza viruses travel across the world in a matter of days or weeks. The anthrax attacks in the United States in 2001,[127] the great influenza pandemic of 1918,[128] and the outbreak of SARS in 2003[129] all illustrate global vulnerability and the societal disruption engendered by such events. Experiences such as these, as well as the West African Ebola epidemic of 2014–16,[109] emphasize the need for robust global public health infrastructure.

Development, security, and public health remain useful frameworks for analyzing world health and necessary health action.[3] Important to recognize is the enormous development and economic progress being made that renders invalid the former binary view of the world's countries as either developed or developing.[130] Demographic, fertility, and health trends are similar across the world but staggered in time. Overall, despite old and new global challenges, there is much reason to be optimistic that the future will be one of safer, healthier, and longer lives.[130]

References

1. Hunter JD, Fineberg HV. Introduction. In: Hunter DJ, Fineberg HV, eds. *Readings in Global Health. Essential Reviews from the New England Journal of Medicine*. New York: Oxford University Press; 2016.
2. Institute of Medicine. *The Future of Public Health*. Washington, DC: National Academy Press; 1988.
3. De Cock KM, Simone PM, Davison V, Slutsker L. The new global health. *Emerg Infect Dis*. 2013;19:1192–7.

4. Quinones S. Dreamland: The True Tale of America's Opiate Epidemic. 2015.
5. National Academies of Medicine. Global Health and Future Role of US. 2017.
6. World Health Organization. Climate change and health. http://www.who.int/en/news-room/fact-sheets/detail/climate-change-and-health. Accessed February 1, 2018.
7. World Economic Forum. The global risks report 2016, 11th edition. http://www3.weforum.org/docs/GRR/WEF_GRR16.pdf.
8. Whitmee S, Haines A, Beyrer C, et al. Safeguarding human health in the Anthropocene epoch: Report of the Rockefeller Foundation-Lancet Commission on planetary health. *Lancet*. 2015; 386(10007):1973–2028.
9. De Cock KM, Mbori-Ngacha D, Marum E. Shadow on the continent—Public health and HIV/AIDS in Africa in the 21st century. *Lancet*. 2002;360:67–72.
10. Commission on the Social Determinants of Health. Closing the gap in a generation: Health equity through action on the social determinants of health. *Final Report of the Commission on Social Determinants of Health*. Geneva: World Health Organization; 2008.
11. Jamison DT, Gelband H, Horton S, eds. *Disease Control Priorities: Improving Health and Reducing Poverty. Volume 9, Disease Control Priorities*. 3rd ed. Washington, DC: World Bank; 2018.
12. Rankin FH. *The White Man's Grave: A Visit to Sierra Leone, in 1834*. London: Richard Bentley; 1836.
13. Staples JE, Monath TP. Yellow fever: 100 years of discovery. *JAMA*. 2008;300:960–2.
14. Kelvin T, Kwok-Yung Y. In memory of Patrick Manson, founding father of tropical medicine and the discovery of vector-borne infections. *Emerg Microbes Infect*. 2012;1(10):e31.
15. The Nobel Prize in Physiology or Medicine 1902. Nobelprize.org. Nobel Media AB 2014. Web. http://www.nobelprize.org/nobel_prizes/medicine/laureates/1902/. Accessed May 4, 2018.
16. Used with permission from Rockefeller Foundation. https://www.rockefellerfoundation.org/.
17. Keating C. *Kenneth Warren and the Great Neglected Diseases of Mankind Programme*. New York: Springer; 2017. DOI: 10.1007/978-3-319-50147-5.
18. Special Programme for Research and Training in Tropical Diseases (TDR): World Health Organization (WHO), United Nations Children's Fund (UNICEF), United Nations Development Programme (UNDP), the World Bank. http://www.who.int/tdr/en/.
19. Hotez PJ. The neglected tropical diseases and the neglected infections of poverty: Overview of their common features, global disease burden and distribution, new control tools, and prospects for disease elimination. In: Eileen R., Choffnes ER, Relman DA, eds. *Rapporteurs. IOM (Institute of Medicine). The Causes and Impacts of Neglected Tropical and Zoonotic Diseases: Opportunities for Integrated Intervention Strategies*, Vol. A7. Washington, DC: The National Academies Press; 2011, pp. 221–37.
20. World Health Organization. Integrating neglected tropical diseases in global health and development. Fourth WHO report on neglected tropical diseases. Geneva, 2017.
21. De Cock KM. Personal view. *BMJ*. 1983;287:1139.
22. Keating C. *Kenneth Warren and the Great Neglected Diseases of Mankind Programme*. New York: Springer International Publishing; 2017.
23. Koplan JP, Bond TC, Merson, et al. Towards a common definition of public health. *Lancet*. 2009;373:1993–5.
24. World Health Organization. Declaration of Alma-Ata. 1978. http://www.who.int/publications/almaata_declaration_en.pdf.
25. Emerging Infections. Microbial threats to health in the United States. In: Lederberg J, Shope RE, Oaks SC., eds. *Institute of Medicine*. Washington, DC: National Academy Press; 1992.
26. The World Bank. *World Development Report 1993. Investing in Health*. New York: Oxford University Press; 1993.
27. Sachs JD. *Investing in Health for Economic Development. Report of the Commission on Macroeconomics and Health*. Geneva: World Health Organization; 2001.
28. Slenczka W, Klenk HD. Forty years of Marburg virus. *J Infect Dis*. 2007;196(Suppl 2):S131–5.
29. Frame JD, Baldwin JM, Gocke DJ, Troup JM. Lassa fever, a new virus disease of man from West Africa. I. Clinical description and pathological findings. *Am J Trop Med Hyg*. 1970;19(4):670–6.
30. Breman JG, Heymann DL, Lloyd G, et al. Discovery and description of Ebola Zaire virus in 1976 and relevance to the West African epidemic during 2013–2016. *J Infect Dis*. 2016;vl(Suppl 3):S93–101.
31. CDC. Pneumocystis pneumonia—Los Angeles. *MMWR*. 1981;30:250–2.
32. Piot P, Taelman H, Minlangu KB, et al. Acquired immunodeficiency syndrome in a heterosexual population in Zaire. *Lancet* 1984;324:65–9.
33. Van de Perre P, Lepage P, Kestelyn P, et al. Acquired immunodeficiency syndrome in Rwanda. *Lancet* 1984;324:62–5.
34. Merson M, Inrig S. *The AIDS Pandemic. Searching for a Global Response*. New York: Springer; 2018.
35. United Nations Development Programme (UNDP): Millennium Development Goals. http://www.undp.org/content/undp/en/home/sdgoverview/mdg_goals.html.
36. The United States President's Emergency Plan for AIDS Relief (PEPFAR). https://www.pepfar.gov/.
37. The United States President's Malaria Initiative (PMI). https://www.pmi.gov/.
38. Foege, WH. *The Fears of the Rich, the Needs of the Poor*. Baltimore, MD: Johns Hopkins University Press; 2018.
39. Muir JA, Farley J, Osterman A, et al. Global health partnerships: Are they working? *Sci Transl Med*. 2016;8(334):334ed4.
40. World Health Organization (WHO). https://www.who.int.
41. United Nations Children's Fund (UNICEF). https://www.unicef.org/.
42. United Nations Population Fund (UNFPA). https://www.unfpa.org/.
43. World Food Programme (WFP). http://www1.wfp.org/.
44. UN Refugee Agency (UNHCR). http://www.unhcr.org/.
45. Sridhar D, Winters J, Strong E. World Bank's financing, priorities, and lending structures for global health. *BMJ*. 2017;358:j3339.
46. Joint United Nations Programme on HIV/AIDS (UNAIDS). http://www.unaids.org/.
47. BMGF 2016 Annual Report. https://www.gatesfoundation.org/Who-We-Are/Resources-and-Media/Annual-Reports/Annual-Report-2016.
48. France D. *How to Survive a Plague: The Inside Story of How Citizens and Science Tamed AIDS*. New York: Alfred A. Knopf; 2016.
49. Médecins Sans Frontières (MSF) International Ebola. http://www.msf.org/en/diseases/ebola.
50. De Cock KM, Centers for Disease Control and Prevention (CDC). Trends in global health and CDC's international role, 1961–2011. *MMWR Suppl*. 2011;60(4):104–11 (Frederic E Shaw, Katrin S Kohl, Lisa M Lee, Stephen B Thacker, Centers for Disease Control and Prevention (CDC). Supplement: Public health then and now: Celebrating 50 years of MMWR at CDC. *MMWR Suppl*. 2011;60(4):2–6).
51. Olivier J, Wodon Q. Faith-inspired health care in sub-Saharan Africa: An introduction to the Spring 2014 issue. *Rev Faith Int Aff*. 2014;12(1):1–7.
52. Xu K., Soucat A., Kutzin J., et al. *New Perspectives on Global Health Spending for Universal Health Coverage*. Geneva: World Health Organization; 2018 (WHO/HIS/HGF/HFWorkingPaper/18.2). Licence: CC BY-NC-SA 3.0 IGO.
53. Institute for Health Metrics and Evaluation (IHME). *Financing Global Health 2017: Development Assistance, Public and Private Health Spending for the Pursuit of Universal Health Coverage*. Seattle, WA: IHME; 2018.
54. Stenberg K, Hanssen O, Edejer TT, et al. Financing transformative health systems towards achievement of the health Sustainable Development Goals: A model for projected resource needs in 67 low-income and middle-income countries. *Lancet Glob Health*. 2017;5(9):e875–87.
55. A/67/L.36. Agenda item 123: global health and foreign policy. In: General Assembly of the United Nations [Internet]. Sixty-seventh United Nations General Assembly, New York, 3–11 September 2012, official documents. Geneva: UNGA; 2013. Available from: https://www.un.org/en/ga/search/view_doc.asp?symbol=A/RES/67/81.
56. Xu K, Evans DB, Carrin G, Aguilar-Rivera AM, Musgrove P, Evans T. Protecting households from catastrophic health spending. *Health Aff (Millwood)*. 2007;26(4):972–83.
57. GBD 2015 Mortality and Causes of Death Collaborators. Global, regional, and national life expectancy, all-cause mortality, and cause-specific mortality for 249 causes of death, 1980–2015: A systematic analysis for the Global Burden of Disease Study 2015. *Lancet*. 2015; 2016(388):1459–544.
58. http://www.unaids.org/en/topic/data.
59. World Malaria Report 2017. Geneva: World Health Organization; 2017. Licence: CC BY-NC-SA 3.0 IGO.
60. Global Tuberculosis Report 2018. Geneva: World Health Organization; 2018. Licence: CC BY-NCSA 3.0 IGO.
61. World Health Organization. Neglected Tropical Diseases. 2017. http://www.who.int/neglected_diseases/diseases/en/.
62. Margolis L, Kotch J. Tracing the Historical Foundations of Maternal and Child Health to Contemporary Times. In: Jonathan B Kotch, eds. *Maternal and Child Health, Programs, Problems and Policy in Public Health*. Burlington, VT: Jones and Bartlett Learning, LLC; 2013, p. 11.
63. Kerber KJ, de Graft-Johnson JE, Bhutta ZA, Okong P, Starrs A, Lawn JE. Continuum of care for maternal, newborn, and child health: From slogan to service delivery. *Lancet*. 2007;370:1358–69.

64. Used with permission from United Nations sustainable development goals. https://www.un.org/sustainabledevelopment/. 2016.
65. United Nations Interagency Group for Child Mortality estimation. *Levels and Trends in Child Mortality Report 2015*. New York: UNICEF; 2015, p. 3. https://www.unicef.org/publications/files/Child_Mortality_Report_2015_Web_9_Sept_15.pdf. Accessed May 3, 2018.
66. WHO, UNICEF, UNFPA. Trends in maternal mortality: 1990 to 2015. Geneva: WHO; 2015, p 16. http://www.who.int/reproductivehealth/publications/monitoring/maternal-mortality-2015/en/. Accessed April 10, 2018.
67. Say L, et al. Global causes of maternal death: A WHO systematic analysis. *Lancet Glob Health*. 2014;2(6):323–33.
68. Partnership for Maternal, Newborn & Child Health. *Strategic Framework 2012–2015*. Geneva: WHO; 2011, p. 20. http://www.who.int/pmnch/knowledge/publications/pmnch_strategic_framework_20111212.pdf. Accessed May 1, 2018.
69. Dieleman JL, Graves C, Johnson E, et al. Sources and focus of health development assistance 1990–2014. *JAMA*. 2015;313(23):2359–68.
70. Piot P, Quinn TC. The AIDS pandemic—A global health paradigm. *N Engl J Med*. 2013;368(23):2210–18.
71. UNAIDS 2017 Fact Sheet. http://www.unaids.org/en/resources/fact-sheet.
72. Cohen MS, Chen YQ, McCauley M, et al. Prevention of HIV-1 infection with early antiretroviral therapy. *N Engl J Med*. 2011;365:493–505.
73. Rodger AJ, Cambiano V, Tina Bruun T, et al. Sexual activity without condoms and risk of HIV transmission in serodifferent couples when the HIV-positive partner is using suppressive antiretroviral therapy. *JAMA*. 2016;316:171–81.
74. INSIGHT START Study Group. Initiation of antiretroviral therapy in early asymptomatic HIV infection. *N Engl J Med*. 2015;373:795–807.
75. WHO. Consolidated guidelines on the use of antiretroviral drugs for treating and preventing HIV infection. Recommendations for a public health approach. Second Edition, 2016. Geneva.
76. De Cock KM, El-Sadr WM. From START to finish: Implications of the START study. *Lancet Infect Dis*. 2016;16:13–14.
77. UNAIDS: 90-90-90—An ambitious treatment target to help end the AIDS epidemic.
78. Kharsany ABM, Karim QA. HIV infection and AIDS in sub-Saharan Africa: Current status, challenges and opportunities. *Open AIDS J*. 2016;10:34–48.
79. United Nations News Report. https://news.un.org/en/story/2017/12/638312-west-and-central-africa-lagging-far-behind-world-hiv-response-warns-unicef. Accessed December 5, 2017.
80. World Health Organization: HIV and Hepatitis Update June 2017. http://www.who.int/hiv/pub/newsletter/hiv-hep_newsletter_jun2017/en/index1.html.
81. Chookajorn T. How to combat emerging artemisinin resistance: Lessons from "The Three Little Pigs." *PLoS Pathog*. 2018;14(4):e1006923.
82. World Health Organization. *Best Buys and Other Recommended Interventions for the Prevention and Control of Noncommunicable Diseases. Updated (2017) Appendix 3 of the Global Action Plan for the Prevention and Control of Noncommunicable Diseases 2013–2020*. Geneva: World Health Organization; 2017.
83. de Martel C, Ferlay J, Franceschi S, Vignat J, Bray F, Forman D, Plummer M. Global burden of cancers attributable to infections in 2008: A review and synthetic analysis. *Lancet Oncol*. 2012;13(6):607–15.
84. Plummer M, de Martel C, Vignat J, Ferlay J, Bray F, Franceschi S. Global burden of cancers attributable to infections in 2012: A synthetic analysis. *Lancet Glob Health*. 2016;4(9):e609–16.
85. Watkins DA, et al. Global, regional, and national burden of rheumatic heart disease, 1990–2015. *N Engl J Med*. 2017;377(8):713–22.
86. Ogoina D, Onyemelukwe GC. The role of infections in the emergence of non-communicable diseases (NCDs): Compelling needs for novel strategies in the developing world. *J Infect Public Health*. 2009;2(1):14–29.
87. Reddy KS, Hunter DJ. Noncommunicable diseases. *N Engl J Med*. 2013;369(26):2563.
88. Remais JV, Zeng G, Li G, Tian L, Engelgau MM. Convergence of non-communicable and infectious diseases in low- and middle-income countries. *Int J Epidemiol*. 2013;42(1):221–7.
89. Bygbjerg IC. Double burden of noncommunicable and infectious diseases in developing countries. *Science*. 2012;337(6101):1499–501.
90. Molyneux D, Sankara DP. Guinea worm eradication: Progress and challenges—Should we beware of the dog? *PLoS Negl Trop Dis*. 2017;11(4):e0005495.
91. Hopkins DR. Disease eradication. *N Engl J Med*. 2013;368:54–63.
92. World Health Organization. *Promoting Mental Health: Concepts, Emerging Evidence, Practice (Summary Report)*. Geneva: World Health Organization; 2004.
93. Ginn S, Horder J. "One in four" with a mental health problem: The anatomy of a statistic. *BMJ*. 2012;344:e1302.
94. Votruba N, Thornicroft G, the FundaMentalSDG Steering Group. Sustainable development goals and mental health: Learnings from the contribution of the FundaMentalSDG global initiative. *Glob Ment Health (Camb)*. 2016;3:e26.
95. WHO: Mental Health included in the UN Sustainable Development Goals. http://www.who.int/mental_health/SDGs/en/.
96. Global Initiative for Essential and Emergency Surgical Health Care (GIEESC). *Emergency and Essential Surgical Care*. Geneva: World Health Organization; November 2008, p. 30. http://www.who.int/surgery/globalinitiative/en/.
97. Bickler SW, Weiser TG, Kassebaum N, et al. Global burden of surgical conditions. In: Debas HT, Donkor P, Gawande A, Jamison DT, Kruk ME, Mock CN, eds. *Essential Surgery: Disease Control Priorities*. Vol. 1. 3rd ed. Washington, DC: The International Bank for Reconstruction and Development/The World Bank; 2015.
98. Rose J, Chang DC, Weiser TG, Kassebaum NJ, Bickler SW. The role of surgery in global health: Analysis of United States inpatient procedure frequency by condition using the global burden of disease 2010 framework. *PLoS One*. 2014;9(2):e89693.
99. Murray CJ, Vos T, Lozano R, et al. Disability-adjusted life years (DALYs) for 291 diseases and injuries in 21 regions, 1990–2010: A systematic analysis for the Global Burden of Disease Study 2010. *Lancet*. 2012;380:2197–223.
100. Meara JG, Leather AJ, Hagander L, et al. Global surgery 2030: Evidence and solutions for achieving health, welfare, and economic development. *Lancet*. 2015;386:569–624.
101. Kim JY. Opening address to the inaugural "The Lancet Commission on Global Surgery" meeting. The World Bank. January 17, 2014. Boston, MA.
102. Resolution WHA68.15. Strengthening emergency and essential surgical care and anaesthesia as a component of universal health coverage. In: *Sixty-eighth World Health Assembly, Geneva, 18–26 May 2015*. Geneva: World Health Organization; 2015.
103. Ologundea R, Maruthappu M, Shanmugarajah K, Shalhoub J. Surgical care in low and middle-income countries: Burden and barriers. *Int J Surg*. 2014;12:858–63.
104. Ghebreyesus TA. All roads lead to universal health coverage. *Lancet Glob Health*. 2017;5:e839–40.
105. Jamison DT, Mosley WH, Measham AR, Bobadilla JL, eds. *Disease Control Priorities in Developing Countries*. New York: Oxford University Press; 1993.
106. Jamison DT, Alwan A, Mock NC et al. Universal health coverage and intersectoral action for health: Key messages from Disease Control Priorities, 3rd edition. *Lancet*. 2018;391(10125):1108–20.
107. WHO and World Bank. *Tracking Universal Health Coverage: 2017 global monitoring report*.
108. Lo TQ, Marston BJ, Dahl BA, De Cock KM. Ebola—Anatomy of an epidemic. Annual Review of Medicine. http://www.annualreviews.org/doi/pdf/10.1146/annurev-med-052915-015604.
109. Arwady MA, Bawo L, Hunter J, et al. Evolution of Ebola virus disease from exotic infection to global health priority, Liberia, mid-2014. *Emerg Infect Dis*. 2015;21:578–84.
110. Brolin Ribacke KJ, Saulnier DD, Eriksson A, von Schreeb J. Effects of the West Africa Ebola virus disease on health-care utilization—A systematic review. *Front Public Health*. 2016;4:222. eCollection 2016.
111. Colavita F, Biava M, Castilletti C, et al. Measles cases during Ebola outbreak, West Africa, 2013–2106. *Emerg Infect Dis*. 2017;23(6):1035–7.
112. Heymann DL, Chen L, Takemi K, et al. Global health security: The wider lessons from the West African Ebola virus disease epidemic. *Lancet*. 2015;385:1884–901.
113. De Cock KM, El-Sadr WM. A tale of two viruses: HIV, Ebola and health systems. *AIDS*. 2015;29:989–91.
114. WHO. Everybody's business: Strengthening health systems to improve health outcomes: WHO's framework. WHO, 2007. http://www.who.int/healthsystems/strategy/everybodys_business.pdf.
115. Bloland P, Simone P, Burkholder B, Slutsker L, De Cock KM. The role of public health institutions in global health system strengthening efforts: The US CDC's perspective. *PLoS Med*. 2012;9:e1001199.

116. Frieden TR, Koplan JP. Stronger national public health institutes for global health. *Lancet.* 2010;376:1721–1722.

117. Frieden TR, Tappero JW, Dowell SF, Hien NT, Guillaume FD, Aceng JR. Safer countries through global health security. *Lancet.* 2014; 383:764–6.

118. Frieden TR, Damon IK. Ebola in West Africa—CDC's role in epidemic detection, control, and prevention. *Emerg Infect Dis.* 2015;21:1897–905.

119. WHO. *International Health Regulations.* 3rd ed. Geneva: World Health Organization; 2005.

120. Peiris M, Anderson LJ, Osterhaus ADME. In: Stohr K, Yuen K, eds. *Severe Acute Respiratory Syndrome.* Hoboken, NJ: Wiley Online Library; 2008.

121. Global Health Security Agenda. https://www.ghsagenda.org/.

122. Pillai SK, Nyenswah T, Rouse E, et al. Developing an Incident Management System to support Ebola response—Liberia, July–August 2014. *MMWR.* 2014;63:930–3.

123. CDC Emergency Operations Center (EOC). https://www.cdc.gov/phpr/eoc.htm.

124. Jamison DT, Summers LH, Alleyne G, et al. Global health 2035: A world converging within a generation. *Lancet.* 2013;382:1898–995.

125. United Nations, Department of Economic and Social Affairs, Population Division. World Population Prospects: The 2017 Revision, Key Findings and Advance Tables. Working Paper No. ESA/P/WP/248, 2017.

126. Theme Issue. Bioterrorism-related anthrax. *Emerg Infect Dis.* 2002;8: 1013–186.

127. CDC. History of 1918 flu pandemic. https://www.cdc.gov/flu/pandemic-resources/1918-commemoration/1918-pandemic-history.htm.

128. Heymann DL, Mackenzie JL, Peiris M. SARS legacy: Outbreak reporting is expected and respected. *Lancet.* 2013;381:779–81.

129. Rosling R. *Factfulness.* New York: Flatiron Books; 2018.

130. Pinker S. *Enlightment Now. The Case for Reason, Science, Humanism and Progress.* UK: Allen Lane; 2018.

CHAPTER 16

Transitions in Global Disease Burden

Awoke Misganaw Temesgen • Christopher J. L. Murray

INTRODUCTION TO TRANSITIONS IN DISEASE BURDEN

A transition in disease burden, the general notion of a shift from communicable to noncommunicable causes of disease and injury, remains a powerful framework for global and regional health policy debates.[1] In 1971, Omran outlined the concept of the epidemiological transition to describe the changing pattern of causes of death that results from sociodemographic development.[2] The epidemiological transition is an extension of the conception of the demographic transition. In the demographic transition, a characteristic evolution occurs in populations over time toward reduced fertility rates, reduced mortality rates, and an older-age distribution of the population. The widely used concept of the epidemiological transition adds the idea that, in addition to these changes, a characteristic change occurs in the contributing causes of death.[1] The epidemiological transition has been broadened to encompass a more general health transition, including both morbidity and mortality. The developments of modern healthcare and medicine drastically reduce infant mortality rates and extend average life expectancy. These factors, coupled with subsequent declines in fertility rates, have catalyzed a transition to noncommunicable diseases (NCDs) as increasingly important causes of health loss. The notion of the epidemiological transition has also been expanded to recognize a transition phase that may lead to a double burden of disease, the growing threat of NCDs as causes of health loss while infectious diseases remain highly prevalent. Too often, the health system may continue to rely heavily on the conventional infectious disease paradigm and be unresponsive to this emerging epidemiological shift.[3]

This chapter describes transitions in disease burden and their determinants, drawing from the Global Burden of Disease (GBD) study and other sources. Disease burden and epidemiological transition measurements should be sufficiently comprehensive to capture the causes of premature death and disability, as well as the major risk factors that underlie disease and injury.[4] GBD is the largest and most comprehensive study to date to measure epidemiological levels and trends worldwide. It is a systematic, scientific effort that uses available data of multiple sources to quantify the comparative magnitude of health loss due to diseases, injuries, and risk factors by age, sex, and geographies for specific points in time. In light of the importance of understanding the concept of disease burden and related issues as a foundation for the material in the subsequent chapters and for all work in global health, we present a brief description of disease burden measurements, and a more detailed discussion of trends by region and disease within the three GBD disease categories of communicable, maternal, neonatal, and nutritional diseases; NCDs; and injuries. We also discuss the implications of these findings for global health programs and policies, and for achievement of the Sustainable Development Goals (SDGs), as well as for mechanisms to improve measurement of disease burden and the highest priorities for future research and training in global health.

MEASURING GLOBAL AND REGIONAL DISEASE BURDEN TRANSITIONS

Measurement of disease burden transitions at global, regional, and country levels and, whenever possible, at subnational locations is useful to compare changing epidemiological patterns against the health system performance, and to identify specific needs for resource allocation in research, policy development, and program decision making.[5] A more macrolevel analysis from the GBD data provides an opportunity to quantify transitions in disease burden and epidemiologic patterns and explore the extent to which transitions are driven by sociodemographic change, reduction in health risks, improvement of health management, or other local factors.[6] The GBD measures premature mortality and disability using a summary measure called disability-adjusted life years (DALYs) across a large number of diseases, injuries, and risk factors that describes global, regional, national, and subnational disease burden transitions and trends in epidemiological patterns, and the effects of recent changes in population health.[5] The GBD results in DALYs and the Socio-demographic Index (SDI)—the geometric mean of income per person, educational attainment in the population older than age 15 years, and total fertility rate that captures the interactions between demographic and socioeconomic change[5]—enable comparative assessments of broad epidemiological patterns across regions and over time, while also making clear how the regions deviate from general patterns.

Readers of this chapter can find detailed GBD methods published in *The Lancet* and elsewhere,[7–10] but we describe the methods briefly to facilitate understanding of the concepts discussed below. The GBD study uses a hierarchy of causes of mortality and morbidity that structure 359 diseases and injuries into four levels of classification to produce levels that are mutually exclusive and collectively exhaustive.[9] In this chapter, we use the first and the second levels that distinguish 3 and 21 broad categories of diseases and injuries, respectively. The first-level categories are: communicable, maternal, neonatal, and nutritional disorders (CMNNDs); NCDs; and injury categories. The second-level categories are: cardiovascular diseases, neoplasms, chronic respiratory diseases, respiratory diseases and tuberculosis, neurological disorders, diabetes and chronic kidney diseases; digestive diseases, maternal and neonatal, unintentional injury, enteric infections, self-harm and violence, transport injury, HIV/AIDS and sexually transmitted infections, neglected tropical diseases and malaria, substance use, nutritional deficiencies, and others. GBD calculates DALYs as the sum of years of life lost (YLLs) and years lived with disability (YLDs) for each cause, location, age group, sex, and year.[5] For all results, GBD reports 95% uncertainty intervals (UIs). The GBD study covers 195 countries and territories.

We summarize the transition of disease burden using World Bank–classified regions and sociodemographic determinants in the regions.

GLOBAL AND REGIONAL DISEASE BURDEN TRANSITIONS

Globally the transition in disease burden has been toward decreasing CMNNDs and increasing NCDs, which clearly shows that a major epidemiological transition unfolded over the past three decades (Fig. 16-1A). Number of DALYs and crude and age-standardized DALY rates for communicable diseases, maternal, neonatal, and nutritional disorders have decreased since 1990. For NCDs, the number of DALYs has increased, crude rates have remained stable, and age-standardized rates have decreased (Fig. 16-1A–C). The difference in trends between Fig. 16-1A and B is caused by population growth, while the difference between Fig. 16-1B and C is the result of changes in the age distribution of the population, implying a demographic transition. This means population increase and aging are keeping the crude rates of DALYs constant, showing that progress in health is shaped by factors beyond the health systems.[5,8,9]

These global trends are driven by region-specific effects, and patterns vary within and between regions, which makes it difficult to develop a single, unified explanation for the epidemiologic transition. Studies have challenged the view of the epidemiological transition as a universal theory of unidirectional change, emphasizing heterogeneity in the pace or quality of the transition in different settings.[11,12] Examining the transition of disease burden within the three broad categories, the global trend reflects the transition that occurred in South Asia during the 1990–2017 period (Table 16-1). For other regions—North America, Latin America and the Caribbean, Europe and Central Asia, East Asia and the Pacific, and North Africa and the Middle East—the transition occurred before 1990. Sub-Saharan Africa has not yet transitioned, but even there CMNNDs are declining and NCDs increasing. The magnitudes of the CMNND decline and the rise of NCDs differ across regions (Table 16-1).

All regions except North America, and Europe and Central Asia have shown large shifts toward increased NCD burden from 1990 to 2017. The increases observed in South Asia, sub-Saharan Africa, North Africa and the Middle East, East Asia and the Pacific, and Latin America and the Caribbean range from 40% to 87%, with the largest increases occurring in the first two regions (Table 16-1). Simultaneously, in South Asia, North Africa and the Middle East, Latin America and the Caribbean, and East Asia and the Pacific, DALYs attributable to CMNNDs declined substantially, ranging from 46% to 63% (Table 16-1). Indeed, sub-Saharan Africa was the only region in which CMNNDs fell less than 20% during this period. In East Asia and the Pacific, for example, CMNNDs showed a rapid, 63% decline, whereas NCDs increased by 42% between 1990 and 2017. A study in the region demonstrated that countries like China have undergone rapid epidemiological changes in the past few decades.[13] In the high- and high-middle-SDI regions (Europe and Central Asia, East Asia and the Pacific, and North America) in 2017 the proportion of NCDs ranged from 78% to 85%, and CMNNDs accounted for a small proportion of disease burden. This shows that NCDs are now leading health problems in populations that have undergone or

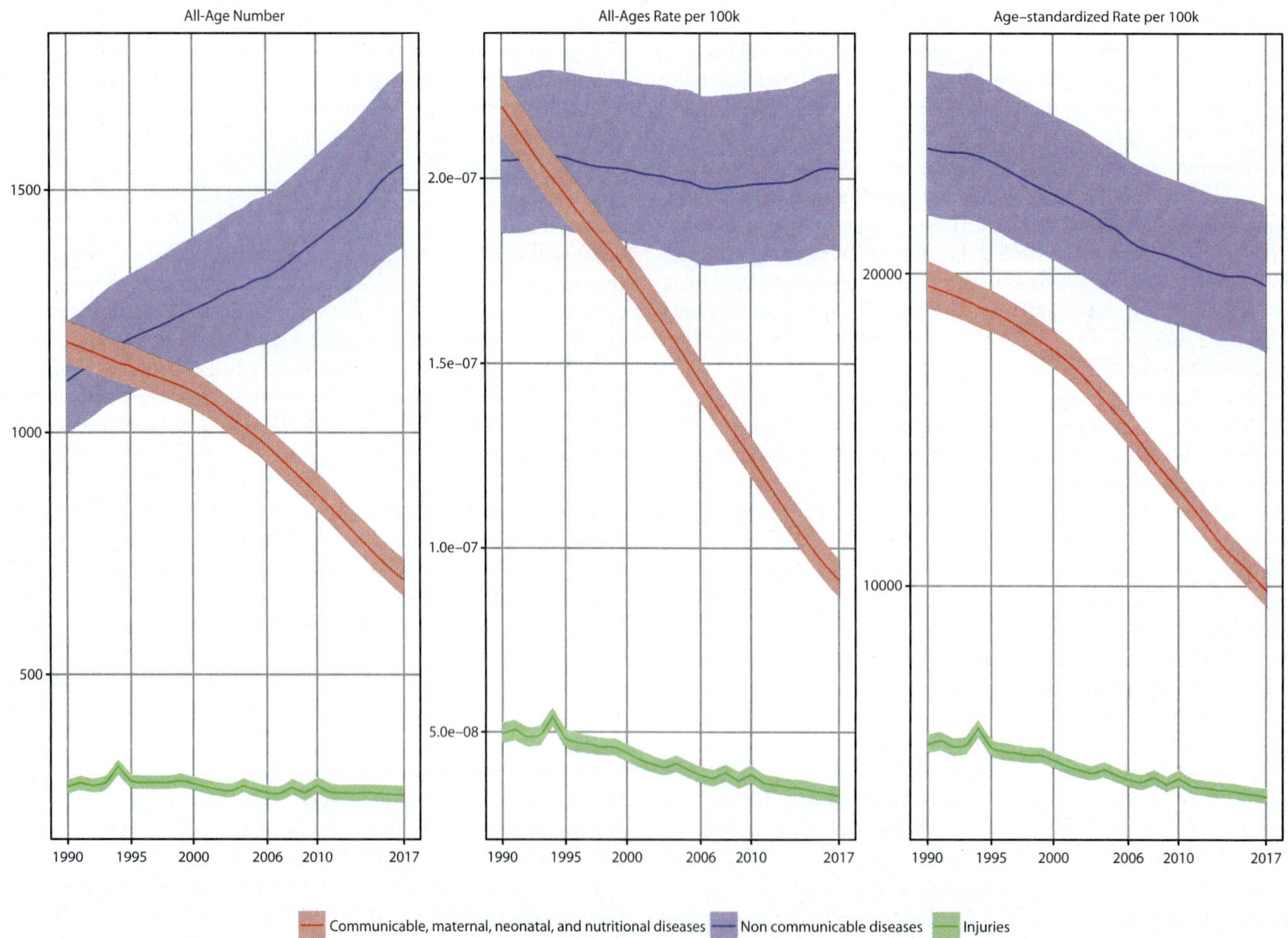

FIGURE 16-1. Trends from 1990 to 2017, by GBD three major categories, in global number of DALYs (A), crude DALY rates (B), and age-standardized DALY rates (C) with 95% uncertainty interval.

TABLE 16-1 PERCENTAGE OF TOTAL DISABILITY-ADJUSTED LIFE YEARS BY BROAD GBD DISEASE CATEGORIES FOR ALL-AGE GROUPS, BOTH SEXES, 2017

	1990			2017			
Regions	Ranks, 1990	Causes, 1990	% Total DALYs	Ranks, 2017	Causes, 2017	% Total DALYs	% Change
Global	1	CMNNDs	46%	1	NCDs	62%	44%
	2	NCDs	43%	2	CMNNDS	28%	−40%
	3	Injuries	11%	3	Injuries	10%	4%
North America	1	NCDs	79%	1	NCDs	85%	7%
	2	Injuries	13%	2	Injuries	10%	−23%
	3	CMNNDs	8%	3	CMNNDs	5%	−33%
Latin America and Caribbean	1	NCDs	50%	1	NCDs	70%	40%
	2	CMNNDs	35%	2	CMNNDs	16%	−56%
	3	Injuries	15%	3	Injuries	15%	−2%
Europe and Central Asia	1	NCDs	75%	1	NCDs	86%	10%
	2	Injuries	13%	2	Injuries	11%	−18%
	3	CMNNDs	12%	3	CMNNDs	7%	−42%
East Asia and Pacific	1	NCDs	55%	1	NCDs	78%	42%
	2	CMNNDs	32%	2	CMNNDs	12%	−63%
	3	Injuries	13%	3	Injuries	10%	−24%
North Africa and Middle East	1	NCDs	45%	1	NCDs	68%	43%
	2	CMNNDs	40%	2	CMNNDS	16%	−60%
	3	Injuries	15%	3	Injuries	16%	11%
South Asia	1	CMNNDs	62%	1	NCDs	55%	87%
	2	NCDs	30%	2	CMNNDs	34%	−44%
	3	Injuries	8%	3	Injuries	10%	24%
Sub-Saharan Africa	1	CMNNDs	74%	1	CMNNDs	63%	−16%
	2	NCDs	19%	2	NCDs	30%	60%
	3	Injuries	6%	3	Injuries	7%	9%

Abbreviations: CMNNDs = communicable, maternal, neonatal, and nutritional diseases; NCDs = noncommunicable diseases.

almost completed the epidemiologic transition.[12] On the other hand, in South Asia, the transition from CMNND burden to NCDs started in 2007. In South Asia and sub-Saharan Africa, there are signs of a protracted transition, with the double burden of communicable diseases and NCDs. Many studies have also recognized regional and national variation in the epidemiological transitions.[11,12,14]

In the two middle-SDI regions, Latin America and the Caribbean, and North Africa and the Middle East, DALYs attributable to NCDs constituted 70% and 68% of the disease burden in 2017, respectively. In contrast, the proportion of CMNNDs and injuries is almost equivalent in both regions at a modest 15–16%.

In South Asia, a low-middle-SDI region, the transition of the disease burden has been dramatic. In 1990, CMNNDs accounted for 62% of the total disease burden, while NCDs accounted for 30%. Between 1990 and 2017, NCDs increased by 87%, causing 55% of the total disease burden by the end of this period; CMNNDs declined by 44%; and injuries increased by 24%. Other studies also showed countries in the South Asia region are experiencing an epidemiological transition, and this is reflected in a growing burden of NCDs.[15,16]

In sub-Saharan Africa, in 1990, three quarters of the disease burden was attributable to CMNNDs which did not show major declines until 2016. However, the proportion of NCDs increased by 60% between 1990 and 2017. Recent mortality studies in Asia and sub-Saharan Africa showed broadly, low- and middle-income regions are rapidly transitioning to lower total mortality and lower infectious disease mortality.[3,17]

Of low- and middle-SDI regions, sub-Saharan Africa and South Asia are currently confronting the most significant challenge because of a continued high burden of communicable diseases in the face of rising burdens of NCDs and in the context of weak and underfinanced health systems in both regions. The transition of the disease burden toward NCDs influences health systems and health financing by affecting population health needs, and the type and level of services demanded. As disease burden shifts, health systems must adapt, expanding or narrowing the scope and scale of services provided and integrated new technologies and approaches. In low- and middle-SDI regions, coping with the current burden of communicable disease and at the same time laying the groundwork for transforming the health system to deal with the impending NCD burden presents a major challenge for policy makers. Even in high-SDI regions, with both significantly more resources and a more stable disease burden dominated by NCDs, policy makers face serious health financing and delivery issues, but have far more financial latitude.

The transition of disease burden and epidemiologic pattern reflects both declines in premature death and increases in disability. In the regions, the decline from CMNNDs has translated primarily to a decline in premature mortality. In contrast, the shift to NCDs is reflected in increases in disability in the regions.[5] Premature

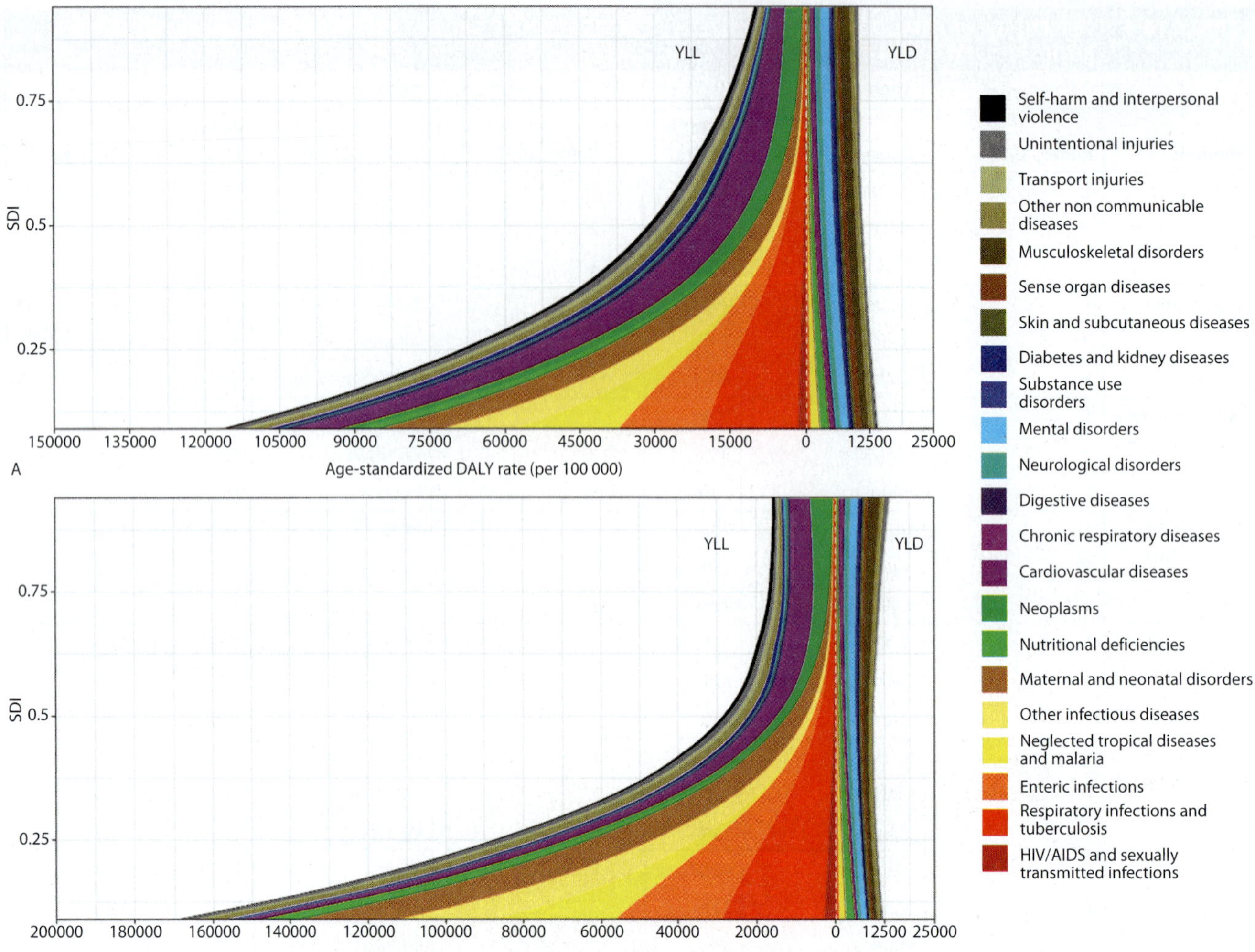

FIGURE 16-2. Expected relationship between age-standardized years of life lost (YLL) and years lived with disability (YLD) rates (per 100,000 people), and Socio-demographic Index (SDI) (A) and all-age YLL and YLD rates (per 100,000 people), and SDI (B) for 21 level two causes of disease burden.

mortality from CMNNDs falls substantially as sociodemographic status increases within the regions (Table 16-1, Fig. 16-2). With higher sociodemographic status, the composition of disease burden shifts toward disabilities associated with NCDs, especially those associated with age-related NCDs such as musculoskeletal disorders, diabetes, and neurological disorders. As sociodemographic status rises, the steady decreases in premature mortality and increases in disability cause the proportion of total DALYs attributable to disabilities to grow.[5]

Globally and regionally, the shift is also visible at a granular, disease-specific level, for example, in six major types of diseases (Fig. 16-3). Cardiovascular disease, neoplasms, and substance use disorders are expanding threats to global health, while the world has made progress on respiratory infections and tuberculosis, and enteric infections between 1990 and 2017.[18] Globally, respiratory infections and tuberculosis, and cardiovascular diseases were leading causes of all-age DALYs in 1990. By 2017, this changed to cardiovascular diseases and neoplasms (Fig. 16-3). Similarly, in South Asia, respiratory infections and tuberculosis, and enteric infections were leading causes of all-age DALY rates in 1990, whereas cardiovascular disease ranked as the leading cause of disease burden, followed by respiratory infections and tuberculosis, and enteric infections in 2017. However, the magnitude and the pattern vary by region. Cardiovascular diseases and neoplasms were increasing causes of all-age DALYs in South Asia, East Asia and the Pacific, Latin America and the Caribbean, North Africa and the Middle East, and sub-Saharan Africa. In contrast, cardiovascular diseases decreased in Europe and Central Asia and exhibited no significant change in North America, while neoplasms were increasing causes of disease burden in North America and showed no significant change in Europe and Central Asia over these years (Fig. 16-4). Substance use has been increasing causes of disease burden for North America, North Africa and Middle East, Europe and Central Asia, and Latin America and Caribbean regions. In North America, the rank shift between 1990 and 2017 was between NCD types. In contrast, respiratory infections and tuberculosis, and enteric infections are still leading causes of all-age DALYs in sub-Saharan Africa, although there has been progress between 1990 and 2017 (Fig. 16-3).

DETERMINANTS OF DISEASE BURDEN TRANSITIONS

In this section we discuss four major drivers of disease burden transitions at global and regional levels. The determinants are sociodemographic determinants, population growth, population aging, and health risk factors. Extending the concept of epidemiological transitions as a function of sociodemographic status, the GBD study has quantified the extent to which sociodemographic status accounts for the transition in disease burden, and has examined the shifts in disease and injury pattern purely expected as a function of changing sociodemographic status. Together, sociodemographic status- and country-specific factors in the regions account for more than 90% of the variance in the disease burden transition.[5,6] The GBD study indicates that sociodemographic determinants of the transition

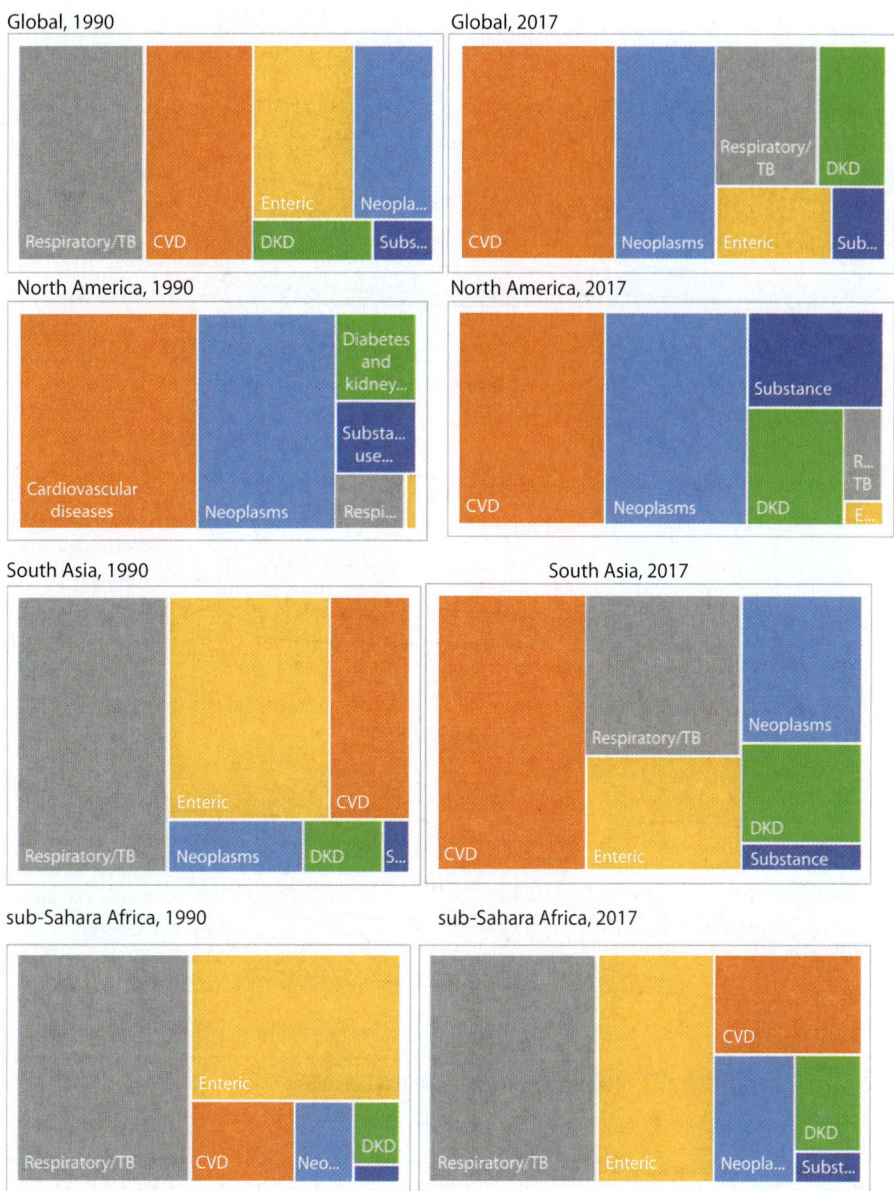

FIGURE 16-3. Global and regional comparison with percent of totally DALYs for all ages and both sexes in 1990 and 2017 for identified six disease types. Abbreviations: CVD = cardiovascular diseases; DKD = diabetes and kidney diseases; enteric = enteric infections; Respiratory/TB = respiratory infections and tuberculosis; Substance = substance use disorders.

encompassing income per person, average years of schooling after age 15 years, and total fertility rate explain more than 50% of the variance for CMNND and some NCD burden between regions and countries between 2006 and 2016. Exposure to health risk factors explains 11% of the decrease in DALYs at the global level, while population aging accounts for 6% of DALYs, and population growth for 12.4%.[5,6]

Sociodemographic Determinants

In the low- and low-middle-SDI regions,[19] sub-Saharan Africa and South Asia, CMNNDs caused the largest disease burden in 1990 and subsequently exhibited the greatest decline from 1990 to 2017, as measured in age-standardized DALYs (Fig. 16-5). These trends were offset by large increases for NCDs in these regions. At all other levels of sociodemographic status, CMNND causes of disease burden were lower than those due to NCDs, and in the high sociodemographic quantiles they were also lower than those due to injuries.[5] When sociodemographic status is low, regions experience higher premature mortality rates mainly from CMNNDs and lower disability rates compared with regions with higher sociodemographic status, which experience proportional premature mortality and disability rates that keep the disease burden constant. Regional developmental agendas in sub-Saharan Africa and South Asia should consider the health and health system impacts of improving income per capita and investments in education and reproductive health in preventing and controlling CMNNDs.

In low- and middle-SDI regions, the peak prevalence of many NCDs occurs at a younger age than in high-SDI regions. The socioeconomic impact of disability and premature death due to NCDs is enormous, since these deaths often affect the main income earner in the household and those who rear children. The health delivery system must be reorganized in order to fight the growing burden of NCDs. Patients with NCDs typically need care over a long period of time, sometimes decades, and this may require technologically advanced equipment which may not be available in these regions. It has been recommended that the management and control of NCDs include clinical management in a primary care setting, population-based interventions on health promotion, and macroeconomic policy.[15,20–22] The task of implementing effective programs to control NCDs in sub-Saharan Africa and South Asia should not be underestimated.

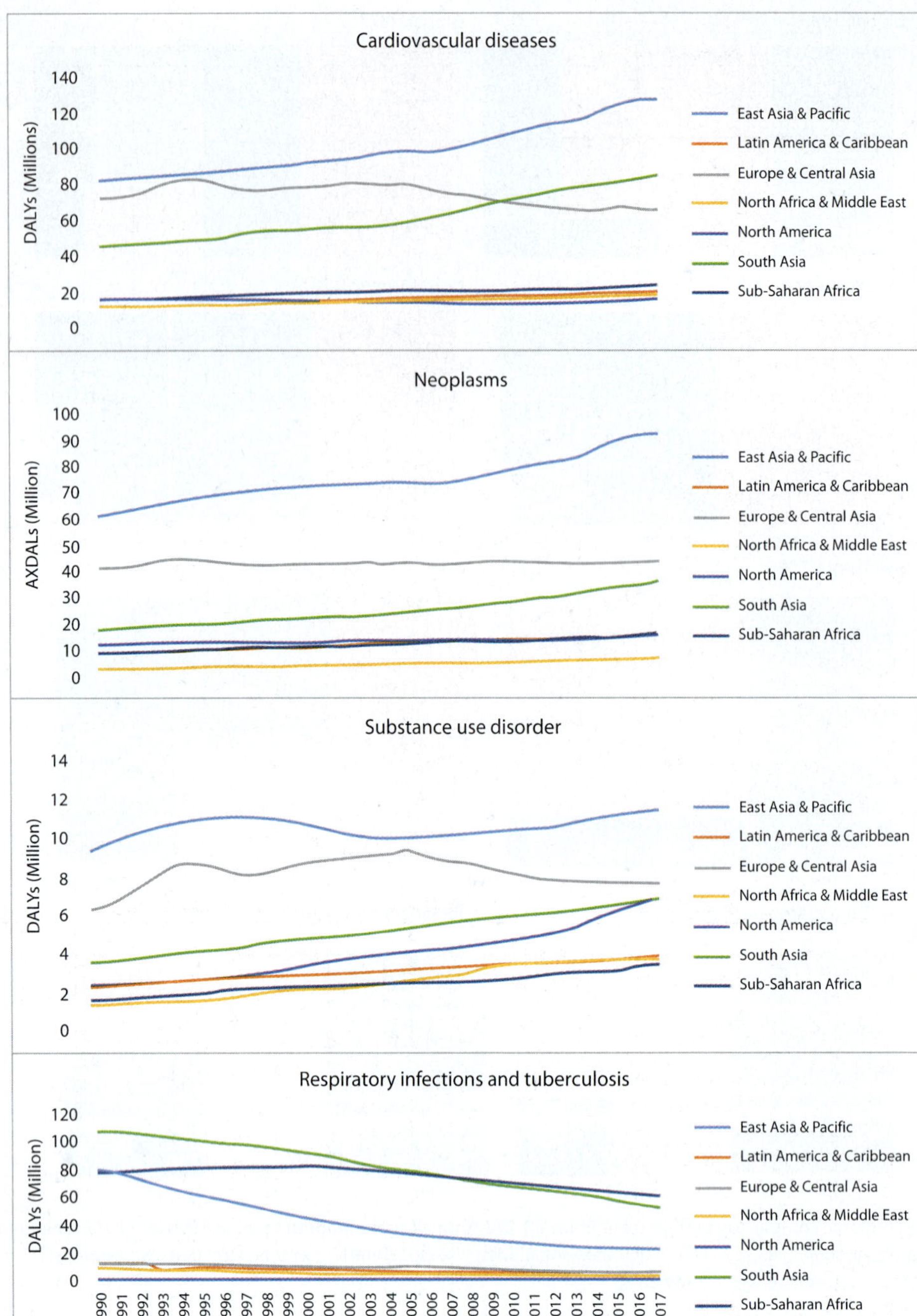

FIGURE 16-4. Regional trends of neoplasms, cardiovascular disease, substance use disorders, and respiratory infections and tuberculosis numbers of all-age DALYs for both sexes from 1990 to 2017.

Population Growth and Aging

Population size and age-structure changes potentiate and accelerate disease burden transitions. Population aging accounts for 14.9% of total deaths globally and population growth for 12.4% of deaths between 2006 and 2016.[5] Demographic changes and the transition in disease burden and epidemiological pattern of regions are closely related, and regions are experiencing varying degrees of these changes. Over recent decades, the reduction in overall disease burden or the total volume of DALYs is limited. This is largely explained by population growth and aging driving up the total number of DALYs. Therefore, demands on health systems are growing. Mortality levels start to decline at the beginning of the demographic transition. This is mainly caused by the reduction in mortality from CMNNDs. As the health transition progresses, fertility levels and the burden of CMNNDs decline, and the average age of the population increases. Thus, eventually, there are more elderly people in the population, and they are more susceptible to NCDs than younger people. The increase in the number of susceptible individuals at older ages increases the overall incidence and prevalence of NCDs, thereby accelerating the epidemiological transition.

There has been a strong shift between 1970 and 2017 toward longer life expectancy worldwide; life expectancy at birth overall increased by 13.5 years for men and 14.8 years for women.[9] The shift was most noticeable in regions at higher levels of SDI status.[23] However, the gap between life expectancy at birth and healthy life expectancy is growing, and indicates that people are not enjoying healthy life years despite their longer lifespan. In high-SDI regions, expanding aging populations are affected by age-related NCDs contributing to transitions in disease burden. Although low-SDI regions are still confronting the health financing issues associated with high-mortality and

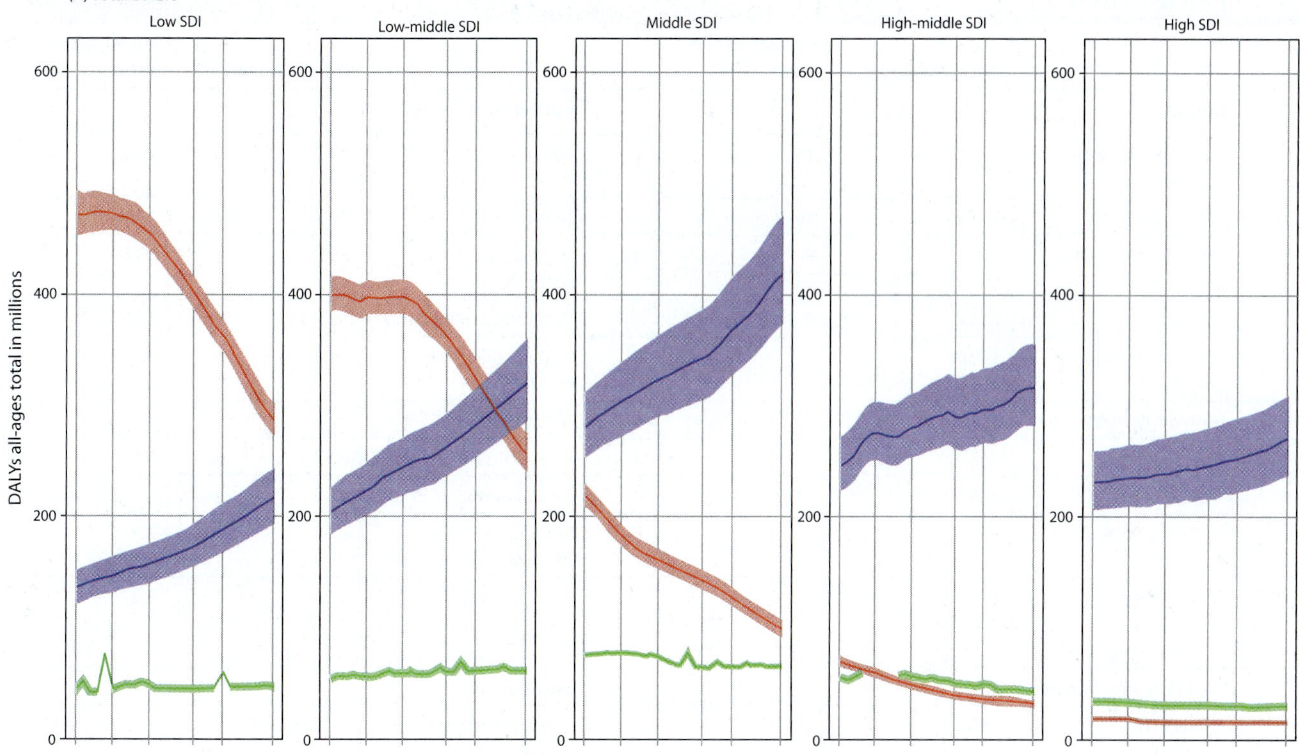

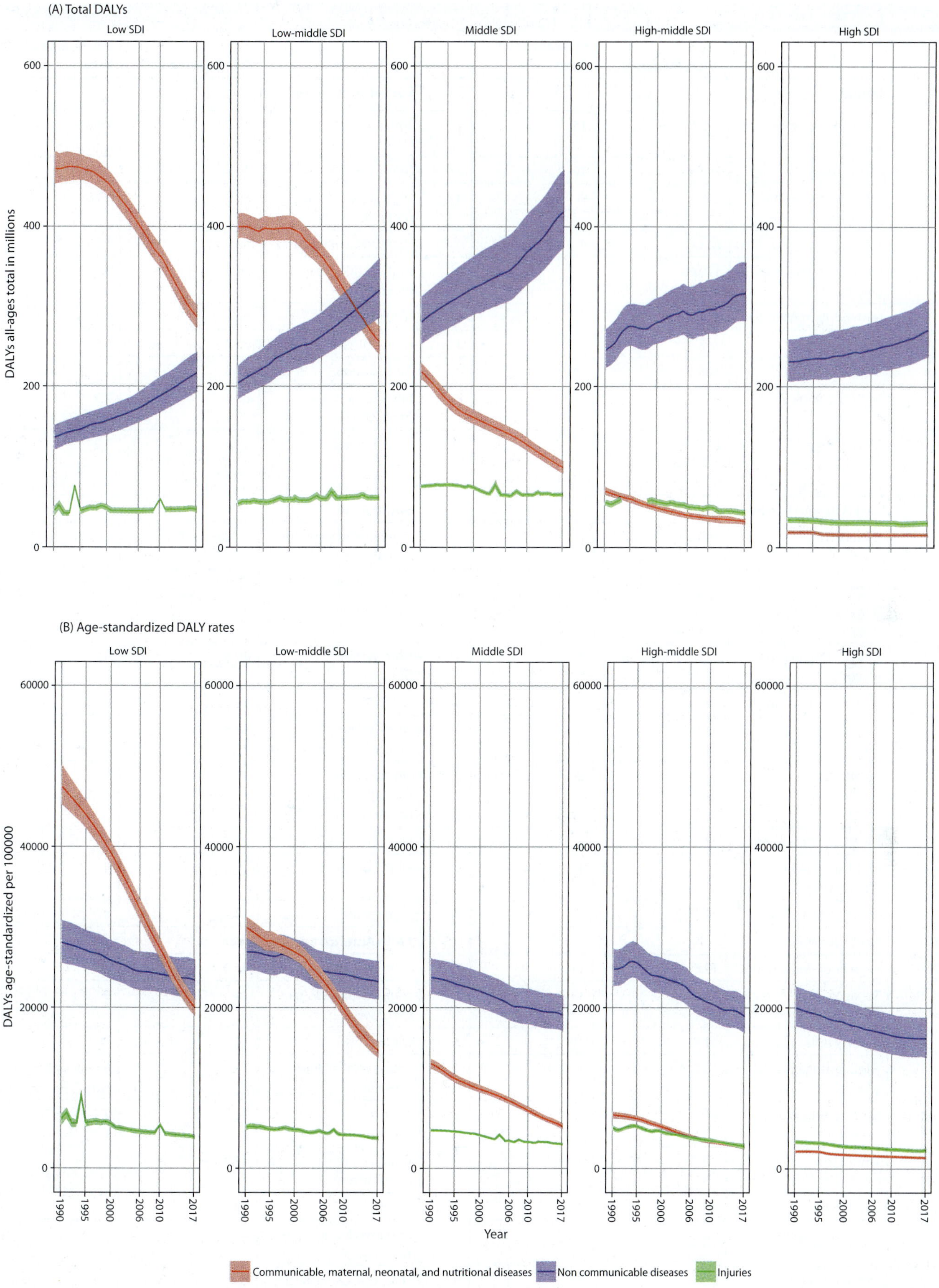

FIGURE 16-5. Trends of total DALYs (A) and age-standardized DALY rates (B) from 1990 to 2017 for GBD communicable, maternal, neonatal, and nutritional disorders; noncommunicable diseases; injuries by sociodemographic quantile with 95% uncertainty interval.

TABLE 16-2 TEN LEADING RISK FACTORS FOR ATTRIBUTABLE DISABILITY-ADJUSTED LIFE YEARS BY REGIONS, GBD 2017

		DALYs (Millions)	*Percentage of Total*			*DALYs (Millions)*	*Percentage of Total*
	Global				**Europe and Central Asia**		
1	Child and maternal malnutrition	326.6	13	1	Tobacco	41.2	14.2
2	Dietary risks	254.5	10	2	Dietary risks	40.6	13.9
3	High systolic blood pressure	218	9	3	High systolic blood pressure	39.6	13.6
4	Tobacco	213.4	9	4	High body-mass index	30	10.3
5	High fasting plasma glucose	170.6	7	5	High fasting plasma glucose	27.8	9.5
6	High body-mass index	147.7	6	6	Alcohol use	24.5	8.4
7	Air pollution	147.4	6	7	High LDL cholesterol	20.2	6.9
8	Alcohol use	108	4	8	Air pollution	11.6	4
9	High LDL cholesterol	94.9	4	9	Impaired kidney function	8.4	2.9
10	Unsafe water, sanitation, and handwashing	84.4	3	10	Occupational risks	8.3	2.8
	East Asia and Pacific				**South Asia**		
1	Dietary risks	100.6	16	1	Child and maternal malnutrition	120.6	19
2	Tobacco	87.2	14	2	Dietary risks	58.4	9
3	High systolic blood pressure	77.9	12	3	Air pollution	49.8	8
4	High fasting plasma glucose	52.8	8	4	High systolic blood pressure	49.6	8
5	High body-mass index	42.6	7	5	Tobacco	40.9	6
6	Air pollution	41.9	7	6	High fasting plasma glucose	38.6	6
7	Alcohol use	31.3	5	7	Unsafe water, sanitation, and handwashing	31	5
8	High LDL cholesterol	28	4	8	High body-mass index	25.3	4
9	Child and maternal malnutrition	27.8	4	9	High LDL cholesterol	24.2	4
10	Occupational risks	23.1	4	10	Alcohol use	23.4	4
	North America				**Latin America and Caribbean**		
1	High body-mass index	12.6	11	1	High body-mass index	15.4	9
2	Tobacco	12.2	11	2	High fasting plasma glucose	15	9
3	Dietary risks	11.4	10	3	Dietary risks	14.4	8
4	High fasting plasma glucose	10.5	10	4	High systolic blood pressure	13.5	8
5	High systolic blood pressure	8.7	8	5	Tobacco	12	7
6	Drug use	7.1	6	6	Child and maternal malnutrition	11.2	7
7	Alcohol use	4.5	4	7	Alcohol use	10.3	6
8	High LDL cholesterol	4.3	4	8	Impaired kidney function	6.1	4
9	Impaired kidney function	3.3	3	9	High LDL cholesterol	6	3
10	Occupational risks	2.9	3	10	Air pollution	5.9	3

(Continued)

TABLE 16-2 TEN LEADING RISK FACTORS FOR ATTRIBUTABLE DISABILITY-ADJUSTED LIFE YEARS BY REGIONS, GBD 2017 (Continued)

		DALYs (Millions)	Percentage of Total			DALYs (Millions)	Percentage of Total
	North Africa and Middle East				**Sub-Saharan Africa**		
1	Dietary risks	13	11	1	Child and maternal malnutrition	146	28
2	High systolic blood pressure	12.2	10	2	Unsafe water, sanitation, and handwashing	44.2	8
3	High body-mass index	11.9	10	3	Unsafe sex	33.6	6
4	Child and maternal malnutrition	11.7	10	4	Air pollution	29.1	6
5	High fasting plasma glucose	10.8	9	5	High systolic blood pressure	15.4	3
6	Tobacco	8.5	7	6	Dietary risks	14.8	3
7	High LDL cholesterol	7.3	6	7	High fasting plasma glucose	14.6	3
8	Air pollution	6	5	8	Alcohol use	12.6	2
9	Drug use	4	3	9	Tobacco	10.2	2
10	Impaired kidney function	3.5	3	10	High body-mass index	9.5	2

high-fertility rates, the proportion of aging individuals in all populations will continue to grow with economic, social, and epidemiological transitions. The future needs of these aging populations must be anticipated, and sustainable health financing schemes must be implemented to ensure that these needs are met over the long term, and that health systems remain functional. Population growth in low- and middle-SDI regions, and aging in high-SDI regions impact the healthcare costs faced by the health system. Regions need to make sure longer life expectancy of their populations translates to healthier life expectancy.

Health Risk Factors that Determine Disease Burden Transition

Studies show that health risk factors for the transition in disease burden include environmental, occupational, metabolic, and behavioral risks. Among risks that are leading causes of disease burden and that indicate risk factor transition, child underweight and stunting, unsafe sanitation, and household air pollution have shown the most significant declines, while metabolic risks, such as body-mass index and high fasting plasma glucose, showed significant increases between 1990 and 2017.[18] NCD burden from neoplasms and cardiovascular diseases are minimally related to SDI status; instead, local factors such as diet, physical activity, and other risk factors have a profound effect. However, with rising SDI status, the proportion of DALYs due to neoplasms and cardiovascular diseases increases because of the decrease in other causes of premature mortality. Some important causes of premature mortality such as neglected tropical diseases, cancers, and intentional injuries are also not strongly correlated with SDI status; rather, they are largely country-specific. Between 1990 and 2017, increasing trends in risk factors such as high systolic blood pressure and failure to reduce significantly risks such as poor diet and smoking have contributed to the growing disease burden from NCDs. Increasing obesity rates in high-income countries are further confirming the epidemiological transition theory as the epidemic of obesity leads to an increase in NCD burden. Decreases in child and maternal malnutrition, unsafe water, and improvements in sanitation and handwashing, and in unsafe sex have contributed to the decline in CMNNDs in the regions.[24]

In 2017, the five leading risk factors in terms of attributable DALYs at the global level were child and maternal malnutrition, dietary risks, high systolic blood pressure, tobacco, and high fasting plasma glucose (Table 16-2). Child and maternal malnutrition; unsafe water, sanitation, and handwashing; unsafe sex; air pollution; and high systolic blood pressure were among the top five attributable causes of DALYs in sub-Saharan Africa. High systolic blood pressure was a common leading risk factor in all regions and high fasting plasma glucose was a leading risk factor in all regions except South Asia and sub-Saharan Africa. Air pollution was a leading risk factor in these two regions (Table 16-2).

Dietary risk factors were among the five leading risks in all regions and the sixth in sub-Saharan Africa, and tobacco was among the five leading risk factors in all regions, the sixth in North Africa and the Middle East, and the ninth in sub-Saharan Africa. Common leading risk factors in terms of attributable DALYs were from metabolic risks. Child and maternal malnutrition remained the leading risk factor in South Asia and sub-Saharan Africa, while dietary risks that are likely true drivers of obesity, high systolic blood pressure, and high fasting plasma glucose[24] resulted in double burdens of undernutrition and overnutrition in the two regions in 2017 (Table 16-2).

IMPLICATIONS OF FINDINGS: GLOBAL AND REGIONAL HEALTH PROGRAMS AND POLICIES

Addressing Leading Risk Factors

The risk factors discussed in this chapter are widespread with major impacts around the globe. Therefore, understanding the role of these risk factors and the potential for interventions to address them is important for developing clear and effective strategies to improve population health at different levels. Reducing or eliminating the ten leading risk factors could reduce nearly three quarter of the disease burden (71% of the DALYs) globally (Table 16-2). Roughly two-thirds or more of the disease burden in sub-Saharan Africa (63%), Latin America and the Caribbean (64%), North America (70%), South Asia (73%), North Africa and the Middle East (74%), East Asia and the Pacific (81%), and Europe and Central Asia (86.5%) could be prevented and controlled if the regions address these ten leading risk factors. Nearly one-fifth (19%) of the disease burden in South Asia is attributable to child and maternal malnutrition, and one-half of the disease burden in sub-Saharan Africa is attributable to three risk factors: child and maternal malnutrition; unsafe water, sanitation, and hand washing; and unsafe sex combined. In low- and low-middle-SDI regions, disease prevention and control efforts must strengthen efforts to address child and maternal malnutrition, unsafe water, inadequate sanitation and hand washing, and unsafe sex, and simultaneously develop systems and strategies to address the growth in behavioral and metabolic risk factors NCDs. This call for action to prevent the dire consequences of the double burden of diseases is a profound challenge both within these countries and for the global health community. Global health programs and policies must reinforce and realize proposed strategies to prevent and control major health risk factors[25] by creating and strengthening approaches to reduce modifiable risk factors and addressing underlying social determinants; increasing national and regional commitments; multisectoral action and partnerships; and monitoring and evaluating risk factor trends and determinants, as well as burden of disease, itself.

Improving Healthcare Practice

Primary healthcare has played a key role in delivering communicable disease prevention and care interventions. In low- and middle-SDI regions, this role could be extended to address the transitions in disease burden and NCDs, as well, within the context of efforts to strengthen health systems by improving primary healthcare delivery. Practical policy directions to improve the primary healthcare response to the problem posed by transitions in disease burden include improving data on communicable disease and NCD; and aligning global and regional response strategies to address disease burden transition with health system strengthening and capitalize on a favorable global policy environment. Implementing these proposals requires action by national and international alliances in mobilizing the necessary investments for improved health of people in low- and middle-SDI countries undergoing disease burden transition.[20]

Addressing Sustainable Development Goals (SDGs) and Sociodemographic Factors

Health inequalities across regions with different sociodemographic levels of development could be addressed, in part, by strengthening and implementing Universal Health Coverage (UHC) strategies.[26,27] Based on projections of past trends from the GBD study, meeting a subset of established SDG targets by 2030 might be possible for some areas of the world, with more than 60% of countries projected to meet targets on under-5 mortality, neonatal mortality, maternal mortality ratio, and malaria. At the same time, on the basis of past trends, much of western and central sub-Saharan Africa is projected to attain very few—if any—defined targets in 2030. Furthermore, at current rates of progress, fewer than 5% of countries are projected to reach 2030 targets for 11 indicators, including childhood overweight, tuberculosis, and road injury mortality. Translation of the global SDG framework into investments and policy remains in its infancy, offering decision makers the opportunity to address both long-standing and emerging health challenges in the SDG era.[26]

Low-SDI regions are struggling under a large burden of CMNNDs, while also confronting increases in the prevalence of NCDs and injuries. The availability of resources to meet these numerous health needs is limited.[28] There is a need to raise levels of international commitment for health and ensure that adequate resources are available for low-income countries to increase spending for essential health services and to meet SDGs. In middle-income countries, some with growing working-age populations, communicable diseases among younger populations will continue to lead to high demands on the health system, while increased life expectancy will heighten demand at the other end of the age spectrum.[14] High-income countries will also have to contend with growing proportions of the population being elderly, and rapidly rising health expenditures. These countries face serious concerns about how a declining working-age population can support the health and the social services demanded by increasing numbers of elderly, as well as the large and growing contingent liabilities of publicly financed health and pension systems.[28]

Addressing Aging Population

As people live longer, they lose more years due to functional health loss. Drawing from GBD empirical characterization of the epidemiological transition on the basis of sociodemographic status, life expectancy, and health, adjusted life expectancy increases linearly with sociodemographic status, and years of functional health loss climb with rising sociodemographic status. Populations around the world are aging rapidly, with some of the fastest changes occurring in low- and middle-SDI countries. Promoting healthy aging, and building systems to meet the needs of older adults, will be sound investments in a future in which older people have the freedom to be and do what they value. There is a need to reinforce strategies to strengthen commitment to action on healthy aging in every country, including developing age-friendly environments; aligning health systems to the needs of older populations; developing sustainable and equitable systems for providing long-term care and improving measurement, monitoring, and research on healthy aging.[29]

Improving Burden of Disease Measurements and Its Translation to Action

Studying disease burden requires bringing together all available epidemiological and demographic data from multiple data sources using a coherent measurement framework, standardized estimation methods, and transparent data sources to allow comparisons of health loss to be made over time and across causes, age–sex groups, and geographies.[1] Based on the context and scope, implementing the following ***CDC-UF*** strategies would improve burden of disease measurements and facilitate translation of the evidence to action. *"C" stands for* ***Capacity*** *building on research, "D" stands for* ***Data*** *quality, availability, and accessibility, "C" stands for* ***Collaboration*** *with local and international research partners, "U" stands for* ***Utilization*** *of evidence to inform policy, and "F" stands for sustainable research* ***Funding****.*

Research system strengthening, training, and infrastructure development: Well-trained human resources and robust research infrastructure in academia, research institutes, and agencies are critical to ensure sustainability of efforts to generate disease burden evidence in developed and developing countries. Burden of disease measurement requires high computational technology and a multidisciplinary research team with advanced training in quantitative and health metrics science. Countries and international research partners need to increase their commitment to strengthening research capacity so as to provide rigorous burden of disease evidence at global, regional, national, and subnational levels.

Improving quality data availability and accessibility: A major challenge in burden of disease measurement has been availability and accessibility of quality data on mortality, cause of death, morbidity and disability, and on demographic, health risk factors, and covariates. Researchers and research institutes must ensure the data collected has maintained its quality, and is shared in usable formats.

Establishing and strengthening research networks and collaborations: Research networking and collaboration are important to obtain strong burden of disease evidence that captures all available data and produces validated estimates at global, regional, national, and subnational levels. Burden of disease study requires experts in different fields, data science knowledge and skills, and epidemiological and context knowledge about the regions and countries. Collaboration with researchers and research institutions helps to generate robust result and facilitate translating the evidence to local and global health policies and strategies.

Improving local and international research funding commitments: A comprehensive burden of disease study is a large undertaking that requires huge funding. To improve disease burden measurements and to support population health with strong evidence, sustainable funding sources are crucial for primary data collection, method and technology development and applications, and dissemination of findings and data sharing to users.

Ensuring evidence to policy translation: In the 21st century, not only generating strong evidence, but also translation to health policies and programs is tremendously important.[30] There is a need to design evidence to policy translation mechanisms and strategies at different levels. In order to effectively provide evidence that will support the development of health policy, a clear understanding of in-country evidence needs of decision makers and the context in which they operate is essential. Institutionalizing the use of evidence in decision making, building commitment to use evidence, including political commitment, as well as buy-in and support from other relevant stakeholder are essential. To use evidence effectively, decision makers must be well-equipped to access and interpret data, and should develop robust institutional mechanisms for utilizing evidence in policy making. Research providers should ensure that they carry out and present work in a way that is responsive to decision-makers' needs and should work with global health advocates to ensure support for the sustainability of using evidence for policy making. Disseminating the practice of evidence-informed policy making within and between countries, and sharing experiences and insights, is a necessary part of improving practices and facilitating broader uptake. Specific activities that are important to sustain evidence utilization include developing and implementing financed national research agendas, trainings especially for low- and middle-income countries; developing methods and technology applications; bringing together researchers, program implementers, and policy makers throughout the process and organizing policy dialogues; working with media to address language and cultural barriers; building incentives and systems; and expand financial and technical support.

References

1. Murray CJL, Barber RM, Foreman KJ, et al. Global, regional, and national disability-adjusted life years (DALYs) for 306 diseases and injuries and healthy life expectancy (HALE) for 188 countries, 1990–2013: quantifying the epidemiological transition. *Lancet.* 2015;386(10009):2145–91.
2. OMRAN AR. The epidemiologic transition: a theory of the epidemiology of population change. *Milbank Q.* 2005;83(4):731–57.
3. Misganaw A, Mariam DH, Araya T. The double mortality burden among adults in Addis Ababa, Ethiopia, 2006–2009. *Prev Chronic Dis.* 2012;9:E84.
4. Lopez AD, Mathers CD. Measuring the global burden of disease and epidemiological transitions: 2002–2030. *Ann Trop Med Parasitol.* 2006;100(5–6):481–99.
5. GBD 2016 DALYs and HALE Collaborators. Global, regional, and national disability-adjusted life-years (DALYs) for 333 diseases and injuries and healthy life expectancy (HALE) for 195 countries and territories, 1990–2016: a systematic analysis for the Global Burden of Disease Study 2016. *Lancet.* 2017;390(10100):1260–1344.
6. GBD 2015 DALYs and HALE Collaborators. Global, regional, and national disability-adjusted life-years (DALYs) for 315 diseases and injuries and healthy life expectancy (HALE), 1990–2015: a systematic analysis for the Global Burden of Disease Study 2015. *Lancet.* 2016;388(10053):1603–58.
7. Foreman KJ, Lozano R, Lopez AD, Murray CJ. Modeling causes of death: an integrated approach using CODEm. *Popul Health Metr.* 2012;10:1.
8. GBD 2017 Causes of Death Collaborators. Global, regional, and national age-sex-specific mortality for 282 causes of death in 195 countries and territories, 1980–2017: a systematic analysis for the Global Burden of Disease Study 2017. *Lancet.* 2018;392(10159):1736–88.
9. GBD 2017 DALYs and HALE Collaborators. Global, regional, and national disability-adjusted life years (DALYs) for 359 diseases and injuries and healthy life expectancy (HALE) for 195 countries and territories, 1990–2017: a systematic analysis for the Global Burden of Disease Study 2017. *Lancet.* 2018;392(10159):1859–1922.
10. GBD 2017 Disease and Injury Incidence and Prevalence Collaborators. Global, regional, and national incidence, prevalence, and years lived with disability for 354 diseases and injuries for 195 countries and territories, 1990–2017: a systematic analysis for the Global Burden of Disease Study 2017. *Lancet.* 2018;392(10159):1789–858.
11. Rivera-Andrade A, Luna MA. Trends and heterogeneity of cardiovascular disease and risk factors across Latin American and Caribbean countries. *Prog Cardiovasc Dis.* 2014;57(3):276–85.
12. Salomon JA, Murray CJL. The epidemiologic transition revisited: compositional models for causes of death by age and sex. *Popul Dev Rev.* 2002;28(2):205–28.
13. Yang G, Wang Y, Zeng Y, et al. Rapid health transition in China, 1990–2010: findings from the Global Burden of Disease Study 2010. *Lancet Lond Engl.* 2013;381(9882):1987–2015.
14. Rivera JA, Barquera S, Campirano F, Campos I, Safdie M, Tovar V. Epidemiological and nutritional transition in Mexico: rapid increase of non-communicable chronic diseases and obesity. *Public Health Nutr.* 2002;5(1A):113–22.
15. Quigley MA. Commentary: shifting burden of disease—Epidemiological transition in India. *Int J Epidemiol.* 2006;35(6):1530–1.
16. Kumar R, Kumar D, Jagnoor J, Aggarwal AK, Lakshmi PVM. Epidemiological transition in a rural community of northern India: 18-year mortality surveillance using verbal autopsy. *J Epidemiol Community Health.* 2012;66(10):890–3.
17. Santosa A, Byass P. Diverse empirical evidence on epidemiological transition in low- and middle-income countries: population-based findings from INDEPTH Network Data. *PLoS One.* 2016;11(5):e0155753.
18. Global Burden of Disease Study 2017. *Global Burden of Disease Study 2017 (GBD 2017) Results.* Seattle, United States: Institute for Health Metrics and Evaluation (IHME); 2017. Available at https://http://vizhub.healthdata.org/gbd-compare/.
19. Global Burden of Disease Study 2015 (GBD 2015). Socio-Demographic Index (SDI) 1980–2015 | GHDx [Internet]. [cited 2018 Oct 7]. Available at http://ghdx.healthdata.org/record/global-burden-disease-study-2015-gbd-2015-socio-demographic-index-sdi-1980%E2%80%932015.
20. Maher D, Smeeth L, Sekajugo J. Health transition in Africa: practical policy proposals for primary care. *Bull World Health Organ.* 2010;88(12):943–8.
21. Council (US) NR. *The Epidemiological Transition in Africa: Are There Lessons from Asia?.* United States: National Academies Press; 2012. Available at https://www.ncbi.nlm.nih.gov/books/NBK114529/.
22. Khalil A. The "epidemiological transmission" and "double-burden of disease": a focus on Africa. *Majmaah J Heal Sci.* 2014;2(2):4.
23. GBD 2016 Mortality Collaborators. Global, regional, and national under-5 mortality, adult mortality, age-specific mortality, and life expectancy, 1970–2016: a systematic analysis for the Global Burden of Disease Study 2016. *Lancet.* 2017;390(10100):1084–1150.
24. GBD 2017 Risk Factor Collaborators. Global, regional, and national comparative risk assessment of 84 behavioral, environmental and occupational, and metabolic risks or clusters of risks for 195 countries and territories, 1990–2017: a systematic analysis for the GBD Study 2017. *Lancet.* 2018;392(10159): 1923–1994.
25. World Health Organization. *Global Action Plan for the Prevention and Control of Noncommunicable Diseases: 2013–2020.* United States: WHO; 2013. Available at http://apps.who.int/iris/bitstream/10665/94384/1/9789241506236_eng.pdf.
26. GBD 2016 SDG Collaborators. Measuring progress and projecting attainment on the basis of past trends of the health-related Sustainable Development Goals in 188 countries: an analysis from the Global Burden of Disease Study 2016. *Lancet.* 2017;390(10100):1423–59.
27. Lim SS, Allen K, Bhutta ZA, et al. Measuring the health-related Sustainable Development Goals in 188 countries: a baseline analysis from the Global Burden of Disease Study 2015. *Lancet.* 2016;388(10053):181–50.
28. Gottret PE, Schieber G. *Health Financing Revisited: A Practitioner's Guide.* Washington, DC: World Bank; 2006:318.
29. WHO. *The Global Strategy and Action Plan on Ageing and Health: 2016–2020.* United States: WHO; 2016. Available at http://www.who.int/ageing/global-strategy/en/.
30. Langlois EV, Daniels K, Akl EA, eds. *Evidence Synthesis for Health Policy and Systems: A Methods Guide.* United States: WHO; 2018. Available at https://www.who.int/alliance-hpsr/resources/publications/Alliance-evidence-synthesis-MethodsGuide.pdf.

CHAPTER

17

Global Environmental Changes Reshaping Health in the 21st Century

Howard Frumkin

We inhabit a different earth than the one our great grandparents inhabited. Over the last two centuries, and especially in the seven or eight decades since World War II, the human condition has changed in unprecedented ways, both reacting to and driving changes in earth systems. These changes have far-reaching implications for human health and well-being. They also demand far-reaching responses—responses that extend the public health paradigm in unprecedented ways.

This chapter begins by introducing the Great Acceleration, a historic transformation of human civilization, featuring rising use of energy and materials, a growing global population, and multiple impacts on earth systems. This transformation ushered in a new geologic epoch, called the Anthropocene, and has pushed some earth systems toward, or perhaps beyond, planetary boundaries. Next, the chapter surveys the human health impacts of these global environmental changes (GECs). Many of these impacts result not from individual environmental changes, but from interactions among them, and with social and economic factors, reflecting the complexity of earth systems and of the many pathways through which they touch human health. Finally, the chapter discusses strategies for protecting human health in the context of GEC.

INTRODUCTION

Some historical context helps set the stage. Roughly 13,000 years ago, the Younger Dryas cooling at the end of the Pleistocene gave way to postglacial warming, marking the beginning of the Holocene. Our ancestors shifted from hunting and gathering to what we recognize as civilization—agriculture and manufacturing, art and culture, and towns and cities. Human well-being improved in countless ways, although there were also costs, such as less diverse diets and less contact with nature.[1]

Recent industrial history provides further context. The current human situation dates back just two or three centuries, when we learned how to unleash vast amounts of energy that had been locked in fossil fuels over geologic time. This ushered in a time of unprecedented growth in population, energy use, manufacturing, agriculture, and travel—indeed, in almost every measure of human activity—called the **Great Acceleration**.[2] These changes are shown in Fig. 17-1.

The Great Acceleration, in turn, changed the planet. Burning fossil fuels and razing forests raised atmospheric concentrations of carbon dioxide and other greenhouse gases (GHGs), altering the climate. Biodiversity diminished as species extinctions accelerated. The pH of oceans fell, as did oxygen levels in many ocean regions. In many parts of the world, nitrogen and phosphorus cycles were profoundly altered, soil degraded, forests extirpated, river flows interrupted, and fresh water supplies depleted. Some of these changes are shown in Fig. 17-2. These impacts are so far-reaching, and so consequential, that they have been recognized as comprising a new geological epoch, the **Anthropocene**.[3,4]

It is possible for these changes to go too far—to transgress limits, and to wreak considerable damage on earth systems, threatening not only human health and well-being, but also the very basis of civilization.[5,6] The image of planetary boundaries shown in (Fig. 17-3)* qualitatively presents this concept.

In addition to the processes shown in (Fig. 17-3)*, for which limits have been posited, other planetary changes also have potential impacts on human health. Examples include urbanization, changes in river systems, and changes in oceans. The following paragraphs describe these GECs.

GLOBAL ENVIRONMENTAL CHANGES

Climate Change

Climate change refers to a wide-ranging set of meteorological and related alterations.[7] A central feature is the increase in mean global surface temperature, largely a function of rising levels of atmospheric GHGs, including carbon dioxide (CO_2), methane, nitrous oxide, and fluorinated gases, and, to a lesser extent, deforestation. The most significant of the GHGs is CO_2 (Fig. 17-4) which derives predominantly from the combustion of the fossil fuels coal, petroleum, and natural gas (with coal the largest contributor). Associated earth system changes include sea-level rise due to the thermal expansion of water and to melting ice; ocean acidification due to absorption of CO_2; diminution of polar ice and of glaciers; changes in storm frequency and severity; changed rainfall patterns (increases in some areas and decreases in others); and more erratic weather. These changes in turn propel a wide variety of changes in other systems, such as shifts in the timing of seasons and in associated plant growth patterns[8,9]; movement of some species as their preferred habitats shift,[10,11] altered insect vector activity,[12–14] and others—many of which have potential impacts on human health.

Biodiversity loss: Biodiversity refers to the variety of life—the number and complexity of species—either at the genetic level, within an ecosystem or on larger spatial scales. It is a complex concept, including functional, genetic, and other dimensions.[15] Biodiversity is essential for robust ecosystem function; when biodiversity declines, ecosystems degrade,[16–18] as do the ecosystem services they provide to humans.[19,20] Biodiversity is currently declining worldwide—a phenomenon that has been dubbed "defaunation"—manifested in both species extinctions and reduced populations of many species.[21] The rate of species extinctions is so high—likely 1000 times background rates[22]—that it represents a mass extinction, the sixth such event

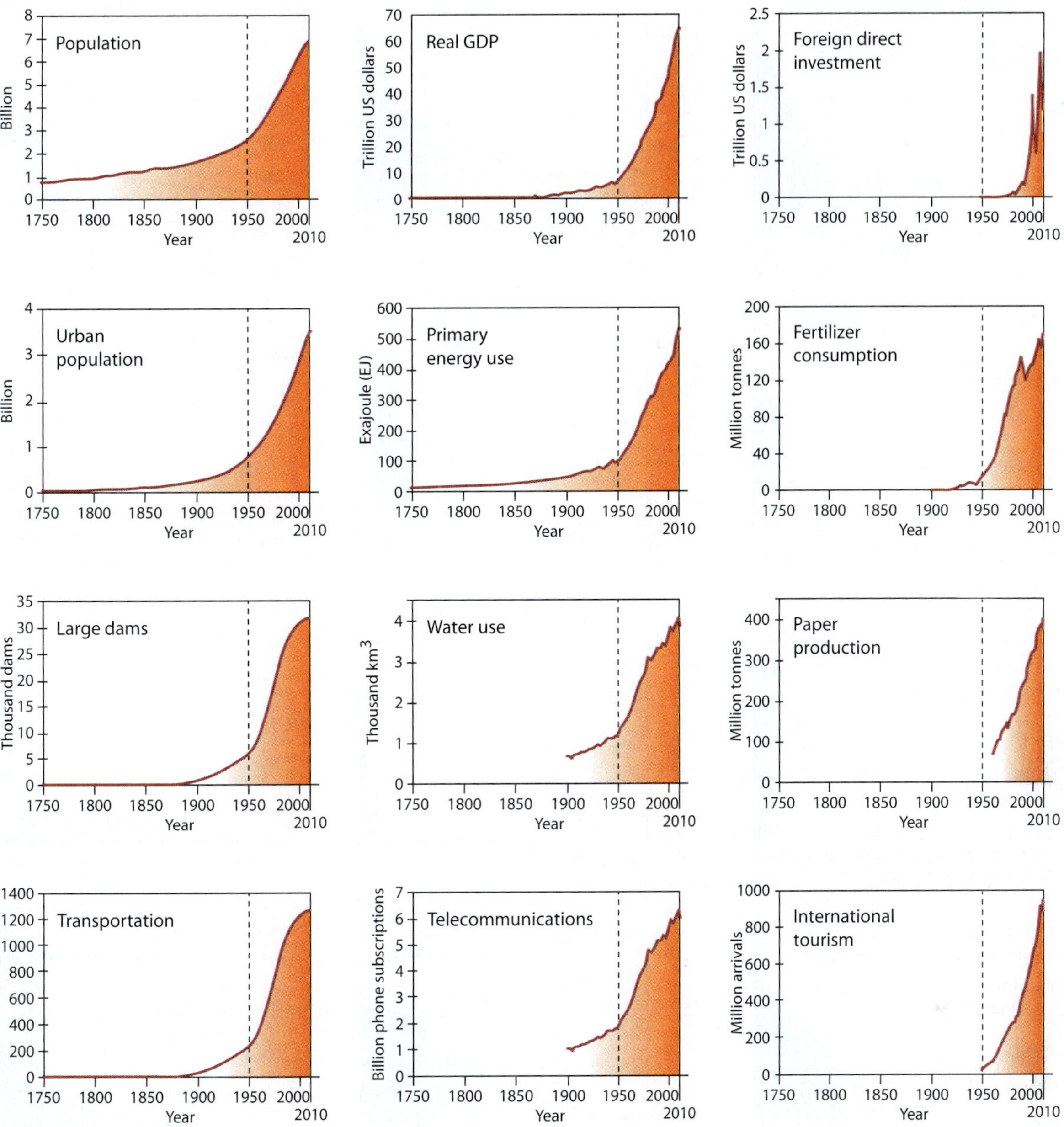

FIGURE 17-1. The Great Acceleration. Trends in globally aggregated indicators of socioeconomic development, 1750–2010. (*Source:* Used with permission from Steffen W, Broadgate WJ, Deutsch L, Gaffney O, Ludwig C. The trajectory of the Anthropocene: The Great Acceleration. *The Anthropocene Review*. 2015;2:81–98.[2])

the last half billion years, and the most devastating since an asteroid wiped out dinosaurs about 66 million years ago.[21,23,24] Among the key drivers are climate change[11] and land use change.[25,26] The 2002 Convention on Biological Diversity, a global agreement, has thus far failed to reduce the rate of species loss.[27] Biodiversity benefits people in diverse ways.[28,29] Conversely, biodiversity loss threatens health[18] through a range of pathways including infectious disease transmission (mediated by altered host or vector abundance; host, vector, or parasite behavior; and/or host or vector condition[30,31]), impaired immunoregulation (perhaps via reduced exposure to "Old Friends," organisms with which humans coevolved and that play a role in immunoregulation[32]), and loss of nutrition.[33,34] Two specific examples of biodiversity loss—pollinator loss and fisheries depletion—are directly relevant to human health because of their impacts on nutrition, as described below.

Chemical Contamination

A hallmark of the Anthropocene has been the production and environmental release of chemical substances. Some of these, such as lead and asbestos, occur naturally, and people have used and released them at low levels for centuries; the industrial era brought a dramatic upscaling of their use. Other substances, such as the many synthetic organic chemicals, began to be produced in the nineteenth and twentieth centuries, with dramatic increases in the second half of the twentieth century. Examples include pesticides; polycyclic aromatic hydrocarbons such as naphthalene and anthracene; halogenated hydrocarbons such as polychlorinated biphenyls, used as coolants and dielectric fluids and polybrominated diphenyl ethers, used as flame retardants; plastics such as polymers of styrene, propylene, and vinyl chloride; plasticizers such as phthalates and bisphenols; and perfluorinated compounds such as perfluorooctanesulfonic acid.

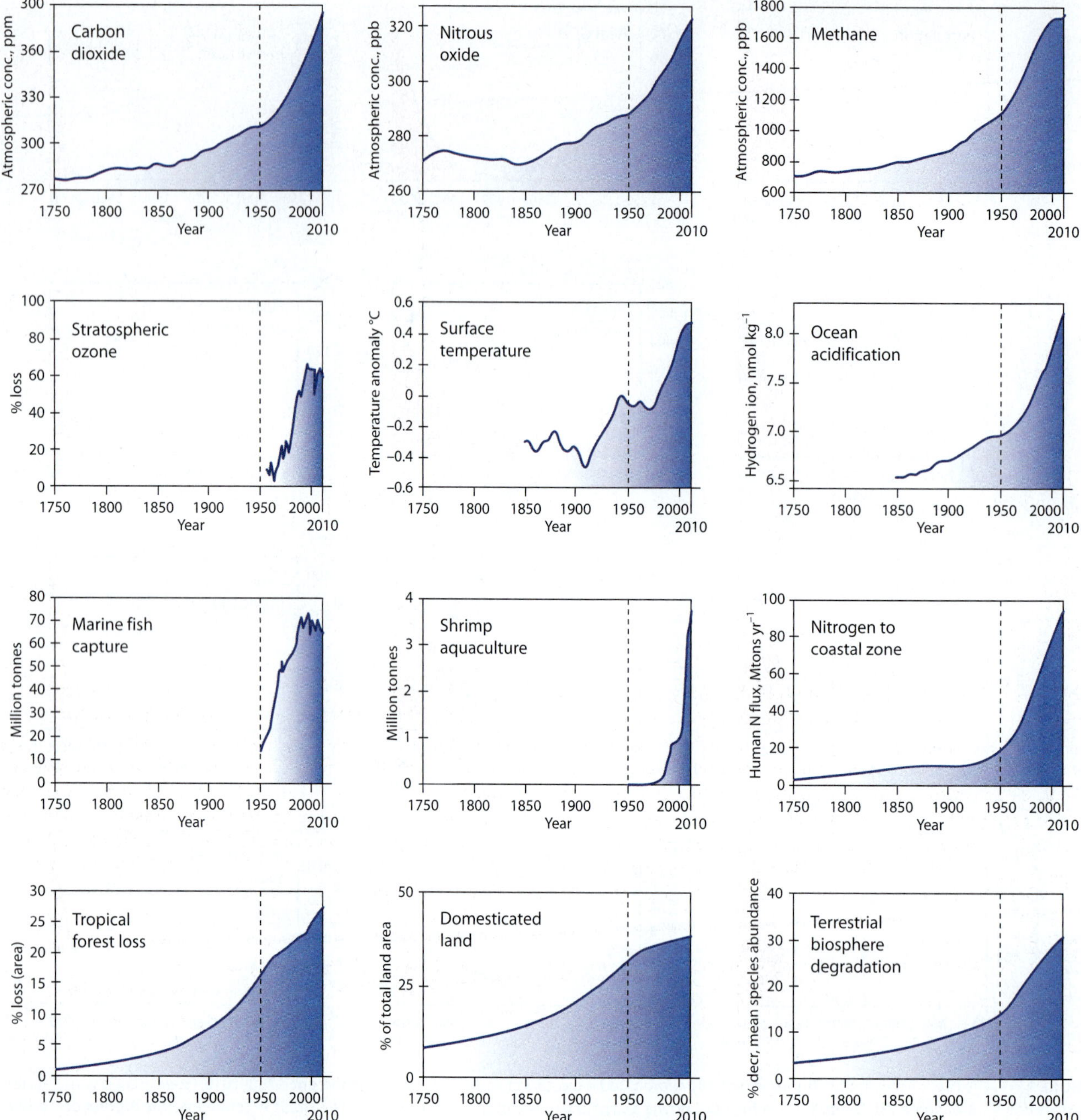

FIGURE 17-2. Trends in the structure and function of earth systems, 1750–2010. (*Source:* Used with permission from Steffen W, Broadgate WJ, Deutsch L, Gaffney O, Ludwig C. The trajectory of the Anthropocene: The Great Acceleration. *The Anthropocene Review*. 2015;2:81–98.[2])

More recently, widespread chemical contamination by pharmaceuticals[35] and nanoparticles[36] has been recognized.

Global contamination by chemicals is far-reaching. For example, persistent organic pollutants (**POPs**) are widely found in fresh water bodies worldwide.[37,38] They are also found in biota, even in places as remote as the Arctic (far from where these substances were ever made or used), especially in marine mammals at high trophic levels of the food web.[39,40] And they are found in humans; biomonitoring has documented body burdens of POPs in substantial proportions of populations tested.[41,42] **Plastics** are another example. Large-scale plastic production began after World War II, and has now reached 300 million metric tons per year, or about 40 kg for each man, woman, and child on earth, accounting for about 4% of global petroleum use.[43] Plastics are extremely persistent; once disposed of, they break down to particles and microplastics and persist in the environment. An estimated 4.8–12.7 million metric tons enter the oceans each year,[44] and much of this is entrained by ocean gyres into massive floating plastic zones. Animals take up this plastic; an estimated 90% of seabirds have plastic in their bodies,[45] and plastic is found in substantial proportions of seafood sold in food markets.[46] In addition to their polymer content, an average of about 7% of plastic consists of other chemicals such as plasticizers and flame retardants.[47] Moreover, plastics efficiently adsorb organic chemicals.[48] Thus, widespread global dissemination of plastic also entails widespread organic chemical exposure. In addition to such planetary-scale exposure, hot spots of chemical exposure occur near sites of chemical manufacturing and use, and at waste sites (Toxic Sites Identification Program, http://www.pureearth.org/projects/toxic-sites-identification-program-tsip/)—a long-term legacy challenge.

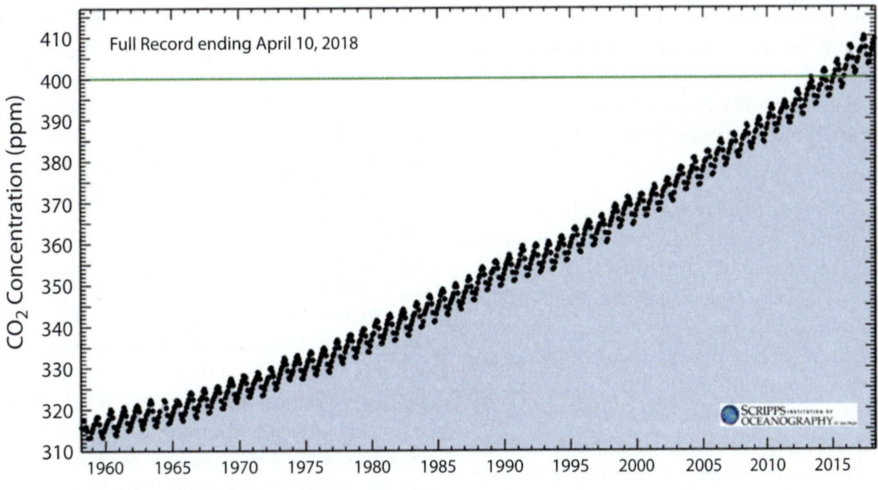

FIGURE 17-4. The Keeling curve, showing atmospheric carbon dioxide (CO_2) concentration as measured at the Mauna Loa Observatory in Hawaii. The CO_2 concentration was about 280 ppm in preindustrial times, and surpassed 400 ppm in 2016. (*Source:* Used with permission from C. D. Keeling, S. C. Piper, R. B. Bacastow, M. Wahlen, T. P. Whorf, M. Heimann, and H. A. Meijer, Exchanges of atmospheric CO_2 and 13CO_2 with the terrestrial biosphere and oceans from 1978 to 2000. I. Global aspects, SIO Reference Series, No. 01-06, Scripps Institution of Oceanography, San Diego, 88 pages, 2001. Retrieved from https://keelingcurve.ucsd.edu/.)

Atmospheric Aerosol Loading

Atmospheric aerosols (or particulate matter, PM) are particles, either liquid or solid, suspended in air. Some aerosols are emitted directly into the atmosphere, from natural sources such as soil dust and sea salt, or from anthropogenic sources such as fuel combustion. Other aerosols form in the atmosphere when precursors such as sulfates and nitrates are chemically converted. Aerosols vary considerably from place to place and across time with respect to particle size, source, chemical composition, concentration, and persistence in the atmosphere.[49] Aerosols are a planetary health issue because they affect both the earth's climate system, through effects on cloud formation and other aspects of the hydrological cycle, and the reflectivity of solar energy arriving at the earth. They are also a direct health issue, with adverse health effects that include cardiovascular and neurologic toxicity, carcinogenesis, and others.[50] Extremely high levels of PM are found in major cities in low- and middle-income countries (LMICs) such as in China[51] and India,[52] where health impacts are severe.[53,54]

Stratospheric Ozone Depletion

The stratosphere, the portion of the atmosphere from 6 to 30 miles (10–50 km) above the earth's surface, contains ozone, which functions to absorb harmful ultraviolet (UV) radiation from the sun. Stratospheric ozone forms from molecular oxygen under the influence of short wavelength UV radiation. It decomposes naturally, but the decomposition is greatly accelerated by halogen radicals such as chlorine and bromine. These are delivered to the stratosphere by anthropogenic chemicals, most notably the chlorofluorocarbons (CFCs).[55] Stratospheric ozone depletion permits more UV-B radiation to arrive at the earth's surface, potentially increasing the risk of cataracts and skin cancer in humans, and potentially altering biogeochemical cycles and terrestrial and damaging marine ecosystems.[56] Stratospheric ozone depletion was scientifically documented in the 1980s, as was the causative role of CFCs. This recognition led to the 1987 Montreal Protocol, which implemented a global phaseout of CFCs—a notable achievement of global environmental governance. Indeed, there is evidence of a slow "healing" of the ozone layer in the upper stratosphere in recent decades.[57] However, evidence also suggests a decline in lower stratospheric ozone concentrations, perhaps a function of climate change.[58]

Ocean Acidification

The world's oceans have absorbed between a quarter and a third of anthropogenic CO_2 emitted into the atmosphere. The dissolved CO_2 reacts with water to form carbonic acid (H_2CO_3) which then dissociates, releasing hydrogen ions to form bicarbonate (HCO_3^-) and carbonate (CO_3^{2-}) ions, and lowering pH of ocean waters. As a result, the pH at the ocean surface has fallen by an estimated 0.1 pH unit from preindustrial levels—equivalent to about a 30% increase in hydrogen ion concentration (since the pH scale is logarithmic)—and this trend is continuing. While the effects of acidification vary across species and locations, coral formation and shell formation by shellfish are threatened, and the biology of some species of zooplankton and algae—key elements of marine food webs—is disrupted.[59] In addition, many fish species are physiologically disrupted, with compromised survival and growth.[60] These problems are compounded by concurrent challenges including nutrient loading, pollution, hypoxia, overfishing, and warming. Potential impacts on human health include reduced dietary protein, iron, vitamin A, and other nutrients from fish.

Other Ocean Alterations

Chemical contamination and acidification are not the only changes affecting the world's oceans. **Oxygen depletion** has been documented in many ocean locations, due principally to climate change. Warmer temperatures decrease oxygen solubility in water, and increase the rate of oxygen consumption through respiration. Moreover, warmer temperatures weaken ocean overturning circulation, reducing the transfer of oxygen from the atmosphere and surface waters into the ocean interior.[61] Along coasts, climate factors also operate to reduce oxygen, but the more important driver is **nutrient loading** (of nitrogen, phosphorus, and organic matter), primarily from agricultural runoff, sewage discharges, and the combustion of fossil fuels. Coastal low-oxygen zones can increase production of nitrous oxide, a potent GHG; reduce eukaryote biodiversity; alter the structure of food webs; and threaten food security and livelihoods. A symptom of altered coastal systems is **harmful algal blooms**, which are becoming more frequent and extensive in many parts of the world.[62,63] Human health impacts include various forms of shellfish poisoning (amnesic, neurotoxic, paralytic, and diarrhetic) and ciguatera fish poisoning, and these health impacts can be compounded by economic impacts on fishing, recreation, and tourism. The combination of nutrient loading, hypoxic water, and algal blooms can trigger major fish die-offs, as has occurred periodically along the Philippine coast.[64,65] These events, too, can threaten local nutrition and livelihoods.

River System Alterations

Human activity has also altered the planet's river systems. More than half of the world's surface water traverses a dam on its way to the oceans,[66] and a current wave of dam construction is projected to double the number of large hydroelectric dams by 2030,[67] leaving almost no free-flowing major river system. In some ways, this is a public health advance; energy poverty is a dangerous predicament, reliable energy is a pillar of health and prosperity, and hydroelectricity is a relatively clean form of power. But dams come at a cost. They affect not just water flow but also fluxes of nitrogen, phosphorus, iron, silica, and sulfur[66]—sometimes with global-scale implications.[68–70] Dammed reservoirs can be significant sources of GHGs.[71] River ecosystems are altered, species composition changes, and fish populations can be seriously compromised.[66] Major dam projects can displace large numbers of people, with attendant risks ranging from infectious disease to depression and anxiety.[72] Changing conditions along rivers can raise the local risk of malaria, schistosomiasis, and other infectious diseases[73–76]; the case of schistosomiasis is discussed below. River alterations can even trigger the formation of toxic materials such as methylmercury.[77] Many of these risks can be managed, but it is clear that alterations in river systems on a planetary scale have implications for human health.

Fresh Water Depletion

The depletion of major aquifers by human water withdrawals is well documented; of the world's 37 largest aquifers, human withdrawals have depleted 21 beyond their tipping points.[78] In some parts of the high plains water system in the United States, principally the Ogallala aquifer, water levels have fallen by over 150 feet since 1950.[79] This will likely aggravate longstanding out-migration from the Great Plains, as wells run dry. In combination with the stresses of climate change,[80] it also likely portends substantial changes in food production patterns. These directly and indirectly affect health and well-being.

Land Changes

Human activities can affect land in at least two ways: by changing land cover and by degrading soil. Land can be characterized according to its dominant biotic and abiotic features and according to its human uses. Examples of **land cover** types include grassland, forest, and wetland, and examples of **land use** categories include agricultural, recreational, and commercial. In 1700, nearly half of the earth's land surface was wild, and most of the remainder (45%) was in a semi-natural state, lightly affected by human habitation and agriculture. By 2000, more than half the earth's land had been appropriated for human use, less than 20% was seminatural, and only a quarter remained wild[81]—a transformation of as much as 50% of the earth's ice-free land surface.[82] Human modifications include deforestation, rangeland expansion, metropolitan expansion, infrastructure development (railroad, road, power lines), hydrological alteration (dams, irrigation, canal construction), agricultural development (crops, livestock), and natural resource extraction (mining, logging, hunting).[83] Forests have been converted to tree plantations or cleared for farming and grazing, grassland has been irrigated to form cropland or overgrazed, and coastal wetlands have given way to urban growth. The need to feed the human population is a major driver; 40% of the earth's ice-free land surface is now in agriculture.[82,84] Globalization of food production and supply has accelerated land use changes far from where products are consumed.[85] But pressure on land also occurs close to markets; a recent analysis suggests that urban expansion will result in a 1.8–2.4% loss of global croplands by 2030, mostly in Asia and Africa, affecting especially fertile croplands.[86] Moreover, some relatively small, but biologically important biomes have been dramatically altered. For example, about 38% of mangrove forests along tropical coasts have been lost, largely to aquaculture—compromising coastal protection, native fish production, and other ecosystem services.[87]

In addition to these direct transformations in land cover and land use, virtually all land has been affected in some way by human activity. Peatland offers an example of such an indirect land change. Peatland covers less than 3% of the earth's surface, much of it in the far north, but plays a critical role in carbon storage. Climate change has resulted in drying of peatlands, permitting smoldering fires that release large amounts of carbon dioxide—a phenomenon that has more than doubled in recent decades.[88] Similarly, boreal forests represent the world's second largest forest biome, and function both as a carbon sink and as the source of over half the world's timber.[89] Drying, pest invasions, and fire, driven by climate change, are displacing and degrading large areas of boreal forest.[90–92] These changes collectively represent major alterations of the world's land, with diverse potential impacts on ecosystem services and on human health.[93]

Soil Loss

Soil is a foundation of many ecosystem functions and services, including agricultural production, carbon storage, and water management,[94,95] with extensive benefits for human health. Soil quantity and quality have been depleted in many parts of the world. With regard to quantity, conventional farming practices, in particular tilling and plowing, allow soil to be lost through erosion and dust formation at rates up to two orders of magnitude faster than it can reform.[96] The United Nations Food and Agriculture Organization estimated in 2015 that soil losses from erosion were reducing global crop yields by 0.3% annually, and would reduce global harvests by 10% by 2050.[97] With regard to quality, such changes as loss of organic matter, nutrient depletion or excess, acidification, and accumulation of salts and/or agrochemicals degrade soil; these follow from overgrazing, overtillage, deforestation, poor land management, harvest of fuelwood, and urbanization.[98] The full extent and nature of soil loss around the world is not well quantified.[98] However, it is clear that reduced soil quantity and quality can threaten human health in various ways. Perhaps most prominently, soil loss is a barrier to the intensified agricultural production needed to feed a growing world population.[99]

Urbanization

Urbanization is not a biophysical change like the other planetary changes described here, but it represents a global shift in both demographic and land use patterns. With more than half of humanity now living in cities—a proportion predicted to reach two-thirds by 2050, as almost all current and future population growth is in cities[100]—the city has become the prototypical human habitat. Megacities of over 10 million people, such as Mexico City and São Paulo, Cairo and Lagos, Karachi and Delhi, and Manila and Jakarta, command much attention, but nearly half the world's urban dwellers live in a growing number of relatively small cities with fewer than 500,000 inhabitants.[100]

Urbanization has emerged with different trajectories, and in different ways, in different places. Europe and the America urbanized relatively early and have plateaued, while rapid urbanization continues in Asia and Africa. In the global south, fast-growing cities confront a range of health and environmental challenges, including deficiencies in basic infrastructure (piped water, sewage, solid waste management, electricity, transportation, housing) and hazardous exposures (extremely poor air quality, noise, and unsafe roadways)—compounding problems of poverty, poor governance, and inadequate social services.[101,102] In wealthy settings in North America, Europe, and Australia, and increasingly in other regions, urban environmental health challenges reflect excessive automobile dependence, with associated urban sprawl, and resulting problems such as poor air quality, sedentary lifestyles, and injury risk.[103] Some problems are common to cities in both wealthy and poor nations, such as extreme social stratification, neighborhoods of concentrated poverty, insufficient greenspace, food deserts, and vulnerability to disasters.

Cities have substantial impacts on planetary systems and vice versa, exemplifying cross-scale relationships.[104,105] Energy and resource flows are concentrated in cities, a phenomenon that increases with prosperity.[106] Accordingly, cities draw energy and materials from, and deposit waste in, places far beyond their borders—a phenomenon termed "urban teleconnections."[107] The concept of urban metabolism was introduced over a half century ago[108]; updated in the context of planetary change, it guides contemporary researchers in quantifying the footprints of cities on their "resource hinterlands."[109,110] Cities also exert direct impacts such as regional warming through the heat island effect.[111] Both distant and proximate impacts stand to increase as cities expand not only demographically but also geographically.[86,112]

Biogeochemical Flows

Nitrogen and phosphorus both cycle through various chemical states in natural systems, processes that are essential to life. Human activity has substantially altered the cycling of both elements.

In the nitrogen cycle, atmospheric nitrogen (N_2) is fixed, or converted to reactive, bioavailable forms such as ammonia (NH_3), which then undergo nitrification to nitrites (NO_2) and nitrates (NO_3). These, in turn, are taken up by living organisms, and incorporated into nucleotides for DNA and RNA, amino acids for proteins, and other essential biological molecules (Fig. 17-5). Nitrogen fixation occurs naturally, carried out primarily by microorganisms, including cyanobacteria and rhizobia associated with the root systems of legumes and certain other plants. Lightning is another mechanism of natural nitrogen fixation. Other microorganisms accomplish the reverse process, denitrification. Over millennia, nitrogen fixation and denitrification remained roughly in balance, maintaining a nitrogen cycle in equilibrium. However, human activities have greatly increased nitrogen fixation on a planetary scale, to the point that anthropogenic nitrogen fixation exceeds natural nitrogen fixation.[113] The quantitatively most important such activity is synthetic fertilizer manufacturing; which dates from the 1913 development of the Haber-Bosch process for synthesizing ammonia. Fertilizer revolutionized agriculture worldwide, and now accounts for over half the nutrients received by the world's crops—but the global efficiency of nitrogen use in agriculture is only about 12%, meaning that most of the biologically available nitrogen applied is lost to the environment.[114] Other human contributions to nitrogen fixation include combustion of fossil fuels and biomass (yielding oxides of nitrogen as byproducts), and large-scale cultivation of leguminous crops. Together, these human activities have substantially altered the nitrogen cycle. Impacts occur from the local scale to the global scale. For example, when fertilizers run off into nearby waterways, excess nitrate accumulation can lead to eutrophication—excessive nutrient enrichment that triggers excessive algal and plant growth. This problem is expected to intensify in regions with high rainfall and heavy nitrogen inputs, such as Southeast Asia, India, and China.[115]

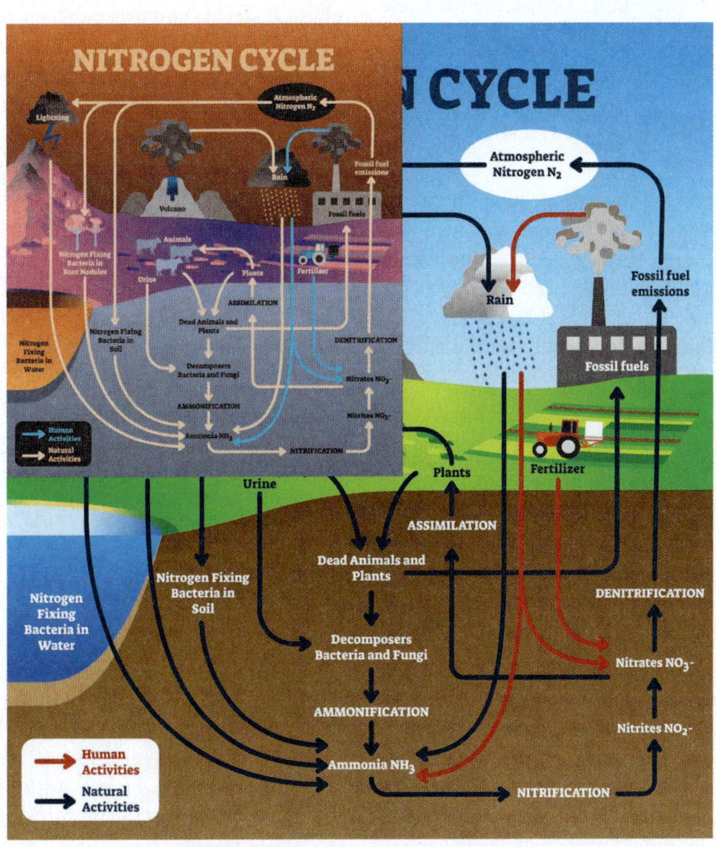

FIGURE 17-5. The nitrogen cycle. (*Source:* VectorMine/Shutterstock.)

Similarly, excess nitrate deposition is associated with soil acidification. Globally, nitrous oxide (N_2O) is a powerful GHG.

Phosphorus is also an essential biological element, a component of nucleic acids, of the phospholipids that comprise cell membranes, of adenosine triphosphate and other components of the cellular energy apparatus, and of bones (in the form of calcium phosphate), among other roles. The phosphorus cycle is substantially slower than the nitrogen cycle. As phosphorus-containing rock weathers, phosphorus leaches into surface water and soil, from which it is taken up by plants, and thence by animals that ingest the plants. The phosphorus thus incorporated into biological material is returned to soil as waste and decomposition products. On a global scale, there is a steady transfer of this phosphorus from rock and soil to water, and eventually to ocean sediments where it accumulates as insoluble calcium phosphate. Globally, seawater contains as much phosphorus as soil.

Human interventions affect phosphorus cycling in at least two important ways. Most importantly, phosphate is mined in large quantities from surface deposits for use in fertilizers. Globally, fertilizer production has reached at least three times the natural rate of phosphorus mobilization.[116,117] As with nitrogen, excessive fertilizer application and inefficient uptake results in considerable runoff of phosphates into waterways, contributing to eutrophication. Rainforest loss also disturbs phosphorus cycling. Rainforest soils contain little or no reserve of phosphorus and other nutrients, so rainforest ecosystems function primarily through nutrient recycling. When rainforests are cut down or burned, rainwater quickly washes away the pool of phosphorus in soil and plants, leaving depleted, unproductive soil[118,119]—a threat to agriculture, and thus to nutrition, in affected areas. Significant changes in the phosphorus cycle may be imminent. First, available phosphorus for use in fertilizers is a finite resource, and "peak phosphorus" may occur during coming decades[120,121]; innovations in phosphorus recovery and reuse will be needed to avoid limitations in agricultural productivity.[122] Second, increased fluxes of carbon and nitrogen relative to phosphorus may alter the balance of these elements in biological processes in ways that are as yet poorly understood.[123]

THE IMPACT OF GLOBAL CHANGES ON HUMAN HEALTH

The Anthropocene is thus marked by a wide range of earth system changes. But these changes have not just spelled disruption and danger. In many ways, the Anthropocene has been good to us. The human population has grown, infant mortality has fallen, and life expectancy has lengthened. We have conquered ancient health scourges such as smallpox, we are close to conquering polio, and we have limited the damage done by many diseases, from leprosy to tuberculosis to syphilis. Violence, while still a widespread problem, has diminished globally.[124]

But the story is not all rosy. Deep disparities persist; the wealthy enjoys far better health than the poor. Infectious diseases—thought by some to be on the way to history books in the decades following World War II, thanks to antibiotics—continue to challenge public health, propelled by globalization, climate change's impact on disease vectors, newly emerging and re-emerging strains of viruses and bacteria, antimicrobial resistance, and other factors. In addition, the Great Acceleration brought with it an epidemiologic transition, in which chronic and degenerative diseases supplanted infectious diseases as leading causes of morbidity and mortality in many parts of the world.[125-127] And GECs now threaten the health gains of the last two centuries in a wide range of ways. There is an irony here: that human health is better than ever, thanks to the gains of the Anthropocene, but looming threats may reverse many of these health gains. This is a core insight of the framework known as Planetary Health. In the words of the Rockefeller Foundation-Lancet Commission on Planetary Health, "we have been mortgaging the health of future generations to realize economic and development gains in the present."[128]

GECs affect virtually every aspect of human health.[128] Drawing the lines from GECs to health is complex; the pathways are both direct and indirect, characterized by positive and negative feedback loops, emergent properties, and surprises. Figure 17-6, showing pathways from climate change to health, hints at this complexity. Heat and weather threaten health directly, through heat waves, extreme weather events, and heat-induced aggravation of air pollution. Other health effects, such as reduced food yields and nutritional content, and increased risk of some infectious diseases, are secondary, mediated by biophysical and ecological changes. Still other health effects are tertiary, mediated through social processes; examples include mental health problems, population displacement, and civil conflict. These effects have been extensively reviewed.[129-132]

The following paragraphs, while not exhaustive, provide key examples of the links between GECs and each major category of global health threat: noncommunicable diseases (NCDs), mental health disorders, developmental disorders, infectious diseases, malnutrition, and traumatic injuries.

Noncommunicable Diseases (NCDs)

Obesity is a risk factor for a wide range of NCDs,[134] including cardiovascular disease,[135,136] diabetes, some cancers,[137] gall bladder disease, and depression.[138] Obesity has become common in both wealthy and low-resource settings worldwide,[139,140] and several GECs play a role. One major contributor is global food system changes, including land use changes, the large-scale production of such dietary components as high-fructose corn syrup, and the increase in caloric intake.[141-143] This phenomenon is especially evident in cities, so urbanization represents a second pathway from GEC to obesity, through reductions in physical activity and urban dietary patterns that center on processed foods.[144,145] A third pathway also relates to food system changes, specifically the industrial production of livestock and poultry, with widespread use of antibiotics. Antibiotics in the food supply may alter the human intestinal microbiome in ways that promote obesity, although further evidence is needed on this point.[146,147] Fourth, certain chemical contaminants, some of these widely distributed in both environmental media and in human tissues, act as obesogens, possibly through early-life endocrine effects.[148,149] A well-documented example is bisphenol A (BPA), a chemical used in the manufacture of polycarbonate plastics and epoxy resins.[150] In both animal experiments and epidemiologic studies, higher BPA levels are associated with increased body weight.

Cardiovascular and Pulmonary Disease

The combustion of fossil fuels not only drives much of climate change, it is also a major contributor to air pollution, and consequently to substantial morbidity and mortality worldwide. Key pollutants include fine PM, ozone, oxides of nitrogen, oxides of sulfur, hydrocarbons, and metals—many of these related to each other through complex atmospheric chemistry. The Global Burden of Disease (GBD) Study estimates that ambient fine particulate matter ($PM_{2.5}$) ranked fifth globally as a mortality risk factor in 2015, accounting for an estimated 4.2 million deaths (7.6% of global deaths) and 103.1 million disability-adjusted life-years (DALYs) (4.2% of global DALYs) in 2015.[151,152] These deaths are not uniformly distributed; the greatest burdens are in China and India (with about 1.1 million annual deaths each), Russia (137,000), Pakistan (135,000), and Bangladesh (122,000). Of note, the World Health Organization estimates of the burden of ambient

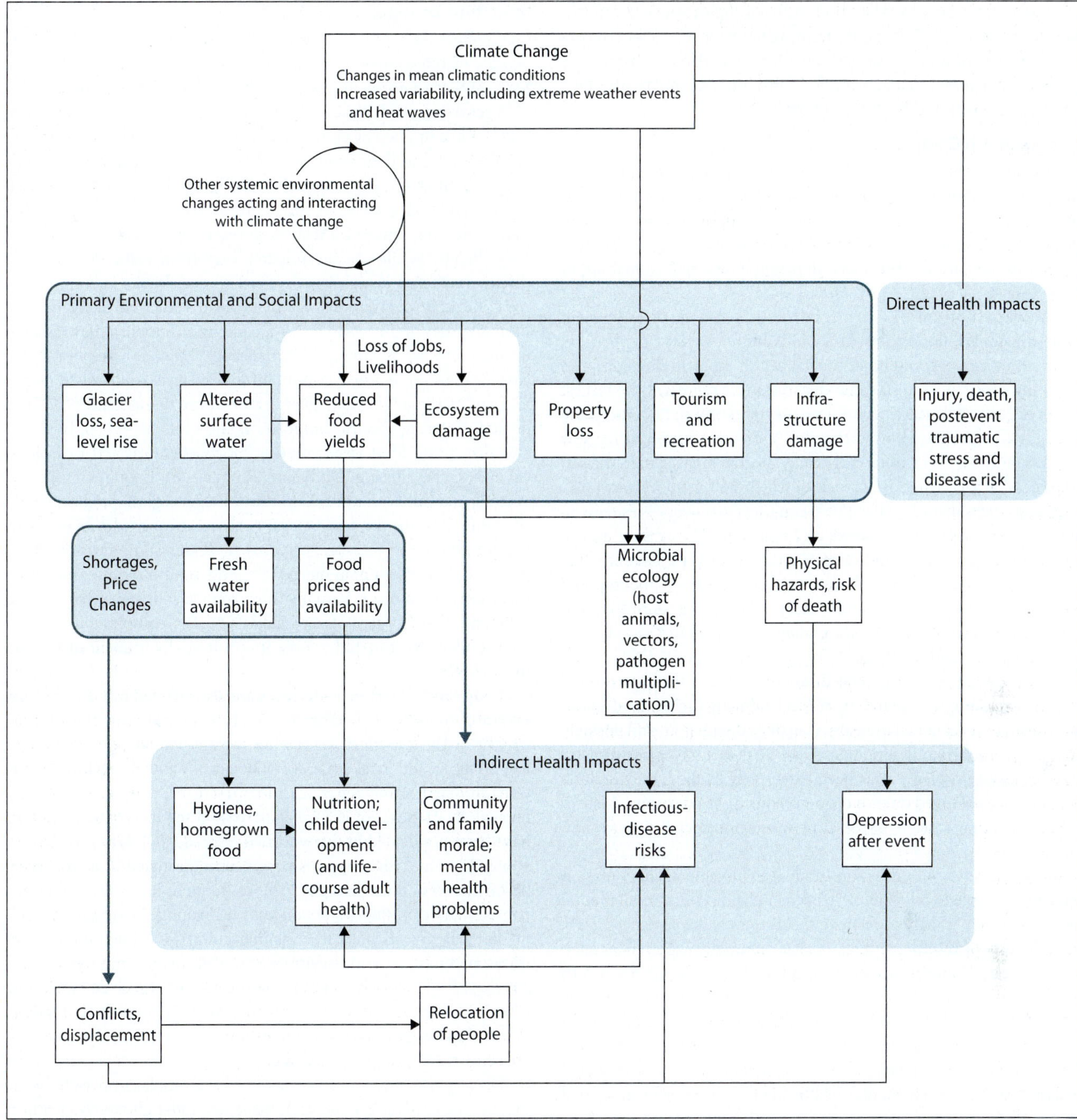

FIGURE 17-6. Pathways from climate change to health. (*Source:* McMichael AJ. Globalization, climate change, and human health. *N Engl J Med.* 2013;368(14):1335–43.[133])

air pollution are somewhat lower than those of the GBD Study: 3 million deaths and 85 million DALYs.[153] Absent a rapid transition toward clean renewable sources of energy, economic growth is projected to increase this burden substantially in some regions, such as Southeast Asia, over coming decades.[154]

The excess deaths from PM exposure are due primarily to NCDs—ischemic heart disease, cerebrovascular disease, chronic obstructive pulmonary disease, and lung cancer—with a small proportion, perhaps one in ten, due to lower respiratory infection.[155] Air pollution exposure, especially to PM, may also contribute to other NCDs, including cardiac arrhythmias.[156] heart failure,[157] type 2 diabetes,[158] neurodevelopmental delay in children, and cognitive decline in older adults.[159]

Ozone is formed from atmospheric precursors—hydrocarbons (methane and volatile organic compounds) and oxides of nitrogen—many of which are combustion products. Like PM, ozone is also associated with excess mortality, although the association is not as strong as for PM.[160] In the GBD data, exposure to ozone caused an additional 254,000 (95% CI 97,000–422,000) deaths and a loss of 4.1 million (95% CI 1.6 million–6.8 million) DALYs from chronic obstructive pulmonary disease in 2015.[151] More recent estimates using updated exposure response relationships suggest at least a fourfold higher burden, with 1.04–1.23 million respiratory deaths in adults attributable to long-term ozone exposures,[161] with the largest increases in attributable mortality in northern India, southeast China, and Pakistan. The association between ozone exposure and mortality seems to relate both to brief high exposures and to long-term exposure.[161,162] Short-term ozone exposure also triggers exacerbations of airways disease (asthma and chronic obstructive pulmonary disease), accounting for substantial numbers of emergency room visits and hospitalizations.[163]

Mental Health Disorders

Mental illness, substance use disorders, and mental distress inflict an enormous burden of suffering globally. GBD data suggest that mental and substance use disorders account for approximately 10.4% of global DALYs and 28.5% of years lived with disability.[164] Although these disorders are multifactorial in origin, GEC may contribute in several ways.

One pathway from GEC to mental health is through disasters such as severe storms, floods, drought, and wildfire. Anxiety, depression, posttraumatic stress, and other mental health problems are common following disasters, and in some circumstances represent the largest health burden.[165] Research conducted several months after Hurricane Katrina, for example, showed that 49.1% of those surveyed in New Orleans, and 26.4% in other hurricane-affected areas, suffered from a DSM-IV anxiety-mood disorder, of which half or more was posttraumatic stress disorder (PTSD).[166] Long-term recovery is the norm, but is not always straightforward; by 2 years after Hurricane Katrina, the prevalence of PTSD and depression in affected populations had actually increased.[167] Similar disease burdens have been documented following other kinds of disasters that are becoming more frequent with climate change, such as typhoons,[168] tornados,[169] floods,[170,171] heat waves,[172,173] and wildfires.[174,175]

Slow-moving environmental disasters may also threaten mental health. For example, research in Australia during the recent decade-long drought revealed an increase in anxiety, depression, and possibly suicidality among rural populations.[176,177] Risk factors for postdisaster mental health problems have been extensively studied; they include personal loss (of loved ones or property) during the disaster, a history of prior trauma, absence of social networks and social support, and others.[166,178,179]

Both acute disasters and more gradual environmental degradation may force people to relocate. Displacement brings substantial mental health impacts.[180,181] These relate to the distress of displacement itself, the difficulty of resettlement, associated traumatic experiences such as sexual and domestic violence, and the absence of mental health services.[182,183]

Environmental degradation may threaten mental health in yet another way: through the disorientation and grief that accompany the loss of familiar, beloved places. This phenomenon has been called "solastalgia."[184,185] Such mental health impacts have been described in Appalachian communities near sites of mountaintop removal for coalmining,[186,187] in fishing communities along the Gulf coast following the 2010 Deepwater Horizon oil spill,[188] and in Alaskan native villages endangered by climate-related changes and confronting cultural and environmental disruption.[189] Rupturing attachments to beloved places can be traumatizing.

Developmental Disorders

Normal human development, from fetal life through early childhood and adolescence, is a delicate balance of physiologic events, which can be perturbed by a wide range of factors. Among these factors are toxic chemicals that have become widespread in the global environment. Interrelated targets include the immune, endocrine, and neurologic systems. For example, neurodevelopmental abnormalities have been reported in association with both POPs[190,191] and particulate air pollution.[192] While evidence is incomplete, and changing diagnostic practices clearly play a role, such exposures may help explain the apparent rise in incidence of such conditions as attention-deficit hyperactivity disorder[193] and autism spectrum disorders.[194]

Infectious Diseases

GECs affect the risk of infectious diseases in many ways. Three categories of infectious disease are illustrative: vector-borne illnesses, food- and waterborne illnesses, and emerging infectious diseases.

Vector-borne disease risk is associated with many aspects of GEC, as exemplified by climate change.[195,196] First, vectors and/or reservoirs may shift their geographic range. Second, vectors, reservoirs, and/or pathogens may respond to changing climate with increased reproductive rates, survival, metabolic activity, and feeding (biting). Third, the prevalence of infection in reservoir or vector populations may change. While specific impacts vary from place to place, and disease incidence is highly influenced by nonclimate factors such as mosquito control programs, vector-borne diseases will likely increase in many parts of the world[197,198]—a conclusion supported by research on such diseases as dengue,[199,200] malaria,[201,202] and the tick-borne diseases Lyme disease, Rocky Mountain spotted fever, and ehrlichiosis.[203]

Land use changes also affect vector-borne disease risk.[204,205] They do so by altering species composition and other aspects of biodiversity, disrupting food webs, altering biogeochemical and hydrological cycles, and altering the dynamics of contact among host species, vectors, and humans. Malaria in the Amazon region, predominantly transmitted by the *Anopheles darlingi* mosquito, provides an example. Deforestation and secondary regrowth under some circumstances promote *A. darlingi* abundance,[206,207] and road-building and settlement expansion bring humans into contact with forest fringes and remnants that act as malaria hotspots.[208] The complex interplay of environment, vector, and people is substantially influenced by land use changes.

Food- and waterborne diseases are also affected by GEC through several pathways. Changes in temperature, rainfall, and other factors may favor the growth or survival of certain pathogens,[209,210] both on a short-term and local scale, as reflected in daily or weekly fluctuations in diarrhea incidence with temperature changes, and in long-term global trends. For example, increasing sea surface temperatures have been implicated in the worldwide spread of *Vibrio* species,[211,212] so much so that these species have been nominated as a "microbial barometer of climate change."[213] More frequent heavy rainfall events contaminate drinking water sources with runoff, increasing the risk of diarrhea[214,215] in both low-income countries with limited water infrastructure[216,217] and wealthier countries with improved infrastructure.[218–220] Widely variable pathogens are involved, including *Campylobacter*, *Cryptosporidium*, norovirus, *Leptospira*, and *Vibrio*. While these organisms have quite different ecological dynamics, all are sensitive to changes in climate.

Dams provide another example of GEC impacts on waterborne disease risk. This is a large-scale issue; as noted above, the world is currently in a dam construction boom. Schistosomiasis exemplifies the potential role of dams in disease ecology. While dams are a relatively clean source of energy, thereby providing health benefits, they can expand the snail vector's habitat (in the aquatic weeds that flourish in reservoirs), prolong the breeding periods (functionally eliminating the dry season that would otherwise reduce snail populations), and prolong human contact with wet environments and, therefore, with snails. A combined analysis of studies from Nigeria, Mali, Cameroon, Côte d'Ivoire, Democratic Republic of the Congo, and Ethiopia found that living near a dam reservoir in endemic areas is associated with more than a doubling of schistosomiasis risk (relative risk 2.4 for *Schistosoma haematobium* and 2.6 for *Schistosoma mansoni*).[76] The Three Gorges Dam was expected to raise the risk of schistosomiasis along some parts of the Yangtze River and to decrease it along others[221]; fortunately, concomitant disease control programs seem to have averted the feared increases.[222,223]

Emerging and re-emerging infectious diseases such as Zika, Ebola, Nipah, Middle East respiratory syndrome, severe acute respiratory syndrome, and H1N1 influenza are driven by many factors, which

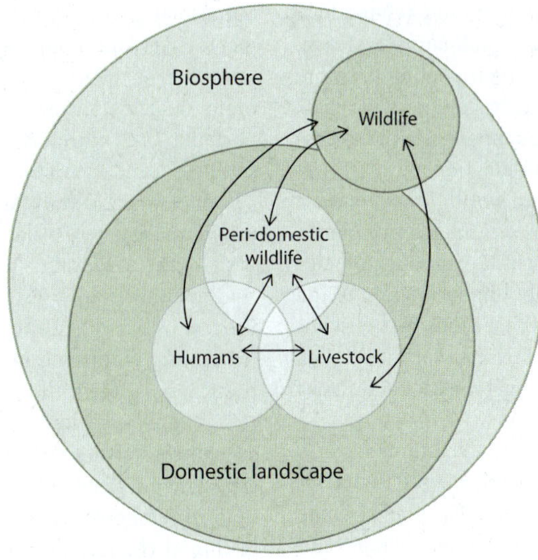

FIGURE 17-7. Pathogen flow at the wildlife–livestock–human interface. Arrows indicate direct, indirect, or vector-borne flow of potential pathogens. (*Source:* Reproduce with Permission from Jones BA, Grace D, Kock R, et al. Zoonosis emergence linked to agricultural intensification and environmental change. *Proc Natl Acad Sci U S A.* 2013;110(21):8399–404.)

are not fully understood. Most such diseases are zoonotic, originating in wild animals, and "jump" to humans through dynamic interactions among wildlife, livestock, and people in the context of rapidly changing environments.[224] Environmental changes can affect reservoir host distribution and density, and the prevalence and intensity of infection, in host species.[225] These relationships are depicted in Fig. 17-7.

When humans expand agriculture and settlements, they encroach on natural ecosystems, alter land cover, and expand ecotones (the transition zones between different biological communities, where different species assemblages mix).[227] This can escalate encounters between humans and wildlife, through activities as diverse as living near forests, growing crops, raising livestock, and hunting bushmeat. For example, the emergence of Kyasanur Forest disease in India followed extensive deforestation in the Western Ghats mountains, with replacement by low vegetation in which the rodents and birds that host the carrier ticks thrive.[228] Intensified livestock production, especially of pigs and poultry, can also promote the emergence and spread of diseases. Concentrated animal feeding operations have been implicated in the emergence of various influenza viruses in recent years,[229] and Nipah virus first emerged in concentrated swine operations in Malaysia.[230] Such processes as deforestation and concentrated livestock production are local phenomena, but they embody global trends, providing new opportunities for genetic diversification, viral and bacterial adaptation, and pathogen spillover.

These risks are amplified by rapid, high-volume global travel—a cardinal feature of modern life that perfectly embodies the Great Acceleration, reflecting the availability of highly available energy (in the form of jet fuel).

Poor Nutrition

Changes in the global food system—conversion of large amounts of forest and grassland to agricultural use; widespread use of fertilizers, pesticides, and herbicides; development and use of high-yield seed strains; extensive pumping of groundwater and diversion of surface waterways for irrigation—have resulted in unprecedented increases in food production. However, there is a "dark side" to this transformation. First, it is unsustainable, due to its heavy resource requirements and environmental impact. Second, increasing prosperity has led to sometimes unwholesome dietary changes.

The global **dietary transition** of recent decades features shifts toward consumption of energy-dense, less diverse, and increasingly processed foods, including animal products, oils and fats, refined carbohydrates, and sugar-sweetened beverages, and behavioral changes such as increased snacking and eating outside the home.[231] These patterns are especially evident in cities, and while they are sometimes considered typical of wealthy societies, they are emerging strongly in LMICs.[232] This dietary pattern, with inadequate intake of fruits, vegetables, nuts, and fiber, has direct implications for NCDs, promoting obesity, cardiovascular disease, diabetes, and some cancers.[231,233–236] It also has environmental impacts that, in turn, may loop back to exert indirect impacts on human health. For example, diets heavy in meat (particularly ruminant meat) require substantially more land, water, and energy throughput to produce than plant-based diets.[237] The United Nations Food and Agriculture Organization (FAO) has estimated that livestock production accounts for 18% of global GHG emissions.[238] Livestock production accounts for the majority of Amazon deforestation, where 70% of deforested land is occupied by pastures, and much of the remainder by feed crops.[239] These land use changes, in turn, contribute to climate change.

A second pathway from GEC to nutrition is the effect of climate change on **agricultural productivity**. Climate change reduces crop yields, particularly at low and mid-latitudes. Compared to a scenario without climate change, crop yields (wheat, rice, and maize) could decline by a median of 0.2% per decade for the rest of the century even as demands increase by an estimated 14% per decade.[240] Climate change could therefore substantially increase the risk of stunting, particularly severe stunting.[241] While stunting in Asia decreased dramatically from 49% in 1990 to 28% in 2010, stunting in Africa plateaued in 1990 at a prevalence of about 40%, suggesting that vulnerability may be highest in Africa.[242] Stunting has serious implications for cognitive development, long-term economic prospects, and subsequent generations.[243]

A recent modeling study of the effects of climate change on crop yield by 2050 suggested a net annual increase of about 529,000 premature deaths (95% CI averaged over all climate scenarios 314,000–736,000) compared with no climate change, mainly as a result of increased NCD mortality.[244] Reductions in fruit and vegetable consumption were the major contributor to increased mortality and most climate-related deaths were projected to occur in South and East Asia. Decreased caloric intake was projected to increase deaths related to undernutrition, but these were approximately balanced by reduced deaths from overweight and obesity.

Another GEC that threatens the food supply is **food-related biodiversity loss**. Two examples are illustrative: pollinators and fish. Pollination by insects is an important form of reproduction for more than 35% of the annual global food production by volume. At least 87 major food crops, and up to 40% of the world's supply of some micronutrients, such as vitamin A, depend on pollination by insects.[245] Pollinators are declining in many parts of the world, probably for a combination of reasons including habitat loss, pesticide use, and parasitic infestation.[246] Pollinator loss can reduce the amount of fruits, vegetables, nuts, and seeds in the diet, contributing to Vitamin A and folate deficiencies. A recent analysis projects that a 50% loss of pollination would cause about 700,000 additional deaths worldwide each year, mostly as a result of increased ischemic heart disease and stroke due to reduced fruit and vegetable consumption.[247]

About 90% of fisheries are now at or beyond maximum sustainable levels of exploitation.[248] Causes include overfishing, ocean acidification, hypoxia, pollution, and nutrient loading. For many human populations, fish are a bedrock dietary source of protein, of micronutrients (often in highly bioavailable form), and of omega-3 fatty acids (mainly from oily fish). Climate change will intensify fisheries depletion.[249] One study projected that more than 10% of the global population could face micronutrient and fatty-acid deficiencies due to fish declines over coming decades, especially in low-and middle-income nations near the equator.[250]

A third pathway from GEC to nutrition is the effect of climate change on the **nutritional content of crops**. A meta-analysis of data on 130 varieties of plants found that elevated CO_2 levels reduced the overall concentration of 25 important minerals in plants, including calcium, potassium, zinc, and iron, by 8% on average.[251] An estimated 138 million (95% CI 120–156) more people, mainly in Africa and South Asia, could be placed at new risk of zinc deficiency by 2050 as a result of elevated CO_2 levels.[252] There is strong evidence that elevated CO_2 levels also reduce protein and increase carbohydrate levels particularly in C3 crops (beans, rice, wheat, potatoes, woody trees). One study found that elevated CO_2 was associated with about a 6% decrease in protein in wheat grains and about an 8% decrease in rice grains but no significant effect in soybeans.[253] Another study focused on rice, the dietary staple for more than two billion people. It found that rising CO_2 levels would result in declines in protein, iron, zinc, and vitamins B1, B2, B5, and B9 (but an increase in vitamin E).[254] The health implications of these changes are under investigation and are likely to depend on the nutritional profile of the affected populations. The rice study, for instance, predicted that nutritional deficits would fall most heavily on people in the poorest of the rice-dependent countries (including Madagascar, Bangladesh, Cambodia, Myanmar, and Laos).[254] A study in the United States showed that the substitution of dietary carbohydrate for dietary protein increased the risk of hypertension, lipid disorders, and 10-year coronary heart disease risk.[255] In low-income countries, if protein intake is low, there may be additional impacts on health.

Traumatic Injuries

Traumatic injuries account for nearly one in ten global deaths each year—more than 5 million of a total of 56 million deaths.[256] A remarkable 85% of these deaths occur in LMICs. The burden of premature mortality, morbidity, and suffering from traumatic injuries is enormous.

Road traffic injuries account for about 1.25 million deaths worldwide each year, or roughly one in four fatal injuries,[257] representing the largest cause of unintentional injury deaths. For every fatal road traffic injury, an estimated 20–50 more people suffer some disability.[257] The conventional analytical approach to road traffic injuries is grounded in the Haddon Matrix, which identifies factors related to host (people), agent (vehicles and equipment), and environment.[258] The "environment" in this context includes not only road design, but also ambient environmental conditions; severe storms bring an increased risk of motor vehicle crashes.[259] Underlying the entire phenomenon of road traffic injuries, however, is the rapid expansion of motor vehicle use over the last century—a defining feature of transportation both within cities and over long-distances, in both wealthy settings[260] and, increasingly, in LMICs.[261] Higher levels of vehicle-miles traveled translate to greater exposure to risk. Accordingly, urban arrangements that promote automobile travel are associated with higher road traffic injury rates.[262,263]

Environmental disasters such as severe storms, floods, and wildfires are increasing due to climate change, and represent another contributor to traumatic injuries and deaths. GEC, and climate change in particular, increase the probability and severity of such events. The risk is highest in low-income settings, and in vulnerable locations such as coastal cities.[264] Such disasters increase the burden of injuries, especially in places with insufficient capacity for disaster preparedness and response. Analyses of disaster risk reduction in the context of climate change have emphasized cross-cutting solutions that build social and physical resilience.[265,266]

Heat increases the risk of injuries. On unusually hot days, rates of interpersonal violence and crime rise,[267–269] and so do workplace injuries.[270,271] With climate change bringing warmer weather, including more extremely hot days in many places, both unintentional and intentional injuries are likely to increase.

PROTECTING HUMAN HEALTH IN THE ANTHROPOCENE

As this chapter has made clear, GECs threaten human health—indeed, the very basis of human civilization—on a vast scale. Protecting human health in the Anthropocene requires solutions on a similarly vast scale. Several points are clear. First, there can be no human health and well-being without a healthy planet. This deceptively simple statement draws on many intellectual and cultural frameworks, from traditional ecological knowledge[272,273] to the more contemporary idea of ecosystem services.[274–276] It needs to be foundational for public health, from the local scale to the global. Second, global public health strategies in the context of planetary health are largely anchored "upstream" from the health sector—in urban planning, transportation, energy, agriculture, and other sectors. This implies that effective global public health action in coming decades will require working with and through other professions and sectors. Third, the best global health strategies will be those that yield benefits not only for health, but also for environmental sustainability, equity, and economics—the concept of cobenefits.[277,278] Fortunately, many of the needed transitions represent just s uch "win-win" solutions.

Clean, Renewable Energy

One of the most effective public health strategies for the twenty-first century, given the far-reaching threats described above, is the transition of energy systems from fossil fuel combustion to clean, renew able sources.[279,280] These include wind and solar power, which have become far more available and less expensive in recent years, hydroelectric power, and tidal and geothermal power, (which are farther from large-scale implementation). Many believe that nuclear power is also part of the needed energy transition, although there is debate on this point.[281,282] This transition—moving beyond burning carbon-based fuels to get power—is known as **decarbonizing** the energy system. In addition to shifting from fossil fuel combustion, "no regrets" measures include energy conservation and efficiency, so that less energy is required to deliver needed services; and the "smart electric grid," a distribution system based on digital technology designed to optimize efficiency and reliability and to reduce waste.

Significant obstacles exist. First, the world's investment in fossil fuel infrastructure is enormous, and abandoning parts of this infrastructure—creating "stranded assets"—poses substantial political and economic challenges. Second, sizeable investments will be needed to create the infrastructure of the clean energy economy. Third, renewable energy technologies pose technical challenges, such as the intermittency of both wind and solar power (many of which can be addressed by innovative technology such as improved battery storage). Fourth, business interests with a stake in fossil fuels wield enormous political influence and have vigorously—and often unscrupulously—fought the needed transition.[283–285] Fifth, LMICs confront urgent problems of energy shortage, and many have focused on rapidly lifting their populations out of energy poverty by the fastest possible means—often fossil fuels.[286]

Fortunately, the transition to clean energy yields extensive benefits for health and well-being (as well as for the economy).[278,287] Chief among these are improvements in air quality, as so much air pollution derives from fossil fuel combustion.[288–290] Additional benefits of decarbonization arise along the fossil fuel life cycle, from reduced injuries and lung disease among coal miners, to reduced risks of breaches of coal ash containment ponds.

The Built Environment: Healthy, Sustainable Buildings

The built environment includes the totality of places designed and created by people, from the small scale of buildings to the large scale of metropolitan areas, including buildings themselves, neighborhoods, and transportation infrastructure. The built environment offers numerous opportunities to address GECs, both optimizing human health and well-being, and promoting environmental sustainability.

Building technology has advanced considerably in recent years. Initial attempts to reduce energy use in buildings, following the oil shocks of the 1970s, relied heavily on reducing outdoor air exchanges; the resulting "tight buildings" were associated with widespread complaints of discomfort and various symptoms, known as "sick building syndrome."[291] A wide range of suspected causes was investigated, including moisture, mold, carbon dioxide, volatile organic compounds, and stress; full understanding of the condition remains elusive. However, emerging "green building" technology that combines efficient heating and cooling with ample supply of fresh air, reduces energy use in the building, minimizes the use of toxic materials in buildings, and provides plenty of daylight and physical activity, among other features, has been associated with improved subjective well-being, academic and work performance, and health.[292,293]

In LMICs, the health implications of indoor air are enormous. An estimated 2.8 billion people worldwide—including more than half of households in Africa and Southeast Asia—heat their homes and cook their food with solid fuels, including wood, crop residues, dung, charcoal, and coal.[294] The resulting indoor air pollution contributes to the burden of respiratory infections, cardiovascular disease, cancer, adverse birth outcomes, and other health problems, and accounts for about 3.5 million deaths each year.[295] Solutions include the provision of cleaner cookstoves, although in many field trials people have been reluctant to abandon traditional cooking methods,[296] and the provision of natural gas or electricity.[297] Reducing the use of solid fuels offers a range of benefits—not only reduced risk of the diseases noted above, but also reduced pressure on forests (thanks to decreased firewood demand), more time and enhanced safety for women (who are spared the need to forage for fuels), and reduced contributions to ambient air pollution.

The Built Environment: Healthy, Sustainable Communities

At the neighborhood scale, a range of strategies has emerged that optimize both human health and environmental sustainability—under such (largely overlapping) names as smart growth, new urbanism, traditional neighborhood development, and livable communities. They are designed to reduce travel demand and automobile dependence, to encourage active transportation (walking and cycling), and to offer amenities such as social interaction and nature contact. The design features that advance these goals include excellent pedestrian and cycling infrastructure, zoning that permits mixed land uses (making homes accessible to schools, stores, workplaces, and other destinations), optimal density (dense enough to reduce travel demand, support mass transit, and achieve efficiencies, but not so dense as to feel overcrowded), vibrant activity centers, community gathering places, and parks and other greenspaces.[298] Places designed in this manner promote health by encouraging routine physical activity, improving air quality, reducing the risk of motor vehicle crashes, reducing noise, and promoting social capital. In addition, by reducing energy and material use, they advance environmental goals.

These principles scale up from the neighborhood level to the metropolitan level. At this larger scale imply relatively compact cities, where overall travel demand is reduced, travel modes other than automobiles are practical, and per capita energy use decreases because of smaller homes (Fig. 17-8). In such cities, mass transit, including buses, light rail, and heavy rail, plays a role. These modes greatly reduce the per capita energy used in travel, and reduce vehicular contributions to air pollution. Transit use decreases the risk of car crash fatalities.[262] Transit use may also promote health through the physical activity involved in walking to and from transit stops[299,300] although research findings on this point have been inconsistent.[301] Emerging developments in urban transportation include ride-sharing, electric vehicles, and autonomous vehicles; the impacts of these innovations remain to be seen.[302–305]

The Food System: From Farm to Table

The global food system has complex, multidirectional relationships with both health and the environment. It is currently failing in several ways. Too many people are hungry, even as increasing numbers of people overconsume calories in the form of calorie-dense, nutrient-poor, and processed foods. Much food is chemically contaminated. Agricultural production methods strain global supplies of water and land, degrade soil quality, promote the emergence and re-emergence of infectious diseases with pandemic potential,[229] contribute to climate change, undermine biodiversity, and expel nutrients, waste, and antibiotics into the environment.[25,307,308] Agriculture is susceptible to climate shocks, both acutely (storms and flooding) and long-term (rising temperatures and CO_2 levels). The challenge is to move toward a food system that operates within planetary limits, delivers ample, healthy food to all, and is resilient to current and projected GECs[309–312]—a system in which success is measured not by tons of yield per hectare, but by people nourished per hectare.[313]

One set of strategies lies with changing agricultural production methods. Sustainable intensification is an approach intended to feed a growing global population, protect farmers, steward resources such as water and soil, and avoid environmental harms.[314,315] Sustainable intensification begins with making existing methods more efficient. For example, farmers can target their use of fertilizer, pesticides, and water to optimize impact while reducing use. Such precision farming can use modern technology, including sensors, detailed soil mapping, GPS and drone mapping, and weather and satellite data. A second aspect of sustainable intensification is substitution of inefficient or harmful methods with alternatives, such as new crop varieties and livestock breeds, biological control agents instead of pesticides, and no-tillage systems. New plant varieties can offer improved conversion of nutrients to biomass, drought tolerance, and/or resistance to pests and diseases. Finally, system redesign can aim for both nutritional and environmental goals (Table 17-1).

An important aspect of environmentally sustainable food systems is the composition of diets. In particular, animal-based food accounts for much of the food system's large carbon footprint due to low feed-conversion efficiencies, enteric fermentation in ruminants, and manure-related emissions.[316] Livestock production also requires substantial bluewater use, cropland and pasture, and nitrogen and phosphorus application. However, in an increasingly prosperous world, the demand for meat has been rising—a trend that not only threatens

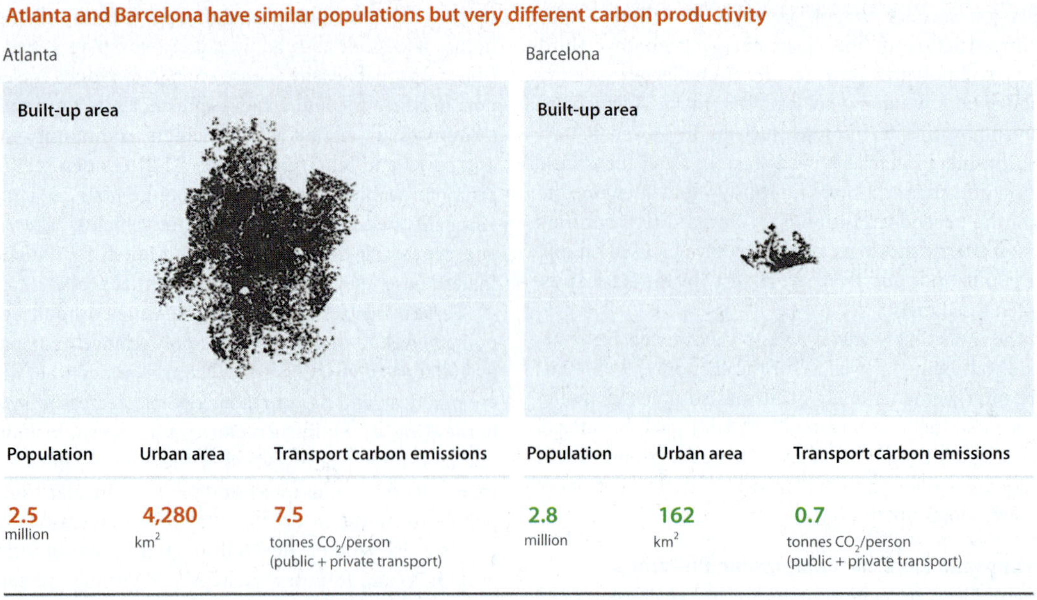

Atlanta and Barcelona have similar populations but very different carbon productivity

	Population	Urban area	Transport carbon emissions
Atlanta	2.5 million	4,280 km²	7.5 tonnes CO_2/person (public + private transport)
Barcelona	2.8 million	162 km²	0.7 tonnes CO_2/person (public + private transport)

FIGURE 17-8. Comparison of Atlanta and Barcelona. The two cities have similar populations, but dramatically different urban areas, with consequent differences in resource and energy use. (*Source:* Reproduced with permission from Global Trends of Urbanization, https://morphocode.com/global-trends-urbanisation/, based on Global Commission on the Economy and Climate. Better Growth, Better Climate: The New Climate Economy Report. Washington DC: World Resources Institute; 2014.)

sustainability, but also brings health risks (some cancers, cardiovascular disease, stroke, diabetes, and other ailments).[316] Dietary patterns that emphasize fruits, vegetables, grains, and nuts, and that limit meat consumption will advance both health and sustainability goals.[312] Innovative sources of dietary protein such as insects[317,318] and artificial (cultured) meat[319] may come to play increasing roles in sustainable diets.

Another important aspect of sustainable food systems is reducing waste. Roughly a third of food that is produced globally goes to waste—in poor settings, close to the point of production, and in wealthy settings, close to the point of consumption.[320] Solutions include improvements throughout the supply chain to reduce loss, food preservation, and changes in consumer behavior.

TABLE 17-1 FOOD SYSTEM REDESIGN FOR SUSTAINABLE INTENSIFICATION

Type of Redesign	Examples
Integrated pest management	Integrated plant and pest management
Conservation agriculture	Zero- and low-till systems; soil conservation and soil erosion prevention; enhancement of soil health
Integrated crop and biodiversity redesign	Organic agriculture; rice-fish systems
Pasture and forage redesign	Management-intensive rotational grazing systems
Trees in agricultural systems	Agroforestry
Irrigation water management	Microirrigation technologies
Intensive small and patch systems	Community farms and allotments

Source: Reproduced with permission from Pretty J, Benton TG, Bharucha ZP, et al. Global assessment of agricultural system redesign for sustainable intensification. *Nature Sustainability*. 2018;1(8):441–6.

Chemicals: The Promise of Green Chemistry

Green chemistry represents a sea change in the goals and operation of the chemical enterprise. The Environmental Protection Agency (EPA) defines green chemistry as "the design of chemical products and processes to reduce and eliminate the use and generation of hazardous compounds." Green chemists seek to design chemicals and processes that serve needed functions, but that minimize harm to people and the environment. The principles of green chemistry appear in Box 17-1.

Far-Reaching Economic Changes

Each of the sets of strategies just discussed—on energy, the built environment, food, and chemicals—is far-reaching but sector-specific. Underpinning all of these is a broader vision of an economic and social transformation that enables and advances health, equity, and sustainability.

At the heart of this broader vision is a transformation in how we convert energy and materials to goods and services, and in how we use the goods and services. The conventional linear economy starts with raw materials, transforms them into useful products, creates waste in the process, and disposes of products when they are no long useful. The **circular economy** has different aspirations. To the extent possible, waste is eliminated; it becomes input for other products or processes. In the words of one scholar, the circular economy "replaces production with sufficiency: reuse what you can, recycle what cannot be reused, repair what is broken, remanufacture what cannot be repaired."[322] Inspiration for the circular economy comes from natural systems, in which waste is nearly unknown. In their 2002 book *Cradle to Cradle: Remaking the Way We Make Things*, architect William McDonough and chemist Michael Braungart described three core principles.[323] First, they wrote, as in nature, everything is a resource for something else. Accordingly, human products should be designed to be disassembled and safely returned to the soil as biological nutrients, or reused in other products. Second, use clean and renewable energy, just as biological systems draw their energy from the sun. Third, celebrate diversity. Just as evolution has yielded an astonishing variety of designs in flora and fauna, human products should strive for diversity and adaptability.

Complementing the circular economy is the **performance economy**—the idea that in many cases people want services more than they want to own products. Companies that provide cotton diapers, or uniforms, and take them back when they need cleaning, exemplify this approach. Who wants to own a cotton diaper? Interface Carpets provide the service of floor covering in this way, as an alternative to selling carpets. Michelin does so with tires, and the Swiss company Elite does so with hotel mattresses, each servicing the product and recovering it for disassembly and reuse at the end of its useful life.[324]

An extension of this idea is the **sharing economy** (also called the collaborative economy). As authors Rachel Botsman and Roo Rogers point out, the average lawn mower is used for 4 hours a year, the average power drill is used for 20 minutes over its entire lifespan, and the average car is idle 22 hours a day, and typically has three unused seats even when it is driven.[325] Such levels of inefficiency represent wasted energy and materials. People can do without owning a car if they use a car share service, without owning a bicycle if they use a bicycle share service, and so on.

These economic models vary greatly, and they are not without critics. But they share the potential to reduce consumption, to reduce energy and materials use, and to reduce waste—protecting health through the many indirect pathways discussed in this chapter—while, ideally, promoting other goals such as social capital and poverty reduction.

Models such as the circular economy, the performance economy, and the sharing economy require new economic paradigms. The field of ecological economics has begun to offer such innovative thinking. Ecological economists view society as embedded in the biosphere, accept the notion of planetary limits to human activity, question the assumption of perpetual growth, take a long-term view of economic activity, and position values such as equity at the center of their thinking—all in contrast to much of conventional economic thinking.[326–329] Ecological economists note that many economically significant costs and services are excluded from ordinary economic calculations—an omission called "externalities"—and urge their inclusion in analyses.

A corollary of this thinking is that conventional economic indicators, such as the gross domestic product, are misguided. Such indicators measure market transactions rather than values-based outcomes such as human well-being, and ignore social costs, environmental impacts, waste and income inequality.[330] One alternative is the genuine progress indicator, which accounts not only for economic activity, but also for such factors as crime and family breakdown, income distribution, and environmental damage.[331] Another alternative is to track progress on the sustainable development goals, either overall, or, in the context of global health, with relation to health.[332]

An example of ecological economics thinking is **doughnut economics**, proposed by economist Kate Raworth[327] (Fig. 17-9). This model combines the idea of planetary boundaries introduced above (Fig. 17-3)* with a focus on social boundaries, defined by human needs. It emphasizes that just as there are upper limits on such environmental harms as ocean acidification, there are lower limits on such human needs as health, education, and political voice. The space between these two sets of limits forms a doughnut, called the safe and just space for humanity, within a regenerative and distributive economy.

Governments around the world have taken steps to implement some of these ideas. At the national level, for example, the government of Wales promulgated a Well-being of Future Generations Act in 2015, which requires public bodies to consider the long-term impact of their decisions, with the goal of preventing such persistent problems as poverty, health inequalities, and climate change (http://futuregenerations.wales/). The government of Bhutan adopted a Gross National Happiness approach which orients national policy toward human well-being. At the local level, many municipal efforts embody principles that advance economic transformation, environmental sustainability, resiliency, health, and equity. For example, in 2017 the city of Jyväskylä, Finland, embraced a circular economy framework for its governance. Other such efforts at the city level are driven by civil society. For example, a network of transition towns (https://transitionnetwork.org/) works toward local transformations based on respecting resource limits, building resilience, promoting health equity, and related values.

BOX 17-1 Twelve Principles of Green Chemistry

1. **Prevention**
   It is better to prevent waste than to treat or clean up waste after it has been created.
2. **Atom Economy**
   Synthetic methods should be designed to maximize the incorporation of all materials used in the process into the final product.
3. **Less Hazardous Chemical Syntheses**
   Wherever practicable, synthetic methods should be designed to use and generate substances that possess little or no toxicity to human health and the environment.
4. **Designing Safer Chemicals**
   Chemical products should be designed to affect their desired function while minimizing their toxicity.
5. **Safer Solvents and Auxiliaries**
   The use of auxiliary substances (such as solvents, separation agents, etc.) should be made unnecessary whenever possible and innocuous when used.
6. **Design for Energy Efficiency**
   Energy requirements of chemical processes should be recognized for their environmental and economical impacts and should be minimized. If possible, synthetic methods should be conducted at ambient temperature and pressure.
7. **Use of Renewable Feedstocks**
   A raw material or feedstock should be renewable rather than depleting whenever technically and economically practicable.
8. **Reduce Derivatives**
   Unnecessary derivatization (use of blocking groups, protection/deprotection, temporary modification of physical/chemical processes) should be minimized or avoided if possible, because such steps require additional reagents and can generate waste.
9. **Catalysis**
   Catalytic reagents (as selective as possible) are superior to stoichiometric reagents.
10. **Design for Degradation**
    Chemical products should be designed so that at the end of their function they break down into innocuous degradation products and do not persist in the environment.
11. **Real-Time Analysis for Pollution Prevention**
    Analytical methodologies need to be further developed to allow for the real-time, in-process monitoring, and control prior to the formation of hazardous substances.
12. **Inherently Safer Chemistry for Accident Prevention**
    Substances and the form of a substance used in a chemical process should be chosen to minimize the potential for chemical accidents, including releases, explosions, and fires.

Source: Adapted from Anastas PT, Warner JC. *Green Chemistry: Theory and Practice*. New York and Oxford: Oxford University Press; 1998.

FUTURE DIRECTIONS

GECs have far-reaching implications for the future of health around the world. These will manifest in at least three areas: practice, research, and training.

Public health practitioners have proposed the idea of "Public Health 3.0"—a re-envisioning of the field that highlights the key role of social and environmental factors in shaping health, implying that cross-sector collaboration and environmental, policy, and systems-level actions are central to public health function.[333] California physician Rishi Manchanda has coined the term "upstreamist" to

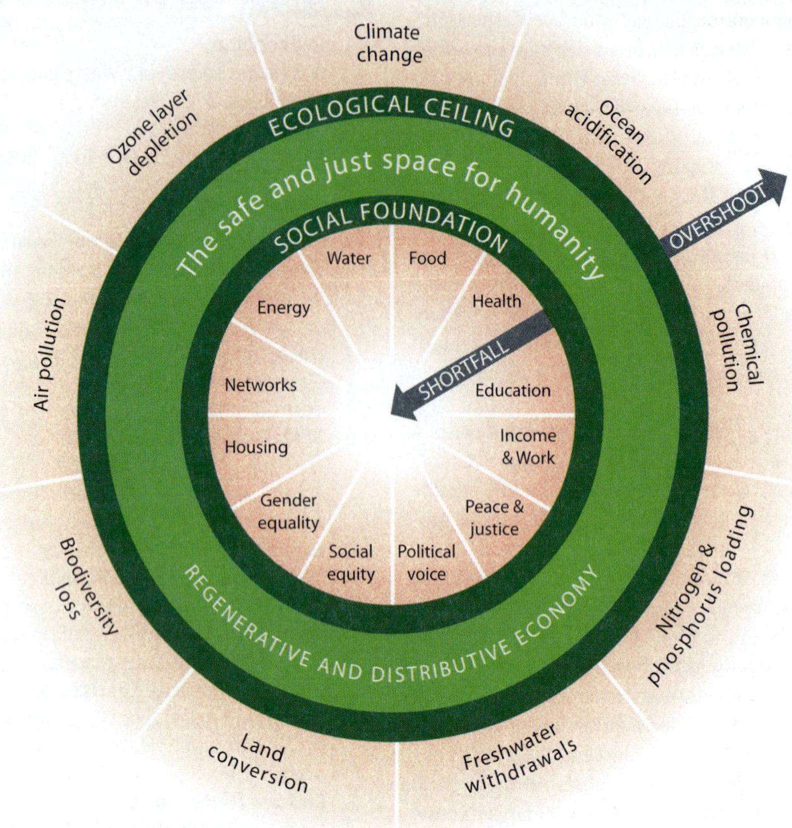

FIGURE 17-9. The doughnut of social and planetary boundaries. (*Source:* Reproduced with permission from Kate Raworth (2021). What on Earth is the Doughnut? Retrieved from https://www.kateraworth.com/doughnut.)

describe health professionals who focus on root causes of illnesses rather than simply on clinical treatment.[334] Machalaba and colleagues[335] have called on health professionals to "transcend silos" in addressing both global health and climate change.

Each of these approaches embodies a mandate for global public health in the Anthropocene. If Planetary Health has roots in such diverse fields as energy policy and agriculture, ecology and urban planning, then health professionals need to be disciplinary and sectoral polyglots—comfortable, if not fluent, with the far-flung fields that increasingly determine the global burden of disease. Health professionals must actively contribute to decisions about how electric power is generated, how people travel, how cities are zoned, and how food is grown—"showing up" when they are invited, inviting themselves when they are not, and insisting on a role when they are shut out. This work must also extend to advocacy—against fossil fuel combustion and automobile-centric transportation systems; for forest conservation, cycling infrastructure, and plant-forward diets. Health professional advocacy was important in implementing potable water supplies and sewer systems in the nineteenth century, and in fighting tobacco and promoting seat belts use in the twentieth century; this same advocacy is needed for Planetary Health in the twenty-first century.

Health research in the Anthropocene must be similarly broad and cross-cutting. How should decisions to build dams be made, and what are the best ways to protect ecosystems and human health when dams are built? How will a changing climate affect the nutrient content of foods, and what crops will be most nutritious and resilient? What agricultural practices and policies most effectively provide nutrition for all? Are there any adverse health effects of wind turbines, and if so how should they be controlled? How should greenspace best be integrated into cities to optimize health, economic development, and ecosystem services? These and countless other questions require deeply interdisciplinary, solutions-oriented, and policy-relevant research.

Finally, health professional training—whether of practitioners or of researchers—needs to reflect the breadth of Planetary Health. Ecology, evolutionary biology, earth sciences, and urban planning—not every health professional can or should study all these fields, but some familiarity for all, and deeper knowledge for some, will equip health leaders of the future to ask the right questions, discover the right answers, and implement the right solutions to protect the health of all people in the Anthropocene.

ACKNOWLEDGMENT

I thank Andy Haines (London School of Hygiene and Tropical Medicine) and Sam Myers (Harvard University), key Planetary Health leaders, for thought partnership over many years and critical review of this chapter.

References

1. McMichael AJ, Woodward A, Muir C. *Climate Change and the Health of Nations: Famines, Fevers, and the Fate of Populations.* Oxford and New York: Oxford University Press; 2017.
2. Steffen W, Broadgate WJ, Deutsch L, Gaffney O, Ludwig C. The trajectory of the Anthropocene: The Great Acceleration. *Anthr Rev.* 2015;2: 81–98.

3. Steffen W, Crutzen PJ, McNeill JR. The Anthropocene: Are humans now overwhelming the great forces of nature? *Ambio*. 2007;36(8):614–21.
4. Steffen W, Grinevald J, Crutzen P, McNeill J. The Anthropocene: Conceptual and historical perspectives. *Philos Trans Royal Soc A*. 2011;369(1938):842–67.
5. Steffen W, Richardson K, Rockstrom J, et al. Planetary boundaries: Guiding human development on a changing planet. *Science*. 2015;347(6223):1259855.
6. Rockström J, Steffen W, Noone K, et al. Planetary boundaries: Exploring the safe operating space for humanity. *Ecology and Society*. 2009;14(2).
7. Stocker TF, Qin D, Plattner G-K, et al. eds. *Climate Change 2013: The Physical Science Basis. Contribution of Working Group I to the Fifth Assessment Report of the Intergovernmental Panel on Climate Change*. Cambridge and New York: Cambridge University Press; 2013.
8. Craufurd PQ, Wheeler TR. Climate change and the flowering time of annual crops. *J Exp Bot*. 2009;60(9):2529–39.
9. Ziska L, Knowlton K, Rogers C, et al. Recent warming by latitude associated with increased length of ragweed pollen season in central North America. *Proc Natl Acad Sci U S A*. 2011;108(10):4248–51.
10. Chen IC, Hill JK, Ohlemuller R, Roy DB, Thomas CD. Rapid range shifts of species associated with high levels of climate warming. *Science*. 2011;333(6045):1024–6.
11. Pecl GT, Araújo MB, Bell JD, et al. Biodiversity redistribution under climate change: Impacts on ecosystems and human well-being. *Science*. 2017;355(6332):eaai9214.
12. Eisen L, Monaghan AJ, Lozano-Fuentes S, Steinhoff DF, Hayden MH, Bieringer PE. The Impact of temperature on the bionomics of Aedes (Stegomyia) aegypti, with special reference to the cool geographic range margins. *J Med Entomol*. 2014;51(3):496–516.
13. Beck-Johnson LM, Nelson WA, Paaijmans KP, Read AF, Thomas MB, Bjørnstad ON. The effect of temperature on Anopheles mosquito population dynamics and the potential for malaria transmission. *PLoS One*. 2013;8(11):e79276.
14. Ewing DA, Cobbold CA, Purse BV, Nunn MA, White SM. Modelling the effect of temperature on the seasonal population dynamics of temperate mosquitoes. *J Theor Biol*. 2016;400:65–79.
15. Naeem S, Prager C, Weeks B, et al. Biodiversity as a multidimensional construct: A review, framework and case study of herbivory's impact on plant biodiversity. *Proc Biol Sci*. 2016;283(1844):20153005.
16. Duffy JE, Godwin CM, Cardinale BJ. Biodiversity effects in the wild are common and as strong as key drivers of productivity. *Nature*. 2017;549:261.
17. Soliveres S, van der Plas F, Manning P, et al. Biodiversity at multiple trophic levels is needed for ecosystem multifunctionality. *Nature*. 2016;536(7617):456–9.
18. Cardinale BJ, Duffy JE, Gonzalez A, et al. Biodiversity loss and its impact on humanity. *Nature*. 2012;486(7401):59–67.
19. Mace GM, Norris K, Fitter AH. Biodiversity and ecosystem services: A multilayered relationship. *Trends Ecol Evol*. 2012;27(1):19–26.
20. Balvanera P, Siddique I, Dee L, et al. Linking biodiversity and ecosystem services: Current uncertainties and the necessary next steps. *BioScience*. 2014;64(1):49–57.
21. Dirzo R, Young HS, Galetti M, Ceballos G, Isaac NJB, Collen B. Defaunation in the Anthropocene. *Science*. 2014;345(6195):401–6.
22. Pimm SL, Jenkins CN, Abell R, et al. The biodiversity of species and their rates of extinction, distribution, and protection. *Science*. 2014;344(6187):1246752.
23. Kolbert E. *The Sixth Extinction: An Unnatural History*. New York: Henry Holt and Company; 2014.
24. Ceballos G, Ehrlich PR, Barnosky AD, García A, Pringle RM, Palmer TM. Accelerated modern human-induced species losses: Entering the sixth mass extinction. *Sci Adv*. 2015;1(5):e1400253.
25. Newbold T, Hudson LN, Hill SL, et al. Global effects of land use on local terrestrial biodiversity. *Nature*. 2015;520(7545):45–50.
26. Newbold T, Hudson LN, Arnell AP, et al. Has land use pushed terrestrial biodiversity beyond the planetary boundary? A global assessment. *Science*. 2016;353(6296):288–91.
27. Butchart SHM, Walpole M, Collen B, et al. Global biodiversity: Indicators of recent declines. *Science*. 2010;328(5982):1164–8.
28. Harrison PA, Berry PM, Simpson G, et al. Linkages between biodiversity attributes and ecosystem services: A systematic review. *Ecosyst Serv*. 2014;9:191–203.
29. Bernstein AS. Biological diversity and public health. *Annu Rev Public Health*. 2014;35(1):153–67.
30. Keesing F, Belden LK, Daszak P, et al. Impacts of biodiversity on the emergence and transmission of infectious diseases. *Nature*. 2010;468(7324):647–52.
31. Pongsiri MJ, Roman J, Ezenwa VO, et al. Biodiversity loss affects global disease ecology. *BioScience*. 2009;59(11):945–54.
32. Rook GA. Regulation of the immune system by biodiversity from the natural environment: An ecosystem service essential to health. *Proc Natl Acad Sci U S A*. 2013;110(46):18360–7.
33. Penafiel D, Lachat C, Espinel R, Van Damme P, Kolsteren P. A systematic review on the contributions of edible plant and animal biodiversity to human diets. *EcoHealth*. 2011;8(3):381–99.
34. Kahane R, Hodgkin T, Jaenicke H, et al. Agrobiodiversity for food security, health and income. *Agron Sustain Dev*. 2013;33(4):671–93.
35. Rosi-Marshall EJ, Royer TV. Pharmaceutical compounds and ecosystem function: An emerging research challenge for aquatic ecologists. *Ecosystems*. 2012;15(6):867–80.
36. Stuart EJE, Compton RG. Nanoparticles-emerging contaminants. In: Moretto LM, Kalcher K, eds. *Environmental Analysis by Electrochemical Sensors and Biosensors: Applications*. New York, NY: Springer; 2015:855–78.
37. Stehle S, Schulz R. Agricultural insecticides threaten surface waters at the global scale. *Proc Natl Acad Sci U S A*. 2015;112(18):5750–5.
38. Malaj E, von der Ohe PC, Grote M, et al. Organic chemicals jeopardize the health of freshwater ecosystems on the continental scale. *Proc Natl Acad Sci U S A*. 2014;111(26):9549–54.
39. Corsolini S, Sara G. The trophic transfer of persistent pollutants (HCB, DDTs, PCBs) within polar marine food webs. *Chemosphere*. 2017;177:189–99.
40. Brown TM, Macdonald RW, Muir DCG, Letcher RJ. The distribution and trends of persistent organic pollutants and mercury in marine mammals from Canada's Eastern Arctic. *Sci Total Environ*. 2018;618:500–17.
41. Porta M, Puigdomenech E, Ballester F, et al. Monitoring concentrations of persistent organic pollutants in the general population: The international experience. *Environ Int*. 2008;34(4):546–61.
42. Pumarega J, Gasull M, Lee DH, Lopez T, Porta M. Number of persistent organic pollutants detected at high concentrations in blood samples of the United States population. *PLoS One*. 2016;11(8):e0160432.
43. Thompson RC, Moore CJ, vom Saal FS, Swan SH. Plastics, the environment and human health: Current consensus and future trends. *Philos Biol Sci*. 2009;364(1526):2153–66.
44. Jambeck JR, Geyer R, Wilcox C, et al. Plastic waste inputs from land into the ocean. *Science*. 2015;347(6223):768–71.
45. Wilcox C, Van Sebille E, Hardesty BD. Threat of plastic pollution to seabirds is global, pervasive, and increasing. *Proc Natl Acad Sci U S A*. 2015;112(38):11899–904.
46. Rochman CM, Tahir A, Williams SL, et al. Anthropogenic debris in seafood: Plastic debris and fibers from textiles in fish and bivalves sold for human consumption. *Sci Rep*. 2015;5:14340.
47. Geyer R, Jambeck JR, Law KL. Production, use, and fate of all plastics ever made. *Sci Adv*. 2017;3(7):e1700782.
48. Lee H, Shim WJ, Kwon JH. Sorption capacity of plastic debris for hydrophobic organic chemicals. *Sci Total Environ*. 2014;470–1:1545–52.
49. McNeill VF. Atmospheric aerosols: Clouds, chemistry, and climate. *Annu Rev Chem Biomol Eng*. 2017;8:427–44.
50. Mukherjee A, Agrawal M. A global perspective of fine particulate matter pollution and its health effects. *Rev Environ Contam Toxicol*. 2018;244:5–51.
51. He MZ, Zeng X, Zhang K, Kinney PL. Fine particulate matter concentrations in urban Chinese cities, 2005–2016: A systematic review. *Int J Environ Res Public Health*. 2017;14(2):191.
52. Singh N, Murari V, Kumar M, Barman SC, Banerjee T. Fine particulates over South Asia: Review and meta-analysis of PM2.5 source apportionment through receptor model. *Environ Pollut*. 2017;223:121–36.
53. Mannucci PM, Franchini M. Health effects of ambient air pollution in developing countries. *Int J Environ Res Public Health*. 2017;14(9):1048.
54. Landrigan PJ, Fuller R, Acosta NJR, et al. The Lancet Commission on pollution and health. *Lancet*. 2018;391:462–512.
55. Rowland FS. Stratospheric ozone depletion. *Philos Trans R Soc Lond B Biol Sci*. 2006;361(1469):769–90.
56. Robinson SA, Erickson DJ 3rd. Not just about sunburn—The ozone hole's profound effect on climate has significant implications for Southern Hemisphere ecosystems. *Glob Chang Biol*. 2015;21(2):515–27.
57. Solomon S, Ivy DJ, Kinnison D, Mills MJ, Neely RR, Schmidt A. Emergence of healing in the Antarctic ozone layer. *Science*. 2016;353(6296):269–74.

58. Ball WT, Alsing J, Mortlock DJ, et al. Evidence for a continuous decline in lower stratospheric ozone offsetting ozone layer recovery. *Atmos Chem Phys.* 2018;18(2):1379–94.
59. Doney SC, Fabry VJ, Feely RA, Kleypas JA. Ocean acidification: The other CO_2 problem. *Ann Rev Mar Sci.* 2009;1(1):169–92.
60. Esbaugh AJ. Physiological implications of ocean acidification for marine fish: Emerging patterns and new insights. *J Comp Physiol B.* 2018;188(1):1–13.
61. Breitburg D, Levin LA, Oschlies A, et al. Declining oxygen in the global ocean and coastal waters. *Science.* 2018;359(6371):eaam7240.
62. Gobler CJ, Doherty OM, Hattenrath-Lehmann TK, Griffith AW, Kang Y, Litaker RW. Ocean warming since 1982 has expanded the niche of toxic algal blooms in the North Atlantic and North Pacific oceans. *Proc Natl Acad Sci U S A.* 2017;114(19):4975–80.
63. Wells ML, Trainer VL, Smayda TJ, et al. Harmful algal blooms and climate change: Learning from the past and present to forecast the future. *Harmful Algae.* 2015;49:68–93.
64. Escobar MTL, Sotto LPA, Jacinto GS, Benico GA, San Diego-McGlone ML, Azanza RV. Eutrophic conditions during the 2010 fish kill in Bolinao and Anda, Pangasinan, Philippines. *J Environ Sci Management.* 2013;35(Special Issue No. 1):29–35.
65. San Diego-McGlone ML, Azanza RV, Villanoy CL, Jacinto GS. Eutrophic waters, algal bloom and fish kill in fish farming areas in Bolinao, Pangasinan, Philippines. *Mar Pollut Bull.* 2008;57(6):295–301.
66. Van Cappellen P, Maavara T. Rivers in the Anthropocene: Global scale modifications of riverine nutrient fluxes by damming. *Ecohydrol Hydrobio.* 2016;16(2):106–11.
67. Zarfl C, Lumsdon AE, Berlekamp J, Tydecks L, Tockner K. A global boom in hydropower dam construction. *Aquat Sci.* 2015;77(1):161–70.
68. Maavara T, Dürr HH, Van Cappellen P. Worldwide retention of nutrient silicon by river damming: From sparse data set to global estimate. *Global Biogeochem Cycles.* 2014;28(8):842–55.
69. Maavara T, Parsons CT, Ridenour C, et al. Global phosphorus retention by river damming. *Proc Natl Acad Sci U S A.* 2015;112(51):15603–8.
70. Maavara T, Lauerwald R, Regnier P, Van Cappellen P. Global perturbation of organic carbon cycling by river damming. *Nat Commun.* 2017;8:15347.
71. Wehrli B. Climate science: Renewable but not carbon-free. *Nat Geosci.* 2011;4:585–6.
72. McDonald-Wilmsen B, Webber M. Dams and displacement: Raising the standards and broadening the research agenda. *Water Altern.* 2010;3(2):142.
73. Zhang X, Peng L, Liu W, et al. Response of primary vectors and related diseases to impoundment by the Three Gorges Dam. *Trop Med Int Health.* 2014;19(4):440–9.
74. Sanchez-Ribas J, Parra-Henao G, Guimaraes AE. Impact of dams and irrigation schemes in Anopheline (Diptera: Culicidae) bionomics and malaria epidemiology. *Rev Inst Med Trop Sao Paulo.* 2012;54(4):179–91.
75. Keiser J, De Castro MC, Maltese MF, et al. Effect of irrigation and large dams on the burden of malaria on a global and regional scale. *Am J Trop Med Hyg.* 2005;72(4):392–406.
76. Steinmann P, Keiser J, Bos R, Tanner M, Utzinger J. Schistosomiasis and water resources development: Systematic review, meta-analysis, and estimates of people at risk. *Lancet Infect Dis.* 2006;6(7):411–25.
77. Calder RS, Schartup AT, Li M, Valberg AP, Balcom PH, Sunderland EM. Future impacts of hydroelectric power development on methylmercury exposures of Canadian indigenous communities. *Environ Sci Technol.* 2016;50(23):13115–22.
78. Richey AS, Thomas BF, Lo M-H, et al. Quantifying renewable groundwater stress with GRACE. *Water Resour Res.* 2015;51(7):5217–38.
79. McGuire VL. USGS: Water-Level and Recoverable Water in Storage Changes, High Plains Aquifer, Predevelopment to 2015 and 2013–15. US Department of the Interior; 2017.
80. Cotterman KA, Kendall AD, Basso B, Hyndman DW. Groundwater depletion and climate change: Future prospects of crop production in the Central High Plains Aquifer. *Clim Change.* 2018;146(1):187–200.
81. Ellis EC, Goldewijk KK, Siebert S, Lightman D, Ramankutty N. Anthropogenic transformation of the biomes, 1700–2000. *Glob Ecol Biogeogr.* 2010;19(5):589–606.
82. Turner BL, Lambin EF, Reenberg A. The emergence of land change science for global environmental change and sustainability. *Proc Natl Acad Sci U S A.* 2007;104(52):20666–71.
83. Foley JA, DeFries R, Asner GP, et al. Global consequences of land use. *Science.* 2005;309(5734):570–4.
84. Lambin EF, Turner BL, Geist HJ, et al. The causes of land-use and land-cover change: Moving beyond the myths. *Global Environ Chang.* 2001;11(4):261–9.
85. Lambin EF, Meyfroidt P. Global land use change, economic globalization, and the looming land scarcity *Proc Natl Acad Sci U S A.* 2011;108(9):3465–72.
86. d'Amour CB, Reitsma F, Baiocchi G, et al. Future urban land expansion and implications for global croplands. *Proc Natl Acad Sci U S A.* 2017;114(34):8939–44.
87. Thomas N, Lucas R, Bunting P, Hardy A, Rosenqvist A, Simard M. Distribution and drivers of global mangrove forest change, 1996–2010. *PLoS One.* 2017;12(6):e0179302.
88. Turetsky MR, Benscoter B, Page S, Rein G, van der Werf GR, Watts A. Global vulnerability of peatlands to fire and carbon loss. *Nat Geosci.* 2014;8:11–14.
89. Astrup R, Bernier PY, Genet H, Lutz DA, Bright RM. A sensible climate solution for the boreal forest. *Nat Clim Change.* 2018;8(1):11–12.
90. Gauthier S, Bernier P, Kuuluvainen T, Shvidenko AZ, Schepaschenko DG. Boreal forest health and global change. *Science.* 2015;349(6250):819–22.
91. Stephens SL, Burrows N, Buyantuyev A, et al. Temperate and boreal forest mega-fires: Characteristics and challenges. *Front Ecol Environ.* 2014;12(2):115–22.
92. Price DT, Alfaro RI, Brown KJ, et al. Anticipating the consequences of climate change for Canada's boreal forest ecosystems. *Environ Rev.* 2013;21(4):322–65.
93. Lawler JJ, Lewis DJ, Nelson E, et al. Projected land-use change impacts on ecosystem services in the United States. *Proc Natl Acad Sci U S A.* 2014;111(20):7492–7.
94. Montgomery DR. *Dirt: The Erosion of Civilizations.* Berkeley, CA: University of California Press; 2007.
95. Montgomery DR. *Growing a Revolution: Bringing Our Soil Back to Life.* 1st ed. New York: W.W. Norton & Company; 2017.
96. Montgomery DR. Soil erosion and agricultural sustainability. *Proc Natl Acad Sci U S A.* 2007;104(33):13268–72.
97. FAO and ITPS. Status of the World's Soil Resources. Rome: Food and Agriculture Organization of the United Nations and Intergovernmental Technical Panel on Soils; 2015.
98. Palm C, Sanchez P, Ahamed S, Awiti A. Soils: A contemporary perspective. *Annu Rev Environ Resour.* 2007;32(1):99–129.
99. Tilman D, Cassman KG, Matson PA, Naylor R, Polasky S. Agricultural sustainability and intensive production practices. *Nature.* 2002;418(6898):671–7.
100. United Nations. World Urbanization Prospects: The 2014 Revision. New York: United Nations Department of Economic and Social Affairs. Population Division; 2015. Report No.: ST/ESA/SER.A/366.
101. Smit W, Hancock T, Kumaresen J, Santos-Burgoa C, Sánchez-Kobashi Meneses R, Friel S. Toward a research and action agenda on urban planning/design and health equity in cities in low and middle-income countries. *J Urban Health.* 2011;88(5):875–85.
102. Satterthwaite D. Editorial: Why is urban health so poor even in many successful cities? *Environ Urban.* 2011;23(1):5–11.
103. Frumkin H, Frank LD, Jackson R. *Urban Sprawl and Public Health: Designing, Planning, and Building for Healthy Communities.* Washington, DC: Island Press; 2004.
104. Wilbanks TJ, Kates RW. Global change in local places: How scale matters. *Climatic Change.* 1999;43(3):601–28.
105. Bai X. Industrial ecology and the global impacts of cities. *J Ind Ecol.* 2007;11(2):1–6.
106. Chavez A, Sperling J. Key drivers and trends of urban greenhouse gas emissions. In: Dhakal S, Ruth M, eds. *Creating Low Carbon Cities.* Cham: Springer International Publishing; 2017:157–68.
107. Seto KC, Reenberg A, Boone CG, et al. Urban land teleconnections and sustainability. *Proc Natl Acad Sci U S A.* 2012;109(20):7687–92.
108. Wolman A. The metabolism of cities. *Sci Am.* 1965;213:179–90.
109. Lenzen M, Peters Greg M. How city dwellers affect their resource hinterland. *J Ind Ecol.* 2010;14(1):73–90.
110. Fry J, Lenzen M, Jin Y, et al. Assessing carbon footprints of cities under limited information. *J Clean Prod.* 2018;176:1254–70.
111. Seto KC, Shepherd JM. Global urban land-use trends and climate impacts. *Curr Opin Environ Sustain.* 2009;1(1):89–95.
112. Seto KC, Guneralp B, Hutyra LR. Global forecasts of urban expansion to 2030 and direct impacts on biodiversity and carbon pools. *Proc Natl Acad Sci U S A.* 2012;109(40):16083–8.

113. Galloway JN, Townsend AR, Erisman JW, et al. Transformation of the nitrogen cycle: Recent trends, questions, and potential solutions. *Science.* 2008;320(5878):889–92.

114. Smil V. Nitrogen cycle and world food production. *World Agric.* 2011;2:9–13.

115. Sinha E, Michalak AM, Balaji V. Eutrophication will increase during the 21st century as a result of precipitation changes. *Science.* 2017;357(6349):405–8.

116. Yuan Z, Jiang S, Sheng H, et al. Human perturbation of the global phosphorus cycle: Changes and consequences. *Environ Sci Technol.* 2018;52(5):2438–50.

117. Elser J, Bennett E. Phosphorus cycle: A broken biogeochemical cycle. *Nature.* 2011;478(7367):29–31.

118. Bringhurst K, Jordan P. The impact on nutrient cycles from tropical forest to pasture conversion in Costa Rica. *Sustain Water Resour Manag.* 2015;1(1):3–13.

119. Maranguit D, Guillaume T, Kuzyakov Y. Land-use change affects phosphorus fractions in highly weathered tropical soils. *Catena.* 2017;149:385–93.

120. Rhodes CJ. Peak phosphorus—Peak food? The need to close the phosphorus cycle. *Sci Prog.* 2013;96(Pt 2):109–52.

121. Scholz RW, Ulrich AE, Eilitta M, Roy A. Sustainable use of phosphorus: A finite resource. *Sci Total Environ.* 2013;461-2:799–803.

122. Cordell D, Rosemarin A, Schroder JJ, Smit AL. Towards global phosphorus security: A systems framework for phosphorus recovery and reuse options. *Chemosphere.* 2011;84(6):747–58.

123. Penuelas J, Poulter B, Sardans J, et al. Human-induced nitrogen-phosphorus imbalances alter natural and managed ecosystems across the globe. *Nat Commun.* 2013;4:2934.

124. Pinker S. *The Better Angels of Our Nature: Why Violence has Declined.* New York: Viking; 2011.

125. Omran AR. The epidemiologic transition. A theory of the epidemiology of population change. *Milbank Mem Fund Q.* 1971;49(4):509–38.

126. Zuckerman MK, Harper KN, Barrett R, Armelagos GJ. The evolution of disease: Anthropological perspectives on epidemiologic transitions. *Global Health Action.* 2014;7:23303.

127. Barrett B, Charles JW, Temte JL. Climate change, human health, and epidemiological transition. *Prev Med.* 2015;70:69–75.

128. Whitmee S, Haines A, Beyrer C, et al. Safeguarding human health in the Anthropocene epoch: Report of The Rockefeller Foundation—Lancet Commission on planetary health. *Lancet.* 2015;386(10007):1973–2028.

129. Smith KR, Woodward A, Campbell-Lendrum D, et al. Human health: Impacts, adaptation, and co-benefits. In: Field CB, Barros VR, Dokken DJ, et al, eds. *Climate Change 2014: Impacts, Adaptation, and Vulnerability Part A: Global and Sectoral Aspects Contribution of Working Group II to the Fifth Assessment Report of the Intergovernmental Panel of Climate Change.* Cambridge and New York: Cambridge University Press; 2014:709–54.

130. Luber G, Lemery J. *Global Climate Change and Human Health: From Science to Practice.* San Francisco, CA: Jossey-Bass; 2015.

131. Levy BS, Patz JA. *Climate Change and Public Health.* New York: Oxford University Press; 2015.

132. Ebi KL, Frumkin H, Hess JJ. Protecting and promoting population health in the context of climate and other global environmental changes. *Anthropocene.* 2017;19:1–12.

133. McMichael AJ. Globalization, climate change, and human health. *N Engl J Med.* 2013;368(14):1335–43.

134. Flegal KM, Kit BK, Orpana H, Graubard BI. Association of all-cause mortality with overweight and obesity using standard body mass index categories: A systematic review and meta-analysis. *JAMA.* 2013;309(1):71–82.

135. Bastien M, Poirier P, Lemieux I, Després J-P. Overview of epidemiology and contribution of obesity to cardiovascular disease. *Progress in Cardiovascular Diseases.* 2014;56(4):369–81.

136. Kivimäki M, Kuosma E, Ferrie JE, et al. Overweight, obesity, and risk of cardiometabolic multimorbidity: Pooled analysis of individual-level data for 120,813 adults from 16 cohort studies from the USA and Europe. *Lancet Public Health.* 2017;2(6):e277–85.

137. Lauby-Secretan B, Scoccianti C, Loomis D, Grosse Y, Bianchini F, Straif K. Body fatness and cancer—Viewpoint of the IARC Working Group. *N Engl J Med.* 2016;375(8):794–8.

138. Mansur RB, Brietzke E, McIntyre RS. Is there a "metabolic-mood syndrome"? A review of the relationship between obesity and mood disorders. *Neurosci Biobehav Rev.* 2015;52:89–104.

139. GBD Obesity Collaborators. Health effects of overweight and obesity in 195 countries over 25 years. *N Engl J Med.* 2017;377(1):13–27.

140. Williams EP, Mesidor M, Winters K, Dubbert PM, Wyatt SB. Overweight and obesity: Prevalence, consequences, and causes of a growing public health problem. *Curr Obes Rep.* 2015;4(3):363–70.

141. Vandevijvere S, Chow CC, Hall KD, Umali E, Swinburn BA. Increased food energy supply as a major driver of the obesity epidemic: A global analysis. *Bull World Health Organ.* 2015;93(7):446–56.

142. Swinburn BA, Sacks G, Hall KD, et al. The global obesity pandemic: Shaped by global drivers and local environments. *Lancet.* 2011;378(9793):804–14.

143. Popkin BM. Relationship between shifts in food system dynamics and acceleration of the global nutrition transition. *Nutr Rev.* 2017;75(2):73–82.

144. Zhai FY, Du SF, Wang ZH, Zhang JG, Du WW, Popkin BM. Dynamics of the Chinese diet and the role of urbanicity, 1991–2011. *Obes Rev.* 2014;15(Suppl 1):16–26.

145. Popkin BM. Urbanization, lifestyle changes and the nutrition transition. *World Dev.* 1999;27(11):1905–16.

146. Leong KSW, Derraik JGB, Hofman PL, Cutfield WS. Antibiotics, gut microbiome and obesity. *Clin Endocrinol (Oxf).* 2018;88(2):185–200.

147. Maruvada P, Leone V, Kaplan LM, Chang EB. The human microbiome and obesity: Moving beyond associations. *Cell Host Microbe.* 2017;22(5):589–99.

148. Darbre PD. Endocrine disruptors and obesity. *Curr Obes Rep.* 2017;6(1):18–27.

149. Nappi F, Barrea L, Di Somma C, et al. Endocrine aspects of environmental "Obesogen" pollutants. *Int J Environ Res Public Health.* 2016;13(8):765.

150. Legeay S, Faure S. Is bisphenol A an environmental obesogen? *Fund Clin Pharmacol.* 2017;31(6):594–609.

151. Cohen AJ, Brauer M, Burnett R, et al. Estimates and 25-year trends of the global burden of disease attributable to ambient air pollution: An analysis of data from the Global Burden of Diseases Study 2015. *Lancet.* 2017;389(10082):1907–18.

152. GBD Risk Factors collaborators. Global, regional, and national comparative risk assessment of 79 behavioural, environmental and occupational, and metabolic risks or clusters of risks, 1990–2015: A systematic analysis for the Global Burden of Disease Study 2015. *Lancet.* 2016;388(10053):1659–1724.

153. WHO. Ambient Air Pollution: A Global Assessment of Exposure and Burden of Disease; 2016.

154. Koplitz SN, Jacob DJ, Sulprizio MP, Myllyvirta L, Reid C. Burden of disease from rising coal-fired power plant emissions in Southeast Asia. *Environ Sci Technol.* 2017;51(3):1467–76.

155. Hoek G, Krishnan RM, Beelen R, et al. Long-term air pollution exposure and cardio- respiratory mortality: A review. *Environ Health.* 2013;12(1):43.

156. Folino F, Buja G, Zanotto G, et al. Association between air pollution and ventricular arrhythmias in high-risk patients (ARIA study): A multicentre longitudinal study. *Lancet Planetary Health.* 2017;1(2):e58–64.

157. Shah AS, Langrish JP, Nair H, et al. Global association of air pollution and heart failure: A systematic review and meta-analysis. *Lancet.* 2013;382(9897):1039–48.

158. He D, Wu S, Zhao H, et al. Association between particulate matter 2.5 and diabetes mellitus: A meta-analysis of cohort studies. *J Diabetes Investig.* 2017;8(5):687–96.

159. Clifford A, Lang L, Chen R, Anstey KJ, Seaton A. Exposure to air pollution and cognitive functioning across the life course—A systematic literature review. *Environ Res.* 2016;147:383–98.

160. Turner MC, Jerrett M, Pope CA 3rd, et al. Long-term ozone exposure and mortality in a large prospective study. *Am J Respir Crit Care Med.* 2016;193(10):1134–42.

161. Malley CS, Henze DK, Kuylenstierna JCI, et al. Updated global estimates of respiratory mortality in adults >/=30 years of age attributable to long-term ozone exposure. *Environ Health Perspect.* 2017;125(8):087021.

162. Atkinson RW, Butland BK, Dimitroulopoulou C, et al. Long-term exposure to ambient ozone and mortality: A quantitative systematic review and meta-analysis of evidence from cohort studies. *BMJ Open.* 2016;6(2):e009493.

163. Ji M, Cohan DS, Bell ML. Meta-analysis of the association between short-term exposure to ambient ozone and respiratory hospital admissions. *Environ Res Lett.* 2011;6(2):024006.

164. Whiteford HA, Ferrari AJ, Degenhardt L, Feigin V, Vos T. The global burden of mental, neurological and substance use disorders: An

analysis from the Global Burden of Disease Study 2010. *PLoS One.* 2015;10(2):e0116820.

165. Goldmann E, Galea S. Mental health consequences of disasters. *Annu Rev Public Health.* 2014;35(1):169–83.
166. Galea S, Brewin CR, Gruber M, et al. Exposure to hurricane-related stressors and mental illness after Hurricane Katrina. *Arch Gen Psychiatry.* 2007;64(12):1427–34.
167. Kessler RC, Galea S, Gruber MJ, Sampson NA, Ursano RJ, Wessely S. Trends in mental illness and suicidality after Hurricane Katrina. *Mol Psychiatry.* 2008;13(4):374–84.
168. Tang TC, Yen CF, Cheng CP, et al. Suicide risk and its correlate in adolescents who experienced typhoon-induced mudslides: A structural equation model. *Depress Anxiety.* 2010;27(12):1143–8.
169. Adams ZW, Sumner JA, Danielson CK, et al. Prevalence and predictors of PTSD and depression among adolescent victims of the Spring 2011 tornado outbreak. *J Child Psychol Psychiatry.* 2014;55(9):1047–55.
170. Fernandez A, Black J, Jones M, et al. Flooding and mental health: A systematic mapping review. *PLoS One.* 2015;10(4):e0119929.
171. Stanke C, Murray V, Amlot R, Nurse J, Williams R. The effects of flooding on mental health: Outcomes and recommendations from a review of the literature. *PLoS Curr.* 2012;4:e4f9f1fa9c3cae.
172. Hansen A, Bi P, Nitschke M, Ryan P, Pisaniello D, Tucker G. The effect of heat waves on mental health in a temperate Australian city. *Environ Health Perspect.* 2008;116(10):1369–75.
173. Hart CR, Berry HL, Tonna AM. Improving the mental health of rural New South Wales communities facing drought and other adversities. *Aust J Rural Health.* 2011;19(5):231–8.
174. Eisenman D, McCaffrey S, Donatello I, Marshal G. An ecosystems and vulnerable populations perspective on solastalgia and psychological distress after a wildfire. *EcoHealth.* 2015;12(4):602–10.
175. McFarlane AC, Van Hooff M. Impact of childhood exposure to a natural disaster on adult mental health: 20-year longitudinal follow-up study. *Br J Psychiatry.* 2009;195(2):142–8.
176. O'Brien LV, Berry HL, Coleman C, Hanigan IC. Drought as a mental health exposure. *Environ Res.* 2014;131:181–7.
177. Guiney R. Farming suicides during the Victorian drought: 2001–2007. *Aust J Rural Health.* 2012;20(1):11–15.
178. Tang B, Liu X, Liu Y, Xue C, Zhang L. A meta-analysis of risk factors for depression in adults and children after natural disasters. *BMC Public Health.* 2014;14(1):623.
179. Rosendal S, Salcioglu E, Andersen HS, Mortensen EL. Exposure characteristics and peri-trauma emotional reactions during the 2004 tsunami in Southeast Asia—What predicts posttraumatic stress and depressive symptoms? *Compr Psychiatry.* 2011;52(6):630–7.
180. Loughry M. Climate change, human movement and the promotion of mental health: What have we learnt from earlier global stressors? In: McAdam J, ed. *Climate Change and Displacement: Multidisciplinary Perspectives.* Portland, OR: Hart Publishing; 2010.
181. Uscher-Pines L. Health effects of relocation following disaster: A systematic review of the literature. *Disasters.* 2009;33(1):1–22.
182. Siriwardhana C, Stewart R. Forced migration and mental health: Prolonged internal displacement, return migration and resilience. *Int Health.* 2013;5(1):19–23.
183. Bustamante LHU, Cerqueira RO, Leclerc E, Brietzke E. Stress, trauma, and posttraumatic stress disorder in migrants: A comprehensive review. *Rev Bras Psiquiatr.* 2018;40(2):220–5.
184. Warsini S, Mills J, Usher K. Solastalgia: Living with the environmental damage caused by natural disasters. *Prehosp Disaster Med.* 2014;29(1):87–90.
185. Albrecht G, Sartore G-M, Connor L, et al. Solastalgia: The distress caused by environmental change. *Australas Psychiatry.* 2007;15(Suppl 1):95–98.
186. Cordial P, Riding-Malon R, Lips H. The effects of mountaintop removal coal mining on mental health, well-being, and community health in Central Appalachia. *Ecopsychology.* 2012;4(3):201–8.
187. Hendryx M, Innes-Wimsatt KA. Increased risk of depression for people living in coal mining areas of central Appalachia. *Ecopsychology.* 2013;5(3):179–87.
188. Austin D, Dosemagen S, Marks B, McGuire T, Prakash P, Rogers B. Offshore Oil and Deepwater Horizon: Social Effects on Gulf Coast Communities. Volume II: Key Economic Sectors, NGOs, and Ethnic Groups. New Orleans: U.S. Department of the Interior. Bureau of Ocean Energy Management; 2014. Contract No.: BOEM 2014-618.
189. Brubaker M, Berner J, Chavan R, Warren J. Climate change and health effects in Northwest Alaska. *Glob Health Action.* 2011;4.
190. Berghuis SA, Bos AF, Sauer PJ, Roze E. Developmental neurotoxicity of persistent organic pollutants: An update on childhood outcome. *Arch Toxicol.* 2015;89(5):687–709.
191. Grandjean P, Landrigan PJ. Neurobehavioural effects of developmental toxicity. *Lancet Neurol.* 2014;13(3):330–8.
192. Volk HE, Lurmann F, Penfold B, Hertz-Picciotto I, McConnell R. Traffic-related air pollution, particulate matter, and autism. *JAMA Psychiatry.* 2013;70(1):71–77.
193. Perera FP, Chang HW, Tang D, et al. Early-life exposure to polycyclic aromatic hydrocarbons and ADHD behavior problems. *PLoS One.* 2014;9(11):e111670.
194. Kalkbrenner AE, Schmidt RJ, Penlesky AC. Environmental chemical exposures and autism spectrum disorders: A review of the epidemiological evidence. *Curr Probl Pediatr Adolesc Health Care.* 2014;44(10):277–318.
195. Metcalf CJE, Walter KS, Wesolowski A, et al. Identifying climate drivers of infectious disease dynamics: Recent advances and challenges ahead. *Proc Biol Sci.* 2017;284(1860):20170901.
196. Liang L, Gong P. Climate change and human infectious diseases: A synthesis of research findings from global and spatio-temporal perspectives. *Environ Int.* 2017;103:99–108.
197. Lafferty KD, Mordecai EA. The rise and fall of infectious disease in a warmer world. *F1000Research.* 2016;5:F1000.
198. Altizer S, Ostfeld RS, Johnson PT, Kutz S, Harvell CD. Climate change and infectious diseases: From evidence to a predictive framework. *Science.* 2013;341(6145):514–9.
199. Naish S, Dale P, Mackenzie JS, McBride J, Mengersen K, Tong S. Climate change and dengue: A critical and systematic review of quantitative modelling approaches. *BMC Infect Dis.* 2014;14:167.
200. Ebi KL, Nealon J. Dengue in a changing climate. *Environ Res.* 2016;151:115–23.
201. Siraj A, Santos-Vega M, Bouma M, Yadeta D, Carrascal DR, Pascual M. Altitudinal changes in malaria incidence in highlands of Ethiopia and Colombia. *Science.* 2014;343(6175):1154–8.
202. Caminade C, Kovats S, Rocklov J, et al. Impact of climate change on global malaria distribution. *Proc Natl Acad Sci U S A.* 2014;111(9):3286–91.
203. Sonenshine DE. Range expansion of tick disease vectors in North America: Implications for spread of tick-borne disease. *Int J Environ Res Public Health.* 2018;15(3):478.
204. Gottdenker NL, Streicker DG, Faust CL, Carroll CR. Anthropogenic land use change and infectious diseases: A review of the evidence. *EcoHealth.* 2014;11(4):619–32.
205. Bauch SC, Birkenbach AM, Pattanayak SK, Sills EO. Public health impacts of ecosystem change in the Brazilian Amazon. *Proc Natl Acad Sci U S A.* 2015;112(24):7414–9.
206. Tucker Lima JM, Vittor A, Rifai S, Valle D. Does deforestation promote or inhibit malaria transmission in the Amazon? A systematic literature review and critical appraisal of current evidence. *Philos Trans R Soc Lond B Biol Sci.* 2017;372(1722):20160125.
207. Stefani A, Dusfour I, Corrêa APS, et al. Land cover, land use and malaria in the Amazon: A systematic literature review of studies using remotely sensed data. *Malar J.* 2013;12(1):192.
208. Barros FS, Honorio NA. Deforestation and malaria on the Amazon frontier: Larval clustering of Anopheles darlingi (Diptera: Culicidae) determines focal distribution of malaria. *Am J Trop Med Hyg.* 2015;93(5):939–53.
209. Hellberg RS, Chu E. Effects of climate change on the persistence and dispersal of foodborne bacterial pathogens in the outdoor environment: A review. *Crit Rev Microbiol.* 2016;42(4):548–72.
210. Sterk A, Schijven J, de Nijs T, de Roda Husman AM. Direct and indirect effects of climate change on the risk of infection by water-transmitted pathogens. *Environ Sci Technol.* 2013;47(22):12648–60.
211. Vezzulli L, Colwell RR, Pruzzo C. Ocean warming and spread of pathogenic vibrios in the aquatic environment. *Microb Ecol.* 2013;65(4):817–25.
212. Vezzulli L, Grande C, Reid PC, et al. Climate influence on Vibrio and associated human diseases during the past half-century in the coastal North Atlantic. *Proc Natl Acad Sci U S A.* 2016;113(34):E5062–71.
213. Baker-Austin C, Trinanes J, Gonzalez-Escalona N, Martinez-Urtaza J. Non-cholera vibrios: The microbial barometer of climate change. *Trends Microbiol.* 2017;25(1):76–84.
214. Carlton EJ, Eisenberg JNS, Goldstick J, Cevallos W, Trostle J, Levy K. Heavy rainfall events and diarrhea incidence: The role of social and environmental factors. *Am J Epidemiol.* 2014;179(3):344–52.

215. Cann K, Thomas DR, Salmon R, Wyn-Jones A, Kay D. Extreme water-related weather events and waterborne disease. *Epidemiol Infect.* 2013;141(04):671–86.
216. Phung D, Huang C, Rutherford S, et al. Association between climate factors and diarrhoea in a Mekong Delta area. *Int J Biometeorol.* 2015;59(9):1321–31.
217. Bhavnani D, Goldstick JE, Cevallos W, Trueba G, Eisenberg JN. Impact of rainfall on diarrheal disease risk associated with unimproved water and sanitation. *Am J Trop Med Hyg.* 2014;90(4):705–11.
218. Kim S, Shin Y, Kim H, Pak H, Ha J. Impacts of typhoon and heavy rain disasters on mortality and infectious diarrhea hospitalization in South Korea. *Int J Environ Health Res.* 2013;23(5):365–76.
219. Chou WC, Wu JL, Wang YC, Huang H, Sung FC, Chuang CY. Modeling the impact of climate variability on diarrhea-associated diseases in Taiwan (1996–2007). *Sci Total Environ.* 2010;409(1):43–51.
220. Drayna P, McLellan SL, Simpson P, Li SH, Gorelick MH. Association between rainfall and pediatric emergency department visits for acute gastrointestinal illness. *Environ Health Perspect.* 2010;118(10):1439–43.
221. Zhu HM, Xiang S, Yang K, Wu XH, Zhou XN. Three Gorges Dam and its impact on the potential transmission of schistosomiasis in regions along the Yangtze River. *Ecohealth.* 2008;5(2):137–48.
222. Zhou YB, Liang S, Chen Y, Jiang QW. The Three Gorges Dam: Does it accelerate or delay the progress towards eliminating transmission of schistosomiasis in China? *Infect Dis Poverty.* 2016;5(1):63.
223. Sun LP, Wang W, Zuo YP, et al. A multidisciplinary, integrated approach for the elimination of schistosomiasis: A longitudinal study in a historically hyper-endemic region in the lower reaches of the Yangtze River, China from 2005 to 2014. *Infect Dis Poverty.* 2017;6(1):56.
224. Allen T, Murray KA, Zambrana-Torrelio C, et al. Global hotspots and correlates of emerging zoonotic diseases. *Nat Commun.* 2017;8(1):1124.
225. Plowright RK, Parrish CR, McCallum H, et al. Pathways to zoonotic spillover. *Nat Rev Microbiol.* 2017;15(8):502–10.
226. Jones BA, Grace D, Kock R, et al. Zoonosis emergence linked to agricultural intensification and environmental change. *Proc Natl Acad Sci U S A.* 2013;110(21):8399–404.
227. Despommier D, Ellis BR, Wilcox BA. The role of ecotones in emerging infectious diseases. *EcoHealth.* 2006;3(4):281–9.
228. Shah SZ, Jabbar B, Ahmed N, et al. Epidemiology, pathogenesis, and control of a tick-borne disease—Kyasanur forest disease: Current status and future directions. *Front Cell Infect Microbiol.* 2018;8:149.
229. Hollenbeck JE. Interaction of the role of Concentrated Animal Feeding Operations (CAFOs) in Emerging Infectious Diseases (EIDS). *Infect Genet Evol.* 2016;38:44–46.
230. Epstein JH, Field HE, Luby S, Pulliam JR, Daszak P. Nipah virus: Impact, origins, and causes of emergence. *Curr Infect Dis Rep.* 2006;8(1):59–65.
231. Popkin BM, Adair LS, Ng SW. Global nutrition transition and the pandemic of obesity in developing countries. *Nutr Rev.* 2012;70(1):3–21.
232. Green R, Milner J, Joy EJ, Agrawal S, Dangour AD. Dietary patterns in India: A systematic review. *Br J Nutr.* 2016;116(1):142–8.
233. Popkin BM. Nutrition transition and the global diabetes epidemic. *Curr Diab Rep.* 2015;15(9):64.
234. Bouvard V, Loomis D, Guyton KZ, et al. Carcinogenicity of consumption of red and processed meat. *Lancet Oncol.* 2015;16(16):1599–600.
235. Larsson SC, Orsini N. Red meat and processed meat consumption and all-cause mortality: A meta-analysis. *Am J Epidemiol.* 2014;179(3):282–9.
236. Anand SS, Hawkes C, de Souza RJ, et al. Food consumption and its impact on cardiovascular disease: Importance of solutions focused on the globalized food system: A report from the Workshop Convened by the World Heart Federation. *J Am Coll Cardiol.* 2015;66(14):1590–614.
237. Wu G, Bazer FW, Cross HR. Land-based production of animal protein: Impacts, efficiency, and sustainability. *Ann N Y Acad Sci.* 2014;1328:18–28.
238. FAO. Livestock's Long Shadow: Environmental Issues and Options Rome: Food and Agriculture Organization; 2006.
239. De Sy V, Herold M, Achard F, et al. Land use patterns and related carbon losses following deforestation in South America. *Environ Res Lett.* 2015;10(12):124004.
240. Porter JR, Xie L, Challinor AJ, et al. Food security and food production systems. In: Field CB, Barros VR, Dokken DJ, et al., eds. *Climate Change 2014: Impacts, Adaptation and Vulnerability Part A: Global and Sectoral Aspects Contribution of Working Group II to the Fifth Assessment Report of the Intergovernmental Panel on Climate Change.* Cambridge and New York: Cambridge University Press; 2014:485–533.
241. Lloyd SJ, Kovats RS, Chalabi Z. Climate change, crop yields, and undernutrition: Development of a model to quantify the impact of climate scenarios on child undernutrition. *Environ Health Perspect.* 2011;119(12):1817–23.
242. de Onis M, Blossner M, Borghi E. Prevalence and trends of stunting among pre-school children, 1990–2020. *Public Health Nutr.* 2012;15(1):142–8.
243. Walker SP, Chang SM, Wright A, Osmond C, Grantham-McGregor SM. Early childhood stunting is associated with lower developmental levels in the subsequent generation of children. *J Nutr.* 2015;145(4):823–8.
244. Springmann M, Mason-D'Croz D, Robinson S, et al. Global and regional health effects of future food production under climate change: A modelling study. *Lancet.* 2016;387(10031):1937–46.
245. Klein A-M, Vaissière BE, Cane JH, et al. Importance of pollinators in changing landscapes for world crops. *Proc Royal Soc B.* 2007;274(1608):303–13.
246. Potts SG, Imperatriz-Fonseca VL, Ngo HT. *The Assessment Report of the Intergovernmental Science-Policy Platform on Biodiversity and Ecosystem Services on Pollinators, Pollination and Food Production.* Bonn: Intergovernmental Science-Policy Platform on Biodiversity and Ecosystem Services (IPBES); 2016.
247. Smith MR, Singh GM, Mozaffarian D, Myers SS. Effects of decreases of animal pollinators on human nutrition and global health: A modelling analysis. *Lancet.* 2015;386(10007):1964–72.
248. FAO. *The State of World Fisheries and Aquaculture.* Rome: Food and Agriculture Organization; 2016.
249. Comte L, Olden JD. Climatic vulnerability of the world's freshwater and marine fishes. *Nature Clim Change.* 2017;7(10):718–22.
250. Golden CD, Allison EH, Cheung WW, et al. Nutrition: Fall in fish catch threatens human health. *Nature.* 2016;534(7607):317–20.
251. Loladze I. Hidden shift of the ionome of plants exposed to elevated CO2 depletes minerals at the base of human nutrition. *eLife.* 2014;3:e02245.
252. Myers SS, Wessells KR, Kloog I, Zanobetti A, Schwartz J. Effect of increased concentrations of atmospheric carbon dioxide on the global threat of zinc deficiency: A modelling study. *Lancet Global Health.* 2015;3(10):e639–45.
253. Myers SS, Kloog I, Huybers P, et al. Increasing CO2 threatens human nutrition. *Nature.* 2014;510(7503):139–42.
254. Zhu C, Kobayashi K, Loladze I, et al. Carbon dioxide (CO2) levels this century will alter the protein, micronutrients, and vitamin content of rice grains with potential health consequences for the poorest rice-dependent countries. *Sci Adv.* 2018;4(5):eaaq1012.
255. Appel LJ, Sacks FM, Carey VJ, et al. Effects of protein, monounsaturated fat, and carbohydrate intake on blood pressure and serum lipids: Results of the OmniHeart randomized trial. *JAMA.* 2005;294(19):2455–64.
256. Mock CN, Smith KR, Kobusingye O, et al. Injury prevention and environmental health: Key messages from disease control priorities. In: Mock CN, Nugent R, Kobusingye O, Smith KR, eds. *Injury Prevention and Environmental Health.* 3rd ed. Washington (DC): The International Bank for Reconstruction and Development/The World Bank; 2017.
257. Bachani AM, Peden M, Gururaj G, Norton R, Hyder AA. Road traffic injuries. In: Mock CN, Nugent R, Kobusingye O, Smith KR, eds. *Injury Prevention and Environmental Health.* 7. Washington, DC: The International Bank for Reconstruction and Development/The World Bank; 2017.
258. Haddon W Jr. A logical framework for categorizing highway safety phenomena and activity. *J Trauma.* 1972;12(3):193–207.
259. Liu A, Soneja SI, Jiang C, et al. Frequency of extreme weather events and increased risk of motor vehicle collision in Maryland. *Sci Total Environ.* 2017;580:550–5.
260. Norton P, Epperson B. *Fighting Traffic: The Dawn of the Motor Age in the American City.* Cambridge, MA: MIT Press; 2009.
261. Wang J, Lin X, Deng W, et al., eds. *Development of a Society on Wheels: Understanding the Rise of Automobile-dependency in China.* New York City, New York: Springer; 2019.
262. Stimpson JP, Wilson FA, Araz OM, Pagan JA. Share of mass transit miles traveled and reduced motor vehicle fatalities in major cities of the United States. *J Urban Health.* 2014;91(6):1136–43.
263. Yeo J, Park S, Jang K. Effects of urban sprawl and vehicle miles traveled on traffic fatalities. *Traffic Injury Prevention.* 2015;16(4):397–403.

264. Banwell N, Rutherford S, Mackey B, Street R, Chu C. Commonalities between disaster and climate change risks for health: A theoretical framework. *Int J Environ Res Public Health.* 2018;15(3):538.

265. Keim ME. Preventing disasters: Public health vulnerability reduction as a sustainable adaptation to climate change. *Disaster Med Public Health Prep.* 2011;5(2):140–8.

266. Banwell N, Rutherford S, Mackey B, Chu C. Towards improved linkage of disaster risk reduction and climate change adaptation in health: A review. *Int J Environ Res Public Health.* 2018;15(4):793.

267. Gamble JL, Hess JJ. Temperature and violent crime in Dallas, Texas: Relationships and implications of climate change. *West J Emerg Med.* 2012;13(3):239–46.

268. Schinasi LH, Hamra GB. A time series analysis of associations between daily temperature and crime events in Philadelphia, Pennsylvania. *J Urban Health.* 2017;94(6):892–900.

269. Anderson CA. Heat and violence. *Curr Dir Psychol Sci.* 2001;10(1):33–38.

270. McInnes JA, Akram M, MacFarlane EM, Keegel T, Sim MR, Smith P. Association between high ambient temperature and acute work-related injury: A case-crossover analysis using workers' compensation claims data. *Scand J Work Environ Health.* 2017;43(1):86–94.

271. Otte im Kampe E, Kovats S, Hajat S. Impact of high ambient temperature on unintentional injuries in high-income countries: A narrative systematic literature review. *BMJ Open.* 2016;6(2):e010399.

272. Gomez-Baggethun E, Corbera E, Reyes-Garcia V. Traditional ecological knowledge and global environmental change: Research findings and policy implications. *Ecol Soc.* 2013;18(4):72.

273. Finn S, Herne M, Castille D. The value of traditional ecological knowledge for the environmental health sciences and biomedical research. *Environ Health Perspect.* 2017;125(8):085006.

274. Bayles BR, Brauman KA, Adkins JN, et al. Ecosystem services connect environmental change to human health outcomes. *EcoHealth.* 2016;13(3):443–9.

275. Lindgren E, Elmqvist T. *Ecosystem Services and Human Health. Oxford Research Encyclopedia, Environmental Science.* Oxford and New York: Oxford University Press; 2017.

276. Ford AES, Graham H, White PCL. Integrating human and ecosystem health through ecosystem services frameworks. *EcoHealth.* 2015;12(4):660–71.

277. Chang KM, Hess JJ, Balbus JM, et al. Ancillary health effects of climate mitigation scenarios as drivers of policy uptake: A review of air quality, transportation and diet co-benefits modeling studies. *Environ Res Lett.* 2017;12(11):113001.

278. Gao J, Kovats S, Vardoulakis S, et al. Public health co-benefits of greenhouse gas emissions reduction: A systematic review. *Sci Total Environ.* 2018;627:388–402.

279. Brown LR, Larsen J, Roney JM, Adams EE. *The Great Transition: Shifting from Fossil Fuels to Solar and Wind Energy.* 1st ed. New York: W.W. Norton & Company; 2015.

280. Smil V. *Energy Transitions: Global and National Perspectives.* 2nd ed. Santa Barbara, CA: Praeger; 2017.

281. Pravalie R, Bandoc G. Nuclear energy: Between global electricity demand, worldwide decarbonisation imperativeness, and planetary environmental implications. *J Environ Manage.* 2018;209:81–92.

282. Morgan MG, Abdulla A, Ford MJ, Rath M. US nuclear power: The vanishing low-carbon wedge. *Proc Natl Acad Sci U S A.* 2018;115(28):7184–9.

283. Oreskes N, Conway EM. *Merchants of Doubt: How a Handful of Scientists Obscured the Truth on Issues from Tobacco Smoke to Global Warming.* New York: Bloomsbury; 2010.

284. Mulvey K, Shulman S. The Climate Deception Dossiers: Internal Fossil Fuel Industry Memos Reveal Decades of Corporate Disinformation. Union of Concerned Scientists; 2015.

285. Brulle RJ. The climate lobby: A sectoral analysis of lobbying spending on climate change in the USA, 2000 to 2016. *Clim Change.* 2018;149(3):289–303.

286. Delina LL. *Accelerating Sustainable Energy Transition(s) in Developing Countries: The Challenges of Climate Change and Sustainable Development.* Abingdon, Oxon and New York: Routledge; 2018.

287. Smith KR, Haigler E. Co-benefits of climate mitigation and health protection in energy systems: Scoping methods. *Annu Rev Public Health.* 2008;29(1):11–25.

288. Li M, Zhang D, Li C-T, Mulvaney KM, Selin NE, Karplus VJ. Air quality co-benefits of carbon pricing in China. *Nat Clim Change.* 2018;8(5): 398–403.

289. Markandya A, Armstrong BG, Hales S, et al. Public health benefits of strategies to reduce greenhouse-gas emissions: Low-carbon electricity generation. *Lancet.* 2009;374(9706):2006–15.

290. Markandya A, Sampedro J, Smith SJ, et al. Health co-benefits from air pollution and mitigation costs of the Paris Agreement: A modelling study. *Lancet Planetary Health.* 2018;2(3):e126–33.

291. Redlich CA, Sparer J, Cullen MR. Sick-building syndrome. *Lancet.* 1997;349(9057):1013–6.

292. Allen JG, MacNaughton P, Laurent JG, Flanigan SS, Eitland ES, Spengler JD. Green buildings and health. *Curr Environ Health Rep.* 2015;2(3): 250–8.

293. Burpee H, Beck DAC, Meschke JS. *Health Impacts of Green Buildings. The Value of Design: Design & Health*; April 22–24, 2014; Washignton, DC: American Institute of Architects; 2014.

294. Bonjour S, Adair-Rohani H, Wolf J, et al. Solid fuel use for household cooking: Country and regional estimates for 1980–2010. *Environ Health Perspect.* 2013;121(7):784–90.

295. Lim SS, Vos T, Flaxman AD, et al. A comparative risk assessment of burden of disease and injury attributable to 67 risk factors and risk factor clusters in 21 regions, 1990–2010: A systematic analysis for the Global Burden of Disease Study 2010. *Lancet.* 2012;380(9859):2224–60.

296. Rosenthal J. The real challenge for cookstoves and health: More evidence. *EcoHealth.* 2015;12(1):8–11.

297. Smith KR. Changing paradigms in clean cooking. *Ecohealth.* 2015;12(1):196–9.

298. Dannenberg AL, Frumkin H, Jackson R. *Making Healthy Places: Designing and Building for Health, Well-Being, and Sustainability.* Washington, DC: Island Press; 2011.

299. Knell G, Durand CP, Shuval K, et al. Transit use and physical activity: Findings from the Houston travel-related activity in neighborhoods (TRAIN) study. *Prev Med Rep.* 2018;9:55–61.

300. Saelens BE, Vernez Moudon A, Kang B, Hurvitz PM, Zhou C. Relation between higher physical activity and public transit use. *Am J Public Health.* 2014;104(5):854–9.

301. Hirsch JA, DeVries DN, Brauer M, Frank LD, Winters M. Impact of new rapid transit on physical activity: A meta-analysis. *Prev Med Rep.* 2018;10:184–90.

302. Pettigrew S. Why public health should embrace the autonomous car. *Aust N Z J Public Health.* 2016;41(1):5–7.

303. Sallis J. Driverless cars could be better or worse for our health—it's up to us 2018. Available from https://theconversation.com/driverless-cars-could-be-better-or-worse-for-our-health-its-up-to-us-87242.

304. Gawron JH, Keoleian GA, De Kleine RD, Wallington TJ, Kim HC. Life cycle assessment of connected and automated vehicles: Sensing and computing subsystem and vehicle level effects. *Environ Sci Technol.* 2018;52(5):3249–56.

305. Graf M. *Assessing the Impact of Ridesharing Services on Public Health and Safety Outcomes.* Milken Institute, CA; 2017.

306. Global Commission on the Economy and Climate. *Better Growth, Better Climate: The New Climate Economy Report.* Washington, DC: World Resources Institute; 2014.

307. Vermeulen SJ, Campbell BM, Ingram JSI. Climate change and food systems. *Annu Rev Environ Resour.* 2012;37(1):195–222.

308. Campbell BM, Beare DJ, Bennett EM, et al. Agriculture production as a major driver of the Earth system exceeding planetary boundaries. *Ecol Soc.* 2017;22(4):8.

309. Godfray HC, Beddington JR, Crute IR, et al. Food security: The challenge of feeding 9 billion people. *Science.* 2010;327(5967):812–8.

310. Gordon LJ, Bignet V, Crona B, et al. Rewiring food systems to enhance human health and biosphere stewardship. *Environ Res Lett.* 2017;12(10):100201.

311. Springmann M, Clark M, Mason-D'Croz D, et al. Options for keeping the food system within environmental limits. *Nature.* 2018;562(7728).

312. Willett W, Rockström J, Loken B, et al. Food in the Anthropocene: The EAT-Lancet Commission on healthy diets from sustainable food systems. *Lancet.* 2019;393(10170):447–92.

313. Cassidy ES, West PC, Gerber JS, Foley JA. Redefining agricultural yields: From tonnes to people nourished per hectare. *Environ Res Lett.* 2013;8(3):034015.

314. Tilman D, Balzer C, Hill J, Befort BL. Global food demand and the sustainable intensification of agriculture. *Proc Natl Acad Sci U S A.* 2011;108(50):20260–64.

315. Pretty J, Benton TG, Bharucha ZP, et al. Global assessment of agricultural system redesign for sustainable intensification. *Nat Sustain.* 2018;1(8):441–6.
316. Godfray HCJ, Aveyard P, Garnett T, et al. Meat consumption, health, and the environment. *Science.* 2018;361(6399):eaam5324.
317. Bessa LW, Pieterse E, Sigge G, Hoffman LC. Insects as human food; from farm to fork. *J Sci Food Agric.* 2020;100(14):5017–22.
318. Sun-Waterhouse D, Waterhouse GIN, You L, et al. Transforming insect biomass into consumer wellness foods: A review. *Food Res Int.* 2016;89(Pt 1):129–51.
319. Stephens N, Di Silvio L, Dunsford I, Ellis M, Glencross A, Sexton A. Bringing cultured meat to market: Technical, socio-political, and regulatory challenges in cellular agriculture. *Trends Food Sci Technol.* 2018;78:155–66.
320. Alexander P, Brown C, Arneth A, Finnigan J, Moran D, Rounsevell MDA. Losses, inefficiencies and waste in the global food system. *Agric Syst.* 2017;153:190–200.
321. Anastas PT, Warner JC. *Green Chemistry: Theory and Practice.* New York and Oxford: Oxford University Press; 1998.
322. Stahel WR. The circular economy. *Nature.* 2016;531(7595):435–8.
323. Braungart M, McDonough W. *Cradle to Cradle: Remaking the Way we Make Things.* 1st ed. New York: North Point Press; 2002.
324. Stahel WR. *The Performance Economy.* New York and Basingstoke, Hampshire, UK: Palgrave MacMillan; 2010.
325. Botsman R, Rogers R. *What's Mine Is Yours: The Rise of Collaborative Consumption.* New York: HarperCollins Business; 2010.
326. Jackson T. *Prosperity Without Growth: Foundations for the Economy of Tomorrow.* 2nd ed. London: Routledge; 2017.
327. Raworth K. *Doughnut Economics: Seven Ways to Think Like a 21st-Century Economist.* London: Random House; 2017.
328. Daly HE, Farley JC. *Ecological Economics: Principles and Applications.* 2nd ed. In: Farley JC, ed. Washington, DC: Island Press; 2011.
329. Costanza R, Cumberland JH, Daly H, Goodland R, Norgaard R, Kubiszewski I. *An Introduction to Ecological Economics.* 2nd ed. Boca Raton, FL: CRC Press; 2015.
330. Costanza R, Kubiszewski I, Giovannini E, et al. Time to leave GDP behind. *Nature.* 2014;505(7483):283–5.
331. Talberth J, Cobb C, Slattery N. *The Genuine Progress Indicator 2006: A Tool for Sustainable Development.* Oakland, CA: Redefining Progress; 2007.
332. Lim SS, Allen K, Bhutta ZA, et al. Measuring the health-related Sustainable Development Goals in 188 countries: A baseline analysis from the Global Burden of Disease Study 2015. *Lancet.* 2017;388(10053):1813–50.
333. DeSalvo KB, O'Carroll PW, Koo D, Auerbach JM, Monroe JA. Public Health 3.0: Time for an upgrade. *Am J Public Health.* 2016;106(4):621–2.
334. Manchanda R. The Upstream Doctors: TED Books; 2013.
335. Machalaba C, Romanelli C, Stoett P, et al. Climate change and health: Transcending silos to find solutions. *Ann Glob Health.* 2015;81(3): 445–58.

Note

*Figure 17-3 can be viewed by opening the table of contents of *Maxcy-Rosenau-Last Public Health & Preventive Medicine* at www.accessmedicine.com.

CHAPTER

18

Global Health Financing: Mechanisms, Trends, and Opportunities

Gavin Yamey • Ipchita Bharali • Sara Fewer • Naomi Beyeler • Jessica Kraus • Marco Schäferhoff • Agnes Soucat • Abdo Yazbeck • Dean Jamison

INTRODUCTION

Global health financing refers to how we generate, allocate, and use funds for health worldwide, from both domestic sources and external sources—including donor assistance for health. There is tremendous variation between countries in the ways in which the health sector is funded, and much debate on the best ways to finance health effectively, efficiently, and equitably. Nevertheless, the evidence points clearly to a number of bedrock principles that all countries must adopt if they are to ensure universal health coverage (UHC), defined as access to quality healthcare for all citizens when they need it without suffering financial hardship.

This chapter aims to capture these key principles as well as the major policy discussions and debates on health financing. While our focus is mostly on low-income countries (LICs) and middle-income countries (MICs), we also discuss lessons learned—both positive and negative—from health financing in high-income countries (HICs).

Why should global health practitioners pay attention to issues of financing? We argue in this chapter that financing matters to global health practice because:

- The uneven distribution of health spending and the low levels of spending in the poorest countries with greatest health needs are an ongoing barrier to global health improvement.[1]
- It will be extremely difficult for LICs and MICs to achieve the health-related Sustainable Development Goals (SDGs) unless they mobilize additional financing for their health sectors.[2]
- Every year, 150 million people worldwide face catastrophic health expenditures—an expenditure of more than 40% of nonfood household expenditure or 10% of overall household expenditure—because they pay for health services.[3] Such impoverishment further increases their vulnerability to ill health.
- Underspending on health is compounded by inefficiency and waste—about 20–40% of all health spending is wasted.[4]
- There is a growing body of evidence suggesting that aid for health has helped to reduce mortality in LICs and MICs. However, it has also had unintended consequences (e.g., governments of LICs and MICs tend to respond to health aid by reducing their own domestic funding of health), levels have stagnated in recent years, many MICs are transitioning away from health aid, and the future of such aid is the subject of much debate.[5]
- HICs and some MICs are facing rapidly rising health costs and unproductive cost escalation, i.e., escalating costs that are not linked to improved healt.h.[6]

This chapter is divided into four sections. In section "The Global Health Financing Landscape," we examine **the status of global health financing**: funding levels, variations in spending between countries, sources of funding, and the size of the global health financing gap. In section "The Role of Health Aid," we look at **the role of health aid**, also known as development assistance for health (DAH), including aid sources and flows, key financing institutions, the impact of DAH on health, and the future of DAH. In section "Domestic Health Financing and Resource Mobilization," we focus on the most important source of health financing: **domestic resources**. We describe the three key roles of governments in health financing—revenue collection, pooling and prepayment, and purchasing—and the linkages between financing, UHC, and health systems strengthening (HSS). We lay out a number of pathways that countries can take to achieve "pro-poor" UHC. Finally, in section "Conclusions: Challenges and Opportunities," we end this chapter by considering **future opportunities and challenges** in the landscape of global health financing. Throughout the chapter, we use case studies to illustrate the issues.

The Global Health Financing Landscape

This section starts (in section "Global Spending on Health") with a data-rich snapshot of the current overall status of global health spending and a brief summary of past and future trends as well as variations across countries. Next, section "Sources of Health Financing" takes a deeper dive into sources of health financing and how they evolve as the development level of countries changes. Finally, section "The Global Health Financing Gap" explores the projected global health financing gap and sets the scene for the sections that follow.

Global Spending on Health

In 2014, according to its Global Health Expenditure Database, the World Health Organization (WHO) estimated that the world spent $7,331,309 million on health which, given the estimated global population size, is equivalent to $1064 per person.[7] Those two numbers, however, hide a staggering gap between what rich and poor countries spend on health. In 2014, countries that belong to the Organisation for Economic Co-operation and Development (OECD), an intergovernmental organization of industrialized and economically developed countries that aims to foster policies to stimulate economic growth, spent $5,906,831 million (over 80% of global health spending) which amounted to $4311 per person. These numbers contrast sharply with health spending in sub-Saharan Africa (SSA) in the same year, which totaled $90,830 million or $110 per person. Figure 18-1 shows the large variations in health spending between countries using the share of the economy allocated to health expenditures. However, this figure arguably hides the real size of the gap. LICs have a smaller sized economy—so spending a smaller percentage of a smaller economy means the absolute amount of spending is *much* lower in LICs than in HICs.

The gap in total and per person spending between developed and developing countries, illustrated above by the numbers for OECD nations and countries in SSA, has implications in obvious and less obvious ways. Clearly, poorer countries, which we know have poorer health outcomes and therefore greater need for healthcare services, are spending far less than wealthier countries where people live longer

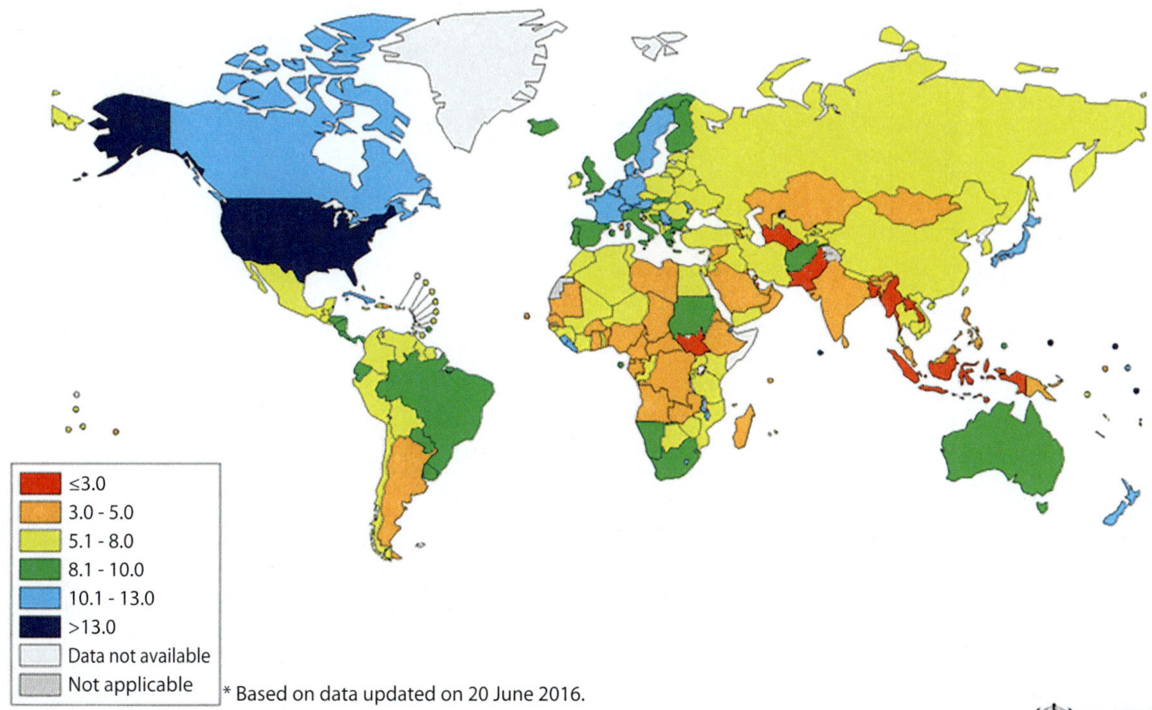
Total expenditure on health
as a percentage of the gross domestic product, 2014*
≤3.0
3.0 - 5.0
5.1 - 8.0
8.1 - 10.0
10.1 - 13.0
>13.0
Data not available
Not applicable
* Based on data updated on 20 June 2016.
The boundaries and names shown and the designations used on this map do not imply the expression of any opinion whatsoever on the part of the World Health Organization concerning the legal status of any country, territory, city or area or of its authorities, or concerning the delimitation of its frontiers or boundaries. Dotted and dashed lines on maps represent approximate border lines for which there may not yet be full agreement.
Data Source: Global Health Obervatory, WHO
Map Production: Information Evidence and Research (IER)
World Health Organization

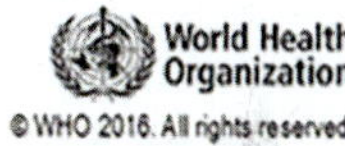
World Health
Organization

FIGURE 18-1. Total expenditure on health as a percentage of gross domestic product (GDP), 2014. (*Source:* Used with Permission from Total expenditure on health as a percentage of gross domestic product. WHO. https://www.who.int/data/gho/data/indicators/indicator-details/GHO/total-expenditure-on-health-as-a-percentage-of-gross-domestic-product.)

and suffer less. Less obvious is that the substantial difference in total spending across HICs and LICs means that health-related research, development of medicines, and development of medical equipment are much more likely to focus on the needs of populations in the better-off countries.[8] Most medical research is influenced by commercial entities, so it is not surprising that they respond more aggressively to demand being generated by wealthier countries. Absent global governance interventions, there are no obvious economic incentives for drug and equipment manufacturers to target research or innovation to the needs of poorer nations.

What Fig. 18-1 shows clearly is that there is a strong association between the income level of nations and their levels of health spending. As national income increases, so does health spending, but unlike most other sectors, health spending appears to grow faster than the economy. Figure 18-2 shows this strong association for OECD countries; it shows that (a) the proportion of national income spent on health goes up with rising income and (b) at any given level of income, that proportion goes up with time (reflecting aging populations and new, costlier health technologies).[9] Research by the International Monetary Fund (IMF) on health expenditures relative to the economy from 1970 to 2008 for two clusters of country, advanced (HICs) and emerging (upper MICs), found clear patterns over time.[10] First, the overall share of health spending relative to the economy grew from 6% in 1970 to over 12% in advanced countries. In emerging countries, it grew from 3% to 5% of the economy in the same time period (1970–2008). In both sets of countries, health spending outgrew the economy. When the data were segmented by public versus private for advanced countries, public spending on health grew faster than private spending on health. This trend implies that populations not only demanded more healthcare as wealth increased, but that they appear to put pressure on governments successfully to increase public spending on health.

Sources of Health Financing

As seen in section "Global Spending on Health" in the IMF's analysis of health finance in advanced and emerging countries, one way to categorize health spending is to simply identify the sources as public or private. Under each of these categories, however, there are different mechanisms for collecting and organizing financing for healthcare. The OECD publishes annual updates on sources of financing for member countries,[11] and identifies four dominant sources.

The first, which typically accounts for over 37% of all health spending in OECD countries, is **general government**, which refers to government-collected revenues or taxes that are not earmarked to a specific sector but in this case provided for healthcare services. The second source, typical accounting for around 35% of all health spending in OECD countries, is funding generated through **employment taxes**, sometimes referred to as social security or social health insurance. The third source, averaging about 20% in OECD countries, is **private out-of-pocket (OOP) spending**, usually paid at the point of contact with health facilities or providers. The fourth and smallest share in OECD nations is funding for healthcare from **private health insurance** arrangements.

Figure 18-3 captures this breakdown by source of financing in all OECD countries. While the data are for 2013 or the nearest year, most years show similar breakdowns (since the overall sources of national health financing do not tend to change quickly in a drastic way). Changes require major reforms that typically take many years to implement. A number of lessons emerge from Fig. 18-3 that provide instructive lessons for developing countries exploring reforms to how they finance healthcare.

First, the wide variations across the OECD countries reflect the reality that there are no globally agreed best practice ways for generating resources for the health sector. The historical reasons for why different countries pursued different ways of financing tend not to

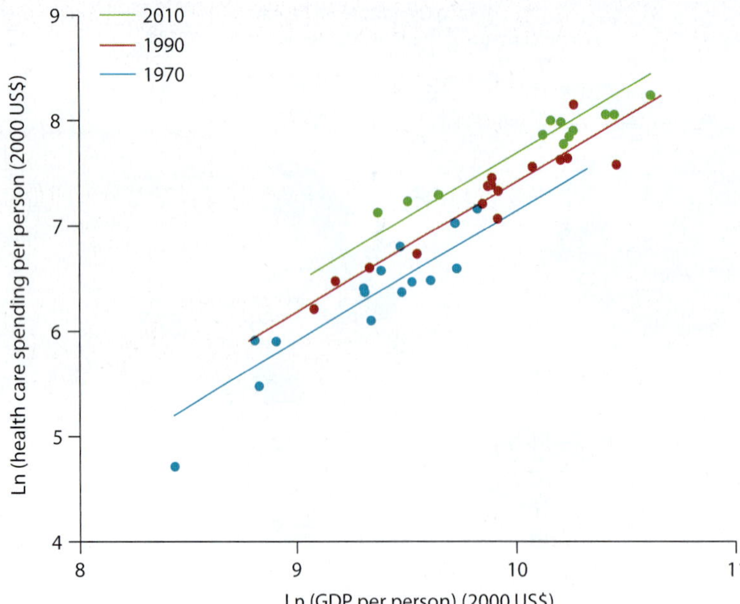

FIGURE 18-2. Relation between income and health spending. This figure presents natural logarithms of GDP per person and healthcare spending per person. (Abbreviation: Ln = logarithm.) (*Source:* Reproduced with Permission from Summers LH, Jamison DT, Alleyne G, et al. Global health 2035: a world converging in a generation. *Lancet* 2013; 382:1898–955.[9])

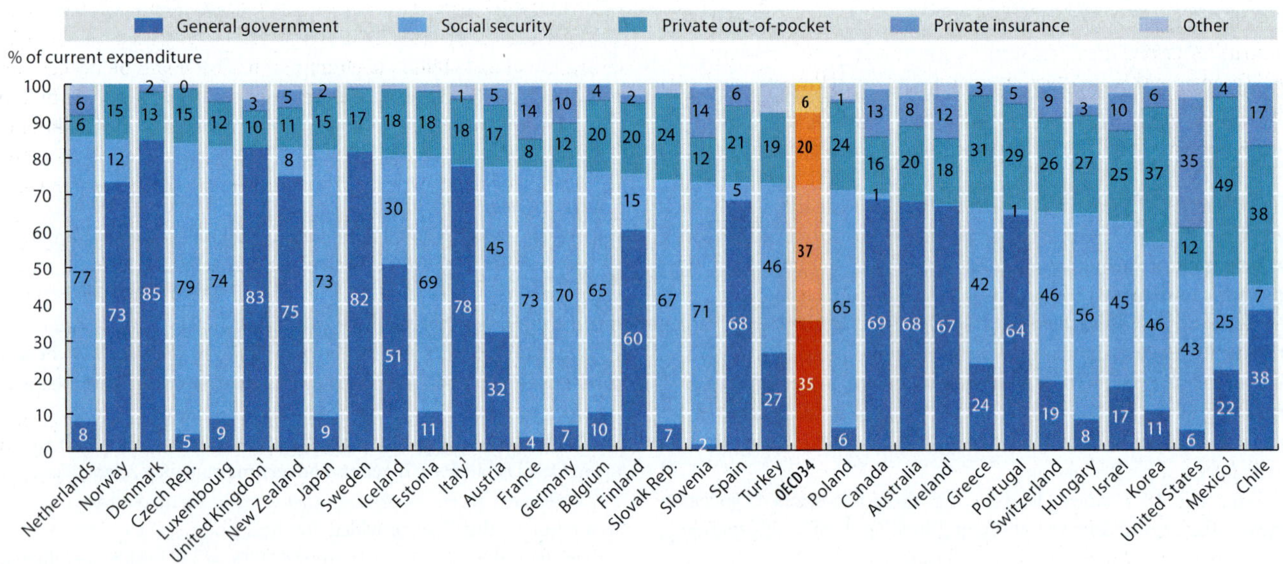

FIGURE 18-3. Sources of financing for health in OECD nations, 2013 or nearest year. (*Source*: Used with Permission from Organisation for Economic Co-operation and Development. OECD.Stat. http://stats.oecd.org/Index.aspx?DataSetCode=SHA.11 *OECD34: average across the 34 OECD nations.*)

be directly related to analysis of efficiency but more likely the results of historic accidents or factors outside the health sector. Second, no country has a "pure" financing model based on a single source of financing. All health sectors have mixed healthcare financing models, though each tends to rely more heavily on one source than the others. Third, the share of private OOP spending appears to be higher for the most recent entrants to the OECD, reflecting a relationship we explore next.

It has been observed empirically for many years that as countries develop—i.e., grow economically—not only does spending on healthcare grow but the composition of the sources of financing changes as well. Table 18-1, created from data in the World Development Indicators database,[11] captures the directionality and patterns of changes along the development spectrum. The table shows standardized measures of health spending, including the share of gross domestic product (GDP) spent on health, total health spending, as well as shares of spending by source of financing.

Three dominant patterns can be seen in Table 18-1. First, it is only LICs that have a significant share of health spending (about a third of all spending) from external sources. That is certainly by design, as donors target their aid to the health sector to countries least able to tackle health needs. Second, the relative share of spending that is private OOP decreases as countries develop. Private OOP spending is regressive, inefficient, and inequitable so policy efforts

TABLE 18-1 COMPOSITION OF HEALTH FINANCING BY INCOME LEVEL, 2014

	HICs	Upper MICs	Lower MICs	LICs
Health expenditure per capita (current U.S.$)	5,266	518.5	92	36.9
Health expenditure, total (% of GDP)	12.3	6.2	4.5	5.7
Health expenditure, public (% of GDP)	7.7	3.4	1.7	2.4
Health expenditure, private (% of GDP)	4.6	2.7	2.8	3.3
Health expenditure, public (% of government expenditure)	17.3	Insufficient data	Insufficient data	Insufficient data
Health expenditure, public (% of total health expenditure)	62.3	55	37.1	42.4
Out-of-pocket health expenditure (% of total expenditure on health)	13.3	32.4	54.9	37.2
Out-of-pocket health expenditure (% of private expenditure on health)	35.4	71.9	87.3	64.5
External resources for health (% of total expenditure on health)	0	0.2%	3.3	33.2

Source: Data from World Bank. World Development Indicators. https://data.worldbank.org/products/wdi.[12]

are always attempting to decrease such spending relative to more efficient sources.[13] Third, as countries develop, government spending on health increases, first by replacing development assistance, then it keeps increasing and replaces some private OOP spending.

The Global Health Financing Gap

In the previous sections, we have discussed how much the world is spending on health and the variations in spending between different countries. A critical next question is: how much *should* it be spending? To answer this question, we must first state the end goal—in other words, if financing is to be increased, what is the ultimate aim?

The Lancet Commission on Investing in Health, an international commission of global health and economics experts, estimated the funding needs to achieve what it called a "grand convergence" in global health.[9] In the Commission's 2013 report, called *Global Health 2035: a world converging within a generation*, the authors defined grand convergence as a universal reduction in deaths from infections [including HIV, tuberculosis (TB), and malaria] and maternal and child health conditions, down to the levels seen today in the best performing MICs (such as China and Costa Rica). Achieving grand convergence by 2035 would be feasible, they found, through aggressive scale up of today's health technologies, strengthening of health systems, and continued development and deployment of new technologies. The estimated cost would be an additional U.S.$70 billion per year, of which about U.S.$45 billion is needed annually in lower MICs and U.S.$25 billion is needed annually in LICs.

This increase would represent a doubling of current funding levels across LICs as a group, and a roughly 20% increase across lower MICs. At the time that the commission published its report in 2013, LICs and lower MICs were on course to add about $10 trillion/year to their annual GDP. If LICs and lower MICs were to devote 1–3% of this growth to health investments, most of the grand convergence could be funded from domestic spending, though the poorest LICs would still require external assistance (DAH).

Going beyond infections and maternal and health conditions alone, Stenberg and colleagues recently estimated the financing gap to strengthen comprehensive service delivery to achieve *all* of the targets in SDG3,[2] the goal to ensure "healthy lives and promote well-being for all at all ages."[14] The target includes reaching "universal health coverage, including financial risk protection, access to quality essential healthcare services and access to safe, effective, quality, and affordable essential medicines and vaccines for all." Stenberg and colleagues developed cost projections for 67 LICs and MICs from 2016 to 2030 that make up 95% of the total population of all LICs and MICs. They modeled two scenarios. The first is what they call a "progress scenario," in which countries advance toward the SDG3 health targets only as much as their health systems capacity allows for, and the second is an "ambitious scenario," in which almost all countries achieve all targets.

Not surprisingly, the researchers find that the financing needed to achieve all SDG 3 targets would be much greater than that needed to reach grand convergence alone. Under the progress scenario, by 2030 an additional $274 billion spending on health would be needed per year, and under the ambitious scenario an additional U.S.$371 billion would be needed annually. About three-quarters of the additional financing would need to go to HSS. Stenberg and colleagues argue that MICs are well equipped to finance the additional investment and so "the financing gap is mostly in low-income countries." Clearly, the lowest income countries will continue to need DAH throughout the SDGs period, especially for HSS, but even in LICs, the authors argue that governments themselves can still fund a universal package of basic services.

In October 2018, The Lancet Commission on Investing in Health revisited its initial *Global Health 2035* report, publishing a new analysis that examined recent progress in global health and projected health and demographic trends to 2035.[15] Three particular findings of this analysis have important implications for global health financing:

- First, recent progress on global TB control has been very disappointing, and a grand convergence on TB will be impossible without a sharp increase in financing for TB control programs and for TB product development. Breakthrough TB technologies will be needed to bend the mortality curve downward. The analysis argued that: "increasing national resources devoted to TB treatment by a factor of 2–3 could help to change the trajectory of TB mortality in countries where the disease remains most important."[15]
- Second, there is a similarly bleak finding when it comes to global noncommunicable disease (NCD) control. For a number of conditions, such as ischemic heart disease, a grand *divergence* in mortality is taking place—some regions of the world are experiencing large rates of decline but other regions experiencing flat or even increasing rates. The prospects for achieving the SDG 3 target on NCDs (a reduction in premature mortality by one third by 2030) seem bleak, says the Commission, unless there are "massive new investments to expand intervention access and improve quality."[15]
- Third, rapidly changing demography will continue to place rising demands on health systems, with enormous implications for health financing—in other words, demography is (financial) destiny. The

Commission argued that most LICs and MICs are facing "historically unprecedented rates of population aging and yet have had neither time nor resources to adapt in the way that HICs have."[15]

The Role of Health Aid

Although progress in improving health in LICs and MICs in the SDGs era will depend heavily on domestic resource mobilization (DRM) by these countries themselves, health aid will continue to play a role—albeit an evolving one. In this section, we explore the nature of the health aid enterprise. We begin, in section "How Health Aid Is Defined," by defining what we mean by health aid. We then examine where such aid comes from and where it flows to (Sources and Flows of Health Aid), then we take a "deep dive" look at the largest, most important global health financing institutions (Key Global Health Financing Institutions). Next, we summarize key evidence on whether health aid "works" and discuss its potential negative and unintended consequences (The Impacts of Health Aid). Finally, we end this section by contemplating the future directions for health aid.

How Health Aid Is Defined

"Health aid," or DAH, is defined as resources that are invested by donors and international agencies with the primary purpose of maintaining or improving health in LICs and MICs.[16] A particularly important category of health aid is official development assistance (ODA) for health, which refers to the official and concessional part of health aid that is supported by public investments.[17] ODA for health does not include private or philanthropic investments (e.g., from the Bill & Melinda Gates Foundation), financing that is less concessional (e.g., financing that is largely given as a loan), resources from donors that do not report to the OECD's financial information system (e.g., health aid from China), or aid to other sectors that deliver health benefits more directly (e.g., water and sanitation or education).

Aid flows for health are unique in that they are used for purposes beyond a funder's borders for countries that have worse economic protection from healthcare costs.[18] Public support for such financing for health, however, is mixed: only about half of the U.S. public says the nation should take a leading or major role in improving the health of people in developing countries.[19]

Sources and Flows of Health Aid

Today's health aid architecture began to take shape after World War II, when international agencies were created at scale to promote social progress and economic growth.[20] With the end of European colonialism, what was known as "tropical medicine" became recognized as "international health," and new international agencies were created that focused on health (Fig. 18-4).[21] The term "global health" is now being used more frequently than "international health" to refer to the work of the health aid community and broader health enterprise (including actions taken by LIC and MIC governments).[22] Global health is a relatively new term that captures the trans-national, multidisciplinary approach to health improvement through tackling challenges that go beyond the boundaries of individual nation states.

Today, global health is one of the largest social sectors of foreign development aid. Following a period of moderate growth and expansion in the 1990s, DAH increased dramatically at the turn of the century.[23] In 2017, $37.4 billion in health aid was disbursed, three times greater than in 2000 and accounting for 22.7% of total health spending in LICs.[23] DAH, however, has remained relatively flat since 2010.[23]

The rise in global health aid between 2000 and 2010, often called the "golden age" or "golden decade" for health aid, corresponded to the launch of the Millennium Development Goals (MDGs). Health was the direct focus of three of the eight MDGs: to reduce child mortality (MDG 4), improve maternal health (MDG 5), and combat HIV/AIDS, malaria and other diseases (MDG 6). A new set of goals, the SDGs, are defining global health priorities and agendas for the 2015–30 period. The SDGs focus on equity (the SDG mantra is "leave no one behind) and, unlike the MDGs, they aim to be relevant to all countries, not only developing countries. One of the goals, SDG 3, focuses directly on health: "ensure healthy lives and promoting well-being for all at all ages." It is estimated that 97 million premature deaths globally could be prevented between now and 2030 if countries expanded health services to reach the SDGs.[2]

Who Are the Major Donors? Health aid is provided through three major sources: national treasuries, private philanthropies, and as debt repayments to international financial institutions.[23] Nearly half of all health ODA is provided by the United States[24]; other major public donors are the United Kingdom and Germany (Fig. 18-5).[23] The Bill & Melinda Gates Foundation is by far the largest single source of private health funding, contributing U.S.$3.3 billion for health in 2017.[23]

Political changes often bring about fluctuations in global health investments. In Australia, for example, the ODA budget became one of the biggest sources of savings to meet austerity measures, leading to declines in health aid.[25] The United States increased its spending on health aid during the tenure of both President George W. Bush and President Barack Obama.[24] Although President Donald Trump's administration proposed large cuts, a bipartisan Congress rejected his proposal and kept U.S. funding for global health mostly intact.[24] Germany, on the other hand, is one of the few countries expected to increase its funding for development and expand its engagement for global health.[26]

Which Health Conditions Receive the Most Aid? Given limited donor financing relative to unmet global health needs, there is much debate on how effective and strategic the current donor investments are, and how and whether DAH can be used more effectively and efficiently (we return to this debate in section "The Impacts of Health Aid"). Donors differ tremendously in terms of the health issues that they support, which channels they use, and to which countries they give health aid.

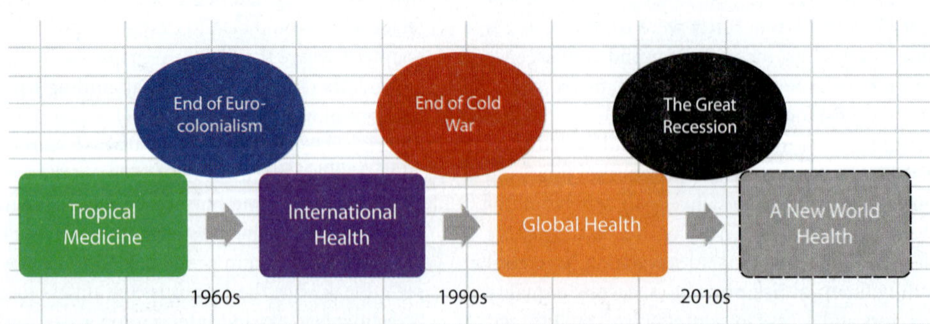

FIGURE 18-4. A historical snapshot of health aid. (Source: From Kharas H. 2009. Development Assistance in the 21st Century, Wolfensohn Center for Development at Brookings, Contribution to the VIII Salamanca Forum, The Fight Against Hunger and Poverty, July 2–4, 2009. https://www.brookings.edu/research/development-assistance-in-the-21st-century/.[21])

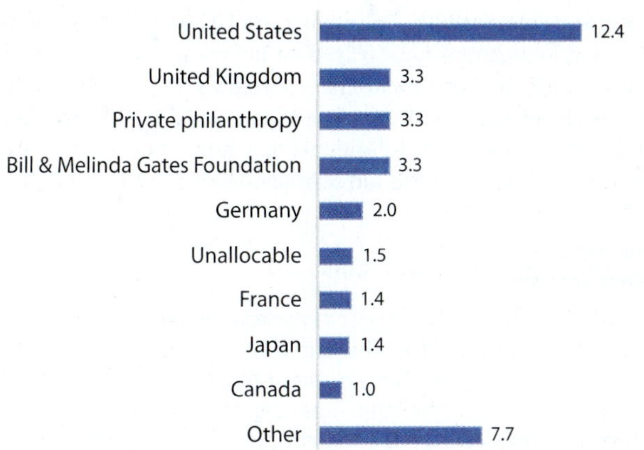

FIGURE 18-5. Amount of DAH (U.S.$ billions) by donor, 2017. (Data for this figure were taken from Institute for Health Metrics and Evaluation (IHME). Financing Global Health 2017: Funding Universal Health Coverage and the Unfinished HIV/AIDS Agenda. Seattle, WA: IHME, 2018.[23])

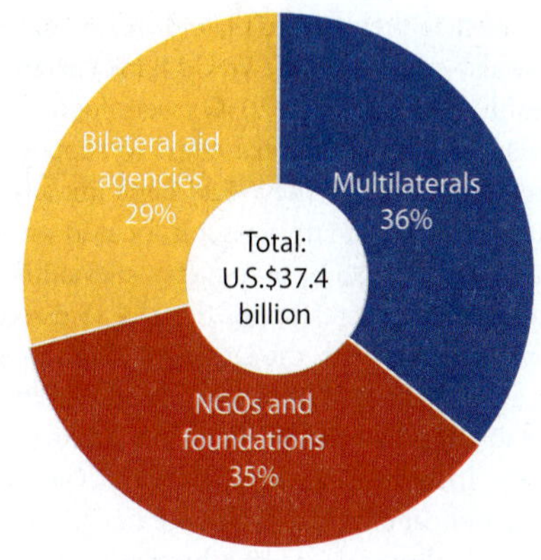

FIGURE 18-6. Global health donor financing across major delivery channels, 2017. (Data for this figure are from Institute for Health Metrics and Evaluation (IHME). Financing Global Health 2017: Funding Universal Health Coverage and the Unfinished HIV/AIDS Agenda. Seattle, WA: IHME, 2018.[23])

Donors largely target their investments to specific health areas that they believe are the most important. During the early 2000s, DAH became increasingly targeted toward the health areas related to MDGs 4–6 (child health, maternal mortality, HIV/AIDS, TB, and malaria).[27] Preliminary data from the Institute for Health Metrics and Evaluation (IHME), a research institute at the University of Washington that produces an annual report on health aid flows, show that in 2017, 31% of DAH went to maternal, newborn, and child health, 24.2% to HIV/AIDS, 7.1% to malaria, and 4.6% to TB.[23]

There are many important factors that should determine the volume of health aid that targets a particular disease, including the proven effectiveness of external assistance in tackling that disease, the comparative advantage of using external versus domestic finance, and the transnational nature of the disease. The burden of disease has not been a major determinant of today's investment decisions by the major donors. For example, NCDs accounted for more than 72.3% of deaths in 2016, but received 2.2% of all health aid.[23] We would argue that aid should be targeted based on its effectiveness, rather than simply being proportional to disease burden. Polio receives the most relative to its burden (U.S.$2454 per disability-adjusted live year, or DALY) and acute respiratory infections receive the least (U.S.$0.58 per DALY).[28] Political scientists such as Jeremy Shiffman have argued that donor investment decisions in global health are closely related to political factors, such as the strength of key actors involved; the power of the ideas they use to frame and portray the issue; and the nature of the political contexts in which they operate.[29]

To Which Channels Does Health Aid Flow? A channel refers to the intermediaries in the flow of funds between donors and recipient countries. Channels include bilateral aid agencies, multilateral organizations, nongovernmental organizations (NGOs), United Nations (UN) agencies, public-private partnerships, and private foundations. In this chapter, we refer to three major channels (i) multilateral aid agencies, (ii) NGOs and foundations, and (iii) bilateral aid agencies (Fig. 18-6). Donor governments largely invest their funds either through bilateral or multilateral aid agencies. NGOs and foundations channel resources mostly from private sources.

Multilateral aid agencies—including UN agencies [e.g., the Joint United Nations Programme on HIV/AIDS (UNAIDS)] and public-private partnerships (e.g., Gavi, the Vaccine Alliance)—pool together resources across donors and disburse them as part of an overall budget of the multilateral organization.[30] In contrast, bilateral aid agencies fund individual countries directly ("bilaterally"); these agencies are often located within ministries of foreign affairs of donor governments.[31] Donors can also provide support to multilaterals that is dedicated to a specific sector or program. This is known as "earmarked" funding to multilaterals and it accounts for 15% of all "bilateral" financing reported here. As shown in Fig. 18-6, overall, about two-thirds of health aid is provided bilaterally or through NGOs and foundations, and about one-third of health aid is provided multilaterally.[23,32]

Financing is ultimately provided to an implementing institution. Major implementing institutions include national ministries of health, national and international NGOs, private sector contractors, and research institutions.[23] Contextual factors and health program objectives often influence which institutions deliver support. Health aid shifted, for example, from NGOs to national ministries once East Timor showed that it had rebuilt its national capacity to manage a district health system.[33] Donors who wish to invest in the development of new health products have also directly supported the launch of several global health partnerships, such as product development partnerships.[34]

To Which Countries and Regions Does Health Aid Flow? Four-fifths of the world's population lives in a country that is eligible to receive health aid (based on data from the World Bank and IHME). Donors differ widely on where they spend their resources. Many donors have a set of priority countries. For example, the Global Fund to Fight AIDS, Tuberculosis and Malaria (the Global Fund) uses a funding allocation methodology that emphasizes higher-burden, LICs.[35] To give another example, Australia focuses its health financing on Southeast Asia and the Pacific, which aligns with the government's overall aid strategy to focus on neighboring, MICs.[25]

Collectively, most financing investments are provided to SSA (32.9%), followed by South Asia (5.0%). The countries in SSA that receive the largest amounts of DAH are Nigeria, Tanzania, Kenya, and Mozambique. The most populous countries in South Asia—India and Pakistan—also receive the most donor financing for health. However, several countries, known as "aid orphans," such as Cameroon, Guinea, and Nigeria, receive very little financing compared to their size, wealth level, and health burden.[36]

Key Global Health Financing Institutions

Multilateral Agencies Multilateral agencies—such as the UN agencies, public-private partnerships, and the multilateral development banks—play a key role in providing strategic guidance, technical support, and funding to health programs and systems around the world. Each multilateral agency has a unique membership and governance structure that represents multiple countries and stakeholders. As a result, these agencies are able to act with a united agenda and pool funding from multiple sources, helping to increase coordination, efficiency, technical specialization, and political and policy support in global health. Such multilateral funds have been shown to be cost-effective (e.g., in supporting global vaccination[37]) and have contributed to saving millions of lives.[38]

Two of the most influential multilateral financing institutions in global health are also the oldest. The World Bank Group (World Bank) and World Health Organization (WHO) were founded in 1944 and 1948, respectively, as part of a global effort to support international cooperation and development. The World Bank initially helped countries rebuild after World War II, but soon focused on infrastructure development and, by the 1960s, on poverty alleviation.[39] The WHO was established during the creation of the UN to direct and coordinate international health. With the launch of the MDGs at the turn of the century, a dynamic, new set of multilateral health agencies was established, notably Gavi and the Global Fund, founded in 2000 and 2002, respectively. Today, the World Bank, WHO, Gavi and the Global Fund lead, partner on, and fund a number of initiatives to advance the SDGs health agenda. Boxes 18-1–18-4 briefly describe each of these four multilateral agencies and their health foci. Figure 18-7 shows the financial contribution that each of them made to health in 2017.

BOX 18-1 The Global Fund to Fight AIDS, Tuberculosis, and Malaria

The Global Fund is a partnership of governments, the private sector, and civil society that provides financial support to HIV, TB, and malaria programs around the world. It is the largest financing institution in global health, investing a total of $32.6 billion from 2002 to 2016.[40] It has raised about 95% of its funds from over 60 country governments, with additional support from foundations, private companies, and innovative financing mechanisms.[41] Donors continue to show their strong support, pledging $12.9 billion for the 2017–19 period during the Fifth Replenishment Conference in Montreal. The Global Fund aims to maximize impact against HIV, TB and malaria, build resilient and sustainable systems for health, promote and protect human rights and gender equality, and mobilize increased resources to scale-up the response across all three diseases. It administers grants through the principles of partnership, country-ownership, performance-based financing, and transparency.

BOX 18-2 The World Health Organization

The WHO provides the largest amount of global health support of all UN agencies, and it functions as the premier agency for leading and stewarding the global health system. It is governed by the World Health Assembly, which consists of delegations from 194 WHO Member States. The WHO facilitates partnerships and global health action; shapes the global health research agenda; sets norms, standards, and policy guidelines that are adopted and implemented worldwide; provides technical support to countries; and monitors global health.[42] In its early years, the WHO conducted mass campaigns against TB, malaria, smallpox, polio, and other communicable diseases.[43] Today, the WHO oversees an expanded portfolio, working with countries to (i) prevent, treat, and care for communicable diseases, (ii) strengthen health systems to achieve UHC, (iii) coordinate a multisector response to NCDs, (iv) address environmental and social determinants of health, and (v) prepare and respond to health emergencies.[42] In recent years, an increasing share of the WHO's funding has been earmarked for special projects,[44] while its core funding in real terms has been in decline. As a result, the WHO's budget is highly constrained and key programs face serious funding challenges. For example, in 2016, the WHO set up a contingency fund for health emergencies in the aftermath of the Ebola outbreak in West Africa, but the fund has fallen very short in reaching its $100 million funding target.[45]

NGOs and Foundations In recent years, NGOs, private philanthropies, and foundations have played an increasing role in channeling global health support. Preliminary estimates suggest that in 2017, **NGOs** channeled $10.6B in support for global health, accounting for about 28% of all DAH disbursed that year.[23] NGOs play a role in both channeling assistance and as implementing institutions. IHME's

BOX 18-3 The World Bank

The World Bank is the largest of the four major multilateral development banks—the other three, all regional development banks, are the African Development Bank, the Asian Development Bank, and the Inter-American Development Bank. The World Bank works to end extreme poverty by 2030 and promote prosperity of the poorest people in every country.[46] It consists of 189 member countries that govern the agency through a Board of Governors and four Boards of Executive Directors.[47] The World Bank provides low-interest loans, zero to low-interest credits, and grants to developing countries to support investments in health and across the development sector. One of the World Bank's comparative advantages is that it works closely with ministries of finance and supports cross-cutting health reforms that are not disease specific, such as HSS.[48] Its specialized staff also provide technical assistance, research, and policy support to countries. The World Bank's leadership in health includes supporting countries to achieve UHC and investing to improve the health of children, adolescent girls, and women.[49] For example, the World Bank hosts the Global Financing Facility, a financing mechanism that supports countries in improving the health and well-being of women, children, and adolescents.[50] The regional development banks also provide financial assistance for health initiatives, typically directly to countries in the form of loans and grants.[51]

BOX 18-4 Gavi, the Vaccine Alliance

Gavi is a public–private partnership that brings together governments, private foundations, UN agencies, the pharmaceutical industry, civil society, and research agencies to increase access to life-saving vaccines for children in lower-income countries.[52] Its strategic goals are to accelerate uptake and coverage of vaccines, strengthen health systems, improve national immunization programs, and ensure quality immunization products at an affordable price.[53] Gavi has transformed the market for vaccines through market shaping, pooling demand from countries, and guaranteeing long-term funding through country co-financing and donor financing mechanisms.[52,53] Through these efforts, for example, Gavi was able to greatly reduce the price of the new pentavalent vaccine (DTP-HepB-Hib). It has developed innovative financing mechanisms, such as the International Finance Facility for Immunization, which uses pledges from donor governments to sell bonds in the capital markets, and the Advance Market Commitment, which leverages committed donor funds to incentivize vaccine development and ensure affordable prices.[54] From 2000 to 2016, Gavi raised a total of $13.9 billion.[55] Gavi also provides technical assistance and grants to countries to fund health system strengthening, vaccine programs, and the immunization supply chain.

Other important UN agencies that provide health support are (from largest to smallest, in terms of their DAH contributions): the UN Children's Fund (UNICEF), the UN Population Fund (UNFPA), the Joint UN Programme on HIV/AIDS (UNAIDS), the Pan American Health Organization (PAHO), and Unitaid.[23]

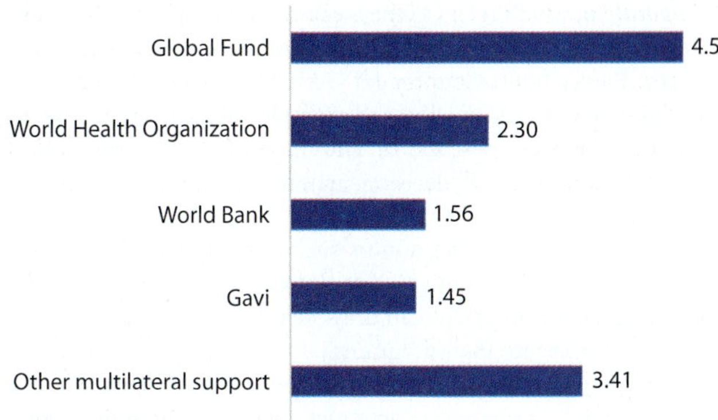

FIGURE 18-7. Multilateral support for global health, US$ billions, 2017. (*Source:* From Institute for Health Metrics and Evaluation (IHME). Financing Global Health 2017: Funding Universal Health Coverage and the Unfinished HIV/AIDS Agenda. Seattle, WA: IHME, 2018.[23])

analysis found that the most important U.S. NGOs for disbursing DAH in 2017 included Management Sciences for Health, Population Services International, and World Vision, Inc.[23] In 2017, the **Bill and Melinda Gates Foundation** provided $3.3B in DAH.[23] The Gates Foundation's funding priorities in global health include newborn and child health, maternal health, family planning, TB, malaria, HIV/AIDS, polio eradication, and HSS.[56] The foundation makes substantial investments in research and development of new vaccines, tools, and diagnostics, and more than half of the foundation's contributions are directed toward multilateral organizations, such as the Global Fund and Gavi. **Bloomberg Philanthropies** is another private foundation with a strong global health focus, and its investments include polio eradication, family planning, maternal health, road traffic injury prevention, tobacco control, and obesity prevention.[57] **The Wellcome Trust** is a U.K.-based charitable foundation that advances science and health research in global health, including by funding development of new vaccines, drugs, and diagnostics as well as biomedical, population health, the impact of environmental change on health, and social science research.[58]

Bilateral Health Agencies As previously mentioned, bilateral funding in global health is direct support from donor governments to recipient countries, typically those that are low- and middle-income. Preliminary estimates suggest that in 2017, the top five bilateral donors to global health were the United States ($5.7B), Germany ($0.9B), the United Kingdom ($0.8B), the European Commission ($0.7B), and Japan ($0.6B).[23] Bilateral donors each have national priorities and strategies in global health, sometimes operating sizeable health programs in recipient countries, delivering health services, providing technical support to health offices, and leading health research. Distinct from multilateral funding agencies, whose principal goal is to achieve stated health objectives, bilateral funding agencies often use DAH to promote multiple objectives, such as improving health outcomes in recipient countries, supporting global development goals, advancing national foreign policy priorities, and pursuing a national security agenda. Below, we briefly describe U.S. bilateral assistance, DAH from other OECD nations, and the role of emerging bilateral donors such as China:

- **The United States government**: three agencies primarily oversee U.S. bilateral funding for health: (i) the *Department of State*, which manages the President's Emergency Plan for AIDS Relief (PEPFAR) through the Office of the Global AIDS Coordinator; (ii) the *Agency for International Development*, which manages the President's Malaria Initiative and the Neglected Tropical Disease program; and (iii) the *Department of Health and Human Services*, which oversees federal agencies including the Centers for Disease Control and Prevention (CDC), National Institutes of Health (NIH), and the Health Resources and Services Administration (HRSA), all of which provide funding and technical assistance to global health efforts. U.S. bilateral health funding supports several priority global health areas including HIV/AIDS, TB, malaria, maternal, newborn, and reproductive health, and neglected tropical diseases. PEPFAR, the lead agency for the U.S. government's HIV/AIDS-related activities, makes up close to two-thirds of all global health spending by the United States.[59] As of 2017, PEPFAR operated in over 50 countries and had committed more than $70 billion since its launch in 2003.[59]
- **Other OECD countries** contribute significant bilateral funding in global health. For instance, the **United Kingdom**, the second-largest bilateral donor, is a leader in funding reproductive healthcare, basic healthcare, medical research, basic nutrition, infectious disease control, health policy and administrative management, and malaria control.[60] **Germany**'s bilateral funding supports basic health infrastructure, infectious disease control, reproductive healthcare, and health policy and administrative management.[61]
- **Emerging donors:** over the past decade a new set of countries—**Brazil, Russia, India, China,** and **South Africa** (the BRICS)—has emerged as increasingly important global health donors (some continue to receive DAH, and so they are simultaneously donors *and* recipients).[62] For example, **China**, now among the top-ten bilateral funders of health in Africa, focuses its health aid on infrastructure, malaria, human resource development, and providing supplies, equipment, and medicines.[63]

The Impacts of Health Aid

Was the sharp rise in health aid that was seen during the MDGs era (the "golden era" for DAH) effective at reducing avertable mortality? In this section, we begin by addressing this question, examining the evidence on whether there is an association between increased DAH investments and reduced death rates. Next, we discuss some of the negative impacts and consequences of DAH, which includes a discussion of the tension between funding "vertical" programs (those that focus narrowly on single priority diseases) versus "horizontal" system-wide strengthening to improve all health services. Finally, we briefly describe some recent approaches to aligning donor-funded, vertical programs with the need for national HSS.

Has Health Aid Been Effective? Successful disease campaigns in past decades, such as smallpox eradication, were very clearly linked to health aid.[64] Yet the impacts of the more recent surge in DAH have received remarkably little research attention. The relative lack of research probably reflects the fact that the surge only began in the year 2000. Nevertheless, a number of recent empirical studies suggest that this surge is likely to have helped in reducing deaths and illness from infectious diseases, and from maternal and child health conditions:

- One study by Bendavid and Bhattacharya found that from 1974 to 2010, each 1% increase in DAH was associated with an increase in life expectancy of 0.24 months and a fall in child mortality by 0.14 deaths per 1000 live births.[65] The strongest association between health aid and health improvements occurred during the golden decade of DAH, from 2000 to 2010. The study found that the improvements linked to health aid are measurable for 3–5 years after aid disbursement. The findings, say the authors, "imply that an increase of $1 billion in health aid could be associated with 364,800 fewer under-5 deaths."
- A study using data from Demographic Health Surveys, also led by Bendavid, compared adult mortality in nine African countries that received DAH for HIV through PEPFAR with 18 African countries that were not PEPFAR focus countries.[66] From 2004 to 2008, all-cause adult mortality fell more in the PEPFAR countries

(adjusted odds ratio of mortality was 0.84 among adults living in PEPFAR focus countries compared with nonfocus countries).

- Jakubowski and colleagues evaluated the impact of the U.S. President's Malaria Initiative.[67] They found that, from 1995 to 2014, population coverage with three key malaria control interventions that PMI funded—insecticide-treated bed nets, artemisinin-based combination therapy, and indoor residual spraying—was greater in PMI countries than in neighboring African countries. They also found that, "after adjusting for baseline differences between countries, overall time trends, other funding sources, and individual characteristics, PMI was associated with 16% annual risk reduction in child mortality."

Negative Impacts and Unintended Consequences of Health Aid The question of whether foreign aid can cause harm, such as by impeding the domestic development efforts of LICs and MICs,[68] has been the subject of fierce debate in recent years. A particularly contentious exchange has been between the health economists Jeffrey Sachs, who lays out the case for aid in his book *The End of Poverty*,[69] and William Easterly, aid skeptic and author of *The White Man's Burden*,[70] though even Easterly acknowledges that DAH for vertical programs has been effective. This broad debate on whether aid harms development is beyond the scope of our chapter. Instead, we briefly summarize three of the most important potential negative impacts or unintended consequences of DAH.

The first is that DAH can lead to a phenomenon called aid substitution, also known as "fungibility," in which a government that receives DAH responds by reducing its own domestic financial contribution to the health sector. The concern about fungibility is that it could mean that DAH does not end up leading to additional health sector resources (economists phrase this as saying that DAH is not "additional" to domestic spending). One study by IHME, for example, found that over the short run, for every dollar that LICs and MICs receive in DAH, they remove $0.44 of their own domestic health spending,[71] though different studies have found lower levels of aid displacement.

While these findings have been troubling to donors, who ultimately wish to see LICs and MICs *increasing* and not decreasing domestic health spending, the policy impacts of substitution will ultimately depend on what happens to the displaced funds. The outcome is likely to be detrimental to development if the displaced funds end up paying for weapons, but helpful if they are used to fund girls' education. There has been very little research on which of these outcomes happens most often, though a recent case study in Tanzania found that "fungibility of external funds may not necessarily be detrimental to Tanzania's development (as evidence suggests the funds displaced may be reallocated to education)."[72]

A second potentially negative consequence of DAH is the lack of overarching governance for the multiple, often overlapping bilateral and multilateral health aid programs. The poor coordination across health aid programs, which Buse and Walt have called the "unruly mélange of external ideas and initiatives,"[73] leads to concerns about "inefficiency, duplication and fragmentation of activities, unclear expectations of different donors' roles, poor accountability, and potential distortion of countries' national health policies."[9] A number of initiatives have been launched aimed at helping to improve donor coordination, such as the Paris Declaration on Aid Effectiveness,[74] which aims to promote donor harmonization with country-led strategies, and the Busan Partnership for Effective Development Cooperation,[75] aimed at fostering donor alignment.

A third concern about the surge in DAH during the golden decade was the potential way in which its focus on vertical programming could have ended up weakening national health systems. Marchal et al, adapting a framework developed by Travis and colleagues,[76] have categorized the negative consequences on health systems into three types[77]:

- *Duplication*, which refers to the creation of multiple parallel, non-integrated systems, such as multiple medicines supply chains. The World Bank's Multi-Country HIV/AIDS Program and PEPFAR, say Marchal and colleagues, are examples of agencies setting up parallel planning, operations, and monitoring systems, which can "undermine local decision-making autonomy and lead to inefficiency."
- *Imbalances,* meaning that donors suck domestic health resources away from national health systems into donor-led programs—for example, donor programs can draw health workers out of general health services into their programs.
- *Interruptions*, which the authors define as "displacement of routine services due to programme activities such as training, fieldwork, administration, and accounting." They give the example of how in Cambodia, donor-driven campaigns on HIV/AIDS, malaria, TB, and birth spacing led to reduced coverage rates of the routine immunization program.

Aligning Donor-funded Vertical Programs with National Health Systems While there are documented examples of donor programs having negative effects on national health systems, a review by the WHO's Maximizing Positive Synergies Collaborative Group also found some evidence that vertical programs can sometimes *benefit* the health system if designed properly.[78] Donor funding for HIV programs, for example, have been used to support wider HSS, including broad training of the health workforce or even—as in Rwanda—supporting health insurance schemes.[79] Moving beyond debates about the advantages of vertical programs versus broad HSS, there is an emerging consensus on "the need to develop ways to more effectively harness disease focused programs, and related funding, to better contribute to strengthening health systems.[80] Two approaches that try to marry vertical with horizontal are the *diagonal approach* and the *T-shaped approach*.

The diagonal approach was first proposed in 2006 by Sepúlveda and colleagues as a way to explain the sharp fall in child mortality in Mexico that began in the 1980s.[81] Their approach refers to incrementally introducing vertical interventions—in this case, child health interventions such as oral rehydration therapy and childhood vaccination—using existing health systems infrastructure. Each new vertical program is built on the success of the prior one, and the programs themselves are used as an entry point to make needed health system improvements.

More recently, in 2016 Takemi put forward the T-shaped approach to HSS that donors could adopt to promote HSS.[82] Echoing the principles of the diagonal approach, the T-shaped approach is defined as "using vertical funding as an entry point to promote health systems strengthening and achieving UHC."[80] Takemi gives the example of how Japan's investments into its successful TB programs in the 1950s and 1960s catalyzed HSS, including the strengthening of surveillance systems.

Nevertheless, these two approaches are unlikely to settle the horizontal versus vertical debate once and for all. Indeed, Shroff and colleagues criticize both the horizontal and T-shaped approach, arguing that (i) neither of the approaches address the negative consequences of disease control programs on national health systems; (ii) both approaches could "catalyze further fragmentation within health systems and undermine national agency and ownership, when programs are funded externally"; and (iii) the experiences of Mexico and Japan cannot easily be extrapolated to other settings.[80]

The Future of Health Aid

Stagnating levels of health aid, economic growth in many LICs and MICs, and a changing distribution of disease burden are creating new challenges and opportunities for the allocation of health aid. Due to economic development, more and more countries will be able to self-finance their domestic health needs and fewer will be dependent on external support (as discussed further in section "Domestic

Health Financing and Resource Mobilization"). Major global financing mechanisms, such as Gavi and the Global Fund, have thus changed their allocation models recently to account for the increased financial capacity of aid recipients.

Most of the world's poor now live in pockets of poverty in MICs, facing high rates of avertable mortality, yet many of these countries now have a national GDP per capita that excludes them from receiving DAH. This situation has been termed "the middle income dilemma."[83] The global burden of HIV, TB, and malaria, for example, falls mostly in MICs—and much of this burden is disproportionately experienced by vulnerable and marginalized subpopulations, including ethnic and cultural groups, refugees, people who inject drugs, and sex workers.[83] The transition of MICs away from DAH raises two critical questions. First, what is the role of donors and the broader international community in a "postaid" world? Second, after donors have withdrawn their direct financial support from MICs, what roles can they still play in helping to improve the health of the poor in the pockets of poverty in MICs?

In its *Global Health 2035* report, which laid out an ambitious investment framework to achieve global health transformation within one generation, the Lancet Commission on Investing in Health (the CIH) considered these questions.[13] Since countries are increasingly able to self-finance the delivery of routine health services, the CIH recommended a radical reorientation of health aid over time toward what it called the "global functions" of DAH. Global functions are characterized by their ability to address transnational issues, and can be categorized into three types:

- *Providing global public goods*, for example, knowledge generation and sharing, development of medical technologies (medicines, vaccines, diagnostics, etc.) for poverty-related and neglected diseases (PRNDs), and policy and implementation research;
- *Tackling negative cross-border regional and global externalities*, for example, pandemic preparedness, tackling antimicrobial resistance (including TB drug resistance), and controlling the cross-border spread of NCD risk factors such as smoking and highly processed foods; and
- *Fostering global health leadership and stewardship*, for example, global consensus building and improving health aid effectiveness.

Global functions are distinct from country-specific support—the latter refers to aid flows aimed at tackling "time-limited problems within individual countries that justify international collective action because of highly constrained national capacity."[84] In 2013, only about one fifth of all DAH was invested in global functions (Fig. 18-8).[83] The CIH argued that as countries transition away from country-specific DAH, an increasing proportion of total DAH should be invested into global functions. The examples of global functions listed above are areas where national governments have significant incentives to "free-ride" and underinvest. In scaling up health aid to global functions, argued the CIH, there should be a major new focus on implementation science, knowledge sharing (including through South-to-South learning), and market shaping.

Strengthening donor support for global functions could have five major benefits:

- First, *every country* benefits from investments in global functions.
- Second, the costs of several global functions are much lower than the costs of inaction. For example, Fan et al. estimate that the economic value of the risk of a severe influenza pandemic is as much as U.S.$570 billion in global losses per year or 0.7% of global income—an economic threat similar to that of global warming.[85]
- Third, the returns on investing in certain global functions, such as product development for PRNDs, are potentially very high. For example, a 70% efficacious vaccine would reduce new HIV/AIDS infections by 44%, leading to large reductions in incidence and potential epidemic control.[86]
- Fourth, investments in global functions may be especially helpful to address the middle-income dilemma. Poor individuals in MICs will benefit from donor support for global functions, such as product development, knowledge sharing, market shaping, and management of cross-border externalities. Countries such as China and India would substantially benefit from collective purchasing of commodities, market shaping to reduce drug prices, and increased international efforts to control multidrug-resistant TB.
- Finally, support for global functions is considered as "nonfungible" (i.e., less prone to aid substitution), and might therefore be a more efficient way for donors to achieve results for poor populations.

While investments in global functions have major benefits, many of them remain significantly underfunded. For example, investments in product development for PRNDs are currently insufficient.[87] A recent study suggests that the annual funding gap is at least $1.5–2.8 billion. The study also shows that the current product pipeline is unlikely to lead to launches of highly efficacious vaccines for HIV, TB, malaria, or hepatitis C.[88] One idea that is gaining traction as a way to mobilize additional funding for product development for PRNDs, and target it toward highly needed products, is a "health investors' platform" aimed at attracting private, philanthropic, and public funders.[89] Such a platform would facilitate pooling and sharing of information on R&D needs, candidate products in the pipeline, estimated development costs and financing gaps, likely markets, and expected health and economic benefits.

Investment is also essential in the management of negative regional and global cross-border externalities. The outbreak of Ebola in West Africa in 2014–16 shone a spotlight on the consequences of neglecting global functions as they relate to infectious disease control. The Commission on a Global Health Risk Framework for the Future calculated that LICs and MICs need an additional $3.4 billion per year to upgrade health systems to prevent infectious disease outbreaks.[90] In addition to these investments, funding is needed for the WHO's pandemic prevention and response capabilities and contingency funds at the WHO and the World Bank.[91]

While the shift in DAH toward global functions will be critical, the poorest countries will still lack the resources to self-finance their health needs and so they will require continued donor support for decades to come. By 2035, there are still likely to be around two dozen LICs, many of which will be fragile or postconflict nations.[13] Emerging donors such as China engage in global health in ways that remain poorly understood, so continued support from traditional donor countries will likely be critical.

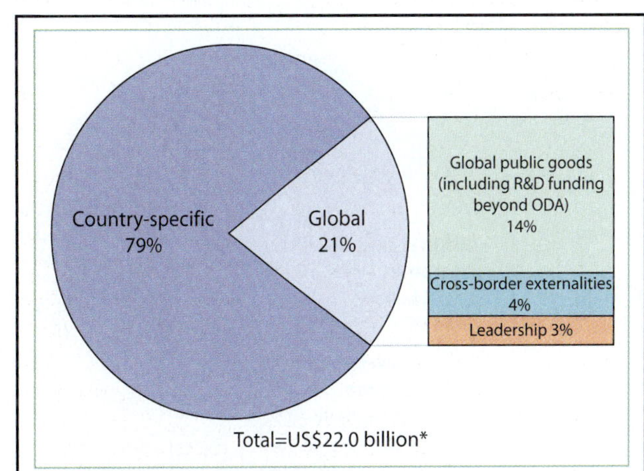

FIGURE 18-8 . Distribution of Official Development Assistance for Health by function in 2013. (*Source*: Reproduced with Permission from Schäferhoff M, Fewer S, Kraus J et al. How much donor financing for health is channeled to global versus country-specific aid functions? *Lancet* 2015;386:2436–41.[83])

Innovations in the global health architecture will be important for both the mobilization of new funding for global functions and the channeling of funding to countries. For example, as mentioned, Gavi launched new models for resource mobilization—the International Finance Facility for Immunization and the Advanced Market Commitment. Another recent innovation is the launch of the World Bank's Pandemic Emergency Facility (PEF), a global insurance mechanism that covers developing countries against the risk of viral pandemic outbreaks.[92] Japan and Germany have provided initial funding to the PEF.

Domestic Health Financing and Resource Mobilization

Given the economic growth of developing countries, their transition away from DAH, and the large price tag for achieving the health SDG targets, domestic health financing by LICs and MICs is now seen as the only viable and sustained way to ensure continued global health improvement. In section "The Global Health Financing Gap," we noted that the cost of reaching the health-related SDGs is estimated at U.S.$371 billion per year by 2030 across 67 LICs and MICs (about $271 per person)[2]; if DAH levels continue to stagnate at around $30 billion/year, over 90% of the financing is going to have to come from domestic resources.E

While the MDGs era was marked by a dramatic rise in DAH, which was associated with sharp declines in mortality from MDG target diseases (discussed in section "The Impacts of Health Aid"), the SDGs era will need to be an era of increasing domestic financing and ownership of health programs. This shift has been characterized as moving "from donorship to ownership."[93] From 1990 to 2011, there has been an extraordinary increase in the GDP of developing countries and a shift in the global population from LIC to MIC status (Fig. 18-9). From 1990 to 2011, the proportion of the global population that lived in LICs fell from almost 6 in 10 to 1 in 10. Previously low-income nations such as Bangladesh, Nigeria, and the Republic of Congo are now MICs. In developing countries, public and private domestic spending far outstrips aid and other external financing (Fig. 18-10).[21] These trends make the achievement of the health SDGs through mostly domestic finance a feasible pathway.

Here in section "How Health Financing Fits into the Health System," we begin by briefly discussing how health financing fits into a country's overall health system. Next, in section "The Critical Functions of Health Financing," we discuss the three major roles of health financing (revenue collection, pooling and prepayment, and purchasing) and how and why they are essential to providing protection against catastrophic medical expenses and achieving UHC. In section "Pro-Poor Pathways to UHC and Financial Protection," we describe "pro-poor pathways" to UHC, proposed by the CIH, which ensure the progressive realization of health coverage—that is, the provision of health and financial protection to the poorest from day one. We end in section "Driving Efficiency and Curbing Unproductive Cost Escalation" by considering ways to drive efficiency in domestic health spending, and to curb unproductive cost escalation.

How Health Financing Fits into the Health System

The WHO's health systems framework sees a functioning health system as having six major *building blocks* and four overall *goals or outcomes* (Fig. 18-11).[94] The mobilization of additional financing is a critical underpinning of HSS, as it helps to ensure adequate investments in the health workforce, medical products and infrastructure (including health information systems), and the scale-up of key health programs and interventions.

What makes for a "good" health financing system? The WHO defines a good system as one that "raises adequate funds for health, in ways that ensure people can use needed services, and are protected from financial catastrophe or impoverishment associated with having to pay them."[94] Indeed, the global momentum toward HSS and UHC is driven as much by a desire to improve health through expanding access to needed, quality health services as by a desire to reduce poverty. In 2005, WHO member states committed to develop and improve their health financing systems to achieve these aims, i.e., to reach UHC.[95]

Reducing reliance on OOP payments for healthcare, which are impoverishing and regressive, is one of the cornerstones of health financing. Direct OOP payments must fall to below 20% of a country's health expenditures in order for the incidence of medical impoverishment to fall to negligible levels.[4] Yet, as shown in Table 18-1, in 2014 the proportion of total health expenditures that came from OOP payments was 37.2% in LICs, 54.9% in lower MICs, and 32.4% in upper MICs.

As we discuss below, reducing OOP expenses can be achieved through using prepaid, pooled public financing mechanisms. Increasing the proportion of health services and interventions that are "prepaid" in this way is one of the three key dimensions of UHC (Fig. 18-12); the other two are increasing the proportion of the population covered and increasing the proportion of all health interventions covered. We refer to these three dimensions of UHC in the rest of this section.

The Critical Functions of Health Financing

The financing building block of a national health system serves three critical functions: collecting revenue, prepayment and risk pooling to provide financial protection, and purchasing of interventions and services.

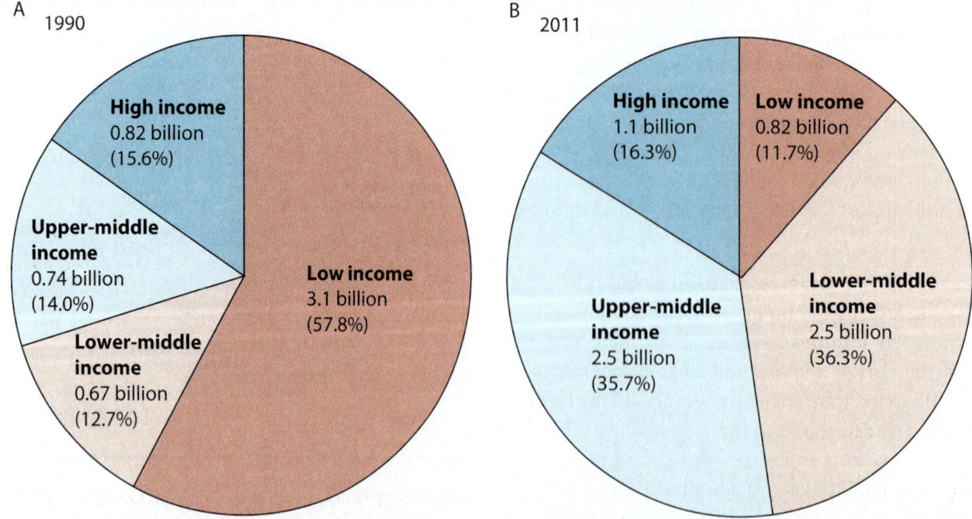

FIGURE 18-9. The movement of populations from low-income to higher income between 1990 and 2011. (*Source*: Reproduced with Permission from Summers LH, Jamison DT, Alleyne G, et al. Global health 2035: a world converging in a generation. *Lancet* 2013; 382:1898–955.[9])

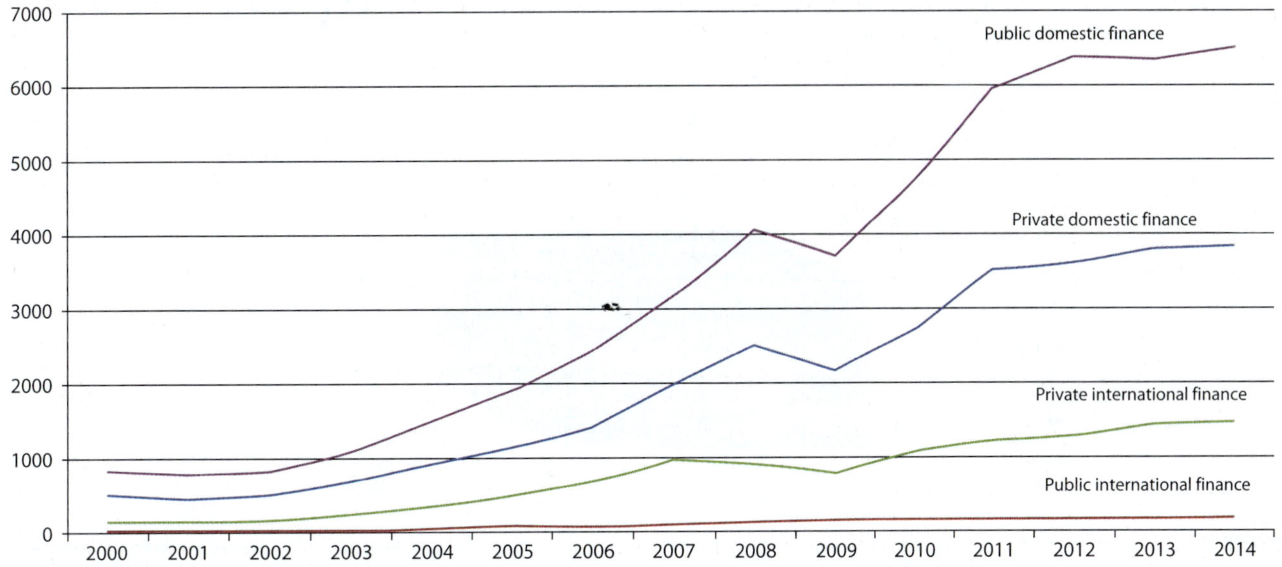

FIGURE 18-10. Financing Trends in Developing Countries, 2000–2014 (in US$, billions, 2013 prices). *Private domestic finance refers to private sector acquisitions, minus disposals, of* assets such as land, buildings, software, transport equipment, and machinery (also known as gross-fixed capital formation). *Private international finance is the sum of foreign direct investment, portfolio equity and bonds, commercial banking and other lending, and personal remittances. Public international finance equals total official flows (official development assistance and other official flows).* (*Source:* From Pablos-Méndez A, Raviglione MC. A new world health era. Glob Health Sci Pract. 2018:1–9.[21])

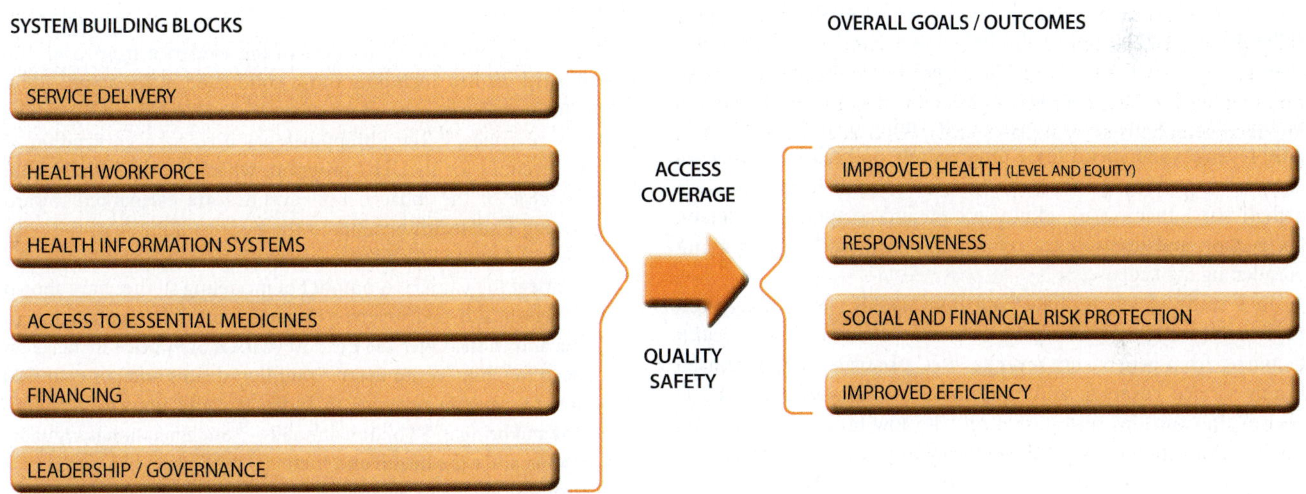

FIGURE 18-11. The WHO health system framework. (*Source:* Used with Permission from WHO. The WHO Health Systems Framework. http://www.wpro.who.int/health_services/health_systems_framework/en/.[94])

Revenue Collection The growing importance of DRM for achieving the SDGs was affirmed in the 2015 Addis Ababa Action Agenda on Financing for Development, which emphasized: "For all countries, public policies and the mobilization and effective use of domestic resources are central to the pursuit of sustainable development. Significant additional domestic resources, supplemented by international assistance, will be critical to realizing sustainable development and achieving the SDGs."[96] Political declarations in support of greater commitment to health financing go back at least 40 years, to the 1978 Alma Ata declaration; they have even included spending targets—most famously, the 2001 Abuja declaration in which African heads of state committed to spending 15% of their national budgets on health.[97] Nevertheless, while LICs and MICs as a whole have steadily increased their overall domestic public spending on health, many countries still fall short of such targets. Ten years after the Abuja declaration, for example, only Rwanda and South Africa had met the 15% target while seven countries had *reduced* their relative contributions of government expenditures to health from 2001 to 2011.[98]

It is clear that UHC is impossible through relying on voluntary private contributions to insurance schemes. As Kutzin says, "no country has attained universal population coverage by relying mainly on voluntary contributions to insurance schemes, whether they are run by nongovernmental organizations, commercial companies, "communities," or governments."[99] Public financing and compulsory contributions, with subsidization for the poor, are the only way to

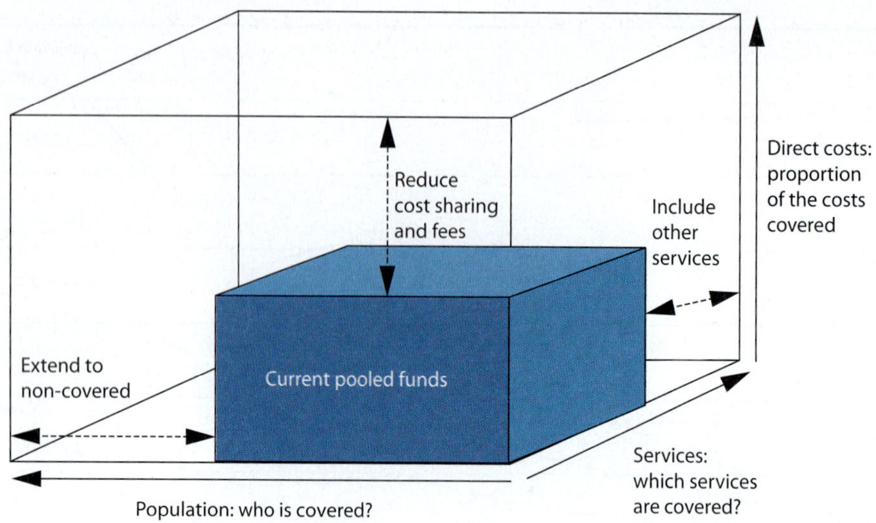

FIGURE 18-12. The UHC cube: three dimensions to consider when going for universal coverage. (*Source*: Reproduced with Permission From World Health Organization. Health Systems Financing: The Path to Universal Coverage. World Health Report 2010.[4])

reach UHC. Without compulsion, the rich and the healthy will opt out—which means there will be insufficient funding to cover the sick and old.[99]

The WHO argues that "all countries have scope to raise more money for health domestically, provided governments and the people commit to doing so."[4] A principal means for doing so is through **general tax revenue.** Improving the efficiency of tax collection is a critical step in improving financing of health and other social sectors. There are now many documented examples of developing countries, such as Brazil, Chile, and Malaysia, reforming their tax systems to raise revenues and spend these progressively on health. Approaches to mobilizing additional domestic finance for health through taxation include strengthening tax administration and compliance, reducing tax evasion and exemptions, reforming overall tax structures and broadening the tax base.[96]

In a study of longitudinal data from 89 LICs and MICs from 1995 to 2011, Reeves and colleagues found that an increase in health financing from general tax revenues was associated with increased health service coverage and financial protection—two key UHC goals.[100] In countries that started off with low tax revenues (under $1000 per person per year), the association was particularly strong: "an additional $100 tax revenue per year substantially increased the proportion of births with a skilled attendant present by 6·74 percentage points (95 % CI 0·87–12·6) and the extent of financial coverage by 11·4 percentage points (5·51–17·2)."

Governments can also raise revenue from compulsory social health insurance contributions—known as **payroll taxes**. However, in many developing countries, most people work outside the formal sector—that is, they are not in formal salaried employment and so are not subject to collection of income or payroll taxes. In this case, general government budget revenues must be used to provide coverage for the informal sector—this was the approach used by Mexico in its UHC scheme, called *Seguro Popular*, and also in Thailand's Universal Coverage Scheme.[99] General government revenues are required in every country worldwide—even in Germany, for example, where health is largely funded by social health insurance, the government "injects general revenues into the system to ensure coverage for those unable to contribute."[99]

Taxing cigarettes, alcohol, sugar-sweetened beverages (SSBs), and fossil fuels can improve public health while also raising additional revenues for health, though the amounts are relatively small compared with general tax revenues. There is ongoing debate about the pros and cons of so-called "earmarking" of this tax revenue for health purposes (i.e., directing it toward health rather than into the nation's overall budget). Some fiscal policy experts argue, for example, that earmarks may be offset by reduced discretionary budget allocations to health, leading to little, if any, overall increase in total public funding for health.[101] Below, we briefly describe all four types of tax:

- *Cigarettes*: There is now overwhelming evidence from over 100 published studies, including those conducted in LICs and MICs, that taxing tobacco can reduce tobacco consumption and generate steady revenues.[102] The Philippines has used tobacco taxation to raise revenues for its UHC program, which is called PhilHealth; about 68% of the tobacco tax revenues are earmarked toward providing PhilHealth benefits to the poorest quintile of the population.[103] Around 30 countries earmark tobacco tax revenues for investment in health.[104] A number of modeling studies have shown the likely health and revenue impacts from tobacco taxation in China and India. Over the next 50 years, a 50% price increase on tobacco in China could avert 20 million deaths and generate $20 billion per year in revenue; in India, it could prevent 4 million deaths and bring in $2 billion annually.[105] Such taxation is arguably pro-poor, since the health and financial protection benefits accrue disproportionately to the poor.[106]
- *Alcohol*: Taxing alcohol can also be an important revenue source and can deter harmful alcohol use. The WHO estimates that increasing taxes to 40% of the retail price across 12 LICs where data are available would lead to (i) a tripling of tax revenues, up to an amount equal to 38% of total health spending in these countries and (ii) a 10% fall in alcohol consumption.[4] In many countries there is still great potential to raise alcohol taxes—alcohol taxes as a share of GDP vary widely, from 0.09% in Nigeria, for example, to 1.05% in Thailand.[13]
- *SSBs*: The consumption of SSBs is associated with increased risk of obesity, and there is emerging evidence that SSB taxes can curb consumption and raise revenue. For example, Mexico introduced a one peso per liter excise tax on SSBs in 2014.[107] An impact evaluation published in 2017 looked at the impact of the tax on SSB consumption and found that purchases of taxed drinks fell by an average of 7.6% over 2 years (5.5% in 2014 and 9.7% in 2015) compared to untaxed drinks the consumption of which increased by 2.1% over the same time period.[107]
- *Fossil fuels*: Taxes on coal, gas, and oil can reduce greenhouse gas emissions and carbon consumption while also raising public revenues.[108] A carbon tax for funding national health insurance has

been considered by a number of governments, including South Africa.[109] Removal of fossil fuel subsidies and reallocation of the revenues to the health sector is another source of health financing—one that also helps to curb NCDs.[13] Many countries, such as Bangladesh, Indonesia, and Pakistan, spend more on subsidies for fossil fuels than they do on public financing of health and education combined.[110]

Risk Pooling and Financial Protection Achieving financial protection, reducing OOP payments, and curbing impoverishing medical expenses requires prepayment and pooling of funds. Countries that have come closest to reaching UHC have used a risk-pooling, prepayment approach, in which the healthy cross-subsidize the poor and the young cross-subsidize the old. Prepaid funds—paid *before* experiencing sickness—are pooled and redistributed to those with the greatest health needs. The result of prepayment and pooling is that financial risk is spread across the population and thus "no individual carries the full burden of paying for healthcare."[111]

Prepayment, pooling, and financial protection were at the heart of the 1948 creation of the United Kingdom's National Health Service (NHS). When the NHS was founded, every household received a leaflet entitled *The New National Health Service*, which noted that the NHS "will relieve your money worries in time of illness."[112]

One major barrier to redistribution is the existence of multiple coverage schemes, known as fragmentation. A "worst case scenario" for fragmentation and inequity is where different social groups are in different schemes.[99] LICs and MICs that started their path to UHC by first launching a health insurance scheme just for workers in the formal sector have run into problems—attention gets focused on those who are already better off, and a two-tier system often results. Reducing fragmentation and bringing more and more people into a single pool promotes efficiency and equity (it can be costly and inefficient to run multiple different small pools).

Strategic Purchasing of Interventions and Services In its influential World Health Report 2000, called *Health Systems: Improving Performance*, the WHO recommended a move away from "passive purchasing" of health services.[113] In passive purchasing, providers are paid through open-ended fee-for-service payments (with no attempt to manage these payments) or they receive a fixed budget from the payer (e.g., publicly funded hospitals get a fixed budget from the government that is unlinked to hospital performance). In its place, the WHO supports "strategic" ("active") purchasing—that is, using data and analysis to purchase services in a way that drives quality, efficiency, and equity.

This theme was taken forward in the World Health Report 2014, called *Health Systems Financing: The Path to Universal Coverage*.[4] Strategic purchasing, argued this report, "can improve quality and efficiency by asking explicit questions about the population's health needs: what interventions and services best meet these needs and expectations given the available resources? What is the appropriate mix of promotion, prevention, treatment, and rehabilitation? How and from whom should these interventions and services be purchased and provided?" In strategic purchasing, payment is linked to provider performance or to the health needs of the population that they serve.[114]

Pro-poor Pathways to UHC and Financial Protection

For countries that have made the policy decision to move toward UHC, one option they could adopt is to try to move simultaneously, in a balanced way, across all three dimensions of the UHC cube (Fig. 18-12). In other words, they could try to increase the proportion of the population covered, the proportion covered through prepaid public finance, and the proportion of health interventions included in the benefits package by the same amount at the same time.

An alternative approach that the CIH endorsed is known as "progressive universalism" or "pro-poor universalism," defined by Gwatkin and Ergo as "a determination to include people who are poor from the beginning."[115] The idea of pro-poor universalism can be traced back to the World Health Report 1999, which proposed a "new universalism."[116] In her forward to this report, Director General Gro Harlem Brundtland wrote that this new universalism recognizes that "if services are to be provided for all then not all services can be provided. The most cost-effective services should be provided first." Pro-poor universalism takes this further by arguing that *interventions that disproportionately benefit the poor* should be provided first.

The CIH laid out two pro-poor pathways, both of which use prepayment and pooling of funds to expand publicly financed insurance:

- The first is *insurance of the entire population with an initially narrow package of interventions and zero user fees* (user fees are defined as "fee-for-service charges at the point of care without the benefit of insurance"). The benefit package initially includes interventions that mostly benefit the poor: essential, highly cost-effective interventions for infections, maternal and child health conditions, and NCDs/injuries. In the most recent edition (the 3rd edition) of *Disease Control Priorities*, a compendium of evidence on the efficacy and program effectiveness of global health interventions, Watkins and colleagues define the components of such an "essential" UHC package.[117] As countries grow economically, they can then expand the package to include additional health services, an approach that Mexico adopted in its path to UHC.[13]
- The second is *public financing of a larger package of interventions to the whole population with some copayment from patients* (though the poorest are exempt from the copayment). Providing a larger benefits package from the outset clearly requires using a wider range of financing mechanisms, including payroll taxes, general taxation revenue, and mandatory insurance premiums and copayments. This is the approach that Rwanda has adopted in its UHC scheme, called *mutuelles de santé*, a community-based national insurance scheme.[118] The Global Fund subsidizes premiums and copayments for the poorest quarter of the population.[118]

While many countries have signaled their intent to expand coverage through a pro-poor approach, there has been little practical guidance available on how to achieve this. To address this gap, in 2015 the Rockefeller Foundation funded the *Bellagio Workshop on Implementing Pro-Poor UHC*.[119] The workshop laid out a set of recommendations to both national governments (e.g., to establish explicit, transparent national decision-making mechanisms) and to the international community (e.g., to support the generation and sharing of knowledge about technical aspects of UHC and the political economy of its implementation).

Driving Efficiency and Curbing Unproductive Cost Escalation

As Kutzkin has argued, "countries cannot simply spend their way to universal health coverage."[99] Raising money, prepayment and pooling, and strategic purchasing must also be accompanied by using resources efficiently (sometimes called "getting more health for the money").

The WHO estimates that at least 20–40% of all resources spent on health are wasted, a conservative estimate—wasted resources that should be directed toward UHC.[4] One of the most common causes of inefficient spending is the failure to use medicines rationally. For example, money is wasted when expensive brand drugs are used instead of cheaper generic versions that are equally effective, or when antibiotics and injections are used needlessly. Other approaches proposed by the WHO to tackling common causes of inefficiency include using incentives to motivate health workers and instituting programs to reduce medical errors.[4]

A related challenge in HICs and some MICs is cost escalation. As the CIH noted, "healthcare costs have been rising rapidly in the past two decades in high-income and many middle-income countries, which puts financial pressure on households and governments."[9] In its

Global Health 2035 report, the CIH reviewed the evidence on ways to curb unproductive cost escalation (i.e., cost escalation with no resulting improvements in health). Examples of promising approaches include: (i) minimizing fee-for-service payments, since these "reward quantity over quality, drive up health costs, and do nothing to promote the use of services such as prevention and patient education, which are high value and low cost"; (ii) single payer approaches, which can greatly reduce administrative costs; and (iii) gatekeeper arrangements, in which patients must see a primary care provider before referral to specialist services.[9]

Conclusions: Challenges and Opportunities

In this chapter, we have laid out mechanisms, trends, obstacles, and opportunities in global health financing. Beginning with a snapshot of current global health spending, sources of such spending, and the likely health financing needs in the SDGs era, we explored the role of both DAH and DRM in meeting these needs. What is clear is that the extremely ambitious health-related SDG targets for 2030—such as ending avertable child deaths, ending HIV, TB, and malaria, and reducing premature deaths from NCDs by 2030—will not be achieved unless there is a massive mobilization of dedicated funding for health.

Our chapter has shown that global health financing is undergoing an extraordinary series of shifts and transitions. Economies of LICs and MICs are growing, accompanied by rising health spending. After a remarkable period of explosive growth in DAH from 2000 to 2010, fueled partly by innovative multilateral financing mechanisms such as Gavi and the Global Fund, and bilateral initiatives such as PEPFAR and PMI, DAH is now stagnant. The global financial crisis and the rise of populist, nationalist, inward-looking governments in countries such as the United States and the United Kingdom have contributed to the flatlining of health aid. All eyes are now on the governments of LICs and MICs—will they step up and channel their economic growth toward the health sector? Will they spend domestic resources effectively and efficiently to save the most lives and promote the most wellbeing possible?

The answers to these questions depend in large part on whether they adopt the bedrock principles of financing UHC. For example, to reduce impoverishment from having to pay OOP medical expenses, we have shown that all countries must use pooling and prepayment. No country can hope to use voluntary private insurance to reach UHC—it is a doomed enterprise. Countries that have come the closest to achieving UHC have done so by using public financing and compulsory enrollment, in which the healthy subsidize the sick and the young subsidize the old. Pro-poor pathways to UHC offer nations the opportunity to achieve equity and both health and financial protection.

The prospects for DRM and greater domestic financing of health in LICs and MICs open up an extraordinary window of opportunity for donors to "reimagine" the future of DAH. When LICs and MICs transition out of external assistance, what then will health aid be for? We have argued that if the total DAH envelope is now stable, at around $30 billion annually, and less and less of this financing is needed by LICs and MICs to support their domestic programs, DAH should increasingly be targeted at global public goods for health and other global functions.

Some of the most critical global health functions are enormously under-funded, including pandemic preparedness, product development for PRNDs, and tackling drug-resistant TB. The time has come for donors, including the emerging BRICS donors, to step up their attention toward these transnational health challenges. Donor funding of global functions such as pooled procurement of medicines and vaccines, and market shaping to reduce the costs of new health technologies is also an important way to help address the "middle income dilemma." Of course, the transition toward global functions does not mean that donors can walk away from direct support to the poorest and most vulnerable populations. Many LICs, especially fragile states, will need this kind of country-specific DAH for decades to come.

Global health financing is evolving from an era of "donorship" to one of "national ownership" in which LICs and MICs should be in the driving seat, protecting their citizens through UHC that will be increasingly financed by themselves. While there are multiple global health challenges ahead—including the rising burden of NCDs, the threat of pandemic flu, and the massive global displacement of people in the face of conflict, climate change, and other threats—there are also reasons to be optimistic that a global health transformation is possible by 2035. These include the economic growth of LICs and MICs, a new global political momentum toward UHC, the prospects of new health technologies, the digital revolution, and the continuing innovations in how global health is financed both internationally and domestically.

References

1. Global Burden of Disease Health Financing Collaborator Network. Evolution and patterns of global health financing 1995–2014: Development assistance for health, and government, prepaid private, and out-of-pocket health spending in 184 countries. *Lancet.* 2017;389:1981–2004.
2. Stenberg K, Hanssen O, Edejer T T-T, et al. Financing transformative health systems towards achievement of the health Sustainable Development Goals: A model for projected resource needs in 67 low-income and middle-income countries. *Lancet Glob Health.* 2017;5(9):e875–87.
3. Xu K, Evans DB, Carrin G, Aguilar-Rivera AM, Musgrove P, Evans T. Protecting households from catastrophic health spending. *Health Aff (Millwood).* 2007;26:972–83.
4. World Health Organization. Health Systems Financing: The Path to Universal Coverage. World Health Report 2010.
5. Bendavid E, Ottersen T, Peilong L, et al. Development assistance for health. In: *Disease Control Priorities,* 3rd ed. Washington, DC: World Bank Group. Part 5, Chapter 16. pp. 299-313. http://dcp-3.org/chapter/2593/donor-assistance-health.
6. Coady D, Clements BJ, Gupta S. *The Economics of Public Health Care Reform in Advanced and Emerging Economies.* Geneva: International Monetary Fund; 2012.
7. World Health Organization. Global Health Expenditure Database. http://apps.who.int/nha/database.
8. Pires Barrenho EA, Miraldo M, Smith PC. Does global drug innovation correspond to burden of disease? The neglected diseases in developed and developing countries. Oct 6, 2017. Available at https://spiral.imperial.ac.uk:8443/handle/10044/1/51581.
9. Summers LH, Jamison DT, Alleyne G, et al. Global health 2035: A world converging in a generation. *Lancet.* 2013;382:1898–955.
10. Fiscal Affairs Department. *Macro-Fiscal Implications of Health Care Reform in Advanced and Emerging Economies.* Washington, DC: International Monetary Fund; 2010. Available at https://www.imf.org/external/np/pp/eng/2010/122810.pdf.
11. Organisation for Economic Co-operation and Development. OECD.Stat. http://stats.oecd.org/Index.aspx?DataSetCode=SHA.
12. World Bank. World Development Indicators. https://data.worldbank.org/products/wdi.
13. Puteh SEW, Almualm Y. Catastrophic health expenditure among developing countries. *Health Syst Policy Res.* 2017;4:1.
14. United Nations. Sustainable Development Goal 3. https://sustainabledevelopment.un.org/sdg3.
15. Watkins DA, Yamey G, Schäferhoff M, et al. Alma Ata at 40 years: Reflections from the Lancet Commission on Investing in Health. *Lancet.* 2018;392(10156):1434–60.
16. Dieleman JL, Graves C, Johnson E, et al. Sources and focus of health development assistance, 1990–2014. *JAMA.* 2015;313(23):2359–68.
17. Organisation for Economic Co-operation and Development. Official Development Assistance—Definition and Coverage. www.oecd.org/dac/stats/officialdevelopmentassistancedefinitionandcoverage.htm.
18. Mills A. Health care systems in low-and middle-income countries. *N Engl J Med.* 2014;370(6):552–7.
19. Kaiser Family Foundation, 2018, Kaiser Health Tracking Poll—January 2018: The Public's Priorities and Next Steps for the Affordable Care Act. www.files.kff.org/attachment/Topline-Kaiser-Health-Tracking-Poll%E2%80%93January-2018.
20. Kharas H. 2009. Development Assistance in the 21st Century, Wolfensohn Center for Development at Brookings, Contribution to the VIII Salamanca Forum, The Fight Against Hunger and Poverty, July 2–4, 2009. https://www.brookings.edu/research/development-assistance-in-the-21st-century/.

21. Pablos-Méndez A, Raviglione MC. A new world health era. *Glob Health Sci Pract.* 2018;6(1):8–16.
22. Brown TM, Cueto M, Fee E. The World Health Organization and the transition from "international" to "global" public health. *Am J Public Health.* 2006;96:62–72.
23. Institute for Health Metrics and Evaluation (IHME). *Financing Global Health 2017: Funding Universal Health Coverage and the Unfinished HIV/AIDS Agenda.* Seattle, WA: IHME; 2018.
24. The Donor Tracker. United States Donor Profile, 2017. https://donortracker.org/sites/default/files/donor_pdfs/DonorTracker_Profile_USA.pdf.
25. The Donor Tracker, Australia Donor Profile, 2017. https://donortracker.org/sites/default/files/donor_pdfs/DonorTracker_Profile_Australia.pdf.
26. Kickbusch I, Franz C, Holzscheiter A, et al. Germany's expanding role in global health. *Lancet.* 2017;390:898–912.
27. Dieleman JL, Schneider MT, Haakenstad A, et al. Development assistance for health: Past trends, associations, and the future of international financial flows for health. *Lancet.* 2016;387:2536–44.
28. Shiffman J. Donor funding priorities for communicable disease control in the developing world. *Health Policy Plan.* 2006;21(6):411–20.
29. Shiffman J, Smith S. Generation of political priority for global health initiatives: A framework and case study of maternal mortality. *Lancet.* 2007;370:1370–9.
30. Gulrajani, N. Bilateral versus multilateral aid channels. Strategic choices for donors. Overseas Development Institute. March 2016. https://www.odi.org/sites/odi.org.uk/files/resource-documents/10393.pdf.
31. McCoy D, Chand S, Sridhar D. Global health funding: How much, where it comes from and where it goes. *Health Policy Plan.* 2009;24(6):407–17.
32. Organisation for Economic Co-operation and Development. Creditor Reporter System, 2018. https://stats.oecd.org/Index.aspx?DataSetCode=CRS1.
33. Alonso A, Brugha R. Rehabilitating the health system after conflict in East Timor: A shift from NGO to government leadership. *Health Policy Plan.* 2006;21(3):206–16.
34. Moran M, Guzman J, Ropars AL, Illmer A. The role of Product Development Partnerships in research and development for neglected diseases. *Int Health.* 2010;2(2):114–22.
35. The Global Fund. Key Populations Action Plan 2015–2017. https://www.theglobalfund.org/media/1270/publication_keypopulations_actionplan_en.pdf.
36. Van de Maele N, Evans DB, Tan-Torres T. Development assistance for health in Africa: Are we telling the right story? *Bull World Health Organ.* 2013;91(7):483–90.
37. Goldie SJ, O'Shea M, Campos NG, Diaz M, Sweet S, Kim SY. Health and economic outcomes of HPV 16, 18 vaccination in 72 GAVI-eligible countries. *Vaccine.* 2008;26(32):4080–93.
38. Komatsu R, Korenromp EL, Low-Beer D, et al. Lives saved by Global Fund-supported HIV/AIDS, tuberculosis and malaria programs: Estimation approach and results between 2003 and end-2007. *BMC Infect Dis.* 2010;10(1):109.
39. World Bank website. History. http://www.worldbank.org/en/about/history.
40. Global Fund. Results Report 2017. https://www.theglobalfund.org/media/6773/corporate_2017resultsreport_report_en.pdf.
41. Global Fund website. Core Pledges and Contributions. https://www.theglobalfund.org/en/financials/.
42. World Health Organization website. About WHO—What we do. http://www.who.int/about/what-we-do/en/.
43. World Health Organization. The Global Guardian of Public Health. May 2016. http://www.who.int/about/what-we-do/global-guardian-of-public-health.pdf?ua=1.
44. World Health Organization website. About WHO—Funding WHO. http://www.who.int/about/finances-accountability/funding/en/.
45. World Health Organization. Public health preparedness and response: Report of the Independent Oversight and Advisory Committee for the WHO Health Emergencies Programme. Jun 2018. http://apps.who.int/gb/ebwha/pdf_files/EB142/B142_8-en.pdf.
46. World Bank website. What We Do. http://www.worldbank.org/en/about/what-we-do.
47. World Bank website. Organization. http://www.worldbank.org/en/about/leadership
48. Sridhar D, Winters J, Strong E. World Bank's financing, priorities, and lending structures for global health. *BMJ.* 2017;358:j3339.
49. World Bank. *The World Bank Annual Report 2017.* Washington, DC: World Bank; 2017.
50. Global Financing Facility. About Us. https://www.globalfinancingfacility.org/introduction.
51. Nelson RM. Multilateral Development Banks: Overview and Issues for Congress. https://fas.org/sgp/crs/row/R41170.pdf.
52. Gavi website. About—Partnership model. http://www.gavi.org/about/gavis-partnership-model/.
53. Gavi. Gavi, the Vaccine Alliance 2016–2020 Strategy. https://www.gavi.org/library/publications/gavi/gavi-the-vaccine-alliance-2016-2020-strategy/.
54. Gavi. How the pneumococcal AMC works. http://www.gavi.org/funding/pneumococcal-amc/how-the-pneumococcal-amc-works/.
55. Gavi website. How our support works. Accessed Mar 22, 2018. http://www.gavi.org/support/process/.
56. Bill & Melinda Gates Foundation website. What we do. https://www.gatesfoundation.org/What-We-Do.
57. Bloomberg Philanthropies website. Our Work—Public Health. https://www.bloomberg.org/program/public-health/#intro.
58. Wellcome Trust website. What we do. https://wellcome.ac.uk/what-we-do.
59. US President's Emergency Plan for AIDS Relief (PEPFAR) website. PEPFAR Funding. https://www.pepfar.gov/documents/organization/252516.pdf.
60. Donor Tracker. United Kingdom Deep Dive Global Health. http://donortracker.org/UK/globalhealth.
61. Donor Tracker. Germany Deep Dive Global Health. https://donortracker.org/germany/globalhealth.
62. Asmus G, Fuchs A, Müller A. 2017. BRICS and Foreign Aid. AidData Working Paper #43. Williamsburg, VA: AidData. https://www.aiddata.org/publications/brics-and-foreign-aid.
63. Shajalal M, Xu J, Jing J, et al. China's engagement with development assistance for health in Africa. *Glob Health Res Policy* 2017;2:24. https://doi.org/10.1186/s41256-017-0045-8
64. Hopkins DR. Disease eradication. *N Engl J Med.* 2013;368:54–63.
65. Bendavid E, Bhattacharya J. The relationship of health aid to population health improvements. *JAMA Intern Med.* 2014;174(6):881–7.
66. Bendavid E, Holmes CB, Bhattacharya J, Miller G. HIV development assistance and adult mortality in Africa. *JAMA* 2012;307:2060–7.
67. Jakubowski A, Stearns SC, Kruk ME, Angeles G, Thirumurthy H. The US President's Malaria Initiative and under-5 child mortality in sub-Saharan Africa: A difference-in-differences analysis. *PLoS Med.* 2017;14(6):e1002319.
68. Moyo D. *Dead Aid: Why Aid Is Not Working and How There Is a Better Way for Africa.* New York: Farrar, Straus and Giroux; 2010.
69. Sachs J. *The End of Poverty: Economic Possibilities for Our Time.* London, England, UK: Penguin Books; 2006.
70. Easterly W. *The White Man's Burden: Why the West's Efforts to Aid the Rest Have Done So Much Ill and So Little Good.* Oxford, UK: Oxford University Press; 2006.
71. Lu C, Schneider MT, Gubbins P, Leach-Kemon K, Jamison D, Murray CJ. Public financing of health in developing countries: A cross-national systematic analysis. *Lancet.* 2010;375:1375–87.
72. Alvarez MM, Borghi J, Acharya A, Vassal A. Is development assistance for health fungible? Findings from a mixed methods case study in Tanzania. *Soc Sci Med.* 2016;159;161–9.
73. Buse K, Walt G. An unruly mélange? Coordinating external resources to the health sector: A review. *Soc Sci Med.* 1997;45(3):449–63.
74. http://www.oecd.org/dac/effectiveness/34428351.pdf.
75. http://www.oecd.org/development/effectiveness/busanpartnership.htm.
76. Travis P, Bennett S, Haines A, et al. Overcoming health-systems constraints to achieve the Millennium Development Goals. *Lancet.* 2004;364:900–6.
77. Marchal B, Cavalli A, Kegels G. Global health actors claim to support health system strengthening—Is this reality or rhetoric? *PLoS Med.* 2009;6(4):e1000059.
78. World Health Organization. Maximizing Positive Synergies Collaborative Group. An assessment of interactions between global health initiatives and country health systems. *Lancet.* 2009;373(9681):2137–69.
79. Farmer P, Garrett L. From "marvelous momentum" to health care for all. *Foreign Affairs* March/April 2007. https://www.foreignaffairs.com/articles/2007-03-01/marvelous-momentum-health-care-all-success-possible-right-programs.
80. Shroff ZC, Ghaffar A, Soucat A. Moving beyond diagonal and T-shaped: Getting the incentives right for the pie and not the slice. *Health Sys Reform.* 2017;3(4):261–67. Available at http://www.tandfonline.com/doi/full/10.1080/23288604.2017.1366964.
81. Sepulveda J, Bustreo F, Tapia R, et al. Improvement of child survival in Mexico: The diagonal approach. *Lancet.* 2006;368:2017–27.

82. Takemi K. Proposal for a T-shaped approach to health system strengthening. *Health Sys Reform.* 2016;2(1):8–10.
83. Schäferhoff M, Fewer S, Kraus J et al. How much donor financing for health is channeled to global versus country-specific aid functions? *Lancet.* 2015;386:2436–41.
84. Jamison DT, Frenk J, Knaul F. International collective action in health: Objectives, functions, and rationale. *Lancet.* 1998;351:514–17.
85. Fan VY, Jamison DT, Summers LH. Pandemic risk: How large are the expected losses? *Bull World Health Organ.* 2018;96:129–34.
86. Harmon TM, Fisher KA, McGlynn MG, et al. Exploring the potential health impact and cost-effectiveness of AIDS vaccine within a comprehensive HIV/AIDS response in low- and middle-income countries. *PLoS One.* 2016;11(1):e0146387.
87. Policy Cures Research G-FINDER survey. http://www.who.int/research-observatory/monitoring/inputs/neglected_diseases/en/.
88. Young R, Bekele T, Gunn A, et al. Developing new health technologies for neglected diseases: A pipeline portfolio review and cost model [version 2; referees: 2 approved, 1 approved with reservations]. *Gates Open Res.* 2018;2:23.
89. Yamey G, Batson A, Kilmarx PH, Yotebieng M. Funding innovation in neglected diseases. *BMJ.* 2018;360:k1182.
90. Commission on a Global Health Risk Framework for the Future. *The Neglected Dimension of Global Security—A Framework for Countering Infectious-Disease Crises.* Washington, DC: National Academies Press; 2016.
91. Yamey G, Schäferhoff M, Aars OK, et al. Financing of international collective action for epidemic and pandemic preparedness. *Lancet Global Health.* 2017;5:e742–4.
92. World Bank. Pandemic Emergency Financing Facility. May 9, 2017. http://www.worldbank.org/en/topic/pandemics/brief/pandemic-emergency-facility-frequently-asked-questions.
93. Oxfam Briefing Paper 51. From donorship to ownership. January 2004. https://www.internationalbudget.org/wp-content/uploads/From-Donorship-to-Ownership-Moving-Towards-PRSP-Roundtable-Two.pdf.
94. WHO. The WHO Health Systems Framework. http://www.wpro.who.int/health_services/health_systems_framework/en/.
95. Resolution WHA58.33. Sustainable health financing, universal coverage and social health insurance. In: Fiftyeighth World Health Assembly, Geneva, 16–25 May 2005. Geneva, World Health Organization, 2005. http:// apps.who.int/gb/ebwha/pdf_fles/WHA58/WHA58_33-en.pdf. Accessed 23 June 2010.
96. UNDESA Briefing Note on the Third international Conference on Financing for Development Action Agenda. http://www.un.org/esa/ffd/wp-content/uploads/sites/2/2015/07/DESA-Briefing-Note-Addis-Action-Agenda.pdf.
97. WHO. The Abuja declaration: Ten years on. 2011. http://www.who.int/healthsystems/publications/abuja_declaration/en/.
98. WHO. *Public Financing for Health in Africa: From Abuja to the SDGs.* Geneva: WHO; 2016. WHO/HIS/HGF/Tech.Report/16.2.
99. Kutzin J. Anything goes on the path to universal coverage? No. *Bull World Health Organ.* 2012;90:867–8.
100. Reeves A, Gourtsoyannis Y, Basu S, McCoy D, McKee M, Stuckler D. Financing universal health coverage—Effects of alternative tax structures on public health systems: Cross-national modelling in 89 low-income and middle-income countries. *Lancet.* 2015;386:274–80.
101. Cashin C, Sparkes S, Bloom D. Earmarking for Health: From Theory to Practice. Health Financing Working Paper No. 5. WHO and R4D, 2017. Available at apps.who.int/iris/bitstream/10665/255004/1/9789241512206-eng.pdf.
102. Chaloupka FJ, Yurekli A, Fong GT. Tobacco taxes as a tobacco control strategy. *Tob Control.* 2012;21:172–80.
103. Chavez JJ, Drope J, Lencucha R, McGrady B. The Political Economy of Tobacco Control in the Philippines. American Cancer Society, Action for Economic Reforms. 2014. https://www.cancer.org/content/dam/cancer-org/research/economic-and-healthy-policy/the-political-economy-of-tobacco-control-philippines-policy-report.pdf.
104. Perucic A-M. Earmarking Tobacco tax revenues. Geneva: WHO. http://www.who.int/health_financing/topics/public-financial-management/D2-S4-Perucic-tobacco-earmarking.pdf.
105. Jha P, Joseph R, Li D, et al. Tobacco Taxes: A Win-Vin Measure for Fiscal Space and Health. Mandaluyong City, Philippines: Asian Development Bank; 2012.
106. Verguet S, Gauvreau C, Mishra S, et al. Tobacco taxation in China: An extended cost-effectiveness analysis. Available at http://www.dcp-3.org/resources/tobacco-taxation-china-extended-cost-effectiveness-analysis.
107. Soares AA. Putting taxes into the diet equation. *Bull World Health Organ.* 2016;94:239–40.
108. UNDP, 2017. Taxes on fuel. http://www.undp.org/content/sdfinance/en/home/solutions/fuel-tax.html.
109. Venter FHJ, Wolvaardt JE. The World Health Organization's mechanisms for increasing the health sector budget. *SAMJ.* August 2016;106(8):771–4. https://www.mm3admin.co.za/documents/docmanager/f447b607-3c8f-4eb7-8da4-11bca747079f/00106253.pdf.
110. International Monetary Fund. *Energy Subsidy Reform: Lessons and Implications.* Washington, DC: International Monetary Fund; 2013.
111. WHO. Health financing for universal coverage. Pooling. http://www.who.int/health_financing/topics/pooling/en/.
112. Central Office of Information. *The new National Health Service. Leaflet Prepared for the Ministry of Health.* London: Central Office of Information; 1948.
113. WHO. The World Health Report 2000: Health Systems—Improving Performance. Geneva: WHO, 2002. http://www.who.int/whr/2000/en/.
114. Mathauer I, Dale E, Meessen B. Strategic Purchasing for UHC: Key Policy Issues and Questions. Health Financing Working Paper No. 8. WHO, 2017. Available at http://apps.who.int/iris/bitstream/handle/10665/259423/9789241513319-eng.pdf?sequence=1.
115. Gwatkin DR, Ergo A. Universal health coverage: Friend or foe of equity? *Lancet.* 2011;377:2160–1.
116. WHO. The World Health Report 1999—Making a Difference. Geneva: WHO, 1999. http://www.who.int/whr/1999/en/.
117. Watkins D, Jamison D, Mills A, et al. Universal health coverage and essential packages of care. DCP3 Volume 9, Chapter 3. Available at http://dcp-3.org/sites/default/files/chapters/DCP3%20Volume%209_Ch%203.pdf.
118. Farmer P, Nutt CT, Wagner CM, et al. Reduced premature mortality in Rwanda: Lessons from success. *BMJ.* 2013;346:f65.
119. Participants at the Bellagio Workshop on Implementing Pro-Poor Universal Health Coverage. Implementing pro-poor universal health coverage. *Lancet Glob Health.* 2016;4:e14–16.

CHAPTER

19

Evaluating Progress in Global Health: Global Health Measures that Build Capacity

Patricia J. Garcia • Nikki Eller • Kesetebirhan Admasu • Dong Roman Xu • Saima Hamid • Chris Elias • Judith N. Wasserheit

INTRODUCTION

It is quite important to deliver effective interventions to individuals and populations. Particularly at the global level, it is necessary to follow those interventions and measure how they work and what effects they have to improve health and promote development. In this chapter, we will discuss why and how we evaluate progress in global health, focusing on the importance of using the process to build local capacity and overcome public health challenges. We will also consider some of the ways in which progress in global health and development is being monitored on the global scale, and how this interacts with metrics of progress in health and development processes at national and local levels.

WHY MEASURE AND EVALUATE PROGRESS IN GLOBAL HEALTH?

Imagine you are the Minister of Health of a country. How would you improve the health of the citizens of your country? You will need to follow four steps (Fig. 19-1):

1. *Define where you are.* You will need to know current levels and trends in disease burden in terms of both morbidity and mortality (e.g., the current child mortality rate and whether it is increasing, decreasing, or remaining stable) and the status of health service infrastructure and capacity to set priorities and goals.
2. *Decide where you want to go.* This involves thinking about what progress in global health would look like and setting specific goals (e.g., reducing child mortality to <25 per 1000 live births).
3. *Close the gap.* Decide how to close the gap between where you are and where you want to be and implement. This requires choosing the best interventions in each priority area (e.g., to reduce child mortality), keeping in mind key considerations such as effectiveness, costs, and feasibility. Implementation by itself is a key step.
4. *Measure and evaluate progress along the way to make sure you reach your goal.* You will need to know how well your interventions are working so that you can refine them, as needed, to reach your goal on time.

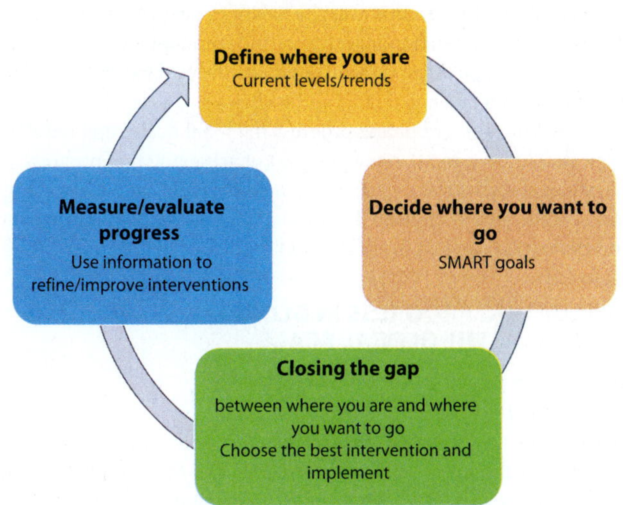

FIGURE 19-1. The cycle of implementation/measurement/evaluation to improve health outcomes.

This is an iterative process. Long-term success depends on countries being empowered to lead the way in setting their own health and development priorities, implementing evidence-based interventions to achieve relevant goals, and establishing systems to assess progress toward their goals. Every step in this process is important, but in this chapter we will focus mainly on step 4: measuring and evaluating progress. However, we are first providing here a more detailed overview of these four steps.

Defining Where You Are

Since data in low- and middle-income countries (LMICs) can be scarce, measuring global health is often a fuzzy process. When data are available, it can be useful to benchmark targeted health conditions and health system metrics to international norms, as benchmarking may reveal gaps that need to be addressed. Countries often conduct their own national assessments to establish baselines for health and development projects. However, because some countries lack the capacity to gather quality data and, especially, to analyze it, and because building that capacity takes time, effort, and fighting local bureaucracy and poor governance, external institutions (global institutions) have tended to conduct their own assessments in parallel. This has both advantages and drawbacks, which we will discuss in the context of the Sustainable Development Goals (SDGs).

The array of institutions monitoring global health includes groups within the United Nations (UN), the World Health Organization (WHO), the Organization for Economic Co-operation and Development (OECD), the World Bank, and the Institute for Health Metrics and Evaluation (IHME). These institutions are able to produce regular reports with far more data than a single country could. They sometimes gather data from scratch, but frequently use the data that countries have collected and analyze it to produce estimates. The WHO Global Health Observatory, for example, tracks 1000 indicators in countries all over the world.[1] However, in recognition of the costs of collecting and processing that much information they have also produced a Global Reference List of 100 Core Health Indicators that they recommend countries focus on.[1] Several of these institutions and philanthropic organizations also formed the Health Data Collaborative in 2016 to help LMICs build national health data capacities.[2] The Collaborative gives countries training and tools to help improve birth and death registration, epidemiologic information, health workforce data, health spending data, and the capacity to analyze and use data. The Collaborative's long-term goals are to work with 60 LMICs by 2024, and to help them transition away from international assistance by 2030.[2] For many countries, all of the different indicators requested by international agencies, donors, and other organizations represent a substantial burden to LMIC health information systems that are often weak and poorly organized.

Information on global health and disease comes from a variety of sources, including health systems, censuses, vital records, disease registries, surveys, scientific studies, and verbal autopsies. The 2005 International Health Regulations laid out the rules for reporting of infectious diseases to public health authorities for surveillance of threats that might reach a global scale.[3] Digital disease detection systems that monitor search engines and social media for disease-related searches and posts have also effectively identified outbreaks, but have yet to be formally integrated into many disease-monitoring systems.[3] But a complete picture of a population's health requires more than just information on infectious diseases (especially as the burden of noncommunicable diseases continues to rise), which is why many governments, NGOs, and other institutions interested in global health conduct regular surveys and studies. The IHME, which produces annual mortality and morbidity statistics at the country level, drew from more than 90,000 data sources to produce their 2017 Global Burden of Disease report.[4] In addition to indicators of health, data on health expenditures and performance are also important for assessing health systems.

Deciding Where You Want to Go

Setting goals in global health is often a part of the political process, as it requires choosing priorities based on shared values, as well as funding and infrastructure to set goals that can be successfully pursued. When data and analytical capacity are available, modeling exercises can help provide an evidence base for current and projected needs, as well as the projected impact of alternative intervention strategies. Often there are internal social, political, and economic factors, as well as external collaborations, institutions, and influences, that set the stage for what stakeholders can do.[5] Stakeholders may include politicians, health workers, patients, people at risk for a health problem, or anybody else who might be affected by a policy or program with a health impact. Stakeholders bring practical, strategic, and technical resources that they use to make decisions and set health policy and goals.[5]

Goals that define global health priorities can be set at different levels, such as local, national, or international, and it is extremely important that goals set at these different levels align. Historically, global health initiatives set at the international or global level have often been poorly coordinated with national health agendas. The International Health Partnership (IHP+) initiative launched by the UN has attempted to address this challenge by developing a tool for joint assessment of national health strategies and plans.[6] Ethiopia has effectively used this tool to coordinate and align the support of development partners to support a single national health strategy. It is also important that stakeholders within each level collaborate, as it takes more than a country's Ministry of Health (MOH) to successfully implement health initiatives.[7]

Another challenge is defining a manageable number of achievable goals. The SMART framework, which stands for Specific, Measurable, Achievable, Relevant, and Time-bound, is a popular way to keep goals realistic.[8] Goals that are overly ambitious or vague are much harder to implement than ones that clearly define what should be done by what date.

Closing the Gap

With a broad range of interventions to choose from, including policy and program options, and needs for prevention and treatment, it can be daunting to decide how to approach a public health challenge. The third edition of Disease Control Priorities (DCP[3]), released in nine volumes between 2015 and 2018, offers policy and program recommendations based on cost-effectiveness research to give decision-makers a starting point.[9] Accompanying estimates of costs, lives saved, and other outcomes give decision-makers the information they need to prioritize and choose interventions best suited for their situations.[9] A study is currently underway to evaluate uptake and effectiveness of the first two DCP editions,[10] and DCP is now working in Ethiopia and the Eastern Mediterranean to facilitate policy discussions.[11]

Although DCP[3] offers great recommendations for effective health interventions, there is often a gap between identifying effective interventions and implementing them on a large scale. Implementation science, described in detail in Chapter 20, offers a framework of rigorous methods to identify and address barriers to getting proven interventions to the people who need them with greater speed, fidelity, efficiency, quality, and coverage. Barriers can exist across the health system, including leadership/governance, healthcare financing, health workforce, medical products/technologies, information and research, and service delivery. Though still a relatively new field, implementation science holds promise for helping translate research into practice at sufficient scale to achieve population health impact and closing the gap between where we are and where we want to be.

Measurement and Evaluation

Measuring global health indicators, such as morbidity and mortality, is necessary but not sufficient for making informed decisions to direct sustainable growth and development. Monitoring involves repeating measurements over time and evaluation takes monitoring to the next level by critically assessing what the measurements mean and by benchmarking them. Evaluation may also be thought of as "critical thinking," or "reasoned judgments of the merit, worth or significance of policies, programs, strategies and systems."[12] Governments can use evaluation to help with budgeting, standardization, strengthening cross-sectoral planning, improving public accountability and performance, building a results framework, and decentralization.[13]

Although evaluation can be an excellent tool for planning and implementation, there are several barriers governments face when incorporating it into routine practice. Governments and individuals may be reluctant to conduct evaluations because they may be perceived as part of audits or inspections.[14] Often, evaluation is given a lower budget priority than health interventions themselves, which means it is frequently cut during times of economic hardship. Another challenge is making sure that decision-makers use the results of an evaluation. It may be helpful to include decision makers in the evaluation design,[14] though this must be balanced against considerations for keeping the evaluation objective or independent.[15] Political problems can also arise based on who conducts the evaluation, a problem we will return to later.

Measuring and evaluating progress in global health and development should be seen as an integral part of achieving that progress, as it enables stakeholders to make informed decisions and direct progress strategically. With local direction and ownership, measurement, and evaluation can be powerful tools for advancing progress.

EVALUATING PROGRESS IN GLOBAL HEALTH ON THE GLOBAL SCALE

Millennium Developmental Goals (MDGs)

Establishing the MDGs

The UN set the first cohesive set of health and development goals intended for use at a global scale at the 2000 UN Millennium Summit. World leaders signed the Millennium Declaration in order to draw global attention and commitment to what were seen as the foremost problems at the time, and to bring political legitimacy and coherence to development goals that had been set at various UN conferences throughout the 1990s.[16] In the year following the summit, a

UN committee working in consultation with 77 countries, the WHO, International Monetary Fund (IMF), World Bank, and various UN agencies worked out a "Road map toward the implementation of the United Nations Millennium Declaration" that formally laid out the MDGs and associated targets and indicators. There was debate from the beginning about whether indicators should be monitored at the global or national level, and how to set equal goals for nations in unequal circumstances. Several more years of technical debates and political negotiations followed before the United States, World Bank, and others really began to coalesce around the MDGs. At the 2005 UN World Summit, governments pledged to align their national goals with those of the MDGs, and three new targets were added to the original 18.[16]

Measuring success with the MDGs: Measuring success toward the MDGs was not easy. The UN chose 1990 as the baseline year for measuring progress, but some countries did not have data from 1990 and so have later baselines.[17] There was also debate over whether progress should be measured at the global or national level, if countries should be judged against themselves over time or against their peers, and whether by absolute progress or rate of progress. Since there is no comparison group at the global scale, some studies have analyzed trends in global development before and after the Millennium Declaration as a way to measure the impact of the MDGs.[17]

Despite these limitations, it would appear progress has been made toward many of the MDGs. An overarching achievement was bringing global attention to the problems of development by clearly articulating goals and targets,[18] and giving international, national, public, and private institutions common goals to work toward. The MDGs also drew attention to the need for better data to measure progress.[17] More specifically, there have been worldwide reductions in the number of people living in extreme poverty (less than $1.90/day in 2011 purchasing power parity), hunger, untreated HIV, and improvements in gender equality, child mortality, and maternal mortality. A good portion of this success was due to advances in China (Box 19-1),[17] though the Chinese government had begun working toward some of the goals years before the Millennium Summit.[19] China was able to achieve much by focusing resources on its poorest and most needy populations, as well as by prioritizing primary healthcare over expensive tertiary or hospital-based care.[19]

An analysis of 10 LMICs (Bangladesh, Cambodia, China, Egypt, Ethiopia, Lao People's Democratic Republic, Nepal, Peru, Rwanda, and Vietnam) that made significant absolute progress toward MDGs 4 and 5a by reducing maternal and child mortality revealed that good governance was key, through consistent and coordinated policies and programs. These countries improved data collection, which helped guide program decisions and accountability, strengthened health system delivery, expanded the health workforce, increased women's education, and improved infrastructure.[20]

Although the countries mentioned so far have been lauded for their success in reducing maternal and child mortality, it is important to recognize that success depends on the metric that is used. The World Bank reported that progress toward the MDGs lagged the most in sub-Saharan Africa (SSA), rural areas, and countries with fragile governments and high levels of conflict,[17] but they reached this conclusion by measuring absolute progress toward the goals. An analysis that instead measured rate of progress toward the goals using the same data found that SSA actually outperformed other regions in terms of how quickly progress was made toward the MDGs.[21]

BOX 19-1 MDG Success in China

China was one of the few countries to achieve MDG 5 by reducing maternal mortality by 75% between 1990 and 2015. The national Chinese government began working to reduce it in 1994, well before the Millennium Declaration, with the Law on Maternal and Infant Healthcare that specified skilled midwives should attend at-home births and write birth certificates. This was accompanied by National Plans of Action to implement the law, and further goals to improve coverage of the tetanus vaccine and the percentage of rural women giving birth at facilities.

In 1999, the National Working Committee on Children and Women within the Chinese MOH partnered with the WHO and the United Nations Children's Fund (UNICEF) to pilot a program aimed at increasing facility births and antenatal visits among rural women. This program successfully expanded over the years, and by 2009, 80% of the funds were still going to the poorest provinces. The program trained midwives and rural health staff to refer women with high-risk pregnancies to hospitals, and outlawed C-sections at smaller facilities. The program also held educational campaigns and gave financial incentives to encourage rural women to give birth at facilities. Introduced in 2003, a voluntary insurance program paid into by families and the government covered 97.5% of farmers by 2012. In 2009, the National Essential Health Services program began covering the costs of five antenatal visits and 42 days of postnatal care for women in rural areas. China also introduced various reforms to improve the health workforce, including increased college enrollments and incentives to attract doctors to rural areas.

Disparities in the maternal mortality rate still exist between urban and rural areas, and between high and low economic strata, and there are concerns that an emphasis on these measures may lead to underreporting. The central Chinese government now faces problems with increased costs of care, overprescribing, and misuse of services. It has the world's highest rates of C-sections and unnecessary ultrasounds (though this is driven largely by urban populations). However, this should not detract from the incredible progress China has achieved.[19]

Critique and Lessons Learned from the MDGs

Though there were many successes, there were also some failures with the MDGs. Politicians, researchers, health professionals, and others have highlighted lessons learned and areas for improvement. Some of the most common critiques include the following:

- *The MDGs were impractical.* There is an inherent tension when setting goals as to whether they should be aspirational or practical, and whether they should be flexible enough to work in different settings or set standards that can be used for benchmarking.[18] The MDGs leaned more toward the aspirational and inflexible side, so many complained that they were not practical or flexible enough for many countries to achieve them.[22]
- *The MDGs did not account for quality.* Some of the MDG indicators used to measure progress in public services like healthcare and clean water account for coverage, but not quality, which can miss meaningful differences. For example, when measuring access to clean water, without measuring quality there is no distinction made between someone who has a sink in their home, and someone who has to share a public tap with hundreds of neighbors.[23]
- *There was not enough input from people from LMICs.* A major concern with the MDGs has been that input was very limited at each stage of the process from the people of the LMICs the goals were intended to serve.[24] Though there was some consultation during the writing of the MDGs, it was not nearly enough. In SSA, much of the financing for development work to reach the MDGs came from donations from high-income countries (HICs), which left the recipient countries vulnerable to financial shocks when the donors decided to cut funding, and gave the donors leverage over policy decisions. Partially due to this lack of inclusion and ownership, for the most part the MDGs were not well integrated into national development plans. For example, the Nigerian government set their own goal called "Vision 2020" to be one of the top 20 world economies by 2020, but had to direct their resources toward the MDGs in order to qualify for foreign aid.[24]

- *The MDGs focus on outcomes instead of process.* The emphasis on development outcomes through targets and indicators rather than the root causes of the outcomes has led to some negative consequences.[25] For example, in some African countries, school lunches and stipends were used to increase enrollment, but without addressing the underlying social and cultural causes of low school attendance, improvements were not maintained when the incentives were taken away.[25]

The Sustainable Development Goals: An Improvement Over the MDGs?

Setting New Goals

As the 2015 deadline for the MDGs approached, the UN worked hard to define new goals for the next 15 years of global health and development: the SDGs. The SDGs needed to address MDG critiques and lessons and to respond to new challenges such as increased globalization through trade, finance, communications, and migration, and shifts toward increased urbanization, older populations, and noncommunicable diseases.[26] The result was 17 goals, broken down into 169 targets, with 230 indicators,[27] up from eight goals, 21 targets, and 60 indicators under the MDGs.[17] Health objectives made up three of the eight MDGs, but were consolidated under one of the 17 goals, SDG 3. Despite the reduced number of goals, the scope of health targets in the SDGs was expanded to include neglected tropical disease, noncommunicable disease, universal health coverage, environmental health, and injuries in addition to maternal health, child health, malaria, tuberculosis, and HIV/AIDS, which made up the MDG objectives.[17] There was also an increased emphasis on the interrelationships between goals, such as the effect of gender and education on health outcomes,[28] reflecting an evolution in understanding of the social determinants of health.

A major change in the SDGs as compared to the MDGs was the attempt to make them more inclusive, both in the planning and execution, and to have "no one left behind."[17] Though the MDGs applied only to LMICs, the SDGs included targets for equality and access that HICs could also strive for, as well as an entire goal focused on revitalizing global partnerships through trade and capacity building for sustainable development. The UN tried hard to include more voices from LMICs in the formulation of the SDGs by consulting with 193 governments and surveying seven million citizens in the "World We Want" project.[17] The Go4Health research consortium conducted focus groups with a number of marginalized populations to inform the writing of the SDGs as well,[29] but as they cautioned, there is a difference between participation and inclusion, and merely soliciting feedback from a wide array of stakeholders did not necessarily mean their input made it into the final drafts.[30]

Another departure from the MDGs was the inclusion of SDG goal 16, which recognized good governance as crucial to advancing development.[31] Although considered in the formulation of the MDGs, it was ultimately left out for political reasons, as it is one thing to encourage a country to improve their health statistics and quite another to tell them to improve their democratic process. However, because "having an honest and responsive government" was highly ranked by the citizens surveyed in the World We Want project, it was included in the SDGs. Goal 16 even implies a need for UN reforms to make governance at the global level more inclusive.[31]

Implementing and achieving SDGs: Figuring out how to implement and achieve the SDGs was for the most part left to the member nations to decide, which allowed the flexibility to adapt the goals to local circumstances, but also left a lot of hard work translating the goals into national priorities and programs. As the 17 SDGs cover quite a lot of ground, choosing where and how to focus efforts, and which indicators to use to measure progress will be crucial.[32] An interesting example of Pakistan's approach to this issue is presented in Box 19-2.

According to the 2017 progress report, based on self-assessments from 43 nations, most countries were still developing implementation plans and frameworks, and many identified low statistical and institutional capacities as key challenges.[34] The report highlighted the diversity of needs and approaches, and only 30% of countries reported on all 17 goals, the rest choosing a subset that they felt were of particular importance. There was general agreement on the need for more disaggregated and localized data, and engagement with subnational levels of government in order to reach the most disadvantaged populations and continue progress toward the goals.[34]

> **BOX 19-2 Identifying What Is Needed to Reach SDG 3 in Pakistan**
>
> Under the leadership of the Federal Ministry of Health and the WHO, Pakistan started a process to identify and address gaps, and to develop implementation plans and monitoring mechanisms to gauge progress for achieving SDG 3 at the country level. They charted Pakistan's rate of progress over the past 15 years and forecasted expected progress for each of the SDG 3 indicators. Next, they identified linkages among SDG 3 targets and the other 16 goals and mapped strategies, legislation, and programs at national and provincial levels to look for gaps and set milestones. Key personnel working in Health, Population, Nutrition, Water, and Sanitation were interviewed as part of a stakeholder analysis to identify integration efforts underway in national and provincial departments, barriers to implementation, and existing elements in program planning and implementation, which could improve local adaptation of SDG 3 targets.
>
> The data analysis showed that Pakistan's current rate of progress for SDG 3 targets is slow. With high maternal and child mortality and rising incidence of communicable diseases, the country is likely to miss global 2030 targets. Other barriers identified were wide provincial variation, and the need for a health survey to collect SDG 3 indicators. Plans were also made to improve multisectoral coordination mechanisms within federal and provincial departments in order to share experiential learning during the implementation of reforms. This analysis and planning process helped catalyze discussions and create awareness of the gaps and changes needed to achieve the targets of SDG 3. Monitoring will help maintain interest and synchronize provincial strategies to achieve the National Health Vision 2025 and the SDGs.[33]

Evaluating the SDGs

In addition to the international agencies such as the UN, WHO, and World Bank that monitor SDG progress, there is a need for countries to conduct their own evaluations of national progress. Although there are some advantages to monitoring the SDGs from a central agency, there are also some advantages to monitoring at national and local levels. Ultimately, coordinated monitoring at multiple levels will be needed, linked with support to increase local capacity.

Advantages to monitoring progress on SDGs and estimates of burden of disease being produced by international or independent organizations include a lower cost of statistical resources and greater perceived objectivity,[35] as well as standardized methods that make it easy to make direct comparisons between countries over time. Countries with limited capacity to collect and analyze data themselves can make use of these estimates. Internationally or independently produced estimates can help guide countries in setting priorities, but the ease of making comparisons is also explicitly intended to hold countries accountable when progress lags.[36] A study of several nations in Africa found that accountability mechanisms were most effective at national and subnational levels, particularly when civil society organizations and citizens got involved, and that adequate data and concrete implementation plans were also important.[37]

National governments can make use of global health estimates for political purposes, such as comparing themselves to peers, monitoring trends over time, and advocating for particular health issues, but they are much less useful for national planning and policy-making.[38] This is partially because estimates at the national level usually do not offer the level of detail needed for program planning, but also because local stakeholders may put more trust in locally produced estimates.[35] Factors that can influence trust in estimates include who paid for them, who produced them and why, how they are communicated, and what other uses they are being put to.[38] Countries that have more robust statistical capacity and hence are more involved in producing estimates in collaboration with international organizations may be more likely to make use of global estimates.[38] Ideally, international organizations work with countries to use local input and measures to inform global ones, and to build local analytical capacity.

Even though many national and international institutions use the same data sources, differences in data cleaning, analytic, and statistical methods can produce different results that can be difficult to reconcile.[36] Stakeholders worry about discrepancies in global health estimates because progress on certain indicators can sometimes determine funding. Ideally, institutions and local health administrators would work together to solve any discrepancies before results are widely published, to avoid confusion or political consequences. The media's preference for globally produced estimates over nationally produced ones may, in part, be due to their perceived objectivity. Indeed, national health administrators may be under political pressure to convey a sense of certainty despite large data gaps or error bars, or may even withhold information to avoid spreading panic or suffering severe containment measures when a high-profile disease such as cholera is detected.[38] It is important to recognize the need for global institutions and national governments to work together, in partnership, to promote sustainable, in-country surveillance and data monitoring, cleaning, and analysis capacity, so that the process of evaluating and monitoring SDG progress can strengthen national systems.

Other Systems that Monitor Global Health and Development at Global, Regional, and National Scales

Although the UN SDGs are probably the most widely used framework for evaluating progress in global health and development, other institutions set goals and monitor progress slightly differently, or on smaller scales. This type of work is complex and ongoing, and some examples help illustrate the need for improved communication and coordination at the different levels. Though far from a comprehensive list, here we give a few examples of goals and evaluation efforts from the World Bank, the African Union, and the South Asian Association for Regional Cooperation, and talk about the process at the national level.

Global Scale

In addition to being a major supporter of the UN SDGs, the World Bank has articulated its own global goals: to reduce the proportion of people living in extreme poverty ($<$\$1.25/day in 2005 constant dollars) to $\leq$3% of the world's population by 2030, and to improve prosperity in the bottom 40% of the population in each of its member countries.[17] While these are very similar to SDGs 1 and 10, differences in wording and indicators make the UN goals slightly more focused on reducing inequality. Though the World Bank's goals explicitly only address poverty, they have made clear in their reports that this will require addressing many of the same needs outlined in the SDGs. They have also acknowledged the need to work together, and are committed to helping the UN particularly with the financing and monitoring of the SDGs.[17]

Regional Scale

Though the World Bank's goals are very similar to the SDGs, the African Union's (AU) Agenda 2063 has a very different timeline and structure.[39] The African Union consists of 55 member nations and was officially launched in 2002, growing out of the Organization of African Unity. They have outlined seven Aspirations to be completed by 2063, with accompanying goals, targets, and indicators and the first 10-year implementation plan. The Aspirations were developed with input from African youth, women, civil society organizations, researchers, government planners, and inter-faith leaders, as well as input from national governments and reviews of past experiences with development projects. The seven Aspirations are:

1. A prosperous Africa based on inclusive growth and sustainable development.
2. An integrated continent, politically united based on the ideals of Pan Africanism and the vision of Africa's Renaissance.
3. An Africa of good governance, democracy, respect for human rights, justice, and the rule of law.
4. A peaceful and secure Africa.
5. An Africa with a strong cultural identity, common heritage, values, and ethics.
6. An Africa whose development is people driven, relying on the potential of African people, especially its women and youth, and caring for children.
7. Africa as a strong, united, resilient, and influential global player and partner.[39]

The Aspirations place less emphasis than the SDGs on material needs, and more on cultural unity and peace, but at the goal and indicator level, there is actually quite a bit of overlap.[40]

Although the UN's SDGs and the AU's Agenda 2063 are separate, the AU produced the Common African Position based on their Aspirations to inform the creation of the SDGs.[40] The UN Development Program (UNDP) estimates that the SDGs and the Agenda 2063 overlap by 89.2% when comparing specific goals and targets.[40] The First 10-Year Implementation Plan for Agenda 2063 includes an explanation of this overlap so that African nations can work toward common goals using common indicators,[39] and at a conference with the United Nations Economic Commission for Africa they agreed to integrate implementation and monitoring so as not to overburden African nations.[41] For accountability purposes, the AU created the African Health Stats website so citizens, governments, and anyone who wants to can compare health indicators across 54 of its member states.[37]

In Asia, the South Asian Association for Regional Cooperation (SAARC) composed of eight member countries, instead of coming up with new goals, has worked to "localize" the MDGs and SDGs and promote international cooperation and collaboration.[42] In 2007, over concerns that the MDGs would not be achieved on time, SAARC's Commission on Poverty Alleviation worked with the UNDP to come up with a subset of SAARC Development Goals, indicators, and a 5-year monitoring plan intended to piggy-back on the systems already in place to monitor the MDGs. The intention of the SAARC Development Goals was to draw attention from national governments to critical areas (livelihood, health, education, and environment), and to advocate for more resources.[42] In 2010, the SAARC Development Fund was established to help finance development programs,[43] and they began collecting and publishing best practices for poverty alleviation to be shared throughout the region. In 2014, SAARC announced they would begin working toward the SDGs, starting by relating them to regional and national development goals and plans.[44]

A number of regional coalitions organized around specific challenges like malaria, zoonotic disease, and health systems strengthening also exist. For example, the African Leader's Malaria Alliance provides a forum for African nations to share best practices for eliminating malaria, and a scorecard that leaders can use to track progress on priority indicators.[45] This scorecard, available as a mobile app, has been so popular that additional indicators in areas such as maternal and child health have been added. The organization also removes indicators when targets are achieved, and recognizes progress through awards of excellence that change with priorities.[45] The Asia Pacific Leaders' Malaria Alliance is a similar organization in Southeast Asia.[46]

Another initiative that is research focused, rather than policy oriented, is the One Health Network—South Asia. Launched by Massey University in New Zealand with support from the World Bank, public health and animal health professionals from seven Asian countries were offered graduate training in epidemiology and biosecurity, and then established research hubs in their home countries. The network has helped improve international research and response to zoonotic disease in the region.[47] As a final example, the Asia Pacific Network for Health Systems Strengthening is a consortium established by nine initial member nations and the World Bank to build capacity for evidence-based health systems and work toward universal health coverage.[48] The network offers courses and holds summits for policymakers and academics to share successes and learn from each other.[48] While these latter two organizations set goals in their mission statements, they are oriented toward knowledge sharing and do not collect data on specific indicators or monitor progress toward them.

These regional organizations help countries that may be facing similar problems, share resources and lessons across borders, and reinforce commitments to development goals. Not all regions have such formal networks though (i.e., Latin America), and ultimately, success in development more often depends on what is being done on smaller scales.

National Scale

Every country has their own process for setting national priorities and health agendas, such as Healthy People in the United States,[49] National Health Objectives in Chile,[50] Healthy China,[51] or National Health Vision 2016–25 in Pakistan.[52] Although the processes differ from country to country, often the broadest level of government sets health priorities and defines indicators, and in many cases leaves implementation up to specialized or regional branches of the government. Many countries also make an effort to solicit feedback from citizens and the healthcare sector when setting priorities, ensure they are addressing the greatest perceived needs, and revisit the agenda every few years.

Once a health agenda has been agreed on and health interventions have been set through policy and programs, continuous evaluation helps countries stay on track. The UN has been a big advocate of incorporating evaluation into global health and development work in recent years through their Evaluation Group, that has established a set of Norms and Standards for Evaluation,[15] as well as an Evaluation Competency Framework to help guide member nations in establishing National Evaluation Policies (NEPs).[53] NEPs define how a government intends to use evaluation to get feedback on their programs and services.

A survey of the status of NEPs in 2015 found a lot of variety among the 109 countries surveyed, with 59 nations practicing some sort of evaluation and 29 having a formal decree or policy requiring that the government conduct evaluations.[14] Some countries with robust evaluation practices, such as Australia and the United Kingdom, do not have a formal NEP, though they do set health goals and monitor progress toward them. All countries have to find a balance between a centralized, standardized evaluation system that may reduce workload and increase comparability between government sectors, and a decentralized system that is flexible enough to respond to local needs. Overall, the survey concluded that a formal NEP was not strictly necessary but helpful for keeping programs and policies effective and up-to-date.[14]

THE ROLE OF TECHNOLOGY IN EVALUATING PROGRESS IN GLOBAL HEALTH

Technology in the form of electronic health information systems can be useful for monitoring and evaluating global health, if the system is organized, connectivity is reliable, and human resources are available to put them to good use. Both physical infrastructure (connectivity, electricity, computers, etc.), and human resources who know how to use the system are critical. A common mistake is to assume that technology is the ultimate solution, when often the process of planning and developing a blueprint of the information structure and determining the use to which data and indicators will be put to is more important. Technology can help improve efficiency, once the processes have been determined and optimized. Technology can be a catalyst for improvements, but without appropriate training and support we risk just digitizing chaos. Since the burden of collecting and entering data into a health information system usually falls on healthcare workers (who are often short-staffed or overworked), it is vital that data collection improve rather than detract from healthcare.[54] In other words, accurate data collection should be a byproduct of service provision. A well-designed electronic medical record system could serve providers to offer better care for their patients as well as serve as a source for health data.

Equally important is that the primary purpose of a technological change should be to improve ease and delivery of healthcare, not just to increase data collection. A group that worked in Bihar, India to develop mobile health applications to be used by maternal and child health workers made improving quality of service their primary goal with data collection a secondary goal.[55] They designed a mobile scheduling assistant that created timelines and reminders for well-child visits for all the patients a health worker was responsible for. During a visit, the app prompted the health worker with questions to ask the patient, and then gave multiple-choice options accompanied by pictures to enter in answers. The app was a success because it made the providers' jobs easier, and allowed them to enter data quickly throughout their visits, rather than leaving it all for the end.[55]

Another good example of an improved health information system comes from Ethiopia, where the MOH improved data collection with help from the United States Agency for International Development's (USAID) Monitoring and Evaluation to Assess and Use Results (MEASURE) program.[56] In 2007, Ethiopian healthcare workers were being asked to collect over 1000 indicators on each patient that visited a healthcare facility in order to satisfy donor agency requests for data. Most of the staff in the statistical departments responsible for processing all of these indicators were health workers who had not performed well at treating patients, and thus were not particularly trained or motivated to work with health information systems. The Ethiopian MOH instituted reforms to help get relevant data to decision-makers and reduced the number of indicators to be reported at the national level to a more manageable 170 that were useful for national level programmatic or policy decisions. The MOH also created a new career Health Information Technician (HIT) to take advantage of data at the facility level to improve planning, quality improvement, and decision-making.[56]

HITs undergo 3 years of training in data recording, analysis, and reporting before they are placed at Ethiopian health facilities.[57] Two years after program implementation, 1736 students enrolled in HIT training.[58] They have since gone on to vastly improve the quality of Ethiopia's health information system.[56] Although HITs are trained to use computers and electronic record systems, for rural areas, the Ethiopian MOH realized a paper-based system was more practical for tracking patients and filling needs in the short term, as it was more easily understood by local staff. With time, rural clinics will also be converted to electronic systems as computer literacy becomes more widespread, a process that has already begun in a number of clinics. So, though technology has played a role in improving Ethiopia's health information systems, investments in human resources have been even more important.[56]

USAID has also helped Pakistan establish a Health Planning, Systems Strengthening and Information Analysis Unit to collect and analyze data for the Ministry of National Health Services and Coordination.[59] The goal of this Unit is to start a national discourse and promote evidence-based policies that will foster innovation and address Pakistan's health needs. An integrated health monitoring system captures data from the provinces, as well as surveys, and indicators and survey results are published in an online dashboard.[60] Progress toward the SDGs is also tracked on the dashboard, and it provides quick and easy access to data for Pakistani decision-makers, international organizations, local medical staff, and anyone else who might be interested.

HOW DO WE BUILD CAPACITY FOR EVALUATION IN GLOBAL HEALTH MOVING FORWARD?

Despite many challenges, we have seen much progress in global health over the past few decades. Moving forward, we must learn from past successes and mistakes to continue building national capacity to evaluate progress in global health and to promote such progress.

Present Challenges

Progress toward better health on a global level will require a lot of work at national and local levels. Evidence shows that countries that were missing the most data on MDG indicators also performed the worst on the MDG goals, even after controlling for statistical capacity and basic infrastructure.[61] Though the lack of data may impede progress toward the MDGs, this data gap may also indicate that these countries did not make the MDGs a priority and were not actively working toward them. The development efforts that will be successful will be those led by locals. LMICs and HICs must forge coequal, mutually beneficial partnerships at every step.[62]

A difficulty that arises in all parts of the world is a resistance to focus on the most vulnerable populations, particularly when they are socially stigmatized. An example of this is populations at high risk of HIV, such as transgender people and injection drug users.[63] Despite all UN member nations agreeing to report on these key populations, as of 2016 only 20 have done so. Without this data, there has been little motivation to act in favor of these groups.[63]

Recent Successes

We see that successful global evaluation efforts engage more with local stakeholders. Although initial monitoring of the HIV epidemic began with a few WHO statisticians in Geneva, in 2003 UNAIDS developed user-friendly software and began conducting international workshops that improved the capacity to produce and use HIV data in LMICs.[64] Another successful project was a collaboration between the IHME and more than 100 institutions (mostly Indian) to produce state-level estimates of disease burden in India. National estimates are totally inadequate for a country as large as India, and this study was partially funded by the Government of India with the intention that it be used to inform their National Health Policy 2017.[65] In contrast, another study estimated child mortality in Africa at a subnational level using sophisticated statistical techniques,[66] but with no African authors or funding involved. It is less certain that this study will be used to inform local decisions.

A great example of a successful collaboration was the reduction of stunting due to chronic malnutrition in children under 5 in Peru from 28% to 13% of children between 2008 and 2016.[67] A collection of 18 national and international organizations headed by UNICEF, CARE Peru, and the Pan American Health Organization brought stunting to national awareness during the 2006 presidential campaign, by getting 10 presidential candidates to sign a commitment to reduce stunting in children under 5 by 5 percentage points in 5 years (The 5-by-5-in-5 Goal). The new president followed through with his commitment and worked with the private sector, NGOs, and different levels of government to set regional targets and implement evidence-based programs to reduce stunting in some of the poorest areas of the country. Three successive presidents have continued the commitment to reducing child nutrition, with the latest goal set by President Kuczynski to reduce chronic malnutrition to 6% of children under 5 by 2021, and reduce anemia to 19%.[67]

CONCLUSION

It is no accident that Peru's success in reducing child stunting, China's success in addressing maternal and child health, and many of the other successes we have seen in global health have followed the four-step process:

1. Know where we are;
2. Decide where we want to go;
3. Decide how to close the gap between where we are and where we want to be; and
4. Measure and evaluate progress along the way to make sure we reach our goals.

Good evaluation requires goals and targets for framing, and relies on processes to collect, clean, and analyze data. The utility of evaluation depends on how closely it feeds back to and is accepted by major stakeholders, who are able to make decisions that affect progress toward the goals and targets.

Although some countries remain unable to collect or process their own health data, collaborations between governments and global agencies should help build sustainable capacity to do so, in addition to focusing on getting data. There has already been tremendous change in many countries, but there are more opportunities to strengthen data and analytic systems, as well as strategic planning, monitoring, and evaluation processes. As the global community concluded while drafting the SDGs, further improvement will depend on our ability to alleviate poverty in the most hard-to-reach places,[26] bringing health improvements to rural and marginalized populations.

References

1. Maurice J. Measuring progress towards the SDGs—A new vital science. *Lancet.* 2016;388(10053):1455–8.
2. Health Data Collaborative—Data for health and sustainable development. Health Data Collaborative. https://www.healthdatacollaborative.org/. Accessed January 4, 2018.
3. Edelstein M, Lee LM, Herten-Crabb A, Heymann DL, Harper DR. Strengthening global public health surveillance through data and benefit sharing. *Emerg Infect Dis.* 2018;24(7):1324–30.
4. Redford S, Alexander L. What data sources go into the GBD? http://www.healthdata.org/acting-data/what-data-sources-go-gbd. Accessed June 26, 2018.
5. Jones CM, Clavier C, Potvin L. Adapting public policy theory for public health research: A framework to understand the development of national policies on global health. *Soc Sci Med.* 2017;177(Suppl C):69–77.
6. Nicod M, Dapaah MB. International Health Partnership and related initiatives (IHP+). Partnerships for the SDGs. https://sustainabledevelopment.un.org/partnership/?p=11941. Accessed June 20, 2018.
7. Nabyonga-Orem J, Ousman K, Estrelli Y, et al. Perspectives on health policy dialogue: Definition, perceived importance and coordination. *BMC Health Serv Res.* 2016;16(Suppl 4):218.
8. SMART criteria. In: *Wikipedia*; 2018. https://en.wikipedia.org/w/index.php?title=SMART_criteria&oldid=846413452.
9. Jamison DT. *Disease Control Priorities*, 3rd edition: Improving health and reducing poverty. *Lancet.* 2018;391(10125):e11–14.
10. Jamison DT, Alwan A, Mock CN, et al. Universal health coverage and intersectoral action for health: Key messages from *Disease Control Priorities*, 3rd edition. *Lancet.* 2018;391(10125):1108–20.
11. DCP3. http://dcp-3.org/. Accessed March 19, 2018.
12. Schwandt T, Ofir Z, Lucks D, El-Saddick K, D'Errico S. *Evaluation: A Crucial Ingredient for SDG Success.* London: The International Institute for Environment and Development; 2016. http://pubs.iied.org/pdfs/17357IIED.pdf. Accessed November 29, 2017.
13. Bamberger M, Segone M, Shravanti R. *National Evaluation Policies for Sustainable and Equitable Development: How to Integrate Gender Equality and Social Equity in National Evaluation Policies and Systems.* Segone M, ed. https://evalpartners.org/sites/default/files/documents/evalgender/NationalEvaluationPolicies_web-single-color%281%29.pdf. Accessed November 29, 2017.
14. Rosenstein B. *Status of National Evaluation Policies Global Mapping Report.* Parliamentarians Forum on Development Evaluation in South Asia with EvalPartners; 2015. http://www.pfde.net/images/pdf/gmrnew.pdf. Accessed November 29, 2017.

15. *Norms and Standards for Evaluation*. New York: United Nations Evaluation Group; 2016. http://www.uneval.org/document/detail/1914. Accessed November 29, 2017.
16. McArthur JW. The origins of the Millennium Development Goals. *SAIS Rev Int Aff.* 2014;34(2):5–24.
17. *Scaling Up Impact: Transitioning from Millennium to Sustainable Development Goals*. The World Bank; 2015. http://ebookcentral.proquest.com/lib/washington/detail.action?docID=4397384 Accessed January 27, 2021.
18. Rosenbaum B. Making the Millennium Development Goals (MDGs) sustainable. *Harv Int Rev*. 2015;37(1):62–64.
19. Gao Y, Zhou H, Singh NS, et al. Progress and challenges in maternal health in western China: A Countdown to 2015 national case study. *Lancet Glob Health*. 2017;5(5):e523–36.
20. Ahmed SM, Rawal LB, Chowdhury SA, et al. Cross-country analysis of strategies for achieving progress towards global goals for women's and children's health. *Bull World Health Organ*. 2016;94(5):351–61.
21. Fukuda-Parr S, Greenstein J, Stewart D. How should MDG success and failure be judged: Faster progress or achieving the targets? *World Dev.* 2013;41(Suppl C):19–30.
22. Vandemoortele J. If not the Millennium Development Goals, then what? *Third World Q*. 2011;32(1):9–25.
23. Satterthwaite D. Guiding the goals: Empowering local actors. *SAIS Rev Int Aff.* 2014;3(2):51–61.
24. Uneze E, Adedeji A. The MDGs' Financing Framework and its implications for the post-2015 Development Agenda: An African perspective. *SAIS Rev Int Aff.* 2014;34(2):103–11.
25. Uneze E, Adedeji A. The MDGs' Financing Framework and its implications for the post-2015 Development Agenda: An African perspective. *SAIS Rev Int Aff.* 2014;34(2):103–11.
26. Scaling Up Impact: Transitioning from Millennium to Sustainable Development Goals. In: *Global Monitoring Report 2015/2016: Development Goals in an Era of Demographic Change*.
27. Yonehara A, Saito O, Hayashi K, Nagao M, Yanagisawa R, Matsuyama K. The role of evaluation in achieving the SDGs. *Sustain Sci*. 2017;12(6):969–73.
28. Edouard L, Bernstein S. Challenges for measuring progress towards the Sustainable Development Goals. *Afr J Reprod Health*. 2016;20(3):45–54.
29. Brolan CE, Hussain S, Friedman EA, et al. Community participation in formulating the post-2015 health and development goal agenda: Reflections of a multi-country research collaboration. *Int J Equity Health*. 2014;13:66.
30. Siddiqui FR. Annotated bibliography on participatory consultations to help aid the inclusion of marginalized perspectives in setting policy agendas. *Int J Equity Health*. 2014;13:124. https://equityhealthj.biomedcentral.com/track/pdf/10.1186/s12939-014-0124-0?site=equityhealthj.biomedcentral.com. Accessed December 12, 2017.
31. Edwards M, Romero S. Governance and the Sustainable Development Goals: Changing the game or more of the same? *SAIS Rev Int Aff.* 2014;34(2):141–50.
32. Biermann F, Kanie N, Kim RE. Global governance by goal-setting: The novel approach of the UN Sustainable Development Goals. *Curr Opin Environ Sustain*. 2017;26:26–31.
33. Hamid S. Localizing the SDG 3 Agenda in Pakistan. July 2018.
34. *Synthesis Report of Voluntary National Reviews 2017*. United Nations: High-Level Political Forum on Sustainable Development; 2017. https://sustainabledevelopment.un.org/content/documents/17109Synthesis_Report_VNRs_2017.pdf. Accessed November 28, 2017.
35. AbouZahr C, Boerma T, Hogan D. Global estimates of country health indicators: Useful, unnecessary, inevitable? *Glob Health Action*. 2017;10(Supp 1):1290370.
36. Maurice J. Measuring progress towards the SDGs—A new vital science. *Lancet*. 2016;388(10053):1455–8.
37. Ten Hoope-Bender P, Martin Hilber A, Nove A, et al. Using advocacy and data to strengthen political accountability in maternal and newborn health in Africa. *Int J Gynaecol Obstet*. 2016;135(3):358–64.
38. Pisani E, Kok M. In the eye of the beholder: To make global health estimates useful, make them more socially robust. *Glob Health Action*. 2017;10(Supp 1):1266180.
39. Used with permission from African Union Commission. Goals & Priority Areas of Agenda 2063. https://au.int/en/agenda2063/goals. Accessed January 23, 2018.
40. *Strengthening Strategic Alignment for Africa's Development Lessons from the UN 2030 Agenda for Sustainable Development*. UNDP Regional Bureau for Africa; 2017.
41. Ninsiima G, Sellami S, Ibrahim IB, Mwangi AW, Kry S, Ahmadi J. *Economic Integration and Development Partnerships: Southern Perspectives*. New Delhi: Research and Information System for Developing Countries; 2017. http://ris.org.in/pdf/Final_ITEC_Report_2017_.pdf#page=43. Accessed June 28, 2018.
42. *SAARC Development Goals (SDGs) 2007–2012: Taking SDGs Forward*. Independent South Asian Commission on Poverty Alleviation; 2007. http://saarc-sec.org/download/publications/TAKING_SDGs_FORWARD_(saarc-sec_20100616032736.pdf. Accessed March 14, 2018.
43. SAARC Development Fund: Regional Integration through Project Funding & Collaboration. About SDF. http://www.sdfsec.org/about-sdf. Published 2016. Accessed March 15, 2018.
44. South Asian Association for Regional Cooperation. http://saarc-sec.org/. Published 2018. Accessed March 14, 2018.
45. The African Leaders Malaria Alliance. ALMA 2030. http://www.alma2030.org/. Accessed November 10, 2018.
46. Asia Pacific Leaders Malaria Alliance Secretariat (APLMA). APLMA. http://aplma.org/. Accessed November 10, 2018.
47. One Health Network South Asia. http://www.onehealthnetwork.asia/. Accessed November 10, 2018.
48. Asia Pacific Network for Health Systems Strengthening. ANHSS. http://www.anhss.org/. Accessed November 12, 2018.
49. Healthy People 2020. https://www.healthypeople.gov/. Accessed March 20, 2018.
50. Aguilera XP, Espinosa-Marty C, Castillo-Laborde C, Gonzalez C. From instinct to evidence: The role of data in country decision-making in Chile. *Glob Health Action*. 2017;10(Suppl 1): 1266176.
51. Healthy China 2030 (from vision to action). WHO. http://www.who.int/healthpromotion/conferences/9gchp/healthy-china/en/. Accessed June 19, 2018.
52. *National Health Vision Pakistan 2016–2025*. Islamabad, Pakistan: Ministry of National Health Services, Regulations and Coordination. http://www.nationalplanningcycles.org/sites/default/files/planning_cycle_repository/pakistan/national_health_vision_2016-25_30-08-2016.pdf. Accessed September 11, 2018.
53. *Evaluation Competency Framework*. New York: United Nations Evaluation Group; 2016. http://www.uneval.org/document/detail/1915. Accessed November 29, 2017.
54. Thomas JC, Silvestre E, Salentine S, Reynolds H, Smith J. What systems are essential to achieving the sustainable development goals and what will it take to marshal them? *Health Policy Plan*. 2016;31(10):1445–7.
55. Krishnan BR. Accurate data collection became a byproduct of service provision. *CARE India*. May 2015. https://www.careindia.org/blog/accurate-data-collection-became-a-byproduct-of-service-provision/. Accessed June 15, 2018.
56. Birhani K. Health Information Strengthening in Ethiopia. November 2017.
57. *Model Curriculum: Health Information Technology (HIT) Level IV*. Ethiopia: Federal TVET Agency; 2016.
58. *Health Information Technicians Training on ARM Report*.
59. *Technical and Management Assistance to Ministry of National Health Services Regulations and Coordination: Federal Component Health System Strengthening*. Islamabad, Pakistan: JSI Research & Training Institute.
60. PHIS—Integrated & Analytical Dashboard. http://nhsrc.pk/. Published 2018. Accessed December 5, 2018.
61. Jacob A. Mind the gap: Analyzing the impact of data gap in Millennium Development Goals' (MDGs) indicators on the progress toward MDGs. *World Dev.* 2017;93(Suppl C):260–78.
62. Pisani E, Kok M. In the eye of the beholder: To make global health estimates useful, make them more socially robust. *Glob Health Action*. 2017;10(sup1):1266180.
63. Davis SLM. The uncounted: Politics of data and visibility in global health. *Int J Hum Rights*. 2017;21(8):1144–63.
64. Mahy M, Brown T, Stover J, et al. Producing HIV estimates: From global advocacy to country planning and impact measurement. *Glob Health Action*. 2017;10(Supp 1):1291169.
65. Dandona L, Dandona R, Kumar GA, et al. Nations within a nation: Variations in epidemiological transition across the states of India, 1990–2016 in the Global Burden of Disease Study. *Lancet*. November 2017;390(10111):2437–60.
66. Golding N, Burstein R, Longbottom J, et al. Mapping under-5 and neonatal mortality in Africa, 2000–15: A baseline analysis for the Sustainable Development Goals. *Lancet*. 2017;390(10108):2171–82.
67. Marini A, Rokx C, Gallagher P. *Standing Tall: Peru's Success in Overcoming Its Stunting Crisis*. Washington, DC: The World Bank; 2017.

APPENDIX 1:

Acronyms used:

AU African Union

GBD Global Burden of Diseases, Injuries, and Risk Factors Study

HIC High-income country

HIT Health Information Technician

IHME Institute for Health Metrics and Evaluation

IMF International Monetary Fund

LMIC Low- and middle-income countries

MDG Millennium Development Goal

MOH Ministry of Health

NEP National Evaluation Policy

NES National Evaluation System

OECD Organization for Economic Co-operation and Development

SDG Sustainable Development Goal

SSA Sub-Saharan Africa

UN United Nations

UNDP United Nations Development Program

UNICEF United Nations Children's Fund

USAID United States Agency for International Development

WHO World Health Organization

CHAPTER

20

Implementation Science: A New Research Paradigm to Accelerate Global Health Impact at Scale

Bryan J. Weiner • Arianna Rubin Means • Melissa Mugambi • Peter Cherutich

The World Health Organization estimates that 13.2 million deaths in 2005 resulted from causes for which proven, low-cost prevention and treatment interventions exist.[1,2] Ten years later, while fewer preventable deaths occurred, still more than 10 million deaths in 2015 were attributed to causes with known, low-cost prevention or treatment options.[1] Since 2005, there have been significant reductions in the excess mortality that low- and middle-income countries (LMICs) experience relative to high-income countries (HICs), particularly due to declining child mortality and deaths due to HIV/AIDS and malaria.[1,2] Yet, despite these reductions in mortality, millions of lives are lost each year from preventable or treatable illnesses and health problems.[1,2]

All women need access to antenatal care in pregnancy, skilled care during childbirth, and care and support in the weeks after childbirth.[3] Nonetheless, millions of women do not receive these lifesaving services. In 2015 alone, an estimated 300,000 women died from preventable causes related to only to pregnancy and childbirth,[4] even though the solutions to prevent or manage life-threatening complications in pregnancy and childbirth are well known.

A similar gap exists in malaria prevention. An estimated 439,000 malaria deaths occurred worldwide in 2015,[1] even though insecticide-treated mosquito nets and indoor spraying of insecticides are known to be effective strategies for preventing and reducing malaria transmission.[5] Although the consequences of contracting malaria are severe, nearly half of the population at risk does not sleep under a treated net, and the proportion of the population at risk benefiting from indoor residual spraying declined from a peak of 5.7% globally in 2010 to 3.1% in 2015.[5]

As these examples attest, the issue is not whether effective health interventions exist, but rather whether effective health interventions are implemented to reach those who would benefit from them. While the knowledge exists to solve many of the world's health problems, a persistent gap remains between knowing what to do (the "know") and putting that knowledge into action (the "do"). It is this gap that the field of implementation science aims to address.

IMPLEMENTATION SCIENCE DEFINED

Implementation science seeks to close the "know-do gap" by systematically identifying and addressing the barriers that hinder access to and use of effective health interventions. Put differently, implementation science involves the systematic study of both the processes used to implement effective health interventions, as well as the contextual factors that affect these processes.[6] As is common in rapidly developing scientific fields, consensus has yet to emerge on the scope of implementation science or its relationship to other emerging fields.[7]

Definitions of implementation science vary from relatively narrow formulations, such as "the study of methods to promote the uptake of research findings into routine healthcare in clinical, organizational or policy contexts,"[8] to broad formulations such as "scientific inquiry into [all] questions concerning implementation."[9] Some definitions of the field include the scientific investigation of the scale of the "know-do gap" or the factors that contribute to its existence[10–12]; other definitions do not.[13–15] Some definitions of the field emphasize the production of generalizable knowledge,[8,16,17] while others emphasize the generation of local solutions.[18–20]

A broad definition of the field suitable for the wide scope and high aspiration of global health, and embraced by the authors of this chapter, is that implementation science asks and answers the fundamental question: how do we get "what works" to people who need it with greater speed, fidelity, efficiency, quality, sustainability, and relevant coverage? This broad definition promotes the systematic application of research methods from diverse disciplines as essential for understanding the context, processes, and outcomes of implementation and, ultimately, scale-up to achieve population-level health benefits. Though not exhaustive, ten research methods and approaches figure prominently in implementation science, as defined here (see Fig. 20-1).

Implementation science overlaps with other emerging or rapidly developing sciences, such as improvement science, program science, and delivery science. As with implementation science, consensus has yet to emerge on the scope and boundaries of these other sciences. While all are concerned with getting "what works" into practice to improve health, there appear to be subtle, yet important differences in their foci. Improvement science, for example, focuses more narrowly on maximizing the learning from improvement efforts and optimizing

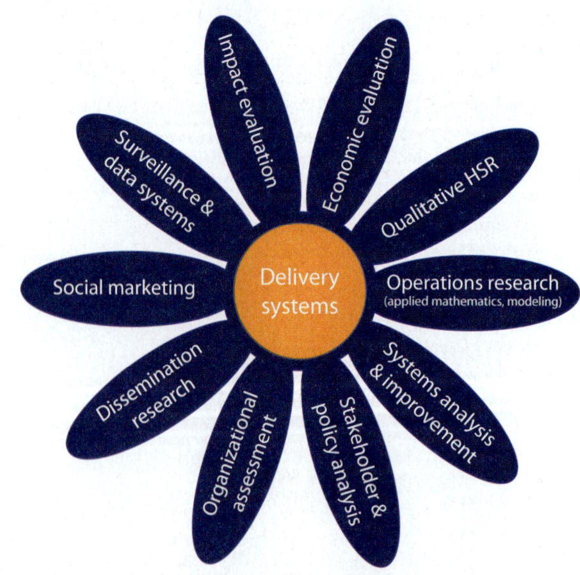
Impact evaluation
Economic evaluation
Surveillance & data systems
Qualitative HSR
Social marketing
Delivery systems
Operations research
(applied mathematics, modeling)
Dissemination research
Systems analysis & improvement
Organizational assessment
Stakeholder & policy analysis

FIGURE 20-1. Implementation science methods flower.

the local benefits of locally generated solutions.[21,22] Program science places greater emphasis on generating research questions by and with program staff and applying scientific knowledge and methods in strategic planning, program implementation, and program management to improve population health.[23] Delivery science focuses broadly on strengthening the capacity of health systems and other societal sectors to implement public policies and demonstrate results.[24] Implementation science's similarities and differences with these other sciences will crystalize as these various fields mature, perhaps leading to a convergence of these fields.

Implementation science differs from clinical or behavioral intervention science in that the latter focuses on establishing the effectiveness of a health intervention, whereas the former focuses on identifying effective methods or strategies for integrating health interventions into routine practice, ideally at large scale. In a sense, implementation science picks up where intervention science leaves off in that it begins with the output of intervention science: an effective health intervention. High-impact science requires a seamless synergy across these two types of researches.

The differences between implementation science and intervention science become apparent when designing clinical trials and implementation trials. Clinical trials evaluate the effectiveness of an intervention thought to improve health outcomes, such as aspirin after myocardial infarction, pre-exposure prophylaxis for the prevention of HIV infection, bed nets, cook stoves, and bike paths. Implementation trials evaluate the effectiveness of an *implementation strategy*, that is, a method or technique to facilitate adoption and integration of an intervention into routine use. An implementation strategy can be a single method, such as task shifting, or a bundle of methods that address multiple implementation barriers (e.g., training to address knowledge and skill barriers, incentives to address motivational barriers, and changing delivery venue to improve access[25]). In clinical trials, the primary outcomes of interest are usually health outcomes, such as mortality, morbidity, functional health status, or quality of life. In implementation trials, the primary outcomes of interest are often indicators of successful implementation, such as adoption of the clinical or policy intervention by healthcare professionals and/or community members, quality of intervention delivery, or sustained delivery of the intervention. Ultimately, these implementation outcomes should be linked to individual or population health outcomes. The key to distinguishing implementation science from intervention science is that the latter focuses on identifying effective interventions to improve health outcomes, whereas the former focuses on ensuring that effective interventions reach those who need them.

Implementation science can be considered a type of health systems research,[26] which is a broader class of research that aims to enhance the efficiency and effectiveness of the health system. Health systems research focuses on issues affecting some or all of the six building blocks of a health system: leadership/governance, healthcare financing, health workforce, medical products/technologies, information and research, and service delivery. Within health systems research, implementation science focuses on issues affecting the delivery of specific health interventions. Health interventions include programs (e.g., Diabetes Prevention Program), practices (e.g., nutritional counseling), principles (e.g., shared decision-making), products (e.g., vaccines), pills (e.g., medications), and policies (e.g., indoor smoking bans) that improve health outcomes, health behaviors, or health-related environments.[27]

EMERGENCE OF IMPLEMENTATION SCIENCE IN THE UNITED STATES

Implementation science is not new. Researchers in the United States have studied the implementation of innovative programs in healthcare organizations since the 1960s,[28] and perhaps even earlier. However, implementation science did not develop into an organized, institutionally supported field of study in the United States until the mid-2000s.

The year 2006 proved a watershed for the emergence of the field of implementation science in the United States. That year, as part of a broader effort to accelerate the medical research process,[29] the National Institutes of Health (NIH) launched the Clinical Translational Science Awards (CTSA) to develop the scientific workforce and programmatic infrastructure needed to conduct translational research.[30] Initially, translational research focused on two "bottlenecks" slowing the speed with which biomedical research discoveries resulted in improvements in health.[14] The first bottleneck (originally labeled "T1") concerned "the transfer of new understandings of disease mechanisms gained in the laboratory into the development of new methods for diagnosis, therapy, and prevention and their first testing in humans."[31] The second bottleneck (originally labeled "T2") concerned "the translation of results from clinical studies into everyday clinical practice and health decision making."[31] Since then, translational research has identified several additional bottlenecks (see Fig. 20-2)[32]; however, the articulation of the T2 bottleneck was crucial for bringing attention and funding to implementation science, which is now, as discussed later, considered "T3" research.

Another major driver of U.S. implementation science was the 2006 Trans-NIH Program Announcement on Dissemination and Implementation Research in Health (DIRH PAR). Previously, the National Cancer Institute and other Institutes and Centers supported dissemination and implementation research through administrative supplements to funded grants.[33] The DIRH PAR represented the first and most significant trans-NIH initiative to encourage investigators to submit research grants to identify, develop, and test "models to disseminate and implement research-tested health behavior change interventions and evidence-based prevention, early detection, diagnostic, treatment, and quality of life improvement services into public health and clinical practice settings."[34] Eight NIH Institutes and Centers participated in the initial DIRH PAR; presently, 16 Institutes and Centers are participating.[35]

The third element to push implementation science further in the United States was the launching of the open-access, peer-reviewed journal, *Implementation Science*, with coeditors from both the United States and the United Kingdom. The journal was the first international scientific outlet dedicated to publishing research on "the scientific study of methods to promote the systematic uptake of research findings and other evidence-based practices into routine practice, and, hence, to improve the quality and effectiveness of health services and care."[36] Now many journals publish implementation science and two new journals specifically focus on implementation science: *Implementation Science Communications* and *Implementation Research and Practice.*

In 2007, the National Institute of Mental Health and the National Cancer Institute cosponsored a technical assistance workshop to offer researchers an opportunity to learn about the purpose of DIRH PAR, hear from successful NIH grantees working in this research area, and get feedback from NIH program staff about submitted concept papers.[37] The next year, the workshop transformed into the NIH Conference on the Science of Dissemination and Implementation to offer the research community the opportunity "to exchange ideas, explore contemporary topics and identify concepts, methods and strategies to build research and organizational capacity for dissemination and implementation science."[38] Still going strong, the 10th Annual Conference on the Science of Dissemination and Implementation in Health took place in 2017.[39]

In 2011, the NIH conducted its first Training Institute for Dissemination and Implementation Research in Health (TIDIRH) to prepare investigators to "conduct research that addresses the complex process of integrating research into policy and practice," and "cultivate interest for D&I research at institutions around the country."[40]

The NIH initiated the TIDIRH to address the limited opportunities that existed at that time for investigators to get in-depth training in dissemination and implementation research.[41] Since the creation of TIDIRH, other research training programs in implementation science have been established, including degree-granting programs. Nevertheless, the TIDIRH continues to provide in-depth training to researchers interested in moving into the field.

In sum, over the past 10 years, implementation science emerged in the United States as an organized, institutionally supported field of study with its own academically based infrastructure, funding mechanisms, scientific journals, research conferences, and training programs. Its emergence in the United States coincided with its emergence in global health, focusing initially on infectious diseases and maternal-child health, and accelerating with the launch of large-scale efforts to combat the high burden of HIV/AIDS in low- and middle-income countries.

EMERGENCE OF IMPLEMENTATION SCIENCE IN GLOBAL HEALTH

Implementation science in global health similarly coalesced as an organized, institutionally supported field of study in the first decade of the new millennium. While nascent implementation science in the United States was largely focused on improving patient-provider interactions in clinical facilities, global implementation science emerged with a predominant focus on improving health service delivery within under-resourced health systems as part of national or transnational initiatives, programs, and policies. In the 1990s, implementation science in global health was indistinguishable from operations research. In 2003, the World Health Organization Special Program for Research and Training in Tropical Diseases (WHO TDR) embraced implementation science as integral to the research process for developing "practical solutions to improve access to efficacious interventions against tropical diseases."[42] In addition to endorsing a conceptual and operational framework for implementation research, WHO TDR outlined how implementation research activities fit within its research program. Through collaborative research grants, WHO TDR began supporting implementation science by, for example, testing microenterprise strategies to improve access to antimalarial drugs in rural Kenya.

In 2008, WHO TDR collaborated with The Global Fund to Fight AIDS, Tuberculosis and Malaria, the United States Agency for International Development (USAID), the Joint United Nations Program on HIV/AIDS (UNAIDS), and The World Bank to develop a framework for operations and implementation research in health and disease control programs. The intent of the framework was to "help researchers and program managers identify the steps needed to set a research question and then work through the steps of research design, implementation, management, and reporting, ultimately leading to the use of the findings to improve health policies and programs in order to attain the desired impact."[43]

The same year, the U.S. President's Emergency Plan for AIDS Relief (PEPFAR) adopted an implementation science framework to inform, guide, and evaluate the expansion of HIV care and treatment.[44] The PEPFAR framework emphasized three components of implementation science: monitoring and evaluation, operations research, and impact evaluation (including modeling and cost-effectiveness analysis). Funding and institutional support for implementation science in global health increased significantly as PEPFAR and other agencies embraced implementation science as a field well positioned to address the "know-do" gap in global health. In 2011, for example, NIH and PEPFAR jointly requested applications for implementation science projects to develop more efficient and cost-effective methods to deliver effective interventions for prevention of maternal-to-child transmission (PMTCT) of HIV.[45]

In its 2008–12 strategic plan, the Fogarty International Center designated implementation science as one of its five priority areas and formulated a goal to support implementation research and training in global health.[46] In 2010, Fogarty convened its first Implementation Science and Global Health meeting to build linkages between implementation science researchers and global healthcare delivery programs. In 2011, Fogarty and the NIH began funding research training programs in global health to expand the scientific workforce in implementation science in sub-Saharan Africa and other parts of the world.[47] Fogarty and the NIH supported 21 programs in 2017 that offered short- or long-term training in implementation science in the sub-Saharan Africa region.[48] In addition, WHO TDR supported seven universities from LMICs in Africa and other parts of the world to offer doctoral-level and masters-level training in implementation science related to infectious diseases.[48]

In 2010, the *Journal of Acquired Immune Deficiency Syndrome (JAIDS)* launched a special section dedicated to implementation and operational research in recognition that "the lessons learned through this research discipline are particularly relevant to guiding best practices in low-resource settings as antiretroviral drug access is expanded."[49] While many other journals publish implementation science articles of relevance to global health, *JAIDS* was the first to create a special section in which implementation scientists could communicate their research findings about the effectiveness of strategies to integrate scientific knowledge, practices, and technologies into clinical care for patients with HIV/AIDS.

Finally, 2013 witnessed the launch of the NIH-PEPFAR PMTCT Implementation Science Alliance to facilitate communication and collaboration among implementation researchers, program implementers, and policy-makers to accelerate the translation of "effective PMTCT interventions into community- and population-level services, programs, and strategies at scale."[50] The Alliance brings together scientists funded through the NIH-PEPFAR Request for Applications described earlier, program implementers and policy-makers from PEPFAR-supported countries, representatives of multilateral institutions (e.g., WHO, UNAIDS, and UNICEF), implementation

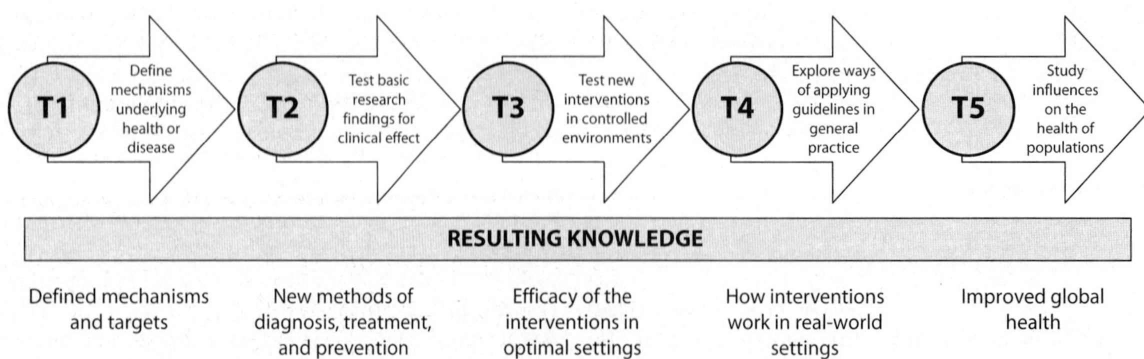

FIGURE 20-2. Translational research bottlenecks. (*Source:* From https://med.nyu.edu/ctsi/what-ctsi.)

science methodologists, and U.S. government representatives and global experts in HIV/AIDS and PMTCT.[51] Through this distinctive research-practice infrastructure, the Alliance is building collaborative capacity for implementation science and addressing scientific, methodological, and practical questions about evidence-based program and policy development for PMTCT. Since then, two additional alliances have formed: the Clean Cooking Implementation Science Network,[52] and the Adolescent HIV Prevention and Treatment Implementation Science Alliance.[53]

IMPLEMENTATION SCIENCE QUESTIONS

As discussed earlier, implementation science asks and answers the fundamental question: how do we get "what works" to people who need it with greater speed, fidelity, efficiency, quality, sustainability, and relevant coverage? Evaluating the effectiveness of implementation strategies for achieving these outcomes is thus a central focus of implementation science. To illustrate, in setting the implementation research agenda for PMTCT, policy-makers, district health workers, academics, implementing partners, and persons living with HIV identified the following questions as key priorities in Zimbabwe[54]:

- What models of service delivery, including nurse-led initiation or other decentralization approaches, can accelerate scale-up and implementation of PMTCT interventions and lifelong antiretroviral therapy by HIV-infected pregnant women or mothers?
- What affordable and sustainable models of service delivery can improve coverage and uptake of effective PMTCT interventions in rural or very rural populations?
- What approaches improve retention of mothers and infants in the continuum of care, including early infant testing and providing infant antiretroviral prophylaxis?

Each question asks about the effectiveness of strategies—including complex strategies such as service delivery models—for improving uptake, coverage, and sustained use of effective interventions to prevent HIV transmission from mother to child. The question of how contextual conditions influence the effectiveness of these strategies is also important, especially for scaling up effective health interventions to new populations or settings. It is important to know, for example, whether the effectiveness of nurse-led initiation of PMTCT varies as a function of client, provider, facility, or community characteristics.

Early in its development, the field of implementation science focused on identifying the barriers and facilitators that affect the adoption and integration of effective health interventions into routine use. As the field matured, attention shifted from descriptive studies of barriers and facilitators of implementation to evaluative studies of strategies for effectively addressing them. However, a pre-implementation assessment of the barriers and facilitators operating in the contexts and settings in which the implementation of a proven health intervention will occur remains important in both research and practice. Such an assessment can, and should, inform the selection of the strategies to be deployed, monitored, and evaluated.

Although questions about the effectiveness of implementation strategies are a central focus of implementation science, the field is also concerned with broader questions that also matter to stakeholders who want to see effective health interventions implemented at scale. For example, as the burden of chronic noncommunicable diseases (NCDs) such as cancer, diabetes, cardiovascular disease, and mental health disorders rises across sub-Saharan Africa, global donors and governments are exploring strategies to integrate NCD and HIV care. NCDs are common among people living with HIV and threaten to undermine HIV treatment outcomes. Stakeholders want to know whether integrating NCD and HIV care—whether through coordination, co-location, or simultaneous delivery of HIV and NCD services to people who need them—is effective in terms of both preventing, detecting, and treating NCDs and achieving and maintaining HIV treatment outcomes. Implementation science can provide the answer to this question. However, these stakeholders want to know more than whether NCD-HIV integration is an effective strategy for getting "what works" in NCD and HIV care to people who need it, when they need it while sustaining or improving the quality of both services and minimizing unintended, adverse effects; they also want to know whether this strategy does so with fidelity, efficiency, quality, and relevant coverage. Implementation science can provide answers to this broader set of questions through the employment of a variety of research disciplines, methods, and approaches (see Table 20-1).[48]

This broader set of implementation science questions can inform stakeholders' efforts to effectively scale up health interventions. Although related in complex ways, implementation and scale-up differ. Scale-up refers to "deliberate efforts to increase the impact of health service innovations successfully tested in pilot or experimental projects so as to benefit more people and to foster policy and program development on a lasting basis."[55] Whereas implementation, and by implication implementation science, focuses on the adoption and integration of effective health interventions in specific settings (e.g., health facilities, schools, and worksites), "going to scale" means increasing geographic coverage from a limited study area to an entire region or a country. As such, scale-up involves implementing effective interventions in dozens, hundreds, or even thousands of settings.

TABLE 20-1 USING YOUR RESEARCH QUESTION TO GUIDE IS METHOD SELECTION

Research Question	Implementation Science Method
What is the effect of IMPLEMENTATION STRATEGY on incidence, morbidity, and mortality at the population level?	Impact evaluation Surveillance and data systems
What is the financial cost of IMPLEMENTATION STRATEGY? What are the most cost-effective models for delivering IMPLEMENTATION STRATEGY?	Economic evaluation
How can we optimize the quality and efficiency of the delivery of the IMPLEMENTATION STRATEGY (including a robust supply chain) within the care setting?	Operations research
How can we improve the fidelity of IMPLEMENTATION STRATEGY?	Systems analysis/quality improvement
What policy changes are necessary for scaling up IMPLEMENTATION STRATEGY? Which stakeholders are critical for obtaining support for IMPLEMENTATION STRATEGY?	Stakeholder/policy analysis
How do we culturally adapt IMPLEMENTATION STRATEGY for different countries, regions, and contexts?	Qualitative methods
How do we increase the reach of IMPLEMENTATION STRATEGY, particularly among marginalized and vulnerable populations?	Dissemination research
How do we create understanding and appeal of DESIRED HEALTH BEHAVIOR?	Social marketing

Source: Adapted from reference 48.

However, scale-up is more than implementation writ large. Going to scale often requires addressing policy, legal, political, regulatory, budgetary, workforce, and supply chain issues; sensitizing and mobilizing communities; aligning donor, governmental, and nongovernmental organization priorities and activities; and other actions that go above and beyond implementation.

IMPLEMENTATION SCIENCE FRAMEWORKS

Implementation science offers a wealth of theories, frameworks, and models for guiding research and practice. In 2012, Tabak et al.[56] identified 61 theories and frameworks, which they collectively called models, for enhancing the dissemination and implementation of evidence-based interventions. Additional theories, frameworks, and models have been developed or introduced since then. Selecting a theory, framework, or model can be challenging, especially for those new to implementation science.[57] Nilsen[58] proposes a taxonomy that distinguishes categories of theories, frameworks, and models based on what he describes as three overarching aims in implementation science:

1. ***Process***—describing or guiding the process of translating research into practice;
2. ***Determinants***—understanding or explaining what influences implementation outcomes; and
3. ***Evaluation***—evaluating implementation success and failure.

Although some theories, frameworks, and models address more than one of these aims, Nilsen's taxonomy provides a useful guide for selecting and applying relevant approaches in implementation research and practice. While theories, models, and frameworks are distinct concepts, these terms are often used interchangeably in implementation science. Hence, those distinctions are not highlighted here. The three main categories of approaches, which align with Nilsen's three overarching aims in implementation science, are process models, explanatory frameworks, and evaluation frameworks.

Process models specify the steps, stages, or phases in the process of translating research into practice, or in the language used in this chapter, the process of implementing evidence-based health interventions. Process models, such as the Knowledge to Action (K2A) Framework[59] and the Canadian Institutes of Health Research (CIHR) Model of Knowledge Translation,[60] depict a linear process, with feedback loops, that begins with research discovery and the production of evidence-based interventions, and moves to the dissemination of those interventions to targeted audiences and the implementation of those interventions in practice. Other process models, such as the Quality Implementation Framework (QIF),[61] the Stetler Model,[62] and the Ottawa Model,[63] provide practical guidance or "how to" advice for planning and execution of implementation efforts. These process models, also called action models or planned action models, are particularly useful for implementation practice because they highlight important tasks that should be considered and prescribe a sequence in which those tasks should be performed. The QIF, for example, specifies four phases: initial considerations regarding the host setting (Phase One), creating a structure for implementation (Phase Two), ongoing structure once implementation begins (Phase Three), and improving future applications (Phase Four). The QIF identifies 14 critical steps or actions believed to constitute high-quality implementation. Phase One steps, for example, include conducting a needs and resources assessment, an assessment of the fit of the evidence-based intervention and the setting, and a capacity or readiness assessment; making decisions about adapting the intervention; obtaining explicit buy-in from critical stakeholders; building organizational capacity; recruiting staff to implement the intervention; and conducting effective staff training. Nilsen observes that process models describe a rational sequence of steps or ideal view of implementation; actual implementation is often nonlinear and messy.

Determinants frameworks describe barriers or enablers, hereafter referred to as determinants, which influence access to or use of evidence-based health interventions and other implementation outcomes discussed later in this chapter. Unlike process models, which describe steps or stages of implementation, determinants frameworks identify factors that hinder or facilitate implementation. Determinants frameworks are useful for assessing the context of implementation and guiding the selection of implementation strategies that overcome barriers or harness enablers. Determinants frameworks are also useful for explaining the level of implementation attained in a specific setting or the variation in implementation attained among multiple settings. The Consolidated Framework for Implementation Research (CFIR) is a widely applied determinants framework in implementation science, with increasing use in the global health context.[64] A "metatheoretical" framework that synthesizes 19 theories and frameworks in dissemination and implementation research, the CFIR includes 37 determinants organized into five domains: intervention characteristics, outer setting, inner setting, individuals involved, and implementation processes. Within the intervention characteristics domain, for example, the CFIR identifies eight determinants: intervention source, evidence strength and quality, relative advantage, adaptability, trialability, complexity, design quality and packaging, and cost. The CFIR's widespread use results from its comprehensiveness, applicability, and flexibility; the authors encourage users to "select constructs from the CFIR that are most relevant for their particular study setting and use these constructs to guide diagnostic assessments of implementation context, evaluate implementation progress, and help explain findings in research studies or quality improvement initiatives."[64] The Theoretical Domains Framework (TDF), another commonly used determinants framework, synthesizes 33 behavior change theories and organizes more than 100 constructs into 14 theoretical domains, such as knowledge, skills, intentions, goals, and social influences.[65] While neither framework hypothesizes causal relationships among determinants, both acknowledge that such relationships exist.

Evaluation frameworks, as the name implies, provide a conceptual structure for evaluating implementation efforts. Unlike determinants frameworks, which identify the factors that influence implementation success, evaluation frameworks identify the metrics for gauging implementation success. In implementation research, determinants frameworks supply possible independent variables, whereas evaluation frameworks supply candidate-dependent variables. The two most commonly used evaluation frameworks in implementation science are Proctor et al.'s Implementation Outcomes Framework (IOF)[66] and RE-AIM.[67] Since the IOF is discussed in a later section, RE-AIM is the focus here. RE-AIM, a well-established framework in implementation science for evaluating the public health impact of health-promotion programs, identifies five dimensions of a program, or intervention, that signal its applicability, scalability, potency, and sustainability in "real-world" settings.[67] Those dimensions are *reach* of the program within the intended target population, *effectiveness* of the program, *adoption* of the program by target settings or staff, *implementation* of the program in terms of the consistency and quality of program delivery, and *maintenance* of program delivery and program effects.[68] As an evaluation framework, RE-AIM is especially suitable for use in global health contexts because it balances traditional concerns about program effectiveness with considerations relevant to implementation and scale-up, such as program coverage (reach) in a targeted population.

Nilsen's taxonomy includes theories derived from other fields such as psychology, sociology, and organization science, which he calls classic theories, as well as theories developed or adapted by researchers for use in implementation science, which he calls implementation theories. Although less comprehensive than determinants frameworks, classic theories and implementation theories offer hypotheses that relate specific aspects of implementation context or process to implementation outcomes. Hence, they are useful for the overarching aim in implementation science of understanding or explaining what influences access to and use of evidence-based health interventions and other implementation outcomes. Moreover, some classic theories and implementation theories identify mechanisms of change, which makes them useful for explaining how or why implementation strategies work.

IMPLEMENTATION STRATEGIES

As described above, a primary focus of implementation science research is to test and evaluate different techniques that can be used to integrate evidence-based practices or interventions into routine public health and clinical practice. These techniques are called implementation strategies. A wide array of implementation strategies have been identified in the literature and by implementation experts.[25,69,70] The Expert Recommendations for Implementing Change (ERIC) study systematically collected input from a wide range of clinical and implementation experts and identified 73 discrete implementation strategies.[70] The ERIC taxonomy allows users to identify single or packages of implementation strategies that may be most appropriate for intervention delivery, providing standardized terminology to allow implementation scientists to compare findings from their work to other research efforts that utilize the same strategy. While the implementation strategies included in the ERIC taxonomy are generated by implementation scientists in high-income settings, the initiative highlights the wide range of implementation strategies available to practitioners, which are described in further detail below. Reviews of implementation strategies have also been undertaken in LMIC settings; however, the evidence base is weaker given that implementation strategies are often inconsistently reported or described with insufficient detail.[26]

Implementation strategies can be organized into five categories based on the relevant actors targeted or involved in the implementation strategy.[26] Many implementation efforts in LMICs involve combinations of strategies in these categories. These categories include those aiming to enhance:

- Government ownership or oversight of health systems;
- The delivery of routine health services within an organization or facility;
- The performance of health service providers or frontline health workers;
- The involvement of households or community members in health service delivery systems; and
- Networks of stakeholders whose cooperation is needed to ensure high-quality health services reach those in need.

1. *Improving government ownership or oversight of health service systems.* Implementation strategies that enhance the ability of governments to perform oversight of health systems via improved policy-making and public financing might include developing evidence-based policies, evaluating existing or potential policies, governance strengthening strategies, public financing incentives, and decentralization of public health services, among others. There are many examples of governance strengthening implementation strategies that have been applied in practice. For example, leadership and management training for MOH personnel working at multiple administrative levels in Zambia was implemented in order to improve healthcare administration and work place climates.[71] Similarly, in Kenya, leadership and management trainings at a facility level were associated with increased coverage of key primary healthcare programs.[72] Additionally, decentralization of health systems is a fundamental component of health sector reform that has been applied in multiple countries throughout the world, with the aim of improving local ownership, governance, and, in effect, population health outcomes.[73,74] However, decentralization should be accompanied by local capacity building to ensure that local entities can assume decentralized responsibilities and functions.[75] This highlights the potential role of implementation scientists in studying factors influencing the effectiveness of decentralization, such as organizational structure and capacity, accountability systems, and stakeholder networks and preferences.
2. *Strengthening the capabilities and performance of health service organizations.* Improving organizational performance of health service delivery is addressed by implementation strategies such as quality performance and assurance strategies, guideline development and adherence promotion, supervisory structures, performance-based financial incentives for teams and individuals, health service integration or reorganization, human resource management, and facility management and supply chain strengthening. A valuable example of an organizational integration implementation strategy is the Integra Initiative, a large 5-year evaluation of an integrated sexual, reproductive health, and HIV intervention implemented in Kenya and Swaziland.[76] The initiative examined effects of facility-level systems integration on staff workload, program costs and cost-effectiveness, intervention acceptability, service coverage, pregnancies, and known HIV status.[76] While quality of care increased in Integra, evaluation of the implementation strategy also highlighted the importance of workload sharing, cross-sector communication, and staff motivation.[77,78]
3. *Strengthening the capabilities and performance of individual providers and frontline workers.* Improving the practices of individual health providers could be addressed by implementation strategies such as providing continuing education and training, enhanced supervision, peer learning and support programs, the development of job aids, and supporting the application of treatment guideline algorithms. For example, training programs for female health workers in India predicated upon the WHO Adolescent Job-Aid booklet appeared to improve health worker knowledge and quality of care for adolescent sexual health issues.[79] Additionally, a systematic review of community health worker supervision practices found that improving supervision quality had a positive impact on coverage of a number of health services, as well as the quality of health services delivered.[80]
4. *Involving households or community members in health service delivery.* Empowering communities and households to participate in health programs or alter their individual health practices may involve implementation strategies such as training community health workers, training community members, social marketing and demand creation, improving participation via community partnerships or community-directed services, strengthening local accountability through joint monitoring or community-based information systems, building local organizational capacity via community mobilization, information education and communication (IEC) campaigns, financial empowerment via in-kind subsidies and microfinancing schemes, and peer support or mentoring programs for healthy behaviors. Onchocerciasis mass drug administration programs provide a relevant example, as they are delivered via community-directed interventions in which communities themselves lead the planning and implementation of intervention delivery.[81] The community-directed implementation strategy has demonstrated success in reaching at-risk populations with high coverage,[82] and has been tested for use in delivering other disease programs such as malaria bed net distribution and vitamin A campaigns in order to increase community coverage and satisfaction.[83]

5. *Supporting networks of stakeholders whose cooperation is needed to ensure high-quality health services.* Supporting public health stakeholder networks may require implementation strategies such as reviewing facilitators and barriers to programs, obtaining broad-based stakeholder support, local adaptation of programs, and stakeholder feedback to inform program modification and management. These implementation strategies may be particularly pertinent in settings where sociocultural or structural challenges inhibit intervention effectiveness. For example, a community-based, cluster-randomized controlled trial of umbilical cord care in Zambia utilized intensive engagement of multilevel stakeholders to ensure that clinical interventions were well received and culturally acceptable to stakeholders including community members and health workers.[84]

The frequency with which different implementation strategies are used in practice appears to vary by implementation phase, health issue, and setting, including health facilities, workplaces, schools, or communities. In a systematic review of HIV interventions targeting adult HIV care in LMICs, authors identified 34 distinct types of interventions predominantly implemented at the provider or community member levels.[85] Common implementation strategies included task shifting, patient outreach, and patient or provider reminders. Yet, a review of implementation strategies to improve provider adherence to cardiovascular disease guidelines in HICs identified a similar overall number of strategies with primary strategies being guideline dissemination, provider education, audit, and feedback (where health professionals are provided a summary of clinical performance to allow them to assess and adjust their performance), and academic detailing.[86] Meanwhile a review of studies aiming to improve clinical practice guideline dissemination and utilization in HICs identified most common implementation strategies to be educational outreach, educational materials, audit and feedback, and provider-targeted reminders.[87] Thus, there is no singular implementation strategy most frequently applied in practice; the salience of different implementation strategies varies greatly by target population, identified implementation barrier, and interventional setting.

Evidence regarding the relative effectiveness or adverse consequences of different implementation strategies in achieving targeted outcomes is sparse. In a review of NCD prevention and management studies in LMICs, intensified team-based care generally led to improvements in medication adherence and hypertension control at the patient/provider level. At the systems-level, implementation strategies addressing universal health insurance coverage appeared to improve hypertension and diabetes control.[88] Another systematic review of implementation strategies to improve primary-care delivery similarly found that the most commonly utilized implementation strategies included those targeting individual providers, including the evaluation of implementation strategies such as audit and feedback or educational meetings and outreach.[89] However, interventions targeting individual providers were associated with small to modest improvements (2–9%) in professional performance or behaviors. Additionally, multifaceted strategies targeting health providers were not necessarily more effective than single strategies alone. The authors of the review concluded, "It remains unclear which implementation strategies are more likely to be effective than others and under what conditions."[89]

There is not an exact science to choosing an appropriate implementation strategy for research or programmatic purposes. However, implementation scientists should consider the specific implementation determinant they are hoping to address, and select relevant strategies accordingly. For example, if healthcare providers in a specific setting continually deviate from treatment guidelines or evidence-based interventions despite having the tools and skills needed to adhere, an implementation strategy may be to conduct audit and feedback across the entire facility regarding health worker guideline adherence to increase self-reflection on clinical decision-making. In Sudan, implementation scientists aimed to reduce inappropriate use of antibiotics through audit and feedback or enhanced audit and feedback interventions targeting prescribers at health facilities.[90] The researchers found that audit and feedback strategies significantly reduced the number of encounters in which antibiotics were prescribed, compared to no intervention. This implementation strategy, delivered at the organizational level, thus provided an opportunity to evaluate targeted improvements to a root determinant of insufficient health service delivery: provider behavior.

Despite an increased appreciation for selecting, naming, and describing implementation strategies with precision, there is significant progress yet to be made in continuing to define a taxonomy of implementation strategies in a global health context, evaluating the influence of implementation strategies on health interventions at different stages of conceptualization, public health practice and health outcomes, and adding clarity to implementation strategies included in the published literature to enhance the ability to replicate the strategies within both research and programmatic settings.[85,91,92]

IMPLEMENTATION OUTCOMES

Interventions that are poorly or partially implemented do not produce expected positive health outcomes.[93] However, even when effectively implemented, interventions still might not produce expected positive health outcomes, if the intervention loses its effectiveness during the process of implementation—for example, if the intervention is adapted in ways that undermine its potency. It is important, therefore, to conceive and evaluate implementation success or failure in terms of outcomes that are distinct from, yet related to, the health outcomes that interventions produce. Proctor et al.[66] define "implementation outcomes" as "the effects of deliberate and purposive actions to implement new treatments, practices, and services." Their Implementation Outcomes Framework identifies eight implementation outcomes (see Table 20-2) and distinguishes them from service delivery outcomes (such as efficiency, timeliness, and patient-centeredness), as well as health outcomes (such as mortality, morbidity, and quality of life). Implementation outcomes serve not only as indicators of implementation success or failure, but also as preconditions for attaining desired service delivery or health outcomes. While implementation outcomes are not the sole focus of implementation science, they play a critical role in implementation science because they serve as indicators of how well an implementation effort is going or how successful such an effort ultimately was.[9] Ultimately, implementation outcomes should be linked to service delivery and health outcomes. It is particularly important to measure and assess the linkages of implementation outcomes to service delivery and health outcomes when health interventions are adapted during implementation, applied to a different population, or delivered in a different setting.

Several points about implementation outcomes merit discussion. First, some of the implementation outcomes listed in Table 20-2, such as acceptability, could apply to a specific intervention, an implementation strategy used to introduce an intervention into a healthcare or community setting, or a broad initiative to implement several interventions at once.

Second, some of these outcomes could be assessed from the perspective of multiple stakeholders or multiple levels of analysis. Appropriateness, for example, can be examined from the point of view of clients or providers; adoption can be analyzed at the individual level (e.g., healthcare providers), the organizational level (e.g., health facilities), or the community or policy level (e.g., cigarettes taxes).

Third, implementation outcomes might be differentially salient to different stakeholders. For example, implementation cost may be most important to policy-makers and administrators, feasibility may

TABLE 20-2 DEFINING IMPLEMENTATION OUTCOMES

Implementation Outcome	Definition[†]	Level of Analysis	Related Terms[‡]
Acceptability	The perception among implementation stakeholders that a given treatment, service, practice, or innovation is agreeable, palatable, or satisfactory	• Individual provider • Individual consumer	Factors related to acceptability (e.g., comfort, relative advantage, credibility)
Adoption	The intention, initial decision, or action to try or employ an innovation or evidence-based practice	• Individual provider • Organization or setting	Uptake, utilization, intention to try
Appropriateness	The perceived fit, relevance, or compatibility of the innovation or evidence-based practice for a given practice setting, provider, or consumer; and/or perceived fit of the innovation to address a particular issue or problem	• Individual provider • Individual consumer • Organization or setting	Relevance, perceived fit, compatibility, perceived usefulness or suitability
Cost	The cost impact of an implementation effort	• Provider or providing institution	Marginal cost, total cost, and numerators for cost-utility, cost-benefit, and cost-effectiveness
Feasibility	The extent to which a new treatment, or an innovation, can be successfully used or carried out within a given agency or setting	• Individual providers • Organization or setting	Practicality, actual fit, trialability
Fidelity	The degree to which an intervention was implemented as it was prescribed in the original protocol, or as it was intended by the program developers	• Individual provider	Adherence, delivery as intended, integrity, quality of program delivery, intensity or dosage of delivery
Penetration	The integration of a practice within a service setting and its subsystems	• Organization or setting	Reach, access, service spread, coverage, or effective coverage (focusing on those who need an intervention and its delivery at sufficient quality, thus combining coverage and fidelity)
Sustainability	The extent to which a newly implemented treatment is maintained or institutionalized within a service setting's ongoing, stable operations.	• Administrators • Organization or setting	Maintenance, continuation, durability, institutionalization, routinization, integration, incorporation

Source: Adapted from references 9[†] and 171[‡].

be most important to direct service providers, and fidelity may be most important to intervention developers.

Fourth, some implementation outcomes may be more important at some stages of implementation than at other stages. Feasibility, for instance, is important early in the process as providers and organizations consider, plan, and introduce new interventions; later, it becomes a "moot point" as the intervention becomes part of routine care.

Fifth, implementation outcomes are themselves interrelated in dynamic, complex ways. Acceptability, appropriateness, and feasibility, for example, are likely associated with adoption, while implementation cost, especially ongoing cost, is likely associated with sustainability.

Finally, reliable, valid, and practical measures do not exist for most of these implementation outcomes,[94] a point discussed further below. Although efforts are underway to develop and test measures of implementation outcomes for use in research and practice, these measures require linguistic and cultural adaptation and additional testing for use in global health contexts.

WHEN TO DO IMPLEMENTATION SCIENCE

Implementation science begins with an efficacious health intervention or intervention package. The translational research pipeline (see Fig. 20-2) outlines the process through which basic science research (T0) becomes research performed on human subjects (T1), and within clinical or other service delivery settings (T2). Implementation science research harnesses evidence regarding intervention efficacy and evaluates these interventions for effectiveness within clinical or other service delivery settings (T3), and with population-level health outcomes (T4). When deciding what evidence to move from T2 to T3 in the translational research pipeline, researchers and policy-makers might consider the strength of evidence supporting a particular intervention by assessing the presence of the intervention in established clinical guidelines or associated networks promoting evidence synthesis, such as the WHO Quality of Care Networks.[95] Additionally, researchers and policy-makers can use Cochrane Collaboration systematic reviews to evaluate the amount and strength of evidence surrounding a specific intervention.[96]

Using these and other data sources, researchers and policy-makers deciding whether or not to engage in stages T3 or T4 of the research pipeline should be able to clearly and unequivocally answer the following questions.[6]

- What is the clinical or public health problem at hand?
- What is the epidemiology of this disease or health status? What are causal factors, associated health outcomes, and relevant efficacious preventative, diagnostic, or therapeutic interventions?
- Why is delivery or receipt of the intervention of interest suboptimal, and what are the observed bottlenecks and gaps in the delivery system?
- If effective interventions for the problem have been established in other settings: What is the situational analysis (i.e., context) that will influence how the effective intervention can be introduced or adapted within the new setting?

Implementation research can be descriptive, interventional, or a combination of both. In descriptive research, implementation scientists may be studying features of a system that act as barriers or facilitators to effective delivery of an intervention. For example, researchers may ask what are potential barriers and facilitators to effective uptake of community-based rapid detection of malaria. In interventional research, implementation scientists will likely be employing specific implementation strategies to improve delivery of an evidence-based intervention (see section on implementation strategies). It should be noted that if researchers are undertaking hybrid research in which both effectiveness and implementation outcomes are of interest,[97] it may be possible that questions third and fourth above would be answered as an integral part of the implementation research undertaken. In this case, implementation science may sometimes begin earlier in the research process, during T2 of the translational research pipeline, in conjunction with clinical or epidemiological research.

HOW TO DO IMPLEMENTATION SCIENCE

Designing Rigorous Implementation Science

As in all research disciplines, it is important for implementation scientists to practice rigorous principles of research design. Within the field of implementation science, explicit identification of implementation components is particularly important to ensure precision in activities and enhance intervention replicability. Implementation strategies can be complex and thus should be clearly defined and described by, at a minimum, the following research features[91]:

1. Actors, or the individuals carrying out the intervention and relevant group characteristics of the individuals;
2. Actions, or the specific activities that will be implemented as part of the intervention;
3. Action targets, or the specific change mechanism hypothesized to be targeted by an implementation strategy; and
4. Dose and temporality, including the timing, frequency, and intensity of the activities that will take place as part of the intervention.

The targeted implementation outcomes should also be explicit and may include both proximal and distal implementation outcomes, should one implementation outcome be expected to precede another. For example, penetration of an intervention within a health system may be a necessary predecessor to intervention sustainability.[66]

Consider a mobile, home-based HIV testing program aimed at increasing HIV testing among adolescents as compared to standard facility-based self-referral programs. The proposed implementation strategy is a restructuring strategy, which involves changing the site of health service delivery (*action*), and may involve task shifting of some health worker responsibilities to lay health workers such as community health workers (*actor*). Transitions to community-based care may increase participation in HIV testing by making the intervention more acceptable to adolescent community-members in HIV endemic areas and thus influencing their individual decision processes (*action target)*. The implementation strategy proposed here would likely take place during an execution stage of the project, as opposed to other potential stages including planning, engaging, or reflecting/evaluating (*temporality)*, although stakeholder engagement should take place in the planning phase.[64] The community-based HIV testing intervention may be targeting the outcome of acceptability (*proximal implementation outcome)* by improving adolescent comfort and satisfaction with intervention delivery and thus demand for convenient HIV testing services (*change mechanism)*. External factors that could influence the effectiveness of the implementation strategy might include the capacity for facility-based health workers to work in communities given their professional responsibilities in health facilities, for adolescents to be available and confident about confidentiality at home for mobile HIV testing, and for health system supervisors to be supportive of change practices, among numerous other contextual factors.

Reporting Upon Rigorous Implementation Science

Recommendations for planning and reporting implementation science have been formalized in guidelines such as Standards for Reporting Implementation Studies of Complex Interventions (STaRI)[98] and the Template for Intervention Description and Replication (TIDieR).[99] These guidelines ask implementation scientists to report upon a range of research features from the study aims that distinguish implementation objectives from intervention objectives to fidelity to the implementation strategy, above and beyond fidelity to the intervention. Additionally, the PRECIS-2 guidelines help authors describe the degree to which a clinical trial is explanatory or pragmatic,[100] while the Medical Research Council (MRC) provides guidance on how to develop and report upon interventions involving multiple interacting components.[101] Adherence to reporting guidelines is helpful for ensuring that implementation research is replicable and core components are easily accessible to other researchers, implementers, or policy-makers.

In addition to the standardized information outlined in these reporting guidelines, it is important for researchers to report upon activities undertaken that were not planned, but were necessary to accommodate implementation realities along the way. This additional information can provide helpful evidence regarding the contextual factors that differentiate implementation of activities across geographies.

Conducting Inclusive Implementation Science

Because implementation science often takes place at the intersection of policy, practice, and research, implementation science requires the involvement of multiple stakeholders, each of whom provides important and distinct perspectives on an implementation issue. Common stakeholders involved in implementation science range from those who benefit from the public health intervention to those who make policy regarding the intervention, including:

- Members of international organizations, such as the WHO;
- Policy-makers in a Ministry of Health, Education, Urban Development, or other relevant offices, and at multiple administrative levels ranging from national to more local levels;
- Financing bodies and regulatory bodies, such as foundations and scientific associations;
- Professional health workers including physicians, nurses, clinical officers, and social workers;
- Lay health workers such as traditional birth attendants and community health workers; and
- Health service beneficiaries, including patients, family members of patients, and communities in which public health efforts are underway.

Stakeholders play key roles during each stage of implementation science planning, execution, and evaluation. Input from a variety of stakeholders can be crucial in ensuring that an intervention is appropriately tailored to a given setting, maximizing the probability of success. Stakeholders can also provide direction and input throughout implementation and during the postimplementation evaluation regarding why an intervention may or may not be working. And finally, stakeholders who will be most affected by the sustaining or scaling of an intervention should participate in informing next steps and it is critical that researchers report findings back to these stakeholders and engage them in reflective processing. Some implementation science tools, such as the quality improvement plan-do-study-act strategy, inherently require involvement from frontline stakeholders to design and carry out interventions aimed at improving healthcare practice. Participatory activities such as this draw from stakeholder knowledge and experience to develop appropriate implementation strategies.[102]

Identification of stakeholders in implementation science can be captured through systematic stakeholder mapping, social marketing segmentation, or other similar methodological approaches.

Additionally, data from interviews, focus groups, surveys, or other data collection techniques can be stratified by stakeholder group to provide information regarding how perspectives from stakeholders may vary. Thus, conducting inclusive implementation science often requires mixed quantitative and qualitative methods of data collection and analysis. A mixed methods approach provides an opportunity to triangulate across data sources and account for multiple perspectives, causal pathways, or types of outcomes.

Lastly, because a large variety of stakeholders are often necessarily involved in implementation research, special ethical considerations must be made. Standard clinical ethical principles apply equally to implementation research; however, because implementation research often targets stakeholders with distinct perspectives on improving health system functioning, who may or may not be direct beneficiaries of implementation research findings, standard consenting procedures and risk communication may require modification.[103]

Conducting Pragmatic Implementation Science

Pragmatic research refers to research that addresses specific practice needs and questions in contexts that are broadly applicable.[104] Pragmatic implementation studies address research questions that evaluate the effectiveness of an implementation strategy in "real-world" practice settings characterized by typical resources, clinical staff, and patient or client mixes.[105] This contrasts with efficacy studies that evaluate the impact of implementation strategies under "ideal" conditions using additional resources, specialized staff, or providers, patients, or clients meeting strict eligibility requirements. When designing pragmatic implementation studies, study comparators represent real-world alternatives or current standards of care, rather than comparators of no treatment or placebo controls.[104] Additionally, the study design or methodological approach used is determined by the implementation question at hand; potential methods often used in pragmatic studies include effectiveness-implementation hybrid trials, randomized or quasi-randomized designs, quality improvement studies, simulation modeling, qualitative data collection, and policy analysis (see Fig. 20-1).

Implementation scientists can take precautions to ensure that the measures and metrics that they select to evaluate key implementation determinants, outcomes, and strategies are also pragmatic in nature. First, the measures should be important to stakeholders, actionable, sensitive to change, and not burdensome to assess. Second, the measures should, to the extent possible, be broadly applicable, useful for benchmarking, psychometrically strong, and grounded in a theory or framework.[106] When implementation science measures are useful and easy to utilize, the indicators may be more easily incorporated into research studies and result in increasingly standardized approaches to measuring key implementation phenomena such as organizational readiness, intervention acceptability, and program sustainability.[107]

"Pragmatic clinical trials" are a specific term for clinical trials that are performed in real-world clinical settings and with highly generalizable patient populations.[108] The goal is to produce clinical evidence at a lower cost and in less time as compared to a standard clinical trial. Study outcomes in pragmatic clinical trials are typically data points captured during routine care, or additional data points easily incorporated within routine care settings. Rather than elucidate biological or social mechanisms of disease, pragmatic clinical trials are intended to inform policy-makers and practitioners regarding the relative advantage of different clinical and public health services. Because implementation science is often less controlled than clinical research, pragmatic trials in implementation science require both clinical, and contextual equipoise, defined as a "genuine uncertainty that the implementation will work in a new context as well as whether the implementation package will work at all."[103] In other words, implementation scientists conducting pragmatic trials conceive, test, and evaluate optimal delivery strategies for efficacious interventions.

Pragmatic trials may have a particularly important role for implementation science conducted in LMICs where the resources needed to deliver efficacious interventions may not be consistently available. For example, while there are international and nationally adapted guidelines to inform the provision of nutritional support for neonates with acute infections, many of these guidelines assume sufficient nurse-to-patient ratios and availability of key material resources such as electric pumps that can deliver low levels of intravenous fluids to small babies. Pragmatic trials would allow implementation scientists in these settings to understand how best to deliver care in facilities where efficacious neonatal interventions from high-resource settings are not directly transferrable, and highly controlled clinical trials would not reflect the realities of everyday practice.[109]

To ensure that implementation science is locally pragmatic when evaluating the delivery of efficacious health interventions developed in HICs, implementation scientists in LMICs must identify opportunities to adapt or prioritize interventions while maintaining fidelity to core mechanisms of action. One example of such an effort was the development of a "translatability scale" to help implementers grade the expected ease of implementing cardiovascular disease practice points and recommendations from higher-resourced settings within resource-limited settings.[110]

Conducting Contextually Relevant Implementation Science

Ensuring that there is appropriate "fit" between an intervention and the practice setting is critical for ensuring pragmatic implementation.[89] As previously described, implementation research does not typically try to control for contextual factors that influence study outcomes, unlike traditional clinical research. Rather, it is well understood that contextual factors such as social, cultural, economic, political, legal, institutional/infrastructural, and environmental characteristics can have a strong moderating influence on the impact of newly introduced evidence-based interventions and thus are important to account for.[6] In any setting, but perhaps particularly in resource-constrained LMICs, there can be tensions between social and economic structures, and individual and collective agency.[111] For example, an evidence-based family planning intervention offering new injectable contraceptives will be implemented quite differently in settings where family planning programming is institutionalized within a government structure as opposed to a setting where there is no government support for family planning. Yet, in either setting, individual and community-level preferences and cultural norms regarding family planning will also undoubtedly influence intervention uptake and sustainability.

The multiple levels at which context influences implementation has been described in the Consolidated Framework for Implementation Research (CFIR) as the "inner setting" and the "outer setting."[64] Although the specific factors that fall within each setting construct may vary across geographies, generally the inner setting includes the structural, economic, political, and cultural contexts within which an implementation process occurs. The outer setting generally includes economic, political, and social contexts within which the implementing organization or entity itself resides. Changes in the outer setting can influence implementation, often mediated through changes in the inner setting. For example, the family planning intervention described above would be influenced by an increase in allocated human resource support from the MOH (i.e., economic context), but this investment would be mediated by the behavior of health providers in health facilities via their acceptance of the new injectable method and associated promotion of the service (i.e., cultural context).

Contextual factors are dynamic, and factors that act as barriers to implementation in one setting may actually facilitate implementation in another.[111] These factors interact with one another and can change over time, producing unpredictable effects that may require continuous adaptation from implementers.[6] Thus, it is important for implementation researchers to fully study and document the implementation context in which their intervention takes place using flexible research methods that can be responsive to changes in policies, programs, and practices. Alexander and Hearld[112] describe a helpful array of methods that can be used to evaluate context. Qualitative methods (e.g., participant observation, document analysis, and key informant interviews) might be useful in gaining insights on contextual factors and how they affect an implementation strategy. Comparative analyses, where the effectiveness of strategies is compared across different contexts, can also provide useful insights. Finally, hierarchical modeling techniques can help quantify the extent to which different contextual levels contribute to implementation effectiveness. When implementation takes place in a particularly complex system, researchers may need to deploy multiple methods or utilize different sources of information to fully study and report upon the implementation context. Ideally, investigating implementation context does not occur simply at study baseline, but iteratively throughout study implementation in order to capture changes to the contextual state over time.

A hallmark of implementation science is ensuring that a proven health intervention maintains its demonstrated effectiveness within a new setting or environment while recognizing that implementation cannot be delivered as a uniform template.[113] Rather the context must inform the way the intervention is introduced. Should researchers seek to understand the transportability of a health intervention, or the ability to use results from one setting to infer the effects of the intervention in another, they can study the mechanism of action through which the implementation strategy influences a targeted outcome and seek to replicate this mechanism of action within the new setting.[85] Involving implementing stakeholders from the new setting in the process of initial implementation research design can be an exceptionally helpful way to adapt an intervention across heterogeneous settings.

Implementation context is not simply a backdrop to an intervention, but rather a key influence on intervention success, and thus context should be understood as a *process* rather than a *place*.[111,114] Context-sensitive implementation is particularly important during the scale-up of evidence-based interventions, as in the South African experience of testing and scaling up PMTCT of HIV programs.[115] Although efficacy studies demonstrated that single-dose nevirapine decreased mother-to-child transmission of HIV by more than 50% and the intervention was fully deployed nationwide in 2002, the intervention appeared to demonstrate surprisingly minimal effectiveness.[116] This finding prompted a number of demonstration projects that used adaptive designs to improve the performance of PMTCT programs by accounting for contextual factors at the local level influencing effective delivery and uptake.[115] These projects allowed the national government to study and adopt new delivery models that drew from systems-engineering quality improvement methods. Along with improved drug regimens, mobile treatment programs, and policy changes that allowed nurses to initiate treatment, the revised context-sensitive South African approach resulted in unprecedented reductions in mother-to-child transmission of HIV.[117]

GAPS AND OPPORTUNITIES IN IMPLEMENTATION SCIENCE

The field of implementation science is growing rapidly, yet it remains a "young" science. The strong demand for implementation science has, to some extent, outpaced the development of theories, measures, and other foundational tools, creating important gaps to be addressed to make implementation science widely applicable and put the field on solid footing. At the same time, as the field seeks to respond to the practical and pressing needs of implementation stakeholders, new opportunities arise for developing and evaluating implementation strategies to address both emergent and persistent problems. To illustrate one gap, many of the theories and frameworks employed in implementation science, such as the CFIR and RE-AIM, were developed by researchers in HICs such as the United States. While implementation scientists have applied these theories and frameworks to study implementation context, processes, and outcomes in global health contexts,[118–123] some adaptation is needed to reflect differences in the health interventions being implemented, and the health system and cultural context in which they are being implemented, especially in LMICs. Health interventions such as ART, mental health treatment, and cancer screening are subject to high levels of stigma and discrimination, an intervention characteristic not reflected in the CFIR. Likewise, the hierarchical structure of health systems in LMICs renders the CFIR's distinction between inner setting and outer setting somewhat ambiguous. Lastly, in collectivist cultures and those in which conformity to hierarchy is accepted and expected, individual motivation and other characteristics of individuals likely play a lesser role in implementation.

Three additional gaps and opportunities in global implementation science merit discussion: measurement, multilevel intervention, and deimplementation.

Measurement

Poor-quality measurement presents a formidable barrier to efforts to advance implementation science. Measurement is the foundation of science. It is difficult, if not impossible, to generate robust, cumulative knowledge if the measures employed in scientific inquiry lack reliability or validity. Reliability in this context refers to the quality of assessment or, put differently, the consistency or repeatability of measurement. Validity refers to the accuracy of assessment or whether a measure really measures what it is supposed to measure.

Reflecting the recent emergence of implementation science as an organized and institutionally supported field of inquiry, the state of measurement in the field is suboptimal. Systematic reviews indicate many of the available measures for assessing implementation context, processes, and outcomes have unknown reliability and validity.[124–128] For example, Chaudoir et al.[127] identified 62 measure constructs thought to predict the implementation of proven health interventions. They observed that organization-level constructs (e.g., management support), provider-level constructs (e.g., attitudes), and intervention-level constructs (e.g., complexity) had the greatest number of measures, whereas structural constructs (e.g., social, political, societal context) and patient-level constructs (e.g., patient needs and preferences) had the least number of measures. Additionally, they observed that for the majority of measures, predictive validity—that is, a statistically significant association with an implementation outcome, such as adoption or fidelity—either had not been examined or was not supported. Similarly, Chor et al.[128] identified 118 measures associated with 27 constructs thought to predict the adoption of proven health or mental health interventions. Measures were unevenly distributed across constructs, with the majority of measures focusing on hypothesized predictors of adoption at the organizational, innovation, and individual staff levels. As with Chaudoir et al.,[127] they observed few measures of patient or client characteristics thought to predict adoption. Moreover, only half of the measures they identified had information available about reliability or validity. Focused reviews of measures for specific constructs reveal a similar pattern. For example, Weiner et al.[125] and Gagnon et al.[129] found many measures of organizational readiness for change, yet few reliable and valid ones.

Poor-quality measurement is not limited to measures of implementation context or process. Lewis et al.[94] identified 108 measures of implementation outcomes used in mental health research. Available measures were unevenly distributed across the eight implementation outcomes described by Proctor et al.[66] Fifty measures assessed acceptability, 19 measures assessed adoption, and the remaining measures assessed the other implementation outcomes, none of which had more than eight measures. Overall, availability of information on reliability and validity across all 104 measures was limited and variable. Forty-six percent of the measures lacked information on four or more of the aspects of reliability and validity examined in the review. Moreover, the level of reliability and validity that measures demonstrated was also limited and uneven. For example, many measures for which information about reliability was available exhibited "good" or "excellent" reliability when raters assessed the level of evidence using a standard rating scale; by contrast, few measures for which information was available about validity exhibit "good" or "excellent" predictive validity.

Systematic reviews of measures have identified two additional measurement issues that merit discussion.[130] First, some measures have different content (e.g., survey questions) even though they purport to measure the same construct, while other measures have the same content even though they purport to measure different constructs. These problems generate concerns about construct validity, that is, concerns about whether measures really measure what they purportedly measure. Preventing or addressing these problems requires explicitly defining constructs, differentiating constructs that are similar conceptually (e.g., receptivity to change and readiness to change), developing items to measure constructs based on such conceptual definitions and distinctions, and evaluating whether these items assess the construct of interest and not related constructs.[131] Second, many measures have not been assessed for, or do not demonstrate, pragmatic quality.[130] Pragmatic measures are important because implementation research takes place in real-world settings. Measures with dozens of items, for example, impose significant burden on survey respondents. Pragmatic measures are also important for encouraging practitioners to use measures to assess implementation context, monitor implementation progress, and evaluate implementation outcomes. Practitioners will not use measures that are not practical, no matter how reliable or valid those measures might be. As noted earlier, pragmatic measures are not only brief, but also important to practitioners, actionable, user-friendly, and sensitive to change.[106]

Although the state of measurement in implementation science is suboptimal, efforts are underway to develop reliable and valid measures of implementation context, processes, and outcomes. For example, researchers have developed reliable, valid measures of attitudes toward evidence-based practice,[132] implementation leadership,[133,134] implementation climate,[135] organizational readiness for implementing change,[136] organizational social context,[137] and implementation outcomes such as acceptability, appropriateness, and feasibility.[138] Further, researchers have identified and operationally defined the practical features of measures that practitioners, themselves, say they value.[107] Measures can now be assessed for practicality using rating scales, providing those looking for measures with additional information beyond that concerning reliability and validity.

More measurement work must be done. Importantly, existing measures and newly developed measures in implementation science need to be linguistically and culturally adapted for use in LMICs, as many of these measures were created in HICs such as the United States. Good measurement practices for adapting measures for cross-cultural use include translating the measure from the source language to the target language (forward translation); translating the translated measure from the target language back to the source language (backward translation); comparing the two translations; using "think aloud" and other cognitive interviewing techniques to assess whether respondents have any difficulty comprehending, interpreting, or responding to the adapted measure; and reassessing the reliability, validity, and practicality of the adapted measure.[139,140] Good measurement practices, such as those described by Hinkin,[141] should also be employed in developing new measures within LMIC contexts so that implementation science can generate robust, cumulative knowledge no matter where it is conducted.

Multilevel Interventions

The deployment and evaluation of multilevel interventions represent another gap and opportunity in implementation science. Increasingly, funders of implementation science have called for research assessing the effectiveness of multilevel intervention packages, that is, interventions that include multiple implementation strategies that target change at two or more levels of a social system (e.g., individuals, groups, organizations, and communities[142–145]). Interest in multilevel interventions has increased with the growing recognition that the barriers and facilitators (i.e., determinants) of access to and use of proven health interventions exist at many levels. For example, determinants at multiple levels influence whether women get cervical cancer screening, including patient knowledge, attitudes, and beliefs; family and social support for screening, staffing, supplies, equipment, and hours of operation of health facilities; and distance or transportation to health facilities. Multilevel interventions should be more effective than single interventions because they address the multiple determinants that promote or inhibit access to and use of proven health interventions. Thus, for example, a multilevel intervention that combines parental nutritional counseling (an individual-level intervention) and school feeding programs (an organization-level intervention) should be more effective than either intervention alone. However, proponents and critics of multilevel interventions acknowledge that more interventions do not necessarily produce more effect.[146,147] In fact, systematic reviews indicate that some multi-component interventions, which include multilevel interventions the components of which frequently target change at different levels, are no more effective than single-component interventions.[69,148–150] This can occur even when the implementation strategies deployed and evaluated at various levels are theory-based, empirically supported, feasible, and acceptable. Poor reporting of the operational details of intervention deployment in research articles makes it difficult to ascertain the extent to which the additional logistical challenges of layering, sequencing, and timing interventions at multiple levels contribute to these disappointing results. However, it is often unclear why specific interventions were selected and combined, suggesting the possibility that poorly conceived design of the multilevel intervention may also play a role. Even well-executed multilevel interventions can produce scattered, redundant, or even contradictory effects without careful thought about how interventions at multiple levels interact in mutually reinforcing ways.

Realizing the promise of multilevel interventions will require advances in three aspects of implementation science. First, researchers and practitioners should select interventions based on a thorough understanding of the determinants of the implementation problem in the specific settings in which the implementation strategies will be deployed. Although seemingly obvious, this is often not done. Researchers evaluating implementation strategies typically recruit healthcare organizations or health professionals into their studies based on their willingness to participate rather than on an assessment of the determinants of the implementation problem; they then deploy and evaluate a predefined implementation strategy that might or might not address the determinants operating in those specific settings. Practitioners engaged in "implementation as usual" are just as likely as researchers to employ favored implementation strategies without first assessing the determinants of the implementation problem.[151] A recently published review identified more than 600 determinants of poor implementation[152]; while this number seems daunting, often only a handful of determinants operate in any given setting at any given time. Several methods for assessing and prioritizing determinants have been identified, evaluated, and compared to one another.[153] No single method seems to outperform the others, as implementation strategies tailored to address determinants identified through these methods appear to be no more effective than untailored implementation strategies.[154] These results suggest either that better methods are needed for assessing and prioritizing determinants or, alternatively, that better methods are needed for selecting and matching implementation strategies to identified determinants.

The second area in which advances are needed is in the understanding of the mechanisms by which implementation strategies work. Knowing how implementation strategies work—that is, how they produce intended effects—is crucial for selecting and matching strategies to identified determinants. Consider the following analogy. Suppose someone wants to hang a picture. She has a nail (a proven intervention for securing pictures to walls). However, she cannot push the nail into the wall with her hands deeply enough to hold the picture (determinant of the implementation problem, depth insufficient to secure the picture to the wall). She needs a better tool (implementation strategy) than her hand to secure the nail in the wall. Of the many tools in her toolbox, she selects a hammer rather than a screwdriver because a hammer applies blunt force on a surface area small enough (mechanism) to secure the nail in the wall. A screwdriver does not do that. As this analogy indicates, selecting the right tool or the right implementation strategy depends on a correct understanding of not only the problem to be solved, but also how a tool or strategy works. Unfortunately, the mechanisms of implementation strategies are poorly understood in no small part because implementation strategies have been treated as "black boxes." More than one-hundred research studies of audit and feedback were conducted before researchers began to inquire how audit and feedback works, that is, how it produces an effect on professionals' behavior.[155] Unfortunately, the mechanisms by which the 73 implementation strategies identified by Powell et al. work remain just as opaque.[156] Recognizing this gap, Lewis et al.[156] have recently proposed methods for theorizing the mechanisms of implementation strategies. As these methods become more widely applied, and the theorized mechanisms revealed as these methods are tested, researchers and practitioners will be better equipped to select and match implementation strategies to identified determinants.

The third area in which advances are needed concerns the causal logic for combining interventions at multiple levels to achieve complementary or synergistic effects. It might seem unnecessary to develop a causal logic for combining interventions at multiple levels if the interventions at each level are selected and matched to determinants at the level in which they operate. However, the causal logic for combining interventions is important because the determinants that operate at different levels are themselves interdependent: they interact and influence each other.[157] This means that the implementation strategies deployed in a multilevel intervention also interact and influence each other. Methods for designing multilevel interventions to produce complementary (e.g., $2 + 2 = 4$) or even synergistic (e.g., $2 + 2 = 5$) effects are still in their infancy. However, Weiner et al.[157] used causal models based on the ideas of mediation and moderation to describe five strategies for combining interventions at multiple levels. Tools from epidemiology, such as directed acyclic graphs, could also be employed to think through the causal logic of multilevel interventions, thereby increasing their effectiveness.

Deimplementation

To date, implementation science as a field has focused almost exclusively on promoting access to and use of effective health interventions. Only recently has attention turned to the problem of deimplementing ineffective or overused practices. Indeed, consensus has yet to develop on terminology; a scoping review of the literature on deadopting "low-value" clinical practices identified 43 unique terms used to describe the process, with "divest" the most frequently used term.[158] Deimplementation can be provisionally defined as "reducing or stopping the use of a health service or practice provided to patients by healthcare practitioners and systems."[159] Deimplementing ineffective or harmful practices can improve outcomes for patients and reduce wasteful healthcare spending. It could also free up time, effort, and resources for health professionals to deliver proven health interventions. Reflecting the nascent state of research into deimplementation, a recently published analysis identified only 20 research grants funded by the NIH and the U.S. Agency for Healthcare Research and Quality between 2000 and 2017[159]; a majority ($N = 11$) were funded between fiscal years 2015 and 2016. Although some efforts to reduce the use of "low-value" practices predate recent emergence of interest in deimplementation, these efforts have focused largely on reducing inappropriate prescribing of antibiotics and other overused drugs.[160] Colla et al.[160] report, based on their systematic review of strategies to reduce "low-value care," that decision support and performance feedback are promising strategies that have a solid evidence base; further, education directed toward health professionals yields changes by itself and when paired with other implementation strategies. However, the authors acknowledged the challenge of defining and measuring "low-value care" in conducting their review of previous published studies, especially with regard to differentiating efforts to reduce "low-value" care from efforts to reduce healthcare utilization generally.

Although it is tempting to think of deimplementation and implementation as two sides of the same coin, Prasad and Ioannidis suggest that this is not likely to be the case.[161] They argue that "evidence wars," on-the-ground realities, and other sociopolitical and economic considerations play an asymmetric role in deimplementation and implementation. Specifically, they propose that deimplementation processes may vary as a function of the type of evidence for and against a practice. For widely adopted practices for which evidence is contradicted by large, high-quality randomized trials, deimplementation efforts are likely to encounter fierce resistance. Proponents of the contradicted practice may publish editorials and marshal counter-evidence by focusing on subgroups of patients who seem to benefit, highlighting lesser clinical endpoints with positive outcomes, or performing additional studies with less scientific rigor. The authors cite examples in which medical societies vigorously contested the results of landmark clinical trials that demonstrated little or no benefit for widespread clinical practices.[161]

Resistance is less likely for ineffective practices than for those for which evidence is subsequently contradicted by large, high-quality randomized trials. As Prasad and Ioannidis note, the former are far more common than the latter. An empirical evaluation of systematic reviews published in the Cochrane Database, for example, found that the existing evidence base was unable to support or refute 49% of clinical practices[162]; a similar assessment found that 48% of American College of Cardiology recommendations are supported by expert opinion only.[163] A logical place to start is to subject these practices to systematic, rigorous evaluation. However, the credibility of such evaluation, and the potential for resistance to emerge in the event of disconfirming findings, depends in large part on the sponsorship and conduct of evaluation by bodies with no real or apparent conflict of interest. Moreover, both the process and the criteria for prioritizing unproven clinical practices for evaluation need to be transparent and acceptable, especially to stakeholders with a vested interest in the continued use of the practice.

Finally, Prasad and Ioannidis propose that preemptive steps be taken to make deimplementation of novel clinical practices efficient, should evidence develop after the practice has been introduced indicating ineffectiveness or harm.[161] In particular, they highlight the role that policy-making bodies, regulatory agencies, and health ministries can play in setting upfront high, evidentiary standards for novel clinical practices, restricting dissemination of such practices while evidence develops, and aligning payment with guidance on acceptable use.

While Prasad and Ioannidis emphasize the role of scientific evidence and sociopolitical context in deimplementation efforts, Wang et al.[164] propose a typology of change that formally couples implementation and deimplementation in the change process. They argue that the processes labeled deimplementation represents four types of change. The first type is reduction or partial reversal in the frequency, breadth, or scale of an existing clinical practice, so that it is provided to only a subgroup of patients who have been demonstrated to realize the greatest benefit of a given intervention. The second type is discontinuation or complete reversal of an existing clinical practice without replacement. In both reduction and discontinuation, no implementation takes place. The third type involves substitution or reversal with a replacement that is a closely related or enhanced and more effective practice. The fourth type is substitution or reversal with unrelated replacement (e.g., substituting physical therapy for opioid prescription for lower back pain). In substitution with related or unrelated replacement, implementation of a new practice is coupled with deimplementation of an old one.

Wang et al.[164] observe that some strategies for implementing new, proven practices—such as clinical decision support, electronic reminders, and educational outreach—also work well for deimplementing outmoded or contradicted ones.[165] However, other strategies appear to work for some types of deimplementation but not others. Persuasive strategies such as provider education, academic detailing, local opinion leaders, and audit and feedback appear to be effective for reduction or partial reversal (e.g., limiting antibiotic prescribing for hospital inpatients[166]), but not for discontinuation or complete reversal (e.g., eliminating advanced imaging for lower back pain[167]). Moreover, policy interventions, such as financial incentives and payment reform, appear to be effective strategies for reducing or discontinuing clinical practices,[168,169] despite limited evidence that they increase health professionals' delivery of proven clinical practices.[170] Wang et al.[164] speculate that variation in the level of cognitive and logistical effort involved in the four types of change that comprise deimplementation, and differences in the relative mixture of learning and "unlearning" each type of change entails, may explain why some strategies work equally well for implementation and deimplementation, while others do not. These authors conclude by noting that coupling the implementation of new, proven practices with the deimplementation of outmoded or contradicted practices could result in an effort-neutral change (in the long term) that overburdened healthcare professionals perceive more favorably than yet another implementation effort that adds to the long list of things to do. This point applies as much to implementation efforts in LMIC contexts as it does to those in HIC.

CONCLUSION

Implementation science addresses a fundamental, pressing problem in global health: how to take affordable, life-saving health interventions that have proven efficacious in earlier phase research studies and implement them at scale in clinical and community settings. Implementation science can accelerate the translation of research into practice and close the "know-do" gap by providing policy-makers, program managers, and other decision-makers with evidence about which strategies for promoting access to and use of proven health interventions are effective and under what conditions. Implementation science can also provide implementers with tools to assess local implementation context, select, and match implementation strategies to contextual conditions, monitor implementation and scale up progress, adjust implementation strategies as needed, and evaluate implementation success. Despite rapidly growing interest in employing evidence-based approaches to implementing effective health interventions, implementation science remains a "young" science. For the field to realize its full potential, effort and resources should be directed toward adapting implementation theories and frameworks for use in global health contexts, strengthening the measurement foundation of the field, developing innovative, yet practical implementation strategies for use in low-resources settings, and applying rigorous research methods to evaluate the effectiveness of these strategies. By engaging implementation stakeholders early and integrating implementation research into the design, planning, and deployment of implementation and scale-up efforts, implementation science can help policy and program decision-makers move from "letting it happen" (or even "hoping it happens") to "making it happen" with greater speed, fidelity, efficiency, quality, sustainability, and relevant coverage.

References

1. *Global Health Estimates 2015: Deaths by Cause, Age, Sex, by Country and by Region, 2000–2015.* Geneva; 2016. http://www.who.int/healthinfo/global_burden_disease/estimates/en/index1.html. Accessed January 28, 2021.
2. Jamison DT, Bremen JG, Measham AR, et al., eds. Cost-effective strategies for the excess burden of disease in developing countries. In: *Priorities in Health.* Herndon, Washington, DC: The International Bank for Reconstruction and Development/The World Bank; 2006. https://www.ncbi.nlm.nih.gov/books/NBK10257/. Accessed January 28, 2021.
3. Lincetto O, Mothebesoane-anoh S, Gomez P, Munjanja S. *Opportunities for Africa's Newborns: Antenatal Care.* Geneva, Switzerland: The World Health Organization Press. 2013.
4. Alkema L, Chou D, Hogan D, et al. Global, regional, and national levels and trends in maternal mortality between 1990 and 2015, with scenario-based projections to 2030: A systematic analysis by the UN Maternal Mortality Estimation Inter-Agency Group. *Lancet.* 2016;387(10017):462–74.
5. World Health Organization. *World Malaria Report 2016.* Geneva: WHO Press 2016.
6. Peters DH, Tran NTNT, Adam T. *Implementation Research in Health: A Practical Guide.* Geneva: WHO Press; 2013, pp. 1–69.
7. Odeny TA, Padian N, Doherty MC, et al. Definitions of implementation science in HIV/AIDS. *Lancet HIV.* 2015;2(5):e178–80.
8. About Implementation Science. Implementation Science. https://implementationscience.biomedcentral.com/about. Accessed April 1, 2017.
9. Peters DH, Adam T, Alonge O, Agyepong IA, Tran N. Implementation research: What it is and how to do it. *BMJ.* 2013;347:f6753.
10. Bhattacharyya O, Reeves S, Zwarenstein M. What is implementation research? *Res Soc Work Pract.* 2009;19(5):491–502.
11. Eccles MP, Armstrong D, Baker R, et al. An implementation research agenda. *Implement Sci.* 2009;4:18.
12. Rabin BA, Brownson RC, Haire-Joshu D, Kreuter MW, Weaver NL. A glossary for dissemination and implementation research in health. *J Public Health Manag Pract.* 2008;14(2):117–23.
13. World Health Organization, UNICEF/UNDP/World Bank/WHO Special Programme for Research and Training in Tropical Diseases. *Implementation Research for the Control of Infectious Diseases of Poverty: Strengthening the Evidence Base for the Access and Delivery of New and Improved Tools, Strategies and Interventions.* Geneva; 2011. http://apps.who.int/iris/bitstream/10665/75216/1/9789241502627_eng.pdf. Accessed January 28, 2021.
14. Woolf SH. The meaning of translational research and why it matters. *JAMA.* 2008;299(2):211–3.
15. Glasgow RE, Eckstein ET, ElZarrad MK. Implementation science perspectives and opportunities for HIV/AIDS research: Integrating science, practice, and policy. *J Acquir Immune Defic Syndr.* 2013;63(Suppl 1): S26–31. http://journals.lww.com/jaids/Fulltext/2013/06011/Implementation_Science_Perspectives_and.5.aspx. Accessed January 28, 2021.
16. Heidari S, Harries AD, Zachariah R. Facing up to programmatic challenges created by the HIV/AIDS epidemic in sub-Saharan Africa. *J Int AIDS Soc.* 2011;14(Suppl 1):S1.
17. Hirschhorn LR, Ojikutu B, Rodriguez W. Research for change: Using implementation research to strengthen HIV care and treatment scale-up in resource-limited settings. *J Infect Dis.* 2007;196(Suppl 3):S516–22.
18. Knapp H, Anaya HD. Implementation science in the real world: A case study of HIV rapid testing. *Int J STD AIDS.* 2013;24(1):5–11.
19. Elzarrad MK, Eckstein ET, Glasgow RE. Applying chronic illness care, implementation science, and self-management support to HIV. *Am J Prev Med.* 2013;44(1 Suppl 2):S99–107.
20. Merson MH, Curran JW, Griffith CH, Ragunanthan B. The president's Emergency Plan for AIDS relief: From successes of the emergency response to challenges of sustainable action. *Health Aff (Millwood).* 2012;31(7):1380–8.
21. Carnegie Foundations for the Advancement of Teaching. Improvement Science in Practice. https://www.carnegiefoundation.org/get-involved/events/improvement-science-in-practice/. Accessed May 1, 2017.
22. The Health Foundation. Evidence Scan: Improvement Science. *Heal Found Heal Scan.* January 2011; 22. http://www.health.org.uk/sites/health/files/ImprovementScience.pdf. Accessed January 28, 2021.

23. Blanchard JF, Aral SO. Program Science: An initiative to improve the planning, implementation and evaluation of HIV/sexually transmitted infection prevention programmes. *Sex Transm Infect.* 2011;87(1):2 LP-3.
24. Kim JY. *Remarks As Prepared for Delivery: World Bank Group President Jim Yong Kim at the Annual Meeting Plenary Session.* Washington, DC: The World Bank; 2012.
25. Powell BJ, McMillen JC, Proctor EK, et al. A compilation of strategies for implementing clinical innovations in health and mental health. *Med Care Res Rev.* 2012;69(2):123–57.
26. Peters DH, El-saharty S, Siadat B, Janovsky K, Vujicic M. *Improving Health Service Delivery in Developing Countries : From Evidence to Action.* Herndon, Washington, DC: World Bank Publications; 2009.
27. Remme JHF, Adam T, Becerra-Posada F, et al. Defining research to improve health systems. *PLoS Med.* 2010;7(11): e1001000.
28. Kaluzny AD, Gentry JT, Glasser JH. Innovation in health care organizations: Review of research and plan of projected studies. *Health Serv Res.* 1968;3(4):316–26.
29. Zerhouni E. MEDICINE: The NIH Roadmap. *Science.* 2003;302(5642): 63–72.
30. National Institutes of Health. Institutional Clinical and Translational Science Award RFA. https://grants.nih.gov/grants/guide/rfa-files/RFA-RM-06-002.html. Published 2006. Accessed January 28, 2021.
31. Sung NS, Crowley WF, Genel M, et al. Central challenges facing the national clinical research enterprise. *JAMA.* 2003;289(10):1278–87.
32. Blumberg RS, Dittel B, Hafler D, von Herrath M, Nestle FO. Unraveling the autoimmune translational research process layer by layer. *Nat Med.* 2012;18:35.
33. Neta G, Sanchez MA, Chambers DA, et al. Implementation science in cancer prevention and control: A decade of grant funding by the National Cancer Institute and future directions. *Implement Sci.* 2015;10(1):1–10.
34. National Institutes of Health. *Dissemination and Implementation Research in Health (R01) Program Announcement.* https://grants.nih.gov/grants/guide/pa-files/PAR-06-039.html. Published 2005. Accessed May 1, 2017.
35. National Institutes of Health. Dissemination and Implementation Research in Health (R01) PAR-16-238.
36. Eccles MP, Mittman BS. Welcome to implementation science. *Implement Sci.* 2006;1:1.
37. National Institute of Mental Health. Dissemination and Implementation Research Workshop: Harnessing Science to Maximize Health. https://www.nimh.nih.gov/news/events/2007/dissemination-and-implementation-research-workshop-harnessing-science-to-maximize-health.shtml. Published 2007. Accessed May 1, 2017.
38. World Health Organization. Conference : Second Annual NIH Conference on the Science of Dissemination and Implementation.
39. AcademyHealth. 10th Annual Conference on the Science of Dissemination and Implementation in Health.
40. Meissner HI, Glasgow RE, Vinson CA, et al. The U.S. training institute for dissemination and implementation research in health. *Implement Sci.* 2013;8:12.
41. Glasgow RE, Vinson C, Chambers D, Khoury MJ, Kaplan RM, Hunter C. National institutes of health approaches to dissemination and implementation science: Current and future directions. *Am J Public Health.* 2012;102(7):1274–81.
42. World Health Organization. *Implementation Research in TDR: Conceptual and Operational Framework.* Geneva; 2016. http://www.who.int/tdr/en/. Accessed January 28, 2021.
43. The Global Fund to Fight AIDS Tuberculosis and Malaria, USAID, World Health Organization, Special Program for Research and Training in Tropical Diseases, UNAIDS, The World Bank. *Framework for Operations and Implementation Research in Health and Disease Control Programs.* Geneva; 2008. http://www.who.int/hiv/pub/operational/or_framework.pdf. Accessed January 28, 2021.
44. Padian NS, Holmes CB, Mccoy SI, Lyerla R, Bouey PD, Goosby EP. Implementation Science for the US President's Emergency Plan for AIDS Relief (PEPFAR). *J Acquir Immune Defic Syndr.* 2011;56(3):199–203.
45. National Institutes of Health. NIH/PEPFAR Collaboration for Advancing Implementation Science in Prevention of Maternal-Child HIV Transmission (PMTCT) (R01) Funding Opportunity Announcement. https://grants.nih.gov/grants/guide/rfa-files/RFA-HD-12-210.html. Published 2011. Accessed January 28, 2021.
46. The John E. Fogarty International Center Advancing Science for Global Health. *Pathways to Global Health Research: Strategic Plan 2008–2012.* Bethesda; 2008. https://www.fic.nih.gov/About/Documents/stratplan_fullversion.pdf. Accessed January 28, 2021.
47. National Institutes of Health. RFA. Limited Competition: Global Health Program for Fellows and Scholars (Global Health Fellows) (R25). https://grants.nih.gov/grants/guide/rfa-files/RFA-TW-11-001.html. Published 2011. Accessed January 28, 2021.
48. Kemp CG, Weiner BJ, Sherr KH, et al. Implementation science for integration of HIV and non-communicable disease services in Sub-Saharan Africa: A systematic review. *AIDS.* 2018;32(Suppl 1):S93–105.
49. New focus area: Implementation and operational research. *J Acquir Immune Defic Syndr.* 2010;54(4):339. http://journals.lww.com/jaids/Fulltext/2010/08010/New_Focus_Area__Implementation_and_Operational.1.aspx. Accessed January 28, 2021.
50. Sturke R, Harmston C, Simonds RJ, et al. A multi-disciplinary approach to implementation science: The NIH-PEPFAR PMTCT Implementation Science Alliance. *J Acquir Immune Defic Syndr.* 2014;67:S163–7.
51. Fogarty International Center. NIH-PEPFAR PMTCT Implementation Science Alliance. https://www.fic.nih.gov/About/center-global-health-studies/Pages/pmtct-prevent-mother-child-transmission-hiv.aspx. Published 2016. Accessed January 28, 2021.
52. Fogarty International Center. Clean Cooking Implementation Science Network (ISN). https://www.fic.nih.gov/About/Staff/Policy-Planning-Evaluation/Pages/clean-cooking-implementation-science-network.aspx. Published 2017. Accessed January 28, 2021.
53. Fogarty International Center. Adolescent HIV Prevention and Treatment Implementation Science Alliance (AHISA). https://www.fic.nih.gov/About/center-global-health-studies/Pages/adolescent-hiv-prevention-treatment-implementation-science-alliance.aspx. Published 2017. Accessed January 28, 2021.
54. Rollins N, Chanza H, Chimbwandira F, et al. Prioritizing the PMTCT implementation research agenda in 3 African countries: Integrating and scaling up PMTCT through implementation research (INSPIRE). *J Acquir Immune Defic Syndr.* 2014;67(Suppl 2):S108–13.
55. Simmons R, Shiffman J. Scaling up reproductive health service innovations: A framework for action. In: Simmons R, Fajans P, Ghiron L, eds. *Scaling Up Health Service Delivery: From Pilot Innovations to Policies and Programmes.* Geneva: World Health Organization; 2007, pp. vii–xvii.
56. Tabak RG, Khoong EC, Chambers DA, Brownson RC. Bridging research and practice: Models for dissemination and implementation research. *Am J Prev Med.* 2012;43(3):337–50.
57. Birken SA, Powell BJ, Shea CM, et al. Criteria for selecting implementation science theories and frameworks: Results from an international survey. *Implement Sci.* 2017;12(1):124.
58. Nilsen P. Making sense of implementation theories, models and frameworks. *Implement Sci.* 2015;10(1):1–13.
59. Wilson KM, Brady TJ, Lesesne C, NWG on Translation. An organizing framework for translation in public health: The Knowledge to Action Framework. *Prev Chronic Dis.* 2011;8(2):A46. http://ovidsp.ovid.com/ovidweb.cgi?T=JS&CSC=Y&NEWS=N&PAGE=fulltext&D=medl&AN=21324260. Accessed January 28, 2021.
60. Canadian Institutes of Health Research. About Knowledge Translation. http://www.cihr-irsc.gc.ca/e/29418.html. Accessed January 8, 2018.
61. Meyers DC, Durlak JA, Wandersman A. The quality implementation framework: A synthesis of critical steps in the implementation process. *Am J Community Psychol.* 2012;50(3–4):462–80.
62. Stetler C. The Stetler Model. In: Rycroft-Malone J, Bucknall T, eds. *Models and Frameworks for Implementing Evidence-Based Practice: Linking Evidence to Action.* Oxford: Wiley-Blackwell; 2010, pp. 51–82.
63. Logan J, Graham I. The Ottawa Model of research use. In: Rycroft-Malone J, Bucknall T, eds. *Models and Frameworks for Implementing Evidence-Based Practice: Linking Evidence to Action.* Oxford: Wiley-Blackwell; 2010, pp. 83–108.
64. Damschroder LJ, Aron DC, Keith RE, Kirsh SR, Alexander JA, Lowery JC. Fostering implementation of health services research findings into practice: A consolidated framework for advancing implementation science. *Implement Sci.* 2009;4(1):1–15.
65. Cane J, O'Connor D, Michie S. Validation of the theoretical domains framework for use in behaviour change and implementation research. *Implement Sci.* 2012;7(1):37.
66. Proctor E, Silmere H, Raghavan R, et al. Outcomes for implementation research: Conceptual distinctions, measurement challenges, and research agenda. *Adm Policy Ment Heal Ment Heal Serv Res.* 2011;38(2):65–76.
67. Glasgow R, Vogt T, Boles S. Evaluating the public health impact of health promotion interventions: The RE-AIM framework. *Am J Public Health.* 1999;89(9):1322–7.
68. RE-AIM.org. Public Health Relevance and Population Health Impact.

69. Allanson ER, Tunçalp Ö, Vogel JP, et al. Implementation of effective practices in health facilities: A systematic review of cluster randomised trials. *BMJ Glob Heal.* 2017;2(2):e000266.
70. Powell BJ, Waltz TJ, Chinman MJ, et al. A refined compilation of implementation strategies: Results from the Expert Recommendations for Implementing Change (ERIC) project. *Implement Sci.* 2015;10(1):21.
71. Mutale W, Vardoy-Mutale A-T, Kachemba A, Mukendi R, Clarke K, Mulenga D. Leadership and management training as a catalyst to health system strengthening in low-income settings: Evidence from implementation of the Zambia Management and Leadership course for district health managers in Zambia. *PLoS One.* 2017;12(7):1–24.
72. Seims LRK, Alegre JC, Murei L, et al. Strengthening management and leadership practices to increase health-service delivery in Kenya: An evidence-based approach. *Hum Resour Health.* 2012;10(1):25.
73. Bossert T. *Health Systems 20/20 Project: Decentralization and Governance in Health.* Bethesda; 2008.
74. Saltman R, Busse R, Figueras J. *Decentralization in Health Care: Strategies and Outcomes (European Observatory on Health Systems and Policies Series).* New York: McGraw-Hill Education; 2006.
75. Tsofa B, Molyneux S, Gilson L, Goodman C. How does decentralisation affect health sector planning and financial management? A case study of early effects of devolution in Kilifi County, Kenya. *Int J Equity Health.* 2017;16(1):151.
76. Warren CE, Mayhew SH, Vassall A, et al. Study protocol for the Integra Initiative to assess the benefits and costs of integrating sexual and reproductive health and HIV services in Kenya and Swaziland. *BMC Public Health.* 2012;12:973.
77. Sweeney S, Obure CD, Terris-Prestholt F, et al. The impact of HIV/SRH service integration on workload: Analysis from the Integra Initiative in two African settings. *Hum Resour Health.* 2014;12:42.
78. Mutemwa R, Mayhew S, Colombini M, Busza J, Kivunaga J, Ndwiga C. Experiences of health care providers with integrated HIV and reproductive health services in Kenya: A qualitative study. *BMC Health Serv Res.* 2013;13(1):18.
79. Archana S, Nongkrynh B, Anand K, Pandav CS. Feasibility and validity of using WHO adolescent job aid algorithms by health workers for reproductive morbidities among adolescent girls in rural North India. *BMC Health Serv Res.* 2015;15(1):400.
80. Hill Z, Dumbaugh M, Benton L, et al. Supervising community health workers in low-income countries—A review of impact and implementation issues. *Glob Health Action.* 2014;7:24085.
81. UNICEF/UNDP/World Bank/WHO Special Programme for Research and Training in Tropical Diseases. *Community-Directed Treatment with Ivermectin: Report of a Multi-Country Study.* Geneva: World Bank; 1996.
82. Sékétéli A, Adeoye G, Eyamba A, et al. The achievements and challenges of the African Programme for Onchocerciasis Control (APOC). *Ann Trop Med Parasitol.* 2002;96(sup1):S15–28.
83. Baron RC, Rimer BK, Breslow RA, et al. Client-directed interventions to increase community demand for breast, cervical, and colorectal cancer screening. A systematic review. *Am J Prev Med.* 2008;35(1 Suppl):S34–55.
84. Hamer DH, Herlihy JM, Musokotwane K, et al. Engagement of the community, traditional leaders, and public health system in the design and implementation of a large community-based, cluster-randomized trial of umbilical cord care in Zambia. *Am J Trop Med Hyg.* 2015;92(3):666–72.
85. Hickey MD, Odeny TA, Petersen M, et al. Specification of implementation interventions to address the cascade of HIV care and treatment in resource-limited settings: A systematic review. *Implement Sci.* 2017;12(1):1–15.
86. Jeffery RA, To MJ, Hayduk-Costa G, et al. Interventions to improve adherence to cardiovascular disease guidelines: A systematic review. *BMC Fam Pract.* 2015;16(1):147.
87. Grimshaw J, Eccles M, Thomas R, et al. Toward evidence-based quality improvement. *J Gen Intern Med.* 2006;21(2):S14.
88. Lee ES, Vedanthan R, Jeemon P, et al. Quality improvement for cardiovascular disease care in low- and middle-income countries: A systematic review. *PLoS One.* 2016;11(6):e0157036.
89. Lau R, Stevenson F, Ong BN, et al. Achieving change in primary care-causes of the evidence to practice gap: Systematic reviews of reviews. *Implement Sci.* 2016;11(1):40.
90. Awad AI, Eltayeb IB, Baraka OZ. Changing antibiotics prescribing practices in health centers of Khartoum State, Sudan. *Eur J Clin Pharmacol.* 2006;62(2):135.
91. Proctor EK, Powell BJ, McMillen JC. Implementation strategies: Recommendations for specifying and reporting. *Implement Sci.* 2013;8(1):1–11.
92. Hoomans T, Severens JL. Economic evaluation of implementation strategies in health care. *Implement Sci.* 2014;9(1):168.
93. Klein KJ, Sorra JS. The Challenge of innovation implementation. *Acad Manag Rev.* 1996;21(4):1055–80.
94. Lewis CC, Fischer S, Weiner BJ, Stanick C, Kim M, Martinez RG. Outcomes for implementation science: An enhanced systematic review of instruments using evidence-based rating criteria. *Implement Sci.* 2015;10(1):1–17.
95. World Health Organization. What is the Quality of Care Network?
96. Higgins JPT, Green S. *Cochrane Handbook for Systematic Reviews of Interventions.* Hoboken, NJ: Wiley; 2011. https://books.google.com/books?id=NKMg9sMM6GUC. Accessed January 28, 2021.
97. Curran GM, Bauer M, Mittman B, Pyne JM, Stetler C. Effectiveness-implementation hybrid designs: Combining elements of clinical effectiveness and implementation research to enhance public health impact. *Med Care.* 2012;50(3):217–26.
98. Pinnock H, Epiphaniou E, Sheikh A, et al. Developing standards for reporting implementation studies of complex interventions (StaRI): A systematic review and e-Delphi. *Implement Sci.* 2015;10(1):42.
99. Hoffmann TC, Glasziou PP, Boutron I, et al. Better reporting of interventions: Template for intervention description and replication (TIDieR) checklist and guide. *BMJ.* 2014;348:g1687.
100. Loudon K, Treweek S, Sullivan F, Donnan P, Thorpe KE, Zwarenstein M. The PRECIS-2 tool: Designing trials that are fit for purpose. *BMJ.* 2015;350:h2147.
101. Craig P, Dieppe P, Macintyre S, Michie S, Nazareth I, Petticrew M. Developing and evaluating complex interventions: The new Medical Research Council guidance. *BMJ.* 2008;337:a1655.
102. Laycock A, Bailie J, Matthews V, Bailie R. Interactive dissemination: Engaging stakeholders in the use of aggregated quality improvement data for system-wide change in Australian indigenous primary health care. *Front Public Heal.* 2016;4:84.
103. Gopichandran V, Luyckx VA, Biller-Andorno N, et al. Developing the ethics of implementation research in health. *Implement Sci.* 2016;11(1):161.
104. Glasgow RE. What does it mean to be pragmatic? Pragmatic methods, measures, and models to facilitate research translation. *Heal Educ Behav.* 2013;40(3):257–65.
105. Zwarenstein M, Treweek S, Gagnier JJ, et al. Improving the reporting of pragmatic trials: An extension of the CONSORT statement. *BMJ.* 2008;337:a2390.
106. Glasgow RE, Riley WT. Pragmatic measures: What they are and why we need them. *Am J Prev Med.* 2013;45(2):237–43.
107. Powell BJ, Stanick CF, Halko HM, et al. Toward criteria for pragmatic measurement in implementation research and practice: A stakeholder-driven approach using concept mapping. *Implement Sci.* 2017;12(1):118.
108. National Institutes of Health. Living Textbook of Pragmatic Clinical Trials. NIH Collaboratory. http://rethinkingclinicaltrials.org/. Accessed December 22, 2017.
109. English M, Karumbi J, Maina M, et al. The need for pragmatic clinical trials in low and middle income settings—Taking essential neonatal interventions delivered as part of inpatient care as an illustrative example. *BMC Med.* 2016;14(1):5.
110. Owolabi M, Miranda JJ, Yaria J, Ovbiagele B. Controlling cardiovascular diseases in low and middle income countries by placing proof in pragmatism. *BMJ Glob Heal.* 2016;1(3):e000105.
111. May CR, Johnson M, Finch T. Implementation, context and complexity. *Implement Sci.* 2016;11(1):141.
112. Alexander JA, Hearld LR. Methods and metrics challenges of delivery-system research. *Implement Sci.* 2012;7(1):15.
113. World Health Organization. In: de Savigny D, Adam T, eds. *Systems Thinking for Health Systems Strengthening.* Albany, Switzerland: World Health Organization; 2009. http://ebookcentral.proquest.com/lib/washington/detail.action?docID=476146. Accessed January 28, 2021.
114. Pfadenhauer LM, Gerhardus A, Mozygemba K, et al. Making sense of complexity in context and implementation: The Context and Implementation of Complex Interventions (CICI) framework. *Implement Sci.* 2017;12(1):21.
115. Edwards N, Barker PM. The importance of context in implementation research. *J Acquir Immune Defic Syndr.* 2014;67:S157–62.
116. Rollins N, Little K, Mzolo S, Horwood C, Newell ML. Surveillance of mother-to-child transmission prevention programmes at immunization clinics: The case for universal screening. *AIDS.* 2007;21(10):1341–7.

117. Barron P, Pillay Y, Doherty T, et al. Eliminating mother-to-child HIV transmission in South Africa. *Bull World Health Organ.* 2013;91(1):70–4.

118. Gimbel S, Rustagi AS, Robinson J, et al. Evaluation of a systems analysis and improvement approach to optimize prevention of mother-to-child transmission of HIV using the consolidated framework for implementation research. *J Acquir Immune Defic Syndr.* 2016;72(Suppl 2):S108–16. http://journals.lww.com/jaids/Fulltext/2016/08011/Evaluation_of_a_Systems_Analysis_and_Improvement.3.aspx. Accessed January 28, 2021.

119. Rodriguez VJ, LaCabe RP, Privette CK, et al. The Achilles' heel of prevention to mother-to-child transmission of HIV: Protocol implementation, uptake, and sustainability. *SAHARA-J J Soc Asp HIV/AIDS.* 2017;14(1):38–52.

120. VanDevanter N, Kumar P, Nguyen N, et al. Application of the consolidated framework for implementation research to assess factors that may influence implementation of tobacco use treatment guidelines in the Viet Nam public health care delivery system. *Implement Sci.* 2017;12(1):27.

121. Warren CE, Ndwiga C, Sripad P, et al. Sowing the seeds of transformative practice to actualize women's rights to respectful maternity care: Reflections from Kenya using the consolidated framework for implementation research. *BMC Womens Health.* 2017;17(1):69.

122. Kramer BJ, Cote SD, Lee DI, Creekmur B, Saliba D. Barriers and facilitators to implementation of VA home-based primary care on American Indian reservations: A qualitative multi-case study. *Implement Sci.* 2017;12(1):109.

123. Orlando LA, Sperber NR, Voils C, et al. Developing a common framework for evaluating the implementation of genomic medicine interventions in clinical care: The IGNITE Network's Common Measures Working Group. *Genet Med.* 2018;20(6):655–63.

124. Emmons KM, Weiner B, Fernandez ME, Tu S-P. Systems antecedents for dissemination and implementation: A review and analysis of measures. *Heal Educ Behav.* 2011;39(1):87–105.

125. Weiner BJ, Amick H, Lee S-YD. Review: Conceptualization and measurement of organizational readiness for change: A review of the literature in health services research and other fields. *Med Care Res Rev.* 2008;65(4):379–436.

126. Allen JD, Towne SD, Maxwell AE, et al. Measures of organizational characteristics associated with adoption and/or implementation of innovations: A systematic review. *BMC Health Serv Res.* 2017;17(1):591.

127. Chaudoir SR, Dugan AG, Barr CHI. Measuring factors affecting implementation of health innovations: A systematic review of structural, organizational, provider, patient, and innovation level measures. *Implement Sci.* 2013;8(1):22.

128. Chor KHB, Wisdom JP, Olin SCS, Hoagwood KE, Horwitz SM. Measures for predictors of innovation adoption. *Adm Policy Ment Health.* 2015;42(5):545–73.

129. Gagnon M-P, Attieh R, Ghandour EK, et al. A systematic review of instruments to assess organizational readiness for knowledge translation in health care. *PLoS One.* 2014;9(12):e114338.

130. Martinez RG, Lewis CC, Weiner BJ. Instrumentation issues in implementation science. *Implement Sci.* 2014;9(1):1–9.

131. Johnston M, Dixon D, Hart J, Glidewell L, Schröder C, Pollard B. Discriminant content validity: A quantitative methodology for assessing content of theory-based measures, with illustrative applications. *Br J Health Psychol.* 2014;19(2):240–57.

132. Aarons GA. Mental health provider attitudes toward adoption of evidence-based practice: The evidence-based practice attitude scale (EBPAS). *Ment Health Serv Res.* 2004;6(2):61–74.

133. Aarons GA, Ehrhart MG, Farahnak LR. The implementation leadership scale (ILS): Development of a brief measure of unit level implementation leadership. *Implement Sci.* 2014;9(1):1–10.

134. Aarons GA, Ehrhart MG, Torres EM, Finn NK, Roesch SC. Validation of the implementation leadership scale (ILS) in substance use disorder treatment organizations. *J Subst Abuse Treat.* 2016;68:31–5.

135. Jacobs SR, Weiner BJ, Bunger AC. Context matters: Measuring implementation climate among individuals and groups. *Implement Sci.* 2014;9(1):1–14.

136. Shea CM, Jacobs SR, Esserman DA, Bruce K, Weiner BJ. Organizational readiness for implementing change: A psychometric assessment of a new measure. *Implement Sci.* 2014;9(1):7.

137. Glisson C, Green P, Williams NJ. Assessing the organizational social context (OSC) of child welfare systems: Implications for research and practice. *Child Abuse Negl.* 2012;36(9):621–32.

138. Weiner BJ, Lewis CC, Stanick C, et al. Psychometric assessment of three newly developed implementation outcome measures. *Implement Sci.* 2017;12(1):1–12.

139. Collins D. Pretesting survey instruments: An overview of cognitive methods. *Qual Life Res.* 2003;12(3):229–38.

140. Vreeman RC, McHenry MS, Nyandiko WM. Adapting health behavior measurement tools for cross-cultural use. *J Integr Psychol Ther.* 2013;1(1):2.

141. Hinkin TR. A brief tutorial on the development of measures for use in survey questionnaires. *Organ Res Methods.* 1998;1(1):104–21.

142. National Institutes of Health. Accelerating Colorectal Cancer Screening and follow-up through Implementation Science (ACCSIS): Coordinating Center (U24). https://grants.nih.gov/grants/guide/rfa-files/RFA-CA-17-039.html. Accessed January 28, 2021.

143. National Institutes of Health. Hypertension Outcomes for T4 Research within Lower Middle-Income Countries (Hy-TREC) (U01). https://grants.nih.gov/grants/guide/rfa-files/RFA-HL-17-014.html. Accessed January 28, 2021.

144. National Institutes of Health. Multilevel Interventions in Cancer Care Delivery: Follow-up to Abnormal Screening Tests. https://grants.nih.gov/grants/guide/pa-files/PA-17-495.html. Accessed January 28, 2021.

145. National Institutes of Health. ImPlementation REsearCh to DEvelop interventions for People Living with HIV (PREClUDE) (U01). https://grants.nih.gov/grants/guide/rfa-files/RFA-HL-18-007.html. Accessed January 28, 2021.

146. Stokols D. Establishing and maintaining health environments: Toward a social ecology of health promotion. *Am Psychol.* 1992;47(1):6–22.

147. Spence JC, Lee RE. Toward a comprehensive model of physical activity. *Psychol Sport Exerc.* 2003;4(1):7–24.

148. Suman A, Dikkers MF, Schaafsma FG, van Tulder MW, Anema JR. Effectiveness of multifaceted implementation strategies for the implementation of back and neck pain guidelines in health care: A systematic review. *Implement Sci.* 2016;11(1):126.

149. Russ LB, Webster CA, Beets MW, Phillips DS. Systematic review and meta-analysis of multi-component interventions through schools to increase physical activity. *J Phys Act Heal.* 2015;12(10):1436–46.

150. Low L-F, Fletcher J, Goodenough B, et al. A systematic review of interventions to change staff care practices in order to improve resident outcomes in nursing homes. *PLoS One.* 2015;10(11):e0140711.

151. Powell BJ, Proctor EK, Glisson CA, et al. A mixed methods multiple case study of implementation as usual in children's social service organizations: Study protocol. *Implement Sci.* 2013;8(1):92.

152. Krause J, Van Lieshout J, Klomp R, et al. Identifying determinants of care for tailoring implementation in chronic diseases: An evaluation of different methods. *Implement Sci.* 2014;9(1):1–12.

153. Wensing M, Oxman A, Baker R, et al. Tailored implementation for chronic diseases (TICD): A project protocol. *Implement Sci.* 2011;6(1):103.

154. Wensing M. The Tailored Implementation in Chronic Diseases (TICD) project: Introduction and main findings. *Implement Sci.* 2017;12(1):5.

155. Foy R, Eccles MP, Jamtvedt G, Young J, Grimshaw JM, Baker R. What do we know about how to do audit and feedback? Pitfalls in applying evidence from a systematic review. *BMC Health Serv Res.* 2005;5 (Table 1):1–7.

156. Lewis CC, Klasnja P, Powell BJ, et al. From confusion to causality: Advancing understanding of mechanisms of change in implementation science. *Front Public Health.* 2018;6:136.

157. Weiner BJ, Lewis MA, Clauser SB, Stitzenberg KB. In search of synergy: Strategies for combining interventions at multiple levels. *J Natl Cancer Inst - Monogr.* 2012;(44):34–41.

158. Niven DJ, Mrklas KJ, Holodinsky JK, et al. Towards understanding the de-adoption of low-value clinical practices: A scoping review. *BMC Med.* 2015;13(1):255.

159. Norton WE, Kennedy AE, Chambers DA. Studying de-implementation in health: An analysis of funded research grants. *Implement Sci.* 2017;12(1):144.

160. Colla CH, Mainor AJ, Hargreaves C, Sequist T, Morden N. Interventions aimed at reducing use of low-value health services: A systematic review. *Med Care Res Rev.* 2016;74(5):507–50.

161. Prasad V, Ioannidis JPA. Evidence-based de-implementation for contradicted, unproven, and aspiring healthcare practices. *Implement Sci.* 2014;9(1):1.

162. El Dib RP, Atallah ÁN, Andriolo RB. Mapping the Cochrane evidence for decision making in health care. *J Eval Clin Pract.* 2007;13(4):689–92.

163. Tricoci P, JM Allen, JM Kramer, RM Califf, SC Smith. Scientific evidence underlying the ACC/AHA clinical practice guidelines. *JAMA.* 2009;301(8):831–41.

164. Wang V, Maciejewski ML, Helfrich CD, Weiner BJ. Working smarter not harder: Coupling implementation to de-implementation. *Healthc (Amst).* 2018;6(2):104–7.

165. Bero LA, Grilli R, Grimshaw JM, Harvey E, Oxman AD, Thomson MA. Getting research findings into practice: Closing the gap between research and practice: An overview of systematic reviews of interventions to promote the implementation of research findings. *BMJ.* 1998;317(7156):465–8.

166. Davey P, Marwick CA, Scott CL, et al. Interventions to improve antibiotic prescribing practices for hospital inpatients. *Cochrane Database Syst Rev.* 2017;2(2):CD003543.

167. Jenkins HJ, Hancock MJ, French SD, Maher CG, Engel RM, Magnussen JS. Effectiveness of interventions designed to reduce the use of imaging for low-back pain: A systematic review. *C Can Med Assoc J.* 2015;187(6):401–8.

168. Swaminathan S, Mor V, Mehrotra R, Trivedi AN. Effect of medicare dialysis payment reform on use of erythropoiesis stimulating agents. *Health Serv Res.* 2015;50(3):790–808.

169. Wang C, Kane R, Levenson M, et al. Association between changes in CMS reimbursement policy and drug labels for erythrocyte-stimulating agents with outcomes for older patients undergoing hemodialysis covered by fee-for-service medicare. *JAMA Intern Med.* 2016;176(12):1818–25.

170. Sabatino SA, Lawrence B, Elder R, et al. Effectiveness of interventions to increase screening for breast, cervical, and colorectal cancers. *AMEPRE.* 2012;43(1):97–118.

171. Proctor E, Silmere H, Raghavan R, et al. Outcomes for implementation research: Conceptual distinctions, measurement challenges, and research agenda. *Adm Policy Ment Heal Ment Heal Serv Res.* 2011;38(2):65–76.

CHAPTER 21

Global Health Systems: What Will It Take to Deliver on the Promise of Health for All?

Wafaa M. El-Sadr • Katherine Harripersaud • Maria Lahuerta • Trisa Taro • Solange Baptiste • Wame Mosime • Yogan Pillay • Ariel Pablos-Mendez • Ilesh Jani • Bereket Alemayehu • Helen de Pinho • Francis Aboagye-Nyame • Stephanie M. Topp • Miriam Rabkin

The health of communities around the world is influenced not only by their disease burden, but by local, regional, and global health systems, which have a profound impact on health promotion and the response to health threats. A focus on health system strengthening has been noted as critical to achieving the goals of global health enabling effective implementation of services and ensuring their sustainability. This chapter describes the various components of health systems and their role in ensuring the health of individuals and populations. It also highlights the interconnectedness of each of the health system "building blocks" including: clinical service delivery, governance and leadership, health financing, human resources for health, laboratory systems, commodities and procurement systems, health information systems (HIS), and community engagement (see Fig. 21-1).

CLINICAL SERVICES DELIVERY

The delivery of high-quality health services is essential to the performance of effective health systems. Health systems are responsible for delivering a broad range of diverse health services including: preventive services such as vaccination; maternal health services such as antenatal and delivery care; curative services such as surgery or management of infectious diseases; and chronic health services for long-term conditions such as HIV and chronic noncommunicable diseases.

The structure and focus of health service delivery is not monolithic, however. Depending on the country, or even the state or province, service delivery may be more generalized *versus*. more specialized; offered at different levels, such as in general practice or primary healthcare clinics *versus* referral hospitals; and via publicly *versus* privately funded and managed institutions. In many low- and middle- income countries (LMICs), decisions affecting the availability, type, level, and degree of specialization of clinical health services have been influenced by trends in thinking within international organizations, most notably the World Health Organization (WHO) and the World Bank (WB). The following section maps these trends over the past half-century and discusses their influence on clinical service delivery in LMICs.

Harnessing the Power of Medical Advances

In the two decades following World War II, there was great optimism that harnessing the power of various medical technologies—including new antibiotics, vaccines, and antimalarial drugs would dramatically improve the health of populations in LMICs. WHO and UNICEF, two of the most influential international health organizations at the time, initiated ambitious disease elimination campaigns that were largely premised on the efficacy of newly available medical technologies. Programs such as the Expanded Program on Immunization (EPI) worked to eradicate polio and eliminate measles and rubella. At the same time, many newly independent nations in Africa and Asia were enthusiastically embracing the idea of providing high-quality healthcare for their citizens, by seeking to establish teaching hospitals and nursing and medical schools modelled in some cases on those of former colonial powers. While these typically urban tertiary-level services consumed a large proportion of health spending, substantial proportions of the populations who lived in rural regions of many of these newly independent nations were not able to access such services. Indeed healthcare for the rural majority in LMICs during the 1950s and 60s was often still delivered by a mix of geographically sparse public clinics, missionary hospitals, and "touring" services based out of urban centers.[1] Less structured care was also informally provided by indigenous and traditional providers, often not imbedded in the regional health system structures.

The Rise of Community-based Health Services

By the 1970s, the thinking about population health in global contexts was broadened beyond a medical and technical focus to include the management of health resources and services. A critical catalyst for this shift was the failure of the eradication campaigns for yaws and malaria, which had faltered once services were integrated into weak primary healthcare services. Globally, morbidity and mortality for rural communities was not improving and, in some cases, had even deteriorated.[2,3] All of these factors led to renewed attention to the importance of *access* to care, using alternative models of health service delivery, such as "barefoot doctors" in China and other community-based health programs in Tanzania, South Africa, Guatemala, and Mexico. These programs provided evidence of the importance of community participation and deepened the appreciation of the social determinants for sustainably addressing population health problems. These changes occurred against a political backdrop in which socialist economies had substantial global influence.

The Declaration of Alma Ata and Comprehensive Primary Healthcare

Throughout the 1970s, a series of WHO technical reports—most notably "Health by the People"—continued to cast a critical eye on previously medicalized health service strategies and stimulated advocacy for a shift in emphasis away from costly curative health services toward more fairly distributed and affordable care, including for preventive services.[4] These principles were synthesized and encapsulated in the Declaration of Alma Ata (launched at the WHO/UNICEF convention—International Conference on Primary Health Care in 1978) which outlined a vision for comprehensive primary healthcare in which nations, irrespective of wealth, were committed to provide health services for all their populations. The principles central to the concept of comprehensive primary healthcare included recognition of and response to the social determinants of health; involvement of all societal sectors in the promotion of health; community participation in planning, implementation, and regulation of primary healthcare; and a focus on achieving equity in health status. Primary healthcare

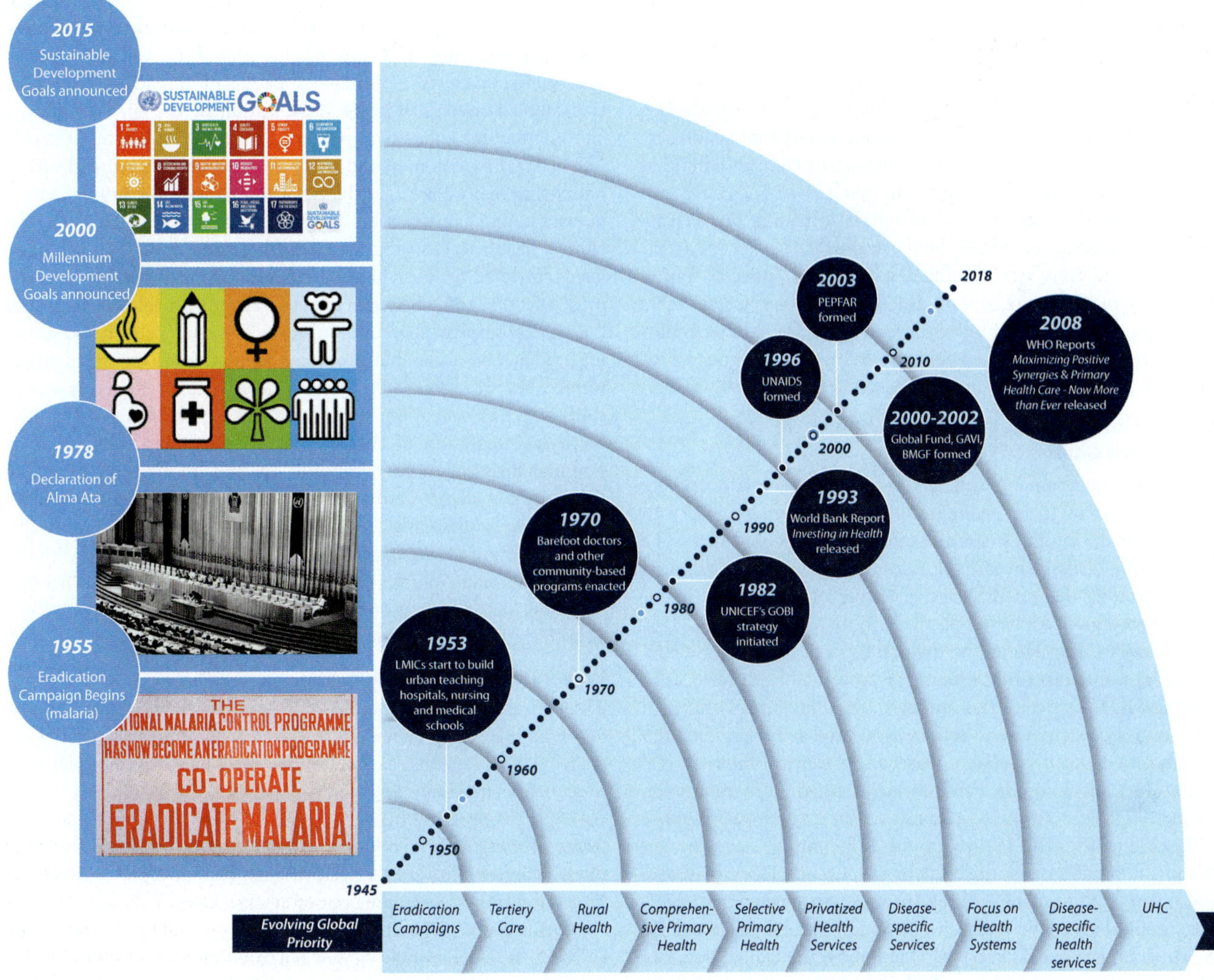

FIGURE 21-1. Health Systems and Evolving Global Priorities

was thus seen as "essential healthcare based on practical, scientifically sound, and socially acceptable methods and technology made universally accessible to individuals and families in the community through their full participation and at a cost that the community and country can afford to maintain at every stage of their development in the spirit of self-reliance and self-determination."[5]

From Comprehensive to Selective Primary Healthcare

Notwithstanding the momentum and sense of common purpose that underpinned the Declaration of Alma Ata with its vision of primary healthcare as a way to achieve "health for all," this was followed by the emergence of fissures in the international community. Some saw the Declaration with its vision for community-oriented services as an attack on the medical establishment and, in particular, on specialized healthcare. Others critiqued the focus on primary healthcare as utopian and lacking in pragmatism. Still others associated the concept of primary healthcare with the then Soviet city, Alma Ata, in which the declaration had been made, viewing it as a veiled attempt to push governments toward "socialized" medicine.

Consequently, just 1 year after the landmark Alma Ata event, "selective" primary healthcare was proposed as an alternative concept to guide international efforts to support clinical service design and delivery in LMICs. The concept of selective—not comprehensive—primary healthcare focused on ensuring more rapid improvements in health outcomes by targeting specific areas of health—notably those affecting children under 5 years of age and women of reproductive age with low-cost medical interventions operationalized as standalone services or interventions.[6] By late 1979, the selective primary healthcare approach had been operationalized by UNICEF, in the form of its large-scale targeted program for Growth Monitoring, Oral Rehydration Therapy, Breastfeeding, Immunization (GOBI), to which family planning, female education and food supplementation (GOBI-FFF) were later added. Such programs became the dominant mode of international service support to low-income countries through the early and mid-1980s, aligning with the agendas of many influential (often medically oriented) stakeholders.

Debt Crises and Structural Adjustment

Following a period in the mid-1970s when commodity prices were high and when many LMICs were encouraged to borrow at low rates from international banks, the 1979 oil crisis helped trigger a global economic recession. Money borrowed by newly independent countries from the International Monetary Fund (IMF), World Bank (WB), and others at the low rates of the early 1970s could not be repaid at the much higher rates incurred in the early 1980s, with a resulting debt crisis. "Structural adjustment" was the strategy developed to help these nations recover from their debt crises. This required that the indebted countries make drastic cuts to public spending—most notably to the health and education sectors—and by decentralizing and privatizing services, where possible, in order to continue to receive loans from the IMF, WB, and other major institutions. In 1987, the WB published its first report dedicated entirely to health—a technical appendix to the structural adjustment policy—which included plans for restructuring health services to enforce fee payment for health services; privatization of health services, and the promotion of private insurance programs.

In 1993, the WB annual report "Investing in Health" further reinforced the Bank's influence on global health, addressing several technical themes including its support for the concept of selective primary healthcare and defining the package of essential health services. Under these influences, the late 1980s and 1990s saw a flood of health sector privatization take place in many lower-income countries, amid broadly crumbling health system infrastructure. Private healthcare markets, based largely on the unregulated sale of pharmaceuticals thrived, thus, contributing to a healthcare "poverty trap" a situation where the poor had diminished access to services.[7] Access to basic services, including proven preventive services and technologies, became increasingly dependent on internationally funded programs such as those initiated by UNICEF and others.

Global Health Initiatives and the Millennium Development Goals

With national governments in many low-income countries lacking domestic resources to invest in health, health service delivery in many nations during the 1990s and into the 2000s continued to be defined by the disease-specific priorities through "vertical" funding streams (funding dedicated to a single issue or disease) by major international organizations. Of particular note, was the rise of HIV-specific funding. Throughout the 1990s, the global spread of the HIV epidemic not only placed devastating pressure on health services in sub-Saharan African countries among others, but directly affected health service capacity due to extensive HIV-related morbidity and mortality among health workers. This led to a series of international organizations (including the newly formed Joint UN Programme on HIV and AIDS—UNAIDS) to advocate for an exceptional response to this emergency. The launch of the Millennium Development Goals in combination with the catalytic effect of the HIV crisis, also led to a burgeoning of new public–private partnerships and philanthropic funders in the global health space. The Global Fund for HIV, Tuberculosis and Malaria (Global Fund), the Global Alliance for Vaccines and Immunization (GAVI), and the Bill and Melinda Gates Foundation were three of the largest players, followed soon by the U.S. bilateral initiative, the landmark President's Emergency Fund for AIDS Relief (PEPFAR), launched in 2003 by President George W. Bush. While varied in focus, all these global health initiatives sought to finance disease-specific services in LMICs and most included HIV among their priorities. By the end of 2017, a remarkable 21.7 million people living with HIV in LMICs had initiated treatment; AIDS deaths were reduced by more than 51% since 2004 and new infections declined by 16% since 2010.[8]

While often prioritizing delivery of clinical health services, global health initiatives in the early 2000s also highlighted the importance of investments in strengthening health system infrastructure, including for the procurement and distribution of commodities, laboratory services, and budgeting, financing, and reporting. Stalled progress toward some of the health-related MDGs reinforced the acknowledgment by policy makers and practitioners of the importance of fundamental health infrastructure, services, and staff. While substantial progress was noted in the response to the HIV epidemic and in under five and maternal mortality, health system limitations were recognized as being at the root of disappointing outcomes for tuberculosis control, integrated management of childhood illness, and the integration of other health services.[9] Thus, overall there was a realization of the need for effective and efficient systems for delivery of health services.

Primary Healthcare Redux

In 2008, WHO launched the "Maximizing Positive Synergies" initiative, intended to ensure that the disease-specific global health initiatives would lead to strengthened health systems.[10] In addition, in 2008 and marking 30 years since the Declaration of Alma Ata, WHO's Annual Report was entitled *Primary Healthcare—Now More than Ever*. Building on a tide of criticisms of the "vertical" service approach characteristic of many global health initiatives, the report critically assessed healthcare organization across high-, middle-, and low-income countries, and noted striking inequalities in access to care, health outcomes, and costs of care both between and within nations. In many countries, the report presented a disturbing picture of crumbling health systems that lacked focus, were inefficient, and clinical health services that were unable to deliver on the most basic needs. It called for a revitalized vision of primary healthcare as the most effective and affordable way to strengthen health systems and the clinical services they underpinned. The report also noted growing evidence to show that programs focused on delivering a single service, like vaccines, could be expanded to deliver others, as well as could serve as a stepping stone for more comprehensive integrated services. Integration of common management functions, such as essential drugs, transport, supervision, and information, could be another early step toward providing integrated and comprehensive care. Unlike in the early 1980s, this "second" call to reorient health systems around the concept of primary healthcare resonated with the concerns of many international and national stakeholders. What had been considered revolutionary three decades earlier, was now viewed as both evidence-based and highly necessary.

Universal Health Coverage

Through the late 2000s and in the buildup to the launch of the Sustainable Development Goals, the concept of "universal health coverage" (UHC) emerged as a defining goal of health service planning in global health. Emerging first in the WHO's 2008 *Primary Health Care: Now More than Ever* report, UHC came to be understood in terms of a tripartite requirement to ensure: (a) fair and equitable physical access to health services, (b) quality of care, and (c) financial protection from catastrophic out-of-pocket costs.

Within the WHO and across most major global health stakeholders, UHC was increasingly viewed as a core strategy for tackling health inequalities globally. In September 2015, the UN General Assembly adopted the 2030 Agenda for Sustainable Development which prioritized UHC as an essential pillar of development. Approximately one-third of countries have UHC, and another third are in the process of implementing UHC, with most of the remainder in Africa only beginning to consider it (exceptions include Rwanda, Ghana, two countries already implementing UHC).[11] Nonetheless, some argued that in a number of LMICs, planning for a broad extension of UHC—and concomitant health systems strengthening—would not be feasible.[12] The need to protect gains made in mitigating or controlling diseases like HIV is also frequently raised as a compelling priority. The future delivery of health services will need to balance addressing these diverse imperatives.

GOVERNANCE AND LEADERSHIP

The delivery of health services necessitates coordinated governance and leadership by engaged stakeholders at each level.

Global Health Actors: WHO, Bilateral Agencies, and Philanthropies

At the global level, WHO's functions include: the establishment of norms and standards; provision of technical support to countries; data collection, reporting, and surveillance of key health conditions. In its early years, WHO focused much of its attention on eradication and control of infectious diseases including malaria, polio, and yaws. At present, its concerns also include global health security and universal health coverage.

From the early part of the twentieth century, philanthropies such as the Rockefeller Foundation engaged in health interventions in LMICs. Since then, the terrain has changed dramatically. Today, the field is populated with a plethora of organizations involved in global health, including the European Union and the African Union, bilateral organizations such as the United States Agency for Development (USAID), the Centers for Disease Control and Prevention (CDC), the United Kingdom's Department for International Development (DFID), the Swedish International Development Agency (SIDA), the Japan International Cooperation Agency (JICA), and more recent entrants such as development cooperation from the governments of China and Brazil, among others. In addition, the late twentieth century and early twenty-first century saw a significant increase in support for global health initiatives by philanthropic organizations. These included the Bill and Melinda Gates Foundation, the Clinton Foundation, and the Bloomberg Foundation, each of which has invested significant amounts of resources into global health. *What Do Governance and Leadership Mean for Health Systems?*

Leadership and governance, also known as "stewardship," has been characterized as:

> ...the role of the government in health and its relation to other actors whose activities impact on health. This involves overseeing and guiding the whole health system, private as well as public, in order to protect the public interest. It requires both political and technical action, because it involves reconciling competing demands for limited resources, in changing circumstances, for example, with rising expectations, more pluralistic societies, decentralization or a growing private sector.[13]

WHO (2014) lists five functions central to governance and leadership at all levels of the health system, from global to local. These are: (1) policy formulation and development of strategic plans; (2) generation and use of information for decision-making; (3) policy implementation, including designing the health system with clear roles and responsibilities for each component of the organization; (4) development of partnerships within and outside the health system; and (5) designing and implementing structures and processes to ensure accountability, including by political representatives and members of civil society.

Governance and Leadership at Country Level

One role of health ministries is to participate in the affairs of the WHO as shareholders—and to ensure, through the World Health Assembly, that ministries of health shape WHO's vision, mission, and policies. The primary role of health ministries, however, is to design and implement policies, legislation, regulations, and health programs within their countries to reduce mortality and morbidity and to ensure equitable access to quality health services on the basis of need.

In order to develop and implement a health system that performs to the expectations of the populations, governance and leadership at national and subnational levels are critical. The government's role is to create the framework and get all sectors of society to play their part in creating a health system that works for everyone. Additionally, the legitimacy of the government and its capacity to plan and allocate equitable resources for health, its ability to deal with any misuse of resources as well as to ensure that any dissatisfaction with services are rapidly addressed are critical to how the government's ability to govern and lead an effective and efficient health system are perceived.

Brinkerhoff and Bossert note that two other sets of actors are key to ensuring proper governance of the health system, in addition to governments.[14] These are health service providers, whether in the public, private for-profit, or private not-for-profit sectors and civil society, including health service users, academics, nongovernmental organizations, and communities at large.[14]

HEALTH FINANCING

An essential component of the health system is sufficient and responsive global health financing and financing of health-related services within countries around the world.

Recent Trends in Global Health Financing

In aggregate, health spending in the world represents 10% of the global economy and the sector is increasing in social and political importance.[15] Official development assistance for health (DAH)—financial and in-kind contributions from high-income countries to LMICs—represents less than one-thousandth of global health spending, yet plays a disproportionate role in global health architecture and governance.[15] DAH grew fivefold between 2000 and 2010, reaching over $30 billion a year between 2010 and 2015.[16] Roughly one-third of the total came from the United States, one-third was designated for Africa and one-third targeted the HIV epidemic. As noted, most of the DAH-financed health initiatives of the early twenty-first century were initially disease-specific "vertically" funded programs; many had substantial impact on targeted outcomes but did not strengthen health systems as a whole. The evolution from the Millennium Development Goals (MDGs) to the Sustainable Development Goals (SDGs) highlighted the importance of investing in health systems, including the technical and governance capabilities required to implement the essential functions of health financing described above.

The great recession following the financial markets crisis of 2008 triggered a shift in the global political economy, and led to a plateauing of DAH[17] as well as a diversifying of donor countries to include China and others. At the same time, economic growth in many low-income countries allowed greater local spending in health. After centuries of flat GDP per capita, the world experienced a fivefold increase in income in the last 50 years: a majority of the countries that were categorized as low income in 2000 are now categorized as middle income. Because total health expenditure is closely correlated with GDP, some countries are moving from having insufficient resources to buy essential life-saving services to surpassing that level (which is approximate $75 USD per capita). This phenomenon is called *the economic transition of health.*[18]

The 2013 Lancet commission on "Global Health 2035: A world Converging within a Generation" documented this historical reduction in poverty, and raised the possibility of a grand convergence in life expectancy between rich and poor countries by 2035. The Report also advocated for the progressive realization of UHC as an efficient and equitable way to achieve desired health outcomes while ensuring financial protection against catastrophic health expenditures. The Report highlighted the critical importance of increasing domestic resource mobilization while implementing key health policy decisions to ensure equitable coverage, high-quality services, and financial protection.[16]

Domestic Resource Mobilization

Although DAH continues to be critical for the decreasing number of low-income countries, domestic resource mobilization is increasingly important for middle-income countries, and the economic transition of health has significant implications for domestic and international health financing. In LMICs lacking robust health financing frameworks, an explosion in demand for health services is often met by unregulated private providers and paid for out-of-pocket. Fee-for-service out-of-pocket spending is inefficient and regressive, and paying health bills is becoming the number one cause of impoverishment in countries without social protection.[19] Out of pocket payments account for 50% of total health expenditures in most African countries, and they reach up to 80% in large South Asian countries, making up 65% in India as of 2016, versus <20% in most member countries of the organization for Economic Cooperation and Development (OECD). It is estimated that over 100 million families suffer catastrophic health expenditures every year.[20]

Thus, the stewardship and financing of health in this era will require many adjustments at national and international levels. Domestically, ministries of health need to manage the whole health sector with savvy policy and regulations rather than aiming to control all health financing and service delivery.

HUMAN RESOURCES FOR HEALTH

It is well established that investments in human capital lead to faster economic growth, and that countries stand to benefit from having a healthy and well-educated workforce.[21,22] Health workers are key to the production of health; without them, achievement of the SDGs, and attainment of UHC will not be possible.

Delivery of healthcare is a complex process. It is highly discretionary and transaction intensive.[23] Countries rely on their health workers to be competent to make the decisions that will protect the health of their populations and to build the resilience of communities and health systems. Effective management of the health workforce is also critically important, as it consumes a significant portion of the health budget—in some instances over 30% is allocated to health workers, who are in turn responsible for managing all other health resources. As efforts are made to contain cost and increase effectiveness, it is important to acknowledge twenty-first-century health challenges related to demographic, epidemiological, and technological changes. These transitions require a transformation in the delivery of services and associated development of a health workforce increasingly being able to manage noncommunicable diseases and injuries, while continuing to contend with the burden of infectious diseases.

Finally, it is important to focus on health workers because they represent the face of the health system. Health systems are regarded as core social institutions, and the "purveyors of a wider set of societal norms and values."[24,25] Thus, how individuals experience their own worth and place in the broader society will be shaped through their interaction with health workers. Based on this experience, they will also make decisions regarding their own and their families' health-seeking behaviors.

Global Vision and Goal for the Health Workforce

Accelerating progress toward UHC and the SDGs requires equitable access to health workers within strengthened health systems. In turn, ensuring universal availability, accessibility, acceptability, coverage, and quality of the health workforce entails action at global, regional, and national levels, including adequate investments to strengthen health systems, and the implementation of effective policies. This is the vision and overall goal of the WHO Global Strategy on Human Resources for Health, adopted by the World Health Assembly in 2016.[26] This strategy provides four objectives: (1) Optimizing performance, quality, and impact of the health workforce through evidence-informed policies on human resources for health; (2) Aligning investment in human resources for health with the current and future needs of the population and of health systems; (3) Building the capacity of institutions at subnational, national, regional, and global levels for effective public policy stewardship, leadership, and governances; and (4) Strengthening data on human resources for health, for monitoring, and ensuring accountability for the implementation of national and regional strategies.

Achievement of these objectives will result in the improved performance and productivity of the health workforce, delivering quality care, where, and when it is required. In other words, a fit-for-purpose and fit-to-practice health workforce.[26]

An essential first step to improving health worker performance and productivity is to understand the current status of the global health workforce, including three critical barriers: the availability of health workers; their quality and competence; and their responsiveness to the needs of the population they serve. Any effort to address these barriers will need to recognize their dynamic interconnectedness. It will require more than a single intervention targeted at a single level of the health system to achieve sustained improvements in the health workforce.

Addressing Availability

There is both an absolute shortage and a maldistribution of health workers. The WHO Global Health Observatory estimates that there were 43 million health workers globally in 2013 (latest data available),[27] including 9.8 million physicians and 20.7 million nurses/midwives.[28] This represents a shortfall of 17.4 million health workers, using a standard threshold of 4.45 skilled health professionals per 1000 population. These shortfalls were not evenly distributed across the globe, with the largest needs-based shortage occurring in the South East Asian and African regions, which had a shortage of 6.9 million and 4.2 million health workers, respectively.

Although WHO projects a 55% increase in the supply of health workers by 2030, demand will continue to outstrip supply, and the global needs-based shortage of health workers is projected to be more than 14 million in 2030.[27] At a national level, efforts to plan for an increase in the number of health workers is often hindered by inadequate human resources information systems (HRIS). The total number of health workers, who they are, and where they are posted is either not known or the information is often outdated.

In addition to these absolute shortages, there is a maldistribution of health workers particularly across urban–rural divides. Currently, about half of the world's population lives in rural and remote areas, and these rural areas are served by only 38% of the total nursing workforce and by less than 25% of the total physicians' workforce.[29] The problem exists across all countries. Failure to attract health professionals to rural areas and retain them in their posts is driven by a number of intersecting factors. Lack of financial incentives, including both inadequate and inconsistent remuneration, is an important factor, but is not the sole factor influencing a health worker's decision to locate to, and remain in a remote area. Other equally important factors include poor living standards, unsafe and inadequate working environments, and insufficient supply of drugs and equipment.[30,31]

Addressing Competency

Even if the right health workers are in place and in adequate numbers, the second set of challenges relates to health workforce quality. Low-performing health workers, and a failure to adhere to standard guidelines and protocols are a major challenge. Although most countries have some form of accreditation and certification, in general there is no or limited proactive surveillance of the quality of practice.[32] Consequently, high-impact interventions are not reaching those most in need.

Gaps in the competencies of health workers are driven by fundamental inadequacies of the health education system, and a failure to respond to the changing population health needs.[32] Curricula are often outdated, static, and largely content focused, rather than competency-based. Practical experience is limited, and largely focused on disease management rather than provision of continuous healthcare. In LMICs, the inability to develop dynamic, relevant training programs is further constrained by chronic underfunding of health training centers in the public sector. As a result, there is an increase in private sector training facilities in many LMICs, raising concerns about accountability, and worsening skill mix imbalances due to an oversupply of particular health cadres.[33] In-service off-site training programs and seminars are often used to address the competency gap, although the evidence has not shown this approach to be very successful.[34,35] There may be a mismatch between training needs and skills required, and in some instances these programs may worsen morale if the selection process for attendance is perceived to be biased.[36,37]

A lack of knowledge and skills is not the only barrier to poor quality of care and low performance.[34] Additional factors include inadequate supervision and feedback, vague and outdated protocols, unclear role definitions, inappropriate skill mix for a given context, and difficult and inadequate working environments.[38]

Addressing Responsiveness

In order for health workers to respond effectively to the needs of the population they must not only be available and competent, they must be motivated to perform at the highest level possible, and able to gain satisfaction from the work they do. Studies examining health worker motivation consistently identify financial incentives as a core motivating factor, but note that they are not the sole or even the most important issue.[39] Equally or more important factors include the failure to provide an adequate career path for health workers, particularly those functioning in rural settings, and lack of support and recognition by supervisors and health managers.[30,40,41] Additional demotivating factors include high workload, lack of equipment and supplies, inadequate practice environments, minimal professional development opportunities, weak regulatory systems that fail to protect health workers, and opaque or absent human resources policies.[39,42,43] This is particularly prevalent in LMICs.

Across all countries job satisfaction is seen to be derived from. the interpersonal relationships that health workers experience in the workplace, the extent to which they have some autonomy over their work, the organizational and management support they receive from their supervisors, and the overall working conditions.[30,40] Health worker experience of disrespect and abuse in the workplace by supervisors, colleagues, and the community, and feeling threatened is not uncommon, with some studies reporting over 50% of nurses feeling unsafe.[44] This has a significant impact on job satisfaction, manifesting in higher absenteeism, and staff turnover, and ultimately affecting retention rates in rural areas.[39,45]

These challenges are compounded by two cross-cutting macrolevel health system challenges. The first relates to the need to strengthen leadership and governance at both global and national level to coordinate and align all sectors associated with the development of the health workforce.[26] The second is the absence of quality country-level health workforce data needed to monitor and plan workforce development.[46] This lack of data undermines any efforts to assume leadership and to hold governments accountable for health workforce development.

Meeting the Challenges

Despite the long list of barriers to the development of an effective global health workforce, there has also been considerable progress over the past decade. Countries have begun to scale-up the production of the health workforce, and efforts have been made to optimize existing health workers.[47–49] New evidence is available that not only indicates what strategies are effective in increasing health worker productivity, but provides insight into how these should be implemented.[34,50]

The WHO Global Strategy on Human Resources for Health argues for a paradigm shift in how to plan, educate, deploy, manage, and reward health workers. In addition to ongoing optimization of existing health workers, the WHO proposes a shift "toward a collaborative primary care approach built on a team based care, and by fully harnessing the potential of technological innovation."[27] This strategy would occur alongside significant proposed investment and reform in the health workforce to address the equity and coverage gaps, at the same time recognizing the health sector as a key economic sector and generator of decent health sector jobs, particularly for women.[51]

LABORATORY SYSTEMS

Laboratory systems are a vital component of the overall health system structure in every country. Laboratory information constitutes key evidence for decision-making in both clinical management and health programs and to the improvement of the quality of patient care and overall service delivery.

Tiered Laboratory Systems

National health laboratory services aim to provide access to timely and quality testing to communities and individuals throughout a country. In order to achieve this goal, laboratory services are usually organized in a tiered network. Higher tier laboratories have more sophisticated infrastructure and specialized human resources to provide referral-testing services for assays that are not cost-effective and/or feasible at the lower tier laboratories. The lower tier laboratories, often in peripheral smaller health facilities, perform rapid tests or simple automated assays.

The determination of the appropriate diagnostic testing menu for each level in a tiered laboratory network requires an analysis of the distribution and magnitude of diseases within the country, as well as of the designated packages of health services provided at the different tiers of the health system. This definition of the testing menu allows the standardization of human resources, diagnostic tests, equipment, and supplies that should be available at each level of the tiered network.

Laboratory-Based Testing and Point-of-Care Testing

The global diagnostic landscape in the last decades has been dominated by complex and relatively expensive laboratory-based technologies. The requirement of sophisticated laboratory infrastructure and highly trained technicians have curtailed universal access to such tests in LMICs. Many individuals remain without access to same-day results for most laboratory tests, instead relying on the transportation of samples and results to and from centralized laboratories. This is impacted by systemic challenges in establishing reliable transportation and communication networks. These limitations often result in long turnaround times for test results, high rates of patient loss to follow-up, and delayed clinical management decisions. Thus, classical laboratory-based diagnostics may not be effective to support ambitious global initiatives such as the UNAIDS 90-90-90 treatment targets for HIV by 2020, the WHO Global Technical Strategy for malaria 2016–30, the WHO End TB Strategy by 2030, and the WHO Roadmap to Control, Eliminate, and Eradicate Neglected Tropical Diseases. Similarly, new and innovative approaches to laboratory service delivery may be required to achieve UHC goals.

Bringing testing services closer to communities and individuals through point of care testing (POCT) technologies is becoming a key element in achieving these global health goals. POCT technologies are often portable, easy-to-operate devices, and instruments, with the potential for same-day diagnosis and initiation of treatment. These technologies may address barriers related to long turnaround times and low result-return rates improving treatment outcomes and patient satisfaction. However, some POCT technologies are not as precise and accurate as conventional laboratory methods. Therefore, training and competency assessment of personnel and continued quality assurance of POCT are critical for successful implementation, and attainment of reliable and accurate results.

The placement of diagnostic tests along a tiered laboratory network requires careful mapping and consideration of a well-balanced mixed platform approach, including both conventional laboratory-based and POCT. This will avoid over or under instrumentation, suboptimal instrument utilization, limits to testing coverage, stockouts of reagents, and fragmented data and quality systems. Some of the key considerations in determining the placement strategy include specimen throughput, required health worker skills, workload, disease prevalence, geographic access, and desired test turnaround time.

Laboratory Quality Systems

Laboratory errors can occur at any of the preanalytic, the analytic, and the postanalytic phases of the quality assurance cycle. The preanalytic phase focuses on specimen collection, processing and transport, and competency assessment. The analytic phase focuses on internal quality control and proficiency testing. The postanalytic phase focuses on data quality management and reporting and result return. Assuring the quality of laboratory testing requires monitoring of this whole cascade of the testing process.

In high-resource countries, laboratory medicine is the foundation of clinical care and disease surveillance and quality assurance is a fundamental component of the practice. It minimizes sample rejection, improves turnaround times, and prevents unneeded diagnostic testing and use of inappropriate treatment. In contrast, in resource-limited settings, laboratory medicine and quality assurance of laboratory service have received less emphasis and limited investment with poor-quality laboratory support leading to suboptimal management of illnesses and disease surveillance. However, with the increased funding for global health in the past decade, many of these countries are currently making great strides in implementing laboratory quality management systems with the goal of accreditation to international standards.

In 2008, the WHO provided leadership through the Lyon Statement on the need for resource-constrained countries to establish practical quality management systems. Several countries across the world launched a program for strengthening laboratory management, the task-based Strengthening Laboratory Management Toward Accreditation (SLMTA) program and the Stepwise Laboratory Quality Improvement Process Toward Accreditation (SLIPTA) with the aim of accelerating national laboratory services toward achieving international accreditation.[52]

Laboratory Systems and the Implementation of the International Health Regulations

The International Health Regulations (IHR) are an international legal instrument that is binding on its 196 signatory countries.[4] The goal of the IHR is to support the global community in detecting, preventing, and responding to acute public health risks that constitute potential cross-border threats. The current version of the IHR was adopted in 2005 and launched in 2007. The IHR (2005) aim "to prevent, protect against, control and provide a public health response to the international spread of disease in ways that are commensurate with and restricted to public health risks, and which avoid unnecessary interference with international traffic and trade"[53]

IHR implementation at country level requires 19 core capacities, divided into four categories: seven capacities in prevention, four in detection, five in response, and three in other issues. Laboratories play a critical role within national efforts to implement the IHR and attain health security.

Evolving Health Needs and Advancing Technologies

Laboratory systems undergo constant change to respond to the evolving needs of health systems and/or to the challenges posed by societal transformations. In the coming years, laboratory systems will need to adapt to challenges such as the demographic transition, the increasing burden of chronic noncommunicable diseases, changing community's expectations and needs, healthcare reforms, and finance constraints.

In parallel, scientific advances in areas such as POCT, personalized medicine, robotics, information management, and mHealth should also create opportunities for innovating laboratory services delivery while increasing cost-efficiency and access to testing. The laboratory systems of the twenty-first century must, increasingly, encompass clinical and public health testing in a comprehensive network of clinical, public health, veterinary, and environmental laboratories.

COMMODITIES AND PROCUREMENT SYSTEMS

Optimally functioning pharmaceutical systems are critical to the successful attainment of health outcomes. Medicines account for 20–30% of global health spending, with even higher figures in LMICs.[54,55] Additionally, medicines are reported to account for 45–57% of out-of-pocket payments.[56] Achieving the goals of global health initiatives such as UHC and the SDGs calls for major expansions in healthcare services and their accompanying medication budgets.

Inadequate access to medications remains one of the leading causes for poor health outcomes and limits the ability of countries to attain their SDGs. Access may be limited by product availability, geographic distribution, cost, or because medicines are delivered through services that do not match patients' cultural or personal preferences. WHO estimates that one-third of the world's population lacks access to essential medicines.[55] In the poorest parts of Africa and Asia, this proportion increases to 50%.[55] In 2017, the Access to Medicines Foundation estimated that 2 billion people lack access to needed medication.[57] By improving access to existing medicines and vaccines, an estimated 10 million lives per year could be saved.[58]

To facilitate improved access to medicines, health supply chain systems aim to ensure the achievement of the six "Rights": the right goods, in the right quantities, in the right condition, delivered to the right place, at the right time, and for the right cost.[59] However, ensuring that commodities are available is a necessary but insufficient condition to ensuring that the commodities contribute to the attainment of the desired health outcomes. Medicines should also be accessible and acceptable to the people that need them and used appropriately so as not to cause harm and to bring about the desired outcomes. Rather than thinking about supply chains in isolation, it is important to consider the "pharmaceutical system" as a whole.

Access to Medicines

At the core of increasing access is the need to provide medical products and services that are safe, efficacious, cost effective, and of high quality. The four aspects of ensuring access to medicines and pharmaceutical services are accessibility, availability, affordability, and acceptability.[60]

- *Accessibility* (geographical) refers to the location of products and services in relation to the location of users. Are products and services located such that users have easy access to them?
- *Availability* refers to the supply of products and services in relation to demand. Are products and services available when users try to access them? If not, demand is not satisfied and positive health outcomes are at greater risk.
- *Acceptability* refers to the characteristics of products and services in relation to the attitudes and expectations of users. Are these characteristics culturally acceptable to users? Do they meet the expectations of users?
- *Affordability* means the price of products and services in relation to the user's ability to pay for them. Are costs in line with user's willingness and ability to pay?

A focus on the recipient of care requires health workers to improve cultural acceptability of medicines and related services. Emphasis must be placed on improving prescribing and dispensing practices and improved patient counselling that will lead to better acceptance of and adherence to the medications. A number of global initiatives have helped to bolster access to affordable medications including The Agreement on Trade-Related Aspects of Intellectual Property Rights (TRIPS) of the World Trade Organization (WTO), implemented in 2005, meant to overcome patent barriers and allow countries to develop and distribute generic medications.[61]

Pharmaceutical Management Challenges

The leading causes of inefficiencies in pharmaceutical systems include poor governance, poor organization, poor coordination, and poor management. Oversight and regulatory authority roles are often fragmented and reside with different agencies and departments, leading to duplication of efforts and conflict. Coordination of development partners and resources is often inadequate, thus hindering holistic strengthening of the system. Funding for the pharmaceutical sector is inadequate and often payments for supplies is delayed, leading to a lack of trust in the procurement system. Countries may lack adequate numbers of appropriately trained and motivated human resources to carry out the needed functions, and staff distribution and utilization is not always optimal, leading to inefficiencies.

A major challenge affecting growth in the sector is the lack of understanding of the linkages and interdependences within the pharmaceutical subsystem of the larger health system, including the inherent supply chain, particularly considering the challenge to maintain cold chain required for vaccinations in some resource-limited settings, and associated quality assurance subsystems in contributing to the achievement of desired health outcomes.

Building Resilient Pharmaceutical Systems

Conflation of pharmaceutical *supply chains* and pharmaceutical *systems* can lead to challenges in oversight and management. A pharmaceutical system consists of all the structures, people, resources, processes, and their interactions within the broader health system that aim to ensure equitable and timely access to safe, effective, quality pharmaceutical products, and related services that promote their appropriate and cost-effective use to improve health outcomes.[62] As Windisch et al. noted, "sustained access to health commodities will depend on the strength of the health system," not solely the strength of the supply chain.[63]

A complex adaptive systems approach to strengthening pharmaceutical system functions is strongly recommended.[64] Governments, ministries of health, regulatory authorities, donors/development partners, academia/educators, pharmaceutical industry, private sector providers (both not for profit and for profit), and technical assistance providers all have a role to play to ensure that a whole system approach is adopted.

The Lancet Commission on Essential Medicines Policies identified five areas that are "crucial to essential medicines policies: paying for a basket of essential medicines, making essential medicines affordable, assuring the quality and safety of medicines, promoting quality use of medicines, and developing new and missing medicines."[65] The readiness of the pharmaceutical system to support UHC efforts is dependent not only on the strength of each pharmaceutical system functional area but also how cohesively these areas work together.[56] Pharmaceutical systems must be designed to provide adequate geographical and service coverage at an appropriate cost to the healthcare system and patients.

The cost of medicines constitutes a large proportion of total healthcare costs as well as out-of-pocket expenditures. Efforts to prevent catastrophic healthcare spending must address the high cost of medicines and out-of-pocket payments by addressing medicine pricing issues and financial barriers to access at the system and individual levels.[56] Appropriate medicines benefits schemes need to be instituted to reduce the burden of out-of-pocket expenditures on medicines, in tandem with robust financial tracking systems to track expenditure and reduce inefficiencies within the pharmaceutical system.[66]

Commensurate attention should be given to quality assurance in pharmaceutical supply systems, so that each medicine reaching a patient is safe, effective, and of acceptable quality. Ensuring continuous availability of quality assured medicines is a challenge for many LMICs. A comprehensive quality assurance program includes both technical and managerial activities.[67] An important component of a country's ability to monitor medicine safety is a national pharmacovigilance system that is supported by the medicine regulatory authority.[68] Regulatory functions are embodied within the responsibilities of national medicines regulatory authorities that have the prerequisite capacity to register medicines in a timely manner and to ensure appropriate quality, safety, and efficacy standards. To perform effectively, national regulatory authorities must have the necessary political support, legal power, human and financial resources, and independence in decision-making.[67]

Availability of an adequate number of skilled workers (e.g., prescribers, laboratory technicians, dispensers, and managers) to provide and support pharmaceutical services is critical to ensuring sustainable access to medicines and other health technologies.

Organization and management systems need to be able to oversee program planning, monitor and evaluate program implementation, and coordinate donor and community participation in pharmaceutical services. Policy and regulatory oversight bodies need to be adequately empowered and resourced to ensure adherence and conformity to the highest standards. Pharmaceutical management information systems that provide information on products, patients, personnel, and infrastructure need to be established and maintained to support evidence-based decision-making. While a number of digital health technologies have been deployed to support access to medicines and pharmaceutical services in support of UHC and the SDGs, the culture of consistently using data for decision-making at all levels is yet to be cultivated and sustained in many LMICs.[69]

Countries need to critically examine the optimal organization of pharmaceutical services that will ensure proper oversight of products, premises, and personnel. National pharmaceutical management systems should take into account the application of innovation and technology, better private sector engagement, and effective workforce development and empowerment toward the goal of ensuring access (availability, affordability, accessibility, acceptability, and quality), patient safety, and appropriate medicine use of pharmaceuticals and other health commodities.

HEALTH INFORMATION SYSTEMS

A well-functioning HIS is one that ensures the production, analysis, dissemination, and use of reliable and timely information on health determinants, health system performance, and health status.[70] A well-functioning HIS is critical to the national health system, providing essential information that enables decision makers—from policy makers to health providers—to make evidence-informed choices for budgeting, health workforce, and responsive service delivery.[71] While sometimes confused with the terms health management information system (HMIS), health informatics or information technology, HIS is an umbrella term that refers to a system composed of the components, producers, users, and other actors that contribute to the production and use of health information.[71]

Types of HIS Data

HIS data can be divided into three main categories, generally overseen by different health institutions (Table 21-1): (1) program data, such as which health services and outreach activities are delivered where, (2) population-based data, including disease surveillance, census data, population-based surveys, and verbal autopsies, and (3) health workforce data, including the number, cadre, and location of health workers.

Program Data

The source of program-level data is most often individual medical records documented in the course of routine service delivery. These typically include information such as demographic information, medical history, visit information, drugs prescribed, and/or laboratory results. In addition to a patient chart or card, individual data may be collected in health registers, such as antenatal care registers or immunization registers, to facilitate monitoring of patients or services. In LMICs, data quality tends to be suboptimal, as health workers are often overburdened and do not have the time, resources, or appropriate training to document the required information accurately.[72]

Health providers and facility managers are generally tasked with aggregating the individual-level data in medical charts or registers to provide periodic reports on the types and numbers of health services delivered. Typically, routine aggregate health data are captured where data are collected, in the health facility, or through community outreach.[73] More than 60 countries worldwide have adopted DHIS2 as their preferred HMIS to manage, compile, and use their health data. Data flow from initial daily data collection (on paper or electronic) at the health facility and community level. Data are then sent to the district level where they are reviewed and inconsistencies sent back to the source for correction. The data are then entered into the national HMIS. Data-quality assurance conducted and data review meetings

TABLE 21-1 CATEGORIES OF HEALTH INFORMATION SYSTEMS (HIS) DATA (EXAMPLES OF DATA SOURCES AND TYPES OF INSTITUTIONS MANAGING THE DATA)

HIS Data Sources	Type	Examples of Data Sources	Types of Institutions Managing the Data
Program (health services and outreach activities)	Routine	Individual health data	MOH, NGOs
		Aggregate health data	MOH, NGOs
	Nonroutine	Health facility assessments	MOH
Population-based	Routine	Disease surveillance	MOH
	Nonroutine	Population-based surveys (e.g., Demographic and Health Survey, AIDS/Malaria indicator survey)	Bureau of statistics
		Vital registration and verbal autopsies	Bureau of statistics
Human resources	Routine	HCW recruitment, placement and retention	MOH, Ministry of Education

are held. The data are then sent to the provincial level where they are aggregated and reviewed routinely and used in program review meetings. From there, data are transmitted to the national level where they are analyzed and compiled for annual reports.[74,75]

In addition to patient-level data, health facility assessments are nonroutine data collected to assess, map, and monitor service availability. The objective of these assessments is to generate reliable and regular information on availability and condition of infrastructure, availability, and condition of medical equipment, availability of health service and headcounts of health workers.

Electronic information systems are capable of bringing together information from a variety of different sources, including information from clinical visits, pharmacy, or the laboratory.[76] If used correctly, electronic systems have the potential to reduce data quality issues by using built-in validation rules and data checks. Additionally, the availability of Internet connectivity in many settings has enabled sharing electronic systems on a cloud or server, making it easier to track patients as they move across facilities. In LMICs, factors that are usually considered in making the switch from paper to electronic medical records include the availability of information technology resources, patient volume, the availability of stable electricity, and Internet access.

Population-Based Data

Population-level data are also needed to complement the data provided by programs, especially to provide information to determine risk, continuity, quality, and coverage of health problems and interventions.[77,78] In contrast to program data, which only provides information on individuals accessing health services, population-level data can provide a more accurate cross section of communities.

Disease surveillance data help to monitor the burden of disease and impact of interventions by measuring occurrence of diseases, certain environmental conditions, and risk factors that need immediate and rapid action to prevent potential outbreaks or epidemics.[79]

Population-based surveys or *household surveys* are mainly conducted to assess prevalence of attitudes, risk behaviors and diseases, and get information about health and social services usage.[80]

Vital events registration captures information on indicators like birth and mortality. According to WHO, a country should have registration of births and deaths coverage >80% for the data to be considered complete and accurate. The systematic documentation of births through the vital registration remains a challenge in many LMICs, and many still rely on household surveys to monitor levels and trends of birth registration. Documentation of deaths is even more problematic, as, only 30% of the world's population live in areas with >90% completeness of death registration through medical certification and coding of the cause of death.[81,82] For this reason, the use of verbal autopsy methods are increasingly being used in low-income countries to ascertain cause of death based on interview with next of kin eliciting information on signs, symptoms, medical history, and circumstances preceding death.

Health Workforce Data

Although usually considered as a separate component of the HIS, a functional HRIS is essential. The HRIS helps to plan for the availability of required health workers of desired quality in the right place, at the right time. A comprehensive HRIS should include all aspects of the healthcare workforce, including registration, deployment, posting, and retention.

The Information Cycle: From Data Sources to Information Use

The information cycle includes multiple steps, such as data collection, data cleaning, data quality, data analysis, information representation, interpretation and use with the ultimate goal of improving health outcomes through data-driven decisions. The most challenging information cycle steps in LMICs are (i) to ensure *data quality*, that is, to achieve consistent, coherent, and nonredundant information systems that provide timely, complete, and accurate information[83,84]; and (ii) to ensure *use of information* by stakeholders, in order to make effective, evidence-based decisions for the provision of health services.[85]

Several reasons have been identified that may lead to suboptimal use of data[86] including: (1) Failure of HIS design to meet and match the needs of the stakeholders, failing to differentiate between wants and needs. (2) Data-quality issues, several health managers, and decision makers fail to use information from the HIS that they have spent reasonable resources (human, financial, and time) due to the perception of poor data reliability, a fact that is exacerbated by limited use of the data, establishing a vicious cycle (as poor use of information leads to poor data quality). (3) Limited capacity to analyze, represent, and use information at both individual and institutional levels. (4) Motives that are beyond information management as such, but are more context and structural related, such as health systems constraints or country related. Finally, in some contexts, political reasons may interfere in information use, particularly when such information does not favor a prevailing argument.

With the expansion of technology looking forward, HIS will move toward triangulation of data and integration of systems through the use of unique identification of clients or the use of biometrics. Additionally, real-time data systems will reduce delays in obtaining data and will allow for rapid review of data for decision-making.

COMMUNITY ENAGEMENT AND ADVOCACY

Well-functioning global health systems are actualized when communities and civil society advocates ensure that care and services are provided in the right way, to the right people, and at the right time. When care and services are not meeting the needs and improving the health outcomes of the recipient of care, communities play a critical role in advocating for change. For example, in confronting the HIV epidemic, advocacy by people living with HIV has brought about dramatic improvements in access to and delivery of antiretroviral therapy (ART).

There is no single definition of community advocacy. However, in its simplest form, it involves community members coming together and taking action. This starts when a community group or groups identify priority issues that affect them, determine what change is needed (e.g., in policies, laws, and services needed to address those priority issues), and then target the individuals, groups, and/or institutions that can influence this change. In practice, almost all community actors who volunteer or identify themselves with a cause-based movement do some type of advocacy work—even if they do not use the word "advocacy."

How Communities Have Engaged with Global Health Systems

Advocacy by communities has been key to action within global health systems around the world. Examples of this can be seen throughout history and in various contexts. Two case studies of successful community advocacy work are described below. In each, success was achieved through demand creation, community monitoring, and policy change:

Case Study: Advocating for Improved Access to HIV Services in Kenya through Community-led Demand Creation

In 2015, Kenya had 897,644 people living with HIV (PLHIV) on ART—approximately 59% of those eligible for ART under treatment guidelines outlined by the WHO at that time. Similar to other countries in East Africa, PLHIV in Kenya had limited information on HIV services. Among the most important of these services is viral load testing—a clinical monitoring test that measures the amount of HIV in the blood. Viral load is used to monitor how well a person's treatment is working, with the goal of ART treatment being to reduce the amount of virus in the blood. In Kenya, knowledge and awareness of viral load testing was low among recipients of care, county health committees, health workers at the facility, and within communities. The same was true for many policy-makers responsible for health as well.

To address this, local community networks organized trainings on viral load testing for PLHIV and government stakeholders. The trainings included health workers, county health committees, and journalists. Activists also used mass media and radio campaigns to raise public awareness and increase pressure on the government to scale-up the use of viral load testing.

As a result of these treatment education and advocacy activities, local community networks were invited to join the Technical Working Group for the development of the new Kenyan HIV Treatment Guidelines, which now includes the latest WHO 2015 recommendations for routine viral load testing. Hence, the national movement of civil society organizations mobilized on the issue of routine viral load testing generated a momentum that continues, to date, to push the national government to provide optimal HIV services, and raise awareness among affected communities to create demand for them. Ongoing advocacy efforts should consider how to link such interventions to programmatic and health outcomes—both qualitative and quantitatively—in order to help substantiate the necessity and effectiveness of community-led action, which is often undervalued and underfunded.

Case Study: Advocating for Increased Access to and Affordability of Hepatitis C Treatment in Argentina

In Argentina, there are an estimated 400,000 people living with hepatitis C (HCV), many of whom have advanced disease and do not have access to the treatment due to its high price. In May 2015, organizations of people with HCV challenged a patent application by a global pharmaceutical company on the drug sofosbuvir, an essential medicine to treat HCV. The proposed patent would have given the company exclusive rights to produce sofosbuvir, granting it a monopoly and allowing for the raising of drug prices. Estimates suggested the patent would have prevented 800,000 people from having access to treatment in Argentina alone.

Using intellectual property-related legal recourses, local organizations filed a patent opposition, highlighting how the pharmaceutical company did not comply with the requirements of Argentine patent law. On December 4, 2017, the National Institute of Industrial Property (INPI) rejected the company's patent application. As a result of the rejected patent, the Ministry of Health of Argentina allowed local producers to develop a generic form of the drug at significantly lower prices. The rejection of the patent was a step forward in protecting local production and procurement of generics and allowing more people to garner the benefits of HCV treatment.

What Does Community Advocacy Look Like?

As illustrated by the case studies above, community advocacy can take many forms depending on the needs of the community and the political and financial context. It can involve a wide range of activities, including participation in decision-making fora; development of position papers on critical issues; organizing petitions signed by community members or public rallies; and working with the media to raise awareness and sway procause public support around issues. In addition, depending on the issue identified, community advocacy can involve action at different levels—community, district, regional, national, and/or global. Stakeholder engagement is an equally important step in the advocacy process, to mobilize attention, action and buy-in from policy makers, community leaders, religious institutions, donor organizations; businesses and corporations, including pharmaceutical companies; trade unions; and global agencies.

The experiences of community advocacy groups around the world show that there are specific factors that contribute to successful advocacy, including the following principles: (1) *Goals should be evidence-based:* Before any advocacy work begins, communities must determine the extent of the problem and have evidence to inform their planning and action, to ensure the work response to the real needs of community members. (2) *Projects should be realistic,* focusing on changes that are possible within the local context and with the resources that are available. Organization, planning, and prioritization are critical. (3) *Initiatives should be owned and operated by community advocates* so that advocates feel committed to and in control of the work. (4) *Activities should be implemented by a group of activists,* so that the work is not dependent on one or two individuals. (5) *Implementation should be creative,* so that it makes the best use of local ideas.

There are many frameworks for the development of an advocacy plan. Where possible, advocates should use planning frameworks that are simple and measurable. This can be guided by taking into account the advocacy cycle. The cycle starts with identifying the issues, gaps, problems, barriers and/or change, prioritizing issues, gaps, problems and barriers, and developing a plan and ending with taking action. And finally, importantly, it is critically important to evaluate the actions taken and distill lessons learned. Working carefully through each step of the advocacy planning cycle is key to successful advocacy.

WAY FORWARD

Achieving the ambitious health goals articulated globally, particularly the SDGs and UHC, requires a focus on strengthening the individual components of health systems as well as understanding how they intertwine to realize compound results.

Clinical services have evolved from focusing on eradication campaigns to revitalizing primary healthcare and embracing UHC. The delivery of these clinical services that emphasize tailored, yet comprehensive integrated approaches, within a UHC framework, necessitates a health system that affords equitable access to skilled health providers and accessible, acceptable, and responsive pharmaceutical supply chains and management systems that are properly funded and governed. Global health actors like the WHO, bilateral organizations, and philanthropies should work together with country-level officials to reliably steward funding that meets, the evolving UHC needs. When not properly managed, this can result in catastrophic health expenditures related to clinical service provision and payment of medications. When properly planned for, pharmaceutical systems can ensure that the right good, right quantities of medications in the right condition and delivered to the right place at the right time for the right cost.

These clinical, governing, and budgeting decisions must be informed by data produced and managed by high-quality laboratory and HIS. Both of these components are constantly evolving the development of new technologies that can facilitate faster and more in-depth reviews of data that are used for decision-making.

All of these components will not be effective if communities and civil society advocates are not engaged at all levels. This component of the health system works to lead the charge for necessary changes and demand generation of essential health services. They help to ensure that these services are provided in the right way, to the right people, and at the right time.

Each of the health system building blocks is essential, yet none can function in isolation. All of the components of the health system described in this chapter are interconnected and each must be optimized on its own and in relation to the other building blocks in order to result in accessible, responsive, efficient, and high-quality health services for all.

References

1. Hall JJ, Taylor R. Health for all beyond 2000: The demise of the Alma-Ata Declaration and primary health care in developing countries. *Med J Aust.* 2003;178(1):17–20.
2. Bennett FJ. Primary health care and developing countries. *Soc Sci Med.* 1979;13a(5):505–14.
3. Benyoussef A, Christian B. Health care in developing countries. *Soc Sci Med.* 1977;11(6–7):399–408.:
4. Newell KW, World Health Organization. In: Newell KW, ed. *Health by the People.* Geneva: World Health Organization; 1975.
5. World Health Organization, WHOEB. Handbook of Resolutions and Decisions of the World Health Assembly and the Executive Board. Volume II, 1973–1984. Geneva: World Health Organization; 1985.
6. Walsh JA, Warren KS. Selective primary health care: An interim strategy for disease control in developing countries. *N Engl J Med.* 1979;301(18):967–74.
7. Whitehead M, Dahlgren G, Evans T. Equity and health sector reforms: Can low-income countries escape the medical poverty trap? *Lancet.* 2001;358(9284):833–6.
8. UNAIDS. Global HIV & AIDS statistics—2018 fact sheet. Geneva. 2018. http://www.unaids.org/en/resources/fact-sheet.
9. Schneider H, Blaauw D, Gilson L, Chabikuli N, Goudge J. Health systems and access to antiretroviral drugs for HIV in Southern Africa: Service delivery and human resources challenges. *Reprod Health Matters.* 2006;14(27):12–23.
10. Samb B, Evans T, Dybul M, et al. An assessment of interactions between global health initiatives and country health systems. *Lancet.* 2009;373(9681):2137–69.
11. Garrett L, Chowdhury AM, Pablos-Mendez A. All for universal health coverage. *Lancet.* 2009;374(9697):1294–9.
12. Poku NK. How should the post-2015 response to AIDS relate to the drive for universal health coverage? *Glob Public Health.* 2018;13(7): 765–79.
13. World Health Organization. Everybody's Business: Strengthening Health Systems to Improve Health Outcomes—WHO's Framework for Action. Geneva, Switzerland; 2007.
14. Brinkerhoff DW, Bossert TJ. Health governance: Principal-agent linkages and health system strengthening. *Health Policy Plan.* 2014;29(6):685–93.
15. World Health Organization. WHO Global Health Expenditure Atlas. Geneva; 2014.
16. Global Burden of Disease Health Financing Collaborator Network. Future and potential spending on health 2015–40: Development assistance for health, and government, prepaid private, and out-of-pocket health spending in 184 countries. *Lancet.* 2017;389(10083):2005–30.
17. Pablos-Mendez A, Raviglione MC. A new world health era. *Glob Health Sci Pract.* 2018;6(1):8–16.
18. Pablos Méndez A TH, de Ferranti D. The cost disease and the economic transition of global health. In: Baumol WJ, ed. *Health Care Costs in Futureworld: Nations Can't Stop the Rising Cost but They Can Afford Them.* New Haven, CT: Yale University Press; 2012.
19. Essue BM, Laba M, Knaul F, et al. Economic burden of chronic ill health and injuries for households in low- and middle-income countries. In: Jamison DT, Gelband H, Horton S, et al, eds *Disease Control Priorities: Improving Health and Reducing Poverty.* Washington, DC: The International Bank for Reconstruction and Development/The World Bank. (c) 2018 International Bank for Reconstruction and Development/ The World Bank; 2017.
20. World Health Organization. Tracking universal health coverage: 2017 Global Monitoring Report—Joint WHO/ World Bank Group Report, December 2017. Geneva; 2017.
21. Jamison DT, Summers LH, Alleyne G, et al. Global health 2035: A world converging within a generation. *Salud Publica Mex.* 2015;57(5):444–67.
22. WHO Commission on Macroeconomics and Health WHO. Macroeconomics and health: Investing in health for economic development: Executive summary/report of the Commission on Macroeconomics and Health. Geneva; 2001.
23. Pritchett L, Woolcock M. Solutions when the solution is the problem: Arraying the disarray in development. *World Dev.* 2004;32(2):191–212.
24. Freedman LP. Achieving the MDGs: Health systems as core social institutions. *Development.* 2005;48(1):19–24.
25. Gilson L. Trust and the development of health care as a social institution. *Soc Sci Med.* 2003;56(7):1453–68.
26. World Health Organization. Global Strategy on Human Resources for Health: Workforce 2030. 2016.
27. WHO. *Global Strategy on Human Resources for Health: Workforce 2030.* Geneva: World Health Organization; 2016. http://www.who.int/hrh/resources/pub_globstrathrh-2030/en/.
28. WHO. Global Health Observatory (GHO) data Geneva: World Health Organization; 2018. http://www.who.int/gho/health_workforce/en/.
29. The World Bank. Rural population (% of total population). In: Revision WUP, editor. 2014.
30. Willis-Shattuck M, Bidwell P, Thomas S, Wyness L, Blaauw D, Ditlopo P. Motivation and retention of health workers in developing countries: A systematic review. *BMC Health Serv Res.* 2008;8:247.
31. Lehmann U, Dieleman M, Martineau T. Staffing remote rural areas in middle- and low-income countries: A literature review of attraction and retention. *BMC Health Serv Res.* 2008;8:19.
32. WHO. Health workforce 2030: Towards a global strategy on human resources for health. 2015.
33. Frenk J, Chen L, Bhutta ZA, et al. Health professionals for a new century: Transforming education to strengthen health systems in an interdependent world. *Lancet.* 2010;376(9756):1923–58.
34. Rowe AK, de Savigny D, Lanata CF, Victora CG. How can we achieve and maintain high-quality performance of health workers in low-resource settings? *Lancet.* 2005;366(9490):1026–35.
35. Potter C, Brough R. Systemic capacity building: A hierarchy of needs. *Health Policy Plan.* 2004;19(5):336–45.
36. Mathauer I, Imhoff I. Health worker motivation in Africa: The role of non-financial incentives and human resource management tools. *Hum Resour Health.* 2006;4:24.
37. Chimwaza W, Chipeta E, Ngwira A, et al. What makes staff consider leaving the health service in Malawi? *Hum Resour Health.* 2014;12(1):17.
38. Improving health worker performance. *Published for the U.S. Agency for International Development by the Quality Assurance Project.* Bethesda, MD: University Research Co., LLC; 2014.
39. Dieleman M, Harnmeijer JW. *Improving Health Worker Performance: In Search of Promising Practices.* Geneva: World Health Organization; 2006.
40. McAuliffe E, Manafa O, Maseko F, Bowie C, White F. Understanding job satisfaction amongst mid-level cadres in Malawi: The contribution of organizational justice. *Reprod Health Matters.* 2009;17(33):80–90.
41. McAuliffe E, Galligan M, Revill P, et al. Factors influencing job preferences of health workers providing obstetric care: Results from discrete

choice experiments in Malawi, Mozambique and Tanzania. *Global Health*. 2016;12(1):86.

42. Bradley S, Kamwendo F, Masanja H, et al. District health managers' perceptions of supervision in Malawi and Tanzania. *Hum Resour Health*. 2013;11:43.
43. McAuliffe E, Daly M, Kamwendo F, Masanja H, Sidat M, de Pinho H. The critical role of supervision in retaining staff in obstetric services: A three country study. *PLoS One*. 2013;8(3):e58415.
44. Boafo IM. The effects of workplace respect and violence on nurses' job satisfaction in Ghana: A cross-sectional survey. *Hum Resour Health*. 2018;16(1):6.
45. Lehmann U, Dieleman M, Martineau T. Staffing remote rural areas in middle and low-income countries: A literature review of attraction and retention. *BMC Health Serv Res*. 2008;8:19.
46. Riley PL, Zuber A, Vindigni SM, et al. Information systems on human resources for health: A global review. *Hum Resour Health*. 2012;10:7.
47. Van Lerberghe W, Matthews Z, Achadi E, et al. Country experience with strengthening of health systems and deployment of midwives in countries with high maternal mortality. *Lancet*. 2014;384(9949):1215–25.
48. Campbell J, Buchan J, Cometto G, et al. Human resources for health and universal health coverage: Fostering equity and effective coverage. *Bull World Health Organ*. 2013;91(11):853–63.
49. WHO. *WHO Recommendations: Optimizing Health Worker Roles to Improve Access to Key Maternal and Newborn Health Interventions through Task Shifting*. Geneva: World Health Organization; 2012.
50. Lobis S, Mbaruku G, Kamwendo F, McAuliffe E, Austin J, Pinho H. Expected to deliver: Alignment of regulation, training and actual performance of emergency obstetric care providers in Malawi and Tanzania. *Int J Gynaecol Obstet*. 2011;115(3):322–7.
51. WHO. *Working for Health and Growth: Investing in the Health Workforce. Report of the High-Level Commission on Health Employment and Economic Growth*. Geneva: World Health Organization; 2016.
52. World Health Organization. WHO Guide for the Stepwise Laboratory Improvement Process Towards Accreditation in the African Region (SLIPTA). Regional Office for Africa, Brazzaville, Republic of Congo; 2015.
53. World Health Organization. Joint external evaluation tool: International Health Regulations Geneva Switzerland; 2005.
54. Etienne C A-BA, Evans DB, editors. The World Health Report: Health Systems Financing: the Path to Universal Coverage. Geneva; 2010.
55. Lu Y HP, Abegunde D, Edeker T. Medicine expenditures. In: World Health Organization, ed. *The World Medicines Situation*. 3rd ed. Geneva, Switzerland: WHO Press; 2010.
56. Eghan K RM. Pharmaceutical Management Considerations for Expanded Coverage of Essential Health Services and Financial Protection Programs. Arlington, VA; 2017.
57. Access to Medicine Foundation. Access to Medicine Foundation. https://accesstomedicinefoundation.org/.
58. Organization WH. Equitable access to essential medicines: a framework for collective action. http://apps.who.int/medicinedocs/pdf/s4962e/s4962e.pdf.
59. USAID Deliver Project TO. *The Logistics Handbook: A Practical Guide for the Supply Chain Management of Health Commodities*. 2nd ed. Arlington, VA; 2011.
60. Bigdeli M, Jacobs B, Tomson G, et al. Access to medicines from a health system perspective. *Health Policy Plan*. 2013;28(7):692–704.
61. Stevens H, Huys I. Innovative approaches to increase access to medicines in developing countries. *Front Med (Lausanne)*. 2017;4:218.
62. Hafner T, Walkowiak H, Lee D, Aboagye-Nyame F. Defining pharmaceutical systems strengthening: Concepts to enable measurement. *Health Policy Plan*. 2017;32(4):572–84.
63. Windisch R, Waiswa P, Neuhann F, Scheibe F, de Savigny D. Scaling up antiretroviral therapy in Uganda: Using supply chain management to appraise health systems strengthening. *Global Health*. 2011;7:25.
64. Peters DH. The application of systems thinking in health: Why use systems thinking? *Health Res Policy Sys*. 2014;12:51.
65. Wirtz VJ, Hogerzeil HV, Gray AL, et al. Essential medicines for universal health coverage. *Lancet*. 2017;389(10067):403–76.
66. Rankin J GM, Eghan K. Management of Medicines Benefit Programs in Low- and Middle-Income Settings: Adapting Approaches from High-Income Countries. Arlington, VA; 2015.
67. Management Sciences for Health. MDS-3: Managing Access to Medicines and Health Technologies. Arlington, VA; 2012.
68. Strengthening Pharmaceutical Systems. Supporting Pharmacovigilance in Developing Countries: The Systems Perspective. Arlington, VA; 2009.
69. Konduri N, Aboagye-Nyame F, Mabirizi D, et al. Digital health technologies to support access to medicines and pharmaceutical services in the achievement of sustainable development goals. *Digit Health*. 2018;4:2055207618771407.
70. Health Metrics Network, World Health Organization. Framework and standards for country health information systems. 2008.
71. Measure Evaluation. Defining Health Information Systems. Health Information Systems Strengthening (HISS) Resource Center. https://www.measureevaluation.org/his-strengthening-resource-center/his-definitions. Accessed January 7, 2018.
72. Heeks R. Information Systems and Developing Countries: Failure, success and local improvisations. *Inf Soc*. 2002;18(2):101–12.
73. Lippeveld T, Sauerborn R, Bodart T, eds. Design and Implementation of Health Information Systems. Washington, DC; 2000.
74. DHIS2 Documentation Team. Dhis2 end user manual 2006. dhis.org.
75. University IaC. DHIS2 In Action 2017. https://www.dhis2.org/inaction.
76. Ross DA, Hinman AR. Public health informatics. In: Wallace RB, ed. *Public Health & Preventive Medicine*. New York: McGraw-Hill; 2008.
77. Heywood A, Rohde J. Using Information for Action: A Manual for Health Workers at Facility Level. Health Information Systems Progran—The EQUITY Project. Cape Town, South Africa; 2001, pp. 21–95.
78. World Health Organization. *Framework and Standards for Country Health Information Systems—Health Metrics Network*. Geneva: World Health Organization; 2008.
79. World Health Organization. 2005. International Health Regulations. http://www.who.int/ihr/about/en/.
80. Johnson TP, ed. *Handbook of Health Survey Methods*. Hoboken, NJ: John Wiley & Sons; 2015.
81. Mahapatra P, Shibuya K, Lopez AD, et al. Civil registration systems and vital statistics: Successes and missed opportunities. *Lancet*. 2007;370(9599):1653–63.
82. Mathers C, Ma Fat D, Inoue M, Rao C. Counting the dead and what they died from: An assessment of the global status of cause of death data. *Bull World Health Organ*. 2005;83:171–7.
83. Chilundo B, Sundby J, Aanestad M. Analysing the quality of routine malaria data in Mozambique. *Malaria J*. 2004;3(1):3.
84. Gimbel S, Micek M, Lambdin B, et al. An assessment of routine primary care health information system data quality in Sofala Province, Mozambique. *Popul Health Metr*. 2011;9:12.
85. Klazinga N, Stronks K, Delnoij D, Verhoeff A. Indicators without a cause. Reflections on the development and use of indicators in health care from a public health perspective. *Int J Qual Health Care*. 2001;13 (No. 6):433–8.
86. Sahay S, Sundararaman T, Braa J. *Public Health Informatics: Designing for Change—A Developing Country Perspective*. New York: Oxford University Press; 2017.

CHAPTER

22 Reproductive Health and Child and Adolescent Health and Development

Alison Drake • Elizabeth Bukusi • David Ross • Maneesh Batra • Donna Denno • Grace John-Stewart

INTRODUCTION

Reproductive health and child and adolescent health and development are inextricably linked. Declines in fertility rates often occur in tandem with economic and educational advancement and are associated with benefits in child health. Infant health (in the first 1000 days since conception) can influence longer-term child, adolescent, and adult health. Maternal nutrition and quality of life influences long-term child outcomes. Child nutrition and infections may alter neurodevelopment and long-term educational and vocational outcomes. Finally, adolescent health may influence adult outcomes and reproductive decision-making as well as next-generation health. Together these intertwined areas contribute a perspective of lifecycle trajectories that addresses outcomes for each population (mothers, infants, children, and adolescents) not in silos—recognizing that each group has distal impact on the other groups and that addressing these relationships at critical windows of risk (preconception adolescence, pregnancy, delivery, neonatal, under-5, and teen years) with tailored interventions could leverage opportunities to improve outcomes of mother-child, adolescent-adult, neonate-child (Fig. 22-1).

Globally, Maternal Child Health (MCH) clinic systems are well established. They provide opportunities for broad coverage of healthcare and public health approaches for populations at-risk and improved maternal child health outcomes. Over the past decades, new interventions have been successfully added to the existing MCH infrastructure. The MCH system can be leveraged to address reproductive and maternal and child health issues, although additional platforms are required to efficiently address adolescent health issues.

In the subsections below we address the different relevant domains in detail: (1) Maternal and reproductive health, (2) Adolescent health, (3) Neonatal health, (4) Infant and child health, and (5) Conclusions, which address cross-cutting approaches to all four populations.

MATERNAL AND REPRODUCTIVE HEALTH

The world's population is currently over 7.6 billion, with an annual growth rate of 1.07%.[1] Population growth rates accelerated to unprecedented levels following World War II, due to the success of public health interventions that resulted in significant declines in mortality. With rising concerns about rapid expansion of the world's population, and impact on economic and social development, an international movement sparked goals of curbing population growth. Efforts focused on achieving demographic targets through reductions in the total fertility rate (TFR), the number of children born per women each year, were largely successful through early family planning programs. TFR declined by 50%, from 6 to 3, between 1974 and 1994.[2]

Human Rights-based Approach to Sexual and Reproductive Health

Progress in decreasing TFR was not universal and unintended pregnancy rates remained high, which made achievement of demographic targets to curb population growth challenging. A fundamental shift from these demographic targets to a human rights-based approach to sexual and reproductive health (SRH) followed the landmark 1994 International Conference on Population and Development (ICPD) conference in Cairo, forming the cornerstone of SRH efforts.

The ICDP goals of universal access to SRH include the ability for individuals to have safe sex, control their own fertility, and have access to services for safe pregnancy, childbirth, and a healthy baby. Realization of these goals has both individual and societal benefits. Allowing women to control their fertility to limit and space their pregnancies increases educational opportunities, earning potential, overall autonomy and wellbeing and improves overall maternal, newborn, and child health. At the societal level, lower fertility rates increase productivity, as more women are able to enter the workforce. Slowing population growth by reducing fertility can also alleviate environmental strains and demands for land use such as crowding, agricultural needs to raise livestock and crops necessary to feed the population, and access to clean and safe sources of water. While the ICPD framework was instrumental in guiding reproductive health policies and family planning programs, international support and funding to drive these goals, and competing needs for funding to combat the HIV epidemic, stalled programmatic impact. Fertility rates remain high in many developing countries, with the highest TFR in sub-Saharan Africa.

Benefits of Decreased Fertility Rates

Reducing TFR by preventing unintended pregnancies and meeting contraceptive needs are high priorities for public health, and critical to the success of the current UN Sustainable Development Goals (SDGs), particularly SDG5 which echoes the ICPD goal of ensuring universal access to ##SRH. Over 300,000 women in developing countries die from preventable pregnancy and childbirth complications each year,[3] including 47,000 maternal deaths attributed to unsafe abortion practices and 21.7 million neonatal deaths during the first month of life.[3-5]

Special Concerns Regarding Adolescent Reproductive Health Outcomes

Adolescent girls are disproportionately at risk of poor maternal and child health outcomes. Pregnancy-related complications are the second leading cause of death among adolescent girls age 15–19, and risks of infant mortality are also high among these young mothers.[6-8] Early marriage and early initiation of sexual activity contribute substantially to fertility rates in LMIC, where 19% of adolescents will

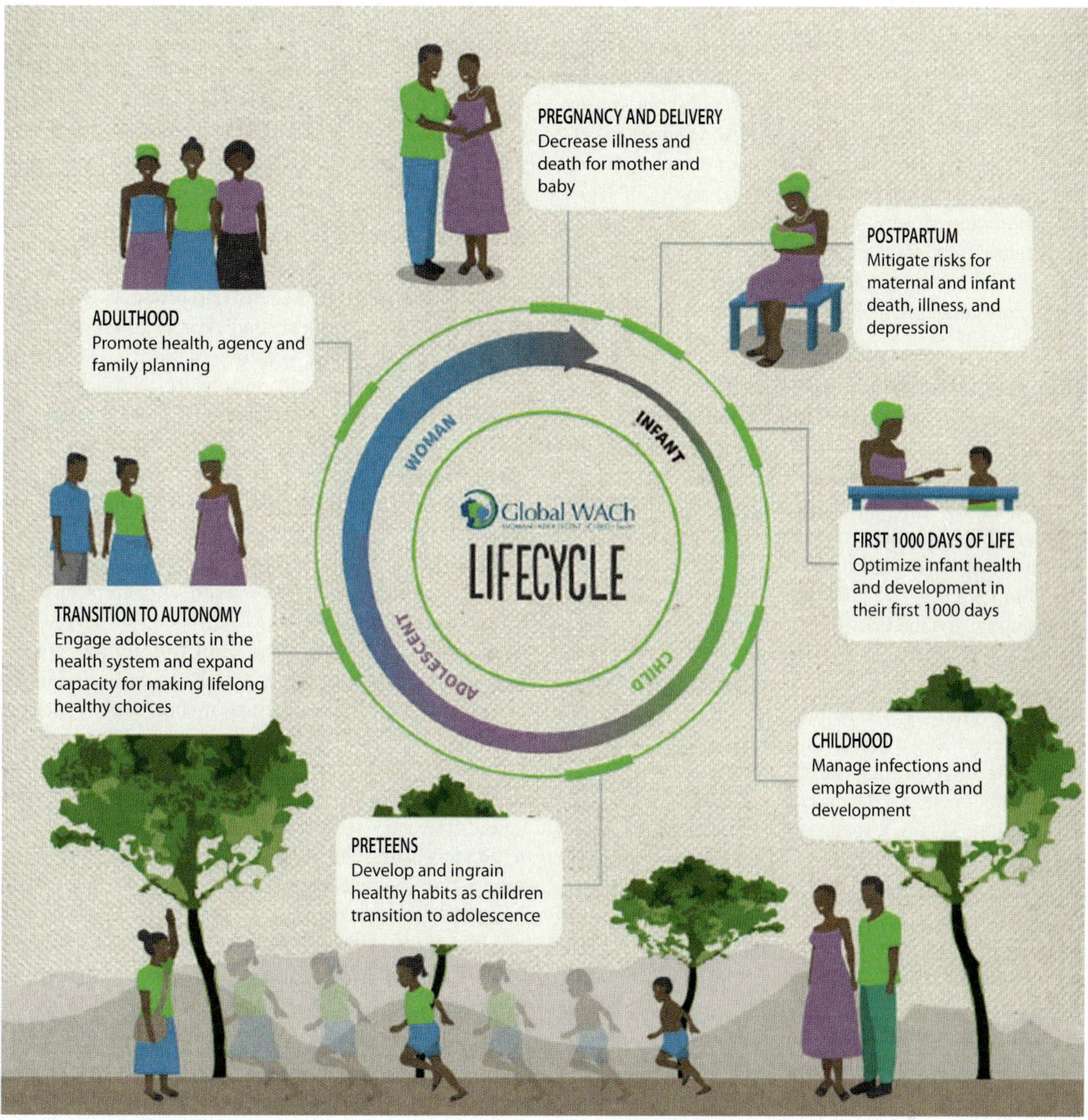

FIGURE 22-1. Using a lifecycle framework to link reproductive, maternal, child, and adolescent health.

become pregnant by age 18. Yet, estimates of adolescent fertility are underreported as girls < 14 years and unmarried adolescent girls are frequently excluded from national surveys from which these estimates data are derived. Adolescent fertility rates declined worldwide from 59 to 51 per 1000 women since 1990; however, most of this decline is attributed to large (50%) reductions in the developed world and only modest declines (8%) in developing regions over the past 25 years.

Programs and policies aimed at delaying early marriage and sexual debut can help reduce adolescent fertility rates and adverse health outcomes resulting from adolescent pregnancy, but efforts to improve the content and quality of SRH for adolescents and provide universal access to family planning are also important. Lack of social support, provider bias, and cultural perspectives on fertility and family planning all contribute to lower utilization of contraceptive use. Provision of high quality, comprehensive sexuality education and SRH services has been shown to be effective in improving ASRH. However, uncoordinated and ineffective delivery, implementation, and duration of these interventions; lack of programmatic coverage and reach; weak SRH curriculum; and inability to address gender inequality beliefs, norms, attitudes, have limited their impact on ASRH outcomes.[9] In addition, youth-friendly health centers (facilities that provide care, activities and counselling tailored to youth and in a youth friendly space) and peer education remain popular components of youth programs despite evidence that suggests they may not be effective if they are not well implemented.[9,10] Future efforts should de-implement ineffective program elements, and implement high fidelity, complementary interventions to holistically address needs for adolescents to maximize benefits.

Family Planning Strategies

Family planning is an effective strategy to mitigate adverse maternal and infant health outcomes resulting from unintended pregnancies (both mistimed and unwanted) for women. Over 40% of the 206 million pregnancies occurring in developing regions each year are unintended.[4] There are diverse family planning methods to help women limit and space pregnancies. These methods include: abstinence, fertility awareness and natural methods [standard days method, 2-day method, withdrawal, and lactational amenorrhea method (LAM)], barrier methods (male and female condoms and diaphragms), short-term hormonal methods (oral contraceptive pills, emergency contraception, injectables, patch, ring), long-acting, reversible contraception [intrauterine device (IUD) and implants], and permanent methods (male and female sterilization). Typical use effectiveness varies substantially by method, with the lowest failure rates for long-acting and permanent methods (<1%), 6–9% for short-term hormonal methods, and > 10% for condoms and all other methods.[11]

Contraceptive method mix, the distribution of methods used, varies substantially by region, with disparities in use driven by a complex combination of cultural beliefs, service delivery models, provider skills, and historical policies and programs. Long-acting and permanent methods are most common in Asia, whereas injectables and oral contraceptive pills are more common in sub-Saharan Africa.[12] Similarly, overall contraceptive prevalence rate (CPR), the proportion of fertile women who are practicing, or whose sexual partners are practicing, any form of contraception, also vary geographically. Globally, CPR has increased from 55% to 64% but gains are disproportionately larger in the Americas and Southeast Asia than in sub-Saharan Africa.

Addressing Target Contraceptive Prevalence Rates

Target CPRs are determined by need for family planning and are context specific. Thus, CPRs are tracked alongside unmet need for family planning, measured as the proportion of women who want to prevent pregnancy and are not, or have male partners and who are not using contraception. Together these metrics help programs and policymakers monitor progress toward improving reproductive health. Annually, 214 million women and girls have unmet need for family planning, accounting for the majority (84%) of unintended pregnancies in developing countries.[13] Unmet need ranges between 4% in East Asia and 24% in sub-Saharan Africa; however there is substantial within-region variation.[14] For example, in 2016 unmet need for family planning exceeded 36% in Benin but was only 13.6% in South Africa.[15] If needs for family planning could be satisfied in developing countries, nearly 76,000 maternal deaths could be averted annually.[4]

Furthermore, every $1 USD spent on family planning saves $2.2 USD on maternal, neonatal, and child healthcare by prevention of unintended pregnancies. Funding and political commitment toward family planning was reinvigorated after the London Summit on Family Planning in 2012, which launched the FP2020 initiative (https://www.familyplanning2020.org/). The goal of this initiative is to reach an additional 120 million contraceptive users by 2020 in 69 of the poorest countries of the world, and accelerate progress on SDG goals toward universal access to family planning. Countries included in FP2020 set individual goals and priorities, with recognition of context-specific needs, to achieve their goals. In addition, growth in the modern contraceptive prevalence rate (mCPR) follows a S-curve. Countries at the low end of the mCPR S-curve will require more substantial changes to infrastructure, changing social norms, and demand creation to catalyze change in contraceptive use, but have the most potential for growth. In contrast, countries with higher mCPR will need to focus efforts on quality, expanding the range of methods and coverage to reach underserved populations, but will have more limited potential for growth. For example, in India where the mCPR rate is 52.1% among married women (38.6% among all women) and unmet need exceeds 20%, it would be useful to increase political commitment to shift the method mix away from permanent methods for birth limiting and expand IUD access to help women space pregnancies.

Risk of HIV/STIs

Vaginal sex without a condom places women at simultaneous risk of pregnancy, HIV, and sexually transmitted infections. Therefore, counselling on condom promotion for women at risk of these infections is warranted, as other methods of contraception provide no protection from HIV or sexually transmitted infection. Using family planning for prevention of unintended pregnancies among women who are infected with HIV or another sexually transmitted infection contributes to reducing mother-to-child transmission risk of these infections. While most family planning methods can safely be used if women are infected with HIV or another sexually transmitted infection, there are some considerations medical providers need to be aware of when prescribing family planning. The WHO Medical Eligibility Criteria describe contraindications to specific family planning methods. For example, women who are HIV infected with advanced clinical disease (WHO stage 3 or 4) are advised not to use the levonorgestrel IUD and women who have pelvic inflammatory disease that may be attributed to a sexually transmitted infection are recommended to not have any type of IUD placed or undergo a tubal ligation until their infection has resolved.[16]

Abortion, Postabortion Care, and Infertility

Access to services for abortion care, postabortion care, and infertility are components of comprehensive reproductive healthcare. Abortion may be medical or surgical; medical abortion is possible in early pregnancy (through the 9th week of gestation) and consists of two medications, mifepristone and misoprostol. Surgical abortion methods depend on pregnancy stage [suction is performed up to 16 weeks gestation and dilation and evacuation (D&E) after 16 weeks gestation]. Many countries have legal restrictions on abortion, which have been not been shown to reduce the number of abortions, and are associated with increased proportion of unsafe abortions.[17] Comprehensive postabortion care may decrease risks associated with unsafe abortion, as well as provide women with contraception to prevent repeat unintended pregnancy.

Infertility in women may result from unsafe abortion practices, but can also be due to other conditions that cause blockage or damage to the fallopian tubes, ovulation disorders, or uterine and cervical abnormalities.[18] In men, infertility is primarily caused by disruptions in testicular or ejaculatory function, hormonal disorders, or genetic disorders.[18] Infertility is defined as not being able to conceive after 1 year of sexual intercourse without a condom. While infertility is difficult to measure, global estimates suggest that 1 in 4 couples in developing countries will experience infertility.[18] Approaches to addressing infertility include expanding access to treatment of sexually transmitted infections, and broadening availability of assisted reproductive technologies to help couples achieve their desired family size.

Maternal Health

Reproductive health includes overall "physical, mental, and societal well-being," not merely the absence of disease or infirmity," for reproductive functions and processes.[19] Maternal health refers to the health of women during pregnancy, labor and delivery, and the postpartum period. During the 25-year period (1990–2015) of the Millennium Development Goals (MDGs), there was an estimated 43.9% decline in maternal mortality rate (MMR) to 216 deaths per 100,000 livebirths. The Sustainable Development Goals (SDGs) target for global MMR by 2030 is less than 70 deaths per 100,000 livebirths, which will require accelerated annual reduction in MMR.[20] Diverse interventions may influence MMR—including improved secondary education for girls, health services for childbirth, access to contraception, training of midwives, treatment for infections such as HIV, mobile health interventions, insurance schemes, and access to transport.[20] These interventions will not only decrease maternal mortality but will also contribute to decreasing maternal morbidity and improving maternal health.

CONCLUSIONS

Continued global investment and commitment to advance the reproductive health agenda will be critical to help women and girls receive access to healthcare services and information to make informed, voluntary decisions about family planning and achieve their desired family size. While current global family planning efforts to increase the number of contraceptive users have resulted in more women and couples across the globe being able to decide if and when to use contraception, achieving universal access to family planning remains a challenge. Strategies to expand the range of methods available to women, integrate service delivery with other health services, and comprehensively address women's reproductive health needs will also be needed. In addition, programs will need to go beyond simple measurement of contraceptive use and include additional indicators of family planning quality and satisfaction with counselling and services received, and method continuation rates, to ensure women are offered the services they need to space and limit their pregnancies.

ADOLESCENT HEALTH

After long being the Cinderella of public health, adolescent health is, at last, coming of age. This is for five main reasons. First, between 1990 and 2015, global neonatal and under-5 mortality rates were halved, resulting in 48 million more children reaching their fifth birthday since 2000, with at least half of this decrease occurring between 2005 and 2015,[14] whereas the global adolescent mortality rate declined by only 12% between 2000 and 2012.[21] Second, there is an increasing global priority given to children and adolescents not just surviving, but also thriving.[22] It is unacceptable for children and adolescents to survive only to live in poverty in unhealthy, unsupportive environments, unable to meet their developmental and health potential.[22] Third, there is a greatly increased global commitment to adolescent health. This is exemplified by the Global Strategy for Women's and Children's Health[23] having been expanded to become the Global Strategy for Women's, Children's and Adolescents' Health (2016–30).[22] Fourth, there is increasing evidence that many interventions can improve adolescent health and can be implemented within programs.[21,24–26] A recent publication called the Global AA-HA! (Accelerated Action for the Health of Adolescents) has summarized the United Nations' guidance related to adolescent health and health programming.[26] Fifth, there is increasing evidence adolescent health is one of the smartest investments that can be made. A recent modelling exercise suggests that an investment of U.S.$4.6 per capita in a package of evidence-based physical, mental and sexual health interventions during adolescence results in a more than tenfold return on investment.[27]

As emphasized throughout this chapter, a lifecourse perspective improves an understanding of what is important to adolescent health. For example, many of the interventions that will have the most profound impact on adolescent health should be implemented before adolescence, such as preconception, periconception and postconception care for young women, and interventions in early childhood related to nutrition, psychosocial development, and vaccination. Similarly, while many of the interventions in adolescence will have short- or medium-term effects during adolescence, at least as many of the effects will occur during adulthood, and some will have effects into the next generation when adolescents become parents themselves.[5,7]

2a. The Burden of Disease and Injury among Adolescents

Globally, more than 3000 adolescents die each day; a total of over 1.4 million per year, largely from preventable causes.[26] Over two-thirds of these deaths occur in African (43%) and Asian (27%) low- and middle-income countries (LMICs).[26] In terms of the overall burden of disease and injury, as measured by disability-adjusted life years (DALYs) lost, some conditions, such as road traffic injury, self-harm, lower respiratory infections, drowning, and unipolar depression are major burdens among all four age/sex groups (10–14 years, 15–19 years, male and female) of adolescents everywhere. However, some adolescent burdens, such as drowning and interpersonal violence only rank highly in males and maternal conditions and anxiety disorders among females, while diarrheal diseases and iron-deficiency anemia are particularly prominent among younger adolescents, and self-harm among older adolescents.[26]

For 10–14 year olds, inadequate handwashing and unsafe water and sanitation are among the leading three health risk factors. Other environmental factors (e.g., air pollution and lead exposure), iron-deficiency anemia, high fasting plasma glucose, high blood pressure, alcohol use, childhood sexual abuse, and unsafe sex also rank highly in this age group. Almost all of these conditions are also leading risk factors among 15–19 year olds. However, risk behaviors such as alcohol and tobacco use, unsafe sex, and, to a lesser extent, drug use are also leading risk factors in the older age group.[26]

Particularly vulnerable adolescents include those living with disabilities or chronic illnesses, those living in remote areas or caught up in social disruption from natural disasters or armed conflicts, and those who are stigmatized and marginalized because of sexual orientation, gender identity, or ethnicity. Adolescent health needs intensify in humanitarian and fragile settings, where they may experience multiple, compounded vulnerabilities simultaneously.[26]

The Global AA-HA! summarized the burden of disease and evidence-based interventions to reduce that burden under seven areas: positive adolescent development; unintentional injuries, such as road traffic injuries and drowning; violence, including collective violence and legal intervention (war), interpersonal and gender-based violence; SRH, including HIV; other communicable diseases, such as acute respiratory infections, diarrhoeal disease and meningitis; non-communicable diseases, nutrition and physical activity; and mental health, substance use and self-harm.[26]

2b. Evidence-based Interventions

Although further research is needed to strengthen and expand the repertoire of evidence-based interventions,[25] effective, evidence-based interventions are available for countries to act now to protect and promote the health of their adolescents.[24–26] Some of these interventions are adolescent specific, such as health promoting schools or human papillomavirus vaccination, while general population interventions must usually be tailored to the specific needs of adolescents in order to reduce adolescent burdens, such as the need for lower blood alcohol limits for adolescent drivers.[26] Often, for adolescents to effectively access general population interventions they will require specific, targeted support.[26]

2c. The Importance of Setting Priorities

There is no single, ideal package of adolescent health interventions that will meet the needs of every country, because the nature, scale and impact of adolescent health needs and resources differ considerably between countries. The Global AA-HA! guidance document advises three key steps in determining what these priority adolescent health interventions should be: a needs assessment, a landscape analysis of what is already being done, followed by the setting priorities, based on financial, health system and political realities.[26]

2d. National Adolescent Health Programming

The Global AA-HA! provides guidance on how to integrate the selected interventions into national programmes.[26] It stresses that, since many of the determinants of adolescent health fall outside the normal remit of the health sector, intersectoral programs are likely to be necessary to make progress in adolescent health involving multiple sectors including education, social protection, telecommunications and mass media, road and transportation, housing and urban planning, energy, environment, and the criminal justice system.[26] With increasing school enrolment, school health programmes provide a growing opportunity to reach adolescents with information, services and care.

Joe Biden, the former U.S. Vice President and now U.S. President-elect has been quoted as saying "Don't tell me what you value. Show me your budget, and I'll tell you what you value."[28] Increasingly, governments and nongovernmental organizations are including specific budgets for adolescent health programs, and this is likely to increase with the recent development of a specific adolescent health module within the OneHealth Tool that many countries use for budgeting.[29]

2e. Monitoring and Evaluation

The Global Strategy for Women's, Children's and Adolescents' Health has agreed to regularly monitor 60 indicators to track national, regional and global progress in women's, children's and adolescents' health.[30] These include 43 indicators that are either adolescent-specific (e.g., the adolescent mortality rate) or include adolescents (e.g., experience of sexual violence). The rapid physical, emotional and social changes and resulting differences in the burden of disease and programmatic needs across the adolescent period make it essential for all adolescent data to be disaggregated by age (5-year age groups) and by sex. It is also essential for adolescent health programmes to monitor the full range of indicators from inputs and processes to outputs, outcomes and impact, since they answer different questions and are useful for different purposes.

2f. Research and Innovation

Compared to younger children, research on adolescent health has been relatively neglected.[25,26] Investments in adolescent health research capacity are urgently needed, especially in low- and middle-income countries where research capacity is weakest but adolescent health needs are greatest.[25] Two recent research priority-setting exercises have identified areas in particular need of research.[31,32] Both exercises showed that priorities have shifted away from basic questions on the prevalence of specific health conditions toward questions about how best to scale-up existing interventions and testing the effectiveness of new ones. Innovation to discover and design adolescent health interventions is also needed, and promising innovations should be fast-tracked to evaluation of their effectiveness.

Ideally, the monitoring, evaluation and research of programmes designed to improve the health of adolescents should include the opinions of adolescents themselves. With increasing age, there is also the increasing potential for adolescents or young people to be engaged as active evaluators rather than only as subjects of the evaluation. This engagement can include adolescents actively and meaningfully participating in the design, implementation, analysis and interpretation of results, and in formulating the recommendations resulting from the programme evaluation. Ideas for how to involve adolescents can be found in the Youth Participation Guide developed by Family Health International and Advocates for Youth.[31,33]

Conclusions

This is an exciting time for adolescent health. Increasingly, adolescent health services and programmes are no longer subsumed under those for children or adults. Instead, adolescent-specific national health strategies and programmes are becoming increasingly common and are expanding from programs with a limited remit, such as adolescent SRH, to comprehensive programs that also include injuries and violence, communicable and noncommunicable diseases, nutrition and physical activity, and mental health, substance use and self-harm, and which span multiple sectors. Most research on adolescent health has been conducted within the last two decades, and several major funders have recently initiated adolescent-specific calls for programme and research proposals.

Even though research and innovation will be essential to build and strengthen the adolescent health programmes of the future, there is sufficient evidence to act now. And there can be no excuses for not doing so, as evidence-based programmes founded on a careful choice of local priorities will harness the triple dividend of benefits for adolescents now, for their future adult lives, and for the next generation,[25,26] with a return on investment to rival that of any public health investment in any age group.[27]

NEONATAL HEALTH

3a. Global Burden of Neonatal Mortality

Newborn mortality rates have seen a less rapid decline over the last two decades than child and maternal mortality rates. While the under-5 mortality rate decreased by approximately 53% between 1990 and 2015, neonatal mortality decreased by 47% to 2.8 million in 2015.[34] As a result, the proportion of childhood deaths attributable to neonatal mortality has been increasing with nearly 45% of childhood deaths occurring in the newborn period in 2015. Without further efforts targeted at improving the situation for newborns, it is estimated that this proportion could exceed 50% by 2030.[34,35]

The vast majority (approximately 99%) of neonatal deaths occur in LMICs and up to two thirds may be preventable.[36] Contributing to the magnitude of the problem are health systems limitations which affect mothers, children and newborns such as: delays in recognition of and reaching appropriate care for neonatal illness, human-resource capacity limitations, insufficient supplies, incomplete coverage of known intervention and prevention modalities, and limited infrastructure to accurately measure mortality.[37–39]

3b. Evidence-based Interventions

According to the WHO, essential care for all newborns irrespective of whether born in a facility or at home, includes thermal care (drying, warming, skin-to-skin, and delayed bathing), hygienic cord and skin care (hand washing, delayed cord care, chlorhexidine), early and exclusive breastfeeding, and neonatal resuscitation if not breathing at birth. Efforts continue to be focused at increasing coverage of essential newborn care, which remains highly variable globally.

Neonatal infections, intrapartum-related complications such as birth asphyxia, and complications from preterm birth remain the leading direct causes of newborn deaths globally.[35] Newborn health and maternal health are intimately related to one another, and as such packaged approaches across the continuum of combined interventions, which involve actions from the community, first-line, regional, referral, and public health levels would be most desirable.

Caring for sick or small newborns is substantially more complicated in low-resource settings where timely access to expensive and advanced care may not be available. Of the approximately 15 million preterm (<37 weeks of gestation) newborns born each year, approximately 2/3 are born in LMICs with the vast majority being born between 32 and 37 weeks of gestation.[40] Approximately 1 million newborns die from direct complications of preterm birth each year. While primary prevention of preterm delivery remains challenging and remains an area of investigation, management of preterm newborns in LMICs has been advancing over the past 15 years. Most notable has been Kangaroo Mother Care (KMC), which is defined as skin-to-skin care, exclusive breast feeding, supportive care of the mother-baby unit, and close follow-up after discharge.[41] With broad coverage, KMC could have the potential to prevent up to 450,000 preterm deaths per year.[37] Further, KMC requires little to no additional costs beyond that of training and implementation.

Birth asphyxia is defined by the WHO as the failure to initiate and sustain spontaneous breathing at the time of birth. While a critical intervention for reducing the prevalence of birth asphyxia is improving access to emergency obstetric care, improving access to a skilled birth attendant with particular attention to newborn resuscitation skills is a promising approach to reducing the number of deaths due to birth asphyxia globally. A large, multicenter trial of newborn resuscitation training for birth attendants conducted in 6 LMICs reported a one third reduction in perinatal deaths.[42] More recently, the Helping Babies Breathe program was developed by the American Academy of Pediatrics and has shown promise in reducing neonatal deaths.[43]

Neonatal infections have remained major causes of newborn mortality globally despite dramatic reductions in infection-related mortality in HICs where body-fluid culture for diagnosis and parenteral antibiotic therapy remain as standard of care. Evidence from LMICs, however, suggest that neonatal infections can be diagnosed and managed in community settings.[44,45] In fact, community-based intervention trials in India and Bangladesh have reported substantial reductions in both overall neonatal mortality and mortality due to sepsis.[46,47]

3c. Need for Prioritization

Without targeted efforts at reducing neonatal mortality and morbidity, further reductions in childhood mortality may be stunted.

Furthermore, reductions in neonatal mortality have been associated with decreased fertility rates, which can lead to improved maternal outcomes as well. Optimizing outcomes for newborns pays dividends across the lifecycle with healthy newborns leading to healthy and thriving children, adolescents and on into adulthood.

INFANT AND CHILD HEALTH

4a. Child Mortality

Each year, millions of children die, the vast majority in poor countries. Tragically, most of these deaths are preventable. Progress is being made: 5.6 million children younger than the age of 5 years died in 2016, down from 12.6 million in 1990.[48] This reduction, while substantial, was insufficient to meet Millennium Development Goal (MDG) 4 (two-thirds reduction in child mortality from 1990 to 2015). The Sustainable Development Goals (SDGs) encompass wider targets. SDG3.2, the target related to child health, calls for ending "preventable deaths of newborns and children under 5 years of age, with all countries aiming to reduce under-5 mortality to at least as low as 25 per 1000 live births" by 2030.[49] Globally, 99% of child deaths occur in low- and middle-income countries (LMICs). A child born in sub-Saharan Africa faces a 1 in 13 chance of dying before his or her fifth birthday compared with 1 in 143 for a child born in the United States and 1 in 189 for high-income countries (HICs) on average. In order to attain the SDG3.2 child mortality reduction target, it is critical to understand the context and causes of childhood deaths, interventions to address these causes, as well as trends in mortality and drivers of these trends.

"Child," as used in this chapter includes persons younger than 5 years of age (excluding neonates who were highlighted previously in this chapter). Children in the 5- to 9-year age group have historically been neglected by the global health community and should be included in health prevention efforts; however, there are currently few age-disaggregated data or interventions focused within this group.

4a. Trends in Child Mortality

There has been a continual decline in rates and numbers of child deaths annually over the intervening decades (Fig. 22-2). However, mortality reductions have been uneven between countries, within countries (with more rapid gains among children from wealthier households, e.g.), and over time. Remarkable gains were made after commencement of data monitoring in the 1960s, followed by a decreased progress starting in the mid-1980s—with stagnating and sometimes increasing mortality rates in some countries—followed by improved U5MR deceleration at the start of this century.

The 4th Millennium Development Goal (MDG4) was based on earlier trends in U5MRs (Fig. 22-2) coupled with data demonstrating that two-thirds of child deaths could be averted with interventions that have proven effectiveness, are available and recommended for wide implementation.[50] In moving to the new SDGs, we can extract lessons learned from the 24 (of 81) LMICs that met MDG4.[51] One example is Malawi, which started with a staggering U5MR of 232 in 1990. By 2013, Malawi was able to achieve MDG4 (2017 U5MR 55.4 per 1000 livebirths) primarily through the scale-up of interventions against the major causes of child deaths (malaria, pneumonia, and diarrhea), programs to reduce child undernutrition, and mother-to-child HIV transmission, and some improvements in the quality of care provided around birth to reduce poor neonatal outcomes.[52] However, it is unclear if Malawi will be able to achieve the SDG3.2 target U5MR of 25 per 1000 livebirths by 2030.

Health is clearly more than survival.[53] The global child health agenda has recently shifted from a "child survival" to a "child thrival" approach. While there are interventions specific to "child thrival" that do not have a major impact on mortality reduction (e.g., early learning and social protection), there is considerable overlap between the key interventions recommended to reduce child mortality and to support child growth and development and reduce long term morbidity and disability. In addition, there is growing evidence early-0life adverse childhood experiences, which could include poverty, abuse,

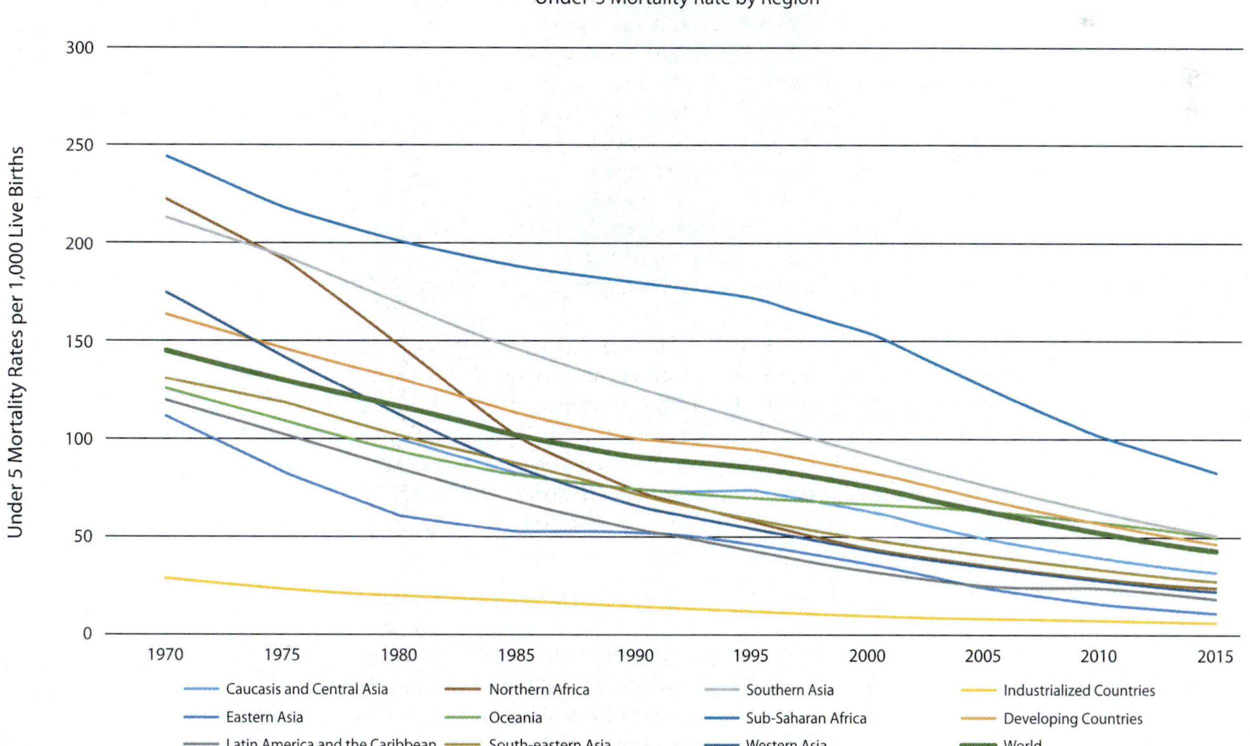

FIGURE 22-2. Under-5 mortality rate by region. (*Source:* Data From UNICEF, Child Mortality Estimates: Country Specific Under-5 Mortality Rates, available from http://data.unicef.org.)

neglect, maternal depression, or parental separation, may result in long-term morbidity.

4b. Major Direct Causes of Child Mortality and Recommended Interventions

Forty-six percent of child mortality occurs in the neonatal period discussed previously in this chapter (Fig. 22-3).[54] Four problems contribute approximately 60% of postneonatal deaths: pneumonia, diarrhea, injuries, and malaria. Undernutrition, defined to include lack of sufficient macronutrients (e.g., protein, calories), micronutrient deficient diets (e.g., vitamin A, zinc, iron), and suboptimal breastfeeding practices) is an *underlying* cause of 45% of all child deaths.[55] Undernutrition increases susceptibility to infections, delays recovery, and is associated with longer-term sequelae.

Pneumonia

Pneumonia is the leading cause of death after the neonatal period, killing more than 700,000 children annually. Pneumococcus (*Streptococcus pneumoniae)* and *Haemophilus influenza* type b (Hib) are the most important etiologies of severe pneumonia in young childhood, causing about half of childhood pneumonia deaths globally.[56,57] Undernutrition leads to impaired immune responses and increased difficulty in clearing secretions due to weakened respiratory muscles. Optimal breastfeeding practices—and adequate micronutrients especially those involved in immune protection such as zinc, are important interventions to prevent respiratory infections.[55,58] Household air pollution is associated with a 1.8-fold risk of contracting pneumonia and is largely caused by burning of solid fuels (e.g., wood, charcoal, dung, crop waste) in dwellings for heat and cooking. These polluting fuels are used by 40% of the world's population. Chimney stoves can reduce household air pollution by half and severe pneumonia by approximately 30%.[59] Hand hygiene (washing with soap) is important for preventing the spread of respiratory infection and requires access to sufficient quantities of water. Vaccinations play a vital prevention role. Secondary bacterial pneumonia is a common sequela of measles and pertussis infections and both are vaccine-preventable. The largest pneumococcus and Hib disease burden is in LMICs.[57] Hib vaccine was first introduced in a LMIC in 1997; 191 countries now incorporate Hib vaccine into national immunization schedules and global coverage is 64% (Fig. 22-4).

Pneumococcal vaccine rollout commenced less than a decade ago in LMICs; it is part of routine schedules in 129 countries and global coverage is 37%.[60] Coverage rates for measles and DPT vaccines are 85% and 86%, below the WHO and UNICEF goal of 90% coverage.[61] Global and national coverage estimates mask disparities in coverage *within* countries. A multicountry analysis demonstrated pro-rich and pro-urban inequities in immunization coverage in most LMICs and pro-male inequities in South-East Asian LMICs.[62] Differences between the wealthiest and poorest quintiles for immunization and other intervention coverage rates as global averages are depicted in Fig. 22-5.

Appropriate antibiotic treatment is critical for reducing case fatality. Prompt and appropriate case management hinges on:

A. Global distribution of deaths among children under age 5, by cause, 2016

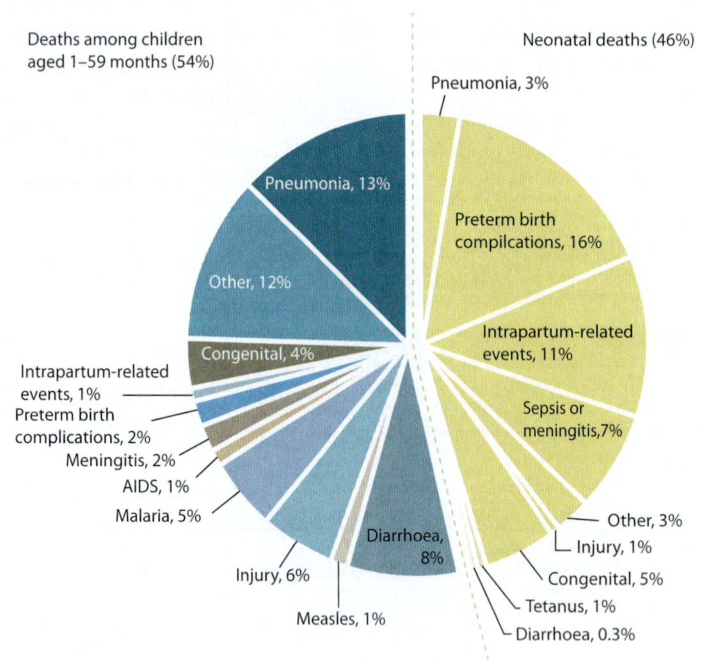

Nearly half of all deaths in children under age 5 are attributable to Undernutrition

B. Global distribution of deaths among newborns, by cause, 2016

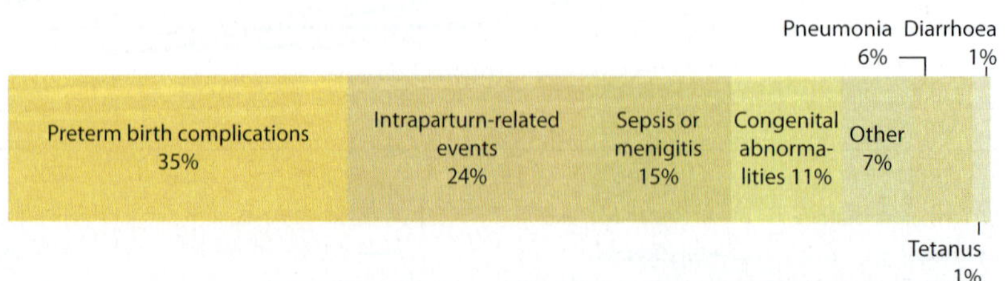

FIGURE 22-3. Infectious diseases and neonatal complications are the leading causes of death among children under age 5. (*Source:* Reproduce with Permission from UNICEF, Unicef. Levels and Trends in Child Mortality Report 2017. UNICEF https://www.unicef.org/reports/levels-and-trends-child-mortality-report-2017. Published October 1, 2017. Accessed January 6, 2021.)

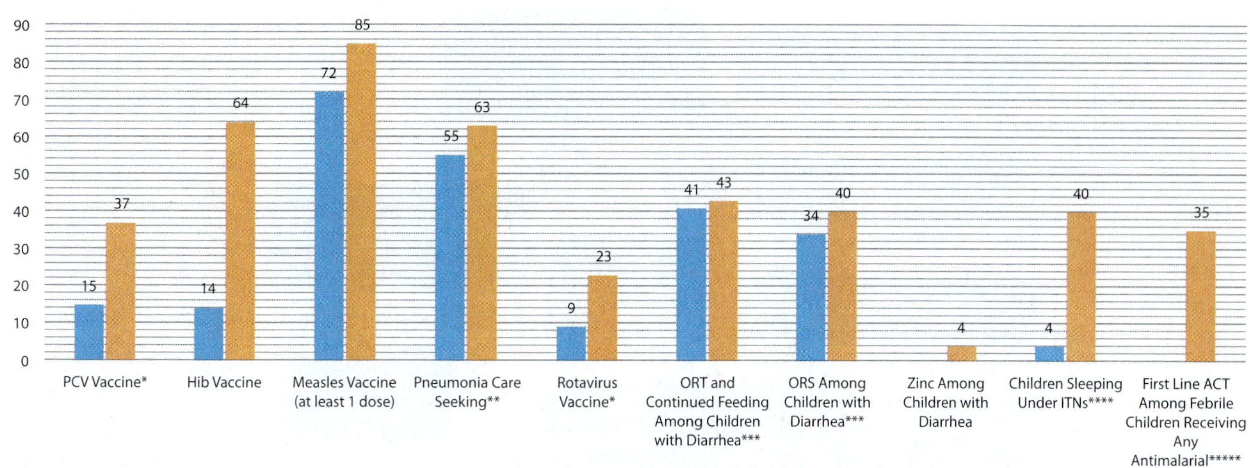

FIGURE 22-4. Global intervention coverage 2000–15. Data represent percent coverage globally except where indicated. (*Sources:* From WHO. Global Immunization Profile, available from http://www.who.int/immunization/monitoring_surveillance/data/gs_gloprofile.pdf?ua=1. Accessed November 24, 2016; UNICEF. Malaria mortality among children under five is concentrated in sub-Saharan Africa, available from https://data.unicef.org/topic/child-health/malaria/#. Accessed November 18, 2016.)

*The 15% and 9% figures in the first blue bars represent data from 2011; widescale adoption into immunization schedules in LMICs commenced more recently, hence 2000 data are not available or negligible.

**Excludes data from China.

***Excludes data from China and India.

****Based on data from sub-Saharan Africa. The 4% figure is data from 2005.

*****Based on data from sub-Saharan Africa.

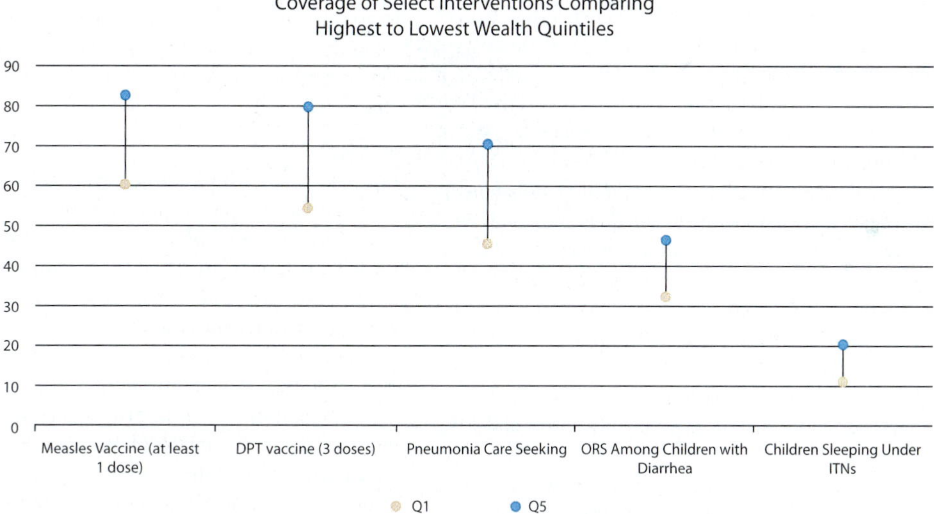

FIGURE 22-5. Coverage of select interventions comparing highest to lowest wealth quintiles. Q1 is the poorest wealth quintile. Q5 is the richest wealth quintile. Data represent percent coverage and are global estimates. (*Source:* Data from From Immunization and ITN data are from Barros AJ et al: Equity in maternal, newborn, and child health interventions in Countdown to 2015: A retrospective review of survey data from 54 countries. *Lancet*. 2012;379(9822):1225–33. The remainders are from UNICEF Data: Monitoring the Situation of Children and Women from data.unicef.org. Accessed November 25, 2016.)

(1) parent/caretaker recognition of symptoms, (2) access to appropriate care without delay, (3) accurate diagnosis and treatment by health workers, and (4) completion of a full therapeutic course of accurate duration and dosage. However, parental recognition that fast breathing and retractions require urgent medical attention is inadequate[63] and less than 65% of children with pneumonia symptoms are taken for appropriate healthcare.[59] Fewer still actually receive antibiotics. Tragically, there has been little improvement in these coverage statistics over the past decade (Fig. 22-4), especially in sub Saharan Africa. Increasingly, programs to train and support lay health workers (LHWs) in diagnosing and treating pneumonia in the communities are being implemented. LHWs trained in pneumonia case management can accurately identify and effectively treat pneumonia.[64] However, in 2010 less than one-third of SSA countries had policies in place to allow LHWs to treat children with pneumonia.[65] Policies and programs conducive to improving access and efforts to educate caregivers on danger signs, in addition to improved coverage of prevention interventions, are critical to reducing the pneumonia burden of disease.

Diarrheal disease

Diarrhea remains the second leading cause of child mortality beyond the neonatal period, causing more than 400,000 child deaths annually. These deaths are almost exclusively in LMICs. It is unlikely that

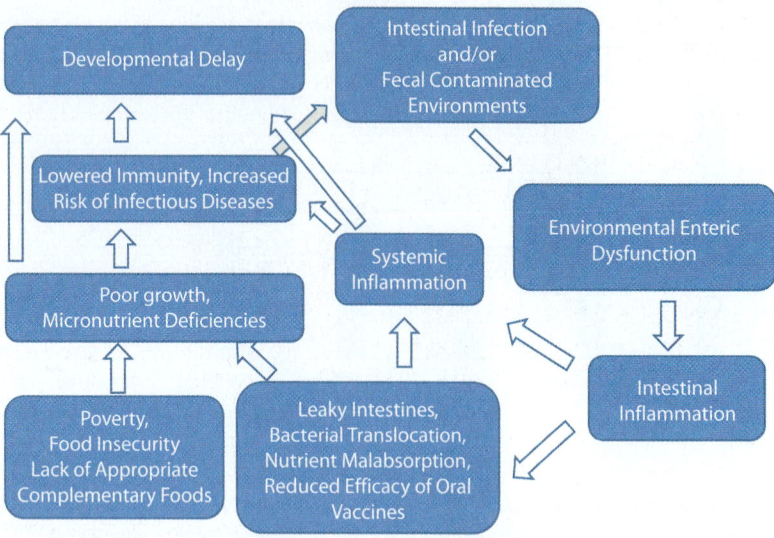

FIGURE 22-6. The vicious cycle of intestinal infection, EED, and undernutrition. (*Source:* Used with Permission from Donna M. Denno, Shadae Paul. Child Health and Survival in a Changing World, *Pediatric Clinics of North America* 64(4): pp:735–754.)

the decline in diarrhea mortality is due to prevention measures as incidence rates have not substantially changed and account for nearly 1.7 billion child episodes annually.[66] The impact of childhood enteric diseases impact on morbidity is increasingly being recognized. Specifically, environmental enteric dysfunction (EED) is prevalent in settings with poor sanitation.[67,68] Recurrent or persistent infection with enteric pathogens or exposure to fecal organisms may trigger the inflammatory response and subsequent EED pathophysiologic cascade. EED may also be caused or exacerbated by micronutrient deficits. EED contributes to undernutrition, itself a risk factor for infectious disease acquisition and mortality; thus, the vicious cycle of malnutrition, infections and EED (Fig. 22-6).

There is much overlap between the interventions to combat pneumonia and diarrhea, such as hand hygiene, adequate nutrition, and improved care seeking and case management. Rotavirus, *Shigella*, *Cryptosporidium*, and enterotoxigenic *Escherichia coli* (ETEC) are important microbiologic causes of moderate-to-severe diarrhea and the latter two organisms plus typical enteropathogenic *E. coli* are predominant causes of mortality.[69] These microbes are spread by fecal-oral route. Improvements in handwashing with soap, sanitation, and water quality could reduce diarrhea risk by 48%, 36%, and 17%, respectively.[70]

At 91%, the 2015 global coverage rate for improved water sources met the MDG7 water target.[59] However, over 663 million people still use unimproved sources; nearly half in SSA and one-fifth in South Asia.[71] This indicator does not describe water security or quality. At least 1.8 billion people worldwide are estimated to drink fecally contaminated water.[72] Only 68% of the world's population has access to improved sanitation facilities.[72] The situation is worse for those living in rural areas, South Asia, and sub-Saharan Africa where coverage is 51%, 47%, and 30%, respectively.[71] Vaccines hold promise for preventing diarrhea due to specific agents. Eighty-four countries have incorporated rotavirus vaccine into routine schedules with 23% coverage globally[60,73] (Fig. 22-4). Vaccines against *Shigella* and ETEC are under development.

Oral rehydration therapy is a cornerstone treatment intervention for diarrhea, which prevents and corrects dehydration and electrolyte losses. A 10- to 14-day course of oral zinc is recommended in treatment of diarrhea in most LMICs.[74] Antibiotics are currently only recommended for dysentery.[69,75] Ongoing studies are investigating the efficacy of an expanded role for antibiotics in the management of diarrhea.[76] ORS has been the cornerstone of diarrhea treatment for decades. Despite this, ORS coverage rates are low and improvements have been sluggish (Figs. 22-4 and 22-5). Zinc treatment was first recommended in 2004, but only three LMIC countries (Bangladesh, Nepal, and Malawi) have coverage rates exceeding 20% and none exceeds 50% coverage. The unacceptable death toll and long-term consequences of enteric diseases are reminders of the work that remains in implementing interventions with proven effectiveness that are already recommended, especially for the most vulnerable children.

Injuries

Injuries are the third leading cause of child mortality beyond the neonatal period and responsible for 336,000 under-5 deaths annually. More than 95% of all injury-related deaths in children occur in LMICs, are largely preventable and disproportionately affect children from poorer households. Ninety percent of child injuries are unintentional; drowning, burns, and fire-related injuries are the leading cause of deaths due to injuries among children under age 5 years. For every death, thousands of children suffer disability from injuries.[77]

Combinations of multidisciplinary approaches have been most effective for reducing child injuries. Examples include: civil and transportation engineers designing and building traffic calming structures (e.g., speed bumps) or barriers to separate pedestrians from traffic, product safety engineers developing tamper-resistant products to prevent poisoning, law enforcement personnel enforcing drunk driving laws, and victim/family advocacy groups serving as powerful change agents. In countries where the greatest child injury reductions have been recorded, combination approaches has been employed based on local epidemiology. For example, in Bangladesh the environmental risk profile translates to drowning as a leading cause of child mortality; researchers and program implementers have focused on drowning prevention by teaching "survival swimming" and safe rescue skills.[78,79]

Malaria

Almost 50% of the world's population lives in malaria endemic areas. Approximately 280,000 children die annually due to malaria, the majority in sub-Saharan Africa. Malaria control requires a multi-pronged approach consisting of both prevention and treatment interventions. Insecticide treated nets (ITNs) are one of the most effective methods of preventing transmission. Regular ITN use in malaria endemic areas has been shown to reduce all-cause child mortality by 17%.[80] Not only do ITNs protect sleeping individuals with a physical barrier against mosquitoes, the insecticide also offers protection to nonusers up to several hundred meters away. ITNs have been provided through free mass distribution with increased use. However, much more progress is required to move current 40% coverage rates to the 80% WHO goals. Rapid diagnostic tests (RDTs) for malaria have transformed malaria diagnosis capacities. However, RDT implementation is lagging; only one-fifth of febrile children treated with an antimalarial were tested for malaria between 2010 and 2014; regions with the highest child malaria-related mortality burden have the weakest coverage.[81] Malaria parasites can quickly develop drug resistance; conventional antimicrobials (e.g., chloroquine, sulfadoxine-pryimethamine) are no longer effective in *P. falciparum* endemic areas. Artemisinin combination therapy (ACT) is the currently recommended first-line drug for uncomplicated malaria in areas characterized by high resistance to conventional therapies. Unfortunately, its use remains too low—only 35% of children treated with an antimalarial for fever in sub Saharan Africa received ACT (Fig. 22-4).

4c. Integrated Approaches to Child Health

WHO and UNICEF developed the Integrated Management of Childhood Illness (IMCI), which focuses on caring for the whole child. IMCI includes treatment algorithms target the most common child mortality causes (excluding injuries) as well as screening and prevention elements, such as monitoring growth and immunization status during sick visits. Effective IMCI implementation includes three components: (1) improving health worker case management skills, (2) improving health practices within families and communities, and (3) improving overall health systems. IMCI evaluations have demonstrated improved clinical performance by health workers by those trained in IMCI. However, the evaluations also showed that less attention has been focused on implementing the family/community and health systems components. To achieve any significant reduction in child mortality through IMCI, full attention to all three components is needed as well as implementation on a larger scale.[82]

Maternal education is arguably the most important determinant of child survival, borne out in many studies. Children whose mothers have no formal education are, on average, 2.8 times as likely to die before their fifth birthday compared to those with mothers with secondary or higher education.[83] While literacy and health literacy are important outcomes of women's education, they do not fully explain the effect on child healthy; agency and decision-making power likely play important roles.[84]

Approximately 10% of the world lives below the international poverty line—$1.90 per day.[85] Relative poverty is defined as large gaps between rich and poor within a society and is associated with worse societal health outcomes. This phenomenon has been demonstrated in both rich and poor countries.[86] Overall, children living in the poorest fifth of households compared to the wealthiest quintile within any given country face a 1.9-fold increased risk of mortality.[87] Unfortunately, income inequality has increased in many countries.[88] Rural residence is another determinant of health—children in rural areas have a 1.7-fold increased risk of dying compared to their urban counterparts. With increasing urbanization, however, urban slum dwellers face survival challenges. Services may not be available in rural areas, but urban slum dwellers may lack *access* due to cost, discrimination and other factors and suffer overcrowded and unsanitary living conditions. Race, ethnicity, and gender are other important determinants.

4d. Conclusions

Of the 79 countries that have U5MRs in excess of the 25 per 1000 target, only 27 will reach SDG3.2 if current rates of progress are sustained.[48,81,89] If SDG3.2 target were met globally, an additional 10 million child lives will be saved between 2017 and 2030.[48,81] New diagnostics, vaccines and medicines have potential to reset the bar on the number of deaths that can be prevented. Assessment of health indicators and coverage rates must be disaggregated to identify and eliminate disparities. Coverage of existing interventions should be scaled up, especially to the poorest and most vulnerable and marginalized populations. Research on implementation strategies is critical to inform scale-up of effective interventions.

OVERALL SUMMARY AND CONCLUSIONS

Reproductive, maternal, neonatal child, and adolescent health are intertwined and can sometimes be addressed by broad interventions that improve outcomes for each of these populations. These interventions includes advocacy for debt relief, health systems improvements, investments in data quality and reporting, and addressing poverty, income, and gender inequalities. Intersectoral investments beyond the health sector contribute to broad health gains in these groups.[89] Current attention is being focused on universal healthcare and pro-poor implementation strategies as a means to accelerate progress.[90,91] Acknowledging the relationships between women, adolescents, and children and using both broad and focused interventions will be necessary for sustained improvements in these populations. Early interventions that led to rapid gains in child survival will need to maintain coverage. At the same time, more complex interventions will be required to attain the SDGs. Leveraging existing platforms such as public sector primary healthcare systems will be useful to deliver some interventions, while novel systems, especially for adolescents, may be required. Tracking data regarding burden of disease in combination with scaling effective interventions was an approach that led to substantial health improvements for women and children in the MDG era. Expanding that approach by broadening intersectoral interventions and tackling the underlying determinants of health will be necessary to meet targets for improvement in reproductive, adolescent, and child health in the SDG era.

References

1. http://www.worldometers.info/world-population/. Worldometers. 2019.
2. UN. World Fertility Patterns. 2015.
3. WHO. Maternal mortality factsheet. https://wwwwhoint/news-room/fact-sheets/detail/maternal-mortality.
4. Guttmacher. Adding it up—Investing in Contraception and Maternal and Newborn Health 2017. https://wwwguttmacherorg/fact-sheet/adding-it-up-contraception-mnh-2017. 2017.
5. WHO. Sexual and reproductive health. https://wwwwhoint/reproductivehealth/topics/unsafe_abortion/en/. 2017.
6. WHO. Health for the world's adolescents. https://wwwwhoint/maternal_child_adolescent/topics/adolescence/second-decade/en/. 2014.
7. Kozuki N, Lee AC, Silveira MF, et al. The associations of parity and maternal age with small-for-gestational-age, preterm, and neonatal and infant mortality: A meta-analysis. *BMC Public Health*. 2013;13(Suppl 3):S2.
8. Finlay JE, Ozaltin E, Canning D. The association of maternal age with infant mortality, child anthropometric failure, diarrhoea and anaemia for first births: Evidence from 55 low- and middle-income countries. *BMJ Open*. 2011;1:e000226.
9. Chandra-Mouli V, Lane C, Wong S. What does not work in adolescent sexual and reproductive health: A review of evidence on interventions commonly accepted as best practices. *Glob Health Sci Pract*. 2015;3:333–40.
10. Chandra-Mouli V, Svanemyr J, Amin A, et al. Twenty years after International Conference on Population and Development: Where are we with adolescent sexual and reproductive health and rights? *J Adolesc Health*. 2015; 56:S1–6.
11. Trussell J. Contraceptive failure in the United States. *Contraception*. 2011; 83:397–404.
12. UN. Trends in Contraceptive Use. http://wwwunorg/en/development/desa/population/publications/pdf/family/trendsContraceptiveUse2015Reportpdf. 2015.
13. Adding it up: Investing in contraception and maternal and newborn health 2017, Fact Sheet. Guttmacher Institute, 2017. Available at https://http://www.guttmacher.org/fact-sheet/adding-it-up-contraception-mnh-2017. Accessed October 11, 2017.

14. UN. Millenium Development Goals Report 2015. http://wwwunorg/en/development/desa/publications/mdg-report-2015html. 2015.
15. FP2020. FP2020. http://wwwfamilyplanning2020org/entities. 2017.
16. WHO. Medical eligibility for contraceptive use. https://apps.who.int/iris/bitstream/handle/10665/181468/9789241549158_eng.pdf;jsessionid=C1D0EACE0BCD9FCCF802926798FA44D1?sequence=1. 2015.
17. Guttmacher. Highly restrictive laws do not eliminate abortion. https://wwwguttmacherorg/infographic/2018/highly-restrictive-laws-do-not-eliminate-abortion. 2018.
18. CDC. Reproductive Health. https://wwwcdcgov/reproductivehealth/infertility/indexhtm.
19. WHO. Framework for health. 2005.
20. Alkema L, Chou D, Hogan D, et al. Global, regional, and national levels and trends in maternal mortality between 1990 and 2015, with scenario-based projections to 2030: A systematic analysis by the UN Maternal Mortality Estimation Inter-Agency Group. *Lancet*. 2016;387:462–74.
21. WHO. Health for the World's Adolescents. A second chance in the second decade. 2014.
22. UN. Every Woman, Every Child. The Global Strategy for Women's, Children's and Adolescents' Health (2016–2030). 2015.
23. UN. United Nations. Global Strategy for Women's and Children's Health. http://wwweverywomaneverychildorg/wp-content/uploads/2016/11/20100914_gswch_en-1pdf. 2010.
24. Catalano RF, Fagan AA, Gavin LE, et al. Worldwide application of prevention science in adolescent health. *Lancet*. 2012;379:1653–64.
25. Patton GC, Sawyer SM, Santelli JS, et al. Our future: A Lancet commission on adolescent health and wellbeing. *Lancet*. 2016;387:2423–78.
26. WHO. Global AA-HA! (Accelerated Action for the Health of Adolescents). Guidance to Support Country Implementation. 2017.
27. Sheehan P, Sweeny K, Rasmussen B, et al. Building the foundations for sustainable development: A case for global investment in the capabilities of adolescents. *Lancet* 2017;390:1792–806.
28. Biden J. Biden's Remarks on McCain's Policies. New York Times. http://www.nytimes.com/2008/09/15/us/politics/15text-biden.html. 2008.
29. WHO. OneHealth Tool. http://wwwwhoint/choice/onehealthtool/en/ (Downloaded 21st November 2017) 2017.
30. WHO. Every Woman, Every Child. Indicator and monitoring framework for the Global Strategy for Women's, Children's and Adolescents' Health. http://wwwwhoint/life-course/publications/gs-Indicator-and-monitoring-frameworkpdf. 2016.
31. Hindin MJ, Christiansen CS, Ferguson BJ. Setting research priorities for adolescent sexual and reproductive health in low- and middle-income countries. *Bull World Health Organ*. 2013;91:10–8.
32. Nagata JM, Ferguson BJ, Ross DA. Research priorities for eight areas of adolescent health in low- and middle-income countries. *J Adolesc Health*. 2016;59:50–60.
33. YouthNet. Youth participation guide: assessment, planning, and implementation. Family Health International, Advocates for Youth. 2005.
34. Liu L, Oza S, Hogan D, et al. Global, regional, and national causes of child mortality in 2000–13, with projections to inform post-2015 priorities: An updated systematic analysis. *Lancet* 2015;385:430–40.
35. Lawn JE, Blencowe H, Oza S, et al. Every Newborn: Progress, priorities, and potential beyond survival. *Lancet*. 2014;384:189–205.
36. Darmstadt GL, Bhutta ZA, Cousens S, Adam T, Walker N, de Bernis L. Evidence-based, cost-effective interventions: How many newborn babies can we save? *Lancet*. 2005;365:977–88.
37. Lawn JE, Kerber K, Enweronu-Laryea C, Cousens S. 3.6 million neonatal deaths—What is progressing and what is not? *Semin Perinatol*. 2010;34:371–86.
38. Bhutta ZA, Das JK, Bahl R, et al. Can available interventions end preventable deaths in mothers, newborn babies, and stillbirths, and at what cost? *Lancet*. 2014;384:347–70.
39. Chang HH, Larson J, Blencowe H, et al. Preventing preterm births: Analysis of trends and potential reductions with interventions in 39 countries with very high human development index. *Lancet*. 2013;381:223–34.
40. Lawn JE, Kinney MV, Belizan JM, et al. Born too soon: Accelerating actions for prevention and care of 15 million newborns born too soon. *Reprod Health*. 2013;10(Suppl 1):S6.
41. Lawn JE, Mwansa-Kambafwile J, Barros FC, Horta BL, Cousens S. 'Kangaroo mother care' to prevent neonatal deaths due to pre-term birth complications. *Int J Epidemiol*. 2011;40:525–8.
42. Carlo WA, Goudar SS, Jehan I, et al. Newborn-care training and perinatal mortality in developing countries. *N Engl J Med*. 2010;362:614–23.
43. Msemo G, Massawe A, Mmbando D, et al. Newborn mortality and fresh stillbirth rates in Tanzania after helping babies breathe training. *Pediatrics*. 2013;131:e353–60.
44. Baqui AH, Saha SK, Ahmed AS, et al. Safety and efficacy of alternative antibiotic regimens compared with 7 day injectable procaine benzylpenicillin and gentamicin for outpatient treatment of neonates and young infants with clinical signs of severe infection when referral is not possible: A randomised, open-label, equivalence trial. *Lancet Glob Health* 2015;3:e279–87.
45. Ganatra HA, Zaidi AK. Neonatal infections in the developing world. *Semin Perinatol*. 2010;34:416–25.
46. Bang AT, Reddy HM, Deshmukh MD, Baitule SB, Bang RA. Neonatal and infant mortality in the ten years (1993 to 2003) of the Gadchiroli field trial: Effect of home-based neonatal care. *J Perinatol*. 2005;25(Suppl 1):S92–107.
47. Baqui AH, El-Arifeen S, Darmstadt GL, et al. Effect of community-based newborn-care intervention package implemented through two service-delivery strategies in Sylhet district, Bangladesh: A cluster-randomised controlled trial. *Lancet*. 2008;371:1936–44.
48. Estimation UNI-aGfCM. Levels & Trends in Child Mortality: Report 2017, Estimates Developed by the UN Inter-agency Group for Child Mortality Estimation. New York; 2017.
49. UN Sustainable Development Goals: 17 Goals to Transform Our World. United Nations. Available at http://www.un.org/sustainabledevelopment/sustainable-development-goals/. Accessed November 23, 2016.
50. Jones G, Steketee RW, Black RE, Bhutta ZA, Morris SS. How many child deaths can we prevent this year? *Lancet*. 2003;362:65–71.
51. World Health Organization, Unicef, United Nations. Levels & trends in child mortality: Report 2015: Estimates developed by the UN Inter-Agency Group for Child Mortality Estimation. 2015.
52. Kanyuka M, Ndawala J, Mleme T, et al. Malawi and Millennium Development Goal 4: A Countdown to 2015 country case study. *Lancet Glob Health*. 2016;4:e201–14.
53. Grad FP. The Preamble of the Constitution of the World Health Organization. *Bull World Health Organ*. 2002;80:981–4.
54. UNICEF. Child Mortality Report 2017. https://datauniceforg/resources/levels-trends-child-mortality/. 2017.
55. Black RE, Victora CG, Walker SP, et al. Maternal and child undernutrition and overweight in low-income and middle-income countries. *Lancet*. 2013;382:427–51.
56. Rudan I, Boschi-Pinto C, Biloglav Z, Mulholland K, Campbell H. Epidemiology and etiology of childhood pneumonia. *Bull World Health Organ*. 2008;86:408–16.
57. Adegbola RA. Childhood pneumonia as a global health priority and the strategic interest of the Bill & Melinda Gates Foundation. Clin Infect Dis. 2012;54(Suppl 2):S89–92.
58. Hambidge KM. Zinc and pneumonia. *Am J Clin Nutr*. 2006;83:991–2.
59. UNICEF Data: Monitoring the Situation of Children and Women. 2016. Accessed at https://data.unicef.org/.
60. Immunization Coverage. WHO, 2016. Available at http://www.who.int/mediacentre/factsheets/fs378/en/. Accessed November 22, 2016.
61. WHO. GIVS—Global Immunization Vision and Strategy 2006–2015. WHO website: Geneva, World Health Organization and United Nations Children's Fund; 2005 October.
62. Restrepo-Mendez MC, Barros AJ, Wong KL, et al. Inequalities in full immunization coverage: Trends in low- and middle-income countries. *Bull World Health Organ* 2016;94:794–805b.
63. Geldsetzer P, Williams TC, Kirolos A, et al. The recognition of and care seeking behaviour for childhood illness in developing countries: A systematic review. *PLoS One*. 2014;9:e93427.
64. Theodoratou E, Al-Jilaihawi S, Woodward F, et al. The effect of case management on childhood pneumonia mortality in developing countries. *Int J Epidemiol*. 2010;39(Suppl 1):i155–71.
65. Gupta GR. Tackling pneumonia and diarrhoea: The deadliest diseases for the world's poorest children. *Lancet*. 2012;379:2123–4.
66. Fischer Walker CL, Perin J, Aryee MJ, Boschi-Pinto C, Black RE. Diarrhea incidence in low- and middle-income countries in 1990 and 2010: A systematic review. *BMC Public Health*. 2012;12:220.
67. Humphrey JH. Child undernutrition, tropical enteropathy, toilets, and handwashing. *Lancet*. 2009;374:1032–5.
68. Keusch GT, Denno DM, Black RE, et al. Environmental enteric dysfunction: Pathogenesis, diagnosis, and clinical consequences. *Clin Infect Dis*. 2014;59:207–12.
69. Kotloff KL, Nataro JP, Blackwelder WC, et al. Burden and aetiology of diarrhoeal disease in infants and young children in developing countries

(the Global Enteric Multicenter Study, GEMS): A prospective, case-control study. *Lancet.* 2013;382:209–22.

70. Cairncross S, Hunt C, Boisson S, et al. Water, sanitation and hygiene for the prevention of diarrhoea. *Int J Epidemio.* 2010;39(Suppl 1):i193–205.
71. UNICEF. 25 Years Progress on Sanitation and Drinking Water. UNICEF; 2015.
72. Key facts from JMP 2015 Report. World Health Organization, 2016. Available at http://www.who.int/water_sanitation_health/monitoring/jmp-2015-key-facts/en/. Accessed November 23, 2016.
73. WHO UNICEF review of national immunization coverage, 1980–2014. WHO, 2013. (Available at http://apps.who.int/immunization_monitoring/globalsummary/wucoveragecountrylist.html. Accessed November 23, 2016.)
74. Zinc for the treatment of diarrhoea: Effect on diarrhoea morbidity, mortality and incidence of future episodes. 2010.
75. Pavlinac PB, Denno DM, John-Stewart GC, et al. Failure of syndrome-based diarrhea management guidelines to detect Shigella infections in Kenyan children. *J Ped Infect Dis.* 2016;5:366–74.
76. Ashorn P. Antibiotics for children with severe diarrhoea (ABCD). Clinical Trialsgov. https://clinicaltrials.gov/ct2/show/NCT03130114. 2017
77. Peden MM, Unicef, World Health Organization. World report on child injury prevention. 2008.
78. Linnan H, Linnan M, Rahman A, Reinten-Reynolds T, Scarr J. Child drowning : Evidence for a newly recognized cause of child mortality in low and middle income countries in Asia. 2012.
79. Linnan M, Rahman A, Scarr J, et al. Child drowning: Evidence for a newly recognized cause of child mortality in low and middle income countries in Asia, Working Paper 2012–07, Special Series on Child Injury No. 2. Florence: UNICEF Office of Research; 2012.
80. Lengeler C. Insecticide-treated bed nets and curtains for preventing malaria. *Cochrane Database Syst Rev.* 2004;2:Cd000363.
81. Committing to Child Survival: A Promise Renewed Progress Report 2015. 2015.
82. Bryce J, Victora CG, Habicht JP, Black RE, Scherpbier RW. Programmatic pathways to child survival: Results of a multi-country evaluation of Integrated Management of Childhood Illness. *Health Policy Plan.* 2005;20(Suppl 1):i5–17.
83. Gakidou E, Cowling K, Lozano R, Murray CJ. Increased educational attainment and its effect on child mortality in 175 countries between 1970 and 2009: A systematic analysis. *Lancet.* 2010;376:959–74.
84. Caldwell J, McDonald P. Influence of maternal education on infant and child mortality: Levels and causes. *Health Policy Educ.* 1982 Mar;2(3–4):251–67.
85. World Bank, International Monetary Fund. Global monitoring report 2015/2016: Development goals in an era of demographic change. 2016.
86. Health WHOCoSDo, World Health O. *Closing the Gap in a Generation: Health Equity through Action on the Social Determinants of Health: Commission on Social Determinants of Health Final Report.* Geneva, Switzerland: World Health Organization, Commission on Social Determinants of Health; 2008.
87. Bucher K, Unicef. *Progress for Children: Beyond Averages: Learning from the MDGS.* New York: UNICEF; 2015.
88. O'Malley J. An equity focus on MDG4 and MDG5. UNICEF; 2015 October.
89. Kuruvilla S, Schweitzer J, Bishai D, et al. Success factors for reducing maternal and child mortality. *Bull World Health Organ.* 2014;92:533–44b.
90. Carrera C, Azrack A, Begkoyian G, et al. The comparative cost-effectiveness of an equity-focused approach to child survival, health, and nutrition: A modelling approach. *Lancet.* 2012;380:1341–51.
91. Victora CG, Barros AJ, Axelson H, et al. How changes in coverage affect equity in maternal and child health interventions in 35 Countdown to 2015 countries: An analysis of national surveys. *Lancet.* 2012;380: 1149–56.

CHAPTER

23 Control and Prevention of Infectious Diseases of Global Significance

Kirkby D. Tickell • Zulfiqar A. Bhutta • Amira M. Khan • Stephen P. Luby • Gillian A. Levine • James A. Litch • Lauren Schwartz • Shamim A. Qazi • Karen L. Kotloff • Ogobara K. Doumbo • Francois Nosten • Jillian Pintye • Nelly Mugo • Ruanne V. Barnbas • Stephen M. Graham • Suman S. Majumdar • Simon J. Brooker • Kebede Deribe • Judd L. Walson

OVERVIEW OF INFECTIOUS DISEASE PREVENTION

This chapter addresses the prevention and control of infectious diseases associated with the greatest burden of global morbidity and mortality. We begin by highlighting overall global progress toward infectious disease control. Subsequent sections focus on the critical role of cross-cutting interventions that decrease host susceptibility and exposure across many infectious diseases, including the optimization of nutritional status and environmental modification through the provision of clean water and improved sanitation. The remainder of the chapter is dedicated to prevention and control strategies for specific syndromes of global importance. The communicable disease sections of this book provide a comprehensive overview of the recommended treatments for specific infectious diseases; this chapter only includes these treatments if they are an essential element of control programs.

Prevention of infectious diseases refers to the avoidance of infection in individuals, while control refers to reduction in the impact of disease across a population. Prevention and control of infectious diseases can be achieved through interventions designed to kill or inactivate a pathogen (such as mass drug administration, MDA), interventions to limit the spread of a vector or reservoir of the pathogen (such as bed net distribution), interventions to reduce underlying host susceptibility (such as management of malnutrition), or interventions targeting modification of the environment to reduce exposure (such as water and sanitation).

Infectious disease prevention and control efforts can be viewed across a spectrum of four categories: control, elimination, eradication, and extinction. Control is defined as reducing the incidence, prevalence, morbidity, or mortality of a condition to locally acceptable levels. This is distinct from elimination (reduction in the incidence of infection to zero within a given geographical area), eradication (permanent reduction in worldwide incidence of an infection to zero), or extinction which implies complete removal of an infectious agent from nature, including no longer being present in any laboratory.[1]

GLOBAL PROGRESS, GOALS, AND TARGETS TOWARD REDUCING MORTALITY AND MORBIDITY DUE TO INFECTIOUS DISEASES

Significant reductions in global morbidity and mortality have been achieved over the past several decades with greatest impact seen in under-5 mortality rates.[2] However, infectious diseases continue to account for a substantial proportion of global deaths.[3] For example, lower respiratory infections, diarrhea, and tuberculosis (TB) continue to be among the top ten drivers of mortality for all ages and sexes and pneumonia and diarrhea remain the leading causes of death for children under 5.[4]

Despite substantial progress made in reducing morbidity and mortality in response to the Millennium Development Goals (MDGs), the health-related targets for MDG 4 (reduce child mortality), 5 (reduce maternal mortality), and 6 (reduce infectious diseases) were not met. Although MDG 4 was not achieved, mortality in the >5 age group declined remarkably during the MDG era (2000–15), with a considerably lower number of children dying in 2015 (5.8 million), as compared to in 1990 (12.7 million).[5] Much of the decline in under-5 mortality rates was attributed to the reduction in infectious disease mortality. Nearly 2.2 million fewer children died from pneumonia, diarrhea, malaria, measles, and AIDS in 2013 as compared to 2000 and the numbers further decreased by 2015 (Table 23-1).[6]

Between 2000 and 2012, measles mortality in children decreased by 80%, diarrheal deaths by 50%, and pneumonia deaths by 40%.[7] Global vaccine coverage increased substantially during the MDG period and is likely a major contributor to these reductions in infection-related deaths. For example, worldwide coverage with three doses of Hib vaccine has reached approximately 70% and hepatitis B vaccine coverage is now 84%.[4] Extensive vaccination efforts have also stopped polio transmission in all but three countries (Afghanistan, Pakistan, and Nigeria). In total, it is estimated that immunization has averted 2.5 million deaths per year in children under-5 between 2000 and 2010.[8]

Although MDG 6, which aimed to "halt and reverse the spread" of HIV, malaria, and other major diseases, was only partially met, extraordinary advancements have been made in the control of HIV.[9] The incidence of HIV has been reduced by 40% and by 2014, 13.6 million HIV-infected individuals had access to antiretroviral (ART) therapy. This compares to just 800,000 with access to ART in 2003. With the successful use of ART, mother-to-child transmission has plummeted; new HIV infections in children decreased by 58% between 2000 and 2014. In addition, malaria and TB incidence rates were 37% and 18% lower in 2015 than in 2000 and malaria and TB mortality rates decreased by 58% and 45%, respectively, in this period.[10]

Building on the progress made toward the MDGs, the Sustainable Development Goals (SDGs) were launched in 2016, with SDG 3 being the consolidated health goal. The goal targets infectious diseases, calling to end the epidemics of AIDS, TB, malaria, and neglected tropical diseases by 2030 and to combat hepatitis, waterborne diseases, and other communicable diseases'. Recognizing that HIV/AIDS and TB continue to account for considerable mortality (1.1 million and 1.4 million deaths in 2015, respectively), the SDGs maintain the focus on these diseases.[4] However, while MDG 6 only focused on HIV, TB, and malaria, the SDG target takes a broader approach, including neglected tropical diseases (NTDs), waterborne diseases (including diarrheal illnesses), and hepatitis.

TABLE 23-1 ESTIMATED NUMBERS OF DEATHS BY INFECTIONS IN NEONATES AND CHILDREN AGED 1–59 MONTHS, AT THE GLOBAL LEVEL IN 2000–15

	2000	2015[a]
Neonates		
Pneumonia	296,000	161,000
Sepsis/Meningitis	532,000	402,000
Tetanus	161,000	34,000
Diarrhea	40,000	18,000
Children (1–59 months)		
Pneumonia	1.4 million	760,000
Meningitis	284,000	115,000
Diarrhea	1.2 million	509,000
Measles	485,000	74,000
Malaria	725,000	306,000
AIDS	220,000	86,000
Pertussis	56,000	54,000

[a]Neonatal sepsis/meningitis, neonatal pneumonia, neonatal tetanus, childhood pneumonia, childhood diarrhea, meningitis, diarrhea, measles, malaria, and AIDS all showed >30% decline in mortality rates from 2000 to 2015.

Source: Adapted from: Liu L, Oza S, Hogan D, et al. Global, regional, and national causes of under-5 mortality in 2000–15: An updated systematic analysis with implications for the Sustainable Development Goals. *Lancet.* 2016;388(10063):3027–35.

Achieving infectious disease specific targets set out in the SDGs will be challenging. The etiology of these diseases results from a complex interplay of many underlying issues, including multiple environmental, socioeconomic, and ecological factors. With the focus shifted to a more integrated and intersectoral approach, the SDGs are ideally poised to achieve the ambitious infectious disease Target 3.3, underpinned by the efforts to realize Universal Health Coverage (UHC). Key evidence-based interventions identified for controlling major childhood infections are summarized in Box 23-1 and illustrate the multisectoral approach needed to address infectious diseases.

Although SDG 3.3 is the only infectious disease specific target, there are several other components of the SDGs, which will contribute to the prevention of infectious diseases. For example, 3.9 (reduction of mortality due to unsafe water, sanitation and hygiene as well as air pollution) and targets within SDG 6 (water and sanitation), SDG 1 (poverty), SDG 4 (education), SDG 7 (clean household energy), and SDG 13 (climate change) are all closely linked to infectious disease control.[11] Given the overall focus of the SDGs on universal health coverage, the potential for delivery platforms targeting inequity and reaching marginalized populations is likely to have significant impact in populations most affected by infectious diseases.

In addition to existing efforts to control and prevent common infectious diseases, there are multiple emerging threats that urgently require novel interventions. Emerging infections pose a significant risk to the health of the global population. Of 335 new infectious diseases catalogued between 1940 and 2004,[12] nearly 60% were of zoonotic origin. Multiple social and environmental factors, including climate change, population growth and movement, urbanization, as well as harmful human behaviors (including war and conflict) all contribute to the threat of emerging infectious diseases.[10] The public health and economic implications of emerging infections (such as Ebola, Zika, and Dengue) have been substantial. The 2014–16 West Africa Ebola outbreak claimed more than 11,000 lives, with nearly 30,000 reported cases, and there is a scientific consensus that Zika virus has resulted in increased incidence of Guillain-Barre syndrome and microcephaly in affected countries.[13] There is a clear need for improved surveillance and novel interventions to deal with these emerging threats.

BOX 23-1 Key Interventions Identified for Control of Major Childhood Infections

Neonatal Infections

Maternal

- Tetanus toxoid immunization
- Maternal infection prevention, screening and management: malaria (IPTp, ITN), syphilis, lower genital tract infections, group B streptococcus, bacterial vaginosis, urinary tract infection, chlamydia, gonorrhea, HIV, toxoplasmosis

Delivery and Intrapartum

- Skilled care at birth and clean birth practices (use of clean birth kits and hand washing with soap)
- Antibiotics for preterm premature rupture of membranes (PPROM)

Newborn Care

- Clean cord care, chlorhexidine cord cleansing if appropriate, clean postnatal practices
- Breast feeding
- Interventions to prevent hypothermia: drying, head covering, skin-to-skin care, and delayed bathing for every newborn baby
- Case management of neonatal sepsis, including oral antibiotics, injection, and hospital-based care

Childhood Pneumonia and Diarrhea

Environmental

- Water, sanitation, and hygiene (WASH)
- Reduce overcrowding and household air pollution

Nutrition

- Breastfeeding promotion
- Preventive supplementation (vitamin A or zinc)

Vaccines

- Measles, *Haemophilus influenzae* type b, pneumococcal infection, rotavirus, cholera

Treatment

- Oral rehydration salt (ORS)
- Continued feeding after diarrhea
- Zinc for diarrhea treatment
- Probiotic use during diarrhea
- Antibiotics and oxygen therapy for pneumonia
- Antibiotics for dysentery

Sources: Bhutta Z, Das J, Walker N, et al. Interventions to address deaths from childhood pneumonia and diarrhoea equitably: What works and at what cost? *Lancet*, 2013;381(9875):1417–29; Bhutta Z, Das J, Bahl R, et al. Can available interventions end preventable deaths in mothers, newborn babies, and stillbirths, and at what cost? *Obstet Gynecol Surv.* 2014;69(11):641–3.

Finally, the emergence of antimicrobial resistance threatens to slow or halt progress in reductions in morbidity and mortality due to infectious diseases. As circulating pathogens increasingly become resistant to commonly available antibiotics, the efficacy of currently recommended treatment approaches is threatened. The World Health Organization warns that the many new antibiotics under development will be insufficient to address the growing number of resistant pathogens, with the greatest risk being of multidrug-resistant TB and resistant gram-negative pathogens.[14] Appropriate and judicious use of antibiotics, development of new antibiotic agents and other novel therapies and improved AMR surveillance are required urgently to address this issue globally. Vaccination against infectious diseases with high rates of AMR, such as typhoid, is also a WHO priority strategy to address the growing threat of AMR.

Despite remarkable progress in reducing morbidity and mortality due to infectious diseases, a large proportion (17%) of all global deaths are still the result of infectious diseases, with the majority of these deaths occurring in younger age groups in Africa, South-east Asia, and the Eastern Mediterranean region.[10,15] Siloed programs targeting single pathogens, or small groups of pathogens, have been relatively successful during MDG era. However, sustaining this remarkable progress in morbidity and mortality reductions may require different approaches in the SDG era. For example, many pathogens share similar transmission pathways, which suggests that cross-cutting environmental modifications, such as improved access to clean water and sanitation, may play an increasingly important role in achieving the SDG targets. In addition, host factors, particularly nutritional status, are also modifiable determinants of many infectious diseases that could be further targeted to reduce the burden of infectious diseases.

UNDERNUTRITION AND INFECTIOUS DISEASE

Undernutrition is among the most prevalent underlying risk factors driving the incidence and severity of many infectious diseases.[16] Over 165 million children are undernourished and over 50% of diarrhea, pneumonia, and measles deaths are associated with undernutrition.[16] Undernourished children are up to 12 times more likely to die from an infectious disease than their well-nourished peers.[16] Undernutrition also affects millions of adults and adolescents,[17] although few programs address malnutrition in these populations outside of disease-specific programs such as in HIV care and treatment programs.

The link between undernutrition and infectious disease is complex and bidirectional. In addition to undernutrition being associated with higher risk of infection and higher mortality, infection also promotes undernutrition through increases in metabolic demand, suppressed appetite, and decreased nutrient uptake and availability.[18–20] This reciprocal relationship between infection and undernutrition is especially important for individuals with chronic infections such as HIV and TB, where infection promotes undernutrition, which in turn increases the risk of opportunistic infection and adverse outcomes.[21,22]

Three forms of undernutrition are particularly important to infectious disease prevention: acute malnutrition, stunting, and specific micronutrient deficiencies.

ACUTE MALNUTRITION

Burden

Acute malnutrition, or wasting, is the most widely recognized form of undernutrition, affecting 52 million children under the age of 5 globally.[16] Children effected by acute malnutrition are often the faces of humanitarian tragedy. However, acute malnutrition is not isolated to famines and warzones: it is endemic in all low- and middle-income countries. Even in emerging economies, such as Brazil and China, 2–2.5% of children are acutely malnourished.[23] Severe acute malnutrition (SAM), the most extreme form of acute malnutrition, is defined by a weight-for-height z-score less than −3, a MUAC under 11.5 cm if 6–60 months old, or the presence of bipedal nutritional edema.[24] Moderate acute malnutrition (MAM) is defined as weight-for-height z-score less than −2 or a mid-upper-arm circumference (MUAC) under 12.5 cm for children 6–60 months old.

Prevention

Guidelines for the management of acutely malnourished children focus on Community Management of Malnutrition (CMAM) programs. These programs reduce the proportion of children with malnutrition who develop a medical complication, including infectious diseases, from approximately 16% down to 2.5%.[25–30] There are four pillars of CMAM programs: community mobilization, outpatient management of SAM without medical complications, inpatient management of SAM with medical complications, and the management of MAM.[31] CMAM programs identify malnourished children through both active and passive screening. During active screening, community health workers conduct door-to-door home visits or organize community mass screenings at child health days. Passive screening occurs when families present to health facilities where nutritional status is assessed. After identification of a child with malnutrition, children without medical complications are managed in the community, with a short course of antibiotics and ready-to-use therapeutic foods for SAM or ready-to-use supplementary foods for MAM.[32] If the child has a medical complication, usually due to infection, they are admitted to hospital for advanced management of their acute illness and initiation of nutritional rehabilitation.

The CMAM approach has the potential to be enormously effective. However, despite the clearly demonstrated effectiveness of CMAM programs, reaching the 52 million acutely malnourished children in need has proven challenging. CMAM is relatively expensive, costing approximately $150 per-child-treated.[33,34] In comparison, a full course of childhood vaccines cost approximately $18 per child in most low- or middle-income countries.[35] These high costs have deterred many countries from implementing full CMAM programs, choosing to either focus on areas of seasonal food insecurity or to forgo a CMAM entirely.[36] Consequently, UNICEF estimates that only 17% of acutely malnourished children participate in CMAM programs.[37] If CMAM coverage reached 90% of children in need globally, as many as 350,000 child deaths could be averted, largely through the prevention of infectious diseases.[38] Failing to prevent these infections before they occur has consequences; while the WHO offers detailed guidance for the management of complicated SAM, inpatient fatality rates between 8% and 24% are common in many settings.[25,26] These high mortality rates underscore the vital importance of preventing infectious diseases among acutely malnourished children through robust management of SAM and MAM in the community.

STUNTING

Burden

Chronic malnutrition, often characterized by stunting, or linear growth faltering (defined by a height-for-age z-score <-2), affects one in three children in sub-Saharan Africa and South Asia.[39] Stunted children are twice as likely to die from pneumonia or diarrhea than better nourished children.[16] The adverse effects of stunting extend into adulthood; stunting is associated with a reduced vaccine efficacy, lower educational attainment, reduced economic output, and higher rates of cardiovascular disease.[16,40]

Prevention

Despite the clear implications of stunting on the global burden of infectious disease, there are currently no internationally accepted guidelines for managing stunting and no widely implemented stunting management programs. Interventions targeting stunting in low-resource settings (including the provision of water, sanitation, and hygiene programs and nutritional supplementation) have largely failed to demonstrate benefit on growth or the incidence of infectious disease.[21–23,42,43] However, stunting does appear to be reversible in some studies. For example, stunted children who move from areas of humanitarian crisis to high-income countries experience dramatic catch-up growth, although the impact of this growth on health and cognitive outcomes is less clear.[44,45]

The exact etiology of stunting is not thoroughly understood, but it is known that poverty, infectious diseases, and poor nutrition combine to suppress growth, delay cognitive development, and increase susceptible to further infection. Exposure to fecal contamination of the environment is common in many low-resource settings and may result in a syndrome of Environmental Enteric Dysfunction (EED). EED is a disorder of the intestinal tract characterized by disruptions in the structure and function of the intestine, resulting in impaired ability to absorb nutrients, increased inflammation, translocation of bacterial products, and chronic immune activation. EED has been associated with stunting, impaired vaccine response, and heightened vulnerability to severe infections.[46,47] There are no currently recommended treatments for EED in international guidelines for stunting management, although significant research into potential interventions targeting this pathway is underway.

MICRONUTRIENT DEFICIENCIES

Burden

Many micronutrient deficiencies are associated with vulnerability to infectious disease and supplementation of specific micronutrients has been successful in reducing mortality in many settings. However, it is important to recognize that there are also specific situations in which micronutrient supplementation may contribute to the severity of infectious disease, most notably the administration of iron during malaria infection.[48] Here we focus on two specific micronutrients, zinc and vitamin A, as supplementation with these micronutrients has been shown to have a particularly important role in minimizing the burden of infectious disease.[49]

Prevention

Vitamin A deficiency affects 90 million preschool children and is associated with diarrhea, respiratory disease, chronic ear infections, and measles.[16,48] Randomized trials of vitamin A supplementation have demonstrated substantial reductions in child mortality, although data are inconsistent and several large vitamin A trials have failed to demonstrate benefit.[41,50,51] Vitamin A supplementation is currently offered to all children aged 6–59 months in populations where the prevalence of night blindness is above 1% or where the prevalence of vitamin A deficiency (serum retinol <0.70 μmol/L) is 20% or higher.[52] Eighty-two countries meet these criteria, largely in central America, sub-Saharan Africa, and South Asia. In these regions, WHO recommends vitamin A be given once between 6 and 12 months of age, often integrated into the childhood vaccination schedule, and every 4–6 months between 12 and 59 months of age.[52] These later doses are typically given during semiannual national campaigns. Currently, 70% of the target population is estimated to receive vitamin A doses.[53] Direct administration of vitamin A is augmented in 54 of the 82 priority countries by additional fortification programs, such as mandatory fortification of vegetable oils with vitamin A.[54]

Although regular zinc supplementation for healthy adults or children is not recommended, there is some evidence that daily zinc supplementation can lead to modest increases in childhood growth, may decrease the incidence of diarrhea and pneumonia, and may lead to small reductions in child mortality. However, data supporting benefit has been inconsistent and has not resulted in widespread implementation, largely because providing daily zinc to large populations of children would be very resource intensive. However, zinc supplementation during episodes of acute diarrhea reduces the duration and severity of the diarrhea and prevents future episodes.[55,56] As a result, the WHO does currently recommend that 14 days of zinc supplementation be given to children with diarrhea, although currently only approximately 5% of children with acute diarrhea globally receive zinc.[49,57,58]

FUTURE DIRECTIONS

Undernutrition has proven to be one of the most intractable problems in global health and continues to be a critical driver of deaths attributed to infectious diseases. The persistence of undernutrition represents a serious obstacle to achieving the Sustainable Development Goals health targets. Many of the tools required to address malnutrition already exist but efforts to scale up delivery of these interventions to the more than 165 million children have not been uniformly successful. Fortunately, there appears to be renewed interest in the prevention and treatment of undernutrition to prevent infectious disease and reduce child mortality. A number of innovative solutions are under development and testing, including food system interventions and therapeutics that optimize enteric function and metabolism.

ENVIRONMENTAL MODIFICATIONS TO INTERRUPT FECAL ORAL DISEASE TRANSMISSION IN RESOURCE-LIMITED SETTINGS

Burden

Environmental modifications that protect community drinking water, food, and the immediate environment from fecal contamination have the potential to markedly reduce population disease burden by interrupting the transmission of a broad array of human pathogens, including bacterial, viral, and protozoal agents that can cause life-threatening infections.

Prevention

Municipal level: Historically, the introduction of centralized water treatment markedly improved community health. In several major U.S. cities between 1900 and 1940, a 40% reduction in overall mortality was observed, half of which was attributed to the introduction of centralized water chlorination and water filtration. In addition, three-quarters of the infant mortality reduction and nearly two-thirds of the child-mortality reduction was attributed to these improvements in water quality.[59]

Sanitation systems have also reduced enteric diseases. London faced recurrent cholera outbreaks until a major civil engineering project installed 100 miles of underground interceptor sewers beginning in the 1850s. These inceptors connected to local sewers and pumped London's sewage past the tidal segment within the Thames so the waste flowed into the ocean.[60]

The civil engineering approaches that proved effective in high-income cities have not been extended to residents living in urban neighborhoods within low-income countries. Even where some municipal water systems exists, intermittent water supply is a characteristic of most municipal water systems in low-income countries.[61] In India, no major city provides water 24 hours a day 7 days a week to all of its residents.[62] All water distribution systems have leaky pipes, even water distribution systems in high-income countries.[63] When water is turned off in a piped network, contaminants that surround the pipe seep into the pipe, so that when water is turned back on these contaminants are pumped through the system.[61,64] Thus, a water distribution system that supplies water intermittently inevitably distributes contaminated water. Since intermittent water distribution systems are characteristically paired with poor sanitary infrastructure, substantial fecal environmental contamination occurs throughout the city. An intermittently functioning water supply efficiently distributes fecal contaminants to community residents.

There are multiple barriers to implementing definitive civil engineering approaches to providing centralized treated drinking water to all residents of low-income country cities. Drinking water infrastructure is expensive to build, to run, to repair, and to maintain. Low-income communities in low-income countries are, by definition, financially constrained, limiting available resources to support such infrastructure. Comprehensive citywide water and sanitation systems require a municipal government that is able to operate, maintain, and collect sufficient revenue to support these complex systems. Many low-income country municipal governments, however, have limited administrative, revenue-generating, and technical capacity.[64] Although governments often claim responsibility for providing essential services, there are often perverse incentives at play, resulting in the provision of limited services to households who then must pay additional fees to secure some basic form of service.[65,66] In the water sector, these fees might pay for an illegal connection or for a tanker truck, whose exclusive contract to operate may include a kickback to ruling politicians.[62,67–69] This exploitative political economy means that the urban poor typically pay 10–100 times more per liter for water than do the wealthier residents in the city.[62]

Rapid population growth combined with critical shortage of available water in many low-income countries also impedes traditional civil engineering approaches. By 2050, the populations of Delhi, Mumbai, Kolkata (India), Dhaka (Bangladesh), Kinshasa (Democratic Republic of Congo), Lagos (Nigeria), and Karachi (Pakistan) are each projected to exceed 30 million people.[70] Even at the current level of service, which leaves many residents without a reliable convenient water supply or a sewer connection, many cities including Chennai, Delhi (India), Lahore (Pakistan), and Dhaka (Bangladesh) are drawing substantially more groundwater from aquifers than is being replenished.[71–74] The combination of population growth and reduction in available water supply progressively reduces water supply per capita.[75] Population growth also requires expansion of sanitation services. Between 1990 and 2010, there was no increase in estimated proportion of households with sewer connection in least developed countries (1990: 12%, 2010: 11%).[76]

The municipal civil engineering approaches to treat water and to remove waste that were developed in high-income water-rich cities are not fit for purpose for water-short low-income country cities. As one example, plummeting per capita water availability in cities of the global south suggest that the 15,000 liters per person per year that water-rich high-income country cities use to move feces from households to waste water treatment plants is unlikely to be available in rapidly growing low-income country cities.[77] Fit for purpose engineered approaches to water supply and sanitation in low-income country municipal contexts would require less resources to build and maintain, less institutional capacity for tariff collection and maintenance, and would deliver safe water to all city residents.

HOUSEHOLD LEVEL PREVENTION

When governments do not provide piped water to households or do not remove fecal waste, household residents take various steps to secure these essential services. Women generally have the responsibility to fetch water and this often requires a substantial amount of time.[78] The amount of time to fetch and carry water also limits the amount of water available in households and encourages households to access water that is closer to the household, even when the water quality is compromised. The farther a household has to walk to fetch water, the more likely children born into the household are to have diarrhea and the more likely they are to die.[79]

Water that is available to low-income communities is often contaminated with human feces and so poses a substantial ongoing risk of person-to-person fecal oral enteropathogen transmission.[80] Even if source water is fairly clean, the process of collecting, carrying, and storing water in the home often introduces fecal contamination from the environment and from hands into drinking water.[81] Many household level approaches can disinfect drinking water including treatment with chlorine, filtration, sunlight, and ultraviolet light.[82] Although these approaches are often used by wealthier households, their cost and the effort to implement them represent substantial barriers to poor households. Fewer than 10% of households in the bottom 40% of the wealth distribution in Southeast Asia and sub-Saharan Africa report treating their drinking water.[83]

Household toilet construction can separate and contain human fecal contamination from the immediate environment. Increased availability of a toilet was a Millennium Development Goal target. In rural areas where the environment has substantial absorptive capacity, well-constructed and maintained latrines can reduce environmental fecal contamination. In dense urban settlements, however, the environment does not have the capacity to absorb and decontaminate the feces from thousands of residents living in each square kilometer. A pit latrine or a latrine with a septic tank can temporarily contain human feces, but a toilet is not a sanitation system. In the absence of a sewer or some other conveyance, residents typically pay to have their latrine/septic tank emptied either manually, or occasionally with a suction pump.[84] Most commonly the contents of these latrines and septic tanks are dumped back into the environment untreated. Only 8% of wastewater in low-income countries is treated before it is returned to the environment.[85] In Dhaka, Bangladesh, 99% of households have access to a toilet but 98% of the feces generated by the 14 million residents of Dhaka are dumped back into the environment untreated,[86] an example of municipal level open defecation.

Although much effort has focused on empowering households to secure safe drinking water and access to a toilet, these interventions have not resulted in the same dramatic improvements in public health that were observed with municipal wide interventions in major cities in Europe and North America in the early twentieth century. Recently, two large randomized trials evaluating household level water and sanitation interventions in Kenya, Bangladesh, and Zimbabwe all failed to demonstrate benefit in reducing diarrhea or improving growth.[87–89] Households who are at greatest risk of death from fecal oral transmission are the poorest households, who have the least education, are at highest risk greatest risk of malnutrition, and whose day-to-day survival is most tenuous.[90] These most vulnerable members of the society are not in a position to assume the substantial responsibility of collecting sufficient drinking water, disinfecting it, and safely separating and removing household wastes.

FUTURE DIRECTIONS

Even in the absence of widespread provision of safe drinking water and safe fecal management, and the lack of improvement in the clinical management of diarrhea,[91] the number of deaths from diarrhea and gastrointestinal infection have decreased markedly in the last few decades.[6,92,93] The causes of this marked decline are incompletely understood, but likely include improved nutrition,[94] reduction in extreme poverty,[95,96] and some improvements in water availability and fecal containment.[97] Nevertheless, in 2016 diarrhea remains the fourth leading cause of years of life lost globally,[92] and as long as a community's food and water supply is contaminated by a fecal stream, residents will commonly become ill from fecal pathogens. New approaches to deliver clean drinking water and sanitary services to settings that are constrained by low-income, poor governance, and limited water availability are sorely needed.

NEWBORN INFECTIONS

Burden

Severe infections account for a quarter of global neonatal (first 28 days of life) mortality, have extremely high case-fatality, and among survivors can also result in substantial developmental delays, neurocognitive impairment, and disability. The risk of severe newborn infection is highest in sub-Saharan Africa and South Asia.[23,98] Newborns acquire infection vertically from the mother in utero, during the perinatal period, or horizontally from exposures in their environment after delivery. Intrauterine or intra-amniotic infections are primary sources of vertically acquired infections, via transplacental exchange of blood and fluids, exposure to pathogens after rupture of membranes and during passage through the birth canal, or through contact with organisms that are part of a healthy bacterial flora and colonize the maternal genital tract. After delivery, hospital-acquired infections can result from contaminated medical supplies and from invasive procedures and in-dwelling medical equipment. Infections with clinical presentation in the first 3 or 7 days of life are defined as early-onset and are most commonly due to fetal or intrapartum exposures. Infections after the first week of life are considered late-onset and generally result from postnatal exposures. Newborn infections are difficult to identify and diagnose and disease progression occurs quickly, making primary prevention extremely important.[99] Estimates suggest that more than 80% of infection-related deaths in newborns could be avoided if the coverage and quality of currently available preventive measures and effective interventions were improved.[100]

Prevention

Routine care from a skilled provider during pregnancy and screening and treatment for maternal infections in pregnancy and the perinatal period have all been demonstrated to prevent infection in the newborn. However, these infection prevention approaches are challenging to implement for births occurring outside of institutional settings or without skilled birth attendant.

The majority of childhood vaccinations are administered after 6 weeks of life, and therefore leave neonates vulnerable to many vaccine-preventable illnesses. Maternal vaccination in or prior to pregnancy may address this early vulnerability via antibody transfer and prevention of vertical transmission, although extent or duration of protection provided by these antibodies is unknown. In some countries, inactivated influenza vaccine, the combined tetanus–diphtheria–acellular pertussis, hepatitis B, and/or hepatitis E vaccine are recommended in pregnancy. Few low- or middle-income countries include these vaccines in routine antenatal care (ANC) programs due to either low burden, insufficient evidence of impact, or the lack of ANC coverage at the appropriate time points for vaccine delivery. Improvements in tetanus toxoid protection in pregnancy have resulted in substantial global declines in newborn tetanus and tetanus-related mortality in the recent decades.[101] Tetanus toxoid injection programs in (and prior to) pregnancy are an example of the benefits of maternal vaccination, and should be part of all routine ANC.[102,103]

The WHO recommends universal syphilis screening and treatment of infected women at the first ANC visit.[104] Screening and treatment for *Chlamydia trachomatis*, *Neisseria gonorrhoeae*, and Herpes Simplex Virus Type 2 (HSV-2) are also recommended.[105,106] Screening for Hepatitis B and C is recommended in specific contexts and among high-risk pregnant women. Among women with active STIs or genital infections, delivery via cesarean section may be recommended to prevent newborn exposure. Prevention of mother-to-child-transmission (PMTCT) of HIV programs are recommended in high-burden settings and can be integrated into routine ANC in all settings. Cotrimoxazole prophylaxis for HIV-infected women may also prevent newborn exposure to other bacterial pathogens with which an HIV-infected woman may be colonized or infected.[107,108] Finally, screening for active TB infection and treatment for TB-infected women is also recommended in high HIV-prevalence settings.

Prophylactic intrapartum antibiotics are recommended for women with known group B Streptococcus (GBS) vaginal or rectal colonization.[109] However, maternal GBS colonization prevalence appears to vary widely and is estimated to account for a smaller proportion of newborn infections in some low-resource settings, including parts of South Asia and sub-Saharan Africa, than in settings such as the United States, although population-level estimates of colonization and etiologies are limited in low-resource settings.[110–115] Universal late-pregnancy GBS screening and targeted prophylactic intrapartum intravenous antibiotic administration (IAP) for colonized women have resulted in substantial declines in early-onset neonatal infection risk.[116–119] However, IAP does not appear to result in a substantial reduction in late-onset GBS infections and GBS screening is not universally recommended as a high-priority intervention. Additionally, IAP requires a well-functioning health system, high ANC coverage with skilled providers in late pregnancy, and high coverage of facility-based delivery with effective communication between ANC and maternity systems, which are often unavailable in low-resource settings.

Maternal malaria infection can harm the mother and increase risk of adverse pregnancy outcomes. Although the burden of neonatal malaria is low, newborns are at risk in high-transmission areas. In malaria-endemic areas insecticide-treated bed nets (ITN), intermittent preventive treatment (IPTp) in pregnancy in high-transmission areas in sub-Saharan Africa, and effective case management (diagnosis and treatment) are recommended.[102]

The prevention and treatment of peripartum infections addresses one of the primary causes of newborn infection and prevents maternal morbidity. Prophylactic intrapartum antibiotics are recommended for women with premature (or prelabor) rupture of membranes (PROM). Women with intra-amniotic infections (chorioamnionitis and endometritis) should also be treated with antibiotics.[109] Induction of labor may be recommended in the case of high maternal risk, and the decision to deliver should be made with consideration of gestational age and fetal status. In addition, screening for genitourinary infection and antibiotic treatment for infection is recommended by WHO in all settings.[102,109]

Whether deliveries occur in the community or at health facility, hygienic and infection-prevention practices during labor, childbirth, and the postnatal period prevent infection. Important measures include frequent and appropriate hand washing with clean water and soap and use of alcohol-containing sanitization solution for health workers and caregivers with contact with women and newborns; conducting the delivery on a clean surface; using a sanitized and cleaned blade to cut the umbilical cord; tying the cord using clean measures and materials; cleaning and drying the newborns with clean towels and wraps following delivery; and wrapping the mother with a clean cloth.[120–124] In health facilities, the WHO recommends cleaning the umbilicus and stump with a clean, dry towel. In births conducted outside of a health facility in high-mortality settings, cord cleaning with chlorhexidine solution is recommended.[109] All newborns should receive topical ocular prophylaxis with tetracycline hydrochloride eye ointment, povidone iodine, or silver nitrate solutions or chloramphenicol eye ointment in both eyes immediately following birth to prevent gonococcal and chlamydial ophthalmia neonatorum, though such localized infections do not generally lead to invasive infections.[105]

Proper sterilization techniques for reusable equipment and supplies such as feeding cups, intubation materials, breathing masks, incubators, as well as proper disposal of one-time use materials such as gloves and syringes are important. In-dwelling catheters, central lines, and intravenous or parenteral feeding lines, when available, are an important source of infection in facilities and measures to limit time with in-dwelling devices and appropriate infection prevention and sterilization practices for insertion, management, and removal help prevent hospital-acquired infections.

Crowding and poor ventilation and inadequate air circulation in health facilities can result in the spread of infection. Avoiding cot and incubator sharing, sterilization of shared equipment, and appropriate infrastructure to support ventilation and air circulation are important.[125,126]

Thermal protection, early, exclusive, and appropriate human milk feeding (breastfeeding preferred when possible), and skin-to-skin contact are recommended for all newborns, but particularly in small or preterm newborns.[125,127–129] Early and exclusive breastfeeding provides newborns with important maternal antibodies which prevent infection and help the newborn immune system control and recover from infectious exposures. Breast milk also has other antimicrobial compounds, which help prevent infections.

Prophylactic antibiotics may prevent infection in newborns born to women with PROM, obstructed or prolonged labor (over 18 hours), or cases of meconium-stained liquor or meconium aspiration. Newborns with suspected or at especially high risk due to prematurity or low birthweight in combination with maternal risk factors for infection may also benefit from prophylactic or early presumptive antimicrobials.[130–132] However, there is debate about the relative benefit of such treatment in light of growing antibiotic resistance, the lack of data on appropriate/effective regimens, a growing literature on the individual consequences of antibiotic exposure, including microbiome disturbances and chronic inflammatory illnesses, and the additional resource requirements of extended hospitalizations for antibiotic administration.[133–137]

The WHO recommends a system-based approach to preventing healthcare-associated infections, which emphasizes the role of national Infection Prevention Committees or leadership teams in developing guidelines and recommendations, organizing and implementing standardized infection prevention trainings and education for health workers, and setting and evaluating performance targets to monitor progress.[138] Facility-based recommendations focus on ensuring infrastructure and resources are available to facilitate infection-prevention and basic water, sanitation, and hygiene services (WASH).

Finally, care in pregnancy to address risk factors for preterm birth and low birthweight and manage maternal complications, indirect risk factors for newborn infection, are important newborn infection prevention strategies. Recommended interventions include nutrition counseling and/or supplementation, prevention of smoking and exposure to air pollution and unclean fuels, prevention and management of hypertension and preeclampsia, management of chronic illnesses including hypertension and gestational diabetes and diabetes mellitus, prevention of domestic violence and adverse occupational exposures, maternal immunization, and the prevention, screening, and treatment of acute maternal infections associated with adverse birth outcomes.[102,139]

Tertiary management can prevent disease dissemination after pathogen acquisition, and slow or stop progression to systemic disease and severe morbidity and mortality. Clean, hygienic care and topical and oral antimicrobials can prevent spread and dissemination of a localized infection. The WHO recommends oral antimicrobial therapy and home-based care for young infants with a localized infection, and encourages follow-up by a trained health worker in the community.[140] Admission to a referral-level facility and intramuscular or parenteral antimicrobial therapy with gentamycin and ampicillin or penicillin as first-line treatment, or intravenous cloxacillin and gentamicin if *Staphylococcus* infection is suspected, is recommended for suspected or confirmed serious bacterial infection.[140,141] Simplified outpatient antibiotic therapy is recommended when inpatient referral-level care is infeasible or unaccepted, with close observation and follow-up by trained health workers.[142]

Facility or community-based postnatal check-ups by trained health workers are also recommended to identify newborns with possible infections for treatment or referral to skilled care, when available. Caregivers should be trained on the danger signs of infection and when to seek care, to encourage early identification and care-seeking for early treatment.[140,141] Supportive care in referral-level health facilities for newborns with infection, including breathing and oxygen support, thermal regulation, and feeding support, can prevent complications of severe infection, when available.[141]

FUTURE DIRECTIONS

Maternal GBS vaccines are currently under development and could be an effective prevention strategy for early and late-onset disease where GBS disease burden is large.[115,143] However, vaccine efficacy is unknown, and an effective program would require high skilled ANC coverage and high vaccine coverage. Other emerging interventions focus on the role of the infant skin and gut microbiome. Limited data indicate that among preterm newborns, supplementation of enteral feeding with lactoferrin may help prevent sepsis, though additional studies are needed to confirm results and inform appropriate dosing and regimens.[144] Among specific high-risk groups including preterm and very low birthweight newborns, enteral probiotics may prevent late-onset infection, but the specific type of probiotic or beneficial bacterial "cocktail" is unknown, and the feasibility and impact in lower-level facilities and among the general newborn population is not well described.[145] Topical emollients such as creams and oils to improve the barrier function and skin integrity of preterm newborns in health facilities and prevent invasive infections in this high-risk group have not demonstrated benefit.[146]

PNEUMONIA

Burden

Infectious pneumonia represents destruction of lung tissue as a result of a pathophysiological response to bacterial, viral, or fungal lower respiratory tract infection. There were 120 million cases of pneumonia among children in 2010 and pneumonia is the leading global cause of death under the age of 5 (approximately 700,000 deaths in 2015) and the third most common cause of death due to infectious disease among adults (2 million deaths in 2015).[93] In addition to mortality, pneumonia is a major cause of morbidity and a common cause for healthcare seeking, placing enormous financial strain on families and healthcare systems.[93] Substantial progress has been made in reducing the burden pneumonia in the past three decades; there was a 22% reduction in pneumonia deaths between 1990 and 2016.[147] If currently available interventions were scaled to reach 80% of their target population, two-thirds of all remaining pneumonia deaths could be prevented.[148] As a result, the WHO have committed to the ambitious target of ending preventable deaths due to pneumonia by 2025.[149]

Many children who do develop pneumonia can be successfully managed in the community with oral antibiotics, parental vigilance, and follow-up visits. Standardized community case management for pneumonia can reduce the case fatality of pneumonia by 70%. Despite this evidence, recent estimates suggest that 62% of children with pneumonia are managed in hospital.[150–152] However, for those children who are severely ill and require advanced management strategies administered in hospital the estimated case fatality ratio is still quite high (6.1%), underscoring the critical importance of pneumonia prevention.[150]

Prevention

The mainstay of the global pneumonia prevention strategy is vaccination, supported by community case management and inpatient therapy for those with severe disease. The *Haemophilus influenzae* type B (Hib) and the pneumococcal conjugate vaccine (PCV) address the two leading causes of death due to pneumonia among children. These two vaccines alone could prevent approximately two-thirds of childhood pneumonia deaths if they reached 90% coverage.[148] However, while Hib has been introduced in 191 countries and 70% of all children globally receive a complete three-dose course, only 134 countries have included PCV in their routine immunizations. In 2016, only 42% of eligible children received PCV.[153]

Influenza vaccination is also likely to reduce pneumonia-associated mortality. In high-income countries, priority groups such as pregnant women and the elderly are targeted with seasonal influenza vaccinations, but uptake is often low. Influenza infection peaks are harder to predict in tropical countries, which have less defined seasons, and cover a large range of latitudes (e.g., China and Brazil), further complicating the timing of national campaigns. Unfortunately, there is little evidence to support how these campaigns should be conducted.[154] Only 64 of 138 low-to-middle-income countries (LMICs) have an influenza vaccination policy, which typically recommended seasonal vaccination for high-risk groups. In Latin America, uptake of influenza vaccination often exceeds overage in high-income countries. However, in Africa and Asia coverage rarely exceeds 1% of the target population and there is little evidence to guide implementation in these countries.[154]

Two further vaccines are important for pneumonia prevention—pertussis and measles. Measles infection drastically increases the risk of both primary measles pneumonia and post measles associated bacterial pneumonia, making high coverage of measles vaccination an important preventive strategy. Pertussis vaccination is traditionally given as part of the diphtheria–tetanus–pertussis (DTP3) or pentavalent vaccine. Despite sustained high global coverage of pertussis vaccination (86% of eligible children in 2016),[155] pertussis continues to cause a significant burden of infection, particularly among neonates too young to receive the vaccine. In response, high-income countries have begun vaccinating mothers at antenatal visits. In these settings, antenatal pertussis vaccination has resulted in an 78% reduction in pertussis infections among neonates, thought to be the result of passive immunity being provided through breast milk.[156] However, this strategy has not been widely implemented in low- and middle-income countries as the cost of vaccination is high and the potential effectiveness is unknown, in part because the burden of neonatal pertussis is not well understood in these settings.[157]

Many nonvaccine interventions are also important to reducing the global burden of pneumonia. As with diarrhea, promoting breastfeeding and reducing childhood malnutrition are important pneumonia prevention strategies. The WHO's the integrated Global Action Plan for Pneumonia and Diarrhoea (GAPPD) policy framework also emphasizes the importance of preventing HIV-infection and providing HIV-infected individuals with daily cotrimoxazole prophylaxis.[149] HIV infection is a particularly important risk factor for pneumonia, as HIV-associated immune suppression increases risk of acquiring both typical and atypical pathogens, such as *Pneumocystis jirovecii* pneumonia (PJP). No vaccine exists for PJP, so prevention efforts focus on reducing the burden of HIV, including providing antiretrovirals to those already infected with HIV and using cotrimoxazole or other agents for PJP prophylaxis.

Air pollution is considered the world's leading environmental cause of mortality, including a substantial burden of air-quality-related respiratory disease. WHO estimates that 4.3 million deaths per year are attributable to household air pollution.[158,159] One-third of the world's population burns biomass to provide heating and cooking facilities in their home.[158] These fires result in particulate pollution that is strongly associated with respiratory disease, particularly among women and young children who have greatest exposure to household fires.[158,160] Cleaner burning stoves may be an important strategy to reduce the burden of pneumonia, and interventions to reduce household air population have demonstrated benefit in reducing levels of population in homes. However, studies evaluating the effect of clean cookstoves on health outcomes have been inconsistent in demonstrating benefit.[161–164] Despite the mixed evidence-base for these interventions, many policy makers and nongovernmental actors have remained passionate advocates for home air pollution reduction interventions.

In addition to indoor air pollution, ambient (outdoor) pollution is also associated with lower respiratory tract infections.[165,166] Overall, 17% of deaths due to lower respiratory tract infections are thought to be attributable to poor outdoor air quality, representing approximately 3 million deaths per year.[159] In 2014, the WHO estimated that 92% of the world's population lived in area with air pollution levels higher than the WHO's air-quality recommendations.[167] Between 2008 and 2013, there was a mean global increase in air pollution ($PM_{2.5}$) of approximately 8% per year. High-income countries in Europe, the Americas, and the western Pacific showed decreases in air pollution during this time, but low- and middle-income countries suffered increases.[167] In response to this challenge, the SDGs incorporate air pollution control as a key indicator in four distinct targets: goal 3.9 (a substantial reduction in death and illnesses due to air pollution), 7.1 (clean energy in homes), 11.2 (access to safe, affordable sustainable transport), and 11.6 (reducing the impact of cities by improving air quality). WHO offers technical support to member states advising on the most cost-effective methods of reducing air pollution, including cleaner transport and power generation, energy efficient housing, and municipal waste management. The value of these policies has been largely proven in high-income countries but it is not clear how effectively they can be integrated into the economic growth strategies of developing countries.[159]

FUTURE DIRECTIONS

Many interventions necessary to prevent pneumonia already exist and the SDGs include ambitious targets for reducing the global disease burden of pneumonia over the next two decades. Gavi, a global alliance for vaccine delivery, led the role-out of PCV vaccination that began in 2010, and global coverage continues to steadily improve with a 6% coverage increase in 2016 alone.[168] This role-out may lead to a profound change in the global epidemiology of lower respiratory tract infection. However, sustaining these gains beyond the impact of this PCV vaccination is likely to become increasingly challenging. Pneumonia deaths are concentrated in hard to reach, vulnerable populations who are often missed by national vaccination campaigns. In addition, widespread adoption of policies and technologies to reduce air pollution are yet to be realized in many settings.

DIARRHEA AND ENTERIC FEVER

Burden

Diarrheal diseases are associated with considerable morbidity and mortality in all age groups, with the greatest burden in sub-Saharan Africa and South Asia. In 2016, there were 1.7 million deaths due to diarrheal diseases among all ages; a disproportionate number of deaths (38%), or 446,000 deaths, occurring among children younger than 5 years of age.[169] Most episodes are caused by infectious agents, with rotavirus, *Cryptosporidium*, *Shigella*, and enterotoxigenic *Escherichia coli* (ETEC) producing heat stable toxin alone or in combination with heat labile toxin appearing to be commonest causes in a recent study of moderate-to-severe diarrhea in seven developing countries.[170]

Enteric fever is a systemic febrile illness caused by *Salmonella enterica* serovar *typhi* and *paratyphi* (causes of typhoid fever) and occasionally by nontyphoidal *Salmonella* strains. An estimated 11–21 million cases and 128,000–161,000 deaths occur from typhoid fever annually, mostly in LMICs.[169,171,172] The highest incidence of these infections occurs in South and Southeast Asia and sub-Saharan Africa, but considerable inter- and intracountry variation exists. The peak age has long been described in school age children (5–14 years), although some recent studies have found a high rate in young children 2–4 years of age.[172–174] Immunocompromised and HIV-infected individuals in Africa are also at risk for an invasive nontyphoidal *Salmonella* infection with a clinical presentation similar to typhoid fever. These infections, which are associated with malaria, hemolytic anemia, and schistosomiasis, have high levels of antimicrobial resistance and mortality.[175] Diarrhea is not a consistent manifestation of enteric fever.

Prevention of Diarrhea

Transmission of diarrheal pathogens and typhoid fever typically occurs through the fecal-oral route. Direct person-to-person transmission predominates when the infectious inoculum is low, for example, *Shigella* spp., while ingestion of contaminated food and water accounts for most remaining transmission. Malnutrition and micronutrient deficiency are important influencers of host susceptibility and play a critical role in determining the severity of disease caused by enteric pathogens. These shared routes of transmission, and common determinants of severity, lead to similar approaches to prevention and control of enteric infections in low-resource settings, with a focus on provision of adequate sanitation and hygiene, micronutrient supplementation, and healthy feeding practices. Development of vaccines is a priority for selected enteric infections associated with a high burden of disease (e.g., rotavirus) or for those with limited treatment options (e.g., typhoid fever). Most prevention and control efforts target infants and children, who experience the highest attack rates and mortality from these diseases.

WHO policy recommendations for prevention diarrheal diseases and typhoid fever rely on high coverage of effective low-cost solutions. GAPPD provides a blueprint for countries to develop, implement, and assess a strategic plan to reduce preventable illness and deaths from pneumonia and diarrhea, two major causes of child mortality, by 2025.[176] WHO recommends activities at the country level to increase coverage of low-cost interventions and scale up access to safe water, sanitation, hygiene, and healthcare. Specific interventions identified for diarrhea prevention include promotion of good health practices (vitamin A supplementation, exclusive breastfeeding for 6 months, and adequate complementary feeding), preventive care [provision of safe drinking water and sanitation (WASH), HIV prevention, and appropriate immunizations], and appropriate case management.

Recommendations for implementation of the GAPPD guidelines are contained within a series of publications related to newborn,[177] child,[178] and adolescent health.[179] There is considerable evidence demonstrating the health benefits of vitamin A, breastfeeding, and adequate nutrition. Vitamin A has been shown to ameliorate the detrimental health effects of diarrheal disease, presumably due to its immunoregulatory properties.[180] A Cochrane review of nine studies concluded vitamin A supplementation was associated with a 12% reduction in mortality related to diarrhea and a 15% reduction in diarrhea incidence.[181] Breastfeeding similarly exhibits protective efficacy against disease and death from diarrhea. A meta-analysis of 18 studies demonstrated that, compared to exclusive breastfeeding for the first 0–5 months of life, partial breastfeeding increased diarrhea incidence by 68% and no breastfeeding increased diarrhea incidence by 165%.[182] The meta-analysis also found that children not breastfeeding during the first 0–5 months of life had a 14.4 (95% CI: 6.1–33.9) times greater risk of all-cause mortality compared to those exclusively breastfed. Additionally, any breastfeeding after 6 months is associated with decreased diarrheal incidence, diarrheal mortality, and all-cause mortality compared to no breastfeeding. Although the mechanisms of action are not completely elucidated, these effects have been attributed to the large variety of biologically active molecules with immunologic and anti-inflammatory properties in human milk, and the beneficial effects of breast milk on the infant microbiome[183,184]; in addition, breastfeeding can reduce the exposure to contaminated fluids and food while providing adequate nutrition.[180] The WHO recommends exclusive breastfeeding until 6 months of age and continued breastfeeding until 2 years of age.[185] Adherence to these recommended practices for exclusive breastfeeding can be improved by community-level educational and promotional interventions.[186]

Improved sanitation and hygiene can reduce transmission of pathogens from the environment and from infected people. Several meta-analyses and systematic reviews have demonstrated that WASH interventions, including various methods to improve water quality, handwashing with soap, and excreta disposal, are able to reduce diarrheal incidence, although the evidence is generally of poor quality and heterogeneity is high.[187,188] Interventions aimed to improve water quality at the point of use (i.e., interrupting so-called "short cycle transmission") appear to be more effective in reducing childhood diarrhea than interventions to improve water supply ("long-cycle transmission"), although as noted earlier in this chapter, several recent randomized trials have failed to demonstrate consistent benefit.[87,88] Effective point-of-use water-quality interventions to prevent diarrhea at the home, school, or workplace include chlorination, flocculation/disinfection, filtration, and solar disinfection.[189] Hand washing with soap[190–192] is also associated with a significant reduction in all-cause diarrhea incidence; however, sustained implementation of these interventions at the public health level can be challenging, so the value of health behavior change programs targeted at communities, schools, or healthcare institutions has been investigated. Hygiene promotion programs shown to be effective in increasing frequency of handwashing include consistent and dynamic educational activities with children such as puppet shows, nursery song videos, and comic books,[193–196] and distribution of hygiene promotion kits for teachers to use.[197]

In 2006, the WHO recommended introduction of rotavirus vaccine into the Expanded Program on Immunization (EPI) in the European Region and the Americas based on efficacy data from these areas. In 2009, this recommendation was extended to all regions of the world based on efficacy studies. Gavi now supports vaccine use in nearly 40 low-income countries. Although efficacy is reduced compared to high-income countries, the vaccine has prevented a substantial number of diarrheal episodes and deaths.

The immune response to measles infection coincides with a short-term decreased immune response against other antigens resulting in an increased susceptibility to secondary bacterial and viral infections.[198] Accordingly, measles infection is associated with an increased risk of diarrhea morbidity and mortality in the acute phase of the disease.[199] Measles vaccination is recommended to prevent both measles and related complications.[176] Reductions in measles incidence as a result of widespread vaccination has contributed to declines in diarrheal mortality observed in recent decades.

The cornerstone of the management of diarrheal diseases is the prevention and treatment of dehydration, accompanied by zinc and continued feeding to shorten illness and maintain nutrition.[176,200] Evidence supports the efficacy of Oral Rehydration Solution (ORS) in the treatment of pediatric diarrhea in low-income countries,[201] while the widespread use of ORS in the WHO Diarrheal Disease Control Program has been credited with saving millions of lives. Currently, low-osmolarity ORS is the formulation of choice[202,203] and should be administered both at home for prevention of dehydration in children with diarrhea and at the health center for those who have "some" dehydration according to WHO criteria.[203,204] Intravenous rehydration is reserved for children with severe dehydration.[203] Zinc supplementation during diarrheal episodes has also been shown to shorten the duration of diarrheal episodes among children in developing countries.[205] In settings where zinc deficiency is prevalent, zinc supplementation helps to restore the mucosal barrier and strengthen antibody and lymphocyte responses against intestinal pathogens.[206] When zinc and ORS are promoted together, use is dramatically increased; one systematic review suggested an 82% increased use of these interventions by mothers for their child's diarrhea treatment.[207] Antibiotics are reserved for children with diarrhea who present with dysentery, SAM, suspected cholera, or enteric fever. Use of antibiotics for other types of diarrhea is not generally recommended given the increasing risk of antibiotic resistance and lack of clear mortality benefit.[208] A renewed focus on prescribing antibiotics only for appropriate indications has led to a significant update to the WHO Model List of Essential Medicines in 2017. Finally, increased use of sensitive and specific diagnostics can assist in appropriate treatment of diarrhea and enteric disease; however, these are rarely available in low-resource settings.

PREVENTION OF ENTERIC FEVER

Given the high burden of disease and increasing antimicrobial resistance, strategies to prevent enteric fever are considered high priority. The sources and modes of transmission of invasive nontyphoidal *Salmonella* in low- and middle-income countries are poorly understood, which limits the ability to prevent infection. Therefore, interventions that focus on diminishing the host susceptibility (e.g., treatment of malnutrition, HIV, elimination of malaria, etc.) are likely to have the most impact. In contrast, contaminated water is a known source of *S. typhi* and *paratyphi* and preventive efforts must also address provision of clean water and sanitation.

Two currently available vaccines, Ty21a oral vaccine (three or four doses, for individuals aged 5 years and older) and Vi capsular polysaccharide vaccine (one dose, for individuals aged 2 years and older) were recommended by WHO in 2008 for programmatic use in high-burden settings but these vaccines are underutilized. Both require booster doses at specified intervals. In 2017, WHO reviewed the evidence for typhoid conjugate vaccines (TCV) and recommended programmatic use of these vaccines for persons in endemic countries over the age of 6 months, accompanied by catch-up vaccination campaigns for children up to 15 years of age.[209] WHO recommended prioritizing introduction in countries with the highest disease burden and growing incidence of drug-resistant typhoid fever. The Vi polysaccharide conjugated to tetanus toxoid (Typbar-TCV®, Bharat Biotech) has been prequalified by WHO and funding was approved by Gavi starting in 2019.

FUTURE DIRECTIONS

The dramatic reductions in mortality from diarrheal diseases seen over the past three decades have been attributed to the widespread uptake of these recommended interventions for diarrhea and enteric disease along with global development and improvements in female literacy. However, the potential public health impact for prevention and control relies on high coverage of interventions with correct, consistent, and sustained use.[176] WHO recommends communication and social mobilization strategies to inform and motivate healthy actions to create a demand for these interventions at the country level. In addition, collaboration with the private sector is also required to maintain consistent supply of vaccines and treatments. Finally, continued monitoring of intervention coverage rates will be required to ensure equitable access to these interventions.[210]

MALARIA

Burden

In most low-income tropical countries, malaria remains a major public health issue and a significant obstacle to economic development. In the 2017 World Malaria Report, the WHO acknowledges progress made in the past decade, but warns against complacency. In 2016, there were 216 million cases of malaria, a slight increase from previous years, with 445,000 malaria attributable deaths.[211] In Africa, the vast majority of these malaria cases are caused by *P. falciparum,* while in South Asia and South Americas, *P. vivax* is the most prevalent parasite. Both parasites are complex organisms, responsible for a disease that is very difficult to control and represents a challenge for National Malaria Programs (NMP) and researchers trying to develop a vaccine. In addition, the negative impacts of environmental and climate changes on malaria transmission in all continents need to be rigorously evaluated in order to develop optimal mitigation strategies.

Between 2001 and 2013, the expansion of malaria interventions contributed to a 47% decline in malaria mortality, averting 4.3 million deaths.[212] The WHO has set even more ambitious targets for 2030, aiming to reduce the incidence of malaria by at least 90%, reduce malaria mortality rates by at least 90%, eliminate malaria in more than 34 countries, and prevent the resurgence of malaria in all malaria-free countries.[212]

Prevention

There are three keys groups of intervention in the WHO recommended strategy for achieving malaria elimination; vector control measures, chemoprophylaxis and treatment, and disease surveillance. Vector control includes universal access to ITNs, or long-lasting insecticidal nets (LLINs), and indoor residential spraying (IRS).[212] The regular mass distribution of free ITN/LLINs largely explains the impressive reductions in the number of malaria cases seen in Africa and WHO encourages all programs to use IRS for the rapid clearance of transmission foci. While the increased coverage with Insecticide Treated Nets (ITNs) largely explains the reduction in the number of cases seen over the past decades in Africa,[213] the widespread vector resistance to the insecticide used in the nets may compromise this strategy in the future. Larval source management is a third vector control strategy, which may be used in addition to ITN/LLINs and IRS. During larval source management the available larval habit (water) is reduced, modified, or treated with biological or chemical agents to prevent the vector's reproduction.

Chemoprophylaxis is the second group of core interventions and includes intermittent preventive treatment of pregnant women (IPTp), intermittent preventive treatment of infants, and seasonal malaria chemoprevention (SMC) for children aged under 5 years. These interventions are recommended for areas of moderate to high transmission in sub-Saharan Africa, and seasonal prophylaxis is reserved for use in the Sahel subregion.[212] SMC in children in Sahel countries and IPTp is still limited by low coverage and effectiveness is compromised by resistance to the antimalarial drug used (sulfadoxine-pyrimethamine SP).[214–216] Finally, the identification and appropriate treatment of malaria-infected individuals is critically important to reducing subsequent infections and reducing transmission.

Many of the obstacles to implementing these interventions in low-resources countries are common to all endemic countries, while others are more specific to certain regions. In virtually all countries where malaria remains a significant health problem, NMPs are constrained by the lack of financial resources. As a consequence, most NMPs rely on external funding from institutions such as the Global Fund, bilateral cooperation agreements, and charities such as the Bill & Melinda Gates Foundation. In 2016, a total of $2.7 billion was invested by governments of endemic countries and international partners, less than half of the $6.6 billion required to meet all targets for that year.[217]

Deficits in human resources capacity, poor infrastructure, and lack of coordination between funding partners mean that the recipient countries can face difficulties to absorb this much-needed funding, creating additional difficulties for NMPs. In addition to these financial and structural barriers, a disease as complex as malaria requires extensive technical support. The WHO mandate is to provide this guidance, but they have been criticized for being slow to recognize and respond to the disastrous consequences of chloroquine resistance in Africa in the 1990s and to the progression of multidrug resistance in Southeast Asia in the 2000s.[218,219]

In Africa, an important limitation to improved malaria control is access to diagnostic tools and effective treatment for all malaria patients. According to WHO, between 2014 and 2016, less than half of African febrile children were seen at a healthcare facility, only half of whom got a malaria test. Of these, only one in five were treated with an artemisinin combination therapy (ACT),[211] the recommended antimalarial. Evidence is also emerging that public health burden of *P. vivax, P. ovale,* and *P. malariae* in sub-Saharan Africa may have underestimated and will require renewed attention.[220]

The rising prevalence of drug resistance among malaria pathogens calls for the urgent development of vaccines. Two candidate malaria vaccines are expected to be available for use in malaria elimination/eradication programs by 2022: RTS, S and whole PfSPZ, but their public health impact as malaria integrated tools for elimination/eradication needs to be further evaluated.

In Southeast Asia, the prevention of malaria by ITNs is much less effective than in Africa, as the vectors biting behaviors are different. Despite this simple evidence, millions of ITNs are being distributed by the Global Fund and others under advice of the WHO. In addition, the major issue facing malaria programs in Southeast Asia is that of drug resistance in *P. falciparum*. Historically resistance to all antimalarial drugs has emerged in this part of the world. Since the late 1950s, the NMPs in this region have adopted a pragmatic approach to malaria, multiplying to point-of-care structures and the village-based approaches, changing from one drug to the next one as resistance progressed: from chloroquine to SP in the 1970s, to mefloquine in the 1980s, and rapidly adopting ACTs in the middle of the 1990s. However, even with the large amount of evidence of their safety and efficacy, ACTs were not recommended for Africa (where chloroquine resistance was causing millions of deaths) before 2006. In 2007, the first evidence of resistance to artemisinin emerged in Cambodia, causing great concerns in the NMPs of the region. Despite numerous meetings, conferences, and elaborate strategic plans, no serious attempts were made to contain the spread of the resistant parasites. By 2015, all countries in the Greater Mekong Subregion were affected. As predicted, resistance to artemisinin has led to the failure of ACTs, with no replacement drug in sight.

In Southeast Asia and in South America, Ministries of Health are also confronted with *P. vivax* malaria, which has a dormant liver stage that complicates detection and treatment. NMPs are advised to use primaquine to eliminate this liver stage, but this medicine must be taken for 14 days and causes hemolysis in patients with G6PD deficiency, an inherited blood disorder that affects up to 20% of people living in these regions.[221] *P. vivax* has also developed resistance to chloroquine in several regions of the Asia-Pacific and Southeast Asia, leaving NMPs with very few options to tackle a parasite that may be more difficult to eliminate than *P. falciparum*.

FUTURE DIRECTIONS

Remarkable progress has been made in the effort to control malaria. However, antimalarial resistance, changes to the global climate, and the logistic, financial, and human resource burden of maintaining this effort undermines the WHO goal to eliminate malaria in more than 34 countries, and these threats may facilitate a resurgence of malaria in populations that have seen dramatic improvements in last decade. Avoiding such a resurgence is critically important to achieving malaria specific and SDG health targets; previous failed elimination efforts have demonstrated that a resurgence among malaria naïve populations is likely to be accompanied by very high case fatality rates and would reverse decades of progress.

HIV

Burden

Over the last decade, combination HIV prevention strategies to both decrease HIV infectiousness and susceptibility have been the mainstay of HIV prevention and control. Globally, 36.7 million people are living with HIV (PLWH); 70% of these know their status, 81% (20.9 million) of those people who know they are infected are on antiretroviral therapy (ART), and 82% of persons on ART are virally suppressed.[222,223] The impact of these extraordinary achievements is evident in the global decrease in HIV-related deaths and rates of mother-to-child-transmission, including among high prevalence countries of sub-Saharan Africa.[224,225] However, HIV incidence remains high among some populations, particularly among adolescent girls and young women.

Prevention

A fundamental principle in the prevention of HIV is the concept of treatment as prevention. UNAIDS current 90-90-90 strategy aims to control the HIV epidemic by 2030 by testing 90% of PLWH, initiating ART among 90% of PLWH tested, and achieving viral suppression among 90% of those on ART.[226] The HIV care continuum has four steps: HIV testing and identification of PLWH, linkage to care and ART initiation, and adherence to ART to achieve viral suppression. High retention at each step is necessary for optimizing efforts toward achieving epidemic control.[227–229]

HIV testing and counselling (HTC) is the first step of HIV treatment and prevention. Routine facility-based HTC or provider-initiated testing and counselling has vastly increased knowledge of HIV status among patients,[230–233] and strengthened PMTCT.[234] However, key populations such sex workers, young adults (especially young women), and men who have sex with men, are disproportionately infected with HIV and have unique barriers to accessing facility-based HTC. Community-based HTC has demonstrated that across multiple modalities (home, mobile, index, key populations, campaign, workplace, and self-testing) community-based HTC can reach priority populations with higher coverage than facility-based HTC.[235–244] Consequently, WHO and UNAIDS strongly recommend implementing community-based HTC for reaching key populations.[245,246]

Current WHO guidelines recommend rapid ART initiation for all people newly diagnosed with HIV, regardless of immune status or CD4 count (a measure of immune deficiency as a result of HIV disease).[247] The rapid initiation of ART following diagnosis, or a "test-and-treat" strategy, is associated with life-saving individual health benefits and is also vital in preventing additional infections.[227,248] Unfortunately, delays with linkage to care are common.[249] In Kenya, the proportion of PLWH linked to care following HIV diagnosis is 42%[250] and it is only 37% in South Africa.[251] Barriers to linkage to care within the resource-limited context include distance from HTC testing sites to ART clinics, long wait times, costs (transportation, lost wages, and childcare), confidentiality concerns, low perceived benefit of ART initiation at time of diagnosis, and infrequent contact with the health system.[236,252] Facilitated linkage (e.g., counsellor follow-up to support linkage) has led to high rates of ART initiation (>75%) in recent studies.[230,253] Similarly, strategies that improve clinic operations and minimize administrative barriers to ART initiation have also demonstrated improvement in ART initiation.[254]

ART adherence and viral suppression reduces HIV-associated morbidity, mortality, and HIV transmission.[255–257] Assessing adherence has proven challenging. Self-reported adherence is often unreliable[258] and laboratory-confirmed drug concentrations are highly effective but too expensive for widespread implementation for routine adherence monitoring.[259–261] Despite the importance of viral suppression to preventing HIV transmission, it is estimated that 70% of PLWH in sub-Saharan Africa are not virally suppressed.[262,263]

Similar to the HIV care continuum, the HIV prevention continuum (Fig. 23-1) builds on HIV testing followed by linkage of HIV-uninfected persons to prevention services, retention in services, and adherence to HIV-prevention strategies.[264]

In addition to identifying HIV-uninfected individuals and starting them on treatment, several additional evidence-based prevention strategies, including biomedical interventions [voluntary medical male circumcision[265–267] and antiretroviral pre-exposure prophylaxis (PrEP)],[234,268,269] behavioral interventions (risk-reduction counseling and condom use), and structural interventions (policies or programs that influence economic security and gender equality) have proven effective at reducing HIV incidence.[270,271]

Prevention services for HIV-uninfected individuals at risk for HIV acquisition require ongoing engagement for as long as risk remains.[264] Even individuals undergoing voluntary medical male circumcision, a one-time biomedical intervention with 60% protective efficacy against HIV for heterosexual males,[265–267] require ongoing risk-reduction counseling and consistent condom use are necessary to further reduce risk.[272,273] Finally, adherence to HIV prevention interventions that involve ongoing use, such as PrEP, is essential for real-world effectiveness.[274] Ultimately, a combination package of prevention interventions that includes structural and behavioral strategies to enhance retention and adherence to the biomedical strategies, is most likely to increase prevention efficacy.[275] While reaching any one individual with the multiple potential strategies proven to prevent

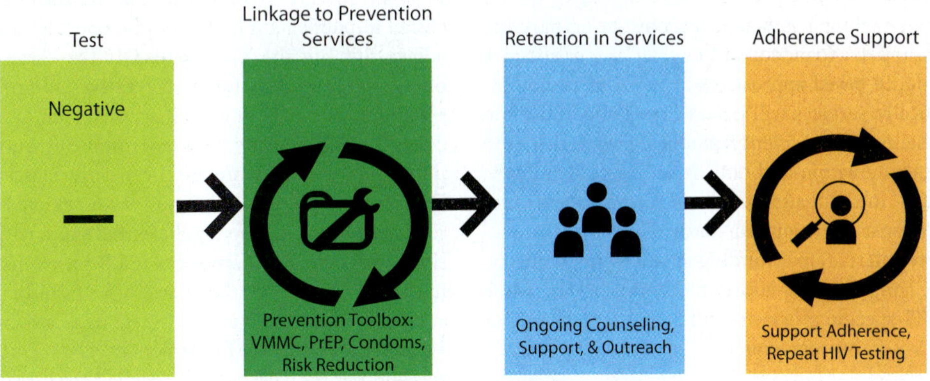

FIGURE 23-1. HIV prevention continuum. (*Source:* Reproduced with permission from McNairy ML, El-Sadr WM. A paradigm shift: Focus on the HIV prevention continuum. *Clin Infect Dis*. 2014;59(Suppl 1):S12–5.[264].)

HIV acquisition is challenging in most settings, ensuring broad population coverage of a package of preventative interventions has been demonstrated to result in successful population level prevention.

STI PREVENTION AND CONTROL IN RESOURCE-LIMITED SETTINGS

Burden

Sexually transmitted infection (STI) control strategies in resource-limited settings are primarily based on behavioral interventions and STI case management. However, STI control efforts have generally not kept pace with the expansion of HIV control interventions. Current global STI control is hampered by asymptomatic infections, lack of scalable diagnostic tests, antimicrobial resistance, and barriers to intervention access, availability, and scale-up.[276,277] Vaccines may offer a new paradigm for STI control, though few options currently exist. In this section, we summarize the current major control and prevention strategies for non-HIV STIs in resource-limited settings.

Prevention

Few primary prevention innovations have been developed for non-HIV STIs. Condom use remains the mainstay of STI risk reduction and condoms are widely and feely available throughout many resource-limited countries. Increasing condom availability also improves condom use,[278,279] although the public health impact of such measures has not been systematically evaluated. Additionally, women are often unable to negotiate condom use within sexual partnerships, suggesting a need for additional female-controlled STI primary prevention strategies.

Human papillomavirus (HPV) is an important vaccine-preventable STI, as infection with some serotypes, particularly HPV types 16 and 18, can lead to the development of cervical or other cancers. Currently, there are two WHO prequalified vaccines that are high efficacious against both HPV types 16 and 18 and are typically administered before the onset of sexual activity. Studies have shown feasibility and acceptability of HPV vaccine administration to adolescent girls in resource-limited countries including Malawi, Rwanda, Tanzania, and Uganda.[280–283] School-based platforms for vaccine delivery have also demonstrated success for HPV vaccine coverage,[280–283] though other approaches for reaching out-of-school youth have been less successful.[282] Challenges to existing STI prevention efforts within resource-limited health systems provide important reasons for advancing additional STI vaccines, although we also note that HPV vaccine uptake in high-income countries has been low.

Prevention through treatment of cases remains critical to STI control. Sensitive diagnostic tests are required for early detection of STIs, both to guide management and to interrupt transmission.[284] However, over 90% of STIs occur in resource-limited settings without access to sensitive diagnostics.[285] As such, syndromic management (based on symptoms) remains the core of STI management. Syndromic management can be effective for urethral discharge in men and for genital ulcer disease.[286–288] However, more robust approaches are needed to control cervical infections in women, especially chlamydia and gonorrhea, because vaginal discharge is a poor proxy for endocervical infection.[286–288] For chlamydia, gonorrhea, and trichomoniasis, affordable point-of-care tests are needed.[289]

Following reports of gonococcal antimicrobial resistance worldwide, WHO urges all countries to systematically monitor gonococcal antimicrobial resistance.[290,291] Current syndromic management approaches can increase unnecessary and incorrect antimicrobial treatment, further confounding this emerging concern.[287] Additionally, widespread adoption of syndromic management strategies without specimen collection for laboratory analysis hampers surveillance of antimicrobial susceptibility.[292] Strengthening surveillance systems will be increasingly important for monitoring STI antimicrobial resistance.

A global action plan for the elimination of mother to child transmission of syphilis was launched in 2007 with a target of reaching 95% coverage of syphilis testing and treatment among pregnant women.[293] Several countries have already adopted universal antenatal syphilis screening using bedside syphilis testing.[294] However, less than one-third of resource-limited countries report antenatal syphilis testing coverage of at least 95% and there are still approximately 1 million new cases of congenital syphilis annually.[295,296] Similar efforts to scale-up treatment and prevention of other STIs during pregnancy have not been implemented and STIs among pregnant women persist as a global maternal-child health challenge.[297,298]

Partner notification and treatment for STIs is recommended to interrupt transmission of infections.[277,299,300] Evidence suggests that patient-oriented partner notification approaches (using index patients to notify their partners, with or without the medication to treat partners)[301] are preferred in resource-limited settings, which is aligned with the WHO recommendation for patient-based notification as the first step within this context.[299,302] Although modelling demonstrations have supported that strategies to increase partner notification for HIV are cost-effective,[303] data for non-HIV STIs are needed and partner notification for most STIs is not systematically addressed by most national programs.

Future Directions in HIV and STI Prevention

Recent scientific advances provide an unprecedented number of effective measures to prevent and control infection with HIV and other STIs.[304] Catalyzed by a strong global consensus that tools now exist to curb the HIV epidemic, UNAIDS established a Fast-Track strategy to end the HIV epidemic by 2030.[305] The ambitious plan was informed by a combination of major scientific breakthroughs and accumulated lessons learned from >20 years of scaling up the global HIV response. Enabling a sufficient response to outpace the epidemic will require rapid, expanded, and targeted use of effective combinations of evidence-based approaches in most-affected communities.[305,306] Specifically, services will need to be client-focused to ensure strong and sustained engagement and utilize new strategies to provide services efficiently within and outside of health facilities[307]; With the "end of AIDS" in sight, additional and sustained resources for the epidemic response are required, particularly in resource-limited settings where international funding supplements domestic investments.[308] Leveraging ongoing efforts to eliminate HIV while also strengthening STI-specific programs will continue to be necessary to control these synergistic epidemics.

TUBERCULOSIS

Burden

Mycobacterium tuberculosis (TB) remains a leading cause of global infectious disease morbidity and mortality, despite being both treatable and preventable. At least one-quarter of the world's population is infected with TB. Many people who are infected with TB never develop active disease, a condition known as latent TB. However, over 10.4 million people with latent TB do progress to active TB disease each year, resulting in over 1.5 million deaths annually.[309,310] Over 90% of cases and more than 95% of TB-related deaths occur in resource-limited settings. The largest proportions of TB cases occur in the WHO Southeast Asian (45%), African (25%), and Western Pacific (17%) Regions.[309] TB most commonly presents as pulmonary disease, which is responsible for ongoing transmission, but can also manifest as extrapulmonary disease in any organ. Risk factors for infection include poverty and overcrowding, living in a TB-endemic community, and being in close contact with a TB case (such as in a household or other at-risk setting including hospitals, HIV clinics, prisons, refugee camps, or migrant worker hostels). While the majority of people infected with *M. tuberculosis* will not develop disease (i.e., active TB), risk factors that increase the likelihood of disease following infection include age (young children, adolescents, and old people), comorbidities such as HIV, diabetes, and malnutrition, or lung disease due to cigarette smoking or work-related exposure such as in miners.

Prevention

The implementation of TB programs in TB-endemic countries has historically been under the stewardship of National Tuberculosis Programmes (NTPs). Programmatic strategies for TB have evolved and expanded over time from "control" to "care and prevention" and now "elimination" with integrated, multisectoral approaches. The initial strategy was endorsed by the WHO in 1994 and recommended the directly observed treatment short-course (DOTS), which focused on reducing transmission by improving case detection and cure, particularly of the most infectious TB cases (i.e., those with sputum smear-positive TB). In 2006, the Stop-TB Strategy was developed to align with the Millennium Development Goals (MDGs) with a broader approach to strengthen health systems and engage all TB care providers to expand and enhance delivery of DOTS and to specifically address TB/HIV, drug-resistant TB and the needs of vulnerable populations such as children.[311] Some progress was made toward the MDGs set for 2015, achieving a halving of TB-related mortality (47% decline since 1990) and reversing the rise in TB incidence (1.4% decline per annum 2000–15). However, a much greater fall in incidence is required to end the TB epidemic.

In 2015, the current WHO End TB Strategy (2016–35) was developed in alignment with the Sustainable Development Goals (SDGs) target of eliminating TB as a public health threat.[312] Achieving this target will require achieving a rate of annual decline of TB incidence to 4–5% by 2020, with a subsequent acceleration of decline to over 10% per annum. The current Global Plan to End TB (2016–20), a costed implementation plan for the End TB Strategy, calls for a "paradigm shift" in the TB response.[313] The commitment to the SDGs offers an opportunity for an integrated response that includes social, economic, and environmental actions, such as in the areas of gender equality, food security, and labor and migration,[314] to complement implementation of biomedical responses described below. The End TB Strategy is built on three pillars: integrated patient-centered TB care *and* prevention; bold policies and supportive systems; and intensified research and innovation.[312] TB prevention and care strategies have been striving to transition from a traditional vertical and siloed approach to a much broader, integrated, and cross-sector approach. However, although the fundamentals remain unchanged, comprehensive approaches have not been applied consistently or widely enough; and have not been backed by needed political will and funding.[315]

Case-Finding and Effective Treatment

Early detection and effective treatment of all individuals with TB, including drug-resistant TB, is critical to stopping transmission. Most NTPs in low- and middle-income countries currently rely on passive case finding with diagnostic tools of inadequate sensitivity for TB and without the ability to detect drug resistance. National prevalence surveys consistently identify a large gap between cases being detected and the actual number of cases in the community—it is estimated that approximately 3 million cases are missed each year.[309] Screening for TB-related symptoms in high-risk groups, such as household contacts or in HIV clinics, with further evaluation of those that screen positive, increases case detection.[316] However, for all presumptive TB cases identified by passive or active case finding, there also needs to be rapid diagnosis and effective treatment in order to interrupt transmission and improve outcomes.

Rapid molecular tests such as Xpert MTB/RIF and recently Xpert MTB/RIF Ultra have the advantage of greater sensitivity and specificity than smear microscopy, as well as much more rapid detection of MDR-TB compared to culture and drug susceptibility testing (the current gold standard).[317,318] There also needs to be decentralization of diagnostics (i.e., point-of-care testing) to reach the most vulnerable populations. This testing must be accompanied by community education, engagement, and an integrated, family-based approach to care.

Effective treatment for TB, linked with patient-centered care in the form of adherence support, socioeconomic, and psychosocial support, is the recommended model of care for optimal management. Early access and adherence to the optimal treatment regimen will result in treatment success in the majority of cases, including those with drug-resistant TB. Improved case detection and treatment provide an opportunity for treating latent TB infection or preventive therapy.

The End TB strategy places far greater emphasis on prevention through the treatment of infection than previous strategies and the coverage of preventive therapy for child contacts in TB-endemic countries was reported in WHO Global TB Report for the first time in 2016, with a minority of countries providing data.[312,319] High-risk populations exposed to drug-susceptible TB, including young child contacts and people living with HIV who do not have active TB, should receive isoniazid preventive therapy (IPT). However, there is a huge policy-practice implementation gap in resource-limited settings and many eligible individuals are not receiving such preventive treatment.[320,321] IPT is cheap, safe, effective, and cost-effective but uptake and adherence are a challenge even in those who are treated, as IPT needs to be taken daily for at least 6 months. Shorter regimens such as 3 months of weekly rifapentine-isoniazid or 3 months of daily rifampicin-isoniazid have equivalent efficacy, less toxicity, and improved adherence, but these are not yet being applied in resource-limited settings.[322–325]

Individuals exposed to MDR-TB are another high-risk group where there is huge potential for treatment of TB infection to dramatically reduce transmission. Although there is some observational evidence of effectiveness of preventive therapy in MDR-TB contacts,[326–328] international guidelines await results of ongoing randomized controlled trials.[322]

For preventive therapy strategies to contribute to a sharper and sustained fall in the incidence of TB over and above case detection and treatment, the population targeted must be dramatically increased. For example, household contact screening will need to include testing and treating for infection of contacts of adolescents and adults, as a limited focus on young children (<5 years) has almost no impact on transmission. Limited evidence from interventions that have tested and treated entire communities have shown marked reductions of TB in those communities sustained over time.[329–331]

NTPs rely heavily on programmatic data for effective monitoring of TB interventions. Successful TB programs are characterized by locally tailored responses that are informed by quality and timely data to guide interventions. A priority for a successful TB program is to strengthen existing health information systems and implement enhanced systems where appropriate, including electronic and mobile platforms. These data systems provide the foundation for continuous quality improvement and operational/implementation research to improve the efficiency, quality, and coverage of programs. The evidence and knowledge that is generated needs to be provided to decision makers to inform policy and practice.

FUTURE DIRECTIONS

Ending the TB epidemic will require not only a sizable increase in the uptake of existing programs but also will necessitate intensifying TB research and innovation.[332] There is ongoing research evaluating treatment regimens for drug-resistant TB and severe forms of TB, such as TB meningitis. These efforts include repurposing of old drugs at higher dosages and testing of recently developed drugs aiming for shorter effective regimens for all age groups. In addition, new regimens that do not include the injectable aminoglycosides, which commonly cause permanent toxicity in the treatment of MDR TB, are under assessment.

NTDS

Burden

Neglected tropical diseases (NTDs) is the term given to a group of (mainly) infectious diseases that are prevalent among populations living in poverty and without adequate access to clean water and sanitation.[333] The World Health Organization identifies 20 diseases and conditions as NTDs, whereas 10 diseases have been identified as priorities in the London Declaration on NTDs—a commitment by global partners to control and eliminate 10 NTDs by 2020.[333] These NTDs are Guinea worm, lymphatic filariasis, onchocerciasis, schistosomiasis, soil-transmitted helminths, visceral leishmaniasis, human African trypanosomiasis, leprosy, and Chagas disease. Table 23-2 summarizes the transmission, morbidity, burden, and global program goals of each NTD.

Prevention

The main intervention strategy against these diseases is either (i) the regular MDA to all people at risk of morbidity and/or infection or (ii) intensified disease management within the primary healthcare system. Both approaches are supported, with varying degree of effectiveness, by vector control, environmental improvement, and health education.

MDA involves treating individuals in a community without determining who is infected. The helminthic NTDs and trachoma can be effectively treated with safe, single-dose drugs, which are donated by pharmaceutical companies as part of their London Declaration commitments.[334] For the soil-transmitted helminthes, a single dose of albendazole or mebendazole is highly effective against *Ascaris* and hookworm, but less effective for *Trichuris*; the addition of other anthelmintics to albendazole has been showed to improve efficacy against *Trichuris*. Praziquantal is effective against all schistosome species. Onchocerciasis is effectively treated using ivermectin, which also kills the microfilariae of lymphatic filariasis, and in countries endemic for onchocerciasis and lymphatic filariasis ivermectin is coadministered with albendazole. In countries where there is no onchocerciasis, lymphatic filariasis is treated using diethylcarbamazine and albendazole. Finally, trachoma can be controlled through repeated doses of the antibiotic, azithromycin.

The practicality of treatment lends itself to a MDA approach whereby all people living in an endemic area are treated without prior diagnosis. The broad-spectrum nature of many anthelmintics allows for the integrated delivery of MDA. There are several key components of a MDA program. A first activity is disease mapping in order to understand the geographical distribution of the disease(s) in question to help target interventions to areas with ongoing transmission (for NTDs targeted for elimination) or highest risk of morbidity (in the case of soil transmitted helminths, schistosomiasis, and trachoma) and to estimate the population requiring treatment and hence drug needs. Using this information, countries submit a periodic request, via WHO, for medicines donated by the pharmaceutical industry. In turn, use of donated drugs and treatment coverage is reported back to WHO.

Co-endemicity of lymphatic filariasis or onchocerciasis and the filarial worm *Loa loa* is an impediment to MDA using ivermectin, owing to the risk of encephalopathy among *L. loa*-infected individuals who receive ivermectin. Efforts are underway to develop methods to rapidly screen individuals to identify and exclude *L. loa*-infected individuals from MDA programs.[335]

Monitoring and evaluation are essential components of MDA programs in order to track progress toward program goals. After a period of regular MDA (5 years for lymphatic filariasis, 10–15 years for onchocerciasis, and 3–5 years for trachoma), mathematical modelling and field studies suggest that transmission can be interrupted and therefore a program should conduct an assessment to evaluate transmission interruption and whether MDA can be stopped.[336] Once MDA has been stopped it is important to conduct posttreatment surveillance for 3–5 years to monitor for recrudescence of transmission. If recrudescence or reintroduction is not detected at the end of the surveillance phase, countries may apply for verification of elimination.

MDA has been highly effective in reducing and interrupting transmission in some settings, and several countries have successfully eliminated lymphatic filariasis, onchocerciasis, and trachoma.[337] In other settings, MDA programs have been less successful, due in part to low MDA coverage, high intrinsic rate of pathogen transmission, or a poorly functioning program.

Potential threats to MDA program include potential selection of drug-resistant parasites as scale-up of program increase drug pressure and decreasing social compliance to MDA, especially as morbidity is eliminated and the incentive to take repeated treatments is lessened. Social mobilization, aimed at increasing compliance and dispelling misconceptions about diseases and treatment, is an essential component of MDA programs.[338,339]

Currently there is no definitive evidence of drug resistance within human parasite populations, but its occurrence in livestock populations warrants careful monitoring in NTD programs. Should resistance be detected, modifications to existing MDA programs may be necessary to ensure continued drug efficacy.

In contrast to the above diseases, there are a variety of NTDs that are managed through intensified disease management. Leishmaniasis, human African trypanosomiasis, and Chagas disease are all caused

TABLE 23-2 BASICS OF NTDS

Disease	Causative Agents	Transmission Route and Control Measures	Principal Morbidity	DALYs in 2016 (Millions)[92]	Program Goal (by 2020 Unless Stated)
Soil-transmitted helminthiases	*Ascaris lumbricoides*, *Trichuris trichiura*, and the hookworms, *Necator americanus* and *Ancylostoma duodenale*	Accidental ingestion of eggs (*Ascaris* and *Trichuris*) or larvae (*A. duodenale*), or through penetration of the skin by infective hookworm larvae in contaminated soil. **Control**: WASH intervention, mass drug administration	Range of symptoms including diarrhea, abdominal pain, growth and cognitive impairment, and anemia.	3.4 (*Ascaris* 1.4, *Trichuris* 0.3, hookworm 1.7	Reduce soil-transmitted helminths morbidity from soil-transmitted helminths in preschool- and school-age children to a level below which it would not be considered a public health problem.
Schistosomiasis	*S. mansoni*, *S. japonicum*, *S. mekongi*, *S. intercalatum* (intestinal) and *S. haematobium* (urogenital)	Exposure to contaminated water in which snail intermediate hosts shed infective larvae which penetrate the skin. **Control**: WASH intervention, mass drug administration, vector control	Intestinal disease: abdominal pain, diarrhea, blood in the stool, hepatic fibrosis leading to portal hypertension. Urogenital disease: hematuria, obstructive uropathy leading to hydronephrosis, bladder cancer.	1.9	Elimination, as a public-health problem from American and Western Pacific Regions and from selected countries in Africa.
Lymphatic filariasis	*Wuchereria bancrofti*, *Brugia malayi*, and *B. timori*	Person-to-person via bites of infected mosquitoes (*Anopheles* and to a lesser extent *Culex* in Africa and the Pacific Islands, but predominantly by *Culex* in Asia). **Control**: Mass drug administration	Hydrocoele, lymphoedema, elephantiasis, and acute episodes of local inflammation involving skin, lymph nodes, and lymphatic vessels often accompany chronic lymphoedema or elephantiasis.	1.2	Global elimination of the disease as a public-health problem and the interruption of transmission.
Onchocerciasis	*Onchocerca volvulus*	Person-to-person by the repeated bites of infected black flies (*Simulium spp.*). **Control**: Mass drug administration	Severe itching, various skin lesions, nodules and blindness.	0.96	Elimination as a public-health and socioeconomic problem.
Trachoma	*Chlamydia trachomatis*	Person-to-person, via direct contact with ocular and nasal discharges from infected individuals, by contact with fomites and, putatively, by eye-seeking flies (e.g., *Musca sorbens*). **Control**: WASH intervention, mass drug administration	Infection is associated with inflammatory changes of the conjunctivae known as "active trachoma." Trachomatous trichiasis, leading to corneal opacification, low vision, and blindness.	0.24	Global elimination of blinding trachoma.
Leprosy	*Mycobacterium leprae*	Via droplets, from the nose and mouth, during close and frequent contacts with untreated cases. **Control**: Intensive disease management	Untreated, leprosy can cause progressive and permanent damage to the skin, nerves, limbs, and eyes.	0.03	Zero disabilities among new pediatric patients and grade-2 disability rate <1 case/million.
Chagas disease	*Trypanosoma cruzi*	Mainly via contact with feces of blood-sucking triatomine bug. Also via blood transfusions, or from a mother to her child during pregnancy. **Control**: Intensive disease management	The acute phases are asymptomatic or have non-specific symptoms. During the chronic phase patients may also be symptom-free but some may progress to clinical forms of the disease (cardiac, digestive, and/or neurological), which can be life threatening if left undiagnosed and untreated.	0.22	Interruption of serological—i.e., transfusion-related transmission.

(*Continued*)

TABLE 23-2 BASICS OF NTDS (*Continued*)

Disease	Causative Agents	Transmission Route and Control Measures	Principal Morbidity	DALYs in 2016 (Millions)[92]	Program Goal (by 2020 Unless Stated)
Human African trypanosomiasis	*T. b. gambiense* (>95% of cases) *T. b. rhodesiense*	Via bites of male and female infected tsetse fly (*Glossina* genus). Mother-to-child, sexual, and accidental laboratory transmission can also occur. **Control**: Intensive disease management and vector control	In the 1st stage, bouts of fever, headaches, joint pains, and itching are the clinical manifestations. In the second stage, changes of behavior, confusion, sensory disturbances, poor coordination, and sleep disturbance. Fatal if untreated.	0.13	Elimination as a public-health problem (<1 case/10,000 persons) in at least 90% of endemic foci and number of cases reported annually reduced below 2000.
Visceral leishmaniasis	*Leishmania donovani* complex in East Africa and the Indian subcontinent and *L. infantum* in Europe, North Africa, and Latin America	Via the bite of infected female phlebotomine sandflies. **Control**: Intensive disease management, vector control	Irregular bouts of fever, substantial weight loss, swelling of the spleen and liver, and anemia. Fatal if untreated.	0.71	Reduction of annual incidence in every sub-district of India to <1 case/10,000 and control in other regions.
Guinea worm	*Dracunculus medinensis*	Ingestion of water contaminated with larvae-infected *Cyclops* spp. (water fleas) **Control**: Intensive disease management, vector control	Severe joint pain during parasite migration and when the worm eventually emerges, intensely painful edema, blister, and an ulcer accompanied by fever, nausea, and vomiting.		Global eradication.

by taxonomically related kinetoplastid protozoan parasites and they can be effectively managed through the primary healthcare system. However, the drugs used for their treatment suffer similar limitations of variable efficacy, toxicity and the need for parenteral administration, and/or lengthy treatment regimens that often require hospitalization.[340] Several simpler, more effective antikinetoplastid drugs are in development.

Infection with *Mycobacterium leprae,* which causes leprosy, is effectively cured using multidrug therapy and the immune-mediated reactions which lead to nerve damage can be managed using oral corticosteroids.

The effective treatment of diseases managed through intensified disease management strategies not only relies on an effective cure, but also correct identification and diagnosis of a case. Diagnosis is typically either clinically based or by use of parasitological and serological tests that require specific laboratory equipment (e.g., ELISA) and have poor sensitivity. In recent years, a range of rapid diagnostic tests (RDTs) have been developed, including immunochromatographic tests using the rK39 antigen for visceral leishmaniasis (VL)[341] and using variant surface glycoprotein antigens for human African trypanosomiasis.[342] Such RDTs have high sensitivity and specificity and can effectively be used at peripheral health centers and during active screening campaigns. However, RDTs are not without their limitations and diagnostic guidelines for intensified disease management diseases can be complex, such that they are not always adhered to during routine clinical practice. There is a need for quality-assurance systems to be in place to guarantee high-quality diagnosis in health facilities and to monitor adherence to diagnostic and treatment guidelines.

The impact of intensified disease management approaches also depends on the effort or effectiveness in finding cases.[343] If there is little effort in finding such cases, then reported diagnoses and cases remain low, but parasite transmission remains unchecked, and the true number of cases is large but unknown. If more effort is placed in case detection, more cases will be found in the first instance, but then eventually transmission will be reduced and the detected and true number of cases will be both low.

Several NTDs are transmitted by vectors and amendable to vector control, which seeks both to reduce the vector populations and to reduce vector-human contact. The principal vector control interventions against NTDs include use of LLINs, indoor residual spraying, and larval source management.[344] The effectiveness of vector control measures depends on the ecology of different vector species and careful attention to the local vector species is required when planning and implementing vector control. Moreover, relying on vector control alone has rarely eliminated transmission of NTDs.

Early onchocerciasis control efforts in West Africa in the 1960s and 1970s were based on insecticide treatment of fast-flowing rivers where the Simuliid blackfly vector breeds. This approach was highly effective, but was expensive, as aircraft were used to deliver the insecticide, and this approach alone was unable to break transmission. Today, onchoceriasis control is mainly based on MDA, but experience in the Americas and select African countries highlight the need for an integrated approach, which includes ground larviciding.

The snail intermediate hosts for schistosomiasis inhabit a variety of water bodies and in specific settings have been effectively controlled with widespread use of molluscicides.[345] However, the range of snail species and the variety of water bodies they prefer, make the large-scale implementation of snail control operationally difficult. An integrated approach of MDA plus with targeted snail control, environmental improvement, and public health education has effectively reduced transmission in China, the Philippines, and Morocco.

Vector control has been a key component of efforts to eliminate human African trypanosomiasis, using trap, and target technologies to control tsetse flies.[346] Indoor residual spraying has contributed to efforts to eliminate VL in India.

In some settings, vector control for other diseases may have resulted in unintended benefits for NTDs. For example, the scale-up of LLINs for malaria control has reduced lymphatic filariasis transmission in several Africa countries, including The Gambia, Kenya, Malawi, and Zambia, where *Anopheles* mosquitoes are the main lymphatic filariasis vector.

Long-term control of soil-transmitted helminths, schistosomiasis, and trachoma requires improvements in WASH in order to break the life cycle of transmission. WASH interventions are diverse, including improved access to water (e.g., water quality and water quantity), sanitation (e.g., access to improved latrines, latrine maintenance, and fecal sludge management), and hygiene practices (e.g., handwashing, soap use, and wearing shoes). Meta-analyses of available data show that WASH access and practices are associated with reduced odds of soil-transmitted helminths, schistosomiasis, and trachoma. However, evidence trial data suggest little or no short-term benefit of WASH intervention on soil-transmitted helminths, schistosomiasis, and trachoma,[347] in part due to low uptake and sustained use of interventions. By contrast, efforts to eradicate Guinea worm have been achieved by implementing preventive measures, focusing on the filtering drinking water and accessing water from improved sources and preventing infected individuals from entering drinking-water sources, supplemented by active surveillance and case containment.[348] Access to WASH services is also critical for management of leprosy and lymphatic filariasis morbidities.

FUTURE DIRECTIONS

Current strategies for the control or elimination of NTDs rely heavily on accurate mapping and surveillance of disease, effective and available drugs for MDA, sensitive field deployable diagnostics, and strong functioning national programs. Improvements in all of these areas are needed to ensure that the morbidity and mortality due to these diseases continues to decline. Given that these diseases affect the most vulnerable populations in the most low-resource settings, the increased attention that these diseases are receiving is welcome. New tools for measuring infection and monitoring control and elimination efforts are being developed. New combinations of therapies are being tested to ensure continued efficacy even if drug resistance becomes an issue and there is a gradual effort to move the global strategy for many of these diseases from control to elimination.

References

1. Dowdle WR. The principles of disease elimination and eradication. *Bull World Health Organ.* 1998;76(Suppl 2):22–5.
2. GBD 2016 Mortality Collaborators. Global, regional, and national under-5 mortality, adult mortality, age-specific mortality, and life expectancy, 1970–2016: A systematic analysis for the Global Burden of Disease Study 2016. *Lancet Lond Engl.* 2017;390(10100):1084–150.
3. Liu L, Oza S, Hogan D, et al. Global, regional, and national causes of child mortality in 2000–13, with projections to inform post-2015 priorities: An updated systematic analysis. *Lancet.* 2015;385:430–40.
4. WHO. The top 10 causes of death. World Health Organization. 2017. http://www.who.int/mediacentre/factsheets/fs310/en/. Accessed December 19, 2017.
5. GBD 2015 Child Mortality Collaborators. Global, regional, national, and selected subnational levels of stillbirths, neonatal, infant, and under-5 mortality, 1980–2015: A systematic analysis for the Global Burden of Disease Study 2015. *Lancet Lond Engl.* 2016;388(10053): 1725–74.
6. UNICEF. Committing to Child Survival: A Promise Renewed. Progress Report 2014. 2014.
7. WHO. Causes of child mortality, 2000–2012. 2012. http://www.who.int/gho/child_health/mortality/mortality_causes_region_text/en/.
8. Centers for Disease Control and Prevention. Morbidity and Mortality Weekly Report (MMWR)—Ten Great Public Health Achievements—Worldwide, 2001–2010. 2011. https://www.cdc.gov/mmwr/preview/mmwrhtml/mm6024a4.htm.
9. United Nations. The Millennium Development Goals Report 2015. http://www.un.org/millenniumgoals/2015_MDG_Report/pdf/MDG%20 2015%20rev%20(July%201).pdf.
10. WHO. Health in 2015: From MDGs, Millennium Development Goals to SDGs, Sustainable Development Goals. 2015. http://apps.who.int/iris/bitstream/10665/200009/1/9789241565110_eng.pdf?ua=1.
11. WHO. Monitoring Health for the SDGs—Chapter 6: SDG Health and Health-Related Targets. 2016. http://www.who.int/gho/publications/world_health_statistics/2016/EN_WHS2016_Chapter6.pdf.
12. Jones KE, Patel NG, Levy MA, et al. Global trends in emerging infectious diseases. *Nature.* 2008;451(7181):990–3.
13. Cao-Lormeau VM, Blake A, Mons S, et al. Guillain-Barre syndrome outbreak associated with Zika virus infection in French Polynesia: A case-control study. *Lancet Lond Engl.* 2016;387(10027):1531–9.
14. WHO. Antibacterial agents in clinical development—An analysis of the antibacterial clinical development pipeline, including tuberculosis. 2017. http://apps.who.int/iris/bitstream/10665/258965/1/WHO-EMP-IAU-2017.11-eng.pdf?ua=1.
15. WHO. Accelerating progress on HIV, tuberculosis, malaria, hepatitis and neglected tropical diseases. A new agenda for 2016–2030. 2015. http://apps.who.int/iris/bitstream/10665/200009/1/9789241565110_eng.pdf?ua=1.
16. Black RE, Victora CG, Walker SP, et al. Maternal and child undernutrition and overweight in low-income and middle-income countries. *Lancet.* 2013;382:427–51.
17. WHO. Malnutrition Fact Sheet. 2017. http://www.who.int/mediacentre/factsheets/malnutrition/en/. Accessed April 18, 2018.
18. Jones KD, Thitiri J, Ngari M, Berkley JA. Childhood malnutrition: Toward an understanding of infections, inflammation, and antimicrobials. *Food Nutr Bull.* 2014;35:S64–70.
19. Prendergast AJ, Humphrey JH. The stunting syndrome in developing countries. *Paediatr Int Child Health.* 2014;34:250–65.
20. Prendergast AJ, Kelly P. Interactions between intestinal pathogens, enteropathy and malnutrition in developing countries. *Curr Opin Infect Dis.* 2016;29(3):229–36.
21. WHO. Guidelines for an Integrate Approach to the Nutritional care of HIV-infected children (6 months–14 years). WHO; 2009.
22. Willumsen J. Nutritional care for HIV-infected children. WHO; 2011. http://www.who.int/elena/titles/bbc/nutrition_hiv_children/en/. Accessed April 18, 2018.
23. UNICEF. Data: Monitoring the Situation of Children and Women. Under-five and infant mortality rates and number of deaths. 2015.
24. World Health Organization. WHO Child Growth Standards and The Identification of Severe Acute Malnutrition in Infants and Children. Geneva: World Health Organization; 2009.
25. Fergusson P, Tomkins A. HIV prevalence and mortality among children undergoing treatment for severe acute malnutrition in sub-Saharan Africa: A systematic review and meta-analysis. *Trans R Soc Trop Med Hyg.* 2009;103:541–8.
26. Hossain M, Chisti MJ, Hossain MI, Mahfuz M, Islam MM, Ahmed T. Efficacy of World Health Organization guideline in facility-based reduction of mortality in severely malnourished children from low and middle income countries: A systematic review and meta-analysis. *J Paediatr Child Health.* 2017;53(5):474–9.
27. Bahwere P, Banda T, Sadler K, et al. Effectiveness of milk whey protein-based ready-to-use therapeutic food in treatment of severe acute malnutrition in Malawian under-5 children: A randomised, double-blind, controlled non-inferiority clinical trial. *Matern Child Nutr.* 2014;10:436–51.
28. Collins S, Dent N, Binns P, Bahwere P, Sadler K, Hallam A. Management of severe acute malnutrition in children. *Lancet.* 2006;368: 1992–2000.
29. Manary MJ, Ndkeha MJ, Ashorn P, Maleta K, Briend A. Home based therapy for severe malnutrition with ready-to-use food. *Arch Child.* 2004;89:557–61.
30. Sandige H, Ndekha MJ, Briend A, Ashorn P, Manary MJ. Home-based treatment of malnourished Malawian children with locally produced or imported ready-to-use food. *J Pediatr Gastroenterol Nutr.* 2004;39:141–6.
31. USAID. Community-based Management of Acute Malnutrition: Technical Brief. 2017. https://www.usaid.gov/what-we-do/global-health/nutrition/technical-areas/community-based-management-acute-malnutrition. Accessed April 18, 2018.
32. UNICEF. *Community-Based Management of Severe Acute Malnutrition : A Joint Statement by the World Health Organization, the World Food Programme, the United Nations System Standing Committee on Nutrition and the United Nations Children's Fund.* Geneva : UNICEF; 2007.
33. Levin C, Brouwer, E. Saving Brains: Literature review of reproductive, neonatal, child and maternal health and nutrition Interventions to mitigate basic risk factors to promote child development. GCC Working Paper Series, GCC 14-08; 2014.

34. International Rescue Committee (IRC). Cost Efficiency Analysis: Treating Severe Acute Malnutrition. 2016.
35. Lydon P, Gandhi G, Vandelaer J, Okwo-Bele JM. Health system cost of delivering routine vaccination in low- and lower-middle income countries: What is needed over the next decade? *Bull World Health Organ.* 2014;92:382–4.
36. UNICEF, Nutrition. Evaluation of Community Management of Acute Malnutrition (CMAM): Global Synthesis Report. 2013.
37. UNICEF. Management of Severe Acute Malnutrition in Children: Working Towards Results At Scale. 2015.
38. Bhutta ZA, Das JK, Rizvi A, et al. Evidence-based interventions for improvement of maternal and child nutrition: What can be done and at what cost? *Lancet.* 2013;382:452–77.
39. World Bank Group. Future of Food: Shaping the Global Food System to Deliver Improved Nutrition and Health. 2016.
40. Kosek MN, Mduma E, Kosek PS, et al. Plasma tryptophan and the kynurenine-tryptophan ratio are associated with the acquisition of statural growth deficits and oral vaccine underperformance in populations with environmental enteropathy. *Am J Trop Med Hyg.* 2016;95(4): 928–37.
41. Awasthi S, Peto R, Read S, et al. Vitamin A supplementation every 6 months with retinol in 1 million pre-school children in north India: DEVTA, a cluster-randomised trial. *Lancet Lond Engl.* 2013;381(9876): 1469–77.
42. Luby SP, Rahman M, Arnold BF, et al. Effects of water quality, sanitation, handwashing, and nutritional interventions on diarrhoea and child growth in rural Bangladesh: A cluster randomised controlled trial. Lancet Glob Health. 2018;6(3):e302–15.
43. Deichsel EL, Tickell KD, Long JE, Jumbe NL, Rowhani-Rahbar A, Walson JL. Challenges in assessing combined interventions to promote linear growth. *Am J Trop Med Hyg.* 2018;98(5):1220–3.
44. Proos LA, Hofvander Y, Wennqvist K, Tuvemo T. A longitudinal study on anthropometric and clinical development of Indian children adopted in Sweden. I. Clinical and anthropometric condition at arrival. *Ups J Med Sci.* 1992;97(1):79–92.
45. Miller BS, Kroupina MG, Mason P, et al. Determinants of catch-up growth in international adoptees from eastern Europe. *Int J Pediatr Endocrinol.* 2010;2010:107252.
46. Becker-Dreps S, Vilchez S, Bucardo F, et al. The association between fecal biomarkers of environmental enteropathy and rotavirus vaccine response in Nicaraguan infants. *Pediatr Infect Dis J.* 2017;36(4):412–6.
47. Parker EP, Ramani S, Lopman BA, et al. Causes of impaired oral vaccine efficacy in developing countries. *Future Microbiol.* 2018;13:97–118.
48. Katona P, Katona-Apte J. The interaction between nutrition and infection. *Clin Infect Dis.* 2008;46(10):1582–8.
49. Darton-Hill I. Zinc Supplementation and growth in children. WHO; 2013. http://www.who.int/elena/bbc/zinc_stunting/en/. Accessed April 18, 2018.
50. Mayo-Wilson E, Imdad A, Herzer K, Yakoob MY, Bhutta ZA. Vitamin A supplements for preventing mortality, illness, and blindness in children aged under 5: Systematic review and meta-analysis. *BMJ.* 2011;343:d5094.
51. Imdad A, Mayo-Wilson E, Herzer K, Bhutta ZA. Vitamin A supplementation for preventing morbidity and mortality in children from six months to five years of age. *Cochrane Database Syst Rev.* 2017 11;3:CD008524.
52. WHO. Vitamin A Supplementation in Infants and Children 6–59 Months of Age. World Health Organization; 2011.
53. UNICEF. Monitoring the Situation of Children and Women: Vitamin A Deficiency. 2018. https://data.unicef.org/topic/nutrition/vitamin-a-deficiency/. Accessed April 18, 2018.
54. Wirth JP, Petry N, Tanumihardjo SA, et al. Vitamin A supplementation programs and country-level evidence of vitamin A deficiency. *Nutrients.* 2017;9(3).
55. Lazzerini M, Ronfani L. Oral zinc for treating diarrhoea in children. *Cochrane Database Syst Rev.* 2013;(1):CD005436.
56. Lamberti LM, Walker CLF, Chan KY, Jian W-Y, Black RE. Oral zinc supplementation for the treatment of acute diarrhea in children: A systematic review and meta-analysis. *Nutrients.* 2013;5(11):4715–40.
57. WHO. Treatment of Diarrhoea: A manual for physicians and other senior health workers. 2007.
58. Unger CC, Salam SS, Sarker MSA, Black R, Cravioto A, El Arifeen S. Treating diarrhoeal disease in children under five: The global picture. *Arch Dis Child.* 2014;99(3):273–8.
59. Cutler D, Miller G. The role of public health improvements in health advances: The twentieth-century United States. *Demography.* 2005;42(1):1–22.
60. Sochan G. Making the city inhabitable: London's sewer system. *Humanit Technol Rev.* 2007;26:27–48.
61. Lee EJ, Schwab KJ. Deficiencies in drinking water distribution systems in developing countries. *J Water Health.* 2005;3(2):109–27.
62. McIntosh AC. Asian water supplies reaching the urban poor: Asian Development Bank and International Water Association; 2003.
63. González-Gómez F, García-Rubio M, Guardiola J. Why is non-revenue water so high in so many cities? *Int J Water Resour Dev.* 2011;27:345–60.
64. Kumpel E, Nelson KL. Comparing microbial water quality in an intermittent and continuous piped water supply. *Water Res.* 2013;47(14): 5176–88.
65. Wade R. The market for public office: Why the Indian state is not better at development. *World Dev.* 1985;13:467–97.
66. Killingsworth JR, Hossain N, Hedrick-Wong Y, Thomas SD, Rahman A, Begum T. Unofficial fees in Bangladesh: Price, equity and institutional issues. *Health Policy Plan.* 1999;14(2):152–63.
67. Davis J. Corruption in public service delivery: Experience from South Asia's water and sanitation sector. *World Dev.* 2004;32:53–71.
68. Hackenbroch K, Hossain S. "The organised encroachment of the powerful"—Everyday practices of public space and water supply in Dhaka, Bangladesh. *Environ Urban.* 2013;25:209–24.
69. Hossain S. The informal practice of appropriation and social control—Experience from a bosti in Dhaka. *Environ Urban.* 2013;25:195–216.
70. Hoornweg D, Pope K. Population predictions for the world's largest cities in the 21st century. *Environ Urban.* 2017;29:195–216.
71. Briscoe J, Qamar U. Pakistan's water economy: running dry. Oxford University Press; 2006.
72. Hoque M, Hoque M, Ahmed K. Declining groundwater level and aquifer dewatering in Dhaka metropolitan area, Bangladesh: Causes and quantification. *Hydrogeol J.* 2007;15:1523–34.
73. Rodell M, Velicogna I, Famiglietti JS. Satellite-based estimates of groundwater depletion in India. *Nature.* 2009;460(7258):999–1002.
74. Srinivasan V, Seto K, Emerson R, Gorelick S. The impact of urbanization on water vulnerability: A coupled human–environment system approach for Chennai, India. *Glob Environ Change.* 2013;23:229–39.
75. World Economic Forum Water Initiative. Water security: The water-food-energy-climate nexus. 2012.
76. Tilmans S, Russel K, Sklar R, Page L, Kramer S, Davis J. Container-based sanitation: Assessing costs and effectiveness of excreta management in Cap Haitien, Haiti. *Environ Urban.* 2015;27:89–104.
77. Winbald U. Towards an ecological approach to sanitation: Swedish International Development Cooperation Agency (SIDA). 1997.
78. Sorenson SB, Morssink C, Campos PA. Safe access to safe water in low income countries: Water fetching in current times. *Soc Sci Med.* 2011;72(9):1522–6.
79. Pickering AJ, Davis J. Freshwater availability and water fetching distance affect child health in sub-Saharan Africa. *Environ Sci Technol.* 2012;46(4):2391–7.
80. Bain R, Cronk R, Hossain R, et al. Global assessment of exposure to faecal contamination through drinking water based on a systematic review. *Trop Med Int Health TM IH.* 2014;19(8):917–27.
81. Wright J, Gundry S, Conroy R. Household drinking water in developing countries: A systematic review of microbiological contamination between source and point-of-use. *Trop Med Int Health TM IH.* 2004;9(1):106–17.
82. Lantagne D, Quick R, Mintz E. Household Water Treatment and Safe: Storage Options in Developing Countries. Woodrow Wilson International Center for Scholars; 2006.
83. Rosa G, Clasen T. Estimating the scope of household water treatment in low- and medium-income countries. *Am J Trop Med Hyg.* 2010;82(2):289–300.
84. Thye Y, Templeton MR, Ali M. A critical review of technologies for pit latrine emptying in developing countries. *Crit Rev Environ Sci Technol.* 2011;41:1793–819.
85. Sato T, Qadir M, Yamamoto S, Endo T, Zahoor A. Global, regional, and country level need for data on wastewater generation, treatment, and use. *Agric Water Manag.* 2013;130:1–13.
86. Peal A, Evans B, Blackett I, Hawkins P, Heymans C. Fecal sludge management: A comparative analysis of 12 cities. *J Water Sanit Hyg Dev.* 2014;4:563–75.
87. SHINE Sanitation, Hygiene, Infant Nutrition Efficacy Project (SHINE, NCT01824940). 2018. https://clinicaltrials.gov/ct2/show/NCT01824940.
88. Luby SP, Rahman M, Arnold BF, et al. Effects of water quality, sanitation, handwashing, and nutritional interventions on diarrhoea and

child growth in rural Bangladesh: A cluster randomised controlled trial. *Lancet Glob Health*. 2018;6(3):e302–15.

89. Null C, Stewart CP, Pickering AJ, et al. Effects of water quality, sanitation, handwashing, and nutritional interventions on diarrhoea and child growth in rural Kenya: A cluster-randomised controlled trial. *Lancet Glob Health*. 2018;6(3):e316–29.
90. Victora CG, Wagstaff A, Schellenberg JA, Gwatkin D, Claeson M, Habicht J-P. Applying an equity lens to child health and mortality: More of the same is not enough. *Lancet Lond Engl*. 2003;362(9379):233–41.
91. Ram PK, Choi M, Blum LS, Wamae AW, Mintz ED, Bartlett AV. Declines in case management of diarrhoea among children less than five years old. *Bull World Health Organ*. 2008;86(3):E–F.
92. GBD 2016 Causes of Death Collaborators. Global, regional, and national age-sex specific mortality for 264 causes of death, 1980–2016: A systematic analysis for the Global Burden of Disease Study 2016. *Lancet Lond Engl*. 2017;390(10100):1151–210.
93. Walker CLF, Rudan I, Liu L, et al. Global burden of childhood pneumonia and diarrhoea. *Lancet Lond Engl*. 2013;381(9875):1405–16.
94. Stevens GA, Finucane MM, Paciorek CJ, et al. Trends in mild, moderate, and severe stunting and underweight, and progress towards MDG 1 in 141 developing countries: A systematic analysis of population representative data. *Lancet Lond Engl*. 2012;380(9844):824–34.
95. Yoshida N, Uematsu H, Sobrado C. Is extreme poverty going to end? An analytical framework to evaluate progress in ending extreme poverty. *Policy Research Working Paper*. Washington, DC: World Bank; 2014.
96. Chen S, Ravallion M. Absolute poverty measures for the developing world, 1981–2004. *Proc Natl Acad Sci U S A*. 2007;104(43):16757–62.
97. WHO. Progress on sanitation and drinking water: 2015 update and MDG assessment: 2015.
98. Garces AL, McClure EM, Perez W, et al. The Global Network Neonatal Cause of Death algorithm for low-resource settings. *Acta Paediatr*. 2017;106(6):904–11.
99. Polin RA, Watterberg K, Benitz W, Eichenwald E. The conundrum of early-onset sepsis. *Pediatrics*. 2014;133(6):1122–3.
100. Bhutta ZA, Das JK, Bahl R, et al. Can available interventions end preventable deaths in mothers, newborn babies, and stillbirths, and at what cost? *Lancet Lond Engl*. 2014;384(9940):347–70.
101. Lawn JE, Blencowe H, Oza S, et al. Every newborn: Progress, priorities, and potential beyond survival. *Lancet Lond Engl*. 2014;384(9938): 189–205.
102. WHO. WHO Recommendations on antenatal care for a positive pregnancy experience. 2016.
103. Demicheli V, Barale A, Rivetti A. Vaccines for women for preventing neonatal tetanus. *Cochrane Database Syst Rev*. 2015;(7):CD002959.
104. WHO. Guidelines on Syphilis Screening and Treatment for Pregnant Women. 2017.
105. WHO. Guidelines on Treatment of *Chlamydia Trachomatis*. 2016.
106. WHO. WHO guidelines for the treatment of *Neisseria gonorrhoeae*. 2016.
107. Lassi ZS, Mansoor T, Salam RA, Das JK, Bhutta ZA. Essential pre-pregnancy and pregnancy interventions for improved maternal, newborn and child health. *Reprod Health*. 2014;11(Suppl 1):S2.
108. Tudor Car L, van-Velthoven MH, Brusamento S, et al. Integrating prevention of mother-to-child HIV transmission (PMTCT) programmes with other health services for preventing HIV infection and improving HIV outcomes in developing countries. *Cochrane Database Syst Rev*. 2011;(6):CD008741.
109. WHO. WHO recommendations for prevention and treatment of maternal peripartum infections. 2015.
110. Johri AK, Lata H, Yadav P, et al. Epidemiology of group B Streptococcus in developing countries. *Vaccine*. 2013;31(Suppl 4):D43–45.
111. Le Doare K, Heath PT. An overview of global GBS epidemiology. *Vaccine*. 2013;31(Suppl 4):D7–12.
112. Melin P, Efstratiou A. Group B streptococcal epidemiology and vaccine needs in developed countries. *Vaccine*. 2013;31(Suppl 4):D31–42.
113. Sinha A, Russell LB, Tomczyk S, et al. Disease burden of group B Streptococcus among infants in sub-Saharan Africa: A systematic literature review and meta-analysis. *Pediatr Infect Dis J*. 2016;35(9):933–42.
114. Cools P, Jespers V, Hardy L, et al. A multi-country cross-sectional study of vaginal carriage of group B Streptococci (GBS) and *Escherichia coli* in resource-poor settings: Prevalences and risk factors. *PLoS One*. 2016;11(1):e0148052.
115. Seale AC, Bianchi-Jassir F, Russell NJ, et al. Estimates of the burden of group B streptococcal disease worldwide for pregnant women, stillbirths, and children. *Clin Infect Dis*. 2017;65(suppl_2):S200–19.
116. Schrag SJ, Verani JR. Intrapartum antibiotic prophylaxis for the prevention of perinatal group B streptococcal disease: Experience in the United States and implications for a potential group B streptococcal vaccine. *Vaccine*. 2013;31(Suppl 4):D20–26.
117. Verani J, McGee L, Schrag S, Division of Bacterial Diseases NCflaRD Centers for Disease Control (CDC). Prevention of perinatal group B streptococcal disease—Revised guidelines from CDC. *MMWR Recomm Rep*. 2010;59(RR-10):1–36.
118. Weston EJ, Pondo T, Lewis MM, et al. The burden of invasive early-onset neonatal sepsis in the United States. *Pediatr Infect Dis J*. 2011;30(11): 937–41.
119. Cagno CK, Pettit JM, Weiss BD. Prevention of perinatal group B streptococcal disease: Updated CDC guideline. *Am Fam Physician*. 2012;86(1): 59–65.
120. Blencowe H, Cousens S, Mullany LC, et al. Clean birth and postnatal care practices to reduce neonatal deaths from sepsis and tetanus: A systematic review and Delphi estimation of mortality effect. *BMC Public Health*. 2011;11(Suppl 3):S11.
121. WHO. WHO Safe Childbirth Checklist Implementation Guide: Improving the quality of facility-based delivery for mothers and newborns. 2015.
122. WHO. WHO Recommendations on postnatal care of the mother and newborn. 2013.
123. Narayanan I, Litch JA, Ram P. Safe and effective infection prevention for inpatient care of newborns. In: Litch JA, Robb-McCord J, Kak L, eds. *Do No Harm Technical Brief Series*. USAID, PCI, Global Alliance to Prevent Prematurity and Stillbirth, American College of Nurse-Midwives; 2017. http://www.everypreemie.org/wpcontent/uploads/2017/06/InfectionPrevention_6.14.17.pdf.
124. WHO. Integrated Management of Pregnancy and Childbirth: Pregnancy, Childbirth, Postpartum and Newborn Care: A Guide for Essential Practice. 2015.
125. WHO. Guidelines on Maternal, Newborn, Child and Adolescent Health: Recommendations on newborn health. 2013.
126. WHO. Standards for Improving Quality of Maternal and Newborn Care in Health Facilities. 2016.
127. WHO. WHO Recommendations on Interventions to Improve Preterm Birth Outcomes. 2015.
128. Salam RA, Mansoor T, Mallick D, Lassi ZS, Das JK, Bhutta ZA. Essential childbirth and postnatal interventions for improved maternal and neonatal health. *Reprod Health*. 2014;11(Suppl 1):S3.
129. WHO. WHO Recommendations on Postnatal Care of the Mother and Newborn. 2013.
130. WHO. Integrated Management of Pregnancy and Childbirth: Pregnancy, Childbirth, Postpartum and Newborn Care: A Guide for Essential Practice. 2015.
131. Polin RA. Management of neonates with suspected or proven early-onset bacterial sepsis. *Pediatrics*. 2012;129(5):1006–15.
132. WHO. Recommendations for Management of Common Childhood Conditions: Evidence for Technical Update of Pocket Book Recommendations: Newborn Conditions, Dysentery, Pneumonia, Oxygen Use and Delivery, Common Causes of Fever, Severe Acute Malnutrition and Supportive Care. 2012.
133. Carstens LE, Westerbeek EAM, van Zwol A, van Elburg RM. Neonatal antibiotics in preterm infants and allergic disorders later in life. *Pediatr Allergy Immunol*. 2016;27(7):759–64.
134. Pitter G, Ludvigsson JF, Romor P, et al. Antibiotic exposure in the first year of life and later treated asthma, a population based birth cohort study of 143,000 children. *Eur J Epidemiol*. 2016;31(1):85–94.
135. Hirsch AG, Pollak J, Glass TA, et al. Early-life antibiotic use and subsequent diagnosis of food allergy and allergic diseases. *Clin Exp Allergy J Br Soc Allergy Clin Immunol*. 2017;47(2):236–44.
136. Simioni J, Hutton EK, Gunn E, et al. A comparison of intestinal microbiota in a population of low-risk infants exposed and not exposed to intrapartum antibiotics: The Baby & Microbiota of the Intestine cohort study protocol. *BMC Pediatr*. 2016;16(1):183.
137. Meropol SB, Edwards A. Development of the infant intestinal microbiome: A bird's eye view of a complex process. *Birth Defects Res Part C Embryo Today Rev*. 2015;105(4):228–39.
138. Storr J, Twyman A, Zingg W, et al. Core components for effective infection prevention and control programmes: New WHO evidence-based recommendations. *Antimicrob Resist Infect Control*. 2017;6:6.
139. Sangkomkamhang US, Lumbiganon P, Prasertcharoensuk W, Laopaiboon M. Antenatal lower genital tract infection screening and treatment programs for preventing preterm delivery. *Cochrane Database Syst Rev*. 2015;(2):CD006178.

140. WHO. Integrated Management of Childhood Illness Chart Booklet. Module 2: The sick young infant. 2014.

141. World Health Organization. *Pocket Book of Hospital Care for Children: Guidelines for the Management of Common Childhood Illnesses*. 2nd ed. Geneva: World Health Organization; 2013.

142. WHO. Guideline: Managing possible serious bacterial infection in young infants when referral is not feasible. 2015.

143. Kim S-Y, Russell LB, Park J, et al. Cost-effectiveness of a potential group B streptococcal vaccine program for pregnant women in South Africa. *Vaccine*. 2014;32(17):1954–63.

144. Pammi M, Suresh G. Enteral lactoferrin supplementation for prevention of sepsis and necrotizing enterocolitis in preterm infants. *Cochrane Database Syst Rev*. 2017;6:CD007137.

145. Dermyshi E, Wang Y, Yan C, et al. The "Golden Age" of probiotics: A systematic review and meta-analysis of randomized and observational studies in preterm infants. *Neonatology.* 2017;112(1):9–23.

146. Cleminson J, McGuire W. Topical emollient for preventing infection in preterm infants. *Cochrane Database Syst Rev*. 2016;(1):CD001150.

147. Institute for Health Metrics and Evaluation. Global Burden of Disease Results Tool. http://ghdx.healthdata.org/gbd-results-tool. Accessed May 1, 2018.

148. Bhutta ZA, Das JK, Walker N, et al. Interventions to address deaths from childhood pneumonia and diarrhoea equitably: What works and at what cost? *Lancet Lond Engl*. 2013;381(9875):1417–29.

149. WHO . Ending Preventable Child Deaths from Pneumonia and Diarrhoea by 2025: The integrated Global Action Plan for Pneumoina and Diarrhoea (GAPPD). WHO/UNICEF; 2013.

150. Nair H, Simões EAF, Rudan I, et al. Global and regional burden of hospital admissions for severe acute lower respiratory infections in young children in 2010: A systematic analysis. *Lancet Lond Engl*. 2013;381(9875):1380–90.

151. Zaidi AKM, Ganatra HA, Syed S, et al. Effect of case management on neonatal mortality due to sepsis and pneumonia. *BMC Public Health*. 2011;11(Suppl 3):S13.

152. Theodoratou E, Al-Jilaihawi S, Woodward F, et al. The effect of case management on childhood pneumonia mortality in developing countries. *Int J Epidemiol*. 2010;39(Suppl 1):i155–71.

153. WHO. Immunization Coverage: Key Facts. WHO; 2018. http://www.who.int/en/news-room/fact-sheets/detail/immunization-coverage. Accessed April 30, 2018.

154. Hirve S. Seasonal Influenza Vaccine Use in Low and Middle Income Countries in the Tropics and Subtropics: A systematic review. WHO. 2015.

155. WHO. Immunization Coverage Fact Sheet. 2017.

156. CDC. Tdap Effectiveness for Infant if Mother Vaccinated during Pregnancy. CDC; 2017. https://www.cdc.gov/pertussis/pregnant/hcp/vaccine-effectiveness.html. Accessed April 30, 2018.

157. Sobanjo-Ter Meulen A, Duclos P, McIntyre P, et al. Assessing the evidence for maternal pertussis immunization: A report from the Bill & Melinda Gates Foundation Symposium on pertussis infant disease burden in low- and lower-middle-income countries. *Clin Infect Dis*. 2016;63(suppl 4):S123–33.

158. WHO. Household air pollution and health: Key facts. 2018. http://www.who.int/mediacentre/factsheets/fs292/en/ Accessed April 30, 2018.

159. WHO. Ambient air pollution: Policy and progress. http://www.who.int/airpollution/ambient/policy-governance/en/. Accessed April 30, 2018.

160. Gordon SB, Bruce NG, Grigg J, et al. Respiratory risks from household air pollution in low and middle income countries. *Lancet Respir Med*. 2014;2(10):823–60.

161. Smith KR, Samet JM, Romieu I, Bruce N. Indoor air pollution in developing countries and acute lower respiratory infections in children. *Thorax*. 2000;55(6):518–32.

162. Smith KR, McCracken JP, Weber MW, et al. Effect of reduction in household air pollution on childhood pneumonia in Guatemala (RESPIRE): A randomised controlled trial. *Lancet Lond Engl*. 2011;378(9804): 1717–26.

163. Quansah R, Semple S, Ochieng CA, et al. Effectiveness of interventions to reduce household air pollution and/or improve health in homes using solid fuel in low- and middle-income countries: A systematic review and meta-analysis. *Environ Int*. 2017;103:73–90.

164. Mortimer K, Ndamala CB, Naunje AW, et al. A cleaner burning biomass-fueled cookstove intervention to prevent pneumonia in children under 5 years old in rural Malawi (the Cooking and Pneumonia Study): A cluster randomised controlled trial. *Lancet Lond Engl*. 2017 14;389(10065):167–75.

165. Nhung NTT, Amini H, Schindler C, et al. Short-term association between ambient air pollution and pneumonia in children: A systematic review and meta-analysis of time-series and case-crossover studies. *Environ Pollut*. 2017;230:1000–8.

166. Nhung NTT, Schindler C, Dien TM, Probst-Hensch N, Perez L, Künzli N. Acute effects of ambient air pollution on lower respiratory infections in Hanoi children: An eight-year time series study. *Environ Int*. 2018;110:139–48.

167. WHO. Ambient air pollution: A global assessment of exposure and burden of disease. WHO; 2016.

168. Gavi. The Vaccine Alliance. Pneumococcal vaccine support. GAVI; 2018. https://www.gavi.org/support/nvs/pneumococcal/.

169 GBD 2016 Causes of Death Collaborators. Global, regional, and national age-sex specific mortality for 264 causes of death, 1980–2016: A systematic analysis for the Global Burden of Disease Study 2016. *Lancet*. 2017;390(10100):1151–210.

170. Kotloff KL, Nataro JP, Blackwelder WC, et al. Burden and aetiology of diarrhoeal disease in infants and young children in developing countries (the Global Enteric Multicenter Study, GEMS): A prospective, case-control study. *Lancet*. 2013;382(9888):209–22.

171. GBD 2016 Disease and Injury Incidence and Prevalence Collaborators. Global, regional, and national incidence, prevalence, and years lived with disability for 328 diseases and injuries for 195 countries, 1990–2016: A systematic analysis for the Global Burden of Disease Study 2016. *Lancet*. 2017;390(10100):1211–59.

172. Antillón M, Warren JL, Crawford FW, et al. The burden of typhoid fever in low- and middle-income countries: A meta-regression approach. Carvalho MS, ed. *PLoS Negl Trop Dis*. 2017;11(2):e0005376.

173. Azmatullah A, Qamar FN, Thaver D, Zaidi AK, Bhutta ZA. Systematic review of the global epidemiology, clinical and laboratory profile of enteric fever. *J Glob Health*. 2015;5(2):020407.

174. Britto C, Pollard AJ, Voysey M, Blohmke CJ. An appraisal of the clinical features of pediatric enteric fever: Systematic review and meta-analysis of the age-stratified disease occurrence. *Clin Infect Dis*. 2017;64(11):1604–11.

175. Crump JA, Sjölund-Karlsson M, Gordon MA, Parry CM. Epidemiology, clinical presentation, laboratory diagnosis, antimicrobial resistance, and antimicrobial management of invasive Salmonella infections. *Clin Microbiol Rev*. 2015;28(4):901–37.

176. WHO. Ending preventable deaths from pneumonia and diarrhoea by 2025. 2013. http://www.who.int/maternal_child_adolescent/news_.

177. WHO Recommendations on Newborn Health. 2017.

178. WHO Recommendations on Child Health. 2017.

179. WHO Recommendations on Adolescent Health. 2017.

180. Das JK, Salam RA, Bhutta ZA. Global burden of childhood diarrhea and interventions. *Curr Opin Infect Dis*. 2014;27(5):451–8.

181. Imdad A, Mayo-Wilson E, Herzer K, Bhutta ZA. Vitamin A supplementation for preventing morbidity and mortality in children from 6 months to 5 years of age. *Cochrane Database Syst Rev*. 2017;12(3):CD008524.

182. Lamberti LM, Fischer Walker CL, Noiman A, Victora C, Black RE. Breastfeeding and the risk for diarrhea morbidity and mortality. *BMC Public Health*. 2011;11(Suppl 3):S15.

183. Cacho NT, Lawrence RM. Innate immunity and breast milk. *Front Immunol*. 2017;8:584.

184. Bäckhed F, Roswall J, Peng Y, et al. Dynamics and stabilization of the human gut microbiome during the first year of life. *Cell Host Microbe*. 2015;17(6):852.

185. WHO. Postnatal care of the mother and newborn 2013. World Health Organization. 2013.

186. Haroon S, Das JK, Salam RA, Imdad A, Bhutta ZA. Breastfeeding promotion interventions and breastfeeding practices: A systematic review. *BMC Public Health*. 2013;13(Suppl 3):S20.

187. Darvesh N, Das JK, Vaivada T, et al. Water, sanitation and hygiene interventions for acute childhood diarrhea: A systematic review to provide estimates for the Lives Saved Tool. *BMC Public Health*. 2017;17(S4):776.

188. Freeman MC, Garn JV, Sclar GD, et al. The impact of sanitation on infectious disease and nutritional status: A systematic review and meta-analysis. *Int J Hyg Environ Health*. 2017;220(6):928–49.

189. Clasen TF, Alexander KT, Sinclair D, et al. Interventions to improve water quality for preventing diarrhoea. *Cochrane Database Syst Rev*. 2015;(10):CD004794.

190. Han AM, Hlaing T. Prevention of diarrhoea and dysentery by hand washing. *Trans R Soc Trop Med Hyg*. 83(1):128–31.

191. Sircar BK, Sengupta PG, Mondal SK, et al. Effect of handwashing on the incidence of diarrhoea in a Calcutta slum. *J Diarrhoeal Dis Res.* 1987;5(2):112–4.
192. Luby SP, Agboatwalla M, Painter J, Altaf A, Billhimer WL, Hoekstra RM. Effect of intensive handwashing promotion on childhood diarrhea in high-risk communities in Pakistan: A randomized controlled trial. *JAMA.* 2004;291(21):2547–54.
193. Watson JA, Ensink JHJ, Ramos M, et al. Does targeting children with hygiene promotion messages work? The effect of handwashing promotion targeted at children, on diarrhoea, soil-transmitted helminth infections and behaviour change, in low- and middle-income countries. *Trop Med Int Health.* 2017;22(5):526–38.
194. Nicholson JA, Naeeni M, Hoptroff M, et al. An investigation of the effects of a hand washing intervention on health outcomes and school absence using a randomised trial in Indian urban communities. *Trop Med Int Health TM IH.* 2014;19(3):284–92.
195. Bieri FA, Gray DJ, Williams GM, et al. Health-education package to prevent worm infections in Chinese schoolchildren. *N Engl J Med.* 2013;368(17):1603–12.
196. Al-Delaimy AK, Al-Mekhlafi HM, Lim YAL, et al. Developing and evaluating health education learning package (HELP) to control soil-transmitted helminth infections among Orang Asli children in Malaysia. *Parasit Vectors.* 2014;7(1):416.
197. Pickering AJ, Davis J, Blum AG, et al. Access to waterless hand sanitizer improves student hand hygiene behavior in primary schools in Nairobi, Kenya. *Am J Trop Med Hyg.* 2013;89(3):411–8.
198. World Health Organization. The Immunological Basis for Immunization Series. Immun Vaccines Biol. Geneva, Switzerland: WHO; 2018
199. Bawankule R, Singh A, Kumar K, Shetye S. Does measles vaccination reduce the risk of acute respiratory infection (ARI) and diarrhea in children: A multi-country study? *PLoS One.* 2017;12(1):1–17.
200. UNICEF/WHO. Diarrhoea: Why children are still dying and what can be done. 2009.
201. Munos MK, Walker CLF, Black RE. The effect of oral rehydration solution and recommended home fluids on diarrhoea mortality. *Int J Epidemiol.* 2010;39(Suppl_1):i75–87.
202. CHOICE Study Group. Multicenter, randomized, double-blind clinical trial to evaluate the efficacy and safety of a reduced osmolarity oral rehydration salts solution in children with acute watery diarrhea. *Pediatrics.* 2001;107(4):613–8.
203. WHO. Pocket Book of Hospital Care for Children: Guidelines for the Management of Common Childhood Illnesses. 2013.
204. WHO IMCI. Integrated Management of Childhood Illness (IMCI) Chart Booklet. Distance Learn Course. 2014;(March):1–76.
205. Lazzerini M, Wanzira H. Oral zinc for treating diarrhoea in children (review). *Cochrane Database Syst Rev.* 2016;(12):CD005436.
206. Shankar AH, Prasad AS. Zinc and immune function: The biological basis of altered resistance to infection. *Am J Clin Nutr.* 1998;68(2 Suppl):447S-63S.
207. Lenters LM, Das JK, Bhutta ZA. Systematic review of strategies to increase use of oral rehydration solution at the household level. *BMC Public Health.* 2013;13(Suppl 3):S28.
208. World Health Organization. *Global Action Plan on Antimicrobial Resistance.* Geneva: WHO Press; 2015, pp. 1–28.
209. Weekly epidemiological record Relevé épidémiologique hebdomadaire. 2017.
210. Fischer Walker CL, Fontaine O, Black RE. Measuring coverage in MNCH: Current indicators for measuring coverage of diarrhea treatment interventions and opportunities for improvement. *PLoS Med.* 2013;10(5):1–6.
211. WHO. World Malaria Report 2017. 2017.
212. WHO. Global Technical Strategy for Malaria 2016–2030. 2015.
213. Bhatt S, Weiss D, Cameron E, et al. The effect of malaria control on *Plasmodium falciparum* in Africa between 2000 and 2015. *Nature.* 2015;526(7572):207–11.
214. Andrews KG, Lynch M, Eckert E, Gutman J. Missed opportunities to deliver intermittent preventive treatment for malaria to pregnant women 2003–2013: A systematic analysis of 58 household surveys in sub-Saharan Africa. *Malar J.* 2015;14:521.
215. Desai M, Gutman J, Taylor SM, et al. Impact of sulfadoxine-pyrimethamine resistance on effectiveness of intermittent preventive therapy for malaria in pregnancy at clearing infections and preventing low birth weight. *Clin Infect Dis.* 2016;62(3):323–33.
216. Thiam S, Kimotho V, Gatonga P. Why are IPTp coverage targets so elusive in sub-Saharan Africa? A systematic review of health system barriers. *Malar J.* 2013;12:353.
217. WHO. Key Points: World Malaria Report 2017. 2017.
218. Imwong M, Hien TT, Thuy-Nhien NT, Dondorp AM, White NJ. Spread of a single multidrug resistant malaria parasite lineage (PfPailin) to Vietnam. *Lancet Infect Dis.* 2017;17(10):1022–3.
219. WHO. Minutes of the Evidence Review Group meeting on the emergence and spread of multidrug-resistant *Plasmodium falciparum* lineages in the Greater Mekong subregion. 2016.
220. Nkumama IN, O'Meara WP, Osier FHA. Changes in malaria epidemiology in Africa and new challenges for elimination. *Trends Parasitol.* 2017;33(2):128–40.
221. Howes RE, Piel FB, Patil AP, et al. G6PD deficiency prevalence and estimates of affected populations in malaria endemic countries: A geostatistical model-based map. *PLoS Med.* 2012;9(11):e1001339.
222. UNAIDS. 90-90-90: An Ambitious treatment target to help end the AIDS epidemic. UNAIDS; 2017.
223. WHO. HIV/AIDS Factsheet. 2017. http://www.who.int/mediacentre/factsheets/fs360/en/.
224. WHO, UNICEF. Global HIV/AIDS Response, epidemic update and health sector progress towards Universal Access, Progress Report. 2011.
225. UNICEF. Children and AIDS, Fifth Taking Stock Report. 2010.
226. UNAIDS. Ending AIDS. Progress towards the 90-90-90 targets. 2017.
227. Gardner EM, McLees MP, Steiner JF, Del Rio C, Burman WJ. The spectrum of engagement in HIV care and its relevance to test-and-treat strategies for prevention of HIV infection. *Clin Infect Dis.* 2011;52(6):793–800.
228. McNairy ML, El-Sadr WM. The HIV care continuum: No partial credit given. *AIDS Lond Engl.* 2012;26(14):1735–8.
229. Barker PM, Mphatswe W, Rollins N. Antiretroviral drugs in the cupboard are not enough: The impact of health systems' performance on mother-to-child transmission of HIV. *J Acquir Immune Defic Syndr.* 2011;56(2):e45–8.
230. Dalal S, Lee C, Farirai T, et al. Provider-initiated HIV testing and counseling: Increased uptake in two public community health centers in South Africa and implications for scale-up. *PLoS One.* 2011;6(11):e27293.
231. Kharsany ABM, Karim QA, Karim SSA. Uptake of provider-initiated HIV testing and counseling among women attending an urban sexually transmitted disease clinic in South Africa—Missed opportunities for early diagnosis of HIV infection. *AIDS Care.* 2010;22(5):533–7.
232. Kennedy CE, Fonner VA, Sweat MD, Okero FA, Baggaley R, O'Reilly KR. Provider-initiated HIV testing and counseling in low- and middle-income countries: A systematic review. *AIDS Behav.* 2013;17(5):1571–90.
233. Yotebieng M, Wenzi LK, Basaki E, et al. Provider-initiated HIV testing and counseling among patients with presumptive tuberculosis in Democratic Republic of Congo. *Pan Afr Med J.* 2016;25:161.
234. WHO. Guideline on When to Start Antiretroviral Therapy and on Pre-Exposure Prophylaxis for HIV. 2015.
235. Genberg BL, Naanyu V, Wachira J, et al. Linkage to and engagement in HIV care in western Kenya: An observational study using population-based estimates from home-based counselling and testing. *Lancet HIV.* 2015;2(1):e20–6.
236. Musheke M, Ntalasha H, Gari S, et al. A systematic review of qualitative findings on factors enabling and deterring uptake of HIV testing in Sub-Saharan Africa. *BMC Public Health.* 2013;13:220.
237. Sekandi JN, Sempeera H, List J, et al. High acceptance of home-based HIV counseling and testing in an urban community setting in Uganda. *BMC Public Health.* 2011;11:730.
238. Lugada E, Millar D, Haskew J, et al. Rapid implementation of an integrated large-scale HIV counseling and testing, malaria, and diarrhea prevention campaign in rural Kenya. *PLoS One.* 2010;5(8):e12435.
239. Chamie G, Kwarisiima D, Clark TD, et al. Uptake of community-based HIV testing during a multi-disease health campaign in rural Uganda. *PLoS One.* 2014;9(1):e84317.
240. Coates TJ, Kulich M, Celentano DD, et al. Effect of community-based voluntary counselling and testing on HIV incidence and social and behavioural outcomes (NIMH Project Accept; HPTN 043): A cluster-randomised trial. *Lancet Glob Health.* 2014;2(5):e267–77.
241. Rosenberg NE, Westreich D, Barnighausen T, et al. Assessing the effect of HIV counselling and testing on HIV acquisition among South African youth. *AIDS Lond Engl.* 2013;27(17):2765–73.
242. Mine M, Chishala S, Makhaola K, Tafuma TA, Bolebantswe J, Merrigan MB. Performance of rapid HIV testing by lay counselors in the field during the behavioral and biological surveillance survey among female sex workers and men who have sex with men in Botswana. *J Acquir Immune Defic Syndr.* 2015;68(3):365–8.

243. Helleringer S, Kohler H-P, Frimpong JA, Mkandawire J. Increasing uptake of HIV testing and counseling among the poorest in sub-Saharan countries through home-based service provision. *J Acquir Immune Defic Syndr.* 2009;51(2):185–93.

244. Tumwebaze H, Tumwesigye E, Baeten JM, et al. Household-based HIV counseling and testing as a platform for referral to HIV care and medical male circumcision in Uganda: A pilot evaluation. *PLoS One.* 2012;7(12):e51620.

245. WHO. Consolidated Guidelines on HIV Testing Services. 2015.

246. UNAIDS. The Gap Report. 2014.

247. WHO. Guideline on when to start antiretroviral therapy and on pre-exposure prophylaxis for HIV. S. 2015.

248. Barnabas RV, van Rooyen H, Tumwesigye E, et al. Initiation of antiretroviral therapy and viral suppression after home HIV testing and counselling in KwaZulu-Natal, South Africa, and Mbarara district, Uganda: A prospective, observational intervention study. *Lancet HIV.* 2014;1(2):e68–76.

249. Siedner MJ, Ng CK, Bassett IV, Katz IT, Bangsberg DR, Tsai AC. Trends in CD4 count at presentation to care and treatment initiation in sub-Saharan Africa, 2002–2013: A meta-analysis. *Clin Infect Dis.* 2015;60(7):1120–7.

250. Medley A, Ackers M, Amolloh M, et al. Early uptake of HIV clinical care after testing HIV-positive during home-based testing and counseling in western Kenya. *AIDS Behav.* 2013;17(1):224–34.

251. Plazy M, Farouki KE, Iwuji C, et al. Access to HIV care in the context of universal test and treat: Challenges within the ANRS 12249 TasP cluster-randomized trial in rural South Africa. *J Int AIDS Soc.* 2016;19(1):20913.

252. Keane J, Pharr JR, Buttner MP, Ezeanolue EE. Interventions to reduce loss to follow-up during all stages of the HIV care continuum in sub-Saharan Africa: A systematic review. *AIDS Behav.* 2017;21(6):1745–54.

253. van Rooyen H, Barnabas RV, Baeten JM, et al. High HIV testing uptake and linkage to care in a novel program of home-based HIV counseling and testing with facilitated referral in KwaZulu-Natal, South Africa. *J Acquir Immune Defic Syndr.* 2013;64(1):e1–8.

254. Fox MP, Rosen S, Geldsetzer P, Barnighausen T, Negussie E, Beanland R. Interventions to improve the rate or timing of initiation of antiretroviral therapy for HIV in sub-Saharan Africa: Meta-analyses of effectiveness. *J Int AIDS Soc.* 2016;19(1):20888.

255. Pineirua A, Sierra-Madero J, Cahn P, et al. The HIV care continuum in Latin America: Challenges and opportunities. *Lancet Infect Dis.* 2015;15(7):833–9.

256. Thompson MA, Mugavero MJ, Amico KR, et al. Guidelines for improving entry into and retention in care and antiretroviral adherence for persons with HIV: Evidence-based recommendations from an International Association of Physicians in AIDS Care panel. *Ann Intern Med.* 2012;156(11):817–33, W-284, W-285, W-286, W-287, W-288, W-289, W-290, W-291, W-292, W-293.

257. Cohen MS, Chen YQ, McCauley M, et al. Antiretroviral therapy for the prevention of HIV-1 transmission. *N Engl J Med.* 2016;375(9):830–9.

258. Simoni JM, Kurth AE, Pearson CR, Pantalone DW, Merrill JO, Frick PA. Self-report measures of antiretroviral therapy adherence: A review with recommendations for HIV research and clinical management. *AIDS Behav.* 2006;10(3):227–45.

259. van Zyl GU, van Mens TE, McIlleron H, et al. Low lopinavir plasma or hair concentrations explain second-line protease inhibitor failures in a resource-limited setting. *J Acquir Immune Defic Syndr.* 2011;56(4):333–9.

260. Gandhi M, Yang Q, Bacchetti P, Huang Y. Short communication: A low-cost method for analyzing nevirapine levels in hair as a marker of adherence in resource-limited settings. *AIDS Res Hum Retroviruses.* 2014;30(1):25–8.

261. Olds PK, Kiwanuka JP, Nansera D, et al. Assessment of HIV antiretroviral therapy adherence by measuring drug concentrations in hair among children in rural Uganda. *AIDS Care.* 2015;27(3):327–32.

262. Rosen S, Fox MP. Retention in HIV care between testing and treatment in sub-Saharan Africa: A systematic review. Bartlett J, ed. *PLoS Med.* 2011;8(7):e1001056.

263. Fox MP, MPA SR. Retention of adult patients on antiretroviral therapy in low- and middle-income countries: Systematic review and meta-analysis 2008–2013. *J Acquir Immune Defic Syndr.* 2015;69(1):98–108.

264. Reproduced with permission from McNairy ML, El-Sadr WM. A paradigm shift: Focus on the HIV prevention continuum. *Clin Infect Dis Off Publ Infect Dis Soc Am.* 2014;59(Suppl 1):S12–5.

265. Weiss HA, Thomas SL, Munabi SK, Hayes RJ. Male circumcision and risk of syphilis, chancroid, and genital herpes: A systematic review and meta-analysis. *Sex Transm Infect.* 2006;82(2):101–9; discussion 110.

266. Gray R, Aizire J, Serwadda D, et al. Male circumcision and the risk of sexually transmitted infections and HIV in Rakai, Uganda. *AIDS Lond Engl.* 2004;18(18):2428–30.

267. Auvert B, Taljaard D, Lagarde E, Sobngwi-Tambekou J, Sitta R, Puren A. Randomized, controlled intervention trial of male circumcision for reduction of HIV infection risk: The ANRS 1265 trial. Deeks S, ed. *PLoS Med.* 2005;2(11):e298.

268. Castel AD, Magnus M, Greenberg AE. Pre-exposure prophylaxis for human immunodeficiency virus: The past, present, and future. *Infect Dis Clin North Am.* 2014;28(4):563–83.

269. Baeten JM, Donnell D, Ndase P, et al. Antiretroviral prophylaxis for HIV prevention in heterosexual men and women. *N Engl J Med.* 2012;367(5):399–410.

270. Parker RG, Easton D, Klein CH. Structural barriers and facilitators in HIV prevention: A review of international research. *AIDS Lond Engl.* 2000;14(Suppl 1):S22–32.

271. Sumartojo E, Doll L, Holtgrave D, Gayle H, Merson M. Enriching the mix: Incorporating structural factors into HIV prevention. *AIDS Lond Engl.* 2000;14(Suppl 1):S1–2.

272. Hayes R, Ayles H, Beyers N, et al. HPTN 071 (PopART): Rationale and design of a cluster-randomised trial of the population impact of an HIV combination prevention intervention including universal testing and treatment—A study protocol for a cluster randomised trial. *Trials.* 2014;15:57.

273. Hayes R, Floyd S, Schaap A, et al. A universal testing and treatment intervention to improve HIV control: One-year results from intervention communities in Zambia in the HPTN 071 (PopART) cluster-randomised trial. *PLoS Med.* 2017;14(5):e1002292.

274. Baeten JM, Haberer JE, Liu AY, Sista N. Preexposure prophylaxis for HIV prevention: Where have we been and where are we going? *J Acquir Immune Defic Syndr.* 2013;63(Suppl 2):S122–9.

275. McNairy ML, Cohen M, El-Sadr WM. Antiretroviral therapy for prevention is a combination strategy. *Curr HIV/AIDS Rep.* 2013;10(2):152–8.

276. Gottlieb SL, Low N, Newman LM, Bolan G, Kamb M, Broutet N. Toward global prevention of sexually transmitted infections (STIs): The need for STI vaccines. *Vaccine.* 2014;32(14):1527–35.

277. Low N, Broutet N, Adu-Sarkodie Y, Barton P, Hossain M, Hawkes S. Global control of sexually transmitted infections. *Lancet Lond Engl.* 2006;368(9551):2001–16.

278. Sandoy IF, Zyaambo C, Michelo C, Fylkesnes K. Targeting condom distribution at high risk places increases condom utilization-evidence from an intervention study in Livingstone, Zambia. *BMC Public Health.* 2012;12:10.

279. Charania MR, Crepaz N, Guenther-Gray C, et al. Efficacy of structural-level condom distribution interventions: A meta-analysis of U.S. and international studies, 1998–2007. *AIDS Behav.* 2011;15(7):1283–97.

280. Watson-Jones D, Baisley K, Ponsiano R, et al. Human papillomavirus vaccination in Tanzanian schoolgirls: Cluster-randomized trial comparing 2 vaccine-delivery strategies. *J Infect Dis.* 2012;206(5):678–86.

281. Mugisha E, LaMontagne DS, Katahoire AR, et al. Feasibility of delivering HPV vaccine to girls aged 10 to 15 years in Uganda. *Afr Health Sci.* 2015;15(1):33–41.

282. Msyamboza KP, Mwagomba BM, Valle M, Chiumia H, Phiri T. Implementation of a human papillomavirus vaccination demonstration project in Malawi: Successes and challenges. *BMC Public Health.* 2017;17(1):599.

283. Binagwaho A, Wagner CM, Gatera M, Karema C, Nutt CT, Ngabo F. Achieving high coverage in Rwanda's national human papillomavirus vaccination programme. *Bull World Health Organ.* 2012;90(8):623–8.

284. Peeling RW. Applying new technologies for diagnosing sexually transmitted infections in resource-poor settings. *Sex Transm Infect.* 2011;87(Suppl 2):ii28–30.

285. Aledort JE, Ronald A, Rafael ME, et al. Reducing the burden of sexually transmitted infections in resource-limited settings: The role of improved diagnostics. *Nature.* 2006;444(Suppl 1):59–72.

286. Chauhan V, Shah MC, Patel SV, Marfatia YS, Zalavadiya D. Efficacy of syndromic management measured as symptomatic improvement in females with vaginal discharge syndrome. *Indian J Sex Transm Dis.* 2016;37(1):28–32.

287. van der Eem L, Dubbink JH, Struthers HE, et al. Evaluation of syndromic management guidelines for treatment of sexually transmitted infections in South African women. *Trop Med Int Health TM IH.* 2016;21(9):1138–46.

288. Zemouri C, Wi TE, Kiarie J, et al. The performance of the vaginal discharge syndromic management in treating vaginal and

cervical infection: A systematic review and meta-analysis. *PLoS One*. 2016;11(10):e0163365.

289. Herbst de Cortina S, Bristow CC, Joseph Davey D, Klausner JD. A systematic review of point of care testing for Chlamydia trachomatis, Neisseria gonorrhoeae, and Trichomonas vaginalis. *Infect Dis Obstet Gynecol*. 2016;2016:4386127.
290. WHO. Global action plan to control the spread and impact of antimicrobial resistance in *Neisseria gonorrhoeae*. 2012. http://apps.who.int/iris/bitstream/10665/44863/1/9789241503501_eng.pdf.
291. Lusti-Narasimhan M, Pessoa-Silva CL, Temmerman M. Moving forward in tackling antimicrobial resistance: WHO actions. *Sex Transm Infect*. 2013;89(Suppl 4):iv57–9.
292. Ndowa FJ, Francis JM, Machiha A, Faye-Kette H, Fonkoua MC. Gonococcal antimicrobial resistance: Perspectives from the African region. *Sex Transm Infect*. 2013;89(Suppl 4):iv11–5.
293. WHO. Global guidance on criteria and processes for validation: Elimination of mother-to-child transmission (EMTCT) of HIV and syphilis. 2014.
294. Swartzendruber A, Steiner RJ, Adler MR, Kamb ML, Newman LM. Introduction of rapid syphilis testing in antenatal care: A systematic review of the impact on HIV and syphilis testing uptake and coverage. *Int J Gynaecol Obstet*. 2015;130(Suppl 1):S15–21.
295. WHO. Antenatal care (ANC) attendees tested for syphilis at first ANC visit data by country. 2015. http://apps.who.int/gho/data/node.main.A1358STI.
296. Kruger C, Malleyeck I. Congenital syphilis: Still a serious, underdiagnosed threat for children in resource-poor countries. *World J Pediatr WJP*. 2010;6(2):125–31.
297. Looker KJ, Magaret AS, May MT, et al. First estimates of the global and regional incidence of neonatal herpes infection. *Lancet Glob Health*. 2017;5(3):e300–9.
298. WHO. Guidelines for the Management of Sexually Transmitted Infections. 2003.
299. Alam N, Chamot E, Vermund SH, Streatfield K, Kristensen S. Partner notification for sexually transmitted infections in developing countries: A systematic review. *BMC Public Health*. 2010;10:19.
300. Cowan FM, French R, Johnson AM. The role and effectiveness of partner notification in STD control: A review. *Genitourin Med*. 1996;72(4):247–52.
301. Golden MR, Anukam U, Williams DH, Handsfield HH. The legal status of patient-delivered partner therapy for sexually transmitted infections in the United States: A national survey of state medical and pharmacy boards. *Sex Transm Dis*. 2005;32(2):112–4.
302. Fenton KA, Peterman TA. HIV partner notification: Taking a new look. *AIDS Lond Engl*. 1997;11(13):1535–46.
303. Sharma M, Smith JA, Farquhar C, et al. Assisted partner notification services are cost-effective for decreasing HIV burden in western Kenya. *AIDS Lond Engl*. 2018;32(2):233–41.
304. Skeen S, Prince B, van Rooyen H, et al. What will it really take to end the HIV epidemic? *AIDS Care*. 2018;30(Suppl 2):1–4.
305. UNAIDS. Fast-Track—Ending the AIDS epidemic by 2030. 2014.
306. Makofane K, Spire B, Mtetwa P. Tackling global health inequities in the HIV response. *Lancet Lond Engl*. 2018;392(10144):263–4.
307. Grimsrud A, Bygrave H, Doherty M, et al. Reimagining HIV service delivery: The role of differentiated care from prevention to suppression. *J Int AIDS Soc*. 2016;19(1):21484.
308. Eisinger RW, Fauci AS. Ending the HIV/AIDS pandemic. *Emerg Infect Dis*. 2018;24(3):413–6.
309. WHO. Global Tuberculosis Report 2017. 2017.
310. Houben RMGJ, Dodd PJ. The global burden of latent tuberculosis infection: A re-estimation using mathematical modelling. *PLoS Med*. 2016;13(10):e1002152.
311. WHO. Stop TB Strategy. 2006.
312. WHO. The End TB Strategy. Global strategy and targets for tuberculosis prevention, care and control after 2015. 2014.
313. The Stop TB Partnership. The Global Plan to End TB, 2016–2020: A Paradigm Shift. 2015.
314. Ortblad KF, Salomon JA, Barnighausen T, Atun R. Stopping tuberculosis: A biosocial model for sustainable development. *Lancet Lond Engl*. 2015;386(10010):2354–62.
315. Das P, Horton R. Tuberculosis—Getting to zero. *Lancet Lond Engl*. 2015;386(10010):2231–2.
316. Yuen CM, Amanullah F, Dharmadhikari A, et al. Turning off the tap: Stopping tuberculosis transmission through active case-finding and prompt effective treatment. *Lancet Lond Engl*. 2015;386(10010):2334–43.
317. Dorman SE, Schumacher SG, Alland D, et al. Xpert MTB/RIF Ultra for detection of Mycobacterium tuberculosis and rifampicin resistance: A prospective multicentre diagnostic accuracy study. *Lancet Infect Dis*. 2018;18(1):76–84.
318. Steingart KR, Schiller I, Horne DJ, Pai M, Boehme CC, Dendukuri N. Xpert(R) MTB/RIF assay for pulmonary tuberculosis and rifampicin resistance in adults. *Cochrane Database Syst Rev*. 2014;(1):CD009593.
319. Graham SM. The management of infection with Mycobacterium tuberculosis in young children post-2015: An opportunity to close the policy-practice gap. *Expert Rev Respir Med*. 2017;11(1):41–9.
320. Rangaka MX, Cavalcante SC, Marais BJ, et al. Controlling the seedbeds of tuberculosis: Diagnosis and treatment of tuberculosis infection. *Lancet*. 2015;386(10010):2344–53.
321. Theron G, Zijenah L, Chanda D, et al. Feasibility, accuracy, and clinical effect of point-of-care Xpert MTB/RIF testing for tuberculosis in primary-care settings in Africa: A multicentre, randomised, controlled trial. *Lancet Lond Engl*. 2014;383(9915):424–35.
322. WHO. Guidelines on the management of latent tuberculosis infection. 2015.
323. Shepardson D, Marks SM, Chesson H, et al. Cost-effectiveness of a 12-dose regimen for treating latent tuberculous infection in the United States. *Int J Tuberc Lung Dis*. 2013;17(12):1531–7.
324. Sterling TR, Villarino ME, Borisov AS, et al. Three months of rifapentine and isoniazid for latent tuberculosis infection. *N Engl J Med*. 2011;365(23):2155–66.
325. Bright-Thomas R, Nandwani S, Smith J, Morris JA, Ormerod LP. Effectiveness of 3 months of rifampicin and isoniazid chemoprophylaxis for the treatment of latent tuberculosis infection in children. *Arch Dis Child*. 2010;95(8):600–2.
326. Bamrah S, Brostrom R, Dorina F, et al. Treatment for LTBI in contacts of MDR-TB patients, Federated States of Micronesia, 2009–2012. *Int J Tuberc Lung Dis*. 2014;18(8):912–8.
327. Seddon JA, Hesseling AC, Finlayson H, et al. Preventive therapy for child contacts of multidrug-resistant tuberculosis: A prospective cohort study. *Clin Infect Dis*. 2013;57(12):1676–84.
328. Seddon JA, Fred D, Amanullah F. *Post-exposure Management of Multidrug-resistant Tuberculosis Contacts: Evidence-based Recommendations. Policy Brief No. 1*. Dubai, United Arab Emirates: Harvard Medical School Center for Global Health Delivery; 2015.
329. Accinelli RA, Romero LR, Garcia RF, Sanchez R. Sustained benefit of community-based tuberculosis interventions after 30 years. *Am J Respir Crit Care Med*. 2015;191(10):1202–3.
330. Comstock GW, Baum C, Snider DEJ. Isoniazid prophylaxis among Alaskan Eskimos: A final report of the bethel isoniazid studies. *Am Rev Respir Dis*. 1979;119(5):827–30.
331. Rendleman NJ. Mandated tuberculosis screening in a community of homeless people. *Am J Prev Med*. 1999;17(2):108–13.
332. Theron G, Jenkins HE, Cobelens F, et al. Data for action: Collection and use of local data to end tuberculosis. *Lancet Lond Engl*. 2015;386(10010):2324–33.
333. WHO. Neglected Tropical Diseases. 2018. http://www.who.int/neglected_diseases/diseases/en/.
334. Uniting To Combat Neglected Tropical Diseases. London Declaration on Neglected Tropical Diseases. 2012. http://unitingtocombatntds.org/wp-content/uploads/2017/11/london_declaration_on_ntds.pdf.
335. Kamgno J, Pion SD, Chesnais CB, et al. A test-and-not-treat strategy for onchocerciasis in *Loa loa*-Endemic areas. *N Engl J Med*. 2017;377(21):2044–52.
336. Hollingsworth TD. Counting down the 2020 goals for 9 neglected tropical diseases: What have we learned from quantitative analysis and transmission modeling? *Clin Infect Dis*. 2018;66(Suppl 4):S237–44.
337. Anon. WHO alliance for the global elimination of trachoma by 2020: Progress report on elimination of trachoma, 2014–2016. *Wkly Epidemiol Rec*. 2018;66(suppl_4):S237–44.
338. Deardorff KV, Rubin Means A, Ásbjörnsdóttir KH, Walson J. Strategies to improve treatment coverage in community-based public health programs: A systematic review of the literature. Pullan RL, ed. *PLoS Negl Trop Dis*. 2018;12(2):e0006211.
339. Krentel A, Gyapong M, Mallya S, et al. Review of the factors influencing the motivation of community drug distributors towards the control and elimination of neglected tropical diseases (NTDs). Friedman JF, ed. *PLoS Negl Trop Dis*. 2017;11(12):e0006065.
340. Barrett MP, Croft SL. Management of trypanosomiasis and leishmaniasis. *Br Med Bull*. 2012;104(1):175–96.

341. Boelaert M, Verdonck K, Menten J, et al. Rapid tests for the diagnosis of visceral leishmaniasis in patients with suspected disease. *Cochrane Database Syst Rev*. 2014;(6):1–119.

342. Bisser S, Lumbala C, Nguertoum E, et al. Sensitivity and specificity of a prototype rapid diagnostic test for the detection of *Trypanosoma brucei gambiense* infection: A multi-centric prospective study. Acosta-Serrano A, ed. *PLoS Negl Trop Dis*. 2016;10(4):e0004608.

343. Medley GF, Turner HC, Baggaley RF, Holland C, Hollingsworth TD. The role of more sensitive helminth diagnostics in mass drug administration campaigns: Elimination and health impacts. *Adv Parasitol*. 2016;94:343–92.

344. Wilson AL, Dhiman RC, Kitron U, Scott TW, van den Berg H, Lindsay SW. Benefit of insecticide-treated nets, curtains and screening on vector borne diseases, excluding malaria: A systematic review and meta-analysis. *PLoS Negl Trop Dis*. 2014;8(10):e3228.

345. King CH, Sutherland LJ, Bertsch D. Systematic review and meta-analysis of the impact of chemical-based mollusciciding for control of *Schistosoma mansoni* and *S. haematobium* transmission. *PLoS Negl Trop Dis*. 2015;9(12):e0004290.

346. Courtin F, Camara M, Rayaisse J-B, et al. Reducing human-tsetse contact significantly enhances the efficacy of sleeping sickness active screening campaigns: A promising result in the context of elimination. *PLoS Negl Trop Dis*. 2015;9(8):e0003727.

347. Freeman MC, Garn JV, Sclar GD, et al. The impact of sanitation on infectious disease and nutritional status: A systematic review and meta-analysis. *Int J Hyg Environ Health*. 2017;220(6):928–49.

348. Biswas G, Sankara DP, Agua-Agum J, Maiga A. Dracunculiasis (guinea worm disease): Eradication without a drug or a vaccine. *Philos Trans R Soc Lond B Biol Sci*. 2013 Aug 5;368(1623):20120146.

CHAPTER

24

Addressing the Growing Burden of Chronic Noncommunicable Diseases

Ala Alwan • Pamela Collins • Rengaswamy Sankaranarayanan • Shekar Saxena

INTRODUCTION

Noncommunicable diseases (NCDs) are responsible for the greatest disease burden worldwide, killing more people than all other causes of death combined and resulting in a devastating impact on health and enormous human suffering. Beyond their health implications, NCDs have a negative social and economic impact and represent a major challenge to sustainable development.

NCDs cover a wide range of conditions. This chapter focuses on the main types responsible for the highest burden, namely cardiovascular diseases (CVDs), diabetes, cancer, chronic respiratory diseases, as well as mental, neurological, and substance (MNS) use disorders.

Despite the progressively increasing magnitude and inequitable distribution, much of the adverse human and social impact caused by NCDs can be averted by applying high-impact, cost-effective prevention, and control strategies implemented through a whole of government approach. The last two decades witnessed a great increase in awareness among policy makers on the pressing need to reduce the NCD burden and a global vision and a road map has been recommended for countries to consider. This chapter reviews the global burden of NCDs and their risk factors, and outlines prevention and control strategies based on evidence and international experience.

BURDEN: MORTALITY, MORBIDITY, AND RISK FACTORS

The prevalence and disease burden of chronic NCDs are steadily increasing worldwide, driven by population growth, ageing, changes in lifestyles and risk factors, alongside achievements in communicable disease control and progress in reducing maternal and child mortality. In 1998, NCDs were estimated by the World Health Organization (WHO) to cause 31.7 million deaths, representing 60% of global mortality. This increased to 38 million (68%) in 2012, and 41 million (71%) in 2016.[1–3] Table 24-1 shows the mortality estimates for 2016.[3] Furthermore, a large proportion of people with NCDs die too young. Almost a quarter of NCD deaths occur prematurely below the age of 60 years, and more than 40% below the age of 70 years.

TABLE 24-1 CAUSES OF DEATHS IN 2016 (WHO GLOBAL HEALTH ESTIMATES)

	NCD Deaths in 2016
Cardiovascular diseases	17.9 million
Cancers	9 million
Chronic respiratory diseases	3.9 million
Diabetes	1.6 million
Mental, neurological, and substance use disorders	2.8 million
Other noncommunicable diseases	5.8 million
All noncommunicable diseases	41 million

Source: World Health Organization: Global Health Estimates. Disease burden by cause, sex and by country. Geneva, 2015. global_burden_disease/estimates/en/index1.html.[3]

Over 80% of deaths due to NCDs are caused by CVDs, diabetes, cancer, and chronic respiratory diseases. Of all NCD deaths in 2016, 17.9 million (45%) were due to CVDs, 9 million (22%) to cancer, 3.9 million (9.5%) to chronic respiratory disease, and 1.6 million (3.9%) to diabetes.[4] An estimated 2.8 million were due to MNS-use disorders.[5] Among CVDs, heart disease and stroke are the main causes, and remain the world's biggest killers.[4,6] Underestimates are likely for diabetes-related deaths since a large proportion of people with diabetes die from cardiovascular complications and are reported as cardiovascular deaths. Similarly, most deaths in people with MNS disorders are attributable to other NCDs. In fact, people with severe mental disorders, in particular, experience a 10- to 20-year shorter life expectancy than the general population.[7,8] Notably, a majority of the more than 800,000 suicides that occur annually are associated with a mental disorder, but these are reported as deaths due to injury and are very likely underestimated in settings where surveillance and reporting are poor or where suicide remains illegal and attempts are a punishable offence.[8] The majority (79%) of suicide deaths also occur in low- and middle-income countries (LMICs), where the majority of the world's population resides.

LMICs are disproportionately affected by mortality associated with NCDs. In 2016, 78% of global deaths due to NCDs occurred in these countries.[4] NCDs are the most frequent causes of death in most countries in the American, Eastern Mediterranean, European, Southeast Asia, and Western Pacific regions. In the African region, there are still more deaths from infectious diseases than from NCDs. Even there, however, the prevalence of NCDs is rising rapidly and NCD-related deaths are projected to exceed deaths due to communicable, maternal, perinatal, and nutritional diseases by 2020. Despite this, public health resources globally are not commensurate with the global burden of NCDs, including MNS disorders.

More than three-quarters of premature deaths from NCDs occur in middle-income countries.

Although mortality from some major NCDs are showing a declining trend in many countries, the total number of deaths due to NCDs continue to increase. For example, there has been a progressive decline in death rates from CVDs and smoking-related cancers in high-income countries over the last four decades. The rates for premature death (30–69 years) from CVDs have declined 28% between 2000 and 2015, more than three times the decrease seen in LMICs.[6] However, despite declining death rates, the number of people dying from NCDs is progressively increasing. Population growth and aging together with improved longevity are major factors in this increase in NCD mortality with an estimated increase of 34% between 2000 and 2015. Deaths from ischemic heart disease (IHD) have been estimated to have increased by 19% globally between 2006 and 2016.[9] As populations age, annual NCD deaths are projected to rise substantially, to 52 million in 2030.[10]

In addition to information about NCD mortality, morbidity data are important for assessing epidemiological trends, and development and evaluation of prevention and control programs. However, for many countries reliable morbidity data and trends are inadequate to assess trends for some of the major NCDs. For cancer, morbidity data are available from population- or hospital-based cancer registries in many countries and data on diabetes and high blood pressure are now increasingly available from population-based surveys conducted over the last few decades. Although disease registries for several other NCDs can provide useful information, complete and consistent data are limited to well-resourced counties or settings.

Global Trends in Cancer

A situational analysis of cancer patterns and trends in incidence is a critical component of cancer control.[11] The International Agency on Research on Cancer (IARC) provides global estimates and a compendium of cancer patterns and crude, age-standardized and age-specific cancer incidence rates for various cancers in different populations/countries.[12] An estimated 18.1 million new cancer cases occurred in 2018, and the Agency estimates that the number will increase to 29.5 million by 2040 (19 million in 2020). The five most common cancers in men are lung, prostate, large bowel, stomach, and liver, and in women breast, large bowel, lung, cervix, and thyroid.[13]

The highest incidence rates for all cancers overall, as well as for lung, colorectal, breast, and prostate cancer, individually, are observed in developed countries.[12] Although high cancer rates are observed in developed countries, mortality is generally plateauing or decreasing for the most common cancer types due to decreased exposure to known risk factors, improved early detection, and better treatment. While mortality rates from these cancers are generally declining in developed countries, they are increasing in LMICs due to increases in smoking, excess body weight, and physical inactivity.[14]

LMICs have the highest incidence rates of stomach, liver, esophageal, oral, and cervical cancer which are largely caused by infectious diseases. On the other hand, incidence rates for breast, lung, large bowel, prostate, and endometrial cancers in several LMICs are on the rise due to increased risk factors levels.

Diabetes

The prevalence of diabetes has been steadily increasing for the past three decades and is growing most rapidly in LMICs where three-quarters of people with diabetes live. It is estimated that there are more than 425 million adults living with diabetes, compared to 108 million in 1980.[15,16] Half of the adults with diabetes are undiagnosed. The age standardized global prevalence of diabetes has risen from 4.7% in 1980 to 8.5% in 2014, reflecting an increase in risk factors, mainly overweight, obesity, and physical inactivity.[1] The prevalence of diabetes ranges from 7.1% in Africa to 13.7% in Eastern Mediterranean countries.[17]

Impaired glucose tolerance and impaired fasting glucose levels are risk markers for future development of diabetes and CVD. People with diabetes have an increased risk of CVD. Diabetes is also a leading cause of end-stage renal disease. Data from a large number of countries indicate that most cases of end-stage renal diseases are caused by diabetes and hypertension.[18] Lower extremity amputations are 10–20 times more common in people with diabetes than in nondiabetic individuals.[19] Diabetes is one of the leading causes of visual impairment and blindness in developed countries.

Chronic Respiratory Diseases

Chronic obstructive pulmonary disease including chronic bronchitis and emphysema is a growing problem in LMICs.[20] Increasing smoking rates and increased exposure to indoor and outdoor air pollution explain the increasing magnitude. Asthma is the most common chronic condition in children. It is estimated there are about 334 million people suffering from asthma worldwide.[21]

Mental, Neurological, and Substance-Use Disorders

MNS-use disorders include depressive disorders, anxiety disorders, schizophrenia, bipolar disorder, epilepsy, dementia, migraines, alcohol use disorders, and substance-use disorders. Distinct from other NCDs, 50% of mental and substance-use disorders observed in adulthood begin by the age of 14, and 75% are present by the age of 24.[22] Depressive and anxiety disorders are the most common. An estimated 268 million people suffer from depression and around 274 million have anxiety disorders. The prevalence increased 13–15% between 2006 and 2015.[23] The rising incidence and prevalence, globally, of substance-use disorders also drives the growing disease burden attributable to MNS disorders. An estimated 7.4 million new cases of drug use disorders emerged in 2016, and the prevalence of these disorders remains high: approximately 62 million people live with these disorders worldwide.[5] The incidence and prevalence of dementia are also rapidly increasing as populations age around the world. There were an estimated 44 million cases in 2016. Other neurological disorders like migraine, Parkinson's disease, and epilepsy also constitute major chronic health problems. As a group, MNS disorders are the leading causes of disability, responsible for an estimated 7% of disability-adjusted life years lost for mental and substance-use disorders and 4% for neurological disorders.

Risk Factors

High levels of common, preventable risk factors are driving much of the increase in NCDs. Four behavioral risk factors are causally linked to CVD, cancers, diabetes, and chronic respiratory diseases. These are tobacco use, harmful use of alcohol, physical inactivity, and unhealthy diet. In turn, these behaviors lead to four key metabolic/physiological changes: elevated blood pressure, overweight/obesity, elevated blood glucose, and elevated blood lipids.

Tobacco use, including smoking and use of smokeless tobacco, is a major risk factor for CVD, diabetes, chronic respiratory disease, and many cancers, including cancers of the oral cavity, pharynx, larynx, lung, esophagus, and pancreas, among other cancers. Those who use smokeless tobacco are at greatest risk for mouth cancer.

The risks to health from tobacco come from both direct tobacco use and exposure to other people's smoke, known as secondhand smoke. In 2015, the overall global rate of current smoking among people aged 15 years and over was 21% and more specifically 39% among men and 6% among women.[24] There are over 1.1 billion smokers worldwide. Although the average rate of current smoking among adults has declined globally from 24% in 2007 to 21% in 2015, it still appears to be increasing in a large number of countries, particularly in the Eastern Mediterranean region and Africa.[25] The declining trend in smoking rates in most high-income countries and some middle-income countries has not translated into fewer smokers because of population growth.[25] In addition to active smokers, there is also a large health burden among those exposed to harm from breathing other people's tobacco smoke. There are also more than 300 million people using smokeless tobacco. Its use is most prevalent in the Southeast Asia region.[26]

Tobacco use is estimated to be responsible for 6 million deaths every year with an additional 890,000 deaths due to exposure to secondhand smoke,[27] and evidence indicates that there is no safe level of exposure to secondhand smoke.[28] If current trends continue, annual tobacco-related deaths are projected to increase to 8 million per year by 2030.[24]

Unhealthy diet and nutritional status are risk factors for CVDs, cancers, and diabetes. Dietary risks are increasing with changing eating patterns, the shift to a global food system with increased availability and marketing of inexpensive processed foods and those rich in refined carbohydrates, sugar, saturated fats, transfats, processed vegetable oils, and salt, as well as increasing global consumption of meat. At the same time, the intake of fruits and vegetables remains low, particularly in LMICs.[29]

Overweight and obesity, resulting from unhealthy dietary trends and physical inactivity, increase the risk of CVDs, cancers, and diabetes. Obesity has been increasing globally and some countries are reporting very high prevalence exceeding 50%. There are no countries reporting significant success in reducing its magnitude.[1] The double burden of obesity coexisting with undernutrition is seen in many countries. Evidence also shows that undernutrition in early life and in utero, which is particularly prevalent among low-income populations, increases the subsequent risk of CVD and diabetes. There is evidence that childhood socioeconomic status is associated with type 2 diabetes and obesity in later life.[10]

Globally, a significant proportion of IHDs is attributed to high lipids. Cholesterol is a major cause of disease burden in both developed and developing countries, and is a risk factor for IHD and stroke. Reduction in serum cholesterol level has been associated with significant reduction in heart disease.[1]

Physical inactivity is also driving the increasing magnitude of NCDs. Mortality estimates indicate that physical inactivity is the fourth leading risk factor globally, causing an estimated 3.2 million deaths around the world.[1] More than 80% of the world's adolescent population is insufficiently physically active.[1] People who are insufficiently physically active have an increased risk of all-cause mortality compared to those who engage in at least 30 minutes of moderate intensity physical activity on most days of the week.[30] Additionally, physical activity lowers the risk of stroke, hypertension, and depression.

In 2010, 23% of adults aged 18 years and over were insufficiently physically active—defined as not meeting the WHO recommendation to do at least 150 minutes of moderate intensity physical activity per week or the equivalent[30] The Middle East and the Americas had the highest prevalence of insufficient physical activity, while the prevalence was lowest in Southeast Asia and Africa. Across all regions, women were less active than men. Current data indicate that there has been no improvement in global levels of physical activity since 2011[31] and the world is not on track to meet the global target for physical activity which is a 10% relative reduction in prevalence of insufficient physical activity by 2025. High-income countries showed an increasing trend in insufficient activity, reporting more than double the prevalence (36.8%) of low-income countries (16.2%) in 2016.[1] The higher levels of activity in LMICs may be explained by high levels of occupational and transport activity in these countries.[32]

The harmful use of alcohol increases the risk of CVD, diabetes, a range of cancers like head and neck, esophagus, liver, large bowel and breast,[33] mental and behavioral disorders, and injuries. Alcohol-related harm can result from both increased alcohol consumption and certain drinking patterns like heavy, episodic drinking. The International Agency on Research on Cancer classified alcohol as a group 1 carcinogen. It is estimated to cause 3.3 million deaths every year, representing 5.9% of all global deaths.[34] In addition to premature mortality, heavy drinking leads to serious social and economic consequences.

The Global Status Report on Alcohol and Health 2014 indicates that individuals 15 years and older drink on average 6.2 L of pure alcohol per year which translates into 13.5 g of pure alcohol per day.[35] However, there are wide variations in alcohol consumption patterns across countries around the world. Adult per capita consumption was highest in the European and American Regions and lowest in the Eastern Mediterranean Region.

Raised blood pressure increases the risk of a variety of noncommunicable conditions, including IHD, stroke, heart failure, and end-stage renal disease. The risk of CVDs increases with increases in blood pressure starting as low as 115/75 mm Hg.[36] Raised blood pressure is currently the top risk for health loss worldwide, and is estimated to have caused 9.4 million deaths worldwide in 2015.[37] Around one-quarter of men and one-fifth of women have raised blood pressure defined as systolic and/or diastolic blood pressure greater than or equal to 140/90 mm Hg.[38] The prevalence of raised blood pressure varies across regions and by country income groups. The prevalence in adults has declined in high-income regions over the last few decades and is also now declining in some middle-income regions. In contrast, it has been stable or increasing in other middle-income and in low-income regions. The highest blood pressure levels have shifted from high-income countries to low-income countries in South Asia and sub-Saharan Africa.[38] Because of the increasing prevalence, population growth, and ageing, the number of adults with raised blood pressure is estimated to have increased from 594 million in 1975 to 1.13 billion in 2015.[38] The public health problem of high blood pressure is compounded by the fact that a major proportion of cases are undetected. Studies show that in many populations more than 50% of people with hypertension are undiagnosed. Around 40% are treated and only one-third of those treated are controlled.[39]

Other Risk Factors

In addition to these four behavioral risk factors and resulting metabolic/physiological risk markers, there are additional risks that are also important in the development of NCDs. Air pollution, both indoor and outdoor, is a major public health problem and one of the key underlying causes for millions of deaths due to IHD, chronic lung diseases, and cancers. Chronic infection is also an important risk factor for some cancers like cervical [*human papillomavirus* (HPV) infection] and stomach (chronic *Helicobacter pylori* infection). Most hepatocellular carcinoma in LMICs is caused by chronic infection with *hepatitis B virus (HBV) or hepatitis C virus (HCV)* or exposure to aflatoxin, whereas in developed countries liver cancer is more often related to cirrhosis with risk factors such as heavy alcohol consumption, fatty liver, obesity, and smoking. High incidence of cholangiocarcinoma caused by liver fluke infection is observed in parts of Southeast Asia, especially in northeast Thailand.[12]

Social exposures can also confer risk. Adverse childhood experiences have been linked to increased risk for depressive and anxiety disorders, cancer, and CVD.[40–42] An intergenerational component of risk has also been reported in which children of parents who suffered numerous adverse childhood experiences display more behavioral health sequelae.[41] Being a victim of violence is also associated with greater risk for mental and substance-use disorders.

NONCOMMUNICABLE DISEASES AND SOCIOECONOMIC DEVELOPMENT

As mentioned before, the magnitude of NCDs is driven by ageing, population growth, effects of rapid and unplanned urbanization, globalization, and marketing of unhealthy lifestyles in the absence of effective prevention and care services.[43] Notably, NCD incidence and prevalence are also influenced by socioeconomic conditions that affect people's exposure to risk factors s and that also have an impact on their health outcomes. Evidence shows that low-income populations have higher levels of several risk factors like tobacco use and harmful alcohol use,[44,45] frequently consume more unhealthy diets, and children in these communities may have a steeper weight gain trajectory from birth.[46,47] The burden of obesity in developing countries is also shifting toward the groups with lower socioeconomic status as countries' income increases.[48] CVDs, diabetes, cancer, and other NCDs, which were once considered health problems affecting mainly affluent populations, are now the leading causes of mortality and disease burden in lower-income communities.

The negative impact of NCDs on socioeconomic development and poverty reduction programs is now widely recognized and is the result of two main mechanisms: loss of productivity and financial risks affecting people with NCDs and their families (Fig. 24-1). Studies from many high-income countries and some LMICs indicate that CVDs including stroke, cancers, chronic respiratory disease,

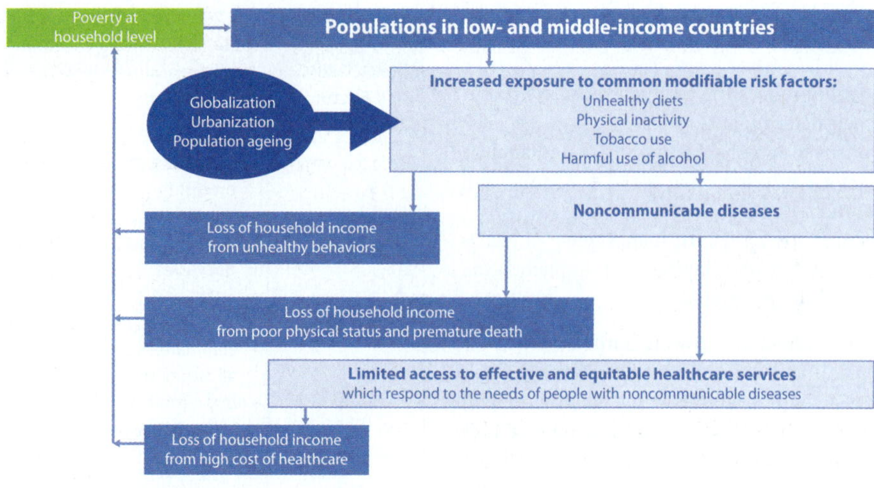

FIGURE 24-1. Poverty contributes to NCDs and NCDs contribute to poverty. (*Source:* Used with permission from World Health Organization, Alwan A, OMS. Global Status Report on Noncommunicable Diseases. 1st ed. Genève, Switzerland: World Health Organization; 2011.)

		Modifiable causative risk factors			
		Tobacco use	Unhealthy diets	Physical inactivity	Harmful use of alcohol
Noncommunicable diseases	Heart disease and stroke	✓	✓	✓	✓
	Diabetes	✓	✓	✓	✓
	Cancer	✓	✓	✓	✓
	Chronic lung disease	✓			

FIGURE 24-2. The four major noncommunicable diseases and major lifestyle-related risk factors.

diabetes, chronic kidney disease, and mental disorders have a large impact on macroeconomic productivity.[49] At the same time, the loss of family income as a result of morbidity, disability, and premature death contributes to poverty. Chronic diseases are also expensive to treat and can impose a substantial impact on households and may lead to further impoverishment. An analysis of 2010 economic data showed that annual direct and indirect costs associated with treatment, care, and lost wages due to mental disorders equaled 2.5 trillion dollars, and estimated that costs will likely increase to 6 trillion by 2030.[50] Public funding for health is only around 50% of current health spending in middle-income countries and less than 30% in low-income countries.[51] Indeed, every year, 100 million people are pushed into extreme poverty because of out-of-pocket health expenses mainly for chronic diseases.[52] In India, about 40% of household expenditures for treating NCDs are financed by households with distress patterns (borrowing and sales of assets).[53] In a systematic review of the global impact of NCDs on households and impoverishment in 16 countries, financial catastrophe due to NCDs was seen in all countries and at different income levels, and occurred in 6–84% of the households depending on the catastrophe threshold.[54] On the other hand, receiving appropriate care is associated with better economic outcomes for individuals and families.[32] Furthermore, at a population level the return on investment for treatment can be high; a recent study demonstrated that implementing a basic package of care for depression and anxiety in a public health system can yield a return of $5.30 USD for every $1 USD investment.[55]

The evidence for the negative impact of NCDs on development is now clear, and the need for concerted government action beyond the health sector is well established. The international community responded in 2015 by integrating the prevention and control of NCDs into the sustainable development goals (SDGs). Governments and development agencies are now challenged to intensify efforts to achieve, by 2030, SDG target 3.4, which calls for a one-third reduction in premature mortality from CVDs, cancers, diabetes, and chronic respiratory diseases, as well as improved mental health and well-being, and SDG 3.5, which calls for strengthening the prevention and treatment of substance abuse.

PREVENTION AND CONTROL STRATEGIES

In 2000, a global strategy for the prevention and control of NCDs was endorsed by the 193 member states of the World Health Assembly.[2] The strategy focuses on the four groups of NCDs which share common risk factors and preventive strategies (Fig. 24-2). As previously noted, the shared risk factors are tobacco use, unhealthy diet, physical inactivity, and the harmful use of alcohol, and these four groups of NCDs also share a major environmental risk factor, air pollution.

The strategy has **three components** implemented through an integrated approach:

- A **prevention** component to reduce the level of exposure to common risk factors and their determinants;
- A **surveillance** component to map NCDs, and track and analyze their behavioral risk factors, as well as their social, economic, and political determinants; and
- A **healthcare** component to strengthen the management of NCDs in national health systems by developing and implementing cost-effective and equitable interventions.

The political necessity to address the growing burden of NCDs is clearly expressed in the United Nations Sustainable Development Goals and by the commitment made by all countries in the political declaration of the high-level meeting of the United Nations General Assembly (UNGA) on the prevention and control of noncommunicable diseases in 2011.[56] Based on the UNGA commitment, the World Health Assembly endorsed a list of high-impact population-based and individual-based intervention "best buys" (Table 24-2) for implementation by countries and a global monitoring framework of nine targets (Box 24-1) to be achieved by 2025. The global targets include one on reduction of premature mortality due to CVDs, cancers, diabetes, and chronic respiratory diseases, which is also endorsed by the SDGs, in addition to six targets on reduction of risk factors and two on health systems interventions.

TABLE 24-2 HIGH-IMPACT, COST-EFFECTIVE INTERVENTIONS FOR NCDS AND THEIR RISK FACTORS

Risk Factor/ Disease	Interventions
Tobacco use	• Increase excise taxes and prices on tobacco products • Implement plain/standardized packaging and/ or large graphic health warnings on all tobacco packages • Enact and enforce comprehensive bans on tobacco advertising, promotion, and sponsorship • Eliminate exposure to secondhand tobacco smoke in all indoor workplaces, public places, public transport • Implement effective mass media campaigns that educate the public about the harms of smoking/ tobacco use and secondhand smoke
Harmful alcohol use	• Increase excise taxes on alcoholic beverages • Enact and enforce bans or comprehensive restrictions on exposure to alcohol advertising (across multiple types of media) • Enact and enforce restrictions on the physical availability of retailed alcohol (via reduced hours of sale)
Unhealthy diet	• Reduce salt intake through the reformulation of food products to contain less salt and the setting of target levels for the amount of salt in foods and meals • Reduce salt intake through the establishment of a supportive environment in public institutions such as hospitals, schools, workplaces, and nursing homes, to enable lower sodium options to be provided • Reduce salt intake through a behavior change communication and mass media campaign • Reduce salt intake through the implementation of front-of pack labelling
Physical inactivity	• Implement community wide public education and awareness campaign for physical activity which includes a mass media campaign combined with other community-based educational, motivational, and environmental programs aimed at supporting behavioral change of physical activity levels
Cardiovascular disease and diabetes	• Drug therapy (including glycemic control for diabetes mellitus and control of hypertension using a total risk approach) and counselling to individuals who have had a heart attack or stroke and to persons with high risk ($\geq$30%) of a fatal and nonfatal cardiovascular event in the next 10 years
Cancer	• Vaccination against human papillomavirus (2 doses) of 9- to 13-year-old girls • Prevention of cervical cancer by screening women aged 30–49
Mental disorders	• Treatment of common conditions like depression, psychotic disorders, and epilepsy • Alcohol prevention measures (see above) • Suicide prevention: reducing access to lethal pesticides

Source: Updated Appendix 3 of the Global Action Plan on noncommunicable diseases. http://www.who.int/nmh/publications/ncd-action-plan/en/; references 133 and 134.

PREVENTION

The evidence base for the prevention of CVD, some cancers, chronic respiratory diseases, diabetes, as well as some MNS is growing. Prevention can be achieved by intervention programs and policies to reduce social and behavioral risk factors and correct metabolic risk factors like high blood pressure, raised blood glucose, overweight and obesity, and high lipids. Interventions to reduce risks require a combination of population-wide and individual-based measures.

Exposure to health risks during early life influences health in later life and increases the risk of CVD, and diabetes.[57] Therefore, implementing interventions throughout the life-course is of critical importance and provides the best chance for prevention. CVDs and the level of several behavioral and physiological risk factors like tobacco use and raised blood pressure are declining in high-income and some middle-income countries.[58] Data are scarce in low and many middle-income countries because of weak health information systems, but most of the recommended prevention interventions are evidence-based, cost-effective, and affordable, and can be implemented even in low-income countries with political commitment, good planning, and community mobilization.

Addressing the same risk factors can prevent diabetes. Evidence from different parts of the world, including China, Finland, India, and the United States, indicates that intensive actions to promote healthy diet, reduce weight, and improve physical activity can prevent or delay the development of diabetes in people with impaired glucose tolerance.[59] Many cancers can also be prevented by reducing the four common risk factors, and chronic obstructive pulmonary disease can be reduced by avoiding exposure to tobacco smoke and indoor and outdoor air pollution.

Tobacco Control Measures

The tobacco epidemic continues around the world because of the aggressive marketing strategies of the tobacco industry and the lack of adequate response. There are large disparities in tobacco use according to socioeconomic status, race, and educational level even in countries where smoking has recently declined significantly.[60] Irrespective of these disparities, tobacco control measures are cost-effective and can reduce tobacco use in all countries implementing them. The evidence base on the cost-effectiveness of tobacco control interventions was the basis for the development of the World Health Organization's Framework Convention on Tobacco Control (WHO FCTC) which became binding law in 2005. It is now considered one of the most rapidly embraced treaties in the United Nations system, with more than 180 parties/countries, covering more than 90% of the world's population.[61] The WHO FCTC combines measures to reduce both the demand and supply of tobacco products as well as other key provisions, including a requirement that parties act to protect public health policies from interference by commercial and other vested interests of the tobacco industry.

BOX 24-1 A Set of Voluntary Global Targets for the Prevention and Control of Noncommunicable Diseases

Mortality:
Target: A 25% relative reduction in overall mortality from cardiovascular diseases, cancer, diabetes, or chronic respiratory diseases.

Behavioral risk factors:
Target: At least a 10% relative reduction in the harmful use of alcohol, as appropriate, within the national context.
Target: A 10% relative reduction in prevalence of insufficient physical activity.
Target: A 30% relative reduction in mean population intake of salt/sodium.
Target: A 30% relative reduction in prevalence of current tobacco use in persons aged 15+ years.

Biological risk factors:
Target: A 25% relative reduction in the prevalence of raised blood pressure or contain the prevalence of raised blood pressure according to national circumstances.
Target: Halt the rise in diabetes and obesity.
Target: At least 50% of eligible people receive drug therapy and counselling (including glycemic control) to prevent heart attacks and strokes. Eligible persons are defined as aged 40 years and over with a 10-year cardiovascular risk ≥30%, including those with existing cardiovascular disease.
Target: An 80% availability of the affordable basic technologies and essential medicines, including generics, required to treat major noncommunicable diseases in both public and private facilities.

Source: https://apps.who.int/iris/bitstream/handle/10665/78617/B132_6-en.pdf?sequence=1&isAllowed=y.

The demand reduction measures include, among other provisions, price and tax measures to reduce tobacco use, interventions to reduce the demand for tobacco, namely: protection from exposure to tobacco smoke through banning of smoking in public places and workplaces, packaging and labelling of tobacco products including health warnings, education and public awareness, bans on tobacco advertising, promotion, and sponsorship, and measures on dependence and cessation. Four of these measures (price and tax increase, health warnings, bans on advertising, and on smoking in public places) are considered highly cost-effective and are included in the list of measures that meet the criteria for inclusion in the WHO recommended list of NCD best buys.[62]

The core supply reduction provisions include addressing illicit trade in tobacco products, reducing sales to and by minors, and supporting transitions from tobacco cultivation to economically viable alternative activities like alternative agricultural crops.

Among the demand reduction measures, raising tobacco taxes is the most effective measure to decrease initiation and increase cessation, especially among young people and the poor.[63,64] Studies indicate that a 10% price increase will reduce overall tobacco use by between 2.5% and 5% in high-income countries.[61] Estimates from low- and middle-income countries suggest even larger reductions in overall consumption. Despite the effectiveness of tobacco taxation, most countries have not met the highest level of achievement (more than 75% of the cigarette retail price), making it the least implemented of the tobacco control measures and the one with least improvement since 2007. WHO indicates that only one in 10 of the world's people live in the 33 countries that levy taxes at the WHO recommended level despite clear evidence that increasing taxes to a sufficiently high level is an extremely effective intervention; it reduces tobacco use and increases government revenues.

The tobacco industry is campaigning aggressively against increased taxation claiming that raising taxes encourages illicit trade, lowers government revenues from taxation, and has a negative impact on the poor. However, these claims are not supported by evidence or international experience.

Among the other proven demand reduction measures, legislating and enforcing smoke-free environments at work and public places can reduce smoking initiation and exposure to secondhand smoke.[65] Health warnings and providing information about the health consequences of tobacco use through mass media campaigns and graphic health warnings on tobacco packages are also effective in reducing demand and consumption.[66] Large graphic warnings that cover at least half of both sides of the package have been shown to be more effective than smaller warnings or those that are limited to text.[67,68] Well-planned and implemented mass media campaigns reduce tobacco use and can reduce secondhand smoke exposure.[69,70] However, as mentioned before, campaigns have to be properly planned, implemented, and sustained over long periods to have the required impact.

A comprehensive set of bans on tobacco advertising, promotion, and sponsorship is another "best buy" that reduces tobacco consumption. Partial bans and voluntary restrictions have little or no effect.[69,71]

Although tobacco cessation treatment is cost-effective in many countries, it did not meet the WHO criteria for a "best buy." However, cessation services in the form of behavioral and pharmacological therapies are recommended whenever possible at the primary-care level.

Tobacco control demand reduction measures have focused primarily on cigarettes, and control of other forms of smoking (e.g., bidi smoking in India, pipe, and cigars) and smokeless tobacco has received comparatively less attention. These should be given priority in many LMICs, particularly in South Asia where tobacco is smoked and chewed in a variety of ways. For instance, in parts of India bidis are smoked more often than cigarettes, yet preventive interventions targeting bidi smoking are practically nonexistent. The complexity of bidi production and sales in the unorganized sector safeguards them from the conventional taxation, price control, and legislation. It is also important to emphasize that while the prevalence of smoking is decreasing, in some LMICs like India, the use of smokeless tobacco is on the rise. Based on the Global Adult Tobacco Survey in India, smokeless chewing forms are the most prevalent forms with 206 million Indians using it.[72]

Needless to say, implementation of the tobacco control measures requires active engagement of nonhealth sectors including finance, trade, industry, and information, in addition to the health sector.

Promoting Physical Activity

Physical inactivity is a major contributor to death and disability from NCDs worldwide.[30,73,74] There is a dose-response relationship for CVD and diabetes with risk reductions routinely occurring at levels of 150 minutes of activity per week.[75,76] Review of evidence indicates that achieving high levels of physical activity can result in significant reduction in the risk of coronary heart disease, stroke, diabetes, breast, and colon cancers.[77] Increasing levels of leisure-time physical activity are associated with lower risks of a large number of cancers beyond colon and breast cancers.[78]

Physical activity can take many different forms like walking, cycling, sports, and other active forms of recreation. It can also occur as part of physical work or daily domestic tasks.

WHO recommends that adults should do at least 150 minutes of moderate-intensity physical activity or at least 75 minutes of vigorous-intensity physical activity throughout the week, or an equivalent combination of moderate- and vigorous-intensity activity. For children and adolescents, the recommendation is to do at least 60 minutes of moderate to vigorous-intensity physical activity daily. Physical activity of amounts greater than 60 minutes daily will provide additional health benefits.

Recognizing these strong links between physical activity, and physical and mental health, in 2013 global health leaders adopted a target of a 10% reduction in levels of physical inactivity by 2025.

Like tobacco control, interventions to increase physical activity at the population level require a multisector approach and a combination of policies aimed at informing, motivating, and supporting individuals and communities to be physically active. In this respect, promoting physical activity and healthy diet through mass media campaigns is a cost-effective and feasible intervention that can be implemented in all countries. Policies should also aim to create a conducive environment like improving road safety, promoting urban planning and design, providing public transport, and facilitating access to recreational and leisure facilities.

Reducing the Harmful Use of Alcohol

Reducing alcohol-related harm is a global priority and is now part of the SDGs. Target 3.5 aims to strengthen the prevention and treatment of substance abuse, including the harmful use of alcohol.[79] Harmful use of alcohol is defined as alcohol per capita consumption (aged 15 years and older) within a calendar year in liters of pure alcohol.[80]

The health impact of the harmful use of alcohol can be reduced by implementing a set of cost-effective interventions that regulate the availability and demand for alcohol.[62] These interventions, which are part of the NCD "best buys" are:

- Increasing excise taxes on alcoholic beverages;
- Enacting and enforcing bans or comprehensive restrictions on exposure to alcohol advertising (across multiple types of media); and
- Enacting and enforcing restrictions on the physical availability of retailed alcohol (via reduced hours of sale).

Other effective interventions (with CEA >$100 per DALY averted) include enacting and enforcing drunk-driving laws and blood alcohol concentration limits via sobriety checkpoints, and providing brief psychosocial intervention for persons with hazardous and harmful alcohol use.

The effectiveness of the above-mentioned interventions depends on their level of enforcement and collaboration of all stakeholders. For example, despite the evidence that alcohol drinking is a major risk factor for multiple NCDs and that 5–6% of cancers globally may be attributed to alcohol drinking, most NCD control initiatives do not adequately address strategies to prevent alcohol abuse.[81–83]

Promoting Healthy Diets

There are still some gaps in the evidence on the relative contribution of certain foods, particularly consumption of total fat and carbohydrates as risk factors for CVDs and other NCDs.[84] However, based on available evidence and current recommendations, an optimal diet includes[85–87]:

- Achieving a balance between energy intake from food and energy expenditure from physical activity to maintain a healthy weight;
- Limiting energy intake from total fats (not to exceed 30% of total energy intake), and shifting fat consumption away from saturated fats (found in fatty meat, butter, palm and coconut oil, cream, cheese, ghee, and lard) to unsaturated fats (found in fish, avocado, nuts, sunflower, canola, and olive oils), and toward elimination of trans fatty acids (found in processed food, fast food, snack food, fried food, frozen pizza, pies, cookies, margarines, and spreads);
- Limiting intake of free sugar to less than 10% of total energy intake which is equivalent to 50 g (or around 12-level teaspoons) for a person of healthy body weight consuming approximately 2000 calories per day. WHO suggests a further reduction to less than 5% of total energy intake for additional health.[88] One intervention is to increase the price of sugar-sweetened drinks. A 20% increase in retail price can result in proportional reductions in consumption[89];
- Limiting refined carbohydrates. Consuming whole grain instead of refined grain products;
- Limiting salt intake to less than 5 g (equivalent to approximately 1 teaspoon) per day;
- Limiting consumption of processed meat and red meat[90];
- Limiting consumption of alcohol beverages; and
- Increasing the consumption of fruits, legumes, whole grains, and nuts to at least 400 g (five portions) of fruits and vegetables a day.

Salt reduction and eliminating the use of industrially produced trans-fatty acids are considered by WHO as a best buy and a good buy, respectively.

Interventions to Reduce Other Risk Factors

Infections are an important cause of cancer. Liver cancer can be prevented by HBV vaccination, HBV and HCV screening of donated blood, organ and tissue products, and infection control in medical practices. In Taiwan, the HBV vaccination program which was introduced in 1984 [and now operates in 185 (95%) countries[91]] has led to more than an 80% decline in liver cancer incidence among young adults.[92] Although new antiviral therapies may prevent chronic infection in those with acute HCV infection and may reduce liver cancer risk in those with chronic HBV or HCV, these interventions remain unaffordable in many high-burden settings despite recent progress made in some countries.[93,94] Chronic *Helicobacter pylori* (*H. pylori*) infection is associated with noncardia stomach cancer, and the steadily declining incidence of stomach cancer in several countries is attributed to less *H. pylori* infection due to improved sanitation and antibiotics, increased availability of fresh vegetables and fruits, and better preservation of foods.

Infection with HPVs causes cervical cancer. HPV16 and HPV18 are responsible for 70–75% of cervical cancers in different regions of the world. Two vaccines, a bivalent and a quadrivalent, targeting HPV16 and 18 are available and have been included in national immunization programs in more than 80 countries.[95] A nine-valent vaccine is also available. The high cost of HPV vaccination has been a major barrier for low- and middle-income countries. Despite substantial evidence on its effectiveness and safety, HPV vaccination implementation is facing resistance and low coverage in part due to misinformation campaigns and negative reporting in the press in some countries.

Nearly two-thirds of the 12.6 million deaths related to environmental exposures each year are due to NCDs, with ambient air pollution contributing to 2.8 million deaths and household air pollution contributing to 3.7 million deaths.[96] Instituting appropriate intersectoral interventions to reduce particulate matter pollution will contribute to reduction of air pollution-related deaths.[97] It is therefore critical for all countries to include evidence-based measures to reduce air pollution as part of the core interventions adopted to improve health and prevent NCDs. The core list of effective interventions includes implementing a national system for air pollution monitoring; actions to discourage the use of kerosene and replacing it with clean household energy sources like liquefied petroleum gas (LPG); halting the use of unprocessed coal as a household fuel; promoting the use of low-emission household energy devices and fuels; building an affordable public transportation system; and adopting and enforcing motor vehicle safety standards.[98]

The prevention of mental and substance-use disorders requires a variety of interventions targeting multiple factors.[99] The prevention of infections (e.g., HIV, meningitis, encephalitis) and micronutrient deficiencies in pregnancy, along with screening and treatment of metabolic disorders like congenital hypothyroidism, can avert developmental disabilities for many children around the world.[100] The prevention of maternal depression, provision of psychosocial stimulation for infants and children, and the delivery of parenting skills training are additional measures that reduce risk of cognitive, affective, attention deficit, and conduct disorders.[99] The passage and implementation of child protection laws should reduce exposure to violence, abuse, and neglect, which also increase risk for mental disorders.

HEALTHCARE

In countries where CVD mortality has been decreasing, the decline has been attributed to both prevention through reductions in major risk factors and treatment.[58,101–104] Different studies provide different estimates of the contribution of primary and secondary prevention in reducing mortality. Some report that more than half of the reduction in mortality from IHDs is attributable to changes in risk factors—especially reduction of tobacco use—while others suggest that between one-third and more than half of the reduction is due to treatment interventions, prominently including hypertension treatment. Irrespective of these estimates, it is clear that the burden of NCDs requires a comprehensive strategy that combines primary prevention and improved healthcare. Increasing access to coronary care units and better treatments for CVDs and diabetes, and improving access to early detection and basic cancer treatment modalities have made it possible for a substantial proportion of people with NCDs to achieve a significant increase in long-term survival.[105]

Like the prevention best buys, many evidence-based, cost-effective, and affordable healthcare interventions can have a major impact in reducing the NCD burden and can be implemented even in low-income countries. These include:

- Drug therapy (including glycemic control for diabetes mellitus and control of hypertension using a total risk approach) and counselling to individuals who have had a heart attack or stroke and to persons with high risk ($\geq$30%) of a fatal and nonfatal cardiovascular event in the next 10 years;
- Low-dose aspirin therapy for acute myocardial infarction;
- Prevention of cervical cancer by screening women aged 30–49, using VIA, or Pap smear (cervical cytology) every 3–5 years, or HPV testing every 5 years and timely treatment of precancerous lesions;
- Screening and brief interventions for alcohol use disorders;
- Cognitive Behavioral Therapy for depression and anxiety disorders; and
- Drug treatment of depression and psychotic disorders.

High-income countries and many middle-income countries will provide access to a wider range of secondary and tertiary care interventions. To improve access to high-impact interventions in low- and middle-income countries, packages covering key health services are recommended by WHO and by the third edition of the Disease Control Priorities as part of actions needed to achieve Target 3.4 of the SDGs (one-third reduction of premature NCD mortality by 2030) and Target 3.8 (achieving UHC).[98,106] The health interventions included in the packages are those that address substantial needs, provide value for money, and are implementable in the context of limited resources. Most of them can be delivered at primary healthcare platforms, supported by effective referral systems for the few specialized services that require a higher level of healthcare.[106,107] For example, the management of cancer will require special efforts to augment services which are nonexistent or deficient in many low and lower-middle income countries like histopathology, radiotherapy, facilities for essential cancer surgery, and access to essential cancer drugs, oral morphine, and palliative care services.

Early detection linked with appropriate treatment and follow-up care is an essential part of effective healthcare for people with NCDs. For example, high blood pressure is the leading risk for death globally. Despite availability of effective and inexpensive treatment, the majority of people with hypertension are undiagnosed. A large proportion of those who are aware of their conditions do not receive healthcare or are inadequately treated. Limited awareness and inadequate control are also common for diabetes, and lead to high rates of complications and premature mortality.

There are two broad approaches to early detection: screening of asymptomatic, apparently healthy general or high-risk populations, and early diagnosis among symptomatic persons. Screening programs for NCDs require well-developed health services, adequately trained providers, high participation of the targeted population, and effective and quality assured testing, diagnosis, and treatment interventions. This means that successful screening programs in high-income countries will not necessarily have the same outcomes in low-resource settings with weak health systems. For example, in cancer, although population-based Pap smear screening programs have led to significant reduction in cervical cancer incidence and mortality in high-income countries, such programs have been less successful in LMICs due to poor organization, inadequate quality assurance, and lack of coverage for testing, diagnosis and treatment.[108] These situations require evaluation of alternative screening approaches such as visual inspection with acetic acid, HPV test-based screening, and novel paradigms such as a single-visit "screen and treat" in which treatment with cryotherapy or thermal coagulation is provided in the screening visit to screen-positive women without clinical evidence of cancer.[109,110] Another cancer-related example is mammography screening for breast cancer. Despite evidence that mammography can reduce breast cancer mortality, it is not feasible in many low- and middle-income countries because of the resources needed and the overdiagnosis and overtreatment associated with this intervention. Evidence is needed from ongoing trials on clinical breast examination before recommending it as a screening method. In the meantime, improving breast awareness and improving access to early diagnosis and treatment in health services is a valuable breast cancer control option in low-resource settings. The second approach for early detection is diagnosis among symptomatic persons by prompt referral, diagnosis, and early treatment.[111] Earlier diagnosis usually results in less aggressive treatments, improved survival, and better quality of life. More than 70% of clinically symptomatic cancer patients in LMICs are diagnosed in advanced clinical stages (stages III and IV).[112] Improved awareness and access to health services can lead to clinical downstaging (diagnosis in earlier clinical stages) and improved survival.[113–116]

Early detection and timely treatment of NCDs require reorientation of health systems that tend to be designed to deliver acute care, and are not equipped to provide effective chronic care in many LMICs. The nature and extent of the health system gaps range from country to country, depending on existing capacity and resources. However, common to most low- and lower-middle-income countries is the lack of adequate preparation and training of the health workforce, lack of adequate and sustainable access to essential medicines and technologies, inefficient information systems, and insufficient finance.[117] In the absence of universal healthcare (UHC) and health insurance schemes, NCDs are expensive diseases to treat, and the patients and their families may have to bear the full costs of their treatment. Without a sustainable *financing* mechanism, the costs of treatment for CVDs, diabetes, and cancers can be devastating for patients and families, eventually leading to severe social inequity. If healthcare is not affordable as in low-resource environments or when basic, prepaid health services are not accessible for certain populations, many people abandon treatment or seek inferior or untested treatments, leading to complications and premature death.

All countries, irrespective of income, can make a difference in addressing these health system gaps by committing to UHC and designing and implementing policies and actions for each gap. Target 3.8 of the SDGs[79] on UHC aims to ensure that all people can obtain the health services they need without suffering financial hardship. As part of the commitment to the SDGs, each country is accountable to develop a vision and a road map for UHC focusing on expanding coverage, establishing effective referral systems, improving health-financing performance, enhancing financial risk protection, and expanding coverage of essential health services, including for NCDs.

SURVEILLANCE

Surveillance for NCDs involves the regular, ongoing collection, analysis, and use of data on the burden, epidemiological characteristics, and outcomes of NCDs to monitor trends over time and provide the basis for policy development, and evaluation of strategies, plans, and intervention programs. NCD surveillance should be an integral part of the national health information system and should ideally encompass three elements: (a) monitoring exposure to risk factors and determinants, (b) measuring morbidity and mortality outcomes, and (c) assessing health system performance.[10,118] Each of the three elements should include a list of tracer indicators adopted by countries according to the characteristics of their disease burden, specific needs and capacity to generate and analyze the required data. Table 24-3 provides a framework for a national NCD surveillance scheme covering the three basic elements.

The core list of risk factors includes tobacco use, physical inactivity, the harmful use of alcohol and unhealthy diet as behavioral risk factors and overweight/obesity, raised blood pressure, raised blood glucose, and raised cholesterol as physiological or metabolic risk factors. Selected social determinants like income and educational level may be included. The information needed to monitor risk factors and determinants is usually obtained from population-based household surveys conducted at regular intervals, usually every 3–5 years, using standardized methods for collecting, analyzing, and disseminating data such as national health interview or health examination surveys or the WHO STEPS survey.[119] Standardized and regularly conducted risk factors surveillance is essential for planning and monitoring trends over time as well as for making comparison across countries or different regions within the same country.

The key indicator for outcomes is cause-specific mortality. For NCDs, the indicator adopted by the United Nations is the mortality rate attributed to CVD, cancer, diabetes, or chronic respiratory disease.[120] Based on a resolution adopted by countries at the World Health Assembly, global monitoring of NCD mortality will focus on premature mortality defined as deaths from these four groups of diseases occurring between the ages of 30 and 70 years.[121] In this respect, a major challenge is that reliable information on cause-specific mortality is not regularly reported by all countries. A large number of countries, particularly in Africa and Asia, do not currently generate reliable or complete data on causes of death.[122] The 2017 World Health Statistics report indicates that "only around 28% of all global deaths are reported to WHO by ICD code (regardless of ICD revision), and even then many such deaths are assigned a garbage code, leaving just 23% of deaths having precise and meaningful information on their cause."[123]

TABLE 24-3	FRAMEWORK FOR NATIONAL NCD SURVEILLANCE
Exposures	• Behavioral risk factors: *tobacco use, physical inactivity, harmful use of alcohol and unhealthy diet.* • Metabolic risk factors: *overweight/obesity, raised blood pressure, glucose, and cholesterol.* • Social determinants: *education, income, access to healthcare.*
Outcomes	• Mortality: *NCD specific mortality.* • Morbidity: *cancer incidence and type (as a core morbidity indicator).*
Health system capacity and response	• Interventions and health system capacity: *infrastructure, policies and plans, access to key healthcare interventions and treatments, partnerships.*

Sources: World Health Organization: Global status report on noncommunicable diseases 2010. Geneva: World Health Organization. 2011[10]; Alwan A, Maclean DR, Riley LM, et al. Monitoring and surveillance of chronic non-communicable diseases: Progress and capacity in high-burden countries. *Lancet.* 2010;376(9755):1861–8.[118])

When reliable data on causes of death are lacking because of coverage or quality gaps, mortality estimates, based on a variety of sources of information, statistical methods, and modeling, are used to monitor mortality trends. However, these can have wide uncertainty ranges for some conditions and regions, and they are no substitute for registering every death through strengthened civil registration and vital statistics systems.[124,125] Interim measures like the use of verbal autopsy methods for cause of death may be considered by countries without well-functioning death registration systems, although interpretation of data to assess cause of death is challenging.[119]

As mentioned before, the basic morbidity information required for policy development is obtained from population-based cancer registries. It is imperative that cancer control plans consider cancer patterns because of the diversity of cancer types in different countries and the potentially different prevention and control strategies. Where population-based cancer registries do not exist, as is the case of many LMICs, hospital-based registries can be used although the information derived is less reliable in describing cancer patterns and trends in defined catchment populations.[10] Valuable information can also be derived from other disease registries like heart diseases, stroke, diabetes, and end-stage renal disease if countries can afford the establishment of registries that are representative of the population studied.

Assessing health system performance and response to NCDs is the third component of the surveillance framework. However, it is challenging in many countries because of scarcity of data. Country capacity can be measured by using indicators on the development and implementation of national policies, prevention strategies and plans, adequacy of infrastructure, and access to essential healthcare interventions. WHO conducts regular global surveys to assess the capacity of countries to respond to NCDs and although some of the reported results and conclusions are not validated through an independent mechanism, some of the findings may be used as indicators of health system response.[126–128]

Measuring coverage with essential health interventions for NCDs is key in assessing health system performance and is equally important in monitoring progress toward universal health coverage. For example, it is reported that, in 2017, half of the world's population did not have full coverage of essential services. This is reflected in the fact that over 1 billion people are estimated to have uncontrolled hypertension.[52] In this case, a preferred indicator for health system performance and for monitoring the service coverage dimension of UHC is effective service coverage. Effective coverage is defined as the proportion of people in need of services who receive services of sufficient quality to obtain potential health gains.[129] A large proportion of countries do not have reliable data to measure effective coverage. Therefore, indicators of service coverage, which is defined as the proportion of people in need of a service that receive it, regardless of quality, are more commonly measured.

Monitoring of coverage with essential NCD health services is part of the SDG indicator 3.8.1 that tracks UHC.[80] It is not practical for countries to include indicators for all preventive and healthcare services that their health systems provide. Instead a limited list of indicators is included in the monitoring framework, focusing on high-impact services for which the required data can be generated and analyzed.[130] In the WHO-World Bank UHC monitoring report, four service coverage indicators have been initially proposed for NCDs based on epidemiological burden, presence of cost-effective interventions, availability of comparable data in most countries, and, whenever possible, a definition that captures effective coverage.

Strengthening NCD surveillance is a priority, particularly for LMICs where health information systems are weak and fragmented, and funding and trained human resources are scarce. Population surveys are rarely conducted at regular intervals, and there are often serious quality gaps in the data generated by these surveys. Also, vital statistics and health system data are deficient.[122,131] Until these constraints are addressed, opportunities for enhancement should focus on strengthening the capacity to generate, analyze, and use data for the core set of indicators in the three surveillance parts mentioned above.

SPECIFIC PREVENTIVE AND CONTROL STRATEGIES

The integrated approach recommended by the global strategy generally applies to all NCDs. However, there are some additional approaches and interventions that need to be specifically considered for specific groups of conditions.

Mental Health Disorders

There is growing evidence for prevention of some mental disorders. Some of the nonspecific macrolevel interventions include attention to nutrition, education, housing, economic stability, and strengthening community networks.[132] More specific interventions include reducing child abuse and neglect, providing mental health and psychosocial support to vulnerable populations including refugees and interventions in the workplace. Reduction in the use of alcohol and psychoactive drugs also prevents mental disorders. Though not all suicides are a result of mental disorders, suicides can be prevented. A recent WHO report summarizes the evidence on this.[133] Specific interventions for suicide prevention include decreasing access to the means to attempt suicide like lethal pesticides and guns as well as identification and treatment of people at high risk of mental disorders.[133]

In the area of healthcare, highly effective interventions exist to treat the majority of MNS-use disorders. Treatment using generic medicines for common conditions like depression, psychotic disorders, and epilepsy is an evidence-based, cost-effective, and affordable approach to reduce the disease burden in all countries. Similarly, low-intensity psychological interventions are available for many mental and substance-use disorders, with the unique advantage of being amenable to be delivered by less trained healthcare providers.[134] It is now clearly accepted that primary-care health professionals can provide basic mental healthcare after training and with support and supervision of specialists.[135] It is also agreed that the treatment of mental disorders must take place in community settings, including in outpatient clinics and short-stay general hospitals and not in long-stay mental hospitals.

CONCLUSIONS AND FUTURE DIRECTIONS

NCDs have emerged as a leading public health problem globally undermining socioeconomic development in all countries and across all socioeconomic groups. The last two decades witnessed an enormous increase in global interest in the prevention and control of NCDs. The development of the global strategy for the prevention and control of NCDs in 2000 and its action plan in 2008[136] increased awareness and commitment for action in countries and in the international health community. Global interest and commitment for containing the progressively increasing burden grew to a higher level with increasing evidence on the negative socioeconomic consequences of NCDs. The impact on sustainable development and the economic cost of inaction led to the high-level meeting of the United Nations General Assembly on NCDs in September 2011, which resulted in the Political Declaration on the Prevention and Control of Noncommunicable Diseases.[56]

The global strategy and the United Nations political declaration emphasize that the prevention and control of NCDs requires an integrated package of core surveillance, primary prevention, and healthcare interventions. Implementing this package can substantially reduce the burden of NCDs.[137] Well planned, politically, and financially supported, these interventions are urgently needed to control the rising burden. While preventive interventions focusing on major risk factors of tobacco use, unhealthy diet, physical inactivity, harmful use of alcohol, environmental air pollution are of paramount importance, systematic investments in improving healthcare infrastructure and addressing health system constraints are equally urgent in most countries. Rapid progress toward UHC in countries, particularly in LMICs, is critical to ensure equitable and affordable access to quality healthcare with financial protection for patients with NCDs.

Extensive international experience and accumulated evidence generated over the last few decades provide important lessons learned which are crucial for accelerating global progress in the global struggle against NCDs. The following summarizes some of these experiences and lessons learned.

1. NCDs are largely preventable and their health and socioeconomic burden can be effectively reduced in all countries by implementing actions to reduce risk factors, improve healthcare, and strengthen surveillance and monitoring.
2. Prevention of risk factors and their determinants is possible through strategies implemented at three levels. First, prevention of the development of risk factors in the first place, from conception to birth and from birth to early life, childhood, and adolescence.[138] Second, reduction of exposure to established risk factors and third, lowering the risk for people who present with clinical signs to prevent further progression of these diseases. In order to achieve the full potential of prevention, it is essential to adopt a comprehensive approach that implements the three strategies.
3. At the population level, exposure to risk factors is seen at different levels. Most people have a moderate level of risk factors, and a smaller proportion of people are at high risk. Taken together, those at moderate risk contribute more to the total burden of disease than those at high risk. For this reason, a comprehensive prevention strategy needs to blend synergistically an approach aimed at reducing risk factor levels in the population as a whole with one directed at high-risk individuals.
4. A priority in generating health gains, reducing risk factors, and improving disease outcomes is to specifically invest in a number of high-impact interventions. Such interventions, sometimes called "best buys," are evidence-based, cost-effective, affordable, culturally acceptable, and can be feasibly implemented in all populations irrespective of socioeconomic status. The best buys can be implemented at the population level or as individual-based measures.[10]
5. Review of prevention programs indicates that the outcome in risk factor reduction depends on the dose or scale of exposure and duration of the interventions. Initiatives of small scale and short duration in delivering interventions result in limited or no positive effects.[139–142] For a substantial health gain and significant reductions in risk and in disease outcomes, delivery of interventions should be of appropriate intensity and sustained over extended periods of time. However, it is important to stress that even modest changes in risk factor levels will have a substantial public health gain.
6. Actions to promote health and prevent disease are not limited to the health sector alone. The role of nonhealth sectors is particularly critical in the prevention of chronic NCDs where most interventions require the involvement and active engagement of other sectors. As the 2000 Global Strategy states "More health gains in terms of prevention are achieved by influencing public policies in domains such as trade, food and pharmaceutical production, agriculture, urban development, social protection, and taxation policies than by changes in health policy alone." Available evidence from the global survey for assessment of national capacity for the prevention and control of NCDs confirms weak multisector coordination. Establishing sustained mechanisms to engage nonhealth sectors is therefore a pressing priority in most countries.[143]
7. Experience indicates that success of prevention programs requires community mobilization, collaboration with civil society organizations, industry, and the private sector and that

effective involvement of industry ranges from positive engagement through voluntary action to regulatory measures taken by the government in the absence of voluntary response.

8. The healthcare needs of people with chronic NCDs are not adequately met by health systems in most LMICs where substantial gaps exist in organizational and financial arrangements of healthcare delivery. Public funding for healthcare is low, and out-of-pocket expenditure is high in many countries, representing a major barrier to access to essential chronic disease interventions.[51] A major challenge is to reorient and strengthen health systems to address inequalities in access and quality of healthcare. Adopting and implementing an essential package of high-impact health services as part of universal health coverage is key.
9. Experience in national prevention initiatives and population-based programs in different countries indicates that although the principles and main strategic directions adopted are generally similar, translation of these directions into practical programs should be based on local circumstances and social and cultural characteristics.[144]
10. Most LMICs have weak health information systems with lack of routine population-based surveillance and they are therefore unable to develop informed policies and plans, which impedes monitoring of trends and progress. An essential requirement for every country is to establish/strengthen a surveillance framework that ensures regular monitoring of key risk factors and determinants, tracking of premature mortality from NCDs, and assessing of health system performance and response.

References

1. World Health Organization. *Global Status Report on Noncommunicable Diseases 2014*. Geneva: World Health Organization; 2014.
2. World Health Organization. Global strategy for the prevention and control of noncommunicable diseases. World Health Assembly. 14-53; 2000. http://www.who.int/nmh/publications/wha_resolution53_14/en/.
3. World Health Organization. Global Health Estimates. Disease burden by cause, sex and by country. Geneva, 2015. global_burden_disease/estimates/en/index1.html.
4. World Health Organization. The top 10 causes of death fact sheet. 2017.
5. Global Burden of Disease 2016. Institute for Health Metrics and Evaluation. Series. Seattle, Washington. 2016.
6. Mathers C, Stevens G, Hogan D, Maganani W, Ho J. *Global and Regional Causes of Death: Patterns and Trends, 2000–15. Disease Control Priorities*, Vol 9. 3rd ed. Washington DC: The World Bank; 2017.
7. Liu NH, Daumit GL, Dua T, et al. Excess mortality in persons with severe mental disorders: A multilevel intervention framework and priorities for clinical practice, policy and research agendas. *World Psychiatry*. 2017;16(1):30–40.
8. Vigo D, Thornicroft G, Atun R. Estimating the true global burden of mental illness. *Lancet Psychiatry*. 2016;3(2):171–8.
9. *The Lancet*. Life, death and disability in 2016. *Lancet*. 2017;390(10100): 1083.
10. World Health Organization. *Global Status Report on Noncommunicable Diseases 2010*. Geneva: World Health Organization; 2011.
11. Selmouni F, Zidouh A, Belakhel L, et al. Tackling cancer burden in low-income and middle-income countries: Morocco as an exemplar. *Lancet Oncol*. 2018;19(2):e93–101.
12. Forman D, Bray F, DH B, et al. *Cancer Incidence in 5 Continents*. Vol X. Lyon: International Agency for Research on Cancer; 2013.
13. International Agency for Research on Cancer. Global Cancer Observatory: Globocan; 2018. http://gco.iarc.fr/.
14. Torre LA, Siegel RL, Ward EM, Jemal A. Global cancer incidence and mortality rates and trends—An update. *Cancer Epidemiol Biomarkers Prev*. 2016;25(1):16–27.
15. World Health Organization. *Global Report on Diabetes*. Geneva: World Health Organization; 2016.
16. International Diabetes Federation. International Diabetes Federation Atlas. 2017.
17. NCD Risk Factor Collaboration. Worldwide trends in diabetes since 1980: A pooled analysis of 751 population-based studies with 4.4 million participants. *Lancet*. 2016;387(10027):1513–30.
18. Saran R, Li Y, Robinson B, Ayanian J, et al. US Renal Data System 2014 Annual Data report: Epidemiology of kidney disease in the United States. *Am J Kidney Dis*. 2015;66(1 Suppl 1):Svii, S1–305.
19. Moxey PW, Gogalniceanu P, Hinchliffe RJ, et al. Lower extremity amputations—A review of global variability in incidence. *Diabet Med*. 2011;28(10):1144–53.
20. Beran D, Zar HJ, Perrin C, Menezes AM, Burney P. Burden of asthma and chronic obstructive pulmonary disease and access to essential medicines in low-income and middle-income countries. *Lancet Respir Med*. 2015;3(2):159–70.
21. Asher I, Pearce N. Global burden of asthma among children. *Int J Tuberc Lung Dis*. 2014;18(11):1269–78.
22. Kessler RC, Angermeyer M, Anthony JC, et al. Lifetime prevalence and age-of-onset distributions of mental disorders in the World Health Organization's World Mental Health Survey Initiative. *World Psychiatry*. 2007;6(3):168–76.
23. Hay S, Abajobir AA, Abate KH. Global, regional, and national disability-adjusted life-years (DALYs) for 333 diseases and injuries and healthy life expectancy (HALE) for 195 countries and territories, 1990–2016: A systematic analysis for the Global Burden of Disease Study 2016. *Lancet*. 2017;390(10100):1260–344.
24. World Health Organization. *WHO Report on the Global Tobacco Epidemic, 2017: Monitoring Tobacco Use and Prevention Policies*. Geneva: World Health Organization; 2017.
25. Global Health Observatory Data. World Health Organization. Series. 2016. http://www.who.int/gho/tobacco/use/en/.
26. Siddiqi K, Shah S, Abbas SM, et al. Global burden of disease due to smokeless tobacco consumption in adults: Analysis of data from 113 countries. *BMC Med*. 2015;13:194.
27. Oberg M, Jaakkola MS, Woodward A, Peruga A, Pruss-Ustun A. Worldwide burden of disease from exposure to second-hand smoke: A retrospective analysis of data from 192 countries. *Lancet*. 2011;377(9760):139–46.
28. World Health Organization. *MPOWER: A Policy Package to Reverse the Tobacco Epidemic*. Geneva: World Health Organization; 2008.
29. Anand SS, Hawkes C, de Souza RJ, et al. Food consumption and its impact on cardiovascular disease: Importance of solutions focused on the Globalized Food System: A report from the workshop convened by the World Heart Federation. *J Am Coll Cardiol*. 2015;66(14):1590–614.
30. World Health Organization. *Global Recommendations on Physical Activity for Health*. Geneva: World Health Organization; 2010.
31. Guthold R, Stevens GA, Riley LM, Bull FC. Worldwide trends in insufficient physical activity from 2001 to 2016: A pooled analysis of 358 population-based surveys with 1.9 million participants. *Lancet Glob Health*. 2018;6(10):e1077–86. Erratum in: *Lancet Glob Health*. 2019;7(1):e36.
32. Guthold R, Louazani SA, Riley LM, et al. Physical activity in 22 African countries: Results from the World Health Organization STEPwise approach to chronic disease risk factor surveillance. *Am J Prev Med*. 2011;41(1):52–60.
33. World Health Organization. Alcohol consumption and ethyl carbamate. *IARC Monogr Eval Carcinog Risks Hum*. 2010;96:3–1383.
34. World Health Organization. *Global Strategy to Reduce the Harmful Use of Alcohol*. Geneva: World Health Organization; 2010.
35. World Health Organization. *Global Status Report on Alcohol and Health 2014*. Geneva: World Health Organization; 2014.
36. Rahimi K, Emdin CA, MacMahon S. The epidemiology of blood pressure and its worldwide management. *Circ Res*. 2015;116(6):925–36.
37. Forouzanfar MH, Liu P, Roth GA, et al. Global burden of hypertension and systolic blood pressure of at least 110 to 115 mm Hg, 1990–2015. *JAMA*. 2017;317(2):165–82.
38. NCD Risk Factor Collaboration. Worldwide trends in blood pressure from 1975 to 2015: A pooled analysis of 1479 population-based measurement studies with 19.1 million participants. *Lancet*. 2017;389(10064):37–55.
39. Chow CK, Teo KK, Rangarajan S, et al. Prevalence, awareness, treatment, and control of hypertension in rural and urban communities in high-, middle-, and low-income countries. *JAMA*. 2013;310(9):959–68.
40. Kelly-Irving M, Lepage B, Dedieu D, et al. Childhood adversity as a risk for cancer: Findings from the 1958 British birth cohort study. *BMC Public Health*. 2013;13:767.
41. Schickedanz A, Halfon N, Sastry N, Chung PJ. Parents' adverse childhood experiences and their children's behavioral health problems. *Pediatrics*. 2018;142(2):e20180023.
42. Lei MK, Beach SRH, Simons RL. Childhood trauma, pubertal timing, and cardiovascular risk in adulthood. *Health Psychol*. 2018; 37(7):613–17.

43. Mayen AL, Marques-Vidal P, Paccaud F, Bovet P, Stringhini S. Socio economic determinants of dietary patterns in low- and middle-income countries: A systematic review. *Am J Clin Nutr*. 2014;100(6):1520–31.
44. Kanjilal S, Gregg EW, Cheng YJ, et al. Socioeconomic status and trends in disparities in 4 major risk factors for cardiovascular disease among US adults, 1971–2002. *Arch Intern Med*. 2006;166(21):2348–55.
45. Allen L, Williams J, Townsend N, et al. Socioeconomic status and non-communicable disease behavioural risk factors in low-income and lower-middle-income countries: A systematic review. *Lancet Glob Health*. 2017;5(3):e277–89.
46. Cameron AJ, Spence AC, Laws R, et al. A review of the relationship between socioeconomic position and the early-life predictors of obesity. *Curr Obes Rep*. 2015;4(3):350–62.
47. de Mestral C, Mayen AL, Petrovic D, et al. Socioeconomic determinants of sodium intake in adult populations of high-income countries: A systematic review and meta-analysis. *Am J Public Health*. 2017;107(4):e1–12.
48. Monteiro C, Moura E, Conde W, Popkin B. Socioeconomic status and obesity in adult populations of developing countries: A review. *Bull World Health Organ*. 2004;82(12):940–6.
49. Chaker L, Falla A, van der Lee SJ, et al. The global impact of non-communicable diseases on macro-economic productivity: A systematic review. *Eur J Epidemiol*. 2015;30(5):357–95.
50. Bloom DE, Cafiero ET, Jane-Llopis E, et al. *The Global Economic Burden of Non-communicable Diseases*. World Economic Forum, Harvard T. H. Chan School of Public Health. September. 2011.
51. World Health Organization. *New Perspectives on Global Health Spending for Universal Health Coverage*. Geneva: World Health Organization; 2017.
52. World Health Organization. *Tracking Universal Health Coverage: 2017 Global Monitoring Report*. World Health Organization, The World Bank. 2017.
53. Engelgau M, Rosenhouse S, El-Saharty S, Mahal A. The economic effect of noncommunicable diseases on households and nations: A review of existing evidence. *J Health Commun*. 2011;16(Suppl 2):75–81.
54. Jaspers L, Colpani V, Chaker L, et al. The global impact of non-communicable diseases on households and impoverishment: A systematic review. *Eur J Epidemiol*. 2015;30(3):163–88.
55. Chisholm D, Sweeny K, Sheehan P, et al. Scaling-up treatment of depression and anxiety: A global return on investment analysis. *Lancet Psychiatry*. 2016;3(5):415–24.
56. United Nations. Political Declaration of the High-level Meeting of the General Assembly on the Prevention and Control of Non-communicable Diseases. United Nations. 66-2; 2012.
57. Barker DJ, Osmond C. Infant mortality, childhood nutrition, and ischaemic heart disease in England and Wales. *Lancet*. 1986;1(8489):1077–81.
58. Ezzati M, Obermeyer Z, Tzoulaki I, et al. Contributions of risk factors and medical care to cardiovascular mortality trends. *Nat Rev Cardiol*. 2015;12(9):508–30.
59. Merlotti C, Morabito A, Ceriani V, Pontiroli AE. Prevention of type 2 diabetes in obese at-risk subjects: A systematic review and meta-analysis. *Acta Diabetol*. 2014;51(5):853–63.
60. National Center for Chronic Disease Prevention and Health Promotion (US) Office on Smoking and Health. The health consequences of smoking—50 years of progress: A report of the Surgeon General. Atlanta, GA: Centers for Disease Control and Prevention (US). 2014.
61. World Health Organization. *WHO Report on the Global Tobacco Epidemic, 2015: Raising Taxes on Tobacco*. Geneva: World Health Organization; 2015.
62. World Health Organization. *Tackling NCDs—WHO Best Buys*. NCD Alliance, World Health Organization; 2017.
63. World Health Organization. *WHO Technical Manual on Tobacco Tax Administration*. Geneva: World Health Organization; 2010.
64. Cancer IAfRo. *Effectiveness of Tax and Price Policies for Tobacco Control*. International Agency for Research on Cancer, 2012.
65. International Agency for Research on Cancer. *Evaluating the Effectiveness of Smoke-Free Policies*. Vol 13. Geneva: World Health Organization; 2009.
66. Hoek J, Wilson N, Allen M, et al. Lessons from New Zealand's introduction of pictorial health warnings on tobacco packaging. *Bull World Health Organ*. 2010;88(11):861–6.
67. Borland R, Wilson N, Fong GT, et al. Impact of graphic and text warnings on cigarette packs: Findings from four countries over five years. *Tob Control*. 2009;18(5):358–64.
68. Hammond D, Fong GT, McNeill A, Borland R, Cummings KM. Effectiveness of cigarette warning labels in informing smokers about the risks of smoking: Findings from the International Tobacco Control (ITC) Four Country Survey. *Tob Control*. 2006;15(Suppl 3):iii19–25.
69. Davis RM, Gilpin EA, Loken B, Viswanath K, Wakefield MA. *The Role of the Media in Promoting and Reducing Tobacco Use*. Bethesda, MD: United States Department of Health and Human Services, National Institutes of Health, National Cancer Institute; 2008.
70. Siegel M. Mass media antismoking campaigns: A powerful tool for health promotion. *Ann Intern Med*. 1998;129(2):128–32.
71. Saffer H, Chaloupka F. The effect of tobacco advertising bans on tobacco consumption. *J Health Econ*. 2000;19(6):1117–37.
72. Gupta P, Arora M, Sinha D, Asma D, Parascondola M. *Smokeless Tobacco and Public Health in India*. New Delhi, India: Ministry of Health & Family Welfare; 2016.
73. Das P, Horton R. Rethinking our approach to physical activity. *Lancet*. 2012;380(9838):189–90.
74. Rocha E. Physical inactivity: Preventable risk factor for cardiovascular disease. In: Andrade J, Pinto F, Arnett D, eds. *Prevention of Cardiovascular Disease*. New York: Springer International Publishing; 2015, pp. 49–58.
75. World Health Organization. *Global Health Risks: Mortality and Burden of Disease Attributable to Selected Major Risks*. Geneva: World Health Organization; 2009.
76. Aune D, Norat T, Leitzmann M, Tonstad S, Vatten LJ. Physical activity and the risk of type 2 diabetes: A systematic review and dose-response meta-analysis. *Eur J Epidemiol*. 2015;30(7):529–42.
77. Kyu HH, Bachman VF, Alexander LT, et al. Physical activity and risk of breast cancer, colon cancer, diabetes, ischemic heart disease, and ischemic stroke events: Systematic review and dose-response meta-analysis for the Global Burden of Disease Study 2013. *BMJ*. 2016;354:i3857.
78. Moore SC, Lee IM, Weiderpass E, et al. Association of leisure-time physical activity with risk of 26 types of cancer in 1.44 million adults. *JAMA Intern Med*. 2016;176(6):816–25.
79. United Nations. *Sustainable Development Goals*. United Nations; 2015.
80. The General Assembly. Work of the Statistical Commission pertaining to the 2030 Agenda for Sustainable Development. United Nations General Assembly. 2017. http://ggim.un.org/documents/A_RES_71_313.pdf.
81. LoConte NK, Brewster AM, Kaur JS, Merrill JK, Alberg AJ. Alcohol and cancer: A statement of the American Society of Clinical Oncology. *J Clin Oncol*. 2018;36(1):83–93.
82. Pelucchi C, Tramacere I, Boffetta P, Negri E, La Vecchia C. Alcohol consumption and cancer risk. *Nutr Cancer*. 2011;63(7):983–90.
83. Henley SJ, Kanny D, Roland KB, et al. Alcohol control efforts in comprehensive cancer control plans and alcohol use among adults in the USA. *Alcohol*. 2014;49(6):661–7.
84. Dehghan M, Mente A, Zhang X, et al. Associations of fats and carbohydrate intake with cardiovascular disease and mortality in 18 countries from five continents (PURE): A prospective cohort study. *Lancet*. 2017;390(10107):2050–62.
85. World Health Organization. *Global Strategy on Diet, Physical Activity and Health*. Geneva: World Health Organization; 2004.
86. American Cancer Society. ACS Guidelines on Nutrition and Physical Activity for Cancer Prevention. [cancer.org]. 2018. https://www.cancer.org/healthy/eat-healthy-get-active/acs-guidelines-nutrition-physical-activity-cancer-prevention.html.
87. World Health Organization. *Fact Sheet on Healthy Diet*. World Health Organization; 2015.
88. World Health Organization. *Guideline: Sugars Intake for Adults and Children*. Geneva: World Health Organization; 2015.
89. World Health Organization. *Fiscal Policies for Diet and the Prevention of Noncommunicable Diseases*. Geneva: World Health Organization; 2016.
90. IARC Working Group on the Evaluation of Carcinogenic Risk to Humans. *IARC Monographs on the Evaluation of Carcinogenic Risks to Humans. Red Meat and Processed Meat*. Lyon: International Agency for Research on Cancer; 2018.
91. World Health Organization. Hepatitis B vaccines: WHO position paper, July 2017—Recommendations. *Vaccine*. 2019 Jan 7;37(2):223–5.
92. Chiang CJ, Yang YW, You SL, Lai MS, Chen CJ. Thirty-year outcomes of the national hepatitis B immunization program in Taiwan. *JAMA*. 2013;310(9):974–6.
93. Webster DP, Klenerman P, Dusheiko GM. Hepatitis C. *Lancet*. 2015;385(9973):1124–35.
94. Lu T, Seto WK, Zhu RX, Lai CL, Yuen MF. Prevention of hepatocellular carcinoma in chronic viral hepatitis B and C infection. *World J Gastroenterol*. 2013;19(47):8887–94.
95. World Health Organization. Human papillomavirus vaccines: WHO position paper, May 2017—Recommendations. *Vaccine*. 2017;35(43): 5753–5.

96. World Health Organization. *Preventing Noncommunicable Diseases by Reducing Environmental Risk Factors*. Geneva: World Health Organization; 2017.

97. World Health Organization. *Ambient (Outdoor) Air Quality and Health*. Geneva: World Health Organization; May 2, 2018.

98. Jamison DT, Alwan A, Mock CN, et al. Universal health coverage and intersectoral action for health: Key messages from Disease Control Priorities, 3rd edition. *Lancet*. 2018;391(10125):1108–20.

99. Patel V, Chisholm D, Parikh R, et al. Global priorities for addressing the burden of mental, neurological, and substance use disorders. In: Patel V, Chisholm D, Dua T, Laxminarayan R, Medina-Mora ME, eds. *Mental, Neurological, and Substance Use Disorders: Disease Control Priorities*, Vol 4. 3rd ed. Washington, DC: The World Bank Group; 2016.

100. Collins PY, Pringle B, Alexander C, et al. Global services and support for children with developmental delays and disabilities: Bridging research and policy gaps. *PLoS Med*. 2017;14(9):e1002393.

101. Unal B, Critchley JA, Capewell S. Explaining the decline in coronary heart disease mortality in England and Wales between 1981 and 2000. *Circulation*. 2004;109(9):1101–7.

102. Tunstall-Pedoe H, Kuulasmaa K, Mahonen M, et al. Contribution of trends in survival and coronary-event rates to changes in coronary heart disease mortality: 10-year results from 37 WHO MONICA project populations. Monitoring trends and determinants in cardiovascular disease. *Lancet*. 1999;353(9164):1547–57.

103. Laatikainen T, Critchley J, Vartiainen E, et al. Explaining the decline in coronary heart disease mortality in Finland between 1982 and 1997. *Am J Epidemiol*. 2005;162(8):764–73.

104. Goldman L, Cook EF. The decline in ischemic heart disease mortality rates. An analysis of the comparative effects of medical interventions and changes in lifestyle. *Ann Intern Med*. 1984;101(6):825–36.

105. Sankaranarayanan R, Swaminathan R, Brenner H, et al. Cancer survival in Africa, Asia, and Central America: A population-based study. *Lancet Oncol*. 2010;11(2):165–73.

106. Stenberg K, Hanssen O, Edejer TT, et al. Financing transformative health systems towards achievement of the health Sustainable Development Goals: A model for projected resource needs in 67 low-income and middle-income countries. *Lancet Glob Health*. 2017;5(9):e875–87.

107. Prabhakaran D, Anand S, Gaziano T, et al. *Cardiovascular, Respiratory and Related Disorders*. Vol 5. 3rd ed. Washington, DC: The World Bank Group; 2017.

108. Sankaranarayanan R. Screening for cancer in low- and middle-income countries. *Ann Glob Health*. 2014;80(5):412–7.

109. Parham GP, Mwanahamuntu MH, Kapambwe S, et al. Population-level scale-up of cervical cancer prevention services in a low-resource setting: Development, implementation, and evaluation of the cervical cancer prevention program in Zambia. *PLoS One*. 2015;10(4):e0122169.

110. Mwanahamuntu MH, Sahasrabuddhe VV, Blevins M, et al. Utilization of cervical cancer screening services and trends in screening positivity rates in a 'screen-and-treat' program integrated with HIV/AIDS care in Zambia. *PLoS One*. 2013;8(9):e74607.

111. Hamilton W, Walter FM, Rubin G, Neal RD. Improving early diagnosis of symptomatic cancer. *Nat Rev Clin Oncol*. 2016;13(12):740–9.

112. Cazap E, Magrath I, Kingham TP, Elzawawy A. Structural barriers to diagnosis and treatment of cancer in low- and middle-income countries: The urgent need for scaling up. *J Clin Oncol*. 2016;34(1):14–9.

113. Devi BC, Tang TS, Corbex M. Reducing by half the percentage of late-stage presentation for breast and cervix cancer over 4 years: A pilot study of clinical downstaging in Sarawak, Malaysia. *Ann Oncol*. 2007;18(7):1172–6.

114. Gadgil A, Sauvaget C, Roy N, et al. Cancer early detection program based on awareness and clinical breast examination: Interim results from an urban community in Mumbai, India. *Breast*. 2017;31:85–9.

115. Ponten J, Adami HO, Bergstrom R, et al. Strategies for global control of cervical cancer. *Int J Cancer*. 1995;60(1):1–26.

116. Sparen P, Gustafsson L, Friberg LG, et al. Improved control of invasive cervical cancer in Sweden over six decades by earlier clinical detection and better treatment. *J Clin Oncol*. 1995;13(3):715–25.

117. Alwan A. *The NCD Challenge: Progress in Responding to the Global NCD Challenge and the Way Forward*. Geneva: World Health Organization; 2017. https://www.who.int/nmh/events/2017/discussion-paper-for-the-ncd-who-meeting-final.pdf.

118. Alwan A, Maclean DR, Riley LM, et al. Monitoring and surveillance of chronic non-communicable diseases: Progress and capacity in high-burden countries. *Lancet*. 2010;376(9755):1861–8.

119. World Health Organization. *Noncommunicable Diseases and Their Risk Factors Accessed*. Geneva: World Health Organization; 2017.

120. SDG indicators Metadata Repository. United Nations, United Nations Statistical Division. Series. https://unstats.un.org/sdgs/metadata/.

121. World Health Assembly. Follow-up to the Political Declaration of the High-level Meeting of the General Assembly on the Prevention and Control of Non-Communicable Diseases. Assembly WH. 66-10; 2013. http://apps.who.int/gb/ebwha/pdf_files/wha66/a66_r10-en.pdf.

122. Mikkelsen L, Phillips DE, AbouZahr C, et al. A global assessment of civil registration and vital statistics systems: Monitoring data quality and progress. *Lancet*. 2015;386(10001):1395–406.

123. World Health Organization. *World Health Statistics 2017: Monitoring Health for the SDGs, Sustainable Development Goals*. Geneva: World Health Organization; 2017.

124. AbouZahr C, de Savigny D, Mikkelsen L, et al. Towards universal civil registration and vital statistics systems: The time is now. *Lancet*. 2015;386(10001):1407–18.

125. World Health Organization. *WHO Methods and Data Sources for Country-level Causes of Death 2000–2012*. Geneva: World Health Organization; 2017.

126. World Health Organization. Assessing national capacity for the prevention and control of NCDs: Report of the 2010 global survey. 2012.

127. Alwan A, Maclean D, Mandil A, World Health Organization. Assessment of national capacity for the prevention and control of noncommunicable diseases: Report of the 2013 global survey. 2001.

128. World Health Organization: Assessing national capacity for the prevention and control of noncommunicable diseases—Report of the 2013 global survey. 2013:1–98.

129. World Health Organization. Tracking universal health coverage: First global monitoring report. June 2015.

130. Boerma T, AbouZahr C, Evans D, Evans T. Monitoring intervention coverage in the context of universal health coverage. *PLoS Med*. 2014;11(9):e1001728.

131. Alwan A, Ali M, Aly E, et al. Strengthening national health information systems: Challenges and response. *East Mediterr Health J*. 2017;22(11):840–50.

132. World Health Organization. *Prevention of Mental Disorders: Effective Interventions and Policy Options*. Geneva: World Health Organization; 2004.

133. World Health Organization. *Preventing Suicide: A Global Imperative*. Geneva: World Health Organization; 2014.

134. Singla DR, Kohrt BA, Murray LK, Anand A, Chorpita BF, Patel V. Psychological treatments for the world: Lessons from low- and middle-income countries. *Annu Rev Clin Psychol*. 2017;13:149–81.

135. World Health Organization. *mhGAP Intervention Guide for Mental, Neurological and Substance Use Disorders in Non-specialized Health Settings: Mental Health Gap Action Programme (mhGAP)*. Geneva: World Health Organization; 2010.

136. World Health Organization. *2008–2013 Action Plan for the Global Strategy for the Prevention and Control of Noncommunicable Diseases: Prevent and Control Cardiovascular Diseases, Cancers, Chronic Respiratory Diseases and Diabetes*. Geneva: World Health Organization; 2009.

137. Alwan AD, Galea G, Stuckler D. Development at risk: Addressing noncommunicable diseases at the United Nations high-level meeting. *Bull World Health Organ*. 2011;89(8):546–546a.

138. Labarthe DR. Prevention of cardiovascular risk factors in the first place. *Prev Med*. 1999;29(6 Pt 2):S72–8.

139. Nissinen A, Berrios X, Puska P. Community-based noncommunicable disease interventions: Lessons from developed countries for developing ones. *Bull World Health Organ*. 2001;79(10):963–70.

140. Schooler C, Farquhar JW, Fortmann SP, Flora JA. Synthesis of findings and issues from community prevention trials. *Ann Epidemiol*. 1997;7(7):S54–68.

141. Ebrahim S, Smith GD. Systematic review of randomised controlled trials of multiple risk factor interventions for preventing coronary heart disease. *BMJ*. 1997;314(7095):1666–74.

142. Borodulin K, Vartiainen E, Peltonen M, et al. Forty-year trends in cardiovascular risk factors in Finland. *Eur J Public Health*. 2015;25(3):539–46.

143. World Health Organization. *Assessing National Capacity for the Prevention and Control of Noncommunicable Diseases: Report of the 2015 Global Survey*. Geneva: World Health Organization; 2016.

144. Puska P. Why did North Karelia-Finland work? Is it transferrable? *Glob Heart*. 2016;11(4):387–91.

CHAPTER

25 Injury Prevention and Trauma Care: Global Perspectives

Paul E. Nevin • James Damsere-Derry • Martha Hijar • Pham Viet Cuong • Charles Mock

INTRODUCTION

Every day, almost 13,000 people lose their lives to injury worldwide. Injuries are a leading cause of death among young people and have an immeasurably pervasive and deleterious impact on society. Among the major causes of injuries are road traffic injuries (RTIs), violence, suicide, burns, drowning, falls, and poisonings. In contrast to their massive burden and preventability, injuries have been largely neglected from the global health agenda. According to the most recent World Health Organization (WHO) estimates, 4.9 million people died in 2015 from injuries (Table 25-1).[1] That's over 70% more than the 2.9 million deaths due to HIV, TB, and malaria combined.[1] Conversely, those three diseases received nearly 36% of global health funding in 2017, while injuries lumped together in an "other health focus areas" category received under 12% of total funding.[2] In addition to being a leading cause of global death, injuries are also a major contributor to global morbidity. Many more people suffer from the long-term physical and psychological consequences of nonfatal injuries than those who lose their lives. Indeed, while accounting for just over 8% of global deaths,[3] injuries contributed 11% of disability-adjusted life years in 2016 (DALYs).[4]

In recent decades, the global burden of injuries has decreased. Transdisciplinary, evidence-based strategies have effectively proven that injuries, when addressed through a public health lens, can be prevented. However, a vast majority of these interventions and subsequent societal benefits are located in high-income countries (HICs). For example, since 1990, DALYs from RTIs in HICs have declined significantly, but in low- and middle-income countries (LMICs), they have increased.[4] There is a clear need for collaboration in global health community to prevent injuries and violence in LMICS, where 90% of the world's injury deaths occur.[5] In this chapter, we outline the burden and risk factors associated with the leading mechanisms of injury globally, with a particular focus on LMICs. We also identify evidence-based strategies for preventing injuries and their applicability in diverse global settings. Greater implementation of proven effective prevention strategies, as well as even a moderate investment in research on injury mechanisms with less well-developed strategies would considerably decrease the unacceptably high burden of injury globally.

TABLE 25-1 2015 GLOBAL INJURY DEATHS[1]

Unintentional Injuries	
Road traffic injuries	1,342,000
Falls	646,000
Drowning	360,000
Burns	180,000
Poisonings	108,000
Exposure to mechanical forces	202,000
Natural disasters	14,000
Other unintentional injuries	675,000
Intentional Injuries	
Suicide	788,000
Interpersonal violence	468,000
Collective violence and legal intervention	156,000
Total:	4,939,000

ROAD TRAFFIC INJURIES

RTIs are a major preventable global health burden. Every year, RTIs claim the lives of more than 1.3 million people[1] and cause nonfatal injuries to up to 50 million people worldwide.[6] RTIs are largest contributor to injury-related DALYs[7] and the leading cause of death among people aged 15–29 years.[8] Younger males are much more likely to be in road traffic incidents than females. Males under age 25 account for almost three-quarters of all road traffic deaths and are about three times more likely to suffer a fatal RTI than their young female counterparts.[8] In addition to the detrimental health impacts, RTIs among such a young population constitute profound economic costs to societies, accounting for economic losses between 3% and 5% of countries' GDP.[6]

The burden of RTIs also disproportionately impacts LMICs experiencing increasing urbanization and motorization. Between 2010 and 2013, 68 countries experienced an *increase* in traffic deaths, 84% of which occurred in LMICs. Over the same time period, 79 countries saw a *decrease* in the number of deaths, but LMICs only accounted for 56% of them.[6] The risk of road traffic death in Africa (26.6 per 100,000 population) is almost triple the risk in Europe (9.3 per 100,000 population).[6] These disparities in RTI burden exist at multiple levels. Among HICs, wealthier countries have lower road traffic death rates than their less-wealthy counterparts[6] and even within individual HICs, individuals from lower socioeconomic status are more likely to be involved in road traffic crashes.[8]

Some of these discrepancies in risk can be attributed to differential rates in the type of road users. All road users are at risk of RTIs, but *vulnerable road users* (pedestrians, bicyclists, and motorcyclists) are at a substantially increased risk of injury compared to motor vehicle occupants.[9] Vulnerable road users account for approximately half of global road traffic deaths (motorcyclists 23%, pedestrians 22%, cyclists 4%).[6] Regional variations in road usage are evident in the burden of RTIs. In Africa, pedestrians account for 39% of road traffic deaths and motorcyclists account for 7%. However, in Southeast Asia, where motorcycles are more frequently used as a family vehicle, motorcyclists account for 34% of road fatalities, with only 13% attributed to pedestrians.[6]

RTIs are preventable and represent an exigent opportunity to save lives and reduce injuries with evidence-based practices and policies. Historically, RTIs have been neglected as a global health priority. Despite representing a burden similar to that of malaria and tuberculosis, road traffic safety was conspicuously missing from the Millennium Development Goals (MDGs).[10] However, this is changing and RTIs are receiving attention and funding more congruent to their cost to society. In 2010, the United Nations (UN) General Assembly declared 2011–20 as the Decade of Action for Road Safety, with WHO subsequently instituting substantial road safety efforts in many countries during this time.[11] The effectiveness of these efforts has been documented in several countries already. For example, an evaluation in Mexico demonstrated a substantial decrease in road traffic deaths, with 10,856 potentially prevented deaths in the 5-year period from 2011 to 2015.[12] Important lessons will likely be learned from more countries when the Decade's efforts are evaluated in 2020. RTIs also figure prominently in the successor to the MDGs, the Sustainable Development Goals (SDGs), including the ambitious target of halving the number of global deaths and injuries from road traffic crashes by 2020 (Sustainable Development Goal 3. Target 3.6).

In an effort to achieve these goals, the WHO released *Save LIVES: A road safety technical package* in 2017 (S-LIVES).[13] The report emphasizes six priority strategies and related evidence-based interventions to reduce RTIs and deaths: **S**peed management, **L**eadership, **I**nfrastructure design and improvement, **V**ehicle safety standards, **E**nforcement of traffic laws, and postcrash **S**urvival. For this chapter, we expand this framework to further explore RTI prevention. Examples of successful interventions for each strategy can be found in Table 25-2.

Speed Management

Speeding is a predominant risk factor for RTIs and contributes to increased crash risk and consequences, particularly for vulnerable road users. A 1 km/h increase in mean vehicle speed leads to a 3% increase in the incidence of crashes and a 4–5% increase in the incidence of road fatalities.[8] A 5% reduction in average speed can lead to a 30% reduction in fatal road crashes.[13] Setting and enforcing national speed limits, particularly in urban environments where there is increased interaction with vulnerable road users, is widely accepted as an essential component of speed reduction strategies. However, of the 180 countries participating in the 2015 *Global status report on road safety*, only 97 had set speed limits of 50 km/h or below in urban areas and only 15% (27 countries) rated their enforcement as "good."[6] In addition to establishing and enforcing speed limit laws, other evidence-based interventions contributing to speed management include building or modifying roads to calm traffic (e.g., roundabouts, chicanes, rumble strips, and road narrowing) and requiring care manufactures to install intelligent speed adaptation (ISA) technology to facilitate drivers' speed choices.[13]

Leadership

Local, national, and international leadership is a key component of successful efforts to reduce the burden of RTIs. Improving road traffic safety requires a multisectoral approach, galvanizing and mobilizing a diverse group of stakeholders, including representatives from health, transportation, education, finance, and police, around specific goals and visions.[13] Important leadership components include establishing an agency specifically focused on road safety; developing, funding, and monitoring a road safety strategy; strengthening data systems to evaluate efforts; and advocating and communicating to the public through education and awareness campaigns.[13] Without strong leadership and endorsement from policy makers and law enforcement leaders, the complex, interdisciplinary efforts necessary to improve road safety are not possible.

Infrastructure Design and Improvement

Poorly designed roads and transportation infrastructure are major contributors to RTIs, particularly when they fail to safely separate vulnerable road users from motor vehicle occupants. The nonprofit organization, international Road Assessment Programme (iRAP), found that half of the roads assessed in LMICs were categorized as highest risk, primarily due to the fact that 84% of the roads did not

TABLE 25-2 EXAMPLES OF EFFECTIVE ROAD SAFETY INTERVENTIONS

Priority Strategy	Intervention	Results	Location
***S**peed management*	Road humps, speed restrictions, and signage installed along 34 primary or secondary school routes	23% reduction in serious pedestrian-vehicle collisions and 68% reduction in fatal collisions[14]	eThekwini, South Africa
***L**eadership*	Multisectoral public education and awareness campaign to reduce traffic injuries and deaths	23.6% decrease in fatal injuries and 25.6% reduction in admission to the ICU saving hospitals 9.3% of their total costs and reducing per patient expenditure by 15.5%[15]	Maringá, Brazil
***I**nfrastructure design and improvement*	School Area Road Safety Assessments and Improvements (SARSAI) program to improve road safety around schools with road humps, bollards, improved sidewalks, crosswalks, increased signage, relocation of school exits, and road safety education	In the year prior to the implementation of SARSAI around 5 primary schools, there were 8 injuries and 1 death. In the year after, there was only 1 injury and no deaths[6]	Dar es Salaam, Tanzania
***V**ehicle safety standards*	Intelligent speed adaptation (ISA) tested in private vehicles to reduce speeding with visual and audio warnings	Significant reductions in mean, maximum, and 85th percentile speed and increased safe driving behavior[16]	Penang, Malaysia
***E**nforcement of traffic laws*	Sobriety check points implemented during high-risk times for drunk-driving incidents Nationwide helmet law required motorcyclists and passengers wear helmets New seatbelt enforcement campaign after 1992 law increased usage rates from 6% to 32%, but declined to 13% by 1995 due to insufficient enforcement	Traffic crashes, injuries, and deaths decreased by 29.9%, 58.7%, and 70.8%, respectively,[17] fivefold increase in helmet usage, 41.4% decrease in head injuries, and 20.8% decrease in deaths[18] From 2004 to 2005, usage rates increased from 22% to 77%[19]	Villa Clara, Cuba Khon Kaen Province, Thailand Buenos Aires, Argentina
*Postcrash **S**urvival*	Emergency care providers dispatched by motorcycle to road traffic crashes	The average response time was 5.18 minutes compared to 11.16 minutes for ambulances[20]	Hanoi, Vietnam

include separated pedestrian walkways.[21] This may partly explain why 90% of the world's traffic deaths occur in LMICs, while accounting for only 54% of the world's vehicles.[6] In addition to aforementioned infrastructure improvements to reduce speeding, there are several highly effective infrastructure solutions that can reduce the burden of RTIs. Priority interventions should focus on providing safe, separate infrastructure for all users (e.g., sidewalks, crosswalks, refuges, overpasses, and separate bicycle and motorcycle lanes). Additional priorities include improving roadside safety with clear zone and collapsible barriers, designing safer intersections, creating vehicle-free or reduced speed zones, creating separate access roads from through-roads, and improving safe public transit routes.[13]

Vehicle Safety Standards

With more than a billion registered automobiles, the world has experienced unprecedented motorization and a proliferation of vehicles in the past decade. LMICs have seen dramatic increases in the number of cars on the road. Between 2005 and 2013, low-income countries saw a 67% increase and middle-income countries experienced an extraordinary 165% increase in their respective shares of total new passenger car registrations in the world.[22] With such an influx in the number of vehicles on the road, assuring their safety is a priority for reducing RTIs. The UN World Forum for Harmonization of Vehicle Regulations establishes voluntary car safety standards and regulations. The S-LIVES report focuses on their seven priority regulations: seat-belts, seat-belt anchorages, frontal impact, side impact, electronic stability control, pedestrian protection, and ISOFIX child restraint anchorage points. Additionally, it recommends the establishment and enforcement of motorcycle regulations including anti-lock brakes and daytime running lights.[13] Unfortunately, vehicles sold in 80% of the world's countries do not currently meet these safety standards.[6] These evidence-based interventions would dramatically decrease the burden of RTIs. If these basic regulations were adopted in just four key countries in Latin America, it would prevent 40,000 deaths and 400,000 serious injuries between 2016 and 2030 and save 143 billion U.S. dollars.[23] Paradoxically, in some countries, vehicles produced for exportation have higher safety standards than those available locally due to disparate regulatory landscapes. The adoption of universal standards would eliminate this inequity.

Enforcement of Traffic Laws

Several behavioral risk factors dramatically increase the likelihood of RTIs: driving under the influence, distracted driving, speeding, and failure to use motorcycle helmets, seat-belts, or child restraints. There is a strong evidence base supporting the establishment and enforcement of laws to discourage these behavioral risks as a highly effective approach to reducing RTIs and deaths. Driving under the influence, or drunk (alcohol-impaired) driving, dramatically increases the risk of RTI and death.[24] Having a blood alcohol concentration (BAC) between 0.02 and 0.05 g/dL is associated with having a three times greater risk of death during a vehicle crash. Between 0.05 and 0.08 g/dL, the risk increases to more than six times that of a sober driver. Above 0.08 g/dL, the risk rises exponentially.[25] Despite being considered best practice, only 47% of all countries have implemented drunk-driving laws based on a BAC limit of 0.05 g/dL and they are much less likely to exist in low-income (13%) and middle-income (43%) countries than in HICs (73%).[6] Enforcement of drunk-driving laws is essential to their success and is more effective when it includes random breath testing checkpoints and public awareness campaigns.[6]

The recent proliferation of mobile telephone use throughout the world has led to a growing burden of distracted driving. A total of 138 countries have laws prohibiting the use of hand-held mobile phones while driving,[13] but their enforcement is inconsistent. Despite evidence that using a phone while driving may be equivalent to or even more dangerous than drunk driving, enforcement is challenging and laws must adapt to evolving technology.[26]

Motorcyclists are vulnerable road users at increased risk for RTIs because they operate in the traffic as large, fast-moving vehicles such as cars, trucks, and busses, but lack their visibility and physical protection. Motorcycle helmets reduce the risk of death by over 40% and the risk of head injury by almost 70%.[27] However, only 44 countries, applying to 1.2 billion people, have laws that meet best practice standards (apply to all drivers and passengers, all roads and engine types, require the helmet to be fastened, and establish helmet standards) and they are disproportionately HICs in Europe.[6] This is worrisome because the burden of motorcycle RTIs is disproportionately in Southeast Asia and Western Pacific regions, with increasing motorcyclists deaths in the Americas.[6] Mandatory helmet laws are highly effective interventions in all settings, including LMICs. Vietnam is a prime example. In 2008, 95% of the 26 million registered vehicles in Vietnam were motorcycles or scooters. A 2007 mandatory helmet use law saw helmet use increase from approximately 30% to 90–99% among adults in four major cities (Hanoi, Ho Chi Minh City, Da Nang, and Can Tho).[28] The first 3 months of the law saw a 16% reduction in the risk of road traffic head injuries and an 18% decrease in the risk of road traffic death.[29] However, usage rates among children remained low with usage rates between 23.3% and 53.8%[28] and represent a need for additional attention. In many countries, helmets with higher safety standards are imported and therefore are more expensive than lower quality helmets produced locally. In response, in 2018, Mexico implemented a new law establishing universal helmet safety standards and labelling requirements for all motorcycle helmets, regardless of manufacturing location.[30] The interdisciplinary law specifically empowers the Ministries and Health and Economy and the Federal Consumer Protection Agency to monitor compliance and promote life-saving helmet usage.

Seatbelts and child restraints are highly effective in reducing the risks of death and injury during traffic crashes. For front seat occupants, seatbelts reduce the risk of death by up to 50% and the risk of injury by up to 45%. For rear seat occupants, fatal and serious injury risk decreases by 25% and minor injury risk by 75%.[24] Enforcement of seatbelt laws is fundamental to the increase in wearing rates. About two-thirds of countries have best practice seatbelt laws that apply to front and rear seat occupants; less than one-third rate their enforcement as "good."[6] Because seatbelts are designed for adults, they are inadequate for children. Proper child restraints are highly effective in saving lives and reducing injuries. Child restraints reduce the risk of death by about 70% in infants and up to 80% in young children.[24,31] Only 17% of the world's population lives in a country with child restraint legislative best practices that include laws based on age, weight, or height for front seat and child restraints and they are much more likely to live in HICs.[6] Enforcement is an ongoing challenge with only 22 countries rating their child restraint law enforcement as "good."[6]

Postcrash Survival

An individual's ability to survive RTIs is highly dependent on emergency response and the strength of the health system in place where a crash occurs. An in-depth look at global trauma care explores this topic in more depth and is presented later in this chapter.

RTIs represent a public health opportunity to greatly reduce global morbidity and mortality. Reducing their burden requires multisectoral approaches involving stakeholders at all levels. Figure 25-1 illustrates the WHO's S-LIVES package of pragmatic strategies, which provide a useful framework for addressing these challenges and reducing the inequity that exists in global RTI burden.

DROWNING

Drowning is the third leading cause of unintentional injury death, killing approximately 360,000 people every year.[32] Due to challenges associated with the collection, classification, and reporting of drowning incidents, current data may considerably underestimate

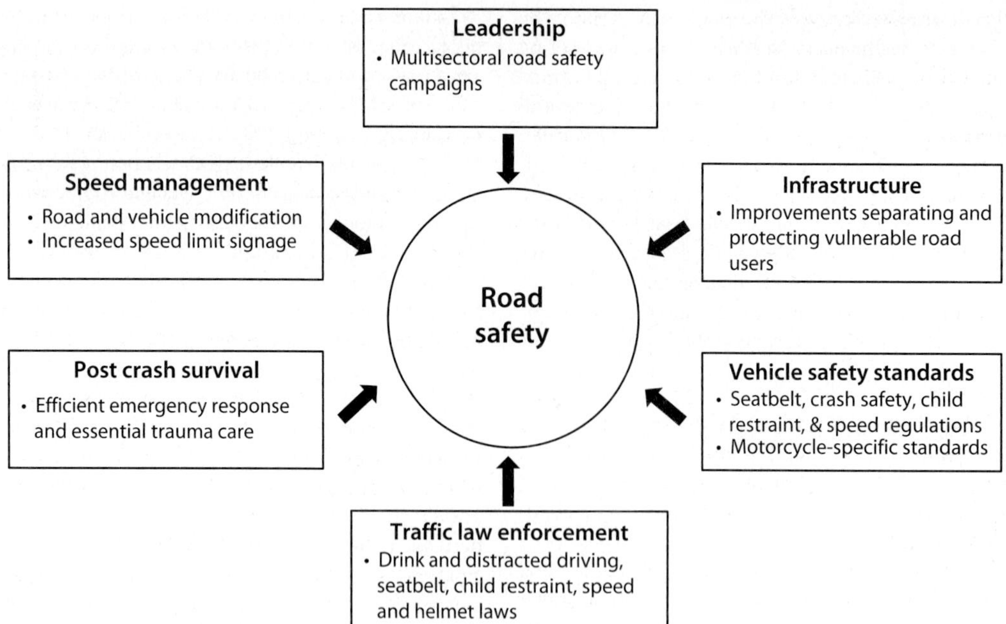

FIGURE 25-1. Effective road safety strategies.

global drowning mortality.[33] These WHO estimates based on the International Classification of Diseases (ICD) 10 only include deaths where drowning is classified as an external cause of death and do not include intentional drownings (homicide or suicide), flood disasters, or water transport incidents, which notably excludes vessels transporting migrants and refugees.[34]

Some studies suggest that drowning rates in LMICs may be four to five times higher than WHO estimates.[35] Facility-based reporting practices in LMICs often preclude drowning deaths where victims are not treated within a national healthcare system from being properly reported.[33] This is important because drowning rates in those countries are more than three times higher than HICs and they disproportionately account for over 90% of all drowning deaths.[34] As with all global health issues, it is important to also identify geographic, age, and gender disparities in global drowning burden. Males are twice as likely to drown as females and over half of all drownings occur in individuals under age 25.[34] Internationally, the highest drowning rates occur in children aged 1–4 years and 5–9 years, respectively.[32] In the Western Pacific Region, drowning is the leading cause of death among children aged 5–14 years.[34]

In 2017, the WHO produced *Preventing drowning: an implementation guide*, which outlines 10 pragmatic and effective approaches countries can implement to reduce drowning. The report acknowledges that the strategies are based on evidence from HICs despite the burden being primarily in LMICs and as such, recommends countries conduct situational assessments to ensure that interventions target relevant, context-specific risk factors.[36] Effective drowning interventions should be multistrategy, based on behavioral theory, and include robust monitoring and evaluation frameworks to inform future policy and practice.[37]

There are evidence-based interventions that can prevent drowning and save lives. However, the majority of these studies have been conducted in HICs. There is limited research showing their effectiveness in LMICs with disparate risk factors. In HICs, most childhood drownings are due to insufficient barriers controlling access to pools.[34] Limiting access with physical barriers such as isolation fencing with self-closing and self-latching gates is highly effective for reducing drownings in those contexts[38] and can be effective in reducing drowning deaths in pools globally. However, in LMICs, drownings more frequently occur in natural water bodies, where it may not be practical to implement covering or fencing to reduce access. In those settings, doorway barriers, playpens, or fenced play areas are affordable interventions to reduce exposure to water and facilitate supervision.[36]

Recently, Bangladesh, where drowning is a leading cause of death among children aged 1–17 years,[39] has seen promising research on preventing drownings. Evidence from studies there indicate that interventions focused on increased supervision and children's swim lessons may reduce drownings in LMIC contexts. The Prevention of Child Injuries through Social-Intervention and Education (PRECISE) program includes two drowning prevention programs targeting children: Anchal (child care) for children aged 1–5 and SwimSafe for children aged 4–12.

Preschool aged children are particularly vulnerable to drowning because they are mobile and may fall into unobstructed water sources. In Bangladesh and other LMICs, this is frequently the case when guardians are busy with other tasks and children are supervised by older siblings.[39] This is especially an issue when lower percentages of children at these ages attend school. To address this risk, the Anchal intervention provided supervised community-based daycare away from water. The intervention reduced the risk of drowning death by 82% and the risk of death from any cause by 44%.[40]

SwimSafe is an education-based intervention that has been specifically designed for risks in LMICs and has been implemented in Bangladesh, Vietnam, and Thailand.[36] In the PRECISE program, water safety, basic swimming, and safe rescue skills were taught to children aged 4–12 in village ponds by locally trained instructors over a 3-week period. The SwimSafe component of the intervention reduced the risk of drowning death by 93%.[40] Despite concerns that teaching swim lessons could potentially increase exposure to and high-risk practices in water, additional research showed that SwimSafe did not increase water exposure or recreational water use.[41] The drowning prevention components of the PRECISE program not only save children's lives but are highly cost-effective, according to WHO criteria, and represent promising strategies in other LMICs.[40]

Personal flotation devices (PFDs), or lifejackets, are designed to keep individuals afloat in open water and are highly effective in preventing drowning in all global contexts. A United States Coast Guard study found that 50% of recreational boating deaths could be prevented by proper PFD use.[42] Laws mandating PFD usage among recreational boaters in Australia increased usage rates from 22% to 63% on small vessels[43] and resulted in a significant decrease in drownings among all recreational boaters.[44] In addition to preventing drownings in recreational boating, regulations mandating PFDs could play an important role in large vessel boating, such as ferries. Between 2000 and 2014, nearly 22,000 people drowned on ferries, with 97% of those deaths occurring in LMICs[45]. Human error, hazardous weather, and overcrowding were common factors associated with the deadly incidents, demonstrating an important impetus for oversight and widespread regulation of large vessels.

The WHO recommends several additional strategies for reducing the global burden of drowning including training bystanders in safe rescue and resuscitation based on guidance from the International Life Saving Federation (ILS), strengthening public awareness, and preventing drowning through disaster risk management.[36] Global climate change will result in more frequent and extreme natural disasters and weather patterns, including flooding, which contributes to an underreported drowning burden. Seventy-five percent of flood deaths are due to drowning, but are not categorized as drowning deaths according to official statistics.[46] Interdisciplinary disaster risk management is essential for preventing flood drownings. Some strategies include land use planning that prohibits housing and infrastructure development in flood-prone areas, managing water through dams and levee systems, establishing early warning systems and ecosystem management plans that conserve natural flood mitigation environments, and investing in flood-resistant infrastructure and insurance schemes.[47]

The burden of global drownings is highly underestimated and routinely neglected, but can be greatly reduced with effective interventions. There is a growing body of evidence on effective prevention interventions in LMICs, but more research is needed to tailor drowning strategies to specific risk factors in local contexts.

FALLS

Falls are the leading nontransport cause of unintentional injury death in the world, killing around 650,000 people each year.[48] Eighty percent of these deaths occur in LMICs, with the Western Pacific and South east Asia regions accounting for 60% of global fall fatalities. Every year, almost 40 million nonfatal falls require medical attention and are responsible for over 17 million DALYs lost.[48] Despite their elevated burden, the true impact of falls is challenging to measure. One of the first steps toward properly assessing falls is the adoption of a universal definition. While researchers tend to focus on the specific falling event (e.g., tripping), seniors and healthcare providers are more likely to reference the preceding causes and subsequent repercussions of the fall.[49] The WHO defines falls as "inadvertently coming to rest on the ground, floor, or other lower level."[50] As such, falls caused by violence, animals, fire, etc. are not included and are instead attributed to their respective causal factor.

Unsurprisingly, age is a major risk factor for falls. The primary high-risk groups for falls are the elderly and young children. The death rate from falls among adults 70 years and older (96.6 per 100,000 population) is dramatically higher than all other age groups, including the next highest group of 50- to 69-year olds (13.5 per 100,000 population).[51] Falls are the leading cause of injury DALY rates among the elderly, with particularly high rates among the aging cohort of individuals with disabilities from previous disasters and wars in Southeast Asia, North Africa, and the Middle East, Andean Latin America, and sub-Saharan African regions.[7] This disproportionate burden of falls in the elderly can be partly attributed to cognitive, sensory, and physical decline associated with aging in environments that are not adapted accordingly.[52] Low bone mass density, which becomes more common as people age and which leads to an increase risk of fracture in a fall, is responsible for a third of global fall deaths.[53] Due to advances in society and health, people are living longer and the world's population is getting older. Each year, the high-risk elder age group becomes larger, continually increasing the toll of falls on society. However, health systems and public health efforts throughout the world are not equally prepared or resourced to address the increased burden of an aging population. As Kalache and Keller state, "industrialized countries became rich before they became old, while developing countries will become old before they become rich."[54]

On the other end of the spectrum is the burden of falls among children. Falling is a normal and natural function of childhood development as they explore their surroundings. Although mortality rates attributed to falls (5.0 per 100,000 population in children under age 5)[55] in children are much lower than in the elderly, nonfatal, but severe falls account for a large portion of years living with disability in the DALY equation as children suffer the impacts of long-term disability throughout the rest of their life. Falls are the most common injury among children in emergency department in most countries, accounting for 25–52% of visits.[35] Fall mortality rates in LMICs are up to three times higher than those in HICs, with the widest gaps in the under 1 age group.[35] It should be noted that variations in fall burden among countries may exist, but the differential statistics may also be influenced by misclassification, such as child abuse being incorrectly documented as a fall.[56] Risk factors for falls among children include younger age, male gender, and low socioeconomic status.[57] Previous studies have indicated that a complex combination of adult supervision, poverty, single parent status, and unsafe environment are important risk factors among child falls.[48]

There are several evidence-based prevention strategies for reducing the burden of falls among the elderly in HICs. For elderly individuals living in the community, group and home-based exercise programs containing balance and strength exercises, including Tai Chi[58] and multifactorial risk assessment and management programs can prevent falls.[59] Home safety improvements, antislip devices, review and reduction of certain medications, cataract surgery, pacemaker insertion, and specialized footwear have also been shown to reduce the burden of falls among the elderly living in the community.[58] In hospitalized patients, strategies including fall-risk assessments, medication management, education, transfer and toileting assistance, equipment and environment modifications, and risk alert mechanisms can prevent falls and reduce fall injuries.[60] While promising, these fall prevention strategies have all been shown to be effective in HICs. There are likely many contexts in LMICs in which these strategies also prevent falls; however, there is currently a dearth of research demonstrating their effectiveness.[61] Competing health demands, insufficient health system infrastructure and resources, and limited presence of systemic geriatric care systems or facilities, placing higher demand on families, may all provide challenges for adapting these interventions to certain LMIC contexts.

Unfortunately, there is a similar lack of evidence of child fall prevention strategies in LMICs.[62] Studies in HICs have shown the effective adoption of prevention strategies, but there is need for additional research on the effect these interventions have on reducing falls or injuries.[63] There are effective intervention strategies to increase use of safety stair gates and decrease use of hazardous baby walkers.[62] Interventions that provide free or subsidized safety equipment (e.g., stair gates), particularly those that also include education, installation, and inspection,[64] appear to be more successful.[65] Increasing urbanization, rural settings, and informal settlements in LMICs may require significant adaptation of existing or the development of new intervention strategies to prevent falls. Further research assessing these interventions in both HICs and LMICs is urgently needed to reduce the burden of the leading cause of injury death after RTIs.

BURNS

Burns, defined as injury to the skin caused by heat or exposure to radiation, radioactivity, electricity, friction, or chemicals, including respiratory harm due to smoke inhalation, cause an estimated 180,000 global deaths annually.[66] Millions more require long-term treatment or suffer from disability, disfigurement, and reduced quality of life from nonfatal burns. Similar to other injuries, the burden of global burns is inequitable. Ninety percent of burns occur in LMICs.[67] The average mortality rate from burns in LMICs is three times higher than in HICs, which also benefit from a ten times higher rate of physicians per 10,000 people.[68] Even in HICs, burns disproportionally impact marginalized racial and ethnic minority communities. In those countries, socioeconomic status accounts for more increased burn risk than other cultural or educational factors.[69] The global burden of burns may be underestimated because there is limited data, particularly from LMICs. To address this gap, the WHO and a network of partners have established a Global Burn Registry to compile burn-related data to improve statistics and inform prevention strategies. This involves a fairly rapid data entry process (5 minute per patient) with submission of the data to WHO, which manages the data and makes collated data available to each participating institution. It has thus far been implemented in 18 countries.[70]

Unlike other mechanisms of injury which disproportionately impact males, females encounter higher burn mortality rates than males. This is mostly attributed to increased female contact with open fire cooking or unsafe cook stoves.[66] In India, over 65% of burn deaths occur in women, primarily between the age of 15 and 34, caused by kitchen accidents, self-immolations, and domestic violence.[71] Men are more likely to encounter burns in the workplace. In addition to women, children are at higher risk for burns, which are the fifth most common cause of nonfatal injuries in children.[66] The intersectionality of risks associated with age and socioeconomic status means that burns disproportionally impact children in low-income settings. The mortality rate of burns in children ages 1–14 is almost eight times higher in LMICs than it is in HICs.[72] A study in Bangladesh found that annually, 173,000 children age 5 and younger suffer from moderate to severe burns.[73] Burns also account for approximately 10% of global child abuse cases.[67]

The majority of burns are preventable. In recent decades, the world has experienced a decrease in burn incidence, but this can be almost entirely attributed to HICs.[68] Some evidence-based prevention strategies that have reduced the burn burden in HICs may be effective in some contexts in LMICs. However, due to disparate risk factors and exposure scenarios, these interventions may not be applicable, particularly in rural, low-income communities that face the highest burden. There is a dearth of burn prevention research in LMICs. A 2016 systematic literature review of burn prevention studies in LMICs found only 11 intervention articles.[74]

Smoke alarms are highly effective at preventing burns. In most HICs, the majority of fatal burns occur in house fires, with many deaths attributed to smoke inhalation.[75] Many victims do not know there is a fire risk until they are unable to escape and become overwhelmed by flames or smoke. There is abundant evidence that smoke detectors reduce the risk of burns from fires, including an 86% decrease in risk of death.[75] Smoke detectors are inexpensive and have the potential to reduce burn incidence, but they must be installed properly and monitored for battery expiration. Education and canvassing campaigns that distribute smoke detectors can increase utilization. One study found that over a 4-year period after a smoke alarm giveaway in a U.S. city, fire-related injuries declined by 80%.[76] Smoke detector evidence is primarily from HICs, but their effectiveness may be applicable in similar contexts throughout LMICs, especially in urban environments.

Scald burns from water are as common as fire-related burns and do not account for a large percentage of burn fatalities, but do contribute to a high proportion of burn injuries, particularly in children.[35] Lowering water temperatures in households is a straightforward intervention to reduce scalding. Multisectoral strategies using legislations, standards, product modification, and education are the most effective. The implementation of one such strategy in Australia, which included reducing the maximum temperature for water in bathrooms to 50°C, greatly decreased the incidence and severity of scalds and saved the health system up to 6.5 million Australian dollars each year.[35] Other evidence-based strategies for reducing the burden of burns in HICs include nonflammable sleepwear, particularly for children, improved electrical safety, sprinkler systems, child-resistant lighters, and safer fireworks.[75] Many of these interventions have potential to be effective in LMICs.

Some interventions have been developed to specifically address risk factors specific to high burn burden contexts in LMICs. In many LMIC households, particularly in rural areas, open fire is used for heat and cooking and represents a significant burn risk. A household randomized trial in Guatemala introduced an improved wood stove with a chimney. Prior to the intervention, the incidence of burns among children aged 18 months or younger was 42.1 per 1000 per year. Following the intervention, the new stoves reduced the rate to 18.1 compared to 35.2 in the control households using open fires.[75] Converting from solid fuel-based cooking and heating to cleaner and safer kerosene or propane-burning stoves has potential to reduce the burden of burns while also improving air quality. Transitioning from traditional floor-level cooking to platform cooking may reduce the risk of burns in children, but further research is needed. The Global Alliance for Clean Cookstoves is currently researching how cookstove design can improve health.

Burns are a highly preventable global injury. Unfortunately, a shortage of data and intervention research clouds our understanding of the burden and solutions to address it in LMICs. Data from the Global Burn Registry and other research can inform policies and strategies to reduce the burn disparity between wealthy and poor populations throughout the world.

POISONING

Every year, unintentional poisoning claims approximately 108,000 lives[1] and nearly 6.6 million DALYs.[77] Globally, unintentional poisonings have declined, but these advancements are not universal. Once again, LMICs bear a disproportionate burden, accounting for 84% of unintentional poisoning deaths.[78] Between 1990 and 2013, South Asia was the only region in the world that did not experience a reduction in its poisoning DALY rates.[7] Intentional self-poisoning, which is also a significant public health burden, has unique risk factors and epidemiology and is covered in the suicide section of this chapter. Much of the research on unintentional poisoning risk factors in LMICs has focused on children, with the most common causes attributed to exposure to medicines, kerosene, and other chemical products.[55] Unsafe storage, a history of previous poisonings, limited adult supervision, hyperactive behavior, low socioeconomic status, and low maternal educational attainment have all been identified as important risk factors for child poisonings in LMICs.[55] In adults, farmers in LMICs suffer disproportionately from poisonings due to exposure to spraying pesticides in agricultural contexts.[79]

There are several evidence-based interventions that show promise for preventing unintentional poisonings. A meta-analysis of studies from HICs found that home safety education interventions led to an increase in safety practices that prevent child injury, including poisoning.[65] Similar prevention strategies may be applicable in LMICs. An education-focused community-based intervention in South Africa used a train-the-trainer model to deploy kerosene safety experts to train local professionals, who then provided educational materials to community members. The intervention led to an increase in kerosene-related knowledge and improvements in kerosene-related safety practices, including proper storage and ventilation.[80] Proper safety warnings and labelling play an important role in educating consumers about the potential danger of poisonous substances. However, a study in Nigeria, found that only 64% of products contained legible product warnings.[81]

The use of child-resistant containers is common practice in HICs and can also be effective in LMICs. A study in South Africa that provided 20,000 households with child-resistant containers found a 47% reduction in kerosene ingestion, the most common cause of accidental child poisoning in the population.[82] In addition to their effectiveness at preventing poisonings, child-resistant container interventions are cost-effective.[83] Sustainable prevention strategies incorporating these findings require buy-in from government policymakers. Unfortunately, in many LMICs, laws requiring the use of child-resistant containers do not exist.[84]

Banning highly toxic pesticides is important for reducing unintentional adult poisonings in agricultural settings. However, many high- and middle-income countries still produce toxic pesticides that are marketed to LMICs, where they are less regulated.[79] Some experts have suggested that, analogous to an Essential Drugs List, a Minimum Pesticides List that identifies safer pesticides for agricultural uses has potential to reduce the harmful effects of highly toxic pesticides.[85]

Poison control centers also play an important role in reducing the burden of poisonings and have been a global health priority for decades. Poison control centers provide important advice on the prevention, diagnosis, and management of poisonings to health providers and the public.[86] Additionally, they play an important role surveilling and compiling data on the existence of and exposure to toxic and hazardous substances. Despite their importance, little progress has been made in establishing new poison centers and as of 2017, only 46% of UN Member States had one.[87]

VIOLENCE

Violence is a major global health problem, claiming the lives of approximately 1.4 million people every year, and causing pervasive physical, reproductive, and mental health issues among survivors.[88] Beyond the proximal suffering of individual victims and their families, violence results in immense distal losses that reverberate throughout communities and society. The WHO defines violence as, "The intentional use of physical force or power, threatened or actual, against oneself, another person, or against a group or community, that either results in or has a high likelihood of resulting in injury, death, psychological harm, maldevelopment or deprivation."[89] Violence is highly correlated with socioeconomic status and inequality. Ninety percent of violence deaths are in LMICs and countries with higher rates of economic inequality have higher mortality rates.[88] Additionally, within countries, violence is disproportionately concentrated among the poorest communities.[88]

Although violence has existed throughout history, it is preventable and the field of public health plays an essential role. Traditionally, violence has come under the purview of law enforcement and criminal justice systems. A public health approach to violence transitions from reactionary responses to the deleterious consequences of the problem to implementing multidisciplinary, evidence-based primary prevention strategies that mitigate the social, behavioral, and environmental factors that precipitate violence.[90] Just as with any other disease, the global health approach to violence prioritizes widespread prevention over individually focused treatment to more extensively reduce the burden on society.

Violence can be categorized as interpersonal, self-directed, or collective, which account for 33%, 56%, and 11% of global violence deaths, respectively.[88] Interpersonal violence is perpetuated by individuals or a small group of individuals; self-directed violence includes suicidal behavior and self-abuse; and collective violence refers to large-scale violence such as war, genocide, terrorism, and economic violence among large groups of people. Collective violence prevention strategies include reducing poverty, inequality, and access to weapons while engaging in and promoting international treaties that protect human rights.[91] This section focuses on evidence-based prevention strategies for interpersonal violence and suicide, which make up almost 90% of violence deaths.

Interpersonal Violence

Interpersonal violence, which can be physical, sexual, or psychological, is the intentional use of force against a person by an individual or group of individuals, including deprivation and neglect.[92] The impact of interpersonal violence extends far beyond the direct death, injury, and disability of discrete incidents. Victims suffer long-term indirect effects including increased risk of infectious diseases, noncommunicable diseases, mental health conditions, reproductive and sexual health problems, and further exposure to violence.[93] Interpersonal violence manifests in many forms, including homicide, child maltreatment, intimate partner violence (IPV), sexual violence, youth violence, and elder abuse. Patterns of interpersonal violence can also be fluid, with new patterns emerging as a result of terrorist acts, drug trafficking, migration, and social and religious tensions.

Annually, there are almost half a million homicides, with males accounting for about 80% of victims.[94] At 32.9 deaths per 100,000 population, the highest homicide rate in the WHO Region of the Americas is 12 times higher than the lowest, the Western Pacific Region.[94] Consistent across regions and country income levels, the burden of homicide disproportionately impacts young adult males aged 15–44 years.[95] When women are victims of homicide, IPV plays a prominent role. Nearly 40% of female homicides are perpetrated by their male intimate partners, while only about 6% of male homicide victims are killed by their female partner.[96] Approximately half of global homicides are committed using guns and around a quarter are carried out using sharp instruments, such as a knives, but this varies widely by region. Firearms are used in 75% of homicides in LMICs in the Americas, but only 25% of homicides in LMICs in Europe.[95] Despite their devastating impact, homicides are only part of the global violence epidemic. For every loss of life due to violence, there are countless more victims suffering from long-term physical, psychological, and social consequences of nonfatal violence and abuse, and women, children, and the elderly disproportionally bear the burden.

Violence against women is a complex phenomenon with serious social repercussions and human rights implications. Women and girls face gender-based violence, which is rooted in gender inequality, in a myriad of ways including: violence by partners and family members; sexual violence, including rape and sexual assault; trafficking for sexual and economic exploitation; femicide (murder because an individual is female, such as with female infanticide, honor killings, dowry-related murder); acid throwing; sexual harassment; female genital mutilation; and child, early, and forced marriage.[97] The impact of gender-based violence is staggering. Globally, one in three women between the ages of 15 and 49 has experienced IPV (physical and/or sexual violence).[98] Over half of all children in the world ages 2–17, about 1 billion children, have experienced physical, sexual, or emotional abuse in the past year.[99]

Interpersonal Violence Prevention Strategies

Public health interventions to prevent violence, particularly in LMICs, require interdisciplinary collaboration between governmental and civil society stakeholders in health, criminal justice, and social services to address underlying risk factors using scientifically credible strategies.[100] Many of the interventions address risk factors that are directly associated with violence, such as access to weapons or alcohol. Others are implemented further upstream to address the social determinants of health that have broad, multiplicative effects on health and well-being, such as improving education and reducing inequality and poverty. The majority of violence prevention evidence comes from HICs. Although these methods have some documented applicability throughout the world, more research is needed in LMICs to prove their effectiveness in lower resource contexts. Considered below are the main categories of violence-prevention strategies.

Violence Against Women

In the last few decades, preventing, sanctioning, and eradicating violence against women has gained space in governmental agendas, including the development of new laws, care centers, and public policies involving civil society. To prevent IPV and sexual violence against women, it is important to address modifiable risk and protective factors in the diverse contexts and settings in which they occur throughout the world. Risk factors associated with IPV and sexual violence include lower education levels; exposure to child maltreatment; harmful substance use; societal norms, including those that promote male sexual entitlement, sexual purity, and family honor; and weak legal sanctions or enforcement.[101]

Upstream intervention strategies preventing child maltreatment, which can reduce future IPV and sexual violence,[102] are addressed later in this chapter. There is also limited, but emerging evidence that interventions treating children and adolescents who have already been subjected to child maltreatment or exposed to IPV may prevent future IPV experiences.[101] School-based education programs enabling children to recognize and avoid potential sexual abuse have also showed preliminary effectiveness.[101] However, there is abundant evidence that school-based interventions addressing dating violence can prevent IPV.[103]

Participatory empowerment interventions that address inequality via microfinance, gender equality, communication, and relationship skills in adults has been shown to be effective in reducing IPV in LMICs. The Intervention with Microfinance for AIDS and Gender Equity, (IMAGE) program in South Africa combines microfinance strategies with skills-based training programs on HIV, gender norms, cultural beliefs, communication, and IPV. Two years after the intervention, there was a 55% decrease in reported acts of IPV.[104] The interdisciplinary approach had multiplicative effects in its female participants and was consistently associated with improved economic well-being, empowerment, and reduced HIV risk behavior.[105] A similar, skills-based training package, *Stepping Stones*, focuses on improving communication and relationship skills in communities. The strategy was originally developed to prevent HIV, but has incorporated violence-prevention components and has been implemented in over 40 LMICs.[101] Men who participated in the program are less likely to commit physical or sexual IPV.[106] In Gambia, couples participating in the program experienced improved communication, reduced quarrelling, and increased acceptance by husbands of their wife's refusal to have sex.[107] Multidisciplinary strategies to prevent IPV have shown potential in a variety of settings, but additional research is needed to validate findings and ensure effectiveness.

Violence Against Children and Youth Violence

With over half of children in the world experiencing violence, implementing strategies that prevent violence against children should be a public health priority in all contexts. In 2016, a major collaboration of global health partners and stakeholders developed the document, *INSPIRE: Seven Strategies for Ending Violence Against Children.*[108] It is an excellent resource for evidence-based prevention strategies for preventing all types of violence among the world's most vulnerable populations, focusing on: (1) **I**mplementation and enforcement of laws; (2) **N**orms and values; (3) **S**afe environments; (4) **P**arent and caregiver support; (5) **I**ncome and economic strengthening; (6) **R**esponse and support services; and (7) **E**ducation and life skills. In this chapter, we focus on the two major forms of violence impacting children: child maltreatment and youth violence.

Child abuse or maltreatment, including physical, emotional, sexual harm, and neglect, has a deep and enduring impact on a child's physical, cognitive, emotional, and social development. Child maltreatment can lead to depression, low self-esteem, poor communication skills, struggling to empathize with others, poor education and economic outcomes, antisocial behavior, and increased likelihood of being a perpetrator or victim of future violence.[109] Primary prevention strategies addressing child maltreatment focus on improving the relationship between children and their parents and caregivers. There is evidence that parenting programs, particularly those that include home visits, improve parental attitude and parenting skills and may thus be effective at preventing child maltreatment.[110] Much of this evidence on parenting programs comes from HICs. The Nurse Family Partnership, in which nurses visit low-income, first-time mothers from pregnancy until 2 years after birth has had very promising results in the United States. Results from three randomized control trials in different U.S. populations found that the intervention led to fewer injuries resulting from abuse or neglect, improved infant emotional and language development, and improved maternal life outcomes, including reduced reliance upon public assistance programs.[111]

Child maltreatment prevention strategies that are effective in HICs may not be applicable in all resource-limited settings of LMICs. However, there is emerging evidence that positive parenting skill interventions may be feasible and effective in LMICs and more research assessing their applicability and impact in low-income contexts is urgently needed.[112] One example of adapting proven interventions is to use lay community health workers in place of more costly, highly trained nurses. A program in South Africa providing support and guidance from previously untrained local lay women to women during pregnancy through 6 months postpartum resulted in a significantly improved mother–infant relationship, when compared to a control group.[113] Similarly, a *Learning Through Play* intervention, that was originally developed in Canada, was adapted to be delivered by community health workers in Pakistan and significantly improved mothers' knowledge and attitudes about infant development.[114]

Child maltreatment is a major risk factor for youth violence, in which children transition from being victims to becoming perpetrators of violence. As children progress through different stages of life, they are influenced by different risk factors for youth violence including delinquency, aggressive behavior, psychological and conduct disorders, poor parental supervision, experiences of inconsistent and harsh discipline, parental involvement in crime, delinquent peers, neighborhood crime, gangs, income inequality, and concentrated poverty.[115] Youth violence prevention strategies address parenting and the development of life skills in children and adolescents through school-based and social development programs.

Positive parenting skills interventions that prevent child maltreatment can also prevent youth violence by addressing similar risk factors.[116] Interventions that include parenting components have been shown to improve many factors associated with youth violence, including mental health, substance use, delinquency, risky sexual behavior, and academic achievement.[117] For example, the Nurse Family Partnership that improved child maltreatment outcomes also saw improvement in the educational and cognitive indicators among children of mothers with poor mental health or low intelligence.[118] More research is needed in LMICs to understand the impact of these interventions on youth violence, but there are some successful examples. A parenting intervention in Burundi providing psychoeducation sessions by lay community counsellors reduced behavior problems among boys living in violence-affected settings.[119]

Life skills are cognitive, emotional, interpersonal, and social skills that enable youth to adapt to the demands of everyday life, fostering self-awareness, self-management, social awareness, relationships, and responsible decision-making.[109] School-based life skills development strategies are effective in reducing youth violence.[115] The *Azulas en Paz*, school-based life skills development intervention in Colombia, reduced aggressive interactions and improved social behavior among participants.[120] The Promoting Alternative Thinking Strategies (PATHS) program is an intensive, multiyear skill-based intervention that has been effective in reducing aggression and disruptive behavior and improving social and emotional skills in HICs.[109] However, high-quality implementation and school support are essential to the success of the intervention. Similar strategies may find challenges in LMICs with lower-resourced schools. Other school-based interventions, including bullying prevention, academic enrichment, dating violence prevention, peer mediation, and after-school or other structure leisure time activities may be effective strategies for preventing youth violence, but more research is needed to evaluate their impact.

Alcohol and Interpersonal Violence

Harmful alcohol use is a major risk factor for violence. Thirty percent of global violence mortality can be attributed to alcohol; in some regions, such as Europe and Central Asia, it is responsible for 56% of violence deaths.[121] Harmful alcohol use is associated with being both a victim and perpetrator of violence and is a preventable risk factor for youth violence, sexual violence, IPV, child maltreatment, and elder abuse.[109] Reducing the harmful use of alcohol is a cross-cutting strategy for preventing violence. Increasing the price of and reducing the availability of alcohol, as well as banning advertising, are proven, cost-effective interventions for preventing violence.[122] In Diadema, Brazil, a new law prohibiting the sale of alcohol between 11:00 pm and 6:00 am, when crime data indicated 60% of murders occurred, led to a 44% reduction in homicides in 3 years.[123] Although much of the evidence comes from HICs, increased alcohol prices have been shown to lead to immediate and long-term reductions alcohol-related mortality.[124] Strategies targeting problem drinkers are also important opportunities to prevent violence. Brief interventions and long-term treatment for problem drinkers have been shown to reduce IPV and child maltreatment.[125] Most of the violence prevention strategies focusing on alcohol are developed in HICs, but there is immediate need for more research in LMICs, where the burden is highest. In low-income populations and LICs, there is a higher disease burden per unit of alcohol consumption than in wealthier populations and countries.[126]

Suicide

Nearly 800,000 people take their own lives each year.[127] Suicide is the second leading cause of death in 15- to 29-year olds globally and three out of every four suicides occur in LMICs.[127] More people lose their lives to suicide than collective or interpersonal violence combined, yet due to stigma surrounding mental health and suicide, it receives far less attention as a major global health problem. Suicide is a global issue, but as seen in Fig. 25-2, the burden varies by age and country-level economic status. In HICs, middle-aged men have much higher suicide rates than their counterparts in LMICs; however, in LMICs, young adults and elderly women have much higher rates of suicide than similar populations in HICs.[128] In HIC, three times more men commit suicide than women, but in LMICs the ratio is closer to two suicides among women for every three in men.[128]

Despite the alarming nature of these global estimates, they may underestimate the true impact of suicides throughout the world. Measuring the burden of suicide requires robust data registries. These registries are important for all public health issues, but can be particularly challenging for suicide, which is such a sensitive and stigmatized topic. Many suicides are not officially reported or are miscategorized. In fact, in many countries, suicide is illegal, creating further challenges for accurately assessing its cost to society. Only 60 of the 172 WHO Member States have sufficient vital registry data and those lacking such infrastructure are predominantly LMICs. As such, the estimates for 112 countries, accounting for 71% of global suicides, are based on modelling methods.[128] These global estimates are helpful for raising awareness and making broad comparisons, but local systems that incorporate important regional and local factors are essential for accurately monitoring suicide trends.[129] It is also important to recognize that LMICs with insufficient infrastructure for documenting suicides likely also suffer from health system deficiencies that may exacerbate the suicide burden. Navigating lower-resourced health systems can be challenging for individuals with low health literacy, particularly those with low mental health literacy.[130] The risk of suicide increases with comorbidity,[131] so access to appropriate and effective healthcare is an essential component of reducing suicide risk.[128]

Preventing Suicide

Just like interpersonal violence, suicide is preventable. There is an urgent need for more research to determine effective prevention strategies, particularly in LMICs, but there is evidence that many lives can be saved when viewing suicide through a public health lens. For suicide prevention, it is important to recognize that suicidal behavior manifests in a cumulative continuum from ideation to plan to attempt.[132] Recognizing individual behaviors and actions at these different stages as risk factors for completed suicide is essential for getting people necessary mental healthcare in time to prevent a completed suicide. The strongest evidence for preventing suicides comes from strategies that reduce access to the lethal means. There is a common misconception that if someone has decided to commit suicide, reducing access to a specific mechanism is ineffective because the individual will simply find an alternative method. However, abundant research has shown that this is not true. Restricting access to lethal means is highly effective for preventing suicide.[133]

Pesticides are used in about one out of every three global suicides,[134] primarily in the rural areas of LMICs in Africa, Central America, Southeast Asia, and the Western Pacific.[128] Reducing access

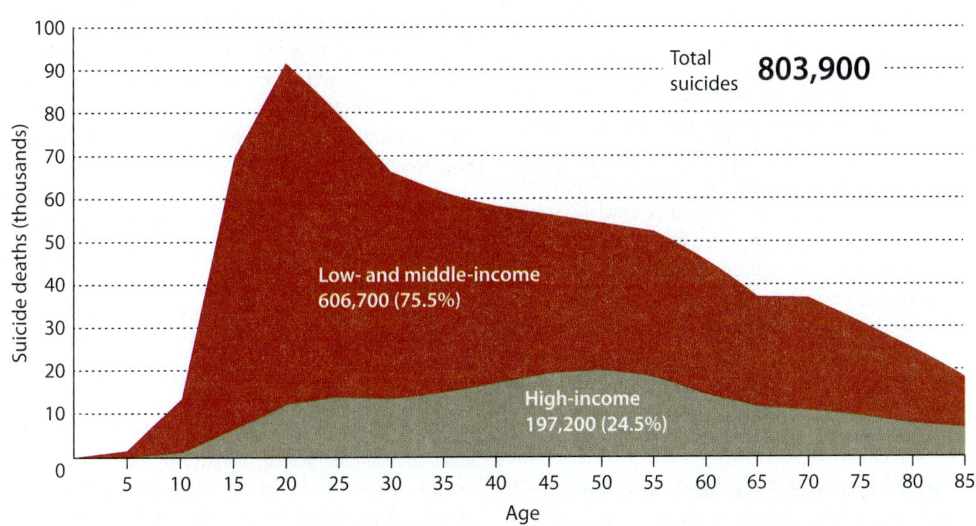

FIGURE 25-2. Global suicides by age and income level of country, 2012. WHO. Preventing Suicide: A Global Imperative. World Health Organization; 2014. With permission.

to highly toxic pesticides can prevent suicides. Restrictions on the import and sale of highly toxic pesticides in Sri Lanka greatly reduced suicides in males and females of all ages and resulted in nearly 20,000 fewer suicides from 1996 to 2005.[135] The expert-recommended Minimum Pesticides List previously identified in the unintentional poisonings section of this chapter also has the potential to reduce suicides from pesticides.[85]

Although the evidence primarily comes from HICs, it is unsurprising that access to firearms is highly correlated with the risk of a completed suicide.[136] Various strategies restricting access to firearms, including firearm control legislation,[137] safe storage requirements,[138] and mandatory waiting periods[139] can prevent suicides in HICs and may have potential in LMIC-contexts. Several studies from HICs have also shown that intervention strategies using physical barriers to reduce access to suicide hotspots, such as bridges, tall buildings, railroads tracks, or isolated locations, are effective in preventing suicides.[140] These interventions are also likely applicable in LMIC contexts where these hotspots are commonly used in suicides.

Similar to its connection to other forms of violence, harmful use of alcohol is strongly associated with suicide in both HICs and LMICs.[141] In 2006, a Russian policy that resulted in fewer alcohol producers and distributors and increased prices, led to a 9% reduction in the suicide rate in males, saving 4000 lives each year.[142] Similar policies have potential to reduce suicides in LMICs, but interventions need to be tailored to the specific alcohol consumption contexts that differ among cultures. In addition to reducing access to lethal means and reducing the harmful use of alcohol, other effective and promising suicide prevention strategies that include: encouraging media to participate in responsible reporting standards related to suicide (to avoid sensationalization, which can lead to "copy cat" suicides); improved care for individuals with mental and substance use disorders; training lay health workers to assess and manage suicidal behavior; and continuing care for people who have previously attempted suicide.[127]

Because suicide is often carried out in spontaneous, acute crisis situations, suicide or crisis hotlines represent an opportunity for preventing suicide in LMICs. Crisis hotlines in the United States have been shown to decrease suicidality during a conversation and even led to decreased hopelessness and psychological pain in subsequent weeks.[143] These hotlines require minimal infrastructure and resources to operate and have potential to prevent suicides in LMIC contexts. Due to limited mental health services in low-resource health systems in Africa and Southeast Asia, nongovernmental organizations currently provide free crisis hotline services.[141] However, more research is needed to understand the effectiveness of crisis hotlines in different global contexts.

Summary

Violence has always existed throughout the world and can never be fully eliminated. However, when viewed through a public health lens, we have the potential to prevent many incidences of violence and greatly reduce its prodigious toll on society. More research and evidence are needed, particularly in LMICs, to validate existing strategies and develop new interventions to prevent violence. The WHO has developed a website database, compiling studies and updating statistics on violence prevalence, consequences, risk factors, and prevention strategy effectiveness. The user-friendly site, http://apps.who.int/violence-info/, is a valuable resource for monitoring and contributing to public health strategies for preventing global violence.

TRAUMA CARE

This chapter is primarily on injury prevention and is oriented toward public health practitioners and researchers. However, trauma care (care of the injured) is an important component of overall efforts to decrease the health burden from injury. In this, there is a role for a wide variety of practitioners, in addition to surgeons, emergency physicians, emergency nurses, and other clinicians. Public health practitioners also have important roles to play, both in advocating for improvements in care in their areas. Oftentimes, they have positions in hospital administrations and in ministries of health/health departments in which they are involved in organizing and planning for trauma care services. It is thus important to note that there is a large amount of avoidable mortality from injury in LMICs and that improvements in organization and planning for trauma care can lower this mortality, even in very resource-constrained environments.

This avoidable mortality is reflected in differing rates of mortality after similar injuries, between high-income countries and LMICs. For example, for people with injuries that were life threatening but salvageable (e.g., injuries to the spleen), one study showed that mortality was six times higher in a low-income site compared with a high-income site.[144,145] Similarly, there is a large burden of disability from extremity injuries in LMICs in comparison to a higher proportion of disability from more difficult to treat neurological injuries in high-income countries. Disability from extremity injuries is eminently amenable to low-cost improvements in orthopedic care and rehabilitation.

Data primarily from high-income countries shows that improving the organization and planning for trauma care services can decrease overall mortality for hospitalized trauma patients by 15–20%. However, it can especially decrease deaths from avoidable causes (e.g., injuries to the spleen, as noted above) by 50%.[146,147] There is often a feeling that similar improvements in trauma care are too expensive or are not feasible in LMICs. However, there are many examples of innovative, affordable, and sustainable improvements in countries at all economic levels. For example, in a city in Mexico, an increase in the number of ambulance dispatch sites combined with improvements in in-service training for ambulance attendants led to a decrease in mortality from 10% to 7% for injured patients transported by that ambulance service. These improvements were associated with a 16% increase in the ambulance service budget, a cost which was sustainable and which has been continued.[148]

Much of the world does not have formal ambulance services which cover most of their populations. Even in these circumstances, progress can still be made by building on the de facto network of first responders who come to the aid of the injured in their locations. For example, a program in landmine-infested postconflict areas of Cambodia and Northern Iraq addressed the high rate of landmine injuries occurring to farmers who were returning to their lands. This program provided 1-day first aid training to thousands of lay people in the remote rural areas, accompanied by more intensive training for a few dozen paramedics living in the larger towns. The program provided basic supplies, but no ambulances or other vehicles. The injured continued to be taken to area hospitals by taxis or private vehicles. Nonetheless, this program resulted in a dramatic decrease in the mortality rate of people with landmine and other injuries: from 40% to 8% after the program was instituted.[148]

Similar improvements are possible in hospital-based care as well. For example, a low-cost trauma quality improvement program in a hospital in Khon Kaen, Thailand identified a high rate of avoidable deaths due to factors such as inadequate resuscitation for patients in shock in the emergency department and delayed surgery for head injuries. The hospital instituted corrective action in the form of increased staffing by senior clinicians in the emergency department at peak times (especially weekend nights), improved communications within the hospital, and better tracking of outcomes in medical records (including identifying and following rates of avoidable deaths). These low-cost measures resulted in a decrease in mortality among all admitted trauma patients from 8% to 5%.[148]

The question then is how to build on such individual success stories and make more progress globally. To do this, the WHO has created several guidelines oriented for LMIC ministries of health and hospitals designed to improve the organization and planning for trauma care. These include:

1. *Prehospital Trauma Care Systems*, which give guidance to ministries of health as to how to initiate and expand on basic ambulance services (as with the example from Mexico noted above); and when such ambulance services are not affordable or feasible in a given area, how to improve prehospital care by building on the network of de facto first responders (as with the example from Cambodia and Iraq noted above).[149]
2. *Guidelines for Essential Trauma Care*, which delineate core trauma care services that every injured person in the world can and should be able to receive, even in the poorest countries. The Guidelines delineate around 200 individual items of human resources (training, staffing) and physical resources (equipment, supplies, infrastructure) that should be in place at facilities along the spectrum ranging from clinics to small hospitals to tertiary care facilities.[147]
3. *Guidelines for Trauma Quality Improvement Programmes*, which provide information on how to set up straightforward methods to monitor and assure the quality of care provided to injured patients, with several types of programs, applicable to countries at all economic levels.[150]
4. Trauma care checklist, which is a simple form that can be used in emergency departments in all countries. It takes 1 minute to administer and is designed to assure that the most important items in the initial evaluation and care of severely injured patients are not overlooked in busy and often confusing emergency department situations.[151]

In conclusion, there are many preventable deaths and disabilities among injured patients in LMICs, which could be averted by affordable, feasible, and sustainable improvements in the organization and planning for trauma care. There are many good examples of such improvements in countries at all economic levels. The resources noted above offer methods for how these improvements can be expanded globally.

SUMMARY

Injury is a leading cause of death and disability globally, accounting for 4.9 million deaths, or 8% of the world's total deaths. The vast majority of these deaths are in LMICs, where conditions are less safe and where medical care once injured is less than optimal. However, for all mechanisms of injury, there are proven successful prevention strategies that have been inadequately applied. In some cases, prevention strategies that have been successful in high-income countries can be applied in LMICs with minimal modifications. In many cases however, there is the need for adapting these to local contexts. For some mechanisms of injury in LMICs, the best prevention strategies still need to be identified.

Despite the vast heterogeneity in burden, milieu, and resources across the world, an evidence-based, public health approach to reducing global injury is supported by reliably consistent principles. Addressing formidable public health challenges requires bold interdisciplinary, multisectoral strategies. Table 25-3 illustrates the

TABLE 25-3 EFFECTIVE INTERVENTIONS FROM A MULTIDISCIPLINARY PERSPECTIVE

Domain of Action	Infrastructure, Built Environment, and Product Design	Laws and Regulation	Advocacy, Education, and Behavior Change
Road Traffic Injuries			
	Road and sidewalk modifications; increased signage; intelligent speed adaptation technology; vehicle and motorcycle helmet safety standards	Increased helmet, seatbelt, child restraint, distracted driving, and drunk driving law implementation and enforcement; vehicle safety standards	Multisectoral education campaigns
Drowning			
	Physical barriers to water	Personal flotation device regulation and enforcement; boat and ferry safety regulation and enforcement; disaster risk management	Swim lessons for children (SwimSafe); community-based daycare and supervision (ANCHAL); safe rescue and resuscitation; public education campaigns
Falls			
	Elderly: home safety improvements, equipment modifications Children: home safety equipment (e.g., stair gates)		Elderly: exercise classes; risk assessment and management programs
Burns			
	Improved cook stoves and systems; smoke detectors; sprinkler systems; nonflammable sleepwear; electrical safety; water temperature regulators		Fire safety campaigns
Poisoning			
	Child-resistant containers	Ban highly toxic pesticides; require product warning labels	Kerosene storage and ventilation safety education; poison control centers
Violence			
	Physical barriers to prevent suicide	Legal protections for women and children; regulating alcohol sales; reducing access to lethal means of suicide	Positive parenting programs with home visits; community health worker perinatal support and guidance; school-based education; microfinance and gender equity; relationship skills classes; psychosocial support for at-risk youth; suicide crisis hotlines

effective intervention strategies presented in this chapter, stratified by different domains of action that must work together to enact real change. From individual behavior change interventions to international regulations, successfully approaching injury globally involves the same principles of multidisciplinary and multisectoral work that are fundamental to all other aspects of global health.

References

1. World Health Organization. *Global Health Estimates: Deaths by Cause, Age, Sex and Country, 2000–2015*. Geneva: WHO; 2015.
2. Institute for Health Metrics and Evaluation (IHME). *Financing Global Health 2017: Funding Universal Health Coverage and the Unfinished HIV/AIDS Agenda*. Seattle, WA. 2018.
3. Naghavi M, Abajobir AA, Abbafati C, et al. Global, regional, and national age-sex specific mortality for 264 causes of death, 1980–2016: A systematic analysis for the Global Burden of Disease Study 2016. *Lancet*. 2017;390(10100):1151–210.
4. Hay SI, Abajobir AA, Abate KH, et al. Global, regional, and national disability-adjusted life-years (DALYs) for 333 diseases and injuries and healthy life expectancy (HALE) for 195 countries and territories, 1990–2016: A systematic analysis for the Global Burden of Disease Study 2016. *Lancet*. 2017;390(10100):1260–344.
5. World Health Organization. Injuries and violence: The facts 2014. 2014.
6. World Health Organization. *Global Status Report on Road Safety 2015*. Geneva: World Health Organization; 2015.
7. Haagsma JA, Graetz N, Bolliger I, et al. The global burden of injury: Incidence, mortality, disability-adjusted life years and time trends from the Global Burden of Disease study 2013. *Inj Prev*. 2016;22(1):3–18.
8. World Health Organization. Road traffic injuries fact sheet. 2017.
9. Peden M, Scurfield R, Sleet D, et al. *World Report on Road Traffic Injury Prevention*. Geneva: World Health Organization; 2004.
10. McMahon K, Ward D. *Make roads safe: A new priority for sustainable development*. FIA foundation for the automobile and society. Commission for global road safety; 2007.
11. Resolution GA. 64/255, Improving global road safety. *United Nations General Assembly, New York*. 2010.
12. Híjar M, Pérez-Núñez R, Salinas-Rodríguez A. Advances in Mexico in the middle of the Decade of Action for Road Safety 2011–2020. *Rev Saude Publica*. 2018;52:67.
13. World Health Organization. Save lives: A road safety technical package. 2017.
14. Nadesan-Reddy N, Knight S. The effect of traffic calming on pedestrian injuries and motor vehicle collisions in two areas of the eThekwini Municipality: A before-and-after study. *S Afr Med J*. 2013;103:621–5.
15. Salvarani CP, Colli BO, Júnior CGC. Impact of a program for the prevention of traffic accidents in a Southern Brazilian city: A model for implementation in a developing country. *Surg Neurol*. 2009;72(1):6–13.
16. Ghadiri SMR, Prasetijo J, Sadullah AF, Hoseinpour M, Sahranavard S. Intelligent speed adaptation: Preliminary results of on-road study in Penang, Malaysia. *IATSS Res*. 2013;36(2):106–14.
17. Guanche Garcell H, Suárez Enríquez T, Gutiérrez García F, Martínez Quesada C, Peña Sandoval R, Sánchez Villalobos J. Impact of a drink-driving detection program to prevent traffic accidents [Villa Clara Province, Cuba]. *Gac Sanit*. 2008;22(4):344–7.
18. Ichikawa M, Chadbunchachai W, Marui E. Effect of the helmet act for motorcyclists in Thailand. *Accid Anal Prev*. 2003;35(2):183–9.
19. Silveira AJ. Seat Belt Use in Buenos Aires Argentina: A 14-Year-Old Struggle. Paper presented at: Road Safety on Four Continents Conference. 2005;13:10.
20. World Health Organization. Post-crash response: Supporting those affected by road traffic crashes. 2016.
21. World Health Organization. *Global Status Report on Road Safety 2013: Supporting a Decade of Action*. Geneva: World Health Organization; 2013.
22. Global NCAP. Democratising Car Safety: Road Map for Safer Cars 2020. 2015.
23. Wallbank C, McRae-McKee, K, Durrell, L, Hynd D. *The Potential for Vehicle Safety Standards to Prevent Deaths and Injuries in Latin America. An Assessment of the Societal and Economic Impact of Inaction*. London: Global NCAP; 2016.
24. Elvik R, Vaa T, Hoye A, Sorensen M. *The Handbook of Road Safety Measures*. Bingley: Emerald Group Publishing; 2009.
25. Killoran A, Canning U, Doyle N, Sheppard L. Review of effectiveness of laws limiting blood alcohol concentration levels to reduce alcohol-related road injuries and deaths. *Final Report London: Centre for Public Health Excellence (NICE)*. 2010.
26. Nevin PE, Blanar L, Kirk AP, et al. "I wasn't texting; I was just reading an email…": A qualitative study of distracted driving enforcement in Washington State. *Inj Prev*. 2017;23(3):165–70:injuryprev-2016-042021.
27. Liu BC, Ivers R, Norton R, Boufous S, Blows S, Lo SK. Helmets for preventing injury in motorcycle riders. *Cochrane Database Syst Rev*. 2008;(1):CD004333.
28. Pervin A, Passmore J, Sidik M, et al. Viet Nam's mandatory motorcycle helmet law and its impact on children. *Bull World Health Organ*. 2009;87(5):369–73.
29. Passmore J, Tu NTH, Luong MA, Chinh ND, Nam NP. Impact of mandatory motorcycle helmet wearing legislation on head injuries in Viet Nam: Results of a preliminary analysis. *Traff Inj Prev*. 2010;11(2):202–6.
30. Estados Unidos Mexicanos. Secretaría de Economía. Secretaría de Salud. Dirección General de Normas. Subsecretaría de Prevención y Promoción de la Salud. Cascos de seguridad para la prevención y atención inmediata de lesiones en la cabeza de motociclistas-Acciones de promoción de la salud-Especificaciones de seguridad y métodos de prueba, información comercial y etiquetado. *NORMA Oficial Mexicana NOM-206-SCFI/SSA2-2018*. 2018.
31. Zaza S, Sleet DA, Thompson RS, Sosin DM, Bolen JC. Reviews of evidence regarding interventions to increase use of child safety seats. *Am J Prev Med*. 2001;21(4, Suppl 1):31–47.
32. World Health Organization. Drowning fact sheet. 2018. http://www.who.int/mediacentre/factsheets/fs347/en/.
33. Linnan M, Rahman A, Scarr J, et al. *Child Drowning: Evidence for a Newly Recognized Cause of Child Mortality in Low and Middle Income Countries in Asia*. Florence: UNICEF Office of Research; 2012.
34. World Health Organization. *Global Report on Drowning: Preventing a Leading Killer*. Greneva: World Health Organization; 2014.
35. Peden M. *World Report on Child Injury Prevention*. Geneva: World Health Organization; 2008.
36. World Health Organization. *Preventing Drowning: An Implementation Guide*. Geneva: World Health Organization; 2017.
37. Leavy JE, Crawford G, Leaversuch F, Nimmo L, McCausland K, Jancey J. A review of drowning prevention interventions for children and young people in high, low and middle income countries. *J Commun Health*. 2016;41(2):424–41.
38. Thompson D, Rivara F. Pool fencing for preventing drowning in children. *Cochrane Database Syst Rev*. 2007;(2):4.
39. Rahman A, Mashreky SR, Chowdhury S, et al. Analysis of the childhood fatal drowning situation in Bangladesh: Exploring prevention measures for low-income countries. *Inj Prev*. 2009;15(2):75–9.
40. Rahman F, Bose S, Linnan M, et al. Cost-effectiveness of an injury and drowning prevention program in Bangladesh. *Pediatrics*. 2012;130(6):e1621–8.
41. Mecrow TS, Linnan M, Rahman A, et al. Does teaching children to swim increase exposure to water or risk-taking when in the water? Emerging evidence from Bangladesh. *Inj Prev*. 2015;21(3):185–8.
42. Cummings P, Mueller B, Quan L. Association between wearing a personal floatation device and death by drowning among recreational boaters: A matched cohort analysis of United States Coast Guard data. *Inj Prev*. 2011;17(3):156–9.
43. Cassell E, Newstead S. Did compulsory wear regulations increase personal flotation device (PFD) use by boaters in small power recreational vessels? A before-after observational study conducted in Victoria, Australia. *Inj Prev*. 2015;21(1):15–22:injuryprev-2014-041170.
44. Bugeja L, Cassell E, Brodie LR, Walter SJ. Effectiveness of the 2005 compulsory personal flotation device (PFD) wearing regulations in reducing drowning deaths among recreational boaters in Victoria, Australia. *Inj Prev*. 2014;20(6):387–92.
45. Golden AS, Weisbrod RE. Trends, causal analysis, and recommendations from 14 years of ferry accidents. *J Public Transport*. 2016;19(1):2.
46. Doocy S, Daniels A, Murray S, Kirsch TD. The human impact of floods: A historical review of events 1980–2009 and systematic literature review. *PLoS Curr*. 2013.
47. World Water Assessment Programme. *The United Nations World Water Development Report 4: Managing Water under Uncertainty and Risk*. Paris: UNESCO; 2012.
48. World Health Organization. Falls Fact Sheet. 2018.
49. Zecevic AA, Salmoni AW, Speechley M, Vandervoort AA. Defining a fall and reasons for falling: Comparisons among the views of seniors, health care providers, and the research literature. *The Gerontologist*. 2006;46(3):367–76.

50. World Health Organization. Falls. http://www.who.int/violence_injury_prevention/other_injury/falls/en/.
51. Mock CN, Nugent R, Kobusingye O, Smith KR. *Disease Control Priorities, (Volume 7): Injury Prevention and Environmental Health*. Washington, DC: World Bank Publications; 2017.
52. Lord SR, Sherrington C, Menz HB, Close JC. *Falls in Older People: Risk Factors and Strategies for Prevention*. Cambridge: Cambridge University Press; 2007.
53. Sànchez-Riera L, Carnahan E, Vos T, et al. The global burden attributable to low bone mineral density. *Ann Rheum Dis*. 2014;73(9):1635–45.
54. Kalache A, Keller I. The greying world: A challenge for the twenty-first century. *Sci Prog*. 2000;83(1):33-54.
55. Norton R, Ahuja RB, Hoe C, et al. Nontransport inintentional injuries. *Injury Prevention and Environmental Health: DCP3*. Washington, DC: The World Bank; 2017, p. 55.
56. Overpeck MD, McLoughlin E. Did that injury happen on purpose? Does intent really matter? *Inj Prev*. 1999;5(1):11–12.
57. Khambalia A, Joshi P, Brussoni M, Raina P, Morrongiello B, Macarthur C. Risk factors for unintentional injuries due to falls in children aged 0–6 years: A systematic review. *Inj Prev*. 2006;12(6):378–81.
58. Gillespie LD, Robertson MC, Gillespie WJ, et al. Interventions for preventing falls in older people living in the community. *Cochrane Database Syst Rev*. 2012;9(11).
59. Chang JT, Morton SC, Rubenstein LZ, et al. Interventions for the prevention of falls in older adults: Systematic review and meta-analysis of randomised clinical trials. *BMJ*. 2004;328(7441):680.
60. Spoelstra SL, Given BA, Given CW. Fall prevention in hospitals: An integrative review. *Clin Nurs Res*. 2012;21(1):92–112.
61. Kalula SZ, Scott V, Dowd A, Brodrick K. Falls and fall prevention programmes in developing countries: Environmental scan for the adaptation of the Canadian falls prevention curriculum for developing countries. *J Safety Res*. 2011;42(6):461–72.
62. Kendrick D, Watson MC, Mulvaney CA, et al. Preventing childhood falls at home: Meta-analysis and meta-regression. *Am J Prev Med*. 2008;35(4):370–9.
63. Young B, Wynn PM, He Z, Kendrick D. Preventing childhood falls within the home: Overview of systematic reviews and a systematic review of primary studies. *Accid Anal Prev*. 2013;60:158–71.
64. Hubbard S, Cooper N, Kendrick D, et al. Network meta-analysis to evaluate the effectiveness of interventions to prevent falls in children under age 5 years. *Inj Prev*. 2015;21(2):98–108.
65. Kendrick D, Young B, Mason-Jones AJ, et al. Home safety education and provision of safety equipment for injury prevention (Review). *Evid Based Child Health*. 2013;8(3):761–939.
66. World Health Organization. Burns Fact Sheet. 2018.
67. Peck MD, Jeschke M, Collins K. In: TWPost, ed. *Epidemiology of Burn Injuries Globally*. Waltham, MA: UpToDate; 2018.
68. Smolle C, Cambiaso-Daniel J, Forbes AA, et al. Recent trends in burn epidemiology worldwide: A systematic review. *Burns*. 2017;43(2):249–57.
69. Peck MD. Epidemiology of burns throughout the world. Part I: Distribution and risk factors. *Burns*. 2011;37(7):1087–100.
70. World Health Organization. Global Burn Registry. http://www.who.int/violence_injury_prevention/burns/gbr/en/. Accessed May 3, 2018.
71. Sanghavi P, Bhalla K, Das V. Fire-related deaths in India in 2001: A retrospective analysis of data. *Lancet*. 2009;373(9671):1282–8.
72. Sengoelge M, El-Khatib Z, Laflamme L. The global burden of child burn injuries in light of country level economic development and income inequality. *Prev Med Rep*. 2017;6:115–20.
73. Mashreky SR, Rahman A, Chowdhury SM, Khan TF, Svanström L, Rahman F. Non-fatal burn is a major cause of illness: Findings from the largest community-based national survey in Bangladesh. *Inj Prev*. 2009;15(6):397–402.
74. Rybarczyk MM, Schafer JM, Elm CM, et al. Prevention of burn injuries in low- and middle-income countries: A systematic review. *Burns*. 2016;42(6):1183–92.
75. World Health Organization. Burn prevention: Success stories and lessons learned. 2011.
76. Mallonee S, Istre GR, Rosenberg M, et al. Surveillance and prevention of residential-fire injuries. *N Engl J Med*. 1996;335(1):27–31.
77. World Health Organization. *Global Health Estimates: DALYs by Cause, Age, Sex and Country, 2000–2015*. Geneva: WHO; 2015, p. 9.
78. World Health Organization. International Programme on Chemical Safety: Poisoning Prevention and Management. 2018. http://www.who.int/ipcs/poisons/en/.
79. Jørs E, Neupane D, London L. Pesticide poisonings in low- and middle-income countries. *Environ Health Insights*. 2018;12:1178630217750876.
80. Schwebel DC, Swart D, Simpson J, Hui S-kA, Hobe P. An intervention to reduce kerosene-related burns and poisonings in low-income South African communities. *Health Psychol*. 2009;28(4):493.
81. Nonyelum SC, Nkem N, Ifeyinwa C-N, Orisakwe OE. Safety warnings and first aid instructions on consumer and pharmaceutical products in Nigeria: Has there been an improvement? *J Pak Med Assoc*. 2010;60(10):801.
82. Krug A, Ellis J, Hay I, Mokgabudi N, Robertson J. The impact of child-resistant containers on the incidence of paraffin (kerosene) ingestion in children. *S Afr Med J*. 1994;84(11):730–4.
83. Norton R, Hyder AA, Bishai D, Peden M. Unintentional injuries. In: Jamison DT, Breman JG, Measham AR, Alleyne G, Claeson M, Evans DB, Jha P, Mills A, Musgrove P, eds. *Disease Control Priorities in Developing Countries*. 2nd ed. Washington, DC: The International Bank for Reconstruction and Development/The World Bank; 2006. Chapter 39.
84. Balan B, Lingam L. Unintentional injuries among children in resource poor settings: Where do the fingers point? *Arch Dis Child*. 2012;97(1):35–8:archdischild-2011-300589.
85. Eddleston M, Karalliedde L, Buckley N, et al. Pesticide poisoning in the developing world—A minimum pesticides list. *Lancet*. 2002;360(9340):1163–7.
86. World Health Organization. International Programme on Chemical Safety: Poisons Centres. 2018. http://www.who.int/ipcs/poisons/centre/en/.
87. World Health Organization. Global Health Observatory (GHO) data: World directory of poisons centres, situation as of September 2017. 2018. http://www.who.int/gho/phe/chemical_safety/poisons_centres_text/en/.
88. World Health Organization. 10 Facts about Violence Prevention. 2017. http://www.who.int/features/factfiles/violence/en/.
89. World Health Organization. World report on violence and health. 2002.
90. Mercy JA, Rosenberg ML, Powell KE, Broome CV, Roper WL. Public health policy for preventing violence. *Health Aff (Millwood)*. 1993;12(4):7–29.
91. World Health Organization. Collective Violence Fact Sheet. 2002.
92. Mercy JA, Hillis SD, Butchart A, et al. Interpersonal violence: Global impact and paths to prevention. *Inj Prev Environ Health*. 803;(11.4): 71.
93. World Health Organization. Preventing violence: A guide to implementing the recommendations of the World Report on Violence and Health. 2004.
94. World Health Organization. *World Health Statistics 2017: Monitoring Health for the SDGs Sustainable Development Goals*. Geneva: World Health Organization; 2017.
95. World Health Organization. Global status report on violence prevention, 2014. 2014.
96. Stöckl H, Devries K, Rotstein A, et al. The global prevalence of intimate partner homicide: A systematic review. *Lancet*. 2013;382(9895):859–65.
97. World Health Organization. Global plan of action to strengthen the role of the health system within a national multisectoral response to address interpersonal violence, in particular against women and girls, and against children. 2016.
98. World Health Organization. *Global and Regional Estimates of Violence Against Women: Prevalence and Health Effects of Intimate Partner Violence and Non-partner Sexual Violence*. Geneva: World Health Organization; 2013.
99. Hillis S, Mercy J, Amobi A, Kress H. Global prevalence of past-year violence against children: A systematic review and minimum estimates. *Pediatrics*. 2016;137(3):e20154079.
100. Mercy JA, Butchart A, Rosenberg ML, Dahlberg L, Harvey A. Preventing violence in developing countries: A framework for action. *Int J Inj Contr Saf Promot*. 2008;15(4):197–208.
101. Butchart A, Garcia-Moreno C, Mikton C. Preventing intimate partner and sexual violence against women: Taking action and generating evidence. 2010.
102. Foshee VA, Reyes M, Wyckoff S. Approaches to preventing psychological, physical, and sexual partner abuse. *Psychological and Physical Aggression in Couples: Causes and Interventions*. Washington, DC: American Psychological Association; 2009, pp. 165–89.
103. Foshee VA, Karriker-Jaffe KJ, Reyes HLM, et al. What accounts for demographic differences in trajectories of adolescent dating violence? An examination of intrapersonal and contextual mediators. *J Adolesc Health*. 2008;42(6):596–604.

104. Pronyk PM, Hargreaves JR, Kim JC, et al. Effect of a structural intervention for the prevention of intimate-partner violence and HIV in rural South Africa: A cluster randomised trial. *Lancet.* 2006;368(9551):1973–83.

105. Kim J, Ferrari G, Abramsky T, et al. Assessing the incremental effects of combining economic and health interventions: The IMAGE study in South Africa. *Bull World Health Organ.* 2009;87(11):824–32.

106. Jewkes R, Nduna M, Levin J, et al. Impact of stepping stones on incidence of HIV and HSV-2 and sexual behaviour in rural South Africa: Cluster randomised controlled trial. *BMJ.* 2008;337:a506.

107. Paine K, Hart G, Jawo M, et al. 'Before we were sleeping, now we are awake': Preliminary evaluation of the Stepping Stones sexual health programme in The Gambia. *Afr J AIDS Res.* 2002;1(1):39–50.

108. World Health Organization. *INSPIRE: Seven Strategies for Ending Violence Against Children.* Geneva: World Health Organization; 2016.

109. World Health Organization. Violence prevention: The evidence. 2010.

110. Wessels I, Mikton C, Ward C, Kilbane T, Alves R. Preventing violence: Evaluating outcomes of parenting programmes. 2013.

111. Olds DL. The nurse–family partnership: An evidence-based preventive intervention. *Infant Ment Health J.* 2006;27(1):5-25.

112. Knerr W, Gardner F, Cluver L. Improving positive parenting skills and reducing harsh and abusive parenting in low-and middle-income countries: A systematic review. *Preve Sci.* 2013;14(4):352–63.

113. Cooper PJ, Tomlinson M, Swartz L, et al. Improving quality of mother-infant relationship and infant attachment in socioeconomically deprived community in South Africa: Randomised controlled trial. *BMJ.* 2009;338.

114. Rahman A, Iqbal Z, Roberts C, Husain N. Cluster randomized trial of a parent-based intervention to support early development of children in a low-income country. *Child Care Health Dev.* 2009;35(1):56–62.

115. World Health Organization. *Preventing Youth Violence: An Overview of the Evidence.* Geneva: World Health Organization; 2015.

116. Farrington DP. Childhood risk factors and risk-focused prevention. *The Oxford Handbook of Criminology.* Vol. 4. Oxford: Oxford University Press; 2007, pp. 602–40.

117. Sandler IN, Schoenfelder EN, Wolchik SA, MacKinnon DP. Long-term impact of prevention programs to promote effective parenting: Lasting effects but uncertain processes. *Ann Rev Psychol.* 2011;62:299–329.

118. Olds DL. Preventing child maltreatment and crime with prenatal and infancy support of parents: The nurse-family partnership. *J Scand Stud Criminol Crime Prev.* 2008;9(S1):2–24.

119. Jordans MJ, Tol W, Ndayisaba A, Komproe I. A controlled evaluation of a brief parenting psychoeducation intervention in Burundi. *Soc Psychiatry Psychiatr Epidemiol.* 2013;48(11):1851–9.

120. Chaux E. Aulas en Paz: A multicomponent program for the promotion of peaceful relationships and citizenship competencies. *Conflict Resolut Q.* 2007;25(1):79–86.

121. Ezzati M, Vander Hoorn S, Lopez AD, et al. Comparative quantification of mortality and burden of disease attributable to selected risk factors. *Global Burden of Disease and Risk Factors,* Vol. 2. Washington, DC: The International Bank for Reconstruction and Development/The World Bank Group; 2006, pp. 241–396.

122. Anderson P, Chisholm D, Fuhr DC. Effectiveness and cost-effectiveness of policies and programmes to reduce the harm caused by alcohol. *Lancet.* 2009;373(9682):2234–46.

123. Duailibi S, Ponicki W, Grube J, Pinsky I, Laranjeira R, Raw M. The effect of restricting opening hours on alcohol-related violence. *Am J Public Health.* 2007;97(12):2276–80.

124. Zhao J, Stockwell T, Martin G, et al. The relationship between minimum alcohol prices, outlet densities and alcohol-attributable deaths in British Columbia, 2002–09. *Addiction.* 2013;108(6):1059–69.

125. Dinh-Zarr TB, Goss CW, Heitman E, Roberts IG, DiGuiseppi C. Interventions for preventing injuries in problem drinkers. *Cochrane Database Syst Rev.* 2004;2004(3):CD001857.

126. Rehm J, Mathers C, Popova S, Thavorncharoensap M, Teerawattananon Y, Patra J. Global burden of disease and injury and economic cost attributable to alcohol use and alcohol-use disorders. *Lancet.* 2009;373(9682):2223–33.

127. World Health Organization. Suicide Fact Sheet. 2018.

128. World Health Organization. *Preventing Suicide: A Global Imperative.* Geneva: World Health Organization; 2014.

129. Bertolote JM, Fleischmann A. A global perspective in the epidemiology of suicide. *Psychology.* 2015;7(2).

130. World Health Organization. *Health Literacy: The Solid Facts 2013.* Copenhagen: WHO Regional Office for Europe; 2014.

131. Nock MK, Hwang I, Sampson NA, Kessler RC. Mental disorders, comorbidity and suicidal behavior: Results from the National Comorbidity Survey replication. *Mol Psychiatry.* 2010;15(8):868–76.

132. Borges G, Benjet C, Medina-Mora ME, Orozco R, Nock M. Suicide ideation, plan, and attempt in the Mexican Adolescent Mental Health Survey. *J Am Acad Child Adolesc Psychiatry.* 2008;47(1):41–52.

133. Yip PS, Caine E, Yousuf S, Chang S-S, Wu KC-C, Chen Y-Y. Means restriction for suicide prevention. *Lancet.* 2012;379(9834):2393–9.

134. Gunnell D, Eddleston M, Phillips MR, Konradsen F. The global distribution of fatal pesticide self-poisoning: Systematic review. *BMC Public Health.* 2007;7(1):357.

135. Gunnell D, Fernando R, Hewagama M, Priyangika W, Konradsen F, Eddleston M. The impact of pesticide regulations on suicide in Sri Lanka. *Int J Epidemiol.* 2007;36(6):1235–42.

136. Anglemyer A, Horvath T, Rutherford G. The accessibility of firearms and risk for suicide and homicide victimization among household members: A systematic review and meta-analysis. *Ann Intern Med.* 2014;160(2):101–10.

137. Mann J, Apter A, Bertolote J, et al. Suicide prevention strategies: A systematic review. *JAMA.* 2005;294(16):2064–74.

138. Caron J. Gun control and suicide: Possible impact of Canadian Legislation to ensure safe storage of firearms. *Arch Suicide Res.* 2004;8(4):361–74.

139. Ludwig J, Cook PJ. Homicide and suicide rates associated with implementation of the Brady Handgun Violence Prevention Act. *JAMA.* 2000;284(5):585–91.

140. Cox GR, Owens C, Robinson J, et al. Interventions to reduce suicides at suicide hotspots: a systematic review. *BMC Public Health.* 2013;13(1):214.

141. Patel V, Chisholm D, Dua T, Laxminarayan R, Vos T. *Disease Control Priorities, (Volume 4): Mental, Neurological, and Substance Use Disorders.* Washington, DC: World Bank Publications; 2016.

142. Pridemore WA, Chamlin MB, Andreev E. Reduction in male suicide mortality following the 2006 Russian alcohol policy: an interrupted time series analysis. *Am J Public Health.* 2013;103(11):2021–6.

143. Gould Madelyn S, Kalafat J, HarrisMunfakh Jimmie L, Kleinman M. An evaluation of crisis hotline outcomes part 2: Suicidal callers. *Suicide Life Threat Behav.* 2010;37(3):338–52.

144. Mock C, Adzotor K, Conklin E, Denno DM, Jurkovich G. Trauma outcomes in the rural developing-world—Comparison with an urban level-I trauma center. *J Trauma.* 1993;35(4):518–23.

145. Mock C, Joshipura M, Arreola-Risa C, Quansah R. An estimate of the number of lives that could be saved through improvements in trauma care globally. *World J Surg.* 2012;36(5):959–63.

146. Mann NC, Mullins RJ, MacKenzie EJ, Jurkovich GJ, Mock CN. Systematic review of published evidence regarding trauma system effectiveness. *J Trauma Acute Care Surg.* 1999;47(3):S25–33.

147. World Health Organization. *Guidelines for Essential Trauma Care.* Geneva: World Health Organization; 2004.

148. Mock C. *Strengthening Care for the Injured: Success Stories and Lessons Learned from Around the World.* Geneva: World Health Organization; 2010.

149. Varghese M, Sasser S, Kellermann A, Lormand J-D, Organization WH. *Prehospital Trauma Care Systems.* Geneva: World Health Organization; 2005.

150. World Health Organization. Guidelines for trauma quality improvement programmes. 2009.

151. World Health Organization. Trauma Care Checklist. http://www.who.int/emergencycare/publications/trauma-care-checklist.pdf. Accessed May 2, 2018.

CHAPTER

26 Global Health Security and Response to Humanitarian Emergencies

Jordan W. Tappero* • Oliver W. Morgan • Chikwe Ihekweazu • Beth P. Bell

Emerging infectious disease outbreaks are inevitable, whether naturally occurring, or due to the inadvertent release of highly pathogenic organisms from laboratories or acts of bioterrorism. Improving preparedness to detect and respond to these outbreaks, thereby limiting their spread and the associated human and economic costs, is the focus of global health security efforts. Humanitarian emergencies, resulting from natural disasters (e.g., earthquakes, tsunamis, floods, and droughts) and civil or military armed conflict also are inevitable and are on the rise.[1] The public health response to these crises is complex, often made even more challenging by their scale and scope, and the associated large-scale population displacements. Epidemics of infectious diseases and humanitarian emergencies are interconnected. The overcrowding, disrupted health services and poor access to food, clean water, and sanitation that occur in the context of humanitarian emergencies increase the risk of infectious disease epidemics.[2,3] Global health security efforts to build stronger capabilities to detect and respond to infectious disease outbreaks create more robust health systems, better able to handle the challenges of humanitarian emergencies. In this chapter, we will discuss both of these profound global health challenges.

GLOBAL HEALTH SECURITY: INTRODUCTION

Outbreaks of infectious disease are among nature's most reliable cruelties. We cannot predict with certainty when or where they will occur, only that it is inevitable that they will, and if not controlled at their source, pose a global threat in both lives lost and economic turmoil.[4,5]

In sub-Saharan Africa in the 1970s and 1980s, widespread, symptomatic HIV infection raged unrecognized for more than a decade, fostering today's costly global pandemic that has killed 35 million people and left another 36.7 million living with a serious infectious disease requiring life-long treatment.[6] In 2003, severe acute respiratory syndrome (SARS) spread from Asia to 29 countries across 3 continents in just 4 months, killing nearly 800[7] and costing an estimated $40 billion before it was contained.[8] In 2009, the emergence of influenza A (H1N1) resulted in the first declaration of a Public Health Emergency of International Concern (PHEIC) under the 2005 International Health Regulations (IHR-2005) and showed the world that it is ill-prepared to respond to a global pandemic threat.[9] In 2012, the Middle East Respiratory Syndrome (MERS) coronavirus emerged in Saudi Arabia,[10] spreading across the Arabian Peninsula and leading to travel-associated cases in Europe, North America, and Asia,[11] including a large nosocomial outbreak in South Korea in 2015.[12,13] In 2014, Ebola emerged for the first time in West Africa, resulting in the world's first regional Ebola epidemic. From 2014 to 2016, Zika virus reached Easter Island from the South Pacific, and soon thereafter marched rapidly from Brazil northwards across the Western Hemisphere[14] with the revelation of birth defects associated with infection in pregnancy. Coronavirus disease 2019 (COVID-19), caused by the newly identified SARS-CoV-2, emerged in Wuhan, China in December, 2019, and by the end of 2020 had spread globally with over 80 million cases reported. Meanwhile, the threat posed by common bacteria that develop resistance to available antibiotics continues to grow.[15]

Both new and previously recognized viral and bacterial pathogens will continue to emerge in new places; today's world of increasing interconnectivity and mobility accelerates this shared global risk. Global transportation and commercial air travel are expanding not only east to west but also north to south, with over 3.6 billion international air passengers in 2016 alone, linking emerging markets to the rest of the world more seamlessly than ever.[16] Changing migration patterns, driven by economic and security factors, and changing land-use patterns, create new exposures among populations and with nature. With this increased connectivity and mobility comes increased risk of infectious disease spread, with the next outbreak only a day's journey away. Climate change further deepens the world's vulnerability, as favorable conditions for the spread of many microbes and vectors increase.

Emerging infectious disease outbreaks are inevitable, but what is not inevitable is for outbreaks to become epidemics, and for regional epidemics to become global pandemics. We can either accept the human and economic costs of periodic epidemics and the threat of a worldwide pandemic or embrace preparedness and response capabilities through investments in global health security. Such investments include assisting countries to reach compliance with the revised World Health Organization (WHO) IHR-2005 through implementation of the Global Health Security Agenda (GHSA) and other improvements, the development of new diagnostics and technologies for the detection and molecular characterization of pathogens, and the enhancement of vaccines and therapeutics for humanitarian crises, including pandemics.

The 2014–2016 West African Ebola epidemic demonstrates the consequences of global health insecurity and shows what, at a bare minimum, is needed to better protect the world.

CASE STUDY: THE 2014–2016 WEST AFRICAN EBOLA EPIDEMIC

Background

Humans can be infected with Ebola virus through direct contact with an infected animal or its carcass or from human-to-human transmission. Outbreaks subsequently arise when human-to-human transmission occurs through direct contact with the blood or body fluids of a symptomatic or deceased infected person. By 2013, Ebola virus, first identified in 1976, had caused more than 25 recognized outbreaks in isolated rural areas across five East and Central African nations, with case fatality ratios ranging from 25% to 90%.[17]

*The views expressed are Dr. Tappero's and not those of the Bill & Melinda Gates Foundation.

These outbreaks were contained in a matter of weeks to a few months by implementing evidence-based clinical and public health measures, including rapid identification of cases and their contacts, isolation of possible cases from family members and communities, supportive care of Ebola patients in Ebola treatment units, and safe burial of all persons who die from infection with Ebola virus.

Detection

In December 2013, Ebola virus emerged for what may have been the first time in West Africa,[18] and spread virtually unnoticed for months in remote, forested areas of southeastern Guinea bordering Liberia and Sierra Leone. In late March 2014, the WHO reported the first cases in West Africa.[19] Within weeks, undetected chains of human-to-human transmission were making their way across the region.

WHO and international partners deployed epidemiologists within days of the initial report to help the affected countries investigate, but the lack of reliable disease surveillance, a public health and healthcare infrastructure devastated by years of conflict, and delayed responses by WHO country and regional authorities[20] hampered efforts to accurately assess the situation and determine the extent of spread. In addition, high population mobility, lack of infection control in healthcare facilities given the absence of gloves, soap, and running water, and longstanding and deeply held funeral practices at odds with safe burial augmented transmission.

By late July 2014, Ebola virus had reached the densely populated capitals of all three nations, the first time the disease had spread widely outside of remote rural areas. On August 8, 2014, WHO's Director General declared the Ebola outbreak to be a PHEIC, only the third such emergency to have been declared.[21]

Response Components

Nearly 40 years of accumulated experience had resulted in a clearly articulated and widely accepted strategy to stop an Ebola virus outbreak, consisting of the measures outlined above. Initially, there were serious challenges to implementation of each of these components in the unfamiliar and complex setting of widespread transmission that included spread to densely populated urban areas. Turning the tide required simultaneously addressing multiple interconnected barriers on many fronts.

Rapid identification of potential cases necessitated laboratory capacity to diagnose Ebola and a reliable reporting system, but there was essentially no Ebola diagnostic capacity in the three affected West African countries where Ebola had not been known to be a threat. Establishing this diagnostic capacity was complicated by Ebola's classification as a Biosafety Level 4 (BSL-4) agent, requiring specialized strict handling both during specimen transport and in the laboratory. The resulting insufficient testing capacity, delays in testing and reporting, and difficulties with optimal laboratory location; all contributed to early trouble stopping the outbreak.[22] Over a period of 25 months laboratorians with Ebola expertise from multiple countries mobilized to establish a network of international field laboratory teams across the three affected countries to provide Ebola diagnostic testing.[23,24]

There were many other components of an effective response that needed to be strengthened. Early on in Monrovia, Liberia, for example, despite the intensified efforts of Medicins Sans Frontieres (MSF) to expand available treatment capacity, the number of available beds was far outstripped by the need. There were not enough trained contact tracing teams to follow contacts of even a small proportion of known cases and many cases remained unidentified because of inadequate surveillance infrastructure. Teams that did identify symptomatic contacts had no available beds in Ebola treatment units to which to refer them for isolation and care, leading some contacts to return to their home villages; this further seeded new transmission hot spots throughout the country. Only four trained and equipped burial teams (out of an estimated need for 32) were available to remove highly infectious corpses. As a result, Ebola cases and deaths grew exponentially, resulting in even more unsafe burials and creating new transmission chains. To turn the tide, each of these interconnected functions was expanded, improved, and integrated, including identifying and training the necessary workforce. Experience controlling the outbreak in St. Paul's Bridge in Monrovia, Liberia in 2015 illustrated the positive effects when cases can be rapidly identified and isolated. Across successive generations of transmission, the average time to detection and isolation fell from 6.0 to 1.5 days, accompanied by a fall in the case reproduction ratio from 5 to 0.[25]

Controlling a complex humanitarian disaster requires an efficient and orderly response, with leadership and coordination at the national level. Each of the three highly affected countries initially had a fractured system to manage the public health emergency. The physical space for daily coordination meetings of national and international advisors and experts was insufficient, and lines of authority were unclear. But by the fall of 2014, with support of international partners, each country had established a national emergency operations center (EOC) with sufficient space and equipment, and a single, national Incident Manager was identified and empowered to report directly to the Office of the President. An incident management system (IMS) was employed to enable the various task forces and partners to bring options and recommendations to the Incident Manager for action.

Even with improvements in response components, the epidemic could not be controlled without engagement, buy-in and mobilization of the community. For example, Ebola patients and their families needed to trust the care offered to them in Ebola treatment units in order to agree to be isolated and treated there. Accurate contact tracing also required cooperation of community members. Participation of religious and other community leaders was vital to addressing the highly sensitive and emotional topic of how to modify traditional burial practices to prevent further transmission. Especially early in the epidemic, myths that Ebola was deliberately being spread by healthcare workers, or that it was a foreign plot were widespread, particularly in populations already distrustful of the government.[26] Therefore, countering and overcoming these beliefs was a high priority. An example of effective community engagement and social mobilization was the Western Area Surge, undertaken in the center and metropolitan area of Freetown, Sierra Leone in December 2014. The Surge was a coordinated effort to increase activities drastically across all areas of the response to halt the rapidly increasing number of cases in the country's capital city. A workforce of many hundreds of Sierra Leoneans was trained in surveillance and all possible patient isolation capacity was made available over a period of few weeks leading up to the surge. Community awareness and mobilization were prioritized by working in each of the area's 69 wards. The massive coordinated effort involved the Ministry of Health and multiple partners with national, local, and community ownership and participation. Ultimately, transmission in the city was reduced dramatically by strengthening capacity of the many key and interrelated components of the response, such as surveillance, active case finding, isolation of sick individuals, contact tracing, testing and treatment capacity, and safe and dignified burial.

While the impact of travel on spread within the three highly affected countries was of great concern, preventing spread to other countries was also a priority. As part of the PHEIC declaration, WHO provided guidance about measures to prevent such spread. Countries with Ebola transmission were advised to implement exit screening at all international airports, land crossings, and seaports for febrile illness consistent with Ebola, and to restrict travel for cases and contacts.[27] Exit screening at all border crossings of the three highly affected countries was attempted and most comprehensively implemented at the airports, where more than 339,000 people were screened.[28] WHO advised against general bans on international travel and did not recommend entry screening. Nonetheless, many countries implemented some form of screening of passengers arriving from the three highly affected countries, including 43 countries that prohibited entry of persons who had departed from a country with widespread transmission.[27] The United States implemented entry screening of arriving passengers from such countries, eventually screening more than 38,000 returning travelers.[28] Ultimately, there were exportations to six additional countries, including the United States, all of which were quickly controlled.

As the PHEIC reached the first-year anniversary (March of 2015), continuous transmission of Ebola virus had been interrupted across Guinea, Liberia, and Sierra Leone. However, throughout year two (April 2015–March 2016), eight additional clusters of Ebola virus disease provided evidence that Ebola virus could persist in the semen of male survivors and be transmitted sexually.[29–32] Sustained maintenance of national capacity to respond to Ebola virus disease clusters in the final year of the epidemic limited the number of generations of viral transmission compared to the first year of the epidemic. In the end, the 2014–2016 West African Ebola epidemic accounted for 28,652 cases and 11,325 deaths.[33]

Other Effects

The Ebola epidemic affected the health sector and the society broadly in the three most severely affected countries. The medical system was overwhelmed early in the crisis, with healthcare facilities closing as many healthcare workers became infected and died, and others did not come to work for fear of becoming infected. Routine health services and public health activities were severely affected. Vaccination coverage declined by an estimated 30% as vaccination campaigns were suspended because of safety concerns.[26,34] Reduced access to healthcare services resulted in reductions in treatment and control of endemic and chronic diseases. One study estimated that a 50% reduction in treatment would have resulted in an additional 10,600 deaths from malaria, tuberculosis, and HIV.[26,35] In countries already with some of the highest rates of maternal and child mortality, there were substantial reductions in the proportion of pregnant women delivering in health facilities.[26]

There were also wider societal impacts. For example, an estimated five million children lost almost a year of education because of school closures.[26] According to 2014 projections from the World Bank, an estimated $2.2 billion was lost in the gross domestic product of the three highly affected countries.[34]

Research and Innovation

Despite extremely challenging circumstances, successful field research was conducted during the epidemic, both to evaluate countermeasures and to study emerging characteristics of Ebola virus. At least three Ebola rapid diagnostic tests (RDTs) were developed, shown to have adequate performance characteristics and authorized for emergency use during the epidemic, including an automated polymerase chain reaction (PCR) device and two dipstick immunoassays that were used safely and effectively by community and primary health workers.[36] A challenging and carefully conducted epidemiologic study elucidated virus persistence in semen to help explain the observed sexual transmission of Ebola virus.[37] Genome sequencing was used in all three countries to understand virus transmission dynamics and the molecular epidemiology.[38–40] In Guinea, a novel and very portable nanopore sequencing instrument generated results in less than 24 hours after receiving an Ebola positive specimen and was used to conduct real-time genomic surveillance and molecular epidemiology.[40]

Since 1976, repeated outbreaks of Ebola virus disease prompted the development of Ebola virus vaccine candidates. During the 2014–2016 West African Ebola epidemic, three vaccine candidates were tested in more than 15 accelerated phase 1 and/or phase 2 vaccine clinical trials, enrolling thousands of participants.[41,42] These vaccines generally elicited good immunogenicity against Ebola virus and no serious adverse events were described.[42] Given the challenges, conducting these trials represented an enormous accomplishment. However, because of these challenges, including the time required to prepare the necessary clinical trial infrastructure and vaccine availability, the trials were begun relatively late in the outbreak.[41,43] Hence, vaccines were not able to be widely deployed and none were licensed.[41] Only one phase 3 trial was conducted, using a recombinant, replication-competent, vesicular stomatitis virus-based vaccine expressing the glycoprotein of a Zaire Ebola virus (rVSV-ZEBOV; Merck & Co with NewLink Genetics Corporation). In an open-label, cluster-randomized ring vaccination of contacts and contacts of laboratory-confirmed cases of Ebola virus disease in Guinea and Sierra Leone, participants received either an immediate or delayed (21 days later) single, intramuscular injection of rVSV-ZEBOV.[44] No cases of Ebola virus disease occurred 10 days or more after vaccination in participants who received immediate vaccination; estimated vaccine efficacy 100% (95% confidence interval: 68.9–100.0; $p = 0.045$).

Similarly, a variety of investigational therapeutic agents were studied during the middle and late stages of the outbreak, largely in uncontrolled clinical trials or in individual patients under compassionate use. These agents were generally chosen either because they had shown promising activity against Ebola virus in vitro or had been demonstrated to reduce mortality in animal challenges, including nonhuman primates.[45] None showed conclusively that any particular investigational agent was superior to supportive care in reducing mortality.[45] Perhaps the most well-known was ZMapp, a cocktail of three monoclonal antibodies against Ebola virus.[42,46] In 2015, a randomized controlled trial of standard of care with and without ZMapp enrolled 71 patients with Ebola virus disease at sites in Guinea, Liberia, Sierra Leone, and the United States. However, enrollment was stopped before reaching the target of 100 participants because the outbreak was waning. The observed posterior probability that ZMapp was superior to standard of care alone was 91.2%, short of the prespecified threshold of 97.5%.[42,45,46] The clinical benefits of individualized supportive care also became clear during the outbreak, with the initial mortality throughout the region of 70% falling to approximately 40% with the application of measures such as better symptom control, treatment of shock, and rapid diagnosis or empirical treatment of concomitant conditions such as malaria and bacterial infections.[47] The combined clinical experience during the outbreak was codified into evidence-based guidelines for supportive care of Ebola patients.[47]

TODAY'S FRAMEWORK FOR GLOBAL HEALTH SECURITY

Strengthening global health security, efforts to prepare for and minimize vulnerability to pandemic and epidemic diseases at national, regional, and global levels, has been driven over decades by the continuing threats of emerging infectious diseases such as HIV, SARS, and pandemic influenza. Its importance is reflected in global frameworks such as the UN Sustainable Development Goals (SDG).[48] These efforts were boosted by the 2014–2016 West African Ebola epidemic, a particularly stark reminder of the importance of enhancing health security. Over 40 targeted examinations of aspects of the Ebola response were published,[49] and a number of commissions, advisory groups, and panels produced reports that aimed to provide a comprehensive assessment and recommendations of priority actions to improve global health security.[49,50] All recognized that infectious disease outbreaks are likely to become more frequent in the future and determined that the world remained tremendously unprepared to address them.[49]

The reports generally agreed on key areas that needed to be strengthened and proposed ways to address identified weaknesses. A major contributor to the slow response was inadequate compliance with the IHR-2005 (see below), including concerns about the validity of many countries' self-reported implementation status and delays in reporting of outbreaks. The reports recognized that strengthening public health as the foundation of the health system and first line of defense was essential, drawing attention to the inadequate core capacities in many countries to detect and respond to infectious disease outbreaks and the need to secure adequate and sustained financing and technical assistance to address these weaknesses.[51] A number of the reports highlighted the importance of accelerating research and development to counter infectious disease threats and addressing knowledge-sharing problems that hamper these efforts. All reports recommended strengthening the WHO and broader UN and humanitarian systems and addressing both operational and institutional problems.[49]

The 2005 Revised International Health Regulations

In 1969, the WHO's IHR were enacted as a collaborative framework to stop the cross-border spread of infectious disease threats such as plague, cholera, yellow fever, and smallpox.[52] The 2003 global SARS outbreak demonstrated that focus on border controls would not stop the spread of disease, and failures to transparently report outbreaks left countries vulnerable to disease importation. Accordingly, in May 2005, the World Health Assembly (WHA) adopted the revised IHR-2005, a legally binding agreement by 196 United Nations member states with the goal to directly address emerging epidemics and other health threats.[53] The IHR-2005 requires countries to strengthen 19 core public health capabilities[54,55] and to report regularly on their progress. These capabilities include eight core public health capacities to improve the speed of detection and response and required reporting of any PHEIC, with real-time dialogue with WHO to determine appropriate actions at borders.[4] Yet, by the 2012 deadline less than 20% of countries reported full compliance with the IHR-2005.[56,57] A 2-year extension to 2014 increased the number of fully compliant countries by only 10%.[3]

Global Health Security Agenda

On February 13, 2014, the United States and 28 partner nations, WHO, the Food and Agricultural Organization (FAO), and the World Organization for Animal Health (OIE) launched the Global Health Security Agenda (GHSA), a collaborative effort dedicated to strengthening global health security by investments in national and regional capacities to prevent, detect, and respond to infectious disease threats, including advancing implementation of the IHR-2005 and other relevant international frameworks and agreements.[5] GHSA envisions a world safe and secure from global health threats posed by infectious diseases, able to prevent or mitigate the impact of naturally occurring outbreaks, as well as accidental or intentional release of dangerous pathogens. GHSA works to leverage host government and donor partner investments to rapidly detect and transparently report such events when they occur, and to respond effectively to limit their spread, ultimately reducing suffering and loss of life and limiting economic impact.

As of October 2018, over 70 nations had joined GHSA (Fig. 26-1). The GHSA consists of an integrated partnership that, in addition to WHO, FAO, and OIE, includes member nations, the World Bank, nongovernmental and other international organizations, development partners, and the private sector. Financial commitments to implement GHSA have been made by the Group of Seven industrialized democracies (G7), Australia, the Republic of Korea, the Nordic countries, and others.[58] The World Bank and a growing list of private partners are also contributing.[3] Individual partner countries are also prioritizing domestic funding for this effort. These commitments were reaffirmed by over 50 GHSA member countries at the September 2016 and the October 2017 GHSA Ministerial Meetings held in Seoul, South Korea and Kampala, Uganda, respectively.

GHSA is a catalyst for worldwide IHR-2005 compliance, established on the principle that every nation must protect its citizens from epidemic health treats. GHSA is a model designed to prevent avoidable epidemics, detect threats early, and respond to them rapidly and effectively at their source,[4,5] consistent with the Institute of Medicine's framework for countering infectious disease crises.[59] The GHSA framework is organized around technical areas, termed "Action Packages," that group the essential health security capabilities of a resilient health system into 11 components (Table 26-1), linked to measurable targets and accompanying milestones to track progress.[3] Each of these targets is important to promote strong, multisectoral capacity to address infectious disease threats.

The most effective prevent, detect, and respond systems are those in use every day engaged in event-based surveillance and program monitoring that can be rapidly scaled up in an emergency. From a public health perspective, real-time, reportable disease surveillance, a national laboratory system, a trained, retained, and adequately paid public health work force, and an EOC with a strong IMS routinely utilized for outbreak response and monitoring of key disease control programs provide the core foundation from which to build other elements. A real-time surveillance system supported by quality and safe laboratory testing allows data for decision making to move rapidly through subdistrict, district, and regional levels to the national level for immediate action. Timely feedback of data down through all administrative levels fosters completeness of reporting. Such feedback ensures that when trained district health officers report a potential threat, it does not mean that the district health office has failed, but rather that it has been successfully watchful. Transparency in reporting must also extend upward from the national Ministry of Health to WHO, FAO, and OIE. In addition to surveillance for specific diseases and infections, surveillance for key syndromes is essential to ensure that health events, such as acute flaccid paralysis (a warning sign of possible resurgent polio virus) or a cluster of deaths among health workers (a harbinger of a viral hemorrhagic fever virus such as Ebola) are reported to international health authorities and promptly investigated.

Many of the factors driving the increasing frequency of emerging infectious diseases, such as demographic changes that bring people into closer contact with animals, and climate change and deforestation, also facilitate transmission of zoonotic and vector-borne infections, those caused by transmission from animals or insect vectors (mosquitoes, ticks, and fleas). It is estimated that 75% of new, emerging infectious diseases in humans are zoonotic in origin.[60] Strengthening surveillance for zoonotic and vector-borne infections in humans can both improve efforts to address endemic diseases and serve as an early warning system for newly emerging or re-emerging infections. Animal surveillance systems generally are weak, especially in low- and middle-income countries, but improving communication between animal and human surveillance systems nonetheless provides another means to track transmission of zoonotic infections.

Antimicrobial resistance is a growing public health threat. Antimicrobials play a crucial role in human and veterinary medicine, but these curative agents are becoming increasingly ineffective as resistant organisms spread around the globe. In March 2015, the United States released its National Action Plan to Combat Antibiotic-Resistant Bacteria; and in May 2015, the WHA adopted the WHO Global Action Plan on Antimicrobial Resistance which calls for countries to develop and implement their own comprehensive national plans. GHSA aims to support development and implementation of these plans, focusing on strengthening surveillance and laboratory capacity, enhancing infection prevention and control, and promoting the prudent use of antibiotics in both the veterinary and human sectors.

Joint External Evaluation (JEE)

The JEE is a voluntary external assessment process that grew out of interest on the part of several bodies in adopting concrete and stringent monitoring procedures to address the recognized shortcomings

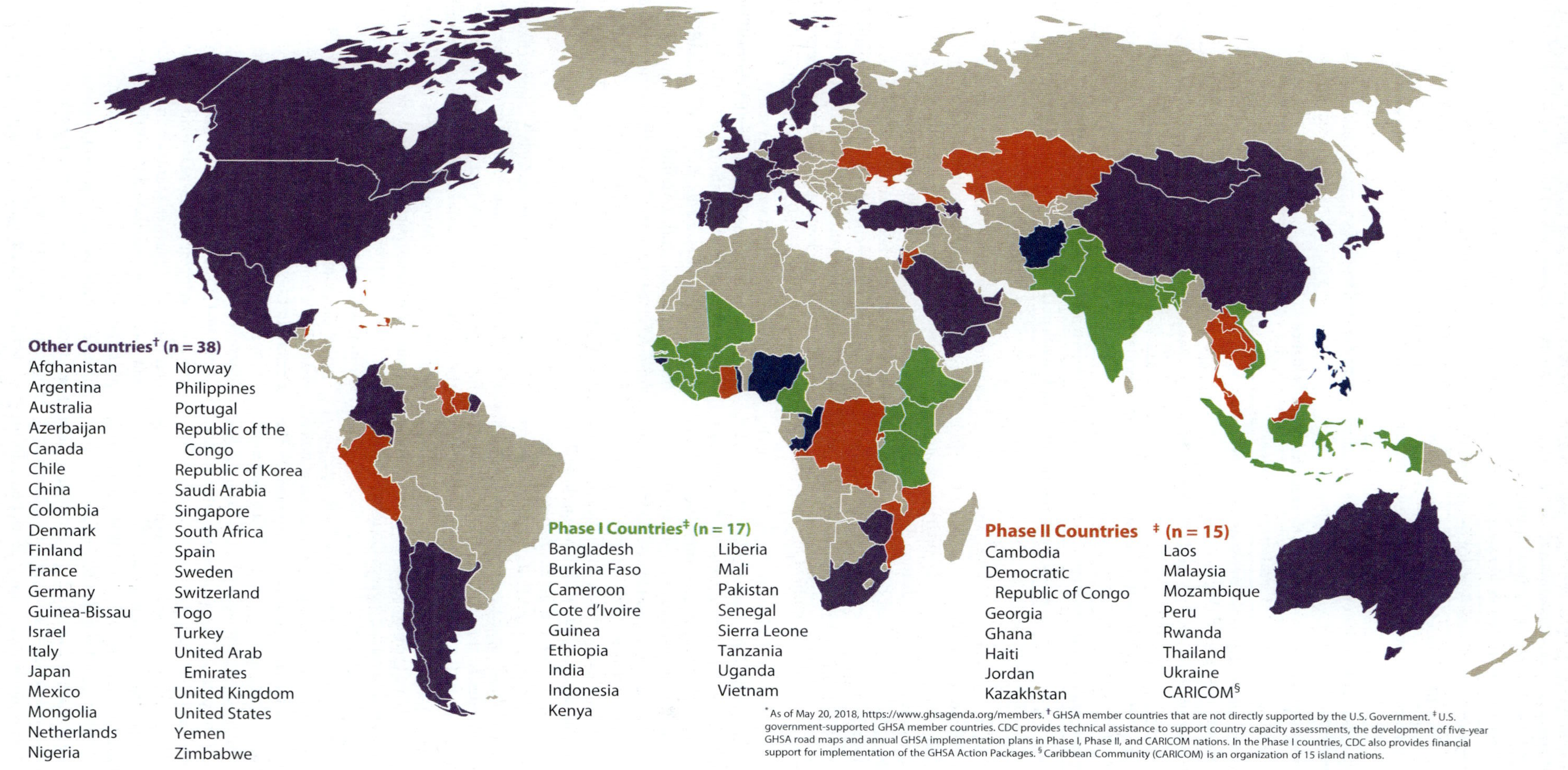

*As of May 20, 2018, https://www.ghsagenda.org/members. † GHSA member countries that are not directly supported by the U.S. Government. ‡ U.S. government-supported GHSA member countries. CDC provides technical assistance to support country capacity assessments, the development of five-year GHSA road maps and annual GHSA implementation plans in Phase I, Phase II, and CARICOM nations. In the Phase I countries, CDC also provides financial support for implementation of the GHSA Action Packages. § Caribbean Community (CARICOM) is an organization of 15 island nations.

FIGURE 26-1. Countries Participating in the Global Health Security Agenda (GHSA), October 2018. (*Source*: Tappero JW, Cassell CH, Bunnell R, et al. US Centers for Disease Control and Prevention and Its Partners' Contributions to Global Health Security. Emerging Infectious Diseases. 2017;23(13). doi:10.3201/eid2313.170946.)

TABLE 26-1 GLOBAL HEALTH SECURITY AGENDA GOALS AND TARGETS

Model	Global Health Security Agenda Targets
PREVENT avoidable outbreaks	Establish surveillance to monitor and slow the spread of **antimicrobial drug-resistant** organisms
	Develop policies and practices that reduce the risk of **zoonotic disease** transmission
	Promote national **biosafety and biosecurity** systems
	Immunize against epidemic prone diseases including 90% coverage of children under the age of one with a measles-containing vaccine
DETECT threats early	Strengthen **national laboratory systems,** including specimen referral networks to cover at least five priority pathogens in at least 80% of the country
	Strengthen interoperable networks for **real-time biosurveillance**
	Surveillance for at least three **priority syndromes**
	Promote practices for rapid, **transparent disease reporting** to WHO, Food and Agricultural Organization, and World Organization for Animal Health
	Train and deploy an effective **public health workforce** including at least one trained field epidemiologist per 200,000 population
RESPOND rapidly and effectively	Develop **emergency operations centers** and functional incident management systems able to operate within 120 minutes of activation
	Promote **multisectoral emergency response**; linkages between public health and law enforcement
	Improve global access to **medical countermeasures and health personnel** during emergencies

of self-assessment and reporting, and to identify gaps and track progress toward clearly defined readiness goals. In 2014, the GHSA Executive Committee called for developing a comprehensive, independently administered monitoring and evaluation framework for GHSA.[53] Soon thereafter, a WHO-sponsored IHR review committee recommended moving from exclusive self-evaluation of IHR compliance to "approaches that combine self-evaluation, peer review, and voluntary external evaluations involving a combination of domestic and independent experts."[55]

In 2015, a GHSA evaluation tool, informed by five previously developed monitoring and evaluation frameworks (WHO IHR Annual Reporting Tool; OIE tool for the Evaluation of Performance of Veterinary Services; CDC's Public Health Emergency Preparedness Performance Measures; Global Immunization Index; the International Atomic Energy Agency Safety Assessment; and the WHO Ebola Virus Preparedness Checklist) was created to track national capacity to address infectious disease threats across 11 core capacities. Informed by the successful implementation of a pilot GHSA evaluation tool, in February 2016 WHO adopted the JEE tool to harmonize independent monitoring for the 11 GHSA targets and IHR compliance efforts across all 19 IHR core preparedness capacities for infectious disease, chemical, radiological, and nuclear threats.[61] The JEE's aim is to determine a country's level of health security capacity, identify gaps, and measure progress going forward. As such, JEEs are a critical part of the all hazards capacity building cycle designed to inform national policy setting, target resources, and track progress. Countries request a JEE through their WHO representative.

The JEE is organized into a set of indicators grouped into categories that generally conform to the GHSA action packages, each scored on a 1–5 scale and depicted in a red/yellow/green-type "dashboard."[62] The external evaluators produce a summary and detailed mission report, provided to the requesting country. Through July 13, 2018, 79 JEE country assessments were completed. Countries can voluntarily make their JEE mission report publicly available on the GHSA and WHO websites.[62] In addition, 28 countries have been scheduled for a JEE in 2018 and 2019, such that at least 103 countries will have completed an externally validated assessment by the May 2019 WHA in Geneva, Switzerland. The United States completed and published its JEE in May 2016 and is actively working to address identified IHR compliance gaps.

Countries that voluntarily receive a JEE mission are active participants in the identification of 60 or more jointly developed priority actions that are ideally utilized to develop a comprehensive national plan of action, including milestones for each year, and identify where external technical support is required by partners. In addition, the national plan of action should prioritize areas for host government financial commitments and highlight financial shortfalls for both current and prospective donors to fill gaps with resources. Country ownership of the national plan of action is essential, requiring commitment from the highest level of government to ensure sustainable domestic resourcing for capacity building. A repeat JEE external assessment is expected within 4–5 years.

To ensure sustainability for the JEE process, a WHO Secretariat for JEEs has been established, supported by a voluntary Alliance for Country Assessments for Global Health Security and IHR Implementation, and a multistakeholder Advisory Group drawn from Alliance members, including countries (69 as of April 2018), nongovernmental organizations, foundations, and multilateral organizations.

GHSA Implementation

Total 2014–2018 funding for GHSA implementation is reported to be over $1.2 billion and many collaborating countries also are supporting implementation of action packages with in-kind contributions.[58] For example, some high-income countries are forming partnerships with specific lower-income countries to assist with implementation of particular action packages. There are many examples of progress in individual countries and specific action packages, but it is too early in the process for a comprehensive assessment.

The U.S. Government committed to invest $1 billion to accelerate GHSA implementation with 31 partnering countries, and the Caribbean Community (CARICOM) comprised of 18 island nations. Among this group of countries, 17 were included in so-called "phase 1," with the objective of achieving all 11 GHSA targets (Table 26-1). The United States also is contributing to baseline JEEs and the development of 5-year road maps and annual implementation plans in all partner countries and CARICOM. Through the second year of implementation (2018), progress has been made in all 17 phase 1 countries against the 11 targets.[63] Examples of early successes include improvements in surveillance for zoonotic diseases, training healthcare workers in infection prevention and control and how to prevent the spread of drug-resistant organisms, and redoubled efforts to increase measles vaccination coverage. Early detection advances have included focused public health workforce training, strengthening surveillance, and improving access to electronic surveillance data. Emergency operation centers have been established and strengthened through exercises and activation for large outbreaks.[63,64]

DIAGNOSTICS AND COUNTERMEASURES

Diagnostics to identify infected patients rapidly, and vaccines and therapeutics to treat them are critical components of any effective epidemic response. The absence of countermeasures for an emerging disease or epidemic not only hampers the response and costs lives, but also can seed panic and fear in the population. As the 2014–2016 West African Ebola epidemic demonstrated, it is generally too late to achieve maximum benefit from these interventions if their development does not begin until after the outbreak has been identified and evaluating intervention efficacy in the context of an ongoing outbreak is very challenging. Compassionate use of unlicensed therapeutics for individual patients can be complicated by potential ethical considerations and does not often generate generalizable information. The importance of increasing the availability of countermeasures for emerging threats was highlighted in a number of post-Ebola commissions and WHO advisory panels.[50]

A number of scientific advances can speed the development of countermeasures to address emerging threats.[65] The advent of next-generation genomic sequencing and related tools has made it possible to quickly identify and characterize unrecognized pathogens. Advances in PCR technology have increased the settings in which diagnostics can be readily deployed to include resource poor settings and broadened the range of options for rapid diagnostic development and deployment. Vaccine platform technology, including viral vectors, virus-like particles, mRNA, and nanoparticles, brings the promise of overcoming the limitations of inactivated vaccines. Furthermore, to the extent that platform technologies are agnostic as to specific pathogens, they can compress the time required for vaccine development because development and manufacture can move forward without waiting for the next epidemic to emerge.[66] Applying a similar rationale in the area of therapeutics has spurred the identification of broad-spectrum antivirals that target common components of a number of viruses. Approaches include RNA polymerase inhibitors, double stranded RNA (dsRNA)-activated caspase oligomerizer (DRACO), and small interfering RNA (siRNA). Monoclonal antibody cocktails also hold considerable promise.[67]

Harnessing these scientific advances to limit illness and death when epidemics emerge will require addressing underlying barriers in countermeasure development and deployment using a number of different approaches. This is true both for developing effective countermeasures before epidemics occur, and for having the research infrastructure in place should clinical trials be necessary in the midst of an epidemic. A barrier to developing countermeasures for pathogens with epidemic potential is the considerable financial risk to private industry, given their poor market potential and the regulatory unknowns.[41] Efforts by funders and international organizations to spur countermeasure development have been fragmented and of insufficient scale. Other systemic weaknesses include poor coordination and confusion about regulatory pathways, and diverse and sometimes conflicting perspectives about ethical considerations in conducting clinical trials, especially in the midst of epidemics. Additional barriers to timely countermeasures research during epidemics include lack of agreement about appropriate clinical trial design, as well as a lack of international norms and standards on sharing data and samples, resulting in few available specimens, limited information sharing, and weak data systems that are not interoperable.

At the 2015 WHA, the member states requested that WHO convene a broad network of experts to develop a research and development blueprint for action to prevent epidemics. The blueprint development process, meant to address many of the recognized weaknesses, was initiated soon thereafter with the objectives of developing and implementing a roadmap for R&D preparedness for known priority pathogens and of enabling an early and efficient roll out of an emergency R&D response.[68]

The WHO blueprint created a list of ten priority pathogens for research and development in public health emergency contexts, using criteria developed by an expert panel, and produced accompanying roadmaps and target product profiles.[69] After the yearly review in February 2018, the list included Crimean Congo hemorrhagic fever virus, Ebola and Marburg viruses, Middle East respiratory syndrome coronavirus and severe acute respiratory syndrome coronavirus, Lassa fever virus, Nipah virus, Rift Valley fever virus, Zika virus, and "disease X," included in an attempt to enable cross-cutting research for a currently unknown disease that might emerge as a human pathogen.[69]

There have been a number of recent developments aimed at increasing the pipeline of countermeasures for diseases of pandemic potential. Both the European Innovative Medicines Initiative and the US Biomedical Advanced Research and Development Authority (BARDA) have invested in these areas.[49] The Coalition for Epidemic Preparedness Innovations (CEPI) is a public-private partnership that aims to "stimulate, finance, and coordinate the development of vaccines against epidemic infectious diseases, especially in cases in which market incentives alone are insufficient."[41] CEPI was launched at the World Economic Forum in Davos in 2017, with initial funding of $620M from the Wellcome Trust, the Bill and Melinda Gates Foundation, the World Economic Forum, and the governments of Norway and India.[41] CEPI includes an ever-expanding group of partners including governments, foundations, and other private and public organizations. CEPI has two objectives: advancing candidate vaccines against high-priority pathogens through phase 2 clinical trials and supporting vaccine platforms that can be rapidly deployed against known and unknown pathogens, with an initial focus on MERS, Lassa, and Nipah viruses. CEPIdx, a similar entity focused on diagnostics was launched in June 2017, but its funding and scope remain unclear.[22]

Using a similar model, in 2016 an initiative was launched to promote innovation in antibiotic research and development to address antibiotic resistance. Termed CARB-X, this initiative is a public-private partnership led by Boston University and supported by BARDA, the National Institutes of Health, and the Wellcome Trust to create a $455 million 5-year global partnership to rejuvenate the pipeline of new antibiotic candidates. As of 2018, CARB-X had invested in 26 companies, with more likely to be added in the near future.[70]

Structures and legal, regulatory, ethical, and scientific procedures that support research and development of countermeasures must also be strengthened. National regulatory authorities have important roles to play to make critical resources such as diagnostics and vaccines available during an emergency and to facilitate eventual licensure. Regulatory authorities in some countries such as the United States, the EU, and Canada have procedures in place that permit use of unapproved countermeasures in the context of a declared emergency (e.g., the Emergency Use Authorization in the United States, as well as procedures that accelerate the regulatory process for licensure, such as the Breakthrough Therapy and Priority Medicines designation of the U.S. Food and Drug Administration (FDA) and Priority Medicines (PRIME) from the European Medicines Agency (EMA)). However, many National Regulatory Authorities (NRA) are weak and underfinanced and lack the necessary expertise to evaluate fully new and highly complex countermeasures. Strengthening collaborations among NRAs building on existing entities such as the African Vaccine Regulatory Forum, is an important step. For example, during the West African Ebola epidemic, with support from WHO and a number of high-income country regulators, the highly affected and neighboring countries were able to fast-track vaccine clinical trials by using joint regulatory and ethical reviews of trial designs and clearing administrative bottlenecks. The WHO Emergency Use Assessment and Listing (EUAL) procedure for diagnostics, vaccines, and therapeutics to be used during a PHEIC, developed during the West African Ebola epidemic, has potential, but needs to be developed further.[71] WHO also developed the Monitored Emergency Use of Unregistered Interventions (MEURI) program to allow for compassionate use or expanded access to unlicensed therapeutics during emergencies.

However, experts recommended that while it is appropriate to provide investigational agents under MEURI, efforts should be made to create the least interference possible with the initiation, conduct, or completion of randomized controlled clinical trials that will allow for the evaluation of investigational therapeutics (http://www.who.int/ebola/drc-2018/notes-for-the-record-meuri-ebola.pdf).

Ethical considerations loom large when undertaking evaluations of vaccines and therapeutics in the context of an emergency, especially where supplies of investigational agents can be very limited. There can be disagreements among investigators about appropriate clinical trial design in outbreak settings. Some question whether it is ethical to undertake randomized controlled trials that might involve withholding untested agents with encouraging preclinical data from some trial participants.[45,46] Others, citing examples from previous epidemics including SARS, 2009 H1N1 influenza, and the West African Ebola epidemic, believe that randomized placebo-controlled trials are needed to truly determine efficacy and to detect adverse effects.[45,72,73] Some investigators point to the benefits of an adaptive randomized trial design in which multiple therapies can be evaluated simultaneously against a shared control group.[73] In the end, there is broad agreement that developing widely accepted protocols that are ready for use when an outbreak strikes is a high priority.[73,74] With this aim in mind, WHO has convened groups of experts to develop innovative clinical trial designs for vaccines and therapeutics for priority pathogens.[74]

Timely sharing of data and specimens during outbreaks is critical for an effective response. FluID, a global platform managed by WHO for influenza data sharing, is a largely successful model that has not yet been replicated for other pathogens.[75] WHO and the Global Research Consortium for Infectious Disease Preparedness (GloPID-R) have initiated efforts to address the many challenges, including a lack of incentives and inadequate infrastructure.[73,76,77] Guides to data sharing have been produced by WHO, GloPID-R's workgroup on data sharing and Chatham House.[74,78,79] Evidence of improvements in this arena was apparent during and following the 2015–2016 Zika outbreak, when multiple online data-sharing platforms and open access information sources were created.[80,81]

Evidence of progress in countermeasure availability for Ebola can be found in the response to two Ebola outbreaks in the Democratic Republic of Congo (DRC) in 2018. In both, the rVSV-ZEBOV vaccine was made available through WHO and used for ring vaccination to assist in controlling the outbreaks (WHO rVSV-ZEBOV).[82,83] On 4 June, an ethics committee in the DRC approved the use of five investigational therapeutics to treat Ebola under the framework of compassionate use/expanded access (MEURI). This was the first time such treatments were made available in the midst of an Ebola outbreak. Clinicians working in the treatment center were charged with making decisions on which drug to use as deemed helpful for their patients and appropriate for the setting. The treatments could be used as long as informed consent was obtained from patients and protocols were followed, with close monitoring and reporting of any adverse events.[84]

Future Needs and Challenges

Much progress has been made in characterizing gaps in global health security and in strengthening efforts to mobilize to address them. However, the needs are broad, deep, and complex, and addressing them in a meaningful way will require large and sustained commitments in many spheres. Our major challenge ahead is to support the long-term investments in political, economic, and human capital needed to truly transform the world's ability to prevent, detect, and respond to infectious disease outbreaks.

RESPONSE TO HUMANITARIAN EMERGENCIES

Introduction

Humanitarian crises (Box 26-1)[85,86] have sudden and long-lasting public health impacts for many people around the world. In 2017, there were 141 million people in 33 countries affected by humanitarian crises.[87] The public health responses to humanitarian crises are often complex, both in terms of scale and urgency, and because of the need to operate in difficult security environments and logistically challenging situations. An effective public health response to humanitarian crises requires a robust approach to collecting data about key epidemiological indicators, as well as interventions and resources available to responding organizations. In some emergencies, completely new public health systems and surveillance mechanisms need to be established. However, in many situations there is an opportunity to strengthen local health systems by adapting humanitarian approaches to leverage local capacities and structures.[30] Notwithstanding, several specific methodologies have been developed specifically to measure important public health indicators in humanitarian crises.

Public health responses to humanitarian crises are conducted by many organizations that include host country government entities, United Nations organizations, nongovernmental organizations, and other public health organizations. There are many specialized humanitarian response agencies such as the United Nations High Commission for Refugees (UNHCR), the World Health Organization (WHO), the United Nations Children's Fund (UNICEF), Medicins Sans Frontieres (MSF), and the International Committee of the Red Cross (ICRC). Coordination of multiple organizations at the global level is led by the Inter-Agency Standing Committee (IASC), which includes key UN and non-UN humanitarian partners. The IASC is chaired by the Emergency Relief Coordinator who serves as the UN Secretary General's representative for major humanitarian emergencies. The IASC is supported by the United Nations Office for the Coordination of Humanitarian Affairs (UNOCHA), which also provides coordination on-the-ground during emergencies. The coordination structure uses a cluster approach, around themes or sectors.[88] The Health Cluster is led by WHO, which provides coordination support to other organizations working in the health sector.

BOX 26-1 Definition of Humanitarian Crises

1. Sudden unplanned displacement of a large proportion of the population away from the place(s) of habitual residence and into any settlement.
2. Direct exposure of a civilian, noncombatant population to new or exacerbated and sustained episodes of armed conflict resulting in reduced access to healthcare, disrupted water supply and sanitation, food insecurity, and/or any other breakdown of critical state functions.
3. A sudden deterioration of nutritional status is impending or has already occurred.
4. Natural or industrial (including nuclear) disaster resulting in temporary homelessness, disruption to critical public services, increased risk of injury and/or exposure to the elements for a substantial proportion of the population.
5. Sudden breakdown of critical administrative and management functions, within the public and/or private sector, due to any reason, resulting in large-scale disruption of public health and/or other critical public functions.

The Sphere Project was initiated in 1997 by several humanitarian NGOs with the aim of establishing minimum standards in four life-saving sectors: water supply, sanitation, and hygiene promotion; food security and nutrition; shelter, settlement, and nonfood items; and health action.[89] The Sphere project is composed of a Humanitarian Charter, four Protection Principles and Core Standards. The protection principles include that all humanitarian agencies should ensure that their actions do not bring further harm to affected people, that their activities benefit those who are most affected and vulnerable, that they contribute to protecting affected people from violence and other human rights abuses, and that they help affected people recover from abuses. The standards have the purpose of improving the quality of humanitarian response based on two core principles: that people affected by humanitarian emergencies have the right to life with dignity and to assistance during a humanitarian emergency; and that all possible actions should be taken to alleviate human suffering resulting from humanitarian emergencies.

Public Health Challenges During Humanitarian Emergencies

Humanitarian crises routinely result in large-scale population displacement, both internally within countries and across borders. These populations are at increased risk for morbidity and mortality associated with overcrowding (e.g., respiratory and diarrheal disease), disruption in health services (e.g., childhood immunizations), and loss of access to food, clean water, and sanitation.[3,90] WHO, United Nations High Commissioner for Refugees (UNHCR), and CDC have defined the epidemiology and public health aspects of humanitarian crises and have identified the importance of surveillance linked to public health interventions to mitigate the health consequences of prolonged displacement.[3,91,92]

Demographic Data

Demographic data are necessary to guide the amount of humanitarian assistance needed and to provide denominators for epidemiological and other indicators. In refugee settings, data may be collected using a census and updated by registration and vital registration data. For populations outside of camps, special demographic surveys methods are required.[93] Important demographic data include the population size, population under 5 years old (population at risk), arrivals and departures, and possibly individuals belonging to vulnerable groups (e.g., unaccompanied minors, elderly, or pregnant women).

Crude Mortality and Under-Five Mortality

Crude mortality rate (CMR) and under-5 mortality rate (U5MR) are usually reported as deaths per 10,000 population per day. Thresholds for mortality that indicate a humanitarian crisis are a CMR of 1 death per 10,000 population per day or an U5MR of 2 per 10,000 per day.[94] Mortality data can be collected from special surveys, health facilities, home visits, graves/cemeteries/burial shrouds, and community leaders.[95] In some circumstances, cause-specific mortality may sometimes be collected using verbal autopsies and health facility data, although this is less common.[96]

Morbidity

In most crisis-affected populations, outbreaks of infectious diseases are a primary concern. Infectious diseases and syndromes that are frequently monitored include diarrhea, acute watery diarrhea, acute respiratory infections, malaria, measles, meningitis, and jaundice. The incidence (new cases per defined population over a specified time period), attack-rate, and case-fatality ratio for these diseases or syndromes are needed to understand the epidemiology and plan appropriate responses. Infectious disease surveillance systems in emergencies use health-facility data and can be supplemented by community-based surveillance approaches.

Maternal, newborn, and child health are also negatively impacted by humanitarian emergencies.[97] A lack of skilled birth attendants and emergency obstetric result in an increase of unsafe deliveries. Women may have more unintended pregnancies and unsafe abortions during emergencies. Emergency situations also result in an increase in pregnancy loss, preterm births, and birth defects. Women and girls may experience increased gender violence and forced or transactional sex.

Increasingly noncommunicable diseases (NCDs) are an important component of morbidity among crisis-affected populations. NCDs that are often a concern in crises include diabetes, hypertension, cardiovascular disease, cancer, and chronic lung disease.[98] Management of NCDs requires specific attention to the requirements and availability of relevant medicines and technologies.

Nutrition

Crisis affected populations may suffer from protein-energy malnutrition and micronutrient deficiencies (vitamin A, iodine, zinc, iron). Malnutrition also increases the impact of communicable diseases. Anthropometric surveys are used to assess nutritional status. Measures include weight for height in Z score according to the WHO standard or National Center for Health Statistics reference. Mid-upper arm circumference (MUAC) is another key measurement. Malnutrition in children aged 6–59 months can be used as a proxy for the population as a whole. Nutritional data are often collected using community surveys (facility-level data are not sufficient on their own). The Standard Monitoring and Assessment of Relief and Transitions (SMART) methodology and the Emergency Nutrition Assessment software are considered standard practice methods for nutritional surveys.[95]

Mental Health

Populations that have experienced humanitarian emergencies are likely to have a high prevalence of mental health needs. The prevalence of depression and posttraumatic disorder may be as high as 15–20% among crisis-affected populations.[99] Effective interventions for crisis-affected populations can be difficult to implement. However, a range of interventions should be considered, including community and family support, focused nonspecialized services, and specialized services.[100] Health centers should have at least one trained professional who can provide some or all services encompassed in psychological first aid.[94]

Vaccination Coverage

It is important to maintain or restore vaccination programs for populations affected by crises. Normally, routine immunization according to the host country Expanded Programme on Immunization (EPI) schedule should be established.[85] Reactive vaccination campaigns with specific antigens may be needed in the event of an outbreak. Implementation of vaccination campaigns and routine immunization programs requires considerable planning and logistics, especially in crisis-affected areas. Estimates of vaccination coverage are essential to evaluate the impact of rapid vaccination interventions and to monitor routine vaccine coverage in crisis-affected populations over the medium to long term. Vaccination coverage should be measured both from administrative (health services) data as well as survey data.[101]

Access to Health Services

Current standards for access to health services are one basic health unit (primary care) per 10,000 population, one health center per 50,000 population, one district hospital per 250,000 population, and >10 inpatient and maternity beds per 10,000 population.[95] In humanitarian emergencies, the Health Services Availability Monitoring System (HeRAMS) is frequently used to assess the availability of health services. This involves establishing a baseline and then updating the information every 3–6 months.

Water Supply and Sanitation

Adequate water supply and sanitation are vital services for public health.[102] In almost every situation, achieving high-quality water supply and sanitation services is challenging. Ensuring access to clean water is critical to prevent outbreaks of waterborne disease. Water treatment involves combinations of storage, aeration, sedimentation, filtration, and disinfection.[103] The minimum quantity of water that must be supplied during a crisis is 15 liters per person per day. Safe water containers should also be made available to avoid household water contamination. Excreta disposal is similarly critical for public health and sufficient toilets (not less than one per 20 persons) and adequate access for men and women, must be made available. Vector control services may be needed to control mosquitos, biting ticks, fleas, rats, and other potential disease vectors. Sufficient solid waste disposal and site drainage are also important considerations for a safe environment.

Public Health Information During Humanitarian Crises

Challenges for Collecting Public Health Information

Humanitarian crises often occur in countries where public health information systems are weak, and postcrisis these systems may have collapsed partially or completely. Without reliable public health information, humanitarian agencies are not able to plan and deliver critical public health services optimally. There are three domains of public health information about crisis-affected populations that must be collected: health status and threats for affected populations; health resources and services availability; and health systems performance.[104] For each domain, a number of health information services or systems should be considered. A review of large conflict-related and natural disaster-related emergencies during 2010–2013 identified major gaps in many core public health information services, particularly during the first 6 months of the crisis.[86] For example, across nine categories of core public health information services (e.g., crude death rate, measles coverage, and mental health assessment), information was available for a maximum of only 5 of 13 large conflict-related crises, and then in only two categories (malnutrition prevalence and epidemic surveillance). There are many challenges that make routine collection of core public health information difficult in emergency settings, including insecurity, poor coordination among responding agencies, limited investment, lack of trained personnel in the field, and lack of consistent tools and methodologies. Key public health information services for humanitarian crises include the following.

Public Health Situation Analysis (PHSA)

A Public Health Situation Analysis (PHSA) is perhaps the most important document following a humanitarian emergency. It should be prepared within a few days of the event. A PHSA should include review of precrisis secondary data about the health status of the affected population; information about availability of health services; and scenario estimates of excess mortality from previous crises of similar typology. The PHSA should be regularly updated during an acute crisis, as more information becomes available and as operational demands require.

Early Warning, Alert, and Response (EWAR)

Populations affected by humanitarian crises are especially at risk of infectious disease outbreaks. It is therefore essential to establish enhance infectious disease surveillance for early warning, alert, and response (EWAR). In essence, EWAR requires the establishment of surveillance for cases of infectious diseases, usually reported from healthcare facilities, and frequently based on syndromes without laboratory confirmation. RDTs, which are available for a growing number of diseases, can be integrated into EWAR reporting. In addition to case reporting, EWAR systems can be used for alert reporting or event-based surveillance, so that disease clusters are reported.

Humanitarian Emergency Settings Perceived Needs Scale (HESPER)

The Humanitarian Emergency Settings Perceived Needs Scale (HESPER) measures the needs of people affected by humanitarian crises by directly soliciting their views.[105] The scale gathers information about the perceived physical, social, and psychological needs of adults, including concerns for their children. Participants rate 26 core items as either serious or not serious. For items with unmet needs, participants rank the three most serious problems. A sum of the items rated as serious produces a total score for each item. The HESPER scale can be used to gather information as part of a rapid assessment or ongoing assessment of a population's needs.

Violence Against Health

Violence against health is tracked using the WHO Surveillance System for Attacks on Health Care (SSA). The objectives of monitoring violence against health are to collect and share reliable data on attacks on healthcare; understand the extent and nature of the problem; generate an evidence base for advocacy; and identify global and context-specific trends. SSA is implemented by WHO through its country offices by identifying SSA information providers, including the protection and health clusters. SSA information providers send to WHO a description of the attack and immediate consequences; date, location, and health resources involved; deaths and injuries; and immediate actions required for re-establishing health services and support to victims. Each report is verified and assigned a level of certainty, ranging from "rumor" for information gleaned from social media, hearsay, or an anonymous source to "confirmed" for corroborated eyewitness or partner organization account. Maintaining the confidentiality of victims and contributors who share information about an attack is an important principle in conducting surveillance for attacks on health. The data collected through the SSA are shared online via a publically available site.

Health Resources Availability Monitoring System (HeRAMS)

HeRAMS is a system for monitoring health facilities, services, and resource availability in emergencies.[106] HeRAMS enables the assessment and monitoring of the status of health facilities and the availability of health services and resources in areas affected by humanitarian crises. The approach is a collaborative process involving all health sector actors responding to a crisis, and it is supported by an online application (https://primewho.org/). HeRAMS can assist in the timely identification of needs and gaps, evidence-based decision making and coordination, efficient planning and implementation of new health services, detailed response monitoring, and advocacy and resource mobilization.

Future Needs and Challenges

Effective public health response to humanitarian crises continues to be a major challenge globally. Despite advances in methods and organizational approaches to collecting data for public health action, generating data for evidence-based decision-making and program development remains inconsistent. With many humanitarian emergencies occurring in difficult and sometimes dangerous settings, it is increasingly challenging to find public health professionals to conduct this work. More than the development of new methods and technologies, the most pressing need for improved public health response is the development of a cadre of public health specialists able to deploy for the extended periods in response to humanitarian crises.

CASE STUDY: HUMANITARIAN CRISIS IN NORTHEAST NIGERIA

Background

Around 2002, an insurgency group called Boko Haram emerged in northeastern Nigeria with uncertain objectives, but loosely interpreted to be against "western education" and what it represented. This group appeared intent on disrupting normal life using extreme violence. Over the succeeding years, using random bombings of public gatherings and schools, first with hidden bombs, and then suicide bombers, they brought great pain and anxiety to the local population. The group subsequently spread across the Lake Chad basin to neighboring countries, including Cameroon, Chad, and Niger. In some of the captured villages, they actually raised their flags in defiance of constituted authority. Beginning in 2016, the Nigerian Military conducted an offensive against Boko Haram, by 2018 regaining much of the territory previously under their control. However, violence and insecurity continued throughout northeastern Nigeria, with occasional attacks on military and civilian infrastructure. A major consequence has been the emergence of large camps for internally displaced people (IDP) in northeastern Nigeria, a phenomenon that had not previously been seen in the country.

Public Health Impact

As of 2018, there were about 8.6 million people in need of humanitarian assistance living in areas previously controlled by Boko Haram. Despite the intervention of the Nigerian Military, much of northeastern Nigeria continued to suffer insecurity, and military escorts were required for movement outside the main towns and urban centers. Access to many areas requiring humanitarian assistance was by air, due to the insecurity of ground transportation. Ongoing violence and threat of kidnapping had intermittently caused the United Nations to suspend humanitarian operations in the region.

According to the International Organization for Migration, by mid-2018 there were nearly 1,920,000 IDP in the six states in northeast Nigeria: Adamawa, Bauchi, Borno, Gombe, Taraba, and Yobe. Nearly four-fifths of the displaced population were women and children. Limited access to food in December 2017 was the major concern for nearly 70% of the people living in northeastern Nigeria, with nearly 3.5 million people in need of nutritional assistance. Global acute malnutrition (GAM) ranged from 10% to 15% across the region. In 2018, 6.9 million people were in need of humanitarian health assistance, with nearly half of all health facilities in the region not functional or destroyed.

Outbreaks of infectious diseases such as cholera, measles, Lassa Fever, hepatitis E, and Yellow Fever have been reported frequently. Malaria, which is endemic in the area, has worse outcomes in the context of poor nutrition and poor access to healthcare facilities. In 2016, three cases of acute flaccid paralysis caused by wild poliovirus were detected among children who had previously lived in Boko Haram controlled areas—the first cases detected in the area in over 2 years. In 2018, Nigeria was one of only three countries in the world that is yet to stop the transmission of wild poliovirus. Additionally, transmission of vaccine-derived polio (cVDPV2) is also ongoing in northeastern Nigeria. A mortality survey conducted in March 2017 in Borno state reported crude mortality to be 0.7 deaths per 10,000 persons per day, and under 5-year-old mortality to be 1.7 deaths per 10,000 persons per day. A PHSA conducted by WHO in January 2018 estimated considerable risks for the population to experience excess mortality, especially related to malnutrition, lack of access to clean water, malaria, meningitis, cholera, and other infectious diseases.

Public Health Response

As of December 2017, there were 45 humanitarian health sector partners, including UN agencies and international NGOs, operating in northeast Nigeria, supporting the States Government to restore access to healthcare services. Almost 60% ($N = 237$) of the health facilities in Borno State were being supported by one or more health partners. Diagnosis of the most relevant diseases with outbreak potential (malaria, measles, and gastroenteritis) was available in more than three-quarters of health facilities, while services related to sexual violence and mental healthcare were available in less than one-third. From January 2017 through November 2017, health sector partners provided 6,372,838 consultations across the supported health facilities in northeastern Nigeria, and 869,889 consultations and 2450 referrals in IDP camps. In 2016, vaccination coverage for measles in northeastern Nigeria ranged from 15% to 58% across administrative areas.

The governments of the states in the northeast of Nigeria, especially Borno State, have invested significantly in rebuilding infrastructure destroyed during the peak of the insurgency, encouraging people to go home. Despite these efforts, the relocation of IDP to their home villages continues to be a challenge with the persisting sense of insecurity in the region. This has the potential to continue for some time because, despite improvements in access to healthcare and other social services, it is difficult to determine when such improvements are sufficient for the country to proceed on its own, even if conditions are not perfect, without putting the population at further risk.

CONCLUSIONS

Multiple characteristics of the modern world will continue to lead to more infectious disease outbreaks, epidemics, and complex humanitarian emergencies of increasing intensity and scope. Heightened awareness of the threat, and redoubled efforts to address it, focusing on prevention, detection, and response, have resulted in some improvements on global and national fronts, but it is clear that the world remains dangerously unprepared. Despite some progress, financing remains a major challenge.[76] Although the GHSA was renewed to 2024, its largest funder, the United States, has not made any financial commitments beyond 2019. No follow-up has been announced to the G7's 2016 commitment to fund capacity building in 76 countries.[76] Furthermore, these commitments represent only a fraction of what is needed, an estimated $4.5 billion annually.[59]

The relatively robust adoption of the JEE mechanism is evidence of recognition of the importance of external, objective, transparent evaluation, and monitoring to enable real progress toward implementation of the IHR-2005. However, meaningful, independent, coordinated, ongoing, and technically competent assessment of overall global capacity to detect and respond to outbreaks remains an urgent priority. The establishment of oversight monitoring boards may help, but these boards must be invested with real authority, and be appropriately resourced. Research and development has received a great deal of attention in recent years, including some creative financing initiatives and efforts by WHO and other groups to develop guidance and address some of the systemic problems such as the need for norms and standards, and data and specimen sharing. New technologic advances hold promise, and some financing is available, particularly in the areas of development of vaccines and antimicrobials. However, countermeasures research must be accelerated further. A 2016 U.S. National Academy of Medicine report estimated the investment gap at $1 billion per year.[49] Experience has repeatedly demonstrated that it is almost impossible to develop countermeasures in the midst of an outbreak in time to influence the course of that outbreak and save lives. Furthermore, prediction of pathogen emergence has been largely unsuccessful. We must redouble efforts to develop diagnostics, vaccines, and therapeutics using multiple research approaches that are as flexible as possible.

Humanitarian crises, rising refugee populations, and large numbers of displaced people are realities of our current world. Caring for these vulnerable populations and managing outbreaks when they occur in these disrupted settings remain major challenges because of security concerns, constraints on access, and the limited number of organizations with the necessary expertise and capacity to act.[76] Building such capacity remains an urgent need.

Advances in technology, and detection and response capacity will have limited effectiveness without a trained workforce. A robust public health workforce, including people with the right types of expertise and appropriate training, remains elusive. Identifying, training, and retaining skilled public health practitioners at all levels of the global public health infrastructure deserve more attention, given its central importance.

The world is only as safe as its most fragile states. We can expect to see an increasing number of emerging infectious disease epidemics and humanitarian emergencies of greater complexity and scope, driven by many changing aspects of the modern world. While awareness of the threat and efforts to address it are growing, the needs are many and complex, and there is a very long way to go. Ensuring global health security, the capacity of every country to find, stop, and prevent health threats, is a global imperative.

References

1. Centers for Disease Control and Prevention. Emergency Management Accreditation Program (EMAP) frequently asked questions (FAQ). Available at https://esp.cdc.gov/sites/ophpr/DEOv2/Documents/One%20Pager_Emergency%20Management%20Accreditation%20Program_20131112.pdf. Atlanta, GA. 2017.
2. Barzilay EJ, Schaad N, Magloire R, et al. Cholera surveillance during the Haiti epidemic—The first 2 years. *N Engl J Med.* 2013;368(7):599–609.
3. Tappero JW, Cassell CH, Bunnell RE, et al. U.S. Centers for Disease Control and Prevention and its partners' contributions to global health security. *Emerg Infect Dis.* 2017;23(13):S5–14.
4. Heymann DL, Chen L, Takemi K, et al. Global health security: The wider lessons from the West African Ebola virus disease epidemic. *Lancet.* 2015;385:1884–901.
5. Frieden TR, Tappero JW, Dowell SF, Hien NT, Guillaume FD, Aceng JR. Safer countries through global health security. *Lancet.* 2014;383(9919):764–6.
6. UNAIDS. Fact Sheet—World AIDS Day 2017. Global HIV Statistics. Available at http://www.unaids.org/sites/default/files/media_asset/UNAIDS_FactSheet_en.pdf. Geneva, Switzerland. 2017.
7. Centers for Disease Control and Prevention. Revised U.S. surveillance case definition for Severe Acute Respiratory Syndrome (SARS) and update on SARS cases—United States and worldwide, December 2003. *MMWR.* 2003;52(49):1202–6.
8. Lee JW, McKibbin WJ. Estimating the global economic costs of SARS. In: Knobler S, Mahmoud A, Lemon S, Mack A, Sivitz L, Oberholtzer K, eds. *Learning from SARS: Preparing for the Next Disease Outbreak: Workshop Summary.* Washington, DC: National Academies Press; 2004.
9. Fineberg HV. Pandemic preparedness and response—Lessons from the H1N1 influenza of 2009. *N Engl J Med.* 2014;370:1335–42.
10. Assiri A, McGeer A, Perl TM, et al. Hospital outbreak of Middle East respiratory syndrome coronavirus. *N Engl J Med.* 2013;369:407–16.
11. Centers for Disease Control and Prevention. Update on the epidemiology of Middle East respiratory syndrome coronavirus (MERS-CoV) infection, and guidance for the public, clinicians, and public health authorities—January 2015. *MMWR.* 2015;64(3):61–62.
12. Ki M. 2015 MERS outbreak in Korea: Hospital-to-hospital transmission. *Epidemiol Health.* 2015;37:e2015033.
13. Cho SY, Kang J-M, Ha YE, et al. MERS-CoV outbreak following a single patient exposure in an emergency room in South Korea: An epidemiological outbreak study. *Lancet.* 2016;388:994–1001.
14. Fauci AS, Morens DM. Zika virus in the Americas—Yet another arbovirus threat. *N Engl J Med.* 2016;374:601–4.
15. Centers for Disease Control and Prevention. About antimicrobial resistance. Available at https://www.cdc.gov/drugresistance/about.html. Atlanta, GA. 2018.
16. Osterholm MT. Global health security—An unfinished journey. *Emerg Infect Dis.* 2017;23 (Suppl):S225–6.
17. Bell BP, Damon IK, Jernigan DB, et al. Overview, control strategies, and lessons learned in the CDC response to the 2014–2016 Ebola epidemic. *MMWR.* 2016;65(Suppl3):4–11.
18. Briand S, Bertherat E, Cox P, et al. The international Ebola emergency. *N Engl J Med.* 2014;371(13):1180–3.
19. Centers for Disease Control and Prevention. Ebola virus disease outbreak—West Africa, 2014. *MMWR.* 2014;63:548–51.
20. Garrett L. Ebola's lessons. How the WHO mishandled the crisis. *Foreign Affairs.* 2015;94(5).
21. World Health Organization. Statement on the first meeting of the IHR Emergency Committee on the 2104 Ebola outbreak in West Africa. Available at http://www.who.int/mediacentre/news/statements/2014/ebola-20140808/en/. Geneva, Switzerland, 2014.
22. Perkins MD, Dye C, Balasegaram M, et al. Diagnostic preparedness for infectious disease outbreaks. *Lancet.* 2017;390(10108):2211–4.
23. Marston BJ, Dokubo E, van Steelandt A, et al. Ebola response impact on public health programs, West Africa, 2014–2017. *Emerg Infect Dis.* 2017;23(13):S25–32.
24. Sealy TK, Erickson BR, Taboy CH, et al. Laboratory response to Ebola—West Africa and United States. *MMWR.* 2016;65(Suppl3):44–49.
25. Nyenswah T, Fallah M, Sieh S, et al. Controlling the last known cluster of Ebola virus disease—Liberia, January–February 2015. *MMWR.* 2015;64:500–4.
26. Elston JWT, Cartwright C, Nkumbi P, Wright J. The health impact of the 2014–15 Ebola outbreak. *Public Health.* 2017;143:60.
27. Rhymer W, Speare R. Countries' response to WHO's travel recommendations during the 2013–2016 Ebola outbreak. *Bull World Health Organ.* 2017;95(1):10–17.
28. Cohen NJ, Brown CM, Alvarado-Ramy F, et al. Travel and border health measures to prevent the international spread of Ebola. *MMWR.* 2016;65(suppl 3):57–67.
29. Mate SE, Kugelman JR, Nyenswah TG, et al. Molecular evidence of sexual transmission of Ebola virus. *N Engl J Med.* 2015;373:2448–54.
30. Marston BJ, Dobubo EK, van Steelandt A, et al. Ebola response impact on public health programs, West Africa, 2014–2017. *Emerg Infect Dis.* 2017;23(Suppl):S25–32.
31. Christie A, Davies-Wayne GJ, Cordier-Lassalle T, et al. Possible sexual transmission of Ebola virus—Liberia, 2015. *MMWR.* 2015;64:479–81.
32. Diallo B, Sissoko D, Loman NJ, et al. Resurgence of Ebola virus disease in Guinea linked to a survivor with virus persistence in seminal fluid for more than 500 days. *Clin Infect Dis.* 2016;63:1353–6.
33. Centers for Disease Control and Prevention. History. 2014–2016 Ebola Outbreak in West Africa. Available at https://www.cdc.gov/vhf/ebola/history/2014-2016-outbreak/index.html. Atlanta, GA. 2017.
34. Centers for Disease Control and Prevention. Cost of the Ebola Epidemic. Available at www.cdc.gov/vhf/ebola/history/2014-2016-outbreak/cost-of-ebola.html. Atlanta, GA. 2016.
35. Parpia AS, Ndeffo-Mbah ML, Wenzel MS, Galvani AP. Effects of response to the 2014–2015 Ebola outbreak on deaths from malaria, HIV/AIDS and tuberculosis, West Africa. *Emerg Infect Dis.* 2016;22(3):433–41.
36. Dhillon RS, Devabhaktuni S, Kelly JD. Deploying RDTs in the DRC Ebola outbreak. *Lancet.* 2018;391(10139):2499–500.
37. Deen GF, Broutet N, Xu W, et al. Ebola RNA persistence in semen of Ebola disease survivors: Final report. *N Engl J Med.* 2017;377:1428–37.
38. Park DJ, Dudas G, Wohl S, et al. Ebola virus epidemiology, transmission, and evolution during seven months in Sierra Leone. *Cell.* 2015;161(7):1516–26.
39. Carroll MW, Matthews DA, Hiscox JA, et al. Temporal and spatial analysis of the 2014–2015 Ebola virus outbreak in West Africa. *Nature.* 2015;524(7563):97–101.
40. Quick J, Loman NJ, Duraffour S, et al. Real-time, portable genome sequencing for Ebola surveillance. *Nature.* 2016;530(7589):228–32.
41. Rottingen JA, Gouglas D, Feinberg M, et al. New vaccines against epidemic infectious diseases. *N Engl J Med.* 2017;376(7):610–13.
42. Cross RW, Mire CE, Feldmann H, Geisbert TW. Post-exposure treatments for Ebola and Marburg virus infections. *Nat Rev.* 2018;17:413–34.
43. Schuchat A, Seward JF, Goldstein ST, Mahon BE. Comment: The Sierra Leone trial to introduce a vaccine against Ebola (STRIVE). *J Infect Dis.* 2018;217(Suppl 1):S1–5.
44. Henao-Restrepo AM, Camacho A, Longini IM, et al. Efficacy and effectiveness of an rVSV-vectored vaccine in preventing Ebola virus disease: Final results from the Guinea ring vaccination, open-label, cluster-randomized trial (Ebola Ca Suffit!). *Lancet.* 2017;389(10068):505–18.
45. Davey RT, Dodd L, Proschan M, et al. The past need not be prologue: Recommendations for testing and positioning the most-promising medical countermeasures for the next outbreak of Ebola virus infection. *J Infect Dis.* 2018;218(suppl_5):S690–7.
46. Baden LR, Rubin EJ, Morrissey S, Farrar JJ, Drazen JM. We can do better—Improving outcomes in the midst of an emergency. *N Engl J Med.* 2017;377(15):1482–4.
47. Lamontagne F, Fowler RA, Adhikari NK, et al. Evidence-based guidelines for supportive care of patients with Ebola virus disease. *Lancet.* 2018;391:700–8.
48. United Nations. Sustainable development goals. Available at https://sustainabledevelopment.un.org/sdgs. New York, NY, 2015.
49. Moon S, Leigh J, Woskie L, et al. Post-Ebola reforms: Ample analysis, inadequate action. *BMJ.* 2017;356:j280.
50. World Health Organization. Extended list of Ebola reviews. Available at http://www.who.int/about/evaluation/extended-list-of-ebola-reviews-may2016.pdf. Geneva, Switzerland, 2016.
51. Gostin LO, Mundaca-Shah CC, Kelley PW. Neglected dimensions of global security: The Global Health Risk Framework Commission. *JAMA.* 2016;15(14):1451–2.

52. World Health Organization. *Health Regulations*. 3rd annotated ed. Geneva: World Health Organization; 1983.

53. Bell E, Tappero JW, Ijaz K, et al. Joint external evaluation—Development and scale-up of global multisectoral health capacity evaluation process. *Emerg Infect Dis*. 2017;23(Suppl):S33–39.

54. Rodier G, Greenspan AL, Hughes JM, Heymann DL. Global public health security. *Emerg Infect Dis*. 2007;13:1447–52.

55. WHO Executive Board, 136th session, EBI136/22 Add.1, 16 January 2015. Implementation of the International Health Regulations (2005). Report of the Review Committee on Second Extensions for Establishing National Public Health Capacities and on IHR Implementation.

56. Hardiman MC. World Health Organization Department of Global Capacities, Alert and Response. World Health Organization perspective on implementation of the International Health Regulations. *Emerg Infect Dis*. 2012;18:1041–6.

57. Fischer JE, Katz R. Moving forward to 2014: Global IHR (2005) implementation. *Biosecur Bioterror*. 2013;11:153–6.

58. Georgetown University Center for Global Health Science and Security. The IHR costing tool. Available at https://tracking.ghscosting.org/#analysis/ghsa/d. Washington, DC, 2017.

59. Sands P, Mundaca-Shah C, Dzau VJ. The neglected dimension of global security—A framework for countering infectious-disease crises. *N Engl J Med*. 2016;374(13):1281–7.

60. Gebreyes WA, Dupouy-Camet J, Newport MJ, et al. The global one health paradigm: Challenges and opportunities for tackling infectious diseases at the human, animal, and environment interface in low-resource settings. *PLoS Negl Trop Dis*. 2014;8(11):e3257.

61. World Health Organization. Joint External Evaluation Tool: International Health Regulations (2005). Available at http://www.who.int/iris/handle/10665/204368. Geneva, Switzerland, 2005.

62. World Health Organization. Joint External Evaluations. Available at http://www.who.int/ihr/procedures/joint-external-evaluations/en/. Geneva, Switzerland, 2018.

63. Global Health Security Agenda: Action packages. Available at https://www.ghsagenda.org/. 2018.

64. Fitzmaurice AG, Mahar M, Moriarty LF, et al. Contributions of the US Centers for Disease Control and Prevention in implementing the Global Health Security Agenda in 17 partner countries. *Emerg Infect Dis*. 2017;23(Suppl):S15–24.

65. Marston HD, Folkers GK, Morens DM, Fauci AS. Emerging viral diseases: Confronting threats with new technologies. *Sci Trans Med*. 2014;6(253):1–6.

66. Marston HD, Paules CI, Fauci AS. The critical role of biomedical research in pandemic preparedness. *JAMA*. 2017;318(18):1757–8.

67. Marston HD, Paules CI, Fauci AS. Monoclonal antibodies for emerging infectious diseases: Borrowing from history. *N Engl J Med*. 2018;378(16):1469–72.

68. World Health Organization. A research and development Blueprint for action to prevent epidemics. Available at http://www.who.int/blueprint/en/. Geneva, Switzerland, 2016.

69. World Health Organization. Methodology for Prioritizing Severe Emerging Diseases for Research and Development. Available at http://www.who.int/blueprint/priority-diseases/RDBlueprint-PrioritizationTool.pdf?ua=1). Geneva, Switzerland, 2017.

70. CARB-X-Combatting Antibiotic Resistant Bacteria: About CARB-X. Available at https://carb-x.org/. 2018.

71. World Health Organization. Regulatory preparedness key to addressing public health emergencies. Available at http://www.who.int/medicines/news/2017/reg_prep_key-to-addressing_ph_emergencies/en/. Geneva, Switzerland, 2017.

72. Cox E, Borio L, Temple R. Evaluating Ebola therapies–The case for RCTs. *N Engl J Med*. 2014;371(25):2350–1.

73. Borio L, Cox E, Lurie N. Combating emerging threats—Accelerating the availability of medical therapies. *N Engl J Med*. 2015;373(11):993–5.

74. World Health Organization. Developing new standards tailored to the epidemic context. Available at http://www.who.int/blueprint/what/norms-standards/en/. Geneva, Switzerland, 2017.

75. World Health Organization. FluID—A global influenza epidemiological data sharing platform. Available at http://www.who.int/influenza/surveillance_monitoring/fluid/en/. Geneva, Switzerland, 2018.

76. Leigh J, Fitzgerald G, Garcia E, Moon S. Global epidemics: How well can we cope? *BMJ*. 2018;362:k3254.

77. Global Research Collaboration for Infectious Disease Preparedness: Data sharing. Available at https://www.glopid-r.org/our-work/data-sharing/. 2016.

78. Global Research Collaboration for Infectious Disease Preparedness: Principles of data sharing in public health emergencies. Available at https://www.glopid-r.org/wp-content/uploads/2018/06/glopid-r-principles-of-data-sharing-in-public-health-emergencies.pdf. 2018.

79. Chatham House, Royal Institute of International Affairs: A guide to sharing the data and benefits of public health surveillance. Available at https://datasharing.chathamhouse.org/. United Kingdom, 2018.

80. University of Oxford. Zika on-line data sharing platform. Available at https://www.wrh.ox.ac.uk/research/zika-online-data-sharing-platform. Oxford, England, 2018.

81. Dye C, Bartolomeos K, Moorthy V, Kieny MP. Data sharing in public health emergencies: A call to researchers. *Bull World Health Organ*. 2016;94:158.

82. Levy Y, Lane C, Piot P, et al. Prevention of Ebola virus disease through vaccination: Where we are in 2018. *Lancet*. 2018;392(10149):787–90.

83. World Health Organization. WHO supports Ebola vaccination of high risk populations in the Democratic Republic of the Congo. Available at http://www.who.int/news-room/detail/21-05-2018-who-supports-ebola-vaccination-of-high-risk-populations-in-the-democratic-republic-of-the-congo. Geneva, Switzerland, 2018.

84. World Health Organization. Treatments approved for compassionate use. Available at http://www.who.int/ebola/drc-2018/treatments-approved-for-compassionate-use/en/. Geneva, Switzerland, 2018.

85. World Health Organization. *Vaccination in Humanitarian Emergencies: Implementation Guide*. Geneva: World Health Organization; 2017.

86. Checci F, Treacy-Wong V, Polonsky J, van Ommeren M, Prudhon C. Public health information in crisis-affected populations: A review of methods and their use for advocacy and action. *Lancet*. 2017;390(10109):2297–313.

87. United Nations Office for Coordination of Humanitarian Affairs: Annual Report 2018. Available at https://www.unocha.org/sites/unocha/files/2017%20annual%20report.pdf. New York, 2018.

88. United Nations Office for Coordination of Humanitarian Affairs: What is the cluster approach? Available at https://www.humanitarianresponse.info/en/about-clusters/what-is-the-cluster-approach. New York, 2018.

89. The Sphere Project. Available at http://www.spherestandards.org/. 2018.

90. Brennan RJ, Nandy R. Complex humanitarian emergencies: A major global health challenge. *Emerg Med (Fremantle)*. 2001;13:147–56.

91. Spiegel PB, Checchi F, Colombo S, Paik E. Health-care needs of people affected by conflict: Future trends and changing frameworks. *Lancet*. 2010;375:341–5.

92. Toole MJ, Waldman RJ. The public health aspects of complex emergencies and refugee situations. *Annu Rev Public Health*. 1997;18:283–312.

93. National Research Council. *Tools and Methods for Estimating Populations at Risk from Natural Disasters and Complex Humanitarian Crises*. Washington, DC: National Academy of Sciences; 2007.

94. The Sphere Project; Humanitarian Charter and Minimum Standards in Humanitarian Response. 2011. Hobbs the Printers, Hampshire, United Kingdom.

95. Standardised Monitoring and Assessment of Relief and Transitions Programme (SMART): Measuring mortality, nutritional status, and food security in crisis situations: SMART methodology, version 1. Available at http://smartmethodology.org/survey-planning-tools/smart-methodology/. 2006.

96. Chandramohan D. Validation and validity of verbal autopsy procedures. *Popul Health Metr*. 2011;9:22.

97. Cooper R. *Maternal, Newborn and Child Health in Emergency Settings. K4D Helpdesk Report*. Brighton, UK: Institute of Development Studies; 2018.

98. Slim S, Hyo-Jeong K, Gojka R, et al. Care of non-communicable diseases in emergencies. *Lancet*. 2017;389: 326–30.

99. Steel Z, Chey T, Silove D, Marnane C, Bryant RA, van Ommeren M. Association of torture and other potentially traumatic events with mental health outcomes among populations exposed to mass conflict and displacement: A systematic review and meta-analysis. *JAMA*. 2009;302:537–49.

100. Inter-Agency Standing Committee (IASC). *IASC Guidelines on Mental Health and Psychosocial Support in Emergency Settings*. Geneva: IASC; 2007.

101. Minetti A, Riera-Montes M, Nackers F, et al. Performance of small cluster surveys and the clustered LQAS design to estimate local-level vaccination coverage in Mali. *Emerg Themes Epidemiol*. 2012;9:6.

102. World Health Organization. *Communicable Disease Control in Emergencies*. Geneva: World Health Organization; 2005.

103. Cairncross S, Feacham R. *Environmental Health Engineering in the Tropics*. 2nd ed. Chichester: Wiley & Sons; 1993.

104. Global Health Cluster. Standards for Public Health Information Services in Activated Health Clusters and Other Humanitarian Health Coordination Mechanisms. 2017.

105. World Health Organization. *The humanitarian Emergency Settings Perceived Needs Scale (HESPER): Manual with Scale*. Geneva: World Health Organization; 2011.

106. Health Resources Availability Monitoring System (HeRAMS). Available at http://www.who.int/hac/herams/en/.

CHAPTER

27 Emerging Technology Innovations in Global Health

Kathryn Kundrod • Sai Paul • Melody Tan • Jennifer Carns • Rebecca Richards-Kortum

INTRODUCTION

In the last 50 years, development of new medical technologies and devices has played an important role in improving health outcomes in high-resource settings. Innovations ranging from the delivery of nasal oxygen, to obstetric ultrasound, to tools for minimally invasive surgery have reduced morbidity and mortality when patients have access. However, access to medical technologies varies widely throughout the world. Most technologies have been designed for high-resource settings and do not work effectively in settings that lack critical infrastructure such as constant, high-quality power, routine maintenance, and regular supply chains. Technologies that are appropriately designed to work in resource-limited settings can increase access to quality healthcare, bringing screening, diagnosis, and treatment closer to patients who face the greatest burdens of disease globally and reducing morbidity and mortality related to preventable and treatable conditions.

An estimated 80% of medical equipment in resource-limited settings is donated from high-resource settings.[1] Most of this equipment cannot function in the challenging environment of a resource-limited setting, and even operational medical devices often have a brief useful lifespan in these settings before being discarded in "equipment graveyards," storage locations for nonfunctional medical equipment in need of repair (Fig. 27-1a). This is the fate of approximately 70% of donated medical equipment in resource-limited settings.[2] Factors reducing the lifespan of medical technologies include harsh environmental conditions, such as open-air settings and the absence of climate control, as well as limitations in infrastructure and in the availability and quality of power and water. The improper use and maintenance of equipment, often due to the limited availability of training and maintenance tools as well as shortages in maintenance staff, can also reduce equipment lifetime. In general, spare parts must be ordered from a distributor and are often unavailable for outdated equipment. Even when affordable spare parts are available, the nearest distributor may be in another country, and the resulting shipping costs, import fees, and taxes can further increase the cost of the part. Furthermore, facilities in remote locations often require travel across poor quality roads and difficult terrain, and many facilities lack a physical street address, additionally complicating supply chain logistics. Similar challenges can affect access to consumables, preventing even functional medical equipment from being used when consumables run out.

Thus, there is an important need to design innovative health technologies that specifically address the challenges of resource-limited settings, as outlined in Table 27-1. New technologies must be robust to environmental and infrastructure challenges and designed for a workflow where staff shortages are common. Supply chain challenges should be addressed early in the design of a technology, and innovative strategies are necessary to address the difficulties in acquiring consumables and spare parts. Technologies must also be implemented in conjunction with strategies to ensure broad access that can be sustained, with consideration given to the cultural and social issues that may impact how a technology is adopted. Figure 27-1 highlights the need for appropriate design and comprehensive planning; in contrast to the oxygen concentrator graveyard in Fig. 27-1a, the Universal Anesthesia Machine (UAM) from Gradian Health Systems is shown in use in Fig. 27-1b. The UAM is an example of a technology designed specifically for the context of resource-limited settings. As discussed in more detail below, these challenges influenced the technical design of the machine to provide a rugged and robust solution including additional power sources. Moreover, Gradian also set up local distribution networks, customizable initial training programs, and appropriate financial models to facilitate sustainable use. This type of comprehensive approach is necessary to ensure the success of health technologies in resource-limited settings.

Although devices and drugs are commonly recognized as health technologies, health innovations include more than just medical devices. The definition of technologies used here also encompasses support systems (spare part depots, clinical laboratories), biological products (vaccines), organizational systems (clinical communication guidelines or systems), and medical and surgical procedures. Figure 27-2 illustrates how health technologies fit into a broader landscape, which includes information communication technologies and technologies for health. Technologies do not need to be material, like devices or drugs, or technologically sophisticated to be impactful; relatively simple and straightforward interventions that are indirectly related to patient care can improve outcomes. For instance, well-designed, culturally sensitive educational brochures or television advertisements can influence population health behaviors. Additionally, technologies can be combined to address health problems more effectively. Devices introduced with innovative organizational systems or supplementary biological products introduced with sustainable support systems will have greater impact in the long term.

INNOVATION, ACCESS, AND SUSTAINABILITY

In this chapter, case studies of emerging technologies centered on medical devices and support systems designed to address important global health needs are presented. Each case study is organized around a three-part framework of *innovation*, *access*, and *sustainability*. *Innovation* addresses the initial conception and design of a new technology, including the context-specific clinical motivation and design criteria required for successful performance. Defining the essential features, user interface, and core technology is part of the innovation process. *Access* is achieved when technology is suitable for implementation in the target environment, which depends on appropriate design, training, education, and/or workflow integration for end users. *Sustainability* involves factors that enable long-term

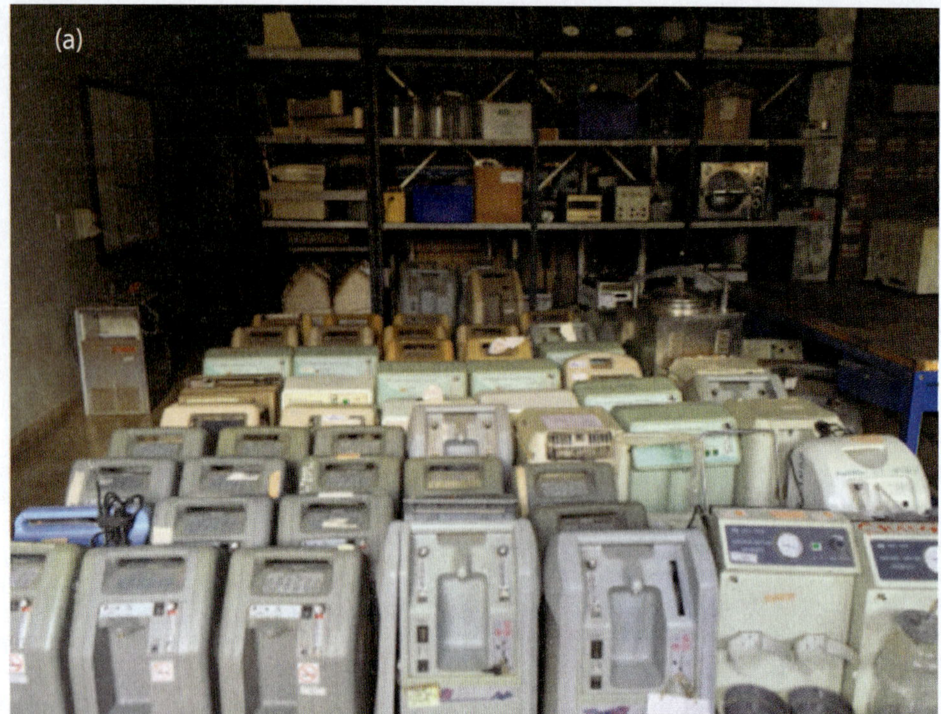

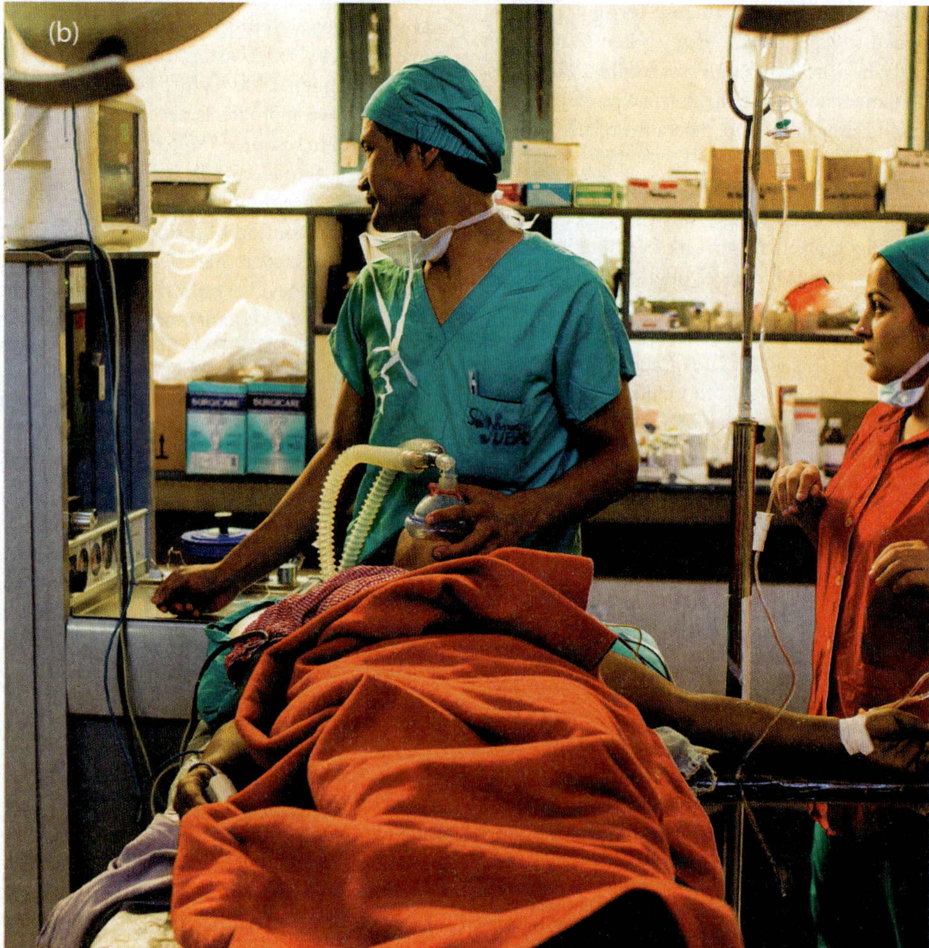

(a) Rice University, (b) Gradian Health Systems.

FIGURE 27-1. Differences in technology lifespans based on appropriate design for resource-limited settings. (a) "Equipment graveyard" filled with discarded oxygen concentrators and other equipment not suitable for resource-limited settings and in need of repair, at Queen Elizabeth Central Hospital in Blantyre, Malawi. (*Source:* Reprinted with permission from Rice University.) (b) The Universal Anesthesia Machine, from Gradian Health Systems, provided with appropriate and sustainable financial models, training, and local maintenance networks, in use in Ghana. (*Source:* Reprinted with permission from Gradian Health Systems.)

TABLE 27-1 CHALLENGES FACING HEALTH TECHNOLOGIES IN RESOURCE-LIMITED SETTINGS

Purchasing and Distribution	Human Resources

Initial technology cost
Cost and availability of spare parts
Cost and availability of consumables
Absence of local distributors
Transportation limitations
  Poor quality of roads
  Lack of physical address for deliveries
Inventory management
	Lack of medical staff
	Lack of maintenance staff
	Lack of specialists
	Lack of training
	Insufficient capacity for patient volume
	Inability to make and maintain patient contact

Infrastructure	**Cultural/Social Factors**

Power outages and/or poor quality
Water outages and/or poor quality
Communications
  Access to telephone
  Access to high-bandwidth Wi-Fi
  Cell phone coverage
Lack of sterilization for medical tools
Inability for providers to physically reach patients
	Lack of awareness of medical resources
	Lack of comprehensive disease management
	Medical misinformation
	Stigmatized illnesses or populations

	Environmental

	Lack of climate control
	  Variable temperature
	  Variable humidity
	Dust

patient impact, such as establishing supply chains to consistently deliver necessary consumables, generating evidence of effectiveness, and ensuring demand for continued support. The cost of a technology and required consumables can be a significant barrier to sustainability. Financial models to support low-cost technologies are discussed in the Conclusion section.

These case studies, presented roughly in the order of most to least mature technologies, have different challenges in the areas of innovation, access, and/or sustainability (Table 27-2). The following questions will be used as a guide through the case studies to better understand each of these concepts.

- *Innovation: How should new approaches to solving clinical and public health challenges be effectively designed?*
- *Access: How do technologies reach the people who need them?*
- *Sustainability: What ensures long-term use and effectiveness of a technology?*

HIV Rapid Diagnostics

Prevention and control of human immunodeficiency virus (HIV) has been a major global health success over the past few decades, and the response to the HIV and acquired immunodeficiency syndrome (AIDS) epidemic has become a model for response to global epidemics.[3] Despite significant advancements in HIV diagnostic testing, some gaps remain. To close these gaps in diagnosis, treatment, and suppression, the United Nations Joint Programme on HIV/AIDS (UNAIDS) established the 90-90-90 goals. This set of goals stated that by 2020, 90% of people living with HIV should receive a diagnosis, 90% of those diagnosed should receive treatment, and 90% of those on treatment should achieve viral suppression.[4] While gaps in screening remain, HIV testing has become possible in traditionally medically underserved regions. For example, between 2005 and 2016, the percentage of people living with HIV in Africa who received a diagnosis increased from 10% to 50%.[5] Three decades of innovation since 1985 have led to accurate and easy-to-use diagnostic tests.[6] Low per-test cost, integration into screening programs, and expanded training for lay health providers allowed resource-limited health systems to access diagnostic tests.[5] Moving forward, HIV self-testing has the potential to expand access even further. Finally, a global coalition of governmental organizations, nongovernmental organizations, and private companies came together to establish distribution channels.[7–9] While gaps remain in HIV diagnostic testing accessibility, HIV diagnostics are an example of what can be achieved when innovation, access, and sustainability are addressed comprehensively to tackle a challenging global health issue.

Innovation

The laboratory-based HIV antibody test, the enzyme-linked immunosorbent assay (ELISA), was first used in 1985 to ensure blood donations did not contain HIV.[6] Because of false positives in the ELISAs, a second laboratory test called a western blot was developed to detect HIV-specific proteins. In 1992, the FDA licensed the first rapid diagnostic test (RDT) for HIV; the test accepted a whole blood sample without the need for sample preprocessing and returned a result in 10 minutes.[10] The RDT used the same detection chemistry as the lab-based ELISA test, but the self-contained, portable format allowed for use outside of centralized lab settings. The portable format was enabled by lateral flow technology. Lateral flow utilizes the wicking properties of paper to automate reagent delivery across "test" and "control" zones on a paper assay. In the case of the HIV RDT, the test zone forms a sandwich assay, similar to ELISA, to detect HIV antibodies or antigen that come from a patient's sample. The control line forms a sandwich using synthetic materials, independent of the composition of the patient's sample. A well-known product that utilizes lateral flow technology is the home pregnancy test, which similarly has a test line that changes color in the presence of human chorionic gonadotropin (hCG) and a control line that changes color regardless of the presence of hCG to indicate the test is functioning properly.

The World Health Organization (WHO) defined criteria for ideal point-of-care tests, such as the HIV RDT (Box 27-1).[11]

While the ASSURED criteria do not set specific target values for each category, they provide test developers a framework for the design goals that a point-of-care diagnostic test should meet. Suggested target values for HIV diagnostics were developed by Wu and Zaman,[11] and their analysis indicates that the HIV RDT performance has met the goals of all ASSURED criteria.

After the introduction of the HIV RDT, public health agencies stressed the importance of widespread screening using the HIV RDT, encouraging additional test development. The HIV RDT has since evolved to incorporate components such as recombinant proteins and synthetic peptides, which are HIV-specific biological elements. HIV test "generations," which are major innovations such as the ability to identify both HIV-1 and HIV-2 viruses that have increased the sensitivity and specificity of the RDT (Fig. 27-3). From the first generation in 1985 to the fifth generation in 2015, sensitivity has increased from 95–98% to 99.5% and specificity has increased from 99% to 100%.[6] With new test generations and treatment developments, guidelines on the use of confirmatory diagnosis using gold standard lab-based tests changed accordingly. For example, a western blot test was required to confirm positive results from a first-generation test. With the introduction of the fourth-generation test, the testing algorithms increased in complexity. A negative result was considered a final result; a positive fourth-generation test would be confirmed by an HIV 1-2 differentiation test. If the differentiation test came up negative, a lab-based nucleic acid test would be required.[6]

HIV RDT technology has become more ubiquitous since their introduction, and the tests are being developed by several companies. As of 2001, the WHO began prequalification of *in vitro* diagnostic products as a validation step for widespread procurement. The prequalification process regulates quality, safety, and efficacy of diagnostics, medicines, vaccines, and medical devices for high-burden diseases through scientific assessment of clinical performance and consistency along with manufacturing site visits.[12] As of November 2018, 18 HIV RDTs have been prequalified for clinical use, with one test (OraQuick HIV Self-Test) approved

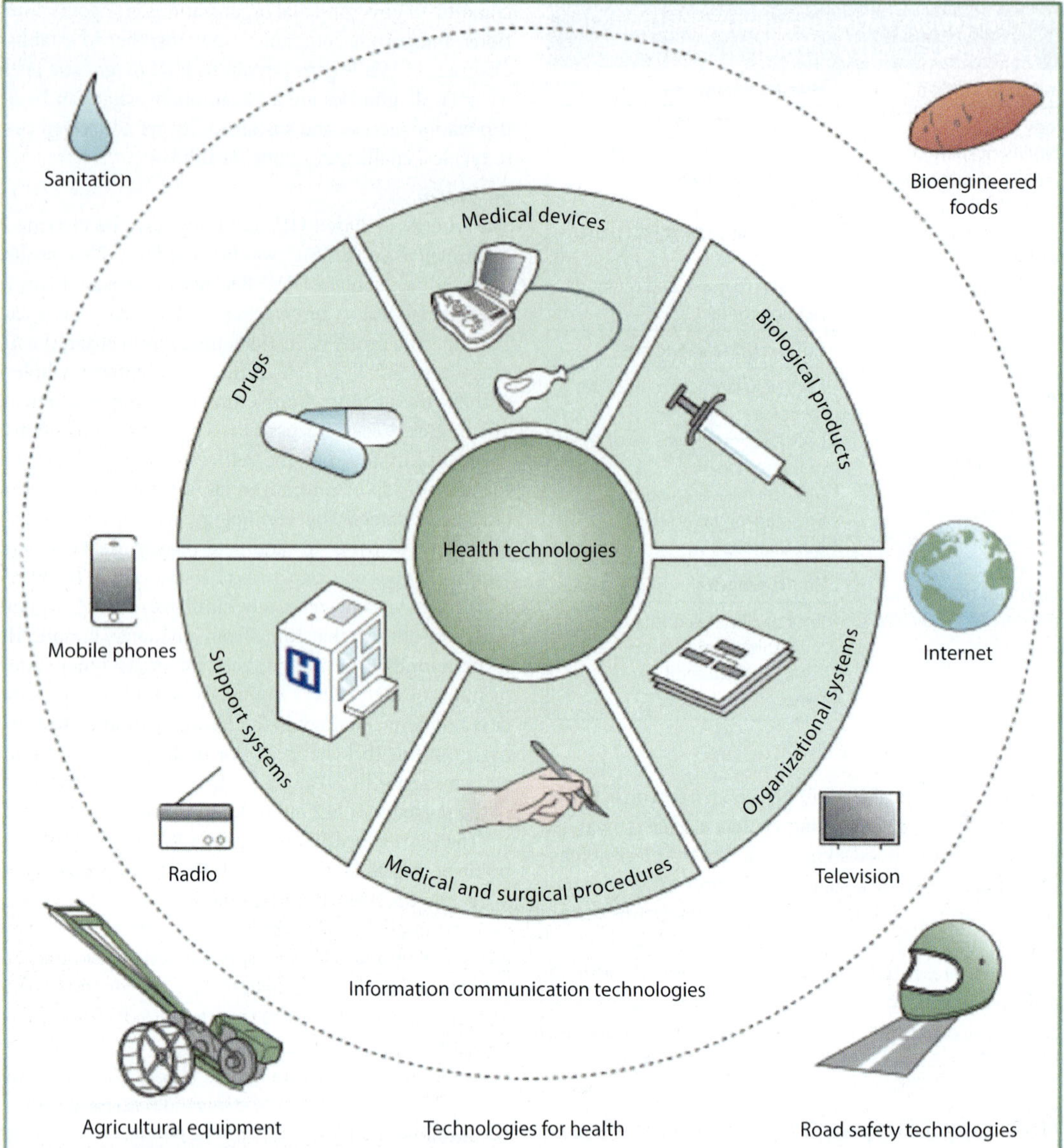

FIGURE 27-2. Overview of types of technologies for global health. (*Source:* Reprinted with permission from Howitt P, Darzi A, Yang G-Z, et al. Technologies for global health. *Lancet.* 2012;380(9840):507–35.[143])

for self-testing[13]; additional self-tests are under development and pursuing prequalification.[14] As of February 2017, The United States Agency for International Development (USAID) had approved 49 HIV RDTs, which include all of the WHO prequalified RDTs and tests that are FDA-approved and only distributed in the United States.[15]

Access

More than 600 million people in 122 low- and middle-income countries (LMICs) received HIV diagnostic testing between 2010 and 2014, demonstrating the widespread increase in access to HIV testing globally. Access has largely been a function of availability and use of RDTs, routine facility-based testing, and expanded training of lay providers along with expanded testing outside of facilities, for example, community-based testing.[5] The expansion of testing has been enabled by the innovation of the HIV RDTs described above.

Global scale-up of HIV testing has resulted in a large increase in people living with HIV (PLHIV) knowing their status. As previously discussed, in Africa this number increased from 10% in 2005 to 50% in 2015.[5] However, gaps in access remain. An estimated 25% of PLHIV globally do not know their status due to a host of factors, including access to testing.[16] Testing among men, young people, and key populations remains low. Key populations—including people who inject drugs intravenously, men who have sex with men, and people who are sex workers, transgender, or imprisoned[17]—account for around 40% of new HIV infections.[5] Low rates of testing among key populations is related to availability, acceptability, stigma, discrimination, and criminalization of behaviors.[5]

HIV self-testing (HIVST) may facilitate greater access by lowering the perceived stigma or discrimination from a provider and by reaching those who may not otherwise get tested.[5] As of July 2017, 40 countries have implemented new policies enabling HIVST implementation, and 48 additional countries have reported HIVST policies are in development.[18] Initially, demand for HIVST took place largely in high-income countries, but HIVST use and demand are growing in LMICs. The Self-Testing Africa (STAR) Initiative is funded by Unitaid, an international organization partnering with the WHO to address HIV/AIDS, tuberculosis, and malaria, along with the Children's Investment Fund Foundation and the Bill and Melinda Gates Foundation. The STAR Initiative has begun generating demand and clarifying public sector distribution and consumer preferences.[18]

TABLE 27-2 OVERVIEW OF TECHNOLOGY CASE STUDIES

HIV Rapid Diagnostics	Helping Babies Breathe	Universal Anesthesia Machine
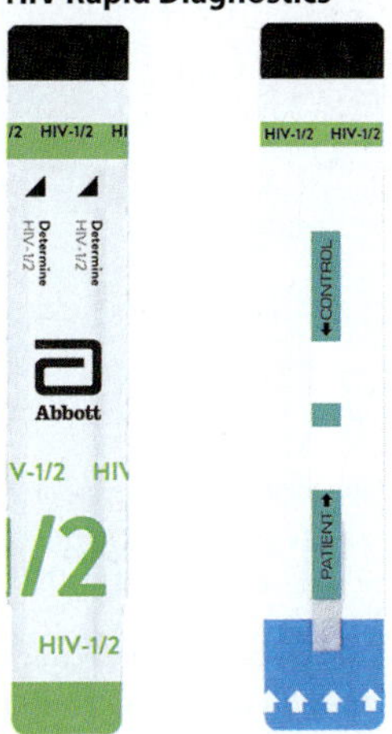 Reproduced with permission of Abbott, © 2021. All rights reserved. Test designed to be used at the point of care to screen for HIV in adults (Alere Determine® HIV ½)	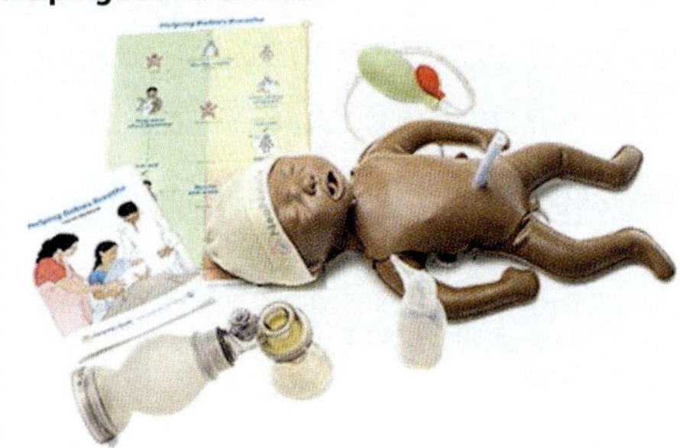 Educational program aimed at standardizing neonatal resuscitation globally (Laerdal Global Health)	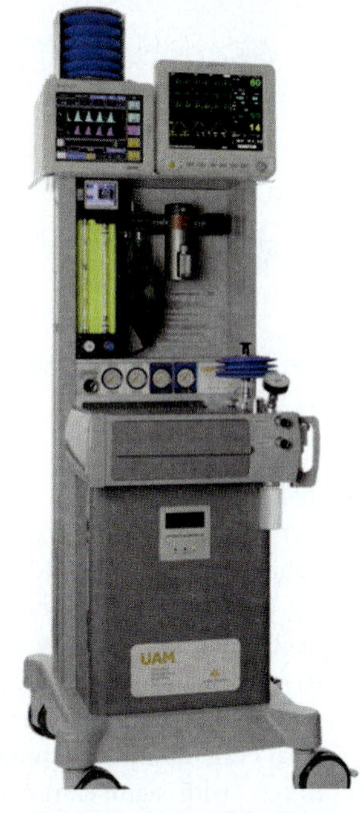 Anesthesia machine with built-in oxygen concentrators, backup power sources, and rugged design for increased capacity to perform surgery (Gradian) Gradian Health Systems
HPV Molecular Screening	**Project ECHO**	**mHealth: Rapid Assay Reader**
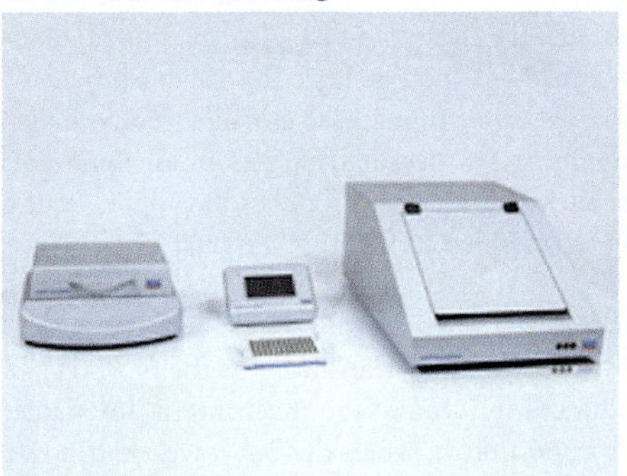 Qiagen LLC HPV DNA molecular screening test developed for use in resource-limited settings; instruments include: a test controller, a luminometer, an orbital shaker, and a magnetic plate holder (careHPV, Qiagen)	 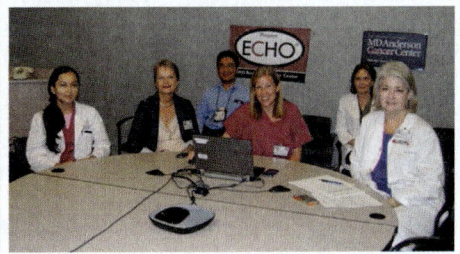 Kathleen Schmeler Program leveraging existing teleconferencing capabilities to facilitate mentorship between specialists and remote healthcare providers (Kathleen M. Schmeler, M.D. Photo from the Project ECHO team at MD Anderson Cancer Center, an ECHO superhub)	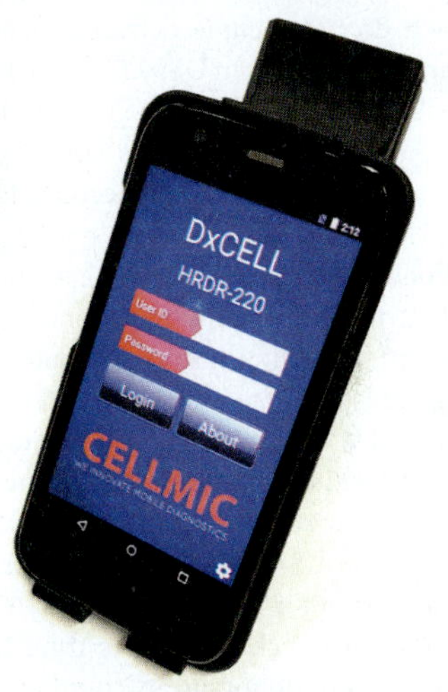 CellMic, LLC Software application and hardware accessory to read rapid diagnostic tests using smartphones (DxCELL, CellMic) CellMic, LLC.

BOX 27-1 WHO ASSURED Criteria for the Ideal Point-of-Care Test

- Affordable
- Sensitive
- Specific
- User-friendly
- Robust and Rapid
- Equipment-free
- Deliverable

Source: Wu G, Zaman MH. Low-cost tools for diagnosing and monitoring HIV infection in low-resource settings. Bull World Health Organ. 2012;90(12):914-920.

Through an initiative by the Bill and Melinda Gates Foundation, the OraQuick® HIV Self Test, widely used in the United States, will be made available at a cost of US$2 per test to 50 LMICs or high HIV burden countries.[18]

Aspects of HIVST that require further innovation and analysis include connecting people who self-test to confirmatory diagnostic testing and treatment, designing products that ensures correct testing procedures by users, clarifying regulatory pathways and guidelines at the country level, and understanding demand and potential for growth.[18]

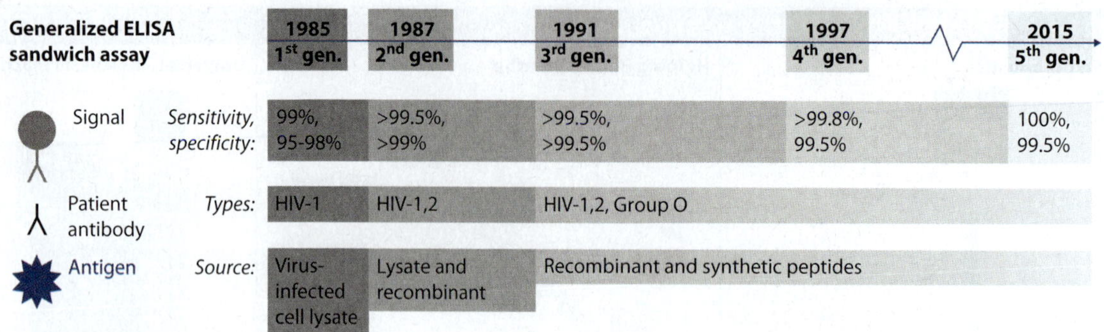

FIGURE 27-3. HIV testing generations. (*Source:* From Alexander TS. Human immunodeficiency virus diagnostic testing: 30 Years of evolution. *Clin Vaccine Immunol.* 2016;23(4):249–53.[6])

Sustainability

One barrier to the long-term impact of HIV tests is the development of a sustainable financing model. Initially, HIV testing was largely funded by international donors. Examples of these early donors include the United States President's Emergency Plan for AIDS Relief (PEPFAR) and the Global Fund, which is a partnership between governments, the private sector, and civil society organizations.[7–9] In 2016, Global Fund donors committed almost US$13 billion to HIV/AIDS projects, with significant contributions coming from private and charitable organizations, middle-income countries, and several African countries.[19] Philanthropic donors, such as the Bill and Melinda Gates Foundation, have also awarded large grants for the development of HIV diagnostics.

Financial support from international aid organizations has kept HIV RDT costs low in resource-limited settings. Ex-works prices, which do not include delivery, distribution, taxes, or commission charges, ranged from US$0.55 to $3.42 in 2016, with over 90% of HIV RDTs procured at prices below US$1.05.[18] The median testing price in 15 studies in LMICs was US$13 per test.[20] In addition, pre- and posttesting counseling can account for a significant portion (38% in the United States) of testing costs.[21] Estimated cost, including cost of goods, healthcare personnel, supply chain costs, and facility costs, of first-time testing in low-income settings is US$8 per test, and follow-up counseling and confirmatory testing for patients who test positive is estimated to cost US$6, while the cost of the test alone is assumed to be US$2.[22] For self-testing, retail prices of HIV tests range from US$22 to US$48 per test in the private sector and US$7.50–15 in the public sector in high-income countries. In LMICs, retail prices range from US$8 to US$16 in the private sector and US$3–6 in the public sector for HIV self-tests.[18]

The current challenge is in transitioning HIV test financing from this group of donors to in-country funding sources to achieve sustainability for the coming decades. Local and central governments are key potential sources of funding. The PEPFAR Sustainable Financing Initiative was started with the goal of working with governments in nine target countries to leverage their domestic resources and share financial responsibility.[23] Other funding could come from implementing user fees, where patients pay a portion of the cost, and other cost-recovery approaches. However, the introduction of user fees in LMICs is controversial, and in some cases, user fees have reduced utilization of health services.[24] For example, a study in Kenya showed worm-prevention treatment uptake decreased from 75% to 19% after fees were introduced, reportedly due to the introduction of cost-sharing.[25] A major limitation for user-fee models is the lack of high-quality evidence on the effects of implementing cost sharing.[24]

There have also been attempts to use innovative funding mechanisms to raise money for HIV testing. One interesting example is the air ticket tax introduced by Unitaid.[26] This is an additional airline tax ranging from US$1 to US$40 per ticket imposed by countries that have agreed to support Unitaid. Participating countries include Cameroon, Chile, Congo, France, Madagascar, Mali, Mauritius, Niger, and Korea. As of 2012, Unitaid raised about US$1.3 billion, about 65% of its revenue, through this tax. Benefits of this mechanism include wide participation from countries and the sustainability of the funding source.[27,28] Another innovative funding mechanism is the Global Fund's Debt2Health program. Through this program, low-income countries can forgo repayment on part of their debt if they invest some amount in their health system through the Global Fund. In 2017, the Spanish government reported that they would forgo €36 million in debts owed to them by Cameroon, the Democratic Republic of Congo, and Ethiopia, in return for these countries investing a total of €15.5 million in Global Fund-supported health programs.[29]

In addition to sustainable financing, vertical integration is necessary to achieve lasting improvements in patient outcomes. This means that access to HIV testing must also be linked to access to treatment and viral load monitoring. The establishment of the UNAIDS 90-90-90 goals aims to increase global access to diagnosis, treatment, and monitoring with stated targets in all three areas of HIV care. Sustainable access to viral suppression is dependent upon success in meeting the established 90-90-90 targets.

Helping Babies Breathe

The birth of a baby involves many transitions as the newborn adapts to life outside of the uterus. One of the most important transitions occurs immediately upon birth, when the baby, who can no longer rely on the placenta for a supply of oxygen, must learn to take in air and breathe within a matter of seconds. While this transition occurs naturally for most babies, as many as 10% of babies fail to initiate and sustain breathing immediately after birth and require assistance.[30] The failure to establish breathing at birth is known as perinatal asphyxia. It is often difficult to reliably predict which pregnancies are at risk for perinatal asphyxia. While in most cases basic resuscitation through the manual compression of a bag and mask is sufficient stimulation for the newborn to commence breathing independently, asphyxia should be identified and acted upon within 1 minute of birth to save the life of the newborn who needs breathing assistance.[31] Delays in resuscitation can result in neurocognitive morbidity or death; furthermore, the incorrect administration of resuscitation (e.g., over inflating the lungs) can injure the newborn. Tragically, a nonbreathing baby in need of resuscitation can be misidentified as a stillbirth, underscoring the need for education to correctly identify when resuscitation is needed. Over the last few decades, educational programs have been developed to address this need, starting with the Neonatal Resuscitation Program (NRP), which was originally developed to standardize resuscitation education across facilities in the United States. However, due to demand, this program was later adapted for use at healthcare facilities globally. Building on the successes of the NRP, the Helping Babies Breathe (HBB) program was developed specifically to address the unique needs for neonatal resuscitation

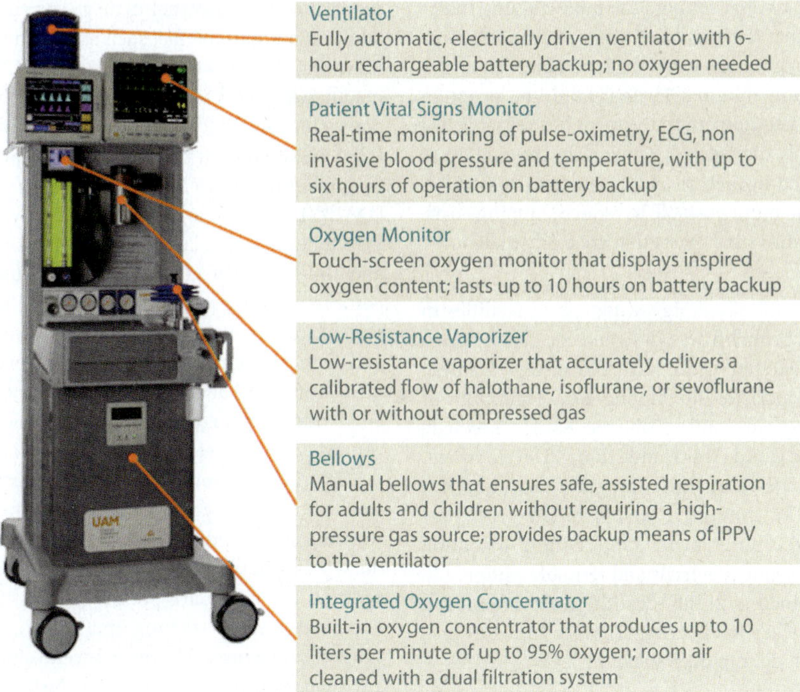
Ventilator
Fully automatic, electrically driven ventilator with 6-hour rechargeable battery backup; no oxygen needed
Patient Vital Signs Monitor
Real-time monitoring of pulse-oximetry, ECG, non invasive blood pressure and temperature, with up to six hours of operation on battery backup
Oxygen Monitor
Touch-screen oxygen monitor that displays inspired oxygen content; lasts up to 10 hours on battery backup
Low-Resistance Vaporizer
Low-resistance vaporizer that accurately delivers a calibrated flow of halothane, isoflurane, or sevoflurane with or without compressed gas
Bellows
Manual bellows that ensures safe, assisted respiration for adults and children without requiring a high-pressure gas source; provides backup means of IPPV to the ventilator
Integrated Oxygen Concentrator
Built-in oxygen concentrator that produces up to 10 liters per minute of up to 95% oxygen; room air cleaned with a dual filtration system
UAM
Gradian Health Systems

FIGURE 27-4. Overview of the Universal Anesthesia Machine (UAM). A ventilator, vital signs monitor, oxygen monitor, low-resistance vaporizer, bellows, and oxygen concentrator are integrated into the UAM. (*Source:* Reprinted with permission from Gradian Health Systems.)

in resource-limited settings. Here, the evolution of the NRP, which laid the groundwork for the development of the HBB program, is discussed.

Development of the NRP began in the 1970s as a standardized educational program established by the American Academy of Pediatrics (AAP) to address neonatal resuscitation in hospitals in the United States, where the infant mortality rate for perinatal asphyxia was 39.9 deaths per 100,000 live births in 1979.[32] The program, which consists of a textbook, posters, and other educational materials, was innovative in many ways. First, it was evidence-based with a structured, self-instructional format. It was also interdisciplinary, including a hands-on approach to focus on skills-based education in addition to traditional knowledge-based education. One of the most significant innovations was a train-the-trainer approach, where workshops were held in centralized locations to educate trainers, who then educated the staff at their home facilities. Since a single regional workshop resulted in dissemination of the program to multiple facilities and institutions, access to the NRP on a regional level within the United States was assisted greatly by the train-the-trainer approach. Access on a global level, however, was far less structured. Soon after the introduction of the NRP in the United States in 1987, the AAP began receiving permission requests to use NRP materials from health professionals in other countries who had been exposed to the program while working in the United States.[33] Consequently, dissemination of NRP training materials was often limited to a localized region or a specific facility. However, in some cases, national groups or societies facilitated the dissemination of NRP materials and trainings at a national level. Examples include the National Neonatology Forum in India, the Perinatal Society of Malaysia, and the Ministry of Health in China.[34–36]

The NRP was successful in many global facilities where it was implemented, with subsequent studies showing a reduction in neonatal mortality at these facilities.[39,40,42–45] In a 2-year prospective study conducted at a hospital in Zhuhai, China from 1993 to 1995, implementation of the NRP resulted in a 63% reduction in early neonatal mortality.[37] A study of 14 teaching hospitals in India showed a decrease in intrapartum-related neonatal mortality from 1.6 per 1000 to 1.1 per 1000 births following implementation of the program in 1990.[38] Building on these successes, the NRP continues to be evaluated and updated approximately every 5 years, with assistance from the International Liaison Committee on Resuscitation (ILCOR), which was formed in 1992 to facilitate cooperation between principal resuscitation organizations worldwide. To date, the NRP course has been taught in over 130 countries, and the textbook has been translated into at least 24 different languages.[41]

Although the NRP was very effective in addressing the resuscitation needs for facility-based births, there were still gaps in neonatal resuscitation unaddressed by the program, especially in LMICs. In particular, studies from the mid- to late-2000s showed that the countries experiencing the highest neonatal mortality burdens did not have sufficient staffing or equipment to perform resuscitation in their healthcare facilities.[42] Furthermore, up to 58–64% of the births in these countries were noninstitutional births occurring outside of health facilities, with approximately 55% of births occurring without a skilled birth attendant present (i.e., nonattended).[43] This motivated the development of a new training program specifically designed to meet these needs: the HBB program.

Innovation

The HBB program, which became available in 2010, was developed to build upon the successful innovations of the NRP but with the needs of resource-limited settings in mind. Rather than focusing on resuscitation guidelines for a well-staffed facility, HBB focused on the needs of a single birth attendant with no or minimal equipment for resuscitation. HBB was innovative in its approach to comprehensive education, focusing not only on basic resuscitation procedures but also on other interventions that have been associated with improving survival in resource-limited settings, including thermal protection of the infant, early breastfeeding, and infection prevention. HBB was also innovative in addressing and attempting to change common mindsets related to neonatal death, such as the idea that neonatal death was inevitable in a resource-limited setting. The HBB training materials adopted a pictorial format that would facilitate education across language barriers and included a low-cost, realistic newborn simulator to facilitate resuscitation training. Furthermore, the program included actual resuscitation equipment in the form of a reusable bag and mask that could be easily disinfected, rather than the single-use disposable devices often used in high-resource settings. This equipment was also designed to be more portable to reduce shipping costs, as it could be broken down into small parts that are easily mailed.

Access

Unlike the NRP, which was initially designed for use in facilities in the United States, the HBB program was designed for global access and was facilitated and accelerated by the HBB Global Development Alliance, a public–private partnership among key organizations including AAP, USAID, Laerdal Foundation, the Eunice Kennedy Shriver National Institute for Child Health and Human Development, Save the Children's Saving Newborn Lives program, and USAID's implementing partners.[44] The innovative design of the HBB program facilitated access to the program by simplifying distribution and transportation of the training materials and reusable equipment. These design factors, combined with the train-the-trainer approach adopted from the NRP, were key in ensuring access to the HBB program, which has now been taught in over 80 countries.[45]

Sustainability

As was the case with the NRP, the train-the-trainer approach adopted by HBB has also been important in the sustainability of the program. Indeed, many early studies demonstrated the need for continued education and refresher trainings to sustain the impact of the program on neonatal outcomes.[46–49] There have been many studies showing decreases in early asphyxia-related morbidity and mortality when these trainings are implemented.[50–53] Furthermore, many studies evaluating the effectiveness of the HBB program have shown a reduction in stillbirths attributed to the correct identification of newborns needing respiratory support who may have previously been misidentified as stillbirths.[51,52,54] Government support, which is essential for the sustainability of this type of program, influenced the design of HBB as it was intended to be a tool to help countries achieve the Millennium Development Goals to reduce childhood mortality set by the United Nations (UN) for 2015.[33] HBB subsequently received emphasis as part of the UN Sustainable Development Goals of ending preventable newborn deaths, as well as the WHO Every Newborn Action Plan to end preventable newborn deaths and stillbirths by 2035.[33,55]

While it is estimated that facility-based basic neonatal resuscitation may avert 30% of intrapartum-related neonatal deaths, and training on a community level may reduce intrapartum-related neonatal deaths by 20%,[42] the ability of the HBB program to improve survival in the long term is yet to be determined. Although many studies have shown a decrease in early asphyxia-related deaths after implementation of the HBB program, some more recent studies have shown little or no impact on overall neonatal mortality, indicating that although more babies are surviving asphyxia-related events, many are not surviving other complications (e.g., infection) that may develop during their stay in the hospital.[51,56] Although HBB's innovative comprehensive approach to neonatal care addressed preventative measures for other common neonatal complications, such as hypothermia and infection, many resource-limited settings remain ill-equipped to deal with these complications when they do develop. As such, there is a continuing need for comprehensive approaches for managing newborn complications, as many newborns in need of additional care experience more than one life-threatening complication that must be addressed to ensure their survival.

Universal Anesthesia Machine

Surgery is often considered a significant challenge in global health, with barriers of expensive and often bulky equipment, high training requirements, infrastructure (e.g., running water and electricity), and additional requirements, such as anesthetics and blood transfusions. However, the need for surgical care in LMICs is significant. In 2010, insufficient access to surgical and anesthesia care was responsible for approximately 16.9 million deaths worldwide, surpassing mortality from HIV/AIDS, tuberculosis, and malaria combined. The Lancet Commission reported that 77.2 million disability-adjusted-life-years (DALYs) could be avoided each year with access to basic surgery.[57] Five billion people lack access to appropriate surgical care globally, and only 3.5% of all surgical procedures occur in the lowest-income countries, inhabited by a third of the world's population.[58] Recent initiatives such as the WHO Global Initiative for Emergency and Essential Surgical Care, Safe Surgery 2020, and Global Surgery 2030 from the Lancet Commission for Global Surgery have heightened attention and promoted research into bringing surgery to resource-limited settings.

Cost is often considered a significant barrier, with modern surgical suites filled with expensive equipment and surgical tools, along with the cost of training specialized surgeons, anesthesiologists, and nurses. Furthermore, accounting for the vast variety of surgical procedures, the irregularity of procedures, and the variable fraction of overhead costs of training and equipment complicate cost calculations of procedures. However, several studies have attempted to present such quantitative analyses, showing favorable cost-effectiveness of surgical care.[59,60] The cost per DALY of caesarean sections and orthopedic surgery were found to be lower than that of ischemic heart disease treatment and multidrug antiretroviral treatment for HIV. The costs of bringing surgical care to resource-limited settings are substantial but proportional to the burden of disease. To create cost-effective and practical programs, the initiatives for global surgery have identified a subset of 44 surgical procedures as essential procedures, including procedures for basic trauma care, emergency obstetric care, general and specialist surgical care, and palliative surgical care. These operations account for 10% of all deaths in LMICs and are among the most cost-effective health interventions.[49] Nevertheless, technological innovations will be essential to bringing a high standard of care to resource-limited settings lacking infrastructure and highly trained staff and physicians, among other factors.

Innovation

The innovation of anesthetics and the anesthesia machine have greatly impacted the surgery landscape, improving the experience for both surgeons and patients. Anesthesia is a vital component of the surgical suite. Anesthesia can be delivered to a specific region (local anesthesia) or to the entire body (total or general anesthesia). Here, the focus is on general anesthesia. General anesthesia can be accomplished by intravenous application or through inhalation. Inhaled anesthesia reaches circulation through the lungs and a major advantage of this technique is more accurate tracking of anesthetic concentration in the blood by comparing the partial pressures of alveolar and pulmonary capillaries and the vaporizer setting, facilitating better drug administration. The concentration of expired anesthesia can also be measured to adjust administration.[61]

While gases are effective as inhaled anesthetics, there are significant risks associated with their toxicity. The amount of anesthetic and oxygen as well as anesthetic vapor delivered simultaneously must be monitored to ensure proper sedation and minimal risks. Modern anesthesia machines include ventilators, suction units, controls for gas and vapor delivery, and displays for patient monitoring. While these machines have become more portable, they still require electricity, medical grade gases, and trained personnel. Furthermore, they are not built for transport through rough terrain or use in harsh conditions. Dr. Paul Fenton developed the Universal Anesthesia Machine (UAM) after seeing the inadequacy of traditional machines in resource-limited settings Fig. 27-4 while he worked at Queen Elizabeth Central Hospital in Blantyre, Malawi. Gradian Health Systems began commercializing the UAM in 2010 and focused on scaling-up use globally.

The UAM is the world's only CE-certified anesthesia machine that can generate its own medical oxygen and, if needed, work without power. It features a built-in, electrically powered oxygen concentrator that can generate up to 95% oxygen at 10 L/min and comes with standard connectors for external oxygen sources such as cylinders and pipelines, as well. In the absence of power and external compressed oxygen, the UAM automatically transitions to draw-over mode, which uses ambient air to deliver anesthesia to the patient. The UAM has options for both automatic and manual ventilation and includes low-resistance vaporizers for halothane, isoflurane, and sevoflurane. The automatic ventilator and monitors for patient vital signs and oxygen output can operate on extended battery backup. The machine is also designed to be robust to heat, humidity, and dust of open-air settings. Replacement components are provided in local spare parts depots for timely, in-country access. Every UAM is supported with a 3-year service warranty carried out by local biomedical technicians, which includes annual preventive maintenance, spare parts, on-demand repairs, and ongoing remote support. The innovation of the UAM is its capability for use without external resources and expensive maintenance.

Access

Partnerships with local organizations, medical providers, and government officials are often considered critical for successful integration of a technology in global health.[62] Fonjungo et al. specify inappropriate design, inconsistent preventative maintenance, and a lack of spare parts and maintenance technicians as major barriers to laboratory equipment maintenance and thus sustainable laboratories and health systems.[63] The technological innovation of the UAM has greatly influenced its accessibility, allowing for use in rural areas without additional resources. Moreover, to facilitate the integration of this surgical equipment into facilities with limited existing surgical capabilities, Gradian provides a standard training with every machine for anesthesia providers and technicians. The 2-day, on-site training includes an orientation on the machine followed by physician-supervised simulations and/or proctored cases.

Depending on the configuration, the cost ranges from US$15,000 to US$25,000. In comparison, conventional anesthesia machines of comparable quality start at approximately US$30,000 and can exceed US$100,000. Gradian works with local organizations and governments as well as donors to support healthcare providers by offering payment plans in cases where the cost of the machine is limiting. The cost includes an initial training as well. After the delivery of a UAM from the local distributor, a Gradian trainer spends several days with local staff, teaching anesthesia providers how to operate the machine clinically. The initial training can also be customized for physicians, nurses, anesthetists, and technicians.

Sustainability

The sustainability of the machine is apparent through its continued use in over 100,000 surgeries since 2011 in over 250 hospitals across 24 countries. A study in Uganda found that only 22% of donated surgical and anesthesia equipment is supported with suitable training.[64] To ensure continued and proper machine performance, Gradian has set up local networks of spare part depots, distributors, and technicians to reduce barriers to continuous and proper use. Regional trainers certified by Gradian train local technicians to ensure regular machine maintenance. In the rare event that an issue requires additional servicing, a master biomedical engineer will be sent in by Gradian.

Working with a donor, the government of Sierra Leone procured 41 machines, and Gradian funded capacity building of nurse-anesthetists through a national train-the-trainer program led by Johns Hopkins University. Funding has also come from international organizations, such as Grand Challenges Canada, who awarded Gradian a $1 million grant to install equipment, train anesthesia providers, and upskill biomedical technicians in four provinces in Zambia as a part of the USAID Saving Lives at Birth program.

Gradian has also explored building capacity through organic growth in Uganda, which has been detailed in a case study by USAID. Uganda was chosen as a candidate to scale-up UAM use due to the high need and likely demand in the country. Although some hospitals were able to support the cost, funding was a major barrier without significant government or nongovernmental organization (NGO) support. Gradian allowed hospitals to pay in installments and, in some cases, offered a subsidized price of US$5000 with the help of a donor. Furthermore, by investing in local infrastructure through effective clinical and technical training and a local distribution partner for installation and ongoing service, the UAM has brought safe anesthetic care to approximately 15,000 patients in 40 operating theaters in Uganda as of October 2016. Their distribution partner now handles everything from sales and marketing to maintenance and repair for the UAM. A local spare parts depot in Kampala, Uganda allows for quick repairs and additional scale-up.[65]

Gradian has demonstrated the importance of following technological innovations with appropriate business models to support usage by the target audience. While technologies such as the UAM undoubtedly improve access to surgery, systems strengthening, such as training programs and establishing distribution networks, will be essential to generating further demand for these technologies and creating sustainable surgical care worldwide.

HPV Molecular Testing

Approximately 500,000 people are diagnosed with cervical cancer each year, and approximately 311,000 deaths result from cervical cancer, with nearly 90% of these deaths occur in LMICs.[66,67] Cervical cancer deaths are expected to rise by almost 25% in the next decade without significant intervention.[68] However, cervical cancer is preventable with effective prevention, screening, and treatment programs.

The vast majority of cervical cancer is caused by the human papillomavirus (HPV), though most HPV infections will never lead to cervical cancer. While over 100 HPV genotypes have been identified, only a subset (13–14 genotypes) are known to be cancer-causing or "high-risk." Cervical cancer prevention can be accomplished in part by administering the HPV vaccine, which protects against high-risk genotypes of HPV.

Screening for cervical cancer and its precursors can be performed using multiple methods: the Papanicolaou (Pap) test, visual inspection by acetic acid (VIA) or Lugol's iodine (VILI), colposcopy, and HPV molecular testing. HPV testing has been an important innovation for cervical cancer screening, though gaps in access remain due to relatively high infrastructure requirements and costs for tests designed to be run at the point of care. When accessible, confirmatory diagnostics are performed most commonly through colposcopy, a microscopy technique for high-magnification visualization of the cervix. After screening and performing confirmatory diagnostics when available, treatment is performed by removing cancerous tissue, commonly through cryotherapy, loop electrosurgical excision procedure (LEEP), cold knife conization, or hysterectomy. Treatment decisions differ according to the stage of cancer at the time of detection or, more commonly in resource-limited settings, according to availability.

The Pap test, which looks for cellular abnormalities in cervical tissue, has been the standard cervical precancer and cancer screening test for decades. During a Pap test, a provider collects a cervical sample, usually with a cervical brush or spatula, from a patient during a gynecologic exam, and the cells from the swab are applied to a slide for reading by a specialist. Because Pap smears must be interpreted by a specialist, samples often must be sent to a centralized lab, leading to long turnaround times for patients to receive their results and often lost to follow-up. Although ideal screening tests are highly sensitive, the Pap test has a low sensitivity (55%) and a high specificity (97%).[69] Pap sensitivity can be as low as 38% and as high as 84% depending on testing conditions.[68] To compensate for low sensitivity, the test's efficacy comes from repeated, regular screening.[70] In the United States, guidelines state that screening among people who are at average risk should occur once every 3 years. When screening programs are successfully implemented, a missed case of precancer may not lead to malignant outcomes due to the slow progression of the disease and the frequency of screenings. However, a person must be able to come back for regular screening to overcome the Pap test's limited sensitivity. When access to care is limited and therefore regular screening is not feasible, cervical cancer incidence and mortality remain high.[71,72]

In resource-limited settings, visual inspection by acetic acid (VIA) or Lugol's iodine (VILI) is often used as an alternative to the Pap test. To perform VIA, a provider applies acetic acid to the cervix, which results in observable changes to the cervical tissue. Ideally, cancerous and precancerous tissue turns white, indicating areas of cervical tissue that require treatment, while noncancerous tissue remains pink. VIA does not require interpretation by a distant specialist and can provide rapid screening results in a few minutes. VIA can range widely in sensitivity (55–96%) and specificity (49–98%),[73] and it leads to overtreatment more commonly than other screening methods.[74] Similarly, VILI is performed by applying Lugol's Iodine to the cervix, and cancerous or precancerous tissue will appear orange in color. VILI has shown a similar wide range of sensitivity (44–98%) and specificity (75–91%).[73] Patient-specific factors that reportedly affect VIA and VILI performance include young age, high parity, premenopausal status, and HPV positivity. Healthcare provider training is also recommended for higher diagnostic accuracy.[73]

In recent years, HPV testing has been introduced into cervical precancer and cancer screening programs. HPV testing is highly sensitive (90.0–97.5%), but has a lower specificity for cervical precancer and cancer (84.2–84.3%) than Pap testing.[75] The role of HPV testing in resource-limited settings is still being evaluated, but WHO guidelines describe several options for appropriate incorporation of HPV testing based on available resources. More specifically, HPV testing can be implemented together with VIA if resources are available to provide the two tests sequentially. Colposcopy should be implemented if the existing screening program meets defined quality indicators (including training, coverage, and follow-up); otherwise, screening should be implemented without a diagnostic follow-up, that is, in a screen-and-treat model. If resources are not available for HPV testing, WHO guidelines recommend VIA screening alone. In any screening program, treatment with LEEP or cryotherapy must be available for the screening to be effective.[76]

Innovation

HPV testing is available in laboratory-based formats in high-resource settings. New HPV testing technologies designed for use in resource-limited settings have the potential to increase global access to high-quality cervical cancer and precancer screening, though the available technologies have significant limitations. Two technologies that aim to lower the cost and complexity of HPV testing, the careHPV test (Qiagen) and the GeneXpert HPV assay (Cepheid), are described here.

The careHPV test was developed to be a cost-effective cervical cancer screening test for use in resource-limited settings.[77] The careHPV test uses the ELISA test format, which is the same test principle utilized in the HIV RDT discussed in the *HIV Rapid Diagnostics* section, to identify the presence of 14 high-risk HPV genotypes. In contrast to the HIV RDT, the sample preparation and testing processes for careHPV require significant instrumentation, infrastructure, and technical skill.

More recently, a high-risk HPV test cartridge was developed for the GeneXpert multianalyte system (subsequently referenced as the Xpert HPV assay). The Xpert HPV assay utilizes qualitative real-time polymerase chain reaction and reports HPV 16 and HPV 18/45 as separate results. Eleven other high-risk types are reported as pooled results across three additional channels. Performance of the Xpert HPV assay is comparable to gold standard technologies used in high-resource settings, such as the Roche cobas assay,[78] and it has shown high sensitivity (89.0–90.4%) and reliability (94.5% agreement between two Xpert results) among women with precancerous lesions.[79] The Xpert HPV assay also may be compatible with self-collected samples.[80] The main limitation of the Xpert HPV assay is high cost, as discussed in the *Sustainability* section.

In addition to commercially available assays, new HPV testing technologies are in preliminary stages of development. Recently, Rodriguez et al. reported development of an HPV test that relies on similar lateral flow technology used in the HIV molecular diagnostic.[81] Lateral flow technology can lower laboratory infrastructure requirements through automating reagent delivery at a low cost and with lower reagent volumes. In contrast to the HIV molecular diagnostic, the workflow presented by Rodriguez et al. includes a 30–45 minute heating step at 63°C to amplify DNA found in HPV 16.[81] This necessitates the use of a heater, which may make the technology prohibitively expensive in some resource-limited settings. However, a single-temperature, battery-powered, and low-cost heater can meet the heating requirements and may expand access to settings in which reliable electricity nor access to a heater are present. While new HPV testing innovations are promising, lateral flow HPV tests are not yet commercially available.

Access

Commercial approaches to developing more affordable HPV molecular tests, such as the careHPV test, are increasing access to HPV testing in some settings. However, cost and infrastructure requirements remain limiting factors, preventing widespread access. The per-test cost of the careHPV test is lowest when all 90 samples, the maximum number of samples, are run together in a batch. Waiting until 90 samples are ready for processing prevents rural and low-volume clinics from running patients' samples in a timely manner. Storing samples for long periods of time until the batch is ready to run can pose problems for sample viability when cold storage is not available or reliable. Additionally, careHPV still requires a high level of user training, and tests require about three hours to complete and must be run in a lab.[75]

The Xpert HPV assay received WHO prequalification, a process described in the *HIV Rapid Diagnostics* section, in December 2017.[82] The Xpert HPV assay may increase access to HPV testing, as the multianalyte GeneXpert platforms are increasingly available in LMICs.[79] Additionally, the Xpert HPV assay requires 1 hour to run and does not require batching; between 1 and 80 samples can be processed at once. The Xpert platform does require a climate-controlled lab.

More recently, self-sampling has shown potential to enable greater access to screening. With this approach, patients self-collect samples outside of a provider's office and send their sample to a centralized testing site, which can increase participation in screening programs. Self-collected swabs have been shown to have comparable molecular test performance to provider-collected swabs when using amplification-based HPV testing, such as Xpert, but not when using hybridization-based HPV testing, such as careHPV.[83–85] Sufficient resources for molecular testing of self-collected swabs, follow-up diagnosis, and treatment are still required to implement self-sampling approaches.

Acknowledging the remaining difficulties of implementing HPV molecular testing, organizations such as PATH have recently advised initiating screening programs with VIA to begin establishing the infrastructure necessary for other screening programs, which will facilitate the introduction of HPV DNA or other molecular tests as they become more affordable.[86]

Sustainability

For HPV molecular diagnostics, procurement and distribution channels are not yet established, and Ministries of Health or providers still need to pay high up-front costs to procure instrumentation.[75] Additionally, even when low per-test costs are achieved through running samples in batches, the cost of HPV molecular testing is still higher than some alternative methods such as VIA. Examples of total testing costs, which vary by setting and resource level, are US$7.50–24.11 for careHPV and US$2.60–19.46 for VIA.[87,88] Example costs for a clinic in a lower-middle income country are US$8.52 for careHPV testing and US$3.52 for VIA testing. In a low-income country, where HPV testing is generally not available, VIA testing costs US$1.60 on average.[88] In addition, the luminometer required to run careHPV tests is too expensive (estimated US$20,000) for many settings.

The actual cost of the Xpert HPV assay will become clearer as the test is scaled up. FIND has negotiated a public sector LMIC price for the Xpert HPV assay of US$14.90 per test, and with instrument costs ranging from US$17,000.[89] Additional costs for patient testing may be substantially higher than the negotiated costs for cartridges and instruments and may vary regionally. For example, cost analyses for a different Xpert assay, which looks for mycobacterium tuberculosis and resistance to rifampicin (MTB/RIF), have indicated that the Xpert-related costs only were US$24.42 per patient in a large study in South Africa,[90] and laboratory costs for Xpert MTB/RIF testing in the United States were US$98.10 per patient.[91] Reducing these prices to a more cost-effective level will be an important factor in sustainability of the Xpert HPV assay.

Establishing supply chains requires a robust body of evidence of efficacy. Increasing evidence is becoming available that indicates HPV molecular testing is the most appropriate screening tool for scale-up in high-resource and in resource-limited settings, which is reflected in recently updated country-level screening policies that focus on HPV screening. Longer-term studies in resource-limited settings are still needed, as most studies published on careHPV implementation have looked solely at clinical outcomes.[92] In addition, the role of HPV vaccination may affect long-term sustainability of HPV molecular testing. HPV vaccination is safe and effective in protecting against nine high-risk HPV genotypes. Universal vaccination must be achieved and sustained for comprehensive protection against cervical cancer. Due to low and disparate global vaccination rates to date,[93,94] cervical precancer and cancer screening remains necessary but the need for screening may diminish as vaccination uptake increases.

Project ECHO

People living in rural areas often face greater challenges accessing health services than their urban counterparts, especially when it comes to accessing specialist care. For example, studies show that more mental health professionals are located in urban, high-population, high-income areas, resulting in a shortage in rural, low-income areas.[95,96] This geographical imbalance is generally also true of other specialties and of the overall distribution of physicians.[97]

Telementoring is one approach that can be used to address this gap. Through telementoring programs, specialists in central medical centers can be connected with remote, typically rural, health providers via teleconferencing or videoconferencing. The specialists provide training and guidance to the remote providers, and the remote providers then provide care to their patients. Telementoring is distinct from telemedicine programs, where patients are still dependent on central specialists for their care. Project Extension for Community Healthcare Outcomes (ECHO) is an example of a novel telementoring program developed to improve access to healthcare for patients in rural and underserved areas.

Innovation

The original Project ECHO model was piloted in 2003 by the University of New Mexico (UNM). Using telementoring, specialists at UNM were able to train rural primary care providers to manage Hepatitis C treatment, which is relatively complex.[98] Project ECHO was designed so that when a new provider is added to the network, ECHO staff first conduct an in-person orientation for staff at the remote site. The orientation covers the conferencing technology and the instruction format for weekly telemedicine clinics. Subsequently, primary care clinicians are organized into learning networks and then go on to meet weekly over videoconference to discuss cases and share information.[99]

Project ECHO is an example of educational and programmatic innovation. Teleconferencing and videoconferencing technologies are not new; however, Project ECHO utilized them in a unique way to equip clinicians with the knowledge and confidence to manage complex medical problems. Project ECHO does not rely on any single specific technology. Instead, its framework can be used with a variety of conferencing technologies, locations, and formats of conveying information (lecture, discussion, case study, etc.) and can be applied to various disease states. This way, participating sites have the freedom to adapt the Project ECHO model to best meet their local needs.

Access

Project ECHO facilitates clinician education and contributes to long-term capacity building, increasing the quality and extent of care that local clinicians can provide patients.[100] In addition to growing capacity, Project ECHO preserves the advantages of allowing patients to see their primary care providers and remain at their community health centers, which can be the most easily accessible and culturally appropriate sites for them to receive care.[99]

In 2011, Arora et al. conducted a prospective cohort study on the outcomes of UNM's Hepatitis C rural patients. The study demonstrated equivalent success between groups treated by specialists at the UNM clinic and by primary care providers at distant ECHO sites, indicating that Project ECHO could effectively extend Hepatitis C treatment to underserved communities in remote areas.[98] Another implementation of Project ECHO in New Mexico targeted the treatment of substance use disorders. The outcome measures of this study focused on the amount of instruction provided by the central site specialists to the ECHO site clinicians, such as the number of hours spent in trainings, patient cases presented, and topics covered.[101] Project ECHO was also applied to other medical conditions including chronic pain management and mental healthcare.[102,103] Baylor St. Luke's Medical Center (Houston, TX) uses ECHO to assist with the management of chronic disease in underserved cities and rural communities in Texas.[104] It should be noted that the outcome measures for many of these studies were related to the amount of instruction provided through mentoring rather than improvements in clinical outcomes.

Project ECHO has primarily been employed in the United States, but there are initiatives to implement it globally through international partnerships. The University of Texas MD Anderson Cancer Center (Houston, TX) has become Project ECHO's first superhub for training other academic centers in oncology care in Texas, Latin America, and Africa.[105] The MD Anderson program started in 2014 with a focus on growing professional capacity for cervical cancer screenings in the medically underserved Rio Grande Valley in South Texas. In 2015, the program was expanded to Latin America with 12 participating countries. Since then, the program has been expanded to Zambia and Mozambique. In addition to teleconferences once or twice a month, there are physician exchanges between MD Anderson and partner sites to facilitate hands-on training. An additional consideration for international partnerships is the reliability of electricity and an Internet connection for teleconferencing. MD Anderson uses ZOOM, a commercially available video conferencing software (available at www.zoom.us), with a free license from UNM/Project ECHO for all participants. ZOOM can be accessed from any smartphone, tablet, or computer, so phone connections can be substituted when electricity is not available. However, MD Anderson providers acknowledge that the need for phone connectivity or electricity is a potential limitation of the program.[106]

Sustainability

The sustainability of Project ECHO has yet to be established. While the program was first launched in 2003, most of the current participating sites have only more recently adopted the model. From a technological perspective, sustainability is not expected to be an issue, at least within the United States, because Project ECHO leverages an existing technology already in common use. Technological sustainability is more of a concern in LMICs, where there is often intermittent electricity, and it may be more difficult to repair and replace equipment. However, Project ECHO does require staff time, which could pose challenges in settings where staff shortages are common. Another consideration is the funding required to support Project ECHO in the long term, which is especially a limitation in resource-limited settings. Arora et al. suggests that the program needs to be integrated into healthcare systems so that funding can be provided through reimbursement mechanisms.[99] Furthermore, structures for scaling-up Project ECHO need to be developed.

The question of sustainability is also important from the perspective of clinical outcomes. Aside from the original study, subsequent studies published on Project ECHO have largely used metrics such as hours of instruction, number of topics covered, and clinician self-assessments as outcomes.[101–103,107] Thus, the extent of Project ECHO's effect on patient health outcomes has not yet been fully established. Furthermore, studies demonstrating increases in clinician knowledge are conducted within a relatively short time frame of the trainings, so the lasting effects of Project ECHO on long-term knowledge acquisition are still unproven. At MD Anderson, the success of the program is being assessed using the following types of measures: (1) process metrics, which include the number of participants, teleconferencing sessions, and cases discussed; (2) provider satisfaction, which is largely self-reported; (3) levels of collaborations, which entails the number of workshops, joint research programs, and observer-ships and trainee exchanges; (4) the number of new providers trained in colposcopy and LEEP; and (5) the number of women undergoing cervical cancer screening and appropriate diagnostic and treatment procedures. Evaluation is still ongoing and results have not yet been reported.[106]

To prove that Project ECHO is effective and sustainable, two outcomes need to be established: (1) that clinicians gain additional knowledge from participating in the program that they retain in the long term, and (2) that increased clinician knowledge translates to improved patient outcomes. Further studies must be conducted at ECHO sites over longer timeframes, and these studies need to measure patient outcomes in addition to instruction provided. Another factor that must be considered for sustainability is treatment financing at ECHO sites, which see fewer patients than central sites. Resources must be available for clinicians to provide care or the knowledge acquired through ECHO will not result in the desired patient outcomes. Overall, the expansion of the ECHO model shows promise in increasing access to treatment for underserved and typically rural populations. However, further studies are required to assess its long-term impact on patient health outcomes.

mHealth: Rapid Assay Reader

Smartphones have extended imaging capabilities previously limited to microscopes and specialized devices with the advancement of onboard optoelectronic image sensors, microprocessors, and improved display resolution. These handheld imaging devices have become ubiquitous and increasingly cost-effective, improving their accessibility in resource-limited and rural settings.[108,109] Researchers in this field, broadly known as "mHealth" or mobile health, have been exploring the combination of smartphones with RDTs. RDTs are low-cost diagnostic tests that are generally visually inspected to determine results; the most well-known RDT example is the home pregnancy test. (*See HIV case study for additional details on this technology.*) However, visual determination of these tests can be unreliable due to user bias, environmental conditions, and material inconsistency, especially at low target concentration levels. Smartphones have the potential to replace traditional expensive and often bulky imaging equipment for more reliable and objective analysis of RDTs with minimal training. In most instances, smartphone cameras (with or without an attachment) capture an image of the RDT and an app interprets the results for the user.

Innovation

The innovation of mHealth solutions lies in bringing the capabilities of large, expensive equipment to the mobile platform. Additionally, while RDTs have improved accessibility of diagnostics globally, mobile readers present a novel auxiliary technology for consistent analysis compared to subjective visual interpretation. Furthermore, smartphones have been used to further improve sensitivity and multiplexing capabilities, through both optimizing image capture and analysis algorithms as well as the implementation of fluorescent markers or microarrays, which are not suitable for visual inspection.[110–112] Data can also be transmitted remotely, expediting real-time disease surveillance and response.[113] Various forms of readers, from scanners to cameras with integrated or separate analysis software, have been previously reported.[114,115] Apart from being portable, familiar, and often already available, smartphones allow for data transmittance and ongoing application development updates via cellular network or Internet connection.

CellMic, LLC has developed a series of rapid assay readers compatible with Bluetooth-enabled smartphones and tablets. These universal readers can read any assay with visual signals (colorimetric, fluorescent, etc.), limited only by the dimensions of their hardware attachment. The first-generation product, DxCELL, comes with an embedded smartphone device, while the forthcoming second-generation product discussed here, DxALL, will come as a compact smart box that can be connected to the user's device via Bluetooth. While DxCELL circumvented challenges in adapting to different devices, CellMic developed DxALL in response to feedback from partners and customers. Without the additional embedded smartphone, DxALL will be offered at a lower price and is expected to better respond to rapidly evolving technology and customer electronics industry. This smart box attachment includes a printed circuit board with several narrow-band LEDs and a lithium-ion battery for optical reflection-mode imaging, so external power is not required. The device is portable, mechanically robust, and improves reliability of RDT results. While improved sensitivity has not been reported by CellMic, objective analysis of faint test lines that result from low target concentrations can improve test interpretation compared to visual discrimination.[116,117] Specific RDTs can be calibrated with the reader using a kit provided by CellMic. Furthermore, the device can be connected to a wireless network for data transfer, spatiotemporal information storage for disease tracking, and printing hard copies for health records. By connecting via Bluetooth, the device is both universal in terms of devices and RDTs.

The first-generation device, DxCELL, was reported in 2012.[118] The prototype weighed only 65 grams and allowed for both reflection and transmission mode imaging. Analysis of captured images occurred on the smartphone but was later moved to the attachment for patient data protection. Analysis was not impacted by irregularities often seen with lateral flow devices, such as manufacturing artifacts. To reduce errors from improper illumination and positioning, additional light sources in the attachment were utilized in place of natural light or smartphone illumination. While the electronics in the attachment were powered by two AAA batteries, an additional design using a USB cable to rely on the smartphone battery was also created to address settings where disposable battery access may be difficult. As an engineering control, two indicator LEDs were used to indicate whether the attachment was successfully powered and whether the RDT was properly loaded. The value of a universal platform was recognized early, as the prototype was validated with malaria, tuberculosis, and HIV RDTs. Each test was also calibrated with the reader to account for differences in control and test line standards and validation mechanisms. As wireless networks may be weak or unreliable in rural settings, the test reports, consisting of the RDT image, patient information, diagnostic result, and additional image information, were stored locally in the absence of connectivity and limited to less than 0.05 megabytes. For reference, standard photos taken on an iPhone 7 range from 1 to 3 megabytes. These design considerations set the foundation for improved accessibility of these readers.

Accessibility

The accessibility of mHealth solutions comes from their pairing with low-cost lateral flow assays as well as the already ubiquitous usage and reduced need for training and maintenance of the mobile platform. They are inherently lightweight and portable, and utilizing the built-in camera and computing capabilities of the user's device reduces cost. Common barriers to emerging technologies in global health, such as establishing local vendor networks and sustainable business models, are mitigated by existing smartphone and RDT vendors and minimal cost of additional equipment. Approximately 585 million people in sub-Saharan Africa lacked consistent access to electricity in 2012, and that figure is expected to rise to 652 million by 2030.[119] In these settings, dependence on electricity for medical care presents obvious challenges. Additionally, while cellphone usage has risen dramatically across Africa, smartphones are less common. A Pew Research Center study found that while roughly 80% of the population across Africa owned a cellphone, only 15% owned a smartphone, compared to 64% in the United States.[120]

Sustainability

Sustainability of mHealth is difficult to assess due to its recent development. In terms of common barriers to sustainable technologies such as maintenance, cost, and transportation, mobile phones inherently have mitigated some of these obstacles. However, there are additional concerns that may limit their continuing use for biological applications, including privacy, universality, and sanitation. Privacy and secure data storage are concerns for all mHealth solutions, as they often depend on smartphone capabilities and user precautions. CellMic's solution of DxALL includes completing data analysis in the attachment and using the user's device only for display and communication of results. While this reduces dependence on device-specific software and hardware specifications, the device's capabilities are not fully utilized and external equipment, such as microprocessors or LEDs, is often required to compensate. If saved to the device, data is kept in application-specific storage and cannot be accessed from the device's hard drive. Furthermore, two-step verification is required to access app data.

The combination of distinct RDTs and separate corresponding readers could quickly become complex for users to navigate, especially for health professionals looking to widen usage. Maintaining readers for different RDTs and across several mobile operating systems, which are constantly being upgraded, can be expensive and time consuming. If readers are only compatible with certain operating systems, devices may need to be purchased exclusively for clinical use, leading to a much more expensive system than intended. CellMic has addressed this issue by creating a universal reader; however, dependency on smartphone software still exists. To reduce downstream effects on users, a change in the application development process for biomedical researchers may be required for more efficient updates.[115] Finally, sanitation guidelines for using personal devices around biological hazards may become necessary to prevent contamination or spread of disease.

Cost can still be a significant barrier in resource-limited settings where infrastructure for devices and electricity needs to be developed. A 2015 study reported the median healthcare spending of all African countries to be US$109 per capita.[99] The cost of a Bluetooth-enabled device can be excessive within these financial constraints. Interestingly, it can be argued that mHealth has gained more traction in high-resource settings for health monitoring and other point-of-care applications. As electronics become cheaper and more ubiquitous, traditional medical devices will continue to evolve and integrate these technologies, especially in resource-limited settings. Electronic devices, such as smartphones, have the potential to serve as the foundation for health system strengthening initiatives, such as data collection and reporting, electronic health records, training and education, and communication with patients.[121] Further research is necessary to understand the possibilities and limitations of these systems.

Case Study Review

These case studies of emerging technologies, each in a different phase of the development and scale-up process, highlight successes as well as remaining challenges in the areas of innovation, access, and/or sustainability (Table 27-3). Even the technologies that are more mature, such as HIV diagnostics, are now facing challenges in access for hard-to-reach populations as well as financial sustainability. Evidence of long-term efficacy is required to determine the sustainable impact of programs like HBB and Project ECHO. Even when programs like HBB are successful in improving survival from one life-threatening condition, they can struggle to reach their full potential in the absence of additional supporting programs to provide comprehensive care for patients who are vulnerable to developing subsequent life-threatening infections or other complications. Even after simplifying more complex technologies, such as the UAM and HPV molecular testing, costs can still present barriers to widespread access. Finally, an early stage technology, like mHealth, requires additional clinical validation before scale-up. In each of these cases, technologies that were appropriately developed for global health applications will need to address continuing challenges in innovation, access, and sustainability.

DISCUSSION

In 2007, the WHO identified the development of appropriate health technologies as a pressing need to solve global health challenges.[2] A major challenge set forth in the Lancet Global Health 2035 Report is to achieve a "grand convergence" in global health to reduce infectious disease, child mortality, and maternal mortality to universally low levels by 2035.[122] Achieving this goal would have enormous public health impact, preventing 10 million deaths every year.[123] To reach this point of convergence, it is critical to invest in global health technologies. This next section connects themes from the case studies and observations from the field of global health technologies to examine ancillary factors that contribute to technology successes. Context-specific design, implementation, scale-up, sustainable financing, policy, and monitoring and evaluation will be discussed.

Context-Specific Design

Global health technology development should be context-specific and meet a clinically defined and/or public health need. While context can be defined in various ways, the WHO categorizes technologies as generally appropriate for use at a health post, health center, district hospital, provincial hospital, or specialized hospital.[124] Many unsuccessful technologies are designed without addressing the challenges of implementation in a specific setting, which can vary greatly between a health post and a specialized hospital (see Table 27-1). Patient populations, including patient volume and capacity of a particular clinic or hospital, can impact the effectiveness of a health

TABLE 27-3 SUMMARY OF CASE STUDIES

HIV Rapid Diagnostic Tests	• **Innovation:** Redesigned laboratory-based HIV test into a format similar to a pregnancy test, allowing for rapid testing outside of clinical laboratories with less provider training • **Access**: Significant increases in screening coverage due to low per-test costs and ease-of-use; gaps in access, particularly among medically underserved and stigmatized groups • **Sustainability**: Screening programs largely funded by nongovernmental and aid organizations; moving toward sustainable financial models
Helping Babies Breathe	• **Innovation**: Evidence-based curriculum and train-the-trainer approach to address resuscitation needs in resource-limited settings; Pictorial format and low-cost, collapsible simulator to facilitate shipping; reusable resuscitation equipment that is easily disinfected • **Access**: Train-the-trainer approach facilitate global access; global dissemination through the Global Development Alliance • **Sustainability**: Adopted by multiple national organizations and governments; preliminary studies have shown short-term improvements in neonatal mortality; further studies needed to establish long-term impact
Universal Anesthesia Machine	• **Innovation**: Rugged design with simple parts for local manufacturing; incorporates an oxygen concentrator, back-up batteries, and hand pump for power; adapted traditional anesthesia machines for resource-limited settings • **Access**: Initial custom training from Gradian encourages proper use and maintenance for physicians, nurses, and technicians • **Sustainability**: Sold at cost to manufacture with options for payment plans and grants; Gradian's local distribution channels and spare part depots improve use and sustainability; external technicians support local distribution channels when needed
HPV Molecular Testing	• **Innovation**: Smaller, less expensive instrumentation for HPV testing • **Access**: New HPV testing technologies have expanded access to highly sensitive cervical cancer screening in resource-limited settings; infrastructure and equipment requirements are limiting • **Sustainability**: Cost remains a limiting factor; evidence that HPV DNA testing is most effective method for cervical cancer screening in resource-limited settings required for government buy-in
Project ECHO	• **Innovation**: Leverages existing videoconferencing technology to provide clinical mentoring by specialists to remote, often rural, nonspecialist providers • **Access**: Telementoring builds healthcare capacity by equipping more clinicians with the knowledge and confidence to manage complex medical problems • **Sustainability**: Sustainability of videoconferencing relatively is well-established; further studies are required to establish the sustainability of the program's impact on long-term clinician education and patient outcomes
mHealth	• **Innovation**: Improves reliability and usability of rapid diagnostic tests and can introduce disease surveillance and patient communication via the smartphone platform without a central laboratory or specialists • **Access**: Leverages the existing familiarity and accessibility of smartphones to improve the use of rapid diagnostic tests • **Sustainability**: Potential for sustainable use with support from developers; progression of smartphone technology may be a barrier if only certain smartphone models or operating systems are compatible

technology. Devices must be robust to dust, humidity, and temperature fluctuations if they are intended for use in open-air hospitals. Similarly, devices must maintain functionality in the presence of low-quality power and water if they are to reach their full potential. The usage of technologies may be limited if they are not intuitive to use and require complex training programs, or if they are difficult to repair and require specialized parts and tools. Since the shipping costs of spare parts or consumables to many destinations can be very expensive, there is a need for innovative designs that leverage resources that are more easily available. Other context-specific criteria can be cultural and often subtle. For example, while 290 million bed nets were supplied between 2008 and 2010 in sub-Saharan Africa, their use was initially limited because the white bed nets resembled funeral shrouds used locally. Changing the color of the nets to green increased their use and significantly improved control of malaria in the region.[59] Finally, medical misinformation, stigma of particular illnesses or populations, and awareness of the availability of medical resources can affect uptake of a particular technology or intervention.

Another potential challenge in the technology development process is maintaining an accurate understanding of the clinical need and priorities for the innovation. One common mistake is designing a product with more features than are required to meet the need, which unnecessarily increases cost and complexity. This can limit utility by making the technology more difficult to use and more expensive to maintain and repair. In other cases, a medical device may be developed for a need that could be more effectively addressed through another approach, such as an educational program, behavior change, or pharmaceutical delivery.[2] For example, with the problem of neonatal hypothermia, innovators should keep in mind that a cheaper or more robust incubator is not the only solution. Kangaroo Mother Care, a method of providing neonatal warming through simple skin-to-skin contact, has been demonstrated to improve neonatal outcomes without device development and the associated complexities of infrastructure requirements and maintenance.[125] While very sick neonates might still require incubators, in many cases, teaching parents how to perform Kangaroo Mother Care is a viable alternative.

Depending on the context and the clinical need, it may be more appropriate to leverage existing infrastructure and technologies rather than deliver a new technology. Technologies that leverage existing infrastructure can circumvent challenges in distribution. For example, the application of smartphones to diagnostic imaging and communication with healthcare professionals leverages existing telecommunication networks to increase healthcare access. Identifying access to landlines, broadband Wi-Fi, and cell coverage in particular locations can help in understanding how technologies that leverage telecommunications infrastructure could be useful. Technologies with familiar features may be easier to use and can reduce the need for additional trainings. For example, the UAM incorporates traditional user interfaces and components, such as oxygen concentrators, along with new technologies required for anesthesia in resource-limited settings. However, distributing a new technology may be necessary in situations where technology used in high-resource settings is completely unsuitable. The HIV RDT is an example of a new technology delivered to expand access to a traditional laboratory test.

Effective innovation begins with identifying needs in specific contexts that can be appropriately addressed by technologies. It is important to consider how a technology will be integrated into the established healthcare landscape early in the development process. Understanding the needs of the medical staff and specialists who work in a particular area can help determine the impact a technology could have. For example, the implementation of a new screening test would have little to no positive impact and would be inappropriate if treatment options are not available or simultaneously introduced.

Finally, ensuring that a technology is designed to integrate into the patient care pathway is important for achieving impact. An example of a comprehensive program that innovators can use to understand technology needs is the UNAIDS 90-90-90 goals. Gaps in reaching these goals exist throughout the full spectrum of HIV diagnosis, treatment, and monitoring[4]; gaps in diagnosis are discussed in more detail in the *HIV Rapid Diagnostics* case study. More broadly, the WHO published its first list of essential medical devices,[126,127] similar to the list of essential medicines.[128] More specific lists of priority medical devices for cancer management[129] and reproductive, maternal, newborn, and child health[130] have also been published.

Implementation

Training is often an essential component to facilitate access to a new technology by ensuring appropriate technology use. In the absence of effective training, technology can be misused and fail to produce the intended results, which can cause providers to abandon the technology. Addressing training requirements within the innovation process by considering ease of use and context-specific resources can help ensure access and sustainability. In some cases, facilitating training is the primary goal of a technology. In others, technologies are designed to be intuitive and simple-to-use, potentially accompanied by a user manual or job aid. As discussed in the *Helping Babies Breathe* case study, educational materials in a simple, pictorial format can circumvent language barriers presented in text-based formats that require translation. For more complex technologies, comprehensive initial trainings, as well as continuing education, are likely to be required. However, even relatively simple technologies, such as the bag and mask for resuscitation included in the Helping Babies Breathe program, have proven to be more effective when refresher training sessions are held.[46–48] These considerations should be factored into the cost of the technology as well as the implementation plan.

There is a need for a streamlined approach to the distribution of medical equipment and the necessary consumables in resource-limited settings. Challenges exist at every level in the distribution chain. Individual countries have unique rules and regulations for the import of equipment that must be addressed. Often, the nearest distributor is in a different country, or even a different continent and shipping costs become prohibitive. Many facilities in resource-limited settings lack a physical street address, which further complicates the distribution process. Designs that eliminate or minimize the cost of consumables may be most sustainable in the face of weak supply chains. For example, paper-based diagnostic tests may reduce the cost of consumables that are currently high in systems like the Xpert HPV assay.[131] Furthermore, most countries have their own regulatory procedures for medical equipment, which can make the integration of new medical equipment challenging, although this process can often be accelerated if the equipment has a CE mark or FDA approval. The difficulties associated with distribution can easily become cost-prohibitive and discourage distributors from operating in areas that are difficult to reach.

Funding mechanisms are often more likely to emphasize technical innovation over simplicity, resulting in complex and costly technologies that are difficult to scale.[131] The ability to afford and support new technologies may be lacking in resource-limited settings, despite need for the technology. Initial investments from nonprofit organizations or other backers can be helpful in building infrastructure for the device, generating revenue for the user to support the purchase, and eventually producing evidence for additional support.[132] Integrated packages of technologies that address focused clinical areas (e.g., surgery or neonatal intensive care) may be easier to scale because they allow implementers to more efficiently navigate implementation barriers for the package as a whole, which may have more noticeable clinical outcomes than when technologies are implemented one at a time.[131] LifeKit by MTTS is an example of generating support for a suite of technologies. LifeKit includes jaundice management, warming systems, and respiratory support machines, among others to treat 75% of the causes of neonatal morbidity and mortality and is in use in 350 hospitals and 25 countries as of March 2018.

Scale-up

Recognizing the success of the Global Alliance for Vaccines Initiative (GAVI), innovators have called for a Global Alliance for Medical Diagnostics Initiative (GAMDI) to coordinate the development, introduction, and utilization of medical diagnostics.[133] Since its inception 16 years ago, GAVI helped create a healthy global vaccine landscape through four guiding principles: product development, health systems strengthening, financing, and market shaping—all critical and unfilled needs for diagnostics and medical technologies in resource-limited settings. Efforts to scale medical technologies in resource-limited settings could be accelerated by adopting similar practices, which have led to the successful scale-up of drugs and vaccines. For example, the Bill and Melinda Gates Foundation recently led the formation of an alliance between 13 pharmaceutical companies, several governments, and other organizations to expedite R&D and delivery of new drugs for ten neglected tropical diseases.[134] Similarly, the Tokyo-based Global Health Innovative Technology Fund (GHIT) is a US$100 million nonprofit fund to promote the development of drugs, vaccines, and diagnostics for infectious diseases.[135] Created as a public–private partnership, GHIT investments are designed to support broad access to resulting products. Although early investments focused on drugs and vaccines, products developed with primary funding from the GHIT will be available in low-income countries under royalty-free licenses. In middle-income countries, GHIT-supported products will be available under licenses prioritizing access for low-income patients.[136]

Technology Policy

The WHO has developed guidelines for medical device policy development, including needs assessment, affordability promotion, and regulation.[137] Policies at local, national, and international levels affect the cost, implementation, and utility of health technologies. Innovations that are simple and accompanied by robust, detailed policies are easier to scale; for example, a very simple antiretroviral therapy (ART) intervention policy led to successful scale-up of ART in Malawi.[138] The policy contained specific, standardized guidelines for training health workers and preparing facilities for ART nationally, allowing for efficient scale-up to both public and private sectors.[139] Finally, it can be difficult to secure financial support for scale-up; often, policymakers are more interested in supporting the introduction of new products than in sustaining and scaling access to existing affordable technologies.[140]

Sustainable Financing

Partnering with funding agencies to build toward financial sustainability is crucial for lasting impact. As an example of an innovative partnership to improve health outcomes, USAID recently joined Merck for Mothers, UBS Optimus Foundation, Hindustan Latex Family Planning Promotion Trust (HLFPPT), Population Services International (PSI), and Palladium to develop the Utkrisht Impact Bond for improving quality of maternal and neonatal healthcare in private facilities in Rajasthan, India. The Utkrisht Impact Bond is a

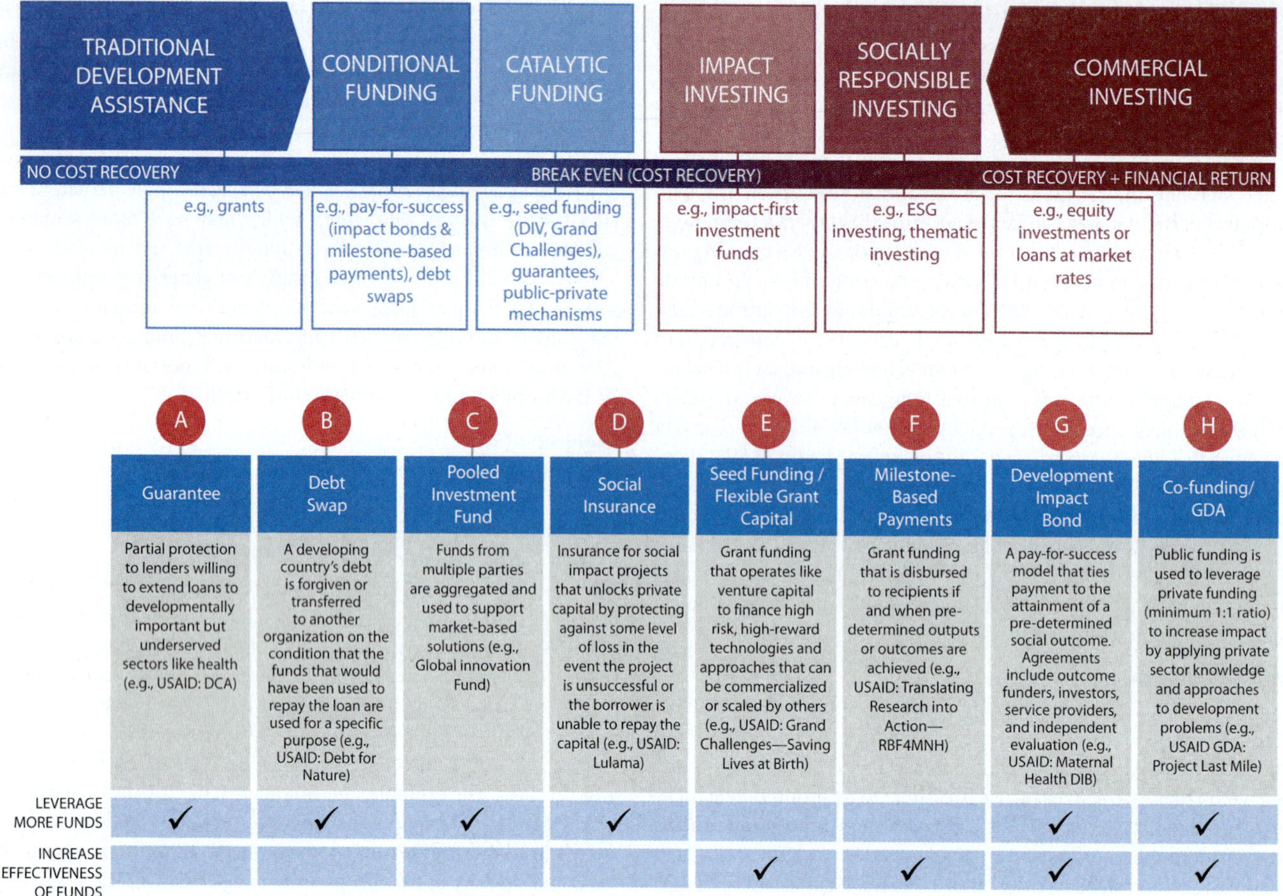

FIGURE 27-5. Financing sources and approaches outlined by USAID. (Top) Spectrum of capital available for global health. The spectrum ranges from public sector grant funding with no expectation of return to private sector financing with an element of cost recovery and a return. (Bottom) Selected nontraditional tools and approaches pursued by USAID and other development organizations to leverage capital for global health across the spectrum of capital. (*Source:* From USAID: Investing for Impact: Capitalizing on the Emerging Landscape for Global Health Financing. 2017. Figure 2)

public–private partnership in which UBS Optimus Foundation provides PSI and HLFPPT with the up-front working capital needed to improve the quality of care in health facilities. If predefined targets are met, USAID and Merck for Mothers will pay back the investment. Palladium is the implementation manager for the impact bond.[141] Funding mechanisms like impact bonds may bring effective global health technologies and services into wider global use. Figure 27-5 illustrates the range of financing available for global health, as well as the innovative, nontraditional financing instruments that USAID and other development organizations can use to leverage this financing for global health activities. As more technologies enter the global health landscape, pushing toward greater access and sustainable financing will be key factors in ensuring that innovations serve to increase health equity globally. More in-depth information on sustainable financing is provided in Chap. 20.

Monitoring and Evaluation

Monitoring and evaluation (M&E) is an important aspect of technology development to address health needs. Several organizations have developed M&E guidelines, which outline indicators and considerations for programs. For example, The Global Fund has developed a monitoring and evaluation toolkit for HIV, tuberculosis, malaria, and health and community systems strengthening. This toolkit includes M&E requirements during a grant life cycle, which global health technology innovators should consider to ensure sustainability.[142]

Following implementation, strong evidence of efficacy and outcomes is needed to garner support and funding to ultimately increase access to and sustainability of the technology. As technologies are shown to be effective, governments and nonprofits are more likely to support their adoption. With government adoption, technologies are more likely to receive additional funding. Financial support is especially important for sustainable access to low-cost technologies developed for global health applications, where profits are often insignificant. M&E provides an understanding of efficiency, effectiveness, impact, and value of an implemented technology for decision makers, ranging from innovators to policymakers. More in-depth information on M&E is provided in Chap. 21.

CONCLUSION

Developing and scaling appropriate technologies for use in resource-limited settings is crucial for improving health outcomes globally. Here, technology development and implementation has been explored in terms of *innovation*, *access*, and *sustainability* through case studies across a wide range of technologies. Through appropriate design, effective partnerships, and innovative strategies to overcome distribution and financing challenges, technology development and scale-up can sustainably improve global health outcomes.

References

1. Bhadelia N. Rage Against the Busted Medical Machines. NPR. 2016. https://www.npr.org/sections/goatsandsoda/2016/09/08/492842274/rage-against-the-busted-medical-machines.
2. Sinha SR, Barry M. Health technologies and innovation in the global health arena. *N Engl J Med.* 2011;365(9):779–82.
3. Piot P, Quinn TC. The AIDS pandemic—A global health paradigm. *N Engl J Med.* 2013;368(23):2210–18.
4. UNAIDS. 90-90-90: An ambitious treatment target to help end the AIDS epidemic. 2014.

5. UNITAID. Technology Landscape: HIV Rapid Diagnostic Tests for Self-Testing, 2nd ed. 2016.
6. Alexander TS. Human immunodeficiency virus diagnostic testing: 30 years of evolution. *Clin Vaccine Immunol.* 2016;23(4):249–53.
7. World Health Organization. Determining costs and financing. 2010.
8. Avert: Funding for HIV and AIDS. 2016. http://www.avert.org/professionals/hiv-around-world/global-response/funding#footnote11_9sh6woi.
9. The Global Fund: Global Fund Overview. 2017. https://www.theglobalfund.org/en/overview/.
10. AIDS.gov: A Timeline of HIV/AIDS. 2016. https://www.hiv.gov/sites/default/files/aidsgov-timeline.pdf.
11. Wu G, Zaman MH. Low-cost tools for diagnosing and monitoring HIV infection in low-resource settings. *Bull World Health Organ.* 2012;90(12):914–20.
12. World Health Organization: WHO Prequalification. 2017. http://www.who.int/topics/prequalification/en/.
13. World Health Organization: WHO list of prequalified in vitro diagnostic products. 2018.
14. UNITAID: Market and Technology Landscape: HIV Rapid Diagnostic Tests for Self Testing, 4th ed. 2018.
15. USAID: USAID List of Approved HIV Rapid Test Kits. 2017. https://www.usaid.gov/sites/default/files/documents/1864/Rapid-Test-Kit-List-February-1-2017-508.pdf.
16. UNAIDS: UNAIDS DATA 2018. 2018.
17. UNAIDS: HIV prevention among key populations. 2016. http://www.unaids.org/en/resources/presscentre/featurestories/2016/november/20161121_keypops.
18. UNITAID: Market and Technology Landscape: HIV Rapid Diagnostic Tests for Self Testing, 3rd ed. 2017.
19. The Lancet HIV. HIV funding key for sustainable development. *Lancet HIV.* 2016;3(11):e499.
20. Johnson C, Dalal S, Baggaley R, et al. *Systematic Review of HIV Testing Costs in High and Low Income Settings.* Geneva: World Health Organization; 2015.
21. Pinkerton SD, Bogart LM, Howerton D, Snyder S, Becker K, Asch SM. Cost of rapid HIV testing at 45 U.S. hospitals. *AIDS Patient Care STDS.* 2010;24(7):409–13.
22. Eaton JW, Johnson CC, Gregson S. The cost of not re-testing: HIV misdiagnosis in the ART "test-and-offer" era. *Clin Infect Dis.* 2017;65(3):522–25.
23. U.S. Agency for International Development: Sustainable Financing Initiative: Controlling the HIV/AIDS Epidemic through Shared Responsibility. 2018. https://www.usaid.gov/what-we-do/global-health/hiv-and-aids/technical-areas/sustainable-financing-initiative.
24. Lagarde M, Palmer N. The impact of user fees on health service utilization in low- and middle-income countries: How strong is the evidence? *Bull World Health Organ.* 2008;86(11):839–48.
25. Kremer M, Miguel E. The illusion of sustainability. *Q J Econ.* 2007;122(3):1007–65.
26. UNITAID: About Us. https://unitaid.eu/about-us/#en.
27. The World Bank, GAVI Alliance: Brief 18: Innovative Financing—Airline Ticket Tax. 2010.
28. UNAIDS: UNITAID: Five years of health innovation brings new approach and new medicines to developing country markets. 2012. http://www.unaids.org/en/resources/presscentre/featurestories/2012/may/20120511unitaid.
29. The Global Fund: Spain, Three African Countries and the Global Fund Launch New Debt2Health Initiative. 2017. https://www.theglobalfund.org/en/news/2017-11-29-spain-three-african-countries-and-the-global-fund-launch-new-debt2health-initiative/.
30. Palme-Kilander C. Methods of resuscitation in low-Apgar-score newborn infants—A national survey. *Acta Pædiatrica.* 1992;81(10):739–44.
31. Kattwinkel J, Perlman JM, Aziz K, et al. 2010 American Heart Association guidelines for cardiopulmonary resuscitation and emergency cardiovascular care, Part 15: Neonatal resuscitation. *Circulation.* 2010;122(18 Suppl 3):S909–19.
32. MacDorman MF, Rosenberg HM. Trends in infant mortality by cause of death and other characteristics. *Vital Heal Stat.* 1993;20(20):1960–68.
33. Niermeyer S. From the Neonatal Resuscitation Program to Helping Babies Breathe: Global impact of educational programs in neonatal resuscitation. *Semin Fetal Neonatal Med.* 2015;20(5):300–8.
34. Boo NY. Neonatal Resuscitation Programme in Malaysia: An eight-year experience. *Singapore Med J.* 2009;50(2):152–9.
35. Deorari AK, Paul VK, Singh M, Vidyasagar D. The National Movement of Neonatal Resuscitation in India. *J TropPediatr.* 2000;46(5):315–7.
36. Xu T, Niermeyer S, Lee HC, et al. Reducing birth asphyxia in China by implementing the Neonatal Resuscitation Program and Helping Babies Breathe initiative. *NeoReviews* 2016;17(8):e425–34.
37. Zhu XY, Fang HQ, Zeng SP, Li YM, Lin HL, Shi SZ. The impact of the Neonatal Resuscitation Program guidelines on the neonatal mortality in a hospital in Zhuhai, China. *Singapore Med J.* 1997;38(11):485–7.
38. Deorari AK, Paul VK, Singh M, Vidyasagar D. Impact of education and training on neonatal resuscitation practices in 14 teaching hospitals in India. *Ann Trop Paediatr.* 2001;21(1):29–33.
39. Vakrilova L, Elleau C, Sluncheva B. French-Bulgarian program "resuscitation of the newborn in a delivery room"—Results and perspectives. *Akush Ginekol (Sofiia).* 2005;44(3):35–40.
40. Carlo WA, McClure EM, Chomba E, et al. Newborn care training of midwives and neonatal and perinatal mortality rates in a developing country. *Pediatrics.* 2010;126(5):1064–71.
41. American Academy of Pediatrics Neonatal Resuscitation Program. https://www.aap.org/en-us/continuing-medical-education/life-support/NRP/Pages/International.aspx.
42. Wall SN, Lee ACC, Carlo W, et al. Reducing intrapartum-related neonatal deaths in low- and middle-income countries—What works? *Semin Perinatol.* 2010;34(6):395–407.
43. Darmstadt GL, Lee ACC, Cousens S, et al. 60 Million non-facility births: Who can deliver in community settings to reduce intrapartum-related deaths? *Int J Gynecol Obstet.* 2009;107:S89–112.
44. Kak LP, Johnson J, McPherson R, Keenan W, Schoen E. Helping Babies Breathe: Lessons Learned Guiding the Way Forward. A 5-Year Report from the HBB Global Development Alliance; 2015.
45. Ersdal HL. Large-scale implementation of Helping Babies Breathe: Lessons Learned Guiding the Way Forward. A 5-Year Report from the HBB Global Development Alliance —What is required? *Paediatr Int Child Health.* 2018;38(1):1–4.
46. Musafili A, Essén B, Baribwira C, Rukundo A, Persson L-Å. Evaluating Helping Babies Breathe: Training for healthcare workers at hospitals in Rwanda. *Acta Paediatr.* 2013;102(1):e34–8.
47. Bang A, Patel A, Bellad R, et al. Helping Babies Breathe (HBB) training: What happens to knowledge and skills over time? *BMC Pregnancy Childbirth.* 2016;16(1):364.
48. Singhal N, Lockyer J, Fidler H, et al. Helping Babies Breathe: Global Neonatal Resuscitation Program development and formative educational evaluation. *Resuscitation.* 2012;83(1):90–6.
49. Ersdal HL, Vossius C, Bayo E, et al. A one-day "Helping Babies Breathe" course improves simulated performance but not clinical management of neonates. *Resuscitation.* 2013;84(10):1422–7.
50. Ashish KC, Wrammert J, Clark RB, et al. Reducing perinatal mortality in Nepal using Helping Babies Breathe. *Pediatrics.* 2016;137(6):e20150117.
51. Goudar SS, Somannavar MS, Clark R, et al. Stillbirth and newborn mortality in India after helping babies breathe training. *Pediatrics.* 2013;131(2):e344–52.
52. Msemo G, Massawe A, Mmbando D, et al. Newborn mortality and fresh stillbirth rates in Tanzania after Helping Babies Breathe Training. *Pediatrics.* 2013;131(2):e353-–60.
53. Rule ARL, Maina E, Cheruiyot D, Mueri P, Simmons JM, Kamath-Rayne BD. Using quality improvement to decrease birth asphyxia rates after 'Helping Babies Breathe' training in Kenya. *Acta Paediatr.* 2017;106(10):1666–73.
54. Bellad RM, Bang A, Carlo WA, et al. A pre-post study of a multi-country scale up of resuscitation training of facility birth attendants: Does Helping Babies Breathe training save lives? *BMC Pregnancy Childbirth.* 2016;16(1):1–10.
55. World Health Organisation. Every Newborn Action Plan. 2014.
56. Wrammert J, A KC, Ewald U, Målqvist M. Improved postnatal care is needed to maintain gains in neonatal survival after the implementation of the Helping Babies Breathe initiative. *Acta Paediatr.* 2017;106(8):1280–5.
57. Meara JG, Leather AJM, Hagander L, et al. Global Surgery 2030: Evidence and solutions for achieving health, welfare, and economic development. *Lancet.* 2015;386:569–624.
58. Sheik Ali S, Jaffry Z, Cherian MN, et al. Surgical human resources according to types of health care facility: An assessment in low- and middle-income countries. *World J Surg.* 2017;41(11):2667–73.

59. Chao TE, Sharma K, Mandigo M, et al. Cost-effectiveness of surgery and its policy implications for global health: A systematic review and analysis. *Lancet Glob Heal.* 2014;2(6):334–45.
60. Mock CN, Donkor P, Gawande A, et al. Essential surgery: Key messages from Disease Control Priorities. *Lancet.* 2015;385:2209–19.
61. Egan TD. Total intravenous anesthesia versus inhalation anesthesia: A drug delivery perspective. *J Cardiothorac Vasc Anesth.* 2015;29(S1):S3–6.
62. Juma C, Yee-Cheong L. Reinventing global health: The role of science, technology, and innovation. *Lancet.* 2005;365(9464):1105–7.
63. Fonjungo PN, Kebede Y, Messele T, et al. Laboratory equipment maintenance: A critical bottleneck for strengthening health systems in sub-Saharan Africa. *J Public Heal Policy.* 2017;33(1):34–45.
64. Elobu AE, Kintu A, Galukande M, et al. Evaluating international global health collaborations: Perspectives from surgery and anesthesia trainees in Uganda. *Surg (United States).* 2014;155(4):585–92.
65. USAID: Ready, Set, Launch: A Country-Level Launch Planning Guide for Global Health Innovations. 2017.
66. World Health Organization. Cervical Cancer. 2019. http://www.who.int/cancer/prevention/diagnosis-screening/cervical-cancer/en/.
67. Bray F, Ferlay J, Soerjomataram I, Siegel RL, Torre LA, Jemal A. Global cancer statistics 2018: GLOBOCAN estimates of incidence and mortality worldwide for 36 cancers in 185 countries. *CA Cancer J Clin.* 2018;68(6):394–424.
68. World Health Organization. Comprehensive Cervical Cancer Control: A Guide to Essential Practice. 2014.
69. Naucler P, Ryd W, Törnberg S, et al: Human Papillomavirus and Papanicolaou Tests to Screen for Cervical Cancer. *N Engl J Med.* 2007;357(16):1589-1597.
70. Safaeian M, Solomon D, Castle PE. Cervical cancer prevention—Cervical screening: Science in evolution. *Obstet Gynecol Clin North Am.* 2007;34(4):739–60.
71. National Institutes of Health. Fact Sheet: Cervical Cancer. 2010.
72. Singh GK, Azuine RE, Siahpush M. Global inequalities in cervical cancer incidence and mortality are linked to deprivation, low socioeconomic status, and human development. *Int J MCH AIDS.* 2012;1(1):17–30.
73. Raifu AO, El-Zein M, Sangwa-Lugoma G, et a.: Determinants of cervical cancer screening accuracy for visual inspection with acetic acid (VIA) and Lugol's iodine (VILI) performed by nurse and physician. *PLoS One.* 2017;12(1):e0170631.
74. Mustafa RA, Santesso N, Khatib R, et al. Systematic reviews and meta-analyses of the accuracy of HPV tests, visual inspection with acetic acid, cytology, and colposcopy. *Int J Gynecol Obstet.* 2016;132(3):259–65.
75. Alfaro K, Arrossi S, Campanera A, et al. Integrating HPV testing in cervical cancer screening programs. 2016.
76. World Health Organization. WHO guidelines for screening and treatment of precancerous lesions for cervical cancer prevention. 2013.
77. Jeronimo J, Bansil P, Lim J, et al. A multicountry evaluation of careHPV testing, visual inspection with acetic acid, and Papanicolaou testing for the detection of cervical cancer. *Int J Gynecol Cancer.* 2014;24(3):576–85.
78. Einstein MH, Smith KM, Davis TE, et al. Clinical evaluation of the cartridge-based GeneXpert human papillomavirus assay in women referred for colposcopy. *J Clin Microbiol.* 2014;52(6):2089–95.
79. Castle PE, Smith KM, Davis TE, et al. Reliability of the Xpert HPV assay to detect high-risk human Papillomavirus DNA in a colposcopy referral population. *Am J Clin Pathol.* 2015;143(1):126–33.
80. Toliman P, Badman SG, Gabuzzi J, et al. Field evaluation of Xpert HPV point-of-care test for detection of human Papillomavirus infection by use of self-collected vaginal and clinician-collected cervical specimens. *J Clin Microbiol.* 2016;54(7):1734–37.
81. Rodriguez NM, Wong WS, Liu L, Dewar R, Klapperich CM. A fully integrated paperfluidic molecular diagnostic chip for the extraction, amplification, and detection of nucleic acids from clinical samples. *Lab Chip.* 2016;16(4):753–63.
82. World Health Organization. WHO Prequalification of In Vitro Diagnostics Public Report: Xpert HPV. 2017. http://www.who.int/diagnostics_laboratory/evaluations/pq-list/hiv-vrl/171221_final_pq_report_pqdx_0268_070_00.pdf.
83. Arbyn M, Smith SB, Temin S, Sultana F, Castle P. Detecting cervical precancer and reaching underscreened women by using HPV testing on self samples: Updated meta-analyses. *BMJ.* 2018;363:k4823.
84. Gupta S, Palmer C, Bik EM, et al. Self-sampling for human Papillomavirus testing: Increased cervical cancer screening participation and incorporation in international screening programs. *Front Public Heal.* 2018;6:77.
85. Polman NJ, Ebisch RMF, Heideman DAM, et al. Performance of human papillomavirus testing on self-collected versus clinician-collected samples for the detection of cervical intraepithelial neoplasia of grade 2 or worse: A randomised, paired screen-positive, non-inferiority trial. *Lancet Oncol.* 2019;20(2):229–38.
86. Jeronimo J, Tsu V, Lamontagne S, et al. Cervical cancer screening and treatment in low-resource settings. *Cervical Cancer Prevention: Practical Experience Series.* Seattle: PATH; 2013.
87. Shi J-F, Chen J-F, Canfell K, et al. Estimation of the costs of cervical cancer screening, diagnosis and treatment in rural Shanxi Province, China: A micro-costing study. *BMC Health Serv Res.* 2012;12(1):123.
88. Campos NG, Sharma M, Kyu AC, et al. Comprehensive Global Cervical Cancer Prevention: Costs and Benefits of Scaling up within a Decade. 2016.
89. FIND. GeneXpert®: Negotiated prices. 2019. https://www.finddx.org/pricing/genexpert/
90. Vassall A, Siapka M, Foster N, et al. Cost-effectiveness of Xpert MTB/RIF for tuberculosis diagnosis in South Africa: A real-world cost analysis and economic evaluation. *Lancet Glob Heal.* 2017;5(7):e710–9.
91. Choi HW, Miele K, Dowdy D, Shah M. Cost-effectiveness of Xpert® MTB/RIF for diagnosing pulmonary tuberculosis in the United States. *Int J Tuberc Lung Dis.* 2013;17(10):1328–35.
92. Cremer M, Maza M, Alfaro K, et al. Scale-up of an human Papillomavirus testing implementation program in El Salvador. *J Low Genit Tract Dis.* 2017;21(1):26–32.
93. Walker TY, Elam-Evans LD, Singleton JA, et al. National, regional, state, and selected local area vaccination coverage among adolescents aged 13–17 years—United States, 2016. *Morb Mortal Wkly Rep.* 2017;66(33):874–82.
94. Bruni L, Diaz M, Barrionuevo-Rosas L, et al. Global estimates of human papillomavirus vaccination coverage by region and income level: A pooled analysis. *Lancet Glob Heal.* 2016;4(7):e453–63.
95. Ellis AR, Konrad TR, Thomas KC, Morrissey JP. County-level estimates of mental health professional supply in the United States. *Psychiatr Serv.* 2009;60(10):1315–22.
96. Thomas KC, Ellis AR, Konrad TR, Holzer CE, Morrissey JP. County-level estimates of mental health professional shortage in the United States. *Psychiatr Serv.* 2009;60(10):1323–28.
97. Dussault G, Franceschini MC. Not enough there, too many here: Understanding geographical imbalances in the distribution of the health workforce. *Hum Resour Health.* 2006;4:12.
98. Arora S, Thornton K, Murata G, et al. Outcomes of treatment for hepatitis C virus infection by primary care providers. *N Engl J Med.* 2011;364(23):2199–207.
99. Arora S, Kalishman S, Dion D, et al. Partnering urban academic medical centers and rural primary care clinicians to provide complex chronic disease care. *Health Aff (Millwood).* 2011;30(6):1176–84.
100. Project ECH.: A Revolution in Medical Education and Delivery: University of New Mexico School of Medicine. 2018. https://echo.unm.edu/.
101. Komaromy M, Duhigg D, Metcalf A, et al. Project ECHO (Extension for Community Healthcare Outcomes): A new model for educating primary care providers about treatment of substance use disorders. *Subst Abus.* 2016;37(1):20–4.
102. Anderson D, Zlateva I, Davis B, et al. Improving pain care with project ECHO in community health centers. *Pain Med.* 2017;18(10):1882–9.
103. Sockalingam S, Arena A, Serhal E, Mohri L, Alloo J, Crawford A. Building provincial mental health capacity in primary care: An evaluation of a Project ECHO Mental Health Program. *Acad Psychiatry.* 2018;42(4):451–7.
104. Project ECHO: Baylor College of Medicine. 2018. https://www.bcm.edu/departments/surgery/divisions/abdominal-transplantation/echo.
105. MD Anderson designated first Project ECHO superhub for oncology | MD Anderson Cancer Center: 2017. https://www.mdanderson.org/newsroom/2017/02/md-anderson-designated-first-project-echo-superhub-for-oncology.html.
106. Lopez MS, Baker ES, Milbourne AM, et al. Project ECHO: A telementoring program for cervical cancer prevention and treatment in low-resource settings. *J Glob Oncol.* 2017;3(5):658–65.
107. Carlin L, Zhao J, Dubin R, Taenzer P, Sidrak H, Furlan A. Project ECHO telementoring intervention for managing chronic pain in primary care: Insights from a qualitative study. *Pain Med.* 2018;19(6):1140–6.
108. Ozcan A. Mobile phones democratize and cultivate next-generation imaging, diagnostics and measurement tools. *Lab Chip.* 2014;14(17):3187–94.

109. Breslauer DN, Maamari RN, Switz NA, Lam WA, Fletcher DA. Mobile phone based clinical microscopy for global health applications. *PLoS One*. 2009;4(7):1–7.

110. Liu G, Mao X, Phillips J A, Xu H, Tan W, Zeng L. Aptamer—Nanoparticle strip biosensor for sensitive detection of cancer cells. *Anal Chem*. 2009;81(24):10013–8.

111. Balsam J, Rasooly R, Bruck HA, Rasooly A. Thousand-fold fluorescent signal amplification for mHealth diagnostics. *Biosens Bioelectron*. 2014;51:1–7.

112. Kozma P, Lehmann A, Wunderlich K, et al. A novel handheld fluorescent microarray reader for point-of-care diagnostic. *Biosens Bioelectron*. 2013;47:415–20.

113. Kumar S, Nilsen WJ, Abernethy A, et al. Mobile health technology evaluation: The mHealth evidence workshop. *Am J Prev Med*. 2013;45(2):228–36.

114. Liu C, Jia Q, Yang C, et al. Lateral flow immunochromatographic assay for sensitive pesticide detection by using Fe_3O_4 nanoparticle aggregates as color reagents. *Anal Chem*. 2011;83(17):6778–84.

115. Yetisen AK, Martinez-Hurtado JL, da Cruz Vasconcellos F, Simsekler MCE, Akram MS, Lowe CR. The regulation of mobile medical applications. *Lab Chip*. 2014;14(5):833.

116. Shekalaghe S, Cancino M, Mavere C, et al. Clinical performance of an automated reader in interpreting malaria rapid diagnostic tests in Tanzania. *Malar J*. 2013;12(1):1–9.

117. Paula Vaz Cardoso L, Dias RF, Freitas AA, et al. Development of a quantitative rapid diagnostic test for multibacillary leprosy using smart phone technology. *BMC Infect Dis*. 2013;13(1):497.

118. Mudanyali O, Dimitrov S, Sikora U, Padmanabhan S, Navruz I, Ozcan A. Integrated rapid-diagnostic-test reader platform on a cellphone. *Lab Chip*. 2012;12(15):2678.

119. Welsch M, Bazilian M, Howells M, et al. Smart and Just Grids for sub-Saharan Africa: Exploring options. *Renew Sustain Energy Rev*. 2013;20:336–52.

120. Poushter J, Bell J, Carle J, et al. Cell Phones in Africa: Communication Lifeline. Pew Research Center. 2015; 1-16.

121. Labrique AB, Vasudevan L, Kochi E, Fabricant R, Mehl G. mHealth innovations as health system strengthening tools: 12 Common applications and a visual framework. *Glob Heal Sci Pract*. 2013;1(2):160–71.

122. Jamison DT, Summers LH, Alleyne G, et al. The Lancet Commissions Global health 2035: A world converging within a generation. *Lancet*. 2013;382:1898--955.

123. Kruk ME, Yamey G, Angell SY, et al. Transforming global health by improving the science of scale-up. *PLoS Biol*. 2016;14(3):e1002360.

124. Medical devices by health care facility: World Health Organization. 2018. http://www.who.int/medical_devices/innovation/health_care_facility/en/index1.html.

125. Lawn JE, Mwansa-Kambafwile J, Horta BL, Barros FC, Cousens S. "Kangaroo mother care" to prevent neonatal deaths due to preterm birth complications. *Int J Epidemiol*. 2010;39(Suppl 1):i144–54.

126. World Health Organization: WHO to develop Essential Diagnostics List. 2017. http://www.who.int/medicines/news/2017/WHO_develop_essential_diagnostics_list/en/

127. *Second WHO Model List of Essential In Vitro Diagnostics*; 2019.

128. World Health Organization: Model List of Essential Medicines: 19th List. 2015.

129. World Health Organization: WHO priority list of medical devices for cancer management. 2017.

130. World Health Organization: Interagency list of medical devices for essential interventions for reproductive, maternal, newborn and child health. 2015.

131. Richards-Kortum R, Oden M. Devices for low-resource health care. *Science*. 2013;342(6162):1055–7.

132. Matthias DM, Taylor CH, Sen D, Metzler M. Local markets for global health technologies: Lessons learned from advancing 6 new products. *Glob Heal Sci Pract*. 2014;2(2):152–64.

133. Mugambi ML, Palamountain KM, Gallarda J, Drain PK. Exploring the case for a global alliance for medical diagnostics initiative. *Diagnostics*. 2017;7(1).

134. Mundel T: Global health needs to fill the innovation gap. *Nat Med*. 2012;18(12):1735.

135. Kirby T. BT Slingsby: Driving forward innovation in global health. *Lancet Infect Dis*. 2015;15(3):274.

136. Slingsby BT, Kurokawa K. The Global Health Innovative Technology (GHIT) fund: Financing medical innovations for neglected populations. *Lancet Glob Heal*. 2013;1(4):e184–5.

137. World Health Organization: Development of medical device policies. 2011. http://apps.who.int/iris/bitstream/handle/10665/44600/9789241501637_eng.pdf;jsessionid=0AF6455A84F0127258079A5856A61640?sequence=1.

138. Yamey G. Scaling up global health interventions: A proposed framework for success. *PLoS Med*. 2011;8(6):e1001049.

139. Harries AD, Zachariah R, Jahn A, Schouten EJ, Kamoto K. Scaling up antiretroviral therapy in Malawi-implications for managing other chronic diseases in resource-limited countries. *JAIDS J Acquir Immune Defic Syndr*. 2009;52:S14–6.

140. Piot P. Innovation and technology for global public health. *Glob Public Health*. 2012;7(Suppl 1):S46–53.

141. USAID: The Maternal and Newborn Health Development Impact Bond. 2018. https://www.usaid.gov/cii/IndiaDIB.

142. The Global Fund. Monitoring and Evaluation Toolkit: HIV, Tuberculosis, Malaria and Health and Community Systems Strengthening. 4th ed. 2011, pp. 1–35.

143. Howitt P, Darzi A, Yang G-Z, et al. Technologies for global health. *Lancet*. 2012;380(9840):507–35.

144. USAID. Investing for Impact: Capitalizing on the Emerging Landscape for Global Health Financing. 2017.

CHAPTER

28 A Trained and Prepared Global Health Workforce Is Required to Achieve Impact*

Rebecca M. Martin • Drew Blakeman

INTRODUCTION

The health workforce is a key cornerstone in health systems, in providing both clinical care and preventive services. In addition, a skilled health workforce is essential for a well-functioning public health infrastructure to respond to disease outbreaks or disasters, and in ensuring that communities demand critical services. Many countries, especially low-income ones, are facing serious shortages of skilled health workers and the geographic distribution, recruitment, and retention of the health workforce are not aligned with the evidence-based needs. To address these challenges so that global health impact is achieved by increasing coverage to health services for communities and ensuring countries are prepared to respond to public health emergencies and health threats, integrated strategies must be developed and implemented to build, support, and sustain the capacity of the global health workforce, while addressing current challenges.

COMPONENTS OF A ROBUST GLOBAL HEALTH WORKFORCE

A workforce capable of contributing to a country's health needs, including its public health system, spans personnel throughout the entire health system and public health sectors. It also includes people working in areas that cut across these sectors, such as those working in veterinary and animal health, community health workers, and biosafety and biosecurity functions. In many cases, staff will be working with counterparts representing other functions on collaborative teams that are able to address complex issues requiring expertise from a number of connected areas.

Health System Workforce

The health system workforce is generally comprised of medical professionals, primarily physicians, nurses, other clinical staff, pharmacists, and other allied health professionals providing primary healthcare services. This health system workforce is on the frontlines, and in addition to providing healthcare services for the sick will often be the first to detect a disease outbreak and initiate community response as it works to create resilient communities. The health system workforce will also be involved with disease-prevention efforts, especially those within health facilities and in the community. By adopting the practice of team-based care, each member of the health workforce can receive training to expand the scope of their duties, for example, nurses taking and recording blood pressures and authorizing prescription refills under physician oversight.

Creating resilient communities requires their engagement in making decisions about their health. Therefore, strong and sustainable relations between communities and the health workforce are required. Training the health workforce on how to engage communities, how to provide health information, how to understand and incorporate the specific social determinants of health in screenings and services, and how to detect and report population-based threats is needed. It is important to understand and analyze the health-related work of all workers in the health system to effectively respond to what is needed now and in the future. There is a need for integrated strategies to address current health workforce needs, including training, retention and recruitment, and geographic distribution to ensure a skilled workforce today and for planning the needed global health workforce for tomorrow.

Public Health Workforce

Although the public health workforce[1] is often called upon to provide healthcare services to individual patients at community-based clinics, its primary concern is with programs designed to promote and protect overall population health. A number of population-based health programs globally have mobilized the public health workforce in various settings, including for prevention and treatment for Human Immunodeficiency Virus (HIV)/AIDS, immunization programs, including vaccination campaigns, and Global Health Security initiatives. For the purposes of this chapter, Global Health Security will be cited frequently as an example of the public health workforce needs and activities to provide a context to the needs. The public health workforce includes epidemiologists, laboratory scientists, biostatisticians, logisticians, supply chain experts, public health managers, and various other support staff with skills necessary for systematic cooperation to meet core competencies relevant to preventing diseases, detecting diseases when and where they occur, and responding to public health emergencies rapidly and efficiently.

Epidemiologists are public health professionals who investigate patterns and causes of disease and injury in humans, often as frontline workers. At the first notification of a possible disease outbreak, they are often deployed to the field, frequently in hazardous conditions, they interview patients, identifying their contacts who may have been exposed, perform basic data analysis, and in coordination with medical staff, determine whether isolation and treatment are indicated. They also facilitate transport of laboratory samples for testing.

Epidemiologists also conduct public health surveillance. This is the continuous and systematic collection, analysis, and interpretation of health-related data needed to plan, implement, and evaluate public health programs and interventions. Surveillance—specifically the capacity to monitor for disease outbreaks—is the foundation for effective prevention, detection, and response and can serve as an

*Disclaimer: The findings and conclusions in this chapter are those of the authors and do not necessarily represent the official position of the Centers for Disease Control and Prevention.

[1] Domestic public health workforce is also addressed in Chapter 46: The Public Health Workforce and in Chapter 9: Public Health Practice

early warning system for impending public health emergencies and detecting threats early.

A skilled workforce equipped with necessary tools is vital for an effective public health surveillance system. Because of the changing epidemiology of diseases and related reporting requirements, combined with opportunities offered by advances in information technology and enhanced public health surveillance, education and training are critical to strengthening surveillance workforce capacity.[1] In addition, with the evolving need for rapid detection and reporting for certain infectious diseases and health conditions, the training and engagement of community health extension workers to conduct community-based surveillance can provide another important level in the public health workforce.

Laboratory scientists, usually working in a reference laboratory, although sometimes deployed into the field, initially test samples to determine what disease agent may be involved in an outbreak. More sophisticated laboratory facilities are able to conduct genomic sequencing to better identify sources of pathogens and possible linkages with other cases. Scientists also develop and test new diagnostics and vaccines before they are deployed as prophylaxis for the general population.

Other public health staff, including biostatisticians with training in epidemiology, collect and analyze data that can be used to determine appropriate interventions and other action. They often have access to more sophisticated systems and analytic tools than do epidemiologists working in the field and can thus perform more robust data analysis that allows conclusions to be drawn and predictions to be made. Biostatisticians also contribute to the design and execution of research studies in collaboration with other statisticians and scientists. Logisticians and supply chain experts are critical for procurement, planning, and executing prevention and response activities, as well as ensuring medical counter measures, for example, vaccines, personal protective equipment, arrive in quality condition and in the right geographic places in the right numbers. Supply chain is also critical for shipping specimens to be tested in laboratories and requires careful management of the conditions. Public health professionals who have proficient management skills, both technical and financial, are imperative to deliver and realize health programs.

Cross-Cutting Functions

Staff in cross-cutting functions include veterinarians and others involved with animal health, which covers wildlife as well as animal husbandry related to farming and livestock. These workers are especially important to Global Health Security programs because of the high and increasing prevalence of zoonotic diseases that jump biological barriers from animals to humans. Most if not all disease epidemics, including the West Africa Ebola Virus Disease (EVD) epidemic, 2014–15, the 2009 H1N1 influenza pandemic, the 2003 SARS pandemic, the 1918–19 Spanish Flu pandemic, and even HIV, are known or likely to have originated in animal populations before crossing to humans, or mutating into pathogens, with the ability for human-to-human transmission.[2] Therefore, it is important that the health workforce be trained in One Health in the context of how animal and human health intersect.[3]

Community health workers are lay staff who most commonly serve the local area in which they live. These are people who have generally not received formal academic or professional training but have been taught to handle specific tasks related to provision of primary healthcare services as a supplement to the professional health workforce. They can be especially valuable members of the healthcare team, especially in areas with shortages of physicians and nurses, as they can assume many of the functions of formally trained staff.

Public health trainees similarly supplement the professional public health workforce. For example, public health professionals enrolled in the CDC Field Epidemiology Training Program (FETP), which operates in more than 60 countries, as of 2018, perform outbreak investigations and contact tracing as they become fully trained as epidemiologists. This training program builds future public health leaders and approximately 80% of fellows that complete the program remain in their countries and work in public health. There are three levels of FETP: Frontline; Intermediate, and Advanced (Fig. 28-1)[4] to ensure there is public health capacity at local, subnational, and national levels. During the West Africa EVD epidemic, 2014, FETP fellows in Lagos, Nigeria were instrumental in performing on-the-ground contact tracing work that prevented an outbreak in that city from spreading throughout the country and region.[5]

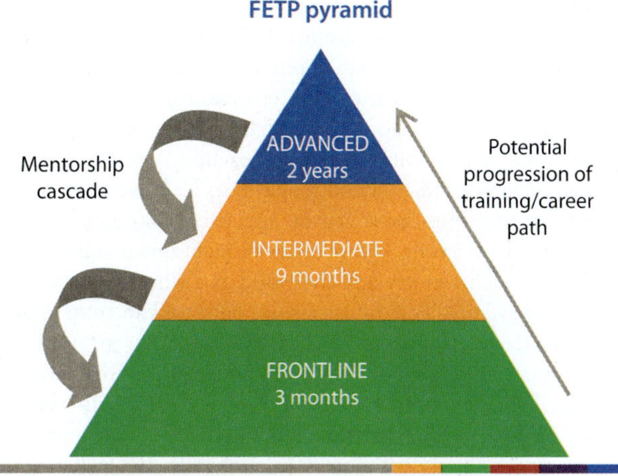

FIGURE 28-1. Field Epidemiology Training Program Pyramid. (*Source:* U.S. Centers for Disease Control & Prevention. Field Epidemiology Training Program (FETP) FactSheet, May 2018.)

Other staffs with training in biosafety and biosecurity functions perform specialty tasks related to biologic agents, often in conjunction with public health laboratories. Whether naturally occurring or intentionally released, as occurred in the release of anthrax in the United States in 2001, biologic agents can be especially lethal and difficult to monitor and track. In addition to identifying biologic agents, personnel with biosafety expertise assist with development of vaccines and other medical countermeasures, and work with law enforcement and political science professionals to identify and track parties who may be responsible for their release.

Global Health Security Tests the Robustness of the Global Health Workforce

The concept of Global Health Security has become increasingly prominent over the past several years.[6] After the global SARS epidemic in 2003, which killed nearly 1000 people and cost more than $40 billion in lost productivity, the world realized that much more needed to be done to prevent the spread of infectious diseases. To address this, in 2005 the World Health Organization (WHO) developed the International Health Regulations (IHR), a binding legal instrument that requires all WHO Member States to take action to prevent and respond to acute public health risks that have the potential to cross borders and threaten people worldwide.[7] However, by 2012, less than a third of countries had met their obligations to strengthen their health security capacity as established by the IHR, and it was clear more was needed to effectively protect the world against infectious disease threats. The Global Health Security Agenda (GHSA), launched in 2014, is a partnership of nearly 50 nations to date, international organizations, and non governmental stakeholders that facilitates collaborative, capacity-building efforts to achieve specific and measurable targets around public health threats, while accelerating achievement of the core capacities required by the IHR and other relevant Global Health Security frameworks.[8]

Even as the GHSA was being announced, Ebola Virus Disease had emerged in a remote forested region of southeastern Guinea, in 2014, and would rapidly explode into an epidemic. The West Africa

EVD epidemic exposed the region's weak surveillance systems and poor public health infrastructure that led to insufficient capacity to effectively prevent, detect, and respond to disease outbreaks—the cornerstones of health security.[9] The epidemic spread rapidly once introduced into densely populated urban centers, which provided unprecedented opportunities for transmission. Ultimately, the EVD epidemic killed more than 11,000 people in six countries over 2 years, primarily in the three most heavily affected countries of Guinea, Liberia, and Sierra Leone, before it was brought under control.[9] It is essential that each country and the world as a whole be better prepared for the eventuality of future disease outbreaks and other public health emergencies. One legacy of the EVD epidemic is that the large-scale mobilization of the healthcare and public health workforce has contributed to long-term sustainability of Global Health Security goals by helping to improve training and enhance preparedness in many countries.[9] There is the need to strengthen the global health workforce in both providing clinical services and ensuring a quality public health infrastructure.

A key component of Global Health Security Agenda implementation is the Joint External Evaluation (JEE), a voluntary, collaborative, and multisectoral process that assesses country capacities to prevent, detect, and rapidly respond to public health risks (Fig. 28-2).[10] The JEE helps countries identify the most critical gaps within their health systems in order to prioritize opportunities for enhanced preparedness and response. Of the 19 separate areas evaluated, four are considered to be core requirements for conducting effective Global Health Security activities—surveillance systems, laboratory capacity, emergency preparedness and response, and human resources.[11]

Workforce development therefore plays a critical role, as it underpins a country's ability to fulfill its Global Health Security obligations. A sufficiently large and trained workforce is needed for all aspects of program development and implementation. Without a trained workforce, programs cannot be effectively managed, and essential on-the-ground work needed to effectively prevent, detect, and respond to disease outbreaks cannot be conducted.[12]

OPPORTUNITIES AND CHALLENGES

There are a number of key opportunities and challenges in building and maintaining a workforce that has sufficient capacity to perform the functions necessary to meet obligations for robust health systems generally and more specifically for Global Health Security as specified in the IHR.

Capacity Building and Strategic Planning

There is a currently a shortfall in trained healthcare, public health, and allied staff that is expected to get progressively worse in coming years unless steps are taken to ensure an ongoing flow of new people to fill these critical positions (Table 28-1).[13] Approximately 40 million new health sector jobs are expected to be created worldwide by 2030, mostly in middle- and high-income countries, but this will leave a projected shortage of 18 million health workers.[14,15]

Only five of 49 low-income countries currently meet the minimum threshold of 23 doctors, nurses, and midwives per 10,000 population.[16] Guidelines also suggest that there should be at least one trained epidemiologist per 200,000 people, a benchmark that many lower income and high populous countries do not meet.[17]

Training, development, and retention of professional workforce in all sectors must be strengthened and expanded to address this expected shortfall.[18] Countries need to implement strategic planning to build the workforce capacity needed to effectively address health challenges of the future and conduct Global Health Security functions, but many lack sufficient national-level planning mechanisms and retention of staff remains a challenge. Ultimately, this is a management issue, and countries and governments will need to address health management, health workforce policies, standardization of processes and clear, and effective guidelines to improve long-term workforce capacity.

Surge Capacity

Even when day-to-day operational needs are adequately staffed, additional workforce capacity will need to be available to handle the additional tasks required during health emergencies. Although some staff

Score	Indicators - Workforce Development		
	D.4.1 Human resources are available to implement IHR core capacity requirements	**D.4.2 Applied epidemiology training program in place such as FETP**	**D.4.3 Workforce strategy**
No Capacity — 1	Country doesn't have multidisciplinary HR capacity required for implementation of IHR core capacities	No FETP or applied epidemiology training program is established	No health workforce strategy exists
Limited Capacity — 2	Country has multidisciplinary HR capacity (epidemiologists, veterinarians, clinicians, and laboratory specialists or technicians) at national level	No FETP or applied epidemiology training program is established within the country, but staff participate in a program hosted in another country through an existing agreement (at Basic, Intermediate and/or Advanced level)	A healthcare workforce strategy exists but does not include public health professions (e.g., epidemiologists, veterinarians, and laboratory technicians)
Developed Capacity — 3	Multidisciplinary HR capacity is available at national and intermediate level	One level of FETP (Basic, Intermediate, or Advanced) FETP or comparable applied epidemiology training program in place in the country or in another country through an existing agreement	A public health workforce strategy exists, but is not regularly reviewed, updated, or implemented consistently
Demonstrated Capacity — 4	Multidisciplinary HR capacity is available as required at relevant levels of public health system (e.g., epidemiologist at national level and intermediate level and assistance epidemiologist (or short course trained epidemiologist) at local level available)	Two levels of FETP (Basic, Intermediate and/or Advanced) or comparable applied epidemiology training program(s) in place in the country or in another country through an existing agreement	A public health workforce strategy has been drafted and implemented consistently; strategy is reviewed, tracked, and reported on annually
Sustainable Capacity — 5	Country has capacity to send and receive multidisciplinary personnel within country (shifting resources) and internationally	Three levels of FETP (Basic, Intermediate, and Advanced) or comparable applied epidemiology training program(s) in place in the country or in another country through an existing agreement, with sustainable national funding	"Demonstrated Capacity" has been achieved, public health workforce retention is tracked and plans are in place to provide continuous education, retain and promote qualified workforce within the national system

FIGURE 28-2. Workforce Development Indicators. (*Source:* Used with Permission from World Health Organization. Joint external evaluation tool: International Health Regulations (2005). Indicators for Workforce Development and Human Resources (animal and human health sectors. 2016. https://apps.who.int/iris/handle/10665/204368. Accessed July 19, 2019.)

Score[5]	Indicators: Human Resources (Animal[1] and Human Health Sectors)			
	D.4.1 An up-to-date multisectoral workforce strategy is in place[2]	D.4.2 Human resources are available to effectively implement 1HR	D.4.3 In-service trainings are available[3]	D.4.4 FETP[4] or other applied epidemiology training program is in place
No capacity — 1	No strategy in place to develop a multisectoral health workforce	Country does not have appropriate human resources[5] capacity in relevant sectors required for epidemic preparedness and control	No continuing professional education (CPE) prigramme through in-service training course is in place	No FETP or applied epidemiology training programme is established
Limited capacity — 1	A strategy to develop healthcare workforce[5] exists but does not include all relevant sectors of public health professions (such as epidemiologist, social scientists, IT specialists, veterinarians/livestock specialists, and community health workers) Basic data on human resources for health are available	Appropriate human resources are available at national level for epidemic preparedness and control	Ad hoc trainings are available for various professions/cadres through disease-specific programs or targeted initiatives	No FETP or applied epidemiology training program is established within the country at the national level, but staff participate in a program hosted in another country through an existing agreement (at any level)
Developed capacity — 3	A multisectoral public health workforce strategy exists, but is not regularly reviewed, updated, or implemented consistently	Appropriate human resources are available in relevant sectors and at national and intermediate levels	Regular trainings, including one Health approach for zoonotic diseases, are available for various professions/cadres through disease-specific program or targeted initiatives	One level of FETP (Basic, Intermediate, or Advanced)[7] or comparable applied epidemiology training program is in place in the country or in another country through an existing agreement
Demonstrated Capacity — 4	A public health workforce strategy[6] has been adopted and implemented consistently, and is reviewed, tracked, and reported on annually	Human resources are available as required in relevant sectors and at relevant levels of the public health system (such as epidemiologist at national and intermediate levels, and assistant epidemiologist (or short course trained epidemiologist) at the local level)	Training plans are developed and regular trainings are conducted by professional bodies or relevant institutions/units to establish skills and competency standards for the workforce at the national level	Two levels of FETP (Basic, Intermediate, and/or Advanced) or comparable applied epidemiology training program(s) are in place in the country or in another country through an existing agreement
Sustainable capacity — 5	Public health workforce retention is tracked and plans are in place to provide continuous education as well as retain and promote a qualified workforce within the national system	Country has capacity to send and receive multidisciplinary personnel within the country (shifting resources) and internationally to assist other countries in developing capacities for epidemic preparedness and control	In-service trainings are regularly conducted at national and subnational levels, and professional bodies or relevant institutions/units regularly review and update training offers	Three levels of FETP (Basic, Intermediate, and Advanced) or comparable applied epidemiology training program(s)[8] are in place in the country or in another country through an existing agreement, with sustainable national funding

FIGURE 28-2. (Continued)

TABLE 28-1 ESTIMATES OF HEALTH WORKER NEEDS-BASED SHORTAGES (MILLIONS) IN COUNTRIES BELOW THE SDG INDEX THRESHOLD BY REGION, 2013 AND 2030

INCOME GROUP	2013				2030				Total Worker % Change
	Physicians	Nurses/ Midwives	Other Cadres	Total	Physicians	Nurses/ Midwives	Other Cadres	Total	
High	0.0	0.1	0.0	0.1	0.0	0.1	0.0	0.1	–7%
Upper middle	0.1	2.6	0.9	3.7	0.2	1.4	0.2	1.8	–50%
Lower middle	1.6	4.3	3.2	9.1	1.2	3.2	2.2	6.6	–28%
Low	0.8	2.0	1.7	4.6	1.0	2.9	2.1	6.1	33%
WHO REGION									
Africa	0.9	1.8	1.5	4.2	1.1	2.8	2.2	6.1	45%
Americas	0.0	0.5	0.2	0.8	0.1	0.5	0.1	0.6	–17%
Eastern Mediterranean	0.2	0.9	0.6	1.7	0.2	1.2	0.3	1.7	–1%
Europe	0.0	0.1	0.0	0.1	0.0	0.0	0.0	0.1	–33%
South east Asia	1.3	3.2	2.5	6.9	1.0	1.9	1.9	4.7	–32%
Western Pacific	0.1	2.6	1.1	3.7	0.0	1.2	0.1	1.4	–64%
World	**2.6**	**9.0**	**5.9**	**17.4**	**2.3**	**7.6**	**4.6**	**14.5**	**–17%**

Note: All values are expressed in millions, rounded to the nearest 100,000. Totals may not precisely add up due to rounding.
Source: Used with Permission from Buchan J, Dhillon IS, Campbell J, eds. *Health Employment and Economic Growth: An Evidence Base*. Geneva: World Health Organization; 2017, p. 15. https://www.who.int/hrh/resources/health_employment-and-economic-growth/en/. Accessed July 19, 2019.

should have emergency response as their primary duty, it is generally not feasible to maintain a sufficiently large and diverse workforce capable of effectively addressing a broad variety of emergency situations. Instead, it is often effective to have a core emergency response workforce augmented by additional staff, based on their specific training, experience, and capabilities, to effectively assist with emergencies as needed when they arise.

Because it may be necessary to assign staff away temporarily from their usual duties, it is important to ensure that day-to-day operations can still be maintained. During the West Africa EVD epidemic, for example, the need to reassign staff to emergency response left many basic healthcare and public health programs understaffed, resulting in many more people becoming ill or dying from avoidable medical conditions that would otherwise have been prevented or treated.[19]

Each country needs to establish an Emergency Operations Center (EOC) to coordinate a rapid and effective emergency response. An EOC is a central command and control facility providing high-level, coordinated strategic decision-making with responsibility for

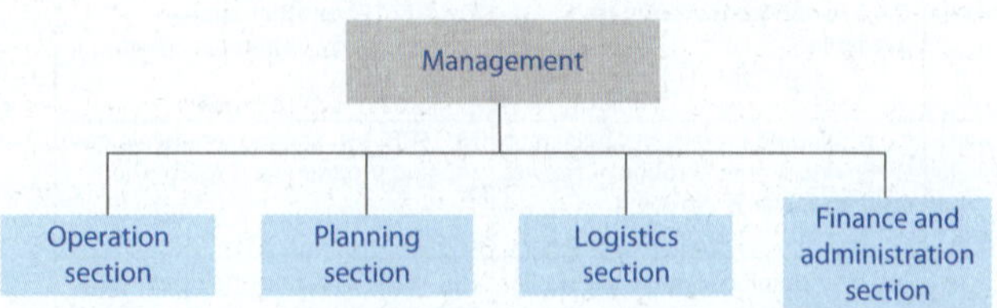

FIGURE 28-3. (*Source:* **Estimated Health Worker Shortages.** Used with Permission from World Health Organization. Incident Management System Model, Framework for a Public Health Emergency Operations Centre. 2015, p.16. https://apps.who.int/iris/bitstream/handle/10665/196135/9789241565134_eng.pdf;sequence=1. Accessed July 22, 2019.)

carrying out emergency preparedness and management functions during an emergency (Fig. 28-3).[20] Individuals staffing the EOC must be sufficiently well trained with the proper authority to carry out necessary actions in response to the emergency. Although many individuals may be assigned for deployment by an EOC during an emergency response, a core staff should always maintain a base level of operational readiness at all times.

A rapid response team (RRT) can also provide surge capacity with minimal impact on day-to-day operations. RRTs are teams of public health experts readily deployable on short notice to provide management and operations expertise as well field-based logistics to support emergency response. They can be a combination of dedicated staff and on-call staff, as is the case with CDC's Global Rapid Response Teams or solely an "on-call" status ready to be deployed from their normally assigned tasks when needed.[21]

International Guidance

As the specialized United Nations agency concerned with international public health, WHO is a central resource for guidance in all the operations of all health system and public health agencies in all countries and regions of the world. The WHO Global Health Workforce Network[22] was established in 2016 as a global mechanism for consultation, dialogue, and coordination on comprehensive and coherent health workforce policies in support of implementation of the ambitious, forward-looking health workforce agenda contained in the Global Strategy on Human Resources for Health[23] and the recommendations of the High-Level Commission on Health Employment and Economic Growth.[14]

The International Association of National Public Health Institutes (IANPHI) links and strengthens the government agencies responsible for public health by leveraging the experience and expertise of its member institutes and exchanging best practices to build robust public health systems.[24] IANPHI provides tools and resources to help countries assess and identify workforce gaps and then develop plans for filling them. Many other nongovernmental organizations (NGOs) also provide guidance and assistance with staffing and training issues.

Human Resources

To be effective, successful delivery of healthcare generally and more specifically during emergencies must be able to obtain and mobilize all necessary resources. Financial capital and political commitment are critical, and generally attract the most attention, but human resources are equally important. Without a sufficiently large and adequately trained workforce that is retained, it will not be possible to implement even the most well-funded and politically popular plans.

In Uganda, for example, training for healthcare workers in health facilities was introduced to improve the accuracy and completeness of vaccine administration data reporting to ensure that all children were being reached by the program. Data improvement teams were deployed to improve data collection, management, analysis, and use in district health offices and health facilities, and to identify gaps in health worker awareness and process implementation. The teams provided on-the-job training to strengthen systems and improve health worker knowledge and skills in maintaining the quality of data necessary for effective vaccination program management.[25]

Adequate support for human resources is necessary to maintain a healthcare and public health workforce with sufficient capacity to effectively perform tasks related to Global Health Security. Many of these are management functions, and include conducting job task analyses across all disciplines, identifying and eliminating administrative inefficiencies, identifying needed equipment and technology and ensuring access to those tools, and adopting strategies to increase workforce retention including providing opportunities for career development and advancement.[26]

Technology Solutions

New technologies have been increasingly developed and implemented that strengthen the ability of a Global Health Security workforce to operate life-saving programs.[27,28] Examples include wireless and mobile computing, which allow epidemiologists and healthcare staff to travel into the field, often to remote communities, to collect data and transmit it to central locations for processing and analysis. New rapid diagnostic tests (e.g., for cholera and malaria) have greatly facilitated faster diagnostics in the field. Laboratory technologies, such as whole-genome sequencing, have become used more widely given advances, and they provide more accurate diagnosis through better identification of pathogens and their source, as well as more rapidly develop new vaccines and other medical countermeasures. However, some of these new technologies often have a steep learning curve, and appropriate training is necessary to receive the full benefit of their use.

Sustainability

It is critical that any advances and improvements in a country's workforce be sustainable over time. There needs to be a mechanism for ongoing personnel recruitment and training to retain the number of skilled workers and their community-based counterparts at required levels, including addressing needs for continuous learning, maintaining core competencies, and retention. Also needed is a strong central coordinating mechanism able to assess current and future workforce needs as well as determine optimal personnel deployment to fulfill Global Health Security obligations.

Integration with Other Programs

Many initiatives related to Global Health Security will involve other healthcare and public health programs, and will often require that the workforce be cross-trained to maximize its effectiveness across multiple functions. This is most apparent with other infectious disease programs, but noncommunicable disease (NCD) programs can also contribute to Global Health Security efforts. Provision of NCD-related services increasingly forms the backbone of health delivery systems, and these existing infrastructures would be essential to contain infectious disease emergencies.[29]

Building on workforce infrastructure that already exists for other programs can save money and time, and ultimately lives, in a public health emergency. For example, programs such as the WHO and CDC-led Global Hearts Initiative can support the Global Health Security objective of threat detection by establishing a mechanism for real-time surveillance and medical workforce development. By developing systems for standardizing hypertension treatment, Global Hearts can contribute to emergency response activities by strengthening medication supply chains.[29]

FETP programs, initially established to improve epidemiology training for infectious diseases, are now also being used to help address the growing NCD burden in many lower-income countries. In the case of cervical cancer, the vast majority of disease is caused by infection with human papillomavirus (HPV), and deploying FETP associates to cervical cancer screening and HPV vaccination efforts integrates with Global Health Security objectives related to surveillance and vaccination.[29]

Partnerships

The global effort to eradicate polio, the Global Polio Eradication Initiative, which was initiated in 1988, is illustrative of how workforce issues can impact a priority public health program. Attaining the goal of reaching and vaccinating every child requires a large global workforce of frontline vaccinators, as well as epidemiologists for surveillance and technical and program staff able to deliver vaccine supplies where needed. Skilled health communicators are needed in communities where there may be resistance to vaccines. A far-reaching effort such as polio eradication, one of the largest public health initiatives in history, also requires skilled program management to ensure that all program components are adequately staffed and performing tasks as expected.[30]

The larger the scale of the program, the more likely that close involvement by partners is needed to ensure delivery of necessary services. The polio eradication effort has enlisted a number of public and private organizations committed to a long-term partnership to ensure that the goal of global eradication is reached. In the context of Global Health Security, partners from within and outside of government will be required to help implement cross-cutting actions across multiple sectors. A centralized mechanism within the ministry of health will need to coordinate partner activities, some of which will involve issues related to workforce composition and training.

MOVING FORWARD

Strengthening and sustaining the global health workforce capacity for global health impact will be essential for the successful implementation of each country's national health program and for countries to be prepared to respond to public health threats and emergencies. Countries that have undergone the JEE process have an accurate idea of their overall health system related to essential public health functions and capacities, including in health workforce development and retention. The detail provided on specific areas where there is currently good capacity as well as those that need further improvement provides a roadmap for country action.[11]

Countries need to develop and implement human resources for health system strategy that is integrated with their comprehensive Global Health Security plan so that they can accelerate their efforts to ensure impact. This is first and foremost a management problem that will most appropriately be addressed by consistently applying human resource best practices that are adapted to meet the particular requirements of a sustainable and resilient health system. Doing this will give countries the health workforce with the necessary skills and qualifications to improve their capacities to prevent diseases and to detect, and respond to ongoing public health challenges and emergent global health threats, both for today and for the future.

References

1. Drehobl PA, Roush SW, Stover BH, Koo D. Centers for Disease Control and Prevention. Public health surveillance workforce of the future. *MMWR Suppl.* 2012;61(3):25–9.
2. Pike BL, Saylors KE, Fair JN, et al. The origin and prevention of pandemics. *Clin Infect Dis.* 2010;50(12):1636–40.
3. Global Forum on Innovation in Health Professional Education; Board on Global Health; Institute of Medicine; National Academies of Sciences, Engineering, and Medicine. Envisioning the Future of Health Professional Education: Workshop Summary. Washington, DC: National Academies Press; April 18, 2016 4, Building a Global Health Workforce. https://www.ncbi.nlm.nih.gov/books/NBK362408.
4. U.S. Centers for Disease Control & Prevention. (2018). Field Epidemiology Training Program (FETP) Fact Sheet, May 2018.
5. Shuaib F, Gunnala R, Musa EO, et al. Ebola virus disease outbreak—Nigeria, July–September 2014. *MMWR Morb Mortal Wkly Rep.* 2014; 63:867–72.
6. Lee JW, McKibbin WJ. Estimating the global economic costs of SARS. In: Knobler S, Mahmoud A, Lemon S, Mac A, Sivitz L, Oberholtzer K, eds. *Learning from SARS: Preparing for the Next Disease Outbreak.* Washington, DC: National Academies Press; 2008, pp. 92–109.
7. International Health Regulations (2005). Third edition. Geneva: World Health Organization, 2016. https://www.who.int/ihr/publications/9789241580496/en.
8. Balajee SA, Arthur R, Mounts AW. Global health security: Building capacities for early event detection, epidemiologic workforce, and laboratory response. *Health Secur.* 2016;14(6):424–32.
9. Marston BJ, Dokubo EK, van Steelandt A, et al. Ebola response impact on public health programs, West Africa, 2014–2017. *Emerg Infect Dis.* 2017;23(13):S25–32.
10. World Health Organization. Joint external evaluation tool: International Health Regulations (2005). 2016.https://apps.who.int/iris/handle/10665/204368. Accessed July 19, 2019.
11. Shahpar C, et al. Protecting the world from infectious disease threats: Now or never. *BMJ Global Health.* 2019;4(4):e001885.
12. No health workforce, no global health security. *Lancet.* 2016;387 (10033):2063.
13. Buchan J, Dhillon IS, Campbell J, eds. *Health Employment and Economic Growth: An Evidence Base.* Geneva: World Health Organization; 2017, p. 15. https://www.who.int/hrh/resources/healthemployment-and-economic-growth/en/. Accessed July 19, 2019.
14. World Health Organization. *Working for Health and Growth: Investing in the Health Workforce. Report of the High-Level Commission on Health Employment and Economic Growth.* Geneva: World Health Organization; 2016. https://www.who.int/hrh/com-heeg/reports/en.
15. Liu, J, Goryakin, Y, Maeda, A, Bruckner, T, Scheffler, R. *Global Health Workforce Labor Market Projections for 2030.* Washington, DC: World Bank Group; 2016. http://documents.worldbank.org/curated/en/546161470834083341/pdf/WPS7790.pdf. Accessed July 19, 2019.
16. World Health Organization. Global Atlas of the Health Workforce. Geneva: World Health Organization; 2019. https://www.who.int/workforcealliance/knowledge/resources/hrhglobalatlas/en.
17. Jones DS, Dicker RC, Fontaine RE, et al. Building global epidemiology and response capacity with field epidemiology training programs. *Emerg Infect Dis.* 2017;23:S158–65.
18. Herrmann J, Blumenstock JS. Global health security: Training a public health workforce to combat international and domestic threats. *J Public Health Manag Pract.* 2014;20 (Suppl 5):S118–9.
19. Brolin Ribacke KJ, Saulnier DD, Eriksson A, von Schreeb J. Effects of the West Africa Ebola virus disease on health-care utilization—A systematic review. *Front Public Health.* 2016;4:222.
20. World Health Organization. Incident Management System Model, Framework for a Public Health Emergency Operations Centre. 2015, p. 16 https://apps.who.int/iris/bitstream/handle/10665/196135/9789241565134eng.pdf;sequence=1. Accessed July 22, 2019.
21. Ariza-Stelling T, Lefevre A, Calles D, et al. Establishment of CDC global rapid response team to ensure global health security. *Emerg Infect Dis.* 2017;23:S203–9.
22. Global Health Workforce Network [web page]. Geneva: World Health Organization, 2019. https://www.who.int/hrh/network/en.
23. World Health Organization. Global Strategy on Human Resources for Health: Workforce 2030. Geneva: World Health Organization; 2016. https://www.who.int/hrh/resources/pubglobstrathrh-2030/en.
24. Pekka P, Jeffrey KP. IANPHI—10 years of collaboration for institutional public health. *Eur J Public Health.* 2017;27(2):192–3.
25. Ward K, Mugenyi K, Benke A, et al. Enhancing workforce capacity to improve vaccination data quality, Uganda. *Emerg Infect Dis.* 2017;23:S85–93.
26. Yeager VA, Wisniewski JM, Amos K, Bialek R. Why do people work in public health? Exploring recruitment and retention among public health workers. *J Public Heath Manag Pract.* 2016;22(6):559–66.
27. Agarwal S, Perry H, Long L, Labrique A. Evidence on feasibility and effective use of mHealth strategies by frontline health workers in developing countries: Systematic review. *Trop Med Int Health.* 2015;20(8): 1003–14.
28. U.S. Centers for Disease Control & Prevention. Success Story: Innovative Mobile Health Initiatives Poised to Transform Tanzania's Tuberculosis HIV Response. 2019. https://www.cdc.gov/globalhivtb/who-we-are/success-stories/success-story-pages/tanzania-mhealth.html. Accessed July 19, 2019.
29. Kostova D, Husain MJ, Sugerman D, et al. Synergies between communicable and noncommunicable disease programs to enhance global health security. *Emerg Infect Dis.* 2017;23:S40–7.
30. Kerr Y, Mailhot M, Williams AAJ, et al. Lessons learned and legacy of the Stop Transmission of Polio program. *J Infect Dis.* 2017;216 (Suppl_1):S316–23.

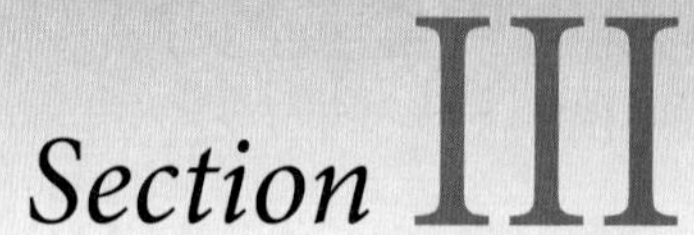

Section Editor
Ana V. Diez Roux

Health Disparities and Vulnerable Populations

CHAPTER 29

The Social Determinants of Health

Paula Braveman

INTRODUCTION

The United States spends far more on medical care than any other nation in the world. Yet its health outcomes have for some time consistently ranked at or near the bottom among affluent nations and even worse than some low-income countries.[1] Furthermore, within the United States, levels of health vary dramatically across states, localities, and different social and economic groups,[2] in patterns that are not explained by differences in medical care. The Scottish physician Thomas McKeown critically examined the widespread assumption that medical care is responsible for the dramatic decline in mortality that occurred in the United States and other affluent countries in the first half of the twentieth century. Using data from the United Kingdom and Wales, he demonstrated for multiple causes of death that the steep reductions in mortality were well under way decades before the availability of effective modalities of modern medicine, such as antibiotics and intensive care units.[3] Substantial disparities in health across different socioeconomic groups are seen even within countries that provide financial access to medical care for the entire population.[4,5] These and numerous other findings have led many observers to question the widely prevalent assumption that medical care is the most important modifiable influence on health.

The term "social determinants of health" has been used primarily to refer to the factors outside of medical care that are important influences on health and at least in theory could be influenced by social policy. There is a prominent exception, however, which may be a source of confusion. The World Health Organization's Commission on the Social Determinants of Health (2005–08) included medical care among the "social determinants." This was presumably out of concern that many resource-poor countries lack even the most rudimentary medical care systems, which, if implemented, could dramatically, rapidly, and at low cost improve the health of their populations; the reasoning may have been that, given that medical care is determined by social policies, it would be a mistake to omit it from the agenda for "social determinants." Outside of this exception, "social determinants of health" have referred to nonmedical factors. In the affluent countries (e.g., western Europe, the United States, Canada, Australia, and Japan), by contrast, medical care has for many decades been far more developed; a focus on the social determinants of health has been in part a response to the tendency for medical care to consume ever-increasing percentages of national budgets in affluent countries, without concomitant improvements in health status.

Despite the mounting evidence of the importance of nonmedical determinants of health, "health" is still often equated with "health-care"; the terms are often used virtually interchangeably. Since the 1960s or 1970s, there has been public awareness of the powerful health effects of health-related behaviors such as diet, exercise, smoking, and alcohol and drug consumption. The major initiatives to improve health in the United States have focused either on improving access to or quality of medical care, or on informing people of the importance of healthy behaviors.

What influences health? Figure 29-1 is a simplified representation of relationships among key factors that shape health; these relationships are supported by extensive literature cited throughout this book. This figure shows both medical care and health-related behaviors as important influences on health. At the same time, the diagram points out that both behaviors and medical care (receipt and quality) are strongly shaped by living and working conditions in homes and neighborhoods; these include such factors as air pollution, proximity of hazardous wastes, lead paint, exposure to crime and domestic violence, social norms, social support, the concentration of liquor stores and fast food outlets, access to transportation, and workplace conditions. The figure shows living and working conditions (represented by the inner of the two arches) influencing health by influencing medical care and behaviors. It also shows that living and working conditions can affect health more directly, without involving either behaviors or medical care; this can occur through the effects of living and working conditions on stress (discussed later in this chapter) and/or how they determine whether one is exposed to toxic substances.

The figure also includes an outer arch, intended to call attention to the fundamental causes of healthy or unhealthy living conditions: the underlying economic and social opportunities and resources available to people, such as education, wealth, power, and racial inequity. These economic and social opportunities and resources largely determine individuals' chances of living and working in healthy social and material conditions, for example, by permitting them to buy or rent homes that are free of health-damaging materials in neighborhoods that have good public schools and safe and pleasant places to exercise; to purchase a nutritious diet; to have rewarding employment with health-promoting working conditions and benefits; and to feel included in society and free from a pervasive threat of crime or arbitrary arrest and incarceration. A rich literature, cited throughout this chapter, supports the relationships depicted in Fig. 29-1. That does not mean that there is complete consensus about the causation of each example that could be cited. It does, however, mean that there is a sizable body of research conducted by respected scholars and published in credible sources, which supports the causal relationships the diagram reflects.

Upstream determinants (the causes of the causes) versus downstream determinants (more visible and immediate causes). The terminology "upstream" or "downstream" is often applied to social determinants of health An upstream determinant is one that is more fundamental or at the root of an issue. A downstream determinant is one that is generally easier to see because it occurs closer to the outcome of interest. Because a downstream determinant is shaped by upstream determinants, addressing it may be relatively futile, since it will continue to occur and have adverse effects on health if the root

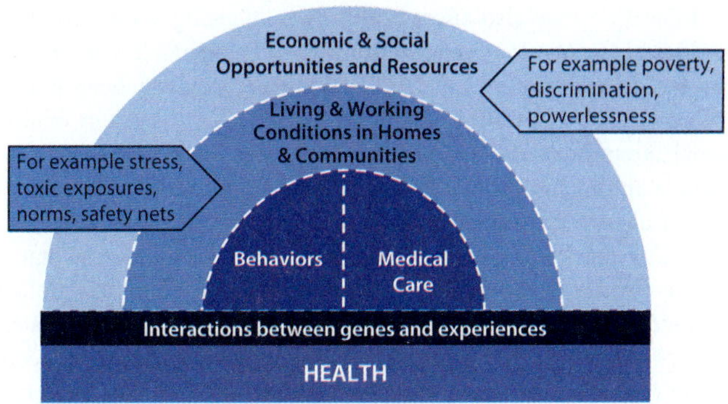

FIGURE 29-1. The social determinants of health. (*Source:* Adapted with permission from Braveman et al. Overcoming Obstacles to Health. Robert Wood Johnson Foundation; 2008, p. 61.)

causes are not dealt with. Imagine a large stream of water, flowing down from its source toward its outlet. In addition, imagine that there is a factory located upstream, near the stream's source, that is continuously dumping toxic chemicals into the stream. People living downstream rely on the stream for their water, including drinking water. Drinking the water is making people sick. A downstream solution is to tell people that the water is contaminated and they should not drink it. What will be the effect of that approach? One can predict that health disparities according to economic resources will widen with the downstream approach, because affluent people will be able to afford buying clean water while low-income people generally will not, and thus will have to continue to drink the poisoned water. The upstream solution would be to ensure that the factory ceases to dump contaminants into the stream.

There are large methodologic challenges inherent in studying the influence of social factors on health. First, the health effects of social factors often do not manifest immediately or soon after they occur; they often become detectable only after several years or decades, for reasons discussed below. Second, studies of the social determinants of health rarely lend themselves to randomization; randomizing people to receive different levels or quality of education, different levels of wealth, or different exposure to racial discrimination would generally be unethical and probably unfeasible. The case for the effects of social factors on health therefore often depends on connecting the dots between evidence from one body of research linking a social factor with an intermediate outcome, and evidence from other studies linking that intermediate outcome with the ultimate health effects.

"Reverse causation?" Critics of the importance of a given social factor for health have often contended that observed relationships—for example, between income and health—actually reflect "reverse causation," that is, that income and health are related because poor health leads to low income rather than vice versa. In many cases—including in the case of income and health—"reverse causation" does indeed occur, for example, when poor health results in loss of income from employment. However, in the case of income and education and many of the other social factors examined in this chapter, research—including studies with longitudinal designs that are not subject to reverse causation—has shown convincingly that reverse causation may contribute to but does not account for the observed strong relationships with health.

The next section explores several social factors thought to play strong and pervasive roles in health. It summarizes research examining the relationships between each factor and health, and refers to the biomedical knowledge that makes the relationships biologically plausible.

HOW DO SOCIAL FACTORS SHAPE HEALTH?[1]

Income, Wealth, and Health

Economic or financial resources include both income (monetary earnings during a specified time period) and wealth (accumulated material assets, such as the value of one's home, household possessions, vehicles and other property, bank accounts, and investments). Economic resources reflect access to material goods and services. Theoretically, wealth may better reflect economic resources overall, but it is more difficult to measure than income and hence less frequently measured in health studies. Among research examining both income and wealth, many (but not all) have found links between wealth and a range of health measures even after considering income.[6–8] Racial/ethnic differences in income markedly underestimate differences in wealth.[9,10]

Reverse causation (income loss due to poor health) occurs but does not fully account for the observed associations of income/wealth and health.[11,12] Many longitudinal studies show that economic resources predict health or its proximate determinants, even after adjustment for education[13–15] (although education is a stronger predictor for other outcomes[16,17] and both are likely to matter).[9,11] Health effects of raising income have been observed in randomized and natural experiments.[11]

Several researchers have observed health effects of income and/or wealth even after controlling for many other relevant factors.[11,18,19] Particularly when other socioeconomic factors are inadequately measured, however, observed links between income/wealth and health may reflect effects of other factors such as educational quality and attainment, childhood socioeconomic circumstances, neighborhood characteristics, physical and psychosocial working conditions, subjective social status, and the stress associated with coping with daily challenges in the face of inadequate economic resources. The health effects of low economic resources may be ameliorated by access to other resources and opportunities; for example, some low-income countries/states (e.g., Cuba, Costa Rica, and Kerala, India) have favorable health indicators that may be explained, despite the prevalence of low income, by long-standing societal investments in education, social safety nets, and/or prevention-oriented healthcare.[20] It is not difficult to imagine how the health impact of low income would be quite different in a setting in which, for example, there were generous subsidies for housing, food, and child care; where high-quality, prevention-oriented medical care was free; and where school quality did not depend on the income level of residents of the surrounding area.

Income inequality (measured at an aggregate level) has repeatedly been linked with health,[21] although a causal link is debated.[22–25] It is not implausible that income inequality could affect health. It could do so by eroding social ties or cohesion.[26] Wilkinson has argued that greater inequality could lead to wealthy and nonwealthy people leading increasingly separate lives, which could produce less empathy on the part of the wealthy for everyone else; less empathy could in turn mean that the wealthy are less willing to support initiatives that benefit society as a whole.[21] It is important to note, however, that it is possible that the link also could be explained by other factors strongly associated with both income inequality and health, such as lack of social solidarity, which could be both a cause and an effect of economic inequality.

Interventions to increase the economic resources of disadvantaged groups have included reform in tax policies and tax credits for low-income working persons such as the Earned Income Tax Credit. There has been increasing interest in building wealth in communities that have historically lacked access to acquiring wealth, for example,

[1] This section of the chapter is based on Braveman P, Egerter S, Williams DR. The social determinants of health: Coming of age. *Annu Rev Public Health*. 2011;32:381–98.

using microloans to start small businesses and education savings accounts for children.

Education and Health

Education—that is, schooling, in contrast to health education—is a powerful determinant of health. Figure 29-2 depicts three interrelated (and sometimes overlapping) pathways through which educational attainment (completed schooling, referred to here simply as "education") is linked with health. It is widely recognized that more education can lead to improved health by increasing a person's knowledge and understanding of health and by increasing the ability to engage in healthy behaviors. This link may be explained in part by literacy, allowing more-educated individuals to understand health information and instructions from medical care providers; this awareness and understanding helps them to make better-informed health-related decisions—including about when and how to seek medical care and negotiate medical care systems—for themselves and their families.[27,28] Greater educational attainment has been associated with engaging in health-promoting behaviors[29] and earlier adoption of health-related recommendations.[30]

A less well recognized but probably even more important way in which education influences health is by shaping employment opportunities; for the vast majority of individuals—apart only from the few individuals who are born into tremendous wealth—employment is the major determinant of income (and hence opportunities for accumulated wealth). Individuals with greater educational attainment experience lower rates of unemployment, which is strongly associated with worse health and higher mortality.[31] Higher educational attainment makes one more likely to have employment with healthier physical and psychosocial working conditions, better health-related benefits, and higher compensation[32] (which determines affordability of health-promoting living conditions).

Education may also affect health by influencing social and psychological factors. More education has been associated with greater perceived control over one's life,[33] which has repeatedly been linked with better health and health-related behaviors.[33–35] Greater educational attainment also is generally associated with higher relative social standing, and subjective social status (an individual's perception of his or her ranking in a social hierarchy) may predict health even after controlling for more objective indicators of social status such as education and income.[36] More education also has been linked with increased social support,[37] which has repeatedly been associated with better physical and mental health.[38,39] Social support appears to buffer the health-damaging effects of stress;[40–42] and to influence health-related behaviors.[38,43] Having socially advantaged social networks enhances access to employment, housing, and other opportunities and resources that influence health.[44]

The quality of one's education is important in addition to the quantity; for example, graduation from an exclusive preparatory school will generally create more opportunities (e.g., for college and subsequently for employment) than graduation from most public high schools. Studies rarely have information on educational quality, however; the number of years of completed schooling or the level of completed schooling are therefore the usual measures of education. The role of educational quality—for example, the employment opportunities, prestige, social networks, and other advantages accompanying a degree from an elite institution—is rarely considered in health studies. The usual measures of educational attainment thus can underestimate health-related differences related to education.[37,45]

While small class sizes, high teacher-to-pupil ratios, and teacher training are widely assumed to be key, there is surprisingly limited consensus in the field of education about what works to improve education, particularly of disadvantaged groups. It is possible that the most effective intervention to improve learning among socially

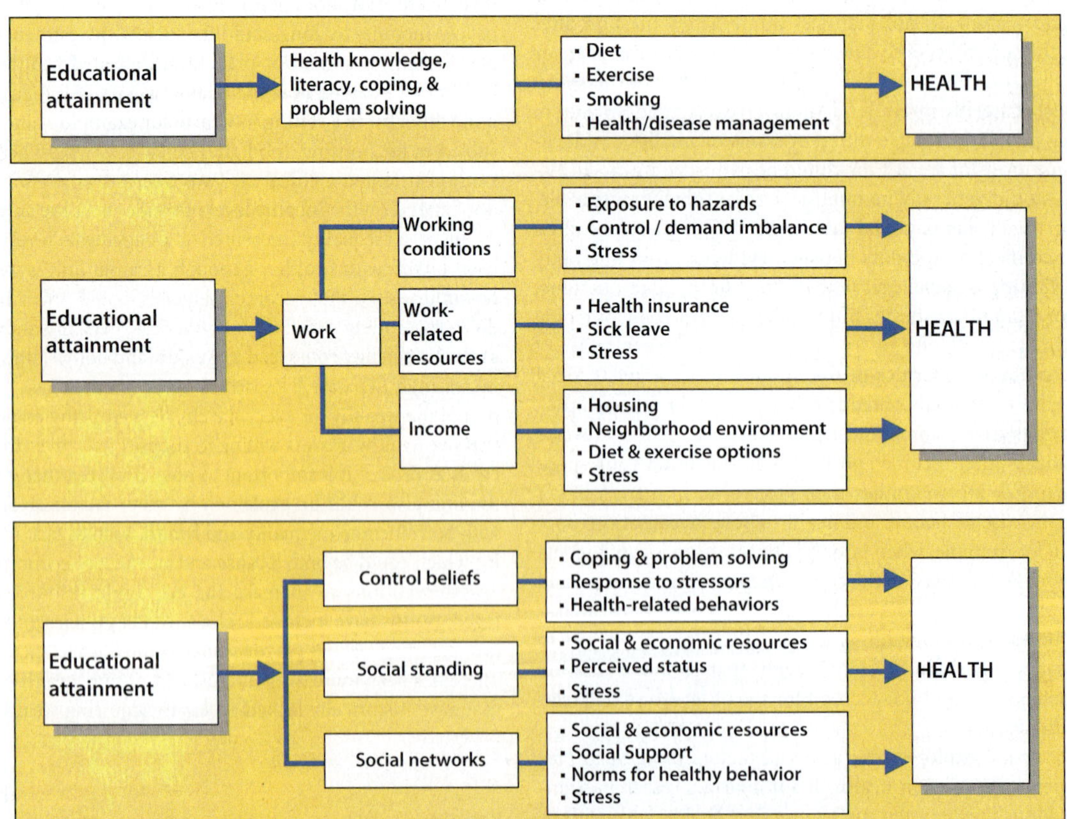

FIGURE 29-2. How could education affect health? (*Source:* Adapted with permission from Egerter, Braveman et al. Education Matters for Health. Robert Wood Johnson Foundation; 2011, p. 5.)

disadvantaged groups is to reduce their disadvantage. For students coming from chaotic, impoverished home situations with little support from adults for their learning, the answer may be that the chaos, poverty, and lack of adult support must be addressed, in order to give any school-based intervention the chance of working.

Neighborhoods and Health

Neighborhoods can influence health through physical conditions such as the quality of air and water and the presence of hazardous substances; housing that exposes residents to lead paint, mold, dust or pest infestation; access to nutritious foods and safe places to exercise; and risk of pedestrian accidents.[58–63] The availability and quality of services in a neighborhood—including schools, transportation, and employment opportunities—also can influence health, for example, by shaping residents' opportunities to earn a livelihood.[64,65] Neighborhoods' physical and service characteristics can exacerbate or mitigate socioeconomic and racial/ethnic disparities in health.

Considerable evidence indicates that health is shaped not only by physical conditions but also by social relationships. For example, neighborhoods where a higher percentage of residents express mutual trust and are willing to intervene for the public good have been shown to have lower homicide rates.[66,67] Conversely, residents of neighborhoods that are less closely knit and have more social disorder have had higher levels of anxiety and depression.[68–70]

Many studies of neighborhoods have lacked information on individuals within the neighborhoods. It is reasonable to question whether associations between neighborhood characteristics and health may primarily reflect characteristics of the individuals living in a neighborhood rather than features of the neighborhoods themselves. Many—but not all—studies have found that neighborhood features are associated with health even after considering residents' individual-level characteristics.[58] Perhaps surprisingly, some—albeit not many—studies have found poorer health among disadvantaged individuals living in relatively advantaged neighborhoods, compared with similarly disadvantaged individuals living in less advantaged neighborhoods.[71,72,73] This may be due to adverse psychological effects of feeling worse-off than one's neighbors; or it may reflect that being disadvantaged while living in a generally disadvantaged neighborhood tends to permit one to have stronger social ties and/or reduced exposure to discrimination because one is part of one's own group.[74]

Interventions to make neighborhoods more health-promoting (or at least less health-damaging) have included a wide range of actions, for example: clean-up of toxic substances; replacement of substandard housing with new housing in good condition; creation of green spaces and bike lanes; community gardens; decreasing the concentration of fast-food outlets, liquor stores, and billboards promoting tobacco and alcohol; and construction of community spaces where residents can gather. They also have included efforts to build wealth, for example, through microloans to start small businesses.

Work and Health

The traditional domain of occupational health and safety has been physical aspects of work. For example, jobs requiring repetitive movements and or high physical workload put workers at higher risk for musculoskeletal injuries and disorders,[75] while physically inactive workers in sedentary jobs are at increased risk of chronic diseases such as diabetes, heart disease, and metabolic syndrome.[76] Workplace physical conditions such as inadequate ventilation, high noise levels, and hazardous chemical exposures can also harm health.

Since the 1990s, however, researchers have also brought attention to the health effects of psychosocial aspects of work. For example, long working hours have been associated with higher rates of stroke and heart disease.[77] Workers in jobs characterized by high demands from supervisors together with low levels of control over their work—for example, over the speed with which they perform tasks or the details of how they perform tasks—or by a perceived imbalance between levels of worker effort and corresponding rewards are at higher risk of poor health.[78,79] Perceived control at work may be a major contributor to socioeconomic differences in health among employed persons.[79–81] Social support at work has also been linked with health[82–84]; employment environments that facilitate mutual support among workers may buffer against the physical and mental health stressors accompanying a job.[85]

Work-related opportunities and resources also can influence health. Employment-related earnings represent most Americans' primary economic resource, shaping health-related decisions made for themselves and their families. In addition, work-related benefits—including medical insurance, paid leave for sickness, childbirth/infant care, or elder care, the flexibility of schedules, workplace wellness programs, and additional child- or elder-care resources and retirement benefits—also could be important. Well-paying jobs are more likely to provide adequate (or any) benefits, greater financial security and ability to afford healthier living conditions. In contrast, the "working poor"—estimated at 7.6 million U.S. workers in 2016[86]—often do not earn enough to cover basic necessities, and are less likely to have health-related benefits.[87,88] Different causal pathways linking work and health may interact to exacerbate social disparities in health: Those who are more socially disadvantaged are more likely to have health-harming (or at least nonhealth-promoting) physical and psychosocial working conditions, in addition to the disadvantaged living conditions associated with lower pay.[89]

Race, Racism, and Health

In the United States and many societies, race or ethnic group is another important social factor influencing health, primarily because of racism. Racism refers not only to overt, intentionally discriminatory actions and attitudes, but also to deep-seated societal structures which—even in the absence of individuals currently intending to discriminate—systematically constrain some individuals' opportunities and resources based on their race or ethnic group.

Racial residential segregation is a key mechanism through which racism produces and perpetuates social disadvantage.[90–93] Racial segregation results in Blacks and Latinos being more likely to reside in disadvantaged neighborhoods with inadequately resourced schools and hence to have lower educational attainment and quality,[91,94] with health effects through pathways discussed above. Racism also is likely to affect health more directly through pathways involving stress; chronic stress related to experiences of racial/ethnic bias, including relatively subtle experiences arising even without consciously prejudicial intent, may contribute to racial/ethnic disparities in health, regardless of one's neighborhood, income, or education.[51,95]

While studies of White people almost invariably show the health improves with increasing education and income, a number of studies have paradoxically observed that health outcomes among more highly educated/higher-income Black people may be worse or not much better than among their less advantaged counterparts.[96–101] More education or income may paradoxically expose Blacks or Latinos to more discrimination because of more contact with (non-Latino) Whites; for example, a college-educated person of color is likely to have a job where most colleagues and coworkers are White, compared with a counterpart with lower educational attainment. In line with an effect of perceived social status, links between race and health also could be shaped by perceptions of how one's race—and its associations with social influence, prestige, and acceptance—affects one's relative place in social hierarchies. Similar associations between discrimination and health as those observed in the United States are being found in other countries.[51]

The most important interventions addressing racism have been enactment and enforcement of laws, including the law that ended slavery, laws abolishing the Jim Crow laws, the Civil Rights Act of 1964, and the Voting Rights Act of 1965. Efforts to reduce racial residential segregation and segregated schools have been important; abolishing school voucher programs would assist with both of the former. Efforts for "affirmative action," that is, actions to correct historical discrimination in school admission or in hiring, have made a contribution but have sometimes been nullified based on accusations that they discriminate against Whites and/or Asians. There are many programs, often worksite based, to promote "cultural competence" or "cultural humility"; their goal is to make people more aware of their unconscious biases and hence less likely to act in a prejudicial manner toward certain social groups.

The Pervasive Role of Stress

Coping with daily challenges can be particularly stressful when one's financial and social (e.g., social support or access to advantageous social networks) resources are limited. Recent biomedical evidence implicates chronic stress in the causal pathways linking many different upstream social determinants with health, through neuroendocrine, inflammatory, immune, and/or vascular mechanisms.[46–48] Chronically stressful experiences—like those associated with social disadvantage, including economic hardship[49,50] and racial discrimination[51]—may trigger the release of cortisol, cytokines, and other substances or processes that can, over time, damage immune defenses, vital organs, and physiologic systems.[47,52] This can lead to more rapid onset or progression of chronic illnesses, including cardiovascular disease,[48] and the bodily wear and tear associated with chronic stress may accelerate aging.[53,54,55,56] The accumulated strain from trying, with inadequate resources, to cope with daily challenges may, over time, lead to more physiological damage than a single dramatically stressful event.[53] A collection of papers by experts from a wide array of disciplines summarizes current knowledge of pathways and biological mechanisms likely to be involved in the health effects of stress and other psychosocial factors—including perceived control, subjective social status, and social support.[57]

Upstream interventions to address stress would consist of efforts to alter the root causes, rather than focus on treatment. Downstream interventions may include training to increase "mindfulness" and help people better manage stress in the short term.

The Importance of Early Childhood Experiences of Social and Economic Advantage or Disadvantage

Among the strongest bodies of evidence for the importance of SDoH is the literature examining the adverse health effects of early childhood (often defined as from birth through age 5) experiences associated with family economic and social disadvantage. Many studies have shown that early experiences affect children's cognitive, behavioral, and physical development,[102–106] which in turn predict health. Differences in children's cognitive, emotional, and behavioral development have been associated with socioeconomically linked differences in children's home environments, including differences in stimulation from parents/caregivers.[50,103,107,108] Biological changes due to adverse socioeconomic conditions in infancy and toddler years appear to become literally "embedded" in children's bodies, determining their developmental capacity.[105] Anatomical differences in children's brain development corresponding to different socioeconomic levels of their families have been observed with brain imaging technology. These are thought to result largely from differences in parental stimulation and positive nurturance that accompany different levels of parental education and income, and can be explained by the effects of the latter.[109,110,111] Some studies have demonstrated that these differences in brain development can be mitigated through interventions.[112–115] Several longitudinal studies following children from early childhood through young adulthood have linked childhood cognitive, emotional, and behavioral development with subsequent adult educational attainment,[116–118,119] which in turn is strongly associated with adult health (discussed above).

Substantial evidence indicates that pathways initiated by childhood adversity can be interrupted. High-quality early childhood

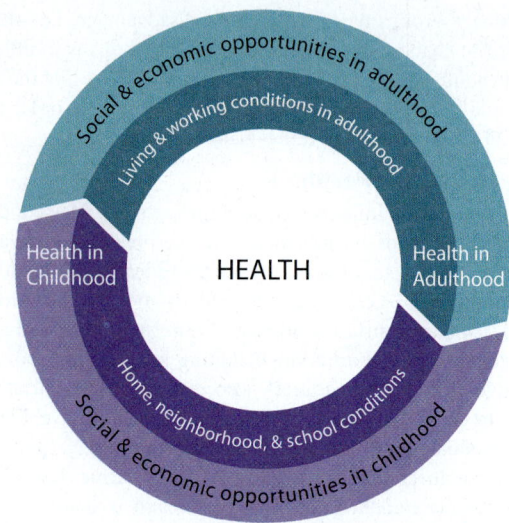

FIGURE 29-3. Experiences and health in one life stage shape experiences and health in later stages. (*Source:* Adapted with permission from Braveman et al. Overcoming Obstacles to Health. Robert Wood Johnson Foundation; 2008, p. 50.)

development interventions—including center-based programs nurturing and stimulating children and supporting and educating parents—have been shown to greatly ameliorate the effects of social disadvantage on children's cognitive, emotional/behavioral, and physical development.[120] The first 5 years of life appear most crucial for development,[106] although opportunities for intervention continue throughout childhood[106] and adolescence.[121]

Early childhood interventions have included center-based early care and education programs such as Early Head Start, the much-studied Carolina Abecedarian Project, and the Perry/High Scope Preschool; home-visiting programs such as the Nurse-Family Partnership; efforts to coordinate early childhood services across programs and even sectors; and supplemental nutrition programs such as WIC and SNAP (mentioned earlier). Tax credits that can significantly boost income for lower-income working families with children, such as the Child Tax Credit and Earned Income Tax Credit, are not generally thought of as early childhood interventions but may be among the most powerful influences.

The Intergenerational Transfer of Social Advantage or Disadvantage and Health

A rich literature examines how differences in social advantage can influence health both over lifetimes and across generations.[122–125] Figure 29-3 is designed to reflect the fact that upstream social factors (such as wealth or belonging to a privileged racial or ethnic group) influence health at each life stage; it also calls attention to the fact that social advantage/disadvantage and health advantage/disadvantage often accumulate over time. Children of socially disadvantaged parents are less healthy and have more limited educational opportunities, both of which diminish their chances for good health and social advantage not only in childhood but also in adulthood. Emerging research on gene-environment interactions suggests that the intergenerational transmission of social advantage and health may be partially explained by epigenetic changes in gene expression, which in turn are passed on to subsequent generations.[126] Epigenetic changes in the body may be induced by stress.[127] Epigenetic changes do not alter one's DNA itself, but they control whether or not a given gene is expressed or suppressed. The science of epigenetics thus turns on its head the whole "nature versus nurture" controversy—that is, whether one's biological inheritance or one's experiences and environment is more important. Both are crucial, and "nature" can be profoundly altered by "nurture."

Interventions to address the intergenerational transfer of social advantage/disadvantage and health include policies and programs to improve early childhood development and education from kindergarten through 12th grade for disadvantaged children; free college; efforts to achieve a "living" (i.e., livable) minimum wage; and efforts to build wealth among communities that have historically lacked access to opportunities to acquire wealth.

CHALLENGES IN ADDRESSING THE SOCIAL DETERMINANTS OF HEALTH

This chapter has focused on making the case for the importance of social factors for health and discussing pathways through which these factors may exert their influence, with limited discussion of interventions. A wide range of interventions to address social determinants of health have been proposed, implemented, and/or evaluated with varying levels of rigor. While it is beyond the scope of this chapter to examine specific interventions in any depth, a few generalizations about interventions can, however, be made here.

The farther upstream a social factor is, the more controversial the proposed solutions will be and, consequently, the greater the resistance will be to addressing them. Upstream social factors include wealth, power, and social inclusion or exclusion (e.g., discrimination based on race or LGBTQ status). Upstream factors are, by definition, at the beginning of long causal chains; they are likely to be deeply embedded in the *status quo.*

Upstream interventions to reduce poverty, for example, could include making taxation more progressive, which would mean the wealthy would pay more and low-income persons would pay less; that is, of course, an approach likely to meet fierce resistance from those who stand to lose should it be implemented. Upstream interventions to reduce poverty also could include raising the minimum wage to levels that provide a "living wage," that is, one that lifts workers out of poverty and enables them to cover basic needs. Generous housing subsidies for low-income families are another example, as is free college, which could reduce intergenerational poverty by making it more feasible for people from low-income families to obtain a college education and in turn the possibility of better-remunerated employment. Some have advocated for universal provision of a basic minimum economic allowance. While the specifics of these upstream approaches vary, each has met with strong resistance from the more socially advantaged groups in society who benefit most from the current *status quo*.

Other proposed antipoverty solutions include expanding eligibility for SNAP, the federal program that provides supplemental nutrition to low-income households, and for WIC, another federal program providing nutritional supplements to pregnant women and young children; both of these programs have repeatedly demonstrated favorable health outcomes.[128,129] Despite their demonstrated effectiveness and the fact that these nutritional supplement programs are not as far upstream as the solutions mentioned above, there are many who oppose them on ideological grounds as handouts that encourage dependency. Although medical care is by definition not a social determinant of health, universal healthcare coverage could be another potentially important part of an antipoverty strategy by preventing impoverishment due to medical expenses. While one could argue that intensive interventions for care and education during infancy through age 5 are less upstream than taxation reform or free college, they could contribute significantly over time to reducing poverty by increasing children's opportunities for success in school and employment as adults. Major business organizations, including the Business Roundtable, have endorsed universal early childhood care and education programs based on their likely contribution to producing a healthy (and therefore productive) future workforce.[130] This support from the business sector for policies on social determinants of health suggests the potential importance of forging alliances that could provide critical support for effecting policy change.

Pessimism is another major challenge. Because the social factors that are farthest upstream are so deeply embedded in the *status quo* and almost always have strong ideological implications, even advocates for the importance of upstream interventions tend to be pessimistic about the possibility of implementing them. This pessimism in turn tends to limit consideration of solutions to more downstream efforts, pursuing the "low-hanging fruit." It is true that short-term opportunities to alter powerful, deeply rooted social and economic structures and institutions affecting public health are often limited; at times, the best one can accomplish in the short term may be a minor or modest downstream reform. Even (or perhaps especially) in those circumstances, however, awareness of the more fundamental causes—the causes of the causes—of poor health and particularly of health disparities remains critical.

Identifying the upstream determinants of a health problem is not merely an academic exercise. If one is unaware of the fundamental causes, unexpected opportunities for solutions may be missed. Sometimes surprises occur and societies make unanticipated and highly consequential progress, as occurred, for example, with the passage of the Civil Rights Act of 1964 and the Voting Rights Act of 1965. Both of these national laws addressed very upstream factors, namely racial discrimination, and both have had profoundly and far-reaching positive influences on U.S. society. Credible evidence, for example, links the Civil Rights Act of 1964 with reduced infant mortality among African Americans.[131] Globally, decades ago, all of the affluent nations other than the United States passed legislation providing universal financial access to medical care and a far more generous social safety net, with far lower rates of poverty (including child poverty) than in the United States. These enormous leaps forward were not confidently predictable at the time.

Failure to develop longer-term strategies that do not lose sight of the ultimate upstream goals. Opportunities to pursue more fundamental determinants may be missed when only short-term strategies are considered. In pursuing downstream solutions that seem more achievable in a short time-frame, strategies can and should be informed and shaped by an understanding of the important causal chains that helps pave the way for subsequent deeper, more upstream efforts. Both downstream and upstream solutions should be pursued, in part because downstream efforts may produce relatively quick positive results that can help energize future efforts for more fundamental change. The strategy for reaching the upstream goal will in many cases require longer-term efforts.

Challenges regarding the strength of the evidence. Another frequently encountered obstacle to addressing upstream social determinants is questioning (or facing questions about) the strength of the evidence on their effects on health. In the first section of this chapter, the large methodologic challenges faced in conducting research on the social determinants of health—particularly the upstream determinants—were briefly noted. These challenges include the long and often complex causal chains involved in the effects of social determinants of health that often play out not across a few years but across decades or longer, making it impossible to measure the main outcomes of interest in the short term. Other research challenges include frequent and important interactions with many other factors, social and not social; and the infeasibility (and, often, lack of ethical acceptability) of conducting randomized experiments to test social determinants of health. These challenges must be kept in mind when reading the literature and assessing its strength.

For decades, there has been a prevalent belief in the fields of health and medicine that only results from randomized trials count as evidence. It is important to remember, however, that randomized designs have weaknesses as well as strengths. One notable weakness of most randomized studies, which tend to be costly and logistically challenging, is that sample sizes and/or compositions are often too limited to generalize results to the general population. In part reflecting increased awareness of the limitations of randomized trials, there has been growing recognition of the compelling existing evidence of the health impact of social factors.[132,133] Researchers need to use the most rigorous research designs possible when studying every research question; however, the range of possible designs will vary with the research question. No single design is appropriate for every question. Although the most rigorous design for examining the effects of upstream social factors on health will typically not be a randomized trial that does not mean that studies of the social determinants of health do not need to be rigorous. Many methods are available to reduce the risk of bias in nonexperimental or quasiexperimental studies, for example, the use of stratification, regression, propensity scores, and instrumental variables.

In summary, intervening to address the social determinants of health requires facing a range of challenges, some concerning knowledge and some primarily political; among these challenges, the most daunting are often political. A commitment to public health would lead those who produce the knowledge, including both researchers and practitioners and decision-makers who innovate and evaluate their experiences, to carefully consider, when they are selecting which questions or issues to study, which knowledge gaps could, if filled, have the greatest impact on creating the political will for upstream policy changes to improve health. Addressing political challenges may not be the sort of activity that motivates most people to pursue careers in public health, but such efforts are indispensable if we are to achieve improvements in the fundamental determinants—the causes of the causes—of health and health equity.

References

1. Woolf SH, Aron LY. The US health disadvantage relative to other high-income countries: Findings from a National Research Council/Institute of Medicine report. *JAMA*. 2013;309(8):771–2.
2. Centers for Disease Control and Prevention. *CDC Health Disparities and Inequalities Report—United States, 2013*. U.S. Department of Health and Human Services, Centers for Disease Control and Prevention; 2013.
3. McKeown T, Record RG, Turner RD. An interpretation of the decline of mortality in England and Wales during the twentieth century. *Popul Stud (Camb)*. 1975;29(3):391–422.
4. Mackenbach JP, Stirbu I, Roskam AJ, et al. Socioeconomic inequalities in health in 22 European countries. *N Engl J Med*. 2008;358(23):2468–81.
5. Mackenbach JP. The persistence of health inequalities in modern welfare states: The explanation of a paradox. *Soc Sci Med*. 2012;75(4):761–9.
6. Pollack CE, Chideya S, Cubbin C, Williams B, Dekker M, Braveman P. Should health studies measure wealth? A systematic review. *Am J Prev Med*. 2007;33(3):250–64.
7. Do DP. The dynamics of income and neighborhood context for population health: Do long-term measures of socioeconomic status explain more of the Black/White health disparity than single-point-in-time measures? *Soc Sci Med*. 2009;68(8):1368–75.
8. Hajat A, Kaufman JS, Rose KM, Siddiqi A, Thomas JC. Long-term effects of wealth on mortality and self-rated health status. *Am J Epidemiol*. 2011;173(2):192–200.
9. Braveman PA, Cubbin C, Egerter S, et al. Socioeconomic status in health research: One size does not fit all. *JAMA*. 2005;294(22):2879–88.
10. Do DP, Frank R, Finch BK. Does SES explain more of the Black/White health gap than we thought? Revisiting our approach toward understanding racial disparities in health. *Soc Sci Med*. 2012;74(9):1385–93.
11. Kawachi I, Adler NE, Dow WH. Money, schooling, and health: Mechanisms and causal evidence. *Ann N Y Acad Sci*. 2010;1186:56–68.
12. Muennig P. Health selection vs. causation in the income gradient: What can we learn from graphical trends? *J Health Care Poor U*. 2008;19(2):574–9.
13. Hoffmann R. Socioeconomic inequalities in old-age mortality: A comparison of Denmark and the USA. *Soc Sci Med*. 2011;72(12):1986–92.
14. Lantz PM, Golberstein E, House JS, Morenoff J. Socioeconomic and behavioral risk factors for mortality in a national 19-year prospective study of U.S. adults. *Soc Sci Med*. 2010;70(10):1558–66.
15. Avendano M, Glymour MM. Stroke disparities in older Americans: Is wealth a more powerful indicator of risk than income and education? *Stroke*. 2008;39(5):1533–40.
16. Herd P, Goesling B, House JS. Socioeconomic position and health: The differential effects of education versus income on the onset versus progression of health problems. *J Health Soc Behav*. 2007;48(3):223–38.
17. Winkleby MA, Jatulis DE, Frank E, Fortmann SP. Socioeconomic status and health: How education, income, and occupation contribute to risk-factors for cardiovascular-disease. *Am J Public Health*. 1992;82(6):816–20.
18. Daly MC, Duncan GJ, McDonough P, Williams DR. Optimal indicators of socioeconomic status for health research. *Am J Public Health*. 2002;92(7):1151–7.
19. Larson K, Halfon N. Family income gradients in the health and health care access of US children. *Matern Child Health J*. 2010;14(3):332–42.
20. Evans RG. Thomas McKeown, meet Fidel Castro: Physicians, population health and the Cuban paradox. *Healthc Policy*. 2008;3(4):21–32.
21. Wilkinson RG, Pickett KE. *The Spirit Level: Why Greater Equality Makes Societies Stronger*. 1st American ed. New York: Bloomsbury Press; 2010.
22. Pickett KE, Wilkinson RG. Income inequality and health: A causal review. *Soc Sci Med*. 2015;128:316–26.
23. Babones SJ. Income inequality and population health: Correlation and causality. *Soc Sci Med*. 2008;66(7):1614–26.
24. Lynch J, Smith GD, Harper S, et al. Is income inequality a determinant of population health? Part 1. A systematic review. *Milbank Q*. 2004;82(1):5–99.
25. Wilkinson RG, Pickett KE. Income inequality and population health: A review and explanation of the evidence. *Soc Sci Med*. 2006;62(7):1768–84.
26. Kawachi I, Kennedy BP. Health and social cohesion: Why care about income inequality? *BMJ*. 1997;314(7086):1037–40.
27. Berkman ND, Sheridan SL, Donahue KE, Halpern DJ, Crotty K. Low health literacy and health outcomes: An updated systematic review. *Ann Intern Med*. 2011;155(2):97–107.
28. Sanders-Phillips K, Settles-Reaves B, Walker D, Brownlow J. Social inequality and racial discrimination: Risk factors for health disparities in children of color. *Pediatrics*. 2009;124 Suppl 3:S176–86.
29. Pampel FC, Krueger PM, Denney JT. Socioeconomic disparities in health behaviors. *Annu Rev Sociol*. 2010;36:349–70.
30. Cutler DM, Lleras-Muney A. Understanding differences in health behaviors by education. *J Health Econ*. 2010;29(1):1–28.
31. Roelfs DJ, Shor E, Davidson KW, Schwartz JE. Losing life and livelihood: A systematic review and meta-analysis of unemployment and all-cause mortality. *Soc Sci Med*. 2011;72(6):840–54.
32. Ma J, Pender M, Welch M. Education Pays 2016: The Benefits of Higher Education for Individuals and Society. College Board; 2016.
33. Mirowsky J, Ross CE. Education, personal control, lifestyle and health—A human capital hypothesis. *Res Aging*. 1998;20(4):415–49.
34. Cobb-Clark DA, Kassenboehmer SC, Schurer S. Healthy habits: The connection between diet, exercise, and locus of control. *J Econ Behav Organ*. 2014;98:1–28.
35. McEachan RRC, Conner M, Taylor NJ, Lawton RJ. Prospective prediction of health-related behaviours with the Theory of Planned Behaviour: A meta-analysis. *Health Psychol Rev*. 2011;5(2):97–144.
36. Demakakos P, Nazroo J, Breeze E, Marmot M. Socioeconomic status and health: The role of subjective social status. *Soc Sci Med*. 2008;67(2):330–40.
37. Mirowsky J. *Education, Social Status, and Health*. New York: Routledge; 2017.
38. Cohen S. Social relationships and health. *Am Psychol*. 2004;59(8):676–84.
39. Berkman LF. Social support, social networks, social cohesion and health. *Soc Work Health Care*. 2000;31(2):3–14.
40. Hostinar CE, Gunnar MR. Social support can buffer against stress and shape brain activity. *AJOB Neurosci*. 2015;6(3):34–42.
41. Gunnar MR, Hostinar CE. The social buffering of the hypothalamic-pituitary-adrenocortical axis in humans: Developmental and experiential determinants. *Soc Neurosci-Uk*. 2015;10(5):479–88.
42. Uchino BN. Social support and health: A review of physiological processes potentially underlying links to disease outcomes. *J Behav Med*. 2006;29(4):377–87.
43. Umberson D, Crosnoe R, Reczek C. Social relationships and health behavior across life the course. *Annu Rev Sociol*. 2010;36:139–57.
44. Campbell KE, Marsden PV, Hurlbert JS. Social resources and socioeconomic status. *Social Networks*. 1986;8(1):97–117.

45. Ross CE, Mirowsky J. Refining the association between education and health: The effects of quantity, credential, and selectivity. *Demography.* 1999;36(4):445–60.
46. Juster RP, McEwen BS, Lupien SJ. Allostatic load biomarkers of chronic stress and impact on health and cognition. *Neurosci Biobehav Rev.* 2010;35(1):2–16.
47. McEwen BS, Gianaros PJ. Central role of the brain in stress and adaptation: Links to socioeconomic status, health, and disease. *Ann N Y Acad Sci.* 2010;1186:190–222.
48. Steptoe A, Marmot M. The role of psychobiological pathways in socio-economic inequalities in cardiovascular disease risk. *Eur Heart J.* 2002;23(1):13–25.
49. Braveman P, Marchi K, Egerter S, et al. Poverty, near-poverty, and hardship around the time of pregnancy. *Matern Child Health J.* 2010;14(1):20–35.
50. Evans GW. The environment of childhood poverty. *Am Psychol.* 2004;59(2):77–92.
51. Williams DR, Mohammed SA. Discrimination and racial disparities in health: Evidence and needed research. *J Behav Med.* 2009;32(1):20–47.
52. Seeman T, Epel E, Gruenewald T, Karlamangla A, McEwen BS. Socio-economic differentials in peripheral biology: Cumulative allostatic load. *Ann N Y Acad Sci.* 2010;1186:223–39.
53. McEwen BS. Protective and damaging effects of stress mediators: Central role of the brain. *Dialogues Clin Neurosci.* 2006;8(4):367–81.
54. Seeman TE, McEwen BS, Rowe JW, Singer BH. Allostatic load as a marker of cumulative biological risk: MacArthur studies of successful aging. *Proc Natl Acad Sci U S A.* 2001;98(8):4770–5.
55. Seeman TE, Singer BH, Rowe JW, Horwitz RI, McEwen BS. Price of adaptation—Allostatic load and its health consequences. MacArthur studies of successful aging. *JAMA Intern Med.* 1997;157(19):2259–68.
56. Oliveira BS, Zunzunegui MV, Quinlan J, Fahmi H, Tu MT, Guerra RO. Systematic review of the association between chronic social stress and telomere length: A life course perspective. *Ageing Res Rev.* 2016;26:37–52.
57. Adler NE, Stewart J. Health disparities across the lifespan: Meaning, methods, and mechanisms. *Ann N Y Acad Sci.* 2010;1186:5–23.
58. Diez Roux AV, Mair C. Neighborhoods and health. *Ann N Y Acad Sci.* 2010;1186:125–45.
59. Booth KM, Pinkston MM, Poston WS. Obesity and the built environment. *J Am Diet Assoc.* 2005;105(5 Suppl 1):S110–7.
60. Giles-Corti B, Donovan RJ. The relative influence of individual, social and physical environment determinants of physical activity. *Soc Sci Med.* 2002;54(12):1793–812.
61. Gordon-Larsen P, Nelson MC, Page P, Popkin BM. Inequality in the built environment underlies key health disparities in physical activity and obesity. *Pediatrics.* 2006;117(2):417–24.
62. Morland K, Diez Roux AV, Wing S. Supermarkets, other food stores, and obesity: The atherosclerosis risk in communities study. *Am J Prev Med.* 2006;30(4):333–9.
63. Sallis JF, Glanz K. The role of built environments in physical activity, eating, and obesity in childhood. *Future Child.* 2006;16(1):89–108.
64. Pastor JM. Geography and opportunity. In: Smelser NJ, Wilson WJ, eds. *America Becoming: Racial Trends and Their Consequences.* Washington, DC: National Academies Press; 2001, pp. 435–68.
65. Williams DR, Collins C. Racial residential segregation: A fundamental cause of racial disparities in health. *Public Health Rep.* 2001;116(5):404–16.
66. Morenoff JD, Sampson RJ, Raudenbush SW. Neighborhood inequality, collective efficacy, and the spatial dynamics of urban violence. *Criminology.* 2001;39(3):517–58.
67. Sampson RJ, Raudenbush SW, Earls F. Neighborhoods and violent crime: A multilevel study of collective efficacy. *Science.* 1997;277(5328):918–24.
68. Kim J. Neighborhood disadvantage and mental health: The role of neighborhood disorder and social relationships. *Soc Sci Res.* 2010;39(2):260–71.
69. Ross CE. Neighborhood disadvantage and adult depression. *J Health Soc Behav.* 2000;41(2):177–87.
70. Cutrona CE, Russell DW, Hessling RM, Brown PA, Murry V. Direct and moderating effects of community context on the psychological well-being of African American women. *J Pers Soc Psychol.* 2000;79(6):1088–101.
71. Pickett KE, Collins JW, Masi CM, Wilkinson RG. The effects of racial density and income incongruity on pregnancy outcomes. *Soc Sci Med.* 2005;60(10):2229–38.
72. Robert SA. Socioeconomic position and health: The independent contribution of community socioeconomic context. *Annu Rev Sociol.* 1999;25(1):489–516.
73. Winkleby M, Cubbin C, Ahn D. Effect of cross-level interaction between individual and neighborhood socioeconomic status on adult mortality rates. *Am J Public Health.* 2006;96(12):2145–53.
74. Williams DR, Mohammed SA, Leavell J, Collins C. Race, socioeconomic status, and health: Complexities, ongoing challenges, and research opportunities. *Ann N Y Acad Sci.* 2010;1186:69–101.
75. da Costa BR, Vieira ER. Risk factors for work-related musculoskeletal disorders: A systematic review of recent longitudinal studies. *Am J Ind Med.* 2010;53(3):285–323.
76. de Rezende LF, Rodrigues Lopes M, Rey-Lopez JP, Matsudo VK, Luiz Odo C. Sedentary behavior and health outcomes: An overview of systematic reviews. *PLoS One.* 2014;9(8):e105620.
77. Kivimaki M, Jokela M, Nyberg ST, et al. Long working hours and risk of coronary heart disease and stroke: A systematic review and meta-analysis of published and unpublished data for 603,838 individuals. *Lancet.* 2015;386(10005):1739–46.
78. de Jonge J, Bosma H, Peter R, Siegrist J. Job strain, effort-reward imbalance and employee wellbeing: A large-scale cross-sectional study. *Soc Sci Med.* 2000;50:1317–27.
79. Karasek RA, Theorell T. *Healthy Work: Stress, Productivity and the Reconstruction of Working Life.* New York: Basic Books; 1990.
80. Kivimaki M, Nyberg ST, Batty GD, et al. Job strain as a risk factor for coronary heart disease: A collaborative meta-analysis of individual participant data. *Lancet.* 2012;380(9852):1491–7.
81. Marmot MG, Bosma H, Hemingway H, Brunner E, Stansfeld S. Contribution of job control and other risk factors to social variations in coronary heart disease incidence. *Lancet.* 1997;350(9073):235–39.
82. Harvey SB, Modini M, Joyce S, et al. Can work make you mentally ill? A systematic meta-review of work-related risk factors for common mental health problems. *Occup Environ Med.* 2017;74(4):301–10.
83. Stansfeld SA, Bosma H, Hemingway H, Marmot MG. Psychosocial work characteristics and social support as predictors of SF-36 health functioning: The Whitehall II study. *Psychosom Med.* 1998;60(3):247–55.
84. Stansfeld S, Shipley M, Marmot M. Work characteristics predict psychiatric disorders: Prospective results from the Whitehall II study. *Occup Environ Med.* 1999;56(5):302–7.
85. Backé EM, Seidler A, Latza U, Rossnagel K, Schumann B. The role of psychosocial stress at work for the development of cardiovascular diseases: A systematic review. *Int Arch Occup Environ Health.* 2012;85(1):67–79.
86. Statistics USBoL. *A Profile of the Working Poor, 2016.* Washington, DC: United States Department of Labor; 2018. Report 1074.
87. Collins SR, Davis K, Doty M, Ho A. *Wages, Health Benefits, and Worker's Health.* New York: Commonwealth Fund; 2004.
88. Heymann J, Boynton-Jarrett R, Carter P, Bond JT, Galinsky E. *Work-Family Issues and Low-Income Families.* New York: Ford Foundation; 2002.
89. Egerter S, Dekker M, An J, Grossman-Kahn R, Braveman P. *Work Matters for Health.* Princeton, NJ: Robert Wood Johnson Foundation; 2008.
90. Williams DR, Priest N, Anderson NB. Understanding associations among race, socioeconomic status, and health: Patterns and prospects. *Health Psychol.* 2016;35(4):407–11.
91. Phelan JC, Link BG. Is racism a fundamental cause of inequalities in health? *Annu Rev Sociol.* 2015;41:311–30.
92. Williams DR, Mohammed SA. Racism and health I: Pathways and scientific evidence. *Am Behav Sci.* 2013;57(8):1152–73.
93. Gee GC, Ford CL. Structural racism and health inequities: Old issues, new directions. *Du Bois Rev.* 2011;8(1):115–32.
94. Orfield G, Frankenberg E, Garces LM. Statement of American social scientists of research on school desegregation to the US Supreme Court in Parents v. Seattle School District and Meredith v. Jefferson County. *Urban Rev.* 2008;40(1):96–136.
95. Nuru-Jeter A, Dominguez TP, Hammond WP, et al. "It's the skin you're in": African-American women talk about their experiences of racism. An exploratory study to develop measures of racism for birth outcome studies. *Matern Child Health J.* 2009;13(1):29–39.
96. Braveman P, Heck K, Egerter S, et al. Worry about racial discrimination: A missing piece of the puzzle of Black-White disparities in preterm birth? *PLoS One.* 2017;12(10):e0186151.
97. Braveman PA, Cubbin C, Egerter S, Williams DR, Pamuk E. Socioeconomic disparities in health in the United States: What the patterns tell us. *Am J Public Health.* 2010;100:S186–96.
98. Braveman PA, Heck K, Egerter S, et al. The role of socioeconomic factors in Black-White disparities in preterm birth. *Am J Public Health.* 2015;105(4):694–702.

99. Colen CG, Geronimus AT, Bound J, James SA. Maternal upward socioeconomic mobility and Black–White disparities in infant birthweight. *Am J Public Health*. 2006;96(11):2032–9.

100. Collins JW, Butler AG. Racial differences in the prevalence of small-for-dates infants among college-educated women. *Epidemiol.* 1997;8(3):315–7.

101. Foster HW, Wu L, Bracken MB, Semenya K, Thomas J, Thomas J. Intergenerational effects of high socioeconomic status on low birthweight and preterm birth in African Americans. *J Natl Med Assoc.* 2000;92(5):213–21.

102. Shonkoff JP, Garner AS, Committee on Psychosocial Aspects of Child and Family Health, et al. The lifelong effects of early childhood adversity and toxic stress. *Pediatrics.* 2012;129(1):e232–46.

103. Bradley RH, Corwyn RF. Socioeconomic status and child development. *Annu Rev Psychol.* 2002;53:371–99.

104. Cohen S, Janicki-Deverts D, Chen E, Matthews KA. Childhood socioeconomic status and adult health. *Ann N Y Acad Sci.* 2010;1186:37–55.

105. Hertzman C. The biological embedding of early experience and its effects on health in adulthood. *Ann N Y Acad Sci.* 1999;896:85–95.

106. Institute of Medicine. *From Neurons to Neighborhoods: The Science of Early Childhood Development.* Washington, DC: National Academies Press; 2000.

107. Guo G, Harris KM. The mechanisms mediating the effects of poverty on children's intellectual development. *Demography.* 2000;37(4):431–47.

108. Yeung WJ, Linver MR, Brooks-Gunn J. How money matters for young children's development: Parental investment and family processes. *Child Dev.* 2002;73(6):1861–79.

109. Noble KG, Houston SM, Brito NH, et al. Family income, parental education and brain structure in children and adolescents. *Nat Neurosci.* 2015;18(5):773–8.

110. Hair NL, Hanson JL, Wolfe BL, Pollak SD. Association of child poverty, brain development, and academic achievement. *JAMA Pediatr.* 2015;169(9):822–9.

111. Fox SE, Levitt P, Nelson CA. How the timing and quality of early experiences influence the development of brain architecture. *Child Dev.* 2010;81(1):28–40.

112. Shonkoff JP. Leveraging the biology of adversity to address the roots of disparities in health and development. *Proc Natl Acad Sci U S A.* 2012;109(Suppl 2):17302–7.

113. Garner AS. Home visiting and the biology of toxic stress: Opportunities to address early childhood adversity. *Pediatrics.* 2013;132(Suppl 2):S65–73.

114. Campbell FA, Pungello EP, Miller-Johnson S, Burchinal M, Ramey CT. The development of cognitive and academic abilities: Growth curves from an early childhood educational experiment. *Dev Psychol.* 2001;37(2):231–42.

115. Barnett WS. Long-term effects of early childhood programs on cognitive and school outcomes. *Future Child.* 1995;5(3):25–50.

116. Rabiner DL, Godwin J, Dodge KA. Predicting academic achievement and attainment: The contribution of early academic skills, attention difficulties, and social competence. *School Psychol Rev.* 2016;45(2):250–67.

117. Campbell FA, Wasik BH, Pungello E, et al. Young adult outcomes of the Abecedarian and CARE early childhood educational interventions. *Early Child Res Q.* 2008;23(4):452–66.

118. Garces E, Thomas D, Currie J. Longer-term effects of Head Start. *Am Econ Rev.* 2002;92:999–1012.

119. Schweinhart L, Barnes HV. *Significant Benefits: The High/Scope Perry Preschool Study Through Age 27.* Ypsilanti, MI: High/Scope Press; 1993.

120. Watamura SE, Phillips DA, Morrissey TW, McCartney K, Bub K. Double jeopardy: Poorer social-emotional outcomes for children in the NICHD SECCYD experiencing home and child-care environments that confer risk. *Child Dev.* 2011;82(1):48–65.

121. Fergus S, Zimmerman MA. Adolescent resilience: A framework for understanding healthy development in the face of risk. *Annu Rev Public Health.* 2005;26:399–419.

122. Larson K, Russ SA, Kahn RS, et al. Health disparities: A life course health development perspective and future research directions. In: Halfon N, Forrest C, Lerner R, Faustman E, eds. *Handbook of Life Course Health Development.* Cham: Springer; 2018, pp. 499–520.

123. Friedman EM, Muennig P. The intergenerational transfer of education credentials and health: Evidence from the 2008 General Social Survey-National Death Index. *J Health Care Poor Underserved.* 2016;27(2):869–90.

124. Galobardes B, Lynch JW, Smith GD. Is the association between childhood socioeconomic circumstances and cause-specific mortality established? Update of a systematic review. *J Epidemiol Commun Health.* 2008;62:387–90.

125. Lynch J, Smith GD. A life course approach to chronic disease epidemiology. *Annu Rev Public Health.* 2005;26:1–35.

126. Kuzawa CW, Sweet E. Epigenetics and the embodiment of race: Developmental origins of US racial disparities in cardiovascular health. *Am J Hum Biol.* 2009;21(1):2–15.

127. Johnstone SE, Baylin SB. Stress and the epigenetic landscape: A link to the pathobiology of human diseases? *Nat Rev Genet.* 2010;11(11):806–12.

128. Lee BJ, Mackey-Bilaver L. Effects of WIC and Food Stamp Program participation on child outcomes. *Child Youth Serv Rev.* 2007;29(4):501–17.

129. Gundersen C, Ziliak JP. Food insecurity and health outcomes. *Health Affair.* 2015;34(11):1830–9.

130. Business Roundtable. *Why America Needs High-Quality Early Care and Education.* Washington, DC: Corporate Voices for Working Families and Business Roundtable; 2009.

131. Almond D, Chay KY, Greenstone M. *Civil Rights, the War on Poverty, and Black-White Convergence in Infant Mortality in the Rural South and Mississippi.* Cambridge, MA: MIT Department of Economics. Working Paper No. 07-04; 2006.

132. Adler N, Bush NR, Pantell MS. Rigor, vigor, and the study of health disparities. *Proc Natl Acad Sci U S A.* 2012;109(Suppl 2):17154–9.

133. Braveman PA, Egerter SA, Woolf SH, Marks JS. When do we know enough to recommend action on the social determinants of health? *Am J Prev Med.* 2011;40(Suppl 1):S58–66.

CHAPTER

30

Race and Ethnic Health Disparities

Sandra S. Albrecht • Kiarri N. Kershaw

INTRODUCTION

Race/ethnic disparities in health remain a persistent challenge in the United States. Though health indicators related to life expectancy, infectious diseases, and infant mortality have improved for most Americans, some race/ethnic minority groups continue to experience a disproportionate burden of preventable disease and death compared with non-Hispanic whites.

National data demonstrate that the U.S. population is becoming more racially and ethnically diverse. According to the 2010 U.S. Census, approximately 36% of the U.S. population belonged to a racial/ethnic minority group. By the year 2060, the United States will be majority-minority, with non-Hispanic whites representing approximately 44% of the total U.S. population.[1] These disparities are not only concerning from an inequities standpoint, but also because of the potential to limit improvements in population health with implications for overall healthcare costs.

The 1985 Heckler Report raised national awareness around the problem of race/ethnic disparities and the disproportionate burden of disease experienced by minorities. In accordance with provisions contained in the Minority Health and Health Disparities Research and Education Act of 2000, the National Institutes of Health began to formally integrate disparities research into its strategic plan. Since then, research on race/ethnic health disparities has increased considerably.

In this chapter, we review the empirical evidence around race/ethnic disparities across a range of health outcomes relevant to preventive medicine and public health. We also discuss the potential factors that contribute to race/ethnic health disparities, and provide an overview of the potential approaches and future directions in this area of research. Although similar disparities persist in many countries around the world, we focus this chapter on a discussion of race/ethnic health disparities specific to the United States given the unique historical social and environmental influences that have contributed to race/ethnic disparities in this country.

OVERVIEW OF RACE/ETHNIC HEALTH DISPARITIES

The term "health disparities" is often defined as a difference in which disadvantaged social groups, such as race/ethnic minorities, who have persistently experienced social disadvantage or discrimination, systematically experience worse health than more advantaged social groups.[2] When these differences in health "are not only unnecessary and avoidable," and are "considered unfair and unjust," they are referred to as health inequities.[3]

Race/Ethnic Definitions

Race/ethnic minority groups in the United States include those individuals who self-identify as Black or African-American, Asian Americans, American Indian or Alaska Native, native Hawaiian or Other Pacific Islander, and Hispanic or Latino populations. Individuals who self-identify as Hispanic or Latino, considered an ethnicity, are persons of Mexican, Puerto Rican, Cuban, South or Central American, or other Spanish culture or origin and may be of any racial category, including white.[4]

Racial and ethnic categories are not static, and have changed considerably over time. Racial categories, in particular, have been included on every U.S. census since 1790, but have changed every decade, reflecting the social and political climate of the times. For example, in 1930, the "one-drop rule" indicated that "a person of mixed White and Negro blood was to be returned as Negro, no matter how small the percentage of Negro blood." It would not be until 2000 that Americans could choose more than one race to describe themselves. Mexicans were counted as their own race in 1930 for the first and only time. Hispanic groups of any kind were not offered as options again until 1970, when the census form began asking about Hispanic origin as a separate question from race. This historical context provides a backdrop for understanding the sociopolitical influences that have contributed to race/ethnic classifications over time. It also provides support against arguments that contend that race/ethnic health disparities are primarily genetic in origin.

Causes of Race/Ethnic Disparities

Race/ethnic health disparities are often thought to be driven by the interplay of biology, behavior, and the social conditions in which individuals live, learn, work, and play. Although some researchers have attributed race/ethnic health disparities to differences in genetic predisposition, this argument assumes that human genetic variation can be differentiated into the standard racial and ethnic categories used in the United States today. However, when considering the socio-political and dynamic nature of race/ethnic categorization in the United States, together with the large body of research that has consistently shown genetic differences between race/ethnic groups to small compared to the genetic variation found *within* race/ethnic groups,[5,6] the totality of the evidence appears to point to nongenetic causes. In this chapter, we focus our discussion of the potential causes of race/ethnic health disparities on nongenetic explanations.

Risks to health do not occur in isolation. The chain of events leading to adverse health outcomes includes both proximal and upstream causes that can accumulate over the life course and that can affect individuals across their life span. Proximal determinants include those factors that act directly or almost directly to cause disease, whereas upstream, or distal, causes are further back in the causal chain (see Fig. 30-1). For the purpose of this chapter, our discussion of the proximal determinants of health focuses on the individual-level factors that have been shown to contribute directly to the development of the various health outcomes for which marked race/ethnic disparities have been demonstrated. These factors are also ones in which some race/ethnic groups disproportionately engage

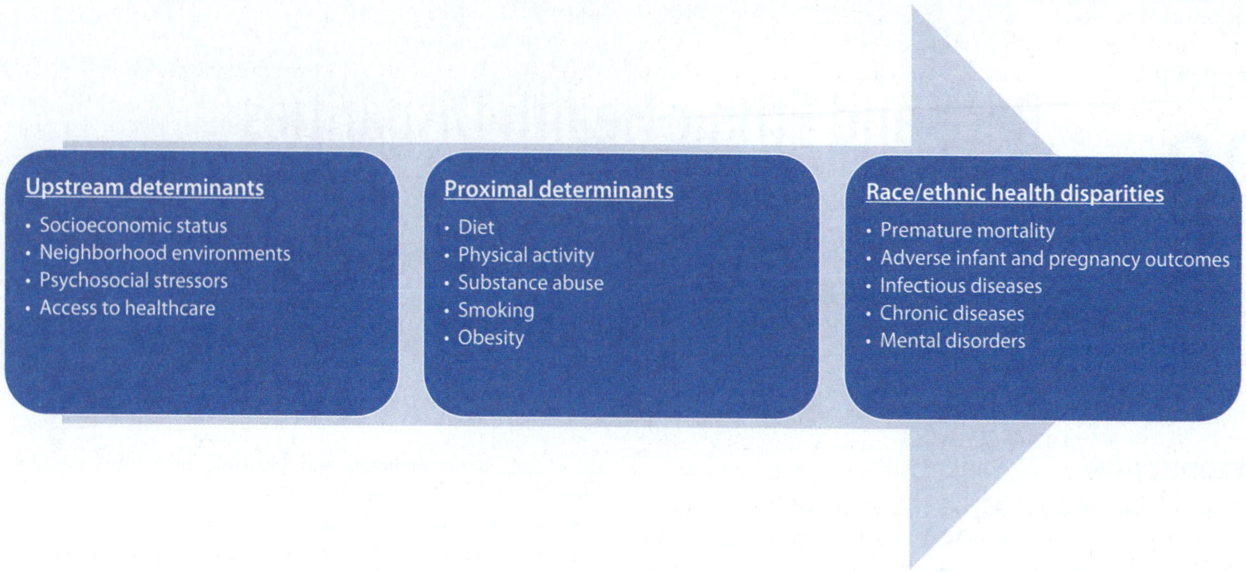

Upstream determinants
- Socioeconomic status
- Neighborhood environments
- Psychosocial stressors
- Access to healthcare

Proximal determinants
- Diet
- Physical activity
- Substance abuse
- Smoking
- Obesity

Race/ethnic health disparities
- Premature mortality
- Adverse infant and pregnancy outcomes
- Infectious diseases
- Chronic diseases
- Mental disorders

FIGURE 30-1. Conceptual model of race/ethnic health disparities.

(e.g., poor diet, smoking, etc.). The upstream factors on which we focus are those that have been deemed "social determinants of health," such as low socioeconomic status (SES), neighborhood environments, psychosocial stressors, and lack of access to care. These factors appear to systematically overburden some minority groups, and have been shown to contribute to race/ethnic disparities across a range of health outcomes.

Although these proximal and upstream determinants of health are reviewed as single factors in their own respective sections in this chapter, it is important to note that to adequately address race/ethnic health disparities, many of these determinants cannot be disentangled or considered in isolation. These determinants are often correlated with each other, they can act at different levels (e.g., individual, community, and society), and they can vary over time. To successfully reduce race/ethnic health disparities will require multilevel approaches that intervene on both the proximal and upstream determinants of health at the same time.

In the section that follows, we will first describe the existing evidence around race/ethnic disparities in adults across a variety of health outcomes, including premature mortality, adverse infant, and pregnancy outcomes, and the most common infectious diseases, chronic diseases, and mental disorders. This illustrates how pervasive health disparities are across a wide breadth of the major outcomes. We follow with a discussion of the proximal and upstream determinants of these disparities, and end with a brief overview of the potential approaches and future directions in this area of research.

RACE/ETHNIC DISPARITIES: BY HEALTH OUTCOME

Premature Mortality

Among both men and women, American Indian and Alaska Natives (AIANs) have the highest rates of premature mortality (defined as death before age 65), and Asian and Pacific Islanders (APIs) have the lowest rates.[7] Based on U.S. death certificate data from 2011 to 2014, the age-standardized AIAN mortality rate per 100,000 for men and women ages 25–39 at the time of death were 442.7 and 240.0, respectively, compared with 165.5 and 86.5 among whites, 60.1 and 30.7 among APIs (the lowest group), and 249.1 and 122.9 among blacks (the next highest group). For these younger adults, the main contributors to the high premature mortality rates seen among AIANs included accidents, chronic liver disease/cirrhosis, and suicide (among men). Accidents were a leading cause of mortality in all race/ethnic groups at this age, but the rate was not as high. Other noteworthy leading causes of premature death in this age group were suicide and self-inflicted injury in white men, and homicide and legal intervention in black men. Black men also had the highest rate of mortality due to diseases of the heart at this age group.

By ages 50–64 mortality rates were similar for blacks (1335 for men and 814.8 for women) and AIANs (1409 for men and 863.1 for women); rates in APIs were still the smallest (407.6 for men and 245.7 for women). The leading causes of premature mortality among adults ages 50–64 were malignant cancers and diseases of the heart for all race/ethnic groups, but the rate of these adverse outcomes was markedly higher among blacks than any other group. Mortality rates for malignant cancers were 361.7 and 268.7 for black men and women, compared with 256.0 and 204.0 for whites, 167.6 and 131.8 for Hispanics, 146.8 and 120.3 among APIs, and 267.5 and 205.3 among AIANs. Heart disease mortality rates were 353.5 in black men and 176.0 in black women. In contrast, rates ranged from a low of 97.7 and 29.3 among API men and women to 293.9 and 117.9 among AIAN men and women, with rates for whites (210.3 and 79.9) and Hispanics (137.8 and 52.3) falling in between. Chronic liver disease/cirrhosis, diabetes mellitus, and accidents were major causes of premature mortality among AIANs ages 50–64.

Adverse Infant and Pregnancy Outcomes

Infants born to non-Hispanic black women have higher rates of preterm birth, small-for-gestational age, and infant mortality than any other race/ethnic group. In 2016, infant mortality rates were 11.4 per 1000 live births among non-Hispanic blacks, 9.4 among AIANs, and 7.4 among Native Hawaiians or other Pacific Islanders.[8] Rates were much lower and similar for infants born to Hispanic, non-Hispanic white, and Native Hawaiian or Asian women (5.0, 4.9, and 3.6 per 1000 live births, respectively).

Patterns of preterm birth were similar by race/ethnicity. Preterm birth rates were highest among non-Hispanic blacks (11.4%) followed by Native Hawaiians or other Pacific Islanders (11.5%) and AIANs (11.4%).[9] Rates were lowest in Asians (8.6%) and similar in non-Hispanic whites (9.0%) and Hispanics (9.5%). This pattern held for both early preterm birth (born prior to 34 weeks of gestation) and late preterm births (born between 34 and 36 weeks of gestation). Among Hispanics, rates were similar by Hispanic origin of mother with the exception of Puerto Ricans who had rates of 11.1%.

Rates of very low birthweight (less than 1500 g) were highest among non-Hispanic blacks (3.0%) and similar among the other groups (ranging from 1.1% among non-Hispanic whites and Asians to 1.5% among Native Hawaiians or other Pacific Islanders).[9] Low birthweight (less than 2500 g) was highest among non-Hispanic blacks as well (13.7%); rates among other groups ranged from 7.0% among non-Hispanic whites to 8.4% among non-Hispanic Asians.

Infectious Diseases

Sexually Transmitted Infections

Blacks have the highest rates of the most common sexually transmitted infections, including chlamydia, gonorrhea, and human papillomavirus (HPV). Chlamydia morbidity rates are highest among blacks than any other race/ethnic group. Data from 2014 show rates in black men and women are 727.7 and 1357.2 per 100,000, respectively.[10] Rates in AIANs (297.1 and 988.9 in men and women, respectively) and Hispanics (202.6 and 546.3) are also higher than those of whites (103.1 and 248.6); rates are lowest in APIs (69.5 and 163.5).

Patterning of gonorrhea is similar to that of chlamydia. Based on data from 2014, gonorrhea morbidity rates are 412.8 per 100,000 in black men and 353.0 in black women.[10] AIANs have the second-highest gonorrhea rates (120.3 in men and 193.7 in women), followed by Hispanics (82.1 in men and 60.5 in women), whites (39.9 in men and 33.7 in women), and APIs (27.9 in men and 13.2 in women).

Over 40% of the U.S. population are infected with some form of the >40 types of HPV. According to NHANES data collected in 2003–06, HPV prevalence is highest in non-Hispanic blacks (59.2%) and lowest in non-Hispanic whites (39.2%; 44.2% in Mexican-Americans and 41.8% in a combined "other" category). The prevalence of high-risk HPV (based on oncogenic potential) is highest in non-Hispanic blacks and lowest in non-Hispanic whites as well (39.6% and 26.9%, respectively). High-risk HPV prevalence fell in the middle for Mexican-Americans and the other race/ethnic group category (30.7% and 28.2%, respectively).

Human Immunodeficiency Virus

The burden of human immunodeficiency virus (HIV) is higher among blacks than any other race/ethnic group.[11] According to the Centers for Disease Control and Prevention, 44% of those who were diagnosed with HIV in 2016 were black compared with 1–2% of all cases among AIANs, Asians, and other Pacific Islanders. Data from 2015 show 24% of all new HIV cases were in Hispanics. These numbers for blacks in particular, but also for Hispanics, are disproportionately larger than their representation in the U.S. population (approximately 12% and 18%, respectively). Surveillance estimates through 2014 indicate 43% of everyone living with HIV was black and 21% were Hispanic. In addition, 16% of blacks and 17% of Hispanics were living with undiagnosed HIV. The higher burden of HIV in this population has been attributed to a variety of factors including the higher rates of other STDs which is associated with increased risk of acquiring and transmitting the disease; stigma, fear, and homophobia; poverty and access to healthcare; and a greater tendency to have sex with partners of the same race/ethnicity.

Hepatitis C

NHANES data indicate Hepatitis C Virus (HCV) RNA prevalence is higher in non-Hispanic blacks than the other race/ethnic groups.[12] HCV RNA prevalence was 2.4% in black men and 0.9% in black women; prevalence ranged from 0.2 to 1.2 in Hispanic, non-Hispanic white, and non-Hispanic Asian men and women. Several local-level studies have shown HCV RNA prevalence is higher in incarcerated and homeless populations, but differences by race in these groups are not generally reported.[13] HCV-related death rates are highest among AIANs (10.8 per 100,000 in 2016), followed by non-Hispanic blacks (7.4 per 100,000). Rates were lowest in APIs (2.1 per 100,000), with non-Hispanic whites, with Hispanics falling in between (4.0 and 5.7 per 100,000, respectively).[14]

Chronic Diseases

Coronary Heart Disease

Coronary heart disease (CHD) prevalence estimates based on NHANES data (2011–14) are similar among non-Hispanic blacks (7.1% in men and 5.7% in women) and non-Hispanic whites (7.7% in men and 5.3% in women).[15] CHD prevalence in Hispanic women (6.1%) is comparable to that of non-Hispanic black and white women; CHD prevalence in Hispanic men is lower than non-Hispanic black and white men, at 5.9%. Asians have the lowest CHD prevalence (5.0% in men and 2.6% in women). Despite these similarities in CHD prevalence among black and white adults, incidence of heart attacks, fatal CHD, and myocardial infarction are all higher among blacks than whites. A study in participants of the Reasons for Geographic and Racial Differences in Stroke (REGARDS) cohort found black–white differences were largely driven by fatal CHD events and that adjustment for traditional cardiovascular disease risk factors (e.g., total cholesterol, systolic blood pressure, and diabetes) largely attenuated all significant associations.[16]

Cancer

Incidence rates of all types of cancer combined are highest among blacks and whites, and lowest among APIs and AIANs (Table 30-1).[17] Among the common cancers, colon and rectum cancer incidence rates are highest among blacks compared with the other race/ethnic groups as are kidney, lung (men only), pancreatic, and prostate (men). Breast cancer incidence rates are similar among black and

TABLE 30-1 NEW CASES OF CANCER BY RACE/ETHNICITY—RATES PER 100,000 PEOPLE

	White	Black	AIAN	API	Hispanic
WOMEN					
Bladder	8.8	6.3	4.3	3.5	4.8
Breast	125.6	123.3	71.2	94.3	93.6
Colon and rectum	32.7	37.5	26.7	25.2	28.0
Kidney and renal pelvis	11.6	12.9	11.5	5.4	12.4
Leukemia	10.6	8.1	6.5	6.0	8.6
Liver and intrahepatic bile duct	4.1	5.6	6.6	6.9	7.8
Lung and bronchus	52.5	46.3	36.7	26.8	24.0
Melanoma	20.5	0.8	5.2	1.3	4.4
Non-Hodgkin lymphoma	15.7	11.5	9.6	10.4	14.3
Pancreatic	10.9	14.6	8.0	8.6	10.0
Thyroid	22.4	13.9	11.0	22.0	21.5
MEN					
Bladder	35.8	18.9	15.3	14.1	17.8
Colon and rectum	42.5	51.1	34.3	33.2	40.5
Kidney and renal pelvis	22.5	25.0	20.2	11.5	21.3
Leukemia	17.5	12.3	9.3	9.0	12.4
Liver and intrahepatic bile duct	11.5	17.5	15.5	19.0	19.2
Lung and bronchus	66.3	75.5	46.1	42.6	35.9
Melanoma	31.3	1.3	6.8	1.4	4.6
Non-Hodgkin lymphoma	22.7	16.0	12.5	15.4	18.5
Pancreatic	14.5	16.8	9.1	9.9	12.4
Prostate	90.2	158.3	49.6	51.0	78.8
Thyroid	7.7	3.9	3.8	7.3	5.7

Data from U.S. Cancer Statistics Working Group. U.S. Cancer Statistics Data Visualizations Tool, based on November 2017 submission data (1999-2015). 2018.

TABLE 30-2 CANCER MORTALITY BY RACE/ETHNICITY—RATES PER 100,000 PEOPLE

	White	Black	AIAN	API	Hispanic
WOMEN					
Bladder	2.2	2.2	1.2	0.9	1.3
Breast	19.8	27.6	12.9	11.8	13.6
Colon and rectum	11.5	15.5	8.7	8.7	8.6
Kidney and renal pelvis	2.4	2.4	2.5	1.1	2.3
Leukemia	4.8	4.2	2.3	2.5	3.5
Liver and intrahepatic bile duct	3.8	4.5	5.0	5.5	6.1
Lung and bronchus	34.9	30.8	22.7	17.1	13.1
Melanoma	1.8	0.2	N/A	0.3	0.5
Non-Hodgkin lymphoma	4.3	3.2	2.9	3.1	3.4
Pancreatic	9.4	12.2	6.6	7.3	7.9
Thyroid	0.5	0.5	N/A	0.7	0.6
MEN					
Bladder	7.9	5.2	2.9	2.8	3.9
Colon and rectum	16.2	23.1	14.6	11.4	14.1
Kidney and renal pelvis	5.8	5.5	5.5	2.6	5.3
Leukemia	8.8	6.8	5.0	4.8	5.5
Liver and intrahepatic bile duct	9.0	13.4	10.2	13.6	12.8
Lung and bronchus	49.9	59.1	32.6	30.0	24.9
Melanoma	4.1	0.5	N/A	0.4	0.9
Non-Hodgkin lymphoma	7.4	5.2	4.1	5.0	5.6
Pancreatic	12.7	14.9	7.0	8.5	9.4
Prostate	17.7	37.5	14.2	9.0	16.0
Thyroid	0.5	0.4	N/A	0.6	0.6

Data from U.S. Cancer Statistics Working Group. U.S. Cancer Statistics Data Visualizations Tool, based on November 2017 submission data (1999-2015). 2018;2018.

white women. Liver cancer incidence is highest among Hispanics, followed by APIs. Bladder cancer and leukemia incidence rates are highest among whites.

Cancer mortality rates are generally highest among blacks (Table 30-2).[17] Data from 2015 show cancer mortality rates per 100,000 people for all types of cancer combined are 226.7 for black men and 152.6 for black women. Rates for white men were 190.1 and for white women were 136.5. Mortality rates were lowest among APIs at 118.9 for men and 87.3 for women. These disparities are consistent across different types of cancer. Black men and women have the highest mortality rates for most common cancers including breast (women), colon and rectal, pancreatic, lung (men only), and prostate (men). Whites have the highest rates of bladder cancer and leukemia. APIs and Hispanics have the highest mortality rates for liver and thyroid cancers.

Stroke

Stroke prevalence is highest among non-Hispanic black men (3.9%) and women (4.0%).[15] Prevalence estimates range from 1% to 3% for all other race/ethnic groups. The available data suggest this is not driven by any particular stroke subtype; blacks have higher incidence rates for ischemic, intracerebral hemorrhagic, and subarachnoid hemorrhagic strokes than whites[15]. The 1-year and 5-year stroke survival rates are worse for older blacks (≥75 years old) than whites, but they are better or similar for younger age groups.

Hypertension

Hypertension prevalence is higher among non-Hispanic blacks than any other race/ethnic group. According to recent NHANES data, hypertension prevalence is 54.9% among non-Hispanic blacks based on the 2017 American Colleges of Cardiology (ACC)/American Heart Association (AHA) Guideline and 41.0% under the JNC7 Guidelines.[18] Hypertension prevalence in non-Hispanic whites went from 33.4% under JNC7 to 47.3% under ACC/AHA; non-Hispanic Asians (24.4–36.7%) and Hispanics (21.1–34.4%) experienced comparable increases under the new guidelines and maintained lower rates than non-Hispanic whites or blacks.

Diabetes

Diabetes prevalence is higher among minority groups than non-Hispanic whites. NHANES data from 2011 to 2014 show age-adjusted diabetes prevalence estimates of 17.7% among non-Hispanic blacks adults, 16.0% among non-Hispanic Asians, and 16.4% among Hispanics, compared with 9.3% among non-Hispanic whites.[19] These disparities by race/ethnicity hold for both diagnosed and undiagnosed diabetes, although Asians have the highest prevalence of undiagnosed diabetes whereas blacks have the highest prevalence of diagnosed diabetes. NHIS data from 2013 to 2015 show diagnosed diabetes prevalence is also high among AIANs at 15.1%.

Data on diagnosed diabetes prevalence are available for a wider array of race/ethnic groups, and they reveal marked variation in the burden of this condition among Asians and Hispanics of different backgrounds.[19] According to NHIS data from 2013 to 2015, diagnosed diabetes prevalence in Asians ranges from a low of 4.3% in Chinese adults (6.2% in men and 2.8% in women) to a high of 11.2% in Asian Indian adults (12.2% in men and 10.0% in women), with Filipino adults falling in between (8.9%; 9.1% in men and 8.9% in women). Diagnosed diabetes prevalence is higher in all included Hispanic groups than in non-Hispanic whites, but estimates are notably higher in Mexicans (13.8%; 14.2% in men and 13.5% in women) and Puerto Ricans (12.0%; 12.2% in men and 11.8% in women) than in Cubans (9.0%; 11.6% in men and 5.9% in women) and Central/South Americans (8.5%; 8.5% in men and 8.8% in women).

Non-Hispanic blacks, Hispanics, and Asians have a lower or similar risk of developing cardiovascular complications of diabetes compared with non-Hispanic whites.[20,21] However, all three minority groups were at higher risk of end-stage renal disease and higher or similar risk of diabetic nephropathy.[21,22] Asians were less likely to have lower extremity amputations than non-Hispanic whites, while risk was higher or similar among blacks and Hispanics. Findings were mixed for diabetic retinopathy and the limited research on racial disparities in diabetic neuropathy suggests similar outcomes across groups. In addition, diabetic retinopathy and neuropathy is not well characterized in Asian or American Indian populations in the United States.

Kidney Disease

According to NHANES, chronic kidney disease prevalence is highest among non-Hispanic blacks and whites (2013–16; 15.9% and 15.6%, respectively).[23] Prevalence is lowest among Mexican-Americans and other Hispanics (12.6% and 11.4%). Although blacks and whites have a similar prevalence of chronic kidney disease, blacks are four times more likely to have end stage-renal disease than whites.[24] Native Americans and Hispanics are twice as likely to have end-stage renal disease; Asians are 1.6 times as likely.

Respiratory Diseases

Based on data from the National Health Interview Survey, asthma prevalence among U.S. adults is highest among Puerto Ricans (9.9% in men and 16.7% in women).[25] Rates are lowest in Mexican-Americans (4.1% and 6.6% in men and women, respectively), and they fall in the middle for non-Hispanic blacks (6.0% and 11.7%) and whites (5.6%

and 10.1%). The prevalence of other major respiratory diseases like emphysema (range from 0.4% in Asians to 1.4% in whites) or bronchitis (from 1.2% in Asians to 3.8% in AIANs) are lowest in Asians and then similar for the other race/ethnic groups.[26]

Alzheimer's Disease

There is not a lot of information available on racial/ethnic disparities in Alzheimer's disease or dementia more broadly. Data from customers of the Kaiser Permanente Northern California healthcare delivery system found the age-adjusted incidence rate of dementia (from 2001 to 2013) was highest among blacks and AIANs (26.6 and 22.2 per 1000 person-years, respectively).[27] Rates were similar among Hispanics, Pacific Islanders, and non-Hispanic whites (19.6, 19.6, and 19.3); they were lowest among Asians at 15.2 per 1000 person-years.

Mental Disorders

Anxiety

According to data from the National Institute of Mental Health's Collaborative Psychiatric Epidemiology Surveys (CPES, 2001–03), the prevalence of DSM-IV social anxiety disorder, generalized anxiety disorder, and panic disorder are higher among whites (12.6%, 8.6%, and 5.1%, respectively) than African Americans (8.6%, 4.9%, and 3.8%), Hispanic Americans (8.2%, 5.8%, and 4.1%), and Asian Americans (5.3%, 2.4%, and 2.1%).[28]

Depression

Racial/ethnic differences in depression prevalence appear to vary by the measure used to determine the outcome. The prevalence of depression, as measured using the Patient Health Questionnaire, is higher among non-Hispanic black men (NHANES 2013–16; 7.1%) than their Hispanic, non-Hispanic white, and non-Hispanic Asian counterparts (6.0%, 5.2%, and 2.2%, respectively).[29] However, differences between black, white, and Hispanic men were not statistically significant. Depression prevalence was similar among Hispanic, white, and black women (10.5–11.0%); it was much lower among Asian women (3.9%). Data from the CPES using the World Mental Health Composite International Diagnostic Interview showed prevalence of 12-month major depression was higher among Mexican Americans, Cubans, and whites (ranging from 8.0% to 8.3%) than African Americans (6.8%).[30] Notably, major depression prevalence was highest among Puerto Ricans (11.9%) and lowest among participants of Asian descent (ranging from 4.2% to 4.6% among Chinese, Filipinos, and Vietnamese).

Schizophrenia

Several studies have shown that blacks are more likely to be diagnosed with schizophrenia than whites. A recent meta-analysis of 14 studies found that blacks were two times more likely to be diagnosed with schizophrenia, regardless of the type of diagnostic instrument used (structured or unstructured interview).[31] There is some evidence suggesting that Hispanics are more likely to be diagnosed with schizophrenia than whites, but the difference is not as large as that seen between blacks and whites.[32]

Trauma

The prevalence of posttraumatic stress disorder (PTSD) is higher in African Americans than other race/ethnic groups. In the CPES, PTSD prevalence was 8.6% among African Americans compared with 6.5% and 5.6% among whites and Hispanics, and 1.6% among Asians.[28] A similar pattern was found using data from the National Epidemiologic Survey on Alcohol and Related Conditions (NESARC, 2004–05).[33]

Summary

Racial/ethnic health disparities are evident across a wide range of health outcomes. With the exception of certain mental disorders and respiratory diseases, outcomes are worse for non-Hispanic blacks than other race/ethnic groups. Outcomes also tended to be worse for AIANs and Puerto Ricans, though less data were available for these groups. The next sections describe proximal and upstream factors that likely contribute to the persistent disparities seen between these groups and whites across a wide array of outcomes.

PROXIMAL DETERMINANTS OF RACE/ETHNIC HEALTH DISPARITIES

Diet

Sugar-Sweetened Beverages

Non-Hispanic black and Hispanic adults are more likely to consume sugar-sweetened beverages than non-Hispanic whites and Asians. According to data from NHANES (2011–14), 8.3% and 8.9% of daily kilocalories in non-Hispanic black men and women, respectively, and 8.1% and 7.4% of daily kilocalories in Hispanic men and women, came from sugar-sweetened beverages.[34] In contrast, 6.4% and 5.4% of daily kilocalories came from sugar-sweetened beverages in non-Hispanic whites and 4.0% and 3.0% came from sugar-sweetened beverages in non-Hispanic Asian men and women.

Data on youth at the same time period show a slightly different pattern. Non-Hispanic black youth (7.9% and 8.9% of total kilocalories in boys and girls, respectively) consumed the most sugar-sweetened beverages and non-Hispanic Asians (3.5% and 3.6%, respectively) consumed the least, but levels for Hispanic boys and girls (7.3% and 6.8%) was lower than those for their non-Hispanic white counterparts (3.5% and 3.6%).[35]

Fruit and Vegetable Intake

According to data from the 2015 BRFSS,[36] blacks and Hispanics (14.3% and 15.7%, respectively) were more likely to meet federal fruit intake recommendations (1.5–2.0 cup equivalents per day) than non-Hispanic whites (11.2%). Blacks (5.5%) were least likely to meet federal vegetable intake recommendations (2.0–3.0 cups per day); percentages were similar for whites and Hispanics (9.5% and 10.5%, respectively).

Data from the 2017 Youth Risk Behavior Survey [37] shows black high school girls (22.3%) were most likely to eat fruit or drink 100% fruit juices three or more times per day compared to all other race/ethnic groups (11.4%, 18.6%, and 13.3% among Asian, Hispanic, and white girls, respectively). Fruit consumption was generally higher among high school boys and still highest among blacks (29.2%, compared with 21.6%, 24.6%, and 19.2% among Asian, Hispanic, and white boys). In contrast to fruit, black high school girls were least likely to eat vegetables one or more times per day (47.4%). Vegetable consumption was highest among Asian and white girls (65.4% and 64.0%, respectively) followed by Hispanic girls (55.2%). As with girls, vegetable consumption was highest among Asian high school boys and lowest among black boys (73.9% vs. 51.5%); Hispanics and whites fell in between the two groups (56.9% and 61.5%, respectively).

Physical Activity

Data from the 2015 National Health Interview Survey show non-Hispanic white adults are more likely to meet the 2008 federal aerobic and strengthening physical activity guidelines than any other race/ethnic group[15]. The guideline for aerobic activity is defined as engaging in $\geq$150 minutes of moderate or 75 minutes of vigorous aerobic leisure-time PA per week (or an equivalent combination), and the guideline from strengthening activity is engaging in leisure time strength training at least twice per week. Only 21.5% (age-adjusted) of all U.S. adults meet these guidelines—23.4% of non-Hispanic whites, 19.8% of non-Hispanic blacks, 19.1% of Asians, 18.9% of AIANs, and 16.8% of Hispanics. More Americans meet the aerobic guidelines (49.0%), but similar disparities remain, particularly among women (50.9% in non-Hispanic whites compared with 35.0% and 41.0% in non-Hispanic blacks and Hispanics).

These patterns of physical activity appear to start in youth. The 2015 Youth Risk Behavioral Surveillance survey defined as engaging in activity that increased their heart rate and made them breathe hard some of the time for at least 60 min/day on all 7 days preceding the survey.[38] The prevalence of this level of activity was fairly low for high school students of all race/ethnic groups, but as with adults, it was highest in non-Hispanic whites (38.5% and 19.5% for boys and girls, respectively). Non-Hispanic black boys and girls had rates of 30.8% and 16.6%; rates for Hispanic boys and girls were 34.2% and 14.7%.

Substance Abuse

Data from the 2017 National Survey on Drug Use and Health show that AIANs have a higher prevalence of past-year alcohol dependence (6.5%) than any other race/ethnic group in the study including non-Hispanic whites, blacks, APIs, Asians, and Hispanics (prevalence range from 1.8% in Asians to 3.0% in whites).[39] Past-year illicit drug use (other than marijuana abuse) is also highest among AIANs (1.8%) than any other race/ethnic group (range from 0.2% to 0.3%). Opioid dependence is highest in AIANs as well (1.9%), followed by APIs and non-Hispanic whites (1.1% and 1.0%, respectively).

Smoking

According to the National Health Interview Survey (2016), smoking prevalence is highest among AIANs at 31.8%.[40] Rates are similar for non-Hispanic blacks and whites, at 16.5% and 16.6%, respectively. Smoking prevalence was 9.0% among Asians and 10.7% among Hispanics in this dataset, but evidence from the 2010–13 National Survey on Drug Use and Health suggest there is considerable variation by subgroup.[40] In this study, smoking prevalence ranged from a low of 7.6% in Chinese and Asian Indian adults to highs of 16.3% and 20.0% in Vietnamese and Korean adults, respectively. Among Hispanics, smoking prevalence ranged from 15.6% in Central and South Americans to 28.5% in Puerto Ricans.

According to 2014 data from the National Youth Tobacco Survey,[41] the prevalence of cigarette use among high school students is highest among non-Hispanic whites (10.8%) followed by Hispanics (8.8%); rates are lowest among non-Hispanic black (4.5%). Data were not available for Asians. Patterns are similar for electronic cigarette use (15.3% among non-Hispanic whites and Hispanics; 5.6% among non-Hispanic blacks). Among middle school students, cigarette and electronic cigarette use was highest among Hispanics (3.7% and 6.2%, respectively) and similar among non-Hispanic whites (2.2% and 3.1%) and non-Hispanic blacks (1.7% and 3.8%). Patterns of cigarette use by race/ethnicity change considerably over the life course.

Obesity

Obesity is patterned by race/ethnicity and gender.[42] Non-Hispanic black women have the highest obesity prevalence of all groups. Recent NHANES data estimates the age-adjusted prevalence in this group to be 55.9%. Estimates are also high for black men (37.4%) and for Hispanics (40.6% in men and 48.9% in women). Obesity prevalence is lowest among non-Hispanic Asians (11.2% in men and 13.6% in women); estimates for whites are close to those seen for black men (36.2% in men and 38.1% in women).

Patterns in childhood and adolescent obesity are similar.[43] Obesity prevalence is substantially higher among Hispanic (28.0% in boys and 23.5% in girls) and non-Hispanic black (19.3% in boys and 25.1% in girls) youth than their non-Hispanic white (14.7% in boys and 13.6% in girls) and Asian (11.2% in boys and 10.1% in girls) counterparts. Age-stratified estimates suggest these patterns emerge in early childhood.[15]

Summary

As with the majority of the diseases, the burden of these proximal factors is heavier for non-Hispanic blacks and AIANs than most other race/ethnic groups. AIANs have higher rates of substance abuse than other race/ethnic groups, which could account for their increased risk of premature mortality due to accidents and cirrhosis/liver disease. In addition, the high level of injection drug use may influence the higher hepatitis C-related mortality rates in this group. The high rates of obesity in non-Hispanic blacks likely represent a major contributor to disparities in stroke and cardiovascular diseases such as hypertensive heart disease and heart failure.

UPSTREAM DETERMINANTS OF RACE/ETHNIC HEALTH DISPARITIES

Socioeconomic Status

SES is a multidimensional construct that incorporates a range of indicators, including, but not limited to, education, income, occupation, and wealth. SES determines access to knowledge, material, and social resources, as well as power and prestige. In the United States, race/ethnicity is highly correlated with SES measures. In the aggregate, Blacks and Hispanics, on average, have lower levels of education than whites, and are more likely to live in poverty.[44] These SES disparities extend to Native Hawaiians/Pacific Islanders (21.5%) and American Indian/Alaskan Natives (17%) who also have lower levels of college graduation than whites (34.2%).[45,46] In contrast, similar data show that Asian-Americans appear to have an SES profile that, on average, is higher than non-Hispanic whites.

A large body of evidence has shown that being of low SES is associated with worse health across a wide range of outcomes.[47] Because some minority groups endure a disproportionate burden of socioeconomic hardship relative to non-Hispanic whites, SES is considered to be a major contributor to health disparities patterned by race/ethnicity. Indeed, a wide range of studies have demonstrated at least a partial attenuation of disparities once SES is accounted for. Nevertheless, race/ethnic disparities in health often still persist across all levels of SES. For example, among college-educated women, blacks have a considerably higher infant mortality rate than whites (11.5 vs. 4.2 per 1000 live births).[48] Another study showed that Blacks had a worse biological risk profile (e.g., blood pressure, other metabolic risk markers, and inflammatory markers) than whites even after adjusting for education and income.[49] In a cohort study of black and white physicians, black physicians had a higher incidence of hypertension, diabetes, and CVD than white physicians.[50]

Several reasons have been posited to explain why race/ethnic health disparities appear to persist even after accounting for SES.[51] One reason relates to the fact that single indicators do not adequately capture the financial constraints faced by some minority groups—also known as the nonequivalence of SES measures across race/ethnic groups. For the same level of education, blacks have poorer financial returns, and are more likely to be unemployed than whites.[52,53] Second, even at higher levels of SES, blacks on average continue to live in racially segregated neighborhoods that are higher in poverty and with fewer health-promoting goods and services.[54,55] This highlights the role of multiple determinants of health acting simultaneously to exacerbate race/ethnic health disparities. Relatedly, psychosocial stressors (discussed further later in this chapter) have also been implicated as factors that can amplify the adverse effects of low SES on health, especially for minorities. For example, experiences of discrimination and internalized racism have been linked to worse health for many minority groups.[56] These psychosocial stressors have been found to persist for minorities even at high levels of SES, which may explain why upward socioeconomic mobility does not appear to confer the same benefits to health as it appears to do for whites.

In sum, although low SES is a major contributor to race/ethnic health disparities, the evidence suggests that the relationship between SES and health may be more complex for minorities, and that other social and environmental factors may be operating in tandem with SES to contribute to poor health.

Neighborhood Environment

A growing body of research suggests that the residential neighborhood environment contributes to a range of health outcomes, including obesity, hypertension, diabetes, mental health, and among others.[57,58] As a result, another factor that has been implicated as a contributor to race/ethnic health disparities relates to characteristics of the neighborhood environments in which many minorities reside. Blacks and Hispanics, in particular, tend to be overrepresented in low-income neighborhoods. With some exceptions, low-income neighborhoods have been associated with limited access to affordable healthy food options and few resources to support physical activity.[59]

Closely linked with neighborhood disadvantage and quite relevant to the experience of many minorities in the United States is residential segregation, a process that sorts individuals into different neighborhoods by race or ethnicity, and which has been implicated as a fundamental cause of health disparities.[60] Residential location determines the availability and quality of economic and social resources including schools, safety, recreational amenities, and public transportation.[60,61] Segregation is largely thought to be the product of housing discrimination and discriminatory lending practices, but it has also been part of the racial/ethnic assimilation process in the United States, especially for immigrants. For Black Americans, segregation increased throughout much of the twentieth century due to a long period of institutional discrimination, leading to constrained opportunities for economic and residential mobility. For Hispanics and other race/ethnic groups with large concentrations of immigrants, such as Asians, the extent of segregation from non-Hispanic whites is much lower than that for Blacks, though Hispanic segregation in particular appears to be on the rise.[62,63] While non-white race/ethnic groups have been subject to discrimination in housing markets, Hispanic and Asian segregation are thought to also reflect the residential preferences of immigrants to live among co-ethnics, facilitating access to social networks and culturally specific resources as they adjust to life in a new country. However, it is unclear whether these structural and social resources are enough to offset the high levels of poverty that tend to characterize these "ethnic enclaves."

Research linking residential segregation to health outcomes for minority residents has been increasing. Although the measurement construct used to characterize segregation has varied across studies (e.g., residential segregation, racial composition, ethnic density, etc.), with a few exceptions, Blacks living in areas with higher levels of Black segregation appear to have a greater prevalence of cardiovascular risk factors than blacks living in less segregated areas.[64] Similar patterns have been demonstrated with other health outcomes. Residing in neighborhoods with more Black segregation has been associated with higher odds of later-stage diagnosis of breast and lung cancers, and higher mortality rates and lower survival rates from breast and lung cancers[65], and it has been associated with a greater prevalence of preterm birth.[66] There are considerably fewer studies of Hispanic segregation and health, and even fewer of Asian segregation, though among the few studies that have been published, results have been mixed. For example, some studies show that living in neighborhoods with greater Hispanic concentration, especially Hispanic immigrants, has been linked to healthier diets,[67–69] and lower prevalence of preterm birth and low birthweight,[70] lower prevalence of obesity, hypertension, and smoking, but also lower levels of physical activity,[64] and poor access to hypertension care and treatment.[71] There is also considerable variation by factors such as gender, country of origin, racial identity, and acculturation.

The influence of residential segregation on health is most likely mediated through built and social environmental characteristics that have also been correlated with socioeconomically disadvantaged neighborhoods. Low-income, Black, and Hispanic communities have been shown to have lower relative availability of healthier dietary alternatives, more liquor stores, and greater advertisement of tobacco, junk food, and sugar-sweetened beverages.[72–74] However, consistent with some of the studies that demonstrate healthier outcomes among individuals living in Hispanic ethnic or immigrant enclaves, there is also evidence of a greater availability of healthier food in these enclaves.[69,75] Nevertheless, in a qualitative study, Hispanics cited inadequate facilities, cost, and neighborhood safety as barriers to physical activity in their communities.[76] Moreover, with respect to access to care, one study showed that counties with a greater proportion of non-English speakers had significantly fewer pharmacies than those with more English speakers.[77] Another study highlighted the problem of pharmacy deserts in minority communities, raising concerns about medication adherence in the populations most burdened by poor health.[78]

In sum, the bulk of the evidence points to the role of structural barriers in neighborhoods and in the wider society that may be contributing race/ethnic disparities across a range of health outcomes.

Psychosocial Stressors

Psychosocial mechanisms such as stress and internalized feelings of inferiority may arise because of socioeconomic deficits (i.e., living in poverty), as well as from adverse interpersonal interactions marked by overt or subtle racism. Psychosocial stress can impact health directly through chronic strain of physiological stress systems that are linked to disease. Through this mechanism, stress can accelerate cellular aging.[79] It can also lead to wear and tear on the body that can dysregulate multiple biological systems and lead to premature illness and mortality.[80] Psychosocial stress can also impact health indirectly because individual facing it may engage in unhealthy behaviors as a coping mechanism. Health behaviors like alcohol, tobacco, and drug use, as well as high-carbohydrate and high-fat diets, are examples of behaviors in which individuals engage to cope with stress.

An example of the type of psychosocial stressor that may be contributing to race/ethnic health disparities includes discrimination. Perceived racial or ethnic discrimination has been associated with a number of different health outcomes,[56] and with unhealthy behaviors,[81] particularly in Blacks. Discrimination is the differential treatment of members (often by race/ethnicity) by both individuals and social institutions. It can amplify the stress individuals experience when they are already of low SES. However it can also offset the benefits of being of higher SES, and has been hypothesized as a contributor to the persistence of race/ethnic health disparities at higher educational and income levels.

Other psychosocial stressors that have been considered in the context of race/ethnic health disparities include factors like goal-striving stress (GSS) and acculturative stress. GSS is the difference between aspiration and achievement. In other words, it is a form of stress that manifests itself when individuals exert high-levels effort to achieve a goal, and yet are unable to attain this goal, especially in the context of structural and psychological obstacles. GSS as a construct has been evaluated in a few studies and has been shown to be associated with greater odds of hypertension, a higher count of physical health problems, and worse mental health in samples of Black study participants.[82–84] Acculturative stress has recently received increased attention in the literature as a stressor relevant for Hispanics and other race/ethnic groups with a high proportion of immigrants, or for individuals who are struggling to adapt to a cultural environment different from the one they had been accustomed to. It has most commonly been examined in the context of mental health outcomes with studies showing greater anxiety and depression among persons experiencing higher levels of acculturative stress.[85,86] Other studies have demonstrated associations with eating disorders[87,88] and problem drinking,[89,90] while another study demonstrated stress-induced alterations in the cortisol-awakening response as a result of acculturative stress in Mexican-Americans.[91]

Psychosocial stressors appear to be a contributor to race/ethnic health disparities as they can lead to engagement in unhealthy lifestyles, and chronically strain physiological stress systems that are linked to disease. Given the body of evidence linking such stressors to poor health, interventions should consider these as one of the targets to address as part of efforts to reduce race/ethnic health disparities.

Access to healthcare

Despite improvements in the screening and diagnosis of a variety of chronic conditions, diseases like hypertension and diabetes remain poorly controlled among minority populations. For example, several studies have shown that Mexican-Americans have worse glycemic control compared with non-Hispanic whites.[40] Similarly concerning disparities are evident between Blacks and whites in terms of control of hypertension.[92] Poor access to care and a lack of health insurance are often cited as important contributors to race/ethnic disparities in management outcomes. It is also a factor that contributes to delayed disease diagnosis, and more advanced disease at diagnosis that is more difficult to treat. Screening and treatment are particularly important for the prevention and control of conditions like cancer, diabetes, and hypertension.

Data from the 2014 National Health Interview Survey indicate that over a quarter of nonelderly Hispanics/Latino adults living in the United States were uninsured, the highest proportion of any race/ethnic group. Although implementation of the Affordable Care Act (ACA) increased health coverage for all race/ethnic groups, Hispanic continued to have the lowest levels of coverage. Some of the reasons are because many some Hispanics work for employers that do not offer health insurance, and also because if they are immigrants, they are less likely to be eligible for public insurance. Lack of insurance has been associated with not having a usual source of care, fewer referrals for procedures, and less access to treatment. Moreover, uninsured individuals are more likely to delay seeking medical care, risking the development of complications that could be avoided with early detection.[93]

Although increasing health insurance coverage and improving access to care are important steps in addressing race/ethnic health disparities, several studies have also shown that disparities continue to persist even after accounting differences in access to care. For example, in an analysis of NHANES data from 1999 to 2002, only 35% of Mexican Americans and 37% of Blacks had adequate glucose control (HbA1C <7.0%) compared with 49% of non-Hispanic whites, even after accounting for health insurance coverage, having a regular provider, and use of diabetes medications.[94]

These studies suggest that broader social factors also likely play a role, and may interact with other patient, provider, and healthcare system-related factors. For example, even for patients with access to care, limited English proficiency may interfere with their ability to achieve management goals for a given health condition. Roughly one-third of Hispanics are not proficient in English,[95] and few healthcare settings provide medical services entirely in Spanish. Hispanic or Latina women were more likely to feel that doctors did not take the time to answer their questions and were more likely to leave the doctor's office without understanding the information they had received.[96] Increasing the number of clinicians who are fluent in Spanish and improving cultural competence among medical staff can contribute to improved communication between the provider and patient, while also improving the health literacy of patients.

In the context of access to care, financial hardship can also create barriers for optimal management of health. Poor adherence to medication and delays in seeking treatment have been strongly linked to cost-related factors, even among patients that have health insurance. As it is, health insurance policies have been trending toward fewer benefits and higher deductibles and co-payments. In large studies of insurance claims data, these high-deductible health insurance policies were linked to increasing trends in emergency room visits and high-severity hospitalizations among diabetes patients, and in delays in seeking care among cancer patients because of high out-of-pocket healthcare costs.[97,98] These trends were most pronounced among low-income individuals, the majority of whom tend to belong to a race/ethnic minority group. As a result, these patterns have implications for exacerbating race/ethnic health disparities in the future.

Finally, limited access to resources to comply with physicians' recommendations regarding diet and physical activity may also modify the effectiveness of healthcare access. As previously noted, a significant proportion of race/ethnic minorities live in high-poverty neighborhoods with poor access to resources to support health eating and an active lifestyle. Many guideline-based recommendations for treatment and management of most health conditions involve health behavior change, in conjunction with pharmaceutical interventions. If resources are not available outside the healthcare system to support a healthy change in diet and an increase in physical activity, then relying on healthcare access alone may be insufficient to address race/ethnic disparities in management outcomes.

Lack of health insurance and poor access to healthcare has been clearly linked to inadequate disease detection, more severe disease, and poor management outcomes for many race/ethnic minority groups. While improving healthcare access should be part of the solution to reduce race/ethnic disparities, the data suggest that this approach may be not enough. Cultural and socioeconomic barriers, such as language, cost, and access to resources, must be overcome, in tandem with increasing healthcare access, to improve management outcomes for race/ethnic minority groups disproportionately burdened by poor health.

APPROACHES TO ADDRESSING HEALTH DISPARITIES/FUTURE DIRECTIONS

The practice of documenting race/ethnic health disparities has proven useful for identifying high-risk groups, and for shedding light on the existence of such inequities in health. However, in the years since the 1985 Heckler Report raised national awareness around the problem of race/ethnic disparities, there has been little success in actually improving the health of minorities in the United States on a large-scale basis. In the following section, we discuss some promising approaches and future directions for addressing race/ethnic health disparities.

Unpacking Heterogeneity within Race/Ethnic Groups

Most research on race/ethnic health disparities tends to compare a range of health outcomes among Blacks, Hispanics, and Asians against non-Hispanic whites. This approach implicitly assumes homogeneity in health risk within race/ethnic groups, despite evidence showing considerable heterogeneity within these groups. Sources of heterogeneity range from factors such as country of origin, immigration history, SES, as well as geographic distribution across the United States, among several others—factors which have been shown to have implications for health. Unpacking within-race/ethnic group heterogeneity in health can help to unravel mechanisms underlying the broader observed disparities. It can also allow for the identification of healthy subgroups within the broader race/ethnic categories to better understand the factors that can promote good health.

A growing number of studies have been conducted demonstrating heterogeneity in risk across a range of health outcomes, especially within Black and Hispanic populations, but increasingly so among Asians. For Blacks, for example, although persistent disparities in hypertension have been reported compared to non-Hispanic whites in the United States, hypertension prevalence among blacks is lower in Caribbean countries. Among blacks in Africa, hypertension prevalence is similar to, or lower, than estimates among whites in the United States.[99] These findings suggest that genetic vulnerability alone does not explain why Blacks are disproportionately burdened by hypertension in the United States, and that other social and environmental factors may be contributing to and/or interacting with genetic predisposition to place some Blacks at high risk for disease.

The Jackson Heart Study (JHS) is another example of a study aimed at unpacking heterogeneity in cardiovascular disease outcomes among U.S. Blacks, specifically those living in Jackson, MS.[100] In the JHS, favorable neighborhood social environments (more social cohesion, less disorder, and less violence) were associated with fewer unhealthy behaviors, like smoking and alcohol consumption.[101] Wealth was also a significant predictor of CVD events in Black women.[102] Taken together, studies such as these highlight the existence of heterogeneity in health risk among Blacks, and help to further refine the ways in which social and environmental factors intersect with biology to contribute to poor (and good) health in some groups.

For Hispanics, this population encompasses substantial diversity within and across ethnic subgroups. With respect to national origin, the largest subgroups, according to the 2010 U.S. Census, are Mexicans (63%), Puerto Ricans (9.2%), Central Americans (7.9%), South Americans (5.5.%), and Cubans (3.5%).[103] Health differences across subgroups are arguably as great as those across race/ethnic groups in the United States. In the Hispanic Community Health Study/Study of Latinos (HCHS/SOL),[104] a cohort study analogous to the JHS, which aims to unpack the sources of heterogeneity in disease within the Hispanic population, Mexican, Puerto Rican, and Dominican subgroups have among the highest diabetes prevalence, while South Americans have the lowest estimates, similar to that of non-Hispanic whites.[105] Similar patterning by subgroups has been reported in HCHS/SOL for other health outcomes.[106] While the exact reasons for these disparities among Hispanics are unknown, explanations are likely related to differences in social and environmental factors, like behaviors retained from the country of origin, migration history, legal status, and even racial composition of these groups (with implications for discrimination).

It is also estimated that just under half of all Hispanics living in the United States are foreign-born. A large body of research has documented better health outcomes, such as fewer cardiovascular risk factors, better maternal and infant health outcomes, better mental health, and lower overall mortality among Hispanic immigrants compared to the U.S.-born, despite high levels of poverty among immigrants.[107–109] Thus, even within a high-risk minority group like Hispanics/Latinos, there are clearly subgroups with considerably better health. Identifying these healthy subgroups among high-risk populations and uncovering the health-promoting characteristics that contribute to better health may serve to benefit other race/ethnic minorities disproportionately living in poverty.

Increasing Community Engagement

There is also increasing recognition of the need to include community and nonacademic partners in research endeavors, especially when it comes to research involving minority populations. Despite the fact that minorities constitute a growing proportion of the U.S. population, they are highly underrepresented in research studies, and there is also evidence of apprehension in terms of engagement with the healthcare system.[110]

One reason for this is because of mistrust in the medical research enterprise which makes some minority groups less inclined to participate in research studies in the first place. Historical gross violations of research ethics, such as those that occurred in the Tuskegee Syphilis Study and elsewhere, have contributed to an unwillingness to participate in research by minorities, especially Blacks.[111,112] There is also evidence of difficulty in recruitment of other minority groups, like Hispanics, because of issues around citizenship and legal status in the United States, in addition to language and cultural barriers.[113,114] This mistrust of the research and healthcare enterprise impedes the ability of researchers and policymakers from fully understanding the barriers to good health in these communities, and it prevents minority communities from benefiting from potentially life-saving interventions. As a result, there has been a call to address the obstacles to recruitment and retention of minority groups in research.[115]

Part of the strategy to improve recruitment is to bring scientific professionals into partnership with affected communities.[116] These strategies can involve community-based participatory research approaches that view participants as partners in planning, conducting, and disseminating research. In addition to this approach, there has been a more general call to include the perspectives of minority communities in helping researchers understand the issues they face. This includes integrating more qualitative approaches to data collection, and acknowledging (rather than dismissing) the intellectual contribution and wisdom that minority voices bring to the research dialogue.

Aside from potential improvements to recruitment and retention, engaging minority communities in research endeavors is also necessary for translating evidence-based interventions in these populations. For a large number of diseases and health outcomes, effective strategies for prevention and treatment already exist or have been proven to work in the context of a randomized clinical trial framework. However when attempts are made to scale-up these interventions or to implement them, especially in minority communities, they appear to be ineffective at reducing the burden of disease or at improving disease management outcomes.[117] The field of implementation science is a burgeoning field that involves investigating ways to improve the translation of evidence-based approaches for the prevention and treatment of diseases. The field incorporates a broader scope than most traditional research—focusing not just on the individual-level, but also on multiple spheres of influence, including the level of provider, healthcare system, community, and policy. Because reducing race/ethnic health disparities involves intervening on multiple determinants at the same time, implementation science is well-suited as an approach for closing the evidence-practice gap for a range of health outcomes impacting minority communities. Moreover, because this research approach requires trans disciplinary research teams that include community and nonacademic partners, this ensures greater engagement with minority communities and a better potential to increase uptake of interventions strategies to reduce race/ethnic health disparities.

Adopting Health in All Policies Approaches

In addition to engaging communities, addressing the wide range of interrelated upstream factors influencing race/ethnic health disparities will require collaborations with sectors outside of the traditional health and medical care ones. Health in All Policies is one approach to promoting cross-sector collaborations.[118] These approaches aim to address social determinants of health by considering the health impacts of decisions made in all sectors and policy areas. This includes economic development, transportation, environmental agencies, schools, and housing departments. Health in All Policies approaches can take many formats but they should all consist of five key elements: (1) promoting health, equity, and sustainability; (2) supporting cross-sector collaboration; (3) creating initiatives that benefit multiple partners; (4) engaging stakeholders; and (5) creating structural or process change.

One way Health in All Policies approaches promote health, equity, and sustainability is by incorporating these factors into specific policies, programs, and processes. Another is to make a consideration of these factors a standard part of government decision-making processes. One example of this is Health Impact Assessments.[119] Health Impact Assessments involve the use of quantitative, qualitative, and participatory techniques to help decision-makers assess the health impacts of policies, plans, and projects across diverse sectors. Broad stakeholder engagement is essential to the success of Health Impact Assessments and other Health in All Policies approaches. As detailed in the previous section, engaging a variety of stakeholders ensures efforts are responsive to community needs.

In addition to stakeholder engagement, cross-sector collaborations are critical to the success of Health in All Policies approaches.

These partnerships have traditionally been led by the health sector, but there is increasing recognition that sustainable, effective collaborations will require more distributed leadership models.[120] A more distributed decision-making model improves equity by promoting broader contributions and engagement. This distributed model also helps collaborators identify initiatives that will benefit multiple partners. This is important for securing support while also ensuring more effective use of scare resources.

The ultimate goal of Health in All Policies approaches is to transform how agencies in different sectors interact with each other and how government decisions are made. This is not easy, as it requires an infrastructure that can sustain cross-sector collaborations and healthy public policy decision-making. Few implementation science studies have examined what makes cross-sector collaborations work and what elements can be replicated to date, but there are a growing number of funding mechanisms available to support these efforts.

CONCLUSION

Race/ethnic disparities exist for nearly every disease included in this chapter. Differences both between and within traditional race/ethnicity groupings were identified, highlighting the need for more research to unpack the sources of heterogeneity. The pervasiveness of these disparities across numerous diseases, particularly among non-Hispanic blacks and AIANs, suggest there are common, upstream factors underlying them that need to be addressed to alleviate the unequal burden of disease facing minority groups in the United States. This chapter highlighted several upstream determinants that could serve as targets for future interventions to address these disparities. Addressing these upstream, root causes of disease at multiple levels has the potential to meaningfully reduce health disparities and promote health equity.

References

1. Colby SL, Ortman JM. Projections of the size and composition of the U.S. population: 2014 to 2060. *Current Population Reports*. Washington, DC: U.S. Census Bureau; 2014, pp. P25-1143.
2. Braveman P. Health disparities and health equity: Concepts and measurement. *Ann Rev Public Health*. 2006;27:167–94.
3. Whitehead M. The concepts and principles of equity and health. *Int J Health Serv*. 1992;22:429–45.
4. Humes K, Jones N, Ramirez R. Overview of race and Hispanic origin: 2010. 2011.
5. Foster MW, Sharp RR. Beyond race: Towards a whole-genome perspective on human populations and genetic variation. *Nat Rev Genet*. 2004;5:790–6.
6. Kittles RA, Weiss KM.Race, ancestry, and genes: Implications for defining disease risk. *Annu Rev Genomics Hum Genet*. 2003;4:33–67.
7. Shiels MS, Chernyavskiy P, Anderson WF, et al. Trends in premature mortality in the USA by sex, race, and ethnicity from 1999 to 2014: An analysis of death certificate data. *Lancet*. 2017;389:1043–54.
8. Division of Reproductive Health and National Center for Chronic Disease Prevention and Health Promotion. Infant Mortality. 2016; 2018.
9. Martin JA, Hamilton BE, Osterman MJK, Driscoll AK, Drake P, Division of vital statistics. Births: Final data for 2016. *Natl Vital Stat Rep*. 2018;67:1–55.
10. US Department of Health and Human Services, Centers for Disease Control and Prevention, National Center for HIV SaTPN and Division of STD/HIV Prevention. Sexually Transmitted Disease Morbidity for selected STDs by age, race/ethnicity and gender 1996–2014.
11. Division of HIV/AIDS Prevention, National Center for HIV/AIDS VH, STD, and TB Prevention, and Centers for Disease Control and Prevention. HIV/AIDS Risk by Racial/Ethnic Groups. 2017; 2018.
12. Centers for Disease Control and Prevention (CDC) and National Center for Health Statistics (NCHS). National Health and Nutrition Examination Survey Data. 2013–2016.
13. Hofmeister MG, Rosenthal EM, Barker LK, et al. Estimating prevalence of hepatitis C virus infection in the United States, 2013–2016. *Hepatology*. 2019;69:1020–31.
14. Centers for Disease Control and Prevention and National Vital Statistics System. Table 4.5: Number and rate of hepatitis C-related deaths, by demographic characteristic and year—United States, 2012–2016. 2012–2016.
15. Benjamin EJ, Virani SS, Callaway CW, et al. Heart disease and stroke statistics—2018 update: A report from the American Heart Association. *Circulation*. 2018;137:e67–492.
16. Safford MM, Brown TM, Muntner P, et al. Association of race and sex with risk of incident acute coronary heart disease events. *JAMA*. 2012;308:1768–74.
17. U.S. Cancer Statistics Working Group. U.S. Cancer Statistics Data Visualizations Tool, based on November 2017 submission data (1999–2015). 2018.
18. Muntner P, Carey RM, Gidding S, et al. Potential US population impact of the 2017 ACC/AHA high blood pressure guideline. *Circulation*. 2018;137:109–18.
19. Centers for Disease Control and Prevention. National Diabetes Statistical Report, 2017. 2017.
20. Shah BR, Victor JC, Chiu M, et al. Cardiovascular complications and mortality after diabetes diagnosis for South Asian and Chinese patients: A population-based cohort study. *Diabetes Care*. 2013;36:2670–6.
21. Lanting LC, Joung IMA, Mackenbach JP, Lamberts SWJ, Bootsma AH. Ethnic differences in mortality, end-stage complications, and quality of care among diabetic patients: A review. *Diabetes Care*. 2005;28:2280–8.
22. Young BA, Maynard C, Boyko EJ. Racial differences in diabetic nephropathy, cardiovascular disease, and mortality in a national population of veterans. *Diabetes Care*. 2003;26:2392–9.
23. United States Renal Data System. Volume 1: Chronic Kidney Disease in the United States. 2018.
24. Nicholas SB, Kalantar-Zadeh K, Norris KC. Racial disparities in kidney disease outcomes. *Semin Nephrol*. 2013;33:409–15.
25. Centers for Disease Control and Prevention. Table 4-1. Current asthma prevalence percent by age, United States: National Health Interview Survey, 2015. 2015; 2018.
26. Centers for Disease Control and Prevention. Table A-2. Selected respiratory diseases among adults aged 18 and over, by selected characteristics: United States, 2016. 2016; 2018.
27. Mayeda ER, Glymour MM, Quesenberry CP, Whitmer RA. Inequalities in dementia incidence between six racial and ethnic groups over 14 years. *Alzheimers Dement*. 2016;12:216–24.
28. Asnaani A, Richey JA, Dimaite R, Hinton DE, Hofmann SG. A cross-ethnic comparison of lifetime prevalence rates of anxiety disorders. *J Nerv Ment Dis*. 2010;198:551–5.
29. Brody DJ, Pratt LA, Hughes J. Prevalence of depression among adults aged 20 and over: United States, 2013–2016. *NCHS Data Brief, no 303*. 2018.
30. González HM, Tarraf W, Whitfield KE, Vega WA. The epidemiology of major depression and ethnicity in the United States. *J Psychiatr Res*. 2010;44:1043–51.
31. Olbert CM, Nagendra A, Buck B. Meta-analysis of Black vs. White racial disparity in schizophrenia diagnosis in the United States: Do structured assessments attenuate racial disparities? *J Abnorm Psychol*. 2018;127:104–15.
32. Minsky S, Vega W, Miskimen T, Gara M, Escobar J. Diagnostic patterns in Latino, African American, and European American psychiatric patients. *Arch Gen Psychiatry*. 2003;60:637–44.
33. Roberts AL, Gilman SE, Breslau J, Breslau N, Koenen KC. Race/ethnic differences in exposure to traumatic events, development of post-traumatic stress disorder, and treatment-seeking for post-traumatic stress disorder in the United States. *Psychol Med*. 2011;41:71–83.
34. Rosinger A, Herrick K, Gahche J, Park S. Sugar-sweetened beverage consumption among U.S. adults, 2011–2014. *NCHS Data Brief*. 2017;(270):1–8.
35. Rosinger A, Herrick K, Gahche J, Park S. Sugar-sweetened beverage consumption among U.S. youth, 2011–2014. *NCHS Data Brief*. 2017;(271):1–8.
36. Lee-Kwan SH, Moore LV, Blanck HM, Harris DM, Galuska D. Disparities in state-specific adult fruit and vegetable consumption—United States, 2015. *MMWR Morb Mortal Wkly Rep*. 2017;66.
37. Centers for Disease Control and Prevention. 1995–2017 High School Youth Risk Behavior Survey Data.
38. Benjamin Emelia J, Muntner P, Alonso A, et al. Heart disease and stroke statistics—2019 Update: A report from the American Heart Association. *Circulation*. 2019;139:e56–66.
39. Substance Abuse and Mental Health Services Administration (SAMHSA). National Survey on Drug Use and Health. *Substance Abuse and Mental Health Services Administration (SAMHSA)'s public online data analysis system (PDAS)*. 2017; 2018.

40. Office on Smoking and Health, National Center for Chronic Disease Prevention and Health Promotion and Prevention. Burden of tobacco use in the US. 2019; 2018.
41. Arrazola RA, Singh T, Corey CG, et al. Tobacco use among middle and high school students—United States, 2011-2014. *Morb Mortal Wkly Rep*. 2015;64:381–5.
42. Hales CM, Fryar CD, Carroll MD, Freedman DS, Aoki Y, Ogden CL. Differences in obesity prevalence by demographic characteristics and urbanization level among adults in the united states, 2013–2016. *JAMA*. 2018;319:2419–29.
43. Skinner AC, Perrin EM, Skelton JA. Prevalence of obesity and severe obesity in US children, 1999–2014. *Obesity (Silver Spring, Md)*. 2016;24:1116–23.
44. Ryan CL and Bauma K. Educational Attainment in the United States: 2015. March 2016.
45. Profile: Native Hawaiians/Pacific Islanders.
46. Profile: American Indian/Alaska Native.
47. Braveman PA, Cubbin C, Egerter S, Williams DR, Pamuk E. Socioeconomic disparities in health in the United States: What the patterns tell us. *Am J Public Health*. 2010;100(Suppl 1):S186–96.
48. Eliminating Racial/Ethnic Disparities in Health Care: What are the Options? October 2008.
49. Crimmins EM, Kim JK, Alley DE, Karlamangla A, Seeman T. Hispanic paradox in biological risk profiles. *Am J Public Health*. 2007;97:1305–10.
50. Thomas J, Thomas DJ, Pearson T, Klag M, Mead L. Cardiovascular disease in African American and white physicians: The Meharry cohort and Meharry-Hopkins cohort studies. *J Health Care Poor Underserved*. 1997;8:270–83; discussion 284.
51. Williams DR, Mohammed SA, Leavell J, Collins C. Race, socioeconomic status, and health: Complexities, ongoing challenges, and research opportunities. *Ann N Y Acad Sci*. 2010;1186:69–101.
52. Kaufman JS, Cooper RS, McGee DL. Socioeconomic status and health in blacks and whites: The problem of residual confounding and the resiliency of race. *Epidemiology*. 1997;8:621–8.
53. Parker K, Horowitz J, Mahl B. On Views of Race and Inequality, Blacks and Whites are Worlds Apart.
54. Acevedo-Garcia D, Osypuk TL, McArdle N, Williams DR. Toward a policy-relevant analysis of geographic and racial/ethnic disparities in child health. *Health Aff (Millwood)*. 2008;27:321–33.
55. Osypuk TL, Galea S, McArdle N, Acevedo-Garcia D. Quantifying separate and unequal: Racial-ethnic distributions of neighborhood poverty in metropolitan America. *Urban Aff Rev Thousand Oaks Calif*. 2009;45:25–65.
56. Williams DR, Mohammed SA. Discrimination and racial disparities in health: Evidence and needed research. *J Behav Med*. 2009;32:20–47.
57. Diez Roux AV, Mujahid MS, Hirsch JA, Moore K, Moore LV. The Impact of neighborhoods on CV risk. *Global Heart*. 2016;11:353–63.
58. Mair C, Diez Roux AV, Galea S. Are neighbourhood characteristics associated with depressive symptoms? A review of evidence. *J Epidemiol Community Health*. 2008;62:940–6, 8 p following 946.
59. Sallis JF, Glanz K. Physical activity and food environments: Solutions to the obesity epidemic. *Milbank Q*. 2009;87:123–54.
60. Williams DR, Collins C. Racial residential segregation: A fundamental cause of racial disparities in health. *Public Health Rep*. 2001;116:404–16.
61. Fischer MJ, Tienda M. Redrawing spatial color lines: Hispanic metropolitan dispersal, segregation, and economic opportunity. In: Tienda M, Mitchell F, eds. *Hispanics and the Future of America*. Washington, DC: The National Academies Press; 2006, pp. 100–37.
62. Iceland J, Nelson KA. Hispanic segregation in metropolitan America: Exploring the multiple forms of spatial assimilation. *Am Sociol Rev*. 2008;73:741–65.
63. Iceland J, Weinberg D, Hughes L. The residential segregation of detailed Hispanic and Asian groups in the United States: 1980–2010.
64. Kershaw KN, Albrecht SS. Racial/ethnic residential segregation and cardiovascular disease risk. *Curr Cardiovasc Risk Rep*. 2015;9(3):10.
65. Landrine H, Corral I, Lee JGL, Efird JT, Hall MB, Bess JJ. Residential segregation and racial cancer disparities: A systematic review. *J Racial Ethn Health Disparities*. 2017;4:1195–205.
66. Salow AD, Pool LR, Grobman WA, Kershaw KN. Associations of neighborhood-level racial residential segregation with adverse pregnancy outcomes. *Am J Obstet Gynecol*. 2018;218:351.e1-351.e7.
67. Dubowitz T, Subramanian SV, Acevedo-Garcia D, Osypuk TL, Peterson KE. Individual and neighborhood differences in diet among low-income foreign and U.S.-born women. *Womens Health Issues*. 2008;18:181–90.
68. Park Y, Neckerman K, Quinn J, Weiss C, Jacobson J, Rundle A. Neighbourhood immigrant acculturation and diet among Hispanic female residents of New York City. *Public Health Nutr*. 2011;14:1593–600.
69. Osypuk TL, Diez Roux AV, Hadley C, Kandula NR. Are immigrant enclaves healthy places to live? The multi-ethnic study of atherosclerosis. *Soc Sci Med*. 2009;69:110–20.
70. Osypuk TL, Bates LM, Acevedo-Garcia D. Another Mexican birthweight paradox? The role of residential enclaves and neighborhood poverty in the birthweight of Mexican-origin infants. *Soc Sci Med*. 2010;70:550–60.
71. Viruell-Fuentes EA, Ponce NA, Alegria M. Neighborhood context and hypertension outcomes among Latinos in Chicago. *J Immigr Minor Health*. 2012;14:959–67.
72. Lee JG, Henriksen L, Rose SW, Moreland-Russell S, Ribisl KM. A systematic review of neighborhood disparities in point-of-sale tobacco marketing. *Am J Public Health*. 2015;105:e8–18.
73. Lovasi GS, Hutson MA, Guerra M, Neckerman KM. Built environments and obesity in disadvantaged populations. *Epidemiol Rev*. 2009;31:7–20.
74. Powell LM, Wada R, Kumanyika SK. Racial/ethnic and income disparities in child and adolescent exposure to food and beverage television ads across the U.S. media markets. *Health Place*. 2014;29:124–31.
75. Grigsby-Toussaint DS, Zenk SN, Odoms-Young A, Ruggiero L, Moise I. Availability of commonly consumed and culturally specific fruits and vegetables in African-American and Latino neighborhoods. *J Am Die Assoc*. 2010;110:746–52.
76. Evenson KR, Sarmiento OL, Ayala GX. Acculturation and physical activity among North Carolina Latina immigrants. *Soc Sci Med*. 2004;59(12):2509–22.
77. Qato DM, Zenk S, Wilder J, Harrington R, Gaskin D, Alexander GC. The availability of pharmacies in the United States: 2007–2015. *PLoS One*. 2017;12:e0183172.
78. Qato DM, Daviglus ML, Wilder J, Lee T, Qato D, Lambert B. 'Pharmacy deserts' are prevalent in Chicago's predominantly minority communities, raising medication access concerns. *Health Aff (Millwood)*. 2014;33:1958–65.
79. Epel ES, Lin J, Wilhelm FH, et al. Cell aging in relation to stress arousal and cardiovascular disease risk factors. *Psychoneuroendocrinology*. 2006;31:277–87.
80. Seeman TE, Crimmins E, Huang MH, et al. Cumulative biological risk and socio-economic differences in mortality: MacArthur studies of successful aging. *Soc Sci Med*. 2004;58:1985–97.
81. Sims M, Diez-Roux AV, Gebreab SY, et al. Perceived discrimination is associated with health behaviours among African-Americans in the Jackson Heart Study. *J Epidemiol Community Health*. 2016;70: 187–94.
82. Cain LR, Glover L, Young B, Sims M. Goal-striving stress is associated with chronic kidney disease among participants in the Jackson Heart Study. *J Racial Ethn Health Disparities*. 2019;6:64–9.
83. Sellers SL, Neighbors HW, Zhang R, Jackson JS. The impact of goal-striving stress on physical health of white Americans, African Americans, and Caribbean blacks. *Ethn Dis*. 2012;22:21–8.
84. Neighbors HW, Sellers SL, Zhang R, Jackson JS. Goal-striving stress and racial differences in mental health. *Race Soc Prob*. 2011;3:51–62.
85. Maldonado A, Preciado A, Buchanan M, Pulvers K, Romero D, D'Anna-Hernandez K. Acculturative stress, mental health symptoms, and the role of salivary inflammatory markers among a Latino sample. *Cultur Divers Ethnic Minor Psychol*. 2018;24:277–83.
86. Preciado A, D'Anna-Hernandez K. Acculturative stress is associated with trajectory of anxiety symptoms during pregnancy in Mexican-American women. *J Anxiety Disord*. 2017;48:28–35.
87. Kwan MY, Gordon KH, Minnich AM. An examination of the relationships between acculturative stress, perceived discrimination, and eating disorder symptoms among ethnic minority college students. *Eat Behav*. 2018;28:25–31.
88. Kroon Van Diest AM, Tartakovsky M, Stachon C, Pettit JW, Perez M. The relationship between acculturative stress and eating disorder symptoms: Is it unique from general life stress? *J Behav Med*. 2014;37: 445–57.
89. Lee CS, Colby SM, Rohsenow DJ, Lopez SR, Hernandez L, Caetano R. Acculturation stress and drinking problems among urban heavy drinking Latinos in the Northeast. *J Ethn Subst Abuse*. 2013;12: 308–20.

90. Conn BM, Ejesi K, Foster DW. Acculturative stress as a moderator of the effect of drinking motives on alcohol use and problems among young adults. *Addict Behav*. 2017;75:85–94.

91. Garcia AF, Wilborn K, Mangold DL. The cortisol awakening response mediates the relationship between acculturative stress and self-reported health in Mexican Americans. *Ann Behav Med*. 2017;51:787–98.

92. Fryar CD, Ostchega Y, Hales CM, Zhang G, Kruszon-Moran D. Hypertension prevalence and control among adults: United States, 2015–2016. *NCHS Data Brief*. 2017:1–8.

93. Davidson JA, Kannel WB, Lopez-Candales A, et al. Avoiding the looming Latino/Hispanic cardiovascular health crisis: A call to action. *Ethn Dis*. 2007;17:568–73.

94. Saydah S, Cowie C, Eberhardt MS, De Rekeneire N, Narayan KM. Race and ethnic differences in glycemic control among adults with diagnosed diabetes in the United States. *Ethn Dis*. 2007;17:529–35.

95. Krogstad JM, Stepler R, Lopez MH. English proficiency on the rise among Latinos. Latino News Briefs; 2015.

96. Julliard K, Vivar J, Delgado C, Cruz E, Kabak J, Sabers H. What Latina patients don't tell their doctors: A qualitative study. *Ann Fam Med*. 2008;6:543–9.

97. Wharam JF, Zhang F, Eggleston EM, Lu CY, Soumerai S, Ross-Degnan D. Diabetes outpatient care and acute complications before and after high-deductible insurance enrollment: A natural experiment for translation in diabetes (NEXT-D) study. *JAMA Intern Med*. 2017;177:358–68.

98. Wharam JF, Zhang F, Wallace J, et al. Vulnerable and less vulnerable women in high-deductible health plans experienced delayed breast cancer care. *Health Aff (Millwood)*. 2019;38:408–15.

99. Cooper R, Rotimi C, Ataman S, et al. The prevalence of hypertension in seven populations of west African origin. *Am J Public Health*. 1997;87:160–8.

100. Sempos CT, Bild DE, Manolio TA. Overview of the Jackson Heart Study: A study of cardiovascular diseases in African American men and women. *Am J Med Sci*. 1999;317:142–6.

101. Wang X, Auchincloss AH, Barber S, et al. Neighborhood social environment as risk factors to health behavior among African Americans: The Jackson Heart Study. *Health Place*. 2017;45:199–207.

102. Gebreab SY, Diez Roux AV, Brenner AB, et al. The impact of life-course socioeconomic position on cardiovascular disease events in African Americans: The Jackson Heart Study. *J Am Heart Assoc*. 2015;4:e001553.

103. Ennis S, Rios-Vargas M, Albert N. The Hispanic Population: 2010. 2011.

104. Sorlie PD, Aviles-Santa LM, Wassertheil-Smoller S, et al. Design and implementation of the Hispanic Community Health Study/Study of Latinos. *Ann Epidemiol*. 2010;20:629–41.

105. Schneiderman N, Llabre M, Cowie CC, et al. Prevalence of diabetes among Hispanics/Latinos from diverse backgrounds: The Hispanic Community Health Study/Study of Latinos (HCHS/SOL). *Diabetes Care*. 2014;37:2233–9.

106. Daviglus ML, Talavera GA, Aviles-Santa ML, et al. Prevalence of major cardiovascular risk factors and cardiovascular diseases among Hispanic/Latino individuals of diverse backgrounds in the United States. *JAMA*. 2012;308:1775–84.

107. Hummer RA, Powers DA, Pullum SG, Gossman GL, Frisbie WP. Paradox found (again): Infant mortality among the Mexican-origin population in the United States. *Demography*. 2007;44:441–57.

108. Calzada EJ, Sales A. Depression among Mexican-origin mothers: Exploring the immigrant paradox. *Cultur Divers Ethnic Minor Psychol*. 2019;25(2):288–98.

109. Alarcon RD, Parekh A, Wainberg ML, Duarte CS, Araya R, Oquendo MA. Hispanic immigrants in the USA: Social and mental health perspectives. *Lancet Psychiatry*. 2016;3:860–70.

110. Pinn VW, Roth C, Bates AC, Wagner R, Jarema K. Monitoring Adherence to the NIH Policy on the Inclusion of Women and Minorities as Subjects in Clinical Research (Comprehensive Report: Fiscal Year 2007 and 2008 Tracking Data). 2009.

111. Corbie-Smith G, Thomas SB, Williams MV, Moody-Ayers S. Attitudes and beliefs of African Americans toward participation in medical research. *J Gen Intern Med*. 1999;14:537–46.

112. Barrett NJ, Ingraham KL, Vann Hawkins T, Moorman PG. Engaging African Americans in research: The recruiter's perspective. *Ethn Dis*. 2017;27:453–62.

113. Martinez IL, Carter-Pokras O, Brown PB. Addressing the challenges of Latino health research: Participatory approaches in an emergent urban community. *J Natl Med Assoc*. 2009;101:908–14.

114. Rosal MC, White MJ, Borg A, et al. Translational research at community health centers: Challenges and successes in recruiting and retaining low-income Latino patients with type 2 diabetes into a randomized clinical trial. *Diabetes Educ*. 2010;36:733–49.

115. Yancey AK, Ortega AN, Kumanyika SK. Effective recruitment and retention of minority research participants. *Annu Rev Public Health*. 2006;27:1–28.

116. Taylor HA, Henderson F, Abbasi A, Clifford G. Cardiovascular disease in African Americans: Innovative community engagement for research recruitment and impact. *Am J Kidney Dis*. 2018;72:S43–6.

117. Mueller M, Purnell TS, Mensah GA, Cooper LA. Reducing racial and ethnic disparities in hypertension prevention and control: What will it take to translate research into practice and policy? *Am J Hypertens*. 2015;28:699–716.

118. Rudolph L, Caplan J, Ben-Moshe K, Dillon L. Health in All Policies: A Guide for State and Local Governments. 2013.

119. National Research Council Committee on Health Impact A. The National Academies Collection: Reports funded by National Institutes of Health *Improving Health in the United States: The Role of Health Impact Assessment*. Washington, DC: National Academies Press, National Academy of Sciences; 2011.

120. Towe VL, Leviton L, Chandra A, Sloan JC, Tait M, Orleans T. Cross-sector collaborations and partnerships: Essential ingredients to help shape health and well-being. *Health Aff (Millwood)*. 2016;35:1964–9.

CHAPTER 31

Connecting Neighborhoods and Health: Methodological Approaches and Substantive Evidence

Dustin T. Duncan • Yazan A. Al-Ajlouni • William C. Goedel • Basile Chaix

NEIGHBORHOODS AND HEALTH: AN INTRODUCTION

The neighborhoods where we live, work, shop, and socialize can influence our health outcomes and health behaviors. In this chapter, we will discuss evidence suggesting that neighborhoods can influence a wide range of health outcomes and health behaviors. Here, as Duncan and Kawachi do in their recent textbook on the topic, we defined "neighborhoods" as "geographical places that can have social and cultural meaning to residents and nonresidents alike and are subdivisions of large places" (p. 1).[1] The purpose of the current chapter is to provide an overview of select methodological and substantive areas in the field of neighborhoods and health research.

We suspect that neighborhoods emerged as an important area of interest for population health research and policies because historical and contemporary research focused on individual-level factors does not fully explain population health outcomes and health disparities. With that said, the field of neighborhoods and health has been in existence for many decades. Louis Rene Villermé, for example, created maps that showed socioeconomic disparities by neighborhood and mortality in Paris as early as 1830. Another one of the earliest (and oft-discussed) investigations of neighborhoods and health is that of John Snow. In 1854, Snow drew a dot map of cases of and deaths from cholera, which identified the source of cholera as the infamous Broad Street pump in the Soho neighborhood in London. This was antithetical to the predominant miasma theory of the time, which suggested that cholera was spread through "bad air." The early research of Snow and Villermé demonstrates that neighborhood health has always been a critical, albeit under-researched area of public health. Not only do neighborhoods serve as the basis of daily life, but they also provide opportunities for important public health interventions. Snow's findings helped foster the eventual consensus that infectious disease outbreaks *are* traceable, and must be targeted at their physical source. Furthermore, Villermé's data on neighborhood—specific mortality rates provided a basis for understanding the syndemic nature of concurrent health outcomes. These historical examples are just two of many that predate the first textbook on the field, published in 2003.[2] Since its publication, there has been an ever-growing number of studies in epidemiology and public health that focus on neighborhoods.

There is a wide range of neighborhood characteristics one can study, including two broad categories: the *built environment* and the *social environment*. The built environment includes all types of physical elements of neighborhood such as access to and attractiveness of destinations (such as parks and stores) and community design features. The location of the Broad Street pump would be an example of a built environment characteristic. The social environment—on the other hand—includes features such as spatial stigma, socioeconomic disadvantage, the social networks of neighbors who can provide social support, collective efficacy, and neighborhood safety.

When connecting built and social environmental characteristics of neighborhoods to health outcomes and health behaviors, conceptual models are often created, which are often referred to as directed acyclic graphs (DAGs) in epidemiology. Figure 31-1 illustrates a conceptual model, with the putative mediator being stress. In this simple figure, neighborhood exposures (i.e., neighborhood stressors) are linked to our sleep health outcome. In particular, individuals exposed to neighborhood stressors experience the highlighted sleep health outcomes explained in the figure, including sleep quality, sleep duration, and sleep problems. Several epidemiological study designs can be employed when examining associations between neighborhoods and health, which can be represented in conceptual models. Because the vast majority of studies connecting neighborhoods to health outcomes rely on cross-sectional designs, many DAGs on neighborhoods to health are often constructed for cross-sectional analyses. For instance, surveys are often employed to measure perceptions of a neighborhood characteristic (such as neighborhood safety) and a health behavior (sleep duration) at the same point in time and as such all analyses are cross-sectional, given the structure of the data. Increasingly, though, longitudinal prospective study designs are being conducted in the neighborhoods and health studies. Examples of complementary designs and methods connecting neighborhoods to health outcomes include examination of a natural experiment as well as use of agent-based models (see Schmidt et al.[3] and Heaton et al4 for further details on these methods).

Now that we have provided a definition of neighborhoods and health as a field and additional background, we will turn to methodological approaches to study neighborhoods. In the next section of the chapter specifically, we discuss the range of quantitative and qualitative methods to study neighborhoods and health, with examples of each method.

QUANTITATIVE AND QUALITATIVE METHODS TO STUDY NEIGHBORHOODS AND HEALTH

It probably comes as no surprise that neighborhoods and health research depends greatly on the ability to measure specific neighborhood exposures—whether it be the built environment or the social environment—before relating these exposures to health outcomes and health behaviors. While the exact neighborhood exposures and health outcomes vary according to the focus of a given study, increased focus on neighborhoods in public health and epidemiology research in tandem with technological advancements have paved the way for the emergence of numerous advanced tools that can be used to measure neighborhood-level variables in research.

Neighborhood health research may use *quantitative methods* (e.g., mathematical and statistical tools to present data and establish

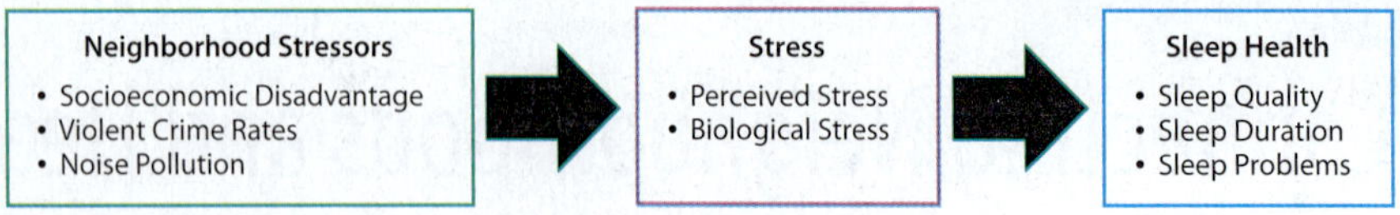

Neighborhood Stressors	→	Stress	→	Sleep Health
• Socioeconomic Disadvantage • Violent Crime Rates • Noise Pollution		• Perceived Stress • Biological Stress		• Sleep Quality • Sleep Duration • Sleep Problems

FIGURE 31-1. Conceptual framework for the influence of neighborhood stressors on sleep health.

TABLE 31-1 QUANTITATIVE AND QUALITATIVE METHODS FOR MEASURING DIFFERENT NEIGHBORHOOD EXPOSURES IN NEIGHBORHOOD HEALTH RESEARCH

Data Collection Methods for Studying Neighborhoods

Quantitative Methods	Qualitative Methods
Self-reported survey	Interviews
Systematic field observations (SFO)	Focus groups
Geographic information systems (GIS)	Ethnographic observations
Web-based geospatial data	Photovoice
Social media and Internet data	Participatory photomapping
Geospatial technologies	Go-along interviews

correlations between variables) or *qualitative methods* (e.g., explanations derived from interviews, focus groups, and observations). Table 31-1 summarizes quantitative and qualitative methods for studying neighborhoods. Objective characteristics such as counts, rates, or density can be easily captured via quantitative measure, whereas qualitative approaches draw conclusions based on information obtained via interviews or observations. There is significant heterogeneity in methodologic approaches even within quantitative and qualitative methods. Each method serves specific purposes that are important in answering different research questions. In some circumstances, one methodological approach might be more appropriate than another.[5] Some emerging research has combined both methods, which is often referred to as "mixed-methods" research.[6] Qualitative methods are useful in generating hypotheses that can be subsequently tested through quantitative data collections and statistical analyses, and are also useful to provide refined interpretations for the statistical associations found through quantitative analysis. This part of the chapter will review quantitative and qualitative methods as they apply to neighborhood health effects research, providing examples where applicable.

QUANTITATIVE METHODS

The number of quantitative studies on neighborhoods and health outweigh the number of qualitative studies on the topic. As discussed earlier, quantitative methods focus on quantifying features and attributes of neighborhoods in order to examine how these features are related to health outcomes in cross-sectional or longitudinal analyses. The most commonly used measurement approaches in neighborhood health research are self-report measures, systematic field observation, as well as geographic information systems and web-based geospatial data. Other approaches that are particularly suitable to neighborhood research, ranging from commonplace approaches that use data from population censuses to characterize the demographic and socioeconomic composition of a neighborhood to more novel methods that leverage social media platforms to characterize public opinion in a neighborhood.

Self-Report Measures

A self-report measure relies on the use of a survey or a questionnaire, in which participants of a study read an item and select a response option. In certain cases free text responses are allowed, which can later be coded and grouped. Items employed in self-report measures can vary, including direct questions, extent of agreement to a specific statement, and expression of opinion regarding a given event. For example, self-report surveys have been utilized in neighborhood health research to measure both perceived physical features (e.g., neighborhood walkability, aesthetics, access to healthy food) and perceived social features (e.g., social cohesion, neighborhood safety). A variety of tools have been developed to collect self-reported data from participants.

An example of self-reported tools for measuring neighborhood social factors include the Project on Human Development in Chicago Neighborhoods (PHDCN), which is a population-based study based in Chicago that aimed to understand the causes and pathways of juvenile delinquency, adult crime, substance abuse, and violence. In this study, informal social control (e.g., the reactions of individuals and groups that bring about conformity to norms and laws) was measured using a five-item Likert-type scale, asking residents about the likelihood that their neighbors could be counted on to intervene in various ways in case of problems in the neighborhood. In another study, the NYC Low-Income Housing, Neighborhoods, and Health Study, neighborhood spatial stigma was measured through the following item: "Overall, what is the reputation of your neighborhood?"[7]

Self-reported surveys have been administered using a variety of methods. Some of these methods, such as pen-and-paper surveys, are considered traditional and have been in use since the earliest studies of neighborhood effects on health. However, other methods to administer surveys have been introduced recently, especially with the emergence of portable technological devices. These include telephone questionnaires, tablets, face-to-face computer-assisted interview (CAPI), and audio computer-assisted self-interview (ACASI) delivered via a desktop computer. For example, telephone-based neighborhood surveys have been conducted, as was done in the Multi-Ethnic Study of Atherosclerosis (MESA) on a separate sample of residents in the neighborhoods of the MESA participants in order to construct neighborhood scales through the ecometric approach corrected from same-source bias.[8] This so-called ecometric approach allows researchers to derive neighborhood-level variables by aggregating the perceptions of neighborhood residents for dimensions for which no administrative or GIS database are available.

While self-reported measures are often reported in a one-time sitting, capturing data on neighborhood environments and health behaviors and outcomes in real-time from participants as they experience their daily lives can allow researchers to minimize certain limitations, such as recall bias. To serve such a purpose, an approach referred to as "ecological momentary assessment" (or EMA) has been utilized in previous research. EMA allows researchers to assess neighborhood conditions, relevant health-related behavior, affect and mood or mental well-being in real-time using text messages or dedicated applications, capturing measurements as they are experienced by participants in their daily lives. In a recent EMA study where participants completed brief smartphone surveys of current negative affect and stressor exposure, severity, and recency, five times daily for 14 days, individuals who reported greater neighborhood violence rated their stressors as more severe.[9] In addition, individuals in this EMA study rating their neighborhood lower in safety or aesthetic quality, or higher in violence, had greater negative affect following stressors.[9]

Systematic Field Observation

Another method to measure neighborhood characteristics is Systematic Field Observation (SFO), which we can categorize into two main methods: (1) sending trained auditors into neighborhoods with a pen and clipboard and, more recently (2) capturing data from video-mounted vehicles.

The first method of SFO includes a series of manual assessments of neighborhood environments. This is usually conducted by trained neighborhood raters, in which a team of raters are sent to a neighborhood at a similar time point to rate characteristics of interest for the research on their presence and quality. SFO has been employed previously in research published in the literature, including measuring neighborhood-level features such as neighborhood disorder in a project that measured 196 census tracts in Chicago.[10,11] These neighborhood-level features were later linked to various health outcomes.[12]

The second method of SFO involves photographic assessments from vehicle-mounted cameras traveling through neighborhoods. This particular method has emerged long after SFO was first established, as it utilizes the use of technology that has developed greatly in the last two decades. The most prominent example of this is Google Street View, which is a technology featured in both Google Maps and Google Earth, providing panoramic views from positions on the street in different neighborhoods. This tool can reflect the characteristics of a neighborhood, allowing researchers to tour through a neighborhood virtually. This has been used previously in neighborhood health research, measuring features of the built environment and neighborhood disorder.[13–15] While this method is not useful in measuring certain neighborhood social factors (e.g., social cohesion, neighborhood safety),[16] neighborhood aesthetics and services proximity (e.g., restaurants, supermarkets, stores) can be reliably assessed with this approach. Several limitations exist to this approach. For example, parked vehicles and sidewalks can be obstacles to a correct assessment of neighborhood characteristics. Additionally, severe weathers (e.g., fog, snow) can influence the applicability of this approach depending on when the photos were taken.

Geographic Information Systems

A geographic information system (GIS) is a framework that allows for organizing layers of geographic information into visualizations, using maps and 3D scenes, and for spatial location analyses. GIS-based approaches have been increasingly used to evaluate neighborhood characteristics, as the databases provided by GIS can be linked to individual participants' health and socioeconomic data. Additionally, researchers can load a single GIS layer or a set of GIS layers to create a customized visualization of data on neighborhood characteristics. Examples of GIS layers include those with locations of park or local supermarkets and fast-food restaurants. This can allow for the measurement of proximity to specific services and/or density in a given neighborhood, as variables processed from GIS data can include both distance metrics and density metrics.[12] For example, Neckernman et al. used GIS measurements to demonstrate that poor neighborhoods had significantly fewer street trees, landmarked buildings, clean streets, and sidewalk cafes.[17] Similarly, these neighborhoods had higher rates of felony complaints, narcotics arrests, and vehicular crashed. Additionally, it is important to note that GIS metrics also allow for the application of a distance decay function; applying higher weights to parks or food outlets (for example) that are closer in proximity to a specific location (e.g., participants' homes). GIS methods are also used to operationalize definitions of neighborhoods of various shapes and sizes around participants' residences[18] and estimate the density and proximity of resources, including recreational facilities[19] and retail food locations.[20] In addition, satellite data (which is often integrated into a GIS system) can characterize urban form and air pollution, among other neighborhood features.

Web-Based Geospatial Data

Web-based geospatial tools (e.g., Walk Score, Park Score, State of Place, US EPA Smart Location, and Google Places) provide a valuable tool for researchers to uniquely quantify various neighborhood-level features. For instance, Walk Score, developed and launched in 2007 by Front Seat Management, allows users to receive numerical score assigned to any address they enter on their website (www.walkscore.com) that measure walkability. This allows researchers to easily quantify neighborhood walkability in various locations rather than undertaking complex calculations using GIS software. The data provided by Walk Score are completely free of charge, accessible to the public, and is being constantly corrected and updated. The way in which a Walk Score® is computed has been explained in detail previously.[21] WalkScore had been used previously in research linking neighborhood walkability to various health outcomes, including obesity and cardiovascular disease risk factors.[22]

Social Media and Internet Data

Analyses of social media and other Internet-sourced data have emerged as a valuable tool for researchers to measure neighborhood-level characteristics. This includes platforms such as Google, Instagram, and Twitter and we briefly discuss one platform in this chapter.

Instagram is a mobile application for photo and video capturing and sharing that has quickly emerged as a prominent social media platform in recent years. This platform allows users to instantaneously share life-moments through photo and video updates that can be associated with specific locations through "tagging." For example, previous research conducted in the United States used Instagram to provide empirical quantitative evidence for understanding dietary choices and nutritional challenges in "food deserts." It demonstrated that Instagram posts geotagged in food deserts indicate consumption of food high in fat, cholesterol, and sugar at a rate higher by 5–17% compared to nonfood desert areas.[23,24] Researchers, however, need to examine the potential measurement error associated with these methods, which could differentially affect the various neighborhoods or groups of people.

In addition to Instagram and other social media platforms, crowdsourcing is considered a valuable tool in measurement of exposures. Crowdsourcing is the practice of obtaining needed services, ideas, or content by soliciting contributions from a large group of people, especially from online communities.[12] This allows researchers to obtain data on neighborhoods, such as neighborhood food stores and neighborhood parks. As an example, Yelp is a free-for-all website with the purpose of helping people finding services in a neighborhood (e.g., restaurants, dry-cleaners, supermarkets) and reviewing them, with the option of including pictures as well. Consequently, this allowed Yelp to be utilized by researchers as a method of measuring features of neighborhoods and neighborhood amenities. Previous research assessed the validity and reliability of Yelp as a method for measuring neighborhood features. For example, Gomez-Lopez et al.[25] compared a Yelp-originating data set of full-line grocery stores in Detroit to a database available from Reference USA and the Detroit Food Map. The findings suggested that Yelp is an even more accurate representation when compared to the official database. Furthermore, Cawkwell et al.[26] used Yelp effectively to measure the number and distribution of hookah bars in New York State. Results showed that hookah bars are clustered near colleges and racial/ethnic minority neighborhoods and showed a significant increase in the number of Hookah bars compared to data published 3 years before. Crowdsourcing applications can also be used in studies where people indicate through the app whether they find a street pleasant, and then surfaces of variations of pleasantness of streets and cities are derived by smoothing the data of many respondents.

Geospatial Technologies

In recent years, geospatial technologies improved drastically. Improvements included the development of wearable devices that allow for the logging of real-time geospatial data. Researchers utilized these devices in neighborhood-health research, including devices like Microsoft's SenseCam[27] (usually worn around the neck), and Memoto (can be clipped into one's clothes). In addition, cameras in the form of glasses can be employed as a measurement tool in neighborhood health research. Perhaps the most two common types of such glasses are Google Glasses (which can also be connected to an image recognition technology; Google Goggles) and glasses often worn during extreme sports (e.g., PiviotHead). These devices allow for photographs of neighborhood conditions as they are experienced by their wearers to create measures similar to those derived from systematic field observation except when using wearable cameras, we can ensure that the participant has indeed been exposed to the neighborhood features shown in the image as they provide a "first-person point-of-view." However, the burden of work related to the manual processing of the image data generated with these tools remains the main barriers to their use. Wearable monitors of noise and air pollutants have also been used to document environmental exposures in residential neighborhoods, either directly worn by study participants or to feed crowdsourcing systems.[28,29]

SUMMARY OF QUANTITATIVE METHODS IN NEIGHBORHOODS AND HEALTH RESEARCH

Quantitative methods are considered appropriate in answering research questions that examine the extent of the effect of an exposure on a health outcome. They provide researchers with powerful tools to present their results and link different exposures and outcomes. However, quantitative methods often fail to underline the pathways under which a specific association occurs, or the "why" that may explain why such an association may occur. Answering such questions is extremely important, especially when attempting to propose intervention methods to address given health issues. This is where the role of qualitative methods comes in; qualitative methodologies can offer the advantage of grounding the exposure within the real-life context, providing insights on the detail and complexity of the true pathways that statistical associations are unable to capture.

QUALITATIVE METHODS

Qualitative methods focus on providing insights to the "qualities" and meanings that are not provided by quantitative measurement, and that cannot be deduced merely from statistical results. In the context of neighborhoods and health research, they predominantly intend to provide qualitative description of what a neighborhood is like, and how participants feel and act toward specific exposures of interest. Similar to quantitative measurements, many approaches and tools can be used in qualitative research. The most commonly used approaches are interviews, focus groups, and observations. Other approaches that are particularly suitable to neighborhood research include photovoice, participatory photomapping, and go-along interviews.

Interviews

Interviews are considered a major tool in qualitative research that involves participants responding to open-ended questions posed by researchers for the purpose of understanding the participants' own lived experiences. Interviews can range from structured set of questions to unstructured conversations between the participant and researcher. The most common form of interview in neighborhood health research is the semistructured interview. In this type of interview, the researcher usually has a predetermined set of topics or "themes" to tackle during the interview but allows for flexibility in the order of question and length of answers. This allows the conversation to be led by what the participant believes to be most relevant. Interview methods are used widely in public health research and neighborhood health research. For example, Clampet-Lundquist and colleagues[30] used interviews to study the dynamics of moving teenagers out of high-risk neighborhoods, showing how girls fare better than boys. Similarly, Keene and colleagues used interviews to study public housing demolition and relocation among older adults in Atlanta.[31] Twenty-five former public housing residents were interviewed, and their narratives were analyzed to focus on the loss of geographically rooted communities of kinship, support, and belonging that many participants, particularly those who have aged in place, attribute to their former developments.

Focus Groups

Another popular method in qualitative research is focus groups. Focus groups involve grouping 6–12 participants with a facilitator, where all participants engage in a group discussion regarding aspects of their neighborhood and their health, and the pathways in which they believe the cause-effect relationship takes place. They offer an advantage over individual interviews in which shared experiences are examined through a group conversation. In the context of neighborhoods and health research, focus groups, bringing participants from same neighborhood, can empower them to speak their minds regarding neighborhood concerns. However, several limitations regarding focus groups exist. This includes difficulty in operating the group, less ability to capture individual experiences in depth, and the requirement of careful attention to the events occurring during the time of focus group conduction. As an example, Frohlich et al. conducted focus groups ($n = 47$) to study neighborhoods and smoking habits among youth.[32] The focus groups ranged in length from 35 to 75 minutes, and included activities such as drawing the perceived territory of the neighborhood. The groups were comprised of boys and girls with a heterogeneity requested within each group (loners, groups of friends, etc.). The authors found that in neighborhoods where there was a high concentration of socioeconomic advantage, residents tended to more heavily discourage smoking, while the opposite was true for more disadvantaged communities.

Ethnographic Observations

Additionally, researchers can employ the ethnographic method of observation, in which researchers engage in daily life in a given neighborhood. While observation methods provide the advantage of capturing how residents interact in their environment firsthand, a major concern regarding this method is that the observer remains an individual who is not a natural resident of a given neighborhood, and thus they are not reflecting the experiences of residents in their assessments.[33] In addition, while this method is very time consuming, spending extended amounts of time in a neighborhood allows observers to develop relationships with residents of a neighborhood, aiding in an accurate reflection of the environment. In 1999, Mullings et al. published a book discussing the findings of observation methods employed in Harlem, New York City.[34] Observation by the team of researchers was used as a method to study the social context of reproduction in Central Harlem, specifically in relation to stress and resilience in the neighborhood.

Photovoice

The above-mentioned methods are categorized as common methods and are widely used across disciplines. Other qualitative methods, however, have been developed to better serve neighborhood health research. For example, photovoice is an approach that uses the aid of photographic content to go along with the interviews. More specifically, often, participants are given cameras to document their neighborhoods. The images and/or videos taken by participants are brought to focus groups (or individuals) and are used to navigate topics and issues of concern regarding neighborhoods. This method allows the participant to feel more connected to the research cause and provide richer material for focus groups and interviews. The photovoice methodology is considered an action-oriented tool: participants document their communities through photography and photonarratives and use these tools to engage in critical dialogue with policymakers and other agents of change.[35] For instance, Wang et al. used photovoice to study neighborhood violence. In this study, 41 youths and adults were recruited and were shown photographs from their neighborhood and were allowed to express their concerns about safety in their neighborhoods. Interestingly, the researchers included policymakers and community leaders in order to provide political will and support for implementing photovoice participants' policy and program recommendations.

Participatory Photomapping

Another technique, referred to as participatory photomapping, builds up on the photovoice methodology. In participatory photomapping, participants generate maps, photos, drawings, and narratives. These are then used to actively interpret one's experience, as presented to the researcher.[36] Dennis et al. employed participatory photomapping to examine the way place contributed to the health of the youth population in Madison, Wisconsin. Participants were instructed to do multiple tasks, including having them study, discuss, and document (e.g., photographs) their neighborhoods. They then engaged in a conversation with the researchers regarding the photographs they have obtained, generating narratives to be used in identifying common theme. GIS data was also used to map out the narratives and common themes identified.

Go-Along Interviews

The go-along interview, as the name suggests, is an interactive method of data collection that involves the researcher interviewing the participant as they walk through the spaces of interest in a participant's neighborhood. This method is considered to be well suited to neighborhood health research as it allows participants to be primed to think about how context affects their lives and provides contextual cues in neighborhoods to direct conversation with researchers.[37,38] Carpiano[37] notes that the go-along interview, as a hybrid of observation and interview, provides an opportunity for the researcher to be led through a "spatialized journey," and to learn "about the local area via the interplay of the respondent's ideas and the researcher's own experience of the respondent's environment" (p. 267). Carpiano et al. demonstrated how go-along interviews can be employed in neighborhood health research by providing the example of studying social capital in Milwaukee, Wisconsin neighborhoods. Another study used go-along interviews among 66 sexual and gender minority adolescents (14–19 years old) in their self-identified communities to explore perceived community attributes, including safe spaces, resources, and supports.[39] In this study, youth chose to walk, use public transportation, and drive to community locations, identifying numerous formal and informal resources in their communities.

SUMMARY OF QUALITATIVE METHODS IN NEIGHBORHOODS AND HEALTH RESEARCH

Qualitative methodologies to neighborhood health research have contributed to our understanding of connections between neighborhoods and health. It provided us with insights that would have not been possible using solely quantitative measurements. These contributions, in the context of neighborhood health research, include exploring the pathway(s) that connect neighborhood features to health outcomes, developing hypotheses, concepts, and theories. Additionally, it allowed for the examination of the meaning of place and the navigation of place (which guided quantitative methods as well). Most importantly, qualitative data gives authentic voice to residents' experiences and concern, which can be very effective when presenting data to policymakers and authority to advocate for action. To date however, quantitative and qualitative research have often remained separate, and researchers will need to develop projects better integrating the two components in order to maximize their interactions. We also note that one can use different study designs for the quantitative and qualitative measurement of neighborhoods for neighborhood health analyses. For example, researchers could collect and analyze longitudinal qualitative neighborhood health data.

NEIGHBORHOODS AND HEALTH: RESEARCH EVIDENCE

Research connecting neighborhoods and health has focused on a vast range of health outcomes, with the first step in such an investigation beginning with conducting a literature review and developing a conceptual model such as the model we discussed previously connecting neighborhoods and sleep health including sleep duration and several sleep problems.[40–43] Early research on neighborhoods and health, broadly speaking, focused on mortality and chronic diseases, such as cardiovascular disease.[1] The next generation of neighborhoods and health research focused on obesity and related cardiovascular risk factors such as hypertension.[44–48] Then, obesity and obesity risk factors (i.e., physical inactivity and diet) were studied, which are the most commonly studied outcomes in neighborhood health research.[49] However, neighborhoods factors have been studied in relation to a wide range of health-related outcomes, including sexually transmitted infections (e.g., HIV),[50–52] mental health (e.g., depression),[53,54] and substance use (e.g., marijuana use).[55]

Table 31-2 highlights several built and social environment characteristics of neighborhoods that are studied in neighborhood health research. In the next section of this chapter, we focus on four neighborhood characteristics that have been linked to health: built environment, food environment, socioeconomic disadvantage, collective efficacy, neighborhood safety, and spatial stigma. For each we describe the neighborhood characteristics (including how it was measured). We then describe one or more example studies linking the specific characteristic to health outcomes. We conclude with a brief discussion on pathways or mechanisms in the relationship of interest in each section, as well as recommendations for future research focusing on the specific domain. Our intent is to provide illustrative examples rather than conduct a comprehensive systematic review. Existing reviews are cited where applicable. We also recognize that we do not discuss all potential neighborhood factors, clinical services in neighborhoods as well as chemical exposures in neighborhoods, for example, are not discussed in this chapter.

Built Environment

The built environment can be considered a foundation for health and wellness. Its structure, whether it be neighborhood layout or availability of amenities, impacts decisions relating to individual and

TABLE 31-2 BUILT AND SOCIAL ENVIRONMENT CHARACTERISTICS OF NEIGHBORHOODS THAT ARE STUDIED IN NEIGHBORHOOD HEALTH RESEARCH

Neighborhood Features	
Physical Features	**Social Features**
Built environment (e.g., walkability, aesthetics)	Neighborhood safety (e.g., neighborhood crime rate, perceived safety)
Food environment (e.g., food desert, proximity to grocery stores)	Social cohesion (e.g., neighbors friendliness, care and comfort from neighbors)
	Spatial stigma (e.g., neighborhood reputation)
	Socioeconomic disadvantage (e.g., neighborhood poverty, neighborhood education level)

population health outcomes. The built environment includes the spatial distribution of urban features related to human activities (as measured with land-use and zoning), road infrastructure, pedestrian infrastructure, traffic, public transport, housing, population density, and various kinds of amenities (e.g., healthcare facilities, recreational and sport facilities). Taking physical activity as an example, a systematic review has highlighted the widespread use of GIS-derived measurements of walkability in urban and suburban neighborhoods and their associations with active transportation (e.g., walking and other modes of physical activity as transportation).[56] The International Physical Activity and Environment Network (IPEN) Adult Study, a multicountry cross-sectional study using a common design and consistent methods, used accelerometer, survey, and GIS data for 6181 participants from 12 cities in 8 countries (Belgium, Brazil, Czech Republic, Denmark, Mexico, New Zealand, the United Kingdom, and the United States) to examine the strength and shape of associations of 11 measures of park access (1 perceived and 10 GIS-based measures) with accelerometer-based moderate-to-vigorous physical activity (MVPA) and four types of self-reported leisure-time physical activity.[57] Results from this study demonstrate that more parks within 1 km from participants' homes were associated with greater leisure-time physical activity and accelerometer-measured MVPA. In addition, participants who lived in the neighborhoods with the most parks did on average 24 minutes more MVPA per week than those living in the neighborhoods with the lowest number of parks. Finally, perceived proximity to a park was positively associated with multiple leisure-time physical activity outcomes. Overall, a large body of research has found that the built environment influences physical activity, including both recreational and transport physical activity.[58] However, the association of these variables with weight-related measures among children and adults has been inconsistent.[56] Using a sample of 485 children in Germany, for example, Gose and colleagues[59] created a walkability index using the weighted *z*-scores of population density, road connectivity, and land-use mix. In multivariate analyses, this index was inversely associated with children's body mass index *z*-scores but did not predict change in BMI over 4 years. On the other hand, in a study among a sample of 49,770 children and adolescents in Massachusetts, Duncan and colleagues[60] found that children who lived in closest proximity to the nearest recreational open space had a lower BMI *z*-score compared to those living farthest away. In addition, living in neighborhoods with fewer recreational open spaces and less residential density, traffic density, sidewalk completeness, and intersection density were associated with an increase in BMI *z*-score over time. These discrepant findings may arise from the variation in the measures used to characterize neighborhoods as more or less walkable. At the time of publication, although there is strong evidence that high densities (of dwellings, services, etc.) make neighborhoods walkable, there is no clear consensus on which exact characteristics are most influential and these may vary across contexts (i.e., cities vs. suburbs, high-income vs. low-income settings).[61]

Food Environment

Another important factor to consider within the built environment category sometimes is the food environment. The distribution of food stores and inequities in access to healthy foods are of particular concern in many countries where the prevalence of obesity is high and increasing and the so-called "food environment" has been widely cited as a promising target for large-scale public health interventions addressing obesity and healthy eating.[62]

A literature review highlighted numerous studies reporting that greater access to grocery stores within neighborhoods was associated with better dietary intake and lower prevalence of obesity among adults.[63] Using cross-sectional data from a sample of 10,763 adult men and women participating in the Atherosclerosis Risk in Communities (ARIC) study, a cohort study designed to investigate the etiology and natural history of atherosclerosis, Morland et al.[64] found that the presence of a supermarket within one's residential neighborhood (defined as a census tract) was associated with a lower prevalence of obesity and overweight. In contrast, greater access to convenience stores and restaurants, including fast food, has been associated with less favorable diet quality and increased prevalence of obesity, although the findings are not consistent.[63] Using data from the Canadian Community Health Survey, Hollands and colleagues found that fast-food density had a positive association with body mass index, where the presence of an additional ten fast-food restaurants per capita corresponded to a weight increase of 1 kilogram.[65]

Much like studies assessing the built environment, the food environment is most often quantified using GIS approaches to provide spatial measures of access to supermarkets, convenience stores, and restaurants. A recent report from the Association of Public Health Epidemiologists in Ontario's Core Indicators Work Group has recommended three key indicators of the food environment: (1) the overall density of food outlets; (2) the relative density of less healthy food outlets; and (3) the proximity of the population to food outlets,[66] although there is significant variation in measures between studies.[67] In addition, there is significant variation in data sources used to characterize food environments, including self-report from neighborhood residents via questionnaire,[68] directories from local departments of health and agriculture,[64] in-situ audits of food stores,[69,70] and novel crowd sourced online sources (e.g., Yelp[71]).

Socioeconomic Disadvantage

Socioeconomic disadvantage (sometimes referred to as neighborhood deprivation) has been associated with a wide range of outcomes like physical activity, diet, obesity, blood pressure, etc. It is the most commonly assessed exposure in studies of neighborhood effects on health[72] and the one that has been historically first considered (i.e., most studies before 2000 focused on neighborhood socioeconomic status as an exposure). This is because it can be most easily measured using publicly available census data that is easily accessible to researchers. Messer and colleagues[73] have proposed a standardized neighborhood deprivation index for the United States to improve consistency across studies. In their initial study, the authors summarized 20 variables available in the federal census using principal components analysis and developed an index of neighborhood deprivation with eight variables, reflecting several community characteristics (e.g., education, employment, housing, occupation, poverty, racial composition, and residential stability). This index was associated with the prevalence of preterm birth and low birth weight across 19 cities and five suburban counties located in four states.

Neighborhood disadvantage is associated with risk of adverse birth outcomes[74] as well as poor health in childhood and adolescence,[75] and adulthood.[76] For example, Janevic and colleagues[77] used a linked hospital discharge and birth database for 517,994 singleton live births in New York City from 1998 and 2002 and examined the association between neighborhood disadvantage, preterm birth, and term low birth weight. The authors defined neighborhood deprivation using a composite index of variables derived from the 2000 decennial federal census and found that the odds of preterm birth for those living in neighborhoods with the highest quartile of deprivation were 1.24 times higher compared to those living in neighborhoods with the lowest quartile of deprivation.

Collective Efficacy

Self-efficacy has been defined as the belief in one's capabilities to organize and execute the courses of action required to manage prospective situations.[78] This concept has been extended to a community level in the form of collective efficacy, or the capacity of a group of people to organize and act as a whole to achieve a common goal.[79] Self-efficacy is crucial to the social environment of a neighborhood which can interact with physical characteristics. The level of collective efficacy can be measured via various proxy variables, such as numbers of vandalism or sports leagues.[80]

In their landmark study using data from the Project on Human Development in Chicago Neighborhoods (PHDCN), Sampson et al.[81] tested the hypothesis that social cohesion within a neighborhood, combined with willingness of residents to intervene on behalf of the common good of the neighborhood, was associated with reduced violence. A community survey was conducted among 8782 residents in all 343 neighborhood clusters to create aggregate resident-reported measures of informal social control and social cohesion (two components of their measure of collective efficacy) as well as measures of witnessed and experienced violence. The researchers applied the so-called ecometric approach alluded to in the first section of the chapter, in order to define such variables of the social environment. Using an adjusted multilevel model, the researchers found that their measure of collective efficacy was associated with lower rates of violence. Further studies have expanded on these findings. Also drawing from a longitudinal study of child and adolescent development conducted as part of PHDCN along with the aforementioned community survey of neighborhood characteristics, Browning and colleagues[82] found that, among a sample of youth in Chicago, the effects of exposure to life-threatening violence (e.g., witnessing a shooting or someone being attacked with a weapon) on the presence of internalizing and externalizing mental health symptoms were only significant for girls who resided in neighborhoods with lower collective efficacy.

Applying a similar ecometric aggregation technique to create a neighborhood-level measure of collective efficacy, Ahern and Galea[83] assessed the association between collective efficacy and major depression in the New York Social Environment Study, a study designed to examine the influence of neighborhood-level exposures on mental health and substance use among a representative sample of residents of 59 community districts in New York City. The authors found that collective efficacy was significantly associated with major depression among older adults (65 years and older), but not among younger adults. Echoing earlier findings from PHDCN and also drawing on data from the New York Social Environment Study, Ahern and colleagues[84] found that higher levels of collective efficacy were associated with a lower prevalence violent victimization. Several other studies have found associations of collective efficacy with a wide range of outcomes in diverse settings, including less-frequent sex worker use among Hispanic/Latino migrant men in Durham, North Carolina[85]; less-frequent heavy drinking among men in rural Mpumalanga, South Africa[86]; lower prevalence depressive symptoms among older adults in metropolitan Rio Grande do Sul, Brazil[87]; and lower body mass index among youth in Los Angeles, California.[88]

Neighborhood Safety

Emerging research in the literature has been focusing extensively on studying the effects of neighborhood safety on various health outcomes. Neighborhood safety is often measured using self-reported measures, yielding a perceived neighborhood safety index. Alternatively, it can be measured using more objective methods such as crime rate or safety complaints by neighborhood residents and then put into a GIS system. In particular, neighborhood safety has been shown to affect physical activity and obesity among different populations.[11,89–94] It is theorized that this relationship occurs due to the fact that the fear of violence and crime discourages individuals to be involved in physical activity, while encouraging different forms of sedentary behaviors. For instance, Bennett et al.,[90] demonstrated that residing in a neighborhood that is perceived to be unsafe at night is a barrier to regular physical activity among individuals, especially women, living in urban low-income housing. It is important to note that low-income populations and racial/ethnic minorities are often more likely to reside in unsafe neighborhoods, thus are considered populations of interest in the context of neighborhood safety health research. Similarly, Duncan et al. examined the relationship between perceived neighborhood safety and overweight status, and found that the perception of neighborhood safety may be associated with overweight status among urban adolescents in certain racial/ethnic groups.[93] Fish et al. reported an association between perceived neighborhood safety and body mass index; a lower perception of safety was associated with a higher body mass index among a sample of adults in Los Angeles.[94] Additionally, Weir et al. showed that parents' perception of neighborhood safety affects children's physical activity. Particularly, increased anxiety regarding neighborhood safety among parents correlated with a decreased level of physical activity for their children.[95] Additionally, neighborhood safety was associated with asthma, which is one of the most common chronic diseases affecting children in the United States.[96] Kopel et al. showed that primary caregivers' perception of neighborhood safety is associated with childhood asthma morbidity among inner-city school children with asthma.[97] In addition, Subramanian et al. found that, among a sample of children aged 0–17 years, participants who perceived their neighborhoods as being never safe were at higher odds for reporting asthma compared to those reporting usually safe.[98]

Spatial Stigma

A wide range of ethnographic studies have shown that low-income inner-city neighborhoods are burdened by "discourses of vilification"[99] and have reputations of being crime-ridden, dangerous, or urban blights, regardless of the reality.[100–102] An emerging body of research suggests that those who reside in socioeconomically marginalized places may be marked by the stigma of place (hereby referred to as "spatial stigma") which, in turn, influences their sense of self, their daily experiences, and their relations with nonresidents of their communities.[103,104] Spatial stigma can include a negative image of the neighborhood in the media, negative perceptions of neighborhood's residents by others, and feelings of judgment by others because they live in a particular neighborhood.

Several qualitative studies have examined spatial stigma and its impacts,[103,104] which helped generate what aspects of spatial stigma may matter; far fewer studies have attempted to quantify the effects of spatial stigma on health. Using data from the NYC Low-Income Housing, Neighborhoods, and Health Study, Duncan and colleagues[7] used a novel four-item scale to assess place-based stigma among a sample of low-income housing residents in New York City to examine the association of this measure with objective measures of body mass index and blood pressure. The investigators found that those who reported living in a neighborhood with a bad reputation were more likely to have higher body mass indexes, higher systolic and diastolic blood pressure, and increased risk of being overweight or obese or having hypertension. In another study with the same sample of low-income housing residents, this research group examined the association between spatial stigma and sleep, finding that a reported negative media perception of the neighborhood was negatively associated with sleep quality and duration.[105] At the time of publishing, we are aware of no other studies quantitatively examining the effects of spatial stigma on health. While this pioneering study considered an individual-level perception of neighborhood stigma, future studies will have to derive neighborhood-level indicators of stigma through the ecometric aggregation strategy discussed above.

FUTURE DIRECTIONS IN NEIGHBORHOOD HEALTH RESEARCH

The existing quantitative and qualitative studies connecting neighborhoods and health have provided a meaningful contribution to the understanding of how neighborhood environments (various characteristics) are important for human health. With that said, there are several promising directions for neighborhood research. First, given the lack of causal inference methods in neighborhoods and health research, we see this is an area that is expanding in recent years, including the natural experiments[3] we previously discussed and the implementation of agent-based methods.[4] Agent-based models use a computational model that contains the algorithms and equations used to encode the behaviors of agents and are representations of these complex systems. A complex system can be operatized as one in which the collective behaviors of the system are a result of dynamic interactions between the individual agents operating within that system. While agent-based models do not directly lend themselves to causal inference, they (can) appreciate the complexity of neighborhood dynamics on health outcomes and health behaviors. This will help future research to consider reverse causation and mechanisms. Combining this design can provide a very detailed mechanism for how exposures are linked to health outcomes, allowing research in the field to efficiently direct intervention policies for best results possible.

Additionally, we can already see different streams of research beginning to converge, which will likely continue in the future. For example, the field is ripe for examining the joint impact of neighborhoods and networks on health, using rigorous methods for both contexts. While there is some existing research on networks and neighborhoods (e.g., see Chen et al.[106]), most studies have yet to apply state-of-the-science methods from the two fields and most of the networks research has focused on social networks. However, there are networks beyond social networks, such as sexual networks and drug-using networks, which may be important for health and well-being. We anticipate that future research will grapple with the issues of modeling neighborhood and network data including modeling approaches for data over time—that is, developing and implementing longitudinal models that account for spatial and network autocorrelation and influences over time. Multiple contexts, beyond social networks and beyond the networks of nonresidential neighborhoods visited, will be a focus of future neighborhoods and health research, including research on integrating neighborhoods with working contexts, neighborhoods and family contexts, as well as neighborhoods and housing conditions. These factors are rarely studied in conjunction; however, they are intrinsically linked.[107,108]

Research on neighborhoods and health will also be advanced by life course neighborhood studies, which are investigations of the differential impact of neighborhood exposures over different stages in the life course (childhood, adolescence, adulthood, etc.). Neighborhood exposures may be more important at some points in the life course than others. For example, among school-aged children, school environments may be most salient. On the other hand, work environments may be most salient for working adults. However, for older adults home neighborhood conditions might be particularly salient, as it has been said that this population is "aging in place." Overall, future research will have to integrate a range of determinants that have often been separately examined, pertaining to the residential and nonresidential neighborhoods, work environments, family environments, and other social networks, as they all evolve over time.

Future research will also continue to examine various biases in the neighborhoods and health literature, including accounting for residential mobility and residential preferences and selective daily mobility (neighborhood selection). Furthermore, we anticipate that future neighborhoods and health research will focus on "downstream" effects. For example, future research may focus on biological stress processes and eventually will become more mainstream. Among a sample of 85 children, a recent cross-sectional study found that neighborhood violence and crime rates were associated with stress biomarkers.[109] A challenge for the future is to integrate into one study, relying as much as possible on objective and dynamic measurements, factors along the entire pathway, including environmental exposures, individual perceptions, behaviors, and biological and health states.

Neighborhoods and health studies that are cross-national are likely to increase, including in less-studied geographic locations, beyond the Unites States, Europe, and Australia (which are locations where the majority of the neighborhoods and health research has been conducted). International comparisons may be complicated. For example, the measurement of neighborhood exposures needs to be consistent and comparable with cross-national research. This may not be the case, as the quality of neighborhood data may differ across geographies. Additionally, future research will examine not only newer neighborhood factors, but also newer locations, including rural areas, which have not been significantly studied to date. While most of the previous research has been conducted in urban locations in the western world, the advancement of the field and increased accessibility of methods will allow researchers to expand the scope of their locations to rural areas in a range of developing contexts. In addition, neighborhoods and health research is needed in nonresidential neighborhoods such as work neighborhoods for adult populations and school neighborhoods for pediatric populations.

CONCLUSIONS AND POLICY IMPLICATIONS OF NEIGHBORHOOD HEALTH RESEARCH

While there is continued research showing that various features of neighborhoods can influence health outcomes and health behaviors, using various quantitative and qualitative methods, there is a need for additional research using emerging methods examining newer neighborhood factors as well as in newer locations and integrating measures from the different components of comprehensive theoretical models. This additional research will help us characterize the associations to guide policy making and behavioral interventions to have real-world impact, including economic policies for restructuring neighborhoods for optimal health. Furthermore, as new policies are put into place based on the findings of neighborhood health research, it is essential to conduct more research evaluating these interventions. This ensures that interventions in place are working toward disrupting the relationship between neighborhood exposures and negative health outcomes studied.

ACKNOWLEDGMENTS

We thank Byoungjun Kim for providing comments on an earlier version of this chapter.

References

1. Duncan DT, Kawachi I. Neighborhoods and health: A progress report. *Neighborhoods and Health*. Oxford: Oxford University Press; 2018, pp. 1–16.
2. Kawachi I, Berkman LF. *Neighborhoods and Health*. Oxford: Oxford University Press; 2003.
3. Schmidt NM, Nguyen QC, Osypuk TL. Experimental and quasi-experimental designs in neighborhood health effects research: Strengthening causal inference and promoting translation. *Neighborhoods and Health*: Oxford: Oxford University Press; 2018, pp. 155–91.
4. Heaton B, El-Sayed A, Galea S. Agent-based models. *Neighborhoods and Health*. Oxford: Oxford University Press; 2018, p. 127.
5. Sale JE, Lohfeld LH, Brazil K. Revisiting the quantitative-qualitative debate: Implications for mixed-methods research. *Qual Quant*. 2002; 36(1):43–53.
6. Padgett DK. *Qualitative and Mixed Methods in Public Health*. SAGE Publications USA, Thousand Oaks, CA Sage Publications; 2011.
7. Duncan DT, Ruff RR, Chaix B, et al. Perceived spatial stigma, body mass index and blood pressure: A global positioning system study among low-income housing residents in New York City. *Geospat Health*. 2016;11(2):399.
8. Mujahid MS, Diez Roux AV, Morenoff JD, Raghunathan T. Assessing the measurement properties of neighborhood scales: From psychometrics to ecometrics. *Am J Epidemiol*. 2007;165(8):858–67.
9. Scott SB, Munoz E, Mogle JA, et al. Perceived neighborhood characteristics predict severity and emotional response to daily stressors. *Soc Sci Med*. 2018;200:262–70.
10. Sampson RJ, Raudenbush SW. Systematic social observation of public spaces: A new look at disorder in urban neighborhoods. *Am J Sociol*. 1999;105(3):603–51.

11. Molnar BE, Gortmaker SL, Bull FC, Buka SL. Unsafe to play? Neighborhood disorder and lack of safety predict reduced physical activity among urban children and adolescents. *Am J Health Promot.* 2004;18(5):378–86.
12. Duncan DT, Goedel WC, Chunara R. Quantitative methods for measuring neighborhood characteristics in neighborhood health research. *Neighborhoods and Health.* Oxford: Oxford University Press; 2018:57.
13. Odgers CL, Caspi A, Bates CJ, Sampson RJ, Moffitt TE. Systematic social observation of children's neighborhoods using Google Street View: A reliable and cost-effective method. *J Child Psychol Psychiatry.* 2012;53(10):1009–17.
14. Rundle AG, Bader MD, Richards CA, Neckerman KM, Teitler JO. Using Google Street View to audit neighborhood environments. *Am J Prev Med.* 2011;40(1):94–100.
15. Marco M, Gracia E, Martín-Fernández M, López-Quílez A. Validation of a Google Street View-based neighborhood disorder observational scale. *J Urban Health.* 2017;94(2):190–8.
16. Caughy MO, O'Campo PJ, Patterson J. A brief observational measure for urban neighborhoods. *Health Place.* 2001;7(3):225–36.
17. Neckerman KM, Lovasi GS, Davies S, et al. Disparities in urban neighborhood conditions: Evidence from GIS measures and field observation in New York City. *J Public Health Policy.* 2009;30(1):S264–85.
18. Chaix B, Merlo J, Evans D, Leal C, Havard S. Neighbourhoods in eco-epidemiologic research: Delimiting personal exposure areas. A response to Riva, Gauvin, Apparicio and Brodeur. *Soc Sci Med.* 2009;69(9):1306–10.
19. Jia P, Cheng X, Xue H, Wang Y. Applications of geographic information systems (GIS) data and methods in obesity-related research. *Obes Rev.* 2017;18(4):400–11.
20. Charreire H, Casey R, Salze P, et al. Measuring the food environment using geographical information systems: A methodological review. *Public Health Nutr.* 2010;13(11):1773–85.
21. Duncan DT. What's your Walk Score®?: Web-based neighborhood walkability assessment for health promotion and disease prevention. *Am J Prev Med.* 2013;45(2):244–5.
22. Méline J, Chaix B, Pannier B, et al. Neighborhood walk score and selected Cardiometabolic factors in the French RECORD cohort study. *BMC Public Health.* 2017;17(1):960.
23. De Choudhury M, Sharma S, Kiciman E. Characterizing dietary choices, nutrition, and language in food deserts via social media. Paper presented at Proceedings of the 19th ACM Conference on Computer-Supported Cooperative Work & Social Computing. 2016.
24. Sharma SS, De Choudhury M. Measuring and characterizing nutritional information of food and ingestion content in instagram. Paper presented at Proceedings of the 24th International Conference on World Wide Web. 2015.
25. Gomez-Lopez IN, Clarke P, Hill AB, et al. Using social media to identify sources of healthy food in urban neighborhoods. *J Urban Health.* 2017;94(3):429–36.
26. Cawkwell PB, Lee L, Weitzman M, Sherman SE. Tracking hookah bars in New York: Utilizing yelp as a powerful public health tool. *JMIR Public Health Surveill.* 2015;1(2):e19.
27. Kelly P, Doherty A, Berry E, Hodges S, Batterham AM, Foster C. Can we use digital life-log images to investigate active and sedentary travel behaviour? Results from a pilot study. *Int J Behav Nutr Phys Act.* 2011;8(1):44.
28. Jarjour S, Jerrett M, Westerdahl D, et al. Cyclist route choice, traffic-related air pollution, and lung function: A scripted exposure study. *Environ Health.* 2013;12(1):14.
29. Dons E, Laeremans M, Orjuela JP, et al. Wearable sensors for personal monitoring and estimation of inhaled traffic-related air pollution: Evaluation of methods. *Environ Sci Technol.* 2017;51(3):1859–67.
30. Clampet-Lundquist S, Edin K, Kling JR, Duncan GJ. Moving teenagers out of high-risk neighborhoods: How girls fare better than boys. *Am J Sociol.* 2011;116(4):1154–89.
31. Keene DE, Ruel E. "Everyone called me grandma": Public housing demolition and relocation among older adults in Atlanta. *Cities.* 2013;35:359–64.
32. Frohlich KL, Potvin L, Chabot P, Corin E. A theoretical and empirical analysis of context: Neighbourhoods, smoking and youth. *Soc Sci Med.* 2002;54(9):1401–17.
33. Keene DE. Qualitative methods and neighborhood health research. *Neighborhood Health Research.* Oxford, UK: Oxford University Press; 2018, pp. 193–215.
34. Mullings L, Wali A. *Stress and Resilience: The Social Context of Reproduction in Central Harlem.* Berlin/Heidelberg, Germany: Springer Science & Business Media; 2001.
35. Wang CC. Youth participation in photovoice as a strategy for community change. *J Commun Pract.* 2006;14(1–2):147–61.
36. Dennis JrSF, Gaulocher S, Carpiano RM, Brown D. Participatory photo mapping (PPM): Exploring an integrated method for health and place research with young people. *Health Place.* 2009;15(2):466–73.
37. Carpiano RM. Come take a walk with me: The "Go-Along" interview as a novel method for studying the implications of place for health and well-being. *Health Place.* 2009;15(1):263–72.
38. Kusenbach M. Street phenomenology: The go-along as ethnographic research tool. *Ethnography.* 2003;4(3):455–85.
39. Porta CM, Corliss HL, Wolowic JM, et al. Go-along interviewing with LGBTQ youth in Canada and the United States. *J LGBT Youth.* 2017;14(1):1–15.
40. Brouillette RT, Horwood L, Constantin E, Brown K, Ross NA. Childhood sleep apnea and neighborhood disadvantage. *J Pediatr.* 2011;158(5):789–95.
41. Spilsbury JC, Storfer-Isser A, Kirchner HL, et al. Neighborhood disadvantage as a risk factor for pediatric obstructive sleep apnea. *J Pediatr.* 2006;149(3):342–7.
42. Duncan DT, Park SH, Goedel WC, et al. Perceived neighborhood safety is associated with poor sleep health among gay, bisexual, and other men who have sex with men in Paris, France. *J Urban Health.* 2017;94(3):399–407.
43. Ruff RR, Ng J, Jean-Louis G, Elbel B, Chaix B, Duncan DT. Neighborhood stigma and sleep: Findings from a pilot study of low-income housing residents in New York City. *Behav Med.* 2018;44(1): 48–53.
44. Ellaway A, Anderson A, Macintyre S. Does area of residence affect body size and shape? *Int J Obes Relat Metab Disord.* 1997;21(4):304–8.
45. Ellaway A, Macintyre S. Does where you live predict health related behaviours?: A case study in Glasgow. *Health Bull.* 1996;54(6):443–6.
46. Hart C, Ecob R, Smith GD. People, places and coronary heart disease risk factors: A multilevel analysis of the Scottish Heart Health Study archive. *Soc Sci Med.* 1997;45(6):893–902.
47. Cubbin C, Hadden WC, Winkleby MA. Neighborhood context and cardiovascular disease risk factors: The contribution of material deprivation. *Ethn Dis.* 2001;11(4):687–700.
48. Roux AVD. Residential environments and cardiovascular risk. *J Urban Health.* 2003;80(4):569–89.
49. Arcaya MC, Tucker-Seeley RD, Kim R, Schnake-Mahl A, So M, Subramanian SV. Research on neighborhood effects on health in the United States: A systematic review of study characteristics. *Soc Sci Med.* 2016;168:16–29.
50. Raymond HF, Chen Y-H, Syme SL, Catalano R, Hutson M, McFarland W. The role of individual and neighborhood factors: HIV acquisition risk among high-risk populations in San Francisco. *AIDS Behav.* 2014;18(2):346–56.
51. Kerrigan D, Witt S, Glass B, Chung S-e, Ellen J. Perceived neighborhood social cohesion and condom use among adolescents vulnerable to HIV/STI. *AIDS Behav.* 2006;10(6):723–9.
52. Bowleg L, Neilands TB, Tabb LP, Burkholder GJ, Malebranche DJ, Tschann JM. Neighborhood context and Black heterosexual men's sexual HIV risk behaviors. *AIDS Behav.* 2014;18(11):2207–18.
53. Latkin CA, Curry AD. Stressful neighborhoods and depression: A prospective study of the impact of neighborhood disorder. *J Health Soc Behav.* 2003:34–44.
54. Kim D. Blues from the neighborhood? Neighborhood characteristics and depression. *Epidemiol Rev.* 2008;30(1):101-–17.
55. Duncan DT, Palamar JJ, Williams JH. Perceived neighborhood illicit drug selling, peer illicit drug disapproval and illicit drug use among US high school seniors. *Subst Abuse Treat Prev Policy.* 2014;9(1):35.
56. Grasser G, Van Dyck D, Titze S, Stronegger W. Objectively measured walkability and active transport and weight-related outcomes in adults: A systematic review. *Int J Public Health.* 2013;58(4):615–25.
57. Schipperijn J, Cerin E, Adams MA, et al. Access to parks and physical activity: An eight country comparison. *Urban For Urban Green.* 2017;27:253–63.
58. Ding D, Gebel K. Built environment, physical activity, and obesity: What have we learned from reviewing the literature? *Health Place.* 2012;18(1):100–5.

59. Gose M, Plachta-Danielzik S, Willié B, Johannsen M, Landsberg B, Müller M. Longitudinal influences of neighbourhood built and social environment on children's weight status. *Int J Environ Res Public Health.* 2013;10(10):5083–96.
60. Duncan DT, Sharifi M, Melly SJ, et al. Characteristics of walkable built environments and BMI z-scores in children: Evidence from a large electronic health record database. *Environ Health Perspect.* 2014;122(12):1359–65.
61. Moudon AV, Lee C, Cheadle AD, et al. Operational definitions of walkable neighborhood: Theoretical and empirical insights. *J Phys Act Health.* 2006;3(s1):S99–117.
62. Khan LK, Sobush K, Keener D, et al. Recommended community strategies and measurements to prevent obesity in the United States. *MMWR Recomm Rep.* 2009;58(7):1–29.
63. Larson NI, Story MT, Nelson MC. Neighborhood environments: Disparities in access to healthy foods in the US. *Am J Prev Med.* 2009;36(1):74–81.
64. Morland K, Roux AVD, Wing S. Supermarkets, other food stores, and obesity: The atherosclerosis risk in communities study. *Am J Prev Med.* 2006;30(4):333–9.
65. Hollands S, Campbell MK, Gilliland J, Sarma S. Association between neighbourhood fast-food and full-service restaurant density and body mass index: A cross-sectional study of Canadian adults. *Can J Public Health.* 2014;105(3):e172–8.
66. Ahalya M, Polsky Jane Y, Éric R, Marc L, Tina M. Geographic retail food environment measures for use in public health. *Health Promot Chronic Dis Prev Can.* 2017;37(10):357.
67. Caspi CE, Sorensen G, Subramanian S, Kawachi I. The local food environment and diet: A systematic review. *Health Place.* 2012;18(5):1172–87.
68. Williams LK, Thornton L, Ball K, Crawford D. Is the objective food environment associated with perceptions of the food environment? *Public Health Nutr.* 2012;15(2):291–8.
69. Baker EA, Schootman M, Barnidge E, Kelly C. Peer reviewed: The role of race and poverty in access to foods that enable individuals to adhere to dietary guidelines. *Prev Chronic Dis.* 2006;3(3):A76.
70. Giskes K, Van Lenthe F, Brug J, Mackenbach J, Turrell G. Socioeconomic inequalities in food purchasing: The contribution of respondent-perceived and actual (objectively measured) price and availability of foods. *Prev Med.* 2007;45(1):41–8.
71. Nguyen Q, Meng H, Li D, et al. Social media indicators of the food environment and state health outcomes. *Public Health.* 2017;148:120–8.
72. Arcaya MC, Tucker-Seeley RD, Kim R, Schnake-Mahl A, So M, Subramanian S. Research on neighborhood effects on health in the United States: A systematic review of study characteristics. *Soc Sci Med.* 2016;168:16–29.
73. Messer LC, Laraia BA, Kaufman JS, et al. The development of a standardized neighborhood deprivation index. *J Urban Health.* 2006;83(6):1041–62.
74. Vos AA, Posthumus AG, Bonsel GJ, Steegers EA, Denktaş S. Deprived neighborhoods and adverse perinatal outcome: A systematic review and meta-analysis. *Acta Obstet Gynecol Scand.* 2014;93(8):727–40.
75. van Vuuren CL, Reijneveld SA, van der Wal MF, Verhoeff AP. Neighborhood socioeconomic deprivation characteristics in child (0–18 years) health studies: A review. *Health Place.* 2014;29:34–42.
76. Algren MH, Bak CK, Berg-Beckhoff G, Andersen PT. Health-risk behaviour in deprived neighbourhoods compared with non-deprived neighbourhoods: A systematic literature review of quantitative observational studies. *PLoS One.* 2015;10(10):e0139297.
77. Janevic T, Stein CR, Savitz DA, Kaufman JS, Mason SM, Herring AH. Neighborhood deprivation and adverse birth outcomes among diverse ethnic groups. *Ann Epidemiol.* 2010;20(6):445–51.
78. Bandura A. *Self-efficacy in Changing Societies.* Cambridge: Cambridge University Press; 1995.
79. Bandura A. Self-efficacy mechanism in human agency. *Am Psychol.* 1982;37(2):122.
80. Putnam RD. Bowling alone: America's declining social capital. *Culture and Politics.* New York: Springer; 2000, pp. 223–34.
81. Sampson RJ, Raudenbush SW, Earls F. Neighborhoods and violent crime: A multilevel study of collective efficacy. *Science.* 1997;277(5328):918–24.
82. Browning CR, Gardner M, Maimon D, Brooks-Gunn J. Collective efficacy and the contingent consequences of exposure to life-threatening violence. *Dev Psychol.* 2014;50(7):1878.
83. Ahern J, Galea S. Collective efficacy and major depression in urban neighborhoods. *Am J Epidemiol.* 2011;173(12):1453–62.
84. Ahern J, Cerdá M, Lippman SA, Tardiff KJ, Vlahov D, Galea S. Navigating non-positivity in neighbourhood studies: An analysis of collective efficacy and violence. *J Epidemiol Community Health.* 2013;67(2):159–65.
85. Parrado EA, Flippen C. Community attachment, neighborhood context, and sex worker use among Hispanic migrants in Durham, North Carolina, USA. *Soc Sci Med.* 2010;70(7):1059–69.
86. Leslie HH, Ahern J, Pettifor AE, et al. Collective efficacy, alcohol outlet density, and young men's alcohol use in rural South Africa. *Health Place.* 2015;34:190–8.
87. Quatrin LB, Galli R, Moriguchi EH, Gastal FL, Pattussi MP. Collective efficacy and depressive symptoms in Brazilian elderly. *Arch Gerontol Geriatr.* 2014;59(3):624–9.
88. Cohen DA, Finch BK, Bower A, Sastry N. Collective efficacy and obesity: The potential influence of social factors on health. *Soc Sci Med.* 2006;62(3):769–78.
89. Loukaitou-Sideris A. Is it safe to walk? 1 neighborhood safety and security considerations and their effects on walking. *J Plan Lit.* 2006;20(3): 219–32.
90. Bennett GG, McNeill LH, Wolin KY, Duncan DT, Puleo E, Emmons KM. Safe to walk? Neighborhood safety and physical activity among public housing residents. *PLoS Med.* 2007;4(10):e306.
91. Carver A, Timperio A, Crawford D. Perceptions of neighborhood safety and physical activity among youth: The CLAN study. *J Phys Act Health.* 2008;5(3):430–44.
92. Carver A, Timperio A, Crawford D. Playing it safe: The influence of neighbourhood safety on children's physical activity—A review. *Health Place.* 2008;14(2):217–27.
93. Duncan DT, Johnson RM, Molnar BE, Azrael D. Association between neighborhood safety and overweight status among urban adolescents. *BMC Public Health.* 2009;9(1):289.
94. Fish JS, Ettner S, Ang A, Brown AF. Association of perceived neighborhood safety on body mass index. *Am J Public Health.* 2010;100(11): 2296–303.
95. Weir LA, Etelson D, Brand DA. Parents' perceptions of neighborhood safety and children's physical activity. *Prev Med.* 2006;43(3):212–17.
96. National AE, Prevention P. Expert Panel Report 3 (EPR-3): Guidelines for the diagnosis and management of asthma-summary report 2007. *J Allergy Clin Immunol.* 2007;120(5 Suppl):S94.
97. Kopel LS, Gaffin JM, Ozonoff A, et al. Perceived neighborhood safety and asthma morbidity in the school inner-city asthma study. *Pediatr Pulmonol.* 2015;50(1):17–24.
98. Subramanian S, Kennedy MH. Perception of neighborhood safety and reported childhood lifetime asthma in the United States (US): A study based on a national survey. *PLoS One.* 2009;4(6):e6091.
99. Wacquant L. Territorial stigmatization in the age of advanced marginality. *Thesis Eleven.* 2007;91(1):66–77.
100. Caldeira TP. *City of Walls: Crime, Segregation, and Citizenship in São Paulo.* Oakland, CA: University of California Press; 2000.
101. Conoley JC, Goldstein AP. *School Violence Intervention: A Practical Handbook.* New York: Guilford Press; 2004.
102. Lobo S. *A House of My Own: Social Organization in the Squatter Settlements of Lima*, Peru. Tucson, AZ: University of Arizona Press; 1982.
103. Keene DE, Padilla MB. Race, class and the stigma of place: Moving to "opportunity" in Eastern Iowa. *Health Place.* 2010;16(6):1216–23.
104. Graham LF, Padilla MB, Lopez WD, Stern AM, Peterson J, Keene DE. Spatial stigma and health in postindustrial Detroit. *Int Q Community Health Educ.* 2016;36(2):105–13.
105. Ruff RR, Ng J, Jean-Louis G, Elbel B, Chaix B, Duncan DT. Neighborhood stigma and sleep: Findings from a pilot study of low-income housing residents in New York City. *Behav Med.* 2018;44(1):48–53.
106. Chen Y-T, Kolak M, Duncan DT, et al. Neighbourhoods, networks and pre-exposure prophylaxis awareness: A multilevel analysis of a sample of young black men who have sex with men. *Sex Transm Infect.* 2019;95(3):228–35.
107. Inagami S, Cohen DA, Finch BK. Non-residential neighborhood exposures suppress neighborhood effects on self-rated health. *Soc Sci Med.* 2007;65(8):1779–91.
108. Oakes JM. The (mis) estimation of neighborhood effects: Causal inference for a practicable social epidemiology. *Soc Sci Med.* 2004;58(10): 1929–52.
109. Theall KP, Shirtcliff EA, Dismukes AR, Wallace M, Drury SS. Association between neighborhood violence and biological stress in children. *JAMA Pediatr.* 2017;171(1):53–60.

CHAPTER

32 Housing and Health

Veronica Eva Helms Garrison • Craig Evan Pollack

INTRODUCTION

Beyond providing basic shelter, the home often comprises the center of people's daily life, a place where people share meals, spend large amounts of time, and engage with family. It may be a place of safety and security or one riddled with precarity and stress. The link between public health and housing is multifaceted. A clean, safe, and decent home is important for individual, family, and community health. Historically, the housing-health connection has focused primarily on homelessness and physical exposures; however, emerging research suggests that the housing-health relationship transcends beyond these two categories. Health is also associated with rental assistance status, housing insecurity, a lack of affordable housing, and neighborhood quality.

Over the past decades, housing has been increasingly recognized as a critical social determinant of health and there have been growing attempts to promote the concept of "housing as a vaccine."[1–4] In this chapter, we discuss the connection between housing and health in four sections:

1. Homelessness;
2. Physical exposures in housing units;
3. Housing affordability and security; and
4. Neighborhood context.

For each section, we describe the scope of the issue, review evidence linking the factor and health, and discuss potential public health and policy solutions to addressing the different exposures. This chapter focuses on established housing-health research. However, it is important to note that some known and emerging issues, such as housing destruction due to natural or man-made causes, housing for certain populations (including disabled populations), and specific health issues related to housing structure type (e.g., high-rise apartments and mobile homes) are not covered in this chapter.

HOMELESSNESS AND HEALTH

Scope: Homelessness

Homelessness can be defined as a state in which a person, family, or household lacks a home, and includes individuals "without permanent housing who may live on the streets; [i]ndividuals who stay in a shelter, mission, single room occupancy facilities, abandoned building or vehicle; [a]nd, individuals in any other unstable or nonpermanent situation."[5] Many definitions of homelessness also include "doubling up," a term used to define circumstances when an individual is forced to stay with friends or family due to an inability to pay for one's own housing unit. When persons who are released from prisons, hospitals, or other institutional do not have a stable housing situation to which they can return, this can also be considered a form of homelessness.[6]

Research on the dynamics of how individuals experiencing homelessness interface with the homeless assistance system reveal a typology of homeless households based on the duration of their homelessness experience. Homeless individuals and families may be categorized as chronically homeless, indicating that they have been homeless for a year or longer; episodically homeless, indicating that they cycle in and out of homelessness; or, transitionally homeless, defined by those who experience homelessness for only a brief period of time (typically less than a month).[7]

Prevalence of Homelessness

Estimating the prevalence of homelessness is difficult for many reasons. Researchers often utilize different parameters to define homelessness, which may make it challenging to compare across estimates. Temporal differences often arise when defining homelessness. For example, point-in-time estimates differ from estimates that capture homelessness over varying durations of time. Finally, some homeless persons may be difficult to locate using traditional survey methods and most jurisdictions do not have a robust surveillance system meant to capture the health of homeless persons.[8–10] Generally, U.S. homelessness prevalence estimates focus on two time frames: point-in-time estimates and annualized counts.

Point-in-Time Prevalence Point-in-time counts represent unduplicated, one-night estimates of homeless persons including sheltered and unsheltered individuals. Every other year, the U.S. Department of Housing and Urban Development (HUD) requires communities to conduct a one-night, point-in-time count during the last week in January. According to HUD's 2017 point-in-time estimates, on any given night, approximately 554,000 persons experience homelessness in the United States.[11] Among homeless individuals, 65% were staying in emergency shelters or transitional housing programs while 35% resided in unsheltered locations.

Annualized Counts During 2016, approximately 1.4 million individuals utilized HUD homeless assistance programs including emergency shelters, transitional housing programs, and/or permanent supportive housing programs.[12] These estimates are conservative because they do not include unsheltered individuals who did not use services.

Another measure that has been utilized to quantify the prevalence of homelessness is 5-year prevalence, defined as the percent of persons homeless at any point during a 5-year period. According to estimates published in 1994, the 5-year prevalence of homelessness in the United States during 1985–90 varied from 3.1% to 4.6% depending on how strict of a definition of homelessness was used.[13] More recent estimates of the 5-year prevalence of homelessness in the United States have not been published.

The broadest definition of homelessness is lifetime prevalence, a metric meant to capture homelessness at any point during an individual's lifetime. According to 1990 estimates, the lifetime prevalence of homelessness varied from 7.4% to 14.0% depending on how strict of a definition of homelessness was used.[13] When compared to four other developed countries, the United Kingdom and United States had the highest lifetime prevalence of homelessness with 7.7% and 6.2% of individual experiencing homelessness, respectively.[14] Recent estimates of the lifetime prevalence of homelessness in the United States have not been published.

Trends over Time

Over the past several decades, several trends in homelessness have emerged in the United States. First, the largest proportion of persons experiencing homelessness has shifted from primarily single men to women, children, and families.[15] Second, when compared to other cities, several jurisdictions such as New York City and Los Angeles experience a disproportionate amount of homeless persons.[16] Third, according to the 2017 point-in-time estimates, homelessness has increased for the first time in 7 years; however, the absolute percent increase between 2016 and 2017 was approximately 1%.[11] The national increase of just under 1% was driven by a 9% increase in unsheltered homelessness, particularly among singles and individuals residing in the west coast.

Evidence Linking Homelessness to Health

Homelessness may both cause poor health and be a consequence of it. For example, if an individual becomes unable to work due to injury or illness, they could potentially lose their job and become homeless. For women and children, domestic violence has also been shown to be a primary cause of homelessness.[17,18] Certain populations, including those with serious mental illness and those with substance abuse, are at particularly high risk of becoming homeless. Prior research suggest that homeless persons with mental illness face increased risk of suicidal behavior, but this may be attributable to the high prevalence of traditional risk factors among this population.[19] In turn, the financial hardship that often leads to homelessness limits resources for health promotion including food and shelter, potentially exacerbating disease and causing premature mortality.[16] Homeless persons have a higher age-adjusted mortality rate.[20] Notably, homeless persons are three to four times likely to die prematurely when compared to the general population.[21]

Below we discuss evidence linking homelessness and specific health conditions and then focus on vulnerable populations who disproportionately suffer adverse health consequences of homelessness and may be at greater risk of homelessness due to their health status.

Association between Homelessness and Adverse Health Outcomes

Homeless individuals are at risk for infectious diseases including tuberculosis, HIV, and hepatitis C virus infection.[22–24] Prior research also suggests that infectious skin conditions such as scabies and body lice are prominent among homeless persons. Other conditions that are prominent among homeless populations include chronic disease, disability, unintentional injury, and violence.[25]

Persons who experience homelessness may have high healthcare utilization both prior to becoming homeless and after becoming homeless. For example, Schanzer et al. conducted a longitudinal study to follow individuals who entered a homeless shelter across a subsequent 18-month period. Results suggest that disease was highly prevalent among newly homeless individuals and study participants reported high utilization of the healthcare system during the year prior to becoming homeless.[20] After becoming homeless, many individuals may be high utilizers of the healthcare system incurring high medical costs. Often, this utilization is linked to high unmet healthcare needs leading to delayed care and care seeking in the emergency department.[26]

Vulnerable Populations

Certain socioeconomic characteristics are associated with an increased risk of homelessness. Generally, homelessness literature tends to review the characteristics of two groups with very different outcomes: homeless singles and homeless families. Literature highlighted below primarily highlights the health of homeless singles. Several groups of people that are often marginalized by society experience disproportionate rates of homelessness, including youth, people with mental and/or substance use illness, veterans, and injection drug users.

Homeless Youth Unaccompanied adolescent homelessness represents a high-risk population. Prevalence estimates suggest that across a 12-month window, the period prevalence of homelessness among U.S. adolescents aged 12–17 years was 4.3% when utilizing the study's broadest definition of homelessness.[27] When examining households with adolescents between 18 and 25 years old, the period prevalence of homelessness was 12.5%.[27] The study also found several disparities in this unique population. While rates were similar among rural and urban counties, youth homelessness rates were higher among adolescent with young parents, ethnic and racial minorities (black and Hispanic), lesbian, gay, bisexual, or transgender youth, and youth who did not finish high school.[27] When compared to adolescents who were not homelessness, homeless youth experienced elevated risk of adverse health behaviors and associated outcomes, including HIV infection and depressive symptoms.[28–31] Notably, one study found that mortality rates for homelessness youth were more than ten times greater when compared to adolescents in the general population.[32]

Elderly Homeless Trends suggest that the U.S. homeless population is aging, resulting in a large portion of homeless elderly persons.[20] This aging trend is consistent with the emergence of increased chronic conditions among homeless persons.[33] The elderly homeless have unique mental and physical health needs.[20]

Homeless Persons with Mental Illness Since the unsuccessful implementation of deinstitutionalization in the mid-1900s, there has been a link between mental illness and homelessness.[34–36] Research suggests that one-quarter to one-third of homeless persons experience serious mental health issues.[37,38] One California study found that among individuals with serious mental illness, the prevalence of homelessness was 15%.[39] The study also found that homeless persons with mental health ailments were more likely to utilize inpatient and emergency medical services.[39] Another study found that homeless adults with mental illness experience high rates of criminal victimization, indicating a critical need for public health professionals, service providers, and law enforcement officials to collaborate to address the unique needs of homeless persons with mental health ailments.[40,41]

Persons with Substance Use Disorders Homeless persons are at an increased risk of experiencing substance use disorders.[42] For example, heavy alcohol use is ten times more prevalent among homeless adults when compared to the general population.[43] Qualitative research suggests that homeless persons utilize alcohol use for social reasons and for reinforcing psychological reasons.[44] Additionally, homeless persons often experience comorbidities associated with serious mental illness and substance use disorders; therefore, it is important for practitioners to recognize how these two health outcomes and behaviors are interrelated.[45]

Homelessness is also associated with injection drug use. One study in Baltimore, Maryland found that homelessness was significantly associated with drug relapse and injection-related risk behaviors.[46] Similarly, a longitudinal cohort study found that homelessness is alarmingly high in persons with a history of injection drug use: 46.7% of study participants reported homelessness.[47] Lastly, tobacco use is widespread among homeless persons. Approximately one-third of homeless person are cigarette smokers.[48] Despite common misconceptions regarding health attitudes, interest in quitting is high among homeless persons but their confidence in their ability to quit is low.[49] When combined with nicotine dependence, psychiatric conditions, and substance use comorbidities, homeless persons face significant challenges associated with reducing tobacco use.[49] In total, tobacco, alcohol, and drugs contribute to a sizable portion of deaths among a sample of homeless persons. In one study, over half (52%) of recorded deaths were substance-attributable.[50]

Veterans Veterans are overrepresented in the general U.S. homeless population.[51] According to point-in-time estimates conducted by the HUD, approximately 50,000 veterans are homeless on any given night.[11] Among a sample of veterans, 8.5% reported lifetime homelessness yet less than one-fifth of these individuals reported utilizing services from the U.S. Department of Veteran Affairs.[52]

A review of the literature found that overall, homeless veterans have high rates of mental illness, physical illness, and substance use disorders.[53] For example, one study found that among a sample of veterans, 19% reported diabetes mellitus.[54] When compared to the general population, homeless veterans face higher rates of morbidity and mortality when compared to the general population.[55] Homeless veterans are also high utilizers of the emergency rooms and have longer lengths of stay when hospitalized, both of which are associated with greater costs.[56] Notably, as the result of targeted programs to address homelessness among veterans, there has been a substantial decline in U.S. veteran homelessness between 2009 and 2015.[57]

Solutions to Address Homelessness

Homelessness can be addressed via a clear solution: increased access to adequate, quality, and affordable housing.[15] However, achieving this solution is complex, frequently requiring consideration of the complex relationship between homelessness and health, and involving multiple partners across sectors. Below, we focus on aspects of the federal government's role in addressing homelessness, the connection to patient-centered healthcare, the role of the housing first approach, and the implementation of permanent supportive housing programs. We further note that many initiatives target specific populations such as "superutilizers" of healthcare as way to bridge housing and health.

Federal Actions to Address Homelessness

Several federal agencies play a key role in homelessness programs. HUD focuses on programs intended to quickly address homelessness among individual and families. Every year, community-based programs funded by HUD serve more than 1 million homeless individuals and families through emergency shelter and transitional and permanent housing programs. The U.S. Department of Health and Human Services (HHS) also serves a critical role in preventing, addressing, and ending homelessness, particularly among youth. Several other agencies seek to address specific needs of homelessness or key subpopulations. For example, the U.S. Department of Veteran Affairs coordinates programs that seek to end homelessness among veterans while the U.S. Department of Education addresses the educational needs of unstably housed children.

The U.S. Interagency Council on Homelessness (USICH) is the federal government's coordinating entity regarding all homelessness initiatives. USICH coordinates activities by working with 19 federal agencies, state and local government, advocacy and non profit organizations, and service providers. The group presented America's strategic plan to end homelessness, entitled *Opening Doors*, to Congress in 2010 and was updated in 2010 and 2015. The plan includes specific objectives around integrating primary and behavioral healthcare. Since the document's launch in 2010, chronic homelessness in the United States has been reduced by 21% and family homelessness by 15%.[57]

Healthcare for the Homeless

Homeless individuals and families experience decreased access to quality healthcare. Initiatives that address healthcare financing and insurance have the potential to reduce homelessness and associated adverse health outcomes.[16] For example, 32 states participated in Medicaid expansion as part of the Affordable Care Act. This expansion provides new insurance options for low-income and homeless persons. When compared to states that did not expand Medicaid, expansion states had increased health coverage rates for homeless persons. Health insurance coverage for homeless persons increased from 45% in 2012 to 67% in 2014.[58] Additionally, along with the Affordable Care Act, new initiatives arose where states requested that the Centers for Medicare and Medicaid approve of publicly funded Medicaid health plans that cover housing costs.[59]

In conjunction with increased access, "patient-centered care" has shown to be an effective approach to promoting positive health outcomes for homeless individuals. Led by the Health Resources and Services Administration (HRSA), more than 250 healthcare for the homeless (HCH) projects utilize patient-centered care strategies.[60] Situated as federally qualified health centers, HCHs feature multidisciplinary teams of healthcare providers that are trained to use targeted care strategies. For example, the Boston Health Care for the Homeless Program pioneered a program where healthcare providers were sent directly to the streets via foot and an overnight van was used to provide needed services to homeless persons.[61] By training staff to be nonjudgmental, consistent, and coordinated, these programs have the potential to engage a difficult to reach population therefore improving rates of preventive and primary care among homeless persons. Continuity and coordination of care across various specialties and sectors is also critical for homeless populations but difficult to achieve.

The colocation of healthcare services near known homelessness hubs (e.g., tent cities and areas with a high density of homeless shelters) has also proven to be effective to promoting health among homeless individuals and families.[62–64] For example, HCH programs often have multidisciplinary teams that contain professionals with expertise in chronic disease management, mental health, and addiction counseling, to name a few. Care coordinators also seek to connect various healthcare and social systems such as clinics, emergency departments, prisons, social services, housing providers, and hospitals.

Housing First Approach

Housing First is an approach that is increasingly being employed to address the needs of homeless individuals. Prior approaches to housing required individuals to achieve predetermined treatment goals before receiving permanent housing. These treatment goals may have included abstinence from drugs or alcohol, mental health treatment, or other program participation. However, these conditions were often challenging for individuals to achieve in the best of circumstances and made more challenging due to homelessness. In contrast, the Housing First model was developed to quickly and successfully connect homeless individuals with permanent housing without the utilization of preconditions. With lower barriers to entry, Housing First then seeks to help individuals maintain housing stability through the use of customized set of supportive services. According to the HUD, Housing First is based on several guiding principles (Box 32-1).[65]

Even though the Housing First model is relatively new, there is strong evidence to suggest the approach is successful in promoting positive outcomes. Specifically, this approach allows program administrators to quickly link participants with a provider that can address urgent physical and mental health needs. When compared to traditional programs, program that utilize Housing First are more successful in harm reduction.[66] Additionally, a randomized trial in five Canadian cities found that the Housing First model improved time in housing after 2 year of follow-up; however, evidence regarding changes in health-related quality of life were inconclusive.[67]

Permanent Supportive Housing

Permanent Supportive Housing (also referred to broadly under the supportive housing umbrella) programs are evidence-based interventions designed to promote the utilization of two simultaneous approaches, supportive housing and supportive wrap-around services, to help homeless persons transition to permanent housing circumstances.[68,69] According to HUD estimates, approximately

BOX 32-1 Principles of Housing First, an Approach to Systematically Address U.S. Homelessness

- Homelessness is first and foremost a housing crisis and can be addressed through the provision of safe and affordable housing.
- All people experiencing homelessness, regardless of their housing history and duration of homelessness, can achieve housing stability in permanent housing. Some may need very little support for a brief period of time, while others may need more intensive and long-term supports.
- Everyone is "housing ready." Sobriety, compliance in treatment, or even criminal histories are not necessary to succeed in housing. Rather, homelessness programs and housing providers must be "consumer ready."
- Many people experience improvements in quality of life, in the areas of health, mental health, substance use, and employment, as a result of achieving housing.
- People experiencing homelessness have the right to self-determination and should be treated with dignity and respect.

The exact configuration of housing and services depends upon the needs and preferences of the population. While the principles of Housing First can be applied to many interventions and as an overall community approach to addressing homelessness, this document focuses primarily on Housing First in the context of permanent supportive housing models for people experiencing chronic homelessness."

Source: U.S. Department of Housing and Urban Development. HUD report – housing first in permanent supportive housing brief.

348,000 people lived in PSH during 2015.[12] Permanent Supportive Housing programs are implemented by mental health authorities and state agency administrators.[70] Services provided can include case management, mental health services, substance use counseling services, independent living skills, vocation services, health services, social activities, and peer support services.

According to the United States Interagency Council on Homelessness, prior research has proven that supportive housing approaches are cost-effective because these programs lower public costs associated with shelters, hospitals, prisons, psychiatric center, and crisis service providers.[71] Often, the Housing First model is used in conjunction with permanent supportive housing.

In addition to public cost-savings, PSH programs have been shown to improve health. For example, a comprehensive review of the evidence regarding the association between permanent supportive housing and mental and substance use disorders found that positive outcomes of permanent supportive housing interventions included reduced homelessness, increased housing stability, and decreased hospitalization and emergency room visits.[68]

PHYSICAL EXPOSURES IN HOUSING UNITS

Scope: Physical Exposures

United States Historical Context

In 1890, Jacob Riis exposed poor living conditions in New York City using photojournalism in "How the Other Half Lives: Studies among the Tenements of New York."[72] This work, depicting dangerous living conditions characterized by overcrowding and poor construction, is often credited with inspiring American housing reforms, including the development of housing and building codes, an important mechanism used to promote population health and safety. In the late nineteenth century and early twentieth century, the first building and housing codes were implemented with the primary goal of improving squalid living conditions for impoverished immigrants and low-income workers.[73] However, poor housing conditions continued to proliferate. The U.S. Census Bureau estimated that in 1940, 45% of households lived in homes without plumbing and several states in the rural south reported a prevalence closer to 80%.[74]

The U.S. Housing Act of 1949, a landmark piece of legislation during the Fair Deal era, sought to improve American housing conditions. As part of the bill's preamble, Congress declared the following goal: "a decent home in a suitable living environment for every American family."[75] President Harry Truman also highlighted this sentiment during his State of the Union address: "Five million families are still living in slums and firetraps. Three million families share their homes with others."[76]

During the second half of the twentieth century, American housing conditions drastically improved. HUD was founded as a cabinet department in 1965 under President Lyndon Johnson. The agency's mission is "to create strong, sustainable, inclusive communities and quality affordable homes for all."[77] Around this time, the percentage of homes without adequate plumbing decreased. Improved living conditions were attributable to a boom in large construction to replace older, dilapidated buildings.[73]

Current Physical Quality of American Housing

The American Housing Survey (AHS) is the most comprehensive nationally representative housing survey in the United States, providing data on housing and neighborhood quality, housing costs, and recent moves for a wide range of housing types. Recent analyses of the AHS utilized three survey years (2005, 2007, and 2009) to analyze more than 100 quality and physical structure variables to examine housing quality and physical adequacy in the United States. Key findings are highlighted below (Box 32-2).[78]

BOX 32-2 Current State of Severely Inadequate Housing in the United States, 2005, 2007, and 2009 American Housing Survey

- Severely inadequate housing is a very strict measure that uses 14 metrics to identify housing units with severe physical inadequacies. To be considered severely inadequate, a unit must contain one of the following: (1) no hot and cold running water; (2) no bathtub or shower; (3) no flush toilet; (4) no plumbing facilities; (5) severe heating/cooling deficiencies[1]; (6) no electricity; (7) exposed wiring, faulty electrical plugs, and frequently blown fuses; or (8) five or more identified structural conditions.[2]
- Severely inadequate housing is very rare in the United States. Less than 2% of occupied housing units in the United States were severely inadequate during the sample timeframe.
- Severely inadequate housing units often do not stay occupied or stay in dilapidated condition over time. Among units identified to be severely inadequate in early survey years, these units either became unoccupied or updated in later survey years. For example, less than 12% of previously inadequate units remained severely adequate in follow-up surveys.
- The severely inadequate housing metric in the American Housing Survey intends to capture the most basic level of quality: physical adequacy. However, the metric fails to capture key components of housing quality that are important to health such as mold, pest infestation, and potential lead hazards.

[1] For example, housing unit was cold for 24 hours or more and the unit experienced more than two breakdowns of the heating equipment that lasted longer than 6 hours.

[2] Structural conditions assessed include: outside water leaks, inside water leaks, holes in the floor, open cracks wider than a dime, a large area of peeling paint, and the presence of rats.

The statistics highlighted in Box 32-2 portray severely inadequate housing, an extreme metric that captures very few U.S. housing units. However, other research confirms that the amount of inadequate housing in the U.S. housing stock is limited.[79] When using a less-extreme metric to assess the physical quality of the U.S. housing stock, an estimated 10 million units are physically inadequate and approximately 20% of vacant single-family homes are physically inadequate.[80]

Evidence Linking Physical Exposures to Health

Physically inadequate housing has been linked with safety hazards and adverse health outcomes.[81] Over the past several decades, health interventions have focused on remediation and modifying physical housing conditions as an approach to improve health.[82] Key physical exposures statistically linked to a range of negative health outcomes include: lead, dampness and mold, disease vector infestations, asbestos, and poor indoor air quality. For each, a brief description of the exposure is followed by key information such as exposure route, prevalence, impact, and policy implications. Additionally, abbreviated discussion is provided for several less common housing-related exposures that can impact health.

Lead

Lead, a naturally occurring dense metal, is a highly poisonous neurotoxin that adversely affects human health.[83] Commonly found in older commercial and housing structures, lead-contaminated house dust was first recognized as a significant health hazard for children by Lockhart Gibson in 1904.[84]

Exposure Route: Lead poisoning occurs when lead builds up in the body.[85] Even small amounts of lead exposure can lead to serious health issues; however, lead contamination is especially serious for children younger than 6 years old because exposure impacts mental and emotional development.[86] In adults, the most common route of exposure is contaminated air, water, or soil while the major source of childhood lead exposure is attributable to lead-based paint and lead-contaminated house dust, both of which are found in older buildings.[87,88]

Exposure Prevalence: Currently, there is no standardized method to measure and collect house dust samples and extrapolate a national prevalence of lead-contaminated house dust. However, the Centers for Disease Control and Prevention estimates that approximately 4 million U.S. households contain children that are likely exposed to high lead levels attributable to lead-contaminated paint.[89] Although lead exposure in adults is less impactful for health when compared to children, lead toxicity remains a concern for U.S. adults. From the early 1970s to the early 2000s, the average adult blood lead level declined from approximately 15 μg/dL to 1–2 μg/dL. Nonetheless, workers in certain industries experience high levels of exposure and certain racial and ethnics groups experience higher blood lead levels, indicating the presence of health disparities.[90]

Impact of Exposure: In children, international pooled analyses from a longitudinal study revealed that environmental lead exposure is significantly associated with intellectual deficits in children.[91] In adults, recent epidemiological and toxicological research suggests that over time, low levels of exposure can damage the heart, kidneys, and brain.[85]

Policy Approach: According to the Environmental Protection Agency (EPA), the Centers for Disease Control and Prevention, and the Office of Lead Hazard Control and Healthy Homes at HUD, lead abatement and lead remediation—two similar but different strategies—represent the best strategies to preventing lead exposure attributable to household lead exposures. Abatement strategies focus on either (1) removing lead from a building or (2) encapsulating lead so it can no longer cause harm. Conversely, remediation strategies seek to address the underlying causes of lead exposure by developing a comprehensive plan to avoid exposure. For example, strategies could include the full removal of all lead painted fixtures and surfaces. Remediation plans often include an abatement strategy.

Dampness and Mold

Molds are fungi that thrive in warm, damp, and humid environments. Mold is found in both indoor and outdoor environments. In housing structures, mold is more common in certain housing areas such as showers, basements, and attics.[92,93]

Exposure Route: Inhalation is considered the primary mechanism of mold exposure. However, many gaps in the literature currently exist and more research is needed to establish the human exposure route for indoor mold. As stated by the Institute of Medicine: "…the entire process of fungal-spore aerosolization, transport, deposition, resuspension, and tracking, all of which determine inhalation exposure, is poorly understood…The significance of exposures to fungi in normal indoor environments through dermal contact and ingestion is also not well understood."[94]

Exposure Prevalence: Currently, there is no national surveillance database that can be used to track the prevalence of dampness and mold in the U.S. housing stock. However, several statistics can be extrapolated to estimate potential exposure prevalence. For example, according to the 2009 American Housing Survey, approximately 10% of homes had water damage from exterior leakage and approximately 8% had water damage attributable to interior leakage.[95] Additionally, an evaluation of grant-funded research and demonstration projects overseen by the HUD's Office of Lead Hazard Control and Healthy Homes found that mold and dampness were the most prevalent hazards identified by grantees.[96]

Impact of Exposure: Several studies suggest a link between adverse respiratory health effects and mold in homes.[97,98] Notably, the Institute of Medicine (IOM) concluded that sufficient evidence exists to establish that exposure to indoor mold is associated with upper respiratory tract symptoms in otherwise healthy individuals. Additionally, individuals with pre-existing asthma experience exacerbated asthma symptoms when exposed to indoor mold. Regarding otherwise healthy children, the IOM found limited evidence regarding a significant relationship between indoor mold exposure and adverse respiratory health effects.[94] Since this comprehensive publication in 2004, the National Institutes of Health has also endorsed a 2012 study that found that indoor household mold was more common in the homes of infants who developed asthma later in childhood.[99]

Policy Approach: Similar to lead, policies and programs that promote remediation of housing-related hazards that contribute to mold and dampness have proven successful.[100,101] To be successful, remediation plans must address the underlying water problem (e.g., leaking roof). Otherwise, the dampness and mold will return. Common remediation strategies for mold and dampness include: reduction of water infiltration, removal of water-damaged materials, and improvements to heating, ventilation, and air-conditioning systems. Additional strategies include educational programs, outreach activities to households with children, and capacity-building initiatives that promote the sustainability of healthy homes projects.

Disease Vectors, Pests, and Infestations

When a home is invaded by insects or pests, individual health is threatened because pests can act as carriers for harmful pathogens and allergens. Pests represent the main source of allergens within residential homes.

Exposure Route: Common disease vectors and pests include: rodents, cockroaches, fleas, flies, termites, fire ants, bed bugs, and mosquitoes. When a housing unit is part of a larger building, a building-wide, small-scale epidemic is possible. Occurrence of pests can be influenced greatly by environmental conditions such as weather. For example, some pests thrive in warm, humid environments while other pests seek out warm housing units during cold winter months.[102]

Exposure Prevalence: When compared to current times, the prevalence of pests was much higher during the 1940s when slums were more common in America. Although much less common today, pest infestations still occur in the United States. However, given that many different categories of pests exist with varying health impacts, prevalence varies by pest. For example, the 1997 American Housing Survey estimated that rats and mice infested approximately 2.7 million housing units. According to a CDC-sponsored survey in two large American cities, approximately 50% of surveyed units reported rat and mice infestation. When considering cockroach infestation, the existence of cockroaches is associated with housing characteristics. For example, housing units with inadequate plumbing, poorly kept open spaces, and poor ventilation are more likely to experience a cockroach infestation.[102]

Impact of Exposure: Given the variance regarding the types of pests that can potentially infest a housing unit, health impacts vary according to the type of pest. Many pests have a parasitic relationship with humans, which can lead to adverse health outcomes. For example, blood parasites and biting insects perforate human skin and can lead to infection. Nowadays, the most common health effect associated with pests is allergies and asthma exacerbations. If an individual is sensitive to allergens, pest infestations can represent a serious health concern. Specifically, mice and cockroaches have been shown to be major drivers of asthma morbidity, especially among inner-city populations.[103–106]

Policy Approach: Integrated pest management techniques, including strategies that ensure regular and adequate maintenance of housing, have proven to be the most successful mechanism for preventing infestations.[107] For example, allergen-reducing environmental interventions include the following approaches: High-Efficiency Particulate Air (HEPA) vacuuming, using dust mite covers on mattresses, carpet removal, and chemical dust mite control.[108–110] Environmental interventions that seek to redress these exposures have been endorsed but do not always lead to a reduction in exposures or asthma symptoms, potentially due to the difficulty of reducing allergens and pollutants in neighborhoods where these exposures are endemic.[109]

Asbestos

Asbestos, a term that refers to six types of naturally occurring mineral fibers, is carcinogenic and can be detrimental to human health.[111]

Exposure Route: No level of asbestos exposure is considered safe for human health. Most persons have inhaled or ingested trace amount of asbestos during their lifetime, but trace amounts rarely cause adverse health outcomes. Most health issues arise when an individual is repeatedly exposed to asbestos over a long period of time. Asbestos disease occurs when an individual inadvertently inhales or ingests microscopic asbestos fibers.[112,113]

Exposure Prevalence: One type of asbestos, chrysotile asbestos, is the most common commercial form of asbestos. This type is strong, resistant, and works well as an insulator; therefore, chrysotile asbestos was commonly used for consumer products before it was phased out in the 1970s due to public health concerns. Notably, asbestos was commonly used to insulate houses, including used for roofing, siding, floor tiles, some types of paint, ironing boards, and heating appliances.[102]

Impact of Exposure: The health impacts of long-term, repeated exposure to asbestos are grave. Occupational studies on exposed workers showed that three conditions are associated with exposure: lung cancer, mesothelioma, and asbestosis.[114]

Policy Approach: Asbestos is a material that is very costly to remove and removal can sometimes exacerbate exposure.[115] Therefore, when handling asbestos exposure in residential homes, it is important to consult the Agency for Toxic Substances and Disease Registry documentation about asbestos entitled "Toxicological Profile for Asbestos."[111]

Indoor Air Quality

Every day, humans are exposed to environmental pollutants. However, recognizing the level of risk associated with environmental pollutant exposure is important. Assessing ongoing exposures in the home is important since most people spent a significant portion of time in their home. Therefore, for most persons, the risk of indoor air pollution exceeds the risk of outdoor pollution.[116]

Exposure Route: Air pollution can enter the home if not enough outdoor air is circulated throughout a home. When outdoor air is introduced in a home, it dilutes emissions from indoor sources that produce pollutants. Additionally, outdoor air circulates to carry indoor pollutants outside (air exchange rate and ventilation). Studies have also shown that high temperatures and humidity can lead to an increased concentration of indoor pollutants. When ventilation is poor in a housing unit, it can lead to poor indoor air quality.[102]

Exposure Prevalence: Indoor air pollutants can be categorized as biologic or chemical. Biological pollutants that impact indoor air quality include: bacteria, molds, viruses, animal dander, cat saliva, dust mites, and pollen. Chemical pollutants include: carbon monoxide, ozone, environmental tobacco smoke (also referred to as secondhand smoke), volatile organic compounds, radon, and pesticides. Over the past decade, several studies have emerged that suggest air in residential homes can be more polluted than outdoor air in large, industrialized cities. Notably, vulnerable persons such as young children, the elderly, and the chronically ill are the most susceptible to indoor air pollutants.[2,117]

Policy Approach: A variety of approaches ranging from education and information dissemination to changing economic incentives around air quality and pollution are likely necessary to address the issue.[118]

Other

Several other less common physical exposures can also impact human health, including thermal comfort, hygiene, dust, lighting, and carbon monoxide, just to highlight a few (Box 32-3).

Solutions to Address Harmful Physical Exposures in Housing Units

As discussed above, policy approaches to address harmful physical exposures in housing units vary greatly according to the type of exposure. Generally, remediation plans that address the underlying causes of risky physical exposures are the most successful. These plans must be coordinated by appropriate entities across various levels of government. Several general strategies to addressing physical exposures in U.S. housing stock are addressed below.

Federal Strategies

At the federal level, HUD has increasingly recognized the important link between the physical infrastructure of housing and population health. HUD oversees the nation's most well-established national healthy homes program and is uniquely positioned to lead the nation's efforts to reduce housing-related hazards. Within HUD, the Office of Lead Hazard Control and Healthy Homes (OLHCHH) provides funds to state and local governments to develop cost-effective ways to protect children and their families from health and safety hazards in their homes. The office's strategic plan highlights four key policy goals: (1) build a national framework for fostering partnerships, (2) create healthy housing through key research including cost-effective methods to address hazards, (3) mainstream a healthy homes approach, and (4) enable communities to create and sustain healthy homes.[119] By collaborating with necessary state and local partners, comprehensive healthy homes programs can be utilized across the country to reduce physical exposure in the U.S. housing stock. For example, many states have a "healthy homes" program office within their Department of Health that addresses and supports livability codes, remediation programs, and lead poisoning prevention programs.

Safety Hazards Assessments

The physical infrastructure of a house can serve as a platform to promote health and wellness for its residents. For a home to be healthy, injury prevention is a necessary concept to address. A home's

BOX 32-3 Abbreviated Discussion of Selected Other Physical Exposures in U.S. Housing

- ***Thermal Comfort***. The term "thermal comfort" has been used to refer to an individual's or household's satisfaction with ambient temperature in a home environment.[191] Often associated with energy consumption, low-income households can struggle to afford adequate heating or cooling.[194] When this occurs, especially among vulnerable populations such as the very young or very old, human health is put at risk.
- ***Hygiene and Sanitation***. A lack of hygiene and proper sanitation equipment is a serious public health concern for developing country, but it is not a prominent problem in the United States. Estimates from the 2015 American Housing Survey estimate that less than 0.01% of surveyed households reported severely inadequate plumbing whereas the 2008–12 American Community Survey indicates that approximately 630,000 occupied homes (0.5% of all U.S. homes) lack complete plumbing facilities.[78]
- ***Dust***. As mentioned previously, exposure to dust mites can lead to adverse health outcomes including asthma and allergies. Dust can be exposed to home via two routes: (1) dust mites and (2) it can be carried inside by shoes or blown through windows and doors.
- ***Lighting***. According to the World Health Organization, having adequate natural and artificial light in a household is a determinant of health but more evidence is needed to determine this relationship.[198] Natural light exposure is associated with vitamin D production, sleep cycle regulation, injury prevention, and mental health.[199] When natural light is not sufficient, artificial light is needed to prevent falls and injuries among the elderly and frail elderly.
- ***Carbon Monoxide***. Carbon monoxide (CO) is a colorless, odorless gas. When humans are exposed, especially in unventilated, indoor environments, CO poisoning occurs. Sudden illness and death is possible. Common symptoms associated with CO exposure are often described as "flu-like." According to the CDC, approximately 400 Americans die every year from unintentional CO poisoning, 20,000 persons visit an emergency room, and 4000 persons are hospitalized.[202–204] Although CO gas is colorless and odorless, poisoning is preventable through the use of carbon monoxide detectors.[206]

structure should be designed to promote safety and avoid risk hazards. One approach to identifying housing hazards is through the use of assessment protocols. Currently, there is no widely accepted standardized set of protocols that can be used to assess multiple health hazards within a home. However, there are several risk-specific protocols that can be used in tandem to conduct hazard assessments and promote public health.[120] HUD developed "Housing-Related Health and Safety Hazard Assessment," a chapter that provides an overview of inspection and assessment methods pertinent to promoting a healthy home. These standards can be used by health professionals to assess home conditions.[121]

Remediation Plans

Once hazards are identified, comprehensive home improvement and remediation plans have the potential to eliminate home health hazards successfully.[82,122] Although these plans are expensive, they remain the most effective approach to promoting health in inadequate housing units. The *Healthy Housing Reference Manual*, published in collaboration by HHS and HUD, serves as a reference manual for public health and housing professionals seeking to create, promote, and maintain healthy housing.[123]

HOUSING AFFORDABILITY

A key component of the link between housing and health is the amount of financial resources families spend on their housing and related expenses (e.g., heating and other utilities). On one hand, higher priced housing may allow greater access to quality housing, safer neighborhoods, and higher performing schools.[124] On the other hand, spending a large proportion of a household's budget on housing costs, especially for low-income families, may stretch financial resources to the breaking point, leaving little money for adequate food, medical care, and other health-promoting resources.[125] Such trade-offs may increase the risk of residential instability and even homelessness as described above. In this section, we discuss the scope of housing affordability and instability, review the evidence linking housing affordability and health, and discuss potential solutions. We highlight issues that are common to both renters and homeowners and note potential differences.

Scope: Housing Affordability

A standard metric for determining whether housing is affordable is based on whether housing costs (typically mortgage or rent plus utility costs) exceed 30% of a families' income.[126] Since housing costs are highly variable based on locality (e.g., market conditions, availability of affordable housing, etc.), rent burden metrics are often calculated using area median income standards that account for geography. According to Joint Center for Housing Studies at Harvard University, nearly one-third of households overall (32.9% or 39.8 million households) and almost half of renters (48.3%) were estimated to be cost-burdened in 2015.[125] Using stricter criteria, 18.8 million households were severely cost-burdened, indicating that they spent over half of their income on housing costs.[125,127]

HUD produces a biannual report to Congress that quantifies housing affordability needs in the United States. The report defines households with "worst case" housing need as "renters with very low incomes—no more than 50% of the Area Median Income (AMI)—who do not receive government housing assistance and who pay more than one-half of their income for rent, live in severely inadequate conditions, or both." The 2017 Worst Case Housing Needs Report stated that in 2015, 8.3 million renter households had worst case housing needs.[127]

The calculation of cost-burden depends both on housing costs and on a families' resources. For housing costs, the supply of affordable housing is severely limited, though the extent of the constraints varies across geographic areas. Low-income families are not only at greater risk of being severely cost-burdened but also have fewer financial resources remaining after paying for housing costs. For example, over 70% of renter households with annual incomes less than $15,000 were severely cost-burdened. Moreover, the proportion of cost-burdened households varies by race/ethnicity: the proportion of cost-burdened black households was 19 percentage points higher than that of white households in 2015.[125] Specifically, for white households, the cost-burdened share was 28%, a number significantly lower than estimates for minority families: 47% for blacks, 44% for Hispanics, and 37% for Asians/others.[125]

Lack of housing affordability impacts renters and homeowners in different ways. For renters, the number of affordable units outstrips the growing demand. One study estimated that for every 100 extremely low-income families, there were only 35 affordable rental units available.[128] Nearly two-thirds of Americans own their own homes (63.6%); however, there are large disparities in home ownership by race/ethnicity and socioeconomic status. The proportion of black families that own their homes has declined over the past decade to 42.2% whereas the proportion of white families is 71.9% leading to a gap of 29.7 percentage points. The proportion of Asians who own homes stands at 55.5% and Hispanics are at 46.0%.[125] Homeowners enjoy tax advantages (including the mortgage interest deduction) and may experience greater wealth accumulation compared to renters.[129] At the same time, they may also experience high housing costs that may have important health ramifications (see section on Foreclosure below).

Evidence Linking Housing Affordability and Health

There are several potential consequences of the lack of housing affordability with respect to health and health promotion, yet untangling these relationships is complex. To the extent that people choose to live in homes with certain characteristics and in particular neighborhoods, it is difficult to isolate causality. Further adding to the complexity, researchers have hypothesized that some families may spend "too little" on housing, consigning them to live in a poor-quality home in an underresourced neighborhood.[124,130,131] In contrast, families who spend more on housing costs may have greater opportunities for health promotion (e.g., better school systems in neighborhoods with higher housing costs). While we recognize these possibilities, we focus on the documented health consequences that households and families face when living in unaffordable homes.

Access to Care for Renters and Homeowners

Overall, adults who have difficulty affording housing costs have been shown to be less likely to have a usual source of medical care and more likely to delay medical care.[132] One study among homeowners and renters in the greater Philadelphia region found living in unaffordable housing was linked to worse self-reported health and higher risks of certain medical conditions (e.g., arthritis but not several other conditions including heart disease, diabetes, asthma, and psychiatric conditions).[133] The same study found that the association between housing affordability and health was stronger among renters when compared to homeowners.[133]

Residential Instability and Housing Insecurity

Families who live in unaffordable housing are at greater risk of residential instability defined as frequent moves. Residential instability has been linked with a range of problems for children and adolescents including cognitive development, behavioral and emotional problems, higher rates of teen pregnancy, lower rates of healthcare continuity, and increased preventable hospitalizations as well as reduced well-being for some adults.[134–138] The number and timing of moves and whether the move involves changing schools is also likely important in the link with cognitive, behavioral, and health outcomes for children.[134,139]

Crowding

Some families that face high housing costs, experience residential crowding, sometimes due to households "doubling up" in their home. In research studies, crowding has been defined according to different criteria, sometimes as the number of persons per rooms, per bedrooms, or the unit square footage per person, and with different thresholds for defining overcrowding (often two persons per bedroom). One study using data from Los Angeles as well as national data found that crowding was linked with poor academic achievement.[140] Among adults, crowding has often, albeit not invariably, been linked with psychological withdrawal and potentially elevated blood pressure.[141–145] Crowding, which reflects a household's socioeconomic status, has been found to co-exist with food insecurity.[146]

Economic Trade-offs: Housing, Food, and Healthcare

More generally, households with high housing costs tend to spend less on food and other household needs. In their annual report, the Harvard University's Joint Center for Housing Studies reported that severely cost-burdened low-income households spent 53% less on food, healthcare, and transportation combined compared to households that were not cost-burdened. Severely cost-burdened, low-income families with children spent less than $300 per month on food compared to nearly $500 per month among those not experiencing housing cost-burdens.[125] The growing literature on food insecurity has shown that children are more than twice as likely to report being in fair or poor health and report higher levels of asthma compared to food secure children.[147] Adults who experience food insecurity also have been found to have worse health problems including poorer self-rated health, mental health problems, diabetes, and hypertension. In another study, infants living in families that faced food insecurity were significantly less likely to be hospitalized if they received housing rental assistance compared to similar families that did not receive assistance.[148]

Moreover, severely cost-burdened low-income families with children and older adult households spend much less on healthcare compared to those not experiencing cost-burden (e.g., $99 per month among low-income older adult households with severe cost-burden vs. $263 per month for those living in affordable housing).[125] High housing costs may cause families to live further away from employment, necessitating longer commute times and leaving less time for exercise or other health-promoting activities. Families who live in unaffordable housing also tend to spend less on child enrichment and have greater cognitive development in children.[130,131]

As another trade-off, some families live in poor quality housing marked by structural issues or system deficiencies.[78]

Eviction and Foreclosure

For renters, evictions may lead to residential instability by forcing them to move. An estimated 900,000 formal eviction judgments were found for 2016.[149] A disproportionate share of evictions have been shown to impact women from predominantly black and Hispanic neighborhoods.[150] Evictions, in turn, make it harder for households to find new homes, often consigning them to poorer quality homes and in worse neighborhoods.

Similarly, homeowners may face foreclosure when they are no longer able to afford their mortgage payments. The dramatic rise in foreclosure starting around 2007 was due to a range of factors including an economic recession, subprime mortgage, and other factors with racial/ethnic minorities disproportionately impacted.[151,152] For some families, in addition to macroeconomic factors, poor health and healthcare-related expenses were a prime cause of foreclosure.[153,154]

With regard to the potential health consequences of foreclosure, one convenience sample found that nearly half of adults in financial counseling for their foreclosure had symptoms of depression with one-third meeting screening criteria for major depression (compared to 13% of people living in poverty nationally).[153] Additionally, findings on increased rates of depression among individuals undergoing foreclosure have been confirmed in longitudinal studies, including those using national samples, and have additionally found decline in health, increase in food insecurity, and increased cost-related medication nonadherence.[155–157]

Solutions to Address Housing Affordability and Health

In this section, we focus on housing assistance programs, which cap the amount of money that families spend on rent and utilities. However, there are several other approaches to address housing affordability that warrant careful policy consideration although these approaches have rarely been investigated with respect to health. For example, changes to municipal zoning codes may allow for more the development of multifamily and smaller units, thereby increasing the supply of affordable housing. As another example, approximately 2.8 million units have been developed through the Low Income Housing Tax Credit (LIHTC). There has been growing interest in targeting these tax credits toward developments that explicitly consider health criteria.[158–160] For example, some health insurance companies have supported the creation of LIHTC developments by providing financing for projects. It is plausible that proposed remedies to address eviction and foreclosure such as providing legal representation to tenants may have spillover effects on health. In addition, finally, with

BOX 32-4 Does Receipt of Rental Assistance Improve Health?

Increasingly, researchers have begun investigating the connection between housing assistance and health by leveraging efforts to link HUD administrative records to other, health-related datasets. Using data from the National Health Interview Survey, researchers have painted a clearer picture of the health characteristics of adults and children living in public and assisted housing, especially when compared to low-income families not in public housing. Because signing up for housing assistance is not random, studies have employed a variety of approaches to address this, including the creation of a group of low-income individuals who are likely on the waitlist for housing assistance. Using this approach, researchers have found:

- Significantly fewer adults receiving housing assistance reported fair or poor heath compared to those who did not (OR 0.77 for living in public housing; OR 0.75 for multifamily housing). Public housing residents were less likely to report serious psychological distress (OR = 0.59).[195]
- Housing assistance was linked with lower rates of uninsurance (31.8% vs. 37.2%) and lower rates of unmet healthcare needs due to cost.[196]

housing affordability fundamentally about housing costs relative to a households' income, efforts to increase household income may be an important component.

Federal Housing Assistance Programs

In 2016, HUD rental assistance programs helped approximately 9.8 million low-income families pay for housing costs.[161] HUD assistance primarily comes from Housing Choice Vouchers, which help family pay for housing in the private market, multifamily programs, including project-based Section 8, and public housing. However, rental assistance is not an entitlement program and the number of families who qualify for housing assistance far outstrips the number that actually receives it: approximately a quarter of very low-income renters eligible for HUD assistance programs actually receive housing assistance.[127] Indeed, because wait lists for rental assistance are so long, many municipalities have closed their waitlist for new households.[162] Several other HUD programs are directed at specific populations including elderly populations, persons living with a disability, people living with HIV and AIDS, and veterans. These populations have unique needs. For example, recently some studies have sought to estimate how the receipt of housing assistance impacts health (Box 32-4).

NEIGHBORHOODS

Scope: Neighborhoods and Health

Homes are situated in neighborhoods, which may exert a powerful influence on health. Neighborhoods vary widely in terms of their composition, structure, and context.[163] The racial, ethnic, and socioeconomic composition of neighborhoods has also been a focus of health and other policy initiatives. Across the United States, 6.1% of census tracts (a proxy for neighborhoods) are characterized by being "extreme poverty neighborhoods" in which 40% of residents have household incomes that fall below the federal poverty limit.[164] These census tracts contain 13.8 million residents, with a disproportionate share being young children and nonwhite persons. Neighborhoods within and across geographic areas have been shown to have high and often increasing levels of segregation (indicating an uneven distribution) by both income and racial/ethnic composition.[165,166] Many health researchers have explored structural characteristics of neighborhoods by focusing on the built and physical environments.[167,168] More broadly, neighborhoods may be situated within cities, suburban areas, and rural geographies, all of which present different policy contexts.

Evidence Linking Neighborhoods and Health

Levels of health behavior, comorbidity, and life expectancy have been shown to vary widely across neighborhoods.[169,170] Similar to studies on housing, the "selection" of households into different neighborhoods is not random and may be correlated with the outcomes under investigation (i.e., health status). Although costly, large-scale social experiments that utilize randomized control trial methodology offer one way to address this methodological challenge (e.g., HUD's Moving to Opportunity Demonstration, see Box 32-5).

Further, studies of neighborhood influences on health have grappled with the appropriate unit of analysis to measure neighborhood effects (including the geographic size and whether to have neighborhoods comport to administratively defined boundaries such as census tracts) and the optimal way to measure neighborhood exposures (which may entail using existing data sources, direct observation, and resident perceived neighborhood quality).[169,171]

Many mechanisms have been posited that link neighborhood environments including physical and social factors with specific health behaviors and outcomes. Specifically, a large body of research has focused on the built environment: neighborhood environment features that may promote physical activity, change dietary patterns, and increase the risk of obesity.[172] For example, access to fresh food varies across neighborhoods and with respect to resident race and socioeconomic status.[173] One study, leveraging a natural experiment of a full service grocery store entering into a neighborhood, found decline in food insecurity, increase in Supplemental Nutrition Assistance Program participation, and fewer new diagnoses of high cholesterol relative to residents of the comparison neighborhood.[174] In another study, the opening of a supermarket in a food "desert" (e.g., an area characterized by limited access to fresh foods) was linked with residents reporting greater perceived availability of produce.[175] Systematic reviews suggest a relationship between the amount of greenspace available in a neighborhood, including parks and recreational spaces with physical activity and obesity.[176,177] Other features of the built environment such as increased housing density, mixed commercial and residential land use have further been linked with physical activity.[178,179]

Neighborhoods characterized by lower socioeconomic status are more likely to have factors thought to harm health and well-being, including greater exposure to violence and presence of environmental toxins. For example, studies that have exploited the timing of neighborhood violence have found that children exposed to recent violence have lower levels of attention, impulse control, and lower academic skills among children as well as distress among their parents.[180,181] Exposure to violence has been linked with biological markers of stress among children.[182,183]

More broadly, social environments differ widely between neighborhoods and have been shown to impact health. Researchers and social epidemiologists have investigated multiple-related concepts including collective efficacy, defined as "social cohesion among neighborhoods combined with their willingness to intervene on behalf of the common good,"[184] and social capital indicating "features of social organization, such as civic participation, norms of reciprocity, and trust in others, that facilitate cooperation for mutual benefit."[185] Studies have found a wide variety of health outcomes including physical health, mental health, and healthcare access, though these features of the neighborhood environments have been conceptualized and measured at a variety of different individual and neighborhood levels which may impact their associations with health.[169,186,187] In addition, residential racial segregation has been linked with health disparities in the United States.[188]

BOX 32-5 Moving to Opportunity for Fair Housing Demonstration Program: Experimental Data on the Link between Neighborhood Poverty and Health

HUD initiated a social experiment, called Moving to Opportunity (MTO) for Fair Housing Demonstration Program, to investigate whether helping families with housing vouchers move to "opportunity" neighborhoods characterized by lower rates of poverty and improved economic outcomes.[193] While prior studies of families that had moved were promising, the concern existed that families who moved were fundamentally different from families who did not (confounding). From 1994 to 1998, HUD's MTO program randomized 4498 low-income families living in public housing within five cities to:

a. A control group,
b. A voucher which required a move to a low-poverty neighborhood (low-poverty voucher), or
c. An unrestricted, traditional Section 8 voucher.

Less than half (48%) of families in the low-poverty voucher group were able to successfully move to a low-poverty neighborhood and many who did move, over time, moved back into higher poverty neighborhoods; 63% of families with the traditional vouchers were able to move with their voucher. Nonetheless, overall experiences of neighborhood poverty were significantly different between study arms. For example, neighborhood census tract poverty rates were approximately 17 percentage points lower for the low-poverty voucher group compared to the control group at 1 year after randomization and 4.9 percentage points lower at 10 years after randomization.

MTO had initially been designed to examine the impact on adult earnings and economic outcomes. For these outcomes, results were largely disappointing. Participation in the labor market was not significantly different between study arms. However, the economic outcomes for children who moved to a low-poverty neighborhood at a young age (<13 years old) were substantial: with higher earnings, increased college attendance, and reduced rates of single parenthood.[200] Though not originally envisioned as a health intervention, MTO resulted in significant differences in health. At the final evaluation (10–15 years following randomization), adults who received a low-poverty voucher were less likely to be obese or have diabetes compared to the control group.[201] The absolute difference between the low-poverty voucher and control group for obesity was 4.6 percentage points (BMI of 35 or more) and for diabetes was 4.3 percentage points. Adults also reported greater overall subjective well-being.[205] The mental health impact on children appeared to vary by gender, with girls reporting lower rates of major depression or conduct disorder whereas boys having higher rates of major depression, conduct disorder, and PTSD.[207] The reasons for these gender-divergent findings have been explored in qualitative work suggesting that this may result from differences in social groups, norms, and where boys and girls tended to spend time.[208]

Overall, the experimental design of MTO provides strong evidence for a link between neighborhood poverty and health. MTO also provides evidence to suggest that, at least for some families, housing mobility programs that help them move with a voucher from high-poverty to opportunity neighborhoods may be a promising health intervention. Several housing mobility programs currently exist across the country, often as a result of settlements from lawsuits claiming that HUD or other entities violated fair housing laws.

BOX 32-6 HOPE VI and the Move to Demolish Severely Distressed Housing

Since 1992, the HOPE VI Program has spent over $6.7 billion to revitalize "severely distressed" public housing projects, defined as homes characterized by extremely poor residents living in dilapidated housing in economically and socially distressed neighborhoods.[192] HOPE VI sought to create mixed-income communities, often replacing high-density, high-rise housing with lower density housing with higher construction standards and better amenities. By attracting higher income residents, developers sought to avoid patterns of mismanagement and disinvestment that had plagued severely distress public housing. Evaluations suggest that such approaches were frequently successful in improving the built environments; however, in deconcentrating poverty, researchers found that a large proportion of households were either unable or did not desire to move back into their redeveloped housing project.

A report by the Urban Institute summarized the mixed success:

> The program has achieved substantial success; it has demolished some of the most distressed and destructive housing environments, replaced them with much higher-quality housing and, in many cases, with mixed-income communities. Many residents who relocated with vouchers are living in higher-quality housing in safer neighborhoods….assistance with relocation and supportive services should be strengthened, and new attention should be given to innovations such as "enhanced vouchers" that would provide long-term counseling and support to vulnerable families in conjunction with housing assistance.[197]

Solutions to Address Neighborhoods and Health

Efforts to address the link between neighborhood environments and health have taken a wide variety of approaches. These include interventions focused on specific neighborhood amenities such as increasing access to healthy food by opening a full-service grocery store and reducing neighborhood violence by restoring blighted or vacant properties.[189] Other efforts have worked to change the broader neighborhood environments by, for example, demolishing distressed public housing (e.g., HOPE VI, see Box 32-6), promoting mixed-income developments, and changing zoning and land-use regulations.[190]

CONCLUSION

Policymakers and practitioners increasingly recognize the impact that homelessness, physical exposures, housing affordability, and neighborhood context can have on individual and community health. To address these factors, advocates have called for a "Health in All Policies" framework, a collaborative approach to "embedding health considerations into decision-making processes across a broad range of sectors."[209] By considering both the intended and unintended health impacts of housing and neighborhood initiatives, this framework hopes to maximize health benefits while reducing harms.[210] At the same time, with payment models that increasingly pay for population health and a growing evidence base around the ways housing and neighborhood factors impact health, healthcare institutions are beginning to consider these issues.[211] New initiatives are being tested around, for example, the best way to collect information on housing instability and link patients to services.[212] While still in its infancy, these approaches to working across sectors hold tremendous opportunities to address the social determinants of health.

References

1. Shaw M. Housing and public health. *Annu Rev Public Health.* 2004;25:397–418.
2. Krieger J, Higgins DL. Housing and health: Time again for public health action. *Am J Public Health.* 2002;92(5):758–68.
3. Bashir SA. Home is where the harm is: Inadequate housing as a public health crisis. *Am J Public Health.* 2002;92(5):733–8.
4. Sandel M. 2014 Housing Opportunity Conference. https://howhousingmatters.org/articles/pediatrician-sees-housing-as-vaccine/. Updated 2015. Accessed January 2018.
5. National Health Care for the Homeless Council. What is the official definition of homelessness? https://www.nhchc.org/faq/official-definition-homelessness. Accessed April 2, 2018.
6. HRSA/Bureau of Primary Health Care. Program assistance letter 99-12, health care for the homeless principles of practice.
7. Kuhn R, Culhane DP. Applying cluster analysis to test a typology of homelessness by pattern of shelter utilization: Results from the analysis of administrative data. *Am J Community Psychol.* 1998;26(2):207–32.
8. Busch-Geertsema V, Culhane D, Fitzpatrick S. Developing a global framework for conceptualising and measuring homelessness. *Habitat Int.* 2016;55:124–32.
9. Minnery J, Greenhalgh E. Approaches to homelessness policy in Europe, the United States, and Australia. *J Soc Issues.* 2007;63(3):641–55.
10. HUD funds communities to establish Homelessness Management Information Systems (HMIS), an administrative data system in which communities record data about households served in HUD's homeless assistance programs. Aggregate statistics from these systems are reported to congress in the annual homeless assessment report (AHAR).
11. The U.S. Department of Housing and Urban Development. The 2017 annual homeless assessment report (AHAR) to congress: Part I. 2017.
12. The U.S. Department of Housing and Urban Development. The 2016 annual homeless assessment report (AHAR) to congress: Part II. 2016.
13. Link BG, Susser E, Stueve A, Phelan J, Moore RE, Struening E. Lifetime and five-year prevalence of homelessness in the United States. *Am J Public Health.* 1994;84(12):1907–12.
14. Toro PA, Tompsett CJ, Lombardo S, et al. Homelessness in Europe and the United States: A comparison of prevalence and public opinion. *J Soc Issues.* 2007;63(3):505–24.
15. Katz MH. Homelessness-challenges and progress. *JAMA.* 2017;318(23): 2293–4.
16. Koh HK, O'Connell JJ. Improving health care for homeless people. *JAMA.* 2016;316(24):2586–7.
17. Rennison CM, Welchans S. Intimate partner violence. *Violence against women.* 2000:1993–98.
18. Breiding MJ. Prevalence and characteristics of sexual violence, stalking, and intimate partner violence victimization—National intimate partner and sexual violence survey, United States, 2011. *MMWR Surveill Summ.* 2014;63(8):1–18.
19. Desai RA, Liu-Mares W, Dausey DJ, Rosenheck RA. Suicidal ideation and suicide attempts in a sample of homeless people with mental illness. *J Nervous Mental Dis.* 2003;191(6):365–71.
20. Schanzer B, Dominguez B, Shrout PE, Caton CL. Homelessness, health status, and health care use. *Am J Public Health.* 2007;97(3):464–9.
21. O'Connell JJ. *Premature Mortality in Homeless Populations: A Review of the Literature.* Nashville, TN: National Health Care for the Homeless Council, Inc.; 2005.
22. Haddad MB, Wilson TW, Ijaz K, Marks SM, Moore M. Tuberculosis and homelessness in the United States, 1994-2003. *JAMA.* 2005;293(22):2762–6.
23. Wolitski RJ, Kidder DP, Fenton KA.HIV, homelessness, and public health: Critical issues and a call for increased action. *AIDS Behav.* 2007;11(6 Suppl):167–71.
24. Beijer U, Wolf A, Fazel S. Prevalence of tuberculosis, hepatitis C virus, and HIV in homeless people: A systematic review and meta-analysis. *Lancet Infect Dis.* 2012;12(11):859–70.
25. Fazel S, Geddes JR, Kushel M. The health of homeless people in high-income countries: Descriptive epidemiology, health consequences, and clinical and policy recommendations. *Lancet.* 2014;384(9953):1529–40.
26. Baggett TP, O'Connell JJ, Singer DE, Rigotti NA. The unmet health care needs of homeless adults: A national study. *Am J Public Health.* 2010;100(7):1326–33.
27. Morton MH, Dworsky A, Matjasko JL, et al. Prevalence and correlates of youth homelessness in the United States. *J Adolesc Health.* 2018;62(1):14–21.
28. Athey JL. HIV infection and homeless adolescents. *Child Welfare.* 1991;70(5):517–28.
29. Bailey SL, Camlin CS, Ennett ST. Substance use and risky sexual behavior among homeless and runaway youth. *J Adolesc Health.* 1998;23(6):378–88.
30. Whitbeck LB, Hoyt DR, Yoder KA. A risk-amplification model of victimization and depressive symptoms among runaway and homeless adolescents. *Am J Community Psychol.* 1999;27(2):273–96.
31. Cauce AM, Paradise M, Ginzler JA, Embry L, Morgan CJ, Lohr Y, Theofelis J. The characteristics and mental health of homeless adolescents: Age and gender differences. *J Emot Behav.* 2000;8(4):230–9.
32. Auerswald CL, Lin JS, Parriott A. Six-year mortality in a street-recruited cohort of homeless youth in San Francisco, California. *PeerJ.* 2016;4:e1909.
33. Hahn JA, Kushel MB, Bangsberg DR, Riley E, Moss AR. BRIEF REPORT: The aging of the homeless population: Fourteen-year trends in San Francisco. *J Gen Intern Med.* 2006;21(7):775–8.
34. Rossi PH. *Down and Out in America: The Origins of Homelessness.* Chicago, IL: University of Chicago Press; 1991.
35. Lamb HR. Deinstitutionalization and the homeless mentally ill. *Hosp Community Psychiatry.* 1984;35(9):899–907.
36. Dear MJ, Wolch JR. *Landscapes of Despair: From Deinstitutionalization to Homelessness.* Princeton, NJ: Princeton University Press; 2014.
37. Sullivan G, Burnam A, Koegel P, Hollenberg J. Quality of life of homeless persons with mental illness: Results from the course-of-homelessness study. *Psychiatr Serv.* 2000;51(9):1135–41.
38. Fischer PJ, Breakey WR. The epidemiology of alcohol, drug, and mental disorders among homeless persons. *Am Psychol.* 1991;46(11):1115–28.
39. Folsom DP, Hawthorne W, Lindamer L, et al. Prevalence and risk factors for homelessness and utilization of mental health services among 10,340 patients with serious mental illness in a large public mental health system. *Am J Psychiatry.* 2005;162(2):370–6.
40. Fitzpatrick KM, La Gory ME, Ritchey FJ. Criminal victimization among the homeless. *Justice Q.* 1993;10(3):353–68.
41. Hiday VA, Swartz MS, Swanson JW, Borum R, Wagner HR. Criminal victimization of persons with severe mental illness. *Psychiatr Serv.* 1999;50(1):62–8.
42. Zlotnick C, Tam T, Robertson MJ.Disaffiliation, substance use, and exiting homelessness. *Subst Use Misuse.* 2003;38(3-6):577–99.
43. Fazel S, Khosla V, Doll H, Geddes J. The prevalence of mental disorders among the homeless in western countries: Systematic review and meta-regression analysis. *PLoS Med.* 2008;5(12):e225.
44. Collins SE, Taylor E, Jones C, et al. Content analysis of advantages and disadvantages of drinking among individuals with the lived experience of homelessness and alcohol use disorders. *Subst Use Misuse.* 2018;53(1):16–25.
45. Gabrielian S, Bromley E, Hellemann GS, et al. Factors affecting exits from homelessness among persons with serious mental illness and substance use disorders. *J Clin Psychiatry.* 2015;76(4):469.
46. Linton SL, Celentano DD, Kirk GD, Mehta SH. The longitudinal association between homelessness, injection drug use, and injection-related risk behavior among persons with a history of injection drug use in Baltimore, MD. *Drug Alcohol Depend.* 2013;132(3):457–65.
47. Song JY, Safaeian M, Strathdee SA, Vlahov D, Celentano DD. The prevalence of homelessness among injection drug users with and without HIV infection. *J Urban Health.* 2000;77(4):678–87.
48. Baggett TP, Anderson R, Freyder PJ, et al. Addressing tobacco use in homeless populations: A survey of health care professionals. *J Health Care Poor Underserved.* 2012;23(4):1650–9.
49. Arnsten JH, Reid K, Bierer M, Rigotti N. Smoking behavior and interest in quitting among homeless smokers. *Addict Behav.* 2004;29(6):1155–61.
50. Baggett TP, Chang Y, Singer DE, et al. Tobacco-, alcohol-, and drug-attributable deaths and their contribution to mortality disparities in a cohort of homeless adults in Boston. *Am J Public Health.* 2015;105(6):1189–97.
51. Fargo J, Metraux S, Byrne T, et al. Prevalence and risk of homelessness among US veterans. *Prev Chronic Dis.* 2012;9:E45.
52. Tsai J, Link B, Rosenheck RA, Pietrzak RH. Homelessness among a nationally representative sample of US veterans: Prevalence, service utilization, and correlates. *Soc Psychiatry Psychiatr Epidemiol.* 2016;51(6):907–16.
53. Weber J, Lee RC, Martsolf D. Understanding the health of veterans who are homeless: A review of the literature. *Public Health Nurs.* 2017;34(5):505–11.

54. Iheanacho T, Rosenheck R. Prevalence and correlates of diabetes mellitus among homeless veterans nationally in the veterans health administration. *J Soc Distress Homeless* 2016;25(2):53–59.

55. Goldstein G, Luther JF, Jacoby AM, Haas GL, Gordon AJ. A taxonomy of medical comorbidity for veterans who are homeless. *J Health Care Poor Underserved*. 2008;19(3):991–1005.

56. O'Toole TP, Buckel L, Bourgault C, et al. Applying the chronic care model to homeless veterans: Effect of a population approach to primary care on utilization and clinical outcomes. *Am J Public Health*. 2010;100(12):2493–9.

57. United States Interagency Council on Homelessness. *Opening Doors: Federal Strategic Plan to Prevent and End Homelessness*. Washington, DC: US Interagency Council on Homelessness; 2015.

58. DiPietro B, Artiga S, Gates A. Early impacts of the Medicaid expansion for the homeless population. 2014.

59. Bamberger J. Reducing homelessness by embracing housing as a Medicaid benefit. *JAMA Intern Med*. 2016;176(8):1051–2.

60. Health Resources and Services Administration. Frequently asked questions about health care for the homeless. 2011.

61. O'Connell JJ, Oppenheimer SC, Judge CM, et al. The Boston health care for the homeless program: A public health framework. *Am J Public Health*. 2010;100(8):1400–8.

62. Blue-Howells J, McGuire J, Nakashima J. Co-location of health care services for homeless veterans: A case study of innovation in program implementation. *Soc Work Health Care*. 2008;47(3):219–31.

63. McGuire J, Gelberg L, Blue-Howells J, Rosenheck RA. Access to primary care for homeless veterans with serious mental illness or substance abuse: A follow-up evaluation of co-located primary care and homeless social services. *Adm Policy Ment Health*. 2009;36(4): 255–64.

64. Blount A. Integrated primary care: Organizing the evidence. *Fam Syst Health*. 2003;21(2):121.

65. U.S. Department of Housing and Urban Development. HUD report—Housing first in permanent supportive housing brief.

66. Tsemberis S, Gulcur L, Nakae M. Housing first, consumer choice, and harm reduction for homeless individuals with a dual diagnosis. *Am J Public Health*. 2004;94(4):651–6.

67. Stergiopoulos V, Hwang SW, Gozdzik A, et al. Effect of scattered-site housing using rent supplements and intensive case management on housing stability among homeless adults with mental illness: A randomized trial. *JAMA*. 2015;313(9):905–15.

68. Rog DJ, Marshall T, Dougherty RH, et al. Permanent supportive housing: Assessing the evidence. *Psychiatr Serv*. 2014;65(3):287–94.

69. United States Department of Housing and Urban Development. Rapid re-housing.

70. Substance Abuse and Mental Health Services Administration. *Permanent Supportive Housing: Building Your Program, HHS pub. no. SMA-10-4509*. Rockville, MD: U.S. Department of Health and Human Services; 2010.

71. United States Interagency Council on Homelessness. Supportive housing. 2017.

72. Riis JA. *How the Other Half Lives: Studies Among the Tenements of New York*. New York, NY: Hill and Wang; 1966.

73. Schwartz AF. *Housing policy in the United States*. New York: Routledge; 2014.

74. U.S. Census Bureau. Historical census of housing tables: Plumbing facilities. 2009.

75. 2 U.S. Code § 1701t. Congressional affirmation of national goal of decent homes and suitable living environment for American families.

76. Harry ST. "Annual message to the congress on the state of the union," January 5, 1949.

77. U.S. Department of Housing and Urban Development. Mission. www.hud.gov/about/mission. Accessed February 12, 2018.

78. U.S. Census Bureau. American housing survey: Housing adequacy and quality as measured by the AHS.

79. Newman S, Holupka S. The quality of America's assisted housing stock: Analysis of the 2011 and 2013 American housing surveys. https://www.huduser.gov/portal/publications/mdrt/Quality-Assisted-Housing-Stock.html. Updated 2017.

80. Emrath P, Taylor H. Housing value, costs, and measures of physical adequacy. *Cityscape*. 2012;1:99–125.

81. Evans GW, Saltzman H, Cooperman, JL. Housing quality and children's socioemotional health. *Environ Behav*. 2001;33(3):389–99.

82. Saegert SC, Klitzman S, Freudenberg N, Cooperman-Mroczek J, Nassar S. Healthy housing: A structured review of published evaluations of US interventions to improve health by modifying housing in the United States, 1990–2001. *Am J Public Health*. 2003;93(9):1471–7.

83. Jaishankar M, Tseten T, Anbalagan N, Mathew BB, Beeregowda KN. Toxicity, mechanism and health effects of some heavy metals. *Interdiscip Toxicol*. 2014;7(2):60–72.

84. Rosner D, Markowitz G, Lanphear B. J. Lockhart Gibson and the discovery of the impact of lead pigments on children's health: A review of a century of knowledge. *Public Health Rep*. 2005;120(3):296–300.

85. Needleman H. Lead poisoning. *Annu Rev Med*. 2004;55:209–22.

86. Centers for Disease Control and Prevention. Screening young children for lead poisoning: Guidance for state and local public health officials. CDC; 1997.

87. Patrick L. Lead toxicity, a review of the literature. Part 1: Exposure, evaluation, and treatment. *Altern Med Rev*. 2006;11(1):2–22.

88. Jacobs DE, Clickner RP, Zhou JY, et al. The prevalence of lead-based paint hazards in U.S. housing. *Environ Health Perspect*. 2002;110(10):599–606.

89. Centers for Disease Control and Prevention. Childhood lead poisoning. https://www.cdc.gov/nceh/publications/factsheets/ChildhoodLeadPoisoning.pdf. Updated 2005. Accessed February 2108.

90. Spivey A. The weight of lead: Effects add up in adults. *Environ Health Perspect*. 2007;115(1):30–6.

91. Lanphear BP, Hornung R, Khoury J, et al. Low-level environmental lead exposure and children's intellectual function: An international pooled analysis. *Environ Health Perspect*. 2005;113(7):894-9.

92. Centers for Disease Control and Prevention. Facts about mold and dampness. https://www.cdc.gov/nceh/publications/factsheets/ChildhoodLeadPoisoning.pdf. Updated 2017. Accessed February 2018.

93. Heseltine E, Rosen J, eds. *WHO Guidelines for Indoor Air Quality: Dampness and Mould*. Denmark: WHO Regional Office Europe; 2009.

94. Institute of Medicine. *Damp Indoor Spaces and Health, Institute of Medicine*. Washington, DC: National Academy Press; 2004.

95. U.S. Census Bureau. *Current Housing Reports, Series H150/09, American Housing Survey for the United States: 2009*. Washington, DC: Government Printing Office; 2009.

96. U. S. Department of Housing and Urban Development, Office of Lead Hazard Control and Healthy Homes. HUD's heathy homes demonstration grantees: A review of evaluation capacity, program administration, and best practices. 2015.

97. Fisk WJ, Lei-Gomez Q, Mendell MJ. Meta-analyses of the associations of respiratory health effects with dampness and mold in homes. *Indoor Air*. 2007;17(4):284-96.

98. Mendell MJ, Mirer AG, Cheung K, Tong M, Douwes J. Respiratory and allergic health effects of dampness, mold, and dampness-related agents: A review of the epidemiologic evidence. *Environ Health Perspect*. 2011;119(6):748-56.

99. Reponen T, Lockey J, Bernstein DI, et al. Infant origins of childhood asthma associated with specific molds. *J Allergy Clin Immunol*. 2012;130(3):639–44.

100. Krieger J, Jacobs DE, Ashley PJ, et al. Housing interventions and control of asthma-related indoor biologic agents: A review of the evidence. *J Public Health Manag Pract*. 2010;16(5 Suppl):11.

101. Kercsmar CM, Dearborn DG, Schluchter M, et al. Reduction in asthma morbidity in children as a result of home remediation aimed at moisture sources. *Environ Health Perspect*. 2006;114(10):1574-80.

102. Centers for Disease Control and Prevention and U.S. Department of Housing and Urban Development. *Healthy Housing Reference Manual (Chapter 4)*. Atlanta, GA: US Department of Health and Human Services; 2006.

103. Gruchalla RS, Pongracic J, Plaut M, et al. Inner city asthma study: Relationships among sensitivity, allergen exposure, and asthma morbidity. *J Allergy Clin Immunol*. 2005;115(3):478-85.

104. Pongracic JA, Visness CM, Gruchalla RS, Evans R, Mitchell HE. Effect of mouse allergen and rodent environmental intervention on asthma in inner-city children. *Ann Allergy Asthma Immunol*. 2008;101(1): 35-41.

105. Ahluwalia SK, Peng RD, Breysse PN, et al. Mouse allergen is the major allergen of public health relevance in Baltimore city. *J Allergy Clin Immunol*. 2013;132(4):830–5.

106. Rosenstreich DL, Eggleston P, Kattan M, et al. The role of cockroach allergy and exposure to cockroach allergen in causing morbidity among inner-city children with asthma. *N Engl J Med*. 1997;336(19): 1356-63.

107. Bonnefoy X. Inadequate housing and health: An overview. *Int J Environ Pollut*. 2007;30(3–4):411-29.

108. Gotzsche PC, Johansen HK, Burr ML, Hammarquist C. House dust mite control measures for asthma. *Cochrane Database Syst Rev*. 2004;(4):CD001187.

109. Morgan WJ, Crain EF, Gruchalla RS, et al. Results of a home-based environmental intervention among urban children with asthma. *N Engl J Med*. 2004;351(11):1068-80.

110. Clougherty JE, Levy JI, Hynes HP, Spengler JD. A longitudinal analysis of the efficacy of environmental interventions on asthma-related quality of life and symptoms among children in urban public housing. *J Asthma*. 2006;43(5):335-43.

111. US Public Health Service and US Department of Health and Human Services. *Toxicological Profile for Asbestos*. Atlanta, GA: Agency for Toxic Substances and Disease Registry; 2001.

112. Murray R. Asbestos: A chronology of its origins and health effects. *Br J Ind Med*. 1990;47(6):361-5.

113. Bourdes V, Boffetta P, Pisani P. Environmental exposure to asbestos and risk of pleural mesothelioma: Review and meta-analysis. *Eur J Epidemiol*. 2000;16(5):411-7.

114. Mossman BT, Bignon J, Corn M, Seaton A, Gee JB. Asbestos: Scientific developments and implications for public policy. *Science*. 1990;247(4940):294-301.

115. Jacobs DE, Kelly T, Sobolewski J. Linking public health, housing, and indoor environmental policy: Successes and challenges at local and federal agencies in the United States. *Environ Health Perspect*. 2007;115(6):976-82.

116. Jones AP. Indoor air quality and health. *Atmos Environ*. 1999;33(28):4535–64.

117. Spengler JD, Sexton K. Indoor air pollution: A public health perspective. *Science*. 1983;221(4605):9-17.

118. Wu F, Jacobs D, Mitchell C, Miller D, Karol MH. Improving indoor environmental quality for public health: Impediments and policy recommendations. *Environ Health Perspect*. 2007;115(6):953-7.

119. U.S. Department of Housing and Urban Development. Leading our nation to healthier homes: The healthy homes strategic plan. https://www.hud.gov/sites/documents/DOC_13701.PDF. Updated 2009.

120. Jacobs DE. A qualitative review of housing hazard assessment protocols in the United States. *Environ Res*. 2006;102(1):13-21.

121. U.S. Department of Housing and Urban Development. Housing-related health and safety hazard assessment. chapter 4. https://www.hud.gov/sites/documents/HHPGM_FINAL_CH4.PDF. Accessed February 2018.

122. Thomson H, Petticrew M, Morrison D. Health effects of housing improvement: Systematic review of intervention studies. *BMJ*. 2001;323(7306):187-90.

123. Centers for Disease Control and Prevention and U.S. Department of Housing and Urban Development. *Healthy Housing Reference Manual*. Atlanta, GA: US Department of Health and Human Services; 2006.

124. Newman S, Holupka CS. Housing affordability and children's cognitive achievement. *Health Aff (Millwood)*. 2016;35(11):2092-9.

125. The Joint Center for Housing Studies. Harvard University. The state of the nation's housing: 2017. http://www.jchs.harvard.edu/sites/default/files/harvard_jchs_state_of_the_nations_housing_2017.pdf. Updated 2017.

126. U.S. Department of Housing and Urban Development. HUD income limits. https://www.huduser.gov/portal/datasets/il.html. Accessed January 2018.

127. U.S. Department of Housing and Urban Development, Office of Policy Development and Research. Worst case housing needs 2017 report to congress.

128. Aurand A, Emmanuel D, Yentel D, Errico E, Pang M. The national low income housing coalition. the gap: A shortage of affordable homes. http://nlihc.org/sites/default/files/gap/Gap-Report_2018.pdf. Updated 2018. Accessed March 2018.

129. The Joint Center for Housing Studies. Harvard University. Update on homeownership wealth trajectories through the housing boom and bust. http://www.jchs.harvard.edu/sites/default/files/2013_wealth_update_mccue_02-18-16.pdf. Updated 2016.

130. Newman SJ, Holupka CS. Housing affordability and child well-being. *Hous Policy Debate*. 2014;25(1):116-51.

131. Newman SJ, Holupka CS. Housing affordability and investments in children. *J Hous Econ*. 2014;24(June):89-100.

132. Kushel MB, Gupta R, Gee L, Haas JS. Housing instability and food insecurity as barriers to health care among low-income Americans. *J Gen Intern Med*. 2006;21(1):71-77.

133. Pollack CE, Griffin BA, Lynch J. Housing affordability and health among homeowners and renters. *Am J Prev Med*. 2010;39(6):515-21.

134. Coley RL, Kull M. Cumulative, timing-specific, and interactive models of residential mobility and children's cognitive and psychosocial skills. *Child Dev*. 2016;87(4):1204-20.

135. Jelleyman T, Spencer N. Residential mobility in childhood and health outcomes: A systematic review. *J Epidemiol Community Health*. 2008;62(7):584-92.

136. Hutchings HA, Evans A, Barnes P, et al. Residential moving and preventable hospitalizations. *Pediatrics*. 2016;138(1):e20152836.

137. Oishi S, Schimmack U. Residential mobility, well-being, and mortality. *J Pers Soc Psychol*. 2010;98(6):980-94.

138. Suglia SF, Duarte CS, Sandel MT. Housing quality, housing instability, and maternal mental health. *J Urban Health*. 2011;88(6):1105-16.

139. Evans GW, Wells NM, Moch A. Housing and mental health: A review of the evidence and a methodological and conceptual critique. *J Soc Issues*. 2003;59(3):475-500.

140. Solari CD, Mare RD. Housing crowding effects on children's wellbeing. *Soc Sci Res*. 2012;41(2):464-–76.

141. Baldassare M. *Residential Crowding in Urban America*. Berkeley, CA: University of California Press; 1979, p. 250.

142. Gove WR, Hughes M, Galle OR. Overcrowding in the home: An empirical investigation of its possible pathological consequences. *Am Sociol Rev*. 1979;44(1):59-80.

143. D'Atri DA. Psychophysiological responses to crowding. *Environ Behav*. 1975;44(1):59-80.

144. Evans GW, McCoy MJ. When buildings don't work: The role of architecture in human health. *J. Environ. Psychol* 1998;18(1):85–94.

145. Paulus PB, McCain G, Cox VC. Death rates, psychiatric commitments, blood pressure, and perceived crowding as a function of institutional crowding. *Environ Psych Nonver Behav*. 1978;3(2):107-16.

146. Cutts DB, Meyers AF, Black MM, et al. US housing insecurity and the health of very young children. *Am J Public Health*. 2011;101(8):1508-14.

147. Gundersen C, Ziliak JP. Food insecurity and health outcomes. *Health Aff (Millwood)*. 2015;34(11):1830-9.

148. Sandel M, et al. Housing as a health care investment affordable housing supports children's health. 2016.

149. Badger E, Bui Q. Research: In 83 million eviction records, a sweeping and intimate new look at housing in America. April 7, 2018.

150. Desmond M. Eviction and the reproduction of urban poverty. *Am J Socio*. 2012;118(1):88-133.

151. Pfeffer FT, Danziger S, Schoeni RF. Wealth disparities before and after the great recession. *Ann Am Acad Pol Soc Sci*. 2013;650(1):98-123.

152. Mian A, Sufi A. *House of Debt: How They (and you) Caused the Great Recession, and How We Can Prevent it from Happening Again*. Chicago, IL: University of Chicago Press; 2015.

153. Pollack CE, Lynch J. Health status of people undergoing foreclosure in the Philadelphia region. *Am J Public Health*. 2009;99(10):1833-9.

154. Houle JN, Keene DE. Getting sick and falling behind: Health and the risk of mortgage default and home foreclosure. *J Epidemiol Community Health*. 2015;69(4):382-7.

155. Alley DE, Lloyd J, Pagan JA, Pollack CE, Shardell M, Cannuscio C. Mortgage delinquency and changes in access to health resources and depressive symptoms in a nationally representative cohort of Americans older than 50 years. *Am J Public Health*. 2011;101(12):2293-8.

156. McLaughlin KA, Nandi A, Keyes KM, et al. Home foreclosure and risk of psychiatric morbidity during the recent financial crisis. *Psychol Med*. 2012;42(7):1441-8.

157. Osypuk TL, Caldwell CH, Platt RW, Misra DP. The consequences of foreclosure for depressive symptomatology. *Ann Epidemiol*. 2012;22(6):379-87.

158. Shi M, Samuels BA, Pollack CE. Low-income housing tax credit: Optimizing its impact on health. *Am J Public Health*. 2017;107(10):1586-8.

159. Bipartisan Policy Center. Building the case: Low-income housing tax credits and health. 2017.

160. Khadduri J. Creating balance in the locations of LIHTC developments: The role of qualified allocation plans. 2013.

161. U.S. Department of Housing and Urban Development. Picture of subsidized housing: 2016. 2016.

162. Leopold J. The housing needs of rental assistance applicants. *Cityscape*. 2012;14(2):275-98.

163. Coulton C. Defining neighborhoods for research and policy. *Cityscape.* 2012;14(2):231-6.

164. Shapiro I, Murray C, Sard B. Basic facts on concentrated poverty. https://s4.ad.brown.edu/Projects/Diversity/Data/Report/report10162013.pdf. Updated 2015. Accessed April 30, 2018.

165. Bischoff K, Reardon S. Residential segregation by income, 1970–2009. https://www.cbpp.org/sites/default/files/atoms/files/11-3-15hous2.pdf. Accessed April 30, 2018.

166. Boustan L. Racial residential segregation in American cities. In: *The Oxford Handbook of Urban Economics and Planning.* Oxford: Oxford University Press; 2011.

167. Northridge ME, Sclar ED, Biswas P. Sorting out the connections between the built environment and health: A conceptual framework for navigating pathways and planning healthy cities. *J Urban Health.* 2003;80(4):556-68.

168. Jackson RJ. The impact of the built environment on health: An emerging field. *Am J Pub Health.* 2003;93(9):1382-4.

169. Diez Roux AV, Mair C. Neighborhoods and health. *Ann N Y Acad Sci.* 2010;1186:125-45.

170. Chetty R, Stepner M, Abraham S, et al. The association between income and life expectancy in the United States, 2001–2014. *JAMA.* 2016; 315(16):1750-66.

171. Weden MM, Carpiano RM, Robert SA. Subjective and objective neighborhood characteristics and adult health. *Soc Sci Med.* 2008;66(6):1256-70.

172. Larson NI, Story MT, Nelson MC. Neighborhood environments: Disparities in access to healthy foods in the U.S. *Am J Prev Med.* 2009;36(1):74-81.

173. Beaulac J, Kristjansson E, Cummins S. A systematic review of food deserts, 1966–2007. *Prev Chronic Dis.* 2009;6(3):A105.

174. Richardson AS, Ghosh-Dastidar M, Beckman R, et al. Can the introduction of a full-service supermarket in a food desert improve residents' economic status and health? *Ann Epidemiol.* 2017;27(12):771-6.

175. Rogus S, Athens J, Cantor J, Elbel B. Measuring micro-level effects of a new supermarket: Do residents within 0.5 mile have improved dietary behaviors? *J Acad Nutr Diet.* 2018;118(6):1037-46.

176. Lachowycz K, Jones AP. Greenspace and obesity: A systematic review of the evidence. *Obes Rev.* 2011;12(5):183.

177. Kaczynski AT, Henderson KA. Environmental correlates of physical activity: A review of evidence about parks and recreation. *Leis. Sci.* 2008;40:S566.

178. Saelens BE, Handy SL. Built environment correlates of walking: A review. *Med Sci Sports Exerc.* 2008;40(7 Suppl):550.

179. Durand CP, Andalib M, Dunton GF, Wolch J, Pentz MA. A systematic review of built environment factors related to physical activity and obesity risk: Implications for smart growth urban planning. *Obes Rev.* 2011;12(5):173.

180. Sharkey PT, Tirado-Strayer N, Papachristos AV, Raver CC. The effect of local violence on children's attention and impulse control. *Am J Public Health.* 2012;102(12):2287-93.

181. McCoy DC, Raver CC, Sharkey P. Children's cognitive performance and selective attention following recent community violence. *J Health Soc Behav.* 2015;56(1):19-36.

182. Shalev I, Moffitt TE, Sugden K, et al. Exposure to violence during childhood is associated with telomere erosion from 5 to 10 years of age: A longitudinal study. *Mol Psychiatry.* 2013;18(5):576-81.

183. Theall KP, Shirtcliff EA, Dismukes AR, Wallace M, Drury SS. Association between neighborhood violence and biological stress in children. *JAMA Pediatr.* 2017;171(1):53-60.

184. Sampson RJ, Raudenbush SW, Earls F. Neighborhoods and violent crime: A multilevel study of collective efficacy. *Science.* 1997;277(5328):918-24.

185. Kawachi I, Kennedy BP, Lochner K, Prothrow-Stith D. Social capital, income inequality, and mortality. *Am J Public Health.* 1997;87(9):1491-8.

186. Kawachi I. Social capital and community effects on population and individual health. *Ann N Y Acad Sci.* 1999;896:120-30.

187. De Silva MJ, McKenzie K, Harpham T, Huttly SR. Social capital and mental illness: A systematic review. *J Epidemiol Community Health.* 2005;59(8):619-27.

188. Williams DR, Collins C. Racial residential segregation: A fundamental cause of racial disparities in health. *Public Health Rep.* 2001;116(5):404-16.

189. Branas CC, South E, Kondo MC, et al. Citywide cluster randomized trial to restore blighted vacant land and its effects on violence, crime, and fear. *Proc Natl Acad Sci U S A.* 2018;115(12):2946-51.

190. Johnson Thornton RL, Greiner A, Fichtenberg CM, Feingold BJ, Ellen JM, Jennings JM. Achieving a healthy zoning policy in Baltimore: Results of a health impact assessment of the TransForm Baltimore zoning code rewrite. *Public Health Rep.* 2013;128(Suppl 3):87-103.

191. Höppe P. Different aspects of assessing indoor and outdoor thermal comfort. *Energy Build.* 2002;34(6):661-665.

192. U.S. Department of Housing and Urban Development. About HOPE VI. https://www.hud.gov/program_offices/public_indian_housing/programs/ph/hope6/about.

193. Sanbonmatsu L, Katz LF, Ludwig J, et al. *Moving to opportunity for fair housing demonstration program: Final impacts evaluation.* U.S. Department of Housing and Urban Development; 2011.

194. Harlan SL, Brazel AJ, Prashad L, Stefanov WL, Larsen L. Neighborhood microclimates and vulnerability to heat stress. *Soc Sci Med.* 2006;63(11):2847-63.

195. Fenelon A, Mayne P, Simon AE, et al. Housing assistance programs and adult health in the United States. *Am J Public Health.* 2017;107(4):571-8.

196. Simon AE, Fenelon A, Helms V, Lloyd PC, Rossen LM. HUD housing assistance associated with lower uninsurance rates and unmet medical need. *Health Aff (Millwood).* 2017;36(6):1016-23.

197. Popkin SJ, Katz B, Cunningham MK, Brown KD, Gustafsaon J, Turnery MA. A decade of HOPE VI: Research findings and policy challenges. *The Urban Institute.* 2004.

198. World Health Organization. Report on the WHO technical meeting on quantifying disease from inadequate housing. 2006.

199. Chepesiuk R. Missing the dark: Health effects of light pollution. *Environ Health Perspect.* 2009;117(1):20.

200. Chetty R, Hendren N, Katz LF. The effects of exposure to better neighborhoods on children: New evidence from the moving to opportunity experiment. *Am Econ Rev.* 2016;106(4):855-902.

201. Ludwig J, Sanbonmatsu L, Gennetian L, et al. Neighborhoods, obesity, and diabetes—A randomized social experiment. *N Engl J Med.* 2011;365(16):1509-19.

202. Iqbal S, Law HZ, Clower JH, Yip FY, Elixhauser A. Hospital burden of unintentional carbon monoxide poisoning in the United States, 2007. *Am J Emerg Med.* 2012;30(5):657-64.

203. Iqbal S, Clower JH, King M, Bell J, Yip FY. National carbon monoxide poisoning surveillance framework and recent estimates. *Public Health Rep.* 2012;127(5):486-96.

204. Centers for Disease Control and Prevention (CDC). Unintentional non-fire-related carbon monoxide exposures—United States, 2001–2003. *Morb Mortal Wkly Rep.* 2005;54(2):36.

205. Ludwig J, Duncan GJ, Gennetian LA, et al. Neighborhood effects on the long-term well-being of low-income adults. *Science.* 2012;337(6101):1505-10.

206. Iqbal S, Clower JH, Hernandez SA, Damon SA, Yip FY. A review of disaster-related carbon monoxide poisoning: Surveillance, epidemiology, and opportunities for prevention. *Am J Public Health.* 2012;102(10):1957-63.

207. Kessler RC, Duncan GJ, Gennetian LA, et al. Associations of housing mobility interventions for children in high-poverty neighborhoods with subsequent mental disorders during adolescence. *JAMA.* 2014;311(9):937-48.

208. Clampet-Lundquist S, Kling JR, Edin K, Duncan GJ. Moving teenagers out of high-risk neighborhoods: How girls fare better than boys. *AJS.* 2011;116(4):1154-89.

209. Rudolph L, Caplan J, Ben-Moshe K, Dillon L. Health in All Policies: A Guide for State and Local Government. http://www.phi.org/resources/?resource=hiapguide. Accessed April 2018. Published 2013.

210. Bostic RW, Thornton RL, Rudd EC, Sternthal MJ. Health in all policies: the role of the US Department of Housing and Urban Development and present and future challenges. *Health Aff (Millwood).* 2012;31(9):2130-7.

211. Burwell SM. Setting value-based payment goals—HHS efforts to improve US health care. *N Engl J Med.* 2015;372(10):897-9.

212. Centers for Medicare & Medicaid Services. Accountable Health Communities Model. https://innovation.cms.gov/initiatives/ahcm/. Accessed May 2018.

CHAPTER

33

Rural America: Public Health Challenges and Opportunities

Janice C. Probst • Jan M. Eberth • Elizabeth Crouch

INTRODUCTION

Rural America is home to approximately 60 million persons, or about 20% of the nation's population.[1] This population is widely distributed, with the U.S. Census Bureau estimating that 97% of the U.S. landmass is rural. The rural economy is critical to the nation. Farm products alone account for about 1% of gross domestic product and 1.4% of national employment, without considering the effects of food processing or other rural industries (2015 data).[2] Culturally and environmentally, rural America is both broad and diverse, with settlement patterns ranging from the dense farms and small towns of the South and Midwest to the far-flung ranches and forested areas of the West, and cultures ranging from Appalachia through communities at the Mexican–American border. Devising public health strategies across this broad sector of the country is complex and requires both detailed local knowledge and national policies that are sensitive to rural differences.

While the population of rural America is equivalent to that of a European nation (e.g., Italy has 59 million residents),[3] rural populations and issues have often been an afterthought within the U.S. health policy community. As a consequence, rural residents experience higher age adjusted mortality rates than their urban peers, a disparity that is particularly acute among rural minority populations. A long history of declining health services availability, coupled with less favorable social determinants of health, is key to this disadvantage. In the sections that follow, we explore how rural America is demarcated from urban America, historic attempts to address service disparities, the current status of health in rural areas, and the outlook for future improvement in rural health.

DEFINING RURAL AMERICA

Rural communities are diverse and varied in their occupational makeup, population density, demographic composition, natural landscapes, and economic stability, which complicates analysis of health and healthcare issues. In addition, understanding "rural America" can be challenged by the variety of definitions used when talking about "rural." The three most commonly used definitions each use a different geographic scale and set of metrics, and consequently include different populations. These include, respectively, Census block classifications, Census tract classifications, and county classifications. There are multiple operational definitions of the rural–urban continuum, most of which have been defined by federal agencies. Common threads across these definitions are population density and geographic isolation, although some definitions like the Rural Urban Commuting Area (RUCA) codes take into consideration other factors like local workplace commuting patterns.

The U.S. Census Bureau defines rurality by exclusion: the spaces and persons not classified as urban are considered rural.[4] Urban is defined by population density, following the concept that rural implies a more dispersed residential pattern. "Urbanized areas" are contiguous blocks and/or tracts with a population density of 500–1000 persons per square mile in each block and a population of 50,000 or more in the total group of blocks. "Urban clusters" are similarly defined at the block level, but the population in the group of contiguous blocks is between 2500 and 49,999 persons. The Census definition is the most finely grained set of criteria currently in use, as it measures at the smallest geographic unit. Defined at the Census block level, 97% of the U.S. landmass is rural, and this area houses 19.3% of the population.[1]

The Census Bureau definition yields only two categories, rural and urban. Researchers and planners frequently wish to make finer distinctions within and between rural and urban areas. Thus, at the Census tract level, the U.S. Department of Agriculture (USDA) defines rurality using RUCA codes.[5] Developed by the University of Washington with sponsorship from the USDA, this coding system characterizes Census tracts based on a combination of population density and work-related commuting patterns. A RUCA version using ZIP Code approximation of Census tracts (ZCTAs), developed by the WWAMI Rural Health Research Center, is also available. RUCA codes classify Census tracts along a 10-point continuum, from metropolitan core areas with work commuting within urbanized areas through rural areas where work commuting is to other rural areas. Additional subcodes for each major code allow for further classification based on work commuting patterns.

RUCAs are particularly helpful when analyzing data from large Western counties, where a classification of "urban" can omit important rural subareas. San Diego County, California, for example, encompasses over 4200 square miles—larger than the states of Rhode Island and Delaware combined. However, only 689 square miles of San Diego County fall within incorporated (urban) areas. RUCA codes distinguish between the urban western part of the county and the more isolated rural eastern areas. The RUCA measure is used by several public health data sets, including the National Survey of Children's Health[6] and the Health Information Trends Survey.[7]

While measures of rurality at the Census block or tract level have the advantage of granularity, they have the disadvantage of changing over time; population growth can cause previous units to be subdivided. Population health metrics are frequently summarized at the county level because populations are large enough for accurate assessment, county boundaries are relatively stable, and counties are local political units with administrative and regulatory responsibilities.

USDA and the Office of Management and Budget (OMB) each provide definitions of rurality at the county level.[8,9] Counties containing an urbanized area of 50,000 or more persons are considered "metropolitan," or urban. Work-related commuting is then used to define "metropolitan statistical areas," economically linked

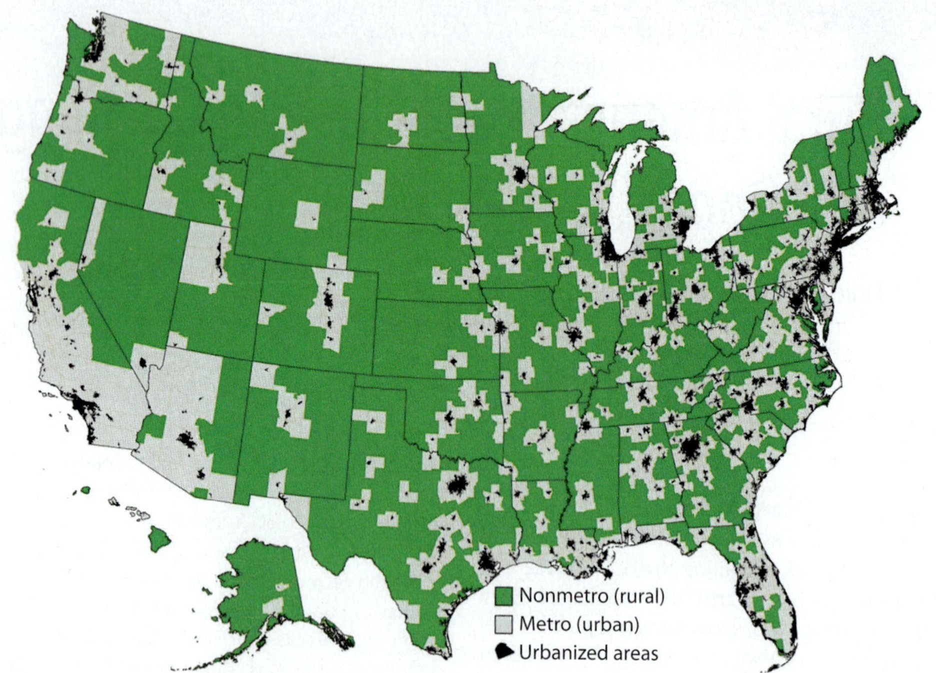

FIGURE 33-1. US Counties by metropolitan/non-metropolitan status, 2013, with identification of urbanized areas. (*Source*: Nonmetropolitan (rural) and metropolitan (urban) counties in the U.S. Usda.gov. https://www.ers.usda.gov/data-products/chart-gallery/gallery/chart-detail/?chartId=62293. Accessed December 28, 2020.)

aggregations of contiguous counties. A county might not contain any urbanized areas with sufficient population to meet the definition of metropolitan, but still be classified as metropolitan based on its economic connection to a larger central county. In the OMB definition, all counties falling in a metropolitan statistical area are considered urban and all other counties, rural. Based on the OMB definition, 72% of the nation's land is rural, housing 46 million persons and 14.6% of the population.[10] Figure 33-1 shows the distribution of U.S. counties by metropolitan/nonmetropolitan status, with urbanized areas within counties also delineated.[11] The degree to which population clusters in large counties may lead to an overstatement of the "urban" population is clearly illustrated in large Western counties.

OMB and USDA also provide a separate classification for nonmetropolitan counties that contain a large town, an urbanized area of between 10,000 and 49,999 residents. These counties are labeled "micropolitan," and adjoining counties can be classified as falling within a "micropolitan statistical area." Generally, "micropolitan" counties are considered rural, because of the small size of their urbanized areas. Some analysts consider only "noncore" counties, that is, those with no towns with more than 10,000 residents, to be rural (e.g.,[12] however, this usage is not common).

Geographic size and population density vary tremendously across counties, with the least populated U.S. county having only 88 persons across 12 square miles (Kalawao County, Hawaii) and the most highly populated U.S. county having more than 10 million people across 4058 square miles (Los Angeles County, California).[13] Several county-level coding systems have been developed that provide finer distinctions than metropolitan/nonmetropolitan for assessing rurality. These include Rural Urban Continuum Codes (nine levels) and Urban Influence Codes (12 levels).[14]

Additional techniques for assessing rural locations include the Index of Relative Rurality, which can be implemented at any measurement level to compare populations within an overall catchment area.[15] The IRR uses four county characteristics to estimate their level of rurality: size, population density, distance to the nearest metropolitan area, and urban settlement as a proportion of the total county.[16] This metric has the advantage of being continuous, ranking all counties from the most to the least rural, which can be useful for statistical analyses. However, it is not yet in broad use for policy purposes, although some analysts have adopted it. Examples include analyses by the Kaiser Family Foundation[17] and by academic researchers.[18]

A listing of a selection of techniques for defining rural is provided in Table 33-1. What all definitions of rural have in common is the concept of low population density—fewer people over more space. In the sections that follow, we will generally be using county-based definitions when providing information about the rural U.S. population. Specifically, the term "urban" will be synonymous with "metropolitan," a county with an urban area of at least 50,000 residents, while "rural" will include all counties that lack any towns or cities of that size or greater. Rural counties will also be characterized as "micropolitan rural," those counties that have a town or city with between 10,000 and 49,999 residents, and "noncore rural," those counties that have no town or urbanized area of 10,000 residents or more.

ECONOMIC AND RACIAL DIVERSITY IN RURAL AMERICA

A typical rural county contains a mix of small towns, manufacturing enterprises, a service sector, and agriculture. While most of the counties classified by the U.S. Department of Agriculture (USDA) as "farming dependent," based on the proportion of income and/or employment associated with that economic sector, are rural (391 out of 444 counties), these represent only about 20% of all rural counties.[14] The next most common category is manufacturing dependent (18%), followed by government dependent (12%), recreation dependent (12%), and mining dependent (9%); the remaining counties are considered nonspecialized. Farming counties are concentrated in the Great Plains, from North Dakota through Texas. Manufacturing counties are most common in the Midwest and South. Mining, a category that includes oil and natural gas, are principally located in Appalachia and in the oil fields of the West. Finally, recreation counties are located in areas where there are amenities such as mountains, lakes, or oceans. Each of these county types differs in employment options for wage earners and is associated with different occupational risks.

In addition to classifying counties by principal industry, the USDA also examines counties from a public policy perspective. Most relevant for public health are the categories for low education

TABLE 33-1 CLASSIFICATION SYSTEMS FOR CHARACTERIZING RURALITY

Organization/Author	Name	Description
County-Level Classifications		
Office of Management and Budget	Metropolitan Statistical Area and Micropolitan Statistical Area	Binary classification (metropolitan/nonmetropolitan) based on population size and adjacency to metropolitan areas; metropolitan (≥50,000 people) vs. nonmetropolitan areas subdivided into micropolitan (≥10,000 people but <50,000 people) and noncore (<10,000 people) counties
Waldorf (Purdue University)	Index of Relative Rurality (IRR)	Continuous (0–1 scale) accounting for population size and distance to closest metropolitan area; can be classified into various levels of rurality
USDA Economic Research Service	Urban Influence Code (UIC)	Ordinal (12 levels); can be categorized into levels such as metropolitan and nonmetropolitan
USDA Economic Research Service	Rural Urban Continuum Code (RUCC) or Beale Codes	Ordinal (10 primary codes) accounting for population density and daily commuting patterns; can be categorized into levels such as metropolitan, micropolitan, small town, and rural areas
National Center for Health Statistics	Urban-Rural Classification Scheme	Ordinal, 6 levels (can be further categorized)
U.S. Census Bureau	Percent Urban	Continuous (0–100%)
Census Tract Classifications		
USDA Economic Research Service	Rural Urban Commuting Area (RUCA)	Ordinal, 10 levels (can be further categorized; e.g., urban codes 1–3 and rural codes 4–10)
ZIP Code Classifications		
WWAMI Rural Health Research Center	ZIP Code Approximation Rural Urban Commuting Area (zRUCA)	Ordinal, 10 levels
USDA Economic Research Service	Frontier and Remote Area (FAR) Codes	Binary classification based on 4 levels of remoteness from an urban area of ≥50,000, ≥25,000–49,999, ≥10,000–24,999, or ≥2500–9999 people
Census Place Classifications		
USDA Business and Industry Loan Program	N/A	Urban: Census Places with >50,000 people and their adjacent and contiguous urbanized areas Rural: All other census places Binary (rural vs. urban)
U.S. Census Bureau	N/A	Urban locations ≥50,000 people, rural locations outside or inside census places (10,000–49,999) Binary (rural vs. urban)[a]
Census Block Classifications		
U.S. Census Bureau (aggregated blocks and/or block groups)	Urban and Rural Areas	Urbanized area/UA: Densely developed territory containing ≥50,000 people Urban cluster/UC: Densely developed territory with ≥2500 people but fewer than 50,000 people Rural: All other territory

(20% or more of adults lack a high school diploma), low employment (less than 65% of working age adults employed), persistent poverty (20% or more residents lived below the Federal poverty level from 1980 through 2011), and persistent child poverty (20% or more children in poverty from 1980 to 2011).[14] The majority of counties in each of these classifications, which are typically associated with high proportions of the population lacking health insurance and with lower levels of health literacy, are rural. Further, many of these counties are concentrated in regions with large minority or other disadvantaged populations, including the historic South, the Southwest, Appalachia, and counties with proportionately large American Indian/Alaska Native (AI/AN) populations.

While the majority of rural residents characterize their race as white, there is a significant minority presence in rural America, reflecting regional history. There are approximately 3.6 million African American residents in rural counties, most of whom (90.4%) live in Southern states. Similarly, approximately 4 million rural residents identify as Hispanic, with 70% of rural Hispanic persons living in states in the Southwestern United States. About 1.7% of rural residents, approximately 1 million persons, identify as AI/AN. A higher proportion of the AI/AN population, about 37%, more live in rural areas than is characteristic of other racial/ethnic groups; much of this population is located in or around tribal lands and reservations. Asian American/Pacific Islander individuals are the smallest rural group, with about 600,000 thousand persons or 1% of the rural population.[19]

Recognizing the racial diversity of rural America is important for countering stereotypes that foster neglect of health inequities in rural areas.[20,21] An analysis by the Centers for Disease Control and Prevention (CDC), restricted to noncore rural counties, only documented disparities in self-reported health status, access to care, and chronic conditions between African American, Hispanic, and AI/AN populations and their white rural counterparts.[12] A "dual disparity" has been recorded by other researchers. Rural minority populations frequently have less favorable social determinants of health and health outcomes than urban minority groups, as well as disparities when compared to white rural residents.[22]

HISTORICAL PERSPECTIVE AND FEDERAL POLICIES AFFECTING HEALTHCARE IN RURAL AMERICA

Policy attention to the health of rural U.S. residents began after the World War II, with the implementation of the Hill-Burton program in 1946. Responding to public perception that the existing distribution of hospitals and physicians did not address public need, the Hill-Burton legislation funded both state-conducted needs assessments and the subsequent construction of hospital and clinic facilities.[23] The program encouraged states to take a public health approach to hospital construction, ensuring that facilities would be placed in areas of need; states were required to give priority to rural areas.[24] A funding algorithm was created that balanced Federal and state contributions based on the relative wealth of each state.[23] A subsequent analysis found that poorer states did indeed received additional support from Hill-Burton.[24] In return for the financial support they received, Hill-Burton funded-facilities were required to provide some free or reduced-cost care to persons who were unable to pay.[25]

Of relevance for race-based health disparities within rural population, the Hill-Burton Act was interpreted to require equity in patient treatment. In much of the South, black patients and physicians were not served by local hospitals in the 1940s[26] and the original version of the Hill-Burton Act allowed "separate but equal" facilities. In 1964, the U.S. Supreme Court ruled that separate facilities violated the 14th Amendment; thus, hospitals receiving Hill-Burton funds had to serve both patients of any race.[27] Subsequently, Medicare and Medicaid both required providers to adhere to the Civil Rights Act of 1964, confirming the requirement for racial equity in care.

Medicare and Medicaid, enacted in 1965, remain disproportionately important to rural residents and healthcare institutions. Among the population younger than 65, employer-sponsored health insurance is less widespread among rural than urban residents (61% vs. 64%). Thus, alternatives such as the Supplemental Children's Health Insurance Program and Medicaid cover proportionately more persons than in urban areas. Subsequent to Medicaid expansion under the Patient Protection and Affordable Care Act, Medicaid has been estimated to provide health insurance coverage for about a quarter (24%) of nonelderly rural residents, versus 22% in urban counties.[17] In addition, rural residents are both more likely to be aged 65 or older, more likely to be disabled, and more likely to live at or below poverty than urban residents.[19]

Because the population they serve is more dependent on Medicare and Medicaid for financial access to care than the urban population, rural healthcare providers are in turn more dependent on these sources for payment. Thus, in the most rural states in the United States physician acceptance of Medicaid remains at about 90%, while in other states it has declined to 71%.[28] Similar differences were found among Medicare patients, with 81% of rural primary-care physicians, versus 72% of those who characterized their practice location as a city, reporting that they were accepting new Medicare patients. In this context, the degree to which Medicare and Medicaid reimbursement levels are sufficient to support rural practitioners assumes particular importance.

Multiple special funding categories have been developed by the Centers for Medicare and Medicaid Services (CMS) to support the accessibility of care in rural communities. The earliest of these programs is the rural health clinic program, established in 1977, which allows private physician offices located in rural areas to receive enhanced reimbursement for services from CMS programs if they meet program specifications. Several programs aimed at retaining general acute-care hospital services in rural communities were instituted in the late 1980s, following a wave of hospital closures subsequent to introduction of the Medicare Prospective Payment System (PPS). Special designations for select types of rural hospital were introduced, which allow for modified forms of reimbursement for Medicare and Medicaid patients. These include Critical Access Hospitals (rural hospitals of 25 beds or less, at least 35 miles from the nearest hospital), Sole Community Hospitals (similar distance requirements but up to 50 beds), Rural Referral Centers (high-volume hospitals drawing patients from substantial distances), Low-Volume Hospitals (rural hospitals with fewer than 200 discharges annually, and several other categories.[29] Similar special funding carveouts exist for other services important to CMS beneficiaries, such as dialysis centers and home healthcare agencies, for which the economics of care delivery vary between rural and urban sites. Rural dialysis facilities often have lower patient volumes than their urban equivalents, while rural home health agencies face longer drive times to reach more dispersed patient caseloads. In addition, CMS has experimented with alternatives to a complete hospital that might allow for retention of some level of care in rural communities, including Frontier Extended Stay Clinics[30] and free-standing emergency rooms.[31]

The Federal Office of Rural Health Policy (FORHP), established in 1987 within the U.S. Department of Health and Human Services, is charged with advising that agency regarding the potential effects of policy changes on rural populations.[32] FORHP funds multiple public health programs of interest for rural residents and providers, including the Black Lung Clinics and Centers of Excellence programs, the Rural Health Opioid program, and Small Rural Hospital Improvement Program. In addition, FORHP supports of State Offices of Rural Health across the country, which serve as focal points for connecting state and local health planners and providers with federal programs and resources.

OTHER KEY POLICY AREAS

Federal influence on health and the social determinants of health goes beyond programs within the U.S. Department of Health and Human Services. Broadly speaking, any and all Federal policies, from interest rates established by the Federal Reserve Board to immigration requirements, are likely to have a larger effect in rural than urban communities. This effect is related to size: rural communities, with smaller and less-diverse economic foundations, are more vulnerable to disruption. The 2008 economic recession, for example, had more severe and lasting economic effects on rural counties.[10] Viewed from a health perspective, four key areas of Federal and state policies influence the quality of rural life: education, housing, infrastructure, and access to capital. Each of these areas is affected by a range of legislation carried out by various government agencies, only a few of which can be highlighted here. Public health planners will wish to contact state personnel in each topic area for detailed and current information.

Education is a key determinant of economic and health-related well-being. Lower educational attainment is associated with higher poverty and unemployment rates at the county level.[33] The quality of local school systems is a key factor for industrial and individual retention in and recruitment to rural counties. Rural schools face many of the same problems that affect inner-city schools: higher levels of poverty in the student body than is the case in suburban schools, together with less academically prepared teachers. In consequence, rural learners lag behind suburban students in student achievement scores. Rural schools are less likely to offer advanced coursework than suburban or urban schools, particularly in the areas of science, technology, engineering, and mathematics. Rural schools also face uniquely rural problems, such as a higher ratio of transportation expenses to other expenses due to the need to transport students for longer distances.[34]

Federal resources for local schools, provided through various titles of the Elementary and Secondary Education Act, target facilities with a high proportion of low-income children.[35] Title I funds are allocated to state agencies through formula-based grants and can be used for instructional programs for low-income children. If 40% or more of students are low income, funding may be used for school-wide programs. Title V of the same Act, the Rural Education Achievement Program, targets small school districts in rural counties. Title I has been criticized both for inadequate Congressional funding and for funding formulas based on absolute numbers of children in need; the latter allocate more dollars to urban than rural schools.[36] Schools are also served by the National School Lunch Program and the National School Breakfast Program, both run by the U.S. Department of Agriculture (USDA), which reimburses schools for meals serviced to qualifying children (up to 185% of the federal poverty level).[37]

Safe and affordable housing is a key need in rural counties, particularly for low-income households. Based on the American Housing Survey, the proportion of dwelling units with severe or moderate inadequacies (problems with plumbing or maintenance, for example) is highest in noncore rural counties (7.0%), followed by micropolitan rural counties (6.3%), central metropolitan counties (5.7%), and suburban metropolitan counties (4.0%).[38] The USDA, through loan programs, assists in the development of single and multifamily housing in rural areas, as well as providing loans for child-care facilities, hospitals, libraries, and other facilities to benefit rural communities.[39] Loans and subsidies are also available from the U.S. Department of Housing and Urban Development (HUD) to help local communities provide housing for at-risk persons.[40] Because housing values vary across communities, both USDA and HUD loans are tied to local-income medians rather than to a uniform federal poverty level. This eligibility criterion may become problematic as rural baby boomers retire and their incomes decrease. These rural senior households, falling at the lower end of the income distribution, may crowd out younger low-income households.[41]

Two infrastructure elements, transportation and broadband, are often inadequate in rural America. Within transportation, road quality and the availability of transit for individuals who do not drive or lack personal vehicles are key issues. Rural roads, due to higher speed limits and fewer safety features, are the location for more than half of all highway fatalities.[42] Rural residents travel further for medical or dental care than do urban residents; the travel burden is particularly acute for rural African American residents.[43] The U.S. Department of Transportation (USDOT) provides funding for roads and transit systems to local and state governments through a grants system. USDOT considers senior citizens, persons with disabilities, persons living in poverty, and households with no vehicle as the focus for rural transit funding. While most rural travel is made using private vehicles, rural transit services provide valuable supports. Rural transit travel is more likely to involve medical care than is travel in a personal vehicle, suggesting the importance of these systems for vulnerable rural persons.[44] Only 70% of rural counties are served by USDOT-funded transit systems; transportation options in other counties for persons needing assistance are not known.[44]

Telemedicine (medical and behavioral health services provided at a distance) and telehealth (applications and information provided to consumers through the Internet) have long been promoted as a way of improving health outcomes in remote rural communities. However, Internet access in rural counties remains problematic. As of 2018, adults in rural counties were less likely than their urban or suburban peers to report using the Internet at all: 78% versus 90% in suburban and 92% in urban counties.[45] While lower Internet use stems in part from lower incomes in rural counties, there are also significant infrastructure gaps that hamper access to broadband by both individuals and businesses. Federal Communications Commission (FCC) data for 2016 showed that 31% of rural residents, and 35% of residents of tribal lands, lacked access to broadband, versus 2% of urban residents.[46] While the FCC has tried to encourage wider distribution of services, the combination of potentially difficult topography (e.g., mountain areas) and a smaller population base have limited the degree to which for-profit firms have extended access to rural counties.[47] In some areas, nonprofit rural electric cooperatives have expanded their role to include to extend broadband to underserved rural communities.[48]

Rural institutions, from hospitals wishing to upgrade facilities through local entrepreneurs wishing to develop a small business, need access to capital. Capital comes in two forms: equity, selling shares of a business enterprise, and debt, loans that must be repaid. For rural health and human services organizations, the ability to incur debt for the financing of expansion, new facilities, and so on can be compromised by a lack of local lenders. Two federal agencies, the Small Business Administration (SBA) and USDA, are key to expanding capital in rural counties. Through a mixture of loans, grants, and loan guarantees, the USDA sponsors the Community Facilities Direct Loan and Grant Program, which supports "essential" services ranging from hospitals to airports to community gardens, as well as multiple small business programs.[49,50] The SBA guarantees loans for small business applicants, including rural locations.[51]

POPULATION HEALTH STATISTICS

Rural Mortality Disparities: Large and Growing

Rural mortality disparities date back to the 1980s, with divergence in mortality rates between rural and urban counties starting in the mid-1980s.[52] As of 2016, age-adjusted death rates for males living in noncore rural counties exceeded those of males in large central metropolitan counties by 22% (995 vs. 812 per 100,000), while death rates for females in the noncore rural counties exceeded large central metropolitan rates by 27% (725 vs. 572 per 100,000; see Table 33-2[53]). In comparison, death rates for males and females in noncore rural counties exceeded those in large central metropolitan counties by

TABLE 33-2 AGE-ADJUSTED DEATH RATES PER 100,000 RESIDENTS, 2016, BY SEX AND RACE/ETHNICITY, BY RESIDENCE

Urbanization level of county of residence:	Gender		Race/Ethnicity					Total
	Female	Male	African American	American Indian/ Alaska Native	Asian/Pacific Islander	White	Hispanic, Any Race	
Large Central Metro	572	812	863	335	387	675	524	680
Large Fringe Metro	585	804	746	382	348	694	460	684
Medium Metro	631	878	900	558	456	740	575	745
Small Metro	660	914	933	655	400	770	537	778
Micropolitan (nonmetro)	706	974	973	705	500	822	577	831
Noncore (nonmetro)	725	995	972	953	410	841	546	854

Sources: Authors' analysis of data from CDC Wonder. Urbanization uses the National Center for Health Statistics 2013 Urbanization Codes, as follows:
Large Central Metro: Counties in a metropolitan statistical area (MSA) of 1 million population that: (1) contain the entire population of the largest principal city of the MSA, or (2) are completely contained within the largest principal city of the MSA, or (3) contain at least 250,000 residents of any principal city in the MSA.
Large Fringe Metro: Counties in MSA of 1 million or more population that do not qualify as large central medium metro counties in MSA of 250,000–999,999 population. Generally meeting the lay definition of "suburban."
Small Metro Counties: Metropolitan counties (population of 50,000 or more in an urbanized area) in MSAs of less than 250,000 total population.
Micropolitan: Nonmetropolitan or rural counties with a population of 10,000 or more, but less than 50,000, living in an urbanized area.
Noncore: Nonmetropolitan counties in which no urbanized area has a population of 10,000 or more.

only 8% and 3%, respectively, in 1999, showing continuing and growing rural disparities.

Differential mortality in rural counties occurs across the life span. Infant mortality is higher in rural counties, with rates of 6.69 infant deaths per 1000 live births, compared to 5.49 infant death rates per 1000 live births in large metropolitan counties (central and fringe counties in a metro area of 1 million or more).[54] Rural counties have lower death rates attributable to low birth weight but higher death rates for congenital malformations, sudden infant death syndrome, unintentional injuries, and postneonatal homicide.[53z] Maternal mortality rates are also higher in rural counties, with rural women having significantly higher death rates related to pregnancy or childbirth than their urban counterparts.[55] In part, disparities in maternal and infant mortality may be attributable to the absence of services in rural counties, resulting in longer travel for care,[56,57] and increases in out-of-hospital births and preterm delivery.[58] More than half of all rural counties lack any hospital obstetric care, with a similar proportion (49%) lacking any obstetrician.[59]

The five leading causes of death in the United States include heart disease, cancer, unintentional injury, chronic lower respiratory disease, and stroke.[60] Deaths due to these five causes are higher in rural than in urban counties, and are declining more slowly, if at all, in rural than in urban counties.[61] The disparities faced by rural populations are illustrated by cancer. Although certain types of cancer occur at higher rates within rural populations,[62] the total *incidence* of all forms of cancer is lower in rural noncore (442.4 per 100,00) and micropolitan (455.0) counties than in small urban (455.7) or large urban (457.3) counties. *Mortality* due to cancer, however, shows the opposite pattern, with noncore rural counties having the highest death rates (180.4 per 100,000), followed by micropolitan rural counties (177.2), small urban counties (165.5) and large urban counties (157.8).[63]

Rural cancer mortality disparities stem from a combination of population behaviors and lack of access to high-quality cancer care. Rural residents are more likely to exhibit behaviors, such as smoking and obesity, that contribute to higher incidence rates for selected cancers.[64] Rural residents are also less likely to receive appropriate screening. Only 58.5% of age-eligible rural adults report receiving any form of colorectal cancer screening, versus 63.2% of urban adults (see ref. 60, Table 72). Higher rates of poverty and reduced access to employer-sponsored health insurance may reduce both timely detection and treatment. Additional barriers are posed by provider shortages in rural communities. Rural residents who receive a colonoscopy for colon cancer screening, for example, are more likely to receive this care from a generalist, rather than a gastroenterologist, than are urban residents.[65] A lack of preventive and screening services may result in lower access to cancer screening, follow-up testing, and treatment and care.[66,67] Later screening results in higher staging of the cancer upon diagnosis.[68] Research has found that rural residents enrolled in clinical trials, which ensure equivalent care across locations, do not experience excess mortality.[69] This suggests that lack of access to appropriate care, rather than unique features of rural life, may underlie mortality disparities.

Suicide, a potentially preventable source of mortality, is the tenth leading cause of death in the United States (see ref. 60, Table 19). Suicide mortality has been persistently higher in noncore rural counties, followed by micropolitan rural counties, than in urban counties. In addition, the rate of increase in suicide deaths is higher in these two types of rural counties than in urban counties.[70] White and AI/AN residents are at highest risk for death from suicide nationally; further, these two groups experience the greatest rural disparities. Thus, the suicide death rate in 2015 was 24.6 per 100,000 population among white residents in rural counties, versus 20.7 in urban counties; among AI/AN residents, the corresponding values were 33.5 per 100,000 in rural counties versus 19.3 in urban counties.[71] Use of firearms as a suicide method was three times as prevalent in rural areas[72]; use of a firearm is more likely to lead to suicide completion than other modes.[73] Rural households are roughly twice as likely to include at least one firearm (58%) as are urban households (29%).[74] Higher rates of suicide in rural areas may be due to greater social isolation, absence of services for mental health or drug abuse treatment, and ready access to firearms.

Higher rates of death from unintentional injuries in rural areas, compared to urban areas, involve both occupational and rural-specific risks. Rural residents are at higher risk for injury due to occupational hazards; logging and agriculture are among occupations with the highest rates of work injury fatalities.[75] Death rates for residential fires are markedly higher in rural areas, possibly due to a combination of older housing stock and greater use of potentially hazardous devices, such as kerosene space heaters.[76] Vehicle crashes in rural areas are more likely to result in death at the scene of the crash or during transport to a hospital than in urban area, due to a combination of higher speeds on rural roads, lower seat belt use, and longer medical transport times.[77,78] Rural residents also face longer times to hospitals, longer waits for emergency medical services due to driving distances, and live further away from advanced trauma centers, which are primarily located in urban areas.[79,80]

Health-Related Quality of Life

The Centers for Disease Control and Prevention (CDC) measure health-related quality of life across several dimensions of self-reported physical and mental health. Across those metrics, rural populations generally report poorer health outcomes. Rural adults are 34% more likely than urban adults to describe their health as only "fair" or "poor" versus "good" through "excellent" (11.8% rural vs. 8.8% urban; age-adjusted estimates for 2015) (see ref. 60, Table 45). A similar rural disparity exists in serious psychological distress during the past 30 days, with 4.3% of rural versus 3.2% of urban adults reporting this problem (see ref. 60, Table 46). Relatedly, rural adults are more likely to experience one or more limitations in basic or complex activities, 22.7% of rural adults versus 15.1% of urban adults (see ref. 60, Table 42). The limitations gap is highest among rural working age residents, those aged 18–64. Among persons in potentially their most productive years, 18.6% of rural residents report limitations, versus 11.5% of urban residents.

The sources of rural disparities in health outcomes are complex and interrelated. As discussed in the sections below, rural populations tend to lag behind their urban peers in healthy behaviors. At the same time, lack of health insurance combined with increasing shortages of healthcare practitioners and facilities in rural communities make it more difficult to deal with adverse health outcomes and to deliver prevention programs that might prevent these outcomes.

Health Behaviors and Related Morbidity in Rural Populations

Behavioral risk factors are one cause of the divergence in morbidity and mortality rates between rural and urban residents. While behavioral differences reflect the differences between urban and rural cultures, behavioral patterns are also a product of the vastly different built environments that surround the two populations, and the relative absence of strong preventive policies and programs in most rural communities. In this section, we address four categories of risk that are higher among rural than urban populations: obesity, the use of tobacco, sexual behaviors and related morbidities, and opioid use.

A combination of poorer nutritional habits and lack of physical activity contribute to the higher rates of obesity observed among rural adults,[81] with a similar pattern present among rural children.[82] An estimated 35.6% of rural adults, and 18.6% of rural children, were obese based on data from the 1999 to 2006 National Health and Nutrition Examination Survey, compared to 30.4% and 15.1%, respectively, among their urban counterparts.[80,81] Rural residents are less likely to have close access to a grocery store.[83] Ironically, given the agricultural nature of many rural counties, rural households are more likely than urban ones to report food insecurity,[84] a risk factor associated with obesity.[85]

The use of tobacco products greatly increases the incidence of heart disease, stroke, cancer, and chronic lower respiratory disease. The prevalence of tobacco use, particularly cigarette smoking, is much higher among rural residents than urban residents.[86] Disparities begin early. An estimated 11.0% of rural adolescents, versus 6.7% of their urban peers, report cigarette smoking, and 7.0% of rural youth, versus 2.9% of urban, report using smokeless tobacco products.[87] Similarly, 25.1% of adults in noncore rural counties and 23.5% of those in micropolitan counties report cigarette smoking, versus 1.61% in the largest urban counties.[64] Regionally, daily smoking and use of smokeless tobacco products are most common in the rural South; however, regional differences are less marked than rural–urban differences within regions.[88]

Fewer preventive programs and lack of alternative activities contribute to high rates of sexually transmitted diseases (STDs) among rural adolescents. Over one-third of rural adolescents report engaging in sexual intercourse before the age of 14 years, with nearly 90% of rural adolescents between the ages of 14–19 reporting sexual activity.[89,90] STD rates are higher among rural African American residents, with particularly higher rates of syphilis, gonorrhea, and chlamydia among Southern, low-income, and rural African-Americans.[91] STD rates are linked in part to higher rates of early sexual behavior among rural African American adolescents.[92] In addition, patients in rural areas may not seek care due to fear of community stigma, allowing the adverse consequences of STDs to proliferate.[93]

Rural young women are more likely to become pregnant than their urban peers, with pregnancy rates among rural adolescents that are 33% higher than urban residents.[94] Factors that may contribute to the higher rate of teen pregnancies in rural areas include lower rates of college enrollment, higher rates of poverty, limited availability of publicly funded reproductive services and counseling, and higher rates of uninsured residents.[93]

The picture for HIV exposure in rural America is mixed. While present HIV prevalence rates are lower in rural than in urban counties, trends suggest that this situation may eventually be reversed. Measured at the national level, the current prevalence of HIV infection among adults and adolescents is lower among rural than urban residents.[95] Rates in urban counties average 379 persons per 100,000 residents, versus 152 across rural counties. The rural Southeast, with its high concentration of minority race, high-poverty populations, represents an exception to the national picture. In South Carolina, for example, HIV prevalence in rural counties exceeds the rate in urban counties (439/100,000 vs. 373/100,000); in Florida, rural and urban rates are nearly equivalent (604/100,000 and 609/100,000, respectively).[96] Rural residents are less likely to report either lifetime or past-year testing for HIV.[97,98] Newer approaches to HIV control, such as pre-exposure medication prophylaxis, are less available in rural than in urban settings.[99,100] A focus on urban populations within the Ryan White enabling legislation may be one factor contributing to reduced availability of both treatment and prevention services within rural counties.[101] A 2015 HIV outbreak in a rural community in Indiana received considerable national attention, but may or may not lead to an improvement in rural prevention and treatment over the long run.[102]

The use of illicit drugs, including opioids, has historically been lower in rural than in urban areas.[103] Survey data from 2012 to 2014 found 6.8% of residents of nonmetropolitan counties reporting any illicit drug use, versus 10.1% in large metropolitan counties and 9.5% in small metropolitan counties.[103] Similarly, a 2014 survey found that 2.8% of adults in urban counties, versus 2.0% of those in rural counties, reported illicit drug dependence or abuse during the past year.[104] The consequences of drug use, however, may be more severe in rural areas. Rates of neonatal abstinence syndrome, an indicator of maternal drug abuse, are higher in rural counties (11.8/1000 births) than in metropolitan counties (4.5/1000 births).[105] Rural overdose drug death rates have increased over time to parallel and, in 2015, exceed, urban rates.[103] The combination of lower use rates but higher death rates stems in part from an absence of both acute and long-term treatment services.[106] Recent changes in federal policy, such as the Comprehensive Addiction and Recovery Act of 2016, have attempted to improve the geographic disparities in providers prescribing buprenorphine for the treatment of opioid use disorder, extending Drug Enforcement Administration (DEA) waivers to nurse practitioners and physician assistants. This has increased the availability of office-based providers to prescribe buprenorphine, but more than half of rural counties still lack a provider.[106]

UNIQUELY RURAL ENVIRONMENTAL AND OCCUPATIONAL HEALTH RISKS

Several occupations concentrated in rural America experience particularly high rates of occupational injury and death. These include logging, mining, and agriculture. Logging is the occupation with the highest rate of fatal injuries (135.9 work injury deaths per 100,000 workers in 2016); farmers and other agricultural workers (23.1 deaths per 100,000) also fall within the ten most dangerous occupational categories.[107]

Oil and gas extraction primarily take place in rural settings. Of 221 counties in the United States characterized as mining-dependent based on income or employment levels, 184 (83%) are rural. At the national level, mining, the overall term for both quarrying and oil and gas extraction, has the third highest death rate among industrial, as distinct from occupational, categories, at 10.1 per 100,000.[107] Pneumoconiosis, a lung disease caused by minute particles of dust, is a risk for persons exposed to coal (coal miner's disease or black lung), or silica (silicosis). It has been estimated that the prevalence of black lung among individuals with 25 years of exposure or more across the United States is 10%. Within miners in Central Appalachia, the estimated prevalence of black lung is 20.6%.[108] Respirable silica dust is an additional hazard of mining, including hydraulic fracking.[109,110]

Agriculture, which relies on an assortment of complex machines from plowing through harvest, comes with a high risk for traumatic injury.[111,112,113] Of concern, the presence of machinery also increases the risk for injury among farm children, both those who are actively engaged in farm work[114] and those who are bystanders.[115] Agriculture is also highly reliant on synthetic pesticides; it is estimated that three-quarters of U.S. pesticide use is associated with farming. Exposures through contact, inhalation, or accidental ingestion are most likely among workers actively engaged in preparing and distributing these chemicals, particularly if they fail to observe appropriate precautions.[116] Again, farm children are at risk, as chemicals can be brought into the home on clothing and footwear.[117]

Air and Water Quality

Environmental exposures within rural communities are varied. Levels of common urban air pollutants are lower in rural counties as a whole, but industrial exposures may lead to high-localized pollution levels. Measured as particulate matter and ozone, air quality becomes better as areas become more rural. The number of days for which ozone levels exceed guidelines set by the Environmental Protection Agency is highest in large urban counties (47.54 days on average per year) and drops to 3.81 days per year in the most rural counties.[118] Particulate matter shows a similar pattern, declining from 12.1 days that exceed EPA thresholds in the most urban counties to 0.95 days per year in the most rural counties.[118]

Within rural communities, agricultural activities are associated with local increases in specific pollutants that may affect health within a smaller radius. Pig farms, for example, are associated with ambient ammonia levels, with adverse effects on children with asthma.[119]

TABLE 33-3 SELECTED METRICS FOR POPULATION HEALTH AND ACCESS TO CARE, 2015

	Metro[a]	Nonmetro[a]
Health-Related Quality of Life		
Serious psychological distress last 30 days (2014–2015)	3.2%	4.3%
At least one basic or complex activity limitation, all adults	15.1%	22.7%
Persons age 18–64 years	11.5%	18.6%
Persons age 65 and older	30.9%	35.6%
Self-reported fair, poor health status, all ages	8.8%	11.8%
4+Chronic conditions (adults)	4.3%	5.8%
Health Insurance Coverage		
Private insurance, all persons under age 65	66.7%	57.8%
Private health insurance through workplace among persons under age 65	58.6%	50.0%
Medicaid coverage among persons under age 65	19.8%	25.4%
No health insurance overage among persons under age 65	10.3%	12.8%
Realized Access to Care		
Delay or nonreceipt of needed services due to cost (all ages)		
Delay or nonreceipt of medical care	9.6%	11.0%
Delay or nonreceipt of prescription drugs	6.7%	8.3%
No healthcare visit to an office or clinic among persons under 18 (2014–15)	8.2%	10.2%
No visit among children under 6 years	5.1%	5.3%
No visit among children age 6 years and older	9.8%	12.6%
Oral healthcare		
Delayed receipt of needed dental care due to cost	11.4%	14.5%
Dental visit in past year		
2 years +	69.4%	60.8%
2–17 years	84.9%	83.3%
18–64 years	65.3%	55.0%
65+	64.6%	54.2%
Emergency department visit in last year		
Among children (age less than 18 years)	4.2%	6.2%
Adults with any visit	18.2%	22.8%
Adults with 2 or more ED visits	6.5%	9.6%
Receipt of Selected Preventive Services among Adults		
Any CRC screening, adults 50–75	63.2%	58.5%
Colonoscopy screening	59.8%	56.5%
Pneumovax	63.4%	64.7%
Flu vaccine	43.4%	41.9%

Note: Values shown as estimated percent of total relevant U.S. population. All estimates are drawn *from Health US 2016* and are age adjusted to the 2000 population.[60] Unless otherwise noted, all estimates pertain to 2015.

[a]"Metro" is defined as a metropolitan county; that is, a county with an urbanized area of 50,000 residents or more as well as any contiguous counties defined as falling within its metropolitan statistical area. "Nonmetro" is all remaining counties; that is, counties that do not have an urbanized area of 50,000 or more residents and are not part of a metropolitan statistical area.

The majority of Americans in both rural and urban counties, about 90%, obtain their water from a public water system.[98] Water quality is poorer in rural systems than in their urban counterparts, with 10% of systems in the most remote rural counties, versus .6% in urban counties, exceeding recommended thresholds for one or more contaminants.[118] Runoff from agricultural chemicals can have adverse effects on small rural water systems, particularly with regard to nitrates and trihalomethanes.[120]

Nationally, 15% of the population, an estimated 13 million households, are estimated to use water from private wells. Private wells are not formally regulated or monitored.[121] A study conducted by the U.S. Geologic Service found that 23% of private wells contained one or more chemicals or contaminants at levels exceeding limits set by the Environmental Protection Agency.[122] While most contaminants come from chemicals naturally occurring in local soil (e.g., radon), nitrate from manmade sources was found in about 4% of wells.[123]

ACCESS TO HEALTH SERVICES AND WORKFORCE CHALLENGES

Rural adults and children are less likely to have private health insurance coverage and, in consequence, are more likely to delay or forego care than their urban peers. Low population density, together with reduced levels of health insurance, reduce the financial viability of local healthcare providers and help perpetuate health workforce shortages in rural communities. We discuss these interrelated issues in this section.

Utilization of Health Services

Overall rural service use, displayed in Table 33-3, illustrates gaps in healthcare coverage and healthcare utilization between rural and urban population. The majority of all Americans under age 65 have some form of private health insurance to provide financial access to care. The proportion with such coverage is higher among urban than rural residents, making Medicaid an important source of coverage for rural populations. Because Medicaid coverage is not available for nondisabled, nonpregnant adults in many states, particularly in the South, a higher proportion of the rural population remains uninsured. The combination of higher rates of poverty with lower rates of health insurance coverage leads to a higher proportion of rural residents reporting that they have delayed, or not received, medical or oral healthcare, which they believed was needed.

Use of preventive services that do not require a substantial technical infrastructure, such as vaccination, does not differ markedly between rural and urban adults. As shown in Table 33-3, rural and urban adults report receipt of pneumovax and flu vaccine at similar rates. Among young children, vaccination rates are slightly lower among rural children for DTaP, polio virus, varicella, PCV, HepA, and rotavirus than their urban counterparts.[124] Differences tend to be larger for relatively new vaccines and those targeted at adolescents. Thus, rural adolescents have lower uptake of meningitis and HPV vaccines than their urban counterparts, while uptake of Tdap is virtually identical.[125] These differences may be due to a variety of factors including parental support and acceptance of vaccination coverage and the lower rates of pediatric care providers in rural areas.[126]

Emergency department use is frequently employed as a measure for inadequate access to other forms of care. Overall, rural residents are more likely to have made an ED visit in the past year and urban residents (Table 33-3). Of note, rural residents are markedly more likely to have made two or more ED visits in the past year, suggesting ongoing access issues that are not resolved or referred to a local provider during an initial visit.

Workforce Shortages

Nationally, only 11% of physician practice in rural America although nearly 20% of the population lives there.[127] Some elements of rurality, such as lower population density and longer travel distance for healthcare, affect nearly all rural residents.[128] Shortages of key personnel, such as physicians, dentists, nurses, and mental health professionals, are common but do not necessarily affect all counties. Below, we discuss how workforce shortages are defined and addressed for rural communities.

At the federal level, the Health Resources and Services Administration (HRSA) of the U.S. Department of Health and Humans Services is responsible for designating health professional shortage areas (HPSAs) and maintains an updated list for these designations.[129] HPSAs are specific to overall disciplines, as a community might lack mental health practitioners but have an adequate supply of primary-care physicians. HPSA designations are important within public health because certain types of grants, at the community level, and loan repayment programs, for individual practitioners, rely on level of HPSA need when defining eligibility criteria.

The HRSA algorithm identifies geographic areas, population groups, or facilities (e.g., prisons) as HPSAs and/or Medically Underserved Area/Populations (MUA/Ps). HPSAs are identified primary-care, dental, and mental health practitioners. Geographic areas comprising an HPSA can be a whole county, groups of counties, or groups of census tracts. Federal regulations stipulate that an area must have a population-to-provider ratio of at least 3500-to-1 to be designated a primary-care HPSA, 5000-to-1 to be designated a dental-care HPSA, and 30,000-to-1 to be designated a mental health HPSA. For particularly vulnerable communities, these thresholds are loosened to 3000-to-1, 4000-to-1, and 20000-to-1, respectively. Additional criteria used to assess community need include the proportion of the population in poverty and travel time to the nearest provider outside the area. In addition, criteria specific to each discipline are taken into consideration: infant health outcomes when designating primary-care shortage areas, whether water systems are fluoridated for dental shortage areas, and elderly to youth ratios and the prevalence of alcohol and drug abuse for mental health shortage areas. Of note, the HPSA designation is not automatically applied; communities must apply for HPSA status. Thus, it is possible that some high-need counties are not represented.

MUA/P designations are based on an "Index of Medical Underservice" that is derived from four criteria: population/provider ratios, proportion of the population below poverty level, percent of the population over age 65, and infant mortality rate.[130] On a 0–100 scale, areas/populations with scores of 62 or less for the IMU qualify for MUA/P designation. Exceptions from this rule can be made that require a state's governor to testify to (and document) the unusual needs of the local population to access needed primary-care services. Medically underserved populations can exist when an overall area has sufficient practitioners, but those do not serve specific populations, such as uninsured persons, persons funded by Medicaid, and specialized groups such as migrant workers or the homeless.

Across the United States, mental health professionals are most likely to be needed, with only 75 of 1976 rural counties (3.8%) being neither partial nor whole-county mental health HPSAs in 2018.[131] Primary care is the next most needed group, with 195 counties (9.9%) that are deemed fully served. Slightly less than a quarter of rural counties (24.4%) are considered adequately served by dental personnel. Conversely, 84.3% of all rural counties are whole-county mental health HPSAs, 32.4% are whole-county primary-care HPSAs, and 21.8% are whole-county dental HPSAs.

Paralleling gaps in primary care, shortages of medical specialists are more common in rural communities. For example, 2016 data from the Area Health Resource File (AHRF) show rural counties have fewer general surgeons (4.5 per 100,000) than their urban counterparts (8.2 per 100,000), with the majority of rural counties having no available general surgeons (52%).[132] Studies have shown the shortage of surgeons in rural areas is due in part to the aging surgeon workforce and associated retirement rate, lower practice satisfaction (e.g., higher on-call requirements), and personal/family issues (e.g., job opportunities for spouse).[133,134,135] Moreover, the ability to provide surgical care is a key contributor to the financial viability of rural hospitals,[136,137] with estimates suggesting that one rural general surgeon will generate $1.4 million for a hospital and 25.9 jobs within the community.[138] Interestingly, a 2006 survey reported that rural surgeon compensation is competitive with their urban counterparts adjusted for the cost of living.[139] The challenge moving forward is competition from large medical centers and metropolitan areas in hiring general surgeons, who are increasingly competing for a smaller pool of candidates.[140]

Data from the AHRF also show a lower density of obstetric and gynecological (OB/GYN) practitioners in rural areas compared to urban areas in 2016 (6.7 per 100,000 women in rural, 15.9 per 100,000 women in urban).[132] Aggregate data conceal the more alarming statistics that 61% of all U.S. counties lack even one OB/GYN. A study of relocation patterns for OB/GYNs between 2005 and 2015 showed that practice relocations were predominately to urban and less socioeconomically deprived counties.[141] The absence of local maternal care providers results in greater drive times for rural women accessing perinatal care. Depending on the level of care needed, the proportion of rural women with access to hospitals providing perinatal care within a 30-minute drive ranged from 61% to 88% (60-minute drive ranged from 80% to 97%); access was most limited for level-III facilities.[142]

The importance of rural OB/GYNs is evident in the adverse outcomes experienced by women in rural communities. Research from the University of Washington Rural Health Research Center found an increasing risk of poor outcomes (e.g., infant mortality) for rural women over the study period 1985–97. Rural women from counties with persistent poverty were particularly affected compared to women from rural counties without persistent poverty.[143]

Finally, there is a lower density of pediatric care providers per 100,000 children under aged 18 years old in rural compared to urban counties (19.0 per 100,000 in rural vs. 55.4 per 100,000 in urban).[132] Almost 58% of rural counties had no pediatrician at all. Fortunately, in many rural areas where access to pediatricians is limited, family physicians are more likely to provide care for children.[144] Pediatric subspecialty care is also a problem for rural areas, particularly those in the Mountain and West North Central areas of the United States.[145]

Recruitment and Retention of Rural Healthcare Practitioners

A detailed literature review classified barriers to rural recruitment of physicians into three categories: lifestyle, practice issues, and competition.[146] Lifestyle issues include fewer social options, lack of career opportunities for spouses, and perceived lower quality of rural school systems.[147] Medical practice issues include long hours and fewer colleagues to handle weekend on-call cases, together with the predominance of government over private health insurance sources in rural communities. Finally, urban systems may have more resources to devote to recruit graduating residents as well as practicing physicians. Despite these disadvantages, there are recruitment strategies that rural communities can pursue.

Studies show that healthcare practitioners raised and/or educated in rural communities are more likely to subsequently practice in similar communities.[148] Practitioners who are inherently motivated to practice in a rural area because of a desire to work in a certain geographic region/small community or related personal preferences are more likely to stay in a rural practice than their colleagues who are practicing on a "return-of-service commitment."[146]

Some practitioners are attracted to rural communities because of the available outdoor activities, such as hunting or fishing.[149] In terms of retention, factors such as owning their practice, having children in the home, and being native to the state increase the likelihood of remaining in practice in a rural Health Professional Shortage Area (HPSA), while being on-call three or more times/week decreased the likelihood of remaining in a rural HPSA.[150] Programs such as loan repayment and rural medical training have been shown to influence provider recruitment, and to a lesser extent, retention.[151,152] Overall, multidimensional programs focusing on improving professional job satisfaction and other nonfinancial objectives were more successful than programs solely focused on financial strategies for recruiting and retaining rural practitioners.

Facility Closures

Rural hospitals occupy an emotional position within the community that differs from facilities in urban centers, where multiple hospitals may compete for physicians and patients. Rural hospitals are more likely to be the single facility in a community and thus both a focus of civic pride and an essential resource for attracting industrial development to the area. Despite this position, however, growing numbers of rural obstetric units and entire hospitals are closing. Nearly 10% of rural counties lost all hospital obstetric services between 2004 and 2014, and another 45% of rural counties had no hospital obstetric services during that time frame at all.[57] Rural counties with greater proportions of minority women and lower median household incomes bore the largest brunt of obstetric losses.

Between January 2010 and August 2018, 87 rural hospitals ceased offering inpatient services.[153] Many of these facilities ceased providing health services of any type altogether. Hospital closures were more common in states that did not expand Medicaid under the Patient Protection and Affordable Care Act, as the proportion of uninsured adults remained higher in those states than in expansion states.[154] The effects of the current wave of hospital closures have not yet been fully studied. Qualitative assessments suggest that community leaders and healthcare providers perceive such closures to adversely affect the health of vulnerable populations, particularly those with transportation difficulties.[155] One quantitative assessment, limited to the Medicare population, found no effects subsequent to closure on hospitalization rates or mortality.[156] On the other hand, a population-based analysis of emergency department closures found such closures to be associated with increased inpatient mortality at neighboring hospitals, suggesting adverse effects from increased distance to care.[157] Free-standing emergency rooms have been suggested as an alternative to hospitals for small communities, but preliminary analyses suggest that these are unlikely to be financially sustainable.[158]

Beyond immediate health effects, rural hospital closure has been associated with a 1.6% increase in local unemployment rates and a 4% decline in per capita income within affected counties.[159] The decline in service ability across rural counties extends to related industries. Between 2003 and 2013, 12.1% of independently owned rural pharmacies closed, leaving 490 communities without any type of retail pharmacy.[160] Because pharmacists are a source of medication guidance for rural residents, this loss can further exacerbate rural–urban health disparities.[161] Continued public health surveillance will be needed to ascertain the degree to which the steady decline in the availability of rural hospitals is linked to the steady increases in rural mortality rates documented in a previous section of this chapter.

ADDRESSING RURAL GAPS: POTENTIAL APPROACHES

Addressing Gaps in Healthcare Service Availability

The presence of healthcare providers, both institutions such as hospitals and practitioners such as physicians, dentists, and advanced practice nurses or dental hygienists, is essential to the availability of prevention and treatment for rural populations. Below, we discuss four possible approaches. Allowing individual practitioners to do more through expansion of scope of practice laws is one way to reach underserved populations. Changes to physician education may help increase retention of these providers in rural communities. Technological solutions that use the Internet to bring care from urban to rural counties are possible, with the caveat that technology changes rapidly. Overarching all of these issues, however, is the question of financing of care. As long as healthcare for rural populations is considered solely as a market-based function, it will remain endangered.

Changes in Scope of Practice Laws

To address physician workforce shortages, some professional organizations have advocated for changes to scope of practice, prescribing, and reimbursement laws for midlevel providers.[162,163] States vary in their licensure and regulatory requirements for nurse practitioners and physician assistants, with some states requiring direct physician oversight and others granting near complete practice autonomy.[164,165] Some of the most restrictive policies are found in the southern United States South Carolina is an example of a state that has increased nurse practitioner ability to prescribe controlled substances (e.g., opioids), as well as the number of nurse practitioners a physician is allowed to supervise (i.e., three to six), but the results of this change have not yet been evaluated.[166]

Accessibility of primary-care services is higher in states allowing midlevel providers to practice at their fullest capacity and/or with higher reimbursement rates than in more restrictive environments.[167,168,169] Research suggests that expanded practice environments are not associated with adverse patient outcomes[170] or reduced quality of care.[171] Retention of these highly qualified professionals in rural areas, however, shares many of the same challenges associated with physician retention, and improved education for rural practice is needed.[172,173]

Changes to Practitioner Education

While midlevel practitioners can supply many forms of office-based primary care, they generally cannot replace physicians in other areas, including hospital care, emergency care, childbirth, and providing coverage after hours.[174] Thus, training physicians who are both willing to practice in rural communities and equipped with a skill set that matches the services they will provide is essential. Programs that can increase the proportion of physicians willing to locate in rural areas include recruiting students with rural backgrounds and placement of students in underserved practice sites during medical education and residency.[175]

Education to prepare physicians for rural practice needs to begin by recognizing differences in services provided between rural and urban physicians. In family medicine, rural physicians are likely to have a broader scope of practice than their urban peers, with less support for activities such as behavioral health.[176] Similar differences occur for general surgery within rural areas.[177] It is uncertain whether placement of learners in rural or underserved settings creates a desire for rural practice, or simply prevents students who entered their career planning on working in underserved settings from changing their minds.[178] Nonetheless, multiple studies have found that learning experiences in rural or other underserved settings during training contributes to subsequent practice in these areas.[179,180,181]

Technological Solutions to Distance and Volume

Internet-based technology has been posed as a means of providing specialized services to small communities that cannot afford to host these services locally. The use of telemedicine, that is, the delivery of clinical services via communications technology, in rural facilities has been demonstrated to reduce costs by reducing unnecessary admissions.[182] The Health Resources and Services Administration, through its Office of the Advancement of Telehealth, works to expand such services through multiple grant programs; some rural-focused philanthropic organizations also underwrite the development of telemedicine networks.[183,184] The Centers for Medicare and Medicaid Services, as a major payor, has also committed to assisting in the broader implementation of telemedicine services as part of its Rural Health Strategy.[185]

As of 2013, only about a third (34.0%) of rural hospitals had one or more telemedicine applications in place, with the most common uses being for radiology and emergency/trauma care.[186] Challenges to the expansion of services include startup costs associated with obtaining necessary equipment, physician licensing when cross-state services are considered, and reimbursement.[187] When appropriately implemented, however, telemedicine programs appear to provide satisfactory specialist services for a range of conditions to rural residents.[188,189,190]

Internet-based technology has also been recommended for telehealth promotion interventions and for interventions to reduce social isolation and loneliness among rural residents. However, technical challenges, principally surrounding access to broadband,[191] underlie the frequent finding that rural populations are less likely to be connected to the Internet.[192] Analysis of the content of social networking connections suggests that there are cultural differences, as well, between rural and urban Internet users. In an early study of social media use, rural residents were found to have smaller networks of "friends," and more restrictive privacy settings, than their urban peers.[193] The way in which rural cultures may influence how and if rural individuals decide to trust and engage with telehealth applications.

Changing the Financing of Rural Healthcare

Given the challenges posed by low population density, it may be infeasible for many rural communities to maintain hospital services, or even physician or nurse practitioner services, within a fee-for-service healthcare economy. "Managed-care" approaches, which typically pay primary-care providers on a per member per month basis, do not address the problem of low patient populations. Similar problems affect rural hospitals, where the high base costs of keeping a facility open are difficult to recoup from a small patient base, even if health insurance were to be more broadly available to rural residents.

What may be needed is a change in perspective, moving healthcare from the category of a discretionary purchased good to a utility. There is precedent for this type of change in the history of rural electrification. In the 1920s, most farms in the United States did not have electricity, in part because farmers were required to pay for installing electric lines, at a cost of $2000–$3000, and subsequently to pay higher rates for electricity delivered over those lines. As of the mid-1930s, only 11% of all farms were connected to electricity. The Rural Electrification Act, passed in 1936, provided federal subsidies for electrification in the form of long-term, low-interest loans to both utilities and individual consumers, with the proviso that individual borrowers would not be liable if a local cooperative defaulted on its loan. By 1960, 97% of all farms were connected to the electric grid.[194]

The Rural Electrification Act was an explicit attempt to improve the quality of rural life when a market solution failed to do so. One of its Congressional supporters noted that rural residents were "growing old prematurely; dying before their time; conscious of the great gap between their lives and the lives of those whom the accident of birth or choice placed in towns and cities."[195] Current innovative budget strategies are recognizing that piecemeal payments may not be an effective approach for services that amount to local utilities, such as hospital. With agreement from all funders, the state of Maryland implemented global budgeting for hospitals in 2014. Under a global budgeting system, each hospital receives a fixed revenue, regardless of the number of patients admitted or services provided. Given the short period of time since program implementation, evidence on its effects is limited and contradictory, with analyses of Medicare claims suggesting that the switch had no effects,[196,197] while a study of emergency department visits across all payors found that the program reduced admissions from hospital emergency departments.[198] No studies have yet explored the long-term effects of the program on health outcomes for rural residents.

Addressing Rural Gaps in the Social Determinants of Health

The discussion of "Other Key Policy Areas," above, focused on several issues: education, safe housing, transportation, broadband, and access to capital funding. Solutions in these areas, particularly education, hold promise for addressing related problems, such as rural poverty, and thus bringing about improvements in the health of rural residents. Unfortunately, there is no "silver bullet" that can be offered to solve any of these issues. However, there is a public health approach that can incorporate them.

The South Carolina Rural Health Action Plan provides an example of a multidisciplinary, multisectoral approach to improving health outcomes in rural communities.[199] Through a year-long process across 2016–17, the South Carolina Office of Rural Health (SCORH) convened more than 70 major stakeholders from the fields of education, housing, economic development, public health, substance abuse, emergency management, and others to define potential methods for improving rural health outcomes. "Stakeholders" were defined as agency heads and others in leadership positions who had the ability to commit their organizations to take action within their areas of responsibility. In addition, "town hall" meetings were convened across rural counties with both good and poor health indicators to obtain input from rural residents. "Town hall" meetings were followed by "sense-making" meetings, during which SCORH staff returned to the communities with summaries of findings, to verify that the staff interpretation accurately reflected community sentiment.

The result of the planning process was a Rural Health Action Plan with more than 50 specific recommendations spread across five focus areas: access to healthcare, education, housing, economic development, and community assets, leadership, and engagement. Action steps are specific and measurable, as in this example from the education category: "Share educational and training facilities between school districts, Technical Colleges, and employment programs within communities so that different populations may take advantage of the same physical space, to the maximum benefit of the resource." Process along all recommendations is tracked annually.

The specific changes needed to improve rural health in South Carolina identified through the SCORH planning process may be markedly different from those in other areas of the country. The process, however, based on broad inclusion of leaders across multiple sectors and feedback to rural residents, is one that is replicable in other communities.

RURAL COMMUNITIES AND THE NEED TO PRESERVE THEM

A former president of the National Rural Health Association frequently laments his inability to come up with a quick comeback when, during a shared cab ride, a Congressman said that if rural people wanted healthcare, they should just move to cities. Only after they had separated did the appropriate response occur to him: "Well, if urban people want food, they should move to the country." This anecdote summarizes, briefly, the issues and dilemmas facing rural populations. America as a nation cannot exist without a rural infrastructure providing food, resources, and energy for internal consumption and for export. At the same time, its urban populations, and policymakers located in urban areas, are not generally conscious of the interconnectedness of the two parts of the nation.

Public health practitioners and policymakers need a focus on place as well as populations when planning health initiatives.[200] Health services and programs developed to serve a population with high Internet connectivity, an abundance of healthcare providers, and ready access to multiple forms of transportation will be ineffective in many rural contexts—and this ineffectiveness will not be the "fault" of rural residents. Recommending that persons take the stairs rather than an elevator,[201] for example, will not be an effective intervention in a community where most facilities, including physician offices, have only a single level.

To address rural health issues, knowledge of actual rural places is needed. Engaging rural residents to define their own approaches to health, healthcare delivery, and the promotion of healthy behavior is one part of developing solutions. However, given the interdependent nature of rural and urban places within the United States, rural populations will also have to become knowledgeable regarding national healthcare policy and advocate for changes when these policies disadvantage rural residents.

References

1. United States Census Bureau. New Census Data Show Differences between Urban and Rural Populations. Release Number CB16-210. https://www.census.gov/newsroom/press-releases/2016/cb16-210.html. Accessed August 27, 2018.
2. Morrison RM, Melton A. Ag and Food Sectors and the Economy. May 2, 2018. https://www.ers.usda.gov/data-products/ag-and-food-statistics-charting-the-essentials/ag-and-food-sectors-and-the-economy. Accessed August 27, 2018.
3. World Population Review. Italy Population 2018. http://worldpopulationreview.com/countries/italy-population/. Accessed August 27, 2018.
4. Ratcliffe M, Burd C, Holder K, Fields A. *Defining Rural at the U.S. Census Bureau. ACSGEO-1, U.S.* Washington, DC: Census Bureau; 2016.
5. U.S. Department of Agriculture. Rural Urban Commuting Area Codes. https://www.ers.usda.gov/data-products/rural-urban-commuting-area-codes/.
6. Health Resources and Services Administration. The National Survey of Children's Health. http://www.childhealthdata.org/learn/NSCH. Accessed August 27, 2018.
7. National Cancer Institute. Health Information National Trends Survey. https://hints.cancer.gov/. Accessed August 27, 2018.
8. Cronmartie J, Parker T. Rural Classifications: Overview. https://www.ers.usda.gov/topics/rural-economy-population/rural-classifications/.
9. U.S. Census Bureau. Metropolitan and Micropolitan. https://www.census.gov/programs-surveys/metro-micro/about.html.
10. U.S. Department of Agriculture. Rural America at a Glance, 2017 Edition. Washington, DC. Economic Information Bulletin 182, November 2017.
11. U.S. Department of Agriculture, Economic Research Service. Nonmetropolitan (rural) and metropolitan (urban) counties in the U.S. https://www.ers.usda.gov/data-products/rural-child-poverty-chart-gallery/rural-child-poverty-chart-gallery/?topicId=14912. 2015.
12. James CV, Moonesinghe R, Wilson-Frederick SM, Hall JE, Penman-Aguilar A, Bouye K. Racial/Ethnic health disparities among rural adults—United States, 2012–2015. *MMWR Surveill Summ.* 2017; 66(23):1–9.
13. US Census Bureau Quick Facts. https://www.census.gov/quickfacts/fact/table/US/PST045217.
14. Economic Research Services, U.S. Department of Agriculture. Rural Classifications. https://www.ers.usda.gov/topics/rural-economy-population/rural-classifications/.
15. Waldorf B. A Continuous Multi-dimensional Measure of Rurality: Moving Beyond Threshold Measures. Selected Paper, Annual Meetings of the Association of Agricultural Economics, Long Beach, CA, July, 2006. http://ageconsearch.umn.edu/handle/21383.
16. Waldorf B, Kim A. *Defining and Measuring Rurality in the US: From Typologies to Continuous Indices.* West Lafayette, IN: Purdue University, Department of Agricultural Economics; April 2015.
17. Foutz J, Artiga S, Garfield R. The Role of Medicaid in Rural America. https://www.kff.org/medicaid/issue-brief/the-role-of-medicaid-in-rural-america/. Accessed April 25, 2017.
18. Cohen SA, Cook SK, Kelley L, Foutz JD, Sando TA. A closer look at rural-urban health disparities: Associations between obesity and rurality vary by geospatial and sociodemographic factors. *J Rural Health.* 2017;33(2):167–79.
19. Probst JC, Ajmal F. Social Determinants of Health among Minority Populations in Rural America. SC Rural Health Research Center Brief, 2019.
20. Illig S. "Rural America" doesn't mean "white America"—Here's why that matters. Vox, April 24, 2017. https://www.vox.com/conversations/2017/4/24/15286624/race-rural-america-trump-politics-media. Accessed August 15, 2018.
21. Kozhimannil KB, Henning-Smith C. Racism and health in rural America. *J Health Care Poor Underserved.* 2018;29(1):35–43.
22. Probst JC, Bellinger J, Walsemann K, Hardin J, Glover S. Higher risk of death in rural blacks and whites than urbanites is related to lower incomes, education, and health coverage. *Health Aff (Millwood).* 2011;30(10):1872–9.
23. Brinker PA, Walker B. The Hill-Burton Act: 1948–1954. *Rev Econ Stat.* 1962;44(2):208–12.
24. Clark LJ, Field MJ, Koontz TL Koontz VL. The impact of Hill-Burton: An analysis of hospital bed and physician distribution in the United States, 1950–1970. *Med Care.* 1980;18(5):532–50.
25. Health Resources and Services Administration. Hill Burton Free and Reduced Cost Health Care. https://www.hrsa.gov/get-health-care/affordable/hill-burton/index.html.
26. Roemer MI. Special health problems of Negroes in rural areas. *J Negro Educ.* 1949;18(3):318–25.
27. Friedman E. U.S. Hospitals and the Civil Rights Act of 1964. *Hospital and Health Networks*, June 2014. https://www.hhnmag.com/articles/4179-u-s-hospitals-and-the-civil-rights-act-of-1964.
28. Paradise J. Data Note: A Large Majority of Physicians Participate in Medicaid. https://www.kff.org/medicaid/issue-brief/data-note-a-large-majority-of-physicians-participate-in-medicaid/. Accessed May 10, 2017.
29. Centers for Medicare and Medicaid Services. Rural Health Resources. https://www.cms.gov/About-CMS/Agency-Information/OMH/equity-initiatives/rural-health/rural-health-resources.html.
30. Centers for Medicare and Medicaid Services. Frontier Extended Stay Clinic Demonstrations. https://innovation.cms.gov/initiatives/Frontier-Extended-Stay-Clinic/.
31. Medicare Payment Advisory Commission. Medicare and the Health Care Delivery Systems, June 2017. Washington, DC.
32. Health Resources and Services Administration, U.S. Department of Health and Human Services. About FORHP. https://www.hrsa.gov/rural-health/about-us/index.html.
33. U.S. Department of Agriculture. Rural Education at a Glance, 2017 Edition. Economic Information Bulletin 171, April, 2017.
34. Lavalley M. Out of the Loop. National School Boards Association Center for Public Education. Alexandria, VA. January 2018.
35. U.S. Department of Education. Programs. https://www2.ed.gov/programs/titleiparta/index.html. Washington, DC. 2015.
36. Dynarski M, Kainz K. Why federal spending on disadvantaged students (Title I) doesn't work. Brookings Institute Report, Washington DC. 2015.
37. U.S. Department of Agriculture. National School Lunch Program (NSLP). https://www.fns.usda.gov/nslp/national-school-lunch-program-nslp. Washington, DC. 2018.
38. Source: Authors' analysis of data from the 2017 American Housing Survey. https://www.census.gov/programs-surveys/ahs/data/interactive/ahstablecreator.html#?s_areas=a00000&s_year=n2017&s_tableName=Table1&s_byGroup1=a1&s_byGroup2=a1&s_filterGroup1=t1&s_filterGroup2=g1&s_show=S. Washington, DC. 2018.
39. U.S. Department of Agriculture. Rural Housing Service. https://www.rd.usda.gov/about-rd/agencies/rural-housing-service. Washington, DC. 2018.
40. U.S. Department of Housing and Urban Development. Rural Housing Stability Assistance Program. https://www.hud.gov/hudprograms/rural-housing. Washington, DC. 2018.
41. Pendall R, Goodman L, Zhu J, Gold A. *The Future of Rural Housing.* Washington, DC: The Urban Institute; 2016.
42. U.S. Department of Transportation. Rural Road Safety Program. https://safety.fhwa.dot.gov/local_rural/. 2018.
43. Probst JC, Laditka SB, Wang J-Y, Johnson AO. Effects of residence and race on burden of travel for care: Cross sectional analysis of the 2001 US National Household Travel Survey. *BMC Health Serv Res.* 2007;7:40.
44. Mattson J. *Rural Transit Fact Book* 2017. Fargo, ND: Upper Great Plains Transportation Institute, Small Urban and Rural Transit Center; 2017.
45. Parker K, Horowitz JM, Brown A, Fry R Cohn D, Igielnik R. *What Unites and Divides Urban, Suburban and Rural Communities.* Washington, DC: Pew Research Center; 2018.
46. Federal Communications Commission. 2018 Broadband Deployment Report. https://www.fcc.gov/reports-research/reports/broadband-progress-reports/2018-broadband-deployment-report. 2018.
47. Keller J. The Agony of Rural America's Inescapable Broadband Gap. https://psmag.com/economics/the-agony-of-rural-americas-inescapable-broadband-gap. 2018.

48. Rogers K. Rural America Is Building High-Speed Internet the Same Way It Built Electricity in the 1930s. Motherboard. https://motherboard.vice.com/en_us/article/ywnz37/electric-coops-internet-america-cooperatives-broadband. 2017.

49. U.S. Department of Agriculture. Community Facilities Direct Loan & Grant Program. https://www.rd.usda.gov/programs-services/community-facilities-direct-loan-grant-program. Washington, DC. 2018.

50. U.S. Department of Agriculture. Programs & Services for Businesses. https://www.rd.usda.gov/programs-services/programs-services-businesses. Washington, DC. 2018.

51. U.S. Small Business Administration. SBA Rural Lending Initiative. https://www.sba.gov/about-sba/sba-initiatives/sba-rural-lending-initiative. 2018.

52. James W, Cossman JS. Long-term trends in Black and White mortality in the rural United States: Evidence of a race-specific rural mortality penalty. *J Rural Health* 2017;33(1):21–31.

53. Authors' Analysis of data from the Centers for Disease Control and Prevention, National Center for Health Statistics. Underlying Cause of Death 1999–2016 on CDC WONDER Online Database, released December, 2017. Data are from the Multiple Cause of Death Files, 1999–2016, as compiled from data provided by the 57 vital statistics jurisdictions through the Vital Statistics Cooperative Program. http://wonder.cdc.gov/ucd-icd10.html. Accessed August 21, 2018.

54. Ely DM, Hoyert DL. Differences between Rural and Urban Areas in Mortality Rates for the Leading Causes of Infant Death: United States, 2013–2015. NCHS Data Brief No. 300, February 2018.

55. Maron, DF. Maternal Healthcare is Disappearing in Rural America. *Scientific American*. February 15, 2017. https://www.scientificamerican.com/article/maternal-health-care-is-disappearing-in-rural-america/. Accessed September 2, 2018.

56. Hung P, Casey MM, Kozhimannil KB, Karaca-Mandic P, Moscovice IS. Rural-urban differences in access to hospital obstetric and neonatal care: How far is the closest one? *J Perinatol*. 2018;38(6):645–52.

57. Hung P, Henning-Smith CE, Casey MM, Kozhimannil KB. Access to obstetric services in rural counties still declining, with 9 percent losing services, 2004–14. *Health Aff (Millwood)*. 2017;36(9):1663–71.

58. Kozhimannil KB, Hung P, Henning-Smith C, Casey MM, Prasad S. Association between loss of hospital-based obstetric services and birth outcomes in rural counties in the United States. *JAMA*. 2018;319(12):1239–47.

59. Rayburn WF, Klagholz JC, Murray-Krezan C, Dowell LE, Strunk AL. Distribution of American Congress of Obstetricians and Gynecologists fellows and junior fellows in practice in the United States. *Obstet Gynecol*. 2012;119(5):1017–22.

60. National Center for Health Statistics. *Health, United States, 2016: With Chartbook on Long-term Trends in Health*. Hyattsville, MD. 2017.

61. Moy E, Garcia MC, Bastian B, et al. Leading causes of death in nonmetropolitan and metropolitan areas—United States, 1999–2014. *MMWR Surveill Summ*. 2017;66(No. SS-1):1–8.

62. Zahnd WE, James AS, Jenkins WD, et al. Rural-urban differences in cancer incidence and trends in the United States. *Cancer Epidemiol Biomarkers Prev*. 2018;27(11):1265–74.

63. Henley SJ, Anderson RN, Thomas CC, Massetti GM, Peaker B, Richardson LC. Invasive cancer incidence, 2004–2013, and deaths, 2006–2015, in nonmetropolitan and metropolitan counties—United States. *MMWR Surveill Summ*. 2017;66(14):1–13.

64. Matthews KA, Croft JB, Liu Y, et al. Health-related behaviors by urban-rural county classification—United States, 2013. *MMWR Surveill Summ*. 2017;66(5):1–8.

65. Eberth JM, Josey MJ, Mobley LR, et al. Who performs colonoscopy? Workforce trends over space and time. *J Rural Health*. 2018;34(2):138–47.

66. MacKinney AC. Access to Rural Health Care—A Literature Review and New Synthesis. Iowa City, IA: Rural Policy Research Institute; 2014. http://www.rupri.org/Forms/HealthPanel_Access_August2014.pdf.

67. Meilleur A, Subramanian SV, Plascak JJ, Fisher JL, Paskett ED, Lamont EB. Rural residence and cancer outcomes in the United States: Issues and challenges. *Cancer Epidemiol Biomarkers Prev*. 2013;22(10):1657–67.

68. Zahnd WE, Fogleman AJ, Jenkins WD. Rural–urban disparities in stage of diagnosis among cancers with preventive opportunities. *Am J Prev Med*. 2018;54(5):688–98.

69. Unger JM, Moseley A, Symington B, Chavez-MacGregor M, Ramsey SD, Hershman DL. Geographic distribution and survival outcomes for rural patients with cancer treated in clinical trials. *JAMA Network Open*. 2018;1(4):e181235.

70. Kegler SR, Stone DM, Holland KM. Trends in suicide by level of urbanization—United States, 1999–2015. *MMWR Morb Mortal Wkly Rep*. 2017;66:270–3.

71. National Healthcare Quality and Disparities Report chartbook on rural health care. Rockville, MD: Agency for Healthcare Research and Quality; October 2017. AHRQ Pub. No. 17(18)-0001-2-EF.

72. Ivey-Stephenson AZ, Crosby AE, Jack SPD, Haileyesus T, Kresnow-Sedacca MJ. Suicide trends among and within urbanization levels by sex, race/ethnicity, age group, and mechanism of death—United States, 2001–15. *MMWR Surveill Summ*. 2017;66(18):1–16.

73. Spicer RS, Miller TR. Suicide acts in 8 states: Incidence and case fatality rates by demographics and method. *Am J Public Health*. 2000:90(12);1885.

74. Igielnik R. Rural and urban gun owners have different experiences, views on gun policy. July, 2017. Pew Research Center. http://www.pewresearch.org/fact-tank/2017/07/10/rural-and-urban-gun-owners-have-different-experiences-views-on-gun-policy/.

75. Bureau of Labor Statistics, U.S. Department of Labor. National Census of Fatal Occupational Injuries in 2016. USDL-17-1667. December 19, 2017.

76. Peek-Asa C, Zwerling C, Stallones L. Acute traumatic injuries in rural populations *Am J Public Health*. 2004;94(10):1689–93.

77. National Center for Statistics and Analysis. Rural/ urban comparison of traffic fatalities: 2015 data. (Traffic Safety Facts. Report No. DOT HS 812 521). Washington, DC: National Highway Traffic Safety Administration. April, 2018.

78. Strine TW, Beck LF, Bolen J, Okoro C, Dhingra S, Balluz L. Geographic and sociodemographic variation in self-reported seat belt use in the United States. *Accid Anal Prev*. 2010;42:1066–71.

79. MacKenzie EJ, Rivara FP, Jurkovich GJ, et al. A national evaluation of the effect of trauma-center care on mortality. *N Engl J Med*. 2006;354(4):366–78.

80. Hsia RYJ, Shen YC. Rising closures of hospital trauma centers disproportionately burden vulnerable populations. *Health Aff (Millwood)* 2011;30(10):1912–20.

81. Trivedi T, Liu J, Probst J, Merchant A, Jhones S, Martin AB. Obesity and obesity-related behaviors among rural and urban adults in the USA. *Rural Remote Health*. 2015;15(4):3267.

82. Liu JH, Jones SJ, Sun H, Probst JC, Merchant AT, Cavicchia P. Diet, physical activity, and sedentary behaviors as risk factors for childhood obesity: An urban and rural comparison. *Child Obes*. 2012;8(5):440–8.

83. Larson NI, Story MT, Nelson MC. Neighborhood environments: Disparities in access to healthy foods in the U.S. *Am J Prev Med*. 2009;36(1):74–81.

84. Coleman-Jensen A, Rabbitt MP, Gregory CA, Singh A. Household Food Security in the United States in 2016, ERR-237, U.S. Department of Agriculture, Economic Research Service. 2017.

85. Gregory CA, Coleman-Jensen A. Food Insecurity, Chronic Disease, and Health Among Working-Age Adults, ERR-235, U.S. Department of Agriculture, Economic Research Service, July 2017.

86. Roberts ME, Doogan NJ, Stanton CA, et al. Rural versus urban use of traditional and emerging tobacco products in the United States, 2013–2014. *Am J Public Health*. 2017;107(10):1554–9.

87. Pesko MF, Robarts AMT. Adolescent tobacco use in urban versus rural areas of the United States: The influence of tobacco control policy environments. *J Adolesc Health*. 2017;61(1):70–6.

88. Roberts ME, Doogan NG, Kurti AN, et al. Rural tobacco use across the United States: How rural and urban areas differ, broken down by census regions and divisions. *Health Place*. 2016;39:153–9.

89. Yan AF, Chiu Y-W, Stoesen CA, et al. STD/HIV-related sexual risk behaviors and substance use among U.S. rural adolescents. *J Natl Med Assoc*. 2007;99:1386–94.

90. Haley T, Puskar K, Terhorst L, et al. Condom use among sexually active rural high school adolescents personal, environmental, and behavioral predictors. *J Sch Nurs*. 2013;29:212–24.

91. Chesson HW, Kent CK, Owusu-Edusei KJr, Leichliter JS, Aral SO. Disparities in sexually transmitted disease rates across the "eight Americas." *Sex Transm Dis*. 2012;39(6):458–64.

92. Milhausen RR, Crosby R, Yarber WL, DiClemente RJ, Wingood GM, Ding K. Rural and nonrural African American high school students and STD/HIV sexual-risk behaviors. *Am J Health Behav*. 2003;27(4):373–9.

93. Crosby RA, Oser CB, Leukefeld CG, Havens JR, Young A. Prevalence of HIV and risky sexual behaviors among rural drug users: Does age matter? *Ann Epidemiol*. 2012;22(11):778–82.

94. Ng AS, Kaye, K. Sex in the (Non) City: Teen Childbearing in Rural America. Washington, DC, The National Campaign to Prevent Teen and Unplanned Pregnancy. 2015.

95. National Center for HIV/AIDS, Viral Hepatitis, STD, and TB Prevention Division of HIV/AIDS Prevention. HIV Surveillance in Urban and Nonurban Areas through 2016. https://www.cdc.gov/hiv/pdf/library/slidesets/cdc-hiv-urban-nonurban-2016.pdf.

96. Rural Health Information Hub. Rural data explorer. https://www.ruralhealthinfo.org/data-explorer?id=193.

97. Ohl ME, Perencevich E. Frequency of human immunodeficiency virus (HIV) testing in urban vs. rural areas of the United States: Results from a nationally-representative sample. *BMC Public Health.* 2011; 11:681.

98. Henderson ER, Subramaniam DS, Chen J. Rural-urban differences in HIV testing among US adults: Findings from the behavioral risk factor surveillance system. *Sex Transm Dis.* 2018;45(12):808–12.

99. Evans M, et al. HIV in a Mostly Rural Area Affected by the Opioid Epidemic—West Virginia, 2017. Presented at Epidemic Intelligence Service conference; April 16–19, 2018; Atlanta. https://www.healio.com/infectious-disease/hiv-aids/news/online/%7B14b892c6-4b93-4fa9-99ee-bc19ac25e9c7%7D/rural-us-counties-with-active-hiv-transmission-lack-prevention-services.

100. Weiss G, Smith DK, Newman S, Wiener J, Kitlas A, Hoover KW. PrEP implementation by local health departments in US cities and counties: Findings from a 2015 assessment of local health departments. *PLoS One.* 2018;13(7):e0200338.

101. Vyavaharkar M, Glover S, Leonhirth D, Probst JC. *HIV/AIDS in Rural America: Prevalence and Service Availability.* Prepared under Grant Award No 1 UIC RH 03711 with the Federal Office of Rural Health Policy, Health Resources and Services Administration. Submitted March 2012.

102. Peters PJ, Pontones P, Hoover KW, et al. HIV infection linked to injection use of oxymorphone in Indiana, 2014–2015. *N Engl J Med.* 2016;375(3):229–39.

103. Mack KA, Jones CM, Ballesteros MF. Illicit drug use, illicit drug use disorders, and drug overdose deaths in metropolitan and nonmetropolitan areas—United States. *MMWR Surveill Summ.* 2017;66(19):1–12.

104. Substance Abuse and Mental Health Services Administration. Behavioral Health Barometer: United States, 2015. HHS Publication No. SMA-16-Baro-2015. Rockville, MD: Substance Abuse and Mental Health Services Administration, 2015.

105. Brown JD, Goodin AJ, Talbert JC. Rural and appalachian disparities in neonatal abstinence syndrome incidence and access to opioid abuse treatment. *J Rural Health.* 2018;34(1):6–13.

106. Andrilla CHA, Moore TE, Patterson DG, Larson EH. Geographic distribution of providers with a DEA waiver to prescribe buprenorphine for the treatment of opioid use disorder: A 5-year update. *J Rural Health.* 2019;35(1):108–12.

107. Bureau of Labor Statistics. National Census of Fatal Occupational Injuries in 2016. Washington, DC, USDL-17-1667. December, 2017.

108. Blackley DH, Halldin CN, Laney AS. Continued increase in prevalence of coal workers' pneumoconiosis in the United States, 1970–2017. *Am J Public Health.* 2018;108:1220–2.

109. Witter RZ, Tenney L, Clark S, Lee S. Newman occupational exposures in the oil and gas extraction industry: State of the science and research recommendations. *Am J Ind Med.* 2014;57(7):847–56.

110. Bang KM, Mazurek JM, Wood JM, White GE, Hendricks SA, Weston A. Silicosis mortality trends and new exposures to respirable crystalline silica—United States, 2001–2010. *MMWR Morb Mortal Wkly Rep.* 2015;64(5):117–9.

111. Landsteiner AM, McGovern PM, Alexander BH, Lindgren PG, Williams AN. Incidence rates and trend of serious farm-related injury in Minnesota, 2000–2011. *J Agromedicine.* 2015;20(4):419–26.

112. Allen DL, Kearney GD, Sheila Higgins S. A descriptive study of farm-related injuries presenting to emergency departments in North Carolina: 2008–2012. *J Agromed.* 2015;20(4):398–408.

113. Gross N, Young T, Ramirez M, Leinenkugel K, Peek-Asa C. Characteristics of work- and non-work-related farm injuries. *J Rural Health.* 2015;31(4):401–9.

114. Larson-Bright M, Gerberich SG, Alexander BH, et al. Work practices and childhood agricultural injury. *Inj Prev.* 2007;13(6):409–15.

115. Williams QLJr, Alexander BH, Gerberich SG, Nachreiner NM, Church TR, Ryan, A. Bystander injury evaluation of children from Midwestern agricultural operations. *J Saf Res.* 2010;41(1):31–7.

116. Damalas CA, Eleftherohorinos IG. Pesticide exposure, safety issues, and risk assessment indicators. *Int J Environ Res Public Health.* 2011;8(5):1402–19.

117. Strong LL, Thompson B, Koepsell TD, Meischke H. Factors associated with pesticide safety practices in farmworkers. *Am J Indust Med.* 2008;51(1):69–81.

118. Strosnider H, Kennedy C, Monti M, Yip F. Rural and urban differences in air quality, 2008–2012, and community drinking water quality, 2010–2015—United States. *MMWR Surveill Summ.* 2017;66(13):1–10.

119. Loftus C, Yost M, Sampson P, et al. Ambient ammonia exposures in an agricultural community and pediatric asthma morbidity. *Epidemiology.* 2015;26(6):794–801.

120. Cox. Trouble in Farm Country: Ag Runoff Fouls Tap Water across Rural America. https://www.ewg.org/tapwater/trouble-in-farm-country.php.

121. U.S. Environmental Protection Agency. Private Drinking Water Wells. https://www.epa.gov/privatewells.

122. DeSimone LA, McMahon PB, Rosen MR, *The quality of our Nation's waters—Water quality in Principal Aquifers of the United States, 1991–2010*: U.S. Geological Survey Circular 1360. 2014.

123. Jones S, Atkin E. Rural America's Drinking Water Crisis. February 12, 2018. The New Republic. https://newrepublic.com/article/147011/rural-americas-drinking-water-crisis.

124. Hill HA, Elam-Evans LD, Yankey D, Singleton JA, Dietz V. Vaccination coverage among children aged 19–35 months—United States, 2015. *MMWR Morb Mortal Wkly Rep.* 2016;65:1065–71.

125. Walker TY, Elam-Evans LD, Singleton JA, et al. National, regional, state, and selected local area vaccination coverage among adolescents aged 13–17 years—United States, 2016. *MMWR Morb Mortal Wkly Rep.* 2017;66:874–82.

126. Shipman SA, Lan J, Chang CH, Goodman DC. Geographic maldistribution of primary care for children. *Pediatrics.* 2011;127:19–27.

127. National Rural Health Association Policy Brief. Physician Assistants: Modernize Laws to Improve Rural Access. Washington, DC. July 2017. https://www.ruralhealthweb.org/NRHA/media/Emerge_NRHA/Advocacy/Policy%20documents/04-09-18-NRHA-Policy-Physician-Assistants-Modernize-Laws-to-Improve-Rural-Access.pdf.

128. Probst JC, Laditka SB, Wang JY, Johnson AO. Effects of residence and race on burden of travel for care: Cross sectional analysis of the 2001 US National Household Travel Survey. *BMC Health Serv Res.* 2007;7:40.

129. Health Resources and Services Administration, U.S. Department of Health and Human Services. Health Professional Shortage Areas. Available at https://bhw.hrsa.gov/shortage-designation/hpsas.

130. Health Resources and Services Administration, U.S. Department of Health and Human Services. Medically Underserved Areas and Populations. https://bhw.hrsa.gov/shortage-designation/muap.

131. Authors' calculations based on data from the Health Resources and Services Administration. https://data.hrsa.gov/data/about.

132. Authors' calculations from the Area Health Resource File. https://data.hrsa.gov/data/download.

133. Doescher MP, Jackson JE, Fordyce MA, Lynge DC. *Variability in surgical practice and patient characteristics in rural and urban US hospital settings.* WWAMI Rural Health Research Center, Final Report #142, February 2015. Seattle, Washington.

134. Shively EH, Shively SA. Threats to rural surgery. *Am J Surg.* 2005;190(2):200–5.

135. Nakayama D, Hughes TG. Issues that face rural surgery in the United States. *J Am Coll Surg.* 2014;219(4):814–18.

136. Doty B, Zuckerman R, Finalyson S, Jenkins P, Rieb N, Heneghan S. General surgery at rural hospitals: A national survey of rural hospital administrators. *Surgery.* 2008;143(5):599–606.

137. Doty B, Zuckerman R, Finlayson S, Jenkins P, Rieb N, Heneghan S. How does degree of rurality impact provision of surgical services at rural hospitals? *J Rural Health.* 2008;24(3):306–10.

138. Eilrich FC, Sprague JC, Whitacre BE, et al. The economic impact of a rural general surgeon and model for forecasting need. September 2010. http://ruralhealthworks.org/wp-content/files/FINAL-General-Surgeon-092210.pdf.

139. Reschovsky JD, Staiti A. Physician incomes in rural and urban America. 2006; Issue Brief No. 92. www.hschange.com/CONTENT/725/. Accessed August 29, 2018.

140. Williams TEJr, Satiani B, Ellison EC. A comparison of future recruitment needs in urban and rural hospitals: The rural imperative. *Surgery.* 2011;150(4):617–25.

141. Xierali M, Nivet MA, Rayburn WF. Relocation of obstetrician-gynecologists in the United States, 2005–2015. *Obstet Gynecol.* 2017;129(3):543–50.
142. Rayburn WF, Richards ME, Elwell EC. Drive times to hospitals with perinatal care in the United States. *Obstet Gynecol.* 2012; 119(3):611–6.
143. Larson EH, Murowchick E, Hart LG. Poor birth outcomes in the rural United States: 1985–1987 to 1995–1997. WWAMI Rural Health Research Center, Project Summary, February 2008. Seattle, Washington.
144. Makaroff LA, Xierali M, Petterson SM, Shipman SA, Puffer JC, Bazemore AW. Factors influencing family physicians' contribution to the child health care workforce. *Ann Fam Med.* 2014;12(5):427–31.
145. Mayer ML. Disparities in geographic access to pediatric subspecialty care. *Matern Child Health J.* 2008;12(5):624–32.
146. Lee DM, Nichols T. Physician recruitment and retention in rural and underserved areas, *Int J Health Care Quality Assurance.* 2014;27(7):642–52.
147. Scammon DL, Williams SD, Li LB. Understanding physicians' decisions to practice in rural areas as a basis for developing recruitment and retention strategies. *J Ambul Care Mark.* 1994;5(2):85–100.
148. Renner DM, Westfall JM, Wilroy LA, Ginde AA. The influence of loan repayment on rural healthcare provider recruitment and retention in Colorado. *Rural Remote Health.* 2010;10(4):1605.
149. Jarman BT, Cogbill TH, Mathiason MA, et al. Factors correlated with surgery resident choice to practice general surgery in a rural area *J Surg Educ.* 2009;66:319–24.
150. Pathman DE, Konrad TR, Dann R, Koch G. Retention of primary care physicians in rural health professional shortage areas. *Am J Public Health.* 2004;94(10):1723–9.
151. Sempowski IP. Effectiveness of financial incentives in exchange for rural and underserviced area return-of-service commitments: Systematic review of the literature. *Can J Rural Med.* 2004;9(2):82–8.
152. Daniels ZM, Vanleit BJ, Skipper BJ, Sanders ML, Rhyne RL. Factors in recruitment and retaining health professionals for rural practice. *J Rural Health.* 2007;23(1):62–71.
153. North Carolina Rural Health Research Program. 87 Rural Hospital Closures: January 2010–Present. http://www.shepscenter.unc.edu/programs-projects/rural-health/rural-hospital-closures/.
154. Lindrooth RC, Perraillon MC, Hardy RY, Tung GJ. Understanding the relationship between Medicaid expansions and hospital closures. *Health Aff (Millwood).* 2018;37(1):111–20.
155. Reif SS, DesHarnais S, Bernard S. Community perceptions of the effects of rural hospital closure on access to care. *J Rural Health.* 1999;15(2):202–9.
156. Joynt KE, Chatterjee P, Orav EJ, Jha AK. Hospital closures had no measurable impact on local hospitalization rates or mortality rates, 2003–11. *Health Aff (Millwood).* 2015;34(5):765–72.
157. Liu C, Srebotnjak T, Hsia RY. California emergency department closures are associated with increased inpatient mortality at nearby hospitals. *Health Aff (Millwood).* 2014;33(8):1323–9.
158. Williams JC, Song PH, Pink GH. Estimated Costs of Rural Freestanding Emergency Departments. NC Rural Health Research Program, Chapel Hill, NC. November 2015.
159. Holmes GM, Slifkin RT, Randolph RK, Poley S. The effect of rural hospital closures on community economic health. *Health Serv Res.* 2006;41(2):467–85.
160. Ullrich F, Mueller KJ. Update: Independently owned pharmacy closures in rural America, 2003–2013. *Rural Policy Brief.* 2014;(2014 7):1–4.
161. Hessler P. Dr. Don: The life of a small-town druggist. The New Yorker. September 26, 2011. https://www.newyorker.com/magazine/2011/09/26/dr-don.
162. American Association of Nurse Practitioners. State Practice Environment. https://www.aanp.org/legislation-regulation/state-legislation/state-practice-environment#hawaii-open. Accessed September 4, 2018.
163. American Association of Physician Assistants. PA Scope of Practice. January 2017. Available at https://www.aapa.org/wp-content/uploads/2017/01/Issue-brief_Scope-of-Practice_0117-1.pdf.
164. Brom HM, Salsberry PJ, Graham MC. Leveraging health care reform to accelerate nurse practitioner full practice authority. *J Am Assoc Nurse Pract.* 2018;30(3):120–30.
165. American Medical Association. Physician assistant scope of practice. 2018. https://www.ama-assn.org/sites/default/files/media-browser/public/arc-public/state-law-physician-assistant-scope-practice.pdf.
166. Wildeman MK. SC nurses given broader prescribing power, greater authority to practice. *The Post and Courier.* August 14, 2018. https://www.postandcourier.com/features/sc-nurses-given-broader-prescribing-power-greater-authority-to-practice/article_fc49370e-9f36-11e8-b000-978ea0de6b64.html.
167. Graves JA, Mishra P, Dittus RS, Parikh R, Perloff J, Buerhaus PI. Role of geography and nurse practitioner scope-of-practice in efforts to expand primary care system capacity: Health reform and the primary care workforce. *Med Care.* 2016;54(1):81–9.
168. Neff DF, Yoon SH, Steiner RL, et al. The impact of nurse practitioner regulations on population access to care. *Nurs Outlook.* 2018;66(4):379–85.
169. Barnes H, Richards MR, McHugh MD, Martsolf G. Rural and nonrural primary care physician practices increasingly rely on nurse practitioners. *Health Aff (Millwood).* 2018;37(6):908–14.
170. Ortiz J, Hofler R, Bushy A, Lin YL, Khanijahani A, Bitney A. Impact of nurse practitioner practice regulations on rural population health outcomes. *Healthcare (Basel).* 2018;6(2):65.
171. Kurtzman ET, Barnow BS, Johnson JE, Simmens SJ, Infeld DL, Mullan F. Does the regulatory environment affect nurse practitioners' patterns of practice or quality of care in health centers? *Health Serv Res.* 2017;52(Suppl 1):437–58.
172. Henry LR, Hooker RS. Retention of physician assistants in rural health clinics. *J Rural Health.* 2007;23(3):207–14.
173. Kippenbrock T, Stacy A, Gilbert-Palmer D. Educational strategies to enhance placement and retention of nurse practitioners in rural Arkansas. *Am Acad Nurse Pract.* 2004;16(3):139–43.
174. Doescher MP, Andrilla CH, Skillman SM, Morgan P, Kaplan L. The contribution of physicians, physician assistants, and nurse practitioners toward rural primary care: Findings from a 13-state survey. *Med Care.* 2014;52(6):549–56.
175. Verma P, Ford JA, Stuart A, Howe A, Everington S, Steel N. A systematic review of strategies to recruit and retain primary care doctors. *BMC Health Serv Res.* 2016;16:126.
176. Skariah JM, Rasmussen C, Hollander-Rodriguez J et al. Rural curricular guidelines based on practice scope of recent residency graduates practicing in small communities. *Fam Med.* 2017 Sep;49(8):594–9.
177. Deal SB, Cook MR, Hughes D, et al. Training for a career in rural and nonmetropolitan surgery—A practical needs assessment. *J Surg Educ.* 2018;75(6):e229–33.
178. Parlier AB, Galvin SL, Thach S, Kruidenier D, Fagan EB. The road to rural primary care: A narrative review of factors that help develop, recruit, and retain rural primary care physicians. *Acad Med.* 2018;93(1):130–40.
179. Ross R. Fifteen-year outcomes of a rural residency: Aligning policy with national needs. *Fam Med.* 2013;45(2):122–7.
180. Ferguson WJ, Cashman SB, Savageau JA, Lasser DH. Family medicine residency characteristics associated with practice in a health professions shortage area. *Fam Med.* 2009;41(6):405–10.
181. MacDowell M, Glasser M, Hunsaker M. A decade of rural physician workforce outcomes for the Rockford Rural Medical Education (RMED) Program, University of Illinois. *Acad Med.* 2013;88(12):1941–7.
182. The National Academies. *The Role of Telehealth in an Evolving Health Care Environment.* Washington, DC: National Academies Press; 2012.
183. Health Resources and Services Administration, Telehealth Programs. https://www.hrsa.gov/rural-health/telehealth/index.html.
184. Stingley S, Schultz H. Helmsley trust support for telehealth improves access to care in rural and frontier areas. *Health Aff (Millwood).* 2014;33(2):336–41.
185. Morse S. Centers for Medicare and Medicaid Services unveils strategy to boost rural telehealth. May 10, 2018. Healthcare Finance. https://www.healthcarefinancenews.com/news/centers-medicare-and-medicaid-services-unveils-strategy-boost-rural-telehealth.
186. Ward MM, Ullrich F, Mueller K. Extent of telehealth use in rural and urban hospitals. *Rural Policy Brief.* 2014;(2014 4):1–4.
187. Merchant KA, Ward MM, Mueller KJ. Hospital views of factors affecting telemedicine use. *Rural Policy Brief.* 2015;(2015 5):1–4.
188. Alanee S, Dynda D, LeVault K et al. Delivering kidney cancer care in rural Central and Southern Illinois: A telemedicine approach. *Eur J Cancer Care (Engl).* 2014;23(6):739–44.
189. Ohl M, Dillon D, Moeckli J et al. Mixed-methods evaluation of a telehealth collaborative care program for persons with HIV infection in a rural setting. *J Gen Intern Med.* 2013;28(9):1165–73.
190. Brown JD, Hales S, Evans TE, et al. Description, utilisation and results from a telehealth primary care weight management intervention for adults with obesity in South Carolina. *J Telemed Telecare.* 2020;26(1-2):28–35.

191. Ferree T. Why Rural America Is Still Not Connected. https://www.broadcastingcable.com/blog/why-rural-america-still-not-connected. Accessed May 8, 2018.

192. Andrew Perrin. "Social Networking Usage: 2005–2015." Pew Research Center. October 2015. http://www.pewinternet.org/2015/10/08/2015/Social-Networking-Usage-2005-2015/.

193. Gilbert E, Karahalios K, Sandvig C. The network in the garden: Designing social media for rural life. *Am Behav Sci.* 2010;53(9):1367–88.

194. U.S. Department of Agriculture. *"Rural Lines—USA: The Story of the Rural Electrification Administration's First Twenty-five Years, 1935–1960."* Washington, DC: U.S. Government Printing Office; January, 1960. https://archive.org/stream/rurallinesusasto811unit_0/rurallinesusasto811unit_0_djvu.txt.

195. National Park Service. Rural Electrification Act. https://www.nps.gov/home/learn/historyculture/ruralelect.htm.

196. Roberts ET, McWilliams JM, Hatfield LA et al. Changes in health care use associated with the introduction of hospital global budgets in Maryland. *JAMA Intern Med.* 2018;178(2):260–8.

197. Roberts ET, Hatfield LA, McWilliams JM et al. Changes in hospital utilization three years into Maryland's global budget program for rural hospitals. *Health Aff (Millwood).* 2018;37(4):644–53.

198. Galarraga JE, Frohna WJ, Pines JM. The impact of Maryland's global budget payment reform on emergency department admission rates in a single health system. *Acad Emerg Med.* 2019;26(1):68–78.

199. South Carolina Office of Rural Health. Rural Health Action Plan. https://scorh.net/rural-health-action-plan/. 2018.

200. Phillips CD, McLeroy KR. Health in rural America: Remembering the importance of place. *Am J Public Health.* 2004;94(10):1661–3.

201. Boreham CA, Wallace WF, Nevill A. Training effects of accumulated daily stair-climbing exercise in previously sedentary young women. *Prev Med.* 2000;30:277e281.

CHAPTER 34

Considering Sexual Orientation, Gender Identity and Expression, and Sex Characteristics in Public Health

Randall Sell • Caroline Voyles

INTRODUCTION

Public health practitioners focus on the health and the threats to health of populations, which can be delineated in various ways using a wide variety of taxonomies. Geography was one of the first classifications used in public health as it conveniently mapped to geographically bound governmental structures that were responsible for the public's well-being.[1] However, taxonomies for classifying individuals have moved beyond geography to include many characteristics of individuals and groups of individuals. Ideally, these taxonomies identify people and clusters of people based upon characteristics that allow us to understand and improve the public's health.

This chapter discusses several interrelated taxonomies that have proven valuable for addressing public health. These include taxonomies based on: (1) sexual orientations, (2) gender identities and expression, and (3) sex characteristics (going forward noted as "SOGIESC").[2,3]

SOGIESC minorities in the United States have been, and in many countries around the world still are frequently arrested, imprisoned and executed for same-sex sexual behavior; arrested for wearing clothing not representative of their biological sex; required to use bathrooms that do not correspond to their gender identity; arrested for dancing together; arrested for publishing and mailing literature not critical of homosexuality; forcibly hospitalized and placed in mental institutions; banned from being represented in literature, plays, and movies; fired from their jobs (e.g., restaurant workers, bankers, school teachers); as students, thrown out of schools and colleges (both public and private); denied parental rights to biological children and adoption rights; denied service in restaurants and bars; banned from serving in the military; denied housing (e.g., rental, homeless shelters); refused the ability to marry, and if intersex, abandoned or killed as infants.[4–10]

Arguments based upon scientific, including public health, research have played a role, often a critical role, in debates about each of these issues. Most fundamentally, the arguments have often concerned whether SOGIESC minorities are inherently ill or defective and deserving of basic rights, or whether they simply represent natural variations of sexuality, gender, and sex characteristics. The stigma and discrimination they often experience fundamentally impacts the health of SOGIESC minorities in ways that have not been adequately assessed or addressed.[11–13]

This chapter provides an overview of SOGIESC terms, how they are defined, and common taxonomies/measures used to sort individuals into SOGIESC categories. This is followed by a review of a few of the pressing public health concerns for SOGIESC minorities, and an introduction to several examples of successful efforts to protect and improve the health of these populations. We then discuss how the study of SOGIESC health requires integrating the concerns of SOGIESC minorities throughout all public health practice, which requires the participation of every discipline currently engaged in public health.

SOGIESC TERMS AND DEFINITIONS

Fundamental to the practice of public health is the monitoring of health and threats to health using epidemiology. Epidemiology requires that populations be clearly and practically defined and that there be valid and reliable measures that can be used to sort persons into categories.

The evolution over the last century of terms, definitions, and measures used to label or describe SOGIESC minorities is complicated and fascinating. It also provides a very useful context for researchers conducting research with SOGIESC populations and for providers serving these populations. This history informs current practice and programming with SOGIESC minorities and can contribute to our understanding of the health status of these populations as well as the ways in which SOGIESC minorities interact with the healthcare system. This chapter focuses on current terms and definitions of these social constructs, while encouraging readers to take a deeper dive into this informative history, which has been described elsewhere.[14–16]

The constructs central to the topics discussed in this chapter are "sexual orientation," "gender identity," "gender expression," and "sex characteristics." We base our discussion on prior work initially developed to create a measure of lesbian, gay, bisexual, transgender, and intersex social inclusion supported by the United Nations Development Programme and the World Bank.[17] This work was informed by conversations with civil society organizations from around the world who work with and represent SOGIESC minority communities.

Sexual Orientation

"Sexual orientation can refer to a self-identity, to attraction to people of the same- and/or different-sex, or sexual behavior with people of the same- and/or different-sex."[17] This definition is helpful but is also open to diverse interpretations. The definition states that sexual orientations can be about an "identity," "sexual behaviors," "sexual attractions," or some combination of these three constructs.[2] This means that understanding the construct of sexual orientation also requires defining and operationalizing these additional constructs. Unfortunately, researchers and service providers working with sexual minorities have not agreed upon such definitions. It is therefore incumbent on anyone working with sexual minorities to explicitly state their working definitions of these constructs and state how these definitions are operationalized in the process of conducting research or providing services.[18]

Because researchers studying these populations do not generally make these definitions explicit, the work of two different researchers (or frequently even two different studies by the same researcher) can be difficult or even impossible to compare.[19] For example, how a research subject gets labeled as "gay," "lesbian," or "bisexual," in one study may be different from how those labels are applied in another study, and these differences are often difficult or impossible to discern from published articles, which rarely provide detailed information in their method sections. Of even more concern, these labels are often applied loosely or uncritically. For example, research subjects are sometimes labeled as sexual minorities because they are sampled from an organization or location frequented by sexual minorities.[19,20]

It should be noted however that sexual orientation is generally operationalized in people's lives based upon their understanding of their own sexual attractions and/or sexual behaviors and how they relate to their identity.[21] For example, a man who is primarily sexually attracted to other men may come to identify as "gay," or a woman primarily sexually attracted to other women as "lesbian." This may occur even if these individuals have never experienced any sexual behavior consequently making actual sexual behavior an unessential component of identity development for some individuals. Because of social pressures, some individuals may only be sexually attracted and have sexual contact with others of the same sex but identify as "straight."[22] This frequent occurrence is often primarily the result of social pressures to not identify as a sexual minority and further demonstrates the discordance that can occur between sexual attractions, sexual behaviors, and sexual minority identities.[23] For other individuals, sexual behavior may play a more important role in defining their identity.

The terms most frequently used to describe sexual orientations in the United States and other English-speaking countries are lesbian, gay, bisexual, and straight.[24] Additional terms include homosexual and heterosexual. In general, the terms "gay" (for men) and "lesbian" (for women) refer to people who have that identity or are primarily attracted to or have sex with people of the same sex; "bisexual" people are those who have that self-identity or who are attracted to or have sex with people of both sexes; and "straight" people are those who have that self-identity or who are primarily attracted to or have sex with people of a different sex. These terms are frequently described in the literature as characterizing the construct of "sexual identity," but a more precise label of the construct is "sexual orientation identity." As it is an identity related to the construct of sexual orientation.

The terms "homosexual" and "heterosexual" are less frequently used as personal identity terms, however, may be used by researchers and clinicians to describe people who have sexual minority identities, same-sex attractions or same-sex behaviors (homosexual), or sexual majority identities, other-sex attractions, or other-sex behaviors (heterosexual). The terms homosexual and heterosexual have a long history in the medical literature and are generally not preferred terms within either sexual minority or sexual majority communities.[25]

Terms used by sexual minorities vary across time and geographic locations. The terms described above are those that have predominated in the United States and some other English-speaking countries. An additional term used in the English-speaking world is the term "queer." Before the 1990s, the term queer was primarily considered a pejorative term and consequently many older sexual minorities have not embraced its recent emergence. The term was actively claimed by the sexual and gender minority activists in the 1990s as a way to take away its power to cause harm. Consequently, many younger people have embraced queer as an identity and descriptive term, which encompasses not just sexual minorities but also people whose gender identity and/or expression does not correspond with their biological sex at birth.[26,27]

Gender Identity

"Gender identity captures whether someone thinks of themselves as male, female, or something else, such as nonbinary."[17] As with the definition of sexual orientation, this definition presents further complications because it utilizes terms that require further definition. The term "gender identity" as well as the terms "male," "female," and "nonbinary" are social constructs whose definitions can be expected to shift over time, to vary across communities, and even vary within small communities defined by geographic location.[28]

A further complication is that gender identity is by definition a self-defined identity. For example, when an individual identifies as "male," their identity is based upon that individual's very personal idea of what "male" is to them. Increasing numbers of individuals are identifying as an "other" gender or as "gender nonbinary."[29] This generally means that the individual does not easily fit within the binary of male or female (as they perceive those constructs) at the moment they are being asked to identify a gender. Many of these individuals express some combination of femininity and masculinity or neither. Consequently, when we group people together who identify as "male," we need to recognize that these "males," while having the same gender identity may have gone through a very different internal process to arrive at that identity. These differences in meanings across individuals can be inconsequential or very significant depending upon how and why gender identity is being assessed.

It should also be noted that all the identities being discussed in this chapter may not only vary over time, but they are also situational meaning that the expression of an identity is contextual.[30] For example, someone may identify as male, female, and/or nonbinary, or even something other than one of these categories, all in the same day depending on the context in which their gender identity is being assessed.

For some individuals their sex assigned at birth may not correspond to their current gender identity. The term "transgender" is often used by researchers and clinicians to describe individuals with such a discordance.[31] The term is also sometimes used by people to describe themselves when their current gender identity and sex assigned at birth do not correspond.[32] These individuals have distinct concerns that need to be examined and addressed.[33]

While some people who fit within the construct of transgender may identify as "transgender," many of these individuals may identify publicly or personally as male *or* female, they may even identify as transgender *and* male, or transgender *and* female. Other terms that are sometimes used as identities are "male to female," commonly abbreviated MTF, or "female to male" commonly abbreviated FTM. These terms are used to denote a transition from an assigned sex at birth to a current gender identity.

The term "cisgender" has been gaining popularity to refer to individuals who are not transgender, that is, individuals whose current gender identity and sex at birth correspond. Various scholars are credited with first using the term cisgender online and in publications in the early to mid-1990s, but the term has been slow to be adopted within public health and other academic communities, as well as the public.[34]

Gender Expression

"Gender expression refers to how people express femininity or masculinity in their appearance, speech, or other behaviors."[17] To understand the concept of gender expression, one needs to also appreciate the constructs of "femininity" and "masculinity," which are constantly shifting over time. These shifts are sometimes rapid, are not uniform across cultures and geographic locations, and can even have noteworthy variations within small communities.[35,36]

Definitions of masculinity and femininity are generally very similar to each other. Femininity refers to qualities usually associated with being a woman, and masculinity is defined as the qualities usually associated with being a man. These definitions are almost always ambiguous about what is meant by the constructs of "woman" or "man" often implying biological sex as the determinant of woman or man status.[37] For public health, it is usually the degree to which a person is perceived by others to be either "masculine" or "feminine," that impacts health outcomes.[38]

It is important to state that a person's internal perception of their masculinity and femininity may not align with others' perceptions of their masculinity and femininity. It is also important to note that masculinity and femininity should not be considered as simple dichotomous constructs.[39] That is, for example, a person is generally not considered as either "masculine" or "not masculine," or "feminine" or "not feminine," but rather some combination of masculinity and femininity.[40]

Most commonly, people perceive masculinity and femininity to be on opposite ends of a bipolar scale. In this conceptualization, to be more masculine, one must be less feminine. As a person moves along the continuum toward masculinity, they depart from femininity.[40] For others, their conceptualization of the constructs of masculinity and femininity are independent of each other. In this instance, a person can be very masculine and very feminine at the same time, or they can be not very masculine and not very feminine simultaneously.[41]

Gender expression is of concern in public health because individuals who do not express their gender in ways that align with their assigned sex at birth may be at risk for discrimination and stigma that can result in negative health outcomes.[42] While, any discordance between gender expression and sex assigned at birth is of concern to sexual and gender minorities (lesbian, gay, bisexual, and transgender people), and has received some attention in these communities, it can also be of importance to sexual and gender majorities (heterosexual or straight, or cisgender people). In fact, because sexual and gender minorities make up such a small percent of the overall population, the discordance between gender expression and assigned sex at birth may be of greater concern (measured by prevalence) to sexual and gender majorities.

The term transgender, which was described above in relationship to its use with gender identity, is also sometimes used to describe individuals whose gender expressions do not match their sex assigned at birth. The term "queer," also described above, is also sometimes used by individuals with any discordance between gender expression and sex at birth. It should be noted that care should be taken in describing someone using these terms, and only done when the terms have been used by the people being described to describe themselves (i.e., as a term of identity), and they have also given permission to use these terms to describe them.

Sex Characteristics

"Sex characteristics refer to biological aspects that relate to sex and are divided into primary and secondary sex characteristics. Primary sex characteristics are those that are present at birth such as chromosomes, gonads, hormones, and outer and inner genitalia. Secondary sex characteristics are those that develop at puberty, such as breasts, facial and pubic hair, the Adam's apple, muscle mass, stature and fat distribution."[17] A person is considered intersex if either they are born with, or during puberty they develop, sex characteristics as described above, that do not align with the typical binary of male or female.

The term intersex is often applied in clinical settings to describe individuals not fitting our common understandings of male and female sex characteristics. This labeling as intersex frequently occurs to very young children and consequently, for many people labeled as intersex, it is not a term of identity. However, for many personal and political reasons some people with such characteristics have begun to publicly identify as "intersex." In many ways, this is similar to the historical adoption of the terms lesbian, gay, bisexual, and transgender.[43] These terms have served many complex and intertwined social and political, as well as very personal purposes.

Another frequent clinical description for intersex people is "disorders of sex development" commonly abbreviated as DSD. This terminology is controversial with many intersex people and their advocates who reject such language because the word "disorder" signifies pathology.[44] All the populations discussed in this chapter have at one time or another been the subject of medical diagnosis and consequently been pathologized.[5] While these clinical diagnoses have arguably allowed for some benefit (e.g., access to mental healthcare, hormones or surgeries) the subjects of these diagnoses have generally rejected such terminology as more harmful than helpful. Consequently, some intersex people and their advocates have replaced the term "disorder" with "difference" describing intersex people as having "differences in sex development" while others have proposed using "variations in sex development."[45,46] In this chapter we will solely use the term intersex which is now more generally understood and accepted then DSD.

One of the primary goals of intersex organizations is preventing unnecessary surgeries on intersex children. Avoiding language that pathologizes intersex people helps with this cause, however, organizations such as InterACT support the autonomy of intersex people to choose the terms they want to use when describing their bodies, and themselves.[47]

Intersex individuals have sometimes been subjected to harmful and unnecessary surgeries and other medical interventions to make their bodies align with society's binary understanding of male or female sex characteristics. The families of these children have often been encouraged by medical professionals to keep this information secret (more than just private) and in many cases not even share the information with the affected child. While intersex organizations support surgeries for children whose lives are in danger, many surgeries are generally unnecessary. These surgeries and interventions frequently result in pain, the loss of sexual function and reproductive capacity, incontinence, and posttraumatic stress disorder among other negative outcomes.[48]

The secrecy of medical professionals and families about intersex conditions has magnified negative health outcomes by supporting internal feelings of shame and stigma. However, perhaps more consequentially, this secrecy prevented the organization and advocacy by intersex people for their own rights. One of the primary rights currently being advocated for is the autonomy of individuals to make their own informed decisions about their own bodies. It was a long-held belief among the medical community that gender was entirely socially constructed, and that a child could easily be raised as either male or female according to family wishes. The medical research that this belief was based upon has now been discredited.[49,50] Further, it is no longer the belief of many that a child has to fit the perfect male–female binary, but rather can freely be some combination of both or neither.[51] There are still many areas in the world where intersex children are abandoned and killed.[52–54]

TAXONOMIES AND MEASURES

Central to understanding the health needs of people based upon SOGIESC categories are the questions and methods used to sort people into categories.[2] This is an inherently fraught process that should be designed to reflect the realities of how people sort themselves into categories in the real world.[30] That is, the taxonomies used to describe sexual orientations, gender identities, gender expressions, and sex characteristics should reflect how people make meaning in their lives. This should be contrasted with efforts by academics or others to construct categories that primarily have meaning externally for those looking in at minority populations.

This process, when done well, involves SOGIESC minority communities in every step from first describing the construct (e.g., sexual orientation or gender identity) to be assessed, to development and testing of measures, testing of methods for collecting data, proper storage of data, proper analysis and interpretation of data, and finally, the reporting and dissemination of findings.[55]

The process of identifying taxonomies and creating measures is obviously a very personal process, as it is with most other demographic characteristic that public health assesses (e.g., race, income). And like many other demographic variables, it is also highly political. For SOGIESC minority communities the collection of data often leads to estimates of population sizes which leads to discussions of importance.[56] Regardless of the sizes of these populations, the collection of SOGIESC data is essential to address the health needs of SOGIESC minorities.

Here we provide an overview of prevailing taxonomies and measures currently in use in public health to study SOGIESC minorities. These taxonomies and measures *need* to constantly evolve as the people and communities they are intended to identify shift and evolve. This evolution should not be used as an excuse to avoid studying SOGIESC minorities by claiming it is too difficult and that perfectly valid measures do not exist. Other demographic categories commonly assessed, such as race, provide similar if not greater challenges.[57]

Sexual Orientation

There have been many attempts to measure sexual orientation in the United States, and hundreds more around the world.[58,59] Persons wanting to assess sexual orientations commonly believe they can create a question or questions on their own to assess this construct.[60] However, like assessing race and ethnicity, researchers should proceed with caution utilizing measures that have been tested for reliability and validity, and field-tested.

One of the most tested questions for assessing sexual orientation in the United States comes from The National Health Interview Survey, which spent several years testing its question in the Questionnaire Design Research Lab of the National Center for Health Statistics at the Centers for Disease Control.[61] The questions resulting from this testing are:

Male respondents are asked:

Which of the following best represents how you think of yourself?

- Gay
- Straight, that is not gay
- Bisexual
- Something else
- I do not know the answer

Female respondents are asked:

Which of the following best represents how you think of yourself?

- Lesbian or gay
- Straight, that is not lesbian or gay
- Bisexual
- Something else
- I do not know the answer

Many important discoveries were made during the testing and development of these questions. For example, many straight or heterosexual people being asked versions of these questions in English had never been asked their sexual orientation, and many did not fully understand what the question was attempting to assess. Many people did not know what the word "heterosexual" meant and some would state that they were "not heterosexual" (confusing it with "homosexual"). The solution was to use the word "straight" rather than heterosexual in the question, however, some heterosexual people were still confused about which category to choose. The investigators found that adding "that is not gay" to clarify the meaning of "straight" increased the validity of the question. For women, the straight/heterosexual response category became "straight, that is not lesbian or gay."

Researchers also found that there was no consistent equivalent to the word "straight" in Spanish-speaking populations in the United States. They found that in the Spanish-language version more valid responses were obtained by keeping the word heterosexual among the response categories.

In the discussion of "sexual orientation" definitions above, we mentioned that sexual orientations can also be assessed using sexual behaviors and sexual attractions. Certain health outcomes commonly investigated in public health are more associated with sexual behaviors such as sexually transmitted infections (STIs) including HIV/AIDS. While other outcomes such as those related to mental health, including depression and suicide attempts, are better assessed using questions assessing sexual attractions. And finally, sexual orientation identity may be more important when examining health outcomes associated with community health such as the adoption of healthy (e.g., condom use by gay men) and unhealthy (e.g., alcohol and other drug use) behaviors.[62]

Researchers have shown that sexual attractions, sexual behaviors, and sexual orientation identity identify overlapping but different populations. For examples of questions on major surveys in the United States assessing sexual attraction, see the National Survey of Family Growth, National Survey on Drug Use and Health, and Population Assessment of Tobacco and Health. Major surveys in the United States using sexual behavior questions to assess sexual orientation are the National Health and Nutrition Examination Survey, National Survey of Family Growth, National Inmate Survey, and in many states the Youth Risk Behavior Survey.[63]

Gender Identity

Most surveys and research projects claim that they assess the construct of "sex," however, most are actually assessing gender identity. This is because "sex" is usually assessed by asking an individual some variation of the question "are you male or female?" Most respondents will accordingly respond by reporting their current gender identity.[64] This simple question provides accurate reports of sex and gender identity for most people whose sex at birth and current gender identity are congruent. However, these questions, by only providing two response categories representing the traditional gender binary, are not adequate for assessing the true diversity of gender identities, or for identifying gender minorities including transgender individuals.[65,66]

A report from the Williams Institute, which brought together experts on gender identity and gender expression, recommends asking two questions to assess gender identity and to determine transgender status (the first question assesses sex assigned at birth, and the second question assesses current gender identity):[67]

What sex were you assigned at birth, on your original birth certificate?

- Male
- Female

How do you describe yourself? (check one)

- Male
- Female
- Transgender
- Do not identify as female, male, or transgender

These questions have only had limited testing or field use and should be subjected to more rigorous examination before widespread adoption.[68] There are numerous variations upon these two questions that are currently being fielded which recognize emerging trends in gender diversity and expression.[69] For example, the University of California added the following questions to all undergraduate applications[70]:

How do you describe yourself? (Mark one answer)

- Male
- Female
- Trans male/Trans man
- Trans female/Trans woman
- Genderqueer/Gender nonconforming
- Different identity

What sex were you assigned at birth, such as on an original birth certificate? (Mark one answer)

- Male
- Female

Simple differences between the Williams Institute and the University of California questions could impact the "accurate" identification of gender minorities. Obvious differences include question ordering and variations in response categories.

The Williams Institute report further recommends using the following question to identify transgender individuals when the two-step process described above cannot be added to a survey.[67] This question is currently in use on the Population Assessment and Tobacco Health Survey, and in numerous states on the Behavioral Risk Factor Surveillance Survey.

> Some people describe themselves as transgender when they experience a different gender identity from their sex at birth. For example, a person born into a male body, but who feels female or lives as a woman. Do you consider yourself to be transgender?
> - Yes, transgender, male to female
> - Yes, transgender, female to male
> - Yes, transgender, gender nonconforming
> - No

These questions, and others currently in the field, provide an opportunity to empirically examine what works for accurately assessing gender diversity.[71] And these explorations will show what value these new questions bring to public health.[72–75] Other major surveys in the United States collecting gender identity data using questions that extend beyond the traditional gender binary include the Health Center Patient Survey, National Adult Tobacco Survey, National Inmate Survey, and National Crime Victimization Survey.

Gender Expression

Taxonomies of gender expression and questions created to reflect these taxonomies, while obviously important for explaining public health outcomes, have rarely been examined in relationship to SOGIESC minority health.[76] Consequently, measures like the Bem Sex-Role Inventory (BSMI), perhaps the most well-known measure of gender expression, are of limited or unknown utility.[77] Further, there is no known (to the authors) surveillance system that currently exists which investigates the relationship between gender expression and health in the United States or elsewhere.

Another challenge with assessing gender expression is that existing measures of gender expression are generally very time and resource intensive. For example, the BSMI has 60 items and other instruments used to measure gender expression such as the Recalled Childhood Gender Identity/Gender Role Questionnaire (23 items), Personal Attitudes Questionnaire (55 items), and the Occupations, Activities, and Traits-Attitudes Measure (75 items) are also too long for routine use.[40,78–80]

The principal public health concern for SOGIESC minorities is the impact of gender nonconformity on health. It is therefore possible to focus the collection of data by limiting the assessment of gender expression to gender nonconformity.[81] A few measures have been developed to specifically identify gender nonconformity. For example, there are the Gender Nonconformity Scale and the Masculine Gender Identity in Female Scale.[82,83] These scales, like the general measures of gender expression described above, are too lengthy for routine use.

To address limitations (including limited validity and reliability testing) of previously developed gender expression measures, and to create a measure that can be used routinely, Wylie et al. produced the following two item tool to assess gender nonconformity.[84]

> A person's appearance, style, or dress may affect the way people think of them. On average, how do you think people would describe your appearance, style or dress?
> - Very feminine
> - Mostly feminine
> - Somewhat feminine
> - Equally feminine and masculine
> - Somewhat masculine
> - Mostly masculine
> - Very masculine
>
> A person's mannerisms (such as the way they walk or talk) may affect the way people think of them. On average how do you think people would describe your mannerisms?
> - Very feminine
> - Mostly feminine
> - Somewhat feminine
> - Equally feminine and masculine
> - Somewhat masculine
> - Mostly masculine
> - Very masculine

This measure, given its recent development by prominent scholars in the field of sex and gender measurement, holds perhaps the most promise of any measure yet advanced. Its primary benefits are its brevity and its focus on identifying gender nonconformity rather than attempting to assess gender expression more broadly.[72] One notable limitation of this measure is, however, that it makes respondents to each question assess masculinity and femininity on a bipolar scale where to be more masculine one has to be less feminine (and vice versa). This does not allow for individuals to simultaneously be very masculine and very feminine (or not very masculine and not very feminine) at the same time.

This bipolarity, which is a trademark of many measures of gender expression (e.g., BSRI), may not reflect the various ways in which gender is expressed.[85] First and foremost, measures should reflect the lived experiences of the people they are created to describe and the traditional binary taxonomy of gender expression, as either feminine or masculine, is not reflective of the world we are living in today. Consequently, important work needs to be conducted examining the measurement of this construct.[86,87]

Sex Characteristics

Public health needs to address the concerns of intersex people who are born with, or during puberty develop, sex characteristics that do not align with the typical male or female binary. Intersex people are often given a specific "diagnosis" and labeled "intersex" by clinicians but also sometimes personally identify as intersex.[88] Consequently, there are two ways of identifying intersex people, diagnosis and/or identity.

Using any of the clinical diagnoses associated with the label "intersex" to identify intersex people is problematic because it promotes the pathologizing of intersex people. Such diagnoses often lead to unnecessary medical interventions upon benign physical variations in sex characteristics.[52]

Intersex organizations such as GATE, which focuses on gender identity, gender expression, and bodily diversity, advocate against the use of the current prevailing terminology, "disorders of sex development," which is used by clinicians and included in the International Classification of Disease 10. Gate prefers "congenital variations of sex characteristics" and is particularly concerned because some of the diagnoses in the ICD 10 "require" treatment.[89] The language change advocated by GATE recognizes that variations in sex characteristics exist and may need to be recognized in clinical settings in some instances; however, the proposed language avoids implying that these variations are "disorders" in need of intervention. Use of the language "differences in sex development also provides alternative nonpathologizing language.

While the use of diagnoses to identify intersex people is highly problematic, the use of various diagnoses in clinical settings is currently the prevailing paradigm for intersex identification and for conducting studies examining the health of intersex people.[90] This is further complicated because, as noted by the Intersex Society of North America (ISNA), it is frequently not a simple diagnosis by a clinician who decides "how small a penis has to be, or how unusual a combination of parts has to be, before it counts as intersex."[88] The ISNA finds that "doctor's opinions about what should count as 'intersex' vary substantially," and they prefer to take the approach of including as intersex "anyone born with what someone believes to be nonstandard sexual anatomy."[88]

As organizations like GATE and ISNA, created in part to advocate for intersex rights, grow and increase in public recognition, intersex people will increase input into the language used to describe themselves. A survey by Johnson et al. of 202 individuals with Androgen Insensitivity Syndrome (AIS) in support groups for people with AIS and their parents, found that only 24% used "disorder of sex development" (DSD) to describe themselves or their children, with most respondents reporting a negative emotional experience related to DSD language. Further, while most (81%) of the respondents had used the specific diagnosis to describe themselves or their children in some setting, most (61%) had also used "Intersex" to describe themselves or their children, and intersex *was the term most preferred* in both clinical settings (55%), and when participating in research studies (67%).[91]

A review by the authors of this chapter of publications using the term "intersex" in PubMed and Google Scholar, from 2014 to 2018, found that the overwhelming majority of articles were case studies of a small number of individuals with similar diagnoses sampled from clinical settings. Few articles sampled outside of clinical settings, such as the Johnson et al. article described above.[16] This is reminiscent of early attempts to study the health of gay men and lesbians who were also sampled at first almost entirely from clinical settings. Samples of gay men and lesbians later came from convenience samples such as gay bars or support groups as was the case in the Johnson et al. study.[16,92] Likewise, the representativeness of samples of intersex people should improve as technologies for identifying and sampling individuals, particularly relatively rare individuals, continues to improve.[93] Until then, the generalizability of findings from case studies is limited.

Finally, it is important to recognize that "intersex" is generally discussed in the literature, in clinical settings, and by some intersex people themselves, as an either or state (e.g., someone is either "intersex" or is "not intersex"). However, as research with intersex people progresses, like with other constructs examined in this chapter, we expect there may not be a simple preferred binary taxonomy. Rather, a taxonomy that allows for more than two distinctions in variations and differences in sex characteristics may arise. In addition, like with the other constructs discussed in this chapter, definitions, measures, and taxonomies of the construct must always strive to reflect the lives of the people they are created to describe.

SOGIESC HEALTH

While the health of SOGIESC minorities has only begun to be examined earnestly in public health, the accumulated knowledge is growing exponentially. Virtually all, if not all, of the health concerns considered within the field of public health are in one way or another relevant to SOGIESC minorities. It is important for everyone working within a public health-related discipline to consider how each SOGIESC minority fits into their work. For example, when studying homelessness or working with homeless populations, it is important to consider what role SOGIESC status may play in creating homelessness and the challenges such status plays in solving the problems of homelessness.

The review here of public health concerns is not comprehensive. Rather, we want this review to highlight the broad range of the public health concerns SOGIESC minorities face. For example, we begin by discussing violence and the complex ways, sometimes unintuitive, that violence impacts the lives of SOGIESC minorities.

In reviewing the literature to the extent possible, we use the language and terminology used in the original publications or reports. For example, if a study is talking about the prevalence of depression among "lesbians," then we report the data here using the term "lesbian." Similarly, if we use the abbreviation LGB, then the research we are discussing explicitly studied lesbians, gays, and bisexuals. If the study also included individuals the authors labeled and discussed as lesbian, gay, bisexual, and transgender, then we would use the acronym LGBT.

Violence

Violence has been framed as a public health issue since at least the early 1990s, with former U.S. Surgeon General C. Everett Koop stating that "the professions of medicine, nursing and the health-related social services must come forward and recognize violence as their issue and one that profoundly affects the public health."[94] Examples of aggressive acts toward sexual and gender minority individuals that are particularly prevalent include intimate partner violence (IPV), anti-LGBTI hate crimes, and bullying.

Intimate Partner Violence. Although studies of IPV in the general population have been frequent in recent decades, relatively few of these have specifically included sexual or gender minorities.[95] Many of the aspects of IPV in heterosexual and SOGIESC minorities may be similar, yet some forms of abuse are specific to sexual and gender minority individuals.[96,97] For example, the threat of being "outed" by a romantic or sexual partner is a unique threat that may be utilized by LGBTI perpetrators of IPV.[97] It is important to develop culturally competent interventions and supports that are not blind to the potential of IPV within these relationships and that take into account the unique challenges that may be present in these cases.

Estimates of rates of IPV for LGBT people vary widely depending on the manner in which IPV and LGBT status are measured in the research study.[95,98,99] While some studies have found that 1% of LGBT individuals reported forced sex perpetration in their current relationships, others have found that more than 97% of LGBT individuals reported any lifetime psychological, physical, or sexual IPV perpetration[100,101]

The National Violence against Women survey found that those with a history of cohabitating with a same-sex partner were more likely to have experienced IPV in their lifetimes compared to those who had only cohabitated with opposite-sex partners.[102] Sexual minority youth have reported higher rates of multiple types of dating violence compared to heterosexual youth, including physical, psychological and cyber dating violence as well as sexual coercion and are more likely to report having experienced abuse overall.[103,104] Transgender individuals may be at greater risk than the general population, as they report experiencing physical abuse in their lifetime at rates similar to or higher than gay and lesbian individuals.[105]

The risk may not be similar across varying subpopulations within the sexual and gender minority umbrella; there is some evidence that bisexual men and women may experience more abuse, particularly regarding the threat of being "outed" by a partner.[104,106] Additionally, girls in same-sex relationships were more likely than boys in same-sex relationships to have experienced IPV compared to their heterosexual counterparts.[107] A similar finding has been found among transgender youth, with female-to-male transgender individuals being more likely to report IPV than male-to-female transgender individuals.[108]

Despite the high prevalence of IPV among sexual and gender minorities, the medical field has been slow to address this issue.[133] Ard and Makadon provide an outline for steps to address IPV among sexual and gender minority patients.[109] Of note, LGB individuals have also been found to report being perpetrators of IPV at higher rates than heterosexuals.[99,103]

Bullying. Bullying has been defined by the Centers for Disease Control and Prevention as "any unwanted aggressive behavior(s) by another youth or group of youths who are not siblings or current dating partners that involves an observed or perceived power imbalance and is repeated multiple times or is highly likely to be repeated."[110] Sexual and gender minority youth have been shown to be more likely to be victims of bullying and peer victimization than heterosexual youth, with over 85% reporting "verbal harassment based on a personal characteristic" such as sexual orientation (70.8%) or gender expression (54.5%) with more than one in five experiencing physical harassment at school.[111–114] The effects of this victimization include negative mental health outcomes as well as academic impacts such as an increased tendency to skip school due to feeling unsafe; additionally, those who report victimization have lower GPAs and less inclination to continue onto postsecondary education.[113–115]

There is evidence that bullying is not uniform among all subpopulations of sexual and gender minorities. Transgender and gender nonconforming youth have been found to be as much as four times as likely to be bullied or harassed in the past year compared to cisgender youth, and bisexual youth are more likely to report being bullied than other sexual minorities.[116,117] Geographical disparities within the United States exist as well; LGBT youth report more bullying in rural areas compared to urban ones and more so in the Midwest and South compared to the Northeast and West.[114] Compounding this finding is rural schools are less likely than urban schools to have supports for sexual and gender minorities, including Gay-Straight Alliance Clubs as well as supportive staff and administrators.[114]

Institutional supports have an impact on the perceived and actual safety of schools for sexual and gender minority youth. Having supportive staff and administrators results in better academic performance and perceived safety among members of this community and those who attend schools with Gay-Straight Alliances or similar student groups are more likely to report a greater sense of belonging and are less likely to report feeling unsafe at schools.[114] Similarly, schools that explicitly include sexual orientation and gender expression in their antibullying policies are associated with a greater number of interventions on the part of staff during anti-LGBTQI bullying incidents and students are more likely to report incidences when they occur.[114]

Despite these demonstrated positive effects, most students attend schools without such supports. It is important for school administrators to continue to implement strategies to prevent peer victimization as part of a comprehensive public health strategy to stop bullying at the institutional level. Parents and clinicians also have a role in preventing bullying and the resulting harms for all youth. Earnshaw et al. outline steps for clinicians providing pediatric care to specifically address LGBT bullying with patients and parents.[118]

Hate Crimes and Hate Violence. The Gay and Lesbian Medical Association (GLMA) has suggested that the "most socially acceptable, and probably the most widespread, form of hate crime…is targeting LGBT people."[99] This statement predates the federal recognition in the United States through the Matthew Shepard Act (2009) that anti-LGBT violence is an official hate crime. Despite the passing of this legislation, bias incidents within the United States against sexual and gender minorities remain a concern, particularly among transgender and gender nonconforming individuals.

The National Coalition of Anti-Violence Programs (NCAVP) reported 77 hate homicides in 2016, including 49 lives lost in the Pulse Nightclub shooting in Orlando. Excluding the mass attack, hate-crime homicides of sexual and gender minorities had increased 17% from the previous year.[119] While homicides are the most extreme example of hate violence, other types of hate-crime events occur, including physical assault, verbal or cyber harassment and threats. The NCAVP report for 2016 describes 1036 sexual and gender minority survivors of hate violence. Of those who reported such events, 58% reported knowing the person who attacked them.[119]

Compounding the frequency of anti-LGBT attacks is the severity of these attacks. Homicides of sexual and gender minorities have been found to be more violent than those which have heterosexual and cisgender victims.[120–123] Further, sexual and gender minority hate crimes victims may be less likely to seek help from law enforcement.[124]

When police are called, police response to anti-LGBT hate violence was not found to be significantly different compared to other violence.[125] Unfortunately, once police arrive, victims may experience further discrimination. The NCAVP study found that 35% of survivors reported that police were indifferent to the incident and 31% were hostile.[119] Black sexual and gender minority survivors of hate violence were more likely to report that they experienced police misconduct, causing victims of violence to perceive police to be unwilling to help, possibly contributing to underreporting of violence by sexual and gender minorities.[119,126]

Cancer

Statistics on cancer among SOGIESC minorities are not routinely collected and there are no large-scale prospective studies of cancer incidence or mortality in these populations.[127,128] However, there is some evidence of increased cancer risk among some SOGIESC minorities. Elevated levels of cancer prevalence are likely at least partially determined by the fact that SOGIESC minorities have demonstrated disparities related to cancer risks.

While Boehmer et al. found no significant differences in overall cancer prevalence between heterosexual and sexual minority women, another study found that bisexual women were more likely to receive a cancer diagnosis than heterosexual women.[129] Both studies found that gay men had significantly higher cancer prevalence than heterosexual or bisexual men.[129,130] Most striking, however, is recent evidence that the disparities in cancer among SOGIESC minorities may widen with age.[129] Below we describe evidence regarding few specific types of cancers.

HIV/AIDS- and HPV-related Cancers. While there are several HIV-related cancers, including Kaposi's sarcoma and non-Hodgkin's lymphoma, an important cancer that affects HIV-positive SOGIESC minorities is anal cancer. HIV-positive men who have sex with men (MSM) are particularly impacted by this disease. Overall, incidence of anal cancer among men who have sex with men who are HIV-positive is estimated to be as much as 80 times higher than men in the general population, a disparity that has seemingly widened since the development of antiretroviral therapy, possibly due to the fact that people are living longer with HIV.[131–134] Among gay men, the rate of anal cancer is 5.1 out of 100,000 for those who are not HIV positive, while, it is 49.5 out of 100,000 for those who are HIV positive.[135] While serostatus accounts for much of the disparity, it cannot account for all of it, as HIV-infected MSM have higher rates of anal cancer than HIV-infected other men and women.[131]

Human papilloma virus (HPV) is also associated with anal cancer, but it is more commonly associated with cervical cancer.[136] Bisexual women are more likely than other women to report a cervical cancer diagnoses and HPV-related cancers are estimated to be more prevalent among transgender individuals than in the general population.[130,137,138] A large number of female-to-male transgender individuals retain their cervixes, necessitating the need for gynecological healthcare. However, this population is less likely to undergo routine cervical cancer screening than cisgender women, potentially delaying necessary treatment and contributing to disparities in health outcomes.[139]

Breast Cancer. SOGIESC minorities have several risk factors related to breast cancer. Evidence regarding incidence of breast cancer among these groups has yet to be collected and examined in ways that can accurately estimate true rates.[140]

Lesbians have higher prevalence of multiple risk factors for breast cancer, including nulliparity, smoking, obesity, and alcohol consumption.[141,142] Despite these disparities, since no cancer registries collect sexual orientation data, it is unclear whether lesbians have a higher incidence of breast cancer than other women.[143] Sexual minority women may, however, experience greater rates of mortality from breast cancer.[144] Perhaps contributing to mortality is that sexual minority women report significantly lower levels of "intentions to participate" in breast cancer screenings compared to heterosexual women[145]; therefore, these women's cancers may progress to a more serious stage with greater risk of death. It has been found that low levels of provider trust, less perceived risk of breast cancer, and negative beliefs about mammography mediated the relationship between sexual orientation and screening intentions.[145] Interventions that specifically address these concerns may increase screening rates and contribute to more sexual minority women surviving the disease.

Transwomen may also have unique risk factors for breast cancer. Exogenous estrogen has been found to be associated with breast cancer in cisgender males and may reflect a risk for transwomen who are undergoing hormone therapy.[146] Progesterone, another possible component in hormone therapy for transwomen, has also been associated with breast cancer risk in postmenopausal women.[147] However, in a cohort study of both male-to-female and female-to-male transgender veterans who had undergone cross-hormone treatment, no differences in breast cancer incidence were found compared to that of the general population.[148] Additional studies are needed to better define breast cancer risk in SOGEISC populations.

Colorectal Cancer. Gay and bisexual men are more likely to receive colorectal cancer screenings than men in the general population.[149] A few reasons that are hypothesized for this difference is that colorectal screenings can be used to diagnose HIV-related malignancies, for which sexual minority men are at greater risk.[149] While heterosexual and sexual minority women have not been found to differ significantly in regards to colorectal screening, more research on how this disease impacts sexual minority women is needed.[150] Among transgender populations, transmen have been shown to have higher odds of sigmoidoscopy/colonoscopy within their lifetime compared to cisgender men and women, while transwomen have been found to have lower odds of up-to-date colorectal cancer screenings.[151]

Prostate Cancer. Although the utility of PSA screening has been a topic of debate, gay and bisexual men have been found to be less likely to receive prostate-specific antigen (PSA) screening for prostate cancer compared to heterosexual men. Black gay and bisexual men have also been found to be less likely to be up-to-date with this test.[149] Findings on actual prostate cancer incidence in sexual minority men have been mixed, however. While one study found no link between sexual orientation identity, anal sex, or history of male partners and prostate cancer risk, others have found that men with frequent or any male partners may be slightly more likely to develop the disease.[152–154]

Transwomen have been found to be more likely to have up-to-date PSA screenings than cisgender men.[151] Gender nonconforming individuals, however, had lower odds of discussing this test with their healthcare provider than cisgender men.[151]

Skin Cancer. Skin cancer incidence has been increasing, particularly nonmelanoma skin cancer.[155] Differences in rates of indoor tanning among SOGIESC minorities have likely contributed to disparities in the rates of skin cancer among various groups. Sexual minority men have been demonstrated to have more twice the risk of reported history of both nonmelanoma skin cancer and melanoma compared to heterosexual men, even after controlling for immunosuppressive conditions such as HIV.[156] Sexual minority women, on the other hand, had half the likelihood of reporting a history of nonmelanoma skin cancer than their heterosexual counterparts.[156] Within this same study, sexual minority men reported much higher rates of indoor tanning compared to heterosexual men, while sexual minority women reported lower rates of this activity compared to heterosexual women.[156] Targeted interventions that address the risks of indoor tanning and the seriousness of various skin cancers for sexual minority men may be warranted to reduce the incidence of this particular disease.

Access to Healthcare and Service Utilization

While access to healthcare encompasses several facets, it has been perhaps most succinctly defined as "the timely use of personal health service to achieve the best possible health outcomes."[157] Structural, personal, and financial factors that extend beyond the simple availability of providers and services may contribute to disparities in access to healthcare.[157] The Office of Disease Prevention and Health Promotion identifies three access-related factors: insurance coverage, utilization of health services, and timeliness of care.[158] While each of these factors may influence SOGIESC minorities' access to healthcare, other factors such as perceived or actual provider stigma and discrimination may influence the timeliness of utilization as well.

Insurance Coverage. Multiple researchers have demonstrated that SOGIESC minorities have reduced likelihood of having health insurance, which is likely to have health implications for utilizing care.[159–161] In a national sample, it was found that female respondents in same-sex relationships were less likely than women in opposite-sex relationships to have health insurance coverage and had 85% increased odds of forgoing medical care due to cost.[161] While this same study found that men in same-sex relationships were less likely than men in opposite-sex relations to have insurance coverage, men in same-sex were equally as likely as men in opposite-sex relationships to have unmet medical needs due to financial issues.[161] In more recent years, significant policy changes within the United States have occurred relating to health insurance coverage for SOGIESC minorities, specifically, the Affordable Care Act (ACA) and same-sex marriage.[162]

Multiple explorations of the effects of the ACA's impact on insurance coverage suggest that it has assisted in reducing the disparities faced by SOGIESC minority communities.[163–165] In the first year of open enrollment of the ACA, the rate of LGBT people with incomes less than 400% of the national poverty level who were uninsured dropped 24%—from one in three in 2013 to one in four in 2014.[164,165] Despite this decline, however, a disproportionate number of LGBT individuals remain without insurance compared to the general population, particularly transgender and gender nonconforming people and people of color.[164,166–168] A reason for this continued disparity may relate to employers' willingness to provide health insurance for SOGIESC minority individuals and couples or for services related to one's SOGIESC status, such as in the case of transition-related care. For those transgender people that do have insurance, however, more is being covered under the ACA. While there have been legal challenges to Health and Human Services' 2016 clarification of the ACA's ban on discrimination based on sex as encompassing gender identity, more and more employers have been offering coverage for these services[169]; in 2017, 79% of the businesses rated by the Human Rights Campaign provided at least one firm-wide insurance plan with transgender-inclusive health coverage with an increase of 103 businesses from the previous year.[170]

While the ACA has supported transgender individuals having coverage for more aspects of their necessary care, same-sex marriage has furthered progress for other individuals within the SOGIESC minority umbrella. Prior to the legalization of same-sex marriage within the United States, it had been shown that partnered SOGIESC minority couples had been less likely to have obtained employer-sponsored health insurance for their same-sex partners.[160,171] The Supreme Court rulings of *Windsor* and *Obergefell* are considered to have increased accessibility to health insurance coverage for same-sex spouses.[162] Following these rulings, federal and state employees who have a spouse of the same sex are guaranteed the same benefits afforded to those in different-sex marriages, although other employers are not required to provide equal benefits if their state or locality does not have additional protections specifically for same-sex couples.[162] While many small employers do not offer insurance coverage for same-sex spouses, one survey found that 93% of employers with 200 or more employees do; since 71% of workers in the United States work for large firms, it appears that more Americans have access to this benefit than do not.[172]

Health Services Utilization. Healthcare utilization has been demonstrated to be a gendered behavior, with cisgender women in the general population being more likely to utilize healthcare services than cisgender men.[173–175] However, sexual orientation may mediate this relationship between accessing healthcare and gender or sex, as sexual minority women have been found to access healthcare less than heterosexual women. This difference is not found among men.[173] Overall, SOGIESC minorities have been found to have lower rates of primary-care utilization, have a lower likelihood of having a usual source of care, and be more likely to report delaying accessing healthcare when it is needed compared to the general population.[160,166]

Perceived or actual stigma or discrimination is one reason that SOGIESC minorities may delay or avoid healthcare. Anticipated, internalized, and enacted stigma scores are negatively correlated with utilization of health services among rural LGBT individuals.[174] While a sample of gay, lesbian, and bisexual veterans was found to utilize services as often as those in the general population, 25% reported avoiding at least one service within the Veterans Health Care Administration because of possible stigma.[176] Another study found that 28% of transgender respondents reported delaying necessary care.[177] This delay cannot be solely contributed to lack of insurance. Despite over 85% of transgender individuals in another sample having health insurance, 31.1% of the sample reported delaying necessary care because they were fearful of discrimination.[178] This delay in care due to fears related to discrimination is associated with poorer physical and mental health.[178]

For those who do choose to access services, many studies suggest that it is not guaranteed that SOGIESC individuals will feel comfortable in disclosing their sexual or gender minority status to their physical or mental healthcare provider for fear of discrimination.[179] Multiple factors, such as race and gender of LGB patients and the gender of one's healthcare provider, have been found to be associated with the likelihood of sexual orientation disclosure.[180] Additionally, the type of provider matters; among cancer patients, 73% had disclosed their LGBT identity to their primary-care physician, while only 47% had disclosed to their surgeons.[181]

Of those who disclose, many do so to correct the provider's heterosexual assumptions, however, suggesting that more cultural competency training that includes the importance of checking one's perceptions of a client's sexual or gender identity is needed.[181,182] In addition to wanting providers to be more educated prior to collecting SO/GI information, transgender patients have suggested that having LGBT-friendly service environments would increase willingness to disclose their sexual orientation or gender identity, although they believed that gender identity would be more important for a provider to know than their sexual orientation.[183]

The fear of discrimination and stigma may be somewhat warranted as it has been demonstrated that healthcare providers have explicit and implicit preferences for those in their own sexual orientation identity group.[184] One national survey found that 19% of transgender clients reported being refused care by a provider.[177] In an exploration of provider attitudes, it was found that providers have more of an attitude of tolerance than acceptance of their LGBT patients, although more recent studies suggest that more providers feel comfortable in serving SOGIESC patients, perhaps related to increasingly more accepting societal attitudes toward these populations.[185–187]

Indeed, a review of nursing students' attitudes over time seems to have shifted in a more positive-leaning direction, although 50% of studies still reported negative views.[188] However, several authors found that providers acknowledge needing more training in sexual and gender minority health topics, as SOGIESC cultural competency training in clinical education has been found to be effective in fostering more positive attitudes toward SOGIESC patients among providers.[186,189,190]

SOGIESC Specific Community Health Centers. One of the strategies that has emerged from with within the SOGIESC community is the development of healthcare centers specifically serving sexual and gender minorities. Within the United States, 63 LGBT community centers provide at least some direct health services, including mental health services, serving hundreds of thousands of people in 2013 alone.[191]

Many of the LGBT community health centers in the United States are clustered on both the East and West coasts and generally align with where same-sex households are more common. Thirteen states have no LGBT community health centers, many of these states located within the center of the country.[192] The development of more health services specifically serving SOGIESC minorities may support greater utilization of services among people within these communities and reduce the need for individuals to delay care due to feelings of shame or fear.

Mental and Behavioral Health

In addition to physical health disparities, SOGIESC minority individuals have been shown to have poorer mental health outcomes compared to the general population in samples from various countries and in multiple age groups.[193–202] Much of these disparities are thought to be the result of minority stress.[198,203–205] Mental health, while an adverse health outcome itself, is also related to chronic disease.[206] Therefore, the prevention and treatment of these types of disorders are important for ensuring productive and healthy lives among SOGIESC minority groups.

Mood and Anxiety Disorders. Meta-analyses of studies relating to sexual minority youth and adults demonstrate a higher likelihood of having a mood disorder such as depression in these groups.[199,204,207] For example, one such review showed sexual minority men and women as being between two and three times as likely as heterosexuals to experience a mood disorder.[204] More recent studies have provided additional evidence for this increased risk, particularly among bisexuals.[208]

While less research has been conducted among older adults, existing studies reveal high rates of depression in sexual and gender minority samples. One large study found that 31% of older LGBT individuals reported current depression.[209] A study focusing on gay men over the age of 50 found a similar finding, with 30% self-reported as being depressed.[210]

Depression is particularly prevalent among transgender adults, with prevalences as high as 50% in some samples.[211–213] Rates of anxiety are also higher than those in the general population at over 40% for both transgender men and women.[212]

Suicidality and Self-Harming Behavior. Self-harming behavior is common among those who are gender minorities, particularly youth. Almost 75% of 14- to 18-year-old transgender boys/men and nonbinary youth in one Canadian sample reported self-harming at least once in the past year and half of the transgender girls/women reported doing so.[214] Among transgender adults in the United Kingdom, 36.8% expressed ever engaging in self-harm.[215] While suicide rates may be higher in those who engage in self-harm than the general population, not all people who do so have suicidal intent and give a variety of reasons for engaging in such behavior.[216,217]

Sexual orientation has also been linked to suicidality among sexual minority youth, with studies finding an average of 28% of sexual minorities reporting a history of suicidality compared to 12% of heterosexuals, with bisexuals being the most at risk.[199] The disparity between sexual minority and heterosexual youth appears to widen as the severity of the suicidal behavior increased; for example, while sexual minority youth are estimated to have approximately two times higher odds of reporting suicidal ideation, suicide attempts had three times higher odds of being reported in sexual minority youth, and attempts necessitating medical attention had an odds ratio of 4.17.[199] As suicidal ideation is found to be more likely among those who have a history of victimization, addressing interpersonal violence is a key aspect of reducing mental health disparities among young people.[202,218]

Some subgroups within the SOGIESC minority umbrella experience suicidality at greater rates. Although LGB people of color have been found to have a similar rate of mental disorders as WHITE LGB people, the rate of serious suicide attempts may be higher among Black and Latinx LGB individuals.[219] Gender minority individuals are also much more likely than the general population to report a lifetime suicide attempt, with rates between 30% and 60% depending on subgroups within this population.[220] Among a sample of older transgender women (ages 40–59), 28% reported a past suicide attempt and 53% had experienced suicidal ideation.[211] While little research has been done with intersex individuals within this area, one pilot study found that a sample of those with DSD had rates of self-harming behavior and suicidality higher than the general population.[221]

Because of limitations of current procedures in identifying the sexual orientation or gender identity of those who have died as a result of suicide, recommendations have been made by the Working Group for Postmortem Identification of SO/GI that may enable further surveillance that can better support and assess suicide prevention efforts for these groups.[222]

Substance Use and Misuse. High rates of substance use and abuse have been observed in SOGIESC minorities; however, different substances are used in different rates by various subgroups. While there is some evidence that alcohol disparities are faced by sexual minority women in the United States,[223] the use of other drugs is more prevalent among sexual minority men,[224] although a more recent study in an Australian sample suggests the use of other drugs may be more common among sexual minority women than in heterosexual women as well.[225] There is some evidence that stigma and discrimination mediates this relationship. One study in the United States found that LGB individuals who reported experience all of three types of discrimination—race, gender, and sexual orientation—had four times greater odds of past-year substance use disorders than those who did not experience any discrimination.[226] High rates of use may place sexual minority individuals at greater risk for disease and injury than their heterosexual peers, furthering disparities in other aspects of public health.

There are multiple findings that suggest that sexual minority women are more likely to engage in heavy drinking than heterosexuals and sexual minority girls are more likely to engage in risky drinking than boys, although this may not be consistent across the globe.[227–229] Within the United States, lesbians and bisexual women have been found to be less likely to abstain from drinking alcohol and have a greater likelihood of reporting dependency or past help-seeking for their drinking.[230] In an Australian sample, "mainly heterosexual" women were more likely than "exclusively heterosexuals" to report at-risk drinking.[231] However, one international study found that it was only in North America that women of different sexual orientations drank differently.[232]

An 2001 study within the United States found that men who have sex with men were more likely than single men in the general population to use stimulants, tranquilizers, hallucinogens, sedatives, and "poppers." Homosexually experienced men were found to be more likely to use cocaine and marijuana daily compared to heterosexual men, although this is not indicative that they have a dependence on either substance.[224,233] While there is a relative lack of research related to transgender people relating to substance abuse, some studies that exist demonstrate that rates of use and of self-reported past treatment for substance use are high among transgender women and that heavy-frequent alcohol use is lower.[234,235] However, much more research is necessary to determine trends among different identities within gender minority population.

Eating Disorders. Eating disorders, such as anorexia nervosa, bulimia nervosa, and binge eating disorder, as well as eating disorders not otherwise specified (EDNOS), have decreased in recent years but remain more common among some subgroups of SOGIESC minorities within the United States.[236] There are a range of symptoms that may be present within these disorders, many of which have been demonstrated to be more prevalent among SOGIESC minorities. One recent meta-analysis demonstrated that sexual minorities overall have a higher likelihood of all eating disorder symptoms.[237] While research is rather limited in terms of actual eating disorder diagnoses by SOGIESC minority status, one study found that sexual minority men and women, as well as men and women unsure of their sexual orientation, had elevated rates of past year eating disorder diagnosis or treatment compared to heterosexuals.[238] Transgender individuals have significantly higher rates of diagnosis than either cisgender heterosexuals or sexual minorities.[238] While the disparities between heterosexual and sexual minority males remained similar from 1999 to 2013, sexual orientation disparities in the use of diet pills, fasting, and purging have widened among females.[236] Exploration as to why disparities are getting worse for some groups and better for others will be critical to address the potentially physically damaging consequences of this mental disorder.

When looking at differences in gender within sexual minority groups in terms of behavior and body dissatisfaction, gay and bisexual men may have a higher prevalence of eating disorders than heterosexual men.[239] Gay men also report significantly more body dissatisfaction than heterosexuals, particularly among those who are affiliated with the gay community.[240] However, lesbians and bisexual women are not found to be more likely to develop eating disorders than heterosexual women although there have been mixed results about sexual minority women and body satisfaction.[239–241]

Within a UK sample of adolescents, sexual minority youth had greater risk for eating disorder symptoms, with sexual minority girls having over twice the odds of binge eating and purging than heterosexual girls when measured at the age of 16 and gay and bisexual boys having 12.5 times the odds of binge eating compared to heterosexual boys.[242]

Reproductive and Sexual Healthcare

Much of the research examining the health disparities facing SOGIESC minorities has focused on STIs, including HIV/AIDS, particularly among men who have sex with men, a focus that is also reflected among research funding from the National Institutes of Health.[243–246] Indeed, HIV/AIDS and other STIs remain a concern for some subpopulations. For example, HIV infections among young MSM of color continue to increase within the United States and it is estimated that transgender people are 49 times more likely to be living with HIV than adults in the general worldwide population.[247–249]

In addition to HIV and other STIs, health screenings related to reproductive health and access to assisted reproductive therapy treatments are important emerging challenges for SOGIESC minorities, particularly as family structures and visibility may change with increasing acceptance of sexual and gender minority identities.

Reproductive Health Screenings. U.S. lesbians are less likely to engage in Papanicolaou (Pap) test screening than heterosexual women.[250] However, one study found that bisexual women are more likely to have a gynecological exam and to do a breast self-examination compared to both heterosexual and lesbian women, suggesting that not all sexual minority women have the same barriers to keeping up-to-date with recommended screenings.[251] Similarly, bisexual African American women living in the U.S. South were more likely to have received a Pap test within the last 3 years than lesbian women.[252]

Female-to-male (FTM) transgender individuals often retain some of their reproductive organs.[253] For FTM patients, a six times higher likelihood of receiving an inadequate Papanicolaou (Pap) test result was found compared to cisgender female patients after accounting for demographic characteristics and time on testosterone. Testosterone use and provider discomfort are thought to at least partially explain why transgender men have this higher likelihood of inadequate results. Additionally, FTM patients are more likely to have multiple inadequate tests and wait as much as five times longer to return for subsequent tests.[254] Indeed, less than one-third of OB/GYNs report being comfortable caring for transmasculine patients, with 11% refusing to perform Pap tests on female-to-male patients.[255]

Pregnancy and Assisted Reproductive Therapies. Many SOGIESC minority individuals and couples have a desire or intention to become parents. In a nationally representative sample within the United States, bisexual women have been found to be more likely to express parenting desires than lesbians, although both groups were less likely to express this desire compared to heterosexual women; among men, whether one's most recent partner was male or female had an impact on expressing desires to parent without having the intention to become one.[256] Within the context of reproductive healthcare as it relates to assisted reproductive therapy and creating biological families, SOGIESC minorities may experience unique challenges compared to cisgender heterosexual individuals.

As recently as 2013 and 2015, the American Society of Reproductive Medicine published committee opinions on SOGIESC minority use of fertility care, stating that there was no sound ethical basis for inequality of treatment related to sexual orientation or gender identity.[257,258] Despite this, not all fertility clinics may be inclusive and welcoming to SOGIESC families. Barriers to care that have been noted from qualitative and quantitative research with sexual minority women seeking or having sought assisted reproductive therapies include unwelcoming fertility clinic staff, fear of provider homophobia, standard clinic forms that are not appropriate for those who are lesbian or bisexual, high cost of obtaining semen and limited donor selections, and legal barriers.[259–261] More research is needed for other SOGIESC minority populations, particularly gay and bisexual men, transgender women, and intersex individuals.

It had previously been assumed that infertility coincided with many DSD conditions; gonadectomy is sometimes performed due to increased risk of germ cell cancers.[262,263] However, recent advances in assisted reproductive therapies have allowed some successes related to harvesting sperm or carrying a pregnancy among those with DSD.[263,264] Others have found promising levels in germ cells in the gonads of those with DSD, particularly at younger ages.[265] Consideration of some ethical challenges (e.g., gonadectomy in general and the preservation of gametes in very young children for future use) are recommended to ensure that the autonomy of such individuals is preserved and that the potential for health and well-being is maximized.[262,263] Additionally, more research is necessary related to the risks associated with removal of the gonads, hormone usage, and fertility treatment outcomes among these individuals at various ages so that DSD children and parents can make the most informed decisions possible.[266]

Pregnancy of and reproductive health services for transgender men have become more prominent in recent scientific literature. Transgender men often have a desire to have children and have the capacity to become pregnant through cryopreservation of gametes.[267,268] However, transition-related procedures and therapies impact fertility either permanently or temporarily. Transgender men who undergo hormone replacement therapy in the form of testosterone may have specific fertility challenges, as it induces amenorrhea, although some do become pregnant even during times that amenorrhea is present.[268,269]

Public opinion is fairly supportive of reproductive options for transgender individuals, with over three-fourths of survey respondents agreeing that "Doctors should be able to help transgender people have biological children."[270] Despite general support of helping trans people parent, only 60% of people reported support for physicians helping transgender men in carrying pregnancies and there was about the same percentage of support for physicians helping transgender minors engage in cryopreservation of gametes before transition.[270] While quantitative support is lacking, qualitative findings suggest that those who proceed to become pregnant may experience psychological challenges and stigma as a male-presenting or gender nonconforming person carrying a baby, such as loneliness and tensions related to their own identity.[271]

Despite the public support of transgender individuals having biological children, physicians may not know how to support or may be personally opposed to trans people doing so. Qualitative findings suggest that many transgender people have negative encounters accessing assisted reproductive services.[272] In response to this negativity, some report advocating for themselves, while others avoid confrontation for fear of being refused services.[272] Another issue pertains to access to contraceptive services. One study found that a majority of the transgender men who were having sex that could result in pregnancy but wanted to avoid becoming pregnant were not using highly effective contraceptive methods or were not using contraception at all.[273] Another cross-sectional survey found that 24% of the pregnancies among testosterone-using transgender men were unplanned.[274]

Various recommendations have been put forth as the result of qualitative and quantitative research with SOGIESC minorities. Recommendations for working with transgender clients include having inclusive forms in which patients can indicate preferred names and pronouns, for providers to use gender-neutral language when working with prospective gender minority patients, and including materials with trans-related content within clinic waiting rooms.[272] Ross et al. proposed ten recommendations following focus groups with their lesbian and bisexual women participants. Examples of these include inviting all parties desired by the patients (including sperm donors or coparents) in the insemination process, minimizing and making consistent the costs related to insemination, providing cues that the provider is welcoming of sexual minority couples, and working toward a universal standard of care across geographic regions, including increasing access for those living outside of rural areas.[259]

Bodily Integrity

The right of autonomy and self-determination over their own bodies, commonly referred to as "bodily integrity," is of particular concern to SOGIESC minorities.[275] Sexual minorities have in many cases been subjected to unwanted and damaging physical interventions (e.g., castration, clitorectomy, lobotomy, drugs), while gender minorities have been denied access to interventions to physically align their sex at birth with their current gender identity.[5,276,277] All of these concerns with bodily integrity are extraordinarily important, but perhaps the most unrecognized concerns are those currently being voiced by intersex people and organizations advocating for intersex rights.

In October 2016, multiple UN Treaty Bodies, Special Rapporteurs on health, torture and violence against women, the Office of the High Commissioner for Human Rights, African Commission on Human and Peoples' Rights, Council of Europe, Office of the Commissioner for Human Rights, Inter-American Commission on Human Rights issued a joint statement condemning human rights violations, a particular concern to intersex people as well as their friends and family[278]:

In countries around the world, intersex infants, children and adolescents are subjected to medically unnecessary surgeries, hormonal treatments and other procedures in an attempt to forcibly change their appearance to be in line with societal expectations about female and male bodies. When, as is frequently the case, these procedures are performed without the full, free, and informed consent of the person concerned, they amount to violations of fundamental human rights.

Parents of children with intersex traits often face pressure to agree to such surgeries or treatments on their children. They are rarely informed about alternatives or about the potential negative consequences of the procedures, which are routinely performed despite a lack of medical indication, necessity, or urgency. The rationale for these is frequently based on social prejudice, stigma associated with intersex bodies, and administrative requirements to assign sex at the moment of birth registration.[278]

The AIS-DSD (Androgen Insensitivity Syndrome—Differences of Sex Development) Support Group is an organization for intersex people (including people with any differences of sex development in addition to those with Androgen Insensitivity Syndrome) and their families.[279] The AIS-DSD advocates for a number of important issues which directly and indirectly facilitate bodily integrity including the complete disclosure of medical information to parents of intersex children; the need for research into the many variations of intersex; support for families and intersex children; and the adoption of specific standards of care for intersex children which consider and protect bodily integrity.[280]

Care must be taken when suggesting any intervention that impacts the bodily integrity of a SOGIESC minority, particularly given the history of atrocities against their bodies. Issues related to bodily integrity and medicine, and public health, and ethics are complex and deserve their own chapter. Any review of the topic of bodily integrity, however, should be led by the voices of those whose bodies are most threatened, which includes many SOGIESC minorities.

SOGIESC HEALTH PROMOTION

While there are many health concerns faced by SOGIESC minorities, there has been an outpouring of efforts to address these concerns. Many of these efforts have come from within SOGIESC minority communities, but increasingly government and large nonprofit agencies are becoming involved. Here we provide a brief introduction to a small sample of these efforts chosen to illustrate the diversity of efforts ranging community-driven (Fenway Health and Trevor Project) to governmental (The Sexual and Gender Minority Research Office of the National Institutes of Health), to large nonprofit organizations (Truth Initiative) to international initiatives (Outright Action International).

Fenway Health

Fenway Health was established in Boston, Massachusetts in the early 1970s under the belief that access to healthcare is not a privilege, but a right.[281] While initially broad in its mission to serve the local community, the organization revised its mission in 1986 to demonstrate its emphasis on providing services to gays and lesbians; it has since expanded yet again to be inclusive of all LGBT individuals.[281] In fiscal year 2018, Fenway Health saw 32,000 patients in its medical, behavioral, dental, and vision services and its helpline for LGBT youth received 2750 calls.[282] It has a wide range of other programs, including addiction recovery, alternative insemination, violence recovery, and pharmacy/medication assistance, reflecting the diverse needs of the local LGBT community.[282]

In addition to providing direct services, Fenway Health also dedicates resources to research and trainings related to providing culturally competent care through its Fenway Institute.[283] Founded in 2001, the Fenway Institute has become a leader in LGBT health and HIV research, advancing knowledge about these topics that inform and influence care to patients beyond those who walk through its doors.[283]

Fenway continues to evolve with the needs of the LGBT community and with medical and public health practice standards, joining forces with other related organizations and having received Patient-Centered Medical Home PRIME Certification in 2016.[282] Its multidisciplinary model, providing comprehensive care to SOGIESC minority individuals, serves as an example to other community health centers seeking to specifically support the health and well-being of these groups.

Truth Initiative

Truth Initiative, formerly known as the American Legacy Foundation, was established in 1999 following the 1998 Master Settlement Agreement related to U.S. tobacco companies, becoming the first national public health organization within the United States dedicated to tobacco control.[284] It is commonly known for its "truth" television ads aimed highlighting facts about tobacco, although this is only part of what the organization does. In addition, Truth Initiative engages in research, youth and community development and empowerment, and the development of digital innovations related to smoking cessation.[284]

As early as 2001, the American Legacy Foundation specifically sought to target tobacco use and its effects within underserved populations, including LGBT communities, through its Priority Populations Initiatives that addressed both smoking prevention and cessation.[284] LGBT populations were selected not only because of the elevated rates of smoking within these communities, but also because of the tobacco industry's history in targeting them through its advertising.[285,286]

Currently, it is unclear whether Truth Initiative's campaigns are effective within SOGIESC communities. Awareness of antitobacco messages in LGBT newspapers was somewhat low in one sample, although this did not specifically ask about Truth campaigns.[287] However, this study also found that current smokers were three times as likely to report seeing antitobacco messages, which suggests that these types of media messages are at least viewed by one population that Truth Initiative may be trying to reach.[287] Holding positive opinions about the "truth" brand was negatively associated with being a smoker and positively associated with quitting intentions among current smokers.[288] Using these findings, the "truth" brand has been estimated to prevent more than 300,000 youth and young adults from smoking in the course of a year.[288] Given the disproportionately high rate of smoking among LGBTQ youth, it is critical to ensure that these messages are seen and liked by this population in order to continue to get the teen smoking rate to zero, as the organization hopes to accomplish.[284]

In 2017, Truth Initiative partnered with the Human Rights Campaign Foundation and the University of Connecticut to launch a comprehensive survey among 8000 LGBTQ youth about smoking, which should continue to shed light on the work that continues to be ahead for these activities.[289]

The Trevor Project

The Trevor Project, an example of a national nonprofit within the United States, is a leader in addressing crisis intervention and suicide prevention for SOGIESC minorities ages 13–24. The organization operates with three strategies—crisis services, life-affirming resources, education, and advocacy—all designed to reduce the incidence of suicide within the SOGIESC youth community. Programs include a telephone lifeline, an online social networking platform, the facilitation of educational workshops, and advocacy to implement policies, as well as other initiatives in support of the various strategies. The services to youth in crisis are virtual via the Internet or telephone; however, cities in various regions of the United States coordinate groups of volunteers to support outreach and fundraising for the various programs. In addition to these activities, the Trevor Project supports research efforts that align with its mission.[290]

Preliminary data suggest that The Trevor Project's services are effective. Over half of youth surveyed who contacted the organization with medium or high-level suicide risk de-escalated to a lower level of risk in the time that they were in contact with one of the counselors.[291] While the effectiveness data are preliminary, the sheer number of crisis contacts also suggests the need for a SOGIESC-specific crisis service. In its 2015 annual report, the organization reported answering over 54,000 calls, texts, and chats, an overall 6.41% increase in crisis contacts over the previous.[292] Of greater concern is that 26% of youth surveyed after using these services reported that they would not have used a different crisis hotline if The Trevor Project did not exist.[291] That some SOGIESC youth are unwilling to utilize other resources may demonstrate mistrust that one's sexual orientation or gender identity may not be affirmed or understood in these more mainstream options.

The Sexual and Gender Minority Research Office of the National Institutes of Health

Within the United States, an example of the federal government's response to SOGIESC minority health disparities lies within the National Institutes of Health (NIH). Part of the Department of Health and Human Services, NIH is the largest funder of biomedical research in the world, and is comprised of 27 institutes and centers as well as the Office of the Director.[293,294] Established in 2015, the Sexual and Gender Minority Research Office (SGMRO) sits within the NIH Division of Program Coordination, Planning, and Strategic Initiatives.[295]

Outlined in its 2016–20 strategic plan are four goals: (1) to expand what is known about sexual and gender minority health through research supported by NIH, (2) to remove barriers to planning, conducting, and reporting of research relevant to these topics, (3) to support the community of researchers who conduct relevant research, and (4) to evaluate progress related to the advancement of SOGIESC minority research.[296,297] Progress toward these goals is published yearly.

Supporting the work of the SGMRO is the SGM Research Coordinating Committee (formerly the LGBT Research Coordinating Committee). Those involved in this committee develop strategies for a research agenda that furthers understanding of disparities and effective interventions related to these groups. Guidance for this strategy has come in part from the Institute of Medicine's (IOM) 2011 report on LGBT health.[141] IOM, NIH, and independent analyses of NIH's funding portfolio have demonstrated improvements since 2011 in the depth and breadth of studies and funding related to SOGIESC minority health and have provided direction as to where progress can continue to be made.[245,246] A strategy that encourages the inclusion of SOGIESC minorities in research questions and study samples will continue to elucidate what health disparities exist, whether they are widening or diminishing, and what is contributing to them. Given its international status regarding health funding, this activity from one governmental entity may have a large effect on SOGIESC minority health worldwide.

OutRight Action International

Initially founded in 1990 as the International Gay and Lesbian Human Rights Commission, OutRight Action International, or OutRight, holds a place at the United Nations Headquarters to advocate for the human rights of LGBTIQ individuals worldwide.[298,299] Its strategies include (1) advocacy to defend and advance LGBTIQ human rights, (2) connecting LGBTIQ activists and allies, (3) research through monitoring conditions for LGBTIQ people around the world, and (4) leveraging resources to build capacity among activists.[300]

OutRight's *Agenda 2030* report assesses how Sustainable Development Goal 3—Ensure Healthy Lives and Promote Well-Being for All at All Ages—relates to health and human rights of LGBTI people and provides recommendations for monitoring and implementation of activities to further this aim.[301] In this document, OutRight emphasizes the importance of community-based organizations in doing this work.[301] However, in many countries, organizations serving LGBTI individuals are not permitted to register as official entities, preventing them from effectively reaching its intended audience; of 194 countries studied, only 56% permit LGBTIQ organizations to legally register as such.[302] This demonstrates the substantial work that still needs to be conducted on a global scale if human rights for SOGIESC minorities are to be acknowledged and consistently supported for all humans regardless of SOCIESC status.

BEST PRACTICES AND NEXT STEPS

Engaging All Academic Disciplines

A fundamental strength of public health is its multidisciplinary nature, which recognizes the need to engage experts with diverse training and skill sets to identify and solve public health problems. It is important for every discipline currently involved in public health practice to consider how their discipline can be used to address the concerns of SOGIESC minorities.

There are numerous examples of cross-disciplinary teams coming together to examine and address a common public health concern. For example, the HIV/AIDS epidemic demonstrated how cross-disciplinary teams, approaches, and methods could be used to understand and address a concern impacting multiple SOGIESC minorities. Physicians and epidemiologists in the United States were the first to recognize the emergence of an epidemic and they played important roles in chronicling the spread of the virus and its impact on public health.[303]

Mental health professionals, including social workers, psychologists, and psychiatrists explored the impact of the virus on people living with HIV as well as those at risk for HIV and their family members.[304,305] Other healthcare providers, notably nurses, played important roles in providing direct patient care and developing treatment protocols, and along with healthcare administrators they proposed healthcare facility policies allowing, for example, same-sex partners to visit and make medical decisions for critically ill partners (who are/were not generally afforded rights equal to spouses).[306]

Anthropologists and sociologists played important roles in adding sociocultural depth to the medical and epidemiological descriptions of HIV/AIDS, and they helped explain the political, social, and economic structures that contributed to the epidemic.[307–309] Historians went to work in the first decade of the epidemic making comparisons with previous epidemics and identifying lessons for how to respond (or not respond), and historical studies of SOGIESC minority communities facilitated a deeper understanding of how communities reacted to the spread of HIV as well as chronicling the capacity of communities to respond to potential, including existential, threats.[43,310]

Simultaneously, economists began to examine the economic cost to individuals and society of HIV/AIDS and political scientists described the impact of the epidemic on political power, representation, and legitimacy.[311,312] Lawyers described how legislation and regulatory policy impacted the spread of the disease and they worked to protect the civil rights of sexual and gender minorities.[313] Further, education professionals developed curriculum to inform the public about HIV, while advertising experts created campaigns to inform the general public as well as at-risk SOGIESC communities.[314]

Many additional disciplines could be added to this discussion (e.g., statisticians, virologists, environmental scientists), but the point is that experts in every discipline involved in addressing public health need to also be involved in addressing the concerns of SOGIESC minorities. To facilitate this process, *we challenge everyone working in public health to ask how SOGIESC minorities might experience or be impacted differentially within your given topic of study.* For example, someone studying autism could ask how SOGIESC minorities differently experience autism and thrive in the systems set up to address the concerns of people with autism. Almost any public health concern could be substituted for the topic of autism in the previous sentence. Please take a moment to do so with your work.

Engaging SOGIESC Minorities

Another strength of public health is the way communities are involved in the production of public health knowledge and efforts to improve the public's health. Rather than examining a population from the outside, public health at its best engages communities in the process of exploring their concerns. This is done through developing community partnerships/relationships involving community members using a range of community-based participatory strategies.[315]

When applied to research, this method is known as "community-based participatory research (CBPR)." CBPR's approach to conducting research is one that equitably involves community members throughout the entire research process.[316] That is, community members are involved in every step of the research process, beginning before any research commences. That is, community members should be involved in identifying the needs of their community and prioritizing what should be the subject of investigation. The research priorities of community members are often not the same priorities as those identified by academic researchers. When any discordance in priorities occurs, priorities identified by the community should be the preferred topics of investigation.[317]

Often what academic researchers find curious or important is not equally curious or important to community members. There has been a long tension between sexual minorities and investigators wanting to identify biological origins for sexual orientations. Over the last century, numerous researchers have explored how hormones, or more recently genetics, could impact sexual attraction, sexual behavior, and sexual orientation identity.[318]

While some community members have argued that discovery of a biological cause for sexual orientations would demonstrate that sexual minorities are not the result of moral failure or some other mental or physical weakness, other community members have argued that such a discovery would lead to efforts to cure and eliminate sexual minorities.

History shows that any causal discovery would lead to attempted cures. Even without any causal evidence, sexual and gender minorities have been subjected (voluntarily or involuntarily) to numerous medical treatments to cure or treat their homosexuality or align their gender identity with their biological sex. An incomplete list of these treatments, all substantiated by publications in scientific journals, include (listed in alphabetical order using the terminology of the authors) aversion therapy, behavior therapy, castration (chemical and surgical), conditioned reaction technique, conditioning, conversion therapy, correction hospitals, covert sensitization, electroshock, group therapy, hysterectomy, incarceration, homoanonymous, hypnosis, lobotomy, LSD, Metrazol, musical analysis, organotherapy, ovariectomy, primal therapy, psychoanalysis, psychotherapy, pudic nerve section, relationship therapy, reparative therapy, sex-hormone medication, sex mutilation, shock treatment, sterilization, suggestive therapy, systematic desensitization, testosterone administration, vasectomy, and vegetotherapy.[5,6,319–330]

The full list of these treatments has yet to be compiled and the negative consequences both historic and lingering may never be fully realized because of the hidden nature and shame associated with this work. This list is provided here because it is important to never forget these atrocities, but also, more importantly, because this list demonstrates what can happen when community members are considered the subjects of research rather than research partners.

SOGIESC minorities should consequently be involved in the identification of research topics and priorities, the selection of research methods including the validation of tools for use with these populations, the identification of subjects, the collection and storage of data, data analysis and interpretation, and the dissemination of findings back to their communities.

Methodological Considerations and Challenges

One of the greatest challenges to studying the health of SOGIESC minorities is creating samples from which data can be collected to produce generalizable findings with a known level of confidence. This is a shared goal of many public health researchers, that is, the desire to produce findings that can be generalized beyond the collected data with some calculable level of confidence (ideally indicated in part by confidence intervals and other statistics).

Importantly, these challenges are not unique to SOGIESC minorities and are common concerns with many if not most topics investigated by public health researchers. This is perhaps because public health researchers are often drawn to the concerns of minority (defined in many ways) populations who are often the subject of discrimination and stigma.

More specifically, stigmatized minority populations often present challenges to public health researchers because they are generally relatively rare (compared to majority populations), stigmatized, and hidden. Fortunately, much has been written about strategies for collecting data and making inferences about populations with these characteristics.[331] There is not enough space to review this literature here, but rather, we want to direct researchers working with rare stigmatized or hidden populations, and SOGIESC minorities, to seek out other publications.[332] Further we want to make it unequivocally clear that research on SOGIESC minorities should never be avoided using methodological challenges as an excuse.[333]

One of the challenges often cited for not collecting data on SOGIESC minorities is a lack of definitions, agreed upon taxonomies, or tools/measures to sort people into SOGIESC categories. These topics, which were addressed in detail above, were legitimate concerns a decade or more ago; however, these concerns can no longer be used as excuses for not conducting research. Measures and definitions of SOGIESC constructs are as well developed as those in other areas including race and ethnicity.

Other concerns that have been raised include reactions of participants to being asked questions about their sexual orientation, gender identity or gender expression, or sex characteristics; sample size and statistical power; and the potentially high cost of collecting data (particularly representative data) given methodological challenges. These concerns have been addressed elsewhere, including by the lead author of this chapter, and we direct readers to publications addressing these issues for further information.[334] Methodological concerns can no longer be used as a reason to avoid work exploring the public health of SOGIESC minority communities.

Developing Leadership

Finally, there is a tremendous lack of leadership within and across countries on SOGIESC minority health including, alarmingly, a lack of leadership on the most basic responsibilities including monitoring health to identify problems and serve as an early warning system. Efforts at addressing SOGIESC minority health have been fragmented targeting single health issues (e.g., HIV, breast cancer, or suicide) and occurring within individual countries (e.g., New Zealand, the United States, and the United Kingdom) rather than spanning them. There is no obvious organizational or governmental source for a coordinated research agenda, the vetting, and dissemination of knowledge and effective interventions, or for the setting of priorities and public policy. Further, there has been little leadership on ethical standards or education content standards in schools of public health, nursing, or medicine.

While this lack of leadership from the top down is discouraging, promising work originating from researchers, many of whom are SOGIESC minorities themselves, and community-based organizations (often created out of a desperate need by community members to respond to health threats not being addressed elsewhere) is rapidly filling a void. It is our hope that this foundation of research and work can eventually support larger efforts to comprehensively address the needs of SOGIESC minorities worldwide.

References

1. Rosen G. *A History of Public Health*. Baltimore, MD: JHU Press; 2015.
2. Sell RL. Defining and measuring sexual orientation: A review. *Arch Sex Behav*. 1997;26(6):643–58.
3. Meyer IH. Why lesbian, gay, bisexual, and transgender public health? *AM J Public Health*. 2001;91(6):856–9.
4. D'emilio J, Freedman EB. *Intimate Matters: A History of Sexuality in America*. Chicago, IL: University of Chicago Press; 1988.

5. Katz J. *Gay American History: Lesbians and Gay Men in the U.S.A.: A Documentary*. New York: Crowell; 1976.
6. Katz J. *Gay/lesbian Almanac: A New Documentary in Which is Contained, in Chronological Order, Evidence of the True and Fantastical History of Those Persons Now Called Lesbians and Gay Men*. 1st ed. New York: Harper & Row; 1983.
7. Duberman MB, Vicinus M, Chauncey G. *Hidden from History: Reclaiming the Gay and Lesbian Past*. Vol 1. New York: Plume; 1990.
8. Marcus E. *Making Gay History*. New York: Harper Collins; 2009.
9. Bérubé A. *Coming Out under Fire: The History of Gay Men and Women in World War II*. Chapel Hill, NC: University of North Carolina Press; 2010.
10. Miller N. *Out of the Past: Gay and Lesbian History from 1869 to the Present*. New York: Vintage; 1995.
11. Meyer IH. Prejudice, social stress, and mental health in lesbian, gay, and bisexual populations: conceptual issues and research evidence. *Psychol Bull*. 2003;129(5):674–97.
12. Bockting WO, Miner MH, Swinburne Romine RE, Hamilton A, Coleman E. Stigma, mental health, and resilience in an online sample of the US transgender population. *Am J Public Health*. 2013;103(5): 943–51.
13. Greenberg JA. Intersex and intrasex debates: Building alliances to challenge sex discrimination. *Cardozo J Law Gend*. 2005;12:99.
14. Dreger AD, Chase C, Sousa A, Gruppuso PA, Frader J. Changing the nomenclature/taxonomy for intersex: A scientific and clinical rationale. *J Pediatr Endocrinol Metabol*. 2005;18(8):729–34.
15. Griffiths DA. Shifting syndromes: Sex chromosome variations and intersex classifications. *Soc Stud Sci*. 2018;48(1):125–48.
16. Johnson EK, Rosoklija I, Finlayson C, et al. Attitudes towards "disorders of sex development" nomenclature among affected individuals. *J Pediatr Urol*. 2017;13(6):608. e601–8.
17. Badgett MVL, Sell RL. *A Set of Proposed Indicators for the LGBTI Inclusion Index*. New York: United Nations Development Programme and World Bank; 2018.
18. Sell RL. Defining and measuring sexual orientation for research. In: *The Health of Sexual Minorities*. New York: Springer; 2007, pp. 355–74.
19. Sell RL, Petrulio C. Sampling homosexuals, bisexuals, gays, and lesbians for public health research: A review of the literature from 1990 to 1992. *J Homosex*. 1996;30(4):31–47.
20. Boehmer U. Twenty years of public health research: Inclusion of lesbian, gay, bisexual, and transgender populations. *Am J Public Health*. 2002;92(7):1125–30.
21. Diamond LM. Development of sexual orientation among adolescent and young adult women. *Dev Psych*. 1998;34(5):1085.
22. Malebranche DJ. Bisexually active Black men in the United States and HIV: Acknowledging more than the "down low." *Arch Sex Behav*. 2008;37(5):810–16.
23. Pathela P, Hajat A, Schillinger J, Blank S, Sell R, Mostashari F. Discordance between sexual behavior and self-reported sexual identity: A population-based survey of New York City men. *Ann Intern Med*. 2006;145(6):416–25.
24. Badgett M. Best practices for asking questions about sexual orientation on surveys. 2009.
25. Foucault M. *The history of sexuality, vol. 2: The use of pleasure*. New York, NY: Vintage; 2012.
26. Duncan LE, Mincer E, Dunn SR. Assessing politicized sexual orientation identity: Validating the Queer Consciousness Scale. *J Homosex*. 2017;64(8):1069–91.
27. Galupo MP, Ramirez JL, Pulice-Farrow L. "Regardless of their gender": Descriptions of sexual identity among bisexual, pansexual, and queer identified individuals. *J Bisex*. 2017;17(1):108–24.
28. Haslanger S. Gender and Social Construction. 2017:299.
29. Tabaac A, Perrin PB, Benotsch EG. Discrimination, mental health, and body image among transgender and gender-non-binary individuals: Constructing a multiple mediational path model. *J Gay Lesbian Soc Serv*. 2018;30(1):1–16.
30. Szreter S, Sholkamy H, Dharmalingam A. *Categories and Contexts: Anthropological and Historical Studies in Critical Demography*. Oxford: OUP; 2004.
31. Collin L, Reisner SL, Tangpricha V, Goodman MJ. Prevalence of transgender depends on the "case" definition: A systematic review. *J Sex Med*. 2016;13(4):613–26.
32. Feinberg L. *Transgender Warriors*. Boston, MA: Beacon Press; 1996.
33. Kenagy GP. Transgender health: Findings from two needs assessment studies in Philadelphia. *Health Soc Work*. 2005;30(1):19–26.
34. Stade RS. The Social Life of Fighting Words. *Confl Soc*. 2017;3(1):108–24.
35. Thompson JrEH, Bennett KM. Masculinity ideologies. In: Levant RF, Wong YJ, eds. *The Psychology of Men and Masculinities*. Washington, DC: American Psychological Association; 2017, pp. 45–74.
36. Sáenz VB, Mayo JR, Miller RA, Rodriguez SL. (Re) defining masculinity through peer interactions: Latino men in Texas community colleges. *J Student Aff Res Pract*. 2015;52(2):164–75.
37. Lehavot K, King KM, Simoni JM. Development and validation of a gender expression measure among sexual minority women. *Psychol Women Q*. 2011;35(3):381–400.
38. Kray LJ, Howland L, Russell AG, Jackman LM. The effects of implicit gender role theories on gender system justification: Fixed beliefs strengthen masculinity to preserve the status quo. *J Pers Soc Psychol*. 2017;112(1):98–115.
39. Bem SL. Gender schema theory: A cognitive account of sex typing. *Psychol Rev*. 1981;88(4):354.
40. Bem SL. The BSRI and gender schema theory: A reply to Spence and Helmreich. *Psychol Rev*. 1981;88(4):369–71.
41. Starr CR, Zurbriggen EL. Sandra Bem's gender schema theory after 34 years: A review of its reach and impact. *Sex Roles*. 2017;76(9–10):566–78.
42. Rivera LM, Dasgupta N. The detrimental effect of affirming masculinity on judgments of gay men. *Psychol Men Masc*. 2018;19(1):102.
43. D'Emilio J. *Sexual Politics, Sexual Communities: The Making of a Homosexual Minority in the United States, 1940–1970*. Chicago, IL: University of Chicago Press; 1983.
44. Davis G. Intersexuality. *The Wiley Blackwell Encyclopedia of Gender and Sexuality Studies*. 2016:1–4.
45. Bakula DM, Mullins AJ, Sharkey CM, Wolfe-Christensen C, Mullins LL, Wisniewski AB. Gender identity outcomes in children with disorders/differences of sex development: Predictive factors. Paper presented at Seminars in Perinatology 2017.
46. Truesdale M, Copp H. Behind the Name: The historical perspective of the pathologizing of atypical sexual development. *J Urol*. 2015;193(4):e588.
47. InterACT. Mission Statement. 2018. https://interactadvocates.org/about-us/mission-history/. Accessed September 8, 2018.
48. Davis G, Evans MJ. Surgically shaping sex: A gender structure analysis of the violation of intersex people's human rights. In: *Handbook of the Sociology of Gender*. New York: Springer; 2018, pp. 273–84.
49. Rosin H. A boy's life. *The Atlantic*. 2008;10727825(302):4.
50. Gaetano P. David Reimer and John Money Gender Reassignment Controversy: The John/Joan Case. 2017.
51. Lykens JE, LeBlanc AJ, Bockting WO. Healthcare experiences among young adults who identify as genderqueer or nonbinary. *LGBT Health*. 2018;5(3):191–6.
52. Carpenter M. The human rights of intersex people: Addressing harmful practices and rhetoric of change. *Reprod Health Matters*. 2016;24(47):74–84.
53. Cheneffusse Ascenzo T. Newborn intersex children and their right to self determination in cosmetic medical interventions. 2017.
54. Bauer M, Truffer D. Intersex genital mutilations. Paper presented at: Human rights violations of children with variations for sex anatomy. NGO report of Germany on the convention on the elimination of all forms of discrimination against women (CEDAW), Zurich 2017.
55. Ridolfo H, Miller K, Maitland A. Measuring sexual identity using survey questionnaires: How valid are our measures? *Sex Res Social Policy*. 2012;9(2):113–24.
56. Gates GJ. How many people are lesbian, gay, bisexual and transgender? 2011.
57. Roth WD. Methodological pitfalls of measuring race: International comparisons and repurposing of statistical categories. *Ethn Racial Stud*. 2017;40(13):2347–53.
58. Wolff M, Wells B, Ventura-DiPersia C, Renson A, Grov C. Measuring sexual orientation: A review and critique of US data collection efforts and implications for health policy. *J Sex Res*. 2017;54(4–5):507–31.
59. Temkin D, Belford J, McDaniel T, Stratford B, Parris D. Improving measurement of sexual orientation and gender identity among middle and high school students. *Child Trends*. 2017;22:1–64.
60. Gonsiorek JC, Sell RL, Weinrich JD. Definition and measurement of sexual orientation. *Suicide Life Threat Behav*. 1995;25 Suppl:40–51.
61. Miller K, Ryan JM. Design, development and testing of the NHIS sexual identity question. 2011.

62. Swartz J, Horn K. A comparative analysis of lifetime medical conditions and infectious diseases by sexual identity, attraction, and concordance: Results from a National US Survey. *Med Res Arch*. 2017;5(8).
63. Wolff M, Wells B, Ventura-DiPersia C, Renson A, Grov C. Measuring sexual orientation: A review and critique of US data collection efforts and implications for health policy. *J Sex Res*. 2017;54(4–5):507–31.
64. Jans M, Wilson BD, Herman JL. Measuring aspects of sexuality and gender: A sexual human rights challenge for science and official statistics. *CHANCE*. 2018;31(1):12–20.
65. Palan KM, Areni CS, Kiecker P. Reexamining masculinity, femininity, and gender identity scales. *Market Lett*. 1999;10(4):357–71.
66. Brenner PS, Bulgar-Medina J. Testing mark-all-that-apply measures of sexual orientation and gender identity. *Field Methods*. 2018;30(4):357–70. 1525822X18795872.
67. Bagett MVL, Baker KE, Conron KJ, et al. Best practices for asking questions to identify transgender and other gender minority respondents on population-based surveys. 2014.
68. Reisner SL, Conron KJ, Tardiff LA, Jarvi S, Gordon AR, Austin SB. Monitoring the health of transgender and other gender minority populations: Validity of natal sex and gender identity survey items in a US national cohort of young adults. *BMC Public Health*. 2014;14(1):1224.
69. Broussard KA, Warner RH, Pope AR. Too many boxes, or not enough? Preferences for how we ask about gender in cisgender, LGB, and gender-diverse samples. *Sex Roles*. 2018;78(9–10):606–24.
70. University of California. Gender Identity and Sexual Orientation Questions. 2018. https://registrar.ucsc.edu/gender-identity/index.html. Accessed September 1, 2018.
71. Rider GN, McMorris BJ, Gower AL, Coleman E, Eisenberg ME. Health and care utilization of transgender and gender nonconforming youth: A population-based study. *Pediatrics*. 2018;141(3):e20171683.
72. Conron KJ, Landers SJ, Reisner SL, Sell RL. Sex and gender in the US health surveillance system: A call to action. *Am J Public Health*. 2014;104(6):970–6.
73. Magliozzi D, Saperstein A, Westbrook L. Scaling up: Representing gender diversity in survey research. *Socius*. 2016;2:2378023116664352.
74. Lindqvist A, Bäck EA, Bäck H, Sendén M, Gothenburg 11–12 June. Measuring gender in surveys. 2018.
75. Reisner SL, Conron KJ, Baker K, et al. “Counting” transgender and gender-nonconforming adults in health research: Recommendations from the Gender Identity in US Surveillance Group. *Transgen Stud Q*. 2015;2(1):34–57.
76. Geist C, Dockendorff K. Gendering Gender: Introducing Gender Image as a Way to Assess Variation in Gender Expression in Survey Research. 2018.
77. Bem SL. The measurement of psychological androgyny. *J Consult Clin Psychol*. 1974;42(2):155.
78. Zucker KJ, Mitchell JN, Bradley SJ, Tkachuk J, Cantor JM, Allin SM. The recalled childhood gender identity/gender role questionnaire: Psychometric properties. *Sex Roles*. 2006;54(7–8):469–83.
79. Spence JT, Helmreich RL, Stapp J. The Personal Attributes Questionnaire: A measure of sex role stereotypes and masculinity-femininity. 1974.
80. Liben LS, Bigler RS, Ruble DN, Martin CL, Powlishta KK. The developmental course of gender differentiation: Conceptualizing, measuring, and evaluating constructs and pathways. *Monogr Soc Res Child Dev*. 2002;67(2):i–viii, 1–147.
81. Gordon AR, Krieger N, Okechukwu CA, et al. Decrements in health-related quality of life associated with gender nonconformity among US adolescents and young adults. *Qual Life Res*. 2017;26(8):2129–38.
82. Phillips G, Over R. Adult sexual orientation in relation to memories of childhood gender conforming and gender nonconforming behaviors. *Arch Sex Behav*. 1992;21(6):543–58.
83. Blanchard R, Freund K. Measuring masculine gender identity in females. *J Consult Clin Psychol*. 1983;51(2):205.
84. Wylie SA, Corliss HL, Boulanger V, Prokop LA, Austin SB. Socially assigned gender nonconformity: A brief measure for use in surveillance and investigation of health disparities. *Sex Roles*. 2010;63(3–4):264–76.
85. Bragg S, Renold E, Ringrose J, Jackson C. ‘More than boy, girl, male, female’: Exploring young people’s views on gender diversity within and beyond school contexts. *Sex Educ*. 2018;18(4):420–34.
86. Glick J, Pollock M, Theall K. Exploring gender expression measurement among gender minorities. Paper presented at *Annals of Behavioral Medicine*. 2018.
87. Green L, Rimes KA, Rahman Q. Beliefs about others’ perceptions—Gender typicality: Scale development and relationships to gender nonconformity, sexual orientation, and well-being. *J Sex Res*. 2018;55(7):837–49.
88. Intersex Society of North America. What is intersex? 2018. http://www.isna.org/faq/what_is_intersex. Accessed September 3, 2018.
89. Carpenter M, Cabral M. Submission by GATE to the World Health Organization: Intersex codes in the International Classification of Diseases (ICD) 11 Beta Draft. 2017.
90. Zainuddin AA, Grover SR, Shamsuddin K, Mahdy ZA. Research on quality of life in female patients with congenital adrenal hyperplasia and issues in developing nations. *J Pediatr Adolesc Gynecol*. 2013;26(6):296–304.
91. Johnson EK, Rosoklija I, Finlayson C, et al. Attitudes towards “disorders of sex development” nomenclature among affected individuals. *J Pediatr Urol*. 2017;13(6):608. e601–8.
92. Sell RL, Petrulio C. Sampling homosexuals, bisexuals, gays, and lesbians for public health research: A review of the literature from 1990 to 1992. *J Homosex*. 1996;30(4):31–47.
93. Sell R, Goldberg S, Conron K. The utility of an online convenience panel for reaching rare and dispersed populations. *PLoS One*. 2015;10(12):e0144011.
94. Koop CE. Foreword. In: Rosenberg ML, Fenley, MA, eds. *Violence in America: A Public Health Approach*. Vol iv. New York: Oxford University Press; 1991.
95. Edwards KM, Sylaska KM, Neal AM. Intimate partner violence among sexual minority populations: A critical review of the literature and agenda for future research. *Psychol Violence*. 2015;5(2):112–21.
96. McClennen JC. Domestic violence between same-gender partners: Recent findings and future research. *J Interpers Violence*. 2005;20(2):149–54.
97. Kulkin HS, Williams J, Bome HF, de la Bretonne D, Laurendine J. A review of research on violence in same-gender couples: A resource for clinicians. *J Homosex*. 2007;53(4):71–87.
98. Howard DE, Wang MQ, Fang Y. Psychosocial factors associated with reports of physical dating violence among US adolescent females. *Adolescence*. 2007;42(166):311.
99. GLMA. Healthy people 2010: Companion document for lesbian, gay, bisexual, and transgender (LGBT) health. Gay and Lesbian Medical Association; 2001.
100. Turell SC. A descriptive analysis of same-sex relationship violence for a diverse sample. *J Family Violence*. 2000;15(3):281–93.
101. Hequembourg AL, Parks KA, Vetter C. Sexual identity and gender differences in substance use and violence: An exploratory study. *J LGBT Issues Counsels*. 2008;2(3):174–98.
102. Tjaden PG. Extent, nature, and consequences of intimate partner violence. National Institute of Justice; 2000.
103. Dank M, Lachman P, Zweig JM, Yahner J. Dating violence experiences of lesbian, gay, bisexual, and transgender youth. *J Youth Adoles*. 2014;43(5):846–57.
104. Freedner N, Freed LH, Yang YW, Austin SB. Dating violence among gay, lesbian, and bisexual adolescents: Results from a community survey. *J Adoles Health*. 2002;31(6):469–74.
105. Langenderfer-Magruder L, Whitfield DL, Walls NE, Kattari SK, Ramos D. Experiences of intimate partner violence and subsequent police reporting among lesbian, gay, bisexual, transgender, and queer adults in Colorado: Comparing rates of cisgender and transgender victimization. *J Interpers Violence*. 2016;31(5):855–71.
106. Walters ML, Chen J, Breiding MJ. The National Intimate Partner and Sexual Violence Survey (NISVS): 2010 findings on victimization by sexual orientation. Atlanta, GA: National Center for Injury Prevention and Control, Centers for Disease Control and Prevention. 2013;648(73):6.
107. Halpern CT, Young ML, Waller MW, Martin SL, Kupper LL. Prevalence of partner violence in same-sex romantic and sexual relationships in a national sample of adolescents. *J Adoles Health*. 2004;35(2):124–31.
108. Reuter TR, Newcomb ME, Whitton SW, Mustanski B. Intimate partner violence victimization in LGBT young adults: Demographic differences and associations with health behaviors. *Psychol Violence*. 2017;7(1):101–9.
109. Ard KL, Makadon HJ. Addressing intimate partner violence in lesbian, gay, bisexual, and transgender patients. *J Gen Intern Med*. 2011;26(8):930–3.
110. Gladden RM, Vivolo-Kantor AM, Hamburger ME, et al. Bullying Surveillance among Youths: Uniform Definitions for Public Health and Recommended Data Elements. 2014.

111. Almeida J, Johnson RM, Corliss HL, Molnar BE, Azrael D. Emotional distress among LGBT youth: The influence of perceived discrimination based on sexual orientation. *J Youth Adoles.* 2009;38(7):1001–14.
112. Friedman MS, Marshal MP, Guadamuz TE, et al. A meta-analysis of disparities in childhood sexual abuse, parental physical abuse, and peer victimization among sexual minority and sexual nonminority individuals. *Am J Public Health.* 2011;101(8):1481–94.
113. Garofalo R, Wolf RC, Kessel S, Palfrey J, DuRant RH. The association between health risk behaviors and sexual orientation among a school-based sample of adolescents. *Pediatrics.* 1998;101(5):895–902.
114. Kosciw JG, Greytak EA, Giga NM, Villenas C, Danischewski DJ. The 2015 National School Climate Survey: The Experiences of Lesbian, Gay, Bisexual, Transgender, and Queer Youth in Our Nation's Schools. Gay, Lesbian and Straight Education Network (GLSEN). 2016.
115. DuRant RH, Krowchuk DP, Sinal SH. Victimization, use of violence, and drug use at school among male adolescents who engage in same-sex sexual behavior. *J Pediatr.* 1998;133(1):113–8.
116. Reisner SL, Greytak EA, Parsons JT, Ybarra M. Gender minority social stress in adolescence: Disparities in adolescent bullying and substance use by gender identity. *J Sex Res.* 2015;52(3):243–56.
117. Russell ST, Everett BG, Rosario M, Birkett M. Indicators of victimization and sexual orientation among adolescents: Analyses from youth risk behavior surveys. *Am J Public Health.* 2014;104(2):255–61.
118. Earnshaw VAP, Bogart LMP, Poteat VPP, Reisner SLS, Schuster MAMDP. Bullying among lesbian, gay, bisexual, and transgender youth. *Pediatr Clin North Am.* 2016;63(6):999–1010.
119. Waters E. Lesbian, Gay, Bisexual, Transgender, Queer, and HIV-Affected Hate Violence in 2016. National Coalition of Anti-Violence Programs (NCAVP); 2016.
120. Gruenewald J. Are anti-LGBT homicides in the United States unique? *J Interpers Violence.* 2012;27(18):3601–23.
121. Gruenewald J, Kelley K. Exploring anti-LGBT homicide by mode of victim selection. *Crim Justice Behav.* 2014;41(9):1130–52.
122. Miller B, Humphreys L. Lifestyles and violence: Homosexual victims of assault and murder. *Qual Sociol.* 1980;3(3):169–85.
123. Comstock GD. *Violence against Lesbians and Gay Men.* Melbourne, Australia: Columbia University Press; 1992.
124. Herek GM, Cogan JC, Gillis JR. Victim experiences in hate crimes based on sexual orientation. *J Soc Issues.* 2002;58(2):319–39.
125. Briones-Robinson R, Powers RA, Socia KM. Sexual orientation bias crimes: Examination of reporting, perception of police bias, and differential police response. *Crim Justice Behav.* 2016;43(12):1688–709.
126. Mallory C, Hasenbush A, Sears B. Discrimination and harassment by law enforcement officers in the LGBT community. 2015.
127. Boehmer U, Clark MA, Timm A, Glickman M, Sullivan M. Comparing sexual minority cancer survivors recruited through a cancer registry to convenience methods of recruitment. *Women's Health Issues.* 2011;21(5):345–52.
128. The Lancet Oncology. Cancer risk in the transgender community. *Lancet Oncol.* 2015;16(9):999.
129. Gonzales G, Zinone R. Cancer diagnoses among lesbian, gay, and bisexual adults: Results from the 2013–2016 National Health Interview Survey. *Cancer Causes Control.* 2018;29(9):845–54.
130. Boehmer U, Miao X, Ozonoff A. Cancer survivorship and sexual orientation. *Cancer.* 2011;117(16):3796–804.
131. Silverberg MJ, Lau B, Justice AC, et al. Risk of anal cancer in HIV-infected and HIV-uninfected individuals in North America. *Clin Infect Dis.* 2012;54(7):1026–34.
132. Frisch M, Biggar RJ, Goedert JJ. Human papillomavirus-associated cancers in patients with human immunodeficiency virus infection and acquired immunodeficiency syndrome. *J Natl Cancer Inst.* 2000;92(18):1500–10.
133. Bower M, Powles T, Newsom-Davis T, et al. HIV-associated anal cancer: Has highly active antiretroviral therapy reduced the incidence or improved the outcome? *J Acquir Immune Defic Syndr.* 2004;37(5):1563-5.
134. D'Souza G, Wiley DJ, Li X, et al. Incidence and epidemiology of anal cancer in the Multicenter AIDS Cohort Study (MACS). *J Acquir Immune Defic Syndr.* 2008;48(4):491–9.
135. Roberts JR, Siekas LL, Kaz AM. Anal intraepithelial neoplasia: A review of diagnosis and management. *World J Gastrointest Oncol.* 2017;9(2):50–61.
136. Grulich AE, Poynten IM, Machalek DA, Jin F, Templeton DJ, Hillman RJ. The epidemiology of anal cancer. *Sex Health.* 2012;9(6):504–8.
137. Robinson K, Galloway K, Bewley S, Meads C. Lesbian and bisexual women's gynaecological conditions: A systematic review and exploratory meta-analysis. *BJOG.* 2017;124(3):381–92.
138. Quinn GP, Sanchez JA, Sutton SK, et al. Cancer and lesbian, gay, bisexual, transgender/transsexual, and queer/questioning populations (LGBTQ). *CA Cancer J Clin.* 2015;65(5):384–400.
139. Gatos KC. A literature review of cervical cancer screening in transgender men. *Nurs Womens Health.* 2018;22(1):52.
140. Meads C, Moore D. Breast cancer in lesbians and bisexual women: Systematic review of incidence, prevalence and risk studies. *BMC Public Health.* 2013;13(1):1127.
141. Graham R, Berkowitz B, Blum R, et al. *The Health of Lesbian, Gay, Bisexual, and Transgender People: Building a Foundation for Better Understanding.* Washington, DC: Institute of Medicine; 2011.
142. Case P, Austin SB, Hunter DJ, et al. Sexual orientation, health risk factors, and physical functioning in the Nurses' Health Study II. *J Womens Health.* 2004;13(9):1033–47.
143. Margolies L, Brown CG. Current State of Knowledge About Cancer in Lesbians, Gay, Bisexual, and Transgender (LGBT) People. *Seminars in Oncology Nursing.* 2018;34(1):3–11.
144. Cochran SD, Mays VM. Risk of breast cancer mortality among women cohabiting with same sex partners: Findings from the National Health Interview Survey, 1997–2003. *J Womens Health.* 2012;21(5):528–33.
145. Hart SL, Bowen DJ. Sexual orientation and intentions to obtain breast cancer screening. *J Womens Health.* 2009;18(2):177–85.
146. Brinton LA, Key TJ, Kolonel LN, et al. Prediagnostic sex steroid hormones in relation to male breast cancer risk. *J Clin Oncol.* 2015;33(18):2041-–50.
147. Fournier A, Berrino F, Riboli E, Avenel V, Clavel-Chapelon F. Breast cancer risk in relation to different types of hormone replacement therapy in the E3N-EPIC cohort. *Int J Cancer.* 2005;114(3):448–54.
148. Brown GR, Jones KT. Incidence of breast cancer in a cohort of 5,135 transgender veterans. *Breast Cancer Res Treat.* 2015;149(1):191–8.
149. Heslin KC, Gore JL, King WD, Fox SA. Sexual orientation and testing for prostate and colorectal cancers among men in California. *Med Care.* 2008;46(12):1240–8.
150. McElroy JA, Wintemberg JJ, Williams A. Comparison of lesbian and bisexual women to heterosexual women's screening prevalence for breast, cervical, and colorectal cancer in Missouri. *LGBT Health.* 2015;2(2):188–92.
151. Tabaac AR, Sutter ME, Wall CSJ, Baker KE. Gender identity disparities in cancer screening behaviors. *Am J Prev Med.* 2018;54(3):385–93.
152. Rosenblatt KA, Wicklund KG, Stanford JL. Sexual factors and the risk of prostate cancer. *Am J Epidemiol.* 2001;153(12):1152–8.
153. Spence AR, Rousseau MC, Parent ME. Sexual partners, sexually transmitted infections, and prostate cancer risk. *Cancer Epidemiol.* 2014;38(6):700–7.
154. Mandel JS, Schuman LM. Sexual factors and prostatic cancer: Results from a case-control study. *J Gerontol.* 1987;42(3):259–64.
155. Rogers HW, Weinstock MA, Harris AR, et al. Incidence estimate of nonmelanoma skin cancer in the United States, 2006. *Arch Dermatol.* 2010;146(3):283–7.
156. Mansh M, Katz KA, Linos E, Chren M, Arron S. Association of skin cancer and indoor tanning in sexual minority men and women. *JAMA Dermatol.* 2015;151(12):1308–16.
157. Institute of Medicine. *Access to Health Care in America.* Washington, DC: The National Academies Press; 1993.
158. ODPHP. Access to Health Services. 2016. https://www.healthypeople.gov/2020/topics-objectives/topic/Access-to-Health-Services#1. Accessed August 31, 2018.
159. Diaz T, Chu SY, Conti L, Nahlen BL. Health insurance coverage among persons with AIDS: Results from a multistate surveillance project. *Am J Public Health.* 1994;84(6):1015.
160. Buchmueller T, Carpenter CS. Disparities in health insurance coverage, access, and outcomes for individuals in same-sex versus different-sex relationships, 2000–2007. *Am J Public Health.* 2010;100(3):489.
161. Heck JE, Sell RL, Gorin SS. Health care access among individuals involved in same-sex relationships. *Am J Public Health.* 2006;96(6):1111–8.
162. Kates J, Ranji U, Beamsderfer A, Salganicoff A, Dawson L. *Health and Access to Care and Coverage for Lesbian, Gay, Bisexual, and Transgender Individuals in the U.S.* Washington, DC: Henry J. Kaiser Family Foundation; 2018.

163. Karpman M, Skopec L, Long SK. Quicktake: Uninsurance rate nearly halved for lesbian, gay, and bisexual adults since mid-2013. Health Reform Monitoring Survey April. 2015.
164. Baker KC, Durso LE, Cray A. Moving the needle: the impact of the Affordable Care Act on LGBT communities. Center for American Progress; 2014.
165. Durso L, Baker K, Cray A. *LGBT Communities and The Affordable Care Act: Findings from a National Survey*. Washington, DC: Center for American Progress; 2013.
166. Gonzales G, Henning-smith C. Barriers to care among transgender and gender nonconforming adults. *Milbank Q.* 2017;95(4):726–48.
167. Gates GJ. In US, LGBT more likely than non-LGBT to be uninsured. 2014.
168. Cooley LA, Hoots B, Wejnert C, Lewis R, Paz-Bailey G, Group NS. Policy changes and improvements in health insurance coverage among MSM: 20 US Cities, 2008–2014. *AIDS Behav.* 2017;21(3):615–18.
169. Baker KE. The future of transgender coverage. *N Engl J Med.* 2017;376(19):1801.
170. HRC. Corporate Equality Index 2018: Rating Workplaces on Lesbian, Gay, Bisexual, Transgender, and Queer Equality. Washington, DC: Human Rights Campaign Foundation; 2018.
171. Ponce NA, Cochran SD, Pizer JC, Mays VM. The effects of unequal access to health insurance for same-sex couples in California. *Health Aff (Millwood).* 2010;29(8):1539–48.
172. Dawson L, Kates J, Rae M. Access to Employer-Sponsored Health Coverage for Same-Sex Spouses: 2017 Update. Henry J. Kaiser Family Foundation; September 25, 2017.
173. Everett BG, Mollborn S. Examining sexual orientation disparities in unmet medical needs among men and women. *Popul Res Policy Rev.* 2014;33(4):553.
174. Whitehead J, Shaver J, Stephenson R. Outness, stigma, and primary health care utilization among rural LGBT populations. *PLoS One.* 2016;11(1):e0146139.
175. Bertakis KD, Azari R, Helms JL, Callahan EJ, Robbins JA. Gender differences in the utilization of health care services. *J Fam Pract.* 2000;49(2):147–52.
176. Simpson TL, Balsam KF, Cochran BN, Lehavot K, Gold SD. Veterans administration health care utilization among sexual minority veterans. *Psychol Servi.* 2013;10(2):223.
177. Grant JM, Mottet LA, Tanis J, Herman JL, Harrison J, Keisling M. National transgender discrimination survey report on health and health care. Washington, DC: National Center for Transgender Equality and the National Gay and Lesbian Task Force. 2010.
178. Seelman KL, Colón-Diaz MJP, LeCroix RH, Xavier-Brier M, Kattari L. Transgender noninclusive healthcare and delaying care because of fear: Connections to general health and mental health among transgender adults. *Transgen Health.* 2017;2(1):17–28.
179. Bjarnadottir RI, Bockting W, Dowding DW. Patient perspectives on answering questions about sexual orientation and gender identity: An integrative review. *J Clin Nurs.* 2017;26(13–14):1814.
180. Klitzman RL, Greenberg JD. Patterns of communication between gay and lesbian patients and their health care providers. *J Homosex.* 2002;42(4):65–75.
181. Kamen CS, Smith-Stoner M, Heckler CE, Flannery M, Margolies L. Social support, self-rated health, and lesbian, gay, bisexual, and transgender identity disclosure to cancer care providers. *Oncol Nurs Forum.* 2015;42(1):44–51.
182. Law M, Mathai A, Veinot P, Webster F, Mylopoulos M. Exploring lesbian, gay, bisexual, and queer (LGBQ) people's experiences with disclosure of sexual identity to primary care physicians: A qualitative study. *BMC Fam Pract.* 2015;16:175.
183. Maragh-Bass AC, Torain M, Adler R, et al. Is it okay to ask: Transgender patient perspectives on sexual orientation and gender identity collection in healthcare. *Acad Emerg Med.* 2017;24(6):655.
184. Sabin JA, Riskind RG, Nosek BA. Health care providers' implicit and explicit attitudes toward lesbian women and gay men. *Am J Public Health.* 2015;105(9):1831–41.
185. Shetty G, Sanchez JA, Lancaster JM, Wilson LE, Quinn GP, Schabath MB. Oncology healthcare providers' knowledge, attitudes, and practice behaviors regarding LGBT health. *Patient Educ Couns.* 2016;99(10):1676–84.
186. Abdessamad HM, Yudin MH, Tarasoff LA, Radford KD, Ross LE. Attitudes and knowledge among obstetrician-gynecologists regarding lesbian patients and their health. *J Womens Health.* 2013;22(1):85–93.
187. Burch A. Health care providers' knowledge, attitudes, and self-efficacy for working with patients with spinal cord injury who have diverse sexual orientations. *Phys Ther.* 2008;88(2):191–8.
188. Lim FA, Hsu R. Nursing students' attitudes toward lesbian, gay, bisexual, and transgender persons: An integrative review. *Nurs Educ Perspect.* 2016;37(3):144.
189. Kitts RL. Barriers to optimal care between physicians and lesbian, gay, bisexual, transgender, and questioning adolescent patients. *J Homosex.* 2010;57(6):730-–47.
190. Strong KL, Folse VN. Assessing undergraduate nursing students' knowledge, attitudes, and cultural competence in caring for lesbian, gay, bisexual, and transgender patients. *J Nurs Educ.* 2015;54(1):45.
191. CenterLink, MAP. 2014 LGBT Community Center Survey Report: Assessing the Capacity and Programs of Lesbian, Gay, Bisexual, and Transgender Community Centers. Denver, CO: Movement Advancement Project; 2014.
192. Martos AJ, Wilson PA, Meyer IH. Lesbian, gay, bisexual, and transgender (LGBT) health services in the United States: Origins, evolution, and contemporary landscape. *PLoS One.* 2017;12(7):e0180544.
193. Chakraborty A, McManus S, Brugha TS, Bebbington P, King M. Mental health of the non-heterosexual population of England. *Br J Psychiatry.* 2011;198(2):143–8.
194. Krueger EA, Meyer IH, Upchurch DM. Sexual orientation group differences in perceived stress and depressive symptoms among young adults in the United States. *LGBT Health.* 2018;5(4):242–9.
195. Valentine SE, Shipherd JC. A systematic review of social stress and mental health among transgender and gender non-conforming people in the United States. *Clin Psychol Rev.* 2018;66: 24–38.
196. Leonard W, Pitts M, Mitchell A, et al. Private lives 2. The second National survey on the health and wellbeing of Gay, Lesbian, Bisexual, Transgender (GLBT) Australians. 2012.
197. Mayock P, Bryan A, Carr N, Kitching K. Supporting LGBT lives in Ireland: A study of the mental health and well-being of Lesbian, Gay, Bisexual and Transgender people. 2009.
198. Scandurra C, Amodeo AL, Valerio P, Bochicchio V, Frost DM. Minority stress, resilience, and mental health: A study of Italian transgender people. *J Soc Issues.* 2017;73(3):563–85.
199. Marshal MP, Dietz LJ, Friedman MS, et al. Suicidality and depression disparities between sexual minority and heterosexual youth: A meta-analytic review. *J Adolesc Health.* 2011;49(2):115–23.
200. Yarns BC, Abrams JM, Meeks TW, Sewell DD. The mental health of older LGBT adults. *Curr Psychiatry Rep.* 2016;18(6):60.
201. Richardson VE, King SD. Mental health for older LGBT adults. *Annu Rev Gerontol Geriatr.* 2017;37(1):59–75.
202. Mustanski BS, Garofalo R, Emerson EM. Mental health disorders, psychological distress, and suicidality in a diverse sample of lesbian, gay, bisexual, and transgender youths. *Am J Public Health.* 2010;100(12):2426–32.
203. Lehavot K, Simoni JM. The impact of minority stress on mental health and substance use among sexual minority women. *J Consult Clin Psychol.* 2011;79(2):159.
204. Meyer IH. Prejudice, social stress, and mental health in lesbian, gay, and bisexual populations: Conceptual issues and research evidence. *Psychol Bull.* 2003;129(5):674.
205. Hatzenbuehler ML, Pachankis JE. Stigma and minority stress as social determinants of health among lesbian, gay, bisexual, and transgender youth: Research evidence and clinical implications. *Pediatr Clin N Am.* 2016;63(6):985.
206. Chapman DP, Perry GS, Strine TW. The vital link between chronic disease and depressive disorders. *Prev Chronic Dis.* 2005;2(1):A14.
207. Lucassen MF, Stasiak K, Samra R, Frampton CM, Merry SN. Sexual minority youth and depressive symptoms or depressive disorder: A systematic review and meta-analysis of population-based studies. *Aust N Z J Psychiatry.* 2017;51(8):774–87.
208. Bostwick WB, Boyd CJ, Hughes TL, McCabe SE. Dimensions of sexual orientation and the prevalence of mood and anxiety disorders in the United States. *Am J Public Health.* 2010;100(3):468.
209. Fredriksen-Goldsen KI, Kim H-J, Emlet CA, et al. The aging and health report: Disparities and resilience among lesbian, gay, bisexual, and transgender older adults. 2011.
210. Shippy RA, Cantor MH, Brennan M. Social networks of aging gay men. *J Mens Stud.* 2004;13(1):107–20.
211. Nuttbrock L, Hwahng S, Bockting W, et al. Psychiatric impact of gender-related abuse across the life course of male-to-female transgender persons. *J Sex Res.* 2010;47(1):12–23.
212. Budge SL, Adelson JL, Howard KA. Anxiety and depression in transgender individuals: The roles of transition status, loss, social support, and coping. *J Consult Clin Psychol.* 2013;81(3):545.

213. Nemoto T, Bödeker B, Iwamoto M. Social support, exposure to violence and transphobia, and correlates of depression among male-to-female transgender women with a history of sex work. *Am J Public Health.* 2011;101(10):1980–8.

214. Veale JF, Watson RJ, Peter T, Saewyc EM. Mental health disparities among Canadian transgender youth. *J Adolesc Health.* 2017;60(1):44–9.

215. Claes L, Bouman WP, Witcomb G, Thurston M, Fernandez-Aranda F, Arcelus J. Non-suicidal self-injury in trans people: Associations with psychological symptoms, victimization, interpersonal functioning, and perceived social support. *J Sex Med.* 2015;12(1):168–79.

216. Cooper J, Kapur N, Webb R, et al. Suicide after deliberate self-harm: A 4-year cohort study. *Am J Psychiatry.* 2005;162(2):297–303.

217. Edmondson AJ, Brennan CA, House AO. Non-suicidal reasons for self-harm: A systematic review of self-reported accounts. *J Affect Disord.* 2016;191:109–17.

218. Bontempo DE, d'Augelli AR. Effects of at-school victimization and sexual orientation on lesbian, gay, or bisexual youths' health risk behavior. *J Adolesc Health.* 2002;30(5):364–74.

219. Meyer I, Dietrich J, Schwartz S. Lifetime prevalence of mental disorders and suicide attempts in diverse lesbian, gay, and bisexual populations. *Am J Public Health.* 2008;98(6):1004–6.

220. Haas AP, Rodgers PL, Herman JL. *Suicide Attempts Among Transgender and Gender Non-Conforming Adults: Findings of the National Transgender Discrimination Survey.* New York, NY: Williams Institute; 2014.

221. Schützmann K, Brinkmann L, Schacht M, Richter-Appelt H. Psychological distress, self-harming behavior, and suicidal tendencies in adults with disorders of sex development. *Arch Sex Behav.* 2009;38(1):16–33.

222. Haas AP, Lane A. Collecting sexual orientation and gender identity data in suicide and other violent deaths: A step towards identifying and addressing LGBT mortality disparities. *LGBT Health.* 2015;2(1):84.

223. Wilsnack SC, Hughes TL, Johnson TP, et al. Drinking and drinking-related problems among heterosexual and sexual minority women. *J Stud Alcohol Drugs.* 2008;69(1):129–39.

224. Woody GE, VanEtten-Lee ML, McKirnan D, et al. Substance use among men who have sex with men: Comparison with a national household survey. *J Acquir Immune Defic Syndr.* 2001;27(1):86–90.

225. Roxburgh A, Lea T, de Wit J, Degenhardt L. Sexual identity and prevalence of alcohol and other drug use among Australians in the general population. *Int J Drug Policy.* 2016;28:76–82.

226. McCabe SE, Bostwick WB, Hughes TL, West BT, Boyd CJ. The relationship between discrimination and substance use disorders among lesbian, gay, and bisexual adults in the United States. *Am J Public Health.* 2010;100(10):1946–52.

227. Talley AE, Hughes TL, Aranda F, Birkett M, Marshal MP. Exploring alcohol-use behaviors among heterosexual and sexual minority adolescents: Intersections with sex, age, and race/ethnicity. *Am J Public Health.* 2014;104(2):295–303.

228. Lehavot K, Williams EC, Millard SP, Bradley KA, Simpson TL. Association of alcohol misuse with sexual identity and sexual behavior in women veterans. *Subst Use Misuse.* 2016;51(2):216–29.

229. Hughes TL, Wilsnack SC, Kantor LW. The influence of gender and sexual orientation on alcohol use and alcohol-related problems: Toward a global perspective. *Alcohol Res.* 2016;38(1):121–32.

230. Drabble L, Midanik LT, Trocki K. Reports of alcohol consumption and alcohol-related problems among homosexual, bisexual and heterosexual respondents: Results from the 2000 National Alcohol Survey. *J Stud Alcohol.* 2005;66(1):111–20.

231. Hughes T, Szalacha LA, McNair R. Substance abuse and mental health disparities: Comparisons across sexual identity groups in a national sample of young Australian women. *Soc Sci Med.* 2010;71(4):824–31.

232. Bloomfield K, Wicki M, Wilsnack S, Hughes T, Gmel G. International differences in alcohol use according to sexual orientation. *Subst Abus.* 2011;32(4):210–19.

233. Cochran SD, Ackerman D, Mays VM, Ross MW. Prevalence of non-medical drug use and dependence among homosexually active men and women in the US population. *Addiction.* 2004;99(8):989–98.

234. Herbst JH, Jacobs ED, Finlayson TJ, McKleroy VS, Neumann MS, Crepaz N. Estimating HIV prevalence and risk behaviors of transgender persons in the United States: a systematic review. *AIDS Behav.* 2008;12(1):1–17.

235. Horvath KJ, Iantaffi A, Swinburne-Romine R, Bockting W. A Comparison of mental health, substance use, and sexual risk behaviors between rural and non-rural transgender persons. *J Homosex.* 2014;61(8):1117–30.

236. Watson RJ, Adjei J, Saewyc E, Homma Y, Goodenow C. Trends and disparities in disordered eating among heterosexual and sexual minority adolescents. *Int J Eat Disord.* 2017;50(1):22–31.

237. Calzo JP, Blashill AJ, Brown TA, Argenal RL. Eating disorders and disordered weight and shape control behaviors in sexual minority populations. *Curr Psychiatry Rep.* 2017;19(8):49-–49.

238. Diemer EW, Grant JD, Munn-Chernoff MA, Patterson DA, Duncan AE. Gender identity, sexual orientation, and eating-related pathology in a national sample of college students. *J Adolesc Health.* 2015;57(2): 144–9.

239. Feldman MB, Meyer IH. Eating disorders in diverse lesbian, gay, and bisexual populations. *Int J Eat Disord.* 2007;40(3):218–26.

240. Beren SE, Hayden HA, Wilfley DE, Grilo CM. The influence of sexual orientation on body dissatisfaction in adult men and women. *Int J Eat Disord.* 1996;20(2):135–41.

241. Austin SB, Ziyadeh N, Kahn JA, Camargo JrCA, Colditz GA, Field AE. Sexual orientation, weight concerns, and eating-disordered behaviors in adolescent girls and boys. *J Am Acad Child Adolesc Psychiatry.* 2004;43(9):1115–23.

242. Calzo JP, Austin SB, Micali N. Sexual orientation disparities in eating disorder symptoms among adolescent boys and girls in the UK. *Eur Child Adolesc Psychiatry.* 2018:1–8.

243. Boehmer U. Twenty years of public health research: Inclusion of lesbian, gay, bisexual, and transgender populations. *Am J Public Health.* 2002;92(7):1125–30.

244. Blondeel K, Say L, Chou D, et al. Evidence and knowledge gaps on the disease burden in sexual and gender minorities: A review of systematic reviews. *Int J Equity Health.* 2016;15(1):16.

245. Coulter RW, Kenst KS, Bowen DJ. Research funded by the National Institutes of Health on the health of lesbian, gay, bisexual, and transgender populations. *Am J Public Health.* 2014;104(2):e105–12.

246. Voyles CH, Sell RL. Continued disparities in lesbian, gay, and bisexual research funding at NIH. *Am J Public Health.* 2015;105(S3):e1–2; Robert WSC, Kenst KS, Bowen DJ, Scout. Coulter et al. respond. Am J Public Health. 2015;105(S3):e2–3.

247. Singh S, Song R, Johnson A, McCray E, Hall H. HIV incidence, prevalence, and undiagnosed infections in U.S. men who have sex with men. *Ann Intern Med.* 2018;168(10):685–94.

248. UNAIDS. Prevention Gap Report. UNAIDS; 2016.

249. Baral SD, Poteat T, Stromdahl S, Wirtz AL, Guadamuz TE, Beyrer C. Worldwide burden of HIV in transgender women: A systematic review and meta-analysis. *Lancet Infect Diss.* 2013;13(3):214–22.

250. Agénor M, Krieger N, Austin SB, Haneuse S, Gottlieb BR. Sexual orientation disparities in Papanicolaou test use among US women: The role of sexual and reproductive health services. *Am J Public Health.* 2014;104(2):e68–73.

251. Kerr DL, Ding K, Thompson AJ. A comparison of lesbian, bisexual, and heterosexual female college undergraduate students on selected reproductive health screenings and sexual behaviors. *Womens Health Issues.* 2013;23(6):e347–55.

252. Agénor M, Austin SB, Kort D, Austin EL, Muzny CA. Sexual orientation and sexual and reproductive health among African American sexual minority women in the U.S. South. *Womens Health Issues.* 2016;26(6):612.

253. Obedin-Maliver J, Makadon HJ. Transgender men and pregnancy. *Obstet Med.* 2016;9(1):4–8.

254. Peitzmeier SM, Reisner SL, Harigopal P, Potter J. Female-to-male patients have high prevalence of unsatisfactory paps compared to non-transgender females: Implications for cervical cancer screening. *J Gen Intern Med.* 2014;29(5):778–84.

255. Unger CA. Care of the transgender patient: A survey of gynecologists' current knowledge and practice. *J Womens Health.* 2015;24(2): 114–18.

256. Riskind RG, Tornello SL. Sexual orientation and future parenthood in a 2011–2013 nationally representative United States sample. *J Fam Psychol.* 2017;31(6):792.

257. Ethics Committee of American Society for Reproductive M. Access to fertility treatment by gays, lesbians, and unmarried persons: A committee opinion. *Fertil Steril.* 2013;100(6):1524–7.

258. Ethics Committee of the American Society for Reproductive M. Access to fertility services by transgender persons: An Ethics Committee opinion. *Fertil Steril.* 2015;104(5):1111–5.

259. Ross LE, Steele LS, Epstein R. Lesbian and bisexual women's recommendations for improving the provision of assisted reproductive technology services. *Fertil Steril.* 2006;86(3):735.

260. Ross LE, Steele LS, Epstein R. Service use and gaps in services for lesbian and bisexual women during donor insemination, pregnancy, and the postpartum period. *J Obstet Gynaecol Can*. 2006;28(6):505–11.

261. Renaud MT. We are mothers too: Childbearing experiences of lesbian families. *J Obstet Gynecol Neonatal Nurs*. 2007;36(2):190–9.

262. Campo-Engelstein L, Chen D, Baratz AB, Johnson EK, Finlayson C. The ethics of fertility preservation for pediatric patients with differences (disorders) of sex development. *J Endocr Soc*. 2017;1(6):638–45.

263. Lee PA, Nordenström A, Houk CP, et al. Global disorders of sex development update since 2006: Perceptions, approach and care. *Horm Res Paediatr*. 2016;85(3):158–80.

264. Guercio G, Costanzo M, Grinspon RP, Rey RA. Fertility issues in disorders of sex development. *Endocrinol Metabol Clin*. 2015;44(4):867–81.

265. Finlayson C, Fritsch MK, Johnson EK, et al. Presence of germ cells in disorders of sex development: Implications for fertility potential and preservation. *J Urol*. 2017;197(3):937–43.

266. Johnson EK, Rosoklija I, Shurba A, et al. Future fertility for individuals with differences of sex development: Parent attitudes and perspectives about decision-making. *J Pediatric Urol*. 2017;13(4):402.

267. Wierckx K, Van Caenegem E, Pennings G, et al. Reproductive wish in transsexual men. *Hum Reprod*. 2012;27(2):483–7.

268. Maxwell S, Noyes N, Keefe D, Berkeley AS, Goldman KN. Pregnancy outcomes after fertility preservation in transgender men. *Obstetr Gynecol*. 2017;129(6):1031–4.

269. Institute of Medicine. *The Health of Lesbian, Gay, Bisexual, and Transgender People: Building a Foundation for Better Understanding*. Washington, DC: The National Academies Press; 2011.

270. Goldman RH, Kaser DJ, Missmer SA, et al. Fertility treatment for the transgender community: A public opinion study. *J Assist Reprod Genet*. 2017;34(11):1457–67.

271. Ellis SA, Wojnar DM, Pettinato M. Conception, pregnancy, and birth experiences of male and gender variant gestational parents: It's how we could have a family. *J Midwifery Womens Health*. 2015;60(1):62–9.

272. James-Abra S, Tarasoff LA, Green D, et al. Trans peoples experiences with assisted reproduction services: A qualitative study. *Human Reprod*. 2015;30(6):1365–74.

273. Cipres D, Seidman D, Cloniger C, Nova C, O'Shea A, Obedin-Maliver J. Contraceptive use and pregnancy intentions among transgender men presenting to a clinic for sex workers and their families in San Francisco. *Contraception*. 2017;95(2):186–9.

274. Light AD, Obedin-Maliver J, Sevelius JM, Kerns JL. Transgender men who experienced pregnancy after female-to-male gender transitioning. *Obstetr Gynecol*. 2014;124(6):1120–7.

275. Morland IJF, Psychology. II. Intimate violations: Intersex and the ethics of bodily integrity. *Fem Psychol*. 2008;18(3):425–30.

276. Stroumsa D. The state of transgender health care: Policy, law, and medical frameworks. *Am J Public Health*. 2014;104(3):e31–8.

277. Katz JN. *The Invention of Heterosexuality*. Chicago, IL: University of Chicago Press; 2007.

278. United Nations. End violence and harmful medical practices on intersex children and adults, UN and regional experts urge. 2016. https://ohchr.org/EN/NewsEvents/Pages/DisplayNews.aspx?NewsID=20739. Accessed September 9, 2018.

279. Zieselman K. Invisible harm. *Narrat Inq Bioeth*. 2015;5(2):122–5.

280. Lee PA, Nordenström A, Houk CP, et al. Global disorders of sex development update since 2006: perceptions, approach and care. *Home Res Paediatr*. 2016; 85(3):158–80.

281. Fenway. Mission & History. 2018. https://fenwayhealth.org/about/history/. Accessed September 9, 2018.

282. Fenway. 2019 Fenway at a Glance. Boston, MA: Fenway Health; 2018.

283. Fenway. The Fenway Institute. 2018. https://fenwayhealth.org/the-fenway-institute/about/. Accessed September 9, 2018.

284. Who We Are and What We Do. 2018. https://truthinitiative.org/about-us. Accessed August 27, 2018.

285. Stevens P, Carlson LM, Hinman JM. An analysis of tobacco industry marketing to lesbian, gay, bisexual, and transgender (LGBT) populations: Strategies for mainstream tobacco control and prevention. *Health Promot Pract*. 2004;5(3_Suppl):129S–34S.

286. Legacy. Tobacco Control in LGBT Communities. 2012.

287. Matthews AK, Balsam K, Hotton A, Kuhns L, Li C-C, Bowen DJ. Awareness of media-based antitobacco messages among a community sample of LGBT individuals. *Health Promot Pract*. 2014;15(6): 857–66.

288. Vallone D, Greenberg M, Xiao H, et al. The effect of branding to promote healthy behavior: Reducing tobacco use among youth and young adults. *Int J Environ Res Public Health*. 2017;14(12):1517.

289. *Truth in Numbers. Every Life Counts. Annual Report 2017*. Truth Initiative; 2017.

290. About the Trevor Project. 2018. https://www.thetrevorproject.org/about/.

291. Preliminary Report Indicates That The Trevor Project's Suicide Prevention Services Are Effective. 2016. https://www.thetrevorproject.org/2016/11/23/preliminary-report-indicates-that-the-trevor-projects-suicide-prevention-services-are-effective/. Accessed August 28, 2018.

292. *The Trevor Project: Together, Saving Young Lives. Annual Report, August 1, 2014–July 31, 2015*. The Trevor Project; 2017.

293. NIH. About NIH. 2018. https://www.nih.gov/about-nih. Accessed September 8, 2018.

294. NIH. Who We Are: Organization. 2017.

295. NIH. Who We Are. 2018. https://dpcpsi.nih.gov/sgmro. Accessed September 7, 2018.

296. NIH. Sexual and Gender Minority Research Office Annual Report FY17. National Institutes of Health; 2017.

297. NIH. NIH FY 2016–2020 Strategic Plan to Advance Research on the Health and Well-being of Sexual and Gender Minorities. 2015.

298. OutRight. United Nations. 2018. https://www.outrightinternational.org/region/united-nations. Accessed September 9, 2018.

299. OutRight. About Us. 2018. outrightinternational.org/about-us. Accessed September 9, 2018.

300. OutRight. Strategic Framework 2020. 2017.

301. OutRight. Agenda 2030 for LGBTI Health and Well-Being. New York, NY: OutRight; 2017.

302. Daly F. The Global State of LGBTIQ Organizing: The Right to Register. New York, NY: OutRight; 2018.

303. Gottlieb MS, Schanker HM, Fan PT, et al. Pneumocystis pneumonia—Los Angeles. *MMWR Morb Mortal Wkly Rep*. 1981;30(21):250–2.

304. Fernandez F, Ruiz P. Psychiatric aspects of HIV disease. *South Med J*. 1989;82(8):999–1004.

305. Shernoff M. Integrating safer-sex counseling into social work practice. *Soc Casework*. 1988;69(6):334–9.

306. Brock RB. On a nursing AIDS task force: The battle for confident care. *Nurs Manag*. 1986;17(3):67–8.

307. Ramin B. Anthropology speaks to medicine: The case HIV/AIDS in Africa. *Mcgill J Med*. 2007;10(2):127.

308. Holland J, Ramazanoglu C, Scott S. AIDS: From panic stations to power relations sociological perspectives and problems. *Sociology*. 1990;24(3):499–518.

309. Rushing WA. *The AIDS Epidemic: Social Dimensions of An Infectious Disease*. New York: Routledge; 2018.

310. Swenson RM. Plagues, history, and AIDS. *Am Scholar*. 1988:183–200.

311. Hellinger FJ. Forecasting the personal medical care costs of AIDS from 1988 through 1991. *Public Health Rep*. 1988;103(3):309.

312. Altman D. Legitimation through disaster: AIDS and the gay movement. 1987.

313. Gostin LO. Public health strategies for confronting AIDS: Legislative and regulatory policy in the United States. *JAMA*. 1989;261(11):1621–30.

314. LaTour MS, Pitts RE. Using fear appeals in advertising for AIDS prevention in the college-age population. *J Health Care Mark*. 1989;9(3):5–14.

315. Hacker K. *Community-Based Participatory Research*. Los Angeles, CA: Sage Publications; 2013.

316. Israel BA, Schulz AJ, Parker EA, Becker AB. Critical issues in developing and following community-based participatory research principles. In: *Community-Based Participatory Research for Health*. San Francisco, CA: Jossey-Bass; 2008.

317. Minkler M. Ethical challenges for the "outside" researcher in community-based participatory research. *Health Educ Behav*. 2004;31(6):684–97.

318. Fausto-Sterling A. *Sexing the Body: Gender Politics and the Construction of Sexuality*. New York: Basic Books; 2000.

319. Daniel FE. Should insane criminals of sexual perverts be allowed to procreate. *Med-Leg J*. 1893;11:275–92.

320. Hughes CH. An emasculated homo-sexual. His antecedent and post-operative life. *Alienist Neurol*. 1914;35:277–80.

321. LeVay S. *Queer Science: The Use and Abuse of Research into Homosexuality*. Cambridge, MA: MIT Press; 1996.

322. Owensby N. Homosexuality and lesbianism treated with metrazol. *J Nerv Ment Dis*. 1940;92(1):65–6.

323. Gayle R. Newdigate Moreland Owensby, M.D. 1882–1952. *Am J Psychiatry*. 1953;109(8):639–40.

324. Terry J. *An American Obsession: Science, Medicine, and Homosexuality in Modern Society*. Chicago, IL: University of Chicago Press; 1999.

325. Werther R, Herzog AW, Lind E. *Autobiography of An Androgyne*. New York: Medico-legal Journal; 1918.

326. Blumer GA. A case of perverted sexual instinct. *Am J Insan* 1882;39: 22–35.

327. Conrad P, Angell A. Homosexuality and remedicalization. *Society*. 2004;41(5):32--9.

328. King M, Smith G, Bartlett A. Treatments of homosexuality in Britain since the 1950s—An oral history: The experience of professionals. *BMJ*. 2004;328(7437):429–32.

329. Smith G, Bartlett A, King M. Treatments of homosexuality in Britain since the 1950s—An oral history: The experience of patients. *BMJ*. 2004;328(7437):427–9.

330. Drescher J. A history of homosexuality and organized psychoanalysis. *J Am Acad Psychoanal Dyn Psychiatry*. 2008;36(3):443–60.

331. McDonald LL, Thompson WJSroesc, designs, parameters tfep. Sampling rare populations. 2004:11–42.

332. Kalton G, Anderson DW. Sampling rare populations. *J R Stat Soc*. 1986:65–82.

333. Lee RM. *Doing Research on Sensitive Topics*. London: Sage; 1993.

334. Sell RL. Challenges and solutions to collecting sexual orientation and gender identity data. *Am J Public Health*. 2017;107(8):1212–4.

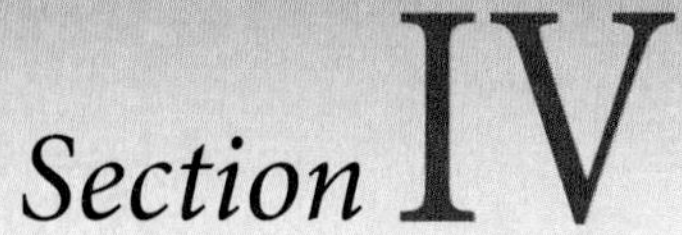

Section Editor
Karen Glanz

Health Behavior, Health Education, and Health Communication

CHAPTER 35

Health Behavior Theories

Karen Glanz • Barbara K. Rimer

Health behavior is central to disease prevention, detection, and treatment management. The leading contributors to disease and death in the United States and globally are behavioral factors, including tobacco use, diet and activity patterns, alcohol consumption, sexual behavior, adherence to medical treatment, and avoidable injuries. Among the most important challenges we face is to understand health behavior and to transform knowledge about behavior into effective strategies for health enhancement. Health behavior research ultimately will be judged by its contributions to improving the behavior and health of populations.[1]

Over the past three decades, experts increasingly have agreed that public health and preventive medicine interventions that are based on social and behavioral science theories are more effective than those lacking a theoretical base. During this period, researchers, practitioners, public health organizations, and funding agencies have come to accept that a theory or theories should be the foundation for well-conceived and effective intervention strategies. The extensive literature in health behavior includes numerous applications of health behavior theory. Thus, we can examine which theories have been most often used over time, and whether use of theory has improved the effectiveness of interventions. Further, systematic reviews and meta-analyses—and systematic reviews of meta-analyses—are available to synthesize the current evidence on theory use and behavior change.[2–4]

This chapter provides an overview of the state-of-the-science of theory use for designing and conducting public health and health promotion interventions. Influential contemporary perspectives stress the multiple determinants and multiple levels of determinants of health and health behavior. We briefly describe selected often-used theories and their key concepts—including the ecological model, health belief model, theory of planned behavior (TPB), transtheoretical model, and social cognitive theory (SCT). This is followed by a review of evidence about patterns and effects of using theory in health behavior intervention research.

EVOLUTION AND TRENDS IN USE OF HEALTH BEHAVIOR THEORIES AND MODELS

The earliest known applications of health behavior theory were the result of social psychologists working in the U.S. Public Health Service in the 1950s trying to understand how to increase participation in programs designed to prevent and detect disease, such as offering chest x-rays to detect tuberculosis.[5] Today, theories have been applied to the development and evaluation of behavioral interventions for many behaviors, for example, adherence to poorly controlled diabetes and hypertension, sun protection and skin self-examination, cancer screening, and oral health promotion (tooth brushing, flossing). Theories have been used to understand and change many behaviors that have emerged more recently or been tied to personal and public health, such as cell phone use while driving, sugar-sweetened beverage consumption, m-health interventions in low- and middle-income countries, promoting HIV serostatus disclosure to sex partners, and climate change risk perceptions. Theory application is also called for in cases where theories have not been used or tested, due to the widely perceived promise of their usefulness.

Theories of health behavior have evolved to reflect an amalgamation of approaches, methods, and strategies from social and health sciences. Collaborations among professionals of different disciplines have led contemporary health behaviors to reflect a blend of perspectives. They draw on the theoretical perspectives, research, and practice tools of such diverse disciplines as psychology, sociology, anthropology, communications, medicine, nursing, economics, and marketing.[1] Health behavior and its close relative in public health—health education/promotion—are also dependent on epidemiology, statistics, and medicine. Today, health behavior, like most disciplines, increasingly is grounded in data science and use of big data and new designs aimed at gaining answers to questions faster.

Theories that gain recognition in a discipline shape the field, help define the scope of practice, and influence the training and socialization of professionals. No single theory or conceptual framework dominates research or practice in contemporary health behavior and health education, but a relatively small number of theories and models are most often used. Sometimes, older theories are given new names with most of the constructs intact.

Over the past three decades, we have reviewed a sample of publications on six different occasions to identify the most often used theories (1988, 1994, 2000, 2005, 2008, and 2019).[1,6] Today, there are tools for reviewing and analyzing published literature that did not exist in the 1980s, most notably online searches on PubMed, Google Scholar, and Web of Science. Simple searches of these databases in mid-2019 attest to the exponential inclusion of health behavior theory in published work: over 18,000 citations on PubMed for "health behavior theory," and more than 3 million hits for the same phrase on Google Scholar. Our most recent updated review of theory use in published research found, similar to a search done a decade ago,[6] that over all, the same theories dominate as did in 2000. As in previous reviews, the most up-to-date review revealed that dozens of theories and models were used, but only a few of them were used in multiple publications or behaviors, and by several authors.

Ten theories or models clearly emerge as the most often used. The first four, and by far the most dominant, are **social cognitive theory**, **the transtheoretical model/stages of change**, **theory of planned behavior**, and the **health belief model**. The remainder of the top ten theories and models are **ecological models/social ecology**, stress and coping, community organization, diffusion of innovations, social support and social networks, and social marketing. Behavioral economics, a blend of economic and psychological

TABLE 35-1 EXAMPLES OF THEORY-BASED INTERVENTION STRATEGIES FOR HEALTH BEHAVIOR CHANGE

Level of Change	Intervention Strategy	Related Theories
Individual	Goal-setting and behavior modification	Social cognitive theory
	Tailoring	Stages of change Health belief model
Interpersonal	Lay health advisors. Community health workers	Social support and Social networks
	Online Support Groups	Social support and Social network
Organizational	Provider reminders and feedback	Social cognitive theory (at the organizational level)
Community	Policy and environmental strategies	Social ecological model

principles, has gained substantial traction in the past decade.[7] The purposes and key constructs/propositions of the **highlighted** theories and models are described briefly in this chapter. These and other theories are also covered elsewhere in this section, in chapters on Health Communications, Social Marketing, Risk Communication, Health Promotion Interventions and Research, and Community-Engaged Research. Selected examples of the application of theoretical constructs in behavior change strategies are shown in Table 35-1.

SOCIAL ECOLOGICAL MODELS

The social ecological model helps to understand factors affecting behavior and provides guidance for developing successful programs through social environments. Social ecological models emphasize multiple levels of influence (such as individual, interpersonal, organizational, community, and public policy). Behaviors both shape and are shaped by the social environment.[8,9]

The principles of social ecological models are consistent with SCT concepts (covered later in this chapter) that suggest initially creating an environment conducive to change is important to making it easier to adopt healthy behaviors. Given the widespread problems of healthy lifestyles in populations, and their role in chronic diseases like diabetes and lung diseases like asthma, more attention is being focused toward increasing the health-promoting features of communities and neighborhoods, especially when there are health inequities. Examples of environmental change strategies for healthful behaviors that are based on social ecological models include reducing exposure to second-hand smoke and high-calorie, high-fat foods in large portions. Changing the healthcare system by giving providers, such as doctors and nurses, reminders, and incorporating brief health counseling in primary care, are other examples of the application of social ecological models to health behavior.

While many public health leaders have highlighted the need to use multilevel models and social ecological frameworks, as one review conducted more than 20 years after the seminal article on these frameworks[8] found, most published articles still describe interventions focused on individual and interpersonal factors.[10] Recent systematic reviews of theory in health behavior also tend to focus on individual level outcomes.[2,3] Indeed, public health practitioners report that they find it challenging to implement complex, multilevel policy, systems, and environmental change interventions due to both cost and the need to collaborate with nontraditional partner organizations.[11] These persistent challenges warrant attention to avoid the embrace of social ecological models being relegated to mere lip-service.

THE HEALTH BELIEF MODEL

The HBM was one of the first theories of health behavior, and remains one of the most widely recognized in the field. The HBM was developed in the 1950s by a group of U.S. Public Health Service social psychologists who wanted to explain why so few people were participating in programs to prevent and detect disease. For example, the Public Health Service was sending mobile x-ray units out to neighborhoods to offer free chest x-rays (screening for tuberculosis).[5] While the service was offered without charge, in a variety of convenient locations, the program had limited uptake. The question was, "Why?"

To find an answer, social psychologists examined what was encouraging or discouraging people from participating in the programs. They theorized that people's beliefs about whether or not they were susceptible to disease, and their perceptions of the benefits of trying to avoid it, influenced their readiness to act.[12]

In ensuing years, researchers expanded upon the HBM constructs and have tested its use across numerous use cases, eventually concluding that six main constructs influence people's decisions about whether to take action to prevent, screen for, and control illness. They showed that people are ready to act if they:

- Believe they are susceptible to the condition (*perceived susceptibility*);
- Believe the condition has serious consequences (*perceived severity*);
- Believe that taking action would reduce their susceptibility to the condition, or its severity (*perceived benefits*);
- Believe the costs of taking action (*perceived barriers*) are outweighed by the benefits;
- Are exposed to cues that prompt action, (e.g., a television ad or a reminder from one's physician to get a mammogram) (*cue to action*); and
- Are confident in their ability to successfully perform an action (e.g., stopping smoking) (*self-efficacy*).

Since health motivation is its central focus, the HBM is a good fit for addressing problem behaviors that evoke health concerns (e.g., cancer screening, influenza vaccinations, high-risk sexual behavior, and the possibility of contracting HIV). Together, the six constructs of the HBM provide a useful framework for designing both short-term and long-term behavior change strategies. When applying the HBM to planning health programs, practitioners should ground their efforts in an understanding of how susceptible the patient, his or her family, or the target population feel to the health problem, whether they believe it is serious, and whether they believe action can reduce the threat at an acceptable cost. Attempting to effect changes in these factors is rarely as simple as it may appear.

High blood pressure screening campaigns often identify people who are at high risk for heart disease and stroke, but who say they have not experienced any symptoms. They do not see the need for medications if they have not experienced symptoms. Because patients do not feel sick, they may not follow instructions to take prescribed medicines or lose weight. The HBM can be useful for developing strategies to deal with noncompliance in such situations. According to the HBM, asymptomatic people may not follow prescribed treatment regimens unless they accept that, though they have no symptoms, they have hypertension (perceived susceptibility). They must understand that hypertension can lead to heart attacks and strokes that could be life threatening (perceived severity). Taking prescribed medication or following a recommended weight loss program will reduce the risks (perceived benefits) without negative side effects or excessive difficulty (perceived barriers). Materials designed to heighten perceived susceptibility while providing reassurance that risk can be lowered without undue side effects can be delivered in a variety of modalities, including print and digital, reminder letters, and/or pill calendars might encourage people to follow their doctors' recommendations (cues to action). For those who have, in the past, had a hard time losing weight or maintaining weight loss, a behavioral contract might help establish achievable, short-term goals to build confidence (self-efficacy).

The health belief model has been critiqued by some authors, who deem it no longer relevant in recent decades. For example, Tanner-Smith and Brown[13] raise concerns that several HBM constructs are weak predictors of behavior, and that the model is not analyzed using methodologically sophisticated approaches. Nevertheless, and perhaps due to the ease of communicating the HBM's core constructs and its intuitively appealing simplicity, the HBM continues to be widely applied. Crude searches of Pubmed and Google Scholar yield about 20,000 citations and more than 700,000 citations in the past decade, respectively. Web of Science citations exceed 10,000 (and thus a citation report over time is not available).

THEORY OF PLANNED BEHAVIOR

Often people's health decisions are influenced by how they view the actions they are considering, and whether they believe important others such as family members or peers would approve or disapprove of their behavior. The theory of planned behavior, which evolved from its predecessor, the theory of reasoned action (TRA), focuses on the relationships between behavior and beliefs, attitudes, subjective norms, and intentions.[14] The concept of perceived behavioral control—which involves the belief about whether one can control his or her performance of a behavior—that is, they may feel motivated if they feel they "can do it," received added attention in TPB. A central assumption of TPB is that "behavioral intentions" are the most important determinants of behavior.[15]

TPB has been applied widely to help understand and explain many types of behavior—not only health-related behaviors. TRA/TPB have been used successfully to predict and explain a wide range of health behaviors and intentions, including smoking, drinking, health services utilization, exercise, sun protection, breastfeeding, substance use, HIV/sexually transmitted disease prevention behaviors and use of contraceptives, mammography, safety helmets, and seatbelts.[14] As predicted, the core constructs of TPB have been found to predict healthy eating such as fruit and vegetable intake and to help explain low-fat milk consumption.[16] Attitudes and behavioral beliefs about health have also been examined within community interventions in schools and communities and found to mediate outcomes of the interventions.[17] The theoretical constructs help explain why some people changed and others did not after exposure to health education programs and communication campaigns.

Although behavioral intentions are central to TPB, there has been some concern that they still are too far-removed to be good predictors of actual behavior. The concept of implementation intentions involves encouraging patients or people receiving an intervention to be very specific about how they would change, including the time frame for change.[14]

Fishbein and colleagues further expanded TRA and TPB to include components from other major behavioral theories, and have proposed use of an integrated behavioral model (IBM).[18] The IBM can be a framework to identify specific belief targets for behavior change interventions in the above conceptualization of experiential and instrumental attitudes, injunctive and descriptive norms, and perceived control and self-efficacy being determined by specific underlying beliefs. Interventions built on one model construct may have effects that further affect the same or other model constructs.[14] While the IBM is a recent expansion of the TPB, it is likely to be more widely used and to have a stronger empirical research base in the coming years.

Like the health belief model, the TPB and the more recent IBM have been criticized for the lack of direct links between the theory and effective behavior change interventions.[19] Despite this criticism, Ajzen—one of the originators of the TRA, TPB, and IBM—asserts that the theory is "alive and well, and not ready to retire,"[15] and a review of recent publications supports this contention. Ajzen notes that a strength of the TBP (and TRA and IBM) has been its openness to evolution over time in response to empirical research; and a weakness of its application has been the lack of sufficient formative research in some studies.[15] The latter issue broadly affects the landscape of applied health behavior theory, as we will come back to again later in this chapter.

THE TRANSTHEORETICAL MODEL AND STAGES OF CHANGE

Long-term behavior change for disease prevention and management involves multiple actions and adaptations over time. Some people may not be ready to attempt changes, while others may already have begun implementing diet modifications. The construct of "stage of change" is a key element of the transtheoretical model of behavior change (TTM), and proposes that people are at different stages of readiness to adopt healthful behaviors or stop harmful ones.[20] The TTM emerged from a comparative analysis of dozens of theories of psychotherapy, in an effort to identify common constructs and themes that helped understand how people changed their behaviors.[20] Readiness to change, or stage of change, has been examined in health behavior research on a variety of topics and found useful in explaining and predicting behavior.

Stages of change is a heuristic model that describes a sequence of steps in successful behavior change: precontemplation (no recognition of need for or interest in change); contemplation (thinking about changing); preparation (planning for change); action (adopting new habits); and maintenance (ongoing practice of new, healthier behavior).[20] People do not always move through the stages of change in a linear manner—they often recycle and repeat certain stages, for example, individuals may relapse and go back to an earlier stage depending on their level of motivation and self-efficacy.

The stages of change model can be used to understand why patients might not be ready to change their behaviors and to improve the success of patient education or other behavior change interventions. Patients can be classified according to their stage of change by asking a few simple questions—in the case of dietary change: are they interested in trying to change their eating patterns, thinking about changing their diet, ready to begin a new eating plan, already making dietary changes, or trying to sustain changes they have been following for some time? By knowing their current stage, a nurse or other health provider can determine how much time to spend with the patient, whether to wait until he or she is more ready to attempt active changes, whether referral for in-depth counseling or case management is warranted, and so on. Knowledge of the patient's current stage of change can also lead to appropriate follow-up questions about past efforts to change, obstacles and challenges, and available strategies for overcoming barriers or obstacles to change.

The transtheoretical model was articulated in the 1980s and gained significant traction in the 1990s. Its enormous popularity led to applications across many behaviors and interventions, and in turn to a number of widely circulated critiques.[21–23] The critiques asserted that the TTM did not work well as a foundation for behavior change programs, that it treated stages as arbitrary categories rather than a continuum, and ultimately that the TTM should be put to rest.[21] A 2019 Web of Science topic search show that publications using the TTM increased to about 100/year in the early 2000s and have continued at a rate of about 120/year from 2005 to the present. Google Scholar shows over 2000 citations to a chapter about TTM published in 2015. It appears that the transtheoretical model continues to be widely respected and used.

SOCIAL COGNITIVE THEORY

SCT, the cognitive formulation of social learning theory that has been best articulated by Bandura,[24,25] explains human behavior in terms of a three-way, dynamic, reciprocal model in which personal factors, environmental influences, and behavior continually interact. SCT synthesizes concepts and processes from cognitive, behavioristic, and emotional models of behavior change, so it can be readily applied to nutritional intervention for disease prevention and management. A basic premise of SCT is that people learn not only through their own experiences but also by observing the actions of others and the results of those actions. Key constructs of SCT that are relevant to health behavior interventions include observational learning, reinforcement, self-control, and self-efficacy.[26]

Principles of behavior modification, which often have been used to promote health behavior change, are derived from SCT. Some elements of behavioral interventions based on SCT constructs of self-control, reinforcement, and self-efficacy include goal-setting, self-monitoring, and behavioral contracting.[12] For habitual behaviors, such as quitting smoking and improving eating patterns, goal setting and self-monitoring seem to be particularly useful components of effective interventions.[17]

Self-efficacy, or a person's confidence in his or her ability to take action and to persist in that action despite obstacles or challenges, seems to be especially important for influencing health behavior change efforts.[25] Health providers can make deliberate efforts to increase patients' self-efficacy using three types of strategies: (1) setting, small, incremental, and achievable goals; (2) using formalized behavioral contracting to establish goals and specify rewards; and (3) monitoring and reinforcement, including patient self-monitoring by keeping records.[1] In group programs, it is possible to easily incorporate activities such as problem-solving discussions, and self-monitoring that are rooted in SCT.

The key SCT construct of reciprocal determinism means that a person can be both an agent for change and a responder to change. Thus, changes in the environment, the examples of role models, and reinforcements can be used to promote healthier behavior. This core construct is also central to social ecological models and in light of the idea that behavior is determined by factors at multiple levels, may be considered more important today than ever before.

HOW HAS THEORY BEEN USED IN HEALTH BEHAVIOR RESEARCH AND PRACTICE? IS IT EFFECTIVE?

Along with the published observations about *which* theories are being used, concerns have been raised about *how* theories are used (or not used) in research and practice.[2,6,27,28] A common refrain is that researchers may not understand how to measure and analyze constructs of health behavior theories[29,30] or that they may pick and choose variables from different theories in a way that makes it difficult to ascertain the role of theory in intervention development and evaluation.[31] Considerable conceptual confusion—among both researchers and practitioners—about interrelationships between related theories and variables has also been observed.[15,32,33] Others have cautioned about the limitations of theory testing because of overreliance on correlational designs,[28] and the paucity of studies that empirically compare more than one theory.[34,35] The difficulty of reliably translating theory into effective interventions to improve clinical effectiveness has led to calls for more pragmatic trials, and increasing attention to the generalizability and translation of interventions into real-world clinical practice[36] and community settings.[37] These are reasonable questions that should encourage us to question *how* we use theory, how we test theory, how we turn theories into interventions, and what conclusions we draw from research.

Use of Theory in Health Behavior Research. Building on our distinctions among the type and degree of theory use,[38] we conducted a review of theory used from 2000 to 2005 that classified articles that employed health behavior theory along a continuum: (1) *informed by theory*: in which a theoretical framework was identified, but no or limited application of the theory was used in specific study components and measures; (2) *applied theory*: in which a theoretical framework was specified and several of the constructs were applied in components of the study; (3) *tested theory*: in which a theoretical framework was specified and more than half the theoretical constructs were measured and explicitly tested, or two or more theories were compared to one another in a study; or (4) *building/creating theory*: in which new or revised/expanded theory was developed using constructs specified, measured, and analyzed in a study.

Of all the theories used in the sample of articles ($n = 69$ articles using 139 theories), 69.1% used theory to inform a study; 17.9% of theories were "applied"; 3.6% were tested; and 9.4% involved building/creating theory.[6] These findings lead us to reaffirm calls by Noar and Zimmerman[34] and Weinstein and Rothman[35] for thorough application and testing of health behavior theories to advance science and move the field forward. Similar observations have been made by Sheeran et al.,[4] Prestwich et al.,[2] and Michie and others[31] also used much more detailed coding schemes for summarizing the use of theory for behavior change interventions and for research to evaluate the outcomes of these interventions, and similarly concluded that most theories are not used fully or in depth.

Use of Theory in Behavioral Interventions and Programs. A further concern relates to the external validity of studies that test theory-based interventions.[39] The difficulty of reliably translating theory into interventions to improve their effectiveness for improving health behavior has led to calls for increased attention to the generalizability and translation of interventions into real-world clinical and public health settings. It is important to ask not only how we use theory, but also how we turn theories into interventions, and how and whether community practitioners are able to implement theory-driven and evidence-based interventions.

Escoffery and colleagues[40] conducted interviews with 59 program development coordinators and 61 recruitment coordinators in National Breast and Cervical Cancer Early Detection Program (NBCCEDP) sites. The main aims of the study were to inventory recruitment and professional development activities of NBCCEDP grantees; to assess the extent to which evidence-based cancer prevention strategies were used; and to understand the bases for and evaluation of these strategies.[41]

The interviews asked respondents if one or more theories were used as a basis for intervention strategies. Responses to open-ended questions were coded by two independent coders. Just under 50% of respondents stated that a theory or theories were used to design the professional development (provider-directed) strategies. The most commonly mentioned theories were adult learning theory, social influence theory, diffusion of innovations, and stages of change. For recruitment, or client-directed strategies, 27% of responding coordinators named one or more theories, including social marketing, stages of change/the transtheoretical model, health belief model, social influence theory, social networks, and peer-to-peer theory. A few people responded by merely listing a concept or term—not a theory; and others said they thought that a theory was used to design the strategy or system, but they did not know what it was called. When asked why particular professional development or recruitment activities were chosen, some of the most common reasons for each were the organization's support, the low cost, and how easy it was to implement the activity.[40]

These findings provide a window to the world of public health practice and indicate that practitioners—in this case, program coordinators—have a moderate level of awareness of theory and theoretical constructs that are used in their interventions. Similar findings were reported recently regarding local health department leaders' experiences planning, implementing, and evaluating complex nutrition and obesity prevention programs for low-income families.[11] The role of theory in program planning and evaluation for these large public health programs is often secondary to practical concerns. This is not surprising, and raises the question of how, and at what level, to integrate theory into large-scale public health programs most effectively.

Are Interventions More Effective if They Are Based on Theory? The empirical question of whether intervention strategies are more effective if they are grounded in theory has been examined in many systematic reviews on various behavioral topics and in several meta-analyses.[42] We reported in an earlier highly cited review article in the *Annual Review of Public Health* that "Increasing evidence suggests that public health and health promotion interventions that are based on social and behavioral science theories are more effective than those lacking a theoretical base."[42] However, the question continues to be examined, with reviews of newly published studies and systematic reviews of meta-analyses. Prestwich and others[2] found that the effectiveness of behavioral interventions grounded in the TTM and SCT were similarly effective, but not more so than interventions developed without an explicit theory base.

Sheeran and others[4] took a different path, and analyzed 204 experiments that tested changes in cognition intended to affect attitudes, norms, and self-efficacy. They found that the included studies resulted in medium-sized changes in intentions and small to medium-sized changes in behavior. Moreover, the effect sizes did not differ systematically in relation to the targeted behavior and methodological rigor of the research. They concluded that this review provides experimental support for predictions based on health behavior theories and supports their role in achieving health behavior change.[4]

Another recent review of published meta-analyses did not find theory-based interventions to be more effective.[3] This review included eight published meta-analyses. Many reviews ($n = 41$) were excluded because they did not conduct meta-analyses on theory versus no theory use.

How, then do we reconcile the conflicting conclusions about the value of health behavior theory? First, different reviews operationalized this question in different ways—so they may each be right, but none provide a full answer to this vexing question. Second, we need to bear in mind the oft-cited concern that applications of theory are often superficial, both with respect to intervention strategies and the research used to test them. And a yes/no conclusion about the utility of health behavior theory may be less meaningful than studies that enable us to discern what works for whom, and under what circumstances.[43]

CONCLUSIONS

There is sufficient evidence from research and practice in public health and preventive medicine to recommend that experts should familiarize themselves with a range of health behavior theories and apply them critically in a variety of settings. This includes applications in clinical settings with individual patients to formulate hypotheses about challenges such as nonadherence as well as developing potential research questions and designing and testing of interventions at a range of levels, including in communities. There are many reasons for both researchers and practitioners to be well versed in the theoretical foundations of health behavior and facile with applying them in their work. Theories are useful during the various stages of planning, implementing, and evaluating interventions. Theories can shape the pursuit of answers to *why? what? how?* Theories can guide the search for *why* people are not following public health and medical advice or not caring for themselves in healthy ways.[1] They can help pinpoint *what* one needs to know before developing and organizing intervention programs. They can provide insight into *how* to shape program strategies to reach people and organizations and make an impact on them. They also help to identify *what* should be monitored, measured, and/or compared in a program evaluation.[38,44,45]

References

1. Glanz K, Rimer BK, Viswanath K, eds. *Health Behavior: Theory, Research, and Practice*. 5th ed. San Francisco, CA: Jossey-Bass; 2015.
2. Prestwich A, Sniehotta FF, Whittington C, et al. Does theory influence the effectiveness of health behavior interventions? Meta-analysis. *Health Psychol.* 2014;33(5):465–74.
3. Dalgetty R, Miller CB, Dombrowski SU. Examining the theory-effectiveness hypothesis: A systematic review of systematic reviews. *Br J Health Psychol.* 2019;24:334–56.
4. Sheeran P, Maki A, Montanaro E, et al. The impact of changing attitudes, norms, and self-efficacy on health-related intentions and behavior: A meta-analysis. *Health Psychol.* 2016;35(11):1178–88.
5. Hochbaum GM. *Public Participation in Medical Screening Programs: A Socio-Psychological Study*. Washington, DC: US Dept. of Health, Education, and Welfare; 1958.
6. Painter JE, Borba CP, Hynes M, Mays D, Glanz K. The use of theory in health behavior research from 2000–2005: A systematic review. *Ann Behav Med.* 2008;35:358–62.
7. Volpp K, Lowenstein G, Asch D. Behavioral economics and health. In: Glanz K, Rimer BK, Viswanath K, eds. *Health Behavior: Theory, Research, and Practice*. 5th ed. San Francisco, CA: Jossey-Bass; 2015, pp. 43–64.
8. McLeroy K, Bibeau D, Steckler A, Glanz K. An ecological perspective on health promotion programs. *Health Educ Q.* 1988;15(4):351–77.
9. Sallis JF, Owen N. Ecological models of health behavior. In: Glanz K, Rimer BK, Viswanath K, eds. *Health Behavior: Theory, Research, and Practice*. 5th ed. San Francisco, CA: Jossey-Bass; 2015:43–64.
10. Golden SD, Earp JA. Social ecological approaches to individuals and their contexts: Twenty years of health education and behavior health promotion interventions. *Health Educ Behav.* 2012;39(3):364–72.
11. Shah HD, Adler J, Ottoson J, Webb K, Gosliner W. Leaders' experiences in planning, implementing, and evaluating complex public health nutrition interventions. *J Nutr Educ Behav.* 2019;51(5):528–38.
12. Glanz K, Rimer BK. *Theory at a Glance: Application to Health Promotion and Health Behavior*. 2nd ed. (monograph). National Cancer Institute, NIH, Public Health Service. US Government Printing Office; 2005; Washington, DC: NIH Publication 05-3896.
13. Tanner-Smith EE, Brown TN. Evaluating the Health Belief Model: A critical review of studies predicting mammographic and pap screening. *Soc Theory Health.* 2010;8(1):95–125.
14. Montano D, Kasprzyk D. Theory of reasoned action, theory of planned behavior, and the integrated behavioral model. In: Glanz K, Rimer BK, Viswanath K, eds. *Health Behavior: Theory, Research, and Practice*. 5th ed. San Francisco, CA: Jossey-Bass; 2015, pp. 95–124.
15. Ajzen I. The theory of planned behaviour is alive and well, and not ready to retire: A commentary on Sniehotta, Presseau, and Araújo-Soares. *Health Psychol Rev.* 2015;9(2):131–7.
16. Booth-Butterfield S, Reger B. The message changes belief and the rest is theory: The "1% or less" milk campaign and reasoned action. *Prev Med.* 2004;39(3):581–8.
17. Glanz K. Current theoretical bases for nutrition intervention and their uses. In: Coulston A, Boushey CJ, eds. *Nutrition in the Prevention and Treatment of Disease*. 2nd ed. Amsterdam, Netherlands: Elsevier Publishers; 2008, pp. 127–38.
18. Fishbein M, Ajzen I. *Predicting and Changing Behavior: The Reasoned Action Approach*. New York: Psychology Press; 2010.
19. Sniehotta FF, Presseau J, Araújo-Soares V. Time to retire the theory of planned behaviour. *Health Psychol Rev.* 2014;8(1):1–7.
20. The transtheoretical model and stages of change. In: Glanz K, Rimer BK, Viswanath K, eds. *Health Behavior: Theory, Research, and Practice*. 5th ed. San Francisco, CA: Jossey-Bass; 2015, pp. 125–48.
21. West R. Time for a change: Putting the transtheoretical (stages of change) model to rest. *Addiction.* 2005;100(8):1036–39.
22. van Sluijs EMF, van Poppel MNM, van Mechelen W. Stage-based lifestyle interventions in primary care: Are they effective? *Am J Prev Med.* 2004;26(4):330–43.
23. Adams J, White M. Why don't stage-based activity promotion interventions work? *Health Educ Res.* 2005;20(2):237–43.
24. Bandura A. *Social Foundations of Thought and Action: A Social Cognitive Theory*. Englewood Cliffs, NJ: Prentice-Hall; 1986.

25. Bandura A. *Self-efficacy: The Exercise of Control.* New York: W.H. Freeman and Company, 1997.
26. Kelder SH, Hoelscher D, Perry CL. How individuals, environments, and health behaviors interact: Social cognitive theory. In: Glanz K, Rimer BK, Viswanath K, eds. *Health Behavior: Theory, Research, and Practice.* 5th ed. San Francisco, CA: Jossey-Bass; 2015, pp. 159–81.
27. Trifiletti LB, Gielen AC, Sleet DA, Hopkins K. Behavioral and social sciences theories and models: Are they used in unintentional injury prevention research? *Health Educ Res.* 2005;20(3):298–307.
28. Weinstein ND. Misleading tests of health behavior theories. *Ann Behav Med.* 2007;33(1):1–10.
29. Marsh KL, Johnson BT, Carey MP. Conducting meta-analyses of HIV prevention literatures from a theory-testing perspective. *Eval Health Prof.* 2001;24(3):255–76.
30. Rejeski WJ, Brawley LR, McAuley E, Rapp S. An examination of theory and behavior change in randomized clinical trials. *Control Clin Trials.* 2000;21(5, Supplement 1):S164–70.
31. Michie S, West R, Campbell R, Brown J, Gainforth H. *ABC of Behaviour Change Theories.* Great Britain: Silverback Publishing; 2014.
32. Rosenstock IM, Strecher VJ, Becker MH. Social learning theory and the health belief model. *Health Educ Q.* 1988;15(2):175–83.
33. Weinstein ND. Testing four competing theories of health-protective behavior. *Health Psychol.* 1993;12(4):324–33.
34. Noar SM, Zimmerman RS. Health behavior theory and cumulative knowledge regarding health behaviors: Are we moving in the right direction? *Health Educ Res.* 2005;20(3):275–90.
35. Weinstein ND, Rothman AJ. Commentary: Revitalizing research on health behavior theories. *Health Educ Res.* 2005;20(3):294–7.
36. Rothwell PM. External validity of randomised controlled trials: "To whom do the results of this trial apply?" *Lancet.* 2005;365(9453):82–93.
37. Rohrbach LA, Grana R, Sussman S, Valente TW. Type II translation: Transporting prevention interventions from research to real-world settings. *Eval Health Prof.* 2006;29(3):302–33.
38. Glanz K, Rimer BK, Lewis FM, eds. *Health Behavior and Health Education: Theory, Research, and Practice.* 3rd ed. San Francisco, CA: Jossey-Bass; 2002.
39. Glasgow RE, Emmons KM. How can we increase translation of research into practice? Types of evidence needed. *Annu Rev Public Health.* 2007;28:413–33.
40. Escoffery C. Inventory and assessment of National Breast and Cervical Cancer Early Detection Programs (NBCCEDP) interventions: Professional development interviews and recruitment interviews. Report to the Centers of Disease Control and Prevention. 2009.
41. Escoffery C, Kegler MC, Glanz K, et al. Recruitment for the National Breast and Cervical Cancer Early Detection Program. *Am J Prev Med.* 2012;42(3):235–41.
42. Glanz K, Bishop DB. The role of behavioral science theory in development and implementation of public health interventions. *Annu Rev Public Health.* 2010;31:399–418.
43. Sheeran P, Klein WMP, Rothman AJ. Health behavior change: Moving from observation to intervention. *Annu Rev of Psychol.* 2017;68:573–600.
44. Glanz K, Rimer BK, Lewis FM, eds. *Health Behavior and Health Education: Theory, Research, and Practice.* 2nd ed. San Francisco, CA: Jossey-Bass; 1996.
45. Glasgow RE, Linnan LA. Evaluation of theory-based interventions. In: Glanz K, Rimer BK, Viswanath K, eds. *Health Behavior: Theory, Research, and Practice.* 4th ed. San Francisco, CA: Jossey-Bass; 2008, pp. 487–508.

CHAPTER 36

Health Communications

Mesfin A. Bekalu • K. Viswanath

Health communication is now considered as critical to understanding and explaining how health behaviors are initiated, changed, and maintained. While communication has always been considered an important mechanism to reinforce or promote health behaviors, transformative developments in information and communication technologies, and their broad and deep penetration make understanding the role of communication central to them. Yet the role of communication is often misunderstood with the assumption that communication has a direct influence on health behaviors. While there are conditions under which that is empirically true, more often communication has a powerful influence on critical antecedents to health behaviors. Understanding the influence of communication on the antecedents and the pathways and mechanisms through which the influence flows is central to studies of health behavior and it is here that health communication theories work in conjunction with health behavior theories.

This chapter will contextualize health communication in social and behavioral change and its potential direct and indirect roles in explaining health behaviors. We will discuss the role of communication as a multilevel phenomenon drawing on the social ecological model[1] as a broad framework and introduce key themes in recent health communication research. These themes include key constructs and hypotheses in health communication and major genres and formats through which health communication has contributed to public health.

HEALTH COMMUNICATION THEORIES

The field of health communication has embraced many theories and models whose roots can be traced to the broader disciplines of communication, social, and behavioral sciences. The decades-old emphasis on evidence-based practice in public health (see Chapter 41 by Mercer) has recently been complemented by the idea that empirical evidence alone is inadequate to direct practice, and that the explanatory and predictive capabilities of theory should be exploited in designing programs and evaluations.[2] Theories, both explanatory and change theories, are helpful to delineate the range of factors that influence and inform the development and implementation of interventions.[3] Specifically, using theory, practitioners and researchers can identify the range of intermediary factors that characterize the link between communication interventions and behaviors.[3]

Below, we will briefly discuss selected communication theories that have been widely used in health particularly in understanding and influencing health behavior at individual and social contextual levels. This is neither meant to be an exhaustive list of theories or models of health communication nor a complete explanation of influence of communication on health behaviors but is meant to be indicative of how communication may influence critical antecedents to health behaviors.

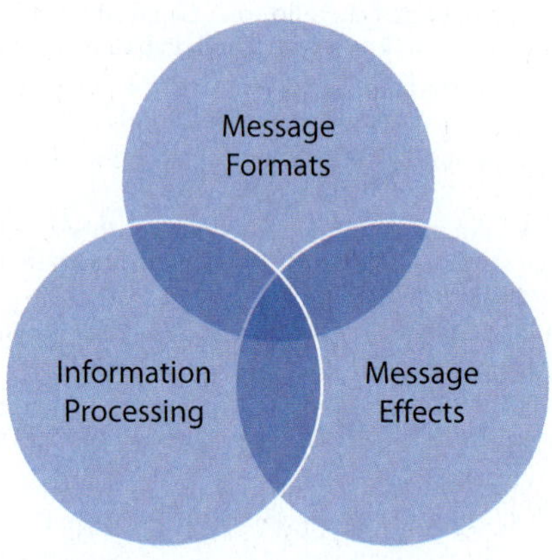

FIGURE 36-1. Three classes of health communication theories.

One challenge facing health communication practitioners and researchers lies in the difficulty of distinguishing between effects that stem from message variability and effects that stem from audience variability.[4] Different theories have been put forward to provide conceptual and analytical frameworks that account for message variability, audience variability, and the resulting communication effects. In strategic communication, the format of a message ("construction") is as crucial, if not more, as its content. Thus, different message formats may be needed for different messages and different audiences. In addition, different messages may require different types and levels of information processing on the part of the message receiver. Information processing may also be affected by various audience-related factors (sociodemographic, cultural, and contextual factors). Figure 36-1 depicts the complex interplay that exists among information processing, message formats, and message effects, and also highlights the interconnectedness of the three.

Message Formats

Message formats refer to the different forms or construction that the content of a given health message can take in order for the message to resonate with the targeted audience. Unlike the content of a message, for example, risk factors for a specific disease condition, message formats focus on how the facts are put together, "constructed," and highlighted or underemphasized depending on the audience. Message formats are useful for tailoring and/or targeting health messages. Messages may be targeted to a subgroup of a population based on the common personal (e.g., values, personality, or preferences) or social [socioeconomic position (SEP) or residential location] characteristics of members of a subgroup or tailored to individuals' characteristics. Message formats in health communication essentially involve the use of empirical evidence that may come through formative research and are also informed by different theories. Below, we will briefly discuss two widely used formats—framing and narratives—to illustrate the role of message formats in health communication.

Message Framing: Framing is a way of organizing messages with an aim to influence perception about how to define and characterize an issue with the goal of persuading a defined audience. Frames are often contested (e.g., issue of abortion as "prochoice" or "prolife") or posed as alternatives. While there are different framing techniques such as temporal[5] and personal/relational,[6] relatively better documentation appears to be available on the relative effectiveness of gain- and loss-framed messages—messages that focus on the benefits of performing a recommended behavior and messages that focus on the costs of failing to perform the behavior, respectively.[7–9] Tracing its tenets to prospect theory,[10] gain versus loss framing has been empirically tested for promoting various health-related behaviors.[11–13] Research on gain versus loss framing has identified differential effectiveness based on the type of health behavior promoted—prevention or detection.[14] Focusing on the risk implications of different types of health behaviors, researchers have proposed a prevention versus detection taxonomy of health behaviors to guide message-framing practices.[14] It has been argued that gain-framed messages should be more effective when people are engaged in deciding whether to adopt a behavior that they perceive as relatively safe and free of undesirable outcomes (e.g., preventing the onset of a health problem), whereas loss-framing should be more effective when individuals are faced with deciding whether to adopt a behavior that they perceive involves some risks of an undesirable outcome (e.g., detecting a health problem). The available empirical evidence, although limited to very few behavioral types, has consistently supported the premise that prevention behaviors would be better promoted by using gain-framed messages.[8] On the contrary, research, albeit limited to cancer screening, has provided support for the proposition that detection behaviors would be better promoted by using loss-framed messages.[8,15] A meta-analytic review of health messages framing research found that gain-framing had small but significant advantage over loss-framing for encouraging prevention behaviors.[12] What was of concern for framing researchers in this meta-analysis was the finding that a significant gain-framed advantage was observed only for dental hygiene behaviors but not for others when the data were examined by behavior type, implying a need for further research in this area.[11]

Narratives: The other widely used message format is narrative versus nonnarrative. Research suggests that compared with the more traditional didactic or factual message format, a narrative format might be more persuasive.[16–18] There is no single definition of narrative universally accepted by researchers. Yet, drawing on themes and concepts that are recurrently used by researchers to describe the term, Kreuter and colleagues define narrative communication as "a representation of connected events and characters that has an identifiable structure, is bounded in space and time, and contains implicit or explicit messages about the topic being addressed."[19] In other words, "a message may be called a narrative if it is a story that contains information about setting, characters, and their motivations."[20] Narrative communication can take different forms: entertainment-education, literature, journalism, testimonials, and story-telling.[19] Specifically, in the context of health communication, researchers have identified five major forms of narratives: "official stories constructed to tell an innocuous version of events or the position of a group, invented stories that are made up or fictional, firsthand experiential stories, secondhand stories of others that we retell, and culturally common stories that are generalized and pervasive in a cultural environment."[17] The theoretical rationale behind the use of narrative communication formats can be summarized in terms of four widely cited hypotheses: transportation, identification, parasocial interaction, and emotion.[21–23]

It is argued that compared to individuals exposed to messages in a non narrative format, those exposed to messages in a narrative format can be drawn into the story and/or transported from the real world into the narrative world, and to the extent they are, they are likely to show effects of the story on their real-world beliefs.[23,24] It is also reasoned that audiences exposed to narratives may identify with story characters, through perceived similarity and wishful identification, and that enhances messages' personal relevance and help overcome perceptions of invulnerability.[23,25] Based on Horton and Wohl's[26] classic notion of parasocial interaction, research on narrative persuasion has also shown that individuals exposed to narratives may engage in a "seeming face-to-face relationship" with story characters that leads to the creation of a unidirectional viewer-character bond which in turn might reduce reactance to message and enhance persuasive effects.[22] Narratives are also theorized to work through emotion.[23] Compared with non narrative messages, narrative messages have the potential to evoke a range of emotions; and messages that elicit emotional reactions are more likely to engender interpersonal conversations through the activation of interpersonal networks that improve message recall.[27,28]

It is argued that due to transportation, identification with characters, parasocial interaction and activation of emotions, messages in a narrative format can result in positive health outcomes as they may reduce resistance and facilitate processing of new or difficult information.[23] A considerable body of health communication research has supported these propositions in cancer prevention—promoting cancer-related outcomes such as HPV vaccine utilization and undergoing cervical and skin cancer screening.[16,25,29–32] In contrast, secular trends show that the entertainment media in general, and movies in particular (forms of narrative communication), have a role in promoting unhealthy behaviors such as smoking and alcohol drinking.[33,34] Research also indicated that the relative persuasiveness of the two formats, narrative and non narrative, depends on different audience-related factors and the specific health behavior being promoted. For instance, a study on processing alcohol education messages among college students found an advantage of non narrative format when the message was congruent with participants' values, and an advantage of narrative format when the message was not congruent (counterattitudinal) with participants' values.[35] Also, a recent meta-analysis found that statistical evidence, a type of non narrative format, had a stronger influence than narrative evidence on beliefs and attitudes, whereas narrative evidence had a stronger influence on intention.[36] This suggested the importance of the match between the specific characteristics of the two formats and those of the outcome—communication effects.

The available literature on the relative effectiveness of narrative versus non narrative formats suggests a need for further research. For example, existing evidence on narrative persuasion does not account for differences in health domain. In a recent study, researchers took issue with the *tacit* assumption that narrative formats are generally more effective than non narratives, and empirically demonstrated that this is not the case at least in public health emergency communication where they found an advantage for a non narrative format in changing knowledge and risk perceptions related to pandemic influenza.[37] They argue that during public health emergencies, such as the outbreak of a deadly influenza, the primary objective of public health professionals is to encourage the public to engage in preventive behaviors against some *imminent threats*. In such a situation, people are less likely to have the time to engage in the kind of message processing required by subtler and elaborate formats such as narratives.[37]

Information Processing

Beyond message formats, there is also the question of how individuals process health messages or health-relevant information, and how that relates to message formats and message effects. Different message formats may engender different styles of information processing and lead to different message exposure outcomes or effects. Below, we will briefly discuss selected information-processing theories that are pertinent to health behavior change.

The elaboration likelihood model (ELM) is a widely studied theory of information processing and behavior change.[38] According to this model, there are two routes to persuasion: the central route and the peripheral route. When a person adopts the central route, s/he takes a logical and conscious thinking to decision-making. This can lead to a *permanent* or long-lasting change in attitude as the individual adopts and elaborates upon the messages' arguments. For this route to be used, the individual should be motivated and have the ability to think about the message. It is reasoned that if a person cares about an issue, then that person engages in conscious processing and elaboration of the information on the issue. On the other hand, if the receiver is not motivated or does not care about the issue, then she or he will use the peripheral route. When this route is used, the individual is somehow swayed by surface characteristics and appeals. Attitude change that results from processing information via the peripheral route is likely to be ephemeral. Here, it might be helpful to look at the threads that weave through the theories of message format, information processing, and communication effects (Fig. 36-1). For example, in line with the propositions of the narrative versus non narrative message format, elaboration likelihood approaches suggest that absorption in a narrative, identification with and response to characters in a narrative, and activation of emotions, should enhance persuasive effects and suppress counterarguing if the implicit persuasive content is counterattitudinal.[39]

The heuristic-systematic model (HSM) is another dual-process model that examines information processing as an antecedent to attitude formation.[40,41] According to HSM, individuals process information using systematic and/or heuristic strategies. Systematic processing takes place when individuals make a judgment by carefully examining, comparing, and relating arguments. In this mode, individuals exert considerable effort in searching information and scrutinizing arguments, maintaining higher standards for the quality of information used in decision-making. In contrast, heuristic processing occurs when individuals are guided by "simple decision rules" to arrive at a judgment about the validity of a message.[40] Simple decision rules might manifest, for example, as agreement with expert opinion, a tendency to agree with perceived social norms, or a willingness to rely on currently available information. It is important to note that decisions made via heuristic processing, as in the ELM, tend to be less stable and less tied to subsequent behavior than decisions reached via systematic efforts. This can have important implications to health communication in terms of the type of message format we choose, the kind of information processing we might want the audience to adopt, and the resulting message effects.

Yet another information-processing theoretical framework is the selective information-processing theory. The assumption that underlies this theory is that the selection and processing of different information is a product of active choice; individuals actively participate in selecting only those stimuli that fulfill their motivational needs.[42] In the context of health communication, audience member's selection and processing of health information should be seen within the broader information environment. Health messages, from planned public communication campaigns to ad hoc programs, enter a crowded media environment filled with messages from competing sources.[43] Health communication practitioners have to capture not only the attention of the public amid such competition, but also motivate them to change health behaviors that are often entrenched or to initiate lifestyle changes that may be new or difficult.[43]

What is less well understood, in the realm of health communication, is how information processing is influenced by structural conditions such as poverty or inequities. Recent work on "scarcity mindset" offers some intriguing insights and hypotheses that are worth exploring.[44] Mullainathan and Shafir argue that "scarcity" (time or money or anything that is perceived in short supply) influences our attention, preferences, choices we make, *deliberations*, and behaviors. If scarcity indeed affects our mental capacity, bandwidth, its influence on how poor people experience cognitive overload and differential attentional allocation in processing information offers some interesting hypotheses worthy of exploration in the future.

Communication Effects

The primary focus of message effect theories is the "acceptance" phase of the communications or "effects" of communication.[45] Selected examples of these theories include the cultivation theory[46] and the knowledge gap hypothesis.[47]

Gerbner's cultivation theory states that heavy viewers of television are more susceptible to media messages and the belief that they are real and valid. One of the important concepts that this theory posits is the concept of *mainstreaming*.[46] In this theory, mainstreaming refers to the power of the media (television, in Gerbner's original propositions) to have similar effects on individuals with high media consumption, regardless of differences in demographic variables. In other words, people from different demographic groups are more likely to have similar belief systems if their media consumption habits are similar. This may have important implications for health communication. These effects of mass media on common world views and belief systems should as posited by cultivation theory, however, must be seen within the wider media ecosystem where digital platforms such as social media networks and personal sites that blend broadcasting with narrowcasting are becoming ubiquitous. In such a case, the breadth to which these common belief systems can be engendered by media and its implications for health communication is question worthy of further research.

On the other hand, the knowledge gap hypothesis states that as the infusion of mass media information into a social system increases, segments of the population with higher socioeconomic status (SES) tend to acquire this information at a faster rate than lower status segments, so that the gap in knowledge between these segments tends to increase rather than decrease.[47] Several early studies on which the knowledge gap hypothesis was based provided empirical support for this hypothesis. However, several other investigations indicated that infusing information into a social system through the mass media did not always create gaps between segments of the population with higher and lower SES, often indicated by educational level; some of these interventions even closed the gap. This inconsistency has led to the exploration of other factors that may be responsible for the differential effects of mass media information campaigns and number of studies have identified various motivational factors, such as concern, attention, salience, and participation, which may be responsible for the knowledge gap phenomenon.[48,49] Studies suggested that motivation can overpower education in predicting knowledge gaps, but other investigators have maintained that the knowledge gap is better predicted by a combination of factors (including group membership, perceived information functionality, motivation, and education) rather than by motivation alone.[50] Overall, over the past decades, this hypothesis has remained a powerful conceptual tool for many investigators who have studied the differential impacts of mass media communication campaigns among different segments of a social system.[51,52] The hypothesis has also given the intellectual ferment for the development of a more recent health-focused model named the *structural influence model* (*SIM*) where structurally induced differential effects of health-related media and messages or communication inequalities (see details below) are hypothesized to go beyond knowledge gaps to include affective and behavioral outcomes.[53]

CONTEXT OF HEALTH COMMUNICATION IN SOCIAL AND BEHAVIORAL CHANGE

Now that we have seen the three main strands of health communication theories (message formats, information processing, and communication effects), it may help to place health communication in

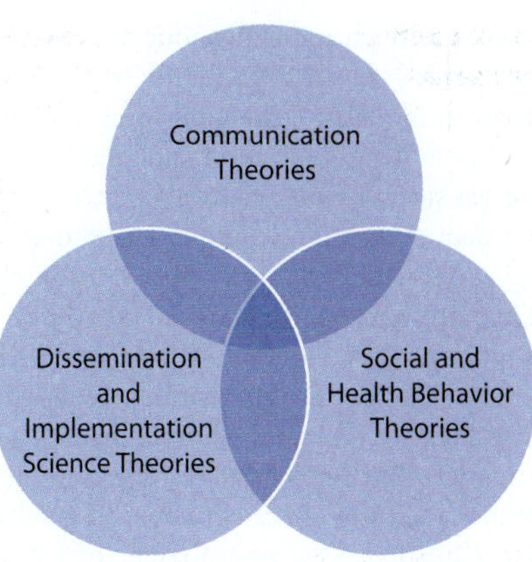

FIGURE 36-2. Three classes of theories that inform behavior change communication (BCC).

the context of planned social change. We argue that three classes of theories inform social and behavioral change: communication theories, social and health behavior theories, and dissemination and implementation theories (Fig. 36-2). Communication theories draw from and contribute to social and health behavior theories, specifically in influencing key mechanisms leading to social and behavioral change. For example, the Integrated Model of Behavior[54] can be used to identify key normative beliefs that could be changed to influence norms, which in turn could lead to promoting desirable behavioral intentions. It is well known that knowing what significant others (peers, family, and friends) do and whether they approve influences a person's beliefs and behaviors. Through strategic communication that promotes or even amplifies what similar others think and how they act, messages can have a powerful effect on an individual or group's perceptions leading to social change. Or communication may promote self-efficacy and skills to ensure that intentions lead to behaviors.[55] A variety of communication theories that discuss message formats such as framing or narratives (discussed above) can inform how to target the beliefs to influence norms.

As shown in Fig. 36-2, dissemination and implementation (D&I) theories are one of the three classes of theories that inform social and behavioral change. D&I theories and models provide a systematic method for understanding, operationalizing, and evaluating the dissemination and implementation of evidence-based interventions that facilitate or promote social and behavioral change. Communication theories also contribute to D&I theories such as when models such as Diffusion of Innovations may identify and target key influentials in a system to persuade others to adapt evidence-informed programs or innovations. There are more than 60 models of D&I theories or frameworks[56] and it is hard to argue that communication is central to all of them. Communication is, nonetheless, essential to promoting the awareness of the evidence-base in easing resistance or promoting legitimacy for change and reinforcing the innovation. Communication and social and behavioral theories may work in tandem with each other to promote the adaption of evidence-base programs. While our main purpose here is to broadly map the three classes of theories within which health communication should be seen, it must be noted that there is an inherent interconnectedness or overlap among these three classes of theories and the boundaries are somewhat porous as work in one class informs the development of work in the other classes of theories.

LEVELS OF ANALYSIS AND HEALTH COMMUNICATION THEORIES

Health communication programs and evaluations may be targeted at factors, processes, and outcomes that operate at just one, or two or more of the following four levels: individual, interpersonal, organizational, and community or sociocultural.[3] Health communication theories may therefore be employed to understand the nature of factors, processes, and outcomes that operate at the four levels and to inform the implementation of strategies to modify or change them.

Individual Level

At the individual level, health communication research may involve the study of communication-specific behaviors such as health information seeking behavior (HISB) and the factors associated with it. Theories may be applied to explore and delineate individual-level demographic (such as age and gender) and psychographic (such as values, opinions, interests, and beliefs) factors that are associated with HISB. Increasing understanding of these factors is important because it provides guidance on how to design effective communication interventions aiming to influence HISB. However, efforts need to go beyond empirically determining the factors associated with HISB. Using an existing theory or formulating one will be helpful to explain why certain social and individual factors influence the health outcome of interest, HISB, for example, and to make predictions about the likelihood of finding the same associations in other contexts and times. Health communication programs targeting factors at the individual level may be informed by most of the widely used behavioral theories such as the health belief model (HBM) and the stages of change (transtheoretical) model. For example, in HBM, individuals' perceptions of *threat, severity, benefits,* and *barriers* are the central constructs that determine the adoption of a recommended health behavior. As such, using HBM, communication efforts may target to modify individual's perceptions so that perceived threat and severity of a given health problem and the benefits of recommended action outweigh perceived barriers to action.[57] Health communication programs targeting individual-level factors may be useful in addressing risk behaviors of individuals such as tobacco, alcohol, and drug addiction. Because the target is an individual behavior, the communication media used in such programs often include one-to-one discussion, telephone calls, emails, and other activities that allow *personal listening* and *response.*[58]

Interpersonal Level

At the interpersonal level, health communication may focus on how two or more people interact and influence one another relevant to health-related outcomes. For example, research in adolescent risk behavior ranging from substance use such as smoking and drinking to sexual initiation has consistently supported the idea that adolescents' adoption of risk behaviors is partly a function of interactions with close peers.[59] Health communication may contribute to influencing the communications among individuals to encourage healthy behaviors or discourage unhealthy behaviors as many antismoking behaviors have done.

A good deal of health communication work addressing factors at the interpersonal level exists in patient-health provider communication where parties interact to create interpersonal relationships, exchange information, and make treatment-related decisions.[60,61] Several theories drawn from health economics and medical sociology have been used to study this type of communication. For example, the principal-agent model posits that the patient-physician communication is characterized by information asymmetry: the physician has more information about the patient's health status and the available treatments, whereas the patient holds better knowledge about how these treatment options fit with her or his lifestyle.[62,63] The latter, of course, is now increasingly under challenge given the advent of patient advocacy movement amplified by health information available on the Internet. Moreover, theories of medical sociology such as paternalism, informed and shared decision models offer important explanatory concepts to the study of patient-provider communication. Paternalism represents a type of interaction in which the doctor, as an expert, decides on the appropriate treatment without involving the patient in the decision-making process. The informed and shared decision models have been proposed as a reaction to the paternalism model and represent some form of patient involvement in the treatment decision-making process. Such models enable us to better understand not only the quantity and quality of communication between a patient and his or her healthcare provider, but also the level and nature of communication outcomes such as patient satisfaction, likelihood of treatment adherence, and thus the resulting health-related outcomes.

Although much of patient-physician communication has changed over the past several decades in the framework of wider healthcare reforms that advocated for a more active, autonomous and thus patient-centered role for the patient, to what extent and how this change manifests itself in the healthcare systems of low- and middle-income countries appears to be worth investigating. Unlike the situation in high-income countries, patient-provider communication may be marred by factors such as shortage of medical personnel (and thus insufficient time for patients), patients' access and use of health information, and other sociocultural and structural conditions.

Overall, unlike the individual-level field of influence, the purpose of health communication programs at the interpersonal level is to understand the factors and processes involved in the interaction among two or more parties and the health-related outcomes that emanate from such interaction among the parties. The focus of change here is not just an individual, but between and among individuals as in the case with improvements in cancer screening or treatment adherence outcomes that result from peer-to-peer or physician-to-patient interpersonal interactions.

Social Media and Social Networks: Related to the interpersonal level of analysis, it is worth remembering that interactions are not always real-life and face-to-face. Online social networks are increasingly complementing and, in some cases, replacing face-to-face interactions. In the United States, about seven-in-ten individuals use social media to connect with one another, receive news content, share information, and entertain themselves.[64] This widespread use may hold promises for strategic communication efforts that seek to promote healthy lifestyles and/or discourage risk behaviors. Social media may provide individuals with a platform that overcomes barriers of distance and time to connect and reconnect with others and thereby expand and strengthen their offline networks.[65] Yet, studies also suggest that social media use is associated with mental health issues such as depression, self-esteem, and "Internet addiction," especially among adolescents and young adults.[66] While further research is needed to characterize how and to what extent social media use results in such health problems, what is happening now with social media use appears to mimic what has happened with television viewership in the 1970s and 1980s, where television has been considered as responsible for shaping, or "cultivating" perceptions of the world as more violent and intimidating than it actually is among heavy viewers.[46]

Notwithstanding, the widespread use of social media or social networking sites over the past decades has brought about a renewed, multidisciplinary research interest into the role of social networks in human health behavior and outcomes. For health communication research, this development has indeed brought about not only a renewed interest but also the need to re-examine and re-evaluate existing assumptions about interpersonal communication, social influence, and the resulting health behavioral outcomes.

Some examples may be helpful here. First, the commonsense conclusion that greater connectivity between individuals within a network's community and between communities would result in greater information sharing and social influence has been challenged by recent data.[67] Going beyond simple simulation of patterns of information transmission, findings from recent big data studies suggest that dense networks may yield less social influence than sparse networks.[67,68] This finding alludes to the fact that information transmission involves much more dynamic and complex processes than what most people assume. Information transmission is not just the same as network models of infection transmission that assume passive exposure is sufficient. Online social networks often rely on communication via social media platforms that is less dynamic and interactive than communication in offline, face-to-face encounters. Social influence as a function of information transmission through a social network requires acceptance on the part of the receiver and the deliberate acts of transmission and retransmission by the sender.[67]

Second, while research in health communication and behavioral sciences has long dealt with "factors" to build theoretical, conceptual, and statistical models, the connectivity property of networks shifts focus from factors to actors.[67] Because actors in a network are connected or interact in some way, what may be of interest for health communication at the interpersonal level of influence are not only the factors associated with each actor, but also the interaction between or among the actors.

Third, in social networks, users may experience and interact with recommendation systems, which are kinds of interpersonal communication that offer new venues of normative influence. These systems may therefore be considered as representations of the world of social influence through pseudointerpersonal forms.[67,69,70] What is more, messages in social media can be narrowcast or broadcast: information may be shared within a small group of network members (narrowcast) or with the entire network members (broadcast). This would require examining how the content of interpersonal communication changes as it moves from traditional personal exchanges to broader audiences.[67] Overall, the *virtual* social network that has tremendously changed the way we interact with each other has brought both challenges and opportunities for health communication practitioners and researchers in studying communication outcomes at the interpersonal level of influence.

Organizational Level

At the organizational level, health communication research may examine how communication among a group of people influences health behavior. Unlike the interpersonal level of analysis, the focus of this level of analysis is communication among a group of people as facilitated or constrained by organizational hierarchies, norms or cultures, and other factors such as the formal and informal communication channels of the organization. It is now widely acknowledged that positive social interactions in organizations are crucial for employees' well-being.[71] People spend a lot of time communicating with their colleagues each day, and this sets an exciting research agenda to explore how such communications are facilitated or constrained by organizational norms, rules and cultures, and influence health behaviors. Health communication programs focusing on this level of analysis may be informed by organizational theories (ranging from Max Weber's theory of fixed structures to the more contemporary poststructuralist theories) as well as behavior change theories (such as the social learning theory, theory of reasoned action and its extension, the theory of planned behavior). These theories may be used to understand how organizational-level communication is associated with health-related behavioral outcomes. For example, research has shown that perceived social influence from co-workers indirectly influences people's health behaviors through their perceived social support from their co-workers, as well as through their organizational socialization.[72] Here, it should be noted that perceived social support or organizational socialization may not be seen only in relation to individuals' interactions (as is the case at the interpersonal level) but in the context of various organizational factors such as organizational norms, communication infrastructure, organizational size, complexity, and the quantity and quality of intraorganizational communication.

Besides drawing from organizational, social, and health behavior theories, health communication programs and evaluations at this level of influence may also be informed by dissemination and implementation models and theories. For example, a new evidence-based behavior change strategy aiming to promote physical activity in an organization could easily be disseminated and implemented through the organization's structural arrangements. Similarly, an evidence-based communication intervention that aims to influence normative beliefs about a given health behavior, for example, vaccination uptake, in an organization can draw on health behavior theories such as the integrated model and be disseminated and implemented using the organization's existing formal and informal communication channels. The focus of health communication programs and evaluations at this level will be the determinants of health behavior at organizational level. Because organization is the level of analysis, communication-induced changes in health-related behaviors and their antecedents are sought and measured at the organizational level. One may study the effects of "naturally occurring" communications in organizations by examining the quality and quantity of information that flows through the formal organizational channels as well as the information that flows through informal communication channels. Similarly, strategic communications such as campaigns can be mounted aiming at changing the determinants of specific health-related behaviors, such as organizational norms or beliefs related to smoking or physical inactivity.

Community and Societal Level

At the community and societal level, health communication addresses how communication contributes to health behavior change within the constraints of the larger community and society.[3] The driving hypothesis underlying this level of analysis is that societal characteristics such as the size of the population, number and range of institutions, and distribution of resources such as wealth, status, and income influence the generation and circulation of messages including on health and the impact of the messages on diverse groups in the system.

One body of work has focused on how community characteristics influence how messages are generated and circulated and how this may influence knowledge and behavior of those exposed to these messages. For example, large communities are heterogeneous, usually have a range of institutions that generate messages (e.g., media, hospitals, and educational institutions) compared to relatively smaller communities. Community size and heterogeneity or degree of community differentiation, in turn, may influence interactions and provide opportunities for learning among different audiences.[73] Here, health communication research and interventions may target the complex interplay among community ties, community integration, community heterogeneity, and health-related media use.

Much of the focus of health communication research and practice at this level has been on mass media communications efforts. Such efforts involve studying or addressing the effects of *intended* strategic communications through the different mass media channels or platforms as well as the *unintended* harmful or beneficial effects of media and messages on health-related outcomes in secular communication contexts such as the news media and the entertainment media. Intended or unintended, mass media messages have the capacity to reach broad cross-section of population and shape public attitudes and beliefs toward health-related behaviors. In strategic communications, mass media can be used to deliver campaign messages or public service announcements to raise awareness or risk perceptions related to pandemics or noncommunicable public health problems such as tobacco or drug use. In secular communication contexts, the news media has the capacity to set and frame public health issues and thereby influence public cognitions and perceptions. Research in agenda-setting and framing theories indicates that mass media have tremendous power not only to set issues on the public agenda but also to frame issues and influence people how to think about them.[74] Similarly, entertainment media (the movies) containing risk behaviors such as smoking, drinking, or violence can influence attitudes and perceptions related to these behaviors through observational learning or modelling. These types of intended or unintended health-related outcomes are sought and addressed at the community or societal level of analysis.

Although health communication at the community or societal level would normally be expected to influence health behavior across the board, communication outcomes are not always uniform across population groups. For example, not all social groups benefit equally from health communication programs. Extensive documentation shows that social groups differ in access to and use of relevant health information—a phenomenon termed as *communication inequalities*.[53] Defined as differences in access and use, attention, retention, and capacity to act on relevant information among social groups, communication inequalities may lead to health disparities and/or exacerbate existing gaps in health-related outcomes among population groups. Health communication programs addressing communication inequalities may draw on the structural influence model of health communication (SIM).[75] The premise of the SIM is that "audiences attend and react to mediated content based on their structural location in the environment and the social roles they play at any given time."[75] This model attempts to encapsulate a body of work that views media and message effects from a more structural or macrosocial perspective. It goes beyond the more conventional reductionist view of media and message effects that focuses on outcomes at the individual level. The model posits that structural antecedents, such as SEP and geography, determine both the information environment and the resources that are available for consumption and suggests that communication may have a role in linking social determinants with health outcomes.[75]

So far, we described the four levels of analysis at which health communication programs and evaluations may be targeted. At each level, different theories may be used to enhance understanding of the factors associated with behavioral outcomes. However, health communication programs and evaluations may also be implemented and evaluated at all four levels. In this case, the social-ecological model stands out as a useful framework to study cross-cutting factors at all levels.[76] According to this model, individual behavior is a product of multiple, overlapping social and environmental influences. It does not only recognize that factors at multiple levels influence behavior but also underscores that influences interact across levels. The model stresses the need to expand interventions into an organized sustainable social movement.

In contextualizing health communication within the broader disciplines of social and behavioral sciences, it may also help to highlight the potential constructs that are amenable to change through health communication efforts. As we pointed out earlier, health communication has seldom been shown to impact health behavior directly, hence our potential constructs that are amenable to change are largely the factors that characterize the link between health communication interventions and behavioral outcomes. We will highlight these factors drawing on the integrative model of behavior (IMB). This model integrates the variables in the most commonly used theories, such as the health belief model, social cognitive theory, and the theory of reasoned action (of which the IMB is an extension).

IMB posits that a behavior is most likely to occur if an individual has a strong intention to perform the behavior, if he or she has the necessary skills and abilities required to perform the behavior, and does not face environmental constraints that would prevent him/her from performing the behavior.[54] According to this model, there are three main determinants of behavior: intention, skills, and environmental constraints. Of these three, previous research has shown that intention can be influenced by targeted health communication efforts.[77,78] Yet, the influence may not be direct. According to IMB, intention to perform a given behavior can be a function of three factors: one's attitude toward the behavior, perceived norms concerning the behavior, and one's self-efficacy with respect to performing the behavior.[54] The model posits that these factors are themselves a function of underlying beliefs regarding the outcomes of the behavior in question, the normative proscriptions of specific referents and specific barriers to (or factors that facilitate) behavioral performance. These, in turn, may be dictated by demographic, personality, attitudinal, and other individual differential variables as well as culture and exposure to media and interventions.[54] Health communication programs may therefore target the underlying beliefs regarding the outcomes of the health behavior in question, the normative proscriptions of specific referents and specific barriers to (or factors that facilitate) behavioral performance. For methodological or measurement reasons, the actual targets will be the manifestations or realizations of these underlying beliefs: attitudes, normative and self-efficacy beliefs—the proximal determinants of intention. Overall, be it through a well-planned, theory-based intervention or an *ad hoc* health communication program, the constructs that are amenable to change through health communication lie largely within the cognitive (awareness and knowledge) and affective (attitudes, emotions, beliefs, and perceptions) domains.

CONCLUSIONS AND FUTURE DIRECTIONS

The aim of this chapter has been to place health communications in its broader context and connect it to population health and health behaviors. The goal here was to provide a selective introduction to various communications constructs and hypotheses and to map communication in relation to studying health behaviors with the argument that communication could influence critical intervening mechanisms leading to behavior change and the various levels at which health communication may play a role.

The broad and deep penetration of information and communication technologies poses an interesting challenge to health communication and health behavior theories. From a philosophy of science perspective, it is not clear how these theories have to be adapted, refined, modified, or even rejected in light of the communication revolutions. Today's communications landscape is characterized by the generation of vast amounts of data or "information" (not necessarily communication) and "proliferation" of delivery platforms through which people are exposed to and access information or communicate with people and systems.[79] Both features have important implications for health communication. For example, the sheer amount of data or information provides a significant challenge to our ability to process the information, make sense of it, and apply it to specific contexts and behaviors. The extent to which these stages of processing, sense-making, and application is influenced by interpersonal, social network, and structural conditions remains to be theorized. Similarly, the large number of delivery platforms and information delivery services have opened up possibilities of reaching the audiences, yet the impact of "always on" nature of communications whether through messaging services or social media on our mental, physical, and social health and well-being is now only beginning to be explored. In addition, the fact that access to most platforms is differential across different SES groups, communication inequalities, calls for more systematic research. It is these knowable yet unexplored questions that make health communications and health behaviors preoccupy our attention over the next decades.

References

1. Sallis JF, Owen N, Fisher EB. Ecological models of health behavior. In: Glanz K, Rimer BK, Viswanath K, eds. *Health Behavior and Health Education: Theory, Research, and Practice*. San Francisco, CA: Jossey-Bass; 2015, pp. 43–64.
2. Green J. The role of theory in evidence-based health promotion practice. *Health Educ Res*. 2000;15(2):125–9.
3. Glanz K, Rimer BK, Viswanath K, eds. *Health Behavior and Health Education : Theory, Research, and Practice*. Vol 5. San Francisco, CA: Jossey-Bass; 2015.
4. Southwell BG. Between messages and people: A multilevel model of memory for television content. *Commun Res*. 2005;32(1):112–40.
5. Bonner C, Newell BR. How to make a risk seem riskier : The ratio bias versus construal level theory. *Judgment and Decision Making*. 2008;3(5):411–6.
6. Ko DM, Kim HS. Message framing and defensive processing: A cultural examination. *Health Commun*. 2010;25(1):61–8.
7. Abhyankar P, O'Connor DB, Lawton R. The role of message framing in promoting MMR vaccination: Evidence of a loss-frame advantage. *Psychol Health Med*. 2008;13(1):1–16.
8. Rothman AJ, Bartels RD, Wlaschin J, Salovey P. The strategic use of gain- and loss-framed messages to promote healthy behavior: How theory can inform practice. *J Commun*. 2006;56.
9. Schneider TR. Getting the biggest bang for your health education buck. *Am Behav Sci*. 2006;49(6):812–22.
10. Tversky A, Kahneman D. The framing of decisions and the psychology of choice. *Science*. 1981;211(4481):453–8.
11. Latimer AE, Salovey P, Rothman AJ. The effectiveness of gain-framed messages for encouraging disease prevention behavior: Is all hope lost? *J Health Commun*. 2007;12(7):645–9.
12. O'Keefe DJ, Jensen JD. The relative persuasiveness of gain-framed and loss-framed messages for encouraging disease prevention behaviors: A meta-analytic review. *J Health Commun*. 2007;12(7):623–44.
13. Bekalu MA, Eggermont S. The relative persuasiveness of gain-framed versus loss-framed HIV testing message: Evidence from a field experiment in Northwest Ethiopia. *J Health Commun*. 2014;19(8):922–38.
14. Rothman AJ, Salovey P. Shaping perceptions to motivate healthy behavior: The role of message framing. *Psychol Bull*. 1997;121(1):3–19.
15. Rothman AJ, Updegraff JA. Specifying when and how gain-and loss-framed messages motivate healthy behavior: An integrated approach. In: Keren G, ed. *Perspectives on Framing*. London: Psychology Press/Taylor & Francis; 2010.
16. Murphy ST, Frank LB, Chatterjee JS, et al. Comparing the relative efficacy of narrative vs nonnarrative health messages in reducing health disparities using a randomized trial. *Am J Public Health*. 2015;105(10):2117–23.
17. Hinyard LJ, Kreuter MW. Using narrative communication as a tool for health behavior change: A conceptual, theoretical, and empirical overview. *Health Educ Behav*. 2007;34(5):777–92.
18. Kreuter MW, Holmes K, Alcaraz K, et al. Comparing narrative and informational videos to increase mammography in low-income African American women. *Patient Educ Couns*. 2010;81(1):S6–14.
19. Kreuter MW, Green MC, Cappella JN, et al. Narrative communication in cancer prevention and control: A framework to guide research and application. *Arch Behav Med*. 2007;33:221–35.
20. Braddock K, Dillard JP. Meta-analytic evidence for the persuasive effect of narratives on beliefs, attitudes, intentions, and behaviors. *Commun Monogr*. 2016;7751(March):1–24.
21. Moyer-Gusé E. Toward a theory of entertainment persuasion: Explaining the persuasive effects of entertainment-education messages. *Commun Theory*. 2008;18(3):407–25.
22. Moyer-Gusé E, Nabi RL. Explaining the effects of narrative in an entertainment television program: Overcoming resistance to persuasion. *Hum Commun Res*. 2010;36(1):26–52.
23. Murphy ST, Frank LB, Chatterjee JS, Baezconde-Garbanati L. Narrative versus nonnarrative: The role of identification, transportation, and emotion in reducing health disparities. *J Commun*. 2013;63(1):116–37.
24. Green MC, Brock TC. The role of transportation in the persuasiveness of public narratives. *J Pers Soc Psychol*. 2000;79(5):701–21.
25. Frank LB, Murphy ST, Chatterjee JS, Moran MB, Baezconde-Garbanati L. Telling stories, saving lives: Creating narrative health messages. *Health Commun*. 2015;30(2):154–63.
26. Horton D, Wohl RR. Mass communication and para-social interaction: Observations on intimacy at a distance, *Psychiatry*. 1956;19:215–29.
27. McQueen A, Kreuter MW, Kalesan B, Alcaraz KI. Understanding narrative effects: The impact of breast cancer survivor stories on message processing, attitudes, and beliefs among African American women. *Heal Psychol*. 2011;30(6):674–82.
28. Ramanadhan S, Nagler RH, McCloud R, Kohler R, Viswanath K. Graphic health warnings as activators of social networks: A field experiment among individuals of low socioeconomic position. *Soc Sci Med*. 2017; 175:219–27.
29. Moran MB, Murphy ST, Frank L., Baezconde-garbanatil L. The ability of narrative communication to address health-related social norms. *Int Rev Soc Res*. 2013;3(2). 131–49.

30. Lemal M, den Bulck JV. Testing the effectiveness of a skin cancer narrative in promoting positive health behavior: A pilot study. *Prev Med (Baltim)*. 2010;51(2):178–81.
31. Borrayo EA, Rosales M, Gonzalez P. Entertainment-education narrative versus nonnarrative interventions to educate and motivate Latinas to engage in mammography screening. *Health Educ Behav*. 2016;44(3):394–402.
32. Stavrositu CD, Kim J. All blogs are not created equal: The role of narrative formats and user-generated comments in health prevention. *Health Commun*. 2014;236(September):1–11.
33. Sargent JD, Morgenstern M, Isensee B, Hanewinkel R. Movie smoking and urge to smoke among adult smokers. *Nicotine Tob Res*. 2009;11(9):1042–6.
34. Bekalu MA, Viswanath K. Smoking portrayal in Ethiopian movies: A theory-based content analysis. *Health Promotion International*, 2019;34(4):687-696.
35. Slater MDM, Rouner D. Value-affirmative and value-protective processing of alcohol education messages that include statistical evidence or anecdotes. *Commun Res*. 1996;23(2):210–35.
36. Zebregs S, van den Putte B, Neijens P, de Graaf A. The differential impact of statistical and narrative evidence on beliefs, attitude, and intention: A meta-analysis. *Health Commun*. 2014;236(August 2014):1–8.
37. Bekalu MA, Bigman CA, McCloud RF, Lin LK, Viswanath K. The relative persuasiveness of narrative versus non-narrative health messages in public health emergency communication: Evidence from a field experiment. *Prev Med*. 2018;111:284–90.
38. Petty RE, Cacioppo JT. The elaboration likelihood model of persuasion. *Adv Exp Soc Psychol*. 1986;19(C):123–205.
39. Slater MD, Rouner D. Entertainment-education and elaboration likelihood: Understanding the processing of narrative persuasion. *Commun Theory*. 2002;12(2):173–91.
40. Trumbo CW. Heuristic-systematic information processing and risk judgment. *Risk Anal*. 1999;19(3):391–400.
41. Chaiken S, Liberman A, Eagly AHH. Heuristic and systematic information processing within and beyond the persuasion context. In: Uleman JS, Bargh JA, eds. *Unintentent Thought*. New York: The Guilford Press; 1989, Chapter 16, pp. 212–52.
42. Dutta MJ. Health information processing from television: The role of health orientation. *Health Commun*. 2007;21(1):1–9.
43. Randolph W, Viswanath K. Lessons learned from public health mass media campaigns: Marketing health in a crowded media world. *Annu Rev Public Health*. 2004;25:419–37.
44. Mullainathan S, Shafir E. *Scarcity: Why Having Too Little Means So Much*. New York: Henry Holt and Company; 2013.
45. Cappella JN. Integrating message effects and behavior change theories: Organizing comments and unanswered questions. *J Commun*. 2006;56(Suppl):S265–79.
46. Gerbner G, Gross L, Morgan M, Signorielli N. Living with television: The dynamics of the cultivation process. *Perspect media Eff*. 1986:17–40.
47. Donohue GA, Tichenor PJ, Olien CN. Mass media and the knowledge gap: A hypothesis reconsidered. *Commun Res*. 1975;2(1):3–23.
48. Viswanath K, Finnegan JR. The knowledge gap hypothesis: Twenty-five years later. *Ann Int Commun Assoc*. 1996;19(1):187–228.
49. Kwak N. Revisiting the knowledge gap hypothesis: Education, motivation, and media use. *Commun Res*. 1999;26(4):385–413.
50. Viswanath K, Kahn E, Finnegan JR, Hertog J, Potter JD. Motivation and the knowledge gap: Effects of a campaign to reduce diet-related cancer risk. *Commun Res*. 1993;20(4):546–63.
51. Niederdeppe J. Beyond knowledge gaps: Examining socioeconomic differences in response to cancer news. *Hum Commun Res*. 2008;34(3):423–47.
52. Slater MD, Hayes AF, Reineke JB, Long M, Bettinghaus EP. Newspaper coverage of cancer prevention: Multilevel evidence for knowledge-gap effects. *J Commun*. 2009;59(3):514–33.
53. Viswanath K, Ramanadhan S, Kontos E. Mass media. In: *Macrosocial Determinants of Population Health*. New York: Springer; 2007.
54. Fishbein M, Yzer M. Using theory to design effective health behavior interventions. *Commun Theory*. 2003;13:164–83.
55. Montaño DE, Kasprzyk D. Theory of reasoned action, theory of planned behavior, and the integrated behavioral model. In: Glanz K, Rimer BK, Viswanath K, eds. *Health Behavior: Theory, Research, and Practice*. San Francisco, CA: Jossey-Bass; 2015, pp. 95–124.
56. Tabak RG, Khoong EC, Chambers DA, Brownson RC. Bridging research and practice: Models for dissemination and implementation research. *Am J Prev Med*. 2012;43(3):337–50.
57. Becker MH, Radius SM, Rosenstock IM, Drachman RH, Schuberth KC, Teets KC. Compliance with a medical regimen for asthma: A test of the health belief model. *Public Health Rep*. 1978;93(3):268–77.
58. Corcoran N. Theories and models in communicating health messages. *Commun Heal Strateg Heal Promot*. 2007:5–31.
59. Maxwell KA. Friends: The role of peer influence across adolescent risk behaviors. *J Youth Adolesc*. 2002;31(4):267–77.
60. Ong LM, de Haes JC, Hoos AM, Lammes FB. Doctor-patient communication: A review of the literature. *Soc Sci Med*. 1995;40(7):903–18.
61. Ha JF, Longnecker N. Doctor-patient communication: A review. *Ochsner J*. 2010;10(1):38–43.
62. Stavropoulou C. The doctor-patient relationship: A review of the theory and policy implications. In: *The LSE Companion to Health Policy*. Cheltenham, UK: Edward Elgar Publishing Limited; 2012, pp. 314–26.
63. Scott A, Vick S. Patients, doctors and contracts: An application of principal-agent theory to the doctor-patient relationship. *Scott J Polit Econ*. 1999;46(2):111–34.
64. Smith A, Anderson M. *Social Media Use 2018: Demographics and Statistics*. 2018. http://www.pewinternet.org/2018/03/01/social-media-use-in-2018/.
65. Lin N. Building a network theory of social capital. In: *Social Capital: Theory and Research*. Oxfordshire, UK: Routledge Press; 2001, pp. 3–30.
66. Kim DA, Benjamin EJ, Fowler JH, Christakis NA. Social connectedness is associated with fibrinogen level in a human social network. *Proc Biol Sci*. 2016;283(1837):1–7.
67. Cappella JN. Vectors into the future of mass and interpersonal communication research: Big data, social media, and computational social science. *Hum Commun Res*. 2017;43(4):545–58.
68. Goel S, Watts DJ, Goldstein DG. The structure of online diffusion networks. *Proc 13th ACM Conf Electron Commer*. 2012;1(212):623–38.
69. Shi R, Messaris P, Cappella JN. Effects of online comments on smokers' perception of antismoking public service announcements. *J Comput Commun*. 2014;19(4):975–90.
70. Walther JB, Jeong-woo J. Communication processes in participatory websites. *J Comput Commun*. 2012;18(1):2–15.
71. Heaphy ED, Dutton JE. Positive social interactions and the human body at work: Linking organizations and physiology. *Acad Manag Rev*. 2008;33(1):137–62.
72. Burke TJ, Dailey SL, Zhu Y. Let's work out: Communication in workplace wellness programs. *Int J Work Heal Manag*. 2017;10(2):101–15.
73. Viswanath K, Randolph Steele W, Finnegan JR. Social capital and health: Civic engagement, community size, and recall of health messages. *Am J Public Health*. 2006;96(8):1456–61.
74. McCombs M. The agenda-setting role of the mass media in the shaping of public opinion. *North*. 2002;2009(05-12):21.
75. Viswanath K, Emmons KM. Message effects and social determinants of health: Its application to cancer disparities. *J Commun*. 2006;56(s1):S238–64.
76. McLaren L, Hawe P. Ecological perspectives in health research. *J Epidemiol Community Health*. 2005;59(1):6–14.
77. Agha S, Van Rossem R. Impact of mass media campaigns on intentions to use the female condom in Tanzania. *Int Fam Plan Perspect*. 2002;28(3):151–8.
78. Bekalu MA, Eggermont S. Exposure to HIV/AIDS-related media content and HIV testing intention: Applying the integrative model of behavioral prediction. *Mass Commun Soc*. 2015;18(2):144–64.
79. Viswanath K, Nagler RH, Bigman-Galimore CA, McCauley MP, Jung M, Ramanadhan S. The communications revolution and health inequalities in the 21st century: Implications for cancer control. *Cancer Epidemiol Biomarkers Prev*. 2012;21(10):1701–8.

CHAPTER

37

Social Marketing: Theory, Practice, and Research

W. Douglas Evans • Jeff French

INTRODUCTION

Social marketing is an approach to policy development and a process for social and behavior change that is growing rapidly. The first two decades of the twenty-first century have seen social programs across the globe expanding and reaching into virtually every aspect of social development including health, environment, energy use, and population management.[1] In particular, social marketing has become a staple of public health programs, with major health policy-making organizations worldwide routinely applying it as a core strategy.

Why has this growth occurred and why has social marketing increasingly come to be applied worldwide? The answer lies in the ability of social marketing to harness technology, increase access to information, and improve social programs that focus on psychological, economic, social, and environmental determinants of societal change. In addition, social marketing is driven by the use of data analytics, evidence, and research to guide the development of social marketing activities.[2]

This chapter explores current trends in social marketing, how new theory and methods are leading to an evolution of research and practice, and briefly examines case studies of social marketing in action. How we encounter social marketing programs (and how often), how we engage with them, and how we experience them *in relation to* competing behavioral alternatives are explored. The chapter also considers other factors, products, and services that are in competition with social marketing objectives, and why it is critically important to understand and tackle these competitive forces.[3] These factors help to explain why people choose and remain loyal to social marketing programs and the brands that represent them, and why they may sometimes decide not to act in ways that public health practitioners would like them to.

The goal of this chapter is to provide a broad overview of social marketing, with particular emphasis on its application in public health. First, we look at theory and strategy in social marketing; research and evaluation methods and growth of the evidence base; corporate social responsibility; and the role of information technology, social media, and mobile phones. Second, we examine the central role of branding as a strategy to change behavior and reframe public perceptions and social norms about behavior. Third, we explore the role of research in developing social marketing efforts and evaluation in assessing intervention effectiveness and efficiency and building the evidence base. Finally, the chapter concludes with discussion of future directions in social marketing, especially the growth of digital health and cocreation of behavior change by citizens and social marketers.

THEORY AND STRATEGY IN SOCIAL MARKETING

There is a growing literature on the evidence underlying social marketing research methods specific to the field, and studies to validate theoretical assumptions and advance theory.[4] These include both quantitative analytic methods and instrumentation and qualitative and special topic methods (e.g., interpersonal research). Communication research methods used in social marketing and theories that underpin it are interdisciplinary in nature, drawing from the social and behavioral sciences, business and marketing, economics and health, and public policy arenas.[5]

Social marketing has been defined as:

> *Social marketing seeks to develop and integrate marketing concepts with other approaches to influence behaviours that benefit individuals and communities for the greater social good. It seeks to integrate research, best practice, theory, participant and partnership insight, to inform the delivery of competition sensitive and segmented social change programmes that are effective, efficient, equitable and sustainable.*[5]

Based on this definition, social marketing is best understood as a comprehensive and strategic approach to facilitating or maintaining social good. It takes a citizen-centered approach in which insights about what matters to people is used to inform the development of effective and efficient social programs that are responsive to the majority of citizens.

This "citizen-centric" approach differentiates social marketing from many other approaches to social policy delivery that are based on a top-down expert-driven solution generation and decision making. The new global consensus social marketing concepts developed through a wide ranging consensus building exercise sponsored by the International Social Marketing Association and now endorsed by all current social marketing associations in 2017 set out a single central principle of social marketing and six core concepts that define its practice. The central social marketing principle is the creation of social and personal good. This is the central purpose of social marketing.[2] To deliver this principle, social marketing applies six core concepts. These six concepts include:

1. Citizen orientation and focus;
2. Setting of explicit social goals;
3. Value proposition delivery via the social marketing intervention mix;
4. Theory, insight, data and evidence-informed audience segmentation;
5. Competition/barrier and asset analysis; and
6. Critical thinking, reflexivity, and being ethical.

Social marketing also applies a wide range of methods that are not unique to public health, and are applied in other approaches to social and behavioral change, for example, the use of systematic planning and evaluation. The social marketing conceptual model identifies a hierarchy of relevance and importance with regard to the key attributes and distinguishing features of social marketing. This helps practitioners to promote and identify good social marketing practices.

These key concepts provide an overarching framework that guides the development of all social marketing strategy, programs, and campaigns.[5] This includes the use of behavioral theory to influence behaviors that affect health; assessing factors that underlie the receptivity of audiences to messages, such as the credibility and likability of the argument; and strategic marketing of messages that aim to change the behavior of target audiences by using the four Ps of marketing—place, price, product, and promotion. These are the four overarching variables that marketing uses to influence intended outcomes, whether they are product purchase or behavior change. Specific examples of predictive theoretical models include the Health Belief Model,[6–9] Theory of Planned Behavior,[10–12] Integrative Model of Behavioral Prediction,[13] and Social Cognitive Theory.[14,15]

Social Marketing as Part of Ecological Approaches

Social marketing applies the six core concepts (described above) to benefit society and the intended audience rather than the marketer or their client.[2] This suggests an ecological component to social marketing in that it seeks to alter social, economic, and environmental factors to bring about change, in addition to supporting and encouraging individual-level change. Social marketing can and should be integrated into multilevel ecological approaches, using intervention strategies based on these six core concepts to support change in community norms, organizational practice, and social policy selection and development.[16] In this way social marketing goes beyond individual-focused health communication and uses multiple interventions at the various ecological levels.[16]

CASE EXAMPLE: Family as an Ecological Level for Nutrition and Physical Activity Promotion

Parents serve as important nutrition and physical activity role models. Their behavior fosters child emulation of eating, exercise, and leisure habits, such as media use.[17,18] Parental modeling can serve as either a risk or protective factor for childhood obesity. To foster beneficial modeling, social marketing can encourage parents to adopt protective behaviors by depicting positive parental role models creating a healthy home environment.[19] Parents who model healthy rather than unhealthy behaviors, such as keeping fruits and vegetables foods in the household instead of junk foods, can lay the foundation for their children to incorporate healthy habits at home and in school and community environments.[20].

Other Ecological Levels of Influence

Further, social marketing can be used to *promote* engagement and positive role modeling of residents, community leaders in the faith and not-for-profit sectors, and local health and healthcare organizations. Community mobilization has long been a major component of social marketing, including coalition building and empowerment of youth to tackle public health challenges such as tobacco control.[21] Youth empowerment at the community level has been used as an intervention component of childhood obesity prevention initiatives.[22]

Policy/society. Social marketing has demonstrated its ability to influence health policy, as exemplified by programs such as the National Cancer Institute's American Stop Smoking Intervention Study (ASSIST).[21] Social marketing can change policy makers' frame of reference for social issues, such as the social acceptability of smoking, contributing to legislation, and policy that changes the environment. Such approaches can be integrated with behavior change strategies aimed at individual citizens and can also be strategically applied in areas such as obesity prevention and smoking.[23]

Figure 37-1 illustrates one way in which a multilevel, ecological approach to social marketing has been conceptualized in relation to obesity.

Social Marketing, Social Modeling, and Behavior Change

Social marketing frequently relies on Social Cognitive Theory (SCT), and thus often uses social modeling as a behavior change strategy.[25] The concept of social modeling has long been understood by psychologists and commercial marketers. In SCT, social modeling plays a central role in social learning and cognition.[14] Social models may

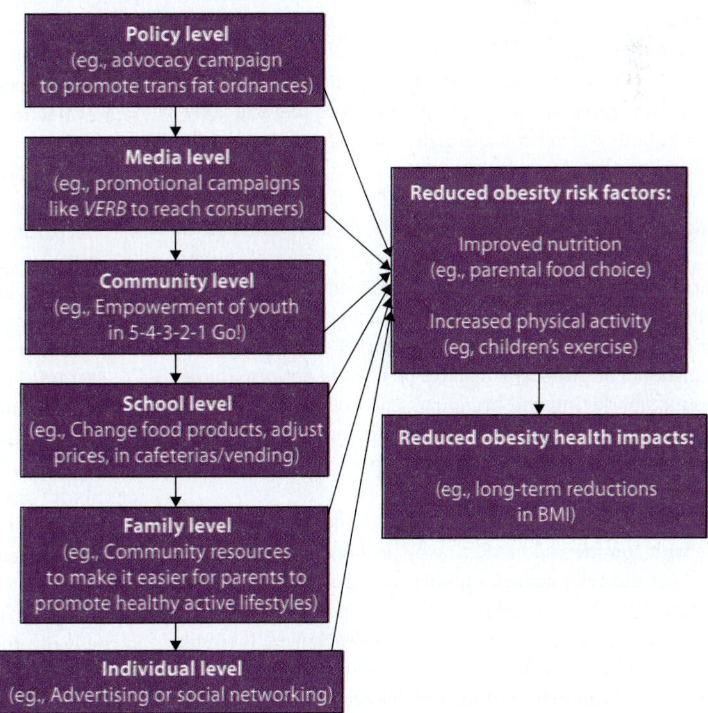

FIGURE 37-1. Obesity prevention social marketing framework. (*Source:* Evans WD, Necheles J, Becker AB, Christoffel KK, Snider J. Social marketing as a childhood obesity prevention strategy. *Obesity.* 2010;18(S1):S23–6.[24]) Adapted with permission from Evans WD, Necheles J, Becker AB, Christoffel KK, Snider J. Social marketing as a childhood obesity prevention strategy. Obesity. 2010;18(S1):S23–6.

embody the ideals promised by an advertisement or more comprehensive marketing campaign.

Idealized and aspirational imagery can be powerful marketing tools to create a social model. Brand marketing often creates an external ideal (i.e., a figure, image, or symbol that embodies socially desirable, idealized brand characteristics). Consider the Marlboro Man riding out on the range, the BMW driver cornering nimbly, or a *VERB* tween creating new active games. Research on "social imagery"—on the process and effects of image formation due to social stimuli such as media and peer influences—shows that formation of social imagery can promote aspiration to obtain or realize an external ideal (i.e., be rugged like the Marlboro Man, or sexy and sporty like the BMW driver).[26] Social marketing uses these same principles to bring about social and behavior change, where the latter are treated as the product—one of the four Ps of marketing noted earlier.

Social modeling has been used to market products and behaviors by making them more appealing than competing products or behaviors.[27] By creating and promoting positive social images of healthy behaviors aimed at countering unhealthy imagery, social marketing efforts can compete for a children and adolescents' time, attention, and behavioral choices. This approach—analysis of the competition and design of competing messages and other forms of support and encouragement—is the stock and trade of commercial marketers, and is the basis of brand development and promotion. In marketing terminology, social marketing can compete with commercial marketing strategies by identifying the "frame of reference" (i.e., the behavioral options in a given social context, such as whether to play or watch TV) and the "point of difference" between behaviors (i.e., how to portray one behavioral option, such as eating fruits and vegetables as more rewarding than another, like eating junk food).[28]

Social marketing campaigns have been developed to compete with commercial marketing and social norms that promote behaviors such as smoking, excessive media use and other sedentary behavior, or consumption of junk and fast foods. For example, the Centers for Disease Control and Prevention's (CDC) VERB: It's What You Do campaign branded children's play as fun, cool, and socially desirable behavior.[29] This branded social marketing campaign portrayed excessive sedentary behavior as dull and boring for the audience of tweens (9–13 years old). The VERB brand's vision was to "free children to play out their dreams."[30] Evaluation of VERB showed that it was effective in promoting awareness and more positive beliefs in the benefits of physical activity, and in promoting more physical activity behaviors in both tween boys and girls who were exposed to the campaign.[30]

Social marketing brands like *5-4-3-2-1 Go!* or the British Broadcasting Corporation's 1999 *Fighting Fat, Fighting Fit* compete in the marketplace of *nutrition and physical activity behavioral options*, not necessarily with a particular branded product or product line, but with the *categories* of nutrition and physical activity (or inactivity) behaviors.[22] Such brands seek to take away "market share" away from the poor nutritional or physically inactive behavioral options. In traditional product marketing and branding, this would represent one product (e.g., Pepsi) increasing its share of a population (e.g., soda drinkers in a market like Chicago) at the expense of a competitor (e.g., Coca-Cola).[27]

Social marketing efforts in a health domain like physical activity compete with commercial marketing by pitting one set of behavioral choices (or lifestyle) against another. For example, the Public Health England "One You" social marketing program depicts people from target demographics making realistic healthy choices. It brands a healthy, active lifestyle as having social and functional benefits greater than those of competing choices such as eating a high-fat diet and being inactive. In essence, the "One You" Brand lifestyle aims to take "market share" away from the behavioral alternatives by providing a more rewarding and valuable set of alternative behaviors.[27]

Branding Behavior Change

Brands build relationships between consumers and products, services, and lifestyle choices by providing beneficial exchanges and adding value. They can be measured through associations that consumers hold for products and services. Through brand promotion, these associations can become established and lead to a long-term relationship, or brand loyalty, between the product or service and consumer. These relationships are the building blocks of marketing and explain much of the success commercial marketers have enjoyed in building the global economy at least since the industrial revolution.[27]

Similarly, "behavioral brands" are the relationships that individuals form with behaviors and lifestyles that embody multiple health behaviors, and can be measured by the associations they form with health behaviors and lifestyles.[31,32] In the health sector in particular, the concept of behavioral branding has become a major component of social marketing campaigns to change a wide range of behaviors from HIV prevention to tobacco use prevention and physical activity promotion.[32] Brands in both the commercial and noncommercial sectors can also apply to organizations, and upstream factors that promote organizational impact and well-being. Health branding—building positive associations with healthy behaviors and lifestyle choices—is a primary strategy by which commercial marketing is applied in social marketing for health.[27]

The purpose of brands and branding is to organize and frame choices[33]—to buy a product, to use a service, or to live a physically active lifestyle or use condoms. Brands use symbols and imagery to organize potential choices and frame the benefits of a particular product, service, or behavior. However, we must always keep in mind that, for the most part, public health programs are voluntary in nature, meaning that prospective "customers" are free to accept or reject the products or services offered to them. As social marketers, success therefore typically hinges on the ability to design products and services that our prospective customers will value and embrace. In this way branding is increasingly a central strategy in the process of creating value for health consumers.

Brand research is critical to strategies to frame consumer choices, and is a good example of social marketing insight and behavioral focus benchmarks. Brand research can occur at the formative stage in design of branded campaigns, and at the campaign implementation stage when the effectiveness of the brand in creating customer associations, relationships, and changing behavior is being evaluated.[32,34]

Brand research serves two functions. First, it is about measuring and evaluating *determinants of brand choice*. Consumers choose to use a category of branded product or behavior (e.g., condoms as a *category* of product) and individual branded *products* within a category (e.g., *Protector Plus* condoms in Zimbabwe) due to market factors such as price, availability, and the brand associations they form with the category or individual product.[35] Brand research is concerned with identifying and analyzing those determinants of brand choice and informing brand managers to improve brand positioning and execution. Thus it represents a kind of formative research.

Second, brand research is concerned with evaluating the outcomes of brand choice. Consumers who use condoms, or individual condom products, will be likely to have different health outcomes than those who do not. What effect do brand choices and utilization of brands (categories or individual products) have on individual-level communication outcomes targeted by campaigns (e.g., specific beliefs targeted by messages) and behavioral outcomes (e.g., the call to action embodied in the campaign)? Brand research, in its evaluation function, is concerned with this question. In particular, it is concerned with the role of brand associations as *mediators* of associated intervention strategies and behavioral outcomes.[31]

Peeling the Brand Onion

Brands and the role of brand research can be explained using the concept of the brand onion.[36] This includes three nested concepts: (1)

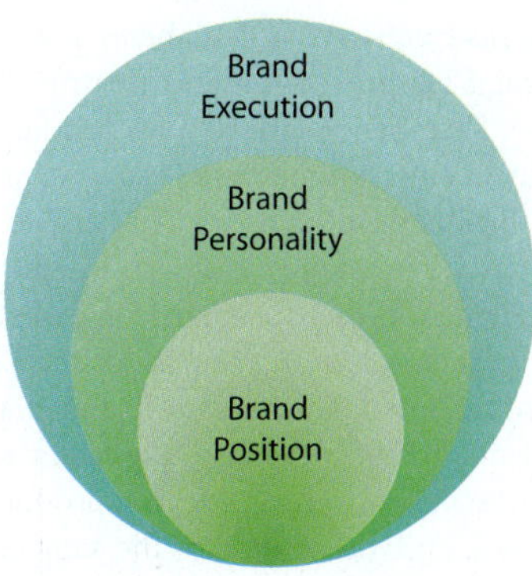

FIGURE 37-2. Brand onion concept. (*Source:* Adapted from Evans WD, Necheles J, Becker AB, Christoffel KK, Snider J. Social Marketing as a Childhood Obesity Prevention Strategy. *Obesity*, 2010;18(S1):S23-S26.[27])

Positioning, (2) Personality, and (3) Execution. Figure 37-2 illustrates the brand onion.

Brand Positioning

Brand positioning is what the marketer wants consumers to know and feel about a product, service, or in social marketing a behavior. A brand's position is what it stands for, the essence of its reputation.[28] Echoing Walter Landor's famous quote—"Products are created in the factory. Brands are made in the mind."—the positioning of a brand represents its life in the minds and hearts of the target audience. Positioning serves as a shortcut for consumer decision making and helps to determine product or behavioral choice.

Brand positioning is often summarized in a "positioning statement." Positioning statements have three basic components:

1. Statement of the target audience;
2. Description of the frame of reference (of choices in which the brand exists); and
3. Point of differentiation (PoD, or benefits) of the brand from competitors including both social (emotional) and functional benefits.

Positioning statements can be framed in terms of the following model or template: "For (target), (brand) is the (frame of reference) that (PoD)." Consider this example from Population Services International's water treatment social marketing program: "Certeza is the simplest water treatment method that leaves your water tasting pleasant and makes it easier to be a good mother."[36]

Brand Personality

What if a brand were to suddenly come alive? What would s/he say and do? How would s/he say and do it? These are the questions to be answered in determining a brand's personality. Brand personality is the expression of the emotional PoD of the brand, the social and emotional features that distinguish the brand and its identity from others. It can be expressed in adjectives like "fun," "sexy," or "serious," like describing a person. These features can shape the tone and sometimes the content of brand promotion and marketing. They can also be measured as brand personality traits in brand research, and represent predictors of brand choice as discussed later in this chapter.[37]

Consider a fictional brand of condoms called "Good Times." The brand personality is young, upbeat, and friendly. How might that personality be expressed in packaging, media, promotional messages, and other features of the personality? These are the factors marketers consider in developing a brand persona.

Or consider a real commercial brand, Marlboro cigarettes. Marlboro has one of the most clearly defined brand personalities in marketing history. The Marlboro man is a rugged individual, a man's man, self-confident, able to get the job done, the strong silent type. Marlboro cigarettes personify these traits and thereby gain identity and credibility with target audience members who value them. Whatever we may think of the health risks of cigarettes, that reputation is the basis for associations Marlboro consumers may form with the brand.

Brand Execution

"The only strategy the consumer experiences is execution." *A.G. Lafley P&G CEO*

Brand execution is how the brand is implemented in the real world. It is the images, colors, symbols, logo, tag lines, shapes, type fonts, language, touch/feel, sound/music, scent, and any other physical manifestations of the brand position and personality used to represent the brand and market it to consumers. It is what the consumer experiences when s/he comes in contact with the brand in the real world and what shapes brand associations. Thus, like personality, it can be measured and evaluated—how did consumers experience the brand execution and what were their reactions?

Or consider symbols. Without even describing a brand in words or more complex images, symbols can represent a brand and convey meaning. The Nike "swoosh" symbol, the iconic Coca-Cola curved bottle, and similar images require no explanation—they represent the brand without any accompanying description.

But widely recognized brands did not become well known simply through good strategy, by strategic positioning, and personality planning. Strong execution, high levels of consumer exposure (i.e., dosage of the marketing efforts), and consistent implementation of a marketing strategy over time produce those results. Thus execution is a critical element in creating brand equity. Measuring and evaluating brands requires assessing implementation (process evaluation), brand equity, and outcomes of exposure to the brand execution.

Like commercial marketing, social marketing campaigns attempt to build brands using these same principles of positioning, personality, and execution. A primary difference between commercial and social marketing lies in the latter's focus on providing benefits to the recipient of the marketing effort, whereas commercial marketing is focused on creating value for the marketer (or owner of the marketing effort) through sales or profit.[4]

SOCIAL MARKETING RESEARCH

There is a growing body of evidence, especially from public health subject areas such as tobacco control, nutrition and physical activity, and HIV/AIDS, to suggest that social marketing can change behavior and is a broadly effective social change strategy that can be applied to modify behaviors across multiple subject areas.[38,39] A recent systematic review published in 2014 by the Task Force on Community Preventive Services of 23 campaigns, in affluent countries, that used products (e.g., bicycle helmets) to promote health and prevent disease and injury concluded that communication and social marketing campaigns using these techniques were effective.[40]

There is also growing evidence that social marketing is effective in programs aimed at other types of behavior change, from increasing environmental conservation to promoting community participation.[41,42] The best evidence of social marketing effectiveness comes from media campaign evaluations, typically studies of large mass media campaigns or laboratory experiments where messages are tested under controlled conditions.[43,44] Recently, however, mobile phones, social media, and other new technologies have been studied as strategies for behavior change as well.[45,46] Some, but not all, of these technologies have been used with a marketing approach (i.e., applying the four Ps of marketing).[4]

Recent evidence reviews indicate that social marketing through mass media is effective in changing health behaviors on a population level. In general, these studies show that social marketing has been effective in changing health behavior such as smoking, physical activity, and condom use, and behavioral mediators such as knowledge, attitudes, and beliefs related to these behaviors.

However, most of these studies have shown relatively small effect sizes of less than 10%.[43]

Snyder found that the average campaign accounted for a range from 5% to 15% of the variation in health risk behavior outcomes but with heterogeneous results, and found that mediated campaigns (i.e., campaigns that bring about behavior change through mediators such as attitudes and beliefs) were effective with small effect sizes.[43] This study found that campaigns with an enforcement component (e.g., seat belt laws) were more effective than those without one. Evans points out that single- or few-time behaviors can be easier to promote than behavior requiring repetition and maintenance over time.[47] Some behaviors that do not require long-term maintenance, or are evaluated only for a short period, such as promoting vitamin A supplements and switching to 1% milk, have shown greater effect sizes, and generally appear to have higher rates of success.[48] Media campaigns have thus been used to modify both complex behaviors, including those involving multiple lifestyle risk factors such as HIV risk behavior, as well as simpler behaviors such as choosing to drink low-fat milk.[47,49]

The most effective mass media campaigns have generally been those with substantial financial resources and those that are supported by on-the-ground backup. Sustained multicomponent programs have the ability to generate high levels of audience exposure and recall or recognition of messages and advertising executions. For example, among the most successful media campaigns to change health behavior have been tobacco counter-marketing campaigns aimed at preventing youth smoking initiation, such as the American Legacy Foundation's *truth* campaign (now renamed the Truth Initiative; https://truthinitiative.org/). Legacy spent several hundred million dollars in the campaign's early years, from 2000 to 2002. Farrelly and colleagues showed that from 1999 to 2002, U.S. youth smoking prevalence declined from 25.3% to 18.0%, and *truth* accounted for approximately 22% of that decline.[50]

This study illustrates how media campaigns can have a big impact on population-level health. For example, in the case of *truth*, the campaign-attributable decline in youth smoking equates to some 300,000 fewer youth smokers, and thus millions of added life years as well as tremendous reductions in healthcare expenditures and other social costs.

There is evidence that media campaigns are effective in targeting other behaviors, such as financial education and literacy. The Media Financial Education project in Kenya aimed to improve knowledge, attitudes, behaviors, and practices for financial capability.[51] This initiative focused on banking, budgeting, savings, and investments to increase levels of financial education in the country. The campaign's primary objective was to encourage people to manage their finances in a sustainable manner more likely to lead to financial security. The basic approach integrated financial education content into an entertaining television program, Makatuno Junction, featuring characters that people could identify with. Outcome evaluation was conducted through a pre and postintervention cross-sectional survey of viewers and nonviewers. Prior to the airing of the episodes involving financial topics, 57% of the baseline survey respondents claimed to have "seen/heard information about the four target financial topics from sources in their environment"—among viewers, this number jumped to 67% after the show. For nonviewers there was no increase in awareness or knowledge, suggesting a potential treatment effect of Makutano Junction.[51]

Evidence for New Technologies and Behavior Change

Randomized trials of text messaging programs have shown behavioral effects among adolescents and adults, minority and nonminority populations, and across nationalities.[52] With mobile phones, the majority of published research has been on short message service, or text messaging. There is evidence that supports text messaging as an effective behavior change strategy in smoking cessation, weight loss, physical activity, and diabetes management, and to a lesser extent for STD prevention and treatment and in treating hypertension.[52–56] There is a relatively new but fast-growing literature on the utility of smartphones and their associated applications (or "apps") for health promotion. A few studies have evaluated the quality of apps for smoking cessation, weight loss, and diabetes self-management, and their usability for diabetes self-management.[57–60] Many of these programs use social marketing principles, but it should also be noted that some utilize media but not the full set of four Ps of marketing.[4] It is also important to recognize that social media marketing efforts (e.g., selling products or promoting causes on Facebook or Twitter) are not the same as social marketing, as they represent the use of a medium rather than a strategic marketing effort.

In summary, media campaigns have been shown to be effective across a wide range of subject matter, with the majority of evidence coming from health and healthcare. Because media campaigns have been effective in contributing to a range of behavior changes—including complex hard-to-change health behaviors and simpler knowledge and awareness raising and consumer choices—the collective evidence suggests that they may be effective in promoting other prosocial behaviors as well, such as environmental conservation and civic participation.[27]

Challenges in Synthesizing Social Marketing Evidence

Assessing the social marketing evidence is complicated by some of the challenges in compiling and synthesizing it. A major limitation of systematic reviews of social marketing, and specific subtopics such as tailored campaigns,[61,62] branding,[32] and the challenge of defining what constitutes marketing strategies, is the absence of well-recognized keywords that can be used to identify relevant literature.[63]

As noted by multiple studies,[63,64] reviews of social marketing evidence have a number of limitations. Methods have not always been systematic, and there is often insufficient information on the search strategy and inclusion criteria. In particular, reviews often fail to state explicitly how social marketing interventions have been defined, and conceptualize social marketing in widely differing ways. For example, in family planning reviews social marketing is often taken to mean, primarily, free distribution of condoms. In others, social marketing is misconstrued as simply social advertising or communications,[65] which represent only the "promotion" P and miss the other three (place, price, and product).

As noted earlier, one key difficulty has been the lack of an agreed and easily operationalized definition of a social marketing intervention. Generic definitions have until recently not been precise enough to help decide whether a specific intervention does or does not qualify as social marketing. One solution to the difficulty is simply to select interventions that are labelled social marketing programs by their managers or evaluators. However, relying solely on the label is problematic. First, it excludes many interventions that are not labelled as social marketing but which appear to incorporate social marketing principles. Second, it includes interventions which, despite their label, are poor examples of social marketing or not social marketing at all. For example, the misperception that social marketing equals advertising means that many interventions which are essentially media campaigns are erroneously described as social marketing.[66] The resulting evidence base, if a search is restricted only to interventions called "Social Marketing," is likely to be limited and flawed.

The basic solution to this problem recognized in recent literature, and applied in the recent systematic review,[63] is to utilize the full set of social marketing benchmark criteria.[38] Programs meeting these criteria represent robust examples of social marketing. The new 2017 global consensus principles of social marketing offer guidance and will further aid this process going forward.

CASE STUDY: Evidence on Social Marketing for Water and Sanitation in Low- and Middle-Income Countries

Recently, there has been growth in social marketing to promote healthy drinking water and sanitation practices, as well as treatments to prevent water-related illnesses such as diarrheal disease.[67,68] However, until recently there were no known efforts to systematically review and assess the extent, nature, and evidence of effectiveness for social marketing in global water and sanitation programs. Evans and colleagues systematically reviewed the published literature on this topic and evaluated the state of practice and evidence in the field.[63] Specifically, they sought to identify (1) the presence or absence of specific social marketing activities in each intervention; (2) the presence or absence of each of marketing considerations including product, pricing, place, and promotional issues; and (3) the outcome of the evaluation conducted in these social marketing interventions. Based on results of this review, the investigators concluded that such interventions needed to incorporate more marketing concepts and techniques, more outcomes research, and more research on the effectiveness of specific intervention strategies and combinations.[63] Table 37-1 illustrates the types of programs and data collected in this review organized around the four Ps of marketing.

First, the investigators identified the types of activities that water and sanitation social marketing interventions efforts have used. There have been widespread efforts to change sanitation practices ranging from personal hygiene to building sanitation infrastructure in villages. Programs have used both individual behavior change and infrastructure improvement schemes to create an environment in which behavior change can occur.

Second, they described the marketing mix used in social marketing in this area. Overall, there is widespread use of each of the four Ps of marketing, with some interventions not having an explicitly reported "price" strategy. This is a strength of the programs reviewed, and it is noteworthy that many use an explicit branding strategy to build long-term relationship with product consumers, such as in Oral Rehydration Therapy (ORT) and Safe Water Systems.

Third, they identified the research evaluation methods, design, and reported impacts from the social marketing efforts. Evaluations were generally well designed under challenging local circumstances and there is consistent evidence of improvements in behavioral mediators (i.e., knowledge, attitudes, beliefs targeted by the social marketing). Virtually all interventions reported on such mediators. Examples included intentions to use water and sanitation products, self-efficacy to use them following interventions such as motivational interviewing and training, and social norms that use of such products was widespread and a preferred practice in the community postintervention. Evidence for behavior change (e.g., use of water purification products) was mixed, with greater successes clustered in Safe Water Systems programs.

This review shares well-known limitations in reviews of social marketing, noted earlier, which stem mainly from variable use of keywords and descriptors for interventions.[62] Not all relevant published studies may have described themselves using social marketing terms, and thus may have been missed by this review. However, we used a variety of search terms and employed expert inputs and knowledge of the field to address this concern. Second, we identified relatively few sanitation-related social marketing interventions. This may be related to the first limitation, and the possibility that social marketing aimed at sanitation appears mainly in the gray literature. However, there is a need to promote these studies and publication of sanitation social marketing interventions.

FUTURE OF SOCIAL MARKETING

One observation is that social marketing research is a dynamic field, its application to a range of social and behavior change challenges expanding as shown in its use a policy development tool and in the published literature on the increasing number of published projects and studies. Applications such as the use of behavioral theory in research, health branding, directly addressing the competition, gaining and applying in-depth audience insight through research, and the other social marketing benchmark criteria (e.g., specific and measureable behavior change targets, use of theory, use of all four Ps of marketing) illustrate this growth. Recent systematic reviews cited earlier suggest that there may be some acceleration in the use of these best practices. Additionally, the growth of major professional associations such as the International Social Marketing Association and

TABLE 37-1 EXAMPLES OF WATER AND SANITATION MARKETING STRATEGIES

	Marketing Mix			
Location	**Product**	**Price**	**Place**	**Promotion**
Water and Sanitation				
Madagascar	Safe Water System ("Sur' Eau")	Subsidized price—$0.30 (46% cost recovery)	• Retail outlets in community • Home visits	• Radio and television spots • Brochures and posters • Community-based sales agents
Western Kenya	Safe Water System ("Klorin")	• Subsidized price ($0.33 for solution; $2.53 for clay pot) • Margins for wholesalers • Sales commission	• Community centers • Schools • Sporting events	• Print media campaigns • T-shirts • Puppet shows, skits, dancers • PHAST methodology used by village health workers • Public product demonstrations
Homa Bay, Kenya	Safe Water System ("WaterGuard")		Maternal and child health clinic	• Nurses at MCH clinic promoted product during appointments
Bobo-Dioulasso, Burkina Faso	• Hand washing • Proper stool disposal		• Health center • Home visits	• Street performance • Posters • School curriculum • Promotional starter kit • Radio spots • House-to-house visit by neighborhood hygiene commission • Discussion groups at health center

Source: Based on Young S, Buszin J, Rai, S, Wallace J. Social Marketing of Water and Sanitation: Systematic Review of Peer-reviewed Literature. *Soc. Sci.* Med, 2014, 110:18-25.[63])

meetings such as the World Social Marketing Conference also attest to the development not only of social marketing as a practice but the research and evidence base.[69]

Social marketing has been most frequently and consistently applied in public health and health behavior change domains such as tobacco control, nutrition, physical activity, HIV/STI prevention, reproductive health, maternal and child health, and related topics. While this focus has spurred the growth of the field, and has yielded many important successes, as noted in the systematic reviews highlighted earlier, it is also important to note the many opportunities to apply social marketing on a host of policy initiatives ranging from transportation to the environment. The breadth of topic areas included in the 2017 World Social Marketing Conference illustrates this expansion of content and reach.[70]

At the same time, many challenges are evident. First and foremost, the true nature of the social marketing evidence base remains somewhat unclear. Systematic reviews such as the one conducted by the Community Guide Task Force provide some insights but are incomplete.[40] Studies such as Evans and colleagues provide further insight and suggest that the evidence is robust and growing.[63] But as discussed earlier in this chapter, problems persist with identifying what studies actually constitute social marketing evidence.[71] These stem mainly from differences in language, lack of consistency in descriptions of social marketing, confusion between straightforward communication campaigns and broader social marketing strategies, and lack of editorial consistency in publishing of social marketing research. They continue to be major issues for academic researchers and groups such as the Community Guide Task Force and National Social Marketing Centre in the United Kingdom to synthesize the evidence.[71]

An important next step in the field is to develop more precise standards for reporting social marketing evidence, increase the quantity and quality of research and evaluation studies published, and educate the social marketing workforce and journal editors on the importance of consistently describing campaigns and social marketing research and evaluation studies. This challenge is not unique to social marketing, but the multidisciplinary and multitopic nature of the field may make it more acute. Consistent use of the new consensus principles and associated terminology will assist with this process and enable social marketing studies to be more easily synthesized and compared to one another. Consistent use of factors such as expressions of absolute percentage point differences in behavior and other outcomes of campaigns are other critical improvements needed to build the evidence base.[72]

What Is the Future Research Agenda?

Based on the investigation of past and present social marketing research in this volume, where is the field headed? Major changes in terms of social marketing implementation have occurred due to digital technologies; cocreation of programs by participants (and the reconceptualizing of the very idea of an "audience"); and the engagement of communities in the process of behavior, systems, and environmental change.[73,74] Given these trends, three areas clearly stand out for the near term development of social marketing research: (1) use of multiple modalities of new media and technologies as platforms not only for campaigns but also research; (2) engagement of participants in the social marketing process, including research activities and evaluation; and (3) attention to and analysis of multiple comorbid conditions that coexist within populations and communities that can be simultaneously addressed by campaigns.

Trends in Research Using New Technologies

Evaluation using social media, mobile devices, and other Internet-connected technologies is already with us and remains at the forefront of future social marketing research. Mobile devices are now a popular and growing channel for providing treatment through support for behavior change and intervention strategies, medication reminders, treatment information, and various other forms of adherence tools targeted to improve health outcomes though healthy behavior adoption.[45,46] While not all of these efforts represent true social marketing (using all four Ps of marketing), many are, and more evidence is needed on their effectiveness. These programs increasingly are evaluated using the same Internet, mobile, and social media technologies through which they are delivered, often in real time.

Engaging Participants in Research

New technologies including the Internet, social media, and mobile phones will potentially expand the reach and effectiveness of public health programs.[45] Some health promotion and disease prevention programs have used social media as delivery channels, such as the Above the Influence substance use prevention program, and its large Facebook presence and efforts to create a social community of youth sharing narratives related to avoidance of marijuana and other drug use.[75] However in public health generally, and drug use prevention in particular, relatively little has been published demonstrating the effectiveness of social media as prevention channels. The U.S. Substance Abuse and Mental Health Services Administration (SAMHSA) has funded a number of state media campaigns for prevention, some of which, including Colorado's *SpeakNow!* Campaign focused on teen drinking prevention, have used social media activities.[75] However, these efforts are in their infancy.

A new social media intervention called *Living the Example (LTE)* aims to train adolescents in branding and advocacy skills in order to promote peer-to-peer advocacy through social networks for substance use prevention. *LTE* is based in part on a previous school-based Shattering the Myth prevention program (http://www.mentorfoundationusa.org/), uses a 6-week, after school curriculum to train youth in branding and peer advocacy using social media. *LTE* trains youth to create persuasive posts using digital media, including video, and in the creative process. The intervention includes a self-expression component where students will learn techniques for expressing their ideas about substance use. Expressive segments are created as videos for social media.

Youth who participate in the social media activities disseminate their videos, photos, and other forms of narratives they create throughout their social media networks using all platforms to which they are current members. They also post to a dedicated project YouTube channel. Researchers document all participant exposure to *LTE* social media metrics captured on the *Hootsuite* social media management platform (https://hootsuite.com) and through survey responses from all participants and control for potential contamination in the analyses. Researchers use the Hootsuite platform to capture social media process (implementation) data. Outcome evaluation surveys in the schools where the youth peer educators are enrolled capture the effects on the secondary audience, the recipients of the messages. The participants both cocreate the intervention and actively participate in the research, process, and outcome evaluation process via multiple digital media modalities.

In a pilot evaluation of *LTE* conducted by Evans and colleagues in 2016, overall youth reported increased intentions to use marijuana [odds ratio (OR) 2.134, $P = .02$] between pre- and posttest.[75] However, youth who reported exposure and receptivity to LTE reported a significant decrease in intentions (OR 0.239, $P = .008$). Investigators observed a similar pattern for sedatives/sleeping pills—an increase in intentions overall (OR 1.886, $P = .07$), but a decrease among youth (some 62% of the sample) who reported exposure and receptivity to LTE (OR 0.210, $P = .02$). They saw the same pattern for use of any drug—an increase in reported intentions overall (OR 2.141, $P = .02$), but a decrease among youth who reported exposure and receptivity to LTE (OR 0.111, $P = .004$). These findings point to the potential for programs like *LTE* to harness the power of peer-to-peer influence for behavior change, opening a new channel for social marketing programs in the digital age.

Comorbid Conditions and Social Marketing

About 19 million new STIs and 40,000 new HIV cases occur each year in the United States. Reducing the burden of HIV/STI infections is a critical public health objective. Strategies need to address risky behaviors associated with infection, a task that is complicated by substance use and abuse.[76] Risk behaviors associated with both public health problems tend to cluster together and increase the likelihood of incidences of HIV/AIDS. Intoxication interferes with decision making and enhances risky sexual behaviors and some substance use (e.g., needle sharing) is directly related to infection.[77] The Monitoring the Future study showing sustained levels of substance use, and the resulting risky sex remains widespread in the United States,[78] making substance use and HIV/STI co-occurring problems.[79] The risk factors associated with both problems are disproportionately high among certain populations, such as young people who frequent bars and nightclubs, where substance use and risky sex are common.[80] But interventions traditionally address single risk factors and not co-occurring problems.

Social marketing by nature is capable of addressing these co-occurring risk factors. Specifically, using a health branding approach, social marketers can create positive brand identification with healthy behaviors among a targeted audience as a behavior change strategy.[27]

Health branding has two important attributes that make it an appropriate strategy for co-occurring behaviors and health risk factors. First, by creating identification with specific healthy behaviors it can address the common risk behaviors for co-occurring problems such as HIV/STI and substance abuse. A second advantage is the ability to target specific high-risk groups with a combined risk profile by promoting benefits of alternative safer behavioral choices (e.g., always carrying a condom when going out, and not using drugs) that underlie the co-occurring conditions.[81] There are examples of effective branding of condom use and specific brands developed through social marketing programs aimed at increasing overall behavior change as opposed to maximizing product sales.[82] For example, recent quasiexperimental and correlational studies have linked drug resistance branding to improved substance abuse attitudes and reduced substance-abuse behavior.[83]

To date, however, there have been no experimental studies addressing co-occurring risk factors for HIV/STI infections and substance abuse or comparing branded and unbranded messages to uncover the added benefits of branding for prevention of HIV/STI and substance use. In addition, we know little about the causal mechanisms through which successful brands operate. There is a need for new research to empirically test health branding as an approach to changing social cognitive determinants of HIV/STI and substance use. The goal of this research would be to develop and compare prevention social marketing strategies and isolate the effects of these strategies, such as branding, on changes in determinants of prevention behavior.

Diffusing Skills in Social Marketing Methods in Public Health

Despite growing evidence showing the effectiveness of social marketing when its full set of proven concepts and practices are applied,[1] as discussed earlier, there has been too little diffusion of the practices of social marketing research in the prevention and health promotion fields. Little has been done to train the healthcare workforce and scientific community to effectively use social marketing research in program development and translation. Continuing with the theme of HIV/STI and substance use programs, prevention practitioners and researchers need a training program to build branding knowledge, skills, aptitude, and resources to support their branding efforts for behavior change.

With the enormous public health burden of HIV/STIs, and other risk behaviors such as substance abuse, effective behavior change strategies are essential. NIH has made major investments in programs to prevent these risk behavior,[84] but translation of effective initiatives into sustained programs with effective delivery and distribution has proven challenging.[85] One reason for this problem is that programs are not adequately marketed, recognized, and appealing to targeted populations who could benefit from them.

This void needs to be filled by expanding the reach and utilization of social marketing strategies in prevention programs. There are two main elements that need to be addressed. First, rigorous research needs to be sponsored and conducted to build the evidence base and establish the effectiveness and cost efficiency of social marketing in multiple subject matter domains using rigorous methods. Second, educational tools need to be developed, tested, and disseminated to increase capacity in the public health and scientific workforce. These factors will be facilitated by more diffusion of research into practice and application of lessons learned to develop improved social marketing programs.

References

1. French J. Business as unusual: The contribution of social marketing to government policymaking and strategy development. Chapter 24. In: Hastings G, ed. *Sage Handbook of Social Marketing*. Thousand Oaks, CA: Sage Publishing; 2013.
2. French J, Gordon R. *Strategic Social Marketing*. London: Sage Publishing; 2015.
3. What Works in Youth HIV Campaigns. https://www.whatworksinyouth-hiv.org/programs/social-media-and-marketing-strategies/strategies-social-marketing-campaigns. Accessed January 18, 2018.
4. Evans WD. *Social Marketing Research Methods for Global Public Health: Methods and Technologies*. New York: Oxford University Press; 2016.
5. Reproduced with permission from iSMA. Global consensus definition of Social Marketing. French J Committee chair. 2014. https://isma.memberclicks.net/assets/Documents_Shared_Website/ESMA,%20AASM,%20SMANA%20iSMA%20 endorsed%20Consensus%20Principles%20and%20Concepts%20paper. pdf. Accessed January 12, 2018.
6. Glanz K, Rimer BK, Viswanath K. *Health Behavior: Theory, Research and Practice*, 5th ed. San Francisco, CA: Wiley & Sons; 2015.
7. Eisen M, Zellman GL, McAlister AL. A health belief model—Social learning theory approach to adolescents' fertility control: Findings from a controlled field trial. *Health Educ Q*. 1992;19:249–62.
8. Rosenstock I. Historical origins of the health belief model. *Health Educ Monogr*. 1974;2(4):328–35.
9. Becker MH. The health belief model and personal health behavior. *Health Educ Monogr*. 1974;2(4):324–508.
10. Ajzen I. From intentions to actions: A theory of planned behavior. In: Kuhl J, Beckmann J, eds. *Action Control: From Cognition to Behavior*. Berlin, Heidelber, New York: Springer-Verlag; 1985, pp. 11–39.
11. Ajzen I. Perceived behavioral control, self-efficacy, locus of control, and the theory of planned behavior. *J Appl Soc Psychol*. 2002;32:665–83.
12. Armitage CJ, Conner M. Efficacy of the theory of planned behavior: A meta-analytic review. *Br J Soc Psychol*. 2001;40:471–99.
13. Fishbein M, Ajzen I. *Predicting and Changing Behavior: The Reasoned Action Approach*. New York: Psychology Press; 2010.
14. Bandura A. *Social Foundations of Thought and Action: A Social Cognitive Theory*. Englewood Cliffs, NJ: Prentice Hall; 1986.
15. Bandura A. The social and policy impact of social cognitive theory. In: Mark M, Donaldson S, Campbell B, eds. *Social Psychology and Evaluation*. New York: Guilford Press; 2011, pp. 33–70.
16. French J. Business as unusual: The contribution of social marketing to government policymaking and strategy development. Chapter 24. In: Hasting G, ed. *Sage Handbook of Social Marketing*. Thousand Oaks, CA: Sage; 2013.
17. Huhman M, Price S, Potter LD. Branding play for children: VERBTM it's what you do. In: Evans WD, Hastings G, eds. *Public Health Branding: Applying Marketing for Social Change*. London: Oxford University Press; 2008.
18. Calvert S. Children as consumers: Advertising and marketing. *Future Child*. 2008;18(1):205–234.
19. Evans WD. Social marketing and children's media use. *Future Child*. 2008;18(1):181–204.
20. Evans WD, Hersey J. Community programs to prevent obesity. In: Golson JG, Keller K, eds. *Encyclopedia of Obesity*. Thousand Oaks, CA: Sage Publications, Inc.; 2008.
21. Evans WD, Ulasevich A, Stillman F, Viswanath V. The ASSIST newspaper tracking system. In: Stillman F, Trochim W, eds. *Evaluation of Project ASSIST: A Blueprint for State-Level Tobacco Control*. Bethesda, MD: National Cancer Institute Press; 2006.

22. Evans WD, Necheles J, Longjohn M, Christoffel K. The 5-4-3-2-1 Go! Intervention: Social marketing for nutrition. *J Nutr Educ Behav.* 2007;39(2 Suppl)(S1):S55–9.
23. Holden DJ, Soloe CS, Messeri P, Evans WD. Lessons learned in implementing youth empowerment programs. In: Haviland L, ed. *Lessons Learned from the Successes of the Tobacco Control Movement.* New York: JSI; 2007.
24. Evans WD, Necheles J, Becker AB, Christoffel KK, Snider J. Social marketing as a childhood obesity prevention strategy. *Obesity.* 2010;18(S1):S23–26.
25. Bandura A. Health promotion by social cognitive means. *Health Educ Behav.* 2004;31(2):143–64.
26. Burton D, Sussman S, Hansen WB, Johnson CA, Flay BR. Image attributions and smoking intentions among seventh grade students. *J Appl Soc Psychol.* 1989;19:656-–64.
27. Evans WD, Necheles J, Becker AB, Christoffel KK, Snider J. Social Marketing as a Childhood Obesity Prevention Strategy. *Obesity,* 2010;18(S1):S23-S26.
28. Tybout A, Sternthal B. Brand positioning. In: Tybout A, Calkins T, eds. *Kellogg on Branding.* New York: John Wiley and Sons, Inc.; 2005.
29. Huhman M, Potter L, Wong F, Banspach S, Duke J, Heitzler C. Effects of a mass media campaign to increase physical activity among children: Year-1 results of the VERB campaign. *Pediatrics.* 2005;116:e247–54.
30. Huhman M, Price S, Potter LD. Branding play for children: VERB™ it's what you do. In: Evans WD, Hastings G, eds. *Public Health Branding: Applying Marketing for Social Change.* London: Oxford University Press; 2008.
31. Evans WD, Price S, Blahut, S. Evaluating the truth® Brand. *J Health Commun* 2005;10(2):181–92.
32. Evans WD, Blitstein J, Vallone D, Post S, Nilsen W. Systematic review of health branding: Growth of a promising practice. *Transl Behav Med.* 2014;5(1):24–36.
33. Keller PA, Harlam B, Loewenstein G, Volpp K. Enhanced active choice: A new method to motivate behavior change. *J. Consumer Psychol.* 2011;21:376–83.
34. Schulz D, Schulz H. Measuring brand value. In: Tybout A, Calkins T, eds. *Kellogg on Branding.* Hoboken, NJ: John Wiley and Sons; 2005.
35. Evans WD, Taruberekera N, Longfield K, Snider J. Brand equity and willingness to pay for condoms in Zimbabwe. *BMC Reproductive Health.* 2011;8:29.
36. Chapman S, Ayers J, LeTouze O, Renard J. Branding and social marketing. In: Evans WD, ed. *Psychology of Branding.* Hauppage, NY: Nova Science Publishers; 2013.
37. Aaker, D. *Building Strong Brands.* New York: Simon & Schuster Inc.; 1996.
38. French J, Blair-Stevens C, McVey D, Merritt R. *Social Marketing and Public Health.* Oxford: Oxford University Press; 2010.
39. Snyder LB, LaCroix JM. How effective are mediated health campaigns? A synthesis of meta-analyses. In: Rice R, Atkin C., eds. *Public Communication Campaigns.* 4th ed. Thousand Oaks, CA: Sage; 2013, pp. 113–29.
40. Robinson, MN, Tansil, KA, Elder, RW, et al. Task Force on Community Preventive Services. Health communication campaigns that include mass media and health-related product distribution: A community guide systematic review. *Am J Prev Med.* 2014;47(3):360–71.
41. The Community Guide (2010). Health Communication and Social marketing: Health Communication Campaigns that Include Mass Media and Health-Related Product Distribution. http://www.thecommunityguide.org/healthcommunication/campaigns.html. Accessed September 1, 2015.
42. The Community Guide. Mass-Reach Health Communication Interventions. 2013. http://www.thecommunityguide.org/tobacco/index.html. Accessed March 27, 2018.
43. Snyder LB. Meta-analyses of Mediated Health Campaigns. In Preiss RW, ed. *Mass Media Effects Research: Advances Through Meta-Analysis.* Hillsdale, NJ: Lawrence Earlbaum Associates; 2002, pp. 357–83.
44. Evans WD, Uhrig J, Davis K, McCormack L. Efficacy methods to evaluate health communication and marketing campaigns. *J Health Commun.* 2009;14(3):244–54.
45. Whittaker R, Matoff-Stepp S, Meehan J, et al. Text4baby: Development and implementation of a national text messaging health information service. *Am J Public Health.* 2012;102:2207–13.
46. Free C, Phillips G, Galli L, et al. The effectiveness of mobile-health technology-based health behavior change or disease management interventions for health care consumers: a systematic review. *PLoS Med.* 2013;10(1):e1001362.
47. Evans WD. How social marketing works in health care. *BMJ.* 2006;322:1207–10.
48. Hornik RC. *Public Health Communication: Evidence for Behavior Change.* Mahwah, NJ: Lawrence Erlbaum Associates; 2002.
49. Agha S. The impact of a mass media campaign on personal risk perception, perceived self-efficacy and on other behavioral predictors. *Aids Care.* 2003;15(6):749–62.
50. Farrelly MC, Davis KC, Haviland ML, Messeri P, Healton CG. Evidence of a dose-response relationship between 'truth' antismoking ads and youth smoking. *Am J Public Health.* 2005;95(3):425–31.
51. The National Social Marketing Centre. Tools and Resources. http://www.thensmc.com/content/tools-resources. Accessed January 24, 2018.
52. Cole-Lewis H, Kershaw T. Text messaging as a tool for behavior change in disease prevention and management. *Epidemiol Rev.* 2010;32(1):56–69.
53. Fjeldsoe BS, Marshall AL, Miller, YD. Behavior change interventions delivered by mobile telephone short-message service. *Am J Prev Med.* 2009;36:165–73.
54. Whittaker R, Borland R, Bullen C, et al. Mobile phone-based interventions for smoking cessation. *Cochrane Database Syst Rev.* 2009;(4):CD006611.
55. Lim MSC, Hocking JS, Hellard ME, et al. SMS STI: A review of the uses of mobile phone text messaging in sexual health. *Int J STD AIDS.* 2008;19(5):287–90.
56. Logan AG, McIsaac WJ, Tisler A, et al. Mobile phone-based remote patient monitoring system for management of hypertension in diabetic patients. *Am J Hypertens.* 2007;20(9):942–8.
57. Franklin VL, Waller A, Pagliari C, et al. A randomized controlled trial of Sweet Talk, a text messaging system to support young people with diabetes. *Diabetes Med.* 2006;23:1332–8.
58. Free C, Knight R, Robertson S, et al. A Randomized Controlled Trial of Mobile (Cell) Phone Text Messaging Smoking Cessation Support: TXT2STOP. Oral Presentation at the Society for Research on Nicotine and Tobacco Annual Meeting, Toronto, Canada. 2011. http://www.srnt.org/index.cfm. Accessed January 24, 2018.
59. Evans WD, Nielsen P, Szekely D, Wallace J, Murray E, Snider J. Initial outcomes from a 4-week follow-up study of the Text4baby program in the military women's population: Randomized controlled trial. *J Med Internet Res.* 2014;16(5):e13.
60. Patrick K, Raab F, Adams M, et al. A text message-based intervention for weight loss: Randomized controlled trial. *J Med Internet Res.* 2009;11(1):1–9.
61. Noar SM, Benac CN, Harris MS. Does tailoring matter? Meta-analytic review of tailored print health behavior change interventions. *Psychol Bull.* 2007;133(4):673–93.
62. Gordon R, McDermott L, Stead M, Angus K. The effectiveness of social marketing interventions for health improvement: What's the evidence? *Public Health.* 2006;120(12):1133–9.
63. Evans WD, Pattanayak SK, Young S, Buszin J, Rai, S, Wallace J. Social marketing of water and sanitation: Systematic review of peer-reviewed literature. *Soc Sci Med.* 2014;110:18–25.
64. Alcalay R, Bell RA. Promoting Nutrition and Physical Activity Through Social Marketing: Current Practices and Recommendations. Prepared for the Cancer Prevention and Nutrition Section, California Department of Health Services, Sacramento, CA. Davis, CA: Center for Advanced Studies in Nutrition and Social Marketing, University of California. 2000.
65. Stead M, Hastings G. Advertising in the social marketing mix: Getting the balance right. In: Goldberg ME, Fishbein MS, Middelstadt SE, eds. *Social Marketing: Theoretical and Practical Perspectives.* 1st ed. Mahwah, NJ: Lawrence Erlbaun Associates; 1997, pp. 29–44.
66. McDermott L, Stead M, Hastings G. What is and what is not social marketing: The challenge of reviewing the evidence. *J Market Manag.* 2005;21(6):545–53.
67. Thevos AK, Olsen SJ, Rangel JM, Kaona FAD, Tembo M, Quick RE. Social marketing and motivational interviewing as community interventions for safe water behaviors: Follow-up surveys in Zambia. *Int Q Community Health Educ.* 2003;21(1):51–65.
68. UNICEF. Social Marketing Approaches to Child Survival. 2010. http://www.unicef.org/supply/files/11_Angus_Spiers_-_PSI_-_Social_Marketing_Approaches_to_Child_Survival.pdf. Accessed January 30, 2018.
69. Freeman MC, Quick RE, Abbott DP, Ogutu P, Rheingans R. Increasing equity of access to point-of-use water treatment products through social marketing and entrepreneurship: A case study in western Kenya. *J Water Health.* 2009;7(3):527–34.
70. Evans WD, Blitstein J, Hersey J, Renaud J, Yaroch, A. Systematic review of public health branding. *J Health Commun.* 2008;13(8):721–41.

71. Centers for Disease Control and Prevention. Gateway to Health Communication and Social Marketing Practice: Research and Evaluation. 2015. http://www.cdc.gov/healthcommunication/research/index.html. Accessed January 24, 2018.
72. Snyder LB, Hamilton MA, Mitchell EW, Kiwanuka-Tondo J, Fleming-Milici F, Proctor D. A meta-analysis of the effect of mediated health communication campaigns on behavior change in the United States. *J Health Commun.* 2004;9(Suppl 1):71–96.
73. Task Force on Community Preventive Services. The Guide to Community Preventive Services: What Works to Promote Health. 2005. http://www.thecommunityguide.org/library/book/Front-Matter.pdf. Accessed January 29, 2018.
74. Lefebvre RC. An integrative model for social marketing. *J Soc Market.* 2011;1(1):54–72.
75. Substance Abuse and Mental Health Services Administration. National Registry of Evidence-based Programs and Practices. 2015. http://www.nrepp.samhsa.gov/. Accessed January 29, 2018.
76. Evans WD, Andrade E, Goldmeer S, Smith M, Snider J, Girardo G. Pilot evaluation of the living the example social media program for prevention. *JMIR Ment Health.* 2017;4(2):e24.
77. Johnston LD, O'Malley PM, Miech RA, Bachman JG, Schulenberg JE. *Monitoring the Future National Survey Results on Drug Use: 1975–2014: Overview, Key Findings on Adolescent Drug Use.* Ann Arbor, MI: Institute for Social Research, The University of Michigan; 2015.
78. Mayer KH, Skeer M, Mimiaga MJ. Biomedical Approaches to HIV Prevention. 2012. http://pubs.niaaa.nih.gov/publications/arh333/195-202.htm. Accessed January 29, 2018.
79. Johnston LD, O'Malley PM, Bachman JG, Schulenberg JE *Monitoring the Future National Survey Results on Drug Use, 1975–2008. Volume I: Secondary School students (NIH Publication No. 09-7402).* Bethesda, MD: National Institute on Drug Abuse; 2009, p. 721.
80. Hipwell A, Stepp S, Chung T, Durand V, Keenan K. Growth in alcohol use as a developmental predictor of adolescent girls' sexual risk-taking. *Prev Sci.* 2012;13(2):118-28.
81. Hecht ML, Lee JK. Branding through cultural grounding: The keepin' it REAL curriculum. In: Evans WD, Hastings G, eds. *Public Health Branding: Applying Marketing for Social Change.* Oxford, UK: Oxford University Press; 2008, pp. 161–79.
82. Tobler NS, Roona MR, Ochshorn P, Marshall DG, Streke AV, Stackpole KM. School-based adolescent drug prevention programs: 1998 Meta-analysis. *J Prim Prev.* 2000;20:275–336.
83. Evans WD, Holtz K, White T, Snider J. Effects of the above the influence brand on adolescent drug use prevention normative beliefs. *J Health Commun.* 2014;19(6):721–37.
84. Lee JK, Hecht ML. Examining the protective effects of brand equity in the *keepin' it REAL* substance use prevention curriculum. *Health Commun.* 2011;26(7):605–14. doi:10.1080/10410236.2011.560797.
85. Fauci AS. Testimony before the Committee on Oversight and Government Reform, U.S. House of Representatives. http://www.hhs.gov/asl/testify/2008/09/t20080916f.html. Accessed January 30, 2018.

CHAPTER 38

Effective and Impactful Risk Communication

William M. P. Klein • Erin M. Ellis

Everyday behaviors and decisions have a dramatic impact on morbidity and mortality[1]; it is estimated, for example, that 30% of all cancers are attributable to tobacco use.[2] The risks of cervical cancer, cardiovascular disease, and car fatalities are reduced greatly by HPV vaccination,[3,4] cholesterol screening,[5,6] and seat belt use,[7] respectively. Consequently, it is important to devise strategies to encourage greater engagement in risk-reducing behaviors and avoidance of risk-increasing behaviors. To that end, researchers have devised several theoretically driven interventions to change attitudes, construct environments, provide resources, strengthen social support, and influence peer norms in ways conducive to healthy and safe behaviors.[8–12]

A key approach to encouraging healthy behaviors and decisions is the effective communication of risk—both at the population level and the individual level. People need to understand how their behaviors influence their health and safety risks, and perhaps most importantly, how current and future behaviors might reduce those risks. This is a major assumption of many models of health behavior such as the Health Belief Model[13] and the Precaution Adoption Process Model.[14] Meta-analyses suggest that risk perceptions are significantly (though modestly) related to health behaviors (e.g., Brewer et al.,[15]); one meta-analysis showed that experimental manipulations of risk perception can have significant effects with moderate effect sizes on health intentions and behaviors.[16] Thus, it is essential to know how to best communicate health risks clearly and effectively. Importantly, one must do so while minimizing the potential for unintended consequences. Consider a study by Stock et al.[17] in which sexually active participants learned about a peer who contracted HIV after just one sexual encounter. Rather than extrapolate from that person's experience to their own by elevating their perceived risk, study participants came to see themselves as even *less* at risk because, they reasoned, if they hadn't been infected yet, they were likely immune. It is also important that risk communications do not elevate risk perceptions so far that recipients become overly anxious and paradoxically less interested in risk reduction.

In this chapter, we review lessons learned from the extensive literature on risk communication. We begin by first identifying the contexts within which risk communication takes place and by then discussing the ways in which people think about and understand risk—an important precursor to considering what types of risk communications will be most effective. We then address how people construe numerical information, and consider implications for communicating risk. This is followed by a consideration of many of the psychological factors (e.g., motivational, emotional) that are present in risk communication contexts—factors that can be as or more important than comprehension when assessing the potential impact of risk communications. Finally, we consider how to strengthen the connection between risk communication and subsequent action, the extent to which communicators of risk information can be trained, and enduring needs for further research in this area.

CONTEXTS AND GOALS OF RISK COMMUNICATION

There are many contexts in which information about risk may be communicated. Healthcare professionals may communicate with patients about how their lifestyle behaviors influence risks for adverse health outcomes, or about the risks involved in treatment options, disease screening procedures (e.g., cancer screening, prenatal screening, and predictive genetic testing), and clinical trial participation.[18,19] Risk communication may occur on a person-to-person level outside clinical settings as well. Family members may communicate with each other about heritable diseases or genetic conditions,[20] and individuals may use online risk calculators and decision aids to estimate their risk for health outcomes such as cancer.[21–23] Beyond these person-to-person contexts, public health communication efforts, including public service announcements, social marketing campaigns, and warning labels, often aim to convey risk information to the public.[24]

Often, the nature of the risk communication will depend on its purpose or goal. A risk communication is sometimes intended to share information that might facilitate an independent choice when there are multiple options and none is objectively superior (i.e., clinical equipoise).[25] In these cases, patients are instructed to make treatment decisions that align with their personal goals and values. More often, a health-related behavior or decision is known to be beneficial or harmful to most people, so the goal of a risk communication is to persuade the audience to change its beliefs and adopt the healthier behavior (e.g., 26). Lastly, the goal of a risk communication may be to fulfill a legal obligation or commercial agenda. For instance, pharmaceutical and tobacco companies are legally mandated to inform consumers about the risks of their products. These risk communication messages may be intentionally or unintentionally difficult to understand. They may be printed in small inconspicuous text, use complex language, and exploit scientific uncertainty.[24,27]

MEASURING AND DEFINING LAY RISK PERCEPTION

In order to design effective risk communications in these various contexts, it is essential to understand how people generally think about risk. Unlike professional risk analysts—who focus on epidemiological, actuarial, archival, and largely numerical data—laypeople's beliefs about risk are influenced by a wide array of cognitive, emotional, and motivational factors. Some of the earliest work on risk perception by Slovic and others (e.g., ref. 28) demonstrated that lay perceptions of population risk were driven largely by two independent dimensions—dread (the perception of uncontrollable, severe outcomes) and knowability (the extent to which people understand the potential hazard and its consequences). As a result, hazards that were high in dread and low in knowability (e.g., nuclear reactors) were viewed as riskier than hazards that were lower in dread and higher in knowability (e.g., food preservatives), even if the objective risk posed by the latter might be higher than that of the former.

A major conclusion from the extensive body of work that followed Slovic's research is that most people have difficulty comprehending and using numerical information, a central skill in comprehending risk. People tend to focus more on frequency than on probability; for example, they might consider an event that occurs 10 out of 100 times to be more likely than an event that occurs 1 out of 10 times.[29] Difficulties with numbers lead small risks to be overestimated and large risks to be underestimated (e.g., ref. 30). One study showed that people generally lump risk into three categories—low risk (below 20%), moderate risk (20–80%), and high risk (over 80%),[31] reflecting more of a "gist" than a comprehension of actual risk.[32] Certain probabilities are imbued with meaning going beyond statistical considerations; for example, reducing a risk from 2% to 1% is less impactful than reducing from 1% to 0% given the psychological reassurance offered by completely eliminating risk,[33] and "50%" can be construed as "uncertain" or tantamount to coin flip with a randomly determined outcome.[34] In general, a large proportion of the population scores poorly on standard tests of numeracy,[35] suggesting that basic risk communications involving numbers may be misunderstood. Unfortunately, simply replacing numbers with verbal labels is not a panacea, given that people generally overestimate the numerical translation of those labels,[36] and given that risk perceptions based on verbal scales are more inconsistent and subject to bias (e.g., ref. 21).

If people are not basing their perceptions of risk on numeric probability estimates, how do they actually think about risk, or perhaps even more importantly, what types of risk perceptions are most predictive of behavior and decision making? Some studies suggest that people often focus on how their risk compares with that of other people ("comparative risk") more than they focus on their absolute risk. Festinger[37] argued that in the absence of objective information, people seek out social comparisons with others to judge their standing on a wide variety of dimensions, comparisons that in turn influence their behavior. Accordingly, several studies have shown that comparative risk—particularly relative to one's peers or "the average person"—is a reliable predictor of health behaviors and decisions, sometimes even more so than absolute risk (e.g., 38). For example, Klein[39] invited participants to imagine that their risk of causing a car accident was 30% or 60% and that this figure was above or below the average among people like them. Strikingly, only comparative standing influenced judgments of driving safety and behavioral intentions; participants who imagined that their 60% risk was below average felt safer and intended fewer behavioral changes than those who imagined that their risk of 30% was above average (see also ref. 40).

In addition to reasoning about their risk toward the end of arriving at absolute or comparative risk perceptions, people also think about risk in affective terms, as foreshadowed by Slovic's[28] early work demonstrating the role of dread. Slovic suggests that people use an "affect heuristic" to judge risk (e.g., ref. 41), coming to think a particular hazard poses more risk if it evokes a negative emotional reaction (see also the "risk as feelings" framework[42]). Indeed, worry about one's chances of experiencing a health outcome is a significant predictor across many studies of health behaviors and decisions,[43] and sometimes even more so than conventional measures of risk perception.[44,45]

Evidence shows that people also have an intuitive or "experiential" perception of personal risk, or what might colloquially be called a "gut intuition" that they will experience an event. In an early demonstration, Weinstein et al.[46] found that a "gut intuition" that one might contract influenza was a better predictor of getting a flu shot than were several other conventional measures of perceived risk. Ferrer et al.[47,48] found that *deliberative* risk perceptions such as absolute and comparative risk, *affective* risk perceptions such as worry, and *experiential* risk perceptions such as gut intuitions were empirically distinguishable and that each explained unique variance in behavioral intentions. (See Table 38-1 for a summary of different types of risk perceptions.)

Finally, it is important to note that people often do not have clearly held *a priori* beliefs about their personal risk. When given the opportunity to respond "don't know" on surveys that ask about perceived risk, many avail themselves of this option. Importantly, such individuals tend to be those at higher risk and in greater need of risk remediation—for example, those of lower socioeconomic status.[49] Even when people provide a response, they may do so with little confidence, prompting some researchers to recommend measuring the conviction with which respondents hold their risk perceptions.[50] And, as noted above, people may think about risk in terms of a few basic categories (small, moderate, and large[31]). Other work suggests that people are averse to thinking about risk itself as being uncertain; for example, people prefer to think their risk is 20% rather than somewhere between 10% and 30%.[51]

TABLE 38-1 DIFFERENT TYPES OF RISK PERCEPTIONS[a]

Type of Risk Perception	Defined	Example Item	Example Application
Deliberative			
Absolute	Logical, rule-based judgments concerning the overall likelihood of developing a disease or illness	How likely is it that you will get [disease] at some point in the future?	A meta-analysis found a consistent relationship between absolute deliberative risk and vaccination.[15]
Comparative	Perceived likelihood of developing disease relative to one's peers or "the average person"	How do you think your chance of developing [disease] in the future compares to the average person of your gender and age?	Women told that their hypothetical risk of breast cancer was above average were more likely to endorse taking a hypothetical breast cancer prevention pill.[40]
Affective	Positive and negative affective responses (e.g., worry, fear) to the possibility of developing a disease	How worried are you about developing [disease] in the future?	Anticipated worry and regret were stronger predictors of vaccination than deliberative risk.[15]
Experiential	Intuitive or gist perception of personal risk; a "gut intuition" that one will experience an event	How easy is it for you to imagine yourself developing [disease] in the future?	Gut intuition that one might contract influenza was a better predictor of getting a flu shot than other perceived risk measures.[46]

[a]See references 47 and 48.

CONVEYING NUMERICAL RISK EFFECTIVELY

Knowing how people appraise risk is the first step to designing effective and impactful risk communications. It is crucial to provide veridical, comprehensible risk information so that it is processed carefully, remembered, and acted upon as intended. We begin by considering implications of cognitive biases in the comprehension of numeric risk information. Our focus here is on *effective* strategies, not necessarily *cost-effective* strategies. Very little work assesses cost-effectiveness of health communications and interventions.[1] Most of the suggestions offered here are largely cost-neutral as they are not resource-intensive and for the most part provide guidance about how basic risk information should be framed and presented.

What numbers are best? The most basic risk communication informs a person that he or she has at a specified percentage risk of experiencing a particular outcome such as a genetically determined disease or of having an infant with a disability. Here we review some key implications of the current literatures on risk perception and risk communication for the types of numerical information one might use in such a context. We also refer the reader to informative and comprehensive summaries by Fagerlin et al.[52] Lipkus,[53] Waters et al.,[54,55] and Fischhoff et al.[24] Suggested practices include the following:

1. *Present risk in comparative terms.* For example, the "Your Disease Risk" calculator provided by the Siteman Cancer Center[56] collects risk information about risk factors for a given health outcome and then informs users of their risk of experiencing that outcome on a comparative scale from "very much below average" to "very much above average." Feedback from this website has been shown to have direct effects on health behaviors and decisions such as engagement in physical activity.[26] Ideally, recipients would receive both absolute and comparative risk, because, as illustrated in the Klein study above, if their comparative risk is low they may not attempt to reduce risk even if it is objectively high.[39]
2. *Avoid use of relative risk.* A reduction from 2% to 1% risk represents a 50% reduction or relative risk. People may anchor on such a large number and believe that a given action will greatly reduce their risk, not understanding that their risk is already low.
3. *Present both percentages and frequencies.* The evidence is mixed on whether people better understand one or the other; percentages are difficult to understand especially when below 1%, and frequencies may be difficult to contextualize; but the evidence for using frequencies is more established (e.g., ref. 57). Most importantly, base rates are important to convey—telling a patient that a certain drug has led to severe side effects in ten patients means something different when the sample of individuals taking the drug is 1000 than when it is 1,000,000. Of note, emphasizing just the numerator increases fear and risk-avoidant behaviors, and decreases comprehension of risk magnitude.[53,58] Using denominators that are factors of 10, as illustrated here, is also recommended. Notably, the risk of most hazards and health problems is rather small; for example, a woman with a 5-year breast cancer risk of 1.67% is considered by the U.S. Food and Drug Administration to be at high risk and therefore eligible for use of tamoxifen as a risk reduction strategy. This presents an interesting conundrum for risk communicators; if ostensibly "high" risk is low in the eyes of recipients—particularly given that their *a priori* risk estimates are higher, they may be unlikely to act on the risk information.
4. *Present multiple risks so that they can serve as context for each other.* Comparing the risk of heart disease to winning the lottery may provide useful context. Moreover, learning about multiple health risks allows one to prioritize resources toward those that need the most attention. Hellwig et al.[59] demonstrated that when people are presented with information about multiple health risks—in this case in the context of genetic sequencing results—they are more attentive to information about those risks and are less likely to be driven largely by their emotional response to the risk information.
5. *Take care when presenting 50% as a risk estimate.* As noted earlier, the interpretation of 50% may be that there is a great deal of uncertainty about one's risk, rather than the correct interpretation that the outcome is half as likely as it is unlikely.
6. *Avoid using the "1 in X" format* (e.g., one in eight women will get breast cancer in their lifetimes). Despite its seemingly intuitive appeal, much evidence suggests that people have trouble understanding this kind of risk estimate.[60,61] People seem to have an easier time understanding proportions that involve denominators that are multiples of 10, as suggested above. Moreover, due to the numerator bias, "1" may convey something different than the equivalent frequency using a denominator that is a multiple of 10.
7. *Use both words and numbers.* It may be useful to contextualize a risk by indicating whether it is high or low—using these terms. Importantly, though, given that people may construe these terms very differently than the risk communicator,[36] it is recommended to use words in addition to—not instead of—numbers in the communication.
8. *Consider the implications of presenting risk ranges (e.g., 20–30%).* People may mistrust point estimates, especially individuals higher in numeracy, knowing that risk estimation is not a perfect science, but other work suggests that people are also averse to ambiguity about risk.[51]

Pictorial approaches to risk communication. The above recommendations concern what kinds of numbers to convey but say little about the format with which to convey them; a growing literature suggests people may often find pictorial representations of risk to be more comprehensible and actionable. Visual aids can improve the comprehension of risk information, increase engagement in the target behavior, reduce the time computational energy, and reduce the effects of other sources of bias such as anecdotes and message framing.[52,62–66] There are several types of graphical displays including bar graphs (useful for making comparisons of risk), pie graphs (useful for showing proportions), and line graphs (useful for showing trends over time[67] for a variant of line graphs: pico-trendlines), as well as heat maps, risk ladders, and pictographs, also known as icon arrays. Here, we focus on pictographs and risk ladders as some of the most commonly used and effective visual aids in risk communication. Examples are displayed in Fig. 38-1A–F.

The choice of graph type and specific visual characteristics often depends on the purpose of the risk communication and whether it is intended to simply inform or to persuade,[68,69] particularly given that visual aids promoting risk comprehension do not necessarily lead to behavior change.[53] The choice should not necessarily be guided by audience ratings or liking, as the graphical formats that doctors and patients rate as liking best do not always produce the most accurate recall of risk information.[68] In one study, doctors were least accurate in their decisions to stop hypothetical clinical trials when they used the graphical format they most preferred (pie charts and bar graphs), and most accurate when they used the graphical format they least preferred (icon arrays and tables).[70]

Studies that have compared the effectiveness of different graph types suggest pictographs are generally best comprehended, are trusted by both high and low numerate individuals, and can reduce the effects of other sources of bias.[52,62–64,66,70–73] Pictographs may be particularly beneficial for individuals with low numeracy and limited language proficiency.[69,72,74,75]

[1] Kaplan RM, Gold M, Duffy S, et al. Economic analysis in behavioral health: Toward application of standardized methodologies. *Health Psychol.* 2019;38(8):672–9.

A

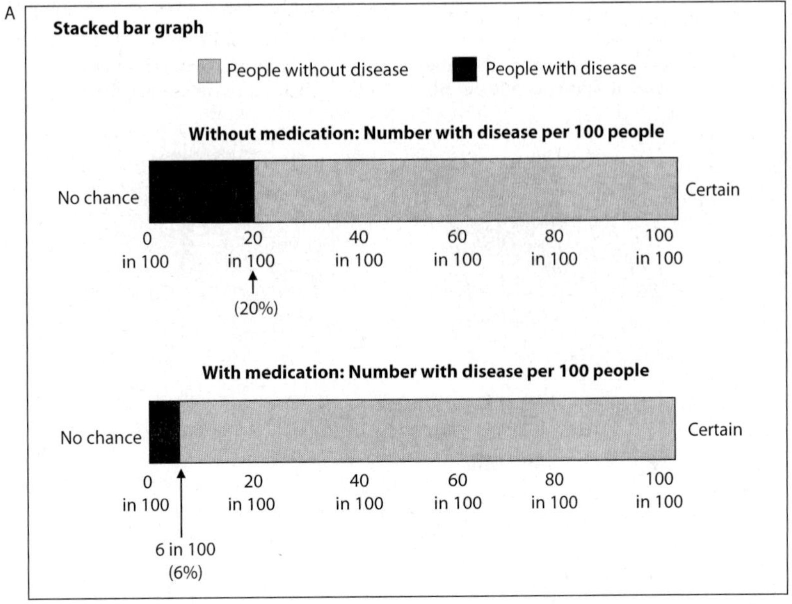

B

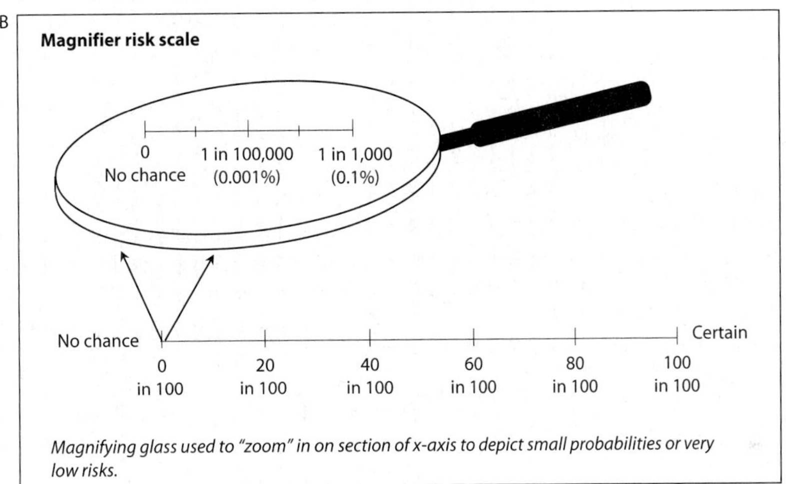

C

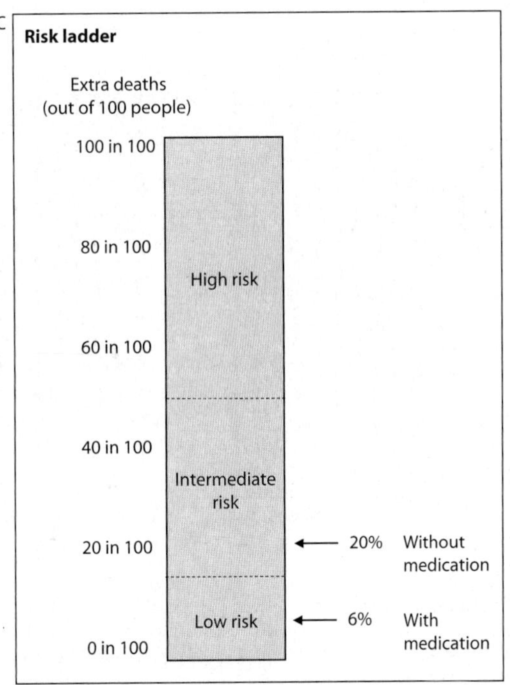

FIGURE 38-1. Continued

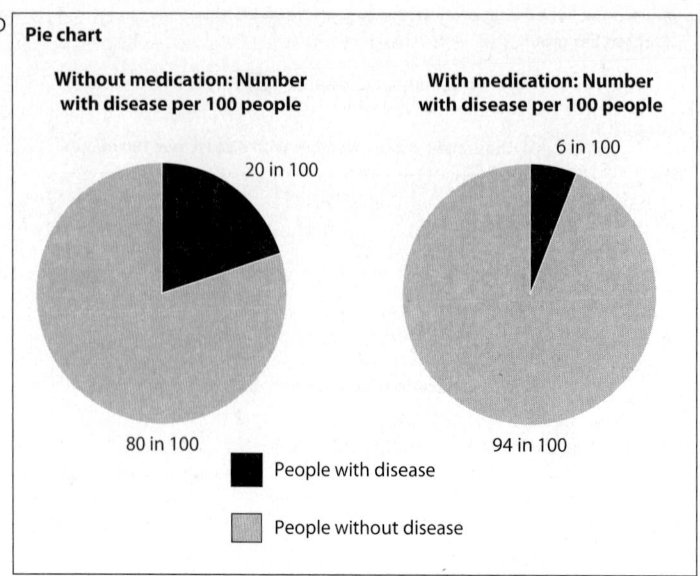

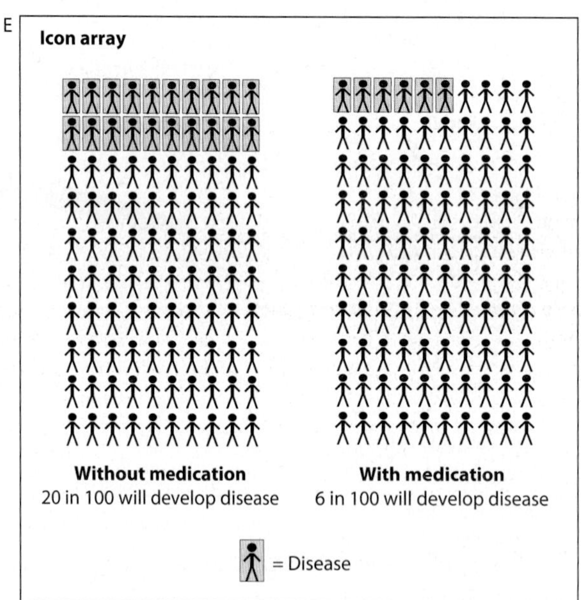

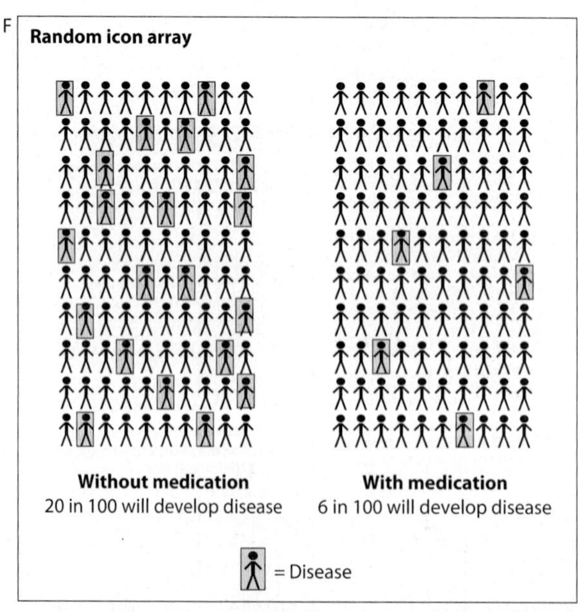

FIGURE 38-1. Six examples (A–F) of graphical formats of risk based on a hypothetical medication that lowers risk for disease from 20 in 100 people to 6 in 100 people.

TABLE 38-2 SELECTED CONSIDERATIONS IN THE FRAMING OF RISK COMMUNICATIONS

Concept	Relevance	Example/Implication
Order	Early and late information in communication remembered more easily	Present most important information at the beginning of the risk communication, and reiterate at the end.
Context	Risk information more impactful if it includes timeline, severity, consequences, and underlying mechanisms or risk-action links	"Your risk of having a myocardial infarction (MI) is 10% in the next 10 years. This is a debilitating condition that can lead to premature death in a matter of hours. You can help prevent an MI with proper nutrition, exercise, medication, and consultation with your physician."
Valence	Gain frames more effective for risk communications regarding health promotion, loss frames more effective for risk communications regarding detection behaviors such as screening	Gain frame: "If you eat more fruits and vegetables, you will feel better"
		Loss frame: "If you don't eat more fruits and vegetables, you will be at higher risk for disease"
Acknowledge *a priori* beliefs about risk	Risk communications should address people's initial beliefs about the health outcome in question, correcting misconceptions and reinforcing accurate beliefs	"Electronic cigarettes are less harmful than conventional cigarettes but nevertheless have their own harms such as disease-causing substances in the flavors used to enhance the sensory experience of electronic cigarettes"
Anecdotal (vs. statistical) information	Personalized narratives can elicit more attention toward and memory for a risk communication	"I got a BRCA1/2 screening test and it was positive, making me talk to my doctor about decreasing my risk"

There is some evidence that recall of risk information is more accurate for pictographs that use anthropomorphic (person-like) icons, such as restroom icons or stick figures, than for those that use blocks, ovals, and asterisks.[76,77] Person-like icons may evoke higher individual concern and personal involvement, thereby increasing motivation to process the information.[76] However, other studies have found no effect of icons on accurate recall of risk level.[78,79]

In pictographs, the number of affected individuals could be displayed scattered throughout the base population in order to convey randomness.[53,54] However, this approach undermines the speed of processing and greater accuracy characteristic of "grouped" pictographs,[53] perhaps because it changes the way the information is visually processed.[68] Random arrays are also rated less favorably than grouped arrays by participants.[54,68] Thus, the benefits of random arrays do not seem to outweigh the drawbacks.

Another type of pictorial representation is a "risk ladder" depicting higher risk on the higher rungs of a ladder.[80] Risk ladders have been used extensively as a means of effectively conveying both absolute and comparative risk information.[53,81] Factors such as the vertical proximity of one's risk estimate on the ladder (independent of numerical risk estimate) and whether comparative risk information is provided influence the effects of risk ladders on comprehension accuracy and behavior change. For instance, nearness to the top of the ladder increases perceived risk, regardless of the numerical estimate that coincides with that location.[80] Providing comparative information within a risk ladder can help individuals—particularly those with low numeracy—to understand their risk,[82] but it can also reduce message acceptance and perceived absolute risk.[83]

Visual aids that are more technologically savvy or visually sophisticated are not necessarily more effective at improving comprehension. Using a virtual reality platform to deliver risk information, Kaphingst et al.[84] found a simpler ladder metaphor (based on a risk ladder) resulted in better comprehension of risk information than a more complex bridge metaphor.[84] Similarly, animated graphs produced lower accuracy than static graphs in one online study,[85] but improved comprehension in another, especially when combined with reflective questions.[86]

Regardless of the format, providing "part-to-whole" information, or information about the denominator (population at risk), as well as the numerator (those affected) is important—consistent with our recommendations above. Otherwise, graphical displays of risk information can produce biased risk estimates. Lastly, individuals who are low in both numeracy and graph literacy may not benefit from visual aids, regardless of their specific characteristics, and may instead require analogies, additional training, or other approaches to conveying the risk information.[69,75]

Beyond numbers and pictures. For risk communication to be maximally persuasive, people often need additional nonnumeric information (see Table 38-2). They may need to understand more about the context within which a risk occurs, including the cause(s) of the risk, timelines, consequences, or the physiological or biological mechanisms through which a risk has its effects.[87,88] This is particularly important for complex and counterintuitive processes, such as drug interactions. Providing this contextual information can increase the credibility and memorability of the message because it provides an explanation and does not expect people to accept a message on faith. Accompanying a risk communication with risk-action links or specific recommended actions or advice to reduce one's risk can also increase self-efficacy and the likelihood of changing one's beliefs and behavior.[53,83,89] Because people have existing beliefs or mental models about risks, it is important to remain consistent with these mental models when providing contextual information,[87] while also countering common misconceptions.[24]

The effectiveness and impact of risk communications will hinge not only on their content but also on their framing. People tend to process and remember information that comes early (primacy effect) and late in a presentation (recency effect). For example, Ubel et al.[90] found that patients using a tamoxifen decision aid were more concerned about side effects when these side effects were presented after (rather than before) the benefits. Some evidence suggests that risk information concerning prevention behaviors such as exercise is more impactful when framed in terms of gains, whereas information concerning detection behaviors such as screening is more impactful when framed in terms of losses.[91] Finally, risk communications that are framed in ways that match people's conventional ways of communicating—by using, for examples, metaphors[92] and narratives[93]—may be more evocative.

PSYCHOLOGICAL FACTORS IN RISK COMMUNICATION

Thoughtful choices about how to communicate numerical risk information are a necessary but not always a sufficient precursor to impactful risk communication. It is also important to pay heed to the many psychological factors that come into play when people are exposed to risk information. Here we focus on examples of motivational and emotional factors in particular.

Motivational Factors. When faced with risk information, people bring many potent motives to the communication context.[94] For example, people tend to hold self-aggrandizing, positive beliefs about themselves on a wide variety of dimensions.[95] They tend to believe that their food choices are healthier than those of their peers[96] and that they are better than average drivers.[97] Not surprisingly, then, people tend to be unrealistically optimistic about their risk,[98] a bias that has been shown to be highly resistant to change.[99] Accordingly, use of numerical information improves when the information produces favorable rather than unfavorable conclusions about oneself and one's risk level.[100] People also actively avoid risk information that may be construed as threatening.[101]

The influence of this self-serving motive has implications for risk communication. Attempting to reduce unrealistic optimism may not be the most prudent approach, considering the resistance of personal risk perceptions to debiasing[99] and some evidence that these exaggerated positive beliefs can have long-term positive health consequences.[102] Instead, strategies that offset defensiveness and the negative effects of this bias may be more effective. One option is to have people reflect on important values ("value affirmation") prior to receiving risk information, which appears to reduce avoidance[103] and promote more objective attention toward and processing of the information (e.g., ref. 104). In one study, when people who were unrealistically optimistic about their colorectal cancer risk were given personalized risk information but also had an opportunity to reflect on an important value in advance, they expressed higher intentions to get a colorectal cancer screening test.[105]

Attempts to make risk communications simple are likely to facilitate greater impact, following a "less is more" approach.[52,106] Given that a single risk communication cannot provide all possible information about a risk, it is important to identify and target the goals that are most important to the target audience. A value-of-information analysis can help to set information priorities by determining the facts that most influence an audience's decision.[24] Participatory designs in which a target audience helps create the communication message can ensure the message resonates with the issues most important to the intended recipients. For instance, these processes may determine that there is one central item, such as fear of a side effect, that drives nearly all decisions. A risk communication message might be adequate if it included just this information; providing any additional information may be distracting. Even risk messages supported by strong evidence can be ineffective if they do not address the audience's concerns and needs. For instance, public health officials have been less effective than vaccine skeptics in communicating vaccination issues that resonated with their audience.[107]

Emotional Factors. In addition to motivational factors, affective or emotional factors can influence the outcomes of a risk communication in several ways. Rather than being universally useful or detrimental, their effects often depend on the fit or congruence between the affect evoked and the goal of the risk communication. For instance, affect-rich outcomes result in more pronounced overweighting of small probabilities compared to outcomes that are less affect-laden,[108] so whether to imbue the outcome with affect, perhaps by using affect-laden images,[109] will depend on if this is a desirable communication outcome. For example, a risk communication may imbue the relatively low probability of developing cervical cancer (8.1 cases per 100,000 women per year) with affect to increase HPV vaccine uptake, but may avoid imbuing the low probability of medication side effects with affect so as not to deter medication uptake.

1. *Effects on information processing.* Emotions are comprised of several dimensions or characteristics that produce predictable and systematic effects on judgment and decision making. For instance, anger and happiness tend to reduce perceptions of risk because they convey a sense of certainty and control, whereas fear is associated with a sense of uncertainty and low controllability, and thus, tends to increase risk perceptions and risk-averse behavior.[110] Fear also can motivate more thoughtful attention to and systematic processing of threat information, particularly information about how to prevent the threat, as well as greater accessibility of the health threat in memory.[111–115] Most research on the role of emotion in risk communication has centered on fear, particularly in the context of fear appeals, or persuasive risk communication messages intended to arouse fear.[89,111,116]

   Research on fear appeals suggests that the fear evoked by a risk communication message can have different effects depending on several factors, and the evidence of whether it is necessary to arouse fear in order for a risk communication to be effective remains equivocal.[116,117] Results from several meta-analyses suggest that fear appeals can motivate behavior change when they also increase self-efficacy and response efficacy, convey personal relevance or susceptibility, and do not convey emotionally laden severity.[89,116] This work underscores the importance of conveying risk-action links, or specific recommended actions or advice on how to reduce one's risk.[88,111]

   Importantly for risk communication, these effects of emotion tend to occur regardless of whether the emotion is *integral* to, or evoked by, the decision at hand, or *incidental* to the decision (i.e., experienced at the time of decision making, but not evoked by it).[110,118] For example, an individual's fearful emotional state may motivate a risk-mitigating health decision, such as getting a colonoscopy, even if the fear is caused by an upcoming job evaluation and not by one's perceived risk of colorectal cancer. The carry-over effects of incidental emotions suggest individuals' emotional state at the time of receiving the risk communication may influence their reactions to it in ways that the risk communicator cannot fully control. However, little work has systematically examined the role of incidental emotions on risk communication effectiveness.
2. *Affect as information.* Several theories of emotion suggest that affect or emotion can serve as information or provide meaning to information that guides decision-making.[41,42,119–122] For instance, negative emotions can serve as warnings even in the absence of cognitive or elaborated processing,[119,120] and, as noted earlier, people's judgments of risk are often based on how they feel about the risk more than what they think about it.[41,42] Affect can also influence the existing knowledge that is most accessible in memory, or call attention to specific new information in a risk communication (e.g., Peters et al.[120]). For instance, graphic warning labels on cigarette packages have been shown to evoke emotions that may influence risk perceptions both by acting as information about risk, and also by calling attention to warning information (i.e., acting as a spotlight).[123,124] Affective reactions may be particularly important when cognitive resources are low,[125,126] and/or when the information is complex and when several types of risk need to be integrated and considered simultaneously.[120] Thus, risk communication messages may benefit particularly from relying on affective content, such as images, when the audience is expected to be distracted, under time constraints, or managing information about competing risks.

   Given the importance of affect in risk perception and judgment, the most usable information in a risk communication may not be objective risk estimates, but rather affectively based gist risk information, or the fear and worry evoked by the health threat. This is particularly important for individuals with low deliberative ability (e.g., low literacy or numeracy) because they tend to rely more on their affective reactions when making risk-related decisions.[120] However, use of affect as a substitute for more deliberative assessments of a risk may not always lead to optimal decision making,[127] so it may be necessary to strategically leverage emotions. For instance, one may want to highlight different types of risk information depending on the predicted effects of emotions. If an audience has preexisting negative feelings about a certain behavioral choice (e.g., medication side effects), they may disproportionately attend to the risks associated with this choice, which may or may not align with the goals of the communication. In addition, if a risk communication is expected to evoke feelings of worry that could elicit defensive processing or avoidance behaviors, acknowledging the affective reaction likely to be evoked by a risk communication may be a useful means of minimizing such reactions.

3. *Social transmission of emotions.* Emotions are also transmitted or transferred between individuals in processes of emotional transmission,[128] contagion,[129] and other phenomena (e.g., refs. 130 and 131). In risk communication, there may be an asymmetrical transmission of emotions whereby the emotions expressed by the message communicator are transmitted to members of the audience.[128] Negative emotions are particularly susceptible to social transmission.[132] Thus, the affect expressed by the communicator may influence a risk communication's effectiveness either directly or in combination with the emotions evoked by the threat and risk information. However, to date, no work has examined such processes.
4. *Anticipated emotions.* People's risk judgments and decisions are often driven by expectations about the future, which could influence how they process a risk communication. Some risk information like HIV screening results or genetic testing for Huntington's disease can be highly consequential. In such cases people are motivated to be prepared for bad news, and thus may "brace" for the impact of such news. This can lead people to become overly pessimistic prior to receipt of risk information,[101] which could influence how they process and respond to the information. Similarly, people make predictions about how they will feel after getting personally relevant information—predictions that are often exaggerated.[133] Weinstein et al.[46] observed that the regret people anticipate experiencing if they contracted influenza without being vaccinated was a stronger predictor than various risk perception measures of subsequent vaccination behavior. Ferrer et al.[134] found that the anticipated affect in response to genetic test results was a greater predictor of deciding to get genetic test results than was current worry about those results. Accordingly, risk communications may be more effective to the extent that they focus not only on the chances of an outcome but also on how one will be able to cope with that outcome.

FROM PROCESSING RISK COMMUNICATIONS TO ACTING ON THEM

Even if people understand their risk and process it nondefensively and accurately, they may not use the information in the desired way. Sometimes, other factors supersede effects of risk information. For instance, HIV risk perceptions are weakly related to condom use behavior[135] partly because condom use decisions are often made in the "heat of the moment." Other times, social support may be necessary to act on the risk information. This is often the case for genetic risk information; receiving genetic test results is much more distressing for individuals who report having insufficient social support.[136–138]

Other times, the message must be accompanied by additional information. For instance, fear appeals only have their desired effects on beliefs and behavioral outcomes when they are accompanied by efficacy messages that increase the audience's belief in its ability to perform the recommended action (i.e., self-efficacy), and/or that this action will mitigate the threat (i.e., response efficacy). Otherwise, they evoke counterproductive defensive reactions.[89] The effectiveness of risk communication messages, including fear appeals, also increases when they are accompanied by protective actions one could take to reduce her/his risk.[53,80] Providing these risk-action links that describe how a protective action reduces one's risk can increase message understanding and response efficacy, thereby increasing perceptions of behavioral control and motivation to engage in the protective behavior.[88] Similarly, one can strengthen implementation intentions, defined as specific actions one will take given certain preconditions (e.g., if I see high-fat food, I will choose something else to eat). Establishing implementation intentions can increase the likelihood of behavior change.[139]

Strategies that have been shown to enhance processing of risk communications may also have the double benefit of strengthening the effects on subsequent behavior. For example, value affirmation opportunities not only increase attention to potentially threatening risk information, but may also increase self-efficacy and lead to behavior change.[140] Social comparison and norm-based information can both increase attention to risk information and tendencies to change behavior.[141]

TRAINING THE RISK COMMUNICATORS

Our focus here has largely been on the content and context of a risk communication, but the impact of such communications is also likely to hinge on the ability of the communicator to understand and work with numbers and risk information. Consider, for example, that much risk communication occurs in a clinical context with healthcare providers conveying risk information to patients. Yet several studies suggest that over half of physicians do not have adequate numeracy levels to understand, interpret, and communicate risk information to their patients.[65,142–145] Although it may seem that physicians' extensive education should prepare them to interpret numeric information,[144] many of the undergraduate and graduate school majors that lead to medical school such as biology and chemistry produce less sophisticated mathematical training than disciplines like psychology and economics.[146] Thus, physicians are not necessarily trained in mathematics or in how to communicate numeric information.

This lack of training may contribute to the rarity with which discussions about risks and benefits occur in clinical contexts; only 8% of patient-provider encounters involve a discussion of risks and benefits.[147] Moreover, physicians' intuitions and preferences regarding the optimal approaches to communicating numeric risk information are often miscalibrated with evidence-based approaches.[70,148] For example, 1 in X formats are used extensively and preferred by physicians,[148,149] but they are more prone to misinterpretation than other formats, leading to subjectively higher and less accurate probability estimates,[60,149,150] especially when not used with a visual aid.[149] As noted earlier, use of percentages or frequencies that utilize the same denominators are recommended instead (i.e., natural frequencies[53,61,150,151]).

Physicians' ability to interpret and communicate risk information improves when visuals aids are used,[65] and when additional training in risk communication skills is provided.[152,153] For instance, trained physicians were more likely to supplement their verbal risk communication with written risk information as well.[152] Patients were also more likely to report changes in the health status and medication side effects when the physician received additional risk communication training.[153] Beyond interventions among practicing physicians, attention to issues of numeracy should also be addressed in medical training.

RESEARCH NEEDS

Although the fields of risk perception and risk communication have advanced greatly and produced several recommended and implementable practices, many questions remain. At the outset we noted that many factors drive health behaviors and decisions, and we need to learn more about how those factors qualify many of the recommendations summarized here. For example, in cases where environmental "nudges"[154] are used to facilitate healthy behavior—such as by making stairs more accessible than elevators—changes in risk perceptions may not be necessary to change behavior, but could influence comparable behavior in other settings not containing the nudge. Moreover, although we know a great deal about how to influence risk perceptions, we know less about how to strengthen the relationship between risk perceptions and behavior[155]; nudges and other factors may be useful in this regard.

A second research need is to understand how new communication media might affect best practices for risk communication. Smart phone technology allows for the collection of multiple sources of information which can be used to undergird a risk communication; for example, someone attempting to lose weight might be given a particular type of tailored risk information about weight gain based on GPS-determined proximity to healthy and unhealthy food sources. Many new communication media are social in nature, introducing a possible role for peers and close others in communicating and acting on risk information. Klein and Ferrer[156] observed that people were more receptive to a risk message when it concerned their close other's risk rather than their own risk, a finding with clear implications for the target of a risk communication. Risk feedback coming from electronic sources may also be just as effective as risk feedback conveyed in conventional counseling settings if it is simple and content-rich, and provides reassurance.[157]

We note also that people's level of risk can change dramatically over time (e.g., as individuals age or as their other risk factors change) in ways they do not comprehend; for example, cancer risk tends to increase as one ages, yet people believe the opposite.[158] Risk also can accumulate exponentially, as is true of the risk of HIV infection as the number of partners increases, yet the notion of an exponential increase is beyond most people's comprehension.[159] Risk itself can also change over time for various reasons. In the case of genetics, as the science evolves, people may learn that they are at high genetic risk for a given disease yet learn later that the information they received is not based on current genetic science. One study suggests that people are not negatively affected by such changes, instead appreciating the changing nature of scientific discovery.[160] In general, we need to know much more about how to incorporate time—and anticipated changes over time—into the communication of risk (see also ref. 52).

Finally, much of the literature discussed here does not pay adequate attention to the many individual differences—personality, demographic, sociocultural, and otherwise—that are certain to qualify the impact of risk communications. Research shows, for example, that optimistic people are more amenable to ambiguous risk communications[161] and that health communications more generally have a greater impact when culturally targeted.[162]

CONCLUSION

Although many factors have an influence on people's health behaviors and decisions, one important factor to consider is the extent to which people feel at risk for health outcomes linked to those behaviors and decisions. Their risk perceptions are multiply determined by a combination of emotional, cognitive, motivational, and other factors. Most importantly, people do not often think about risk in strictly numerical terms, and when faced with numerical risk information, may have trouble comprehending and acting on it. Accordingly, effective and impactful risk communications are going to be those that acknowledge people's difficulty with numerical information as well as the many other influences that hover over the processing of these risk communications. For example, reporting absolute and comparative risk rather than relative risk, using comprehensible pictorial representations of risk, capturing the recipient's emotional state, and providing resources to reduce one's risk are potentially useful strategies. To the extent that risk communications "go beyond" the numbers and pay attention to how people think and reason, and to the extent that such communications are integrated into theoretically driven interventions that consider other influential factors, they can go a long way toward optimizing public health.

References

1. Willett WC. Balancing life-style and genomics research for disease prevention. *Science*. 2002;296(5568):695–8.
2. Lortet-Tieulent J, Sauer AG, Siegel RL, et al. State-level cancer mortality attributable to cigarette smoking in the United States. *JAMA Intern Med*. 2016;176(12):1792–8.
3. Munoz N, Bosch FX, Castellsagué X, et al. Against which human papillomavirus types shall we vaccinate and screen? The international perspective. *Int J Cancer*. 2004;111(2):278–85.
4. Schiffman M, Castle PE, Jeronimo J, Rodriguez AC, Wacholder S. Human papillomavirus and cervical cancer. *Lancet*. 2007;370(9590):890–907.
5. Record NB, Onion DK, Prior RE, et al. Community-wide cardiovascular disease prevention programs and health outcomes in a rural county, 1970–2010. *JAMA*. 2015;313(2):147–55.
6. Stone NJ, Robinson J, Lichtenstein AH, et al. 2013 ACC/AHA guideline on the treatment of blood cholesterol to reduce atherosclerotic cardiovascular risk in adults: A report of the American College of Cardiology/American Heart Association Task Force on Practice Guidelines. *J Am Coll Cardiol*. 2014; 63(25 Pt B):2889–934.
7. Sauber-Schatz EK, West BA, Bergen G. Vital signs: Restraint use and motor vehicle occupant death rates among children aged 0–12 years—United States, 2002–2011. *MMWR Morb Mortal Wkly Rep*. 2014;63(5):113–8.
8. Hardeman W, Johnston M, Johnston D, Bonetti D, Wareham N, Kinmonth AL. Application of the theory of planned behaviour in behaviour change interventions: A systematic review. *Psychol Health*. 2002;17(3):123–58.
9. Hoey LM, Ieropoli SC, White VM, Jefford M. Systematic review of peer-support programs for people with cancer. *Patient Educ Couns*. 2008;70(3):315–37.
10. Mayne SL, Auchincloss AH, Michael YL. Impact of policy and built environment changes on obesity-related outcomes: A systematic review of naturally occurring experiments. *Obes Rev*. 2015;16(5):362–75.
11. Shaya FT, Chirikov VV, Mullins CD, et al. Social networks help control hypertension. *J Clin Hypertens (Greenwich)*. 2013;15(1):34–40.
12. Sheeran P, Maki A, Montanaro E, et al. The impact of changing attitudes, norms, and self-efficacy on health-related intentions and behavior: A meta-analysis. *Health Psychol*. 2016;35(11):1178–88.
13. Becker MH, Janz NK. The health belief model applied to understanding diabetes regimen compliance. *Diabetes Educ*. 1985;11(1):41–7.
14. Weinstein ND, Sandman PM. Predicting homeowners' mitigation responses to radon test data. *J Soc Issues*. 1992;48(4):63–83.
15. Brewer NT, Chapman GB, Gibbons FX, Gerrard M, McCaul KD, Weinstein ND. Meta-analysis of the relationship between risk perception and health behavior: The example of vaccination. *Health Psychol*. 2007;26(2):136–45.
16. Sheeran P, Harris PR, Epton T. Does heightening risk appraisals change people's intentions and behavior? A meta-analysis of experimental studies. *Psychol Bull*. 2014;140(2):511–43.
17. Stock ML, Gibbons FX, Beekman JB, Gerrard M. It only takes once: The absent-exempt heuristic and reactions to comparison-based sexual risk information. *J Pers Soc Psychol*. 2015;109(1):35–52.
18. Epstein RM, Alper BS, Quill TE. Communicating evidence for participatory decision making. *JAMA*. 2004;291(19):2359–66.
19. Paling J. Strategies to help patients understand risks. *Br Med J*. 2003;327(7417):745–8.
20. Forrest K, Simpson SA, Wilson BJ, et al. To tell or not to tell: Barriers and facilitators in family communication about genetic risk. *Clin Genet*. 2003;64(4):317–26.
21. Damman OC, Bogaerts NMM, van den Haak MJ, Timmermans DRM. How lay people understand and make sense of personalized disease risk information. *Health Expect*. 2017;20(5):973–83.
22. Elwyn G, Kreuwel I, Durand MA, et al. How to develop web-based decision support interventions for patients: A process map. *Patient Educ Couns*. 2011;82(2):260–5.
23. Waters EA, Sullivan HW, Nelson W, Hesse BW. What is my cancer risk? How internet-based cancer risk assessment tools communicate individualized risk estimates to the public: Content analysis. *J Med Internet Res*. 2009;11(3):e33.
24. Fischhoff B, Brewer NT, Downs JS, eds. *Communicating Risks and Benefits: An Evidence-Based User's Guide*. Silver Spring, MD: U.S. Department of Health and Human Services, Food and Drug Administration; 2012.
25. Elwyn G, Edwards A, Kinnersley P, Grol R. Shared decision making and the concept of equipoise: The competences of involving patients in healthcare choices. *Br J Gen Pract*. 2000;50(460):892–9.
26. Fowler SL, Klein WM, Ball L, McGuire J, Colditz GA, Waters EA. Using an internet-based breast cancer risk assessment tool to improve social-cognitive precursors of physical activity. *Med Decis Making*. 2017;37(6):657–69.

27. Michaels D, Monforton C. Manufacturing uncertainty: Contested science and the protection of the public's health and environment. *Am J Public Health*. 2005;95(S1):S39–48.
28. Slovic P. Perception of risk. *Science*. 1987;236(4799):280–5.
29. Denes-Raj V, Epstein S. Conflict between intuitive and rational processing: When people behave against their better judgment. *J Pers Soc Psychol*. 1994;66(5):819–29.
30. Johnson EJ, Tversky A. Affect, generalization, and the perception of risk. *J Pers Soc Psychol*. 1983;45(1):20–31.
31. Cameron LD, Sherman KA, Marteau TM, Brown PM. Impact of genetic risk information and type of disease on perceived risk, anticipated affect, and expected consequences of genetic tests. *Health Psychol*. 2009:28(3):307–16.
32. Reyna VF, Brainerd CJ. Fuzzy-trace theory and framing effects in choice: Gist extraction, truncation, and conversion. *J Behav Decis Mak*. 1991;4(4):249–62.
33. Pope RE. The delusion of certainty in Savage's sure-thing principle. *J Econ Psychol*. 1991;12(2):209–41.
34. Bruine de Bruin WB, Fischhoff B, Millstein SG, Halpern-Felsher BL. Verbal and numerical expressions of probability: "It's a fifty–fifty chance." *Organ Behav Hum Decis Processes*. 2000;81(1):115–31.
35. Lipkus IM, Samsa G, Rimer BK. General performance on a numeracy scale among highly educated samples. *Med Decis Making*. 2001;21(1):37–44.
36. Berry D, Raynor T, Knapp P, Bersellini E. Over the counter medicines and the need for immediate action: A further evaluation of European Commission recommended wordings for communicating risk. *Patient Educ Couns*. 2004;53(2):129–34.
37. Festinger L. A theory of social comparison processes. *Hum Relat*. 1954;7:117–40.
38. Blalock SJ, DeVellis BM, Afifi RA, Sandler RS. Risk perceptions and participation in colorectal cancer screening. *Health Psychol*. 1990;9(6):792–806.
39. Klein WM. Objective standards are not enough: Affective, self-evaluative, and behavioral responses to social comparison information. *J Pers Soc Psychol*. 1997;72(4):763–74.
40. Fagerlin A, Zikmund-Fisher BJ, Ubel PA. "If I'm better than average, then I'm ok?": Comparative information influences beliefs about risk and benefits. *Patient Educ Couns*. 2007;69(1):140–4.
41. Slovic P, Finucane ML, Peters E, MacGregor DG. The affect heuristic. *Eur J Oper Res*. 2007;177(3):1333–52.
42. Loewenstein GF, Weber EU, Hsee CK, Welch N. Risk as feelings. *Psychol Bull*. 2001;127(2):267–86.
43. Consedine NS, Magai C, Krivoshekova YS, Ryzewicz L, Neugut AI. Fear, anxiety, worry, and breast cancer screening behavior: A critical review. *Cancer Epidemiol Biomarkers Prev*. 2004;13(4):501–10.
44. Dillard AJ, Ferrer RA, Ubel PA, Fagerlin A. Risk perception measures' associations with behavior intentions, affect, and cognition following colon cancer screening messages. *Health Psychol*. 2012;31(1):106–13.
45. Janssen E, van Osch L, de Vries H, Lechner L. Measuring risk perceptions of skin cancer: Reliability and validity of different operationalizations. *Br J Health Psychol*. 2011;16(Pt 1):92–112.
46. Weinstein ND, Kwitel A, McCaul KD, Magnan RE, Gerrard M, Gibbons FX. Risk perceptions: Assessment and relationship to influenza vaccination. *Health Psychol*. 2007;26(2):146–51.
47. Ferrer RA, Klein WMP, Persoskie A, Avishai-Yitshak A, Sheeran P. The tripartite model of risk perception (TRIRISK): Distinguishing deliberative, affective, and experiential components of perceived risk. *Ann Behav Med*. 2016;50(5):653–63.
48. Ferrer RA, Klein WMP, Avishai-Yitshak A, Jones K, Villegas M, Sheeran P. When does risk perception predict protection motivation? A person-by-situation analysis. *PLoS One*. 2018;13(3):e0191994.
49. Waters EA, Hay JL, Orom H, Kiviniemi MT, Drake BF. "Don't know" responses to risk perception measures: Implications for underserved populations. *Med Decis Making*. 2013;33(2):271–81.
50. Taber JM, Klein WM. The role of conviction in personal risk perceptions: What can we learn from research on attitude strength? *Soc Personal Psychol Compass*. 2016;10(4):202–18.
51. Han PKJ, Moser R, Klein WMP. Perceived ambiguity about cancer prevention recommendations: Relationship to perceptions of cancer preventability, risk, and worry. *J Health Commun*. 2006;11(0 1):51–69.
52. Fagerlin A, Zikmund-Fisher BJ, Ubel PA. Helping patients decide: Ten steps to better risk communication. *J Natl Cancer Inst*. 2011;103(19):1436–43.
53. Lipkus IM. Numeric, verbal, and visual formats of conveying health risks: Suggested best practices and future recommendations. *Med Decis Making*. 2007;27(5):696–713.
54. Waters EA, McQueen A, Cameron LD. Perceived risk and health risk communication. In: Hamilton HE, Chou WYS, eds. *The Routledge Handbook of Language and Health Communication*. London: Routledge; 2014, pp. 47–60.
55. Waters EA, Fagerlin A, Zikmund-Fisher BJ. Overcoming the many pitfalls of communicating risk. In: Diefenbach MA, Miller-Halegoua S, Bowen DJ, eds. *Handbook of Health Decision Science*. New York: Springer; 2016, pp. 265–77.
56. Siteman Cancer Center website. https://siteman.wustl.edu/prevention/ydr.
57. Hoffrage U, Lindsey S, Hertwig R, Gigerenzer G. Communicating statistical information. *Science*. 2000;290(5500):2261–2.
58. Stone ER, Bruine de Bruin W, Wilkins AM, MacDonald Gibson J. Designing graphs to communicate risks: Understanding how the choice of graphical format influences decision making. *Risk Anal*. 2017;37(4):612–28.
59. Hellwig LD, Biesecker BB, Lewis KL, et al. The ability of patients to distinguish among genomic variant sub-classifications. *Circ Genom Precis Med*. 2018;11(6):e001975.
60. Sirota M, Juanchich M, Kostopoulou O, Hanak R. Decisive evidence on a smaller-than-you-think phenomenon: Revisiting the "1-in-X" effect on subjective medical probabilities. *Med Decis Making*. 2014;34(4):419–29.
61. Zikmund-Fisher BJ. Time to retire the 1-in-X risk format. *Med Decis Making*. 2011;31(5):703–4.
62. Fagerlin A, Wang C, Ubel PA. Reducing the influence of anecdotal reasoning on people's health care decisions: Is a picture worth a thousand statistics? *Med Decis Making*. 2005:25(4):398–405.
63. Feldman-Stewart D, Brundage MD, Zotov V. Further insight into the perception of quantitative information: Judgments of gist in treatment decisions. *Med Decis Making*. 2007;27(1):34–43.
64. Garcia-Retamero R, Cokely ET. Communicating health risks with visual aids. *Curr Dir Psychol Sci*. 2013;22(5):392–9.
65. Garcia-Retamero R, Cokely ET, Wicki B, Joeris A. Improving risk literacy in surgeons. *Patient Educ Couns*. 2016;99(7):1156–61.
66. Zikmund-Fisher BJ, Ubel PA, Smith DM, et al. Communicating side effect risks in a tamoxifen prophylaxis decision aid: The debiasing influence of pictographs. *Patient Educ Couns*. 2008;73(2):209–14.
67. Fagerlin A, Valley TS, Scherer AM, Knaus M, Das E, Zikmund-Fisher BJ. Communicating infectious disease prevalence through graphics: Results from an international survey. *Vaccine*. 2017;35(32):4041–7.
68. Ancker JS, Senathirajah Y, Kukafka R, Starren, JB. Design features of graphs in health risk communication: A systematic review. *J Am Med Inform Assoc*. 2006;13(6):608–18.
69. Garcia-Retamero R, Okan Y, Cokely ET. Using visual aids to improve communication of risks about health: A review. *Sci World J*. 2012;2012:562637.
70. Elting LS, Martin CG, Cantor SB, Rubenstein EB. Influence of data display formats on physician investigators' decisions to stop clinical trials: Prospective trial with repeated measures. *BMJ*. 1999;318(7197):1527–31.
71. Garcia-Retamero R, Galesic M, Gigerenzer G. Do icon arrays help reduce denominator neglect? *Med Decis Making*. 2010;30(6):672–84.
72. Hawley ST, Zikmund-Fisher BJ, Ubel P, Jancovic A, Lucas T, Fagerlin A. The impact of the format of graphical presentation on health-related knowledge and treatment choices. *Patient Educ Couns*. 2008;73(3):448–55.
73. Smit AK, Keogh LA, Hersch J, et al. Public preferences for communicating personal genomic risk information: A focus group study. *Health Expect*. 2016;19(6):1203–14.
74. Galesic M, Garcia-Retamero R, Gigerenzer G. Using icon arrays to communicate medical risks: Overcoming low numeracy. *Health Psychol*. 2009;28(2):210–16.
75. Garcia-Retamero R, Galesic M. Who profits from visual aids: Overcoming challenges in people's understanding of risks. *Soc Sci Med*. 2010;70(7):1019–25.
76. Kreuzmair C, Siegrist M, Keller C. Does iconicity in pictographs matter? The Influence of iconicity and numeracy on information processing, decision making, and liking in an eye-tracking study. *Risk Anal*. 2017;37(3):546–56.
77. Zikmund-Fisher BJ, Witteman HO, Dickson M, et al. Blocks, ovals, or people? Icon type affects risk perceptions and recall of pictographs. *Med Decis Making*. 2014;34(4):443–53.
78. Gaissmaier W, Wegwarth O, Skopec D, Müller A-S, Broschinski S, Politi MC. Numbers can be worth a thousand pictures: Individual differences in understanding graphical and numerical representations of health-related information. *Health Psychol*. 2012;31(3):286.
79. Stone ER, Yates JF, Parker AM. Effects of numerical and graphical displays on professed risk-taking behavior. *J Exp Psychol Appl*. 1997;3(4):243.

80. Sandman PM, Weinstein ND, Miller P. High risk or low: How location on a "risk ladder" affects perceived risk. *Risk Anal.* 1994;14(1):35–45.

81. Lipkus IM, Hollands JG. The visual communication of risk. *J Natl Cancer Inst Monogr.* 1999;(25):149–63.

82. Keller C, Siegrist M, Visschers V. Effect of risk ladder format on risk perception in high- and low-numerate individuals. *Risk Anal.* 2009;29(9):1255–64.

83. Janssen E, Ruiter RAC, Waters EA. Combining risk communication strategies to simultaneously convey the risks of four diseases associated with physical inactivity to socio-demographically diverse populations. *J Behav Med.* 2018;41(3):318–32.

84. Kaphingst KA, Persky S, McCall C, Lachance C, Beall AC, Blascovich J. Testing communication strategies to convey genomic concepts using virtual reality technology. *J Health Commun.* 2009;14(4):384–99.

85. Kasper J, van de Roemer A, Pöttgen J. et al. A new graphical format to communicate treatment effects to patients—A web-based randomized controlled trial. *Health Expect.* 2017;20(4):797–804.

86. Okan Y, Garcia-Retamero R, Cokely ET, Maldonado A. Improving risk understanding across ability levels: Encouraging active processing with dynamic icon arrays. *J Exp Psychol Appl.* 2015;21(2):178–94.

87. Cameron LD. Illness risk representations and motivations to engage in protective behavior: The case of skin cancer risk. *Psychol Health.* 2008;23(1):91–112.

88. Cameron LD, Marteau TM, Brown PM, Klein WMP, Sherman KA. Communication strategies for enhancing understanding of the behavioral implications of genetic and biomarker tests for disease risk: The role of coherence. *J Behav Med.* 2012;35(3):286–98.

89. Witte K, Allen M. A meta-analysis of fear appeals: Implications for effective public health campaigns. *Health Educ Behav.* 2000;27(5):591–615.

90. Ubel PA, Smith DM, Zikmund-Fisher BJ, et al. Testing whether decision aids introduce cognitive biases: Results of a randomized trial. *Patient Educ Couns.* 2010;80(2):158–63.

91. Gallagher KM, Updegraff JA. Health message framing effects on attitudes, intentions, and behavior: A meta-analytic review. *Ann Behav Med.* 2011;43(1):101–16.

92. Spina M, Arndt J, Landau MJ, Cameron LD. Enhancing health message framing with metaphor and cultural values: Impact on Latinas' cervical cancer screening. *Ann Behav Med.* 2018;52(2):106–15.

93. McQueen A, Kreuter MW, Kalesan B, Alcaraz KI. Understanding narrative effects: The impact of breast cancer survivor stories on message processing, attitudes, and beliefs among African American women. *Health Psychol.* 2011;30(6):674–82.

94. Klein WMP, Cerully JL. Health-related risk perception and decision-making: Lessons from the study of motives in social psychology. *Soc Personal Psychol Compass.* 2007;1(1):334–58.

95. Dunning D, Heath C, Suls JM. Flawed self-assessment implications for health, education, and the workplace. *Psychol Sci Public Interest.* 2004;5(3):69–106.

96. Scherer AM, Bruchmann K, Windschitl PD, et al. Sources of bias in peoples' social-comparative estimates of food consumption. *J Exp Psychol Appl.* 2016;22(2):173.

97. Horswill MS, Waylen AE, Tofield MI. Drivers' ratings of different components of their own driving skill: A greater illusion of superiority for skills that relate to accident involvement. *J Appl Soc Psychol.* 2004;34(1):177–95.

98. Shepperd JA, Waters EA, Weinstein ND, Klein WMP. A primer on unrealistic optimism. *Curr Dir Psychol Sci.* 2015;24(3):232–7.

99. Weinstein ND, Klein WM. Resistance of personal risk perceptions to debiasing interventions. *Health Psychol.* 1995;14(2):132–40.

100. Mata A, Sherman SJ, Ferreira MB, Mendonça C. Strategic numeracy: Self-serving reasoning about health statistics. *Basic Appl Soc Psychol.* 2015;37(3):165–73.

101. Melnyk D, Shepperd JA. Avoiding risk information about breast cancer. *Ann Behav Med.* 2012;44(2):216–24. doi:10.1007/s12160-012-9382-5.

102. Persoskie A, Ferrer RA, Nelson W, Klein WMP. Pre-cancer risk perceptions predict post-cancer subjective well-being: Domain-specific optimism and long-term resilience. *Health Psychol.* 2014;33(9):1023–32.

103. Howell J L, Shepperd JA. Reducing information avoidance through affirmation. *Psychol Sci.* 2012;23(2):141–5.

104. Klein WMP, Harris PR. Self-affirmation enhances attentional bias toward threatening components of a persuasive message. *Psychol Sci.* 2000;20(12):1463–7.

105. Klein WMP, Lipkus IM, Scholl SM, McQueen A, Cerully JL, Harris PR. Self-affirmation moderates effects of unrealistic optimism and pessimism on reactions to tailored risk feedback. *Psychol Health.* 2010;25(10):1195–208.

106. Peters E, Klein WMP, Kaufman A, Meilleur L, Dixon A. More is not always better: Intuitions about effective public policy can lead to unintended consequences. *Soc Issues Policy Rev.* 2013;7(1):114–48.

107. Downs JS, de Bruin WB, Fischhoff B. Parents' vaccination comprehension and decisions. *Vaccine.* 2008;26(12):1595–607.

108. Rottenstreich Y, Hsee CK. Money, kisses, and electric shocks: On the affective psychology of risk. *Psychol Sci.* 2001;12(3):185–90.

109. Keller C, Siegrist M, Gutscher H. The role of the affect and availability heuristics in risk communication. *Risk Anal.* 2006;26(3):631–39.

110. Lerner JS, Keltner D. Beyond valence: Toward a model of emotion-specific influences on judgement and choice. *Cogn Emot.* 2000;14(4):473–93.

111. Cameron LD, Chan CKY. Designing health communications: Harnessing the power of affect, imagery, and self-regulation. *Soc Personal Psychol Compass.* 2008;2(1):262–82.

112. Cameron LD, Diefenbach MA. Responses to information about psychosocial consequences of genetic testing for breast cancer susceptibility: Influences of cancer worry and risk perceptions. *J Health Psychol.* 2001;6(1):47–59.

113. Forgas JP. Affect and information processing strategies: An interactive relationship. In: Forgas JP, ed. *Feeling and Thinking: The Role of Affect in Social Cognition. Studies in Emotion and Social Interaction*, second series. New York: Cambridge University Press; 2000, pp. 253–80.

114. Liberman A, Chaiken S. Defensive processing of personally relevant health messages. *Pers Soc Psychol Bull.* 1992;18(6):669–79.

115. Shackman AJ, Sarinopoulos I, Maxwell JS, Pizzagalli DA, Lavric A, Davidson RJ. Anxiety selectively disrupts visuospatial working memory. *Emotion.* 2006;6(1):40–61.

116. Ruiter RAC, Kessels LTE, Peters G-JY, Kok G. Sixty years of fear appeal research: Current state of the evidence. *Int J Psychol.* 2014;49(2):63–70.

117. de Hoog N, Stroebe W, de Wit JBF. The impact of vulnerability to and severity of a health risk on processing and acceptance of fear-arousing communications: A meta-analysis. *Rev Gen Psychol.* 2007;11(3):258–85.

118. Lerner JS, Keltner D. Fear, anger, and risk. *J Pers Soc Psychol.* 2001;81(1):146.

119. Damasio AR, Everitt BJ, Bishop D. The somatic marker hypothesis and the possible functions of the prefrontal cortex [and discussion]. *Philos Trans R Soc Lond B Biol Sci.* 1996;351(1346):1413–420.

120. Peters E, Lipkus I, Diefenbach MA. The functions of affect in health communications and in the construction of health preferences. *J Commun.* 2006;56:S140–62.

121. Schwarz N, Clore GL. Mood as information: 20 years later. *Psychol Inq.* 2004;14(3–4):296–303.

122. Zajonc RB. Feeling and thinking: Preferences need no inferences. *Am Psychol.* 1980;35(2):151–75.

123. Evans AT, Peters E, Shoben AB, et al. Cigarette graphic warning labels increase both risk perceptions and smoking myth endorsement. *Psychol Health.* 2018;33(2):213–34.

124. Evans AT, Peters E, Strasser AA, Emery LF, Sheerin KM, Romer, D. Graphic warning labels elicit affective and thoughtful responses from smokers: Results of a randomized clinical trial. *PLoS One.* 2015;10(12):e0142879.

125. Finucane ML, Alhakami A, Slovic P, Johnson SM. The affect heuristic in judgments of risks and benefits. *J Behav Decis Mak.* 2000;13(1):1–17.

126. Shiv B, Fedorikhin A. Heart and mind in conflict: The interplay of affect and cognition in consumer decision making. *J Consum Res.* 1999;26(3):278–92.

127. Kahneman D. A perspective on judgment and choice: Mapping bounded rationality. *Am Psychol.* 2003;58(9):697.

128. Larson RW, Almeida DM. Emotional transmission in the daily lives of families: A new paradigm for studying family process. *J Marriage Fam.* 1999;61(1):5–20.

129. Bolger N, DeLongis A, Kessler RC, Wethington E. The contagion of stress across multiple roles. *J Marriage Fam.*1989;51(1):175–83. doi:10.2307/352378.

130. Butler EA. Temporal interpersonal emotion systems. *Pers Soc Psychol Rev.* 2011;15(4):367–93.

131. Butler EA, Randall AK. Emotional coregulation in close relationships. *Emot Rev.* 2013;5(2):202–10.

132. Thompson A, Bolger N. Emotional transmission in couples under stress. *J Marriage Fam.* 1999;61:38–48.

133. Wilson TD, Gilbert DT. Affective forecasting: Knowing what to want. *Curr Dir Psychol Sci.* 2005;14(3):131–4.

134. Ferrer RA, Taber JM, Klein WMP, Harris PR, Lewis KL, Biesecker LG. The role of current affect, anticipated affect, and spontaneous self-affirmation in decisions to receive self-threatening genetic risk information. *Cogn Emot.* 2015;29(8):1456–65.

135. Gerrard M, Gibbons FX, Bushman BJ. Relation between perceived vulnerability to HIV and precautionary sexual behavior. *Psychol Bull.* 1996;119(3):390–409.

136. Esplen MJ, Madlensky L, Aronson M, et al. Colorectal cancer survivors undergoing genetic testing for hereditary non-polyposis colorectal cancer: Motivational factors and psychosocial functioning. *Clin Genet.* 2007;72(5):394–401.

137. Gritz ER, Peterson SK, Vernon SW, et al. Psychological impact of genetic testing for hereditary nonpolyposis colorectal cancer. *J Clin Oncol.* 2005;23(9):1902–10.

138. Vernon SW, Gritz ER, Peterson SK, et al. Correlates of psychologic distress in colorectal cancer patients undergoing genetic testing for hereditary colon cancer. *Health Psychol.* 1997;16(1):73–86.

139. Gollwitzer PM. Implementation intentions: Strong effects of simple plans. *Am Psychol.* 1999;54(7):493–503.

140. Harris PR, Epton T. The impact of self-affirmation on health cognition, health behaviour and other health-related responses: A narrative review. *Soc Personal Psychol Compass.* 2009;3(6):962–78.

141. Lipkus IM, Klein WMP. Effects of communicating social comparison information on risk perceptions for colorectal cancer. *J Health Commun.* 2006;11(4):391–407.

142. Abdel-Kader K, Dew MA, Bhatnagar M, et al. Numeracy skills in CKD: Correlates and outcomes. *Clin J Am Soc Nephrol.* 2010;5(9):1566–73.

143. Anderson BL, Schulkin J. Physicians' perceptions of patients' knowledge and opinions regarding breast cancer: Associations with patient education and physician numeracy. *Breast Care.* 2011;6(4):285–88.

144. Anderson BL, Schulkin J. Physicians' understanding and use of numeric information. In: Anderson BL, Schulkin J, eds. *Numerical Reasoning in Judgments and Decision Making about Health.* Cambridge, England: Cambridge University Press; 2014, pp. 59–79.

145. Sheridan SL, Pignone M. Numeracy and the medical student's ability to interpret data. *Eff Clin Pract.* 2002;5(1):35–40.

146. Fong GT, Krantz DH, Nisbett RE. The effects of statistical training on thinking about everyday problems. *Cogn Psychol.* 1986;18(3): 253–92.

147. Braddock IC, Edwards KA, Hasenberg NM, Laidley TL, Levinson W. Informed decision making in outpatient practice: Time to get back to basics. *JAMA.* 1999;282(24):2313–20.

148. Sirota M, Juanchich M, Petrova D, Garcia-Retamero R, Walasek L, Bhatia S. Health professionals prefer to communicate risk-related numerical information using "1-in-X" ratios. *Med Decis Making.* 2018;38(3):366–76.

149. Pighin S, Savadori L, Barilli E, Cremonesi L, Ferrari M, Bonnefon JF. The 1-in-X effect on the subjective assessment of medical probabilities. *Med Decis Making.* 2011;31(5):721–9.

150. Zikmund-Fisher BJ. Continued use of 1-in-X risk communications is a systemic problem. *Med Decis Making.* 2013;34(4):412–3.

151. Schwartz A, Zikmund-Fisher BJ. Time to retire the 1-in-X risk format. *Med Decis Making.* 2011;31(5):703–4.

152. Elwyn G, Edwards A, Hood K, et al. Achieving involvement: Process outcomes from a cluster randomized trial of shared decision making skill development and use of risk communication aids in general practice. *Fam Pract.* 2004;21(4):337–46.

153. Rickles NM, Svarstad BL, Statz-Paynter JL, et al. Improving patient feedback about and outcomes with antidepressant treatment: a study in eight community pharmacies. *J Am Pharm Assoc.* 2006;46(1):25–32.

154. Thaler RH, Sunstein CR. *Nudge: Improving Decisions About Health, Wealth, and Happiness.* New Haven, CT: Yale University Press; 1999.

155. Sheeran P, Webb TL. The intention–behavior gap. *Soc Personal Psychol Compass.* 2016;10(9):503–18.

156. Klein WMP, Ferrer RA. On being more amenable to messages that threaten close others (vis-à-vis the self). *Pers Soc Psychol Bull.* 2018;44(10):1411–23.

157. Biesecker BB, Lewis KL, Umstead KL, et al. Web platform vs, in-person genetic counselor for return of carrier results from exome sequencing: A randomized clinical trial. *JAMA Intern Med.* 2018;178(3):338–46.

158. Taber JM, Klein WMP, Lewis KL, Johnston JJ, Biesecker LG, Biesecker BB. Reaction to clinical reinterpretation of a gene variant by participants in a sequencing study. *Genet Med.* 2018;20(3):337–45.

159. Linville PW, Fischer GW, Fischhoff B. AIDS risk perceptions and decision biases. In: Pryor G, Reeder GD, eds. *The Social Psychology of HIV Infection.* Hillsdale, NJ: Erlbaum; 1993, pp. 5–38.

160. Taber JT, Klein WMP, Suls J, Ferrer RA. Lay awareness of the relationship between age and cancer risk. *Ann Behav Med.* 2017;51(2):214–25.

161. Han PKJ, Klein WMP, Lehman T, Killam B, Massett H, Freedman AN. Communication of uncertainty regarding individualized cancer risk estimates: Effects and influential factors. *Med Decis Making.* 2011;31(2):354–66.

162. Kreuter MW, McClure SM. The role of culture in health communication. *Annu Rev Public Health.* 2004;25:439–55.

CHAPTER 39

Health Literacy: An Update

Rima E. Rudd • Oana R. Groene • D. Maria Navarro • Susan Reid

INTRODUCTION AND OVERVIEW

Literacy, the foundation of education, sheds light on the well-established pathway between education and health outcomes. However, literacy had not been a consideration in most health studies, programs, or practices in industrialized nations until recently because literacy concerns were generally associated with developing nations. In the early 1990s, findings from international surveys of adult literacy conducted in 22 industrialized nations indicated that literacy is problematic in these technologically sophisticated nations with consequences for the economy, daily life, and civic engagement.[1] These findings inspired health researchers to examine the influence of literacy on health outcomes. Within the first decade of research, links between the literacy skills of patients and their health outcomes were firmly established.[2] As a result, health literacy emerged as a new variable for health studies—offering insight into health outcomes and health disparities and generating interest among health researchers, practitioners, and policy makers.

Over the past two decades, the definition of health literacy has evolved, new component factors have emerged, and new measures have been developed. Studies indicate that health literacy considerations can improve strategic efforts in clinical care by improving dialogue and discussion between and among health professionals and between health professionals and patients with concrete implications for health outcomes. Health literacy in the public health arena is informing programs and evaluation studies in health communication, health promotion, disease prevention, care management, environmental health, and preparedness. Examination of institutional and system level characteristics that support or impede health literacy are informing health policy initiatives in many countries.

BACKGROUND

Rigorous surveys of adult literacy skills were initiated in the 1990s among member countries of the Organization for Economic Cooperation and Development (OECD) to examine the population's readiness to participate in sophisticated technological and complex social and economic environments. Findings from the first wave of international adult literacy surveys[1,3] as well as those from subsequent surveys[4,5] indicated that large percentages of the population of most industrialized nations have limited literacy and math skills. This means that a significant proportion of adults have difficulty using commonly available materials to accomplish everyday tasks with accuracy and consistency. These everyday tasks relate to activities undertaken for civic engagement, participation in the workforce, family, health, economics, and community as well as for problem solving and use of technology. Assumptions that universal schooling yields high or even adequate population skill levels were shown to be faulty. Literacy was indeed found to be a significant issue in most industrialized nations. This realization spurred interest among health researchers examining a wide variety of health outcomes.

Population-based measures of health literacy further strengthened interest from the health sector. The Health and Adult Literacy Survey (HALS) and the National Assessment of Adult Literacy (NAAL) focused on health-related items and tasks linked to the adult literacy surveys. Analyses indicated that about half of U.S. adults, including both those without a high school diploma and those who completed high school, have limited health literacy skills.[6–8] Similar results were found for several other countries that applied the HALS analysis to their adult literacy surveys such as Australia,[9] Canada,[10] and the Netherlands.[11] The European Health Literacy Survey (HLS-EU), a questionnaire focused on self-perceived health literacy, found that close to half the population in participating countries of the EU reported problematic or inadequate levels of health literacy.[12] These population measures yielded similar and problematic findings that health literacy is linked to a variety of social factors. Data analyses from each of these studies indicate that population groups with lower socioeconomic status and of lower social standing within any given country (due to minority or immigrant status, for example) have lower health literacy skills and/or perceived more difficulty with health-related activities and communications.

In the United States, health literacy studies began in the late 1990s shortly after the published results of the first wave of adult literacy surveys (NALS and IALS) and have now firmly established a link between people's literacy skills and their health outcomes. Research indicates that people with limited literacy skills are less likely to engage in health promotion action or disease prevention initiatives, and are less likely to have success with chronic disease management. They are more likely to report poor health and more likely to die at an earlier age than are those with stronger literacy skills.[2,13] Consequently, health literacy has emerged as a new variable for analyses of health outcomes and health disparities and as a new consideration in efforts to redress inequities.

EXPANDING CONCEPT

The term health literacy was formally defined by Nutbeam in the World Health Organization's 1998 Health Promotion Glossary as the cognitive and social skills, which determine the motivation and ability of individuals to gain access to, understand, and use information in ways which promote and maintain good health.[14] Nutbeam later noted that health literacy is an evolving concept and expanded his original definition to offer a more nuanced understanding of various levels of health literacy.[15] In so doing, Nutbeam offered a more proactive concept of health literacy as an asset contributing to personal and community well-being rather than a deficit to be measured. He proposed that *functional health literacy* is linked to basic skills and focuses on one's ability to understand and act on health information. *Communicative or interactive health literacy*, on the other hand, is linked to higher-level skills and focuses on interactions with health information and health professionals as individuals seek, evaluate, and use health information. *Critical health literacy*, building on these skills adds analytic, strategic, and social skills to contribute to knowledge development and use information to influence personal and community life.[16]

In the United States, additional perspectives from the education and literacy fields added to an evolving concept of health literacy. The U.S. 2003 Health Communication Objectives,[17] the 2004 health literacy report from the National Academies of Science,[18] and the 2010 National Action Plan to Improve Health Literacy[19] all suggested that health literacy be understood as an interaction or exchange rather than as a characteristic or ability of individuals. As a result, the lens of health literacy inquiry has shifted from a sole focus on an examination of people's literacy skills and links to health outcomes to include the equally important contributing factors of the clarity and complexity of health information, the communication skills of health and healthcare professionals, and the literacy-related characteristics of health institutions and health systems.[20,21] Increasingly now, attention is being given to the skills of the reader and the quality/complexity of the text, to the skills of the listener as well as the skills of the speaker/communicator, along with the facilitating or inhibiting factors in the immediate environment. Figure 39.1 illustrates the interrelated variables that are increasingly being recognized as core components of health literacy.

Health researchers, practitioners, and policy makers are recognizing that health literacy cannot be defined, measured, or ameliorated when attention is paid to only one part of these complex interactions. These insights are forging new paths of inquiry and broadening the scope of proposed remedial practices.

ADDRESSING KEY COMPONENTS OF HEALTH LITERACY

New developments in health literacy are emerging because of a broader conceptualization of health literacy and an expanded scope of interest. As a result, health literacy inquiries and evaluation studies now include not just patients but members of the lay public as well as a variety of health practitioners. Researchers are taking a closer look at health professionals' ability to communicate complex ideas including math and are providing more in-depth examinations of health information prepared for the public.

Situational analyses are leading to the identification of barriers and facilitating factors found in health and healthcare institutions and systems that support or inhibit patient navigation as well as professionals' norms and actions. In addition, while most health literacy inquiries to date have focused on the clinical encounter, new studies are taking place outside of healthcare settings. The literature indicates a growing interest in health literacy for preparedness and disaster

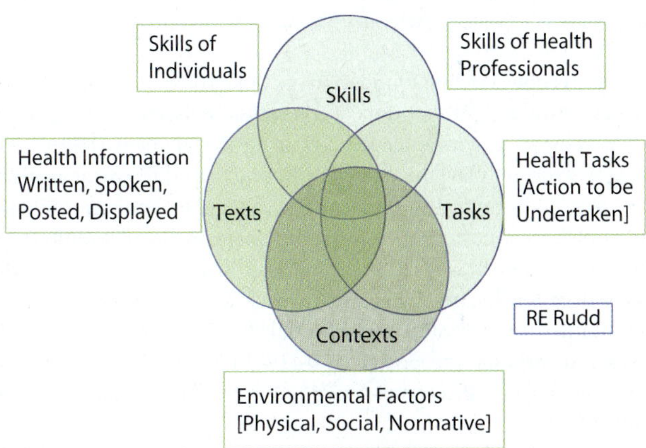

FIGURE 39-1. Components of health literacy.

management as well as for science literacy and environmental health literacy. To update health literacy developments, we address skill development, information quality, and institutional attributes as well as outline emerging areas of interest.

Skills of the Public

A continuing examination of patients' health literacy skills is evident in the abundance of measurement tools developed to examine a wide range of skills including speaking, listening, and math skills.[22] In addition, many health promotion and health education programs are including attention to health literacy and are designed to increase health literacy across an array of health issues and activities.[23]

A new segment of the public has emerged in the European Union with a strong articulation of patients' rights and responsibilities and a desire for these rights to be protected by the health system itself. Not so much as passive recipients but through their own involvement as rights holders with duties. In addition, The Patient Advocacy Forums recognize that others, particularly those who care for people who are ill, are also involved in care discussions and management, often on a collective level. Patient advocacy or the representation and defense of patients has evidenced a good deal of interest in health literacy to make health information more widely accessible. Simultaneously, the forums seek to ensure that patients and advocates have access to statements of their rights as well as of their responsibilities. Linked organizations, such as Eurodis, the organization focused on rare disease patient organizations, are grappling with plain language materials to support active patient involvement.[24,25]

Most recently emerging as a key issue in health literacy discussions is the problem of math-related expectations and demands—involving calculations and numeric concepts. People grapple with numbers in myriad health-related activities including shopping, checking weather charts, and using food or medicine labels. In healthcare situations, they are expected to understand a test result or vital sign measure in the context of a normal range. They are challenged to undertake risk/benefit analysis for critical decisions. Several researchers, such as Apter and colleagues[26] found that numeracy skills of both patients and providers are associated with health outcomes. Consequently, we need to recognize that activities in clinical encounters that involve hearing, reading, or discussion of numbers may be fraught with difficulties, errors, or misconceptions. Numbers are important for health action and for health decisions but frequently get in the way for many adults and confound rather than provide assistance.[27,28]

Skills of Health Professionals

With more balanced examinations of key players in the information-exchange process, additional critical variables can be analyzed and influences on health outcomes can be more thoroughly understood. Unfortunately, the abilities or competencies of those who provide information in healthcare and public health have yet to be rigorously measured with a health literacy lens and the possible contributions to health outcomes are currently unknown.

Several studies have begun to assess health literacy awareness and practice in dentistry, nursing, and pharmacy.[29–31] Coleman and colleagues have been examining needed health literacy competencies in medicine.[32] Evidence suggests that health literacy is partially addressed in medical education in the United States but that there is no consistent approach to content, methodology, or evaluation of such teaching. In U.S. studies, training interventions have been found to improve knowledge, broaden health professionals' understanding of and attitudes toward health literacy, improve self-reported confidence in medication counselling, increase effectiveness in using teach back, and improve ability to use illustrations and plain language when communicating with patients.[33,34]

In a review of professional education, Wills notes that health literacy also is partially addressed in professional schools in the European Union.[35] In England, for example, Groene noted that stakeholders in medical education demonstrated little familiarity with the health literacy concept and did not see merit to address it in an overcrowded curriculum. The study also demonstrated substantial variability in different levels of health literacy-related competencies between groups of GP trainees. Many were knowledgeable about consequences of low health literacy and were able to recognize a warning sign of low health literacy; however, most overestimated numeracy and literacy levels of the English population. Trainees were cognizant about the preferred way of checking for patients' understanding but did not generally understand that navigation and activation represented a shared responsibility between patients and providers.[36]

Johnson and colleagues looked at numeracy among health professional trainees and questioned whether physicians are being prepared for evidence-based medicine.[37] Training in numeracy communication and in the benefits and problems related to various mathematical displays may assist all who communicate health-related numbers and numerical concepts. At the same time, researchers are providing guidance for action. For example, public health and healthcare professionals are being encouraged to do the math for the reader or patient,[26] to provide numbers along with words,[38] to consider the value of different types of graphic representation,[39] and to provide visual as well as verbal explanations of risk.[40]

In addition, a new health literacy issue has emerged related to the skills of health professionals. The multilayered problem of specialized professional language is coming to light for the dissemination of information—among specialists and between researchers/scientists and practitioners. For example, Goto and colleagues discovered that in the aftermath of the nuclear reactor disaster in Fukushima, public health nurses were losing the trust of the community members they long served. Part of the problem was that the nurses did not themselves understand the scientific data they were given and could only offer answers to critical questions using the same scientific terms they were offered untranslated.[41,42]

Quality of Health Information

As noted above, early definitions of health literacy focused on people's ability to access and use health information. While this remains an important consideration, the "accessibility" of health information is emerging as critical to an understanding of links between health literacy and health outcomes. The demand side of the literacy exchange includes health materials designed to help the public understand and use health information, follow directions, consider options, and respond to calls to action. Examinations of these materials over time and across an array of health topics, have found that they are not broadly accessible.

For almost five decades now, researchers have been reporting on the reading level of health materials, tools, and messages designed for public use—primarily related to informed consent, health information, directions, preparations, and self-care. In general and across various health topics, findings indicated a mismatch between the documented literacy skills of the public and the literacy demands of the health materials. While the early health literacy studies included examinations of the difficulty of health texts, these efforts were not integrated into the studies of links between health literacy and health outcomes. Furthermore, the focus was primarily on the "readability score" of health information—a relatively superficial examination of word and occasionally, sentence length.

The current literature shows evidence of efforts to assess health materials in more comprehensive ways and to examine information posted online as well. As shown in Table 39.1, new tools, such as the CDC Health Literacy Index[43] and the AHRQ PEMAT[44]—both inspired by the early work of Doak et al. and their SAM tool,[45] are readily available online to help researchers and practitioners assess health materials with a focus on clarity, vocabulary and sentence structure, organization, data displays, and an articulation of action steps. Furthermore, the PMOSE/IKIRSCH tool[46] developed for educators to examine the difficulty of displays, such as lists, graphs, and charts, is increasingly being cited in health materials assessment studies. The categories-of-interest and scoring emphasis in all of the tools also offer insight for the design and development of health materials.

Educators use the term "texts" to refer to written materials as well as talk and posting. Critical health information is also delivered in the dialogue and discussions that take place in the clinical encounter as well as in the public arena. Several years ago, Nouri and Rudd found a paucity of studies that included attention to literacy-related issues in the clinical encounter.[47] Roter, best known for in-depth analysis of practitioner/patient exchange, did include literacy analyses, for example, in genetic testing discussions.[48] In addition, Roter offers a conceptual approach for capturing the oral literacy demand in healthcare dialogue, provides reviews of several studies that support the predictive validity of the framework, and proposes ways to both diminish literacy demand and support more effective healthcare exchanges.[49]

Public health and mass communication for emergency preparedness and recovery efforts are increasingly including attention to health literacy issues. Critical analyses conducted through a health literacy lens have highlighted communication errors and are leading to proactive efforts to include health literacy expertise in the development of public health messages[50,51] and to better prepare health practitioners to communicate with the public.

Health communication efforts coupled with health literacy insights are now more attentive to the quality of numeric information, as is noted above, and tools are under scrutiny as well. A variety of document tools such as medicine or nutrition labels help people simplify daily routines such as self-care and shopping. In addition, tools can be customized; for example, a simple tape marker on a peak flow meter used by a person with asthma can offer a signal for immediate action.

Finally, attention is being given to the materials development processes. The components of rigorous formative research to be undertaken in the production of materials have long been well articulated in health education and health communication literature,[52] but we lack evidence that such processes are regularly followed. Furthermore, there is no indication that such processes or assessment reports are required by any institutional review boards. Consequently, regulations related to the design of both print and eHealth materials may be called for. Integration of health literacy insights with professional training for those responsible for the development and design of health texts can be beneficial to the public and help set standards for review boards.

Health Environments

When the context is highlighted as a key component of health literacy, various institutional and system factors related to literacy can be identified, measured, and considered in analyses of health outcomes. This process can also yield insight and spark impetus for needed change.

There is now a strong foundation for this approach. Rudd and colleagues introduced the notion of a healthcare literacy environment and developed a workbook for capturing key elements and developing a strategic plan for change.[53] Ratings are offered for navigation, print communication, the oral exchange, technology, policies, and protocols followed by suggestions for action and examples of efficacious change. Several researchers are using this tool to assess a variety of healthcare environments such as dental services within community health centers and hospitals.[54,55] The Universal Tool Kit developed through and posted by AHRQ includes mechanisms for assessing clinical offices and similarly offers strategies and tools for change.[56]

In 2012, the National Academy of Medicine [formerly IOM] Roundtable on Health Literacy introduced the notion of institutional

TABLE 39-1 SELECTED TOOLS FOR ASSESSMENTS OF HEALTH MATERIALS

Tool	Measure	Focus	Key Elements	Type of Material	Insights
SMOG	Grade-level score	Number of multisyllabic words Length of sentences	Number of words with more than 2 syllables in 30 sentences	Prose	Avoid long words and complex sentences
PMOSE/ IKIRSCH	Grade-level score	Format	Density of items Complexity of structure	Lists, charts, graphs	Examine format to reduce density and complexity
SAM	Score based on suitability [match with intended audience's needs]	Organization, writing style, appearance, and appeal	Content Literacy demand Graphics Layout Learning stimulation Cultural appropriateness	Prose	Be attentive to a wide variety of design and organizational issues that ease the reading and comprehension processes
PEMAT	Score based on *understandability* and *actionability*	Ease of reading Focus on taking action	*Understandability* • Word choice and style • Use of numbers • Organization • Layout and design • Use of visual aids *Actionability*	Prose and audiovisuals	Focus on clarity of message and on action steps
CDC INDEX	Score based on clarity of main message and call to action	Content, organization Writing and numeracy elements, science, clear action	Identified audience Main message Call to action Information design State of the science	Prose	Know the intended audience Focus on primary message Highlight action steps

attributes and set out a list of ten attributes necessary for the development of health literacy.[57] These attributes include the leadership making health literacy integral to the mission of the organization and integrated into planning, evaluation, patient safety, and quality improvement. It focuses on the institutional responsibility for preparing the workforce as well as on its responsibility for providing information and enhancing the engagement of patients, family member, and the community it serves. This publication has garnered international interest and, as a result, a variety of practitioners, managers, and policy makers are engaged in discussions of needed cultural adaptations or modifications for use in their institutions.[58]

Health Policies

Visions of a health-literate society have been described for the United States in the 2004 Institute of Medicine report[18] and for Canada in 2008.[59] U.S. Government goals related to health literacy were first articulated through the 2000 goals and objectives for Healthy People 2010[17,60] and later in the 2010 National Health Literacy Action Plan.[19] The goals set forth include actions that can be taken by public and private agencies, institutions, and professional groups. They include the development and dissemination of health and safety information; efficacious changes in healthcare systems that improve access to information, care, and decision-making; educational enhancements; partnership development; support for research; and the dissemination of evidence-based health literacy practices and interventions. These goals to improve health literacy have implications for healthcare systems and for the economy as well.[61]

The National Academy of Medicine's Health Literacy Round Table workshop on international work highlighted several governmental initiatives.[58] Soon thereafter, one of the most elaborate efforts was undertaken in New Zealand. The initial impetus for New Zealand to explore health literacy was the Ministry of Health's focus on the need to reduce inequalities and inequities for Māori (New Zealand's indigenous people). Health literacy was deemed critical to achieving the outcomes outlined in the Maori Health Strategy, He Korowai Oranga Ministry of Health as well as for other areas such as health equity, person and family-centered care and cultural competence. This decision led to the development of the Framework for Health Literacy.[62] In the same year, the Ministry also published Health Literacy Review: A Guide[63] to support the development of an action plan for becoming a health-literate organization, the provision of health-literate services, and strong health literacy leadership. In addition, the posting of a guide for healthcare organizations seeking to review and improve care. A health literacy navigator[64] set out the leadership and management actions, knowledge and skills required by the health system, health organizations, workforce, and individuals and families. It also described system and service attributes of an envisioned health literate health system with the goal of establishing health literacy as a core business at all levels of the health system leading to improved health outcomes and reduced health costs.

CONCLUSIONS

As is noted above, findings from health literacy studies are influencing professional education, clinical practice, health education and promotion efforts, and institutional as well as system level policies. Research insights are re-invigorating efforts to promote and perhaps require the implementation of well-established guidelines for rigorous formative research, with an emphasis on pilot testing health information materials with members of the intended audience. A new perspective has turned the focus of attention on those of us responsible for communicating health information—making us more attentive to the language, structure, and content of our communication and program efforts.

The promulgation of assessment tools for examining written and posted health materials and the calls for regular use of "teach-back" in clinical encounters are based on a new focus on the communication skills of public health and healthcare professionals and the need to take responsibility for clear communication. Consequently, health and healthcare professionals are being asked to closely examine our assumptions about and expectations for clients, patients, and community members and be critically attuned to the burdens we inadvertently place on those seeking information, involvement, and care. The premise is that changes in texts, in communication practices, as well as in the characteristics of health institutions and systems could improve health literacy and influence health outcomes.

Developments to date include new initiatives being forged both within healthcare environments and in the broader community, outside of the clinical encounter. Here, a health literacy perspective can be brought to bear on a diverse set of programs addressing topics such as water quality, emergency response, food safety, air quality, and preparedness. Evaluation studies can examine efficacious change and outcomes in terms of civic engagement, community action, policy developments, and health outcomes.

The current focus on health literacy as an interaction brings new variables to the fore for consideration and analysis and can offer new insights for our understanding, our research design, and our practice. This calls for health outcome studies that consider the skills of the lay public as well as the complexity of health materials and tools and the communication skills of scientists, researchers, and practitioners in health and healthcare. In addition, we need to factor into our analyses of the characteristics of institutions and systems that facilitate or stymie access to information, engagement, and decision-making. Health literacy studies to date have not simultaneously addressed or measured these factors in analyses of health literacy contributions to health outcomes.

However, what is needed first and foremost are validated measures of these new variables. This offers opportunities for researchers to develop and test an array of tools. While there are well over 100 tools to assess the health literacy skills of patients,[22] we do not yet have a standard tool to assess the communication skills of those who deliver health information. We also need to fill the gaps in current assessments of health materials with tools that measure the numeracy demand in health information. Furthermore, we must more closely examine forms and questionnaires used in research and in healthcare encounters to understand the ease or difficulty of their use. Finally, we need to more widely use existing processes for identifying the literacy-related physical and social characteristics of public health and healthcare settings that constrain or facilitate access, engagement, and care. Measures of these important variables and an understanding of their contribution to health outcomes can inform professional training, practice in the clinical encounter, partnerships and programs in the community, and policy development. These tools could then support the strategy first articulated in Kurt Lewin's *Force Field Analysis*—a theoretical guideline for promoting change by focusing first on identifying and then eliminating barriers to change so that facilitating factors can establish a momentum without hindrances.[65]

As health literacy researchers recalibrate definitions and develop new measures for each of the component parts, many of the previous research and practice gaps of health literacy studies can be addressed. Findings from research studies can inform the challenges to remove literacy-related barriers from the various local, state, regional, and national public health efforts to support and encourage the capacity of communities. This is turn, can further strengthen health education, health promotion, and disease prevention activities.

References

1. Tuijnman A, Kirsch I, Murray S. Jones S. *Literacy, Economy and Society: Results of the First International Adult Literacy Survey*. Ottawa, CA: Statistics Canada; 1995.
2. DeWalt DA, Berkman ND, Sheridan S, Lohr KN, Pignone MP. Literacy and health outcomes—A systematic review of the literature. *J Gen Intern Med*. 2004;19:1228–39.
3. Kirsch IS. *Adult Literacy in America: A First Look at the Results of the National Adult Literacy Survey*. Washington, DC: US Government Printing Office, Superintendent of Documents (Stock No. 065-000-00588-3); 1993.
4. Desjardins R, Murray TS, Tuijnman AC. *Learning A Living: First Results of the Adult Literacy and Life Skills Survey*. Ottawa, CA: Statistics Canada; 2005.
5. Desjardins R, OECD colleagues. *OECD Skills Outlook 2013: First Results from the Survey of Adult Skills*. Paris, France: OECD Publications; 2013.
6. Rudd RE, Kirsch I, Yamamoto K. *Literacy and Health in America. Policy Information Report. Educational Testing Service*. Princeton NJ: ETS Publications; 2004.
7. Rudd RE. Health literacy skills of US adults. *Am J of Health Behav*. 2007;31(Suppl 1), S8–18.
8. Kutner M, Greenberg E, Jin Y, Paulsen C. *The Health Literacy of America's Adults: Results From the 2003 National Assessment of Adult Literacy (NCES 2006-483). U.S. Department of Education*. Washington, DC: National Center for Education Statistics; 2006.
9. Australia Barber MN, Staples M, Osborne RH, Clerehan R, Elder C, Buchbinder R. Up to a quarter of the Australian population may have suboptimal health literacy depending upon the measurement tool: Results from a population-based survey. *Health Promot Int*. 2009;24(3):252-61.
10. Murray TS, Rudd RE, Kirsch I, Yamamoto, K, Grenier, S. *Health Literacy in Canada. Initial Results from the International Adult Literacy and Skills Survey*. Ottawa: Canadian Council on Learning; 2007.
11. van der Heide I, Wang J, Droomers M, Spreeuwenberg P, Rademakers J, Uiters E. The relationship between health, education, and health literacy: Results from the Dutch adult literacy and life skills survey. *J Health Commun*. 2013;18(Suppl1):172–84.
12. Sorensen, K, Pelikan JM, Rothlin F, et al. Health literacy in Europe: Comparative results of the European health literacy survey (HLS-EU). *Eur J Public Health*. 2015;25(6):1053–8.
13. Berkman ND, Sheridan SL, Donahue KE, Halpern DJ, Crotty K. Low health literacy and health outcomes: An updated systematic review. *Ann Intern Med*. 2011;155:97–107.
14. Nutbeam D. Health promotion glossary. *Health Promot Int*. 1998;13(4):349–64.
15. Nutbeam D. The evolving concept of health literacy. *Soc Sci Med*. 2008;67(12), 2072–8.
16. Nutbeam D. Health literacy as a public health goal: A challenge for contemporary health education and communication strategies into the 21st century. *Health Prom Int*. 2000;15(3):259–67.
17. Rudd RE. *Health Literacy Objectives in U.S. Department of Health and Human Services, Office of Disease Prevention and Health Promotion. National Action Plan to Improve Health Literacy*. Washington, DC: USDHHS; 2003.
18. Kindig DA, Panzer AM, Nielsen-Bohlman L, eds. *Health Literacy: A Prescription to End Confusion*. Washington, DC: National Academies Press; 2004.
19. Baur CBaur C (senior editor). *U.S. Department of Health and Human Services. National Action Plan to Improve Health Literacy*. Washington, DC: USDHHS; 2010.
20. Rudd RE. Improving Americans' health literacy. *N Engl J Med*. 2010;363(24):2283–5.
21. Pleasant AR, Rudd RE, O'Leary C, et al. *Considerations for A New definition of Health Literacy*. Discussion Paper. Washington, DC: National Academy of Medicine; 2016.
22. Health Literacy Toolshed. http://www.healthliteracy.bu.edu.
23. National Academies of Sciences, Engineering, and Medicine. *Community-Based Health Literacy Interventions: Proceedings of a Workshop*. Washington, DC: The National Academies Press; 2018.
24. EU Patient Advocacy. *EPF Background Brief: Patient Empowerment*. Brussels: European Patients Forum; 2015.
25. EU Eurodis or Active Citizenship Network. European Charter of Patients' Rights. Rome, IT. 2002.
26. Apter AJ, Paasche-Orlow MK, Remillard JT, et al. Numeracy and communication with patients: They are counting on us. *J Gen Int Med*. 2008;23(12):2117–24.
27. Ancker JS, Kaufman D. Rethinking health numeracy: A multidisciplinary literature review. *J Am Med Inform Assoc*. 2007;14(6):713–21.
28. Rudd RE. *Numbers Get in the Way. Commentary, National Academy of Medicine*, Washington, DC: The National Academies Press; 2016.
29. Maybury C, Horowitz AM, Yan AF, Green KM, Wang MQ. Maryland dentists' knowledge of oral cancer prevention and early detection. *J Calif Dent Assoc*. 2012;40(4):341–50.
30. Cafiero, M. Nurse practitioners' knowledge, experience, and intention to use health literacy strategies in clinical practice. *J Health Commun*. 2013;18(Suppl 1):70–81.
31. Devraj R, Gupchup GV. Knowledge of and barriers to health literacy in Illinois. *J Am Pharm Assoc*. 2012;52(6):183-93.
32. Coleman CA, Hudson S, Maine LL. Health literacy practices and educational competencies for health professionals: A consensus study. *J Health Commun*. 2013;4(18 sup1):82–102.
33. Coleman C. Teaching health care professionals about health literacy: A review of the literature. *Nurs Outlook*. 2011;59:70–8.
34. Green JA, Gonzaga AM, Cohen ED, Spagnoletti CL. Addressing health literacy through clear health communication: A training program for internal medicine residents. *Patient Educ Couns*. 2014;95 (1):76–82.

35. Wills J. Where is health literacy in the education of health professionals? In: Proceedings of the 22nd IUHPE world conference on health promotion, Curitiba, Brazil. 2016.
36. Groene OR, Wills J, Crichton N, Rowlands G, Rudd R. The health literacy dyad: The contribution of future GPs in England. *Educ Prim Care.* 2017;28(5):274–81.
37. Johnson TV, Abbasi A, Schoenberg ED, et al. Numeracy among trainees: Are we preparing physicians for evidence-based medicine. *J Surg Edu.* 2014;71(2):211–5.
38. Peters E, Hibbard J, Slovic P, Dieckmann N. Numeracy skill and the communication, comprehension, and use of risk-benefit information. *Health Aff (Willwood).* 2007;26(3):741–8.
39. Ancker JS, Senathirajah Y, Rita Kukafka R, Starren JB. Design features of graphs in health risk communication: A systematic review. *J Am Med Informat Assoc.* 2006;13(6):608–18.
40. Fagerlin A, Zikmund-Fisher BJ, Ubel PA. Helping patients decide: Ten steps to better risk communication. *J Natl Cancer Inst.* 2011;103(19):1436–43.
41. Goto A, Rudd RE, Lai AY, Yoshida-Komiya H. Health literacy training for public health nurses in Fukushima: A case study of program adaptation, implementation, and evaluation. *Japan Med Assoc J.* 2014;57(3):146–3.
42. Goto A, Lai AL, Kumagai A, et al. Collaborative processes of developing a health literacy toolkit: A case from Fukushima after the nuclear accident. *J Health Commun.* 2018;23(2):200–6.
43. Baur C, Prue C. The CDC Clear Communication Index is a new evidence-based tool to prepare and review health information. *Health Promot Pract.* 2014;15:629–37.
44. Shoemaker SJ, Wolf MS, Brach C. Development of the Patient Education Materials Assessment Tool (PEMAT): A new measure of understandability and actionability for print and audiovisual patient information. *Patient Edu Couns.* 2014;96(3):395–403.
45. Doak CC, Doak LG, Root JH. *Teaching Patients with Low Literacy Skills.* 2nd ed. Philadelphia, PA: Lippincott-Raven Publishers; 1996. www.hsph.harvard.edu/healthliteracy.
46. Mosenthal PB, Kirsch IS. A new measure for assessing document complexity: The PMOSE/IKIRSCH document readability formula. *J Adolesc Adult Lit.* 1998;41(8):638–57.
47. Nouri SS, Rudd RE. Health literacy in the "oral exchange": An important element of patient–provider communication. *Patient Edu Couns.* 2015;98(5):565-71.
48. Roter DL, Erby LH, Larson S, Ellington L. Assessing oral literacy demand in genetic counseling dialogue: Preliminary test of a conceptual framework. *Soc Sci Med.* 2007;65:1442–57.
49. Roter DL. Oral literacy demand of health care communication: Challenges and solutions. *Nurs Outlook.* 2011;59(2):79–84.
50. Fischhoff B. The science of science communication. *PNAS.* 2013;110 (Suppl 3):14033–9.
51. Rudd RE, Comings JP, Hyde J. Leave no one behind: Improving health and risk communication through attention to literacy. *J Health Commun.* 2003;8(Suppl 1):104–15.
52. National Cancer Institute. Making Health Communication Programs Work: A Planner's Guide. Bethesda, MD: U.S. Dept. of Health and Human Services, Public Health Service, NIH, Office of Cancer Communications, National Cancer Institute; 2002.
53. Rudd RE, Anderson JE. *The Health Literacy Environment of Hospitals and Health Centers. Partners for Action: Making Your Healthcare Facility Literacy-Friendly.* Cambridge, MA: National Center for the Study of Adult Learning and Literacy (NCSALL); 2006. www.hsph.harvard.edu/healthliteracy.
54. Horowitz AM, Maybury C, Kleinman DV, et al. Health literacy environmental scans of community-based dental clinics in Maryland. *Am J Public Health.* 2014;104(8):e85–93.
55. Oelschlegel S, Graveel KL, Tester E, Heidel RE, Russomanno J. Librarians promoting changes in the health care delivery system through systematic assessment. *Med Ref Serv Q.* 2018;37(2):142–52.
56. DeWalt DA, Callahan LF, Hawk VH, et al. *Health Literacy Universal Precautions Toolkit. AHRQ Publication No. 10-0046-EF.* Rockville, MD: Agency for Healthcare Research and Quality; 2010.
57. Brach C, Dreyer B, Schyve P, et al. *Attributes of a Health Literate Organization. Roundtable on Health Literacy.* Washington, DC: National Academies of Science; 2012.
58. Roundtable on Health Literacy; Board on Population Health and Public Health Practice; Institute of Medicine. *Health Literacy: Improving Health, Health Systems, and Health Policy around the World: Workshop Summary. Roundtable on Health Literacy.* Washington, DC: National Academies of Science; 2013.
59. Rootman I, Gordon-El-Bihbety D. *A Vision for a Health Literate Canada: Report of the Expert Panel on Health Literacy.* Ottawa, CA: Canadian Public Health Association; 2008.
60. Online Archive site. https://www.healthypeople.gov/2010/.
61. Koh HK, Berwick DM, Clancy CM, et al. New federal policy initiatives to boost health literacy can help the nation move beyond the cycle of costly 'crisis care'. *Health Aff (Willwood).* 2012;31(2):434–41.
62. New Zealand Ministry of Health. A Framework for Health Literacy. 2015. https://www.health.govt.nz/publication/framework-health-literacy.
63. New Zealand Ministry of Health. *Health Literacy Review: A Guide.* Wellington: Ministry of Health; 2015.
64. New Zealand Health Literacy Navigator. https://www.healthnavigator.org.nz/clinicians/h/health-literacy/.
65. Lewin K. *Field Theory in Social Science.* New York: Dorwin Cartwright Publishers; 1951.

CHAPTER

40 Health Promotion Interventions and Research

Jennifer B. Unger • Kim D. Reynolds • Donna Spruijt-Metz

Health promotion interventions focus on keeping people healthy rather than treating them after they become sick. This can be achieved in several ways, including helping people become more motivated to change their behavior and modifying the environment to make it more conducive to health-promoting behaviors. The field of health promotion is based on the assumptions that people's behaviors impact their health outcomes that people can change their health-related behaviors when they have the necessary knowledge, resources, motivation, and skills, as well as a supportive environment, and that interventions can provide or increase their knowledge, resources, motivation, and skills. The goal of health promotion interventions is to empower people to modify their behavior to optimize their health. Many of the risk and protective factors for health and disease outcomes are behaviors that can be modified, including diet, physical activity, tobacco, alcohol, and other substance use, sexual behaviors, and screening.[1] Because optimal health involves the performance of multiple healthy behaviors and the avoidance of multiple unhealthy behaviors, health promotion interventions often emphasize broad lifestyle changes rather than modification of a single behavior. The design of behavioral interventions involves a series of decisions including operationalization of the goals of the intervention (e.g., prevent substance use, increase physical activity, increase condom use), the target population (e.g., adults, adolescents, a specific ethnic group), the way in which the intervention will be delivered (e.g., mass media, in person, online), and the design of the specific intervention messages and activities.

The process of modifying health behaviors proceeds via several steps. First, the interventionist must define precisely which behaviors need to be modified. For example, to prevent obesity, an interventionist might decide to encourage participants to increase their physical activity, decrease their sedentary behavior, increase their vegetable intake, decrease their sugar intake, or improve all of these behaviors. It is essential to determine which behaviors the intervention will target, so that intervention messages can be designed to encourage individuals to modify those particular behaviors. The target behavior should be operationalized as concretely as possible (e.g., "walk 10,000 steps per day" rather than "get more exercise").

The next step is to understand the conditions that facilitate or hinder performance of the target behaviors and determine which of these are modifiable. For example, if people are not engaging in physical activity because they lack knowledge of the benefits of physical activity, an intervention could teach them about the benefits of physical activity. However, if they already know the benefits of physical activity but lack a safe place to exercise or friends to exercise with, teaching them about the benefits of physical activity is unlikely to change their behavior. A possible solution might be to increase the safety of the neighborhood, but that is probably not under the interventionist's control. In this case, a possible intervention strategy might be to work with local institutions such as schools or churches to provide group exercise classes in safe locations.

Theories of health behavior are useful for identifying the personal, interpersonal, and environmental factors that facilitate or hinder the performance of healthy behaviors.[2] Chapter 35 this section of the book[3] outlines the predominant theories that describe the predictors of health behaviors. These theories offer insights about how to encourage people to improve their health behaviors. Several of these theories involve modifying individuals' knowledge, attitudes, motivation, perceived social norms, and/or self-efficacy to perform health-promoting behaviors. Other theories also advocate altering social contexts and environments, although that typically requires more resources.

After using theory to identify some factors that might be facilitating or hindering healthy behaviors, a researcher will conduct etiological research, based on theory, to decide which of these factors are most strongly associated with performance of health behaviors in a particular population. This indicates which risk and protective factors need to change to cause individuals to practice healthier behaviors. Some program planners conduct this etiological research themselves by collecting new data, whereas others look to the extensive body of literature about known risk and protective factors. For example, a program planner who conducts a literature search on the known risk and protective factors for unprotected sex among Hispanic adolescents will find numerous articles. If the health behavior or the target population has not been widely documented in the literature, the program planner must conduct this etiological research before developing interventions.

The next step is to design interventions that effectively modify the most important risk and protective factors. These are often called mediators because they represent an intermediate step in the causal chain from the intervention to behavior change.[4] For example, an intervention to prevent unprotected sex could give young women opportunities to practice negotiating condom use with their partners. The increased condom negotiation skills and self-efficacy that they gain from this experience are the mediating variables. It is expected that improvements in these mediating variables will lead to improvements in health-related behaviors (e.g., less unprotected sex), which ultimately will lead to improvements in health outcomes (fewer sexually transmitted diseases and unintended pregnancies). This chapter describes classic and emerging strategies for delivering interventions to their intended audiences. It discusses decisions that health promotion professions typically make during the planning and development of health promotion interventions: selecting the target population, determining the extent to which the target population will be involved in the process, choosing the modality by which the intervention will be delivered, deciding whether the intervention will be adaptive or static, and considering innovative intervention strategies.

SELECTING THE TARGET POPULATION

Targeted and Tailored Interventions

For interventions to have the largest population health impact and cost-effectiveness, they are typically directed toward the people who need them most. These target populations can be defined by their demographic characteristics (e.g., adolescents and young adults have the highest risk for experimenting with tobacco), by their health status (e.g., overweight people high a higher risk of developing diabetes), or by other factors. Interventions can vary in the breadth of their target audience. General-audience interventions are directed at the broadest possible audience and typically deliver advice that is relevant to most people (e.g., physical activity is beneficial, smoking is harmful). Targeted interventions are relevant to a subgroup of the population, based on shared demographic characteristics or behaviors. For example, messages about mammography are targeted to middle-aged women, whereas messages about not sharing needles are targeted to intravenous drug users. Tailored interventions adapt the health education messages to the characteristics, needs, and interests of individuals. For example, a smoking cessation intervention could assess participants' readiness and motivation for smoking cessation and most salient barriers to cessation, and each participant could receive intervention modules to address their specific challenges and move them to the next stage of readiness.[5] Tailored interventions are often, although not always, more effective than generic nontailored interventions at producing changes in attitudes and behavior.[6,7]

Family and Social Network Interventions

Some interventions focus on the entire family as the target for behavior change. This strategy is especially useful in situations where parents are partially, but not completely, in control of their children's behaviors. For example, parents are responsible for the food that they provide to their children, but ultimately their children must develop healthy eating habits and make healthy food choices autonomously. Therefore, intervening with parents and their children is a useful approach to help parents provide a variety of healthy foods and encourage children to make healthful food choices. An example of a family intervention is NEEDS for Tots.[8] This program trains preschool teachers to lead classroom activities that encourage children to try new foods and participate in enjoyable family mealtimes. The preschool teachers also give the parents worksheets and activities to practice at home, such as offering multiple healthy food choices and implementing pleasant family mealtimes. Intervening with both the children and their parents reinforces the messages and helps the entire family to improve their mealtime habits.

Social networks extend beyond family and include friends, classmates, colleagues, and professionals such as doctors and clerics, and other people who play a role in a person's social environment. Social networks also can include online communities, organizations, and political entities or other units that form a social structure that connects people to each other. Research has increasingly shown that our social networks impact our health and health behaviors.[9] A recent review shows strong evidence for behavior change and maintenance in social networks interventions on various health-related behaviors, as opposed to concentrating predominantly on the individual.[10]

INVOLVEMENT OF THE TARGET POPULATION

Health promotion programs can vary in the extent to which the target population is involved in the planning and delivery of the intervention. Traditionally, most health promotion interventions have been initiated, developed, delivered, and evaluated by people who are not members of the target population (e.g., university researchers, health department personnel). This can create barriers to effective health promotion if well-meaning outsiders do not really understand the sociocultural conditions that influence health behaviors, if the interventionists do not understand how to navigate the existing social structures in the population to gain entry and acceptance, and/or if the target population does not trust that the interventionists have their best interests in mind. Involving members of the target population in the intervention can help to overcome these barriers. (See chapter 42 later in this section, on Community Engaged Research.[11])

Hiring Members of the Target Population as Group Leaders or Health Educators

The effectiveness of a health promotion intervention can depend on who delivers the intervention. In addition to being competent, knowledgeable individuals with good communication skills, people who deliver interventions also should be trusted role models for the target population. Trusted role models are typically similar to the target population in some way, such as race/ethnicity, gender, age, sexual orientation, or health behaviors. Often health educators are people who have already mastered a behavior or navigated a developmental stage that the target population is still learning. For example, interventions for adolescents can be taught by college students, and interventions for drug users can be taught by ex-drug users. Recruiting members of the target population to deliver the intervention can increase community acceptance of the intervention. Social network interventions[10] analyze the structure of the social network to identify members who would serve as good role models for the group. For example, in a closed system such as a school or workplace, the interventionist can survey the entire group to determine which individuals within the social network are well liked and respected. These individuals can be recruited as group leaders to deliver the intervention to their peers. Social network analysis also can be used to segment the target population into naturally occurring groups (e.g., groups of friends in a school) and select the group leader for each group based on that person's level of influence within the group.[10]

Community-Based Participatory Research

Recruiting members of the target community to deliver the intervention is a first step toward obtaining community trust in the program, but this still does not guarantee that the community will be strongly invested in the program or will find it useful. Members of the target population also can be involved at all stages of the intervention, including determining which health issues and behaviors the intervention should address, designing the intervention, implementing the intervention, and evaluating its effects. (For more on this, see also chapter 42.)

Most health promotion interventions use a traditional top-down structure, in which the interventionist is the expert and the participants are the learners. However, members of the target population often have unique insights about the barriers to healthy behaviors in their communities. Often these barriers are basic unmet needs for transportation, food, and personal hygiene items, which might not even occur to researchers.[12] Often, the health behavior identified by the interventionist is not the most pressing concern in the community. For example, if an interventionist comes to a community intending to increase physical activity, she might find that community members are not exercising in local parks because they are worried about violence and crime. They might not be interested in a physical activity program, but they might be interested in a program that provides activities to youth to deter them from crime and provides better lighting in the parks to discourage criminal activity. This intervention, in addition to reducing crime in the parks, might have an added benefit of increasing physical activity.

Community-based participatory research (CBPR) is a collaborative process that engages community members and academic researchers as equal partners in common effort to understand and improve the health and well-being of the community. CBPR capitalizes on the unique strengths, experiences, and ways of knowing of academic researchers and community members. For example, academic researchers have expertise in theories of health promotion, intervention strategies used in other populations, research design, and formal evaluation methods. Community members have expertise in the specific health priorities and barriers to health behavior change in their communities, as well as the most effective ways to communicate with community members. When academic researchers and community members combine their expertise and work together to combine knowledge with action, CBPR interventions have the potential to achieve social change, improve health outcomes, and achieve health equity.[13,14]

An example of a CBPR approach is Communities for Healthy Living.[15] This childhood obesity prevention program established a partnership between academic researchers and a community-based organization that administered a Head Start program. The team first established a community advisory board consisting of parents and grandparents of children in Head Start, community-based organization professionals, and health service professionals. This community advisory board participated in all decision-making for the project, including naming the project, hiring the project coordinator, developing operating guidelines, and convening meetings. The community advisory board and the academic research partners worked together to educate each other about scientific knowledge of the causes and consequences of childhood obesity and the specific causes and consequences of childhood obesity observed in the community. Parents participated in an initial needs assessment, contributed to intervention development, and received training as intervention facilitators to deliver the intervention. This approach ensured that the community was invested in the program and that the program was responsive to the community's needs and unique risk factors for childhood obesity. The program also increased community capacity and parent empowerment by training the parents as health educators, increasing the likelihood that the program would continue after the formal grant support ended.

MODALITIES OF HEALTH PROMOTION INTERVENTIONS

Interventions can be delivered through several different modalities. Modalities are the vehicles, or channels, through which interventions are transmitted from the interventionist to the participants. Interventions can be delivered in person (either one-to-one or in groups), through print materials such as pamphlets, through mass media broadcasts, or through interactive media such as social media or texting. Depending on the modality selected, interventions can be one way, such as a public service announcement on television, or interactive, such as an intervention engaging in a text or social media conversation with a client. When choosing a modality for an intervention, it is essential to consider the breadth of the target population, the ways in which they feel comfortable receiving information, and the cost-efficiency of various modalities.

Mass Media

Mass media provide a cost-efficient vehicle for delivering health promotion interventions to wide, heterogeneous audiences. Mass media include broadcast media (e.g., television, radio), digital media (websites, social media), print media (pamphlets, magazines, newspapers), and outdoor media (e.g., billboards, ads on bus shelters, signs at sports stadiums). Exposure to mass media messages can inform the public about the importance of health issues, give them a framework for thinking about these issues, explain specific health-promoting behaviors, and encourage positive attitudes and emotions toward health-promoting behaviors.[16–18] The effectiveness of a particular message depends on numerous factors: the characteristics of the message (e.g., the information that the message conveys about the disease or health behavior); the source (e.g., the credibility and likeability of the spokesperson); the channel (e.g., television, radio, magazines, billboard, Internet); and the receiver (e.g., the characteristics of the people viewing or hearing the message, including their demographic characteristics, health status, and awareness of health issues). For a mass media message to change people's behavior, people must notice the message, pay attention to it, understand it, remember it, retrieve the information from memory at the appropriate time, and use the information conveyed to select new behaviors.[19] The advantage of mass media is that it can reach a large number of people quickly. The disadvantage is that it is difficult to create messages that are relevant and memorable to all members of the target population.

The California Tobacco Control Program[20] is an example of a mass media intervention for health promotion. This long running, highly publicized statewide media campaign disseminates anti-tobacco messages through various communication channels, including television, radio, print media, billboards, and websites. The campaign's ads vary in intended target audience (e.g., adolescents, adult smokers, specific ethnic groups) and in the tobacco-related issue addressed (e.g., preventing youth access to tobacco, encouraging smokers to call a quitline, portraying the tobacco industry as manipulative). The statewide media campaign has reached the vast majority of California youth and adults and has maintained its high visibility for over 20 years. Although most statewide tobacco control programs have historically used traditional media such as television, radio, and billboards, many state tobacco control programs are increasingly expanding to new media platforms such as websites and social media.[21] The California Tobacco Control Program's website allows smokers to register online for telephone counseling, download fact sheets, and access digital information and local resources for quitting smoking.[22] The California Tobacco Control Program and other large-scale mass media campaigns have been effective in decreasing smoking prevalence among adults.[23]

Mass media health education campaigns can be more effective if they establish a unique "brand" associated with the campaign's messages. Branding is a marketing strategy that tailors the language, tone of voice, messaging, product delivery, and visual media to promote and identify the brand. Branding can help make healthy behaviors more personally compelling and culturally relevant for a target audience. For example, the truth® antitobacco campaign[24] encourages adolescents and young adults to join a social movement to refute the tobacco industry's claims. Campaign advertisements are delivered on television shows and social media that are popular among youth, with a common branded theme of intelligent, attractive youth resisting the tobacco industry's attempts to manipulate them into smoking. (See also Chapter 36 on Health Communication.[25])

Classes and Curricula

School-based curricula provide an ideal modality to deliver health promotion interventions because students are already gathered in a setting where they are accustomed to learning new information and skills. Schools are also a good setting to deliver and evaluate multisession curricula because students arrive at the same classroom every day, resulting in fewer missed lessons and more complete follow-up data. In addition, school-based health education curricula occur at an ideal developmental period, because most health-risk and health-protective behaviors begin to emerge during childhood and adolescence. However, gaining entry into schools to deliver and evaluate interventions can be very difficult because schools have limited amounts of classroom time and typically need to devote most of that time to teaching basic skills. Therefore, other school-related settings such as after-school programs are often more welcoming to health promotion interventionists.

Some school-based curricula focus on one health issue such as obesity prevention. Numerous school-based programs have been effective in increasing physical activity, improving dietary intake, and reducing body mass index (BMI) among children and adolescents.[26] These programs typically provide multiple sessions of didactic instruction about diet and exercise, opportunities for physical activity during the school day, and family activities to improve diet and exercise behaviors. An example of an effective intervention to reduce obesity in children is Planet Health.[27,28] Planet Health is a school-based interdisciplinary curriculum focused on improving the health and well-being of sixth- to eighth-grade students while building and reinforcing skills in language, arts, math, science, social studies, and physical education. Through classroom and physical education activities, Planet Health aimed to increase activity, improve dietary quality, and decrease inactivity, with a particular focus on decreased TV viewing. Evaluations of Planet Health have demonstrated reductions in TV viewing, increases in fruit and vegetable consumption, lowered BMI, and reductions in disordered eating symptoms such as binging, purging, and using diet pills.[29]

Other curricula are not specific to one health behavior or health outcome; they teach broader positive youth development skills that are expected to lead to healthier decisions across multiple domains.[30] Because schools have limited time to deliver health curricula, they are often more accepting of curricula that teach more general decision-making skills that are applicable to multiple issues. A wide range of behaviors has been targeted by curricula (e.g., violence, stress, substance use, diet, exercise habits). There are four main caveats to using a classroom curriculum: (a) both teachers and administrators need to be supportive, (b) instructors must be properly trained, (c) the curriculum needs to be appropriate (developmentally, culturally, behaviorally) for the target group, and (d) the curriculum chosen should be known to be effective unless it is being delivered as part of an intervention study.

Online Interventions

Online interventions, delivered on a computer, tablet, or smartphone, have become increasingly popular. The content can include didactic information, knowledge and skills assessments, and role-play activities with avatars to practice skills. Online interventions also can provide opportunities for self-monitoring. For example, online interventions to promote weight control have provided platforms for participants to record their dietary intake and receive feedback about their calorie consumption.[31] These data can be linked to output from accelerometers on a wristband, pedometer, or smartphone to monitor physical activity. Participants can receive automatic feedback on their behaviors and can track their progress over time.[32]

Social media includes interactive online platforms through which individuals and groups can share information, news, links, photos, or videos within a virtual network. Over two-thirds of U.S. adults use social media.[33] The barriers to using social media are low because most social media platforms are freely available and can be accessed at any time of day from any Internet-connected device including mobile phones, tablets, or computers. Social media interventions to improve health behaviors have used forums, blogs, Facebook, Twitter, YouTube, and chat rooms, sometimes combined with interactive games.[34] Social media can be used to recruit participants through targeted ads, to connect participants in online support groups, to inspire competition among participants with online games and contests, and to contact participants online for follow-up assessments. These interventions are less expensive to implement than in-person interventions and are not geographically limited, so they can reach people in rural areas and people with limited mobility or transportation.

Mobile and Digital Health Interventions

Mobile phones are useful for delivering reminders to practice healthy behaviors, because most participants carry their mobile phones with them and check them repeatedly throughout the day. The intervention can be in the form of an app that participants install on their phones, or the intervention can simply send text messages to the participants' phones. Text messaging is an ideal way to deliver health promotion messages because use of cellular phones is becoming ubiquitous in the United States and worldwide. The text messaging functionality exists on most cellular phones, including smartphones as well as cheaper, simpler phones that do not access the Internet. Text messaging allows health promotion messages to be delivered to participants instantly and frequently. Text messaging and other forms of mobile interventions can be delivered in the context of people's daily lives, when and where they are most needed or most likely to be acted upon.[35]

The use of mobile phones to deliver health promotion messages has increased substantially in the past decade. A recent systematic review of review articles[36] found 89 studies published between 2009 and 2014. Most of these studies found that text-messaging interventions were effective in improving diabetes self-management, weight loss, physical activity, smoking cessation, and medication adherence for antiretroviral therapy. Text messaging interventions have been used with diverse populations including cardiovascular disease patients,[37] adolescents and adults,[38] and racial/ethnic minorities.[39]

It is unclear whether text message interventions need to be tailored to the participant's personal characteristics. A meta-analysis of the impact of tailored text messages on health behaviors revealed that messages tailored to the participant's personal psychosocial factors (e.g., self-efficacy, motivation) were significantly more effective in changing health behaviors than those without tailoring.[40] However, another meta-analysis of text message interventions[41] concluded that tailored or targeted text messages were not more effective than generic text messages.

Other technologies, such as wearable or deployable sensors, are increasingly being used to intervene in the context of people's everyday lives. These are often used in concert with smartphones or Internet/telemedicine-based interventions. These technologies can (1) communicate information about adherence to the health professional; (2) identity times and places that are high-risk for nonadherence; and (3) provide immediate feedback to participants to help them improve their adherence.[42] Wearable sensors (such as step counters) and deployable sensors (such as cameras or air pollution detectors) can provide information on people's behavior and the context in which their behavior takes place. These clues can provide real- or near-time information that can be used to help participants improve their behavior, for instance, providing immediate feedback if a person has been sitting at their desk for more than 30 minutes. Geographical positioning systems found in wearable devices and smartphones can provide information on contexts that are important for health promotion, for instance helping to understand where and when a person is most likely to be physically active. They can provide important information for disease prevention, such as communicating with sensors that are deployed to detect particulate matter and providing warning systems for asthmatic patients. Advances in deployable sensors have led to the development of "smart" or sensor-enabled institutions, workplaces, homes, and vehicles that will enable much deeper understanding of human behavior in real time and in context. Data being accrued now is leading to new dynamic models of human behavior and new types of interventions.[43] These new interventions are beginning to take into account social and environmental surroundings as well as personal factors such as mood and availability to respond to an intervention.

When implementing interventions that involve targeted electronic media, it is important to gauge participants' preference for and comfort with various forms of electronic communication. Some people prefer text messages, whereas others might prefer emails or more traditional communication methods such as personal phone calls or mailed postcards. Instead of choosing the same communication method for all participants or making assumptions about people's preferences, it is useful to ask participants which type of communication they prefer.[44]

ADAPTIVITY

Interventions can vary in adaptivity. An adaptive intervention is one that changes over time in response to the client's progress in changing behavior. For example, a smoking cessation intervention can begin by increasing motivation and self-efficacy to quit smoking, and then after the client quits, the intervention can shift to providing strategies to avoid relapse. Static interventions, in contrast, provide the same sequence and timing of information and activities to all participants regardless of the extent to which they master the skills in the previous sessions.[5]

Adaptive interventions are based on the premise that some participants will improve their behavior after a brief, inexpensive intervention, whereas others will need more intensive interventions to change their behavior. Adaptive interventions use decision rules to determine which intervention components to deliver at which times.[45] For example, all participants could first receive a brief educational session. Some participants will change their behavior based on this low-intensity intervention; these participants would then receive no further intervention or a brief follow-up booster intervention. The participants who do not change their behavior in response to the initial low-intensity intervention could be routed to a higher-intensity intervention such as individualized motivational counseling. Therefore, participants receive the treatment they need, but patients who respond to low-intensity treatment do not receive more treatment than they need.[46]

Some adaptive interventions involve only one or two decision rules. Participants who respond to a low-intensity intervention might receive no additional interventions, whereas participants who do not respond to the low-intensity intervention would be routed to a more intensive intervention. These "stepped care" protocols have been used in clinical practice for decades to avoid overtreating patients when a lower-intensity treatment would suffice.[47] However, adaptive interventions might be even more effective if they adapt according to these decision rules multiple times per day. For most behaviors, the likelihood of making healthy or unhealthy choices fluctuates throughout the day. For example, former smokers typically report specific times when they have more cravings to smoke, such as early morning, when drinking alcohol, or when in the presence of smokers.[48] In other situations, such as interacting with children or playing sports, they might experience fewer cravings. Adaptive interventions can/should be combined with ecological momentary assessment to deliver specific intervention components based on frequent measurements of individuals' recent behavior and emotional states. A just-in-time adaptive intervention (JITAI) adapts the characteristics of the intervention (e.g., the type, timing, and intensity) over time according to the participant's changing emotional state and social context. The goal of JITAIs is to deliver the right type of support at the time and context in which the participant needs it most and is most likely to be receptive to it.[49]

An example of a JITAI is Smart-T,[48] a smartphone app for smoking cessation that delivers messages tailored to the participant's risk for relapse, which can fluctuate throughout the day depending on the participant's emotional state and social-environmental factors. After participants quit smoking, the app prompts them five times per day to assess their risk of relapse, which is calculated based on their self-reported urge to smoke, stress, recent alcohol consumption, interaction with smokers, motivation to quit, and cigarette availability. The app then delivers customized messages based on the most imminent risk factors for relapse, helping participants to manage negative emotions, get out of situations that encourage smoking, or seek social support.

INNOVATIVE INTERVENTION STRATEGIES

Narrative Interventions

Rather than just presenting factual information, some interventions use narratives to deliver health education and encourage viewers to practice healthier behaviors.[50] Narrative health education, or entertainment-education, presents realistic stories of characters making decisions about their health behaviors. When viewers become immersed in an engaging story, they become cognitively and affectively engaged and are more likely to change their real-world beliefs and behaviors to match those modeled in the story. Even when viewers know the story is fictional, they still become immersed in the story and become less likely to counterargue against the messages. They meet likeable characters who validate their own ambivalence about changing behavior but ultimately overcome that ambivalence and role model healthy behaviors. Immersion into the story and identification with the characters increase persuasion.[51]

An example of a narrative health promotion intervention is The Tamale Lesson.[52] This 11-minute video was developed to increase cervical cancer screening among Hispanic women. The video tells the story of a Hispanic family preparing for the youngest daughter's quinceañera or 15th birthday celebration. The gathering of women in the kitchen making tamales provides a setting for a candid conversation among women of multiple ages and generations. One young woman discloses to her sister that she has been diagnosed with HPV. As the story unfolds, the protagonist shares facts about HPV, its relation to cervical cancer, and the importance of Pap tests in detecting cervical cancer. The protagonist convinces her female relatives to go to a clinic to have their first Pap test. In a 6-month longitudinal study, Tamale Lesson was more effective than a didactic video with the same content in improving cervical cancer knowledge and attitude, as well as receiving or scheduling a Pap test.[52]

Motivational Interviewing

Motivational interviewing (MI) is a collaborative counseling technique aimed at helping people increase their motivation and readiness to make behavioral changes.[53] MI counselors use nonjudgmental, empathetic encouragement to create a positive interpersonal collaboration that is conducive to self-examination, understanding, and change. One of the goals of MI is to evoke intrinsic motivation for change. The counselor encourages the client to explore how their current health-related behaviors might conflict with their health goals, to evaluate their own reasons for and against behavior change, to discover behavior change strategies that are personally relevant, and to convince themselves that they can make changes. Core strategies in MI include agenda setting and eliciting change talk. In agenda setting, clients determine the goals for change so that they are active and willing participants. Eliciting change talk involves having participants generate self-motivational statements and is based on the premise that people are more likely to act on plans they develop themselves.[54]

MI interventions can be particularly effective for populations who are at a low level of readiness to change their behavior, and can be tailored to individual needs and circumstances including making them developmentally appropriate. Additionally, MI can be used to tailor interventions for cultural competence because the client sets the goals rather than the clinician. MI has been used in dietary and physical activity interventions for the general population and for patients with chronic disease, smoking cessation, substance abuse prevention, medical adherence in diabetes, psychosis, and other chronic illnesses, increasing screening, suicide prevention, and HIV-risk prevention.[55-62]

Policy Interventions

Policy change is another important tool for health promotion. The "Health in All Policies" initiative[76] encourages policymakers to develop policies that enhance health, well-being, and equity. New policies cause people to alter their behavior almost immediately, regardless of whether or not they have been convinced of the necessity of changing their behavior. For example, when communities implement restaurant smoking bans, the restaurant owners immediately prohibit smoking in their establishments (or risk paying a fine), and their patrons refrain from smoking (or risk being asked to leave the restaurant). In this way, nonsmokers in the restaurant are immediately protected from exposure to second hand smoke, even before the smoking patrons and restaurant owners have changed their attitudes about smoking in restaurants. Over time, the public observes the lack of smoking in restaurants, and smoking in restaurants becomes viewed as an unacceptable behavior.[63] In the long term, this may encourage smokers to quit or reduce their smoking so that they can dine comfortably in nonsmoking restaurants. In the short term, the policy protects restaurant staff and other customers from exposure to secondhand smoke. Smoke-free policies have recently extended to multiunit housing, parks, and other places where children are likely to be present, directly reducing children's exposure to smoke.[64] Policies also can decrease smoking behavior by taxing cigarettes, thereby making them more expensive.[65]

Policies also have been used to provide consumers with the information they need to practice healthier behaviors. For example, the United States requires food manufacturers to list the ingredients and nutrient content of packaged foods. Several U.S. states require restaurants to list the calorie counts of their foods on menus.[66] These policies ensure that consumers have information about their food options, but it is also essential for the consumers to know how to read food labels and to have the numeracy skills to understand calorie counts and portion sizes.[66]

Built Environment Interventions

The built environment usually includes not only the physical structure of the cities, towns, and rural settings in which we live but also legal- and policy-level determinants of behavior. Improving neighborhood walkability, quality of parks and playgrounds, and providing adequate active transport infrastructure is likely to generate positive impacts on activity in children and adults.[67] Intervention strategies that include the built environment have substantial potential to impact an entire population, rather than just select individuals. Supportive built environments can also support individual-level behavior change. For example, making more fresh fruits and vegetables available in the home, at work, and in convenience stores may help some who have recently decided to change their diet to eat more fruits and vegetables.[68] Environmental and policy approaches can continue to influence behavior over time without requiring continued and active intervention by public health professionals. For example, building neighborhoods with sidewalks and safe street crossings will increase the frequency of walking even if a health-promotion program is never delivered to people who live in those neighborhoods.[69] Simple interventions such as posting signage to encourage people to use stairways have been effective to increase physical activity. In addition, urban design that fosters physical activity has been a focus of great interest for addressing the ongoing epidemic of obesity as well as increasing quality of life. Interventions to encourage walking can be more effective when the neighborhood is aesthetically attractive.[70] Simple modifications to the built environment such as dimming the lights and reducing use of electronic screens at night can lead to improved sleep and circadian rhythms, which can reduce the risk of numerous diseases.[71]

In addition to changing the built environment to improve people's behavior, people can choose to move to built environments that provide more opportunities for healthy behaviors and/or fewer opportunities for risky behaviors, if they have the resources to move. In the Moving to Opportunity study, one of the few studies that randomized participants to move to higher socioeconomic status neighborhoods or remain in low socioeconomic status neighborhoods, moving to an improved built environment resulted in lower risk for substance use and mental health problems among girls.[72] However, boys did not benefit equally from the relocation intervention.

The Community Preventive Services Task Force[73] now recommends alterations to transportation systems and land use to increase street connectivity, sidewalk and trail infrastructure, bicycle infrastructure, public transit infrastructure and access, mixed land use environments, and access to parks and recreational facilities. The development of theories of environmental influence and of intervention strategies using the environment are emerging areas of research. Physicians and other professionals should be aware of the important role that various elements of the built environment may play on the formation of health behaviors, risk for disease, and their use in the formulation of solutions to ongoing health-related problems.

Caveat

When implementing any health-related intervention, it is important to do no harm. Health promotion interventions can potentially have harmful consequences. For example, interventions to encourage behavior change can lead to feelings of failure, self-blame, low self-efficacy, and stigma among participants who do not change their behavior successfully.[74] Participating in behavioral interventions can separate participants from their social support networks if they are forced to abstain from social events that include unhealthy menus, alcohol, or excessive sedentary behavior.[74] Health promotion interventions also can impose additional burden on the staff who must implement complex procedures, potentially leading to staff stress and burnout.[75] It is important to assess potential unintended effects and prevent or mitigate them.

CONCLUSION

The development of behavioral interventions is an art as well as a science. This chapter has provided some issues to consider when selecting or designing interventions. Numerous interventions are available to clinicians and health service agencies. It is important to use interventions that are effective and appropriate for the target population, both in content and in modality of delivery. When selecting health promotion interventions, service providers should consider the characteristics of the target population, including their existing level of knowledge, skills, and self-efficacy to change behavior, as well as the modalities of program delivery that would be most useful to them. Of course, this must be balanced with the capacity of the organization to deliver services. Implementation of high-quality, evidence-based interventions can potentially educate diverse populations about health-risk and health-protective behaviors and motivate them to practice healthier behaviors. Ultimately, this can lead to improved health outcomes and quality of life for a significant portion of the population.

References

1. Johnson NB, Hayes LD, Brown K, Hoo EC, Ethier KAI. CDC National Health Report: Leading causes of morbidity and mortality and associated behavioral risk and protective factors. *MMWR Suppl.* 2014;63(4):3–27.
2. Glanz, K, Rimer BK, Viswanath, K, eds. *Health Behavior: Theory, Research and Practice.* 5th ed. San Francisco, CA: Jossey-Bass; 2015.
3. Glanz chapter, this volume.
4. Liu J, Ulrich C. Meditation analysis in nursing research: A methodological review. *Contemp Nurse.* 2016;52(1):125–9.
5. Piper ME, Schlam TR, Cook JW, et al. Toward precision smoking cessation treatment I: Moderator results from a factorial experiment. *Drug Alcohol Depend.* 2017;171:59–65.
6. Hartmann-Boyce J, Lancaster T, Stead LF. Print-based self help interventions for smoking cessation. *Cochrane Database Syst Rev.* 2014;6:CD001118.
7. Jones M, Ross B, Cloth A, Heller L. Interventions to reach underscreened populations: A narrative review for planning cancer screening initiatives. *Int J Public Health.* 2015;60(4):437–47.
8. Ruder EH, Lohse BA. NEEDs for tots: A teacher-ready and parent-friendly curriculum focuses on principles of the Satter division of responsibility in feeding. *J Nutr Educ Behav.* 2017;49(4):357–59.
9. De La Haye K, Robins G, Mohr P, Wilson C. Obesity-related behaviors in adolescent friendship networks. *Soc Networks.* 2010;32(3):161–7.
10. Hunter RF, De La Haye K, Badham J, Valente T, Clarke M, Kee F. Social network interventions for health behaviour change: A systematic review. *Lancet.* 2017;390:47.
11. Parker chapter, this volume.
12. Massengale KEC, Erausquin JT, Old M. Health, social, and economic outcomes experienced by families as a result of receiving assistance from a community-based diaper bank. *Matern Child Health J.* 2017;100(2):1985–94.

13. Jull J, Giles A, Graham ID. Community-based participatory research and integrated knowledge translation: Advancing the co-creation of knowledge. *Implement Sci.* 2017;12(1):150.
14. Tremblay MC, Martin DH, Macaulay AC, Pluye P. Can we build on social movement theories to develop and improve community-based participatory research? A framework synthesis review. *Am J Community Psychol.* 2017;59(3–4):333–62.
15. Jurkowski JM, Green Mills LL, Lawson HA. Engaging low-income parents in childhood obesity prevention from start to finish: A case study. *J Community Health.* 2013;38(1):1–11.
16. Carson KV, Ameer F, Sayehmiri K, et al. Mass media interventions for preventing smoking in young people. *Cochrane Database Syst Rev.* 2017;6(6):CD001006.
17. Momin B, Neri A, McCausland K, et al. Traditional and innovative promotional strategies of tobacco cessation services: A review of the literature. *J Community Health.* 2014;39(4):800–9.
18. Robinson MN, Tansil KA, Elder RW, et al. Community preventive services task force. Mass media health communication campaigns combined with health-related product distribution: A community guide systematic review. *Am J Prev Med.* 2014;47(3):360–71.
19. Lundgren, RE, McMakin, AH, eds. *Risk Communication: A Handbook for Communicating Environmental, Safety, and Health Risks.* 5th ed. Hoboken, NJ : Wiley-IEEE Press; 2013.
20. Roeseler A, Burns D. The quarter that changed the world. *Tob Control.* 2010;19:3–15.
21. Emery S, Aly EH, Vera L, Alexander RL Jr. Tobacco control in a changing media landscape: How tobacco control programs use the internet. *Am J Prev Med.* 2014;46(3):293–6.
22. Lee YO, Momin B, Hansen H, et al. Maximizing the impact of digital media campaigns to promote smoking cessation: A case study of the California tobacco control program and the California smokers' helpline. *Calif J Health Promot.* 2014;12(3):35–45.
23. Bala MM, Strzeszynski L, Topor-Madry R. Mass media interventions for smoking cessation in adults. *Cochrane Database Syst Rev.* 2017.
24. Vallone D, Greenberg M, Xiao H, et al. The effect of branding to promote healthy behavior: Reducing tobacco use among youth and young adults. *Int J Environ Res Public Health.* 2017;14(12):1517.
25. Vishwanath chapter, this volume.
26. Brown EC, Buchan DS, Baker JS, Wyatt FB, Bocalini DS, Kilgore L. A systematised review of primary school whole class child obesity interventions: Effectiveness, characteristics, and strategies. *Biomed Res Int.* 2016;2016:4902714.
27. Blaine RE, Franckle RL, Chuang E, et al. Using school staff members to implement a childhood obesity prevention intervention in low-income school districts: The Massachusetts childhood obesity research demonstrations. *Prev Chronic Dis.* 2017;14:1–14.
28. Carter, J, Wiecha, JL, Peterson, KE, Nobrega S, Gortmaker SL. *Planet Health: An Interdisciplinary Curriculum for Teaching Middle School Nutrition and Physical Activity.* 2nd ed. Illinois: Windsor, CA: Human Kinetics Pub; 2007.
29. Austin SB, Spadano-Gasbarro JL, Greaney ML, et al. Effect of the planet health intervention on eating disorder symptoms in Massachusetts middle schools. *Prev Chronic Dis.* 2012;9:1––10.
30. Taylor RD, Oberle E, Derlak JA, Weissberg RP. Promoting positive youth development through school-based social and emotional learning interventions: A meta-analysis of follow-up effects. *Child Dev.* 2017;88(4):1156–71.
31. Raaijmakers LC, Pouwels S, Berghuis KA, Nienhuijs SW. Technology-based interventions in the treatment of overweight and obesity: A systematic review. *Appetite.* 2015;95:138–51.
32. Abril EP. Tracking myself: Assessing the contribution of mobile technologies for self-trackers of weight, diet, or exercise. *J Health Commun.* 2016;21(6):638–46.
33. Greenwood S, Perrin A, Duggan M. Social Media Update 2016. Pew Research Center.
34. Nour M, Yeung SH, Patridge S, Allman-Farinelli M. A narrative review of social media and game-based nutrition interventions targeted at young adults. *J Acad Nutr Diet.* 2017;117(5):735–52.
35. Spruijt-Metz D, Wen CK, O'Reilly G, et al. Innovations in the use of interactive technology to support weight management. *Curr Obes Rep.* 2015;4(4):510–19.
36. Hall AK, Cole-Lewis H, Bernhardt JM. Mobile text messaging for health: A systematic review of reviews. *Annu Rev Public Health.* 2015;36(1):393–415.
37. Adler AJ, Martin N, Mariani J, et al. Mobile phone text messaging to improve medication adherence in secondary prevention of cardiovascular disease. *Cochrane Database Syst Rev.* 2017;4(4):CD011851.
38. Kazemi DM, Borsari B, Levine MJ, Li S, Lamberson KA, Matta LA. A systematic review of the mHealth interventions to prevent alcohol and substance abuse. *J Health Commun.* 2017;22(5):413–32.
39. Boland VC, Stockings EA, Mattick RP, McRobbie H, Brown J, Courtney RJ. The methodological quality and effectiveness of technology-based smoking cessation interventions for disadvantaged groups: A systematic review and meta-analysis. *Nicotine Tob Res.* 2016;20(3):276–85.
40. Head KJ, Noar SM, Iannarino NT, Grant Harrington N. Efficacy of text messaging-based interventions for health promotion: A meta-analysis. *Soc Sci Med.* 2013;97:41–8.
41. Armanasco AA, Miller YD, Fjeldsoe BS, Marshall AL. Preventive health behavior change text message interventions: A meta-analysis. *Am J Prev Med.* 2017;52(3):391–402.
42. De Leon E, Fuentes LW, Cohen JE. Characterizing periodic messaging interventions across health behaviors and media: Systematic review. *J Med Internet Res.* 2010;16(3):93.
43. Spruijt-Metz D, Hekler E, Saranummi N, et al. Building new computational models to support health behavior change and maintenance: New opportunities in behavioral research. *Transl Behav Med.* 2015;5(3):335–46.
44. Finkelstein SR, Liu N, Jani B, Rosenthal D, Poghosyan L. Appointment reminder systems and patient preferences: Patient technology usage and familiarity with other service providers as predictive variables. *Health Informatics J.* 2013;19(2):79––90.
45. Collins LM, Nahum-Shani I, Almirall D. Optimization of behavioral dynamic treatment regimens based on the sequential, multiple assignment, randomized trial (SMART). *Clin Trials.* 2014;11(4):426–34.
46. Kidwell KM, Hyde LW. Adaptive interventions and SMART designs: Application to child behavior research in a community setting. *Am J Eval.* 2015;37(3):344–63.
47. Van Straten A, Hill J, Richards DA, Cuijpers P. Stepped care treatment delivery for depression: A systematic review and meta-analysis. *Psychol Med.* 2015;45(2):231–46.
48. Hebert ET, Stevens EM, Frank SG, et al. An ecological momentary intervention for smoking cessation: The associations of just-in-time, tailored messages with lapse risk factors. *Addict Behav.* 2017;78:30–35.
49. Nahum-Shani I, Smith SN, Spring BJ, et al. Just-in-time adaptive interventions (JITAIs) in mobile health: Key components and design principles for ongoing health behavior support. *Ann Behav Med.* 2016;52(6):446–62.
50. Hinyard LJ, Kreuter MW. Using narrative communication as a tool for health behavior change: A conceptual, theoretical, and empirical overview. *Health Educ Behav.* 2007;34(5):777––92.
51. Green MC, Clark JL. Transportation into narrative worlds: Implications for entertainment media influences on tobacco use. *Addiction.* 2013;108(3):477–84.
52. Murphy ST, Frank LB, Chatterjee JS, et al. Comparing the relative efficacy of narrative vs nonnarrative health messages in reducing health disparities using a randomized trial. *Am J Public Health.* 2015;105(10):2117–23.
53. Tuccero D, Railey K, Briggs M, Hull SK. Behavioral health in prevention and chronic illness management: Motivational interviewing. *Prim Care.* 2016;43(2):191–202.
54. Magill M, Apodaca TR, Borsari B, et al. A meta-analysis of motivational interviewing process: Technical, relational, and conditional process models of change. *J Consult Clin Psychol.* 2017;86(2):140–57.
55. Borrello M, Pietrabissa G, Ceccarini M, Manzoni GM, Castelnuovo G. Motivational interviewing in childhood obesity treatment. *Front Psychol.* 2015;6:1732.
56. Bus K, Peyer KL, Bai Y, Ellingson LD, Welk GJ. Comparison of in-person and online motivational interviewing-based health coaching. *Health Promot Pract.* 2018;19(4):513–21.
57. Ekong G, Kavookjian J. Motivational interviewing and outcomes in adults with type 2 diabetes: A systematic review. *Patient Educ Couns.* 2016;99(6):944–52.
58. Hoy J, Natarajan A, Petra MM. Motivational interviewing and the transtheoretical model of change: Under-explored resources for suicide intervention. *Community Ment Health J.* 2016;52(5):559–67.
59. Miller SJ, Foran-Tuller K, Ledergerber J, Jandorf L. Motivational interviewing to improve health screening uptake: A systematic review. *Patient Educ Couns.* 2017;100(2):190–8.
60. Samdal GB, Eide GE, Barth T, Williams G, Meland E. Effective behaviour change techniques for physical activity and healthy eating in overweight and obese adults; systematic review and meta-regression analyses. *Int J Behav Nutr Phys Act.* 2017;14(1):42.

61. Schaefer MF, Kavookjian J. The impact of motivational interviewing on adherence and symptom severity in adolescents and young adults with chronic illness: A systematic review. *Patient Educ Couns.* 2017;100(12):2190–9.

62. Spencer JC. Wheeler SB. A systematic review of motivational interviewing interventions in cancer patients and survivors. *Patient Educ Couns.* 2016;99(7):1099–105.

63. Jacobs M, Alonso AM, Sherin KM, Koh Y, Dhamija A, Lowe AL, ACPM Prevention Practice Committee. Policies to restrict secondhand smoke exposure: American college of preventive medicine position statement. *Am J Prev Med.* 2013;45(3):360–7.

64. Bartholomew KS. Policy options to promote smokefree environments for children and adolescents. *Curr Probl Pediatr Adolesc Health Care.* 2016;45(6):146–81

65. Henriksen L, Andersen-Rodgers E, Zhang X, et al. Neighborhood variation in the price of cheap tobacco products in California: Results from healthy stores for a healthy community. *Nicotine Tob Res.* 2017;19(11):1330–7.

66. Levine DI. The curious history of the calorie in U.S. policy: A tradition of unfulfilled promises. *Am J Prev Med.* 2017;52(1):125–9.

67. Smith M, Hosking J, Woodward A, et al. Systematic literature review of built environment effects of physical activity and active transport—An update and new findings on health equity. *Int J Behav Nutr Phys Act.* 2017;14(1):158.

68. Gordon-Larsen P. Food availability/convenience and obesity. *Adv Nutr.* 2014;5(6):809–17.

69. Carlin A, Perchoux C, Puggina A, et al. The physical environmental determinants of physical activity behaviour: A "determinants of diet and physical activity" (DEDIPAC) umbrella systematic literature review. *PLoS One.* 2017;12(8):e0182083.

70. Perez LG, Kerr J, Sallis JF, et al. Perceived neighborhood environmental factors that maximize the effectiveness of a multilevel intervention promoting physical activity among Latinas. *Am J Health Promot.* 2017;32(3):334–43.

71. Ball LJ, Palesh O, Kriegsfeld LJ. The pathophysiologic role of disrupted circadian and neuroendocrine rhythms in breast carcinogenesis. *Endocr Rev.* 2016;37(5):450–66.

72. Schmidt NM, Glymour MM, Osypuk TL. Housing mobility and adolescent mental health: The role of substance use, social networks, and family mental health in the moving to opportunity study. *SSM Popul Health.* 2017;3:318–25.

73. Community Preventive Services Task Force. Recommendation for built environment interventions to increase physical activity. *MMWR Morb Mort Wkly Rep.* 2017;66(17):460.

74. Devine CM, Barnhill A. The ethical and public health importance of unintended consequences: The case of behavioral weight loss interventions. *Public Health Ethics.* 2018;11(3):356–61.

75. Gugglberger L, Flaschberger E, Teutsch F. 'Side effects' of health promotion: An example from Austrian schools. *Health Promot Int.* 2017;32(1):157–66.

76. Pepin D, Winig BD, Carr D, Jacobson PD. Collaborating for health: Health in All policies and the law. *J Law Med Ethics.* 2017;45(1_Suppl):60–4.

CHAPTER 41

Evidence-Based Community Interventions

Shawna L. Mercer*

Many public health professionals and other stakeholders are charged with improving health in their communities, often despite having limited time or resources for doing so. Evidence-based community interventions are an important part of the toolbox for improving public health.[1] The term "evidence-based community interventions" is sometimes used indiscriminately; however, it createsmisunderstanding and potentially leads to the use of interventions that will not achieve their intended outcomes. To ensure understanding of what exactly constitutes an evidence-based community intervention, this chapter will begin by considering the composite parts of the term. It will then discuss the value of using evidence-based community interventions, and identify how they fit into community health improvement planning and decision making. The final section of this chapter will identify where readers can find information about evidence-based community interventions.

WHAT CONSTITUTES A COMMUNITY?

The traditional definition of "community" has been a group of people, with some common ties, living in the same geographic or geopolitical area, such as a neighborhood, town, or county.[2] Within the field of public health, community is typically understood more broadly to also include other groups of people who share common interests or characteristics (e.g., age, race, ethnicity, religion, or culture), or who participate together in activities within a particular setting (e.g., work, school, or a recreational setting).[3–5] A community therefore consists of a population group along with the place, venue, unit, or virtual platform where the population group's activity takes place.[3] Communities may be as diverse as states, counties, neighborhoods, rural areas, health systems, worksites, places of worship, schools, the military, specific racial ethnic groups, and online groups, among others. Those involved in developing and evaluating community interventions need to pay close attention to whether interventions may work better or differently in some communities than others.

WHAT IS AN INTERVENTION AND WHAT TYPES OF INTERVENTIONS CAN BE USED IN COMMUNITIES TO IMPROVE HEALTH?

The wide range of types of communities is matched by the diverse types of interventions that can be used within communities. Interventions are actions taken to improve a situation or to have some other intended effect on an outcome of interest.[6] In public health, community interventions focus on changing the behavior of individuals, or helping individuals to maintain desired behaviors, with the ultimate goal of improving the health and well-being of as many people as possible within that community. Community interventions can aim to change behavior directly, or they can aim to change it indirectly by creating conditions that encourage behavior change. The socio ecologic model posits that behavior is determined by factors or conditions across five levels.[7] Community interventions can focus on one or more of these five levels—(a) the intrapersonal level (aiming to directly change characteristics of individuals such as knowledge and behavior); (b) interpersonal (aiming to effect individual-level behavior change by changing how individuals interact with each other); (c) institutional (intervening on organizations and institutions to which an individual belongs); (d) community (intervening on relationships between organizations and institutions within a community, and on community networks); and (e) public policy (intervening at the level of policies and laws that govern communities).[7,8] Intervening at multiple levels may be necessary for both initial and sustained behavior change.[9]

To effect change at one or more levels of the socioecological model, community interventions can be divided into the following four basic types:

1. Informational and educational interventions. These interventions consist of materials (e.g., a pamphlet), tools (e.g., a website or application), services (e.g., an educational campaign), and programs designed to provide information or to educate. Such interventions may be as relatively straightforward as providing a short informational document or as intensive as a multisession education program. These interventions typically operate at the intrapersonal level.
2. Behavioral and social interventions. These interventions consist of programs and services that involve behavior change strategies built on theories and principles from the behavioral and social sciences.[10] These programs and services may contain educational components in addition to behavior change strategies. Examples of such interventions are programs that help to build skills and self-efficacy, or that provide coaching and counseling. These interventions typically operate at intrapersonal and interpersonal levels.
3. Environmental and policy interventions. These interventions aim to change aspects of the physical or built (i.e.,

* At the time that this chapter was written, Shawna Mercer was Director of the Guide to Community Preventive Services (The Community Guide) and Chief of The Community Guide Branch; Division of Public Health Information Dissemination; Center for Surveillance, Epidemiology, and Laboratory Services; Centers for Disease Control and Prevention. The findings and conclusions in this chapter are those of the author and do not necessarily represent the official position of the Centers for Disease Control and Prevention (CDC).

human-made) environment, policies within an organization, or policies at the local, state, or federal level. These two types of interventions are grouped together because environmental interventions often involve changing policies. Examples include built environment interventions to increase physical activity (e.g., combining transportation system interventions with land use and environmental design)[11] and organizational policies to increase sun protection measures in childcare centers (e.g., more shade structures, required use of sunscreen).[12] Environmental and policy interventions typically operate at one or more of institutional, community, and public policy levels of the socioecological model.

4. Health system interventions. These interventions aim to change one or more aspects of the health system. Health system interventions include interventions focused on bringing more people to the point of care (e.g., providing transportation, child care, or language translation services), strengthening the way care or services are delivered (e.g., employing community health workers or team-based care), and influencing provider behavior (e.g., using provider assessment and feedback, or reminders to providers to encourage their patients to undergo preventive screenings) (all examples are from The Community Guide).[13] Many health system interventions, especially those that operate in healthcare systems, connect closely with and support the delivery of evidence-based clinical interventions—that is, clinical preventive services and other clinical interventions that are typically delivered by primary care and other clinicians.[14–16] Health system interventions operate at one or more of interpersonal, institutional, community, or public policy levels. Note that some systematic review groups include both public health system interventions and healthcare system interventions in this category of health system interventions (e.g., The Community Guide[13]). Other systematic review groups include only public health system interventions in the health system category and categorize healthcare system interventions with clinical interventions (e.g., Cochrane[14]).

Many community interventions focus directly on improving health outcomes such as preventing or controlling disease, disability and injury, or addressing risk factors for disease, disability, and injury. Other community interventions aim to improve health in the future by first addressing the social determinants of health—that is, by trying to improve conditions that influence health risks and outcomes in the places where people live, work, learn, worship, and play.[17,18] Social determinants of health may include such things as lower education levels, poverty, inadequate housing, and unsafe neighborhoods. Evaluating the effectiveness of community interventions focused on social determinants of health involves assessing whether the interventions are effective in improving both the social determinants of health and, ultimately, health. For example, high school completion programs have been found to increase academic achievement which, in turn, is linked with long-term health.[19,20] Using community interventions that are effective in improving social determinants of health can also have a meaningful influence on health equity.[21,22]

In sum, community interventions consist of programs, services, policies, and systems that seek to increase or maintain health-enhancing behaviors and ultimately improve the health of entire communities.[23] In this regard, they make a substantial contribution to population health in its concern with the health outcomes of whole groups of individuals and its quest to improve the health of entire populations.[24] Community interventions can do this either through (a) supporting or extending clinical interventions or (b) operating entirely within a public health framework, with a focus on one or more of addressing the social determinants of health, helping people to achieve better health, reducing health disparities, or achieving health equity in the communities where they live, learn, work, worship, and play.

WHAT DOES IT MEAN THAT A COMMUNITY INTERVENTION IS EVIDENCE-BASED?

When trying to decide what intervention to use to address a particular public health challenge in their community, public health professionals might consider a number of different sources of evidence about what to do (see Fig. 41-1) (adapted from refs. 25 and 26). All of these sources of evidence can provide different types and amounts of important information to assist in decision making (this is discussed further in the section entitled "How do evidence-based community interventions fit into evidence-based or evidence-informed decision making?"). However, as discussed below, community interventions are typically considered to be evidence-based only when high-quality research and evaluation studies show them to be effective.

Public health professionals might reflect on their own previous experience or use word of mouth to find out informally how others approached a public health challenge in their community. Both of these sources of evidence can provide valuable information about things to consider when selecting and implementing a particular intervention.[1] However, using the same intervention may not lead the public health professional to the same outcome if the current situation differs in important ways from their own past experience or from the past situations faced by their colleagues. For example, different population subgroups might react differently to the same intervention, or the intervention might not be able to be executed the same way in a different setting with different personnel and resources. It is also possible that factors other than the intervention might have been partially or fully responsible for the positive outcome in the previous situations. For example, another intervention could have been delivered at the same time that was actually responsible for the changes, or the intended outcome could have already been increasing in the population and therefore would have been erroneously attributed to the intervention. If one is relying on subjective anecdotal evidence of what happened in another situation, information is limited about whether the intervention itself was actually responsible for the outcome and whether one will receive the same outcome if the current situation differs in some known or unknown way.

Objective sources of evidence that can more reliably help a user determine whether a community intervention is effective in causing the desired outcome include research studies and program evaluations, in which those receiving an intervention are compared to a control or comparison group that does not receive the intervention, or where other study design features are employed that increase one's confidence that the intervention itself is responsible for the change.[27,28] Note, however, that if only one well-designed research study or program evaluation is found, evidence is still limited. The main conclusion that can be drawn from one study or evaluation is that the intervention caused the outcome under the conditions that existed within that study.

Locating multiple high-quality research studies or program evaluations that come to similar conclusions can further increase confidence in whether the intervention caused the outcome. It is possible,

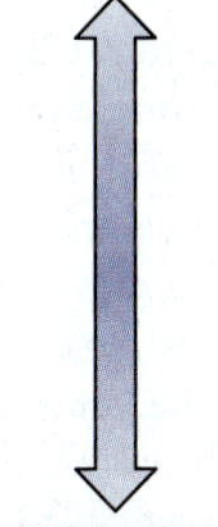

FIGURE 41-1. Different forms of evidence.

however, that additional studies or evaluations exist that were not located, and they may have found different results. The strongest type of evidence, therefore, comes from a systematic review that considers all available studies of the intervention's effectiveness. A systematic review uses formal and systematic methods to search for and identify all relevant studies, assess their quality, and critically appraise and summarize the evidence from all included studies.[29-31] A systematic review provides an overall assessment of effectiveness and typically examines how effectiveness changes if there are differences from study to study in the way the intervention is structured and delivered, or to whom it is delivered. A meta-analysis—which involves statistically pooling, analyzing, and summarizing the results—may also be undertaken if the studies included in a systematic review are homogenous enough to permit such analyses.[32,33] However, such homogeneity is relatively rare for studies of real-world community interventions, in which there is considerable variation from one study to another in things such as intervention components and execution, study sample, and setting.

Good-quality systematic reviews and meta-analyses carefully define the intervention they are studying, identify the essential elements of the intervention versus other components that may or may not be present, and stipulate inclusion and exclusion criteria. This clear delineation is particularly important when assessing community interventions because of the substantial variation typically encountered in how community interventions are structured and delivered from study to study, as well as how the interventions are used in different communities.

Another type of review that can be helpful to developers of community interventions is a narrative review. A narrative review summarizes the evidence qualitatively, providing interpretation and critique.[34,35] The ultimate aim of a narrative review is to secure a deeper understanding of the intervention, its context, and other aspects of the situation.[34,35] Types of narrative reviews include hermeneutic reviews (which focus on increasing theoretical understanding), realist reviews (with a focus on understanding which interventions produce specific outcomes in some situations but not in others), and meta-narrative reviews (which focus on trying to understand how concepts and ideas have been viewed by different researchers and academic disciplines over time).[35] Many narrative reviews are systematic in searching for and critically assessing all available evidence.

All of the forms of evidence shown in Fig. 41-1 and discussed above can help decision makers to understand an intervention and how it can be used. Community interventions are considered to be evidence-based; however, only if high-quality research and evaluation studies show them to be effective in achieving their intended outcomes.[36] Systematic reviews and meta-analyses provide the strongest evidence as to the effectiveness of community-based interventions because their rigorous and systematic processes summarize and interpret all included evidence, help to reduce bias in interpretation, and improve the power and precision of results.[29,36,37]

WHAT CHALLENGES ARE FACED WHEN ASSESSING THE EFFECTIVENESS OF COMMUNITY INTERVENTIONS?

Two challenges in particular stand out among the numerous challenges that are faced when trying to evaluate whether a community intervention is evidence-based. First, it may not always be possible to evaluate a community intervention using a randomized controlled trial (RCT) or through devising an appropriate control group. For example, when evaluating the effectiveness of a law, it is typically not possible to randomly assign some people to follow the law and others to not follow the law. In other cases, it may not be ethical to withhold certain services from some participants. There may also be considerable differences between the kinds of people who would agree to participate in a study versus the target population as a whole. To adequately assess the effectiveness of community interventions, therefore, usually involves using a wide range of study designs in addition to RCTs—including interrupted time series designs, other quasiexperimental designs, cross-sectional studies, and other designs.[1,27] This, in turn, requires careful consideration of the suitability of the study design, what biases might accompany the use of each design, and how triangulation may be employed to determine what can be learned from each different type of design.[1,27,29]

A second challenge stems from the fact that individual studies of the effectiveness of a community intervention, as well as all systematic reviews, assess internal validity—that is, whether the intervention is responsible for the outcome under the conditions set forth in the study or evaluation.[28] Yet, what user audiences really want to know is whether they can achieve similar outcomes in their particular community, with their specific populations, settings, resources, and circumstances. The strongest sources of information about whether something will work across a range of communities, therefore, are systematic reviews that also look at external validity—that is, whether the intervention works across, and is applicable to, various populations, settings, and situations, and with different types or amounts of resources.[27,28] There is particular value to a systematic review that shows an intervention to be effective across different studies where there is variation in the way the intervention is structured and delivered. This is because intervention developers can then have confidence that, even if they adapt or fit the intervention to their community, they can expect to see similar effectiveness to what was seen in the systematic review, as long as they keep their intervention consistent with what the systematic review describes as the essential parts of the intervention.

Given both of these challenges, systematic reviews that permit the inclusion of practice-based evidence as well as research-based evidence can yield additional insights.[43] This is because practice-based evidence involves evaluating community interventions implemented in practice—that is, in real-world circumstances under real-world conditions.

HOW DOES CALLING AN INTERVENTION EVIDENCE-BASED FIT WITH THE CONCEPTS OF BEST AND PROMISING PRACTICES?

Part of getting to the place where community interventions are identified as evidence-based is to ensure that community interventions can be devised, developed, and tested in multiple situations to determine their effectiveness. It is therefore valuable to consider where an intervention exists along an evidence continuum. This continuum has been described as consisting of four levels: (1) emerging practices, (2) promising practices, (3) leading or likely effective practices, and (4) best practices.[38-40] Emerging practices have been described as newer practices that have a plausible theoretical basis and preliminary evidence of impact through field-based summaries or early evaluations. These interventions need more evaluation to determine whether their effectiveness can be replicated. Promising practices include practices that demonstrate some evidence of effectiveness through unpublished, non–peer-reviewed intervention evaluations. Leading practices, or likely effective practices, include practices that show growing evidence of effectiveness assessed through peer-reviewed studies or through a nonsystematic review of published intervention evaluations. Best practices include practices that have been identified as effective through systematic reviews of research and evaluation studies.

There is value in determining where along the continuum the evidence for a particular community intervention is, so that one can understand how much confidence to have at a given time in the intervention's effectiveness, and also to identify worthy candidates to move along the continuum through additional research and evaluation. Researchers, evaluators, and funders of research and evaluation can make major contributions to developing the evidence base for community interventions by thinking of the continuum as a pipeline, and seeking to stimulate flow through the pipeline by identifying or devising novel interventions, and then actively fostering the refinement and testing of those interventions. Emerging, promising, and leading community interventions may benefit from undergoing evaluability assessment to determine whether they are ready for various types of evaluation and how their readiness may be improved.[41,42] Establishing best practices may be further facilitated if those who are working to identify promising and leading practices engage with systematic review groups when they uncover interventions that they think may have enough high-quality data on effectiveness to undergo systematic review. Finally, thinking in terms of a pipeline serves as a reminder that it is important to assess whether new data about effectiveness becomes available, and whether best practices remain as such, or whether circumstances or context may cause them to become less effective over time.

WHAT IS THE VALUE OF USING EVIDENCE-BASED COMMUNITY INTERVENTIONS AND HOW CAN THEY BE USED?

Using a community intervention that is evidence-based provides decision makers with confidence that they will receive a similar outcome if they implement the intervention in similar situations. This can be particularly valuable when resources are scarce or limited. This is because decision makers can concentrate their available resources on trying to ensure that the evidence-based intervention is implemented as fully as possible rather than also having to try to devise an intervention de novo, or having to come up with a second intervention if a nonevidence-based intervention did not achieve the intended outcome. Starting with an evidence-based intervention will also typically shorten the time until the intervention is ready to be implemented.

Information about evidence-based community interventions can help public health professionals engage with people in healthcare settings by identifying how community interventions can support the delivery of effective clinical services. It can also help public health professionals explain to those in other governmental agencies—like education, social services, and transportation—how collaborating on certain community interventions might help all of them achieve their respective aims.

Information on evidence-based community interventions can be used to plan, modify, and evaluate programs, services, policies, and systems; strengthen applications for programmatic funding; and justify why current evidence-based initiatives should be maintained. One important piece of information that is typically provided in a systematic review relates to what size (or magnitude) of an effect decision makers should expect to see if they implement the evidence-based community intervention that is the subject of the systematic review. Since the effect size provided in a systematic review is calculated on the basis of all of the effect sizes from the individual research and evaluation studies included in the systematic review, decision makers can have confidence that the effect size they would see would be similar. Knowing what they can expect to achieve if they use a particular intervention can help decision makers set realistic goals or determine how far they will be able to go toward achieving a goal that others have set for them.

Finally, many systematic reviews of the effectiveness of community interventions also identify evidence gaps. Filling these evidence gaps has the potential to make a significant impact on public health. Researchers and program evaluators can use the evidence gaps as a source of ideas and develop studies to answer outstanding questions. Furthermore, they can strengthen their funding applications by identifying how they are seeking to fill important evidence gaps. Agencies and organizations that fund research and evaluation can play a particularly important role in strengthening the evidence base when they highlight evidence gaps as priority areas within their funding announcements, thereby encouraging targeted research and evaluation by multiple researchers and evaluators.[23]

HOW DO EVIDENCE-BASED COMMUNITY INTERVENTIONS FIT INTO EVIDENCE-BASED OR EVIDENCE-INFORMED DECISION MAKING?

When legislators, public health and healthcare professionals, and other community decision makers are trying to figure out what community interventions might provide the best fit for their community, evidence from research and evaluation is rarely complete enough to be the sole factor in their decision making.[44] Yet, scientific evidence is often missing from the decision-making process altogether. Bringing evidence-based community interventions to the decision-making process is one of the aims of evidence-based public health.[1,25] Evidence-based public health has been defined as the process of integrating science-based interventions alongside community preferences to improve the health of populations.[1,45] The goal is to have information about evidence-based community interventions included as part of the mix of factors that are considered—so that decision makers can identify community interventions that have been successful in other communities and can explore whether one or more of these interventions might be appropriate for their specific community. Some people call this process evidence-based decision making and others call it evidence-informed decision making.[1,44–46]

Evidence-based or evidence-informed decision making in public health involves distilling and disseminating the best available information from research, practice, and experience, and using it to inform, implement, evaluate, and improve public health practice and policy.[1,46–48] A practical model of evidence-based decision making specifies that four sources of information need to be integrated into the decision process: (1) the best available research and evaluation evidence about a community intervention (e.g., its effectiveness, applicability to different populations and settings, cost and cost-effectiveness, and implementation), (2) information about community health issues and the local environmental and organizational context (e.g., how the intervention might fit with other existing and planned initiatives and policies; how the cultural context might influence an intervention's acceptability and feasibility, and the balance between fidelity and adaptation that is needed for the intervention to be implemented effectively), (3) existing resources including practitioner expertise (e.g., the availability, amount, and types of personnel, financial, and other resources), and (4) population characteristics, needs, values, and preferences (e.g., considering the specific populations that live in the community and maintaining a commitment to shared decision making in public health and healthcare) (Fig. 41-2).[49]

WHAT ARE IMPORTANT DRIVERS OF THE CURRENT INTEREST IN USING EVIDENCE-BASED COMMUNITY INTERVENTIONS?

Within public health and healthcare, there are a number of important drivers for why communities are searching for and implementing community interventions. First, many state and local health departments are undergoing or considering voluntary national public health accreditation through the Public Health Accreditation Board.[50] As part of the accreditation and re-accreditation processes, health departments must conduct a community health assessment and develop a community health improvement plan.[51] Second, not-for-profit hospitals that wish to keep their charitable or tax-exempt status under section 501(c)(3) of the Federal Internal Revenue Code must demonstrate their community benefit by conducting a community health needs assessment every 3 years and adopting an implementation strategy that addresses identified needs.[52,53] Third, many communities are galvanized or required to implement community

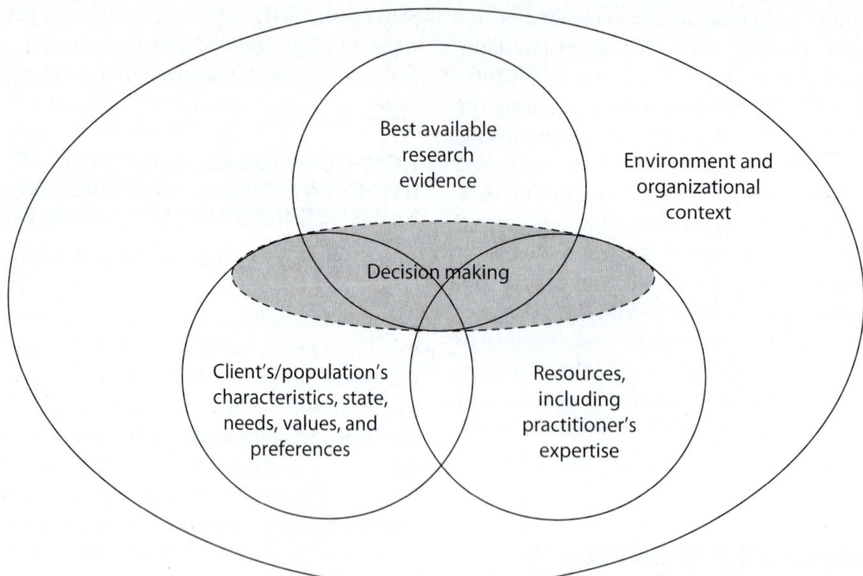

FIGURE 41-2. Transdisciplinary model of domains that influence evidence-based (also called evidence-informed) decision making Reproduced with Permission from Satterfield JM, Spring B, Brownson RC, et al. Toward a transdisciplinary model of evidence-based practice: A transdisciplinary model of evidence-based practice. Milbank Q. 2009;87(2):368-390..

interventions as a result of where they rank in comparison with other communities in the annual America's Health Rankings of states[54] or the annual U.S. County Health Rankings.[55] Fourth, many communities are encouraged or required to set public health goals in accordance with the U.S. national Healthy People initiative[56] or with state or local expectations, and they need to implement community interventions to achieve those goals. Fifth, policymakers and funders are typically requiring greater accountability, often specifically encouraging or requiring use of evidence-based interventions because of the likelihood that they will result in the intended outcome.[57–60]

A number of community health planning frameworks and models have been developed to assist health professionals and communities with these various types of community health improvement planning. Each of these planning models includes steps that involve identifying community needs and selecting and implementing interventions to meet those needs. Models and frameworks that can be used for a variety of purposes across a broad range of settings and situations include the PRECEDE—PROCEED Framework,[61] Intervention Mapping,[62] Community Health Assessment aNd Group Evaluation (CHANGE),[63] and Health Impact Assessments.[64] Models and frameworks specifically targeted to needs of health departments include State Health Improvement Planning (SHIP) Guidance and Resources[65] and Mobilizing for Action through Planning and Partnerships (MAPP).[66] Frameworks to assist charitable hospitals with their community benefit requirements include the Community Health Assessment Toolkit[67] and Assessing and Addressing Community Health Needs.[68] Finally, communities that are working to achieve Healthy People objectives may benefit from using Mobilize, Assess, Plan, Implement, and Track (MAP-IT).[69]

WHERE CAN I FIND INFORMATION ABOUT EVIDENCE-BASED COMMUNITY INTERVENTIONS?

Many individual researchers and research teams have published, and continue to publish, systematic reviews, meta-analyses, and narrative reviews of community interventions—often as part of building a body of work related to a specific topic or research question. A large number of these reviews are of high quality. Yet, completing a high-quality systematic review is very time consuming and requires special training, and most researchers typically only want to do reviews in their area of interest or responsibility. As a result, there are always more community interventions whose effectiveness needs to be evaluated than there are individual researchers that can do this work. Additionally, there are increasing expectations that reviews of community interventions be consistent with evolving international standards and that reviews include, or be combined with, information that maximizes their usefulness for nontechnical, "real-world" audiences (e.g., refs. 1, 39, 46, and 70–75). Moreover, all of this information needs to be relatively easy to locate for nontechnical, real-world audiences who are increasingly expected by funders and others to use evidence-based approaches (e.g., refs. 57–60). As a result, a number of organizations, agencies, and groups produce systematic reviews and meta-analyses and other related information. Additionally, other groups compile information from existing systematic reviews and other sources into clearinghouses or repositories. A number of the most prominent producers and compilers of evidence-based community interventions are discussed below.

Groups that Produce Systematic Reviews to Identify Evidence-Based Community Interventions

Major systematic review groups that include evidence-based community interventions are discussed below. These systematic review groups evaluate the effectiveness of community-based interventions to determine which are evidence-based. One of these systematic review groups is focused entirely on community interventions, whereas other groups include community interventions among the types of interventions that they assess. Given the many community interventions whose effectiveness needs to be assessed, a number of these groups actively seek to build on each other's work rather than to duplicate efforts. Many of the groups also collaborate on reviews and methods work. Relevant features of these groups are shown and compared in Table 41-1.[13–15,23,29,70,71,76–83]

The Guide to Community Preventive Services (The Community Guide)

The Community Guide[13] is entirely dedicated to evidence-based community interventions (Table 41-1). It consists of two principal components—(1) systematic reviews that assess all available evidence on the effectiveness of community interventions and (2) recommendations and other findings about the effectiveness of the community interventions, which are made by the Community Preventive Services Task Force (CPSTF) on the basis of the systematic reviews.[29,84] The CPSTF is a nonfederal, independent, nonpartisan panel of experts in public health research, practice, and policy, which was established

TABLE 41-1 FEATURES OF MAJOR SYSTEMATIC REVIEW GROUPS THAT IDENTIFY EVIDENCE-BASED COMMUNITY INTERVENTIONS

Systematic Review Group	Purpose	Subset of Included Topics that Contain Evidence-Based Community Interventions	Consideration of (1) Applicability, External Validity? (2) Implementation? (3) Economic Information? (4) Effects on Disparities, Health Equity?	Formal Recommendations About the Effectiveness of Community Interventions?
The Guide to Community Preventive Services (The Community Guide)	• Identify evidence-based community interventions for improving health and reducing disease, disability, and injury • Help communities select and implement interventions that meet their needs • Identify evidence gaps	All 22 public health topic areas related to • Prevention and control of diseases, disabilities and injuries • Improving risk factor status • Addressing health issues in particular settings • Addressing health equity and the social determinants of health	(1) Structured, systematic process to assess applicability (a) To different setting (b) To different population (c) With different intervention characteristics (e.g., dose, duration, deliverer) (2) Considerations for Implementation— (3) information gleaned from the literature and experience (4) Systematic Economic Reviews for community interventions with evidence of effectiveness, assessing (a) Cost (b) Cost effectiveness (c) Cost benefit, return on investment (5) Formal process for considering disparities and health equity for all reviews	Recommendations made by the statutorily mandated Community Preventive Services Task Force, with input from stakeholders • Recommend—strong evidence of effectiveness • Recommend—sufficient evidence of effectiveness • Insufficient evidence to recommend for or against • Recommend against—sufficient evidence of ineffectiveness or harm • Recommend against—strong evidence of ineffectiveness or harm
Cochrane	• Identify evidence-based interventions in healthcare by conducting SRs of the available evidence • Make the evidence accessible to user audiences	(a) Cochrane Public Health Review Group: 10 topic areas that aim to improve health and related outcomes at the population level by addressing the social, economic, and financial determinants of health (b) Other Cochrane topic-specific Review Groups: some reviews, mostly at the individual level	(1) Systematic, structured processes for examining the (a) Population (b) Intervention (2) Considered in many of the community intervention-relevant reviews (3) Considered in some of the community intervention-relevant reviews (4) Considered in many of the community intervention-relevant reviews	No
Campbell Collaboration	Identify and disseminate information about evidence-based interventions in social, behavioral, and educational areas	Some relevant views in the following Campbell focal areas: • Education • Crime and justice • Social welfare • Disability • Business and management • Knowledge translation and implementation • Nutrition • International development	(1) Often considered in many of the community intervention-relevant reviews (2) Considered in many of the community intervention-relevant reviews (3) Considered in some of the community intervention-relevant reviews (4) Considered in many of the community intervention-relevant reviews	No

National Institute for Health and Care Excellence (NICE)	Provide national (United Kingdom) guidance and advice to improve health and social care	• Conditions and diseases • Lifestyle and wellbeing • Population groups • Service delivery, organization and staffing • Settings	(1) Applicability to the (a) Question (b) People affected by the guideline (c) Setting (2) Considered in some of the community intervention-relevant reviews (3) Systematic economic review assessing (a) Cost utility (b) Cost-effectiveness (c) Cost consequences (d) Cost benefit (e) Cost minimization (4) Considered in most of the community intervention-relevant reviews	Recommendations developed by independent committees, including professionals and lay members, and consulted on by stakeholders for • Actions that must be taken • Actions that should be taken • Actions that could be taken • Actions that should not be taken
Washington State Institute for Public Policy (WSIPP)	Research public policy issues of interest to policymakers in the legislature and (Washington) state agencies	• Children's services • Criminal justice • Employment and welfare • Education • Health care • Mental health • Prevention • Substance abuse • Transportation	(1) Considered in some of the community intervention-relevant reviews (2) Considered in some of the community intervention-relevant reviews (3) Systematic economic reviews of benefit-cost/return on investment, also assess risk of investment (4) Considered in some of the community intervention-relevant reviews	No
HIV/AIDS Prevention Research Synthesis Project	Help Human Immunodeficiency Virus (HIV) prevention planners and providers in the United States to select interventions that are appropriate for their community	HIV prevention interventions in the following categories: • Structural interventions • Interventions supporting linkage to, retention in, and re-engagement in HIV care • Medication adherence interventions • Risk reduction interventions	(1) Considered in many of the community intervention-relevant reviews (2) Considered in some of the community intervention-relevant reviews (3) Considered in some of the community intervention-relevant reviews (4) Considered in many of the community intervention-relevant reviews	No

in 1996 and is statutorily mandated to make recommendations for a range of decision makers.[23] The U.S. Centers for Disease Control and Prevention (CDC) is mandated to provide support for the ongoing operations of the CPSTF.

To adequately understand the evidence as well as the needs of real-world practitioners and policymakers, each Community Guide systematic review is conducted by a team of systematic review methods and subject matter experts from governmental agencies, academia, and policy and practice settings. Community Guide reviews include research-based evidence as well as practice-based evidence.[43] In addition to evaluating overall effectiveness of a community intervention, all Community Guide systematic reviews also use a structured process to assess (a) whether the findings are applicable (i.e., external validity) to different settings and populations and (b) whether effectiveness differs with variations in the way the intervention is structured and delivered (e.g., dose and duration of the intervention and type of individual delivering the intervention). The reviews also consider potential harms and other benefits as well as whether the interventions could promote health equity. The CPSTF considers all of this information when making its recommendations.

To date, the CPSTF has issued more than 230 recommendations about effective community interventions and other findings (i.e., recommendations against ineffective or harmful community interventions and findings of insufficient evidence to recommend for or against an intervention) related to 22 public health topics. These topics include prevention and control of a wide range of diseases, disabilities, and injuries; improving risk factor status; addressing health issues in particular settings (such as the worksite or schools); and addressing health equity and social determinants of health. For all community interventions recommended by the CPSTF, the associated Community Guide systematic review identifies factors to consider when implementing the intervention. Additionally, since economic information is one of the main pieces of information sought by user audiences, a systematic economic review is conducted for many interventions that receive a Task Force recommendation of effectiveness. These systematic economic reviews look at cost, cost benefit and return on investment, and cost effectiveness.[71,76]

To facilitate public health planning, Community Guide topics are coordinated with the U.S. Healthy People[85] topic areas. Additionally, when an intervention relates to a Healthy People objective, this information is provided on the Community Guide website in the Considerations for Implementation section for that intervention, and Healthy People refers people to the intervention in The Community Guide.[39,86] The Community Guide website also provides a Crosswalk tool[87] to assist health departments that are seeking U.S. national accreditation. This Crosswalk identifies evidence-based interventions from The Community Guide whose implementation could help health departments to document conformity with Public Health Accreditation Board domains, standards, and measures.[88] Finally, the Community Guide website also notes when CPSTF-recommended community interventions support or extend the delivery of clinical interventions recommended by the U.S. Preventive Services Task Force[16] or increase the use of vaccines recommended by the Advisory Committee on Immunization Practices.[89]

Cochrane Reviews

A number of evidence-based community interventions are included in Cochrane (formerly known as the Cochrane Collaboration, Table 41-1). Cochrane is a nonprofit, nongovernmental organization formed in 1993 to identify evidence-based interventions in healthcare by conducting systematic reviews of the available evidence and undertaking various efforts to make the evidence accessible to user audiences.[77] A very large international network of thousands of researchers, clinicians, and others work to support the mission of Cochrane. Researchers and other contributors from more than 120 countries undertake systematic reviews for Cochrane, working under the auspices of Cochrane Review Groups that ensure the reviews are consistent with Cochrane methodologic standards and provide technical assistance. The protocols for Cochrane reviews, as well as the reviews themselves, are posted in the Cochrane Library, also known as the Cochrane Database of Systematic Reviews.[14]

Most of the systematic reviews of community interventions included in Cochrane have been conducted under the auspices of the Cochrane Public Health Review Group.[78] This Review group was registered in 2008, succeeding the Cochrane Health Promotion and Public Health Field, which functioned from 1996 through early 2008.[90,91] The Cochrane Public Health Review Group focuses on interventions that aim to improve health and related outcomes at the population level by addressing the social, economic, and financial determinants of health.[79] The intent is that the reviews will also contribute to strengthening health equity. The Cochrane Public Health Review Group classifies its reviews into ten areas: (1) income distribution and financial interventions, (2) education, (3) public safety, (4) housing and the built environment, (5) employment and the work environment, (6) social networks and support, (7) food supply and access, (8) transport, active transport, and physical activity, (9) the natural environment, and (10) systems for health. At the time of writing, 27 reviews had been completed through the Cochrane Public Health Review Group, and 30 additional review protocols had been registered. To facilitate careful consideration of how interventions might perform in different settings and with different populations, Cochrane reviews employ the PICO(T) framework, looking carefully at the population, intervention, comparator, outcomes, and study design.[70]

Other community interventions included in the Cochrane Library are evaluated by topic-specific Cochrane Review Groups. This is most common among Review Groups that include health promotion among their foci. Most of the community interventions within topic-specific Cochrane Review Groups are at the level of the individual (the first level of the socioecological framework).[7]

The Campbell Collaboration

The Campbell Collaboration is a nonprofit, nongovernmental organization that aims to identify and disseminate information about evidence-based interventions in social, behavioral, and educational areas (Table 41-1).[80] Created in 2000, the Campbell Collaboration is a sister organization to Cochrane. Similar to Cochrane, investigators from many countries around the world conduct systematic reviews for Campbell. Investigators work under the auspices of the Campbell Collaboration's Coordinating Groups, which provide technical assistance and ensure that the systematic reviews meet Campbell's methodologic standards. The protocols for Campbell reviews, and the reviews themselves, are posted in the Campbell Library.[81]

Systematic reviews of community interventions with relevance for public health are undertaken by investigators associated with most of the areas of emphasis for the Campbell Collaboration including education, crime and justice, social welfare, disability, business and management, knowledge translation and implementation, nutrition, and international development. Many of these reviews are specifically relevant to supporting evidence-informed policymaking.

National Institute for Health and Care Excellence

The United Kingdom's (UK) National Institute for Health and Care Excellence (NICE) provides guidance and advice to improve health and social care through conducting systematic reviews and technology assessments, making evidence-based guidelines and recommendations, and helping to ensure that health and social care professionals have easy and quick access to reliable information (Table 41-1).[15] NICE was originally established in 1999 to examine how to reduce variation in the quality and availability of care and treatments provided through the UK's National Health Service. Early on, its scope expanded to also include public health, and, in 2013, it was statutorily mandated to also develop guidance for social care.

NICE operates independently of government but is accountable to the UK Department of Health and Social Care. NICE currently has over 70 guidelines in the areas of public health and social care.

Washington State Institute for Public Policy

The Washington State Institute for Public Policy (WSIPP) was created in 1983 by the legislature of the U.S. State of Washington to research public policy issues of interest to policymakers in the legislature and state agencies (Table 41-1).[82] The research typically consists of systematic reviews of the effectiveness or cost-benefit of various policy-relevant topics. The institute is nonpartisan and typically conducts its systematic reviews in response to specific questions from the legislature. WSIPP reports have identified evidence-based community interventions in the areas of children's services, criminal justice, employment and welfare, education, healthcare, mental health, prevention, substance abuse, and transportation.

Prevention Research Synthesis Project

The Prevention Research Synthesis (PRS) Project, developed by the U.S. CDC, aims to help Human Immunodeficiency Virus (HIV) prevention planners and providers in the United States to select interventions that are appropriate for their community (Table 41-2).[83] It does this by conducting systematic reviews to identify evidence-based interventions (EBIs) and best practices for (HIV) prevention. In addition to publishing its reviews, the resulting EBIs are listed in their Compendium of Evidence-Based Interventions and Best Practices for HIV Prevention.[92] The compendium classifies interventions into the following groups: structural interventions; interventions supporting linkage to, retention in, and re-engagement in HIV care; medication adherence interventions; and risk-reduction interventions.

Repositories and Clearinghouses of Evidence-Based Community Interventions

Compilers of evidence-based community interventions include clearinghouses and repositories of information about community interventions. Some of these databases are focused solely on interventions that have been assessed using systematic reviews and meta-analyses (highest quality evidence) while others also include interventions that fall into the equivalent of emerging, promising, or leading practices categories. Some of these compilers do extensive searches of the literature for reviews relevant to their purposes and identify reviews that are produced by individual groups of researchers as well as reviews completed under the auspices of major systematic review groups. With the increased focus on using evidence and addressing the social determinants of health, the number of repositories and clearinghouses is growing. Some of the most prominent repositories and clearinghouses are described below. Some of these repositories and clearinghouses themselves include, or consist entirely of, other repositories and clearinghouses. Relevant features of these repositories and clearinghouses are shown and compared in Table 41-2.[39,75,85,93-100]

Health Evidence

Health Evidence is a repository of systematic reviews of the effectiveness of public health interventions in the areas of prevention, health protection, and health promotion (Table 41-2).[93] Established in 2005, Health Evidence searches seven electronic databases and also performs hand searches of the Cochrane library and other evidence services to identify relevant systematic reviews, meta-analyses, and metasyntheses (i.e., syntheses of multiple systematic reviews or meta-analyses).[94] All seven of the databases have been searched from 1995 to present and searches are updated monthly. Each systematic review and meta-analysis included in the repository undergoes a formal quality assessment and this information is provided to users alongside the review. Health Evidence includes a large number of systematic reviews of community interventions. Health Evidence also contains information and tools to help the public health workforce and policymakers search for reviews. The site also includes a checklist and other products to help people work through the various steps of an evidence-informed decision-making process.

What Works for Health—County Health Rankings and Roadmaps

County Health Rankings and Roadmaps (CHR&R)[55] ranks all counties in the United States annually on a range of factors that relate to and can influence health. The annual rankings are intended to catalyze change in communities.[101] To support such change, CHR&R also includes a Roadmaps component, which consists of guidance and tools to help communities take action and determine who to partner with, as well as What Works for Health—a database of evidence-informed programs and policies that communities can use to bring about change (Table 41-2).[95] What Works for Health includes programs and policies related to the four groupings of factors used by CHR&R for the county rankings—namely, health behaviors, clinical care, social and economic factors, and the physical environment. Each intervention is assigned an evidence rating of scientifically supported, some evidence, expert opinion, insufficient evidence, mixed evidence, or evidence of ineffectiveness. Interventions are also assessed in terms of their likely effect on racial/ethnic, socioeconomic, geographic, or other disparities.

Results First Clearinghouse Database

The Results First Clearinghouse Database[96] aims to help policymakers at all levels of government identify evidence-based programs and use this information to make data-driven budget decisions (Table 41-2).[75] The Database includes information from nine national research clearinghouses that address the areas of child welfare, juvenile justice, criminal justice, social policy and programs, education, substance abuse, health, and mental health. For each intervention, the Database uses the ratings established by the individual clearinghouse and assigns the intervention a color from the Results-First color coding system, which attempts to create a common language between the individual rating systems. This allows policymakers to readily see where the intervention falls on a spectrum of five levels from highest rated (green) to second highest rated (yellow) to mixed effects (blue) to no effects (gray) to negative effects (red). Interventions can also be given an insufficient evidence classification, which has no corresponding color, and indicates there is currently not enough evidence to determine impact. Results First also works with policymakers in many states to support their use of evidence-based policymaking.[59]

Healthy People Evidence-Based Resources

Healthy People,[85] an initiative of the U.S. Office of Disease Prevention and Health Promotion, has provided science-based 10-year goals and objectives for each decade since 1990 to galvanize people at federal, state, and local levels to improve the health of Americans. For the Healthy People 2020 cycle, a database of Evidence-Based Resources[97] was added to assist people in identifying strategies they could use to attain specific Healthy People goals and objectives (Table 41-2). Included interventions cover the full spectrum of Healthy People. Each intervention is assigned a rating of 1–4 based on the strength of the evidence, considering all of effectiveness, feasibility, reach, sustainability, and transferability.[39,40] As previously described, a crosswalk exists between Healthy People and The Community Guide whereby the Healthy People Evidence-Based Resources database identifies interventions determined to be effective by the Community Preventive Services Task Force, and the Community Guide website identifies which Healthy People goals and objectives relate to a particular community intervention in the Considerations for Implementation section for that intervention.

Research-Tested Intervention Programs

The U.S. National Cancer Institute aims to assist program planners and public health practitioners through its Cancer Control P.L.A.N.E.T.—Plan, Link, Act, Network with Evidence-based Tools[102] and the associated Research-Tested Intervention Programs (RTIPs)—a searchable database of evidence-based cancer control and cancer survivorship

TABLE 41-2 FEATURES OF REPOSITORIES AND CLEARINGHOUSES THAT IDENTIFY EVIDENCE-BASED COMMUNITY INTERVENTIONS

Repository or Clearinghouse[a]	Purpose	Subset of Included Topics Relevant to Evidence-Based Community Interventions	Sources of Relevant Systematic Reviews Included in the Repository or Clearinghouse	Sources of Other Relevant Evidence Included—Emerging, Promising, Leading Practices; Individual Studies	Ratings of the Evidence? (1) Assessment of the Quality of Included Evidence? (2) Other Formal Ratings or Recommendations?
Health Evidence	Help public health find and use best evidence in practice	27 topics related to diseases, disabilities, and injuries including • Risk factors • Life stages • Specific settings • Social determinants of health	• Electronic search of seven bibliographic databases • Hand search of Cochrane Library and various evidence sources	Not included	(1) Quality Assessment Tool (a) Strong (total score 8–10) (b) Moderate (total 5–7) (c) Weak (total 4 or less) (2) High-level syntheses, with recommendations, for topics with numerous reviews
What Works for Health—County Health Rankings and Roadmaps	Identify policies and programs that are a good fit for a community's priorities, especially after they review their county's health rankings	• Health behaviors • Clinical care • Social and economic factors • Physical environment	• Systematic reviews from four relevant sources considered as gold standard evidence: • The Community Guide • Cochrane • Campbell Collaboration • Health Evidence • Systematic reviews that are included in one or more other repositories and clearinghouses from which What Works for Health compiles evidence (see next column)	• Evidence from other repositories and clearinghouses from governmental and private organizations that assess programs and policies and assign their own ratings: • Best Evidence Encyclopedia • Blueprints for Healthy Youth Development • The California Evidence-Based Clearinghouse for Child Welfare (CEBC) • Public Health Law Research (PHLR) • What Works Clearinghouse • Youth.gov • Individual studies from the published and grey literature	(1) Evidence ratings of (a) Scientifically supported (b) Some evidence (c) Expert opinion (d) Insufficient evidence (e) Mixed evidence (f) Evidence of ineffectiveness (2) Likely effect on disparities (a) Racial/ethnic (b) Socioeconomic (c) Geographic (d) Other
Results First Clearinghouse Database	Help policymakers at all levels of government identify evidence-based programs and use this information to make data-driven budget decisions	• Crime and delinquency • Child and family well-being • Education • Employment and job training • Mental health • Public health • Sexual behavior and teen pregnancy • Substance use	• Systematic reviews that are included in one or more of the nine national repositories and clearinghouses from which Results First compiles its evidence (see next column)	• Evidence from nine national repositories and clearinghouses that assess programs and policies and assign their own ratings including • Blueprints for Healthy Youth Development (Blueprints) • California Evidence-Based Clearinghouse for Child Welfare (CEBC) • CrimeSolutions.gov • Substance Abuse and Mental Health Services Administration's National Registry of Evidence-based Programs and Practices (NREPP) • Research-Tested Intervention Programs (RTIPs) • Social Programs That Work • Teen Pregnancy Prevention (TPP) Evidence Review • What Works for Health • U.S. Department of Education's What Works Clearinghouse (WWC)	(1) Applies color-coding to the clearinghouses' individual rating systems, aiming to create a common language (a) Highest rated (b) Second-highest rated (includes promising practices) (c) Mixed effects (d) No effects (e) Negative effects (f) Insufficient evidence (includes RTIPs' ratings of 2.9 and below and What Works for Health's "expert opinion") (2) No

Healthy People Evidence-Based Resources	Provide evidence-based resources that can help meet Healthy People's 10-year national objectives for improving the health of all Americans	Many of the Healthy People Topics that are used to categorize the national objectives for improving the health of Americans—42 topics for Healthy People 2020	• Systematic reviews from relevant sources considered as gold standard evidence including • The Community Guide • Cochrane • Other relevant systematic reviews identified by subject matter experts	Other evidence identified by subject matter experts associated with each Healthy People Topic area	(1) Evidence ratings of (a) Proven (The Community Guide, Cochrane, or similar authoritative group) (b) Likely Effective (c) Promising (d) Emerging (2) No
Research-Tested Intervention Programs (RTIPS)	Provide a searchable database of evidence-based cancer control intervention programs and program materials so program planners and practitioners have ready access to research-tested materials	• Cancer Screening • Breast • Cervical • Colorectal • Prostate • Diet/Nutrition • HPV Vaccination • Informed Decision Making • Obesity • Physical Activity • Public Health Genomics • Sun Safety • Tobacco Control	• Does not directly include systematic reviews • RTIPS programs that relate to systematic reviews from The Community Guide and other major systematic reviews groups are identified as such	• Database includes cancer control programs that are tested in one or more research studies, and that have program materials available for use by others • Voluntary; programs may request to be considered for inclusion and must meet eligibility criteria	(1) Rating System for interventions and program materials (a) Research Integrity (based on scientific rigor) (b) Intervention Impact (both Population Reach and Effect Sizes) (c) Dissemination Capability (d) RE-AIM framework (i) Reach (ii) Effectiveness or efficacy (iii) Adoption (iv) Implementation consistency, costs, and adaptations (v) Maintenance (2) No
Evidence-Based Practices Resource Center—Substance Abuse and Mental Health Services Administration (SAMHSA)	Provide communities, policymakers, clinicians, and others with information and tools to help them incorporate evidence-based practices in their community or clinical setting	Substance abuse prevention, treatment, and recovery practices	• Provides links to systematic review groups including • The Community Guide • Prevention Research Synthesis Project • Systematic reviews that are included in one or more other repositories and clearinghouses from which the Evidence-Based Practices Resource Center compiles evidence (see next column)	• Evidence from other repositories and clearinghouses from governmental and private organizations including • Prevention Research Synthesis Project • Blueprints for Healthy Youth Development • Suicide Prevention Resource Center • Social Programs that Work • CrimeSolutions.gov • Program Directory Search at Youth.gov • Model Programs Guide at the Office of Juvenile Justice and Delinquency Prevention • RTIPS • Teen Pregnancy Prevention Evidence Review • What Works Clearinghouse • Evidence-Based Practices for Substance Use Disorders	(1) Not by the Resource Center itself, although quality may be assessed by the systematic review groups and repositories that are included in the Resource Center (2) No

[a]As shown across the columns, many of the repositories and clearinghouses themselves include other repositories and clearinghouses.

programs (Table 41-2).[98] RTIPS identifies high-quality programs that are specific examples of the type of evidence-based community interventions included in The Community Guide and other systematic reviews, or that are otherwise deemed to be of adequate quality to be included. RTIPs are a voluntary system and candidate programs must meet certain criteria to be considered. Eligible programs are reviewed and rated on research integrity, intervention impact, dissemination capability, and components of the RE-AIM Framework (i.e., reach, effectiveness, adoption, implementation, and maintenance).[99] Also available for each included program are program materials developed by the researchers. This information can help users to figure out how to adapt the intervention for use in their specific setting and may provide specific instructions for developing and implementing the intervention. When a program included in RTIPS is a specific instance of an intervention that is recommended by the CPSTF and included in The Community Guide, this is noted on both the RTIPS and Community Guide websites.

Substance Abuse and Mental Health Services Administration—Evidence-Based Practices Resource Center

The U.S. Substance Abuse and Mental Health Services Administration (SAMHSA) has established an Evidence-Based Practices Resource Center[100] to provide communities, policymakers, clinicians, and others with tools and information that can help them incorporate evidence-based substance abuse prevention, treatment, and recovery practices in their community or clinical setting (Table 41-2). The Center includes resources such as systematic evidence reviews, summaries of systematic reviews, clinical practice guidelines, consensus guidelines, toolkits, resource guides, and treatment improvement protocols. SAMHSA's Center for the Application of Prevention Technologies (CAPT)[103]—a companion initiative—provides training and technical assistance focused on strengthening substance abuse prevention systems and the behavioral health workforce. Although CAPT's first responsibility is to support SAMHSA-funded grantees, CAPT materials, models, and tools are also available for use by others at local, regional, and state levels. CAPT helps users implement a prevention planning process that involves incorporating data in strategic planning, selecting and implementing evidence-based community interventions, and collaborating with behavioral health providers. CAPT also provides professional development for the behavioral health workforce.

HOW CAN I SELECT FROM AMONG THE AVAILABLE SOURCES OF EVIDENCE-BASED COMMUNITY INTERVENTIONS?

A number of the issues discussed in this chapter can serve as a checklist of questions that potential users can ask to help them decide which sources might include evidence-based community interventions that could be useful for their particular setting, population, and situation, and how much confidence they can have that they will achieve similar outcomes. Each question below is accompanied by a short discussion. More detail on each issue is provided earlier in this chapter and in Tables 41-1 and 41-2.

Does the Source Contain Community Interventions That Are Related to My Specific Area of Interest?

Some systematic review groups and repositories are topic-specific while others cover a range of topics. Both types can be perused to see if they include many, a few, or no evidence-based community interventions that could be used to address a specific issue if interest. Importantly, some of the repositories stipulate that they do not necessarily include all of the evidence-based community interventions that are available from the underlying systematic review groups and repositories from which they select interventions, and they recommend that users go directly to the underlying source if they cannot find the type of intervention for which they are searching.

Does the Source Assess the Quality of the Evidence about the Effectiveness of the Community Intervention?

All systematic review groups discussed in this chapter and in Table 41-1 assess the quality of the existing evidence about community interventions as a fundamental part of their methods. In comparison, the repositories and clearinghouses differ with respect to whether and how they address the quality of the underlying evidence (Table 41-2). Some perform their own assessments of the quality of the underlying evidence; some refer users to quality assessments produced by the underlying sources of evidence included in the repository; and others do not specifically discuss the quality of the evidence. Potential users can have greater confidence that the community intervention will lead to the intended outcome as the quality of the studies showing its effectiveness increase.[29–31,36,37]

Does the Source Assess the Strength of the Evidence for the Effectiveness of the Community Intervention?

All of the systematic review groups discussed in this chapter and shown in Table 41-1 assess the strength of the evidence for the effectiveness of community interventions. Community interventions that are identified as evidence-based by such systematic review groups are typically considered to have the strongest evidence of effectiveness. In comparison, many of the repositories and clearinghouses discussed in this chapter and shown in Table 41-2 rate the community interventions that they include on an evidence continuum, with those identified through systematic reviews being labeled as the highest rated or strongest evidence, or as best practices. Some repositories and clearinghouses leave it to users to locate evidence about the strength of the evidence. In general, the stronger the evidence for a community intervention, the more confidence users can have that the intervention will be effective in new situations that are similar to those that were studied.[29–31]

Does the Source Permit the Inclusion of Evidence from a Range of Study Designs?

When the effectiveness of a community intervention cannot be assessed using RCTs, or RCTs do not enable adequate assessment of external validity, the use of other study designs may be particularly beneficial. Yet, when different study designs are used, assessments of the quality and strength of the evidence become even more important—to ensure consideration of biases that might not be able to be accounted for with certain study designs and to see how different studies taken together may provide more complete information.[1,27–29] Most of the sources of evidence discussed in this chapter include a range of study designs so this may be more of an issue when considering other sources, and individual systematic reviews.

Does the Source Assess Applicability to Different Settings, Populations, and Situations?

Users can gain greater confidence that a community intervention will be effective for their specific population, setting, and situation if the systematic review group or repository indicates that the intervention was found to be effective across a range of populations, settings, and situations.[1,27,28] Most of the systematic review groups discussed in this chapter and included in Table 41-1 provide information on whether the community intervention has been found to be effective in different settings and populations, and some also specifically highlight what happens to effectiveness when the intervention is delivered in different ways by different deliverers. Some of the repositories and clearinghouses specifically include this information (Table 41-2).

CONCLUSION

Subsequent to earlier calls to increase the evidence base for community health,[104,105] the number of community interventions identified as evidence-based has increased substantially in recent years. Evidence-based community interventions play a critical role in improving health and wellness, reducing health disparities, addressing the social determinants of health, and supporting health equity in the communities where people live, work, learn, worship, and play. Information about evidence-based community interventions serves as an important input into evidence-based (or evidence-informed) decision making, thereby enabling health professionals and communities to consider robust information about effective community interventions alongside information about their organizational and environmental context, available resources, and population needs and preferences in order to identify what will work best for their community. They also support community health improvement planning at federal, state and provincial, and local levels in support of many public health initiatives including public health department accreditation, U.S. charitable hospital community benefit requirements, state and county health rankings, strategic planning around Healthy People and other goal-setting initiatives, and responding to funding announcements that require use of evidence-based approaches.

Areas deserving of future work related to evidence-based community interventions include identifying more effective interventions across more areas of public health, strengthening practice-based evidence to increase its inclusion in systematic reviews, encouraging evaluation and further refinement of emerging and promising community interventions, increasing practitioner and policymaker skills around evidence-based decision making, and strengthening implementation of evidence-based community interventions.

References

1. Brownson RC, Baker EA, Leet TL, Gillespie KN, True WR. *Evidence-Based Public Health*. 2nd ed. New York: Oxford University Press; 2011.
2. Willis CL. Definitions of community, II: An examination of definitions of community since 1950. *South Sociologist*. 1977;9:14–19.
3. Goodman RA, Bunnell R, Posner SF. What is "community health"? Examining the meaning of an evolving field in public health. *Prev Med*. 2014; 67(Suppl 1):S58–61.
4. Green LW, Mercer SL. Participatory research: Can public health researchers and agencies bridge the push from funding agencies and the pull from communities? *Am J Public Health*. 2001;19(12):1926–9.
5. MacQueen KM, McClellan E, Metzger DS, et al. What is community? An evidence-based definition for participatory public health. *Am J Public Health*. 2001;91(12):1929–38.
6. Merriam-Webster Dictionary: Merriam-Webster, Incorporated. 2018. https://www.merriam-webster.com/dictionary/intervention. Accessed April 21, 2018.
7. McLeroy, KR, Bibeau D, Steckler A, Glanz K. An ecological perspective on health promotion programs. *Health Educ Q*. 1988;15(4):351–77.
8. Sallis JF, Owen N, Fisher EB. Ecological models of health behavior In: Glanz K, Rimer BK, Viswanath K, eds. *Health Behavior and Health Education: Theory, Research, and Practice*. 4th ed. San Francisco, CA: Jossey-Bass; 2008, pp. 465–85.
9. Golden SD, Earp JL. Social ecological approaches to individuals and their contexts: Twenty years of health education and behavior health promotion interventions. *Health Educ Behav*. 2012;39(3):364–72.
10. Glanz K, Rimer BK, Viswanath K, eds. *Health Behavior and Health Education: Theory, Research, and Practice*. 5th ed. San Francisco, CA: Jossey-Bass; 2015.
11. The Community Guide: Physical Activity: Built Environment Approaches Combining Transportation System Interventions with Land Use and Environmental Design. 2016. https://www.thecommunityguide.org/findings/physical-activity-built-environment-approaches. Accessed July 22, 2016.
12. The Community Guide: Skin Cancer: Child Care Center-Based Interventions. 2013. https://www.thecommunityguide.org/findings/skin-cancer-child-care-center-based-interventions. Accessed July 22, 2018.
13. The Community Guide. https://www.thecommunityguide.org. Accessed May 28, 2018.
14. Cochrane Library. https://www.cochranelibrary.com/. Accessed August 19, 2018.
15. NICE—National Institute for Health and Care Excellence. https://www.nice.org.uk/. Accessed August 19, 2018.
16. U.S. Preventive Services Task Force. https://www.uspreventiveservicestaskforce.org/. Accessed January 15, 2019.
17. Marmot M, Commission on social determinants of health: Achieving health equity: From root causes to fair outcomes. *Lancet*. 2007;370(9593):1153–63.
18. World Health Organization: What are social determinants of health? 2018. http://www.who.int/social_determinants/sdh_definition/en/. Accessed August 3, 2018.
19. Community Preventive Services Task Force: Health Equity: High School Completion Programs. 2013. https://www.thecommunityguide.org/findings/health-equity-high-school-completion-programs. Accessed August 3, 2018.
20. Wilson SJ, Tanner-Smith EE, Lipsey MW, Steinka-Fry K, Morrison J. Dropout prevention and intervention programs: Effects on school completion and dropout among school-aged children and youth. *Campbell Syst Rev*. 2011. http://campbellcollaboration.org/lib/project/158/. Accessed August 3, 2018.
21. Braveman P. Health disparities and health equity: Concepts and measurement. *Annu Rev Public Health*. 2006;27:167–94.
22. Williams DR, Costa MV, Odunlami AO, Mohammed SA. Moving upstream: How interventions that address the social determinants of health can improve health and reduce disparities. *J Public Health Manag Pract*. 2008;14(Suppl):S8–17.
23. Community Preventive Services Task Force: Guiding Community Health Outcomes through Evidence: 2014–2015 Annual Report to Congress, Federal Agencies and Prevention Stakeholders, including a Special Update on Recommendations to Prevent Cancers. 2015. https://www.thecommunityguide.org/sites/default/files/assets/2015-congress-report-full_0.pdf. Accessed June 3, 2018.
24. Kindig D, Stoddart G. What is population health? *Am J Public Health*. 2003;93(3):380–3.
25. Brownson RC, Fielding JE, Maylahn CM. Evidence-based public health: A fundamental concept for public health practice. *Annu Rev Public Health*. 2009;30:175–201.
26. Chambers D, Kerner J. Closing the gap between discovery and delivery. Dissemination and Implementation Research Workshop: Harnessing Science to Maximize Health. Rockville, MD, May 26, 2007. https://cancercontrol.cancer.gov/IS/pdfs/DIPAROrientWebPosting082806.pdf. Accessed May 29, 1918.
27. Mercer SL, DeVinney BJ, Fine LJ, Green LW, Dougherty D. Study designs for effectiveness and translation research: Identifying trade-offs. *Am J Prev Med*. 2007;33(2):139–54.
28. Shadish W, Cook T, Campbell D. *Experimental and Quasi-Experimental Designs for Generalized Causal Inference*. Boston, MA: Houghton Mifflin; 2002.
29. Briss PA, Zaza S, Pappaioanou M, et al. Developing an evidence-based Guide to Community Preventive Services—Methods. *Am J Prev Med*. 2000;18(Suppl 1):35–43.
30. Cooper H, Hedges LV, Valentine JC, edsCooper H, Hedges LV, Valentine JC, eds. *The Handbook of Research Synthesis and Meta Analysis*. 2nd ed. New York: Russell Sage Foundation; 2009.
31. Higgins J, Green S. *Cochrane Handbook for Systematic Reviews of Interventions*. Version 5.1. 2011. https://training.cochrane.org/handbook. Accessed July 29, 2018.
32. Deeks JJ, Higgins JPT, Altman DG. Cochrane Statistical Methods Group: Analysing data and undertaking meta-analyses. In: Cooper H, Hedges LV, Valentine JC, eds. *The Handbook of Research Synthesis and Meta Analysis*. 2nd ed. New York: Russell Sage Foundation; 2009.
33. Haidich AB. Meta-analysis in medical research. *Hippokratia*. 2010;14(Suppl 1):29–37.
34. Greenhalgh T, Robert G, Macfarlane F, Bate P, Kyriakidouc O, Peacock R. Storylines of research in diffusion of innovation: A meta-narrative approach to systematic review. *Soc Sci Med*. 2005;61(2):417–30.
35. Greenhalgh T, Thorne S, Malterud K. Time to challenge the spurious hierarchy of systematic over narrative reviews? *Eur J Clin Invest*. 2018;48:e12931.
36. Des Jarlais D, Lyles C, Crepaz N, The TREND Group. Improving the reporting quality of nonrandomized evaluations: The TREND statement. *Am J Public Health*. 2004;94(3):361–6.
37. Woolf SH, George JN. Evidence-based medicine: Interpreting studies and setting policy. *Hematol Oncol Clin North Am*. 2000;14(4):761–84.
38. Brennan L, Castro S, Brownson RC, Claus J, Orleans CT. Accelerating evidence reviews and broadening evidence standards to identify effective, promising, and emerging policy and environmental strategies for prevention of childhood obesity. *Annu Rev Public Health*. 2011;32:199–223.
39. Secretary's Advisory Committee on National Health Promotion and Disease Prevention Objectives for 2020: Evidence-based clinical and

public health: Generating and applying the evidence. Washington, DC: U.S. Department of Health and Human Services. 2010. https://www.healthypeople.gov/sites/default/files/EvidenceBasedClinicalPH2010.pdf. Accessed August 18, 2018.

40. Spencer LM, Schooley MW, Anderson LA, et al. Seeking best practices: A conceptual framework for planning and improving evidence-based practices. *Prev Chronic Dis.* 2013;10:E207.
41. Patton MQ. *Utilization-Focused Evaluation: The New Century Text.* Thousand Oaks, CA: Sage; 1997.
42. Wholey JS. Evaluability assessment. In: Wholey JS, Hatry HP, Newcomer KE, eds. *Handbook of Practical Program Evaluation.* San Francisco, CA: Jossey-Bass; 2004, pp. 33–62.
43. Vaidya N, Thota AB, Proia KK, et al. Practice-based evidence in Community Guide systematic reviews. *Am J Public Health.* 2017;107(3):413–20.
44. Culyer AJ, Lomas J. Deliberative processes and evidence-informed decision making in healthcare: Do they work and how might we know? *Evid Policy.* 2006;2(3):357–71.
45. Kohatsu ND, Robinson JG, Torner JC. Evidence-based public health: An evolving concept. *Am J Prev Med.* 2004;27(5):417–21.
46. Ciliska D, Thomas H, Buffett C. An Introduction to Evidence-Informed Public Health and a Compendium of Critical Appraisal Tools for Public Health Practice. National Collaborative Center for Methods and Tools. https://www.nccmt.ca/uploads/media/media/0001/01/b331668f85b-c6357f262944f0aca38c14c89c5a4.pdf. 2008 (links revised and updated in 2010). Accessed July 29, 2018.
47. Jacobs JA, Clayton PF, Dove C, et al. A survey tool for measuring evidence-based decision-making capacity in public health agencies. *BMC Health Serv Res.* 2012:12:57.
48. National Collaborating Centre for Methods and Tools: A Model for Evidence-Informed Decision Making in Public Health. https://www.nccmt.ca/about/eiph. Accessed July 30, 2018.
49. Satterfield JM, Spring B, Brownson RC, et al. Toward a transdisciplinary model of evidence-based practice. *Milbank Q.* 2009;87(2):368–90.
50. Public Health Accreditation Board: What is Public Health Department Accreditation? https://www.phaboard.org/what-is-public-health-department-accreditation/. Accessed January 16, 2019.
51. Public Health Accreditation Board: Guide to National Public Health Department Initial Accreditation. June 2015. https://www.phaboard.org/wp-content/uploads/2018/11/Guide-to-Accreditation-final_LR2.pdf. Accessed January 16, 2019.
52. Internal Revenue Service: Additional Requirements for Charitable Hospitals; Community Health Needs Assessments for Charitable Hospitals; Requirement of a Section 4959 Excise Tax Return and Time for Filing the Return: 2015 Addendum. https://www.irs.gov/irb/2015-05_IRB#TD-9708. February 2, 2015. Accessed January 15, 2019.
53. Rubin DB, Singh SR, Young GJ. Tax-exempt hospitals and community benefit: New directions in policy and practice. *Annu Rev Public Health.* 2015;36:545–57.
54. United Health Foundation: America's Health Rankings. https://www.americashealthrankings.org/. 2018. Accessed May 28, 2018.
55. County Health Rankings and Roadmaps. http://www.countyhealthrankings.org/. 2018. Accessed January 15, 2019.
56. Office of Disease Prevention and Health Promotion: About Healthy People. https://www.healthypeople.gov/node/5840. Accessed August 19, 2018.
57. Bipartisan Policy Center: A Prevention Prescription for Improving Health and Health Care in America. https://bipartisanpolicy.org/wp-content/uploads/2017/01/BPC-Prevention-Prescription-Report.pdf. Washington, DC, May 2015. Accessed August 1, 2018.
58. Commission on Evidence-Based Policymaking: The Promise of Evidence-Based Policymaking. September 2017. https://www.cep.gov/content/dam/cep/report/cep-final-report.pdf. Accessed August 1, 2018.
59. Pew-MacArthur Results First Initiative: Evidence-Based Policymaking: A Guide for Effective Government. Pew-MacArthur Results First Initiative, November 2014. http://www.pewtrusts.org/-/media/assets/2014/11/evidencebasedpolicymakingaguideforeffectivegovernment.pdf. Accessed June 21, 2018.
60. Results for America: A 2016 Policy Playbook—Invest in What Works: How to Solve Our Nation's Great Challenges. Results for America Invest in What Works Policy Series, March 2015. http://results4america.org/wp-content/uploads/2015/03/2015-3-26-2016-Policy-Playbook-FINAL.pdf. Accessed August 1, 2018.
61. Green LW, Kreuter MW. *Health Program Planning—An Educational and Ecological Approach.* 4th ed. Boston, MA: McGraw Hill; 2005.
62. Bartholomew LK, Parcel GS, Kok G, Gottleib NH, Fernandez ME. *Planning Health Promotion Programs: An Intervention Mapping Approach.* 3rd ed. San Francisco, CA: Jossey-Bass; 2011.
63. Centers for Disease Control and Prevention: Community Health Assessment aNd Group Evaluation (CHANGE) Action Guide: Building a Foundation of Knowledge to Prioritize Community Needs. U.S. Department of Health and Human Services, Atlanta, GA. 2010. https://www.cdc.gov/nccdphp/dch/programs/healthycommunitiesprogram/tools/change/pdf/changeactionguide.pdf. Accessed June 15, 2018.
64. Dannenberg AL, Bhatia R, Cole BL, et al. Growing the field of health impact assessment in the United States: An agenda for research and practice. *Am J Public Health.* 2006;96(2):262–70.
65. Association of State and Territorial Health Officials: Developing a State Health Improvement Plan: Guidance and Resources. June 2015. http://www.astho.org/Accreditation-and-Performance/Developing-a-State-Health-Improvement-Plan-Guidance-and-Resources/Home/. Accessed August 19, 2018.
66. National Association of City and County Health Officials: Mobilizing for Action through Planning and Partnerships (MAPP). https://www.naccho.org/programs/public-health-infrastructure/performance-improvement/community-health-assessment/mapp. Accessed August 19, 2018.
67. Association for Community Health Improvement: Community Health Assessment Toolkit. 2017. www.healthycommunities.org/assesstoolkit. Accessed August 19, 2018.
68. Catholic Health Association of the United States: Assessing and Addressing Community Health Needs. 2015. https://www.chausa.org/communitybenefit/assessing-and-addressing-community-health-needs. Accessed August 19, 2018.
69. Office of Disease Prevention and Health Promotion: Healthy People 2020 Program Planning. https://www.healthypeople.gov/2020/tools-and-resources/Program-Planning. Accessed August 19, 2018.
70. Armstrong R, Hall BJ, Doyle J, Waters E. 'Scoping the scope' of a Cochrane review. *J Public Health.* 2011;33(1):147–50.
71. Chattopadhyay SK, Jacob V, Mercer SL, et al. Community Guide cardiovascular disease economic reviews: Tailoring methods to ensure utility of findings. *Am J Prev Med.* 2017;53(6)(Suppl 2):S155–63.
72. Glasgow RE, Lichtenstein E, Marcus AC. Why don't we see more translation of health promotion research to practice? Rethinking the efficacy-to-effectiveness transition. *Am J Public Health.* 2003;93(8):1261–7.
73. Green LW, Glasgow RE, Atkins D, Stange K. Making evidence from research more relevant, useful, and actionable in policy, program planning, and practice: Slips "twixt cup and lip." *Am J Prev Med.* 2009;37(6)(Suppl 1):S187–91.
74. Leviton LC. Generalizing about public health interventions: A mixed-methods approach to external validity. *Ann Rev Public Health.* 2017;38:371–91.
75. Pew-MacArthur Results First Initiative: Results First Clearinghouse Database User Guide. Pew-MacArthur Results First Initiative, June 2015. https://www.pewtrusts.org/-/media/assets/2015/06/results_first_clearinghouse_database_user_guide.pdf. Accessed June 21, 2018.
76. Carande-Kulis VG, Maciosek MV, Briss PA, et al. Methods for systematic reviews of economic evaluations for the Guide to Community Preventive Services. *Am J Prev Med.* 2000;18(1)(Suppl 1):75–91.
77. Cochrane. https://www.cochrane.org/. Accessed August 19, 2018.
78. Cochrane Public Health. https://ph.cochrane.org/. Accessed August 19, 2018.
79. Waters E, Petticrew M, Priest N, Weightman A, Harden A, Doyle J. Evidence synthesis, upstream determinants and health inequalities: The role of a proposed new Cochrane Public Health Review Group. *Eur J Public Health.* 2008;18(3):221–3.
80. Campbell Collaboration. https://campbellcollaboration.org/. Accessed August 19, 2018.
81. Campbell Library. https://campbellcollaboration.org/library.html. Accessed August 19, 2018.
82. Washington State Institute for Public Policy. https://www.wsipp.wa.gov/. Accessed January 15, 2019.
83. Centers for Disease Control and Prevention: HIV/AIDS Prevention Research Synthesis Project. https://www.cdc.gov/hiv/dhap/prb/prs/. Accessed July 19, 2018.
84. Zaza S, Wright-de Aguero L, Briss PA, et al. Data collection instrument and procedure for systematic reviews in the Guide to Community Preventive Services. *Am J Prev Med.* 2000;18(1)(Suppl 1):44–74.
85. Office of Disease Prevention and Health Promotion: HealthyPeople.gov. https://www.healthypeople.gov. Accessed August 19, 2018.

86. Office of Disease Prevention and Health Promotion: Search Healthy People 2020 Evidence-Based Resources. https://www.healthypeople.gov/2020/tools-resources/Evidence-Based-Resources. Accessed August 19, 2018.

87. The Community Guide: PHAB Crosswalk. https://www.thecommunityguide.org/crosswalk. Accessed August 19, 2018.

88. Mercer SL, Banks SM, Verma P, Solomon Fisher J, Corso LC, Carlson V. Guiding the way to public health improvement: Exploring the connections between The Community Guide's evidence-based interventions and health department accreditation standards. *J Public Health Manag Pract.* 2014;20(1):104–10.

89. Advisory Committee on Immunization Practices (ACIP). https://www.cdc.gov/vaccines/acip/index.html. Accessed January 15, 2019.

90. Cochrane Public Health Group Registered! Cochrane Public Health Review Group Newsletter. May 2008. https://ph.cochrane.org/sites/ph.cochrane.org/files/public/uploads/PHRGNewsletterMay2008.pdf. Accessed January 15, 2019.

91. Proposed registration of a Cochrane-Campbell Public Health Review Group. August 12, 2007. https://ph.cochrane.org/sites/ph.cochrane.org/files/public/uploads/Overview_Transition.pdf. Accessed January 15, 2019.

92. Centers for Disease Control and Prevention: Compendium of Evidence-Based Interventions and Best Practices for HIV Prevention. https://www.cdc.gov/hiv/research/interventionresearch/compendium/index.html. Accessed July 19, 2018.

93. Health Evidence. https://www.healthevidence.org. Accessed August 13, 2018.

94. Dobbins M, DeCorby K, Robeson P, Husson H, Tirilis D, Greco L. A knowledge management tool for public health: Health-evidence.ca. *BMC Public Health.* 2010;10:496.

95. County Health Rankings and Roadmaps: What Works for Health. http://www.countyhealthrankings.org/take-action-to-improve-health/what-works-for-health. Accessed August 13, 2018.

96. Pew: Results First Clearinghouse Database. https://www.pewtrusts.org/en/research-and-analysis/data-visualizations/2015/results-first-clearinghouse-database. Accessed August 19, 2018.

97. Office of Disease Prevention and Health Promotion: Search Healthy People 2020 Evidence-Based Resources. https://www.healthypeople.gov/2020/tools-resources/Evidence-Based-Resources. Accessed August 13, 2018.

98. National Cancer Institute: Research-Tested Intervention Programs (RTIPs). https://rtips.cancer.gov/rtips/index.do. Accessed August 19, 2018.

99. Glasgow RE, Vogt TM, Boles SM. Evaluating the public health impact of health promotion interventions: The RE-AIM Framework. *Am J Public Health.*1999;89(9):1322–7.

100. Substance Abuse and Mental Health Services Administration: Evidence-Based Practices Resource Center. https://www.samhsa.gov/ebp-resource-center. Accessed January 15, 2019.

101. Remington PL, Booske BC. Measuring the health of communities—How and why? *J Public Health Manag Pract.* 2011;17(5):397–400.

102. National Cancer Institute: Cancer Control P.L.A.N.E.T.—Plan, Link, Act, Network with Evidence-Based Tools. https://cancercontrolplanet.cancer.gov/planet/index.html. Accessed August 19, 2018.

103. Substance Abuse and Mental Health Services Administration: CAPT—Center for the Application of Prevention Technologies. https://www.samhsa.gov/capt/. Accessed January 15, 2019.

104. Truman BI, Smith-Akin CK, Hinman AR, et al. The Task Force on Community Preventive Services. Developing the Guide to Community Preventive Services—Overview and rationale. *Am J Prev Med.* 2000;18(1)(Suppl 1):18–26.

105. Rimer BK, Glanz K, Rasband G. Searching for evidence about health behavior and health education interventions. *Health Educ Behav.* 2001;28(2):231–48.

CHAPTER

42 Community-Engaged Research*

Edith A. Parker • Barbara Baquero • Paul A. Gilbert • Jason D. Daniel-Ulloa

INTRODUCTION

Since the 1990s, the emphasis on engaging communities, patients, and other stakeholders in clinical, public health, and translational sciences research has grown tremendously. While this emphasis on engaged research began primarily in public health, the number and type of biomedical and clinical researchers implementing engaged research are increasing spurred by research-funding initiatives from agencies such as the Patient Centered Outcomes Research Initiative (PCORI),[1] the National Institutes of Health (NIH),[2] and the Centers for Disease Control and Prevention (CDC).[3]

Community-engaged research (CEnR) has been referred to by many different names [e.g., community-based participatory research (CBPR),[4,5] tribal participatory research,[6] participatory action research or action research,[7] community-participatory partnered research,[8] community-owned and -managed research[9]], which reflect variations in approaches and level of involvement in the research. Recently, researchers have begun to use CEnR as an inclusive term to describe any type of engaged research focused on health improvement, regardless of the degree or type of engagement.[10,11]

HISTORICAL ROOTS OF CEnR RESEARCH

Engaging the intended beneficiaries of research in the research process is not new; it has existed for many years in different disciplines. Wallerstein and colleagues note two traditions, the Northern and Southern, which contribute to today's CBP approach. Named for their origins in the northern and southern hemispheres, respectively, both traditions reject a (post) positivist view of reality.[12] Rather than presuming a single underlying truth that scientists could discover with the correct tools, these traditions hold that knowledge is socially constructed. Thus, any truth is created through interactions and is specific to a time and a place. To understand a phenomenon, you must engage and interact with the persons who experience that phenomenon as partners in the research exploration.

The northern tradition involved a utilization-focused research approach, such as the work of psychologist Kurt Lewin and his action research involving a cycle of planning, action and investigating the results of the action.[12] The southern tradition arose in the early 1970s from Marxist critiques of underdevelopment, Catholic liberation theology, and the drive to improve the practice of adult education and development among populations vulnerable to the impact of globalization. This tradition is perhaps best represented by Paulo Freire, whose approach to research was to engage community members as participants in the inquiry instead of as subjects of the research study.[12]

An additional influence for health sciences research is the southern tradition, with roots in the work of Drs. Sidney and Emily Kark and colleagues at the Institute of Family and Community Health and the Department of Social, Preventive and Family Medicine in the Natal Medical School in Durban, South Africa.[13] The Karks are recognized for their contribution to the development of the community-oriented primary care (COPC) movement as well as other innovations, which have influenced current-day preventive medicine and public health in this country. The Karks and their colleagues established a community health center in Pholela, Natal, which included a focus on social determinants of disease as well as a public health outreach program. Clinic staff included doctors, nurses, and health educators who worked with community members to address health, sanitation, and nutrition problems. Their practice-based experiences led to the understanding that community members should be engaged early in the process for practice development as well as research endeavors, and that appropriate research programs should respond to community needs.[13] The influence of Guy Steuart, one of the Karks' colleagues, can be seen in many aspects of CBPR, including recognition of community as the unit of identity[14]; the importance of community participation and control[15]; and the initial steps for developing a partnership for action, which he referred to as a "community diagnosis." To undertake a "community diagnosis," the professional works with community members to assess their own strengths and problems, which they subsequently address together.[16,17]

In the 1990s, research-funding agencies and foundations began to support engaged research. Several factors were responsible for this move. One was the emergence of the human immunodeficiency virus/acquired immunodeficiency syndrome (HIV/AIDS) epidemic and resulting pressure from activists to influence the initiation of clinical trials in the late 1980s and early 1990s. This stimulated increased recognition of the importance of engaging intended beneficiaries in research.[18] The National Institute of Allergy and Infectious Diseases (NIAID) was one of the first NIH agencies to mandate community engagement in clinical trials through establishment of Community Advisory Boards beginning in 1990. Reflecting on that time period, Anthony Fauci, head of NIAID, noted that one of the most productive decisions he made was to respond to activists' demands, which resulted in modification of clinical trials to become more user-friendly, and an accelerated drug approval process (while retaining proper attention to safety) through activist engagement with the Food and Drug Administration (FDA).[19]

* This chapter is a product of the University of Iowa Prevention Research Center for Rural Health and the University of Iowa Institute for Clinical and Translational Science and supported by the Centers for Disease Control and Prevention under Cooperative Agreement Number U48DP005021 and the National Center for Advancing Translational Sciences of the National Institutes of Health under Award Number U54TR001356. The content is solely the responsibility of the authors and does not necessarily represent the official views of the National Institutes of Health or the Centers for Disease Control and Prevention.

Another impetus was concern about the relevance of public health research and practice in relationship to community health needs. The Kellogg Foundation began the community-based public health (CBPH) initiative in 1990, funding seven schools of public health to work collaboratively with local health departments in forming research partnerships with people in the communities they serve.[20] From these seven community-academic partnerships, many other CBPR collaborations and research projects emerged, as did the Kellogg-funded Community Health Scholars postdoctoral training Program, which sought to train future researchers in the methods of CBPR.[21] Also in the mid-1990s, the CDC began to mandate community-engaged research in two of its funded academic public health research initiatives. The first, the Urban Research Center initiative, began in 1995 with three funded centers that were mandated to partner with communities in a CBPR approach.[22] The second, the Prevention Research Centers initiative, had been in existence since 1985, but in the 1998 Request for Applications, the CDC first mandated that applicants demonstrate community engagement in their research. Initially, the Centers were required to create advisory boards or committees as a method for community engagement, but through the years, community engagement with the Centers evolved into more of a CBPR approach.[23]

In the late 1990s, various NIH agencies began to fund and support community-engaged research, particularly CBPR, due to concerns about health inequities. For example, in the 1990s, the National Institute for Environmental Health Sciences (NIEHS) began funding initiatives that required demonstrated collaboration between environmental health scientists and members of community organizations, such as the Environmental Justice: Partnerships for Communication grants and the Centers for Children's Environmental Health initiatives. NIEHS was the first NIH institute to release a specific funding request for CBPR research, requiring a community-academic partnership in which the community partner contributed substantially to the overall research process, including the identification of the project's focus issue.[24] The National Center on Minority Health and Health Disparities introduced their Excellence in Partnerships for Community Outreach, Research on Health Disparities and Training (EXPORT) grant funding opportunities in 2002, which focused on understanding and eliminating racial- and ethnic-related health disparities and required that academic institutions actively collaborate with community-based partners.[25]

In 2006, NIH began the Clinical and Translational Science Awards (CTSAs) which sought to speed the translation of scientific discoveries to clinical practice, (often referred to as the "bench to bedside" process) by providing funding for infrastructure (both intellectual and physical) to conduct clinical and translational science. The CTSA program is now administered by the National Center for Advancing Translational Sciences (NCATS). Community engagement has been a core area since the beginning of the CTSA, however the core description in the original Request for Applications (RFA) opened with this sentence, "Community outreach could foster collaborative partnerships and enhance public trust in clinical and translational research, facilitating the recruitment of research participants from the community," which suggested a more narrow view of engagement as facilitating recruitment.[26] By 2012, community engagement, as well as other previously required key functions, were no longer required components due to the desire of NCATS to offer flexibility to the individual CTSAs to build upon their strengths.[27] In their review of the CTSA program in 2013, an Institute of Medicine (IOM) committee recommended that the CTSA program should ensure involvement of stakeholders (i.e., patients, family members, healthcare providers, clinical researchers, and other community stakeholders) across the continuum of clinical and translational research. The stakeholders were to be involved in setting priorities and making decisions across all phases of clinical and translational research and in the leadership and governance of the CTSA program, and not just to enhance recruitment strategies.[27] More recently, Request for Funding Announcements (RFAs) have reflected these recommendations and expanded the ways and extent of community engagement in the CTSAs.

More recently, PCORI (the Patient-Centered Outcomes Research Institute) was established and funded as part of the 2010 Patient Protection and Affordable Care Act, with the purpose of funding comparative effectiveness research to help patients and providers better choose treatment options and make more informed decisions around clinical care.[1] Influenced by the potential for engaged approaches such as participatory action research and CBPR to improve the relevance and use of research, PCORI mandates engaged approaches in their funded projects.[28] Engagement focuses on patient partners (including patients, family members, and caregivers and the organizations representing them) and stakeholder partners (defined as clinicians, researchers, purchasers, payers, healthcare industry, healthcare systems, policy makers, and training institutions). Among the engagement principles of PCORI are reciprocal partnerships (e.g., roles and decision making are defined collaboratively); partnership guidelines (e.g., fair compensation and reasonable and thoughtful requests for time); co-learning (e.g., researchers help patients and other stakeholders to understand the research process, team learning about patient-centeredness and stakeholder engagement); and transparency-honesty-trust (e.g., inclusive decision making).[28]

CONTINUUM OF ENGAGEMENT IN RESEARCH

An important aspect of CEnR is the concept of an engagement continuum, ranging from the most participatory and engaged research endeavors at one end, such as CBPR, to minimal participation by the community at the other end, such as a research study that counts focus groups with potential participants on recruitment methods as engagement. Balazs and Morello-Frosch present a useful continuum depicting a range of engagement from involvement as a study participant (described as "helicopter science," in which the researcher drops in, collects the data, and then leaves) to research partner, (described as CBPR in which the engagement involves full partnership in research, protocol design, fundraising, data ownership and leveraging the study results, and the partnership for social change).[29] The authors suggest that the most benefit to the rigor of the research comes when community members participate as full partners in the research.

The Community Engagement Key Function Committee of the CTSA[30] adapted an engagement continuum in which the less participatory end includes "outreach" (defined by "some" community involvement, such as providing the community information), followed by "consult" (more involvement such as getting feedback from the community), "involve" (better community involvement such as communication flowing both ways), "collaborate" (community involvement with partnerships formed to address each aspect of the project from development to solution), and "shared leadership" (defined as strong bidirectional relationship, with final decision making at the community level). Wallerstein and colleagues note a concern that this continuum offers outreach as a possible type of engagement, which could reinforce a unidirectional, rather than bidirectional, perspective.[12]

Not surprisingly, definitions of CEnR differ based on their levels of engagement. CBPR is defined as a partnership approach to research that equitably involves, for example, community members, organizational representatives, and researchers in *all* aspects of the research process and in which all partners contribute expertise and share decision making and ownership.[4] Israel and colleagues suggest the following guiding principles of a CBPR approach: acknowledges community as the unit of identity; builds on strengths and resources within the community; facilitates a collaborative and equitable partnership in all phases of research; promotes co-learning and capacity-building among all partners; integrates and achieves a balance between knowledge generation and intervention; emphasizes health problems of local relevance; involves systems development through a cyclical process; disseminates findings and knowledge gained to all partners, involving all partners in the dissemination process; and requires a long-term process and commitment to sustainability.[31]

The NIH CTSA Consortium[30] and the Institute of Medicine (IOM)[27] adopted a definition of community engagement originally articulated by CDC and the Agency for Toxic Substances and Disease Registry (ATSDR), a federal agency that was created by the Superfund Law in 1980 to engage directly with communities around evaluating any harmful health effects related to natural and man-made hazardous exposures. ATSDR deals daily with the challenge of responding to community concerns with scientific knowledge that may not directly address or support the identified community concerns.[32] Both CDC and ATSDR were interested in giving guidance to community engagement. The definition of community engagement jointly developed by CDC and ATSDR is, "the process of working collaboratively with and through groups of people affiliated by geographic proximity, special interest, or similar interest or similar situations to address issues affecting the well-being of those people."[33] This definition is more general in nature and is applicable to public health practice as well as research.

Another definition of CEnR is any research that provides communities with influence in the research process beyond assistance with recruitment of participants.[10]

Definitions of "community" also vary among the types of CEnR research. For example, CBPR researchers consider community as the unit of identity and characterize community as consisting of emotional connections to other members, shared values and norms, mutual influence, common interests, and joint commitment to shared needs; thus, community may be geographically centered such as a neighborhood or may be geographically dispersed, such as persons who share a characteristic (e.g., race or sexual identity).[31] The IOM committee reviewing the CTSA initiative proposed a more expansive definition of "community" as the people who seek and provide healthcare as well as those persons and organizations in communities who are working to improve the health of populations. Thus, "community" may include stakeholders connected to clinical and translational research, including patients and families, community organizations, disease advocates, physicians, nurses, dentists, nutritionists, social workers, and many others.[27] This definition has been adopted by the CTSA initiative in their funding opportunity announcements, in which they define community as including "all stakeholders connected to clinical and translational research. Communities may include but are not limited to nonprofit or industry entities engaged in translational research, and might include disease advocacy groups, local health providers, community-based organizations, and other national or local communities."[34]

WHY CEnR?

While the reasons for emphasizing community engagement in research are many and may differ based on the type of research and level of engagement, an existing common thread is a dissatisfaction with the often-limited impact of biomedical and clinical research on improving the health of patients, communities, and populations. Increasing engagement in research is seen as a strategy to improve the impact of research.

Researchers who emphasize CBPR share concerns about the increasing inequities in health among populations and the inability of a (post) positivist approach to address those inequities without addressing the issue of power.[12,35] Additionally, they share concerns about the historical exclusion of communities from influence in "paternalistic" research processes; the failure of past interventions to improve health (both community and clinical) and the lack of sustainability of initiatives that are proven to be effective; and the question of relevance of, direct benefit from, and even sometimes harm resulting from research endeavors for some communities.[14,36,37]

Clinical and translational researchers share concerns about the slow pace or lack of dissemination, implementation, and adoption of research findings into clinical practice[38,39]; limitations of the medical model to fully consider a patient's social, environmental, and cultural context and thus to understand health if communities and patients are not engaged[40]; relevance of research questions and the transparency of research activities[39]; cultural appropriateness of clinical research protocols; and successful enrollment and retention of research participants.[27] Furthermore, many researchers share concerns about ethical violations in research and see community engagement as one strategy to safeguard against such risks.[14,27,36,37]

Depending on the degree and extent of engagement, a community-engaged approach is thought to address many of these concerns by developing partnerships with communities that can better allow for: identification of community needs and priorities; community input and data on relevant research questions; development of context and culturally appropriate interventions that better address issues of health disparities; more safeguards to ensure ethical approaches to research; an increased likelihood of translation of results; increased relevance and applicability of research to the concerned communities; trust building in the community for research and researchers; improved participant recruiting and retention; and improved rigor, relevance, and reach of science[14,29,36,37,41]

Given the recent emergence of external funding for CEnR, systematic reviews are just now beginning to be published. Several systematic reviews have found evidence to support the effectiveness and impacts of CEnR, though more specifically CBPR, while others have found more mixed results (see Table 42-1). In a Cochrane review of community coalition-driven interventions that employed CEnR approaches to reduce health disparities among racial and ethnic minority populations, Anderson and colleagues[42] found that community system-level change strategies produced small, inconsistent effects and that broad health and social care system-level strategies (e.g., targeting accessibility of services or policies and procedures to improve quality of care) had consistently positive small effects. They found that interventions that involved lay community health outreach workers or group-based health education led by professional staff have produced fairly consistent positive effects on health behaviors and health status. The authors note, however, the low level of certainty of their findings, noting the characteristics of the evidence base and especially research design limitations (e.g., 67% of the studies were nonrandomized).

In a systematic review of the impact of community engagement on health and health inequalities among disadvantaged populations, Cyril and colleagues[43] found that 21 of 24 studies that met the inclusion criteria for the review had positively impacted health behaviors, public health planning, health service access, health literacy, and a range of outcomes. More than half of the studies (58%) were rated to have good methodology, 71% of the studies were judged to have good community involvement in research, and 42% achieved high levels of community engagement. Components that facilitated health outcomes included real power-sharing, collaborative partnerships, bidirectional learning, incorporating the voice and agency of the communities in the research protocol and the use of bicultural health workers for intervention delivery.[43]

Cook and colleagues[44] conducted a systematic review of CBPR to address health disparities in Environmental and Occupational Health research in the United States and found that in 14 of the 20 studies reviewed, CBPR led to community-level action to improve the health and well-being of the community members.

TABLE 42-1 REVIEWS OF COMMUNITY-ENGAGED RESEARCH

Paper and Focus	Design	Inclusion Criteria	Findings
Anderson and colleagues To assess effects of community coalition-driven interventions in improving health status among racial and ethnic minority populations	• Cochran review with systematic search for studies published 1990–3/31/2014; no pooled effects across intervention types.	• Studies of Community coalitions with at least one racial or ethnic minority group representing the focal population and at least two community public or private organizations.	• 58 studies included. • Broad-scale community system-level change strategies led to little or no difference in measures of health behavior or health status (very low-certainty evidence). • Broad health and social care system-level strategies leads to small beneficial changes in measures of health behavior or health status in large samples of community residents (very low-certainty evidence). • Lay community health outreach worker interventions led to beneficial changes in health behavior measures of moderate magnitude in large samples of community residents (very low-certainty evidence). • Lay community health outreach worker interventions may lead to beneficial changes in health status measures in large samples of community residents; however, results were not consistent across studies (low-certainty evidence). • Group-based health education led by professional staff resulted in moderate improvement in measures of health behavior (very low-certainty evidence) or health status (low-certainty evidence).
Cyril and colleagues To examine the impact of Community Engagement (CE) on health and health inequalities; which methodological approaches maximize the effectiveness of CE, and components of CE that are acceptable, feasible, and effective among disadvantaged populations.	• Systematic review. • Assessment of study quality using CONSORT and STROBE guidelines. • CE model and actual community involvement assessed using IAP2 Public Participation Spectrum and involvement in each aspects of the study. • Studies from January 1995 to June 2015.	• Studies that: include CE in a health intervention study with disadvantaged populations (DP); used CE to develop health programs for DP; evaluated CE as an intervention component. • Studies were excluded if they did not measure impact; did not describe CE model used; and were letters, opinion pieces, review articles or theses.	• 24 studies met inclusion criteria. Of those, 11 used an experimental design, 2 were quasiexperimental, 2 were longitudinal, 4 were qualitative, and 5 were mixed methods. • 8 studies reported positive impacts on health behaviors. • 6 studies reported positive impacts of CE on health outcomes. • 3 studies reported increased awareness and knowledge of health issues • 2 studies demonstrated increased participation in screening programs. • 4 studies reported community-level changes (e.g., community empowerment, community-level health initiatives, public health planning, use of public parks). • 58% of the included studies were rated as of good quality. • 71% of the studies showed good community involvement in the research. • 42% of the studies achieved high levels of community engagement in the CE models. • Factors facilitating the effectiveness of CE models included partner input in intervention design, shared learning between academic and community partners, and bridging people on research teams.
Cook and colleagues To examine extent to which CBPR integrates action to effect community-level change and to ascertain factors that facilitate such integration.	Medline search for studies published before 2008.	Original articles in English; CBPR-PAR study conducted in the United States; studies that investigated the effect of environmental or occupational risk factors on health or intervention studies.	• 33 articles reporting on 20 studies met inclusion criteria. • 10 of 20 studies were initiated by affected communities. • Variety of roles for community members, from consultation to more extensive roles (e.g., defining research questions). • Research quality of observational studies may not rate high on research design rigor. • 14 of 20 studies demonstrated action to improve well-being of community members' health; nine of these 14 studies were ones initiated by the affected communities.

(Continued)

TABLE 42-1 REVIEWS OF COMMUNITY-ENGAGED RESEARCH (*Continued*)

Paper and Focus	Design	Inclusion Criteria	Findings
De Las Nueces and colleagues To examine the effectiveness of current community-based participatory research (CBPR) clinical trials involving racial and ethnic minorities.	Systematic review in PubMed and CINAHL from January 2003 to May 2010.	• All English language clinical trials in English-speaking North America that employed CBPR.	• 19 articles met inclusion criteria; 13 of these were RCTs. • Of the 17 articles with a control group, 13 reported a significant difference in outcomes among the intervention group when compared with controls (though 4 of these did not adjust for baseline differences). • Community involvement was mentioned mostly in relationship to recruitment of subjects (84%) and delivery of intervention (84%) with less community involvement for interpretation of findings (21% for quantitative findings) or in disseminating findings (47%)
O'Mara and colleagues To evaluate the effectiveness of public health interventions that engage the community on a range of health outcomes across diverse health issues.	Reviewed database of primary studies compiled from systematic reviews and additional articles since 1990. • Conducted a random effects meta-analysis of health outcomes, behavior and related constructs, and a narrative summary of community outcomes.	• RCTs and non-RCTs; only studies in OECD countries; studies in which community engagement was the main approach.	• 131 studies met inclusion criteria. • The overall effect size for health behavior outcomes was $d = .33$ (95% CI .26, .40). • The interventions were also effective in increasing positive health consequences ($d = .16$, 95% CI .06, .27); health behavior self-efficacy ($d = .41$, 95% CI .16, .65); and perceived social support ($d = .41$, 95% CI .23, .65). • Examination of role of different models of community engagement on intervention effectiveness yielded insufficient evidence.
Milton and colleagues To explore the population impact of initiatives which sought to engage communities in addressing social determinants of health.	Systematic Review using NICE methods of articles since 1990.	• Study referenced community engagement in relation to the planning, design, delivery, or governance of initiatives to address selected determinants of health (e.g., social capital, built empowerment, substance abuse prevention). • Studies excluded if: targeted individual rather than community; focused on screening programs, healthcare setting, or secondary prevention; happened outside of the United Kingdom.	• 14 papers included in the direct impact review representing 13 studies. • Studies represented varying levels/methods of engagement, but analysis unable due to sample size and other factors to provide information on relative impact of each of the methods/levels. • No evidence of positive impact on population health or quality of services but outcomes related to well-being at the community level (e.g., social capital, social cohesion), as well as housing improvements and crime reductions were reported.

Abbreviations: CINAHL = Cumulative Index of Nursing and Allied Health Literature; CBPR = Community-based participatory research; CEnR = Community-engaged research; CONSORT = Consolidated Standards of Reporting Trials; IAP2 = International Association for Public Participation; NICE = National Institute for Health and Care Excellence, United Kingdom; OECD = Organization for Economic Co-operation and Development; PAR = Participatory Action Research; RCT = Randomized controlled trial; STROBE = Strengthening the Reporting of Observational studies in Epidemiology.

In a systematic review of clinical trials employing a CBPR approach, De Las Nueces and colleagues[45] reviewed 19 articles that met the inclusion criteria. They found that 13 of the 17 studies reporting control group design also reported a significant difference in behavioral and clinical outcomes among the intervention group compared to the control group. The authors noted very high success rates in recruiting and retaining minority participants and achieving significant intervention effects.

O'Mara and colleagues[46] undertook a meta-analysis to examine the effectiveness of community-engaged public health interventions with disadvantaged groups. They found solid evidence that community engagement interventions have a positive impact on a range of health outcomes across various conditions.

Milton and colleagues[47] performed a systematic review of the impact of community engagement on health and social outcomes. They found no evidence of positive impacts on health or quality of life from projects with community engagement approaches, but did note that there were positive impacts on housing, crime, social capital, and community empowerment initiatives.

Anecdotal examples are also emerging of how PCORI-type engagement positively impacts the course of research. Woolf and colleagues[48] describe how engaging with patients in a study resulted in patients challenging project objectives, identifying problematic wording of research materials, and adding important topics, all of which contributed to improved readability for a lay audience, sensitivity to patient issues, and creative suggestions for how to administer questionnaires.

Wallerstein and colleagues[12] note that methodologies and/or Cochran Review criteria may be too limited or inappropriate for engaged research, as they might not capture the results of CBPR studies—for example, policy studies that might be better suited to a case study approach. Others have suggested that methodological developments are needed to better evaluate complex, multifaceted interventions employing engaged approaches,[47] as well as facets of community engagement itself.[47,49] Finally, issues might also exist with word count limitations for journal articles, making it difficult to report both the study results as well as a thorough description of the type and extent of engagement methods used. That said, there are several initiatives currently underway focused on development of new methods and approaches to evaluating CEnR, including CBPR.[11,12,50,51]

HOW DOES "ENGAGEMENT" TAKE PLACE IN TRANSLATIONAL RESEARCH? EXAMPLES OF CEnR IN RESEARCH

Engaged approaches have been used with a range of research designs and methods to explore a variety of health topics,[31,52] suggesting that CEnR approaches are not limited to certain diseases, study types, or research methods. In addition, there are examples of engaging communities and/or other stakeholders in all stages of research, from identifying the topic for research, to developing the research questions and designing the research study, to analyzing and interpreting the data and research results, to participating in the dissemination of the research in more traditional (publications and conference presentations) and lay venues (community forums, community and organizational newsletters). However, the process of community engagement in research may differ based on the level of engagement, definition of community, and stage and type of translational research.

While different conceptualizations of the translational science continuum currently exist, for the purposes of this chapter, we adopt the conceptual model of translational research referred to by the IOM CTSA review committee.[27] This model consists of a continuum from T0 (zero) to T4 and connects basic research findings with clinical decision making to community and public health interventions in order to effect health improvements more broadly. The earliest stage, T0, focuses on basic science research, such as preclinical and animal studies that seek to define mechanisms, targets, and lead molecules. T1 focuses on the translation of T0 basic science findings to humans, and consists of proof-of-concept Phase 1 clinical trials focused on new methods of diagnosis, treatment, and prevention. T2 focuses on further translation to patients and may consist of Phase 2 clinical trials and Phase 3 clinical trials in which controlled studies lead to effective care. T3 focuses on translation to practice and includes Phase 4 clinical trials and clinical outcomes research that hope to lead to delivery of recommended and timely care to the right patient. T4 focuses on translation to community and includes population-level outcomes research, such as community-wide diabetes intervention projects that might employ a CBPR approach.

With the increasing emphasis on engaged research, there has also been an increase in resources to guide researchers and communities through an engaged research process. These include several books focused on CBPR and/or participatory action research in health, online resources created by NIEHS, PCORI, NCATS, and the individual awardees of these institutes and materials developed by groups such as Campus Community Partners for Health (https://www.ccphealth.org). For example, PCORI's "Engagement in Health Research Literature Explorer" (https://www.pcori.org/literature/engagement-literature) is a searchable list of publications on engagement in health research. With acknowledgment of these existing resources and our limited ability to provide in this chapter an exhaustive description of how to engage stakeholders in all aspects of research, we present here some selected examples of engagement across the continuum of T0–T4 research.

Engagement in T0-T1 Research—As noted by NCATS, most CEnR has taken place in the T3 and T4 stages of translational research, with fewer examples of and experience with identifying and involving communities from the early research stages and throughout the translational continuum.[34] In its review of the CTSA, the IOM[27] highlighted the role that disease advocacy organizations have played in basic research through identifying research areas, providing financial resources and specimens to support the research and "putting a human face" on the diseases studied (p. 117). Examples of this type of engagement include the Genetic Alliance, which focuses on advocacy for access to quality care and research around genetic diseases, and the Cystic Fibrosis Foundation, which partners with researchers to advance discoveries around the treatment of cystic fibrosis. In another example, Callard and colleagues[53] argue for the involvement of "service users," such as patients/consumers *before* a psychiatric drug or therapy is developed (in the T1 phase). The service users can share their lived experience regarding which symptoms of the psychiatric diagnosis are most troubling rather than having the researcher simply draw on scientific and clinical expertise vis-à-vis the type of medication that is likely to produce the most therapeutic value for the end-user.

Promising strategies to facilitate engagement of T0–T1 researchers with community stakeholders have emerged in recent years. Kost and colleagues[38] describe a research navigation program created to foster research pairing basic science with community-driven scientific aims, thus covering many levels of translational research. In this program, a research navigator serves as a matchmaker between basic mechanistic science researchers and individuals representing the aims and health priorities of communities to then develop projects that integrate T0 science with early translational (T1–T2) and T3–T4 research. Joosten and colleagues[54] describe the community-engagement studio, which was developed to facilitate project-specific input from community and patient stakeholders for investigators interested in input on research design, implementation, and dissemination. This approach can be used for any level of translational research.

Engagement in T2–T3 Research—With the advent of PCORI, more examples of engagement in T2 and T3 research are available. For example, a PCORI-funded study explored how patients approach decisions about cancer screening through use of an online module that asked questions about their stage of readiness for screening, primary concerns, and preferred approach to decision making. Once a patient completed this information, he/she could choose to have this information forwarded to their electronic medical record. Surveys were administered to the patients and their clinicians after the visit to see how well this information was addressed by the clinician in the patient's visit. To develop the module, both patient and clinician stakeholders were engaged using different methods. In the first year of the study, patient engagement consisted of ten focus groups about cancer screening concerns, online discussions and in-person meetings involving a working group of 46 patients reviewing drafts of the modules, and participating in cognitive testing of wording (13 patients participating) and usability testing of prototypes (7 patients). In addition, a 14-member patient advisory board met monthly to oversee the project. Clinicians were also engaged in the project as a 14-member working group, which met monthly to assist in planning the intervention and the implementation of the intervention. As mentioned earlier, the study investigators noted study improvements that were a result of the engagement of patients and clinicians.

For T2 and T3 research, much emphasis on CEnR is on engaging physicians in research. Often that engagement comes through Practice-Based Research Networks (PBRNs) which help to translate T1 and T2 research into effective everyday clinical practice. PBRNs use participatory methods that engage practicing clinicians and their patients in identifying the problems arising in daily practice that create a gap between recommended care and actual care. They then provide the space and context to test system improvements in primary care to address those problems.[55] The role of physicians in the research might be as a participant in the research, principal or coinvestigator on the study, or recruiter of participants in the research.

Engagement in T4 Research—Given a long historical connection to CBPR, there are more examples of engagement in T4 research, many of which involve engagement of community stakeholders throughout the research process.[35,36] The Community Action Against Asthma (CAAA) partnership is a long-standing CBPR partnership that has undertaken several different research projects focused on the environmental causes of asthma.[56,57] CAAA is primarily focused on T4 research, though some subprojects were more T0 in nature. CAAA began in 1998 in response to the community-identified issue of childhood asthma related to environmental causes. The project is guided by a Steering Committee (SC) of community organizations and these members have been involved in all aspects of the research process, such as hiring of project staff (including research scientists), development of funding proposals, development of the all study protocols (including data collection questionnaires), development of the community health worker interventions, selection of participant incentives, recruitment strategies, interpretation of data findings, and serving as coauthors on publications and conference presentations.[58,59] SC members did not participate directly in the statistical analysis for the project but summary tables of data were shared with them as the data analysis was produced. The SC met monthly for 2 hours and their member organizations were given a stipend to defer costs of employee's participation.

Two important elements for CEnR at any level of translational research are provision for evaluation and assessment of the engagement experience (i.e., the process and the outcome)[60,31] and provision of the necessary resources (e.g., training for community members on research methods; training for researchers on partnership/engaged methods of research; reimbursement to community members for their time and travel expenses).[61]

CHALLENGES IN CEnR

Challenges of a CEnR approach include partnership-related issues, methodological issues and broader social, political, economic, institutional, cultural, or ethical issues.[35] Partnership issues may include, for example, difficulty in establishing trust and respect among all partners[62]; inequitable distribution of power and control and conflicts over funding[14]; and the time-consuming nature of the process for all involved in establishing a partnership and implementing the research project in an engaged fashion.[14] Tensions may arise when grants are not funded especially if the academic partners and community partners have not discussed this possibility and how they will handle it, should it arise. Methodological challenges may include questions of scientific quality of the research by researchers[14] [e.g., if a randomized controlled trial (RCT) design is not used] or concerns of fairness to the community by community partners (if a RCT design is used and a potentially beneficial intervention is withheld from the community).[44] Tensions may also arise if the research does not support the hypotheses posited by the researchers and/or communities, though having established a level of trust in the partnership may help to alleviate this challenge. Broader societal issues may also present challenges, such as existing structural racism which provides power and privilege to white members in a CEnR partnership but that can be consciously or unconsciously reproduced by any person in a CEnR partnership[63] to the detriment of the partnership. Another societal concern is that disease advocacy groups may draw research funding away from research on diseases that affect disadvantaged groups, as an analysis of NIH funding patterns suggests may be happening.[64] Institutional issues may include Human Subject review boards who do not fully understand CEnR research and can thus serve as barrier to implementation of the research project.[65]

Other challenges to CEnR are related to its expansion as a recognized approach to research. With the growth in attention to CEnR, modifications have been applied over time that deviate from the original philosophies and approaches of CBPR. For some, these modifications are troublesome, go against the spirit and rationale of CBPR, and may lessen the impact of an engaged approach. Trickett[66] notes that CBPR has developed as a "worldview" with central tenets (e.g., community as the unit of identity; community involvement in decision making throughout the process; a constructivist philosophy of science) that cannot be altered. He suggests that using CBPR selectively to accomplish predetermined goals (such as translating findings of controlled trials into real-world community application) limits local control and involvement of communities to carrying out the science devised by others.

Others note the potential risks of a partially engaged approach. Wallerstein and colleagues raise concerns about the danger of manipulation or cooptation of the community to rubberstamp researchers' decisions if a more limited definition and extent of community engagement is used.[12]

Ethical considerations of using a partially engaged approach are also present. For example, the National Academy of Sciences, in their report on the "Ethical Considerations for Research on Housing—Related Health Hazards Involving Children" noted the importance of community-researcher discussions to share and review the proposed research protocol in order to identify concerns and risks that researchers and even IRBs might miss.[67]

Those supporting less than full engagement suggest that any level of engagement is better than none and can enhance areas of research, such as recruitment or protocol design. In addition, a CBPR approach might not be possible for all types of research, such as a clinical trial when the topic of research has already been decided. Finally, there is a lack of empirical evidence about the overall effectiveness, cost-benefit, and cost-effectiveness of full versus partial engagement in research, thus limiting our knowledge of whether approaches that involve less engagement than CBPR are less effective than full engagement in research.

Given the philosophical aspects of this debate, a total resolution is not possible at this time. However, as more CEnR at all levels of engagement is undertaken, knowledge of best practices and most effective and ethical approaches in translational research will increase. This increase may well inform our knowledge of the impact of limiting the extent of engagement in research.

CONCLUSION

In the last 20 years, CEnR has evolved from a sometimes marginalized research approach, such as the early years of CBPR when concerns were raised about the rigor of the research, to a recognized and reputable approach promoted by NIH and other funding agencies. Growing evidence suggests that it is an effective approach for enhancing research and achieving health outcome results. While much remains to be learned about the latest incarnation of engaged research, CEnR, and its application to all phases of translational research, many suggest that the time for engagement has come. As *The Economist* magazine reported in the obituary of Joseph Marie Albert Lange, a prominent HIV researcher who died in the crash of Malaysian Airlines flight MH17 over Ukraine on July 17, 2014 "Instead of closeting themselves away in laboratories, he insisted that researchers like him should talk to the people whom their work was intended to benefit. He recognized what medical researchers often miss: that patients, even those participating in experiments, are not 'subjects,' but partners."[68]

References

1. Selby JV, Beal AC, Frank L. The Patient-Centered Outcomes Research Institute (PCORI) national priorities for research and initial research agenda. *JAMA*. 2012;307(15):1583–4.
2. Ahmed SM, Palermo AG. Community engagement in research: Frameworks for education and peer review. *Am J Public Health*. 2010;100(8):1380–7.
3. Harris JR, Riley PL, Kreuter M, Simoes EJ. The prevention research centers directors: Reflections covering two decades of leadership. *Am J Prev Med*. 2017;52(3S3):S211–3.

4. Israel BA, Eng E, Schulz AJ, Parker EA. *Methods in Community-Based Participatory Research for Health*. San Francisco, CA: Jossey-Bass; 2005.
5. Minkler M, Wallerstein N. *Community Based Participatory Research for Health*. San Francisco, CA: Jossey-Bass; 2003.
6. Fisher PA, Ball TJ. Tribal participatory research: Mechanisms of a collaborative model. *Am J Community Psychol*. 2003;32(3–4):207–16.
7. Fals-Borda O, Rahman MA. *Action and Knowledge: Breaking the Monopoly with Participatory Action Research*. New York: Intermediate Technology Publications/Apex; 1991.
8. Jones L, Wells K. Strategies for academic and clinician engagement in community-participatory partnered research. *JAMA*. 2007;297(4):407–10.
9. Heaney CD, Wilson SM, Wilson OR. The West End Revitalization Association's community-owned and -managed research model: Development, implementation, and action. Progress in community health partnerships: Research, education, and action. *Prog Community Health Partnersh*. 2007;1(4):339–49.
10. Anderson EE, Solomon S, Heitman E, DuBois JM, Fisher CB, Kost RG, et al. Research ethics education for community-engaged research: A review and research agenda. *J Empir Res Hum Res Ethics*. 2012;7(2):3–19.
11. Oetzel JG, Villegas M, Zenone H, White Hat ER, Wallerstein N, Duran B. Enhancing stewardship of community-engaged research through governance. *Am J Public Health*. 2015;105(6):1161–7.
12. Wallerstein N, Duran B, Oetzel JG, Minkler M. *Community-Based Participatory Research for Health: Advancing Social and Health Equity*. 3rd ed. Hoboken, NJ: Jossey-Bass & Pfeiffer Imprints, Wiley; 2017.
13. Yach D, Tollman SM. Public health initiatives in South Africa in the 1940s and 1950s: Lessons for a post-apartheid era. *Am J Public Health*. 1993;83(7):1043–50.
14. Israel BA, Schulz AJ, Parker EA, Becker AB. Review of community-based research: Assessing partnership approaches to improve public health. *Annu Rev Public Health*. 1998;19:173–202.
15. Steuart GW. Social and behavioral change strategies. 1985. *Health Educ Q*. 1993;Suppl 1:S113–35.
16. Steckler AB, Dawson L, Israel BA, Eng E. Community health development: an overview of the works of Guy W. Steuart. *Health Educ Q*. 1993;Suppl 1:S3–20.
17. Eng E, Strazza K, Rhodes SD, Griffith D, Shirah K, Mebane E. Insiders and outsiders assess who is "The Community." In: Israel BA, Eng E, Schulz AJ, Parker EA, eds. *Methods for Community-Based Participatory Research for Health*. 2nd ed. San Francisco, CA: Jossey-Bass; 2013, pp. 133–60.
18. Kagan JM, Rosas SR, Siskind RL, et al. Community-researcher partnerships at NIAID HIV/AIDS clinical trials sites: Insights for evaluation and enhancement. *Prog Community Health Partnersh*. 2012;6(3):311–20.
19. Fauci A. After 30 Years of HIV/AIDS, Real Progress and Much Left to Do. *The Washington Post*. Washington, DC; 2011.
20. Brownson RC, Riley P, Bruce TA. Demonstration projects in community-based prevention. *J Public Health Manag Pract*. 1998;4(2):66–77.
21. Belone L, Griffith DM, Baquero B. Academic positions for faculty of color. In: Wallerstein N, Duran B, Oetzel JG, Minkler M, eds. *Community-Based Participatory Research for Health*. 3rd ed. San-Francisco, CA: Jossey-Bass; 2017, pp. 265–71.
22. Higgins D, Metzler M. Implementing community-based participatory research centers in diverse urban settings. *J Urban Health*. 2001;78(3):488–94.
23. Hawkins-Cox D, Harris JR, Brownson RC, Ammerman A, Gray BS. The Prevention Research Centers Program: Researcher-community partnerships for high impact results. In: Gullota TP, Bloom M, eds. *Encyclopedia of Primary Prevention and Health Promotion*. New York: Springer Science+Business Media, preprinted with permission; 2014.
24. O'Fallon LR, Dearry A. Community-based participatory research as a tool to advance environmental health sciences. *Environ Health Perspect*. 2002;110 (Suppl 2):155–9.
25. Chau TS, Islam N, Tandon D, Ho-Asjoe H, Rey M. Using community-based participatory research as a guiding framework for health disparities research centers. *Prog Community Health Partnersh*. 2007;1(2):195–205.
26. NIH. Institutional Clinical and Translational Science Award RFA-RM-06-002. 2005.
27. IOM. *The CTSA Program at NIH: Opportunities for Advancing Clinical and Translational Research*. Washington, DC: The National Academies Press; 2013.
28. Sheridan S, Schrandt S, Forsythe L, Hilliard TS, Paez KA, Advisory Panel on Patient Engagement. The PCORI engagement rubric: Promising practices for partnering in research. *Ann Fam Med*. 2017;15(2):165–70.
29. Balazs CL, Morello-Frosch R. The three R's: How community based participatory research strengthens the rigor, relevance and reach of science. *Environ Justice*. 2013;6(1):10.
30. McCloskey DJ. *Principles of Community Engagement*. 2nd ed. Bethesda, MD: National Institute of Health, NIH Publication No. 11-7782, Clinical and Translational Science Awards Community Engagement Key Function Committee Task Force on the Principles of Community Engagement; 2011.
31. Israel BA, Eng E, Schulz AJ, Parker EA. *Methods for Community-Based Participatory Research for Health*. 2nd ed. San Francisco, CA: Jossey-Bass; 2013.
32. Little PC. Negotiating community engagement and science in the federal environmental public health sector. *Med Anthropol Q*. 2009;23(2):94–118.
33. CDC. *Principles of Community Engagement*. 1st ed. Atlanta, GA: CDC/ATSDR Committee on Community Engagement; 1997, p. 7.
34. NCATS. PAR-18-464 Clinical and Translational Science Award (U54 Clinical Trial Optional). Department of Health and Human Services; 2017.
35. Israel BA, Schulz AJ, Parker EA, Becker AB. Review of community-based research: Assessing partnership approaches to improve public health. *Annu Rev Public Health*. 1998;19:173–202.
36. Minkler M, Wallerstein N. *Community-Based Participatory Research for Health: From Process to Outcomes*. 2nd ed. San Francisco, CA: Jossey-Bass; 2008.
37. Horowitz CR, Robinson M, Seifer S. Community-based participatory research from the margin to the mainstream: Are researchers prepared? *Circulation*. 2009;119(19):2633–42.
38. Kost RG, Leinberger-Jabari A, Evering TH, et al. Helping basic scientists engage with community partners to enrich and accelerate translational research. *Acad Med*. 2017;92(3):374–9.
39. Concannon TW, Fuster M, Saunders T, et al. A systematic review of stakeholder engagement in comparative effectiveness and patient-centered outcomes research. *J Gen Intern Med*. 2014;29(12):1692–701.
40. Barkin S, Schlundt D, Smith P. Community-engaged research perspectives: Then and now. *Acad Pediatr*. 2013;13(2):93–7.
41. Freeman E, Seifer SD, Stupak M, Martinez LS. Community engagement in the CTSA program: Stakeholder responses from a national Delphi process. *Clin Transl Sci*. 2014;7(3):191–5.
42. Anderson LM, Adeney KL, Shinn C, Safranek S, Buckner-Brown J, Krause LK. Community coalition-driven interventions to reduce health disparities among racial and ethnic minority populations. *Cochrane Database Syst Rev*. 2015;(6):CD009905.
43. Cyril S, Smith BJ, Possamai-Inesedy A, Renzaho AM. Exploring the role of community engagement in improving the health of disadvantaged populations: A systematic review. *Glob Health Action*. 2015;8:29842.
44. Cook WK. Integrating research and action: A systematic review of community-based participatory research to address health disparities in environmental and occupational health in the USA. *J Epidemiol Community Health*. 2008;62(8):668–76.
45. De las Nueces D, Hacker K, DiGirolamo A, Hicks LS. A systematic review of community-based participatory research to enhance clinical trials in racial and ethnic minority groups. *Health Serv Res*. 2012;47(3 Pt 2):1363–86.
46. O'Mara-Eves A, Brunton G, Oliver S, Kavanagh J, Jamal F, Thomas J. The effectiveness of community engagement in public health interventions for disadvantaged groups: A meta-analysis. *BMC Public Health*. 2015;15:129.
47. Milton BA, Attree P, French B, Povall S, Whitehead M, Popay J. The impact of community engagement on health and social outcomes: A systematic review. *Commun Dev J*. 2012;47(3):316–34.
48. Woolf SH, Zimmerman E, Haley A, Krist AH. Authentic engagement of patients and communities can transform research, practice, and policy. *Health Aff (Millwood)*. 2016;35(4):590–4.
49. Cottrell E, Whitlock E, Kato E, et al. *Defining the Benefits of Stakeholder Engagement in Systematic Reviews*. Rockville, MD: Agency for Healthcare Research and Quality (US); 2014.
50. Eder MM, Carter-Edwards L, Hurd TC, Rumala BB, Wallerstein N. A logic model for community engagement within the Clinical and Translational Science Awards consortium: Can we measure what we model? *Acad Med*. 2013;88(10):1430–6.
51. Ray KN, Miller E. Strengthening stakeholder-engaged research and research on stakeholder engagement. *J Comp Eff Res*. 2017;6(4):375–89.
52. Viswanathan M, Ammerman A, Eng E, et al. Community-based participatory research: Assessing the evidence. *Evid Rep Technol Assess (Summ)*. 2004(99):1–8.

53. Callard F, Rose D, Wykes T. Close to the bench as well as at the bedside: Involving service users in all phases of translational research. *Health Expect*. 2012;15(4):389–400.

54. Joosten YA, Israel TL, Williams NA, et al. Community engagement studios: A structured approach to obtaining meaningful input from stakeholders to inform research. *Acad Med*. 2015;90(12):1646–50.

55. Westfall JM, Fagnan LJ, Handley M, et al. Practice-based research is community engagement. *J Am Board Fam Med*. 2009;22(4):423–7.

56. Parker EA, Israel BA, Robins TG, et al. Evaluation of community action against asthma: A community health worker intervention to improve children's asthma-related health by reducing household environmental triggers for asthma. *Health Edu Behav*. 2008;35(3):376–95.

57. Parker EA, Israel BA, Williams M, et al. Community action against asthma—Examining the partnership process of a community-based participatory research project. *J Gen Intern Med*. 2003;18(7):558–67.

58. Israel BA, Parker EA, Rowe Z, et al. Community-based participatory research: Lessons learned from the Centers for Children's Environmental Health and Disease Prevention Research. *Environ Health Perspect*. 2005;113(10):1463–71.

59. Edgren KK, Parker EA, Israel BA, et al. Community involvement in the conduct of a health education intervention and research project: Community Action Against Asthma. *Health Promot Pract*. 2005;6(3):263–9.

60. Hicks S, Duran B, Wallerstein N, et al. Evaluating community-based participatory research to improve community-partnered science and community health. *Prog Community Health Partnersh*. 2012;6(3):289–99.

61. Gesell SB, Klein KP, Halladay J, et al. Methods guiding stakeholder engagement in planning a pragmatic study on changing stroke systems of care. *J Clin Transl Sci*. 2017;1(2):121–8.

62. Lucero JE, Wright KE, Reese A. Trust development in CBPR partnerships. In: Wallerstein N, Duran B, Oetzel JG, Minkler M, eds. *Community-Based Participatory Research for Health Advancing Social and Health Equity*. San Francisco, CA: Jossey-Bass; 2017, pp. 61–71.

63. Muhammad M, Garzon C, Reyes A, the West Oakland Environmental Indicators Project. Understanding contemporary racism, power, and privilege and their impacts on CBPR. In: Wallerstein N, Duran B, Oetzel JG, Minkle M, eds. *Community-Based Participatory Research for Health*. 3rd ed. San Francisco, CA: Jossey-Bass; 2017, pp. 47–59.

64. Best RK. Disease politics and medical research funding: Three ways advocacy shapes policy. *Am Sociol Rev*. 2012;77(5):780–803.

65. Morello-Frosch R, Brown P, Brody JG. Democratizing ethical oversight of research through CBPR. In: Wallerstein N, Duran B, Oetzel JG, Minkler M, eds. *Community-Based Participatory Research for Health*. 3rd ed. San Francisco, CA: Jossey-Bass; 2017, pp. 215–25.

66. Trickett EJ. Community-based participatory research as worldview or instrumental strategy: Is it lost in translation(al) research? *Am J Public Health*. 2011;101(8):1353–5.

67. Lo B, O'Connell ME, National Research Council (U.S.). *Committee on Ethical Issues in Housing-Related Health Hazard Research Involving Children Youth and Families. Ethical Considerations for Research on Housing-related Health Hazards Involving Children*. Washington, DC: National Academies Press; 2005.

68. Joep Lange Obituary. *The Economist*. July 24, 2014.

CHAPTER

43

A Comprehensive Approach to Planning Public Health Programs and Policies

Laura Linnan • Maija Leff

INTRODUCTION

A myriad of planning and evaluation approaches exist. Many have been applied to public health applications exclusively, while others are used in business, education, politics, and the social sciences. Most of the systematic planning models include some focus, in large or small part, on evaluation as a component inextricably linked to planning. The purpose of this chapter is to first give a brief review of several of the more traditional public health planning models, their history, and their typical use. Then, a new community-engaged planning, implementation, and evaluation approach developed by faculty at the University of North Carolina Gillings School of Global Public Health is described, along with its potential strengths and limitations.

TRADITIONAL PLANNING MODELS

Table 43-1 offers a brief summary of planning models[1–12] that have been widely used in public health. The first is PRECEDE-PROCEED. Previously, a small team led by the lead author conducted a survey to assess the familiarity with and use of planning models as part of the required training of public health educators. Results revealed that, while educators were aware of many different types of planning models, PRECEDE-PROCEED was taught by 88% of respondents at both the graduate and undergraduate levels.[13] This model is used with community-based health promotion and today is recognized for its community-engaged process. The next two, PATCH and Healthy People 2010 Toolkit, were developed by government officials to assist local or state governments with a strategic planning process that would enable them to link to national benchmarks and tailor local efforts. The Total Quality Improvement (TQI) approach to planning emerged from the healthcare field, where practitioners were eager to find ways to plan and evaluate improvements in the quality of healthcare delivered in their organizations using a data-driven approach. Still others, such as MATCH and Intervention Mapping, were created to provide guidance on the planning of multilevel interventions designed to improve public health. These examples are provided to illustrate both the similarities and differences of some commonly utilized planning models.

The remainder of this chapter will describe in detail a new planning and evaluation approach. This approach is data-informed, accommodates processes to assist with planning and evaluation, promotes engagement with key stakeholders at all steps in the process, offers guidance for prioritizing from among multiple options, and includes an iterative set of steps that would offer ongoing monitoring and improvement. It also accommodates both programmatic and policy interventions.

A COMMUNITY-ENGAGED PLANNING, IMPLEMENTATION, AND EVALUATION APPROACH

Figure 43-1 includes key steps in this community-engaged planning, implementation, and evaluation approach. Step 1 refers to understanding and prioritizing health problems. Step 2 includes identifying, analyzing, and prioritizing health programs and policy options. Step 3 includes developing policies, programs, and related strategies. Step 4 involves adoption and implementation of priority programs and policies. It is noteworthy that both an inner component (e.g., engaging and communicating with key stakeholders) and an outer component of the circle (e.g., evaluation and reporting) represent continuous, ongoing, iterative aspects of this planning approach.

Engaging and Communicating with Key Stakeholders

Evidence suggests that engaging stakeholders early and often in a planning effort provides valuable input, creates co-ownership of the effort, builds capacity, makes the best use of community strengths, minimizes limitations, and creates a strong foundation of trust. For example, when planning worksite-based health programming for employees, it is desirable to mobilize an employee health and safety committee comprised of a diverse, representative sample of workers and managers from as many departments, shifts, and types of workers as possible. By engaging with these key stakeholders early and throughout the planning process, one might learn what type of programs are of greatest interest to workers, when the programs should be offered, and how to best ensure high participation in programs.

Appropriate stakeholder input requires taking care to understand and honor the wisdom, traditions, and history of key stakeholders. The timing of when and how often input is solicited, the manner or methods used to communicate with stakeholders, and, being intentional about who is/is not engaged in key discussions are important aspects of engaging with stakeholders. Engaging stakeholders demonstrates respect that will serve all steps of the planning, implementation, and evaluation process. Specifically, stakeholder input as programs/policies are identified and prioritized builds ownership of the intervention initiatives. Yet it is helpful to have ongoing stakeholder engagement to ensure that programs and policies are implemented with integrity and if necessary, to take corrective action during the implementation process. Once programs/policies are implemented, stakeholder engagement can help make sense of the results with insights that would not otherwise be available. In summary, program planners are likely to benefit at all stages when partners are fully engaged. Corbie-Smith and colleagues[14] emphasize how various consensus development methods support ethically driven guidelines for engaged research. One example of long-term partnership with owners, stylists/barbers, and their customers developing a wide array of chronic disease prevention interventions illustrates how engaging key stakeholders has helped evolve two decades of effective programs in beauty salons and barbershops in North Carolina.[15]

Evaluation and Reporting

Like stakeholder engagement, evaluation is specified as a continuous process in this planning-implementation-evaluation approach. Planning and evaluation efforts are truly inextricably linked. In fact, it

TABLE 43-1 OVERVIEW OF SELECTED PUBLIC HEALTH PLANNING MODELS

Model	Developers	Year	Description	Typical Use
PRECEDE-PROCEED[1]	Green, Kreuter, and associates	1974 (PRECEDE), 1992 (PROCEED added)	PRECEDE-PROCEED is a two-part planning, intervention, and evaluation model. PRECEDE was introduced first as a planning approach where a community identifies and prioritizes quality-of-life issues of greatest importance and then links those to potential health-related outcomes. Planners then work backward, conducting an epidemiological assessment to identify what behaviors and environmental conditions determine the quality-of-life issue. Next, an inventory of predisposing, enabling, and reinforcing factors that are associated with the behavioral and environmental determinants are established. These factors, or "precursors," are the conditions that an intervention aims to directly act on. Priorities are established both within and among these categories of factors by considering their importance and changeability. In the final planning stage, planners identify evidence-based interventions or best practices that could be used to impact the precursors, and consider how administrative, regulation, and policy context will constrain or support different intervention options. In PROCEED, the planners implement and evaluate the intervention. Evaluation has three components: process evaluation (to ensure the intervention is carried out according to plan), impact evaluation (to monitor whether environmental and behavioral determinants are changing), and outcome evaluation, to track whether the overall health and quality-of-life priorities are improved. Taken together, PRECEDE-PROCEED is a robust, time-tested planning, implementation, and evaluation approach recognized for its community-engaged process.	Planning for community-based health promotion and health education.
Planned Approach to Community Health (PATCH)[11]	The Centers for Disease Control and Prevention (CDC)	1983	PATCH is a planning approach which aims to promote effective community health education that addresses local-level health priorities. As such, it is a model that emphasizes building capacity for health at the state and local level. PATCH planning has the following characteristics: First, planners organize local stakeholders who participate actively in the collection and review of local health data to inform a planning process. Next, stakeholders collectively set objectives and standards of success; and then design and implement strategies to meet objectives (e.g., community mobilization, health education, and mass media). Throughout the process, planners engage in continuous monitoring of problems, and intervention strategies to evaluate progress and detect the need for change, and they secure the support of national and local public health infrastructure systems.	PATCH originated as a cooperative program of technical assistance by the CDC. It was used by state-level and local-level public health agencies to identify and intervene on local health issues while receiving technical support and resources from the federal level.
Healthy People 2010 Toolkit[12]	Public Health Foundation	1999	The Healthy People 2010 planning toolkit leads the planner through seven "action areas" for building a statewide public health plan: building leadership support and developing the planning team, identifying and securing resources for planning, identifying, and engaging community partners, setting health priorities and establishing objectives, measuring baseline indicators and measuring progress, sustaining the planning process, and communicating health goals and objectives. The focus on the HP 2010 toolkit is to build the capacity of an organization to effectively plan. Therefore, compared to other planning models, there is a greater focus on defining what resources are required for the planning process itself. For example, the toolkit includes resources for creating the planning team, securing funding from governmental and community stakeholders, writing planning partnership agreements, selecting data sources, setting priorities, and other practical steps in a large, multistakeholder planning process.	The toolkit was designed to be used by states, territories, and tribes to help prepare Healthy People 2010 plans.

(*Continued*)

TABLE 43-1 OVERVIEW OF SELECTED PUBLIC HEALTH PLANNING MODELS (*Continued*)

Model	Developers	Year	Description	Typical Use
Total Quality Improvement (TQI); over time, evolved into Continuous Quality Improvement (CQI)[3–5]	Deming, applied to health promotion by Kaluzny, McLaughlin, and Simpson, as well as Kahan and Goodstadt	1981	Quality improvement provides a framework for planning and monitoring improvements in health services. Originally designed by Deming to improve manufacturing processes (1981), it places a heavy emphasis on statistical or data-driven monitoring of products to detect unacceptable levels of variance in product quality. Kahan and Goodstadt (1999) describe a variant of Quality Improvement to be used with health promotion initiatives. In this 11-step , the process is to (1) define goals of the intervention for all constituents, (2) translate these into desired outcomes, (3) set measurable objectives and identify measurement tools, (4) identify the processes/interventions currently being used to achieve these outcomes, (5) review research/gray literature and data to pinpoint processes/interventions that come closest to achieving the objectives, (6) plan to implement one of these new processes/interventions, (7) implement, (8) document implementation process, (9) monitor results, (10) make changes to the process/intervention according to results, and (11) continue to cycle through steps 4–10.	Originally designed to improve quality in manufacturing; public health interventions often take place in healthcare settings.
Multi-Level Approach to Community Health (MATCH)[9]	Simons-Morton, Simons-Morton, Parcel, and Bunker	1988	MATCH identifies factors at multiple levels of influence and expects a planner to design an intervention at three important levels: individual, organizational, and governmental. There are four phases in MATCH planning: (1) Select health goals; (2) Plan the intervention (e.g., this step identifies the individuals/groups who have the authority to create change at each of the three levels); (3) intervention implementation; and (4) evaluation (including process, impact, and outcome).	MATCH was developed to assist communities in the planning and evaluation of community programs.
Intervention Mapping[8]	Bartholomew, Parcel, and Kok	1998	Intervention Mapping was designed in the late 1990s to meet a need for planning strategies that specifically addressed intervention design, as opposed to needs assessment or evaluation. There are five steps in the process: (1) Specify the immediate desired outcomes of an intervention ("proximal program objectives"). The planner works backward from the ultimate health outcome that is envisioned, listing behaviors, and environmental conditions that must change ("performance objectives") to facilitate a change in health. Determinants of these behaviors/environmental conditions are then identified, and objectives established for prioritized determinants (these are the proximal program objectives); (2) After setting proximal program objectives for each determinant, the planner selects theory-based intervention methods and practical strategies; (3) Design and organize the program by operationalizing the strategies and deciding on the channel that will be used to deliver the strategies, pilot test and refine program materials; (4) Create an intervention adoption and implementation plan; and (5) Design evaluation instruments and a timeline.	Developing, implementing, sustaining, and evaluating theory-based health promotion programs

is difficult to talk about planning without considering how to evaluate the process and outcomes associated with the policies and programs that are being planned and implemented. Many planning models have a "built-in" evaluation component.[4,5,8,9,11,12] For example, Green and Kreuter, developers of the PRECEDE planning model, quickly added a PROCEED component that included process, impact, and outcome evaluation components aligned with each planning step.[1]

While most planning models have incorporated evaluation, there are independent evaluation models that might be particularly useful to consider. One compelling evaluation approach that could be linked to planning efforts is Glasgow's, Vogt's, and Boles's RE-AIM approach.[16] Originally, RE-AIM was used to evaluate interventions, allowing planners to compare different interventions using five constructs: *reach*, reflecting participation among representative groups of individuals; *effectiveness*, or the expected outcomes associated with the intervention; *adoption* of the intervention by a representative number of organizations; *implementation* of the intervention with fidelity, with minimal negative outcomes; and *maintenance* of the intervention effects among individuals and/or settings where it has been adopted. As applied to the example of weight loss interventions, for example, when evaluating whether online weight-loss classes or bariatric surgery would be a more fitting intervention in a given setting, a RE-AIM evaluation would help planners see that while bariatric surgery may produce the most effective weight loss (e.g., produce the greatest amount of weight loss = high rating on effectiveness), it is only available to individuals who can pay for it

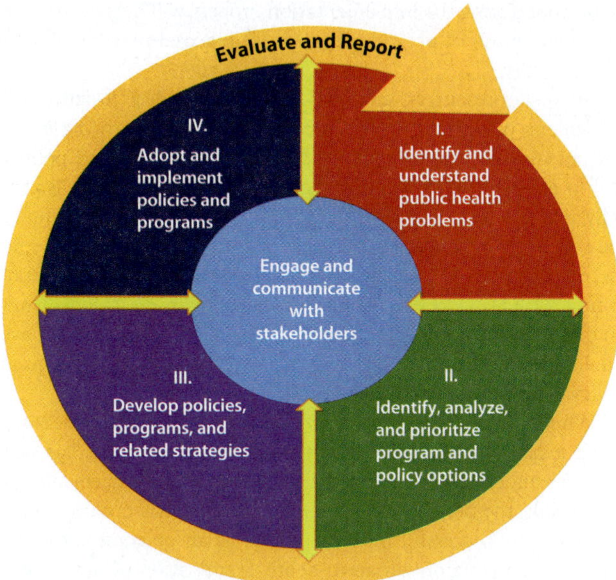

FIGURE 43-1. A comprehensive planning-implementation-evaluation approach.

and meet a certain weight category (low reach). In addition, it can only be delivered at certain types of health clinics by highly skilled surgeons (reduces implementation rating and potential adoption). On the other hand, online weight-loss classes have produced modest weight loss (moderate effectiveness), are available to all but those without access to Internet (moderate to high reach), are not costly and once developed are consistently offered without specialized staffing (moderate to high implementation and potential adoption rating). Thus, planners have useful types of information to compare the goals of the program with the needs of a potential community or group. If the planner worked in a hospital and had primary responsibility for helping morbidly obese patients with comorbid conditions lose weight, she might consider bariatric surgery over online weight-loss programs. In a worksite with employees of mixed weights, who want easy, convenient access to weight-loss opportunities and do not require major weight loss, the online programs may be perfect. In any decision to prioritize among program or policy options, RE-AIM constructs and comparisons can be extremely helpful. An increasing number of intervention studies are reporting on these RE-AIM constructs,[17] enabling planners to make data-based comparisons.

Outcome evaluation typically considers effectiveness of an intervention on a health outcome or a behavioral outcome, but when one wants to understand how or why a particular outcome occurred, we use process evaluation.[18] There are times when a well-planned intervention does not achieve its intended outcomes. In these cases, we need to understand if it was a failure of the intervention or a failure of how the intervention was implemented. Implementation science has embraced the study of how, when, and under what conditions interventions are best implemented.[19] Any good planning approach should attend to outcome and process measures that will yield the best understanding of whether, how, and why an intervention was (or was not) effective.

Stakeholder engagement in the evaluation effort and use of mixed methods are highly desirable as part of a comprehensive evaluation effort. Talking with the intended beneficiaries of an intervention during the planning process can help shape an intervention to the actual needs and interests of a target population. Evidence-based interventions often need to be adapted for new populations so planners will benefit from interviews or focus groups that offer insights from the perspective of the intended beneficiaries. Mid-course corrections can sometimes be made with input from key stakeholders, and certainly at the end of an intervention as part of a continuous quality improvement process. When combined with survey data or other more quantitative data, planners will benefit from a rich set of perspectives to help make informed decisions at the planning, implementation, and evaluation stages. For example, a review of emergency room data at the midpoint of a community-based intervention designed to reduce injuries due to falls may help planners make mid-course corrections if the number of falls increases despite exposure to the intervention. Further corrections might be possible if the quantitative data from hospital records was supplemented with qualitative interview data with individuals admitted to the emergency room suffering an injury due to a fall. These mixed methods approaches can yield powerful, valuable data to improve both implementation and intervention outcomes.

Reporting results of outcome and process evaluation efforts to stakeholders is also critical. Too often, planners and evaluators collect data but either provide no feedback to participants or they provide incomplete, insufficient, or misleading information about program processes or results. Clear, understandable reporting of insights about the program plans, implementation, and/or evaluation are considered essential and iterative components of the planning approach. For participants who have low levels of literacy, visual representation of data can be used. Not only is the type of reporting important, but the timeliness of reporting, and who tells the story should be considered. Thus, both stakeholder engagement and evaluation and reporting factors into all aspects of the planning, implementation, and evaluation phases. Next, the specific steps in a comprehensive planning-implementation-evaluation approach will be described.

THE PLANNING AND IMPLEMENTATION APPROACH

Identify and Understand Public Health Problems

To effectively begin a planning process, gather and review available data about the public health problem(s) facing a particular community or group. Ideally, this would be accomplished with the community or intended beneficiaries so there is a shared understanding of the number and type of public health problems to be addressed. Sometimes, a planner will have funding to address a particular public health problem which will eliminate the need to prioritize among public health problems, but other times planners will have an opportunity to work with community members to prioritize which public health issue to address. In cases where a public health problem is already prioritized (and in all cases), the planner should use interviews or focus groups to understand the perspective of different constituent groups with regard to the public health problem(s). Next, planners take available data and community perspectives to prioritize which public health problem to address.

During this part of the planning process, it is worthwhile to begin to gather information about assets and/or strengths that might exist in the community to address the prioritized public health problem. Too often, planners only consider the "needs" of a community, which is a deficit-based approach. Instead, community members often appreciate the opportunity to talk about strengths that planners can build on to most effectively address the priority public health issue. In addition, it is useful for planners to create a theory of the public health problem—to answer why this problem exists and the underlying causes of the problem. Again, community perspective on the causes of the problem will typically add insights that are essential for successfully addressing the problem. A visual representation of the underlying causes, checked with community members, is an excellent way to have an ongoing dialogue with intended beneficiaries about foundational causes and potential solutions.

Identify, Analyze, and Prioritize Program and Policy Options

Once the public health problem and its underlying causes are explicated, planners review the evidence-based intervention literature to clarify policy or programmatic interventions to address the underlying causes, and the prioritized public health problem. Next, planners should create an inventory of programs, policies, and/or other strategies that have been effective in addressing this problem. Using available data, planners rate the evidence for each program or policy intervention on key variables such as importance, changeability, effectiveness, addressing the public health problem, timeliness of producing public health change, cost, and/or community benefit. Once again, it is valuable to take this inventory and invite community members to rate the strategies on selected variables, discuss the results, and then prioritize intervention methods. As in the first step, planners then use the ratings to prioritize from among the identified policies, programs, and other strategies. Typically, a multilevel intervention to address the prioritized public health problem is planned.

Once intervention strategies are prioritized, it is useful to create a visual representation of how prioritized policies or programs will create positive outcomes will reduce or eliminate the priority public health problem. To do this well, engage with intended beneficiaries to confirm and gain consensus on the programs, policies, and other strategies that make up a "solution map." During these conversations, it is always helpful to check back with the community to make sure all relevant assets and strengths have been exposed. Assets or strengths include key partnerships, people with specialized expertise, available funding for programs, marketing, services, or participant incentives.

Develop Policies, Programs, and Related Strategies

Once relevant, evidence-based policy or programmatic interventions are identified, planners may find that important gaps exist. Planners can consult with established sources of evidence reviews, such as the CDC Guide to Community Preventive Services,[20] NCI-funded Cancer Control Planet,[21] or the Substance Abuse and Mental Health Services Administration's Evidence-Based Practices Resource Center[22] to identify potential evidence-based interventions. Where no relevant evidence-based programs or policies exist, planners may need to either adapt an existing program/policy that has worked for a different population or setting or health issue, or, develop a new interventions altogether. If a planner does an adaptation, using ADAPT-ITT[23] or some other recognized adaptation approach will maximize efficiency. Excellent examples of adapted interventions exist, as do reminders about the care that is required to ensure fidelity when an adaptation is enacted.[24]

Once policies and programs are in place, at this stage the interventions would benefit from stakeholder engagement to ensure that the prioritized solutions (programs, policies/other strategies) benefit from all available input, and that available assets, strengths, and resources are fully mobilized prior to implementation. Stakeholders can help adapt and/or otherwise tailor existing or adapted evidence-based programs to "fit" the community. Consider how the programs or policies are promoted, described, implemented, and evaluated. Whenever possible, pretest approaches. Moreover, pilot test interventions before widespread launch to be sure that tailoring or adaptation really works. One of the many benefits of pilot or feasibility testing is to identify potential unintended consequences of prioritized programs, policies, or other strategies. Even at this early phase, planning for sustainability of effective programs or policies is warranted. While beyond the scope of this chapter, several seminal papers have emphasized key characteristics of programs and policies that must be accounted for when planning for sustainability.[25–27]

Adopt and Implement Programs, Policies, and Related Strategies

Until recently, the successful implementation of evidence-based policy and programmatic interventions was underappreciated. The field of implementation science has emerged over the past decade to help shine a light on the importance of thoughtful implementation strategies and related measurement.[28] Engaged stakeholders before and during the implementation process will help ensure successful adoption of prioritized interventions and may help ensure sustainability.

Adequate resources and expertise are needed to effectively implement prioritized interventions. These are clearly necessary, but not sufficient for success. Leadership that includes the political will to adopt new programs or policies, and enforce them is critically important. Leadership is typically required from the "top" of the governing organization, but leadership can also come from middle management and/or the intended beneficiaries in a grassroots groundswell of stakeholder support. While grassroots support works on initial program or policy adoption, to make these efforts last over time, and get the ongoing resources needed to sustain a program/policy, top-level support must be cultivated.

While implementation is clearly a process that can be measured along a pathway to intended outcomes, more attention has been given to understanding the actual mechanisms of implementation. As a result, the field of implementation science has evolved studies that consider successful implementation as an outcome measure.[28] Planners can certainly do an in-depth examination of intervention implementation and decide which measures are most appropriate given the evaluation questions to be answered. It is essential to gather feedback from those who are responsible for implementing selected programs, policies, and other strategies, as well as those who participate or interact with them directly. At minimum, planners should strive to clarify with data whether the policies and programs are implemented according to plans, with fidelity, and gather information on participant responsiveness to the interventions. Effective documentation of program and policy implementation will be a crucial component of the continuous quality-improvement process. All data collected at this stage should be shared with key stakeholders, reviewed carefully, and discussed so that corrective actions may be taken early on to ensure successful implementation, and assist with plans for sustainability.

STRENGTHS

The planning approach reviewed in this chapter incorporates lessons learned and key strategies from a selected review of widely used public health planning models. This approach is both community-engaged and data-driven, which offers great promise for increasing participation among intended beneficiaries, adoption among organizations, ownership from all key stakeholders that helps bring resources and other support to the interventions, and provides a strong foundation for long-term success and potential sustainability.

This approach can work for planning both policy and programmatic interventions. Clearly, there are nuances associated with policy change that cannot be overlooked (e.g., more emphasis on political realities of who is in power at local, state, or national levels which dramatically affects the likelihood of adoption or the lack of political will to take on policy change). Yet, a planning approach that fully engages all key stakeholders, and uses data and stakeholder input to drive decision making, holds the greatest promise of success.

In addition to stakeholder engagement, utilizing mixed methods all along the process of planning, implementing, and evaluating programmatic and policy interventions is an important strength of this approach. A continuous quality improvement process can occur if evaluation, feedback, and reporting occurs throughout all phases of the planning approach. Another strength is the emphasis on taking an inventory of strengths/assets of key stakeholders, as well as what already exist in support of a planned program or policy change. This step—often overlooked—identifies strengths that serve as a foundation from which to build capacity and trust among key stakeholders. It would be unfortunate to spend time and resources developing a program that already existed in a community. This can happen unless an effort is made to find out what type of programs or resources exist and make use of them as part of the planning process. Sometimes a program needs a minor adaptation or some additional resources to fill an important gap. An inventory of assets/strengths is critical for building community capacity to effect change.

Finally, there is no one-size-fits-all intervention "solution" to complex public health problems, and this planning approach can accommodate multiples intervention solutions. Quite often, intervention solutions occur at multiple levels such that programs or policies at the individual, group, community, and policy levels may combine to produce the best health outcomes. For example, to reduce the incidence of lung cancer, interventions might be implemented with individual smokers (e.g., evidence-based smoking cessation classes and/or use of nicotine replacement medications); peer support from family members of smokers; and worksite-based and public policies that create smoke-free places. Taken together, the combined effect of these multilevel interventions make it more likely that smoking rates will drop over time.

LIMITATIONS

Alongside a number of considerable strengths, there are several potential limitations associated with this approach. First, the type of stakeholder engagement advocated for takes time and commitment. In some cases, there is an urgency to a planning approach that makes it difficult to fully engage stakeholders at all stages of the process. Moreover, it is not always possible to engage all key stakeholders in the planning process. It is useful to ask—who does *not* have a voice about this issue? Even when there is commitment to stakeholder engagement, it may not be possible to hear from all stakeholders. This can create important gaps in the planning effort that are very difficult, if not impossible, to fill. Another limitation is that resource-limited communities may not be able to fully engage in a planning process. If people do not have time or ability to get involved in planning, this introduces gaps in the planning approach, and/or constraints on successful implementation. Another risk of this planning approach is the risk that consensus cannot be reached when attempting to prioritize among potential interventions. If consensus cannot be established, the risk of diluting the strength of an intervention or approach to intervening is worrisome. Conflict can deplete resources, motivation, and passion for taking on needed change. Another challenge of this approach occurs when one is attempting to plan to address a new or emerging public health problem where there is very little or no evidence established about interventions that might be effective. In these cases, planners can use the planning approach but investigate interventions that are "similar"—either effective for different audiences, organizations, or health issues. Often, this will require adaptation of an intervention, which can introduce concerns about outcome effectiveness. Even more important in these circumstances to document each step in the implementation process and all evaluation results.

Sometimes early in the planning process planners identify a social determinant of health such as institutional racism or gender discrimination as a priority public health problem. These historical determinants of poor health[29] introduce new, additional challenges into the planning and implementation approach. The approach to plan, implement, and evaluate an intervention to address social determinants can be specified using this approach, but the evidence for interventions effective in addressing these root cause issues is still emerging. Other limitations may include identifying partners with expertise or resources to allocate for data collection, management, and/or reporting; overall costs associated with planning; and the potential for unanticipated negative consequences of the planning or implementation approach. It is possible that unanticipated positive consequences or spillover benefits can occur as well; however, the identified limitations are real and challenging to overcome.

SUMMARY

This chapter outlined a data-driven, continuous quality improvement, fully engaged planning, implementation, and evaluation approach that can be applied for both programmatic and policy interventions. The approach merges many key principles from selected planning models that UNC Gillings School of Global Public Health faculty have incorporated into the school's core, foundational training requirements for MPH students. This approach benefits from critically important principles of community engagement, community organization and social action, as well as utilization-focused evaluation that engages community at all places along the planning-implementation-evaluation process.

Accrediting agencies responsible for overseeing the training of public health professionals in schools and programs of public health, like the Council on Education in Public Health (CEPH), require students to master specific competencies related to program planning and evaluation. These skills in planning and evaluation are required in more/less depth for all three degree levels (bachelor's, master's, and doctoral) and may include the ability to assess population needs and capacities, to apply awareness of cultural values in the intervention design and implementation process, and to select evaluation methods for the intervention.[30] Hopefully, the approach detailed in this chapter will prove useful to practitioners as well as faculty who are training the next generation of public health researchers and practitioners. Not without challenges, this approach has been adopted for use in our practice-based work, engaged scholarship, and training programs.

ACKNOWLEDGMENTS

I would like to extend heartfelt thanks to members of the Gillings MPH Core Development Team (Karine Dube, DrPH, Elizabeth French, MA, Shelley Golden, PhD, MPH, Pamela Lee, MA, Alex Lightfoot, EdD, Jackie MacDonald Gibson, PhD, Aimee McHale, JD, MSPH, Yesenia Merino, MPH, Jane Monaco, DrPH, Melanie Studer, MHSA, Varsha Subramanyam, MPH, Aviya Williams, MS, Courtney Woods, PhD, Karin Yeatts, PhD) whose deliberations and creative, innovative thinking has led to the ideas presented in the description of key principles presented in this comprehensive planning and evaluation approach. Special thanks to Aimee McHale, JD, MSPH for her contributions to our collective thinking on planning and evaluating policy change—an important focus of our intervention planning work.

References

1. Green LW, Kreuter MW. CDC's planned approach to community health as an application of PRECEED and an inspiration for PROCEED. *J Heal Educ.* 1992;23(3):140–7.
2. Green LW. Toward cost-benefit evaluations of health education: Some concepts, methods, and examples. *Health Educ Monogr.* 1974;2(1_suppl):34–64.
3. Deming WE. Improvement of quality and productivity through action by management. *Natl Product Rev.* 1981;1(1):12–22.
4. Kaluzny AD, McLaughlin CP, Simpson K. Applying total quality management concepts to public health organizations. *Public Health Rep.* 1992;107(3):257–264. http://www.ncbi.nlm.nih.gov/pubmed/1594734. Accessed June 22, 2018.
5. Kahan B, Goodstadt M. Continuous quality improvement and health promotion: Can CQI lead to better outcomes? *Health Promot Int.* 1999;14(1):83–91.
6. Center for Community Health and Development. Other Models for Promoting Community Health and Development | Section 2. PRECEDE/PROCEED. Community Tool Box. https://ctb.ku.edu/en/table-contents/overview/other-models-promoting-community-health-and-development/preceder-proceder/main. Published 2018. Accessed June 22, 2018.
7. Green LW, Kreuter MW. *Health Promotion Planning: An Educational and Environmental Approach.* 2nd ed. Mountain View, CA: Mayfield; 1991.
8. Bartholomew LK, Parcel GS, Kok G. Intervention mapping: A process for developing theory and evidence-based health education programs. *Heal Educ Behav.* 1998;25(5):545–63.

9. Simons-Morton DG, Simons-Morton BG, Parcel GS, Bunker JF. Influencing personal and environmental conditions for community health: A multilevel intervention model. *Fam Community Health.* 1988;11(2):25–35. http://www.ncbi.nlm.nih.gov/pubmed/10288523. Accessed June 22, 2018.
10. Committee on Valuing Community-Based Non-Clinical Prevention Programs, Board on Population Health and Public Health Practice, Institute of Medicine. *An Integrated Framework for Assessing the Value of Community-Based Prevention.* Washington, DC: National Academies Press; 2012.
11. Kreuter MW. PATCH: Its origin, basic concepts, and links to contemporary public health policy. *J Heal Educ.* 1992;23(3):135–9.
12. Public Health Foundation. Healthy People 2010 TOOLKIT: A Field Guide to Health Planning. https://www.healthypeople.gov/2010/state/toolkit/. Published 2002. Accessed June 22, 2018.
13. Linnan LA, Regan-Sterba K, Lee A, Breny-Bontempi J, Crump C. Planning models in health education: Current status and recommendations for teaching and practice. *Health Promot Pract.* 2005;6(3):308–19.
14. Corbie-Smith G, Wynn M, Richmond A, et al. Stakeholder-driven, consensus development methods to design an ethical framework and guidelines for engaged research. Young B, ed. *PLoS One.* 2018;13(6):e0199451.
15. D'Angelo H, Owens-Ferguson Y, Thomas S. Health education and community building in African American barbershops and beauty salons: An innovative approach to addressing health disparities. In: Minkler M, ed. *Community Organizing and Community Building for Health and Welfare.* 3rd ed. New York: Rutgers Press; 2012.
16. Glasgow RE, Vogt TM, Boles SM. Evaluating the public health impact of health promotion interventions: The RE-AIM framework. *Am J Public Health.* 1999;89(9):1322–7.
17. Gaglio B, Shoup JA, Glasgow RE. The RE-AIM framework: A systematic review of use over time. *Am J Public Health.* 2013;103(6):e38–46.
18. Linnan L, Steckler A. Process evaluation for public health interventions and research: An overview. In: Linnan L, Steckler A, eds. *Process Evaluation for Public Health Interventions and Research.* San Francisco, NC: Jossey-Bass; 2002, pp. 1–23.
19. Colditz G, Emmons K. The promise and challenges of dissemination and implementation research. In: Brownson R, Colditz G, Proctor E, eds. *Dissemination and Implementation Research in Health: Translating Science to Practice.* 2nd ed. New York: Oxford University Press; 2017, pp. 1–18.
20. The Community Preventive Services Task Force. The Guide to Community Preventive Services (The Community Guide). https://www.thecommunityguide.org/. Accessed June 22, 2018.
21. Division of Cancer Control and Population Sciences at the National Cancer Institute. Cancer Control P.L.A.N.E.T. https://cancercontrolplanet.cancer.gov/planet/. Accessed June 22, 2018.
22. Substance Abuse and Mental Health Services Administration. Evidence-Based Practices Resource Center. https://www.samhsa.gov/ebp-resource-center. Accessed June 22, 2018.
23. Wingood GM, DiClemente RJ. The ADAPT-ITT Model. *JAIDS J Acquir Immune Defic Syndr.* 2008;47(Suppl 1):S40–6.
24. Allen JD, Linnan LA, Emmons KM. Fidelity and its relationship to implementation effectiveness, adaptation, and dissemination. In: *Dissemination and Implementation Research in Health: Translating Science to Practice.* New York: Oxford University Press; 2012, pp. 281–304.
25. Shediac-Rizkallah MC, Bone LR. Planning for the sustainability of community-based health programs: Conceptual frameworks and future directions for research, practice and policy. *Health Educ Res.* 1998;13(1):87–108.
26. Scheirer MA. Linking sustainability research to intervention types. *Am J Public Health.* 2013;103(4):e73–80.
27. Scheirer MA, Dearing JW. An agenda for research on the sustainability of public health programs. *Am J Public Health.* 2011;101(11):2059–67.
28. Brownson R, Colditz G, Proctor E, eds. *Dissemination and Implementation Research in Health: Translating Science to Practice.* 2nd ed. New York: Oxford University Press; 2017.
29. Marmot M, Friel S, Houweling T, Taylor S, Commission on Social Determinants of Health. Closing the gap in a generation: Health equity through action on the social determinants of health. *Lancet.* 2008;327(9650):1661–9.
30. Council on Education for Public Health. *ACCREDITATION CRITERIA: SCHOOLS OF PUBLIC HEALTH and PUBLIC HEALTH PROGRAMS.* Silver Spring; 2016. https://ceph.org/assets/2016.Criteria.pdf. Accessed June 22, 2018.

CHAPTER 44

Health Impact Assessment: A Tool for Promoting Healthier Communities

Katherine Hirono • Andrew L. Dannenberg

WHAT IS HEALTH IMPACT ASSESSMENT?

Many sectors outside of health, such as transportation, housing, education, energy, and criminal justice, have substantial impacts on health. There is a need for methods to facilitate communication between decision makers in those sectors and public health professionals. One such method is health impact assessment (HIA), a systematic process that examines a proposed policy, plan, program, or project for potential positive and negative health impacts, and offers recommendations to promote favorable and mitigate adverse health outcomes (Box 44-1). Unlike other forms of evaluation designed to examine impacts after implementation, HIA seeks to inform proposed policies and projects before decisions are made. HIAs are designed to improve decisions from a health perspective, not to assess community health needs, nor to stop projects from moving forward.

BACKGROUND

HIA has its origins in environmental impact assessment (EIA), which uses a similar process to examine the potential environmental impacts of a proposed decision. The conduct of EIAs in the United States is based on the National Environmental Policy Act (NEPA) of 1969[4] that was designed "to promote efforts which will prevent or eliminate damage to the environment and biosphere and stimulate the health and welfare of man"(4, p. 4321) and to "assure for all Americans safe, healthful, productive and aesthetically and culturally pleasing surroundings"(4, p. 4331).[8] While NEPA could be used to examine health impacts of projects and policies, in practice, health has received relatively little attention in most EIAs. For example, EIAs commonly estimate the change in air quality (an environmental impact) resulting from a proposed policy or project, but rarely estimate the associated change in respiratory disease rates (a health impact) that could be expected from that change in air quality.[9] The use of EIAs, combined with a growing understanding of the influence of broader social, economic, and environmental factors on health outcomes,[10] has led to the development of HIA as a separate tool. Published in 1999, the "Gothenburg Consensus Paper" is one of the first internationally recognized standards for HIA.[11] Since then, there have been dozens of guidance documents and practice standards published in various countries throughout the world.[1,12–15] Over 400 HIAs were conducted in the United States between 1999 and 2017.[16]

THE USE OF HIA FOR HEALTHY PUBLIC POLICY

There has been growing recognition in the field of public health that to improve population health and reduce health disparities, there is a need to improve decisions that occur outside of routine health-focused decision processes.[3,17,18] This includes decisions about policies and programs that affect transportation, housing, social welfare, energy, education, employment, and other social determinants of health.[19] HIA can help to inform decisions in nonhealth sectors, by predicting the potential health impacts of decisions in these sectors and offering recommendations to mitigate harms and improve benefits for health.[20] Factors that contribute to successful HIAs are discussed in the "Effectiveness of HIA" section below.

A key component of healthy public policy (Box 44-2) is consideration for health equity. Inequities in health are largely caused by the unequal distribution of social, environmental, and political resources.[21] HIAs focus on the potential impacts of decisions on particular groups within a population to determine the distribution of those impacts (see, e.g., Box 44-4: Case Study 2). HIAs provide recommendations to narrow the gap in existing health disparities and to reduce the potential for proposed policies to lead to new health inequalities.

HIA can be adapted to fit within usual policymaking timelines, structures, and processes.[22] HIA can be used to inform public policies in three key ways.[23] First, it can be used when policies are being formed to help weigh alternatives and consider policy options (see, e.g., Box 44-3: Case Study 1). Second, HIA can be used in the development of strategic policy, helping to include consideration of population health and equity in policy decisions. Third, HIA can be used to inform the implementation of a decision. Including HIA within policy formation is a strategy to ensure that public policies do as much as possible to improve the social determinants of health and health inequalities.

BOX 44-1 Health Impact Assessment Definition

"HIA is a systematic process that uses an array of data sources and analytic methods and considers input from stakeholders to determine the potential effects of a proposed policy, plan, program, or project on the health of a population and the distribution of those effects within the population. HIA provides recommendations on monitoring and managing those effects."[1]

BOX 44-2 Definition of Healthy Public Policy

"Healthy public policy is characterized by an explicit concern for health and equity in all areas of policy and by accountability for health impact. The main aim of healthy public policy is to create a supportive environment to enable people to lead healthy lives. Such a policy makes healthy choices possible or easier for citizens. It makes the social and physical environments health enhancing."[3]

BOX 44-3 Case Study 1—Healthier Lives, Stronger Families, Safer Communities: How Increasing Funding for Alternatives to Prison Will Save Lives and Money in Wisconsin, 2012

Facing overcrowded prisons, in 2007 Wisconsin piloted Treatment Alternatives and Diversion (TAD) programs in seven counties where low-risk, nonviolent offenders could attend drug and alcohol treatment court, day reporting centers, or mental health treatment in lieu of going to prison. Because the number of eligible offenders far outnumbered the available slots in TAD programs, WISDOM, a grassroots organization, and Human Impact Partners, a nonprofit HIA consulting group, conducted an HIA on the potential health impacts on offenders, their families, and their communities if the state were to substantially increase funding for TAD. A University of Wisconsin evaluation showed TAD programs were saving the state $1.93 in criminal justice costs for every $1.00 spent. The HIA included literature review, secondary data, key informant interviews, and information from counties with TAD programs and from alternative courts in other states. The HIA examined the health and social impacts of substance use, mental health, physical health, recidivism, stress, family structure, poverty, housing, and social cohesion on the offender, their family, and their community. The HIA demonstrated that alternatives to prison lowered recidivism and supported better health outcomes for the offender and for their children and families. If more parents were eligible for TAD programs, their children would be less likely to enter foster care, have less educational disruption, and have fewer behavioral problems. The HIA recommended expanded funding for TAD and priority for services to parents. There was wide media coverage and pledges of support from legislators. Because of the HIA, state legislators increased annual TAD funding from $1 million to $4 million to help keep more than 2000 people out of prison.

Source: Adapted from Hom et al.[6]

BOX 44-4 Case Study 2: HB 2800: Oregon Farm to School and School Garden Policy HIA, Oregon, 2011

In 2011, the Oregon House of Representatives considered farm to school and school garden legislation that proposed two new programs: reimbursements for school meals incorporating Oregon food products, and grants for school gardens and agricultural education. With foundation funding, a local public health organization, Upstream Public Health, conducted an HIA on this proposed legislation. Improving the variety and nutritional content of school meals has clear health benefits, but this HIA also explored potential results of economic changes and brought a specific focus on low-income children, children of color, and rural communities. Using literature review, analysis of existing data, economic analysis of food procurement, and substantial stakeholder input, the HIA examined health effects from changes in employment, diet and nutrition, school garden education, environmental health, and social capital. Key decisions throughout the HIA process were informed by two advisory committees that included technical experts, advocates, and representatives of affected population groups. There were three primary recommendations. First, schools should only be reimbursed for food produced or processed in Oregon (as opposed to packaged or packed in Oregon) to maximize local economic benefits. Second, education program grants should be provided preferentially to schools serving students from low-income households, students of color, or those living in food deserts. Third, the education grants should be awarded to programs with multiple farm-to-school elements that include local food procurement, nutrition and garden education, local food and nutrition promotion, and community involvement. After the HIA authors testified during a House committee hearing, the original bill was amended, fully incorporating two of the HIA recommendations and partially incorporating the third recommendation, and the amended bill passed in April 2011.

Source: Adapted from Cowling K, Lindberg R, Dannenberg AL, Neff RA, Pollack KM. (2017).[7]

HIA AND OTHER FORMS OF IMPACT ASSESSMENT

As a type of impact assessment, HIA can either be conducted as a stand-alone process, or integrated into other forms of impact assessment. Common types of impact assessment include EIA, social impact assessment (SIA), and equity-focused health impact assessment.[24] As an integrated process, HIA can be included within a standard EIA or SIA process as a standalone report (see, e.g., U.S. Environmental Protection Agency, 2009[25]). Otherwise, it can be incorporated throughout the process to create an Integrated Impact Assessment.[26]

HIA VALUES AND STAKEHOLDER ENGAGEMENT

HIA is informed by five key principles[11]:

1. Democracy,
2. Equity,
3. Sustainable development,
4. Ethical use of evidence, and
5. Comprehensive approach to health.

Each of these core principles helps to underpin why and how an HIA should be conducted. Democracy means that the HIA should involve the populations who are likely to be impacted by the decision, and to provide them with a means to participate in the decision-making process. HIAs both predict potential impacts and consider the distribution of impacts within a population. By considering equity, HIAs seek to predict health impacts that are unfair and avoidable,[27] especially within vulnerable populations. HIAs seek to promote sustainable development by assessing both short- and long-term impacts of a proposal. HIAs incorporate ethical use of evidence by using a wide range of evidence, including lay person perspectives, to inform recommendations, not to support or oppose a proposal (see, e.g., Box 44-5: Case Study 3). HIAs should also maintain ethical standards by being scientifically based and having a high level of transparency. Lastly, HIA uses a comprehensive approach to health by considering impacts that may be caused by the social, economic, and environmental determinants of health (see, e.g., Box 44-3: Case Study 1).

Because both democracy and equity are core HIA values, there is a strong emphasis on incorporating stakeholder engagement into HIA practice. A stakeholder is considered anyone who may be interested in the outcome of a decision, including decision makers, local community members, health departments, academic institutions, and community-based organizations. Community members and other stakeholders can help to prioritize data and recommendations, identify overlooked or underresearched impacts, and shape communication of the findings.[28] Involving stakeholders in all steps of the HIA can help improve the HIA findings and recommendations, and has benefits to participants such as increased civic agency and empowerment.[29]

STEPS OF HIA

Similar to other forms of impact assessment, an HIA typically follows a six-step process: screening, scoping, assessment, recommendations, reporting, and monitoring and evaluation (Fig. 44-1). The HIA steps will usually be carried out by an individual HIA practitioner, or more

BOX 44-5 Case Study 3: Healthy Vinton/Vinton Saludable Health Impact Assessment, Texas, 2014

The University of Texas El Paso in collaboration with the Border Environmental Cooperation Commission and Pan American Health Organization conducted a health impact assessment on a proposed water and sanitation improvement project in the border town of Vinton, Texas. Vinton has high levels of unemployment and poverty with limited infrastructure, including water supply. Part of the community connects to two private suppliers who draw from local wells, while the other part is connected to the public water supply. Private water supplies are commonly contaminated with arsenic and industrial pollutants. Domestic shallow wells are also commonly contaminated, and many households rely on failing septic tanks and cesspools for wastewater collection and treatment. Previous water and sanitation projects had been voted down by city council based on the high cost of implementation. The HIA collected primary data, including tap water samples, household surveys, focus groups, and key informant interviews. Impacts examined included gastrointestinal illnesses such as giardiasis, dysentery, and hepatitis; fire safety; and opportunities for economic and community development. The HIA found that water and sanitation improvement projects should connect Vinton to the El Paso Water Utilities. The results of the HIA were presented to the Texas Water Development Board to show how poor water quality can harm public health. As a result of the HIA, Vinton received $2.7 million to design a new water system, and was promised an additional $27 million for the new system implementation.

Source: Adapted from Hargrove W, Juarez-Carillo P. (2014).[5]

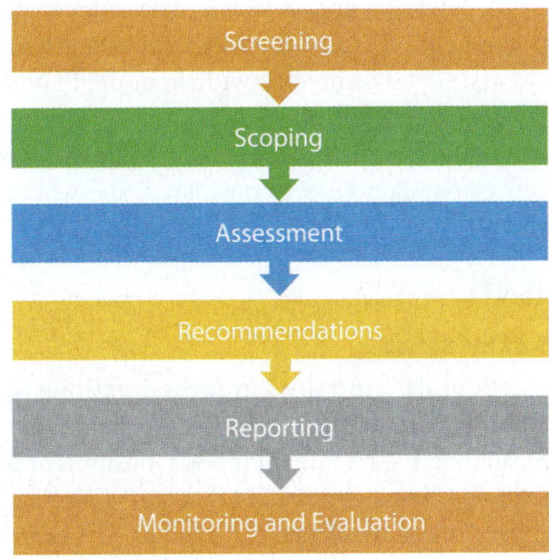

FIGURE 44-1. The steps of HIA.

commonly, an HIA team. HIA teams are usually four to six people from either the same or various organizations who contribute various skills and expertise to conduct an HIA, and may also include community members or decision makers. It is useful to have some formal public health training when conducting an HIA, but it is not a requirement, and many HIAs have been conducted by nonhealth organizations (see, e.g., Box 44-3: Case Study 1). There is no formal qualification or licensing to be an HIA practitioner, and most individuals or teams will learn how to conduct an HIA through a process of learning-by-doing.

SCREENING

During screening, the HIA practitioner articulates the decision to be informed and the rationale for why the HIA will add value to the process; provides a preliminary judgment of potential health impacts; estimates the time and resources needed to complete the HIA; describes the decision-making context including who the decision makers are and how the HIA will inform the decision; and recommends whether or not the HIA should proceed.[1] In some cases, an HIA may not be the best tool to inform a decision, and other approaches such as a health note, checklist, or audit may be more appropriate.[30]

SOME KEY QUESTIONS TO ANSWER DURING SCREENING:

Is there Sufficient Information about the Proposal to Conduct an HIA?

For the HIA to proceed there must be meaningful documentation about the proposal and decision-making process. This helps clarify when the decision will occur and how much time is available to conduct the HIA. Timing is important; an HIA should not be conducted too early when few details about a proposal are available, nor too late when the decision process can no longer incorporate recommended changes into the proposal.

How Will the Decision Potentially Affect Health?

The potential impacts of the decision are determined in the assessment step, but an initial judgment of whether the decision may affect health is made in the screening step. For example, a proposed public housing development may have implications for income and overcrowding which are both related to health. The mechanisms by which these determinants will affect the population, and other health impacts, are determined during the assessment. In contrast, building a utility line across an uninhabited stretch of desert may have environmental impacts, but is unlikely to have major human health impacts.

How Will the HIA Add Value to the Decision-Making Process?

For some decisions that will have impacts on health, decision makers may be unwilling to consider input and recommendations from an HIA. In such cases, an advocacy group may or may not be able to use HIA results to try to influence the decision makers. In other cases, the potential health impacts of a decision may be well known to the decision makers, and the HIA may not add value. For example, a new park or trail is inherently favorable to health, although an HIA might influence its design to provide better accommodation for persons with disabilities.

Are Vulnerable Populations Likely to Be Impacted by the Decision?

Because reducing health disparities is an important goal of HIAs, it is especially valuable to conduct HIAs for decisions that are likely to impact vulnerable populations.

STAKEHOLDER INVOLVEMENT IN SCREENING

Stakeholders can participate in the screening step by helping to identify potential health impacts, opportunities to inform the decision, and local vulnerable populations. Stakeholders may also identify potential funding opportunities and other resources, such as staff time, from within their own organizations and communities.

SCOPING

Scoping is used to identify which potential health impacts deserve consideration and to create a plan for conducting the HIA. Examining the parameters of the project in advance can help to save time, resources, and subsequent work.

Health Pathways

Because HIAs are often limited in time and resources, not all potential health impacts can be assessed. Scoping enables the practitioner to determine which health impacts should be assessed based on the available evidence, resources, and level of importance. One approach

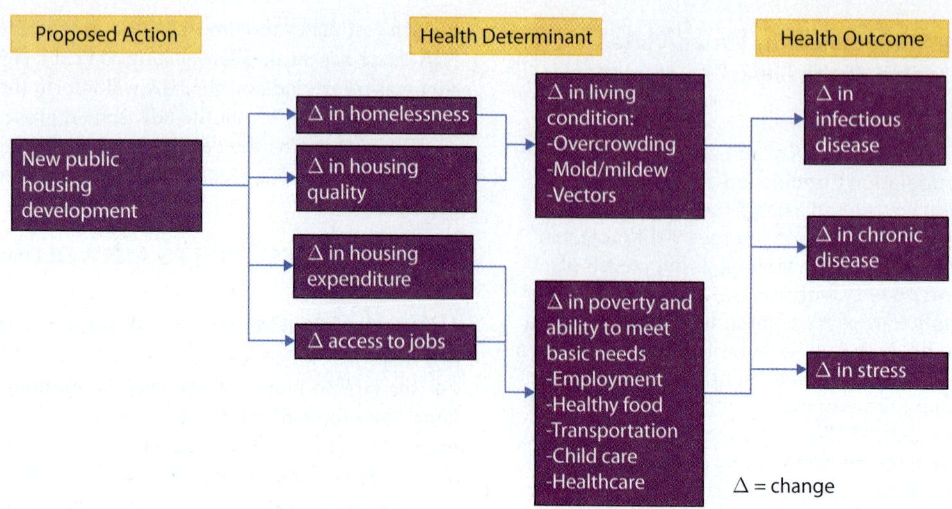

FIGURE 44-2. Health Pathway Diagram example. (*Source:* Adapted from San Francisco Department of Public Health. Baseline Conditions Assessment of HOPE SF Redevelopment: Sunnydale. 2010. http://www.pewtrusts.org/~/media/assets/2010/09/sunnydalepublichousingredevelopment.pdf. Accessed 30 Jan, 2018.[31])

for determining potential health impacts is to develop a logic framework that traces the pathway of a decision from impacts on social, environmental, and economic determinants to changes in health outcomes (Fig. 44-2, adapted from ref. 31). Another approach is to develop a table that allows for a rapid appraisal of all potential ways in which a decision may affect health.[1]

Potentially Affected Populations

Another purpose of scoping is identification of the populations likely to be affected by the proposed project or policy (see, e.g., Box 44-4: Case Study 2). Of particular importance is how the impacts of a decision might be distributed within a population such as by gender, race, age, disability, socioeconomic status, education level, or geography. Defining these populations helps ensure the collection of appropriate data during the assessment phase of the HIA.

Depth of HIA

HIAs can vary widely in the amount of time and resources required and in the depth of health impacts considered. Desktop or rapid HIAs may use existing evidence to assess a few health impacts qualitatively and may be conducted within a few weeks. Intermediate or comprehensive HIAs will consider more health impacts, larger or more varied populations, may collect primary data, and may require months to several years to complete (see, e.g., Box 44-5: Case Study 3).

HIA Team and Stakeholder Involvement

A formal HIA project team should be developed at the scoping stage. This can include public health professionals, academics, and other stakeholders and community members. The project team is responsible for conducting all stages of the process and should be limited to a handful of key members. Forming a steering committee can help to provide the project team with needed resources and guidance, and a diversity of perspectives and skills. The steering committee can be larger than the project team and may involve academics with expertise in specific subject areas or methodologies, representatives of community-based organizations, decision makers, project proponents, and community members (see, e.g., Box 44-4: Case Study 2).

Scoping should include the development of a stakeholder engagement plan. For rapid HIAs, there is limited time to do in-depth engagement, while comprehensive HIAs can involve robust engagement strategies. Ideally, all elements in an HIA, including stakeholder engagement, are conducted in a manner consistent with best practice guidelines.[28]

Data Sources, Methods, and Research Questions

Once the potential health impacts have been determined, the appropriate research questions, methodologies, and data sources need to be identified. The types of data sources and methods that can be used will depend on the amount of time and resources allocated to the HIA. The available evidence will vary with the topic and scope of the HIA.

Role of Stakeholders in Scoping

Stakeholders can play a critical role in developing the scope of an HIA. Input from a diverse range of stakeholders can help to elucidate potential health pathways and available data sources. Community stakeholders can help prioritize the most important health impacts for the HIA to assess.[28] Stakeholders with an in-depth understanding of the decision-making process, such as decision makers, can help determine where the HIA can add the most value in terms of which health impacts or populations are considered, and what type of evidence is used.

ASSESSMENT

Typologies of Evidence

Potential sources of data in HIA can include existing scientific literature (i.e., academic journals), public sector data (national health surveys or census data), government reports, business or professional reports and surveys, local news sources, expert opinions, and community members' views. Evidence collected as part of the HIA process is called primary data, while existing evidence used in an HIA is called secondary data (i.e., academic publications, governmental reports, previously completed health surveys). Deciding which type of data sources to use depends on the time, skills, and resources available, and on the questions the HIA is seeking to answer.[32]

Baseline Health Profile

Before predicting how a decision will impact a population, it is necessary to establish a baseline profile of the health and social conditions of that population. This profile should identify relevant health, economic, social, and environmental trends and factors. The profile should identify the health status of the overall population and its subpopulations. Determining these differences can help to identify populations who may be more vulnerable to the impacts of a proposed change.[1] Data sources that may be used to create a baseline profile include census data, population, and behavior surveys such as the Behavioral Risk Factor Surveillance Survey (https://www.cdc.gov/brfss/index.html), hospital records, or other government reports. Indicators included in the baseline profile may include general demographic characteristics, health status of the affected population, indicators of health behavior such as smoking rates and alcohol use, environmental conditions, and other social conditions such as employment status, crime statistics, education levels, quality of housing, and transportation infrastructure.

It may be difficult to create a comprehensive health profile for local populations under consideration when insufficient data are available at the local level. Proxies may be used when needed data are not available or disease rates are too small to calculate. For example, rather than determining the rates of lung disease in a small community, relevant proxies such as smoking rates and ambient air pollution can be used.[1] Some comprehensive HIAs may collect baseline data, particularly when existing evidence is not available, such as in rural communities in the developing world.

Use of Evidence

Assessment can rely on both qualitative and quantitative evidence (see, e.g., Box 44-5: Case Study 3). In some cases, evidence can be quantified or input into models to create predicted outcomes. For example, increases in rates of pedestrian-vehicle injury may be predicted based on modeling of injuries related to land use and traffic patterns.[33] In other cases, qualitative data, such as key informant interviews or community focus groups, can be used to help determine the direction if not the magnitude of the potential changes associated with a decision. Not all evidence should be given equal weight. This is particularly important to address when data are speculative or different evidence conflicts. For example, some community members may indicate they think a transit route should be in a specific location where it helps them personally, with little knowledge of the impact of that transit route on overall community travel patterns. In other cases, available data may relate to the overall community, but not be sufficiently localized to highlight impacts on specific vulnerable populations within the community.

Characterizing Evidence

Health impacts may be characterized based on a set of indicators, such as the following:

- Direction: whether the impact is beneficial or harmful to health. In some cases, the direction of the impact may be unclear, or beneficial to some persons and harmful to others. Differential impacts should be indicated as part of the characterization of distribution.
- Intensity: the level of severity of the impact (i.e., minor, moderate, fatal).
- Magnitude: the number of people expected to be impacted.
- Timing: the timeframe in which the impact will occur (i.e., short, medium, or long term) and the duration of the anticipated impact (i.e., some impacts may only occur during the construction phase of a project while others might last indefinitely).
- Likelihood: the probability that the potential impact will occur.
- Certainty: the level of confidence in the prediction, based on the strength of the evidence.
- Distribution: the distribution of an effect within a population according to spatial boundaries, or within specific populations. Understanding how an impact affects different population groups is the basis for assessing health equity. Differential impacts may be assessed according to characteristics such as age, gender, ethnicity/race, socioeconomic status, locational disadvantage, and disability.

To characterize each impact, many HIAs use an assessment matrix (see, e.g., Haigh et al.[34]). In addition to the indicators above, the matrix should describe the impact and the causal pathway for that impact, the sources of data for each impact, and the weight assigned to the data. When possible, an overall rating of importance may be assigned to each effect (see, e.g., The Sequoia Foundation[35]).

The Role of Stakeholders in Assessment

Stakeholders can play a critical role in the assessment step. They can serve to identify potential evidence, assist in the data collection process, and serve as sources of evidence via stakeholder interviews or focus groups. Stakeholders can also help to characterize the data. Particularly when there may be limited evidence for the prediction, or when predictions conflict, stakeholders can help to prioritize sources of data, weigh the evidence, or provide additional insight relevant to local communities.

RECOMMENDATIONS

The goal of the recommendations step is to develop a set of evidence-based recommendations that will mitigate identified negative health impacts and optimize potential positive impacts. The output of this step will be a set of recommendations that correspond to the findings of the assessment.

HIAs are designed to provide specific recommendations to improve the decision about a proposed project or policy, rather than providing an overall assessment of whether or not the proposal should move forward (see, e.g., Box 44-4: Case Study 2). Each recommendation should describe the impact it is aiming to improve, a rationale for the recommendation based on the evidence developed in the HIA, and who is responsible for and the timing of its implementation.

The Role of Stakeholders in Recommendations

Developing HIA recommendations is a key opportunity for the involvement of stakeholders. Involving decision makers in this step will help to ensure that the recommendations are written to be practical, sufficiently specific, and politically feasible. For example, a recommendation to "make the proposal more equitable to all senior citizens" is too vague to be implemented, whereby a recommendation to increase the specific percent of project resources used to build facilities needed by seniors is specific and practical.

Community members can also play an important role at this stage. They can help to prioritize which recommendations are most important to the community, which will be useful in the HIA reporting step. Involving the HIA Steering Committee in the development of recommendations will help to ensure that stakeholders have input into this stage and create ownership and buy-in for the recommendations.

REPORTING

The goal of this stage is to communicate the findings and recommendations of the HIA to decision makers, stakeholders, and community members. A communications plan is ideally designed during the scoping step of the HIA. HIA reporting is generally best done with multiple formats designed for their specific audiences. For example, a one-page executive summary may be used by decision makers, a detailed HIA report is valuable to project staff, and a press release may be prepared for use by the media. When developing communication outputs, it is important to think about the intended audience in terms of levels of literacy (including technical literacy), language, use of jargon, and style of presentation.

Various guidance documents exist for developing HIA reports.[36–38] It is important to be transparent about the HIA process and to detail every stage (while not being so long as to be unreadable).

The HIA report should detail the HIA process and outcomes including:

- The decision the HIA is seeking to inform and rationale for undertaking the HIA (Screening step);
- The plan for undertaking the HIA (Scoping step);
- The baseline health profile;
- A summary of the evidence collected;
- Characterization of impacts—this should be presented in summary form and may include the assessment matrix;

- Recommendations;
- Reporting plan;
- Monitoring and evaluation plan; and
- The role of stakeholders (stakeholder engagement plan).

The Role of Stakeholders in Reporting

Stakeholders can be useful in creating a communication plan by identifying the appropriate communication strategy for each audience. Stakeholders may also be able to identify opportunities for presenting the findings of the HIA. For example, an HIA might be presented at a City Council meeting in the form of a formal presentation to decision makers and communicated to local community members via handouts or social media.

MONITORING AND EVALUATION

Monitoring and evaluation is the sixth step in the conduct of an HIA. These are related but distinct activities. *Monitoring* refers to the development and conduct of an implementation plan for following up on the recommendations of the HIA. A complete HIA report should include the implementation plan and should document stakeholder engagement in the development of that plan. Monitoring includes proposing indicators, actions, responsible parties, and a timeline for such implementation.[38] The activities of implementation typically occur after the HIA report is complete and may be conducted by staff different from those who wrote the HIA report. For example, in the Hawaii Agricultural Plan HIA,[39] the change in Hawaii Island's farm and ranch employment (indicator) would be monitored by the Hawaii State Departments of Agriculture and Labor (responsible parties) from 2012 to ongoing (timeline).

Evaluation of HIA is important to assess the outcomes of the HIA, improve methods, identify positive and negative unintended consequences, and justify requests for future resources. Three types of evaluation can be conducted on HIAs: process, impact, and outcome.[1] A *process* evaluation examines the process followed in conducting an HIA compared to the practitioner's intended plan or to established guidelines for HIA practice.[38] An *impact* evaluation examines the impacts of an HIA on specific decisions and other events; such information is valuable to those who decide whether to conduct HIAs. For example, an impact evaluation of the Clark County (Oregon) Bicycle and Pedestrian Master Plan HIA found that eight of the 11 HIA recommendations were fully adopted and the other three were partially adopted.[40] The third type, *outcome* evaluation, examines changes in health status or health determinants due to the HIA, but is rarely conducted.

The Role of Stakeholders in Monitoring and Evaluation

Decision makers can play a key role in helping to develop a monitoring plan. As in the recommendations stage, they will be able to identify who is responsible for implementing the proposed recommendation, and therefore who will be responsible for monitoring that change over time. Members of the steering committee, who are based in the affected community, can also help to track the impacts of the HIA, and impacts of the decision over time, and keep decision makers accountable to what they have agreed to change.

THE EFFECTIVENESS OF HIA

Effectiveness of HIAs can be categorized into four categories[41]: *Direct* (leads to changes in decision), *General* (raises awareness but no specific changes in decision), *Opportunistic* (favorable decision would have been made anyway), and *Ineffective* (HIA ignored in decision). In practice, these categories may be difficult to use when different aspects of a single HIA fall into multiple categories.

Based on impacts in approximately 200 individual HIAs, one report synthesized the key findings, success factors, and challenges from five large HIA impact evaluation studies from the United States, Europe, Australia, and New Zealand.[42] This report found that major impacts of HIA include directly influencing some decisions, improving collaboration among stakeholders, increasing awareness of health issues among decision makers, and giving community members a stronger voice in local decisions. Factors that contribute to successful HIAs include engaging stakeholders, timeliness, policy, and systems support for conducting HIAs, having persons with appropriate skills on the HIA team, obtaining the support of decision makers, and providing clear feasible recommendations. Challenges that may reduce HIA success include poor timeliness, underestimation of time and resources needed, difficulty in accessing relevant data, use of jargon in HIA reports, difficulty in involving decision makers in the HIA process, and absence of a requirement to conduct HIAs.

CHALLENGES IN HIA PRACTICE

There are a number of challenges and research opportunities related to the conduct of HIAs.[42] First, funding, time, and capacity to conduct HIAs are major challenges because HIAs have not been institutionalized into routine public health practice in most places. There is some flexibility within each HIA step that allows HIAs to be scaled to the resources, time, and capacity available.

Second, further work is needed to document the value of HIA in promoting equity and reducing health inequities. Such work requires identifying appropriate indicators of equity that are likely to be affected by decisions and for which changes can be measured.

Third, because the impacts of HIAs are complex, no simple answer exists for policymakers and funders who ask how HIAs make a difference in decision making. HIAs are more likely to make a difference in decision making and potentially improve health if they have the characteristics described above for successful HIAs, such as engaging stakeholders, timeliness, and offering practical recommendations. HIAs may be more effective in some sectors than in others.

Fourth, unlike EIAs, most HIAs conducted in the United States have been voluntary, meaning that decision makers are neither required to seek the conduct of an HIA nor required to consider its recommendations if an HIA is done. This situation is unlikely to change in an antiregulatory environment.

Fifth, HIAs range from rapid desktop analyses to comprehensive studies that require substantial time and resources. Further work could lead to guidelines on the depth and breadth of HIAs needed for projects and policies in various contexts.

Sixth, the importance of an implementation and monitoring plan in the recommendations of an HIA is often underemphasized by HIA practitioners. Further work could establish best practices to routinely create such plans in HIAs and facilitate follow-up of these plans.

HIA AROUND THE WORLD

Internationally, substantial work in HIA began in the early 1990s, primarily in Europe.[9] This, combined with the World Health Organization's (WHO) promotion of HIA as a tool to promote health and health equity,[10,11,43] led to the uptake of HIA practice in various countries around the world.[44] Europe and the United Kingdom are host to several WHO Collaborating Centers for Health Impact Assessment.[45] HIA practice has also been promoted widely in Oceania, with Australia developing a national framework for the integration of HIA into EIA.[46] In Asia, there has also been formalization of HIA practice with countries like Mongolia[47] incorporating HIA in their rules and regulations for conducting EIA, and China incorporating HIA into their action plans on environment and health.[48] There are both nascent and established HIA programs in countries such as Canada,[49] Thailand,[50] South Korea,[51]

New Zealand,[52] and Scotland.[53] There is also increasing promotion of the use of HIA in Southeast Asia,[54] Africa,[55] the Middle East,[56] and Latin America.[57]

The first reported HIA conducted in the United States was in 1999 on a living wage ordinance in San Francisco, California.[58] The use of HIA in the United States has grown since then,[59] with 419 HIAs completed or in progress as of January 2018.[16] Interest in HIA has also spurred the development of established HIA programs,[60] academic research,[9] university courses,[61] training programs,[9] and the establishment of a professional society dedicated to HIA.[62] While HIA is not federally mandated in the United States, there have been efforts to institutionalize the practice. Organizations like the National Prevention Council,[63] U.S. Department of Health and Human Services,[64] Centers for Disease Control and Prevention,[65] and U.S. Environmental Protection Agency[66] have provided guidance and support for the use of HIA.

FUTURE DIRECTIONS FOR THE FIELD

As a relatively new field, HIA is continually adapting to current public health research and priorities. Some organizations have established HIA programs and advocated for further institutionalization of HIA practice. The Minnesota Department of Health established a program to conduct HIAs throughout the State, provide training and technical assistance on HIA, and has facilitated a Minnesota HIA Coalition that supports the incorporation of health in decision making.[67] The Alaska state health department has established a state level HIA program and considers HIA as "one aspect of a 'best practices' approach to responsible development in Alaska."[68] In Wales, the government established an HIA support unit as part of its strategy to improve health and equity.[69] In 2017, the Welsh government passed the Public Health (Wales) Bill which included a requirement for HIA, making it a statutory process for all public bodies (local authorities, health boards, etc.) in Wales.[70] As policymakers see the value from the evidence and recommendations created from the HIA process, more HIA programs and policies may be established throughout the world.

Interest in HIA has also been included as part of growing support for the Health in All Policies (HiAP)[2] approach to reducing health disparities and promoting health (Box 44-6). HIA has been promoted as a tool that can help to address the integration of HiAP.[71] The state of California initiated work on this approach with the formation of a multiagency Health in All Policies Task Force based on an executive order from the governor in 2010.[72] The South Australian Government established an HiAP approach which includes a health lens analysis, similar to HIA.[73] As countries adopt HiAP frameworks, HIA may be implemented and adapted as part of these approaches to improving health and equity.

CONCLUSION

The primary purpose of using health impact assessment as a tool in decision making is to increase the awareness of health impacts in other sectors, so that such impacts are routinely considered in all decisions that affect people. Eventually it may be possible to achieve healthy outcomes without needing to conduct a formal HIA on every proposed individual policy and project. Should that occur, such an accomplishment would be due in large part to the success of the hundreds of HIAs that have been and are now being done.

BOX 44-6 Health in All Policies Definition

"Health in all policies is an approach to public policies across sectors that systematically takes into account the health implication of decisions, seeks synergies, and avoids harmful health impacts in order to improve population health and health equity."[2]

References

1. National Research Council. *Improving Health in the United States: The Role of Health Impact Assessment.* Washington, DC: National Academies Press; 2011.
2. World Health Organization, Ministry of Social Affairs and Health Finland. The Helsinki Statement on Health in all Policies. Paper presented at The 8th Global Conference on Health Promotion2013; Helsinki, Finland.
3. World Health Organization. *Adelaide Recommendations on Healthy Public Policy.* Adelaide, South Australia, April 5–9, 1988.
4. National Environmental Policy Act of 1969.
5. Hargrove W, Juarez-Carillo P. *Health Vinton/Vinton Saludable HIA demonstration project final report.* Center for Environmental Resource Management, University of Texas El Paso; 2014.
6. Hom E, Dannenberg A, Farquhar S, Thornhill L. A systematic review of health impact assessments in the criminal justice system. *Am J Crim Justice.* 2017;42(4):883–908.
7. Cowling K, Lindberg R, Dannenberg A, Neff R, Pollack K. Review of health impact assessments informing agriculture, food, and nutrition policies, programs, and projects in the United States. *J Agric Food Syst Commun Dev.* 2017;7(3):139–57.
8. Wernham A, Bhatia R. Integrating human health into environmental impact assessment: An unrealized opportunity for environmental health and justice. *Environ Health Perspect.* 2008;116:991–1000.
9. Dannenberg AL. A brief history of health impact assessment in the United States. *Chronicles Health Impact Assess.* 2016;1(1):1-8.
10. World Health Organization. The Ottawa charter for health promotion: First International Conference on Health Promotion, Ottawa, November 21, 1986.
11. WHO European Centre for Health Policy. Health impact assessment: Main concepts and suggested approach. The Gothenburg Consensus Paper. Brussels: WHO Regional Office for Europe; 1999.
12. Hebert KA, Wendel AM, Kennedy SK, Dannenberg AL. Health impact assessment: A comparison of 45 local, national, and international guidelines. *Environ Impact Assess Rev.* 2012;34:74–82.
13. Ewan C, Ewan CE. *National framework for environmental and health impact assessment.* National Health and Medical Research Council; 1993.
14. Abrahams D, Den Broeder L, Doyle C, et al. EPHIA-European policy health impact assessment: A guide. International Health Impact Assessment Consortium Liverpool: IMPACT, University of Liverpool. 2004.
15. Harris P, Harris-Roxas B, Harris E, Kemp L. *Health Impact Assessment: A Practical Guide.* Sydney, Australia: Centre for Health Equity Training, Research and Evaluation, Part of the UNSW Centre for Primary Health Care and Equity, UNSW; 2007.
16. Health Impact Project. Data Visualization: HIA in the United States. 2015. http://www.pewtrusts.org/en/multimedia/data-visualizations/2015/hia-map. Accessed January 29, 2018.
17. World Health Organization. *The Ottawa Charter for Health Promotion: First International Conference on Health Promotion,* Ottawa, November 21, 1986.
18. World Health Organization. The Bangkok charter for health promotion in a globalized world. 2006.
19. Dahlgren G, Whitehead M. *Policies and Strategies to Promote Social Equity in Health.* Stockholm: Institute for Future Studies; 1991.
20. World Health Organization. Closing the Gap in a Generation: Health Equity through Action on the Social Determinants of Health: Commission on Social Determinants of Health Final Report. World Health Organization. 2008.
21. Marmot M, Bell R. Fair society, healthy lives. *Public Health.* 2012;126:S4–10.
22. Kemm J. Health impact assessment: A tool for healthy public policy. *Health Promot Int.* 2001;16(1):79–85.
23. Harris P, Sainsbury P, Kemp L. The fit between health impact assessment and public policy: Practice meets theory. *Soc Sci Med.* 2014;108:46–53.
24. Simpson S, Mahoney M, Harris E, Aldrich R, Stewart-Williams J. Equity-focused health impact assessment: A tool to assist policy makers in addressing health inequalities. *Environ Impact Assess Rev.* 2005;25(7–8):772–82.
25. U.S. Environmental Protection Agency. Red Dog Mine Extension—Aqqaluk Project: Supplemental Environmental Impact Statement—3.13 Health. 2009.
26. Bond R, Curran J, Kirkpatrick C, Lee N, Francis P. Integrated impact assessment for sustainable development: A case study approach. *World Dev.* 2001;29(6):1011–24.
27. Whitehead M. The concepts and principles of equity and health. *Int J Health Serv.* 1992;22(3):429–45.

28. Stakeholder participation working group of the 2010 HIA of the Americas Workshop. *Guidance and best practices for stakeholder participation in health impact assessments: Version 1*. Oakland, CA. 2012.
29. Human Impact Partners, Group Health Research Institute. Community participation in health impact assessments: A national evaluation. Seattle, WA. 2016.
30. Quigley R, Cavanagh S, Harrison D, Taylor L, Pottle M. *Clarifying Approaches to: Health Needs Assessment, Health Impact Assessment, Integrated Impact Assessment, Health Equity Audit, and Race Equality Impact Assessment*. London: Health Development Agency; 2005.
31. San Francisco Department of Public Health. Baseline Conditions Assessment of HOPE SF Redevelopment: Sunnydale. 2010. http://www.pewtrusts.org/~/media/assets/2010/09/sunnydalepublichousingredevelopment.pdf. Accessed January 30, 2018.
32. Petticrew M, Roberts H. Evidence, hierarchies, and typologies: Horses for courses. *J Epidemiol Commun Health*. 2003;57(7):527–9.
33. Wier M, Weintraub J, Humphreys EH, Seto E, Bhatia R. An area-level model of vehicle-pedestrian injury collisions with implications for land use and transportation planning. *Accid Anal Prev*. 2009;41(1):137–45.
34. Haigh F, Harris P, Chok NN, Coffey J, Thornell M. *Villawood East Master Plan: Health Impact Assessment Report*. Sydney, Australia: Centre for Health Equity Training, Research and Evaluation, part of the Centre for Primary Health Care and Equity, UNSW; 2013.
35. The Sequoia Foundation. A health impact assessment of the proposed Cabin Creek Biomass Energy Facility in Placer County, California. 2012. http://ucanr.edu/sites/swet/files/176217.pdf.
36. Fredsgaard MW, Cave B, Bond A. *A Review Package for Health Impact Assessment Reports of Development Projects*. Leeds, UK: Ben Cave Associates, Ltd; 2009.
37. Spicket J, Katscherian D. *A Guide for the Evaluation of Health Impact Assessments Carried Out within the EIA Process*. WHO Collaborating Centre for Environmental Health Impact Assessment; 2014.
38. Bhatia R, Farhang L, Heller J, et al. Minimum elements and practice standards for Health Impact Assessment, Version 3. 2014.
39. Kohala Center. Health Impact Assessment of 2010 Hawai'i County Agriculture Development Plan. 2012.
40. Clark County Public Health. Evaluation of health impact assessment: Clark County bicycle and pedestrian master plan. 2011.
41. Wismar M, Blau J, Ernst K, Figueras J. *The Effectiveness of Health Impact Assessment: Scope and Limitations of Supporting Decision-Making in Europe*. Brussels: European Observatory on Health Systems and Policies; 2007.
42. Dannenberg AL. Effectiveness of health impact assessments: A synthesis of data from five impact evaluation reports. *Prev Chronic Dis*. 2016;13(E84).
43. World Health Organization. The Jakarta Declaration on Leading Health Promotion into the 21st Century. 1997.
44. Harris-Roxas B, Viliani F, Bond A, et al. Health impact assessment: The state of the art. *Impact Assess Proj Apprais*. 2012;30(1):43–52.
45. World Health Organization. WHO Collaborating Centres on HIA. http://www.who.int/hia/network/cc/en/. Accessed January 29, 2018.
46. National Health and Medical Research Council. *National Framework for Environmental and Health Impact Assessment*. Canberra: Commonwealth of Australia; 1994.
47. WHO Representative Office Mongolia. Country programme on extractive industries and health. 2014. http://www.wpro.who.int/mongolia/mediacentre/releases/country_programme_on_extractive_industries_and_health/en/. Accessed January 29, 2018.
48. People's Republic of China. National Environmental Action Plan 2007–2015. http://www.china.org.cn/english/environment/238275.htm. Accessed January 29, 2018.
49. National Collaborating Centre for Healthy Public Policy, Institut National de Santé Publique Québec. Health Impact Assessment. 2010; http://www.ncchpp.ca/54/Health_Impact_Assessment.ccnpps. Accessed January 29, 2018.
50. Phoolcharoen W, Sukkumnoed D, Kessomboon P. Development of health impact assessment in Thailand: Recent experiences and challenges. *Bull World Health Organ*. 2003;81(6):465–7.
51. Kim D, Kim J. Health impact assessment in healthy cities in Korea: Working Paper 2011–02. Korea Institute for Health and Social Affairs; 2011.
52. Canterbury District Health Board Community and Public Health. Health in All Policies. 2018. https://www.cph.co.nz/your-health/health-in-all-policies/. Accessed January 31, 2018.
53. NHS Health Scotland. Scottish health and inequalities impact assessment network. 2014. http://www.healthscotland.com/resources/networks/shian.aspx. Accessed January 31, 2018.
54. Caussy D, Kumar P, Sein UT. Health impact assessment needs in south-east Asian countries. *Bull World Health Organ*. 2003;81:439–43.
55. O'Mullane M. *Integrating Health Impact Assessment with the Policy Process: Lessons and Experiences from Around the World*. Oxford: Oxford University Press; 2013.
56. Fakhri A, Harris P, Maleki M. Proposing a framework for health impact assessment in Iran. *BMC Public Health*. 2015;15(1):335.
57. Kwiatkowski R. The role of health impact assessment in advancing sustainable development in Latin America and the Caribbean. *J Environ Health*. 2015;77(8):16.
58. Bhatia R, Katz M. Estimation of health benefits from a local living wage ordinance. *Am J Public Health*. 2001;91(9):1398–402.
59. Dannenberg AL, Bhatia R, Cole BL, Heaton SK, Feldman JD, Rutt CD. Use of health impact assessment in the U.S.: 27 Case studies, 1999–2007. *Am J Prev Med*. 2008;34(3):241–56.
60. Society of Practitioners of Health Impact Assessment Working Group. Building regional capacity for health impact assessment: Mapping regional resources.
61. Pollack KM, Dannenberg AL, Botchwey ND, Stone CL, Seto E. Developing a model curriculum for a university course in health impact assessment in the USA. *Impact Assess Proj Apprais*. 2015;33(1):80–5.
62. Society of Practitioners of Health Impact Assessment. SOPHIA: Society of Practitioners of Health Impact Assessment. https://hiasociety.org/. Accessed January 31, 2018.
63. National Prevention Council. National Prevention Strategy: America's plan for better health and wellness. Office of the Surgeon General; 2011.
64. Healthy People 2020. Evidence-Based Resource Summary. 2018. https://www.healthypeople.gov/2020/tools-resources/evidence-based-resource/transportation-health-impact-assessment-toolkit. Accessed January 31, 2018.
65. Centers for Disease Control and Prevention. Health impact assessment. 2016. https://www.cdc.gov/healthyplaces/hia.htm. Accessed January 31, 2018.
66. U.S. Environmental Protection Agency. The health impact assessment (HIA) resource and tool compilation: A comprehensive toolkit for new and experience HIA practitioners in the U.S. 2016.
67. Minnesota Department of Health. Health impact assessment (HIA). 2017. http://www.health.state.mn.us/divs/hia/. Accessed January 31, 2018.
68. Reproduced with permission from Alaska Department of Health and Social Services. Alaska Health impact assessment (HIA) program. 2015. http://dhss.alaska.gov/dph/Epi/hia/Pages/default.aspx. Accessed January 31, 2018.
69. Public Health Network CYMRU. Welcome to the Wales Health Impact Assessment Support Unit. 2018. http://www.health.state.mn.us/divs/hia/. Accessed January 31, 2018.
70. Public Health (Wales) Act 2017.
71. American Public Health Association. Promoting health impact assessment to achieve health in all policies. 2012.
72. California Department of Public Health. Health in all policies (HIAP). 2018. https://www.cdph.ca.gov/Programs/OHE/Pages/HIAP.aspx#. Accessed March 13, 2018.
73. Government of South Australia. *The South Australian Approach to Health in All Policies: Background and Practical Guide*. Rundle Mall, South Australia: Department of Health; 2011.

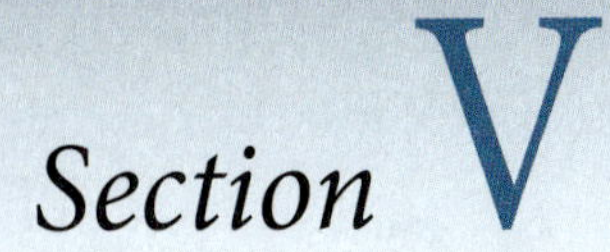

Section Editor
Paul Halverson

Healthcare and Public Health Systems

CHAPTER

45 Structure and Function of the Public Health System in the United States

Thomas Quade • Kailey Love • William Riley

OVERVIEW

Public health is defined as "the efforts organized by society to protect, promote, and restore the people's health...directed to the maintenance and improvement of the health of all the people through collective or social actions."[1] The *public health system* is a complex network of organizations working together collectively to assure conditions in which society can be healthy.[2,3] This system includes a wide array of government agencies, private organizations, public health departments, community health centers, healthcare systems, advocacy groups, the media, and social service agencies. The governmental role to protect the public's health is represented by *public health agencies* at several levels of responsibility: federal, tribal, state, territorial, and local.[4]

Public health contributes tremendous value to society. Its prevention efforts are responsible for 25 years of the nearly 30-year improvement in life expectancy at birth in the United States over the past century. This is based on evidence that only about 5 years of the 30-year improvement are the result of medical care.[5] Public health approaches carry significant potential for future contributions as well, since almost half of all deaths in the United States are premature and result from preventable causes.[6] This chapter will review the structure and function of public health in the United States. (Also see Chap. 9: Public Health Practice in the United States.)

THE STRUCTURE OF PUBLIC HEALTH

Public health is practiced in a variety of settings by a variety of professionals. Although community-based organizations and health systems contribute to the practice of public health, it is typically associated with a constellation of activities at the federal, state, and particularly, local levels. Unlike many community-based organizations, only official public health agencies have statutory responsibility for the health status of the populations they serve. Legal authority for this responsibility is based on a variety of federal, state, and local ordinances, including the granting of police powers.

The structure and function of modern public health in the United States has accelerated dramatically following a 1988 IOM report that described the public health system as being in disarray, with no coherent vision or mission.[2] Adding to this impetus were the threats of terrorism and the expanding role of public health in addressing social determinants of health in an era of increasing social disparity. Previous approaches to illness and health have been replaced with a new understanding of the complex relationship between social issues, cultural factors, genetics, behavior, illness care, and prevention. Today, public health spans almost all health discipline, relying upon the three core functions of public health: Assessment, Policy Development, and Assurance.

Public Health's Three Core Functions

It has been over 30 years since the IOM identified the three core functions for governmental public health departments: Assessment, Policy Development, and Assurance.[2] These core functions are described below.

Assessment. Every public health agency should regularly and systematically collect, assemble, analyze, and make available information on the health of the community, including statistics on health status, community health needs, and epidemiologic and other studies of health problems.

Policy Development. Every public health agency should exercise its responsibility to serve the public interest in the development of comprehensive public health policies by promoting the use of the scientific knowledge base in decision making about public health and by leading in developing public health policy.

Assurance. Public health agencies should assure their constituents that services necessary to achieve agreed upon goals are provided, either by encouraging actions by other entities, by requiring such action through regulation, or by providing services directly. They should also involve key policy makers and the public in determining a set of high-priority personal and community-wide health services that governments will guarantee to every member of the community, including subsidization of direct provision of personal healthcare.

The three core functions of public health do not include individual-care services. While it is a core function of public health to ensure equity and access, this does not involve service delivery. Nevertheless, some public health agencies provide clinical-care services such as primary-care clinics, home healthcare, and vaccinations.[3]

The Ten Essential Services

The U.S. Department of Health and Human Services convened a workgroup in 1994 to determine how public health activities could be more clearly described. This workgroup developed the Ten Essential Services in 1995 to more clearly define the services communities needed in order to achieve the three core functions of public health.[7] Those Ten Essential Services include:

1. Monitor health status to identify community health problems.
2. Diagnose and investigate health problems and health hazards in the community.
3. Inform, educate, and empower people about health issues.
4. Mobilize community partnerships to identify and solve health problems.
5. Develop policies and plans that support individual and community health efforts.
6. Enforce laws and regulations that protect health and ensure safety.
7. Link people to needed personal health services and ensure the provision of healthcare when otherwise unavailable.
8. Ensure a competent public health and personal health workforce.

9. Evaluate effectiveness, accessibility, and quality of personal and population-based health services.
10. Research for new insights and innovative solutions to health problems.

These Ten Essential Services have become the central focal point for many public health activities, including evaluating the capacity of communities to assess their capacity for healthfulness, defining a public health research agenda, and providing a framework for determining the workforce competencies required to deliver them well. The relationships of the essential services to the IOM's three core functions are illustrated below in Fig. 45-1.[7,8]

National Public Health Performance Standards

The National Public Health Performance Standards (NPHPS) were developed by the Centers for Disease Control and Prevention (CDC) for both the state-level public health system as well as the local public health system to operationalize the Ten Essential Services.[8] The NPHPS are designed to assist governmental public health agencies in assessing and improving their public health systems. Initially intended to describe the work of local health departments, they have subsequently been recognized as a compilation of services that need to be available in communities for populations to be as healthy as possible. In addition to assessing the activities engaged by health departments, the NPHPS also include activities of many other individuals, groups, agencies, and institutions. This broadens the concept of public health to include everyone involved in efforts to improve health status.

Public Health Accreditation

The Public Health Accreditation Board (PHAB)[9] is a nonprofit entity formed in 2007 to implement and oversee national public health department accreditation. The PHAB is based on the belief that the best way to improve population health status is to improve the performance of public health departments. The PHAB accreditation process is based on the national public health performance standards and dedicated to continuous quality improvement (QI). QI in public health is defined as a distinct management process using a set of QI tools and techniques to ensure that public health departments consistently meet their community's health need and improve the health status of their populations.[10]

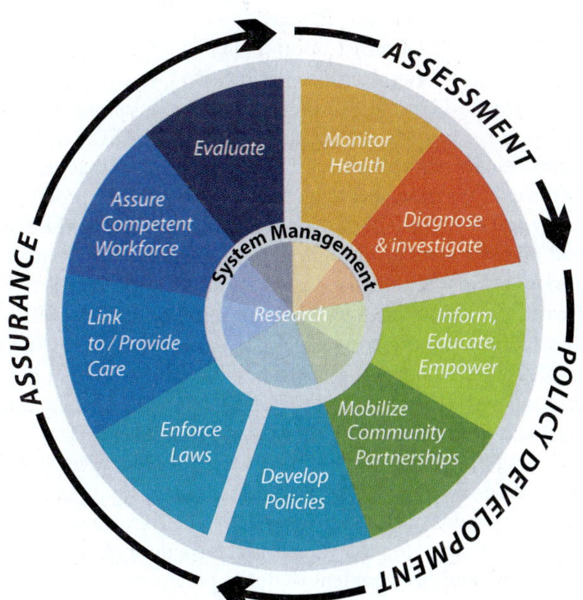

FIGURE 45-1. Ten essential services. (*Source:* Carson City: Health and Human Services. The Ten Essential Public Health Services. Reproduced with permission from Carson City: Health and Human Services. The Ten Essential Public Health Services. Retrieved from http:// gethealthycarsoncity.org/home/the-10-essential-public-health-services/.[8])

Health departments may become accredited by successfully completing a peer review process. The PHAB accreditation process consists of 12 domains and over 32 standards based on a self-assessment with a peer-reviewed process involving the degree to which the health department conforms to the set of standards and measures that are matched to the Ten Essential Services. Currently, over 223 state, tribal, and local health departments are accredited which serve a population of over 214 million persons, constituting 66% of the U.S. population.[9,11] PHAB continuously engages in a process to assure that the standards and measures reflect and facilitate the evolution of best practices.

The Role of Public Health Professional Associations

Public Health Associations play a key role in the development of public health professionals. Continuing education is required in many public health professions and highly recommended wherever it is not required due to the nature of the work, the technology, and the continual policy landscape changes. Additionally, it provides an excellent opportunity to fill one of the notable gaps in public health education: leadership development. Public health leaders are frequently promoted from positions within public health organizations, often with few leadership experiences or opportunities to learn effective leadership skills. However, professional development can be nurtured through professional associations. The primary professional associations are described below.

- **American Public Health Association (APHA)**
  The American Public Health Association (APHA) is the largest of all of the public health associations and is the most diverse in its membership as it advances the work of public health practitioners, educators, researchers, and policy advocates. It has 54 local affiliates and represents the voices of approximately 50,000 combined affiliate, organizational, and individual members. Founded in 1872, it also the longest history of the public health associations. The APHA is a highly respected source of public health policy information.
- **Association of State and Territorial Health Officials (ASTHO)**[35]
  All 50 states, the District of Columbia, and 8 U.S. territories have a governmental public health agency with a chief health official. The Association of State and Territorial Health Officials (ASTHO) supports public health officers at the state and territorial levels to advance the public's health and well-being.
- **National Association of County and City Health Officials (NACCHO)**
  The National Association of County and City Health Officials (NACCHO) was formed in 1994 when the National Association of County Health Departments (the national association for directors of county health departments) and the United States Conference of Local Health Officers (the national professional association for directors of city health departments) merged. NACCHO is an important contributor to the development of strategies and tools for public health practice and an important force in the development of national public health policy. NACCHO has state-level affiliated associations, referred to as State Association of Country and City Health Officials (SACCHO) though locally they may be called something else, for example, Association of Health Commissioners.
- **National Association of Local Boards of Health (NALBOH)**
  Most local health departments are governed by a board of health. Because they are typically citizen boards appointed by elected officials, a large majority of board of health members have little or no background in the health sciences and have relied on the health department they represent to inform them about the discipline of public health and their responsibilities to it. The National Association of Local Boards of Health (NALBOH) was formed in 1992 to provide training for local board of health members.

NALBOH has state-level associations in many states that are comprised of local boards of health.

- **National Network of Public Health Institutes (NNPHI)**
  The National Network of Public Health Institutes (NNPHI) serves as a central hub aiding more than 40 public health institutes across the country. These public health institutes are nonprofit organizations that advance public health practice, largely through convening, training, and other capacity building efforts. They also make systematic improvements in population health through policy development and dissemination.
- **National Environmental Health Association (NEHA)**
  A large portion of the mandated regulatory work done in health departments is in environmental health and performed by Registered Sanitarians who serve as the health inspector. The National Environmental Health Association (NEHA) is the national public health practice association that provides credentialing, continuing education, and training resources for its members. NEHA publishes a peer-reviewed journal, *Journal of Environmental Health*. Many states have state-level environmental health associations that are also involved in state-level policy development and advocacy efforts as well as workforce continuing education.
- **Association of Public Health Nurses (APHN)**

The Association of Public Health Nurses (APHN) began as the Association of State and Territorial Directors of Nursing in 1935 and served as an advisory group of state health department nurses. The APHN is an affiliate of ASTHO and a forum to exchange ideas and opportunities for networking among public health nurses at all levels. The APHN provides continuing education units (CEUs) for public health nursing credentialing as well as engages in policy development and advocacy for the public's health.

The Role of the Federal Government

The federal government has a central role in the public health system, with the Department of Health and Human Services (DHHS) serving as the main federal authority in health. Federal government powers derive from two areas in the U.S. Constitution: (1) the power to protect the public's health and safety through the commerce clause, and (2) the power to tax and spend for the general welfare.[12] These federal activities fall into two major categories. The first category includes *direct functions* such as assessment, policy making, resource development, knowledge transfer, and financing. The second category consists of *contracted functions*, which are primarily to the states and territories, and local communities.[13]

The federal responsibility to protect the health of the public has evolved significantly over time. Today, the federal government performs a crucial role in six main areas of population health. These six areas are: (1) policy making, (2) finance, (3) public health protection, (4) collection and dissemination of information about U.S. health and healthcare delivery systems, (5) capacity building for population health, and (6) direct management of services.[3] The federal government authorizes the expenditure of federal funds, sets taxes on products to promote healthy use or discourage unhealthy use, and regulates business and persons whose activities may affect interstate commerce. Decisions by the judicial branch can also impact federal policy in many ways that affect health, such as upholding governmental power to protect people's health, setting conditions on the receipt of public funds, and upholding a woman's right to reproductive privacy.[3]

The Department of Health and Human Services

Public health-related activities and responsibilities are scattered throughout the federal government, but the principle federal agency for health-related programs is the Department of Health and Human Services (DHHS). DHHS is involved in policy making, financing of public health activities, public health protection, collection and dissemination of information, capacity building, and direct management of services.[3]

The Public Health Service (PHS) is the agency within DHHS responsible for the public health of the American people through a number of health agencies. The PHS originated as the Marine Hospital Service in the late 1700s to meet the needs of Merchant Marine seamen.[14] The Service was later renamed the Public Health Service when it took on new responsibilities, most notably providing states with expertise to deal with major infectious disease epidemics.[15] The PHS consists of eight major operating agencies listed below.

- **Agency for Healthcare Research and Quality (AHRQ)**[16]
  The Agency for Healthcare Research and Quality's (AHRQ) mission is to produce evidence to make healthcare safer, higher quality, more accessible, equitable, and affordable, and to work within the U.S. Department of Health and Human Services and with other partners to make sure that the evidence is understood and used.
- **Agency for Toxic Substances and Disease Registry (ATSDR)**[17]
  The Agency for Toxic Substances and Disease Registry (ATSDR) is charged with carrying out the health-related responsibilities related to federal laws concerned with the release of toxic substances into the environment. It directs programs designed to protect workers and the general public from exposure to hazardous substances. The ATSDR collects, analyzes, and disseminates data relating to serious diseases resulting from exposure to toxic or hazardous substances; maintains listing of areas either close to the public or restricted in use because of toxic contamination; and helps the Environmental Protection Agency to identify hazardous waste substances requiring regulation. It also works with private and public healthcare organizations to provide medical care and testing to individuals who may have been exposed.
- **Centers for Disease Control and Prevention (CDC)**[18]
  The Centers for Disease Control and Prevention (CDC) was established in 1973 and is responsible for the prevention and control of diseases as well as responding to public health emergencies. In consultation with state and local healthcare authorities, the CDC develops and administers national programs to help prevent and control the spread of communicable and preventable diseases and to prevent chronic disease. The agency also directs and enforces quarantine activities and provides consultation to other nations on the control of preventable diseases.
- **Food and Drug Administration (FDA)**[19]
  The Food and Drug Administration (FDA) was formed in 1970 and charged with protecting the health of the nation against unsafe foods, drugs, medical devices, and cosmetics. The FDA carries out its mission through a number of centers and offices that perform a large variety of tasks, including testing and evaluating products for safety and effectiveness; developing standards ensuring the quality and nutritional value of foods; and testing and labeling medical devices before they are made available for use by the public.
- **Health Resources and Services Administration (HRSA)**[20]
  The Health Resources and Services Administration (HRSA) is responsible for addressing the access, quality, and cost of healthcare. HRSA works with states and communities to help deliver healthcare to underserved areas and groups with special needs, including migrant workers, mothers and children, homeless people, immigrant populations, and individuals living in rural areas. HRSA also administers the National Organ Transplant Act, serving as a resource for individuals seeking information about the availability and procurement of donor organs and bone marrow. A number of bureaus within HRSA provide additional services including the Bureau of Primary Health Care to recruit professionals to health professional shortage areas. HRSA also operates the Maternal and Child Health Bureau (MCH) to develop federal policies to improve healthcare service delivery to mothers, children, and infants.

- **Indian Health Service (IHS)**[21]
 The Indian Health Service (IHS) is responsible for providing federal health services to American Indians and Alaska Natives. The responsibility to provide members of federally recognized tribes health services is based on Article I, Section 8 of the U.S. Constitution. The IHS goal is to raise the health status for Indian people and provide a comprehensive health service delivery system for approximately 2 million American Indians and Alaska Natives who belong to 566 federally recognized tribes in 35 states. Health services provided include medical, dental, and environmental health programs.
- **National Institutes of Health (NIH)**[22]
 The National Institutes of Health (NIH) is the principal biomedical research agency of the federal government, with a number of institutes that conduct research in specific areas, including: (1) The National Cancer Institute, which has made the cure of cancer a national goal; (2) The National Heart, Lung, and Blood Institute, which conducts research into the uses of blood and the management of blood resources, administers programs for the prevention and treatment of hypertension, stroke, respiratory illnesses, and sickle cell anemia; (3) Other institutes to conduct research in the areas of alcohol and drug abuse, mental health, communication and neurological disorders, and aging; and (4) Operating the National Library of Medicine (NLM) the nation's chief source of medical information which makes medical research databases such as MEDLINE and TOXLINE available to the public.
- **Substance Abuse and Mental Health Services Administration (SAMHSA)**[23]

The Substance Abuse and Mental Health Services Administration (SAMHSA) is the agency within the U.S. Department of Health and Human Services that leads public health efforts to reduce the impact of substance abuse and mental illness on America's communities. People suffering from either substance use and mental disorders, or both, because of their illness are often excluded from the current healthcare system. The gap in service to this population unnecessarily jeopardizes the health and wellness of people and causes a ripple effect in costs to American communities.

The Public Health Service Commissioned Corps The PHS also includes the U.S. Public Health Service Commissioned Corps, consisting of more than 6700 public health professionals dedicated to delivering the nation's public health programs.[24] The Commissioned Corps is one of America's seven uniformed services, which fulfills essential public health roles within the nation's federal government agencies and programs. Officers are assigned to all of the PHS Agencies and to a number of agencies outside of PHS, including the Bureau of Prisons, U.S. Coast Guard, and the Environmental Protection Agency.[25]

In addition, there are significant activities related to public health that occur outside of DHHS in other parts of the executive branch. Examples include the Women, Infants, and Children Program (WIC) run by the Department of Agriculture (the largest public health program in the country in terms of dollars spent), the many pollution and contamination control programs run by the Environmental Protection Agency (EPA), the workplace safety programs run by the Occupational Safety and Health Administration (OSHA) which is part of the Department of Labor, and the healthcare and public health services provided to active-duty military personnel by the Department of Defense.

The State Public Health Role

The U.S. Constitution designates the state government as the principal entity responsible for protecting the public's health.[2] Every state and eight territories have an agency with responsibility for public health activities.[26,35] States and their local subdivisions discharge their primary responsibility for health through laws and regulations concerning public health matters in their jurisdiction.[3]

The IOM describes the duties of the state health department as[2]:

- Assessment of the health needs in the state based on statewide data collection;
- Assurance of an adequate statutory base for health activities in the state;
- Establishment of statewide health objectives, delegating power to locals as appropriate and holding them accountable;
- Assurance of appropriate organized statewide effort to develop and maintain essential, personal, educational, and environmental health services; provision of access to necessary services; and solution of problems inimical to health;
- Guarantee of a minimum set of essential health services; and
- Support of local service capacity, especially when disparities in local ability to raise revenue and/or administer programs require subsidies, technical assistance, or direct action by the state to achieve adequate service levels.

The 50 states and 8 territories have developed agencies to fulfill these responsibilities. There is substantial variability in the organizational structures of these agencies. In some cases, the State Health Agency (SHA) is a cabinet-level office reporting directly to the governor. In other circumstances, the SHA functions are subsumed as part of a larger administrative organization, which often includes social services functions as well as health. SHAs are frequently led by political appointees who often have no substantive health expertise. These individuals report to their governors and are cabinet-level officers. (See Chap. 7: Public Health Surveillance.)

State Health Agency Activities

The activities of SHAs vary considerably. For example, state Medicaid programs typically do not report to the SHA.[2] Rather, Medicaid management is the responsibility of the state welfare agency. In fact, the group receiving the largest amount of public health services is women and children. Women and children also receive a substantial portion of Medicaid expenditures, thus providing opportunity for synergy between these two governmental functions. Environmental health was traditionally a part of the SHA's responsibility until the 1960s. At that point, growing concern about environmental degradation led interest groups and policy-makers to give special attention to many environmental issues. The federal government created the Environmental Protection Agency (EPA) in response to those same concerns and most states followed the federal lead by creating a state environmental protection agency separate from the SHA. Although most major environmental concerns are dealt with by state environmental protection agencies, most SHAs have retained responsibility for some environmental health issues, including food service, recreation facility inspections, and investigation of chronic disease clusters that might have an environmental etiology.

THE LOCAL PUBLIC HEALTH ROLE

Local health departments (LHDs) are the governmental entities closest to the community and citizens in every community, no matter how small or remote, should receive protection from a local public health delivery system.[2] Similar to the state health departments, the LHDs are responsible for implementing the three core functions and Ten Essential Services of public health. The LHD *assessment function* is to develop or collect information to analyze and understand the health status of their community.[2] The *policy development function* is to develop public health policies based on the best available scientific knowledge while the *assurance function* is to ensure that necessary services are provided.[2] With a majority of the U.S. population now served by accredited health departments, the minimum basic services delivered by local health departments have better standardization.

There are approximately 2800 local public health departments in the United States, and 40% serve less than 25,000 people while the majority (55%) of LHDs employ fewer than 25 FTEs.[11] The organizational relationships between the state and local health departments vary considerably. In five states the LHDs are units of the state government while in 27 states the LHDs are units of the local government. The remaining 18 states have more than one type of governance for the LHDs. Leadership at the local level is more stable than it is in SHAs. In 2016, approximately one in four top executives in LHDs had been in office 11 or more years. In general, the smaller jurisdictions have the longest tenure and the largest health departments experience turnover rates comparable to those in SHAs. Approximately 16% of LHD directors have doctoral degrees, and 46% have a master's degree. The larger LHDs are more likely to have doctoral-level top executives. Among those serving more than 500,000 people, 49% of the LHDs are led by someone with a doctoral degree.

Services

Despite the recommendation that a group of essential public health services be tendered by every LHD, the evidence shows that there is great disparity in services offered. Most LHDs report that they offer clinical preventive services, such as adult immunizations (90%), childhood immunizations (88%), tuberculosis testing (84%), HIV testing and counseling (62%), and blood lead testing (61%).[27]

The growing trend in states to provide Medicaid managed-care arrangements has moved paying clients out of health departments into the private sector without reducing the need for care for the growing numbers of uninsured. This threatens the viability of healthcare access for the medically disenfranchised, challenging both the private and public sectors to develop collaborative arrangements to assure continued access to personal health services.

In general, environmental issues are more clearly identified as the responsibility of the health department at the local level than they are at the state level. Most LHDs enforce state environmental laws (restaurant inspections, trailer park inspections, etc.), regulate private water and sewage systems, and enforce other local environmental ordinances. Confusion does sometimes occur when LHDs receive environmental complaints about problems when jurisdiction for dealing with those problems lies with other agencies. In these cases, it is the job of the LHD to coordinate the response and assure that the state or federal agency with jurisdiction follows through on investigation and resolution of the problem. Among the most common environmental health services provided by LHDs are food safety education (77%) and public health nuisance abatement (76%).[27]

THE FUNCTION OF GOVERNMENTAL PUBLIC HEALTH

The previous section reviewed the core functions, essential services, performance standards, accreditation, and the three levels of governmental public health. This section reviews selected topics related to functioning of public health departments including funding, leadership, and determinants of population health.

Public Health Funding

Funding for governmental Public Health departments is very low, especially in comparison to overall health expenditures. Public health funding for all federal, state, and local health departments was $82.1 billion in 2015 (federal $12.1 billion, state $28.6 billion, and local $41.4 billion).[28,29] This amount constitutes approximately 2.5% of total national health expenditures of $3.3 trillion.[28]

Funding for the three levels of governmental public health varies considerably. All *federal*-level funding is from federal sources while *state*-level funding is from both state and federal sources. Approximately 50% of state health agency funding flows from the federal government, primarily the United States Department of Agriculture (USDA) and, to a lesser extent, from the CDC.[29] At the *local* level, there are four major sources of funding: local taxes, state grants, federal grants, and fees for service. Over time, there have been a significant shift in the portion of support at the local level coming from each area. In addition, the average per person expenditure varies by the size of the LHD. The mean expenditure per person per year by departments serving 25,000 or fewer individuals in 2016 was $68.[11] For LHDs' serving populations greater than 1,000,000, the mean expenditure per person per year was $44.[11] These are small numbers given the range of responsibilities assumed by these agencies and in comparison to healthcare expenditures that are over $10,000 per person per year.[11,34]

Determinants of Health and Healthcare Expenditures

There is a substantial mismatch between the factors that affect the health of the population and where healthcare expenditures are made in our nation. Of the primary factors that affect the population health: (1) health behaviors such as nutrition, exercise, and smoking; (2) the influence of genetics on health such as cystic fibrosis; (3) environmental factors including air quality and clean water; and (4) the healthcare delivery system,[30] the most important impact on health is personal behaviors (50%), while the least important impact is the healthcare system (10%). In contrast, however, the three main categories of expenditure are: (1) access to healthcare delivery (such as physician and hospital ser-vices, drugs, and health insurance administration; (2) other costs such as research and capital expenditures; and (3) governmental public health expenditures. This represents a basic paradox in the healthcare system. While health behaviors have the greatest impact on health, very little healthcare expenditures are dedicated to pre-vention. The healthcare system is focused on treating persons after the occurrence of disease or injury, rather than health promotion and disease prevention.

Social Determinants of Health

The relationship between healthcare expenditures and the factors that affect health has been expanded in the last two decades to include the concept of the Social Determinants of Health (SDOH).[31] SDOH are conditions in the environments where people live, work, and play that affect a wide range of health, quality-of-life outcomes, and risks.[5] Resources that enhance quality of life can have a significant influence on population health outcomes. Examples of these resources include safe and affordable housing, access to education, public safety, availability of healthy foods, local emergency/health services, and environments free of life-threatening toxins.[11] Figure 45-2 shows five key social determinants of health developed by Health People 2020.[32] These five key areas include: Economic Stability, Education, Social and Community Context, Health and Health Care and Neighborhood, and Built Environment. The SDOH model expands the relationship between healthcare expenditures and health habits by emphasizing that healthy habits are determined in large part by the environment that we live and that the healthy choices we make are influenced in a significant way by the options that are available.

Setting National Health Priorities

The first national health objectives were issued in 1979 by the Surgeon General of the United States in the report *Healthy People: The Surgeon General's Report on Health Promotion and Disease Prevention*.[33] This report laid out a series of goals for mortality reductions to be achieved in the United States for the next 10-year period. The most recent report, *Healthy People 2020*, was issued by the CDC and documents the shift toward the pursuit of health equity and a focus on social and environmental characteristics that influence the population's access to health. The vision of Healthy People 2020 is to have a society in which all people live long, healthy lives. The four overarching goals of *Healthy People 2020* are: (1) attain high-quality, longer lives free of preventable disease, disability, injury, and premature death; (2) achieve health equity, eliminate disparities, and improve the health of all groups; (3) create social and physical environments that promote good health for all; and (4) promote quality

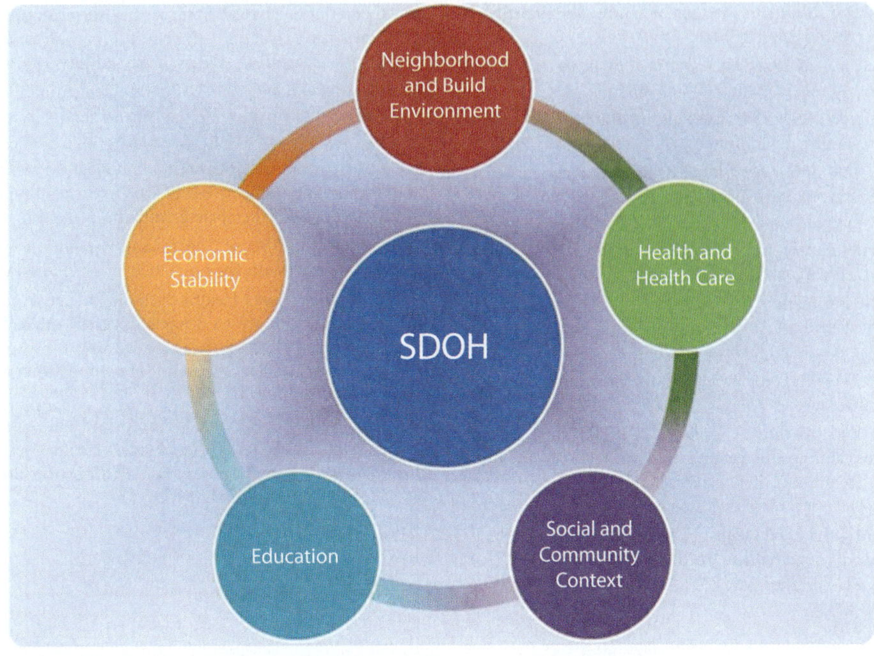

FIGURE 45-2. Social determinants of health. (*Source:* Office of Disease Prevention and Health Promotion. Health People: 2020 Topics and Objectives. https://www.healthypeople.gov/2020/topics-objectives/topic/social-determinants-of-health.[32])

of life, healthy development, and healthy behaviors across all life stages.[33] Healthy People 2020 is the federal government's prevention agenda for building a healthier nation. It is a statement of national health objectives designed to identify the most significant preventable threats to health and to establish national goals to reduce these threats. The CDC is currently preparing Healthy People 2030.

Setting Local Health Priorities

Setting local objectives is a very important step in preparing for an ordered process of allocating resources where the impact is likely to be greatest. Local priorities flow from national objectives and are translated into action at the local level. The value in identifying local actionable priorities is as much in the process of doing so as it is in targeting limited local resources to improve the health of the local population. The process of setting local priorities is informed by macrolevel data, such as the Healthy People documents. It is guided by the state-level priorities identified in the various State Health Improvement Plans (SHIPS). The SHIPs are similarly informed by the input upward from the local health districts. Local policies, systems, and environmental changes are the erectors and the dismantlers of the barriers that stand between a population and its opportunity to achieve its own optimal health. The public health system consisting of the local health department and the vast network of organizations must be involved in recognizing the opportunities, of identifying the priorities, and sustaining the local investment in the pursuit of population health at the community level.

ACKNOWLEDGMENTS

The editor and authors recognize the contributions of previous authors of this chapter: F. Douglas Scutchfield and C. William Keck.

References

1. Reproduced with permission from Last JM. *A Dictionary of Epidemiology*. 2nd ed. New York: Oxford University Press; 1988.
2. Institute of Medicine, Committee for the Study of the Future of Public Health. *The Future of Public Health*. Washington, DC: National Academy Press; 1988.
3. Institute of Medicine, Committee on Assuring the Health of the Public in the 21st Century. *The Future of the Public's Health in the 21st Century*. Washington, DC: National Academy Press; 2003.
4. Gostin LO. *Public Health Law and Ethics: A Reader*. Berkeley, CA: University of California Press; 2010.
5. Bunker JP, Frazier HS, Mosteller F. Improving health: Measuring effects of medical care. *Milbank Q.* 1994;72:225–58.
6. Mokdad AH, et al. Actual causes of death in the United States, 2000. *JAMA*. 2004;291:1238–45.
7. Scutchfield FD, Keck CW. *Concepts of Public Health Practice. Principles of Public Health Practice*. 2nd ed. Albany, NY: Delmar Publishers Inc; 2003, pp. 6–7.
8. Reproduced with permission from Carson City: Health and Human Services. The Ten Essential Public Health Services. http://gethealthy-carsoncity.org/home/the-10-essential-public-health-services/. Accessed July 30, 2018.
9. Public Health Accreditation Board. Accreditation Background. http://www.phaboard.org/about-phab/public-health-accreditation-background/. Accessed July 30, 2018.
10. Riley WJ, Moran JW, Corso LC, Beitsch LM, Bialek R, Cofsky A. Defining quality improvement in public health. *J Public Health Manag Pract*. 2010;16(1):5–7.
11. Public Health Accreditation Board. Standards and Measures for Initial Accreditation. http://www.phaboard.org/accreditation-process/public-health-department-standards-and-measures/. Accessed July 30, 2018.
12. Gostin LO. *Public Health Law and Ethics: A Reader*. Berkeley, CA: University of California Press; 2010.
13. Hanlon JJ, Pickett G. *Public Health: Administration and Practice*. St. Louis, MO: C.V. Mosby; 1984.
14. U.S. Marine Hospital. http://www.marinehospital.org/past.htm. Accessed July 30, 2018.
15. Fee E. History and development of public health. In: Scutchfield FD, Keck CW, eds. *Principles of Public Health Practice*. Albany, NY: Delmar Publishers Inc; 2003, pp. 11–30.
16. Agency for Healthcare Research and Quality. 2018. Mission and Budget. https://www.ahrq.gov/cpi/about/mission/index.html. Accessed July 17, 2018.
17. Agency for Toxic Substances and Disease Registry. 2018. https://www.atsdr.cdc.gov/about/index.html. Accessed July 17, 2018.
18. Centers for Disease Control and Prevention. 2018. About the CDC. https://www.cdc.gov/about/organization/cio.htm. Accessed July 17, 2018.
19. U.S. Food & Drug Administration. 2018. FDA: What We Do. https://www.fda.gov/aboutfda/whatwedo/. Accessed July 18, 2018.
20. Health Resources & Services Administration. 2018. About HRSA. https://www.hrsa.gov/about/index.html. Accessed July 17, 2018.

21. Indian Health Service. 2018. About HIS. https://www.ihs.gov/aboutihs/?-mobileFormat=true. Accessed July 18, 2018.
22. National Institutes of Health. 2018. NIH: What We Do. https://www.nih.gov/about-nih/what-we-do. Accessed July 17, 2018.
23. Substance Abuse and Mental Health Services Administration. 2018. About SAMHSA. https://www.samhsa.gov/about-us. Accessed July 17, 2018.
24. Surgeon General. 2018. U.S. Public Health Service Commissioned Corps. https://www.surgeongeneral.gov/corps/index.html. Accessed July 18, 2019.
25. Medical Definition of USPHS (United States Public Health Service). 2018. https://www.medicinenet.com/common_medical_abbreviations_and_terms/article.htm#c_-_medical_abbreviations. Accessed July 17, 2018.
26. National Public Health Performance Standards. http://www.astho.org/Programs/Accreditation-and-Performance/National-Public-Health-Performance-Standards/. Accessed July 30, 2018.
27. National Profile of Local Health Departments. http://nacchoprofilestudy.org/. Accessed July 31, 2018.
28. Centers for Medicare and Medicaid Services. 2018. National Health Expenditure Data: Historical. https://www.cms.gov/Research-Statistics-Data-and-Systems/Statistics-Trends-and-Reports/NationalHealthExpendData/NationalHealthAccountsHistorical.html. Accessed July 19, 2018.
29. Association of State and Territorial Health Officials. 2016. Astho Profile Survey. http://www.astho.org/Profile/Volume-Four/2016-ASTHO-Profile-Top-Findings/. Accessed July 19, 2018.
30. Centers for Disease Control and Prevention. National Center for Health Statistics: Health Expenditures. https://www.cdc.gov/nchs/fastats/health-expenditures.htm. Accessed July 31, 2018.
31. Healthy People. 2018. Social Determinants of Health. https://www.healthypeople.gov/2020/topics-objectives/topic/social-determinants-of-health. Accessed July 20, 2018.
32. Office of Disease Prevention and Health Promotion. Health People: 2020 Topics and Objectives. https://www.healthypeople.gov/2020/topics-objectives/topic/social-determinants-of-health. Accessed July 31, 2018.
33. Centers for Disease Control and Prevention. Health People 2020. https://www.cdc.gov/dhdsp/hp2020.htm. Accessed July 31, 2018.
34. Peterson-Kaisers Health System Tracker. How does health spending in the U.S. compare to other countries? https://www.healthsystemtracker.org/chart-collection/health-spending-u-s-compare-countries/#item-relative-size-wealth-u-s-spends-disproportionate-amount-health. Accessed July 30, 2018.
35. Association of State and Territorial Health Officials. 2017. Astho Profile of State and Territorial Public Health. http://www.astho.org/Profile/Volume-Four/2016-ASTHO-Profile-of-State-and-Territorial-Public-Health/. Accessed July 19, 2018.

CHAPTER 46

The Public Health Workforce

Valerie A. Yeager

INTRODUCTION

The wide range of activities subsumed under the rubric of public health practice is provided by a large and diverse workforce. Assessing the size and composition of the public health workforce facilitates information necessary to identify workforce gaps, forecast trends and needs, and guide workforce development policies. In sum, enumerating the public health workforce is a crucial step toward strengthening the workforce infrastructure. Despite the value in enumerating the public health workforce, this is no easy task as there is no standard system of monitoring the public health workforce or standard worker title or classification scheme. Further, public health includes diverse employment settings (federal, state, and local) entailing highly varied roles and disciplines across these settings. In the most recent effort to enumerate governmental public health workers in the United States, an estimated 290,988 were identified in federal, state, and local public health agencies.[1] This chapter presents insights about the makeup of the governmental public health workforce and its disciplines, public health practice settings and evolving system changes, educational backgrounds of the workforce and training programs, and ongoing challenges for the public health workforce. (See Chapter 9: Public Health Practice in the United States.)

THE DISCIPLINES OF PUBLIC HEALTH

The two largest groups of professionals identified in public health practice are public health nurses (47,270) and environmental health professionals (23,838).[1] In addition to these two professions, physicians, health educators, laboratory scientists, epidemiologists, and public health officials are most likely to be mentioned as important contributors to public health. In the early history of public health, it was professionals with an environmental focus, including engineers, who made some of the most striking contributions, assuring that drinking water was safe, sewage systems installed, and waste products appropriately handled. As the specific causes of diseases became known in the first half of the twentieth century, physicians with public health training became more prominent, and measures of disease prevention such as isolation of infected persons, tracing of individual contacts, and vaccination became important public health tools. The complete list of professions associated with public health practice includes all of those associated with medical care (dentist, pharmacist, physical and occupational therapist, psychologist, social worker), others less frequently seen in patient-care settings (occupational health and industrial hygiene, law, veterinary medicine), and many with important analytic and data skills (biostatistics, economics, informatics). Much like the healthcare workforce, the public health workforce is overwhelmingly professional (individuals with baccalaureate or higher degrees), enriched by a wide range of technicians (in laboratory, environment, and informatics, to name a few areas) and critical support staff in administrative, data entry, and other tasks.

The professions in public health are supported by an impressive array of technicians and paraprofessionals as well. Laboratory technicians, dental technicians, computer technicians, community outreach workers, and environmental technicians are all represented. In addition, because much of public health depends on documentation and communication, there is a rich array of administrative and data management support staff. One of the complications in both describing and studying the public health workforce is that any one individual can often be described by several labels: the discipline in which he or she has formal training, the job title assigned by the employing agency, the functional activity in which the majority of time is spent, and the program in which this takes place. For example, an MD might be hired as a public health program specialist and spend the majority of time planning and conducting outbreak investigations in the sexually transmitted disease control program. Or a laboratory technician may be hired as an investigator and spend the majority of time visiting community-based laboratories to support a quality assurance program in lead testing. Nearly 87,000 workers or 30% of the governmental workforce could not be assigned to one of the 14 general public health worker categories presented in Table 46-1.[1] This speaks to the range of expertise and activities under the umbrella of governmental public health. Keep in mind that the governmental public health workforce is only part of the public health workforce, thus most efforts at enumerating the public health workforce are limited because public health activities are spread across multiple nongovernmental organizations as well as private organizations and other governmental agencies at all levels of government.

What unites all of these groups is the common attention to the health of populations, rather than individuals. The specific functions any one worker may be asked to fulfill are often not specific to the discipline in which he or she was trained, but rather a service to the community to which the world view of that discipline can contribute. For example, in developing a community-wide health education program on reduction of tobacco use, physicians, health educators, environmental health specialists, nurses, and media specialists might all be employed under the programmatic title, "A Clean Indoor Air Team," and would pool their various perspectives into a single programmatic effort that might eventually be carried out in a community through the media, volunteers, hospital staff, and public health nurses.

Nurses provide one example of the diversity of public health work and workers. For over a hundred years, public health nurses have been working in support of the health of the population, applying their expertise in clinical services and social and public health science.[2] This effort has taken many forms, and led practitioners from crowded urban tenements to isolated farms to suburban workplaces, from healthy children to tubercular workers to the elderly seeking to maintain their independence. While it is difficult to say that there is a "typical" public health nurse, there are commonalities across many

TABLE 46-1 PUBLIC HEALTH WORKER OCCUPATIONS BY LEVEL OF GOVERNMENT

Occupational Category	Local Public Health Agency	State Public Health Agency	Federal Public Health Agency	Total (%)
Administrative/clerical personnel	35,000	14,559	6,085	55,644 (19%)
Behavioral health professional	4,000	1,839	895	6,734 (2%)
Emergency preparedness staff	2,900	810	–	3,720 (1%)
Environmental health worker	13,300	4,618	5,920	23,838 (8%)
Epidemiologist	1,800	2,476	–	4,276 (2%)
Health educator	5,100	1,572	43	6,715 (2%)
Laboratory worker	2,000	5,699	5,685	13,384 (5%)
Nutritionist	5,000	1,276	223	6,499 (2%)
Public health dental worker	2,600	356	443	3,399 (1%)
Public health informatics specialist	2,100	729	–	2,829 (1%)
Public health manager	10,100	3,296	4,998	18,394 (6%)
Public health nurse	29,191	12,286	5,793	47,270 (16%)
Public health physician	2,100	791	6,700	9,591 (3%)
Public information specialist	2,100	174	–	2,274 (1%)
Uncategorized worker	30,200	35,960	20,271	86,431 (30%)
Total	147,491 (50%)	86,411 (30%)	57,056 (20%)	290,988 (100%)

Source: Reproduced with permission from Beck AJ, Boulton ML, Coronado F. Enumeration of the governmental public health workforce, 2014. *Am J Prev Med.* 2014;47 (5 Suppl 3):S306-S313. doi:10.1016/j.amepre.2014.07.018.

agencies of different sizes, serving diverse communities. Public health nurses were historically employed to work in those public health programs that require some contact with individuals, especially if that contact involves some aspects of "hands-on" clinical practice. This includes the staffing of immunization clinics, sexually transmitted disease and tuberculosis control programs, child and maternal health services, senior health promotion programs, and workplace health clinics. Nurses are also found in epidemiology programs, and working to assure the quality of day-care centers, hospitals, and long-term care facilities through licensing and certification. In large health departments, a nurse might work exclusively in one or two program areas, and even in a limited part of the jurisdiction served. In many middle sized and most small departments, the nurse must be a generalist, moving day-to-day and hour-by-hour from program to program. Much of the apparent specialization and narrow targeting of work efforts is driven by the current approach to funding of public health, in which dollars are tied to very defined activities and population groups, rather than being available for more broad-based efforts to work with a population group or community to improve health overall.

While increased support has been growing for addressing the social determinants of health in recent years, public health professionals have long understood that protecting the public's health requires attention to individual and family circumstances, social and economic factors, and the full experience of the local community. The individual experiencing illness and seeking care may be the most visible evidence of the need for public health in a community, though individual medical care in response to symptoms is not central to public health practice. However, where there are large numbers of individuals uninsured or lacking primary care, public health departments often have physicians, physician assistants, nurse practitioners, and public health nurses to provide personal-care services. There is no indication that this care has automatically been provided in ways that differ in content or focus from that provided in any other ambulatory care practice. However, many health department-based primary-care programs are different in their focused attention on prevention, the special community needs of the populations seeking care, and to the potential for building new, better systems of care and prevention (such as patient-centered medical homes).

As health departments have long been a source of primary care and prevention for the uninsured or other vulnerable populations, especially in the South, they have often supported the services by quietly riding on the economic coattails of Medicaid or other special funding sources. A maternal child health-focused public health nurse or child health physician generating up to two-thirds or three-fourths of salary costs through billable services may well be supported to invest the remaining one-third to one-fourth of time in improved community health systems. Absent the Medicaid resource, the health department may be unable to find the resource to continue these professionals even half time. Making the case for a community-funding base for this shift is an important challenge to public health across the country. The challenge is to ask the correct question, which is "how will I assure that care and necessary services are available to those who lack it?," not "how can I be sure that I am still here to give care?" In the rush to downsize government and control spending for health and illness services, many fear that policy makers will inadvertently eliminate important community-based programs, such as health promotion to increase activity and reduce obesity. This issue may become less and less relevant as public health agencies continue to divest primary-care programs from their list of organizational responsibilities as they increasingly partner with the outside organizations to meet their communities' direct healthcare needs they once tackled internally.

WHERE IS PUBLIC HEALTH PRACTICED?

The field of public health can be distinguished from other areas of health-related practice by the combined impact of three foci: prevention, community, and systems. While none of these is unique to public health, the combination is a particularly powerful one. Prevention is, of course, the historic defining feature of public health. As causal links and antecedents of disease have been understood, public health practitioners have taken steps to reshape exposure patterns or strengthen resistance or eliminate causes of diseases. The earliest efforts were directed at infectious conditions, both before and after the introduction of protective immunizations and effective antibiotic treatment. More recently, prevention has extended to noninfectious diseases such as cancer and heart disease, and to injury, both unintentional and intentional. The expanding science base for prevention practice has supported provision of services in a variety of settings (home, school, workplace, health clinic) using multiple media (brochures, audio and video recordings, games, drama, targeted direct messaging, and social media) and multiple reinforcers (public policy on tobacco control). Emerging approaches such as harm reduction (seeking to achieve at least some movement toward more healthful choices even if full prevention of risk is not feasible) also play a part.

Some prevention activities are directly provided to specific individuals, such as immunizations or prenatal care. Many others are provided to people at the population group or community level. In either case, public health is differentiated from the vast majority of health and illness-care practice by the use of settings other than hospitals and doctors' offices as the site of intervention. Schools and work sites, store-front clinics, neighborhood events, homes, and shopping malls have also been used to assure that services and messages are available to people at the times and places where they will have the greatest impact in promoting health. The term *community* may well be overused; the fact that a health-related service is outside the four walls of a hospital does not make it a community service. Changes in medical and nursing practice have meant that many procedures previously requiring a hospital operating room or nursing-care unit are performed in clinics or homes.

For the public health worker, all activities are done in the context of community. Community means more than place, and may not occur in a single place. It also means relationship, whether one is considering an official geopolitical community, a neighborhood, or a community of affinity such as an advocacy or professional group. One widely used statement about public health in America[4] captures the importance of relationships in the vision of "healthy people in healthy communities."

Related to the concept of community is that of systems, the notion that any one component of the community is tied in some way to all others, so that changes in any one component will lead sooner or later to some changes elsewhere. A focus on both prevention and community from a systems perspective pushes the practitioner to consider how the system relationships may be developed or strengthened, or how illness-fostering, noncommunity system elements may be reduced. Working with this perspective means that any work with an individual can be the source of data regarding the functioning of systems within the community, and lead to intervention at additional levels to promote healthy change. No one person can simultaneously work at all levels (individual, family, neighborhood, community-wide system), so the system of workers collaborating to assure that needed information flows among those performing different functions is an additional important part of the systems view. Further, efforts to inform system change and understand system effectiveness and efficiencies is being informed by the important work of the Public Health Services and Systems Research field that has gained momentum over the last two decades.

Given all of the above, it is impossible to define the public health workforce by the name on the employing agency door, though the largest concentration is employed by official governmental public health agencies (local, regional, state, or federal). Some community programs such as nonprofit community health centers and migrant health centers work with the community to improve health in ways that are clearly public health practice, but these employees are often not included in the enumeration of the public health workforce. The total number of public health workers reported is also deceptive in that the workers are not spread evenly in relation to the population. The last enumeration effort to report state-level data found differences in the ratio of public health workers to the population that ranged from 37/100,000 in Pennsylvania to 566/100,000 in South Carolina, all while the national average at the time (year 2000) was 158/100,000.[5] While this suggests there is variation in the assurance to the citizens that their health is being protected, caution should be exercised, as these variations are caused in part by state and local decisions to locate public health activities outside of identifiable governmental public health agencies, by varying degrees of reliance on public health for clinical services, and on the lack of a standardized system for routine reporting on the public health workforce.

DEGREES AND CREDENTIALS

Because of the myriad skills needed in the field, entry routes to public health practice have historically not included formal training in public health. For example, many experts in social dynamics of the populations most vulnerable to HIV infection (gay men, sex workers, injecting drug users) entered public health practice during the early years of the AIDS epidemic. As programs matured and workers considered promotions and career development, many of these have added public health training (formal or informal) and can now be found working in a wide range of programs. Still, recent surveys indicated that approximately 17% of the governmental public health workforce has a formal public health degree.[3]

For the largest professional group, nurses, the picture can be most confusing. Nurses with the same legal credential to practice may have widely differing educations. Again, historically, neither the associate degree nor diploma education included public health as a required curriculum component. Basic education about public health nursing practice is included in the baccalaureate curriculum, and some public health systems have attempted to reserve the job title "public health nurse" for baccalaureate graduates only. Whatever their entry education, nurses employed to work in public health agencies or other entities with a focus on public health and the community must master at least some content about population perspectives on health, epidemiology, health behavior, and environmental influences on health.[5,6]

Advanced education for practice in communities is at least as confusing as entry-level education. Some public health nurses have studied in schools of public health, others in schools of nursing; some have degrees in both fields. Some physicians in public health practice are board certified in preventive medicine, but many others are pediatricians, obstetricians, or infectious disease specialists. As with entry-level education, the degrees and job titles alone do not identify whether the physician or nurse is practicing public health or not. The answer to that question must be sought in questions of focus and goal.

In a historic report, the Institute of Medicine (now the National Academy of Medicine) considered the confusing picture of education for public health practice in *Who Will Keep the Public Healthy?*[6] and provided guidance for the field of public health education. Since then, the field of public health has changed. For example, the number of schools and programs of public health have increased substantially and the number of graduates from baccalaureate public health programs went from 1469 graduates in 2004 to 6464 in 2012.[7] The IOM report suggested that schools of public health should concentrate their efforts on training those headed toward leadership positions, while expanding continuing education for the workforce generally, and working collaboratively with other schools (e.g., medicine, nursing, law) to improve the public health content included in their regular curricula. Now that undergraduate programs in public health have grown substantially, new strategies must be developed to recruit these graduates into appropriate roles in governmental public health.[8] This is particularly important given that approximately 38% of the existing public health workforce reported intentions to leave the workforce or retire by 2020.[3] With regard to masters-level public health trainees, the IOM report suggested that the content of public health education at the graduate level be grounded in an ecological view of health (including a focus on social determinants of health), emphasize practice, and work toward competency not only in the five classic areas of public health education (biostatistics, epidemiology, environmental health, social and behavioral science, and management) but in eight areas that have emerged as critical in the twenty-first century: cultural competency, communication, community-based participatory research, ethics, genomics, global health, informatics, and policy and law.

Many public health workers are credentialed by an association or entity representing a single profession, such as public health nursing, preventive medicine, health education, or environmental health. Many others bring skills for which there is no specific national credential, such as epidemiology, public health law, or public health leadership. Years of work and planning went into the development of the Certified in Public Health (CPH) exam as a single basic public health certification that could be used by any public health professional as an assurance of competency in the field. The American Public Health Association, the Association of State and Territorial Health Officials, the National Association of County and City Health Officials, the National Association of Local Boards of Health, and the U.S. Department of Health and Human Services (namely, the Centers for Disease Control and Prevention and the Health Resources and Services Administration) were all actively involved in the development of the CPH exam. Although the exam has been available for over a decade, it has not been adopted widely with ongoing questions regarding the value of the exam in the context of its cost to the individual, duplicate credentials for public health workers from existing specialties, and whether passing the CPH exam makes a difference in getting hired into public health governmental service.

CURRENT CHALLENGES

Two of the most prominent challenges to the public health workforce today are those associated with shrinking budgets that results in fewer public health positions—either resulting from attrition and the elimination of vacant positions—and simultaneously expanding expectations for those workers that remain. This is further complicated by the impending retirement or loss of some 38% of the workforce who indicated planning to leave their agencies over the next couple years. These intentions were disproportionately among higher-level managers and leaders, which may translate to extraordinary losses to institutional memory and experience. Recruiting graduates from baccalaureate and master-level public health programs cannot fill such a void, even if successfully recruiting these individuals were likely (reports indicate that they historically primarily take jobs outside of governmental public health practice).[7] Some of the challenges to recruiting trained individuals into governmental public health positions relates to the long-held requirements that specific positions be filled by nurses and other licensed patient-care professionals. As public health shifts away from direct care activities that relied on nursing skills, agencies have their work cut out for them in revising policies and requirements that may be limiting who they can recruit.

A continuing feature of public life in the United States is concern that government has gotten "too big," and that a goal for all elected officials is to substantially reduce the presence of government. This is easily translated into a reduction in the size of governmental agencies, the major expense of which is usually the workforce. Public health programs and activities have never been designed as entitlements, that is, services to which people are assured access by virtue of some identifying feature (e.g., Medicare for those over 65, Medicaid for those on Aid to Families with Dependent Children, Social Security to workers over 65). Each public health program is reauthorized and refunded year to year, or at best, in a 5-year cycle (which directly relates to the high numbers of employees hired on fixed external contracts rather than as full time equivalent, permanent public health employees).

The nationwide attention to emergency preparedness and the threats of deliberately caused disease outbreaks such as the anthrax events of late 2001 have been helpful in raising the profile of public health as a part of the community safety net, needing general revenue support to be ready to respond if needed. Unfortunately, the appropriations process at national and state levels has not made this new revenue additive. In many cases, agencies are the same size as before or smaller. Recent reports indicated losses of over 60,000 full time equivalents at the local and state levels since the Great Recession of 2009.[9] Unfortunately, these losses mean the now smaller workforce is being asked to assume more active roles in emergency preparedness and community response, while continuing the long-standing array of other public health services.

ACKNOWLEDGMENT

The editor and author recognize the contributions of Kristine M. Gebbie, the previous author of this chapter.

References

1. Beck AJ, Boulton ML, Coronado F. Enumeration of the governmental public health workforce, 2014. *Am J Prev Med*. 2014;47(5S3):S306–13.
2. Thompson ME, Keeling AA. Nurses' role in the prevention of infant mortality in 1884-1925: health disparities then and now. *J Pediatr Nurs*. 2012 Oct;27(5):471–8. doi: 10.1016/j.pedn.2011.05.011. Epub 2011 Jul 16. PMID: 22920658; PMCID: PMC3428594.
3. Sellers K, Leider JP, Harper E, et al. The Public Health Workforce Interests and Needs Survey: The first national survey of state agency employees. *J Public Health Manag Pract*. 2015;21(suppl 6):S13–27.
4. Public Health Functions Steering Committee. Public Health in America Statement, Fall, 1994.
5. Health Resources and Services Administration. *Enumeration 2000*. New York: Columbia University School of Nursing; 2000. Available at http://publichealth.jbpub.com/turnock/3e/chapterOutline/phworkforce2000.pdf.
6. Pope AM, Snyder MA, Mood LH, eds.Pope AM, Snyder MA, Mood LH, eds. *Nursing Health and Environment*. Washington, DC: National Academy Press; 1995.
7. Leider JP, Castrucci BC, Plepys CM, Blakely C, Burke E, Sprague JB. Characterizing the growth of the undergraduate public health major: U.S., 1992–2012. *Public Health Rep*. 2015;130(1):104–13.
8. Yeager VA, Beitsch LM, Hasbrouck, L. A mismatch between the educational pipeline and public health workforce: Can it be reconciled? *Public Health Rep*. 2016; 131:507–9.
9. National Association of County and City Health Officials (NACCHO). Understand the Changing Public Health Landscape: Findings from the 2017 Forces of Change Survey. Available at https://www.naccho.org/uploads/downloadable-resources/2017-Forces-of-Change-Main-Report1.pdf.

CHAPTER

47 Health Policy Development

Leslie M. Beitsch • Samantha Goldfarb

There are many different avenues for influencing policy development for public health and preventive medicine. In addition to policy decisions made by the U.S. Congress, as the legislative branch of the federal government, public policy decisions affecting preventive medicine and public health are also made in a variety of ways, including the following: (1) at the federal level in the executive branch (i.e., the Department of Health and Human Services, the Centers for Disease Control and Prevention, the Surgeon General's Office, the Food and Drug Administration, etc.); (2) at the state level in both the executive (i.e., the governor's office and state health department) and legislative branches; (3) at the city and local levels of governments; and (4) in the private sector in private associations, representing healthcare organizations and professionals, among health plans and employers, hospitals and healthcare settings, and finally within practice settings.

There are two policy-making trends that are noteworthy among groups. First, there are priorities that differ based on the level of government—for example, the federal government spends more money on the elderly (e.g., Medicare, Social Security), while state/local governments spend more on children (e.g., Medicaid). This can be problematic given differences in administrative oversight, which ultimately results in a patchwork system of coverage and generosity.[1] Second, there is wide variation in how policies are funded—some are funded through mandatory budget requirements while others are based on appropriations. In 1995, the unfunded mandate reform was passed which limits the ability of the federal government to mandate programs that state and local governments would be responsible to fund. This devolution of federal responsibility, therefore, left many programs and policies up to state discretion, which results in discrepancies based on state/local values and priorities.[1]

AGENDA SETTING

The process of agenda setting is instrumental for initiating the policy-development process.[2,3] The formal policy agenda is defined as those issues on the forefront that policy makers plan to address in the near term. Critically then, the first step in any policy-development process is to get an issue on the formal policy agenda. Policy makers rarely develop their own bills due to time constraints; this places them at the mercy of evaluating ideas from every angle typically backed by lobbyists, analysts, and special interest groups who passionately dictate what they should do and how it should be accomplished.[1] Therefore, two of the most commonly used strategies for getting an issue on the policy agenda include: gaining *inside access* to decision makers in the policy arena, and organizing an *outside initiative* through grass-roots mobilization or coalition building to call the issue to the attention of policy makers.[2] These agenda-setting strategies can be used separately or together, in combination. Both have been used successfully to influence the policy agenda setting for public health and preventive medicine.

Using Inside Access Strategies to Influence Policy-Making

During the 103rd Congress (which was then debating dramatic health reform which ultimately was not embraced), effective inside access was achieved by state and local public health officials who met individually with their elected representatives in Congress to discuss the importance of securing stable and adequate funding for the core functions of public health under a reformed healthcare system. Public health officials, both as constituents and leaders in their state and communities, bring credibility and lend importance to an issue, and can facilitate translation of public health issues in terms that make them locally relevant to individual elected representatives.[4] This includes disseminating the information in ways that meet policy makers' needs, perhaps through development of a short brief or webinar addressing the issue. A mutual sharing of knowledge and relationship building with policy makers is critical in this process.[1]

Using Outside Initiative Strategies to Influence Policy-Making

As a prominent example, the National Breast Cancer Coalition and other women's groups organized a massive and effective post-card-writing campaign at the grassroots level across the country highlighting the importance of covering mammography screening as a health insurance benefit as part of healthcare reform before the 103rd Congress. U.S. senators and representatives reported receiving hundreds of postcards from their constituents calling their attention to this issue. Legislators of all political perspectives care deeply about how an issue affects their constituents, and will pay more attention to an issue if it comes from the grassroots level. These strategies are essential in advancing issues pertaining to preventive medicine and public health given that policy makers are often forced to make rapid decisions about the best solutions to complex problems with the trade-off being who to cover and at what cost.[1]

The state of Washington is often a model for how states may proceed, in the absence of reforms at the federal level, to fill the policy vacuum with effective public health initiatives. Washington coalesced key public health stakeholders and engaged in productive planning to successfully formulate public health policy—with tangible results. Washington State developed its own Public Health Improvement Plan in 1994, and revised it again in 2017. It was a collaborative effort with state legislature oversight and was subsequently enacted into law.[5] Currently, Oregon and Ohio have taken similar approaches to improve their statewide public health systems. The original Washington State plan was developed by the Department of Health and a Public Health Improvement Plan Steering Committee, representative of a broad coalition of public health and healthcare organizations in the state. The coalition included: representatives of the Department of Health, the state medical association, the association of community clinics, consumers, public health nursing directors, state legislators, schools of public health, labor unions, the state nurses' association, local public health officials, the hospital association, the healthcare purchasers' association, and the Indian Health Service. The purpose of the plan was to help achieve three goals—stabilization of healthcare costs, assurance of universal access to healthcare, and improvement of population health. The plan included comprehensive recommendations for public health capacity, finance and governance of the public health system, and standards and strategies for addressing key public health problems. It served as the blueprint for state legislation enacted to reform Washington State's public health system, and served as a model for other states. The breadth of the external coalitions participating with a unified voice added strength to the message conveyed to policy makers and elected officials.

Open Policy Windows Framework

The open policy windows framework suggests that when policy opportunities (termed "windows") are open, policy makers are willing to invest the time, energy, and political capital necessary because their efforts are more likely to pay off. These windows are considered open when three conditions for social change converge: (1) problems are recognized, (2) policy solutions are available, and (3) political climate supports change.[1]

DIFFICULTIES IN GETTING PUBLIC HEALTH AND PREVENTIVE MEDICINE ON THE POLICY AGENDA

Public health and preventive medicine have had varying success in increasing awareness of the value and benefits of increasing access to preventive care until recent years. Their voice has been bolstered by relying on a growing scientific evidence base that demonstrates the effectiveness and relative cost-effectiveness of many preventive services on health outcomes during a time of rapidly escalating healthcare costs. However, the relative importance of public health and preventive medicine in health policy development over the last decade is illustrated by estimates that less than 3% of total health expenditures in the United States are spent on population-based public health and prevention programs.[6,7] There are many reasons for this neglect, including the bias toward the medical model in health policy development. Nonetheless, considered altogether, there is major growth potential for public health and prevention policy advocacy as society moves toward greater emphasis on population health.

Theory of Paradox

The theory of paradox provides a conceptual framework for moving beyond seemingly antithetical viewpoints to recognizing the validity and utility of each in order to frame policies that foster compromise. For this to happen, two conditions must occur. First, there needs to be a push in the ignored direction, which is to recognize preventive medicine and public health as a parallel right to medical care and treatment. Second, there must be simultaneous pursuit of two or more virtually opposing but valid policy goals. As more policy solutions are presented, the chances of achieving comprehensive solutions to complex problems significantly increase. For example, are there certain health conditions for which preventive medicine provides greater benefits than treatment, and vice versa?[1]

Incremental Policy Development: Adding Prevention Benefits to the Medicare Program

Perhaps the best example of how policy developments for preventive medicine proceeds incrementally are the efforts over recent decades to add preventive services benefits to the Medicare program. The amendments to the Social Security Act, which authorized the Medicare program in 1965, included a provision (Section 1862) that prohibits reimbursement for any preventive care. The original Medicare program was based on the Blue Cross and Blue Shield programs operating at that time, where preventive care was not considered medically necessary. Since preventive care is neither high cost nor unpredictable, it did not fit within the then prevalent notion of a health insurance model designed to spread risk.

Between 1965 and 1980, over 350 bills were introduced into the U.S. Congress proposing to add preventive care benefits under Medicare before one bill finally passed adding the pneumococcal vaccine as a covered benefit. Only incrementally, and within the context of huge budget reconciliation bills, were additional screening and immunization benefits added to the Medicare program since that time—that is, until the passage of the Affordable Care Act. Most benefits added were those supported by sound research demonstrating not only their efficacy, but also their relative cost-effectiveness. The pneumococcal vaccine was shown to be cost saving to the Medicare program, while mammography and Pap smears were added later only when studies from the Office of Technology Assessment showed that they were relatively cost effective.[8] Since that time, large gains have been realized in increasing access to preventive care under the Medicare program. Some early additions of covered preventive services are depicted in Table 47-1. For example, since 1992 coverage has been added for (a) a "welcome to Medicare physical"; (b) cardiovascular screening for cholesterol, HDL, and triglycerides; (c) pelvic exam; (d) colon cancer screening including fecal occult blood, flexible sigmoidoscopy, colonoscopy, and barium enema; (e) prostate cancer screening including a digital rectum exam and PSA test (not currently recommended); (f) hepatitis B vaccine; (g) bone mass measurement; (h) diabetes screening and management including fasting plasma glucose test, diabetes glucose monitors, test strips and lancets, and self-management training; (i) glaucoma screening tests; and (j) smoking cessation treatments including counseling for smoking and tobacco use and coverage of tobacco treatment medications under the new Part D prescription drug benefit. Table 47-1 describes coverage, for whom, at what costs, and with what restrictions when the additions were included under Medicare.

Key Factors Influencing Health Insurance Coverage of Preventive Care

The key factors associated with successful policy development for adding prevention benefits in the Medicare program include an incremental approach of adding only a few benefits at a time, with a well-documented evidence base of effectiveness and cost-effectiveness of the preventive service, coupled with sponsorship and leadership by key policy makers. Factors associated with failure include lack of active support from beneficiaries and health professionals, projected increases in costs to the medical care system associated with adding the benefit, and competing priorities on the formal policy agenda.

PREDICTING THE OUTCOMES AND DESIGNING SUCCESSFUL STRATEGIES FOR PREVENTION POLICY

One of the most useful models for predicting the likely success or failure of proposed policies, and one that is also useful to facilitate the design of more effective strategies for influencing the policy-making process, is the well-established James Q. Wilson model of concentrated and diffuse cost and benefits (Table 47-2).[9] To apply Wilson's model to a particular policy, one must first identify the intended effects of the policy—that is, who will benefit from the policy and who will bear the costs. In each case, one must also assess if the benefits and costs are concentrated or diffuse. Concentrated costs are those imposed on a well-organized, relatively small number of individuals or groups where the cost will be strongly felt. An example of a concentrated cost would be a tax policy requiring hospitals to contribute to a pool to support local public health activities. A diffuse cost, in contrast, is one where the cost burden is widely distributed among a large group of relatively unorganized individuals or groups, where the impact of the cost is relatively small. Compared with the more concentrated hospital tax, an example of a diffuse cost would be a small increase in individuals' income tax or on insurance premiums to pay to support public health activities. Policies that rely on concentrated costs are typically more difficult

TABLE 47-1 PREVENTIVE SERVICES COVERED UNDER THE MEDICARE PROGRAM, MARCH 2006

Preventive Service	Services Covered	Cost-Sharing Required	Restrictions	Definition of High Risk
Welcome to Medicare physical	Preventive physical exam, medical history, blood pressure, weight, height, vision test, electrocardiogram, immunizations, review of health, education, and counseling needs	Must first meet $124 Plan B deductible; 20% of the Medicare-approved amount above the deductible	Once in a lifetime	
Cardiovascular screening	Screening for cholesterol-level, HDL, and triglycerides after 12-hour fasting	None	Every 5 years	
Breast cancer screening	Screening mammograms	20% of Medicare-approved amount with no Plan B deductible	Every 12 months for women age 40 and older, with one baseline mammogram for women ages 35–39	
Cervical and vaginal cancer screening	Pap test; pelvic exam	None for the Pap lab test; 20% of the Medicare-approved amount with no Part B deductible for Pap test collection and pelvic exam	Every 24 months	
Colon cancer screening	Fecal occult blood test	None	Every 12 months for people age 50 and older	Had colon cancer before; close relative with colorectal polyps or colorectal cancer; history of polyps; inflammatory bowel disease
	Flexible sigmoidoscopy	20% of Medicare-approved amount after the yearly Part B deductible; 25% if done in a hospital	Every 24 months	
	Screening colonoscopy	20% of Medicare-approved amount after the yearly Part B deductible; 25% if done in a hospital	Every 24 months if high risk; once every 10 years if low risk, but not within 48 months of screening sigmoidoscopy	
	Barium enema	20% of Medicare-approved amount after the yearly Part B deductible	May be used instead of sigmoidoscopy or colonoscopy. Every 24 months if high risk; every 48 months if low risk	
Prostate cancer screening	Digital rectal exam	20% of Medicare-approved amount after the yearly Part B deductible	Every 12 months for men 50 and older	
	Prostate specific antigen (PSA) test	None	Every 12 months for men 50 and older	
Vaccines	Influenza	None	Once per year in fall or winter	
	Pneumococcal	None	Once in a lifetime	
	Hepatitis B	20% of the Medicare-approved amount after the yearly Part B deductible	Persons at high risk for hepatitis B	Persons with hemophilia, ESRD, immunosuppression
Bone mass screening	Bone mass measurement test	20% of Medicare-approved amount after the yearly Part B deductible	Every 24 months	
Diabetes screening	Fasting plasma glucose test	None	Up to two screenings per year for individuals at high risk; requires physician referral	Persons with high blood pressure, dyslipidemia, obesity, or history of high blood sugar
	Diabetes glucose monitors, test strips and lancets	20% of Medicare-approved amount after the yearly Part B deductible		
	Self-management training	20% of Medicare-approved amount after the yearly Part B deductible		
Glaucoma test	Glaucoma eye exam			

(*Continued*)

TABLE 47-1 PREVENTIVE SERVICES COVERED UNDER THE MEDICARE PROGRAM, MARCH 2006 (*Continued*)

Preventive Service	Services Covered	Cost-Sharing Required	Restrictions	Definition of High Risk
Glaucoma test	Glaucoma eye exam	20% of Medicare-approved amount after the yearly Part B deductible	Every 12 months for persons at high risk	Persons with diabetes, a family history of diabetes, African American and over 50 years
Smoking and tobacco use cessation	Four counseling cessations per quit attempt. Defined as face-to-face patient contact of either intermediate (greater than 3–10 minutes) or intensive (greater than 10 minutes)	20% of Medicare-approved amount after the yearly Part B deductible	Two attempts per year for high-risk persons or eight counseling sessions per year May receive another eight sessions during a second or subsequent year after 11 months	Persons who use tobacco and have a tobacco-related disease or take therapeutic agents affected by tobacco use
	Tobacco cessation medications prescribed by a physician (e.g., nicotine replacement therapy, Zyban)	Part of Medicare Part D drug benefit; cost-sharing varies by plan		

TABLE 47-2 JAMES Q. WILSON MODEL OF CONCENTRATED AND DIFFUSE COST AND BENEFITS

	Concentrated Benefits	Diffuse Benefits
Concentrated costs	(±) Alternating victories. Equally matched battles between organized interest groups.	(–) A losing policy. Organized opposition with opponents. Little organized support. Need to reframe policy effects to get out of this box.
Diffuse costs	(+) A winning policy. Organized support with little organized opposition.	(±) Incremental policy development, without strong, organized support or opposition.

Source: Data from Wilson JQ. *The Politics of Regulation*. New York: Basic Books, 1980, pp. 357–94.

to adopt, as the group targeted to bear the cost is likely to organize strong opposition to the policy and will, depending upon political power, be successful in defeating it. However, when the benefits are also concentrated and the group which will benefit is equally well organized and prepared to support the policy proposal, a more positive outcome is likely. In this case, the victories are likely to be alternating. Policies that have concentrated benefits and diffuse costs are proven winners, given well-organized proponents, while those bearing the concentrated cost are not. Policies that have both diffuse benefits and costs proceed incrementally without strong or well-organized support or opposition.

Taking this theoretical framework and translating it into successful policy development for public health and preventive medicine, it is best to conceptualize proposed new policy and its impacts as having diffuse costs and concentrated benefits. Conversely, in trying to defeat a proposed policy, it is wise to frame the policy's effects as having concentrated costs. The existential challenge for public health is rooted in the fact that most public health programs, by definition, have diffuse benefits, making it very difficult to organize sufficient political support for them successfully.

IMPORTANCE OF PROBLEM DEFINITION IN POLICY DEVELOPMENT

Another critical dimension for influencing the policy agenda is how a particular problem is defined.[10] During periods of budget constraint, programs that are seen as cost saving or relatively inexpensive are particularly popular among policy makers.[3] If reforming and/or increased investment in public health and preventive medicine are portrayed as contributing toward lowering healthcare costs, advocates may be more successful in capturing the attention of policy makers.[11] In contrast, if public health is viewed as contributing toward increasing government expenditures and enlarging the role of government, it will be difficult to get the attention of policy makers in a political environment that seeks to reduce the role and size of government.

THE ROLE OF EVIDENCE-BASED GUIDELINES FOR PREVENTIVE MEDICINE POLICY: THE U.S. PREVENTIVE SERVICES TASK FORCE REPORT

One of the greatest influences on health insurance policy for preventive medicine was the 1989 release of the U.S. Preventive Services Task Force Report, which established national guidelines for clinical preventive services.[12] The report was prepared for the Department of Health and Human Services, and the Task Force recommendations were based on a rigorous review of the scientific evidence on the efficacy and effectiveness of 169 clinical preventive services. This report has been highly influential because the recommendations were grounded in health services research demonstrating the effects of preventive medicine, and its recommendations were developed by an independent task force, unassociated with any specific special interest, professional group, or government. Well-designed clinical trials demonstrating the effectiveness and cost-effectiveness of specific preventive care measures are one of the most powerful tools for influencing purchaser and health plan decision makers to pay for and cover preventive medicine services.

The Task Force work is continuously updated and its deliberations on the evidence of specific services are regularly published in highly visible peer reviewed literature. The Task Force Report has also had an influence in the development of quality measures to assess the performance of health plans. The National Committee for Quality Assurance (NCQA) defined seven of its nine quality measures in its Health Plan Employer Data and Information Set (HEDIS) 2.0 (now known as the Healthcare Effectiveness Data and Information Set), based on the recommendations for specific screening and immunization services in the U.S. Preventive Services Task Force Report.[13] Employers, as purchasers of healthcare, as well as insurers, have also relied on the U.S. Preventive Services Task Force Report to define standard benefits packages to be offered by health plans and to define performance standards for assessing the performance of health plans and the quality of care delivered to their employees.[10] Currently all A and B grade recommendations are health insurance covered services without cost to the beneficiary by virtue of the Affordable Care Act.

THE IMPORTANCE OF POPULATION-BASED DATA AND GOALS FOR PUBLIC HEALTH POLICY: HEALTHY PEOPLE 2000 AND BEYOND

One of the leading advances furthering public health policy formulation in the last three decades has been the development and release of the *Healthy People 2000* and its successors, providing goals and objectives for the nation.[14] It not only documents the current health status of the U.S. population, but it establishes population-based goals for improving population health. *Healthy People 2000* provided the foundation for establishing data systems at the national, state, and local levels for collecting and reporting on population data. Regular reports on progress have served as the benchmark to measure the influence of public health programs and healthcare policies on the nation's health. The goals and objectives were developed between 1987 and 1990 using an extensive consultative and hearings process by the U.S. Public Health Service in partnership with the National Academy of Science and the Institute of Medicine.[15] Similar processes have been carried forward with *Healthy People 2010, 2020*, and now the current development of *Healthy People 2030* in its planning stages.

The impact of the *Healthy People* goals and objectives has been far reaching. Congress has enacted laws that incorporate the objectives, and most states issued their own *Healthy People 2000* plans, while continuing to do so with each new decade. Equally significant, *Healthy People* has instigated the building of coalitions to improve public health and reporting systems to monitor the health status of the population.[14] Paralleling the federal and state actions, *Healthy People* has also been widely adopted at the local level and by private and voluntary agencies. Even the quality measures for health plans developed by the National Committee for Quality Assurance were based in part on the *Healthy People 2000* objectives to reward health plans for keeping populations healthy.[16]

NEW OPPORTUNITIES FOR POLICY DEVELOPMENT IN AN ERA OF ACCOUNTABILITY

Perhaps the greatest opportunity for policy development that promotes public health and preventive medicine is the recent shift toward defining the problems in the healthcare systems as ones of quality and accountability. Quality and "value" in the healthcare system are increasingly defined as maintaining and improving the health of the population; as such, monitoring changes in the health status of the population is necessary to ensure quality and accountability, with public health and preventive medicine becoming important partners in the solution. The fields of public health and preventive medicine offer expertise and experience in community-based prevention programs and population-based data collection and can take a leadership role in policy development in these areas.

One early hallmark of this shift toward increased accountability is the aforementioned development of HEDIS measures by NCQA. The majority of the quality measures in HEDIS 2.0, 2.5, 3.0, and so forth (HEDIS 2015, 2016, 2017, 2018, 2019) address provision of clinical preventive services in accordance with the current U.S. Preventive Services Task Force recommendations. Health maintenance organizations (HMOs) all over the country are being evaluated against these measures, and their performance is being published in report cards made available to employers and the general public. The trend is toward employers requiring that HMOs guarantee their performance in meeting quality standards by placing a percentage of their premium at risk via penalties, or alternatively, offering incentives for better performance outcomes.[11] Building requirements for collecting data, meeting performance standards, and adding economic incentives for performance guarantees into the contracts between HMOs and purchasers (including private employers, state Medicaid agencies, and federal Medicare contracts) are among the most effective policy tool currently available for increasing appropriate provision of preventive care to the insured population.

ADDITIONAL PUBLIC POLICY TOOLS FOR PROMOTING PREVENTION AND PUBLIC HEALTH

There are many additional policy tools that are effective in promoting population health. Taxation of unhealthy products (e.g., cigarettes, alcohol, sugary drinks), regulation of individual and industry behaviors that will promote health and prevent disease (e.g., regulating helmet use and industrial environmental pollution), and public health education (e.g., media campaigns promoting good nutrition and physical activity) are all important and effective tools that can contribute toward a more impactful healthcare system that promotes and maintains health.[17] It is essential that policy for preventive medicine and public health be developed at all applicable levels (i.e., national, state, local, and institutional), and be based on a comprehensive evidence-based model. These policies should seek to influence the medical care system, communities, and governmental policies to promote population health and prevent disease.[17]

ACKNOWLEDGMENT

The editor and authors recognize the contributions of previous author of this chapter: Helen Schauffler.

References

1. Bogenschneider K. *Family Policy Matters: How Policymaking Affects Families and What Professionals can Do*. New York: Routledge; 2014.
2. Cobb R, Ross JK, Ross MH. Agenda building as a comparative political process. *Am Polit Sci Rev*. 1976;70(1):126–38.
3. Kingdon JW. *Agendas, Alternatives, and Public Policies*. New York: Harper Collins; 1984.
4. Scutchfield FD, Keck CW. *Principles of Public Health Practice*. Boston, MA: Cengage Learning; 2009.
5. Washington State Department of Health. State Health Improvement Plan. 2017; https://www.doh.wa.gov/Portals/1/Documents/1200/2017%20SHIP%20Annual%20Report.pdf.
6. Beitsch LM, Brooks RG, Menachemi N, Libbey PM. Public health at center stage: New roles, old props. *Health Aff (Willwood)*. 2006;25(4):911–22.
7. U.S. Department of Health and Human Services. *For a Healthy Nation: Returns on Investment in Public Health*. Washington, DC: U.S. Department of Health and Human Services; 1994.
8. Schauffler HH. Disease prevention policy under Medicare: A historical and political analysis. *Am J Prev Med*. 1993;9(2):71–7.
9. Wilson JQ. *The Politics of Regulation*. New York: Basic Books; 1980, pp. 357–94.
10. Schauffler HH, Rodriguez T. Exercising purchasing power for preventive care. *Health Aff (Willwood)*. 1996;15(1):73–85.
11. Omen G. *Prevention: Benefits, Costs and Savings*. Washington, DC: Partnership for Prevention; 1994.
12. U.S. Preventive Services Task Force. *Guide to Clinical Preventive Services: An Assessment of the Effectiveness of 169 Interventions*. Baltimore: Williams & Wilkins; 1989.
13. National Committee on Quality Assurance. Health Plan Employer Data and Information Set (HEDIS). Version 2.0. Washington, DC; 1993.
14. U.S. Public Health Service. *Healthy People 2000: National Health Promotion and Disease Prevention Objectives*. Washington, DC: U.S. Department of Health and Human Services; 1990.
15. McGinnis JM, Lee PR. Healthy people 2000 at Mid Decade. *JAMA*. 1995;273(14):1123–9.
16. Stone DA. *Policy Paradox and Political Reason*. Glenview, IL: Scott Foresman & Co; 1988.
17. Schauffler HH, Faer M, Faulkner L, Shore K. Health promotion and disease prevention in health care reform. *Am J Prev Med*. 1994;10(5 Suppl):1–31.

CHAPTER 48

Understanding Revenue and Delivery Models in the United States Healthcare System

Nir Menachemi • Casey P. Balio

INTRODUCTION

The U.S. healthcare system has frequently experienced change and reform to how care is delivered and how services are reimbursed. These changes are frequently induced by new policies that govern how health services are paid for by governmental insurance programs including Medicare and Medicaid. Collectively, these policies influence revenue and delivery models that have historically included fee-for-service, prospective payment models, and managed-care models. More recently, reimbursement policies have resulted in updated revenue and delivery models including integrated delivery systems (IDSs), bundled payments, and accountable-care organizations.

To many observers, the recent pace and intensity at which change is occurring appears to be greater than usual. For example, the United States is experiencing increases in the number of physician employees (as opposed to independent practitioners), practice consolidation into larger groups, information technology adoption, a consumerism movement in healthcare, high deductible health plans, and a focus on population health management each of which make it challenging for health providers and administrators to adapt to the evolving environment. All of this change can be challenging to fully appreciate and understand. However, a grounding in the historical health financing milestones that have led us to today can aid the reader to better understand how and why these changes are occurring. Further, understanding the historic content that has influenced revenue and delivery models will allow the reader to anticipate further changes that may affect the U.S. healthcare system.

Thus, the purpose of the current chapter is to briefly describe important attributes of the U.S. healthcare system and to highlight key historical milestones that have affected how care is reimbursed; and thus how care is delivered. Changes to the U.S. healthcare system are typically motivated by improving quality, reducing costs, and/or improving access to care.[1] At least one of these three goals, which are together known as the "iron triangle," are frequently the subject of health policy interventions included in any healthcare reform initiatives. To illustrate this, we organize our historical discussion by decade starting with the 1960s and illustrate lessons learned for each era in terms of affecting the components of the iron triangle at the societal level. In our description, we will discuss how each payment reform, throughout the decades, has affected revenue and delivery models. Figure 48-1 summaries these major changes that occurred by decade. We will conclude the chapter with recommendations pertinent to health administrators and public health practitioners.

1960s

In 1965, President Truman signed the historic Social Security Amendments Act that created Medicare and Medicaid. In the decades prior, health insurance coverage was becoming increasingly common for Americans who primarily received such coverage via their employers.[2–5] For a variety of reasons and market forces, federal policies encouraged employers to offer medical coverage in order to receive tax deductions for both the employer and the employee. This made the United States unique in the world in terms of making the employer the primary vehicle from which health insurance is obtained. Medicare and Medicaid were, in part, an attempt to make health coverage available to individuals less likely to have an employer (e.g., the retired elderly and the jobless poor, respectively). The enactment of Medicare and Medicaid ultimately increased access to healthcare for many Americans; and in turn resulted in the federal government becoming the de facto largest health coverage provider in the nation. Medicaid was established to provide coverage for low-income or disabled individuals and is jointly funded through national and state funds. Because Medicaid is administered at the state level, eligibility, coverage, and applications differ by state.

Medicare eligibility, for most Americans, begins at age 65. Medicare hospital coverage, which like today, made up the largest proportion of Medicare expenses at the time,[6] was primarily financed through a new payroll tax on American workers. Importantly life expectancy in 1965 was 66.8 years for men and 73.7 years for women[7] suggesting that Medicare coverage was not expected to be long term for the typical individual living at the time. Nevertheless, economists and political commentators noted that the federal government, especially through Medicare, had no safeguards against the ill consequences of "moral hazard."[8–10] Moral hazard, in this context, is the tendency of individuals to over utilize services when they are financially shielded from the consequences of this over utilization.[8–10] In other words, if an insurance company or other payer covers the costs of medical care, a patient (and perhaps the provider) may desire a maximum amount of services including those with marginal or no value, thus affecting the overall cost of care without improving the quality. Recall that cost and quality (together with access) are the main components of the iron triangle.

1970s

The decade of the 1970s had two relevant milestones: the RAND Health Insurance Experiment (HIE), and the Health Maintenance Organization (HMO) Act of 1973. The RAND HIE was the largest most comprehensive social science experiment ever performed in the United States with the explicit intention of trying to understand how moral hazard affects healthcare utilization, medical outcomes, and overall health.[11] Separately, the HMO Act was a deliberate attempt to increase the proliferation of HMOs, a revenue and delivery model that focused on aligning physician and patient behavior on cost containment and improvements in quality including health outcomes.[12,13] In an effort to combat moral hazard, HMOs used several strategies including gatekeeper models, capitation payments, selective contracting, and prior authorization requirements to accomplish

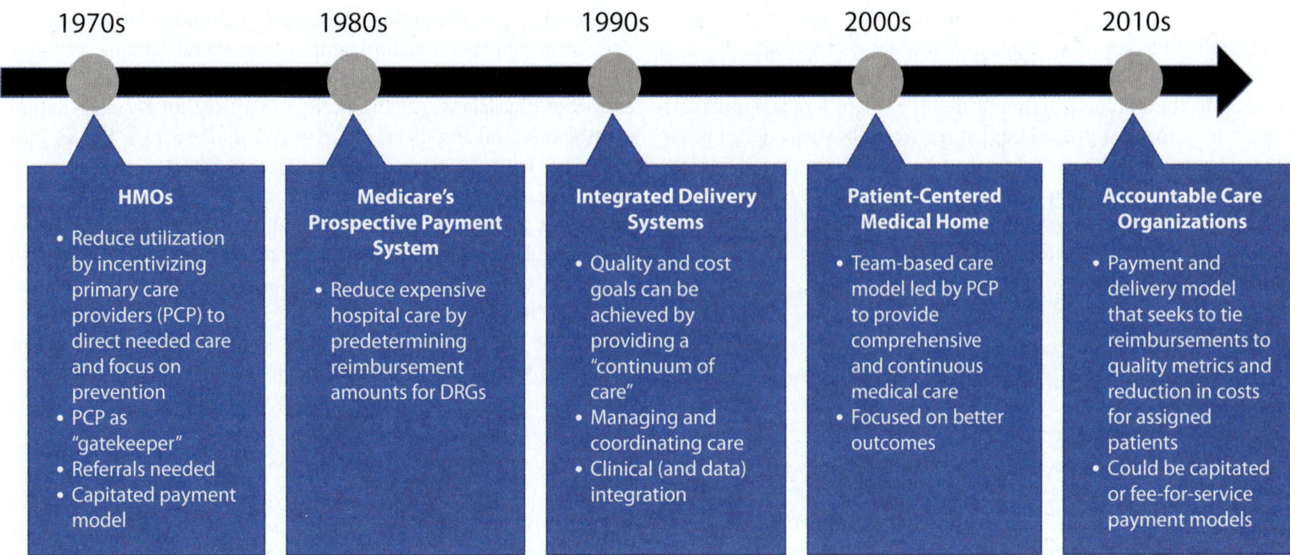

FIGURE 48-1. Major revenue and delivery models brought upon by U.S. reimbursement policies by decade.

their goals.[14–16] HMOs were relatively unique at the time because they were structured as prepaid plans, or capitated plans, which unlike the traditional fee-for-service plans were not incentivized to provide more services.[17] The term "health maintenance" refers to the fact that by changing the incentive structure, these plans would focus more on prevention and overall health, as opposed to potentially unnecessary or avoidable medical care. The Act required employers to give their employees a choice for coverage in an HMO plan if such a plan was available in their market. This resulted in rapid increases in HMO organizations nationally.[12,18]

The RAND HIE was concerned with the impact of patient cost sharing (e.g., copayment and coinsurance rates) on utilization, quality, and overall health status. The RAND HIE found that cost sharing, in a dose-response manner, reduced spending for health services relative to a comparison group of patients who received free care. The reduction in spending came from less use of care (medical visits and hospital admissions) but not the cost of care once it was utilized.[11,19,20] Moreover, cost sharing did not have a detrimental impact on overall health status except for the sickest and poorest patients suggesting that for most individuals moral hazard could be controlled with cost-sharing.

HMOs used various tactics to control costs or affect quality—each with varying levels of success. For example, HMOs used a gatekeeper model that required patients to receive referrals from primary care prior to accessing more expensive specialty care; and capitation reimbursement strategies that attempt to limit physician-induced demand for care common in fee-for-service models (fee-for-service models reimburse providers a set fee for each service they provide for a given patient). Research on the impact of the gatekeeper[21,22] and capitation models find that these strategies are only moderately effective at controlling costs. HMOs were more successful at reducing costs by using selective contracting which is a competitive strategy that strengthens the HMOs market power.[23–26] Selective contracting is the creation of a preferred provider network comprised of physicians and hospitals willing to accept lower reimbursements in exchange for access to the HMOs patient population. Overall, evidence suggests that HMO were generally effective at reducing costs without adversely affecting quality mainly by gaining local market power.[27,28] The impact of focusing on prevention within HMOs was more difficult to assess because of the frequency at which patients change health plans. For the investments in prevention to yield financial returns, an individual would need to stay enrolled with the same plan for many years.

Keep in mind how each policy change (e.g., the HMO Act of 1973) ultimately influences how care is delivered and paid for. Each change in practice is then studied so that researchers can determine which strategies used by providers most influenced cost, quality, or access. This research is then helpful when the next round of policy changes are being contemplated because in many cases, future policies have taken into consideration the lessons learned from previous attempts to reform practice.

1980s

As a result of continued growing concerns that the federal government was responsible for increasing the over use of medical services (e.g., moral hazard), and using taxpayer funds to pay for it, the Prospective Payment System (PPS) was implemented. Prior to the PPS, Medicare reimbursed hospitals on a cost-based retrospective basis.[29] This meant that after a given hospitalization, a hospital would bill Medicare for the costs incurred for the care provided to a given Medicare recipient. This suggested that hospital revenue could be increased simply by increasing the costs required to care for patients. Not surprisingly, much variation existed in lengths of stay and hospital resources provided from one patient to the next. The PPS system implemented a new reimbursement model based on diagnostic-related groups (DRGs).[30] Under PPS, hospitals would receive a single fixed payment per case-type to accommodate every service provided during an inpatient stay. Case-types were determined based on a DRG system, which determined an a priori reimbursement amount for a given condition. This new payment model encouraged hospitals to be better stewards of resources because any costs incurred above what was expected would reduce the amount left over in Medicare's payment to the hospital.[30] Because physicians make admission and discharge decisions, which ultimately influence hospital resource expenditures, the relationship between hospitals and physicians under PPS became more complex.[31]

Critics of the PPS were concerned that this new policy would financially ruin hospitals because many of their costs would not be covered.[32,33] Critics also worried that PPS incentives would lead patient to be discharged too soon due to financial, not health, concerns.[33] Scientific evaluations of the PPS found that Medicare costs per capita were lowered by 3.7% due mainly to a 5.3% reduction of per capita admission.[34] This suggests that hospitals after PPS tended to be for sicker patients and/or that less sick patients were forgoing inpatient care. In addition, researchers found that there was no decline in quality of care and in fact mortality rates improved.[35] Taken together, this suggests that the PPS may have helped to reduce some moral hazard.

Simultaneously, researchers noted that during the 1980s, corresponding to the implementation of the PPS, there was a significant increase in outpatient procedures, which were not subjected to prospective payments.[36] It is not clear if the shift to outpatient surgeries was due to reimbursement pressures, evolving surgical techniques improvements in technology, or some combination of these factors. Either way, Medicare costs during the 1980s were curbed.

1990s

At this point, the ubiquity of HMOs, who used selective contracting, resulted in disgruntled hospitals and physicians who perceived HMO tactics as meddlesome and threatening.[37] HMOs were able to negotiate lower reimbursement rates with providers in part by threatening exclusion from their proprietary-care networks and large patient bases.[38] To combat the perceived aggressive behaviors of HMOs, hospitals and doctors formed IDSs in many markets. IDSs were single legal entities made up of providers representing the full continuum of care including outpatient services (both physician and nonphysician services), acute care (emergency and inpatient services), long-term care (postacute services including skilled nursing), and hospice care to patients.[39] While IDSs and HMOs share many similarities; and some early HMOs were in fact IDSs, the IDS movement in the 1990s was driven by providers whereas the HMO of the 1970s were driven by payers and providers. IDSs in the 1990s were typically formed when hospitals systems purchased or partnered with physician practices and postacute care providers through vertical integration. Vertical integration is when an organization acquires or merges with another organization that is either before or after them in the continuum of care. In contrast, horizontal integration occurs when an organization acquires or merges with another organization of the same type, for example, when two hospitals merge.

The consolidated entity known as the IDS gained significant negotiating power against HMOs in many markets because of their ability to cover the full continuum of care and the fact that they represented many physicians and services in that market. Besides having more leverage in HMO reimbursement negotiations, IDSs had multiple other theoretical benefits as well.[38–40] For example, an IDS has greater economies of scale and scope (than individual providers) that could result in reducing overhead costs, obtaining better deals from suppliers, and/or the ability to obtain cheaper capital (similar to some HMOs). Moreover, quality and the coordination of care should, theoretically, be better if a single entity, rather than fragmented providers, was responsible for the full continuum of care. Ultimately the benefits of IDSs to providers stem from structural integration (e.g., forming a new legal entity thus gaining immediate negotiating power with HMOs) and functional integration (e.g., aligning all providers in the IDS and improving coordination of care)[41]; the latter of which proved more difficult in the 1990s.[41,42]

Functional integration requires getting all providers across the full continuum of care to effectively coordinate services and if facilitated by getting all of the information systems to seamlessly transfer health data from one setting to the other within the IDS. Most IDSs never achieved functional integration for several reasons including: (1) management's failure to deal with the natural independent mindedness of physicians, (2) the predominant fee-for-service environment that served as a disincentive to coordinate care or reduce costs (note that fee-for-service implicitly incentivizes a higher volume of services in order to increase revenue), and (3) the skeptical nature of physicians who lacked trust in IDS administrators who focused on measuring productivity, financial outcomes, technological shortfalls (of information systems at the time), and other managerial metrics that were not previously common in the practice of medicine.[42,43] Ultimately, the costs of forming IDSs, especially pertaining to purchasing physician practices, and the inability to achieve functional integration resulted in a lack of realized benefits.[42] Many IDSs sold the physician practices they purchased back to the physicians.[44,45]

2000s

In the early part of the first decade of the new millennium, a full backlash against managed care resulted in the evolution of many HMOs into Preferred Provider Organizations (PPOs).[46–48] PPOs dropped certain tactics that providers disdained especially if research evidence suggested these tactics we ineffective at reducing costs or improving quality. As such, PPOs were perceived as less aggressive against patients and providers to limit consumer and medical choice. A description of how HMOs, PPOs, and traditional indemnity insurance plans differ with respect to premiums, choice of providers, services covered, and payer ability to assure quality of care is presented in Table 48-1.

Despite the changes to managed-care practices, healthcare costs continued to rise,[49] and the looming threat of a large number of Baby Boomers retiring and becoming eligible for Medicare, coupled with the increase in life expectancy[50] caused projections of forthcoming Medicare trust fund insolvency.[51,52] The Medicare trust fund was the government account that paid for hospital care within the program. Given that Medicare hospital coverage was funded by a payroll tax, the large expected reductions in payroll tax revenue (when Baby Boomers retire) and the simultaneous expected health services utilization of Baby Boomers becoming Medicare eligible resulted in a fiscal challenges for the program.[53] Furthermore, given that the average Medicare recipient was now living significantly longer than in the 1960s when Medicare was enacted, reform was needed to reduce healthcare costs especially in the Medicare program. Similarly, the increase in life expectancy had the potential to strain Medicaid budgets because these programs frequently pay for a large component of nursing home care.

A variety of new revenue and delivery models, known as alternative payment models (APMs), were identified that had promise in reducing costs, improving coordination of care and improving quality. Among these models were Patient Centered Medical Homes (PCMH), which are focused on primary care; bundled payments which are focused on hospital care; and Accountable Care Organizations (ACOs), which are focused on all healthcare utilization.[54] PCMH are a way of organizing primary care that emphasizes care coordination and communication in an effort to improve quality and reduce costs.[55,56] In many ways, the

TABLE 48-1 DIFFERENCES ON VARIOUS ATTRIBUTES BY HEALTH INSURANCE PLAN TYPE

Plan Type	Patient Premiums	Patient Deductibles	Patient Choice of Provider	Services Covered	Payer Ability to Assure Quality
Traditional (indemnity)	High	Low	Not limited	All prevention, and a wide range of other services	Low
PPO	Moderate	Low or high	Somewhat limited	All prevention, and a more limited list of other services	Moderate
HMO	Lowest	Low	Very limited	All prevention, and a wide range of other service	High

PCMH is a modern version of the HMO gatekeeper model re-envisioned from the perspective of the physician rather than the payer.[56] Bundled payments are agreements whereby hospitals and postacute care providers agree to receive and share a single payment for an "episode of care" that requires improved coordination across clinical settings. In many ways, bundled payments are an evolved version of PPS that now also includes providers other than just the hospital. ACOs are groups of doctors, hospitals, and other providers, who voluntarily come together to provide coordinated care to Medicare and other patients—and are at financial risk for patient outcomes.[57,58] ACOs are effectively modern IDSs[39] that do not have to integrate by ownership and can instead do so by contracts and or local relationships.

In 2009, in the midst of the largest economic downturn in modern history, the Affordable Care Act was passed and signed into law. Although the Act included many provisions to increase access to care including through insurance mandates, removing out-of-pocket costs associated with preventive services, and an elimination of preexisting conditions clauses; the reforms to Medicare payments have been the most disruptive changes to how providers practice. These payment reforms known as value-based purchasing required Medicare to begin abandoning traditional fee-for-service reimbursement models and move toward APMs. Whereas fee-for-service may incentivize quantity of care (including by inducing moral hazard), APMs focus on the value of care by holding providers accountable for the outcomes, and associated costs, of patients under their care, thereby addressing the cost and quality goals of the iron triangle. Importantly, evidence from the PPS of the 1990s suggested that Medicare costs can be curbed by limiting potential moral hazard by forcing providers to provide care within a predetermined reimbursement rate.[34,59]

2010s

The Affordable Care Act was politically and legally controversial. Legal challenges to the law that were decided by the U.S. Supreme Court focused on the individual mandates (which required citizens to have insurance coverage), Medicaid expansions (which forced state eligibility rules for Medicaid to be more generous and cover more individuals), and whether the government can force employers to offer contraception as a preventive service in private health plans. The individual mandates were determined to be constitutional because the government is allowed to influence consumer participation in the health insurance market through the ability to levy a tax on those who do not obtain coverage. Medicaid expansion was deemed unconstitutional because it required states to share in the cost of the increased coverage. However, rather than invalidate the entire Act, the court decided that each state can opt into the expansion if they choose. Lastly, the court determined that the government cannot force employers to offer contraception in private health plans; but failed to invalidate the entire Act.

Importantly, the value-based purchasing tenets of the Affordable Care Act, while resisted by providers, did not receive much political or legal challenge. In fact, the Republican led congress that was elected 2 years after the passing of the Affordable Care Act passed the Medicare and CHIP Reauthorization Act (MARCA) of 2015 which was signed into law by President Obama. In other words, MACRA, which strengthened Medicare's commitment to value-based purchasing was enacted with bipartisanship. MACRA directs Medicare to accelerate efforts to reduce fee-for-service payments and instead begins shifting physician and hospital reimbursements toward APMs and other shared-risk payment models. Shared-risk payment models require "skin in the game" among providers who are held accountable for patient outcomes including costs. In other words, providers can lose reimbursement if they do not reduce costs and/or improve quality. Through individual mandates, Medicaid expansions, and value-based purchasing, the ACA attempts to address all three goals of the healthcare iron triangle.

In order to be successful in APMs or any shared-risk payment model, a focus on cost reduction (including by preventing unnecessary expensive utilization) is paramount. Models of care that improve coordination within an IDS, focus on prevention, and attempt to improve care including by better utilizing community and clinical resources are collectively known as population health management (PHM). PHM, which is rooted in the practice of public health in the context of healthcare delivery, is now considered necessary to be successful under value-based purchasing arrangements in the U.S. healthcare system. The PHM Framework[60] includes conducting health assessments of a given population, risk stratifying individuals based on their known proclivity to have certain diseases or outcomes, and then developing tailored interventions designed to (1) keep healthy individuals well, (2) aggressively manage risks for at-risk individuals, and (3) provide the appropriate care coordination or disease case management for those requiring extensive clinical utilization. PHM is only in its infancy in the current U.S. healthcare system. Early evidence shows most ACOs have seen minor cost savings,[61–63] reduced utilization,[63] and mixed evidence on quality,[62] although ACOs in higher spending areas or with higher benchmarks are more likely to see savings.[61]

In response to the large amount of change in the market, many physicians consolidated into larger group practices,[64] or become employees of hospitals and health systems in part to shield themselves from regulatory and market forces.[65] Thus, the current changes brought upon by changing reimbursement policies are continuing to affect revenue and delivery models in the United States. Separately, change is occurring for patients as well. An increased focus on consumerism in healthcare has emphasized the importance of the patient experience and patient satisfaction. Concomitantly, the focus on consumerism has increased expectations that patients become more financial responsible for their healthcare decisions. High-deductible health plans are insurance products with high patient cost-sharing in exchange for lower premiums. Such plans incentivize patients to see lower cost providers and to potentially forgo care that may not be needed.[66] Thus, high-deductible health plans represent a revenue and delivery model that aims to influence patient behaviors as opposed to providers.

The Trump Administration

President Donald Trump's campaign was focused on a few major platforms, including the repeal and replacement of the Affordable Care Act. After his inauguration in 2017, he supported several failed bills in Congress each of which attempted to repeal or replace major provisions of the Act.[67–69] Nevertheless, President Trump signed into law the Tax Cuts and Jobs Act of 2017, which effectively repealed the tax penalty of the individual mandate of the Affordable Care Act. Specifically, while Americans are still required to maintain health insurance coverage, there is now no penalty (e.g., no tax) for failing to do so. As such, it is expected that more Americans will forgo coverage, which will in turn result in increased premiums because those dropping out will cause an increase in the remaining risk pool.[70] Separately, the Trump Administration has enacted several policies consistent with campaign promises to disrupt the Affordable Care Act. For example, the administration cut the open-enrollment advertisement budget that encourages individuals to gain coverage through the Affordable Care Act insurance market exchanges from $100 million to $10 milion.[71] Moreover, the open-enrollment period on Healthcare.gov was shortened from 3 months to 45 days.[72]

CONCLUSIONS

Reforms to the U.S. healthcare system have attempted to reduce costs, improve quality, and/or improve access to care for many decades. Each attempt at affecting revenue and delivery models does so by changing reimbursement or other policies within Medicare,

Medicaid, or the federal government. While there may be political disagreements regarding how to accomplish the goals of the triple aim,[73] a set of underlying facts cannot be ignored. Namely, the United States spends more per capita on healthcare than any other nation in the world, quality of care in the United States is subpar compared to comparable nations, and many Americans are uninsured and do not have access to the care they need. Moreover, the continued transition of Baby Boomers into Medicare is causing financial stains on the system that is financed by payroll taxes as conceived in the 1960s.

What can be expected next? One can anticipate a continued focus on quality, costs, and the patient experience. These three concepts, which are similar to the iron triangle, are now being called the triple aim of the U.S. healthcare system.[73] Health services delivery organizations are going to be expected to develop improved PHM skills; and innovation in doing so will likely result in financial rewards from payers. As Medicare solidifies its commitment to APMs, history suggests that other payers will soon follow.[74] Indeed, major private payers are increasing a focus on value-based reimbursement models to incentivize health systems to reduce costs and/or improve quality of care. Overall, changes in reimbursement policies that are increasingly stressing population health are effectively forcing health systems to think more like public health professionals. In essence, health systems will be financially rewarded when they are able to prevent disease or slow disease progression, facilitate patients' access to the lowest cost and most appropriate setting for care, and mobilize community resources that enable patients to address the social determinants of health that exacerbate their healthcare utilization.

References

1. Kissick WL. *Medicine's Dilemmas: Infinite Needs versus Finite Resources.* New Haven: Yale University Press; 1994.
2. Skolnik AM. Employee-benefit plans, 1954–60. *Soc Sec Bull.* 1962;25:5.
3. Follmann JF. The growth of group health insurance. *J Risk Insur.* 1965;32(1):105–12.
4. Holland DM, National Bureau of Economic Research. *Private Pension Funds; Projected Growth.* New York: National Bureau of Economic Research; distributed by Columbia University Press; 1966.
5. Scofea LA. The development and growth of employer-provided health insurance. *Mon Labor Rev.* 1994;117(3):3–10.
6. De Lew N.Medicare: 35 Years of service. *Health Care Financ R.* 2000;22(1):75–103.
7. National Center for Health Statistics. *Vital Statistics of the United States, 1965.* Washington, DC: National Center for Health Statistics; 1967.
8. Pauly MV. Medicare drug coverage and moral hazard. *Health Aff (Millwood).* 2004;23(1):113–22.
9. Pauly MV. The economics of moral hazard: Comment. *Am Econ Rev.* 1968;58(3):531–7.
10. Hall CP. Deductibles in health insurance: An evaluation. *J Risk Insur.* 1966;33(2):253–63.
11. Brook RH, United States. Department of Health and Human Services, Rand Corporation, Rand Health Insurance Experiment. *The Effect of Coinsurance on the Health of Adults: Results from the Rand Health Insurance Experiment.* Santa Monica, CA: Rand; 1984.
12. Gruber LR, Shadle M, Polich CL. From movement to industry—The growth of HMOs. *Health Aff (Millwood).* 1988;7(3):197–208.
13. Dorsey JL. The Health Maintenance Organization Act of 1973 (P.L. 93-222) and prepaid group practice plans. *Med Care.* 1975;13(1):1–9.
14. Lyles A, Palumbo FB. The effect of managed care on prescription drug costs and benefits. *Pharmacoeconomics.* 1999;15(2):129–40.
15. Langwell KM. Structure and performance of health maintenance organizations: A review. *Health Care Financ Rev.* 1990;12(1):71–9.
16. Ellwood PM, Jr., Anderson NN, Billings JE, Carlson RJ, Hoagberg EJ, McClure W. Health maintenance strategy. *Med Care.* 1971;9(3):291–8.
17. Luft HS. Assessing the evidence on HMO performance. *Milbank Mem Fund Q Health Soc.* 1980;58(4):501–36.
18. Gold MR. HMOs and managed care. *Health Aff (Millwood).* 1991;10(4): 189–206.
19. Newhouse JP, United States. Department of Health and Human Services, Rand Corporation. *Some Interim Results from a Controlled Trial of Cost Sharing in Health Insurance.* Santa Monica, CA: Rand Corp.; 1982.
20. Lohr KN, Brook RH, Kamberg CJ, et al. Use of medical care in the Rand Health Insurance Experiment. Diagnosis- and service-specific analyses in a randomized controlled trial. *Med Care.* 1986;24(9 Suppl):S1–87.
21. Martin DP, Diehr P, Price KF, Richardson WC. Effect of a gatekeeper plan on health services use and charges: A randomized trial. *Am J Public Health.* 1989;79(12):1628–32.
22. Forrest CB, Reid RJ. Passing the baton: HMO's influence on referrals to specialty care. *Health Aff (Millwood).* 1997;16(6):157–62.
23. Melnick GA, Zwanziger J, Bamezai A, Pattison R. The effects of market structure and bargaining position on hospital prices. *J Health Econ.* 1992;11(3):217–33.
24. Zwanziger J, Melnick GA, Bamezai A. The effect of selective contracting on hospital costs and revenues. *Health Serv Res.* 2000;35(4):849–67.
25. Mobley LR. Effects of selective contracting on hospital efficiency, costs and accessibility. *Health Econ.* 1998;7(3):247–61.
26. Robinson JC, Phibbs CS. An evaluation of Medicaid selective contracting in California. *J Health Econ.* 1989;8(4):437–55.
27. Miller RH, Luft HS. Does managed care lead to better or worse quality of care? *Health Aff (Millwood).* 1997;16(5):7–25.
28. Cutler DM, McClellan M, Newhouse JP. How does managed care do it? *Rand J Econ.* 2000;31(3):526–48.
29. Guterman S, Dobson A. Impact of the Medicare prospective payment system for hospitals. *Health Care Financ Rev.* 1986;7(3):97–114.
30. Iglehart JK. Medicare begins prospective payment of hospitals. *N Engl J Med.* 1983;308(23):1428–32.
31. Glandon GL, Morrisey MA. Redefining the hospital-physician relationship under prospective payment. *Inquiry.* 1986;23(2):166–75.
32. Mayes R. The origins, development, and passage of Medicare's revolutionary prospective payment system. *J Hist Med Allied Sci.* 2007;62(1):21–55.
33. Iglehart JK. Early experience with prospective payment of hospitals. *N Engl J Med.* 1986;314(22):1460–4.
34. Sloan FA, Morrisey MA, Valvona J. Effects of the Medicare prospective payment system on hospital cost containment: An early appraisal. *Milbank Q.* 1988;66(2):191–220.
35. Kahn KL, Rogers WH, Rubenstein LV, et al. Measuring quality of care with explicit process criteria before and after implementation of the DRG-based prospective payment system. *JAMA.* 1990;264(15):1969–73.
36. Duffy SQ, Farley DE. Patterns of decline among inpatient procedures. *Public Health Rep.* 1995;110(6):674–81.
37. Hilzenrath DS. Backlash builds over managed care. *Washington Post*; 1997.
38. Bazzoli GJ, Dynan L, Burns LR, Yap C. Two decades of organizational change in health care: What have we learned? *Med Care Res Rev.* 2004;61(3):247–331.
39. Hwang W, Chang J, Laclair M, Paz H. Effects of integrated delivery system on cost and quality. *Am J Manag Care.* 2013;19(5):e175–84.
40. Walston SL, Kimberly JR, Burns LR. Owned vertical integration and health care: Promise and performance. *Health Care Manage Rev.* 1996;21(1):83–92.
41. Byrne MM, Ashton CM. Incentives for vertical integration in healthcare: The effect of reimbursement systems. *J Healthc Manag.* 1999;44(1):34–44; discussion 45-36.
42. Budetti PP, Shortell SM, Waters TM, et al. Physician and health system integration. *Health Aff (Millwood).* 2002;21(1):203–10.
43. Gillies RR, Zuckerman HS, Burns LR, et al. Physician-system relationships: Stumbling blocks and promising practices. *Med Care.* 2001;39(7 Suppl 1):I92–106.
44. Lake T, Devers K, Brewster L, Casalino L. Something old, something new: Recent developments in hospital-physician relationships. *Health Serv Res.* 2003;38(1 Pt 2):471–88.
45. Weil TP. Divesting losers: Chipping away at integrated delivery systems. *Physician Exec.* 2002;28(3):44–51.
46. Cooper PF, Simon KI, Vistnes J. A closer look at the managed care backlash. *Med Care.* 2006;44(5):4–11.
47. Mechanic D. The managed care backlash: Pserceptions and rhetoric in health care policy and the potential for health care reform. *Milbank Q.* 2001;79(1):35–54; 32 p preceding VI.
48. Draper DA, Hurley RE, Lesser CS, Strunk BC. The changing face of managed care. *Health Aff (Millwood).* 2002;21(1):11–23.
49. Glied S, Ma S, Solis-Roman C. Where the money goes: The evolving expenses of the US Health Care System. *Health Aff (Millwood).* 2016;35(7):1197–203.
50. Chetty R, Stepner M, Abraham S, et al. The association between income and life expectancy in the United States, 2001–2014. *JAMA.* 2016;315(16):1750–66.

51. Budetti PP. Health reform for the 21st century? It may have to wait until the 21st century. *JAMA*. 1997;277(3):193–8.
52. Miller T. Increasing longevity and Medicare expenditures. *Demography*. 2001;38(2):215–26.
53. Lubitz J, Beebe J, Baker C. Longevity and Medicare expenditures. *N Engl J Med*. 1995;332(15):999–1003.
54. Shay PD, Mick SS. Post-acute care and vertical integration after the Patient Protection and Affordable Care Act. *J Healthc Manag*. 2013;58(1):15–27; discussion 27-18.
55. Assurance NCFQ. *Benefits of NCQA Patient-Centered Medical Home Recognition*. Washington, DC: NCQA; 2016.
56. Crabtree BF, Nutting PA, Miller WL, Stange KC, Stewart EE, Jaen CR. Summary of the National Demonstration Project and recommendations for the patient-centered medical home. *Ann Fam Med*. 2010;8(Suppl 1): S80–90; S92.
57. McClellan M, McKethan AN, Lewis JL, Roski J, Fisher ES. A national strategy to put accountable care into practice. *Health Aff (Millwood)*. 2010;29(5):982–90.
58. Fisher ES, Shortell SM. Accountable care organizations accountable for what, to whom, and how. *JAMA*. 2010;304(15):1715–16.
59. Ellis RP, McGuire TG. Hospital response to prospective payment: Moral hazard, selection, and practice-style effects. *J Health Econ*. 1996;15(3):257–77.
60. Care Continuum Alliance. Outcomes Guidelines Report Volume 5. Washington, DC; 2010.
61. McWilliams JM, Chernew ME, Landon BE, Schwartz AL. Performance differences in year 1 of pioneer accountable care organizations. *New Engl J Med*. 2015;372(20):1927–36.
62. McWilliams JM, Hatfield LA, Chernew ME, Landon BE, Schwartz AL. Early performance of accountable care organizations in Medicare. *New Engl J Med*. 2016;374(24):2357–66.
63. Nyweide DJ, Lee W, Cuerdon TT, et al. Association of pioneer accountable care organizations vs traditional Medicare fee for service with spending, utilization, and patient experience. *JAMA*. 2015;313(21):2152–61.
64. Muhlestein DB, Smith NJ. Physician consolidation: Rapid movement from small to large group practices, 2013–15. *Health Aff (Millwood)*. 2016;35(9):1638–42.
65. Burns LR, Goldsmith JC, Sen A. Horizontal and vertical integration of physicians: A tale of two tails. *Adv Health Care Manag*. 2013;15:39–117.
66. Agarwal R, Mazurenko O, Menachemi N. High-deductible health plans reduce health care cost and utilization, including use of needed preventive services. *Health Aff (Millwood)*. 2017;36(10):1762–8.
67. The Henry J. Kaiser Family Foundation. Summary of the American Health Care Act. Kaiser Family Foundation; 2017.
68. The Henry J. Kaiser Family Foundation. Summary of the Better Care Reconciliation Act of 2017. The Henry J. Kaiser Family Foundation; 2017.
69. The Henry J. Kaiser Family Foundation. Summary of Graham-Cassidy-Heller-Johnson Amendment. The Henry J. Kaiser Family Foundation; 2017.
70. Congressional Budget Office. Repealing the Individual Health Insurance Mandate: An Updated Estimate. Congressional Budget Office; November, 2017.
71. Jost T. CMS cuts ACA advertising by 90 percent amid other cuts to enrollment outreach. Health Affairs Blog. 2017.
72. Shafer PD, Stacie. Looking ahead to 2018: Will a shorter open enrollment period reduce adverse selection in exchange plans? Health Affairs Blog. 2017.
73. Berwick DM, Nolan TW, Whittington J. The triple aim: Care, health, and cost. *Health Aff (Millwood)*. 2008;27(3):759–69.
74. Tunis SR. Why Medicare has not established criteria for coverage decisions. *N Engl J Med*. 2004;350(21):2196–8.

CHAPTER

49 Implementing Public Health Programs

W. Oscar Fleming • Rohit Ramaswamy

CHALLENGES IN ACHIEVING PUBLIC HEALTH OUTCOMES

The root causes and manifestations of public health challenges reflect the diversity and complexity of human life as well as our living and working environments. For example, tobacco use can have effects on the tobacco user (primary), those nearby through second-hand smoke (secondary), and the immediate environment through accumulation of nicotine and other carcinogens (tertiary). Working to prevent and reduce the health impacts of tobacco use requires a diverse range of interventions. These might include clinical and behavioral interventions with the user in addition to broadly targeted efforts to change social attitudes toward tobacco use and raise awareness of the risks of environmental tobacco exposure for young children. This example is mirrored in many other challenges public health seeks to address, such as obesity, opioid abuse, injury prevention, maternal and infant mortality, among others. In summary, many common public health problems require complex, multifaceted interventions.

Further adding to the complexity are the populations and systems involved. There is a great diversity of cultures within and between national borders and regions, and a rapidly evolving shared culture as our world becomes more connected and urbanized. This variation leads to many ways of understanding and valuing health as well as a wide range of systems to promote health and well-being. The legacy of human history and the impact of a rapidly evolving context have immediate and long-term effects on how interventions are perceived and utilized in various settings. As a result, not only do public health interventions need to be have multiple components, but their delivery also has to be tailored and responsive to the characteristics of each setting.

In the face of such complexity, there is a need to develop evidence based multilevel interventions for public health.[1] In the last several decades, a sustained focus on quality and outcomes has expanded the availability of evidence-based public health programs that have demonstrated some effectiveness (e.g., improved child well-being) through research and evaluations.[2,3] These programs seek to influence key factors that affect the public's health.[4] For example, Trauma Focused Cognitive Behavioral Therapy (TF-CBT) and the Positive Parenting Program (Triple P) are programs with different approaches seeking to achieve a common outcome of improved child well-being and reduced maltreatment.[5,6] TF-CBT is a therapeutic intervention for children and parents delivered by a trained clinicians designed to prevent and address posttraumatic stress, depression, and behavioral challenges.[6] Triple P is a system of parenting education programs delivered by professionals and lay people alike designed to have broad community coverage.[7]

Many of these interventions are widely available on registries and websites and promoted and funded by Federal, state, and private agencies.[8–11] The strength of the evidence of effectiveness varies and is often depicted along a continuum running from ineffective through promising to proven. Notwithstanding their proliferation and promotion, there are many areas for which we do not have proven public health interventions. In response, there is ongoing investment in research to identify new interventions to fill gaps in our knowledge and intervention arsenal.

The need for effective interventions in various contexts is only one part of the puzzle. To realize the intended improvement in the public's health, at scale, effective interventions must be *implemented as intended* across a diverse range of delivery contexts and levels.[12,13] This means that public health interventions must be widely disseminated and accessible to potential users. Furthermore, our public health systems must be prepared and able to effectively select, introduce, and sustain the programs to realize the intended outcomes.

Recent reviews of the state of practice have identified a significant time lag between the demonstration of program effectiveness in research settings and their wide spread use in public health settings.[14] There is also a lack of knowledge about how exactly the results achieved in controlled research environments need to be adapted across diverse contexts. Evaluation of the implementation of well-established, public health interventions, such as the surgical safety checklist have demonstrated no significant impact at scale, possibly due to poor or inconsistent implementation.[15] Therefore, evidence of effectiveness in one setting is not enough to ensure successful outcomes when implementation takes place.[16] In short, many public health interventions are taking too long to reach the intended beneficiaries and are not realizing the promised effects.

There are many factors contributing to this situation, including poor knowledge of local contexts, inadequate attention to adaptation, entrenched workforce behavior and organizational cultures and the absence of translational supports to help integrate emerging evidence successfully and quickly into practice contexts. Parallel to the ongoing focus on better evidence-based interventions, the field of Implementation science has evolved in response to implementation challenges. As a field, implementation science involves both implementation research and practice.

Eccles and Mittman define implementation research as: *Implementation research is the scientific study of methods to promote the systematic uptake of research findings and other evidence-based practices into routine practice, and, hence, to improve the quality and effectiveness of health services. It includes the study of influences on healthcare professional and organisational behavior.*[13] Implementation practice supports the use of implementation research with the aim of improving implementation processes in real-world settings. The goals of implementation science include significantly reducing the time required to bring effective public health interventions into widespread use; expanding the capacity of public health actors to support and sustain high-quality use of these interventions; and, finally, creating enabling organizational and policy environments that promote the systematic implementation of effective interventions in the field.

In summary, as there continues to be an increased emphasis on the use of interventions that have demonstrated effectiveness to address the complex public health challenges of today, there is the need for public health professionals trained in implementation science capable of using a range of evidence from multiple disciplines to analyze and address probable facilitators and barriers to successful and sustainable delivery of these interventions to populations. These specialists must also be able to engage counterparts in the public health system, including consumers, agency leaders and staff, and policy makers, in the design of appropriate and feasible roadmaps for practice change and to ensure that the necessary capacity and infrastructure is in place to support the programs effective delivery. Yet, while this need is well recognized, there is still uncertainty and inconsistency in defining the key elements and concepts of implementation science. In the following section, these are further described.

WHAT IS NEEDED FOR SUCCESSFUL IMPLEMENTATION?

Fixsen and colleagues have synthesized a broad range of implementation related research to identify key factors that can be addressed to increase the quality and outcomes of implementation efforts.[17] The findings are organized into several frameworks known as the Active Implementation Frameworks. The following section briefly summarizes these frameworks and provides some examples of their application in real world public health contexts.

Usable Innovations

To be most useful for practitioners, public health interventions must be well defined.[18] This means that there should be a clear description of the intended beneficiaries. Relevant principles and values underpinning the intervention should also be articulated. The primary elements of the intervention, often called the core components, should be clearly specified and operationalized so that they are teachable, learnable, observable, and doable.[19] Well-defined interventions include methods for assessing performance fidelity and quality. While it may not be realistic to expect to find this level of detail in published effectiveness studies, program developers who provide support for implementation, can often provide this information. The successful selection of programs and their alignment with a specific context involves the host agency or system, consumers, the program developer and/or purveyor, and relevant funding agencies and policy makers to maximize contextual fit and feasibility. With this information, leaders and teams can make informed, contextualized decisions about program selection.

Implementation Stages

The nature of implementation practice varies over time. The Active Implementation Stages framework codifies this evolution into four stages: *Exploration, Installation, Initial implementation, and Full implementation.* Exploration involves the active assessment of possible interventions against the identified needs of a selected population or community and the careful appraisal of the capacity of the public health system to successfully introduce the interventions. The stage ends with the selection of one or more interventions, where the installation stage begins. During installation, public agencies are putting in place the necessary infrastructure to support the selected intervention. This includes recruiting hiring and preparing staff, preparing support systems (e.g., a data system), adapting policy, procuring necessary materials, and raising awareness in the community for the coming change. The installation stage is often skipped or under attended to, often to the detriment of the new intervention.

When the new intervention is initiated (e.g., the first new family receives the intervention), the initial implementation stage has begun. Intervention practitioners are trying out new skills and are often at risk of reverting to business as usual. Active and ongoing support for practice change and system enhancement is often key in this stage. Intentional use of quality improvement methods can drive rapid learning and facilitate adaptations to improve the fit between the intervention and the host community. Initial outcomes are typically slow to be seen and inconsistent but with ongoing support and improvement programs can realize increasing quality. When programs realize consistent fidelity with a majority of implanting staff, a site moves into full implementation. In this stage, attention turns to sustaining fidelity, ongoing and often incremental improvement, and considerations of scale up.

The stages are not linear. Changing circumstances, such as a change in community conditions, can necessitate a return to an earlier stage. Furthermore, implementing sites within a single system may be at different stages at the same time. Nonetheless, stages can be useful in helping focus attention on identifying and selecting the right strategies for the work at hand.

Implementation Drivers

The implementation drivers address the critical infrastructure (i.e., the people, materials, polices, and other resources) required to deliver the program as intended. The drivers are addressed over time through the implementation stages described above. Ideally, the infrastructure necessary to effectively deliver an intervention is well understood and thoroughly explored before a selection decision is finalized. Once an intervention is selected, the focus of implementation shifts to building and improving this infrastructure. Attending to the drivers is critical, as many programs fail due to underdevelopment of the supportive infrastructure required for success.[20]

The implementation drivers (Fig. 49-1) are organized into three domains. *Competency* drivers relate to recruiting, preparing, and coaching staff and service providers to support and deliver the selected intervention, with fidelity. *Organizational* drivers related to robust data systems, management practice and policy, and work with external partners and stakeholders to help create the enabling context for the program's success. Finally, *Leadership* drivers, which encompass diverse leadership skills and actions needed at multiple levels within systems to ensure sustained resources and commitment to achieving effective implementation at adequate scale to influence the prioritized outcomes for the populations in need.

Implementation Teams

Implementation teams represent one approach to organizing the public health workforce to effectively employ implementation strategies to deliver evidence-based programs.[21–23] A synthesis of core elements of 25 implementation frameworks revealed that 68% (17) of the frameworks included in the review mentioned implementation

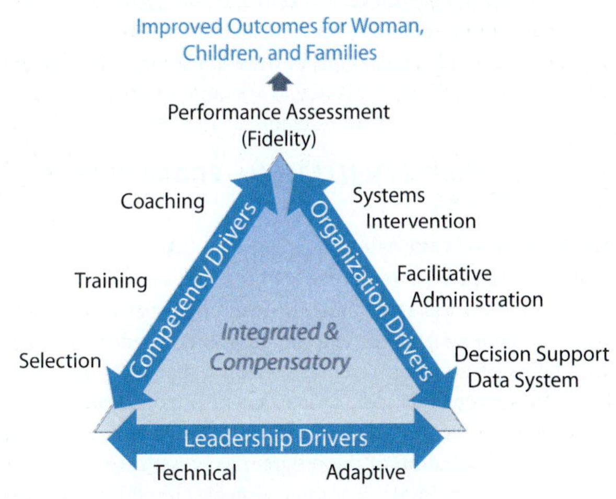

FIGURE 49-1. Implementation drivers.

teams as a critical factor of success.[24] Roles for an implementation team include engaging with organizational and community stakeholders, developing implementation plans, providing coaching and technical assistance, evaluating processes, providing supportive feedback, and fostering organizational learning.

Despite finding broad inclusion of teams in many frameworks, Meyers et al. noted that empirical evidence supporting the use of teams was limited and largely based on case studies.[24] There have been few empirical studies of the use of teams in complex public health settings. Instead, the literature has largely focused on the role of individual practitioners.[25–28]

The relatively small number of studies of implementation teams limits understanding of how teams' function and with whom, as well as the critical facilitators of and barriers to their success. Without operationalized workforce strategies that fit with and are feasible for our public service systems, the growing body of EBPs will remain largely "on the shelf" with limited impact for children, families and society at large.

Improvement Cycles

The selection and introduction of a new program into a complex system typically necessitates considerable practice change to ensure the host system can successfully integrate the new practices required. While some practice change can be foreseen, many unforeseen changes will arise as programs are adopted into increasing diverse contexts. Through intentional and systematic quality improvement efforts, real-world feedback can be captured and used to incrementally improve infrastructure to increase the likelihood for high fidelity practice and community impact.[29] Implementation Science and Quality Improvement (or Improvement Science) have existed and evolved as discrete and separate fields but need to be understood as integral to one another. Quality Improvement approaches focus on developing solutions to improve the processes and systems that surround a specific program or service. There are a variety of quality improvement methods but at the core of each is a basic cycle, the Plan-Do-Study-Act (PDSA) cycle that teams use to identify and test possible solutions to identified gaps in quality. Multiple improvement cycles are used to test and refine the proposed solution.

PDSA cycles have great relevance for supporting implementation. Because context and setting influence the quality of implementation, merely developing an implementation strategy does not guarantee that it will work in the context in which the improvement activities take place. Implementation teams need to systematically test and develop feasible and effective implementation strategies that are context appropriate using the iterative PDSA cycles. As we develop and test these implementation strategies, it may become necessary to redesign the intervention in a way that facilitates implementation. QI and implementation science are, therefore, interrelated fields whose tools can be used synergistically to create the best improvement intervention that is most effectively implemented in its setting.

Metz et al. provide an example of the application of implementation theory and methods in service to systemic improvement in the context of county child welfare systems (see Box 49-1).[30]

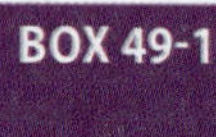

BOX 49-1 Active Implementation Frameworks for Successful Service Delivery: Catawba County Child Well-Being Project

In 2007, the National Implementation Network (NIRN) partnered with the Catawba County (North Carolina) Department of Social Services and The Duke Endowment to expand services and supports for children and families served by the child welfare system, focused on improving foster youth's transition to adulthood. A continuum of evidence-based or informed postcare services for children and families in permanent placements were selected, developed, and implemented. The Active Implementation Frameworks were used to promote successful program operations and implementation. Investing in the development of active implementation teams and cross-sector leaders was a key aspect of the early successes demonstrated in Catawba County. Implementation teams engaged in the development and installation of implementation drivers to provide the infrastructure for change. Assessments of the implementation drivers provided critical information for action planning to strengthen this infrastructure and improve fidelity over time. Project results provide promising data for the use of the AIFs to promote high-fidelity implementation of empirically supported treatments and innovations.

Source: Adapted from Metz et al.

SUPPORTING IMPLEMENTATION—FRAMEWORKS AND STRATEGIES

Implementation Frameworks

Over the last 20 years, a number of implementation researchers have developed frameworks that define the many steps between the identification of appropriate and feasible programs to address a public health challenge and the improvement of related outcomes in the field.[31,32] These steps include: (1) assessment of contextual determinants likely to influence the successful uptake of selected programs; (2) systematic adaptation of the program to be sensitive to the context; (3) selection of implementation strategies to address identified determinants; (4) development of individual, organizational, and systemic implementation capacity; and (5) measurement of both implementation and service outcomes to guide continuous quality improvement.[33]

The Consolidated Framework for Implementation Research (CFIR) is a commonly used framework to categorize barriers to implementation.[34,35] As its title suggests, CFIR consolidates aspects of nineteen other frameworks to present a unified set of determinants. The framework includes five domains: *Intervention Characteristics, Inner Setting, Outer Setting, Characteristics of the Individual,* and *Process.* Under each domain a series of constructs are identified and described (Table 49-1).

The inclusion of multiple domains and the breadth of determinants within these domains support thorough analysis of the implementation context. For a specific public health intervention, the nature of the context and available resources factor into the prioritization of specific determinants for action. For example, the implementation of a program such as Triple-P at a community health center might require the analysis of individual (family and provider) and organizational (clinic) factors that affect implementation. However, the implementation at the county level might require an analysis of the external environment for implementation, for example, the relationship between the different county agencies and nonprofit organizations responsible for funding and supporting the implementation. These might all focus on one level (e.g., the inner setting) or cut across domains (e.g., inner setting and characteristic of the intervention). Tools and resources for the CFIR have been developed to support the careful measurement of determinants to inform implementation actions.

Another type of implementation framework seeks to define the specific steps to be taken to prepare for implementation, to build capacity, to measure progress and to improve the quality of specific implementation efforts. These process frameworks typically integrate actions such as: (1) identifying the assessment needs and context, (2) evidence appraisal and selection; (3) implementation capacity building and infrastructure development; and (4) performance assessment and quality improvement. Other cross-cutting elements like effective data use and communication may be integrated as well.

The Quality Implementation Framework (QIF) is an example of a process framework.[24] Like the CFIR, the QIF integrates elements from

TABLE 49-1 DOMAINS AND CONSTRUCTS FROM THE CONSOLIDATED FRAMEWORK FOR IMPLEMENTATION RESEARCH[34]

Domain/Construct	Description
I. INTERVENTION CHARACTERISTICS	
A. Intervention source	Perception of key stakeholders about whether the intervention is externally or internally developed
B. Evidence strength and quality	Stakeholders' perceptions of the quality and validity of evidence supporting the belief that the intervention will have desired outcomes
C. Relative advantage	Stakeholders' perception of the advantage of implementing the intervention versus an alternative solution
D. Adaptability	The degree to which an intervention can be adapted, tailored, refined, or reinvented to meet local needs
E. Trialability	The ability to test the intervention on a small scale in the organization, and to be able to reverse course (undo implementation) if warranted
F. Complexity	Perceived difficulty of implementation, reflected by duration, scope, radicalness, disruptiveness, centrality, and intricacy and number of steps required to implement
G. Design quality and packaging	Perceived excellence in how the intervention is bundled, presented, and assembled
H. Cost	Costs of the intervention and costs associated with implementing that intervention including investment, supply, and opportunity costs
II. OUTER SETTING	
A. Patient Needs and Resources	The extent to which patient needs, as well as barriers and facilitators to meet those needs are accurately known and prioritized by the organization
B. Cosmopolitanism	The degree to which an organization is networked with other external organizations
C. Peer Pressure	Mimetic or competitive pressure to implement an intervention, typically because most or other key peer or competing organizations have already implemented or in a bid for a competitive edge
D. External Policy and Incentives	A broad construct that includes external strategies to spread interventions including policy and regulations (governmental or other central entity), external mandates, recommendations and guidelines, pay-for-performance, collaboratives, and public or benchmark reporting
III. INNER SETTING	
A. Structural characteristics	The social architecture, age, maturity, and size of an organization
B. Networks and communications	The nature and quality of webs of social networks and the nature and quality of formal and informal communications within an organization
C. Culture	Norms, values, and basic assumptions of a given organization
D. Implementation climate	The absorptive capacity for change, shared receptivity of involved individuals to an intervention and the extent to which use of that intervention will be rewarded, supported, and expected within their organization
1. Tension for change	The degree to which stakeholders perceive the current situation as intolerable or needing change
2. Compatibility	The degree of tangible fit between meaning and values attached to the intervention by involved individuals, how those align with individuals' own norms, values, and perceived risks and needs, and how the intervention fits with existing workflows and systems
3. Relative priority	Individuals' shared perception of the importance of the implementation within the organization
4. Organizational incentives and rewards	Extrinsic incentives such as goal-sharing awards, performance reviews, promotions, and raises in salary and less tangible incentives such as increased stature or respect
5. Goals and feedback	The degree to which goals are clearly communicated, acted upon, and fed back to staff and alignment of that feedback with goals
6. Learning climate	A climate in which: (a) leaders express their own fallibility and need for team members' assistance and input; (b) team members feel that they are essential, valued, and knowledgeable partners in the change process; (c) individuals feel psychologically safe to try new methods; and (d) there is sufficient time and space for reflective thinking and evaluation
E. Readiness for implementation	Tangible and immediate indicators of organizational commitment to its decision to implement an intervention
1. Leadership engagement	Commitment, involvement, and accountability of leaders and managers with the implementation
2. Available resources	The level of resources dedicated for implementation and ongoing operations including money, training, education, physical space, and time
3. Access to knowledge and information	Ease of access to digestible information and knowledge about the intervention and how to incorporate it into work tasks
IV. CHARACTERISTICS OF INDIVIDUALS	
A. Knowledge and beliefs about the intervention	Individuals' attitudes toward and value placed on the intervention as well as familiarity with facts, truths, and principles related to the intervention
B. Self-efficacy	Individual belief in their own capabilities to execute courses of action to achieve implementation goals

(Continued)

TABLE 49-1 DOMAINS AND CONSTRUCTS FROM THE CONSOLIDATED FRAMEWORK FOR IMPLEMENTATION RESEARCH[34] (*Continued*)

Domain/Construct	Description
I. INTERVENTION CHARACTERISTICS	
C. Individual stage of change	Characterization of the phase an individual is in, as he or she progresses toward skilled, enthusiastic, and sustained use of the intervention
D. Individual identification with organization	A broad construct related to how individuals perceive the organization and their relationship and degree of commitment with that organization
E. Other oersonal attributes	A broad construct to include other personal traits such as tolerance of ambiguity, intellectual ability, motivation, values, competence, capacity, and learning style
V. PROCESS	
A. Planning	The degree to which a scheme or method of behavior and tasks for implementing an intervention are developed in advance and the quality of those schemes or methods
B. Engaging	Attracting and involving appropriate individuals in the implementation and use of the intervention through a combined strategy of social marketing, education, role modeling, training, and other similar activities
1. Opinion leaders	Individuals in an organization who have formal or informal influence on the attitudes and beliefs of
2. Formally appointed internal implementation leaders	Individuals from within the organization who have been formally appointed with responsibility for implementing an intervention as coordinator, project manager, team leader, or another similar role
3. Champions	"Individuals who dedicate themselves to supporting, marketing, and 'driving through' an [implementation], overcoming indifference or resistance that the intervention may provoke in an organization
4. External change agents	Individuals who are affiliated with an outside entity who formally influence or facilitate intervention decisions in a desirable direction
C. Executing	Carrying out or accomplishing the implementation according to plan
D. Reflecting and evaluating	Quantitative and qualitative feedback about the progress and quality of implementation accompanied with regular personal and team debriefing about progress and experience

Source: Adapted with permission from Damschroder, L.J., Aron, D.C., Keith, R.E. et al. Fostering implementation of health services research findings into practice: a consolidated framework for advancing implementation science. Implementation Sci 4, 50 (2009). https://doi.org/10.1186/1748-5908-4-50.

multiple separate frameworks to create a unified guide for implementation efforts. The QIF is divided into four phases, each comprising supporting strategies. Table 49-2 provides a summary of the QIF.

CFIR and the QIF are just two of the many frameworks that lay out the breadth of the conceptual and practical issues included in the scope of implementation science. These frameworks address, in varying degrees, the process of translating research into practice, the evaluation of implementation efforts, and the critical factors influencing implementation practice and results. Reflecting the complexity of public health, these frameworks also typically encompass a range of determinants at multiple levels of a system.[36]

Implementation Strategies

Implementation strategies are "methods or techniques used to enhance the adoption, implementation or sustainability of a…program or practice."[20] These strategies address multiple levels (e.g., service delivery, organizational, system, and policy) and involve diverse actors (e.g., policy makers, consumers, service providers, funders, managers).[37] The range of actors highlights the fact that responsibility for implementation extends well beyond direct service providers.[38] Implementation strategies can be used, alone (discrete) or in concert (multifaceted) to build capacity, address emergent challenges and facilitate progress through the stages of implementation.[37] Examples include the identification and support of internal champions, providing ongoing and high-quality training, promoting service uptake with consumers, and informing local opinion leaders. Table 49-3 defines three types of strategy and provides examples of each.

To date, the core features of most strategies (i.e., its essential elements) and guidelines for their effective use have been inadequately described and tested, limiting their widespread use.[39] Expanded evaluation of strategies in real-world contexts needs been prioritized in order to increase generalizability and uptake.[17,40–44] Given the range of actors implicated, it is also necessary to define potential users for the implementation strategy and how the public health workforce can be organized and supported to do so successfully. Guidelines for specifying strategies address the need for clarifying the core elements of the strategy, such as the intended actor or user, and classify strategies by their purpose, such as scale up.[39,45]

TABLE 49-2 THE QUALITY IMPLEMENTATION FRAMEWORK

Phase one: Initial considerations regarding the host setting
Assessment strategies 1. Conducting a needs and resources assessment 2. Conducting a fit assessment 3. Conducting a capacity/readiness assessment
Decisions about adaptation 4. Possibility for adaptation
Capacity-building strategies 5. Obtaining explicit buy-in from critical stakeholders and fostering a supportive community/organizational climate 6. Building general/organizational capacity 7. Staff recruitment/maintenance 8. Effective preinnovation staff training
Phase two: Creating a structure for implementation structural features for implementation
9. Creating implementation teams 10. Developing an implementation plan
Phase three: Ongoing structure once implementation begins
Ongoing implementation support strategies 11. Technical assistance/coaching/supervision 12. Process evaluation 13. Supportive feedback mechanism
Phase four: Improving future applications
14. Learning from experience

TABLE 49-3 TYPES AND EXAMPLES OF IMPLEMENTATION STRATEGIES[46]

Type	Definition	Example
Discrete	Individual approaches to addressing implementation barriers	• Training • Technical assistance • Funding
Multifaceted	Two or more discrete strategies used together	• Training combined with follow-on coaching • Organizational needs assessment and data sharing agreements with external partners
Blended	The interweaving of several discrete strategies addressing multiple levels and barriers to change, often organized in protocols or as branded implementation interventions	• Availability, Responsiveness, and Continuity (ARC) model • The Institute for Healthcare Improvement's Framework for Spread

Tailoring of strategies

Just as interventions need to be adapted to the context where they are to be used, implementation strategies must be tailored to best fit the context where they will be used. Guidance for this work is only beginning to emerge, though research in this area has been prioritized. Key challenges to strategy selection and tailoring include the currently limited empirical literature, the infrequent use of theory and conceptual models in implementation strategy research, and the breadth of contexts in which evidence based and other interventions are used.[47] While tailored strategies have been shown to be effective in influencing practice change, the evidence base is not robust. Tools and resources have been developed to guide the assessment of contextual factors that influence implementation.[48,49] Research into tailoring methods is a priority and has included the study of such methods as concept mapping, group model building, and intervention mapping.[50] Recommendations to advance the evidence base include improving the specifications of methods used to select and tailor strategies, to clearly describe the strategies used, and use logic models to clearly explain how the strategies are intended to work.[50]

OTHER CONSIDERATIONS FOR SUCCESSFUL IMPLEMENTATION

Evaluating Implementation Quality

Even with the systematic use of implementation frameworks, and the development of tailored strategies, it is important to evaluate and improve the quality of implementation and to make changes as the implementation is taking place. This process evaluation is a critical feature of the implementation process that is not usually an area of emphasis in the development of evidence-based interventions. The RE-AIM framework (Reach, Effectiveness, Adoption, Implementation, Maintenance) and PRECEDE-PROCEED (Predisposing, Reinforcing and Enabling Constructs in Educational Diagnosis and Evaluation-Policy, Regulatory, and Organizational Constructs in Educational and Environmental Development) were both developed to evaluate public health programs. Both frameworks identify specific aspects of implementation that should be evaluated along with program aspects and outcomes.

Policy and Funding Support

Policy makers and funding agencies play an important role in assuring effective use of proven interventions.[38,51] Prioritizing support for high-quality implementation of public health interventions is a key component of this. To make this happen, policy makers and funders should understand and appreciate their role in the context of the larger system. Rather than standing apart from the practitioners they fund, funders can be "at the table" so that feedback from implementation can inform polices and future contracts and agreements.

In addition, policy makers and funders can make intentional choices to change how they fund programs. Rather than fund programs solely based on long-term outcome, funders can support implementation by ensuring communities and implementers have the time and resources necessary to prepare for implementation and set performance objectives related to implementation quality.

Finally, funding agencies and policy makers can promote learning through quality improvement. Establishing an enabling environment that values learning and accepts the potential for failures and context driven adaptation can reduce the rigidity that often leads to promising programs having less than desired impact due to poor implementation.

The experience of child welfare reform in New York City highlights how multiple actors are part of a give and take in a shared effort to improve implementation across a complex system.[52] Beginning 2011, New York City Administration for Children's Services (ACS) has been working to expand the use of evidence based and informed practice models in prevention services continuum. The initiative's goals included improving family functioning and child well-being, reducing repeat maltreatment, and preventing placement in foster care. As of 2015, one in four families was served by an evidence based/informed practice model, and work continues to expand the system wide reach of these programs.

ACS administrators, multiple practice model developers and purveyors, and child welfare service providers worked together to identify, select, introduce, and adapt 11 models. Key lessons drawn from the success of the ongoing effort include the sustained and collaborative partnership supported by robust communication and feedback loops, as well as the intentional use of implementation science to provide a framework to guide collective efforts.

Addressing Equity Issues

According to Healthy People 2020, *health equity* will be achieved when every person has the opportunity to "attain his or her full health potential" and no one is disadvantaged from achieving this potential because of social position or other socially determined circumstances.[53] Health inequities are "…disparities in health between social groups who have different levels of underlying social advantage/disadvantage," which "put groups of people who are already socially disadvantaged at further disadvantage with respect to their health." Health inequities are not only unnecessary and avoidable but, in addition, are considered unfair and unjust.[54]

Attention to implementation science or lack thereof can influence equity. Communities and populations with increased burden of disease have a greater potential to benefit from the introduction of proven programs that respond to identified health risks and are delivered effectively, at scale, over time. However, without implementation science, despite best intentions, the emphasis on evidence-based public health has as much potential to exacerbate inequities as to improve health equity. Implementation science is needed to make sure that strategies for implementation are developed for all settings, not only those with higher resources. If the implementation does not address the additional challenges in poorer and vulnerable settings and attempts a one-size-fits-all approach, the uptake of these programs will be lower and weaker in communities that are less resourced. Intentional use of implementation science methods to guide program selection and delivery can address barriers to program selection and delivery in these settings. Furthermore, implementation capacity developed to address one public health challenge can be leveraged to support efforts to address other public health issues, thus realizing a greater return on investment.

Workforce Capacity

Unfortunately, successfully introducing and sustaining EBPs within complex public health systems remains a challenge.[55-60] because public health interventions are fragmented across various human service systems (e.g., child welfare, public health, education) and are not well aligned with local needs, resulting in service gaps and disparities. Human service agencies vary in their ability to effectively utilize evidence-based programs and to engage in collaborative networks through which these programs can achieve broader impact.[61] For example, public health departments are often central players in creating, supporting, and sustaining collective efforts to improve child well-being. However, their capacity to utilize evidence-based implementation methods to support collective action varies considerably.[62]

Implementation science has only recently emerged as a topic of study within the range of human service fields that produce public health professionals. While many universities and higher learning institutions are expanding their efforts and integrating a focus on both implementation research and practice, there is a great unmet need for implementation-informed public health practitioners.[63] In addition to expanded preservice training, intentional efforts to build implementation know how in the active workforce must be prioritized. For this to be done, accessible methods and tools in plain language are needed, as are the human and financial resources to support this work. Exemplary efforts, such as the investments in workforce capacity by the National Institutes for Health (e.g., implementation researchers) and the Substance Abuse and Mental Health Service Agency (e.g., behavioral health service implementers), must be expanded in other agencies that work closely with the public health workforce, including the Health Resources and Services Administration and the Centers for Disease Control.

CONCLUSION

As our world becomes more complex, and more and more populations are faced with the increasing impacts of diseases that reflect our modern lifestyles and the changing environment, there is a growing need to advance the science of public health and to find tested, researched interventions that work across multiple levels of the socio-ecological model. However, the same complexity that emphasizes this also illuminates the need for tested, researched, implementation strategies that work across multiple levels and contexts. The newly emergent field of implementation science is in the process of developing conceptual frameworks and formulating research questions and methods to meet this need, but much is still unknown. As they advance together, systematic intervention development to generate usable interventions, and rigorous implementation research to identify implementation strategies have the potential to realize effective and sustainable outcomes worldwide.

References

1. Resnicow K, Page SE. Embracing chaos and complexity: A quantum change for public health. *Am J Public Health*. 2008;98(8):1382–9.
2. NIRN. Glossary | NIRN Project site.
3. EPIScenter. Defining Evidence Based Programs | EPISCenter.
4. Van Scoyoc A, Wilen JS, Daderko K, Miyamoto S. Multiple aspects of maltreatment: Moving toward a holistic framework. In: Daro B, Huang LA, Cohn Donnelly A, Powell BJ, eds. *Advances in Child Abuse Prevention Knowledge*. Vol. 5. New York: Springer US; 2015, pp. 21–41.
5. Sanders MR. Triple P-positive parenting program as a public health approach to strengthening parenting. *J Fam Psychol*. 2008;22(4):506–17.
6. de Arellano MAR, Lyman DR, Jobe-Shields L, et al. Trauma-focused cognitive-behavioral therapy for children and adolescents: Assessing the evidence. *Psychiatr Serv*. 2014;65(5):591–602.
7. Sanders MR. Adopting a public health approach to the delivery of evidence-based parenting interventions. *Can Psychol Can*. 2010;51(1): 17–23.
8. Blueprints for Healthy Youth Development—Center for the Study and Prevention of Violence—Institute of Behavioral Science.
9. SAMHSA. National Registry of Evidence-based Programs and Practices. https://www.samhsa.gov/nrepp. Published 2017. Accessed February 7, 2017.
10. TITLE V MATERNAL AND CHILD HEALTH SERVICES BLOCK GRANT TO STATES PROGRAM, Guidance and Forms—blockgrant-guidance.pdf.
11. Focusing on Evidence-Based Interventions for Children.
12. IOM (Institute of Medicine) and NRC, (National Research Council). *New Directions in Child Abuse and Neglect Research*.; 2014.
13. Eccles MP, Mittman BS. Welcome to implementation science. *Implement Sci*. 2006;1(1).
14. Institute of Medicine. *Improving the Quality of Health Care for Mental and Substance-Use Conditions*. Washington, DC: National Academies Press; 2006.
15. Urbach DR, Govindarajan A, Refik S, Wilton AS, Baxter NN. Introduction of surgical safety checklists in Canada. *N Engl J Med*. 2014; 370(11):1029–38.
16. Wandersman A, Alia K, Cook BS, Hsu LL, Ramaswamy R. Evidence-based interventions are necessary but not sufficient for achieving outcomes in each setting in a complex world: Empowerment evaluation, getting to outcomes, and demonstrating accountability. *Am J Eval*. 2016; 37(4).
17. Fixsen DL, Naoom SF, Blase KA, et al. Implementation research: A synthesis of the literature. *Univ Sout Florida, Nationeal Implement Res Netw*. 2005;169:181–204.
18. Michie S, Fixsen D, Grimshaw JM, Eccles MP. Specifying and reporting complex behaviour change interventions: The need for a scientific method. *Implement Sci*. 2009;4:40.
19. Fixsen D, Blase K, Metz A, Van Dyke M. Statewide implementation of evidence-based programs. *Except Child*. 2013;79(2):213–30.
20. Saldana L, Chamberlain P, Wang W, Brown CH. Predicting program start-up using the stages of implementation measure. *Adm Policy Ment Heal Ment Heal Serv Res*. 2012;39(6):419–25.
21. Aarons GA, Fettes D, Hurlburt M, et al. Collaboration, negotiation, and coalescence for interagency-collaborative teams to scale-up evidence-based practice. *J Clin Child Adolesc Psychol*. 2014;6(2):915–28.
22. Hurlburt M, Aarons GA, Fettes D, Willging C, Gunderson L, Chaffin MJ. Interagency collaborative team model for capacity building to scale-up evidence-based practice. *Child Youth Serv Rev*. 2014;39:160–8.
23. Saldana L, Chamberlain P. Supporting implementation: The role of community development teams to build infrastructure. *Am J Community Psychol*. 2012;50(3–4):334–46.
24. Meyers DC, Durlak JA, Wandersman A. The quality implementation framework: A synthesis of critical steps in the implementation process. *Am J Community Psychol*. 2012;50(3–4):462–80.
25. Flaspohler P, Duffy J. Unpacking prevention capacity: An intersection of research-to-practice models and community-centered models. *Am J Community Psychol*. 2008;41:182–196.
26. Wandersman A, Duffy J, Flaspohler P, et al. Bridging the gap between prevention research and practice: The interactive systems framework for dissemination and implementation. *Am J Community Psychol*. 2008;41(3–4):171–81.
27. Wandersman A, Chien VH, Katz J. Toward an evidence-based system for innovation support for implementing innovations with quality: Tools, training, technical assistance, and quality assurance/quality improvement. *Am J Community Psychol*. 2012;50(3–4):445–59.
28. Leeman J, Calancie L, Hartman MA, et al. What strategies are used to build practitioners' capacity to implement community-based interventions and are they effective?: A systematic review. *Implement Sci*. 2015;10:80.
29. Ramaswamy R, Reed J, Livesley N, et al. Unpacking the black box of improvement. Int J Qual Health Care. 2018; 30: 15–9.
30. Metz A, Bartley L, Ball H, Wilson D, Naoom S, Redmond P. Active implementation frameworks for successful service delivery: Catawba county child wellbeing project. *Res Soc Work Pract*. 2015;25(4):415–22.
31. Metz A, Bartley L. Active implementation frameworks for program success: How to use implementation science to improve outcomes for children. *Zero Three*. 2012;32(4):11–8.
32. Meyers DC, Katz J, Chien V, Wandersman A, Scaccia JP, Wright A. Practical implementation science: Developing and piloting the quality implementation tool. *Am J Community Psychol*. 2012;50(3–4):481–96.
33. Nilsen P. Making sense of implementation theories, models and frameworks. *Implement Sci*. 2015;10(1):1–13.
34. Damschroder LJ, Aron DC, Keith RE, Kirsh SR, Alexander JA, Lowery JC. Fostering implementation of health services research findings into practice: A consolidated framework for advancing implementation science. *Implement Sci*. 2009;4(50):40–55.

35. Kirk MA, Kelley C, Yankey N, Birken SA, Abadie B, Damschroder L. A systematic review of the use of the consolidated framework for implementation research. *Implement Sci.* 2015;11(1):72.

36. McKibbon KA, Lokker C, Wilczynski N, et al. A cross-sectional study of the number and frequency of terms used to refer to knowledge translation in a body of health literature in 2006: A tower of Babel? *Implement Sci.* 2010;5(1):16.

37. Powell BJ, Waltz TJ, Chinman MJ, et al. A refined compilation of implementation strategies: Results from the expert recommendations for implementing change (ERIC) project. *Implement Sci.* 2015;10(1):21.

38. Raghavan R, Bright CL, Shadoin AL. Toward a policy ecology of implementation of evidence-based practices in public mental health settings. *Implement Sci.* 2008;3:26.

39. Proctor EK, Powell BJ, McMillen JC. Implementation strategies: Recommendations for specifying and reporting. *Implement Sci.* 2013;8:139.

40. Proctor E. Implementation science and child maltreatment: Methodological advances. *Child Maltreat.* 2012;17(1):107–12.

41. Lobb R, Colditz G. Implementation science and its application to population health. *Annu Rev Public Health.* 2013;34(1):235–51.

42. Martinez RG, Lewis CC, Weiner BJ. Instrumentation issues in implementation science. *Implement Sci.* 2014;9(1):118.

43. Roland D, Oliver A, Edwards ED, Mason BW, Powell CVE. Use of paediatric early warning systems in Great Britain: Has there been a change of practice in the last 7 years? *Arch Dis Child.* 2014;99(1):26–29.

44. Powell BJ, McMillen JC, Proctor EK, et al. A compilation of strategies for implementing clinical innovations in health and mental health. *Med Care Res Rev.* 2012;69(2):123–57.

45. Leeman J, Birken SA, Powell BJ, Rohweder C, Shea CM. Beyond " implementation strategies ": Classifying the full range of strategies used in implementation science and practice. *Implement Sci.* 2017; 12: 125.

46. Powell BJ, McMillen JC, Proctor EK, et al. A compilation of strategies for implementing clinical innovations in health and mental health. *Med Care Res Rev.* 2012;69(2):123–57.

47. Waltz TJ, Powell BJ, Chinman MJ, et al. Expert recommendations for implementing change (ERIC): Protocol for a mixed methods study. *Implement Sci.* 2014; 9(1):39.

48. Flottorp SA, Oxman AD, Krause J, et al. A checklist for identifying determinants of practice : A systematic review and synthesis of frameworks and taxonomies of factors that prevent or enable improvements in healthcare professional practice. *Implement Sci.* 2013; 8(1):35.

49. Wensing M. Methods to identify implementation problems. In: *Methods to Identify Implementation Problems.* Edinburgh, Scotland: Elsevier; 2005, pp. 109–20.

50. Powell BJ, Beidas RS, Lewis CC, et al. Methods to improve the selection and tailoring of implementation strategies. *J Behav Heal Serv Res.* 2017;44:177–94.

51. Metz A, Albers B. What does it take? How federal initiatives can support the implementation of evidence-based programs to improve outcomes for adolescents. *J Adolesc Heal.* 2014;54(3 Suppl.):S92–6.

52. Clara F, García KY, Metz A. Implementing Evidence-Based Child Welfare: The New York City Experience; 2017.

53. Ayers J, Bloyd J, Fink B. DRAFT FOUNDATIONAL PRACTICES FOR HEALTH.

54. Braveman P, Gruskin S. Defining equity in health. *BMJ.* 2003; 57(4):254–8.

55. Haines A, Kuruvilla S, Borchert M. Briding the implementation gap between knowledge and action for health. *Bull World Health Organ.* 2004;82(10):724–32.

56. Committe and Crossing the Quality Chasm: Adaptation to Mental Health and Addicitive Disorders. *Improving the Quality of Health Care for Mental and Substance-Use Conditions.* Washington, DC: National Academies Press; 2006.

57. Oakleaf M, Are they learning ? Are we ? Learning outcomes and the academic library. *Libr Q.* 2011; 81(1): 61–82.

58. Institute of Medicine. *Crossing the Quality Chasm: A New Health System for the 21st Century.* Washington, DC: National Academies Press; 2001.

59. Lanier P, Maguire-jack K, Mienko J, Panlilio C. In: Daro D, Cohn Donnelly A, Huang LA, Powell BJ, eds. *Advances in Child Abuse Prevention Knowledge.* New York: Springer International Publishing; 2015.

60. Lanier P, Jonson-Reid M, Stahlschmidt MJ, Drake B, Constantino J. Child maltreatment and pediatric health outcomes: A longitudinal study of low-income children. *J Pediatr Psychol.* 2010;35(5):511–22.

61. Lang JM, Campbell K, Shanley P, Crusto CA, Connell CM. Building capacity for trauma-informed care in the child welfare system: Initial results of a statewide implementation. *Child Maltreat.* 2016;21(2):113–24.

62. Lovelace KA, Aronson RE, Rulison KL, Labban JD, Shah GH, Smith M. Laying the groundwork for evidence-based public health: Why some local health departments use more evidence-based decision-making practices than others. *Am J Public Health.* 2015;105:S189–97.

63. Kroelinger CD, Rankin KM, Chambers DA, Diez Roux AV, Hughes K, Grigorescu V. Using the principles of complex systems thinking and implementation science to enhance maternal and child health program planning and delivery. *Matern Child Health J.* 2014;18(7):1560–4.

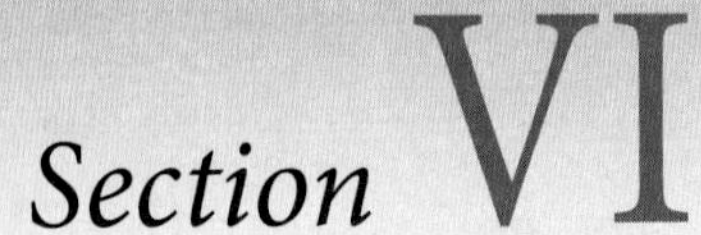

Section VI

Section Editors
Patrick Remington and Maria Mora Pinzon

Noncommunicable and Chronic Conditions

CHAPTER

50 Screening for Early and Asymptomatic Conditions

Robert B. Wallace

DEFINITION OF SCREENING

The typical natural history of many diseases and conditions suggests that at some point in the life course their biological onset occurs, during or after conception, and progresses at varying rates until it become clinically evident. This interval may be short, such as for neonatal hearing loss, or long-term, as in Alzheimer's disease. Some diseases may never become clinically manifest and thus afford little clinical harm. This may occur for various reasons including biological variation, often not well understood, or the occurrence of competing clinical events, or possibly natural or clinically mediated environmental modification (called "primary prevention"). Important to the discussion here, the harms of nascent diseases and conditions also may be mitigated, deferred or eliminated by the early and asymptomatic detection of disease; that is, disease screening (also called "secondary prevention"). However, even when an overt clinical illness is already present, "tertiary prevention" can offer rehabilitative and other clinical interventions that may deter disease progression and help return the patient to a healthier state.

Disease screening activities usually take two general forms: (a) screening for biological disease antecedents that are part of known biobehavioral pathogenetic pathways to overt disease, such as abnormal blood cholesterol or blood pressure levels; or (b) screening directly for metabolic, physiological, behavioral, or anatomic markers of the disease itself, such as serological levels of a biomarker secreted by a tumor or a series of clinical symptom reports indicative of an emerging mental illness. In addition, preliminary screening might be conducted for factors that indicate increased risk of disease occurrence, irrespective of whether they are part of the pathogenetic mechanism. This highlights the fact that screening may be done in stages, for instance by screening first for general disease susceptibility and/or risk, such as for certain demographic, anatomic or behavioral characteristics. After the disease is detected, this would in turn be followed by provision of clinically appropriate treatment(s) to cure or to prevent the progression of pathophysiological processes that would otherwise cause overt clinical manifestations and individual harm. Thus, some screening tests may also be diagnostic tests, although staged screening is becoming more common to narrow the indications for the use of diagnostic procedures. This may be seen as greater adherence to the trend in "precision medicine," although this concept can be somewhat controversial.[1] Disease screening may be applied to community (e.g., mass screening), as well as clinical populations, depending on the effectiveness and emergent nature of the situation, but there is little point in screening if follow-up resources to address findings are not available.

The term "disease screening" should be used with clarity, as it may be part of a larger, comprehensive health maintenance or health surveillance program, and so the general definition of disease screening may not fit all situations. In addition, since many generally healthy individuals will have some at least temporary symptoms and feelings of ill-health at various times, the criterion that screened patients be "asymptomatic" must always be considered. When symptom reports matter, their presence may change the yield and characteristics of a screening test. Further, with increasing biological understanding of disease pathogenesis and outcomes, more screening tests are emerging through modern genetics and molecular biology, requiring clinicians to remain conversant with the meaning and consequences of a positive or negative test. While it has often been true of many screening tests, the movement toward molecular and genetic testing suggests that a positive test could possibly lead to increased risk for several different medical conditions that might require clinical evaluation and diagnosis, because, for example, a certain gene variant may be associated with more than one distinct clinical condition.

In general, disease screening is applied to populations with a relatively low prevalence rate of the conditions of interest. However, because of the increasing number and types of effective screening tests that have been developed, screening burdens in primary care and other clinical settings may be increasing. More research is needed to determine the most efficient and effective ways to conduct "bundled" or "multiphasic" screening, particularly in primary care, where care delivery challenges remain. In addition, the diagnosis of one disease in an individual patient may lead to additional screening procedures, such as for environmental or other toxic substance exposures in the home or workplace that are known to cause the illness in question, or the screening for relevant conditions in family members of the index patient.

THE ASSESSMENT OF SCREENING TESTS

If a test is being considered for use in screening, some general criteria that aid in selecting and applying an appropriate test were posited many years ago by Wilson and Jungner.[2] These included:

a. The disease should be common enough to warrant a search for its risk factors or latent stages because screening for excessively rare diseases may result in unacceptable cost-benefit ratios;
b. The morbidity or mortality (i.e., burden of suffering) of the untreated target condition should be substantial;
c. An effective preventive intervention or therapy must exist and should yield a more beneficial outcome when applied to the presymptomatic rather than to the symptomatic stage;
d. The screening test should be acceptable to the population and logistically suitable for general, routine application; and
e. Other criteria for an effective screening test exist,[3] such as maintenance of test accuracy over time and freedom from screening-related adverse health effects.

Even with concerted application of these screening criteria, major pitfalls may cause an erroneous assessment of a screening program's value. An example is *lead time bias*, the interval between presymptomatic disease detection by a screening test and symptom onset.[4,5] If the natural history of a disease is variable or not thoroughly understood during the presymptomatic and early symptomatic stages, a screening test may identify a presymptomatic condition earlier and increase the interval to overt morbidity but not change the ultimate outcome. *Length bias* occurs when there is a correlation between the duration of disease latency and the natural history of the symptomatic phase.[4,5] If the mild form of a disease has a longer latency and is hence more easily found on screening than are more severe, progressive forms of the disease, the screening test may appear falsely beneficial. These and other potential biases have been identified[3] and must be considered in test evaluation. See Maxim et al.[3] for further resources on this topic.

In general, the validity and utility of a screening test depends on the scientific evidence base to justify the screening particular intervention. Evaluation of screening tests begins with a careful and thorough systematic review of the relevant scientific literature, which may or may not adequately support a decision. Ultimately, however, the decision to recommend a screening test in a clinical guideline is subjective. The process should include transparency, peer review, and broad stakeholder consultation. The value of many screening tests may be proven only through one or more comprehensive, credible randomized clinical trials, but important ancillary approaches are extremely helpful, including adherence to a conceptual framework that organizes and addresses most dimensions of the screening process. An important summary of these methods is available from the work of the U.S. Preventive Services Task Force.[6]

In approaching the quantitative assessment of a given screening test, various measures are used such as sensitivity, specificity, predictive values, and receiver-operator characteristics, discussed further below. Additional measures that are often important include procedure cost-effectiveness, individual and public acceptability of the test activity, and financing the procedure within the health system context. Many of the techniques employed in quantitative test assessment are similar to other, general mathematical approaches to evaluation methods used in both clinical and preventive medicine, such as in clinical decision-making, diagnostic test assessment, and discrimination and calibration of clinical prediction models.[3,7,8] The principal evaluative characteristics of a screening test, sensitivity and specificity, test characteristics that can apply to any laboratory or diagnostic test data as well as other information collected from the medical history and physical examination.

In the context of a screening test, *sensitivity* is the proportional detection of individuals with the disease of interest in the tested population, expressed as follows:

$$\text{Senstivity (\%)} = \frac{\text{True positives}}{\text{True positives} + \text{False negatives}} \times 100$$

True positives are individuals with the disease and whose test result is positive. False negatives are individuals whose test result is negative despite having the disease. *Specificity* is the proportional detection of individuals without the disease of interest, expressed as follows:

$$\text{Specificity (\%)} = \frac{\text{True negatives}}{\text{True negatives} + \text{False positives}} \times 100$$

True negatives are individuals without the disease and whose test result is negative. False positives are those who have a positive test result but do not have the disease. Sensitivity is limited by the proportion of cases missed by the test (false negatives) and specificity is limited by the proportion of noncases found to be positive (false positives). Ideally, a test would have a 100% sensitivity and specificity, but few if any tests have achieved this. Unfortunately, sensitivity and specificity are often inversely related. This relationship has been expressed as the receiver operating characteristic (ROC)[4] of a numerically continuous test result. The ROC allows optimal specification of test sensitivity and specificity. The sensitivity, or true-positive ratio, is displayed along the ordinate, and the specificity, or false-positive ratio, is exhibited on the abscissa. As the sensitivity increases, so does the false-positive ratio in most instances. When a ROC has been established for a test, any one of several sensitivity and specificity combinations may be evaluated for suitability in test application and contrasted with potential alternate tests. Further information on the application of ROC curves, and the accompanying "C-statistic," is available.[9]

Sensitivity and specificity values from the literature are most applicable to populations and test conditions similar to those under which the values were established. However, it is possible that test properties may differ according to mode of administration (e.g., telephone vs. mail questionnaire), or by the demographic or related features of the target population, and thus, further generalization or extrapolation of these values can be inaccurate. For example, it has been suggested that the use of estrogenic hormone therapy among postmenopausal women may decrease the sensitivity and specificity of mammographic screening for breast cancer.[10]

Whereas the operating characteristics of a test are of major help in selecting a screening test, the predictive value of a test is a major aid in interpretation of a result. The *predictive value* of a *positive test* is the proportion of all individuals with positive tests who have the disease and is expressed as follows:

$$\text{Positive Predictive Value (\%)} = \frac{\text{True positives}}{\text{True positives} + \text{False positives}} \times 100$$

The predictive value of a negative test is the proportion of all individuals with negative tests who are nondiseased. This is expressed as follows:

$$\text{Negative Predictive Value (\%)} = \frac{\text{True negatives}}{\text{True negatives} + \text{False negatives}} \times 100$$

Predictive values are dependent on both the operating characteristics and the prevalence of the disease in the target population.[9] For any given set of operating characteristics, the positive predictive value is directly related to prevalence, and the negative predictive value is inversely related to prevalence. Therefore, in screening situations where the prevalence is relatively low, the operating characteristics must be very high to avoid low positive predictive values. In most screening situations for serious fatal conditions, such as cancer, the test or test sequence offering the highest sensitivity ordinarily will be preferred. This has the effect of finding as many cases as possible but may correspondingly increase the number of false positives. The effect of sensitivity, specificity, and prevalence on predictive values has been clearly demonstrated.

Cost-effectiveness is especially important in screening programs because of the number of asymptomatic individuals who must be evaluated for the relatively small number of diseased cases. There is value in formal cost-effectiveness analysis,[11] which should be undertaken as part of program evaluation. The program's or test's value must include an assessment of all costs and a realistic appraisal of effectiveness. Positive predictive values are often well below 50% for many initial screening situations, so that secondary diagnostic evaluation is nearly always required to eliminate false positives, adding substantially to program cost.

As noted above, exhaustive reviews of the efficacy of clinically applicable screening programs, largely those conducted in primary care, have been conducted by the U.S. Preventive Services Task Force and several other disciplinary, specialty and international groups, with recommendations offered in part with consideration of cost-effectiveness. On the other hand, public or mass screening may have inherent advantages from the standpoint of efficiency. The tests and procedures selected for use are often highly standardized and may be administered more inexpensively than they can in clinical or more specialized settings, and generally they can be applied without the need for direct physician supervision. To enjoy the efficiency of mass screening, such programs must be carefully organized and managed. Individual recipients of both normal and abnormal test results must be carefully considered, and assisted in working through test findings. Those with abnormal test results must have a properly organized follow-up evaluation protocol, and those with normal results should be informed of the predictive value of a normal test to avoid false reassurance. Even with the inherent efficiency of mass screening, many such programs must still be focused on populations with sufficient disease or risk factor prevalence to maximize program efficiency.

An important issue in applying screening programs is the clinical context where patients have active clinical problems unrelated to the targeted illness being screened. For example, a screening test or program conducted on a new ambulatory clinic visit or at hospital admission could be problematic for some screening activities. Comprehensive clinical screening with routine physical examinations or other clinical or laboratory tests remains controversial, largely because there is often little evidence in the scientific literature concerning the efficacy or effectiveness of standard screening tests in the face of substantial acute or chronic comorbid illness. For example, does routine screening mammography maintain its effectiveness in persons with liver failure or cholesterol screening in the face of an active carcinoma? These are questions yet to be adequately addressed by careful research. In the past, so-called "multiphasic" screening programs have been proposed and implemented for persons being admitted to the hospital. Now, many screening activities are being conducted on hospital admission, such as carriage of microorganisms that are important causes of nosocomial infections, the presence of malnutrition or a positive HIV serology, or risk of falls or other safety hazards. As with all screening tests, the properties of these tests in the hospital setting should be thoroughly evaluated and understood.

The conceptual framework noted above, promulgated by the U.S. Preventive Services Task Force, for evaluating screening tests also considers another important issue: the role of screening tests in causing psychological distress or other adverse effects. There are several examples in the literature of patient distress associated with screening tests, such as occurs among patients awaiting the results of a test or when clinical actions are uncertain, while a "false positive" test is being evaluated; an important example is screening mammography.[12] Health professionals must be aware of the potential for such circumstances, and approach them with skillful program management, and high quality counselling services.

References

1. Joyner MJ. Precision medicine, cardiovascular disease and hunting elephants. *Prog. Cardiovasc Dis.* 2016;58(6):651–60.
2. Wilson JMG, Jungner G. *Principles and Practice of Screening for Disease. Public Health Paper No. 34.* Geneva: World Health Organization; 1968.
3. Maxim D, Niebo R, Utell M. Screening tests: A review with examples. *Inhal Toxicol.* 2014;26(13):811–28.
4. Pelikan S, Moskowitz M. Effects of lead time, length bias, and false negative assurance on screening for breast cancer. *Cancer.* 1993;71:1998–2005.
5. Swets JA. Measuring the accuracy of diagnostic systems. *Science.* 1988;240:1285–93.
6. Krist AH, Wolff T, Mabry-Hernandez IR, Bibbins-Domingo K. Advancing the United States preventive services task force methods: Important considerations in making evidence-based guidelines *Am J Prev Med.* 2018;54(Suppl 1):A1–S103.
7. Moskowitz CS. Using free-response receiver operating characteristics curves to assess the accuracy of machine diagnosis of cancer. *JAMA.* 2017;318(22):2250–1.
8. Alba AC, Agoritsas T, Walsh M, et al. Discrimination and calibration of clinical prediction models. Users' guides to the medical literature. *JAMA* 2017;318(14):1377–84.
9. Pencina MJ, D'Agostino RB Sr. Evaluating discrimination of risk prediction models. The "C Statistic." *JAMA* 2015;314(10):1063–4.
10. Laya MB, Larson EB, Taplin SH, et al. Effect of estrogen replacement therapy on the sensitivity and specificity of screening mammography. *J Natl Cancer Inst.* 1996;88:643–9.
11. Gold MR, Siegel JE, Russell LB, Weinstein MC, eds. *Cost Effectiveness in Health and Medicine.* New York: Oxford University Press; 1996.
12. Rosenbaum L. Invisible risks, emotional choices—Mammography and medical decision-making. *N Engl J Med.* 2014;371(16):1549–52.

CHAPTER

51 Cancer

Leslie K. Dennis • Charles F. Lynch • Heidi E. Brown • Christina M. Laukaitis • Stephanie Lashway • Elaine M. Smith

Cancer and its associated issues have an important impact on public health practice that is global. Worldwide cancer is among the top causes of death. Cancer is a major health concern in both developed and developing countries. Cancer etiology studies describe cancer within different populations along with identifying the causes of cancer. Cancer prevention takes this a step further and looks at ways to reduce or eliminate some of the risk factors for cancer. The public health approach is to prevent cancer.

Cancers or neoplasms are diseases characterized by abnormal proliferation of cells. If the proliferating cells invade surrounding tissues and spread through lymphatics or blood vessels, the resultant tumor is malignant; if they do not, it is benign. Some benign neoplasms may be fatal, including histologically benign brain tumors that grow and displace normal brain tissue in the confined space of the skull, and hepatocellular adenomas that rupture and cause bleeding into the peritoneal cavity. Some benign tumors such as intestinal polyps are considered premalignant lesions and confer a high risk of progression to malignancy. The term cancer usually implies a malignant or invasive tumor.

DESCRIPTIVE EPIDEMIOLOGY

Classification

Cancers are classified according to their organ or tissue of origin (site or topography code) and histological features (morphology code). A number of classification schemes have been developed, the most recent and widely used of which appears in Chap. 2 of the *International Classification of Diseases,* 10th revision (ICD-10), which is largely a topography code,[1] and the *International Classification of Diseases for Oncology,* 3rd edition (ICD-O), which contains an expanded version of the topography code in ICD-9 as well as a detailed morphology code.[2]

Sources of Incidence and Mortality Rates

Mortality rates are calculated from death certificate records and population census data. Mortality rates from various countries have been compiled periodically.[3] Cancer mortality rates for the United States are published by the United States' National Cancer Institute (NCI) and Centers for Disease Control and Prevention (CDC).[4–6]

Population-based cancer registries, which have been established in many countries, provide information on incidence rates. These have been compiled in Cancer in Five Continents, which is jointly published periodically by the International Agency for Research on Cancer (IARC) and the International Association of Cancer Registries (IACR).[7] In the United States, the best source of cancer incidence rates is the Surveillance, Epidemiology, and End Results (SEER) program of the NCI, which supports a network of 18 population-based cancer registries throughout the country. Results from this program are published annually and more detailed monographs are published periodically[4,8,9] and available online (https://seer.cancer.gov/). Both incidence and mortality statistics for the United States are summarized for the lay public and projected rates are published annually by the American Cancer Society.[10]

A North American Association of Central Cancer Registries (NAACCR) was established in 1987, and beginning in 1991, the CDC made funds available to individual states for cancer registration. The cost of collecting high-quality data on a sufficiently large proportion of all cases in a defined population is considerable; however, utilization of these data for research or cancer control purposes justifies cancer registration efforts. Since 2011, NAACCR has over 140 members including registries in all 50 states, all Canadian provinces, and all major cancer surveillance organizations in North America. NAACCR provides age-adjusted cancer incidence statistics for the United States and Canada by cancer site, race ethnicity, sex, and age groups that can be queried for the most recent 5-year data available along with stage information.[11]

Magnitude of the Cancer Problem

In the aggregate, cancer is second only to heart disease as a cause of death in the United States and accounts for about 23% of all deaths.[10] However, in Hispanics, Asian Americans, women age 40–79, men age 45–79 and in 22 states, it is the leading cause of death.[10] In 2015, approximately 158.5 deaths from cancer occur per 100,000 people per year, compared with about 168.5 per 100,000 from heart disease, 37.63 per 100,000 from cerebrovascular diseases, 41.6 per 100,000 for chronic lower respiratory diseases, and 43.2 per 100,000 from accidents.[12] Based on U.S. incidence and mortality rates for 2012–14, the lifetime probabilities of developing invasive cancer have been estimated to be 39.7% in men and 37.6% in women; the lifetime probabilities of dying of cancer are estimated at 22.0% in men and 18.8% in women.[4] The National Cancer Institute estimated that care for cancer survivors accounted for an estimated $137.4 billion in medical-care costs in the United States in 2010 including initial and continuing care along with care the last year of life.[13]

Relative Importance of Specific Neoplasms

The importance of a malignancy can be judged by the number of years of life lost due to its occurrence in a population. This measure reflects the incidence of the cancer, the fatality rate in those who develop it, and the age at which the cancer tends to occur, resulting in more weight to childhood cancers than overall mortality rates; because of economic implications, it can be of value in setting priorities for research and prevention. In order of estimated years of life lost, the 10 most important cancers in the United States are lung, colon and rectum, female breast, pancreas, liver and intrahepatic bile duct, leukemia, brain and other nervous system, non-Hodgkin's lymphoma, prostate, and ovary.[4]

The estimated age-standardized incidence rates of all cancers vary among the various regions of the world, and the cancers of most importance in developing countries are different from those in developed countries such as the United States. In order by numbers of cases, the 10 most common cancers across the globe in 2015 are those of the breast, lung and bronchus, colon and rectum, prostate, stomach, liver, non-Hodgkin's lymphoma, leukemia, bladder, and cervical.[14]

The most common cancers in men are those of the prostate, lung, and colon and rectum; the cancers causing the most deaths in the United States are lung, colon and rectum, prostate, and pancreas.[10] In women, breast cancer is by far the most common neoplasm, followed by cancers of the lung, and colon and rectum.[10] However, because of the more favorable survival of women with breast than lung cancer, mortality rates of female lung cancer exceed those for female breast cancer in the United States then they are both followed by colon and rectum, and pancreatic cancer mortality.[10] In Europe in 2012 similar to the United States, the three cancers with the highest mortality are lung, colon, and rectum, and female breast, respectively.[3] But in 40 countries in Europe, the fourth highest mortality is from stomach cancer.[3]

Time Trends

Since 1990, mortality rates for most cancer sites have been declining in the United States. Incidence rates have not shown a similar declining pattern, supporting the concept that increasing screening and improved therapies are contributing more to the declining mortality. Figure 51-1, A and B, shows trends in age-adjusted incidence rates for various cancers in the United States from 1973 to 2013 for men and women, respectively.[10] Figure 51-2, A and B, shows trends in mortality rates for the most common cancers in the United States from 1973 to 2013, for men and women of all ages.[10]

Breast and prostate cancer incidence increased dramatically in the 1980s and early 1990s as a result of mammography and prostate-specific antigen (PSA) screening, respectively; however prostate cancer incidence started dropping around 2008 with the recommendation by the U.S. Preventive Services Task Force to no longer screen with PSA.[4,15] There have been declines in mortality rates for breast cancer starting in the early 1990s and for prostate cancer at the end of the 1990s. A report evaluating the reduction of breast cancer mortality in the United States from 1975 to 2000 concluded that both screening mammography and treatment primarily contributed to the reduction.[16]

The reason for the marked decline in rates of stomach cancer (not shown) is unknown but may be related to treatment of bacteria *Helicobacter pylori (H. pylori)* as the cause of stomach ulcers. The striking increase among females from 1973 to 1993 in rates of lung cancer deaths is largely due to cigarette smoking.

The 5-year relative survival rates of newly diagnosed cancer patients for all races across all cancer sites in the United States have increased from 53% in 1980s to 66% in 2007–13.[10] Table 51-1 shows the 5-year survival rates for men and women from 2007 to 2013. Cancers of the prostate, thyroid, skin, and breast have the highest survival rates in adults. The lowest survival rates are for cancers of the pancreas, lung, esophagus, liver, brain and other nervous systems, and stomach.

Temporal trends in survival from cancer in children are most encouraging. From 1974 to 2013, 5-year survival rates in children under age 15 increased for all sites. From 2007 to 2013, 5-year survival rates were 92% for acute lymphocytic leukemia, 66% for acute myeloid leukemia, 75% for brain and other nervous system, 90% for non-Hodgkin's lymphoma, 98% for Hodgkin's disease, 77% for cancers of the bone and joints, and 85% for all cancer sites combined.[4,10] There has been little change in the incidence of these neoplasms in children, thus reductions in mortality have resulted in prolonged survival due primarily to improved therapy.

Age

Cancer is primarily a disease of older adults. With some notable exceptions (e.g., cancers of the uterine cervix, testis, some leukemia subtypes, and cancers with strong infectious causes), there is an exponential increase in incidence rates with age. The median age at which cancer was diagnosed from 2010 to 2014 was 66.0 for males and 65.0 for females, while the median age at death was 72.0 for males and 73.0 for females.[4] However, several cancers can develop in childhood or as an adult. Only Acute lymphocytic leukemia has a median age at diagnosis under 30 at age 15.[4]

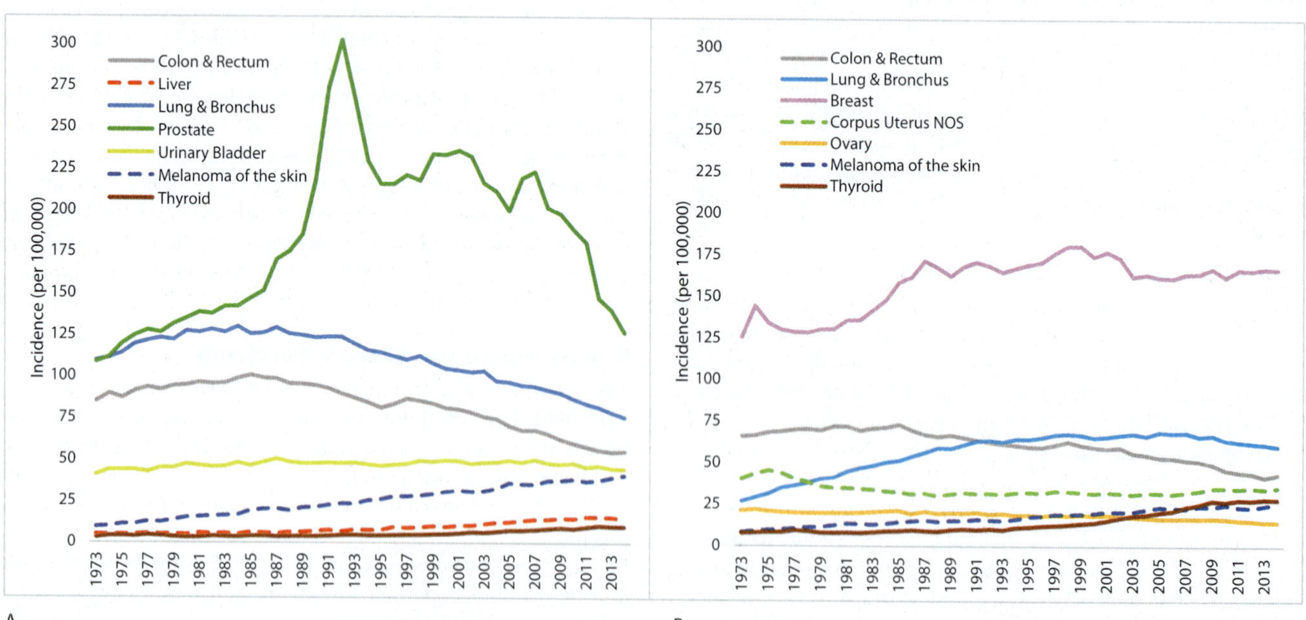

FIGURE 51-1. Surveillance, Epidemiology, and End Results Program (SEER) site-specific cancer incidence rates by year and gender for adults (aged 15+) A. Males, B. Females. [*Source:* Surveillance Research Program, National Cancer Institute SEER*Stat software (www.seer.cancer.gov/seerstat) version 8.3.4. Surveillance, Epidemiology, and End Results (SEER) Program (www.seer.cancer.gov) SEER*Stat Database: Incidence—SEER 9 Regs Research Data, Nov 2016 Sub (1973–2014) <Katrina/Rita Population Adjustment>—Linked To County Attributes—Total U.S., 1969–2015 Counties, National Cancer Institute, DCCPS, Surveillance Research Program, released April 2017, based on the November 2016 submission].

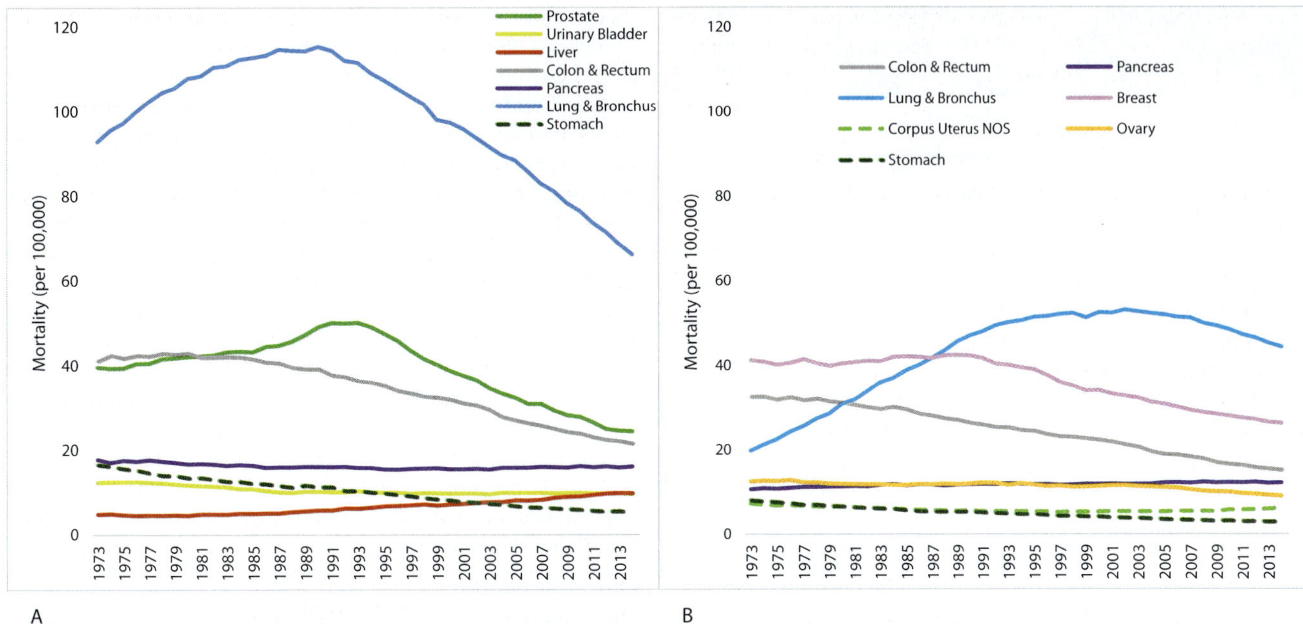

FIGURE 51-2. Surveillance, Epidemiology, and End Results Program (SEER) site-specific cancer mortality rates by year and gender for adults (aged 15+) A. Males, B. Females. [*Source:* Epidemiology, and End Results (SEER) Program (www.seer.cancer.gov) SEER*Stat Database: Mortality—All COD, Aggregated With State, Total U.S. (1969–2014) <Katrina/Rita Population Adjustment>, National Cancer Institute, DCCPS, Surveillance Research Program, released December 2016. Underlying mortality data provided by NCHS (www.cdc.gov/nchs)].

Cancers most probably arise from DNA-damaged cells that are capable of mitotic division and differentiation. In adults, most cancers are carcinomas that arise from basal epithelial cells of ectodermal or endodermal origin. In children, most cancers are of mesodermal origin and consist largely of leukemias and lymphomas that arise from hematopoietic and lymphoid stem cells and sarcomas that probably develop from undifferentiated cells of embryonal origin.

Incidence rates for the most common childhood cancers in the United States are shown in Fig. 51-3.[4,10] The mortality rates for even the most frequent cancers in children are many times lower than the rates of comparable tumors for all ages (Fig. 51-3), which largely reflect rates in adults. The highest mortality rate from cancer in children used to be for acute lymphocytic leukemia but as can be seen in the figure the mortality rates have decreased significantly for this cancer. While the mortality of brain and other nervous system cancers in children has also been decreasing, it is now the leading cause of cancer deaths in the United States among children.

Sex

Most major cancers occur more frequently in men than in women, exceptions being carcinomas of the breast, thyroid, and gallbladder.[4] Smoking-related cancers, described in detail subsequently, occur more frequently in men, in large part because of their earlier and greater exposure to tobacco smoke. Some other cancers, such as carcinomas of the bladder and mesotheliomas, are more frequent in men, at least in part because of their greater occupational exposure to various chemical carcinogens and asbestos, respectively. Other cancers that occur more frequently in men include the lymphomas and leukemias, bones and joint, oral cavity and pharynx, stomach, kidney, pancreas, rectum, salivary gland, and liver. The reasons for the excess of these cancers in males are uncertain. Women may be less exposed to whatever environmental factors contribute to their development. For example, males overall have higher rates of melanoma likely due to more sun exposure, but under age 50 women have higher rates, likely related to increase artificial ultraviolet (UV) tanning in recent decades.[4]

Geography and Migration Studies

Within different countries, incidence and mortality rates of all cancers vary considerably from one geographic region to another. Migrants or their descendants, tend to eventually develop most cancers at rates more similar to those in their country of adoption than to those in their country of origin, suggesting an important role for environmental risk factors in most cancers.[16] In the United States, the patterns of cancer occurrence in recent immigrants reflect the cancer patterns in their countries of origin and become less distinct as these groups become more acculturated with the passage of time. The frequency of occurrence of many cancers also varies among racial groups residing in the same country. This variation may be due to factors related to their distinct cultural patterns, social behavior, or economic status, but in some instances may be due to genetic differences among the races.

Some cancers appear to be related to a "Western" lifestyle. Cancers that tend to occur at lower rates in developing countries and migrants from these countries than in lifelong residents of such areas as North America and Western Europe include cancers of the colon and rectum, which may be related to diets rich in animal products. Cancers of the prostate, ovary, corpus uteri, and breast have to some extent been related to high consumption of meats and fats, have also been associated with endocrinological and reproductive factors.

Other cancers occur more frequently in developing countries and in migrants from these countries. For example, compared to white populations of the United States and Western Europe, migrants from Asian countries have higher rates of:

(1) Stomach cancer, related to infection with *H. pylori*;
(2) Liver cancers caused partially by hepatitis B and C viruses;
(3) Cancers of the nasopharynx, caused in part by the Epstein-Barr virus (EBV)[17,18];
(4) Oropharyngeal and oral cavity cancers, which are related to human papillomaviruses (HPV) in addition to tobacco use and alcohol consumption; and
(5) Cancer of the uterine cervix, where HPV is considered necessary for its development.

TABLE 51-1 AVERAGE 5-YEAR RELATIVE SURVIVAL RATES (2008–12 CASES) BY PRIMARY SITE AND SEX FOR ALL AGES ALL RACES, SEER 18 AREAS COMBINED

	Ages 15+	
	5-Year Relative Survival (%)[a]	
Site	Male	Female
Oral cavity and pharynx	63.5	66.7
Esophagus	18.5	18.9
Stomach	28.9	34.8
Colon and rectum	64.3	65.3
Liver and IBD(a)	16.7	17.2
Pancreas	8.3	8.0
Larynx	62.0	59.2
Lung and bronchus	15.3	21.4
Melanoma of the skin	89.7	94.3
Breast	84.1	89.8
Cervix uteri	–	67.0
Corpus and uterus, NOS	–	81.3
Ovary(b)	–	46.9
Prostate	98.5	–
Testis	95.5	–
Urinary bladder	78.4	73.3
Kidney and renal pelvis	73.4	75.0
Brain and ONS(a)	27.2	29.4
Thyroid	95.7[b]	98.9[b]
Hodgkin lymphoma	85.0	87.0
Non-Hodgkin lymphoma	69.3	73.0
Myeloma	49.7	50.2
Leukemia	59.1	56.3
Acute lymphocytic	43.0	40.1
Chronic lymphocytic	83.6	82.7
Myeloid and Monocytic	38.2	39.4
All sites	66.6	67.2

Sources: Incidence data from SEER 18 areas (San Francisco, Connecticut, Detroit, Hawaii, Iowa, New Mexico, Seattle, Utah, Atlanta, San Jose-Monterey, Los Angeles, Alaska Native Registry, Rural Georgia, California excluding SF/SJM/LA, Kentucky, Louisiana, New Jersey, and Georgia excluding ATL/RG). Mortality data are from the NCHS public use data file for the total United States. Surveillance, Epidemiology, and End Results (SEER) Program (www.seer.cancer.gov) SEER*Stat Database: Incidence—SEER 18 Regs Research Data+ Hurricane Katrina Impacted Louisiana Cases, Nov 2016 Sub (2000–14) <Katrina/Rita Population Adjustment>—Linked To County Attributes—Total U.S., 1969–2015 Counties, National Cancer Institute, DCCPS, Surveillance Research Program, released April 2017, based on the November 2016 submission.

[a]Rates are based on follow-up of patients through 2014.

[b]The relative cumulative rate increased from a prior interval and has been adjusted.

Cancers that are strongly related to smoking or tobacco use occur with a frequency commensurate with the smoking habits in the population. Thus, cancers of the lung, larynx, bladder, kidney, and pancreas have tended to occur more frequently in developed than developing countries, but rates of these neoplasms are increasing in developing countries where more widespread cigarette smoking has accompanied economic changes.

Race

The United States, unlike many other countries often stratifies cancer data by race. The overall incidence and mortality rates and the ratio of mortality to incidence in various racial and ethnic groups in the United States for 2010–14 are shown in Table 51-2.[4] Comparing 1998–2003 data with data from 1988 to 1992, rates in all racial/ethnic groups have increased with the possible exception of American Indian/Alaska Natives, which have the lowest cancer rates. However, comparing 2010–14 data with 1998–2003 we see rates for American Indian/Alaska Natives as the only rates that have increased for both men and women (a small increase is also seen in Hispanic women). Cancer among men in other racial/ethnic groups is lower than rates for 1998–2003. Variations in overall cancer incidence reflect the mix of cancers in the different groups. Variations in mortality are due to differences in both incidence and survival. The differences in the ratio of mortality to incidence rates provide a rough indicator of differences in overall survival from cancer. These are a reflection of both the types of cancer that predominate in the different groups and the level of utilization of screening and treatment services by their members. Less-advantaged groups have the highest ratios of mortality to incidence, clearly indicating that improvement of services could have an impact on the cancer burden in these populations.

Cancer Disparities

The National Cancer Institute (NCI) defines "cancer health disparities" as adverse differences in cancer incidence, prevalence or deaths along with differences in cancer survivorship, and burden of cancer or related health conditions that exist among specific population groups in the United States. While improvements in diagnosis and treatment of cancers have improved among all populations, some disparities remain. Table 51-2 reports the incidence and mortality rates for all cancer combined by racial group. Differences in incidence can reflect different lifestyle factors. A higher ratio of mortality to incidence often suggests a lack of early diagnosis and/or treatment. The high ratio in American Indian/Alaska Native males is of concern, as is the somewhat higher ratio in Blacks (males and females). Whereas Asian or Pacific Islanders have ratios similar to non-Hispanic Whites and Hispanics have the lowest ratio. When specifically comparing change in death rates between Whites and Blacks (see SEER Figure 1.10), for many of the cancers for which death rates are decreasing, they have decreased more in Blacks but are still higher in Blacks (cervix, stomach, larynx, colon and rectum, prostate, lung and bronchus) with a few with higher death rates in Whites (oral cavity and pharynx, esophagus, kidney, and renal pelvis).[4] For female breast, the decrease is higher and mortality remains lower among Whites. This higher mortality or lower survival among Black women has been affected by lack of medical coverage, early detection barriers, unequal access to cancer treatments. Recent research indicates that aggressive breast cancer tumors are more common in young African American or Black women and Hispanic Latino women living in low SES areas (Bauer et al., 2007).[19] However subsequent research within these California patients found that in Los Angeles, women with lower SES were less likely to receive adjunct radiation therapy (Parise 2012).[20] More aggressive breast cancer is less responsive to standard treatments creating poorer survival rates (Carey et al., 2006).[21]

Additional information on cancer health disparities and efforts to reduce them can be found at https://www.cancer.gov/about-nci/organization/crchd or by searching for "NCI cancer disparities."

ETIOLOGY AND PRIMARY PREVENTION

Criteria for Causality

Primary cancer prevention is prevention of the initial development of a neoplasm or its precursor. This can be accomplished only if one or more causes of the neoplasm are known, and it is achieved by reducing or preventing exposure to the causative agent or enhancing exposure to the protective agent. A harmful agent is considered causal if reducing or removing a population's exposure to it results in a decrease in the amount of disease occurring in that population; a protective agent is considered truly beneficial if increasing or

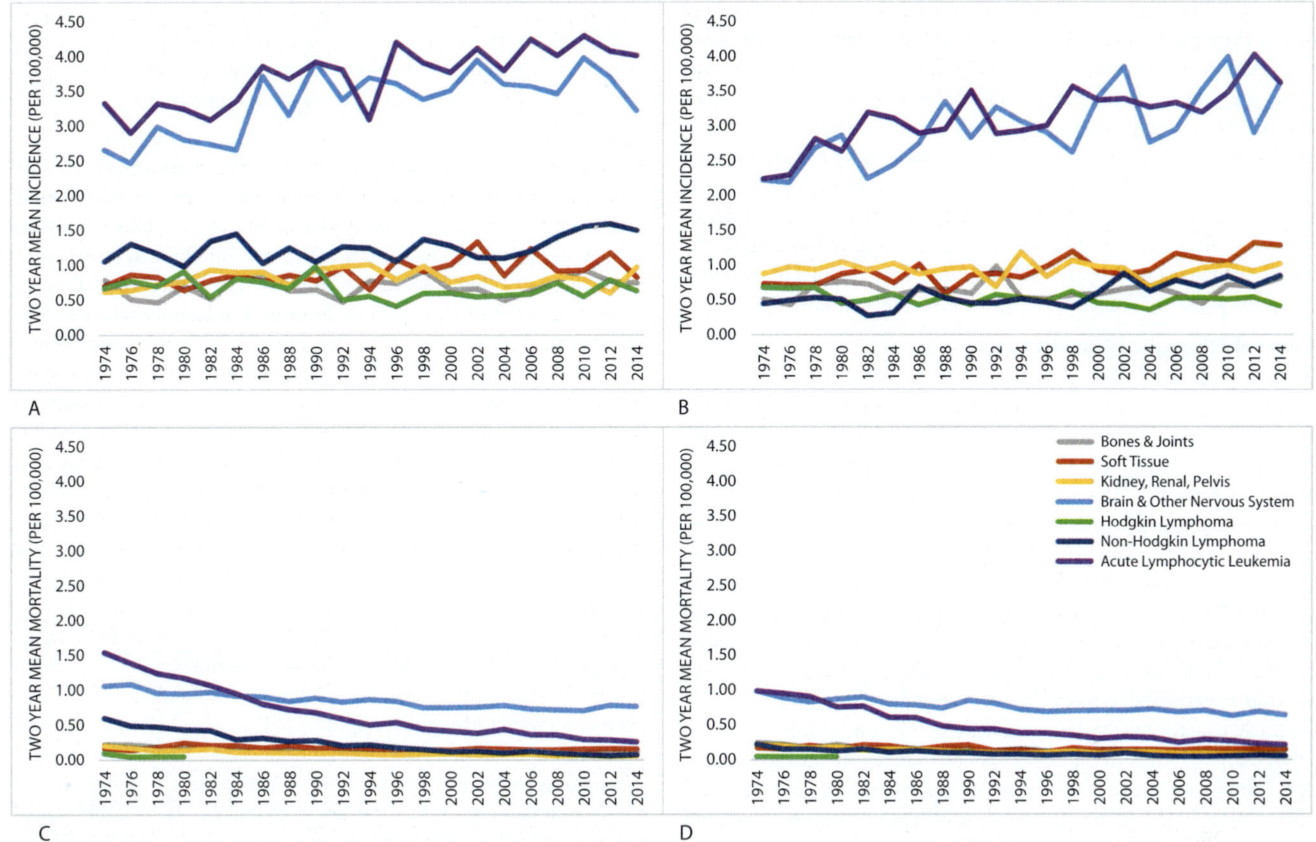

FIGURE 51-3. Surveillance, Epidemiology, and End Results Program (SEER) site-specific cancer incidence and mortality rates by year and gender in children (0–14 years). A. Males incidence, B. Females incidence, C. Males mortality, D. Females mortality. [*Source:* Incidence—Surveillance, Epidemiology, and End Results (SEER) Program (www.seer.cancer.gov) SEER*Stat Database: Incidence—SEER 9 Regs Research Data, Nov 2016 Sub (1973–2014) <Katrina/Rita Population Adjustment>—Linked To County Attributes—Total U.S., 1969–2015 Counties, National Cancer Institute, DCCPS, Surveillance Research Program, released April 2017, based on the November 2016 submission. Mortality—Surveillance, Epidemiology, and End Results (SEER) Program (www.seer.cancer.gov) SEER*Stat Database: Mortality—All COD, Aggregated With State, Total U.S. (1969–2014) <Katrina/Rita Population Adjustment>, National Cancer Institute, DCCPS, Surveillance Research Program, released December 2016. Underlying mortality data provided by NCHS (www.cdc.gov/nchs)].

TABLE 51-2 AGE-ADJUSTED INCIDENCE AND MORTALITY RATES OF ALL CANCERS COMBINED IN RACIAL AND ETHNIC GROUPS IN THE UNITED STATES, 2010–14*

	Men			**Women**		
2010–14						
Race/Ethnic Group	**Incidence**[a]	**Mortality**[a]	**Ratio**	**Incidence**[a]	**Mortality**[a]	**Ratio**
American Indian/Alaska Native[b]	331.4	184.0	0.56	308.9	129.3	0.42
Asian or Pacific Islander	308.6	122.7	0.40	296.1	88.8	0.30
Black	549.7	247.3	0.45	397.4	161.8	0.41
White	497.1	199.8	0.40	421.5	141.9	0.34
Hispanic[c]	373.2	142.6	0.38	323.3	97.7	0.30

Source: Howlader N, Noone AM, Krapcho M, et al., eds. SEER Cancer Statistics Review, 1975–2014, National Cancer Institute. Bethesda, MD, https://seer.cancer.gov/csr/1975_2014/, based on November 2016 SEER data submission, posted to the SEER website, April 2017.

*Rates are per 100,000 and age-adjusted to the 2000 U.S. standard population (19 age groups—Census P25-1130).

[a]Incidence source: SEER 18 areas (San Francisco, Connecticut, Detroit, Hawaii, Iowa, New Mexico, Seattle, Utah, Atlanta, San Jose-Monterey, Los Angeles, Alaska Native Registry, Rural Georgia, California excluding SF/SJM/LA, Kentucky, Louisiana, New Jersey, and Georgia excluding ATL/RG). Mortality source: U.S. Mortality Files, National Center for Health Statistics, Centers for Disease Control and Prevention.

[b]Rates for American Indian/Alaska Native are based on the CHSDA(Contract Health Service Delivery Area).

[c]Hispanic is not mutually exclusive from Whites, Blacks, Asian/Pacific Islanders, and American Indians/Alaska Natives. Incidence data for Hispanics are based on NAACCR Hispanic Identification Algorithm (NHIA) and exclude cases from Hawaii, Seattle, and Alaska Native Registry. Mortality data for Hispanics exclude deaths from Maine, Massachusetts, New Hampshire, and North Dakota.

expanding a population's exposure to it results in a decrease in the amount of disease occurring in that population.

To determine whether an agent is a cause of a particular disease in humans, information from all relevant studies must be assessed critically. In making such an assessment, evidence for causality is strengthened if Hill's criteria listed near the end of Chapter 4: Epidemiology and Public Health are met. Additional criteria include evidence that risk is reduced following a reduction in exposure.

Attempts to determine whether an agent is carcinogenic in humans must often be made without information on all of these criteria, using whatever evidence is available. Investigators must examine existing evidence to identify additional questions that should be addressed by further studies, physicians must assess available evidence to be able to give their patients adequate advice, and public officials must assess the evidence to determine needs for laws and regulations to limit exposure. Each must weigh the evidence for a causal relationship and consider the consequences of falsely implicating a substance as being carcinogenic when it is not and of failing to identify as carcinogenic a substance that is. All must also be willing to alter their opinions as results of additional investigations become available. Errors of judgment can be minimized by a clear understanding of basic epidemiologic principles and by careful examination of available evidence using the above-referenced criteria for assessing causality.

General Etiological Considerations

At the cellular level, cancer is a genetic disease. The development of a cancer appears to involve a multistep accumulation of genetic damage, leading eventually to the development of abnormal cells with a selective advantage over normal cells, and finally to an incipient tumor that acquires the ability to invade surrounding tissue.[22] The molecular epidemiology of cancer involves the use of molecular techniques in epidemiologic studies to provide new insights.[23] For each organ site, a tumor is the end result of multiple genetic aberrations that may be caused by multiple agents, and the same endpoint may be reached via different pathways. As a result, multiple risk factors are observed for all cancers, and only a small proportion of individuals who are exposed to most known carcinogens develop cancer. For example, a factor may increase cancer risk if it contributes directly to DNA damage, alters the ability of the cell to recognize or repair damage, inhibits apoptosis, encourages cell proliferation, enhances vascularization of the incipient tumor, or otherwise confers a selective advantage to that clone of cells. Similarly, agents that inhibit tumor development might act by reducing epithelial absorption of carcinogens, inhibiting the enzymatic activation of procarcinogens, enhancing the metabolic destruction of carcinogenic agents, promoting DNA repair, or causing cell differentiation or apoptosis and thereby reducing the number of stem and intermediate cells susceptible to the effects of carcinogens.

Most of the genes in which mutations appear to play a mechanistic role in carcinogenesis are categorized as either oncogenes or tumor suppressor genes, or are involved directly in DNA repair. Most identified oncogenes are mutated forms of genes (proto-oncogenes) that code for proteins involved in signal transduction, the regulation of gene expression, or growth-regulating mechanisms such as growth factors or growth factor receptors; overexpression of these genes results in enhanced cell proliferation. As an example, KRAS is a proto-oncogene that acts as an on/off switch for cell signaling. When it functions in a normal manner, it controls cell proliferation, but when it is mutated, cells can proliferate continuously, which can lead to the development of cancer. KRAS mutations are found at high rates in leukemias, colorectal, lung, and pancreatic cancers. Most known tumor suppressor genes function as negative regulators of cell proliferation. The tumor suppressor gene p53, for example, is mutated in a majority of epithelial tumors. Other contributors to the carcinogenic process probably include genes affecting angiogenesis, metastasis, and other components of the process such as the ability to evade or disable the immune response.

The latent period between exposure to some agent and the development of a neoplasm is dependent in part on the mechanism by which the agent operates. For example, mesothelioma follows exposure to asbestos only decades after exposure; the same is true of breast cancers following radiation to the chest, suggesting that these agents act early in the carcinogenic process. On the other hand, endometrial cancers can occur within 2 years of exposure to exogenous estrogens, suggesting a late-stage effect of these hormones. Reticulum cell sarcomas have developed within just months of exposure to immunosuppressive drugs in persons with renal transplants. A single exposure may act at one or more points in the progression to neoplasia, and its mechanism of action may vary across cancer sites. For example, epidemiologic evidence suggests that tobacco acts early in the carcinogenesis of esophageal and gastric adenocarcinoma, late in pancreatic tumors, and at both early and late stages in lung tumors.

Tobacco

Tobacco use is the single largest preventable cause of cancer (and other diseases) and premature death in the United States.[24] Use of tobacco is responsible for about 31% of all cancer deaths worldwide in men aged 30–69 and for 6% in women for these ages, which is more than all other known causes of cancer combined.[24] Tobacco increases the risk of cancers of the lung, oral and nasal cavities, esophagus, stomach, liver, pancreas, large intestine, kidney, bladder, cervix, and myeloid leukemia.[10,24,25] Table 51-3 shows the estimated proportion of cases that would be prevented in the absence of tobacco use (the population-attributable risk percent), and the estimated annual number of deaths worldwide and in the United States attributable to tobacco.[10,14,24–26] Population-attributable risks for tobacco are dependent on the proportion of people in the population who use tobacco, the relative risk (RR) of the particular cancer in users of tobacco, and the presence of other causes of the cancers of interest in the population. Estimates of population-attributable risks thus vary among populations, and the values for the United States are different from values for other parts of the world (and the global estimates are more prone to error). The highest tobacco-related cancer incidence rates have been observed in Mongolia, Republic of Korea, and China.[27] Overall, these estimates outline the importance of cancer prevention through eliminating smoking in populations. Cigarette smoking is responsible for most cancers of the oral cavity, esophagus, larynx, and lung.[26] In addition to the major cancer sites mentioned above for which the associations with tobacco are well established, a growing body of evidence implicates cigarette smoking as a contributor to the risk of colon and rectal cancers along with ovary (mucinous carcinoma cell type).[24,26] There is little or no evidence of an association with cutaneous melanoma and conflicting evidence for prostate cancer.

TABLE 51-3 CANCER DEATHS ATTRIBUTABLE TO SMOKING: WORLDWIDE AND U.S. ESTIMATES[a]

Cancer Site	Smoking Population Attributable Fraction	2015 Deaths Worldwide	Smoking Population Attributable Fraction	2017 Deaths in U.S.[b]
Lung and bronchus	70	1,205,400	86	134,048
Oral cavity	42	115,248	71	6,887
Larynx	69	72,806	69	2,516
Esophagus	42	184,380	71	11,140
Bladder	28	52,640	41	6,917
Pancreas	22	90,552	30	12,927
Liver	14	113,470	29	8,387
Stomach	13	106,456	25	2,740
Colorectal	7	58,240	7	3,518
Leukemia	9	31,815	17	4,165
Cervical, uterus	2	4,572	11	463
All cancer	21	1,840,566	29	174,267

[a]Estimated smoking population attributable fraction and worldwide death rates based on Danaei et al., 2005 accept for larynx and colorectal cancer are from Whiteman & Wilson, 2016.[25,26]

[b]Based on 2017 U.S. death rates estimated by the American Cancer Society (Siegel et al., 2017).[10]

Risks of a variety of neoplasms are also increased in users of other forms of tobacco. Compared to nonsmokers, risk in pipe and cigar smokers is approximately doubled for lung cancer, increased fourfold for cancer of the larynx, and doubled or tripled for neoplasms of the esophagus, oral cavity, pharynx, and bladder. Pipe smoking approximately triples one's risk of lip cancer, and chewing tobacco or using snuff results in a fourfold increase in the risk of oral cancer.[28]

Secondhand smoke and environmental tobacco smoke also significantly increase the risk of lung cancer.[24] Secondhand smoke contains more than 50 carcinogens and there is no risk-free level of exposure. Thus, passive smoking may account for the majority of the lung cancer not due to smoking, residential radon, or industrial exposures. The 2006 Surgeon General's report found that millions of Americans are still exposed to secondhand smoke in their homes and workplaces despite substantial progress in tobacco control.[24] Secondhand smoke also causes premature death and disease in children and adults who do not smoke.[24] Separating nonsmokers from smokers, ventilating buildings, and cleaning air cannot eliminate exposure to nonsmokers; only eliminating smoking in indoor spaces will do so.

In the United States and worldwide sales of electronic cigarettes (e-cigarettes) increase more than 15-fold in 15 years.[29] Electronic cigarettes are devices that typically deliver nicotine, flavoring, and other additives to users via inhaled aerosol.[30] Such devices are referred to as "e-cigs," "vapes," "vape pens," "mods," and "e-hookahs" to name a few. The overall impact on public health remains unclear.[31] Children appear to be a main target with over 7000 flavors of e-cigarettes including fruit and candy flavors.[29] One concern is toxicity if children drink the viles that the e-cigarette refills come in due to the flavoring attraction.[31] Additionally since e-cigarettes are not currently regulated in the United States, we do not know all the chemicals in these products. Further research is needed to understand this and examine any impact on cancer incidence and mortality, including any effect of burning tobacco sensation that is replaced by the nicotine and other unknown chemicals in these e-cigarettes.

Alcohol

The risk of several human neoplasms is clearly associated with alcohol consumption, especially for cancer of the oral cavity and pharynx, larynx, esophagus, and breast with liver and colorectal being probable.[25,32,33] Globally, alcohol contributes 3.5–5% of all cancer deaths.[33] Alcohol consumption results in an estimated 20,000 cancer deaths annually in the United States.[34] Risk of hepatocellular carcinomas is increased in heavy drinkers as alcohol-related liver disease is a risk factor,[35] but the extent to which part of this is due to the unusually high prevalence of hepatitis B and C in alcoholics is unknown. If alcohol is a cause of liver cancer, it is an uncommon complication of its use, because these tumors are rare in countries such as the United States where exposure to alcohol is common.

Cancer risk is typically increased only in those tissues that come in direct contact with undigested alcohol. Risk is thus increased for squamous cell carcinomas of the mouth (buccal cavity and pharynx), esophagus, and supraglottic larynx, but not, for example, of the lung or bladder. Esophageal, oral, and laryngeal squamous cell cancers are all also related to smoking, and most studies show the effect of smoking on the risk of these tumors to be greater in drinkers than in nondrinkers. Alcohol thus appears to modify the carcinogenic effect of tobacco smoke.[27] The effect of alcohol on these neoplasms may also be greater in individuals with marginal nutritional status than in better-nourished individuals. In the United States, alcohol and tobacco account for about 80% of these cancers.

Adenocarcinomas of the lower esophagus, gastroesophageal junction, and gastric cardia have also been consistently associated with alcohol use, but the relationship is not as strong as for the squamous cell carcinomas of the upper aerodigestive tract. Risks of cancer of the distal stomach, and pancreas, have not been consistently related to alcohol use, but observed associations between heavy drinking and pancreatic cancer warrant further study. An association between alcohol intake and breast cancer has been observed in multiple investigations, even after controlling for known risk factors for breast cancer; while this relationship is not well understood, a consensus group suggests that 4–9% of breast cancers may be caused by alcohol consumption.[25]

Approximately 5% of all cancer deaths worldwide and 4% of cancer deaths in the United States can be attributed to alcohol use.[25] Most alcohol-related neoplasms develop as a result of smoking as well as drinking, and cessation of smoking would have nearly the same impact on the occurrence of these neoplasms as cessation of drinking. A review article found that the risk of laryngeal and pharyngeal cancers was reduced with alcohol drinking cessation but the cessation may take over 35 years to reduce the elevated risks of cancer to that of nondrinkers.[36]

Industrial Exposures

In 1972, the IARC in Lyon, France, initiated a series of monographs on the evaluation of carcinogenic risks to humans. As of 2006, 88 multidisciplinary committees of experts have reviewed the published literature on approximately 900 suspect chemicals, industrial processes, drugs, radiation exposures, and infectious agents and classified them as to their likely carcinogenicity in animals and humans. Of the over 800 chemical and industrial processes evaluated, the available evidence was considered sufficient to clarify over 35 agents and groups of agents, mixtures, or industrial processes with exposure circumstances as carcinogenic to humans (Group 1).[37–41] These chemical and industrial processes have been most strongly and consistently associated with lung, bladder, and skin cancer in addition to a few others for some specific agents. Over 50 other chemicals, mixtures, and exposure circumstances were judged to be probably carcinogenic to humans (Group 2A); over 200 others were considered possibly carcinogenic to humans (Group 2B). The remaining chemicals, mixtures, and exposure, circumstances were considered not classifiable as to their carcinogenicity to humans (Group 3). Estimates of the global burden of occupational cancer are in the 2–4% range.[42–44] More information on such exposures are described in later in this book in Section VII on Environmental and Occupational Health.

Asbestos. Mesothelioma as well as lung, laryngeal, or ovarian cancers are caused by asbestos. It is most closely associated with mesothelioma. The World Health Organization estimates that 125 million people globally are currently exposed to asbestos in the workplace, and that 107,000 die each year from mesothelioma, lung cancer, or asbestosis.[68] The time period from initial exposure to mesothelioma development is typically 20–40 years. In the United States during 1999–2015, a total of 45,000 malignant mesothelioma deaths were reported, increasing from 2479 in 1999 to 2597 in 2015. This increasing number was unexpected based on past projections.[69] Asbestos-related diseases remain a major public health problem worldwide. Although most high exposure to asbestos has occurred in the workplace, such exposure can also occur outside the workplace, for example, from home renovation of older insulation and ceiling and floor tiles. Outside-the-workplace exposure to other carcinogens can also occur such as aflatoxin, arsenic, and benzene.

Environmental Pollution

Numerous efforts have been made to assess the impact of ambient air pollution on lung cancer risk.[25,45,46] Although rates of lung cancer are higher in urban than in rural areas, smoking is also more prevalent in urban areas. Primarily from large cohort studies in Europe and the United States, there are now results supporting air pollution as a risk factor for lung cancer. One report estimates 5% of lung cancers worldwide are attributable to urban air pollution with this risk rising to 7% in low- and middle-income countries.[25] As defining what is in air pollution is difficult since it is affected by local climate, IARC has specifically classified exposure to diesel exhaust emissions as carcinogenic in humans (Group 1).[46] More recent studies of diesel exhaust include mathematical modeling of wind patterns and testing within communities near major highways.

Ionizing Radiation

Radiation is the process by which energy is emitted or transferred in the form of particles or waves. Electromagnetic radiation is a form of energy all around us and spans a wide range of wavelengths and frequencies. It includes radio waves, microwaves, infrared, ultraviolet radiation (sunlight), x-rays, and gamma rays. Radiation that has enough energy to knock electrons off atoms and molecules, converting them to ions, is considered ionizing radiation. Since ionizing radiation is caused by these unstable atoms, it tends to be more of a health threat to humans. Nonionizing radiation is considered less harmful except if the amount of heat energy transfers is large such as sunlight or other ultraviolet radiation or microwaves to whatever is being cooked in them.

Ionizing radiation can cause a variety of human neoplasms.[47] Most of the evidence for this comes from studies that followed individuals exposed to moderate or high doses from nuclear explosions, medical treatments, and occupational sources. Exposures have been both external and internal. IARC has identified radionuclides (plutonium-239, radium-224, radium-226, radium-228, radon-222, and thorium-232) and their decay products as well as phosphorus-32, radioiodines, α-particle-emitting radionuclides, and β-particle-emitting radionuclides, in addition to x- and gamma (γ)-radiation, and neutrons, as carcinogenic to humans.[48–52]

All humans are exposed to natural radiation. Primary sources of natural radiation include inhalation (mainly radon gas), ingestion, cosmic rays, and terrestrial gamma rays.[53] Approximately half of all ionizing radiation received by individuals in the United States comes from natural background sources. Radium is found in soil where it decays to a naturally occurring radioactive gas, radon-222, which can seep into houses and accumulate under conditions of poor ventilation.[50,54] Radon is a naturally occurring gas that is colorless, odorless, and tasteless. It is found everywhere as it is produced from the decay of naturally occurring uranium in the soil. Overall, radon gas is the greatest contributor to natural radiation exposure, accounting for about 50% of the total average annual effective dose. Radon-222 progeny, primarily plutonium-218 and plutonium-214, are the likely cause of lung cancer in uranium miners, and with recent data, it is felt that residential radon-222 progeny contribute appreciably to the population's lung cancer burden.[50,51] Residential radon gas is the most important cause of lung cancer after smoking. It is estimated to cause between 3% and 14% of all lung cancers in a given country (3–20% of lung cancer deaths), depending on the national average radon level and smoking prevalence.[55,56] In the United States, radon is estimated to cause about 21,000 lung cancer deaths per year.[57] Manmade sources of radiation also exist and include medical uses of radiation, atmospheric nuclear testing, nuclear power production, and occupation activities. In developed countries, medical uses of radiation are the largest source of manmade exposure and, on average, amount to about 50% of the 240 mrem global average level of natural exposure.[53]

Studies of individuals who have received total body radiation from external sources have shown that some organs are more susceptible to the carcinogenic effects of radiation than others. In the atomic bomb survivors in Japan, there were large increases in rates of carcinomas of the anatomically exposed thyroid and mammary glands and of leukemias arising from the highly susceptible cells of the bone marrow; lesser increases in rates of lymphomas and carcinomas of the stomach, esophagus, and bladder were observed; and risks of cancer at other sites were either not altered or the increases were too small to measure with certainty. Risk of leukemia was also increased in early radiologists who took few precautions to reduce their general exposure to radiation and probably also in individuals exposed *in utero* to x-rays from pelvimetry.

Cancer survivorship has been increasing to where cancer survivors now constitute 4.8% of the U.S. population in 2016.[58] This is a high-risk group for second cancers, which now account for 16% of all cancer incidence (excluding nonmelanoma skin cancers).[59] These second cancers represent a serious side effect of treatment with radiation and chemotherapy. Most types of cancer can be caused by exposure to ionizing radiation.[60]

External sources of radiation directed at specific sites have resulted in a variety of neoplasms. Breast cancer was induced in women treated with x-rays for a variety of benign breast conditions and in women who received multiple fluoroscopies of the chest in conjunction with pneumothorax treatment of tuberculosis. Individuals treated with x-rays for ankylosing spondylitis have had increased rates of leukemia and lung cancer and, like the atomic bomb survivors, lesser increases in rates of lymphomas and cancers of the stomach and esophagus. An increased risk of lung cancer has been observed in women who received radiation following mastectomy for breast cancer and radiotherapy for Hodgkin's disease. Children treated with x-rays for tinea capitis and enlarged thymus have developed leukemia and neoplasms of the salivary and thyroid glands. Those treated for an enlarged thymus have also had an increased risk of leukemia, and those with tinea capitis developed more brain tumors than expected. Public health concerns may increase as computed tomography (CT) scans, which have higher radiation doses than dental radiography or screening mammography, have increased 20-fold since 1980.[61]

Internal exposures to radiation have likewise resulted in increased risks of cancer at specific sites. Inhalation of radioactive dusts contributed to the increased rates of lung cancer in the atomic bomb survivors, and inhalation of radon and its decay products resulted in elevated rates of lung cancer in miners of uranium, iron, and fluorspar. Radium inadvertently swallowed by radium-dial watch painters and administered for treatment of ankylosing spondylitis was concentrated in osseous tissues and caused high rates of bone cancers. Individuals exposed to iodine-131 (I-131) in fallout from a hydrogen bomb test and in emissions from the nuclear power plant accident at Chernobyl subsequently had increased rates of thyroid cancer. The radiopaque contrast material thorotrast that was used to x-ray the liver has resulted in hepatic cancers, as well as leukemias and lung carcinomas. Women receiving cervical radium implants and other forms of pelvic radiation for a variety of gynecological conditions have had increased rates of cancers of the rectum, vagina, vulva, ovary, and bladder, as well as leukemia.

The results of most studies show a linear increase in risk of neoplasms with the amount of radiation received over a wide range of observed doses, with a possible decrease in the slope of the dose-response curve at very high levels of exposure. These observations are based primarily on studies of individuals who received from tens to hundreds of rads. Doses commonly received today are orders of magnitude lower, and it is uncertain whether the dose–response curve should be linearly extrapolated to these low levels to provide an estimate of the associated risk. There may be a threshold level below which radiation does not induce neoplasms, perhaps because mechanisms of DNA repair are adequate. If so, linear extrapolation would overestimate the risk at low levels of radiation. Conversely, chronic exposure to low levels of radiation might be more carcinogenic, rad for rad, than acute exposure at a higher dose. If so, linear extrapolations would underestimate the risk of low doses. Since there is little evidence for the latter possibility, most authorities believe that it is reasonable, as well as prudent, to assume a linear, nonthreshold dose–response relationship. Experimental studies have documented that a single alpha particle can provide permanent damage to a cell.[52] This finding supports the biologic plausibility of the linear, nonthreshold relationship.

It is difficult to accurately estimate the number of cancers attributable to radiation from all sources experienced by the general population.[62] Nevertheless, available knowledge indicates that reducing medical exposures and residential (indoor) radon will have the most impact toward reducing population exposure and radiogenic cancer risk.

Nonionizing Radiation

Nonionizing radiation, in contrast to ionizing radiation, is electromagnetic radiation that does not have sufficient energy to remove electrons to form an ion (charged particle). Nonionizing radiation includes ultraviolet (UV) radiation, visible light, infrared, and microwave and radio frequencies. Among these, the major carcinogen is UV radiation which comes from the sun or artificial sources such as tanning beds or booths.

UV Radiation. Sunlight is a cause of nonmelanoma skin cancers (squamous and basal cell carcinomas), as evidenced by the observations that these tumors tend to occur on exposed parts of the body, risk increases with the amount of sun exposure, and incidence rates are greater in light-skinned than in dark-skinned individuals. However, these skin cancers are rarely deadly, and routine data on nonmelanoma skin cancer are not collected by cancer registries in the United States since the number of nonmelanoma skin cancers is greater than all other cancers combined. An estimated 4.3 million cases of basal cell and squamous cell skin cancer are treated in the United States.[63]

The relationship of cutaneous malignant melanomas to sunlight is more complicated.[64,65] Various types of sun exposure have been reported to be associated with melanoma, ranging from severe sunburns, occupational activities, vacation sun exposure, beach activities, other recreational activities, cumulative or chronic sun exposure, and early migration to sunny places. Incidence rates for cutaneous melanoma are highest in individuals with little natural skin pigmentation, often with intermittent sun exposure such as sunburns or sunny vacations.[64,65] Investigation of migrants to Australia provided evidence that sun exposure at an early age or long-term exposure may be of particular importance.[64] Early UV exposure is of concern with the expanding popularity of tanning beds and booths. Current evidence suggests an increase in melanoma risk among tanning bed users. Modern tanning bed units have UV levels comparable to tropical sunlight and irradiate almost 100% of the skin, which is assumed to be two to ten times more skin surface area than sunlight exposure.[66] Incidence rates have been increasing as younger populations expose more of their bodies to such units, especially among women. In the white U.S. population, incidence rates of melanomas of the skin have dramatically increased over the last few decades, due in part to changes in diagnostic criteria and enhanced awareness of the importance of early evaluation of melanotic lesions. Melanoma increases with age (the mean age at diagnosis is about 64 for 2010–14,[4] but individuals can develop melanoma at any age including childhood and adolescence. This is why dermatologists warn against sun exposure and sunburns during childhood; however, sunburns at any age are important risk factors for melanoma.[67] While the relationship between cutaneous melanoma and specific types of sun exposure is complex, the American Cancer Society estimates that nearly all skin cancers are related to UV radiation (even familial cancers that are likely related to genetic factors and UV radiation).[63] Almost 90% of melanomas are estimated to be caused by UV radiation according to the Surgeon General's report.[63] All individuals, but particularly those with light skin who burn easily, should be encouraged to avoid excessive direct exposure to intense sunlight (midday) and to use sunshades and sunscreens.

Electric and Magnetic Fields (EMFs). Use of electronic devices has increased exponentially over the past few decades. Studies have focused public attention on the possible association between exposure to EMFs, particularly from electric power lines and cellular telephones, and risk of cancer. Based on methodological concerns and limited experimental evidence, no clear relationships between EMF and chronic disease have been established.[70,71] However, an association is observed most consistently in studies of childhood leukemia in relation to postnatal exposures above 0.4 microT.[70,71] Similarly, a relationship between cellular telephone use and glioma has been observed in several studies.[72] Study of EMF is made particularly difficult by our inability to identify and accurately measure the relevant exposure. A number of reviews of the subject have been published.[70,71,73,74] In 2011, the IARC classified radiofrequency electromagnetic field (RF-EMF) as possibly carcinogenic to humans.[72] Recent reviews and meta-analyses showed association between mobile phone use and risk of intracranial tumors: glioma and acoustic neuroma.[75–77]

Ionizing and nonionizing radiation are discussed more in-depth later in this book.

Sex Hormones and Reproductive Factors

Sex Hormones. Sex steroid hormones have been associated with an increased risk of most reproductive cancers, including breast, endometrium, ovary, cervix, prostate, and testis. This section will evaluate endogenous and exogenous hormonal risks as well as other reproductive factors, many of which also are linked indirectly to potential hormonal alterations.

In evaluating the effects of exogenous female sex hormones on the risk of neoplasms in women, it is important to categorize these substances according to their estrogenic or progestogenic pharmacological effect. At one end of the spectrum are the pure progestational agents, such as depot-medroxyprogesterone acetate (DMPA), which is used as a long-acting injectable contraceptive in many countries and to treat malignant and benign proliferative disorders of the endometrium. Other progestational contraceptives include the "mini-pill" which is an OC, the injectable contraceptive, norethindrone, and subcutaneous implants, such as Norplant. At the other end of the spectrum are the pure estrogen preparations. Between the two ends of the estrogen-progestin spectrum are the sequential OCs, which contained only estrogen in pills taken for 2 weeks of a cycle followed by a weak progestin of short duration and which had a net estrogenic effect, and the more commonly used combined OCs with an estrogen and a progestin in each pill, and therefore a net pharmacological effect more progestational than the sequential pills. More recent products differ from these older formulations in dosage and in types of estrogens and progestins contained and are referred to as biphasic and triphasic OCs. Because of the breakthrough bleeding side effect of the biphasic formulations, these are not widely used.

The most common are the conjugated "natural" estrogens (e.g., Premarin), used largely to treat or prevent symptoms and conditions associated with menopause, and the nonsteroidal synthetic estrogen, DES (diethylstilbestrol), to prevent early miscarriage. Those used during peri- and postmenopause to reduce menopausal side effects and osteoporosis include estrogen replacement therapy (ERT) and estrogen/progestin hormone replacement therapy (HRT). More recent formulations have been marketed with reduced hormonal formulations yet having similar beneficial effects with fewer adverse side effects.

Breast Cancer. Although some studies, including a clinical trial, of breast cancer in women given DES for threatened abortion show no evidence of an increased risk of cancer,[78,79] a larger investigation showed a 40% increase risk with a latency period of 20 years after DES exposure.[80] The effect of combined OCs on risk of breast cancer has been evaluated in a number of large cohort and case-control studies as well as in meta-analyses[81] and the risk is increased by about 25% in current users and declines to that of never users about 10 years after cessation of use.

The RR estimate in women who ever used OCs is estimated to be 1.1. Tumors tend to be more localized in users than in nonusers, suggesting enhanced surveillance in recent and current users as an explanation for the increased risk. Even if this is a causal phenomenon, use of OCs result in few additional cases of breast cancer because most current and recent users of OCs are young women with a low background rate of this disease.[82] Among those who last used OCs less than 10 years ago, and for more than 5 years, the risk was shown to increase approximately 13%.[81] Recent and current users of a progestational agent had increased breast cancer risk but not after 5 years since last use, and an overall RR of 1.1 for ever use.[83] A case-control analysis of OC use and breast cancer subtypes in the African American Breast Cancer Epidemiology and Risk Consortium showed that only parous, but not nulliparous, women had greater risk regardless of recency or duration of OCs.[84] In the largest study to date, among 1.8 million Danish women ages 15–49 enrolled in the Danish Sex Hormone Registry Study with no prior history of cancer, thromboembolism, or infertility treatment, more detailed findings suggest the importance of separately evaluating all types of OCs and routes of hormonal delivery.[82] Current or recent use of combination hormonal contraceptives also was associated with risks between 1.0 and 1.6 but similar exposure and duration among progestin-only intrauterine systems also carry a higher risk of breast cancer compared to those who had never used hormonal contraceptives for $>$ 1 year (RR = 1.2). This includes use of non-OC steroid hormones: patch (norgestimate), vaginal ring (etonogesterel), which also have higher risks.

Studies of breast cancer in relation to ERTs given at menopause have shown an increased risk in women particularly among those who are current users of ERTs for 5 years or longer (RR = 1.2–1.4).[85] A small increase in risk with years of use beyond 5 years has been observed in most studies, with a decline in risks to that of nonusers from 2 to 5 years after cessation of use.[86] A collaborative reanalysis of 51 studies[87] on this issue found that during or shortly after use, there was a RR of 1.02 for each year of use for those with 1–4 years of use, and 1.03 for those with more than 5 years of use.

The association between risk of breast cancer among users of estrogen plus progestin and prior use of OCs has been evaluated in a number of follow-up studies.[88-90] The addition of a progestin to ERTs increases the risk by an additional 10% over that of ERT users or a 40% greater risk than among never HRT users. Relatively short-term combined estrogen plus progestin HRT use increases incident breast cancers which are diagnosed at a more advanced stage compared with placebo use.[88] The AARP study showed an increased risk among all ER+ tumors in HRT especially among users of $\geq$ 10 years (RR = 2.4, 2.1–2.8).[91] Risk was slightly higher when progestins were prescribed continuously rather than sequentially ($\leq$15 days/mo). In a U.S. cohort population, risk was pronounced among women reporting use of HRT (OR = 3.5), both OCs and HRT (OR = 2.6), or OCs and long-term HRT use (OR = 3.9).[90] Among postmenopausal women there was no effect of OC use, but risk was modestly elevated among HRT users of more than 5 years under age 65 (OR = 1.4). These results emphasize that timing of exogenous hormone use is important.

Tamoxifen, which has antiestrogenic properties in the breast, and raloxifene, a selective estrogen receptor modulator, have been shown to reduce the risk of breast cancer in the contralateral estrogen receptor positive breast of a woman who receives these adjuvant therapies for primary breast cancer. Recent studies have verified that risk of breast cancer recurrence among early stage (T1, estrogen receptor positive/ER+) after stopping adjuvant hormonal therapy, continue over a 20-year follow-up.[92] The risk of recurrence was found to be strongly associated with baseline TN status, ranging from 10% to 41%. The risk of recurrence was associated with the baseline breast cancer TN status.

Among the limited studies of breast cancer and endogenous sex steroid hormones (produced by the body), data indicate elevated risk for women in the top quintile of total estradiol (RR = 1.9), or free estradiol (RR = 2.7) after adjustment for BMI and other risk factors.[93-96]

Endometrial Cancer. The risk of endometrial cancer is increased twofold or more in women who took sequential OCs and who were not monitored for endometrial hyperplasia.[85,97,98] In contrast, risk of cancer remains significantly decreased (RR = 0.5) for 20 years or longer in users of combination OCs[99] compared to never users. The reduction in risk is even lower among those who used the progesterone-only OCs and in users of DMPA[100] because of their net progestational effect on the endometrium.

Those who received estrogens for menopausal conditions, primarily as ERTs, also are at significantly greater risk of endometrial cancer. Tamoxifen, which is used as an adjuvant therapy for breast cancer, has an estrogenic effect on the uterus and has also been shown to increase the risk of endometrial cancer.[101] To reduce the risk of endometrial cancer in users of drugs containing estrogens, a progestin is often included, either continuously with the estrogen or cyclically for a specified number of days each month, and this has been shown to markedly reduce the risk of endometrial cancer to that of never users. Several case-control studies have shown an increased total and bioavailable estrogens and decreased plasma levels of sex hormone binding globulin in postmenopausal women who develop endometrial cancer as compared to healthy controls.[102,103] In premenopausal women, one epidemiologic study showed a decrease in total and bioavailable estradiol. It has further been suggested that in this group of women it is lower progesterone rather than higher estrogen that increases the risk of premenopausal endometrial cancer. Additional evidence of the effects of endogenous hormones on cancer development comes from the increased risk in polycystic ovarian syndrome, a disease that is characterized by low progesterone levels in women who have normal estrogen levels. In both pre- and postmenopausal women, obesity and chronic hyperinsulinemia are associated with changes in total and bioavailable sex steroid levels, especially estrogen. In sum, there are few if any studies that have used a prospective design to directly examine endogenous hormonal levels well in advance of malignancy.

Ovarian Cancer. Risk of epithelial ovarian cancer in women who have ever used combined OCs is approximately 50% of that of never users, and the risk decreases with duration of use.[104] A further reduction in risk is seen in the progesterone-only OCs. The benefit of either type of OC persists 10–20 years after use has been discontinued. The benefit includes women with a family history of ovarian cancer and those with a mutation in the BRCA1 or BRCA2 gene.[105,106] Furthermore, the reduced risk is similar in parous and nulliparous women without known infertility. A single study has shown no effect of DMPA on risk of ovarian cancer, thus the association is unclear to date. Several large cohort and case-control studies have shown an increased risk of ovarian cancer among either ERT (RR = 1.6) or HRT (RR = 1.2) as well as a significant duration effect (RR = 1.3–1.8).[107,108] The Health-AARP study of postmenopausal hormone use in more than 92,500 women examined whether the association between long-term estrogen plus progestin hormone replacement therapy (>10 yrs) showed an increased risk of ovarian cancer.[108] Findings reiterated previous investigations that long-term use of unopposed estrogens significantly increased the risk (RR = 2.2) of this cancer and estrogen plus progestin also is associated with a significantly increased risk of ovarian regardless of estrogen/progestin regimen, sequential (RR = 1.6) or continuous (RR = 1.4).[109]

In contrast, the Breast Cancer Detection Demonstration Project cohort follow-up study showed no increased risk ovarian cancer with either ever or duration in HRT use of 4 years or more, whereas risk was elevated in ERT users (RR = 1.8–3.2).[110] Studies of endogenous hormones associated with ovarian cancer are limited and rely on indirect evidence such as the protective effects of pregnancies and OC use, which suppress pituitary gonadotropin secretion and increased risk among women with polycystic ovarian syndrome, who are known to have elevated circulating luteinizing hormones (LH). However, these findings are contradicted by the lack of an increase in risk among those with an early age at menopause and with twin pregnancies, both of which are associated with an increase in gonadotropin levels; in the lack of an increase in ovarian cancer after menopause which is associated with increasing LH and follicle stimulating hormone; and in the increased risk with ERT use and obesity. Research also has shown a lack of association between circulating androgens and ovarian cancer risk in postmenopausal women, but an increased risk is seen with androstendione and dehydroepiandrosterone in premenopausal women. Despite the link between insulin and insulin-like growth hormones (IGF-I) receptor and activation of intracellular signaling pathways and its effects on metabolism of other hormones, studies to date do not support its involvement with ovarian cancer. Likewise, IGF-I, which has been associated with increased risk of other reproductive cancers, breast and prostate, did not show evidence of an association in the only epidemiologic investigation of risk based on prediagnostic data to date.[111] In summary, although evidence is accumulating regarding endogenous hormones associated with ovarian cancer, additional investigations particularly among prospective study designs are required.

Cervical and Vaginal Cancers. Studies of HRTs and risk of cervical cancer are limited but suggest an increased risk in users (RR = 2.3–2.7) and with increasing duration in use.[112,113]

DES was prescribed between 1938 and 1971 to treat up to 5 million women in the United States for threatened abortion. Approximately 80% of the female offspring exposed to DES in utero have been found to have glandular epithelium resembling that of the endometrium, and presumably of Müllerian origin, in the vagina or cervix. This is referred to as adenosis. A small portion of women with this condition have developed clear cell adenocarcinomas of the vagina or (less frequently) the cervix in their teens or twenties especially if their mother took DES early in pregnancy.[114] The risk of clear cell carcinoma is between 1.4/1000 and 1/10,000 among exposed women.[115] This represents a high proportion of neoplasms in this age group, including virtually all vaginal cancers. Women exposed in utero to DES with vaginal or cervical adenosis should be followed carefully for the development of clear cell carcinoma. These neoplasms represent the first documented instances of transplacental carcinogenesis in humans. In some countries, DES has been used as a "morning after" pill to prevent pregnancy or to treat menopausal symptoms.

Vulvar Cancer. Although endogenous hormones have not been evaluated in the development of vulvar cancer, few studies have examined the association between this reproductive tumor and sex steroid hormones. In the follow-up AARP study of women (n = 201,469) for risks associated with this tumor, after controlling for confounders, current users of OC showed an increased risk of squamous intraepithelial neoplasia grade 3 (VIN3) and in SCC type among current OC users, but not invasive cancer regardless of histologic type. Among those with SCC histologic type only, VIN3 risk increased in past and current users of hormone replacement therapy whereas level of risk was similar regardless of length of time used.[116] Based on what is known about HPV-related cervical cancer and the age-related curve among VIN3 cases in the AARP study, exposure to exogenous hormones among those with HPV, which was not evaluated in this study, their effects on transcriptional regulatory regions of HPV DNA which have been shown to be up regulated by the viral genes, may provide an explanation why incidence of CIN3 was elevated in the 40- to 65-year-old age range. Although one prior study showed greater vulvar cancer risk associated with early menopause,[117] neither AARP nor other studies have.[118] The Coffey et al. study[117] however combined early natural and surgical menopause together. *Liver cancer:* Combined OCs have clearly been shown to cause benign hepatic cell adenomas and focal nodular hyperplasia. These are highly vascular tumors that can rupture, bleed into the peritoneal cavity, and cause death. Fortunately, they are a rare complication of OC use, occurring at a rate of less than 3 per 100,000 women-years in women under 30 years of age. Case-control studies conducted in developed countries have shown that primary hepatocellular carcinomas are also rare complications of OC use.[119] Some of these studies, plus investigations conducted largely in developing countries, provided evidence that this adverse effect is not mediated by enhancing the influence of other factors such as hepatitis B or C on risk.

Colorectal Cancer. Data collected about lifestyle, medical history, diet, etc. along with blood samples, from the Nurses' Health Study, the Women's Health Study, the Health Professional Follow-Up Study, and the Physicians' Health Study II were evaluated for the association between endogenous sex steroid hormones and colorectal cancer risk.[120] Based on these combined data, there appears to be an association between levels of sex hormones and colorectal cancer risk in men and an inverse association between the ratio of estradiol to testosterone and colorectal cancer in postmenopausal women. Other studies of exogenous hormones show that OC ever or new users (RR = 0.4–0.7) compared to never users[121–123] as well as in HRT current or ever users (RR = 0.3–0.5) is not protective against colorectal cancer.[122] Studies of malignant melanoma from case-control, cohort studies, and a meta-analysis failed to confirm earlier reports that risk of malignant melanoma is increased by use of OCs.[99] Compared to never users, those who used OCs for greater than 1 year showed no excess risk (RR = 0.82–1.15), nor for duration, age first used, recency, or latency effects.[124] Isolated reports of associations between OCs and pituitary adenomas, choriocarcinomas, gallbladder carcinomas, and thyroid tumors have also appeared, but these observations have not been convincingly confirmed by epidemiological investigations.[99]

Prostate Cancer. Both prostate and testicular cancers in males have been associated with endogenous sex hormones with the primary hypothesis that androgens are causally related to prostate cancer etiology. Although there have been a number of studies that have investigated the role of androgens, few have had an adequate sample size, serum taken prior to cancer development and diagnosis, or controlled for confounding, especially age-related, known changes in serum hormone levels that may not reflect current cancer risk. In the one prospective study that addressed these issues, the Physicians' Health Study showed that risk of prostate cancer was greater with increasing testosterone quartile levels (RR = 1.0–2.4), and decreased with increasing sex hormone binding globulin (RR = 1.0–0.4) and estradiol regardless of comparative quartile level (RR = 0.5).[125] Based on 11 randomized controlled trials and nonplacebo-controlled investigations of men with a history of prostate cancer, there is no evidence that testosterone (replacement) therapy (TRT) is causally related to prostate cancer.[126] There also was no increased risk in men with hypogonadism, or PIN.[127] The relation between prostate cancer risk and total serum testosterone is unclear. Several studies have shown that increasing testosterone to supraphysiologic levels does not increase serum PSA significantly.[128–130] The theory is that once androgen receptors in the prostate are saturated, increasing testosterone no longer has an effect on androgen level. Further, this saturation point has been shown to occur at physiologic testosterone levels and linked to a rise in PSA level. A U.S. 15-year follow-up study of men diagnosed with any prostate-related condition found neither a 1-year nor a 5-year average of testosterone was significantly associated with prostate cancer risk.[131] However, faster age-related reductions did significantly affect the risk of prostate cancer.

Testicular Cancer. It has been hypothesized that initial hormonal exposure levels in utero and excess estrogen or insufficient androgens lead to testicular cancer. Maternal exogenous estrogen use during pregnancy has been associated with both cryptochordism, a significant risk factor for testicular cancer, and subsequent development of testicular cancer in offspring. In addition, risk is greater in male offspring of women having their first child as compared to multiparous women, consistent with plasma estrogen levels, which are noted to be higher in primiparous women.[132] Although it has been suggested that maternal exposure to DES leads to increased testicular cancer risk, there is insufficient evidence to support this claim.[133] Among the testicular cancer risk factors, it appears that late age at puberty is linked to a significant decrease (~50%) in risk of testicular cancer, supporting a hormonal influence in its etiology.[134,135]

Infectious Agents

An estimated 15% of new cancer cases are attributable to infection.[17] This includes cancers resulting from infection with bacteria, viruses and even parasites, thought the latter are primarily in developing countries. Worldwide, two million new cancer cases, 92% of all infection-attributable cancers, were attributable to four infectious agents: *H. pylori*, human papillomavirus (HPV), and the hepatitis and viruses, HBV and HCV.[17] That infectious agents cause an increasing number of cancers opens up novel opportunities for the development of prevention and treatment strategies as well as new challenges in implementing them.[136]

Bacteria. It is estimated that *H. pylori* infects the gastric mucosa of about half of the world population,[137] and though only 1–3% of individuals with *H. pylori* infections develop gastric cancer,[138] over 89.0% of noncardia gastric adenocarcinomas have been attributed to infection with *H. pylori*.[17] Gastric cancer is the third leading cause of cancer deaths worldwide. Based on 2012 estimates, there were 951,000 new cases of gastric cancer worldwide.[139] Though more commonly associated with developing countries in Asia where about 50% of gastric cancer cases occur and *H. pylori* prevalence rates may reach as high as 80% in certain populations,[140] the relationship between *H. pylori* and gastric cancer is also of potential importance in developed countries. This pathogen has been associated with both intestinal and diffuse histologic types, and most strongly with the development of noncardia tumors.[141] The mode of transmission for *H. pylori* infection remains unclear with evidence suggesting an oral-fecal route.[142] As a result of the association between noncardia gastric cancer and *H. pylori*, the malignancy can be prevented or produce resolution of premalignant lesions by use of antibiotic therapy.

Viruses. Human papillomavirus (HPV) is the next most common oncogenic infectious agent after *H. pylori*. HPV is a necessary, but not sufficient, cause of cervical cancer and is associated with a high proportion (60–85%) of vulvar, vaginal, penile, and anal cancer sites. HPV is transmitted primarily through sexual contact and invades the tissues by epithelial microtears. The most prevalent and oncogenic types are HPV 16 and 18, which account for about 66.2% of invasive cervical cancer in the United States.[143] Other, less prevalent types that cause genital cancers are HPV 31, 33, 35, 39, 45, 51, 52, 56, 58, 59, 68, 73, and 82. Although the prevalence of genital HPV infection in adults 18–59 years of age during 2013–14 was 45.2% in the United States, infections usually are cleared or become latent and undetectable.[144] In individuals for whom infection persists for a prolonged time, intraepithelial lesions are likely to develop, some of which eventually progress to invasive carcinomas. The factors responsible for progression to anogenital malignancies include hormonal factors (e.g., steroid contraceptives), chemical factors (e.g., cigarette smoking), and immunodeficiency [e.g., human immunodeficiency virus (HIV) infection, immunosuppression for renal transplantation].

In contrast, HPV is an independent risk factor for 25% of head and neck cancers and does not require other major risk factors, such as tobacco and alcohol, for malignancy to develop. HPV types associated with head and neck cancers are limited primarily to HPV 16, 18, 31, and 33, and both younger age and male gender are more likely to be infected with the virus in the oral tissues.

A quadrivalent HPV vaccine targeting types 6, 11, 16, and 18 has been available since 2006 and is recommended for females aged 9–13 (up to age 26 if not vaccinated previously) and males 11–12 (up to age 21 if not vaccinated previously).[145,146] Two additional vaccines exist. A bi-valent (types 16 and 18) for girls and women was approved in 2010. The nine-valent (against HPV types 6, 11, 16, 18, 31, 33, 45, 52, and 58) vaccine was approved in 2014, replacing the quadrivalent HPV vaccine.[147] Vaccine uptake is low in the United States, with only 43.4% of U.S. adolescents (13–17 years) surveyed up-to-date with the recommended HPV vaccination series in 2016, while 60.4% had received at least one vaccine dose.[148] Prevalence of HPV types 6, 11, 16, and 18 has decreased significantly in females 14–24 years (the ages most likely to benefit from the vaccine) from the prevaccine to early postvaccine era, while the prevalence in females aged 25–34 years did not change significantly.[149] Similarly, there was a significant decrease in cervical lesions associated with HPV types 16 and 18 in females aged 15–19 between 2007 and 2014.[150] More time and research are needed to observe if HPV vaccination decreases the incidence of its associated cancers.

The hepatitis viruses, B and C, are causative agents in liver cancer and HCV also in non-Hodgkin's lymphomas. Worldwide, liver cancer is the second leading cause of cancer death (GLOBCAN: http://globocan.iarc.fr/old/FactSheets/cancers/liver-new.asp). In the United States, cases of liver and intrahepatic bile duct cancer have been increasing at about 3% a year for the last decade, making it the fastest growing cancer.[4] Treatment has also improved, with U.S. 5-year survival rates increasing to 16.8% in 2009 compared with 3.0% in 1975.[4] While other risk factors include heavy alcohol use, nonalcoholic fatty liver disease, diabetes, and obesity, this cancer can develop in individuals who are chronic carriers of HBV or HCV. In parts of Africa, Asia, and the Pacific, HBV is endemic with most infections occurring during childhood, and 90% of HCC are infected with HBV. Transmission of HBV or HCV is through contact with infected bodily fluids. In high-risk areas, perinatal transmission of HBV from mother to child at or soon after birth, before immune competence is fully developed, results in the child becoming a chronic HBV carrier and at higher risk of subsequently developing HCC. In areas with lower prevalence of HBV, most infections are acquired horizontally in early adulthood through intravenous drug use or unprotected sex. Less commonly, contaminated surgical instruments and donor organs and medical personnel who are in frequent contact with infected blood products are at high risk if not vaccinated against HBV.

Vaccination for HBV was first approved in the United States in 1981, resulting in a decline in acute HBV infection.[151] However, current HBV vaccination coverage rates among U.S. adults at least 19 years old remain low at 24.5%.[152] Currently, there is no vaccine to protect against HCV. Although blood transfusions were once a significant route of transmission, improved diagnostic tests, greater screening, and vaccination against HBV have dramatically reduced the risk of acquisition of HBV.

Epstein-Barr virus (EBV), a herpes virus, has been etiologically associated with Burkitt's lymphoma, nasopharyngeal carcinomas, and Hodgkin's disease, though the faction of cancers attributable to EBV infection varies greatly across regions.[17] Primary EBV is usually asymptomatic in humans and exists as a latent infection, which is seroprevalent in over 90% of the adult population worldwide. However, only a small proportion of individuals infected with EBV develop these neoplasms and the worldwide distribution of them is different. Thus, it is apparent that other factors are essential in conjunction with EBV for these tumors to develop. Almost all individuals with Burkitt's lymphoma or nasopharyngeal carcinomas have antibodies against EBV, compared with lower percentages in unaffected persons, and antibody titers are higher in the diseased cases. Endemic Burkitt's lymphoma, which occurs in equatorial Africa, is associated with EBV in 95% of cases, whereas EBV is only associated with 1–3% of sporadic Burkitt's lymphoma cases, which occur in Western Europe and the Americas.[153] EBV is associated with the undifferentiated nasopharyngeal carcinomas type, which is detected primarily in men over age 40 years of age, regardless of geographic location. Although the neoplasm is rare, the incidence is very high in Asian and Alaskan native populations with rates between 25 and

50/100,000 compared to less than 1/100,000 in Caucasian populations.[154] In Singapore, where Chinese, Malays, and Indians live in close proximity and share similar dietary and social habits, the incidence of nasopharyngeal carcinomas is 18.5, 3.1, and 0.9 per 100,000 in males, respectively, suggesting that genetic rather than environmental exposures are important to the development of this tumor. EBV also contributes to the development of Hodgkin's disease. The virus causes infectious mononucleosis, and those with a history of infectious mononucleosis have a two- to threefold increase in risk of Hodgkin's disease but not EBV-negative HL. Compared to nondiseased individuals, cases of Hodgkin's disease have a higher prevalence of antibodies against EBV and higher antibody titers. However, EBV DNA or gene products can be demonstrated in only half of cases, and only 30–40% of cases have anti-EBV antibodies, suggesting either the existence of causal pathways not including EBV or loss of EBV infection after tumor development. In immunodeficient patients such as those receiving transplants or having AIDS (acquired immunodeficiency syndrome), there also is an increased incidence of EBV-associated Hodgkin's disease.[155]

Human Herpesviridae (HHV-8) is the causative agent of Kaposi's sarcoma. Once very rare, in the early 1980s a more aggressive form of Kaposi's sarcoma associated with immune deficiency was seen in AIDS patients and was one of the first indications of the AIDS epidemic. As the incidence rate of AIDS dropped in the United States in the 1990s, so also did that of Kaposi's sarcoma,[156] though it remains the most common cancer among those living with HIV/AIDS.[157] In parts of Africa where HIV and HHV-8 seroprevalence is high, Kaposi's sarcoma accounts for a significant proportion of all cancers. For example, 24% in Mozambique, 27% in Uganda, and 35% in Zimbabwe, and in South Africa, where Kaposi's sarcoma is the most common neoplasm among HIV positive children with rising incidence.[157] It is worth noting the HIV alone is not the direct cause of cancers, though it may work as a factor in combination with other factors.

As its name indicates, human T-lymphotropic virus, HTLV-1, is associated with the development of adult T-cell leukemias and lymphomas.[17] The cancer is more prevalent in some areas of Japan, the South Pacific, the Caribbean, and Africa where the virus is endemic, but is of less significance in the nonendemic United States. The population seropositivity level remains unclear as most studies have examined selective, high-risk groups.[158] While most infections remain asymptomatic, about 10% of infected individuals become symptomatic[159] with a lifetime chance around 3% of developing adult T-cell leukemia.[160] Transmission is believed to occur through cell-to-cell contact of virus-infected cells during the exchange of bodily fluids (e.g., breast milk, semen, blood transfusions, and contaminated needles of drug users).

Parasites. In 1994, an IARC working group[161] judged that *Schistosoma haematobium* was a definite cause of squamous cell bladder cancer (Group 1), that the liver flukes *Opisthorchis viverrini* and *Clonorchis sinensis* were definitely (Group 1) and probably (Group 2) causes of cholangiocarcinomas of the liver, respectively. Schistosomiasis affects more than 200 million people, primarily in the Middle East and parts of Africa, and humans are the host for the blood fluke, which infects them through the skin exposed to water containing the infective larvae. The eggs elicit granulomas that cause disease in the urogenital system. *O. viverrini* infects humans who eat undercooked fresh-water fish and the adult parasite lives within the intrahepatic bile ducts. The highest incidence of cholangiocarcinoma in the world is in Thailand where the parasite is endemic and the vast majority of these cases are caused by this fluke.

The implications of infectious causes for cancers expand the repertoire of disease prevention strategies. These include the development of vaccines and use of antibiotics as described above, but also to intervene and block transmission of the infection. Beyond these established associations, there is evidence that the list of cancers with infectious causes will continue to grow.[136]

Obesity, Nutrition, and Physical Activity

Reasons for the large international differences in the incidence of most cancers are unknown, but studies of the changes in cancer rates among migrants have clearly shown that they are largely due to variation in environmental factors, not in genetic predisposition or susceptibility to carcinogens. Correlational studies have been conducted to identify factors that vary across countries in accordance with variations in the rates of various cancers. These studies have shown a variety of dietary components to be related to a number of different neoplasms. To investigate these associations further, many case-control studies and several large cohort studies have been conducted,[162–168] a variety of laboratory investigations have been performed to elucidate possible mechanisms for observed epidemiological findings, and randomized trials of dietary supplements or modifications have been conducted or are under way.[169–177]

Overview of Risk. When reviewing preventable lifestyle and environmental factors related to cancer, a consensus group examined major dietary issues and physical activity.[25] They found evidence that low fruit and vegetable intake are associated with cancer of the colon and rectum, stomach, lung, and esophagus.[25] However, low fruit and vegetable consumption is related to high dietary fat intake, along with obesity, and possibly physical inactivity. Being overweight or obese (high body mass index, BMI) have been associated with cancer of the breast (postmenopausal), colon and rectum, corpus uteri, endometrium (uterus), esophagus, gallbladder, kidney, and ovary.[25,26] Obesity is likely also related to physical inactivity which has been associated with breast, colorectal, and endometrial cancers.[25] The lack of independence among these factors makes understanding true causal associations difficult.

Carcinogenic Mechanisms. Food items may be contaminated by preformed carcinogens. Aflatoxins produced by fungi that can grow in grains and other crops in warm, moist climates have been linked to liver cancers in some parts of the world.[42] In China, mutagens have been detected in fermented pancakes and vegetable gruels, and these have been related to both esophageal cancer in humans and neoplasms of the gullet in chickens; and nasopharyngeal carcinomas have been related to consumption of salted fish and fermented food during infancy.[42]

Carcinogens may be formed in the body by bacteria.[42] Nitrites may be ingested in small amounts with preserved meats and fish or formed in larger quantities from dietary nitrates, either spontaneously before being eaten or in the presence of bacteria in the body; and carcinogenic *N*-nitroso compounds may then be produced from ingested amines and nitrites by bacteria in the stomach of people with chronic gastritis, in the bladder of individuals with urinary tract infection, or in the normal colon and mouth to produce cancers of the stomach, bladder, colon, and esophagus, respectively. Smoked and cured foods, charcoal-broiled meats, and some fruits and vegetables from contaminated areas may contain carcinogenic polycyclic aromatic hydrocarbons.

A high-fat diet may increase bile production and produce an environment in the large bowel conducive to the growth of bacteria capable of forming carcinogens, and perhaps steroid hormones, from bile salts. Production of such substances provides one plausible explanation for the observed associations between a high-fat diet and cancers of the colon, breast, and prostate. A meta-analysis of 83 studies showed an inverse association between adherence to a Mediterranean diet and cancer mortality along with a small decrease in breast cancer risk.[163] Another review showed that the Mediterranean diet reduces the risk and mortality of prostate cancer.[164] Two meta-analyses examined associations between dietary inflammatory index and cancer with both finding an association with colorectal cancer and one also finding an association with breast and lung cancer.[165,178]

When examining red and processed meat consumption, reviews have found associations with bladder cancer,[166] gastric cancer among case-control studies (but not among cohort studies),[167] and pancreatic cancer among case-control studies.[168]

Obesity. Globally, obesity is an epidemic with an estimated 110 million children and adolescents in 2013, and 640 million adults in 2014, being obese. Obesity has doubled in children since 1980 and increased sixfold in adults since 1975. Excess body fat has also been linked to several cancer types including those previously mentioned (postmenopausal breast, colon and rectum, corpus uteri, endometrium, esophagus, gallbladder, kidney, and ovary) along with a recent meta-analyses also finding evidence for gastric cardia, renal cell carcinoma, liver, pancreas, thyroid, multiple myeloma, and meningioma.[179] Here, the RRs were highest for uterus and esophageal adenocarcinoma when comparing the highest BMI category versus normal BMI. Historically, tumor promotion by excess endogenous estrogens was considered as a possible mechanism for endometrial and postmenopausal breast cancers. Early menarche and late menopause, risk factors for breast and endometrial cancers, have been directly or indirectly related to overnutrition and more recently hormones in meat. In postmenopausal women, estrogens are derived from androgens produced by the adrenal gland. This reaction takes place in adipose tissue and is enhanced in obese women. However, as other cancers have been associated with increasing BMI in the past decade, it is suggested that obesity associated metabolic and adipose tissue changes may contribute to cancer.[180]

Bias in Dietary Studies. Epidemiological studies of diet and cancer are difficult to perform and evaluate for a variety of reasons. One common problem in all epidemiological approaches is that many individual dietary constituents are highly correlated. For example, diets that are poor in animal protein are also likely to be poor in animal fat and high in carbohydrates and fiber. Additionally, food frequency questionnaires vary in the type of nutrients emphasized through kinds of foods listed, number of foods listed (do they include ethnic foods and/or restaurants), methodology for food selection, definitions of food groups, nutrients in databases, instructions given to responders relative to serving-size estimations, format for completing the questionnaire (self-administered or clinician-administered), and methodology for quality control (method of contacting the respondent to resolve items left blank). Under such circumstances, it is difficult to determine which of the interrelated dietary constituents (if any) is responsible for observed variations in risk. Another difficulty is that diet many years prior to the development of a neoplasm may be of the greatest etiological relevance and diets may change over time. Such information is difficult (although not impossible) to obtain in case-control studies. Cohort studies can theoretically overcome this problem, but must include large numbers of subjects and must be continued for decades and hence require large commitments of time and money. Despite these methodological problems, results of recent research strongly suggest that dietary factors contribute to the etiology of a variety of neoplasms. Some of the more likely mechanisms are briefly summarized in the following paragraphs.

Physical Activity. Increased physical activity is associated with decreased risk of breast, colon, and prostate cancers.[181] Although the epidemiologic evidence is not completely consistent, regular exercise appears to reduce the risk of breast cancer, perhaps because of the effects of physical activity on body weight. There is also evidence that exercise exerts an independent effect on the risk of colon cancer, possibly by decreasing stool transit time and therefore the duration of exposure to carcinogens in the gut. Related to physical inactivity (and obesity) is the growing body of research around sedentary behavior. Sedentary behavior is associated with colorectal cancer, endometrial, ovarian, breast, and prostate cancer risk.[182,183] Sedentary behavior may be associated with health outcomes independent of physical activity.[182]

Protective Dietary Constituents. Dietary constituents may also protect against cancer. Diets high in fresh fruits and raw vegetables have been associated with decreased risks of carcinomas of virtually all sites within the gastrointestinal and respiratory systems, the uterine cervix, and (less consistently) other tissues. Foods rich in retinol (preformed vitamin A) have also been associated with reduced risks of some epithelial cancers. Levels of many of the potentially protective micronutrients are highly correlated in human diets, making it difficult to determine which micronutrients are most strongly associated with reduced risks, and the specific substances in fruits and vegetables responsible for the apparent protective effects have therefore not been conclusively identified. It is likely that different micronutrients or combinations of micronutrients operate at different sites, and a variety of protective mechanisms have been suggested. For example, the reduced risks of stomach and esophageal carcinomas may be due to inhibition by vitamin C of *N*-nitroso compound formation; vegetables of the *Brassicaceae* family have been hypothesized to induce activity of mixed-function oxidases, which may detoxify ingested carcinogens responsible for colon cancer development; and vitamins C, E, and β-carotene quench free radicals that cause oxidative damage to DNA. Evidence that vitamin B6 may reduce cancer risk was seen in a recent meta-analysis.[184]

Dietary fiber may increase the bulk of the bowel contents, dilute intraluminal carcinogens, and enhance transit time through the gut. These mechanisms would reduce contact of the colonic mucosa with carcinogens and explain the inverse association between dietary fiber and the risk of colon cancer. Certain plant foods also contain phytoestrogens. These weak estrogens may reduce the risk of hormonally mediated cancers by binding competitively to estrogen receptors and thereby exerting antiestrogenic effects. However, more recently, it is becoming apparent that microbiome influence cancer risk. Probiotics and/or prebiotics (fiber that is soluble or fermentable) can increase levels of an endogenous histone deacetylase inhibitor and diminish tumorigenesis.[185]

Although the evidence that a diet high in fruits and vegetables decreases cancer risk has been used as one rationale for marketing vitamin supplements, there is no evidence that such supplements are protective against any neoplasm, and some evidence that they may even be harmful. For example, a number of studies have linked high fruit and vegetable intake, as well as high serum β-carotene levels, with a reduced risk of lung cancer, but clinical trials of β-carotene supplementation in individuals at high risk of lung cancer found *increased* lung cancer rates among supplemented patients.[176] These findings serve as a reminder that our current understanding of the constituents of fruits and vegetables, and their mechanisms of action, is incomplete. Current knowledge suggests that better outcomes are associated with diets lower in meats and animal fats and higher in fiber, fresh fruits, and vegetables, including: citrus fruits with high levels of vitamin C, vegetables of the *Brassicaceae* or Cruciferae family (such as cauliflower, cabbage, garden cress, bok choy, broccoli, brussel sprouts, and similar green leafy vegetables), and vegetables rich in β-carotene (carrots, sweet potatoes, winter squash, spinach, and kale along with fruits like cantaloupe and apricots). Smoked, charred, or cured meats would be avoided or used in moderation, as would alcoholic beverages. This diet would probably reduce the risk of cancers, risks of cardiovascular and cerebrovascular diseases. There is little evidence that supplementation of a prudent diet with vitamins would have a beneficial effect on cancer risk.

Genetic Factors

The study of cancer genetics has exploded in the past decade. The recognition that some families suffer an excess burden of cancer led to the mapping of cancer predisposition genes for the breast/ovarian and Lynch cancer syndromes.[186,187] Hereditary cancer syndromes are now thought to be responsible for 5–10% of cancer[188] and identifying a syndrome changes recommended screening for breast, ovarian,

TABLE 51-4 COMMON FAMILIAL CANCER SYNDROMES

Syndrome	Gene	Cancer
Retinomablastoma	RB	Retinomablastoma, osteoscarcoma
Li-Fraumeni	P53	Breast, sarcoma, leukemia, brain
Familial breast, ovarian cancer syndrome	BRCA1/ BRCA2	Breast, ovary
Ataxia telangiectasia	ATM	Breast
WAGR	WT2/WT1	Wilms' tumor
Familial adenomatious polyposis/Gardner's syndrome	APC	Colon
Hereditary Nonpolyposis Colorectal Cancer (HNPCC)	MSH2, MLH1, pPMS1, -hPMS2	Colon, uterus
Multiple endocrine neoplasia type 1	MEN1	Carcinoids, pancreas, parathyroid, pituitary
Von Hippel-Lindau	VHL	Renal cell carcinoma, hemangioblastoma

colon, renal skin, and endocrine cancers.[189] Work over the past three decades has identified dozens of genes that, when mutated, more than double cancer risk (Table 51-4). These moderately and highly penetrant genes contribute to the more than 50 inherited cancer syndromes.[189] There are many more genes that increase cancer risk only a few percentage points, or that may cause someone to be susceptible to cancer in response to an environmental exposure (Table 51-4). These lower penetrance genes are more difficult to identify, and whether or how to change the care of a patient who carries a mutation in one of them is less clear.[190]

Key characteristics of hereditary cancer syndromes include an earlier age of cancer diagnosis than sporadic cancer, bilateral or multiple primary occurrences of cancer in the same person, and clustering of cancer within a family.[191] Familial retinoblastoma, a classical example of hereditary cancer risk, arises because an individual inherits a germline mutation in one allele of the *Rb* gene, which is then followed by a somatic mutation in the other allele.[192] Somatic mutations at both alleles of the gene are required to cause the more common sporadic cases of retinoblastoma. Children with hereditary *Rb* are often born with eye tumors, while children develop sporadic retinoblastomas by age 3. In contrast, in the *Li-Fraumeni syndrome*, a germline TP53 mutation is associated with a greater incidence of rhabdomyosarcoma, sarcoma, adrenocortical carcinoma, brain tumors, breast cancer, leukemia, or adenocortical carcinomas as either a child or adult.[193] In both cases, Knudson's two hit hypothesis for the genetic cause of cancer is fulfilled.[192] The hereditary nature of the first hit in genetic cancer syndromes explains the earlier-than-typical onset of cancer.

Inherited *BRCA1* and *BRCA2* mutations strongly increase risk of breast and ovarian cancer, although the actual risk is likely lower than early estimates of 80% lifetime risk of breast and 25–60% risk of ovarian cancer.[194] Furthermore, there is significant variability in cancer risk among *BRCA1/2* mutation carriers and other factors can modify the *BRCA1/2* breast cancer risk, including genes at other loci (such as those involved in hormone or carcinogen metabolism), reproductive history, and exogenous exposures such as OCs. Overall, about 1/300 (0.3%) of women in the general population carry a mutation in *BRCA1* or *BRCA2*, but about 3% of women with breast cancer and 10% of women with ovarian cancer have a mutation in one of these genes.[195] There are founder mutations common in some populations. Among healthy women of Ashkenazi Jewish ancestry, 1/40 carries a mutation and 40% of Ashkenazi women with ovarian cancer have a *BRCA1* or *BRCA* mutation.[196,197] Women with *BRCA1/2* gene mutations are screened for cancer differently than women in the general population. They start breast cancer screening in the mid-1920s and add ovarian cancer screening by the 1930s. Medications and surgery can also be used to reduce cancer risk.[198] However, mutations in *BRCA1/2* explain only about half of families with hereditary breast and ovarian cancer, while newly identified genes explain many of the unexplained families. More than 30 additional genes have been implicated in breast or ovarian cancer, and most of these interact with *BRCA1/2* in detecting and repairing damage to DNA.[199] As of 2017, the American National Comprehensive Cancer Network (NCCN) has issued clinical guidelines to change the breast or ovarian cancer prevention care of women with mutations in 17 of those genes,[198] mostly by screening earlier and offering preventive surgery or medication. Additional actionable genes include: *ATM, BRIP1, CDH1, CHEK2, NBN, NF1, PALB2, PTEN, RAD51C, RAD51D, STK11, TP53*, and the mismatch repair genes also responsible for *Lynch syndrom*e (see below).

About 10% of colorectal cancers can be attributed to known heritable germline mutations.[200] Familial adenomatous polyposis (FAP) is an autosomal dominant syndrome presenting with hundreds to thousands of adenomatous colorectal polyps that are caused by mutations in the *APC* gene.[201] Adenomas typically develop in the mid-teens in these patients, and colorectal cancer is almost certain if this condition is untreated. *Lynch syndrome* (hereditary nonpolyposis colorectal cancer [HNPCC]) is an autosomal dominant disorder characterized by early onset of colorectal cancer with microsatellite instability. Mutations in mismatch repair genes (*MLH1, MSH2, PMS1, and PMS2*) cause *Lynch syndrome* and lead to a lifetime colon cancer risk of up to 85% in these individuals, endometrial cancer risk of about 40% for women, and elevation of ovarian, renal and other gastrointestinal organs.[202] Again, there are treatment guidelines for cancer screening and prevention in people with FAP and HNPCC involving early and frequent endoscopic monitoring of the gastrointestinal tract, uterine and ovarian cancer screening, as well as preventative surgery.[203]

Other genes that increase cancer risk and change how a patient is cared for include *WT1* and *WT2*, which are associated with Wilms' tumor, also called nephroblastoma, in children. Only about 2% of children with Wilms' tumor have a family history of this and about 10% is associated with de novo germline *WT1* mutations or epigenetic imprinting effects seen only in the affected child.[204] Those with bilateral tumors generally have a germline mutation of the gene and tumors arise only if a second event occurs with loss of function of the remaining normal allele. Children identified to have a risk of Wilms tumor should receive intensive screening through early childhood.

MEN1 (multiple endocrine neoplasia type 1) syndrome is a hereditary condition caused by mutations in the gene of the same name that is characterized by the presence of neuroendocrine tumors. It is inherited in an autosomal dominant pattern and has a high penetrance characterized by the occurrence of tumors of the parathyroid glands, endocrine pancreas, and anterior pituitary gland.[205] Individuals with Von Hippel Lindau are at risk for the development of tumors of renal carcinoma, as well as cancers of the pancreas, adrenal glands, brain, spine, eye, and ear.[206] Again, there are screening protocols for both disorders to identify tumors at an early treatable stage.

Although only a small proportion of cancers appear to be caused by inherited mutations at single loci, it is increasingly clear that less-penetrant genetic factors also play an important role in tumors. A mutation in a single copy of either *MUTYH or ATM* confer a slightly increased risk of cancer, while having mutations in both copies of either gene causes a person to have a large increase in risk or a different phenotype altogether. People with a single *MUTYH* mutation have a slight increase in colon cancer risk, while people with mutations in both copies have a syndrome often indistinguishable from FAP.[207,208] Similarly, women with a single *ATM* mutation have double the average risk of breast cancer, whereas people with the autosomal recessive syndrome ataxia-telangiectasia have an increased cancer risk but are more easily recognized by neurodegeneration beginning in childhood.[209–211]

Genetic variation can also explain why some individuals exposed to known carcinogens develop cancer; others with similar exposure do not. A number of types of genes could modify risk. First, there are genes involved in the metabolism of environmental carcinogens that can modulate exposure to potentially mutagenic occurrences. One of these groups includes inherited polymorphisms in genes that code for enzymes affecting the ability of the body to metabolize or detoxify carcinogens or potential carcinogens. These include those that code for the glutathione *S*-transferases (GST), cytochrome P-450 enzymes (CYP), and *N*-acetyltransferases (NAT). Some of the presumed high-risk genotypes are highly prevalent and may contribute substantially to the overall cancer risk within populations. Growth regulation effects associated with bioavailable steroid hormones can be modified by several of the CYP inherited genotypes, which may affect those with *BRCA1/2* mutations. Among Caucasians, 40–50% have the glutathione *S*-transferase M1 (*GSTM1*) null genotype, which may confer a 10–50% increased risk of lung and bladder cancer and other tumors.[212,213]

CANCER CONTROL AND PREVENTION

Overview of Known Causes of Cancer

Globally, a new diagnosis of cancer affected an estimated 14.1 million people in 2012 and was responsible for 8.2 million deaths, making it the second leading cause of death.[3] The United States contributed 590,000 deaths to this total.

There is increasing data about preventive factors for cancer. Globally, about one-third of deaths from cancer are due to five leading factors: obesity, low fruit and vegetable intake, lack of physical exercise, tobacco use, and alcohol use. Tobacco use is the most important of these factors, contributing to 22% of cancer deaths.[214] In 2015, four out of five smokers were residing in a low- to middle-income country and increasingly the burden of disease from tobacco is concentrated in these countries.[215]

In the United States, recent reports indicate that more than half of incident cancers could be prevented by applying knowledge we already have.[216,217] Colditz et al. reported a potential reduction in the cancer burden of 55% by applying the preventive knowledge we have to tobacco, obesity, diet, physical inactivity, occupation, viruses, family history, alcohol, reproductive factors, radiation/sunlight, pollution, and prescribed drugs.[216] Among these, tobacco was the most important followed by obesity and physical inactivity (Fig. 51-4).[216] A recent assessment of smoking-attributable cancer deaths in U.S. adults 35 years of age and older found 168,000 deaths could have been averted from cancer in 2011 over many different sites including lung, larynx, esophagus, oral cavity and pharynx, bladder, liver and intrahepatic bile duct, stomach, kidney and renal pelvis, cervix, colorectum, pancreas, and myeloid leukemia.[218] Lung and larynx had the highest attributable percentages (over 75%), but these percentages exceeded 40% of more for esophagus, oral cavity and pharynx, and bladder in both men and women.

Comprehensive Cancer Control

In the United States in 1998, the Centers for Disease Control and Prevention initiated a nationwide comprehensive cancer control (CCC) effort. Comprehensive cancer control was defined as an integrated and coordinated approach to reducing cancer incidence, morbidity and mortality through prevention, early detection, treatment, rehabilitation, and palliation.[219] The CCC approach brought together key partners and organizations to develop a plan in each state and territory to reduce the number of community members with cancer. Cancer researchers and practitioners in federal agencies, public health departments, research centers, medical practices, advocacy groups, and other settings were engaged in an ongoing effort to first develop, and thereafter implement, a comprehensive approach to cancer prevention and control in their geographic areas.[220] As of 2017, all 50 states, the District of Columbia, 6 U.S. Pacific Island jurisdictions and Puerto Rico, and 8 tribes and tribal organizations had produced 63 plans. This nationwide effort emphasizes the implementation of evidence-based cancer prevention and cancer strategies at the community level.

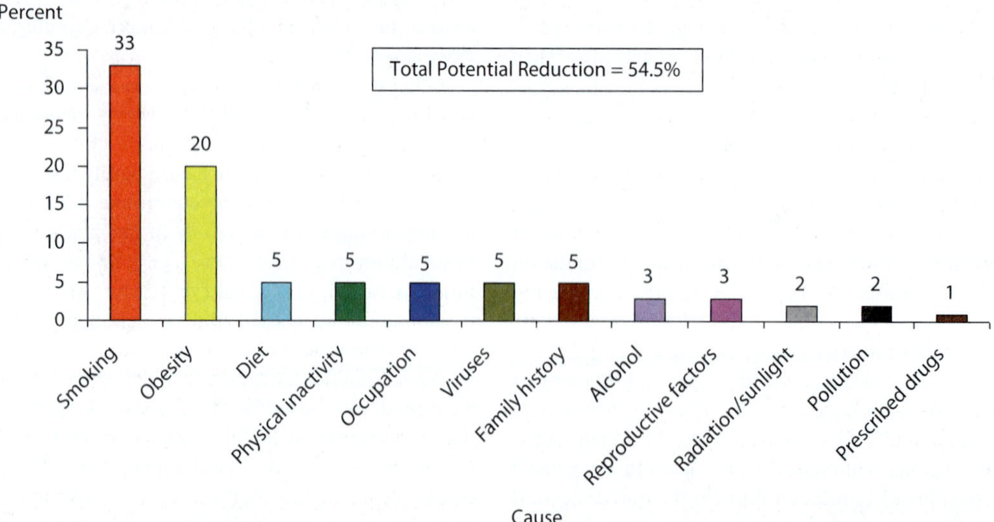

FIGURE 51-4. Potential reduction of cancer burden in United States. (*Source:* Adapted from Colditz GA, Wolin KY, Gehlert S. Applying what we know to accelerate cancer prevention. *Sci Transl Med.* 2012;4.)

In 2010, the CDC established six priorities for its funded CCC programs that include the following[221,222]:

- Emphasizing primary prevention of cancer—stopping cancer before it starts;
- Helping people find cancer early by getting screened as recommended;
- Supporting people who have been diagnosed with cancer through treatment and beyond;
- Helping put policies in place to make sure cancer control measures are there for places that need it most;
- Promoting access to quality healthcare for all people that respects and incorporates cultural traditions, including those in communities with a higher burden of cancer; and
- Evaluating policies and programs to see if they work well.

Goals for Cancer Reduction

The leading health indicators in *Healthy People* 2020 comprise 26 indicators organized under 12 topics.[223] Nine of the 12 topics are highly related to cancer include access to health services; clinical preventive services; environmental quality; nutrition, physical activity, and obesity; oral health; reproductive and sexual health; social determinants; substance abuse; and tobacco. These indicators affect cancer by reducing the number of new cancer cases as well as the illness, disability, and death caused by cancer. Regarding the overall cancer death rate, the objective is a 10% improvement from 179.3 per 100,000 in 2007–09 to 161.4 in 2020. To achieve this, 10% improvements are targeted for death rates for lung, breast, uterine, oropharyngeal, prostate, and melanoma cancers, and a 15% improvement for colorectal cancer.[223]

In 2014, the National Roundtable set a goal to increase colorectal cancer screening rates to 80% by 2018. Achieving this goal would avert 277,000 new cancers and 203,000 CRC deaths from 2013 through 2030.[224]

In 1996, the Board of Directors of the American Cancer Society (ACS) set a goal to reduce cancer mortality by 50% from its peak mortality in 1990 by the year 2015. This goal was not met, but cancer mortality in 2015 was 26% lower than in 1990.[225]

Strategies for Primary Prevention Efforts

Lifestyle choices are major risk factors for cancer. In 2017, the ACS had the following recommendations for individual choices to reduce cancer occurrence and stay healthy[226]:

1. Stay away from tobacco; if you smoke, get help quitting; keep your children tobacco free; create a smoke-free workplace.
2. Drink no more than 1 drink per day for women or 2 per day for men.
3. Eat a healthy diet, with emphasis on plant foods; limit processed meat and red meat; each at least 2.5 cups of vegetables and fruits daily; select whole grain rather than refined grain products; choose foods and drinks that allow for a healthy weight.
4. Be as lean as possible throughout life without being underweight; avoid excess weight gain; limit intake of high-calorie foods and drinks.
5. Be physically active and limit sedentary behavior; for adults, get at least 150 minutes of moderate intensity or 75 minutes of vigorous intensity activity each week; for children and adolescents, get at least one hour of moderate or vigorous intensity activity each day.
6. Be safe in the sun; protect yourself by slipping on a shirt, using sunscreen and applying it properly, wearing a hat, and wearing sunglasses to protect your eyes; seek shade; avoid tanning beds and sun lamps; protect children from the sun.
7. To assist with these recommendations, the ACS recommends public, private, and community organizations work together at the national, state, and local levels to apply policy and environmental changes; these changes need to increase access to affordable, healthy foods in communities, places of work, and schools; decrease access to and marketing of foods and drinks with low nutritional value, particularly to youth; and provide safe, enjoyable, and accessible environments for physical activity in schools and workplaces, and for transportation and recreation in communities.

   For sexually transmitted diseases (STDs) the Centers for Disease Control and Prevention recommend[227]:

8. Educate yourself about STDs and take control; consider abstinence (the most reliable way to avoid infection is not to have sex); get vaccinated for hepatitis B and, if eligible, for HPV; reduce the number of sexual partners; use condoms; practice mutual monogamy (be sexually active with only one person).

   For other carcinogenic substances:

9. Support efforts to reduce exposures to known carcinogens in the workplace. The continuing occurrence of mesothelioma deaths, particularly among younger populations, underscores the need for maintaining efforts to prevent asbestos exposure and for ongoing surveillance to monitor temporal trends.
10. Support efforts to identify and reduce exposures outside the workplace to known carcinogens such as arsenic and asbestos.
11. Mitigate elevated residential radon levels; use radiation prudently for medical use.

Cancer-related Clinical Preventive Services

The United States Preventive Services Task Force (USPSTF) is a volunteer, independent panel of national experts who make evidence-based recommendations about clinical preventive services that address primary and secondary prevention. The USPSTF was created in 1984 and since 1998, the U.S. Congress has authorized that the Agency for Healthcare Research and Quality convene the USPSTF, and provide its members with ongoing scientific, administrative, and dissemination support.

The USPSTF assigns letter grades to their recommendations based on the strength of evidence and the balance of benefits to harms. These recommendations only apply to people who have no signs or symptoms of the disease or condition under consideration, and address only services offered in the primary-care setting or services referred by a primary-care provider. The USPSTF does not consider the costs of a preventive service when determining a recommendation grade. The grade definitions are as follows[228]:

- Grade A—USPSTF recommends the service. There is high certainty that the net benefit is substantial.
- Grade B—USPSTF recommends the service. There is high certainty that the net benefit is moderate or there is moderate certainty that the net benefit is moderate to substantial.
- Grade C—USPSTF recommends selectively offering or providing this service to individual patients based on professional judgment and patient preferences. There is at least moderate certainty that the net benefit is small.
- Grade D—USPSTF recommends against this service. There is moderate to high certainty that the service has no net benefit or that harms outweigh the benefits.
- Grade I—USPSTF concludes that the current evidence is insufficient to assess the balance of benefits and harms of the service.

Primary Preventive Services

As of December 2017, the cancer-related primary prevention services that the USPSTF recommends with a grade of A or B including the following[228]:

- Alcohol misuse screening and behavioral counseling;
- Sexually transmitted diseases counseling;
- Skin cancer counseling;
- Tobacco use counselling and intervention;

- Breast cancer: medications for risk reduction;
- Obesity screening;
- BRCA-related cancer in women screening;
- Hepatitis B and C screening; and
- HIV infection screening.

The USPSTF defers to the CDC's Advisory Committee for Immunization Practices (ACIP) for recommendations regarding cancer-related vaccinations. In 2017, these vaccines included hepatitis B and HPV.[229] The USPSTF and ACIP recommendations address several of the major risk factors for cancer.

The American Academy of Family Physicians (AAFP) has a Commission on Health and Public Science (CHPS) that reviews recommendations released by the USPSTF and makes recommendations to AAFP Board of Directors. In their July 2017 recommendations the AAFP gave a grade of A or B (analogous to the USPSTF grading scheme) to each of the cancer-related primary prevention services that the USPSTF recommended.[230] This is typical as the AAFP usually agrees with the USPSTF. Similarly, the American Academy of Pediatrics has recommendations for preventive pediatric healthcare that cover infancy through adolescence, and includes cancer-related recommendations for alcohol, smoking, BMI, HIV, cervical dysplasia, and immunizations/vaccines.[231]

Secondary Preventive Services

Secondary preventive services involve cancer screening. Again, more detail can be found in Chapter 50: Screening for Early and Asymptomatic Conditions.

In 2012 under the Affordable Care Act, a USPSTF screening recommendation grade of A or B required that commercial payers both cover and pay for the screening. As of 2017, the USPSTF recommended screening with a grade of A or B for female breast cancer, cervical cancer, colorectal cancer, and lung cancer.[232] In addition, USPSTF screening guidelines were under review for cervix, ovary, pancreas, and prostate cancers. The USPSTF approach to making recommendations regarding cancer screening is displayed in Fig. 51-5, using pancreatic cancer as an example. Answers to several key questions are sought.

Many professional organizations have evidence-based recommendations about the use of cancer screening tests. These include the American Cancer Society,[233] the National Comprehensive Cancer Network,[234] and the American College of Physicians,[235] among others. These organizations generally agree with the USPFTF recommendations, but can vary on some details. The USPFTF recommendations will be used herein as an example.

Breast Cancer Screening

Breast cancer is the most commonly diagnosed nonskin cancer in women in the United States. In 2017 for breast cancer screening, the USPSTF[236] gave a grade B recommendation for screening mammography every other year for women aged 50–74 years. For women aged 40–49 years the grade recommendation was C, meaning that women who placed a higher value on the potential benefit than the potential harms could choose to begin every other year screening between the age of 40 and 49 years. The USPSTF considers the evidence insufficient (Grade of I) to recommend screening mammography for women aged 75 years and older, or among all women to assess the benefits and harms of digital breast tomosynthesis (DBT) as a primary breast cancer screening method. The USPSTF also considers the evidence insufficient to recommend additional screening for women with dense breast tissue who, after a negative screening mammogram, receive breast ultrasonography, magnetic resonance imaging, DBT, or other methods.

These recommendations apply to asymptomatic women aged 40 years and older who do not have a pre-existing breast cancer or a previously diagnosed breast lesion, and who are not at high risk for breast cancer because of a known underlying genetic mutation or a history of chest radiation at a young age.

Cervical Cancer Screening

In 2017 for cervical cancer screening, the USPSTF[236] gave a grade A recommendation for cervical cancer screening in women ages 21–65

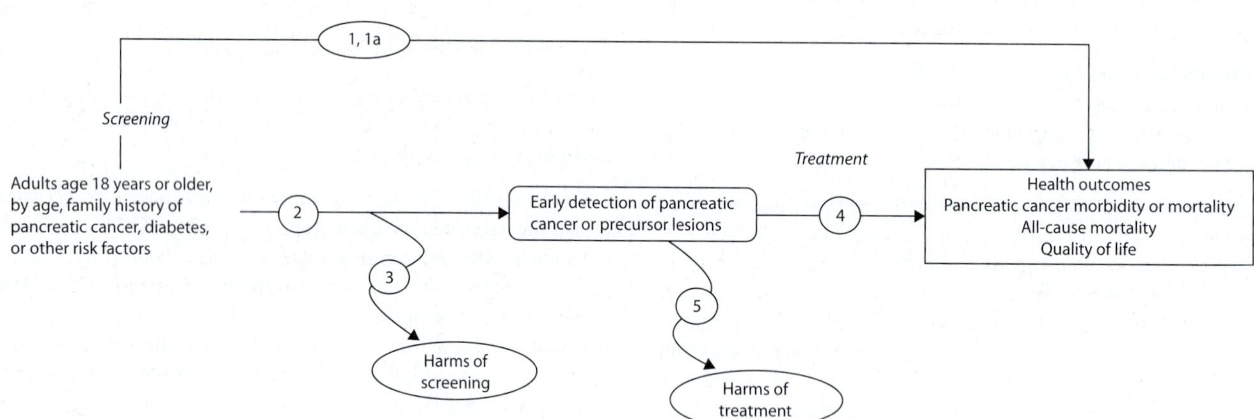

1. Does screening for pancreatic adenocarcinoma improve cancer morbidity or mortality or all-cause mortality?
    a. Does screening effectiveness vary by clinically relevant subpopulations (e.g., by age group, family history of pancreatic cancer, personal history of new-onset diabetes, or other risk factors)?
2. What is the diagnostic accuracy of screening tests for pancreatic adenocarcinoma?
3. What are the harms of screening for pancreatic adenocarcinoma?
4. Does treatment of screen-detected or asymptomatic pancreatic adenocarcinoma improve cancer mortality, all-cause mortality, or quality of life?
5. What are the harms of treatment of screen-detected pancreatic adenocarcinoma?

FIGURE 51-5. United States Preventive Services Task Force (USPSTF) view of screening: Pancreatic cancer as example. (*Source:* Reproduced with permission from .S. Preventive Services Task Force. Pancreatic Cancer: Screening. September 2017. Retrieved from https://www.uspreventiveservicestaskforce.org/usptsf/document/draft-research-plan/pancreatic-cancer-screening..)

years via the Pap smear (cytology) every 3 years or, for women age 30–65 years who want to lengthen the screening interval, screening with a combination of cytology and HPV testing every 5 years. The USPSTF recommends against screening (Grade of D) for cervical cancer with HPV testing, alone or in combination with cytology, in women younger than age 30 years; and recommends against screening in (1) for women younger than age 21 years; (2) in women older than 65 years who have had adequate prior screening and are not otherwise at high risk of cervical cancer; and (3) in women who have had a hysterectomy with removal of the cervix, and who do not have a history of a high-grade precancerous lesion or cervical cancer.

These recommendations do not apply to women who have received a diagnosis of a high-grade precancerous cervical lesion or cervical cancer, women with in utero exposure to diethyl-stilbestrol, or women who are immunocompromised (such as women with an HIV diagnosis). In 2017, the USPSTF had a draft recommendation statement to modify the grade A recommendation "for cervical cancer screening in women age 21–65 years via the Pap smear (cytology) every 3 years" to "screening for cervical cancer every 3 years with cervical cytology alone in women ages 21–29 years."[237]

Colorectal Cancer Screening

Colorectal cancer is the third most commonly diagnosed nonskin cancer in the United States and the second leading cause of cancer mortality. In 2016, the USPSTF updated their recommendations for colorectal cancer screening[238] and recommended screening beginning at age 50 years and continuing until age 75 years with a Grade of A. They gave a grade of C for screening adults aged 76–85 years, stating this should be an individual decision that accounts for the patient's prior screening history and overall health. The USPSTF acknowledged there are several tests available for colorectal cancer screening. These included stool-based tests (guaiac-based fecal occult blood test (gFOBT, fecal immunochemical test (FIT), and FIT-DNA), direct visualization tests (flexible sigmoidoscopy alone or in combination with FIT, colonoscopy, and CT-directed colonography), and serology tests such as SEPT9 methylated DNA test. In a review of these tests,[120] the USPSTF found that use of any of these tests is better than not being screened at all. They recommended the conduct of more research to determine the relative benefits and harms of each test.

Lung Cancer Screening

Lung cancer is the leading cause of cancer mortality in the United States. In 2013, the USPSFT updated their lung cancer screening recommendation.[239] They recommended annual screening with low-dose computed tomography (LDCT) in adults aged 55–80 years who have a 30 pack-year smoking history and currently smoke or have quit within the past 15 years. Their assigned grade was B. This recommendation updated their 2004 recommendation, in which they concluded that the evidence was insufficient to recommend for or against screening for lung cancer in asymptomatic persons with LDCT, chest radiography, sputum cytologic evaluation, or a combination of these tests. The primary reason for the updated recommendation was findings from the National Lung Screening Trial, a well-conducted, controlled clinical trial.[240] The USPSTF continued to acknowledge that smoking cessation remained the most important intervention to decrease lung cancer incidence and mortality.

Prostate Cancer Screening

Prostate cancer is the most commonly diagnosed nonskin cancer in men in the United States. In 2008, the USPSTF found insufficient evidence (Grade of I) that PSA testing for prostate cancer improved health outcomes for men younger than 75 years.[15] They recommended against screening for prostate cancer in men 75 years and older (Grade of D). In 2012, recent research studies were reviewed and the USPSTF updated their recommendation against PSA testing for prostate cancer screening to include men of all ages.[241] This recommendation was met with considerable controversy, but did result in decreased PSA testing, although this widely varied between states.[242] In 2017, the USPSTF has again reviewed the recent evidence and has produced a draft recommendation that clinicians inform men ages 55–69 years about the potential benefits and harms of PSA testing for prostate cancer screening. The Grade was C indicating that the decision about PSA testing should be an individual decision. In the draft recommendation, the USPSTF continued to recommend against PSA screening in men 70 years and older (Grade of D).[243]

Screening for Other Cancers

As of 2017, the research data the USPSTF has reviewed for oral, skin, and bladder cancers are insufficient (Grade of I) to recommend for or against screening. The USPSTF recommends against screening (Grade of D) for ovarian, pancreatic, testicular, and thyroid cancers.[244] The recommendations for ovarian and pancreatic cancers are currently under review.

Evidence-based Initiatives for Cancer Prevention and Control at the Population Level

Although cancer prevention and control rely on multiple individual behaviors, it is important to consider the programs and policies that facilitate these behaviors. Two initiatives that collect information on evidence programs are: *The Guide to Community Preventive Services: What Works to Promote Health?* (https://www.thecommunityguide.org/), which provides systematic reviews of selected population-based interventions, and the Cancer Control P.L.A.N.E.T. (https://cancercontrolplanet.cancer.gov/planet/), which provides data and resources to program staff, public health officials, and researchers to design, implement, and evaluate evidence-based programs. The National Comprehensive Cancer Control Program also provides plans that are specific to states and are based on data collected about people living there. These plans provide strategies that are anticipated to work and create a plan for action for them.

Cancer Survivorship

There are more than 15.5 million invasive cancer survivors in the United States as of January 1, 2016. This number is expected to rise to 20.3 million by January 1, 2026.[245] The CDC and the LIVESTRONG Foundation are leading a public health effort to address the issues faced by this growing number of cancer survivors, and developed A National Action Plan for Cancer Survivorship: Advancing Public Health Strategies.[246]

Cancer survivors face physical, psychological, social, spiritual, and financial issues. These can be present at diagnosis, during treatment, and thereafter. The National Action Plan emphasizes collaborative, community-based activities that can reduce the burden of cancer on survivors. Goals of this plan for cancer survivors include the following: (1) preventing secondary cancers and the recurrence of cancer whenever possible; (2) promoting appropriate disease management following diagnosis and treatment to better ensure a maximum number of years of healthy life; (3) minimizing preventable pain, disability, and psychosocial distress; and (4) assisting in accessing family, peer, community support, and other resources to better cope with their cancer.

The primary outcome of this plan has been to establish a greater awareness of the issues cancer survivors face and to get organizations to take action. The CDC's National Comprehensive Cancer Control Program is an example of an organization that is addressing cancer survivorship goals of the National Action Plan with one of its six priorities addressing people who have been diagnosed with cancer through treatment and beyond. As another example, the American Society of Clinical Oncology (ASCO) has provided clinical practice guidelines for fatigue[247] and chronic pain,[248] two common physical symptoms of the cancer survivor. Palliative care, another important issue for the cancer survivor, has also been given attention.[249] ASCO has also endorsed the ACS survivorship care guidelines for prostate cancer[250] and for head and neck cancer.[251] These types of action are essential to improving the lives of cancer survivors and their loved ones, a rapidly growing segment of the population.

References

1. World Health Organization. International J Cancer Statistical Classification of Diseases and Related Health Problems. 10th ed. Geneva: World Health Organization; 1992.
2. World Health Organization. International Classification of Diseases for Oncology: ICD-O. 3rd ed. Geneva: World Health Organization; 2000.
3. Ferlay J, Steliarova-Foucher E, Lortet-Tieulent J, et al. Cancer incidence and mortality patterns in Europe: Estimates for 40 countries in 2012. *Eur J Cancer*. 2013;49(6):1374–403.
4. Howlader N, Noone AM, Krapcho M, et al. *SEER Cancer Statistics Review, 1975–2014*. Bethesda, MD: National Cancer Institute; 2017.
5. Jemal A, Ward EM, Johnson CJ, et al. Annual Report to the Nation on the Status of Cancer, 1975–2014, featuring survival. *J Natl Cancer Inst*. 2017;109(9):djx030.
6. U.S. Cancer Statistics Working Group. *United States Cancer Statistics: 1999-2014 Incidence and Mortality Web-based Report*. Atlanta: U.S. Department of Health and Human Services, Centers for Disease Control and Prevention, National Cancer Institute; 2017.
7. Cancer incidence in five continents. *IARC Sci Publ*. 2002;(155):1–781.
8. Bleyer A, O'Leary M, Barr R, et al. *Cancer Epidemiology in Older Adolescents and Young Adults 15 to 29 Years of Age: Including Seer Incidence and Survival, 1975–2000*. Bethesda, MD: National Cancer Institute; 2006.
9. Pinheiro PS, Morris CR, Liu L, et al. The impact of follow-up type and missed deaths on population-based cancer survival studies of Hispanics and Asians. *JNCI Monographs*. 2014:210–7.
10. Siegel RL, Miller KD, Jemal A. Cancer Statistics, 2017. *CA Cancer J Clin*. 2017;67(1):7–30.
11. NAACCR. Fast Stats: An interactive tool for quick access to key NAACCR cancer statistics. North American Association of Central Cancer Registries; 2017. www.naaccr.org. Accessed 11-1-2017 2017.
12. National Center for Health Statistics (US). *Health, United States, 2016: With Chartbook on Long-term Trends in Health*. Hyattsville, MD: National Center for Health Statistics; 2017.
13. National Cancer Institute. Cancer Trends Progress Report. Bethesda, MD: National Cancer Institute, National Institute of Health. Department of Health and Human Services; 2017.
14. Fitzmaurice C, Collaboration G, Allen C, et al. Global, regional, and national cancer incidence, mortality, years of life lost, years lived with disability, and disability-adjusted life-years for 32 cancer groups, 1990 to 2015: A systematic analysis for the global burden of disease study. *JAMA Oncol*. 2017;3(4):524–48.
15. U.S. Preventive Services Task Force. Screening for prostate cancer: U.S. Preventive Services Task Force recommendation statement. *Ann Intern Med*. 2008;149(3):185–91.
16. Berry DA, Cronin KA, Plevritis SK, et al. Effect of screening and adjuvant therapy on mortality from breast cancer. *N Engl J Med*. 2005;353(17):1784–92.
17. Plummer M, de Martel C, Vignat J, et al. Global burden of cancers attributable to infections in 2012: A synthetic analysis. *Lancet Global Health*. 2016;4(9):E609–16.
18. Parkin DM. The global health burden of infection-associated cancers in the year 2002. *Int J Cancer*. 2006;118(12):3030–44.
19. Bauer KR, Brown M, Cress RD, et al. Descriptive analysis of estrogen receptor (ER)negative, progesterone receptor (PR)-negative, and HER2-negative invasive breast cancer, the so-called triple-negative phenotype—A population-based study from the California Cancer Registry. *Cancer*. 2007;109(9):1721–8.
20. Parise CA, Bauer KR, Caggiano V. Disparities in receipt of adjuvant radiation therapy after breast-conserving surgery among the cancer-reporting regions of California. *Cancer*. 2012;118(9):2516–24.
21. Carey LA, Perou CM, Livasy CA, et al. Race, breast cancer subtypes, and survival in the Carolina Breast Cancer Study. *JAMA*. 2006;295(21):2492–502.
22. Nowell PC. The clonal evolution of tumor cell populations. *Science*. 1976;194(4260):23–8.
23. Chen YC, Hunter DJ. Molecular epidemiology of cancer. *CA Cancer J Clin*. 2005;55(1):45–54.
24. Schottenfeld D, Beebe-Dimmer JL, Buffler PA, et al. Current perspective on the global and United States cancer burden attributable to lifestyle and environmental risk factors. *Annu Rev Public Health*. 2013;34 (34):97–117.
25. Danaei G, Vander Hoorn S, Lopez AD, et al. Causes of cancer in the world: Comparative risk assessment of nine behavioural and environmental risk factors. *Lancet*. 2005;366(9499):1784–93.
26. Whiteman DC, Wilson LF. The fractions of cancer attributable to modifiable factors: A global review. *Cancer Epidemiol*. 2016;44:203–21.
27. Lee YC, Hashibe M. Tobacco, alcohol, and cancer in low and high income countries. *Ann Glob Health*. 2014;80(5):378–83.
28. United States Advisory Committee to the Surgeon General, United States. Public Health Service. The health consequences of using smokeless tobacco: a report of the Advisory Committee to the Surgeon General. Bethesda, MD: U.S. Dept. of Health and Human Services, Public Health Service; 1986.
29. Allen JG, Flanigan SS, LeBlanc M, et al. Flavoring chemicals in e-cigarettes: Diacetyl, 2,3-pentanedione, and acetoin in a sample of 51 products, including fruit-, candy-, and cocktail-flavored e-cigarettes. *Environ Health Perspect*. 2016;124(6):733–9.
30. U.S. Department of Health and Human Services. E-Cigarette Use Among youth and Young Adults, A Report of the Surgeon General. Atlanta, GA: US Department of Health and Human Services, Centers for Disease Control and Prevention, National Center for Chronic Disease Prevention and Health Promotion, Office on Smoking and Health; 2016.
31. Chatham-Stephens K, Law R, Taylor E, et al. Notes from the field: Calls to poison centers for exposures to electronic cigarettes—United States, September 2010–February 2014. *MMWR*. 2014;63(13):292–3.
32. Malhotra J, Praud D, Boffetta P. Changes in the trend of alcohol-related cancers: Perspectives on statistical trends. *Chem Res Toxicol*. 2015;28(9):1661–5.
33. Roswall N, Weiderpass E. Alcohol as a risk factor for cancer: Existing evidence in a global perspective. *J Prev Med Public Health*. 2015;48(1): 1–9.
34. Nelson DE, Jarman DW, Rehm J, et al. Alcohol-attributable cancer deaths and years of potential life lost in the United States. *Am J Public Health*. 2013;103(4):641–8.
35. Welzel TM, Graubard BI, Quraishi S, et al. Population-attributable fractions of risk factors for hepatocellular carcinoma in the United States. *Am J Gastroenterol*. 2013;108(8):1314–21.
36. Kiadaliri AA, Jarl J, Gavriilidis G, et al. Alcohol drinking cessation and the risk of laryngeal and pharyngeal cancers: A systematic review and meta-analysis. *PLoS One*. 2013;8(3):e58158.
37. IARC Working Group on the Evaluation of Carcinogenic Risks to Humans. Formaldehyde, 2-butoxyethanol and 1-tert-butoxy-2-propanol. *IARC Monogr Eval Carcinog Risks Hum*. 2006;88:1–478.
38. IARC. Chromium, nickel and welding. *IARC Monogr Eval Carcinog Risks Hum*. 1990;49:1–648.
39. IARC. Occupational exposures to mists and vapours from strong inorganic acids and other industrial chemicals. Working Group views and expert opinions, Lyon, 15–22 October 1991. *IARC Monogr Eval Carcinog Risks Hum*. 1992;54:1–310.
40. IARC. Overall evaluations of carcinogenicity: an updating of IARC Monographs volumes 1 to 42. *IARC Monogr Eval Carcinog Risks Hum Suppl*. 1987;7:1–440.
41. IARC. Some organic solvents, resin monomers and related compounds, pigments and occupational exposures in paint manufacture and painting. *IARC Monogr Eval Carcinog Risks Hum*. 1989:1–442.
42. Peto J. Cancer epidemiology in the last century and the next decade. *Nature*. 2001;411(6835):390–5.
43. Doll R, Peto R. The causes of cancer: quantitative estimates of avoidable risks of cancer in the United States today. *J Natl Cancer Inst*. 1981;66(6):1191–308.
44. Doll R. Epidemiological evidence of the effects of behaviour and the environment on the risk of human cancer. *Recent Results Cancer Res*. 1998;154:3–21.
45. Cohen AJ. Outdoor air pollution and lung cancer. *Environ Health Perspect*. 2000;108:743–50.
46. Vineis P, Forastiere F, Hoek G, et al. Outdoor air pollution and lung cancer: Recent epidemiologic evidence. *Int J Cancer*. 2004;111(5):647–52.
47. Boice J, Land C, Preston D. Ionizing radiation. In: Schottenfeld D, Fraumeni J, eds.Schottenfeld D, Fraumeni J, eds. *Cancer Epidemiology and Prevention*. New York: Oxford University Press; 1996, p. 319–54.
48. IARC. IARC Working group on the evaluation of carcinogenic risks to humans: Ionizing radiation, Part I, X- and gamma- radiation and neutrons. Lyon, France, 26 May–2 June, 1999. *IARC Monogr Eval Carcinog Risks Hum*, 2000;75 Pt 1(PT 1):1–448.
49. IARC. Ionizing radiation, part 2: Some internally deposited radionuclides. Views and expert opinions of an IARC working group on the evaluation of carcinogenic risks to humans. Lyon, 14–21 June, 2000. IARC Monogr Eval Carcinog Risks Hum, 2001;78(Pt 2):1–559.

50. Krewski D, Lubin JH, Zielinski JM, et al. A combined analysis of North American case-control studies of residential radon and lung cancer. *J Toxicol Environ Health-Part a-Current Issues*. 2006;69(7–8):533–97.
51. Darby S, Hill D, Deo H, et al. Residential radon and lung cancer—Detailed results of a collaborative analysis of individual data on 7148 persons with lung cancer and 14208 persons without lung cancer from 13 epidemiologic studies in Europe. *Scand J Work Environ Health*. 2006;32 Suppl 1:1–83.
52. National Research Council (U.S.). *Committee on Health Risks of Exposure to Radon. Health Effects of Exposure to Radon*. Washington, DC: National Academy Press; 1999.
53. UNSCEAR. The United Nations Scientific Committee on the Effects of Atomic Radiation. *Health Phys*. 2000;79(3):314.
54. Robertson A, Allen J, Laney R, et al. The cellular and molecular carcinogenic effects of radon exposure: A review. *Int J Mol Sci*. 2013;14(7):14024–63.
55. WHO. WHO Handbook on Indoor Radon: A Public Health Perspective. Geneva: World Health Organization; 2009.
56. Kim SH, Hwang WJ, Cho JS, et al. Attributable risk of lung cancer deaths due to indoor radon exposure. *Ann Occup Environ Med*. 2016;28:8.
57. EPA. *EPA Assessment of Risks from Radon in Homes*. Washington, DC: U.S. Environmental Protection Agency, Office of Radiation and Indoor Air; 2003.
58. Bluethmann SM, Mariotto AB, Rowland JH. Anticipating the "Silver Tsunami": prevalence trajectories and comorbidity burden among older cancer survivors in the United States. *Cancer Epidemiol Biomarkers Prev*. 2016;25(7):1029–36.
59. Travis LB, Rabkin CS, Brown LM, et al. Cancer survivorship—Genetic susceptibility and second primary cancers: Research strategies and recommendations. *J Natl Cancer Inst*. 2006;98(1):15–25.
60. Van Leeuwen FE, Travis LB. Second cancers. In: DeVita VT, Hellman S, Rosenberg SA, et al., eds.DeVita VT, Hellman S, Rosenberg SA, et al., eds. *Cancer, Principles & Practice of Oncology*. Philadelphia, PA: Lippincott Williams & Wilkins; 2001, pp. 2939–64.
61. Brenner DJ, Hall EJ. Current concepts—Computed tomography—An increasing source of radiation exposure. *N Engl J Med*. 2007;357(22):2277–84.
62. Brenner DJ, Doll R, Goodhead DT, et al. Cancer risks attributable to low doses of ionizing radiation: Assessing what we really know. *Proc Natl Acad Sci U S A*. 2003;100(24):13761–6.
63. U.S. Department of Health and Human Services. *The Surgeon General's Call to Action to Prevent Skin Cancer*. Washington, DC: U.S. Dept of Health and Human Services, Office of the Surgeon General; 2014.
64. Armstrong BK. Epidemiology of malignant melanoma: Intermittent or total accumulated exposure to the sun? *J Dermatol Surg Oncol*. 1988;14(8):835–49.
65. Armstrong BK, Kricker A, English DR. Sun exposure and skin cancer. *Australas J Dermatol*. 1997;38 Suppl 1:S1–6.
66. Wester U, Boldemann C, Jansson B, et al. Population UV-dose and skin area—Do sunbeds rival the sun? *Health Phys*. 1999;77(4):436–40.
67. Dennis LK, Vanbeek MJ, Beane Freeman LE, et al. Sunburns and risk of cutaneous melanoma: Does age matter? A comprehensive meta-analysis. *Ann Epidemiol*. 2008;18(8):614–27.
68. (WHO) WHO. Asbestosis: elimination of asbestos-related diseases. Fact sheet No. 343. 2014.
69. Mazurek JM, Syamlal G, Wood JM, et al. Malignant mesothelioma mortality—United States, 1999–2015. *MMWR*. 2017;66(8):14–8.
70. Feychting M, Ahlbom A, Kheifets L. EMF and health. *Annu Rev Public Health*. 2005;26:165–89.
71. Ahlbom A, Cardis E, Green A, et al. Review of the epidemiologic literature on EMF and health. *Environ Health Perspect*. 2001;109:911–33.
72. Baan R, Grosse Y, Lauby-Secretan B, et al. Carcinogenicity of radiofrequency electromagnetic fields. *Lancet Oncol*. 2011;12(7):624–6.
73. Washburn EP, Orza MJ, Berlin JA, et al. Residential proximity to electricity transmission and distribution equipment and risk of childhood leukemia, childhood lymphoma, and childhood nervous system tumors: Systematic review, evaluation, and meta-analysis. *Cancer Causes Control*. 1994;5(4):299–309.
74. Heath CW, Jr. Electromagnetic field exposure and cancer: A review of epidemiologic evidence. *CA Cancer J Clin*. 1996;46(1):29–44.
75. Bortkiewicz A, Gadzicka E, Szymczak W. Mobile phone use and risk for intracranial tumors and salivary gland tumors—A meta-analysis. *Int J Occup Med Environ Health*. 2017;30(1):27–43.
76. Yang M, Guo WW, Yang CS, et al. Mobile phone use and glioma risk: A systematic review and meta-analysis. *PLoS One*. 2017;12(5):e0175136.
77. Carlberg M, Hardell L. Evaluation of mobile phone and cordless phone use and glioma risk using the Bradford Hill viewpoints from 1965 on association or causation. *Biomed Research Int*. 2017;2017:9218486.
78. Colton T, Greenberg ER, Noller K, et al. Breast cancer in mothers prescribed diethylstilbestrol in pregnancy. Further follow-up. *JAMA*. 1993;269(16):2096–100.
79. Vessey MP, Fairweather DVI, Normansmith B, et al. A randomized double-blind controlled trial of the value of stilbestrol therapy in pregnancy—Long-term follow-up of mothers and their offspring. *Br J Obstet Gynaecol*. 1983;90(11):1007–17.
80. Greenberg ER, Barnes AB, Resseguie L, et al. Breast-cancer in mothers given diethylstilbestrol in pregnancy. *N Engl J Med*. 1984;311(22):1393–8.
81. Collaborative Group on Hormonal Factors in Breast Cancer. Breast cancer and hormonal contraceptives: Collaborative reanalysis of individual data on 53 297 women with breast cancer and 100 239 women without breast cancer from 54 epidemiological studies. Collaborative Group on Hormonal Factors in Breast Cancer. *Lancet*. 1996;347(9017):1713–27.
82. Morch LS, Skovlund CW, Hannaford PC, et al. Contemporary hormonal contraception and the risk of breast cancer. *N Engl J Med*. 2017;377(23):2228–39.
83. Skegg DC, Noonan EA, Paul C, et al. Depot medroxyprogesterone acetate and breast cancer. A pooled analysis of the World Health Organization and New Zealand studies. *JAMA*. 1995;273(10):799–804.
84. Bethea TN, Rosenberg L, Hong CC, et al. A case-control analysis of oral contraceptive use and breast cancer subtypes in the African American Breast Cancer Epidemiology and Risk Consortium. *Breast Cancer Res*. 2015;17:13.
85. Nelson HD. Assessing benefits and harms of hormone replacement therapy—Clinical applications. *JAMA*. 2002;288(7):882–4.
86. Ewertz M. Hormone therapy in the menopause and breast cancer risk—A review. *Maturitas*. 1996;23(2):241–6.
87. Collaborative Group on Hormonal Factors in Breast Cancer. Breast cancer and hormone replacement therapy: Collaborative reanalysis of data from 51 epidemiological studies of 52,705 women with breast cancer and 108,411 women without breast cancer. Collaborative Group on Hormonal Factors in Breast Cancer. *Lancet*. 1997;350(9084):1047–59.
88. Chlebowski RT, Hendrix SL, Langer RD, et al. Influence of estrogen plus progestin on breast, cancer and mammography in healthy postmenopausal women—The Women's Health Initiative Randomized trial. *JAMA*. 2003;289(24):3243–53.
89. Dumeaux V, Fournier A, Lund E, et al. Previous oral contraceptive use and breast cancer risk according to hormone replacement therapy use among postmenopausal women. *Cancer Causes Control*. 2005;16(5):537–44.
90. Shantakumar S, Terry MB, Paykin A, et al. Age and menopausal effects of hormonal birth control and hormone replacement therapy in relation to breast cancer risk. *Am J Epidemiol*. 2007;165(10):1187–98.
91. Brinton LA, Richesson D, Leitzmann MF, et al. Menopausal hormone therapy and breast cancer risk in the NIH-AARP diet and health study cohort. *Cancer Epidemiol Biomarkers Prev*. 2008;17(11):3150–60.
92. Pan HC, Gray R, Braybrooke J, et al. 20-Year risks of breast-cancer recurrence after stopping endocrine therapy at 5 years. *N Engl J Med*. 2017;377(19):1836–46.
93. Toniolo PG, Levitz M, Zeleniuchjacquotte A, et al. A prospective-study of endogenous estrogens and breast-cancer in postmenopausal women. *J Natl Cancer Inst*. 1995;87(3):190–7.
94. Key TJ, Appleby PN, Reeves GK, et al. Body mass index, serum sex hormones, and breast cancer risk in postmenopausal women. *J Natl Cancer Inst*. 2003;95(16):1218–26.
95. Dorgan JF, Longcope C, Franz C, et al. Endogenous sex hormones and breast cancer in postmenopausal women: Reanalysis of nine prospective studies. *J Natl Cancer Inst*. 2002;94(8):606–16.
96. Colditz GA. Relationship between estrogen levels, use of hormone replacement therapy, and breast cancer. *J Natl Cancer Inst*. 1998;90(11):814–23.
97. Cook L, Weiss N, Doherty J. Endometrial cancer. In: Schottenfeld D, Fraumeni J, eds.Schottenfeld D, Fraumeni J, eds. *Cancer Epidemiology and Prevention*. New York: Oxford University Press; 2006.
98. Weiss N. Epidemiology of endometrial cancer. In: Lilienfeld A, ed. *Reviews in Epidemiology*. New York: Elsevier; 1983.
99. Prentice RL, Thomas DB. On the epidemiology of oral contraceptives and disease. *Adv Cancer Res*. 1987;49:285–401.
100. WHO. Depot-medroxyprogesterone acetate (DMPA) and risk of endometrial cancer. The WHO Collaborative Study of Neoplasia and Steroid Contraceptives. *Int J Cancer*. 1991; 49(2):186–90.

101. Curtis RE, Boice JD, Jr., Shriner DA, et al. Second cancers after adjuvant tamoxifen therapy for breast cancer. *J Natl Cancer Inst.* 1996;88(12):832–4.
102. Kaaks R, Lukanova A, Kurzer MS. Obesity, endogenous hormones, and endometrial cancer risk: A synthetic review. *Cancer Epidemiol Biomarkers Prev.* 2002;11(12):1531–43.
103. Zeleniuch-Jacquotte A, Akhmedkhanov A, Kato I, et al. Postmenopausal endogenous oestrogens and risk of endometrial cancer: Results of a prospective study. *Br J Cancer.* 2001;84(7):975–81.
104. Riman T, Nilsson S, Persson I. Review of epidemiological evidence for reproductive and hormonal factors in relation to the risk of epithelial ovarian malignancies—Reply. *Acta Obstet Gynecol Scand.* 2005;84(10):1024–5.
105. Modan B, Hartge P, Hirsh-Yechezkel G, et al. Parity, oral contraceptives, and the risk of ovarian cancer among carriers and noncarriers of a BRCA1 or BRCA2 mutation. *N Engl J Med.* 2001;345(4):235–40.
106. Narod SA, Risch H, Moslehi R, et al. Oral contraceptives and the risk of hereditary ovarian cancer. *N Engl J Med.* 1998;339(7):424–8.
107. Garg PP, Kerlikowske K, Subak L, et al. Hormone replacement therapy and the risk of epithelial ovarian carcinoma: A meta-analysis. *Obstet Gynecol.* 1998;92(3):472–9.
108. Trabert B, Wentzensen N, Yang HP, et al. Ovarian cancer and menopausal hormone therapy in the NIH-AARP diet and health study. *Br J Cancer.* 2012;107(7):1181–7.
109. Santen RJ, Allred DC, Ardoin SP, et al. Postmenopausal hormone therapy: An endocrine society scientific statement. *J Clin Endocrinol Metab.* 2010;95(7 Supple 1):s1–66.
110. Lacey JV, Mink PJ, Lubin JH, et al. Menopausal hormone replacement therapy and risk of ovarian cancer. *JAMA.* 2002;288(3):334–41.
111. Lukanova A, Lundin E, Toniolo P, et al. Circulating levels of insulin-like growth factor-I and risk of ovarian cancer. *Int J Cancer.* 2002;101(6):549–54.
112. Lacey JV, Brinton LA, Barnes WA, et al. Use of hormone replacement therapy and adenocarcinomas and squamous cell carcinomas of the uterine cervix. *Gynecol Oncol.* 2000;77(1):149–54.
113. Smith EM, Ritchie JM, Levy BT, et al. Prevalence and persistence of human papillomavirus in postmenopausal age women. *Cancer Detect Prev.* 2003;27(6):472–80.
114. Herbst AL, Ulfelder H, Poskanzer DC. Adenocarcinoma of the vagina. Association of maternal stilbestrol therapy with tumor appearance in young women. *N Engl J Med.* 1971;284(15):878–81.
115. Melnick S, Cole P, Anderson D, et al. Rates and risks of diethylstilbestrol-related clear-cell adenocarcinoma of the vagina and cervix—An update. *N Engl J Med.* 1987;316(9):514–6.
116. Brinton LA, Thistle JE, Liao LM, et al. Epidemiology of vulvar neoplasia in the NIH-AARP Study. *Gynecol Oncol.* 2017;145(2):298–304.
117. Coffey K, Gaitskell K, Beral V, et al. Past cervical intraepithelial neoplasia grade 3, obesity, and earlier menopause are associated with an increased risk of vulval cancer in postmenopausal women. *Br J Cancer.* 2016;115(5):599–606.
118. Newcomb PA, Weiss NS, Daling JR. Incidence of vulvar carcinoma in relation to menstrual, reproductive, and medical factors. *J Natl Cancer Inst.* 1984;73(2):391–6.
119. Thomas D. Exogenous steroid hormones and hepatocellular carcinoma. In: Tablr E, DiBiceglie A, Purcell R, eds.Tablr E, DiBiceglie A, Purcell R, eds. *Etiology, Pathology, and Treatment of Hepatocellular Carcinoma in North America.* Houston: Gulf Publishing Company; 1990, pp. 77–89.
120. Lin JS, Piper MA, Perdue LA, et al. Screening for colorectal cancer updated evidence report and systematic review for the US Preventive Services Task Force. *JAMA.* 2016;315(23):2576–94.
121. Fernandez E, La Vecchia C, Franceschi S, et al. Oral contraceptive use and risk of colorectal cancer. *Epidemiol.* 1998;9(3):295–300.
122. Hannaford P, Elliott A. Use of exogenous hormones by women and colorectal cancer: Evidence from the Royal College of General Practitioners' Oral Contraception Study. *Contraception.* 2005;71(2):95–8.
123. Martinez ME, Grodstein F, Giovannucci E, et al. A prospective study of reproductive factors, oral contraceptive use, and risk of colorectal cancer. *Cancer Epidemiol Biomarkers Prev.* 1997;6(1):1–5.
124. Karagas MR, Stukel TA, Dykes J, et al. A pooled analysis of 10 case-control studies of melanoma and oral contraceptive use. *Br J Cancer.* 2002;86(7):1085–92.
125. Gann PH, Hennekens CH, Ma J, et al. Prospective study of sex hormone levels and risk of prostate cancer. *J Natl Cancer Inst.* 1996;88(16):1118–26.
126. Shabsigh R, Crawford ED, Nehra A, et al. Testosterone therapy in hypogonadal men and potential prostate cancer risk: A systematic review. *Int J Impot Res.* 2009;21(1):9–23.
127. Rhoden EL, Morgentaler A. Testosterone replacement therapy in hypogonadal men at high risk for prostate cancer: Results of 1 year of treatment in men with prostatic intraepithelial neoplasia. *J Urol.* 2003;170(6 Pt 1):2348–51.
128. Klap J, Schmid M, Loughlin KR. The relationship between total testosterone levels and prostate cancer: A review of the continuing controversy. *J Urol.* 2015;193(2):403–13.
129. Schenk JM, Till C, Hsing AW, et al. Serum androgens and prostate cancer risk: Results from the placebo arm of the Prostate Cancer Prevention Trial. *Cancer Causes Control.* 2016;27(2):175–82.
130. Warburton D, Hobaugh C, Wang G, et al. Testosterone replacement therapy and the risk of prostate cancer. *Asian J Andr*ol. 2015;17(6):878–81.
131. Wang K, Chen XG, Bird VY, et al. Association between age-related reductions in testosterone and risk of prostate cancer-An analysis of patients' data with prostatic diseases. *Int J Cancer.* 2017;141(9):1783–93.
132. English PB, Goldberg DE, Wolff C, et al. Parental and birth characteristics in relation to testicular cancer risk among males born between 1960 and 1995 in California (United States). *Cancer Causes Control.* 2003;14(9):815–25.
133. Strohsnitter WC, Noller KL, Hoover RN, et al. Cancer risk in men exposed in utero to diethylstilbestrol. *J Natl Cancer Inst.* 2001;93(7):545–51.
134. Coupland CAC, Chilvers CED, Davey G, et al. Risk factors for testicular germ cell tumours by histological tumour type. *Br J Cancer.* 1999;80(11):1859–63.
135. Weir HK, Kreiger N, Marrett LD. Age at puberty and risk of testicular germ cell cancer (Ontario, Canada). *Cancer Causes Control.* 1998;9(3):253–8.
136. Casper C, Fitzmaurice C. Infection-related cancers: Prioritising an important and eliminable contributor to the global cancer burden. *Lancet Global Health.* 2016;4(9):E580-1.
137. Brown LM. Helicobacter pylori: Epidemiology and routes of transmission. *Epidemiol Rev.* 2000;22(2):283–97.
138. Wroblewski LE, Peek RM, Wilson KT. Helicobacter pylori and gastric cancer: Factors that modulate disease risk. *Clin Microbiol Rev.* 2010;23(4):713–39.
139. Colquhoun A, Arnold M, Ferlay J, et al. Global patterns of cardia and non-cardia gastric cancer incidence in 2012. *Gut.* 2015;64(12):1881–8.
140. Fock KM, Ang TL. Epidemiology of Helicobacter pylori infection and gastric cancer in Asia. *J Gastroenterol Hepatol.* 2010;25(3):479–86.
141. Munoz N. Is Helicobacter pylori a cause of gastric cancer? An appraisal of the seroepidemiological evidence. *Cancer Epidemiol Biomarkers Prev.* 1994;3(5):445–51.
142. Bui D, Brown HE, Harris RB, et al. Serologic evidence for fecal oral transmission of Helicobacter pylori. *Am J Trop Med Hyg.* 2016;94(1):82–8.
143. Saraiya M, Unger ER, Thompson TD, et al. US assessment of HPV types in cancers: Implications for current and 9-valent HPV vaccines. *J Natl Cancer Inst.* 2015;107(6):djv086.
144. McQuillan G, Kruszon-Moran D, Markowitz LE, et al. *Prevalence of HPV in Adults Aged 18–69: United States, 2011–2014. NCHS Data Brief, No 280.* Hyattsville, MD: National Center for Health Statistics; 2017.
145. Hanson CM, Eckert L, Bloem P, et al. Gavi HPV programs: Application to implementation. *Vaccines.* 2015;3(2):408–19.
146. Centers for Disease Control and Prevention (CDC). Recommendations on the use of quadrivalent human papillomavirus vaccine in males—Advisory Committee on Immunization Practices (ACIP), 2011. *MMWR.* 2011;60(50):1705–8.
147. Petrosky E, Bocchini JA, Hariri S, et al. Use of 9-valent human papillomavirus (HPV) vaccine: Updated HPV vaccination recommendations of the Advisory Committee on Immunization Practices. *MMWR.* 2015;64(11):300–4.
148. Walker TY, Elam-Evans LD, Singleton JA, et al. National, regional, state, and selected local area vaccination coverage among adolescents aged 13–17 years—United States, 2016. *MMWR.* 2017;66(33):874–82.
149. Markowitz LE, Liu G, Hariri S, et al. Prevalence of HPV after introduction of the vaccination program in the United States. *Pediatrics.* 2016;137(3):e20151968.
150. Flagg EW, Torrone EA, Weinstock H. Ecological Association of human papillomavirus vaccination with cervical dysplasia prevalence in the United States, 2007–2014. *Am J Public Health.* 2016;106(12):2211–8.
151. Centers for Disease Control and Prevention. Hepatitis B—Vaccination of Adults. 2017. www.cdc.gov/hepatitis/hbv/vaccadults.htm. Accessed November 13, 2017.
152. Williams WW, Lu PJ, O'Halloran A, et al. Surveillance of vaccination coverage among adult populations—United States, 2014. *MMWR Surveill Summ.* 2016;65(1):1–36.

153. Brady G, MacArthur GJ, Farrell PJ. Epstein-Barr virus and Burkitt lymphoma. *J Clin Pathol.* 2007;60(12):1397–402.
154. Goldsmith DB, West TM, Morton R. HLA associations with nasopharyngeal carcinoma in Southern Chinese: A meta-analysis. *Clin Otolaryngol.* 2002;27(1):61–7.
155. Dolcetti R, Boiocchi M, Gloghini A, et al. Pathogenetic and histogenetic features of HIV-associated Hodgkin's disease. *Eur J Cancer.* 2001;37(10):1276–87.
156. Curtiss P, Strazzulla LC, Friedman-Kien AE. An update on Kaposi's sarcoma: Epidemiology, pathogenesis and treatment. *Dermatol Ther.* 2016;6(4):465–70.
157. Robey RC, Bower M. Facing up to the ongoing challenge of Kaposi's sarcoma. *Curr Opin Infect Dis.* 2015;28(1):31–40.
158. Cook LBM, Taylor GP. HTLV-1 and HTLV-2 prevalence in the United States. *J Infect Dis.* 2014;209(4):486–7.
159. Watanabe T. Current status of HTLV-1 infection. *Int J Hematol.* 2011;94(5):430–4.
160. Gonzalez-Alcaide G, Ramos JM, Huamani C, et al. Human tlymphotropic virus 1 (htlv-1) and human t-lymphotropic virus 2 (htlv-2): Geographical research trends and collaboration networks (1989–2012). *Rev Inst Med Trop Sao Paulo.* 2016;58:11.
161. IARC. Schistosomes, liver flukes and Helicobacter pylori. IARC working group on the evaluation of carcinogenic risks to humans. Lyon, 7–14 June 1994. *IARC Monogr Eval Carcinog Risks Hum.* 1994;61:1–241.
162. Dennis LK, Snetselaar LG, Smith BJ, et al. Problems with the assessment of dietary fat in prostate cancer studies. *Am J Epidemiol.* 2004;160(5):436–44.
163. Schwingshackl L, Schwedhelm C, Galbete C, et al. Adherence to mediterranean diet and risk of cancer: An updated systematic review and meta-analysis. *Nutrients.* 2017;9(10):1063.
164. Capurso C, Vendemiale G. The mediterranean diet reduces the risk and mortality of the prostate cancer: A narrative review. *Front Nutr.* 2017;4:38.
165. Shivappa N, Godos J, Hebert JR, et al. Dietary inflammatory index and colorectal cancer risk—A meta-analysis. *Nutrients.* 2017;9(9):1043.
166. Al-Zalabani AH, Stewart KFJ, Wesselius A, et al. Modifiable risk factors for the prevention of bladder cancer: A systematic review of meta-analyses. *Eur J Epidemiol.* 2016;31(9):811–51.
167. Zhao ZW, Yin ZF, Zhao QC. Red and processed meat consumption and gastric cancer risk: A systematic review and meta-analysis. *Oncotarget.* 2017;8(18):30563–75.
168. Zhao ZW, Yin ZF, Pu ZS, et al. Association between consumption of red and processed meat and pancreatic cancer risk: A systematic review and meta-analysis. *Clin Gastroenterol Hepatol.* 2017;15(4):486–93.
169. Taylor PR, Greenwald P. Nutritional interventions in cancer prevention. *J Clin Oncol.* 2005;23(2):333–45.
170. Corte-Real J, Guignard C, Gantenbein M, et al. No influence of supplemental dietary calcium intake on the bioavailability of spinach carotenoids in humans. *Br J Nutr.* 2017;117(11):1560–9.
171. Mayne ST, Cartmel B, Baum M, et al. Randomized trial of supplemental beta-carotene to prevent second head and neck cancer. *Cancer Res.* 2001;61(4):1457–63.
172. Mayne ST, Ferrucci LM, Cartmel B. Lessons learned from randomized clinical trials of micronutrient supplementation for cancer prevention. *Annu Rev Nutr.* 2012;32:369–90.
173. Christen WG, Gaziano JM, Hennekens CH, et al. Design of physicians' health study II—A randomized trial of beta-carotene, vitamins E and C, and multivitamins, in prevention of cancer, cardiovascular disease, and eye disease, and review of results of completed trials. *Ann Epidemiol.* 2000;10(2):125–34.
174. Wang L, Sesso HD, Glynn RJ, et al. Vitamin E and C supplementation and risk of cancer in men: Posttrial follow-up in the Physicians' Health Study II randomized trial. *Am J Clin Nutr.* 2014;100(3):915–23.
175. Wright ME, Groshong SD, Husgafvel-Pursiainen K, et al. Effects of beta-carotene supplementation on molecular markers of lung carcinogenesis in male smokers. *Cancer Prev Res.* 2010;3(6):745–52.
176. Omenn GS, Goodman GE, Thornquist MD, et al. Effects of a combination of beta carotene and vitamin A on lung cancer and cardiovascular disease. *N Engl J Med.* 1996;334(18):1150–5.
177. Ferlay A, Bernard L, Meynadier A, et al. Production of trans and conjugated fatty acids in dairy ruminants and their putative effects on human health: A review. *Biochimie.* 2017;141:107–20.
178. Fowler ME, Akinyemiju TF. Meta-analysis of the association between dietary inflammatory index (DII) and cancer outcomes. *Int J Cancer.* 2017;141(11):2215–27.
179. Lauby-Secretan B, Scoccianti C, Loomis D, et al. Body fatness and cancer—Viewpoint of the IARC Working Group. *N Engl J Med.* 2016;375(8):794–8.
180. Goodwin PJ, Stambolic V. Impact of the obesity epidemic on cancer. *Ann Rev Med.* 2015;66:281–96.
181. Friedenreich CM, Orenstein MR. Physical activity and cancer prevention: Etiologic evidence and biological mechanisms. *J Nutr.* 2002;132(11):3456S–64S.
182. de Rezende LFM, Lopes MR, Rey-Lopez JP, et al. Sedentary behavior and health outcomes: An overview of systematic reviews. *PLoS One.* 2014;9(8):e105620.
183. Lynch BM. Sedentary behavior and cancer: A systematic review of the literature and proposed biological mechanisms. *Cancer Epidemiol Biomarkers Prev.* 2010;19(11):2691–709.
184. Mocellin S, Briarava M, Pilati P. Vitamin B6 and cancer risk: A field synopsis and meta-analysis. *J Natl Cancer Inst.* 2017;109(3):1–9.
185. Bultman SJ. The microbiome and its potential as a cancer preventive intervention. *Semin Oncol.* 2016;43(1):97–106.
186. Lynch HT, Lynch PM, Lanspa SJ, et al. Review of the Lynch syndrome: History, molecular genetics, screening, differential diagnosis, and medicolegal ramifications. *Clin Genet.* 2009;76(1):1–18.
187. Welcsh PL, Schubert EL, King MC. Inherited breast cancer: An emerging picture. *Clin Genet.* 1998;54(6):447–58.
188. Nagy R, Sweet K, Eng C. Highly penetrant hereditary cancer syndromes. *Oncogene.* 2004;23(38):6445–70.
189. Lindor NM, McMaster ML, Lindor CJ, et al. Concise handbook of familial cancer susceptibility syndromes—Second edition. *J Natl Cancer Inst Monogr.* 2008;(38):1–93.
190. Shiovitz S, Korde LA. Genetics of breast cancer: A topic in evolution. *Ann Oncol.* 2015;26(7):1291–9.
191. Robson ME, Storm CD, Weitzel J, et al. American Society of Clinical Oncology policy statement update: Genetic and genomic testing for cancer susceptibility. *J Clin Oncol.* 2010;28(5):893–901.
192. Knudson AG, Jr. Mutation and cancer: Statistical study of retinoblastoma. *Proc Natl Acad Sci U S A.* 1971;68(4):820–3.
193. Varley JM. Germline TP53 mutations and Li-Fraumeni syndrome. *Hum Mutat.* 2003;21(3):313–20.
194. Chen SN, Parmigiani G. Meta-analysis of BRCA1 and BRCA2 penetrance. *J Clin Oncol.* 2007;25(11):1329–33.
195. Nelson HD, Pappas M, Zakher B, et al. Risk assessment, genetic counseling, and genetic testing for BRCA-related cancer in women: A systematic review to update the U.S. Preventive Services Task Force recommendation. *Ann Intern Med.* 2014;160(4):255–66.
196. Roa BB, Boyd AA, Volcik K, et al. Ashkenazi Jewish population frequencies for common mutations in BRCA1 and BRCA2. *Nat Genet.* 1996;14(2):185–7.
197. Satagopan JM, Boyd J, Kauff ND, et al. Ovarian cancer risk in Ashkenazi Jewish carriers of BRCA1 and BRCA2 mutations. *Clin Cancer Res.* 2002;8(12):3776–81.
198. NCCN Clinical Practice Guidelines in Oncology. Genetic/Familial High-Risk Assessment: Breast and Ovarian. In: Network NCC, ed., 2017.
199. Walsh T, Lee MK, Casadei S, et al. Detection of inherited mutations for breast and ovarian cancer using genomic capture and massively parallel sequencing. *Proc Natl Acad Sci U S A.* 2010;107(28):12629–33.
200. Ai-Sukhni W, Aronson M, Gallinger S. Hereditary colorectal cancer syndromes: Familial adenomatous polyposis and Lynch syndrome. *Surgical Clin North Am.* 2008;88(4):819–44.
201. Lynch HT, Snyder C, Davies JM, et al. FAP, gastric cancer, and genetic counseling featuring children and young adults: A family study and review. *Fam Cancer.* 2010;9(4):581–8.
202. de la Chapelle A. The incidence of Lynch syndrome. *Fam Cancer.* 2005;4(3):233–7.
203. NCCN Clinical Practice Guidelines in Oncology. Genetic/Familial High-Risk Assessment: Colorectal. 2017.
204. Ruteshouser EC, Huff V. Familial Wilms tumor. Am J Med Genet C Semin Med Genet. 2004;129C(1):29–34.
205. Geerdink EA, Van der Luijt RB, Lips CJM. Do patients with multiple endocrine neoplasia syndrome type 1 benefit from periodical screening? *Eur J Endocrinol.* 2003;149(6):577–82.
206. Linehan WM, Zbar B. Focus on kidney cancer. *Cancer Cell.* 2004;6(3):223–8.
207. Win AK, Hopper JL, Jenkins MA. Association between monoallelic MUTYH mutation and colorectal cancer risk: A meta-regression analysis. *Fam Cancer.* 2011;10(1):1–9.

208. Win AK, Cleary SP, Dowty JG, et al. Cancer risks for monoallelic MUTYH mutation carriers with a family history of colorectal cancer. *Int J Cancer.* 2011;129(9):2256–62.
209. Ahmed M, Rahman N. ATM and breast cancer susceptibility. *Oncogene.* 2006;25(43):5906–11.
210. Renwick A, Thompson D, Seal S, et al. ATM mutations that cause ataxia-telangiectasia are breast cancer susceptibility alleles. *Nat Genet.* 2006;38(8):873–5.
211. Thompson D, Duedal S, Kirner J, et al. Cancer risks and mortality in heterozygous ATM mutation carriers. *J Natl Cancer Inst.* 2005;97(11):813–22.
212. Yu Y, Li X, Liang C, et al. The relationship between GSTA1, GSTM1, GSTP1, and GSTT1 genetic polymorphisms and bladder cancer susceptibility: A meta-analysis. *Medicine (Baltimore).* 2016;95(37):e4900.
213. Liu H, Ma HF, Chen YK. Association between GSTM1 polymorphisms and lung cancer: An updated meta-analysis. *Genet Mol Res.* 2015;14(1):1385–92.
214. GBD 2015 Risk Factors Collaborators. Global, regional, and national comparative risk assessment of 79 behavioural, environmental and occupational, and metabolic risks or clusters of risks, 1990–2015: A systematic analysis for the Global Burden of Disease Study. *Lancet.* 2016;388(10053):1659–1724.
215. U.S. National Cancer Institute and World Health Organization. *The Economics of Tobacco and Tobacco Control. National Cancer Institute Tobacco Control Monograph 21.* Bethesda, MD: U.S. Department of Health and Human Services, NIH, NCI and Geneva, CH: WHO; 2016.
216. Colditz GA, Wolin KY, Gehlert S. Applying what we know to accelerate cancer prevention. *Sci Transl Med.* 2012;4(127):127rv4.
217. Emmons KM, Colditz GA. Realizing the potential of cancer prevention—The role of implementation science. *N Engl J Med.* 2017;376(10):986–90.
218. Siegel RL, Jacobs EJ, Newton CC, et al. Deaths due to cigarette smoking for 12 smoking-related cancers in the United States. *JAMA Intern Med.* 2015;175(9):1574–6.
219. Abed J, Reilley B, Butler MO, et al. Comprehensive cancer control initiative of the Centers for Disease Control and Prevention: An example of participatory innovation diffusion. *J Public Health Manag Pract.* 2000;6(2):79–92.
220. Given LS, Black B, Lowry G, et al. Collaborating to conquer cancer: A comprehensive approach to cancer control. *Cancer Causes Control.* 2005;16:3–14.
221. National Comprehensive Cancer Control Program.
222. Centers for Disease Control and Prevention. National Comprehensive Cancer Control Program. 2017.
223. DHHS. *Healthy People 2020.* Washington, DC: U.S. Department of Health and Human Services, Office of Disease Prevention and Health Promotion; 2017.
224. Meester RGS, Doubeni CA, Zauber AG, et al. Public health impact of achieving 80% colorectal cancer screening rates in the United States by 2018. *Cancer.* 2015;121(13):2281–5.
225. Byers T, Wender RC, Jemal A, et al. The American Cancer Society challenge goal to reduce US cancer mortality by 50% between 1990 and 2015: Results and reflections. *CA Cancer J Clin.* 2016;66(5):359–69.
226. American Cancer Society. Stay Healthy. 2017.
227. Centers for Disease Control and Prevention. How you can prevent sexually transmitted diseases. 2017.
228. United States Preventive Services Task Force. Methods and Processes, Grade Definitions after 2012. 2017.
229. Centers for Disease Control and Prevention. Vaccine recommendations and guidelines of the ACIP.
230. American Academy of Family Physicians. Summary of Recommendations for Clinical Preventive Services, July 2017.
231. American Academy of Pediatrics. Recommendations for Preventive Pediatric Health Care.
232. United States Preventive Services Task Force. Published Recommendations.
233. Smith RA, Andrews K, Brooks D, et al. Cancer screening in the United States, 2016: A review of Current American Cancer Society guidelines and current issues in cancer screening. *CA Cancer J Clin.* 2016;66(2):96–114.
234. National Comprehensive Cancer Network. NCCN Guidelines for Detection, Prevention & Risk Reduction. 2017.
235. American College of Physicians. Clinical Guidelines and Recommendations. https://www.acponline.org/clinical-information/guidelines.
236. United States Preventive Services Task Force. Final Recommendation Statement—Breast Cancer: Screening. 2017.
237. United States Preventive Services Task Force. Draft Recommendation Statement—Cervical Cancer: Screening. 2017.
238. US Preventive Services Task Force, Bibbins-Domingo K, Grossman DC, et al. Screening for colorectal cancer: US Preventive Services Task Force recommendation statement. *JAMA.* 2016;315(23):2564–75.
239. Moyer VA, US Preventive Services Task Force. Screening for Lung cancer: US preventive services task force recommendation statement. *Ann Intern Med.* 2014;160(5):330–8.
240. Aberle DR, Adams AM, Berg CD, et al. Reduced lung-cancer mortality with low-dose computed tomographic screening. *N Engl J Med.* 2011;365(5):395–409.
241. Moyer VA. U. S. Preventive Services Task Force. Screening for prostate cancer: US Preventive Services Task Force recommendation statement. *Ann Intern Med.* 2012;157(2):120–34.
242. Vetterlein MW, Dalela D, Sammon JD, et al. State-by-state variation in prostate-specific antigen screening trends following the 2011 United States Preventive Services Task Force Panel update. Urology. 2018;112: 56–65.
243. United States Preventive Services Task Force. Draft Recommendation Statement—Prostate Cancer: Screening. 2017.
244. United States Preventive Services Task Force. Published Recommendations. 2017.
245. American Cancer Society. *Cancer Treatment & Survivorship Facts & Figures 2016–2017.* Atlanta, GA: American Cancer Society; 2016.
246. Lance Armstrong Foundation and Centers for Disease Control and Prevention. A National Action Plan for Cancer Survivorship: Advancing Public Health Strategies. 2004.
247. Bower JE, Bak K, Berger A, et al. Screening, assessment, and management of fatigue in adult survivors of cancer: An American Society of Clinical Oncology Clinical Practice guideline adaptation. *J Clin Oncol.* 2014;32(17):1840–50.
248. Paice JA, Lacchetti C, Bruera E. Management of chronic pain in survivors of adult cancers: ASCO Clinical Practice Guideline summary. *J Oncol Pract.* 2016;12(8):757–62.
249. Ferrell BR, Temel JS, Temin S, et al. Integration of palliative care into standard oncology care: American Society of Clinical Oncology Clinical Practice guideline update. *J Clin Oncol.* 2017;35(1):96–112.
250. Resnick MJ, Lacchetti C, Bergman J, et al. Prostate cancer survivorship care guideline: American Society of Clinical Oncology Clinical Practice guideline endorsement. *J Clinic Oncol.* 2015;33(9):1078–85.
251. Nekhlyudov L, Lacchetti C, Davis NB, et al. Head and Neck Cancer Survivorship Care Guideline: American Society of Clinical Oncology Clinical Practice guideline endorsement of the American Cancer Society Guideline. *J Clin Oncol.* 2017;35(14):1606–21.

CHAPTER

52

Cardiovascular Disease

Russell V. Luepker • Margaret Nolan

INTRODUCTION

Cardiovascular diseases (CVDs) involving the heart and blood vessels are public health concerns around the world, particularly coronary or ischemic heart disease (CHD), hypertensive heart disease, and rheumatic heart disease. CHD remains the leading cause of adult death worldwide (Fig. 52-1), although its incidence differs widely and the mortality ascribed to it is changing (Fig. 52-2). While deaths from CVD have fallen substantially in industrialized nations, they are rising dramatically in others particularly in the developing world.[1] Age-adjusted U.S. deaths ascribed to CVD declined dramatically for men and women during the first decade of the twenty-first century, (Figs. 52-3 and 52-4). After 2011, however, this rate of decline in CVD mortality began to slow,[2] most markedly for deaths from cerebrovascular disease. Though the exact reasons for this slowing are still unclear, population-level risk factors, such as obesity and diabetes, have continued to rise.[3,4]

Deaths ascribed to hypertensive heart disease have diminished over recent decades in many industrialized countries.[5] In West Africa, Latin America, and East Asia, however, the high prevalence still found in hospitals and clinics indicates the continued worldwide importance of hypertension.

Rheumatic fever and rheumatic valvular heart disease remain public health concerns in many developing countries and are still seen among disadvantaged peoples in affluent nations. Cardiomyopathies, often of unknown or infectious origin, constitute a common cause of heart disease in many regions, particularly Africa and Latin America. In the United States, as the "Baby Boomer" generation ages, the prevalence of illegal substance use among adults ages 50–65 has increased dramatically over the past decade, raising additional concerns about the cardiovascular effects of drugs and alcohol in this age group.[6] Finally, congenital heart disease continues to contribute to the heart disease burden among youth and adults of all countries.

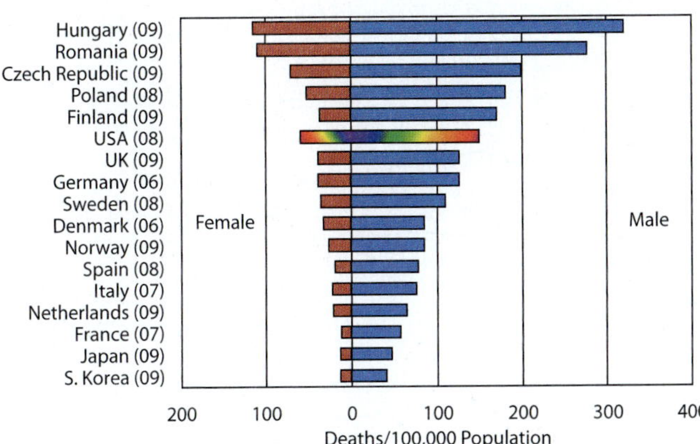

FIGURE 52-1. Age-adjusted death rates for coronary heart disease by country and sex, ages 35–74, 2006–09. (*Source:* National Heart, Lung, and Blood Institute. Morbidity and mortality chart book on cardiovascular, lung, and blood diseases. Bethesda, Maryland: NIH Publication; 2012.)

The worldwide public health potential for primary prevention of most CVD is established by several salient facts: (a) the large population differences in CVD incidence and death rates; CVD is rare in some countries and common in others; (b) dynamic national trends in CVD deaths, both upward and downward; (c) rapid changes in CVD risk among migrant populations; (d) the identification of modifiable risk characteristics for CVD among and within populations; and (e) the positive results of preventive trials.

The following chapter expands on these CVDs, their trends, and the magnitude of burden on populations. The population-wide factors associated with risk of these diseases are described. Because the majority of CVD is caused by social, cultural, and economic factors, public health approaches are central to prevention and control strategies.

CORONARY HEART DISEASE

CHD is the leading cause of adult deaths in many industrial societies. Much about its causes and prevention has been learned from diverse research methods, including clinicopathological observations, laboratory-experimental studies, population studies, and clinical trials. The evidence of causation from all these disciplines is congruent. As a result, several ubiquitous cultural characteristics described below are now established as powerful influences on population risk of CHD. These influences and risk factors appear to be safely modifiable for individuals and for entire populations.[7–9]

The sum of evidence suggests that there is widespread human susceptibility to atherosclerosis and, consequently, that CHD is maximally exhibited when the environment is unfavorable. These ubiquitous susceptibilities, exposures, and behaviors lead eventually to the mass precursors of CHD found among so many people in high-incidence societies. The rationale and the potential for preventive practice, as well as for public policy in prevention, are based on several well-established relationships: between risk factor levels and CHD, between health behaviors and risk factor levels, and between culture and mass health behaviors.

Epidemiology of CHD

Summarized here are the salient observations about CHD:

- Population comparisons show large differences in trends in CHD incidence and mortality rates (Fig. 52-2) and in the extent of its underlying vascular disease, atherosclerosis.
- Population differences in the mean levels and distributions of CHD risk characteristics (particular lipid levels) are strongly correlated with population differences in CHD rates.

- Within populations, several risk characteristics (blood cholesterol, blood pressure levels, diabetes, smoking, alcohol, and other drug use) are strongly and continuously related to future individual risk of a CHD event.
- Population differences in average levels of CHD risk characteristics are already apparent in youth. Individual values of children tend to "track" into adult years.
- There are significant differences in mortality within the United States with a distinct excess across the Ohio River Valley (Fig. 52-5).
- CHD risk characteristics and incidence in migrants rapidly approach levels of the adopted culture.
- Trends in CHD mortality rates, both upward and downward, occur over relatively short periods of 5–10 years. These trends tend to be associated with changes in medical care and case-fatality rates as well as with trends in incidence and in population distributions of risk characteristics.
- The rapid decrease in age-adjusted CHD mortality rates in the United States is shared by men and women, by whites and non-whites, and by younger and older age groups (Fig. 52-4), but has begun to plateau.
- The decrease in age-adjusted CHD mortality rates in the United States is associated with an even greater decrease in death rates from stroke. This leads to increases in lifespan. Moreover, in the last decades there has been a lesser decrease in non-CVD deaths and in deaths from all causes (Fig. 52-6).
- Randomized clinical trials find a direct effect of CHD risk factor lowering on subsequent disease rates. Preventive trials also establish that levels of risk factors, and their associated health behaviors, can be significantly and safely modified.
- The epidemiological evidence is congruent with clinical, animal and laboratory findings about the causes and mechanisms of atherosclerosis, the process that underlies the clinical manifestations of CHD.

Role of Diet

Dietary Fats

There is considerable evidence that habitual diet in populations, a culturally determined characteristic, has an important influence on the mean levels and distribution of blood lipoproteins and, therefore, on the population risk and potential for prevention of CHD. Several dietary factors influence individual and population levels of low-density lipoproteins (LDLs) in the blood, a leading pathogenetic factor in atherosclerosis. These include foods that increase LDL and cholesterol such as saturated fats, trans fats, dietary cholesterol, and calorie excess. Other foods including vegetables, fruits, fiber, and alcohol may lower harmful cholesterol. Many experts consider that the cholesterol-raising properties of some habitual diets are essential to the development of mass atherosclerosis, leading in turn to high rates of CHD. Where average total blood cholesterol level in a population is low (less than 200 mg/dL, or 5.2 mmol/L), CHD is

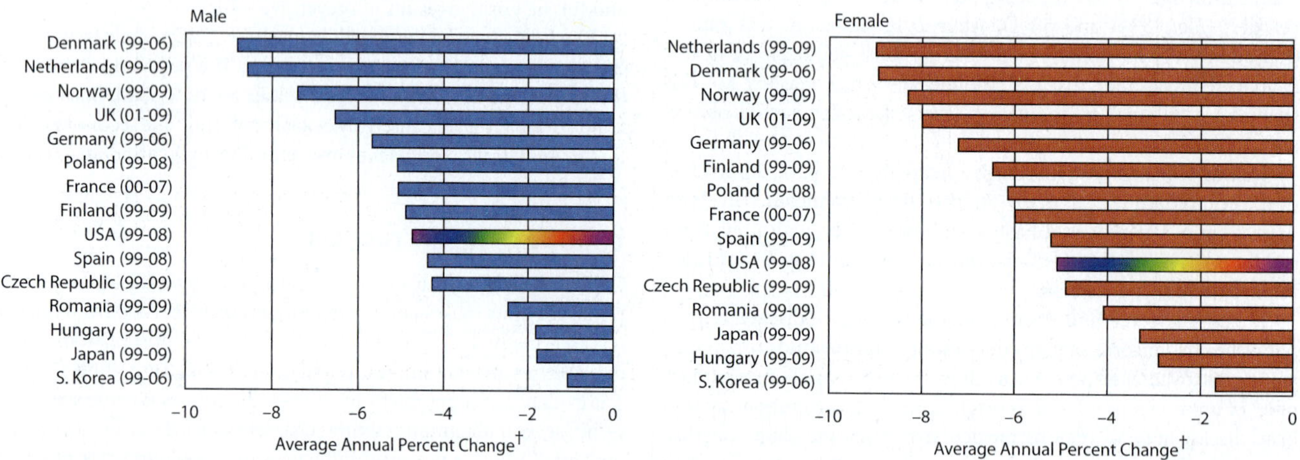

FIGURE 52-2. Change in age-adjusted death rates for coronary heart disease in males and females by country, ages 35–74, 1999–2009. (*Source:* National Heart, Lung, and Blood Institute. Morbidity and mortality chart book on cardiovascular, lung, and blood diseases. Bethesda, Maryland: NIH Publication; 2012.)

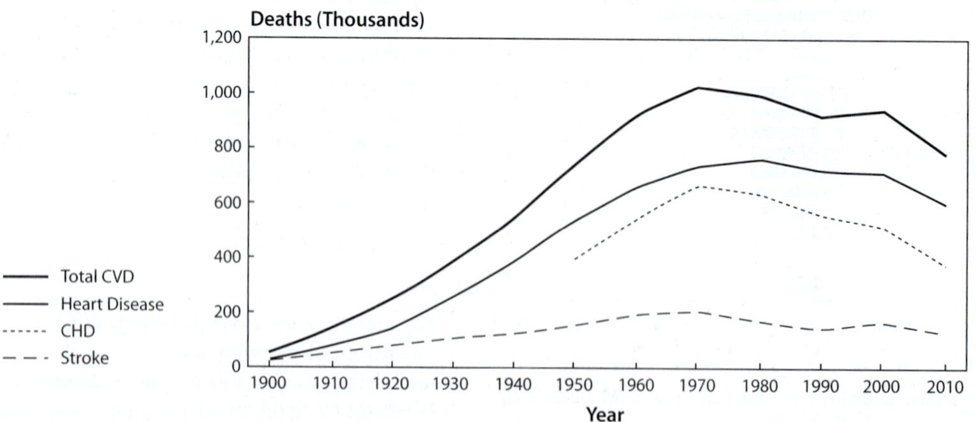

FIGURE 52-3. Death from cardiovascular diseases, the United States, 1900–2010 (*Source:* National Heart, Lung, and Blood Institute. Fact Book. Bethesda, MD: NIH Publication; 2012.)

uncommon, irrespective of population levels of smoking and hypertension. From this evidence, there is now a consensus about the leading population causes of CHD and general acceptance of policy recommendations that lead toward a gradual, universal change in the habitual diets of populations in which CHD rates are high.

Epidemiological studies comparing stable, rural agricultural societies find a strong relationship between habitual diet, average blood cholesterol levels, and incidence of CHD.[10–12] For example, diets of populations with a high incidence of CHD are characterized by relatively high saturated fatty acid (greater than 15% of daily calories) and cholesterol intake and low carbohydrate intake (under 50%). Diets in populations with a low CHD incidence are characterized mainly by low saturated fatty acid intake (less than 10% of calories) and high carbohydrate intake but widely varying

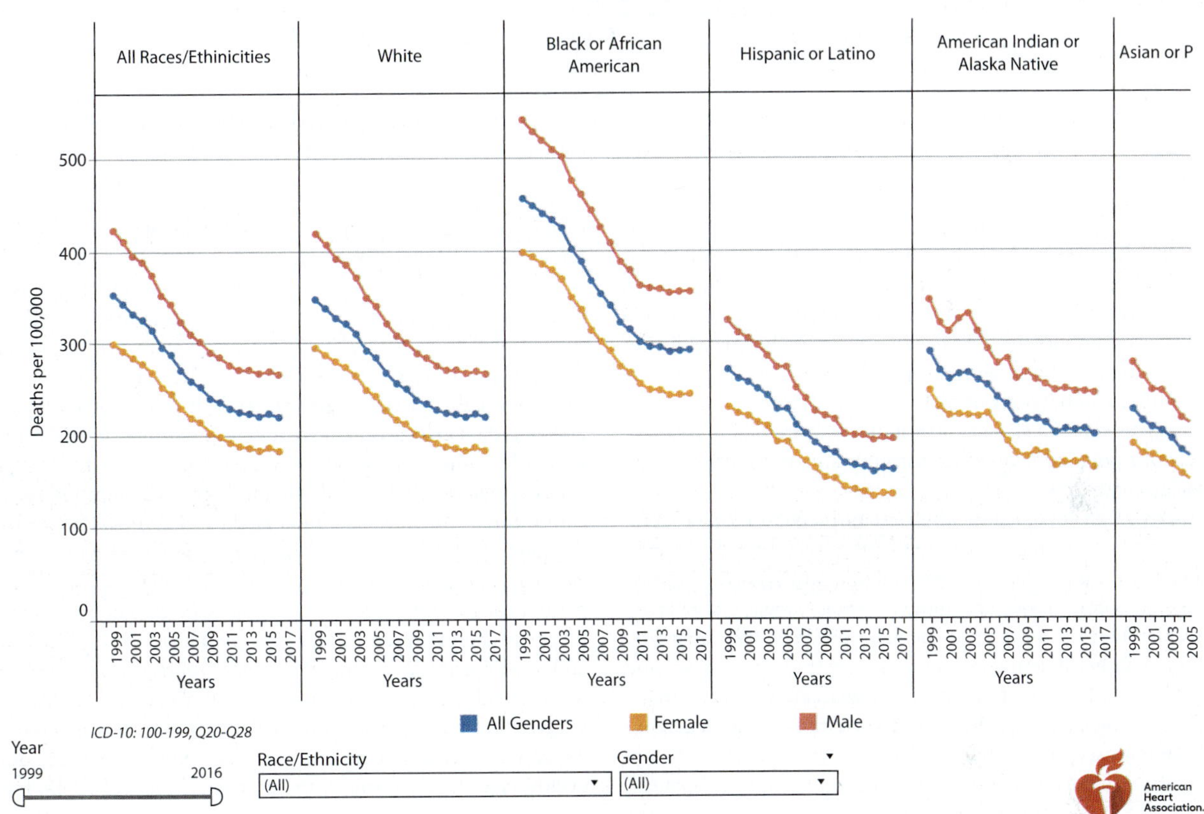

FIGURE 52-4. Age-adjusted death rates for cardiovascular disease by race/ethnicity and sex, the United States, 1999–2016. (*Source:* Reproduced with permission from American Heart Association. Center for Health Metrics and Evaluation (CHME). Data Visualizations. https://aha2017chme.wpengine.com/data-visualization/. Accessed January 2, 2020.)

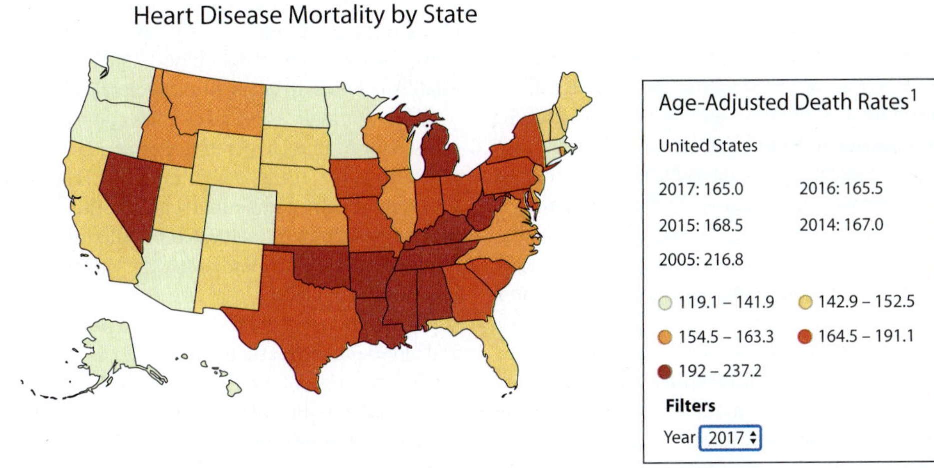

FIGURE 52-5. Age-adjusted death rates for coronary heart disease by state, the United States, 2017. (*Source:* Centers for Disease Control and Prevention. Available at: https://www.cdc.gov/nchs/pressroom/sosmap/heart_disease_mortality/heart_disease.htm.)

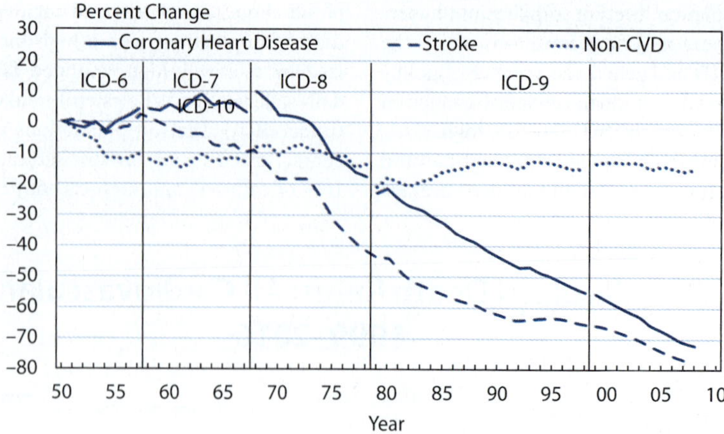

FIGURE 52-6. Change in age-adjusted death rates for cardiovascular and noncardiovascular diseases, the United States, 1950–2008. (*Source:* National Heart, Lung, and Blood Institute. Morbidity and mortality chart book on cardiovascular, lung, and blood diseases. Bethesda, MD: NIH Publication 2012.)

total fat intake (varying mainly in the proportion of monounsaturated fatty acid calories).[12] Most of the difference in mean population levels of serum total (and LDL) cholesterol can be accounted for by measured differences in fatty acid composition of the habitual diet. Moreover, population CHD rates can be predicted, with precision over time, by average population blood cholesterol levels.[13] Cross-cultural comparisons of diet versus postmortem findings of atherosclerosis reveal a strong correlation between habitual dietary fat intake of a population and the frequency and extent of advanced atherosclerotic lesions.[14]

Studies of migrant populations indicate the predominance of sociocultural influences, including diet, in trends of risk and CHD among migrants. For example, Japanese who migrate to California become taller, heavier, more obese, and more sedentary; their diet changes dramatically; they eat more meat and dairy products, saturated fatty acids and cholesterol, and consume less complex carbohydrate and less alcohol than their counterparts in the Nagasaki-Hiroshima area.[15] They develop higher risk profiles and disease rates within a generation. With few exceptions, migrant Hawaiian Japanese have risk factor values intermediate between mainland and California Japanese, and the CHD rate in migrants generally parallels their mean values for risk factor levels.

The rapid evolving national trends in CHD deaths are another indication of the predominance of culture in the population causes and prevention of CHD, as disease occurrence changes more rapidly than any genetic characteristics. Nevertheless, systematic explanatory studies of trends in CHD mortality are very recent, and current attempts to estimate the relative contribution of cultural versus medical care contributions are challenging.[16–20] In a number of countries on an upward slope of CHD mortality, smoking and calorie and fat consumption are increasing and physical activity is decreasing. In many other industrial countries, including the United States, decreasing CHD mortality rates parallel significant reductions in average risk characteristics and improved cardiac care.[16,17,19,20,21] Standardized measurements of risk and disease trends are not generally available for comparisons among countries, but the public health implications of these simultaneous trends in behaviors, risk, disease rates, and medical care are immense.

Another feature of diet, the relative excess of calorie intake over expenditure, influences health through the metabolic maladaptations of hyperlipidemia, hyperinsulinism, and hypertension.[22] Defined as the metabolic syndrome,[23] this caloric imbalance occurs in sedentary cultures and results in mass obesity. With or without mass obesity, however, high salt intake and low potassium intake in populations appear to encourage the wide exhibition of hypertensive phenotypes. Other cations (e.g., magnesium, calcium) may also be significant dietary influences on population levels of blood pressure, while alcohol intake is clearly involved (see below).

Anthropology and paleontology provide insights into the probable effects of rapid cultural change, including modern diets, from the lifestyle to which humans adapted during earlier periods of evolution. Until 500 or so generations ago, all humans were hunter-gatherers. The habitual eating pattern likely involved alternating scarce and abundant calories and a great variety of foods. It surely included lean wild game and usually a predominance of plant over animal calories, a relatively low sodium and high potassium intake, and of course there was universal breast feeding of infants. Observations of the eating patterns among extant hunter-gatherer tribes confirm the varied nature and the adequacy (or near adequacy) of such an eating pattern for growth and development, as well as for the potential of longevity and the absence of mass phenomena such as atherosclerosis and hypertension.[24–26] Although modern humans can scarcely return to such subsistence economies, the anthropological observations suggest that current metabolic maladaptations derived from affluent eating and exercise patterns imposed rapidly on a very different evolutionary legacy result in the mass precursors of CVDs found in modern society.[25]

Several well-conducted cohort studies have provided evidence of diet-CHD relationships within societies in which CHD risk is high.[27–30] With particular care to reduce variability and increase validity of individual dietary intake assessments, all of these studies were able to demonstrate small but significant and often independent prediction of CHD risk based on specific nutrient intake or other dietary characteristics. In our view, this evidence is less persuasive than the powerful synergism of diet, blood lipid levels, and CHD risk so firmly established over 40 years, but it is clearly confirmatory.

With this logic, habitual diet has come to be considered the necessary factor in mass hypercholesterolemia and, thus, in the mass atherosclerosis that leads to high rates of CHD. The population data are, however, equally compatible with another idea, that all three of the major risk factors (i.e., elevated population averages of blood cholesterol, blood pressure, and smoking) are essential for a high population burden of CHD.

The relationship of habitual diet to population levels of blood lipids and blood pressure, and to CHD rates, is largely congruent with clinical and experimental observations. First, experimental modification of diet has a predictable effect on group blood lipid levels. When calories and weight are held constant in controlled diet experiments and diet composition is varied, the largest dietary contributions to serum total and LDL cholesterol levels are (a) the proportion of calories consumed as saturated fatty, trans fatty acids, and dietary cholesterol, all of which raise cholesterol levels, and (b) polyunsaturated fatty acids, which have a cholesterol lowering effect. The role of monounsaturates is debated, with some suggesting a neutral effect while others a cholesterol-lowering effect.[31–34] Although this is debated, these clinical experiments confirm the broader relation found between long-term habitual diet and population mean levels of blood lipids.[10,11]

Animal experiments are not addressed here but are relevant to the human diet-CHD relationship in that lesions resembling the human plaque are produced by dietary manipulations of blood lipoprotein levels; the fatty components of these animal plaques are reversible with dietary manipulations to lower blood lipoprotein levels.[35,36]

Plasma cholesterol-lowering preventive trials, which tend to complete the overall evidence for causation, indicate the feasibility and safety of changing risk factors and demonstrate the actual lag times between such change and its effect on CHD rates.[23] The synthesis of results of all these trials and their implications for the public health are central because carrying out the "definitive diet-heart trial" is thought to be very difficult in a diverse affluent society. However, a clinical trial in Spain compared a Mediterranean diet supplemented with olive oil or nuts to a control low fat diet. In this large trial of adults at high risk but with no CVD history, lower rates of major CVD endpoints were observed in both treatment arms, compared with the low-fat control arm.[37]

Proteins

International vital statistics on deaths correlated with national food-consumption data indicate that, as with fat consumption, strong ecologic correlations exist between animal protein intake and death rates from CHD, but there is little evidence that this association is causal. Anitschkow[38] found originally that it was dietary lipid rather than protein that resulted in hyperlipidemia and atherosclerosis in his experimental rabbits. Controlled metabolic ward studies in men under isocaloric conditions, with fat intake held constant while protein intake was varied between 5% and 20% of daily calories, found no change in blood cholesterol level (University of Minnesota, unpublished data).

Neither clinical, experimental, nor epidemiological evidence is now sufficient to attribute a specific effect of dietary protein on either blood lipid levels or CHD risk. The overall importance of the consumption of meats from domesticated animals and of fatty milk products is therefore thought to rest mainly in their fatty acid content rather than their protein content, at least with respect to CHD risk.

Carbohydrates

There is generally a positive association between population intake of refined sugars and CHD mortality and a negative relationship between complex carbohydrates and CHD mortality. Although these diet components are seriously confounded with other dietary factors that are strongly associated with carbohydrate intake, the effect of certain fibers, including the pectins in fruit, bran fiber, and the guar gum of numerous vegetables and legumes, on blood sugar and on blood lipid regulation has attracted interest. This is particularly so now that the fatty acid effects are well delineated; yet they fail to explain all of the observed population differences in blood lipids or all the lipid changes seen during experiments involving different nutrient composition.

More important, however, is that plausible mechanisms of atherogenesis are not established for sugars. The relationship between consumption of sugar-sweetened beverages and risk of weight gain and Type II diabetes as risk factors for CVD is robust.[39,40] More recently, diet soda consumption has also been implicated as an independent risk factor for diabetes, suggesting that sweet beverage consumption may be a complex factor associated with other risk behaviors.[41] The broader issue of plant foods (fruits, vegetables, pulses, legumes, and seeds), their complex carbohydrates, protein, other nutrients, and fibers is nevertheless of great public health interest because their consumption may affect the risk of cancers as well as of CVD.

The summary view is that the different amounts of sugars consumed in "natural diets" around the world do not account for the important differences found in population levels of blood lipids and their associated CHD risk.

Alcohol

The effects of alcohol on CHD risk are complex and conflicting, with increasing risk for some risk factors, but a potential decrease in risk for moderate levels of consumption. Positive correlations between alcohol consumption and blood pressure levels found for individuals in population studies appear to be dose related and independent of body weight and smoking habits.[42,43] Evidence is also consistent with respect to the positive relationship of alcohol consumption to blood high density lipoprotein (HDL) cholesterol level and of change in alcohol consumption to change in HDL cholesterol level. Substitution of alcohol for carbohydrates in a mixed U.S. diet results in a rise in HDL, mainly the HDL_3 subfraction, one that may not be strongly related to CHD risk.[44]

Experimentally, myocardial metabolism and ventricular function are affected by relatively small doses of alcohol. In addition, neurohormonal links are established between alcohol-stimulated catecholamine excretion and myocardial oxygen requirements. These effects could act as contributory factors to the clinical manifestations of ischemia.

The epidemiological evidence from longitudinal studies about the relation of alcohol to CHD risk is, however, conflicting.[45–47] Inverse relationships of alcohol intake and CHD are found in some studies, whereas a U-shaped, linear, or no relationship is found in others. Positive relationships, when found, are usually independent of tobacco, obesity, and blood pressure levels.[47,48]

Reasons for these inconsistent findings in the alcohol–coronary disease relationship may involve the poor (self-report) measurement for alcohol intake as well as misclassification of the cause of death among heavy drinkers who are known to die of sudden, unexplained causes. Moreover, there are many confounding factors, including blood pressure levels, cigarette smoking, and diet all associated with alcohol use.

Preventive practice with respect to alcohol is, therefore, based on its social and public health consequences rather than on any possible direct effect, favorable or otherwise, on CVD risk. A major concern about regular alcohol use is, however, its enhancement of overeating, underactivity, and smoking, along with its intrinsic caloric density. Given these several relationships, public health recommendations for alcohol are not yet indicated in any quantity as a "protective measure" for heart diseases.

Salt

Salting of food, primarily for preservation, began with civilization and trade. Now salting is based mainly on acquired taste and is likely a "new" phenomenon in an evolutionary sense. Moreover, the mammalian kidney probably evolved in salt-poor regions where the predominantly plant and wild game diet was likely very low in sodium and rich in potassium. Thus, survival of humans and other mammals in salt-poor environments may have rested on an evolutionarily acquired and exquisite sodium-retaining mechanism of the kidney. The physiological need for salt under ordinary circumstances is approximately only 1–2 grams of sodium chloride per day. It is hypothesized that this mechanism is now overwhelmed by the concentrated salt presented to modern humans in preserved meats and pickled foods, in many processed foods, and in the strong culturally acquired taste for salt.[25,49]

Clinical, experimental, and epidemiological links between salt intake and hypertension are increasingly well forged.[49,50] Marked sodium depletion dramatically reduces blood pressure in persons with severe hypertension. Sodium restriction enables high blood pressure to be controlled with lower doses of antihypertensive drugs. In many patients, salt restriction may result in adequate control of mild to moderate hypertension without drugs.[51] Weight reduction and salt restriction appear to be independently important in lowering high blood pressure.[51] In summary, a culture with high salt consumption appears to encourage maximal exhibition of an inherent human susceptibility to hypertension. Because potassium tends to reduce the blood pressure-raising effects of sodium, the sodium-potassium ratio of habitual diets also may be important in the public health.[52]

Surveys consistently find strong relationships between average population blood pressure and salt intake.[50,53,54] High blood pressure is usually prevalent in high-salting cultures, irrespective of the prevalence of obesity. In contrast, hypertension is usually absent in low-salting cultures, despite frequent obesity. Moreover, rapid acculturation to greater salt intake among South Pacific islanders who migrate to industrialized countries is associated with an increased frequency of hypertension and elevated mean blood pressure.[55] Even within high-salting cultures, when special efforts are made to reduce the measurement error for blood pressure and to characterize individual sodium intake with maximum precision, significant individual salt–blood pressure correlations are usually found.[55,56]

Despite all this evidence, neither preventive practice nor public health policy on reduction of salting is well advanced. This may be due in part to professional skepticism, based perhaps on the relatively weak individual correlations of salt intake and blood pressure. Admittedly, modification of salt intake by traditional dietary counseling has not been very successful. However, when interventions are attempted in a supportive and systematic way, change in salting behavior is readily achievable.[57] In the United States, wider education has significantly and widely influenced food processing and marketing of products with lower salt content, and a great deal of voluntary public health action has been taken by food companies.

Current U.S. national dietary goals recommend no more than 4.5–6.0 grams of salt daily.[58] For individuals, this is achievable by not salting foods at the table, by adding no salt in cooking, and by avoidance of salt-rich foods, particularly canned, processed, and pickled foods. Despite the absence of a strong policy, preventive practice and public health approaches to reduced salt consumption are increasing. Significant public health effects of such population changes might be expected in high-salting societies, in light of trends in blood pressure and stroke observed in Japanese populations.[59]

Blood Lipoproteins

Clinical, experimental, and epidemiological evidence of the relationship between certain blood lipoproteins, atherosclerosis, and incidence of CHD is strong, consistent, and congruent. Because much knowledge is available, we present here only a summary of what we regard as the salient facts in this relationship, along with a few key references.23

- Associations are consistently strong between mean population levels of total serum cholesterol and measured CHD incidence.[10,11]
- Associations are variable between mean population levels of fasting serum triglycerides and coronary disease rates.[60,61]
- Total serum cholesterol levels at birth have similar means and ranges in many cultures.[62]
- Average levels and distributions of total serum cholesterol differ widely for populations of school-age children.[62] They tend to parallel the differences found in adult population distributions of blood lipid levels, that is, means and distributions are found to be elevated in youth when they are elevated in adult populations.[62]
- Means and distributions of total serum cholesterol of migrants rapidly approach those of the adopted country, whether higher or lower than the country of origin.[15]
- Blood lipids measured in cohorts of healthy adults followed over time show consistently positive relationships, usually with a continuously rising individual risk of CHD according to the entry levels of total serum cholesterol (and LDL), at least until late middle age.[8,63,64]
- Computation of the population risk attributable to blood cholesterol levels indicates that the majority of excess CHD cases occur in the central segment of the population distribution, that is, 220–310 mg/dL, whereas only 10% derive from values above 310.[7,65]
- In healthy cohorts, a strong inverse relationship between individual HDL cholesterol level and its ratio to total cholesterol is found with subsequent CHD risk. It is relatively stronger at older ages and within populations that have a relatively high CHD risk overall.[36,61,66]
- Large-scale experiments indicate the feasibility and apparent safety of blood cholesterol lowering from moderate changes made in dietary composition, with and without weight loss.[9,34,67]
- Clinical trials of lipid lowering alone in middle-age, high-risk populations indicates a reduction of CHD risk according to the degree and duration of exposure to the lowered cholesterol level.[9,68–70] Further, clear evidence has emerged that a class of lipid-lowering agents, the "statins" can reduce the risk of further CHD morbidity and mortality when coronary disease is already clinically apparent.[71–73]
- There has probably been a significant drop, of approximately 10–15%, in the U.S. mean total serum cholesterol level in 20 years, which is partly explained by changes in composition of the habitual diet during this period.[8,74,75]

Consensus from these facts has resulted in a vigorous population strategy of reduction in blood lipid level in the United States. Major recommendations are now in place for a change in eating patterns among North Americans.[34] Moreover, the U.S. National Cholesterol Education Program and more recently the American College of Cardiology/American Heart Association guidelines have apparently increased both public and professional awareness and has improved the medical practice of lowering blood cholesterol.[23,76–81]

Overweight and Obesity

Whatever the physiological or social disadvantages of obesity and overweight, their relationship to CVD risk and mortality remains interesting and difficult to dissect. From a clinical perspective, extreme obesity is associated with manifest physical limitations and a propensity for many disabilities and illnesses. Beyond this, however, associations with CVDs are not consistent throughout most of the distribution of relative weight or skin-fold measurements.[82]

Overweight and weight gain tend to raise risk factor levels, and correction of the many metabolic disorders that accompany obesity is prompt and substantial when weight loss is achieved, with or without an increase in physical activity. When weight loss is carried out primarily through increased physical activity, appetite is generally "self-regulated" and body fat is lost, lean body mass is better maintained, insulin activity is lowered, glucose tolerance is improved, LDL and very low-density lipoprotein (VLDL) levels are lowered, HDL level is raised, and cardiovascular efficiency is enhanced. As we shall review here, however, the status of obesity and weight gain and loss as risk factors for CVD is complex.

Obesity is arbitrarily considered to be present when the fat content of the body is greater than 25% of body mass in men and 30% in women. Overweight is equally arbitrarily chosen as greater than 130% relative weight, according to life insurance build and mortality tables, or on a body mass index (kg/m^2) greater than 59. "Ideal weight" criteria are often based on standards associated with the lowest mortality risk in life insurance experience. The prevalence of overweight (and obesity) in U.S. adults is variously estimated from 20% to 70%, depending on the measurement used and the definition chosen, as well as by age, sex, and race classification.[83]

A most salient fact about overweight in the United States is that average weight and relative body weight are increasing in all race and sex groups, according to national health surveys.[84] Obesity rose from

30.5% in 1999–2000 to 39.8% in 2015–16.[85] (Fig. 52-7). The prevalence of extreme overweight is increasing at a greater rate than is average weight.[85] This trend affects all gender and major ethnic groups.

The causes of mass obesity in populations are only partly understood. Widespread abundance, availability, and low cost of calorie-dense foods, along with many environmental cues to appetite, encourage overeating in relation to physiologic need. These environmental "facilitators" act on an apparently widespread genetic susceptibility to obesity. This, in turn, may be an evolutionary legacy from hunter-gatherer lifestyles. Moreover, there are other factors that enhance excess calorie intake relative to need. For example, dietary fat is more efficiently stored as adipose tissue than is carbohydrate under conditions of excess calorie intake.[34] Refined sugars have less satiety value than the complex carbohydrates of fruits and vegetables. In addition, alcohol is cheap and available in many societies.

One major cause of mass obesity in Western populations appears to be the increase of relative sedentariness. Americans are, on average, heavier now than they were earlier in this century when, in fact, they consumed significantly more calories per day.[34] The stable, rural, laboring populations that consume (and expend) more energy are, in turn, the leaner populations.[10] Unfortunately, however, sedentariness in populations is largely confounded with calorie density and other differences in eating patterns.

Comparisons among and within populations in the Seven Countries Study illustrate the complexity of the relationship of overweight and obesity to CHD and to death from all causes.[10,11] Among populations, CHD incidence is not correlated with any measure of obesity or overweight. The population distributions of skin-fold obesity are, however, strikingly different. They almost fail to overlap, for example, between the highest skin-fold values found among Serbian farmers and the lowest values among sedentary U.S. rail clerks.[10] Obesity is, therefore, a mass phenomenon and is apparently strongly determined by (a) the average energy expenditure of the population and (b) the composition (caloric density) of the diet.

Within populations, the picture is highly variable. In East Finns, with high CHD rates, incident CHD cases are evenly distributed across the entry distribution of skin-fold fatness and overweight. In another population with a high CHD incidence—U.S. railroad workers—the relationship between skin-fold obesity and CHD death is weakly positive, in contrast to an insignificant and opposite relationship for relative body weight. In another population with a high CHD incidence, consisting of rural Dutch men, there is a strongly positive linear relationship between CHD incidence and overweight and obesity throughout the wide range of values found there. Among men from the southern Mediterranean regions of Italy, Greece, and Yugoslavia, there is a U-shaped relationship between overweight or obesity and CHD risk, as well as with deaths from all causes. There the thinnest individuals as well as the heaviest and fattest have the higher disease rates; lowest disease risk is found for those with intermediate weight values.[10,11]

Multivariate analysis in the Seven Countries Study, used to adjust for the many confounding variables related alike to body mass and to CHD, shows no consistent relationship of 10-year CHD incidence with either relative weight or fatness.[11] In most of these populations, there is a tendency for CHD incidence to be slightly higher in the upper than in the lower half of the fatness distributions, but this tendency disappears when other variables are simultaneously considered. Similarly, except for men at the extremes of the distribution, within generally high-incidence and overweight U.S. populations, there is little relationship between obesity or overweight and risk of CHD or death in men.

Within populations, several other longitudinal studies, including the Framingham Heart Study,[86] the Evans County Study,[87] and the Manitoba Study,[88] suggest that an independent contribution of relative weight to risk in a society with high CHD incidence may be reflected only in very long-term CHD risk. In Framingham, in addition, weight gain since youth is a risk predictor for CHD.[86] Finally, in the Evans County Study, initial overweight and weight gain over time are also strongly related to the 7-year incidence of new hypertension.[87]

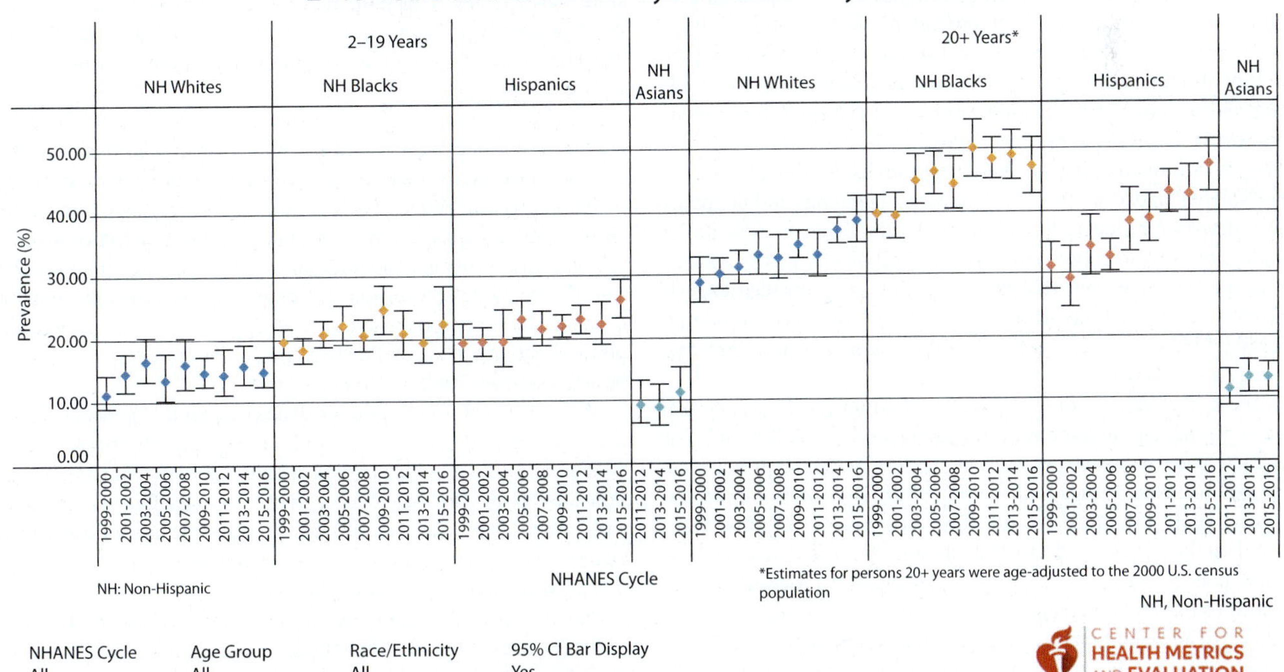

FIGURE 52-7. Trends in the prevalence of obesity in the United States among persons 2–19 years and 20+ years by race/ethnicity: NHANES, the United States, 1999–2000 through 2015–16. (*Source:* Reproduced with permission from American Heart Association. Center for Health Metrics and Evaluation (CHME). Data Visualizations. https://aha2017chme.wpengine.com/data-visualization/. Accessed January 2, 2020).

The ability to distinguish CVD risk according to the body distribution of obesity, usually measured as the ratio of waist to hip circumference (WHR), is also relevant.[89] WHR is positively related to risk of CHD, premature death, noninsulin-dependent diabetes mellitus, and cancers in women, as well as to established CVD risk factor levels. The finding that several diseases correlate better with fat distribution than with general measures of overweight or obesity has raised hypotheses about possible separate metabolic entities and about the pathogenesis, risk, and treatment of obesity.[90,91]

Results of autopsy studies are inconclusive. The International Atherosclerosis Project concluded that the degree and severity of atherosclerosis were not consistently associated with overweight and obesity.[92]

Finally, a major gap exists in our knowledge of the effect of weight reduction on disease risk in a relatively overweight society at high risk from combined CHD risk factors. This hugely confounded question, as well as the effects of weight cycling, remains to be clarified.[93]

In summary, obesity and overweight are centrally involved with the many metabolic maladaptations related to diabetes mellitus, hypertension, blood lipids, and probably atherogenesis. It is central to the metabolic syndrome.[23] These maladaptations are particularly amenable to correction by weight loss, with or without increased physical activity. The epidemiological evidence indicates, however, that relative body weight and obesity have a different disease-related significance in different populations and cultures. This may be due in part to different composition of the diets by which individuals and populations become obese, as well as to coexisting elevated distributions of other CVD risk characteristics. In most societies with high CHD incidence in which the issue has been systematically studied, the independent relationship between overweight, obesity, and CHD risk is seen mainly at the extremes of relative weight and over the longer term. Inconsistent disease associations and the obvious and dramatic declines in CVD deaths in the United States over the last 40 years, despite the clearly increased average U.S. body mass, indicate the primary importance for population CVD risk of factors other than overweight and obesity.

Physical Inactivity

Two primal human activities are the obtaining and consuming of food. Only since the advent of agriculture, and more recently of urbanization and industrialization, has the sustained subsistence activity of humans changed dramatically. In affluent industrial societies with automated occupations, motorized transport, and sedentary leisure, reduced energy expenditure is one of the more profound changes in human behavior. Aside from its likely importance as a fundamental departure from evolutionary adaptations and its apparently determining effect on mass obesity, the evidence specifically linking physical activity to chronic and CVD disease risk is difficult to obtain and interpret. A definitive, long-term controlled experiment on habitual activity with respect to CVD risk is not considered feasible.[94] Here is a brief synthesis of the evidence relating habitual activity to CHD risk.

The caliber of the coronary arteries at autopsy is larger in very active people, but limitations of design, method, feasibility, and cost have prevented a satisfactory study of the effect of exercise training on changes in coronary angiograms or functional measures of ischemia. Clinical trials of cardiac rehabilitation after myocardial infarction, including the effects of exercise training, are difficult. A meta-analysis found that cardiac prevention and rehabilitation programs in the context of risk factor management reduced CVD mortality and morbidity.[95] In addition to fatal and morbid outcomes, there is a growing consensus on the benefits of physical activity among patients with clinically significant CVDs including myocardial infarction, angina pectoris, peripheral vascular disease, and congestive heart failure. Symptom reduction, improved exercise tolerance and functional capacity, and improvement in psychological well-being and quality of life are among the benefits.[96] Exercise also improves lipids and blood pressure and helps control obesity.[97]

The major source of information about the role of physical activity in the primary prevention of CHD is indirect, from observational studies. These usually involve attempts to identify the confounding effects of lifestyle characteristics other than physical activity.[97] A review by Powell and colleagues[98] concluded that the majority of observational studies meeting their criteria found a significant and graded relationship between physical inactivity and the risk of first CHD event and that studies with a stronger design were more likely to show an effect. These authors calculated a median risk ratio of 1.9, that is, a 90% excess risk of CHD among physically inactive persons.

A subset of 16 studies from the review of Powell et al that measured individual levels of physical activity was added to studies from the Multiple Risk Factor Intervention Trial (MRFIT) and U.S. railroad workers.[97,99,100] All 18 studies showed that habitual physical activity was inversely related to death from CHD or death from all causes. The more recent studies adjusted for confounding risks and this adjustment usually diminished, but did not abolish, the risk associated with physical inactivity. Several studies found that the relation was largely explained by the level of physical fitness, in that the gradient of risk with the level of physical activity largely disappeared when measures of fitness were controlled. In a cohort study, fitness measured by a maximal exercise treadmill test predicted all-cause mortality for men and women, independently of other risk characteristics.[99,101]

The duration, frequency, and intensity of physical activity that may be protective against CHD remain, nevertheless, at issue. Recent studies suggest that an energy expenditure of 150–300 kcal daily, in activity of moderate intensity such as walking and working around the house, is associated with lower risk, as is a moderate amount of vigorous physical activity.[97,99,100,102] Anthropologic observations suggest that healthy farmers and herdsmen rarely work at a pace that leads to shortness of breath or exhaustion. Systematic observations in the Seven Countries Study indicate that even a substantial amount of regular, vigorous physical activity does not necessarily protect an individual or a population from CVD risk, particularly if other risk factors such as mass hypercholesterolemia are prevalent. In that study, farmers and loggers in eastern Finland were found to be the most physically active of men, and yet they had the highest rates of CHD; there was little less risk among the more physically active within that population.[10,11]

The interpretation of these many observations is that habitual, current physical activity very likely protects against coronary death.[97] A basic uncertainty that remains is whether the apparent benefit is due to physical activity itself or to its effect on other risk factors. People tend to exercise if they are able to and if they feel good when they exercise. Those who do not exercise may have subclinical or clinical disease. Fitness, a component strongly determined by constitution, may be a major contributor to an apparently protective effect of physical activity. It is possible that fitness determines both who will be active and who will be protected from CHD.

At least two other pieces of evidence suggest that genetics are not the major operant. Any protective effect of having once been a college athlete, and thus presumably genetically superior, disappears with time after graduation, whereas current physical activity is associated with lower risk.[103] Moreover, it seems that genetic factors are likely to be less important to participation in moderate exercise than to participation in vigorous exercise, but both carry a lower risk of CHD.

Finally, safety should be the foremost consideration both in prescribing exercise for individuals and in making recommendations for the public health. Several studies have found an excess risk of primary cardiac arrest during and shortly after strenuous exercise in all subjects, regardless of their level of habitual physical inactivity, despite a much lower overall risk of sudden coronary death in habitually active subjects.[104,105] They concluded that the reduced risk of sudden death due to regular physical activity was greater than the excess risk of sudden death during vigorous activity. This view, important for the public health, would be small comfort, however, to the families of those stricken while running. The evidence suggests that brisk walking or other moderately vigorous activity is the more reasonable exercise prescription, at least for sedentary and middle-aged people who have not maintained their fitness from youth.[97]

Diabetes and Hyperglycemia

Since the insulin era began, enabling persons with diabetes to survive, a strong relationship between Type 1 (insulin-dependent) diabetes and atherosclerosis risk has emerged. Most who die with diabetes succumb to advanced atherosclerosis. In addition, there are important mechanistic interrelations between insulin-glucose regulation, lipoprotein and uric acid metabolism, obesity and hypertension, on the one hand, and atherosclerosis on the other. Unfortunately, the prevalence of Type 2 diabetes in the U.S. population is rising associated with increasing obesity with an estimated 30.3 million diagnosed and undiagnosed adult diabetics in 2017.[106] The long-term effects of this trend are unknown but it may undermine the advances in CVD prevalence and mortality.

The association of clinical diabetes mellitus with CHD and atherosclerotic manifestations is documented clinically, pathologically, and epidemiologically.[107,108] It is thought that hyperinsulinemia, hypoglycemic episodes, or both in treated diabetics, coupled (formerly) with the common prescription of a high-fat, low-carbohydrate low-fiber diet, increases vascular complications. Cross-cultural comparisons suggest that the risk of atherosclerosis and CVD in diabetic patients is indeed related to factors other than the glucose-insulin disorder itself. For example, apparently low rates of atherosclerosis exist in diabetic eastern Jews, Chinese, and Southwest American Indians.[107,108] The Pima Indians of Arizona are thought to be an example of the theoretical "thrifty genotype," that is, a population only recently (in evolutionary terms) exposed to calorie abundance, that frequently (50% of adults) develops an obese, diabetic phenotype but nevertheless manifests little CVD.[109]

In longitudinal studies among cohorts, clinical diabetes mellitus is associated with excess CHD risk and severity of CHD, and many studies confirm the excess of fatal myocardial infarction in women with diabetes.[110] The excess risk among diabetics is not always differentiated by the degree of hyperglycemia or the degree of control. Much of the excess CHD risk in diabetics is, in fact, accounted for by associated risk variables.[107,108] More severe atherosclerosis, diabetic cardiomyopathy, and a hypercoagulable state are also thought to contribute to the excess risk of diabetes.[108] Finally, in most autopsy studies, coronary artery disease and the frequency and severity of myocardial infarction are greater in diabetics than in control subjects.[108,111]

In healthy persons, glucose intolerance alone is weakly and inconsistently associated with CVD risk.[109,112] However, high insulin activity was found to be a significant independent predictor of coronary events in cohorts studied in Australia, France, and Finland,[108] and it has also been proposed as a cause of excess atherosclerosis in Asian migrants.[112]

Diabetic treatment by the control of blood glucose levels is the mainstay of therapy. However, the role of glucose control in the reduction of cardiovascular and other complications has been controversial. The University Group Diabetes Program (UGDP) reported an increased rate of myocardial infarction with the use of first-generation sulfonyl ureas despite effective blood glucose control.[113] These effects are not seen with later agents.[114] The Diabetes Control and Complications Trial (DCCT) studied "tight" glucose control in insulin-dependent diabetics. Findings included significant reduction in retinopathy, microalbuminuria, and clinical neuropathy. Elevated LDL cholesterol levels were also reduced with tight control.[115] Cardiovascular and peripheral vascular disease were also reduced, but did not reach significance.[116] A meta-analysis of clinical trials of the hypoglycemic drug rosiglitazone found increases in myocardial infarction and cardiovascular death.[112] These observations led the Food and Drug Administration to offer guidelines for including cardiovascular outcomes in glucose lowering medications in 2008. Since then there have been a number of trials of high-risk type 2 diabetic patients with SLGT-2, DPP4 inhibitors and GLP-1 receptor agonist classes. These have confirmed cardiovascular safety and some may even lower CVD risk.[117]

In summary, the relationship between diabetes, atherosclerosis, and coronary disease is well established among persons with clinical diabetes living under the conditions of affluent Western culture. Data from other cultures suggest, however, that other factors, such as physical activity, body weight, blood pressure, blood lipid levels, dietary composition, and smoking habits, greatly affect the risk of CHD among diabetics. This, plus evidence that the metabolic disorders of middle-age persons with diabetes can be significantly improved through exercise and modified by diet and weight loss, provide a sound rationale for preventive practice. More study of these complex issues is needed to develop an effective preventive approach to non-insulin-dependent diabetes mellitus itself.

Elevated Blood Pressure: Hypertension

It is estimated that hypertension contributes to more than one-half of adult deaths in the United States.[118] It is a strong and independent risk factor for CHD and stroke, and there are plausible mechanisms for its effects on atherosclerosis and vascular disease. Patients with CHD have higher average blood pressure than control subjects. Experimental atherosclerosis induced in animals is directly related to pressure levels within the arterial system. In cohort studies, elevated blood pressure is positively, continuously, and independently related to CHD risk, according to increasing levels of systolic or diastolic blood pressures. The relationship of elevated blood pressure to risk of cerebrovascular hemorrhage and congestive heart failure is even stronger than the relationship to risk of CHD and thrombotic stroke.

The preventive potential for hypertension control is illustrated by drug trials that have demonstrated a significant decrease in rate of stroke and heart failure. The Systolic Hypertension in the Elderly Project (SHEP) demonstrated the importance of systolic blood pressure control in this group.[119] Results of other trials suggest that CHD risk is lowered by control of hypertension, but most have had insufficient power to study this question.[120] The ALLHAT study treated hypertension with diuretics and more recent antihypertensive drugs with CHD as an endpoint. There was no placebo group. They found thiazide-type diuretics to be superior to more modern agents for combined CVD, stroke and heart failure.[121] More recently, the Randomized Trial of Intensive versus Standard Blood-Pressure Control (SPRINT) found that reducing systolic blood pressure to a target of 120 mm Hg resulted in lower rates of fatal and nonfatal major cardiovascular events and death from any cause.[122]

Blood pressure control has greatly improved in the United States in the last 40 years, according to surveys showing a substantial decrease in the proportion of hypertensive persons unidentified or not under control.[58,123,124] These trends have occurred in parallel with downward trends for both CHD and stroke mortality, although a direct relationship cannot be established. In fact, the mortality rate from stroke was diminishing long before safe and effective antihypertensive therapy was widely used. Moreover, stroke death rates in the United States fell during the 1950s and 1960s, when CHD death rates were rising sharply.[16]

Estimated changes in death rates for CHD and stroke, based on models of hypertension control, suggest a large potential for the prevention of CVD. Primary prevention of hypertension would likely have even more impressive effects on the public health.

Present challenges to preventive practice lie mainly in more effective control of elevated blood pressure in the elderly, among persons living in poverty, and in finding the ideal combination of drug and hygienic management for correction of mild or borderline levels of high blood pressure. The larger public health challenge lies in improvement of population wide correlates of hypertension, such as physical inactivity, overweight, and high salt and alcohol intake. Such primary preventive and public health approaches promise to minimize the exhibition of high blood pressure, since human populations are apparently widely susceptible.

Tobacco Smoking

The broader relationship of tobacco to disease and health is detailed elsewhere in this text Chapter 166: Tobacco Use and Tobacco Use Disorder. In the past, clinical evidence of a direct relationship between cigarette smoking and coronary disease was anecdotal. Experimentally, ischemic pain, angiographic coronary spasm, and electrocardiographic findings are now demonstrated during smoking in patients with compromised coronary circulation.[125]

For individuals living within societies with a high CHD incidence, smoking is consistently found to be a strong and independent risk factor for myocardial infarction and sudden death.[126] The risk is continuous from persons who have never smoked, to ex-smokers, to those who smoke even in small amounts and is also related to duration of the habit.[127] Interactions with other risk factors are also important, as indicated by the weak association of smoking with CHD risk in low-risk societies.[10,11] For example, the observed incidence of CHD in populations that do not have a base of relative mass hypercholesterolemia is much lower than the risk predicted with multiple regression equations derived from U.S. or northern Europe data. The Japanese, for example, with a heavy prevalence of smoking and substantial amounts of hypertension, but without hypercholesterolemia, show much less coronary heart disease than would be predicted.[10,11]

As is the case with serum cholesterol level, most of the CHD cases attributable to smoking derive from the central part of the distribution, that is, light and moderate smokers; the prevalence of heavy smokers is low. A 17% population-attributable risk fraction for smoking and CHD deaths in the United States was estimated (conservatively) in the Carter Report.[128] Smoking is particularly significant in CHD risk among women.[129]

Smoking cessation is associated with lower CHD rates according to years of cessation.[130] While those who have never smoked have the best disease experience, long-term quitters approximate their rates, and even temporary quitters have a better risk experience than persistent smokers.[131] Improvement in the prognosis of survivors of myocardial infarction who quit smoking also tend to confirm the harmful cardiovascular effects of cigarettes and supports the potential for CHD prevention by reduction of tobacco use.[127,132]

The recent advent of electronic cigarettes (e-cigarettes) presents a potential new public health problem. They are touted as safer than regular cigarettes and a method for smoking cessation. However, they are increasingly marketed by tobacco companies and may be a gateway to tobacco use among youth. There is limited evidence of CVD effects given the recency of these devices but there is reason to postulate adverse outcomes from the nicotine and other chemicals inhaled.[133]

Synthesis of this evidence, therefore, suggests that cigarette smoking is neither a primary nor a necessary factor in determining population rates of CHD. It is, rather, a strong and independent risk factor for CHD and vascular disease among individuals living in high-incidence populations where there is a significant background of coronary and peripheral atherosclerosis.

Mechanisms presumed to be important in CHD include the physicochemical effects of tobacco, that is, increased heart rate and myocardial contractility and greater myocardial oxygen demand due to raised catecholamine levels, decreased oxygen-carrying capacity of the blood, elevated fibrinogen levels, and platelet-aggregating effects. Other possible mechanisms include elevated fasting blood glucose levels and white blood cell-counts and lower HDL levels, all found among smokers.[125]

A public health policy to foster so-called "safer cigarettes," at least with respect to lowering CVD risk, is not supported by the evidence of persistent high exposure to gas-phase toxins in "low-yield" cigarette users.[125] Moreover, the promotion and adoption of Western-type cigarettes and smoking patterns in developing countries augurs ill for the future CVD risk in those populations. In contrast, smoking prevalence has decreased substantially in the United States, where large numbers of educated adults, in particular, have stopped smoking.[134] This is attributed to increased community awareness of the health need to stop smoking, to social pressure and legislation for "clean indoor air" and "smoke-free" environments, increased taxation and to a greater access to the support and skills needed for quitting. The downward U.S. trend in smoking is not as evident, however, among lower socioeconomic groups and heavy smokers.[135]

Under "ideal" supportive circumstances, such as that given high-risk participants in the MRFIT, smoking cessation success rates approximate 40% in the first year, with maintenance of this rate for up to 4 years among volunteer participants. Thus, a long-standing medical pessimism about helping patients stop smoking might be replaced by optimism for cessation programs that are systematically applied. Moreover, communitywide educational and legislative efforts are increasingly effective.[136,137] The results of all these efforts and the population trends downward in smoking frequency provide a rational basis for more public programs and for a more focused national policy to reduce cigarette smoking and tobacco production. It is equally possible that the currently declining rate of cigarette smoking will level off, unless educational programs and wider social support for nonsmoking reach the lower socioeconomic classes and heavy smokers. In addition, despite the effectiveness of these broad policy and clinical interventions, declines in smoking have not been the same across all levels of social and economic status, resulting in significant disparities in smoking and smoking-related CHD in the United States today.

Hemostatic Factors

For decades, arguments have existed about the relative predominance of the role of classical risk factors versus thrombosis in the pathogenesis of atherosclerosis and CHD. A more unified theory now joins the effects of diet and blood lipids, physical activity and smoking, and diabetes and insulin levels to atherosclerosis and to thrombosis. The interaction between chronic arterial wall disease and the blood properties leading to clot formation continues to be a major subject for research as it becomes clear that a critical fixed obstructive lesion is not necessary for myocardial infarction. In fact, thrombi forming on so-called "soft plaques," which rupture account for a significant proportion of acute events.[138] The components of the coagulation system found so far to be of major interest are platelets and fibrin and they aggregate when cell walls are damaged and develop fibrin platelet masses, and platelet aggregation.[139,140]

Of the several hemostatic variables measured with respect to subsequent CHD risk, fibrinogen has received the most attention. Several investigators conclude that an elevated fibrinogen level is likely to be causally associated with CHD but that its elevation overall may be due primarily to smoking.[139]

As for primary prevention of CHD events with low-level anticoagulation, such as with small doses of aspirin, this appears now to be established for nonfatal myocardial infarction in adults, particularly between ages 50–59 with at least a 10% risk of 10-year CVD mortality.[141,142]

Physical Environment

It is increasingly apparent that modern industrialized society developed an environment not conducive to good health.[143] Communities are built without parks, playgrounds, libraries, nearby stores, sidewalks, or public transit. The result is dependence on personal automobiles and social isolation. These environments may actually promote chronic diseases such as CHD. There is increasing understanding of the effects of these practices and attempts to promote healthier community designs.

The weather, particularly the influx of cold fronts and rapid falls in barometric pressure, has been correlated with new hospital admissions for coronary events and sudden death.[144] Reasonable preventive practice includes advice to avoid exposure, in particular the combination of isometric work and cold, and to use light face masks to maintain a favorable personal air temperature and humidity.

Similarly, atmospheric inversions and air pollution are related to hospitalization and death rates from pulmonary and CVDs, particularly in the elderly. These observations are increasingly linked to specific environmental pollution agents including nitrogen, sulfur dioxide, ozone, lead, and particulate matter.[145] Most recently fire particles ($PM_{2.5}$) < 2.5 μm have received attention. The result of combustion, they easily reach the alveoli. Experimental data suggests they may play a role in the acute onset of CVDs particularly among those with atherosclerosis.

Social Support

Several prospective population-based studies have established social support or "social connectedness" as a factor associated with reduced risk of death. Two large studies—one from Finland[146] and one from Sweden[147]—examined CVD disease risk. The pattern of results suggests a relationship between social support and mortality, at least in men. Whether this is a causal relationship or is attributable to a confounding variable such as baseline health or to personality characteristics such as hostility is unclear, and this line of investigation might well be continued.

Attempts have been made to change psychosocial characteristics experimentally and to measure CHD risk factors and disease changes. Recently, the enhancing recovery in coronary heart disease patients (ENRICH) trial tested cognitive behavioral therapy and antidepression medications postmyocardial infarction to increase social support and decrease depression. The trial showed no difference in the endpoint of recurrent myocardial infarction and death.[148]

Gender and Estrogens

The excess risk of CHD and atherosclerosis in men at earlier ages is documented throughout affluent Western society. The sex differential is much less prominent, however, in nonwhite populations and in areas where the overall incidence is relatively low.[149] The particular susceptibility of men is only partly explained by their higher risk factor configurations between the ages of 25 and 60. On the other hand, the relative protection from CHD among premenopausal women is thought to be related to hormones, although the effect of early oophorectomy, menopause, or estrogen replacement therapy explains these differences. In countries with a high incidence of CHD, where there is relative mass hyperlipidemia much more of the plasma cholesterol is carried in the HDL fraction in women. Recent experimental evidence concerning mechanisms of LDL and HDL function, related to cell receptors and lipid transport in and out of the arterial wall, confirm this particular biological difference as a likely cause for some of the sex difference in CHD risk.

In contrast, women have a proportionately greater risk of angina pectoris than of myocardial infarction or sudden death. While they have less severe atherosclerosis in the coronary arteries, the sex difference is not as apparent in cerebral, aortic, and peripheral vessels. Survival of women after myocardial infarction is poorer in-hospital, although this is balanced by greater out-of-hospital death for men.

Finally, trends in CHD deaths in the United States indicate that the age-specific decline in mortality is proportionately greater in women than in men.[16] Similarly, the rise in CHD death rates among women in Eastern Europe, where CVD deaths overall are increasing rapidly, is proportionately greater in women and in young women.[150]

The excess risk of thromboembolism, stroke, and myocardial infarction in women taking oral contraceptives (OCs), and the interaction of OCs with age and smoking, are well established. Young women taking OCs have systematically higher serum lipid levels, higher blood pressure, and impaired glucose tolerance compared with control subjects.[151]

Numerous epidemiologic studies evaluated the use of postmenopausal estrogen in the primary prevention of CVD.[152] Meta-analysis suggested a relative risk of 0.50–0.65 for coronary artery disease in estrogen users.[153] These data exemplify the danger of extrapolating observational studies to therapeutic lesions. When randomized studies of hormone replacement therapy were initially performed the Heart and Estrogen/Progestin Replacement Study (HERS) and the Women's Health Initiative (WHI) trial, no benefit and potential harm was observed.[154,155] More recent analyses that have stratified WHI findings by age, and the Early Versus Late Intervention Trial (ELITE) of estradiol therapy at varying ages of initiation, suggest that starting estrogen within 5–10 years after menopause is a critical component of its cardioprotective effects, while minimizing adverse effects. Long-term follow-up studies of the WHI are ongoing, but are suggestive of cardioprotection when initiated in this window.[156,157]

In summary, the sex differential for atherosclerosis and CVD events and their time trends is not completely explained on the basis of known effects of hormones on the level of risk factors. More study of gender difference is needed.

Genetic Factors

Much current work is opening up the understanding of host–environment relationships. The relative contribution of genes to disease risk of populations can be exaggerated, however, by studies of gene effects when limited to homogeneous, high-risk cultures where exposure is great and universal. Most of the lack of understanding, and much of the difficulty in identification of susceptible persons, lies in the unavailability of specific genetic markers for CVD and the incapacity of family studies to discriminate intrinsic components without such markers.[158] Findings of the gene loci for apolipoprotein regulation hold great promise of an improved understanding of individual differences in blood lipoproteins and their response to diet. There is, for example, evidence of the genetic inheritance of LDL subclasses HDL, apo-B, and apo-E.[148] A substantial proportion of the variation in apo-B levels (43%) may be explained by a major locus.[159] A major gene controlling LDL subclasses may account for much of the familial aggregation of blood lipids and CHD risk.[160]

Most intrinsic blood lipoprotein regulation, however, is clearly polygenic and strongly interactive with the environment, especially with composition of the habitual diet. Controlled experiments in metabolically normal people suggest that there is a normal distribution of individual blood lipid responses to a known dietary change.[161]

The rare major gene effects that cause extreme manifestations of the hyperlipidemias are increasingly well characterized, but they account for only a small fraction of the mass phenomenon of hypercholesterolemia found in affluent cultures. Thus, most atherosclerotic complications and most of the excess CHD events in the general population cannot be attributed to major gene effects. Nevertheless, gene-culture interactions remain important to preventive practice for better detection and individualized therapy of patients who have elevated blood lipid values.

Genetic control of CVD risk factors other than blood lipids is even less well known.[162] For example, not yet identified are genetic traits that might affect individual sensitivity to salt intake, to the atherogenic effect of cigarette smoking, or to the regulation of blood insulin and glucose levels, arterial wall enzymes, or personality type. There has been growing research on the genetics of hypertension. Markers have been discovered in a disease, which is most likely polygenic.[163]

The public health view that a favorable environment assures minimal expression of phenotypic risk provides the rationale for a population approach to prevention. This rationale has not been effectively challenged, but neither has it been universally accepted.

Combined Risk Factors

Clinical, laboratory, and epidemiological studies of CVD risk factors have been oriented mainly toward determining individual causal roles for each factor. CVDs are clearly related, however, in both individuals and communities, to multiple factors operating together over time. Multiple-factor risk is firmly established and actually is quantified for both CHD and stroke. Based mainly on Framingham and Pooling Project analysis, a consistent, independent, and at least additive contribution is found for each of the major risk factors: cigarette smoking, arterial blood pressure, and total serum cholesterol level.[63] The risk ratio between highest and lowest categories for combined risk within populations is approximately eight- to tenfold, in contrast to the risk ratio for single risk factors, which is approximately two- to fourfold.

Prediction regressions derived from follow-up experience in European men, with the use of four major risk factors at baseline, when applied to men in the United States, show the multiple-risk concept to be "universal." That is, the regressions define a continuum of CHD risk among individual U.S. men in a society that has quite different CHD rates overall.[164] The slope of the relationship (regression) between the combined risk factors and disease, however, is much steeper in the United States than in the European population. At any given level of multiple risk, U.S. rates are twice those in Europe. This cultural difference in the "force" of risk factors indicates that a sizable influence on population differences in CHD risk remains unknown, although lifelong exposure to CHD risk is not captured in a single measure. Another indication of the combined force of risk factors comes from studies of low risk groups within industrialized populations. Those with low lipids, normal blood pressure, nonsmokers, nonobese, and without diabetes have very low CHD and stroke rates.[165–167] Nevertheless, since these few risk factors operate universally and explain a substantial part of individual and population risk differences, public health action on that part of the difference now explained is both promising and indicated.

Still another interpretation of the evidence of combined risk of CHD is that the synergism between risk characteristics leads to a major potential for preventive effects in the population by achieving relatively small shifts in the means and distributions of the multiple risk factors. This does not exclude the possibility of a population threshold for risk factors, below which population risk is remote. That is indicated by the relative scarcity of mass atherosclerosis and CHD in societies in which average serum total cholesterol levels are less than 200 mg/dL. Nor does it exclude the concept of necessary versus contributory causes. In the absence of the presumed necessary factor (i.e., mass hypercholesterolemia), population risk is negligible. It may be that the departures from perfect prediction, found with the use of multiple regression analysis, are due in part to their failure to include the duration of exposure to, or the directionality of, a particular risk level.

RHEUMATIC HEART DISEASE

Rheumatic fever and rheumatic heart disease remain important worldwide public health problems.[168] They are particular problems where poverty, overcrowding, malnutrition, and inadequate medical care are found.[169–175] Even in industrialized societies, a relatively high prevalence of rheumatic fever persists in pockets of poverty, and outbreaks have been reported in affluent areas.[176–181] Despite that rheumatic fever is demonstrably preventable and rheumatic heart disease has declined dramatically in most industrialized nations, this condition remains a major public health problem internationally.

For more than 80 years it has been known that group A streptococcus infection underlies initial and recurrent attacks of rheumatic fever (see Chapter 155). The immunologic mechanisms and circumstances by which infection with this organism produces rheumatic fever and rheumatic heart disease and acute and chronic glomerulonephritis are well understood.[182] In some surveys, as many as 3% of patients develop rheumatic fever after known streptococcal infections.[183] As many as 50% of those who have once had rheumatic fever will, if untreated, experience attacks after a subsequent streptococcal infection. This suggests that host factors significantly determine susceptibility. Age is also an obvious factor, for example, infants do not develop rheumatic fever even though they are susceptible to streptococcal infection. Such differences in susceptibility are clearly developmental, such as the variation with age, but others may have a genetic basis. The tendency of rheumatic fever to cluster in families, however, may be explained by shared environment as well as genes.

A worldwide decrease in acute rheumatic fever incidence is observed since the early twentieth century. This trend has been attributed to improved living conditions, the use of antibiotics for strep pharyngitis and possibly shifting strep serotypes. Recent increases observed in Mexico and the Western Pacific may be the result of improved detection.[184,185] While the incidence of acute rheumatic fever is decreasing, the prevalence of rheumatic heart disease appears to be increasing worldwide. This may be the result of improved detection with echocardiography and advances in medical and surgical treatments leading to improved survival.[184,186]

The diagnosis of acute rheumatic fever is made principally from clinical findings with the revised Jones criteria (see Chap. 155). These may be insensitive, however, to detect mild cases, particularly in Western countries where clinical patterns have changed so that arthritis is often the only presenting manifestation. Chorea, subcutaneous nodules, and erythema marginatum are now rarely seen. Diagnosis may be complicated by the lack of a preceding sore throat or an apparent infection.

Current recommendations by the American Heart Association for the primary prevention of acute rheumatic fever and rheumatic heart disease and prophylaxis for bacterial endocarditis in those with known rheumatic valve disease are published elsewhere.[187]

CONGENITAL HEART DISEASE

Malformations of the cardiovascular system are among the more frequently occurring congenital defects. They result from developmental errors caused by inherent defects in the genetic material of the embryo, environmental factors, or both and account for almost one-third of congenital anomalies.[188–192]

Family studies suggest that the offspring of parents with congenital heart disease have malformation rates ranging from 1.4% to 16.1%.[193] Identical twins are both affected 25–30% of the time. While these and other findings of familial aggregation suggest genetic factors, common environment may also play a role.[192] Noncardiac inherited disorders also produce cardiovascular defects; these include Marfan's syndrome, Friedreich's ataxia, glycogen storage disease, and Down's and Turner's syndromes.

Maternal viral infections during pregnancy are estimated to cause up to 10% of all congenital cardiac malformations. Rubella in the first 2 months of pregnancy is associated with congenital malformations in about 80% of live births and is thought to account for 2–4% of all congenital heart disease. Subclinical Coxsackie virus infections may be related to congenital heart disease. Acute hypoxia, residence at high altitudes, high carboxyhemoglobin levels, and uterine vascular changes from cigarette smoking are other potential causes.[191] Maternal x-ray exposure results in an increased incidence of Down's syndrome and possibly other congenital defects.[190] Maternal metabolic defects, such as diabetes mellitus and phenylketonuria, are associated with increased incidence of congenital heart defects.

Data on the true incidence of congenital heart disease are limited. The chief sources of information are birth certificate and hospital birth data.[189] Birth certificate data usually underestimate the true rate as the defect may not be discovered until later. It is estimated that there are 36,000 births with congenital heart disease in the United States and 1.5 million worldwide annually.[8,194] Incidence is estimated at 8 per 1000 births including stillbirths and planned abortions.[8] The common congenital malformation, bicuspid aortic valve, is rarely discovered until later adult life with an estimated incidence of 13.7 per 1000 births.[8] Most are correctable by modern medical and surgical methods, including cardiac transplantation; it is estimated that only one child per 1000 cannot be helped by such approaches.[195] As a result, infant mortality from congenital CVD has fallen steadily (Fig. 52-8). As with other conditions, mortality among black youth has fallen less than for whites. The correction of congenital defects by surgical and other interventions is an important factor in increasing survival. Patients who have been repaired live into adulthood presenting new challenges in their care and increased mortality compared to unaffected adults.[194,196,197]

Although the overall incidence of congenital heart disease has apparently remained stable, the distribution of types of defects may be shifting. This includes unexplained increases in ventricular septal defects and patent ductus arteriosus. A decline in the number of infants born with rubella-caused defects may be explained by vaccination programs.[198]

Primary prevention of congenital heart disease includes the following established measures[199]:

1. Genetic counseling of potential parents and families with congenital heart disease;
2. Rubella immunization programs;
   a. Identification of susceptible women of childbearing age by serologic examination,
   b. Immunization of susceptible women,
   c. Avoidance of pregnancy for 2 months after rubella vaccination,
3. Avoidance of exposure to viral diseases during pregnancy;
4. Administration of all usual vaccines to all children to eliminate reservoirs of infection;
5. Avoidance of radiation during pregnancy;
6. Avoidance of exposure to gas fumes, air pollution, cigarettes, alcohol, pesticides, herbicides, and high altitude during the first trimester of pregnancy; and
7. Avoidance of drugs of any kind during the first trimester of pregnancy, especially drugs of known or suspected teratogenic potential.

CARDIOMYOPATHIES AND MYOCARDITIS

Cardiomyopathies are a broad group of cardiac diseases that involve the heart muscle. Although less common in industrialized nations, they are estimated for 30% or more of heart disease deaths in some developing countries.[200] Cardiomyopathies are of diverse etiology and classification systems have evolved as knowledge has increased. Originally, they classified by the functional results of their effects on the myocardium: dilated or congestive, hypertrophic and restrictive. Subsequently, in 1995, the WHO recommended classification by the pathophysiology: dilated, hypertrophic, restrictive, arrhythmogenic right ventricular and unclassified.[201] Increased data about etiology has resulted in three major categories: genetic, acquired, and mixed or unknown.[202,203]

Some cardiomyopathies are diagnosed in their acute phase, where inflammation of the myocardium is common (myocarditis). While myocarditis is particularly difficult to categorize, diagnosis has been facilitated by the widespread use of endomyocardial biopsy. These techniques have suggested that an inflammatory reaction is more common than was previously suspected. Identified causes include infectious, metabolic, toxic, allergic, and genetic factors.[204] Myocarditis and cardiomyopathy may be mild and undetected but also can be rapidly fatal with progressive heart failure.

In industrialized nations, cardiomyopathies appear to be increasing in prevalence, although it is unclear whether there is an actual increase or an increase in professional awareness and improved diagnostic techniques.[205] The latter include use of the echocardiogram, Doppler flow studies, and catheter-based endomyocardial biopsy. Surveillance of Olmsted County, Minnesota, found an incidence of idiopathic dilated cardiomyopathy of 6 per 100,000 person years. Overall prevalence was 35.3 per 100,000 population.[206] Mortality from cardiomyopathy in the United States varies by age, race, and sex (Fig. 52-9). Mortality is higher in blacks than whites and greater in men than women. Mortality increases with age, suggesting the pattern of a chronic condition.

Alcohol abuse is an important cause of cardiomyopathy, accounting for approximately 8% of all cases in the United States.[205,207] Alcohol causes myocardial damage by several mechanisms.[208,209] These include (a) a direct toxic effect, (b) effects of thiamine deficiencies, and (c) effects of additives such as cobalt in alcoholic beverages. Abstinence from alcohol may halt or even reverse the cardiomyopathy.[210]

Another major cause of cardiomyopathy in industrialized countries is viral infection, particularly Coxsackie B virus, echovirus, influenza, and polio,[211] often beginning as a viral myocarditis. Subclinical viral disease is thought to be more common than was

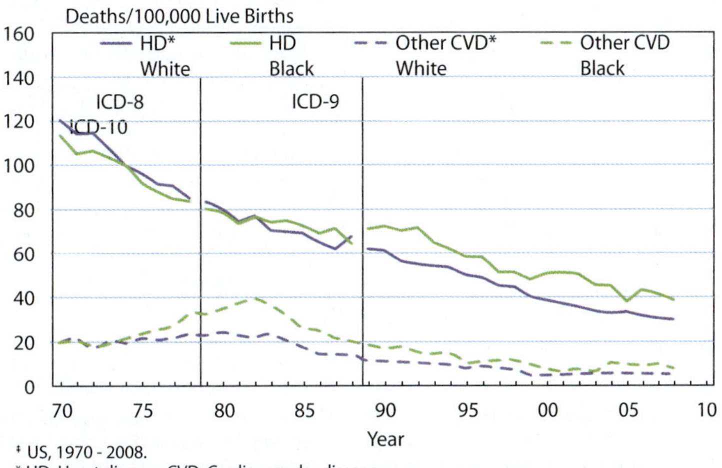

FIGURE 52-8. Infant mortality from congenital malformations of the circulatory system by race, the United States, 1970–2008. (*Source:* National Heart, Lung, and Blood Institute. Morbidity and mortality chart book on cardiovascular, lung, and blood diseases. Bethesda, MD: NIH Publication;2012.)

previously suspected, with most patients recovering without damage. More severe forms, however, result in dilated cardiomyopathy and death due to congestive heart failure or arrhythmias. Recent research has suggested an autoimmune component and indicated that immunosuppressive therapy may be helpful in modifying the disease.[212] However, clinical trials have shown no benefit for corticosteroids.[213]

Hypertrophic cardiomyopathy (HCM) is another cause of death.[214] Largely undetected until the advent of echocardiographic techniques, it is becoming increasingly clear that this condition can be fatal and be managed with pharmacologic therapy.[214] An Italian registry for HCM found a majority of patients were male (62%) and 89% were New York Heart Association class I–II. Most were in their fourth to sixth decade of life. Cardiovascular mortality was 1% per year, mainly due to heart failure.[215] The genetic origins of this condition are recognized.[203,216] In South and Central America, trypanosomiasis (Chagas' disease) is endemic; an estimated 20 million people are afflicted.[217] Extensive chronic myocarditis with heart failure may be observed years after the initial infection with the trypanosome. An acute infectious phase, characterized by fulminant and fatal myocarditis, occurs mainly in children. In most cases, however, an average of 20 years passes before Chagas' cardiomyopathy becomes clinically apparent. An autoimmune process may play some role in the disease.[218] Diagnosis is made by means of serologic study or a xenodiagnostic test. Although antiparasitic agents, such as nitroimidazole derivatives, can alter the acute infestation, there is little evidence that they are effective for the cardiomyopathy.[200]

There is increasing awareness of cardiomyopathy in Africa where it is suspected to be higher than reported based on autopsy studies.[219] Unfortunately, there are few data on etiology and prevalence.

PREVENTIVE STRATEGIES

Most of CVD is preventable with public health approaches. A population approach to CVD prevention has been formally outlined by the World Health Organization.[7] It embraces both the systematic practice of screening and education for high risk, where national priorities can afford such practices, and broad public health policy and programs in health promotion for communities.

Strategies for preventive practice are now widely available. Community-based strategies, programs, and materials are becoming available. National programs are under way in blood pressure control, diet and blood lipids, and smoking. Finally, health promotion resource centers are now established for training in the design and dissemination of preventive programs. The student and the health worker are referred to these sources: the Centers for Disease Control and Prevention, Atlanta, GA (https://www.cdc.gov/heartdisease/prevention.htm); and the National Heart Lung and Blood Institute, Bethesda, MD (www.nhlbi.nih.gov).

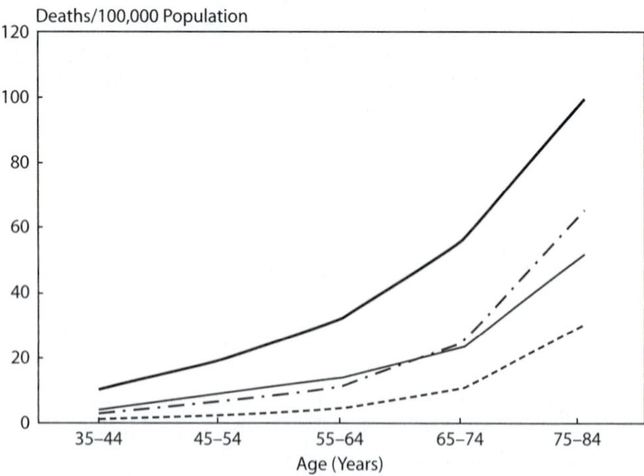

FIGURE 52-9. Death rates for cardiomyopathy by age, race, and sex, the United States, 2008. (*Source:* National Heart, Lung, and Blood Institute. Morbidity and mortality chart book on cardiovascular, lung, and blood diseases. Bethesda, MD: NIH Publication; 2012.)

References

1. Roth GA, Huffman MD, Moran AE, et al. Global and regional patterns in cardiovascular mortality from 1990 to 2013. *Circulation.* 2015;132(17):1667–78.
2. Sidney S, Quesenberry CP, Jaffe MG, et al. Recent trends in cardiovascular mortality in the United States and public health goals. *JAMA Cardiol.* 2016;1(5):594–9.
3. Ogden CL, Carroll MD, Kit BK, Flegal KM. Prevalence of childhood and adult obesity in the United States, 2011–2012. *JAMA.* 2014;311(8):806–14.
4. CDC's Division of Diabetes Translation. National Diabetes Surveillance System. Long-term trends in diabetes. http://www.cdc.gov/diabetes/statistics/slides/long_term_trends.pdf. Published October 2014. Accessed March 20, 2016.
5. World Health Organization. World Health Statistics. https://apps.who.int/iris/handle/10665/332070. 2017.
6. Kuerbis A, Sacco P, Blazer DG, Moore AA. Substance abuse among older adults. *Clin Geriatr Med.* 2014;30(3):629–54.
7. World Health Organization. Prevention of Coronary Heart Disease: Report of a WHO Expert Committee. WHO Technical Report Series, No. 678. Geneva; 1982.
8. Benjamin EJ, Blaha MJ, Chiuve SE, et al. American Heart Association Statistics Committee and Stroke Statistics Subcommittee. Heart disease and stroke statistics—2017 Update: A report from the American Heart Association. *Circulation.* 2017;135(10):E146–603.
9. The Multiple Risk Factor Intervention Trial Research Group. Mortality after 16 years for participants randomized to the Multiple Risk Factor Intervention Trial. *Circulation.* 1996;94(5):946–51.
10. Keys A. Coronary heart disease in seven countries. *Circulation.* 1970;(Suppl I):41–2.
11. Keys A. *Seven Countries: Death and Coronary Heart Disease in Ten Years.* Cambridge, MA: Harvard University Press; 1979.
12. Gordon T, Garcia-Palmieri MR, Kagan A, Kannel WB, Schiffman J. Differences in coronary heart disease in Framingham, Honolulu and Puerto Rico. *J Chronic Dis.* 1974;27(7–8):329–44.
13. Rose G. Incubation period of coronary heart disease. *Br Med J.* 1982;284:1600–1.
14. McGill HCJr.McGill HCJr., ed ed. *Geographic Pathology of Atherosclerosis.* Baltimore: Williams & Wilkins; 1968.
15. Marmot MG, Syme SL, Kagan A, et al. Epidemiologic studies of coronary heart disease and stroke in Japanese men living in Japan, Hawaii and California: Prevalence of coronary and hypertensive heart disease and associated risk factors. *Am J Epidemiol.* 1975;102(6):514–25.
16. Higgens MW, Luerpker RV. Trends and determinants of coronary heart disease mortality: International comparisons. *Int J Epidemiol.* 1989;18(Suppl 1):S1–2.
17. McGovern PG, Jacobs DRJr, Shahar E et al. Trends in acute coronary heart disease mortality, morbidity, and medical care from 1985 through 1997: The Minnesota Heart Survey. *Circulation.* 2001;104(1):19–24.
18. Tunstall-Pedoe H, Kuulasmaa K, Tolonen H, et al. In: Tunstall-Pedoe H, ed. *With 64 Other Contributors for the WHO MONICA Project, in MONICA Monograph and Multimedia Sourcebook.* Geneva: World Health Organization; 2003.
19. Luepker RV. Falling coronary heart disease rates: A better explanation? (Editorial). *Circulation.* 2016;133(1):8–11.
20. Stern MP. The recent decline in ischemic heart disease mortality. *Ann Intern Med.* 1979;91(4):630–40.
21. Luepker, RV. Epidemiology of atherosclerotic disease in population groups. In: Pearson TA, Criqui MH, Luepker RV, Oberman A, Winston M, eds. *Primer in Preventive Cardiology.* Dallas, TX: American Heart Association; 1994, pp. 1–10.
22. Elmer PJ. Obesity and cardiovascular disease: Practical approaches for weight loss in clinical practice. In: Pearson TA, Criqui MH, Luepker RV,

Oberman A, Winston M, eds. Primer in Preventive Cardiology. Dallas, TX: American Heart Association; 1994, pp. 189–204.

23. Grundy SM, Cleeman JI, Merz CN, et al. Implications of recent clinical trials for the National Cholesterol Education Program Adult Treatment Panel III Guidelines. *Circulation*. 2004;110(2):227–39.
24. Truswell AS. Diet and nutrition of hunter-gatherers. *Ciba Found Symp*. 1977;49:213–21.
25. Blackburn H, Prineas RJ. Diet and hypertension: Anthropology, epidemiology, and public health implications. *Prog Biochem Pharmacol*. 1983;19:31–79.
26. Eaton SB, Konner M. Paleolithic nutrition: A consideration of its nature and current implications. *N Engl J Med*. 1985;312(5):283–9.
27. Shekelle RB, Shryock AM, Paul O, et al. Diet, serum cholesterol, and death from coronary heart disease: The Western Electric study. *N Engl J Med*. 1981;304(2):65–70.
28. Kromhout D, de Lezenne Coulander C. Diet, prevalence and 10-year mortality from coronary heart disease in 871 middle-aged men: The Zutphen study. *Am J Epidemiol*. 1984;119(5):733–41.
29. McGee DL, Reed DM, Yano K, Kagan A, Tillotson J. Ten-year incidence of coronary heart disease in the Honolulu Heart Program: Relationship to nutrient intake. *Am J Epidemiol*. 1984;119(5):667–76.
30. Kushi LH, Lew RA, Stare FJ, et al. Diet and 20-year mortality from coronary heart disease: The Ireland-Boston Diet-Heart Study. *N Engl J Med*. 1985;312(13):811–8.
31. Keys A, Grande F, Anderson JT. Bias and misrepresentation revisited—"Perspective" on saturated fat. *Am J Clin Nutr*. 1974;27(2):188–212.
32. Hegsted DM, McGandy RB, Myers ML, Stare FJ. Quantitative effects of dietary fat on serum cholesterol in man. *Am J Clin Nutr*. 1965;17(25):281–95.
33. Ascherio A, Hennekens CH, Buring JE, et al. Trans-fatty acids intake and risk of myocardial infarction. *Circulation*. 1994;89(1):94–101.
34. Mattson FH, Grundy SM. Comparison of effects of dietary saturated, monounsaturated, and polyunsaturated fatty acids on plasma lipids and lipoproteins in man. *J Lipid Res*. 1985;26(2):194–202.
35. St. Clair RW. Atherosclerosis regression in animal models: Current concepts of cellular and biochemical mechanisms. *Prog Cardiovasc Dis*. 1983;26(2):109–32.
36. Clarkson TB, Bond MG, Bullock BC, McLaughlin KJ, Sawyer JK. A study of atherosclerosis regression in Macaca mulatta: V. Changes in abdominal aorta and carotid and coronary arteries from animals with atherosclerosis induced for 38 months and then regressed for 24 or 48 months at plasma cholesterol concentrations of 300 or 200 mg/dL. *Exp Mol Pathol*. 1984;41(11):96–118.
37. Estruch R, Ros E, Salas-Salvadó J, et al. Primary prevention of cardiovascular disease with a Mediterranean diet. *N Engl J Med*. 2013;368:1279–90.
38. Anitschkow N. *Experimental Atherosclerosis in Animals, in Arteriosclerosis*. Cowdry EVCowdry EV, ed. New York: Macmillan; 1983, p. 271.
39. de Koning L, Malik VS, Kellogg MD, et al. Sweetened beverage consumption, incident coronary heart disease, and biomarkers of risk in men. *Circulation*. 2012;125(14):1735–41.
40. Fung TT, Malik V, Rexrode KM et al. Sweetened beverage consumption and risk of coronary heart disease in women. *Am J Clin Nutr*. 2009;89(4):1037–42.
41. Gardener H, Moon YP, Rundek T, Elkind MSV, Sacco RL. Diet soda and sugar-sweetened soda consumption in relation to incident diabetes in the Northern Manhattan study. *Curr Dev Nutr*. 2018;2(5):nzy008.
42. Wallace RB, Lynch CF, Pomrehn PR, Criqui MH, Heiss G. Alcohol and hypertension: Epidemiologic and experimental considerations. The Lipid Research Clinics Program. *Circulation*. 1981;64(3 Pt 2):III:41–7.
43. Dyer AR, Stamler J, Paul O, et al. Alcohol, cardiovascular risk factors and mortality: The Chicago experience. *Circulation*. 1981;64(3):20–7.
44. Haskell WL, Camargo CJr, Williams PT, et al. The effect of cessation and resumption of moderate alcohol intake on serum high density lipoprotein subfractions. *N Engl J Med*. 1984;310(13):805–10.
45. Ellison RC. Balancing the risks and benefits of moderate drinking. *Ann N Y Acad Sci*. 2002;957:1–6.
46. Djoussé L, Ellison RC, Beiser A, Scaramucci A, D'Agostino RB, Wolf PA. Alcohol consumption and risk of ischemic stroke: The Framingham Study. *Stroke*. 2002;33(4):907–12.
47. Li JM, Mukamal KJ. An update on alcohol and atherosclerosis. *Curr Opin Lipidoly*. 2004;15(6):673–80.
48. Haseeb S, Alexander B, Baranchuk A. Wine and cardiovascular health: A comprehensive review. *Circulation*. 2017;136(15):1434–48.
49. Kare MR, Fregly MJ, Bernard RA, eds.Kare MR, Fregly MJ, Bernard RA, eds. *Biological and Behavioral Aspects of Salt Intake*. New York: Academic Press; 1980.
50. Freis ED. Salt, volume and the prevention of hypertension. *Circulation*. 1976;53(4):589–95.
51. Appel LJ, Champagne CM, Harsha DW, et al. Effects of comprehensive lifestyle modification on blood pressure control: main results of the PREMIER clinical trial. *JAMA*. 2003;289(16):2083–93.
52. Meneely GR, Battarbee HD. High sodium–low potassium environment and hypertension. *Am J Cardiol*. 1976;38(6):768–85.
53. Gleibermann L. Blood pressure and dietary salt in human populations. *Ecol Food Nutr*. 1973;2(2):143–56.
54. Intersalt: An international study of electrolyte excretion and blood pressure: Results for 24 hour urinary sodium and potassium excretion. Intersalt Cooperative Research Group. *BMJ*. 1988;297(6644):319–28.
55. Joseph JG, Prior IA, Salmond CE, Stanley D. Elevation of systolic and diastolic blood pressure associated with migration: The Tokelau Island Migrant Study. *J Chronic Dis*. 1983;36(7):507–16.
56. Kesteloot H, Vuylsteks M, Costenoble A. Relationship between blood pressure and sodium and potassium intake in a Belgian male population group. In: Kesteloot K, Joossens J, eds. *Epidemiology of Arterial Blood Pressure*. The Hague: Nijhoff; 1980, pp. 345–51.
57. Appel LJ, Brands MW, Daniels SR, et al. Dietary approaches to prevent and treat hypertension: A scientific statement from the American Heart Association. *Hypertension*. 2006;47(2):296–308.
58. Chobanian AV, Bakris GL, Black HR, et al. The Seventh Report of the Joint National Committee on Prevention, Detection, Evaluation, and Treatment of High Blood Pressure: The JNC 7 report. *JAMA*. 2003;289(19):2560–72.
59. Shimamoto T, Komachi Y, Inada H, et al. Trends for coronary heart disease and stroke and their risk factors in Japan. *Circulation*. 1989;79(3):503–15.
60. Hulley SB, Rosenman RH, Bawol RD, Brand RJ. Epidemiology as a guide to clinical decisions. The associations between triglycerides and coronary heart disease. *N Engl J Med*. 1980;302:1383–9.
61. NIH Consensus Conference. Triglyceride, high density lipoprotein, and coronary heart disease. NIH Consensus Development Panel on Triglyceride, High-Density Lipoprotein, and Coronary Heart Disease. *JAMA*. 1993;269(4):505–10.
62. Conference on Blood Lipids in Children. Optimal levels for early prevention of coronary artery disease. *Prev Med*. 1983;12:725–7.
63. The Pooling Project Research Group. Relationship of blood pressure, serum cholesterol, smoking habits, relative weight and ECG abnormalities to incidence of major coronary events: Final report of the Pooling Project. *J Chronic Dis*. 1978;31(4):201–306.
64. Stamler J, Wentworth D, Neaton JD. Is the relationship between serum cholesterol and risk of premature death from coronary heart disease continuous and graded? Findings in 356,222 primary screenees of the Multiple Risk Factor Intervention Trial (MRFIT). *JAMA*. 1986;256(20):2823–8.
65. Blackburn H. The concept of risk. In: Pearson TA, Criqui MH, Luepker RV, Oberman A, Winston M, eds. *Primer in Preventive Cardiology*. Dallas, TX: American Heart Association; 1994, pp. 25–41.
66. Gordon T, Castelli WP, Hjortland MC, Kennel WB, Dawber TR. High density lipoprotein as a protective factor against coronary heart disease. *Am J Med*. 1977;62(5):707–14.
67. The National Diet-Heart Study Final Report. *Circulation*. 1968;37 (3 Suppl):I1–428.
68. Frick MH, Elo O, Haapa K, et al. Helsinki Heart Study: Primary-prevention trial with gemfibrozil in middle-aged men with dyslipidemia. Safety of treatment, changes in risk factors, and incidence of coronary heart disease. *N Engl J Med*. 1987;317(20):1237–45.
69. Shepherd J, Cobbe SM, Ford I, et al. Prevention of coronary heart disease with pravastatin in men with hypercholesterolemia. West of Scotland Coronary Prevention Study Group. *N Engl J Med*. 1995;333(20):1301–7.
70. Randomized trial of cholesterol lowering in 4444 patients with coronary heart disease: The Scandinavian Simvastatin Survival Study (4S). *Lancet*. 1994;344(8934):1383–9.
71. Kjekshus H, Pedersen TR. Reducing the risk of coronary events: Evidence from the Scandinavian Simvastatin Survival Study (4S). *Am J Cardiol*. 1995;76(9):64C–8C.
72. Pfeffer MA, Sacks FM, Moye LA, et al. Cholesterol and recurrent events: A secondary prevention trial for normolipidemic patients. CARE Investigators. *Am J Cardiol*. 1995;76(9):98C–106C.

73. Ridker PM, Danielson E, Fonseca FA, et al. Rosuvastatin to prevent vascular events in men and women with elevated c-reactive protein. *N Engl J Med*. 2008;359(21):2195–207.
74. Johnson CL, Rifkind BM, Sempos CT, et al. Declining serum total cholesterol levels among US adults. The National Health and Nutrition Examination Surveys. *JAMA*. 1993;269(23):3002–8.
75. Arnett DK, Jacobs DRJr, Luepker RV, Blackburn H, Armstrong C, Class SA. Twenty-year trends in serum cholesterol, hypercholesterolemia, and cholesterol medication use: The Minnesota Heart Survey, 1980–1982 to 2000–2002. *Circulation*. 2005;112(25):3884–91.
76. Expert Panel on Detection, Evaluation, and Treatment of High Blood Cholesterol in Adults. Executive summary of the third report of the National Cholesterol Education Program (NCEP) Expert Panel on detection, evaluation, and treatment of high blood cholesterol in adults (Adult Treatment Panel III). *JAMA*. 2001;285(19):2486–97.
77. Goodman DS, Hulley SB, Clark LT, et al. Report of the National Cholesterol Education Program Expert Panel on detection, evaluation, and treatment of high blood cholesterol in adults. *Arch Intern Med*. 1988;148(1):36–69.
78. National Cholesterol Education Program. Second report of the Expert Panel on detection, evaluation, and treatment of high blood cholesterol in adults (Adult Treatment Panel II). *Circulation*. 1994;89(3):1333–445.
79. National Cholesterol Education Program. Report of the Expert Panel on population strategies for blood cholesterol reduction: Executive summary. National Heart, Lung and Blood Institute, National Institutes of Health. *Arch Intern Med*. 1991;151(6):1071–84.
80. American Academy of Pediatrics. National Cholesterol Education Program: Report of the Expert Panel on Blood Cholesterol Levels in Children and Adolescents. *Pediatrics*. 1992;89(3 Pt 2):525–84.
81. Stone NJ, Robinson JG, Lichtenstein AH, et al. 2013 ACC/AHA guideline on the treatment of blood cholesterol to reduce atherosclerotic cardiovascular risk in adults: A report of the American College of Cardiology/American Heart Association Task Force on Practice Guidelines. *Circulation*. 2014;129(25 Suppl 2):S1–45.
82. Barrett-Connor EL. Obesity, atherosclerosis and coronary heart disease. *Ann Intern Med*. 1985;103(6 Pt 2):1010–9.
83. CDC/National Center for Health Statistics. https://www.cdc.gov/nchs/fastats/obesity-overweight.htm.
84. Ogden CL, Carroll MD, Fryar CD, Flegal KM. Prevalence of Obesity Among Adults and Youth: United States, 2011–2014. NCHC Data Brief No. 219, November 2013.
85. Hales CM, Carroll MD, Fryar CD, Ogden CL. Prevalence of Obesity Among Adults and Youth: United States, 2015–2016. NCHS Data Brief. No. 288, Oct. 2017.
86. Hubert HB, Feinleib M, McNamara PM, Castelli WP. Obesity as an independent risk factor for cardiovascular disease: A 26-year follow-up of participants in the Framingham Heart Study. *Circulation*. 1983;67(5):968–77.
87. Tyroler HA, Heyden S, Hames CG. In: Paul O, ed. *Weight and Hypertension: Evans County Studies of Blacks and Whites, in Epidemiology and Control of Hypertension*. New York: Grune & Stratton; 1975.
88. Rabkin SW, Mathewson FA, Hsu PH. Relation of body weight to the development of ischemic heart disease in a cohort of young North American men after a 26 year observation period: The Manitoba Study. *Am J Cardiol*. 1977;39(3):452–8.
89. Larsson B, Svardsudd K, Welin L, Wilhelmsen L, Bjorntorp P, Tibbin G. Abdominal adipose tissue distribution, obesity, and risk of cardiovascular disease and death: 13-Year follow up of participants in the study of men born in 1913. *Br Med J*. 1984;288(6428):1401–4.
90. Donahue RP, Abbott RD, Bloom E, Reed DM, Yano K. Central obesity and coronary heart disease in men. *Lancet*. 1987;1(8537):821–4.
91. Bjorntorp P. The associations between obesity, adipose tissue distribution and disease. *Acta Med Scand Suppl*. 1988;723:121–34.
92. Montenegro MR, Solberg LA. Obesity, body weight, body length, and atherosclerosis. *Lab Invest*. 1968;18(5):594–603.
93. Lissner L, Bengtsson C, Lapidus L, et al. Body weight variability and mortality in the Goteborg prospective studies of men and women. In: Bjorntorp P, Rossner S, eds. *Proceedings of the European Congress of Obesity*. London: John Libbey; 1989, pp. 55–60.
94. Taylor HL, Buskirk ER, Remington RD. Exercise in controlled trials of the prevention of coronary heart disease. *Fed Proc*. 1973;32(5):1623–7.
95. van Halewijn G, Deckers J, Tay HY, van Domburq R, Kotseva K, Wood D. Lessons from contemporary trials of cardiovascular prevention and rehabilitation: A systematic review and meta-analysis *Int J Cardiol*. 2017;232:294–303.
96. Blackburn H, Jacobs DRJr. Physical activity and the risk of coronary heart disease. *N Engl J Med*. 1988;319(18):1217–9.
97. Physical activity and cardiovascular health. NIH Consensus Development Panel on physical activity and cardiovascular health. *JAMA*. 1996;276(3):241–6.
98. Powell KE, Thompson PD, Caspersen CJ, Kendrick JS. Physical activity and the incidence of coronary heart disease. *Annu Rev Public Health*. 1987;8:253–87.
99. Leon AS, Connett J, Jacobs DRJr, Rauramaa R. Leisure-time physical activity levels and risk of coronary heart disease and death: The Multiple Risk Factor Intervention Trial. *JAMA*. 1987;258(17):2388–9,.
100. Slattery ML, Jacobs DRJr, Nichaman MZ. Leisure time physical activity and coronary heart disease death: The U.S. Railroad Study. *Circulation*. 1989;79(2):304–11.
101. Blair SN, Kohl HW3rd, Paffenbarger RSJr, Clark DG, Cooper KH, Gibbons LW. Physical fitness and all-cause mortality: A prospective study of healthy men and women. *JAMA*. 1989;262(17):2395–401.
102. Paffenbarger RSJr, Wing AL, Hyde RT. Physical activity as an index of heart attack risk in college alumni. *Am J Epidemiol*. 1978;108(3):161–75.
103. Paffenbarger RSJr, Hyde RT, Wing AL, Steinmetz CH. A natural history of athleticism and cardiovascular health. 1984;*JAMA*. 252(4):491–5.
104. Siscovick DS, Weiss NS, Fletcher RH, Lasky T. The incidence of primary cardiac arrest during vigorous exercise. *N Engl J Med*. 1984;311(14):874–7.
105. Mittleman MA, Maclure M, Tofler GH, Sherwood JB, Goldberg RJ, Muller JE. Triggering of acute myocardial infarction by heavy physical exertion: protection against triggering of regular exertion. Determinants of Myocardial Infarction Onset Study Investigators. *N Engl J Med*. 1993;329(23):1677–83.
106. Centers for Disease Control and Prevention. National Diabetes Statistics Report, 2017. Atlanta, GA: Centers for Disease Control and Prevention, U.S. Department of Health and Human Services; 2017. https://www.cdc.gov/diabetes/pdfs/data/statistics/national-diabetes-statistics-report.pdf. Bethesda, MD, 2017.
107. West KM. *Epidemiology of Diabetes and Its Vascular Lesions*. New York: Elsevier; 1978, pp. 375–402.
108. Pyorala K, Laakso M, Uusitupa M. Diabetes and atherosclerosis: An epidemiologic view. *Diabetes Metab Rev*. 1987;3(2):463–524.
109. Knowler WC, Bennett PH, Hamman RF, Miller M. Diabetes incidence and prevalence in Pima Indians: A 19-fold greater incidence than in Rochester, MN. *Am J Epidemiol*. 1978;108(6):497–505.
110. Barrett-Connor E, Wingard DL. Sex differential in ischemic heart disease mortality in diabetics: A prospective population-based study. *Am J Epidemiol*. 1983;118(4):489–96.
111. Stamler R, Stamler J, Lindberg HA, et al. Asymptomatic hyperglycemia and coronary heart disease in middle-aged men in two employed populations in Chicago. *J Chronic Dis*. 1979;32(11–12):805–15.
112. Hughes LO. Insulin, Indian origin and ischemic heart disease. *Int J Cardiol*. 1990;26(1):1–4.
113. The University Group Diabetes Program. A study of the effects of hypoglycemic agents on vascular complications in patients with adult onset diabetes. V. Evaluation of pheniformin therapy. *Diabetes*. 1975;24(Suppl1):65–184.
114. United Kingdom Prospective Diabetes Study (UKPDS). 13: Relative efficacy of randomly allocated diet, sulphonylurea, insulin, or metformin in patients with newly diagnosed non-insulin dependent diabetes followed for three years. 1995;*Br Med J*. 310(6972):83–8.
115. Diabetes Control and Complications Trial Research Group. Nathan DM, Genuth S, Lachin J, et al. The effect of intensive treatment of diabetes on the development and progression of long-term complications in insulin-dependent diabetes mellitus. *N Engl J Med*. 1993;329(14):977–86.
116. Nissen SE, Wolski K. Effect of rosiglitazone on the risk of myocardial infarction and death from cardiovascular causes. *N Engl J Med*. 2007;356(24):2457–71.
117. Schnell O, Rydén L, Standl E, Ceriello A, D&CVD EASD Study Group. Updates on cardiovascular outcome trials in diabetes. *Cardiovasc Diabetol*. 2017;16(1):128.
118. Bundy JD, Mills KT, Chen J, Li C, Greenland P, He J. Estimating the association of the 2017 and 2014 hypertension guidelines with cardiovascular events and deaths in US adults: an analysis of national data. *JAMA Cardiol*. 2018;3(7):572–581.
119. Prevention of stroke by antihypertensive drug treatment in older persons with isolated systolic hypertension. Final results of the Systolic Hypertension in the Elderly Program (SHEP). SHEP Cooperative Research Group. *JAMA*. 1991;265(24):3255–64.

120. Hypertension Detection and Follow-Up Group. The effect of treatment on mortality in "mild" hypertension: Results of the Hypertension Detection and Follow-Up Program. *N Engl J Med.* 1982;307(16):976–80.

121. Furberg CD, Wright JT, Davis BR, et al. Major outcomes in high-risk hypertensive patients randomized to angiotensin-converting enzyme inhibitor or calcium channel blocker vs diuretic: The Antihypertensive and Lipid-Lowering Treatment to Prevent Heart Attack Trial (ALLHAT). *JAMA.* 2002;288(23):2981–97.

122. SPRINT Research Group. Wright JTJr, Williamson JD, Whelton PK, et al. A randomized trial of intensive versus standard blood-pressure control. *N Engl J Med.* 2015;373(22):2103–16.

123. Luepker RV, Steffen LM, Jacobs DRJr, Zhou X, Blackburn H. Trends in blood pressure and hypertension detection, treatment and control 1980–2009: The Minnesota Heart Survey. *Circulation.* 2012;126(15):1852–7.

124. U.S. Department of Health and Human Services. *Morbidity and Mortality 2012 Chart Book on Cardiovascular, Lung and Blood Diseases.* Washington, DC: National Institutes of Health; 2012.

125. McGill HCJr. Potential mechanisms for the augmentation of atherosclerosis and atherosclerotic disease by cigarette smoking. *Prev Med.* 1979;8(3):390–403.

126. Filion KB, Luepker RV. Cigarette smoking and cardiovascular disease: Lessons from Framingham. *Global Heart.* 2013;8(1):35–41.

127. Wilhelmsen L. Coronary heart disease: Epidemiology of smoking and intervention studies of smoking. *Am Heart J.* 1988;115(1 Pt 2):242–9.

128. Amler RW, Dull HBAmler RW, Dull HB, eds. *Closing the Gap: The Burden of Unnecessary Illness.* New York: Oxford University Press; 1987.

129. Willett WC, Green A, Stampfer MJ, et al. Relative and absolute excess risks of coronary heart disease among women who smoke cigarettes. *N Engl J Med.* 1987;317(21):1303–9.

130. Doll R, Hill AB. Mortality in relation to smoking: Ten years' observations of British doctors. *Br Med J.* 1964;1(5395):1399–410.

131. Friedman GD, Petitti DB, Bawol RD, Siegelaub AB. Mortality in cigarette smokers and quitters: Effect of base-line differences. *N Engl J Med.* 1981;304(23):1407–10.

132. Aberg A, Bergstrand R, Johansson S, et al. Cessation of smoking after myocardial infarction: Effects on mortality after ten years. *Br Heart J.* 1983;49(5):416–22.

133. Bhatnagar A. E-cigarettes and cardiovascular disease risk: Eevaluation of evidence, policy implications, and recommendations. *Curr Cardiovasc Risk Rep.* 2016;10(24):1–10.

134. Filion KB, Steffen LM, Duval S, Jacobs DRJr, Blackburn H, Luepker RV. Trends in smoking among adults from 1980 to 2009: The Minnesota Heart Survey. *Am J Public Health.* 2012;102(4):705–13.

135. Luepker RV, Rosamond WD, Murphy R, et al. Socioeconomic status and coronary heart disease risk factor trends: The Minnesota Heart Survey. *Circulation.* 1993;88(5 Pt 1):2172–9.

136. Luepker RV, Murray DM, Jacobs DRJr, et al. Community education for cardiovascular disease prevention: Risk factor changes in the Minnesota Heart Health Program. *Am J Prev Med.* 1994;84(9):1383–93.

137. Public Health Service, Office on Smoking and Health. *Report of the Surgeon General. Reducing the Health Consequences of Smoking: Twenty-Five Years of Progress.* Rockville, MD: U.S. Department of Health and Human Services; 1989.

138. Farb A, Tang AL, Burke AP, Sessums L, Liang Y, Virmani R. Frequency of active coronary lesions, inactive coronary lesions and myocardial infarction. *Circulation.* 1995;92(7):1701–9.

139. Meade TW. Clotting factors and ischemic heart disease. In: Meade TW, ed. *The Epidemiological Evidence from Anti-coagulants in Myocardial Infarction: A Reappraisal.* New York: John Wiley & Sons; 1984.

140. Libby P, Simon DI. Inflammation and thrombosis: The clot thickens. *Circulation.* 2001;103(13):1718–20.

141. Ridker PM, Cushman M, Stampfer MJ, Tracy RP, Hennekens CH. Inflammation, aspirin, and the risk of cardiovascular disease in apparently healthy men. *N Engl J Med.* 1997;336(14):973–9.

142. Bibbins-Domingo K, U.S. Preventive Services Task Force. Aspirin use for the primary prevention of cardiovascular disease and colorectal cancer: U.S. Preventive Services Task Force recommendation statement. *Ann Intern Med.* 2016;164(12):836–45.

143. Jackson RJ. The impact of the built environment on health: An emerging field. *Am J Public Health.* 2003;93(9):1382–4.

144. Beard CM, Fuster V, Elveback LR. Daily and seasonal variation in sudden cardiac death, Rochester, Minnesota, 1950–1975. *Mayo Clin Proc.* 1982;57(11):704–6.

145. Brook RD, Rajagopalan S, Pope CAIII, et al. Particulate matter air pollution and cardiovascular disease: An update to the scientific statement from the American Heart Association. *Circulation.* 2010;121(21):2331–78.

146. Kaplan GA, Salonen JT, Cohen RD, Brand RJ, Syme SL, Puska P. Social connections and mortality from all causes and from cardiovascular disease: Prospective evidence from Eastern Finland. *Am J Epidemiol.* 1988;128(2):370–80.

147. Orth-Gomer K, Johnson JV. Social network interaction and mortality: A six year follow-up study of a random sample of the Swedish population. *J Chronic Dis.* 1987;40:949–57.

148. Berkman LF, Blumenthal J, Burg M, et al. Writing Committee for the ENRICHD Investigators: Effects of treating depression and low perceived social support on clinical events after myocardial infarction: The Enhancing Recovery in Coronary Heart Disease (ENRICHD) Randomized Trial. *JAMA.* 2003;289:3106–16.

149. McGill Jr HC, Stern MP. In: Paoletti R, Gotto Jr AM eds. *Sex and Atherosclerosis, in Atherosclerosis Reviews.* New York: Raven Press, Vol. 4. 1979, pp. 157–242.

150. Demirovic J. Recent trends in coronary heart disease mortality among women in Yugoslavia. *CVD Epidemiol Newslett.* 1988;44:96–7.

151. Wahl P, Walden C, Knopp R, et al. Effect of estrogen/progestin potency on lipid/lipoprotein cholesterol. *N Engl J Med.* 1983;308(15):862–7.

152. Grady D, Rubin SM, Petitti DB, et al. Hormone therapy to prevent disease and prolong life in postmenopausal women. *Ann Intern Med.* 1992;117(2):1016–37.

153. Stampfer MJ, Colditz GA. Estrogen replacement therapy and coronary heart disease: A quantitative assessment of the epidemiologic evidence. *Prev Med.* 1991;20(1):47–63.

154. Hulley S, Grady D, Bush T, et al. Randomized trial of estrogen plus progestin for secondary prevention of coronary heart disease in postmenopausal women: Heart and Estrogen/progestin Replacement Study (HERS) Research Group. *JAMA.* 1998;280(7):605–13.

155. Rossouw JE, Anderson GL, Prentice RL, et al. Risks and benefits of estrogen plus progestin in healthy postmenopausal women: Principal results from the Women's Health Initiative Randomized Controlled Trial. *JAMA.* 2002;288(3):321–33.

156. Naftolin F, Friedenthal J, Nachtigall R, et al. Cardiovascular health and the menopausal woman: The role of estrogen and when to begin and end hormone treatment. *F1000Res.* 2019;8:F1000 Faculty Rev-1576.

157. Hodis HN, Mack WJ, Henderson VW, et al. Vascular effects of early versus late postmenopausal treatment with estradiol. *N Engl J Med.* 2016;374(13):1221–31.

158. Austin MA, King MC, Bawol RD, Hulley SB, Friedman GD. Risk factors for coronary heart disease in adult female twins: Genetic heritability and shared environmental influences. *Am J Epidemiol.* 1987;125(2):308–18.

159. Hasstedt SJ, Wu L, Williams RR. Major locus inheritance of apolipoprotein B in Utah pedigrees. *Genet Epidemiol.* 1987;4(2):67–76.

160. Austin MA, King MC, Vranizan KM, Newman B, Krauss RM. Inheritance of low-density lipoprotein subclass patterns: Results of complex segregation analysis. *Am J Hum Genet.* 1988;43(6):838–46.

161. Jacobs DRJr, Anderson JT, Hannan P, Keys A, Blackburn H. Variability in individual serum cholesterol response to change in diet. *Arteriosclerosis.* 1983;3:349–56.

162. Hunt SC, Hasstedt SJ, Kuida H, Stults BM, Hopkins PN, Williams RR. Genetic heritability and common environmental components of resting and stressed blood pressures, lipids, and body mass index in Utah pedigrees and twins. *Am J Epidemiol.* 1989;129(3):625–38.

163. Dominiczak AF, Brain N, Charchar F, McBride M, Hanlon N, Lee WK. Genetics of hypertension: Lessons learnt from Mendelian and polygenic syndromes. *Clin Experiment Hypertens.* 2004;26(7–8):611–20.

164. Keys A, Aravanis C, Blackburn H, et al. Probability of middle-aged men developing coronary heart disease in five years. *Circulation.* 1972;45(4):815–28.

165. Stamler J, Stamler R, Neaton JD, et al. Low risk-factor profile and long-term cardiovascular and noncardiovascular mortality and life expectancy: Findings of the 5 large cohorts of young adults and middle-aged men and women. *JAMA.* 1999;282(21):2012–8.

166. Daviglus ML, Stamler J, Pirzada A, et al. Favorable cardiovascular risk profile in young women and long-term risk of cardiovascular and all-cause mortality. *JAMA.* 2004;292(13):1588–92.

167. Daviglus ML, Liu K, Pirzada A, et al. Favorable cardiovascular risk profile in middle age and health-related quality of life in older age. *Arch Intern Med.* 2003;163(20):2460–8.

168. Carapetis JR, Steer AC, Mulholland EK, Weber M. The global burden of group A streptococcal diseases. *Lancet Infect Dis.* 2005;5(11): 685–94.

169. Strasser T. Rheumatic fever and rheumatic heart disease in the 1970s. *Public Health Rev.* 1976;5:207–34.

170. World Health Organization. *Intensified Program: Action to Prevent Rheumatic Fever/Rheumatic Heart Disease. WHO Document WHO/ CVD/84.3.* Geneva: World Health Organization; 1984.

171. Zhimin W, Yubao Z, Lei S, et al. Prevalence of chronic rheumatic heart disease in Chinese adults. *Int J Cardiol.* 2006;107:356–9.

172. Bar-Dayan Y, Elishkevitz K, Goldstein L, et al. The prevalence of common cardiovascular diseases among 17-year-old Israeli conscripts. *Cardiology.* 2005;104(1):6–9.

173. Hanna JN, Heazlewood RJ. The epidemiology of acute rheumatic fever in Indigenous people in north Queensland. *Aust N Z J Public Health.* 2005;29(4):313–7.

174. Ahmed J, Mostafa Zaman M, Monzur Hassan MM. Prevalence of rheumatic fever and rheumatic heart disease in rural Bangladesh. *Trop Doct.* 2005;35(3):160–1.

175. Zuehlke, LJ, Engel ME, Watkins D, Mayosi BM. Incidence, prevalence and outcome of rheumatic heart disease in South Africa: A systematic review of contemporary studies. *Int J Cardiol.* 2015;199:375–83.

176. Veasy LG, Tani LY, Hill HR. Persistence of acute rheumatic fever in the intermountain area of the United States. *J Pediatr.* 1994;124(1):9–16.

177. Hoffman JI. Congenital heart disease: Incidence and inheritance. *Pediatr Clin North Am.* 1990;37(1):25–43.

178. Zangwill KM, Wald ER, Londino AVJr. Acute rheumatic fever in western Pennsylvania: A persistent problem into the 1990s. *J Pediatr.* 1991;118(4 Pt 1):561–3.

179. Carapetis JR, Currie BJ. Rheumatic fever in a high incidence population: The importance of monoarthritis and low grade fever. *Arch Dis Child.* 2001;85(2):223–8.

180. Giannoulia-Karantana A, Anagnostopoulos G, Kostaridou S, Georgakopoulou T, Papadopoulou A, Papadopoulos G. Childhood acute rheumatic fever in Greece: Experience of the past 18 years. *Acta Paediatr.* 2001;90(7):809–12.

181. Kurahara DK, Grandinetti A, Galario J, et al. Ethnic differences for developing rheumatic fever in a low-income group living in Hawaii. *Ethn Dis.* 2006;16(2):357–61.

182. Wannamaker LW, Matsen JMWannamaker LW, Matsen JM, eds. *Streptococci and Streptococcal Diseases: Recognition, Understanding, and Management.* New York: Academic Press; 1972.

183. Gordis L, Lilienfeld A, Rodriguez R. Studies in the epidemiology and preventability of rheumatic fever. II. Socio-economic factors and the incidence of acute attacks. *J Chronic Dis.* 1969;21(9):655–66.

184. Seckeler MD, Hoke TR. The worldwide epidemiology of acute rheumatic fever and rheumatic heart disease. *Clin Epidemiol.* 2011;3:67–84.

185. Fernando L, Pamela S, Alejandra L. Cardiovascular disease in Latin America: The growing epidemic. *Prog Cardiovasc Dis.* 2014;57(3):262–7.

186. Essop R, Peters F. Contemporary issues in rheumatic fever and chronic rheumatic heart disease. *Circulation.* 2014;130(24):2181–8.

187. Gerber MA, Baltimore RS, Eaton CB. Prevention of rheumatic fever and diagnosis and treatment of acute streptococcal pharyngitis: A scientific statement from the American Heart Association Rheumatic Fever, Endocarditis, and Kawasaki Disease Committee of the Council on Cardiovascular Disease in the Young, the Interdisciplinary Council on Functional Genomics and Translational Biology, and the Interdisciplinary Council on Quality of Care and Outcomes Research: Endorsed by the American Academy of Pediatrics. *Circulation.* 2009;119(11):1541–51.

188. Elliot RS, Edwards JE. Pathology of congenital heart disease. In: Hurst JW, ed. *The Heart.* New York: McGraw-Hill; 1978.

189. van der Linde D, Konings EE, Slager MA, et al. Birth prevalence of congenital heart disease worldwide: A systematic review and meta-analysis. *Am Coll Cardiol.* 2011;58(21):2241–7.

190. Nora JJ. Etiologic factors in congenital heart diseases. *Pediatr Clin North Am.* 1971;18(4):1059–74.

191. Alberman ED, Goldstein H. Possible teratogenic effect of cigarette smoking. *Nature.* 1971;231(5304):529–30.

192. Rose V, Gold RJ, Lindsay G, Allen M. A possible increase in the incidence of congenital heart defects among the offspring of affected parents. *J Am Coll Cardiol.* 1985;6(2):376–82.

193. Ferencz C. Offspring of fathers with cardiovascular malformations. *Am Heart J.* 1986;111(6):1212–3.

194. Perloff JK, Warnes CA. Challenges posed by adults with repaired congenital heart disease. *Circulation.* 2001;103(21):2637–43.

195. Bailey NA, Lay P. New horizons: Infant cardiac transplantation. *Heart Lung.* 1989;18(2):172–8.

196. Williams RG, Pearson GD, Barst RJ, et al. Report of the National Heart, Lung, and Blood Institute Working Group on research in adult congenital heart disease. *J Am Coll Cardiol.* 2006;47(4):701–7.

197. Greutmann M, Tobler D, Kovacs AH, et al. Increasing mortality burden among adults with complex congenital heart disease. *Congenit Heart Dis.* 2015;10(2):117–27.

198. NHLBI Working Group on Heart Disease Epidemiology: Report. NIH Report 79-1667. Washington, DC: Government Printing Office, 1979.

199. Congenital Heart Disease Study Group. Primary prevention of congenital heart disease. In: Wright IS, Fredrickson DT, eds. *Cardiovascular Diseases, Guidelines for Prevention and Care. Reports of the Inter-Society Commission for Heart Disease Resources.* Washington, DC: Government Printing Office; 1972, p. 116.

200. World Health Organization. *Cardiomyopathies: Report of a WHO Expert Committee. WHO Technical Report Series, No. 697.* Geneva: World Health Organization; 1984.

201. Richardson P, Mckeena W, Bristow M, et al. Report of the 1995 World Health Organization/International Society and Federation of Cardiology Task Force on the definition and classification of cardiomyopathies. *Circulation.* 1996;93(5):841–2.

202. Maron BJ, Towbin JA, Thiene G, et al. Contemporary definitions and classification of the cardiomyopathies: An American Heart Association Scientific Statement. *Circulation.* 2006;113(14):1807–16.

203. McKenna WJ, Maron BJ, Thiene G. Classification, epidemiology, and global burden of cardiomyopathies. *Cir Res.* 2017;121(7):722–30.

204. Myocarditis and related disorders. Proceedings of the International Symposium on Cardiomyopathy and Myocarditis. *Heart Vessels Suppl.* 1985;1:1320.

205. Shabetai R. Cardiomyopathy: How far have we come in 25 years, how far yet to go? *J Am Coll Cardiol.* 1983;1(1):252–63.

206. Gillum RF. Idiopathic cardiomyopathy in the United States, 1970–1982. *Am Heart J.* 1986;111(4):752–5.

207. Okada R, Wakafuji S. Myocarditis in autopsy. *Heart Vessels Suppl.* 1985;1:23–9.

208. Rubin E. Alcoholic myopathy in heart and skeletal muscle. *N Engl J Med.* 1979;301(1):28–33.

209. Alexander CS. Cobalt-beer cardiomyopathy: A clinical and pathologic study of twenty-eight cases. *Am J Med.* 1972;53(4):395–417.

210. Regan TL, Haider B, Ahmed SS, Oldwurtel H, Ettinger PO, Lyons MM. Whiskey and the heart. *Cardiovasc Med.* 1977;2:165–170.

211. Levine HD. Virus myocarditis: A critique of the literature from clinical, electrocardiographic and pathologic standpoints. *Am J Med Sci.* 1979;277(2):132–43.

212. McAllister HAJr. Myocarditis: Some current perspectives and future directions. *Tex Heart Inst J.* 1987;14(4):331–4.

213. Parrillo JE, Cunnion RE, Epstein SE, et al. A prospective, randomized, controlled trial of prednisone for dilated cardiomyopathy. *N Engl J Med.* 1989;321(16):1061–8.

214. Wigle ED. Hypertrophic cardiomyopathy 1988. *Mod Concepts Cardiovasc Dis.* 1988;57(1):1–6.

215. Cecchi F, Olivotto I, Betocchi S, et al. The Italian registry for hypertrophic cardiomyopathy: A nationwide survey. *Am Heart J.* 2005;150(5): 947–54.

216. Ahmad F, Seidman JG, Seidman CE. The genetic basis for cardiac remodelling. *Annu Rev Genomics Hum Genet.* 2005;6:185–216.

217. Hagar JM, Rahimtoola SH. Chagas' heart disease. *Curr Probl Cardiol.* 1995;20(12):825-–924.

218. World Health Organization. *Report of the WHO Consultation on Cardiomyopathies: Approaches to Prevention and Early Detection. WHO Document, WHO/CVD/85.6.* Geneva: World Health Organization; 1985.

219. Silwa K, Damasceno A, Mayosi BM. Epidemiology and etiology of cardiomyopathy in Africa. *Circulation.* 2005;112(23):3577–83.

CHAPTER

53

Diabetes and Other Metabolic Disorders

Rachel G. Miller • Lingshu Xue • Diego Tamez • Janice C. Zgibor

INTRODUCTION

Diabetes and other metabolic disorders, such as thyroid disease, Chushing's syndrome, and polycystic ovary syndrome (PCOS) are important chronic diseases both in terms of the number of persons affected and the considerable associated morbidity and early mortality. In this review, we will focus on the epidemiology and public health implications of diabetes, with an additional section for a brief discussion of thyroid disease, Cushing's syndrome, and PCOS.

DIABETES

Diabetes is a chronic disease in which there is a deficiency in the action of the hormone insulin. This may result from a quantitative deficiency of insulin, an abnormal insulin level, resistance to its action, or a combination of deficits. Two major forms of the disease are recognized: type 1 diabetes (formerly referred to as insulin-dependent or juvenile diabetes) which comprises about 10% of all cases, and type 2 diabetes (formerly referred to as noninsulin-dependent or adult-onset diabetes), which accounts for about 90% of the cases. Type 2 diabetes may occasionally occur as a result of other diseases such as acromegaly and Cushing's syndrome. Metabolic disorders such as hemochromatosis, can also cause the disease. Diabetes can also be drug induced, for example, by steroids and possibly by the thiazide diuretics and oral contraceptives. Finally, diabetes may occur secondary to disease processes directly affecting the pancreas, such as cancer or chronic pancreatitis, which destroys the insulin-producing beta cells in the pancreatic islets (of Langerhans). However, these are relatively rare causes of diabetes.

In addition to these primary and secondary types of diabetes, two further classifications of abnormalities of glucose tolerance are of note. Gestational diabetes occurs during pregnancy but typically remits shortly after delivery. Impaired glucose tolerance (IGT) or impaired fasting glucose (IFG), now termed "prediabetes," are conditions in which blood glucose is elevated but not high enough to be classified as diabetes. Nonetheless, these conditions may carry some increased risk of large vessel (e.g., coronary heart) disease.[1] Both gestational diabetes[2] and prediabetes[3] carry an increased risk for the subsequent development of type 2 diabetes. The types of diabetes and clinical stages are outlined in Fig. 53-1.

Diagnosis

The diagnosis of type 1 diabetes is fairly straightforward. Type 1 diabetes often, though by no means always, has its onset in childhood. Classically, the child will have symptoms of excessive thirst (polydipsia), excessive urination (polyuria), and weight loss. In a child with high blood glucose, these symptoms almost invariably point to type 1 diabetes. These patients lose virtually all capacity to produce insulin and without treatment they develop severe metabolic disturbances, including ketoacidosis and dehydration, which can lead to death. As death from ketoacidosis is largely preventable, the continuing though small number of deaths from this cause represents a challenge to our preventive health services.[4,5] In an international study, wide variations in mortality from acute diabetes complications were noted, with high rates in Japan and low rates in Finland.[6] This variation was thought to reflect disease incidence (low in Japan and high in Finland) and resulting availability of skilled healthcare.

Type 2 diabetes usually presents in adulthood. In the past, the terms noninsulin-dependent, adult- or maturity-onset, and mild diabetes have been used. These terms are somewhat misleading, since type 2 diabetes may present in youth and the complications may be far from mild. People with type 2 diabetes, however, produce some insulin, although its secretion is often delayed, and there is usually some resistance to its action in the peripheral tissues. This resistance is often associated with elevated concentrations of insulin, particularly in newly recognized cases. However, concentrations are now recognized to be low in many type 2 diabetes subjects, especially after accounting for obesity and using more specific assays.[7] In type 2 diabetes, the diagnosis is often based on the presentation of one of the complications, rather than on the basis of classic symptoms. Such complications can be macrovascular (accelerated atherosclerosis with coronary artery, peripheral vascular, or cerebrovascular manifestations), microvascular (with disease of the small vessels in the kidneys or the eyes), or neuropathic (which may take the form of a variety of neurological syndromes). In addition, the disease may also be recognized as a result of routine screening for elevated blood glucose or by the presence of glucose in the urine. Some cases, however, may be diagnosed because of classic symptoms.

According to the 2017 American Diabetes Association (ADA) guidelines, people are diagnosed with type 2 diabetes if they have (1) fasting plasma glucose (FPG) $\geq$ 126 mg/dL (7.0 mmol/L); (2) 2-hour plasma glucose (2-h PG) $\geq$ 200 mg/dL (11.1 mmol/L) after a 75-gram oral glucose tolerance test (OGTT); or (3) HbA1c $\geq$ 6.5% (48 mmol/mol).[8] The most recent addition to the diagnostic criteria is the HbA1c. When using HbA1c, it should be standardized to the Diabetes Control and Complications Trial reference assay.[8]

There are differences in the criteria for diagnosis of type 2 diabetes between the American Diabetes Association and the World Health Organization (Table 53-1). The controversy surrounding these tests is based on the fact that these diagnostic tests may identify somewhat different populations.[8,9] Data from the Cardiovascular Health Study in older Americans suggests that IGT is more predictive of CVD than its fasting corollary IFG.[10] Additionally, the efficacy trials for the prevention of type 2 diabetes used IGT as their measure of glucose intolerance, and not IFG or HbA1c.[8] Because of differences in the criteria for the diagnosis of type 2 diabetes, estimates of the prevalence and temporal trends of type 2 diabetes are difficult, if not impossible, to evaluate. Furthermore, the different criteria for type 2 diabetes used

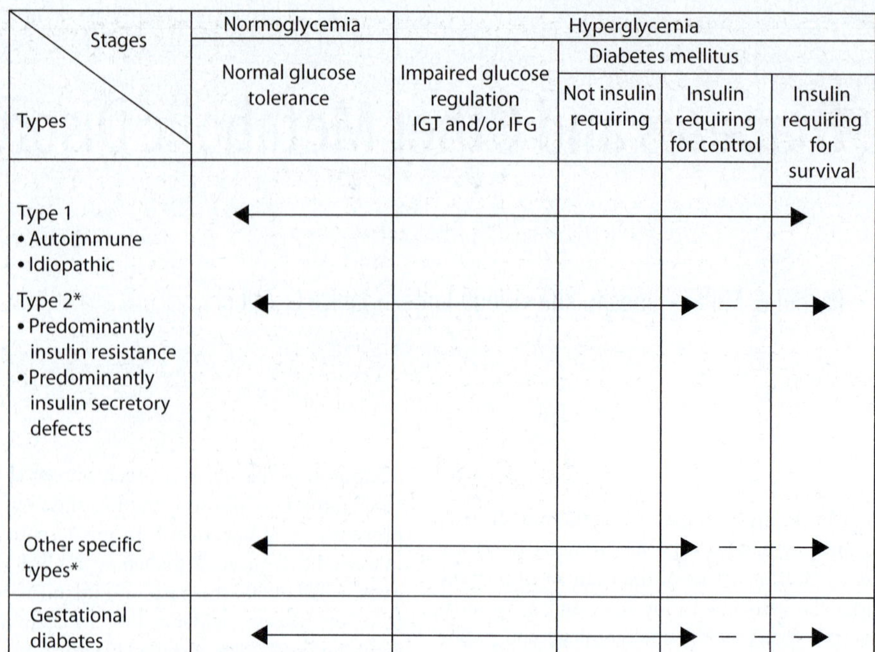

FIGURE 53-1. Disorders of glycemia: etiological types and clinical stages. In rare instances patients in these categories (e.g., Vacor Toxicity, Type 1 presenting in pregnancy, etc.) may require insulin for survival. (Source: Adapted with Permission from Classification Of Diabetes Mellitus 2019, World Health Organization.)

TABLE 53-1 CRITERIA FOR THE CLASSIFICATION OF TYPE 2 DIABETES*†

Diabetes	Impaired Glucose Tolerance	Impaired Fasting Glucose
FPG≥126 mg/dL (7.0 mmol/L)§ OR 2-h PG ≥ 200 mg/dL (11.1 mmol/L) during an OGTT‡ OR HbA1c ≥6.5% (48 mmol/mol)+ OR Classic symptoms of hyperglycemia or hyperglycemic crisis, a random plasma glucose ≥ 200 mg/dL (11.1 mmol/L)	FPG 100–125 mg/dL (5.6 and 6.9 mmol/L)	2-h 140–199 mg/dL (7.8 and 110 mmol/L)

*In the absence of unequivocal hyperglycemia, repeat testing
†Prediabetes = impaired fasting glucose or impaired glucose tolerance.
‡Following 75 g or oral glucose load.
§Fast = no caloric intake for ≥ 8 hours.
+ The test should be performed in a laboratory using methods that is National Glycohemoglobin Standardization Program (NGSP) certified and standardized to the Diabetes Control and Complications Trial (DCCT) assay.

by different research groups and countries make geographical comparisons difficult.

Heterogeneity in Primary Diabetes

Although the two different primary types of diabetes have been described, the classification of diabetes into these groups is not simple. For example, children classified with type 1 diabetes may actually have Maturity-Onset Diabetes (MODY),[11,12] which is characterized by an autosomal dominant pattern of inheritance and a low frequency ketoacidosis. Children in such families, however, are often treated with insulin, although they do not depend on insulin for their survival and actually have type 2 diabetes. Since MODY is uncommon, accounting for < 5% of all type 2 diabetes cases, this section will focus on type 1 diabetes and type 2 diabetes. Similarly 5–10% of adults with presumed type 2 diabetes, have evidence of autoantibodies seen in type 1 diabetes, and may have an incomplete form of type 1 diabetes, sometimes called LADA (latent autoimmune diabetes of adulthood).[13]

Type 1 Diabetes

Descriptive Epidemiology. Type 1 diabetes is caused by the autoimmune destruction of the beta cells of the pancreas, and represents approximately 10% of all cases with diabetes. At present, lifelong insulin therapy is the only treatment for the disease. Without exogenous insulin injections, individuals with type 1 diabetes will not survive. Although the prevalence of type 1 diabetes is < 1% in most populations, the geographic variation in incidence is enormous, ranging from < 1/100,000 per year in many Asian countries to approximately 58/100,000 per year in Finland (Fig. 53-2).[14] The only chronic childhood disorder more prevalent than type 1 diabetes is asthma. It has been estimated that approximately 40 million people worldwide, mostly children and young adults, have type 1 diabetes.[15]

The incidence of type 1 diabetes is increasing worldwide at a rate of about 3% per year.[16] This trend appears to be most dramatic in the youngest age groups, and is completely unrelated to the current increase in type 2 diabetes in children. More children with beta cell autoantibodies, a hallmark of type 1 diabetes, are being diagnosed with the type 1 diabetes around the world each year. Although the peak age at onset is at puberty, type 1 diabetes can also develop in adults. Epidemiologic studies have revealed no significant gender differences in incidence among individuals diagnosed before age 15.[17] However, after age 25, the male-to-female incidence ratio is approximately 1.5. Significant differences have also been reported depending on socioeconomic and urban-rural status, however, results have been conflicting.[18,19] Higher incidence of type 1 diabetes has been linked to higher socioeconomic status, and, albeit less consistently, with residence in lower population density areas. While type 1 diabetes incidence tends to be greater in the northern hemisphere compared to the southern, there is also a notable seasonal variation in the incidence of type 1 diabetes in many countries from both hemispheres, with lower rates in the warm summer months, and higher rates during the cold winter.[20]

Genetic Susceptibility. First-degree relatives have a higher risk of developing type 1 diabetes than unrelated individuals from the

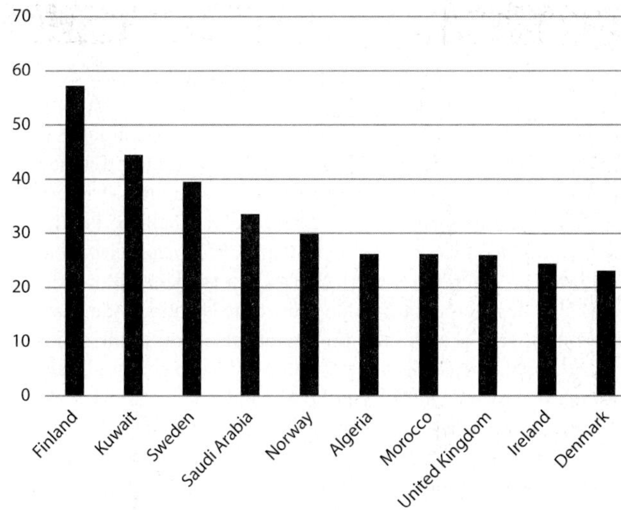

FIGURE 53-2. Type 1 diabetes incidence < 20 years of age, per 100,000 population per year, top ten countries. (Source: International Diabetes Federation. *IDF Diabetes Atlas,* 8th ed. Brussels, Belgium: International Diabetes Federation, 2017.)

TABLE 53-2 SEVERAL TYPE 1 DIABETES SUSCEPTIBILITY GENES

Gene	Locus	Variant	Estimated RR[a]
HLA-DQB1	6p21.3	*0201 and *0302	3–45
INS	11p15. 5	Class I	1–2
CTLA4	2q31–35	Thr17Ala	1–2
PTPN22	1p13	Arg62Trp	1-2

[a]RR = relative risk.

general population (approximately 6% vs. < 1%, respectively).[21] These data suggest that genetic factors are involved with the development of the disease. At present, there is evidence that more than 50 regions of the genome may be involved in genetic susceptibility to type 1 diabetes.[22] However, it has been confirmed in genome-wide association studies that none of the candidates identified have a greater influence on type 1 diabetes risk than that conferred by genes in the HLA (Human Leukocyte Antigens) region of chromosome 6.[23,24] This region contains several hundred genes known to be involved in immune response. Those most strongly associated with the disease are the HLA class II genes (i.e., HLA-DR, DQ, DP). These molecules are involved in the processing of antigens from inside the cell to its surface in order to stimulate an immune response. However, it has become apparent that neither genetic nor environmental risk factors alone contribute to the development of type 1 diabetes. Rather, it is clear that gene-environmental interactions are involved.

A. *IDDM1.* The HLA class II genes, also referred to as insulin-dependent diabetes mellitus 1(IDDM1), contribute approximately 40–50% of the heritable risk for type 1 diabetes.[25] When evaluated as haplotypes, DQA1*0501-DQB1*0201 and DQA1*0301-DQB1*0302 are most strongly associated type 1 diabetes in Caucasian populations. They are in linkage disequilibrium with DRB1*03 and DRB1*04, respectively. Specific DRB1*04 alleles also modify the risk associated with the DQA1*0301-DQB1*0302 haplotype. Other reported high-risk haplotypes for type 1 diabetes include DRB1*07-DQA1*0301-DQB1*0201 among African-Americans, DRB1*09-DQA1*0301-DQB1*0303 among Japanese, and DRB1*04-DQA1*0401-DQB1*0302 among Chinese. DRB1*15-DQA1*0602-DQB1*0102 is protective and associated with a reduced risk of type 1 diabetes in most populations. Recent reports suggest that other genes in the central, class I, and extended class I regions may also increase type 1 diabetes risk independent of HLA class II genes.[26,27]

Individuals with two high-risk DRB1-DQA1-DQB1 haplotypes have a significantly higher type 1 diabetes risk than individuals with no high-risk haplotype. The type 1 diabetes risk among those with only one susceptibility haplotype is also increased, but the effect is more modest. As shown in Table 53-2, relative risk estimates range from 10 to 45 and 3 to 7, respectively, for these groups, depending on race.[21] In terms of absolute risk, Caucasian individuals with two susceptibility haplotypes have an approximately 6% chance of developing type 1 diabetes through age 35 years. However, this figure is substantially lower in populations where type 1 diabetes is rare (i.e., < 1% among Asians). Recent studies have also suggested that HLA-associated factors may increase risk of type 1 diabetes through their association with beta cell autoantibodies. HLA factors have been associated with both the type of autoantibody to first appear[28] and the age at autoantibody seroconversion, with high risk haplotypes associated with a younger age at seroconversion.[29,30] In addition to *IDDM1*, two other genes are now known to influence type 1 diabetes risk.[22] These include insulin (INS), *cytotoxic T lymphocyte-associated 4* (CTLA-4), and protein tyrosine phosphatase nonreceptor type 22 (PTPN22).

B. *INS.* The *INS* gene, located on chromosome 11p15.5, has been designated as *IDDM2.* Positive associations have been observed with a nontranscribed variable number of tandem repeat (VNTR) in the 5' flanking region.[31,32] There are two common variants. The shorter class I variant predisposes to type 1 diabetes (approximate relative increase: 1–2), whereas the longer class III variant appears to be dominantly protective. The biological plausibility of these associations may relate to the expression of insulin mRNA in the thymus. Class III variants appear to generate higher levels of insulin mRNA than class I variants. Such differences could contribute to a better immune tolerance for class III-positive individuals by increasing the likelihood of negative selection for autoreactive T-cell clones. The effect of *INS* appears to vary by ethnicity, with lesser effects in non-Caucasian populations.[33]

C. *CTLA-4.* The *CTLA-4* gene is located on chromosome 2q31–35,[34] where multiple type 1 diabetes genes may be located. CTLA-4 variants have been associated with type 1 diabetes, as well as other autoimmune disease. *CTLA-4* negatively regulates T-cell function. However, impaired activity, which has been associated with the Thr17Ala variant, may increase type 1 diabetes risk. Overall, the relative increase in risk for the CTLA-4Ala17 variant has been estimated as approximately 1.5.

D. *PTPN22.* The *PTPN22* gene is located on chromosome 1p13 and encodes protein tyrosine phosphatase nonreceptor type 22, which is involved in T cell activation.[35] The C1858T single nucleotide polymorphism has been associated with other autoimmune diseases, including rheumatoid arthritis, systemic lupus erythematosus, and Graves' disease.

Environmental Risk Factors. The epidemiological patterns described above suggest that environmental factors contribute to the etiology of the type 1 diabetes. In particular, the recent temporal increase in type 1 diabetes incidence points to a changing global environment rather than variation in the gene pool, which require the passage of multiple generations. Twin studies also provide evidence for the importance of environmental risk factors for type 1 diabetes. Type 1 diabetes concordance rates for monozygous twins are higher than those for dizygous twins (approximately 30% vs. 10%, respectively).[36] However, most monozygous twin pairs remain discordant. Thus, type 1 diabetes cannot be completely genetically determined.

Environmental risk factors are thought to act as either "initiators" or "accelerators" of beta cell autoimmunity, or "precipitators" of overt symptoms in individuals who already have evidence of beta cell destruction.[37]

They also may function by mechanisms that are directly harmful to the pancreas, or by indirect methods that produce an abnormal immune response to proteins normally present in cells. The type 1 diabetes environmental risk factors that have received most attention are viruses, infant nutrition, and hygiene.

A. *Viruses.* Enteroviruses, especially Coxsackie virus B (CVB), have been the focus of numerous ecologic and case-control studies.[38] CVB infections are frequent during childhood and are known to have systemic effects on the pancreas. Recent prospective studies are helping to elucidate the role of viruses to the etiology of type 1 diabetes. A meta-analysis of cohort and case-control studies found a clinically significant association between a history of enterovirus infection and type 1 diabetes.[38] Recently, investigators from The Environmental Determinants of Type 1 Diabetes in the Young (TEDDY) study reported that a higher rate of respiratory infections is associated with increased risk of autoantibody seroconversion in children at high risk for developing type 1 diabetes.[39] Other viruses, including mumps, cytomegalovirus, rotavirus, and rubella, have also been associated with the disease.[40] Additionally, maternal viral infections have been associated with an increased future risk of type 1 diabetes in the developing fetus.[41,42]

B. *Nutrition.* Another hypothesis that has been the subject of considerable interest relates to early exposure to cow's milk protein and the subsequent development of type 1 diabetes. The first epidemiologic observation of such a relationship was by Borch-Johnsen et al., who found that type 1 diabetes children were breast-fed for shorter periods of time than their nondiabetic siblings or children from the general population.[43] The authors postulated that the lack of immunologic protection from insufficient breast feeding may increase risk for type 1 diabetes later during childhood. It was also postulated that shorter duration of breast feeding may indirectly reflect early exposure to dietary proteins that stimulate an abnormal immune response in newborns. Most recently, it has been hypothesized that the protective effect of breast feeding may be due, in part, to its role in gut maturation.[44] Breast milk contains growth factors, cytokines, and other substances necessary for the maturation of the intestinal mucosa. Breast-feeding also protects against enteric infections during infancy, and promotes proper colonization of the gut. Interestingly, enteroviral infections can also interfere with gut immunoregulation, which may explain the epidemiologic associations between viral infections and type 1 diabetes. Other potential dietary triggers include early introduction of cereals, which has been associated with increased risk of islet autoimmunity, particularly in children with the high-risk HLA genotypes.[45]

C. *Hygiene.* The role of hygiene in the etiology of type 1 diabetes is also currently being explored, with mixed results.[46–49] It has been hypothesized that delayed exposure to microorganisms due to improvements in standard of living hinders the development of the immune system, such that it is more likely to respond inappropriately when introduced to such agents at older (compared to younger) ages. This explanation is consistent with recent reports indicating that factors such as day care attendance,[46] sharing a bedroom with a sibling, and contact with pets are protective against type 1 diabetes.[47] Further studies are needed to determine if improved hygiene can explain the temporal increase in the incidence of type 1 diabetes worldwide.

Treatment and Prevention of Type 1 Diabetes. At the present time, there is no way to prevent type 1 diabetes. Lifelong insulin administration, either by injection or insulin pump, is currently the only available treatment for the disease. However, promising research is underway to develop an "artificial pancreas," which is a closed-loop system comprising a sensor to measure blood glucose levels and a wirelessly connected insulin pump to deliver the necessary amount of insulin, as determined by a computer algorithm.[50] Although a cure for type 1 diabetes is currently unavailable, several large multinational investigations have been designed to evaluate a variety of primary and secondary disease interventions. The tested interventions have included prophylactic nasal insulin [Diabetes Prediction and Prevention Project (DIPP) in Finland],[51] oral and injected insulin [Diabetes Prevention Trial-1 (DPT-1) in the United States],[52] as well as high doses of nicotinamide [European Nicotinamide Diabetes Intervention Trial (ENDIT)],[53] the avoidance of cow's milk exposure during the first six months of life [trial to reduce in genetically at-risk (TRIGR) in Finland, the United States, and other countries],[54] and delayed introduction of gluten-containing foods (BABYDIET).[55] These investigations have focused on "prediabetic" individuals identified from families with at least one child with type 1 diabetes. DIPP, TRIGR, and BABYDIET used HLA-DQB1 screening and recruited only individuals at increased genetic risk. The remaining trials recruited relatives with evidence of beta cell autoimmunity as a preclinical marker for disease. To date, none of these interventions have prevented or delayed the onset of type 1 diabetes.[51–55] More recently, it has been hypothesized that early exposure to antigens, in this case, insulin, may induce immune tolerance and prevent autoimmunity. Thus, a pilot trial (Primary Oral Insulin Trial (Pre-POINT) in Germany, Austria, the United States, and the United Kingdom) studied the immune response to high-dose oral insulin compared to placebo in children with increased genetic risk.[56] Pre-POINT identified children with two first-degree relatives with type 1 diabetes and HLA haplotype DR4-DQB1*0302 or DR4-DQB1*0302 and who were autoantibody negative. The investigators found evidence of an immune response to oral insulin, supporting the possibility of preventing autoimmunity though immune tolerance induction and further study is underway. Finally, *Type 1 Diabetes TrialNet* is a collaborative network of clinical centers and experts in diabetes and immunology under which new intervention strategies are being planned.[57] It is ultimately hoped that through genetic testing, individuals at high risk for type 1 diabetes could be identified prior to the onset of the disease—at a time when primary prevention strategies could be safely administered. It is most likely that such predictive genetic testing would be offered to families with an affected individual before it was made available to the general population.

Type 2 Diabetes

Epidemiology. Type 2 diabetes is more difficult to define than type 1 diabetes. The rates among and within countries vary dramatically, partially depending on the specific classification criteria used for type 2 diabetes. The most recent data from the International Diabetes Federation (IDF) estimates the worldwide prevalence to be 424 million people or 8.8% of adults age 20–79. The prevalence is expected to increase to 629.6 million by 2045.[15] Globally, costs are estimated to be $727 billion on healthcare—or one for every eight dollars spent on healthcare.[15] The prevalence of type 2 diabetes increases with age, with the highest prevalence among those age > 60 years. There is little difference by sex. There is approximately twofold difference in the number of cases in urban versus rural areas. The United States ranks third behind India and China with 30.3 million peoples having type 2 diabetes.[15,58] The prevalence of type 2 diabetes also varies by race and ethnicity. The age-adjusted prevalence of diagnosed and undiagnosed diabetes 2011–14 was higher among Asians, non-Hispanic Blacks, Native Americans, and Hispanics.[58] Globally, the prevalence is higher among indigenous populations.[59,60] This increase in prevalence is likely due to westernization of diets resulting in higher rates of obesity.[60]

Risk Factors. A pattern of increasing rates of obesity in the population parallels the increasing prevalence of type 2 diabetes worldwide.[15,61] In the United States, for example, the prevalence of obesity among adults, defined as a Body Mass Index (BMI) of greater than 30 kg/m^2, has increased from 12% in 1991 to 19.8% in 2000, to 36% according to data from 2011 to 2014.[62] The highest prevalence for obesity was reported in Mississippi at 25.9% in 2001. A corresponding increase is reported in diabetes prevalence was also observed.[58] Interestingly, within a country such as the United States, one generally finds an inverse relationship between obesity and socioeconomic class,[58] with higher rates of type 2 diabetes in lower socioeconomic groups.[59] However, a risk factor associated with higher socioeconomic status is decreased physical activity. As socioeconomic status increases, the overall level of physical activity generally declines, especially that related to work. Further, lower rates of physical activity are found in ethnic minorities.[60] Thus, at the same time that caloric intake is increasing, physical activity is decreasing, leading to an increased prevalence of obesity within the population. A more recently researched risk factor for obesity is time spent sedentary. This is not necessarily the lack of physical activity. Sedentary behavior may include screen time, sitting while driving or commuting, and sitting while reading or participating in other seated activities.[63] One review found that there may be a dose–response relationship between where increased television viewing time is positively associated with weight. Sedentary time may also be associated with insulin resistance.[63] Currently physical activity guidelines in the United States for those age 18–64 recommend 150 minutes of moderate-intensity aerobic activity like brisk walking every week or 75 minutes of vigorous-intensity aerobic activity like jogging or running, and strength training, working all major muscle groups, on 2 or more days per week.[64] Only one in five adults meet these recommendations.[65]

Nutrition plays a role in both diabetes risk and prevention. The goals of nutrition should be to maintain a healthy weight, incorporate nutrient-dense foods in appropriate portion sizes. Cultural sensitivity around dietary recommendations is crucial for adoption of healthy eating behaviors.[66]

Genetic Factors. While family history plays a significant role in the risk for developing type 2 diabetes, we still know little about specific genotypes associated with the disease. This is likely because of the complexity identifying specific genes association with type 2 diabetes combined with the complexity of the gene environment interactions.[67] Currently, only a few genes have been identified through linkage and candidate gene studies. In genome-wide association studies (GWAS) several genes have been identified in possibly playing a role in the heritability of type 2 diabetes. *TCF7L2* is the most promising of this group. This gene may play a role in type 2 diabetes by "decreasing insulin secretion from beta cells perhaps by altering the action of incretins that modulate the insulin response to meals.[67–69] While other genes have been identified in GWAS studies their mechanism in conferring risk for diabetes is not well understood, although research indicates it may be through insulin secretion, or results could not be replicated in other populations.[67] Increased interest in epigenetics were gene expression in response to environmental circumstances may exist for two to three generations. There are times of increased susceptibility where the environment can have the biggest influence on development. It is during this time that genetic programming can be modified and susceptibility to disease increases.[70] The best example of this is the intrauterine nutrition and birthweight.[67] As the current science exists, the role of genetics in the risk of type 2 diabetes accounts for a small portion of diabetes risk.

Diabetes Prevention. The development of type 2 diabetes is a two-stage process, with the first stage being resistance to insulin's action (likely exacerbated by obesity and physical inactivity) and the second stage being failure of the pancreas to increase insulin secretion enough to overcome this resistance. This theory receives support from a number of reports including one from the Pima Indians, which showed differing predictive values of fasting and post challenge insulin values for developing type 2 diabetes consistent with a hyperinsulinemic phase followed by eventual insulinopenia.[71]

The efficacy of lifestyle interventions to prevent type 2 diabetes is well studied. These trials applied sound methods for implementing diabetes prevention strategies, and will be briefly reviewed. The focus of these trials was lifestyle modification including weight loss and increased physical activity. The Da Qing study[72] followed 577 subjects with IGT from local clinics. Subjects were randomized at the clinic level to diet, exercise, diet and exercise, or a control group and followed for 6 years. Intervention groups experienced a significantly lower incidence of type 2 diabetes compared to controls (31%, 46%, 42%, and 67.7%, respectively). A lower incidence of diabetes was also seen in those with lower BMIs. Similar to the Da Qing trial, the Finnish Diabetes Prevention Study[73] examined whether the onset of type 2 diabetes could be prevented through lifestyle modification in subjects with IGT. Five hundred twenty-two subjects were randomized to an intervention group that received individualized counseling aimed at weight reduction, dietary fat reduction, saturated fat reduction, increased dietary fiber, and increased physical activity. The trial demonstrated that lifestyle changes significantly reduced the risk of diabetes in middle-aged, overweight subjects. After a modest (4.7%) weight loss, those in the intervention group experienced a 58% reduction in incidence of diabetes over a mean follow-up of 3.2 years. Moreover, blood pressure, triglycerides, and high-density lipoprotein cholesterol levels also improved significantly. The study to prevent noninsulin-dependent diabetes mellitus (STOP-NIDDM) trial[74] randomized 714 (IGT) subjects to acarbose and 715 subjects to a control group. After a mean follow-up of 3.3 years, compared to controls, there was a 25% relative risk reduction in the incidence of diabetes. Finally, in the Diabetes Prevention Program (DPP)[75] 3234 subjects with IGT were randomized to placebo, metformin (850 mg twice daily), or intensive lifestyle modification. The lifestyle modification consisted of weekly one-on-one counseling for a 16-week curriculum during the first 24 weeks of the study. Subsequent visits were held about once per month. The goal of the lifestyle arm was 7% weight loss and 150 minutes per week of physical activity. Intensive lifestyle modification reduced the incidence of type 2 diabetes in persons at high risk by 58% in comparison to the metformin study group in which incidence was reduced by 31%. The DPP has also shown that these interventions reduce the incidence of new metabolic syndrome by 41% (lifestyle) and 17% (metformin) compared with placebo.[76]

The efficacy of the diabetes prevention studies is clear, the effectiveness studies translating the findings of these studies to the "real world" have also demonstrated promising results. One of the challenges of implementing these prevention programs at the community level is cost. The CDC conducted a systematic review for the Community Preventive Services Task force in 2015.[77] Twenty-eight studies were included. Costs were expressed in 2013 dollars. The median program cost per participant was $653, with the group-based programs being most cost effective. Some additional challenges include reaching disadvantaged populations, sustainability, and delivery methods that increase access. As insurance coverage for these programs increases, these barriers may be overcome.

Screening

The recent emphasis on diabetes prevention has prompted a growing number of blood glucose screenings. The purpose of screening is to identify asymptomatic individuals who may have diabetes; however, screening is not the same as diagnosis as screening is conducted in asymptomatic people, and the effectiveness of diagnosing an asymptomatic individual is still controversial. A systematic review by the U.S. Preventive Service Task Force in 2014 concluded that while there are effective treatments to delay the progression to type 2 diabetes, screening did not reduce mortality. Recently two randomized controlled trials were released that investigated the effectiveness of screening for type 2 diabetes in asymptomatic individuals and reduced mortality. These were from the ADDITION Study Europe but focused specifically on the Danish population.[78,79] One study showed no reduction in mortality in the screened population compared with the general Danish population[78]; however, the other[79] showed a significant reduction in adjusted all-cause mortality, cardiovascular mortality, cancer mortality, and diabetes-related mortality. There was also a significant reduction in cardiovascular events. These studies were not without limitations including inadequate control groups or lack of randomization.[80] Screening in the community setting outside a healthcare setting may not be completely effective because of the possibility of inadequate follow-up after a positive test, or repeat testing in those who are negative. Therefore, this type of screening is currently not recommended.[8] Criteria for screening by a healthcare professional or within the healthcare setting for prediabetes and diabetes in asymptomatic adults include[81]:

1. Overweight (BMI ≥ 25 kg/m² or ≥ 23 kg/m² in Asian Americans) and have one or more additional risk factors;
   a. Physical inactivity,
   b. First-degree relative with diabetes,
   c. High-risk race/ethnicity (e.g., African American, Hispanic/Latino, Native American, Asian American, Pacific Islander),
   d. History of CVD,
   e. Hypertension (≥140/90 mm Hg or on therapy for hypertension),
   f. HDL cholesterol level < 35 mg/dL (0.90 mmol/L) and/or a triglyceride level > 250 mg/dL (2.82 mmol/L), and
   g. Women with PCOS.
2. Patients with prediabetes (A1C ≥5.7% [39 mmol/mol], IGT or IFG) should be tested yearly;
3. Women who were diagnosed with GDM should have lifelong testing at least every 3 years;
4. For all other patients, testing should begin at age 45 years; and
5. If results are normal, testing should be repeated at a minimum of 3-year intervals, with consideration of more frequent testing depending on initial results and risk status.

DIABETES-RELATED MORBIDITY AND MORTALITY

Prior to the introduction of insulin in 1922 by Banting and Best, life expectancy of patients with type 1 diabetes was about 1–2 years. After the development and widespread use of insulin, there was a dramatic increase in life expectancy for patients with type 1 diabetes. Suddenly those with type 1 diabetes could lead relatively normal lives. However, 20–30 years later the long-term sequelae of type 1 diabetes began to become evident.

Both type 1 diabetes and type 2 diabetes patients are at risk for these long-term complications. Complications come mainly from disorders of the circulation, either macrovascular, including accelerated atherosclerosis resulting in stroke, heart, and peripheral vascular disease, or microvascular disorders of the kidney and retina, as well as neuropathy. The complications appear to be similar for both type 1 diabetes and type 2 diabetes, although the prevalence may be somewhat higher in type 1 diabetes mainly due to longer diabetes duration in those with type 1. The relationships with age and duration also vary between the two types of diabetes, partly because of the younger age of onset of type 1 diabetes (which leads to complications at a younger age) and the difficulty of determining the onset of type 2 diabetes (which means complications are often present at the onset of known disease). However, careful analysis controlling for these time-dependent variables suggests that the incidence of the microvascular complications is remarkably similar by true duration.[82]

Mortality in Type 1 Diabetes

Compared to people without diabetes, mortality rates are estimated to be two- to fourfold higher in type 1 diabetes[83,84] and approximately twofold higher in type 2 diabetes,[85] with cardiovascular disease as the leading cause of death. In a systematic review of 23 population-based cohorts, type 1 diabetes was associated with excess mortality worldwide; however, the magnitude of excess risk varied widely.[86] More recently, data from the Scottish Linkage Registry[84] and the Swedish National Diabetes Register[87] have also shown increased mortality associated with type 1 diabetes, with a more marked excess observed in women, particularly for deaths due to cardiovascular causes. Despite this continued excess risk of mortality, there are signs of improvement. The Allegheny County diabetes registry has shown an improvement in survival, relative to the general population, by diagnosis cohort (1965–69, 1970–74, 1975–79).[88] When cause-specific mortality was examined, declines in deaths due to renal disease, cardiovascular disease, and acute complications were noted.[89] There were, however, differential results by race, where African-Americans had significantly higher mortality rates for deaths due to the same causes. In the Pittsburgh Epidemiology of Diabetes Complications study, a 15-year increase in life expectancy was observed in the cohort diagnosed between 1965 and 1980, compared to the group diagnosed between 1950 and 1964, with the life expectancy of the more recently diagnosed cohort approaching that of the general U.S. population.[90] The reasons for these observed improvements in survival are not well established, but there is evidence that the changes in diabetes treatment regimens may be at least partially responsible. Recent data from the Diabetes Control and Complications Trial (DCCT) and its associated Epidemiology of Diabetes Interventions and Complications (EDIC) follow-up study have demonstrated that, after a mean of 27 years of follow-up, the overall risk of mortality in those who had received intensive insulin therapy in the original DCCT trial portion of the study was reduced compared to those who received conventional therapy.[91] Good glycemic control is strongly associated with decreased microvascular disease, particularly the development of albuminuria, which has emerged as the risk factor, which may best account for the excess mortality associated with type 1 diabetes.[92,93] Thus, the incorporation of intensive insulin therapy into clinical practice following the results of the DCCT may explain much of the improvements in mortality seen in the observational data.

Mortality in Type 2 Diabetes

Diabetes is the seventh leading cause of death in the United States representing a death rate of 23.2 deaths per 100,000 or 3% of individuals in the general population of the United States.[94] The prevalence of diabetes continues to increase parallel to the increase in obesity. While mortality rates for people with diabetes decreased, they paralleled the decreased mortality among those without diabetes; therefore, mortality rates for people with diabetes remain relatively stable. All-cause mortality rates are two to three times higher among people with diabetes compared with those who do not have diabetes. Cardiovascular disease is the leading cause of death and people with diabetes are twice as likely to have CVD. Trends in mortality attributable to type 2 diabetes are somewhat difficult to compare due to changing definitions of diabetes, agreement of definitions worldwide, and methods of ascertainment of mortality data. Most mortality data in the United States is obtained from death certificates. The inconsistencies in reporting diabetes as a cause of death lead to underestimates of mortality. Data from cohort studies provide the most robust estimates of mortality. Cohort studies do not rely on death certificates alone, but rather adjudicate causes of death from medical records or family members. There are sex-specific differences in diabetes mortality. In the Framingham study, women experienced a threefold risk increased risk and men a twofold increased risk compared to nondiabetic participants. There are also difference by race and ethnicity where deaths are higher in non-Hispanic black, Hispanic, and non-Hispanic American Indian populations compared to non-Hispanic whites.[94]

Eye Disease (Retinopathy)

Diabetic retinopathy occurs when there are specific changes in the appearance of the retina, and is the leading cause of blindness among 20–74 years olds.[95] There are two types of diabetic retinopathy—proliferative and nonproliferative. Nonproliferative retinopathy is an early stage of the complication. Microaneurysms may leak fluid into the retina leading to swelling if the macula. This results in blurred vision, although some people may be asymptomatic in the early stages. Proliferative retinopathy is the more advanced form. During this stage, new small blood vessels begin to grow. Because they are weak, they may leak blood-clouding vision. There may also be retinal detachment or glaucoma. The prevalence of diabetic retinopathy increases with longer duration of diabetes. Hispanics and African Americans with diabetes are more likely to develop retinopathy. Hypertension and hyperlipidemia also increase risk.[96]

Epidemiology. The prevalence of diabetic retinopathy is highly related to diabetes duration for both type 1 and type 2 diabetes. After 20 years of diabetes, virtually 100% of those with type 1 diabetes[97] and approximately one-third to two thirds (depending on the source) of those with type 2 diabetes,[97–99] show some evidence of damage to the retina. Among those with type 2 diabetes, those using insulin have a higher prevalence of retinopathy compared with those who do not use insulin.[97] A higher proportion of people with type 2 diabetes have retinopathy present at diagnosis compared with type 1 diabetes likely due to the onset of diabetes occurring 4–7 years prior to diagnosis.[100]

As diabetic retinopathy can be detected before it threatens vision, blindness due to diabetic retinopathy can be prevented in many cases. There are several risk factors in the causal pathway of retinopathy. These include diabetes duration, hyperglycemia, hypertension, dyslipidemia, and obesity.[95] Women who have diabetes and become pregnant should be particularly vigilant and participate in eye exams at the recommended frequency for pregnant women.[101] The best prevention against the onset of retinopathy is controlling risk factors.[96] Clinical guidelines provide the recommended frequency of comprehensive dilated eye exams. According to the 2017 Standards of Medical Care[102] for people with type 1 diabetes, should have a comprehensive dilated eye exam within 5 years after the onset of diabetes. In people with type 2 diabetes, a comprehensive dilated eye exam should be conducted at the time of diagnosis. If there is no retinopathy present, exams should be conducted every 2 years provided the patient has good glycemic control. Otherwise, dilated retinal examinations should be conducted every year. It is thus important that patients and physicians be educated about the need for frequent eye examinations and that adequate clinical treatment for diabetic retinopathy be available in the community.

Renal Disease (Nephropathy)

Epidemiology. Diabetic renal disease is a major cause of morbidity and mortality among those with diabetes.[103] Diabetes is currently the leading cause of treatment for end-stage renal disease (ESRD), accounting for 44% of the 120,688 new ESRD cases during 2014.[104] According to the 2014 data, 238,376 people with diabetes have ESRD and are living on chronic dialysis or with a kidney transplant. Diabetes increases the risk of renal failure 17- to 20-fold. Recent data suggest that over 80% of people with type 1 diabetes will eventually have some degree of renal damage (i.e., including those with microalbuminuria—a more modest degree of abnormal urinary albumin excretion that is predictive of more advanced disease), with $> 70\%$ developing clinically significant proteinuria and renal disease.[105] End-stage renal disease rates remain high, with $> 25\%$ of persons with type 1 diabetes eventually developing the condition. The relative risk of mortality from renal disease for persons with diabetes compared to the general population is highest for those in the 15- to 44-year age group, consistent with a higher prevalence and severity in type 1 diabetes.[106] However, it is clear that mortality is increased even at earlier stages of nephropathy, with both the FinnDiane and Pittsburgh EDC studies demonstrating that all excess mortality in type 1 diabetes can be attributed to increased albuminuria.[92,93]

Prevalence rates are somewhat lower in type 2 diabetes overall, partly because the later age of onset means many patients may have died from heart disease before there has been sufficient duration to develop renal disease. Despite recent advances in the diagnosis and treatment of renal failure in diabetes, the problem has not been resolved.

Prevention. The presence of microalbuminuria appears to predict the subsequent development of diabetic nephropathy and end stage renal failure.[107] Of particular note is the value of ACE inhibitors and angiotensin receptor blockers in slowing the progression of renal disease.[108] The effect of ACE inhibitors appears to be independent of any blood pressure lowering effect. Hypertension, which may be primary or secondary to the renal disease, accelerates the development of renal failure. Lipid disturbances may also predict the development of microalbuminuria.[109] The major predictor, however, of the development of early diabetic renal disease is poor glycemic control.[110,111] The value of an intensive therapy regimen was also clearly demonstrated in the DCCT (54% reduction).[112] Interestingly, in type 1 diabetes, insulin resistance is emerging as a powerful predictor of nephropathy[113] as well as coronary artery disease (CAD), which may explain their association. Further, much attention is being paid to the genetic susceptibility to nephropathy, as there is clearly a major genetic component.[114]

Nerve Disease (Neuropathy)

Epidemiology. Another major complication of diabetes is neuropathy, which affects many organ systems. The major consequences of diabetic neuropathy are pain, weakness, and loss of sensation. Parallel disorders of the autonomic nervous system may lead to problems of sexual function and urinary and gastrointestinal abnormalities. The two major classifications of neuropathy are distal symmetrical polyneuropathy (DSPN) and cardiovascular autonomic neuropathy (CAN).[115] Estimates of the prevalence of either type of neuropathy are complicated by the variety of measurement modalities. Additionally, the onset of these abnormalities can precede the diagnosis of diabetes by several years. As an example, neuropathic changes may be present among more than 10% of people at diagnosis with approximately half developing DSPN over time.[115] Approximately 11–25% of people with prediabetes have peripheral neuropathy.[116] Later manifestations of DSPN may include foot ulceration. A likely result of loss of sensation.

CAN manifests as a reduction in heart rate variability, and is associated with increased mortality or CVD among those with diabetes.[117] CAN causes a delay in the perception of pain; therefore, the patient may be asymptomatic resulting in a silent or unrecognized myocardial infarction (MI).[117] In a meta-analysis, the prevalence of MI among those with diabetes was twice as high in those with CAN compared to those without CAN (1.96 95%CI: 1.53–2.51),[118] supporting further investigation of CAN as a risk factor for unrecognized MI. CAN may also be present in the prediabetic state and is often present at diagnosis.[119,120] Other manifestations of autonomic neuropathy include disturbances of the gastrointestinal system and the urogenital system.[115]

Prevention. It has long been recognized that strict control of blood glucose may improve neural function, for example, peripheral nerve conduction. The evidence in type 1 diabetes is much clearer than for type 2 diabetes.[115] In the DCCT/EDIC study, intensive glycemic control reduced the risk of DSPN and CAN by 64% and 45%, respectively ($p < 0.01$), compared with conventional therapy. These differences remained at the 13-/14-year follow-up in EDIC.[121] Strategies that control risk factors for diabetes complications such as blood pressure and lipid control, in addition to glycemic control may be the best strategy for prevention of this group of complications. Certain medications may provide symptomatic relief for DSPN; however, the evidence thus far is short term.[122]

Macrovascular Disease and Atherosclerosis

The most convincing epidemiological evidence for increased cardiovascular disease in diabetes comes from large-scale prospective studies, many of which were primarily designed to study cardiovascular disease in the general population. Studies like Framingham[123] and the Cardiovascular Health Study[124] have demonstrated that diabetes (uniquely defined in Framingham as "glucose intolerant") is associated with a greatly enhanced risk and that cardiovascular disease is the leading cause of death in those with diabetes.[125,126] Diabetes leads to a greater than normal risk for all manifestations of atherosclerosis, including coronary, cerebrovascular, and peripheral vascular disease.[123,127] The latter is so common in diabetes that nearly 40% of all lower extremity amputations in the United States occur in persons with diabetes.[128] In the general population women have a lower risk of CHD than men, but this advantage is lost in women with diabetes, who have rates approaching those of men.[129,130] A meta-analysis suggests that a reduction in the gender differential for CHD in diabetes is true for CHD mortality but not for morbidity.[131] The survival of diabetic patients, especially women, after a cardiac event also appears to be less than that seen in the general population. The reasons for the greater excess risk in women is unknown, but it has been suggested that women with diabetes may have less favorable cardiovascular risk profiles or are less likely to receive treatment for blood pressure or high cholesterol compared to men.[129,132]

When it occurs, atherosclerosis is often more extensive in diabetic than in nondiabetic subjects,[133,134] although not all studies show a clear relationship between blood sugar and CVD. For example, in the UKPDS, HbA1c was a borderline predictor of MI and intensive therapy had only a borderline ($p = 0.052$) 16% reduction in CHD events.[135] In more recent trials, Action to Control Cardiovascular Risk in Diabetes study (ACCORD),[136] Action in Diabetes and Vascular Disease trial (ADVANCE),[137] and Veterans Affairs Diabetes Trial (VADT)[138] intensive insulin therapy did not reduce the risk of nonfatal MI, stroke, or CVD death. The reasons for the absence of benefit in preventing cardiovascular events and mortality in these studies is unclear, but may be explained by several factors, including long duration of diabetes, established cardiovascular events, or levels of CVD risk factors at baseline. Divergent opinions also are apparent in terms of the role of blood sugar in the nondiabetic range. Early studies failed to show a relationship between blood glucose levels in the nondiabetic range and CVD[139]; however, recent meta regression analysis and pooled analyses show a relationship in the normal glucose range.[140,141] Recently, investigators from the Epidemiology of Diabetes Interventions and Complications Study (follow-up of the DCCT) have demonstrated a long-term benefit of early intensive glycemic control on the incidence of CVD in type 1 diabetes. Among 1375 patients, the number of incident CVD events in those intensively treated during the DCCT was reduced compared to those on conventional therapy (46 compared to 98 events).[142] More recent data from the Swedish National Diabetes Register has shown a strong association between glycemic control and CVD mortality.[87]

The IGT stage is often characterized by hyperinsulinemia and insulin resistance. In the Paris study, in multivariate analyses, insulin concentration rather than diabetic IGT status was the stronger predictor of CHD.[143] A further factor linked with hyperinsulinemia is central adiposity, which was discussed earlier as a risk factor for the development of diabetes.[144–147] Central adiposity is also a risk factor for CVD independent of obesity,[148] a finding most clearly shown in women. Consequently a male type of fat deposition (if found in women) may be associated with hyperinsulinemia[149] and thus may provide a marker for a metabolic derangement predisposing to both diabetes and CVD generally, and the relatively poorer cardiovascular prognosis of diabetic women. This association of central adiposity with insulin resistance and the metabolic syndrome is thought to be the prime basis of the excess CVD in type 2 diabetes and glucose intolerance and also has been proposed as a leading feature of CVD in type 1 diabetes.[150–153]

As lipoproteins are altered in diabetes, it is tempting to hypothesize that these changes account for the increased CVD risk seen in diabetes. Many studies,[123,125,144,154,155] have shown that serum cholesterol levels relate to CVD risk in those with diabetes in a way similar to that seen in the general population. However, total and LDL cholesterol levels are not greatly elevated in many diabetics, so the role of cholesterol in explaining the *increased* risk in diabetes is limited.[156] Data from the Multiple Risk Factor Intervention Study (MRFIT), which screened over 360,000 men for CVD risk factors and subsequently followed them for mortality, suggest men with type 2 diabetes had rates three times higher than nondiabetics all along the cholesterol curve.[157] In type 1 diabetes, as indicated earlier, it appears that the major determinant of CVD risk is proteinuria,[114] although recent risk factor engines also suggest that hypertension, white blood cell count, HDLc, non-HDLc, triglycerides, diabetes duration, and smoking are associated with incident CAD events.[158–161]

If cholesterol concentration itself has a limited role, other lipid measures may be of greater importance to diabetes. There is evidence that triglyceride level is an independent risk factor for CVD in both type 1 and type 2 diabetes.[162,163] Furthermore, alterations in HDL concentration and a shift toward a more atherogenic lipoprotein composition occur in diabetes, which may further increase cardiovascular risk.[164] Insulin itself, beyond its effect on the lipids, can have direct effects on the arterial wall that promote atherogenicity.[165,166] Hyperinsulinemia has also been related to blood pressure elevation.[167–169] The importance of insulin is also shown by its demonstration as an independent risk factor for CVD in some,[170–173] but not all,[174–176] prospective studies of men in the general population, however distinguishing insulin effects per se from hyperinsulinemia representing insulin resistance is difficult.[177]

Many studies have demonstrated altered hemostatic factors including platelets and fibrinogen, which may provide yet another mechanism for the enhanced CVD risk in diabetes.[178] Finally, the haptoglobin (Hp) genotype has emerged as a potentially important CVD risk factor in diabetes and may help to explain the increased risk of CVD in the presence of hyperglycemia.[179] Thus it is abundantly clear that those with diabetes have severe handicaps to face in terms of cardiovascular risk above and beyond the lipoprotein disturbances.

Diabetes Care

While the last two decades provided an explosion of technology and treatment options for people with diabetes, achievement of therapeutic goals remains a challenge. In the United Stated, only 18% achieve treatment goals for HbA1c, blood pressure, and LDLc.[180] Reasons for this can be attributed to system, provider, and patient factors. Diabetes care remains challenging in the current healthcare environment in the United States. The health system remains fragmented and is poorly designed to coordinate care. While more health systems are adopting electronic health records, they may not communicate with each other and do little to solve the fragmentation issue.

The future of diabetes care must be integrated and patient centered where care is coordinated to meet the needs of the patient and is delivered by a team of providers. These providers can include but is not limited to the physician, diabetes educator, behavioral specialist, social worker, and a community health worker. Care should be accessible to patients. Barriers around access may include physical, financial, psychosocial, health beliefs or culture, and psychological.[181–183] The social determinants of health also need to be considered as one of the complexities of treatment. The World Health Organization defines the social determinants of health as *the conditions in which people are born, grow, work, live, and age, and the wider set of forces and systems shaping the conditions of daily life.*[184] These factors provide the context in which people must care for their diabetes and may be critical variables in the pathway to improved outcomes in people with diabetes.

SUMMARY AND FUTURE

The release of the results of the DCCT and UKPDS more than 20 years ago have put beyond question, the value of intensive therapy to lower blood glucose levels in terms of the so called triopathy of type 1 and type 2 diabetes complications (retinopathy, nephropathy, and neuropathy). As intensive therapy with insulin also increases the risk of severe hypoglycaemia[185] and is difficult to translate into general practice, it would seem prudent to also focus on other CVD risk factors (e.g., hypertension and hyperlipidemia) to prevent these complications in type 2 diabetes. Studies examining cardiovascular events among people with type 2 diabetes demonstrate that controlling these risk factors can directly impact the occurrence of both new[186–190] and repeat events.[191–193] While major clinical trials, ACCORD,[136] ADVANCE,[137] and VADT,[138] have found that intensive insulin therapy did not reduce the risk of nonfatal MI, stroke, or CVD death, several new trials have shown promising results for other glucose-lowering therapies, including SGLT-2 inhibitors and GLP-1 receptor antagonists[194] Several additional trials of glucose-lowering therapies and CVD outcomes are underway and promise to provide greater insight.

While the evidence for the prevention of diabetes and its complications is clear, translation into the community of diabetes care providers and patients remains challenging. The goal of prevention is to improve short- and long-term outcomes as well as the economic consequences of a disease. Models of chronic illness care that focus on a multilevel approach to primary and secondary prevention are necessary in order to prevent the morbidity and mortality associated with diabetes.

THYROID DISORDERS

Hypothyroidism

Hypothyroidism is defined as thyroid hormone deficiency, which results in the inability to meet the metabolic demands of the body.[195] Its diagnosis is primarily based on biochemical tests, which measure the level of thyroid stimulating hormone and free thyroxine levels in the blood.[196] The diagnosis is made when high level of thyroid stimulating hormone is above the reference range and levels of free thyroxine levels are below the reference range.[196] Clinically, it can have a myriad of symptoms based on the degree of thyroid dysfunction and length of time with the dysfunction. Common clinical symptoms include goiter, depression, dry skin, weakness, weight gain, memory impairment, bradycardia, macroglossia, menorrhagia, myalgias, proximal muscle weakness, hair loss, and edema.[195] Hypothyroidism can also present without clinical manifestations, in which case it is termed subclinical hypothyroidism.[197] Laboratory findings in such case present an elevated thyroid-stimulating hormone with normal free thyroxine levels in the blood.[195]

Epidemiology. Hypothyroidism is a relative common condition, affecting approximately 1 in 300 Americans in the general population.[195] However, there is controversy on the definition for hypothyroidism, as the presence of an elevated Thyroid Stimulating Hormone (TSH) level can result in subclinical hypothyroidism, which as the name specifies, no clinical symptoms of overt thyroid disease are present. Due to such discrepancies, the prevalence of hypothyroidism in the United States can range from 0.3% to 3.7% and from 0.2% to 5.3% in Europe.[196] The prevalence of hypothyroidism is affected by age, with a higher prevalence in populations older than 60 years old, as well as higher in females than in males and in Caucasians.[195,196] Dietary iodine also has an effect in the prevalence of hypothyroidism, which is higher in both, populations with iodine deficiency and in populations with iodine excess.[196]

Causes. As thyroid function is regulated as part of the hypothalamic-pituitary axis, its causes can be due to dysfunctions at different levels of thyroid regulation. It can be defined as primary, secondary, and tertiary.[196] Primary hypothyroidism refers to dysfunction of the thyroid gland, whereas secondary hypothyroidism refers to dysfunction of the pituitary gland and impaired production and secretion of thyroid-stimulating hormone. Tertiary hypothyroidism refers to dysfunction of the hypothalamus, thus affecting the production of thyrotropin-releasing hormone.

The most common cause of primary hypothyroidism worldwide is iodine deficiency; however, in areas of adequate iodine intake, autoimmune disease is the most common cause, such as most of the United States.[196]

Hyperthyroidism

Hyperthyroidism is defined as excess thyroid hormone production and secretion. It can be classified as overt hyperthyroidism, in which there are low level of TSH concentration and high concentrations of thyroid hormones, or subclinical hyperthyroidism, in which there is a normal TSH concentration with raised levels of thyroid hormone concentration.[198] Clinical manifestations result from symptoms due to amplification of catecholamine signaling and include: palpitations, heat intolerance, diaphoresis, tremor, stare, lid lag, anxiety, disturbed sleep, weight loss, sweating, and polydipsia.[199]

Epidemiology. The prevalence of hyperthyroidism in the United States is 1.3%. It increases with age and is more frequent in women.[198] Data on ethnic differences is scarce; however, it seems to be more frequent in whites than in other races.[198] Mild hyperthyroidism is also reported to have a higher incidence in iodine deficient areas if compared to iodine sufficient areas and decrease after the introduction of universal salt iodization programs.[198]

Causes. In iodine sufficient areas, the most common cause is Grave's Disease.[199] Grave's disease is an autoimmune disease thought to be multifactorial, resulting in thyroid stimulating antibodies activate TSH receptors resulting in thyroid hormone synthesis.[199] Female sex, history of autoimmune disease, smoking, and psychological stress are risk factors for Grave's disease.[198,199] Other common causes include toxic adenoma, which is the second most common cause in the United States and the most common cause in older individuals living in iodine-deficient areas.[198] The condition results from nodules arising due to frequent replication of clonogenic cells resulting in a somatic activation of TSH receptors. If a single nodule arises, the condition is called toxic adenoma.[199] Other less common causes include thyrotropin-induced thyrotoxicosis, trophoblastic tumors, gestational hypothyroidism, pituitary secreting adenomas, metastatic follicular thyroid cancer, and struma ovarii.

Screening and Diagnosis of Thyroid Disease

The initial screening test for diagnosis of thyroid disease is measuring serum TSH levels, which reference ranges have been statistically defined. Screening for thyroid disease has been a topic of controversy. The U.S. Preventive Services Taskforce found insufficient evidence for recommending routine screening for thyroid disease in asymptomatic results in the detection of subclinical hypothyroidism in many adults but citing poor evidence that treatment of subclinical hypothyroidism results in improvement of clinically important outcomes.[200] The American Academy of Family Physicians recommends screening in asymptomatic adults with risk factors for thyroid disease such as history of autoimmune disease, history of head or neck irradiation, goiter, family history of thyroid disease, history of iodine, or other drugs that can influence thyroid function. The American Thyroid Association and the American Association of Clinical Endocrinologists recommend screening in patients that are at increased risk of thyroid disease, such as persons with autoimmune diseases including type 1 diabetes, family history of thyroid disease, history of thyroid radiation or thyroid surgery, and can be considered in persons above 60 years of age.[201] If hyperthyroidism is suspected, in the United States, the American Thyroid Association and the American Association of Clinical Endocrinologists recommend a thyroid radioactive iodine uptake test. If iodine uptake test is contraindicated or unavailable, thyroid receptor antibodies can be measured.[198]

Treatment

Treatment for hypothyroidism consists of thyroid hormone replacement. For hyperthyroidism, it depends in the cause. There are three options for Grave's disease, and risk versus benefits should be considered before treatment. Treatment options include antithyroid medications (propylthiouracil or methimazole), radioactive ablation therapy, or surgery.[199] Radioactive ablation or surgery are the preferred methods for definite treatment in toxic multinodular goiter as these patients rarely go into remission with drug therapy.[198]

CUSHING'S SYNDROME

It is a metabolic condition that results from chronic exposure of excess glucocorticoids. The source of steroids can be exogenous or endogenous.[202] It can present with a variety of clinical features such as obesity, weight gain, round face, hirsutism, acne, supraclavicular/dorsocervical fat pads, facial plethora, violaceous striae, osteopenia, decreased linear growth in children, muscle weakness, and atrophy.[203] Neuropsychiatric manifestations include psychosis, depression, cognitive dysfunction, short-term memory loss, and emotional liability. Metabolically it also can result in hypertension, glucose intolerance, hyperlipidemia, hepatic steatosis, and nephrolithiasis. Sexual manifestations such as decrease libido and menstrual irregularity can also be present.[202]

Epidemiology. The estimated incidence of Cushing's syndrome is 0.2–5.0 per million people per year with a prevalence of 39–79 per million with a female to male ratio of 3:1.[203] The estimated standard mortality ratio is 3.8.[202] Mortality in Cushing's syndrome is increased, with a standard mortality ratio between 2.0 and 4.0, with cardiovascular deaths being the most common.[202]

Causes. Cushing 'syndrome can be divided in exogenous and endogenous causes. The most common form being due to administration of supra physiologic doses of exogenous steroids.[202] Endogenous Cushing's syndrome is further divided into ACTH (adrenocorticotrophic hormone) dependent and ACTH independent, with ACTH dependent accounting for about 80%.[203] Of the ACTH dependent, pituitary adenomas are the most common, and when that is the cause of the syndrome, it is named Cushing's disease. Nonpituitary tumors account for 5–10%.[203] ACTH-independent Cushing's syndrome account for 15–20% with most of them being unilateral adrenal adenomas, and rarely adrenocortical carcinomas.[202] Other causes of ACTH-independent Cushing's syndrome include bilateral macro and micro nodular adrenal hyperplasia and McCaune-Albright syndrome (fibrous dysplasia of the bone, café-au-lait skin spots, precocious puberty that can also present with hyperthyroidism, growth hormone excess, and Cushing's syndrome).[204]

Screening and Diagnosis. As described above, there are no guidelines for screening for Cushing's syndrome. The diagnosis should be based on clinical presentation with signs and symptoms suggestive of Cushing's syndrome. A complete list of the patient's medication should be reviewed to look for exogenous steroids, as that is the most common cause. In patients with clinical sings compatible with Cushing's syndrome, a 24-hour urine free cortisol level test should be measured. 60 μg/day is used as the cutoff value.[203] If the 24-hour urine free cortisol test is positive, the next step would be measurement of plasma corticotrophin to distinguish between ACTH-dependent and ACTH-independent Cushing's syndrome. If the plasma corticotrpin is not measurable, then non–ACTH-dependent Cushing's syndrome should be suspected, and a CT or MRI of the adrenal glands should be done next. A measurable plasma corticotropin suggests ACTH-dependent Cushing's syndrome, warranting a measurement of central-plasma to peripheral-plasma corticotropin via petrosal sinus sampling. A ratio of three or more suggests a eutopic cause and should be followed by a CT or MRI of the pituitary and hypothalamus. A ratio less than three indicates an ectopic cause and a CT or MRI of the chest should follow. Despite still being used as a test to differentiate ACTH-dependent and ACTH-independent Cushing's syndrome, the dexamethasone suppression test only has a positive predictive value of 0.4% and should no longer be used.[203]

Treatment. In the case of Cushing's syndrome due to exogenous use of systemic steroids, discontinuation of such steroids should be the first line of treatment. In the case of Cushing's disease, transphenoidal tumor resection is the optimum initial treatment.[205] However, such procedure has an initial remission rate of 60–80% and a relapse rate of up to 20% in 10 years.[206] After pituitary tumor resection, patients will need glucocorticoid replacement. Medical therapy is an option in cases acute complications of hypercortisolism, surgical pretreatment, for unresectable or metastatic tumors, or in the case of occult ectopic ACTH secreting tumors. Medical agents used include glucocorticoid receptor antagonists, steroidogenesis inhibitors, and tumor directed drugs.[205] Pituitary radiotherapy is a second line therapy for recurrent disease after trans sphenoidal tumor resection or as a first-line therapy for nonsurgical candidate, and it has shown to result in a 50–83% remission from 6 to 60 months after treatment, however pituitary hormone deficiency is a consequence after 2 years in on third of patients.[205] Unilateral cortisol secreting adenomas can be treated with unilateral adrenalectomy.[205] In patients with bilateral macronodular adrenal hyperplasia or primary pigmented nodular adrenocortical disease can be treated with bilateral adrenalectomy.[205] Ectopic ACTH secreting tumors should be surgically resected, followed by glucocorticoid and mineralocorticoid replacement.[203]

POLYCYSTIC OVARY SYNDROME

PCOS is a disorder of exclusion that presents with irregular menses, hypogonadism, and ovulatory dysfunction.[207,208] It is considered the most common cause of anovulatory infertility[207] with 90–95% of women presenting with anovulatory infertility having PCOS.[208] It's clinical presentation hast most women presenting with oligomenorrhea, prolonged erratic menstrual bleeding, and amenorrhea.[208] Symptoms of androgen excess can present with hirsutism, occurring in up to 70% of women with the disease and with severe acne. Obesity is present in 50–80% of women with PCOS and glucose intolerance in 30–35%.[207]

Epidemiology. The prevalence of PCOS varies depending on which one of the three main diagnostic criteria is used: Rotterdam, National Institute of Health (NIH), or the Androgen Excess and PCOS Society. Each set of criteria vary on the combinations of hyperandrogenism, ovulatory dysfunction, and polycystic ovarian morphologic features.[207] Using the NIH criteria, the prevalence is estimated at 4–8% of women of reproductive age, however, if using the Rotterdam criteria, the estimate can be up to 17.8%.[208] PCOS has been associated with a higher prevalence other metabolic disorders such as glucose intolerance, type, 2 diabetes mellitus, dyslipidemia, hypertension, bipolar disorder, depression, anxiety, and eating disorders.[208] It is estimated, that due to anovulation, obesity and insulin resistance, which in turn provokes prolonged estrogen mediated mitogenic stimulation of the endometrium without enough progesterone for endometrial differentiation, women with PCOS are at 2.7 higher risk of developing endometrial cancer than women without PCOS.[207]

Causes. Given that up to 80% of women with this disorder are obese, part of the causes for PCOS are considered environmental factors leading to obesity.[207] However, the exact cause of the disease is unknown, with mechanisms suggesting complex involving insulin resistance, abnormalities with ovarian steroidogenesis and follicular development manifesting in anovulation and androgen excess.[207]

Diagnosis. The diagnosis of PCOS is one of exclusion and is based on clinical presentation of symptoms of hyperandrogenism, which levels can be measured by laboratory tests, ovulatory dysfunction, and polycystic ovarian morphologic features that can be confirmed by ultrasound. Three main criteria for the diagnosis of PCOS have been established, and are the Rotterdam Criteria, the Androgen Excess Society and the National Institutes of Health/National Institute of Child Health and Human Disease. Each criteria differs in the combination of the three main features required for the disease. The NIH criteria requires evidence of ovulatory dysfunction and hyperandrogenism, but lack of polycystic ovarian morphology does not exclude the diagnosis in the presence of the former two features.[207] The Rotterdam criteria allows for the diagnosis of PCOS in the absence of measured hyperandrogenemia or clinical features of hyperandrogenism if oligo-ovulation or anovulation with polycystic ovaries are present.[208] The Androgen Excess Society requires the presence of hyperandrogenism with the combination of ovulatory dysfunction, or presence of polycystic ovaries.[207]

Treatment. Treatment for PCOS can include nonpharmacologic such as weight management and lifestyle modifications, and pharmacologic approaches. Treatment goals are targeted toward management of clinical features of hyperandrogenism and ovarian dysfunction. The pharmacological first line of treatment involves combined estrogen-progestin oral contraceptives.[207] In addition, Clomiphene can be used for management of ovulatory failure, continued progestin therapy for endometrial protection. Spironolactone can be used for antiandrogenic treatment.[208]

References

1. Fuller JH, Shipley MJ, Rose G, Jarrett RJ, Keen H. Coronary-heart-disease risk and impaired glucose tolerance. The Whitehall study. *Lancet.* 1980 Jun 28;1(8183):1373–6.
2. O'Sullivan J. Quarter century of glucose intolerance: Incidence of diabetes mellitus by USPHS, NIH, and WHO criteria. In: Eschwege E, ed. *Advances in Diabetes Epidemiology.* Amsterdam: Elsevier Biomedical Press; 1982, pp. 123–31.
3. Jarrett RJ, Keen H, McCartney P. Worsening of diabetes with impaired glucose tolerance: Ten-year experience in the Bedford and Whitehall Studies. In: Eschwege E, ed. *Advances in Diabetes Epidemiology.* Amsterdam: Elsevier Biomedical Press; 1982, pp. 95–102.
4. Orchard TJ. From diagnosis and classification to complications and therapy: DCCT part II? *Diabetes Care.* 1994;17(4):326–38.
5. Holman RC, Herron CA, Sinnock P. Epidemiologic characteristics of mortality from diabetes with acidosis or coma, United States, 1970–78. *Am J Public Health.* 1983;73(10):1169–73.
6. Laporte RE. Diabetes Epidemiology Research International Mortality Study Group. Major cross-country differences in risk of dying for people with IDDM. *Diabetes Care.* 1991;14:49–54.
7. Temple RC, Carrington CA, Luzio SD, et al. Insulin deficiency in non-insulin-dependent diabetes. *Lancet.* 1989;1(8633):293–5.
8. American Diabetes Association. Classification and diagnosis of diabetes. Diabetes care. 2016;39(Supplement 1):S13–22.
9. Unwin N, Shaw J, Zimmet P, Alberti KGMM. Impaired glucose tolerance and impaired fasting glycaemia: The current status on definition and intervention. *Diabet Med.* 2002;19(9):708–23.
10. Smith NL, Barzilay JI, Shaffer D, et al. Fasting and 2-hour postchallenge serum glucose measures and risk of incident cardiovascular events in the elderly: The cardiovascular health Study. *Arch Intern Med.* 2002;162(2):209.
11. Møller AM, Dalgaard LT, Pociot F, Nerup J, Hansen T, Pedersen O. Mutations in the hepatocyte nuclear factor-1alpha gene in Caucasian families originally classified as having Type I diabetes. *Diabetologia.* 1998;41(12):1528–31.
12. Lehto M, Wipemo C, Ivarsson S-A, et al. High frequency of mutations in MODY and mitochondrial genes in Scandinavian patients with familial early-onset diabetes. *Diabetologia.* 1999;42(9):1131–7.
13. Zimmet PZ, Tuomi T, Mackay IR, et al. Latent autoimmune diabetes mellitus in adults (LADA): The role of antibodies to glutamic acid decarboxylase in diagnosis and prediction of insulin dependency. *Diabet Med.* 1994;11(3):299–303.
14. Patterson C, Guariguata L, Dahlquist G, Soltész G, Ogle G, Silink M. Diabetes in the young—A global view and worldwide estimates of numbers of children with type 1 diabetes. *Diabetes Res Clin Pract.* 2014;103(2):161–75.
15. International Diabetes Federation. Diabetes Atlas [Internet]. 8th ed. Brussels, Belgium: International Diabetes Federation; 2017. Available at http://www.diabetes.org.
16. Vehik K, Dabelea D. The changing epidemiology of type 1 diabetes: Why is it going through the roof? *Diabetes Metab Res Rev.* 2011;27(1):3–13.
17. Kyvik KO, Nystrom L, Gorus F, et al. The epidemiology of Type 1 diabetes mellitus is not the same in young adults as in children. *Diabetologia.* 2004;47(3):377–84.
18. Borchers A, Uibo R, Gershwin M. The geoepidemiology of type 1 diabetes. *Autoimmun Rev.* 2010;9(5):A355–65.
19. Liese AD, Puett RC, Lamichhane AP, et al. Neighborhood level risk factors for type 1 diabetes in youth: The SEARCH case-control study. *Int J Health Geogr.* 2012;11:1.
20. Moltchanova EV, Schreier N, Lammi N, Karvonen M. Seasonal variation of diagnosis of Type 1 diabetes mellitus in children worldwide. *Diabet Med.* 2009;26(7):673–8.
21. Dorman J, Bunker C. HLA-DQ locus of the human leukocyte antigen complex and type 1 diabetes mellitus: A HuGE review. *Epidemiol Rev.* 2000;22(2):218–27.
22. Cooper JD, Howson JMM, Smyth D, et al. Confirmation of novel type 1 diabetes risk loci in families. *Diabetologia.* 2012;55(4):996–1000.
23. Rich SS, Akolkar B, Concannon P, et al. Current status and the future for the genetics of type I diabetes. *Genes Immun.* 2009;10(SUPPL. 1):S128–31.
24. Pociot F, Lernmark Å. Genetic risk factors for type 1 diabetes. *Lancet.* 2016;387(10035):2331–9.
25. Hirschhorn JN. Genetic epidemiology of type 1 diabetes. *Pediatr Diabetes.* 2003;4(2):87–100.
26. Nejentsev S, Reijonen H, Adojaan B, et al. The effect of HLA-B allele on the IDDM risk defined by DRB1*04 subtypes and DQB1*0302. *Diabetes.* 1997;46(11):1888–92.
27. Lie BA, Todd JA, Pociot F, et al. The predisposition to type 1 diabetes linked to the human leukocyte antigen complex includes at least one non-class II gene. *Am J Hum Genet.* 1999;64(3):793–800.
28. Törn C, Hadley D, Lee HS, et al. Role of type 1 diabetes—Associated SNPs on risk of autoantibody positivity in the TEDDY study. *Diabetes.* 2015;64(5):1818–29.
29. Krischer JP, Lynch KF, Schatz DA, et al. The 6 year incidence of diabetes-associated autoantibodies in genetically at-risk children: The TEDDY study. *Diabetologia.* 2015;58(5):980–7.
30. Ziegler AG, Rewers M, Simell O, et al. Seroconversion to multiple islet autoantibodies and risk of progression to diabetes in children. *JAMA.* 2013;309(23):2473–9.
31. Pugliese A, Zeller M, Fernandez A, et al. The insulin gene is transcribed in the human thymus and transcription levels correlated with allelic variation at the INS VNTR-IDDM2 susceptibility locus for type 1 diabetes. *Nat Genet.* 1997;15(3):293–7.
32. Bennett ST, Wilson AJ, Esposito L, et al. Insulin VNTR allele-specific effect in type 1 diabetes depends on identity of untransmitted paternal allele. *Nat Genet.* 1997;17(3):350–2.
33. Undlien DE, Hamaguchi K, Kimura A, et al. IDDM susceptibility associated with polymorphisms in the insulin gene region A study of blacks, Caucasians and orientals. *Diabetologia.* 1994;37(8):745–9.
34. Anjos S, Polychronakos C. Mechanisms of genetic susceptibility to type I diabetes: Beyond HLA. *Mol Genet Metab.* 2004;81(3):187–95.
35. Steck A, Rewers M. Genetics of Type 1 diabetes. *Clin Chem.* 2011;57(2):176–85.
36. Tuomilehto J. The emerging global epidemic of type 1 diabetes. *Curr Diab Rep.* 2013;13(6):795–804.
37. Maahs D, West N, Lawrence J, Mayer-Davis E. Epidemiology of type 1 diabetes. *Endocrinol Metab Clin North Am.* 2010;39(3):481–97.
38. Yeung W-CG, Rawlinson WD, Craig ME. Enterovirus infection and type 1 diabetes mellitus: Systematic review and meta-analysis of observational molecular studies. *BMJ.* 2011;342:d35.
39. Lonnrot M, Lynch K, Elding Larsson H, et al. Respiratory infections are temporally associated with initiation of type 1 diabetes autoimmunity: The TEDDY study. *Diabetologia.* 2017;60(10):1931–40.
40. Beyerlein A, Donnachie E, Ziegler A-G. Infections in early life and development of Celiac disease. *Am J Epidemiol.* 2017;186(11):1277–80.
41. Rešić Lindehammer S, Honkanen H, Nix WA, et al. Seroconversion to islet autoantibodies after enterovirus infection in early pregnancy. *Viral Immunol.* 2012;25(4):254–61.
42. Viskari H, Knip M, Tauriainen S, et al. Maternal enterovirus infection as a risk factor for type 1 diabetes in the exposed offspring. *Diabetes Care.* 2012;35(6):1328–32.
43. Borch-Johnsen K, Mandrup-Poulsen T, Zachau-Christiansen B, et al. Relation between breast-feeding and incidence rates of insulin-dependent diabetes mellitus. A hypothesis. *Lancet.* 1984;324(8411):1083–6.

44. Vaarala O. Is the origin of type 1 diabetes in the gut? In: *Immunology and Cell Biology*. New York: Nature Publishing Group; 2012, pp. 271–6.
45. Norris JM. Infant and childhood diet and type 1 diabetes risk: Recent advances and prospects. *Curr Diab Rep*. 2010;10(5):345–9.
46. McKinney PA, Parslow R, Gurney K, Law G, Bodansky HJ, Williams DRR. Antenatal risk factors for childhood diabetes mellitus, a case-control study of medical record data in Yorkshire, UK. *Diabetologia*. 1997;40(8):933–9.
47. Marshall AL, Chetwynd A, Morris JA, et al. Type 1 diabetes mellitus in childhood: A matched case control study in Lancashire and Cumbria, UK. *Diabet Med*. 2004;21(9):1035–40.
48. Cardwell CR, Carson DJ, Patterson CC. No association between routinely recorded infections in early life and subsequent risk of childhood-onset Type 1 diabetes: A matched case-control study using the UK General Practice Research Database. *Diabet Med*. 2008;25(3):261–7.
49. Mustonen N, Siljander H, Peet A, et al. Early childhood infections precede development of beta-cell autoimmunity and type 1 diabetes in children with HLA-conferred disease risk. *Pediatr Diabetes*. 2018;19(2):293–9.
50. Thabit H, Hovorka R. Coming of age: The artificial pancreas for type 1 diabetes. *Diabetologia*. 2016;59(9):1795–805.
51. Kupila A, Sipilä J, Keskinen P, et al. Intranasally administered insulin intended for prevention of type 1 diabetes—A safety study in healthy adults. *Diabetes Metab Res Rev*. 2003;19(5):415–20.
52. The Diabetes Prevention Trial-Type 1 Study Group. Effects of oral insulin in relatives of patients with type 1 diabetes: The diabetes prevention trial-type 1. *Diabetes Care*. 2005;28(5):1068–76.
53. Gale EAM, Bingley PJ, Emmett CL, Collier T, European Nicotinamide Diabetes Intervention Trial (ENDIT) Group. European Nicotinamide Diabetes Intervention Trial (ENDIT): A randomised controlled trial of intervention before the onset of type 1 diabetes. *Lancet*. 2004;363(9413):925–31.
54. Knip M, Virtanen SM, Becker D, Dupré J, Krischer JP, Åkerblom HK. Early feeding and risk of type 1 diabetes: Experiences from the trial to reduce insulin-dependent diabetes mellitus in the genetically at risk (TRIGR). *Am J Clin Nutr*. 2011;94(6 Suppl):1814S–20S.
55. Hummel S, Pflüger M, Hummel M, Bonifacio E, Ziegler A-G. Primary dietary intervention study to reduce the risk of islet autoimmunity in children at increased risk for type 1 diabetes: The BABYDIET study. *Diabetes Care*. 2011;34(6):1301–5.
56. Bonifacio E, Ziegler A-G, Klingensmith G, et al. Effects of high-dose oral insulin on immune responses in children at high risk for type 1 diabetes. *JAMA*. 2015;313(15):1541.
57. Type 1 Diabetes Trial Net [Internet]. Available at www.trialnet.org.
58. Prevention C for DC and. National Diabetes Statistics Report, 2017. Atlanta, GA: Department of Health and Human Services; 2017.
59. Murdock D, Salit J, Stoffel M, et al. Longitudinal study shows increasing obesity and hyperglycemia in micronesia: Increasing obesity and hyperglycemia in micronesia. *Obesity*. 2013;21:E421–7.
60. WHO | Pacific islanders pay heavy price for abandoning traditional diet [Internet]. 2017. Available at http://www.who.int/bulletin/volumes/88/7/10-010710/en/.
61. Nguyen NT, Nguyen X-MT, Lane J, Wang P. Relationship between obesity and diabetes in a US adult population: Findings from the National Health and Nutrition Examination Survey, 1999–2006. *Obes Surg*. 2011;21(3):351–5.
62. Ogden CL, Carroll MD, Fryar CD, Flegal KM. Prevalence of Obesity Among Adults and Youth: United States, 2011–2014. *NCHS Data Brief*. 2015;219:1–8.
63. The Sedentary Behaviour and Obesity Expert Working Group. Sedentary Behaviour and Obesity: Review of the Current Scientific Evidence [Internet]. 2010. Available at https://www.gov.uk/government/uploads/system/uploads/attachment_data/file/213745/dh_128225.pdf.
64. How much physical activity do adults need? | Physical Activity | CDC [Internet]. 2017 Nov. Available at https://www.cdc.gov/physicalactivity/basics/adults/index.htm.
65. Facts about Physical Activity | Physical Activity | CDC [Internet]. 2017. Available at https://www.cdc.gov/physicalactivity/data/facts.htm.
66. American Diabetes Association. Lifestyle management. *Diabetes Care*. 2017;40(Supplement 1):S33–43.
67. Ali O. Genetics of type 2 diabetes. *World J Diabetes*. 2013;4(4):114.
68. Gjesing AP, Kjems LL, Vestmar MA, et al. Carriers of the TCF7L2 rs7903146 TT genotype have elevated levels of plasma glucose, serum proinsulin and plasma gastric inhibitory polypeptide (GIP) during a meal test. *Diabetologia*. 2011;54(1):103–10.
69. Schäfer SA, Tschritter O, Machicao F, et al. Impaired glucagon-like peptide-1-induced insulin secretion in carriers of transcription factor 7-like 2 (TCF7L2) gene polymorphisms. *Diabetologia*. 2007;50(12):2443–50.
70. Skinner KS. Environmental epigenetic transgenerational inheritance and somatic epigenetic mitotic stability. *Epigenetics*. 2011;6(7):838–42.
71. Saad MF, Knowler WC, Pettitt DJ, Nelson RG, Mott DM, Bennett PH. The natural history of impaired glucose tolerance in the Pima Indians. *N Engl J Med*. 1988;319(23):1500–6.
72. Pan X-R, Li G-W, Hu Y-H, et al. Effects of diet and exercise in preventing NIDDM in people with impaired glucose tolerance: The Da Qing IGT and diabetes study. *Diabetes Care*. 1997;20(4):537–44.
73. Lindstrom J, Louheranta A, Mannelin M, et al. The Finnish Diabetes Prevention Study (DPS): Lifestyle intervention and 3-year results on diet and physical activity. *Diabetes Care*. 2003;26(12):3230–6.
74. Chiasson J-L, Gomis R, Hanefeld M, et al. The STOP-NIDDM Trial: An international study on the efficacy of an alpha-glucosidase inhibitor to prevent type 2 diabetes in a population with impaired glucose tolerance: Rationale, design, and preliminary screening data. *Diabetes Care*. 1998;21(10):1720–5.
75. Knowler WC, Barrett-Connor E, Fowler SE, et al. Reduction in the incidence of Type 2 diabetes with lifestyle intervention or metformin. *N Engl J Med*. 2002;346(6):393–403.
76. Orchard TJ, Temprosa M, Goldberg R, et al. The effect of metformin and intensive lifestyle intervention on the metabolic syndrome: The Diabetes Prevention Program Randomized Trial. *Ann Intern Med*. 2005;142(8):611.
77. Li R, Qu S, Zhang P, et al. Economic evaluation of combined diet and physical activity promotion programs to prevent type 2 diabetes among persons at increased risk: A systematic review for the Community Preventive Services Task Force. *Ann Intern Med*. 2015;163(6):452.
78. Simmons RK, Griffin SJ, Witte DR, Borch-Johnsen K, Lauritzen T, Sandbaek A. Effect of population screening for type 2 diabetes and cardiovasular risk factors on mortality and cardiovascular events: A controlled trial among 1,912,392 Danish adults. *Diabetologia*. 2017;60(11):2183–91.
79. Simmons RK, Griffin SJ, Lauritzen T, Sandbaek A, Sandbæk A. Effect of screening for type 2 diabetes on risk of cardiovascular disease and mortality: A controlled trial among 139,075 individuals diagnosed with diabetes in Denmark between 2001 and 2009. *Diabetologia*. 2017;60(11):2192–9.
80. Simmons D, Zgibor JC. Should we screen for type 2 diabetes among asymptomatic individuals? Yes. *Diabetologia*. 2017;60(11):2148–52.
81. American Diabetes Association. Classification and diagnosis of diabetes. *Diabetes Care*. 2018;41(Suppl 1):S13–27.
82. Knuiman MW, Welborn TA, Mccann VJ, Stanton KG, Constable IJ. Prevalence of diabetic complications in relation to risk factors. *Diabetes*. 1986;35:1332–9.
83. Eeg-Olofsson K, Cederholm J, Nilsson PM, et al. Glycemic control and cardiovascular disease in 7,454 patients with type 1 diabetes: An observational study from the Swedish National Diabetes Register (NDR). *Diabetes Care*. 2010;33(7):1640–6.
84. Livingstone SJ, Looker HC, Hothersall EJ, et al. Risk of cardiovascular disease and total mortality in adults with type 1 diabetes: Scottish registry linkage study. *PLoS Med*. 2012;9(10):e1001321.
85. Lind M, Garcia-Rodriguez LA, Booth GL, et al. Mortality trends in patients with and without diabetes in Ontario, Canada and the UK from 1996 to 2009: A population-based study. *Diabetologia*. 2013;56(12):2601–8.
86. Morgan E, Cardwell CR, Black CJ, McCance DR, Patterson CC. Excess mortality in Type 1 diabetes diagnosed in childhood and adolescence: A systematic review of population-based cohorts. *Acta Diabetol*. 2015;52(4):801–7.
87. Lind M, Svensson A-M, Kosiborod M, et al. Glycemic control and excess mortality in type 1 diabetes. *N Engl J Med*. 2014;371(21):1972–82.
88. Secrest AM, Becker DJ, Kelsey SF, LaPorte RE, Orchard TJ. All-cause mortality trends in a large population-based cohort with long-standing childhood-onset type 1 diabetes: The Allegheny County type 1 diabetes registry. *Diabetes Care*. 2010;33(12):2573–9.
89. Secrest AM, Becker DJ, Kelsey SF, Laporte RE, Orchard TJ. Cause-specific mortality trends in a large population-based cohort with long-standing childhood-onset type 1 diabetes. *Diabetes*. 2010;59(12):3216–22.
90. Miller RG, Secrest AM, Sharma RK, Songer TJ, Orchard TJ. Improvements in the life expectancy of type 1 diabetes: The Pittsburgh Epidemiology of Diabetes Complications study cohort. *Diabetes*. 2012;61(11):2987–92.
91. The Diabetes Control and Complications Trial/Epidemiology of Diabetes Interventions and Complications (DCCT/EDIC) Research Group. Association between 7 years of intensive insulin treatment of type 1 diabetes and long-term mortality. *JAMA*. 2015;313(1):45–53.

92. Groop P-H, Thomas MC, Moran JL, et al. The presence and severity of chronic kidney disease predicts all-cause mortality in type 1 diabetes. *Diabetes*. 2009;58(7):1651–8.

93. Orchard TJ, Secrest AM, Miller RG, Costacou T. In the absence of renal disease, 20 year mortality risk in type 1 diabetes is comparable to that of the general population: A report from the Pittsburgh Epidemiology of Diabetes Complications Study. *Diabetologia*. 2010;53(11):2312–9.

94. Rosenquist KJ, Fox CS, Cowie CC, et alRosenquist KJ, Fox CS, Cowie CC, et al, eds. CSS. Mortality trends in type 2 diabetes. In: *Diabetes in America*. 3rd ed. Bethesda, MD: National Institutes of Health; 2017, pp. 36.1–36.14. (NIH Pub No 17-1468).

95. Lee R, Wong TY, Sabanayagam C. Epidemiology of diabetic retinopathy, diabetic macular edema and related vision loss. *Eye Vis (Lond)*. 2015 Dec 3;2(1): 17. Available at http://www.eandv.org/content/2/1/17.

96. American Optometric Association. Diabetic Retinopathy [Internet]. St Louis, MO; 2017 Dec. Available at https://www.aoa.org/patients-and-public/eye-and-vision-problems/glossary-of-eye-and-vision-conditions/diabetic-retinopathy.

97. Klein B. Epidemiology of ocular functions and diseases in persons with diabetes. In: Cowie CC, Casagrande SS, Menke A, et al., eds. *Diabetes in America*. 3rd ed. Bethesda, MD: National Institutes of Health; 2017, pp. 21.1–21.49.

98. Voigt M, Schmidt S, Lehmann T, et al. Prevalence and progression rate of diabetic retinopathy in type 2 diabetes patients in correlation with the duration of diabetes. *Exp Clin Endocrinol Diabetes*. 2018;126(9):570–6.

99. Park S, Rhee SY, Jeong SJ, et al. Features of long-standing Korean type 2 diabetes mellitus patients with diabetic retinopathy: A study based on standardized clinical data. *Diabetes Metab J*. 2017;41(5):393.

100. Harris MI, Klein R, Welborn TA, Knuiman MW. Onset of NIDDM occurs at least 4–7 yr before clinical diagnosis. *Diabetes Care*. 1992;15(7):815–9.

101. The Diabetes Control and Complications Trial Research Group. Effect of pregnancy on microvascular complications in the diabetes control and complications trial. *Diabetes Care*. 2000;23(8):1084–91.

102. American Diabetes Association. Standards of medical care in diabetes—2013. *Diabetes Care*. 2017;36(Suppl 1):S11–66.

103. Krolewski AS, Skupien J, Rossing P, Warram JH. Fast renal decline to end-stage renal disease: An unrecognized feature of nephropathy in diabetes. *Kidney Int*. 2017;91(6):1300–11.

104. Saran R, Robinson B, Abbott KC, et al. US Renal Data System 2016 Annual Data Report: Epidemiology of kidney disease in the United States. *Am J Kidney Dis*. 2017;69(3): A7–8.

105. Costacou T, Orchard TJ. Cumulative kidney complication risk by 50 years of type 1 diabetes: The effects of sex, age, and calendar year at onset. *Diabetes Care*. 2018;41(3):426–33.

106. Geiss LS, Herman WH, Teutsch SM. Diabetes and renal mortality in the United States. *Am J Public Health*. 1985;75(11):1325–6.

107. Papadopoulou-Marketou N, Chrousos GP, Kanaka-Gantenbein C. Diabetic nephropathy in type 1 diabetes: A review of early natural history, pathogenesis, and diagnosis. Diabetes Metab Res Rev. 2017; e2841.

108. American Diabetes Association. Standards of medical care in diabetes—2017. *Diabetes Care*. 2017;40(Suppl 1).

109. Tolonen N, Forsblom C, Thorn L, et al. Lipid abnormalities predict progression of renal disease in patients with type 1 diabetes. *Diabetologia*. 2009;52(12):2522–30.

110. Lloyd CE, Becker D, Ellis D, Orchard TJ. Incidence of complications in insulin-dependent diabetes mellitus: A survival analysis. *Am J Epidemiol*. 1996;143(5):431–41.

111. Stratton IM, Adler AI, Neil HA, et al. Association of glycaemia with macrovascular and microvascular complications of type 2 diabetes (UKPDS 35): Prospective observational study. *BMJ*. 2000;321(7258):405–12.

112. Diabetes Control and Complications Trial/Epidemiology of Diabetes Interventions and Complications Research Group. Effect of intensive therapy on the microvascular complications of type 1 diabetes mellitus. *JAMA*. 2002;287(19):2563–9.

113. Orchard TJ, Chang Y-F, Ferrell RE, Petro N, Ellis DE. Nephropathy in type 1 diabetes: A manifestation of insulin resistance and multiple genetic susceptibilities? Further evidence from the Pittsburgh Epidemiology of Diabetes Complication Study. *Kidney Int*. 2002;62(3):963–70.

114. Orchard TJ, Costacou T. Cardiovascular complications of type 1 diabetes: Update on the renal link. *Acta Diabetol*. 2017;54(4):325–34.

115. Pop-Busui R, Boulton AJ, Sosenko JM. Peripheral and autonomic neuropathy in diabetes. In: *Diabetes in America*. 3rd ed. Bethesda, MD: National Institute of Diabetes and Digestive and Kidney Diseases, National Institutes of Health; 2018, pp. 1–20.

116. Vinik A, Ullal J, Parson HK, Casellini CM. Diabetic neuropathies: Clinical manifestations and current treatment options. *Nat Clin Pract Endocrinol Metab*. 2006;2(5):269–81.

117. Juhani Airaksinen KE, Juhani Koistinen M. Association between silent coronary artery disease, diabetes, and autonomic neuropathy. Fact or fallacy? *Diabetes Care*. 1992;15(2):288–92.

118. Vinik AI, Ziegler D. Diabetic cardiovascular autonomic neuropathy. *Circulation*. 2007;115(3):387–97.

119. Niakan E. Silent myocardial infarction and diabetic cardiovascular autonomic neuropathy. *Arch Intern Med*. 1986;146(11):2229.

120. Papanas N, Vinik AI, Ziegler D. Neuropathy in prediabetes: Does the clock start ticking early? *Nat Rev Endocrinol*. 2011;7:682–90.

121. Martin CL, Albers JW, Pop-Busui R, Group for the DR. Neuropathy and related findings in the Diabetes Control and Complications Trial/Epidemiology of Diabetes Interventions and Complications Study. *Diabetes Care*. 2014;37(1):31–8.

122. Dy SM, Bennett WL, Zhang A, et al. Preventing Complications and Treating Symptoms of Diabetic Peripheral Neuropathy. Rockville, MD: AHRQ Comparative Effectiveness; 2017; Report No.: 17-EHC005-EF.

123. Kannel W, McGee D. Diabetes and glucose tolerance as risk factors for cardiovascular disease: The Framingham Study. *Diabetes Care*. 1979;2(2):120–6.

124. Smith NL, Barzilay JI, Kronmal R, Lumley T, Enquobahrie D, Psaty BM. New-onset diabetes and risk of all-cause and cardiovascular mortality: The cardiovascular health study. *Diabetes Care*. 2006 Sep 1;29(9):2012–7.

125. Barrett-Connor E, Wingard D. Sex differential in ischemic heart disease mortality in diabetics: A prospective population-based study. *Am J Epidemiol*. 1983;118:489–96.

126. Panzram G. Mortality and survival in type 2 (non-insulin-dependent) diabetes mellitus. *Diabetologia*. 1987;30:123–31.

127. Donahue R, Orchard T. Diabetes mellitus and macrovascular complications. *Diabetes Care*. 1992;15:1141–55.

128. Ziegler-Graham K, MacKenzie EJ, Ephraim PL, Travison TG, Brookmeyer R. Estimating the prevalence of limb loss in the United States: 2005 to 2050. *Arch Phys Med Rehabil*. 2008;89(3):422–9.

129. Huxley R, Barzi F, Woodward M. Excess risk of fatal coronary heart disease is associated with diabetes in men and women: Meta-analysis of 37 prospective cohort studies. *BMJ*. 2006;332:73–8.

130. Kalyani RR, Lazo M, Ouyang P, et al. Gender differences in diabetes and risk of incident coronary artery disease in healthy young and middle-aged adults. *Diabetes Care*. 2014;37(3):830–8.

131. Orchard TJ. The impact of gender and general risk factors on the occurrence of atherosclerotic vascular disease in non-insulin-dependent diabetes mellitus. *Ann Med*. 1996;28(4):323–33.

132. Wexler D, Grant R, Meigs J, Nathan D, Cagliero E. Sex disparities in treatment of cardiac risk factors in patients with type 2 diabetes. *Diabetes Care*. 2005;28:514–20.

133. Dabelea D, Kinney G, Snell-Bergeon JK, et al. Effect of type 1 diabetes on the gender difference in coronary artery calcification: a role for insulin resistance? The Coronary Artery Calcification in Type 1 Diabetes (CACTI) Study. *Diabetes*. 2003;52(11):2833–9.

134. Raggi P, Cooil B, Ratti C, Callister T, Budoff M. Progression of coronary artery calcification and occurrence of myocardial infarction in patients with and without diabetes mellitus. *Hypertension*. 2005;46:238–43.

135. Turner R. Intensive blood-glucose control with sulphonylureas or insulin compared with conventional treatment and risk of complications in patients with type 2 diabetes (UKPDS 33). *Lancet*. 1998;352(9131):837–53.

136. Accord Study Group. Effects of intensive blood pressure control in type 2 diabetes mellitus. *N Engl J Med*. 2010;362:1575–85.

137. The ADVANCE Collaborative Group. Intensive blood glucose control and vascular outcomes in patients with type 2 diabetes. *N Engl J Med*. 2008;358(24):2560–72.

138. Duckworth W, Abraira C, Moritz T, et al. Glucose control and vascular complications in veterans with type 2 diabetes. *N Engl J Med*. 2009;360(2):129–39.

139. International Collaborative Group. Joint discussion. *J Chronic Dis*. 1979;32:829–37.

140. Gao W, Qiao Q, Tuomilehto J. Post-challenge hyperglycaemia rather than fasting hyperglycaemia is an independent risk factor of cardiovascular disease events. *Clin Lab*. 2004;50:609–15.

141. Ford ES, Zhao G, Li C. Pre-diabetes and the risk for cardiovascular disease. A systematic review of the evidence. *J Am Coll Cardiol*. 2010;55(13):1310–7.

142. Nathan DM, Cleary PA, Backlund J-YC, et al. Intensive diabetes treatment and cardiovascular disease in patients with type 1 diabetes. *N Engl J Med.* 2005;353(25):2643–53.

143. Eschwege E, Richard JL, Thibult N, et al. Coronary heart disease mortality in relation with diabetes, blood glucose and plasma insulin levels. The Paris Prospective Study, ten years later. *Horm Metab Res Suppl.* 1985;15:41–6.

144. Ohlson LO, Larsson B, Svardsudd K, et al. The influence of body fat distribution on the incidence of diabetes mellitus. 13.5 Years of follow-up of the participants in the study of men born in 1913. *Diabetes.* 1985;34(10):1055–8.

145. McKeigue PM, Shah B, Marmot MG. Relation of central obesity and insulin resistance with high diabetes prevalence and cardiovascular risk in South Asians. *Lancet.* 1991;337(8738):382–6.

146. Vazquez G, Duval S, Jacobs DR, Silventoinen K. Comparison of body mass index, waist circumference, and waist/hip ratio in predicting incident diabetes: A meta-analysis. *Epidemiol Rev.* 2007;29: 115–28.

147. Qiao Q, Nyamdorj R. Is the association of type II diabetes with waist circumference or waist-to-hip ratio stronger than that with body mass index. *Eur J Clin Nutr.* 2010;64:30–4.

148. Després J-P. Body fat distribution and risk of cardiovascular disease: an update. *Circulation.* 2012;126(10):1301–13.

149. Peiris AN, Mueller RA, Smith GA, Struve MF, Kissebah AH. Splanchnic insulin metabolism in obesity. Influence of body fat distribution. *J Clin Invest.* 1986;78(6):1648–57.

150. Orchard TJ, Olson JC, Erbey JR, et al. Insulin resistance-related factors, but not glycemia, predict coronary artery disease in type 1 diabetes: 10-Year follow-up data from the Pittsburgh Epidemiology of Diabetes Complications Study. *Diabetes Care.* 2003;26(5):1374–9.

151. Soedamah-Muthu SS, Chaturvedi N, et al. Risk factors for coronary heart disease in type 1 diabetic patients in Europe: The EURODIAB Prospective Complications Study. *Diabetes Care.* 2004;24(2):530–7.

152. Kilpatrick ES, Rigby AS, Atkin SL. Insulin resistance, the metabolic syndrome, and complication risk in type 1 diabetes: "Double diabetes" in the diabetes control and complications trial. *Diabetes Care.* 2007;30(3):707–12.

153. Cleland SJ, Fisher BM, Colhoun HM, Sattar N, Petrie JR. Insulin resistance in type 1 diabetes: What is "double diabetes" and what are the risks? *Diabetologia.* 2013;56:1462–70.

154. Haffner SM, Stern MP, Hazuda HP, Rosenthal M, Knapp JA, Malina RM. Role of obesity and fat distribution in non-insulin-dependent diabetes mellitus in Mexican Americans and non-Hispanic whites. *Diabetes Care.* 1986;9(2):153–61.

155. Turner RC, Millns H, Neil HAW, et al. Risk factors for coronary artery disease in non-insulin dependent diabetes mellitus: United Kingdom prospective diabetes study (UKPDS: 23). *BMJ.* 1998;316(7134):823–8.

156. Orchard T. Dyslipoproteinemia and diabetes. *Endocrinol Metab Clin North Am.* 1990;19:361–80.

157. Stamler J, Vaccaro O, Neaton JD, Wentworth D. Diabetes, other risk factors, and 12-yr cardiovascular mortality for men screened in the multiple risk factor intervention trial. *Diabetes Care.* 1993;16(2):434–44.

158. Zgibor JC, Ruppert K, Orchard TJ, et al. Development of a coronary heart disease risk prediction model for type 1 diabetes: The Pittsburgh CHD in Type 1 Diabetes Risk Model. *Diabetes Res Clin Pract.* 2010;88(3):314–21.

159. Cederholm J, Eeg-Olofsson K, Eliasson B, Zethelius B, Gudbjörnsdottir S. A new model for 5-year risk of cardiovascular disease in Type1 diabetes; from the Swedish National Diabetes Register (NDR). *Diabet Med.* 2011;28(10):1213–20.

160. Soedamah-Muthu SS, Vergouwe Y, Costacou T, et al. Predicting major outcomes in type 1 diabetes: A model development and validation study. *Diabetologia.* 2014;57(11):2304–14.

161. Vistisen D, Andersen GS, Hansen CS, et al. Prediction of first cardiovascular disease event in type 1 diabetes: The steno T1 risk engine. *Circulation.* 2016;133(11):1058–66.

162. Laakso M, Zimmet P, Alberti K, et al. Cardiovascular disease in type 2 diabetes from population to man to mechanisms: The Kelly West Award Lecture 2008. *Diabetes Care.* 2010;33(2):442–9.

163. Nathan DM, Bebu I, Braffett BH, et al. Risk factors for cardiovascular disease in type 1 diabetes. *Diabetes.* 2016;65(5):1370–9.

164. Verges B. Pathophysiology of diabetic dyslipidaemia: Where are we? *Diabetologia.* 2015;58:86–99.

165. Stout RW, Bierman EL, Ross R. Effect of insulin on the proliferation of cultured primate arterial smooth muscle cells. *Circ Res.* 1975;36(2):319–27.

166. Porta M, La Selva M, Molinatti P, Molinatti GM. Endothelial cell function in diabetic microangiopathy. *Diabetologia.* 1987;30:601–9.

167. Modan M, Halkin H, Almog S, et al. Hyperinsulinemia. A link between hypertension obesity and glucose intolerance. *J Clin Invest.* 1985;75(3):809–17.

168. Donahue RP, Orchard TJ, Becker DJ, Kuller LH, Drash AL. Sex differences in the coronary heart disease risk profile: A possible role for insulin. The Beaver County Study. *Am J Epidemiol.* 1987;125(4):650–7.

169. Ferrannini E, Buzzigoli G, Bonadonna R, et al. Insulin resistance in essential hypertension. *N Engl J Med.* 1987;317(6):350–7.

170. Ducimetiere P, Eschwege E, Papoz L, Richard JL, Claude JR, Rosselin G. Relationship of plasma insulin levels to the incidence of myocardial infarction and coronary heart disease mortality in a middle-aged population. *Diabetologia.* 1980;19(3):205–10.

171. Pyorala K. Relationship of glucose tolerance and plasma insulin to the incidence of coronary heart disease: Results from two population studies in Finland. *Diabetes Care.* 1979;2(2):131–41.

172. Welborn TA, Wearne K. Coronary heart disease incidence and cardiovascular mortality in Busselton with reference to glucose and insulin concentrations. *Diabetes Care.* 1979;2(2):154–60.

173. Després JP, Lamarche B, Mauriège P, et al. Hyperinsulinemia as an independent risk factor for ischemic heart disease. *N Engl J Med.* 1996;334(15):952–7.

174. Ferrara A, Barrett-Connor EL, Edelstein SL. Hyperinsulinemia does not increase the risk of fatal cardiovascular disease in elderly men or women without diabetes: The Rancho Bernardo Study, 1984–1991. *Am J Epidemiol.* 1994;140(10):857–69.

175. Orchard TJ, Eichner J, Kuller LH, Becker DJ, McCallum LM, Grandits GA. Insulin as a predictor of coronary heart disease: Interaction with apolipoprotein E phenotype A report from the multiple risk factor intervention trial. *Ann Epidemiol.* 1994;4(1):40–5.

176. Welin L, Eriksson H, Larsson B, Ohlson LO, Svärdsudd K, Tibblin G. Hyperinsulinaemia is not a major coronary risk factor in elderly men—The study of men born in 1913. *Diabetologia.* 1992;35(8):766–70.

177. Kim SH, Reaven GM. Insulin resistance and hyperinsulinemia. *Diabetes Care.* 2008 Jul 1;31(7):1433–8.

178. Jax TW, Peters AJ, Plehn G, Schoebel F-C. Hemostatic risk factors in patients with coronary artery disease and type 2 diabetes—A two year follow-up of 243 patients. *Cardiovasc Diabetol.* 2009;8(1):48.

179. Costacou T, Levy AP. Haptoglobin genotype and its role in diabetic cardiovascular disease. *J Cardiovasc Transl Res.* 2012;5:423–35.

180. Casagrande SS, Fradkin JE, Saydah SH, Rust KF, Cowie CC. The prevalence of meeting A1C, blood pressure, and LDL goals among people with diabetes, 1988–2010. *Diabetes Care.* 2013;36(8):2271–9.

181. Zgibor JC, Songer TJ. External barriers to diabetes care: Addressing personal and health systems issues. *Diabetes Spectr.* 2001;14(1):23–8.

182. Zgibor JC, Simmons D. Barriers to blood glucose monitoring in a multiethnic community. *Diabetes Care.* 2002;25(10):1772–7.

183. Simmons D, Weblemoe T, Voyle J, Prichard A, Leakehe L, Gatland B. Personal barriers to diabetes care: Lessons from a multi-ethnic community in New Zealand. *Diabet Med.* 1998;15(11):958–64.

184. WHO. Social Determinants of Health [Internet]. 2017. Available at http://www.who.int/social_determinants/en/.

185. The Diabetes Control and Complications Trial Research Group. The effect of intensive treatment of diabetes on the development and progression of long-term complications in insulin-dependent diabetes mellitus. *N Engl J Med.* 1993;329(14):977–86.

186. Downs JJR, Clearfield M, Weis S, et al. Primary prevention of acute coronary events with lovastatin in men and women with average cholesterol levels results of AFCAPS/TexCAPS. *JAMA.* 1998;279(20):1615–22.

187. Elkeles RS, Diamond JR, Poulter C, et al. Cardiovascular outcomes in type 2 diabetes: A double-blind placebo-controlled study of bezafibrate: The St. Mary's, Ealing, Northwick Park diabetes cardiovascular disease prevention (SENDCAP) study. *Diabetes Care.* 1998;21(4):641–8.

188. Koskinen P, Mänttäri M, Manninen V, Huttunen JK, Heinonen OP, Frick MH. Coronary heart disease incidence in NIDDM patients in the Helsinki heart study. *Diabetes Care.* 1992;15(7):820–5.

189. UK Prospective Diabetes Study Group. Efficacy of atenolol and captopril in reducing risk of macrovascular and microvascular complications in type 2 diabetes: UKPDS 39. BMJ. 1998; 317(7160):713–20.

190. Hansson L, Zanchetti A, Carruthers SG, et al. Effects of intensive blood-pressure lowering and low-dose aspirin in patients with hypertension: Principal results of the hypertension optimal treatment (HOT) randomised trial. *Lancet.* 1998;351(9118):1755–62.

191. Goldberg RB, Mellies MJ, Sacks FM, et al. Cardiovascular events and their reduction with pravastatin in diabetic and glucose-intolerant myo-

cardial infarction survivors with average cholesterol levels: Subgroup analyses in the Cholesterol and Recurrent Events (CARE) Trial. *Circulation.* 1998;98(23):2513–9.

192. Tonkin A, Alyward P, Colquhoun D, et al. Prevention of cardiovascular events and death with pravastatin in patients with coronary heart disease and a broad range of initial cholesterol levels. *N Engl J Med.* 1998;339(19):1349–57.
193. Pyörälä K, Pedersen TR, Kjekshus J, Faergeman O, Olsson AG, Thorgeirsson G. Cholesterol lowering with simvastatin improves prognosis of diabetic patients with coronary heart disease: A subgroup analysis of the Scandinavian Simvastatin Survival Study (4S). *Diabetes Care.* 1997;20(4):614–20.
194. Schnell O, Rydén L, Standl E, Ceriello A. Updates on cardiovascular outcome trials in diabetes. *Cardiovasc Diabetol.* 2017;16(1):128.
195. Gaitende DY, Rowley KD, Sweeney LB. Hypothyroidism an update. *Am Fam Physician.* 2012;86 (3):244–51.
196. Chaker A, Bianco AC, Jonklaas J, Peeters RP. Hypothyroidism. *Lancet.* 2017;390:1552–62.
197. Bello F, Bakari G. Hypothyroidism in adults: A review and recent advances in management. *J Diabetes Endocrinol.* 2012;3(5):57–9.
198. De Leo S, Lee SY, Braverman LE. Hyperthyroidism. *Lancet.* 2016;388: 906–18.
199. Kravets I. Hyperthyroidism: Diagnosis and treatment. *Am Fam Physician.* 2016;93(5):363–73.
200. LeFebre ML. Screening for thyroid dysfunction: U.S. Preventive Task Force Recommendation statement. Ann Intern Med. 2015;162(9):641–51.
201. Ross DS, Burch HB, Cooper DS, et al. 2016 American Thyroid Association Guidelines for Diagnosis and Management of Hyperthyroidism and Other Causes of Thyrotoxicosis. *Thyroid.* 2016; 26(10):1343–1421.
202. Sharma ST, Niemann LK, Feelders RA. Cushing's syndrome: Epidemiology and developments in disease management. *Clin Epidemiol.* 2015;7:281–93.
203. Loriaux DL. Diagnosis and differential diagnosis of Cushing's syndrome. *New Engl J Med.* 2017;376(15):1451–9.
204. Dumitresco CE, Collins MT. McCaune-Albright syndrome. *Orphanet J Rare Dis.* 2008;3(12):1–12
205. Lacroix A, Feelders RA, Stratakis CA, Niemann L. Cushing's syndrome. *Lancet.* 2015;386:913–27.
206. Buliman A, Tataranu LG, Mirica A, Dumitrache C. Cushing's disease: A multidisciplinary overview of the clinical features, diagnosis and treatment. *J Med Life.* 2016;9(1):12–18.
207. McCartney CR, Marshall JC. Polycystic ovary syndrome. New Engl J Med. 2016;375(1):54–64.
208. Sirmans SM, Pate KA. Epidemiology, diagnosis, and management of polycystic ovary syndrome. *Clin Epidemiol.* 2014;6:1–13.

CHAPTER

54

Genitourinary Disorders

Yahya Jan • Maria C. Mora Pinzon • Sana Waheed

KIDNEY DISEASES

The full spectrum of renal disease can range from a rapid decline in renal function manifesting as acute kidney injury (AKI), a more gradual worsening of renal function known as chronic kidney disease (CKD) or a complete failure of the kidneys leading to end-stage renal disease (ESRD).

Chronic Kidney Disease

CKD is defined as abnormalities of kidney structure or function, which persist for greater than 3 months. The function of the kidney is assessed by glomerular filtration rate (GFR) and a persistent decline in GFR to less than 60 mL/min/ 1.73 m^2 characterizes someone as having kidney disease.[1,2] CKD can also be a result of structural damage to the kidney with manifestations like albuminuria, hematuria, and tubular damage causing loss of electrolytes or damage detected on imaging or pathology. CKD is divided into stages based on GFR as shown in Fig. 54-1.[1] Moreover the degree of albuminuria predicts the risk for disease progression as described in Fig. 54-1.[1]

Burden of Chronic Kidney Disease and End-stage Renal Disease

The prevalence of CKD worldwide is estimated to be between 11% and 13%,[3] and to be 14.8% among adults in the United States with 14.8%.[4] The prevalence of CKD varies based on gender and race with women and African Americans having a higher prevalence.[5] With the increase in the prevalence of diabetes and increasing age of the population, the incidence of CKD is expected to increase further as diabetes is the leading cause of CKD.[6]

Not only is CKD a prevalent problem but these patients have multiple other comorbidities. It has been estimated that 40% of individuals with CKD also have diabetes and 32% have hypertension.[4] One of the major causes of morbidity and mortality in the CKD population is cardiovascular disease (CVD). Studies have shown a 10–47% incidence of CVD in patients with CKD and lower eGFR and increased albuminuria are independent predictors of CVD in this patient population.[7-11] As a result of these comorbidities, the quality of life and life expectancy for most of these patients are is quite low and patients on dialysis have a much higher mortality rate compared to the general Medicare population.[6]

Moreover, renal replacement therapy (i.e., dialysis and kidney transplantation) is expensive procedures and Centers for Medicare and Medicaid Services extends coverage to all patients with ESRD who require dialysis or transplantation. This accounts for 7.1% of the overall Medicare paid claims cost, for less than 1% of the total Medicare population.[6]

Presentation of Kidney Disease

Most symptoms of CKD do not appear till late in the disease process, which has historically caused a delay in the diagnosis of CKD. The presence of certain medical conditions, such as hypertension and diabetes mellitus, increase the risk for a patient to develop kidney disease. This high-risk population should be screened for the presence of kidney disease and a simple urinalysis can be used to detect protein or blood in the urine. GFR can actually be measured by doing a 24-hour urine collection but more commonly equations like the Modification of Diet in Renal Disease or Chronic Kidney Disease Epidemiology (CKD-EPI) are used to estimate the GFR based on the serum creatinine level.[12] Occasionally kidney disease can manifest with symptoms like blood in the urine, flank pain, swelling of legs, and nonspecific symptoms like fatigue.

Although specific interventions for many diseases are not yet available, progressive renal damage may be slowed by certain interventions, thereby avoiding or delaying the development of ESRD and need for renal replacement therapy. Control of coexisting or secondary hypertension, blockade of the renin/angiotensin/aldosterone system in patients with proteinuria and in diabetics, and strict control of blood glucose levels are of proven value.[13-15] Other strategies to improve outcomes in patients with kidney disease include control of hyperlipidemia, control of obesity, reduction of left ventricular hypertrophy, cessation of tobacco use, and improved nutritional status including a low-sodium diet.[16]

SPECIFIC RENAL DISEASES

Diabetic Renal Disease

Diabetic nephropathy is the leading cause of ESRD in the United States, accounting for approximately 44% of all patients on dialysis.[6,13] With the increasing prevalence of type 2 diabetes in the general population, it is predicted that 58% of all prevalent ESRD patients in 2030 will have diabetes as their primary diagnosis. Approximately 40% of diabetic have some manifestation of diabetic kidney disease ranging from mildly increased albuminuria to ESRD.[17] On the other hand, up to 30% of patients with type 2 diabetes and chronic kidney disease do not have diabetic nephropathy, but instead some other pathology, most commonly vascular disease.[18]

The pathogenesis of diabetic nephropathy is not yet fully understood. Hyperglycemia is the initiating factor leading to advanced glycosylation end-products, transforming growth factor-β, and endothelins accumulate in the extracellular matrix leading to the decline of renal function in diabetics.[19] Initially, there is an increase in the glomerular filtration rate which leads to the development of proteinuria and glomerular hypertension and over time the glomerular capillary lumina are obliterated and the glomerular filtration rate eventually declines.

The most important early clinical marker of diabetic nephropathy is moderately increased albuminuria, which corresponds to a urinary albumin excretion rate of 30–300 mg/day or 20–200 mcg/min.[20] Unfortunately, albuminuria is not an early marker for diabetic nephropathy. Irreversible kidney damage has already occurred by the time albuminuria is detected, and it is a risk factor for increased overall mortality. Identification of diabetics with moderately increased

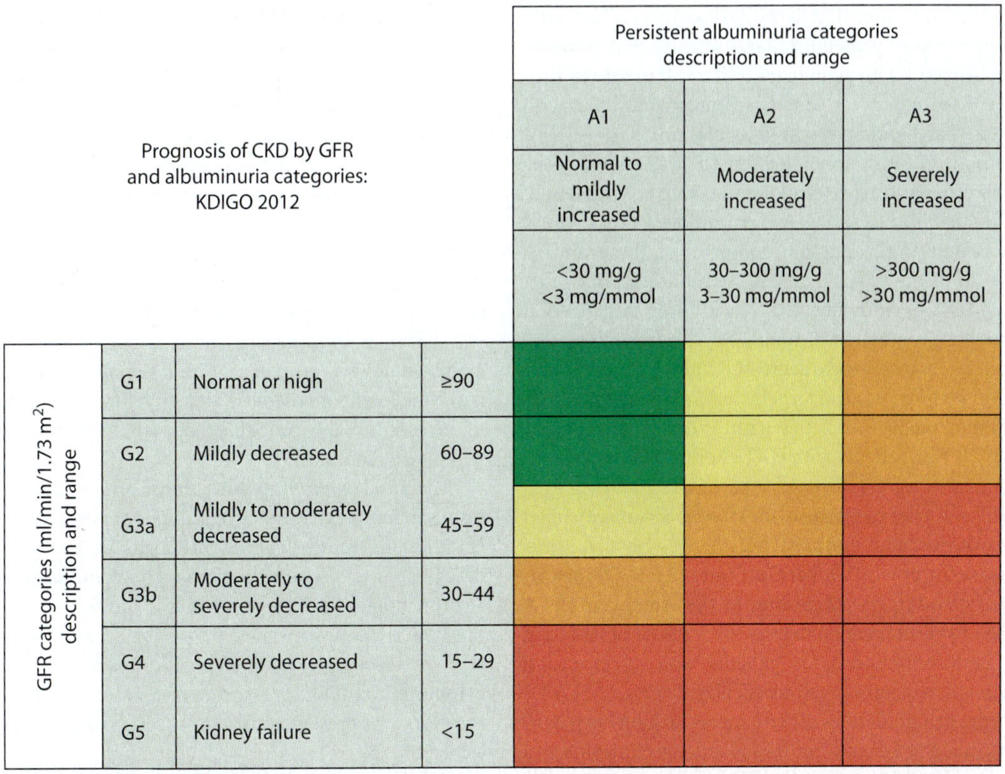

Prognosis of CKD by GFR and albuminuria categories: KDIGO 2012				Persistent albuminuria categories description and range		
				A1	A2	A3
				Normal to mildly increased	Moderately increased	Severely increased
				<30 mg/g <3 mg/mmol	30–300 mg/g 3–30 mg/mmol	>300 mg/g >30 mg/mmol
GFR categories (ml/min/1.73 m²) description and range	G1	Normal or high	≥90			
	G2	Mildly decreased	60–89			
	G3a	Mildly to moderately decreased	45–59			
	G3b	Moderately to severely decreased	30–44			
	G4	Severely decreased	15–29			
	G5	Kidney failure	<15			

FIGURE 54-1. Risk of CKD disease progression-based on GFR and albuminuria. Some patients with CKD have further progression of their disease and reach a diagnosis of ESRD, requiring some form of renal replacement therapy like peritoneal dialysis, hemodialysis, or renal transplantation. (*Source:* Reproduced with permission from *Kidney Int Suppl*. 2013;3:5–14.)

albuminuria is important because they progress to diabetic nephropathy (excretion of > 300 mg of protein per 24 hours) and eventually ESRD, and treatment to reduce albuminuria appears to delay this progression.[21]

Several major clinical trials have provided guidance for therapy in diabetics to prevent diabetic nephropathy and the complications associated with it. Treatment of overt diabetic nephropathy with an angiotensin-converting enzyme (ACE) inhibitor in patients with type 1 and type 2 diabetes has been shown to delay (but not totally halt) the rate of deterioration of renal function. This effect is independent of the effect of ACE inhibition on the treatment of blood pressure.[22]

The Diabetes Control and Complications Trial (DCCT) has demonstrated the beneficial effects of intensive insulin therapy on reducing the risk of diabetic nephropathy. Since then several other trials have supported this finding, including the United Kingdom Prospective Diabetic Study, which demonstrated the benefit of intensive insulin therapy in type 2 diabetics.[23,24] More recently pancreatic transplantation has been shown to stabilize the progression of diabetic kidney disease at several stages.[25]

Hypertension is also more common in diabetics with moderately increased albuminuria, especially in patients with type 2 diabetes, and is both a predictor and a consequence of nephropathy in type 2 diabetes. Hypertension has been shown to increase the rate at which diabetic nephropathy progresses and antihypertensive therapy has been shown to slow its course.[26]

Since the course of diabetic nephropathy can be altered by proper treatment, it is recommended that diabetics should be screened annually for albuminuria.[17] If albuminuria is present and persists, ACE inhibitor or angiotensin receptor blocker therapy is appropriate in both normotensive and hypertensive patients. Glycemic control and blood pressure should be monitored on a regular basis and the blood pressure goal should be less than 130/80 mm Hg in the setting of moderately and severely increased albuminuria.[1] In addition, moderately increased albuminuria is frequently associated with elevated levels of cholesterol and triglycerides, so dietary restriction of cholesterol and weight reduction should be emphasized.

While significant advances have been made in the approach to patients with diabetic nephropathy, we await the results of ongoing basic science research studies and clinical trials, which will increase the knowledge and improve the management of diabetic nephropathy, hopefully eliminating or at least significantly reducing the requirement for renal replacement therapy with its attendant comorbidity in this population.

Hypertensive Renal Disease

Hypertension is the second most common cause of CKD accounting for approximately 30% of the prevalent ESRD patients with African Americans having a greater predisposition toward developing hypertension associated kidney disease.[6] Hypertension can be both the cause and effect of CKD and sustained blood pressure elevations can cause progression of kidney disease.[27]

Additional risk factors for nephropathy in hypertensive persons include the degree of systolic hypertension, the presence of diabetes, male sex, increasing age, and high normal serum creatinine levels.

Primary hypertensive renal disease can be of two kinds. The more common, sometimes called "nephrosclerosis" is a form of chronic renal insufficiency associated with long-standing blood pressure elevation. The second, a form of AKI associated with malignant hypertension, is now rare where treatment of hypertension is widespread.

Although widespread treatment of hypertension has reduced other hypertensive morbidities, its effect on hypertensive renal disease is still not clear. Two regional studies in the United States showed that renal damage can progress in some treated hypertensive persons despite adequate blood pressure control[28,29] and the community-based Hypertension Detection and Follow-up Program confirmed this phenomenon.[30] The African-American Study of Kidney

Disease and Hypertension looked at 1094 African-Americans with long-standing hypertension, proteinuria, and unexplained progressive renal disease. There was no significant difference in rate of progression of kidney disease between blood pressure groups, although it should be noted that blood pressure was controlled to at least 140/90 or less in both groups. An ACE inhibitor was shown to be more effective than other antihypertensives in slowing progression of renal disease.[30] The inability to show an effect of lower target blood pressures may be related to the length of follow-up in these studies. Long-term follow-up of the participants in the modification of diet in renal disease (MDRD) study suggest that a lower target blood pressure may slow the progression of nondiabetic kidney disease in patients with moderately to severely decreased kidney function and proteinuria.[31] Blood pressure control targets vary based on guidelines published by different medical societies with as many as eight different guidelines.[2,9,32–36] In patients with CKD, both extremes of high and low blood pressures were associated with increased mortality.[37] Results of the SPRINT trial has shown that lower BP is associated with improved cardiovascular mortality but there is no consensus from Kidney Disease Improving Global Outcomes (KDIGO) regarding optimal BP control targets. According to the American Heart Association (AHA) hypertension guidelines 2017 a goal of less than 130/80 mm Hg is recommended for patients with hypertension regardless of their atherosclerotic cardiovascular disease (ASCVD) risk score.[38] Even though guidelines differ in areas lacking large randomized control trial, the general consensus among clinicians is a goal blood pressure of < 140/90 mm Hg. This is also a recommendation endorsed by the Eighth Joint National Committee, which was based on long-term randomized control trials among patients with HTN. Guidelines from KDIGO were based on expanded evidence base specifically related to HTN and kidney disease progression and recommended a blood pressure of < 130/80 mm Hg for patients with CKD and moderate to severe albuminuria with or without diabetes.[39]

Glomerulonephritis

The term glomerulonephritis encompasses several syndromes in which injury to the glomerulus is the common underlying disorder and they can manifest with variable degrees of hematuria and/or proteinuria, red blood cell casts, hypertension, edema, oliguria/anuria, and renal insufficiency. The glomerulonephritides are further classified into nephrotic and nephritic syndromes, nephrotic syndromes present with proteinuria as their main clinical manifestation whereas nephritic syndromes are characterized by hematuria and AKI.

Glomerulonephritis is the third most common cause of ESRD in the United States, behind diabetes and hypertension.[6] Pathological diagnosis relies on a renal biopsy.

Nephrotic Syndromes: Nephrotic syndromes are characterized by > 3.5 grams/day of proteinuria, hypoalbuminemia and edema. The major morphological categories of nephrotic syndrome are

1. minimal change disease,
2. focal segmental glomerular sclerosis,
3. membranous glomerulonephritis, and
4. membranoproliferative glomerulonephritis.

Even though each subtype can afflict subjects of all ages, minimal change disease is the most common lesion in children, whereas adults are more prone to have membranous glomerulonephritis focal segmental glomerular sclerosis. Membranous glomerulonephritis is the most common cause of nephrotic syndrome worldwide and may be a primary disorder or may be associated with infections such as hepatitis B or C or malignancies. Minimal change disease has the best prognosis, with remission usual before adulthood.

The incidence of focal segmental glomerular sclerosis has increased significantly in the last two decades and is frequently secondary to or associated with other diseases, including infections. It is now the most common primary glomerulopathy underlying ESRD in the United States.[40] Immune complex mediated membranoproliferative glomerulonephritis is frequently associated with hepatitis C but other infections and/or tumors may also cause a lesion of MPGN. The treatment depends on the underlying cause of glomerulonephritis and immunosuppressive agents may be needed in some cases in addition to ACE inhibitors or angiotensin receptor blockers, which are a mainstay of treatment in nephrotic syndromes to reduce proteinuria.[41,42]

Risk factors for progression of various forms of nephrotic syndrome include elevated serum creatinine, hypertension, male gender, age > 50, renal biopsy evidence of glomerular sclerosis and/or interstitial fibrosis, and the persistence of heavy proteinuria. Progression is slowed down if protein excretion remains mild or falls toward normal, whether spontaneously or with treatment. With progressive proteinuria, it is highly probable that patients with nephrotic syndromes will progress to ESRD.

Nephritic Syndromes: While most of the nephritic syndromes are immune complex mediated (e.g., lupus nephropathy, IgA nephropathy, cryoglobulinemic vasculitis, and postinfectious glomerulonephritis), other patterns of glomerular injury include formation of antibodies against glomerular components like the basement membrane (as is the case in antiglomerular basement membrane disease). Another class of diseases causing nephritic syndrome are antineutrophilic cytoplasmic antibodies associated vasculitis, which can be localized to the kidney or present with generalized systemic manifestations.

1. *IgA nephropathy* is considered to be the most common form of glomerulonephritis in the world.[43] It is more common in the western Pacific rim where incidence in older patients is reported to be increasing,[44] while in Europe and the United States, lower prevalence rates have been reported. There is familial clustering of IgA deposits in the kidney.[45] Most patients present with microscopic or macroscopic hematuria. In 30–40% of patients, there may be proteinuria usually associated with microscopic hematuria, and in < 10% of patients there is AKI, edema, and hypertension on presentation. IgA nephropathy usually has an indolent course with about 25–30% of patients reaching ESRD within 20–25 years.[44] Patients who present with hypertension, heavy proteinuria or an elevated creatinine are at higher risk for progression to ESRD. Randomized clinical trials have demonstrated the benefit of ACE inhibitors or angiotensin receptor blockers in the reduction of proteinuria. The use of immunosuppressive drugs has not shown a clear benefit in the treatment of IgA nephropathy.[46]
2. *Post infectious Glomerulonephritis.* The epidemiology and pathogenesis of postinfectious glomerulonephritis are well defined.[47] It is characterized by the onset of hematuria, proteinuria, hypertension, and sometimes oliguria and renal insufficiency, typically 2–3 weeks after a streptococcal throat infection or a skin infection. Treatment is often supportive with the use of antiproteinuric drugs and good blood pressure control.
3. *Lupus nephritis* can be seen in association with systemic lupus or with isolated renal involvement. The damage within the kidney is immune complex mediated and the serum complement levels are often low which can help in diagnosis. The treatment of lupus nephritis depends on the extent of renal involvement but often includes use of immunosuppressive medications.
4. *Antiglomerular Basement Membrane (anti-GBM) disease and antineutrophil cytoplasmic antibody associated (ANCA) vasculitis* often present with rapid deterioration of kidney disease in the setting of hematuria and there can be pulmonary involvement in some cases. Use of immunosuppressive drugs with or without plasmapheresis remain the mainstay of treatment.

Autosomal Dominant Polycystic Kidney Disease

Autosomal dominant polycystic kidney disease (PKD) is the most common genetic renal disorder and the fourth most common single cause of ESRD in the United States.[6] Patients with PKD constitute about 4.4% of patients requiring renal replacement therapy.[48] The disease is characterized by fluid-filled cysts in the kidney, which can compress surrounding tissue leading to renal insufficiency and eventually ESRD. It occurs in every one of 400–2000 live births, and an estimated 500,000 people have the disease in the United States.[49] Approximately 10% of patients have a new mutation with no family history of PKD.

PKD is a systemic disease with cyst development and a variable clinical course. Cysts can also occur in the liver, pancreas, seminal vesicles, and arachnoid. Other serious complications include changes in vasculature, especially intracranial aneurysms that are five times more common in the general population and has significant morbidity and mortality. Abnormalities in the regulation of cell growth, epithelial fluid secretion, and extracellular matrix metabolism contribute to the clinical problems associated with PKD. Renal manifestations of PKD include hematuria, urinary tract infections, flank pain, nephrolithiasis, hypertension, and the most serious, renal failure. At risk individuals can be diagnosed by ultrasound, CT, or MRI which can detect multiple cysts. The sensitivity of these tests is not very high when used in patients under 20–25 years of age although ultrasound has been shown to be fairly sensitive and well standardized for patients > 30 years. Genetic testing can now establish the genotype in approximately 60% of individuals with PKD. If a mutation can be identified within a single family member, then testing can be used to determine if relatives carry that mutation and have PKD. Genetic counselling is very important for patients with this disorder.[50]

Renal Disease and Illicit Drugs

Drug abuse is being recognized more frequently as a cause of renal disease and has great social and economic impact. In 2009, approximately 22 million or 8.7% of American population were thought to have used illicit drugs.[51] A majority of illicit drug use was marijuana, but there is use of other drugs like cocaine, heroin, hallucinogens, inhalants, and prescription drugs[52] and a significant positive and independent association between illicit drug use and risk for mild kidney function decline has been demonstrated.[53] In 2008 American Heart Association published a statement of negative effects of cocaine on cardiovascular health.[54] Methamphetamines have been associated with acute reversible kidney injury from acute tubular necrosis related to hypotension, rhabdomyolysis, disseminated intravascular coagulation, and hyperpyrexia.[55–58]

Heroin use is associated with focal segmental glomerulosclerosis and membranoproliferative glomerulonephritis; however, no causal pathways have been established due to confounding factors.[59] Cocaine use has been reported in the literature to have caused AKI,[60,61] kidney infarction,[62] and malignant hypertension.[63] Chronic use of cocaine has been reported to have caused tubular injury in animals[64] and arterial disease in humans. Some studies have[53,65,66] shown associations between illicit drug use and kidney disease ranging from mild renal impairment[53] to ESRD.[65,66] Cocaine exerts its effects on the kidney by changes in renal hemodynamics, glomerular matrix, and induction of renal atherogenesis.

Renal deposition of amyloid, associated with chronic inflammation and infection, occurs in skin poppers.[67] Proteinuria and sometimes renal failure is diagnosed at an average age of 41 years, 10 years older than FSGS patients. In a New York City autopsy series, 5% of addicts and 26% of addicts with suppurative skin infections had unsuspected renal amyloidosis.[68]

Other renal diseases related to drug abuse include immune-complex glomerulonephritis associated with infectious endocarditis or hepatitis B antigenemia, membranoproliferative glomerulonephritis and cryoglobulinemia associated with hepatitis C, necrotizing vasculitis related most strongly to amphetamine abuse, tubular dysfunction and occasionally AKI in solvent sniffers, and AKI due to muscle breakdown due to some drugs.

Treatment of addicts with ESRD is often complicated by noncompliance, communicable diseases like hepatitis B, hepatitis C, and HIV/AIDS, and, with continued drug abuse, infection, and clotting of vascular access and recurrence of disease in kidney transplants. Such problems accentuate dilemmas about responsibility for personal health and allocation of limited resources.

Renal Disease and the Human Immunodeficiency Virus

The understanding of renal disease associated with human immunodeficiency virus (HIV) infection continues to evolve. HIV disease can be associated with AKI and can lead to chronic kidney disease. Historically HIV disease has been associated with a specific histopathological pattern of disease known as HIV-associated nephropathy. Patients with this disorder usually have nephrotic range proteinuria accompanied by renal insufficiency which progresses fairly rapidly to ESRD.[69] On exam, there is frequently no significant peripheral edema or hypertension, and the kidneys are normal to enlarged in size despite being highly echogenic. This may be contrasted to heroin-associated nephropathy in which hypertension is frequently present, the kidneys are small, and progression to ESRD is a slower process. Although it is not always possible to distinguish HIV-associated disease from other forms of glomerulosclerosis, the following pathological findings are felt to be very suggestive of HIV nephropathy and include focal to global glomerulosclerosis, collapse of the glomerular tuft, severe tubulointerstitial fibrosis with some inflammation, microcyst formation, tubular degeneration, and characteristic tubuloreticular inclusions.[70]

Other than HIV-associated nephropathy, HIV can be associated with an immune complex mediated process in the kidney, which is called HIV-associated immune complex kidney disease. Both of these disorders are more frequent in individuals of African ancestry.[69] Compared to HIV-associated nephropathy, HIV immune complex kidney disease patients have more exposure to antiretroviral therapy exposure, lower viral loads, and higher CD4 cell counts.[71–74] Moreover, immune complex kidney disease is less likely to progress to ESRD than HIV-associated nephropathy.[73]

AKI is also more frequently seen in HIV infected individuals than in non-HIV-infected individuals,[75] and HIV is an independent risk factor for AKI in hospitalized and community living individuals.[69] Among hospitalized patients, kidney injury occurs two to three times the rate of noninfected individuals[75] and incidence ranges from 6% to 18%. Patients who are HIV positive and develop AKI due to acute tubular necrosis tend to be younger than the non-HIV positive patient with acute tubular necrosis, and frequently the acute tubular necrosis is associated with sepsis. Studies suggest that the incidence of AKI is 10-fold lower after the initial 3 months of HIV care.[76]

Much of the acute tubular necrosis associated with HIV disease is preventable if patients receive adequate volume support prior to use of nephrotoxic agents or during episodes of hypovolemia and if attention is paid to medication/antibiotic dosing.[77]

There is no specific cure for HIV nephropathy but the use of ACE-I and ARBs can be helpful in reducing the degree of proteinuria. There has been a decrease in overall morbidity and mortality due to HIV disease with the introduction of highly active antiretroviral therapy since the mid-1990s.[78]

Thrombotic Microangiopathy

Several disease processes like thrombotic thrombocytopenic purpura, hemolytic uremic syndrome—both classic and atypical and malignant hypertension result in worsening of renal function by causing thrombotic microangiopathy in the kidney. The renal pathologic lesions include edematous intimal expansion of arteries, fibrinoid necrosis of arterioles, and edematous subendothelial expansion in glomerular capillaries.[79]

Classic hemolytic uremic syndrome is typically seen in children in the setting of *E. coli* infection. Treatment involves supportive therapy with red blood cell transfusions, control of hypertension and dialysis if necessary. Apheresis may be helpful in more severe cases with central nervous system involvement. The prognosis for typical childhood hemolytic uremic syndrome is usually good. Atypical hemolytic uremic syndrome is a disorder of complement dysregulation and complement inhibitors like Eculizumab can be helpful in treatment. Thrombocytopenic purpura is a disorder, which presents with the classic triad of microangiopathic hemolytic anemia, thrombocytopenia, and AKI and occurs as a result of a deficiency of a certain metalloproteinase and plasmaphresis is the mainstay of treatment for these patients.

Acute kidney injury: Acute kidney injury refers to rapid deterioration of kidney function. There are various classifications for characterizing AKI based on serum creatinine and urine output. The Kidney Disease Improving Global Outcomes (KDIGO) guidelines defines AKI as an increase in serum creatinine by >= 0.3 mg/dL within 48 hours or increase in serum creatinine to 1.5 times baseline which is presumed to have occurred within the last 7 days or a urine volume of less than 0.5 mL/kg/hr for 6 hours.[80] Most cases of AKI are classified as either prerenal, intrarenal, or postrenal. Prerenal is mostly caused by poor oral intake, vomiting, diarrhea, shock, or diuretics resulting in dehydration and decreased circulatory volume. When AKI is due to either progression of prerenal cause to actual damage to the kidney or due to an intrinsic pathology of the kidney, it is classified as intrarenal. Postrenal AKI refers to when it is secondary to obstruction in the urinary tract most commonly due to kidney stones, prostate enlargement (BPH), or prostate cancer. AKI is more common in patients with underlying chronic kidney disease, 15.7% versus 5.3% in patients with normal renal function.[81] The majority of cases of AKI in the hospitalized patients are either caused by a prerenal etiology or acute tubular necrosis. About 70% of acute tubular necrosis cases are attributed to systemic infection and hypotension.[82] The long-term prognosis for these patients depends on their pre-existing renal function, severity of renal insufficiency and degree of oliguria/anuria.[83]

AKI in the intensive care unit (ICU) setting is also very common. Nearly all of these patients have had multiple renal insults, and it is frequently seen in the context of multiorgan failure. Survival is significantly reduced in these patients, especially in the presence of multiorgan failure.

Despite increasing awareness of the etiology of AKI and advancing technology, the mortality of AKI has not decreased significantly over the last several decades. Even mild episodes of AKI are associated with increases in morbidity and mortality. A multicenter observational study of 17,126 ICU patients in Austria showed a mortality of 62.8% in patients requiring renal replacement therapy compared to 38.5% in matched controls without AKI.[84] The exact reason for the above is not clear, and may be related to distant biochemical and histologic effects of renal ischemia on cardiac function and other organ systems yet to be elucidated. While short-term survival is low for patients with AKI in the ICU, the long-term outcomes in patients who survive to hospital discharge are much better. Of the patients who survived to hospital discharge among 979 critically ill patients with AKI requiring renal replacement therapy, 6-month survival was 69% and 5-year survival 50%.[85] Treatment options for AKI are limited and consist of blood pressure support, optimization of cardiac function, and treatment of underlying conditions including sepsis and limiting nephrotoxic agents.

END-STAGE RENAL DISEASE (ESRD)

The term ESRD refers to permanent failure of kidneys requiring renal replacement therapy with either dialysis or transplantation. As of December 2013, there were over 660,000 persons with ESRD in the United States—an increase of 68% since 2000.[6] The same racial trends as CKD are seen with ESRD, with the prevalence of ESRD being 3.7 times higher in African Americans than Caucasians.[6] Of the patients being treated for ESRD in 2014, 63.7% of all cases were receiving hemodialysis, 6.8% were receiving peritoneal dialysis, and 29.2% had a functioning kidney transplant.[6] In 2014 about 17,107 kidney transplants were performed in the United States which included 5537 came from living donors.[86] In the year 2015 alone, there were over 100,000 new patients to the ESRD program. The trends of number of patients with ESRD by cause from the year 2013–15 are shown in Table 54-1.

There have been several advancements in the treatment of ESRD patients, which have included high flux dialyzers, use of biocompatible membranes, automation of peritoneal dialysis, use of vitamin D derivatives for treatment of renal osteodystrophy, and genetically engineered erythropoietin for treatment of anemia reducing the need for blood transfusions.

Several efforts are underway to improve the quality of life for patients undergoing dialysis and to improve the quality metrics for dialysis patients so better care can be provided to this patient population.

THE FUTURE

Diagnosis and new therapeutic approaches remain a big area of interest currently both in clinical medicine as well as basic science research. In addition to the decrease in the death rate from hypertensive renal disease, renal infections, and renal congenital abnormalities, the incident rate for ESRD caused by diabetes has begun to stabilize, and that for ESRD caused by glomerulonephritis has begun to decline.

While progress has been made, the number of patients' age 45–64 years reaching ESRD continues to increase in a linear fashion. Thus, the cost of providing care has continued to increase. Based on expenditures in 2014 Medicare fee-for-service spending for beneficiaries with ESRD was 32.8 billion, accounting for 7.2% of the overall Medicare paid claims costs.[6] For westernized societies who have already made a large commitment to life support for subjects with irreversible renal failure, supporting the funding for these programs will continue to be a challenge. For all societies, the challenge remains to better understand the factors that contribute to ESRD. The public health perspectives of many of these diseases remain poorly defined and the distributions and natural histories of many remain obscure. While progress has been made in identifying specific prevention and treatment strategies, many diseases continue to lack specific strategies, and the prevalence of ESRD will continue to increase.

Epidemiological and health services research in renal and urinary tract diseases continues to expand. In the United States the American Society of Nephrology, United States Renal Data Services, Dialysis Outcome and Practice Patterns Study, National Institute of Diabetes and Digestive and Kidney Diseases have collated existing data on rates, morbidities, mortalities, resource utilization, and costs. They are supporting studies on diabetic renal disease, hypertension, progressive glomerular sclerosis, progression of renal failure, urinary tract obstruction, prostatic hyperplasia, prostatic cancer screening,

TABLE 54-1 TRENDS IN INCIDENT ESRD PATIENTS BASED ON THE CAUSE OF ESRD

Cause of ESRD	2013	2014	2015
Diabetes	52,514	54,151	56,269
Hypertension	34,391	34,553	34,762
Glomerulonephritis	9,016	9,148	9,209
Cystic disease	2,548	2,580	2,835
Other urologic cause	1,413	1,466	1,477
Other/Missing/Unknown cause	18,278	19,135	19,562

Source: Adapted from USRDS annual data report.

and urinary incontinence. They have also established research initiatives in interstitial cystitis, HIV-associated renal disease, the genetic basis of PKD, and renal disease and hypertension in minorities. To prevent or delay kidney damage, the National Kidney Foundation has established a free screening program for individuals at increased risk for developing kidney disease with the goals of raising awareness about kidney disease, providing free testing and encouraging people "at risk" to visit a doctor and follow the recommended treatment plan.[87] Educational information and support is also being provided. The well-established United States Renal Data System continues to provide valuable longitudinal data on patients with ESRD.

Scientists around the world in the United States, Italy, Singapore, and Sweden are working on developing a wearable artificial kidney, which would provide an option for patient requiring dialysis and awaiting transplant. A lot of advances have been made with, developments of lightweight, wearable dialysis systems feasible. These advances include the miniaturization of sensors and pumps[88]; small, long-lasting batteries[89–91] ultrapermeable membranes that reduce dialyzer size[88,92,93]; and new filtration materials to cleanse and reuse dialysate solutions without the need for large quantities of purified water.[94] Main components of a wearable kidney include dialysis membrane, dialysate regeneration, vascular access, patient monitoring, power source, and pumping system. One such system is the Wearable Artificial Kidney made by a technology firm in California, has published results from two clinical trials in humans, which offer a lot of promise. No wearable artificial kidney has received regulatory approval for marketing in the United States. In the United States, the FDA accepted the Wearable Artificial Kidney system for the Expedited Access Pathway program.[95] This program is intended to improve clinical data collection and reduce the time to regulatory approval for innovative technologies that serve important clinical needs.[94]

Anemia in ESRD patients remain an important risk factor for cardiovascular and other comorbidities in ESRD. Currently treatments options include erythropoietin and derivatives, which are IV or subcutaneous medications required frequently. This is both a source of discomfort and also has high-economic burdens. New medications on the horizon include Hypoxia inducible factor inhibitors, which are oral medications that help stimulate intrinsic bone marrow cells and affects iron metabolism to improve hemoglobin. They are currently undergoing trials and are expected to be approved for use by 2019.

Mesenchymal stem cell-based therapy is a model of tissue regeneration approach that holds the potential capability of treating renal failure. Use of bone marrow-derived mesenchymal stem cells is commonly performed and has safety data that shows feasibility. However, using new sources of stem cells with more therapeutic capability is encouraging. Scientists are doing studies to detect the presence of a multipotent mesenchymal stem cell population residing in human kidney. Mesenchymal stem cell trials are underway in patients with AKI, CKD, diabetic nephropathy, focal segmental glomerulosclerosis, and for systemic lupus erythematosis. During injury, these cells can differentiate into myofibroblasts, which can help with tissue repair. Mesenchymal stem cells represent a new front for stem cell therapy in a variety of inflammatory diseases. The application of mesenchymal stem cells is thought to be due to their ability to migrate to the sites of injury, differentiate into different cell types, and exert paracrine effect that modulate the immune and inflammatory response.

The results of these initiatives should invigorate the practice of nephrology, guide judicious apportionment of limited resources, support formulation of rational health policy, and improve the overall outcomes for patients with renal and urinary tract disease

GENITOURINARY TRACT DISEASES

Urinary Tract Infections

Urinary tract infections (UTIs) are one of the most common types of infection encountered in clinical medicine. They account for approximately 8.3 million physician visits and necessitate or complicate over 1 million hospital admissions annually in the United States.[96] The estimated annual cost of UTIs is $1.6 billion for evaluation and treatment.[97,98] Uncomplicated UTIs are most frequent in young, healthy, sexually active women with normal urinary tracts, and it is estimated that 40–50% of women will have a UTI in their lifetime. UTIs are also common in preschool girls, in postmenopausal women, and in elderly men and women, especially those who are institutionalized and those with indwelling urinary catheters. UTIs in older men are often associated with urinary retention due to BPH, urethral strictures, calculi, and debilitating illness and are thus designated as complicated and more difficult to treat.

Most infections are localized to the bladder and urethra, but some involve the kidneys and renal pelvis (pyelonephritis), or the prostate. UTIs rarely lead to renal damage or AKI unless they are associated with diabetes, pregnancy, reflux, obstruction, or neurogenic bladder.

Most UTIs in young women are new events, are uncomplicated, and caused by *E. coli* and other bowel organisms that enter the bladder through the short female urethra. Subjects with recurrent UTIs have increased density of bacterial receptors on epithelial cell surfaces in the vagina and bladder. Intercourse, diaphragm use, and failure to void after intercourse all increase risk. Women who have closely spaced recurrent infections with the same organisms or who have pyelonephritis should be evaluated for urinary tract abnormality, as should men with persistent infection. Complicated UTIs are frequently caused by non-*E. coli* pathogens such as *Enterococcus* and *Klebsiella* species.

In the presence of symptoms, white cells and bacteria in a clean-void midstream specimen of urine usually indicate a UTI. The usual bacterial count considered diagnostic on urine culture is $> 100{,}000$ CFU/mL, but many patients have lower counts, including half of those with cystitis and most patients with urethral syndromes. Such symptomatic infections should be treated by antimicrobials.

Screening for bacteriuria in symptom-free persons is not cost effective and may lead to inappropriate treatment, drug reactions, and selection of resistant organisms. Treatment of asymptomatic bacteriuria is not generally recommended, except in pregnant women, diabetics, and children with vesicoureteral reflux.

UTIs are the leading form of nosocomial infection and are especially common in nursing homes.[99] Spread can be reduced by separation of catheterized patients from others who are debilitated or catheterized, and by washing the hands after patient contact. For subjects who require temporary catheterization, risks of infection can be reduced by aseptic insertion, curtailed duration of catheterization, and meticulous care of the patient and the drainage system. However, infection remains very common in persons with chronic indwelling catheters and in patients who undergo urinary catheterization during a hospital stay. About 15–25% of hospitalized patients receive a urinary catheter during their hospital stay and the most important risk factor for developing a UTI is the prolonged use of a urinary catheter.[99]

Nephrolithiasis (Kidney Stones)

Nephrolithiasis has been recognized since antiquity and continues to be a major cause of morbidity. The prevalence of kidney stones in the United States in 8.8% with higher prevalence in men compared to women.[100] Risk factors for development of a stone include male sex, Caucasian race, obesity, hypertension, diet high in animal protein and salt but low in calcium and fluid, hot climate or occupation, and family history of kidney stones.[101] The initial stone usually presents in the third to fifth decade and up to 50% will have a recurrent stone within 5 years. Geographic variations in incidence may be attributable to temperature and sunlight exposure as well as limited access to beverages. Urinary stone disease is relatively uncommon in underdeveloped countries where bladder stones predominate.

Most kidney stones (75–85%) contain calcium, primarily in the form of calcium oxalate. The remaining stones contain uric acid, struvite, cystine, and/or small amounts of other compounds. The content of the stone may give clues to the underlying physiological problem, especially in the case of stones without calcium. Disorders associated with stone disease include primary hyperparathyroidism, renal tubular acidosis, enteric hyperoxaluria, sarcoidosis, cystinuria, and urinary tract infection or obstruction. Risk factors associated with calcium stone formation include low urinary volume, hypercalciuria, hyperoxaluria, hypocitraturia, and hyperuricosuria.[102]

Most patients present with flank pain radiating into the groin, which is abrupt in onset and frequently severe. Gross or microscopic hematuria, dysuria, frequency, nausea, and vomiting can be present. Occasionally, patients will have an ileus. Diagnosis is confirmed by ultrasound or CT scan with a noncontrast CT being the imaging of choice for these patients. Most kidney stones pass spontaneously, and the patient can be supported with analgesics and increased water intake. Urological intervention may be required including endoscopic "basket" removal, extracorporeal shock-wave lithotripsy, endoscopic lithotripsy with ultrasonic, electrohydraulic, or laser probes, open pyelolithotomy, and percutaneous nephrolithotomy. These procedures have reduced the costs, morbidity, and hospitalization rates compared with open surgery, which is rarely used anymore.

Given the high rate of recurrence in the patients, the primary objective of therapy is to prevent the formation of recurrent stones. Patients are asked to strain their urine for stone collection and composition analysis. Maintaining calcium intake helps prevent absorption of oxalate and outweighs the risk associated with high calcium intake. Oxalate restriction, reduction of animal protein intake, thiazide diuretics, and other agents may also be recommended depending on the patient's underlying medical condition and the cause of stone formation.

Urinary Incontinence

Urinary incontinence is defined as involuntary leakage of urine.[103] There are several types of incontinence, the most commons are[103]: (1) stress incontinence (loss of urine with physical exertion), caused by sphincter dysfunction; (2) urinary urge incontinence (sudden urge to urinate elicited by a stimuli, such as running water), it has an idiopathic origin or is due to hyperreflexia of the detrusor muscle, and it can be associated with overactive bladder; and (3) mixed (stress and urge combined)

The principal risk factor is vaginal delivery, other described factors are age, body mass index, hormonal status, ethnicity, and family history.[104]

According to statistics from National Health and Nutrition Examination Survey (NHANES), urinary incontinence affects more than half of women and more than a quarter of men aged 65 years old and over.[105] The annual direct cost of urinary incontinence in the United States (in 1995 dollars) was estimated as $16.3 billion annually,[106] although, a more recent study including only the cost of urge incontinence, estimates that the total cost in 2007 was $65.9 billion, with projected costs of $82.6 billion in 2020.[107]

Even though urinary incontinence is common, many individuals do not seek treatment, and consider it a normal part of the aging process, resulting in lower self-esteem, depression, and social isolation, which highlights the importance of eliminating the stigma associated with it.[103]

Diagnosis of incontinence involves physical examination, thorough history, and urinalysis to rule out other causes of urinary symptoms like urinary tract infections. Standardized surveys such as Urinary Distress Inventory and the Incontinence Impact Questionnaire can help to assess the severity of the symptoms, and evaluate treatment results. Urodynamic studies are available to evaluate lower urinary tract function, and are recommended in the diagnosis of patients with complex conditions, in those that have failed previous therapy, those with an underlying neurologic condition, and those with pelvic organ prolapse considering surgery.

Although urinary incontinence is a widespread problem, there is limited evidence regarding strategies that can used to prevent it. Some studies suggest that pelvic floor muscle training during pregnancy can prevent incontinence in the short term.[108] Pelvic floor muscle training (with or without biofeedback) has also been described as a treatment option to control symptoms and possible prevent progression of urinary incontinence.[103] Other strategies for management of symptoms are behavioral therapy, avoiding caffeine and alcohol, minimizing fluids. Surgical management is also available, with cure rates ranging 60–100%, variations are due to the surgical technique. Pharmacologic therapy is available for urge incontinence symptoms.[103]

Endometriosis

Endometriosis is defined as abnormal growths of endometrial tissue in locations other than the uterine lining.[109] It is estimated to be present in 11% of women in the reproductive age[110] and its prevalence increases to 30–45% on infertile women or those with chronic pain.[109,111] However, its exact prevalence is unknown because direct visualization through surgery is required for its diagnosis. Endometriosis is one of the leading cause of gynecologic hospitalization in the United States,[109]and it is estimated that its annual direct and indirect costs in the United States is $69.4 billion [112]

Clinical manifestations of the diseases vary from asymptomatic, to severe debilitating pelvic pain, although the most common complains are infertility, dysmenorrhea, and pelvic pain, which is most commonly associated with menstruation, but can be constant or present as dyspareunia.

Since risk factors and pathophysiology of the disease are not well defined, there are no preventive strategies. Treatment depends on the extent of the disease and fertility concerns. Nonsteroidal anti-inflammatory medications are useful in the management of pain. Hormonal therapy can be used to interrupt the cycles, and prevent bleeding of the endometriotic tissue. Surgical treatment is recommended for patients with severe disease or those who want to preserve fertility.[109]

Benign Prostatic Hyperplasia

BPH is extremely common in older men. It has been reported that BPH can be found in 88% of autopsies in men $\geq$ 80 years of age, and that nearly 50% of men $\geq$ 50 years of age have symptoms compatible with BPH.[113] Three men in ten may ultimately require surgery. While it frequently causes morbidity, it is rarely responsible for death.

The cause of BPH is not known. Necessary conditions are the presence of androgens and aging. No associations with socioeconomic factors, sexual behavior, use of tobacco or alcohol, or other diseases have been consistently demonstrated, and there is no firm evidence that BPH is a precursor of prostate cancer.[114]

In BPH subjects, a period of rapid prostate enlargement occurs, usually after the age of 50, followed by stabilization. The natural history of symptoms can vary greatly, many subjects have mild symptoms for years, with no change, and many do not require surgical intervention. Clinical symptoms result from variable compression of the bladder outlet, and include storage symptoms with increased frequency, nocturia, urgency, and urinary incontinence. It can also lead to voiding symptoms, which includes slow urinary stream, splitting or spraying urinary stream, hesitancy, and straining to void and terminal dribbling, and the potential for infection, complete obstruction, and bleeding. Age, urinary flow rate, and prostate volume are risk factors for acute urinary retention. Evaluation consists of rectal examination, blood chemistry studies, urinalysis and culture, measurement of residual urine volume after voiding, cystourethroscopy, urodynamic evaluation, and imaging or contrast studies of the kidneys and ureters.

Many patients can be observed while monitoring for progression. Alpha-adrenergic blocking agents and 5-alpha reductase inhibitors have been shown to delay progression of the symptoms and when used in combination may have a greater effect. Alpha reductase inhibitors may reduce the size of the prostate and when used alone or in combination with alpha-adrenergic blocking agents in some studies have been shown to reduce the incidence of acute urinary retention.[115] For more severe symptoms, prostatectomy is the standard of care. Indications for surgery vary, need better definition, and should be weighed against the comorbidities, complications, outcomes, and costs. Firm indications are acute urinary retention, hydronephrosis, recurrent urinary infections, severe hematuria, severe outflow obstruction, and urgency incontinence. Persistence of symptoms and impotence can result from surgery in a significant minority of subjects. Newer procedures are being developed including the use of prostatic stents, balloon dilatation of the prostate, laser prostatectomy, and microwave hyperthermia.

Prostate Cancer

Prostate cancer is a disease of aging men and is an important public health problem in the United States as well as throughout the world. It is the most commonly diagnosed cancer in men except for nonmelanoma skin cancer in the United States and is the second leading cause of male cancer deaths.[116] Estimated number of incident prostate cancer cases in 2019 were 174,650 with estimated 31,620 deaths in 2019.[117]

Prostate cancer accounts for 15.3% of all cancers in men in developed countries and 4.3% in developing countries.[118] The incidence, prevalence, and mortality rates from prostate cancer increase with age, particularly after 50 years of age. The incidence of prostate cancer has been increasing since the 1990s with the widespread use of PSA as a screening tool. Following PSA testing introduction it peaked in 1992 and 1995 and had risen approximately at a rate of approximately 1% per year. Historically the incidence of prostate cancer is higher in African Americans than in whites in the United States.[119] Associations with venereal disease, sexual activity, and smoking have been proposed but not proven. Studies have been conflicting regarding vasectomy, but more recent studies have not found evidence for an association. Additional possible risk factors include elevated testosterone levels, a high intake of dietary fat, and other dietary habits.

Several genetic mutations/deletions and polymorphisms may be associated with an increased risk for prostate cancer, but no single prostate cancer gene has been identified. These findings may support increased attention to screening in certain populations such as African Americans.

Screening for prostate cancer has been a topic of debate over the years and the most recent United States Preventive Services Task Force recommendations from 2017 have made a category C recommendation for men aged 55–69 to undergo prostate cancer screening by checking prostate specific antigen annually based on an individual's preference after discussing the risks and benefits of screening. They do not recommend screening in patients older than 70 years of age.[120]

Most patients diagnosed with early-stage prostate cancer do not have symptoms attributable to the cancer. Patients typically present with lower urinary tract symptoms, which may be related to obstruction (urgency, nocturia, frequency, and hesitancy) from an enlarged prostate gland causing bladder-neck obstruction. These symptoms are very similar to those seen with BPH. Other less common signs and symptoms include back pain from vertebral metastases and new onset of impotence. A few patients have symptoms related to urinary retention caused by bladder-neck obstruction, bilateral hydronephrosis from periaortic lymph node enlargement, or spinal cord compression from epidural extension. Rarely, patients present with an enlarged supraclavicular node or elevation of liver tests. Today an increasing number of patients present with any of the small, well-differentiated carcinomas remain confined to the prostate and are only detected at autopsy (latent or autopsy cancers). The majority of tumors never become active, but how to predict which will become so has not been determined. It is estimated that the average lifetime risk of developing prostate cancer in an American male is 17% while the risk of dying from prostate cancer is only 3%.[116] Management of prostate cancer may include watchful waiting, hormonal therapy, prostatectomy, and radiation therapy depending on the stage of the cancer. Treatment considerations should include age, life expectancy, comorbid conditions, side effects, and costs. Urinary incontinence, impotence, and radiation morbidity comprise the treatment-related adverse effects. The Prostate Cancer Prevention Trial looked at the use of finasteride, a 5-alpha reductase inhibitor that prevents conversion of testosterone to dihydrotestosterone, as a chemopreventive agent. While it prevented or delayed the number of cancers and reduced urinary tract symptoms, it also was associated with an increased risk for high-grade prostate cancer.[121] Currently, there are ongoing trials looking at similar agents as well as chemotherapy for various stages of diagnosed prostate cancer. Multiple clinical trials are currently underway which should help identify the best method of screening, as well as chemo preventive therapies and therapies for the various stages of prostate cancer.

Cervical Cancer

Cervical cancer is the twenty-first century most common cancer in the United States, yet it is the fourth most common cancer among women worldwide. It is estimated, that 12,820 new cases will be diagnosed in 2017 in the United States and there will be 4.210 deaths for the same period.[122] The overall 5-year survival rate for cervical cancer is 67%; however, survival approaches 92% for cervical cancers detected in situ [123]

The primary risk factor for cervical cancer is infection with human papillomavirus virus (HPV),[124] other risk factors are: cigarette smoking, five or more pregnancies, partners with greater than six other sexual partners.[125]

Primary prevention of cervical cancer is achieved thorough vaccination against HPV, which has been associated with a 64% decreases on HPV prevalence among females 14–19 years, and a 43% decrease among those 20–24 years old in the United States since 2007.[126] In Europe, HPV vaccination has been associated with a decrease of cervical cancer cases.[127]

The USPSTF recommends screening for cervical cancer in women age 21–65 years with cytology (Pap smear) every 3 years or, for women age 30–65 years, screening with a combination of cytology and HPV testing every 5 years.[128]

Endometrial Cancer

Endometrial cancer is the fourth most common cancer in women in the United States and the most commonly diagnosed gynecologic cancer.[129] In 2017, it is expected that 61,380 women in the United States will be diagnosed with endometrial cancer, and 10,920 will die from the disease.[123] Approximately, 3% of women will be diagnosed with endometrial cancer in their lifetime. The overall 5-year survival is 81.3%, and this rate has been stable over the last 10 years, but there are variation according to race, African-American women are more likely to die of the disease than their white counterparts (3.8 deaths per 100,000 person vs. 2.1 deaths per 100,000).

The principal clinical manifestation of the disease if abnormal vaginal bleeding, most commonly postmenopausal. Risk factors for the disease include: administration of exogenous unopposed estrogens, obesity, diabetes, nulliparity, and family history. Prevention of the disease includes the addition of progesterone to the hormonal regimen, and surveillance of women at high risk of the disease. There is no screening test recommended for women at average risk [130]

Bladder Cancer

Bladder cancer is the most common cancer of the urinary tract. According to estimations, bladder cancer will be responsible for 79,030 new cases and 16,870 deaths in the United States in 2017. The overall 5-year survival rate is 77%.[123]

The incidence rate of bladder cancer is almost four times higher among men than women, and two times higher among whites than blacks.[130] Cigarette smoking is the best established cause of bladder cancer. Bladder cancer risk for a current smoker is approximately three times that of a nonsmoker.[131] Other risk factors are associated with occupational exposures to dye, rubber, leather, paint, and aluminum industries.

Primary prevention is associated with smoking cessation. No screening protocol is recommended at this time.

References

1 Levin A, Stevens PE, Bilous RW, et al. Improving global outcomes (KDIGO) CKD work group. KDIGO 2012 clinical practice guideline for the evaluation and management of chronic kidney disease. *Kidney Int.*, 2013;3:1–150.

2. Andrassy KM. Comments on 'KDIGO 2012 clinical practice guideline for the evaluation and management of chronic kidney disease'. *Kidney Int.* 2013;84(3):622–3.

3. Hill NR, Fatoba ST, Oke JL, et al. Global prevalence of chronic kidney disease—A systematic review and meta-analysis. *PLoS One.* 2016;11(7):e0158765.

4. NHANES. National Health and Nutrition Examination Survey 2012.

5. NIH. National Institute of Diabetes and Digestive Health and Kidney Diseases Website. 2016.

6. USRDS. United States Renal Data System. 2016 USRDS annual data report: Epidemiology of kidney disease in the United States. National Institutes of Health, National Institute of Diabetes and Digestive and Kidney Diseases, Bethesda, MD, 2016. 2016.

7. Iimori S, Naito S, Noda Y, et al. Anaemia management and mortality risk in newly visiting patients with chronic kidney disease in Japan: The CKD-ROUTE study. *Nephrology (Carlton).* 2015;20(9):601–8.

8. Martinez-Castelao A, Gorriz JL, et al. Baseline characteristics of patients with chronic kidney disease stage 3 and stage 4 in Spain: The MERENA observational cohort study. *BMC Nephrol.* 2011;12:53.

9. Ritchie J, Rainone F, Green D, et al. Extreme elevations in blood pressure and all-cause mortality in a referred CKD population: Results from the CRISIS study. *Int J Hypertens.* 2013;2013:597906.

10. Shah R, Matthews GJ, Shah RY, et al. Serum fractalkine (CX3CL1) and cardiovascular outcomes and diabetes: Findings from the chronic renal insufficiency cohort (CRIC) study. *Am J Kidney Dis.* 2015;66(2):266–73.

11. Yuan J, Zou XR, Han SP, et al. Prevalence and risk factors for cardiovascular disease among chronic kidney disease patients: Results from the Chinese cohort study of chronic kidney disease (C-STRIDE). *BMC Nephrol.* 2017;18(1):23.

12. Florkowski CM, Chew-Harris JSC. Methods of estimating GFR—Different equations including CKD-EPI. *Clin Biochem Rev.* 2011;32(2):75–9.

13. The Diabetes Control and Complications (DCCT) Research Group. Effect of intensive therapy on the development and progression of diabetic nephropathy in the diabetes control and complications trial. *Kidney Int.* 1995; 47(6):1703–20.

14. Klahr S, Levey AS, Beck GJ, et al. The effects of dietary protein restriction and blood-pressure control on the progression of chronic renal disease. Modification of diet in renal disease study group. *N Engl J Med.* 1994;330(13):877–84.

15. Pedrini MT, Levey AS, Lau J, Chalmers TC, Wang PH. The effect of dietary protein restriction on the progression of diabetic and nondiabetic renal diseases: A meta-analysis. *Ann Intern Med.* 1996;124(7):627–32.

16. Striker G. Report on a workshop to develop management recommendations for the prevention of progression in chronic renal disease. *J Am Soc Nephrol.* 1995;5(7):1537–40.

17. KDOQI clinical practice guidelines and clinical practice recommendations for diabetes and chronic kidney disease. *Am J Kidney Dis.* 2007;49 (2 Suppl 2):S12–154.

18. Kramer HJ, Nguyen QD, Curhan G, Hsu CY. Renal insufficiency in the absence of albuminuria and retinopathy among adults with type 2 diabetes mellitus. *JAMA.* 2003;289(24):3273–7.

19. Mogyorosi A, Ziyadeh FN. Update on pathogenesis, markers and management of diabetic nephropathy. *Curr Opin Nephrol Hypertens.* 1996;5(3):243–53.

20. Messent JW, Elliott TG, Hill RD, Jarrett RJ, Keen H, Viberti GC. Prognostic significance of microalbuminuria in insulin-dependent diabetes mellitus: A twenty-three year follow-up study. *Kidney Int.* 1992;41(4):836–9.

21. Parving HH, Lehnert H, Brochner-Mortensen J, Gomis R, Andersen S, Arner P. The effect of irbesartan on the development of diabetic nephropathy in patients with type 2 diabetes. *N Engl J Med.* 2001;345(12):870–8.

22. Lewis EJ, Hunsicker LG, Bain RP, Rohde RD. The effect of angiotensin-converting-enzyme inhibition on diabetic nephropathy. The collaborative study group. *N Engl J Med.* 1993;329(20):1456–62.

23. UK Prospective Diabetes Study Group. Tight blood pressure control and risk of macrovascular and microvascular complications in type 2 diabetes: UKPDS 38. *BMJ.* 1998; 317(7160):703–13.

24. Nathan DM, Genuth S, Lachin J, et al. The effect of intensive treatment of diabetes on the development and progression of long-term complications in insulin-dependent diabetes mellitus. *N Engl J Med.* 1993;329(14):977–86.

25. Fioretto P, Steffes MW, Sutherland DE, Goetz FC, Mauer M. Reversal of lesions of diabetic nephropathy after pancreas transplantation. *N Engl J Med.* 1998;339(2):69–75.

26. Clark CMJr, Lee DA. Prevention and treatment of the complications of diabetes mellitus. *N Engl J Med.* 1995;332(18):1210–7.

27. Bakris GL, Williams M, Dworkin L, et al. Preserving renal function in adults with hypertension and diabetes: A consensus approach. National kidney foundation hypertension and diabetes executive committees working group. *Am J Kidney Dis.* 2000;36(3):646–61.

28. Rostand SG, Brown G, Kirk KA, Rutsky EA, Dustan HP. Renal insufficiency in treated essential hypertension. *N Engl J Med.* 1989;320(11):684–8.

29. Tierney WM, McDonald CJ, Luft FC. Renal disease in hypertensive adults: Effect of race and type II diabetes mellitus. *Am J Kidney Dis.* 1989;13(6):485–93.

30. Shulman NB, Ford CE, Hall WD, et al. Prognostic value of serum creatinine and effect of treatment of hypertension on renal function. Results from the hypertension detection and follow-up program. The hypertension detection and follow-up program cooperative group. *Hypertension.* 1989;13(5 Suppl):I80–93.

31. Sarnak MJ, Greene T, Wang X, et al. The effect of a lower target blood pressure on the progression of kidney disease: Long-term follow-up of the modification of diet in renal disease study. *Ann Intern Med.* 2005;142(5):342–51.

32. Mancia G, Fagard R, Narkiewicz K, et al. 2013 Practice guidelines for the management of arterial hypertension of the European society of hypertension (ESH) and the European society of cardiology (ESC): ESH/ESC task force for the management of arterial hypertension. *J Hypertens.* 2013;31(10):1925–38.

33. Go AS, Bauman MA, Coleman King SM, et al. An effective approach to high blood pressure control: a science advisory from the American heart association, the American college of cardiology, and the centers for disease control and prevention. *Hypertension.* 2014;63(4):878–85.

34. James PA, Oparil S, Carter BL, et al. 2014 evidence-based guideline for the management of high blood pressure in adults: Report from the panel members appointed to the eighth joint national committee (JNC 8). *JAMA.* 2014; 311(5):507–20.

35. Krause T, Lovibond K, Caulfield M, McCormack T, Williams B. Management of hypertension: Summary of NICE guidance. *BMJ.* 2011;343:d4891.

36. Weber MA, Schiffrin EL, White WB, et al. Clinical practice guidelines for the management of hypertension in the community: A statement by the American society of hypertension and the international society of hypertension. *J Clin Hypertens (Greenwich).* 2014;16(1):14–26.

37. Kovesdy CP, Bleyer AJ, Molnar MZ, et al. Blood pressure and mortality in U.S. veterans with chronic kidney disease: A cohort study. *Ann Intern Med.* 2013;159(4):233–42.

38. Carey RM, Whelton PK, Committee AAHGW. Prevention, detection, evaluation, and management of high blood pressure in adults: Synopsis of the 2017 American college of cardiology/American heart association hypertension guideline. *Ann Intern Med.* 2018;168(5):351–8.

39. Becker GJ, Wheeler DC, Zeeuw DD, et al. Kidney disease: Improving global outcomes (KDIGO) blood pressure work group. KDIGO clinical practice guideline for the management of blood pressure in chronic kidney disease. *Kidney Int.* 2012; 2:337–414.

40. Kitiyakara C, Eggers P, Kopp JB. Twenty-one-year trend in ESRD due to focal segmental glomerulosclerosis in the United States. *Am J Kidney Dis.* 2004;44(5):815–25.

41. Cattran D. Management of membranous nephropathy: When and what for treatment. *J Am Soc Nephrol.* 2005;16(5):1188–94.

42. Kramer BK, Schweda F. Ramipril in non-diabetic renal failure (REIN study). Ramipril efficiency in nephropathy study. *Lancet.* 1997; 350(9079):736; author reply -7.

43. van Paassen P, van Breda Vriesman PJ, van Rie H, Tervaert JW. Signs and symptoms of thin basement membrane nephropathy: A prospective

regional study on primary glomerular disease—The limburg renal registry. *Kidney Int.* 2004;66(3):909–13.

44. Barratt J, Feehally J. IgA nephropathy. *J Am Soc Nephrol.* 2005;16(7):2088–97.
45. Suzuki K, Honda K, Tanabe K, Toma H, Nihei H, Yamaguchi Y. Incidence of latent mesangial IgA deposition in renal allograft donors in Japan. *Kidney Int.* 2003;63(6):2286–94.
46. Rauen T, Eitner F, Fitzner C, et al. Intensive supportive care plus immunosuppression in IgA nephropathy. *N Engl J Med.* 2015;373(23):2225–36.
47. B R-I. Diseases of the Kidney. 4th ed. Chap. 63. Boston. 1986.
48. Harris PC, Torres VE. Polycystic kidney disease. *Annu Rev Med.* 2009;60:321–37.
49. Gabow PA. Autosomal dominant polycystic kidney disease. *N Engl J Med.* 1993;329(5):332–42.
50. J G. "Dangerfield's disorders": Rise to the forefront. Nephsap. 2005.
51. Substance abuse and Mental health services administration. Results from the 2009 National survey on Drug Use and Health: Volume 1. Summary of National findings (NSDUH Series H-38A, HHS publication No. SMA 10-4586), Rockville, MD. 2010.
52. Akkina SK, Ricardo AC, Patel A, et al. Illicit drug use, hypertension, and chronic kidney disease in the US adult population. *Transl Res.* 2012;160(6):391–8.
53. Vupputuri S, Batuman V, Muntner P, et al. The risk for mild kidney function decline associated with illicit drug use among hypertensive men. *Am J Kidney Dis.* 2004;43(4):629–35.
54. McCord J, Jneid H, Hollander JE, et al. Management of cocaine-associated chest pain and myocardial infarction: A scientific statement from the American Heart Association Aacute Cardiac Care Committee of the council on clinical cardiology. *Circulation.* 2008;117(14):1897–907.
55. Fahal IH, Sallomi DF, Yaqoob M, Bell GM. Acute renal failure after ecstasy. *BMJ.* 1992;305(6844):29.
56. Ginsberg MD, Hertzman M, Schmidt-Nowara WW. Amphetamine intoxication with coagulopathy, hyperthermia, and reversible renal failure. A syndrome resembling heatstroke. *Ann Intern Med.* 1970;73(1):81–5.
57. Henry JA, Jeffreys KJ, Dawling S. Toxicity and deaths from 3,4-methylenedioxymethamphetamine ("ecstasy"). *Lancet.* 1992;340(8816):384–7.
58. Kendrick WC, Hull AR, Knochel JP. Rhabdomyolysis and shock after intravenous amphetamine administration. *Ann Intern Med.* 1977;86(4):381–7.
59. Jaffe JA, Kimmel PL. Chronic nephropathies of cocaine and heroin abuse: A critical review. *Clin J Am Soc Nephrol.* 2006;1(4):655–67.
60. Herzlich BC, Arsura EL, Pagala M, Grob D. Rhabdomyolysis related to cocaine abuse. *Ann Intern Med.* 1988;109(4):335–6.
61. Roth D, Alarcon FJ, Fernandez JA, Preston RA, Bourgoignie JJ. Acute rhabdomyolysis associated with cocaine intoxication. *N Engl J Med.* 1988;319(11):673–7.
62. Sharff JA. Renal infarction associated with intravenous cocaine use. *Ann Emerg Med.* 1984;13(12):1145–7.
63. Thakur V, Godley C, Weed S, Cook ME, Hoffman E. Case reports: Cocaine-associated accelerated hypertension and renal failure. *Am J Med Sci.* 1996;312(6):295–8.
64. Barroso-Moguel R, Mendez-Armenta M, Villeda-Hernandez J. Experimental nephropathy by chronic administration of cocaine in rats. *Toxicology.* 1995;98(1–3):41–6.
65. Norris KC, Thornhill-Joynes M, Robinson C, et al. Cocaine use, hypertension, and end-stage renal disease. *Am J Kidney Dis.* 2001;38(3):523–8.
66. Perneger TV, Klag MJ, Whelton PK. Recreational drug use: A neglected risk factor for end-stage renal disease. *Am J Kidney Dis.* 2001;38(1):49–56.
67. Neugarten J, Gallo GR, Buxbaum J, Katz LA, Rubenstein J, Baldwin DS. Amyloidosis in subcutaneous heroin abusers ("skin poppers' amyloidosis"). *Am J Med.* 1986;81(4):635–40.
68. Menchel S, Cohen D, Gross E, Frangione B, Gallo G. AA protein-related renal amyloidosis in drug addicts. *Am J Pathol.* 1983;112(2):195–9.
69. Campos P, Ortiz A, Soto K. HIV and kidney diseases: 35 Years of history and consequences. *Clin Kidney J.* 2016;9(6):772–81.
70. Humphreys MH. Human immunodeficiency virus-associated glomerulosclerosis. *Kidney Int.* 1995;48(2):311–20.
71. Booth JW, Hamzah L, Jose S, et al. Clinical characteristics and outcomes of HIV-associated immune complex kidney disease. *Nephrol Dial Transplant.* 2016;31(12):2099–107.
72. Foy MC, Estrella MM, Lucas GM, et al. Comparison of risk factors and outcomes in HIV immune complex kidney disease and HIV-associated nephropathy. *Clin J Am Soc Nephrol.* 2013;8(9):1524–32.
73. Kumar N, Perazella MA. Differentiating HIV-associated nephropathy from antiretroviral drug-induced nephropathy: A clinical challenge. *Curr HIV/AIDS Rep.* 2014;11(3):202–11.
74. Naicker S, Rahmanian S, Kopp JB. HIV and chronic kidney disease. *Clin Nephrol.* 2015;83(7 Suppl 1):32–8.
75. Wyatt CM, Arons RR, Klotman PE, Klotman ME. Acute renal failure in hospitalized patients with HIV: Risk factors and impact on in-hospital mortality. *AIDS.* 2006;20(4):561–5.
76. Kalim S, Szczech LA, Wyatt CM. Acute kidney injury in HIV-infected patients. *Semin Nephrol.* 2008;28(6):556–62.
77. Rao TK, Friedman EA. Outcome of severe acute renal failure in patients with acquired immunodeficiency syndrome. *Am J Kidney Dis.* 1995;25(3):390–8.
78. Mocroft A, Ledergerber B, Katlama C, et al. Decline in the AIDS and death rates in the EuroSIDA study: An observational study. *Lancet.* 2003;362(9377):22–9.
79. Remuzzi G, Ruggenenti P. The hemolytic uremic syndrome. *Kidney Int.* 1995;48(1):2–19.
80. Clinical practice guidelines for acute kidney injury 2012. Available at https://kdigo.org/wp-content/uploads/2016/10/KDIGO-2012-AKI-Guideline-English.pdf.
81. Nash K, Hafeez A, Hou S. Hospital-acquired renal insufficiency. *Am J Kidney Dis.* 2002;39(5):930–6.
82. Mehta RL, Pascual MT, Soroko S, et al. Spectrum of acute renal failure in the intensive care unit: The PICARD experience. *Kidney Int.* 2004;66(4):1613–21.
83. Hou SH, Bushinsky DA, Wish JB, Cohen JJ, Harrington JT. Hospital-acquired renal insufficiency: A prospective study. *Am J Med.* 1983;74(2):243–8.
84. Metnitz PG, Krenn CG, Steltzer H, et al. Effect of acute renal failure requiring renal replacement therapy on outcome in critically ill patients. *Crit Care Med.* 2002;30(9):2051–8.
85. Morgera S, Kraft AK, Siebert G, Luft FC, Neumayer HH. Long-term outcomes in acute renal failure patients treated with continuous renal replacement therapies. *Am J Kidney Dis.* 2002;40(2):275–9.
86. OPTN. http://optn.transplant.hrsa.gov/. 2016.
87. National Kidney Foundation Keep Healthy. Available at https://www.kidney.org/keephealthy.
88. Armignacco P, Lorenzin A, Neri M, Nalesso F, Garzotto F, Ronco C. Wearable devices for blood purification: Principles, miniaturization, and technical challenges. *Semin Dial.* 2015;28(2):125–30.
89. Ronco C, Davenport A, Gura V. The future of the artificial kidney: Moving towards wearable and miniaturized devices. *Nefrologia.* 2011;31(1):9–16.
90. Rosner MH, Ronco C. Remote monitoring for the wearable artificial kidney. *Contrib Nephrol.* 2011;171:243–7.
91. Yee J. Rise of the small machines: Salvation. *Adv Chronic Kidney Dis.* 2013;20(6):449–51.
92. Burgin T, Johnson D, Chung H, Clark A, McGrath J. Analytical and finite element modeling of nanomembranes for miniaturized, continuous hemodialysis. *Membranes (Basel).* 2015;6(1).
93. Johnson DG, Khire TS, Lyubarskaya YL, et al. Ultrathin silicon membranes for wearable dialysis. *Adv Chronic Kidney Dis.* 2013;20(6):508–15.
94. Topfer L-A. Wearable artificial kidneys for end-stage kidney disease. In: CADTH Issues in Emerging Health Technologies. Ottawa (ON): Canadian Agency for Drugs and Technologies in Health; 2017, p. 150.
95. Institute E. U.S Clinical trial data announced on wearable artifical kidney prototype. *Health Technol Trends* 2015;27(11):1–3.
96. Burt CW, Schappert SM. Ambulatory care visits to physician offices, hospital outpatient departments, and emergency departments: United States, 1999–2000. *Vital Health Stat.* 2004;13(157):1–70.
97. Foxman B. Epidemiology of urinary tract infections: Incidence, morbidity, and economic costs. *Am J Med.* 2002;113 Suppl 1A:5s–13s.
98. Foxman B. Epidemiology of urinary tract infections: Incidence, morbidity, and economic costs. *Dis Mon.* 2003;49(2):53–70.
99. Center for Disease Control: Catheter Associated Urinary Tract Infection. Available at https://www.cdc.gov/hai/ca_uti/uti.html.
100. Scales CD, Jr., Smith AC, Hanley JM, Saigal CS. Prevalence of kidney stones in the United States. *Eur Urol.* 2012;62(1):160–5.
101. Curhan GC, Willett WC, Rimm EB, Stampfer MJ. A prospective study of dietary calcium and other nutrients and the risk of symptomatic kidney stones. *N Engl J Med.* 1993;328(12):833–8.

102. Pak CY. Etiology and treatment of urolithiasis. *Am J Kidney Dis.* 1991;18(6):624–37.

103. Tarnay CM. Urinary incontinence & pelvic floor disorders. In: DeCherney AH Nathan L, Laufer N, Roman AS, eds. *CURRENT Diagnosis & Treatment: Obstetrics & Gynecology*. 11th ed. New York: McGraw-Hill; 2013.

104. Danforth KN, Townsend MK, Lifford K, Curhan GC, Resnick NM, Grodstein F. Risk factors for urinary incontinence among middle-aged women. *Am J Obstet Gynecol.* 2006;194(2):339–45.

105. Gorina Y, Schappert S, Bercovitz A, Elgaddal N, Kramarow E. Prevalence of incontinence among older Americans. *Vital Health Stat.* 3. 2014(36):1–33.

106. Wilson L, Brown JS, Shin GP, Luc KO, Subak LL. Annual direct cost of urinary incontinence. *Obstet Gynecol.* 2001;98(3):398–406.

107. Coyne KS, Wein A, Nicholson S, Kvasz M, Chen CI, Milsom I. Economic burden of urgency urinary incontinence in the United States: A systematic review. *J Manag Care Pharm.* 2014;20(2):130–40.

108. Bazi T, Takahashi S, Ismail S, et al. Prevention of pelvic floor disorders: International urogynecological association research and development committee opinion. *Int Urogynecol J.* 2016;27(12):1785–95.

109. Sarajari S, Muse KNJr, Fox MD. Endometriosis. In: DeCherney AH NL, Laufer N, Roman AS, eds. *CURRENT Diagnosis & Treatment: Obstetrics & Gynecology*. 11th ed. New York: McGraw-Hill; 2013.

110. Buck Louis GM, Hediger ML, Peterson CM, et al. Incidence of endometriosis by study population and diagnostic method: The ENDO study. *Fertil Steril.* 2011;96(2):360–5.

111. Mounsey AL, Wilgus A, Slawson DC. Diagnosis and management of endometriosis. *Am Fam Physician.* 2006;74(4):594–600.

112. Simoens S, Dunselman G, Dirksen C, et al. The burden of endometriosis: Costs and quality of life of women with endometriosis and treated in referral centres. *Hum Reprod.* 2012;27(5):1292–9.

113. Napalkov P, Maisonneuve P, Boyle P. Worldwide patterns of prevalence and mortality from benign prostatic hyperplasia. *Urology.* 1995;46(3 Suppl A):41–6.

114. Chang RT, Kirby R, Challacombe BJ. Is there a link between BPH and prostate cancer? *Practitioner.* 2012;256(1750):13–6, 2.

115. McConnell JD, Roehrborn CG, Bautista OM, et al. The long-term effect of doxazosin, finasteride, and combination therapy on the clinical progression of benign prostatic hyperplasia. *N Engl J Med.* 2003;349(25):2387–98.

116. Jemal A, Siegel R, Ward E, et al. Cancer statistics, 2006. *CA Cancer J Clin.* 2006;56(2):106–30.

117. Howlader N, Noone A, Krapcho M, Miller D, Brest A, Yu M, et al. SEER Cancer Statistics Review, 1975–2016, National Cancer Institute. Bethesda, MD, https://seer.cancer.gov/archive/csr/1975_2016/, based on November 2018 SEER data submission, posted to the SEER web site, April 2019.

118. Gronberg H. Prostate cancer epidemiology. *Lancet.* 2003;361(9360):859–64.

119. Farkas A, Schneider D, Perrotti M, Cummings KB, Ward WS. National trends in the epidemiology of prostate cancer, 1973 to 1994: Evidence for the effectiveness of prostate-specific antigen screening. *Urology.* 1998; 52(3):444–8; discussion 8-9.

120. US Preventive Services Task Force. 2017. Available at https://www.uspreventiveservicestaskforce.org/uspstf/recommendation/prostate-cancer-screening.

121. Thompson IM, Goodman PJ, Tangen CM, et al. The influence of finasteride on the development of prostate cancer. *N Engl J Med.* 2003;349(3):215–24.

122. National Cancer Institute. Bethesda M. SEER (Statistics, Epidemiology and End Results) Cancer Stat Facts: SEER Cancer Stat Facts Cervix Uteri Cancer. http://seer.cancer.gov/statfacts/html/cervix.html.

123. National Cancer Institute. Bethesda MboNSds. SEER Cancer Statistics Review, 1975–2014 2017. Available at http://seer.cancer.gov/csr/1975_2014/.

124. Schiffman M, Castle PE, Jeronimo J, Rodriguez AC, Wacholder S. Human papillomavirus and cervical cancer. *Lancet.* 2007;370(9590):890–907.

125. Bosch FX, de Sanjose S. Chapter 1: Human papillomavirus and cervical cancer—Burden and assessment of causality. *J Natl Cancer Inst Monogr.* 2003;(31):3–13.

126. Markowitz LE, Liu G, Hariri S, Steinau M, Dunne EF, Unger ER. Prevalence of HPV after introduction of the vaccination program in the United States. *Pediatrics.* 2016;137(3):e20151968.

127. Basu P, Banerjee D, Singh P, Bhattacharya C, Biswas J. Efficacy and safety of human papillomavirus vaccine for primary prevention of cervical cancer: A review of evidence from phase III trials and national programs. *South Asian J Cancer.* 2013;2(4):187–92.

128. Force. USPST. Final Update Summary: Cervical Cancer September 2016. Available at https://www.uspreventiveservicestaskforce.org/uspstf/recommendation/cervical-cancer-screening.

129. Department of Health and Human Services CfDCaP, and National Cancer Institute. U.S. Cancer Statistics Working Group. United States Cancer Statistics: 1999–2014 Incidence and Mortality Web-based Report. Atlanta (GA): 2017. Available at http://www.cdc.gov/uscs.

130. Society. AC. Cancer Facts & Figures 2017 2017. Available at https://www.cancer.org/content/dam/cancer-org/research/cancer-facts-and-statistics/annual-cancer-facts-and-figures/2017/cancer-facts-and-figures-2017.pdf.

131. Al-Zalabani AH, Stewart KF, Wesselius A, Schols AM, Zeegers MP. Modifiable risk factors for the prevention of bladder cancer: A systematic review of meta-analyses. *Eur J Epidemiol.* 2016;31(9):811–51.

CHAPTER

55

Gastrointestinal and Liver Disorders

Adnan Said • Arnold Wald

INTRODUCTION

Gastrointestinal and liver diseases are a prevalent group of disorders, and include chronic and acute conditions that are infectious, metabolic, autoimmune, and result from a complex interplay of environmental and genetic influences. In this chapter, we discuss two of the most prevalent gastrointestinal and liver disorders that occur globally, nonalcoholic fatty liver disease (NAFLD) and irritable bowel syndrome (IBS).

NONALCOHOLIC FATTY LIVER DISEASE

Introduction and Definitions

Nonalcoholic fatty liver disease is a chronic liver disease characterized by fat infiltration in the liver (steatosis). It is closely related to obesity and the metabolic syndrome of diabetes, hyperlipidemia, and hypertension.[1] The liver injury can progress to varying degrees of severity over several years, varying from mild liver disease in most, to cirrhosis and liver cancer in a significant minority. By many estimates it is the most prevalent cause of chronic liver disease in the United States and worldwide.[2]

NAFLD comprises a spectrum of liver disease spanning from nonalcoholic fatty liver (NAFL) to nonalcoholic steatohepatitis (NASH) and cirrhosis (Fig. 55-1). NAFL signifies presence of isolated hepatic steatosis without evidence of liver cell (hepatocellular) injury and carries minimal-risk of progression to cirrhosis. NASH signifies steatosis with inflammation and hepatocyte injury and has a higher likelihood of progress to cirrhosis, liver failure, and liver cancer. Although NASH is clearly the more progressive form of the disease, emerging data suggest that NAFL may not be completely benign and itself can progress to NASH in around 25% of patients over a 2-year follow-up period.[3]

Epidemiology of NAFLD

Incidence of NAFLD

Although there are no true population-based incidence data for NAFLD in the United States, a study based on liver enzyme levels in veterans under the age of 45 has shown an increase in incidence from 2% to 4% between 2003 and 2011.[4] True population incidence of NAFLD (based on imaging studies) has been reported from Asia (China and Japan) and Israel with NAFLD incidence reported as 28/1000 person-years from Israel, 34 per/1000 person-years from China and 87 per 1000 person-year from Japan.[2] One of the few reported studies regarding incidence is a prospective, observational study from Japan. Using ALT levels and ultrasonography of the liver in patients without significant alcohol use, they found that at baseline, 812 of 4401 (18%) participants had NAFLD. During the mean follow-up period of 414 days (SD, 128), the authors observed 308 new cases (10%) of NAFLD among 3147 participants who were disease-free at baseline.[5]

NAFLD Prevalence

The determination of population prevalence of NAFLD has been challenging due to need for an invasive liver biopsy for definitive diagnosis. Using elevated liver enzymes as a surrogate for NAFLD (after excluding other liver diseases by serologic testing and history) is associated with poor sensitivity as well as poor specificity. As many as 30% of NAFLD patients may have normal liver enzymes even when advanced liver disease is present.

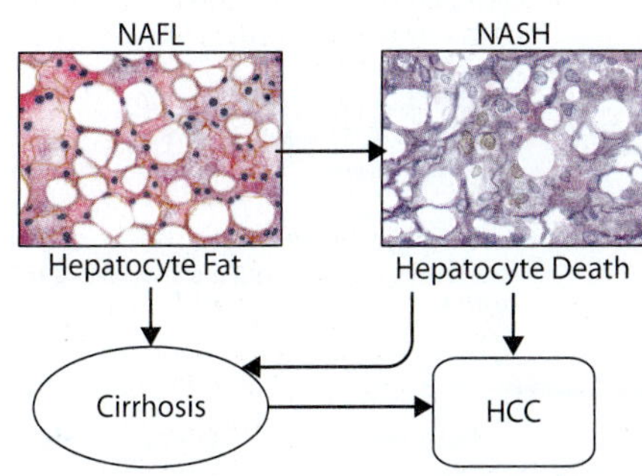

FIGURE 55-1. The histologic and clinical spectrum of nonalcoholic fatty liver disease (NAFLD).

Over the last two decades improvement in imaging technology and the ability to utilize these modalities in population-based studies has greatly improved the ability to detect liver steatosis and thereby glean a more accurate picture of NAFLD prevalence without the need for liver biopsy.[6]

In the United States Browning et al.[7] performed a population study of 2287 participants in the Dallas Heart Study (DHS) by evaluating for liver steatosis (fat) by proton nuclear magnetic resonance spectroscopy (H-MRS) and found 31% met their criteria for NAFLD. Of these patients, 79% were found to have a normal ALT level underlying the importance of imaging for more accurate diagnosis.

Although the prevalence of alcohol and infectious hepatitis has remained stable, the prevalence of NAFLD has been rising globally as well as in the U.S. adult and pediatric population, in parallel with the epidemic of obesity and metabolic syndrome. From 2000 to 2015, the worldwide prevalence of NAFLD increased from 20% to 27%.[2] A recent study using data from the U.S. National Health and Nutrition Examination Survey found that NAFLD prevalence doubled between the survey periods of 1988–94 and 2005–08 from 5.5% to 11%.[8]

The global prevalence of NAFLD is estimated at 25% according to a recent systematic review with the highest prevalence reported in South America (31%) and the Middle East (32%) followed by Asia (27%), the United States (24%), Europe (23%), and Africa (14%). The data for these prevalence studies with the largest number of patients comes from North America , Asia and Europe with lower numbers from the Middle East, Africa, and South America (Fig. 55-2).[2]

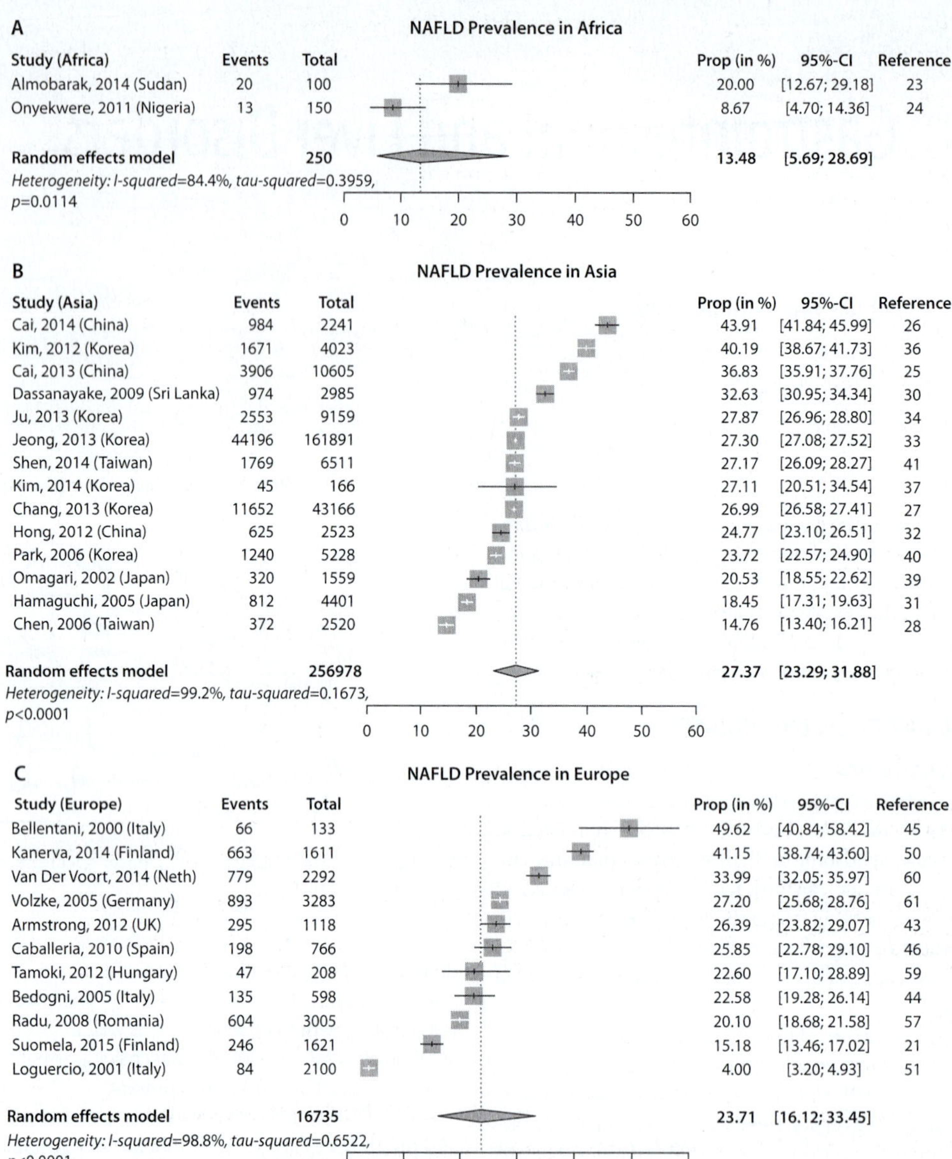

FIGURE 55-2. Global Prevalence of NAFLD. (*Source:* Used with permission from Younossi ZM, Koenig AB, Abdelatif D, Fazel Y, Henry L, Wymer M. Global epidemiology of nonalcoholic fatty liver disease-meta-analytic assessment of prevalence, incidence, and outcomes. *Hepatology.* 2016;64(1):73–84.[2])

Ethnic variation has been demonstrated with the Hispanic population being at the highest risk of fatty liver disease and blacks being at the lowest risk when compared to non-Hispanic whites. Asians also appear to be at decreased risk. Browning et al.[7] found the prevalence of NAFLD was highest in Hispanic Americans (45%), followed by non-Hispanic Whites (33%) and African-Americans (24%) a difference in prevalence by race and ethnicity that has been confirmed by other studies as well.[9] A major contribution to this racial/ethnic difference can be explained by genetic variation, particularly a single nucleotide polymorphism (SNP) in a gene (PNPLA3) that is involved in triglyceride (lipid) hydrolysis in the liver and the ethnic prevalence of which mirrors the ethnic differences in frequency of NAFLD.[10] These racial and ethnic differences are influenced by cultural susceptibility in diet and lifestyle patterns but persist independent of body mass index (BMI), demographic, and metabolic factors.[11,12]

NAFLD prevalence also increases with age, with a peak incidence reported in the sixth decade of life. The range of prevalence however is fairly narrow increasing from 22% to 30% between ages 30 and 70. Very few studies report on NAFLD prevalence after age 70.

Pediatric NAFLD is increasingly identified as a healthcare problem on the rise paralleling childhood obesity trends although population data are sparse. An autopsy study of 742 children (ages 2–19) who died of unnatural causes used liver histology (biopsy) as the gold standard and demonstrated a NAFLD prevalence of 9.6% adjusted for age, sex, race, and ethnicity. There was a pronounced age-related increase of liver fat (steatosis) ranging from 0.7% for ages 2–4 up to 17.3% for ages 15–19 years.[13] In children with obesity, the prevalence of NAFLD was 38%. In a meta-analysis of pediatric NAFLD, the general pediatric population prevalence has been reported at 7.6%.[14]

Differences in sex prevalence of NAFLD also exist. Earlier reports of persons with NAFLD showed a female preponderance to the condition; however, more recent studies in Japanese, Italian, and U.S. populations have consistently found men to be at increased-risk.[11,15,16]

NASH Prevalence

True prevalence of NASH the progressive subset of NAFLD, is difficult to assess in the general population since the diagnosis of NASH still depends on a liver biopsy. The prevalence of NASH is estimated to be 3–5% in the United States with estimates varying from 1.5% to 6.5%.[17] It is higher in patients with NAFLD who have indications for liver biopsy such as symptoms or elevated liver enzymes; the prevalence of NASH in these NAFLD patients is around 60%. In studies

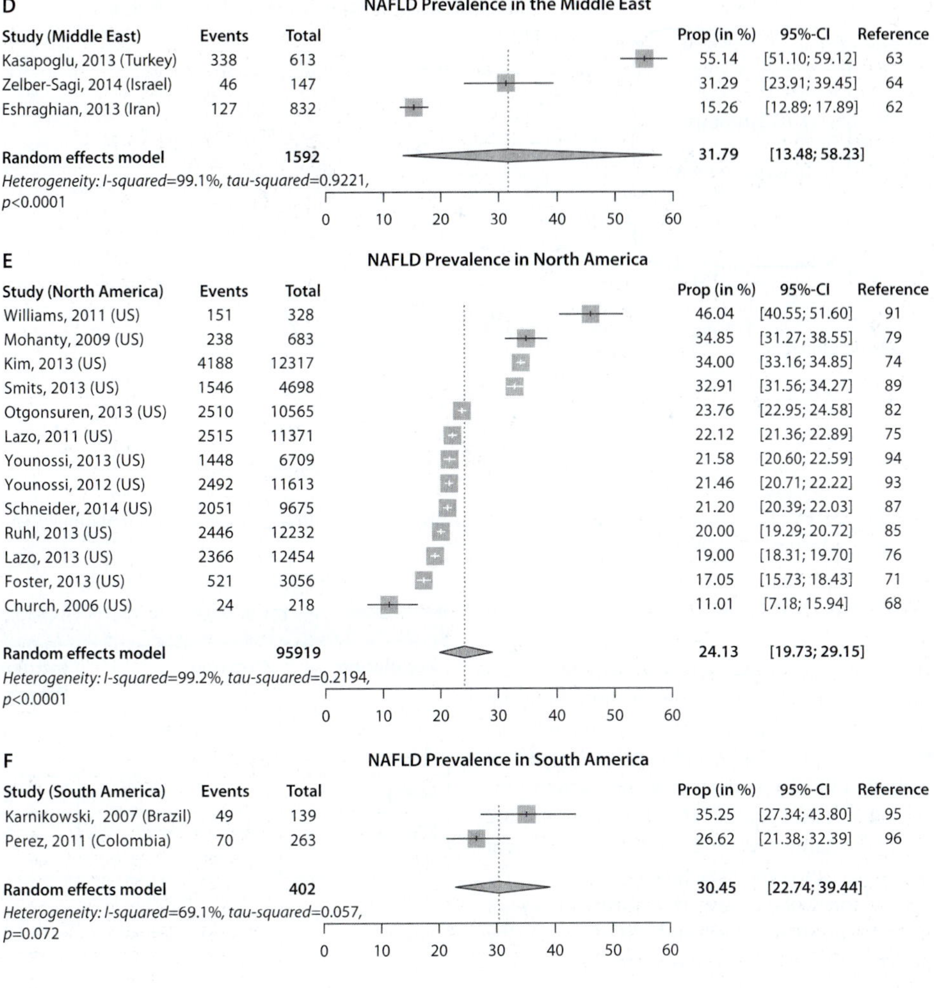

FIGURE 55-2. (Continued)

where biopsies were routinely done without a clinical indication the prevalence of NASH among NAFLD varied from 7% in Asia to 30% in North America.[2]

NASH is an increasingly common reason for decompensated cirrhosis and liver cancer. Over their lifetime 5–15% of patients with NAFLD progress to cirrhosis and currently, it is the second most common indication for liver transplantation in the United States after chronic hepatitis C and on track to becoming the most common by 2020.[18] In the U.S. general population, NAFLD is the most rapidly increasing reason for developing liver cancer.[19]

In higher-risk populations such as patients with diabetes, the prevalence of NAFLD is higher varying from 33% to 70%. In patients with morbid obesity, the prevalence of NAFLD exceeds 75% and has been reported as high as 95%.[2,20]

Causality and Risk Factors NAFLD

Pathophysiology NAFLD is a complex disease that has genetic predispositions and is affected by various environmental factors. NAFLD is regarded as the hepatic manifestation of the metabolic syndrome (presence of at least three of the following: abdominal obesity, hypertriglyceridemia, low high-density lipoprotein levels, hypertension, and high-fasting glucose levels). Obesity (defined as waist circumference > 102 cm in men or > 88 cm in women or simplified to BMI ≥ 30) and diabetes are two of the primary associated-risk factors for NAFLD.[1]

Underpinning the rising prevalence of these associated conditions and NAFLD are societal and individual trends in unhealthy eating habits (proliferation of high-caloric processed foods, and diets with a high content of sugar, corn syrup, and fat) and decreased physical activity levels. The industrialization of food production as well as deficiencies in neighborhood planning with poor walkability and public transport system availability are partly to blame for this epidemic.

Being overweight in childhood and adolescence, especially weight gain during school years, is a significant-risk factor for development of NAFLD by late childhood and adulthood.

Several genetic-risk factors have been reported, with nonsynonymous SNPs in two genes in particular, PNPLA3 (patatin-like phospholipase domain-containing protein 3) and TM6SF2 (transmembrane 6 superfamily member 2), being the most consistently validated. The prevalence of the PNPLA3 SNP is highest in the Hispanic population and leads to the higher prevalence of NAFLD in this population. I148M PNPLA3 genetic mutation has consistently been shown to be the most common genetic determinant of NAFLD.[10]

Alcohol intake and obesity have been shown to act synergistically in increasing the risk of liver disease development.[21] The effect of more moderate alcohol consumption on NAFLD is unclear currently and will require more study of cumulative lifetime alcohol consumption. There are population data suggesting that low levels of alcohol use (one or fewer drinks per day), wine in particular, may be associated with lower risk of developing NAFLD compared to those who drink more or not at all. Environmental factors such as acculturation, education level, healthcare use, and income might have a role in modifying background genetic predisposition though they have not been shown to be independent-risk factors.

NASH, which has a higher chance of progression to fibrosis and cirrhosis, is independently associated with factors including Diabetes, age, BMI, as well as with genetic polymorphisms in PNPLA3.

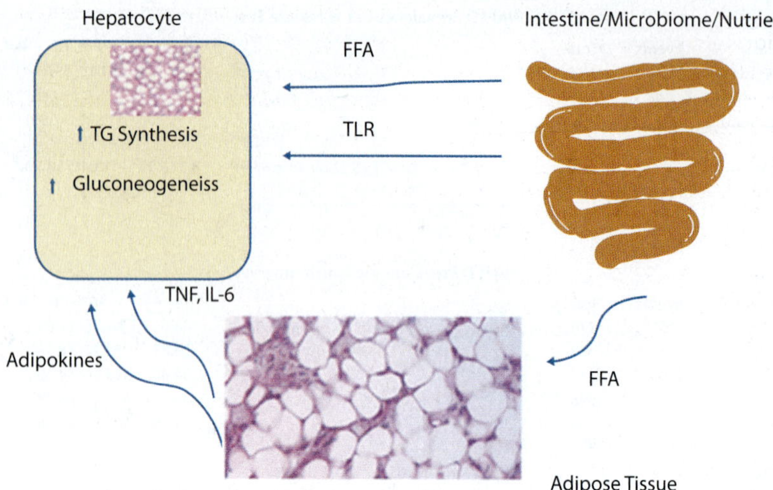

FIGURE 55-3. Pathophysiology of NAFLD. An interaction between intestine, adipose tissue, and hepatocytes. (Abbreviations: FFA = free fatty acids; IL = interleukin; TNF = tumor necrosis factor; TLR = Toll-like receptor.)

At a pathophysiologic level, NAFLD is associated with insulin resistance and oxidative stress.[22] The hallmark finding of NAFLD is accumulation of triglyceride (TG) in the cytoplasm of hepatocytes (Fig. 55-3). This is caused by an imbalance between lipid build up [fatty acid uptake and de novo lipogenesis (DNL)] and removal [mitochondrial fatty acid oxidation (FAO) and export as a part of very low-density lipoprotein (VLDL) particles]. Further factors contributing to transition from a healthy liver to NAFLD include adipose tissue dysfunction, hepatic insulin resistance, dysbiosis of the gut microbiome, toxic metabolites, and genetic factors.

The pathophysiology of nonalcoholic fatty liver disease involves a complex interplay of interactions between visceral adipose tissue, the liver, and the intestine. The role of gut microbiota and the influence that diet plays in modulating this microbiome also sends signals to the liver that influence lipid and carbohydrate metabolism as well as fat information.[23]

Clinical Significance and Outcomes in NAFLD

NAFLD patients are typically asymptomatic until the condition progresses to cirrhosis. It is often found incidentally on abdominal imaging including ultrasound, CT, or MRI (hepatic steatosis). An enlarged liver (hepatomegaly) may be the presenting symptom is some patients. Vague right upper abdominal discomfort, malaise, and/or fatigue can occur in patients with NASH but is very nonspecific.

Blood chemistry can show mild to moderate elevations in aspartate aminotransferase (AST) and alanine aminotransferase (ALT); however, even advanced NAFLD can present with normal liver enzyme levels in up to 30% of individuals with NAFLD.

Impact on Population Health

Patients who are older and have type 2 diabetes are at higher-risk for NASH and cirrhosis. In patients with NASH the risk of developing cirrhosis has been estimated to be around 20% over 10 years and end stage liver 8% over that time period [24]

In a global epidemiology study, in patients with NASH the incidence of hepatocellular carcinoma was 0.44 per 1000 person-years. Liver specific and overall mortality was 0.77 per 1000 person-years and 11.77 per 1000 person-years in NAFLD, but in NASH was higher at 15.44 per 1000 (liver specific) and 25.6 per 1000 person-years (overall mortality). The adjusted hazard ratio for NAFLD liver-related mortality was 2.6 (0.9–7.4) for overall mortality, it was 1.04 (1.03–1.04).[2]

In patients with diabetes, a community-based study has shown increased-risk of mortality associated with the diagnosis of NAFLD. In the Rochester epidemiology project 116 of 337 diabetic subjects were diagnosed with NAFLD. Overall 29% of patients died and independent predictors of mortality was presence of NAFLD (HR 2.2, 95% CI 1.1–4.2), presence of heart disease and duration of diabetes.[25]

TABLE 55-1 CAUSES OF MORTALITY IN NAFLD

Population	Outcome	Incidence Rate Per 1000 Person-Years (95% CI)
NAFLD	CVD-specific mortality	4.79 (3.43–6.7)
NAFLD	HCC	0.44 (0.29–0.66)
NAFLD	Liver-specific mortality	0.77 (0.33–1.77)
NAFLD	Overall mortality	15.44 (11.73–20.34)
NASH	Advanced fibrosis	67.95 (46.84–98.56)
NASH	HCC	5.29 (0.75–37.56)
NASH	Liver-specific mortality	11.77 (7.1–19.53)
NASH	Overall mortality	25.56 (6.29–103.8)

Source: Adapted from Younossi ZM, Koenig AB, Abdelatif D, Fazel Y, Henry L, Wymer M. Global epidemiology of nonalcoholic fatty liver disease-meta-analytic assessment of prevalence, incidence, and outcomes. *Hepatology.* 2016;64(1):73–84.[2]

What do Patients with NAFLD Die from? (Table 55-1)[2]

In a community study of over 7 year of follow-up from Minnesota, NAFLD patients were shown to have excessive risk of mortality compared to population-based age and sex-matched controls (SMR 1.34, 1.003–1.76).[26] In population database studies (NHANES) between 1988 and 1994 NAFLD was associated with higher mortality due to cardiovascular disease, nonhepatic malignancy, and liver disease.[27]

Given the commonality of risk factors for NAFLD and cardiovascular disease, cardiac disease is the leading cause of mortality in these patients. However, the development of NAFLD is associated with increased cardiovascular mortality independent of associated metabolic conditions. A meta-analysis of observational studies also confirmed the increased risk of CVD in NAFLD (OR 1.64, 1.26–2.13) and in NASH as well (OR 2.58, 1.78–3.75).[28]

Obesity, diabetes, and metabolic syndrome are also risk factors for carcinogenesis and a multitude of cancers are increased in patients with NAFLD including liver cancer, breast cancer, kidney cancer, and colon cancer among others. Liver disease mortality from cirrhosis and liver cancer is then the third most common-risk of mortality in NAFLD.[26]

Patients with diabetes, older age, and cirrhosis have the highest mortality rates in NAFLD. As opposed to isolated steatosis (NAFL), patients with NASH have higher risk of progressing to cirrhosis and therefore subsequent complications of cirrhosis including variceal hemorrhage, ascites, encephalopathy, and liver failure. In a study with NASH-related cirrhosis, liver cancer occurred at a cumulative incidence of 2.4% over a 3 year and 12.8% over a 7-year follow-up. [29]

Hepatocellular carcinoma in NASH like in most other chronic liver diseases occurs predominantly in the setting of cirrhosis. NAFLD associated hepatocellular carcinoma is the third most common cause of hepatocellular carcinoma in the United States. Given the high burden of NAFLD and NASH, the number of patients with NAFLD- and NASH-related hepatocellular carcinoma will continue to increase and the incidence of NAFLD associated hepatocellular carcinoma is increasing the fastest at 9% annual incidence rate increase.[19]

Direct Healthcare Costs and Quality of Life

There is paucity of robust economic data for patients with NAFLD. The data that is present indicate increasing healthcare resource utilization and costs associated with NAFLD. Furthermore, the data suggest that the costs of NAFLD may be mostly mediated through the presence of metabolic conditions but the impact of NAFLD on liver-related outcomes is expected to grow. The presence of advanced liver disease leads to increased morbidity and mortality as well as increased healthcare costs both in the outpatient and hospital setting.[30]

Health-Related Quality of Life (HR-QOL) was assessed in adults with NAFLD who were enrolled in the Nonalcoholic Steatohepatitis Clinical Research Network (NASH-CRN) multicenter study. SF-36 was used as the HR-QOL measurement tool, and the scores were compared with the U.S. population normative scores (norm score = 50). There were a total of 713 subjects with NAFLD with over 62% of the patients being female (male = 269, female = 444). The mean age of subjects was young at 48.3 years. Over 60% of the patients had definite NASH, with 28% having bridging fibrosis or cirrhosis. Almost 30% of the patients had diabetes. Results indicated that the patients with NAFLD had worse physical component scores (PCS, mean = 45.2) and mental component scores (MCS, mean = 47.6) when compared with the U.S. population norm score or with patients without any chronic illnesses (PCS = 55.8 and MCS = 52.5). Furthermore, patients who had progressed to NASH reported lower PCS scores compared with patients with only NAFLD (44.5 vs. 47.1, $p = 0.02$; respectively). Subjects with cirrhosis had significantly lower PCS results compared with all others (38.4 vs. no cirrhosis 47.6). MCS did not differ between patients whether they had NASH or by degree of fibrosis when compared with the general population.[31]

Diagnosis of NAFLD

Patients with unsuspected hepatic steatosis detected on imaging (Ultrasound or CT) or who have abnormal liver chemistries should be worked up for NAFLD. These patients should be assessed for metabolic-risk factors (obesity, diabetes mellitus, or dyslipidemia).[32]

NAFLD is confirmed by the presence of hepatic steatosis (fat) on imaging or liver biopsy in the absence of alternative explanations for the steatosis. Studies that have diagnosed NAFLD-based on elevated liver enzymes without confirmation of steatosis on imaging or biopsy are fraught with inaccuracies. Not only are elevation of liver enzymes nonspecific but they are also frequently normal in patients with NAFLD including those with advanced liver disease.

Although associated with obesity, NAFLD is a diagnosis of exclusion as there are other causes of fat infiltration in the liver, prevalent among them alcohol excess, chronic hepatitis C infection and medications that can cause fat deposition in the liver. These conditions are easily screened for by history and serologies. Alcohol excess that can cause liver disease is typically defined as greater than 21 standard drink of alcohol per week in men and greater than 14 drinks per week in women.[33]

Routine screening for NAFLD in high-risk groups attending primary care, diabetes, or obesity clinics is not advised at this time, but there should be a high-index of suspicion for NAFLD and NASH in patients with type 2 diabetes. This is primarily due to gaps in our knowledge regarding the natural history of NAFLD and treatment outcomes in NAFLD discovered by screening.

It is essential to emphasize that a diagnosis of NAFLD includes the determination of whether progressive liver disease, NASH, and fibrosis, are present in order to tailor treatment and monitoring.

Liver Biopsy

Currently, the gold standard for establishing a diagnosis of NAFLD and staging fibrosis is liver biopsy. In NAFLD liver histology typically shows steatosis graded as mild (<33% of hepatocytes involved), moderate 33–66% or severe (>66% steatosis). Other findings seen in NASH include lobular inflammation and hepatocyte ballooning indicative of hepatocyte injury as well as varying degrees of fibrosis from none (stage 0) to cirrhosis (stage 4 fibrosis).[32]

Liver biopsy has inherent limitations because of sampling error, intraobserver and interobserver variability. It is costly and also carries risks including a mortality risk of up to 0.14% following the procedure, pain, intraperitoneal bleeding, and infection. As a result, it is not practical for screening millions of at-risk individuals and for repeated assessments.

Noninvasive Testing in NAFLD

Noninvasive approaches to diagnosis of NAFLD are used widely and include imaging of the liver, liver stiffness testing, and biological marker testing.[6]

Hepatic Steatosis

Abnormal hepatic steatosis is defined by a liver fat content of $\geq$ 5%. MRI-based techniques (MRI PDFF or MR Spectroscopy), provide an accurate estimate of liver fat content. They are however expensive, time consuming and not widely accessible. Conventional ultrasonography remains the most commonly used imaging modality to diagnose hepatic steatosis. It is wide availability and low in cost, but has limited accuracy compared with MRI, especially in obese individuals.

Transient elastography-based techniques are increasingly utilized to diagnose steatosis and estimate the degree of hepatic fibrosis. Fat and fibrosis affects shear wave propagation through tissue and this property can be used to measure liver attenuation (steatosis) and velocity (fibrosis) utilizing a Fibroscan machine. This machine uses an ultrasonic probe placed over the skin in the right upper quadrant to produce shear waves of 50 MHz that pass through the liver. Measurements of shear wave attenuation called Controlled Attenuation Parameter (CAP) assess for presence and grade of hepatic steatosis. CAP has been shown to be less accurate that MRI-PDFF in diagnosing steatosis, but is cheaper and a point of care quantitative modality.[6]

Currently there are many widely available serum-based diagnostic panels for NAFLD that utilize a mix of serum tests and other demographic, anthropometric measures that are combined in validated single measurements for diagnosis of NAFLD. Examples include Fatty Liver Index (triglycerides, BMI, GGT, waist circumference) and NAFLD Liver Fat Score (Metabolic syndrome, type 2 diabetes mellitus, fasting insulin, ALT, AST). These panels have been found to have sensitivities and specificities in the 70% range and show reasonable accuracy for predicting steatosis.

Assessing NASH and Fibrosis

There are no clinical signs or symptoms that differentiate steatosis from NASH. Various diagnostic panels for predicting nonalcoholic steatohepatitis include NASH test and Apoptosis panel (CK18 fragments, soluble Fas, and Fas ligand).[6] None of these biomarkers has found clinical utility thus far in distinguishing NASH from isolated steatosis

Assessing Fibrosis

Fibrosis is a sign of the stage of liver disease. Fibrosis stage 4 (F4) is categorized as cirrhosis and F0-F1 is considered none-minimal fibrosis. Clinical decision aids such as NAFLD fibrosis score[34] (biomarkers evaluated: age, glucose level, BMI, platelet count, albumin, and AST/ALT ratio) or fibrosis-4 index (FIB-4- biomarkers measured include age, AST/platelet count, ALT) utilize a combination of serum and clinical variables to predict the presence of advanced fibrosis or cirrhosis.[35,36] These tests are most useful in distinguishing patients who may have cirrhosis from those without fibrosis and thus may aid in clinical decision making including whether to perform a liver biopsy or make a referral to a liver specialist (in patients with test indicating advanced fibrosis).

Imaging-based techniques such as vibration controlled transient elastography (Fibroscan) or MRI-based elastography can be used to identify those at low or high-risk for advanced fibrosis (bridging fibrosis or cirrhosis) with more accuracy than serum markers. The drawbacks to these methods include cost and availability (MRE) and limited utility in obesity, and acute inflammation (Fibroscan).[37]

Treatment and Prevention of NAFLD

Treatment of NAFLD entails treatment of the liver disease as well as of the associated metabolic syndrome (obesity, diabetes, hyperlipidemia, and hypertension).

Lifestyle Modifications in NAFLD

Lifestyle modifications are integral in the treatment of NAFLD at any stage and are the principal intervention for patients with isolated steatosis and NASH without fibrosis. Patients are advised to lose $\geq$ 7% of body weight if overweight or obese (3–5% weight loss will improve steatosis, 7–10% is needed to improve histopathological features of NASH and fibrosis).[23]

This weight loss is best achieved gradually (losing no more than 1–2 lbs. per week) and sustained through a combination of diet and exercise. Basic principles of diet include reducing calories (by at least 30% or by 750–1000 kcal/day for an average U.S. adult) and reducing consumption of simple carbohydrates and saturated fat. Reduction of sugar-sweetened beverages and of fructose-enriched food and drinks is recommended. In general, using fresh fruits and vegetable and lean meats and minimizing processed foods is recommended.

Although many different diets have been studied and shown to be beneficial (e.g., Mediterranean diet), studies have also shown that any diet that follows the basic principle noted above and results in weight loss achieves the benefits of reversing NASH.[38]

Significant alcohol use can exacerbate steatohepatitis and limiting consumption of alcohol ($\leq$ 1 drink/day for women and $\leq$ 2 drinks/day for men) is recommended. A preponderance of epidemiologic data also shows that consumption of coffee (two or more cups) per day is associated with reduced prevalence of NAFLD. If coffee is consumed, it should be caffeinated and addition of sweetened syrups, sugar and large servings of milk/other calories may negate any beneficial effects.[23]

Recommendations for physical activity include at least 150–200 minutes of moderate to vigorous intensity physical activity per week (examples are moderate jogging, weight training, and sports such as tennis, swimming, or biking). For patients that do not exercise a gradual build up to this level is recommended. Limited data suggest that the combination of diet and exercise may be more beneficial than either in isolation.[33]

Fatigue-related to chronic liver disease impacts physical functioning in patients with NAFLD. The impact of NASH treatment on HR-QOL has not been fully described. In a study from Australia, researchers studied a group of 35 patients with CLD and the impact of a 3-month diet and exercise program on clinical outcomes and HR-QOL (SF-36). The study did show moderate clinical improvement. In the group of patients who lost weight, PCS and MCS scores after the initial 3-month intervention significantly increased (p = 0.0001 and p = 0.004, respectively) with the majority of the health domains comparable to the population norms. In patients who had maintained their weight loss at 15 months, both the PCS and MCS remained significantly higher than their baseline scores (p = 0.005 and p = 0.003, respectively), while for the patients who regained weight, their PCS and MCS scores decreased and were no different than at baseline.[39]

Pharmacotherapeutics in NAFLD

Currently there are no pharmacologic agents that have an FDA indication specifically for NAFLD or NASH. There are however pharmacological treatments aimed at different components of metabolic syndrome that can be used off label for NAFLD-related liver disease-based on controlled trials studies and published guidelines. These agents when used for NAFLD should generally be limited to those with biopsy-proven NASH and fibrosis.

Pioglitazone is an insulin-sensitizing agent used in diabetes (PPAR Gamma agonist) and can be used to treat patients with and without type 2 diabetes with biopsy-proven NASH. It has been shown to improve histologic changes in NASH including steatosis, ballooning, and inflammation but not fibrosis.

For nondiabetic adults with biopsy-proven NASH, *Vitamin E* administered at a daily dose of 800 IU/day can be used as well and can cause similar histologic improvements as Pioglitazone.

It must be noted that trials of these agents in NASH were generally limited to 24 months or less and longer-term benefits are not known. Consideration to side effects must also be given; pioglitazone can cause weight gain. Vitamin E has some concerns regarding increase all-cause mortality, and in a large trial increased-risk of prostate cancer.[40]

Patients with NAFLD are at high-risk for cardiovascular morbidity and mortality and aggressive modification of CVD risk factors should be considered in all NAFLD patients. Statins can be used to treat dyslipidemia in patients with NAFLD, NASH, and NASH cirrhosis, but should be avoided in patients with decompensated cirrhosis.[41,42] Metformin can be used for diabetes including in patients with NAFLD; however, it has no beneficial effects specifically on NASH.

There are numerous pharmacologic agents in phase 1 and phase 2 trials and a few in phase 3 trials for NAFLD. Some of these agents work on glucose or lipid metabolism in the liver whereas other are antifibrotic or antioxidant. [43]

Foregut bariatric surgery can be considered in otherwise eligible obese individuals with NAFLD or NASH, though it is not an established option to specifically treat NASH. Case series have shown improvement in histologic markers of NASH in patients after bariatric surgery.[41]

Prevention

Preventative efforts, just as the first line treatment, are focused on reducing obesity and the metabolic syndrome. Prevention of NAFLD is imperative and is a societal challenge that includes changes in nutrition, neighborhood planning, and health education starting an early age, ideally in school-age children.

IRRITABLE BOWEL SYNDROME

Introduction and Definitions

IBS is a chronic functional disorder of the gastrointestinal tract characterized by chronic abdominal pain and altered bowel habits in the absence of an organic disease. In the absence of a biologic disease marker, the diagnosis has traditionally been based on a cluster of symptoms. The earliest was the so-called "Manning criteria,"[44] which was based most stringently on the presence of three or more characteristic symptoms (Box 55-1). Subsequently, there have been various iterations of IBS criteria created by the Rome study groups,[45] which are currently used for research purposes (Box 55-2). When evaluating the relevant literature for IBS, it is important to note that various studies have used different criteria, which may result in variable data concerning prevalence, incidence, and cost considerations.

From a clinical standpoint, subtypes of IBS have been defined as follows:

- IBS with constipation (IBS-C): Patient reports that abnormal bowel movements are usually constipation (types 1 and 2 in the Bristol Stool Form Scale; BSFS).
- IBS with diarrhea (IBS-D): Patient reports that abnormal bowel movements are usually diarrhea (types 6 and 7 in the BSFS).

BOX 55-1 Manning Criteria for IBS

- Looser stools with onset of pain
- More frequent bowel movements at onset of pain
- Visible distension
- Feeling of distension
- Mucus per rectum
- Feeling of incomplete emptying (often)

Strict criteria > 3 of above
Less strict criteria > 2 of above

Source: Adapted from Manning AP, Thompson WG, Heaton KW, Morris AF. Towards positive diagnosis of the irritable bowel. *Br Med J.* 1978;2(6138):653–4.[44]

BOX 55-2 Rome III Criteria[1] for IBS

Recurrent abdominal pain or discomfort at least 3 days per month in the last 3 months associated with two or more of the following:

1. Improvement with defecation
2. Onset associated with change in stool frequency
3. Onset associated with change in form of stool

Source: Adapted from Longstreth GF et al. Functional bowel disorders. In: *Rome III: The Functional Gastrointestinal Disorders.* 3rd ed. McLean VA: Degnan Assoc Inc.; 2006.[45]

[1] Criterion fulfilled for the last 3 months with onset of symptoms at least 6 months prior to diagnosis

- Mixed IBS (IBS-M): Patient reports that abnormal bowel movements are usually both constipation and diarrhea (more than one-fourth of all the abnormal bowel movements are constipation and more than one-fourth are diarrhea) over at least a 3-month period of time.
- Unclassified IBS (IBS-U): Patients who meet diagnostic criteria for IBS but cannot be accurately categorized into one of the other three subtypes.[46]

This review will discuss the epidemiology, pathophysiology, impact on population health and the treatment of this common disorder. As IBS is not associated with increased mortality, the emphasis of this review will be on morbidity and the associated economic impact of IBS in the adult population.

Epidemiology

Prevalence of IBS

There have been numerous cross-sectional surveys conducted that have reported the prevalence of IBS in the community. The majority of these studies have used accepted diagnostic criteria, and some have used more than one definition within the same population.[47] In one meta-analysis, 23 studies used the Manning criteria, 24 used Rome I criteria, 36 used Rome II criteria, and 5 used Rome III criteria. Twelve studies used a symptom questionnaire to define IBS and in five of these, there had been validation before using them. Prevalence was noted to be higher when three or more of the Manning criteria were used (14%, CI 95%: 10.0–17.0%) and lowest when Rome I criteria were used (8.8%, 95% CI: 6.8–11.2%). The prevalence of IBS according to country is shown in Fig. 55-4.[47] The disparity in prevalence of IBS by country was not solely related to the diagnostic criteria employed.

The majority of studies did not report the predominant stool pattern in IBS. Of the 14 that recorded only three IBS subtypes, 35% were IBS-C, 40% were IBS-D, and 23% were IBS-M. Of the nine that included IBS-U subtypes as well, there was a more even distribution, ranging from 22 to 24% mean prevalence for each of the four subgroups. In general, the pooled prevalence was higher in women than in men (14%; range 11–16% vs. 9%; range 7.3–10.5%) with significant heterogeneity between studies. There appeared to be no relationship between socioeconomic status in the four studies, which reported it and no strong influence of age as well.

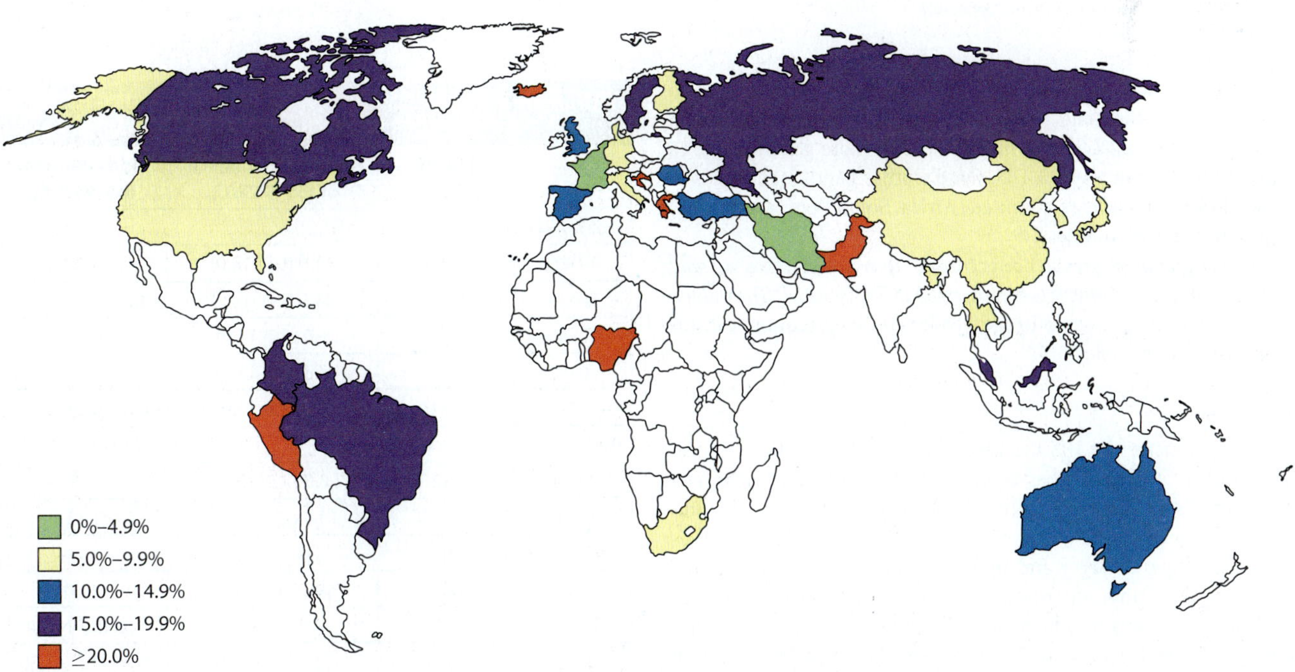

FIGURE 55-4. Prevalence of IBS according to country. (*Source:* Used with permission from Lovell RM, Ford AC. Global prevalence of and risk factors for irritable bowel syndrome: A meta-analysis. *Clin Gastroenterol Hepatol.* 2012;10(7):712–21 e714.[47])

TABLE 55-2 PREVALENCE OF IBS ACCORDING TO MANNING, ROME I, AND ROME II CRITERIA BY COUNTRY

Country	Manning Criteria (%)	95% CI	Rome I Criteria (%)	95% CI	Rome II Criteria (%)	95% CI
United States	16.0	14.0–18.0	9.0	6.0–12.0	7.0	6.0–7.0
Canada	No studies	N/A[a]	13.0	12.0–16.0	18.0	7.0–33.0
United Kingdom	19.0	15.0–24.0	10.0	8.0–11.0	10.0	7.0–14.0
Sweden	19.0	13.0–26.0	14.0	8.0–20.0	13.0	9.0–18.0
Holland	6.0	4.0–9.0	No studies	N/A[a]	No studies	N/A[a]
France	2.0	2.0–3.0	3.0	1.0–5.0	2.6	0.3–7.2
Finland	10.0	9–11.0	6.0	5.0–6.0	5.0	4.0–6.0
Iceland	31.0	28.0–33.0	No studies	N/A[a]	No studies	N/A[a]
Russia	No studies	N/A[a]	19.0	17.0–22.0	No studies	N/A[a]
Germany	No studies	N/A[a]	6.0	0.2–18.9	12.0	10.0–14.0
Spain	No studies	N/A[a]	14.0	10.0–18.0	No studies	N/A[a]
Italy	No studies	N/A[a]	7.0	6.0–9.0	7.0	6.0–8.0
Romania	No studies	N/A[a]	14.0	11.0–19.0	No studies	N/A[a]
Croatia	No studies	N/A[a]	18.0	24.0–32.0	No studies	N/A[a]
Turkey	No studies	N/A[a]	No studies	N/A[a]	11.0	6.0–16.0
Iran	No studies	N/A[a]	No studies	N/A[a]	9.0	6.0–13.0
Nigeria	No studies	N/A[a]	No studies	N/A[a]	32.0	27.0–36.0
Bangladesh	No studies	N/A[a]	8.0	7.0–10.0	8.0	6.0–9.0
Pakistan	No studies	N/A[a]	No studies	N/A[a]	28.0	4.0–62.0
Singapore	5.0	0.9–12.3	10.0	9.0–12.0	9.0	7.0–10.0
South Korea	15.0	12.0–19.0	9.0	6.0–12.0	6.0	2.0–11.0
China	10.0	8.0–13.0	2.4	0.3–6.3	5.0	4.0–6.0
Japan	No studies	N/A[a]	No studies	N/A[a]	6.0	5.0–7.0
Malaysia	No studies	N/A[a]	No studies	N/A[a]	16.0	13.0–18.0
Peru	24.0	21.0–28.0	No studies	N/A[a]	No studies	N/A[a]
Brazil	No studies	N/A[a]	No studies	N/A[a]	17.0	12.0–33.0
Australia	14.0	13.0–15.0	8.0	2.0–17.0	7.0	6.0–8.0
Israel	No studies	N/A[a]	No studies	N/A[a]	3.0	2.0–4.0

Source: Used with permission from Lovell RM, Ford AC. Global prevalence of and risk factors for irritable bowel syndrome: A meta-analysis. *Clin Gastroenterol Hepatol.* 2012;10(7):712–21 e714.[47] Note: N/A, not applicable.
[a]No studies.

It is important to note that the meta-analysis was restricted to those based on the general population and excluded those based on convenience samples. This makes the data more generalizable to community individuals with IBS. On the other hand, many areas of the world were sparsely represented (Africa, South Asia, Australasia) or absent (Central America).

The geographical prevalence according to Manning, Rome I and Rome II criteria by country is summarized in Table 55-2.[47] The pooled prevalence of IBS according to age, gender and socioeconomic status is summarized in Table 55-3.[47]

TABLE 55-3 POOLED PEVALENCE OF IBS ACCORDING TO AGE, GENDER, AND SOCIOECONOMIC STATUS

	No. of Subjects	Pooled Prevalence of IBS (95% CI)	Odds Ratio for IBS (95% CI)
Age band (*y*)			
<30	6909	11.0 (6.0–18.0)	1.00
30–39	7247	11.0 (7.0–16.0)	1.04 (0.85–1.87)
40–49	7543	9.6 (6.0–14.0)	0.86 (0.59–1.24)
50–59	5434	7.8 (5.0–11.1)	0.68 (0.40–1.17)
≥60	5540	7.3 (4.3–11.0)	0.63 (0.38–1.04)
Gender			
Male	78,913	8.9 (7.3–10.5)	1.00
Female	83,330	14.0 (11.0–16.0)	1.67 (1.53–1.82)
Socioeconomic status			
High	866	14.0 (9.0–19.0)	1.00
Medium	1732	14.0 (8.0–22.0)	1.02 (0.72–1.44)
Low	2663	13.0 (7.0–22.0)	0.99 (0.71–1.36)

Source: Used with permission from Lovell RM, Ford AC. Global prevalence of and risk factors for irritable bowel syndrome: A meta-analysis. *Clin Gastroenterol Hepatol.* 2012;10(7):712–21 e714.[47]

Incidence

The natural history of IBS has been studied on a number of occasions and its prevalence has been reported to remain stable over short periods of time[48–50] with resolution of symptoms in some individuals matched by the onset of new symptoms in others over 1–2-year follow-ups. A larger and more extended study of the natural history of IBS symptoms was carried out in Northern England by Ford and associates in adults aged 50–59 years at the time of follow-up.[51] Subjects were chosen for dyspepsia but not for symptoms of IBS. Information was extracted from primary care records and 3873 (46%) of the original sample completed IBS symptom data at both baseline and follow-up. Of this group, 214 (5.5%) had IBS at baseline compared to 686 (18%) at the 10-year follow up. Of the 3659 individuals without IBS at baseline, 15% developed new onset of symptoms meeting IBS criteria at 10 years, giving a linear incidence of 1.5% per year using Manning criteria. Using multivariate logistic regression, lower quality of life at baseline, dyspepsia at baseline, and female gender were significantly associated with new onset IBS.

Among the individuals with IBS at baseline, 67% had persistent IBS at the 10-year follow-up. Of the patients who had IBS symptoms at any time in the study, 17% had consulted a primary-care physician for symptoms of IBS on one or more occasions and 4% had consulted in the last year of follow-up. The median number of consultations during the 10-year follow-up was one (range 1–14). Using multivariate logistic regression, H pylori infection and any dyspepsia-related consultation were significantly associated with IBS consultation whereas female gender and NSAID use were of borderline statistical significance. To summarize, in this study from the United Kingdom, poor quality of life at baseline was a strong predictor of new onset IBS but not of IBS-related consultation; the latter appeared to be more strongly related to consultation for other functional GI disorders.

Contemporaneous with the above study, a 12-year longitudinal population-based study from Olmstead County in the United States surveyed 1365 adults (90% Caucasian) for functional gastrointestinal symptoms.[52] Between the initial and final surveys, the point prevalences for IBS were stable (8.3% and 11.4%, respectively). Among persons with symptoms at baseline, 20% had similar symptoms, 40% had no symptoms, and 40% had different symptoms at follow-up. Thus, although the prevalence of functional GI symptoms was stable over time, the turnover of symptom status was high. Of interest, the new onset rate of IBS-D was higher than IBS-C and IBS-M (4.2% vs. 1.6%; 1.3%). As with the UK study, complete resolution of symptoms occurred in approximately 40% and the numbers of persons who reported new onset of symptoms exceeded those reporting the disappearance of symptoms.

A Biopsychosocial Model of Functional GI Disorders such as IBS

The ability to study causality in a disorder with no biological disease markers is fraught with difficulties. This is certainly the case with IBS as a representative of functional GI disorders. Many hypotheses have been advanced and found wanting. The current conceptual model is the biopsychosocial construct, as shown in Fig. 55-5.[46]

The figure indicates that predeterminants such as early life experiences together with psychosocial factors may interact with altered gut physiology via the brain-gut axis. This concept infers that these factors are bidirectional and mutually interactive and therefore, influence both the clinical presentation of the disorder and the clinical outcomes. Among the physiological processes that may lead to GI symptoms are abnormal gut motility, visceral hypersensitivity, immune dysregulation, inflammation and barrier dysfunction, the intestinal microbiome, diet, and the brain-gut axis. No one factor alone accounts for the symptoms of IBS and all must be considered in the management of affected patients. This becomes apparent when considering treatment approaches (see below).

Impact on Population Health

Although there is little or no mortality associated with IBS, symptoms are long lasting and there are no curative therapies available. As a chronic illness, the economic impact of this disorder is considerable. The economic costs may be broken down into (1) direct healthcare costs that are driven by symptoms, diagnostic testing, medical consultations, and treatments, and (2) effects on work productivity and daily activity impairment. In addition, to be factored in is the presence of comorbidities on this population and how these may influence healthcare and economic costs.

Indirect Costs and Impact

In a 2015 survey conducted by the American Gastroenterological Association, [53] IBS patients reported that their symptoms interfered with work productivity on an average of 9 days per month and missed work on average of 2 days per month. Indirect costs (i.e., loss of work and reduced productivity) have been estimated to be up to $20 billion dollars annually in the United States with an estimated annual cost per patient of $9933 (in 2012 US dollars). [54,55]

In a recent study of indirect costs of IBS, impairment experienced at work (presenteeism) accounted for approximately 75% of the total annual indirect costs for respondents with IBS, far in excess of absenteeism from work.[56] Compared to controls, IBS respondents missed significantly more work (5.1% vs. 2.9%), experienced higher levels of presenteeism (17.9% vs. 11.3%) and had greater overall work productivity loss (20.7% vs. 13.2%) and higher daily activity impairment.[56] These findings are consistent with an earlier systematic review of IBS in the United States, Canada, and the United Kingdom.[57]

Direct Healthcare Costs

Almost 30 years ago, it was estimated that up to 25% of all visits to gastroenterologists in the United States were for IBS with additional others for other functional GI disorders.[58] This accounted for 3.5

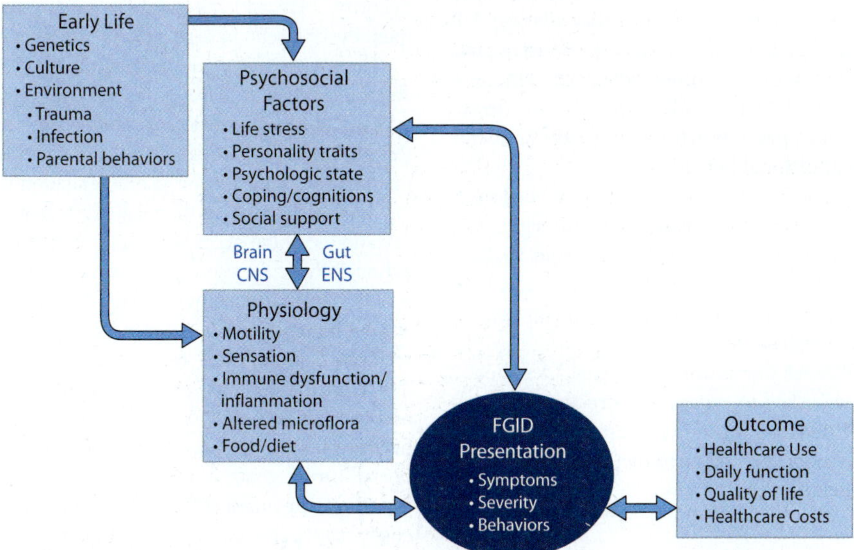

FIGURE 55-5. Biopsychosocial conceptual model. (*Source:* Used with permission from Drossman DA. Functional Gastrointestinal Disorders: History, Pathophysiology, Clinical Features and Rome IV. *Gastroenterology.* 2016.[46])

million visits to healthcare practitioners in 1991 and undoubtedly is much higher today. Earlier studies showed that IBS patients made twice as many health visits per year as did age matched controls and that 78% of the excess visits were for nongastrointestinal complaints.[59] A subsequent analysis of this phenomenon suggests that comorbidity in IBS may be a consequence of the psychological trait for somatization, defined as the tendency to amplify the intensity and overinterpret the significance of any somatic sensation.[60] This excess comorbidity is the primary determinant of excess healthcare costs associated with IBS although it does not apply to all patients with IBS. In addition, there are no comorbid disorders that are uniquely associated with IBS, thus decreasing the chances that they may be a consequence of shared pathophysiology.

Given the high-economic impact due to healthcare utilization among IBS patients, recent attempts to identify factors leading to high utilizers have been made. The investigators used the Andersen model as a conceptual framework for accessing healthcare services[61] which holds that a decision to use healthcare is related to (1) predisposition to use services; (2) ability to use services; and (3) need for services. The important conclusion was that the decisions to use healthcare are not simply influenced by symptom-specific factors but by a variety of lifestyle and (most importantly) economic factors such as health insurance coverage.[62]

Treatment of IBS

A validated standardized algorithm for the treatment of IBS does not exist. Treatment, therefore, depends upon the type and severity of symptoms and the nature of associated psychosocial issues in an individual patient. A strong guiding principle is that a robust patient-healthcare provider relationship is an important determinant of outcome and reduction of healthcare utilization. Treatments may generally be divided into dietary and lifestyle modifications, pharmacologic agents, and behavioral therapies, all of which have been validated by randomized and controlled studies.

Dietary Modifications

Although fiber supplements are widely recommended for IBS, a meta-analysis of seven high-quality studies failed to find significant benefit, although some benefits might occur with soluble (psyllium) vs. insoluble (bran) fiber in IBS-C. Unfortunately, fiber supplements may exacerbate symptoms such as abdominal bloating and discomfort.[63] Other dietary interventions such as gluten-free and low FODMAP (fermentable oligo-, di-, and monosaccharides, and polyols) diets have become increasingly popular. Several studies support the benefit of gluten-free diets in a subset of IBS patients in the absence of celiac disease.[64] It remains uncertain whether the clinical benefits are a consequence of gluten withdrawal, elimination of other wheat proteins and highly fermentable short-chain fatty acids or a placebo effect.[65] Adding a gluten-free diet to patients who are already on a low FODMAP diet offers no additional benefits.

There is accumulating evidence from prospective controlled studies that dietary FODMAP restriction is associated with significant symptom improvement in many patients with IBS (Table 55-4). It appears that restriction of both fructose and fructans is most beneficial. Significant symptom improvement was noted in IBS patients compared to a standard Australian diet.[66]

Response to a low FODMAP diet is usually assessed after about 2 weeks. Responders are then asked to engage in a structured reintroduction of restricted foods to allow the individual to tailor his or her diet. It is optimal to involve a properly trained dietician or nutritionist in the care of these patients.[67]

Pharmacologic Agents

Pharmacologic approaches to IBS may be divided into medications for IBS-C, patients with IBS-D, and for any patient with IBS in order to ameliorate abdominal pain (Table 55-5).

TABLE 55-4 LOW FODMAP DIET

Avoid or Reduce These Foods			
Fructose	**Lactose**	**Oligos**	**Polyols**
Fruits: Apple, mango, pear, watermelon, juice, dried fruit	Milk: milk from cows/goats/sheep, custard, ice cream, yogurt, eggnog	Vegetables: Beets, broccoli, brussels sprouts, cabbage, fennel, garlic, onion, chicory root	Fruits: Apricot, avocado, blackberry, cherry, nectarine, peach, plum, prune, fig
Other: Asparagus, honey, high fructose corn syrup, molasses	Cheese: Soft, un-ripened cheese	Other: Barley, beans, chickpeas, couscous, inulin, lentils, pistachios, rye, soy milk, wheat (pasta, bread), veggie burgers	Vegetables: Cauliflower, corn, mushroom, sweet potato Sweeteners: Ending in "ol" (e.g., xylitol, sorbitol), isomalt and sucralose (Splenda)

TABLE 55-5 PHARMACOLOGIC AGENTS FOR IBS

IBS-C	IBS-D	IBS-All
Linaclotide	Rifaximin	TCAs
[a]Plecanatide	Loperamide	Dicyclomine; oil of peppermint
Lubiprostone	Alosetron	
PEG-3350	[a]Eluxadoline	

[a]No guidelines have been issued in these recently released drugs.

Most drugs work through different pathophysiologic mechanisms. For example, for patients with IBS-C, Linaclotide, Plecanatide, and Lubiprostone increase intestinal chloride and water secretion to combat constipation whereas PEG does so through a hyperosmolar effect. For IBS-D, rifaximin is an antibiotic, loperamide is a μ-opioid agonist, alosetron works through the serotonin 3 receptor, and eluxadoline has effects on all three opioid receptors in the gut (mu, kappa, and delta). Tricyclic agents (TCAs) presumably work via central neurochemical changes and antispasmodics (dicyclomine, encapsulated oil of peppermint) work largely through peripheral anticholinergic pathways. The large and diverse number of drugs are indicative of the lack of fundamental understanding of IBS. Moreover, few drugs are effective in the majority of IBS patients and there is no more than a 10–15% improvement over placebo in most studies, which have been published.

The AGA guidelines incorporated the Grading of Recommendations Assessment, Development and Evaluation (GRADE) methodology and best practices as outlined by the Institute of Medicine.[68] Recommendations are either strong or conditional (weak). The evidence that provides the basis for recommendation is rated high, moderate, or low quality. Because of the relatively recent release of plecanatide and eluxadoline, these drugs were not incorporated into present guidelines although they have been approved for use in IBS by the FDA.

Of the pharmacologic agents for IBS-C, linaclotide received a strong recommendation with high-quality evidence, lubiprostone received a conditional recommendation on moderate-quality evidence, and PEG was given a conditional recommendation-based on weak evidence (27). The first two agents showed modest benefit over placebo whereas there is no data to support the use of PEG. For all three agents, adverse effects were relatively few and diarrhea is perhaps the major side effect. Both linaclotide and lubiprostone are costly (as are eluxadoline and plecanatide) and may involve high-out-of-pocket expenses for patients.

For IBS-D, both rifaximin and alosetron received conditional recommendations based on moderate quality evidence.[69] The latter is approved by the FDA only for women who have failed all other treatments. There is a very small risk (approximately 1 case/1000 patient years) for ischemic colitis. Although loperamide has very low-quality evidence to support its use, it can be very effective if used in a proactive fashion.

The case for TCAs and antispasmodics is based on low-quality evidence but both agents can be very effective for abdominal pain and, in the case of TCAs, for reducing diarrhea in IBS patients.[69]

Behavioral Therapy for IBS

For patients with unrelenting IBS symptoms, cognitive behavioral therapy and gut directed hypnosis have been found to be beneficial.[70] Such therapies should be performed by experienced and well-trained behavioral specialists who are an integral part of the medical team, which treats patients with functional GI disorders.

References

1. Moore JB. Non-alcoholic fatty liver disease: The hepatic consequence of obesity and the metabolic syndrome. *Proc Nutr Soc.* 2010;69(2):211–20.
2. Younossi ZM, Koenig AB, Abdelatif D, Fazel Y, Henry L, Wymer M. Global epidemiology of nonalcoholic fatty liver disease-Meta-analytic assessment of prevalence, incidence, and outcomes. *Hepatology.* 2016;64(1):73–84.
3. Wong VW, Wong GL, Choi PC, et al. Disease progression of non-alcoholic fatty liver disease: A prospective study with paired liver biopsies at 3 years. *Gut.* 2010;59(7):969–74.
4. Kanwal F, Kramer JR, Duan Z, Yu X, White D, El-Serag HB. Trends in the burden of nonalcoholic fatty liver disease in a United States cohort of veterans. *Clin Gastroenterol Hepatol.* 2016;14(2):301–8.e1–2.
5. Hamaguchi M, Kojima T, Takeda N, et al. The metabolic syndrome as a predictor of nonalcoholic fatty liver disease. *Ann Intern Med.* 2005;143(10): 722–8.
6. Younossi ZM, Loomba R, Anstee QM, et al. Diagnostic modalities for non-alcoholic fatty liver disease (NAFLD), non-alcoholic steatohepatitis (NASH) and associated fibrosis. *Hepatology.* 2018;68(1): 349-60.
7. Browning JD, Szczepaniak LS, Dobbins R, et al. Prevalence of hepatic steatosis in an urban population in the United States: Impact of ethnicity. *Hepatology.* 2004;40(6):1387–95.
8. Younossi ZM, Stepanova M, Afendy M, et al. Changes in the prevalence of the most common causes of chronic liver diseases in the United States from 1988 to 2008. *Clin Gastroenterol Hepatol.* 2011; 9(6):524–30 e521; quiz e560.
9. Rich NE, Oji S, Mufti AR, et al. Racial and ethnic disparities in nonalcoholic fatty liver disease prevalence, severity, and outcomes in the United States: A systematic review and meta-analysis. *Clin Gastroenterol Hepatol.* 2018;16(2):198–210 e192.
10. Romeo S, Kozlitina J, Xing C, et al. Genetic variation in PNPLA3 confers susceptibility to nonalcoholic fatty liver disease. *Nat Genet.* 2008;40(12): 1461–5.
11. Ruhl CE, Everhart JE. Determinants of the association of overweight with elevated serum alanine aminotransferase activity in the United States. *Gastroenterology.* 2003;124(1):71–9.
12. Ruhl CE, Everhart JE. Epidemiology of nonalcoholic fatty liver. *Clin Liver Dis.* 2004;8(3):501–19, vii.
13. Schwimmer JB, Deutsch R, Kahen T, Lavine JE, Stanley C, Behling C. Prevalence of fatty liver in children and adolescents. *Pediatrics.* 2006; 118(4):1388–93.
14. Anderson EL, Howe LD, Jones HE, Higgins JP, Lawlor DA, Fraser A. The prevalence of non-alcoholic fatty liver disease in children and adolescents: A systematic review and meta-analysis. *PLoS One.* 2015;10(10):e0140908.
15. Shen L, Fan JG, Shao Y, et al. Prevalence of nonalcoholic fatty liver among administrative officers in Shanghai: An epidemiological survey. *World J Gastroenterol.* 2003;9(5):1106–10.
16. Bellentani S, Tiribelli C, Saccoccio G, et al. Prevalence of chronic liver disease in the general population of northern Italy: The dionysos study. *Hepatology.* 1994;20(6):1442–9.
17. Sherif ZA, Saeed A, Ghavimi S, et al. Global epidemiology of nonalcoholic fatty liver disease and perspectives on US minority populations. *Dig Dis Sci.* 2016;61(5):1214–5.
18. Kim WR, Lake JR, Smith JM, et al. OPTN/SRTR 2013 Annual Data Report: Liver. *Am J Transplant.* 2015;15 Suppl 2:1–28.
19. Said A, Ghufran A. Epidemic of non-alcoholic fatty liver disease and hepatocellular carcinoma. *World J Clin Oncol.* 2017;8(6):429–36.
20. Williams CD, Stengel J, Asike MI, et al. Prevalence of nonalcoholic fatty liver disease and nonalcoholic steatohepatitis among a largely middle-aged population utilizing ultrasound and liver biopsy: A prospective study. *Gastroenterology.* 2011;140(1):124–31.
21. Boyle M, Masson S, Anstee QM. The bidirectional impacts of alcohol consumption and the metabolic syndrome: Cofactors for progressive fatty liver disease. *J Hepatol.* 2018;68(2):251–67.
22. Sanyal AJ. Mechanisms of disease: Pathogenesis of nonalcoholic fatty liver disease. *Nat Clin Pract Gastroenterol Hepatol.* 2005;2(1):46–53.
23. Diehl AM, Day C. Nonalcoholic steatohepatitis. *N Engl J Med.* 2018; 378(8):781.
24. Hossain N, Afendy A, Stepanova M, et al. Independent predictors of fibrosis in patients with nonalcoholic fatty liver disease. *Clin Gastroenterol Hepatol.* 2009;7(11):1224–9, 1229 e1221–2.
25. Adams LA, Harmsen S, St Sauver JL, et al. Nonalcoholic fatty liver disease increases risk of death among patients with diabetes: A community-based cohort study. *Am J Gastroenterol.* 2010;105(7):1567–73.
26. Adams LA, Lymp JF, St Sauver J, et al. The natural history of nonalcoholic fatty liver disease: A population-based cohort study. *Gastroenterology.* 2005;129(1):113–21.
27. Ong JP, Pitts A, Younossi ZM. Increased overall mortality and liver-related mortality in non-alcoholic fatty liver disease. *J Hepatol.* 2008;49(4): 608–12.
28. Targher G, Byrne CD, Lonardo A, Zoppini G, Barbui C. Non-alcoholic fatty liver disease and risk of incident cardiovascular disease: A meta-analysis. *J Hepatol.* 2016;65(3):589–600.
29. White DL, Kanwal F, El-Serag HB. Association between nonalcoholic fatty liver disease and risk for hepatocellular cancer, based on systematic review. *Clin Gastroenterol Hepatol.* 2012;10(12):1342–59 e1342.
30. Younossi ZM, Henry L. Economic and quality-of-life implications of non-alcoholic fatty liver disease. *Pharmacoeconomics.* 2015;33(12):1245–53.
31. David K, Kowdley KV, Unalp A, et al. Quality of life in adults with nonalcoholic fatty liver disease: Baseline data from the nonalcoholic steatohepatitis clinical research network. *Hepatology.* 2009;49(6):1904–12.
32. Torres DM, Harrison SA. Diagnosis and therapy of nonalcoholic steatohepatitis. *Gastroenterology.* 2008;134(6):1682–98.
33. Chalasani N, Younossi Z, Lavine JE, et al. The diagnosis and management of non-alcoholic fatty liver disease: Practice guideline by the American association for the study of liver diseases, American college of gastroenterology, and the American gastroenterological association. *Hepatology.* 2012;55(6):2005–23.
34. Angulo P, Hui JM, Marchesini G, et al. The NAFLD fibrosis score: A noninvasive system that identifies liver fibrosis in patients with NAFLD. *Hepatology.* 2007;45(4):846–54.
35. Kim BK, Kim DY, Park JY, et al. Validation of FIB-4 and comparison with other simple noninvasive indices for predicting liver fibrosis and cirrhosis in hepatitis B virus-infected patients. *Liver Int.* 2010;30(4):546–53.
36. Sterling RK, Lissen E, Clumeck N, et al. Development of a simple noninvasive index to predict significant fibrosis in patients with HIV/HCV coinfection. *Hepatology.* 2006;43(6):1317–25.
37. Tsai E, Lee TP. Diagnosis and evaluation of nonalcoholic fatty liver disease/nonalcoholic steatohepatitis, including noninvasive biomarkers and transient elastography. *Clin Liver Dis.* 2018;22(1):73–92.
38. Fan JG, Cao HX. Role of diet and nutritional management in non-alcoholic fatty liver disease. *J Gastroenterol Hepatol.* 2013;28 Suppl 4:81–7.
39. Hickman IJ, Jonsson JR, Prins JB, et al. Modest weight loss and physical activity in overweight patients with chronic liver disease results in sustained improvements in alanine aminotransferase, fasting insulin, and quality of life. *Gut.* 2004;53(3):413–9.
40. Said A, Akhter A. Meta-Analysis of randomized controlled trials of pharmacologic agents in non-alcoholic steatohepatitis. *Ann Hepatol.* 2017; 16(4):538–47.
41. Chalasani N, Younossi Z, Lavine JE, et al. The diagnosis and management of nonalcoholic fatty liver disease: Practice guidance from the American association for the study of liver diseases. *Hepatology.* 2018;67(1):328–57.
42. Sanyal AJ, Chalasani N, Kowdley KV, et al. Pioglitazone, vitamin E, or placebo for nonalcoholic steatohepatitis. *N Engl J Med.* 2010;362(18): 1675–85.
43. Younossi ZM, Loomba R, Rinella ME, et al. Current and future therapeutic regimens for non-alcoholic fatty liver disease (NAFLD) and non-alcoholic steatohepatitis (NASH). *Hepatology.* 2018;68(1):361–71.
44. Manning AP, Thompson WG, Heaton KW, Morris AF. Towards positive diagnosis of the irritable bowel. *Br Med J.* 1978;2(6138):653–4.
45. Longstreth GF, Thompson WG, Chey WD, Houghton LA, Mearin F, Spiller RC. Functional bowel disorders. In: *Rome lll: The Functional Gastrointestinal Disorders.* 3rd ed. McLean, VA: Degnan Assoc Inc.; 2006.

46. Drossman DA. Functional gastrointestinal disorders: History, pathophysiology, clinical features and Rome IV. *Gastroenterology.* 2016; S0016-5085(16):00223-7.

47. Lovell RM, Ford AC. Global prevalence of and risk factors for irritable bowel syndrome: A meta-analysis. *Clin Gastroenterol Hepatol.* 2012;10(7): 712–21 e714.

48. Agreus L, Svardsudd K, Nyren O, Tibblin G. Irritable bowel syndrome and dyspepsia in the general population: Overlap and lack of stability over time. *Gastroenterology.* 1995;109(3):671–80.

49. Mearin F, Baro E, Roset M, Badia X, Zarate N, Perez I. Clinical patterns over time in irritable bowel syndrome: Symptom instability and severity variability. *Am J Gastroenterol.* 2004;99(1):113–21.

50. Williams RE, Black CL, Kim HY, et al. Stability of irritable bowel syndrome using a Rome II-based classification. *Aliment Pharmacol Ther.* 2006;23(1):197–205.

51. Ford AC, Forman D, Bailey AG, Axon AT, Moayyedi P. Irritable bowel syndrome: A 10-yr natural history of symptoms and factors that influence consultation behavior. *Am J Gastroenterol.* 2008;103(5):1229–39; quiz 1240.

52. Halder SL, Locke GR, 3rd, Schleck CD, Zinsmeister AR, Melton LJ, 3rd, Talley NJ. Natural history of functional gastrointestinal disorders: A 12-year longitudinal population-based study. *Gastroenterology.* 2007;133(3):799–807.

53. http://www.gastro.org/press_releases/ibs-in-america-survey-highlights-physical-social-and-emotional-impact.http://www.gastro.org/press_releases/ibs-in-america-survey-highlights-physical-social-and-emotional-impact.

54. Hulisz D. The burden of illness of irritable bowel syndrome: Current challenges and hope for the future. *J Manag Care Pharm.* 2004;10(4): 299–309.

55. Nellesen D, Yee K, Chawla A, Lewis BE, Carson RT. A systematic review of the economic and humanistic burden of illness in irritable bowel syndrome and chronic constipation. *J Manag Care Pharm.* 2013;19(9): 755–64.

56. Buono JL, Carson RT, Flores NM. Health-related quality of life, work productivity, and indirect costs among patients with irritable bowel syndrome with diarrhea. *Health Qual Life Outcomes.* 2017;15(1):35.

57. Inadomi JM, Fennerty MB, Bjorkman D. Systematic review: The economic impact of irritable bowel syndrome. *Aliment Pharmacol Ther.* 2003;18(7):671–82.

58. Everhart JE, Renault PF. Irritable bowel syndrome in office-based practice in the United States. *Gastroenterology.* 1991;100(4):998–1005.

59. Levy RL, Whitehead WE, Von Korff MR, Feld AD. Intergenerational transmission of gastrointestinal illness behavior. *Am J Gastroenterol.* 2000; 95(2):451–6.

60. Whitehead WE, Palsson OS, Levy RR, Feld AD, Turner M, Von Korff M. Comorbidity in irritable bowel syndrome. *Am J Gastroenterol.* 2007; 102(12):2767–76.

61. Andersen RM. Revisiting the behavioral model and access to medical care: Does it matter? *J Health Soc Behav.* 1995;36(1):1–10.

62. Gudleski GD, Satchidanand N, Dunlap LJ, et al. Predictors of medical and mental health care use in patients with irritable bowel syndrome in the United States. *Behav Res Ther.* 2017;88:65–75.

63. Rao SS, Yu S, Fedewa A. Systematic review: Dietary fibre and FODMAP-restricted diet in the management of constipation and irritable bowel syndrome. *Aliment Pharmacol Ther.* 2015;41(12):1256–70.

64. Biesiekierski JR, Newnham ED, Irving PM, et al. Gluten causes gastrointestinal symptoms in subjects without celiac disease: A double-blind randomized placebo-controlled trial. *Am J Gastroenterol.* 2011;106(3): 508–14; quiz 515.

65. Skodje GI, Sarna VK, Minelle IH, et al. Fructan, rather than gluten, induces symptoms in patients with self-reported non-celiac gluten sensitivity. *Gastroenterology.* 2018;154(3):529–39 e522.

66. Halmos EP, Power VA, Shepherd SJ, Gibson PR, Muir JG. A diet low in FODMAPs reduces symptoms of irritable bowel syndrome. *Gastroenterology.* 2014;146(1):67–75 e65.

67. Eswaran S, Farida JP, Green J, Miller JD, Chey WD. Nutrition in the management of gastrointestinal diseases and disorders: The evidence for the low FODMAP diet. *Curr Opin Pharmacol.* 2017;37:151–7.

68. *Institute of Medicine (US) Committee on Standards for Developing Trustworthy Clinical Practice Guidelines. Clinical Practice Guidelines We Can Trust.* Washington DC: National Academies Press (US); 2011.

69. Weinberg DS, Smalley W, Heidelbaugh JJ, Sultan S, Amercian Gastroenterological Association. American Gastroenterological Association Institute Guideline on the pharmacological management of irritable bowel syndrome. *Gastroenterology.* 2014;147(5):1146–8.

70. Radziwon CD, Lackner JM. Cognitive behavioral therapy for IBS: How useful, how often, and how does it work? *Curr Gastroenterol Rep.* 2017;19(10):49.

CHAPTER

56

Respiratory Diseases

David B. Coultas • Katherine A. Artis • Jonathan M. Samet

Globally life expectancy has increased to 71.8 years in 2015, from 61.4 years in 1980,[1] contributing to the growing burden of disability associated with chronic diseases.[2] Among these chronic conditions respiratory diseases are a major contributor to both morbidity (Table 56-1) and mortality (Table 56-2) at all ages worldwide. Moreover, the burden of disability from all respiratory diseases has increased (Table 56-1), partly attributable to improved survival among children and adolescence and population growth among regions with higher sociodemographic indicators (SDIs) based on higher incomes, higher educational attainment, and reduced fertility rates.[3] In 2015, asthma and chronic obstructive pulmonary disease (COPD) were ranked 11th and 14th among the leading causes of disability worldwide.[2]

Of the 55.8 million global deaths in 2015, about 16% were attributed to respiratory diseases[1] (Table 56-2). Although the absolute total number of deaths increased by 14.1% since 1990 and 4.1% since 2005, over the past 30 years the overall and most disease-specific death rates have declined.[1] For respiratory diseases, between 2005 and 2015, absolute numbers and mortality rates have varied (Table 56-2). The number of deaths and death rates declined for lower respiratory tract infections, neonatal preterm birth complications, and asthma. In contrast, the number and disease-specific mortality rates declined for lung cancer, COPD, and pneumoconiosis. And only interstitial lung diseases (ILDs) had both an increase in total number of deaths and mortality rate.

Of the ten leading causes of death worldwide, the disease-specific distributions vary considerably by countries and regions ranked by SDI.[1] While lower respiratory tract infections are ranked number three in the top-ten causes of death worldwide, among countries with low- and low-middle SDI they are consistently ranked number one. In countries with higher SDI (i.e., high, high-middle, and middle), lower respiratory tract infections are consistently ranked among the fifth or sixth leading causes of death. Neonatal preterm birth complications are not among the top ten causes of death among countries with high-middle or high SDI, but are ranked fifth or sixth among middle-, low-middle, and low-ranked countries. Of the chronic diseases, COPD ranks number ten globally, and ranks number four, seven, eight, and ten among middle, high-middle-, high-, and low-middle-ranked countries, respectively. Finally, lung cancer ranks number three and four among high- and high-middle-ranked countries.

The respiratory system, which includes the lungs and the upper airway that joins the trachea to the larynx, is exposed to a wide range of potentially injurious agents (Table 56-3). On average, adults inhale

TABLE 56-1 GLOBAL PREVALENCE AND YEARS LIVED WITH DISABILITY (YLD) FROM RESPIRATORY DISEASES AND ALL CONDITIONS, 2015

Condition	Prevalence (×1000)	% Change between 2005 and 15	YLD (×1000)	% Change between 2005 and 15
Neonatal preterm birth complications	41,855	+10.6	5,091	+4.4
Lower respiratory infection	8,987	+5.1	540	+4.9
Lung cancer	3,300	+37.7	514	+31.1
Chronic respiratory disease	514,626	+12.1	30,466	+11.8
COPD	174,483	+17.1	12,047	+16.2
Asthma	358,198	+9.5	15,899	+9.4
Pneumoconiosis	2,406	+30.3	474	+26.6
Interstitial lung diseases	1,916	+25.8	235	+25.7
All conditions	–		792,005	+15.1

Abbreviation: ASR = age standardized ratio.
Source: From GBD disabilities 2016.[2]

TABLE 56-2 GLOBAL NUMBER OF DEATHS AND AGE-STANDARDIZED MORTALITY RATES FROM RESPIRATORY DISEASES, 2015

Condition	Deaths (×1000)	% Change 2005–15	Age-Standardized Mortality Rate (per 100,000)	% Change 2005–15
Neonatal preterm birth complications	806	−25.9	11	−29.8
LRI	2,736.7	−3.2	41.6	−19.5
Lung cancer	1,722.5	+20.1	26.6	−8.1
Chronic respiratory disease	3,795.5	+2.3	61.0	−22.8
COPD	3,188.3	+2.8	51.7	−22.9
Asthma	397.1	−11.7	6.1	−31.3
Pneumoconiosis	36.1	+13.2	0.6	−14.4
ILD	121.8	+51.5	2.0	+14.1
All deaths	55,792.9	+4.1	850.1	−17.1

Source: From GBD 2016.[1]

TABLE 56-3 MECHANISMS OF LUNG INJURY AND EXAMPLES OF INJURIOUS AGENTS AND ASSOCIATED DISEASES

	Example	
Mechanism of Injury	**Agent**	**Disease**
Infection	Respiratory syncytial virus	Bronchiolitis
	Streptococcus pneumonia	Pneumonia
Carcinogenesis	Cigarette smoke	Lung cancer
	Asbestos	Mesothelioma
Immunologic	Thermophilic actinomycetes	Hypersensitive pneumonitis
Inflammation	Cigarette smoke	COPD
	Oxides of nitrogen	Silo-fillers' lung
Fibrogenesis	Asbestos	Asbestosis
	Coal dust	Coal workers' pneumoconiosis
Other	Plicatic acid	Western red cedar workers' asthma
	Cotton dust	Byssinosis
	Diactyl	Obliterative bronchiolitis

about 5 L of air per minute; with exercise, the amount may increase 20-fold or more. With 10,000–20,000 L of air inhaled daily, agents present even in low concentrations may be toxic. The respiratory system is equipped with a remarkably effective system of defense mechanisms against inhaled particles and gases. Disease may result, however, if an acute exposure overwhelms the defenses (e.g., toxic gas inhalation), if an agent is particularly toxic even at low concentrations (e.g., toluene diisocyanate, plicatic acid), if exposure is sustained (e.g., cigarette smoking, diacetyl), or if the exposed person is particularly susceptible (e.g., asthmatics).

The major risk factors for respiratory diseases include outdoor and indoor air pollution, occupational exposures, infectious agents, and health-related behaviors (e.g., smoking) (Table 56-4). Over the past 25 years, the distribution and burden of these risk factors have been changing worldwide varying with population growth, ageing, and prevalence of exposures.[4] Thus prioritization and targeting of risk factors for prevention will vary with population demographics and patterns of exposures in the population.

Despite global declines in cigarette smoking over the past 25 years (28.4% for men and 34.4% for women), it remains one the major causes of respiratory disease morbidity and mortality.[5] In 2015, the prevalence of daily smoking worldwide was estimated at 25.0% for men and 5.4% for women. Moreover, 6.4 million deaths, 11.5% of all deaths worldwide were attributed to smoking, and of these a majority are attributed to respiratory diseases (Table 56-2). Additionally, the majority of deaths associated with smoking were found in four countries (the United States, India, China, Russia). Progress in curbing smoking prevalence has varied by geography, SDI (low and middle countries), and gender (women).

Of environmental risk factors, the greatest threats to respiratory health are ambient air pollution,[6,7] climate change,[8] and emerging infections.[9-11] Ambient air pollution was the fifth-ranking mortality risk factor in 2015, contributing to 7.6% of global deaths and 4.2% of disability-adjusted life-years.[6,7] Health effects associated with climate change include worsening air pollution (i.e., ozone, $PM_{2.5}$, wild fire smoke), heat stress, extreme weather conditions, sand storms, and aeroallergens.[12] Currently the most susceptible are already experiencing the adverse consequences of heat stress with rising temperatures (e.g., elderly women with pulmonary diseases).

At the population level, prevention of respiratory diseases has traditionally been addressed through policies and regulations to minimize exposures to toxic agents, immunizations, and screening. However, at the global level recent pandemics have prompted multicountry, interdisciplinary collaborations to create a global infectious disease surveillance system, which has the potential to identify and address the complex environmental, cultural, political, economic, and behavioral factors that contribute to pandemics of severe lower respiratory tract infections.[9-11]

In addition, with the advent of "precision medicine" (i.e., prevention and treatment strategies that take individual variability into account) offers potential new opportunities for individual prevention that are rapidly expanding. This is possible as our understanding of the complex mechanisms that determine susceptibility to development of acute and chronic respiratory tract injury including biological, social, behavioral, and environmental factors.[13] This understanding has been possible through large-scale biologic, clinical, population, and environmental databases and computational tools.[13] While there are current examples of this in respiratory medicine (e.g., screening for cystic fibrosis), the full potential for precision medicine for disease prevention will require substantial research and resources to effectively deliver.[14,15]

Opportunities for prevention of respiratory diseases starts with the periods of lung development in utero and growth among newborns, children, and adolescents, which are critical in determining susceptibility for future development of chronic respiratory diseases such as asthma and COPD in adulthood.[16,17] A number of exposures *in utero* may adversely affect lung development and future risk of chronic respiratory diseases (e.g., maternal smoking).[17,18] Moreover, development of the respiratory microbiome immediately after birth may affect respiratory tract development and risk for respiratory tract infections[19] and COPD.[20]

PEDIATRIC RESPIRATORY DISEASES

Overall, among children and adolescents 19 years of age and younger, there were 7.26 million deaths worldwide in 2015, and 80% occurred among children younger than 5 years of age.[3] During the past 25 years overall mortality declined, however, the relative declines have been less among developed countries, which now accounts for about 75% of all deaths compared to 1.6% for the most developed countries.[3] Neonatal preterm birth complications and lower respiratory tract infections were the top-two leading causes of death, which have also declined dramatically between 1990 and 2015. Despite the overall improvement in mortality, because of improved survival and population growth, the burden of disability from all causes among children and adolescents increased 4.3% from 1990 to 2015.[3]

Respiratory Distress Syndrome

Respiratory distress syndrome (RDS) in the newborn results primarily from surfactant deficiency associated with lung immaturity and preterm birth (i.e., < 37 weeks gestation).[16] Because of surfactant deficiency, the lung does not effectively exchange oxygen and carbon dioxide after birth, and positive pressure ventilation is frequently required to maintain life. A frequent complication of preterm birth is bronchopulmonary dysplasia (BPD) or chronic lung disease of infancy defined as need for any oxygen and/or positive-pressure ventilation support.[21] As survival for preterm infants has improved since the original description of BPD 50 years ago, the criteria for diagnosing BPD has been evolving to better predict future respiratory morbidity.[21,22]

Neonatal preterm birth complications are the most common cause of mortality worldwide among children.[3] In addition, while the mortality rate has declined, preterm birth complications are the leading

TABLE 56-4 RISK FACTORS AND MORTALITY AND DISABILITY ADJUSTED LIFE YEARS (DALY) ATTRIBUTED TO RESPIRATORY DISEASES

Risk Factor	Deaths (×1000)	% Change 2005–15	DALY (×1000)	% Change 2005–15
Air pollution				
All causes	6,485	+0.3	167,290	−10.5
Ambient particulate air pollution	4,241	+7.8	103,066	−4.2
LRI				
Lung cancer	675	−8.3	28,360	−26.6
COPD	283	+25.7	6,209	+20.1
Ambient ozone pollution	864	+3.2	16,848	+2.6
COPD				
Residential radon	254	+22.7	4,116	+16.6
Lung cancer				
Household air pollution from solid fuels	64	+19.7	1,386	+14.3
All causes	2,854	−13.0	85,644	−20.3
LRI	729	−19.5	36,883	−30.3
Lung cancer	149	−6.3	3,439	−9.6
COPD	657	−15.3	13,373	−14.3
Occupational exposures				
All causes	1,086	+14.2	63,615	+13.9
Occupational lung carcinogens				
Asbestos	155	+31.6	2,314	+23.4
Diesel exhaust	120	+30.8	2,657	+29.8
Second-hand smoke	96	+14.7	2,113	+13.6
Mesothelioma	23	+47.2	410	+37.3
Occupational particulate matter, gases, fumes	354	+6.0	8,729	+4.6
COPD				
Occupational asthmagens	42	-16.9	2,621	-4.8
Asthma				
Tobacco smoke				
All causes	7,165	+4.2	170,889	−2.0
Smoking				
LRI	350	+5.4	7,044	−1.1
Lung cancer	1,175	+15.8	24,140	+9.4
COPD	1,427	+5.3	26,443	+2.4
Asthma	45	−17.6	2,024	−9.0
ILD	17	+37.2	302	+24.1
Second-hand smoke				
All causes	886	+0.2	25,212	−15.9
LRI	183	−23.0	10,103	−35.6
Lung cancer	29	+32.6	691	+29.0
Smoking all causes	6,402	+4.7	148,623	+1.0
Childhood and maternal malnutrition				
All causes	1,414	−38.0	172,120	−30.7
LRI (nonexclusive breastfeeding)	208	−35.7	17,928	−35.7
LRI (childhood underweight)	110	−47.5	9,416	−47.4
LRI (childhood wasting)	535	−37.9	45,989	−37.8
LRI (childhood stunting)	155	−45.1	13,335	−45.0
LRI (Zinc deficiency)	24	−41.4	2,056	−41.2
Alcohol and drug use				
All causes	2,750	+6.0	111,365	+2.4

(*Continued*)

TABLE 56-4 RISK FACTORS AND MORTALITY AND DISABILITY ADJUSTED LIFE YEARS (DALY) ATTRIBUTED TO RESPIRATORY DISEASES (*Continued*)

Risk Factor	Deaths (×1000)	% Change 2005–15	DALY (×1000)	% Change 2005–15
TB	126	−13.9	4,725	−14.1
LRI	106	+13.6	2,355	+3.3
Diet low in fruits				
All causes	2,924	+7.8	75,590	+5.5
Lung cancer	207	+20.1	4,391	+13.8
High BMI				
All causes	3,960	+19.5	120,132	+22.0
Low physical activity				
All causes	1,605	+18.9	34,603	+17.4
All deaths	32,234	+4.9	1,015,470	−5.6

Source: From: GBD 2017.[4]

BOX 56-1 Risk Factors for Preterm Delivery

Maternal demographic characteristics

- Young or advanced maternal age
- Black race
- Low socioeconomic status

Unhealthy lifestyle

- Tobacco use
- Substance use
- Low or high prepregnancy body mass index

Pregnancy history

- Short interpregnancy interval
- Previous preterm delivery
- Multiple gestations

Pregnancy complications

- Placental abruption or previa
- Intrauterine infection
- Polyhydramnios
- Oligohydramnios

Maternal medical disorders

- Asthma
- Obesity
- Hypertension
- Diabetes
- Thyroid disease

Mental health

- Psychological or social stress
- Depression

Fertility treatments

- Assisted reproductive technology (ART)
- Non-ART fertility treatments

Source: Shapiro-Mendoza CK BW, Henderson Z, James A, Howse JL, Iskander J, Thorpe PG. CDC grand rounds: public health strategies to prevent preterm birth. MMWR 2016;65(32):826-830.

cause of disability-adjusted life years (DALY) (Tables 56-1 and 56-2). Furthermore, despite the overall decline in mortality there is marked variation by country and region related to SDI ranging from 1.7 per 100,000 to 72.3 per 100,000 among the highest and lowest regions, respectively.[3]

The decline in mortality has been partly attributed to improvements in obstetric and neonatal care in developed countries, particularly among extremely premature neonates (i.e., 23–24 weeks' gestation).[23,24] Mortality, commonly the result of RDS, is inversely related to each additional week of gestation, ranging from 44.2% at 23 weeks to 1.8% at 36 weeks gestation.[24] Moreover, there are racial and ethnic disparities in mortality. In the United States, black infants have the highest preterm-related mortality (4.9 per 1000 live births) compared to American Indian or Alaska Natives (2.0), Hispanics (1.8), whites (1.6), and Asian/Pacific Islanders (1.5).[25]

Worldwide neonatal preterm birth complications are the tenth leading cause of years lived with disability(YLD).[3] And morbidity among premature new-borns who survive RDS is also strongly associated with duration of gestation, with or without the diagnosis of BPD.[26–28] For example, home oxygen use among infants discharged from the neonatal intensive care unit, an indicator of respiratory impairment varies inversely with gestation duration (56% at 23–28 weeks, 25% at 29–33 weeks, and 10% at 34–36 weeks of gestation).[26] Respiratory disease diagnosed within the first 2 years of life, associated with respiratory medications, emergency visits, and hospitalizations; occurs in 45% diagnosed with moderate or severe BPD.[28] Risk factors for BPD and subsequent respiratory morbidity include maternal smoking, lower birth weight, white race, maternal smoking, and pre-existing maternal hypertension.[28]

Prevention of premature birth represents the most effective method for reducing morbidity and mortality associated with RDS and BPD.[25,29] Among the numerous risk factors for preterm delivery (Box 56-1), optimizing access to prenatal care is the highest priority to prevent tobacco and substance use and improve maternal health.[25] Moreover, because prematurity is frequently associated with poor socioeconomic conditions contributing to geographic and racial/ethnic disparities, policies, and resources to improve access to prenatal care offers a feasible solution for primary prevention. In contrast, secondary prevention of preterm delivery with antenatal corticosteroids and surfactant replacement only provide partial solutions, for the prevention of RDS and its complications.[30]

Cystic Fibrosis

Cystic fibrosis is the most common lethal genetic disease in whites of Northern European descent, estimated to occur in about 1 in 3000–4000 live births.[31] The disease occurs less frequently in other racial and ethnic groups in the United States with estimates of 1 in 4000–10,000 Hispanic births; 1 in 15,000–20,000 African American births; and less commonly among American Indian/Alaska Native and Asian births.[31] Cystic fibrosis is transmitted as an autosomal recessive trait, and the heterozygote frequency in persons of Northern European descent is about 1 in 25.[32]

More than 2000 mutations of the cystic fibrosis transmembrane conductance regulator (CFTR) gene on chromosome 7 have been characterized since the gene was identified in 1989, and one mutation (delta F508) accounts for about two-thirds of all CF alleles worldwide.[33,34] The CFTR gene mutations result in an inability of epithelial cells to secrete chloride ions and the production of an abnormally thick mucus, and impaired binding and killing of bacteria.[33] This defect affects the lungs, intestines, and exocrine glands and may result in diverse clinical manifestations, but patients invariably develop COPD from repeated infections that destroy lung tissue.[33] Pulmonary involvement has been reported in over 90% of all patients with cystic fibrosis and accounts for the majority of hospital admissions and deaths.[31] The prognosis for patients with cystic fibrosis has improved markedly since cystic fibrosis was first described in 1938.[33] Among developed countries, the median survival is now more than 40 years, with Canada reporting a median survival of 51 years during the period 2009–13.[34] The improved survival has resulted in an overall increase in prevalence, with adults with cystic fibrosis now out-numbering children.[35] Among European countries projected estimates are that by 2025, the prevalence of cystic fibrosis will increase by 50%, with a 75% and 20% increase among adults and children, respectively.[35] Moreover, the projected changes vary with gross national income per capita, an indicator of public health and healthcare system resources for screening and for providing comprehensive management.[36]

The improved prognosis of cystic fibrosis has been associated with the expansion of early detection with screening[37] and comprehensive multidisciplinary healthcare.[31,33] Evidence of improved health outcomes associated with screening from patient registries and cost-effectiveness has contributed to the growing adoption of new-born screening worldwide.[37] For example, for the period 1988–2010, data from the Australian cystic fibrosis registry has demonstrated improved outcomes associated with the early diagnosis of cystic fibrosis.[38] The details of the comprehensive multidisciplinary healthcare of cystic fibrosis is beyond the scope of this review and has been discussed extensively elsewhere.[31,33] Moreover, universal access to healthcare is associated with improved survival among Canadian patients compared to patients living in the United States.[34]

Respiratory Tract Infection

Overall, respiratory viruses are responsible for most childhood respiratory tract infections.[39,40] The predominant clinical syndromes include colds (infections of the upper respiratory tract), epiglottitis (infection of the epiglottis), croup or laryngeotracheobronchitis (infection of the larynx and large airways), bronchiolitis (infection of the small airways), and pneumonia (infection of the lung tissues). Rhinoviruses are most closely associated with colds, parainfluenza viruses with croup, respiratory syncytial virus with bronchiolitis, and various viruses, including respiratory syncytial virus and the parainfluenza viruses with pneumonia.[39,40] In less-developed countries, measles and whooping cough (*Bordatella pertusis*) may be important causes of severe respiratory tract infection.[3] *Mycoplasma* and *Chlamydia* are relatively infrequent causes of childhood respiratory infections.[40] Birth cohort surveillance has shown that during the first year of life children experience 1.8 respiratory tract infections annually, 95% of these episodes are upper respiratory infections, and over 60% are attributed to viruses.[40] Children up to 5 years of age experience an average of about five upper respiratory tract infections per year.[41]

Worldwide, in 2015 about 2.74 million deaths were attributed to lower respiratory tract infections,[42] but over the past 25 years the number of deaths and disability associated with lower respiratory tract infections among children and adolescents has declined 65% and 81%, respectively.[3] However, among children under 5 years of age from developing countries they remain a major cause of mortality accounting for about 90% of deaths in children and adolescents in 2015.[3,42] Mortality rates are highest in countries of sub-Saharan Africa (215.1 per 100,000) and lowest among high-income countries (3.4 per 100,000), with a relative difference between the highest and lowest mortality rates of over 800%.[42] These deaths are most often the result of respiratory failure associated with bronchiolitis and pneumonia. And most worldwide mortality among children under 5 years of age is attributed to bacteria with pneumococcal pneumonia and *H. influenza* type b accounting for 64.1% of deaths, followed by RSV and influenza accounting for 6.6% of deaths.[42]

Although respiratory tract infections are a much less frequent cause of death among children and adolescents from developed countries, they are a major source of morbidity.[3,42] Worldwide, most morbidity occurs among children younger than 5 years of age, with an estimated 101.8 million episodes of lower respiratory tract infections, resulting in 60.6 million DALY.[42] Hospitalizations for severe lower respiratory tract infections are indicated because of respiratory distress, hypoxemia, and increased risk for apnea associated with viral infections (RSV 25%, influenzae 10%) and bacteria (*Streptococcus pneumoniae* 18.3%, *H. influenzae* type B 4.1%).[39,43,44] Moreover, respiratory tract infections in childhood are associated with long-term sequelae, including loss of lung function after severe episodes of lower respiratory tract infection, the development of asthma, the development of bronchiectasis, and an increased risk of developing COPD in adulthood.[17,45,46]

Many risk factors for respiratory tract infections have been identified and successful efforts to address them have resulted in declines in morbidity and mortality worldwide.[42] Improvements in morbidity indicators in developing countries has been associated with improved childhood nutrition and reduced household and ambient air pollution.[42] Early initiation and exclusive breast feeding is associated with reduced neonatal mortality.[47] Effective vaccines are available for a limited number of bacteria (e.g., *S. pneumoniae, H. influenzae*) and viruses (e.g., influenza) that cause respiratory tract infections.[42] The reduction in lower respiratory tract infection morbidity has been associated with *H. influenza B* vaccine.[42] The persistence of poor socioeconomic conditions, low maternal education, indoor air pollution from biomass fuel burning and second-hand smoke exposure, severe malnutrition, and other chronic diseases largely explains the high global variation in morbidity and mortality from respiratory tract infections.[48] However, available evidence is lacking on effectiveness of antibiotics in reducing mortality among children at high risk for lower respiratory tract infections,[49] and may partly explain a decline in antibiotic trials to prevent lower respiratory tract infections,[50] or of technology to rapidly detect viral infections to improve outcomes.[39,51] Innovative, multipronged approaches to address these complex risk factors for respiratory tract infections will be required to close these wide gaps between countries in morbidity and mortality.

The ongoing search for improved vaccines and new prevention strategies will be necessary for the primary prevention of known and emerging infectious agents that cause respiratory tract infections. Moreover, the limited effectiveness of antiviral agents[52] and growing antibiotic resistance[53] are partly contributing to the search for more effective vaccines.[54,55] Similarly, at the global level recent pandemics have initiated international collaborations to investigate and develop interventions for the complex environmental, cultural, political, economic, and behavioral factors that contribute to emerging infections causing severe lower respiratory tract illnesses.[9,10,56] At the individual level, growing evidence suggests the potential to tailor interventions to boost host defenses against respiratory tract infections based on variations in genotype[54] and lung microbiome phenotype.[19,57]

Asthma

Asthma is a chronic condition characterized by airway inflammation and hyper-responsiveness; reversible airflow obstruction; and episodic wheezing, cough, and dyspnea.[58] Asthma results from a number

TABLE 56-5 RISK FACTORS AND STRENGTH OF EVIDENCE FOR CHILDHOOD ASTHMA

	Strong	Mild-Moderate	Insufficient
FAMILIAL/PRENATAL			
Parental and sibling history of asthma	X		
Male gender		X	
Race/ethnicity			
• African-American		X	
• Hispanic		X	
• Native American		X	
• Asian		X	
ETS		X	
Maternal			
• Age (younger and older)		X	
• Weight gain, obesity during pregnancy		X	
• Stress			
• UTI			
• Use of antibiotics		X	
• Paracetamol		X	X
• Folate, vitamin D status during pregnancy		X	
• Diet (nutrients, vitamins		X	X
PERINATAL			
Birth caesarean section		X	
Preterm delivery		X	
Birth weight		X	
Neonatal hyperbilirubinemia			X
POSTNATAL			
Older siblings at home (protective)		X	
Viral infections		X	
Overweight or obesity		X	
Mold and fungi		X	
Air pollution		X	
ETS		X	
Farm environment		X	
Endotoxin		X	
Allergens		X	
BCG vaccination			X
Breast feeding			X
Diet and nutrients			X
Menarche			X
Toxins			X
Antibiotics			X
Probiotics			X
GERD			X

Sources: From Castro 2016, Geier 2017, Wu 2017.

of genetic variations and environmental exposures in early childhood, and the phenotypic expression of the disorder is heterogeneous.[45,59,60] Numerous investigations of the occurrence of asthma in children have been conducted worldwide, and data from cross-sectional and longitudinal investigations indicate a wide range in the prevalence and incidence of childhood asthma.[3,61,62] These differences may be partly explained by a number of factors including environmental differences between countries, methods used to define asthma (e.g., parental reports of wheeze, physician-diagnosed asthma), translation and meaning of wheeze, access to care, and physician diagnostic patterns.[62] Therefore, results must be interpreted with caution, understanding the potential implications of various definitions and methods. For example, the natural history of wheezing illness compared to physician-diagnosed asthma are not the same.[59,62]

Worldwide asthma is the most common chronic condition among children.[3] Global estimates of the prevalence and YLD among children and adolescence (<19 years of age), and changes in these metrics between 1990 and 2015, were recently reported by the Global Burden of Disease Child and Adolescent Health Collaboration.[3] Multiple population surveys were utilized and the definition of asthma used was a reported diagnosis of asthma by a physician with wheezing in the past 12 months.[3] And while there was a global increase in age-standardized asthma prevalence and YLD from 2005 to 2015 (Table 56-1), among children and adolescents the average prevalence of asthma and YLD declined by 5.3% and 5.1%, respectively.[3] These declines were greatest among middle-, high-middle-, and high-SDI countries. However, during this period, prevalence and YLD increased in low- and low-middle-SDI countries. Moreover, asthma is associated with a large financial burden, with an estimated annual cost in 2015 of about $6 billion annually among school-aged children in the United States.[63]

Many risk factors have been identified for asthma that are associated with the prenatal, perinatal, and postnatal periods of development including familial/personal characteristics, lifestyle, and environmental factors[18] (Table 56-5). Among these risk factors, family history of asthma among parents and siblings is consistently associated with the development of asthma providing strong evidence for the role of genetics.[18,47] In addition, while genetic susceptibility and gene-environment interactions play a major role in controlling the biological mechanisms in response to environmental exposures, including allergic sensitization, inflammation, and bronchial hyperreactivity, understanding these complex mechanisms continues to be an active area of investigation.[54,59,64] Moreover, growing evidence suggests that environmental exposures alter gene activity in the development of asthma, independent of DNA sequence termed epigenetic mechanisms.[64]

Other prenatal factors, including demographic, pregnancy-related complications, and environmental exposures have been associated with mild-moderate increased risk for the development of asthma (Table 56-5). In a large U.S. cohort of over 1 million infants, the risk for asthma was slightly increased among males (odds ratio 1.7), racial and ethnic minorities (odds ratios 1.1–1.7), and younger maternal age.[65] However, in other populations older maternal age has been associated with an increased risk for childhood asthma.[66] Maternal health, pregnancy-related complications, and associated *in utero* exposures may increase risk for asthma including maternal weight gain and obesity, stress, antibiotic and paracetamol use, and pre-eclampsia[67] (Table 56-5). However, evidence from cohort and intervention studies is needed to establish a causal link for these factors.

In contrast, environmental tobacco smoke exposure, including maternal smoking during the prenatal period, has been consistently demonstrated in observational and intervention studies. In addition, while there is evidence of exposure to allergens *in utero*, there is no evidence for an increased risk of asthma associated with these exposures.[68] Similarly, there is insufficient or conflicting evidence on the

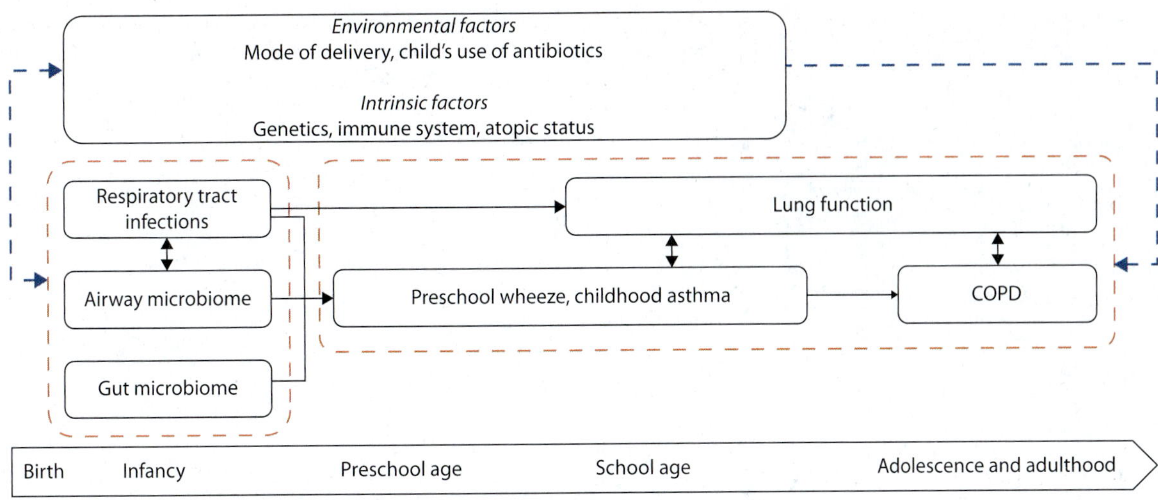

FIGURE 56-1. Pathways leading from respiratory tract infections and the microbiome in early life, to chronic obstructive respiratory diseases across the life course, and influencing factors. (Abbreviation: COPD = chronic obstructive pulmonary disease.) (*Source:* Reproduced with Permission from van Meel ER, Jaddoe VWV, Bønnelykke K, de Jongste JC, Duijts L. The role of respiratory tract infections and the microbiome in the development of asthma: A narrative review. Pediatr Pulmonol. 2017;52(10):1363–1370.)

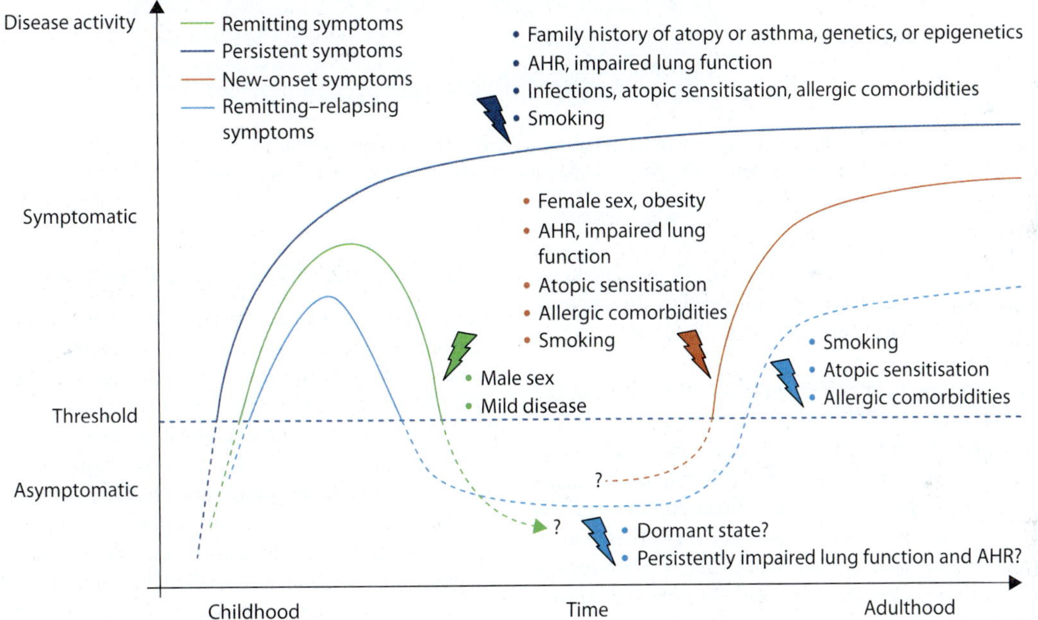

FIGURE 56-2. Determinants of disease course across asthma transitions and ages. (*Source:* Used with Permisison. Fuchs O, Bahmer T, Rabe KF, von Mutius E. Asthma transition from childhood into adulthood. The Lancet Respiratory Medicine 2017;5(3):224–234.)

role of maternal diet, including vitamin or mineral supplementation, in childhood asthma.[18,69]

During the perinatal/new-born period the risk of childhood asthma has been associated with the type of delivery and birth outcomes[67] (Table 56-5), which include delivery by caesarean section, preterm delivery, and low birth weight (<2500 grams). The airway microbiome is likely altered in newborns delivered by caesarean section compared to vaginal delivery, and different patterns of airway colonization are associated with increased risk of asthma[41,70] (van Meel 2017-use figure 1) (Fig. 56-1). In observational studies, neonatal hyperbilirubinemia is associated with childhood asthma, but evidence is considered insufficient to establish causality and will require longitudinal and intervention studies.

During the postnatal period of infancy and early childhood, lower respiratory tract infections and exposures to other airborne environmental agents together comprise the largest group of risk factors (Table 56-5) (Fuch's figure 2) (Fig. 56-2). Severe lower respiratory tract infections, including hospitalization for RSV bronchiolitis,[18,71] are associated with the highest risk. Among infants, airway colonization with *S. pneumoniae, H. influenzae, Moraxalla catarrhalis* are at increased risk for asthma.[71] In contrast, a lower risk of asthma is consistently associated with exposure to indoor aeroallergens during infancy (e.g., house dust mite, cockroach, cat), bacterial components (e.g., endotoxin), and specific fungi[72] in urban[73,74] and farming environments.[75–78] However, increased risk is associated with self-reports of home dampness and mold exposure in later childhood.[18,79]

In contrast to the protective effect of inhaled organic dusts during infancy, indoor and outdoor air pollution increase the risk of asthma.[18] Exposure to environmental tobacco smoke is independently associated with wheezing illness and asthma.[80,81] Similarly, exposure to outdoor air pollution comprised of multiple airway irritants (e.g., particulates, nitrogen oxides, sulfur dioxide) from automobile and other sources of combustion-related pollution is associated with increased asthma risk.[18,82,83]

In addition to inhaled exposures, nutrition-related factors during infancy and early childhood including breastfeeding, types of food eaten, and obesity may influence the development of asthma.[18] Breastfeeding is a protective factor for asthma that may be greatest

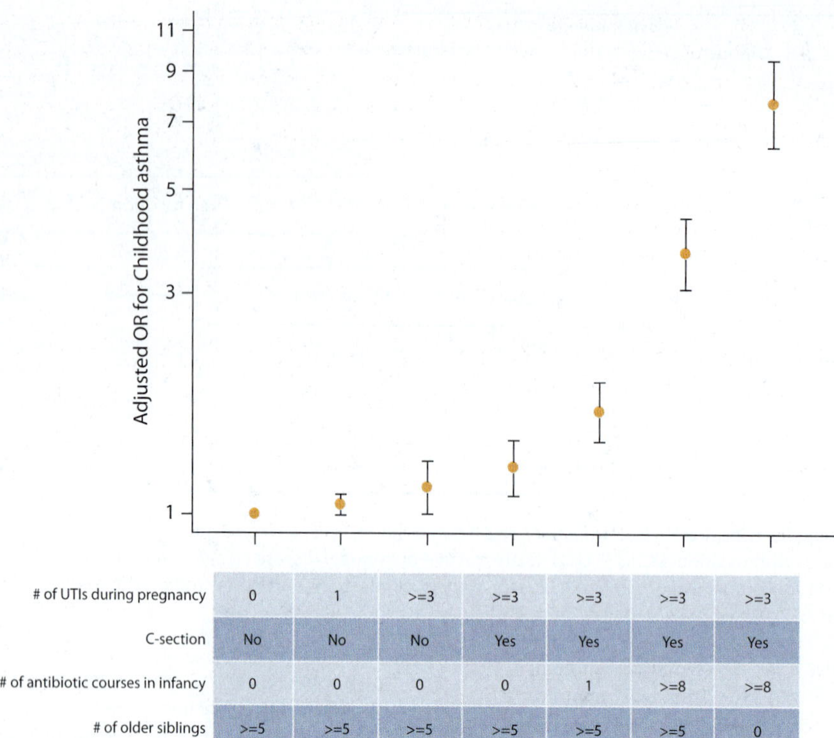

# of UTIs during pregnancy	0	1	>=3	>=3	>=3	>=3	>=3
C-section	No	No	No	Yes	Yes	Yes	Yes
# of antibiotic courses in infancy	0	0	0	0	1	>=8	>=8
# of older siblings	>=5	>=5	>=5	>=5	>=5	>=5	0

FIGURE 56-3. Adjusted odds ratios (AOR) for childhood asthma in various scenarios of cumulative exposure. (*Source:* Used with Permission. Wu P, Feldman AS, Rosas-Salazar C, et al. Relative Importance and Additive Effects of Maternal and Infant Risk Factors on Childhood Asthma. *Plos One* 2016;11(3):e0151705.)

among children with a family history of atopy.[18] Higher intake of vegetables, fruit, and fish intake have a protective effect. In addition, childhood overweight and obesity are consistently associated with an increased risk for asthma.[18]

Taken together, the multiple risk factors for asthma during the pre-, peri-, and postnatal periods highlights the complex gene-environment mechanisms in the development of asthma, which suggests that primary prevention will require multifaceted interventions targeting specific exposures and times during these different periods of development.[58,84] Moreover, exposures during each of these developmental periods is associated with a cumulative dose-response increase in risk of asthma[85] (Wu 2016-figure 4) (Fig. 56-3). Growing evidence supports a lower occurrence of asthma with multifaceted interventions (e.g., avoidance of house dust mite, pets, environmental tobacco smoke, day care until after the first year of life, delay of solid foods, and encouragement of breast feeding)[84] particularly within the first year of life.[86,87] Future opportunities for primary prevention include prevention of lower respiratory tract infections (e.g., RSV vaccine)[71] or preventing alterations of the respiratory and/or gastrointestinal microbiome that increase susceptibility to respiratory tract infections (e.g., minimize antibiotic utilization during pregnancy and infancy).[41]

Most preventive strategies for asthma have been directed at secondary and tertiary prevention with pharmacologic and other interventions to lessen morbidity and mortality.[58] The use of inhaled corticosteroids and bronchodilators greatly reduces morbidity from asthma. Many nonpharmacological interventions have also been examined, including patient and family education, environmental control, immunizations, allergen immunotherapy, physical training, chest physiotherapy, and education. These multifaceted interventions likely contribute to the worldwide decline in childhood asthma morbidity and mortality.[3] Moreover, as knowledge of the complex gene-environment interactions in the development of asthma continues to grow, opportunities to further tailor interventions will come available for all levels of prevention.[88]

ADULT RESPIRATORY TRACT DISEASES

Among adults the global prevalence, disability, and number of deaths from chronic respiratory diseases has increased over the past 10 years, but average mortality rates have declined between 2005 and 2015 (Tables 56-1 and 56-2). The growing prevalence and number of deaths is largely the result of population growth and deaths attributed to smoking, air pollution, occupational exposures, and lifestyle factors (i.e., overweight/obesity, low physical activity) (Table 56-4). Moreover, the overall decline in mortality rate has contributed to the increase in the number of years living with disability (Table 56-1).

While there has been an overall decline in worldwide mortality rates for chronic respiratory diseases,[1] there are wide variations between and within countries.[1,89] For example, lung cancer and COPD are relatively infrequent contributors to years of life lost in countries with low compared to higher SDI.[1] Moreover, within the United States, regional mortality from chronic respiratory diseases varies widely, with mortality rates in 2014, for COPD at the county level ranging from 9.9 deaths/100,000 to 152.3 deaths/100,000, with the highest mortality is found in the Appalachian region of the southeast.[89]

Lower Respiratory Tract Infections

Deaths from lower respiratory tract infections are highest among the very young and the elderly. Of the 2.74 million worldwide deaths from lower respiratory tract infections, about 46% occur among adults 70 years of age and older.[42] The major clinical syndromes of lower respiratory tract infections among adults are acute bronchitis, influenza, and pneumonia. Major risk factors are smoking and COPD. Smoking cessation and immunizations for influenza and pneumococcal pneumonia are the major prevention strategies to prevent death.

Asthma

Globally asthma is the most common chronic condition with an estimated prevalence of nearly 360 million, but a relatively infrequent cause of death accounting for only about 0.1% of prevalent cases.[90] Globally, between 1990 and 2015, asthma prevalence increased 12.6%

due to population growth. However, the relative changes in prevalence and number of deaths varied widely by country SDI status, with 94.8% and 22.1% increases in prevalence and number of deaths among low-SDI countries, respectively, compared to 13.8% and 53.2% declines among highest-SDI countries. In contrast, changes in age-standardized prevalence and mortality rates were more consistent worldwide declining on average 17.7% and 58.8%, respectively.

The decline in mortality is associated with an increase in asthma morbidity measured by YLD and DALY.[90] In 2015, asthma ranked 23rd globally in DALY among 315 causes. Moreover, asthma results in a large economic burden associated with direct healthcare expenditures for medications and hospitalizations, and indirect costs associated with lost productivity. These costs vary widely between countries and regions within countries.[91–94]

These variations in asthma prevalence, disability, and mortality are likely attributable to population differences in the many complex gene-environment mechanisms involved in the development of asthma as well as differences in healthcare access and quality (Fuchs 2017-figure 2) (Fig. 56-2). While asthma is the most common chronic condition of childhood, the time course and transition to adulthood is highly variable, and only 3–5% of children have persistent asthma symptoms into adulthood.[45] Risk factors associated with persistence are family history of asthma, childhood allergy, early life respiratory tract infections, active smoking starting in adolescence, and impaired lung function.[45,95]

Other risk factors for asthma in adults include personal characteristics, lifestyle, and environmental exposures. Among adolescents and adults, asthma is more common among females compared to children, where asthma is more common among males.[45] This difference may be explained by differences in airway geometry and increased bronchial hyperresponsiveness among adult females compared to males. However, the higher incidence in older women may partly be explained by physician bias in labelling obstructive lung disease in women as asthma rather than COPD. Asthma may be misdiagnosed, often because of lack of spirometric testing, in about 30% of individuals with physician-diagnosed asthma.[96]

A number of lifestyle characteristics and environmental exposures have been investigated as potential factors contributing to the rising occurrence of asthma in adults including obesity, smoking, and environmental/occupational exposures.[45] A consistent finding in children and adults has been the association between increasing weight and increased risk for asthma.[97] While active or involuntary smoking worsens asthma symptoms, evidence for new-onset asthma has been inconsistent,[98] and the inconsistency may be partly attributed to methodological differences between studies.

While early life exposures to a farming environment is associated with decreased risk for childhood asthma, it has not been found among adults,[99] and is more likely a cause of occupational asthma.[100] Workplace exposures may cause new-onset asthma through different mechanisms (i.e., immunologic sensitization, airway irritants), or exacerbate pre-existing asthma.[100] Globally about 10% of asthma burden are attributed to occupational exposures and about 8% to smoking.[90] However, the population attributable risk for occupational exposures has ranged from 5% to 30% depending on the methods used to define asthma and exposure.[100,101]

As discussed previously, emerging evidence suggests that the potential for primary prevention of asthma starts in early childhood through multifaceted interventions. However, except for occupational asthma,[100] there is little evidence that targeting other risk factors associated with new-onset adult asthma, including lower respiratory tract infections, obesity, or atopic sensitization are effective for primary prevention of adult-onset asthma. Replacement of agents known to cause occupational asthma,[102] or prompt recognition and avoidance are the main strategies for prevention of occupational asthma.[100]

Like children, the control of asthma is primarily accomplished by optimizing management with inhaled corticosteroids, combined with long-acting bronchodilators when appropriate, and avoidance of triggers.[58,103] While difficult to control and death from asthma are uncommon,[60] the highest rate of asthma-related deaths occur in older (>65 years of age) females, African Americans, and Hispanics.[104] However, the overall decline in mortality from asthma worldwide (Table 56-1), particularly among high-income countries, suggests that access to healthcare and optimizing asthma management has been effective.[90]

Chronic Obstructive Pulmonary Disease

Compared to asthma, the worldwide prevalence of COPD is about half as common (Table 56-1), but has an age-standardized mortality rate eightfold higher (Table 56-2).[90] Globally, between 1990 and 2015, COPD prevalence increased 44.2% due to population growth and ageing. However, the relative changes in prevalence varied widely by country SDI, with the greatest increases in prevalence among middle-(104.8%) and low-middle-SDI (74.3%) countries, and the smallest increase among high SDI countries (35.3%).

In 2015, COPD was the third leading cause of death worldwide after cardiovascular diseases and cancers.[1] Changes in numbers of deaths between 1990 and 2015, was greatest among low-(68.8%), low-middle- (51.5%), and high-SDI (31.6%) countries, whereas deaths from COPD declined among high-middle- (−11.1%) and middle-SDI (−3.4%) countries.

COPD ranked eighth in disability adjusted life years in 2015, accounting for 2.6% of the global burden of disease among 315 causes.[90] COPD results in a large economic burden associated with direct healthcare expenditures for medications and hospitalizations and indirect costs associated with lost productivity.[105,106] Moreover, the increasing prevalence of COPD will create growing demand for healthcare services.[107,108] These costs vary widely between countries and regions within countries.[106,109,110] Smoking, ambient particulate air pollution, household air pollution, occupational particulates, ozone, and second-hand smoke explain over 70% of DALY worldwide.[90] Smoking has the greatest contribution among high SDI countries (54.8%) and environmental and occupational risks have a relatively low contribution (7.0%).[90] Whereas the reverse is found among low-SDI countries where smoking contribution is relatively low (7.9%) and environmental and occupational risks contributions are substantially higher (40.4%).[90]

COPD is a clinically applied term for persistent and generally symptomatic obstruction to airflow within the lungs.[106] However, the phenotypic expression is heterogeneous. The lungs of most persons with COPD display a mixture of emphysema, enlargement and destruction of the air spaces, and inflammation and narrowing of the smaller airways, although emphysema or airway abnormalities may predominate. Emphysema reduces the driving pressure for airflow, and the airway abnormalities increase the resistance to airflow. Moreover, chronic airway remodeling in patients with asthma may result in irreversible loss of lung function,[111] and have features of asthma and COPD, which is associated with poorer prognosis.[112]

The natural history of COPD generally follows a slow but progressive course that offers a lengthy time window for intervention. The results of epidemiological studies suggest that impaired lung growth from smoking during childhood and adolescence[17] and sustained loss of ventilatory function beyond that expected from aging alone causes clinically evident COPD. The rate of decline in smokers tends to increase with the amount smoked, and smoking cessation results in a slower rate of decline compared with that in smokers unable to quit.[113,114]

In developed countries, 80–90% of COPD is attributed to smoking.[106,114] However, only 15–20% of smokers develop COPD, which suggests genetic variations affecting susceptibility to toxic effects of cigarette smoke and other environmental exposures.[115] Moreover, only about 1% of cases of COPD, distinguished by severe emphysema, occur in smokers and nonsmokers with a genetic deficiency of alpha-1-antitrypsin, a substance that defends against injury by proteolytic enzymes. Growing evidence supports an increased risk for COPD among heterozygote MZ alpha-1-antitrypsin genotype.[116] Occupational agents can also contribute to the development of COPD.[117,118] Other postulated risk factors for COPD include maternal smoking during pregnancy, premature birth and BPD, childhood respiratory tract infection, and hyperresponsiveness of the airways of the lung.[17] Moreover, there is emerging evidence for a role of the lung microbiome in the development of COPD.[20]

Clinicians make the diagnosis of COPD in patients with sufficient chronic airflow obstruction to result in shortness of breath and limitation of exercise capacity. In epidemiological studies, COPD is considered to be present if lung function tests demonstrate a specified degree of impairment or if a physician's diagnosis is reported. Although prevalence can be readily assessed with the use of these criteria, a physician's diagnosis alone may result in substantial diagnostic misclassification because the symptoms of COPD are nonspecific, spirometry is underutilized, or variations in spirometric criteria of airflow obstruction all may contribute to under and overdiagnosis of COPD.[119–122]

The single-most important strategy for the prevention of COPD is to never start smoking or quit at a young age.[123] Other prevention strategies include minimizing indoor and outdoor air pollution, and occupational exposures.[103] The slow evolution of COPD provides an opportunity to identify and to target for intervention the smokers in whom the disease is developing. With sustained smoking, lung function among smokers declines at a more rapid rate.[113,114] Lung function testing of chronic smokers can identify individuals whose function has dropped below the range of normal values but not yet reached the degree of impairment associated with frank COPD. However, screening for asymptomatic airflow obstruction has not been recommended as an effective preventive strategy.[124]

Acute Respiratory Distress Syndrome

First described in the late 1960s, the clinical syndrome of acute respiratory distress syndrome (ARDS) is characterized by increased lung permeability, edema, and inflammation in response to and occurring within 7 days of a "direct" or "indirect" lung insult.[125,126] Examples of direct lung insults include pneumonia, aspiration of gastric contents, pulmonary contusion, inhalation injury and near drowning. Indirect lung insults are serious systemic illnesses (such as nonpulmonary sepsis, trauma, pancreatitis, drug overdose) that trigger the lung injury response despite originating outside the lungs.[125] Both direct and indirect insults lead to a common presentation of bilateral opacities on chest imaging and acute hypoxemic respiratory failure often requiring mechanical ventilator support.[126] Though a necessary treatment, mechanical ventilation is increasingly recognized as a risk factor that can potentiate the original lung injury. Despite significant improvements over time, ARDS remains a lethal disease with an in-hospital mortality rate of 45%.[127] Additionally, survivors suffer from high rates of prolonged cognitive and physical function impairments as well as mood disorders including depression and posttraumatic stress disorder.[128]

Estimates of the incidence of ARDS range from 20 to 86 cases per 100,000.[129] The wide range may be in part be explained by a clinical definition that has evolved over time. However, it may also be an underestimate of the true incidence as the definition includes imaging and blood gas criteria that are not widely available in low-income countries and a significant number of clinicians fail to recognize ARDS even when all criteria are met.[125]

Despite decades of research, there are no effective pharmacologic therapies to reverse ARDS once already established, and treatment largely consists of supportive care and reducing additional ventilator-induced lung injury.[130] Hence, there is new focus on strategies to prevent ARDS through primary and secondary prevention strategies. Examples of primary prevention efforts include vaccination to reduce the incidence of influenza and pneumococcal pneumonia and standardized anesthesia practices to avoid perioperative aspiration events.[130] Not all patients with risk factors for lung injury (e.g., pneumonia, sepsis, pancreatitis) will go on to develop ARDS.[131] Secondary prevention strategies involve preventing additional iatrogenic lung injury such as avoidance of unnecessary blood transfusions and use of lung protective ventilation to avoid a "second hit" that triggers ARDS in an at-risk patient.[130]

Pulmonary Thromboembolism

Venous thromboembolism includes deep vein thrombosis (DVT) and pulmonary embolism (PE).[132] PE is a common consequence of DVT, whereby a blood clot travels from the deep vein where it originated and lodges in one or more pulmonary arteries. Depending on the degree of resultant right heart strain and the individual's ability to compensate for this physiologic stress, patients with PE present on a spectrum of trivial symptoms to fatal cardiovascular collapse.[132]

PE is a common medical illness with available estimates of incidence ranging from 29 to 78 per 100,000 person-years, increasing with advanced age.[133] Of these individuals, many will suffer recurrences, develop chronic pulmonary hypertension or experience reduced exercise tolerance, poorer quality of life and decreased life expectancy.[132,134] Incidence of PE appears to be increasing over time though it remains unclear whether this is due to widespread access to improved diagnostic imaging with computed tomography (CT) pulmonary angiography or a true increase in disease occurrence.[134,135]

Once diagnosed with pulmonary angiography, PE patients are risk-stratified into low-, medium-, and high-risk groups, which carry short-term mortality rates of $< 1\%$, 5–15%, and up to 50%, respectively.[132] However, PE mortality appears to be declining both in the United States and worldwide.[134,136] A 30-year nationwide population-based cohort in Denmark over the period of 1980–2011 suggests that the observed PE mortality reduction is primarily explained by dramatic improvements in historic 30-day mortality rates.[134] A number of patient characteristics have been associated with increased mortality including obesity, increasing age, being male and black, and associated comorbid conditions (e.g., trauma, cancer).[134]

Identification of venous thromboembolism risk factors is key to both diagnosis and prevention of PE. Risk factors are categorized as inherited (e.g., genetic mutations causing coagulation disorders) or acquired (e.g., prolonged immobilization causing venous stasis, trauma causing endothelial damage).[132,137] Acquired risk factors are further subgrouped into those that arise from a temporary condition (e.g., pregnancy, indwelling catheters, air travel) and those that are chronic (e.g., inflammatory conditions such as malignancy).[132,137] In 40–50% of PE events, no predisposition is identified, highlighting the difficulty in suspecting PE as a diagnosis. In some cases, the patient has not yet been diagnosed with their predisposing chronic disease. Other "idiopathic" PE cases may be explained by diseases whose association with PE is underrecognized (e.g., inflammatory bowel disease), or a combination of recently recognized "minor" PE risk factors such as obesity, advanced age, smoking, hypertension, and certain infectious or endocrine illnesses.[137]

The current primary prevention strategy for PE includes uniformly administering mechanical or pharmacologic thromboprophylaxis to specific groups of individuals known to be at high risk for venous thromboembolism (e.g., hospitalized medical patients, patients undergoing major orthopedic surgery).[138] Current recommendations have been reviewed elsewhere and balance the individual's risk of thrombosis with that of bleeding complications from the prevention agent.[138]

Interstitial Lung Diseases

The ILDs, also referred to as diffuse parenchymal lung diseases, are a heterogeneous group of disorders comprising more than 200 entities, many of which are rare with no known cause.[139] ILDs result from injury to and abnormal healing of the distal lung parenchyma causing common clinical symptoms and characteristic radiographic and histologic patterns.[140] Many ILDs cause irreversible lung damage leading to disability (Table 56-1) and death (Table 56-1). From 2005 to 2015, the global number of deaths from ILD has increased by 51%.[1] This trend is even more pronounced in the United States, where over the period of 1980–2014, ILD deaths increased from 2.7 to 5.5 per 100,000 population, with certain geographic areas sustaining mortality rates up to 15 per 100,000 population.[89]

The true prevalence and incidence of ILD is difficult to ascertain due to evolving ILD classification systems, changing diagnostic strategies, different epidemiologic data sources (e.g., administrative databases, population-based studies and registries) and the paucity of studies evaluating collective ILD epidemiology rather than that of individual diseases.[139] In one United States population-based study, the overall ILD prevalence was higher in men compared with that in women, at 81 per 100,000 and 67 per 100,000, respectively.[141] The overall incidence was 32 per 100,000/year among men and 26 per 100,000/year among women.[141] Relatively similar rates were observed in more recent population cohorts in Denmark,[142] France,[143] and Turkey.[144] With the widespread use of chest CT imaging, there is a growing population of patients with "subclinical ILD," or incidentally discovered radiographic interstitial lung abnormalities in the absence of disease symptoms.[145] This may be an opportunity for earlier ILD diagnosis. Alternatively, since not all interstitial lung abnormalities represent an active process that will progress to clinical disease, this may also lead to overdiagnosis.

ILDs are grouped into five major clinical categories including those associated with connective tissue disease (CTD-ILD), drug and treatment-related (e.g., radiation-induced pneumonitis), primary or unclassified (e.g., sarcoidosis, lymphangioleiomyomatosis), occupational/environmental and the idiopathic interstitial pneumonias [e.g., idiopathic pulmonary fibrosis (IPF), nonspecific interstitial pneumonia].[140,146] The most common ILDs are IPF, sarcoidosis, hypersensitivity pneumonitis, CTD-ILD, drug induced, and pneumoconiosis, with wide variation in the relative distribution according to sampled populations.[143,144,147–150] In a U.S. ILD cohort, "unclassifiable ILDs," or those in which no specific diagnosis can be assigned despite best diagnostic efforts, represented 10% of the overall cohort, highlighting the challenges of definitive ILD subtyping.[151] Of the ILDs, IPF is the most lethal, with a median survival of only 2.5–3.5 years.[152]

Both endogenous and environmental factors have been proposed as determinants of ILDs. Epigenetic processes, where environmental exposures lead to DNA modifications and pathologic gene expression in susceptible individuals, are increasingly recognized as a likely explanation for the mechanism of IPF.[153] The environmental exposures causing some ILDs are known (e.g., silicosis, asbestosis) and can be successfully eliminated through governmental and occupational regulation.[101] However, the etiology of most ILDs remains unknown, limiting disease prevention efforts. A recent prospective cohort of healthy adults followed over 10 years demonstrated that subclinical ILD detected on CT scans was associated with self-reported occupational exposure to vapors/gas, dust, and fumes.[154] Indeed, multiple studies support the hypothesis that IPF is a heterogeneous disease caused and worsened by inhalation of a variety of airborne environmental and occupational particulates,[155] including air pollution.[156] While awaiting additional studies that more conclusively reveal specific associations between environmental agents and ILD, prevention should focus on policies that eliminate inhaled particulate matter. Additionally, some idiopathic ILDs are classified as smoking related,[157] suggesting yet another justification of tobacco reduction efforts.

Sleep Apnea

The obstructive sleep apnea (OSA) syndrome is characterized by excessive daytime sleepiness and episodes of upper airway collapse during sleep causing cessation (apneas) or reduction of breathing flow (hypopneas).[158] Recurrent apneas and hypopneas cause fragmented sleep and can result in repetitive hypoxia and inappropriate sympathetic nervous system activation.[159] OSA has been independently associated with automobile and occupational accidents,[160] decreased quality of life, and may in part cause or contribute to the severity of common chronic diseases including hypertension, heart failure, coronary artery disease, cardiac arrhythmias, stroke, diabetes, and chronic obstructive lung disease.[159] OSA is also associated with increased cardiovascular mortality.[161]

The prevalence of moderate to severe OSA in the general population is estimated at 6–17%[162] and has significantly increased over the last several decades.[163] The prevalence is higher among men, obese persons, and increases substantially with age.[162] Thus, sleep apnea can be expected to pose a greater public health burden on aging and increasingly obese communities.

Given the association between obesity and OSA, weight reduction is a means of both preventing and reducing the severity of OSA, but offers limited improvement unless body weight is substantially reduced.[158] For moderate to severe sleep apnea, continuous positive airway pressure through a face or nasal mask is the main treatment modality.[158] Treatment improves daytime sleepiness and overall quality of life but the long-term impact on important medical co-morbidities such as cardiovascular disease remains unclear.[158]

CONCLUSIONS

Respiratory diseases are common causes of morbidity and mortality worldwide, and many of these diseases can be prevented. Because the occurrence of the various respiratory diseases varies widely in different geographic locations, epidemiological data are important for development of prevention strategies. Over the past 25 years, there has been substantial declines in mortality for many of the respiratory diseases. However, this has been associated with increases in prevalence and disability associated with chronic respiratory diseases. Moreover, in addition to tobacco smoking, which continues to be a major cause of avoidable respiratory disease from the prenatal period through adulthood, air pollution and occupational exposures are a growing cause for concern.

REFERENCES

1. GBD 2015 Mortality and Causes of Death Collaborators. Global, regional, and national life expectancy, all-cause mortality, and cause-specific mortality for 249 causes of death, 1980–2015: A systematic analysis for the global burden of disease study 2015. *Lancet.* 2016;388:1459–544.
2. GBD 2015 Disease and Injury Incidence and Prevalence Collaborators. Global, regional, and national incidence, prevalence, and years lived with disability for 310 diseases and injuries, 1990–2015: A systematic analysis for global burden of disease study 2015. *Lancet.* 2016;388:1545–602.
3. Global Burden of Disease Child and Adolescent Health Collaboration. Child and adolescent health from 1990 to 2015: Findings from the global burden of dieases, injures, and risk factors 2015 study. *JAMA Pediatr.* 2017;171:573–92.
4. GBD 2015 Risk Factors Collaborators. Global, regional, and national comparative risk assessment of 79 behavioural, environmental and occupational, and metabolic risks or clusters of risks, 1990–2015: A systematic analysis for the global burden of disease study 2015. *Lancet.* 2016;388:1659–724.
5. GBD 2015 Tobacco Collaborators. Smoking prevalence and attributable disease burden in 195 countries and territories, 1990–2015: A systemic analysis from the global burden of disease study 2015. *Lancet.* 2017;389:1885–906.
6. Cohen AJ, Brauer M, Burnett R, et al. Estimates and 25-year trends of the global burden of disease attributable to ambient air pollution: An analysis of data from the global burden of diseases study 2015. *Lancet.* 2017;389(10082):1907–18.
7. Landrigan PJ, Fuller R, Acosta NJR, et al. The Lancet Commission on pollution and health. *Lancet.* 2018;391(10119):462–512.
8. Watts N, Adger WN, Ayeb-Karlsson S, et al. The Lancet countdown: Tracking progress on health and climate change. *Lancet.* 2017;389(10074):1151–64.
9. Degeling C, Johnson J, Kerridge I, et al. Implementing a One Health approach to emerging infectious disease: Reflections on the socio-political, ethical and legal dimensions. *BMC Public Health.* 2015;15(1):1307.

10. Hill-Cawthorne GA, Sorrell TC. Future directions for public health research in emerging infectious diseases. *Public Health Res Pract.* 2016;26(5):2651655.

11. Paules CI, Eisinger RW, Marston HD, Fauci AS. What recent history has taught us about responding to emerging infectious disease threats. *Ann Intern Med.* 2017;167(11):805.

12. Bayram H, Bauer AK, Abdalati W, et al. Environment, global climate change, and cardiopulmonary health. *Am J Respir Crit Care Med.* 2017;195(6):718–24.

13. Collins FS, Varmus H. A new initiative on precision medicine. *N Engl J Med.* 2015;372(9):793–5.

14. Parikh RB, Schwartz JS, Navathe AS. Beyond genes and molecules—A precision delivery initiative for precision medicine. *N Engl J Med.* 2017;376(17):1609–12.

15. Greene JA, Loscalzo J. Putting the patient back together—Social medicine, network medicine, and the limits of reductionism. *N Engl J Med.* 2017;377(25):2493–9.

16. Stocks J HA, Sonnappa S. Early lung development: Lifelong effect on repiratory health and disease. *Lancet Respir Med.* 2013;1:748–2.

17. Martinez FD, Drazen JM. Early-life origins of chronic obstructive pulmonary disease. *N Engl J Med.* 2016;375(9):871–8.

18. Castro-Rodriguez JA, Forno E, Rodriguez-Martinez CE, Celedón JC. Risk and protective factors for childhood asthma: What is the evidence? *J Allergy Clin Immunol.* 2016;4(6):1111–22.

19. Man WH, de Steenhuijsen Piters WAA, Bogaert D. The microbiota of the respiratory tract: Gatekeeper to respiratory health. *Nat Rev Microbiol.* 2017;15(5):259–70.

20. Sze M, Hogg J, Sin D. Bacterial microbiome of lungs in COPD. *Int J Chron Obstruct Pulmon Dis.* 2014;9: 229–38.

21. Isayama T, Lee SK, Yang J, et al. Revisiting the definition of bronchopulmonary dysplasia. *JAMA Pediatr.* 2017;171(3):271.

22. Poindexter BB, Feng R, Schmidt B, et al. Comparisons and limitations of current definitions of bronchopulmonary dysplasia for the prematurity and respiratory outcomes program. *Ann Am Thorac Soc.* 2015;12(12):1822–30.

23. Stoll BJ, Hansen NI, Bell EF, et al. Trends in care practices, morbidity, and mortality of extremely preterm neonates, 1993–2012. *JAMA.* 2015;314(10):1039.

24. Manuck TA, Levy PT, Gyamfi-Bannerman C, Jobe AH, Blaisdell CJ. Prenatal and perinatal determinants of lung health and disease in early life. *JAMA Pediatr.* 2016;170(5):e154577.

25. Shapiro-Mendoza CK, Barfield WD, Henderson Z, James A, Howse JL, Iskander J. Thorpe PG. CDC grand rounds: Public health strategies to prevent preterm birth. *MMWR.* 2016;65(32):826–30.

26. Lagatta JM, Clark RH, Brousseau DC, Hoffmann RG, Spitzer AR. Varying patterns of home oxygen use in infants at 23–43 weeks' gestation discharged from United States neonatal intensive care units. *J Pediatr.* 2013;163(4):976–82.e2.

27. Islam JY, Keller RL, Aschner JL, Hartert TV, Moore PE. Understanding the short- and long-term respiratory outcomes of prematurity and bronchopulmonary dysplasia. *Am J Respir Crit Care Med.* 2015;192(2):134–56.

28. Morrow LA, Wagner BD, Ingram DA, et al. Antenatal determinants of bronchopulmonary dysplasia and late respiratory disease in preterm infants. *Am J Respir Crit Care Med.* 2017;196(3):364–74.

29. Stringer J, Stringer E, Smid M. A worldwide epidemic: The problem and challenges of preterm birth in low- and middle-income countries. *Am J Perinatol.* 2016;33(03):276–89.

30. Sweet DG, Carnielli V, Greisen G, et al. European consensus guidelines on the management of respiratory distress syndrome—2016 Update. *Neonatology.* 2017;111(2):107–25.

31. Sanders DB, Fink AK. Background and epidemiology. *Pediatr Clin North Am.* 2016;63(4):567–84.

32. Ioannou L, McClaren BJ, Massie J, et al. Population-based carrier screening for cystic fibrosis: A systematic review of 23 years of research. *Genet Med.* 2013;16(3):207–16.

33. Elborn JS. Cystic fibrosis. *Lancet.* 2016;388(10059):2519–31.

34. Stephenson AL, Sykes J, Stanojevic S, et al. Survival comparison of patients with cystic fibrosis in Canada and the United States. *Ann Intern Med.* 2017;166(8):537.

35. Burgel P-R, Bellis G, Olesen HV, et al. Future trends in cystic fibrosis demography in 34 European countries. *Eur Respir J.* 2015;46(1):133–41.

36. Schwarz C, Hartl D. Cystic fibrosis in Europe: Patients live longer but are we ready? *Eur Respir J.* 2015;46(1):11–2.

37. Castellani C, Massie J, Sontag M, Southern KW. Newborn screening for cystic fibrosis. *Lancet Respir Med.* 2016;4(8):653–61.

38. Coffey MJ, Whitaker V, Gentin N, et al. Differences in outcomes between early and late diagnosis of cystic fibrosis in the newborn screening era. *J Pediatr.* 2017;181:137–45.e1.

39. Wishaupt JO, van der Ploeg T, de Groot R, Versteegh FGA, Hartwig NG. Single- and multiple viral respiratory infections in children: Disease and management cannot be related to a specific pathogen. *BMC Infect Dis.* 2017;17(1):62.

40. Kumar P, Medigeshi GR, Mishra VS, et al. Etiology of acute respiratory infections in infants. *Pediatr Infect Dis J.* 2017;36(1):25–30.

41. van Meel ER, Jaddoe VWV, Bønnelykke K, de Jongste JC, Duijts L. The role of respiratory tract infections and the microbiome in the development of asthma: A narrative review. *Pediatr Pulmonol.* 2017;52(10):1363–70.

42. GBD 2015 LRI Collaborators, Troeger C, Forouzanfar M, et al. Estimates of the global, regional, and national morbidity, mortality, and aetiologies of lower respiratory tract infections in 195 countries: A systematic analysis for the Global Burden of Disease Study 2015. *Lancet Infect Dis.* 2017;17(11):1133–61.

43. Lafond KE, Nair H, Rasooly MH, et al. Global role and burden of influenza in pediatric respiratory hospitalizations, 1982–2012: A systematic analysis. *PLoS Med.* 2016;13(3):e1001977.

44. Shi T, McAllister DA, O'Brien KL, et al. Global, regional, and national disease burden estimates of acute lower respiratory infections due to respiratory syncytial virus in young children in 2015: A systematic review and modelling study. *Lancet.* 2017;390(10098):946–58.

45. Fuchs O, Bahmer T, Rabe KF, von Mutius E. Asthma transition from childhood into adulthood. *Lancet Respir Med.* 2017;5(3):224–34.

46. Dratva J, Zemp E, Dharmage SC, et al. Early life origins of lung ageing: Early life exposures and lung function decline in adulthood in two European cohorts aged 28–73 years. *PLoS One.* 2016;11(1):e0145127.

47. Khan SJ, Dharmage SC, Matheson MC, Gurrin LC. Is the atopic march related to confounding by genetics and early-life environment? A systematic review of sibship and twin data. *Allergy.* 2018;73(1):17–28.

48. Sonego M, Pellegrin MC, Becker G, Lazzerini M. Risk factors for mortality from acute lower respiratory infections (ALRI) in children under five years of age in low and middle-income countries: A systematic review and meta-analysis of observational studies. *PLoS One.* 2015;10(1):e0116380.

49. Onakpoya IJ, Hayward G, Heneghan CJ, Onakpoya IJ. Antibiotics for preventing lower respiratory tract infections in high-risk children aged 12 years. *Cochrane Database Syst Rev.* 2015;(9):CD011530.

50. Ruopp M, Chiswell K, Thaden JT, Merchant K, Tsalik EL. Respiratory tract infection clinical trials from 2007 to 2012. A systematic review of ClinicalTrials.gov. *Ann Am Thorac Soc.* 2015;12(12):1852–63.

51. Gill PJ, Richardson SE, Ostrow O, Friedman JN. Testing for respiratory viruses in children. *JAMA Pediatr.* 2017;171(8):798.

52. McCloskey B, Dar O, Zumla A, Heymann DL. Emerging infectious diseases and pandemic potential: Status quo and reducing risk of global spread. *Lancet Infect Dis.* 2014;14(10):1001–10.

53. Zumla A, Hui DS, Al-Tawfiq JA, Gautret P, McCloskey B, Memish ZA. Emerging respiratory tract infections. *Lancet Infect Dis.* 2014;14(10):910–11.

54. Larkin EK, Hartert TV. Genes associated with RSV lower respiratory tract infection and asthma: The application of genetic epidemiological methods to understand causality. *Future Virol.* 2015;10(7):883–97.

55. Adegbola RA, DeAntonio R, Hill PC, et al. Carriage of Streptococcus pneumoniae and other respiratory bacterial pathogens in low and lower-middle income countries: A systematic review and meta-analysis. *PLoS One.* 2014;9(8):e103293.

56. Breiman RF, Van Beneden CA, Farnon EC. Surveillance for respiratory infections in low- and middle-income countries: Experience from the centers for disease control and prevention's global disease detection international emerging infections program. *Int J Infect Dis.* 2013;208(suppl 3):S167–72.

57. Quinn RA. Integrating microbiome and metabolome data to understand infectious airway disease. *Am J Respir Crit Care Med.* 2017;196(7):806–7.

58. Global Initiative for Asthma. Global Strategy for Asthma Management and Prevention, 2017.

59. Martinez FD, Vercelli D. Asthma. *Lancet.* 2013;382(9901):1360–72.

60. Israel E, Drazen JM, Reddel HK. Severe and difficult-to-treat asthma in adults. *N Eng J Med.* 2017;377(10):965–76.

61. Ellwood P, Asher MI, Billo NE, et al. The Global Asthma Network rationale and methods for Phase I global surveillance: Prevalence, severity, management and risk factors. *Eur Respir J.* 2017;49(1):1601605.

62. Uphoff EP, Bird PK, Antó JM, et al. Variations in the prevalence of childhood asthma and wheeze in MeDALL cohorts in Europe. *ERJ Open Res.* 2017;3(3):00150–2016.

63. Sullivan PW, Ghushchyan V, Navaratnam P, et al. The national cost of asthma among school-aged children in the United States. *Ann Allergy Asthma Immunol.* 2017;119(3):246–52.e1.
64. DeVries A, Vercelli D. Epigenetic mechanisms in asthma. *Ann Am Thorac Soc.* 2016;13(Suppl 1):S48–50.
65. Geier DA, Kern JK, Geier MR. Demographic and neonatal risk factors for childhood asthma in the USA. *J Matern Fetal Neonatal Med.* 2019;32(5):833–7.
66. Kashanian M, Mohtashami SS, Bemanian MH, Moosavi SAJ, Moradi Lakeh M. Evaluation of the associations between childhood asthma and prenatal and perinatal factors. *Int J Gynaecol Obstet.* 2017;137(3):290–4.
67. Rusconi F, Gagliardi L. Pregnancy complications and wheezing and asthma in childhood. *Am J Respir Crit Care Med.* 2018;197(5):580–8.
68. Prescott SL. Maternal allergen exposure as a risk factor for childhood asthma. *Curr Allergy Asthma Rep.* 2006;6:75–80.
69. Wolsk HM, Chawes BL, Litonjua AA, et al. Prenatal vitamin D supplementation reduces risk of asthma/recurrent wheeze in early childhood: A combined analysis of two randomized controlled trials. *PLoS One.* 2017;12(10):e0186657.
70. Bisgaard H HM, Buchvald F, Loland L, et al. Childhood asthma after bacterial colonization of the airway in neonates. *N Engl J Med.* 2007;357:1478–95.
71. Feldman AS, He Y, Moore ML, Hershenson MB, Hartert TV. Toward primary prevention of asthma. Reviewing the evidence for early-life respiratory viral infections as modifiable risk factors to prevent childhood asthma. *Am J Respir Crit Care Med.* 2015;191(1):34–44.
72. Mueller-Rompa S, Janke T, et al. Identification of fungal candidates for asthma protection in a large population-based study. *Pediatr Allergy Immunol.* 2017;28(1):72–8.
73. Lynch SV, Wood RA, Boushey H, et al. Effects of early-life exposure to allergens and bacteria on recurrent wheeze and atopy in urban children. *J Allergy Clin Immunol.* 2014;134(3):593–601.e12.
74. O'Connor GT, Lynch SV, Bloomberg GR, et al. Early-life home environment and risk of asthma among inner-city children. *J Allergy Clin Immunol.* 2018;141(4):1468–75.
75. Ege MJ, Mayer M, Normand A-C, et al. Exposure to environmental microorganisms and childhood asthma. *N Engl J Med.* 2011;364(8):701–9.
76. Genuneit J. Exposure to farming environments in childhood and asthma and wheeze in rural populations: A systematic review with meta-analysis. *Pediatr Allergy Immunol.* 2012;23(6):509–18.
77. Stein MM, Hrusch CL, Gozdz J, et al. Innate Immunity and asthma risk in Amish and Hutterite farm children. *N Eng J Med.* 2016;375(5):411–21.
78. Feng M, Yang Z, Pan L, et al. Associations of early life exposures and environmental factors with asthma among children in rural and urban areas of Guangdong, China. *Chest.* 2016;149(4):1030–41.
79. Tischer C, Chen CM, Heinrich J. Association between domestic mould and mould components, and asthma and allergy in children: A systematic review. *Eur Respir J.* 2011;38(4):812–24.
80. U.S. Department of Health and Human Services. *The Health Consequences of Involuntary Exposure to Tobacco Smoke: A Report of the Surgeon General.* Atlanta, GA: U.S. Department of Health and Human Services, Centers for Disease Control and Prevention, Coordinating Center for Health Promotion, National Center for Chronic Disease Prevention and Health Promotion, Office on Smoking and Health; 2006.
81. Blaisdell RJ, Broadwin RL, Vork KL. Developing asthma in childhood from exposure to second-hand tobacco smoke—Insights from a meta-regression. *Environ Health Perspect.* 2007;115(10):1394–400.
82. Gasana J, Dillikar D, Mendy A, Forno E, Ramos Vieira E. Motor vehicle air pollution and asthma in children: A meta-analysis. *Environ Res.* 2012;117:36–45.
83. Gehring U, Wijga AH, Hoek G, et al. Exposure to air pollution and development of asthma and rhinoconjunctivitis throughout childhood and adolescence: A population-based birth cohort study. *Lancet Respir Med.* 2015;3(12):933–42.
84. Maas T, Kaper J, Sheikh A, et al. Mono and multifaceted inhalant and/or food allergen reduction interventions for preventing asthma in children at high risk of developing asthma. *Cochrane Database Syst Rev.* 2009;(3):CD006480.
85. Wu P, Feldman AS, Rosas-Salazar C, et al. Relative importance and additive effects of maternal and infant risk factors on childhood asthma. *PLoS One.* 2016;11(3):e0151705.
86. Scott M, Roberts G, Kurukulaaratchy RJ, Matthews S, Nove A, Arshad SH. Multifaceted allergen avoidance during infancy reduces asthma during childhood with the effect persisting until age 18 years. *Thorax.* 2012;67(12):1046–51.
87. Gehring U, de Jongste JC, Kerkhof M, et al. The 8-year follow-up of the PIAMA intervention study assessing the effect of mite-impermeable mattress covers. *Allergy.* 2012;67(2):248–56.
88. Guilleminault L, Ouksel H, Belleguic C, et al. Personalised medicine in asthma: From curative to preventive medicine. *Eur Respir Rev.* 2017;26(143):160010.
89. Dwyer-Lindgren L, Bertozzi-Villa A, Stubbs RW, et al. Trends and patterns of differences in chronic respiratory disease mortality among US counties, 1980–2014. *JAMA.* 2017;318(12):1136–49.
90. GBD 2015 Chronic Respiratory Disease Collaborators, Soriano JB, Abajobir AA, et al. Global, regional, and national deaths, prevalence, disability-adjusted life years, and years lived with disability for chronic obstructive pulmonary disease and asthma, 1990–2015: A systematic analysis for the Global Burden of Disease Study 2015. *Lancet Respir Med.* 2017;5(9):691–706.
91. Bahadori K, Doyle-Waters MM, Marra C, et al. Economic burden of asthma: A systematic review. *BMC Pulm Med.* 2009;9(1):24.
92. Ismaila AS, Sayani A, Marin M, Su Z. Clinical, economic, and humanistic burden of asthma in Canada: A systematic review. *BMC Pulm Med.* 2013;13:70.
93. Fletcher M, Jha A, Dunlop W, et al. Patient reported burden of asthma on resource use and productivity across 11 countries in Europe. *Adv Ther.* 2015;32(4):370–80.
94. Mukherjee M, Stoddart A, Gupta RP, et al. The epidemiology, healthcare and societal burden and costs of asthma in the UK and its member nations: Analyses of standalone and linked national databases. *BMC Med.* 2016;14(1):113.
95. Chan JYC, Stern DA, Guerra S, Wright AL, Morgan WJ, Martinez FD. Pneumonia in childhood and impaired lung function in adults: A longitudinal study. *Pediatr.* 2015;135(4):607–16.
96. Aaron SD, Vandemheen KL, FitzGerald JM, et al. Reevaluation of diagnosis in adults with physician-diagnosed asthma. *JAMA.* 2017;317(3):269.
97. Forno E, Han Y-Y, Libman IM, Muzumdar RH, Celedón JC. Adiposity and asthma in a nationwide study of children and adults in the United States. *Ann Am Thorac Soc.* 2018;15(3):322–30.
98. Verlato G, Nguyen G, Marchetti P, et al. Smoking and new-onset asthma in a prospective study on Italian adults. *Int Arch Allergy Immunol.* 2016;170(3):149–57.
99. House JS, Wyss AB, Hoppin JA, et al. Early-life farm exposures and adult asthma and atopy in the Agricultural Lung Health Study. *J Allergy and Clin Immunol.* 2017;140(1):249–56.e14.
100. Tarlo SM, Lemiere C. Occupational asthma. *N Eng J Med.* 2014;370(7):640–9.
101. Cullinan P, Muñoz X, Suojalehto H, et al. Occupational lung diseases: from old and novel exposures to effective preventive strategies. *Lancet Respir Med.* 2017;5(5):445–55.
102. Rosenman KD, Beckett WS. Web based listing of agents associated with new onset work-related asthma. *Respir Med.* 2015;109(5):625–31.
103. Abramson MJ, Koplin J, Hoy R, Dharmage SC. Population-wide preventive interventions for reducing the burden of chronic respiratory disease. *Int J Tuberc Lung Dis.* 2015;19(9):1007–18.
104. Skloot GS, Busse PJ, Braman SS, et al. An official American Thoracic Society workshop report: Evaluation and management of asthma in the elderly. *Ann Am Thorac Soc.* 2016;13(11):2064–77.
105. Singh JA, Yu S. Utilization due to chronic obstructive pulmonary disease and its predictors: A study using the U.S. National Emergency Department Sample (NEDS). *Respir Res.* 2016;17(1):1.
106. Global Strategy for Diagnosis, Management and Prevention of COPD 2017 Update.
107. Gershon A, Thiruchelvam D, Moineddin R, Zhao XY, Hwee J, To T. Forecasting hospitalization and emergency department visit rates for chronic obstructive pulmonary disease. A time-series analysis. *Ann Am Thorac Soc.* 2017;14(6):867–73.
108. Khakban A, Sin DD, FitzGerald JM, et al. The projected epidemic of COPD hospitalizations over the next 15 years: A population based perspective. *Am J Respir Crit Care Med.* 2017;195(3):287–91.
109. Ford ES, Murphy LB, Khavjou O, Giles WH, Holt JB, Croft JB. Total and state-specific medical and absenteeism costs of COPD among adults aged 18 years in the United States for 2010 and projections through 2020. *Chest.* 2015;147(1):31–45.
110. Ehteshami-Afshar S, FitzGerald JM, Doyle-Waters MM, Sadatsafavi M. The global economic burden of asthma and chronic obstructive pulmonary disease. *Int J Tuberc Lung Dis.* 2016;20(1):11–23.
111. Pascual RM, Peters SP. Airway remodeling contributes to the progressive loss of lung function in asthma: An overview. *J Allergy Clin Immunol.* 2005;116(3):477–86.

112. Woodruff PG, van den Berge M, Boucher RC, et al. American Thoracic Society/National Heart, Lung, and Blood Institute Asthma—Chronic obstructive pulmonary disease overlap workshop report. *Am J Respir Crit Care Med.* 2017;196(3):375–81.

113. Anthonisen NR, Connett JE, Kiley JP, et al. Effects of smoking intervention and the use of an inhaled anticholinergic bronchodilator on the rate of decline of FEV1. *JAMA.* 1994;272(19):1497.

114. US Department of Health and Human Services. *The Health Consequences of Smoking: 50 Years of Progress. A Report of the Surgeon General.* Atlanta, GA: US Department of Health and Human Services, Centers for Disease Control and Prevention, National Center for Chronic Disease Prevention and Health Promotion, Office on Smoking and Health; 2014.

115. Lee SD, Kim WJ. Candidate genes for COPD: Current evidence and research. *Int J Chron Obstruct Pulmon Dis.* 2015;10:2249–55.

116. Silverman EK. Risk of lung disease in PI MZ heterozygotes. Current status and future research directions. *Ann Am Thorac Soc.* 2016;13(Suppl_4):S341–5.

117. Blanc PD, Menezes AMB, Plana E, et al. Occupational exposures and COPD: An ecological analysis of international data. *Eur Respir J.* 2008;33(2):298–304.

118. Doney BC, Henneberger PK, Humann MJ, et al. Occupational exposures to vapor-gas, dust, and fumes in a cohort of rural adults in Iowa compared with a cohort of urban adults. *MMWR.* 2017;66(21):1–5.

119. Collins BF, Feemster LC, Rinne ST, Au DH. Factors predictive of airflow obstruction among veterans with presumed empirical diagnosis and treatment of COPD. *Chest.* 2015;147(2):369–76.

120. van Dijk W, Tan W, Li P, et al. Clinical relevance of fixed ratio vs lower limit of normal of FEV1/FVC in COPD: Patient-reported outcomes from the CanCOLD cohort. *Ann Fam Med.* 2015;13(1):41–8.

121. Lamprecht B, Joan BS, Michael S, et al. Determinants of underdiagnosis of COPD in national and international surveys. *Chest.* 2015;148(4):971–85.

122. Quaderi S, Hurst JR. One-off spirometry is insufficient to rule in or rule out mild to moderate chronic obstructive pulmonary disease. *Am J Respir Crit Care Med.* 2017;196(3):254–6.

123. Services USDoHaH. The Health Benefits of Smoking Cessation; 1990.

124. Siu AL, Bibbins-Domingo K, Grossman DC, et al. Screening for chronic obstructive pulmonary disease. *JAMA.* 2016;315(13):1372.

125. Thompson BT, Chambers RC, Liu KD. Acute respiratory distress syndrome. *N Eng J Med.* 2017;377(19):1904–5.

126. Ferguson ND, Fan E, Camporota L, et al. The Berlin definition of ARDS: An expanded rationale, justification, and supplementary material. *Int Care Med.* 2012;38:1573–82.

127. Maca J, Jor O, Holub M, et al. Past and present ARDS mortality rates: A systematic review. *Respir Care.* 2016;62(1):113–22.

128. Herridge MS, Moss M, Hough CL, et al. Recovery and outcomes after the acute respiratory distress syndrome (ARDS) in patients and their family caregivers. *Int Care Med.* 2016;42(5):725–38.

129. Villar J, Blanco J, Kacmarek RM. Current incidence and outcome of the acute respiratory distress syndrome. *Curr Opin Crit Care.* 2016;22(1):1–6.

130. Yadav H, Thompson BT, Gajic O. Fifty years of research in ARDS. Is acute respiratory distress syndrome a preventable disease? *Am J Respir Crit Care Med.* 2017;195(6):725–36.

131. Hudson LD, Milberg JA, Anardi D, Maunder RJ. Clinical risks for development of the acute respiratory distress syndrome. *Am J Respir Crit Care Med.* 1995;151(2):293–301.

132. Giordano NJ, Jansson PS, Young MN, Hagan KA, Kabrhel C. Epidemiology, pathophysiology, stratification, and natural history of pulmonary embolism. *Tech Vasc Interv Radiol.* 2017;20(3):135–40.

133. Heit JA. Epidemiology of venous thromboembolism. *Nat Rev Cardiol.* 2015;12(8):464–74.

134. Sogaard KK, Schmidt M, Pedersen L, Horvath-Puho E, Sorensen HT. 30-Year mortality after venous thromboembolism: A population-based cohort study. *Circulation.* 2014;130(10):829–36.

135. Huang W, Goldberg RJ, Anderson FA, Kiefe CI, Spencer FA. Secular trends in occurrence of acute venous thromboembolism: The worcester VTE study (1985–2009). *Am J Med.* 2014;127(9):829–39.e5.

136. Horlander KT, Mannino DM, Leeper KV. Pulmonary embolism mortality in the United States, 1979–1998. *Arch Intern Med.* 2003;163(14):1711.

137. Riva N, Donadini MP, Ageno W. Epidemiology and pathophysiology of venous thromboembolism: Similarities with atherothrombosis and the role of inflammation. *Thromb Haemost.* 2014;113(6):1176–83.

138. Granziera S, Cohen AT. VTE primary prevention, including hospitalised medical and orthopaedic surgical patients. *Thromb Haemost.* 2015;113(6):1216–23.

139. Demedts M, Wells AU, Antó JM, et al. Interstitial lung diseases: An epidemiological overview. *Eur Respir J.* 2001;18(Suppl 32):2S–16S.

140. Interstitial Lung Disease, 5th ed. Shelton, CT: People's Medical Clearing House; 2011.

141. Coultas DB, Zumwalt RE, Black WC, Sobonya RE. The epidemiology of interstitial lung diseases. *Am J Respir Crit Care Med.* 1994;150(4):967–72.

142. Kornum JB, Christensen S, Grijota M, et al. The incidence of interstitial lung disease 1995–2005: A Danish nationwide population-based study. *BMC Pulm Med.* 2008;8(1):24.

143. Duchemann B, Annesi-Maesano I, Jacobe de Naurois C, et al. Prevalence and incidence of interstitial lung diseases in a multi-ethnic county of Greater Paris. *Eur Respir J.* 2017;50(2):1602419.

144. Musellim B, Okumus G, Uzaslan E, et al. Epidemiology and distribution of interstitial lung diseases in Turkey. *Clin Respir J.* 2014;8(1):55–62.

145. Doyle TJ, Hunninghake GM, Rosas IO. Subclinical interstitial lung disease. *Am J Respir Crit Care Med.* 2012;185(11):1147–53.

146. American Thoracic Society/European Respiratory Society International Multidisciplinary Consensus Classification of the Idiopathic Interstitial Pneumonias. *Am J Respir Crit Care Med.* 2002;165(2):277–304.

147. Thomeer MJ, Costabe U, Rizzato G, Poletti V, Demedts M. Comparison of registries of interstitial lung disease in three European Countries. *Eur Respir J.* 2001;32(Suppl):114s–8s.

148. Singh S, Collins BF, Sharma BB, et al. Interstitial lung disease in India. Results of a prospective registry. *Am J Respir Crit Care Med.* 2017;195(6):801–13.

149. Patterson KC, Shah RJ, Porteous MK, et al. Interstitial lung disease in the elderly. *Chest.* 2017;151(4):838–44.

150. Storme M, Semionov A, Assayag D, et al. Estimating the incidence of interstitial lung diseases in the Cree of Eeyou Istchee, northern Québec. *PLoS One.* 2017;12(9):e0184548.

151. Ryerson CJ, Urbania TH, Richeldi L, et al. Prevalence and prognosis of unclassifiable interstitial lung disease. *Eur Respir J* 2013;42(3):750–57.

152. Ley B, Collard HR, King TE. Clinical course and prediction of survival in idiopathic pulmonary fibrosis. *Am J Respir Crit Care Med.* 2011;183(4):431–40.

153. Helling BA, Yang IV. Epigenetics in lung fibrosis. *Curr Opin Pulm Med.* 2015;21(5):454–62.

154. Sack CS, Doney BC, Podolanczuk AJ, et al. Occupational exposures and subclinical interstitial lung disease. The MESA (Multi-Ethnic Study of Atherosclerosis) air and lung studies. *Am J Respir Crit Care Med.* 2017;196(8):1031–9.

155. Taskar VS, Coultas DB. Is idiopathic pulmonary fibrosis an environmental disease? *Proc Am Thorac Soc.* 2006;3(4):293–8.

156. Winterbottom CJ, Shah RJ, Patterson KC, et al. Exposure to ambient particulate matter is associated with accelerated functional decline in idiopathic pulmonary fibrosis. *Chest.* 2018;153(5):1221–8.

157. Margaritopoulos GA, Harari S, Caminati A, Antoniou KM. Smoking-related idiopathic interstitial pneumonia: A review. *Respirology.* 2016;21(1):57–64.

158. Balachandran JS, Patel SR. Obstructive sleep apnea. *Ann Intern Med.* 2014;161(9):ITC1.

159. Farrell PC, Richards G. Recognition and treatment of sleep-disordered breathing: an important component of chronic disease management. *J Transl Med.* 2017;15(1):114.

160. Terán-Santos J, Jimenez-Gomez A, Cordero-Guevara J. The association between sleep apnea and the risk of traffic accidents. *N Eng J Med.* 1999;340(11):847–51.

161. Loke YK, Brown JWL, Kwok CS, Niruban A, Myint PK. association of obstructive sleep apnea with risk of serious cardiovascular events: A systematic review and meta-analysis. *Circ Cardiovasc Qual Outcomes.* 2012;5(5):720–8.

162. Senaratna CV, Perret JL, Lodge CJ, et al. Prevalence of obstructive sleep apnea in the general population: A systematic review. *Sleep Med Rev.* 2017;34:70–81.

163. Peppard PE, Young T, Barnet JH, Palta M, Hagen EW, Hla KM. Increased prevalence of sleep-disordered breathing in adults. *Am J Epidemiol.* 2013;177(9):1006–14.

CHAPTER 57

Musculoskeletal Disorders

Erin Hammer • M. Alison Brooks • Christie M. Bartels

Globally, musculoskeletal conditions including arthritis and back pain affect 1.5 billion people.[1] They are the second greatest cause of global disability,[1] and in the United States, arthritis and musculoskeletal conditions are the leading cause of disability and physician visits.[2,3] Among U.S. community dwelling adults, 55.4 million people have doctor diagnosed arthritis and musculoskeletal disorders and 23.7 million of those people experience activity limitations, a figure greater than any other disease category (Fig. 57-1).[2–4]According to the 2012 National Health Interview Survey, age adjusted rates for musculoskeletal conditions may be as high as 54% of Americans, compared to 31% and 28% for cardiovascular and respiratory conditions, respectively.[5] Ambulatory visits for arthritis and rheumatic conditions exceed 100 million annually (Table 57-1), and the total U.S. economic cost for musculoskeletal disease was estimated to be $213 billion in 2011.[5] Indirect costs from lost earnings and services represent a particularly high proportion of this cost, since many people are affected during their most productive years.

DISORDERS PRIMARILY OF ADULTS

Low Back and Neck Pain

Between 75% and 85% of people experience low back pain at some time during their lives.[6] One study asked adults to recall the last 3 months, and estimated that 59 million patients self-report low back pain and 30 million report neck pain.[7] Annually, 25% of adults report episodes of back pain which accounted for 53.8 million physician visits in 2012.[5] Most episodes improve within a few weeks, but recurrences are common, and low back pain often becomes a chronic problem with intermittent, usually mild, exacerbations. In a small proportion of cases, the pain becomes constant and severe, and such cases account for a high proportion of the cost; one study found that 25% of the cases accounted for 90% of the costs.[8]

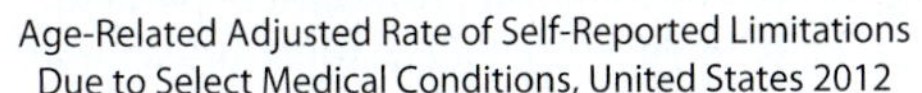

Age-Related Adjusted Rate of Self-Reported Limitations
Due to Select Medical Conditions, United States 2012

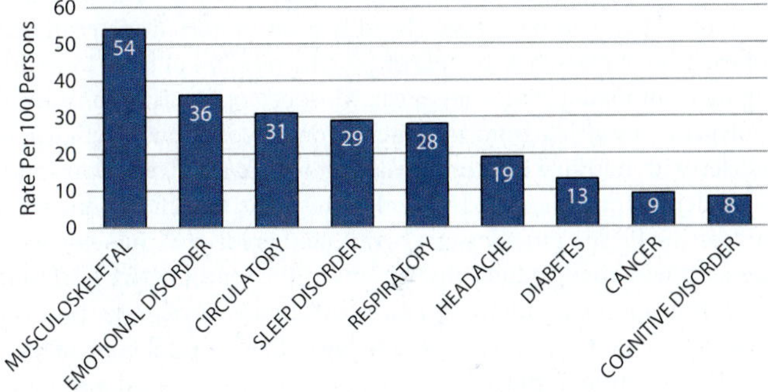

FIGURE 57-1. Estimated number of persons in the United States in 2012 with limitation of activity attributable to specific disease categories. (*Source:* Adapted at https://www.cdc.28gov/nchs/nhis/nhis_2012_data_release.htm.)

It is likely that the different conditions comprising the category "low back pain" (e.g., sprains and strains, disc herniations, spinal stenosis, spondylosis, and spondylolisthesis, facet abnormalities) have different causes. However, the category "low back pain" is generally considered either mechanical or inflammatory. Early in care of mechanical low back pain, techniques, such as magnetic resonance imaging and computerized tomography, are not particularly helpful in most instances because of the low correlation between symptomatology and the abnormalities seen on imaging.[9] For this reason, several professional organizations listed imaging in early low back pain (less than 6 weeks duration) as a target for "Choose Wisely" stewardship campaigns.[10]

Low back pain is more common in people who do heavy manual work than in those whose work is sedentary. Jobs that involve heavy lifting (e.g., of objects weighing 25 lbs or more) are associated with an increase in risk for back pain. Components of lifting that appear to increase the risk for both herniated disc and low back pain, in general, include frequent lifting of heavy objects while bending and twisting the body, holding heavy objects away from the body while lifting, and failing to bend the knees while lifting.[11–13] Several studies have found a modest association between cigarette smoking and low back pain and between smoking and herniated disc, possibly related to decreased diffusion of nutrients into the intervertebral disc.[14] Motor vehicle driving and exposure to other forms of whole body vibration are detrimental to the spine.[12,15–18] Some evidence suggests that height is a risk factor for low back pain, that weight has little or no effect, and that a narrow spinal canal increases the risk, at least for lumbar disc herniation.[19,20] Among possible psychological risk factors, the strongest evidence is for low social support in the workplace and low job satisfaction.[21]

There is significant potential for the prevention of low back pain. One useful approach is the modification of factors in the work place.[7] Training and educational programs implemented among postal workers[22] and nurses[23] have not reduced the frequency of low back problems. Rather, redesigning jobs to minimize bending and twisting motions and the amount of weight lifted may be more likely to decrease the number of back injuries and also may allow an injured worker to return to work sooner. Wearing lumbar supports in some high-risk occupations is sometimes used for primary prevention, but the limited available evidence suggests that it is probably not effective.[24]

Exercises to strengthen back and abdominal muscles and to improve overall fitness can decrease the incidence and duration of low back pain.[25] Other possible methods of primary prevention include cessation of smoking, moving around in situations requiring prolonged exposure to one position, and vibration dampening. Use of

TABLE 57-1 2011 U.S. AMBULATORY VISITS WITH ARTHRITIS AND RHEUMATIC CONDITIONS

Condition	Estimated No. of Visits
Joint pain	35,344,300
Osteoarthritis	21,740,100
Gout	4,979,500
Rheumatoid arthritis	5,246,600
Spondylarthropathies	5,466,600
Diffuse connective tissue diseases	2,430,300
Other rheumatic conditions	28,826,700

Source: Adapted from Helmick CG, Watkins-Castillo SI. *Ambulatory Care Visits in The Burden of Musculoskeletal Diseases in the United States*. US Bone and Joint Initiative. 2014. Rosemont, IL. (Data: 2011 Healthcare Cost and Utilization Project). Available at http://www/boneandjointburden.org/2014-report/ivc20/ambulatory-care-visits.

TABLE 57-2 OUTCOMES OF RANDOMIZED TRIAL OF BED-REST FOR 2 DAYS, BACK EXERCISES VS. NORMAL ACTIVITIES AS TOLERATED IN ACUTE LOW BACK PAIN

Outcome Measure	Bed Rest ($N = 59$)	Exercises ($N = 41$)	Normal Activities ($N = 62$)
Number of sick days	9.2	7.2	4.7
Intensity of pain (11-point scale)	2.1	1.8	1.3
Ability to work (11-point scale)	7.7	7.8	8.5
Lumbar flexion (modified Schober)	6.3	6.0	6.6
Oswestry back-disability index (0–100; higher numbers indicate worsening disability)	11.8	10.8	7.4

Source: Modified from Malmivaara A, Häkkinen U, Aro T, et al. The treatment of acute low back pain—Bed rest, exercises, or ordinary activity? *N Engl J Med*. 1995;332:351–5.

motor vehicles with adjustable seat positioning and good lumbar support, reducing the amount of time professional drivers must drive, and improving the ergonomic properties of their driving situation may also be beneficial.[18,26]

Most back pain improves without any specific therapy. The Centers for Disease Control and Prevention recommends physical therapy, exercise, and nondrug options for chronic pain stating, "Clinicians should consider opioid therapy only if expected benefits for both pain and function are anticipated to outweigh risks to the patient."[27] Predictors of disability from low back pain include long duration of the pain; a history of previous low back pain, disability, and hospitalizations; low educational level and employment grade; psychosocial factors such as dissatisfaction with the job and low social support on the job; heavy physical demands on the job; heavy smoking; whether insurance payments are being received; the perception of fault; and whether a lawyer has been retained.[28–30]

Of considerable importance in tertiary prevention for many people with acute low back pain is a continuation of normal activities to the extent tolerated, minimization of bedrest, and a prompt return to work (Table 57-2).[30,31] Ergonomic redesign or activity moderation (e.g., limits for lifting, burdening or prolonged sitting or standing) may facilitate return to work.[32] Because surgical treatment is often unsatisfactory, conservative approaches such as core strengthening exercises, physical therapy, and chronic back pain classes incorporating behavioral and physical rehab are frequently used for tertiary prevention.[25,33,34]

Between 60% and 70% of the population report neck pain at some time during their lives.[35] As with low back pain, neck pain can be caused by a variety of sources, and recurrences are common. Compared with low back pain, limited research exists regarding the causes of neck pain. Previous neck pain and low back pain are strong predictors.[36,37] Awkward postures, and poorly designed workspaces appear to be associated with mild neck pain. For instance, frequent use of computers with a fixed screen and keyboard height that requires a bent neck can cause neck pain.[38,39] Some evidence indicates that heavy lifting, cigarette smoking, frequent aquatic diving from a board, motor vehicle driving, and exposure to other sources of whole-body vibration increase the risk for neck pain in general or prolapsed cervical intervertebral disc in particular.[40–42] There have been a few reports that repetitive motions, forceful exertions, prolonged neck flexion, or specific arm and trunk motions relate to risk for neck or neck/shoulder pain.[36,39,43] Several psychological factors, including mental or psychological stress, have also been associated with the development of neck pain.[39,44,45]

Little research has been undertaken on the primary prevention of neck pain or on ways to reduce the likelihood of disability among those with neck pain. Encouraging workers using computers to take frequent breaks appears to enhance recovery from neck and upper-limb disorders[46] and might reduce the likelihood of developing neck pain.[47]

Osteoporosis

Osteoporosis, characterized by low bone mass and microarchitectural deterioration of bone tissue leading to enhanced bone fragility and a consequent increased risk of fracture,[48] is present in 10.2 million U.S. adults.[49] Fractures of the hip, vertebrae, and distal radius in the forearm are particularly common. Aging is a leading risk factor, and women are affected four times more often than men.[50] Although osteoporosis may occur secondarily to such conditions as hormonal defects, connective tissue disorders, or certain drug therapies, such as corticosteroids, most cases are idiopathic.

Males have higher baseline bone mass than females, and American Blacks have higher bone mass than non-Hispanic whites, Hispanic whites, and Asian-Americans.[51] After about age 40–50 years, bone mass is lost in both men and women of all racial and ethnic groups, but a particularly rapid decrease occurs in women in the years around and following menopause. It has been estimated that a white woman of age 50 has a 17% chance of fracturing a hip, a 16% chance of fracturing a distal forearm, and a 16% chance of having a clinically diagnosed vertebral fracture during the remainder of her lifetime.[52] One year mortality following a hip fracture is estimated to be 14–58%, making primary osteoporosis prevention important.[53]

Bone mass in later adulthood, when osteoporotic fractures are most common, depends on peak bone mass in young adulthood and rate of subsequent bone loss. Heredity is an important determinant of early bone mass, but the role of genetics on rates of bone loss with aging or in menopause is less clear. Most osteoporosis is considered polygenic, resulting from the interaction of common polymorphic alleles with multiple environmental factors.[54] Weight, physical activity, calcium intake, and possibly other nutrients also affect bone mass across the lifespan to a lesser extent than heredity.[55,56] In some adolescents and young adults, disruptions of the reproductive hormone axis from anorexia, intense athletic activity, and use of progestin-only injectable contraceptives can lead to lower than normal bone mass.[57]

The relatively rapid rate of bone loss in middle-aged and older women has been related to a decrease in estrogen production. Women who have had an oophorectomy have earlier loss of bone mass than other women. On the average, the lower the endogenous estrogen concentration around the time of menopause, the higher the rate of bone loss.[58] Thin women less than 130 pounds are at higher risk than obese women, partly because of their lower estrogen production, lower concentration of circulating estrogens, and the decreased mechanical bone loading.

In the adult years, low dietary calcium consumption is modestly associated with lower bone mass, and calcium supplementation affords some protection.[59,60] The role of other dietary constituents is less clear. It is known that prolonged immobilization may result in loss of bone mass. Weight bearing exercise programs have been shown to have a modest protective effect against loss of bone mass in the lumbar spine and probably the hip as well.[61] Whether exercise reduces the risk for fractures is unclear.[62] Cigarette smoking after menopause increases the risk for osteoporosis and hip fracture.[63] Heavy, alcohol consumption[64] and corticosteroid use[65] are associated with lower bone mass and an increased risk for fracture at all ages, while use of thiazide diuretics is associated with increased bone mass and decreased risk of hip fracture.[58]

Given the large contributions of modifiable risk factors in the etiology of osteoporosis, the potential for prevention is significant. Recommended prevention strategies start with measures to promote adequate bone mass at an early age, such as adequate intake of calcium and vitamin D through diet or sunlight, sufficient physical activity, and not smoking. However, the U.S. Preventive Services Task Force concluded evidence was insufficient to recommend calcium and vitamin D supplementation in healthy premenopausal women and asymptomatic men.[66] In other subgroups, randomized trials indicate that supplemental calcium affords protection against loss of bone mass.[59] Vitamin D formulations can have a positive effect on bone mass, and reduce the frequency of fractures among those with prior fractures, osteoporosis, or vitamin D deficiency.[67,68] Randomized trials have shown that exercise programs involving aerobic activity, weight bearing activity, resistance exercises, and endurance and strength training result in less loss of bone mass.[61,66,69,70]

When lifestyle or nonpharmacologic interventions are inadequate or 10-year risk for hip or other major fracture are high, pharmaceutical agents may also be recommended to prevent or slow loss of bone mass.[71] Although menopausal hormone therapy with estrogen alone or estrogen with progestin protects against loss of bone mass and the occurrence of fractures while it is taken, it is no longer recommended for prevention because of the conclusion by the Women's Health Initiative[72] that its long-term risks outweigh its long-term benefits. Bisphosphonates, such as oral alendronate or IV zoledronate, prevent or slow loss of bone mass and prevent fractures.[73,74] Trials with oral etidronate show less robust protection against fractures.[74] The selective estrogen receptor modulator raloxifene (Evista) has been shown to slow loss of bone mass and to reduce the occurrence of vertebral fractures, but not to reduce the risk for nonvertebral fractures, including hip fracture.[75] Calcitonin may reduce somewhat the likelihood of new vertebral fractures in women who cannot take the other agents.[76] Teriparatide, a recombinant human parathyroid hormone that acts through increasing bone formation, reduces the risk for vertebral and nonvertebral fractures. It is approved for up to 2-year use in patients at high risk for fracture including those who fail bisphosphonates,[76] and other new agents are emerging. In summary, the usefulness of pharmaceutical agents in the treatment of osteoporosis and osteoporotic fractures or prevention of glucocorticoid induced osteoporosis[77] in women is clear, while all are advised to use supportive measures to maintain bone health.

Providers screen healthy perimenopausal and postmenopausal women for high fracture risk by measuring their bone mineral density by dual energy x-ray absorptiometry. The U.S. Preventive Services Task Force recommends screening women who are 65 and older or with fractures, osteoporosis, or whose 10-year fracture risk equals or exceeds a 65-year-old woman.[70] For example, screening is recommended in persons on prolonged glucocorticoids or seizure medications, with medical problems predisposing to low bone density (e.g., celiac), or those with prior low trauma factures.[70] Likewise, screening may be augmented with online risk calculation tools such as the U.S. fracture risk-assessment (FRAX) tool, available at http://www.shef.ac.uk/FRAX/.

Reducing the likelihood of falls among both women and men with osteoporosis may be an important way to prevent fractures. Risk factors for falls include increasing age, female sex, functional limitations (including problems with balance and gait and poor muscle strength), arthritis, depression, orthostatic hypotension, cognitive impairment, visual impairment, various other chronic illnesses, and use of multiple prescription medications.[78,79] Several strategies have demonstrated in randomized controlled trials to reduce the likelihood of falling among older adults.[80]

Whether a fracture results from a fall and the site of the fracture will depend on such factors as the orientation of the fall, a person's ability to initiate protective responses, and the presence of shock absorbers, such as a person's fat, and bone strength.[79,81,82] A history of falls, a recent increase in the number of falls, and previous fractures are predictive of hip fracture,[83] with a pelvic fall doubling risk of a new fall. Architectural and geometrical properties of bone also affect the likelihood of a fracture.[84,85] Randomized trials in nursing homes or other populations at high risk for hip fracture have shown that institutions with programs in which hip protectors are provided have reduced risks for hip fracture, although compliance is poor.[86]

Osteoarthritis

Osteoarthritis (also called OA or degenerative joint disease), affects 27 million Americans and is characterized by focal loss of articular cartilage with proliferation and remodeling of subchondral bone.[7] Manifestations include pain and stiffness accompanied by loss of function, most often in weight bearing joints like knees and hips. The presence and severity of osteoarthritis in most population studies have been classified using radiographic criteria defined in the Atlas of Standard Radiographs of Arthritis.[87] These criteria include osteophytes, bony spurs, joint space narrowing, subchondral cysts, and bony remodeling. Newer imaging technologies characterize other important attributes of the disease processes, including bone marrow edema and irregularities of articular cartilage.[88,89]

Idiopathic osteoarthritis may affect single joint groups (commonly the knees, hands, feet, hips, and spine) or may present as generalized osteoarthritis, characterized by involvement of three or more joint groups and typically affecting perimenopausal and postmenopausal women.[90] Secondary osteoarthritis follows the occurrence of traumatic, congenital, developmental, or systemic disorders involving the joints.

The etiology of osteoarthritis is multifactorial and associated with systemic factors, including obesity, aging, gender, smoking, and heritability. Obesity is known to increase the risk for osteoarthritis of several joints.[91,92] Even in middle age, obesity is associated with more than a twofold increase in knee osteoarthritis.[93] The prevalence and severity of osteoarthritis increases with age and obesity, and rates are rising.[7,94] Under age 45, the age-specific prevalence is higher in men than women, while over age 55, the age-specific prevalence is greater in women than men. Women have a greater number of joints involved and more frequently report morning stiffness, joint swelling, and nocturnal pain.[95] The more common occurrence of Heberden's nodes (distal finger joint nodules) in women is believed to be related to a single autosomal gene that is dominant in women and recessive in men.[96] Heritability estimates from twin studies range from 0.39 to 0.65 and are independent of known risk factors including obesity.[97] Studies have demonstrated linkage of a polymorphism of the type II collagen gene (Col2A1), a collagen found in cartilage, with generalized osteoarthritis.[98]

Repetitive joint trauma associated with athletic or occupational activity can predispose to osteoarthritis. For instance, high prevalence is found in the elbows and knees of miners,[99] in the fingers of cotton pickers,[100] in the hips of farmers,[101] and in the fingers, elbows, and knees of dock workers.[102] Jobs requiring a great deal of knee bending, squatting, kneeling, stair climbing, heavy lifting, and mechanical loading increase the risk for knee osteoarthritis.[94]

The knee is among the commonly affected joints. Radiographic evidence of knee osteoarthritis, defined as grade two or greater, is estimated to be present in about 30% of people over the age of 65 years, and of those with radiographic evidence, one-third are symptomatic.[103] One study reported that in women aged 40–55, the prevalence is 15%.[104] Disabling symptoms in the knee occur in about 10% of persons older than age 55, and of these, about one quarter are severely disabled.[105] On a population basis, the magnitude of the disability from knee osteoarthritis is considered to be as great as heart disease, and greater than the disability from any other medical condition among the elderly.[106] A World Health Organization report predicts that knee osteoarthritis will become the fourth most important global cause of disability in women and eighth most important cause in men.[103] Studies in persons with radiologic evidence of knee osteoarthritis have identified the following factors to be predictive of knee pain: severity of radiographic changes, presence of morning stiffness, crepitus on passive range of motion, and a depressed mood.[107]

In addition to obesity, other nonoccupational risk factors for osteoarthritis of the knee include knee injury, prior surgery including meniscectomy, and also the presence of Heberden's nodes.[108] Several studies have noted an inverse association between osteoporosis and osteoarthritis of the knee and hip.[109] A history of unilateral knee injury has been strongly associated with ipsilateral but not contralateral osteoarthritis of the knee.[94] Recreational, low-impact physical activity, including running, does not appear to be associated with knee osteoarthritis in most people, but elite athletes and recreational runners who already have abnormal or injured joints are at increased risk for osteoarthritis.[110] Osteoarthritis of the hip is more weakly associated than the knee with obesity, hip injury, and Heberden's nodes but is strongly associated with developmental disorders that may affect the shape of the hip joint, including developmental dislocation of the hip and slipped capital femoral epiphysis (SCFE).[109]

Osteoarthritis of the knee is associated with decreased survival in persons aged 55 and older.[104] Likely explanations for this observation include the association of obesity with osteoarthritis and mortality, and possibly the adverse effects of treatment with nonsteroidal anti-inflammatory drugs (NSAIDs). Finally, osteoarthritis of the knee, especially with concomitant pain, often results in long-term activity and mobility limitation.[107]

Primary prevention of osteoarthritis is possible by preventing the potentially modifiable risk factors mentioned above, including obesity, repetitive joint usage, and trauma. Weight loss can lower risk for the development of osteoarthritis and probably slows disease progression.[111] Early treatment of conditions such as developmental dislocation of the hip, slipped epiphysis, and various other developmental and acquired bone and joint disorders may curtail the development of, or limit the extent of, osteoarthritis. In other cases, injury prevention may reduce osteoarthritis. For example, 70% of persons with anterior cruciate ligament injuries treated surgically with a patellar tendon graft developed radiological evidence of osteoarthritis within 7 years.[112]

Intervention strategies aimed at controlling the symptoms of pain, stiffness, and the functional limitations associated with osteoarthritis have been organized into a set of clinical recommendations (Table 57-3).[113] Recommendations incorporate a combination of nonpharmacological and pharmacological modalities. Nonpharmacological modalities include exercise programs and physical therapy, weight loss, and wedged insoles, frequently accompanied by a pharmacological intervention. Educational and self-management activities as well as supervised exercise can help.[114–116] "High-quality evidence supports exercise to improve pain and function in hip and knee OA."[117]

TABLE 57-3 RECOMMENDATIONS FOR MANAGEMENT OF OSTEOARTHRITIS

Nonpharmacologic	Pharmacologic
Recommended Strongly:	Conditionally Recommended:
1. Cardiovascular or land-based exercises	1. Acetaminophen
2. Aquatic exercise	2. Oral/topical NSAIDS (+/- topical salicylates)
3. Weight loss	3. Tramadol
Conditionally Recommended:	4. Intrarticular steroids (knee and hips only)
1. Self-management programs	5. Topical capsaicin (hands only)
2. Manual therapy combined with supervised exercise	Conditionally Not Recommended:
3. Instructions on using thermal agents	1. Glucosamine
4. Walking aids	2. Chondroitin sulfate
5. ADL management and assistive devices	
6. Joint protection technique education	No Recommendation:
7. Medially directed patellar taping (knee OA)	1. Opioids
8. Medially wedged insoles (if lateral knee OA)	2. Duloxetine
9. *Acupuncture, tai chi, transcutaneous electrical stimulation (if moderate to severe knee OA)	3. Hyaluronates

Abbreviations: ADL = activities of daily living; NSAIDS = nonsteroidal anti-inflammatory drugs; OA = osteoarthritis.

Source: Data from Hochberg MC, Altman RD, April KT, et al. American College of Rheumatology 2012 recommendations for the use of non-pharmacologic and pharmacologic therapies in osteoarthritis of the hand, hip, and knee. *Arthritis Care Res (Hoboken)*. 2012;64(4):465–74.

Acupuncture, Tai Chi, and transcutaneous electrical stimulation may be effective for moderately severe knee osteoarthritis.[113]

If medication is used, acetaminophen (paracetamol) is generally the first choice rather than NSAIDs because of its better overall gastrointestinal system safety profile.[118] The use of therapeutic agents for osteoarthritis has become more complex in regard to weighing the benefits from relief of pain and disability versus the possibility of adverse events. There is support for the use of NSAIDs with a gastroprotective agent to reduce the risk of duodenal and gastric ulcers.[119] Alternatives to NSAIDs include COX 2 selective inhibitors.[120] Studies on slow-acting agents for osteoarthritis, including glucosamine sulfate, or chondroitin sulfate, have been largely negative, and hyaluronic acid injections have an unclear role.[113,121,122] Joint replacement has become the intervention of choice for individuals with severe pain and disability refractory to nonsurgical treatment.[119,123] The success of total hip replacement has been long recognized, and total knee replacement is also safe and effective in reducing pain and improving function and quality of life.[123] Total hip replacement offers better return of function than knee replacement in comparative studies.[124]

Rheumatoid Arthritis

Rheumatoid arthritis is a chronic inflammatory autoimmune disease, characterized by proliferative synovitis that results in bony erosion and destruction of articular cartilage that can cause articular deformities. The clinical symptoms include stiffness, pain, and swelling of multiple joints, most commonly the small joints of the hands and wrists.[125] It can be associated with extra-articular manifestations including vascular, pulmonary, and eye disease complications although most of these are declining with modern treatment.[126] The clinical course can vary and early treatment is critical. Persistent rheumatoid arthritis is associated with progressive disability[127,128] and earlier mortality.[129] Although some studies suggest that, overall, the disease course may be more benign,[130] other studies indicate that the impact of inflammation on the vasculature is substantial. The use of treatments to control inflammation (e.g., methotrexate, anti-TNF agents) improve quality of life, functioning, and vascular risk.[129,131]

The lifetime incidence of rheumatoid arthritis is ~1.0%, with an annual incidence of 25–50/100,000.[132] Prevalence is estimated at 1.5 million.[133] Several classification systems have evolved over time from the 1958 American Rheumatism Association (ARA) criteria[134] to the 2010 criteria of the American College of Rheumatology (ACR).[125] A study using data from the Third National Health and Nutrition Examination Study (NHANES III) compared rheumatoid arthritis prevalence estimates in persons over the age of 60 using three different rheumatoid arthritis classifications and estimated prevalence at ~2%.[3]

In NHANES III, the prevalence of rheumatoid arthritis was approximately 1.5 times greater in older women than older men[3]; others estimate 3:1 females to males. Prevalence increased with age, with 1.6–1.9% affected in the 60–70 year age range compared to 2.5–2.8% in persons 70–80, suggesting more rheumatoid arthritis in older birth cohorts.[132] In the Olmsted County, Minnesota, the incidence of severe extra-articular manifestations was 1 per 100 person-years of follow-up; approximately 15% of rheumatoid arthritis patients had these manifestations.[135]

Several Native American tribes have particularly high prevalence of rheumatoid arthritis, including the Yakima of central Washington State and the Mille-Lac Band of Chippewa in Minnesota. Asians, including Japanese and Chinese, appear to have lower prevalence than Whites.[136]

Genetic and environmental factors including smoking have an important etiologic role in rheumatoid arthritis.[137] The disease exhibits some familial aggregation but only a 30% concordance rate in monozygotic twins. Studies have demonstrated a strong association between the class II major histocompatibility antigen HLA-DR4 and rheumatoid arthritis; in whites, the relative risk for this association exceeds 4.0.[138,139] Further, the HLA-DR4 subtype has been associated with the extra-articular manifestations.[137] Smokers with two copies of HLA-DRB1, called "the shared epitope," have 36 times the risk of developing RA compared to controls.[140] HLA-DR1, HLA-DR4, and HLA-DR10 are all associated with rheumatoid arthritis.[141] These alleles encode a common amino acid sequence in the antigen-binding cleft. It is thought that these HLA-DR alleles influence presenting self-peptides to immune cells creating autoimmunity. Other genetic markers of immunologic status are being investigated.[142] The role of infectious agents as etiologic factors in rheumatoid arthritis has been extensively explored, with links.[143]

Declining rheumatoid arthritis incidence among women, but not men, was noted between 1960 and 2000; these findings were consistent with a protective effect of oral contraceptives[144] and decline in smoking. A meta-analysis confirmed a protective effect of oral contraceptive use on the development of rheumatoid arthritis, with a pooled relative risk of 0.70.[145] The Nurses' Health Study and other epidemiologic reports have suggested that smoking, obesity, dental disease, and low consumption of fish may increase incidence of rheumatoid arthritis, which might be targets for prevention.[146,147] Rheumatoid arthritis is associated with premature mortality.[136] Causes of death that are more frequent in persons with rheumatoid arthritis include cardiovascular, respiratory, infectious diseases, and gastrointestinal disorders.[148,149] Persistent synovitis and inflammation, the presence of rheumatoid factor, extra-articular involvement, functional losses, low levels of education, and the HLA-DR4 epitope have been associated with increased mortality and excess disability.[150,151]

Disability is a major concern among persons with persistent rheumatoid arthritis, although modern treatments may be reducing disability. A meta-analysis found that physical demands of the job, older age, low functional capacity, and lower educational attainment are factors that predict work disability.[152]

Methods of primary prevention or screening for rheumatoid arthritis are not common, although serologic markers including rheumatoid factor or cyclic citrullinated peptides may be present long before onset.[153] First-line medical therapy during diagnostic evaluation may use anti-inflammatory NSAIDS, which are analgesic, and lead to improvement in pain and swelling. However, there is no evidence that they affect the underlying disease process. It is now recommended that disease modifying antirheumatic drugs (DMARDS), biologics, or small molecule immunomodulatory therapies that may modify the course of the disease be initiated early in persons with persistent synovitis.[154,155] Such therapies include use of DMARDS, such as hydroxychloroquine, an antimalarial drug, sulfasalazine, or methotrexate, as monotherapy or combined as "triple therapy," which was as effective as newer biologic agents.[156] Older DMARDs (intramuscular gold, D-penicillamine, azathioprine, and cyclosporin A) have largely been replaced by new biologic therapies targeting tumor necrosis factor alpha, interleukin-6, CTLA-4 or CD-20, and small molecules targeting JAK kinase.[138] These agents have dramatically improved function, radiographic outcomes, and prognosis in rheumatoid arthritis but have also led to dramatically increased drug costs. Brief oral or intramuscular corticosteroids have a role in management of the rheumatoid arthritis patient as an adjunct to remittive therapy[155] but should not be continued long term.

Other Inflammatory Rheumatic Diseases

Spondylarthropathies are a family of inflammatory arthritis conditions that include ankylosing spondylitis, reactive arthritis, psoriatic arthritis, arthritis associated with inflammatory bowel disease (ulcerative colitis or Crohns), juvenile spondylarthropathy, or undifferentiated spondylarthropathy.[157] "Spondylo" refers to shared clinical features including involvement of the axial spine and the sacroiliac joints at the junction of the spine and pelvis. Younger onset (<45 years often), NSAID response, morning stiffness, and relief with activity can distinguish these conditions from far more common mechanical back pain.[158] These conditions often share genetic predisposition with HLA-B27 positivity. Scientists think molecular mimicry is the method by which HLA-B27 associates with risk of spondyloarthropathies. Approximately 15% of US Caucasians are HLA-B27 positive with variation by ethnicity. Gene environment interactions include triggering reactive arthritis by invasive gastrointestinal or genitourinary infections like Salmonella, Shigella, Yersinia, or Chlamydia in some but not all HLA-B27 positive hosts, and 60% concordance for ankylosing spondylitis among monozygotic twins. Treatment consists of first line NSAIDS which are disease modifying, physical therapy and in some cases, biologic therapies.[159]

Systemic Lupus Erythematosus (called SLE or lupus) is a classic multiorgan, autoimmune connective tissue disease that often affects young women, outnumbering men 9:1.[160] Lupus affects U.S. blacks three times more often than white patients, and increased rates are noted in other racial and ethnic minorities as well.[161] Lupus can affect nearly any organ system. Significant lupus complications include kidney failure, nervous system involvement, and early stroke, heart attacks, and mortality. Kidney failure and early mortality disproportionately impact black patients, making lupus a health disparities area. Hydroxychloroquine, an antimalarial drug with immune modulation features, is a mainstay for treatment. It has been shown to reduce new organ involvement and prolong life.[161,162] Glucocorticoids and other immunosuppressive agents are used in more severe cases. Few opportunities for prevention exist for these conditions, given the limited understanding of their etiology and lack of association with modifiable risk factors.

Foot Disorders in Older Adults

About three-fourths of fully active older adults complain of painful feet.[163,164] In a survey in which feet were professionally examined in a sample of community-dwelling older adults,[165] the prevalence of foot disorders was higher still; 75% for toenail disorders, 60% for lesser toe deformities, 58% for corns and calluses, 37% for bunions, and 36% for signs of fungal infection, cracks/fissures, or maceration between toes.

Foot pain, especially if chronic and severe, can be a significant cause of disability.[166,167] In addition, even slight deformities of the foot can lead to impaired proprioception, mechanical problems, changes in gait and balance, and pain, resulting in increased risks for falls[168] and foot fracture.[169] The prevalence and severity of foot conditions increase with age, as the aging process can result in neuropathy, ischemia, and atrophy of the planter fat pad, skin, and nails.[170] Chronic conditions such as diabetes, peripheral vascular disease, and inflammatory and osteoarthritis often involve the feet.[170] Obesity has also been reported to be a risk factor for foot pain.[167] Articular and skeletal disorders of the feet may result from congenital abnormalities, degenerative disease, aging, infections, neoplasms, and trauma,[171] as well as from osteoarthritis, rheumatoid arthritis, and less commonly, gout. Improperly fitting shoes and other stresses on the foot can lead to deformities including bunions (hallux valgus), hammer, and claw toes.

Prevention at all levels includes appropriate treatment of diseases that can involve the feet, the wearing of proper shoes, wearing socks or stockings, bathing the feet frequently, avoidance of obesity, protection against infection and trauma to the feet, and proper care of toenails.[172] Once foot problems occur, soft, well-padded shoes or pads should be worn to relieve pressure in sore areas. In most instances, these simple methods can reduce much of the discomfort associated with foot problems. In some cases, rest, application of heat and cold, specific exercises, and use of special corrective shoes may be needed.[171] Almost half of all people with foot disorders are not receiving care for the problem.[172]

Paraplegia and Quadriplegia

Paraplegia and quadriplegia refer to conditions rendering one unable to use the lower limbs or upper and lower limbs, respectively. The most common cause of paraplegia and quadriplegia in Western countries is vertebral fractures and dislocation from trauma. Complete transection of the spinal cord results in paralysis of all muscles supplied by motor neurons below the level of the lesion and in the loss of skin sensation in all areas supplied by sensory neurons below the lesion. Because neurons in the central nervous system do not regenerate, both motor and sensory paralysis is permanent.

The effect on the patient, family, and friends is immediate and enormous. Most affected individuals were previously independent and must learn to cope with partial or complete paralysis, loss of sensation in major parts of the body, loss of voluntary control over body functions including bowel and bladder dysfunction, and loss of sexual function. The patient's work, marriage, family, and social relationships are likely to be substantially altered.[173]

In the United States, nearly 282,000 people are disabled with spinal cord injuries, with 17,000 new cases occurring each year[174] Spinal cord injuries occur most frequently in persons ages 15–40 years, are three to four times more common in males than females, and are more frequent in blacks than whites.[175,176,157] In developed countries, motor vehicle accidents, especially those involving motorcycles, are by far the leading cause of these injuries. One U.S. study[177] found that among those whose spinal cord injury occurred as a result of being in a motor vehicle, 70% were involved in a vehicle rollover, 39% were ejected from the vehicle, and only 25% reported using seatbelts. In another study,[178] drugs and alcohol had been used before the injury in at least 25% of cases. Other major causes are falls (especially in the elderly); sports and recreational activities such as diving in shallow water, gymnastics and contact sports; violence and self-inflicted injuries.[175,176,178,179] In developed countries, the proportion of spinal cord injuries attributable to sports and recreational activities has increased in recent years, while the proportion of work-related accidents has decreased in many countries as safer work practices have been implemented. In developing countries, other common causes vary and violence has become more common in recent years.[175]

The most important primary prevention measures in developed countries are those that reduce the likelihood of motor vehicle accidents and lessen the risk of injury if accidents do occur. These measures include: drunk driving laws; speed limits; and use of seat belts, head rests, airbags, or helmets. Prevention of falls in the elderly and safety measures in occupational and recreational settings are also important. For instance, in high school and collegiate football, rules banning "spearing" or initial contact with the top of the helmet when making a tackle have markedly reduced the frequency of permanent cervical quadriplegia.[180] In Canada, a decline in the number of major spinal cord injuries has been noted in ice hockey following the implementation of education and rules changes.[181] In developing countries, education on safe tree climbing and carrying heavy objects is needed.[175]

The number of survivors with paraplegia and quadriplegia has greatly increased because of medical and surgical advances. Since most of those injured are in their late teens and early adult years, enormous costs and very long-term severe disability ensue. Lifetime costs per patient generally range from about $1.1 to $2.6 million.[174] In addition to psychological problems, the greatest difficulties are in self-care, locomotion, obtaining employment, and medical complications. Common medical complications include urinary tract infections, pressure sores, cardiac and vascular problems, and autonomic dysreflexia.[182] Patient education and good nursing care can reduce the likelihood of many of these complications.[175]

The object of tertiary prevention is to return the affected person to maximum physical and social functioning. Accordingly, in addition to specialists in orthopedic and neurological surgery, other specialists that should be involved in therapy of these patients include occupational and physical therapists, psychiatrists, orthotics specialists, urologists, and vocational counsellors. Long leg braces, crutches, and gait training may help highly motivated paraplegics with low-level lesions return to walking and may even enable them to become self-supporting. Because many paraplegics drive cars and work, wheelchair accessibility is increasingly important.[183] Sexual counselling also may be helpful.

DISORDERS PRIMARILY OF CHILDREN

Adolescent Idiopathic Scoliosis

Scoliosis, or abnormal lateral curvature of the spine associated with rotation of the vertebrae, is the most common cause of spinal deformity in North American children.[184] Of the various forms of scoliosis, the most common is adolescent idiopathic scoliosis (AIS). About 2–3% of children develop curves of 10° or more before growth ceases, and about 2–3 per 1000 children develop curves of 30° or more.[185,186] Children with AIS are more likely than their unaffected peers to develop spinal osteoarthritis and report more back and neck pain in adulthood, while lung and heart complications appear to be limited to more severe forms of the disease such as early-onset scoliosis.[187,188] Further curve progression rarely takes place in adults.[189]

AIS is most frequently diagnosed around the ages of 11–14 years in girls and 14–16 years in boys. Mild curves of less than 15° are found with almost equal frequency in both sexes, but girls are ten times more likely than males to progress to curves in excess of 30°.[190]

Once girls have reached menarche, their risk for developing scoliosis is reduced.[191] Although surgical series have indicated that scoliotic curves are most common at the thoracic level, screening programs identifying children who do not necessarily seek medical care have found that the peak frequency is at the thoracolumbar level.[192]

The risk for AIS in first-degree relatives is about three to four times higher than in other children.[193] Twin studies indicate a genetic etiology for both the development and progression of scoliosis.[194] The mode of inheritance is uncertain, but research suggests that some cases might be due to X chromosome mutations or X-linked polymorphism of estrogen receptor genes.[195,196] Little is known of other risk factors for development of the disease. Some evidence suggests that prepubertal standing height, sitting height, recent increase in sitting height, and early age at gain in sitting height are predictive,[197] and that children who are skeletally more mature, taller, and leaner at the onset but not at the end of puberty are most likely to be affected.[191,198] These observations suggest that the scoliotic spine grows faster and earlier than the normal spine.[191,198,199] Impaired visual and vestibular functioning, defects in proprioceptive postural control, asymmetric muscle activity, unequal leg length, high concentrations of calcium in paraspinal muscles, collagen disorders, and defects of the elastic fiber system may be etiologically involved, but evidence is not conclusive, suggesting that there are likely many factors that contribute to the development and progression of AIS.[198,200,201]

Scoliotic curves progress in around two-thirds of patients before skeletal maturity, though the degree of curve progression is dependent on a variety of factors.[202] Skeletal maturity assessed by the Risser sign, the ossification stage of the iliac apophysis, predicts progression risk.[202] Other risk factors for progression are doubled as opposed to single curves, thoracic as opposed to curves at lower levels, curves of greater magnitude at presentation (>25°), absence of a sacral tilt, limb length inequality, early chronological age, and female sex.[203-205]

Because the etiology of AIS is variable and no modifiable risk factors have been identified, primary prevention is not feasible. Efforts have been focused instead on secondary prevention—that is, the early detection of the disease. The traditional screening test for scoliosis has been the forward-bend test, in which the child's back is examined while he or she bends forward from the waist. The rotation that accompanies the lateral curvature in scoliosis results in posterior prominence of the ribs on the concave side of the curvature, so that a "rib hump" is often apparent on forward bending. The forward-bend test has good specificity but fairly low sensitivity. The inclinometer (scoliometer), which measures trunk asymmetry as an indicator of trunk rotation, has been reported to have high sensitivity and fairly good specificity, but results can be distorted by patient obesity.[206-208] There are also a number of smartphone applications that provide reliable, valid measurements of the degree of scoliosis.[209,210] Most school screening programs use the forward-bend test.

In the United States, school screening programs identify large numbers of children with possible spinal curvatures and have been legislated in 21 states. Positive screening tests are followed up with radiographic examination for more definitive diagnosis. Curves of over 5° are monitored by serial radiographs every few months. Should a curve progress to 25°, treatment is generally indicated to try to prevent further progression. Braces are most commonly used for curves of 25°–45°, while surgery to correct at least part of the deformity and to halt further progression is often indicated for curves of 45° or greater, particularly in growing children.[211]

School screening programs for scoliosis are widespread, but there is minimal evidence that these programs affect patient-centered outcomes.[212-214] First, it is uncertain that school screening programs have brought about a reduction in the prevalence of severe deformities or the number of operations needed.[215] Treatment with bracing has been shown to reduce the progression of the curvature, but there is inadequate evidence to demonstrate an association with long-term outcomes. In addition, while the sensitivity of many of the screening tests is high, the false positive rate is also high, which leads to costly referral for radiographs, examinations, and greater medical expense and anxiety.[190] Because of the mixed evidence for the efficacy and utility of screening for scoliosis, there is no consensus across recommendations. The U.S. Preventive Services Task Force was unable to recommend for or against routine screening of adolescents for scoliosis in its updated 2018 recommendations.[215] In contrast, the American Academy of Orthopaedic Surgeons, Scoliosis Research Society, Pediatric Orthopaedic Society of North America, and American Academy of Pediatrics have endorsed a joint statement that screening should be performed as part of preventive medical visits for females at age 10 and 12 years, and males once at age 13 or 14 years.[216]

Slipped Capital Femoral Epiphysis

SCFE, in which the epiphysis of the head of the femur is displaced posteriorly and inferiorly off the diaphysis, is primarily a disease of adolescents. SCFE is strongly associated with the future development of osteoarthritis, particularly in those when severe.[217] It is closely related to the adolescent growth spurt and does not occur once the epiphysis is closed. Incidence of SCFE varies between populations and geographical region. In the United States, incidence per 100,000 children aged 8–15 years old ranges from 17.2 in the Northeast, 7.7 in the Midwest, and 2.1 in the Southwest.[218] The mean age at diagnosis has dropped over the last 20 years corresponding with trends in earlier onset of puberty. Average age of onset of SCFE has decreased to 11.2 years in girls and 12.0 years in boys.[218] SCFE is about 1.5 times more common in males than in females.[219]

Incidence of SCFE varies between races and appears to be highest in African American children with an incidence of 24.6 cases per 100,000 children, nearly four times higher than for Caucasian children.[219] Children of Hispanic and Asian descent also have higher incidence than Caucasians with incidence rates of 15.8 and 10.1, respectively. In most studies in northern latitudes, symptoms begin more frequently in spring and summer than in fall and winter.[220,221]

A large proportion of children with slipped epiphysis are markedly overweight[222,223]; about half are at or above the 95th percentile for their age (Fig. 57-2). Obese children have increased femoral retroversion, which could increase the shear forces leading to epiphyseal failure.[224-226] Familial aggregation of cases has been reported,[227] but it is not clear whether this aggregation is primarily attributable to inherited characteristics or to common environmental factors.

SCFE has been attributed to other factors that weaken the epiphyseal plate, which occurs during periods of rapid growth.[228]

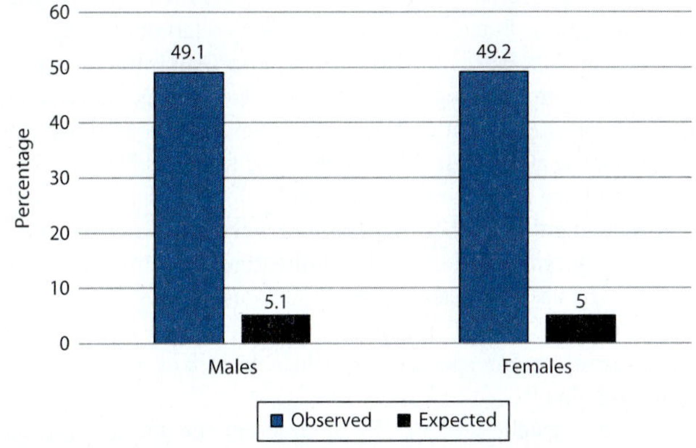

FIGURE 57-2. Percentage of children with slipped epiphysis with weights at or above 95th percentile for their age. (*Source:* Adapted from Kelsey JL, Acheson RM, Keggi KJ. The body builds of patients with slipped capital femoral epiphysis. *Am J Dis Child.* 1972;124:276–81.)

Animal experiments indicate that a deficit of sex hormones relative to growth hormone widens of the epiphyseal plate and reduces the shear force necessary to displace the epiphysis.[229] Children with the unusual combination of being overweight and undergoing slow maturation appear to be at high risk, and clinical suspicion should heighten if they present with hip pain. Additionally, children with endocrinopathies such as hyper or hypothyroidism, hyperparathyroidism, and hypopituitarism and pediatric cancer survivors with a history of total body irradiation are more at risk for developing SCFE.[230,231]

Because SCFE is associated with the development of osteoarthritis, there is great interest in prevention of its development. The only known means of primary prevention is avoidance of obesity in adolescents. No screening tests for slipped epiphysis exist, but the diagnosis should be suspected in adolescents who have a limp and hip or knee discomfort, especially if there is restriction of internal rotation of the hip. Radiographic examination with two views should be performed immediately to confirm the diagnosis.

In one long-term follow up study, 41% of children who have a SCFE developed the condition in the contralateral hip, though this may be higher in African American children.[218,232] MRI at the time of diagnosis of the primary SCFE does not predict future contralateral slip.[233] Prophylactic pinning of the asymptomatic contralateral hip should be considered in children with a slipped epiphysis.[234,235] At a minimum, the contralateral hip should be carefully monitored, especially for those whose first SCFE occurred at an early age.[223,236] Slippage that is stable or mild when treated early by hip pinning has a favorable prognosis, whereas late diagnosis or severe displacement is more likely to result in early onset of osteoarthritis of the hip and permanent disability despite treatment.

Fractures in Children

Each year about 1 in 20–25 children fracture or dislocate a bone.[237,238] One-third of children fracture at least one bone before 17 years of age.[239] In childhood, fracture incidence rates increase until about ages 11 years in females and 14 years in males,[239] with males at higher risk throughout childhood and adolescence.[239–242] In one series,[241] over one-half of childhood fractures occurred while the child was at play, participating in a sport, or in a traffic accident. In another series,[242] 36% of childhood fractures occurred during sports and leisure-time activities. The bones most frequently fractured in children are the hand, radius and ulna, skull and face, clavicle, foot and ankle, and humerus.

Fractures of the phalanges of the hands often occur during contact sports, skating, playing, and fighting, while fractures of the distal forearm tend to result from a fall on an outstretched hand, particularly during ball games, and bicycle, playground, or skateboard accidents. Carpal and metacarpal hand fractures most often result from fights, falls, and sports. Fractures of the clavicle (collarbone) frequently occur during falls, ball games, or contact sports. Ankle fractures most often result from bicycling or motor biking, falls, ball games, skating, skiing, or playing.[241] Tall and obese children, as well as those who smoke, may be at elevated risk for childhood fractures.[243,244]

The primary prevention of fractures in children depends mainly upon reducing the number of sports and recreational injuries, automobile and bicycle accidents, falls, child-battering injuries, and other traumas. The use of impact absorbing surfaces in playgrounds could reduce the frequency of fractures at many sites, and wearing wrist guards during certain sports could reduce the risk of fractures of the radius and ulna.[242]

Fractures usually heal rapidly in children; the younger the age, the more rapid the healing. However, if the growth plate is involved in the fracture, growth in that bone may be adversely affected, particularly if a crushing injury has occurred. Other complications are rare but may include infection, delayed union, nonunion, avascular necrosis, and malunion. Prevention of these complications involves thorough cleansing of an open (compound) fracture and competent initial treatment of the fracture.

Overuse Injuries

Over 60 million boys and girls participate in youth sports in the United States, including nearly 8 million high school students.[245,246] There are many benefits to participation in youth sports including, higher self-esteem, lower risky substance use, and lower cardiovascular disease risk factors including obesity.[247–249] However, children and adolescents who engage in organized sports are also at risk for developing overuse musculoskeletal injuries. Approximately 25% of high school athletes sustain an overuse injury every year, due to repetitive loading of bones, ligaments, tendons, and soft tissues.[250,251]

Common overuse injuries include tendinopathies, bone stress injuries, physeal growth plate injuries, and injuries to the chondral surfaces of long bones. Shoulder tendinopathies including those of the rotator cuff and biceps are common in overhead athletes such as baseball players and swimmers.[250] Repetitive overhead motion and activation of the stabilizing muscles around the shoulder can cause a cyclic pattern of muscle inflammation, pain, and dysfunction that can lead to chronic changes in the tendon.[252] Lower extremity tendinopathies of the patellar and Achilles tendons are common in explosive, jumping sports such as basketball and volleyball.[253]

Athletes who compete in sports that require repetitive impact, such as runners, are at elevated risk of developing bone stress injuries.[254] These injuries can occur in the long bones of the leg, pelvis, and feet when the microtrauma of impact exceeds the body's ability to heal. If untreated, the initial weakness in the bone can lead to frank fracture. Female athletes, particularly those that suffer from the Female Athlete Triad (menstrual irregularity, low energy availability, and low bone mineral density) are particularly at risk for developing bone stress injuries.[255,256]

Physes, or growth plates, are responsible for the growth of long bones and are vulnerable to injury in youth and adolescent athletes.[257] Repetitive loading, torsional, or shearing forces can cause disruption of the chondrocytes of the physis and lead to premature closure of growth plates or growth discrepancy.[258] Common locations of this injury include the proximal humeral physis in baseball (Little Leaguer's shoulder), volleyball, and swimming athletes and the distal radial physis in gymnasts.[257] Apophysitis, or inflammation of the growth centers that establish the contour of bones, are prevalent overuse injuries. These frequently occur at the tibial tubercle (Osgood-Schlatter disease), inferior patella (Sinding-Larsen-Johansson syndrome), calcaneus (Sever's disease), and medial epicondyle of the humerus (Little Leaguer's elbow).[259–262] Diagnosis of physeal injuries is made with radiographs of the affected limb, and it can be helpful to compare to the contralateral side to assess for widening of the physis.[257] Apophyseal sites tend to be the weakest aspect of the muscle-tendon-bone unit and are prone to acute avulsion fractures with resisted explosive motion.[263]

Children and adolescents are at risk of developing overuse injuries during times of rapid growth and with high training volume.[251] Quantifying how much physical activity is "too much" is challenging, but measures of early sports specialization can clarify this issue. Highly specialized athletes are those that train > 8 months per year, choose a single main sport, and quit all sports to focus on one sport.[264] High levels of sports specialization are associated with increased risk of developing overuse injuries Table 57-4.[265]

Several groups have made recommendations to prevent overuse injuries in youth athletes. For example, Major League Baseball has responded to the epidemic of upper extremity injuries in youth athletes by instituting pitch counts limits by age.[266] Additionally, it has been recommended that children should not participate in sports more hours per week than their age. (A 12 years old should be involved in organized physical activity less than 12 hours per week.)[267] In most cases, intense single-sport specialized training should be delayed until late adolescence.[268]

TABLE 57-4 LOWER EXTREMITY INJURIES BY SPORTS SPECIALIZATION LEVEL IN HIGH SCHOOL ATHLETES

	Total, *n*	Injured, *n* (%)	Cox Hazard Ratio (95% CI)	*P* Value
Primary sports specialization level				
Low	831	24 (2.9)	Reference	---
Moderate	366	27 (7.4)	2.61 (1.34–5.07)	0.005
High	183	20 (10.9)	4.74 (2.04–11.05)	<0.001

Source: Adapted from McGuine TA, Post EG, Hetzel SJ, Brooks MA, Trigsted S, Bell DR. A prospective study on the effect of sport specialization on lower extremity injury rates in high school athletes. *Am J Sports Med.* 2017;45(12):2706–12.

Developmental Dysplasia of the Hip

Developmental dysplasia of the hip (DDH) encompasses a spectrum of findings from mild instability of the femoral head to frank displacement out of the acetabulum. Because many dislocations occur immediately after birth or occasionally later during the first year of life, the term "developmental dysplasia of the hip" is now frequently used instead of the older term "congenital dislocation of the hip."[269] DDH may be categorized as dislocated, located but unstable, or simply dysplastic.[269] Without prompt treatment, the affected leg may be shorter, the child may limp, gait abnormalities may develop, surgery may be required, and osteoarthritis of the hip is likely in early adulthood.

The incidence of DDH varies considerably between ethnic groups. Frequencies ranging from 1 per 1000 to 10 per 1000 births have been reported in most North America, Western Europe, Israel, Australia, and New Zealand to 10 per 1000 to 123 per 1000 in Navajo, Apache, and Cree-Ojibwa people of North America.[270] In the Sámi of Scandinavia and in children from Hungary, northern Italy, Brittany, and the Faroe Islands, incidence of DDH is similarly elevated. DDH is rare among Black people in Africa, the West Indies, or among Chinese living in Hong Kong.[198] Although the frequency of dysplasia or dislocation of the hip has been rising, much of the apparent rise may be attributable to more extensive screening at birth and increased awareness by physicians.

Girls have a nearly four times greater odds of developing DDH than boys.[271] Breech presentation in utero compared to vertex increases the odds by around five times due to persistent upward pressure of the greater trochanter.[244] Ligamentous and capsular laxity are also probably predisposing factors.[272] A positive family history also increases the odds of developing DDH by nearly six times. Both hereditary and environmental factors contribute to the familial excess.[273,274] On average, infants with DDH have had longer gestation periods than other infants and are considerably more likely to have been born by breech delivery than other infants.[274,275] In most areas, a greater than expected number of cases are encountered in children born in late fall and winter than in summer.[275]

No feasible methods of primary prevention are known. In regard to secondary prevention, clinical examination of newborn infants for DDH is recommended.[276] Two screening tests have generally been used: the Ortolani and the Barlow. The Ortolani test involves placing the hip in flexion and gently adducting and then abducting the hip. The test is considered positive if a palpable jerk and audible clunk are heard as the head of the femur returns to the acetabulum. Some practitioners also consider an audible click to constitute a positive test. In the Barlow test, gentle downward pressure is exerted over the lesser trochanter with the hip in flexion and adduction; the unstable hip shifts from the acetabulum, and a sensation similar to the Ortolani sign is produced. About half of the hips noted to be unstable immediately after birth become stable within a few days[277]; thus, these tests are often repeated for the first 6 months of life. Despite recommendations for their routine use, the sensitivity and specificity of screening by the Ortolani and Barlow tests is poor.[278–280] In one study, only one-third of genuine cases were detected, and the ratio of false positives to true positives was 10 to 1.[278] The question has arisen as to whether the screening procedures may, themselves, induce hip dislocation.[281,282]

Definitive diagnosis of DDH relies on imaging with radiography or ultrasonography. In recent years, ultrasound, which provides a defined image of the bony and cartilaginous neonatal hip, has become widely available for screening for developmental dysplasia/dislocation of the hip. Although it was initially believed that it might alleviate some of the problems with the Barlow and Ortolani tests,[283,284] its use in routine screening of all infants has not been found to be cost effective. Among its limitations are its high cost, the large proportion of hips testing positive on screening that develop normally, and the tendency of some cases to occur after the neonatal period.[285–288]

Diagnostic radiography is most useful in detecting hip asymmetry, subluxation, and hip dislocation between 4 and 6 months of age after the femoral head secondary ossification centers have formed.[276] Ultrasonography is thought to be superior to radiography, especially in the first 3 months of life, due to the absence of radiation to the pelvis.

A 2013 Cochrane Review and the U.S. Preventive Services Task Force found insufficient evidence to promote universal screening with ultrasound as it did not appear to prevent adverse outcomes.[289,290] The American Academy of Orthopaedic Surgeons found moderate evidence to support imaging with ultrasound before 6 months of age for infants with the following risk factors: breech presentation, positive family history, positive Ortolani or Barlow exam, parental concern, history of improper swaddling, or suspicious or inconclusive physical exam.[291]

Early detection of DDH allows for referral to an orthopedic specialist to ensure appropriate treatment. Infants with a stable exam but evidence of DDH on ultrasound can be observed with serial examinations.[291] Infants with clinical instability are treated with braces, splints, or harnesses for 2–4 months. If diagnosed after the neonatal period, surgery is generally required and is associated with worse prognosis.[292]

CONCLUSION

Musculoskeletal conditions are highly prevalent as inherited and acquired conditions, and their response to primary and secondary prevention varies. Some methods of primary prevention are possible for back disorders, osteoporosis, osteoarthritis, foot disorders, paraplegia and quadriplegia, slipped epiphysis, and fractures. Given the public health burden from musculoskeletal disorders and the association with modifiable risk factors, greater focus should be given to primary prevention; especially efforts to promote lifelong healthy diets and physical activity, and to prevent cigarette smoking, obesity, and injuries.

Screening for scoliosis, congenital dislocation of the hip, and osteoporosis are widely available. Although the tests for scoliosis and congenital dislocation of the hip are widely used at present, questions regarding their efficacy remain unresolved.

Secondary and tertiary prevention are more frequently used for musculoskeletal disorders in adults, yet there is limited success beyond reconstructive joint surgery. Given their high prevalence and chronicity, it is not surprising that musculoskeletal disorders have significant effects on quality of life and high individual and societal costs. Improving the quality of life of affected individuals and developing screening strategies remain important, but preventing musculoskeletal injuries and disorders from occurring is also key.

ACKNOWLEDGMENTS

The authors thank Jennifer L. Kelsey and Mary Fran Sowers for their contributions on previous versions of this chapter and thank Amanda Perez for administrative support.

References

1. Global Burden of Disease Study. Global, regional, and national incidence, prevalence, and years lived with disability for 301 acute and chronic diseases and injuries in 188 countries, 1990-2013: A systematic analysis for the Global Burden of Disease Study 2013. *Lancet.* 2015;386(9995):743–800.
2. Centers for Disease Control and Prevention. Arthritis-Related Statistics. 2017. Available at https://www.cdc.gov/arthritis/data_statistics/arthritis-related-stats.htm. Accessed November 18, 2017.
3. Helmick CG, Felson DT, Lawrence RC, et al. Estimates of the prevalence of arthritis and other rheumatic conditions in the United States. Part I. *Arthritis Rheum.* 2008;58(1):15–25.
4. Praemer A, Furner A, Rice DP. *Musculoskeletal Conditions in the United States.* 2nd ed. American Academy of Orthopaedic Surgeons; 1999.
5. The Burden of Musculoskeletal Diseases in the United States. Musculoskeletal Diseases. 2014. Available at http://www.boneandjointburden.org. Accessed November 18, 2017.
6. Andersson GB. Epidemiology of low back pain. *Acta Orthop Scand Suppl.* 1998;281:28–31.
7. Lawrence RC, Felson DT, Helmick CG, et al. Estimates of the prevalence of arthritis and other rheumatic conditions in the United States. Part II. *Arthritis Rheum.* 2008;58(1):26–35.
8. Snook SH. Low back pain in industry. In: White AA, 3rd, Gordon SL, eds. *Symposium on Idiopathic Low Back Pain.* St. Louis, MO: CV Mosby; 1982.
9. Deyo RA, Weinstein JN. Low back pain. *N Engl J Med.* 2001;344(5): 363–70.
10. American Academy of Family Physicians. Imaging tests for lower-back pain: You probably don't need an x-ray, CT scan, or MRI. *Choosing Wisely.* 2012. Available at https://www.aafp.org/family-physician/patient-care/clinical-recommendations/all-clinical-recommendations/cw-back-pain.html. Accessed November 18, 2017.
11. Kelsey JL, Githens PB, White AA, 3rd, et al. An epidemiologic study of lifting and twisting on the job and risk for acute prolapsed lumbar intervertebral disc. *J Orthop Res.* 1984;2(1):61–6.
12. Liira JP, Shannon HS, Chambers LW, Haines TA. Long-term back problems and physical work exposures in the 1990 Ontario Health Survey. *Am J Public Health.* 1996;86(3):382–7.
13. Hoogendoorn WE, Bongers PM, de Vet HC, et al. Flexion and rotation of the trunk and lifting at work are risk factors for low back pain: Results of a prospective cohort study. *Spine (Phila Pa 1976).* 2000;25(23):3087–92.
14. Leboeuf-Yde C. Smoking and low back pain. A systematic literature review of 41 journal articles reporting 47 epidemiologic studies. *Spine (Phila Pa 1976).* 1999;24(14):1463–70.
15. Kelsey JL, Githens PB, O'Conner T, et al. Acute prolapsed lumbar intervertebral disc. An epidemiologic study with special reference to driving automobiles and cigarette smoking. *Spine (Phila Pa 1976).* 1984;9(6):608–13.
16. Pope MH, Magnusson M, Wilder DG. Kappa Delta Award. Low back pain and whole body vibration. *Clin Orthop Relat Res.* 1998(354):241–8.
17. Lings S, Leboeuf-Yde C. Whole-body vibration and low back pain: A systematic, critical review of the epidemiological literature 1992–1999. *Int Arch Occup Environ Health.* 2000;73(5):290–7.
18. Krause N, Rugulies R, Ragland DR, Syme SL. Physical workload, ergonomic problems, and incidence of low back injury: A 7.5-year prospective study of San Francisco transit operators. *Am J Ind Med.* 2004;46(6):570–85.
19. Heliovaara M. *Epidemiology of Sciatica and Herniated Lumbar Intervertebral Disc.* Finland: Social Insurance Institution, Research Institute for Social Security, Rehabilitation Research Centre; 1988.
20. Leboeuf-Yde C. Body weight and low back pain. A systematic literature review of 56 journal articles reporting on 65 epidemiologic studies. *Spine (Phila Pa 1976).* 2000;25(2):226–37.
21. Hoogendoorn WE, van Poppel MN, Bongers PM, Koes BW, Bouter LM. Systematic review of psychosocial factors at work and private life as risk factors for back pain. *Spine (Phila Pa 1976).* 2000;25(16):2114–25.
22. Daltroy LH, Iversen MD, Larson MG, et al. A controlled trial of an educational program to prevent low back injuries. *N Engl J Med.* 1997;337(5):322–8.
23. Lagerstrom M, Hansson T, Hagberg M. Work-related low-back problems in nursing. *Scand J Work Environ Health.* 1998;24(6):449–64.
24. Jellema P, van Tulder MW, van Poppel MN, Nachemson AL, Bouter LM. Lumbar supports for prevention and treatment of low back pain: A systematic review within the framework of the Cochrane Back Review Group. *Spine (Phila Pa 1976).* 2001;26(4):377–86.
25. Lahad A, Malter AD, Berg AO, Deyo RA. The effectiveness of four interventions for the prevention of low back pain. *JAMA.* 1994;272(16):1286–91.
26. Porter JM, Gyi DE. The prevalence of musculoskeletal troubles among car drivers. *Occup Med (Lond).* 2002;52(1):4–12.
27. Dowell D, Haegerich T, Chou R. CDC guideline for prescribing opioids for chronic pain—United States, 2016. *MMWR Morb Mortal Wkly Rep.* 2016;65(1):1–49. Available at https://www.cdc.gov/mmwr/volumes/65/rr/pdfs/rr6501e1.pdf. Accessed November 18, 2017.
28. Tubach F, Leclerc A, Landre MF, Pietri-Taleb F. Risk factors for sick leave due to low back pain: A prospective study. *J Occup Environ Med.* 2002;44(5):451–8.
29. Deyo RA, Diehl AK. Psychosocial predictors of disability in patients with low back pain. *J Rheumatol.* 1988;15(10):1557–64.
30. Cats-Baril WL, Frymoyer JW. Identifying patients at risk of becoming disabled because of low-back pain. The Vermont Rehabilitation Engineering Center predictive model. *Spine (Phila Pa 1976).* 1991;16(6):605–7.
31. Malmivaara A, Hakkinen U, Aro T, et al. The treatment of acute low back pain—Bed rest, exercises, or ordinary activity? *N Engl J Med.* 1995;332(6):351–5.
32. Loisel P, Abenhaim L, Durand P, et al. A population-based, randomized clinical trial on back pain management. *Spine (Phila Pa 1976).* 1997;22(24):2911–8.
33. Hall H, Iceton JA. Back school. An overview with specific reference to the Canadian Back Education Units. *Clin Orthop Relat Res.* 1983;(179):10–17.
34. Lonn JH, Glomsrod B, Soukup MG, Bo K, Larsen S. Active back school: Prophylactic management for low back pain. A randomized, controlled, 1-year follow-up study. *Spine (Phila Pa 1976).* 1999;24(9):865–71.
35. Cote P, Cassidy JD, Carroll L. The Saskatchewan Health and Back Pain Survey. The prevalence of neck pain and related disability in Saskatchewan adults. *Spine (Phila Pa 1976).* 1998;23(15):1689–98.
36. Smedley J, Inskip H, Trevelyan F, Buckle P, Cooper C, Coggon D. Risk factors for incident neck and shoulder pain in hospital nurses. *Occup Environ Med.* 2003;60(11):864–9.
37. Croft PR, Lewis M, Papageorgiou AC, et al. Risk factors for neck pain: A longitudinal study in the general population. *Pain.* 2001;93(3):317–25.
38. Yu IT, Wong TW. Musculoskeletal problems among VDU workers in a Hong Kong bank. *Occup Med (Lond).* 1996;46(4):275–80.
39. Korhonen T, Ketola R, Toivonen R, Luukkonen R, Hakkanen M, Viikari-Juntura E. Work related and individual predictors for incident neck pain among office employees working with video display units. *Occup Environ Med.* 2003;60(7):475–82.
40. Kelsey JL, Githens PB, Walter SD, et al. An epidemiological study of acute prolapsed cervical intervertebral disc. *J Bone Joint Surg Am.* 1984;66(6):907–14.
41. Magnusson ML, Pope MH, Wilder DG, Areskoug B. Are occupational drivers at an increased risk for developing musculoskeletal disorders? *Spine (Phila Pa 1976).* 1996;21(6):710–17.
42. Krause N, Ragland DR, Greiner BA, Fisher JM, Holman BL, Selvin S. Physical workload and ergonomic factors associated with prevalence of back and neck pain in urban transit operators. *Spine (Phila Pa 1976).* 1997;22(18):2117–26; discussion 2127.
43. Ariens GA, van Mechelen W, Bongers PM, Bouter LM, van der Wal G. Physical risk factors for neck pain. *Scand J Work Environ Health.* 2000;26(1):7–19.
44. Leclerc A, Niedhammer I, Landre MF, Ozguler A, Etore P, Pietri-Taleb F. One-year predictive factors for various aspects of neck disorders. *Spine (Phila Pa 1976).* 1999;24(14):1455–62.
45. Ariens GA, van Mechelen W, Bongers PM, Bouter LM, van der Wal G. Psychosocial risk factors for neck pain: A systematic review. *Am J Ind Med.* 2001;39(2):180–93.
46. van den Heuvel SG, de Looze MP, Hildebrandt VH, The KH. Effects of software programs stimulating regular breaks and exercises on work-related neck and upper-limb disorders. *Scand J Work Environ Health.* 2003;29(2):106–16.
47. McLean L, Tingley M, Scott RN, Rickards J. Computer terminal work and the benefit of microbreaks. *Appl Ergon.* 2001;32(3):225–37.
48. Who are candidates for prevention and treatment for osteoporosis? *Osteoporos Int.* 1997;7(1):1–6.
49. Wright NC, Looker AC, Saag KG, et al. The recent prevalence of osteoporosis and low bone mass in the United States based on bone mineral density at the femoral neck or lumbar spine. *J Bone Miner Res.* 2014;29(11):2520–6.
50. The Burden of Musculoskeletal Diseases in the United States. Osteoporosis and Related Conditions: Current Prevalence by Demographics. 2014.

Available at http://www.boneandjointburden.org/2014-report/va1/current-prevalence-demographics. Accessed November 2, 2015.

51. Villa ML, Nelson L, Nelson D. Race, ethnicity and osteoporosis. In: Marcus R, Feldman D, Kelsey J, eds. *Osteoporosis*. 2nd ed. San Diego, CA: Academic Press; 2001, pp. 569–84.
52. Melton LJ, 3rd, Chrischilles EA, Cooper C, Lane AW, Riggs BL.Perspective. How many women have osteoporosis? *J Bone Miner Res*. 1992;7(9):1005–10.
53. Schnell S, Friedman SM, Mendelson DA, Bingham KW, Kates SL. The 1-year mortality of patients treated in a hip fracture program for elders. *Geriatr Orthop Surg Rehabil*. 2010;1(1):6–14.
54. Peacock M, Turner CH, Econs MJ, Foroud T. Genetics of osteoporosis. *Endocr Rev*. 2002;23(3):303–26.
55. Bonjour JP, Rizzoli R. Bone acquisition in adolescence. In: Marcus R, Feldman D, Kelsey J, eds. *Osteoporosis*. Vol. 1. San Diego, CA: Academic Press; 2001, pp. 621–38.
56. Specker BL, Namgung R, Tsang RC. Bone mineral acquisition in utero, during infancy, and throughout childhood. In: Marcus R, Feldman D, Kelsey J, eds. *Osteoporosis*. Vol. 1. 2nd ed. San Diego, CA: Academic Press; 2001, pp. 599–620.
57. Sowers M. Premenopausal reproductive and hormonal characteristics and the risk for osteoporosis. In: Marcus R, Feldman D, Kelsey J, Rosen CJ, eds. *Osteoporosis*. Vol. 1. 3rd ed. San Diego, CA: Academic Press; 2001, pp. 861–77.
58. Cauley JA, Salamone LM. Postmenopausal endogenous and exogenous hormones, degree of obesity, thiazide diuretics, and risk of osteoporosis. In: Marcus R, Feldman D, Kelsey J, eds. *Osteoporosis*. San Diego, CA: Academic Press; 2001, pp. 741–69.
59. Shea B, Wells G, Cranney A, et al. Calcium supplementation on bone loss in postmenopausal women. *Cochrane Database Syst Rev*. 2004;(1):CD004526.
60. Cumming RG. Calcium intake and bone mass: A quantitative review of the evidence. *Calcif Tissue Int*. 1990;47(4):194–201.
61. Wallace BA, Cumming RG. Systematic review of randomized trials of the effect of exercise on bone mass in pre- and postmenopausal women. *Calcif Tissue Int*. 2000;67(1):10–18.
62. Karlsson M. Does exercise reduce the burden of fractures? A review. *Acta Orthop Scand*. 2002;73(6):691–705.
63. Law MR, Hackshaw AK. A meta-analysis of cigarette smoking, bone mineral density and risk of hip fracture: Recognition of a major effect. *BMJ*. 1997;315(7112):841–6.
64. Kanis JA, Johansson H, Johnell O, et al. Alcohol intake as a risk factor for fracture. *Osteoporos Int*. 2005;16(7):737–42.
65. Kanis JA, Johansson H, Oden A, et al. A meta-analysis of prior corticosteroid use and fracture risk. *J Bone Miner Res*. 2004;19(6):893–9.
66. Force USPST, Grossman DC, Curry SJ, et al. Vitamin D, calcium, or combined supplementation for the primary prevention of fractures in community-dwelling adults: US Preventive Services Task Force Recommendation Statement. *JAMA*. 2018;319(15):1592–9.
67. Papadimitropoulos E, Wells G, Shea B, et al. Meta-analyses of therapies for postmenopausal osteoporosis. VIII: Meta-analysis of the efficacy of vitamin D treatment in preventing osteoporosis in postmenopausal women. *Endocr Rev*. 2002;23(4):560–9.
68. Avenell A, Mak JC, O'Connell D. Vitamin D and vitamin D analogues for preventing fractures in post-menopausal women and older men. *Cochrane Database Syst Rev*. 2014;(4):CD000227.
69. Howe TE, Shea B, Dawson LJ, et al. Exercise for preventing and treating osteoporosis in postmenopausal women. *Cochrane Database Syst Rev*. 2011;(7):CD000333.
70. Force USPST. Screening for osteoporosis: U.S. preventive services task force recommendation statement. *Ann Intern Med*. 2011;154(5):356–64.
71. Qaseem A, Forciea MA, McLean RM, Denberg TD, Clinical Guidelines Committee of the American College of Physicians. Treatment of low bone density or osteoporosis to prevent fractures in men and women: A clinical practice guideline update from the American College of Physicians. *Ann Intern Med*. 2017;166(11):818–39.
72. Rossouw JE, Anderson GL, Prentice RL, et al. Risks and benefits of estrogen plus progestin in healthy postmenopausal women: Principal results from the women's health initiative randomized controlled trial. *JAMA*. 2002;288(3):321–33.
73. Cummings SR, Black DM, Thompson DE, et al. Effect of alendronate on risk of fracture in women with low bone density but without vertebral fractures: Results from the Fracture Intervention Trial. *JAMA*. 1998;280(24):2077–82.
74. Byun JH, Jang S, Lee S, et al. The efficacy of bisphosphonates for prevention of osteoporotic fracture: An update meta-analysis. *J Bone Metab*. 2017;24(1):37–49.
75. Ettinger B, Black DM, Mitlak BH, et al. Reduction of vertebral fracture risk in postmenopausal women with osteoporosis treated with raloxifene: Results from a 3-year randomized clinical trial. Multiple Outcomes of Raloxifene Evaluation (MORE) Investigators. *JAMA*. 1999;282(7):637–45.
76. Zizic TM. Pharmacologic prevention of osteoporotic fractures. *Am Fam Physician*. 2004;70(7):1293–300.
77. Buckley L, Guyatt G, Fink HA, et al. American College of Rheumatology guideline for the prevention and treatment of glucocorticoid-induced osteoporosis. *Arthritis Care Res (Hoboken)*. 2017;69(8):1095–110.
78. Tinetti ME. Clinical practice. Preventing falls in elderly persons. *N Engl J Med*. 2003;348(1):42–49.
79. Schwartz AV, Capezuti E, Grisso JA. Falls as risk factors for fractures. In: Marcus R, Feldman D, Kelsey J, eds. *Osteoporosis*. 2nd ed. San Diego, CA: Academic Press; 2001, pp. 795–807.
80. Stevens JA, Burns E. CDC Compendium of Effective Fall Interventions: What Works for Community-Dwelling Older Adults, 3rd Edition. 2015. Available at https://www.cdc.gov/homeandrecreationalsafety/falls/compendium.html. Accessed November 18, 2017.
81. Cummings SR, Nevitt MC. A hypothesis: The causes of hip fractures. *J Gerontol*. 1989;44(4):M107–111.
82. Keegan TH, Kelsey JL, King AC, Quesenberry Jr CP, Sidney S. Characteristics of fallers who fracture at the foot, distal forearm, proximal humerus, pelvis, and shaft of the tibia/fibula compared with fallers who do not fracture. *Am J Epidemiol*. 2004;159(2):192–203.
83. Schwartz AV, Nevitt MC, Brown Jr BW, Kelsey JL. Increased falling as a risk factor for fracture among older women: The study of osteoporotic fractures. *Am J Epidemiol*. 2005;161(2):180–5.
84. Faulkner KG, Cummings SR, Black D, Palermo L, Gluer CC, Genant HK. Simple measurement of femoral geometry predicts hip fracture: The study of osteoporotic fractures. *J Bone Miner Res*. 1993;8(10):1211–17.
85. Singh M, Nagrath AR, Maini PS. Changes in trabecular pattern of the upper end of the femur as an index of osteoporosis. *J Bone Joint Surg Am*. 1970;52(3):457–67.
86. Parker MJ, Gillespie LD, Gillespie WJ. Hip protectors for preventing hip fractures in the elderly. *Cochrane Database Syst Rev*. 2004;(3):CD001255.
87. Council for International Organizations of Medical Sciences. *The Epidemiology of Chronic Rheumatism: Atlas of Standard Radiographs of Arthritis*. Vol. 2. Oxford: Blackwell Scientific Publications; 1963.
88. Sowers MF, Hayes C, Jamadar D, et al. Magnetic resonance-detected subchondral bone marrow and cartilage defect characteristics associated with pain and X-ray-defined knee osteoarthritis. *Osteoarthritis Cartilage*. 2003;11(6):387–93.
89. Myers SL, Dines K, Brandt DA, Brandt KD, Albrecht ME. Experimental assessment by high frequency ultrasound of articular cartilage thickness and osteoarthritic changes. *J Rheumatol*. 1995;22(1):109–16.
90. Altman R, Asch E, Bloch D, et al. Development of criteria for the classification and reporting of osteoarthritis. Classification of osteoarthritis of the knee. Diagnostic and Therapeutic Criteria Committee of the American Rheumatism Association. *Arthritis Rheum*. 1986;29(8):1039–49.
91. Carman WJ, Sowers M, Hawthorne VM, Weissfeld LA. Obesity as a risk factor for osteoarthritis of the hand and wrist: A prospective study. *Am J Epidemiol*. 1994;139(2):119–29.
92. Davis MA, Ettinger WH, Neuhaus JM. The role of metabolic factors and blood pressure in the association of obesity with osteoarthritis of the knee. *J Rheumatol*. 1988;15(12):1827–32.
93. Lachance L, Sowers M, Jamadar D, Jannausch M, Hochberg M, Crutchfield M. The experience of pain and emergent osteoarthritis of the knee. *Osteoarthritis Cartilage*. 2001;9(6):527–32.
94. Nguyen US, Zhang Y, Zhu Y, Niu J, Zhang B, Felson DT. Increasing prevalence of knee pain and symptomatic knee osteoarthritis: Survey and cohort data. *Ann Intern Med*. 2011;155(11):725–32.
95. Acheson RM, Chan YK, Clemett AR. New Haven survey of joint diseases. XII. Distribution and symptoms of osteoarthrosis in the hands with reference to handedness. *Ann Rheum Dis*. 1970;29(3):275–86.
96. Stecher RM. Heberden's nodes; a clinical description of osteo-arthritis of the finger joints. *Ann Rheum Dis*. 1955;14(1):1–10.
97. Spector TD, Cicuttini F, Baker J, Loughlin J, Hart D. Genetic influences on osteoarthritis in women: A twin study. *BMJ*. 1996;312(7036):940–3.
98. Palotie A, Vaisanen P, Ott J, et al. Predisposition to familial osteoarthrosis linked to type II collagen gene. *Lancet*. 1989;1(8644):924–7.

99. Lawrence JS. Rheumatism in coal miners. III. Occupational factors. *Br J Ind Med.* 1955;12(3):249–61.

100. Lawrence JS. Rheumatism in cotton operatives. *Br J Ind Med.* 1961;18:270–6.

101. Croft P, Coggon D, Cruddas M, Cooper C. Osteoarthritis of the hip: An occupational disease in farmers. *BMJ.* 1992;304(6837):1269–72.

102. Partridge RE, Duthie JJ. Rheumatism in dockers and civil servants. A comparison of heavy manual and sedentary workers. *Ann Rheum Dis.* 1968;27(6):559–68.

103. Harvard School of Public Health, World Health Organization, World Bank. *The Global Burden of Disease.* Vol. 1. Geneva: World Health Organization; 1996.

104. Sowers M, Lachance L, Hochberg M, Jamadar D. Radiographically defined osteoarthritis of the hand and knee in young and middle-aged African American and Caucasian women. *Osteoarthritis Cartilage.* 2000;8(2):69–77.

105. Peat G, McCarney R, Croft P. Knee pain and osteoarthritis in older adults: A review of community burden and current use of primary health care. *Ann Rheum Dis.* 2001;60(2):91–7.

106. Guccione AA, Felson DT, Anderson JJ, et al. The effects of specific medical conditions on the functional limitations of elders in the Framingham Study. *Am J Public Health.* 1994;84(3):351–8.

107. Hochberg MC, Lawrence RC, Everett DF, Cornoni-Huntley J. Epidemiologic associations of pain in osteoarthritis of the knee: Data from the National Health and Nutrition Examination Survey and the National Health and Nutrition Examination-I Epidemiologic Follow-up Survey. *Semin Arthritis Rheum.* 1989;18(4 Suppl 2):4–9.

108. Cooper C, McAlindon T, Snow S, et al. Mechanical and constitutional risk factors for symptomatic knee osteoarthritis: Differences between medial tibiofemoral and patellofemoral disease. *J Rheumatol.* 1994;21(2):307–13.

109. Felson DT. Epidemiology of hip and knee osteoarthritis. *Epidemiol Rev.* 1988;10:1–28.

110. Lane NE. Exercise: A cause of osteoarthritis. *J Rheumatol Suppl.* 1995;43:3–6.

111. Felson DT, Zhang Y, Anthony JM, Naimark A, Anderson JJ. Weight loss reduces the risk for symptomatic knee osteoarthritis in women. The Framingham study. *Ann Intern Med.* 1992;116(7):535–9.

112. Pinczewski LA, Deehan DJ, Salmon LJ, Russell VJ, Clingeleffer A. A five-year comparison of patellar tendon versus four-strand hamstring tendon autograft for arthroscopic reconstruction of the anterior cruciate ligament. *Am J Sports Med.* 2002;30(4):523–36.

113. Hochberg MC, Altman RD, April KT, et al. American College of Rheumatology 2012 recommendations for the use of nonpharmacologic and pharmacologic therapies in osteoarthritis of the hand, hip, and knee. *Arthritis Care Res (Hoboken).* 2012;64(4):465–74.

114. Petrella RJ, Bartha C. Home based exercise therapy for older patients with knee osteoarthritis: A randomized clinical trial. *J Rheumatol.* 2000;27(9):2215–21.

115. Deyle GD, Henderson NE, Matekel RL, Ryder MG, Garber MB, Allison SC. Effectiveness of manual physical therapy and exercise in osteoarthritis of the knee. A randomized, controlled trial. *Ann Intern Med.* 2000;132(3):173–81.

116. Mazzuca SA, Brandt KD, Katz BP, Chambers M, Byrd D, Hanna M. Effects of self-care education on the health status of inner-city patients with osteoarthritis of the knee. *Arthritis Rheum.* 1997;40(8):1466–74.

117. Fransen M, McConnell S, Harmer AR, Van der Esch M, Simic M, Bennell KL. Exercise for osteoarthritis of the knee. *Cochrane Database Syst Rev.* 2015;1:CD004376.

118. Abramson SB. Et tu, acetaminophen? *Arthritis Rheum.* 2002;46(11):2831–5.

119. Jordan KM, Arden NK, Doherty M, et al. EULAR Recommendations 2003: An evidence based approach to the management of knee osteoarthritis: Report of a task force of the Standing Committee for International Clinical Studies Including Therapeutic Trials (ESCISIT). *Ann Rheum Dis.* 2003;62(12):1145–55.

120. Bjordal JM, Ljunggren AE, Klovning A, Slordal L. Non-steroidal anti-inflammatory drugs, including cyclo-oxygenase-2 inhibitors, in osteoarthritic knee pain: Meta-analysis of randomised placebo controlled trials. *BMJ.* 2004;329(7478):1317.

121. Runhaar J, Rozendaal RM, van Middelkoop M, et al. Subgroup analyses of the effectiveness of oral glucosamine for knee and hip osteoarthritis: A systematic review and individual patient data meta-analysis from the OA trial bank. *Ann Rheum Dis.* 2017;76(11):1862–9.

122. Singh JA, Noorbaloochi S, MacDonald R, Maxwell LJ. Chondroitin for osteoarthritis. *Cochrane Database Syst Rev.* 2015;1:CD005614.

123. Bellamy N, Campbell J, Robinson V, Gee T, Bourne R, Wells G. Viscosupplementation for the treatment of osteoarthritis of the knee. *Cochrane Database Syst Rev.* 2006;(2):CD005321.

124. Ethgen O, Bruyere O, Richy F, Dardennes C, Reginster JY. Health-related quality of life in total hip and total knee arthroplasty. A qualitative and systematic review of the literature. *J Bone Joint Surg Am.* 2004;86-A(5):963–74.

125. Aletaha D, Neogi T, Silman AJ, et al. 2010 Rheumatoid arthritis classification criteria: An American College of Rheumatology/European League Against Rheumatism collaborative initiative. *Arthritis Rheum.* 2010;62(9):2569–81.

126. Bartels CM, Bell CL, Shinki K, Rosenthal A, Bridges AJ. Changing trends in serious extra-articular manifestations of rheumatoid arthritis among United State veterans over 20 years. *Rheumatology (Oxford).* 2010;49(9):1670–5.

127. Westhoff G, Listing J, Zink A. Loss of physical independence in rheumatoid arthritis: Interview data from a representative sample of patients in rheumatologic care. *Arthritis Care Res.* 2000;13(1):11–22.

128. Barrett EM, Scott DG, Wiles NJ, Symmons DP. The impact of rheumatoid arthritis on employment status in the early years of disease: A UK community-based study. *Rheumatology (Oxford).* 2000;39(12):1403–9.

129. Boers M, Dijkmans B, Gabriel S, Maradit-Kremers H, O'Dell J, Pincus T. Making an impact on mortality in rheumatoid arthritis: Targeting cardiovascular comorbidity. *Arthritis Rheum.* 2004;50(6):1734–9.

130. Gabriel SE. Update on the epidemiology of the rheumatic diseases. *Curr Opin Rheumatol.* 1996;8(2):96–100.

131. Roubille C, Richer V, Starnino T, et al. The effects of tumour necrosis factor inhibitors, methotrexate, non-steroidal anti-inflammatory drugs and corticosteroids on cardiovascular events in rheumatoid arthritis, psoriasis and psoriatic arthritis: A systematic review and meta-analysis. *Ann Rheum Dis.* 2015;74(3):480–9.

132. Uhlig T, Kvien TK. Is rheumatoid arthritis disappearing? *Ann Rheum Dis.* 2005;64(1):7–10.

133. Myasoedova E, Crowson CS, Kremers HM, Therneau TM, Gabriel SE. Is the incidence of rheumatoid arthritis rising?: Results from Olmsted County, Minnesota, 1955–2007. *Arthritis Rheum.* 2010;62(6):1576–82.

134. Ropes MW, Bennett GA, Cobb S, Jacox R, Jessar RA. 1958 Revision of diagnostic criteria for rheumatoid arthritis. *Bull Rheum Dis.* 1958;9(4):175–6.

135. Turesson C, O'Fallon WM, Crowson CS, Gabriel SE, Matteson EL. Occurrence of extraarticular disease manifestations is associated with excess mortality in a community based cohort of patients with rheumatoid arthritis. *J Rheumatol.* 2002;29(1):62–7.

136. Kelsey JL, Hochberg MC. Epidemiology of chronic musculoskeletal disorders. *Annu Rev Public Health.* 1988;9:379–401.

137. Turesson C, Weyand CM, Matteson EL. Genetics of rheumatoid arthritis: Is there a pattern predicting extraarticular manifestations? *Arthritis Rheum.* 2004;51(5):853–63.

138. del Junco D, Luthra HS, Annegers JF, Worthington JW, Kurland LT. The familial aggregation of rheumatoid arthritis and its relationship to the HLA-DR4 association. *Am J Epidemiol.* 1984;119(5):813–29.

139. Goldstein R, Arnett FC. The genetics of rheumatic disease in man. *Rheum Dis Clin North Am.* 1987;13(3):487–510.

140. Bang SY, Lee KH, Cho SK, Lee HS, Lee KW, Bae SC. Smoking increases rheumatoid arthritis susceptibility in individuals carrying the HLA-DRB1 shared epitope, regardless of rheumatoid factor or anti-cyclic citrullinated peptide antibody status. *Arthritis Rheum.* 2010;62(2):369–77.

141 Weyand CM, Goronzy JJ. Inherited and noninherited risk factors in rheumatoid arthritis. *Curr Opin Rheumatol.* 1995;7(3):206–13.

142. McInnes IB, Schett G. The pathogenesis of rheumatoid arthritis. *N Engl J Med.* 2011;365(23):2205–19.

143. Albani S, Carson DA. Etiology and pathogenesis of rheumatoid arthritis. In: Koopman WJ, ed. *Arthritis and Allied Conditions.* Vol. 1. 13th ed. Baltimore, MD: Williams & Wilkins; 1997, pp. 979–92.

144. Kay CR. The Royal College of General Practitioners' oral contraception study: Some recent observations. *Clin Obstet Gynaecol.* 1984;11(3):759–86.

145. Spector TD, Hochberg MC. The protective effect of the oral contraceptive pill on rheumatoid arthritis: An overview of the analytic epidemiological studies using meta-analysis. *J Clin Epidemiol.* 1990;43(11):1221–30.

146. Sparks JA, Chen CY, Jiang X, et al. Improved performance of epidemiologic and genetic risk models for rheumatoid arthritis serologic phenotypes using family history. *Ann Rheum Dis.* 2015;74(8):1522–9.

147. Sparks JA, Iversen MD, Yu Z, et al. Disclosure of personalized rheumatoid arthritis risk using genetics, biomarkers, and lifestyle factors to

motivate health behavior improvements: A randomized controlled trial. *Arthritis Care Res (Hoboken)*. 2018;70(6):823–33.

148. Avina-Zubieta JA, Choi HK, Sadatsafavi M, Etminan M, Esdaile JM, Lacaille D. Risk of cardiovascular mortality in patients with rheumatoid arthritis: A meta-analysis of observational studies. *Arthritis Rheum*. 2008;59(12):1690–7.
149. Sparks JA, Chang SC, Liao KP, et al. Rheumatoid arthritis and mortality among women during 36 years of prospective follow-up: Results from the nurses' health study. *Arthritis Care Res (Hoboken)*. 2016;68(6):753–62.
150. Alarcon GS. Epidemiology of rheumatoid arthritis. *Rheum Dis Clin North Am*. 1995;21(3):589–604.
151. Pincus T, Callahan LF. Formal education as a marker for increased mortality and morbidity in rheumatoid arthritis. *J Chronic Dis*. 1985;38(12):973–84.
152. de Croon EM, Sluiter JK, Nijssen TF, Dijkmans BA, Lankhorst GJ, Frings-Dresen MH. Predictive factors of work disability in rheumatoid arthritis: A systematic literature review. *Ann Rheum Dis*. 2004;63(11):1362–7.
153. Rantapaa-Dahlqvist S, de Jong BA, Berglin E, et al. Antibodies against cyclic citrullinated peptide and IgA rheumatoid factor predict the development of rheumatoid arthritis. *Arthritis Rheum*. 2003;48(10):2741–9.
154. Singh JA, Furst DE, Bharat A, et al. 2012 Update of the 2008 American College of Rheumatology recommendations for the use of disease-modifying antirheumatic drugs and biologic agents in the treatment of rheumatoid arthritis. *Arthritis Care Res (Hoboken)*. 2012;64(5):625–39.
155. Weinblatt ME. Treatment of rheumatoid arthritis. In: Koopman WJ, ed. *Arthritis and Allied Conditions*. Baltimore, MD: Williams & Wilkins; 1997, pp. 1131–41.
156. O'Dell JR, Mikuls TR, Taylor TH, et al. Therapies for active rheumatoid arthritis after methotrexate failure. *N Engl J Med*. 2013;369(4):307–18.
157. Rheumatology ACo. Spondyloarthritis. 2013. Available at https://www.rheumatology.org/Practice-Quality/Clinical-Support/Clinical-Practice-Guidelines/Axial-Spondyloarthritis.
158. Rudwaleit M, van der Heijde D, Landewe R, et al. The development of Assessment of SpondyloArthritis international Society classification criteria for axial spondyloarthritis (part II): Validation and final selection. *Ann Rheum Dis*. 2009;68(6):777–83.
159. Ward MM, Deodhar A, Akl EA, et al. American College of Rheumatology/Spondylitis Association of America/Spondyloarthritis Research and Treatment Network 2015 Recommendations for the treatment of ankylosing spondylitis and nonradiographic axial spondyloarthritis. *Arthritis Rheumatol*. 2016;68(2):282–98.
160. Centers for Disease Control and Prevention. Systemic Lupus Erythematosus (SLE). Available at http://www.cdc.gov/arthritis/basics/lupus.htm. Accessed 23 June 2016.
161. Lim SS, Bayakly AR, Helmick CG, Gordon C, Easley KA, Drenkard C. The incidence and prevalence of systemic lupus erythematosus, 2002–2004: The Georgia Lupus Registry. *Arthritis Rheumatol*. 2014;66(2):357–68.
162. Bertoli AM, Vila LM, Apte M, et al. Systemic lupus erythematosus in a multiethnic US Cohort LUMINA XLVIII: Factors predictive of pulmonary damage. *Lupus*. 2007;16(6):410–17.
163. Evanski PM. The geriatric foot. In: *Disoders of the Foot and Ankle*. Philadelphia, PA: WB Saunders;1982, pp. 964–78.
164. Elton PJ, Sanderson SP. A chiropodial survey of elderly persons over 65 years in the community. *Public Health*. 1986;100(4):219–22.
165. Dunn JE, Link CL, Felson DT, Crincoli MG, Keysor JJ, McKinlay JB. Prevalence of foot and ankle conditions in a multiethnic community sample of older adults. *Am J Epidemiol*. 2004;159(5):491–8.
166. Benvenuti F, Ferrucci L, Guralnik JM, Gangemi S, Baroni A. Foot pain and disability in older persons: An epidemiologic survey. *J Am Geriatr Soc*. 1995;43(5):479–84.
167. Leveille SG, Guralnik JM, Ferrucci L, Hirsch R, Simonsick E, Hochberg MC. Foot pain and disability in older women. *Am J Epidemiol*. 1998;148(7):657–65.
168. Tinetti ME, Speechley M, Ginter SF. Risk factors for falls among elderly persons living in the community. *N Engl J Med*. 1988;319(26):1701–7.
169. Keegan TH, Kelsey JL, Sidney S, Quesenberry Jr CP. Foot problems as risk factors of fractures. *Am J Epidemiol*. 2002;155(10):926–31.
170. Robbins JM. Recognizing, treating, and preventing common foot problems. *Cleve Clin J Med*. 2000;67(1):45–7, 51-42, 55-46.
171. Helfand AE. At the foot of South Mountain. A 5-year longitudinal study of foot problems and screening in an elderly population. *J Am Podiatry Assoc*. 1973;63(10):512–21.
172. Edelstein JE. Foot care for the aging. *Phys Ther*. 1988;68(12):1882–6.
173. Smart CN, Sanders CR. *The Costs of Motor Vehicle Related Spinal Cord Injuries*. Washington, DC: Insurance Institute for Highway Safety; 1976.
174. National Spinal Cord Injury Statistical Center. Spinal Cord Injury (SCI): Facts and Figures at a Glance. 2016. Available at https://msktc.org/lib/docs/Data_Sheets_/SCIMS_Facts_and_Figures_2017_August_FINAL.pdf. Accessed November 18, 2017.
175. Ackery A, Tator C, Krassioukov A. A global perspective on spinal cord injury epidemiology. *J Neurotrauma*. 2004;21(10):1355–70.
176. Stover SL, Fine PR. The epidemiology and economics of spinal cord injury. *Paraplegia*. 1987;25(3):225–8.
177. Thurman DJ, Burnett CL, Beaudoin DE, Jeppson L, Sniezek JE. Risk factors and mechanisms of occurrence in motor vehicle-related spinal cord injuries: Utah. *Accid Anal Prev*. 1995;27(3):411–5.
178. Woodruff BA, Baron RC. A description of nonfatal spinal cord injury using a hospital-based registry. *Am J Prev Med*. 1994;10(1):10–14.
179. Sekhon LH, Fehlings MG. Epidemiology, demographics, and pathophysiology of acute spinal cord injury. *Spine (Phila Pa 1976)*. 2001;26 (24 Suppl):S2–12.
180. Torg JS, Vegso JJ, Sennett B, Das M. The National Football Head and Neck Injury Registry. 14-Year report on cervical quadriplegia, 1971 through 1984. *JAMA*. 1985;254(24):3439–43.
181. Tator CH, Provvidenza CF, Lapczak L, Carson J, Raymond D. Spinal injuries in Canadian ice hockey: Documentation of injuries sustained from 1943–1999. *Can J Neurol Sci*. 2004;31(4):460–6.
182. Krassioukov AV, Furlan JC, Fehlings MG. Medical co-morbidities, secondary complications, and mortality in elderly with acute spinal cord injury. *J Neurotrauma*. 2003;20(4):391–9.
183. Sutton RA, Bentley M, Castree B, Mattinson R, Pattinson J, Smith R. Review of the social situation of paraplegic and tetraplegic patients rehabilitated in the Hexham Regional Spinal Injury Unit in the north of England over the past four years. *Paraplegia*. 1982;20(2):71–9.
184. Winter RB, Lovell WW. Spinal problems in pediactric orthopedics. In: Morrissy RT, ed. *Lovell and Winter's Pediatric Orthopedics*. Vol. 2. 3rd ed. Philadelphia, PA: Lippincott; 1990, pp. 670–702.
185. Shands AR, Jr., Eisberg HB. The incidence of scoliosis in the state of Delaware; a study of 50,000 minifilms of the chest made during a survey for tuberculosis. *J Bone Joint Surg Am*. 1955;37-A(6):1243–9.
186. Morais T, Bernier M, Turcotte F. Age- and sex-specific prevalence of scoliosis and the value of school screening programs. *Am J Public Health*. 1985;75(12):1377–80.
187. Topalis C, Grauers A, Diarbakerli E, Danielsson A, Gerdhem P. Neck and back problems in adults with idiopathic scoliosis diagnosed in youth: An observational study of prevalence, change over a mean four year time period and comparison with a control group. *Scoliosis Spinal Disord*. 2017;12:20.
188. Weiss HR, Karavidas N, Moramarco M, Moramarco K. Long-term effects of untreated adolescent idiopathic scoliosis: A review of the literature. *Asian Spine J*. 2016;10(6):1163–9.
189. Agabegi SS, Kazemi N, Sturm PF, Mehlman CT. Natural history of adolescent idiopathic scoliosis in skeletally mature patients: A critical review. *J Am Acad Orthop Surg*. 2015;23(12):714–23.
190. Dunn J, Henrikson NB, Morrison CC, Nguyen M, Blasi PR, Lin JS. Screening for adolescent idiopathic scoliosis: A systematic evidence review for the U.S. Preventive Services Task Force. 2017. file:///C:/Users/acperez/Downloads/adolescent-scoliosis-draft-er.pdf. Accessed November 18, 2017.
191. Hazebroek-Kampschreur AA, Hofman A, van Dijk AP, van Ling B. Determinants of trunk abnormalities in adolescence. *Int J Epidemiol*. 1994;23(6):1242–7.
192. Brooks HL, Azen SP, Gerberg E, Brooks R, Chan L. Scoliosis: A prospective epidemiological study. *J Bone Joint Surg Am*. 1975;57(7):968–72.
193. Wynne-Davies R. Familial (idiopathic) scoliosis. A family survey. *J Bone Joint Surg Br*. 1968;50(1):24–30.
194. Kesling KL, Reinker KA. Scoliosis in twins. A meta-analysis of the literature and report of six cases. *Spine (Phila Pa 1976)*. 1997;22(17):2009–14; discussion 2015.
195. Wu J, Qiu Y, Zhang L, Sun Q, Qiu X, He Y. Association of estrogen receptor gene polymorphisms with susceptibility to adolescent idiopathic scoliosis. *Spine (Phila Pa 1976)*. 2006;31(10):1131–6.
196. Justice CM, Miller NH, Marosy B, Zhang J, Wilson AF. Familial idiopathic scoliosis: Evidence of an X-linked susceptibility locus. *Spine (Phila Pa 1976)*. 2003;28(6):589–94.
197. Nissinen M, Heliovaara M, Seitsamo J, Poussa M. Trunk asymmetry, posture, growth, and risk of scoliosis. A three-year follow-up of Finnish prepubertal school children. *Spine (Phila Pa 1976)*. 1993;18(1):8–13.

198. Kelsey JL. *Epidemiology of Musculoskeletal Disorders (Monographs in Epidemiology and Biostatistics)*. Oxford: Oxford University Press; 1982.

199. Nissinen M, Heliovaara M, Ylikoski M, Poussa M. Trunk asymmetry and screening for scoliosis: A longitudinal cohort study of pubertal schoolchildren. *Acta Paediatr*. 1993;82(1):77–82.

200. Keessen W, Crowe A, Hearn M. Proprioceptive accuracy in idiopathic scoliosis. *Spine (Phila Pa 1976)*. 1992;17(2):149–55.

201. Miller NH. Cause and natural history of adolescent idiopathic scoliosis. *Orthop Clin North Am*. 1999;30(3):343–52.

202. Bunnell WP. The natural history of idiopathic scoliosis before skeletal maturity. *Spine (Phila Pa 1976)*. 1986;11(8):773–6.

203. Tan KJ, Moe MM, Vaithinathan R, Wong HK. Curve progression in idiopathic scoliosis: Follow-up study to skeletal maturity. *Spine (Phila Pa 1976)*. 2009;34(7):697–700.

204. Dickson RA, Stamper P, Sharp AM, Harker P. School screening for scoliosis: Cohort study of clinical course. *Br Med J*. 1980;281(6235):265–7.

205. Lonstein JE. Natural history and school screening for scoliosis. *Orthop Clin North Am*. 1988;19(2):227–37.

206. Margalit A, McKean G, Constantine A, Thompson CB, Lee RJ, Sponseller PD. Body mass hides the curve: Thoracic scoliometer readings vary by body mass index value. *J Pediatr Orthop*. 2017;37(4):e255–60.

207. Grossman TW, Mazur JM, Cummings RJ. An evaluation of the Adams forward bend test and the scoliometer in a scoliosis school screening setting. *J Pediatr Orthop*. 1995;15(4):535–8.

208. Cote P, Kreitz BG, Cassidy JD, Dzus AK, Martel J. A study of the diagnostic accuracy and reliability of the Scoliometer and Adam's forward bend test. *Spine (Phila Pa 1976)*. 1998;23(7):796–802; discussion 803.

209. Balg F, Juteau M, Theoret C, Svotelis A, Grenier G. Validity and reliability of the iPhone to measure rib hump in scoliosis. *J Pediatr Orthop*. 2014;34(8):774–9.

210. Qiao J, Xu L, Zhu Z, et al. Inter- and intraobserver reliability assessment of the axial trunk rotation: Manual versus smartphone-aided measurement tools. *BMC Musculoskelet Disord*. 2014;15:343.

211. El-Hawary R, Chukwunyerenwa C. Update on evaluation and treatment of scoliosis. *Pediatr Clin North Am*. 2014;61(6):1223–41.

212. Sox HC Jr, Berwick DM, Berg AO, et al. Screening for adolescent idiopathic scoliosis. Review article. US Preventive Services Task Force. *JAMA*. 1993;269(20):2667–72.

213. Williams JI. Criteria for screening: are the effects predictable? *Spine (Phila Pa 1976)*. 1988;13(10):1178–86.

214. Goldberg CJ, Dowling FE, Fogarty EE, Moore DP. School scoliosis screening and the United States Preventive Services Task Force. An examination of long-term results. *Spine (Phila Pa 1976)*. 1995;20(12):1368–74.

215. U.S. Preventative Services Task Force. Draft Recommendation Statement: Adolescent Idiopathic Scoliosis: Screening. 2017. Available at https://www.uspreventiveservicestaskforce.org/uspstf/document/draft-recommendation-statement/adolescent-idiopathic-scoliosis-screening. Accessed November 18, 2017.

216. American Academy of Orthopedic Surgeons and Scoliosis Research Society. Position Statement—Screening for the Early Detection for Idiopathic Scoliosis in Adolescents. 2015. Available at https://www.srs.org/about-srs/news-and-announcements/position-statement---screening-for-the-early-detection-for-idiopathic-scoliosis-in-adolescents. Accessed November 18, 2017.

217. de Poorter JJ, Beunder TJ, Gareb B, et al. Long-term outcomes of slipped capital femoral epiphysis treated with in situ pinning. *J Child Orthop*. 2016;10(5):371–9.

218. Loder RT, Skopelja EN. The epidemiology and demographics of slipped capital femoral epiphysis. *ISRN Orthop*. 2011;2011:486512.

219. Lehmann CL, Arons RR, Loder RT, Vitale MG. The epidemiology of slipped capital femoral epiphysis: An update. *J Pediatr Orthop*. 2006;26(3):286–90.

220. Loder RT. A worldwide study on the seasonal variation of slipped capital femoral epiphysis. *Clin Orthop Relat Res*. 1996(322):28–36.

221. Brown D. Seasonal variation of slipped capital femoral epiphysis in the United States. *J Pediatr Orthop*. 2004;24(2):139–43.

222. Kelsey JL, Acheson RM, Keggi KJ. The body build of patients with slipped capital femoral epiphysis. *Am J Dis Child*. 1972;124(2):276–81.

223. Loder RT. The demographics of slipped capital femoral epiphysis. An international multicenter study. *Clin Orthop Relat Res*. 1996(322):8–27.

224. Tucker J, Moore M, Rooy J, Wright A, Rothschild C, Werk LN. Reliability of common lower extremity biomechanical measures of children with and without obesity. *Pediatr Phys Ther*. 2015;27(3):250–6.

225. Galbraith RT, Gelberman RH, Hajek PC, et al. Obesity and decreased femoral anteversion in adolescence. *J Orthop Res*. 1987;5(4):523–8.

226. Pritchett JW, Perdue KD. Mechanical factors in slipped capital femoral epiphysis. *J Pediatr Orthop*. 1988;8(4):385–8.

227. Rennie AM. Familial slipped upper femoral epiphysis. *J Bone Joint Surg Br*. 1967;49(3):535–9.

228. Weiner D. Pathogenesis of slipped capital femoral epiphysis: Current concepts. *J Pediatr Orthop B*. 1996;5(2):67–73.

229. Morscher E. Strength and morphology of growth cartilage under hormonal influence of puberty. Animal experiments and clinical study on the etiology of local growth disorders during puberty. *Reconstr Surg Traumatol*. 1968;10:3–104.

230. Witbreuk M, van Kemenade FJ, van der Sluijs JA, Jansma EP, Rotteveel J, van Royen BJ. Slipped capital femoral epiphysis and its association with endocrine, metabolic and chronic diseases: A systematic review of the literature. *J Child Orthop*. 2013;7(3):213–23.

231. Mostoufi-Moab S, Isaacoff EJ, Spiegel D, et al. Childhood cancer survivors exposed to total body irradiation are at significant risk for slipped capital femoral epiphysis during recombinant growth hormone therapy. *Pediatr Blood Cancer*. 2013;60(11):1766–71.

232. Jerre R, Billing L, Hansson G, Wallin J. The contralateral hip in patients primarily treated for unilateral slipped upper femoral epiphysis. Long-term follow-up of 61 hips. *J Bone Joint Surg Br*. 1994;76(4):563–7.

233. Wensaas A, Wiig O, Hellund JC, Khoshnewiszadeh B, Terjesen T. Magnetic resonance imaging at primary diagnosis cannot predict subsequent contralateral slip in slipped capital femoral epiphysis. *Skeletal Radiol*. 2017;46(12):1687–94.

234. Bhattacharjee A, Freeman R, Roberts AP, Kiely NT. Outcome of the unaffected contralateral hip in unilateral slipped capital femoral epiphysis: A report comparing prophylactic fixation with observation. *J Pediatr Orthop B*. 2016;25(5):454–8.

235. Schultz WR, Weinstein JN, Weinstein SL, Smith BG. Prophylactic pinning of the contralateral hip in slipped capital femoral epiphysis: Evaluation of long-term outcome for the contralateral hip with use of decision analysis. *J Bone Joint Surg Am*. 2002;84-A(8):1305–14.

236. Hurley JM, Betz RR, Loder RT, Davidson RS, Alburger PD, Steel HH. Slipped capital femoral epiphysis. The prevalence of late contralateral slip. *J Bone Joint Surg Am*. 1996;78(2):226–30.

237. National Center for Health Statistics. Current Estimates From the National Health Interview Survey, United States, 1987. *Vital and Health Statistics Data From the National Health Survey Series 10, No 166*. 1988.

238. Rivara FP, Calonge N, Thompson RS. Population-based study of unintentional injury incidence and impact during childhood. *Am J Public Health*. 1989;79(8):990–4.

239. Cooper C, Dennison EM, Leufkens HG, Bishop N, van Staa TP. Epidemiology of childhood fractures in Britain: A study using the general practice research database. *J Bone Miner Res*. 2004;19(12):1976–81.

240. Naranje SM, Erali RA, Warner WC, Jr., Sawyer JR, Kelly DM. Epidemiology of pediatric fractures presenting to emergency departments in the United States. *J Pediatr Orthop*. 2016;36(4):e45–48.

241. Landin LA. Fracture patterns in children. Analysis of 8,682 fractures with special reference to incidence, etiology and secular changes in a Swedish urban population 1950–1979. *Acta Orthop Scand Suppl*. 1983;202:1–109.

242. Lyons RA, Delahunty AM, Kraus D, et al. Children's fractures: A population based study. *Inj Prev*. 1999;5(2):129–32.

243. Kim SJ, Ahn J, Kim HK, Kim JH. Obese children experience more extremity fractures than nonobese children and are significantly more likely to die from traumatic injuries. *Acta Paediatr*. 2016;105(10):1152–7.

244. Jones DH. The early diagnosis of congenital dislocation of the hip joint. *Br J Clin Pract*. 1965;19:443–9.

245. National Council of Youth Sports. Report on Trends and Participation in Organized Youth Sports. 2008. Available at http://www.ncys.org/pdfs/2008/2008-ncys-market-research-report.pdf. Accessed November 18, 2017.

246. The National Federation of State High School Associations. 2016–17 High School Atheletics Participation Survey. 2017. Available at http://www.sportsdestinations.com/management/marketing-sponsorships/high-school-sports-participation-2016-2017-13281. Accessed November 18, 2017.

247. Oosterhoff B, Kaplow JB, Wray-Lake L, Gallagher K. Activity-specific pathways among duration of organized activity involvement, social support, and adolescent well-being: Findings from a nationally representative sample. *J Adolesc*. 2017;60:83–93.

248. McCabe KO, Modecki KL, Barber BL. Participation in organized activities protects against adolescents' risky substance use, even beyond development in conscientiousness. *J Youth Adolesc.* 2016;45(11):2292–306.
249. Hebert JJ, Klakk H, Moller NC, Grontved A, Andersen LB, Wedderkopp N. The prospective association of organized sports participation with cardiovascular disease risk in children (the CHAMPS Study-DK). *Mayo Clin Proc.* 2017;92(1):57–65.
250. Schroeder AN, Comstock RD, Collins CL, Everhart J, Flanigan D, Best TM. Epidemiology of overuse injuries among high-school athletes in the United States. *J Pediatr.* 2015;166(3):600–6.
251. DiFiori JP, Benjamin HJ, Brenner JS, et al. Overuse injuries and burnout in youth sports: A position statement from the American Medical Society for Sports Medicine. *Br J Sports Med.* 2014;48(4):287–8.
252. Paz DA, Chang GH, Yetto JM, Jr., Dwek JR, Chung CB. Upper extremity overuse injuries in pediatric athletes: Clinical presentation, imaging findings, and treatment. *Clin Imaging.* 2015;39(6):954–64.
253. Simpson M, Rio E, Cook J. At what age do children and adolescents develop lower limb tendon pathology or tendinopathy? A systematic review and meta-analysis. *Sports Med.* 2016;46(4):545–57.
254. Fernandez WG, Yard EE, Comstock RD. Epidemiology of lower extremity injuries among U.S. high school athletes. *Acad Emerg Med.* 2007;14(7):641–5.
255. Thein-Nissenbaum JM, Rauh MJ, Carr KE, Loud KJ, McGuine TA. Menstrual irregularity and musculoskeletal injury in female high school athletes. *J Athl Train.* 2012;47(1):74–82.
256. Barrack MT, Gibbs JC, De Souza MJ, et al. Higher incidence of bone stress injuries with increasing female athlete triad-related risk factors: A prospective multisite study of exercising girls and women. *Am J Sports Med.* 2014;42(4):949–58.
257. Caine D, DiFiori J, Maffulli N. Physeal injuries in children's and youth sports: Reasons for concern? *Br J Sports Med.* 2006;40(9):749–60.
258. Hosseinzadeh P, Milbrandt T. The normal and fractured physis: An anatomic and physiologic overview. *J Pediatr Orthop B.* 2016;25(4):385–92.
259. Circi E, Atalay Y, Beyzadeoglu T. Treatment of Osgood-Schlatter disease: Review of the literature. *Musculoskelet Surg.* 2017;101(3):195–200.
260. Forrester RA, Eyre-Brook AI, Mannan K. Iselin's disease: A systematic review. *J Foot Ankle Surg.* 2017;56(5):1065–9.
261. Greiwe RM, Saifi C, Ahmad CS. Pediatric sports elbow injuries. *Clin Sports Med.* 2010;29(4):677–703.
262. Arnold A, Thigpen CA, Beattie PF, Kissenberth MJ, Shanley E. Overuse physeal injuries in youth athletes. *Sports Health.* 2017;9(2):139–47.
263. McKinney BI, Nelson C, Carrion W. Apophyseal avulsion fractures of the hip and pelvis. *Orthopedics.* 2009;32(1):42.
264. Myer GD, Jayanthi N, Difiori JP, et al. Sport specialization, Part I: Does early sports specialization increase negative outcomes and reduce the opportunity for success in young athletes? *Sports Health.* 2015;7(5):437–42.
265. McGuine TA, Post EG, Hetzel SJ, Brooks MA, Trigsted S, Bell DR. A prospective study on the effect of sport specialization on lower extremity injury rates in high school athletes. *Am J Sports Med.* 2017;45(12):2706–12.
266. Major League Baseball Pitch Smart. Guidelines for Youth and Adolescent Pitchers. http://m.mlb.com/pitchsmart/pitching-guidelines. Accessed October 25, 2017.
267. Myer GD, Jayanthi N, DiFiori JP, et al. Sports specialization, Part II: Alternative solutions to early sport specialization in youth athletes. *Sports Health.* 2016;8(1):65–73.
268. Jayanthi N, Pinkham C, Dugas L, Patrick B, Labella C. Sports specialization in young athletes: Evidence-based recommendations. *Sports Health.* 2013;5(3):251–7.
269. Mooney JF, 3rd, Emans JB. Developmental dislocation of the hip: A clinical overview. *Pediatr Rev.* 1995;16(8):299–303; quiz 304.
270. Loder RT, Skopelja EN. The epidemiology and demographics of hip dysplasia. *ISRN Orthop.* 2011;2011:238607.
271. de Hundt M, Vlemmix F, Bais JM, et al. Risk factors for developmental dysplasia of the hip: A meta-analysis. *Eur J Obstet Gynecol Reprod Biol.* 2012;165(1):8–17.
272. Carter C, Wilkinson J. Persistent joint laxity and congenital dislocation of the hip. *J Bone Joint Surg Br.* 1964;46:40–5.
273. Record RG, Edwards JH. Environmental influences related to the aetiology of congenital dislocation of the hip. *Br J Prev Soc Med.* 1958;12(1):8–22.
274. Gunther A, Smith SJ, Maynard PV, Beaver MW, Chilvers CE. A case-control study of congenital hip dislocation. *Public Health.* 1993;107(1):9–18.
275. Robinson GW. Birth characteristics of children with congenital dislocation of the hip. *Am J Epidemiol.* 1968;87(2):275–84.
276. Shaw BA, Segal LS, Section On O. Evaluation and Referral for Developmental Dysplasia of the Hip in Infants. *Pediatrics.* 2016;138(6).
277. Sharrard WJW. *Pediatric Orthopaedics and Fractures.* Vol. 1. Oxford: Blackwell Scientific Publications; 1993.
278. Knox EG, Armstrong EH, Lancashire RJ. Effectiveness of screening for congenital dislocation of the hip. *J Epidemiol Community Health.* 1987;41(4):283–9.
279. Leck I. An epidemiological assessment of neonatal screening for dislocation of the hip. *J R Coll Physicians Lond.* 1986;20(1):56–62.
280. Holen KJ, Tegnander A, Bredland T, et al. Universal or selective screening of the neonatal hip using ultrasound? A prospective, randomised trial of 15,529 newborn infants. *J Bone Joint Surg Br.* 2002;84(6):886–90.
281. Jones DA. Neonatal hip stability and the Barlow test. A study in stillborn babies. *J Bone Joint Surg Br.* 1991;73(2):216–8.
282. Moore FH. Examining infants' hips—Can it do harm? *J Bone Joint Surg Br.* 1989;71(1):4–5.
283. Macfarlane A. Screening for congenital dislocation of the hip. *Br Med J (Clin Res Ed).* 1987;294(6579):1047.
284. Berman L, Klenerman L. Ultrasound screening for hip abnormalities: Preliminary findings in 1001 neonates. *Br Med J (Clin Res Ed).* 1986;293(6549):719–22.
285. Patel H, Canadian Task Force on Preventive Health Care. Preventive health care, 2001 update: Screening and management of developmental dysplasia of the hip in newborns. *CMAJ.* 2001;164(12):1669–77.
286. Hernandez RJ, Cornell RG, Hensinger RN. Ultrasound diagnosis of neonatal congenital dislocation of the hip. A decision analysis assessment. *J Bone Joint Surg Br.* 1994;76(4):539–43.
287. Rosendahl K, Markestad T, Lie RT. Ultrasound screening for developmental dysplasia of the hip in the neonate: The effect on treatment rate and prevalence of late cases. *Pediatrics.* 1994;94(1):47–52.
288. Homer CJ, Baltz RD, Hickson GB, Miles PV. Clinical practice guideline: Early detection of developmental dysplasia of the hip. Committee on Quality Improvement, Subcommittee on Developmental Dysplasia of the Hip. American Academy of Pediatrics. *Pediatrics.* 2000;105(4 Pt 1):896–905.
289. Shorter D, Hong T, Osborn DA. Cochrane review: Screening programmes for developmental dysplasia of the hip in newborn infants. *Evid Based Child Health.* 2013;8(1):11–54.
290. U.S. Preventative Services Task Force. Developmental Hip Dysplasia: Screening. 2006. Available at https://www.uspreventiveservicestaskforce.org/Page/Document/UpdateSummaryFinal/developmental-hip-dysplasia-screening. Accessed November 18, 2017.
291. Mulpuri K, Song KM, Goldberg MJ, Sevarino K. Detection and nonoperative management of pediatric developmental dysplasia of the hip in infants up to six months of age. *J Am Acad Orthop Surg.* 2015;23(3):202–5.
292. Cunningham KT, Moulton A, Beningfield SA, Maddock CR. A clicking hip in a newborn baby should never be ignored. *Lancet.* 1984;1(8378):668–70.

CHAPTER 58

Diseases of the Nervous System

Richard K. Crawford • James C. Torner

INTRODUCTION

Diseases of the nervous system (DNS) are etiologically diverse, giving rise to myriad conditions both acute and chronic in nature. Neurological disorders may have an insidious onset or have symptoms that are nonspecific, making classification difficult. Early stages of some disorders are characterized by a variable presentation or by subtle signs and symptoms that are difficult to detect or that go unrecognized until function is impaired. Their occurrence may be at birth, which may confer a lifelong disability, or may occur in middle or late life, which may result in progressive disability and death. Some disorders in children may be developmental and may go undetected until the children reach the age at which deficits are assessed. Hence, recognition, diagnosis, and progression of neurological symptoms may affect the true magnitude and observed onset of neurological disorders.

Diagnoses of neurological disorders requires recognition of symptoms, and confirmation with a neurological examination tailored to symptoms and to onset. Diagnostic tests have changed with advances in imaging and electrophysiological testing. Diagnostic clarity has been enhanced by the use of structural imaging techniques [e.g., computerized tomography (CT) and magnetic resonance imaging (MRI)], as well as functional neuroimaging, which utilize surrogates of neuronal activity (e.g., blood oxygenation, glucose metabolism, electrical activity) to facilitate the visualization of brain. Some of the functional studies available are functional magnetic resonance imaging (fMRI), positron emission tomography (PET), and electroencephalography (EEG). Additionally, cognitive tests developed by neuropsychologists have aided in the diagnosis of cognitive decline. Hence, the evaluation of incidence and prevalence over time is difficult due to changing diagnostic criteria and the likelihood of changing classifications and inclusion of milder or early-onset disease, for example, in multiple sclerosis (MS). Epidemiologic trends are impacted by advances in technology and shifting diagnostic practices and one should be mindful of this when assessing the literature.[1]

The Global Burden of Disease Study (GBD), conducted by the Institute for Health Metrics and Evaluation (IHME), highlights the tremendous morbidity and mortality of neurologic disease and the increasing importance this constellation of conditions has on healthcare costs, services, and policy. Disability Adjusted Life Years (DALYs) are one estimate of the magnitude or burden of disease and while the total estimated DALYs decreased globally by 31% to 32,711 per 100,000 from 1990 to 2017, the DALYs attributed to DNS increased by 14%. This higher morbidity, as well improvements in management of communicable diseases, maternal and neonatal care, and unintentional injuries, has led to diseases of the nervous system rising from 15th in 1990 to the 9th leading cause of DALYs in 2017 (1278–1454 per 100,000).[2] Global and U.S. estimates of DALYs from GBD2017 for diseases of the nervous system are listed in Table 58-1. In May of 2019, member states of the World Health Organization agreed to adopt the International Statistical Classification of Diseases (ICD-11), to go into effect in 2022, which reclassifies stroke as neurological rather than cardiovascular.[3,4] Accounting for this new classification makes diseases of the nervous system the leading global cause of mortality and the third leading cause of DALYs.[5,6] As is delineated in Table 58-1a–b, the leading causes of disability are similar globally as they are in United States, with the exception of meningitis being more prominent globally, and Parkinson's being among the top five causes in the United States. Women in the United States have rates of DALYs 37% higher than males, compared to a 4% difference globally. Prominent gender disparities, greater morbidity due to diseases of the nervous system in women compared to men, are also evident in high sociodemographic index (SDI) countries, but are less substantial in low SDI countries.[6] This may partially explain the observation that, as life expectancy is increasing, those years are spent in poorer health and this burden is greatest among women.[2,7] Increased nonfatal health loss reflects both success in terms of diminishing rates of premature death, but also failure in terms of maintaining healthcare for diseased and injured individuals.[8] This increase in disability is expected to continue, partly because of the projected increase in the number of individuals reaching the age at which they are at risk of onset for many of these disorders. It is increasingly evident that differential access to care, economic inequality, imbalanced risk factor profiles, and increasing disability needs can and do challenge the ability of health systems to achieve equitable health outcomes in the face of complex and resource-draining diseases and injuries. Addressing such lapses in health equity can pose a burden to underresourced healthcare systems and economies.[2,9]

GLOBAL AND U.S. MORTALITY, INCIDENCE, AND PREVALENCE OF NEUROLOGICAL DISORDERS

Table 58-2 outlines estimates for the leading global causes of mortality among neurological disorders and changes in these rates from 2000 to 2017. As with morbidity estimates above, gender-specific rates are also included. Table 58-3 includes 2017 mortality data for the United States from CDC Wonder for neurological conditions identified by the current ICD10 classification, as the newly adopted ICD-11 will not be implemented until 2022. With the exception of cerebrovascular conditions, Alzheimer's disease, and Parkinson's disease, mortality estimates are relatively low. Cerebrovascular disease remains a major cause of death with an age-adjusted rate of 37.59 per 100,000 persons, although this has been declining across both genders and all races groups. In contrast, age-adjusted rates of death from progressive neurological disorders such as Parkinson's disease and Alzheimer's disease have increased, likely due to both improved diagnostic accuracy and an aging population.

TABLE 58-1 GLOBAL AND U.S. ESTIMATES OF DALYS FROM GLOBAL BURDEN OF DISEASE PROJECT, 2017

(a) Global					
Cause	**DALY Rate**[a]	**% Total (2017)**	**% Change (2000–17)**	**Female Rate**[a]	**Male Rate**[a]
Alzheimer's disease	399.47	1.22	36.05	495.65	304.01
Epilepsy	193.63	0.59	-15.47	183.5	208.1
Meningitis	266.62	0.82	-48.47	247.69	285.41
Migraine	618.36	1.88	5.27	785.56	452.4
Motor neuron disease	11.5	0.04	21.20	9.74	13.24
Multiple sclerosis	14.2	0.04	4.62	17.79	10.63
Parkinson's disease	73.03	0.22	31.79	62.89	83.1
Stroke	1728.32	5.29	-4.89	1573.12	1882.35
Other neurological	51.9	0.16	4.50	48.18	55.60
(b) United States					
Cause	**DALY Rate**[a]	**% Total (2017)**	**% Change (2000–17)**	**Female Rate**[a]	**Male Rate**[a]
Alzheimer's disease	785.85	2.54	21.23	975.87	589.87
Epilepsy	128.05	0.41	5.19	128.65	127.43
Meningitis	19.48	0.06	-42.48	17.53	21.49
Migraine	740.16	2.38	0.18	1010.30	461.54
Motor neuron disease	61.27	0.20	31.24	52.01	70.81
Multiple sclerosis	62.80	0.20	12.38	83.59	41.37
Parkinson's disease	126.78	0.41	28.45	94.81	159.74
Stroke	1103.46	3.57	-2.07	1142.38	1063.32
Other neurological	74.43	0.24	11.31	67.10	70.81

Source: Institute for Health Metrics and Evaluation (IHME). GBD Compare Data Visualization. Seattle, WA: IHME, University of Washington, 2018. Available at http://vizhub.healthdata.org/gbd-compare.[a]Per 100,000.

TABLE 58-2 GLOBAL ESTIMATES OF DEATHS FROM GLOBAL BURDEN OF DISEASE PROJECT, 2017

Cause	**Deaths**[a]	**Death Rate**[b]	**% Total Death Rate (2017)**	**% Change (2000–17)**	**Female Rate**[b]	**Male Rate**[b]
Alzheimer's disease	2,514.62	32.91	4.49	47.33	43.32	22.58
Epilepsy	130.24	1.7	0.23	-19.84	1.44	1.97
Meningitis	288.02	3.77	0.51	-44.80	3.52	4.02
Migraine	n/a	n/a	n/a	n/a	n/a	n/a
Motor neuron disease	34.07	0.45	0.06	33.36	0.39	0.50
Multiple sclerosis	20.7	0.27	0.04	10.09	0.32	0.22
Parkinson's disease	340.64	4.46	0.61	39.44	3.87	5.04
Stroke	6,167.29	80.72	11.02	-2.22	78.64	82.78
Other neurological	53.95	0.71	0.10	9.65	0.63	0.78

[a]In thousands.
[b]Per 100,000.
Source: Institute for Health Metrics and Evaluation (IHME). GBD Compare Data Visualization. Seattle, WA: IHME, University of Washington; 2018. Available at http://vizhub.healthdata.org/gbd-compare.

The last national assessment by National Ambulatory Medical Care Survey (NAMCS) specific to neurology was in 2010, which examined the roughly 14 million visits to neurologists that were reported by respondents.[10] The rate of visits was 2.9 per 100 persons per year. In 2010, the top four diagnoses were migraine, Parkinson's disease, headache, and epilepsy. About 60% of visits were related to routine follow-up for a chronic condition, 11% for a flare-up of a chronic condition, and 24% of the visits for new problems.[11]

The magnitude of neurological disorders worldwide and in the United States is wide ranging in incidence, prevalence, morbidity, and mortality as well as across ages and etiologies. The remainder of the chapter describes several neurological disorders that are an increasing public health problem including some where the etiology is yet to be identified.

CEREBRAL PALSY

Cerebral palsy (CP) is a group of nonprogressive motor impairment syndromes that arise during brain development and is recognized early in life as the child develops.[12] CP is the second highest reason for hospitalization of child neurological impairment (15.6% vs. 52.2% Epilepsy).[13] CP is the most common motor disability in childhood and is classified based on the extremities involved (monoplegia,

TABLE 58-3 U.S. DEATH RATES FROM NEUROLOGICAL DISORDERS, 2017

ICD10	Disorder	Deaths	Rate per 100,000
G00–G03	Meningitis	615	0.16
G04	Encephalitis	403	0.10
G10	Huntington's disease	1108	0.28
G12.2	Motor neuron disease	5,723	1.98
G20	Parkinson's disease	31,754	8.37
G30	Alzheimer's disease	121,404	31.04
G35	Multiple sclerosis	4,312	1.09
G40–G41	Epilepsy	2,679	0.76
G47	Sleep disorders	1,138	0.29
G61	Guillain-Barre and other polyneuropathies	693	0.17
G70	Myasthenia gravis and other myoneural disorders	1,271	0.32
G71	Muscular dystrophy and other primary disorders of muscles	1,341	0.36
G80	Cerebral palsy	2,026	0.59
G81–G83	Plegias and other paralytic syndromes	1,092	0.28
G91	Hydrocephalus	835	0.22
G00–G99	Neurological disorders	216,353	55.9
C70–C72	Brain pathology	12,830	4.45
M46–M51	Spinal disorders	500	0.17
Q00–07	Congenital malformations of the nervous system	1,277	0.44
F01	Vascular dementia	16,247	4.14
F03	Unspecified dementia	101,934	25.87
I60–I69	Cerebrovascular disease	146,383	37.59

Source: https://wonder.cdc.gov.

hemiplegia, diplegia, or quadriplegia) as well as the neurological dysfunction (spastic, athetotic, hypotonic, dystonic, or combined). The most common form is spastic CP which is present in about 77% of prevalent cases. The presence of other neurological disabilities, such as intellectual disability, seizure disorders, and vision impairment are more common in persons with CP with rates of 40%, 35%, and 15%, respectively.[14–16] A similar association has been observed between CP and autism spectrum disorders (ASDs) where the prevalence of ASD is approximately 6.9% in children with CP, 18.4% among those with nonspastic CP, compared to 1% in the general population.[16]

The CDC tracks CP through the Autism and Developmental Disabilities Monitoring (ADDM) Network in four regions including: northern and central Alabama; metropolitan Atlanta, Georgia; metropolitan St. Louis, Missouri; and south-eastern Wisconsin. In 2008, the ADDM CP Network included nearly 150,000 8-year-old children, constituting roughly 4% of U.S. population of 8-year-olds, and identified 451 children with CP. This rate of 2.8–3.4 per 1000 has remained relatively stable since 1996 with rates ranging from 3.1 to 3.6 per 1000.[16,17] The same study also reports higher prevalence in Black children compared to Whites, and in males compared to females, both with prevalence ratios of 1.5:1. Rates were similar between Hispanic and non-Hispanic White children. The Surveillance of Cerebral Palsy in Europe (SCPE) has reported rates from 1.16 to 2.08 per 1000 live births; however, caution is necessary when making comparisons between prevalence estimates derived from live births and those from census counts of children during a specified time.[16,18–20] Challenges to comparing rates also include differences in the case definition over time and between countries and, because CP is developmental, it may present in a variety of forms and severities and may disappear with growth. Case ascertainment may require surveillance using multiple sources. The Disabilities Education Act allows surveillance through special education programs in school systems. In Atlanta, over 90% of children with developmental disabilities could be identified through education sources.[21] These collective factors may make prevalence a better measure than incidence. Prematurity is the most important risk factor with weight at birth the surrogate measure. A study from the ADDM Network found that the prevalence of CP was substantially higher among children born weighing less than 1500 grams (59.5 per 1000 live births) and between 1500 and 2499 grams (6.2 per 1000 live births) compared to children weighing 2500 grams or more (1.1 per 1000).[14] Similarly, data from Sweden noted prevalence per 1000 live births to be 43.7 for children born at 28–31 weeks, 6.1 for those born between 32 and 36 weeks, and 1.4 for those with greater than 37 weeks gestation.[22] Risk factors for CP can be broken down into three main categories of events that disrupt the developing brain including predisposing intrauterine factors, acute peripartum events, and those occurring in the neonatal period.[23,24] Predisposing intrauterine factors include multiple gestation, intrauterine growth restriction, congenital malformations (most commonly microcephaly and cardiac followed by musculoskeletal and urinary), infection resulting in inflammation, thrombophilia, or untreated maternal hypothyroidism.[23,25,26] The most common peripartum events associated with CP are placental abruption, chorioamnionitis, and birth asphyxia.[27,28] Neonatal period events that have been identified include hemorrhage, sepsis, and periventricular leukomalacia.[29,30] Injury during the perinatal and postnatal periods such as intrauterine exposure to heavy metals, neonatal hyperbilirubinemia, and exposure to benzyl alcohol may be related to CP occurrence.[31]

Genetic factors may play role in CP occurrence and several studies have reported positive familial history and genetic risk in CP children. Twins are at higher risk, but they share a common pregnancy and birthing process and much of the risk may be attributed to lower birthweight.[32] As many as one-third of children with CP may lack traditional risk factors. For many of these children, a genetic basis to their condition is suspected although the underlying genetic basis is likely complex.[33] Most of the risk factors for CP are in the prenatal period; however, thus far, improvements in obstetric and neonatal care and an increasing frequency of obstetric interventions have not been shown to decrease the incidence of CP.[34,35] Among full-term infants, abnormalities of coagulation such as factor V Leiden and antiphospholipid antibodies have been associated with CP.[36,37]

Prevention strategies include targeting risk factors such as preterm birth, targeting the disease process itself through the use of magnesium sulfate in preterm deliveries as protection from cerebral hemorrhage, and postexposure treatment of the affected neonate such as cooling those with birth asphyxia.[23,38] Another important area of prevention is acquired CP, which is caused by brain damage occurring more than 28 days after birth. This may account for up to 10% of prevalence estimates with the most common causes being due to brain injury from motor vehicle accidents, falls, and child abuse, as well as brain infections including meningitis.[21] In addition to mitigating morbidity, bolstering prevention efforts are also valuable from an economic perspective as costs associated with chronic diseases are high. For instance, among children enrolled in Medicaid in 2005, annual medical costs for those with CP were $16,721, ten times higher than those without CP or intellectual disability, and the CDC estimates that the lifetime cost to care for someone with CP is nearly 1 million dollars.[39,40]

SEIZURE DISORDERS

Seizures are alterations in consciousness associated with an above-normal discharge of neurons of the brain. Seizures can be classified based on etiology as acute symptomatic (provoked) seizures and unprovoked seizures. The term epileptic seizure is used to distinguish a seizure caused by abnormal neuronal from a nonepileptic event such as a psychogenic seizure. Unprovoked, recurrent seizures are considered epilepsy which have numerous causes, each reflecting underlying brain dysfunction.[41] Groups of clinical characteristics that consistently occur together such as seizure type, age of onset, EEG findings, triggering factors, genetics, prognosis, and response to an antiepileptic drugs is referred to as an epilepsy syndrome.[42] In 2017, the International League Against Epilepsy (ILAE) proposed a revised classification which has been increasingly adopted. The objective is to increase the accuracy and precision of seizure diagnoses by simplifying the language and shifting away from the terms simple versus complex, partial versus generalized, and primary versus secondary as they were often used incorrectly. Instead, the emphasis is more specific to where the seizure begins (focal, generalized, or unknown) and the level of awareness.[43] Generalized seizures are assumed to be accompanied by impaired awareness and all types are also further defined by motor symptoms. The origin of the seizure is important because it affects the choice of medication, the possibility of surgical intervention, and overall prognosis. Knowledge of the patient's awareness is relevant to assessing their safety during the seizure.

Epilepsy occurs mostly in the young and the elderly, with approximately 75% of epilepsy beginning in childhood reflecting the heightened susceptibility of the developing brain.[42,44] Six population-based studies reported increased standardized mortality ratios for those with epilepsy, ranging between 1.6 and 9.3.[45] The population study from Rochester, Minnesota, spanned a 50-year period and also provided insight into incidence; the cumulative incidence for epilepsy was 3.0%, unprovoked seizures were 4.1%, and any convulsive disorder approached 10%. The overall age-adjusted incidence in the study was 44 per 100,000 person-years.[44] Data from CDC Wonder reflects an increase in the age-adjusted mortality rate from 0.48 to 0.76 per 100,000 from 2002 to 2017 and the Global Burden of Disease Projects estimates epilepsy to be the fourth leading neurological cause of disability in the United States after stroke, dementia, and migraines. In 2008, the CDC reported data from the 2005 Behavioral Risk Factor Surveillance System, indicating that 1.65% of noninstitutionalized adults from 19 states reported that they had ever been told by a doctor that they had epilepsy or seizure disorder (i.e., a history of epilepsy) and 0.84% reported having active epilepsy. The report indicated that persons with active epilepsy have two- to threefold increase in mental and physical unhealthy days and a fourfold increase in activity limitations.[46]

Although the cause of epilepsy in many patients is unknown, seizures can be the result of almost any insult that perturbs brain function. These insults include acquired causes and can be related to the development of definable brain lesions such as after a stroke or traumatic brain injury, infectious diseases including neurocysticercosis, brain tumors, CNS degenerative diseases, and autoimmune diseases.[47,48] The World Health Organization estimates that 25% of epilepsy globally, is preventable by addressing the above risk factors.[49] There have been models of epilepsy in animals without evidence of neurodegeneration, such as febrile seizures, suggesting that neuronal death is not required for epileptogenesis.[50] Prolonged febrile seizures are related to increased epilepsy risk although it is unclear if this association holds in the absence of genetic or acquired predisposing factors. Febrile seizures occur in 2–6% of children, with approximately 15% being prolonged.[50]

The role of genetic mutations is becoming more robust with more than 500 genes having been identified as causing or contributing to the development of epilepsy.[51,52] Other factors where a relationship has been observed, but without a direct causal pathway, are medical conditions such as asthma, hypertension, and opiate use disorder. Similarly, comorbid mood disorders such as depression and anxiety are more prevalent in patients with epilepsy compared to the general population.[53] Positive family history has also been associated with development of epilepsy and twin studies have shown a higher concordance for monozygotic compared to dizygotic twins.[54] Over 70% of patients with epilepsy are able to achieve remission with proper antiepileptic medication therapy; however, more than 80% of those with epilepsy live in developing countries where three-quarters or more are inadequately treated.[49,55,56] Numerous reasons are highlighted for this treatment gap including inadequate health delivery systems, lack of trained personnel, lack of essential drugs, stigma, and traditional beliefs and practices that often do not consider epilepsy as a treatable condition.[56] The stigma is exacerbated by and perpetuates inadequate public health funding in developing countries. Individuals fear going outside of their homes unaccompanied and what people might think of them if they were to have a seizure in public.[57] The stigma has been observed to manifest itself in numerous ways such as children with epilepsy being banned from school, adults who are barred from marriage, and denial of employment even when seizures would not render the work unsuitable or unsafe.[58]

HEADACHES

Headache is the most common neurological disorder globally and in the United States. Global prevalence estimates of active headache disorders among adults to be 42% for tension-type, 11% for migraine, and 3% for chronic daily headache.[59] The Global Burden of Disease Project estimates that headaches are the 12th leading cause overall for disability-adjusted life years and the 8th leading cause among women with roughly 85% of the total burden being attributed to migraines.[6] In the United States, the National Headache Foundation estimates over 150 million workdays are lost annually due to the pain and associated symptoms of migraine and costs employers over 30 billion dollars due to missed work and reduced productivity. Headache is one of the most common symptoms prompting people to seek medical care and is reflected in data from the National Hospital Ambulatory Medical Care Survey which consistently ranks headaches as the fourth or fifth most common reason to present to the emergency department.[60] Similarly, among neurology clinic visits in 2010, migraines were the most common diagnosis and, among primary-care visits in 2016, headaches were the most common neurologic complaint.[10,11]

Primary headache disorders constitute nearly 98% of all headaches and include migraine, tension headache, and trigeminal autonomic cephalgias (TAC, including cluster headache); however, secondary headaches from another disorder such as brain tumor, stroke, or vasculitis are important to recognize as they are serious and may be life threatening.[61] Diagnosis is based on clinical presentation including a detailed history and physical exam with additional investigation rarely being required. In regards to new headaches, patients are often concerned about a brain tumor; however, focal neurological deficits or seizure are more likely presenting symptoms. The 1-year risk of a malignant brain tumor was found to be 0.045% among patients presenting to the primary care with a new onset of headache while headaches may be the sole presenting symptom in 3–4% of tumors at a later stage.[62,63] Nevertheless, brain imaging is warranted in patients with *new* headaches is the setting of high-risk features such as age older than 50, presence of cancer, immunosuppression, or concomitant fever or Lyme disease.[64] There are also a number of red-flag symptoms as well as specific features suggesting a secondary headache source which should prompt further investigation, including imaging.

Classification criteria are established by the International Headache Society and the third edition of the International Classification of Headache Disorders was finalized in 2018.[65] The sections on tension-type headaches and trigeminal autonomic cephalgia remain largely unchanged.[66] Tension-type headaches typically consist of bilateral, are pressing or tightening in quality and of mild to moderate intensity, lasting minutes to days. The pain does not typically worsen with routine physical activity and is not associated with nausea, although photophobia or phonophobia may be present.[67] Cluster headaches are the archetypal TAC which, as a group, are primary headaches with a common clinical phenotype consisting of trigeminal pain with autonomic signs, which may include lacrimation, rhinorrhea, and miosis.[68] New diagnostic criteria have been included for migraine with aura that better distinguish it from transient ischemic and chronic migraine, which was in the appendix of previous versions, has now been included in the main body of the classification.[66] Classically, migraines last 4–72 hours and are characterized by moderate to severe pain with pulsating quality which is aggravated by routine physical activity and associated with nausea and/or photophobia and phonophobia. In adults, 60–70% are unilateral compared to predominantly bilateral in children and adolescents. Among those diagnosed with migraines, 30–40% are accompanied by an aura lasting minutes to an hour. Over 90% of auras include visual symptoms, although other sensory, speech, or motor symptoms may be present and while auras most commonly precede the migraine, they may also occur during or after it. The visual disturbance can be variable and include fortification spectra, sparkling or shimmering colored dots and blobs, and scotoma.[69] There is increasing evidence that this phenomenon is due to cortical spreading depression (or depolarization) although the mechanism(s) have yet to be fully elucidated.[69,70] There is also a category for "other" types of primary headaches which include primary cough, primary exercise, primary headache associated with sexual activity, primary thunderclap, primary stabbing, nummular, and others.

The incidence of migraine depends on gender, age, and type with the highest rates seen in young adult women, particularly for migraines with aura. Data from the 2015 National Hospital Interview Survey describes that the overall prevalence of migraine or severe headache was 15.3%, it was more than twice as common in females as in males, 20.7% and 9.7%, respectively, with the highest overall prevalence of migraine seen in those aged 18–44 years at 17.9%. Prevalence is seen to decrease with age and reported by 15.9% among those aged 45–64, 7.3% in 65–74 years old, and 5.1% in those over 75 years of age.[60] The increased prevalence of migraine in women compared to men is generally found to be restricted to the reproductive years and thought to be due to cyclic variation in estrogen. The male-to-female ratio in the United States is similar to that Europe and Africa, although the exact percentages differ.[71] This is consistent with studies of headaches in childhood where no gender differences in prevalence were identified before the age of 7.[72] A review of 37 studies of headaches in childhood found that prevalence increases with age and range from 2.7% to 10%.[73,74] Data from the United States National Health Interview Survey (NHIS) suggest little change in the combined prevalence of migraines or severe headaches from 2005 to 2015 which increased from 15.1% to 15.4%.

The higher concordance of migraines in monozygotic compared to dizygotic twins suggests a familial risk, but this may be overestimated due to biases in ascertainment.[75] Other contributing factors include ingestion of some foods (those with tyramine, including chocolate and aged cheeses) or alcoholic beverages (red wines, particularly). Psychosocial characteristics also appear to be associated with headache occurrence. These include characteristics of perfectionism, inflexibility, and hypochondriasis, as well as anxiety and depression. Stress and psychosocial events are also likely to be important. While a tremendous source of morbidity, the consequences of migraine are not viewed as life-threatening; however, migraine may be associated with hypertension, atherosclerotic heart disease, and stroke.[76] Substantial variation in migraine prevalence with socioeconomic factors such as income and insurance status as well as by race have also been identified.[60,77] In their analysis of the NHIS data, they note the highest prevalence in those below the poverty threshold (21.7%) and with annual family income of less than $35,000 (19.9%). Among those under the age of 65, the prevalence was 26.0% in Medicaid beneficiaries, compared to 17.1% and 15.1% in those without insurance or with private insurance, respectively. This survey of over 100,000 persons and 40,000 households also identified a higher burden of migraines or severe headaches in American Indians with a prevalence of 18.4% compared to 16.2%, 15.4%, and 11.3%, in Blacks, Whites, and Asians, respectively.

NEUROTOXIC DISORDERS

Classic heavy metal exposures and solvents have led to neurological disorders, similarly, occupational exposures to industrial chemicals have also been associated with acute neurological diseases.[78,79] Pesticides have been observed in several human studies to be related to neurological symptoms; a meta-analysis of retrospective case-control studies found among patients with neurological symptoms the combined odds ratio of having been exposed was 1.94 (CI = 1.49–2.53).[80] Organophosphorus insecticides are recognized by their neurotoxic effects, which include paralysis.[81]

Implications of chemicals for chronic diseases are being evaluated. For Parkinson's disease, the ingestion of 1-methyl-4-phenyl tetrahydropyridine (MPTP) results in Parkinsonism symptoms, and similar compounds such as paraquat and rotenone have caused Parkinsonism in animals.

Among those with Parkinson's disease, several studies have identified an increased odds of having been exposed to chemicals in herbicides, insecticides, alkylated phosphates, organochlorines, and wood preservatives.[82–85] The Agricultural Health Study reported that organic solvent exposure was related to depression among agricultural producers.[86]

Alzheimer's disease has been speculated to be potentially of neurotoxic origin, but studies have not been conclusive, including the role of aluminium.[87] This is likely partly due to the multifactorial and highly variable presentation of the disease and further research is needed.

MULTIPLE SCLEROSIS

MS is one of the demyelinating diseases and is characterized by white matter lesions.[88] Classification of MS is dependent on clinical criteria that feature multiple lesions in the CNS separated in multiple locations and symptomatic attacks. Clinical presentation is highly variable, symptoms may include sensory, visual, and motor dysfunction. The spectrum of MS ranges from benign disease to rapidly fatal cerebral demyelination. The disease is generally progressive and is characterized by clinical remissions and exacerbations.[89] Diagnosis of MS has been aided by the use of MRI which may detect early lesions.[90]

Onset of MS occurs between ages 15 and 65 years. The median ages at onset for cases identified in Rochester, Minnesota were 34 years for men and 32 years for women.[91] Women had an incidence of 7.7 per 100,000, and 3.4 per 100,000 for men. MS shows a north-south geographical distribution, where the northern hemisphere has distinct high-risk zones for MS. This has been observed in the United States and Europe. High-risk areas have prevalence rates of MS of greater than 50 per 100,000; low-risk areas have less than 5 per 100,000. The north-south gradient is still apparent with a higher prevalence in North America compared to South America.[92] Prevalence appears to be increasing over time. Ethnic differences may exist, but few studies have been done.

Studies among migrants suggest that persons who move from an area of high prevalence to one of low prevalence take on the risk level of their new environment. The country (latitude) and the age of migration appear to an important determinant in MS risk.[93–95] Migration before early adolescence (before age of 15) shifts the risk to the new country. With migration after age 15, the individual has the risk of the former country. Studies of the Faroe Islands by Kurtzke, identified a minimum exposure time of 2 years was necessary to confer susceptibility.[96–98]

The causes of MS are still unknown. The hypothesis is that gene and environmental factors are necessary for MS occurrence. Ecological studies have shown associations with low temperature, plants, soil, industrialization, meat consumption, certain types of meat, and dairy foods.[99] Ethnic background may play a role since the highest rates are in areas populated by those with a northern European/Scandinavian background. Clusters of MS have been reported in Canada, Norway, and Florida. Epidemics have occurred in the Faroe Islands and in Iceland with no cases of MS apparent before 1945 followed by peaks in 1945, 1955, and 1965.[96–98] Infectious agents have been studied extensively, but no single agent has yet been identified. Measles virus and canine distemper virus has received the most attention. Case-control studies have demonstrated a relationship with dog ownership. Infection may also be related to immunologic changed to increase susceptibility. Other factors that have been investigated with conflicting results include trauma, and exposure to trace elements and heavy metals, such as zinc and lead. Cigarette smoking may exacerbate the MS symptoms. Studies have demonstrated an increased risk in long-term smokers.[100]

A possible role for genetic factors in the etiology of MS has also been investigated, supported by the familial aggregation of MS reported in several studies.[101] Familial aggregation may be due to shared environment or genetic susceptibility. Twin studies have generally found a greater concordance for MS among monozygotic twins than among dizygotic twins. The risk to family members is low with 4% for siblings and 2–4% for children depending on gender. Since northern Europeans have a higher frequency of HLA-DR2, haplotype studies of HLA in MS have been the most consistent.[102] Further candidate genes are peptide transporter genes and genes encoding tumor necrosis factor.

Changes in diagnostic studies may lead to improved ascertainment but few longitudinal, population-based databases exist. Survival is longer for women than men. Approximately 75% of MS patients will survive 25 years or more.[103] The rate of progression and disability is variable. Many patients, even with progression, remain ambulatory for many years. There is currently no definitive therapy for MS that affects the ultimate course of the disease but steroid or ACTH therapy is used for acute exacerbations. Beta-interferon and azathioprine may be helpful in preventing relapses but data on rate of progression are inconclusive.

PARKINSON'S DISEASE

Parkinson's disease (PD) is the second-most common neurodegenerative disorder affecting 2–3% of the population $\geq$ 65 years of age.[104] PD is a progressive neurologic disorder of unknown etiology, characterized by motor symptoms such as bradykinesia, resting tremor, rigidity, and postural reflex. These symptoms are the manifestation of neuronal loss in the substantia nigra causing striatal dopamine deficiency. This finding along with intracellular inclusions containing aggregates of α-synuclein are the neuropathological hallmarks of PD.[105] Misdiagnosis with depression and multiple system involvement leads to variable case determinations. Clinical criteria can only lead to a diagnosis of probable PD, while a definite diagnosis requires postmortem confirmation. Clinicopathological studies have shown that in 80–90% of the cases the clinical diagnosis of PD was confirmed at autopsy.[106] PD may occur with dementia in 10–40% of cases.[107,108] It is not currently possible to predict which patients will progress to Parkinson's disease with dementia (PDD), but clinicopathological findings are quite similar to dementia with Lewy bodies suggesting they are part of a continuum of the same disease process rather than two distinct entities. While motor symptoms still present first, as in PD, those who progress to PDD may experience cognitive impairment, REM sleep disorder, memory problems, fatigue, anxiety, autonomic dysfunction, and visual hallucinations.[109]

A systematic review of 25 incidence studies illustrated that worldwide incidence estimates of PD range from 5 to > 35 new cases per 100,000 individuals yearly.[110] This is probably due to methodological differences and, in general, incidence studies may be affected by underdiagnosing of PD, especially among the most elderly. Prevalence estimates of PD vary significantly as well, but it is considered to be rare prior to the age of 50, and that the disease affects approximately 1% of those over the age of 65 and 3–4% over the age of 85.[108,111] It appears both incidence and prevalence are increasing, but, as age is the most significant risk factor, it is unclear if it is higher than what would be expected in an aging population.[112] The number of people with PD is expected to double between 2005 and 2030 in part due to improvement in healthcare and longer survival as identified in one 20-year study.[113,114] Many studies have identified rates up to twice as high in men although some report only slightly increased risk and one found no gender differences.[115]

Treatment of PD is anchored on augmenting nigrostriatal dopaminergic transmission employing both pre- and postsynaptic targets in conjunction with dopamine agonists such as L-DOPA.[116] Nonmotor symptoms become increasingly prevalent over the course of the illness causing substantial burden on quality of life for both the patient and caregivers.[115] Modifying disease progression and further delaying disability are the key unmet needs to be addressed by current and future research efforts. Gene-based therapies and targeting the aggregation and transport of α-synuclein are areas on ongoing experimental therapeutics.[116] Deep brain stimulation has been effective to mitigate motor symptoms, particularly in younger patients who retain a good response to individual doses of levodopa in the absence of cognitive impairment or active psychosis.[117] Most epidemiological studies suggest that PD reduces life expectancy with mortality hazard ratios between 1.5 and 2.7.[108] Dementia in those patients who progress to PDD may be largely responsible for the reduced life expectancy, as mortality risk is only moderately increased in those who do not develop dementia.[118]

The etiology of PD continues to be largely unknown. Monogenic or familial PD caused by pathogenic mutations in genes account for 5–10% of cases with nearly 20 genes being implicated in either recessive or dominant patterns of inheritance.[104] Twin studies also suggest a predominance of environmental over genetic etiologies.[119] Age continues to be the greatest risk factor and it is likely that development of PD is a multifactorial process involving both environmental and lifestyle factors.[115] PD may be partially precipitated by exposure to toxins (e.g., carbon monoxide or manganese), drugs (e.g., phenothiazides), traumatic or vascular lesions of the brain, or tumors.[120] Etiological studies using a variety of case ascertainment methods have suggested that rural residence, farming, well-water drinking, and herbicide/pesticide exposure are related to PD.[120] Infectious agents have been evaluated, particularly focusing on the epidemic of 1918; however, no agents or relationships have been found. A meta-analysis of caffeine consumption identified marked protective effects of caffeine consumption which may be unique to men.[121] The specific mechanism is unclear, but this relationship is supported by animal models where caffeine against MPTP-induced Parkinsonism.[122] Numerous studies have reported a lower risk of PD among cigarette smokers. Various explanations for this observation have been proposed, but whether the inverse association between cigarette smoking and risk of PD has a biological significance or a behavioral relationship remains controversial.[123] PD remains an increasing problem with the advancing age of the global population.

DEMENTIAS

Dementia is a clinically and etiologically heterogeneous set of syndromes characterized by impairment across multiple domains such as memory, reasoning, judgment, calculation, abstraction, and language that interfere with everyday functioning such as activities of daily living and social activities, which is distinct from normal aging, and cannot be explained by delirium or major psychiatric disorder. Mild cognitive impairment (MCI) is considered an early stage of dementia; it is diagnosed when individuals show a lower performance in one or more cognitive domains that is greater than would

TABLE 58-4 DEMENTIA PREVALENCE IN NORTH AMERICA ACCORDING TO AGE

Age Group (years)	Prevalence (%)
60–64	0.8
65–69	1.7
70–74	3.3
75–79	6.5
80–84	12.8
≥85	30.1

be expected for the patient's age and educational background, but do not meet the criteria for dementia. The rate of progression of MCI to dementia is uncertain.[124]

A Delphi Consensus Study estimated dementia prevalence for 5-year age bands, in men and women combined, across all 14 WHO regions. Rates in North America are shown in Table 58-4. Regional prevalence estimates for those older than age 60 were 1.6% in Africa, 4.0% in China and Western Pacific regions, 4.6% in Latin America, 5.4% in Western Europe, 6.4% in North America, and 3.9% worldwide.[125] The study also projected substantially higher increases in prevalence in developing countries relative to North America and Western Europe. The World Health Organization reports that 60% of those with dementia reside in low- and middle-income countries, a proportion which is anticipated to continue rising as the developing nations' share of the worldwide population over 65 will increase from 59% to 71% by 2030.[126] Globally, the number of people living with dementia is expected to increase from 50 million to 130 million by 2050.[127] In 2010, the global cost of dementia care was estimated at $604 billion, and it is estimated to increase to $1 trillion by 2030.[128] Due to varied definitions and methodologies used across countries and WHO regions, estimating the overall burden is difficult, as prevalence and incidence estimates are hampered by diagnostic challenges and lack of pathological confirmation.[129,130] Of all chronic diseases, dementia is one of the most important contributors to dependence and disability.

Alzheimer's disease (AD) is the most common form of dementia, accounting for 50–60%, and is followed by vascular dementia (VaD) and dementia with Lewy bodies (DLB), representing roughly 25% and 15–20% of cases, respectively.[131–133] While there is substantial variation across studies, it is agreed that age is the most significant risk factor and it is estimated that over 90% of dementia occurs in those older than 65 years of age.[134]

The epidemiology of the dementias poses a growing public health challenge; although there are no medications that modify the disease, an estimated 30% of dementia cases may be attributable to potentially modifiable risk factors.[127] According to the U.S Preventive Services Task Force, there is inconclusive evidence to recommend screening of cognitive impairments in the population older than 65 years; however, if dementia is suspected, patients should undergo evaluation using a validated tool (e.g., Mini-Cog), and, if the results are abnormal, further evaluation is warranted.[124,135]

The Alzheimer's Association developed a practice guideline to facilitate clinical evaluation of AD and other dementias in primary and specialty care clinics; it consists of 20 recommendations for primary- and specialty-care settings developed for the evaluation of cognitive behavioral syndrome (CBS) and AD dementia clinical spectrums. The recommendations outline a tiered utilization structure of assessments and tests based on a given individual profile, including presentation and risk factors to: (1) establish the presence and characteristics of the CBS; (2) investigate possible causes and contributing factors to arrive at an etiologic diagnosis(es) based on established disease criteria; and (3) appropriately educate, communicate findings, and disclose the syndromic and etiologic diagnosis(es) to ensure ongoing management, care, and support.[136]

Alzheimer's Disease

AD is characterized by an insidious onset and progressive course of cognitive decline with memory impairment being the most common initial symptom. Visuospatial deficits are also often present early in the disease course while, typically, behavioral symptoms and impairment in language occur later. Neuropathological findings which define AD as a unique neurodegenerative disease include extracellular aggregates of β-amyloid and intracellular hyperphosphorylated-tau deposits, also called neurofibrillary tangles. It is primarily these two proteins which serve as the basis for CSF biomarkers in AD.[137]

The rates of progression from amnestic MCI to AD have been reported at 10–15% per year and up to 60% in 3 years when in the setting of both amyloid and neuronal injury biomarkers (tau or imaging evidence).[138,139] Multiple cohort studies have demonstrated over 80–85% of those with a diagnosis of probable AD have pathological findings consistent with AD on autopsy.[140–142] However, the incidence of many pathologies increases with age and additional vascular and/or neurodegerative pathologies were found in most of those cases. Some degree of additional pathology on autopsy has been identified in up to 95% of those diagnosed with Alzheimer's dementia and in 35% the primary pathology was other than AD.[143,144] Most commonly, these include cerebrovascular findings such arteriosclerosis (or small vessel disease SVD) and stroke (including cortical and subcortical microinfarcts and lacunar strokes), lewy bodies (intracellular α-synuclein aggregates), and TDP-43 (TAR DNA-binding protein—one of the clinicopathologic correlates of frontotemporal dementia and ALS).[141,145] This obscures syndromic classifications and makes it difficult to assess the relative importance of any specific pathology and the ability to ascribe to it cognitive and functional decline. Numerous longitudinal studies provide evidence of the importance of the cumulative result of neurodegenerative and vascular pathologies.[146,147] Mixed pathology has also been identified as doubling the risk of dementia compared with only degenerative lesions.[148] It has been suggested that the utility of biomarkers diminishes with age due to overlapping neuropathology and due to the substantial increase in asymptomatic AD neuropathology beyond 70 years of age, such that they may be most useful in diagnosing early-onset AD (EOAD) or in evaluating atypical presentations.[145]

In EOAD, clinical symptoms present between the ages of 30 and 60 and are estimated to account for 1–5% of all AD.[149] While the majority of AD is sporadic, there are several genes displaying a familial pattern of inheritance that have been implicated in 10–20% of EOAD. The most common autosomal dominant genes are APP, PSEN1, and PSEN2, resulting in the overproduction of amyloid.

The most prominent changes visible on structural neuroimaging (MRI or CT) is hippocampal atrophy in the medial temporal lobes, progressing to the temporal neocortex, and then to all neocortical association areas.[150] The average life expectancy after a diagnosis of AD depends heavily on the level of impairment at diagnosis and subsequently may range from 3 to 20 years.[151,152] Some of the variability in outcomes also seems likely to result from the complicated nature of mixed overlapping pathologies and variable phenotypes.

Age and family history of the disease in a first-degree relative are the strongest epidemiological risk factors for AD. For instance, those who are 85 and older have 14 times the incidence of AD compared with persons age 65–69, and having at least one first-degree relative with dementia confers a relative risk of 3.5 times higher, compared with those without a family history. Other risk factors, in addition to cerebrovascular disease and its contributing causes of hypertension and diabetes, include head trauma, chronic inflammation, obstructive sleep apnea, education level, number of siblings, nonsuburban residence, maternal age at birth, hypothyroidism, and apolipoprotein E4 genotype.[153,154]

Regarding race/ethnicity, African Americans have increased risk of dementia, followed by American Indian/Alaska Native, Hispanic/Latinos, Pacific Islanders, Whites, and Asian-Americans. According to Mayeda et al., the cumulative 25-year risk at age 65 was 38%, 35%, 32%, 25%, 30%, and 28%, respectively.[155] These disparities might be influenced by increased presence of comorbidities. Other differences in outcomes exist by race/ethnicity; for example, Whites have the highest mortality rate and shortest survival among races, while Asian Americans have the longest survival.[156] The causes of racial differences in Alzheimer's death rates might be the result of competing causes of mortality; compared with non-Hispanic Whites, non-Hispanic Blacks have higher mortality rates from cardiovascular disease at younger ages.[157]

The diagnostic criteria for AD have changed over the last few years, creating a point of caution when comparing data across databases and countries. In 2011, the National Institute on Aging and Alzheimer's Association (NIA-AA) released an updated version of their diagnostic criteria, largely to differentiate the disease into three distinct stages, including preclinical, MCI, and dementia.[158] In 2019, the NIA-AA published their guidance on diagnostic criteria of AD for research purposes, which includes the role of imaging in each of the stages as well as the use of biomarkers.[159] The preclinical stage is the presence of laboratory or imaging biomarkers in the absence of cognitive deficits and, is itself, divided into three stages. Progression through this stage is less clear given the lack of longitudinal studies built on this relatively newly defined diagnostic framework, but this approach may foster a better understanding of the sequence of events leading to cognitive impairment associated with AD.[160-162] Concerns have been expressed over the use of biomarkers in the evaluation of AD due to potential misuse, leading to increased expenditures, treatment, and labeling of patients who may not develop cognitive impairment.[143]

In the current absence of compelling disease modifying treatment, there has been substantial interest in addressing risk factors suggesting that interventions targeting these factors could perhaps delay or prevent the onset of dementia. There is increasing evidence that intensive blood pressure control reduces risk of MCI; participants in the Systolic Blood Pressure Intervention Trial (SPRINT, $n = 9361$) were randomized to SBP target of $<$ 120 mm Hg (intensive treatment) versus $<$ 140 mm Hg (standard treatment). After a median follow up of 3.26 years, the researchers found a statistically significant lower rate of new cases of MCI (19%; $p = 0.01$) in the intensive blood pressure treatment group. The combined outcome of MCI plus probable all-cause dementia was lower (15%; $p = 0.02$) in the intensive versus standard treatment group.[163] However, MCI was not the primary outcome of the study, and the trial was terminated early, which limits our capacity to evaluate long-term effects of this intervention.

Since the vast majority of people with dementia live in low- and middle-income countries, future interventions should preferably be accessible and affordable to implement across a wide range of healthcare systems, as many countries have limited diagnostic tools, no access to clinical trials, and limited to no specialized doctors and researchers.[127]

Creutzfeldt-Jakob Disease (CJD)

CJD is a rapidly progressive neurodegenerative disease resulting from the conformational conversion of a normal nonpathogenic cellular prion protein into an abnormal misfolded pathological form. There are three major types of CJD: sporadic CJD (sCJD), genetic or familial CJD (fCJD), and acquired or variant CJD (vCJD). In the United States the incidence is from 250 to 300 new cases per year.[164] Approximately 85–90% of CJD cases occur sporadically affecting 1–1.5 people per million annually.[165] About 90% of patients die within 1 year progressing experiencing failing memory, behavioral changes, lack of coordination and visual disturbances progressing to mental deterioration, involuntary movements, blindness, weakness of extremities, and coma. Familial cases account for about 10% of CJD cases worldwide and over 20 causative mutations have been identified.[166] The peak incidence of sCJD occurs between 55 and 75 years of age, whereas fCJD typically presents before age 55. No obvious environmental risk to disease has been recognized for sCJD or fCJD.[165] The least common, vCJD commonly occurs even younger, in the late teens or young adulthood.[166] In the mid-1980s, bovine spongiform encephalopathy (BSE) emerged in the United Kingdom in cattle and vCJD has been linked to ingestion of beef tainted with BSE. Compared to sCJD, disease progression is slightly slower, with a mean duration of 14.5 months.[167] While late stage sCJD and vCJD are clinically indistinguishable, earlier in the course, vCJD is typically dominated by neuropsychiatric symptoms such as anxiety, depression, and withdrawal. The first 10 vCJD cases were reported in April 1996 in the United Kingdom.[168] As of April 2015, 229 vCJD cases have been reported from seven European (the United Kingdom, France, Spain, Republic of Ireland, Netherlands, Italy, and Portugal) and five non-European countries or regions (the United States, Canada, Saudi Arabia, Japan, and China-Taiwan), with 177 cases being reported from the United Kingdom. Since 2006, the annual deaths from vCJD have dramatically reduced and none have been reported since 2014.[169] All vCJD patients to date have been homozygous for methionine at the polymorphic codon 129 of the human prion protein gene.[170] The threat to continually emerging prion strains in livestock is uncertain and as there are still no specific therapeutic and prophylactic interventions available for prion diseases, active surveillance of human prion diseases is critical for disease control and prevention.[165]

STROKE

Stroke is among the leading causes of mortality and morbidity globally and in the United States. In 2016, an estimated 5.5 million deaths are attributed to stroke worldwide, the second leading cause, with approximately 142,000 occurring in the United States making it the fifth leading cause.[171] While the age-adjusted incidence and mortality has been declining in high-income countries for decades, the absolute number of people affected by stroke continues to increase rapidly throughout the world. In fact, there is no country with a decreasing burden in absolute terms.[172] Globally, from 1990 to 2010, age-adjusted incidence was largely unchanged, but embedded within that was a 68% increase in total incidence.[173] Prevalence rate increased by 15% paired with an 84% increase in the total number of people living with stroke. Over that period, DALYs and deaths increased by 12% and 26% in absolute terms, but their rates both decreased by approximately 25%. The reduction in rates are likely multifactorial including improved prevention and management of stroke, particularly in high-income countries, as well as increasing life expectancy and global population growth.[174] There is also a divergence between low- and middle-income countries (LMIC) and high-income countries (HIC) where a 12% increase occurred in LMIC compared to a 12% decrease in HIC.[173] Overall, LMIC bear a disproportionate amount of the burden of stroke including 60% of incident ischemic and 83% of hemorrhagic events. Similarly, 64% of the DALYs due to ischemic strokes and 86% of the DALYs due to hemorrhagic strokes were borne by LMIC.[175] An even more granular examination reveals substantial geographic variation in stroke burden reflecting that while enhanced stroke prevention efforts and care are needed broadly, there may be benefit to region-specific strategies.[176,177]

Roughly 80% of strokes are ischemic due to either thrombosis, embolism, or systemic hypoperfusion and 20% are due to hemorrhage, either intracerebral or subarachnoid. About 20–25% of patients presenting with a stroke syndrome have a stroke mimic; most commonly seizures, syncope, sepsis, peripheral vestibulopathy, and toxic or metabolic encephalopathy.[174] Transient ischemic attacks (TIA) have classically been defined as a transient reduction in cerebral blood flow precipitating focal neurologic deficits which resolve within 24 hours. However, as our understanding continues to evolve through advances in neuroimaging, there is clear risk of permanent tissue even when symptoms resolve within minutes. This has prompted a movement toward a tissue-based, rather than time-based definition of TIA.[178] This means a TIA would be defined by neuroimaging findings consistent with a lack a permanent tissue damage rather than a by symptom resolution within a somewhat arbitrary 24 hours. The tissue-based reclassification may decrease incidence of TIAs by 30% with a concomitant increased incidence in strokes by 7%.[179] In settings where sensitive neuroimaging is available, this may improve risk stratification due to enhanced predictive value for a subsequent cerebrovascular event. A multicenter study of 12 international sites in developed countries identified the 7-day incidence of stroke after tissue positive findings to be 7.1% in contrast to 0.4% among tissue negative patients.[180] Whereas, in India, a study utilizing the time-based definition of TIA report the 7-day risk of to be as high as 11% and a 24–29% incidence over 5 years.[181]

The National Health and Nutrition Survey estimates a prevalence of 2.5% in the United States for 2016. The Behavioral Risk Factor Surveillance System (BRFSS) estimated a similar prevalence in 2016, including 2.9% among males and 2.8% among females.[171] Rates vary by ethnicity with the lowest rates seen in Asian/Pacific Islanders (1.2%) and Hispanics (2.3%) and compared to non-Hispanic Blacks (4.7%) and American Indian/Alaska Natives (5.3%). Most strokes occur in individuals over the age of 65. Among those less than 40 years of age in the United States, stroke prevalence is just 0.5%, rising to more than 6% in 60–79 years olds and roughly 13.5% in those older than 80.[176] The Global Burden of Disease Project estimates that 90% of the stroke risk could be attributed to modifiable risk factors such as hypertension, hyperglycemia, hyperlipidemia, obesity, and renal dysfunction with 74% being tied to behavioral risk factors, such as smoking, sedentary lifestyle, and an unhealthy diet.

EMERGING NEUROLOGICAL CONDITIONS

There is an increasing awareness of the neurological consequences of emerging infectious diseases. The largest outbreak to date of the Ebola virus occurred in 2013–16 in west Africa, predominantly affecting Guinea, Sierra Leone, and Liberia (over 28,000 cases).[182,183] The central nervous system may be a reservoir for Ebola virus. A case of meningoencephalitis 9 months after initial recovery from acute Ebola virus disease has been described.[184] On neurologic examination, survivors were observed to have a higher prevalence of abnormal reflexes (1.4%), tremor (0.9%), speech abnormalities (0.7%), and cranial nerve abnormalities (0.7%).[185]

In 2015, there was a large epidemic of Zika virus in Brazil. The neurological consequences included an increase in the occurrence of microcephaly in newborns and its long-term sequelae.[186] A significant increase in Guillain-Barré syndrome (GBS) incidence has been observed. GBS presents with generalized muscle weakness, facial palsy, and inability to walk. Acute myelitis, encephalitis, meningoencephalitis, and chronic inflammatory demyelinating polyneuropathy have also been described.[187]

Acute flaccid myelitis (AFM) is a serious paralytic disease first described in 2014. AFM is characterized by the presence of fever or respiratory symptoms and the acute onset of limb weakness, predominantly involving the upper limbs.[188] Neuroinvasive enteroviruses have been identified as causes of sporadic cases of AFM, including EV-D68 and EV-A71.[189] Significant impairment remains, with only 10% showing complete recovery.

CONCLUSION

The increasing prevalence of chronic neurological conditions is due to the aging of the population, effective treatments, and longer survival. This has profound impacts on the magnitude of disability and impairment in the population and will have more as the number of people with chronic conditions increase. There are still many neurological conditions that public health screening or prevention await further research. The exciting findings of genetic predisposition aided with environment interaction studies are important for future research in determining causation and risk. The emerging consequences of systemic infections is important indicators of neurosusceptibility and long-term effects. The need for public health and clinical services will continue to grow as the neurological disease burden increases.

References

1. Håberg AK, Hammer TA, Kvistad KA, et al. Incidental intracranial findings and their clinical impact; the HUNT MRI study in a general population of 1006 participants between 50–66 years. *PLoS One.* 2016;11(3):e0151080.
2. Kyu HH, Abate D, Abate KH, et al. Global, regional, and national disability-adjusted life-years (DALYs) for 359 diseases and injuries and healthy life expectancy (HALE) for 195 countries and territories, 1990–2017: A systematic analysis for the Global Burden of Disease Study 2017. *Lancet.* 2018:1859–922.
3. Shakir R, Norrving B. Stroke in ICD-11: The end of a long exile. *Lancet.* 2017;389(10087):2373.
4. Royo-bordonada MÁ. Revising the ICD : Stroke is a brain disease revising the ICD. *Lancet.* 2016;388(10059):2475–6.
5. Roth GA, Abate D, Abate KH, et al. Global, regional, and national age-sex-specific mortality for 282 causes of death in 195 countries and territories, 1980–2017: A systematic analysis for the Global Burden of Disease Study 2017. *Lancet.* 2018;392(10159):1736–88.
6. Institute for Health Metrics and Evaluation—University of Washington. Global Burden of Disease Compare | IHME Viz Hub. https://vizhub.healthdata.org/gbd-compare/. Published 2019. Accessed July 14, 2019.
7. Dicker D, Nguyen G, Abate D, et al. Global, regional, and national age-sex-specific mortality and life expectancy, 1950–2017: A systematic analysis for the Global Burden of Disease Study 2017. *Lancet.* 2018; 392: 1684–735.
8. GBD 2017 Disease and Injury Incidence and Prevalence Collaborators. Global, regional, and national incidence, prevalence, and years lived with disability for 354 diseases and injuries for 195 countries and territories, 1990–2017: A systematic analysis for the Global Burden of Disease Study 2017. *Lancet.* 2018;392:1789–858.
9. Spencer S. Global Burden of Disease 2010 study: A personal reflection. *Glob Cardiol Sci Pract.* 2013;2013(2):15.
10. Rui P, Okeyode T. National Ambulatory Medical Care Survey: 2016 National Summary Tables. 2019. Available at https://www.cdc.gov/nchs/data/ahcd/namcs_summary/2016_namcs_web_tables.pdf.
11. CDC. National Ambulatory Medical Care Survey Factsheet-Neurology. *NAMCS.* 2010;6:35–6. Available at http://www.cdc.gov/nchs/data/ahcd/NAMCS_2010_factsheet_neurology.pdf.
12. Kuban KCK, Leviton A. Cerebral palsy. *N Engl J Med.* 1994;330:188–95.
13. Berry JG, Poduri A, Bonkowsky JL, et al. Trends in resource utilization by children with neurological impairment in the United States inpatient health care system: A repeat cross-sectional study. *PLoS Med.* 2012;9(1):e1001158.
14. Winter S, Autry A, Boyle C, Yeargin-Allsopp M. Trends in the prevalence of cerebral palsy in a population-based study. *Pediatrics.* 2004;110(6):1220–5.
15. Braun KVN, Understanding cerebral palsy: The power of population-based surveillance. *Dev Med Child Neurol.* 2017;59(7):676–77.
16. Christensen D, Van Naarden Braun K, Doernberg NS, et al. Prevalence of cerebral palsy, co-occurring autism spectrum disorders, and motor functioning—Autism and developmental disabilities monitoring network, USA, 2008. *Dev Med Child Neurol.* 2014;56(1):59–65.
17. Durkin MS, Benedict RE, Christensen D, et al. Prevalence of cerebral palsy among 8-year-old children in 2010 and preliminary evidence of trends in its relationship to low birthweight. *Paediatr Perinat Epidemiol.* 2016;30(5):496–510.
18. Sellier E, Surman G, Himmelmann K, et al. Trends in prevalence of cerebral palsy in children born with a birthweight of 2,500 g or over in Europe from 1980 to 1998. *Eur J Epidemiol.* 2010;25(9):635–42.
19. Arneson CL, Durkin MS, Benedict RE, et al. Prevalence of cerebral palsy: Autism and developmental disabilities monitoring network, three sites, United States, 2004†. *Disabil Health J.* 2009;2(1):45–8.
20. Johnson A. Prevalence and characteristics of children with cerebral palsy in Europe—surveillance of cerebral palsy in Europe (SCPE). *Dev Med Child Neurol.* 2002;44:633–40.

21. Boyle CA, Yeargin-Allsopp M, Doernberg NS et al. Prevalence of selected developmental disabilities in children 3–10 years of age: The Metropolitan Atlanta Developmental Disabilities Surveillance Program. *MMWR*. 1996;45(SS-2):1–14.
22. Pakula AT, Van Naarden Braun K, Yeargin-Allsopp M. Cerebral palsy: Classification and epidemiology. *Phys Med Rehabil Clin N Am*. 2009;20(3):425–52.
23. Stavsky M, Mor O, Mastrolia SA, Greenbaum S, Than NG, Erez O. Cerebral palsy—Trends in epidemiology and recent development in prenatal mechanisms of disease, treatment, and prevention. *Front Pediatr.* 2017;5(February):1–10.
24. Stanley F, Blair E, Albert E. *Cerebral Palsies: Epidemiology and Causal Pathways*. London: Mac Keith Press; 2000.
25. Rankin J, Cans C, Garne E, et al. Congenital anomalies in children with cerebral palsy: A population-based record linkage study. *Dev Med Child Neurol*. 2010;52(4):345–51.
26. Grether J, Nelson K. Maternal infection and cerebral palsy in infants of normal birth weight. *Clin Pediatr (Phila)*. 2007;37(7):456.
27. Wu YW, Colford JM. Chorioamnionitis as a risk factor. *J Am Med Assoc*. 2000;284(11):1417–24.
28. Nelson KB. Thrombophilias, perinatal stroke, and cerebral palsy. *Clin Obstet Gynecol*. 2006;49(4):875–84.
29. Nelson K, Ellenberg JH. Antecedents of cerebral palsy. *N Engl J Med*. 1986;315:81–6.
30. Blair E, Stanley FJ. Intrapartum asphyxia: A rare cause of cerebral palsy. *J Pediatr*. 1988;112(4):515–9.
31. Benda GI, Hiller JL, Reynolds JW. Benzyl alcohol toxicity: Impact on neurologic handicaps among surviving very low birth weight infants. *Pediatrics*. 1986;77(4):507–12.
32. Nelson KB, Ellenberg JH. Childhood neurological disorders in twins. *Paediatr Perinat Epidemiol*. 1995;9(2):135–45.
33. Fahey MC, Maclennan AH, Kretzschmar D, Gecz J, Kruer MC. The genetic basis of cerebral palsy. *Dev Med Child Neurol*. 2017;59(5):462–9.
34. Lethbridge-Çejku M, Rose D, Vickerie J. Summary health statistics for U.S. adults national health interview survey, 2004. *Vital Heal Stat 10*. 2006;10(228):1–164.
35. Emond A, Golding J, Peckham C. Cerebral palsy in two national cohort studies. *Arch Dis Child*. 1989;64(6):848–52.
36. Nelson KB, Grether JK. Potentially asphyxiating conditions and spastic cerebral palsy in infants of normal birth weight. *Am J Obstet Gynecol*. 1998;179(2):507–13.
37. Johnston M V., Harum KH, Hoon Jr. AH, Kato GJ, Casella JF, Breiter SN. Homozygous factor-V mutation as a genetic cause of perinatal thrombosis and cerebral palsy. *Dev Med Child Neurol*. 1999;41(11):777–80.
38. Nelson KB, Grether JK. Can magnesium sulfate reduce the risk of cerebral palsy in very low birthweight infants? *Obstet Gynecol Surv*. 1995;50(8):573–5.
39. Kancherla V, Amendah DD, Grosse SD, Yeargin-Allsopp M, Van Naarden Braun K. Medical expenditures attributable to cerebral palsy and intellectual disability among Medicaid-enrolled children. *Res Dev Disabil*. 2012;33(3):832–40.
40. CDC. Economic costs associated with mental retardation, cerebral palsy, hearing loss, and vision impairment—United States, 2003. *MMWR Morb Mortal Wkly Rep*. 2012;53(3):57–9.
41. Shorvon SD. The causes of epilepsy: Changing concepts of etiology of epilepsy over the past 150 years. *Epilepsia*. 2011;52(6):1033–44.
42. Stafstrom CE, Carmant L. Seizures and epilepsy: An overview for neuroscientists. *Cold Spring Harb Perspect Biol*. 2015;7(5):1–19.
43. Fisher RS, Cross JH, French JA, et al. Operational classification of seizure types by the International League Against Epilepsy: Position paper of the ILAE Commission for Classification and Terminology. *Zeitschrift fur Epileptol*. 2018;31(4):272–81.
44. Hauser WA, Annegers JF, Rocca WA. Descriptive epidemiology of epilepsy: Contributions of population-based studies from Rochester, Minnesota. *Mayo Clin Proc*. 2009;71(6):576–86.
45. Hitirisa N, Mohanraj R, Norriec J, Brodiea MJ. Mortality in epilepsy. *Epilepsy Behav*. 2007;10:363–76.
46. Kobau R, Zahran H, Thurman DJ, Zack MM, Henry TR, Schachter SC PP. Epilepsy surveillance among adults—19 States. *Beha MMWR Surveill Summ*. 2008;57(6):1–20.
47. WAHauser. Epidemiology of epilepsy. In: Gorelick PB, Alter M, eds. *Handbook of Neuroepidemiology*. New York: Marcel Dekker, Inc.; 1994, pp. 315–56.
48. Annegers JF, Rocca WA. Causes of epilepsy: Contributions of the rochester epidemiology project. *Mayo Clin Proc*. 1996;71(6):570–5.
49. World Health Organization. Epilepsy—Prevention. https://www.who.int/news-room/fact-sheets/detail/epilepsy. Published 2019.
50. Dube CM, Ravizza T, Hamamura M, et al. Epileptogenesis provoked by prolonged experimental febrile seizures: Mechanisms and biomarkers. *J Neurosci*. 2010;30(22):7484–94.
51. McTague A, Howell KB, Cross JH, Kurian MA, Scheffer IE. The genetic landscape of the epileptic encephalopathies of infancy and childhood. *Lancet Neurol*. 2016;15(3):304–16.
52. Monteiro GC, Aroca ILZ, Margarit BP, Herán IS. Epilepsy. *Med*. 2019;12(72):4222–31.
53. Shackleton DP, Kasteleijn-Nolst Trenité DGA, de Craen AJM, Vandenbroucke JP, Westendorp RGJ. Living with epilepsy: Long-term prognosis and psychosocial outcomes. *Neurology*. 2003;61(1):64–70.
54. Kaneko S Okada M, Iwasa H et al. Genetics of epilepsy: Current status and perspectives. *Neurosci Res*. 2002;44:11–30.
55. Sander L. The epidemiology of the Epilepsies revisited. *Curr Opin Neurol*. 2003;16:165–70.
56. de Boer HM, Mula M, Sander JW. The global burden and stigma of epilepsy. *Epilepsy Behav*. 2008;12(4):540–6.
57. De Boer H. "Out of the Shadows": A global campaign against epilepsy. *Epilepsia*. 2002;43:7–8.
58. Pahl K, de Boer HG. Epilepsy and rights. In: *Atlas: Epilepsy Care in the World*. Geneva: World Health Organization; 2005, pp. 72–73.
59. Stovner LJ, Hagen K, Jensen R, et al. The global burden of headache: A documentation of headache prevalence and disability worldwide. *Cephalalgia*. 2007;27(3):193–210.
60. Burch R, Rizzoli P, Loder E. The prevalence and impact of migraine and severe headache in the United States: Figures and trends from government health studies. *Headache*. 2018;58(4):496–505.
61. Ahmed F. Headache disorders: Differentiating and managing the common subtypes. *Br J Pain*. 2012;6(3):124–32.
62. Kernick D, SStapley, PJGoadsby, Hamilton W. What happens to new-onset headache presented to primary care? A case-cohort study using electronic primary care records. *Cephalalgia*. 2008; 28(11):1188–95.
63. Kurtzke JF. Neuroepidemiology. *Ann Neurol*. 1984;16(3):265–77.
64. Bajwa ZH, Wootton RJ, II. Evaluation of headache in adults. In: Post TW, ed. *UpToDate*. Waltham, MA: UpToDate; 2019.
65. Vincent M, Wang S. Headache Classification Committee of the International Headache Society (IHS) The International Classification of Headache Disorders, 3rd edition. *Cephalalgia*. 2018;38(1):1–211.
66. Olesen J. The international classification of headache disorders. *Lancet Neurol*. 2018;17(5):396–7.
67. Jensen RH. Tension-type headache—The normal and most prevalent headache. *Headache Curr*. 2018;58(2):339–45.
68. Benoliel R. Trigeminal autonomic cephalalgias. *Br J Pain*. 2012;6(3):106–23.
69. Harriott AM, Takizawa T, Chung DY, Chen SP. Spreading depression as a preclinical model of migraine. *J Headache Pain*. 2019;20(1):45.
70. Cui Y, Kataoka Y, Watanabe Y. Role of cortical spreading depression in the pathophysiology of migraine. *Neurosci Bull*. 2014;30(5):812–22.
71. Woldeamanuel YW, Andreou AP, Cowan RP. Prevalence of migraine headache and its weight on neurological burden in Africa: A 43-year systematic review and meta-analysis of community-based studies. *J Neurol Sci*. 2014;342(1):1–15.
72. Annequin D, Tourniaire B, Massiou H. Migraine and headache in childhood and adolescence. *Pediatr Clin N Am*. 2000;47(3):617–31.
73. Straube A, Andreou AP. Primary headaches during lifespan. *J Headache Pain*. 2019;20(35).
74. Albers L, von Kries R, Heinen F, Straube A. Headache in school children: Is the prevalence increasing? *Curr Pain Headache Rep*. 2015;19(3):4.
75. Lipton R, Stewart W. Migraine in the United States: A review of use. *Neurology*. 1993;43(3):6–10.
76. Couch J, Hassanein R. Headache as a risk factor in atherosclerosis-related diseases. *Headache*. 1989;29:49–54.
77. Blackwell D, Villarroel M. Tables of summary health statistics for U.S. adults: 2017 National health interview survey. National Center Health Statistics. 2018.
78. White R, Proctor S. Solvents and neurotoxicity. *Lancet*. 1997;349:1239–43.
79. Landrigan PJ, Kreiss K, Xintaras C, et al. Clinical epidemiology of occupational neurotoxic disease. *Neurobehav Toxicol*. 1980;2:43–8.

80. Priyadarshi A, Khuder SA, Schaub EA, et al. A meta-analysis of Parkinson's disease and exposure to pesticides. *Neurotoxicology.* 2000;21:435–40.

81. Senanayake N, Karalliedde L. Neurotoxic effects of organophosphorus insecticides. *N Engl J Med.* 1987;316:761–3.

82. Semchuck KM, Love EJ LR. Parkinson's disease and exposure to agricultural work and pesticide chemicals. *Neurology.* 1992;42:1328–35.

83. Butterfield PG, Valanis BG, Spencer PS et al. Environmental antecedents of young-onset Parkinson's disease. *Neurology.* 1993;43:1150–8.

84. Seidler A, Hellenbrand W, Robra BP et al. Possible environmental, occupational and other etiologic factors for Parkinson's disease: A case-control study in Germany. *Neurology.* 1996;46:1275–84.

85. Gorell JM, Johnson CC, Rybicki BA, et al. The risk of Parkinson's disease with exposure to pesticides, farming, well water, and rural living. *Neurology.* 1998;50:1346–50.

86. Siegel M, Starks SE, Sanderson WT, Kamel F, Hoppin JA, Gerr F. Organic solvent exposure and depressive symptoms among licensed pesticide applicators in the Agricultural Health Study. *Int Arch Occup Env Heal.* 2017;90(8):849–8.

87. Colomina MT, Peris-Sampedro F. Aluminum and Alzheimer's disease. *Adv Neurobiol.* 2017;18:183–97.

88. McFarlin D, McFarland H. Multiple sclerosis. Parts 1 and 2. *NEJM.* 1982;307:1183–8, 1246–51.

89. Thompson AJ, Hutchinson A, Brazil J et al. A clinical and laboratory study of benign multiple sclerosis. *QJ Med.* 1986;58:69–80.

90. McDonald I. Diagnostic methods and investigation in multiple sclerosis. In: Compston A, ed. *McAlpine's Multiple Sclerosis.* 3rd ed. New York: Churchill Livingstone; 1988, pp. 251–79.

91. Wynn DR, Rodriguez M, O'Fallon WM, et al. A reappraisal of the epidemiology of multiple sclerosis in Olmsted County, Minnesota. *Neurology.* 1990;40:780–6.

92. Evans C, Beland SG, Kulaga S, et al. Incidence and prevalence of multiple sclerosis in the Americas: A systematic review. *Neuroepidemiology.* 2013;40(3):195–210.

93. Alter M, Leibowitz U, Speer J. Risk of multiple sclerosis related to age at immigration to Israel. *Arch Neurol.* 1966;15(3):234–7.

94. Dean G. Annual incidence, prevalence, and mortality of multiple sclerosis in white South-African-born and in white immigrants to South Africa. *Br Med J.* 1967;2(5554):724–30.

95. Jr SS, Blizzard L, Otahal P, Van Der Mei I, Taylor B. Latitude is significantly associated with the prevalence of multiple sclerosis : A meta-analysis. *J Neurol Neurosurg Psychiatry.* 2011;82(10):1132–41.

96. Kurtzke JF, Hyllested K Multiple sclerosis in the Faroe Islands I. Clinical and epidemiological features. *Ann Neurol.* 1979;5:6–21.

97. Kurtzke JF, Hyllested K Multiple sclerosis in the Faroe Islands II. Clinical update, transmission, and the nature of MS. *Neurology.* 1985;36:307–28.

98. Kurtzke JF, Hyllested K Multiple sclerosis in the Faroe Islands III. An alternative assessment of the three epidemics. *Acta Neurol Scand.* 1987;76:317–39.

99. Granieri E. Exogenous factors in the etiology of multiple sclerosis. *J Neurovirol.* 2000;6(Supp. 2):S141–6.

100. Hernan M, Olek M, Ascherio A. Cigarette smoking and incidence of multiple sclerosis. *Am J Epidemiol.* 2001;154:69–74.

101. Weinshenker B. Epidemiology of multiple sclerosis. *Clin Neurol.* 1996;14:291–308.

102. Compston A. Genetic suspectibility to multiple scelerosis. In: Compston A, ed. *McAlpine's Multiple Sclerosis.* 3rd ed. New York: Churchill Livingstone; 1998, pp. 101–42.

103. Poser C. The epidemiology of multiple sclerosis: A general overview. *Ann Neurol.* 1994;36(S2):S180–93.

104. Del Rey NL-G, Quiroga-Varela A, Garbayo E, et al. Advances in Parkinson's disease: 200 Years later. *Front Neuroanat.* 2018;12(December):1–14.

105. Radhakrishnan DM, Goyal V. Parkinson's disease: A review. *Neurol India.* 2018;66(Suppl S):26–35.

106. Litvan I, Bhatia K, Burn D. Movement Disorders Society Scientific Issues Committee report: SIC Task Force appraisal of clinical diagnostic criteria for Parkinsonian disorders. *Mov Disord.* 2003;18:467–86.

107. Aarsland D, Tandberg E, Larsen JP, Cummings JL. Frequency of dementia in Parkinson disease. *Arch Neurol.* 1996;53:538–42.

108. De Lau LML, Breteler MMB. Epidemiolohy of PD. *Lancet Neurol.* 2006;5(6):525–35.

109. "Davis Phinney Foundation." The Difference Between Lewy Body Dementia, Parkinson's Disease and Alzheimer's Disease. Available at https://www.davisphinneyfoundation.org/blog/difference-lewy-body-dementia-parkinsons-disease-alzheimers-disease/. Published 2019.

110. Twelves D, Perkins KSM, Counsell C. Systematic review of incidence studies of Parkinson's disease. *Mov Disord.* 2003;18(1):19–31.

111. de Rijk M, Launer LJ, Berger K, et al. Prevalence of Parkinson's disease in Europe: A collaborative study of population-based cohorts. *Neurology.* 2000;54(11 Supp):S21–3.

112. Tysnes OB, Storstein A. Epidemiology of Parkinson's disease. *J Neural Transm.* 2017;124(8):901–5.

113. Lix LM, Hobson DE, Azimaee M, Leslie WD, Burchill C, Hobson S. Socioeconomic variations in the prevalence and incidence of Parkinson's disease: A population-based analysis. *J Epidemiol Community Health.* 2010;64(4):335–40.

114. Calabrese VP, Dorsey ER, Constantinescu R, et al. Projected number of people with Parkinson disease in the most populous nations, 2005 through 2030. *Neurology.* 2007;69(2):223–4.

115. Kim SD, Allen NE, Canning CG, Fung VSC. Parkinson disease. *Handb Clin Neurol.* 2018;159:173–93.

116. Poewe W, Seppi K, Tanner CM, et al. Parkinson disease. *Nat Rev Dis Primers.* 2017;3:1–21.

117. Connolly BS, Lang AE. Pharmacological treatment of Parkinson disease: A review. *JAMA.* 2014;311(16):1670–83.

118. Levy G, Tang MX, Louis ED et al.. The association of incident dementia with mortality in PD. *Neurology.* 2002;59:1708–13.

119. Wirdefeldt K, Gatz M, Reynolds CA, Prescott CA, Pedersen NL. Heritability of Parkinson disease in Swedish twins: A longitudinal study. *Neurobiol Aging.* 2011;32(10):1923.e1–8.

120. Tanner CM, Chen B, Wang W. Environmental factors in the etiology of Parkinson's disease. *Can J Neurol Sci.* 1987;14:419–23.

121. Hernán MA, Takkouche B, Caamaño-Isorna F, Gestal-Otero JJ. A meta-analysis of coffee drinking, cigarette smoking, and the risk of Parkinson's disease. *Ann Neurol.* 2002;52(3):276–84.

122. Munoz DG, Fujioka S. Caffeine and Parkinson disease. *Neurology.* 2018;90(5):205–6.

123. Mayeux R, Tang MX, Marder K et al. Smoking and Parkinson's disease. *Mov Disord.* 1994;9:207–12.

124. Lin J, O'Connor E, Rossom R, Perdue L, Ekstrom E. Screening for cognitive impairment in older adults: A systematic review for the U.S. Preventive Services Task Force. *Ann Intern Med.* 2013;159(9):601–12.

125. Ferri CP, Prince M, Brayne C, et al. Global prevalence of dementia: A Delphi consensus study. *Lancet.* 2005;366(9503):2112–7.

126. Qiu C. Epidemiology of Alzheimer's disease: Occurrence, determinants, and strategies toward intervention. *Dialogues Clin Neurosci.* 2009;11(2):111–28.

127. Eggink E, Moll van Charante EP, van Gool WA, Richard E. A population perspective on prevention of dementia. *J Clin Med.* 2019;8(6):834.

128. Prince M, Albanese E, Guerchet M, Al . E. World Alzheimer report 2014. Dementia and risk reduction: An analysis of protective and modifia-ble risk factors. Alzheimer's Disease International. 2014. Available at https://www.bmj.com/content/350/bmj.h3029.

129. Prince M, Knapp M, Guerchet M, et al. Dementia UK: Second Edition. *Alzheimer's Soc.* 2014.

130. Launer LJ. Statistics on the burden of dementia : Need for stronger data. *Lancet Neurol.* 2018;18(1):P25–27.

131. Lobo A, Launer L, Fratiglioni L. Prevalence of dementia and major subtypes in Europe: A collaborative study of population-based cohorts. Neurologic Diseases in the Elderly Research Group. *Neurology.* 2000;54:S4–9.

132. Burns A. Dementia—Clinical review. *BMJ.* 2009;338:b75.

133. Zaccai J, McCracken C, Brayne C. A systematic review of prevalence and incidence studies of dementia with Lewy bodies. *Age Ageing.* 2005;34(6):561–6.

134. Stephan B, Birdi R, Tang E, Cosco T, Robinson L. Secular trends in dementia prevalence and incidence worldwide: A systematic review. *J Alzheimers Dis.* 2018;66:653–80.

135. Falk N, Cole A, Hospital F, Medicine F, Park W. Evaluation of suspected dementia. *Am Fam Physician.* 2018;97(6):398–405.

136. Atri A, Hendrix J, Carrillo M, Dickerson B. First practice guidelines for clinical evaluation of Alzheimer's disease and other dementias for primary and specialty care. Alzheimer's Association International Conference 2018. 2018. https://www.alz.org/aaic/downloads2018/Sun-clinical-practice-guidelines.pdf.

137. Anoop A, Singh PK, Jacob RS, Maji SK. CSF biomarkers for Alzheimer's disease diagnosis. *Int J Alzheimers Dis.* 2010;2110:606802.

138. Vos SJB, Kornhuber J, Wiltfang J, et al. Prevalence and prognosis of Alzheimer's disease at the mild cognitive impairment stage. *Brain.* 2015;138(Pt 5):1327–38.

139. Petersen RC, Smith GE, Waring SC. Mild cognitive impairment clinical characterization and outcome. *Arch Neurol.* 1999;56:303–8.
140. Kapasi A, DeCarli C, Schneider JA. Impact of multiple pathologies on the threshold for clinically overt dementia. *Acta Neuropathol.* 2017;134(2):171–86.
141. James BD, Wilson RS, Boyle PA, Trojanowski JQ, Bennett DA, Schneider JA. TDP-43 stage, mixed pathologies, and clinical Alzheimer's-type dementia. *Brain.* 2016;139(11):2983–93.
142. Matthews F, Arthur A, Barnes L. A two-decade comparison of prevalence of dementia in individuals aged 65 years and older from three geographical areas of England: Results of the cognitive function and ageing study I and II. *Lancet.* 2013;382:1405–12.
143. Hachinski V. Dementia: Paradigm shifting into high gear. *Alzheimer's Dement.* 2019;15(7):985–94.
144. Jellinger KA, Attems J. Prevalence and impact of vascular and Alzheimer pathologies in Lewy body disease. *Acta Neuropathol.* 2008:427–36.
145. Elahi FM, Miller BL. A clinicopathological approach to the diagnosis of dementia. *Nat Rev Neurol.* 2017;13(8):457–76.
146. Schneider J, Bennett D. Where vascular meets neurodegenerative disease. *Stroke.* 2010;41(10):144–6.
147. Akoudad S, Wolters FJ, Viswanathan A, et al. Cerebral microbleeds are associated with cognitive decline and dementia: The Rotterdam Study. *JAMA Neurol.* 2016;73(8):934–43.
148. Reza M, Avan A, Cipriano LE, Munoz DG, Sposato LA, Hachinski V. Concomitant vascular and neurodegenerative pathologies double the risk of dementia. *Alzheimer's Dement.* 2018;14(2):148–56.
149. Reitz C, Way R, Cb C. Epidemiology of Alzheimer disease. *Nat Rev Neurol.* 2012;7(3):137–52.
150. Johnson KA, Fox NC, Sperling RA, Klunk WE. Brain imaging in Alzheimer disease. *Cold Spring Harb Perspect Med.* 2012;2(4):a006213.
151. Scarmeas N, Tang MX, Schupf N. Survival in Alzheimer disease: A multiethnic, population-based study of incident cases. *Neurology.* 2008;71(19):1489–95.
152. Larson EB, Shadlen M, Wang L, Mccormick WC, Bowen JD, Teri L. Survival after initial diagnosis of Alzheimer disease. *Ann Intern Med.* 2004;140(7):501–9.
153. Sloane PD, Zimmerman S, Suchindran C, et al. The public health impact of alzheimer's disease, 2000–2050: Potential implication of treatment advances. *Annu Rev Public Health.* 2002;23(1):213–31.
154. Hachinski V, Einhäupl K, Ganten D, et al. Preventing dementia by preventing stroke: The Berlin manifesto. *Alzheimer's Dement.* 2019;15(7):961–84.
155. Glymour MM, Quesenberry CP, Whitmer RA. Inequalities in dementia incidence between six racial and ethnic groups over 14 years. *Alzheimers Dement.* 2016;12(3):216–24.
156. Mayeda ER, Glymour MM, Quesenberry CP, Johnson JK, Pérez-Stable EJ, Whitmer RA. Survival after dementia diagnosis in five racial/ethnic groups. *Alzheimers Dement.* 2017;13(7):761–9.
157. Taylor C, Greenlund S, McGuire L, Lu H, Croft J. Deaths from Alzheimer's Disease—United States, 1999–2014. *MMWR Morb Mortal Wkly Rep.* 2017;66:521–6.
158. McKhann GM, Knopman DS, Chertkow H, et al. The diagnosis of dementia due to Alzheimer's disease: Recommendations from the National Institute on Aging-Alzheimer's Association workgroups on diagnostic guidelines for Alzheimer's disease. *Alzheimer's Dement.* 2011;7(3): 263–9.
159. Alzheimer's Disease Diagnostic Guidelines. National Institute on Aging. Available at https://www.nia.nih.gov/health/alzheimers-disease-diagnostic-guidelines. Published 2019. Accessed February 8, 2019.
160. Sperling RA, Aisen PS, Beckett LA, et al. Toward defining the preclinical stages of Alzheimer's disease : Recommendations from the National Institute on Aging-Alzheimer's Association workgroups on diagnostic guidelines for Alzheimer's disease. *Alzheimer's Dement.* 2011;7(3): 280–92.
161. Morris JC, Blennow K, Froelich L, et al. Harmonized diagnostic criteria for Alzheimer's disease : Recommendations. *J Intern Med.* 2014;275(3):204–13.
162. Jack JrCR, Liu E, Luis J, Montine T, Phelps C. NIA-AA research framework: Toward a biological definition of Alzheimer's disease. *Alzheimers Dement.* 2018;14(4):535–62.
163. SPRINT MIND Investigators for the SPRINT Research Group, Williamson J, Pajewski N, Auchus A, et al. Effect of intensive vs standard blood pressure control on probable dementia: A randomized clinical trial. *JAMA.* 2019;12(321):553–61.
164. Belay E, Schonberger L. The public health impact of prion diseases. *Annu Rev Public Heal.* 2005;26:191–212.
165. Chen C, Dong XP. Epidemiological characteristics of human prion diseases. *Infect Dis Poverty.* 2016;5(1):1–10.
166. Brown K, Mastrianni JA. The prion diseases. *J Geriatr Psychiatry Neurol.* 2010;23(4):277–98.
167. Heath CA, Cooper SA, Murray K, et al. Diagnosing variant Creutzfeldt–Jakob disease: A retrospective analysis of the first 150 cases in the UK. *J Neurol Neurosurg Psychiatry.* 2011;82:646–51.
168. Will RG. Acquired prion disease: iatrogenic CJD, variant CJD, kuru—Hľadať Googlom. 2003:255–65.
169. Diack A, Head M, McCutcheon S, Boyle A, Will R. Variant CJD: 18 years of research and surveillance. *Prion.* 2014;8(4):286–95.
170. Belay E. Transmissible spongiform encephalopathies in humans. *Annu Rev Microbiol.* 1999;53:283–314.
171. Benjamin EJ, Muntner P, Alonso A, et al. Heart Disease and Stroke Statistics-2019 Update: A Report From the American Heart Association. Vol. 139; 2019.
172. Feigin VL, Norrving B, George MG, Foltz JL, Roth GA, Mensah GA. Prevention of stroke: A strategic global imperative. *Nat Rev Neurol.* 2016;12(9):501–12.
173. Hankey GJ. Stroke. *Lancet.* 2017;389(10069):641–54.
174. Gibson LM, Whiteley W. The differential diagnosis of suspected stroke: A systematic review. *J R Coll Physicians Edinb.* 2013;43:114–48.
175. Krishnamurthi RV, Feigin VL, Forouzanfar MH, et al. Global and regional burden of first-ever ischaemic and haemorrhagic stroke during 1990–2010. *Lancet Glob Heal.* 2013;1(5):e259–81.
176. Fisher M. Stroke and TIA: Epidemiology, risk factors, and the need for early intervention. *Am J Manag Care.* 2008;14(Suppl. 7):5–7.
177. Wroblewska L, Kitada T, Endo K, et al. Stroke prevention worldwide—What could make it work? *Neuroepidemiology.* 2016;33(8):839–41.
178. Easton JD, Saver JL, Albers GW, et al. Definition and evaluation of transient ischemic attack: A scientific statement for healthcare professionals from the American heart association/American stroke association stroke council; council on cardiovascular surgery and anesthesia; council on cardio. *Stroke.* 2009;40(6):2276–93.
179. Khare S. Risk factors of transient ischemic attack: An overview. *J Midlife Heal.* 2016;7(1):2–7.
180. Giles MF, Albers GW, Amarenco P, et al. Early stroke risk and ABCD2 score performance in tissue-Vs time-defined TIA: A multicenter study. *Neurology.* 2011;77(13):1222–8.
181. Khadilkar S. Neurology: The scenario in India. *J Assoc Physicians India.* 2012;60:42–4.
182. Lo TQ, Marston BJ, Dahl BA, De Cock KM. Ebola: Anatomy of an epidemic. *Annu Rev Med.* 2017;68:359–70.
183. Briand S, Bertherat E, Cox P, et al. The international Ebola emergency. *N Engl J Med.* 2014;371:1180–3.
184. Jacobs M, Rodger A, Bell DJ, et al. Late Ebola virus relapse causing meningoencephalitis: A case report. *Lancet.* 2016;388:498–503.
185. Group TPIS. A longitudinal study of Ebola sequelae in Liberia. *N Engl J Med.* 2019;380:924–93.
186. Araujo AQ, Silva MT, Araujo AP. Zika virus-associated neurological disorders: A review. *Brain.* 2016;139(8):2122–30.
187. Souza I, Barros-Aragão F, Frost PS, Figueiredo CP, Clarke JR Late neurological Consequences of Zika virus infection: Risk factors and pharmaceutical approaches. *Pharmaceuticals.* 2019;12:60.
188. Lopez A, Lee A, Guo A et al. Vital signs: Surveillance for acute flaccid myelitis—United States, 2018. *MMWR Morb Mortal Wkly Rep.* 2019;68:608–14.
189. Dyda A, Stelzer-Braid S, Adam D, Chughtai AA, MacIntyre CR The association between acute flaccid myelitis (AFM) and enterovirus D68 (EV-D68)—What is the evidence for causation? *Euro Surveill.* 2018;23(3).

CHAPTER

59 Visual Disorders

Luxme Hariharan • Ellery Lopez Starr • Renata Garcia • Jason A. Penniecook • Jeff Pettey • Eric Hanson • Priya Morjaria • Josie Noah • Danny Haddad • Olachi J. Mezu-Ndubuisi • Kevin L. Winthrop • Camila V. Ventura • Van Charles Lansingh

INTRODUCTION

Visual disorders such as uncorrected refractive error (URE), cataract, glaucoma, diabetic retinopathy, and retinopathy of prematurity (ROP) are leading public health problems worldwide, causing significant morbidity and dramatically affecting the lives of hundreds of millions of people daily. Overall, 75–80% of the causes of blindness and visual impairment (VI) are avoidable or treatable with early detection, evidence-based screening, and timely treatment. More specifically, for 2015, it was estimated that 81.2% of the blindness is preventable or treatable.[1] Unfortunately, 90% of avoidable blindness disproportionately affects the most vulnerable communities including the poor, women, children, the elderly, and people living in rural areas.[1,2]

In recent years, there has been an international *"call to action"* to break down barriers to eye health and to improve equity in eye care across all communities and age groups. In 2013, all Member States of the World Health Organization (WHO) signed, *Universal eye health: a global action plan 2014–19*.[3] For the past 5 years, the global community has been committed to reduce the prevalence of blindness and VI and to increase eye-care coverage among the most vulnerable populations. While there has been much progress and innovation in the early detection and treatment of visual disorders over the years, currently many blindness prevention and control strategies are still implemented in disease-specific silos that work independently of other vision and public health programs. However, in order to successfully eliminate avoidable blindness worldwide, and to effectively address visual disorders in a timely, systematic, and sustainable fashion, it is imperative that existing silos are torn down and replaced with effective bridges that integrate vision into existing public health programs and infrastructure in a horizontal and vertical manner across multiple sectors.[3,4] Successful eye-care integration needs to start at the primary health level and needs to be implemented simultaneously to the strengthening of health systems. For this to occur, intersectoral, multistakeholder synergistic collaboration among governments, non-for-profit organizations, academic institutions, schools, hospitals, research centers, the United Nations, and socially minded programs of the private sector, is not only optimal but in fact essential.

Additionally, local and global blindness prevention and treatment programs should be successfully embedded within current health and legal systems, with collaborative and inclusive policies to have the most sustainable, lasting, and cost-effective impact. These policies must address the multifaceted causes of blindness and VI across ages, diseases, and regions. They also require creative, innovative multipronged and interdisciplinary solutions based on collaborative synergy among ophthalmologists, optometrists, nurses, public health experts, community health workers, school system leaders, pediatricians, neonatologists, hospital leadership, policy experts, legislators, nonprofits, government programs, private sector, and academic institutions. This collaborative and partnership approach should also emphasize advocacy for high-quality, affordable, and sustainable blindness prevention and treatment programs and universal eye health coverage for all patients regardless of their age, demographic or geographic location.[3]

The implementation of the most recent WHO global action plan has come to an end, making it an opportune time for the medical and the public health community at large to reflect on the lessons learned, progress made toward comprehensive and universal eye health coverage, and the ongoing challenges and barriers that still exist. The aim of the following chapter on visual disorders is to shed light on what is most useful to further empower public health practitioners and preventive medicine physicians interested in creating mechanisms to prevent blindness and to form a united front with eye-care professionals to strengthen eye-care integration. The chapter utilizes a public health and health systems-based approach to take readers on a journey from the front of eye (the anterior segment) to the back of the eye (the posterior segment) and discusses childhood visual disorders, infectious diseases affecting the eye and the clinical pathology of visual disorders. Two best practice approaches in vision and public health that demonstrate successful health system integration leading to blindness reduction and prevention in both children and adults are also highlighted.

Key Definitions of Blindness and Visual Impairment

In order to solve any public health problem effectively, it is imperative to first define the problem clearly. Global vision experts classify the degree of VI as mild, moderate, severe, "blindness," " presbyopia," and "low vision," although specific definitions can vary by region, by country, and by institution.[5]

Table 59-1 summarizes VI classifications used in prior studies of the World Health Organizations (WHO) and the Global Burden of Disease (GBD) research group. These categories are based on visual acuity (VA) measured using the metric system and the American Snellen VA system, and they have been used in the past by programs and in GBD epidemiological studies of blindness and VI. In contrast, Table 59-2 contains the 2018 updated definitions of the International Classification of Disease (ICD)-11 guidelines. Definitions shown in Table 59-2 will be the baseline definitions used for future GBD studies. In Table 59-2, VA levels are measured using the metric system, the decimal system, and the American Snellen system. According to the ICD-11 definition, the VA in binocular VI should be measured with both eyes open with ocular correction, if needed. For characterizing monocular VI, VA should be measured one eye at a time with ocular correction, if needed[6]

The United States (U.S.) National Eye Institute (NEI) defines blindness as a VA level of 20/200 or worse with best available correction. The NEI defines VI as the best corrected VA less than (20/40) in the better-seeing eye (excluding those who were categorized as

TABLE 59-1 DEFINITIONS OF VISION IMPAIRMENT (VI)

Category of Vision Impairment (VI)	Definition
Mild vision impairment (MVI)	Worse than 6/12 (20/40) but 6/18 (20/60) or better
Moderate and severe VI (MSVI)	Worse than 6/18 (20/60) but 3/60 (20/200) or better
Blindness	Worse than 3/60 (20/200)
Presbyopia	Near vision worse than N6 or N8 at 40 cm and best corrected visual acuity ≥ 6/12 (20/40)
Functional Low Vision	Worse than 6/18 or 20/60 but greater than or equal to light perception in the better eye that is untreatable and uncorrectable

[a]6/12 indicates measurement using the metric system, while 20/40 represents the American Snellen System, in which case Presenting Snellen Visual Acuity in the Better Eye (20/40) means that a person sees at 20 ft what they should see at 40 ft.

TABLE 59-2 ICD-11 CLASSIFICATION OF VISION IMPAIRMENT (VI) AND BLINDNESS

Category	Presenting Distance Visual Acuity	
	Worse than:	Equal to or Better Than:
No vision impairment		6/12 5/10 (0.5) 20/40
1) Mild vision impairment	6/12 5/10 (0.5) 20/40	6/18 3/10 (0.3) 20/70
2) Moderate vision impairment	6/18 3/10 (0.3) 20/70	6/60 1/10 (0.1) 20/200
3) Severe vision impairment	6/60 1/10 (0.1) 20/200	3/60 1/20 (0.05) 20/400
4) Blindness	3/60 1/20 (0.05) 20/400 No light perception	1/60 1/50 (0.02) 5/300 (20/1200) or counts fingers (CF) at 1 meter
6) Blindness	1/60 1/50 (0.02) 5/300 (20/1200)	Light perception
7) Blindness	No light perception	

[a]6/12 indicates measurement using the metric system, while 20/40 represents the American Snellen System.

TABLE 59-3 PREVALENCE OF ADULT VISION IMPAIRMENT AND AGE-RELATED EYE DISEASES IN AMERICA

Estimated Number of Cases by Vision Problem Age ≥ 40	
Age-related macular degeneration[a]	2,069,403
Cataract	24,409,978
Diabetic retinopathy	7,685,237
Glaucoma	2,719,379

[a]Age-related macular degeneration, age 50 and older.
Source: Based on 2010 U.S. Census populations. Total Population ≥ 40 = 142,648,393. Last Reviewed: April 2016.

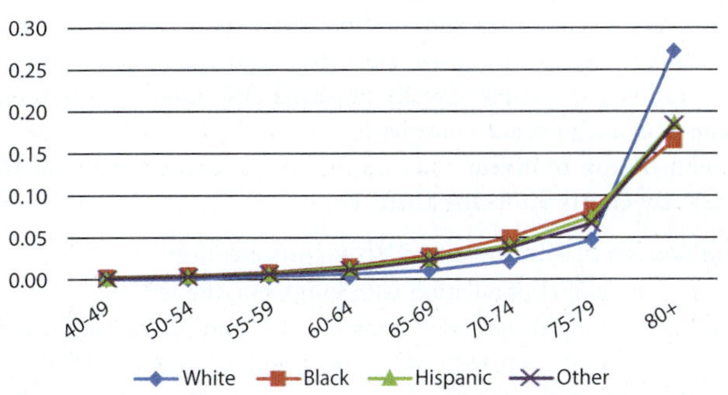

FIGURE 59-1. The National Eye Institute (NEI) 2010 United States prevalence rates of all visual impairment (VI). Courtesy: National Eye Institute, National Institutes of Health (NEI/NIH)

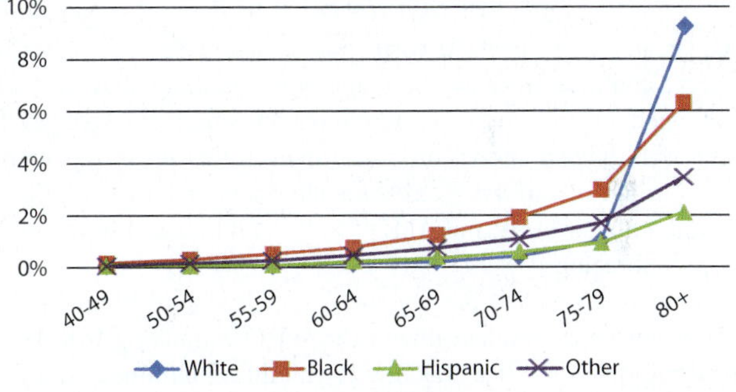

FIGURE 59-2. The National Eye Institute (NEI) 2010 United States prevalence rates of blindness. Courtesy: National Eye Institute, National Institutes of Health (NEI/NIH)

being blind by the U.S. definition). The NEI category "All Vision Impairment" includes both low vision and blindness.[7] Table 59-3 demonstrates the prevalence of adult VI and age-related eye diseases in America from the NEI in 2010. Figures 59-1 and 59-2 show the prevalence according to age, and race/ethnicity.

Overall, the slight variations in definitions, terminology, and measurements of blindness and VI across the globe and institutions is a main challenge of implementing uniform screening and treatment strategies and programs worldwide.

Magnitude, Prevalence, and Causes of Blindness and Visual Impairment

Previously, the WHO periodically published global data of blindness and VI.[8] The Global Burden of Disease (GBD) dataset is now considered the standard global dataset, given that it utilizes a more precise methodology and includes more complete data and is updated every 5 years.[1,5,9–13] The most recent 2015 GBD study was a systematic review and meta-analysis of blindness and VI data from 288 population-based studies from 98 countries, including 61 new studies from 35 countries, that were published between 1980 and 2015.[5] Hierarchical models were used to estimate the 2015 prevalence (by age, country, and sex) of mild visual impairment (MVI), moderate or severe vision impairment (MSVI), blindness, and functional presbyopia as defined in Table 59-1. This study updated the 2010 global, regional, and country-level blindness and vision impairment prevalence estimates for 2015, with the inclusion of functional presbyopia estimates for the first time and more precise data (individual-level data for many studies).[5]

Among the 7 billion people alive in 2015, 36 million people were estimated to be blind, whereas 216 million people had MSVI.[5] This study also revealed that the global age-standardized all-age prevalence of blindness decreased from 0.75% [80% uncertainty interval (UI): 0.25–141] in 1990 to 0.48% [80% UI: 0.17–0.87] in 2015, and that the global age-standardized all-age prevalence of MSVI decreased from 3.83% (80% UI: 1.66–6.42) to 2.90% (UI: 1.314.80). Furthermore, functional presbyopia affected an estimated 1094.7 million (80% UI: 581.1–1686.5 million) people aged 35 years and older and 666.7 million (80% UI: 364.9–997.6 million) being aged 50 years or older. The estimated number of people with blindness increased by 17.9%, from 30.6 million in 1990 to 36.0 million in 2015. The number of people with MSVI also increased by 35.5%, from 159.9 million in 1990 to 216.6 million in 2015. In 2015 in high-income countries and Eastern and Central Europe, the age-standardized prevalence rates of blindness, MSVI, MVI, and presbyopia were 0.15% (UI 80%: 0.06–0.26), 1.27% (80% UI: 0.55–2.17), 1.27 (80% UI 0.40–2.43), and 18.58 (UI 80%: 5.47–34.60), respectively.[10]

While there was an overall reduction in the age standardized prevalence of blindness and VI from 1990 to 2015, the increased growth and aging of the global population caused an increase in the total number of people visually impaired and blind. Furthermore, there was a significant contribution from uncorrected presbyopia, demonstrating an urgent and immense need to scale screening and treatment efforts across the board.

The Causes of Blindness and Visual Impairment

Among the global population with blindness, the leading causes of blindness among all ages were cataract, URE, and glaucoma.[1] Among the global population with MSVI the leading cause was URE, followed by cataract, age-related macular degeneration (AMD), glaucoma, corneal opacity, diabetic retinopathy, and trachoma.[1] Among adults aged 50 years and older, the leading causes of blindness were cataract (35.15%), URE (20.28%), and glaucoma (8.49%). The leading causes of MSVI for this age group were URE (52.34%), cataract (25.15%), and AMD (4.38%).

In adults aged 50 years and older in 2015, cataract and URE combined contributed to 55% of blindness and 77% of VI.[1] Thus, preventable vision loss due to cataract (treated with cataract surgery) and URE (treated with spectacle correction, contact lenses, or refractive surgery) continue to cause the majority of blindness and MSVI in adults aged 50 years and older. World regions varied markedly in the causes of blindness and vision impairment in this age group, with a lower burden of cataract (<22% for blindness and 14.1–15.9% for VI) and a higher burden of AMD (>14% of blindness) in the high-income subregions.[1,5,14]

At the other end of the age spectrum, childhood blindness has a lower absolute prevalence; with the WHO estimating that 4% of global blindness in 2010 was due to childhood blindness and corneal opacities, with the former affecting approximately 1.6 million children.[8] Although the overall prevalence is low, in terms of "years of blindness," a child going blind in early childhood and surviving to 50 years of age (as an example) has many years of disability.[8] Therefore, in terms of "years of blindness," the burden of childhood blindness ranks second to cataract blindness in adults and merits to be addressed as a global priority in public health ophthalmology.

Current Geographic Distribution: Globally and in North America

Importantly, since 1990, the trends in global blindness have transitioned from infections (such as river blindness and Trachoma) and nutrition-related causes (such as vitamin A deficiency) of blinding eye diseases to those of a chronic nature (such as diabetic retinopathy and glaucoma) that generally stem from noncommunicable disorders. This change is referred to as an "epidemiological transition"[1] (Table 59-4).

The United States

The 2015 GBD study lists the leading causes of blindness and VI in the U.S. and Canada. The principal cause of blindness in the United States and Canada is cataract (20.13%), followed by AMD (15.85%) glaucoma (13.45%), URE (13.08%), and diabetic retinopathy (4.33%). The leading cause of MSVI in these countries is URE (49.53%), followed by cataract (14.39%), AMD (10.86%), diabetic retinopathy (4.55%), and glaucoma (3.56%).

According to the NEI, in the United States the most prevalent causes of VI and blindness in the United States are AMD, cataract, glaucoma, and diabetic retinopathy.[6] Top causes in children include refractive error, amblyopia ("lazy eye"), and strabismus.[6] By 2050, the NEI estimates that the prevalence of AMD, glaucoma, cataract, and diabetic retinopathy will double for each disease[6] (Fig. 59-3).

Risk Factors and Social Determinants for Blindness and Vision Impairment

Social and biological determinants play a role in increasing the risk of blindness and VI from avoidable causes. These include: being a women, increasing age (directly), lower education, lower income (inversely), geographic differences (greater in rural settings, greater with increased distance from a health center and finally depending on the regional economic development), and in some diseases race, although the effect may be confounded by other social variables (e.g., glaucoma has an increased risk in people with Hispanic or African heritage).[1,2,5] Special attention to disparities should be given when planning to address avoidable blindness, by focusing efforts on those that are the most vulnerable. For example, a recent study in Ophthalmology by Naidoo et al. found that: "People with myopia who are older and live in a rural area of a less-developed country are less likely to have adequate optical correction."[15]

Additionally, the 2015 GBD Study revealed that visual and hearing impairment together with other sense organ deficits were among the most common causes of disability years in the global population aged 65 years and older worldwide.[9,16,17] This was especially true in South Asia where the prevalence of blindness and MSVI was among the highest, compared to other world regions[5,17]). Blindness and VI at all ages due to diabetic retinopathy [odds ratio (OR): 2.52 (1.48–3.73)] and cataract [OR 1.21 (1.17–1.25)] were more common among women, whereas blindness and VI due to glaucoma [OR: 0.71 (0.57–0.86)] and corneal opacity [OR: 0.54 [(0.43–0.66)] were more common among men, with no sex difference related to AMD [OR: 0.91 [(0.70–1.14)].[1,2,5]

In summary, approximately 75–80% of Blindness and VI is avoidable with timely screening and low cost interventions such as glasses or cataract surgery. Approximately 90% of individuals with these conditions live in low- and middle-income countries and blindness disproportionally affects the most vulnerable communities (including women, children, elderly, and rural populations). For these reasons, the public health and eye-care community must work together to conquer blindness.

The Direct and Indirect Cost of Blindness

Eliminating avoidable blindness is one of the most cost effective ways of fighting poverty worldwide. The direct costs of blindness and VI vary based on the socioeconomic development of the country and the region including both health providers and patient's out-of-pocket costs.[18] For example, direct costs include inpatient and outpatient services, medicines, diagnostics, eye exams (especially for those with MSVI), home aids for the elderly population with VI, and others services, costs of health professionals, eye-care work force, and medical costs, in addition to research. Indirect costs are costs that are not burdened on the health system but instead are costs to the individual and society. These include, for example, government transfer payments (such as welfare costs), visual aids, productivity loss, and caretakers' costs (and losses).[18]

Screening Guidelines: Unites States and Globally

The early detection of blindness and VI is critical for effective treatment therefore standardized screening programs are extremely important. The United States the Preventive Services Task Force

TABLE 59-4 2019 GLOBAL PREVALENCE TABLE OF SPECIFIC CONDITIONS

	Uncorrected Refractive Error (%)	Cataract (%)	Glaucoma (%)	Age-related Macular Degeneration (%)	Diabetic Retinopathy (%)	Corneal Opacity(%)	Trachoma (%)	Other (%)
China	18.7	0.2	0.3	0.9	0.9	0.7	Not available	2.9
East Asia (includingChina)	12.9	43.6	7.1	5.3	0.5	4.3	1.8	24.6
India and others (South Asia)	36.4	36.6	5.8	2.4	0.2	2.4	0.0	16.1
Asia excluding China and India (Avg of high income and southeast Asia)	**12.9**	**32.7**	**10.3**	**11.0**	**2.2**	**3.4**	**0.1**	**27.6**
High-income Asia Pacific	13.1	20.3	13.5	16.7	3.9	2.4	0.0	30.1
Southeast Asia	12.6	45.0	7.0	5.2	0.6	4.4	0.1	25.1
Australia and others (Australasia)	13.1	19.7	13.5	16.5	4.5	2.4	0.0	30.4
Europe (Avg of regions)	**12.9**	**26.0**	**13.9**	**19.8**	**2.8**	**4.3**	**0.0**	**20.3**
Central Europe	12.9	28.2	13.8	18.6	2.4	4.9	0.0	19.2
Eastern Europe	12.8	24.9	13.8	21.7	3.7	4.8	0.0	18.4
Western Europe	13.1	24.8	13.8	19.2	2.4	3.3	0.0	23.4
Central Asia and Russia	12.9	25.9	14.2	14.0	3.6	3.6	0.0	25.9
North Africa and Middle East	12.3	28.1	6.9	3.2	1.4	4.5	2.6	41.0
Central sub-Saharan Africa	12.7	43.6	14.1	5.2	0.5	4.0	0.3	19.6
East sub-Saharan Africa	12.2	44.7	11.7	3.2	0.2	3.8	7.0	17.3
West sub-Saharan Africa	12.4	43.6	13.3	4.0	0.4	3.9	3.4	19.2
Southern sub-Saharan Africa	12.4	35.2	15.5	11.8	1.6	4.1	0.5	19.1
USA and Canada	13.1	20.1	13.5	15.9	4.3	2.4	0.0	30.8
Latin America and Caribbean (Avg of regions)	**12.8**	**24.2**	**10.6**	**6.0**	**1.3**	**1.8**	**0.0**	**41.8**
Caribbean	12.6	25.7	9.6	5.6	0.8	1.7	0.0	44.0
Andean Latin America	12.6	27.5	9.4	3.8	0.4	1.6	0.0	44.7
Central Latin America	12.7	24.0	10.0	6.2	1.0	1.6	0.0	44.6
Southern Latin America	13.0	21.7	13.6	14.3	3.5	2.4	0.0	31.5
Tropical Latin America	12.9	21.9	10.5	7.4	1.3	1.5	0.0	44.5
Oceania	47.6	34.6	1.4	2.1	0.3	1.6	0.0	12.3
World	20.3	35.2	8.5	5.9	1.1	3.2	1.0	24.9

Source: Adapted from Bourne RRA, Flaxman SR, Braithwaite T, et al. Magnitude, temporal trends, and projections of the global prevalence of blindness and distance and near vision impairment: A systematic review and meta-analysis. *Lancet Glob Health.* 2017;5:e888–97.

(USPSTF), recommends vision screening at least once in all children aged 3–5 years to detect amblyopia and/or its risk factors.[19] For older adults, the USPSTF concludes that the current evidence is insufficient to assess the balance of benefits and harms of screening for impaired VA.[20] The International Council of Ophthalmology (ICO) has global guidelines for screening, treatment, and rehabilitation for each separate visual disorder including diabetic retinopathy, cataract, glaucoma, and AMD (http://www.icoph.org/). These guidelines are prepared and distributed to serve a supportive and educational role for eye-care professionals worldwide, and aim to improve the quality of eye care for patients. Examples of the such guidelines include the following:

(1) ICO Guidelines for Diabetic Eye Care: In 2013, the ICO published ICO Guidelines for Diabetic Eye Care with recommendations for screening and evaluating people with diabetes for potentially blinding eye problems. The Guidelines also provide instructions for treating those with diabetic retinopathy and other ocular complications of diabetes. They represent a technical consensus from the ICO Task Force on Diabetic Eye Care, and an extensive review of diabetic eye-care guidelines collected from around the world.

(2) ICO Guidelines for Glaucoma Eye Care: These address screening in low, middle, and high resource settings, which differentiate the guidelines from what already exists.

(3) ICO Clinical Guidelines: for other conditions such as eye disease in leprosy (initial evaluation and management), ocular HIV/AIDS-related diseases, trachoma.

Further clinical guidelines can be found at the American Academy of Ophthalmology Preferred Practice Pattern® Guidelines (www.aao.org/ppp).

The Most Common Eye Diseases: NEI Looks Ahead

Between 2010 and 2050, the estimated number of people affected by the most common eye diseases will double.

AGE-RELATED MACULAR DEGENERATION

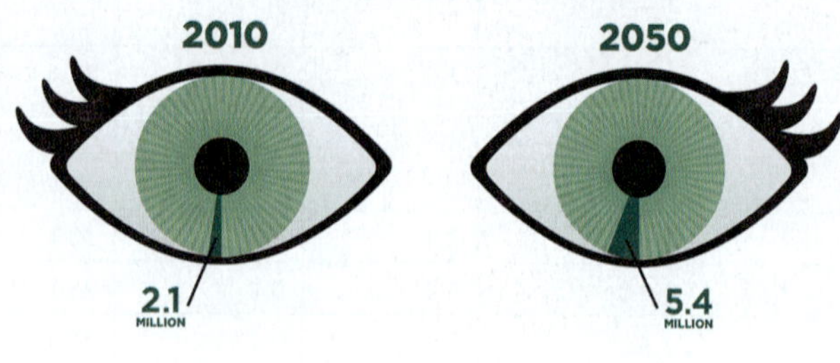

CATARACT

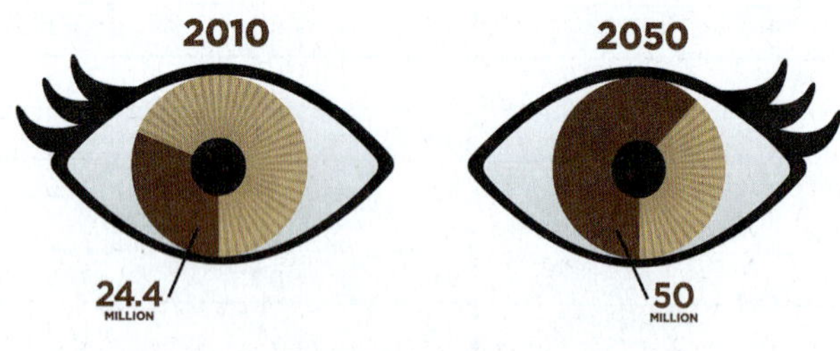

DIABETIC RETINOPATHY

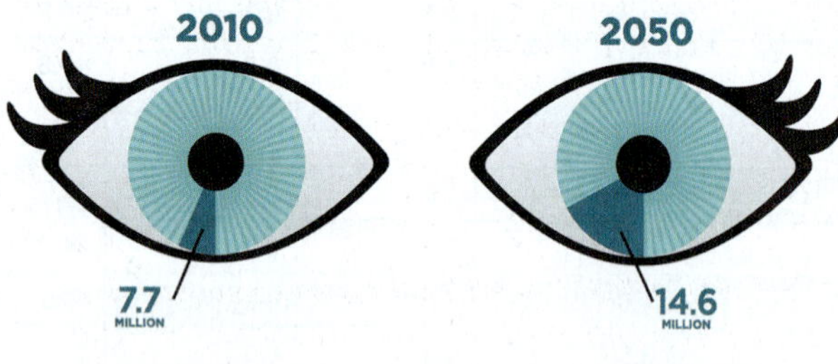

GLAUCOMA

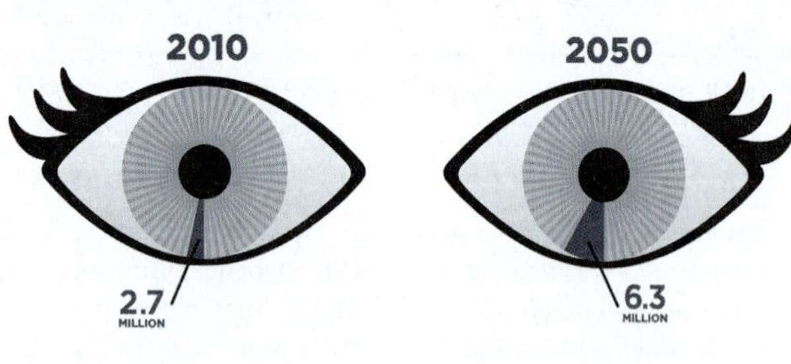

Each eye represents a total of 80 million people, the estimated number of Americans who will be 65 and older in 2050, the population most affected by these diseases.

For more information on eye disease, visit **http://nei.nih.gov/health**.

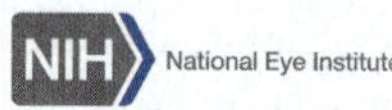

FIGURE 59-3. The National Eye Institute (NEI) most common eye diseases in 2010 and 2050, a look ahead. Courtesy: National Eye Institute, National Institutes of Health (NEI/NIH)

ANTERIOR SEGMENT DISORDERS OF THE EYE

Uncorrected Refractive Errors

According to the WHO, more than 1.22 billion people are visually impaired simply because they do not have access to a pair of spectacles. Thus, they are living their lives daily with blurred vision unnecessarily unable to fulfill their full visual potential.

Refractive errors are described as an ocular condition that occurs due to the discrepancy between the axial length of the eye and the refractive power of the lens. Thus, when parallel light enters the eye, it is does not focus on the retina. UREs cause blurred vision in the affected eye and can vary in severity.

The most common type of refractive errors are: myopia (short sightedness), hyperopia (long sightedness), and astigmatism. In addition, presbyopia is a type of refractive error that occurs due to the physiological changes in the eye due to age. With myopia, the light rays entering the eye focus in front of the retina, and objects up close appear to be clear whereas objects in the distance cannot be seen clearly (Fig. 59-4).

Myopia is the most common form of refractive error and usually starts around the age of 9–10 years and progresses in severity throughout adolescence. Hyperopia is characterized by difficulty seeing objects up close, the light rays entering the eye focus behind the retina. Hyperopia is common in younger children and usually resolves around the age of 10 years. Astigmatism affects all age groups and does not change with age. It causes distorted vision because of an irregular shaped cornea. Presbyopia occurs in adults and is the universal cause of near vision impairment due to the ageing process.

Refractive errors cannot be prevented but for most cases, a simple and cost-effective solution to correcting refractive errors is spectacles. Refractive errors are easily diagnosed by an eye-care professional. However, the proportion of people with corrected refractive errors is variable due to availability, affordability, accessibility, and awareness of services.

Based on data from the Vision Loss Expert Group, refractive error is the second leading cause of blindness and the leading cause of moderate or severe vision impairment.[1] Data from population-based studies estimate there are 7.4 million people who are blind and 116.3 million people who are visually impaired due to UREs. An estimated 1094 million (80% UI 581–1686 million) people worldwide are affected by presbyopia, of which 244 million people are uncorrected or under corrected amongst people aged over 50 years.[21] Presbyopia is a significant burden on economic productivity. It has an impact on quality of life and economic sustainability in people of prime working capability and older persons. Presbyopia does not just affect the population in high-income settings due to its impact on reading and writing, but it also hinders the ability to complete other near vision tasks such as sewing, cooking, sorting grains, etc., which can affect people in low-and middle-income countries.[1,5]

The proportion of VI due to UREs in children is as high as 97.1% in China.[22] Globally there is an increasing incidence of myopia in what is now known as an "epidemic." There is correlation of environmental factors related to urbanization such as prolonged close work and lack of time spent outdoors thought to be responsible.[23] UREs have wider consequences on a child's academic performance, visual functioning, behavioral development, and quality of life. Given the significant impact of UREs on pediatric vision, it is important that when planning for services, identification of persons that require refractive correction is efficient, that appropriate personnel perform the refractions, and that the spectacles provided are affordable and cosmetically acceptable.[14]

In summary, UREs affect people of all ages, gender, and cultural settings. Its public health significance is substantial in both children and adults. All services for the provision of eye healthcare must include an effective way of detecting and correcting refractive errors keeping

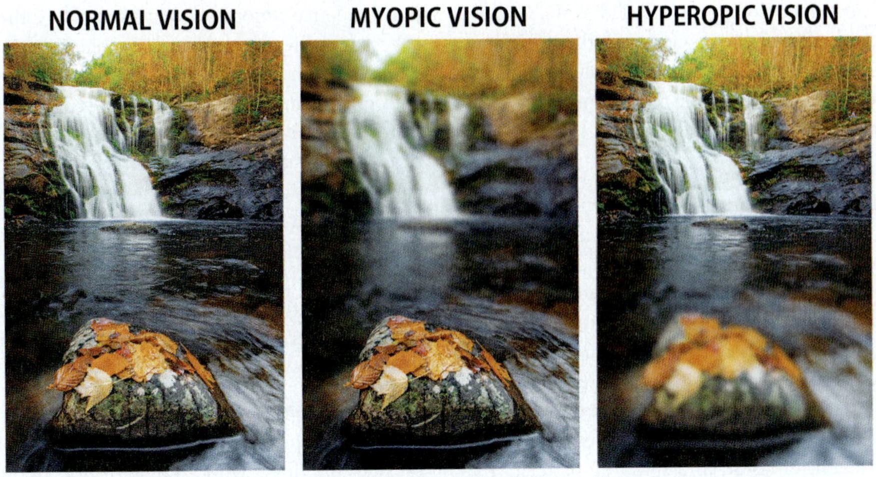

NORMAL VISION MYOPIC VISION HYPEROPIC VISION

FIGURE 59-4. A visual graphic of a patient's view (visual images) of specific refractive errors. *Source*: Madan Patange/Shutterstock.

in mind the challenges of different requisites for provision of services for children and adults in both high- and low-resource settings.

Cataract

Cataracts remain the primary cause of blindness globally (33%), and the second most common cause of MSVI after URE.[1,5] Updated data from the Vision Loss Expert Group of the 2015 Global Burden of Disease study estimates 12.6 million people worldwide are blind from untreated cataracts. Primarily a process of aging, cataracts occur when the eye's natural lens undergoes conformational changes resulting in progressive opacification of the lens and decreased vision. In its most common form (senile cataracts), this gradually blinding process is associated with an increase in the weight and thickness of the lens, and a decrease in lens accommodation as new layers of cortical fibers harden the lens nucleus.[1,5]

The prevalence of cataract within an age demographic doubles for each decade after 40 years, and given unrestrained population growth, particularly in developing countries, as well as an aging global population, the number of cataract blind is expected to increase.[24] Cataracts are generally not amenable to primary prevention, but can be treated effectively with surgical extraction and implantation of a synthetic replacement lens. Screening is done for adults when patients exhibit visual symptoms and the quality of life is affected usually over the age of 65. In the pediatric population, according to recent published guidelines from the American Academy of Pediatrics (AAP), the American Academy of Ophthalmology (AAO), and the American Association of Pediatric Ophthalmology and Strabismus (AAPOS), screening to identify congenital and acquired cataract is recommended through the "Red Reflex" or "Bruchner" test during the neonatal exam, pediatric well child visits, birth urine metabolite screenings, and evidence-based childhood vision screening programs.

Both Pediatric and Adult cataract surgery techniques and technologies have been greatly refined in the last 20–30 years, allowing increased efficiency, improved outcomes, and quicker recovery times. The prevailing technology used for cataract surgery in the developed world, phacoemulsification, uses ultrasound technology to break apart the cataractous, opacified lens in the eye and then aspirates the emulsified pieces so that an artificial lens can be implanted. The entire procedure can be performed through a small, 2.2 mm incision in as little as 5 minutes, start to finish.[25]

Despite such innovations, lack of access to well-trained ophthalmologists and significant cost barriers hinder people in low- and middle-income countries from reaching existing, cost-effective treatments.[26] Awareness and cultural acceptance have also complicated efforts to improve access to care, with studies in Nepal and Kenya showing utilization rates of less than 70% even when patients are provided free surgery and transportation.[24,26] Contrarily, in wealthier nations with greater access to surgery and higher health literacy, demand for cataract surgery has extended to portions of the population who would not even qualify as visually impaired by WHO standards.[24,25]

Although the primary risk factor for cataract is age, cataract formation often occurs earlier in life in developing nations. In India, for example, the average age for visually significant cataracts to develop is 14 years earlier than in the United States. Other than age, environmental, physical, and nutritional risk factors have also been associated with earlier onset or progression of cataracts.[24] These include exposure to UV-B light, diabetes, high blood pressure, corticosteroid therapy, smoking, alcohol, protein energy malnutrition, and dehydration.[27] While these risk factors indicate a relationship between cataracts and oxidative damage, and suggest dietary antioxidant therapy could offer protective factors, studies have not born out a definitive relationship. Consequently, the main preventive measures remain reducing UV-B exposure and smoking cessation.[24]

Current international efforts are focused primarily on closing the substantial human resource gap and developing national eye-care plans that function in coordination with other public health initiatives. Properly trained eye-care personnel producing high-quality and high-volume cataract surgery is a primary need in order to halt and eventually reduce the rising backlog of cataract.[26] Nowhere is this need highlighted more starkly than in Africa, where there are 2.9 ophthalmologists per 1 million people; yet two-thirds of these are concentrated in urban centers, relegating many regions to only one ophthalmologist for every 1–3 million people. Data support the inference that adequate well-trained doctors and eye-care teams are inextricably linked to the quality of services rendered. In addition, quality, producing excellent outcomes, in turn generates patient awareness and demand for these services, irrespective the environment.[26]

Additional efforts are being directed into development of infrastructure, supply chains, and care delivery systems that support well-trained ophthalmologists and maximize efficiencies. Institutions in India and Nepal have established themselves as epicenters for both training of eye-care personnel from other, underdeveloped countries and for innovation of low-cost intraocular lenses and surgical equipment necessary for cataract surgery.[28] Additionally, innovation by Dr. Sanduk Ruit from Nepal of a suture less surgical technique, termed Manual Small Incision Cataract Surgery (MSICS), represented a momentous step forward for global cataract care.[29,30] This surgical technique reduced the material cost of cataract surgery to less than $25 USD, obviated the need for expensive, high technology equipment, but still provides equivalent outcomes and complication rates to phacoemulsification technology. Not only did MSICS reduce the cost of surgery while providing equal outcomes, this technique also became foundational infrastructure for high-volume surgical systems and cost-recovery models that offer real promise for overcoming the burden of cataract blindness globally.[29]

Glaucoma

Glaucoma is characterized as a progressive optic neuropathy that primarily results in peripheral vision loss that is not defined solely by high eye pressure a common misperception in the general medical community. Although in the past, elevated intraocular pressure (IOP) was considered the cause and part of the definitive diagnosis of the disease, the exact pathophysiology of the disease continues to be controversial and elusive. The characteristic visual field loss that describes glaucoma has remained constant, however, for over a century, with progressive damage of optic nerve fibers causing a loss of vision from peripheral to central vision in a spiraling pattern. This damage is related to changes in vascular perfusion of the optic nerve head and is worsened by elevated IOP. The peripheral vision loss characteristic of advanced glaucoma is particularly debilitating in the developing world as it greatly inhibits a one's ability to safely navigate one's surroundings.

While glaucoma is considered a leading cause of blindness worldwide, the current and projected disease burden estimates might be inaccurate due to the lack of accessible, inexpensive, and accurate screening tests for the early detection of glaucoma. Current estimates suggest that around 65 million people are affected with glaucoma worldwide, and expected to increase to 76 million by 2020, and 111.8 Million by 2040.[31] The number of people with moderate to severe vision loss or overt blindness secondary to glaucoma is estimated at 7.0 million in the latest data, and a proportional increase is expected by 2020.[1] Most of the patients affected by glaucoma are in the developing world.[32,33]

The two main types of Glaucoma include Primary Angle Closure (PACG) and Primary Open Angle (POAG), which refer to the anatomy of the anterior segment angle of the eye. The overwhelming majority of cases of PACG are in Asia and Asian-descent populations, while POAG is distributed throughout the world, with high rates in populations of African descent. The rate of occult glaucoma is roughly equal to that of detected disease even in developed nations, making it a further public health challenge.

Like cataract and AMD, glaucoma prevalence rates increase dramatically over the age of 65, making it another of the visual disorders affecting the older adults of the world's population. However, in contrast to cataract, blindness, and visual loss from glaucoma are permanent without any effective treatment to significantly restore visual function. Available surgical and medical therapies work through lowering of intraocular pressure, which only results in a slowing of the progressive visual field loss and optic nerve damage.

Patients are frequently diagnosed late when substantial permanent visual loss has already occurred. Clearly, glaucoma is a prime target for early intervention measures; unfortunately, making an early diagnosis is problematic, especially when characteristic field loss, often not noticeable until 80% or more of the optic nerve is permanently damaged, is now considered the definitive diagnostic tool. Other measurements of optic nerve head signs, such as cup-to-disc ratios, cup asymmetry, and splinter hemorrhages, provide useful supplemental information, but lack sensitivity and specificity. According to the USPSTF, current evidence is insufficient to assess the balance of benefits and harms of screening for POAG in adults.[34]

While epidemiologic studies of POAG are limited by their differing disease definitions, small sample sizes, and questionable sampling methods, they suggest a number of risk factors for the development of POAG, with or without elevated IOP (sometimes called "normal or low-tension glaucoma"). Age is the most common risk factor, the incidence among adults $>$ 60 years old is seven times larger than the incidence among $<$ 40 years-old. Other risk factors include: (1) race, studies have shown that blacks have four times greater risk than whites in both the United States and the United Kingdom, and with most glaucoma in blacks occurring at a younger age; (2) family history of glaucoma, with approximately 13–26% of cases having a genetic component; (3) diabetes (via increased IOP); (4) myopia; and (5) hypertension. Other inconsistent associations include smoking, atherosclerotic diet; and protective effects from vitamin B12, ω-3 fatty acid, magnesium, and exercise.[35]

In summary, Glaucoma has significant basic science, diagnostic, and treatment challenges that make it a serious public health problem with disproportionately severe consequences for the developing world.

Corneal Disease

In the developing world, corneal diseases from scarring are a major cause of blindness with a range of infectious and inflammatory etiologies and nearly 80% are avoidable.[36–38] Leading causes differ depending on the infrastructure, socioeconomic status, and access to care in each country.[38,39] While worldwide corneal blindness also predominantly effects an aging population, in the developing countries corneal blindness impacts a large population of working age individuals.[38,40]

The most widely used procedure to restore sight in corneal blindness is corneal transplantation.[37] In 2012, nearly 185,000 corneal transplants were performed globally. The United States leads with 199.10 per 1,000,000 corneal transplants per capita (or nearly 64,000 corneal transplants per year), while India, which bears the largest burden of corneal blindness, had a rate of 22.10 per 1,000,000 corneal transplants per capita (or nearly 25,000 corneal transplants per year).[37]

Of 116 countries in the Gain et al survey, only three performed more than 10,000 transplants annually, 21 performed between 1001 and 10,000 corneal transplants, and the remaining 92 countries provided fewer than 1000 corneal transplants a year.[37] Corneal Transplants are dependent on access to corneal tissue, which must be procured from donors following death.

Depending on the indication for surgery, outcomes are varied, and are particularly poor in cases of active infection or other comorbidities.[38] The lifetime follow-up care requirement for transplants is an additional burden to patients and care providers, with distance, age, and gender being leading risk factors for lack of adherence to recommended treatment protocol.[41] However, with early treatment, improved ocular health, and sight restoration are possible.

An appropriate legislative framework must be in place to ensure that access to donors is both ethical and effective, and that the development and implementation of eye banking programs is established at the national and regional level.[42]

The United States, New Zealand, Australia, as well as several other countries, have established government policy maintaining donor registries and mandating referral of death to organ, eye, and tissue banks, which has resulted in higher rates of donation in these countries. In India, while no donor registry or required referral exists at the national level, individual eye banks have established Hospital Corneal Recovery Programs (HCRP), which allow trained counselors to gain consent from families to recover tissue. If this program were to be institutionalized as a national policy, India could meet its need with less than 1% of all annual deaths, or approximately 75,000 donors.[38] Developing supportive policy is critical to develop self-sustainability in corneal tissue supply in countries who currently have back-logs of patients.[38,39]

Timely access to care is particularly critical for patients who suffer from corneal abrasions caused by eye trauma. Symptoms of corneal abrasions include pain, tearing, and red eyes posttrauma, which should prompt immediate evaluation by an eye-care specialist. Studies in Southeast Asia have demonstrated that when antimicrobial ointment is applied within 18 hours of injury, only 4% of patients went on to develop corneal ulcers.[43–46] Prevention, through public education campaigns, and trained community health workers in the diagnosis and first aid treatment of eye injury can significantly reduce the number of persons requiring a corneal transplant.[43] For patients requiring corneal transplantation, access to qualified transplant providers remains a barrier in many geographies, including Africa, Latin America, and Asia, where there are few opportunities to train in corneal subspecialty. There are also many trained corneal surgeons who do not have the institutional support to do keratoplasty or who lack access to tissue and instruments. Steps need to be taken to address these barriers to ensure more surgical care providers.

To summarize, eliminating corneal blindness requires a systemic approach that addresses two key issues: first, ensuring patients have access to competent, timely care, and second, ensuring eye banks and surgeons have access to donors. Integrating policy, prevention, human resource development, community outreach, and a well-established eye banking system into National Eye Health Plans will allow progress to be made in countries currently bearing the largest burden of corneal blindness.

INFECTIOUS DISEASE AND THE EYE

Trachoma

Trachoma, unlike the above visual disorders, is an infectious disease, concentrated in poor and rural areas of the world, with the highest burden among women and children.[47,48] Globally, much progress has been made to reach the goal of elimination of trachoma as a public health problem. From 1990 to 2015, VI reduced from 4.4 million to about 2.0 million cases, out of which irreversible blindness was reduced from 0.9 million to 0.4 million worldwide.[1] While no longer a leading cause of blindness worldwide (trachoma represented some 15% of global blindness as recently as 1990), it remains the leading infectious cause. Globally, 142.6 million people live in endemic areas that warrant annual treatment with donated Zithromax® (Azithromycin, Pfizer Inc, New York, NY, USA). Its cost is estimated at U.S. $2.9 billion a year in productivity loss due to vision loss, increasing if economic costs of loss productivity due to trichiasis (corneal scarring) is included.[49]

Chlamydia trachomatis, the causative microorganism, causes an inflammation in the conjunctiva of the eye, resulting in the formation of follicles which scar, predominantly, the upper eyelid until it turns inward with the lashes rubbing the eye, gradually leading to irreversible blindness.[50]

The World Health Organization's Global Alliance for the Elimination of Trachoma by the year 2020 (GET2020) has the goal of eliminating trachoma as a public health problem by the year 2020. Through the implementation of the SAFE strategy, Surgery, Antibiotics, Facial Cleanliness and Environmental Improvements, much progress has been achieved since the launch in 1998. This comprehensive strategy combines prevention at the primary level by the improvement of living standards and hygiene in endemic areas, as proper face-washing with clean water is protective and mass drug distribution of azithromycin, donated by Pfizer, to entire populations of endemic districts, with morbidity management of surgery of those that are suffering of trichiasis and at immediate risk of blindness.[47–51]

As of the end of 2018, eight countries (Cambodia, Ghana, Islamic Republic of Iran, Lao People's Democratic Republic, Mexico, Morocco, Nepal, and Oman) have been officially validated as having eliminated trachoma as a public health problem, while a further five countries (China, Gambia, Iraq, Myanmar, and Togo) have reported achieving the elimination prevalence targets.[48] Nevertheless, 50 years of global public health efforts to eliminate trachoma has emphasized that, without improvement in the sanitation, water, population densities, economies, and attention to literacy and cultural appropriateness in public education programs, secondary interventions will not be successful in completely controlling the disease.[47,50]

Onchocerciasis

In endemic regions of Africa, the Arabian Peninsula, and the Americas, Onchocerciasis, or "River Blindness," is the second leading infectious cause of blindness.[1] Of those currently infected, nearly 100% are in Africa. While the dermatologic effects of onchocerciasis are more common than eye disease among those infected (6 million people), the VI associated with the disease, which is irreversible, can be devastating and represents an important public health challenge within endemic regions.[1]

The disease, caused by the parasite *Onchocerca volvulus,* is spread by the Simulian black fly, which lives in and around fast-flowing rivers in endemic areas. The adult worms (macrofilariae) can live in a human for about 15 years, but it is the larvae (microfilariae) that cause the pathology. An adult female can release up to 1000 microfilariae per day. When these larvae die, the immunological reaction and associated inflammation result in the eye pathology. Unfortunately, onchocerciasis is a public health example where development projects have sometimes assisted in the proliferation of the disease by increasing vector breeding sites (near fast-flowing rivers or streams). Mectizan® (Ivermectin, Merck & Co., Inc., Kenilworth, NJ, USA) is a microfiliaricidal drug, which kills the microfilaria, which prevent the ultimate pathology and the transmission of *O. volvulus,* in addition, it has a temporary sterilizing impact, allowing a treatment regime of 6–12 months. Merck & Co., Inc., has donated Mectizan® for the elimination of onchocerciasis since 1988. More recently small-scale efforts have utilized doxycycline that targets endosymbiotic Wolbachia sp. that live within *O. volvulus* worms and are necessary for worm reproduction and survival. The use of both doxycycline and ivermectin can effectively shorten Onchocerca worm life span and prevent both new infection and new eye disease among the population.[52] However, the longer duration of treatment with doxycycline, and its side effects, has made this treatment not suitable for public health implementation.

Currently, large-scale elimination and control efforts exist both in Africa and Latin America. In Latin America, this campaign has delivered twice yearly ivermectin to over one million persons at risk for infection for many years, resulting in the elimination of the parasite and eye disease from all endemic foci except one foci remaining within the Amazon rainforest.[52,53] This area involves approximately 50,000 indigenous residents where transmission occurs cross-border between Brazil and Venezuela. Current efforts to intensify ivermectin delivery to this region are being coordinated by the Onchocerciasis Elimination Program for the Americas and local ministries of health. Within Africa, the African Program for Onchocerciasis Control (APOC) operated for 20 years until 2015 also using mass-drug administration with ivermectin to eliminate Onchocerciasis from some regions while controlling disease spread in others. Current efforts at elimination are now being bundled with other elimination campaigns targeting neglected tropical diseases such as schistosomiasis, intestinal helminthiasis, trachoma, and lymphatic filariasis. Over 194 million people were treated with Mectizan® in 2018. In South America, the disease has been eliminated in four countries (Brazil, Columbia, Ecuador, and Mexico), with still small focus left at the border between Brazil and Venezuela, and in Africa, Togo was the first country to have been validated to have eliminated onchocerciasis, and Chad, Mali, Niger, Senegal, and Uganda are also close to elimination.[53]

AIDS and the Eye

AIDS is an increasing world health problem, and more than 200,000 individuals are affected by it in the United States. Because of its overall increasing prevalence, it has also become a significant cause of visual morbidity. Between 40% and 70% of all AIDS patients exhibit ocular disease, and postmortem examinations have found evidence of ocular disease in greater than 95% of cases.[54,55] AIDS may involve the eye directly by causing a microangiopathy, characterized by the presence of cotton wool spots, or by opportunistic infection, or neoplastic and neuro-ophthalmologic manifestations. Anterior segment manifestations include common diseases, such as molluscum contagiosum, as well as rare diseases, such as microsporidial keratitis and Kaposi's sarcoma. The most common posterior segment opportunistic infection is cytomegalovirus (CMV) retinitis. It affects between 5% and 40% of AIDS patients. CMV rarely causes retinal disease unless the CD4 count falls below 50 cells/mm^3. CMV viral load has also been found to play a key role in predicting CMV retinitis. Initially, CMV retinitis may be asymptomatic or present with trivial symptoms. Hence, screening this population is important to identify patients requiring initiation of therapy. Studies have been shown that antivirals for CMV in prolong the life of AIDS patients. Finally, CMV retinitis predisposes patients to retinal detachments (24% among those with retinitis at 1 year). For patients with CMV retinitis in remission, maintenance therapy is continued to prevent reactivation of CMV retinitis. Once the CD4 count of a patient recovers, however, maintenance therapy can safely be discontinued.

In recent years, the more widespread use of highly active antiretroviral therapy (HAART) strategies against HIV have successfully diminished the incidence of CMV and other opportunistic infections associated with AIDS. Such therapy helps maintain CD4 counts above the threshold where infections such as CMV retinitis occur. However, it should be noted that ocular inflammatory disease ("immune-recovery uveitis") can sometimes occur due to the immune reconstitution that occurs with successful HAART.[56]

Zika Virus and the Eye

Before 2015, the Zika virus (ZIKV) was considered an inoffensive virus, responsible for causing mild symptoms such as fever, pruritic rash, arthralgia, and malaise in 20% of the infected population.[57] It was not until October of 2015 that severe birth defects were related to ZIKV bringing alarm to international entities including the World Health Organization (WHO) as it spread rapidly throughout the Americas.[58]

The most obvious birth defect linked to the ZIKV was microcephaly, reported in up to 91% of cases.[59] However, later reports have shown that the distinctive features of the congenital Zika syndrome (CZS) are: (1) microcephaly, (2) brain abnormalities, (3) ocular findings, including retinal, optic nerve, and other structural anomalies (microphthalmia, iris coloboma, lens subluxation, cataract, glaucoma), and (4) congenital contracture, including unilateral or bilateral clubfoot and arthrogryposis multiplex, pronounced early hypertonia or spasticity with extrapyramidal symptoms.[60,61]

The first study that reported the ocular findings in the CZS was published in January 2016 by Ventura et al.[62] The study described focal pigmentary changes and the well-defined chorioretinal scar in the macular region of three affected infants, showing the immense tropism of the virus for the retina. Nowadays, these ocular manifestations are considered a hallmark of this new entity and may be present in up to 55% of the children with CZS.[63–65] In addition to the retinal findings, optic nerve manifestations have been described including optic nerve pallor, optic nerve hypoplasia, and increased disc cupping. Moreover, vascular abnormalities, iris coloboma, lens subluxation, congenital glaucoma, and microphthalmia, despite being less prevalent, have also been reported in the literature, broadening even more the ophthalmologic spectrum of the CZS.[63,66–69]

As for the ocular manifestations related to the acquired Zika infection (AZI), they are considered rare and usually evolve to complete visual recovery. In the literature, the most common ocular manifestation of AZI is nonpurulent conjunctivitis.[57,70] However, hypertensive anterior uveitis, unilateral maculopathy, and bilateral posterior chorioretinitis have been described.[71–74]

By December 2015, the Ministry of Health (MoH) estimated 440,000–1,300,000 cases of ZIKV infection in Brazil, and since then, 42 countries are experiencing their first outbreak if ZIKV with ongoing mosquito-borne transmission.[75]

The impact of CZS on the visual development will certainly vary depending on severity of the CNS damage. However, according to Ventura et al. infants with CZS regardless of ocular manifestations present with VI.[76] Thus, early detection of the ophthalmologic findings in infants with CZS should be done during the critical period when there is plasticity of the visual system. This period provides a window of opportunity for neuronal activity responsible for vision to be routed from the damaged areas of the visual pathways and primary visual cortex to other areas of the brain responsible for visual function.[77]

Ocular assessment requires a multidisciplinary team including comprehensive ophthalmic examination, visual function, visual milestones (performed by ophthalmologists), and functional vision assessment (assessed by therapists).[76,77] It is essential to treat for other known causes of VI including refractive errors, anisometropia, hypoaccommodation, amblyopia, and strabismus. The most recent study by Ventura et al. studied the immediate response to overcorrection in babies with hypoaccommodation and showed that 62% improved in the examination room.[78]

It is not clear what will be the long-term impacts of CZS on vision and overall development over the years. In fact, many questions remain about the future of surviving children affected by CZS as they transition from infancy to childhood. The best strategy to answer them is by providing continued monitoring and follow-up with careful physical examinations and developmental evaluations. This close support will also help detect early complications and avoid sequelae.

POSTERIOR SEGEMENT AND THE EYE

Diabetic Retinopathy

Diabetic retinopathy is an ocular complication of diabetes mellitus that is caused by the damaged of the blood vessels of the retina. The most important public health intervention to prevent Diabetic Retinopathy is tight blood glucose control with the HBA1C less than 7% and well as routine dilated retinal exams.[79–81]

Pathophysiology

Although defects in neurosensory function have been demonstrated in patients with diabetes mellitus before the onset of vascular lesions, the early clinical manifestations of diabetic retinopathy include the formation of microaneurysms and intraretinal hemorrhages. Microvascular damage leads to retinal ischemia, cotton-wool spotting, increase in intraretinal hemorrhages, venous abnormalities, and intraretinal microvascular abnormalities. In this stage, the increase in vascular permeability can produce retinal edema; if it is located in the center of the macula can produce a significant decrease in central vision. The proliferative stage is the result of ischemia secondary to the closure of arterioles and venules with secondary proliferation of new vessels in the optic nerve, retina, iris, and anterior chamber angle. These new vessels lead to tractional retinal detachment and neovascular glaucoma. Vision may be lost in this stage as a result of lack of capillary perfusion or edema of the macula, vitreous hemorrhage and distortion or traction retinal detachment.[79–81]

Diabetic retinopathy is the leading cause of new cases of legal blindness among working-age Americans and represents one of the leading causes of blindness in this age group.[82,83] The prevalence of diabetic retinopathy in adults of 40 years or more with diabetes in the United States is 28.5% and worldwide it is 34.6%, that is, 93 million people have some degree of diabetic retinopathy. The prevalence of vision-threatening diabetic retinopathy is 4.4% in the United States, and 10% worldwide.[84,85] The number of Americans aged 40 or older with diabetic retinopathy is expected to triple between 2005 and 2050, from 5.5 million to 16 million.[82]

The duration of diabetes is one of the most important risk factors for the development of diabetic retinopathy.[86] After 5 years, approximately 25% of patients with diabetes mellitus type 1 will have diabetic retinopathy, while after 15 years, 80% of patients will have some degree of diabetic retinopathy. In the Los Angeles Latino Eye Study (LALES) and in Proyecto VER (Vision, Evaluation and Research), 18% of participants with diabetes over 15 years of age had proliferative diabetic retinopathy.[86–88]

Among patients with type 2 diabetes mellitus older than 30 years with a disease duration of less than 5 years, 40% of patients who use insulin and 24% of those who do not use insulin have clinical findings of diabetic retinopathy. These percentage increase to 84% and to 53%, respectively, when the duration of diabetes has been documented for a maximum of 19 years. Proliferative diabetic retinopathy develops in 2% of patients with type 2 diabetes who have diabetes for less than 5 years and in 25% of patients with diabetes for 25 years or more.[86]

Glycemic control is the key modifiable risk factor associated with the development of diabetic retinopathy. There is general agreement that the duration of diabetes and the severity of hyperglycemia are the main risk factors for developing retinopathy. Once retinopathy is present, the duration of diabetes seems to be a less important factor than glycemic control in predicting progression from the earliest stages to the later stages of retinopathy.[89,90] It is recommended that an HbA1c of 7% or lower be the target for glycemic control in most patients. The intensive management of hypertension may delay the progression of retinopathy, but the data are inconclusive. Large studies have suggested that the management of serum lipids can reduce the progression of retinopathy and the need for treatment.[91,92] The results of multiple studies have shown the importance of controlling the values of adequate glycemic control, serum lipid levels and blood pressure in patients with type 2 diabetes mellitus.[89,92]

Patients with normal retina or mild diabetic retinopathy should be examined every year[86] because, 5–10% of patients without retinopathy will develop diabetic retinopathy within 1 year, or the existing retinopathy will worsen in a similar percentage.[93–95] Laser treatment, fundus photographs and fluorescein angiography are not necessarily indicated.[96] Patients with mild-moderate nonproliferative diabetic retinopathy without clinically significant macular edema should be monitored every 6–12 months, laser treatment and fluorescein angiography are not indicated in this group of patients, fundus color photographs and Ocular Coherence Tomography (OCT) of macula can be used to determine baseline in these patients for future comparisons.[96] For patients with mild nonproliferative diabetic retinopathy, the incidence of clinically significant macular edema at 4 years or macular edema that is not clinically significant is approximately 12%. For moderate nonproliferative diabetic retinopathy, the risk increases to 23% for patients with type 1 or 2 diabetes.[97]

In cases of severe nonproliferative diabetic retinopathy and proliferative diabetic retinopathy without high-risk characteristics, the recommendations for treatment are similar to one another. Half of patients with severe nonproliferative diabetic retinopathy will develop proliferative diabetic retinopathy within 1 year, and 15% will have proliferative diabetic retinopathy with high-risk characteristics. For patients with very severe nonproliferative diabetic retinopathy, the risk of developing proliferative diabetic retinopathy within 1 year is 75%. Additionally, 45% will become proliferative diabetic retinopathy with high-risk characteristics in this same period of time.[97] Therefore, these patients should be re-examined within 2–4 months.[96] The ETDRS suggested panretinal photocoagulation should not be recommended for eyes with mild or moderate nonproliferative diabetic retinopathy, as long as follow-up could be maintained. When retinopathy is more severe, laser treatment should be considered and should not be delayed when the eye is in high-risk proliferative stage.[98]

Further analysis suggest that laser treatment before the development of proliferative diabetic retinopathy with high risk characteristics is appropriate in patients with type 2 diabetes mellitus, because it reduced the risk of severe vision loss or vitrectomy by 50% in patients treated early.[99] Laser treatment generally induces regression of retinal neovascularization.[98,99]

RETINAL VASCULAR DISEASE

Retinal Vein Oclussions

Retinal vein occlusions (RVOs) are the second most frequent retinal vascular disorder associated with visual loss.[100] Occurs when there is a total or partial obstruction of a vein in the retina and is classified by the location of the obstruction. If the obstruction is behind the head of the optic nerve it is known as central retinal vein occlusion (CRVO), occlusion at the major bifurcation is determined to be a hemiretinal vein occlusion (HRVO), and any obstruction within a tributary is a branch retinal vein occlusion (BRVO).[100–102]

Worldwide prevalence of any type of retinal venous occlusion is 0.52% (CI 4.40–5.99), the prevalence of BRVO is 0.44% (CI: 4.40–5.99), while the prevalence of CRVO is 0.08% (CI: 0.61–0.99). Prevalence increases with age, but does not differ by gender.[103] Atherosclerosis is a risk factor associated with all types of RVO, but may be secondary to other processes such as inflammation, vasospasm, or compression. The main risk factors for BRVO include systemic arterial hypertension, atherosclerosis, and diabetes. Other associations such as thrombophilia have been described.[104,105]

Patients with RVOs may have diminished VA due to several complications caused by the interruption of blood flow, including macular edema, macular ischemia, optic neuropathy, vitreous hemorrhage, or tractional retinal detachment.[100] Decreased vision, flashes, or floaters can be subtle especially if the severity is mild or the distribution of area affected does not involve the macula.

The aim of the treatment is to reduce the complications of a RVO to minimize the loss of vision secondary to macular edema and the complications associated with neovascularization. Diagnosis is made with a retinal exam and fluorescein angiography of the retinal vessels. In cases of iris neovascularization or retinal neovascularization, the best treatment is peripheral panretinal photocoagulation.[106,107] The laser does not usually improve the VA, but it decreases the risk of progression to iris neovascularization and may prevent neovascular glaucoma.[102] Recent studies suggest that intravitreal steroids (triamcinolone, fluocinolone, dexamethasone in prolonged release devices) and the use of intravitreal anti-VEGF (bevacizumab, ranibizu-mab, aflibercept, pegaptanib) may be effective in the treatment of macular edema improving VA.[106,107]

Macular Degenerations and Dystrophies

Macular diseases are a major cause of decreased VA worldwide. This includes hereditary retinal diseases such as dystrophies, and multifactorial degenerations such as AMD. Studies in molecular genetics have allowed us to map many hereditary macular dystrophies and in many cases, define the specific gene that causes them. Progress has been made in understanding the pathophysiological mechanisms of these diseases with many ongoing trials with the aim of determining whether a pharmacological therapy can reverse or at least arrest the natural course of these disorders. In addition, good results have also been obtained in the treatment of complications typical of hereditary dystrophies, such as cystoid macular edema and choroidal neovascularization (CNV).[108]

AMD is a disorder characterized by localized morphological changes at the level of the retinal pigment epithelium (RPE), including: intermediate-sized drusen, hypopigmentation or hyperpigmentation of the RPE, reticular pseudodrusen, geographic atrophy (GA), CNV, polypoid choroidal vasculopathy, or retinal angiomatous proliferation.[109] It is the leading cause of blindness in people over 50 years old in developed countries, affecting approximately 196 million people in 2020, and expected to increase to 288 million in 2040. In people between 45 and 85 years, the global prevalence of any type of AMD is

8.7%, early AMD 8.0%, and advanced AMD 0.4%. The early form of this disease is more common in individuals of European descent than in Asians, while the prevalence in late phases did not differ significantly.

Clinically, the disease is divided into two well-defined forms: The "wet" form represents 20% of cases of AMD. Its main characteristic is the development of CNV with fluid exudation, RPE detachment, hemorrhage, scarring and severe, and irreversible visual loss if not treated in a timely manner. The "dry" form is characterized by a progressive degeneration of the pigment epithelium of the retina that leads to the death of photoreceptors in the same area. The most serious manifestation of this form is GA.[110]

The pathophysiology of AMD is poorly understood and probably multifactorial. The proposed mechanisms have included oxidative stress and atherosclerosis. Studies have shown allelic variants of genes that code for the alternative pathway of complement, particularly CHF (complement factor H). Mutations in chromosome 1q31, HTRA1 in 10q26 (Tyr402His) and a gene called LOC387715 in 10q increase the risk that a patient presents AMD.[111]

The risk factors with strong association for progression to advanced stages are: age over 65 years, cigarette consumption, previous cataract surgery, and family history of AMD in advanced stages. The risk factors with less association to progression to advanced stages are: increase in body mass index, hypertension, positive history of cardiovascular disease, increase in plasma levels of fibrinogen and diabetes mellitus. The factors that do not present an association or are not conclusive are: gender, positive history of cerebrovascular disease, triglycerides, and serum C-reactive protein. The darker pigmentation of the iris has been described as protective factor.[110]

The treatment of macular degeneration related to age depends on the stage. Modifiable risk factors must be targeted identified to reduce the risk of AMD. Antioxidant vitamins and minerals are currently used to delay the progression of the disease in advanced stages.[109] According to the results of important studies such as AREDS, the use of these supplements in early stages is not justified. In early AMD only 1.3% of patients progressed to advanced stages in the following 5 years. Management with anti-VEGF drugs has become the treatment of choice for neovascular forms of AMD since the use of these agents has shown better visual and anatomical results than other therapeutic modalities like thermal laser photocoagulation and photodynamic therapy.

Retinitis Pigmentosa

Retinitis pigmentosa is the term given to a group of hereditary diseases that have as characteristic the degeneration of cones and rods and the deposit of pigment. Most cases have Mendelian inheritance; however, studies have reported up to 40% of sporadic cases. Most patients have the nonsyndromic form in which case the disease is confined to the eye, with the prevalence of 1:4000, which represents 80% of patients. Meanwhile, 20–30% of patients have associated nonocular diseases (syndromic retinitis pigmentosa).[108,112]

The most frequent phenotype is rod-cone dystrophy. Typical ocular fundus findings include pallor of the optic nerve, stenosis of arterioles, and pigmentary deposits most commonly located in the periphery of the retina. In early stages, night blindness is the main symptom, vision can be normal or abnormal, in the electroretinogram a decrease in the amplitude of the b-wave will be observed in scotopic conditions and variable visual field defects can be observed. In advanced stages of the disease, there is a significant compromise of the visual field with a nonrecordable electroretinogram.[113]

The syndromes most commonly associated with retinitis pigmentosa are Usher syndrome and Bardet-Biedl syndrome. Usher syndrome accounts for approximately 14% of cases of retinitis pigmentosa and mutations in at least 11 genes are responsible for this disease.[108] This syndrome is characterized by deafness and gradual loss of vision. Hearing problems are due to a defect in the inner ear, which can sometimes also affect the vestibular system. It is classified according to the degree of deafness, at the time of appearance of symptoms and if there is a condition of the vestibular system: Patients with type I are deaf at birth and have serious balance problems from an early age. Vision problems usually start at 10 years old and lead to blindness. Type II is characterized by moderate to severe deafness and normal balance. Vision problems begin in early adolescence and worsen more slowly than in type I, patients with type III are born with normal hearing, deterioration occurs during the first decade with progressive worsening during follow-up. Bardet-Biedl syndrome occurs in about 1 in 150,000. It is characterized by typical retinitis pigmentosa with obesity, mental retardation or mild psychomotor retardation, postaxial polydactyly, hypogenitalism, and renal anomalies.[114]

The monitoring of patients is important to monitor the progression of the disease and recognize and treat associated complications. It is ideal to identify inheritance patterns to determine prognosis and to perform genetic counseling. Gene therapy is surely a promising point considering the results obtained in animal models.

CHILDHOOD BLINDESS AND VISUAL DISORDERS

While 40–60% of blindness in children is avoidable or treatable to prevent blindness or to restore sight, many areas have limited resources to specifically address eye conditions in children.[115] In addition, there is often suboptimal coordination and collaboration of existing organizations that work to implement effective vision screening programs and timely treatment.[115–117]

The significant burden that childhood blindness and vision impairment places on society extends beyond blindness alone. Childhood visual disorders can also have significant social and economic impacts on education, productivity, families, and communities worldwide. For example, 80% of learning is through vision; therefore, children who are visually impaired are often unable to develop normally, nor fully realize their academic and social ambitions, especially if they lack access to quality and timely visual rehabilitation or disability services.[115–117] Furthermore, the impact of blindness in children is often greater than adults, as one study highlights the number of "blind years" due to all causes of blindness in children is almost equal to the number of "blind years" due to cataract in adults.[118] Clearly avoidable childhood blindness is a global health priority that both Ministries of Health and Finance should collaboratively address and jointly prioritize on political agendas.

The prevalence and causes of childhood blindness vary widely across the globe reflecting socioeconomic development, coverage of specific control measures, and access to high quality eye care.[115] For example, in wealthier nations VI is predominantly from URE, amblyopia ("lazy eye"), central nervous system disorders, genetic retinal dystrophies strabismus (eye muscle misalignment), and diseases of the optic nerve. In poorer countries, corneal scarring secondary to largely preventable conditions such as measles, vitamin A deficiency, the use of harmful traditional eye remedies and ophthalmia neonatorum are the main causes of blindness. In middle-income countries with the rise in premature births and the varying development of neonatal care infrastructure, there is a higher incidence of blindness from ROP. Other significant causes worldwide include cataract, glaucoma, congenital abnormalities, and hereditary retinal dystrophies.[119] One study estimates that in almost half of the children who are blind today, the underlying cause could have been prevented, or the eye condition treated to preserve vision or restore sight.[116] These differing causes of childhood blindness are also highly dependent on the availability of primary healthcare and tertiary eye-care services, accessible instruments, and effective vision screening programs. The major causes have changed significantly over the last 20 years secondary to improved socioeconomic development; greater coverage of and access to public health interventions such as measles immunization and vitamin A supplementation, as well as improved access to eyecare services for children.

Ample evidence supports that vision screening is the best way to detect potential visual problems early in children. Effective and evidence-based vision screening in children is particularly important, as visual problems in children can largely go undetected because there are often no symptoms and the children do not complain since they think it is the norm. Fortunately, timely vision screening implemented through evidence-based screening methods can help detect vision problems. In the developed world, one in every 20 children has a visual problem including 5–10% of preschoolers and 25% of school-aged children.[120,121] In the developing world, these numbers are often unknown because of limited measuring tools, limited published studies and limited standardized programs.

A child's visual system is unique from an adult's, since their visual pathways are continually developing and are malleable to interventions until age 10 years old. Thus, timely interventions in a child, such as glasses, can mitigate permanent visual loss from common treatable conditions such as refractive error and amblyopia.[122] Unfortunately, in developing countries particularly, only a minority of children receive effective vision screening that could detect their refractive error or amblyopia risk at an age when treatment can have the best outcome. Early detection and timely treatment is critical for preventing permanent vision loss. Timeliness of screening is crucial as the effectiveness of amblyopia therapy declines starting at age 5 years old. In addition to identifying children who may benefit from early interventions (such as glasses) to improve or correct vision, screening and ophthalmic evaluation can also help to identify vision threatening conditions such as retinal anomalies, cataracts, glaucoma, life-threatening retinoblastoma, and neurological disorders. In the United States, the USPSTF recommendations include screening at least once in all children aged 3–5 years to detect amblyopia or its risk factors.[19]

It is often difficult in lower middle-income countries (LMICs) to set up preschool screening for young children; therefore, services for prevention and detection of blinding eye diseases should become an integral component of services for mothers and preschool age children through such programs as the WHO Integrated Management of Neonatal and Childhood illness.

The control of childhood blindness is a priority of WHO's and the International Association for the Prevention of Blindness (IAPB) Vision 2020 global initiative.[119] The VISION 2020 priorities established by the initiative for blindness prevention are the following:

1. To reduce the global prevalence of childhood blindness from 0.75 per 1000 children to 0.4 per 1000 children.
2. To eliminate corneal scarring caused by vitamin A deficiency, measles, or ophthalmia neonatorum.
3. To eliminate new cases of congenital rubella syndrome.
4. All children with congenital cataracts to receive appropriate surgery, with immediate and effective optical correction, in suitably equipped specialist centers.
5. All babies at risk of ROP to have retinal examination, by a trained observer, 6–7 weeks after birth. Laser treatment to be provided for all those with treatable disease.
6. All school children to receive a simple vision screening examination, with glasses provided for all those with significant refractive error. This should be effectively integrated into school programs."

In addition to this initiative, many nongovernmental organizations have made the elimination of avoidable childhood blindness a priority in their organizational missions, through effective screening methods, innovative technology, telemedicine outreach, and through development of well-equipped tertiary eye centers.[123–125]

Other strategies to eliminate avoidable causes of blindness in children include implementing effective public health policies, advocacy initiatives, and legislation specifically addressing the causes. These additional tools may augment traditional medical and surgical methods to eliminate avoidable causes of blindness in children. For example, effective legislation and policies passed at the local and country levels can enforce proper vision screenings in schools, screenings for ROP, and access to timely treatment effectively embedded into healthcare systems. This multipronged approach to prevent vision loss from avoidable causes will have a greater impact than focusing purely on developing clinical and surgical services.[126]

Global programs that appropriately prioritize childhood blindness prevention by utilizing multiple, varied, and interdisciplinary strategies are key to ensuring that the future of our children's eyesight is protected.

Xerophthalmia

Xerophthalmia is one of the preventable causes of blindness in children in developing countries characterized by cornea scarring from vitamin A deficiency. In this case, the micronutrient deficiency leads to irreversible blindness in the young.[127] Within this category of children, a difficulty exists in estimating consistent rates and impact secondary to a high rate of mortality from malnutrition and measles. Other children show primarily signs of clinical xerophthalmia, from eye dryness to ulceration. Current recommendations include exclusive breast-feeding for the first 4–6 months of life and complementing diets with food items high in vitamin A.[126] Preventive interventions include programs to distribute high doses of vitamin A to infants and children in areas with high rates of micronutrient deficiency, which has been largely successful through organizations such as UNICEF and in countries such as India.[115,116] In the case of xerophthalmia, the nutritional deficiency leading to blindness also represents an increased risk for other childhood illnesses and mortality particularly due to measles and other infectious diseases. Although on the decline, vitamin A deficiency still remains a public health issue as does the control of measles by immunization, since epidemics are still occurring in countries with low immunization coverage.[116]

Retinopathy of Prematurity

ROP is a multifactorial disorder of abnormal retinal vascular development in premature infants exacerbated by prolonged use of supplemental oxygen for their lung immaturity.[128,129] Despite current management strategies, ROP remains one of the leading causes of childhood blindness worldwide, affecting about 1300 children each year.[130] The most significant risk factors for ROP are lower gestational age at birth and prolonged use high levels of oxygen.[131,132] Additional risk factors for ROP include inadequate postnatal nutrition, poor postnatal weight gain, sepsis, and bacteria in the blood stream.[133–136]

Between 85% and 90% of low-birth weight children exposed to oxygen will demonstrate some evidence of ROP, though relatively few infants suffer severe VI.[136] It is estimated that only 6% of infants reach a stage of ROP requiring treatment.[137] Long-term complications of ROP for a child visual system include: myopia, strabismus, color deficits, visual field defects, macular dragging, and retinal detachment.[138]

Sight-threatening ROP requires urgent treatment; therefore, its rates reflect the overall level of care infants receive.[139–142] Vision loss from ROP can largely be avoided by interventions that reduce preterm birth, high-quality neonatal care, and early detection of sight-threatening retinopathy with prompt, laser treatment.

Since oxygen is the most controllable risk factor in ROP, judicious monitoring of oxygen saturations in premature infants receiving supplemental oxygen has become the standard of care in most neonatal intensive care units, but its clinical application has been limited due to concerns of an increased risk of mortality despite a reduction in severe ROP amongst participants in a randomized clinical trial that compared lower range of oxygen saturations (85–89%) to a higher range (91–95%).[143,144]

ROP Pathophysiology

Exposure to high concentrations of oxygen interferes with the process of retinal blood vessel development (neovascularization) in premature infants. With preterm birth, the infant is cut off from placental blood supply of critical proteins and growth factors like insulin-like growth factor-1 (IGF-1), exacerbated by exposure to the developing retinal blood vessels to hyperoxia, which downregulates vascular endothelial growth factor (VEGF), leading to cessation of retinal vessel growth.[145] As the infant matures after birth, retinal hypoxia develops leading to neovascularization, vitreous hemorrhage, which if untreated, could progress to tractional retinal detachment by fibrovascular proliferation resulting in visual morbidity.[146,147]

ROP Screening Recommendations

Current recommendations call for infants below 1500 g birth weight and less than 30 weeks gestation at birth to be carefully screened at specific intervals starting from four to 6-week postnatally using dilated retinal exams.[148] While, cryotherapy for patients reduced the risk for retinal detachment by 50% among those who reached a well-described threshold disease, there were long-term structural and functional deficits following treatment.[149] The final report from the cryotherapy for ROP study showed the rate of retinal detachment after 10 years was still 4.4% in treated patients (156). These patients will need lifetime ophthalmologic monitoring and care. Laser photocoagulation has recently supplanted cryotherapy as the primary means of treatment of threshold ROP.[57] The Early Treatment for ROP (ETROP) study has addressed guidelines for earlier treatment of ROP than threshold level using laser photocoagulation to improve outcomes.[148]

Studies examining vitamin E as a prevention strategy for ROP have raised caution, because while it reduced the risk of severe ROP, it increased the risk of sepsis.[150] In the past decade, intravitreal bevacizumab, a monoclonal antibody against VEGF has been increasingly explored as an off-label treatment of proliferative ROP, but concerns of repeat treatments due to its short half-life and systemic absorption with lack of long-term safety and efficacy has restricted its clinical application.[151] However, a recently reported 2-year follow-up study did not show any difference in medical or neurodevelopment outcomes in the cohort of infants treated with bevacizumab compared to laser therapy.[152]

In the early twenty-first century approximately 50–60,000 children aged 0–15 were blind from ROP worldwide with high numbers in Latin America.[153,154] The increase in the number of infants becoming blind from ROP was due to higher survival of preterm infants as neonatal intensive care expanded in many LMICs, inadequate e control of known risk factors, and suboptimal coverage of screening and treatment.[153]

Over the last two decades many LMICs have developed programs for ROP control, although many have incomplete coverage and poor coordination. In a recent review of ROP services in 11 countries in Latin America and the Caribbean the following were associated with higher program coverage: national guidelines; policies for prevention, detection, and treatment of ROP; legislation that mandates eye examination of all preterm infants; and national data collection instruments.[155] However, studies examining the role and impact of these factors have been limited.

Ongoing clinical and molecular research in potential mechanisms regulating abnormal retinal vascular recovery following oxidative stress will be critical to the development of new, safe, and effective therapeutic strategies that will preserve long-term visual function.

Childhood Visual Disorders Conclusions and Summary

In order to effectively eliminate avoidable childhood blindness and VI globally it is imperative to fully develop the continuum of care, from community health through primary, secondary, and tertiary care, with referral systems between these levels, and access to evidence-based screening, treatment, vision rehabilitation, and special education services for children. Furthermore, there are unique and context specific needs at each level of care depending on the socioeconomic development level of the country and the specific childhood visual disorder. Therefore, programs should be uniquely tailored in the specific context they apply through multidisciplinary teams, avoiding a "one size fits all" approach.

BEST PRACTICE CASE STUDIES: SPOTLIGHT ON PERU AND ARGENTINA

Two examples that effectively highlight the reduction of blindness from a program successfully embedded in the healthcare and legal system with local advocacy and partnerships across multiple stakeholders was demonstrated addressing: (1) avoidable adult blindness from Cataract in Peru and (2) avoidable childhood blindness from ROP in Argentina. Both examples address different visual conditions affecting different age groups; however, the strategies and factors leading to success in each case were similar. These key factors include: (1) sustainable funding, (2) a persistent driving and uniting force, and (3) national advocacy.

Best Practice Example: Cataract Blindness Reduction in Peru

In Peru, a combined, partnership, and integrated public health approach was successfully used to decrease blindness from cataract. The partnership between the International Agency for the Prevention of Blindness (IAPB) and its NGO partners, PAHO (Pan-American Health Organization) and the PAAO (Pan-American Association of Ophthalmology) resulted in a concerted "Prevention of Blindness Plan" for all the countries in Latin America, helping to develop and equip new stakeholders and eye health providers. The Funding in Peru was provided by the Clinton Foundation, the Carlos Slim Foundation, IAPB, and the Peruvian MoH. This was a success story since the number of people blind from cataracts throughout the country decreased significantly. Using Cataract Surgical Rate (CSR) as one of the key indicators as an example of success, the country was able to increase the CSR rate from 761 in 2005 up to 1130 in 2013, leaving fewer blind from cataract.[156,157]

The primary strategic objective of this initiative in the region surrounding Cañariaco, Peru was to provide free cataract surgeries to those in need. Presurgery questionnaires discovered that individuals visually impaired by cataracts were significantly poorer, less productive, and had a reduced quality of life than postsurgery patients. Since the inception of the cataract project in July 2009, the initiative has completed more than 20,000 cataract surgeries and held regional cataract campaigns resulting in surgeries in all 24 regions of Peru.[156]

The country also conducted a countrywide Rapid Assessment of Avoidable Blindness (RAAB) study in 2014, which enabled them to further monitor the results of interventions with a solid baseline indicator. It also was used to determine if the target of 25% reduction in the prevalence of blinding cataract was feasible, as called for by the WHO 2014–2019 Global Action Plan.[158]

Best Practice Example: ROP Blindness Reduction in Argentina

While ROP is a largely avoidable cause of blindness in children globally, there continues to be a rise in ROP in middle-income countries throughout Latin America, Eastern Europe, and South Asia.[126] This rise is secondary to a combination of increased survival of preterm infants, resource-scarce medical environments, and lack of policies, training, and human resources. However, Argentina is an example of country in Latin America where rates of ROP blindness have declined and ROP programs have been successfully and effectively embedded within the health and legal system.[126]

A recent study published in Health Policy and Planning in 2018, described the activities and stakeholders, including MoH and UNICEF, involved in the process, from recognition of an epidemic of ROP blindness to the development of national guidelines, policies, and legislation

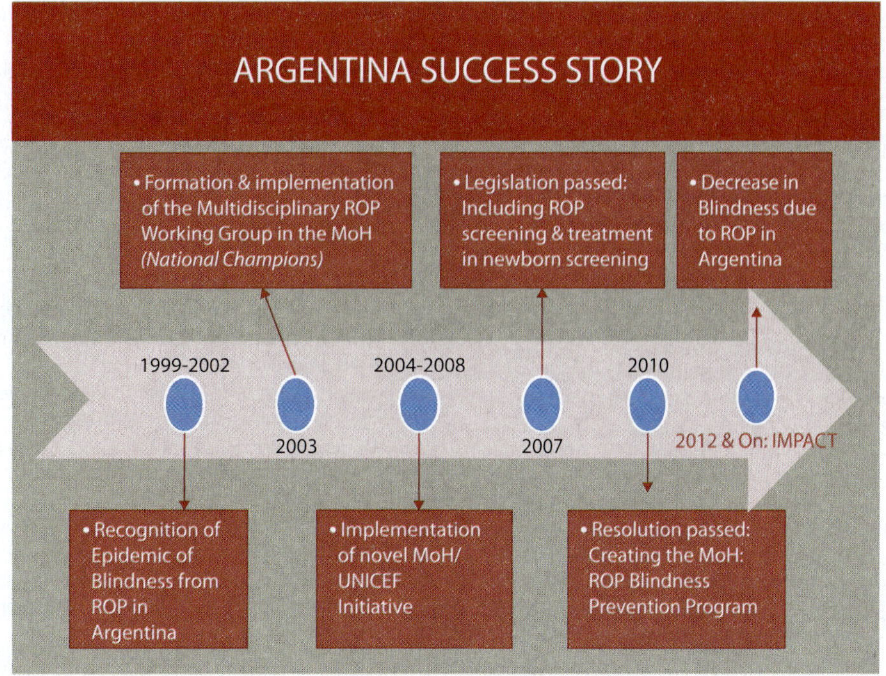
ARGENTINA SUCCESS STORY
• Formation & implementation of the Multidisciplinary ROP Working Group in the MoH (National Champions)
• Legislation passed: Including ROP screening & treatment in newborn screening
• Decrease in Blindness due to ROP in Argentina
1999-2002
2004-2008
2010
2003
2007
2012 & On: IMPACT
• Recognition of Epidemic of Blindness from ROP in Argentina
• Implementation of novel MoH/ UNICEF Initiative
• Resolution passed: Creating the MoH: ROP Blindness Prevention Program

FIGURE 59-5. Overview timeline of key milestones and events in Argentina from 1999 to the present.

for control.[126] The methods of the study included a "retrospective mixed methods case study with data collected on rates of severe ROP from 13 neonatal intensive care units from 1999 to 2012, and on the proportion of children blind from ROP in nine blind schools in seven provinces." Additionally, legislative document review, focus group discussions, and key informant interviews were conducted with neonatologists, ophthalmologists, neonatal nurses, parents, MoH officials, clinical societies, legislators, and UNICEF officials in seven provinces.[126]

The study demonstrated that by 2012, ROP had declined as a cause of blindness in children in schools for the blind, and there were declining rates of severe ROP needing treatment in the NICUs visited. The factors that played a significant role in this decline included: national advocacy, coordination by the MoH, persistence, funding, leadership, legislation, and international collaboration. As a result, Argentina was one of the first countries to draft and enact legislation and to work with UNICEF on ROP blindness prevention, which played a key catalytic role in instigating the MoH resolution and decreasing childhood blindness. The key lessons learned and challenges faced in Argentina can potentially be scaled LMIC in Latin America and beyond.

Key Take Away Messages and Lessons Learned from The Argentina Study include (Fig. 59-5)[126]

- "Persistence and advocacy by a group of national professionals, legislation instigated by a mother of a blind child, and catalytic action by PAHO set the agenda for policy change for the control of visual loss from ROP in Argentina."
- "The following agencies collaborated to implement the national program for ROP: the MoH, UNICEF Argentina, professional societies and an international nongovernment organization."
- "Further case studies with cross-country synthesis and analysis could be used to explore agenda setting and the role and impact of legislation in other countries in the region."

CONCLUSIONS

Although the global prevalence of blindness and VI has continuously decreased since 1990, the increase in population and the aging demographics have resulted in an increase in the number of people with visual disorders overall. The top three causes of blindness worldwide are cataract, URE, and glaucoma, while the top three causes of VI are (URE), cataract, and AMD, supporting the ongoing epidemiological transition from infectious diseases to chronic, noncommunicable disease causes. Given the increase in the population with vision loss, it is imperative that the global health community unite across all levels and actors to establish accessible and affordable comprehensive eye-care systems and deploy the adequate workforce to be able to cover the expected demand of these visual disorders.

The Challenges and the Future

One of the main persistent challenges in blindness prevention and treatment programs is ensuring that national health policies, legislation, prevention strategies, and programs have sound monitoring and evaluation systems to continually evaluate effectiveness, efficiency, and impact. It is clear that strong national leadership, advocacy, collaboration, persistence, funding, and commitment are necessary to strengthen health systems for effective blindness prevention and control. Key national leaders and international partnerships can make a significant impact in prioritizing blindness on global health agendas. Consequently, it is critical diverse actors and players across the public health and the eye-care arenas work together to set effective policies for blindness prevention globally. This is vital to continue to break silos and to build bridges to prevent and control avoidable blindness and VI across the United States and globally for future generations to come.

References

1. Flaxman SR, Bourne RRA, Resnikoff S, et al. Global causes of blindness and distance vision impairment 1990–2020: A systematic review and meta-analysis. *Lancet Glob Health*. 2017;5:e1221–34.
2. Bourne RRA, Stevens GA, White RA, et al. Causes of vision loss worldwide, 1990–2010: A systematic analysis. *Lancet Glob Health*. 2013;1:e339–49.
3. World Health Organization. Universal eye health: A global action plan 2014–2019. 2013.
4. Blanchet K, Gilbert C, de Savigny D. Rethinking eye health systems to achieve universal coverage: The role of research. *Br J Ophthalmol*. 2014;98:1325–8.
5. Bourne RRA, Flaxman SR, Braithwaite T, et al. Magnitude, temporal trends, and projections of the global prevalence of blindness and distance and near vision impairment: A systematic review and meta-analysis. *Lancet Glob Health*. 2017;5:e888–97.

6. ICD-11 for Mortality and Morbidity Statistics. Available at https://icd.who.int/browse11/l-m/en#/http%3a%2f%2fid.who.int%2ficd%2fentity%2f1103667651.
7. Statistics and Data. Available at https://nei.nih.gov/eyedata/blind.
8. Pascolini D, Mariotti SP. Global estimates of visual impairment: 2010. *Br J Ophthalmol.* 2012;96:614.
9. Nangia V, Jonas JB, George R, et al. Prevalence and causes of blindness and vision impairment: Magnitude, temporal trends and projections in South and Central Asia. *Br J Ophthalmol.* 2018;103:871–7.
10. Bourne RRA, Jonas JB, Bron AM, et al. Prevalence and causes of vision loss in high-income countries and in Eastern and Central Europe in 2015: Magnitude, temporal trends and projections. *Br J Ophthalmol.* 2018;102:575–85.
11. Kahloun R, Khairallah M, Resnikoff S, et al. Prevalence and causes of vision loss in North Africa and Middle East in 2015: Magnitude, temporal trends and projections. *Br J Ophthalmol.* 2019;103:863–70.
12. Keeffe J, Taylor HR, Fotis K, et al. Prevalence and causes of vision loss in Southeast Asia and Oceania: 1990–2010. *Br J Ophthalmol.* 2014;98:586–91.
13. Leasher JL, Braithwaite T, Furtado JM, et al. Prevalence and causes of vision loss in Latin America and the Caribbean in 2015: Magnitude, temporal trends and projections. *Br J Ophthalmol.* 2019;103:885--93.
14. Stevens GA, White RA, Flaxman SR, et al. Global prevalence of vision impairment and blindness. *Ophthalmology.* 2013;120:2377–84.
15. Naidoo KS, Fricke TR, Frick KD, et al. Potential lost productivity resulting from the global burden of myopia: Systematic review, meta-analysis, and modeling. *Ophthalmology.* 2019;126:338–46.
16. Collaborators GDalIaP. Global, regional, and national incidence, prevalence, and years lived with disability for 310 diseases and injuries, 1990–2015: A systematic analysis for the Global Burden of Disease Study 2015. *Lancet.* 2016;388:1545–602.
17. Jonas JB, George R, Asokan R, et al. Prevalence and causes of vision loss in Central and South Asia: 1990–2010. *Br J Ophthalmol.* 2014;98:592–8.
18. Taylor HR, Pezzullo ML, Keeffe JE. The economic impact and cost of visual impairment in Australia. *Br J Ophthalmol.* 2006;90:272–5.
19. Grossman DC, Curry SJ, Owens DK, et al. Vision screening in children aged 6 months to 5 years: US Preventive Services Task Force recommendation statement. *JAMA.* 2017;318:836–44.
20. Siu AL, Bibbins-Domingo K, Grossman DC, et al. Screening for impaired visual acuity in older adults: US Preventive Services Task Force recommendation statement. *JAMA.* 2016;315:908–14.
21. Frick KD, Joy SM, Wilson DA, Naidoo KS, Holden BA. The global burden of potential productivity loss from uncorrected presbyopia. *Ophthalmology.* 2015;122:1706–10.
22. He M, Huang W, Zheng Y, Huang L, Ellwein LB. Refractive error and visual impairment in school children in rural Southern China. *Ophthalmology.* 2007;114:374–82.e371.
23. Pan C-W, Ramamurthy D, Saw S-M. Worldwide prevalence and risk factors for myopia. *Ophthalmic Physiol Opt.* 2011;32:3–16.
24. Brian G, Taylor H. Cataract blindness—Challenges for the 21st century. *Bull World Health Organ.* 2001;79:249–56.
25. Singh A, Strauss GH. High-fidelity cataract surgery simulation and third world blindness. *Surg Innov.* 2014;22:189–93.
26. Akin JS, Guilkey DK, Hazel, Denton E. Quality of services and demand for health care in Nigeria: A multinomial probit estimation. *Soc Sci Med.* 1995;40:1527–37.
27. Krumpaszky HG, Klauss V. Title Page/Contents/Foreword. In: *Epidemiology of Blindness and Eye Disease.* Basel: S. Karger AG; 1996, p. ii-6.
28. Ruit S, Paudyal G, Gurung R, Tabin G, Moran D, Brian G. An innovation in developing world cataract surgery: Sutureless extracapsular cataract extraction with intraocular lens implantation. *Clin Exp Ophthalmol.* 2000;28:274–9.
29. Ruit S, Tabin G, Chang D, et al. A prospective randomized clinical trial of phacoemulsification vs manual sutureless small-incision extracapsular cataract surgery in Nepal. *Am J Ophthalmol.* 2007;143:32–8.e32.
30. Gogate P, Kulkarni S, Krishnaiah S, et al. Safety and efficacy of phacoemulsification compared with manual small-incision cataract surgery by a randomized controlled clinical TrialSix-week results. *Ophthalmology.* 2005;112:869–74.
31. Tham YC, Li X, Wong TY, Quigley HA, Aung T, Cheng CY. Global prevalence of glaucoma and projections of glaucoma burden through 2040: A systematic review and meta-analysis. *Ophthalmology.* 2014;121:2081–90.
32. Thomas R. Glaucoma: Problems in the developing world. World blindness and its prevention. In: Pararajasegaram R, Rao GN, eds. *Beijing: Proceedings of the Sixth General Assembly of the International Agency for the Prevention of Blindness.* Vol. 6. September 5–10, 1999, pp. 175–9.
33. Thomas R. Glaucoma in developing countries. *Indian J Ophthalmol.* 2012;60:446–50.
34. Moyer VA. Force USPST: Screening for glaucoma: U.S. Preventive Services Task Force recommendation statement. *Ann Intern Med.* 2013;159:484–9.
35. Tielsch JM. The epidemiology and control of open angle glaucoma: A population-based perspective. *Annu Rev Public Health.* 1996;17:121–36.
36. WHO Action Plan for the Prevention of Avoidable Blindness and Visual Impairment 2009–2013. Available at https://www.who.int/blindness/ACTION_PLAN_WHA62-1-English.pdf.
37. Gain P, Jullienne R, He Z, et al. Global survey of corneal transplantation and eye banking. *JAMA Ophthalmol.* 2016;134:167–73.
38. Oliva MS, Schottman T, Gulati M. Turning the tide of corneal blindness. *Indian J Ophthalmol.* 2012;60:423–7.
39. Wang H, Zhang Y, Li Z, Wang T, Liu P. Prevalence and causes of corneal blindness. *Clin Exp Ophthalmol.* 2014;42:249--53.
40. Dandona L, Dandona R, Naduvilath TJ, et al. Is current eye-care-policy focus almost exclusively on cataract adequate to deal with blindness in India? *Lancet.* 1998;351:1312–16.
41. Tabin GC, Gurung R, Paudyal G, et al. Penetrating keratoplasty in Nepal. *Cornea.* 2004;23:589–96.
42. International Council of Ophthalmology. Donation, Processing, Allocation, Advocacy, and Legislation Supporting Human Corneal Tissue for Ocular Transplant. 2017.
43. O'Brien KS, Lietman TM, Keenan JD, Whitcher JP. Microbial keratitis: A community eye health approach. *Community Eye Health.* 2015;28:1–2.
44. Srinivasan M, Upadhyay MP, Priyadarsini B, Mahalakshmi R, Whitcher JP. Corneal ulceration in south-east Asia III: Prevention of fungal keratitis at the village level in south India using topical antibiotics. *Br J Ophthalmol.* 2006;90:1472–5.
45. Upadhyay MP, Karmacharya PC, Koirala S, et al. The Bhaktapur eye study: Ocular trauma and antibiotic prophylaxis for the prevention of corneal ulceration in Nepal. *Br J Ophthalmol.* 2001;85:388–92.
46. Whitcher JP, Srinivasan M. Corneal ulceration in the developing world—A silent epidemic. *Br J Ophthalmol.* 1997;81:622–3.
47. Taylor HR, Burton MJ, Haddad D, West S, Wright H. Trachoma. *Lancet.* 2014;384:2142–52.
48. World Health Organization. WHO Alliance for the Global Elimination of Trachoma by 2020: Progress report on elimination of trachoma, 2018. *Wkly Epidemiol Rec.* 2019;94:317–28.
49. Frick KD, Basilion EV, Hanson CL, Colchero MA. Estimating the burden and economic impact of trachomatous visual loss. *Ophthalmic Epidemiol.* 2003;10:121–32.
50. West SK. Trachoma: New assault on an ancient disease. *Prog Retin Eye Res.* 2004;23:381–401.
51. World Health Organization. WHO Alliance for the Global Elimination of Trachoma by 2020: Progress report on elimination of trachoma, 2014–2016. *Wkly Epidemio Rec.* 2017;92:359–68.
52. The Carter Center: Eye of the Eagle. Vol. 18. Atlanta, GA; 2017.
53. The Carter Center: Eye of the Eagle—Summer 2017. Vol. 18. Atlanta, GA; 2017.
54. Jabs DA, Green WR, Fox R, Polk BF, Bartlett JG. Ocular manifestations of acquired immune deficiency syndrome. *Ophthalmology.* 1989;96:1092–9.
55. Pepose J. Ophthalmic manifestations of HIV infection. *Curr Topics in AIDS.* 1989:191–206.
56. Wohl DA, Kendall MA, Owens S, et al. The safety of discontinuation of maintenance therapy for cytomegalovirus (CMV) retinitis and incidence of immune recovery uveitis following potent antiretroviral therapy. *HIV Clin Trials.* 2005;6:136–46.
57. Duffy MR, Chen T-H, Hancock WT, et al. Zika virus outbreak on Yap Island, federated states of Micronesia. *N Engl J Med.* 2009;360:2536–43.
58. The history of Zika virus. Available at https://www.who.int/emergencies/zika-virus/timeline/en/.
59. Cuevas EL, Tong VT, Rozo N, et al. Preliminary Report of Microcephaly Potentially Associated with Zika Virus Infection During Pregnancy—Colombia, January–November 2016. *MMWR Morb Mortal Wkly Rep.* 2016;65:1409–13.
60. Moore CA, Staples JE, Dobyns WB, et al. Characterizing the pattern of anomalies in congenital Zika syndrome for pediatric clinicians. *JAMA Pediatr.* 2017;171:288.
61. Moura da Silva AA, Ganz JSS, da Silva Sousa P, et al. Early growth and neurologic outcomes of infants with probable congenital Zika virus syndrome. *Emerg Infect Dis.* 2016;22:1953–6.

62. Ventura CV, Maia M, Bravo-Filho V, Góis AL, Belfort R. Zika virus in Brazil and macular atrophy in a child with microcephaly. *Lancet.* 2016;387:228.

63. de Paula Freitas B, de Oliveira Dias JR, et al. Ocular findings in infants with microcephaly associated with presumed Zika virus congenital infection in Salvador, Brazil. *JAMA Ophthalmol.* 2016;134:529.

64. Ventura CV, Maia M, Travassos SB, et al. Risk factors associated with the ophthalmoscopic findings identified in infants with presumed Zika virus congenital infection. *JAMA Ophthalmol.* 2016;134:912.

65. Yepez JB, Murati FA, Pettito M, et al. Ophthalmic manifestations of congenital Zika syndrome in Colombia and Venezuela. *JAMA Ophthalmol.* 2017;135:440.

66. de Miranda HA, Costa MC, Frazão MAM, Simão N, Franchischini S, Moshfeghi DM. Expanded spectrum of congenital ocular findings in microcephaly with presumed Zika infection. *Ophthalmology.* 2016;123:1788–94.

67. Ventura CV, Maia M, Ventura BV, et al. Ophthalmological findings in infants with microcephaly and presumable intra-uterus Zika virus infection. *Arq Bras Oftalmol.* 2016;79(1):1–3.

68. de Paula Freitas B, Zin A, Ko A, Maia M, Ventura CV, Belfort R. Anterior-segment ocular findings and microphthalmia in congenital Zika syndrome. *Ophthalmology.* 2017;124:1876–8.

69. de Paula Freitas B, Ko AI, Khouri R, et al. Glaucoma and congenital Zika syndrome. *Ophthalmology.* 2017;124:407–8.

70. Ventura CV, Ventura LO, Bravo-Filho V, et al. Optical coherence tomography of retinal lesions in infants with congenital Zika syndrome. *JAMA Ophthalmol.* 2016;134:1420.

71. Rasmussen SA, Hayes EB. Public health approach to emerging infections among pregnant women. *Am J Public Health.* 2005;95:1942–4.

72. Maharajan MK, Ranjan A, Chu JF, et al. Zika virus infection: Current concerns and perspectives. *Clin Rev Allerg Immunol.* 2016;51:383–94.

73. Sarno M, Sacramento GA, Khouri R, et al. Zika virus infection and stillbirths: A case of hydrops fetalis, hydranencephaly and fetal demise. *PLoS Negl Trop Dis.* 2016;10:e0004517.

74. França GVA, Schuler-Faccini L, Oliveira WK, et al. Congenital Zika virus syndrome in Brazil: A case series of the first 1501 livebirths with complete investigation. *Lancet.* 2016;388:891–7.

75. Satterfield-Nash A, Kotzky K, Allen J, et al. Health and development at age 19–24 months of 19 children who were born with microcephaly and laboratory evidence of congenital Zika virus infection during the 2015 Zika virus outbreak—Brazil, 2017. *MMWR Morb Mortal Wkly Rep.* 2017;66:1347–51.

76. Ventura LO, Ventura CV, Lawrence L, et al. Visual impairment in children with congenital Zika syndrome. *J AAPOS.* 2017;21:295–9.e292.

77. Brandão AdO, Andrade GMQ, Vasconcelos GC, Rossi LDdF, Saliba GR. Instruments for evaluation of functionality in children with low vision: A literature review. *Arq Bras Oftalmol.* 2017;80(1):59–63.

78. Ventura LO, Lawrence L, Ventura CV, et al. Response to correction of refractive errors and hypoaccommodation in children with congenital Zika syndrome. *J AAPOS.* 2017;21:480–4.e481.

79. Patz A, Smith RE. The ETDRS and Diabetes 2000. *Ophthalmology.* 1991;98:739–40.

80. The Diabetes Control and Complications Trial Research Group. The effect of intensive diabetes treatment on the progression of diabetic retinopathy in insulin-dependent diabetes mellitus. The Diabetes Control and Complications Trial. *Arch Ophthalmol.* 1995;113:36–51.

81. Diabetic Retinopathy PPP—Updated 2017. American Academy of Ophthalmology; 12/1.

82. Willis JR, Doan QV, Gleeson M, et al. Vision-related functional burden of diabetic retinopathy across severity levels in the United States. *JAMA Ophthalmol.* 2017;135:926.

83. Powers M, Greven M, Kleinman R, Nguyen QD, Do D. Recent advances in the management and understanding of diabetic retinopathy. *F1000Research.* 2017;6:2063.

84. Kempen JH, O'Colmain BJ, Leske MC, et al. The prevalence of diabetic retinopathy among adults in the United States. *Arch Ophthalmol.* 2004;122:552–63.

85. Zhang X, Saaddine JB, Chou CF, et al. Prevalence of diabetic retinopathy in the United States, 2005–2008. *JAMA.* 2010;304:649–56.

86. Klein R. The Wisconsin epidemiologic study of diabetic retinopathy. II. Prevalence and risk of diabetic retinopathy when age at diagnosis is less than 30 years. *Arch Ophthalmol.* 1984;102:520.

87. Varma R, Torres M, Peña F, Klein R, Azen SP. Prevalence of diabetic retinopathy in adult Latinos. *Ophthalmology.* 2004;111:1298–306.

88. West SK, Klein R, Rodriguez J, et al. Diabetes and diabetic retinopathy in a Mexican-American population: Proyecto VER. *Diabetes Care.* 2001;24:1204–9.

89. Davis MD, Fisher MR, Gangnon RE, et al. Risk factors for high-risk proliferative diabetic retinopathy and severe visual loss: Early Treatment Diabetic Retinopathy Study Report #18. *Invest Ophthalmol Vis Sci.* 1998;39:233–52.

90. White NH, Sun W, Cleary PA, et al. Prolonged effect of intensive therapy on the risk of retinopathy complications in patients with type 1 diabetes mellitus: 10 Years after the Diabetes Control and Complications Trial. *Arch Ophthalmol.* 2008;126:1707–15.

91. Klein R, Sharrett AR, Klein BEK, et al. The association of atherosclerosis, vascular risk factors, and retinopathy in adults with diabetes. *Ophthalmology.* 2002;109:1225–34.

92. van Leiden HA, Dekker JM, Moll AC, et al. Blood pressure, lipids, and obesity are associated with retinopathy: The Hoorn study. *Diabetes Care.* 2002;25:1320–5.

93. Klein R, Knudtson MD, Lee KE, Gangnon R, Klein BEK. The Wisconsin epidemiologic study of diabetic retinopathy: XXII the twenty-five-year progression of retinopathy in persons with type 1 diabetes. *Ophthalmology.* 2008;115:1859–68.

94. Klein R. The Wisconsin epidemiologic study of diabetic retinopathy. X. Four-year incidence and progression of diabetic retinopathy when age at diagnosis is 30 years or more. *Arch Ophthalmol.* 1989;107:244.

95. Kriska AM, LaPorte RE, Patrick SL, Kuller LH, Orchard TJ. The association of physical activity and diabetic complications in individuals with insulin-dependent diabetes mellitus: The epidemiology of diabetes complications study—VII. *J Clin Epidemiol.* 1991;44:1207–14.

96. American Academy of Ophthalmology Retina/Vitreous Panel. Preferred Practice Pattern®Guidelines. Diabetic Retinopathy. San Francisco, CA: American Academy of Ophthalmology; 2017.

97. Early Treatment Diabetic Retinopathy Study Research Group. Early photocoagulation for diabetic retinopathy. ETDRS report number 9. Early Treatment Diabetic Retinopathy Study Research Group. *Ophthalmology.* 1991;98:766–85.

98. The Diabetic Retinopathy Study Research Group. Indications for photocoagulation treatment of diabetic retinopathy: Diabetic Retinopathy Study Report no. 14. The Diabetic Retinopathy Study Research Group. *Int Ophthalmol Clin.* 1987;27:239–53.

99. Ferris F. Early photocoagulation in patients with either type I or type II diabetes. *Am J Ophthalmol.* 1997;123:576.

100. Ip M, Hendrick A. Retinal vein occlusion review. *Asia Pac J Ophthalmol (Phila).* 2017;7(1):40–5.

101. Buehl W, Sacu S, Schmidt-Erfurth U. Retinal vein ccclusions. *Dev Ophthalmo.* 2010;46:54–72.

102. Pulido JS, Flaxel CJ, Adelman RA, Hyman L, Folk JC, Olsen TW. Retinal Vein Occlusions Preferred Practice Pattern® Guidelines. *Ophthalmology.* 2016;123:P182–208.

103. Rogers S, McIntosh RL, Cheung N, et al. The prevalence of retinal vein occlusion: Pooled data from population studies from the United States, Europe, Asia, and Australia. *Ophthalmology.* 2010;117:313–9.e311.

104. O'Mahoney PRA. Retinal vein occlusion and traditional risk factors for atherosclerosis. *Arch Ophthalmol.* 2008;126:692.

105. The Eye Disease Case-control Study Group. Risk Factors for Branch Retinal Vein Occlusion. The Eye Disease Case-control Study Group. *Am J Ophthalmol.* 1993;116;286–96.

106. Jonas JB, Monés J, Glacet-Bernard A, Coscas G. Retinal vein occlusions. *Dev Ophthalmol.* 2017;58:139–67.

107. The Central Vein Occlusion Study Group. A randomized clinical trial of early panretinal photocoagulation for ischermic central vein occlusion. The Central Vein Occlusion Study Group N report. *Ophthalmology.* 1995;102:1434–44.

108. Battaglia Parodi M, La Spina C, Corradetti G, Berchicci L, Petruzzi G, Bandello F. Retinal hereditary and degenerative/dystrophic diseases (non-age-related macular degeneration). *Dev Ophthalmol.* 2016;55:205–11.

109. American Academy of Ophthalmology Retina/Vitreous Panel: Preferred Practice Pattern®Guidelines. Age-Related Macular Degeneration. San Francisco, CA: American Academy of Ophthalmology; 2015.

110. Velez-Montoya R, Oliver SCN, Olson JL, Fine SL, Quiroz-Mercado H, Naresh M. Current knowledge and trends in age-related macular degeneration. *Retina.* 2014;34:423–41.

111. Wang G, Dubovy SR, Kovach JL, et al. Variants at chromosome 10q26 locus and the expression of HTRA1 in the retina. *Exp Eye Res.* 2013;112:102–5.

112. Hartong DT, Berson EL, Dryja TP. Retinitis pigmentosa. *Lancet.* 2006;368:1795–809.
113. Zhang Q. Retinitis pigmentosa: Progress and perspective. *Asia Pac J Ophthalmol (Phila).* 2016;5:265–71.
114. Priya S, Nampoothiri S, Sen P, Sripriya S. Bardet–Biedl syndrome: Genetics, molecular pathophysiology, and disease management. *Indian J Ophthalmol.* 2016;64:620.
115. Universal eye health: a global action plan 2014–2019. Available at https://www.who.int/blindness/AP2014_19_English.pdf?ua=1.
116. Rahi JS, Gilbert EC. Epidemiology and the worldwide impact of visual impairment in children. In: Lambert SR, Lyons CJ, eds. *Taylor and Hoyt's pediatric ophthalmology and strabismus.* London: Elsevier; 2016.
117. Thylefors B. A global initiative for the elimination of avoidable blindness. *Indian J Ophthalmol.* 1998;46:129--30.
118. Gilbert C, Foster A. Childhood blindness in the context of VISION 2020—The right to sight. *Bull World Health Organ.* 2001;79:227–32.
119. World Health Organization: Vision 2020: The Right to Sight: Global Initiative for the Elimination of Avoidable Blindness. 2007.
120. World Health Organization, Blindness and Deafness Unit & International Agency for the Prevention of Blindness: Preventing blindness in children: Report of a WHO/IAPB scientific meeting, Hyderabad, India, 13–17 April 1999; 2000.
121. Gilbert C, Rahi J, Quinn G. *The Epidemiology of Eye Disease.* London: Arnold Publishers; 2003.
122. Rahi JS, Gilbert CE, Foster A, Minassian D. Measuring the burden of childhood blindness. *Br J Ophthalmol.* 1999;83:387–8.
123. Gilbert C, Foster A, Négrel AD, Thylefors B. Childhood blindness: A new form for recording causes of visual loss in children. *Bull World Health Organ.* 1993;71:485–9.
124. Gogate P, Gilbert C, Zin A. Severe visual impairment and blindness in infants: Causes and opportunities for control. *Middle East Afr J Ophthalmol.* 2011;18:109–14.
125. Kong L, Fry M, Al-Samarraie M, Gilbert C, Steinkuller PG. An update on progress and the changing epidemiology of causes of childhood blindness worldwide. *J AAPOS.* 2012;16:501–7.
126. Hariharan L, Gilbert CE, Quinn GE, et al. Reducing blindness from retinopathy of prematurity (ROP) in Argentina through collaboration, advocacy and policy implementation. *Health Policy Plan.* 2018;33:654–65.
127. Resnikoff S, Pascolini D, Etya'ale D, et al. Global data on visual impairment in the year 2002. *Bull World Health Organ.* 2004;82:844–51.
128. Patz A, Payne J. Retinopathy of prematurity. In: Duane TD, ed. *Clinical Ophthalmology.* Vol. 3. Philadelphia: Harper & Row; 1983, pp. 1–19
129. Patz A. Symposium on retrolental fibroplasia. Summary. *Ophthalmology.* 1979;86:1685–9.
130. Steinkuller PG, Du L, Gilbert C, Foster A, Collins ML, Coats DK. Childhood blindness. *J AAPOS.* 1999;3:26–32.
131. Brown BA, Thach AB, Song JC, Marx JL, Kwun RC, Frambach DA. Retinopathy of prematurity: Evaluation of risk factors. *Int Ophthalmol.* 1998;22:279–83.
132. Flynn JT. Acute proliferative retrolental fibroplasia: Multivariate risk analysis. *Trans Am Ophthalmol Soc.* 1983;81:549–91.
133. Wallace DK, Kylstra JA, Phillips SJ, Hall JG. Poor postnatal weight gain: A risk factor for severe retinopathy of prematurity. *J AAPOS.* 2000;4:343–7.
134. VanderVeen DK, Martin CR, Mehendale R, Allred EN, Dammann O, Leviton A. Early nutrition and weight gain in preterm newborns and the risk of retinopathy of prematurity. *PLoS One.* 2013;8:e64325.
135. Tolsma KW. Neonatal bacteremia and retinopathy of prematurity. *Arch Ophthalmol.* 2011;129:1555.
136. Flynn JT. Retrolental fibroplasia. *Arch Ophthalmol.* 1977;95:217.
137. Cryotherapy for Retinopathy of Prematurity Cooperative Group. Multicenter Trial of Cryotherapy for Retinopathy of Prematurity. Preliminary results. Cryotherapy for Retinopathy of Prematurity Cooperative Group. *Arch Ophthalmol.* 1988;106:471.
138. Stephenson T, Wright S, O'Connor A, et al. Children born weighing less than 1701 g: Visual and cognitive outcomes at 11–14 years. *Arch Dis Chil Fetal Neonatal Ed.* 2007;92:F265–70.
139. Zin AA, Magluta C, Pinto MF, et al. Retinopathy of prematurity screening and treatment cost in Brazil. *Rev Panam Salud Publica.* 2014;36:37–43.
140. Manja V, Lakshminrusimha S, Cook DJ. Oxygen saturation target range for extremely preterm infants: A systematic review and meta-analysis. *JAMA Pediatr.* 2015;169:332–40.
141. Fielder AR, Gilbert C, Quinn G. Can ROP blindness be eliminated? *Biol Neonate.* 2005;88:98–100.
142. Darlow BA, Ells AL, Gilbert CE, Gole GA, Quinn GE. Are we there yet? Bevacizumab therapy for retinopathy of prematurity. *Arch Dis Child Fetal Neonatal Ed.* 2013;98:F170–4.
143. Blencowe H, Lawn JE, Vazquez T, Fielder A, Gilbert C. Preterm-associated visual impairment and estimates of retinopathy of prematurity at regional and global levels for 2010. *Pediatr Res.* 2013;74:35–49.
144. SUPPORT Study Group of the Eunice Kennedy Shriver NICHD Neonatal Research Network, Carlo WA, Finer NN, et al. Target ranges of oxygen saturation in extremely preterm infants. *N Engl J Med.* 2010;362:1959–69.
145. Smith LEH, Shen W, Perruzzi C, et al. Regulation of vascular endothelial growth factor-dependent retinal neovascularization by insulin-like growth factor-1 receptor. *Nat Med.* 1999;5:1390–5.
146. James S, Lanman JT. History of oxygen therapy and retrolental fibroplasia. Prepared by the American Academy of Pediatrics, Committee on Fetus and Newborn with the collaboration of special consultants. *Pediatrics.* 1976;57:591–642.
147. Palmer E. Retinopathy of prematurity. *Focal Points: Clinical Modules for Ophthalmologists.* Vol. 11. San Francisco, CA: American Academy of Ophthalmology; 1993.
148. Good WV, Group ETfRoPC. Final results of the early treatment for retinopathy of prematurity (ETROP) randomized trial. *Trans Am Ophthalmol Soc.* 2004;102:233–48.
149. Palmer EA, Hardy RJ, Dobson V, et al. 15-year outcomes following threshold retinopathy of prematurity: Final results from the multicenter trial of cryotherapy for retinopathy of prematurity. *Arch Ophthalmol.* 2005;123:311–8.
150. Brion LP, Bell EF, Raghuveer TS. Vitamin E supplementation for prevention of morbidity and mortality in preterm infants. *Cochrane Database Syst Rev.* 2003;(4):CD003665.
151. Mintz-Hittner HA, Kennedy KA, Chuang AZ. Efficacy of intravitreal bevacizumab for stage 3+ retinopathy of prematurity. *N Engl J Med.* 2011;364:603–15.
152. Kennedy KA, Mintz-Hittner HA. Medical and developmental outcomes of bevacizumab versus laser for retinopathy of prematurity. *J AAPOS.* 2018;22:61–5.e61.
153. Gilbert C. Retinopathy of prematurity: A global perspective of the epidemics, population of babies at risk and implications for control. *Early Hum Dev.* 2008;84:77–82.
154. Gilbert C, Fielder A, Gordillo L, et al. Characteristics of infants with severe retinopathy of prematurity in countries with low, moderate, and high levels of development: Implications for screening programs. *Pediatrics.* 2005;115:e518–25.
155. Arnesen L, Durán P, Silva J, Brumana L. A multi-country, cross-sectional observational study of retinopathy of prematurity in Latin America and the Caribbean. *Rev Panam Salud Publica.* 2016;39:322–9.
156. OPS/OMS Perú—Plan Nacional de Salud Ocular y Prevención de la Ceguera en fase de revisión. Lima, Peru; 2013.
157. Clinton Giustra Ocular Health | Candente Copper Corp. Available at https://www.candentecopper.com/shared-value/community-initiatives/clinton-giustra-ocular-health/.
158. Campos B, Cerrate A, Montjoy E, et al. Prevalencia y causas de ceguera en Perú: encuesta nacional. *Revista Panamericana de Salud Pública.* 2014;36:283–9.

CHAPTER 60

Oral Health

Greg Nycz • Terri Kleutsch • Aloksagar Panny • Amit Acharya • Ingrid Glurich

HISTORICAL OVERVIEW OF ORAL AND DENTAL PUBLIC HEALTH

In 1840, the Baltimore College of Dental Surgery was founded as the world's first dental school, establishing the *Doctor of Dental Surgery* degree. Twenty-six years later, Harvard University Dental School, the first dental school with a University affiliation began to offer the *Dentariae Medicinae Doctorae* degree, thus establishing the current paradigm of dental education and the practice of dentistry as an autonomous domain, completely detached from the medical education and the practice of medicine.[1] Over time, these domains evolved into two distinct industries, artificially detaching oral and systemic health in a manner that does not emulate the biological reality. The separation of dentistry and medicine had important repercussions that continue to affect public health and healthcare delivery both in the United States and globally.

Notably, dental public health is a relatively new addition to the field of public health. Prominent milestones affecting dental healthcare delivery can be identified in United States history and illustrate some of the outcomes attributable to the autonomous evolution of dentistry and medicine. While medical insurance availability can be traced back to the official establishment of health insurance in the early 1930s by the New York State Insurance Commissioner to cover medical expenses, dental expense coverage continued as a fee-for-service model until as late as 1954, when California introduced the first dental insurance plans. Inclusion of dental insurance to partially cover cost of services first began to gain some traction in the 1970s when the United Automobile Workers Union began incorporating employer-based plans as a collective bargaining agreement component.[2] However, large proportions of the population continued to have no access to dental insurance, with low-income populations who could not afford out-of-pocket costs disproportionately affected.

A series of congressional acts including: (a) establishment of the first community health center through the Economic Opportunity Act in 1965, (b) the 1977 Rural Health Initiative, and (c) establishment of Federally Qualified Health Centers under Medicare and Medicaid in 1989 and 1990, respectively, provided some aid to assist the low-income public with access to affordable medical care.[3] However, none of these initiatives supported comprehensive dental-care services. It was not until 2000, when Surgeon General David Satcher published his report "*Oral Health in America*" that public awareness was raised to what Dr. Satcher coined as "the silent epidemic" in referencing the largely insidious and pervasive national oral health crisis that had become established.[4] Dr. Satcher provided stark statistics with respect to high prevalence of dental caries in pediatric populations and poor dental health in the elderly and raised awareness to large access disparities for large subpopulations of Americans. Disparities in the access to dental-care services were most pronounced in dental professional shortage areas and further exacerbated by low Medicaid reimbursement rates, which were causing dentists to reduce or exclude services to Medicaid patients and children enrolled in the Children's Health Insurance Program (CHIP).

Following the Surgeon General's report, community health centers were encouraged with supplemental funding opportunities to include provision of primary dental care as a component of their services to their local communities. Oral health indicators were incorporated into Healthy People 2010 and Healthy People 2020 to track progress in addressing oral disease, including an increase federally qualified health center programs addressing oral healthcare and tracking of utilization of this access annually.[5] The Institute of Medicine Report published 10 years after Dr. Satcher's original report, suggested that little improvement was documented and that barriers to oral healthcare access persisted especially among underserved and vulnerable populations including children, racial and ethnic minorities, the poor, elderly, rural-dwelling, and special needs patients.[6] This conclusion was validated by a 2017 systematic analysis of the global, regional, and national prevalence, incidence, and evaluation of disability adjusted life years (DALY) surrounding oral disease across 195 nations which reported no improvement in oral health outcomes across the 25-year time frame between 1990 and 2015. The study reported an increase in untreated dental conditions from 2.5 billion to 3.5 billion people globally, with an associated 64% increase in DALY lost to oral diseases.[7] In a 2015 analysis, economic impact of the increased burden in oral disease in 2010 was projected at U.S.$442 billion in direct and indirect cost with direct cost of treatment projected at U.S.$298 billion annually, accounting for an estimated 4.6% of global health expenditures.[8] In 2016, the FDI World Dental Federation established a universal definition of oral health, which more holistically defines attributes and factors contributing to oral health. This definition recognizes the multidimensional biopsychosocial nature of oral health and ability to complete oral-associated functions without craniofacial pain or disease. Moreover, core elements of oral health encompassed oral health/disease status, physiological and psychosocial functionality.[9]

Notably, a growing evidence base supported by systematic review and meta-analyses of the scientific literature supports that oral diseases increase the risk for, or contribute directly to promotion of, systemic diseases. Oral diseases such as periodontal disease, an infectious process of the gums that promotes systemic inflammation, have been implicated as contributory factors driving a myriad of chronic conditions including dysglycemia and diabetes progression,[7-9] rheumatoid arthritis,[10-12] chronic renal disease,[13-15] increased risk for cardiovascular and cerebrovascular disease,[16] adverse pregnancy outcomes,[17] and among other conditions. Since oral disease represents a modifiable disease highly amenable to prevention and treatment during early stages of development, the growing recognition of links between oral and systemic disease is trending toward "reintegrating" the mouth into the body relative to healthcare delivery and adoption of new models involving integrated medical-dental healthcare delivery. Alternative models for addressing dental disparities are currently being explored, with emphasis specifically targeting prevention, early detection, and treatment of oral disease. Evolution of these alternative delivery models are expected to affect oral and dental public health delivery models in the future.

OVERVIEW OF THE GOALS OF DENTAL PUBLIC HEALTH: ASSESSMENT OF POPULATION ORAL HEALTH, POLICY DEVELOPMENT, AND SERVICE DELIVERY

Dental public health was envisioned as a nonclinical dental specialty designed to apply scientific approaches and principles to population-based oral healthcare delivery to assess healthcare needs and efficacy of oral health delivery services to achieve optimal oral health in a population-specific manner. As a specialty component of the overarching public health infrastructure officially recognized by the American Dental Association in the early 1950s,[21] dental public health encompasses population-based oral healthcare delivery with an emphasis on population surveillance to inform disease prevention strategies and policy, health promotion, and service delivery. To achieve these goals, important foci include:

- Epidemiological surveillance of population-based oral health and disease;
- Community health education, disease prevention and promotion of oral health through public health initiatives such as water fluoridation projects and school-based sealant placement programs;
- Assessment of extent of regional dental-care delivery and provision of access for all segments of the population;
- Monitoring extent of community access to dental care and adequacy of size of the workforce;
- Policy development to support access for all segments of the population including disparity populations; and
- Measuring extent of access by disparity populations to inform service and policy surrounding sustainment or growth of the dental safety net.

To accomplish its tasks, the dental public health infrastructure encompasses collaborative ties across a broad spectrum of constituents including:

- Federal, state, and local governmental entities and agencies;
- Educational entities spanning academic schools of dentistry, dental hygiene and public health, schools of medicine, nursing and other allied healthcare fields, community-based educational programs such as Headstart, primary and secondary schools, trade and vocational education programs, dental training and residency programs and the National Inter-Professional Oral Health Initiative that is promoting cross-disciplinary care[22];
- Key workforce constituents including primary-care providers spanning both dental and medical healthcare provision (e.g., in determining barriers to dental-care access and workforce concerns), environmental workforce including public waterworks (e.g., in conjunction with water fluoridation), school leadership (e.g., in conjunction with school-based community sealant placement programs), health boards, and community health center directors (e.g., in conjunction with healthcare delivery to disparity population healthcare delivery and assessment of population needs) as well as community members (e.g., in assessing access to care and monitoring self-reported health status);
- Healthcare industry: insurance industry, medical and dental healthcare administrators, dental practices in various settings and community health centers; and
- Research: central to its function is the conduct and monitoring of oral health-related research across multiple domains including, but not limited to: population health epidemiology defining extent of disease and trends in efficacy of interventions to address disease, health services research surrounding definitions of cost of healthcare delivery, literature defining clinical best practices, evidence-based research surrounding definition of best practices, quality metrics surrounding dental healthcare delivery; research surrounding service delivery to disparity populations and identification of barriers and opportunities to improve access for the population as a whole and for specific subpopulations (e.g., elderly, children, disabled, and institutionalized individuals); monitoring strength of the evidence surrounding links between oral and systemic health and disease and opportunities for building collaborations between medical and dental providers and development of innovations in healthcare delivery and educational materials to improve health literacy at the level of the population and providers across the interdisciplinary divide.

Key constituencies involved in defining dental public health infrastructure and direction include the Association of State and Territorial Dental Directors, American Association of Public Health Dentistry, American Public Health Association, the Medicaid/Children's Health Insurance Program (CHIP), Dental Association, and the National Network for Oral Health Access. The stated mission of the Association of Public Health Dentistry, also reflected by the other associations, includes:

- "Promotion of effective efforts in disease prevention, health promotion and service delivery;
- Education of the public, health professionals and decision-makers regarding the importance of oral health to total well-being; and
- Expansion of the knowledge base of dental public health and fostering competency in its practice."[21]

The collective objective is to establish equitable dental healthcare access and service delivery to all segments of the population with the goal of improving oral health, activating patients to participate in establishment of good oral health, comparing delivery models across different population settings, designing and implementing effective programs and improving competency of dental public health to improve care delivery and population health.

Tools, Indices, and Tracking Approaches Utilized in Public Health Dentistry

Tools to measure oral health parameters have been developed to support uniform assessment of disease in order to accomplish disease surveillance across established oral health measures. Measures are designed for use in tracking incidence, prevalence, and severity of a disease.

Table 60-1 summarizes common indices used in oral health assessment.[23]

Measurements of periodontal health are made using probes with standardized predefined markings (in millimeters) (e.g., World Health Organization probe) to ensure measurement precision. The study design will define the number of teeth, sites per tooth, and partial or full mouth assessment specifying number of teeth to be examined per oral quadrant and will determine optimal index for the study. Periodontal measures may include bleeding on probing, periodontal pocket depth, clinical attachment loss, alveolar bone loss, and number of missing teeth. Probing is generally performed at six sites per tooth for assessment of presence of periodontitis (Table 60-2).

Dental caries assessment is generally performed using a mouth mirror and explorer. Surveillance is ideally performed in a defined population sample with a defined population denominator to support epidemiological evaluation.

Additional Dental Public Health Indicators

Population health surveillance further measures indicators that will provide an overview of population behaviors relative to oral health maintenance and provide a high-level assessment of changes in

TABLE 60-1 COMMON INDICES USED IN ORAL HEALTH ASSESSMENT IN DENTAL PUBLIC HEALTH SETTINGS[a]

Periodontal Health Assessment Indices	Dental Caries Indices
Plaque control record	Decayed, Missing and Filled Teeth (DMFT)1 Index
Navy Plaque Index	WHO Modification of DMF2 Index
Quigley-Hein Plaque Index	Significant Caries Index (SiC)
Turesky-Gilmore-Glickman Modification of the Quigley-Hein Plaque Index	Dental Caries Index for deciduous teeth (DMFT1 and DMFS3)
Patient Hygiene Performance Index (PHP Index)	Mixed dentition
Gingival Index (GI)	WHO Index for dental caries
Calculus Surface Index	International Caries Detection and Assessment System (ICDAS)[76]
Periodontal Index (PI)	PUFA [Pulpal Involvement (P/p), Ulceration Caused by Dislocated Tooth Fragments (U/u), Fistula (F/f), and Abscess (A/a)] Index
Community Periodontal Index (CPI)	Caries Assessment Spectrum and Treatment (CAST) Index
Periodontal Disease Index (PDI)	
The Navy Periodontal Disease Index (NPDI)	**Fluorosis Index**
Gingival Bleeding Index (GBI)	Tooth Surface Index of Fluorosis (TSIF)
Papillary-Marginal-Attached Gingival Index	Dean's Fluorosis Index
Gingival Bone Count Index	Community Fluorosis Index
Community Periodontal Index of Treatment Needs (CPITN)	Developmental Defects of Enamel Index
Russell's Periodontal Index.	Fluorosis Risk Index
National Institute of Dental and Craniofacial Research (NIDCR) protocol	Thylstrup-Fejerskov Index of Fluorosis (TF)
Periodontal Screening and Recording Index	

[a]A slide share of many of these indices can be found online at: Nenava D. Dental indices. https://www.slideshare.net/darpannenava/dental-indices.[23]
Note: DMF[2] index = decayed, missing, filled index. DMFT[1] index = decayed, missing, filled teeth index. DMFS[3] index = decayed, missing, filled surfaces (where tooth has four to five surfaces evaluated dependent on tooth type for a total of 128 surfaces across 28 teeth).

population health over time. Oral health indicators[24] selected for tracking include:

- Edentulism in adults >/= 65 years of age;
- Adults >/= 65 years of age with >/= six missing teeth;
- Visit to dentist or dental clinic among adults >/= 18 years of age;
- Frequency of dental visits in children and adolescents aged 1–17 years;
- Frequency of dental visits in children and adolescents aged 1–17 years for preventive dental care;
- Rates of adults age 18–64 with no tooth loss;
- Oral health services administered at Federally Qualified Health Centers;
- Survey of populations provided with optimally fluoridated drinking water; and
- Number of women receiving preventive dental care before pregnancy.

TABLE 60-2 SUMMARY OF CDC-AAP CARE DEFINITIONS FOR POPULATION-BASED PERIODONTITIS SURVEILLANCE

Level of PD	Measures and Definitions
None	No measures positive for presence of PD
Mild	>/= 2 interproximal sites exhibiting • CAL >/= 3 mm • PPD >/= 4 mm (not on same tooth) or 1 site with PPD >/= 5 mm
Moderate	>/= 2 interproximal sites exhibiting • CAL >/= 4 mm (not on same tooth) • PPD >/= 5 mm (not on same tooth)
Severe	>/= 2 interproximal sites exhibiting • CAL >/= 6 mm (not on same tooth) • and >/= 1 site with PPD >/= 5 mm

Abbreviations: PD = periodontal disease; CAL = clinical attachment loss; PPD = periodontal pocket depth.
Source: Adapted from Eke PI, Page RC, Wei L, Thorton-Evans G, Genco RJ. Update of the case definitions of population-based surveillance of periodontitis. *J Periodontol.* 2012;83:1449–54.[86]

Traditionally, data emanate from the Behavioral Risk Factor Surveillance System but must be interpreted with caution. Notably, the population in which surveillance data are collected is not representative of healthcare access rates acquired when compared to State or other national surveillance data surrounding these indicators in high disparity populations. Currently, projected goals for oral health indicators set by Healthy People 2020 were based on nationally representative Medical Expenditure Panel Survey data annually supplied by Agency for Healthcare Research and Quality since 1966, which provide estimates of healthcare access, cost and source of payment, insurance coverage and care quality for the noninstitutionalized U.S. civilian population.[25]

OVERVIEW OF ORAL PUBLIC HEALTH INITIATIVES

Primary Prevention of Dental Caries

Fluoridation of Drinking Water

The public drinking water fluoridation program has been lauded by the CDC as one of its most successful public health achievements in the twentieth century.[26] The program was launched based on prevailing evidence of the capacity of fluoride to make dentition less susceptible to caries. Fluoride was shown to exert caries-inhibitory activity mainly in posteruptive phases of tooth development and had a proven track record for increasing resistance of teeth to dental decay and caries progression.[66] Fluoridation involves controlled addition of fluoride up to an optimal concentration with the goal of reducing rates of dental caries incidence.[27,28] The optimal level for fluoridation of drinking water was determined by the Department of Health and Human Services is 0.7 parts per million.[29] The CDC has continued to monitor the community water fluoridation programs as an objective for Healthy People 2020.[30]

The Community Preventive Task Force in 2013[31] continued to recommended fluoridation of community water supplies to promote caries prevention following review of the evidence surrounding efficacy for caries prevention and lack of evidence of fluorosis, a potential adverse effect associated with exposure to too much fluoride. Fluoridation of public water supplies has been estimated to reduce childhood dental caries incidence by between 18% and 40%[4] and its inclusion in tooth dentifrices positively impacts on rate of cariogenesis. School-based public health initiatives involving fluoride varnish application or polymer sealant placement in the pediatric population to deter caries formation in this population have further been targeted to reduce the burden of disease in this subpopulation as discussed below.[32]

School-based Dental Sealant Programs

In an attempt to protect permanent teeth following eruption, dental sealants are applied to chewing surfaces of permanent molars and premolars especially in the pits and fissures where they act as physical barrier preventing bacterial growth that can lead to dental decay.[33] Based on Center for Disease Control (CDC) surveillance estimates, sealants could prevent up to 80% of caries in school-aged children.[34] School-based sealant programs were piloted and implemented to provide sealants to children from low-income families where especially high rates of caries have been documented. Studies have also reported a reduction in the prevalence of childhood dental caries in states implementing school-based sealant programs.[35,36] As a follow-up initiative, the CDC developed the Sealant Efficiency Assessment for Locals and States (SEALS) program to capture, store and analyze the data from school-based sealant programs. These data are expected to support interstate comparisons surrounding efficacy of their programs and inform development of best practices.[37]

Primary-Care and Integrated-Care Delivery

Integrating oral health screening of pediatric patients by pediatric providers for the purpose of early caries intervention is being phased into pediatric and Med-Peds primary healthcare settings in order to promote good oral health and educate parents about the importance of early childhood caries prevention as primary and permanent teeth erupt. Physicians conduct oral health screening including caries scans at well-child visit, triaging pediatric patients to dental homes as needed. A prototype of a screening form developed for use during a well child visit is shown in Fig. 60-1.[38]

Physicians also monitor whether the child has exposure to fluoridated drinking water and conduct dietary counseling and education on caries prevention with parents. Effectiveness of this integrated-care delivery model in delimiting caries disease burden in this population is being monitored.[39,40]

Updated CAMBRA*** Caries Risk Assessment Form for Patients Aged 0 to 5 (January 2019)
(Refer to the second page of this form for instructions for use.)

Patient name: Reference number:
Provider name: Date:

Caries risk component	Column 1	Column 2	Column 3
Biological or environmental risk factors*		Check if Yes**	
1. Frequent snacking (more than three times daily)			
2. Uses bottle/nonspill cup containing liquids other than water or milk			
3. Mother/primary caregiver or sibling has current decay or a recent history of decay (see high-risk description on next page)			
4. Family has low socioeconomic/health literacy status			
5. Medications that induce hyposalivation			
Protective factors**			Check if Yes**
1. Lives in a fluoridated drinking water area			
2. Drinks fluoridated water			
3. Uses fluoride-containing toothpaste at least two times daily—a smear for ages 0–2 years and pea sized for ages 3–6 years			
4. Has had fluoride varnish applied in the last six months			
Biological risk factors — clinical exam*		Check if Yes**	
1. Cariogenic bacteria quantity — **Not currently available**			
2. Heavy plaque on the teeth			
Disease indicators — clinical exam	Check if Yes**		
1. Evident tooth decay or white spots			
2. Recent restorations in last two years (new patient) or the last year (patient of record)			
	Column 1 total	Column 2 total	Column 3 total
Yes in Column 1 indicates high risk **Yes in columns 2 and 3: Consider the caries balance as illustrated on next page**			

Final overall caries risk assessment category (check) determined as per guidelines on next page

HIGH ☐ **MODERATE** ☐ **LOW** ☐

***Biological and environmental risk factors are split into a) question items, b) clinical exam.**
****Check the "yes" answers in the appropriate column. Shading indicates which column to place the appropriate "yes."**

FIGURE 60-1. Caries risk assessment forms.[38] Adapted with permission from the California Dental Association. Copyright © 2007, 2011, 2019.

Dental Public Health Initiatives for Reducing Periodontitis

Public Health Initiatives to Support Tobacco Cessation

Smoking increases risk for periodontitis and development of lesions on the oral mucosa.[41] Study data indicated a dose-response effect of tobacco consumption where the prevalence and severity of periodontitis is directly proportional to the number of cigarettes consumed and time period/years of smoking.[41,42] Community-based tobacco cessation programs targeting high-risk individuals and communities are an important public health initiative for prevention of periodontitis.[43,44] The National Tobacco Control Program created by the CDC in 1999 provides funding and technical support to all the states in the United States for planning and implementing tobacco cessation initiatives[45] An example of a tool targeting education to support smoking cessation was creation of "SmokefreeTXT," a text-based cessation service utilizing text messaging by the National Cancer Institute to provide support, tips, and advice to teens trying to quit smoking.[46]

A growing evidence base supported by systematic review and meta-analysis continue to define a growing number of oral-systemic relationships between periodontitis and exacerbation of chronic systemic health conditions. Moreover, improvement in population surveillance defining periodontitis prevalence found that rates of periodontitis had historically been underestimated and have achieved epidemic proportions.[47] Despite this evidence base and potentially because of challenges associated with tracking compliance with improved dental hygiene practices across a defined population, public health programs to reduce population levels of periodontitis are currently lacking.[48] Among recommendations made by the CDC for potential future public health initiatives surrounding reduction of periodontitis prevalence were:

1. educating health professionals and the public about the relationship between periodontal and cardiovascular diseases;
2. restructuring benefits for public programs to provide infection control services to Medicaid and Medicare recipients;
3. advocating for medical insurance coverage of periodontal services; and
4. establishing a surveillance program to monitor periodontal disease trends in the population and identify high-risk groups to target with intervention programs.[48]

Healthy People 2020 did issue an objective to reduce the proportion of adults aged 45–74 years with moderate or severe periodontitis.[49]

Public Health Initiatives Targeting Oral Cancer Reduction

Improving Oral Cancer Outcomes

Healthy People 2000[50] originally proposed 17 oral cancer objectives to promote reduction in rates of oral cancer. Surveillance data were then tracked to measure progress on achieving the defined objectives. The final CDC report showed a slight improvement in oral cancer mortality rates between 1990 and 2000, albeit not in minority populations. Since smoking is a key established risk factor promoting emergence of oral cancer, six additional key objectives focused on reduction in tobacco exposure and smoking were included:

- Reduce smoking prevalence to < 15% among individuals 20 years of age
- Reduce smoking initiation in children and youth so that < 20% become smokers by age 20.
- Reduce smokeless tobacco use by males aged 12–14 years to a prevalence of < 4%.
- Increase > 75% the proportion of primary care and oral healthcare providers who routinely advise cessation and provide

assistance and follow-up for their patients with primary tobacco exposure.

- Reduce deaths due to cancer of the oral cavity and pharynx to < 10.5 per 100,000 men aged 45–74 years and 4.1 per 100,000 women aged 45–74 years.
- Increase > 40% the proportion of people aged > 50 years with a primary-care provider visit in the preceding year who have received oral examinations during one such visit.[50]

Surveillance data will be tracked to measure progress on achieving the defined objectives.

The current Healthy People 2020[49] objective (OH-6) has targeted an increase in the proportion of oral and pharyngeal cancers detected at the earliest possible stage. Updates to baseline improvements as 2017 have set the current target at 35.9%. Reduction in heavy drinking was an additional objective as it is also a known risk factor for oral cancer.

Human Papilloma Virus Vaccination

Human papilloma virus (HPV) represents an additional risk factor especially for nonsmokers and two of three persons with oropharyngeal cancers test positive for HPV.[51] Some states are currently advancing initiatives to advance rates of HPV vaccination through school vaccine programs or campaigns. Since HPV serotype 16, which has been most commonly associated with oral cancers, is included in the vaccine, it has been posited that rates of oral cancer attributed to HPV may also be reduced in the future and early evidence is validating this hypothesis.[51,52]

Addressing Public Health Challenges: Access Challenges and Oral Health Disparities across the Lifespan

The dental public health sector is further tasked with improving provision of equitable dental healthcare access to include disparity populations. Solving the growing healthcare access crisis is a further priority on the dental public health agenda. Notably, access to dental care is substantially lower among disparity population in comparison to access suggested by the Center for Disease Control's (CDC) Behavioral Risk Factor Survey System survey data.[53] Access to dental healthcare for disparity populations is associated with numerous barriers.

The largest barrier to access to dental care remains cost and lack of coverage for access to care across different age groups. Foremost, low-income adults have low rates of commercial dental insurance coverage through the workplace. Prior to passage of the Affordable Care Act, Medicaid offered no coverage for childless adults. Access for childless adults meeting the definition of 138% of the federal poverty level who represent 75% of the estimated 16.6 million Medicaid-eligible U.S. population, was facilitated through Medicaid expansion options made available at the state level and adopted by some states.[54] A study by Singhal et al. (2017)[55] suggested that while there was an increase in number of childless adults with access to dental visits in states adopting expanded Medicaid benefits, there was a decrease in number of annual visits for adults with children who previously had some access but who were likely competing for access to limited slots set aside in dental practices for Medicaid patients due to poor reimbursement rates and failure to expand the dental workforce providing care to Medicaid patients. As of 2017, 38 states and the District of Columbia had opted to adopt some elements of the Medicaid expansion options with only 16 states offering more comprehensive benefits, while 19 states continue to provide no adult Medicaid coverage leaving adults with no access. No dental coverage is offered through Medicare-only absent procurement of supplemental dental benefits purchased by the individual.[55]

A second barrier to dental access encountered by low-income and other disparity populations is insufficient dental health workforce. In 2016, approximately 49 million people were residents of 5000 regions designated as dental professional shortage areas aligning with predilection of dentists to practice in nonrural areas and curtailment of services to the Medicaid and special needs populations.[56] In the throes of the burgeoning dental access crisis in the years leading up to, and following, the Affordable Care Act, States continue to look to Community Health Center infrastructure to serve as a safety net in addressing dental access gaps for disparity populations. States have been working through the Community Health Center infrastructure, which has been tasked to assist with establishment of dental-care access for disparity populations. Community Health Centers have been proactive in addressing the oral health crisis. Service delivery data showed that in 2014, over 22.5 million individuals, 46% of whom were Medicaid beneficiaries and 28% of whom were uninsured, gained access through Community Health dental access initiatives nationwide.[57] However, the increased capacity for dental access afforded to the Medicaid population by the Affordable Care Act also created a challenge for Community Health Centers who flagged workforce recruitment, retention, and insufficient reimbursement at their top challenges.[58] The Affordable Care Act provided support for expansion of access through Community Health Centers by awarding billions in funding to the Health Center Trust Fund and National Health Service Corp, which is tasked with provision of medical and dental providers to underserved areas over the next 5 years.

To address the issue of dental provider shortage areas and increase capacity to promote preventive initiatives such as the school-based sealant programs, some states have expanded provider scope of practice to permit hygienists to practice independently without the requirement for supervision by a dentist.[56] Further, expansion of the dental workforce is being achieved in three States by incorporating a newly established practitioner, the Dental Therapist, a mid-level provider, who represents the counterpart to the Physician Assistant provider in the medical domain. To expand dental access to the Medicaid population, some States require that, at minimum, half of the case load of Dental therapists must include Medicaid recipients[59] A third alternative being adopted by some States is a Tele-dentistry approach which supports remote consultation by patients with registered dental practioners who can apply technology to examine the patient remotely, develop treatment plans and triage the patient for care to the most appropriate participating provider.[56] A need to update dental public health competencies has also been highlighted in order to keep abreast of the changing landscape in oral healthcare delivery in the dental public health arena and that expansion of the role of the dental public health and workforce are required to support and analyze effectiveness of changes to access and service delivery policy.[60,61]While provisions for dental care for children living in poverty are included under Medicaid and Children's Health Insurance Program (CHIP), access for pediatric patients from low-income families is lower than for children whose families have dental insurance coverage. This situation is partially attributable to poor reimbursement rates associated with Medicaid expansion, which deters dental providers from providing care to low-income populations.[62] In many instances, these patients seek care in emergency rooms and urgent-care departments in medical settings, which are not equipped to deliver appropriate dental care and only address acute symptoms rather than the underlying cause. Comparative cost analysis found that seeking emergency care was associated with tenfold higher cost compared to cost of preventive care delivered in the dental setting so that such access to care is not cost effective.[63]

In addition, poor dental health may have profoundly negative repercussions on the quality of life for these individuals, potentially impacting their capacity to function at work or school, obtain employment due to unsightly dental health, may negatively influence social life and impact negatively on their self-image and mental status.[64] Dental issues often result in dietary restriction and may have further ramifications on overall health. For individuals living in regions of the United States that are designated as dental shortage areas, access barriers are further magnified.

Vulnerable populations including the elderly, especially those that are institutionalized, face significant difficulties in accessing dental care. Given that in these populations risk and prevalence of dental disease is already high due to comorbidities, polypharmacy, declining immune-competence and dietary restrictions associated with poor oral health, quality of life may be profoundly impacted. Persons with physical and mental disabilities may also encounter access issues because dental offices may be ill equipped or practitioners poorly trained to deliver care appropriately, leading to additional barriers to access.[65] Access is also often denied to individuals who are HIV positive. Similarly, uninsured veterans may also encounter access disparities.

As the landscape of oral public health access continues to change, attention is being drawn to ethical considerations surrounding continued observation of persistence of access disparity especially for low-income populations and across race and ethnicity.[66,67] Themes continually cross-cutting resolution of oral health disparities include: (1) the need to develop and deliver care to patients in a more medical-dental integrated manner, (2) overhauling the traditional dental educational curriculum to include attention to cultural competency, greater emphasis on prevention and health literacy promotion across the lifespan, and (3) advocacy by the public health sector to promote adequate access and coverage for care more holistically for all members of the population.[66–68]

OVERVIEW OF FREQUENTLY ENCOUNTERED ORAL DISEASE IN THE PRIMARY-CARE DENTAL SETTING

The final section of this chapter provides a description of the common diseases of the oral cavity in order to have a more complete overview of the oral and dental health conditions with highest impact on the population and of highest relevance to the public health sector.

Odontogenic Infection: Dental Caries, Pulpitis, Periapical Abscess

Pathophysiology

Dental caries (commonly referred to as "cavities" or "tooth decay"), the leading cause of odontogenic infection, represent disruption of the protective enamel and dentin which surrounds and protects the underlying the tooth pulp, (the living tissue found in the interior of the tooth) from cariogenic microbes in the oral environment, and exposing it to colonization and infection.[69] Dental caries affects individuals across the entire age spectrum. The disease is transmissible, with transmission of cariogenic pathogens occurring from parent to child in the first year of life. Environmental factors that potentiate cariogenic potential are multifactorial and include diet, constituency of the resident microbial flora, genetically programmed host defense mechanisms, and hygiene practices.

Cariogenesis is promoted when dietary carbohydrates deposited in enamel attract colonization by pathogenic populations of acid-loving bacterial species including *Streptococcus* species, *S. mutans* and *S. salivarius, Lactobacilli* species and *Veillonella* species (among others), which produce an acidic environment consequential to sugar metabolism. Left untreated, the caries lesion may progress from an early white spot lesion to cavitation, resulting ultimately in destruction and loss of the tooth. Unchecked tooth decay incrementally progresses and is characterized by breakdown of dentin and enamel consequential to microbial acid production. Eventually the protective layers surrounding the pulp are breached. Persistence of microbes on the tooth surface and introduction to the pulp stimulates inflammatory response to microbes presence and increases potential for periapical abscess formation within the pulp. Drainage associated with inflammatory processes may further result in fistula formation. Advancing disease may be associated with substantial dental pain associated with inflammation and swelling, and severely affect quality of life. Less frequently, odontogenic infection that spreads to the dental pulp may also originate from an abscess in the gums, generally requiring management with antibiotic treatment. With aging, root caries may also increase in frequency, occurring in the presence of gum recession and root exposure or when periodontal disease separates the gum from the tooth, permitting root exposure. Such caries require immediate treatment to prevent tooth loss.

Epidemiology

Public health surveillance of oral health and disease is essential for monitoring rates of disease incidence and prevalence across populations to inform interventional and preventive strategies and their relative efficacy in disease management and control. Surveillance of caries prevalence in public health is largely assessed applying the decayed, missing, filled (DMF) index. A systematic review of the global burden of untreated caries published in 2015 reported untreated caries in permanent teeth as the most prevalent condition worldwide, affecting over 2.4 billion individuals and the tenth most prevalent condition in children, with an estimated 621 million children affected.[70] Oral disease surveillance has identified three prevalence peaks: childhood (6 years), young adult (25 years), and elderly (70 years).[70] In the United States, caries is the most prevalent condition in children age 6–19 years, and nine out of ten adults age > 20 years show evidence of root decay.[71]

The disease is largely preventable with patient education, relatively low-cost hygiene interventions, and support of public health initiatives including fluoridation of public drinking water that target disease control. The Centers for Disease Prevention and Control (CDC) continues to issue recommendations for twice daily brushing of teeth with a fluoride toothpaste, cleaning between teeth (flossing or with use of a interdental cleaner), and annual dental visit for an oral examination inclusive of assessment for dental decay and professional cleaning.[72] Other public health initiatives underway to curb caries include fluoridation of drinking water, fluoride prophylaxis, sealant placement programs in community settings, and interdisciplinary patient screening to identify at-risk patients.

Rampant Caries Including Early Childhood Caries and Rates Detected in Older Children

Environmental factors facilitating cariogenesis vary across the age spectrum and public health approaches need to address management and interventional approaches in an age-appropriate manner. For example, early childhood caries, (also designated "nursing bottle caries" or "baby bottle tooth decay"), represent a subset of rampant caries seen in infants and toddlers. Containment of early childhood caries is being targeted by implementation of clinical practice guidelines recommending early childhood caries risk assessment by pediatricians of infants prior to the age of 1 year and their establishment in a dental home.[73] Since transmission of cariogenic pathogens may pass from mother to child, attention to maternal oral health beginning in the prenatal period and throughout early childhood is important in: (1) establishing a healthy oral microbiome in the infant and (2) instilling knowledgeability surrounding dietary practices that promote cariogenesis.

Implementation of early oral health education and practices holds high potential for procuring cost-effective caries interventions with added long-term benefits of improving baseline oral and systemic health and potential for sustainment across the lifespan in patients appropriately activated to participate in maintenance of dental and oral health. Following establishment of permanent dentition in the mouth of children and as they transition into adulthood, provision of access to prophylactic interventions such as fluoride varnishes, sealants become important in maintaining dental integrity challenged by environmental exposures.

Health of permanent teeth can be influenced by patterns of disease reflected in primary dentition as observed in a longitudinal follow-up study in pediatric population that identified early childhood caries as a risk factor for caries development in permanent teeth.[74]

Notably, a 2017 study reported that, in comparison to the global average for decayed-missing-filled index measure of 2.0 in 12-year-old children, the rate in the United States was 1.2, leaving room for improvement.[75] Stagnated progress in addressing oral disease in children is also cited in the 50-state report issued by the PEW Charitable Trusts in 2015,[78] which indicated that only 11 states had achieved the Healthy People 2010 goal of application of sealants to permanent molars of 50% of 8 years olds. Further, 78% of the states and District of Columbia had failed to establish dental sealant programs in most of their "high needs" schools defined by 50% of enrolled children qualifying for the school lunch program. With release of Healthy People 2020, the health indicator target for sealant placement in children 6–9 years of age had been lowered by half to 25.9% from the Healthy People 2010 target of 50%, closely aligning to actual achievement rates and deincentivizing promotion of this preventive intervention. Within the same temporal period, the CDC's report on Children's Oral Health cited that the rate of untreated tooth decay in youth aged 5–19 years living in poverty was double that of children not living in poverty (25% vs. 11%, respectively), with significant negative impact on the children's quality of life and potentially, overall health.[77] Oral health literacy interventions beyond the dental domain are required to raise awareness across all sectors regarding the importance of addressing oral disease across the entire lifespan. Lack of such recognition in the policy sector is noted in the observation that twelve states and the District of Columbia had not submitted sealant placement data to the National Oral Health Surveillance System in the previous 5 years leading up to release of the PEW report.[78]

Caries and the Aging Population

Risk factors for oral diseases, including caries in the aging population, are multifactorial and represent additional challenges for the public health arena. Among key contributory factors are:

Access barriers to dental care due to changes in insurance status and lack of provision for dental health service coverage associated with national healthcare policies provided to the adult Medicare-eligible population. For elderly individuals institutionalized due to health status, access to professional oral healthcare may be very limited.

Changing health status associated with development of conditions requiring increased pharmacological intervention. Pharmacological exposures may result in dry mouth (xerostomia), an oral condition characterized by reduced salivary flow. Because saliva bathes the teeth with antimicrobial substances, reduced salivary flow increases susceptibility to cariogenesis, introducing new challenges to achieving caries prevention.

Changing health status necessitating dietary changes. Capacity to absorb and use nutrients essential to oral health may also occur with changes in health status. Moreover, altered health status may result in limited capacity of the elderly to maintain oral health hygiene practices.

Assessment of oral health quality of life continue to document significantly poorer health outcomes and quality of life across low socio/economic status, racial, and ethnic status.[79,80]

Disparities are also noted for dental-care delivery to older adults, as documented by higher rates of tooth decay, periodontal disease, and tooth loss, especially among poor elderly and in racial and ethnic minority populations.[81,82]

A 2015 systematic review and meta-analysis[70] surrounding global trends in the burden of untreated caries cautioned that while emphasis placed on reducing burden of disease in pediatric populations especially in developed countries may have made some inroads in that subpopulation, an increase in rates of untreated caries in adults 25 years of age or older was observed when good oral hygiene practices were not maintained across the lifespan. Factors influencing adherence to good oral health practices are multifaceted and age-appropriate programs to reinforce and support compliance with preventive care may be required across the lifespan to ensure maintenance of healthy dentition and oral cavity tissues.

Diagnosis, Management, and Prevention

International Caries Detection and Assessment Criteria were developed as the standard for caries diagnosis and are the clinical practice guidelines defining criteria currently in use for diagnosis of caries in the United States and globally.[76] Caries treatment involves removal of decay and elimination of any potential microbial presence prior to restoration of the tooth surface, selecting among a variety of materials to lay reestablish an inert barrier to protect the tooth pulp from further microbial assault. Public health initiatives have included fluoridation of public drinking water as a deterrent to dental caries. The public health sector continues to monitor prevalence of fluorosis, white deposits on teeth induced as a consequence of excessive fluoride exposure.

From a public health perspective, a major focus in curtailing odontogenic infection should be on prevention, since these diseases are largely preventable. Attention should be placed on: (1) assuring that communities have appropriate water fluoridation, (2) educating primary-care providers on the importance of early detection and prevention of early childhood caries, and (3) education of parents surrounding the importance of early institution of good oral health practice and a dental home. Following establishment of permanent dentition in the mouth of children and as they transition into adulthood, provision of prophylactic interventions such as fluoride varnishes and sealants is key in maintaining dental integrity challenged by environmental exposures. Oral health literacy should be promoted among patients, using interdisciplinary providers to emphasize the importance of good oral hygiene, dietary habits, and negative impacts of smoking on oral health. Oral health prevention and control programs have contributed to the steady decline in edentulism in the population over age 60 years, as noted over time across six national cross sectional surveys conducted across five decades between 1957 and 2012. However, special emphasis is still required in targeting disparity populations where rates of disease remain disproportionately high.[83]

Periodontal Diseases

Pathophysiology

Periodontal disease represents a spectrum of diseases initiated by infectious processes whose presentation may be modified by systemic factors and conditions. The spectrum of gum disease ranges from a mild, self-limited form of disease called gingivitis, to periodontitis, a condition that advances in severity and establishes chronicity in the absence of good hygienic practices and professional management.

Gingivitis Gingivitis represents the milder, more self-limited form of gum disease. The condition is most commonly induced by deposition of dental plaque, which causes a localized inflammatory response manifesting as inflamed, swollen gum tissue and may be associated with bleeding. Over 90% of the population exhibits gingivitis.[84] Gingivitis resolves readily in response to oral hygiene practices (brushing, flossing, use of mouth rinses with antimicrobial activity) and professional dental cleaning. In the absence of good hygiene, dental plaque development on tooth surfaces progresses to periodontitis, a more serious form of gum disease.

- Pregnancy-associated gingivitis: is a form of gingivitis characterized by inflammation and gum overgrowth that arises in response to hormonal changes occurring during pregnancy rather than being induced by plaque. The condition is generally self-limited, with resolution occurring postpartum but requires management which may include gum debridement and close monitoring of plaque levels to ensure that good oral hygiene practice is being applied.[84]

Generally, establishment and maintenance of good oral health in pregnant women is vital to the future oral and systemic health of the infant since the oral microbiome of the mother plays an important role in determining the composition of the oral and systemic microbiomes of the infant (including the intestinal microbiome) that become established at, and after, birth.[85] Microbiome transference has important implications for establishment of the immune system of the infant and future disease susceptibility.

Plaque-induced Periodontitis Periodontitis is a serious condition caused by presence of periodontal pathogens in biofilms, which form on dental surfaces when oral hygiene is not effectively practiced. The condition can ultimately result in tooth loss due to progressive deterioration of gum integrity and damage to underlying bone structure supporting the tooth caused by infectious/inflammatory processes depositing at the margin of the tooth and gum line. Failure to effectively remove plaque buildup results in plaque mineralization and formation of dental calculus (also termed tartar). Calculus formation effectively walls off periodontal pathogens in a protective, permissive niche where microbial presence and metabolic products sustains chronic inflammatory processes responding to the microbial presence. Tissue destruction resulting from bacterial presence and inflammatory host response contribute to a deepening of the periodontal pockets below the gingival margin separating the tooth from the gum tissue support, resulting in tooth mobility. Moreover, periodontal destruction extends to deeper tissues, eventually impacting also the bone underlying the tooth. Ensuing bone loss further destabilizes the tooth resulting eventually in tooth loss. Dental professionals diagnose, classify, and track changes in disease severity based on measurements that define extent to pathology. Periodontal measures include pocket depth measures, clinical attachment loss, documentation of bleeding on probing of the inflamed gingival tissue, and radiographic validation of bone loss (see Table 60-1).[86]

Epidemiology of Periodontal Disease

As with nearly all oral diseases that do not have an underlying genetic component, these conditions are largely preventable with good oral hygiene practices including annual professional assessment of gum health. However, although gum disease is largely preventable, periodontitis has achieved epidemic proportions globally with far-reaching consequences creating a public health challenge, which remains to be addressed in the United States and globally. Approximately 65 million individuals or 47% of the U.S. population are estimated to have periodontitis with higher prevalence noted in Hispanic and Black populations.[87] Prevalence of periodontitis among individuals > 65 years of age is estimated to exceed 70%.[87]

Risk Factors for Periodontitis with Special Significance to Dental Public Health

- Disparity populations especially those with limited access to oral healthcare are at highest risk and include low-income, under or uninsured, elderly, institutionalized and individuals with disabilities that affect their ability to access professional care or engage in oral hygiene care. Capacity to pay for care continues as a barrier to accessing dental care. While the overall rate in 2015 for the proportion of the population with dental coverage was 71.4%, stark differences exist across the lifecycle in dental coverage: 87.9% for those under 21, 72.4% for those aged 21–64, and only 38.4% for those 65 and older.[88] A growing body of evidence is validating connections between periodontitis and chronic systemic disease conditions impacting on large sectors of the population. In some instances, as with periodontitis and uncontrolled diabetes mellitus, disease exacerbation has been shown to be bidirectional with inflammatory mechanisms associated with elevations in blood sugars contributing to risk for periodontitis.[89] Systematic review of the literature has further demonstrated reductions in blood sugar levels resulting from amelioration of periodontitis.[11,90]
- Gingival hyperplasia, a condition commonly encountered in the dental setting, may be attributable to genetic factors or more commonly, pharmaceutical exposure, manifesting as an adverse drug event. Management may include surgical debridement of excess gingival tissue to increase efficacy of oral hygiene and removal of oral plaque. Prevalence of drug-induced gingival overgrowth varies by drug, ranging widely from 20% to 80%. Rates as high as 70% and 80%, respectively, have been reported for phenytoin and cyclosporine.[91] Xerostomia (dry mouth), another potential adverse event arising from pharmaceutical exposures, is also a risk factor for periodontitis and other oral conditions, is explored in more detail below.

Management and Disease Prevention

Periodontitis, once established, generally requires professional intervention and involves scaling and root planning to eliminate plaque and requires periodic follow-up with a dental professional to monitor for recurrence. Periodontitis is largely preventable and responsive to good oral hygiene practices including twice daily brushing, flossing, and use of antiseptic mouth rinses. Professional dental cleaning and oral examinations at least once yearly or as recommended by the dental professional is advocated for maintaining good periodontal health. Cessation of smoking should be encouraged.

Dry Mouth (Xerostomia)

Overview

Xerostomia is characterized by reduced salivary flow which deprives the oral cavity of protective factors contained in saliva that deter induction of oral disease by microbial opportunists across the spectrum of tissue found in the oral cavity. While dry mouth is less frequently encountered in younger individuals < 50 years of age consequential to injury or diseases impacting functional capacity of the salivary gland, it occurs more frequently in the age group > 50 years of age as an adverse drug event secondary to pharmaceutical exposure to classes of pharmaceutical agents known to impact salivary flow.[92] A recent systematic review (2017) released a comprehensive compendium of medications inducing xerostomia and including level of evidence supporting the association.[93]

Epidemiology and Diagnosis

Prevalence estimates of the condition remain somewhat controversial, with studies citing a lack of standardized guideline for diagnosis. Further, prevalence is posited to vary across populations.[94] A 2012 systematic review estimated a range of xerostomia prevalence at 5.5–39% in the general population, 17–40% in community dwelling elderly, and 20–72% on institutionalized elderly. Across the population impacted by chronic systemic conditions including diabetes, Parkinson's disease, cancer or in patients with physical disabilities, rates of hypo-salivation and xerostomia prevalence are projected to approach 100% ranging in severity from mild to severe. Notably, this study further reported that prevalence rates varied depending on whether unstimulated versus stimulated salivary flow was assessed.[95]

Pathological Impacts

Reduction in salivary flow and its antibacterial activity has broad implications on oral health, enabling higher incidence of dental caries, periodontal disease, and oral mucosal infection induced by a variety of microbial agents (bacterial, viral, or fungal). In addition, reduction in salivary flow may contribute to dysphagia (difficulty in swallowing) and malnutrition. Oral or dental pain associated with infectious processes and difficulty in swallowing may restrict intake of a balanced diet.

Management and Prevention

Because of its prevalence, public health emphasis again needs to be on education and interdisciplinary-care management. This condition is often underdocumented in health records. Creation of improved capacity for interdisciplinary tracking of pharmaceutical exposures and clinical decision support tools to assist providers in identifying patients at high risk for xerostomia based on medication exposures, especially patients exposed to polypharmacy, represent important public health initiatives with high potential to improve overall oral health of patients. Active ascertainment of onset of dry mouth with the patient is essential and education of the public surrounding the potential impact of dry mouth on oral health represents an additional interventional target, which could be supported by medical and dental providers as well as pharmacists. In high-risk patients, salivary flow rate assessment may be undertaken and appropriate interventions such as use of mouth rinses that stimulate saliva production should be recommended to mitigate the condition and restore adequate salivary content in order to preserve overall oral health.

Oral Cancer

Epidemiology

Oral cancer ranks among the ten most common malignancies worldwide with 90% of cases diagnosed as oral squamous cell carcinomas with highest incidence in developed countries.[96] Based on latest SEER data from 2007 to 2013, rates of incident cases and death have remained largely unchanged although an increasing rate of 0.6% has been noted across the past 10 years.[97] Rates of new cancers were estimated at 11.2 per 100,000 person years and mortality rate of 2.5 per 100,000 person years. Oral cancer has an overall 5-year survival rate of 65%, ranking among it among major cancers with the lowest survival rates.[97,98] Notably, early detection of oral cancer is associated with a 5-year survival rate of 84% but rates of oral cancer detection at early stages are low, estimated at only 30%.[98] Frequency of diagnosis occurs with aging, with an average age at diagnosis of 64 years. Oral cancer represents approximately 3% of all new emergent cancer in 2017 with nearly 50,000 new cases and 9700 deaths, representing 1.6% of cancer-related mortality. Disease prevalence in 2014 was estimated at approximately 347,000 individuals affected by oral/oropharyngeal cancer in the United States, with prevalence in males two- to threefold higher irrespective of race/ethnicity.[98]

Little is known about pathogenesis and progression of oral cancer and to date, no biomarkers have been identified to assist with detection or facilitate screening for the condition. The latest guidelines last issued in November of 2013 by the United States Preventive Services Task Force found that the current evidence base did not support evaluation of the benefit-to-harm balance associated with oral cancer screening in asymptomatic adults in the general population. Thus, recommendation for such screening is currently precluded.[99] However, because oral cancer is associated with high survival rates if detected early, and this cancer occurs with very high frequency in individuals with tobacco and alcohol exposures, the American Society of Clinical Oncology recommends that the subset of individuals habitually exposed to these substances should routinely seek a simple oral cancer evaluation from dental and medical providers.[98]

Risk Factors

Oral cancer is largely preventable because leading risk factors are generally modifiable. Major risk factors include smoking, heavy drinking and human papilloma virus infection, often a sexually transmitted disease. Nearly 90% of individuals diagnosed with oral cancer have a history of tobacco exposure (cigarettes, chewing tobacco, or snuff) and risk increases with duration and frequency of tobacco use and approximately 75–80% of persons diagnosed with oral cancer have a history of heavy alcohol consumption.[100] Combined tobacco and alcohol exposures are posited to compound risk of oral cancer. In patients with oral-pharyngeal cancers 85–90% test positive for HPV 16,[101] a serotype also associated with cervical cancer.

Individuals with lichen planus are also at moderately increased risk for oral cancer. Lichen planus is a relatively common noncontagious, noncancerous, cell-mediated immune condition associated with inflammation of the skin and mucous membranes of unknown etiology potentially involving autoimmune mechanisms,[102] and has been associated with hepatitis C infection.[103] Occurring most commonly in middle-aged individuals, this condition can manifest as painful, erythematous, erosive, or bullous lesions ("white spot" lesions) on mucous membranes of the mouth, mimicking oral cancer lesions and must be closely monitored for malignant transformation. To lower risk in these patients, dental professionals will identify any potential physiological triggers, eliminate any potential sources of dental irritation, and treat topically with steroids. Additional autoimmune-mediated, mucomembranous oral diseases including pemphigus vulgaris, mucous membrane pemphigoid, discoid lupus erythematosus and erythema multiforme, may present with oral lesions that must be differentiated from oral cancer.[104] Management of mucosal lesions is important to prevent further microbial infection of lesions especially by organisms such as viruses associated with mutagenic potential.

Kaposi's sarcoma is a type of cancer that can impact mucous membranes including those of the oral cavity. While this cancer is relatively rare, it may be encountered in patients infected with HIV or in recipients of kidney transplants. This form of cancer tends to manifest as abnormal, raised, purplish bumps below the mucous membranes in the mouth as a consequence of compromised immune responsiveness and in HIV-infected patients. A role for an additional virus Herpesvirus 8 (HHV-8) in the immune compromised host is posited and this cancer may progress quickly with high mortality rates.[105]

Diagnosis and Management

Although early diagnosis is associated with 83% survival rate if detected early, oral cancer is often first diagnosed in later stages of the disease contributing to the high mortality of the disease.[98] Tumor, lymph node metastasis staging is used to grade stage prior to treatment. In early stages, oral cancer may manifest as red or white initially painless lesions, swelling or thick patches on oral mucosal surfaces, most frequently occurring on the tongue, floor of the mouth or lips. In the throat area, they may cause sore throat, hoarseness, and difficulty with chewing, swallowing, or speaking. Pain in the ear and mobile teeth not originating from other dental conditions are additional symptoms. Persistence of such lesions for more than 2 weeks requires evaluation by a dental professional and evaluation of mucosal scrapings (versus biopsy) to determine diagnosis.[106] Optimal treatment to date includes surgery, radiation therapy (external beam radiotherapy, brachytherapy) combined with chemotherapy adjuvant therapy.[96]

Prevention

Outside of oral examination by dental professionals, no biomarkers have been defined to date to permit screening of at-risk patients for oral cancer. From a public health perspective, the current best approach for oral cancer reduction is patient and provider education on risk factors that promote oral cancer and emphasis on reduction of high-risk behaviors including tobacco use and heavy drinking to minimize cancer risk. Vaccines currently available for HPV should be encouraged, since early evidence indicates that these vaccines may be effective at reducing oral cancer risk.[107]

Nonbacterial Oral Infection

Viral Infection

Viruses are among the spectrum of microbial entities that colonize the oral cavity, often without causing disease. Viral presence may, however, also cause pathology in the oral cavity in some instances, significantly impacting oral health and causing diseases with important public health implications. Families of viruses with known associations to oral disease are briefly reviewed in Table 60-3.

- Human Papilloma virus (HPV): This DNA virus can be detected in mucosal scrapings of 95% of individuals with good oral health.[106] As discussed in the previous section, HPV represents a sexually transmitted disease which increases risk for oral and cervical cancer in association with infection by certain HPV serotypes that possess mutagenic potential (e.g., HPV serotype 16, 18). Public health initiatives are needed to both educate and promote vaccination in appropriate populations to minimize risk for both oral and systemic cancers associated with HPV infection.
- Human herpes virus: Human herpes viruses (HHV) encompass a family of complex double-stranded DNA viruses and include the following viruses with potential for induction of oral pathology: Herpes simplex (HSV) 1 and 2, Varicella zoster virus, Epstein Barr virus (EBV), and HHV 8, generally in immunocompromised patients.[108] These viruses set up chronic colonization of the human host across their lifetime, with potential for emergence as pathogens if the host becomes immunocompromised. HHV 1 and 2 are associated with ulcer formation orolabial herpes presenting as an ulcer on oral mucosal surfaces. Varicella, the causal agent of chicken pox and herpes zoster, may also cause the vesicular rash on the oral mucosa. EBV colonizes adults, and along with CMV may cause mononucleosis. The main oral condition caused by EBV is hairy leukoplakia, a rare condition seen only in immunosuppressed patients which presents as "hairy" white lesions on the along the edge of the tongue and must be distinguished from oral cancer. HHV 8 is also associated with pathogenesis of Kaposi sarcoma, a skin cancer which also presents on the mucosa in the oral cavity in patients immunosuppressed patients and patient with acquired immunodeficiency disease (AIDS).

Potential association of HHV viral infection, especially CMV and EBV in potentiating periodontal disease has been posited in the last decade, but literature remains controversial.[109] Strongest evidence is associated with a case report of disease attenuation in a patient with severe refractory periodontitis following antiviral treatment to reduce the viral load of EBV detected in periodontal pockets along with periodontal pathogens. Since EBV and CMV replicate in leukocytes, it was hypothesized leukocytes infected by viruses are recruited to the periodontal tissues during the inflammatory response and acted as co-pathogens in sustaining periodontitis.[110]

Moreover, viral load may be indicative of viral pathogenicity. In instances where viral co-infection is posited, determination of viral presence and load is recommended. Approaches to clinical assessment of viral load in the oral cavity include virus-specific quantitative polymerase chain reaction assay, microarray analysis or pyrosequencing. If high viral load relative to what is normally present in the healthy oral cavity is present, intervention with antiviral agents might be considered in the context of periodontal or other oral infections associated with detection of high viral loads.

- Human Enterovirus: Enteroviruses are members of the single-stranded RNA picornavirus family and include human entero viruses and Coxsackie virus. Oral manifestations of entero-viral infections impact mainly the pediatric population and may cause hand, foot and mouth disease which manifests as membranous papulovesicular lesions presenting often in association with fever. Coxsackie virus Type A16 and Enterovirus 71 are most frequently associated with these infections although other HEV have been associated with this condition. Herpangioma, a rare condition also mainly affecting children, is a similar condition whose symptomology includes formation of oral ulcers and blisters.[108]

- Human immunodeficiency virus (HIV) and oral manifestations:

HIV is a retrovirus that infects lymphocytes, specifically CD4T cells, resulting in dysregulation of the immune response and loss in capacity to respond effectively to microbial challenge. HIV promotes an increasingly permissive environment for emergence of unchallenged opportunistic infection in the absence of antiretroviral therapeutic intervention. Oral manifestations of HIV infection are symptomatic of compromised mucosal immune response mechanisms, innate and acquired immune response capacity, leading to oral disease and promotion of systemic inflammatory disease. While oral transmission of HIV is possible, it is believed to occur at very low frequency through the oral cavity due to multifactorial host defense mechanisms present within the oral cavity.[111] However, oral disease may emerge as a secondary presentation in the individuals infected by HIV. Common oral diseases consequential to HIV infection include oropharyngeal candidiasis (including erythematous or pseudomembranous presentations), oral wart formation, oral ulceration, angular stomatitis (swollen red patches at the corner of the mouth), melanotic hyperpigmentation, and hairy leukoplakia.[113] An estimated 70–90% of individuals infected with HIV are projected to present with oral mucosal infections over the course of their infection.[112] Appearance of oral manifestations (most frequently oral candidiasis) associated with HIV infection and increased severity of presentation frequently occur as CD4 counts approach $< 200/\mu l$ and often herald progression to AIDS. Oral disease manifestations of HIV are however, highly responsive to therapy, most resolving within 3 months and hairy leukoplakia within 5 months. Individuals with HIV infection are also susceptible to malignant diseases induced by HHV including HHV-8-associated Kaposi's sarcoma and Epstein Barr virus-associated malignancies (e.g., non-Hodgkin's lymphoma).

Notably, a unique presentation of periodontal disease is associated with HIV infection.[113] Termed linear gingival erythema, presentation includes a bright red band of tissue at the gingival margin, bleeding on probing and painful inflammation. Microscopically, gram negative anaerobes, enteric bacteria, and yeast cells (likely candida) will be visible. Left untreated, this presentation is associated with accelerated periodontal destruction. Required treatment includes debridement and administration of antibiotics followed by use of antibacterial and antifungal rinses.[113] Necrotizing ulcerative periodontal disease is another aggressive painful disease associated with severe immunosuppression encountered in the context of HIV infection. Presentation includes soft tissue necrosis, spontaneous bleeding, deep pocket formation attributable to accelerated periodontal destruction, which frequently extends into the underlying periodontal tissue, causing interproximal bone loss. Patients with this condition may also be febrile, exhibit lymphadenopathy and mixed infection by periodontal pathogens and *Candida albicans*. Treatment involves debridement, scaling, and pseudomembrane removal with chlorhexidine.[114] Posttreatment includes oral hygiene with antibacterial rinses and systemic antibiotic prescription if systemic symptomology is present. Patients must also be counseled surrounding dietary improvement and vitamin supplementation, healthy habits, and smoking cessation if the patient is a smoker.[114]

Improved access to combination antiviral therapy and resultant improvement in immune response is associated with substantive reduction in rate of HIV oral disease. Guidelines for the prevention and treatment of opportunistic infections in HIV-infected adults and adolescents have been created to keep dental and medical providers abreast of available treatment options and the latest research surrounding their efficacy. Guidelines offer recommendations for management of patients with HIV and the myriad co-pathologies impacting this subpopulation.[115] For example, a sampling of several updates in 2017 with relevance to oral health included recommendations for (1) inclusion of isavuconazole as an option for uncomplicated esophageal candidiasis; (2) issuance of updated guidelines on antiviral treatment and drug interaction.[116]

TABLE 60-3 OVERVIEW OF INFECTIOUS AGENTS OF THE ORAL CAVITY

Bacteria	Disease	Virus	Disease	Fungus	Disease
Periodontal pathogens	Periodontitis	Human Papilloma virus	Oral cancer	Candida species	Thrush, mucosal erytheman, denture stomatosis; median rhomboid glottis; hyperplastic candidiasis; angular cheilitis; chronic mucocutaneous candidiasis; HIV-associated candidiasis
Cariogenic pathogens	Caries	Human Herpes virus Epstein Barr virus Varicella Zoster Human Herpes virus (serotype 8)	Oral ulcers Oral leukoplakia Mucosal rash Kaposi's sarcoma	Aspergillus species	Aspergillosis
		Human Entero virus	Pediatric foot and mouth disease	Cryptococcus neoformans	Ulcerations, nodules, granulomas, leukoplakia-like lesions
		Human immune-deficiency virus	Erythematous or pseudomembranous presentations, oral wart formation, oral ulceration, angular stomatitis, melanotic hyperpigmentation; hairy leukoplakia; linear gingival erythema; necrotizing ulcerative periodontitis	Histoplasma capulatum	Histoplasmosis (granulomatous lesions)
				Blastomyces dermatiditis	Blastomycosis; verrrucal lesions, draining lesions, radiolucent lesions in the maxilla or mandible
				Mucorales species	Oral mucormycosis (ulcers)

Fungal Infections

Fungal infections occurring in the oral cavity occur most frequently in individuals challenged by diminished immune response capacity associated with illness or treatment that diminishes immune competency in regulating opportunistic infection (e.g., chemotherapy and radiation). Fungal infections of significance to oral health were summarized in a review (Krishnan, 2012) and key points are highlighted below.[117]

Candidiasis Currently eight species belonging to the Candida genus have emerged as the most common agents of oral candidiasis. Factors predisposing to emerging of candidiasis include:

- Pharmacological agents that suppress the immune system, cause xerostomia or impact normal flora, which keep colonizing Candida in check, facilitate emergence of the Candida infection, and are important factors in increasing emergence of Candida as an oral pathogen. Pharmacological exposures associated with candidiasis emergence include: corticosteroids, prolonged wide-spectrum antibiotic exposure, antiproliferative drugs (chemotherapy), psychotropic drugs, and drugs associated with xerostomia induction.
- Systemic diseases are associated with impaired capacity of immune response to suppress emergence of opportunistic infection. Included among these conditions are poorly controlled diabetes mellitus, hyper- or hypothyroidism, Addison's disease and Sjogren's syndrome, autoimmune conditions, HIV infection, cancer, and cancer treatment including radiation and chemotherapy. The elderly are also at increased risk in the subpopulation experiencing loss of immune function attributable to aging especially in combination with poor oral hygiene, poor diet, and presence of other chronic systemic disease that may require polypharmacy for disease management, heightening risk for xerostomia.

Oral candidiasis can manifest as a spectrum of clinical presentations including:

- Pseudomembranous candidiasis (thrush): is the most common presentation of Candida infection and manifests as white patches of consisting of cellular and fungal debris which are removable by wiping.
- Erythematous candidiasis: presents as localized erythematous (red) patches on oral mucosa and may be symptomatic (often, a burning sensation) or asymptomatic. This presentation is most common in the context of prolonged wide-spectrum antibiotic or steroid exposure.
- Denture stomatitis (also referred to as chronic atrophic candidiasis): this condition impacts membranous tissue exposed to dental prosthesis and is classified across three grades of severity that can be differentiated by characteristics of the lesions where type one presents as localized erythema, type II a more diffuse erythema covering larger membranous surfaces exposed to dental prosthesis and type III presents as a granular or papillary form. Denture stomatitis is attributable to poor oral and denture hygiene. Carious lesions may provide a harbor for candida species and restoration of carious lesions should be undertaken to eliminate potential niches, which may host fungi. Other factors that predispose to this condition include bacterial infection, mal-fitting prostheses that irritate the membranes, and allergic reaction to prosthetics.
- Median rhomboid glossitis (also termed central papillary atrophy or chronic multifocal candidiasis): erythematous presentation on the posterior surface of the tongue or hard palate.
- Hyperplastic candidiasis: appears as a nonremovable white plaque surrounded by erythematous tissue and may resemble leukoplakia, a premalignant condition from which it must be differentiated. Lesional appearance may be opaque or translucent, slightly raised, and occur as single or multiple patches, often localized to the buccal mucosa. Biopsy is recommended to achieve accurate diagnosis by demonstrating presence of fungal hyphae.
- Angular cheilitis: is fungal infection at the corners of the lips causing erythematous, crusty, fissured lesions. The condition may

involve multimodal (bacterial and fungal) infection and may be associated with nutritional deficiencies including iron and vitamins B12 and C, and high diets high in carbohydrate content.

- Chronic mucocutaneous candidiasis: this form of candidiasis presents as a hyperplastic lesion and does not respond well to topical antifungal treatment. A genetic component involving defects in cellular immune response may underlie the condition. This candidiasis may be associated with endocrinopathies and autoimmune conditions and iron deficiency anemia.
- HIV associated candidiasis: candida infection is the most common secondary infection in patients with HIV and in this population most commonly presents as either pseudomembranous, erythematous, or hyperplastic candidiasis. An additional fungal infection that may be seen mainly in individuals with HIV infection in the United States is Coccidioidomycosis.

Other Clinically Signification Fungal Infections In addition to candida genus, other clinically important fungal conditions associated mainly with opportunistic infection in immunocompromised individuals, which may be associated with oral cavity involvement. An overview of these infections is provided in Table 60-3.

Diagnosis and Management

Differential diagnosis of oral fungal infection involves histological and microscopic examination of scrapings or biopsy treated with differential staining to distinguish characteristic features of the fungal infection, culturing to demonstrate fungal growth on differential media, serotyping, immuno-assay, or polymerase chain reaction-based assay to achieve speciation. A thorough medical history review to determine underlying factors that may be promoting fungal infection to mitigate these factors is essential. Review of pharmacological exposure, nutritional status, other underlying comorbidities, immune status, and use and condition of any oral appliances, salivary gland function and adequacy of salivary production assessment should be considered. Antifungal therapy is applied commensurate with medical history, tolerability, oral symptomology, anticipated capacity for patient compliance and fungal pathogen. Treatment may be topical applying polyene or azole-based antifungal agents or miconazole gel, be administered by oral suspensions of nystatin, or amphotericin lozenges. Refractory lesions may be treated systemically with ketoconazole, fluconazole, itraconazole, or amphotericin, but first line use of these agents is discouraged to prevent emergence of drug resistance.[117]

PREVENTION, TRENDS, AND FUTURE DIRECTIONS

Foremost, conceptualizing oral disease as preventable and modifiable has enormous capacity to improve oral and overall health in the United States in a cost-effective manner. The dental public health sector must realign its priorities, broaden its partnerships with medicine and health educators, and redouble its efforts for primary prevention, and the provision of timely, affordable access to dental healthcare for all segments of the population, including creation of more effective payer and coverage models to address oral health coverage deficits particularly in the elderly population. Priority dental public health foci include:

- Re-examination of oral health access across time in the framework of annually collected CMS Early and Periodic Screening, Diagnostic and Treatment (EPSTD) data whose purpose is to assess effectiveness of EPSDT service to Medicaid and CHIP populations[118];
- Implementation of effective screening and prevention of early childhood caries across the medical/dental sector;
- Improving dental health literacy to help patients to be active participants in establishing and maintaining oral health across their lifespan;
- Creation/implementation of alternative integrated medical-dental-care delivery models to bridge the traditionally siloed models for medical and dental healthcare delivery (e.g., National Inter-Professional Oral Health Initiative)[22] and associated payer models;
- Establishment of dental-quality tracking metrics to assess and maximize quality of dental healthcare delivery;
- Re-evaluation/amendment of traditional dental healthcare education to create a dental workforce that is responsive to the changing healthcare delivery landscape and positioned for facile engagement of more integrated models of healthcare delivery across all sectors of the population;
- Expansion of programs that amplify the pool of dental professional workforce with mid-level training (e.g., dental hygienists and dental therapists)[119] to provide an expanded workforce for provision of preventive and basic dental-care services to underserved populations such as those residing in dental shortage areas; and
- Increasing access to healthcare services offered at community health centers and other safety net providers.

References

1. American Dental Association History of Dentistry Timeline. Available at http://www.ada.org/en/about-the-ada/ada-history-and-presidents-of-the-ada/ada-history-of-dentistry-timeline. Accessed March 28, 2018.
2. Garla BK, Satish G, Divya KT. Dental insurance: A systematic review. *J Int Soc Prev Community Detn*. 2014;4(Suppl 2):S73–7.
3. Taylor J. The fundamentals of Community Health Centers. National Health Policy Forum. Aug 31, 2004. https://www.nhpf.org/library/background-papers/BP_CHC_08-31-04.pdf. Accessed April 27, 2018.
4. Satcher D. Surgeon General, Department of Health and Human Services. Oral Health in America: A report of the Surgeon General. https://www.nidcr.nih.gov/DataStatistics/SurgeonGeneral/Report/ExecutiveSummary.htm. Accessed March 23, 2018.
5. Office of Disease Prevention and Health Promotion. Health People 2020 Leading Health Indicators: Progress Update March, 2014. https://www.healthypeople.gov/2020/leading-health-indicators/Healthy-People-2020-Leading-Health-Indicators%3A-Progress-Uate. Accessed April 3, 2018.
6. Institute of Medicine and National Research Council. Improving access to oral health care for vulnerable and underserved populations. 2011. https://www.hrsa.gov/sites/default/files/publichealth/clinical/oralhealth/improvingaccess.pdf. Accessed April 3, 2018.
7. Kassebaum NJ, Smith AGC, Bernabé E, et al. Global, regional, and national prevalence, incidence, and disability-adjusted life years for oral conditions for 195 countries, 1990–2015: A systematic analysis for the global burden of diseases, injuries, and risk factors. *J Dent Res*. 2017;96:380–7.
8. Listl S, Galloway J, Mossey PA, Marcenes W. Global economic impact of dental diseases. *J Dent Res*. 2015;94:1355–61.
9. Glick M, Williams DM, Kleinman DV, Vujicic M, Watt RG, Weyant RJ. A new definition for oral health developed by the FDI World Dental Federation opens the door to a universal definition of oral health. *Br Dent J*. 2016;221:792–3.
10. Borgnakke WS, Ylostalo PV, Taylor GW, Genco RJ. Effect of periodontal disease on diabetes: Systematic review of epidemiologic observational evidence. *J Clin Periodontol*. 2013;40(suppl 14):S135–52.
11. Wang T, Jen I, Chou C, Lei YP. Effect of periodontal therapy on metabolic control in patients with type 2 diabetes mellitus and periodontal disease: A meta-analysis. *Medicine (Baltimore)*. 2014;93(28):e292.
12. Corbella S, Francetti L, Taschierri S, De Siena F, Fabbro MD. Effect of periodontal treatment on glycemic control of patients with diabetes: A systematic review and meta-analysis. *J Diabetes Invest*. 2013;4:502–9.
13. Konig MF, Abusleme L, Reinholdt J, et al. *Aggregatibacter actinomycetemcomitans*–induced hypercitrullination links periodontal interaction to autoimmunity in rheumatoid arthritis. *Sci Transl Med*. 2016 December 14;8(369):369ra176.
14. Leech MT. The association between rheumatoid arthritis and periodontitis. *Best Prac Res Clin Rheumatol*. 2015;29:189–201.
15. Koziel J, Mydel P, Potempa J. The link between periodontal disease and rheumatoid arthritis: An updated review. *Curr Rheumatol Rep*. 2014;16:408.
16. Zhang J, Jiang H, Sun M, Chen J. Association between periodontal disease and mortality in people with CKD: A meta-analysis of cohort studies. *BMC Nephrol*. 2017;18:269.
17. Wahid A, Chaudrhry S Ehsan A et al. Bidirectional relationship between chronic kidney disease and periodontal disease. *Pak J Med Sci*. 2013;29:211–5.

18. Lee C-F, Lin C-L, Lin S-Y et al. Surgical treatment for patients with periodontal disease reduces risk of end-stage renal disease: A nationawide population-based retrospective cohort study. *J Periodontol.* 2014;85:50–6.
19. Almeida APCPSC, Fagundes NCF, Maia LC, Lima RR. Is there an association between periodontitis and atherosclerosis in adults? A systematic review. *Curr Vasc Pharmacol.* 2018;16(6):569–82.
20. Corbella S, Taschieri S, Del Fabbro M, Francetti L, Weinstein R, Ferrazzi E. Adverse pregnancy outcomes and periodontitis: A systematic review and meta-analysis exploring potential association. *Quintessence Int.* 2016;47:193–204.
21. American Dental Association. Dental Public Health 2012. Available at http://www.ada.org/~/media/ADA/Member%20Center/FIles/dph_educational_module.pdf?la=en. Accessed April 16, 2018.
22. National inter-professional oral health initiative. Clinicians for oral health. 2017. https://www.niioh.org/.
23. Nenava D. Dental indices. https://www.slideshare.net/darpannenava/dental-indices.
24. Centers for Disease Control and Prevention. Indicator definitions-Oral health. Jan 2015. https://www.cdc.gov/cdi/definitions/oral-health.html. Accessed April 3, 2018.
25. Office of Disease Prevention and Health Promotion: HealthPeople.gov. Medical Expenditure Panel Survey. https://www.healthypeople.gov/2020/data-source/medical-expenditure-panel-survey. Accessed April 23, 2018.
26. Centers for Disease Control and Prevention. Achievements in public health, 1900–1999: Fluoridation of drinking water to prevent dental caries. *MMWR.* 1999;48:933–40.
27. De Almeida Lde F, Cavalcanti YW, Valença AM. In vitro antibacterial activity of silver diamine fluoride in different concentrations. *Acta Odontol Latinoam.* 2011;24(2):127–31.
28. Carey CM. Focus on fluorides: Update on the use of fluoride for the prevention of dental caries. *J Evid Based Dent Pract.* 2014;14 Suppl:95–102.
29. Centers for Disease Control and Prevention. Optimal fluoride levels in drinking water. 4/19/2015. https://www.cda.org/news-events/revised-optimal-fluoride-level-in-drinking-water-released. Accessed April 17, 2018.
30. HealthyPeople.gov. Healthy People 2020: Dental caries (cavities): Community water fluoridation. 2013. https://www.healthypeople.gov/2020/tools-resources/evidence-based-resource/dental-caries-cavities-community-water-fluoridation. Accessed April 12, 2018.
31. Community Preventive Services Task Force. Oral Health, preventing dental caries, community water fluoridation: Task Force findings and rationale statement (last updated 1/23/2017). https://www.thecommunityguide.org/sites/default/files/assets/Oral-Health-Caries-Community-Water-Fluoridation_3.pdf. Accessed April 13, 2018.
32. Lam A, Chu CH. Caries management with fluoride varnish in children in the US. *NY State Dent J.* 2011;77:38–42.
33. Ahovuo-saloranta A, Forss H, Walsh T, Nordblad A, Mäkelä M, Worthington HV. Pit and fissure sealants for preventing dental decay in permanent teeth. *Cochrane Database Syst Rev.* 2017;7:CD001830.
34. American Dental Association. CDC reports backs school-based sealant programs. Oct 18, 2016. http://www.ada.org/en/publications/ada-news/2016-archive/october/cdc-report-backs-school-based-sealant-programs20161018t153255. Accessed April 13, 2018.
35. Leonard JR, Bowman BA, Mensah GA. Impact of targeted, school-based dental sealant programs in reducing racial and economic disparities in sealant prevalence among schoolchildren—Ohio, 1998–1999. *MMWR Morb Mortal Wkly Rep.* 2001;50(34):736–8.
36. Gooch BF, Griffin SO, Gray SK, et al. Preventing dental caries through school-based sealant programs: Updated recommendations and reviews of evidence. *J Am Dent Assoc.* 2009;140(11):1356–65.
37. Centers for Disease Control and Prevention. Sealant efficiency assessment for locals and states (SEALS). Updated November 15, 2017. https://www.cdc.gov/oralhealth/dental_sealant_program/seals.htm. Accessed April 3, 2018.
38. Council on Clinical Affairs. Guidelines on caries risk assessment and management for infants, children, and adolescents. Reference Manual: Clinical Practice Guidelines (Revised). Vol. 37; 2014, pp. 132–9.
39. Bernstein J, Gebel C, Vargas C, et al. Integration of oral health into the well-child visit at federally qualified health centers: Study of 6 clinics, August 2014–March 2015. *Prev Chronic Dis.* 2016;13:E58.
40. Douglass JM, Clark MB. Integrating oral health into overall health care to prevent early childhood caries: Need, evidence, and solutions. *Pediatr Dent.* 2015;37(3):266–74.
41. Tomar SL, Asma S. Smoking-attributable periodontitis in the United States: Findings from NHANES III. National health and nutrition examination survey. *J Periodontol.* 2000;71:743–51.
42. Kibayashi M, Tanaka M, Nishida N, et al. Longitudinal study of the association between smoking as a periodontitis risk and salivary biomarkers related to periodontitis. *J Periodontol.* 2007;78:859–67.
43. Curry SJ, Emery S, Sporer AK, et al. A national survey of tobacco cessation programs for youths. *Am J Public Health.* 2007;97(1):171–7.
44. Asvat Y, Cao D, Africk JJ, Matthews A, King A. Feasibility and effectiveness of a community-based smoking cessation intervention in a racially diverse, urban smoker cohort. *Am J Public Health.* 2014;104 Suppl 4:S620–7.
45. Centers for Disease Control and Prevention. National tobacco control program. Aug 30, 2016. https://www.cdc.gov/tobacco/stateandcommunity/tobacco_control_programs/ntcp/index.htm. Accessed April 3, 2018.
46. National Institutes of Health. NCI launches smoking cessation support for teens. Dec 12, 2011. https://www.nih.gov/news-events/news-releases/nci-launches-smoking-cessation-support-teens. Accessed April 3, 2018.
47. Glurich I, Nycz, G, Acharya A. Status update on translation of integrated primary dental-medical care delivery for management of diabetic patients. *Clin Med Res.* 2017;15:21–32.
48. Beck J. Public health implications of chronic periodontal infection in adults. Centers for disease control and prevention, Division of Oral Health, National Center for Chronic Disease Prevention and Health Promotion July 13, 2013. https://www.cdc.gov/OralHealth/archive/conferences/periodontal_infections08.htm. Accessed April 23, 2018.
49. Office of Disease Prevention and Health Promotion: Healthy People 2020 objectives: Oral Health. https://www.healthypeople.gov/2020/topics-objectives/topic/oral-health/objectives. Accessed April 23, 2018.
50. National Center for Health Statistics. Healthy People 2000 Final Review. Hyattsville, Maryland: Public Health Service. 2001. Library of Congress Catalog Card Number 76-641496. https://www.cdc.gov/nchs/data/hp2000/hp2k01.pdf. Accessed April 27, 2018.
51. Palfrey S. New initiatives to improve HPV vaccination rates. *Hum Vaccin Immunother.* 2016;12:1594–8.
52. Gillison ML, Broutian T, Graubard B, et al. Impact of HPV vaccination on oral HPV infections among young adults in the U.S. ASCO Abstr # 153036 June 2017, Chicago Ill ASCO University Meeting abstract June 5, 2017. https://meetinglibrary.asco.org/record/153036/abstract. Accessed April 17, 2018.
53. Grantsmakers in Health Returning the mouth to the body: Integrating oral health and primary care. Issue Brief #40, September 2012, Washington DC. http://www.gih.org/files/FileDownloads/Returning_the_Mouth_to_the_Body_no40_September_2012.pdf. Accessed April 19, 2018.
54. Garfield R, Damico A. The Coverage Gap: uninsured poor adults in the states that do not expand Medicaid. Henry J Kaiser Family Foundation, 2016. https://www.kff.org/medicaid/issue-brief/the-coverage-gap-uninsured-poor-adults-in-states-that-do-not-expand-medicaid/. Accessed April 25, 2018.
55. Singhal A, Damiano P, Sabik L. Medicaid adult dental benefits increase use of dental care but impact of expansion on dental service use was mixed. *Health Aff (Millwood).* 2017;36(4):723–32.
56. Hinton E, Paradise J. Access to dental care in Medicaid: Spotlight on non elderly adults. Kaiser Commisiion on Medicaid and the uninsured. March 2016.
57. Shin P, Sharac J, Zur J, Rosenbaum S, Paradise J. Health Center Patient Trends, enrollment activities and service capacity: Recent experience in Medicaid Expansion and non-expansion states. Henry J Kaiser Family Foundation Report, 2015. https://www.kff.org/medicaid/issue-brief/health-center-patient-trends-enrollment-activities-and-service-capacity-recent-experience-in-medicaid-expansion-and-non-expansion-states/view/footnotes/. Accessed April 26, 2018.
58. Rosenbaum S, Pardise J, Markus A, et al. Community Health Centers: Recent growth and the role of ACA. Henry J Kaiser Family Foundation Report, Jan 2017. https://www.kff.org/medicaid/issue-brief/community-health-centers-recent-growth-and-the-role-of-the-aca/. Accessed April 26, 2018.
59. Yalowich R, Corso C. Enhancing oral health access through safety net partnerships: a primer and resource guide for Medicaid Agencies. Washington DC, National Academy for State Health Policy, Aug 2015. https://nashp.org/wp-content/uploads/2015/08/Enhancing-Oral-Health-Primer-for-Medicaid-Agencies.pdf. Accessed April 26, 2018.
60. Weintraub JA, Rozier RG. Updated competencies for the dental public health specialist: Using the past and present to frame the future. *J Public Health Dent.* 2016;76:S4–10.

61. Tomar S. An assessment of the dental public health infrastructure in the United States. *J Public Health Dent.* 2006;66:5–16.
62. MacDougall H. Dental disparities among low income American Adults: A social work perspective. *Health Soc Work.* 2016;41:208–10.
63. Pew Center on the States. (2012, February 1). A costly dental destination: Hospital care means states pay dearly. http://www.pewtrusts.org/~/media/assets/2012/01/16/a-costly-dental-destination.pdf. Accessed April 26, 2018.
64. Otto M. *Teeth: The Story of Beauty, Inequality, and the Struggles for Oral Health in America.* New York: New Press; 2017.
65. Mouradian WE, Corbin SB. Addressing health disparities through dental-medical collaborations, Part II. Cross cutting themes in the care of special populations. *J Dent Educ.* 2003;67:1320–6.
66. Naidoo S. Ethical considerations in community oral health. *J Dent Educ.* 2015;79(5 Suppl):S38–44.
67. Lee JY, Divaris K. The ethical imperative of addressing oral health disparities: A unifying framework. *J Dent Res.* 2014;93:224–30.
68. Mouradian WE, Berg JH, Somernab MJ. Addressing health disparities through dental-medical collaborations, Part I. The role of cultural competency in health disparities: Training of primary care medical practitioners in childen's oral health. *J Dent Educ.* 2003;67:860–8.
69. Featherstone JD Dental caries-a dynamic process. *Aust Dent J.* 2008;53:286–91.
70. Kassenbaum NJ, Bernabe E, Dahiya M, Bhandari B, Murray CJ, Marcenes W. Global burden of untreated caries: A systematic review and metaregression. *J Dent Res.* 2015;94:650–8.
71. Dye, BA, Tan S, Smith V, Lewis BG, et al. Trends in oral health status, Untied States 1988–1994 to 1999–2004. *Vital Health Stat 11.* 2007;(248):1–92.
72. Centers for Disease control and prevention. Hygiene related diseases: Dental caries (tooth decay). September 2016. https://www.cdc.gov/healthywater/hygiene/disease/dental_caries.html. Accessed April 26, 2018.
73. American Academy for Pediatrics Section on Pediatric Dentistry and Oral Health. Policy statement: Preventive Oral Health Intervention for Pediatricians. *Pediatrics.* 2008;122:1387–94.
74. Llena C, Calabuig E. Risk factors associated with new caries lesions in permanent molars in children: A 5-year historical cohort follow-up study. *Clin Oral Investig.* 2018;22(3):1579–86.
75. Santosh ABR, Ogle OE, Williams D, Woodbine EF. Epidemiology of oral and maxillofacial infections. *Dent Clin N Am.* 2017;61:217–33.
76. Dikmen B Icdas II criteria: International caries detection and assessment system. *J Instanb Univ Fac Dent.* 2015;49:63–72.
77. Centers for Disease Control. Children's Oral Health Nov 2014. https://www.cdc.gov/oralhealth/children_adults/child.htm. Accessed April 23, 2018.
78. The PEW Charitable Trusts report. States stalled on dental sealant program, Apr 2015. http://www.pewtrusts.org/~/media/assets/2015/04/dental_sealantreport_final. Accessed April 24, 2018.
79. Huong DL, Park M. Socieconomic and racial/ethnic oral health disparities among US older adults: Oral health quality of life and dentition. *J Public Health Dent.* 2014;75:85–92.
80. Griffen SO, Jones JA, Brunson D, Griffin PM, Bailey WD. Burden of oral disease among older adults and implications for public health priorities. *Amer J Public Health.* 2012;102:411–8.
81. Griffen SO, Jones JA, Brunson D, Griffin PM, Bailey WD. Burden of oral disease among older adults and implications for public health priorities. *Amer J Public Health.* 2012;102:411–8.
82. Friedman PK, Kaufman LB, Karpas SL. Oral health disparity in older adults. *Dent Clin N Am.* 2014;58:757–70.
83. Slade GD, Akinkugbe AA, Sander AE. Projections of US edentulism prevalence following 5 decades of decline. *J Dent Res.* 2014;93:959–65.
84. Wilder RS, Moretti AJ. Gingivitis and periodontitis in adults: Classification and dental treatment. Updated April 17, 2017. https://www.uptodate.com/contents/gingivitis-and-periodontitis-in-adults-classification-and-dental-treatment. Accessed April 18, 2018.
85. Gilbert SF. A holobiont birth narrative: The epigenetic transmission of the human microbiome. *Front Genet.* 2014 Aug 19;5:282.
86. Eke PI, Page RC, Wei L, Thorton-Evans G, Genco RJ. Update of the case definitions of population-based surveillance of periodontitis. *J Periodontol.* 2012;83:1449–54.
87. Eke PI, Dye BA, Wei L et al. Update on prevalence of periodontitis in adults in the United States: NHANES 2009–2012. *J Periodontol.* 2015;86:611–22.
88. Manski RJ, Rohde F. Dental Services: Use, Expenses, Source of Payment, Coverage and Procedure Type, 1996–2015: Research Findings No. 38. November 2017. Agency for Healthcare Research and Quality, Rockville, MD. https://meps.ahrq.gov/data_files/publications/rf38/rf38.pdf. Accessed April 26, 2018.
89. Casanova L, Hughes FJ, Preshaw PM. Diabetes and periodontal disease: A two-way relationship. *Br Dent J.* 2014;217:433–7.
90. Sgolastra F, Severino M, Pietripaoli D, Gatto R, Monaco A. Effectiveness of periodontal treatment to improve metabolic control in patients with chronic periodontitis and type 2 diabetes: A meta-analysis of randomized controlled trials. J Periodontol. 2013;84:958–73.
91. Ramirez-Ramiz A, Brunet-LLobet L, Lahor-Soler E, Mirnada-Rius J. On the cellular and molecular mechanisms of drug-induced overgrowth. *Open Dent J.* 2017;11:420–35.
92. Tan ECK, Lexomboon D, Sandborgh-Englund G, Haasum Y, Johnell K. Medications that cause dry mouth as an adverse effect in older people: A systematic review and metaanalysis. *J Am Geriatr Soc.* 2018;66(1):76–84.
93. Wolff A, Joshi RK, Ekstrom J, et al. A Guide to medications inducing salivary gland dysfunction, xerostomia, and subjective sialorrhea: A systematic review sponsored by the World Workshop on Oral Medicine. *Drugs R D.* 2017;17:1–28.
94. Orellana MF, Lagravere MO, Baychuk DG, Majore PW, Flores-Mir C. Prevalence of xerostomia in population-based samples: A systematic review. *J Public Health Dent.* 2006;66:152–8.
95. Liu, B, Dion MR, Jurasic MM, Gibson G, Jones JA. Xeerostomia and salivary hypofunction in vulnerable elders: Prevalence and etiology. *Oral Surg Oral Med Oral Pthol Oral Radiol.* 2012;114:52–60.
96. Rivera C. Essentials of oral cancer. *Int J Clin Exp Pathol.* 2015;8:11884–94.
97. National Cancer Institute. Surveillance, epidemiology and end results program. Cancer Stat Facts: Oral cavity and pharynx cancer. https://seer.cancer.gov/statfacts/html/oralcav.html. Accessed April 18, 2018.
98. Cancer.Net. Oral and Oropharyngeal cancer statistics 7/2016. https://www.cancer.net/cancer-types/oral-and-oropharyngeal-cancer/statistics. Accessed April 18, 2018.
99. US Preventive Service Task Force: Oral Cancer Screening Recommendation summary, Nov 2013. https://www.uspreventiveservicestaskforce.org/Page/Document/UpdateSummaryFinal/oral-cancer-screening1. Accessed April 27, 2018.
100. Illinois Department of Public Health. Oral Cancer, 2008. http://www.idph.state.il.us/cancer/factsheets/oralcancer.htm. Accessed April 18, 2018.
101. Anderson KS, Dahlstrom KR, Cheng JN, et al. HPV16 antibodies as risk factors for oropharyngeal cancer and their association with tumor HPV and smoking status. *Oral Oncol.* 2015;51:662–7.
102. Halonen P, Jakobsson M, Heikinheimo O, Riska A, Gissler M, Pukkala E. Cancer risk of *Lichen planus*: A cohort study of 13,100 women in Finland. *Int J Cancer.* 2017;142:18–22.
103. Al-Shamiri HM, Tarakji B, Shugaa-Addin B. Hepatitis C virus infection in oral lichen planus: A systematic review and meta-analysis. *Aust Dent J.* 2016 Sep;61:282–7.
104. Feller L, Ballyram R, Khammissa RA, Altini M, Lemmer J. Immunopathogenic oral diseases: An overview focusing on pemphigus vulgaris and mucous membrane pemphigoid. *Oral Health Prv Dent.* 2017;15:177–82.
105. Mesri EA, Cesarman E, Boshoff. Kaposi's sarcoma herpesvirus/human herpesvirus-8 (KSH/HHV8), and the oncogenesis of Kaposi's sarcoma. *Nat Rev Cancer.* 2010;10:707–19.
106. Furrer VE, Benitez MB, Furnes M, Lanfranchi HE, Modesti NM. Biopsy vs superficial scraping: Detection of human papillomavirus 6, 11, 16, 18 in potentially malignant and malignant oral lesions. *J Oral Pathol Med.* 2006;35:338–44.
107. Kim SM. Human papilloma virus in oral cancer. *J Korean Assoc Oral Maxillofac Surg.* 2016;42:327–36.
108. Grinde B, Olsen I. The role of viruses in oral disease. *J Oral Microbiol.* 2010 Feb 12;2. doi: 10.3402/jom.v2i0.2127.
109. Slots J. Herpesviral-bacterial synergy in the pathogenesis of human periodontitis. *Curr Opin Infect Dis.* 2007;20:278–83.
110. Sunde PT, Olsen I, Enersen M, Grinde B. Patient with severe periodontitis and subgingival Epstein-Barr virus treated with antiviral therapy. *J Clin Virol.* 2008;42:176–8.
111. Shugars DC, Sweet SP, Malamud D. Kazmi SH, Page-Shafer K, Challacombe SJ. Saliva and inhibition of HIV-1 infection: Molecular mechanisms. *Oral Dis.* 2002;8:169–75.

112. Heron SE, Elahi S. HIV infection and compromised mucosal immunity: Oral manifestations and systemic inflammation. *Front Immunol.* 2017;8:241.

113. Baccaglini L, Atkinson CC, Patton LL, Glick M, Ficarra G, Peterson DE. Management of oral lesions in HIV-positive patients. *Oral Surg Oral Med Oral Pathol Oral Radiol Endodontol.* 2007:103(suppl 1):S50.e1–23.

114. Todescan S, Atout RN. Managing patients with necrotizing ulcerative periodontitis. *J Can Dent Assoc.* 2013;79:d44. http://www.jcda.ca/article/d44.

115. US Department of Health and Human Services. AIDSinfo. Guidelines for the prevention and treatment of opportunistic infections in HIV-infected adults and adolescents. https://aidsinfo.nih.gov/guidelines/html/4/adult-and-adolescent-opportunistic-infection/0. Accessed April 24, 2018.

116. US Department of Health and Human Services: AIDSinfo Guidelines for the Use of Antiretroviral Agents in Adults and Adolescents Living with HIV. https://aidsinfo.nih.gov/guidelines/html/1/adult-and-adolescent-arv-guidelines/367/overview. Accessed April 24, 2018.

117. Krishnan PA. Fungal infections of the oral mucosa. *Indian J Dent Res.* 2012;23:650–9.

118. Medicaid.gov. Early and Periodic Screening, Diagnostic and Treatment. https://www.medicaid.gov/medicaid/benefits/epsdt/index.html. Accessed April 12, 2018.

119. WK Kellogg Foundation: What is a dental therapist? https://www.wkkf.org/what-we-do/healthy-kids/oral-health/what-is-a-dental-therapist. Accessed April 17, 2018.

CHAPTER

61

Health Promotion and Disability Prevention in Older Persons

Alexis M. Eastman

Increased risk of disease, disability, and death are well-known hazards of old age. While disease incidence and death are the conventional indices of a society's health status, functional disability is perhaps the most consequential index when dealing with health in old age. This chapter defines the character and magnitude of disability in old age, reviews preventive and therapeutic approaches to specific and general causes of disability among the elderly, and examines the role of healthcare organizations in facilitating the delivery of such services.

DIMENSIONS OF THE PROBLEM

Concept and Measurement of Disability

Conceptually, disability has been classified by the World Health Organization as part of a continuum of stages of disease impact that include:[1,2]

- *Impairment.* The loss or abnormality of psychological, physiological, or anatomical integrity at the level of specific organ systems.
- *Disability/Activity Limitation.* The inability to perform an activity within the range considered normal for a human being, hence a functional limitation experienced at the level of the person as a whole.
- *Handicap/Participation Restriction.* A disadvantage resulting from an impairment or disability which if not addressed, limits an individual's ability to participate in society.

Collectively this continuum has been referred to as the "disablement model." While each stage of the model has specific assessment tools and interventions, which are discussed throughout this chapter, the key overarching principles in the intervention for all three stages are holistic patient-centered evaluation, multidisciplinary coordination, and longitudinal care.

A wide variety of systems have been developed for measuring functional ability/disability.[3] The best known of these are the Activities of Daily Living (ADL) and the Instrumental Activities of Daily Living (IADL) indices. The ADL index, first introduced by Katz and colleagues, classifies limitations in six fundamental, sociobiological functions of daily living: bathing, dressing, toileting, transferring from bed or chair, continence, and feeding.[4] Lawton and others broadened the scope with the IADL concept which incorporates measures of more complex adaptive or self-maintaining functions: cooking, medication management, telephone use, transportation, housekeeping, money management, and grocery shopping.[5] In addition to screening and care planning for individual patients, these measurement systems have been very useful for describing the disability status of the elderly population, estimating community and institutional service needs, and evaluating outcomes of interventions designed to limit disability.

The concept of "preclinical disability" focuses on identifying stages in the natural history of functional loss, which precede the onset of overt ADL or IADL dependencies. This phenomenon was originally measured in terms of adaptive modifications in the performance of common tasks such as doing housework or getting out of bed.[6] Physiologic and performance measures of lower extremity function have also been shown to be powerful predictors of future onset of frank disability across diverse older populations.[7]

In the last 30 years, there has been an increased focus on a complex of physiologic deteriorations characterized as "frailty," which identifies older persons at high risk of decline in functional status and is a predictor of poor health outcomes in almost all medical interventions. There are a myriad of different assessment tools for frailty, and ongoing discussion as to what determines frailty. Currently, there are two dominant paradigms of frailty:

1. Frailty as an accumulation of deficits, including symptoms, signs, diseases, and disabilities. In this paradigm, frailty is characterized as a form of accelerated aging.[8]
2. Frailty as a biologic syndrome of decreased physiologic reserve. In this paradigm, frailty is characterized as a syndrome with distinct pathophysiology.[9]

Currently, the most utilized measures of frailty include at least three of the following attributes: unexplained weight loss, poor grip strength, self-reported exhaustion, slow walking speed, and low physical activity.[10]

Magnitude of Aging and Disability

The aging or *graying* of populations is occurring in all parts of the world, most profoundly in developed nations, as illustrated in estimates compiled by the United Nations (Fig. 61-1). Driven by a combination of increasing average life expectancy and decreasing birth rates, this "longevity revolution" will result in ever-increasing numbers of persons over 60 years of age and over 80 years of age among whom functional disability is most prevalent.

Almost 40% of Americans over the age of 65 living both in the community and in nursing homes have at least one disability. Among community dwelling disabled elderly, the most common ADL dependencies include bathing and transferring, while dependence on assistance with eating is least common. Shopping and meal preparation are the most common IADL dependencies. All domains of ADL and IADL limitation increase dramatically with age and are generally more prevalent in women than men.[11]

There is a strong association between ADL limitation and the presence of chronic medical conditions. With few exceptions such as stroke and hip fracture, it has been difficult to establish direct cause and effect relationships between specific diseases or combinations of diseases and the onset of disability. Nonetheless, it is reasonable to presume that a substantial amount of disability is attributable to physical and physiological impairments resulting from specific chronic diseases.[12,13] In turn, the prevention of such impairments and consequent disability would be largely dependent on the success

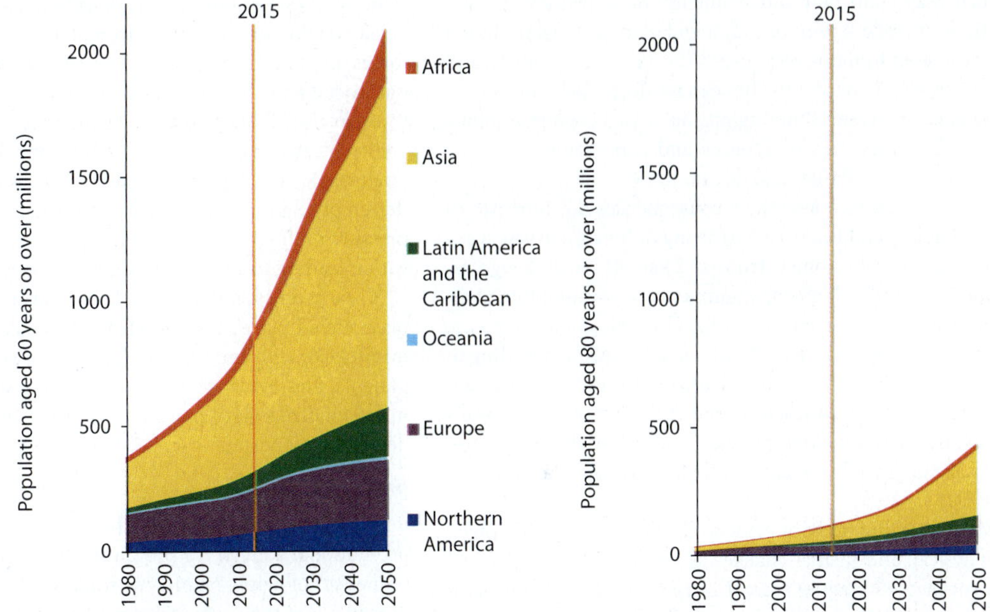

FIGURE 61-1. Percentage of population 60 years and over and 80 years and over in different regions of the world. UN data and predictions 1950–2025. [*Source:* From United Nations, Department of Economic and Social Affairs, Population Division (2015). World Population Ageing 2015 (ST/ESA/SER.A/390.)]

with which major chronic diseases are prevented or controlled using techniques reviewed in other chapters in this volume. A substantial amount of disability in old age may also be explained and potentially prevented by health-promotion activities, with attention to lifestyle, physical, psychological, environmental, and social support factors, which increase the risk of functional decline among older persons.[14] Comprehensive strategies of health promotion, multidisciplinary assessment and rehabilitation, and environmental adaptation are the key preventive approaches to positively address such factors.

A further dimension of the societal impact of disability in old age is the strong relationship between functional impairment and use of health services. A 1995 study from the Medicare Current Beneficiary Survey found that the aggregate annual physician, pharmaceutical, hospital, and long-term-care expenditures incurred by older persons was an additional $26.1 billion for each decrease in ADL ability from baseline, and it is likely that this figure has increased substantially in the past two decades.[15]

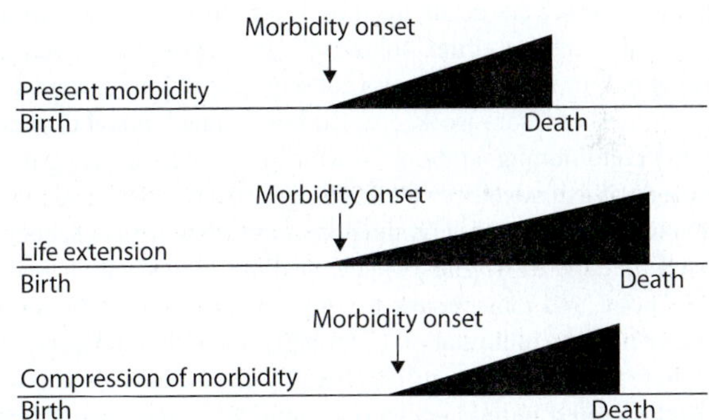

FIGURE 61-2. Conceptual relationship between age and percentage of the population remaining free of the respective stages in the natural history of chronic disabling disease.

Secular Trends

Increasing life expectancy in old age has led to several forecasts on the anticipated burden of disability. At one extreme is Fries's "compression of morbidity" thesis, which, with reference to Fig. 61-2, argues that age of onset of disabling chronic disease among the elderly is being postponed to a greater degree than life expectancy is expanding.[16] Under these circumstances, age-specific prevalence and aggregate years of disability before death would be expected to diminish. At the other extreme is the "failure of success" thesis promulgated by Gruenberg[17] and others, which argues that increase in life expectancy among the elderly is largely the result of advances in life-sparing medical treatments of existing disease, which, with reference to Fig. 61-2, results in increase in the average duration of certain chronic disabling diseases and would result in expanded future need for chronic-care services. Others have suggested that increased life expectancy reflects a combination of both phenomena, resulting in delayed age of onset of chronic disease and disability but not substantially reducing the overall health service burden.[18]

Various longitudinal population studies to empirically assess trends in the burden of disability among older persons are ongoing in the United States and elsewhere.[19] Common to such studies is a quest to identify and quantify determinants of disability-free aging, variably referred to as "active life expectancy"[20] or "successful aging."[21] Among these, the National Long-Term Care Survey (NLTCS), a longitudinal study involving very large sequential cohorts of older Americans, has documented an annual decline of 0.6–2.2% in the prevalence of chronic disability between 1982 and 2004, translating into a roughly similar population of older persons with chronic disabilities (7.1 vs. 6.9 million) despite a 34.6% increase in the population of older persons in that same time.[22]

HEALTH PROMOTION AND DISEASE AND DISABILITY PREVENTION

In considering approaches to prevention of disability in the aging population, as well as in the aging individual, it is useful to bear in mind several factors that are involved in the occurrence of disability. These include the contributions to disability attributable to biologic changes of aging, pathologic disease processes, and disuse or deconditioning. Also important are the contributions to the prevention or reversal of disability attributable to health promotion and therapeutic, rehabilitative, and environmental interventions.

Impairments and Losses

Old age is associated with increased occurrence of a wide array of physiological, physical, psychological, and social impairments or losses, which may contribute independently or collectively to disabilities. These include autonomic dysregulation (e.g., labile blood pressure), decreased immune response, reduced visual, auditory, and olfactory acuity, loss of muscle and bone mass, decreased proprioception and balance, increased skin fragility, decreased cognitive ability, nutritional deficiencies, loss of spouses and companions, reduced income, and loss of social roles and of autonomy.

Some of these changes and their consequences are intrinsic to the biology of aging, and lead to a narrowing of functional reserve, a phenomenon known as "homeostenosis." Examples include age-related decline in the individual's maximum oxygen consumption (VO_2 max), a fundamental index of capacity for physical activity; decrease in muscle mass (sarcopenia); modifications of lens protein leading to cataract formation; decrease in bone density with resultant osteoporosis and heightened risk of fracture; and stiffening of arterial walls causing increased systolic blood pressure and risk of disabling cerebrovascular accident while concomitantly increasing orthostasis and risk of falls.[23]

However, a growing body of evidence indicates that many physiological, physical, and mental changes as well as virtually all social changes associated with aging are not intrinsic to the aging process but are due to potentially modifiable extrinsic or self-induced factors.

Disuse/Deconditioning

The first level of preventable extrinsic factors in functional decline is discontinuation of usual activity referred to as "disuse" or "deconditioning."[24] This may occur insidiously as older persons withdraw from usual activities either voluntarily in response to a sense of "growing old" or involuntarily as a consequence of intercurrent acute illness, retirement from work, etc. The best studied model of general disuse/deconditioning, and one to which older persons are particularly prone, is extended bed rest. Prolonged bed rest may lead to a litany of physiologic adaptations and potentially disabling consequences as listed in Table 61-1. The physiological and structural changes in muscle, bone, and joint tissues are of particular concern because of their contribution to limitation of mobility and risk of falls and fractures. Rate of decrease in muscle strength may be as high as 5% per day in the bedfast individual, with leg muscles losing strength faster than arm muscles. Disuse osteoporosis results from both cessation of bone synthesis and increased resorption and tends to predominantly affect weight-bearing bones. Immobility and loss of weight-bearing forces on joints contribute to changes in both periarticular and articular tissue structure, which may lead to joint contractures.

Also contributing directly or indirectly to bed-rest-induced disability are atelectasis and other pulmonary changes that predispose to pneumonia, slowing of peristalsis with resulting constipation, bladder emptying difficulties leading to urinary incontinence, sustained pressure on fragile skin leading to pressure sores, and sensory deprivation leading to an array of negative affective and cognitive effects.

Clearly an essential principle is to avoid bed rest except as truly necessitated by medical problems. Instances of the latter should be minimized, with emphasis on progressive mobilization of bed-bound patients, and evidence supports early physical therapy intervention in hospitalized older patients to shorten hospitalization length and decrease posthospital-care needs.[25,26]

TABLE 61-1 COMPLICATIONS OF BEDREST

Cardiovascular	Decreased cardiac output, contributing to decreased aerobic capacity
	Orthostatic intolerance
	Venous thrombophlebitis
Respiratory	Atelectasis
	Relative hypoxemia
	Pneumonia
Musculoskeletal	Muscle atrophy and loss of strength
	Decreased muscle oxidative capacity, contributing to decreased aerobic capacity
	Bone loss (osteoporosis)
Gastrointestinal	Constipation
Genitourinary	Incontinence
	Renal calculi
Skin	Pressure sores
Functional	Impaired ambulation
Psychological	Sensory deprivation

Source: Reproduced with permission from Harper CM, Lyles YM. Physiology and complications of bed rest. *J Am Geriatr Soc.* 1988;36(11):1047–1054. doi:10.1111/j.1532-5415.1988.tb04375.x.

Physical Activity

Regular physical exercise is perhaps the single most important health promotional activity for preventing many of the dysfunctional consequences of aging. Numerous studies have demonstrated that older persons, like their younger counterparts, can significantly increase physical fitness, as reflected in VO_2 max, by engaging in regular aerobic exercise. Furthermore, there is clear experimental evidence involving older subjects that progressive resistance training can both retard and reverse losses of muscle mass and strength and bone density, reduce falls, improve physical function and decrease frailty in older adults.[27] Additionally, progressive resistance training improves gait speed, stair climbing, rising from a chair, and other significant physical tasks following participation in exercise programs without any adverse events.[28]

The application of such experimental observations to preventing disability is captured in the concept of "threshold levels" as follows:

> Strength, aerobic power and other indices of physical ability change on continuous scales whereas functional and quality of life changes are quantal. Thus a very small strength gain may be accompanied by a considerable functional improvement if it takes the patient from being just unable to transfer independently to being just able to do so. This also applies in reverse: A gradual loss of strength may not be apparent until the patient is suddenly unable to perform a crucial function.[29]

Despite the demonstrated benefits of regular physical activity, the majority of older Americans live essentially sedentary lives, which prompted the Public Health Service in the late 1990s to set a national goal of reducing to less than 25% the proportion of persons over age 65 who engage in no leisure time physical activity. The Surgeon General's recommendations call for 30 minutes a day of moderate activity which may consist of walking, gardening, cycling, swimming, and other and which must be sustained for benefits to accrue. More recent recommendations add strengthening, flexibility and balance training, and support having an individualized formal activity plan to achieve the necessary level of physical activity.[30]

EARLY INTERVENTIONS AND REHABILITATION

One of the targets of Healthy People 2020 was to increase the proportion of older adults who are up to date on the core set of clinical preventive services.[31] In order to achieve this, in 2011 several federal agencies released a report titled "Enhancing Use of Clinical Preventive Services Among Older Adults: Closing the Gap,"[32] where they examine the clinical preventive services recommended for older adults, current gaps, measures, and possible interventions to improve the uptake of these services in diverse communities. Table 61-2 illustrates the key preventive services with gaps in uptake and recommended interventions

TABLE 61-2 SUMMARY OF INTERVENTIONS FOR KEY GAPS IN PREVENTIVE HEALTH SCREENING

Featured services	Client-Oriented Interventions	Provider- and System-Oriented Interventions
Influenza and pneumococcal vaccination	• Home visits to increase vaccination coverage • Multi-component interventions for expanding access in health care settings • Reduced client out-of-pocket costs • Client reminder and recall systems • Multi-component interventions that include education	• Provider assessment and feedback • Provider reminder systems • Standing orders
Breast cancer screening	• Client reminders • Small media • One-on-one education, tailoring information to each person's needs • Reduced structural barriers • Reduced out-of-pocket costs	• Provider assessment and feedback • Provider reminder and recall systems
Colorectal cancer screening	• Client reminders for colorectal cancer screenings by fecal occult blood testing (FOBT) • Small media • Reduced structural barriers.	• Provider assessment and feedback • Provider reminder and recall systems
Diabetes screening	Reviewed only for diabetes control • Diabetes self-management education in community gathering places	Reviewed only for diabetes control • Case management interventions to improve glycemic control • Disease management programs
Lipid disorder screening	Not reviewed	Not reviewed
Osteoporosis screening	Not reviewed	Not reviewed
Smoking cessation counselling	• Reduced client out-of-pocket costs for cessation therapies • Multi-component interventions that include telephone support	• Increased unit price of tobacco products • Mass media campaigns when combined with other interventions • Provider reminders when used alone or with provider education

Source: From Centers for Disease Control and Prevention, Administration on Aging, Agency for Healthcare Research and Quality, and Centers for Medicare and Medicaid Services. Enhancing Use of Clinical Preventive Services Among Older Adults. Washington, DC: AARP, 2011.[32]

However, despite the best efforts of health promotion and disability prevention, most older persons will develop one or more potentially disabling medical conditions. Under these circumstances the goals of healthcare are early medical or surgical intervention, rehabilitation, and continuing supportive or palliative care to limit disability and provide for highest level of independence of individuals and their caregivers. Components of such tertiary prevention include both specific interventions for individual disabling conditions and provision of comprehensive geriatric medicine services.

SELECTED DISABLING CONDITIONS

Falls and Fractures

According to the CDC, approximately 20–30% of community dwelling elderly persons and up to half of nursing home residents fall every year. In the United States, falls are the leading cause of traumatic brain injury in older persons, cause 95% of hip fractures and are associated with $31 billion in direct medical costs annually. Hip fractures have an associated 20–40% 1-year mortality and death rates from falls have steadily risen since 2005 (Fig. 61-3).

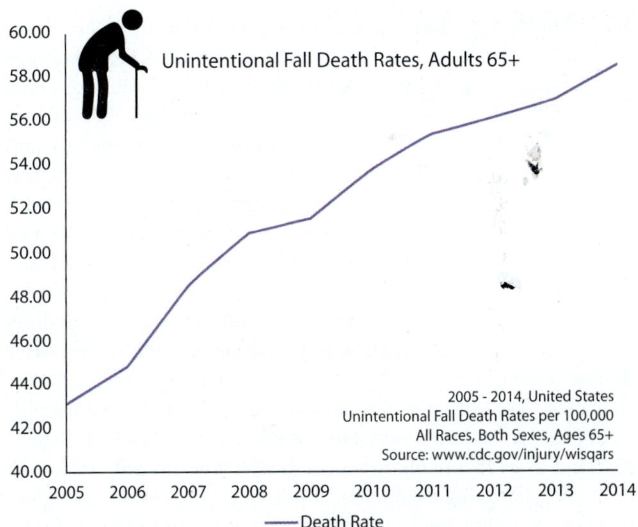

FIGURE 61-3. Unintentional fall death rates, adults over 65 years old, since 2005. (*Source:* From https://www.cdc.gov/homeandrecreationalsafety/falls/adultfalls.html.)

More than a million fractures occur in older persons in the United States each year, the three most common sites being vertebrae, proximal hip, and distal forearm (Colles' fracture). The principle contributing factor is osteoporosis or loss of bone mass, a progressive natural process that begins in the fourth or fifth decade of life and renders aging individuals increasingly susceptible to fracture associated with relatively minor trauma. Osteoporosis is accentuated in women following menopause, and age-specific risks of osteoporotic fractures are markedly higher among older women versus men (Fig. 61-4). Osteoporosis is significantly retarded by oral bisphosphonates and subcutaneous denosumab, somewhat retarded by postmenopausal estrogen replacement therapy, improved by teriparatide and probably slowed by regular exercise and supplemental calcium and vitamin D intake throughout adulthood.[33]

Risk of falling increases with the number and type of chronic disabling conditions present and medications being taken. Visual and proprioceptive abnormalities, musculoskeletal and neurological diseases, depression and dementia, and hypotension-inducing conditions (biologic and iatrogenic) are particularly important. Assessment for frailty and physical screening tools such as the Berg

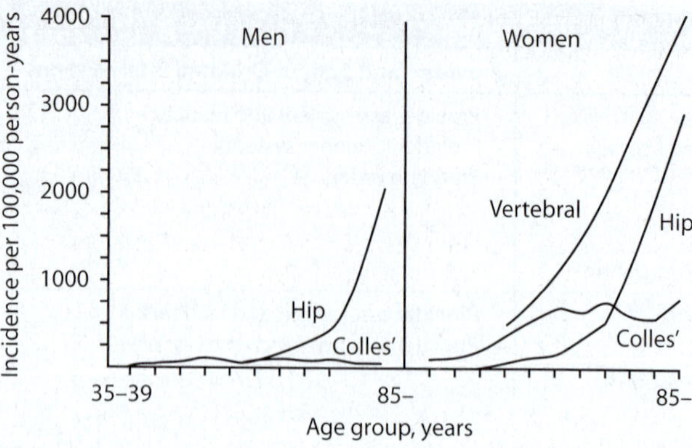

FIGURE 61-4. Incidence rates for the three common osteoporotic fractures (Colles', hip, and vertebral) in men and women, plotted as a function of age at the time of the fracture. (*Source:* Reproduced with permission from Riggs BL, Melton LJ 3rd. Involutional osteoporosis. *N Engl J Med.* 1986;314(26):1676–1686. doi:10.1056/NEJM198606263142605.)

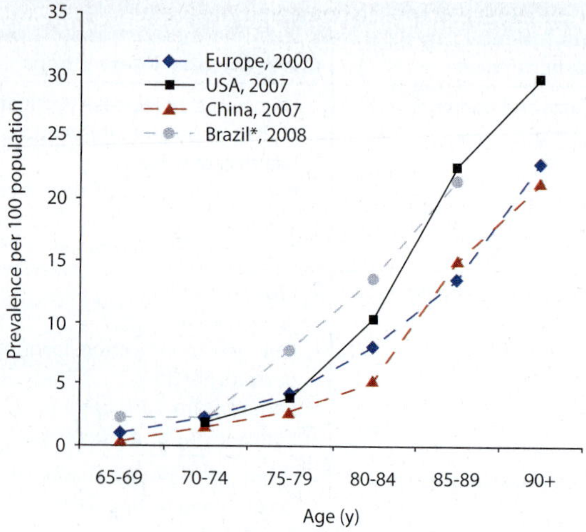

FIGURE 61-5. Age-specific prevalence of Alzheimer's disease (per 100 population) across continents and countries. *Prevalence of all types of dementia. (*Source:* Reproduced with permission from Qiu C, Kivipelto M, von Strauss E. Epidemiology of Alzheimer's disease: occurrence, determinants, and strategies toward intervention. Dialogues in Clinical Neuroscience. 2009;11(2):111–128.)

Balance Scale, Timed Up and Go, and five times Sit to Stand tests are the most evidence-supported measures of future falls risk.[34,35]

Currently, interventions that target multiple risk factors (e.g., medications, home safety, strength, and balance) are most effective in preventing falls both in nursing homes and in community-dwelling populations.[36,37] The USPSTF recommends exercise or physical therapy and vitamin D supplementation to prevent falls in community-dwelling adults aged 65 years or older who are at increased risk for falls. No single recommended tool or brief approach can reliably identify older adults at increased risk for falls, but several reasonable and feasible approaches are available for primary-care clinicians, including the screening tests mentioned above.[38]

Sensory Impairment—Hearing and Vision

The 2001–08 U.S. National Health Survey Supplement on Aging established prevalence rates of hearing impairment of 63% at age 70–79, rising to 84% at 80+ years of age among community-dwelling men and 48% and 75% among women at the same ages.[39] Prevalence of significantly impaired vision, including blindness, among men and women is approximately 18% at age over 70. In addition to potentially profound limitations in an individual's ability to communicate with others, impairments in both of these sensory systems are associated with significant limitations in performing traditional ADL and IADL functions as well as with depression and cognitive difficulty.[40]

Early detection and therapeutic intervention may reverse or delay sensory impairments attributable to certain specific degenerative disease processes, such as visual loss due to diabetic retinopathy or glaucoma. The American Academy of Ophthalmology recommends a comprehensive vision evaluation every 1–2 years after the age of 65,[41] and as of this publication, the USPSTF is currently reviewing its hearing screening recommendations. In large measure, the task of reducing disability due to sensory loss focuses upon either restoring the lost sense as in surgical treatment of senile cataract or prosthetic treatment in presbycusis or in adaptive devices, such as specialized magnifiers and lights in low vision disorders. Cataract surgery with lens implantation has been shown to improve physical function as well as vision.[42] Hearing aids, voice amplifying devices, and lip reading represent the mainstays of hearing rehabilitation, which, if used effectively, can reverse physical and particularly psychosocial disability associated with hearing loss.

Depression and Dementia

Mental and psychological disability among the elderly are major societal concerns, particularly in long-term care institutions. Depression and dementia constitute the most prominent forms of affective and cognitive disorders encountered in old age. Both conditions may result from multiple causes, and while generally not directly preventable, the impact of depression and dementia on affected individuals or their caregivers may be alleviated through judicious intervention.

Major depression, found in some 5% of older persons in the community, and clinically significant depressive symptoms, found in 8–16% are associated with increased risk of physical disability. Rates are higher in recently hospitalized patients (37%) and depression is often comorbid with cognitive impairment.[43] The USPSTF recommends depression screening for all adults, provided there are adequate systems in place for accurate diagnosis, treatment, and follow-up.[44] Both the PHQ-9 and the Geriatric Depression Screen are validated for older patient populations and cognitive behavioral therapy, antidepressant medication, and electroconvulsive therapy are all effective in treating late-life depression and its disabling effects. Best results appear to be achieved through collaborative-care management involving mental health and primary-care practitioners working together.[45]

Broadly defined by the DSM-V as "Multiple cognitive deficits, which include memory impairment and at least one of the following: aphasia, apraxia, agnosia, or disturbance in executive functioning" with an associated social or occupational dysfunction, Major Neurocognitive Disorder (formerly "dementia") is a disabling mental condition, well known to aging societies, which increases dramatically in prevalence from 14% at age 70 to 37% or above at age 90.[46] (Fig. 61-5). The most common pathologic subtypes of dementia are Alzheimer's disease and multi-infarct dementia. A small percent of cases of potentially reversible "pseudodementias" occur secondary to treatable causes including hypothyroidism, subdural hematoma, drug toxicity, and others.

Cognitive screening is now part of the Medicare Annual Wellness Visit for all older adults. However, the National Institute recommends that screening be limited to older adults who notice cognitive changes or who have caregivers who notice cognitive changes, when the medical provider notices cognitive changes, and all persons over the age of 80.[47] Screening tools such as the Animal Fluency Test, Mini-COG, GP-COG, Mini-Mental Status Exam (proprietary), St Louis University Mental Status Exam, and Montreal Cognitive Assessment are all validated tools for clinical practice. The benefits of early detection include identifying disease states that mimic dementia (pseudodementia) for appropriate treatment, managing comorbidities that impact cognition, eliminating medications with cognitive side effects, initiating therapies to slow cognitive decline, and ensuring the patient has appropriate support and resources to maintain independent function and plan for future cognitive decline.[48]

There are several drugs, mainly cholinesterase inhibitors, that show modest effects in slowing cognitive decline in dementia,[49] and there is ongoing research into the positive effects of diet, physical and mental exercise for prevention and treatment of dementia. Additionally, there is growing evidence that controlling risk factors, such as physical inactivity, diabetes, depression, excessive alcohol use, and tobacco use may significantly reduce dementia incidence.[50]

A variety of intervention strategies have been developed with the twin goals of maintaining independence and dignity for dementia patients and providing social and psychological support for their caregivers.[51] These invariably involve a multidisciplinary approach. Patient care includes continuing attention to basic medical and nursing needs with emphasis on adequate nutrition, assistance with toileting and grooming, and prevention or early treatment of minor infections and skin breakdown. Regularly scheduled exercise training may help to maintain patient function and may help slow cognitive decline.[52] Support for caregivers in the community includes counselling and education about the natural course and management of dementia, particularly the highly stressful memory loss and aberrant behavior; assistance with obtaining legal, financial, and safety advice; and provision of temporary relief through day care or short-term residential respite care. To ensure appropriate and effective care for patients with advanced disease, often accompanied by wandering and agitation, special memory-care facilities have been widely and successfully introduced in the United States and elsewhere.[53]

In addition to the burden suffered directly by patients and their caregivers, Alzheimer's and related disorders pose an immense monetary cost, estimated by the Alzheimer's Association in 2017 at some $259 billion annually in the United States.

Stroke

Stroke or cerebrovascular disease comprises a heterogeneous group of pathological entities all of which carry a high risk of residual disability. While age-specific stroke mortality rates have declined dramatically, and levels of disability among survivors of incident stroke have improved in recent decades,[54] stroke remains the fourth leading cause of death and the most severely disabling condition of old age. Among acute stroke survivors, 30–40% become dependent in self-care, with most functional recovery occurring within 3–6 months poststroke; over 50% experience significant depression and social isolation, and 20–30% are institutionalized for continuing care.[55] Globally, 90% of the stroke burden is due to modifiable behavioral, metabolic and environmental risk factors. Air pollution is of particular risk in low- and middle-income nations.[56] Randomized trials have found that hospital-based special stroke units, which combine acute medical-nursing expertise and multidisciplinary rehabilitation, yield decreased mortality and in some instances decreased long-term disability and institutional placement when compared to stroke management on general medical units.[57] The use of thrombolytic therapy in acute ischemic stroke significantly lowers rates of poststroke disability in patients treated within 3–4.5 hours of onset of stroke.[58]

Parkinson's Disease

Parkinson's disease is a progressive degenerative condition resulting largely from deficiency of the neurotransmitter substance dopamine in the midbrain and causing generalized movement and postural abnormalities. Disabling manifestations include resting tremor, shuffling gait and increased falls, autonomic instability, and increased risk of dementia. Increasingly common with aging, the prevalence is estimated at 500–1000 per 100,000 over age 60, with more than half of prevalent cases being over 70 years of age.[59] Conventional treatment to ameliorate manifest disability in Parkinson's disease consists of one of a variety of dopamine replacement regimens plus physical therapy, though these become increasingly ineffective as the disease progresses. Deep brain stimulation has become the main surgical intervention for controlling some of the disabling effects of Parkinson's disease.[60]

Heart Failure and Chronic Obstructive Pulmonary Disease

Heart failure and chronic obstructive pulmonary disease (COPD) constitute the two most common disabling chronic cardiopulmonary conditions of old age. From a public health perspective, the impact of both conditions on society at large in the United States and elsewhere is manifest by increasing mortality and morbidity rates for both conditions among older persons since the 1980s. From a clinical perspective, impact of these conditions on patient functional status and quality of life has been shown to be partially controllable through use of selected medical and rehabilitative interventions as well as palliative care.[61]

Heart failure is the most common reason for hospitalization among persons over age 65 in the United States, Coordinated Transitions of Care (C-TraC) programs, inpatient Acute Care of the Elderly (ACE) and Hospital Elder Life Programs (HELP), Geriatric Evaluation and Management clinics, Hospital at Home services, and Long-Term Care intervention programs.

Geriatric Strategies

Comprehensive geriatric assessment represents the core clinical activity of geriatric medicine. Practiced in inpatient and outpatient settings by geriatricians, nurses, social workers, rehabilitation therapists, and others working in collaboration, geriatric assessment is a multidimensional, multidisciplinary process which identifies medical, social, and functional needs, and the development of an integrated/coordinated care plan to meet those needs.[62] While there are many models of comprehensive geriatric assessment depending on the healthcare setting, they all share common key features:

- Specialty expertise in aging;
- Multidimensional evaluation of medical, functional, mental, social, and environmental needs (may include screening for polypharmacy, falls risk, nutrition, socioeconomic needs, elder abuse, psychologic or cognitive status, or other setting-appropriate screens);
- Coordinated multidisciplinary care;
- Patient-centered-care plans;
- Care plan delivery, including rehabilitative and multidimensional components; and
- Iterative evaluation of care plan.[63]

Meta-analyses of community-dwelling and hospitalized older adults show that the odds of surviving and living in their own homes are generally more favorable for those managed by comprehensive geriatric assessment programs, especially if those programs include medical recommendation implementation and extended ambulatory follow-up.[64,65]

The need for progressive geriatric care is particularly evident in the acute hospital sector where older patients not only constitute the largest constituency of admissions, but also are at particularly high risk of experiencing decline in physical and mental function.[66] Such strategies have been incorporated into hospitals in various ways across developed nations. The simplest approach involves referral for consultation by a multidisciplinary geriatrics team. Other strategies include a special hospital-based or affiliated unit to which patients are transferred for geriatric rehabilitation following acute care on a medical or surgical service, or a designated part of an inpatient medical service as an acute geriatric admitting unit.

Among the documented successes of hospital-based geriatric programs, three prototypic experiences are illustrative.

The first of these is an early model based at the Sepulveda Veterans Administration Medical Center in Los Angeles, which comprised a 15-bed geriatric unit operated by a full-time medical, nursing, and social work team, with part-time participation by rehabilitation therapists and others. In a randomized trial, older hospitalized patients transferred to the geriatric unit, when compared with controls managed on a general medical unit, over a 1-year follow-up, experienced significantly lower mortality, a reduced likelihood of nursing home admission, fewer overall acute hospital and nursing home days, significantly greater improvement in functional status and morale, and lower average cost of care.[67] At 3 years of follow-up, the benefit in mortality and quality of life was preserved.[68]

The second experience involved a collaborative orthogeriatric rehabilitation unit developed at Sheba Medical Centre in Tel HaShomer, Israel. Since 1998, ongoing studies have randomized elderly hip fracture patients admitted from the emergency department to either the regular orthopedic surgery service or a specialized orthogeriatric unit with a multidisciplinary service headed by a geriatrician. In a trial of 320 patients, median length of hospital stay was shorter, and odds of successful postoperative rehabilitation were higher in the orthogeriatric unit patients.[69]

A third prototypic experience exemplifies that consultative comprehensive geriatrics assessment can be an effective tool in hospital care of older patients. Designed to target delirium, a high-risk outcome that increases mortality and functional decline, a parallel group study in the Leuven University hospitals in Belgium randomized older patients with hip fracture to usual care or usual care with a comprehensive geriatric assessment consultative team. The multidisciplinary team of a physician, nurse, social worker, physical therapist, and occupational therapist, evaluated the patient and made recommendations regarding care to the primary team. Incidence of delirium and cognitive dysfunction at discharge was half as likely in the group receiving geriatric assessment, though there was no difference in length of delirium nor 1-year survival rates.[70] An emerging model of virtual comprehensive geriatric assessment using telemedicine and electronic health records may provide access to geriatric assessment for underserved communities in the future.[71]

Comprehensive Health Services

Successful provision of geriatric assessment, rehabilitation, and continuing care with a preventive orientation is most likely to occur in a comprehensive healthcare program in which the various elements discussed earlier are linked together under one system of financing. Such systems have been developed in Great Britain, Scandinavian countries, and a number of other societies with national health programs. In the United States, fragmentation among healthcare payors and an excessive reliance on costly institutional services (acute hospitals and nursing homes) has left many gaps in the provision of services, which could prevent or alleviate disability and dependency in old age. A limited number of projects, including the PACE and GRACE models discussed as well as PACT programs in the Veteran's Administration health services,[72] have developed model comprehensive programs for older persons in the United States, but sustainable funding remains a concern.[73] The emerging Patient Centered Medical Home, modelled on the principles of comprehensive geriatric evaluation, utilizes innovative-care delivery strategies for maintaining maximal functional well-being among both older persons living in the community as well as younger community-dwelling persons with chronic conditions and has been adopted by many health systems in the United States.[74] At such time that a national health program should evolve, these model experiences will provide the evidence to draw upon in ensuring financing for progressive comprehensive services for society's oldest and most vulnerable members.

Advance-Care Planning

In the last decade, advance-care planning has arisen as an important method for ensuring a person's values guide their medical care. It usually comprises a conversation or a series of conversations about potential future medical decisions, preferences for treatments that prolong life, cardiopulmonary resuscitation preferences, and general values with respect to quality of life. Additionally, patients are given counselling on how to communicate these values to caregivers and loved ones, and they are codified in some form of advanced directive. Ideally, these conversations are held far in advance of a medical crisis and can be used to help guide management in those times.[75] Many organizations and professional societies provide training in how to successfully hold effective advance-care planning conversations, though to date, evidence is limited as to the success of any one particular approach.[76] Despite limited evidence as to approach for conversations, advance-care planning is associated with lower healthcare costs in the final week of life, less ICU utilization, reduced hospitalizations in heart failure patients, and decreased aggressive interventions in the last month of life. More importantly, advance-care planning is associated with increased likelihood of death outside the hospital, improved perceived quality of death and fewer reported concerns about the quality of healthcare interactions.[77–81] As the goal of patient-centered care becomes more prevalent, advance-care planning is an important addition to the concept of comprehensive care for older adults.

Additional resources

Albert SM. *Public Health and Aging. An Introduction to Maximizing Function and Well-Being*. New York: Springer; 2004.

Halter JB, Ouslander JG, Studenski S, et al. eds. *Hazzard's Geriatric Medicine and Gerontology*, 7th ed. New York: McGraw-Hill; 2017.

References

1. International Classification of Impairments, Disabilities and Handicaps (ICIDH). Geneva, World Health Organization; 1980.
2. International Classification of Impairments, Disabilities and Handicaps (ICIDH) Beta-2 Draft. Geneva, World Health Organization; 1999.
3. Andresen EM, Rothenberg BM, Zimmer JG. *Assessing Health Status among Older Adults*. New York: Springer; 1997.
4. Katz S, Ford AB, Moskowitz RW, et al. Studies of illness in the aged. The index of ADL. *JAMA*. 1963;185:914–9.
5. Lawton MP, Brody EM. Assessment of older people: Self-maintaining and instrumental activities of daily living. *Gerontologist*. 1969;9:179–86.
6. Fried LP, Herdman SJ, Kuhn KE, et al. Preclinical disability: Hypotheses about the bottom of the iceberg. *J Aging Health*. 1991;3:285–300.
7. Guralnik JM, Ferrucci L, Pieper CF, et al. Lower extremity function and subsequent disability: Consistency across studies, predictive models, and value of gait speed alone compared with the short physical performance battery. *J Gerontol A Biol Sci Med Sci*. 2000;55(4):M221–31.
8. Rockwood K, Mitniski A. Frailty In relation to the accumulation of deficits. *J Gerontol A Biol Sci Med Sci*. 2007;62(7):722–7.
9. Fried LP, Tangen CM, Walston J, et al. Frailty in older adults: Evidence for a phenotype. *J Gerontol A Biol Sci Med Sci*. 2001;56(3):M146–57.
10. Ferrucci L, Guralnik J, Studenski S, et al. Designing randomized trials aimed at preventing or delaying functional decline and disability in frail older persons: A consensus report. *J Am Geriatr Soc*. 2004;52:1–10.
11. Wan H, Larsen LJ. U.S. Census Bureau, American Community Survey Reports, ACS-29, Older Americans With a Disability: 2008–2012, U.S. Government Printing Office, Washington, DC, 2014.
12. Boult C, Kane RL, Louis TA, et al. Chronic conditions that lead to functional limitation in the elderly. *J Gerontol*. 1994;49:M28–36.
13. Wang L, van Belle G, Kukull WB, Larson EB. Predictors of functional change: A longitudinal study of nondemented people aged 65 and older. *J Am Geriatr Soc*. 2002;50:1525–34.
14. Stuck A, Walthert J, Nikolaus T, et al. Risk factors for functional status decline in community-living elderly people: A systematic review of the literature. *Soc Sci Med*. 1999;48:445–9.
15. Guralnik J, Alecxih L, Branch LG, Weiner JM. Medical and long-term care costs when older persons become more dependent. *Am J Public Health*. 2002;92:1244–5.
16. Fries JF, Bruce B, Chakravarty E. Compression of morbidity 1980–2011: A focused review of paradigms and progress. *J Aging Res*. 2011;2011:261702.
17. Gruenberg EM. The failures of success. *Milbank Mem Fund Q*. 1977;55:3–24.
18. Manton KG. Changing concepts of morbidity and mortality in the elderly population. *Milbank Mem Fund Q*. 1982;60:183–244.
19. Freedman V, Martin L, Schoeni R. Recent trends in disability and functioning among older adults in the United States: A systematic review. *JAMA*. 2002;288:3137–46.
20. Katz S, Branch LG, Branson MH, et al. Active life expectancy. *N Engl J Med*. 1983;309:1218–24.

21. Rowe JW, Kahn RL. Human aging: Usual and successful. *Science.* 1987;237:143–9.
22. Manton KG. Recent declines in chronic disability in the elderly U.S. population: Risk factors and future dynamics. *Annu Rev Public Health.* 2008;29:91–113.
23. Boss GR, Seegmiller JE. Age-related physiological changes and their clinical significance. *West J Med.* 1981;135(6):434–40.
24. Bortz WM. Disuse and aging. *JAMA.* 1982;248:1203–8.
25. Hartley PJ, Keevil VL, Alushi L, et al. Earlier physical therapy input is associated with a reduced length of hospital stay and reduced care needs on discharge in frail older inpatients: An observational study. *J Geriatr Phys Ther.* 2019;42(2):E7–14.
26. de Morton N, Keating JL, Jeffs K. Exercise for acutely hospitalized older medical patients. *Cochrane Database Syst Rev.* 2007;(1):CD005955.
27. Waters D, Baumgartner R, Garry P, Vellas B. Advantages of dietary, exercise-related, and therapeutic interventions to prevent and treat sarcopenia in adult patients: An update. *Clin Interv Aging.* 2010;5:259–70.
28. Liu CJ, Latham NK. Progressive resistance strength training for improving physical function in older adults. *Cochrane Database Syst Rev.* 2009;2009(3):CD002759.
29. Young A. Exercise and physiology in geriatric practice. *Acta Med Scan Suppl.* 1986;711:227–32.
30. Nelson ME, Rejeski WJ, Blair SN, et al. Physical activity and public health in older adults: Recommendation from the American College of Sports Medicine and the American Heart Association. *Circulation.* 2007;116(9):1094–105.
31. https://www.healthypeople.gov/2020/topics-objectives/topic/older-adults/objectives.
32. Centers for Disease Control and Prevention, Administration on Aging, Agency for Healthcare Research and Quality, and Centers for Medicare and Medicaid Services. Enhancing Use of Clinical Preventive Services Among Older Adults. Washington, DC: AARP, 2011.
33. Qaseem A, Forciea MA, McLean RM, Denberg TD. Treatment of low bone density or osteoporosis to prevent fractures in men and women: A clinical practice guideline update from the American College of Physicians. *Ann Intern Med.* 2017;166:818–39.
34. Lusardi MM, Fritz S, Middleton A, et al. Determining risk of falls in community dwelling older adults: A systematic review and meta-analysis using posttest probability. *J Geriatr Phys Ther.* 2017;40(1):1–36.
35. Cheng MH, Chang SF. Frailty as a risk factor for falls among community dwelling people: Evidence from a meta-analysis. *J Nurs Scholarsh.* 2017;49:529–36.
36. https://www.uspreventiveservicestaskforce.org/uspstf/document/RecommendationStatementFinal/falls-prevention-in-older-adults-interventions.
37. Phelan EA, Aerts S, Dowler D, Eckstrom E, Casey CM. Adoption of evidence-based fall prevention practices in primary care for older adults with a history of falls. *Front Public Health.* 2016;4:190.
38. Gillespie LD, Gillespie WJ, Robertson MC, Lamb SE, Cumming RG, Rowe BH. Interventions for preventing falls in elderly people. *Cochrane Database Syst Rev.* 2003;4:CD000340.
39. Lin FR, Niparko JK, Ferrucci L. Hearing loss prevalence in the United States. *Arch Intern Med.* 2011;171(20):1851–2.
40. Crews JE, Campbell VA. Vision impairment and hearing loss among community-dwelling older Americans: Implications for health and functioning. *Am J Public Health.* 2004;94(5):823–9.
41. Feder RS, Olsen TW, Prum BEJr, et al. Comprehensive Adult Medical Eye Evaluation Preferred Practice Pattern(*) guidelines. *Ophthalmology.* 2016;123(1):P209–36.
42. Applegate WB, Miller ST, Elam JT, et al. Impact of cataract surgery with lens implantation on vision and physical function in elderly patients. *JAMA.* 1987;257:1064–6.
43. Taylor WD. Depression in the elderly. *N Engl J Med.* 2014;371:1228–36.
44. Siu AL, The US Preventive Services Task Force (USPSTF). Screening for depression in adults: US Preventive Services Task Force recommendation statement. *JAMA.* 2016;315(4):380–7.
45. Unutzer J, Katon W, Callahan C, et al. Collaborative care management of late-life depression in the primary care setting. *JAMA.* 2002;288:2836–45.
46. Plassman BL, Langa KM, Fisher GG, et al. Prevalence of dementia in the United States: The aging, demographics, and memory study. *Neuroepidemiology.* 2007;29(1-2):125–32.
47. Barnes DE, Beiser AS, Lee A, et al. Development and validation of a brief dementia screening indicator for primary care. *Alzheimers Dement.* 2014;10(6):656–65.e1.
48. Weimer DL, Sager MA. Early identification and treatment of Alzheimer's disease: Social and fiscal outcomes. *Alzheimers Dement.* 2009;5(3):215–26.
49. Trinr N, Hoblyn J, Mohanty S, et al. Efficacy of cholinesterase inhibiters in the treatment of neuropsychiatric symptoms and functional impairment in Alzheimer disease. A meta-analysis. *JAMA.* 2003;289:210–6.
50. Schiepers OJG, Köhler S, Deckers K, et al. Lifestyle for brain health (LIBRA): A new model for dementia prevention. *Int J Geriatr Psychiatry.* 2018;33:167–75.
51. Mace NL, Rabins PV. *The 36-Hour Day: A Family Guide to Caring for Persons with Alzheimer Disease.* Baltimore: Johns Hopkins University Press; 2011.
52. Law LL, Barnett F, Yau MK, Gray MA. Effects of combined cognitive and exercise interventions on cognition in older adults with and without cognitive impairment: A systematic review. *Ageing Res Rev.* 2014;15:61–75.
53. Park-Lee E, Sengupta M, Harris-Kojetin LD. Dementia special care units in residential care communities: United States, 2010. NCHS data brief, no 134. Hyattsville, MD: National Center for Health Statistics, 2013.
54. Barker WH, Mullooly JP. Stroke in a defined elderly population, 1967–1985. A less lethal and disabling but no less common disease. *Stroke.* 1997;28:284–90.
55. Dombovy ML. Rehabilitation and the course of recovery after stroke. In: Whisnant JP, ed. *Stroke: Populations, Cohorts, and Clinical Trials.* Oxford: Butterworth Heinemann; 1993, pp. 218–37.
56. Feigen VL, Roth GA, Parmar P, et al. Global burden of stroke and risk factors in 188 countries, during 1993–2010: A systematic analysis for the Global Burden of Disease Study 2013. *Lancet Neurol.* 2016;15:913–24.
57. Stroke Unit Trialists' Collaboration. Organised inpatient (stroke unit) care for stroke. Cochrane Database of Systematic Reviews 2013, Issue 9.
58. Lansberg MG, O'Donnell MJ, Khatri P, et al. Antithrombotic and thrombolytic therapy for ischemic stroke: Antithrombotic therapy and prevention of thrombosis, 9th ed: American College of Chest Physicians Evidence-Based Clinical Practice Guidelines. *Chest.* 2012;141(2 Suppl):e601S–36S.
59. Pringsheim T, Jette N, Frolkis A, Steeves TD. The prevalence of Parkinson's disease: A systematic review and meta-analysis. *Mov Disord.* 2014;29:1583–90.
60. Pahwa R, Factor SA, Lyons KE, et al. Practice parameter: Treatment of Parkinson disease with motor fluctuations and dyskinesia (an evidence-based review): Report of the Quality Standards Subcommittee of the American Academy of Neurology. *Neurology.* 2006;66:983–95.
61. Singer AE, Goebel JR, Kim YS, et al. Populations and interventions for palliative and end-of-life care: A systematic review. *J Palliat Med.* 2016;19(9):995–1008.
62. Parker SG, McCue P, Phelps K, et al. What is comprehensive geriatric assessment (CGA)? An umbrella review. *Age Aging.* 2018;47(1):149–55.
63. Ellis G, Gardner M, Tsiachristas A, et al. Comprehensive geriatric assessment for older adults admitted to hospital. *Cochrane Database Syst Rev.* 2017;9(9):CD006211.
64. Stuck AE, Siu AL, Wieland D, et al. Comprehensive geriatric assessment a meta-analysis of controlled trials. *Lancet.* 1993;342:1032–6.
65. Ellis G, Whitehead MA, O'Neill D, Langhorne P, Robinson D. Comprehensive geriatric assessment for older adults admitted to hospital. *Cochrane Database Syst Rev.* 2011;(7):CD006211.
66. Graf C. Functional decline in hospitalized older adults. *Am J Nurs.* 2006;106(1):58–67.
67. Rubenstein LZ, Josephson KR, Wieland GD, et al. Effectiveness of a geriatric evaluation unit: A randomized clinical trial. *N Engl J Med.* 1984;311:1664–70.
68. Rubenstein LZ, Josephson KR, Harker JO, et al. The Sepulveda GEU Study revisited: Long-term outcomes, uses of services, and costs. *Aging (Milano).* 1995;7(3):212–7.
69. Adunsky A, Lusky A, Arad M, Heruti RJ. A comparative study of rehabilitation outcomes of elderly hip fracture patients: The advantage of a comprehensive orthogeriatric approach. *J Gerontol.* 2003;58:M542–7.
70. Deschodt M, Braes T, Flamaing J, et al. Preventing delirium in older adults with recent hip fracture through multidisciplinary geriatric consultation. *J Am Geriatr Soc.* 2012;60:733–9.
71. Malone ML, Vollbrecht M, Stephenson J, et al. Acute care for elders (ACE) tracker and e-geriatrician: Methods to disseminate ACE concepts to hospitals with no geriatricians on staff. *J Am Geriatr Soc.* 2010;58(1):161–7.
72. Engel PA, Spencer J, Paul T, Boardman JB. The geriatrics in primary care demonstration: Integrating comprehensive geriatric care into the medical home: Preliminary data. *J Am Geriatr Soc.* 2016;64(4):875–9.
73. Day H, Eckstrom E, Lee S, et al. Optimizing health for complex adults in primary care: Current challenges and a way forward. *J Gen Intern Med.* 2014;29(6):911–4.

74. Tuepker A, Kansangara D, Skaperdas E, et al. "We've not gotten even close to what we want to do": A qualitative study of early patient-centered medical home implementation. *J Gen Intern Med.* 2014;29(Suppl 2):614–22.

75. Struck BD, Brown EA, Madison S. Advance care planning in the outpatient geriatric medicine setting. *Prim Care.* 2017;44(3):511–8.

76. Myers J, Cosby R, Gzik D, et al. Provider tools for advance care planning and goals of care discussions: A systematic review. *Am J Hosp Palliat Care.* 2018;35(8):1123–32.

77. Zhang B, Wright AA, Huskamp HA, et al. Health care costs in the last week of life: Associations with end-of-life conversations. *Arch Intern Med.* 2009;169(5):480–8.

78. Khandelwal N, Kross EK, Engelberg RA, Coe NB, Long AC, Curtis JR. Estimating the effect of palliative care interventions and advance care planning on ICU utilization: A systematic review. *Crit Care Med.* 2015;43(5):1102–11.

79. Kernick LA, Hogg KJ, Mellerick Y, Murtagh FEM, Djahit A, Johnson M. Does advance care planning in addition to usual care reduce hospitalisation for patients with advanced heart failure: A systematic review and narrative synthesis. *Palliat Med.* 2018;32(10):1539–51.

80. Starr LT, Ulrich CM, Corey KL, Meghani SM. Associations among end-of-life discussions, health-care utilization, and costs in persons with advanced cancer: A systematic review. *Am J Hosp Palliat Care.* 2019;36(10):913–26.

81. Teno JM, Gruneir A, Schwartz Z, Nanda A, Wetle T. Association between advance directives and quality of end-of-life care: A national study. J Am Geriatr Soc. 2007;55(2):189–94.

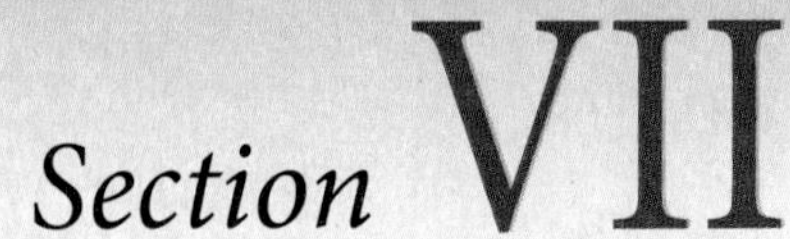

Section Editors
Jonathan Samet and Ana Navas-Acien

Environmental and Occupational Health

CHAPTER 62

Environmental and Occupational Exposures: Sources, Characteristics, Consequences, and Control

Jonathan M. Samet • Ana Navas-Acien

INTRODUCTION

This chapter introduces the range of environmental and occupational agents that affect human health, providing a foundation for the more focused chapters that follow. The significance of the environment for human health has long been recognized; writing in *On Airs, Waters, and Places*, Hippocrates commented around 400 BC that:

> Whoever wishes to investigate medicine properly, should proceed thus: in the first place to consider the seasons of the year, and what effects each of them produces for they are not at all alike, but differ much from themselves in regard to their changes. Then the winds, the hot and the cold, especially such as are common to all countries, and then such as are peculiar to each locality. We must also consider the qualities of the waters, for as they differ from one another in taste and weight, so also do they differ much in their qualities. (Part 1, Page 1)[1]

Here, Hippocrates considered physical location, climate, and water. Today's construct would be far broader and more embracing, considering not only the natural determinants of the environment but those related to human activities as they affect exposures of people and the health of ecosystems. In today's world, the sources of exposures are not only visible and local, but also invisible and global. In low- and middle-income countries and sometimes in high-income countries, sources of pollution can be identified by tell-tale smoke from factories and powerplants, motor vehicles, trash burning and waste incinerators, and biomass and heating oil burning.[2] Water and food pollution are also global threats, both from naturally occurring (e.g., arsenic in ground water) and anthropogenically generated (e.g., synthetic pesticides) agents. People may be inhaling pollution that has been generated in other countries and reaches them via a global journey, or ingesting long-lasting chemicals that persist in the environment, such as perfluorooctanoic acid (PFOA) and other per- and polyfluoroalkyl substances (PFAS). Persistent chemicals can travel long distances from water, soil, and waste pollution into food and bioaccumulate; they are also distributed globally through food packaging and industrial food production.

Construed broadly, environmental exposures include not only physical, biological, and chemical agents, but also the psychosocial stressors sustained in the places where people live and work, for example, the stress of living in a mega-city.[3] In addressing the overall health of populations, the totality of exposures needs consideration with an understanding of how they may act together. Thus, environmental health is broad and holistic and the cumulative load of environmental exposures is a key driver of population health. These environmental exposures comprise both involuntarily sustained exposures to pollutants, but also those consequent to personal actions and societal-level drivers. These exposures are one element of the array of factors driving health of individuals and populations, some reflecting the broad set of social determinants of health, including involuntarily imposed exposures that are externalities of polluting industries, and some reflecting the behaviors and choices of individuals.

In the twenty-first century, workplaces remain a critical venue for exposures that impact health. Many hazards are well known, including occupational carcinogens, for example, asbestos and radon progeny, dusts that cause lung disease, for example, coal dust and silica, toxic and irritating gases, for example, formaldehyde, and neurotoxicants, for example, lead and pesticides. Some exposures are inherent to particular occupations, for example, herbicides and agricultural workers, while some extend across diverse occupations and workplaces, for example, inducers of occupational asthma. In higher-income countries, workplace standards and practices control some exposures to levels that are considered to convey acceptable risk. Many occupational standards, however, are outdated or not properly implemented and too many cases of avoidable occupational disease continue to occur, such as coal workers' pneumoconiosis and silicosis.[4,5]

Looking globally, exposures to occupational agents persist at injury- and disease-causing levels. This persistence reflects the transfer of much "dirty" industry, such as steel production, ship-breaking, and recycling of electronic wastes, to low- and middle-income countries from high-income countries. New technologies, for example, electric car batteries and solar panels require a complex mix of metals, resulting in new extensive mining in Africa, Asia, and other regions with health implications for the miners and nearby communities. The scope of the resulting occupational exposures is uncertain, but a substantial burden of disease has been estimated for occupational exposures in low- and middle-income countries.[2]

For the purposes of monitoring, research, and control, assessments of exposure in the general environment and in workplaces are approached with a focus on particular sources, for example, powerplants or groundwater, or agents, for example, coal dust or smoke from biomass combustion. In many instances, research and control were motivated by catastrophic epidemics of disease, such as asbestosis in asbestos-exposed workers[6] and Minamata disease from methylmercury exposure in Japan,[7] or by extraordinary episodes of pollution with tragic consequences, such as the London Fog of 1952—an air pollution episode that caused at least 10,000 deaths over several weeks (see these and other historic environmental and occupational disasters in Box 62-1).[8] Emerging environmental health problems may also be identified through biomonitoring, now possible through analyses of blood or other biosamples collected in surveys or for other purposes. For example, blood lead levels in U.S. children have been tracked for decades; the monitoring documented the beneficial impact of removing lead from gasoline and the persistence of unacceptably high blood lead levels in some children, especially in disadvantaged communities related to drinking water

BOX 62-1 Historic Pollution Episodes with Tragic Consequences

- **1912: Itai-itai (*It Hurts-It Hurts*) Disease**: Mass cadmium poisoning (bone deformities, anemia, and kidney failure) occurring in Toyama Prefecture, Japan due to zinc mining polluting the Jinzū River, which was used for rice fields, drinking water, and other needs by the local population.
- **1924: Asbestosis:** The first case of asbestosis was published in the medical literature in 1923 but it was not until 1931 that asbestosis was recognized on a medical and judicial basis. Several tens of millions of workers have been exposed to asbestos in the United States alone, with thousands of cases of mesothelioma being diagnosed each year.
- **1935: Gauley Bridge Disaster:** Around 1500 workers, most of them African American, died of silicosis due to serious silica pollution and lack of protection during tunnel construction in Gauley Bridge, West Virginia.
- **1952: London Fog:** Severe air pollution event affecting London from December 5 to 9, 1952 causing at least 4000 deaths during those days.
- **1956: Minamata Disease:** Neurological disease caused by severe methylmercury poisoning first described in 1956. The outbreak was related to the release of contaminated wastewater from a chemical factory into Minamata Bay, Japan, which continued from 1932 to 1968 and the bioaccumulation of methylmercury in seafood that was consumed by the local population.
- **1958: Antofagasta Arsenic Outbreak:** A population with more than 130,000 inhabitants in Northern Chile was exposed to arsenic in drinking water at 900 µg/L for 12 years resulting in increased cancer and cardiovascular risk, especially for those exposed during early life.
- **1976: Seveso Accident:** Accident in a chemical manufacturing plant in Italy resulting in the highest known exposure to 2,3,7,8-tetrachlorodibenzo-p-dioxin (TCDD) in general populations. Exposed population suffered from chloracne (skin lesions), increased cancer risk, and increased cardiovascular risk, and lower sperm counts.
- **1982: Bhopal Accident:** Accident at a pesticide plant in India resulted in the release of 45 tons of methyl isocyanate. Thousands died in hours. Other health effects were blindness, organ failure, and birth defects affecting half a million people.
- **1986: Chernobyl Accident:** Worst nuclear-power-plant disaster in history. Large amounts of radiation were released into the atmosphere affecting large parts of Europe and resulting in thousands of death from acute radiation syndrome and cancer.

contamination and lead paint in old housing. In 1999, the Centers for Disease Prevention and Control (CDC) substantially expanded the national biomonitoring program, with hundreds of environmental chemicals assessed annually in representative samples of the noninstitutionalized U.S. population, in the National Health and Nutrition Examination Survey (NHANES).[9]

Research on environmental and occupational agents typically incorporates three approaches: (1) basic research on the mechanisms by which an agent might cause injury and disease; (2) toxicology testing involving in vitro systems, animals, and in some instances humans to assess short-term and long-term consequences of exposure; and (3) epidemiological studies of exposed populations to characterize the health consequences of exposures, including clinical disease. Each approach has well-known strengths and limitations. Mechanistic research is fundamental, but probing for mechanisms pushes ever deeper as scientific methods advance, as with today's omics methodologies. A full mechanistic understanding is not necessary, however, for implementation of control measures. Toxicological approaches, particularly those involving animals, may have uncertain relevance for humans, and experimental exposures of people to agents can only examine short-term effects and cannot pose unacceptable and permanent risks. There is a trend away from assessing toxicity in animal models and increasing reliance on various methods for in vitro testing of compounds.[10]

Epidemiological research is subject to the well-known problems of confounding by other factors and bias from measurement problems and the selection of the study population. However, only epidemiological studies provide information on health risks directly from exposed people. Beyond these three principal lines of investigation, natural experiments based on documented changes in exposures (e.g., strict air pollution control during the Beijing Olympic Games in 2008,[11] or arsenic remediation in Atofagasta, Chile[12]) provide unique opportunities to investigate the health impacts of reducing exposures and to "validate in reverse" the findings of epidemiologic studies directed at characterizing how risk increases with exposure. Randomized clinical trials based on exposure prevention or mitigation, are also possible, although such trials are typically expensive and challenging to carry out (e.g., the RESPIRE trial in Guatemala, which involved randomization to a low-emission cooking stove to reduce exposure to household air pollution[13]). Natural experiments and randomized trials, when possible, can be useful for developing and assessing the impact of preventive interventions.

The findings of research on the hazard posed by an agent, that is, is there an adverse effect, in combination with an understanding of the distribution of exposure and of potential interventions and their effectiveness are the foundation for evidence-based environmental management and regulation.[14] Together, hazard and exposure (what are the levels of exposure and who is exposed) determine the risk to a population. An assessment of risk is often a starting point for controlling a hazard by providing understanding of the risk posed and its distribution among groups within the population.[14] In some regulatory contexts, a comprehensive risk assessment may be required.

Most occupational and environmental health problems are managed at the local, state, or national levels through regulations and other policy measures. Some environmental problems might require interventions other than regulation and policy measures, either because of lack of authority to regulate (e.g., private wells in the United States are not regulated) or because regulation is unlikely to be successful (e.g., the generally unachievable European food safety standard for arsenic in rice[15,16]). In the presence of regulation, monitoring may be requisite to assurance compliance and to support enforcement. Exposure monitoring can be useful also in the absence of regulation, to identify more highly exposed population subgroups in need of interventions. As a general principle, the intent of regulations is to protect against exposures that lead to an unacceptable likelihood of adverse effects. For most agents, regulation takes place at the national level, but for some agents, global agreements are needed, such as the Vienna Convention for the Protection of the Ozone Layer targeting chlorofluorocarbons and the UN Framework Convention on Climate Change.[17,18]

SOURCES OF CONTAMINATION

The sources of exposure are myriad, described by a matrix that includes locations and the media into which the pollutants are emitted and by which people are exposed. Exposure media can be grouped into air, water, and food along with delivered energy—ionizing and nonionizing radiation, heat, and noise, for example. The circumstances of exposure may also be critical, for example, light exposure at night has been classified as carcinogenic by the International Agency for Research on Cancer (IARC).[19,20] Viewed across the environments where people spend time, sources are myriad and many go unrecognized by the people exposed. Some sources can be far removed, even residing in other countries, and unrecognized by the exposed individuals. For example, homeowners may not recognize that stored paints and solvents in garages may be contaminating the air in the home or that radon, a colorless, odorless, and invisible gaseous carcinogen may be present at high levels. Similarly, lead sources in homes, including drinking water from lead pipes, lead paints, and lead-containing dust, may not be recognized.

Outdoor sources of airborne pollutants can be conveniently classified as stationary, powerplants and industry, and mobile—vehicles, airplanes, and boats. Sources of water pollution, from the human exposure perspective, can be classified as affecting drinking water (central water systems or private wells) or recreational water (beaches, lakes, and rivers). These sources can be contaminated by industrial and municipal waste and storm-water runoff, which can be a source of drinking water and recreational water; soil and food may be contaminated by waste and storm water as well. Soil pollution can also be a relevant direct source of exposure for children and for people involved in certain occupations and leisure time activities, such as gardening. Soil pollution is also a major source of food contamination.

CONCEPTS OF EXPOSURE

Overview

In approaching occupational and environmental health problems, an understanding of how potentially hazardous agents come into contact with people is critical, along with the extent of the contact.[3] The general terminology refers to the *source(s)* from which contaminant emissions originate; *concentration(s)* of the agent in the media (i.e., air, water, and food) through which human contact occurs; *exposure(s) measures* that integrate concentration and the time spent at the particular concentration; *route* of exposure (inhalation, ingestion, dermal, mucosai, parenteral, transplacental); and *dose(s)* referring to the amount of material entering into the body and reaching target organs. These concepts have long been employed but have been updated as the field of exposure sciences has advanced.

For example, for an airborne contaminant, the strength of emissions from the sources can be measured, for example, emissions of particles or nitrogen oxides. The emissions contaminate the surrounding air with the pollutants at concentrations that depend on a variety of physical and meteorological factors. Exposure occurs when people inhale the contaminated air. Exposure is calculated for air pollutants as the product of the pollutant concentration in the place(s) where time is spent with the amount of time spent in that place. For example, a person working outdoors at a concentration of particulate matter (PM) less than 2.5 microns in aerodynamic diameter (so-called $PM_{2.5}$) of 100 μg/m^3 for 8 hours would have an exposure of 800 μg/m^3-hrs.

The concept of total personal exposure is central to characterizing the risks of environmental contaminants whether in workplaces or general environmental contexts.[3] For inhaled pollutants, total personal exposure to a pollutant reflects the concentrations in the various places where time is spent, weighted by the time spent in each. The time domain for consideration of exposure depends on the dynamics of the underlying processes of injury; for some exposures, for example, carbon monoxide, a brief timeframe is relevant for some adverse health effects while for others, for example, air pollution and cancer, a longer time domain is appropriate. For contaminated food and water, total personal exposure would reflect the total intake across foods and beverages. For some agents, for example, lead, exposure could be sustained by several media, inhaling air contaminated by lead from industrial processes and lead dust, drinking lead-containing water, and eating lead-contaminated foods or paint chips (e.g., through pica, which is common in children).

For environmental chemicals present in multiple media and incorporated into the body through different routes (e.g., inorganic and organic chemicals), biomarkers of the original compound and its metabolites, if available, are critical to assess total personal exposure and are often used as markers of internal dose. For chemicals that are not quickly excreted from the body (e.g., metals such as cadmium and lead, and persistent organic chemicals), information on cumulative exposure and the resulting body burden is relevant to risk for long-term health effects. Cumulative exposure for some agents of this type can be assessed through biomarkers with long half-life. For chemicals with short half-lives in the body, assessing cumulative exposure is more challenging and requires full knowledge of different sources of exposure, the concentrations of the agent in the source/media, and the duration of exposure. For example, for cumulative exposure to arsenic in water, information is needed on all drinking water sources to which a person has been exposed over the lifetime, the arsenic concentrations in each water source, and the years of exposure to each water source (often reported as μg/L-years). Cumulative exposure data are important as risk assessment is often conducted assuming lifetime exposure to a particular concentration.

The microenvironmental model is a useful construct for inhaled agents. A microenvironment is a place where time is spent that has a particular pollutant concentration profile during the time spent there; for example, a motor vehicle represents a microenvironment during time spent commuting. A microenvironment with a high concentration of pollution, such as an urban street "canyon" (i.e., a street hemmed in by buildings), could make a substantial contribution to total exposure, even if only a brief time were spent there. This model is useful for considering the numerous microenvironments relevant to air pollution and associated risks to health, and how characteristics of the environment determine exposures. The residence is particularly important because most people spend the majority of time at home, and there are indoor sources of air pollution and the pollutants in outdoor air penetrate into homes. In urban areas, the air contaminants in the home include those generated by indoor sources, such as cooking and smoking of tobacco, and the penetration of outdoor air pollutants indoors, including pollutants such as particles and carbon monoxide generated by local traffic. The streets, which may have "hot spots" of air pollution generated by traffic or industrial sources, are another key and distinct microenvironment.

The microenvironment model is also useful for water pollution, as people drink water in different settings, at home and work and in the homes of others and also consume bottled water. They can be exposed to water pollution through different activities beyond drinking water such as cooking, washing teeth, showering, and bathing, and through recreational activities. The contribution of food pollution to exposure to environmental agents is particularly challenging to assess, given the complexities of food consumption patterns, the variable chemical concentrations in different foods and even in the same foods, and the difficulties of accurately assessing food intake both on average (through food frequency questionnaires) and recently (through dietary recalls). For that reason, a comprehensive assessment of intake of contaminated food is particularly challenging, and often we need to rely on biomarkers, with the caveats that the same agents may be present in other sources distinct from food.

The timing of exposure across the life course is highly influential in susceptibility to injury and the extent of injury and also long-term implications. Age at first exposure is particularly critical. Exposure in early life (*in utero* and during the first years of life) can affect risk for adult-onset disease, in particular diabetes and cardiovascular disease but also cancer and other health outcomes. This concept is known as the *Developmental Origin of Health and Disease* (DOHAD).[21] Depending on the agent and the timing of exposure, the health consequences can be different. Especially sensitive periods are known as "windows of susceptibility," including pregnancy, early development, adolescence, and other periods. Other concepts connected with the timing of exposure include the time since first and last exposure (which are useful for exposures with finite durations) and latency (which might require lagging to identify the critical timing of exposure for disease development).

A GENERAL EXPOSURE MODEL

Figure 62-1 presents a general schema of exposure that is integrative in setting out sources and their drivers, time-activity patterns of people, and the exposures that result.[3] Moving through the diagram, the left-most side sets out sources, including the upstream drivers of exposures, that is, factors determining the types of sources, their locations, the intensity and duration of exposures, and the control measures used. Construed broadly, the upstream drivers reach across the range of social determinants of health; for example, in many urban locales, industrial sources are located more densely in poorer neighborhoods as are heavily trafficked roadways, increasing exposures to noise and air pollution.

Moving to the right, contact with the agent and the intensity of exposure are driven by what is released into the environment and how people interact with the environment, as determined by time-activity patterns, that is, the places where people spend time and the amount of time spent in these locations and corresponding microenvironments. Pollution concentrations in some locations may be temporally and spatially dynamic, such as on the sidewalks of busy streets where stalled traffic may result in "hot spots" that may be cleared by wind. For water exposures, concentrations can be constant over time (e.g., naturally occurring contaminants in groundwater such as arsenic) but highly heterogeneous spatially, with completely different concentrations in adjacent wells in the same localized geographic area.

The concept of exposure (the diagram's middle) has been broadened to encompass contact of people with agents, whether external to the body or internally incorporated. Examples of external exposures include noise and radiation while lead is an exposure that is internally incorporated. As captured by the diagram, environmental agents enter the body and interact with critical receptors in various organs that drive processes leading to injury, ill health, and disease. Here, the dose refers to the materials reaching the targeted receptors. Some stressors act more generally, such as psychological stress, which may affect health through the various mechanisms underlying the stress response. At the far right, "outcomes" refers to the consequences of pollutant exposures, comprising a broad array of adverse effects, some transitory, for example, exacerbation of asthma or increased coughing, and some long-term and irreversible, for example, development of lung cancer.

The concept of the "exposome" has been proposed to capture the breadth of exposures and the need to characterize them across the life course in order to fully understand how the environment affects health.[3] The characterization of the exposome draws on emerging measurement methods, such as metabolomics, in combination with the long-standing approaches described above. While still aspirational, the concept of the exposome is a useful reminder of the need to integrate the totality of environmental exposures to fully characterize how the environment affects health.

METHODS FOR EXPOSURE ASSESSMENT

The assessment of environmental exposures for research, monitoring, or control purposes can be challenging due to multiple sources; variation in intensity, duration, and frequency of exposure; the diversity of exposures and their frequent presence as elements of complex mixtures; the impact of human behavior on exposures; timing of exposures and of their consequences over time; and technical and laboratory challenges along with measurement error and misclassification.[3] These problems are well known and typically considered carefully in developing exposure measurement strategies and in interpreting and applying the results.

There are multiple approaches to assess exposures, such that an exposure assessment strategy is tailored to be fit for its purpose. For example, to assess the beneficial impact of an environmental policy, documenting that the environmental concentration of the agent has declined may be sufficient. To assess the health effects of a particular agent in an epidemiological study, a comprehensive strategy might be needed to estimate total personal exposure at the individual level. For risk assessment, more complex modeling of exposure–dose relationships might be needed, along with a description of exposure at the population level.

Approaches for exposure assessment (Table 62-1) can be classified as methods that quantify personal exposure (through personal monitoring, biomonitoring, or questionnaires/diaries), methods that quantify exposure in the environments (water, air, food) of the residence, community, or site of activity (environmental measures), and indirect methods that do not directly assess the agent of interest (e.g., job title, community of residence, duration of exposure, distance from exposure). In addition, exposure models and dose (toxicokinetic) models

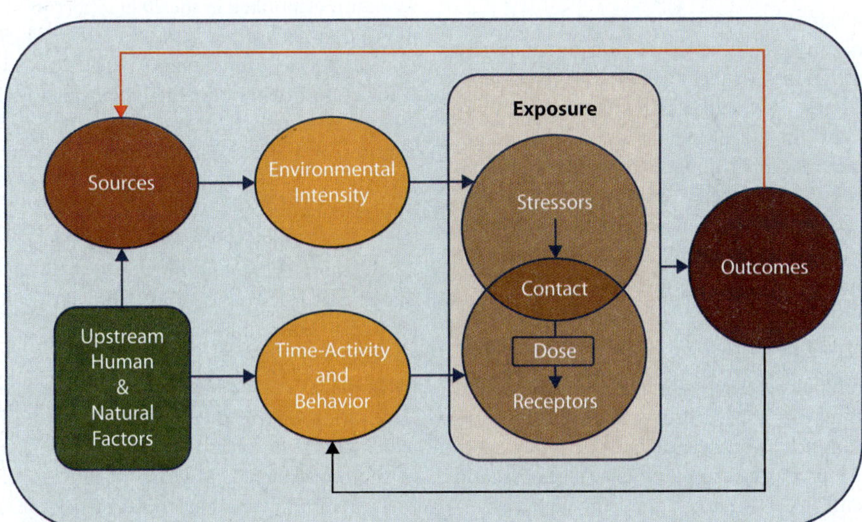

FIGURE 62-1. Conceptual framework showing the core elements of exposure science as related to humans and ecosystems. (*Source:* Reproduced with permission from National Research Council, Committee On Human And Environmental Exposure Science In The 21st Century, Board on Environmental Studies and Toxicology, Division on Earth and Life Studies. Exposure science in the 21st century: a vision and a strategy. Washington, D.C.: National Academies Press; 2012.[3])

TABLE 62-1 METHODS FOR EXPOSURE ASSESSMENT

Goal of Exposure Assessment	Method
Quantify personal exposure	• Personal monitoring • Biomonitoring • Questionnaires/diaries
Quantify exposure in the environment	• Water, air, food monitoring in different environments (home, work, leisure time, community, site of activity)
Indirect methods	• Job title, community of residence, duration of exposure, distance from exposure, etc.
Modeling approaches	• Exposure models (e.g., air pollution models) • Dose models, also called toxicokinetic models (e.g., PBPK)

are also useful to estimate exposures and doses. Over time, such models have become increasingly sophisticated and comprehensive as relevant data sets have become larger and more far-reaching and computing power has grown rapidly. For example, global models for estimating concentrations of PM air pollution are now widely utilized; they integrate available monitoring and source data with satellite and meteorological data. More generally, models of environmental exposures may combine environmental monitoring, questionnaire data, and other information to estimate exposure levels in the environment. A mathematical or statistical model is then developed that has a structure based in understanding of the underlying processes. If possible, a model should be validated against actual data and its sensitivity to key assumptions assessed to gain understanding of the uncertainty in the estimates.

Dose models, also called toxicokinetic models or compartmental models, may also be used to estimate internal doses delivered to key target sites. They are formulated mathematically using systems of differential equations, with one equation representing each of the compartments in the system (generally an organ/tissue, e.g., blood, liver, or kidney). Multicompartmental models are called physiologically based pharmacokinetic models (PBPK). Parameters represent absorption potential, blood flow rates, organ volumes, and other system components. These models are often used in risk assessment.

MECHANISMS OF INJURY

Environmental and occupational agents can cause injury and disease in virtually every organ system. The resulting health problems and diseases are covered in specific chapters in this section. Broadly, the disease-causing processes can be classified as (1) inflammation and oxidative stress; (2) sensitization; (3) carcinogenesis; (4) teratogenesis; and (5) psychological stress. Within these broad categories, there are diverse mechanisms and there are overlaps among the categories. For example, there are multiple hallmarks of a carcinogen and inflammation is considered as a nonspecific driver of carcinogenesis. Immune sensitization can occur through different components of the immune system. An understanding of possible mechanisms is fundamental to developing research approaches and also to consideration of disease prevention and control.

Adverse Outcomes

The range of adverse health outcomes relevant to environmental and occupational agents is extensive and reflective of the broad array of exposures and the multiplicity of processes by which they cause adverse effects. The injury processes caused by environmental and occupational agents extend to all organ systems. The adverse outcomes of environmental and occupational exposures are extensive, extending to essentially all organ systems. The outcomes range from subtle indications of injury detected through biomarkers to overt disease and death. The list is encompassing and includes diseases related specifically to particular exposures, for example, silica and the lung disease silicosis, and also multifactorial diseases, including cardiovascular diseases and metabolic diseases. Environmental and occupational agents may also accelerate age-related declines of organ function, including loss of lung function with aging and neurocognitive decline.

With the availability of biomarkers and sensitive measures of structure and function that can find indication that injury is in progress as well as early changes, for example, lung function testing, heart rhythm monitoring, and CT imaging of organs, questions have been raised, particularly in the regulatory context, as to what constitutes an "adverse health effect."[22] This question has been repeatedly raised around the health consequences of outdoor air pollution and guidance has been elaborated. For example, ground-level ozone causes transient reduction of lung function in some susceptible individuals at concentrations common in cities in the United States. In rulemaking, the significance of such transient changes has been discussed extensively, leading to the issuance of guidance by the major scientific societies concerned with respiratory health.[22]

Assessing Risks

Risk assessment often plays a foundational role in determining the necessity of implementing prevention and control measures, the stringency of such measures, and the targeting of strategies. The current general approach for risk assessment in the United States was defined decades ago in a landmark 1983 report of the National Research Council, widely known as "the Red Book" (National Research Council (NRC) and Committee on the Institutional Means for Assessment of Risks to Public Health, 1983). The Red Book described four elements to a risk assessment:

- Hazard identification: Is a hazard posed by the exposure?
- Exposure assessment: What is the distribution of the exposure?
- Dose-response assessment: How does risk vary with exposure (or dose)?
- Risk characterization: What is the extent of the risk to the population and what are the uncertainties in the characterization of risk?

Thus, a full quantitative risk assessment provides an understanding of whether an occupational or environmental agent poses a hazard and how the resulting risk is distributed within the exposed population. Since the 1983 Red Book, the formalism of risk assessment has been elaborated to more fully account for stakeholder engagement and to assure that the questions addressed are those needing to be answered for regulatory, policy, and other purposes. Most recently, this framework was elaborated in the 2009 report from the National Academies of Science: *Science and Decisions: Advancing Risk Assessment.*[14]

Globally, environmental exposure assessments, evidence on the association of environmental exposures with health outcomes, and data on disease burden have been combined to estimate how much disease can be prevented by reducing or eliminating environmental exposures. This information is critical for decision-making and implementation by healthcare providers, policy makers, and public health practitioners. The World Health Organization (WHO), in its 2016 report *Preventing disease through healthy environments* estimated that in 2012, 12.6 million deaths globally, representing 23% (95% confidence interval 13–34%) of all deaths, were attributable to the environment.[23] To account for years of life lost due to mortality as well as years of productive life lost due to disability, the WHO also uses a metric called Disability Adjusted Life Years (DALYs), which combines years lived with disability considering the severity of the impairment and years of life lost. The WHO has estimated that 22% (95% confidence interval 13–32%) of the disease burden, summarized in DALYs, is attributable to modifiable environmental exposures.[23] The WHO used several approaches including comparative risk assessment (CRA) methods, epidemiologic data, transmission pathways, and expert judgment derived data to estimate these figures. CRA methods include detailed exposure and exposure-risk information data and are considered the highest level of evidence. In a separate global effort, the Institute for Health Metrics Evaluation (IHME) has estimated that disease caused by all forms of pollution was responsible for 9 million premature deaths in 2015 (16% total mortality) and 268 million DALYs (254 million years of life lost and 14 million years lived with disability).[24] These efforts by WHO and IHME are thus consistent that pollution is a major cause of disease, disability, and premature mortality, while differences between estimates can be explained by different definitions of pollution/environmental exposures, which was broader for WHO.[2]

Susceptibility and Vulnerability

The concepts of susceptibility and vulnerability are also critical to public health and occupational and environmental agents. While the terms are sometimes used interchangeably, we consider susceptibility to represent increased risk at a particular level of exposure among those who are susceptible compared with those who are not. Vulnerability refers to an increased likelihood of exposure or of higher exposure compared with those who are not vulnerable. Numerous factors are potential determinants of susceptibility: the presence of underlying chronic diseases, such as asthma or diabetes, genetic factors, and other exposures that act synergistically with an agent, example, cigarette smoking, and radon progeny. Among beryllium-exposed workers, genetics are a strong determinant of risk for chronic beryllium disease.[25]

The concept of vulnerability is closely tied to environmental justice, a higher burden of environmental exposures for those with less favorable socioeconomic circumstances. The Environmental Protection Agency defines environmental justice as: "Environmental justice is the fair treatment and meaningful involvement of all people regardless of race, color, national origin, or income, with respect to the development, implementation, and enforcement of environmental laws, regulations, and policies."[26] It is directed at reducing the burden of exposures that affects particular populations, often driven by socioeconomic status, race, or ethnicity. An extensive literature documents disparities in environmental exposures.[27–30]

Summary

Myriad environmental and occupational exposures affect human health, and may also harm ecosystems, indirectly harming public health. This chapter provides a general framework for considering how such exposures affect human health, reviewing foundational concepts of exposure, response, hazard and risk, and vulnerability and susceptibility. Subsequent chapters in this section build on this introduction.

References

1. Hippocrates. *On Airs, Waters, and Places*. 400 BC.
2. Landrigan PJ, Fuller R, Acosta NJR, et al. The Lancet Commission on pollution and health. *Lancet*. 2018;391(10119):462–512.
3. National Research Council, Committee On Human And Environmental Exposure Science in the 21st Century, Board on Environmental Studies and Toxicology, Division on Earth and Life Studies. *Exposure Science in the 21st Century: A Vision and a Strategy*. Washington, DC: National Academies Press; 2012.
4. Blackley DJ, Halldin CN, Laney AS. Continued increase in prevalence of coal workers' pneumoconiosis in the United States, 1970–2017. *Am J Public Health*. 2018;108(9):1220–2.
5. Mazurek JM, Wood JM, Schleiff PL, Weissman DN. Surveillance for silicosis deaths among persons aged 15–44 Years—United States, 1999–2015. *MMWR Morb Mortal Wkly Rep*. 2017;66(28):747.
6. Becklake MR. Exposure to asbestos and human disease. *N Engl J Med*. 1982;306(24):1480–2.
7. Yorifuji T, Tsuda T, Takao S, Harada M. Long-term exposure to methylmercury and neurologic signs in Minamata and neighboring communities. *Epidemiology (Cambridge, Mass)*. 2008;19(1):3–9.
8. Logan WP. Mortality in the London fog incident, 1952. *Lancet*. 1953;1(6755):336–8.
9. Prevention CfDCa. National Report on Human Exposure to Environmental Chemicals. 2017; Prevention of Childhood Lead Toxicity | From the American. Accessed October 8, 2019.
10. National Academies of Sciences Engineering and Medicine. Division on Earth and Life Studies, Board on Environmental Studies and Toxicology, Committee on Incorporating 21st Century Science into Risk-Based Evaluations. Using 21st Century Science to Improve Risk-Related Evaluations. Washington, DC: National Academies Press; 2017.
11. Rich DQ, Liu K, Zhang J, et al. Differences in birth weight associated with the 2008 Beijing Olympics air pollution reduction: Results from a natural experiment. *Environ Health Perspect*. 2015;123(9):880–7.
12. Roh T, Steinmaus C, Marshall G, Ferreccio C, Liaw J, Smith AH. Age at exposure to arsenic in water and mortality 30–40 years after exposure cessation. *Am J Epidemiol*. 2018;187(11):2297–305.
13. Smith KR, McCracken JP, Weber MW, et al. Effect of reduction in household air pollution on childhood pneumonia in Guatemala (RESPIRE): A randomised controlled trial. *Lancet*. 2011;378(9804):1717–26.
14. National Research Council. *Science and Decisions: Advancing Risk Assessment*. Washington, DC: National Academies Press; 2009.
15. Panel EC. Scientific opinion on arsenic in food. *EFSA J*. 2009;7(10):1351.
16. European Food Safety Authority. Dietary exposure to inorganic arsenic in the European population. *EFSA J*. 2014;12(3):3597.
17. United Nations. Vienna Convention for the Protection of the Ozone Layer. In. Vol. 1513. Vienna: United Nations; 1985:293.
18. United Nations. United Nations Framework Convention on Climate Change. 2019. https://unfccc.int/. Accessed January 24, 2019.
19. Ward EM, Germolec D, Kogevinas M, et al. Carcinogenicity of night shift work. *Lancet Oncol*. 2019;20(8):1058–9.
20. International Agency for Research on Cancer. *Painting, Firefighting, and Shiftwork*. Lyon, France: International Agency for Research on Cancer; 2010.
21. Wadhwa PD, Buss C, Entringer S, Swanson JM. Developmental origins of health and disease: Brief history of the approach and current focus on epigenetic mechanisms. *Semin Reprod Med*. 2009;27(5):358–68.
22. Thurston GD, Kipen H, Annesi-Maesano I, et al. A joint ERS/ATS policy statement: What constitutes an adverse health effect of air pollution? An analytical framework. *Eur Respir J*. 2017;49(1):1600419.
23. Prüss-Üstün A, Wolf J, Corvalán C, Bos R, Neira M. *Preventing Disease through Healthy Environments: A Global Assessment of the Burden of Disease from Environmental Risks*. Geneva: World Health Organization; 2016.
24. GBD 2015 Risk Factors Collaborators. Global, regional, and national comparative risk assessment of 79 behavioural, environmental and occupational, and metabolic risks or clusters of risks, 1990–2015: A systematic analysis for the Global Burden of Disease Study 2015. *Lancet*. 2016;388(10053):1659–724.
25. Balmes JR, Abraham JL, Dweik RA, et al. An official American Thoracic Society statement: Diagnosis and management of beryllium sensitivity and chronic beryllium disease. *Am J Respir Crit Care Med*. 2014;190(10):e34–59.
26. U.S. Environmental Protection Agency. Environmental Justice. 2019; https://www.epa.gov/environmentaljustice. Accessed December 11, 2019.
27. Brulle RJ, Pellow DN. Environmental justice: Human health and environmental inequalities. *Annu Rev Public Health*. 2006;27:103–24.
28. Taylor DA. Is environmental health a basic human right? Environ Health Perspect. 2004; 112(17):A1006–9.
29. Lee C. Environmental justice: Building a unified vision of health and the environment. *Environ Health Perspect*. 2002;110(suppl 2):141–4.
30. Cole LW, Foster SR. *From the Ground up: Environmental Racism and the Rrise of the Environmental Justice Movement*. Vol. 34. New York: NYU Press; 2001.

CHAPTER

63 Exposures and Their Assessment, Including General and Occupational Environments

Kirsten Koehler • Ana M. Rule • Lesliam Quirós-Alcalá

WHAT IS EXPOSURE ASSESSMENT?

An exposure assessment is a comprehensive evaluation of how an individual or a population comes into contact with one or more potentially hazardous agents or stressors of concern. The agent or stressor can be any biological, chemical, or physical entity that can cause or induce an adverse response and will hereafter be referred to as an "agent." The exposure is thus the concentration or amount of the agent that comes into contact with a host over a relevant time scale. When defining an exposure, it is important to define three dimensions of exposure: (1) the exposure level (i.e., the concentration or intensity); (2) the duration of the exposure (i.e., how long someone is exposed to the agent); and (3) the frequency of exposure (i.e., how often the exposure occurs over some time scale of interest). It is common to think of "exposure" only in terms of the exposure level or concentration, but in order to appropriately characterize an agent's potential health effects, all three dimensions must be considered over an appropriate time scale. The appropriate time scale depends on the pathogenesis and natural history of the health outcome of concern. For example, for an acute response (e.g., allergic response such as dermal irritation or asthma exacerbation), the time scale of exposure may be short (minutes to days), but for chronic health effects (e.g., cancer), the time scale may be much longer (years to decades). Additionally, for some agents, the timing of when exposures occur should be considered. Exposures during critical windows of development, including during the preconception, prenatal, and childhood or adolescence periods may merit particular attention as these could result in long-lasting health impacts. For example, exposures to organophosphate (OP) pesticides during the prenatal period, have been linked to poorer cognition and behavior problems in children. Gestational age and dose are important determinants for potential adverse effects in the offspring.[1]

To appropriately characterize total exposure, it is necessary to consider all possible routes of exposure: inhalation, direct (e.g., contaminated foods, breastmilk, beverages) and indirect (e.g., hand-to-mouth activity) ingestion, skin or mucosal absorption, injection, and the transplacental route (in the case of a fetus). It is common to consider these routes separately, due to different sources of the agent or different activities undertaken by an individual that result in exposure to a given agent. A complete estimation of exposure would include all routes (i.e., aggregate exposure); however, methods of exposure assessment are most advanced for inhalation exposures and will be the focus of much of this chapter.

Domains of Exposure

Once the dimensions and possible routes of exposure have been determined, an exposure assessment can be planned. Exposures can be assessed in two domains: ecological or population level, or personal, that is, for an individual. Each approach has strengths and weaknesses, depending on the context and the purpose. Ecological estimates involve exposure assessment that is done for groups of people based on a common location, activity, or source. Such assessments are typically accomplished through area environmental monitoring that is intended to be representative of exposures for individuals in the target population. For example, in the United States, each state is required to monitor air pollutants to characterize exposures for those individuals living in the states who are exposed to air pollution.

Personal exposures, on the other hand, are assessed with consideration of the microenvironmental model, giving consideration to where people spend time and the concentrations of pollutants of interest in the various microenvironments, that is, places having particular characteristics and concentrations of agents. One approach is to make direct measurements of exposure by having individuals carry personal sampling equipment as they go about their daily tasks. Such personal exposures to air pollutants are often considered the "gold standard" because the estimates account for the specific activities undertaken by the individual. However, because each individual's activities (and the exposure level associated with each activity) tend to vary from day to day, the variability in exposures among repeated measures for a single individual can be as large or larger than the variability observed between individuals.

There are also cost considerations. Personal exposure assessment is generally more resource intensive and expensive compared to ecological estimates and may be unfeasible for assessing exposures among large populations. Ecological estimates are often preferable when estimates of exposures are needed for large numbers of people. These estimates are more likely to be expressed as simply the exposure level, without careful consideration of the frequency or duration of exposure, as these parameters would vary between individuals. One approach is to carry out nested personal sampling within a larger population to more fully characterize exposure and to have validation data available for the population-level estimates. Biomarkers of exposure (see below) can be another informative approach for characterizing both individual- and population-level exposures.

Exposome

An emerging concept in the field of exposure assessment is the exposome: the idea that the totality of human environmental exposures (i.e., nongenetic), both internal and external, from conception to death can be assessed.[2–4] The exposome is intended to conceptually complement the human genome. The goal of exposome projects is to measure the cumulative imprint of environmental influences and the associated biological responses throughout the lifespan using an array of tools.[3,5–8] It is envisioned that exposome measurements would include exposures from the environment, diet, behavior (e.g., psychosocial stressors that may be independent risk factors for adverse effects and physical activity), and endogenous processes. To measure all cumulative exposures will require bringing together many different technologies and measurement methods, which should encompass: (1) the internal exposome including the microbiome, and markers of inflammation and oxidative stress, (2) the external exposures including chemical, physical, and biological agents arising from indoor and outdoor environments, including occupational and lifestyle factors, and (3) the social, economic, ecological, and psychological factors that can affect risks and outcomes for chronic diseases.[9] A holistic exposome assessment would likely use advanced and novel technologies including metabolomics, proteomics, epigenetics, and transcriptomics, in addition to the more commonly considered exposure assessments discussed in this chapter, potentially resulting in thousands of measurements per person. Analytical and statistical methods to use high-density exposome data for human health studies are in development.

WHY CONDUCT AN EXPOSURE ASSESSMENT?

Exposure is often measured to assess compliance with a governmental regulation. However, exposure may also be assessed for research purposes to evaluate whether there is a health concern in an occupational group or target community (e.g., general population; susceptible groups of concern defined by select characteristics such as age or race; communities in close proximity to an exposure source of concern).

Environmental Compliance

In the United States, some environmental contaminants are regulated by the Environmental Protection Agency (US EPA). For air pollution, the Clean Air Act of 1970 called for evidence-based National Ambient Air Quality Standards (NAAQS) that are set for six criteria pollutants: carbon monoxide, lead, nitrogen dioxide, ozone, particulate matter (PM) (now regulated in two size fractions), and sulfur dioxide. These standards are based on the full scope of scientific evidence on the health effects of exposure to each pollutant. Primary standards are intended to provide public health protection, extending to sensitive populations such as pregnant women, children, and older adults. Secondary standards provide public welfare protection, such as protecting visibility, animals, or crops. States are required to conduct central-site monitoring to ensure that concentrations of each criteria pollutant remain below regulated levels. Monitoring is conducted at least once every 6 days for all criteria air pollutants in every county (except those with a waiver). Monitors can be located according to six general site types[1]: to measure the highest concentrations expected to occur in the area[2]; to measure typical concentrations in the area[3]; to determine the impact of a specific source or source category[4]; to determine background levels[5]; to determine the impact of regional pollution transport to the area; or[6] to measure impacts on visibility, vegetation damage, or welfare-based impacts.

In 1990 following an amendment of the Clean Air Act, US EPA initiated a comprehensive law to significantly reduce emissions of hazardous air pollutants or HAPs. These air pollutants include 187 chemicals that are known or suspected to cause serious health effects, including cancer, reproductive effects or birth defects, or because they cause adverse environmental effects. There are two tiers of regulations for HAPs. For some, regulations are based on technological feasibility of controls, or maximal available control technology. For others, the levels are set using a risk-based approach, if technology-based standards are found to not provide an adequate margin of safety.[10] As of 2019, air toxics are monitored at 27 sites nationally, with most sites monitoring at least 100 chemicals.

In 2005, the World Health Organization (WHO) published air quality guidelines providing global guidance on recommended ambient pollution levels for PM, ozone, nitrogen dioxide, and sulfur dioxide. These recommendations were based on a review of the accumulated scientific evidence on the health effects of exposure to air pollution constituents. Countries are not required to show compliance with these recommended levels and, in the United States, current NAAQS levels are generally higher than those recommended by WHO. Nevertheless, the WHO guidelines represent the only globally reaching values for those countries without resources to develop their own guidelines. The WHO guidelines also offer targets for low- and middle-income countries with concentrations well above the guideline values.

WHO has also published recommendations for indoor air-quality levels. Indoor air quality is not typically regulated in the United States except by the Occupational Safety and Health Administration (OSHA) for worker exposures to some chemicals and particles (see Section 2.2). The EPA does offer a guideline concentration for indoor radon.

Currently, the US EPA also regulates 90 contaminants in drinking water in six categories: micro organisms, disinfectants, disinfection byproducts, inorganic chemicals, organic chemicals, and radionuclides. As with air pollutants, there are two categories of standards. Primary standards are developed to protect public health and secondary standards protect against cosmetic effects (e.g., skin or tooth discoloration) and aesthetic effects (e.g., water taste, odor, and color).

Occupational Compliance

In the United States, exposures to occupational agents are regulated by OSHA for most workers or by the Mine Safety and Health Administration (MSHA) for miners. OSHA was established in 1971 and regulates occupational agents by setting permissible exposure limits (PELs). The majority of the current PELs are still at the same levels as when they were adopted shortly after 1971, and OSHA acknowledges that many of these PELs are not adequate to protect worker health. OSHA currently has 470 PELs for chemical agents regularly used in industrial settings. Lists of all PELs and methods for sampling of chemical agents are available through the OSHA website.[11] For many agents, compliance is assessed through personal exposure assessment, not through area sampling (as is common for environmental compliance). PELs are established for time-weighted average (TWA) exposures and cannot be exceeded in any 8-hour work shift of a 40-hour work week. Based on available resources, industrial hygienists responsible for ensuring worker health and safety at their workplace will typically combine workers into similar exposure groups (SEGs); that is, groups of workers expected to have similar exposure levels based on similar tasks and working locations. Monitoring is then conducted on a subset of workers within the SEGs expected to be most highly exposed.

The National Institutes of Occupational Safety and Health or NIOSH also publishes Recommended Exposure Limits (RELs). Some RELs are the same as the OSHA PELs while others tend to be more protective (i.e., lower exposure levels). The American Conference of Governmental Industrial Hygienists (ACGIH) also publishes occupational exposure limits referred to as Threshold Limit Values or TLVs. Similar to the PELs, the TLVs are airborne concentrations of chemical agents to which nearly all healthy workers can be repeatedly exposed on a daily basis for a working lifetime without experiencing adverse health effects. However, TLVs, unlike PELs, are updated more frequently based on the most current scientific literature. Therefore, TLVs are often much more protective than PELs; it is not unusual that a safe level for a TLV for an airborne agent is an order of magnitude lower than the levels set by the OSHA promulgated PEL. While not a legally enforceable standard, many industries or companies choose to meet the TLV to ensure their workers are protected. As with PELs, TLVs, and RELs are published as 8-hour TWAs and measurements should be collected as personal exposures during a full work shift (nominally 8 hours).

ACGIH, NIOSH, and OSHA publish Short-Term Exposure Limits (STELs), which are measured for 15-minute exposures and are relevant for chemical agents known to have acute toxicity, including irritants and asphyxiants. ACGIH also publishes Biological Exposure Indices (BEI) that provide guidance to industrial hygienists for interpreting biomonitoring results. BEI's represent levels of an agent in a specified biological media (e.g., urine, blood) that is most likely to be present both in healthy workers and in those exposed to the contaminant at exposure levels at the TLV. One important issue to note is that PELs and TLVs may not be protective of vulnerable populations, including pregnant women, women of reproductive age, children, and individuals with pre-existing conditions, as these exposure limits and guidelines are based on healthy individuals and do not take into account potential windows of susceptibility. Additionally, while TLVs are more frequently updated to reflect the most current science, updates are not conducted on all chemicals and of necessity rely on the studies available at the time of update.

Research

Exposures may also be assessed to determine whether they are linked to adverse health effects. Research can be completed on environmentally exposed or occupationally exposed individuals and the methods for the exposure assessment will likely differ depending on the target populations and resources available. It is also critical to consider the appropriate time scale of exposure for the health concern in relation to the temporal aspects of the underlying pathogenetic process. For example, it would not be reasonable to collect exposures on a single day if the health effect of concern has a long latency period, like cancer, unless there is a basis for assuming that the exposure measured on a single day is typical of the individual's exposures over years to decades. For example, arsenic levels in drinking water from the same water source are generally stable over time. Thus, a single measure may provide a good estimate of long-term exposure for an individual who has used this water source for a long period of time or even lifetime. A carefully designed exposure assessment can minimize exposure misclassification (i.e., the assignment of individuals to the wrong exposure group) and reduce the potential for bias in epidemiologic studies.

DESIGNING AN EXPOSURE ASSESSMENT

There are many decisions that need to be made to ensure that the right data are collected for the appropriate purpose prior to conducting an exposure assessment. The first consideration is to decide which agent or agents will be assessed. Concentrations of different agents emitted from the same source may be highly correlated. Measuring multiple agents will increase costs and may not provide additional useful information if the exposures are highly correlated; a "signature" or surrogate contaminant might be more informative. It is also important to consider the appropriate time course of exposure, in relation to the health effect under consideration. Important questions to consider are: Is the exposure assessment duration directly relevant to the health effect? Are the exposures measured representative of "typical" exposures? Are short-duration, high-level exposures (i.e., peaks) relevant? Figure. 63-1 provides a summary of the key decisions to make when designing an exposure assessment. Ultimately, the process for exposure assessment should be tailored to the goals of the assessment and study.

Designing an exposure assessment strategy requires careful consideration of a number of factors. For example, when deciding what kind of air sampling equipment to use for a specific agent, there may be a need to consider whether active or passive sampling is appropriate. Active sampling requires the use of a pump to draw an agent (chemical or biological) through a sample collection media or sensing zone of an instrument. Using an active approach results in a simple calculation of concentration (i.e., amount per unit volume) because the mass of the contaminant can be assessed through analysis of the media, and the flow rate and time are known to determine the volume of air sampled. If personal samples are sought, the sampling pump must be sufficiently small and lightweight to be worn, battery-operated, and not interfere with daily tasks or personal protective equipment that may be needed in an occupational setting to perform a particular task. Passive sampling relies on diffusion for the agent to reach the sampling media or sensing zone. Passive sampling is most common for gases because they diffuse rapidly. Passive sampling can be done for PM when a sensor is used, but is not appropriate for gravimetric sampling, where PM must be collected on a filter media using a pump. Determining the airborne concentration from a passive sample requires knowledge of the temperature and humidity of the air to determine the diffusion of air to the sampling media or sensing zone. An advantage of passive sampling is that the sampling costs are often low, requiring less instrumentation; however, the total sampling costs will depend on the analytical cost as well.

Another consideration is whether cumulative samples (also called "integrated") will be collected (i.e., sample is collected onto media for off-line analysis of single or multiple agents) or whether a sensor will be used for a continuous exposure assessment. Sensors exist for many air pollutants, but not all agents of interest, and limits of detection can vary dramatically between different sensors (both for sensors made by different manufacturers for the same agent and for different agents). However, some sensors can provide high temporal resolution information on exposure levels, which may be needed for understanding acute health impacts or how exposures vary under different exposure scenarios. Sensors also often rely on indirect methods to determine concentration, which can lead to reduced accuracy. Cumulative samples provide less temporal resolution, but since a sample is captured on media for direct measurement, the measures typically have higher accuracy and precision.

Quality Control/Quality Assurance for Exposure Data

When designing an exposure assessment, quality control and quality assurance processes are requisite to ensure that accurate data are collected. First, a written Standard Operating Procedure (SOP) is developed before sampling begins and is followed precisely by all study staff to ensure that proper sampling is conducted and that all samples are collected in the same manner. The SOP includes details on pre- and postsampling instrument calibration when applicable, sample handling, flow rates, sample transport, data recording procedures,

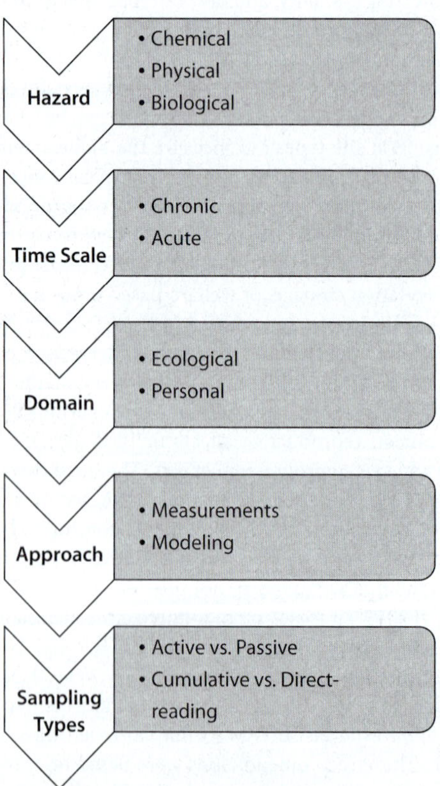

FIGURE 63-1. Flow chart of key decisions that must be made when designing an exposure assessment.

and storage procedures to maintain sample integrity. It should be sufficiently detailed to assure replicability of all procedures.

For any methods involving collection of a physical sample on a sample media, it is crucial to collect blank and duplicate samples. Blank samples are treated identically to any other sample, except that no air, for example, is pulled through the media. This means that samples are set-up, transported, stored, and analyzed identically to any other field sample. The field blanks can be used to determine the limit of detection (LOD) for the samples. It is common to have 10–20% of total samples collected be blanks. Depending on the analysis method, labs may also evaluate lab blanks, which are treated similarly to the samples, except they are not transported to the field. Collecting both field and lab blanks can help to determine whether samples are being contaminated during transport, sample collection, and/or during analysis. Duplicates, identical samples set up alongside the primary sample, should also be collected at a rate of 10–20%. Duplicates can be used to evaluate the precision of the method. Although it may not be possible to collect blanks with sensors, duplicates should still be collected, unless only a single sensor is available. Depending on the cost of analyses, blanks and duplicates can add substantial cost to an exposure assessment, but should not be overlooked.

Error in Exposure Measurements

All measurements are subject to uncertainty. Quantifying the uncertainty on measurements is important to ensure that appropriate inferences are made from the data. Measurement error can be thought of as having two components: random error and systematic error. Random error is related to the precision of a measurement and can be assessed by repeated measurements of the same condition. Systematic error is the difference between a measurement and the true value (accuracy) and can only be assessed through calibration of the measuring device. It is critical to follow manufacturer recommendations for calibrations (either in lab or by returning the device to the manufacturer) to minimize the potential for systematic bias. In some cases, it is possible to conduct "zero" and "span" checks prior to deploying a device, which can be useful to evaluate whether a device is out of calibration (devices are subject to drift, component failures, clogging of flow systems, and dirtying of sensors). For a device that measures airborne concentrations of an agent, a zero check involves measuring air that is free of the agent of interest to evaluate the response and correct, if necessary. A span check involves measuring air at a known concentration to evaluate the response of the device. For gaseous agents, this can be accomplished by purchasing a compressed air mixture at a desired concentration. For PM, establishing a span is more complicated and often not feasible in the field; however, a "spike test" can be generated using simple means (i.e., shaking clothes) to ensure that the device is responding. Alternately, in some cases it may be possible to compare a measurement with a "gold standard" for some period of time to evaluate the accuracy of the measurement.

QUANTITATIVE EXPOSURE ASSESSMENT

The objective of quantitative exposure assessment is to measure (quantify) the amount of an agent that can potentially reach people. The amount of agent that reaches a subject depends on the concentration at the boundary of exposure (mouth, nostrils, skin, etc.), as well as a series of exposure dimensions such as frequency and duration of exposure. Exposure factors are typically assessed in the form of questionnaires or observations, or can be derived from literature sources and adjusted for site-specific conditions and/or specific populations.[12] There are three major categories of agents: physical, chemical, and biological.

Sampling Approaches

Physical Agents

Physical agents are factors within the environment that can harm the body without necessarily touching it. The most important physical agents are noise, heat, vibration, height (slips, trips, and falls), fire and explosion, radiation, and pressure. The physical agents that are routinely sampled and quantified (most commonly in occupational settings) are noise, heat, and radiation. We will briefly discuss noise as an example; other physical agents and the respective exposure assessments are discussed elsewhere.[13]

Vibrations that are detected by the human ear are classified as sound. The term "noise" is used to indicate unwanted sound. Noise is measured in decibels (dB), which is the unit of sound pressure levels. There are several metrics to measure sound pressure, and the most useful is the A-weighted pressure levels (dBA), which closely match the perception of loudness by the human ear. Decibels are measured using noise dosimeters on a logarithmic scale, which means that a small change in the number of decibels results in a large change in the amount of noise and the potential for damage to a person's hearing.

OSHA's PEL for noise is 90 dBA for all workers for an 8-hour day. The OSHA standard uses a 5 dBA exchange rate. This means that when the noise level is increased by 5 dBA, the amount of time a person can be exposed to a certain noise level to receive the same dose is cut in half. Both ACGIH and NIOSH have recommended that all worker exposures to noise be controlled to a lower level than required by the PEL. ACGIH and NIOSH recommend a level equivalent to 85 dBA for 8 hours to minimize occupational noise induced hearing loss. Additionally, NIOSH recommends a 3 dBA exchange rate (instead of 5 dBA, as recommended by OSHA) so that every increase by 3 dBA halves the recommended amount of exposure time.

Since 1981, OSHA has required employers to implement a Hearing Conservation Program when workers are exposed to 85 dBA or higher TWA over an 8-hour work shift. Hearing Conservation Programs require employers to measure noise levels, provide free annual hearing exams and free hearing protection, provide training, and conduct evaluations of the adequacy of the hearing protectors in use, unless engineering or administrative changes are made that reduce worker noise exposure to less than the 85 dBA.[14]

Noise dosimeters to measure exposure typically log the 8-hour average and peak values, provide A-weighted results, and most currently have the option to choose between 5 and 3 dBA exchange rate. Noise dosimeters log real-time information that can be downloaded to a computer for fast assessment of noise exposure, and to evaluate if a process needs to be modified or the exposure time reduced.

Chemical Agents

Quantifying exposure to chemical agents involves measuring the concentration of the chemical in the environment. The method used to measure exposure depends on the physical state of the chemical (solid, liquid, gas) and how the chemical enters the body (air, water, food). This chapter focuses on assessment of airborne agents entering the body through the inhalation route.

Particulate Matter Aerosols are defined as stable suspensions of fine solid or liquid particles in air. The particles in the air are called PM and have been shown to have independent health effects from the gases that are also present in air. PM is ubiquitous and sources of PM can be both anthropogenic and natural. Particle size, often defined as aerodynamic diameter, is the most important parameter for characterizing and describing the behavior of and exposure to aerosols; particle behavior (e.g., how long they stay suspended in air, how they follow air streams, and the mechanisms and sites of deposition in the upper airway and lung) varies greatly with particle size.

Understanding the particle size characteristics of aerosols can help to determine penetration into specific regions of the respiratory tract, and which sampling strategy is best for quantifying human exposure. A typical ambient aerosol is composed of three modes or size fractions and spans 5 orders of magnitude (Fig. 63-2). The smallest particles, sometimes referred to as the nucleation mode, can be as small as several nanometers in diameter. The second mode is often called the accumulation mode. It contains particles in the range of several hundred nanometers. These particles tend to stay suspended and are not efficiently removed from the atmosphere; hence, the particles "accumulate" in the atmosphere. These particles are primarily from anthropogenic origin, often derived from combustion processes. The largest particles in the aerosol mix are typically derived from mechanical disintegration of a parent material producing a dust or spray with diameters up to several hundred micrometers (mechanical mode). These larger particles are composed of crustal elements such as metals, silicon, calcium, as well as biological particles such as allergens and pollens. Mechanical mode particles stay suspended for hours to days in the air, and do not travel long distances under normal atmospheric conditions. The smallest particles typically dominate the number concentration of particles (Fig. 63-2A) and the large mode of particles dominates the particle mass due the cubic relationship between particle diameter and mass (Fig. 63-2B). Particle size ranges for several common particle types are shown as bars in Fig. 63-2A.

Sampling Strategies for Airborne Particulate Matter For health and regulatory purposes, sampling methods collect certain size fractions while excluding others, depending on the pollutant and health effect of interest. The fraction of interest depends on the context for the measurement. The five common sampling metrics for PM are shown in Fig. 63-2B (read values off the right y-axis). These metrics are sometimes characterized by their cut-point diameter, that is, the diameter for which 50% of the particles are sampled, and 50% of the particles are removed from the air stream prior to collection or analysis.

For current regulatory purposes, the EPA defines ambient particles into two size fractions: coarse PM and fine PM. EPA defines the coarse fraction as containing particles between 2.5 and 10 μm that deposit in the thoracic region of the respiratory tract and can have local irritating as well as systemic effects. The fraction of all particles smaller than 10 μm are called PM_{10}. Coarse particles settle out of the atmosphere relatively quickly, within hours to days. The fine fraction, referred to as $PM_{2.5}$, is composed of particles smaller than 2.5 μm in

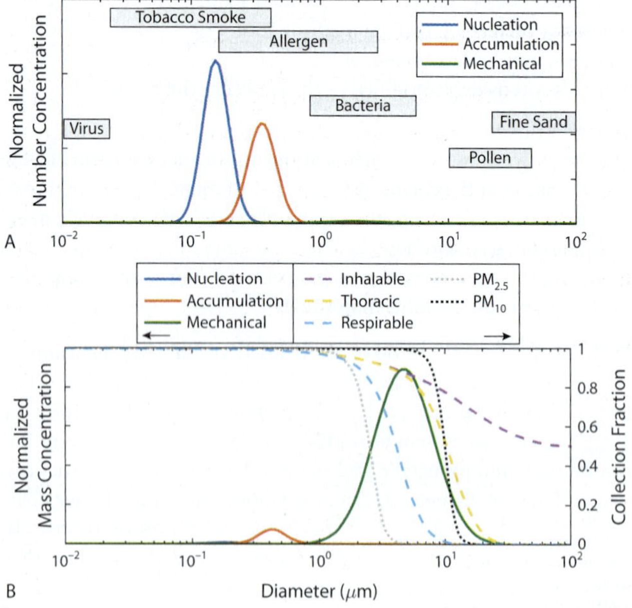

FIGURE 63-2. (A) Normalized number concentration for the three modes of aerosol commonly found in the environment. The number of particles in the Mechanical mode is so small it is barely visible on the plot. Overlaid on the plot are size ranges for common particle types. (B) Normalized mass concentration for the three modes of aerosol. The nucleation mode contributes almost negligibly to particle mass and is barely visible on the plot. Particle sampling metrics correspond to the collection fraction denoted on the right and y-axis.

aerodynamic diameter. The 2.5 μm cut-point was established as the minima between the typically anthropogenically derived particles in the accumulation aerosol mode from the generally naturallyderived particles in the mechanical aerosol mode. This size fraction contains particles that can penetrate to the alveolar region of the lung. Fine particles are typically generated by combustion processes and are mostly composed of carbon, sulfur, and heavy metals. Fine particles can stay suspended days or weeks and travel long distances from the sources, undergoing chemical and physical transformation.

In occupational settings, three particle size fractions have been established for exposure assessment. The inhalable fraction contains particles that can penetrate the nose and mouth and includes particles as large as 100 μm. The thoracic fraction has a cut-point at 10 μm, and is the only metric with a cut-point used by the EPA. The respirable fraction has a cut-point at 4 μm and represents the fraction of particles able to penetrate into the lungs.

The ultrafine fraction is composed of particles smaller than 0.1 μm. This size fraction is also sometimes referred to as nanoparticles (particularly when particles are engineered to have specific properties). Ambient ultrafine particles are primarily generated from combustion sources. The ultrafine fraction contributes negligibly to mass-based metrics of PM exposures because of the small mass of these tiny particles. However, the ultrafine fraction is of health concern because the particle counts are far higher than in the larger size fraction, the particles penetrate deep into the lungs, and can translocate across the lung and be transported through the blood to other parts of the body. At present, neither the US EPA nor OSHA have regulations specific to the ultrafine fraction of particles.

Size Selection Particle size selection of an air sampler depends on the physical characteristics of the sampler and the air flow at which the sample is collected. PM samplers are designed and precision-machined to collect certain size fractions (i.e., those described above and in Fig. 63-2B) of the size distribution by accelerating particles into a nozzle and removing some particles from the airstream. Sometimes we are interested in analyzing the larger, removed particles, sometimes we collect the smaller particles that pass through. There are several physical principles that can be used to separate particles from an air stream depending on the particle size of interest (shown graphically in Fig. 63-3): (A) gravitational settling is most important for particles larger than ~100 um; (B) impaction is most important for particles between 0.3 μm and 100 μm; (C) diffusion is most important for particles smaller than 0.1 μm; (D) interception can be used for all particles sizes when collecting particles on a filter, when particles are intercepted by the filter material; and (E) electrostatic forces are typically only used in industrial operations to remove particles from being exhausted into ambient air and are more effective for smaller particles, but can be effective at all sizes with large enough electrostatic forces.[15] These same processes (with the exception of electrostatic forces) also govern how particles deposit in the human respiratory tract.

The most common size-selective devices used to assess exposure to PM are inertial impactors and cyclones (see schematics in Fig. 63-4). In both cases, particles larger than a desired cut size (i.e., 2.5 μm) are removed from the air stream while particles smaller than the cut size remain in the air stream for subsequent analysis (i.e., measured via electronic detection in real time or collected on a filter for later laboratory evaluation). An impactor accomplishes this separation by directing air toward a plate that forces a 90° turn in the air flow; only particles below the cut size are able to make this turn and stay in the air flow. A cyclone accomplishes the separation by sending the flow cyclonically through a cone and again, only particles below the cut size are able to make the turns to stay in the air flow.

Sample Analysis PM samples can be analyzed by weighing the mass collected (gravimetric analysis), by performing chemical analyses on the collected mass to determine PM composition (metals, organics, biological), or by optical methods to determine particle count, shape, certain compositions (i.e., asbestos), and size distribution.

Gases and Vapors A gas is a state of matter. It refers to a substance that has a single defined thermodynamic state at room temperature (e.g., oxygen, nitrogen dioxide). A vapor is the gaseous form of a substance that coexists as both a gas and a solid or liquid at normal temperature and pressure (e.g., mercury, benzene). Because both gases and vapors behave similarly in air, and the principles used for quantifying them are the same, they are considered here as a single category for exposure assessment purposes.

Sampling Strategies for Gases and Vapors There are two methods for collecting gases and vapors: (1) active (with the use of a sampling pump) and (2) passive, based on diffusion, which involves the spread of particles through the air by Brownian motion from a region of higher concentration to one of lower concentration. There are three basic properties of gases that are useful for quantifying the concentration of gases and vapors: (1) solubility, (2) vapor pressure, and (3) reactivity. Lastly, there are two types of collection media: (1) absorbents are liquids in which a gas or vapor dissolves by bubbling (impingers); and (2) adsorbents (or sorbents), which are solid substances with large surface area where gas molecules are deposited (activated carbon or silica gel). Active sampling is typically used to collect samples by absorption, whereas diffusion creates its own air movement and is the main principle driving passive sampling. Adsorption can be used in passive or active modes.

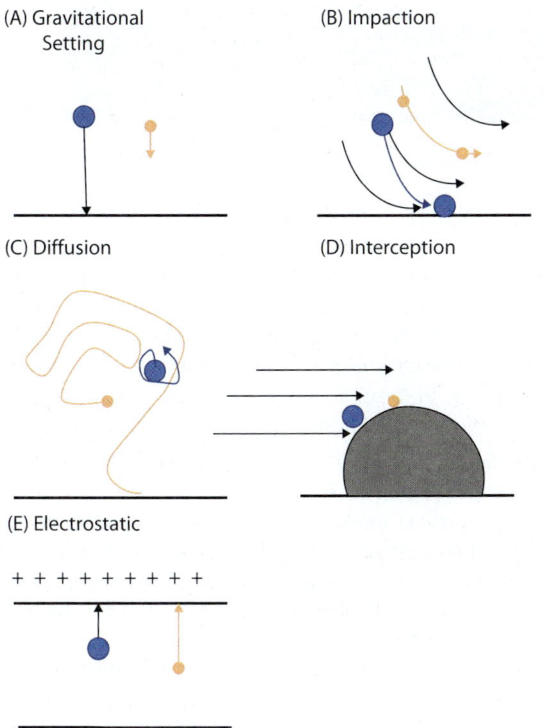

FIGURE 63-3. Mechanisms of particle separation from an air stream: (A) gravitational settling; (B) impaction; (C) diffusion; (D) interception; and (E) electrostatic forces.

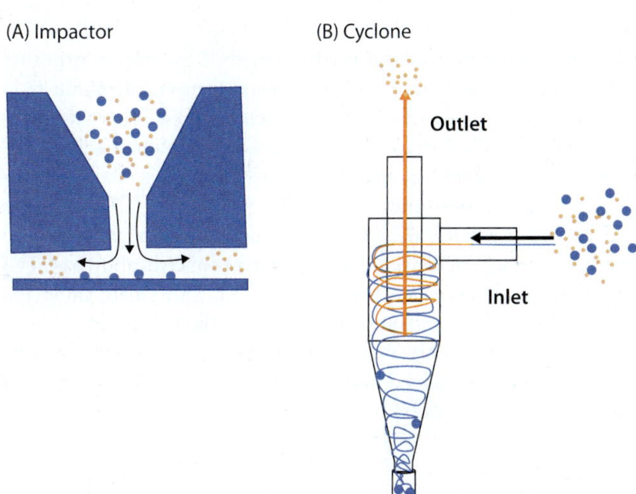

FIGURE 63-4. Schematic of the operation of (A) impactor and (B) cyclone.

Another strategy for collecting a sample to evaluate gas or vapor concentrations is called a grab sample, which involves bringing a determined volume of air into an inert container for later analysis. The most common containers are stainless steel vacuum cylinders (Summa cannisters), flasks under negative pressure, and Tedlar bags (Fig. 63-5).

Finally, there are many direct-reading instruments that can perform sampling and analysis simultaneously, as described in the following section.

Sample Analysis If a gas or vapor has been collected by absorption or adsorption, the molecules need to be desorbed (or extracted) from the sampling media (i.e., liquid, charcoal) before analysis in the lab. Once desorbed, the gas molecules can be analyzed in the same way as gases collected using grab samples, typically with gas chromatography, which separates the different molecules in a sample for identification and uses a series of calibration curves to quantify concentrations. Both NIOSH and EPA have a comprehensive list of validated methods for analysis of gases and vapors.[16,17]

There are also multiple direct-reading instruments for gases and vapors. Some instruments can identify multiple gases simultaneously and others are designed for a specific gas. The main methods used for gas analysis are: spectroscopic (based on light absorption), electrochemical, and photoionization detectors (PIDs).

Spectroscopic methods are based on the principle that different gas molecules absorb light at different wavelengths or frequencies. Instruments that use spectroscopic methods are the most sensitive and precise, which is why they are used as reference methods, and are also the most expensive. Spectroscopic methods used to measure the criteria air pollutant gases include: ultraviolet light for ozone, infrared for CO, fluorescence for SO_2, and chemiluminescence for NO_2.

Electrochemical (EC) sensors measure concentrations of a target gas by oxidizing or reducing the gas at an electrode and measuring the resulting current, which is directly proportional to the gas concentration. Electrochemical sensors are inexpensive, small, and easy to integrate with electronics in a portable device. Some commercially available devices integrate multiple EC sensors into one single instrument. However, the shelf-life of the sensor is only a few years and can be reduced to a few months with exposure to high concentrations of the target gas. Other disadvantages are potential interferences in the presence of other gases and relative humidity and that they are less sensitive compared to spectroscopic methods.

PIDs operate with a high-energy ultraviolet lamp that ionizes gases present in the air. Ionized molecules carry an electrical charge that is measured by a detector and converted to a concentration. PIDs are typically used to detect total volatile organic compounds (VOCs); they are portable and easy to use, but do not provide gas identification and cannot detect semivolatile compounds.

Biological Agents

Biological aerosols are airborne particles of biological origin, that is, particles that are living or originate from living organisms. Bioaerosol sizes span several orders of magnitude, from viruses that measure a few nanometers (Fig. 63-2) to pollen or allergens that can measure

(A) Summa Canister

(B) Tedlar bag

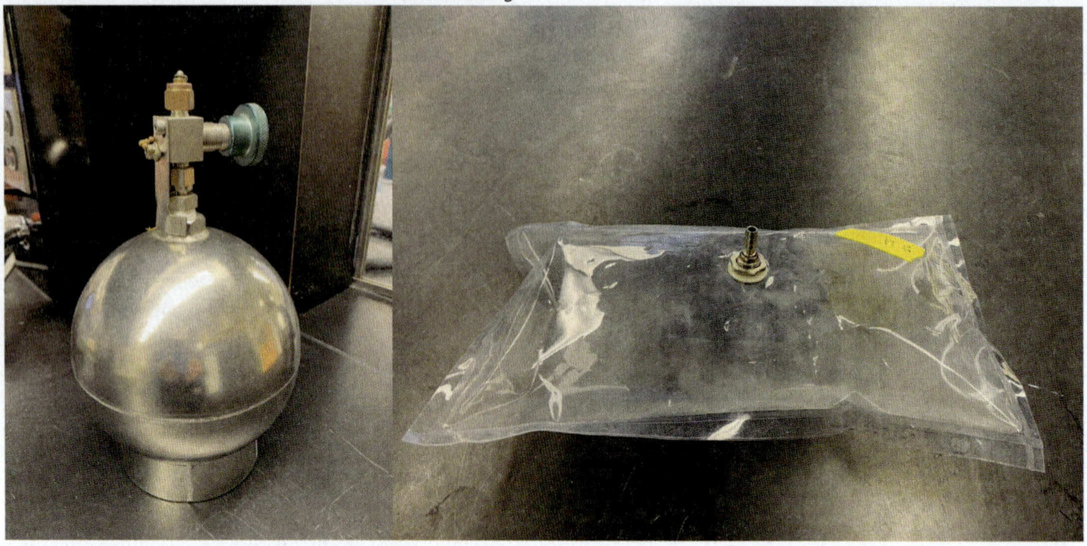

FIGURE 63-5. Pictures of (A) Summa canister and (B) Tedlar bag. *Source*: (A-B) Ana María Rule, PhD.

tens of micrometers. Biological aerosol agents are a concern from such well-known sources as agriculture, hospitals, and municipal waste management, but also from resistant and new strains of known pathogens, such as avian and swine flu, and emerging problems such as the coronavirus causing SARS (severe acute respiratory syndrome) and MRSA (multidrug resistant *Staphylococcus aureus*).

The main health effects are infections, allergic responses, and toxic reactions that can be localized or systemic, and their impact on public health spans from disability, loss of healthy years, to mortality. However, to date, exposures to biological agents are not regulated by federal agencies. Establishing regulatory thresholds has been challenging since bioaerosols are mixtures of different microorganisms (many nonpathogenic), there are high background concentrations, and there is huge interindividual response variability.

Sampling strategies for bioaerosols use the same principles as those described for PM (impaction, centrifugal motion). The type of bioaerosol of concern determines the size fraction to be sampled. In addition, environmental factors such as temperature, moisture, and UV light, as well as the collection medium, affect microorganism viability, which is important for some analysis types. Most sample collection media are liquid or gels that provide a suitable environment to preserve biological integrity of the sample. General limitations include desiccation of organisms during sampling, overgrowth in high concentration environments, and competition of different organisms, which requires the use of selective media.

The most common analysis methods include culture (basic enumeration of colonies and further molecular identification), microscopy, molecular techniques such as immunoassays and polymerase chain reaction, and chemical analysis such as gas chromatography. There are a few direct reading instruments available, but infrequently used, based on ultraviolet properties of microorganisms and portable gas chromatographs.

Modeling Approaches

In addition to physical sampling of agents, another approach commonly used in exposure assessment is modeling and may complement the use of direct measurements and other data, when available. For example, studies designed to evaluate how chronic exposures vary over space may rely on modeling to estimate exposures as a function of location. The within-city spatial variation is, in many cases, larger than the between-city variation.[18] As such, monitoring to capture the small-scale variability in pollutant concentrations may not be feasible. Instead, spatial prediction models can assign exposures to individuals based on high-resolution modeled pollutant concentrations for the region and individuals' home addresses or postal codes. Two common modeling approaches include chemical transport modeling and land-use regression (LUR).[18] Other modeling approaches may be used to estimate concentrations in indoor spaces, in locations where collecting measurements is not feasible, or for estimation of exposures that occurred at an earlier time point.[19]

Chemical Transport Modeling

Chemical transport models are mathematical models that predict air pollutant concentrations by evaluating emissions, transport, and chemical reactions that take place in each grid cell of a given spatial domain.[20] These models are data and computationally intensive. The model requires information, at each grid box, on emissions, meteorology (temperature, humidity, wind), and chemical reactions (as a function of temperature and humidity) to complete the calculations. Advanced models, like the Community Multi-scale Air Quality Model (CMAQ) developed by the US EPA are freely available,[21] but require substantial training to use appropriately. These models can provide high quality estimates of exposures over fine spatial and temporal domains. However, the precision of the estimates may depend on the size of the grids (where finer grids will require more computational power) and the accuracy of the emissions data.

Land-use Regression

LUR modeling is increasingly used as a method to improve exposure estimation for populations,[22] with less computational demands than chemical transport models. Simple models may rely on proximity to sources, such as the distance to large roadways, to estimate exposure.[23] LUR is a more widely applied method, which seeks to reduce exposure misclassification and capture more variability.[22,24] Covariates such as land-use, traffic density, meteorology, and geography are used to predict the spatial distribution of pollutant concentration based on a training dataset, typically from an intense measurement campaign (usually 1–2 weeks, 15–100 sites) to develop the LUR model. Often, hundreds of variables are included as potential predictors, but usually only a handful are retained in the final model. The approach involves simple linear regression:

$$z_j = \beta_o + \sum_{i=1}^{n} \beta_i X_{i,j} + \varepsilon_j \text{ Equation 1}$$

where Z_j is the concentration at site j, $X_{i,j}$ are the n predictors of concentration evaluated at each site, the β's are the regression coefficients, and ε_j is the residual error, which may contain spatial correlation structure. LURs are computationally efficient, but depend on the accuracy of the training dataset. Although some methods are being developed for time-varying LUR from hourly to daily resolution, 25 LURs are more commonly used for chronic exposures from seasonal to annual timescales.[18]

Remote Sensing Approaches

Remote sensing, the acquisition of information about an object without making physical contact, as through satellites or high-flying aircraft, is another approach for exposure assessment. The World Health Organization Global Burden of Disease estimated the burden of disease attributable to air pollution in 2010 and has done so for subsequent years up to 2017.[26] To do so, exposure estimates were required for the entire globe, including areas that have limited or no routine monitoring for air pollution. Satellite measures of aerosol optical depth (estimated as the extinction of light through the entire atmosphere by particles) were combined with chemical transport modeling (see Chemical Transport Modeling) and monitoring data, where available, to estimate exposures over the entire globe at 0.1×0.1 resolution.[27] Remote sensing is gaining popularity even in places like the United States that operate monitoring networks for air pollution. For example, some researchers have included aerosol optical depth measured from satellites as a covariate to improve the predictiveness of LUR models.[28] Additionally, remote sensing can be used to assess land-use, of which a number of metrics have been recently linked with public health. For example, exposure to greenspace has been linked with health benefits, including stress reduction, improved birth outcomes, and reduced crime rates, among other benefits.[29,30]

Other Modeling Approaches

A number of models can be used to estimate concentrations in indoor spaces, relying on different assumptions and data requirements. Several models are described briefly below (see ref. 19 for more detailed descriptions).

Saturation Vapor Pressure Model: Uses the ideal gas law to assume that the concentration in air can be predicted from the saturation concentration (i.e., the maximum possible quantity of a substance that can dissolve in a standard volume of a specific solvent under standard conditions of temperature and pressure) of an agent in air. This model tends to overestimate exposures by assuming that the chemical is continuously open to the air and that there is no ventilation.

Well-Mixed Room Model: This model assumes that the concentration can be calculated from a known generation rate of the agent, the volume of the room, and the ventilation parameters of the room. The model assumes the generation rate is either constant or follows known behaviors such as decreasing exponentially.

Near-Field, Far-Field Model: This model accounts for the fact that rooms may not be well mixed, and instead may have a region near the source with higher concentrations (i.e., the "near-field") surrounded by a region with lower concentration (i.e., the "far-field"). As will the well-mixed room model, it is assumed that the generation rate is known and that ventilation parameters are known, but also that there is a known air exchange between the near- and far-field.

BIOMONITORING

Human biomonitoring assesses exposures to chemicals and their adverse effects through the measurement of biomarkers in biological specimens. Biomarkers are also used to assess susceptibility to respond to a specific agent.

The exposure biomarkers can include the chemicals themselves, their metabolites, or reaction products.[31] Biomarkers may be measured in many biological media, including blood, urine, saliva, nails, hair, teeth, exhaled breath, human milk, semen, amniotic fluid, cord blood, placenta, and meconium. The appropriate biological media may depend on the agent of interest. For example, exposure to lead is routinely assessed by measuring lead in blood, while exposure to select pesticides, like OPs and pyrethroids, can be accessed via measurement of specific and nonspecific urinary metabolites. Specific metabolites are those that arise from exposure to unique compounds while nonspecific metabolites reflect exposure to multiple compounds.

Biomonitoring is an integral component of exposure assessment both for surveillance activities and for research, and many environmental and occupational epidemiologic studies evaluate environmental exposures, as measured through biomarkers, to adverse health effects. Biomonitoring can also provide essential information for identifying emerging environmental agents that need to be further monitored and studied with regard to potential health risks in specific population subgroups or areas.[32] For example, biomonitoring data from the National Health and Nutrition Examination Survey (NHANES)—a survey on a representative sample of the U.S. general population—indicates that, among the U.S. general population, women and African Americans have elevated exposures to chemicals commonly found in personal care products.[31] However, one drawback of using biomarkers is that they reflect aggregate exposures from all routes, which can make it difficult to assess the source of exposure. Another limitation is that biomarker concentrations can be affected by pharmacokinetic and metabolic factors and by disease status, including early disease. Therefore, environmental monitoring in exposure assessment complements biomonitoring and can provide insights into the sources as well as major routes and pathways of exposure to environmental contaminants.

Types of Biomarkers

In general, there are three distinct types of biomarkers, including biomarkers of exposure, effect, and susceptibility. Each provides unique information that can be useful for exposure assessment and can further inform risk assessments and epidemiologic studies.

Biomarkers of Exposure: A biomarker of exposure refers to a chemical, its metabolite, or the product of an interaction between a chemical and a given target molecule or cell that arises from an environmental exposure and is measured in the human body.[32] Examples of biomarkers of exposure include the measurement of benzene in exhaled breath, cotinine in blood or urine to assess exposure to secondhand smoke exposure, metals in deciduous teeth to assess prenatal exposures, and dialkylphosphate (DAP) urinary metabolites to assess exposure to OP pesticides. DAPs are nonspecific biomarkers of exposure, which provide a good integrated measure of cumulative exposure to several OP pesticides; however, because they are nonspecific it is challenging to determine which parent compounds gave rise to the DAPs in an individual's urine sample.[32,33] This holds true for other nonspecific urinary metabolites.

Biomarkers of Effect. The International Programme on Chemical Safety defines a biomarker of effect as a measurable biochemical, physiologic, behavioral, or other alteration in the body that, depending on the magnitude, can be recognized as associated with a possible health impairment or disease.[34] Biomarkers of effect may be used directly in the hazard identification and in the dose-response assessment phases of a risk assessment.[35] For example, acetylcholinesterase (AChe) inhibition has been used as a biomarker of effect on the nervous system following exposure to OP and carbamate pesticides in both occupational and environmental studies. AChe is a key enzyme in the central nervous system responsible for terminating nerve impulses by catalyzing the hydrolysis of the neurotransmitter acetylcholine. As a specific molecular target of OP and carbamate pesticides, AChe activity and its inhibition are recognized to be human biological markers of pesticide poisoning among farmworkers.[36]

Biomarkers of Susceptibility. A biomarker of susceptibility is defined as an indicator of an inherent or acquired ability of an organism to respond to the challenge of exposure to a specific environmental agent. In other words, biomarkers of susceptibility reflect intrinsic characteristics or factors that may make certain individuals more sensitive to the potential adverse effects of a given environmental agent by modifying an individual's response to these exposures. For example, paraoxonase 1 or PON1 activity has been used as a biomarker of susceptibility to OP pesticides. PON1 is an enzyme that can detoxify the -oxon derivatives of some OP pesticides that can also act as an antioxidant. Studies have reported that individuals with low PON1 activity may be more susceptible to the potential health effects of OP pesticides due to decreased metabolic capacity toward OP -oxons and lower antioxidant defenses when compared to individuals with average or high PON1 activity.[37]

Biological Matrix Selection

Selection of an appropriate biological matrix for biomonitoring depends heavily on the physicochemical properties of the chemical of interest as these determine metabolism and excretion routes. However, advances in analytical techniques with very low limits of quantitation have expanded the possibilities and enabled the use of noninvasive matrices with relatively low concentration of xenobiotics (i.e., exogenous chemicals foreign to a living organism such as pharmaceuticals, pesticides, and other pollutants) in biomonitoring studies.[38] Two of the most widely used biological matrices are blood and urine.

Blood is commonly used to measure persistent and bioaccumulative chemicals such as brominated flame retardants, certain metals, and polychlorinated biphenyls. Because blood is in constant contact with the whole organism and in equilibrium with tissues and organs where some chemicals may deposit, blood is often preferred for selected chemicals. However, venipuncture is invasive, compromising willingness to provide samples. A less-invasive alternative to venipuncture is collection of dry blood spot (DBS) samples in which drops of whole blood are collected on filter paper from a simple finger prick. This approach can be useful in research settings with limited resources (e.g., remote rural areas, developing countries, limited or no access to refrigeration for sample storage). DBS has been used in environmental population studies and advancements in technology will likely minimize constraints and current limitations associated with this matrix (e.g., issues with limits of detection and reliance on conversion of single analyte measurements to corresponding plasma or serum values).[39]

Other matrices that can be used to assess exposure to persistent and bioaccumulative chemicals include umbilical cord blood, placenta, and human milk. Variability in serum lipid concentrations in these matrices for lipophilic compounds (i.e., compounds that can bioaccumulate in adipose tissue), such as brominated flame retardants, is accounted for by expressing results as "concentration of chemical per gram of serum lipids." Umbilical cord blood may also be used to provide information on environmental exposures during the gestational period to both the mother and the fetus,[40] a life stage that is characterized by high vulnerability to environmental exposures.

Urine is most useful for analysis of nonpersistent chemicals that are rapidly metabolized and excreted such as environmental phenols (e.g., bisphenol A, parabens) and phthalates. However, one limitation of using urine as a matrix for nonpersistent chemicals with short-half lives is that multiple samples per individual are usually required to properly characterize exposure given the wide variability of urinary excretion rates among individuals, and great temporal variability in urine composition within individuals. To try to account for differences in urine dilution in spot urine samples, urinary concentrations of parent compounds or their metabolites are often corrected for creatinine, specific gravity, or osmolality. Alternative methods, which are difficult to implement both in surveillance and in epidemiologic research include the collection of 24-hour urine samples or first morning voids. Urinary biomarker concentrations usually reflect recent rather than chronic exposures. Metabolites measured in urine may also reflect exposure to the parent compounds that are metabolized in the body, the breakdown products (metabolites) themselves if these are present in the environment and are not further metabolized in the body prior to excretion, or a combination of both. For example, DAP metabolites have been widely used to assess exposure to organophosphorous pesticides (OPs); however, studies have shown that DAPs may also be present in food and house dust and, if excreted unchanged, urinary DAP concentrations may reflect exposure to the parent OPs, the DAPs themselves, or both.[33,41] Another metabolite with a challenging interpretation in certain populations is dimethylarsinate (DMA). While DMA is a major metabolite of inorganic arsenic, which is highly toxic, it is also a major metabolite of arsenosugars and arsenolipids, which are found in seafood and have markedly lower toxicity compared to inorganic arsenic.[42] Still, urinary biomarkers are widely used in biomonitoring and epidemiologic studies.

Other matrices that have been used in biomonitoring and epidemiologic studies include human hair, nails, and deciduous teeth. Human hair may be used to measure long-term exposure to trace elements like arsenic or to organic chemicals such as nicotine; however, external deposition of chemicals in hair may alter results.[43] Nails, particularly toenails, can also be used as biomarkers for most trace elements and may be used as an integrated measure of exposures occurring for several weeks that took place over several previous months. In recent years, deciduous teeth (i.e., milk teeth or primary teeth) have been used to assess exposure to metals during the gestational period. Deciduous teeth start developing toward the end of the first trimester forming new layers on a daily basis. These layers capture traces of chemicals that the fetus may be exposed to, serving as a record of fetal exposure to chemicals during critical windows of development.[44] Saliva may also be used to assess exposure to low molecular weight compounds like cotinine, select trace elements, and organic solvents, though some limitations mainly related to sensitivity are reported.[45] Exhaled breath is also used to assess exposure to select inhaled contaminants like VOCs and certain metals (e.g., manganese); however, the information obtained from this matrix is mostly limited to target tissues in the respiratory system.

Advantages and Disadvantages of Current Biomarkers for Monitoring Environmental Exposures

As outlined in Table 63-1, biomarkers have several advantages and disadvantages. One of the advantages of biomarkers is that they can be used to confirm absorption of many xenobiotics in the body. They also serve as an integrated measure of exposure, reflecting exposure from all possible sources and routes, including ingestion, inhalation, and dermal absorption. In addition, recent advances in analytical sensitivity, methodologies, and instrumentation allow for the detection of chemicals in different matrices at very low concentrations. Biomarkers can also be useful for testing and validating exposure models especially when the results of modeling predictions are compared to the estimated internal doses measured in exposed individuals. Moreover, biomonitoring can help public health professionals assess exposure trends over time, allowing them to identify emerging chemicals of concern and to evaluate whether a given public health intervention or policy designed to mitigate exposure is effective. For example, when products are reformulated, restricted from select consumer products, or completely phased out from the market, biomonitoring can help confirm whether these changes resulted in reduction of human exposures. Biomarkers can also be useful for identifying environmental health disparities and identifying potential vulnerable subgroups based on factors such as gender, race/ethnicity, age, occupation, physical and lifestyle factors, and location of residence or job.

Despite these advantages, there are some disadvantages of conventional biomonitoring for assessment of exposures. For one, it is not always possible to define the specific sources or pathways of exposure given that biomarkers integrate exposure from several routes and pathways. In addition, unless toxicological and epidemiological studies have defined toxicity and the dose-response curve, it may not be possible to define the toxic dose of a given chemical in humans with

TABLE 63-1 ADVANTAGES AND DISADVANTAGES OF TRADITIONAL BIOMARKERS FOR MONITORING EXPOSURES

ADVANTAGES	DISADVANTAGES
• Confirms absorption of the agents or xenobiotics into the human body • Serves as an integrated measure of exposure from all routes and all sources • Analytical techniques available allow for the measurement of very low concentrations of many chemical substances • Helps to test and validate exposure models • Provides accurate and precise measurements of biologically persistent chemicals • Useful for establishing baseline values, evaluating temporal exposure trends, and evaluating efficiency of exposure mitigation interventions and policies. • Useful for identifying environmental health disparities and highly exposed vulnerable subgroups • Can be used in epidemiological studies in combination with health data to examine associations between the body burden of pollutants and their health effects and to test research hypotheses	• Not always possible to define specific sources or pathways of exposure given it integrates exposure from several routes and pathways • Not always able to define the toxic dose • Susceptible to inferior analytical methods which may limit ability to adequately interpret results • Meaningful reference or clinically relevant levels are not always available • Analysis is limited to available analytical methods • Laboratory analysis of samples may be costly and time-consuming • Participants may be unwilling to provide samples if collection procedures are invasive • May only reflect transient exposures and multiple samples may be necessary to properly characterize exposure

sufficient certainty. Biomarker measurements can also be affected by contamination, which may limit interpretation of results. For example, because many chemicals of interest may be present in every day consumer products, including laboratory supplies and equipment, it is possible that samples could be contaminated during the collection or sample processing. Consequently, rigorous collection and laboratory procedures are key to ensure interpretable results, in addition to having samples analyzed in labs accredited by reputable third parties to ensure the technical competence of the laboratory conducting the sample analysis. Another disadvantage of biomarkers is that for many pollutants, population reference levels are not available. Moreover, lack of toxicologic and epidemiologic data for many chemicals makes it nearly impossible to discern whether levels observed in a given population should be considered safe or of potential concern. It is also possible that the degree of risk is population- or individual-dependent. Additionally, analyses are limited to available methods and corresponding limits of quantification, and some methods are costly and time consuming, limiting the number of analyses that can be conducted. Lastly, as indicated previously, measures in some media (e.g., urine) may only reflect recent exposures and multiple samples per individual may be necessary to properly characterize exposures due to the potential for high intraindividual variability.

Ethical Considerations When Conducting Human Biomonitoring

There are several ethical issues that should be considered prior to the collection of human biological specimens especially when samples are collected from vulnerable populations, including children. For example, it is important to obtain informed consent from individuals prior to the collection of their biological specimens, including informed consent from parents or caregivers when children are underage, as well as assent from the children themselves. Adequate provisions for obtaining informed consent from adults and child assent prior to collecting any biological specimens should be considered and implemented. Additionally, when obtaining biological specimens in research settings all collection protocols will need to be reviewed by an internal review board to ensure that sample collection follows ethical principles. Other issues that should be considered by researchers and discussed with individuals providing specimens include how privacy of individuals will be maintained, who may access these samples once the initial target agents of interest are measured, ensuring that individuals providing samples understand the purpose of the biomonitoring and how these results will be used, whether individuals who were minors when they provided the sample will need to be re consented if their samples are used in the future, whether there are any risks and benefits involved from the provision of samples, and whether and how the biomonitoring results will be returned and communicated to individuals. Other considerations have been described in detail elsewhere.[32,46,47]

INDIRECT METHODS OF EXPOSURE ASSESSMENT

Complementary to or in the absence of environmental (i.e., area or personal environmental exposure assessment via direct or modeling approaches) or human biomonitoring data (see Section VI), there are several instruments or indirect methods that can help with exposure assessment of environmental exposures both in occupational and research settings. Some examples of such methods include questionnaires, time-activity diaries and ecological momentary assessments, job exposure matrices, and professional judgment.

Questionnaires

Questionnaires are routinely used in both occupational and environmental epidemiology studies to complement exposure assessment. Questionnaires are not only useful for capturing information at the individual-level, including demographic characteristics like age, gender, occupation, and general lifestyle behaviors that may affect exposures to agents, but they may also be used to query individuals on exposures in different settings, including at home and the workplace (both in current time and in the past). Ideally, questionnaires would be used in combination with environmental or human biomonitoring data; however, the use of environmental and biomonitoring data may be limited by the resources available. Questionnaires are still useful when no other methods of exposure assessment are available and allow environmental and occupational health professionals to collect information on the presence or absence of exposure to an agent, as well as other key exposure factors or domains, including duration, frequency and time of exposure. They are particularly important for assessing past exposures if environmental measures are not available or biomarkers do not have sufficiently long half-lives. However, a major shortcoming is that questionnaires rely on self-report, which could lead to exposure misclassification and bias in assessing exposure–disease relationships. Prior to designing and administering questionnaires, careful consideration should be given to the length of the questionnaire, details of what is being asked, logistics of administration (interviewer-administered vs. self-administered questionnaire), cultural sensitivity to the target population, participation, completion rate, and costs involved. Additionally, the framing and wording of any questionnaire can affect the responses provided and inferences that may be drawn from such responses. In general, standardized validated questions/questionnaires should be used whenever possible to support inferences and allow for comparisons across studies; such questionnaires are available for a variety of domains. It is also important to note that recall bias could be an issue that could also lead to exposure misclassification. This may occur when those who have the disease or outcome of interest are more likely to report exposures or events that could be related to the exposure-disease relationship compared to those who do not have the disease or outcome of interest. It is also possible that individuals may not recall past exposure-related events if the period of interest occurred some time ago. However, recall of exposures may be enhanced by careful formatting of questions. For example, one could ask an individual to recall certain occupations and then go back and detail exposures for these occupations during their lifetime. This can include a checklist of specific jobs, tasks, materials, and other workplace exposures to minimize differential recall. In general, overly detailed questions and jargon should be avoided. Additionally, it is critical that questions are clear and elicit the information needed to reduce any reporting bias among respondents and reduce respondent fatigue.[48]

Time-Activity Diaries and Ecological Momentary Assessments

A time-activity diary is a technique that has been used to collect individual-level data on human behavior in an open-ended format on an activity-by-activity basis. Individuals keep these diaries for a predetermined time period of interest and record information on their activities (ideally, in real time). Most studies that use time-activity diaries include other facets of each reported activity as well, including location of activity. Data from time-activity diaries may also be used as benchmarks to identify whether the activity patterns of high-risk groups deviate from the rest of the population. The data extracted from time-activity diaries can be used to identify high- and low-risk populations, without further information on factors such as point sources of exposure and proximity to exposure sources. They may also be used to model general activity or exposures within various microenvironments. However, in some cases, they may not be as useful; for example, when modeling pollutant effects that are hard to detect over short periods, such as over a day or week.[49] Recent technological advances have paired time-activity diaries with global positioning systems (GPSs) devices to pair known locations with reported activities.[50] Time-activity diaries may also be employed as a mobile phone-based application that prompts participants to report their information, which may reduce recall bias.[51]

Another approach to capture time-activity and behavioral information involves ecological momentary assessments or EMAs. EMA is a technique whereby individuals complete brief surveys about their moods, behaviors, and social interactions in real time, typically with a mobile device, which could also have a sensor to monitor exposures to a given agent. EMA facilitates collection of "momentary" data in real time and in a person's natural environment, helping to reduce survey recall bias. They could also be used as a tool to study factors that influence exposure-related behaviors in real-world contexts. GPS may be used in conjunction with EMAs to produce georeferenced responses and observations related to an individual's activities. For example, this technique could be used in a study of place effects on the use of substances of emerging concern like e-cigarettes, where activity space data could be used to assess a person's exposures to environmental risks, including neighborhood disadvantage, or the locations of stores selling e-cigarette products, to develop statistical models of the effect of such exposures on substance use and related outcomes.[52,53] This data could complement chemical exposure data and help inform potential exposure mitigation interventions. It should be noted that EMAs first emerged in the field of clinical psychology, and its use in environmental health studies to date is limited.

Job Exposure Matrix (JEM)

A job exposure matrix is a tool commonly used by occupational health professionals and in occupational epidemiology studies. It is an efficient method used to assign exposure estimates in a population and may be the only means available for exposure assessment when only job title and industry are available on the population of interest as it may not be possible or feasible to contact the target population. The JEM provides a simple and systematic approach with which to convert coded occupational data, such as industry or job title, into a matrix of potential exposures to agents or other risk factors, eliminating the need to assess individual exposures in detail. Two major advantages of using JEMs include cost and minimized differential information bias. Assessing exposures to individuals by title, for example, is less costly than assessing exposures on an individual basis. Additionally, because the JEM does not distinguish between diseased and nondiseased individuals, the use of JEMs can reduce differential information bias, which may result when evaluating exposures for individuals. JEMs provide exposure rankings that are not subject to recall bias. However, nondifferential exposure misclassification may still occur as variability of exposure within occupational classes in different workplaces, locations, or over time is not usually considered. In addition, JEM categories are not always comparable across studies, can be demanding to develop, and are highly dependent on the occupational health professional expert assigning the rankings.[54]

Professional Judgment

Accurate professional judgment can be useful in integrating limited occupational and environmental monitoring data. However, inaccuracies in judgment could also lead to inadequate levels of protection in occupational health settings or wasting resources on other workers. In fact, it has been estimated that in occupational settings, professional judgment tends to underestimate exposures, although focused training seems to remove this bias substantially.[55] There are also several factors that can impact the validity and reliability of professional judgment in exposure assessment. Some of these factors include the expertise of the individual assessing exposure and whether the focus is on a broad class or a specific agent(s). Still, expert exposure estimates can be more accurate than self-reports and giving the assessor access to data to improve exposure estimates (e.g., subject reported exposure data, work conditions, and measurement data) could improve reliability and validity of the data collected.

ANALYSIS METHODS FOR EXPOSURE DATA

When designing an analysis plan for exposure data, there are a number of considerations to ensure statistically appropriate results. The value of a comprehensive exploratory data analysis cannot be underestimated.[56] An exploratory data analysis can help identify the distributions of the data, important variables, missing data, outliers, and anomalies. A note about outliers: simply because a value is outside the expected range does not mean that it is not valid. As will be discussed below, it is not uncommon for exposure levels to vary over multiple orders of magnitude. Data should not be excluded simply because the value appears to be high without having an explanation for the value. It is important to check why a given value may be an outlier (e.g., is a data entry error or comes from an instrument malfunction) to determine whether this value should be excluded.

Distributions of Exposure Data

Although many statistical methods require that data are normally distributed, exposure data are not typically normally distributed. Instead, data are most commonly log-normally distributed because exposures cannot be less than zero, most values are low, and a wide range of exposure values is typically collected. A distribution is characterized by a measure of the central tendency and a measure of the spread of the data. Normal distributions are typically described using the mean and the standard deviation. Although the mean, median, and mode are the same for a normal distribution, these central tendency measures are different for a lognormal distribution (see example lognormal distribution in Fig. 63-6). The geometric mean and the median better represent the central tendency, and the geometric standard deviation the spread in a lognormal distribution. It is common to report the geometric mean (μ_g) among n exposure measures (A_n) for lognormally distributed data:

$$\mu_g = \sqrt[n]{A_1 A_2 A_3 \ldots A_n} \quad \text{Equation 2}$$

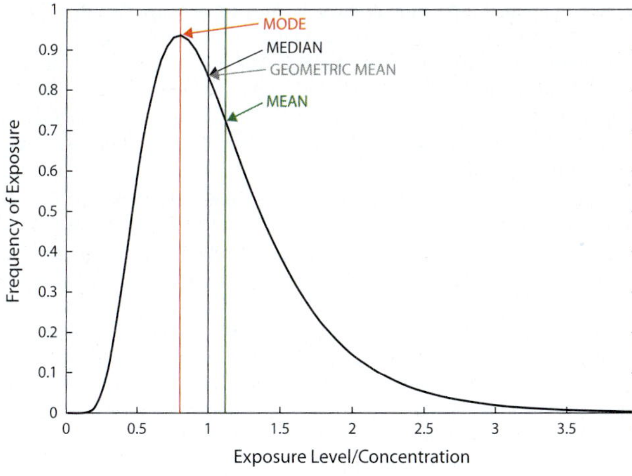

FIGURE 63-6. A lognormal distribution indicating measures of central tendency (mode, median, geometric mean, and mean).

Similarly, it is common to report the geometric standard deviation:

$$\sigma_g = exp\sqrt{\frac{\sum_{i=1}^{n}\left(in\frac{A_i}{\mu_g}\right)^2}{n}} \quad \text{Equation 3}$$

To use exposure measurement data for many statistical analyses, it is often necessary to log transform exposure data, resulting in a distribution that is approximately normally distributed. An advantage of log-transformation of highly skewed data is that this transformation results in a variable that is less affected by outliers and influential points. If the data are not lognormally distributed, other transformations may be considered. When sample sizes are small, the likelihood of measuring high-level exposures decreases, but does not necessarily mean that high-level exposures are not possible.

Missing and Censored Data

Exposure data can be missing for many reasons: equipment may fail, there may be logistical challenges with a site or a participant, a participant may refuse to answer a question, or samples may be physically lost or damaged during transport or analysis. Data may also be censored, most commonly when measures are below the LOD or limit of quantification. When conducting data analysis, it is critical to perform a comprehensive exploratory data analysis to understand the degree and pattern (if any) of missingness. The data analyst should evaluate whether missingness is different by demographics or other variables. The goal is to determine if the data is either missing at random, meaning that the probability of missingness depends only on the observed measurements, or missing completely at random, meaning the probability of missingness for any given variable is independent of observed measurements, or not missing at random. When data is either missing at random or missing completely at random, the impact on results should be minimal, but if not, then the probability of a measurement being missing depends on an unobserved variable, which may confound the association between exposure and health outcome.

Two statistical approaches may be used to analyze a data set with missing observations: listwise deletion or imputation. In listwise deletion, any entries with missing observations are excluded and analysis is conducted on the remaining dataset. While this approach is simple, it can be problematic, especially when values are not missing at random. Alternately, imputation approaches may use values of known observations to replace the missing values with substituted values. Mean substitution, in which missing values are replaced with the mean of the existing observations, is common in many fields, but is not recommended for exposure data. This is especially true when observations are missing because the values were below the LOD. Replacing values below the LOD with the mean value of observations above the LOD will clearly result in a bias toward higher exposures. Instead, it is common to substitute missing values with the value of the LOD divided by two or the LOD divided by the square root of two (especially when the data is lognormally distributed); these methods will generally yield unbiased estimates of the mean when the detection frequency is above 50% (DF $>$ 50%).[57] More advanced statistical approaches including the Central Limit Theorem, regression-based or Monte Carlo-based approaches, or Maximum Likelihood Estimation can be used, but may not perform any better than the simpler substitution approaches unless the proportion of data missing is high ($>$50%) for lognormally distributed data.[57] When relying on substitution or other imputation approaches for missing data, data analysts should conduct sensitivity analyses to evaluate whether a data analysis choice has resulted in a meaningful impact on the results. Another option for modeling exposures when detection frequencies are low (e.g., DF $<$ 60%) is to dichotomize exposure (detected versus not detected) as this may still provide useful data regarding whether a given agent should be further studied in relation to a given outcome.

Correlation Within Exposure Data

Exposure data can be correlated in time, space, among repeated measures of an individual, between individuals, between pollutants, or in other ways. When considering a statistical analysis approach, it is important to evaluate whether a statistical test requires independent measurements, and whether that is an appropriate assumption given the data collection strategy. More advanced statistical methods including linear mixed models (LMMs) or generalized estimating equations (GEEs) that can account for the correlation among repeated exposure measurement data explicitly to account for nonindependence and correlation within and between observations. GEE is often used when one is interested in making inferences at the population level.[58] Typically, GEE cannot account for multiple levels of correlation. LMM, on the other hand, can explicitly account for multiple levels of correlation (e.g., workers within departments, departments within a company, company within an industry) and allow you to examine both the population-level effects and the individual effects.[59]

EMERGING TECHNOLOGIES FOR EXPOSURE ASSESSMENT

Measurement of Environmental Exposures

New approaches are being developed to reduce the cost, size, and power requirements for monitoring, particularly in the realm of personal monitoring. Low-cost sensor technology has exploded in popularity for assessing both personal exposures to air pollutants and for operating a high density of networks of ambient air pollution monitors. Many low-cost sensors are now available for PM and a number of trace gases. Over the last decade, many low-cost sensors were sold as only the sensor, without any electronics to power, interpret or data log the result. Increasingly, some of these sensors are now being incorporated into off-the-shelf monitors that have been engineered for ease of use by researchers and the public. One limitation with these sensors is that they often have higher limits of detection and lower accuracy than traditional sampling approaches. Furthermore, users may find that they require substantial effort to calibrate and may require frequent calibrations (on the order of days to months).

Measurement of Biological Responses

Humans are exposed to multiple chemicals at any given time and emerging "-omics" techniques provide some promise to assess the totality of exposures and their potential effects. These "-omics" techniques are based on high-throughput methods that allow for the assessment and measurement of response modulation at different scales in humans. One such technology includes metabolomics, which entails the study of small molecules that result from metabolism (metabolites). Through untargeted biomonitoring approaches like metabolomics, thousands of metabolites can be monitored with a relatively small biospecimen sample volume for the cost of a single traditional biomonitoring analyses for a given panel of chemicals.[60,61] Metabolomics can help scientists have a better understanding of the physiological state of an organism in response to different stimuli, including exposures to environmental contaminants. In response to chemical exposures, metabolites originating endogenously or exogenously may be created and recent studies indicate that metabolomics may enhance our understanding of the exposome (i.e., the measure of all the exposures of an individual over the course of a lifetime and how these exposures impact to health).[38] Notwithstanding, this field is still emerging and is not without its own challenges, but may be an important component of future exposome projects.

CONCLUSIONS

The field of exposure science is constantly evolving as new technologies and methods emerge. Exciting advances are being made to reduce the cost and size of sampling equipment while maintaining high quality measures and low limits of detection. Although some of these methods may not be approved for assessing compliance with regulatory limits, such advances will increase the amount of exposure data that can be collected for epidemiologic analysis. A general trend toward higher resolution exposure assessment, both in the measurement and modeling realms can minimize exposure error and improve our ability to detect relationships between exposures and human health. In this chapter, we have summarized the reasons to conduct an exposure assessment, important exposure assessment design considerations for sampling and analyzing data and listed some common approaches for exposure assessment. Altogether, these approaches can lead us toward a more holistic assessment of the exposome.

References

1. Sagiv SK, Bruno JL, Baker JM, et al. Prenatal exposure to organophosphate pesticides and functional neuroimaging in adolescents living in proximity to pesticide application. *Proc Natl Acad Sci U S A.* 2019;116(37):18347–56.
2. Council NR. *Exposure Science in the 21st Century: A Vision and a Strategy.* Washington, DC: The National Academies Press; 2012.
3. Wild CP. The exposome: From concept to utility. *Int J Epidemiol.* 2012;41(1):24–32.
4. Rappaport SM. Implications of the exposome for exposure science. *J Expo Sci Environ Epidemiol.* 2011;21(1):5–9.
5. Wild CP. Complementing the genome with an "exposome": The outstanding challenge of environmental exposure measurement in molecular epidemiology. *Cancer Epidemiol Biomarkers Prev.* 2005;14(8):1847–50.
6. Wild CP. Environmental exposure measurement in cancer epidemiology. *Mutagenesis.* 2009;24(2):117–25.
7. Wild CP. Future research perspectives on environment and health: The requirement for a more expansive concept of translational cancer research. *Environ Health.* 2011;10(Suppl 1):S15.
8. Rappaport SM, Smith MT. Epidemiology. Environment and disease risks. *Science.* 2010;330(6003):460–1.
9. van Tongeren M, Cherrie JW. An integrated approach to the exposome. *Environ Health Perspect.* 2012;120(3):A103–4;author reply A104.
10. Environmental Protection Agency: Hazardous Air Pollutants. https://www.epa.gov/haps 2018.
11. Occupational Safety and Health Administration: Permissible Exposure Limits—Annotated Tables. https://www.osha.gov/dsg/annotated-pels/index.html. 2019.
12. Environmental Protection Agency. *Exposure Factors Handbook: 2011 Edition.* Washington, DC: U.S. Environmental Protection Agency; 2011.
13. Centers for Disease Control: Hazards & Exposures. https://www.cdc.gov/niosh/topics/hazards.html. 2017.
14. Occupational Safety and Health Administration: Occupational Noise Exposure. https://www.osha.gov/SLTC/noisehearingconservation/. 2019.
15. Hinds WC. *Aerosol technology : Properties, Behavior, and Measurement of Airborne Particles.* 2nd ed. New York: Wiley; 1999.
16. Environmental Protection Agency: Collection of Methods. https://www.epa.gov/measurements-modeling/collection-methods. 2017.
17. Centers for Disease Control: NIOSH Manual of Analytical Methods (NMAM). https://www.cdc.gov/niosh/nmam/default.html. 2018.
18. Jerrett M, Arain A, Kanaroglou P, et al. A review and evaluation of intraurban air pollution exposure models. *J Expo Anal Env Epid.* 2005;15(2):185–204.
19. Ramachandran G. *Occupational Exposure Assessment for Air Contaminants.* Boca Raton, FL: Taylor & Francis; CRC Press; 2005.
20. Zhang Y, Bocquet M, Mallet V, Seigneur C, Baklanov A. Real-time air quality forecasting, part I: History, techniques, and current status. *Atmos Environ.* 2012;60:632–55.
21. Wyat Appel K, Napelenok S, Hogrefe C, et al. Overview and Evaluation of the community Multiscale Air Quality (CMAQ) Modeling System Version 5.2. 2018; Cham.
22. Briggs DJ, Collins S, Elliott P, et al. Mapping urban air pollution using GIS: A regression-based approach. *Int J Geogr Inf Sci.* 1997;11(7):699–718.
23. English P, Neutra R, Scalf R, et al. Examining associations between childhood asthma and traffic flow using a geographic information system. *Environ Health Perspect.* 1999;107(9):761–7.
24. Hoek G, Beelen R, de Hoogh K, et al. A review of land-use regression models to assess spatial variation of outdoor air pollution. *Atmos Environ.* 2008;42(33):7561–78.
25. Dons E, Van Poppel M, Kochan B, Wets G, Int Panis L. Modeling temporal and spatial variability of traffic-related air pollution: Hourly land use regression models for black carbon. *Atmos Environ.* 2013;74:237–46.
26. Cohen AJ, Brauer M, Burnett R, et al. Estimates and 25-year trends of the global burden of disease attributable to ambient air pollution: An analysis of data from the Global Burden of Diseases Study 2015. *Lancet.* 2017;389(10082):1907–18.
27. Brauer M, Amann M, Burnett RT, et al. Exposure assessment for estimation of the global burden of disease attributable to outdoor air pollution. *Environ Sci Technol.* 2012;46(2):652–60.
28. Liu Y, Paciorek CJ, Koutrakis P. Estimating regional spatial and temporal variability of PM(2.5) concentrations using satellite data, meteorology, and land use information. *Environ Health Perspect.* 2009;117(6):886–92.
29. Fong KC, Hart JE, James P. A review of epidemiologic studies on greenness and health: Updated literature through 2017. *Curr Environ Health Rep.* 2018; 5(1):77–87.
30. Egorov A, Mudu P, Braubach M, Martuzzi M. Urban green spaces and health: A review of evidence. Copenhagen: WHO Regional Office for Europe; 2016.
31. Calafat AM, Ye X, Wong LY, Bishop AM, Needham LL. Urinary concentrations of four parabens in the U.S. population: NHANES 2005–2006. *Environ Health Perspect.* 2010;118(5):679–85.
32. WHO Regional Office for Europe. Human biomonitoring: Facts and figures. Copenhagen, 2015.
33. Quiros-Alcala L, Bradman A, Smith K, et al. Organophosphorous pesticide breakdown products in house dust and children's urine. *J Expo Sci Environ Epidemiol.* 2012;22(6):559–68.
34. Nordberg M, Duffus J, Templeton DM. Glossary of terms used in toxicokinetics (IUPAC Recommendations 2003). *Pure Appl Chem.* 2004;76(5):1032–82.
35. World Health Organization. The International Programme on Chemical Safety (IPCS)—Biomarkers and risk assessment: Concepts and principles. Geneva, Switzerland, 1993. http://www.inchem.org/documents/ehc/ehc/ehc155.htm.
36. Lionetto MG, Caricato R, Calisi A, Giordano ME, Schettino T. Acetylcholinesterase as a biomarker in environmental and occupational medicine: New insights and future perspectives. *Biomed Res Int.* 2013;2013:321213.
37. Huen K, Bradman A, Harley K, et al. Organophosphate pesticide levels in blood and urine of women and newborns living in an agricultural community. *Environ Res.* 2012;117:8–16.
38. Dennis KK, Marder E, Balshaw DM, et al. Biomonitoring in the era of the exposome. *Environ Health Perspect.* 2017;125(4):502–10.
39. Sharma A, Jaiswal S, Shukla M, Lal J. Dried blood spots: Concepts, present status, and future perspectives in bioanalysis. *Drug Test Anal.* 2014;6(5):399–414.
40. Smolders R, Schramm K-W, Nickmilder M, Schoeters G. Applicability of non-invasively collected matrices for human biomonitoring. *Environ Health-Glob.* 2009;8(1):8.
41. Lu C, Bravo R, Caltabiano LM, et al. The presence of dialkylphosphates in fresh fruit juices: Implication for organophosphorus pesticide exposure and risk assessments. *J Toxicol Environ Health A.* 2005;68(3):209–27.

42. Navas-Acien A, Francesconi KA, Silbergeld EK, Guallar E. Seafood intake and urine concentrations of total arsenic, dimethylarsinate and arsenobetaine in the US population. *Environ Res*. 2011;111(1):110–18.

43. Orloff K, Mistry K, Metcalf S. Biomonitoring for environmental exposures to arsenic. *J Toxicol Environ Health B Crit Rev*. 2009;12(7):509–24.

44. Andra SS, Austin C, Arora M. The tooth exposome in children's health research. *Curr Opin Pediatr*. 2016;28(2):221–7.

45. Michalke B, Rossbach B, Goen T, Schaferhenrich A, Scherer G. Saliva as a matrix for human biomonitoring in occupational and environmental medicine. *Int Arch Occup Environ Health*. 2015;88(1):1–44.

46. Perovich LJ, Ohayon JL, Cousins EM, et al. Reporting to parents on children's exposures to asthma triggers in low-income and public housing, an interview-based case study of ethics, environmental literacy, individual action, and public health benefits. Environ Health. 2018;17(1):48.

47. Manno M, Sito F, Licciardi L. Ethics in biomonitoring for occupational health. *Toxicol Lett*. 2014;231(2):111–21.

48. Nieuwenhuijsen MJ. Design of exposure questionnaires for epidemiological studies. *Occup Environ Med*. 2005;62(4):272–80.

49. NRC. *Human Exposure Assessment for Airborne Pollutants: Advances and Opportunities*. Washington, DC: National Academy of Sciences; 1991.

50. Koehler K, Good N, Wilson A, et al. The Fort Collins commuter study: Variability in personal exposure to air pollutants by microenvironment. *Indoor Air*. 2019;29(2):231–41.

51. Donaire-Gonzalez D, Valentin A, de Nazelle A, et al. Benefits of mobile phone technology for personal environmental monitoring. *JMIR Mhealth Uhealth*. 2016;4(4):e126.

52. Mennis J, Mason M, Coffman DL, Henry K. Geographic imputation of missing activity space data from ecological momentary assessment (EMA) GPS positions. *Int J Environ Res Public Health*. 2018;15(12):2740.

53. Shiffman S, Stone AA, Hufford MR. Ecological momentary assessment. *Annu Rev Clin Psychol*. 2008;4:1–32.

54. Kauppinen TP, Mutanen PO, Seitsamo JT. Magnitude of misclassification bias when using a job-exposure matrix. *Scand J Work Environ Health*. 1992;18(2):105–12.

55. Ramachandran G. Toward better exposure assessment strategies—The new NIOSH initiative. *Ann Occup Hyg*. 2008;52(5):297–301.

56. NIST: Exploratory Data Analysis. http://www.itl.nist.gov/div898/handbook/eda/eda.htm 2013.

57. Hewett P, Ganser GH. A comparison of several methods for analyzing censored data. *Ann Occup Hyg*. 2007;51(7):611–32.

58. Hubbard AE, Ahern J, Fleischer NL, et al. To GEE or not to GEE: Comparing population average and mixed models for estimating the associations between neighborhood risk factors and health. *Epidemiology*. 2010;21(4):467–74.

59. Rappaport S, Kupper L. *Quantitative Exposure Assessment*. El Cerrito, CA: Stephen Rappaport; 2008.

60. Johnson JM, Yu T, Strobel FH, Jones DP. A practical approach to detect unique metabolic patterns for personalized medicine. *Analyst*. 2010;135(11):2864–70.

61. Jones DP. Sequencing the exposome: A call to action. *Toxicol Rep*. 2016;3:29–45.

CHAPTER

64

Basic Toxicology and Mode of Action of Toxic Substances

David L. Eaton • Rachel M. Shaffer

FUNDAMENTAL CONCEPTS OF TOXICOLOGY

Types of Toxic Substances

Toxicology is defined as "*the study of the adverse effects of chemicals on living organisms, and the assessment of the probability of their occurrence.*"[1] Chemical substances—either natural or manmade—that can cause adverse effects on biological organisms are referred to as "toxicants." Those chemicals substances that are not normally produced within the body are often referred to as "xenobiotics."

Toxicology is more relevant than ever to public health: the number of manmade chemicals continues to increase, and exposures occur even before conception (affecting oocytes and sperm). Some chemicals are persistent in the environment, raising concern about the consequences of exposure across the life course and for future generations. In addition, with the large numbers of chemicals in the environment, predicting hazards to take preventive steps has proved challenging. This chapter provides an introduction to principles of toxicology, covering the diverse physiological processes by which toxicants are handled in the body and how they cause adverse effects.

There are numerous ways to classify chemicals into "categories" relevant to public health, including (1) by use (i.e., pesticides, food additives, pharmaceuticals, cosmetics, and industrial chemicals), (2) by route of exposure (e.g., air pollutants, drinking water contaminants, food contaminants, and dermal contaminants), (3) by primary "target organ"/toxic effect (liver toxicants, neurotoxicants, nephrotoxicants, lung toxicants, carcinogens, mutagens, and teratogens), and (4) by source (natural products, metals/elements, combustion products, and industrial/environmental contaminants). It is beyond the scope of this chapter to detail each of these potential categories, but a brief review of this classification by source is perhaps most relevant from a public health perspective. Other chapters in this volume will provide more detail for specific classes of chemicals and our sources of exposure to potentially toxic substances.

(1) *Natural Products (Toxins)*

Although the term "toxin" is often (incorrectly) used to describe any substance that can produce adverse effects, this term actually refers to a specific subset of toxicants that are produced by biological organisms, such as plants, animals, fungi, and microbiota. Indeed, several such natural products are among the most toxic substances known to humankind. Aflatoxins, a family of mycotoxins produce by the mold, *Aspergillus flavus* that frequently infects corn, peanuts, and other dietary staples, is a highly potent hepatotoxic (damaging to the liver) and hepatocarcinogenic (causing liver cancer) chemical.[2] Aflatoxins contribute significantly to the global burden of hepatocellular carcinoma, especially in developing countries where storage of corn and peanuts is often under conditions that do not prevent mold growth.

However, when used under the appropriate dose, route of exposure, and frequency, many natural products have been developed into successful pharmaceuticals and related treatments. For example, botulinum toxin Type A, produce by the bacterium *Clostridium botulinum* and related species, is the most acutely lethal substance ever identified. Yet, forms of botulinum toxin are useful therapeutically to treat certain neuromuscular conditions, as well for cosmetic purposes (e.g., "BoTox" injections to reduce facial wrinkles).[3]

Another example is a highly prescribed anticoagulant. During the 1920s–1930s, many cattle in the mid-west mysteriously died from what appeared to be internal bleeding. The deaths were eventually associated with the consumption of moldy "sweet clover" hay.[4] In the early 1940s, scientists discovered that a natural product present in sweet clover, called "coumarin," was metabolized by the molds growing on the hay to 3,3′-methylene-bis(4-hydroxycoumarin), or dicoumarol, that prevented blood from clotting. Subsequent research led to the discovery of a variant form that was even more potent and rapidly acting than dicoumarol. This compound, called "Warfarin," was initially developed into an effective rodenticide.[3] In the early 1950s, warfarin was developed into a clinically useful anticoagulant drug, Coumadin. Even though newer anticoagulant drugs have been developed, warfarin is still widely prescribed to prevent clotting in people at high risk for thrombotic heart disease and stroke.

(2) *Metals, Metalloids, and other Trace Elements*

Although metals and other potentially toxic elements are naturally occurring, they are not technically considered "toxins" since they are not produced by biological agents. [However, there are often "organic" forms of some elements (e.g., methyl mercury) that are formed by biological processes.] Exposures to metals come mainly through inhalation and ingestion, with higher absorption rates through inhalation as compared to ingestion.

The toxicity of metals is determined by many factors. The toxic effects of a metal or other trace element often result from binding and displacement of a different essential element in the active site of an enzyme, thereby altering its normal function. For example, superoxide dismutase (SOD) is an enzyme that plays a critical role in protecting cells from oxidative damage from endogenously produced hydrogen peroxide. One important form of SOD requires zinc and/or copper to function properly. Cadmium is a toxic metal similar to zinc but without any essential function in the body. It has high binding affinity for an endogenous protein called "metallothionein" (MT), which functions physiologically as a storehouse for zinc and is essential for maintaining intracellular redox status. Cd has much higher affinity than Zn for MT, resulting in a decrease in intracellular stores of Zn. Although it was initially thought that Cd inhibited SOD directly, recent research suggests that Cd indirectly affects SOD by preventing MT-Zn from maintaining SOD function.[5]

In other instances, the ionic characteristic of the metal/element favors binding to reduced sulfhydryl groups that are often present in the active site of many enzymes. Such complexation, that is, formation of enzyme-metal complexes, may lead to loss of function of a variety of enzymes and thus to a wide range of toxic effects.

Some metals can have different valence states. The valence state of specific metal ions determines the toxicological effects. For example, trivalent arsenic (As^{+3}) is highly toxic, linked to both acute and chronic effects in multiple organ systems, as well as carcinogenicity, while the toxicity of pentavalent arsenic (As^{+5}) is lower. As^{+5}, however, is reduced to As^{+3} in the human body before undergoing methylation and further detoxification. Therefore, the valence state of metals in the environment is not considered for monitoring and regulation.[6] Although the specific mode of action of arsenic toxicity and carcinogenesis is not completely understood, these effects may result from trivalent As complexation with a variety of different enzymes, including some enzymes involved in DNA repair.[7] Iron is another element with toxicity varying by valence state. Ferric iron (Fe^{+2}), when complexed with heme proteins (i.e., hemoglobin and myoglobin) avidly binds to molecular oxygen (O_2), whereas oxidized iron (Fe^{+3}) is unable to bind to O_2. Thus, exposure to chemicals such as nitrates and nitrites in drinking water that oxidize heme iron (from the +2 to the +3 state) can lead to methemoglobinemia and subsequent tissue hypoxia, especially in newborn infants.[8] Cyanide ion (CN^-) is another example of a substance that can interact with heme iron in the oxidized state. The potent and rapid toxic effects of CN^- can be somewhat ameliorated by therapeutic generation of methemoglobinemia via oxidation of heme iron intravenous infusion of a solution of $NaNO_2$ or by inhalation of amyl nitrite. Rather than binding to intracellular cytochrome C oxidase, the CN^- is complexed with the oxidized iron in circulating methemoglobin to form cyanomethemoglobin. The subsequent slow release of CN^- from the oxidized iron in hemoglobin can then be enzymatically detoxified via complexation with sulfur to form the relatively nontoxic thiocyanate ion.

(3) *Combustion Byproducts*

Oxidation of hydrocarbons present in organic matter (coal, petroleum products, wood and other plant materials, etc.) can result in the formation of a wide variety of toxic substances. For example, carbon monoxide (CO) is produced from the incomplete combustion of petroleum products. CO has an affinity for reduced iron in hemoglobin that is about 200 times greater than molecular oxygen, and thus relatively low concentrations of CO in breathing air can result in serious, often fatal cellular hypoxia.[9] Other potentially toxic combustion byproducts include polyaromatic hydrocarbons (PAHs). PAHs are highly lipophilic and rapidly absorbed into the body following oral or inhalation exposure to PAHs. Because of their high lipophilicity, PAH elimination from the body requires biotransformation to more water-soluble forms [see section "Metabolism (Biotransformation)"]. Some biotransformation products, particularly certain arene oxides such as benzo(a)pyrene-diol-epoxide (BPDE), are highly reactive electrophilic intermediates that can bind to nucleophilic sites in proteins and DNA, thereby disrupting normal cellular function. BPDE and certain other PAH oxides are highly mutagenic and carcinogenic via covalent adduction to DNA. Although there are many other potentially toxic substances that are formed when organic materials—both natural and synthetic—undergo combustion, CO and PAHs represent the most common toxic byproducts of combustion. Cigarette smoke is one of the most prevalent forms of potentially continuous, long-term exposure to combustion byproducts. There are over 7000 different chemicals identified in cigarette smoke, including CO, various oxides of nitrogen (NO_X), and hundreds of different PAHs.[10]

(4) *Synthetic Organic Chemicals with Industrial/Environmental Exposures*

With the passage of the Toxic Substances Control Act (TSCA) in 1976, the U.S. Environmental Protection Agency (EPA) established an "inventory" of tens of thousands of chemicals potentially available for use in commerce. Most synthetic chemicals in widespread use and for which extensive human exposures are likely (e.g., pesticides, food additives and contaminants, drugs) have not been subject to sufficient toxicological testing to characterize potential hazards. The insufficiency of testing was recognized more than 50 years ago following numerous environmental and occupational chemical disasters, such as the widespread distribution of dioxin-contaminated waste oil in Times Beach Missouri, and community exposures to improperly disposed chemical wastes ("Love Canal").

The National Toxicology Program (NTP) was established as part of the National Institute of Environmental Health Sciences (NIEHS) in 1978 to facilitate toxicity testing of chemicals of potential public health concern. The National Academies of Science (NAS) completed an evaluation of the state of knowledge of toxicity testing of chemicals in 1982 to facilitate prioritization of the thousands of chemicals in commerce with little or no toxicity information.[11] At that time, the committee estimated that for the highest production volume chemicals (>1 million lbs/yr) only about 20% of the chemicals had some toxicity data available. After 50 years of the NTP, substantial improvements have been made, but even within the NTP, somewhat less than 1000 "top priority" chemicals have been subjected to 2-year chronic toxicity/carcinogenicity testing.[12] More recently, in response to the 2016 Frank R. Lautenberg Chemical Safety for the 21st Century Act, EPA published a new TSCA inventory in 2019 that listed 40,655 chemicals that were currently in active commerce in the United States.[13] The 2016 amendments and reauthorization of TSCA continue to emphasize the importance of toxicity testing for new chemicals introduced into commerce in the United States, but large gaps in knowledge of the potential human health and environmental impacts of thousands of chemicals used in commerce in the United States remain a significant public health concern.

Basic Concepts of the "Dose–Response Relationship" and Its Importance to Toxicology and Public Health

Introduction to Concepts of Dose

The term "dose" sounds simple, but there are different concepts of dose that are important in toxicology. The "administered dose" (or "applied dose") is the amount of toxicant that is utilized in an experimental toxicology study. The "internal dose" (or "absorbed dose") is the amount of toxicant that is actually absorbed into the organism. An even more refined concept is that of "target organ dose" (or "biologically effective dose"), which refers to the amount of the toxicant that reaches the target site and causes adverse effects. It is important to distinguish between these concepts of dose in evaluating toxicological studies and understanding dose–response relationships; the target organ dose or biologically effective dose is the most relevant toxicologically.[14]

A long-held paradigm in toxicology was first presented in the mid-seventeenth century by the physician/scientist/philosopher, Paracelsus, who stated *"All substances are poisons; there is none which is not. The dose differentiates a poison from a remedy."* While this may hold in many scenarios, gains in scientific understanding of how xenobiotics—both natural and manmade—are handled by the body have challenged this precept. From a public health perspective, the risk of an adverse event at different doses is critical to deciding on the need for preventive measures and the steps to be taken to reduce risks.

The "route" of exposure affects the likelihood and extent of an adverse outcome following an exposure to a toxic substance. For substances of occupational and environmental health concern, there are three common routes of exposure: oral (usually ingestion, through food or water, although pica and soil ingestion are common in children); inhalation (breathing in vapors or airborne particles); and dermal (direct contact with the skin). Less common routes include direct injection (e.g., tattoos) and mucosa (e.g., tampons and other products). The transplacental route is important for fetal exposures. For substances that enter the body through oral ingestion, the extent of absorption (bioavailability) is dependent on numerous factors. The important processes of "absorption, distribution, metabolism, and excretion (ADME) of toxicants" are discussed in more detail in section "Absorption, Distribution, Metabolism (Biotransformation), and Excretion (ADME)."

Dose–Response Relationships

Toxicologists have classically recognized two fundamentally different types of "dose–response relationships." The first is the individual dose–response relationship, which describes the specific response of an individual organism to increasing doses of a chemical. This individual dose–response relationship is also often referred to as a "graded dose–response relationship," since the response is measured over continuous dose levels. It should be noted that each specific biological effect of a chemical, for example, carcinogenicity and immunotoxicity, might have a different dose–response relationship. The individual, or "graded" dose response curve is shown in Fig. 64-1A. For certain substances, such as essential trace metals and vitamins, having too small of dose can actually be toxic (e.g., a vitamin deficiency), illustrated by the ascending line on the left hand of Fig. 64-1A. For some toxicants, there are doses below which the toxic substance has no evident toxic effect, the so-called "threshold of safety" in Fig. 64-1A.

The second major type is a population or quantal dose–response relationship, which describes the distribution of individual responses over an entire population (Fig. 64-1B). In this scenario, individuals are classified as either responders or nonresponders for each given dose. However, because individuals within a population will have some variability in their susceptibility to a toxicant, there may not be meaningful population thresholds, in contrast to what might be identified in an individual dose-response curve.[15]

Shapes of Population-Based Dose-Response Curves

The traditionally assumed shape of dose-response curves is monotonic, with increasing doses causing unidirectional changes in response (either an increase or decrease in toxic effect).

Most toxic substances have multiple molecular targets that contribute to an adverse response, and each specific molecular response will have its own dose–response relationship. If the response being measured is a complex and nonspecific outcome (e.g., a general adverse outcome such as death, body weight change, food consumption, number of tumors, or number of offspring with birth defects), it is likely that there are multiple molecular events that contribute to the observed outcome, and each has its own "dose–response" relationship. Thus, different dose–response relationships may be applicable. Since the form of the dose–response relationship has critical implications for public health, toxicological research often has the goal of characterizing the dose-response with sufficient precision for decision-making. This goal demands carefully designed studies. If only three or four doses are used in a study, the true shape of the dose–response relationship cannot be fully characterized over a wide range of doses.

Nonmonotonic dose–response relationships may occur in circumstances where a toxic substance has an effect at low doses that is not evident at higher doses, and/or imparts a "stimulatory" effect at low doses, a concept referred to as "hormesis" (Fig. 64-2). Although the low dose "stimulatory" effect has often been identified as a "beneficial" effect, this is not always the case. Hormesis was first described for ionizing but also may pertain to some other chemical responses, and remains controversial.[16] In these circumstances, a plot of response over a wide range of doses results in a "U-shaped" dose-response curve, conceptually similar to the individual dose–response curve for essential trace elements and nutrients (Fig. 64-1). Hormetic responses, by definition, have unique quantitative features that describe the magnitude and width of the low-dose stimulatory response.[14,16] An example is the substantial epidemiological evidence demonstrating that moderate alcohol consumption reduces the incidence of some types of coronary heart disease,[17] whereas chronic relatively high-dose alcohol consumption clearly increases the risk of liver cirrhosis and liver cancer, as well as cancer of the esophagus.[18]

Some toxicants, including endogenous hormones and synthetic endocrine-disrupting chemicals (EDCs) that act via hormone receptors, may also show bi- or even multiphasic (i.e., nonmonotonic) adverse responses (Fig. 64-2). This distinction means that the high-dose exposures often utilized in traditional toxicity testing could potentially underestimate the risk posed by EDCs at the lower doses often encountered in the environment. Such a response has been described for multiple chemicals, including natural hormones such as 17B-estradiol, pharmaceuticals such as diethylstilbestrol (DES), and synthetic chemicals such as bisphenol A (BPA) and phthalates.[19] In response to studies suggesting very low-dose and nonmonotonic effects of BPA and other EDCs, multiple organizations, including the Environmental Protection Agency (EPA) and the Food and Drug Administration (FDA), established an extensive toxicological evaluation of BPA, called CLARITY-BPA,[20,21] to re-evaluate the essential

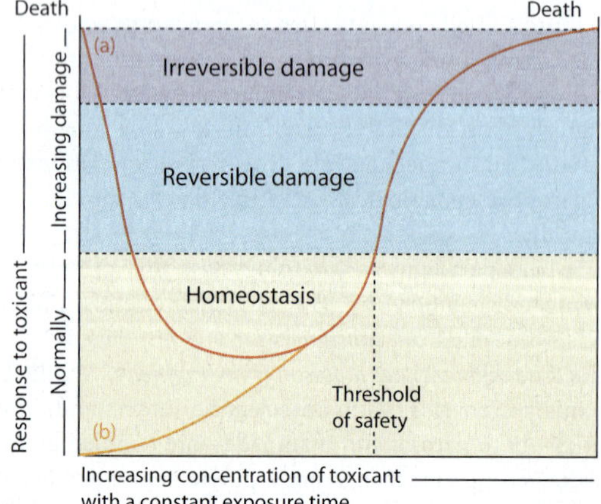

FIGURE 64-1. Classical dose–response relationships. (*Source:* From Eaton DL, Gilbert SG. Principles of Toxicology. In: CD Klaasen, ed. *Casarett and Doull's Toxicology. The Basic Science of Poisons*, 8th ed. Chap. 22. New York: McGraw Hill Medical, pp. 13-48.[14])

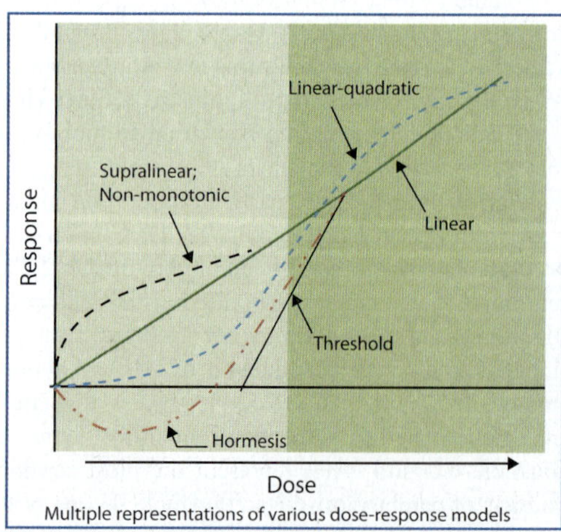

FIGURE 64-2. Multiple representations of dose–response relationships.

assumptions underlying chemical testing procedures, especially for chemicals that may act as modulators (agonists or antagonists) of endocrine pathways.

Absorption, Distribution, Metabolism (Biotransformation), and Excretion (ADME)

Absorption

For a chemical substance to produce systemic toxicity (toxicity in one or more parts of the body, distant from the site of contact), it must first be absorbed into the bloodstream and circulated to target tissues. This path can be completed via any of the three common "routes of exposures": ingestion (oral), inhalation (pulmonary), and dermal. Administration of chemicals via direct injection (parenteral routes of exposure: intravenous, intramuscular, intradermal, or others) is an important route of exposure for pharmaceuticals but generally not relevant to the discussion of occupational/environmental exposures.

Absorption depends on a variety of factors, including (a) the concentration of the substance at the site of contact, (b) the lipid solubility of the substance, (c) the thickness of the barrier between the surface and the underlying blood supply, (d) the extent of blood flow to the region (which determines the rate of removal of the substance once it has crossed the barrier, and (e) the total surface area available for absorption. The extent of absorption of a toxic substance is a key determinant of its "bioavailability." Bioavailability refers to the fraction of the "exposed dose" that reaches the systemic circulation and depends both upon the extent of absorption and the amount that might be removed by the liver following oral absorption into the portal circulation (blood flowing from the gut to the liver).

The relative rates of absorption across the GI tract, lung, and skin can be substantially different because of the different values for the parameters discussed above. For example, absorption across the skin is generally very slow and often incomplete because of the relatively low surface area of exposure, the relatively great distance of diffusion and a low permeability coefficient, compared to those for the GI tract and the lung. The skin is composed of multiple cell layers of squamous cells, including the keratinized outer layer, the epidermis. The presence of keratin (a protein) provides a substantial protective barrier to simple diffusion of many lipid-soluble substances. Disruption of the barrier posed by the skin can greatly facilitate the dermal absorption of most toxic substances. Thus, abrasions and/or cuts on the surface of the skin can result in much greater systemic bioavailability of a substance that contacts the skin.

In contrast to the skin, the GI tract and the lung provide both large surface areas and minimal diffusion distances; therefore, absorption of lipid-soluble substances can occur very rapidly and completely. The rate and extent of absorption of toxic substances following oral exposure is influenced by a variety of biological and physical factors, such as pH and surface area. Substances that are weak organic acids or bases exist in different ionic forms, depending on the pKa of the substance and the pH of the GI tract. For weak organic acids with pKa's in the range of 2.5–3.5, absorption will be higher in the acid pH of the stomach, relative to the small intestine. However, although much more of the weak organic acid will exist in the protonated, lipid-soluble form in the stomach compared to the intestine, the much greater surface area of the small intestine, coupled with longer contact time, greatly facilitates absorption in the small intestine. For weak organic bases, little absorption generally occurs in the stomach because most of the molecules are in the protonated, charged (and thus nonlipid soluble) form because of the acidity of the stomach. The presence of stomach acid and digestive enzymes in the GI track can also greatly alter absorption of some substances, particularly peptides and small proteins, which are generally hydrolyzed to amino acids. This is the primary reason why most "biologic" drugs cannot be administered orally. Finally, insoluble organic matter in the gut can also bind to and sequester some toxic substances, greatly reducing bioavailability following ingestion. This is the clinical basis for administering "activated charcoal" in some poisonings, which can be lifesaving in some circumstances.

Absorption of inhaled toxic substances across the lung can be very rapid, approaching the rate of intravenous administration for highly lipid-soluble substance. Nicotine is a well-known example; it enters the lung on small particles and quickly moves from sites of absorption into the circulation. Metal exposure through inhalation can also result in almost complete metal absorption from air into the blood stream, in contrast to absorption through ingestion, which is more variable. For most toxic gases, inhalation is the primary route of exposure. The rate of absorption is influenced not only by the lipid solubility, but also by the "blood:gas partition coefficient," which is a measure of the relative solubility of the gas in blood vs. inhaled air. For gaseous substances that bind to components of the blood, absorption can be very rapid and complete. The relative efficacy of many anesthetics used clinically is determined in large part by their blood:gas partition coefficients. In addition, the concentration of the gas in the inhaled air is another crucial determinant of exposure via inhalation. Consequently, respiratory protection and good occupational hygiene practices can greatly reduce the extent of exposure and potential adverse health effects from airborne chemicals in the workplace.

Distribution

Once absorbed into the systemic circulation, chemicals can be distributed throughout the body. The rate of distribution depends on blood flow, rate of diffusion into cells of a certain organ or tissue, and affinity of the chemical for different organs or tissues. Chemicals absorbed into the bloodstream will initially be distributed to the most highly perfused tissues, which include the brain, heart, lungs, and liver. The rate of diffusion from the systemic circulation into cells is dependent in large part on the lipid solubility of the substance, often described as the "octonol:water partition coefficient," or $\log K_{ow}$. Chemicals with a high $\log K_{ow}$ (e.g., >1) will rapidly diffuse across cell membranes and distribute initially to highly perfused tissues. Thus, for example, inhalation of high concentrations of many organic solvents can have rapid effects on CNS function, resulting initially in CNS stimulation (e.g., the "high" that results from glue sniffing), but subsequently CNS depression, leading potentially to narcosis and death. Other highly lipid soluble chemicals with long biological half-lives (e.g., DDT, PCBs, dioxins) will initially distribute in highly perfused organs, but over time will redistribute to fat tissues. Thus, adipose tissue will ultimately have the highest concentrations, followed by liver and brain, which also contain relatively high amounts of lipids.

Although passive diffusion is the predominant way that most chemicals cross cellular membranes, some substances may serve as substrates for membrane transport processes and be concentrated in specific tissues. Liver, kidney, lung, and intestinal cells have both active influx and efflux transporters, and consequently specific "target organ" toxicity may result from accumulation of specific substances that are actively transported into the tissue. Transporters are important for some metals. For example, cadmium absorption through the gastrointestinal tract has been related to the activation of iron transporters.[22] For metalloids, aquaporins have shown to be important for intracellular transport of arsenic, in particular in its trivalent form.[23]

Another important determinant of distribution is protein binding. Some substances can bind to plasma proteins, such as albumin, with relatively high affinity. This binding hinders hepatic first pass clearance (see below) and increases distribution in the body. Many pharmaceutical drugs bind to plasma proteins such that 98+% of the drug is bound, with only a small (e.g., <2%) available in the "free," unbound form. Only the unbound fraction is available to diffuse into tissues and exert its pharmacological effects. Exposure to another substance, such as another drug or xenobiotic that binds to the same protein in the blood can result in displacement of the bound molecules, potentially greatly exaggerating the pharmacological or toxicological effect.

There are also barriers that alter the distribution of chemicals to tissues in the body. For example, the "blood-brain barrier" (BBB) is highly effective at keeping many drugs and chemicals from reaching the brain and interfering with brain function. The BBB consists of specialized tight junctions in the brain endothelium as well as glial cell projections that wrap around capillaries in the brain. This barrier prevents water-soluble chemicals from diffusing between cells in the endothelium, protecting neurons from exposure. However, because these barriers are largely composed of lipid bilayers in the membranes, the BBB is ineffective in preventing lipid-soluble chemicals from entering the brain. The testes also contain specialized processes to prevent most chemicals from coming in contact with sperm-forming cells, but, like the BBB, this barrier function is not completely effective, especially for lipid-soluble substances. The BBB is also not fully mature during early life, resulting in a period of particular risk from exposure to neurotoxic chemicals.

Metabolism (Biotransformation)

In classical pharmacology, the recognition that most drugs are rapidly eliminated from the body formed the basis for "drug metabolism" as an important concept in both pharmacology and toxicology. Although the term drug metabolism is still widely used, a more appropriate term is "biotransformation," the basic enzymatic processes that result in biological modification (transformation) of the chemical structure of a molecule.

Biotransformation of xenobiotics is among the most important concepts in toxicology, because genetic differences in biotransformation capability contribute greatly to both interindividual and species differences in toxicity. There are two fundamental biological purposes for biotransformation: (1) to make lipid-soluble compounds water soluble so that they can be eliminated via excretion from the body, and (2) to alter the chemical structure of both endogenous and exogenous chemicals in order to reduce or eliminate their biological activity (including potential toxicity).

Although the majority of biotransformation of both endogenous and exogenous chemicals in the body occurs in the liver, most tissues in the body have some capacity for biotransformation. Indeed, specific "target organ toxicity" (this section) is often the result of specific biotransformation of a substance in that tissue that leads to the tissue-specific toxicity. The process of xenobiotic biotransformation is generally complex and multistep—that is, a single "parent" molecule may end up in many different chemical forms, each referred to as a "metabolite." While the fundamental purpose of biotransformation is to reduce biological effects, including toxicity, of a foreign substance, sometimes a chemical is converted to one or more intermediate forms that is/are more reactive (and thus more toxic) than the "parent" molecule. For instance, reduction of As^{5+} into As^{3+} results in the generation of a more reactive, highly toxic compound before further methylation results in lower toxicity arsenic compounds.

The process of biotransformation is often divided into different general "phases": phase I metabolism/biotransformation refers to the first action of the body on a chemical, which is usually an oxidation reaction for lipophilic substances (hydrocarbons) but can also be hydrolysis reactions if the substances contain ester or amide bonds. Phase II reactions refer to the process in which a product of phase I metabolism is further altered, usually by the addition of a highly water-soluble endogenous molecule that imparts large changes in both the structure and water solubility of the phase I metabolite. These are called "conjugation reactions" and require endogenous cofactors to donate a part of their structure (such as a sulfate, sugar, or amino acid component). Finally, the highly water-soluble conjugated metabolite can be eliminated in the urine and/or bile (and subsequently feces). However, because these final conjugated metabolites are water soluble and cannot readily diffuse across cellular membranes, specific membrane transport processes are used to move the conjugate from the intracellular space where it was formed into urine or bile. This final step is often referred to as "Phase III metabolism."

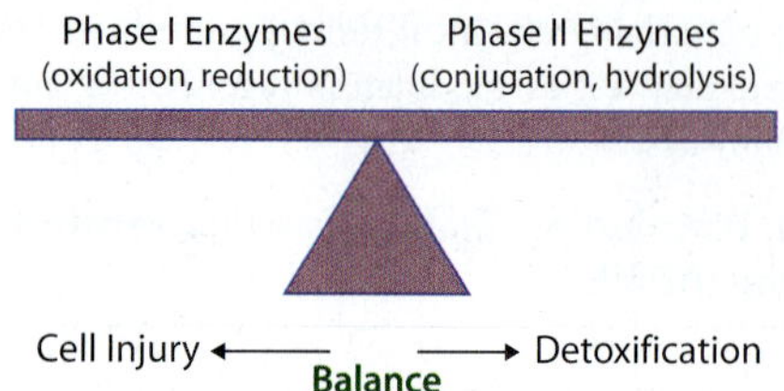

FIGURE 64-3. Multistep process of xenobiotic activation and detoxification.

The rates of each biotransformation reaction can differ dramatically, and thus it is the overall balance of activation to detoxification that is a predominant determinant of toxicity of a xenobiotic at a specific dose (Fig. 64-3). The relative balance between activation and detoxification is often dose dependent, such that the ratio of specific metabolites at low doses may be substantially different than at high doses. Further, many xenobiotic biotransformation enzymes are inducible by other exposures (diet, drugs, occupational and environmental chemicals), and there are common genetic differences (polymorphisms) in many biotransformation genes, which can contribute to substantial interindividual variability.

For chemicals absorbed via the GI tract following ingestion, nearly all of the absorbed material passes into the portal circulation and through the liver prior to distribution to other tissues in the body. The liver thus works as an "in-line" metabolic filter for any substance that is absorbed from the small intestine and stomach. Through the "first pass effect," the liver can remove much of the absorbed material before it enters the systemic circulation.

Phase 1 Oxidation/Reduction Reactions For lipophilic hydrocarbons such as most petroleum products and many drugs, pesticides and persistent environmental contaminants, oxidation is the critical first step in eliminating the substance from the body. Most phase 1 oxidation reactions are catalyzed by one or more members of the multigene family of enzymes referred to collectively as "Cytochromes P450" (CYPs). CYPs are heme-containing proteins that bind molecular oxygen via the heme iron. They have a second catalytic site that recognizes and binds a wide range of organic molecules. Once the substrate (xenobiotic) is bound to the catalytic site, the CYP enzyme obtains two electrons from NADP(H) via another enzyme, cytochrome P450 reductase. The catalytic function of the enzymes is to split molecular oxygen (O_2), inserting one an atom of oxygen, usually in the form of a hydroxyl group (-OH) into the structure of the molecule, with the other atom released as water. The oxidized substrate now has a reactive moiety (the hydroxyl group or epoxide) for subsequent conjugation (the hydroxyl group) or hydrolysis of the epoxide to form a dihydrodiol.

There are approximately 60 different CYP genes in the human genome. Many of these play important physiological roles in the synthesis and degradation of specific endogenous molecules, including hormones. A subset of CYPs has broad substrate specificity and are able to metabolize a wide range of drugs and other xenobiotics. In the human liver, the primary CYP enzymes responsible for the oxidation of xenobiotics, in order of relative amounts, are: CYP3A4 and 5 (29%) CYP2C8 and 9 (18%), CYP4F2 and 3 (15%), CYP1A2 (13%), CYP2E1 (7%), CYP2A6 (4%), CYP2D6 (1–2%), and CYP2B6 (0.2%) (the remaining approximately 13% are distributed among numerous other CYP genes) (Fig. 64-4). Genetic polymorphisms in CYP enzymes are very common, and there are large interindividual differences in expression of specific CYP genes in liver and other tissues that can contribute to interindividual differences in susceptibility to toxic substances. Differential susceptibility needs to be taken into account when standards and other measures are proposed to mitigate adverse effects.

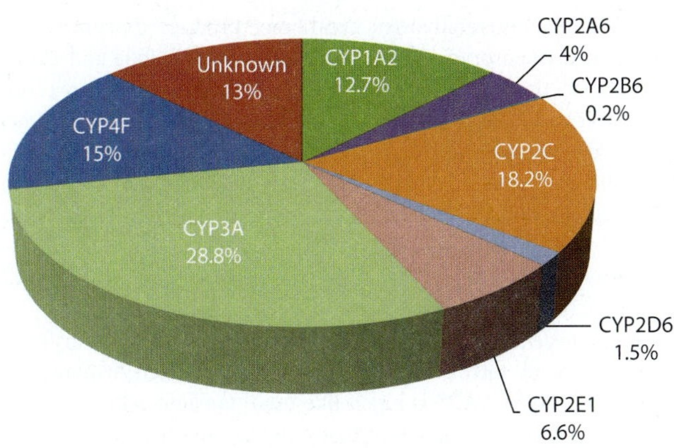

FIGURE 64-4. Revised human liver P450 pie. The inset figure depicts the percentage contributions of individual P450 enzymes based on the immunoquantification performed by Shimada et al. (1994). The larger figure shows the revised P450 pie with CYP4F contributing to 15% of the total hepatic P450s. (*Source:* Adapted with permission from Michaels S, Wang MZ. *Drug Metab Dispos* 2014; 42:1241–1251.)

Because different CYP enzymes have different affinities for a wide variety of xenobiotics, the rates of biotransformation of a specific xenobiotic can vary greatly between one species and another, and between individuals within a population, depending of the kinetic characteristics of the specific enzymes involved in biotransformation. A classic example of the importance of CYP oxidation in the activation and detoxification of xenobiotics is that of the biotransformation of the potent liver toxin and carcinogen, aflatoxin B1 (AFB1). In human liver, CYP1A2 acts as a "high affinity, but low capacity" catalyst for the formation of two oxidation products of AFB1, one to the highly reactive and carcinogenic product, AFB 8,9-epoxide (AFBO), and the other to a much less toxic product, AFM1. However, human CYP3A4, which is the most prevalent of all CYP enzymes in the liver, also oxidizes AFB1 to the toxic AFBO, and to another oxidation product, AFQ1, which is nontoxic. Kinetically, CYP3A4 acts as a high capacity, but low-affinity enzyme. Thus, at high concentrations (e.g., >10 uM) of AFB1 in *in vitro* experiments with human liver tissue, CYP3A4 appears to be the predominant human CYP in forming the toxic AFBO metabolite. However, at lower concentrations (e.g., <0.5 uM) that would be seen following dietary exposures to AFB1, CYP1A2 becomes the predominant CYP enzyme in activating AFB to AFBO.[24]

In addition to CYP enzymes, there are many other families of enzymes that can participate in the phase 1 oxidation and/or reduction of xenobiotics. The "Flavin-Dependent Monooxygenases," or FMOs, function in the oxidation of so-called "heteroatoms" such as sulfur and nitrogen. These enzymes also contain a heme unit that binds molecular oxygen but use FAD(H)2 rather than NAD(P)H as the electron donor. An example of a toxicologically important FMO-mediated oxidation reaction is the metabolism of the dietary breakdown product, trimethylamine (TMA). TMA is a substrate for FMO oxidation. TMA is a highly odiforous compound, with the smell of "rotten fish." Fortunately, it is quickly oxidized by FMO3 to TMA-Oxide (TMAO), which has no odor. A genetic deficiency in FMO3 leads to a condition called "Fish-Odor Syndrome" (trimethylaminuria), in which TMA is secreted in sweat as well as urine, producing a body odor resembling rotten fish.[25]

Dehydrogenase enzymes catalyze oxidation reactions for short chain alcohols, such as methanol, ethanol, and propanol. An example of an important dehydrogenase enzyme is alcohol dehydrogenase, which catalyzes the oxidation of ethanol to acetaldehyde. Acetaldehyde is toxic, but it is quickly further oxidized to acetic acid by aldehyde dehydrogenase (ALDH). Acetic acid is nontoxic and is used in the citric acid cycle to generate adenosine triphosphate (ATP). However, if acetaldehyde is not quickly eliminated, consumption of ethyl alcohol can lead to moderate or potentially serious toxicity, including vascular dilation resulting in "flushing reactions," headaches, nausea, and vomiting. A genetic deficiency in ALDH is common in certain Asian populations, and carriers of this variant allele often avoid alcohol consumption because of the unpleasant reactions that can occur. This enzyme pathway has also been leveraged for drug treatment: a drug that inhibits ALDH, "Antabuse" (disulfuram) has been developed and used to treat alcoholism by inducing an "avoidance" reaction to alcohol consumption.

Numerous other oxidase enzymes exist in the body. For example, monoamine oxidase (MAO), which can exist in two forms, MAO-A and MAO-B, are present in many tissues throughout the body. These enzymes function physiologically in the oxidation of the primary, secondary, and tertiary amines such as neurotransmitters epinephrine, norepinephrine, dopamine, and serotonin, as well as many drugs.

Phase 1 Hydrolysis Reactions Another key phase 1 reaction is hydrolysis. Many drugs, and some environmental pollutants, exist as esters or amides, and are subject to o-hydrolysis via the addition of water across the ester or amide bond. The resulting products are an acid and an alcohol (from esters) and an amine and alcohol (from amides). For example, the neurotransmitter acetylcholine is hydrolyzed by the enzyme acetylcholinesterase (AChE). This critically important enzymatic reaction quickly eliminates acetylcholine from synaptic spaces following its release in response to cholinergic nerve stimulation. Organophosphorous pesticides, such as malathion, parathion, and chlorpyrifos, and the nerve gas agents Sarin and Tabun, are effective inhibitors of AChE activity. High exposure can result in acute cholinergic crisis, that is, a toxic accumulation of acetylcholine, leading to paralysis and respiratory failure. The consequences of long-term, lower-level exposure to cholinesterase inhibitors are not well defined, although findings of several studies have suggested that permanent neurological deficits could result.[26]

Other enzymes, such as the carboxylesterases, also function to hydrolyze a wide variety of exogenous esters. The widely used local anesthetic, procaine, is quickly hydrolyzed via a carboxylesterase to an inactive form. Because there are carboxylesterase enzymes that circulate in blood, procaine is a quite short-acting anesthetic. The amide form, procainamide, is hydrolyzed much more slowly and thus is a much longer acting local anesthetic.

From a toxicological perspective, hydrolysis of epoxides via enzymes called epoxide hydrolases (EH) is a very important hydrolytic reaction. Many chemicals that show carcinogenic activity do so through oxidation to a reactive epoxide intermediate. If not quickly hydrolyzed to the diol (or conjugated to an endogenous nucleophile such as glutathione) by an EH, the electrophilic epoxide can bind to nucleophilic sites on DNA and proteins to form adducts, leading to mutations. There are two basic forms of EH: one is located in the endoplasmic reticulum of the cell and thus is called "microsomal epoxide hydrolase (mEH)," whereas the second form exists primarily in the cytosol of the cell and hence is called cytosolic or "soluble epoxide hydrolase (sEH)." mEH is the more important of the two enzymes, as it is active in hydrolyzing a wide variety of potentially toxic and carcinogenic epoxides. For example, the polyaromatic hydrocarbon (PAH), benzo(a)pyrene (BaP), present in tobacco smoke and soot, tars and oils derived from combustion of petroleum products and other organic materials, is a potent carcinogen. The carcinogenic activity of BaP occurs via initial oxidation of CYP1A1 to form BaP-7,8-epoxide. This unstable and reactive intermediate is hydrolyzed to the dihydrodiol. Although this would appear to be a detoxification reaction, the BaP-7,8-dihydrodiol is further oxidized by CYP1A1 to from BaP-7,8-dihydrodiol-9,10-epoxide (BPDE). If not further hydrolyzed by mEH or conjugated with glutathione, BPDE can bind to DNA, forming a relatively stable BPDE-DNA adduct that can result in mispairing during DNA replication and introduction of mutations, a key step in carcinogenesis.

Other esterases and amidases can also play important roles in biotransformation of xenobiotics. For example, an enzyme called "paraoxonase" (PON) is involved in the hydrolysis of certain organophosphorous pesticides to nontoxic forms. Genetic polymorphism in the PON1 gene has been implicated in differential susceptibility to poisoning from certain organophosphorous pesticides.[27]

Phase 2 Conjugation Reactions Once a xenobiotic has a "functional group" (such as a hydroxyl, carboxylic acid, primary or secondary amine, and free thiol group) further biotransformation can occur, resulting in the addition of a polar, endogenous molecule. The major classes of phase 2 conjugation enzymes are: glutathione-S-transferases (GSTs), glucuronosyl transferases (UGTs), sulfotransferases (SULTs), N-acetyl transferases (NATs), and methyltransferases (MTs). Other enzymes can also utilize certain amino acids in transferase reactions.

i. *Glutathione S-Transferases:* GSTs mediate the transfer of the tripeptide, glutathione (g-glutamyl-cystenyl-glycine) to an electrophilic site on a molecule, which is usually an epoxide or reactive nitrogen atom. In humans, there are five major functional classes of GSTs: alpha (GSTA; 5 genes), mu (GSTM; 2 genes), theta (GSTT 2 genes), pi (GSTP 2 genes), and zeta (GSTZ; one gene). GSTs are soluble enzymes, meaning that they are not membrane bound and exist in the cytosolic fraction of cells. There are two microsomal forms of GST (mGSTs) but their role in glutathione conjugation of xenobiotics is relatively minor. Alpha class GSTs represent the major forms found in liver, and to a lesser extent, other tissues.

   Mu class GSTs are particularly interesting because of the presence of a major genetic polymorphism in GSTM1, in which approximately 50% of most racial/ethnic groups are homozygous null for GSTM1; in other words, 50% of the population are missing both functional alleles of GSTM1 and thus have no GSTM1 activity (GSTM1-null). Most of the remainder of the population has one functional allele (hemizygous), but 2–3% of people are homozygous for the active allele. GSTM1 is involved in the detoxification of numerous reactive epoxides, including epoxides of benzo(a) pyrene (BPDE) and aflatoxin B1 (AFBO), formed by CYP oxidation. Individuals who are GSTM1-null have been shown to be at higher risk for a variety of cancers linked to environmental and occupational exposures. For example, smokers who are GSTM1-null exhibit a 20–50% increased risk for lung and bladder cancer, compared to GST-positive populations.[28] Likewise, individuals who are GSTM1 null are at ~1.5-fold increase risk of liver cancer if chronically exposed to aflatoxin B1 in their diets, compared to those who are GSTM1-positive.[29]

   Glutathione conjugates of xenobiotics are taken up either by the liver or the kidney, where subsequent enzymatic processes remove both the glutamate and glycine amino acids, leaving only the cysteine complexed with the xenobiotic via the sulfhydryl group. The cysteine is usually quickly conjugated via N-acetylation to yield N-acetylcysteine-xenobiotic conjugate, which is rapidly eliminated in urine and/or bile.

ii. *UDP-Glucuronyl Transferases (UGTs):* UGTs are a family of enzymes with the catalytic function of transferring a molecule of glucuronic acid (an oxidized form of glucose) from the donor molecule, UDP-glucuronic acid, to a substrate (such as a xenobiotic). UGTs can perform this transfer to substrates with hydroxyl groups, carboxylic acids, and primary amines in their structures. The glucuronic acid moiety imparts a high level of water solubility as well as major structural changes that generally eliminate the potential toxic characteristics of the parent molecule.

   Some UGTs are involved in endogenous metabolism and thus play physiological roles. For example, UGT1A enzymes conjugate bilirubin, a potentially toxic breakdown product of heme, to bilirubin-diglucuronide, which is secreted into the bile and eliminated in the feces. Genetic polymorphisms of UGTs involved in bilirubin conjugation can result in mild (Gilbert's syndrome; ~70% reduction in UGT-bilirubin activity) to severe (Crigler-Najjar syndrome; >90% reduction in UGT-bilirubin activity) effects. Glucuronide conjugation represents one of the most common forms of xenobiotic conjugation, and often plays an important role in reducing or eliminating the toxic properties of oxidized products of CYP and FMO oxidation.

iii. *Sulfotransferases (SULTs):* SULT enzymes catalyze the transfer of an "activated" form of sulfate that is in phosphoadenosylphosphosulfate (PAPS). PAPS is much like the important cellular energy molecule ATP, but has a terminal sulfate, rather than a phosphate, moiety. As with glucuronide conjugation, sulfate conjugation produces a highly water-soluble form of the molecule that can be readily eliminated through membrane transport processes.

   Although most sulfate conjugates are stable and represent effective detoxification processes, there are numerous examples for which sulfate conjugation actually results in a reactive intermediate that is the ultimate toxic form of the molecule. For example, the plant toxin, aristolochic acid, is metabolized initially to an N-oxide that is then conjugated via SULT enzymes. The sulfate conjugate serves as a good substrate for renal transporters in the proximal tubules, and thus is taken from the blood and concentrated in the kidney for elimination in the urine. However, the sulfate conjugate is chemically unstable, and rearranges in the kidney to re-form the N-oxide, which binds to key proteins in the renal proximal tubular cells, causing potentially serious kidney disease.[30]

iv. *N-Acetyltransferases (NATs).* As the name suggests, NATs transfer an acetate group, in the form of Acetyl-CoA, to the recipient substrate. Substrates for NAT enzymes are principally primary and secondary amines. There are only two NAT genes in humans, NAT1 and NAT2. These enzymes are structurally very similar and have overlapping substrate specificity, although there are also important differences. However, although seemingly a simple family with only two members, these enzymes are highly polymorphic with more than two dozen different allelic variants, many of which affect catalytic activity. Thus, people carrying different functional variants are often classified as "slow," "intermediate," "rapid," and "ultrarapid" metabolizers, depending upon the specific allelic variants they carry. Some drugs are eliminated primarily via N-acetylation, and thus there can be a wide range in interindividual effectiveness due to enzyme activity. For example, the antihypertensive drug, hydralazine, is quickly eliminated in ultrarapid NAT2 metabolizers, and normal pharmacological doses are ineffective. Conversely, slow NAT2 metabolizers may have serious adverse reactions to a normal therapeutic dose because of the slow elimination. Because both NAT1 and NAT2 are involved in the biotransformation of a variety of environmental carcinogens (mostly aromatic amines and N-nitroso compounds), including both "activation" and "detoxification" reactions, polymorphisms in NAT1 and NAT2 may cause differential susceptibility to carcinogenic responses to these compounds following long-term occupational and/or environmental exposures.

v. *Amino Acid Conjugation.* Although less commonly involved in the biotransformation of xenobiotics than the previously discussed conjugation reactions, some carboxylic acids, such as benzoic acid, and certain potentially toxic hydroxylamines can be conjugated with amino acids such as glycine and serine. For example, benzoic acid is conjugated with glycine, resulting in the formation of hippuric acid. Aspirin (acetylsalicylic acid) is also primarily metabolized via hydrolysis to salicylic acid, most of which is then conjugated with glycine and eliminated in the urine. Since the primary xenobiotic substrates for amino acid conjugation are carboxylic acids, amino acid conjugation often "competes" with glucuronic acid conjugation (facilitated by UGTs, as discussed above). In general, amino acid conjugation acts like a "high-affinity, low-capacity" system, whereas glucuronide conjugation acts more like a "low affinity, high capacity" system. Thus, at relatively low doses, amino acid conjugation of carboxylic acid xenobiotics may predominate, while glucuronide conjugation predominates at higher doses.

Excretion Like the liver, the kidney plays a critical role in the elimination of potentially toxic xenobiotics from the body. Because a major function of the kidney is the filtration of the blood to remove unwanted waste products (e.g., urea, excess sodium and chloride ions, excess glucose), it can participate in the elimination of toxic substances that have been absorbed into the blood. Excretion by the kidney is primarily a physical process. There are two central ways that the kidney removes toxic substances from the bloodstream: (1) by filtration and elimination in the urine, and (2) by active secretion into the urine, with subsequent elimination in the urine. Filtration can be an effective means of eliminating water-soluble xenobiotics, but it has little value for elimination of lipid-soluble chemicals, because 99+% of the water in the filtrate formed in the glomerulus is reabsorbed in the remaining parts of the nephron. As water is reabsorbed, the concentration of solutes in the tubular fluid increases, and the solutes move down their concentration gradients. The primary "barrier" to diffusion in the nephron is lipid bilayers in the cells making up the distal tubule and collecting ducts, and thus lipid-soluble materials simply diffuse back into the interstitial fluid of the kidney, where the capillary network collects the solutes as well as the reabsorbed water. However, water-soluble substances, including nearly all conjugated xenobiotics (glucuronides, sulfates, N-acetylated chemicals, including those derived from glutathione) are not able to diffuse across the cell membranes and are concentrated and eliminated in the urine. However, for many xenobiotics, including many conjugates, additional elimination occurs via active transport processes across the cell wall that can move water-soluble substances from the blood through the kidney cells and into tubular fluid, against a concentration gradient.

Target Organ/Tissue Toxicity

Many toxic substances often have marked toxic effects on only one or a few specific organs or tissues, which is usually determined based on specific molecular targets unique to a particular tissue, and/or because of organ/tissue-specific biotransformation. Below we provide a brief summary of the major target organs for toxicity and the primary relevant mechanisms, with the recognition that (1) often times the "target organ" is primary site of toxicity, but usually not the only one, and (2) the "target organ" can vary by both dose and route of exposure. For example, corrosive substances, such as strong acids and bases, may exert their toxic effects at the site of contact, such that inhalation exposure results in lung damage, while oral exposure results in oral/gastrointestinal damage, and skin (dermal) exposure results in epidermis and dermis damage.

The Nervous System

Overall, the nervous system (brain, spinal cord, peripheral sensory and motor neurons, autonomic nervous system) is a major target for many toxic substances, both from single, acute exposures, and from repeated, chronic exposures. The primary reasons that the nervous system is a frequent target of toxicity relate to the complexity of its functions (e.g., the wide variety of different receptors and activating ligands/neurotransmitters that can be disrupted by chemicals), the high level of blood flow to the brain and spinal cord (about 15% of cardiac output), and the high demand for glucose as the predominant source of energy.

There are several common modes of action for chemicals causing acute toxic effects on the nervous system, including (1) interference with neurotransmitter function, (2) cytotoxicity to neurons and/or other cells in the nervous system, (3) interference with axonal function and myelination, and (4) effects on ion transport across neuronal membranes. In many instances, a single neurotoxic substance may act via multiple different modes of action, depending on the extent and rate of exposure and other variables.

a. Interference with neurotransmitter function can result when a chemical acts as either an agonist or antagonist to a particular neuroreceptor, or via inhibition of breakdown or reuptake of neurotransmitters. Numerous plant and animal toxins also target the nervous system via modulation of neurotransmitter function. For example, the plant alkaloids atropine and scopolamine bind to and block the binding of acetycholine to cholinergic receptors. Not surprisingly, atropine is an effective antidote to poisoning with organophosphorous pesticides because it can attenuate the overstimulation of cholinergic receptors that result from the accumulation of acetylcholine following AChE inhibition.
b. Other drugs and chemicals can affect nervous system function by causing direct cytotoxicity to neurons in the brain and/or peripheral nervous system. An example of this mode of action is the "street use" of an illicit synthetic form of heroin called MPTP (1-methyl-4-phenyl-1,2,3,6-tetrahydropyridine). Even relatively brief periods of use of MPTP produce an irreversible form of brain damage almost indistinguishable from Parkinson's disease.[31] MPTP is metabolized in the brain to a reactive molecule called MPP+, which is a good substrate for membrane transporters of the neurotransmitter, dopamine. Thus, MPP+ is selectively taken into dopaminergic neurons, where it reacts with critical proteins in the cell and causes specific loss of these neurons. Numerous metals, such as lead and mercury, alter nervous system function in subtle and not fully understood, likely as the result of metal complexation with neuronal proteins and subsequent alteration of function, including neuronal cell death/disfunction.[32] This is especially important for exposures to the developing nervous system during fetal and early life. Many EDCs may influence neurodevelopment in related ways because of the role that hormonal signaling plays in development of the nervous system during fetal and neonatal life.
c. Some chemicals can produce toxicity that damages the axon and/or the myelination processes critical to axonal function. For example, the organic solvent, N-hexane, is biotransformed into a reactive metabolite called 2,5-hexane dione. This metabolite is selectively toxic to long axons, causing a "dying back" type of neuropathy associated with both sensory and motor neuron dysfunction.
d. Still other neurotoxic agents act by altering the flux across ion channels in the neuron. For example, local anesthetics such as lidocaine produce their anesthetic effects by blocking sodium channels in sensory neurons. But these same drugs (i.e., lidocaine, procainamide) and other sodium channel blockers (e.g., quinidine, phenytoin) have found use in the treatment of cardiac arrhythmias and as anticonvulsants. Several potent marine toxins, including saxitoxin (Red Tide) and tetrodotoxin (from Pufferfish), can cause serious toxicity and even death via inhibition of sodium channels in motor neurons.

Liver

Like the nervous system, the liver represents a very common target for toxic substances for the following reasons: (1) its anatomic location and role in metabolism, receiving nearly all of the blood flow from the small intestine and stomach; (2) the permeable nature of the hepatic structure (hepatocytes are in nearly direct contact with plasma, since the capillary endothelium lacks tight junctions), which allows xenobiotics to be quickly taken into the liver, resulting in high intracellular concentrations; and (3) the presence of the highest concentration of biotransformation enzymes of any tissue in the body. As discussed above, biotransformation is somewhat of a "double-edged sword": the primary purpose is transform lipid-soluble toxic chemicals to water-soluble nontoxic metabolites, but in the process, highly toxic reactive intermediates may be formed. If protective pathways designed to eliminate the toxic metabolite are overwhelmed, the liver may be subject to toxic effects of the metabolites.

Perhaps the best example of this is the widely used over-the-counter analgesic, acetaminophen (APAP). When ingested, APAP is quickly absorbed in the intestine and delivered to the liver via the portal circulation. APAP rapidly diffuses into the liver, where it undergoes biotransformation by a variety of competing pathways. One of these pathways, oxidation of APAP to a reactive quinoneimine intermediate (NAPQI) via CYP2E1, represents a relatively small fraction of total metabolism at therapeutic doses, and the small amount of NAPQI is quickly detoxified via glutathione conjugation. However, at large doses (>10 tablets, ~4000 mg), a higher proportion of the dose goes to NAPQI, and the intracellular glutathione used to detoxify the NAPQI is quickly depleted. As a result, NAPQI binds to numerous endogenous proteins, disrupting normal hepatocellular function and leading to potentially fatal hepatotoxicity.

In experimental toxicology and pharmacology, where large doses of the agent of interest are given, hepatotoxic effects are relatively common.[33] The question for risk assessment is whether such effects occur at doses that might be encountered in nonexperimental conditions, such as environmental/occupational exposures.

Kidney

As discussed above, the kidney plays an important role in the elimination of xenobiotics by both filtration and active transport into renal tubular fluid for elimination via urinary excretion. However, the kidney can also be a target organ for toxicity. Numerous substances, such as cadmium (Cd) and mercury salts, are highly toxic to the kidney. In the case of Cd, the kidney is the primary site of chronic toxicity following long-term, low-level exposure to Cd, usually through dietary or occupational exposures, and through smoking, which is the main source of Cd for general populations. Following oral absorption, Cd is rapidly taken into the liver, where it is bound to a low molecular weight, sulfhydryl-rich protein called metallothionein (MT).[34] The expression of the MT protein is induced in the liver following repeated exposures to Cd as well as a variety of other metals. The metal-MT complex serves to protect the liver from the metal binding to other critical sulfydryl groups on proteins. The Cd-MT complex is eliminated from the liver into the bloodstream, where it is then filtered and actively taken back into the kidney cells via transporters designed to reabsorb small biologically important peptides and proteins. Once in the kidney, the MT-Cd complex is slowly degraded by intracellular proteases, releasing the Cd into proximal tubule cells in the kidney. Over many years, the accumulating Cd alters renal function and may cause frank renal failure.

Similarly, mercury salts are concentrated in the kidney and also perturb renal function and cause renal tubular nephrosis. There are numerous other examples of kidney-specific toxicity that occur as a consequence of concentration of the xenobiotic or its hepatic metabolite in kidney cells. Other notable environmental chemicals that have somewhat selective toxicity toward the kidney include the phytotoxin aristolochic acid (the cause of "Balkan Endemic Nephropathy") and several halogenated hydrocarbons. Numerous drugs have also been shown to selectively target the kidney, including several aminoglycoside antibiotics, cyclosporin, some Nonsteroidal anti-inflammatory compounds, and the chemotherapeutic agent, Cisplatin.[35]

Skin

Dermatological reactions represent one of the most common types of adverse responses following environmental and workplace exposures to a variety of substances. Dermatological reactions are generally one of two types: (1) irritant contact dermatitis and/or (2) allergic contact dermatitis. The former is representative of responses to dermal contact with corrosive agents, such as strong acids or bases. However, many other chemicals can exhibit nonspecific irritation effects on the skin, including the production of rashes that are not immunologically derived.

Allergic contact dermatitis results from a delayed T-cell hypersensitivity reaction. Upon first exposure, some chemicals penetrate the epidermis, then act as immunogenic haptens by complexing with certain carrier proteins, where they are processed by resident macrophages (Langherhans cells). The Langherhans cells then present the processed hapten-peptide complex to T-helper cells in regional lymph nodes, stimulating the release of inflammatory cytokines and proliferation of the sensitive T-helper cells. Over several weeks, an immune response is generated through memory T-cells that enter the systemic circulation. As literally thousands of chemicals have been shown or suspected of causing allergic dermatitis, this pathway represents a major source of occupational injury and illness. Allergic reactions to chemicals can be highly variable, however, and usually only a small percent of workers develop allergic contact dermatitis following exposures. Yet for those who do become sensitized, even small amounts of exposure can induce an allergic response. Patch testing can be used to identify specific chemical allergens in individuals.

Some chemicals can also induce photosensitivity and/or phototoxicity with resulting development of serious skin rashes following exposure to the sensitizing agent and ultraviolet light. Some polyaromatic hydrocarbons, psoralens and psoralen derivatives, dyes such as acridine orange, and numerous drugs have been associated with the development of phototoxicity.

Finally, occupational exposures to certain polychlorinated hydrocarbons, including chlorinated dibenzodioxins, dibenzofurans, and naphthalenes, have been associated with the development of "chloracne" a severe and potentially disabling form of acne eruptions on the skin. Typically, comedomes and cysts develop behind the ears and around the eyes, shoulders, back and genitalia. This can be associated with both hyperpigmentation and the development of excess hair in unusual places (hypertrichosis).

Respiratory System

The respiratory tract is comprised of the upper respiratory tract (regions above the neck) and the lower respiratory tract (airway passages below the neck, and the lung). The respiratory system is a frequent target organ following inhalation exposures to a wide variety of toxic substances, including gases, solvents and corrosive vapors, and particulates. Adults inhale about 10,000 liters of air per day, so substantial amounts of contaminants, even at seemingly low concentrations, may reach the lung.

An important determinant of toxicity is the site of deposition of the toxicants. Key factors affecting deposition include solubility, diffusivity, and reactivity of the chemical as well as breathing rate of the affected individual. For example, highly soluble gases such as SO_2 cannot penetrate deeply and thus mostly cause irritation to the nose and upper respiratory tract. By contrast, less soluble gases such as ozone can penetrate deep into the lung, causing toxicity to the key airway exchange structures (alveoli). For particles, size is an important determinant of deposition. Particles > 10 um in diameter are mostly deposited in the nose, while smaller particles can penetrate more deeply into the respiratory tract. Chronic exposures to certain kinds of particulate matter, such as asbestos fibers (asbestosis), silica (silicosis), and carbon particles (black lung disease), can result in specific diseases with pulmonary fibrosis as the underlying pathology following years of exposure.

Asthma is one of the most common environmental-related conditions of the respiratory system. The disease is characterized by inflammation and reversible narrowing of the airways due to increased reactivity to irritants. Inhaled agents may exacerbate asthma, for example, secondhand tobacco smoke, or causes asthma, for example, isocyanates. Examples of xenobiotics linked to asthma development or exacerbation include the isocyanates, ozone, and NO_2.

Some chemicals target the lung specifically, even if exposures are not via inhalation. For example, following oral or dermal exposure to the herbicide paraquat, the compound is slowly redistributed to the lung, where active transport concentrates it in the alveolar epithelium. Paraquat is a bipyridyl compound that readily undergoes redox cycling in the presence of high oxygen concentrations. Once this process begins, oxygen free radicals are generated at a rate that exceeds the ability of antioxidant defense mechanisms, such as SOD, to detoxify them. Lung damage and subsequent development of extensive pulmonary edema. Death usually ensues within a week to a month following exposure.

Cardiovascular System

The cardiovascular system is comprised of the heart and a large network of vasculature including arteries, capillaries, and veins. Toxicants may cause toxicity to the heart (cardiotoxicity) through several mechanisms, including disruption of ion homeostasis. Proper cardiac function depends on tightly controlled ion channels and related ion homeostasis. Xenobiotics that change this ion balance—either by blocking the calcium (Ca^{2+}), potassium (K^+), or sodium (Na^+) channels or by interfering with the sodium/potassium-ATPase that is necessary for ion transport, may cause cardiotoxicity, manifesting as disruptions to normal heart rhythms. Several heavy metals, solvents, and halogenated hydrocarbons are suspected to exert cardiotoxicity through these pathways.[36] Other potential mechanisms of cardiotoxicity include changes to coronary blood flow, oxidative stress, and apoptosis.

The vascular system is responsible for delivering oxygen and nutrients to tissues and organs throughout the body and also serves to remove waste products from metabolism. Because xenobiotics that enter the body through all routes of absorption come in contact with vascular cells on their way to other sites of the body, the blood vessels of the vascular system are at high risk for toxic injury. Key mechanisms of vascular injury include: (1) changes in membrane structure and function; (2) oxidative stress, which results in changes to gene regulation and decreased antioxidant defenses; (3) activation of vessel toxicants; and (4) accumulation of toxicant in the vascular system cells. The consequences of vascular system injury include atherosclerosis, thrombosis, and changes in blood pressure.

There are many chemicals that exert toxicity on the vascular system—and in particular on the endothelial cells that line the surface of the vessels. For example, cigarette smoke, which is comprised of thousands of compounds, has been linked to decreases in vasodilation, increases in inflammatory cytokines (associated with endothelial cell injury), and membrane lipid peroxidation. The primary hypothesized mechanism for these changes is oxidative stress, including free-radical mediated reductions in nitric oxide (NO).[37,38]

Immune System

The immune system is composed of a series of balanced, complex, multicellular, and physiological mechanisms that function to preserve the integrity of the host. Functionally, the immune system distinguishes "self" tissues (organs and cells) from foreign ("nonself") materials (e.g., bacteria, viruses, transformed cells) and then utilizes one or more of its specialized, complex systems to neutralize and/or eliminate the foreign materials. The immune system operates as a continuum, and perturbation to the system by xenobiotics may lead to altered immune competence. Changes leading to enhanced responsiveness (or failure to recognize self) can progress to autoimmune disease or hypersensitivity, while decreased ability to recognize (or neutralize/eliminate) foreign material can lead to immunosuppression and illness.[39] Substances are considered immunotoxic when they adversely affect normal immune system operations.

Primary lymphoid organs (bone marrow, thymus) produce and support production of immune cells (e.g., B and T cells). Secondary lymphoid organs (spleen and lymph nodes) filter antigens from the blood and body fluids; other secondary lymphoid tissues are associated with the skin, mucosal laminal propria, gut, bronchioles, and nasal cavity.[39] Functionally the mammalian immune system is comprised of two divisions: (1) innate immunity, which is nonspecific in nature, involves responses by neutrophils, macrophages, natural killer (NK) cells, and dendritic cells (DCs); and (2) acquired (or adaptive) immunity, which is characterized by specificity and immunological memory and subdivided into (a) humoral immunity, which depends on production of antigen-specific antibody B cells and their subsequent interactions with other cells of the immune system and (b) cell-mediated immunity (CMI), which encompasses acquired immunity not dependent on antibody involvement. Many different types of assays have been used to assess immune system status following exposure to different test articles. In general, these assays evaluate various aspects of immune response (e.g., antibody production or resistance to infection) of control animals compared to responses in groups of animals previously treated with different concentrations of test article.

Some diseases are caused by the immune response to occupational exposures. Berylliosis, resulting from the metal beryllium, is a paradigmatic example. This disease was first described in the 1940s; today, exposure persists in several industries. The immunopathogenesis of the disease is well understood, including how beryllium activates the immune system and an assay for beryllium sensitization is available.[40]

Reproductive System (Male and Female)

The reproductive system is the set of organs that plays a role in sexual reproduction (Fig. 64-5). The key steps that must be coordinated by these organs for successful sexual reproduction include release of an egg at the correct time in the reproductive cycle, fertilization of the egg by sperm cells, transport of the fertilized egg to the uterus, implantation of the early embryo into the wall of the uterus, formation of the placenta and support of the developing child; birth of the fetus, and care of the infant.

Reproductive toxicants are chemical, biological, or physical agents that adversely affect the sexual function and fertility of males and females at any of these stages (Fig. 64-6). These phases of the reproductive cycle occur throughout human life, ranging from prenatal development, infancy, puberty, and lactation. All stages of the reproductive cycle have the potential to be disrupted by xenobiotics, with lifelong consequences for fertility. As will be discussed further in the context of developmental toxicity, the timing of an exposure has an important effect on its ultimate toxicity.

A prototypical example of male reproductive toxicity is testicular dysgenesis syndrome (TDS), which has been observed in both rodents and humans. TDS is comprised of the following four associated conditions: testicular germ cell cancer, cryptorchidism, hypospadias, and low sperm count/poor semen quality. The origins of TDS are in the early fetal development period.[41] External genital organs are identical in males and females until the ninth week of gestation, and normal masculinization of genitalia is stimulated by fetal testicular androgens. Given the hormonal dependence of these developmental changes, the male reproductive tract is highly sensitive to endocrine disruption. Exposure to antiandrogens, such as phthalates, during critical periods of male reproductive development has been linked to TDS.[42] A related example is that of anogenital distance (AGD). Male rats exhibit longer AGD than females; there are analogous differences in humans.[43] Male AGD is linked to fertility.[44] In developing males, exposure to xenobiotics that disrupt normal testosterone concentrations—either by acting as androgen receptor antagonists or by inhibiting normal testosterone synthesis—can result in shortening of the AGD. By contrast, in developing females, exposure to androgen results in lengthening of the AGD.[45] These changes exemplify how disruptions to normal reproductive system development during critical periods can have lifelong consequences for sexual reproduction.

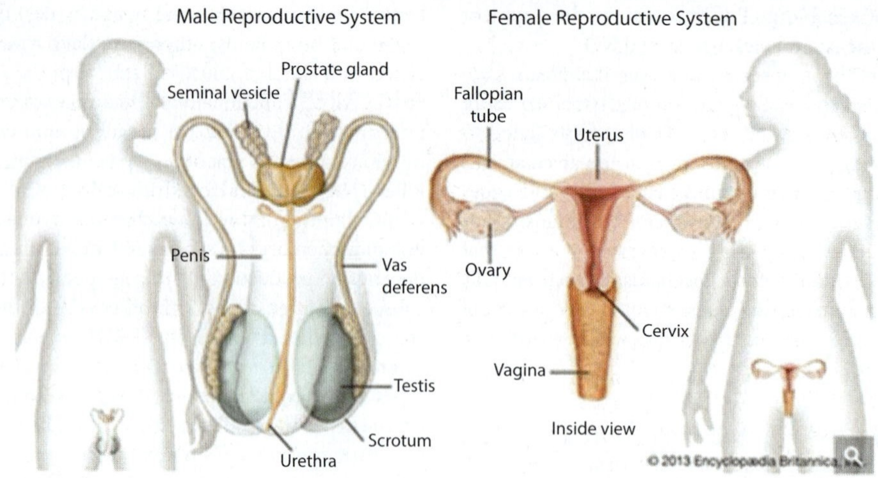

FIGURE 64-5. Organs and structures of the male and female reproductive systems. (*Source*: https://www.britannica.com/science/human-reproductive-system. © Encyclopaedia Britannica, Inc.)

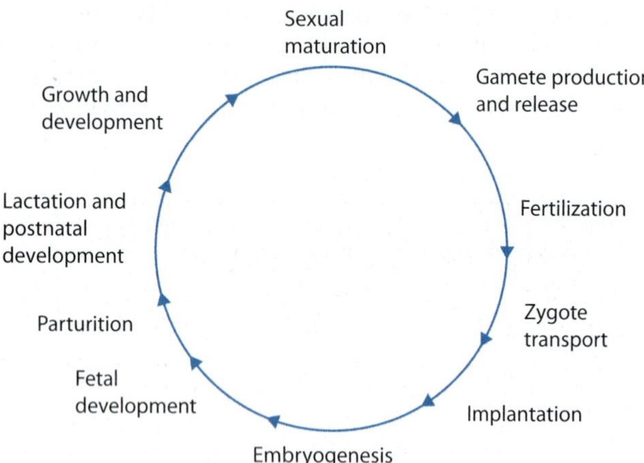

FIGURE 64-6. A schema of the reproductive cycle. (*Source:* Reproduced with permission from Foster PMD, Gray LE. Toxic Responses of the Reproductive System. In Casarett and Doull's Toxicology. The Basic Science of Poisons, 8th ed. CD Klaasen, ed, Chap. 21, pp. 861-906. McGraw Hill Medical, New York.

Basic Mechanisms/Modes of Action

There are myriad ways that xenobiotics can cause toxicity. Among the many potential "modes of action" (or, "mechanisms of action"), there are two broad categories that are highly relevant to most drugs and chemicals: one is through activation of receptors, and the other is through metabolism in the body to reactive intermediates that can cause oxidative stress and/or bind to DNA and cause genetic damage.

Toxic Responses via "Receptor-Ligand" Interactions

One of the most common mechanisms/modes of action by which toxicants exert effects is through receptor-ligand interactions. A large percentage of genes in the human genome encode specific proteins called "receptors," which work through highly complex and integrated networks of chemical and electrical signals. Receptors can be visualized as locks that remain in the "off" position, until another molecule, either endogenous or exogenous, interacts in a very specific way with the receptor (Fig. 64-7). These molecules that bind to receptors are referred to as "ligands." There are two possible outcomes when a ligand interacts with its specific (sometimes called "cognate") receptor: it can either turn the receptor to the "on" position, or it can bind to and block the receptor without turning it on. If a ligand acts via the first process—switching the receptor to the "on" position, the ligand is referred to as an "activating ligand," or an "agonist." Ligands

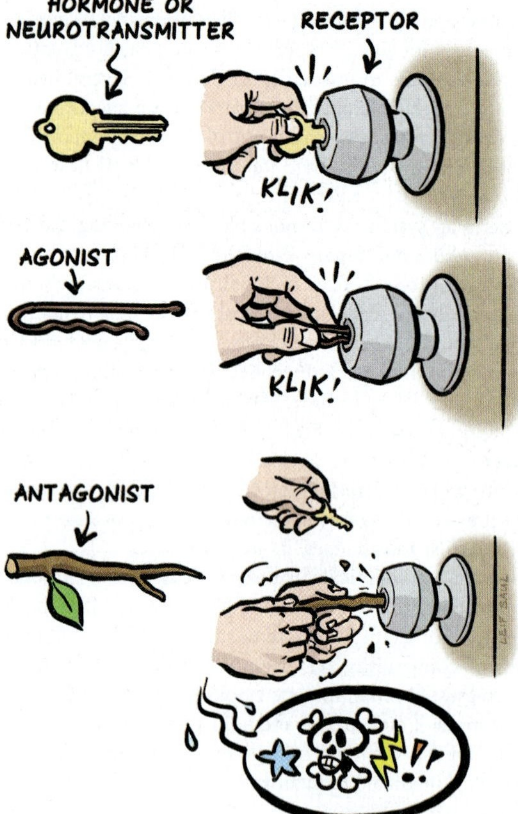

FIGURE 64-7. Conceptual model of ligand receptor interactions. **(© Leif Saul.)**

that bind to their cognate receptor but do not activate it are referred to as "antagonists." By binding to but not activating the receptor, they prevent other endogenous ligands from binding to and activating that receptor.

Histamine and antihistamines exemplify this type of interaction. Histamine is released from mast cells in response to an environmental signal, such as allergenic pollens, proteins, and insect venom. When histamine is released, it binds very specifically to histamine receptors, of which there are several (H1, H2, and H3). Antihistamines are antagonist ligands to H1, H2, and/or H3 receptors, blocking the histamine from binding to the receptor. Antihistamines represent a very useful class of molecules in the treatment of many allergies.

Hormones, such as estrogen, testosterone, glucocorticoids, and thyroid hormone, are also activating ligands to specific receptors. For example, estrogen binds to the estrogen receptor(s), testosterone binds to the testosterone receptor, and thyroid hormone binds to the thyroid hormone receptor. When these hormones bind to their cognate receptors, they trigger a series of downstream events, often including changes in the expression of numerous different genes and/or the activation of a series of complex signal transduction pathways.

Exogenous chemicals also have the potential to interact with these receptors. Chemicals that produce biological effects by interfering with hormone signaling pathways are frequently called "endocrine disrupting chemicals" (EDCs), or simply "endocrine disruptors." For example, the molecule diethylstilbestrol, or DES, is very potent agonist of the estrogen receptor, disrupting normal estrogen signaling. It was prescribed to women between 1938 and 1971 to prevent miscarriage and other pregnancy complications. Daughters of women who took DES during pregnancy were found to be at elevated risk of a rare vaginal cancer.

Environmental estrogen exposure also occurs from a wide range of plant-derived phytoestrogens.[46] Some of these chemicals, such as genestein, are potent estrogen agonists and occur at relatively high concentrations in soy and certain other plants. Other environmental pollutants, such as breakdown products of the pesticides, DDT methoxychlor, and some environmental contaminants such as bisphenol A, also act as estrogen receptor agonists.[20,21]

In a similar manner, some chemicals can act as blocking ligands (antagonists). For example, the drug, tamoxifen, which is widely used in the treatment of estrogen-responsive breast cancer, is useful in treating breast cancer because it blocks the interaction of estrogen with the estrogen receptor, which is required for the growth of breast cancer cells.

Both agonist and antagonist ligands can interfere with normal endocrine signaling. When the lock is opened (i.e., the agonist binds to and activates the receptor) a series of downstream events is initiated. These events usually involve changes in the way that other genes in a cell are turned on or off, a process called "transcriptional regulation," because the information in the gene is transcribed into messenger RNA, which in turn is used to make a functional protein (referred to as "translation") (Fig. 64-8).

EDCs have two possible ways of interfering with normal endocrine signaling—one is referred to as a "direct" effect, in which the molecule interacts directly with the endocrine receptor, either as an agonist, or an antagonist. Some chemicals can also modify endocrine pathways in an "indirect" way via changing the way hormones in the body are broken down (metabolized) (Fig. 64-8). Exposure to high doses of some common occupational and environmental chemicals and other ligands of "environmental response genes," such as AhR, CAR and PXR, can increase the expression (i.e., turns on the genes, referred to as "enzyme induction") of several enzymes in the body that are responsible for breaking down estrogen and other hormones.

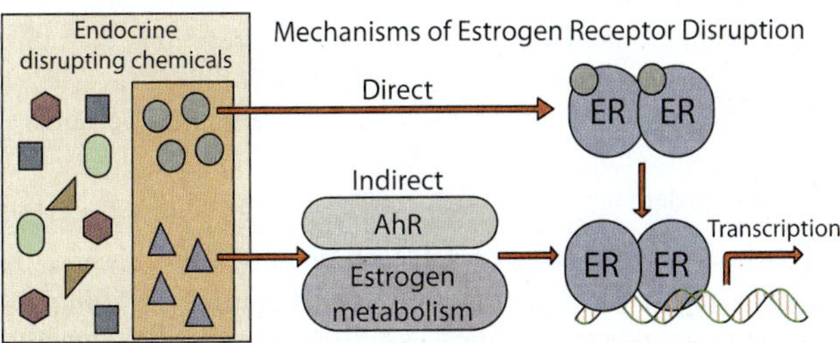

FIGURE 64-8. Direct and indirect mechanisms of endocrine disruption by exogenous chemicals. (*Source*: Based on from Shanle EK, Xu W. Endocrine disrupting chemicals targeting estrogen receptor signaling: Identification and mechanisms of action. *Chem Res Toxicol.* 2011;24(1):6–19.)

In any given cell that expresses particular receptors, there are billions of receptor molecules, existing in either an "on" (agonist is bound to the receptor) or "off" (no agonist is bound to the receptor, or it is occupied by an antagonist ligand) position.

The magnitude of the biological response that occurs following ligand activation of a particular receptor type (e.g., estrogen receptor, AhR, CAR, etc.) is a function of the percent of total receptors occupied at the same time. In other words, there is a dose–response relationship between ligand concentration and the number of receptors that are occupied (Fig. 64-9).

Dose–response relationships for receptor-mediated responses may vary in shape. Some are very steep, meaning that, at the low dose end of the curve, there is no measurable biological response in an individual until the dose becomes high enough to occupy a significant percentage of all of the receptors in a particular cell. Once the concentration of chemical in the tissue reaches a level adequate to occupy a significant percentage of receptors, further increases in dose/concentration cause dramatic increases in the magnitude of response. In other words, there are clear "thresholds" at the lower end of the dose range. However, for chemicals that act as ligands of endogenous receptors where agonist actions are already at biologically active concentrations, which includes many EDCs, there is no apparent threshold, since the concentration of activating ligand is already above the apparent "threshold" concentration. Because of the importance of specific hormonal signals at precise timepoints of development, for example, even small concentrations of some EDCs can lead to negative downstream consequences.[14,21]

Another important concept in understanding the toxicology of molecules that act via specific receptor-mediated pathways is that of "potency." While multiple different chemicals might have the ability to interact with the same receptor, they may differ drastically in how much of the chemical it takes to cause a biologically relevant activation of the receptor. This is one of the most important concepts in the pharmacology of drugs that are designed to interact with specific receptors, since the effective dose is dependent upon both the amount of chemical administered (the dose) and how potent it is in interacting with the receptor. For example, there are multiple different steroid drugs that are widely used to treat inflammation and

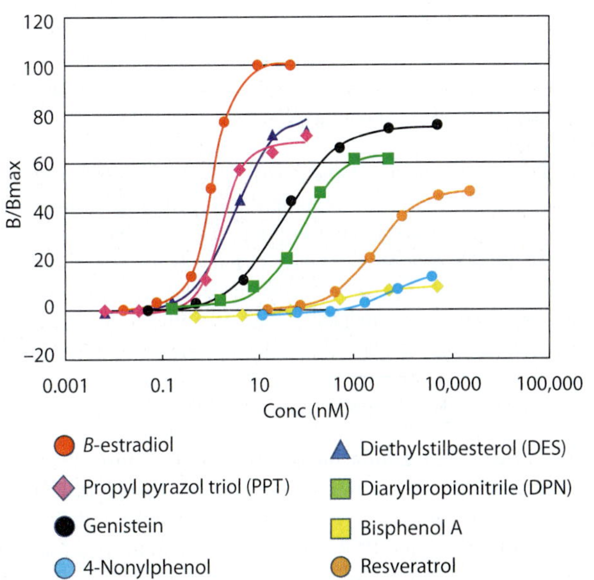

FIGURE 64-9. Dose–response relationship for activation of the estrogen receptor by different activating ligands. (*Source*: Adapted with permission from Fujikura Kasei Co., Ltd. Product: EnBio RCAS for Estrogen receptor alpha. Available at: https://www.cosmobio.co.jp/connections/p_ku_e_view.asp?PrimaryKeyValue=12914&selPrice=1.)

a variety of other human conditions by altering the glucocorticoid receptor. These are frequently referred to as "steroids" in the lay literature, but there are actually very specific forms of steroid molecules that interact specifically with one type of the glucocorticoid receptor. Drugs like prednisone, dexamethasone, and hydrocortisone all interact with and activate glucocorticoid receptor(s), but the "equally effective doses" for each of these are: hydrocortisone, 20 mg; dexamethasone, 0.75 mg; and prednisone, 5 mg. Thus, even though they act the same way (activate the corticosteroid receptor), it takes about 27 times more hydrocortisone than dexamethasone to cause the same effect (dexamethasone is 27 times more potent than hydrocortisone). So, too, different forms of the same class of environmental chemical can have vastly different potency in causing an effect through a receptor.

Examples of Important "Receptor-Ligand Interactions in Toxicology"

The Aryl Hydrocarbon Receptor The best studied of all ligand-receptor interactions and the associated adverse responses is that of dioxins and dioxin-like compounds interacting with the Aryl hydrocarbon Receptor (AhR). The prototypical chlorinated dioxin is 2,3,7,8-tetrachlorodiobenzo(p)dioxin, or TCDD. There are dozens of different dioxin congeners, but TCDD is by far the most toxic. Chlorinated dioxins were a byproduct of the production of certain herbicides and other commercial products that utilized trichlorophenol in their synthesis. TCDD is formed through dimerization of two molecules of 3,4,5-trichlorophenol. It is best known as the toxic contaminant in Agent Orange, an herbicide formulation that contained equal parts of 2,4,5-T and 2,4-D, two herbicides widely used in agriculture, utility and roadside rights-of-way, forestry and home use weed control. The recognition of the potent toxic effects of TCDD, as well as its presence in Agent Orange and other trichlorophenol-based products, did not occur until the mid-1960s. An industrial accident at a trichlorophenol manufacturing facility occurred in Seveso, Italy in 1976 and resulted in widespread environmental contamination with dioxins.

Certain congeners of the widespread environmental contaminant polychlorinated biphenyls (PCBs) are considered "dioxin-like" because they can interact with and activate the AhR. Among the 209 possible PCB molecules (congeners), there are 12 forms that can interact with and activate the rodent (rat and mouse) AhR. These 12 forms are known as dioxin-like PCBs (DL-PCBs). Although all 12 forms have some ability to activate the rodent AhR, they differ in their potency toward the human AhR, which is an important consideration when using carcinogenesis bioassay studies in rodents to predict human risk.

PCBs produce many of their toxic effects via interacting with and activating the nuclear receptor, AhR. AhR is an example of a "ligand-activated nuclear transcription factor." When the ligand activates the Ah receptors, a series of biological events occur that may ultimately result in toxic effects, including liver cancer. When a sufficient number of dioxin-like molecules bind to the AhR, additional molecules in the cell (called cofactors) attach, and the complex is transported into the nucleus of a cell, where it recognizes specific regions of DNA, called "dioxin response elements" (DREs).

"Constitutive Androstane Receptor" (CAR) and "Pregnane X-Receptor" (PXR) Numerous drugs and some xenobiotics found in the environment are effective agonists of either PXR and/or CAR.[47] Like the AhR, CAR and PXR are ligand-activated nuclear transcription factors. CAR and PXR have been labeled as "master xenobiotic receptors" because of their important role in regulating the expression of multiple different genes involved in xenobiotic biotransformation. Although CAR and PXR are distinct nuclear transcription factors, they have overlapping regulation in terms of both ligands and target genes.[48] Both seem to be involved in the expression of multiple CYP genes, especially CYP3A4, multidrug resistant transporters (MRPS), some UDPGTs. Because of the important role played by certain CYPs, UDPGTs, MDRs, and other enzymes involved in biotransformation of endogenous hormones (i.e., estrogen, testosterone, thyroid hormone), drugs and chemicals that modify expression of these genes have been implicated as potential EDCs.

Toxic Responses from Oxidative Stress

Formation of Reactive Oxygen Species (ROS) Although one of the primary purposes of biotransformation is to rid the body of xenobiotics, in so doing the body can actually make the chemical *more* toxic, not less. As discussed above, biotransformation can result in the formation of reactive intermediates that can bind to proteins and DNA in the cell where they were generated. Sometimes the "reactive intermediate" molecules can also stimulate the generation of more reactive molecules in the body, causing a multiplying cascade of additional reactive intermediates. Usually these reactive intermediates involve the generation of forms of oxygen that themselves are highly reactive ("oxygen radicals"), such as superoxide anion, hydrogen peroxide, and the hydroxyl radical. This process referred to as "oxidative stress." These free radicals can interact with all classes of biomolecules in the body.

The body is well equipped with protective pathways to deal with these reactive forms of oxygen, since they can be generated by normal endogenous processes in the body, including oxidative phosphorylation and P450 metabolism. However, with high levels of oxidative stress, these protective pathways can be overwhelmed, resulting in serious adverse effects, including organ failure and death. In fact, oxidative stress is linked to multiple chronic diseases, including cancer, heart disease, lung disease, renal disease, and some neurological diseases.

Antioxidant Response Pathways The body employs antioxidants, which can be either enzymatic or nonenzymatic, as defense mechanisms against oxidative stress. Enzymatic antioxidants, including SOD, glutathione peroxidase (GSHPx), and catalase (CAT), work by breaking down and eliminating free radicals from the body. For example, SOD can interact with the superoxide radical (O_2-), transforming this highly reactive species into the less reactive molecular oxygen (O_2) and hydrogen peroxide (H_2O_2). However, as noted above, hydrogen peroxide is a potent oxidizer capable of generating oxygen radicals and must be further degraded by catalase enzymes with the presence of cofactors such as copper and zinc.

Nonenzymatic antioxidants, including vitamin C, vitamin E, beta-carotene, and glutathione, work by interfering with free radicals and related chain reactions in the body. For example, vitamin E can donate a hydrogen (H) atom to free radicals to nullify them.

Cell and Tissue Damage via Oxidative Stress

(1)Oxidative damage to cell membranes

Free radicals can cause serious damage to cellular membranes, which contain abundant polyunsaturated fatty acids (PUFAs) through the process of lipid peroxidation. In this process, the reactive free radicals sequester electrons from the lipids of cell membranes, stimulating free radical chain reactions that affect the PUFAs that make up cell membranes. If these processes are not terminated by antioxidants, cell membranes may be damaged and/or ruptured.

(2)Oxidative damage to DNA

Free radicals can damage DNA through several mechanisms, including single or double strand DNA breaks; purine, pyrimidine, or deoxyribose modifications; and DNA cross-links. Perhaps the most important consequence of oxidative damage to DNA is the production of the mutagenic 8-hydroxydeoxyguanosine (8-OHdG) adduct, which is formed through the oxidation of guanine at the C8 position. Oxidative damage to DNA is very common, occurring extensively on a daily basis in nearly every cell in the body. Fortunately, the vast majority of this potential DNA damage is repaired by highly effective DNA repair processes.[49] Important DNA repair pathways include (1) direct reversal, in which cellular enzymes directly remove the DNA damaging adducts; (2) excision repair, in which an incorrect or damaged base or nucleotide is removed and replaced; and (3) double-stranded break repair, in which whole chromosomes are put back together after double-strand breaks. However, if an oxidized base in DNA goes unrepaired, or is repaired incorrectly, it can introduce a base pair change in DNA sequence, potentially result in a mutation that is then passed down to all "daughter cells" following normal DNA replication during cell division.

Mitochondrial DNA is particularly susceptible to oxidative damage. This enhanced susceptibility is due to several factors, including (1) proximity to the electron transport system, which generates ROS; (2) lack of protection by histones; and (3) limited DNA repair capacity.

Nonorgan Directed Toxicity

Mutagenesis

Mutations result when the normal sequences of bases in a strand of DNA are altered in such a way that the genetic code is changed. Mutations can occur in either of two general cells types: germ cells (eggs in females, sperm in males), or somatic cells (all other cells in the body). Mutations in germ cells can result in heritable changes in DNA that can be passed on to future generations following reproduction. Mutations in somatic cells are passed on to future cells derived from the mutated somatic cell but are not passed from one generation to the other. However, mutations in somatic cells can have numerous adverse consequences, including cell and tissue injury and death, development of tumors (carcinogenesis), development of abnormalities during embryonic and fetal development, or development of birth defects following in utero exposure.

There are multiple different ways that mutations can be introduced into a gene. The most common is a "base pair" alteration, in which a nucleotide (A, C, T, or G) is changed. If the change in the nucleotide results in change in the codon (three-base pair sequence that codes for specific amino acids during translation), it is referred to as a "missense mutation" and will result in a change in protein structure. A change in nucleotide sequence that introduces a "stop codon" in the gene sequence can result in the complete lack of a functional protein, referred to as a "nonsense" mutation. These are just two of many ways in which the sequence of DNA can be altered to introduce mutations.

Another mechanism for mutagenesis is "cross-linking." For example, ultraviolet (UV) radiation forms thymine-thymine dimers on strands of DNA, either by connecting two adjacent thymine nucleotides on the same strand (intrastrand cross link) or by cross-linking two thymine nucleotides on each of the complimentary strands of DNA. Crosslinking can result in incorrect strand separation during DNA synthesis, either halting synthesis, or potentially inserting incorrect base pairs into the newly synthesized DNA.

As discussed above, oxidative damage to DNA is the most common form of DNA damage that can lead to mutations. Many chemicals can be biotransformed into reactive forms that bind directly to DNA, forming "bulky" DNA adducts. If left unrepaired, or repaired incorrectly, such bulky DNA adducts can lead to introduction of mutations.

The vast majority of mutations that occur in the human genome are of no consequence, either because they do not alter the biological function of a protein; the mutation is in a nonfunctional part of an intron or intergenic DNA; or DNA repair processes correct the damage. However, over time, and following exposures to wide variety of mutagens, not all DNA damage is repaired correctly, leading to an increase in a variety of diseases. Although cancer is the most widely recognized consequence of somatic mutations, many other diseases of aging, such as Alzheimer's disease and atherosclerotic cardiovascular disease are partly due to the accumulation of somatic mutations over time.

Carcinogenesis

In the field of chemical carcinogenesis, there are three broad processes that contribute to the development of cancer: (1) initiation (a stable, heritable change that turn a "normal cell" into a "precancerous cell"), (2) promotion (the precancerous cell is stimulated to divide into a small population of precancerous cells), and (3) progression (additional genetic changes are acquired that allow the precancerous cells to acquire additional characteristics of cancer cells, including spreading to other tissues [metastasis]) (Fig. 64-10).

While this three-stage process is an over-simplification of very complicated biology, it is a useful paradigm to start with, since it is well ingrained in regulatory philosophy of chemical carcinogens.[50] Chemicals that can cause the initial genetic changes are called "initiators," and chemicals that can enhance the growth of initiated cells (in both the "promotion" and "progression" stages) are called "Promoters."

Initiation Initiators are chemicals that trigger initial genetic changes. Some examples of chemicals classified as initiators include polycyclic hydrocarbons and nitrosamines. Because initiators act directly to damage DNA, they are often referred to as "genotoxic carcinogens." There are multiple different ways a chemical can damage DNA and introduce mutations: (1) it can directly interact with and bind to DNA; (2) it can be metabolized in the body to a reactive form that can then interact with and bind to DNA; or (3) it can directly or indirectly generate high levels of "oxidative stress," which itself can cause DNA damage. Alternatively, a chemical can interfere with normal DNA repair processes, allowing "background DNA damage" to go unrepaired.

The vast majority of DNA damage that occurs is repaired by a host of different DNA repair processes, including repair of the altered

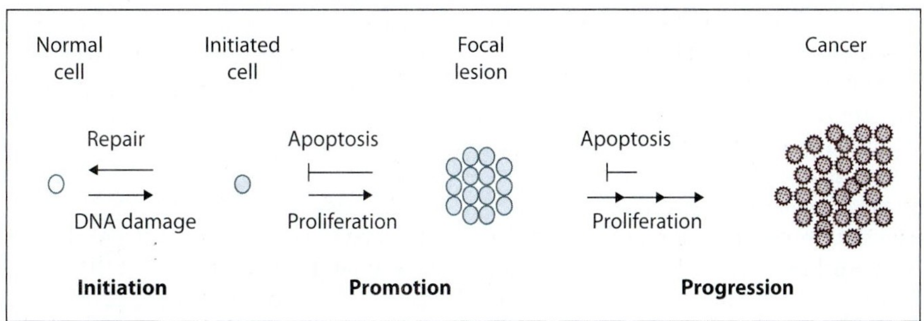

FIGURE 64-10. The multistage process of chemical carcinogenesis. (*Source:* Adapted with permission from Klaunig KE. Chemical Carcinogenesis, In *Casarett and Doull's Toxicology*. The Basic Science of Poisons, 8th ed. CD Klaasen, ed, Chap. 8, pp. 393-444. McGraw Hill Medical, New York..[53])

base prior to DNA replication, and/or immediately following DNA replication by "postreplication repair." If an alteration in a base pair is corrected through either of these processes, it is not a considered mutation, as it is not passed to the next generation of cells. Mutations, by definition are stable, heritable changes in DNA that become "fixed" in the genome.

In general, the process of going from a "normal cell" to a cancerous cell requires multiple mutations in different genes. Mutations must "turn on" certain genes, called "oncogenes," that are normally turned off, and they also must "turn off" certain other genes, called "tumor suppressor genes" that function to control the rate of cell division in cells. Subsequent additional mutations are needed that allow precancerous cells (those with activated oncogenes and inhibited tumor suppressor genes) to become cancers. It has been estimated that most cancers require four to ten or more mutations for a normal cell to become a cancerous cell.[51]

Promotion In the second stage of carcinogenesis, called "promotion," there is selective expansion of initiated cells into a preneoplastic lesion. In general, promotion is thought to be a reversible event.

Xenobiotics that trigger these changes are called "promotors." Promotors are not considered mutagenic and are not able to trigger tumor formation on their own, but they are able to alter the normal cell cycle by increasing cell proliferation and inhibiting apoptosis. Therefore, in contrast to initiators, promoters are most often classified as nongenotoxic, since they do not act directly to damage DNA.

Progression The third stage of carcinogenesis is progression, which involves the conversion of the preneoplastic lesion into a neoplasm. During this process, additional DNA damage, including chromosomal aberrations and translocations, results in mutations that cause altered cell cycle regulation. As a result, the cells grow dramatically, overwhelming nearby normal cells. Chemicals that contribute to the progression stage are typically clastogenic (causing chromosomal abnormalities). In contrast to the first two stages of carcinogenesis described above, progression to either benign or malignant neoplasms is irreversible.

DEVELOPMENTAL TOXICITY/TERATOGENESIS

It is estimated that less than half of all human conceptions result in the birth of a normal infant.[52] Much of this is attributed to spontaneous abortions/miscarriages that occur early in pregnancy (i.e., first trimester). However, another cause of abnormal pregnancy can be due to developmental abnormalities originating during the fetal period. Teratogens, which cause malformations/abnormalities of the embryo, are an important class of xenobiotics that may interfere with this process of normal and healthy development, resulting in developmental toxicity. Examples of known teratogens include thalidomide, ethanol, lead, and chlorinated dioxins, among others. More broadly, developmental toxicity encompasses toxicity that occurs during any stage of development of an organism, including preconception, conception, prenatal development, and postnatal development until puberty. Common mechanisms of developmental toxicity include mutations, chromosomal breakage, changes in mitosis, changes in energy availability, membrane alterations, and enzyme inhibition.

One of the most important determinants of developmental toxicity is the period in which exposure occurs. Early life development proceeds with specifically timed signaling pathways that control particular cellular changes (such as implantation and organogenesis). All of these changes make the fetus uniquely susceptible to toxicants. Interference from exogenous exposures during critical periods of sensitivity can derail these normal processes, resulting in serious and lifelong consequences. Because of the strong link between timing of exposure and toxic effect, researchers are often able to pinpoint the period in which exposure occurred based on the observed malformation. For example, ethylenethiourea (ETU), a fungicide breakdown product, produces specific malformations in the rat embryo depending on the timing of exposure. Exposure during days 10–11 produces eye malformations, while exposure during days 11–15 produces cleft palate.[53]

An important and, unfortunately very common, example of developmental toxicity is the case of fetal alcohol spectrum disorder. Ethanol (alcohol) readily crosses the placenta, and therefore blood alcohol can rapidly reach equilibrium between the mother and fetus. Exposure to ethanol during organogenesis in early pregnancy can interfere with neural cell proliferation and stimulate apoptosis in neural crest cells. As a consequence, the infant is born with characteristic facial structures and often neurodevelopmental deficiencies.

Developmental toxicity can result in not only structural deficits but also functional deficits (such as attention deficit hyperactivity disorder) that might not be detected until later infancy or childhood. There is also growing concern about developmental-related reproductive alterations (such as decreased sperm count), often caused by EDC exposure, that are not apparent until puberty or adulthood. Hormones are crucial in many of the critical periods of development described above, and therefore the embryo is particularly sensitive to chemicals with hormonal agonist or antagonist activity. Common mechanisms of developmental toxicity involving the endocrine system include interference or activation of steroid receptor ligands, changes to steroid hormone metabolizing enzymes, or changes in endogenous release of hormones. As discussed earlier, DES is an example of a potent, hormonally active developmental toxicant.

Mixtures in Toxicology: A Major Challenge for Today and the Future

Much of this chapter has provided examples of how individual toxic substances can act on biological systems to produce adverse effects. Much of what we have learned about the toxic effects of specific chemicals comes from studies in laboratory animals. Yet, in contrast to these controlled laboratory settings, humans are not exposed to only one chemical at a time. Indeed, there are thousands of chemicals present in our diet, the air we breathe, the water we drink, and the lifestyles we follow.

The consequences of these joint exposures may be different than single exposures. For example, multiple chemicals with the same "mode of action" may act additively to cause adverse effects even if exposure to each chemical alone would cause no effect. Alternatively, one chemical may cause no adverse effects at a certain dose but may induce biological changes that increase the susceptibility to another chemical, a process referred to as "potentiation." For example, there are a number of plant toxins, chemicals used in industry, pesticides (e.g., thiocarbamate) and a number of pharmaceutical agents which are relatively nontoxic on their own. However, they act as inhibitors of the enzyme ALDH, which is critical in the metabolism of numerous endogenous and exogenous aldehydes, such as formaldehyde and acetaldehyde.[54] If someone receives a dose of an ALDH inhibitor and is subsequently exposed to a moderate, but generally "nontoxic" dose of an alcohol, significant adverse effects associated with the accumulation of the aldehyde of that alcohol can occur.

Sometimes, the joint effects of two chemicals in combination are much greater than would be expected based on simple additivity; this scenario is referred to as "synergy." For example, both aflatoxin B1 and hepatitis B virus (HBV) are important risk factors for liver cancer. Epidemiological studies in regions of the world where both of these risk factors are present have demonstrated strong synergism between these two risk factors. In several studies, liver cancer risk was elevated about two- to threefold from dietary AFB exposure alone, about 12- to 15-fold from HBV alone, but the two risk factors together increased liver cancer risk more than 60-fold.[55]

Because of the challenges in designing chemical interaction studies (how many, and which ones? What doses? How long? What outcomes to assess?), mixtures studies seem almost intractable. Yet numerous studies have been completed and progress has been made in designing such studies, often using epidemiological parameters of multiple human exposures.[56] Mathematical approaches for assessing risks of multiple exposures to pesticides have been proposed,[57] but the wider application of such approaches to the myriad of potential mixtures remains elusive, a major challenge in the field of toxicology, and an area of active research.

Summary

There are myriad contaminants in the environment and in workplaces that may harm individuals across a population. Whether and how they harm health depends on the physiological processes by which they are handled in the body and the mechanisms by which they cause injury. Some agents target particular organs and time windows while others have more general consequences. The complex pathway from exposure to disease may be hard to chart, complicating efforts to anticipate toxicity from new and existing agents and to characterize risk and population impact. Nonetheless, the science of toxicology, especially with the many new molecular tools that allow detailed determination of modes of action of toxic substances, holds promise for improving public health by identifying human-relevant hazards for both existing and new chemicals. Early identification of potential hazards and risks allows for interventions to reduce or eliminate exposures and protect public health.[58]

References

1. Klaassen CD, ed.Klaassen CD, ed. *Cassarett and Doull's Toxicology: The Basic Science of Poisons*, 9th ed. New York: McGraw Hill; 2019.
2. Rushing BR, Selim MI. Aflatoxin B1: A review on metabolism, toxicity, occurrence in food, occupational exposure, and detoxification methods. *Food Chem Toxicol.* 2019;124:81–100.
3. Naumann M, Jankovic J Safety of botulinum toxin type A: A systematic review and meta analysis. *Curr Med Res Opin.* 2004;20(7):981–90.
4. Lim GB. Warfarin: From rat poison to clinical use. *Nat Rev Cardiol.* 2017 Dec 14. Online ahead of print.
5. Polykretis P, Cencetti F, Donati C, Luchinat E, Banci L. Cadmium effects on superoxide dismutase 1 in human cells revealed by NMR. *Redox Biol.* 2019;21:101102.
6. National Research Council. *Critical Aspects of EPA's IRIS Assessment of Inorganic Arsenic: Interim Report.* Washington, DC: The National Academies Press; 2013. https://doi.org/10.17226/18594.
7. Sage AP, Minatel BC, Ng KW, et al.Oncogenomic disruptions in arsenic-induced carcinogenesis. *Oncotarget.* 2017;8(15):25736–55.
8. Ward MH, Jones RR, Brender JD, et al. Drinking water nitrate and human health: An updated review. *Int J Environ Res Public Health.* 2018;15:1557.
9. Pan, KT, Leonardi GS, Croxford B. Factors contributing to CO uptake and elimination in the body: A critical review. *Int J Environ Res Public Health.* 2020;17:528.
10. U.S. Department of Health and Human Services. *The Health Consequences of Smoking—50 Years of Progress: A Report of the Surgeon General.* Atlanta, GA (2014): U.S. Department of Health and Human Services, Centers for Disease Control and Prevention, National Center for Chronic Disease Prevention and Health Promotion, Office on Smoking and Health.
11. National Research Council. *Toxicity Testing: Strategies to Determine Needs and Priorities.* Washington, DC: The National Academies Press; 1984. https://doi.org/10.17226/317.
12. NTP (National Toxicology Program). *Report on Carcinogens*, 14th ed. Research Triangle Park, NC: U.S. Department of Health and Human Services, Public Health Service; 2016. https://ntp.niehs.nih.gov/go/roc14.
13. https://www.epa.gov/newsreleases/epa-releases-first-major-update-chemicals-list-40-years.
14. Eaton DL, Gilbert SG. Principles of toxicology. In: Klaassen CD, ed. *Casarett and Doull's Toxicology. The Basic Science of Poisons*, 8th ed. Chap. 22. New York: McGraw Hill Medical; 2013, pp. 13–48.
15. National Research Council. *Science And Decisions: Advancing Risk Assessment.* Chap. 5. Washington, DC: The National Academies Press; 2009, pp. 130–1.
16. Baldwin J, Grantham VJ. Radiation hormesis: Historical and current perspectives. *Nucl Med Technol.* 2015;43(4):242–6.
17. Yoon S, Jung J, Lee S, et al. The protective effect of alcohol consumption on the incidence of cardiovascular diseases: Is it real? A systematic review and meta-analysis of studies conducted in community settings. *BMC Public Health.* 2020;20(1):90.
18. Bagnardi V, Rota M, Botteri E, et al. Alcohol consumption and site-specific cancer risk: A comprehensive dose–response meta-analysis. *Br J Cancer.* 2015;112:580–93.
19. Vandenberg LN, Colborn T, Hayes TB, et al. Hormones and endocrine-disrupting chemicals: Low-dose effects and nonmonotonic dose responses. *Endocr Rev.* 2012;33(3):378–455.
20. National Toxicology Program. *NTP Research Report on the CLARITY-BPA Core Study: A Perinatal and Chronic Extended-Dose-Range Study of Bisphenol A in Rats. NTP RR 9.* Research Triangle Park, NC: National Toxicology Program. (9); 2018, pp. 1–221.
21. Prins GS, Patisaul HB, Belcher SM, Vandenberg LN. CLARITY-BPA academic laboratory studies identify consistent low-dose Bisphenol A effects on multiple organ systems. *Baso Clin Pharm Tox.* 2019;125(S3):14–3.
22. Min KS, Sano E, Ueda H, et al. Dietary deficiency of calcium and/or iron, an age-related risk factor for renal accumulation of cadmium in mice. *Biol Pharm Bull.* 2015;38(10):1557–63.
23. Mukhopadhyay R, Bhattacharjee H, Rosen BP. Aquaglyceroporins: Generalized metalloid channels. *Biochim Biophys Acta.* 2014;1840(5):1583–91.
24. Gallagher, EP, Kunze KL, Stapleton PL, Eaton, DL. The kinetics of aflatoxin B1 oxidation by human cDNA-expressed and human liver microsomal cytochromes P450 1A2 and 3A4. *Toxicol Applied Pharmacol.* 1996;141(2):595–606.
25. Krueger SK, Williams DE. Mammalian flavin-containing monooxygenases: Structure/function, genetic polymorphisms and role in drug metabolism. *Pharmacol Ther.* 2005;106(3):357–87.
26. Jokanović M. Neurotoxic effects of organophosphorus pesticides and possible association with neurodegenerative diseases in man: A review. *Toxicology.* 2018;410:125–31.
27. Costa LG, Giordano G, Cole TB, Marsillach J, Furlong CE. Paraoxonase 1 (PON1) as a genetic determinant of susceptibility to organophosphate toxicity. *Toxicology.* 2013;307:115–22.
28. Carlsten C, Sagoo GS, Frodsham AJ, Burke W, Higgins JP. Glutathione S-transferase M1 (GSTM1) polymorphisms and lung cancer: A literature-based systematic HuGE review and meta-analysis. *Am J Epidemiol.* 2008;167(7):759–74.
29. Shen YH, Chen S, Peng YF, et al. Quantitative assessment of the effect of glutathione S-transferase genes GSTM1 and GSTT1 on hepatocellular carcinoma risk. *Tumour Biol.* 2014;35(5):4007–15.
30. Chang SY, Weber EJ, Sidorenko VS, et al. Human liver-kidney model elucidates the mechanisms of aristolochic acid nephrotoxicity. *JCI Insight.* 2017;2(22):e95978.
31. Langston JW. The MPTP story. J Parkinsons Dis. 2017;7(Suppl 1):S11–9.
32. Caito S, Aschner M. Neurotoxicity of metals. *Handb Clin Neurol.* 2015;131:169–89.
33. Kullak-Ublick GA, Andrade RJ, Merz M, et al. Drug-induced liver injury: Recent advances in diagnosis and risk assessment. *Gut.* 2017;66(6):1154–64.
34. Klaassen CD, Liu J, Diwan BA. Metallothionein protection of cadmium toxicity. *Toxicol Appl Pharmacol.* 2009;238(3):215–20.
35. Schnellman, RG. Toxic responses of the kidney. In: CDKlaasen, ed. *Casarett and Doull's Toxicology. The Basic Science of Poisons*, 8th ed. Chap. 8. New York: McGraw Hill Medical; 2013, pp. 665–90.
36. Cosselman KE, Navas-Acien A, Kaufman JD. Environmental factors in cardiovascular disease. *Nat Rev Cardiol.* 2015:12(11):627–42.
37. Messner B, Bernhard D. Mechanisms of endothelial dysfunction and early atherogenesis. *Arterioscler Thromb Vasc Biol.* 2014;34:509–15.
38. Ambrose JA, Barua RS. The pathophysiology of cigarette smoking and cardiovascular disease. *J Am Coll Cardiol.* 2004;43(10):1731–7.
39. Kaplan BLF, Sulentic CEW, Holsapple MP, Kaminski NE. Toxic responses of the immune system. In: CDKlaasen, ed. *Casarett and Doull's Toxicology. The Basic Science of Poisons*, 8th ed. Chap. 12. New York: McGraw Hill Medical; 2013, pp. 559–638.
40. Fontenot AP, Falta MT, Kappler JW, Dai S, McKee AS. Beryllium-induced hypersensitivity: Genetic susceptibility and neoantigen generation. *J Immunol.* 2016;196(1):22–7.
41. Sharpe RM, Skakkebaek NE. Testicular dysgenesis syndrome: Mechanistic insights and potential new downstream effects. *Fertil Steril.* 2008;89(2 Suppl):e33–8.
42. Fisher JS. Environmental anti-androgens and male reproductive health: Focus on phthalates and testicular dysgenesis syndrome. *Reproduction.* 2004;127(3):305–15.

43. Swan SH, Main KM, Liu F, et al. Decrease in anogenital distance among male infants with prenatal phthalate exposure. *Environ Health Perspect.* 2005;113(8):1056–61.

44. Eisenberg ML, Hsieh MH, Walters RC, Krasnow R, Lipshultz LI. The relationship between anogenital distance, fatherhood, and fertility in adult men. *PLoS One.* 2011;6(5):e18973.

45. Hotchkiss AK, Lambright CS, Ostby JS, Parks-Saldutti L, Vandenbergh JG, Gray JrLE, Prenatal testosterone exposure permanently masculinizes anogenital distance, nipple development, and reproductive tract morphology in female Sprague-Dawley rats. *Toxicol Sci.* 2007;96(2):335–45.

46. Rietjens IMCM, Jochem Louisse J, Karsten Beekmann K. The potential health effects of dietary phytoestrogens. *Br J Pharmacol.* 2017; 174(11):1263–80.

47. Oladimeji PO, Chen T. PXR: More than just a master xenobiotic receptor. *Mol Pharmacol.* 2018:93(2):119–27.

48. Toporova L, Balaguer P. Nuclear receptors are the major targets of endocrine disrupting chemicals. *Mol Cell Endocrinol.* 2019;502:110665.

49. Davies KJA. Oxidative stress, antioxidant defenses, and damage removal, repair, and replacement systems. *IUBMB Life.* 2000;50:279–89.

50. Klaunig KE. Chemical carcinogenesis. In: CDKlaasen, ed. *Casarett and Doull's Toxicology. The Basic Science of Poisons*, 8th ed. Chap. 8. New York: McGraw Hill Medical; 2013, pp. 393–444.

51. Martincorena I, Raine KM, Gerstung M, Dawson KJ, Haase K, Van Loo P, et al. Universal patterns of selection in cancer and somatic tissues. *Cell.* 2017;171(5):1029–41.e21.

52. Schardein JL. *Chemically Induced Birth Defects.* 3rd ed. New York: Marcel Dekker; 2000.

53. Ruddick JA, Khera KS. Pattern of anomalies following single oral doses of ethylenethiourea to pregnant rats. *Teratology.* 1975;12(3):277–81.

54. Koppaka V, Thompson DC, Chen Y, et al. Aldehyde dehydrogenase inhibitors: A comprehensive review of the pharmacology, mechanism of action, substrate specificity, and clinical application. *Pharmacol Rev.* 2012;64(3):520–39.

55. Wild CP, Montesano R. A model of interaction: Aflatoxins and hepatitis viruses in liver cancer aetiology and prevention. *Cancer Lett.* 2009;286(1):22–8.

56. Hernández AF, Tsatsakis AM. Human exposure to chemical mixtures: Challenges for the integration of toxicology with epidemiology data in risk assessment. *Food Chem Toxicol.* 2017;103:188–93.

57. Goumenou M, Tsatsakis A. Proposing new approaches for the risk characterisation of single chemicals and chemical mixtures: The source related hazard quotient (HQ_S) and hazard index (HI_S) and the adversity specific hazard index (HI_A) *Toxicol Rep.* 2019:6:632–6.

58. Toxicology in the 21st Century: https://tox21.gov.

CHAPTER 65

Research Approaches in Environmental and Occupational Health

Jonathan M. Samet • Ana Navas-Acien

INTRODUCTION

Research on occupational and environmental agents is undertaken to address several general questions, all needing to be answered as the basis for policies, regulations, and other interventions to mitigate exposures with adverse health impacts:

- Does the agent cause adverse health effects?
- How does risk vary with exposure levels?
- Who is exposed, how are people exposed, and why are people exposed?
- What groups may be differentially susceptible to the exposure?
- How can exposures and their related health effects be reduced or eliminated?

The answers to these questions come from research that is based in toxicology, including animal bioassays, in vitro experiments, and brief human exposures for some agents, in epidemiological studies of exposed populations, and in exposure assessments. Intervention studies to reduce exposures are a less frequent approach, but randomized trials have been carried out to assess possibly beneficial interventions and quasiexperimental designs have been used to assess the consequence of policy measures. Mechanistic understanding and evaluation of the impacts of interventions also provide answers to these key questions. In a general framework, we seek to understand the path from sources of exposure to adverse health effects (Fig. 65-1).

Research is often triggered by concerns about adverse health effects resulting from environmental or occupational exposures. Sentinel events, such as the rare lung disease bronchiolitis obliterans in popcorn workers handling the flavoring diacetyl[1] or skin hyperkeratosis following chronic exposure to arsenic in water[2] provide a warning by being uncommon and relatively specific. The finding of exposure through biomonitoring may be another trigger, bringing recognition that populations are exposed, as has occurred over the last several decades with the detection in blood samples of per- and polyfluoroalkyl substances that contaminate water and food.[3] Research also extends to the mechanisms by which agents cause disease; mechanistic understanding contributes to reducing uncertainties related to interpreting the findings of epidemiological studies and of bioassays, helping to support the extension of toxicological research to humans, gauging the plausibility of associations found in epidemiological studies, and informing the modeling of exposure-response relationships. Ideally, decision-making is based in integration of information from these various lines of research so that the weight of evidence on the key questions above can be determined and the critical uncertainties characterized.

This chapter provides an overview of the research methods used to address environmental and occupational agents. While there are commonalities, worker populations are by nature selected from the general population and research on the general population is inherently challenged by the heterogeneity of groups within the population. The chapter covers toxicological approaches, which have increasingly shifted away from animal bioassays and exposures of humans to *in vitro* methods, and epidemiological methods that involve individual- and population designs, including multilevel studies. The topic of exposure assessment is covered separately in Chapter 63. The role of experimental designs, including natural experiments and quasiexperiments is covered briefly. Approaches to integrating research findings for decision-making, including causal inference and risk assessment, are covered in other chapters.

The evidence from observational epidemiological studies, when available, and toxicological studies is complementary. Epidemiological studies assess the consequences of exposures sustained in the "real world" and individuals exposed may cover the full spectrum of susceptibility—from the fetus to the elderly. The exposures reflect those sustained across the course of a lifespan, whether to a brief, high-level concentration of an agent, for example, particulate matter air pollution during a short-period of time,[4] or to long-term exposure to a carcinogen, for example, exposure to secondhand tobacco smoke[5] or to arsenic in drinking water.[6] Epidemiological studies of environmental and occupational agents are challenged to assess exposure with accuracy and to contend with the consequences of other factors that may confound the associations of the exposures of interest with health outcomes. Toxicological studies have the advantage of assessing adverse health effects of an agent that is delivered under controlled circumstances in experiments that limit the effects of other factors. However, the agents used in experimental settings may differ from those involved in population exposures and substantial uncertainty is inevitable in generalizing from animal experiments to human populations. Understanding of mechanisms gained in toxicological studies may facilitate the bridging from toxicological studies to the findings of epidemiological studies.

TOXICOLOGICAL APPROACHES

Overview

Toxicological approaches, in contrast to epidemiological approaches, involve the direct exposure of a responsive biological system to the agent(s) of interest; the system may be in vivo, involving a living organism, whether animal or human, or in vitro, involving cells, molecules, and artificial organs or organoids. Toxicological testing has the advantage of assessing the potential for an agent to cause injury with control of the dose and of other factors that may influence the response. It can be used to deepen understanding of mechanisms by which an agent causes injury, thus giving insights into dose-response and the potential for prevention. Toxicological assays have the disadvantage of not necessarily representing the circumstances of "real-world" exposures and the complex mixtures to which people are exposed, such as urban air pollution. Additionally, there is the

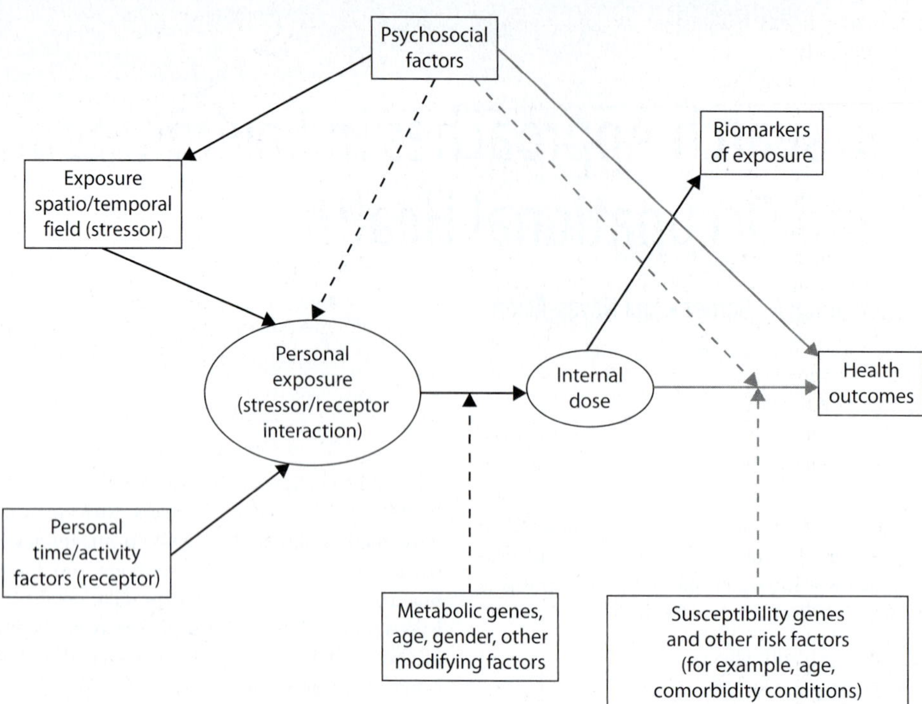

FIGURE 65-1. General framework for the path from exposure to health outcomes. (*Source*:. National Research Council. 2012. Exposure Science in the 21st Century: A Vision and a Strategy. https://doi.org/10.17226/13507. Reproduced with permission from the National Academy of Sciences, Courtesy of the National Academies Press, Washington, D.C.[7].)

unavoidable uncertainty associated with extending findings from a toxicological model to the circumstances of human exposure.

Toxicological assays have been a critical element in the suite of approaches used to assay the toxicity of environmental and occupational agents.[7] The approaches have changed over time, as methodologies have evolved for delivering agents and assessing outcomes. Societal factors have also had a prominent role, limiting exposures to human volunteers to be brief and without lasting effects, and increasingly restricting use of animals for toxicity testing. As a result, there is a move toward using in vitro bioassays for screening for toxicity and follow-up animal bioassays only if warranted. Expense also limits the use of animal bioassays.

One consequence of the high cost of testing agents, particularly chemicals, for their toxicity is exposure of people to thousands of agents for which information on potential risks is lacking or uncertain. In Europe, the European Union's REACH initiative (Registration, Evaluation, Authorization, and Restriction of Chemicals) requires prospective registration of new chemicals and submission of information on safety and risk by manufacturers.[8] The safety evaluation is based in high throughput cell assay systems that provide information on whether an agent activates a pathway that leads to injury, for example, oxidative stress or DNA damage. In the United States, prospective registration of new chemicals is not required, and a risk assessment process may be implemented following the registration and commercialization of the chemical if there is a basis for concern.[9]

Human Toxicology

For some agents, the potential for risk is assessed through controlled exposures of human volunteers to the agent. Such exposures must be ethical by not posing an unacceptable risk, and any consequences of exposure need to be reversible. Participants need to be recruited as informed volunteers and without any coercion. This type of study has been referred to as a "clinical" study. The design has the advantage of a controlled exposure and the potential to collect data on toxicity, for example, biomarkers, that might not be available in a general population context.

For example, the clinical study design has been widely used to assess the short-term consequences of exposure to specific air pollutants, including gases (carbon monoxide, ozone, nitrogen dioxide, and sulfur dioxide), particles, and mixtures (diesel exhaust). Numerous studies have been carried out on the effects of ozone on the lung, for example.[10,11] In a series of studies carried out by the U.S. Environmental Protection Agency and others, volunteers inhaled ozone at concentrations measured in polluted areas and their lung function was tracked with documentation of a short-term drop in some, susceptible individuals. Some protocols incorporated exercise to increase the dose and some included bronchoscopy to directly measure the inflammatory response in the lung.[12] One study assessed whether there was particular sensitivity among older persons.[11] For several major air pollutants regulated under the Clean Air Act, the findings of such human exposure studies have figured prominently in the standard-setting process, for example, for carbon monoxide and ozone.

Human volunteer studies have also been carried out for other agents, for example, pesticides using markers for the effects of pesticides and symptoms as outcomes.[13] Clinical studies have also been conducted to assess absorption and excretion patterns after exposure to a known dose of a known toxic chemical. For instance, studies with experimental radiolabeled arsenic in the 1970s were critical in showing that arsenic is eliminated through the urine in three phases.[14] Such research raises complex ethical questions, particularly when carried out by manufacturers for regulatory purposes.[13] There is also a long history of testing of agents for warfare in members of the military under circumstances that have raised retrospective questioning of the ethics of the exposures.[15]

Animal Bioassays

Animal bioassays have been a mainstay of the assessment of the risks of environmental and occupational agents for decades. Such studies have the strengths of (1) complete control of the exposures delivered; (2) homogeneity of the animals included with regard to species and strain; (3) control of potential confounding factors; (4) the opportunity to make observations at any time point; and (5) the availability of tissues for pathology and molecular studies. A wide range of species have been used, including primates, dogs, and rodents. In recent decades, much primate research has ended and current research tends to use rodents, particularly mice that are well-characterized genetically. Additionally, specialized strains that carry genes conveying susceptibility can now be produced. Humanized mouse models are also starting to be developed to better investigate the impact of environmental exposures in a more appropriate genetic framework.[16,17] More efficient animal models are becoming widely used. The zebrafish embryo model has emerged as a high-throughput tool for investigating the effects of environmental exposures.[18] Key to their increasing use are the advances in our understanding of the evolutionary conservation of genomic, biochemical and developmental features between zebrafish and humans, including their utility to study potential mechanisms for environmental toxicity during development and its connections to adult onset disease.[19]

Not surprisingly, a key concern is the relevance of animal bioassays for risk to humans. For some outcomes, mechanisms that produce disease are known to not be relevant to humans, for example, some kidney cancers in male rats are related to the accumulation of a low-molecular weight protein that does not appear to be relevant for humans.[20] Additionally, the array of results from a bioassay may not be coherent with differing observations in different species, for example, rats and mice, or in males and females. Recent bioassays of the effects of radiofrequency electromagnetic radiation, the type of radiation emitted by cell phones, are illustrative. In the bioassay carried out by the National Toxicology Program of the National Institute for Environmental Health Sciences, male and female rats and mice were exposed to radiation intended to mimic exposure from 2G and 3G devices.[21–23] With regard to the occurrence of cancer, the results were positive in male rats, but not in female rats and the findings in male and female mice were equivocal. In male rates, schwannomas of the heart were observed, an exceedingly rare tumor in people. Differences in susceptibility by species and sex have no ready explanation and could be related to complex gene–environment interactions or hormone–environment interactions, for instance.

Nonetheless, animal bioassays are still a workhorse for assessing the risks of environmental and occupational agents. The National Toxicology Program tests agents that are considered important for public health using rigorous protocols; nominations can be made. Almost universally, toxicity testing is done with adherence to Good Laboratory Practice (GLP), a system intended to assure the quality of data.[24]

In Vitro Methods

In vitro methods involve use of various cellular and molecular systems to explore the potential of compounds to cause injury in ways that could lead to disease. The sophistication of these methods has evolved substantially such that agents can now be tested in large numbers using robotic systems that can apply a range of concentrations to different cellular assays. The read-out from these systems is typically the RNA transcriptome, providing insight into the pathways that have been activated. A seminal 2007 report from the National Research Council, *Toxicity Testing in the 21st Century*, proposed a paradigm for chemical toxicity testing that involved initial assessment with high throughput assays and follow-up animal bioassays as needed.[7] The possibilities for more specific testing have been advanced by the development of organoids, that is, "organs on a chip," that can bring greater organ specificity and relevance to results of *in vitro* tests.[25,26]

In interpreting the findings of high throughput testing, emphasis is placed on patterns of response that indicate that a pathway has been activated that is known to lead to injury, so-called "adverse outcome pathways."[27] Systems have been proposed for determining if such activation has occurred and linking the pathways to particular adverse effects. Schema for using the results of high throughput testing in practice have been developed by a committee of the National Academies of Science, Engineering, and Medicine.[7]

ENVIRONMENTAL EPIDEMIOLOGY

Overview

Environmental epidemiology comprises the methods used to investigate the effects of environmental agents, as exposures occur to human populations. For many agents, the results of epidemiological studies have driven policies and regulations intended to protect the public health. Notable examples include outdoor air pollution,[4,28] childhood lead exposure,[29] and arsenic in drinking water.[30] Viewing the cigarette as an environmental agent, epidemiological studies provided convincing evidence on the consequences of active smoking from 1950 on while reports on the adverse consequences of secondhand smoke exposure were published from the early 1980s on.[5]

Studies on environmental agents draw on the array of epidemiological designs. Studies may be initiated specifically to address the consequences of one or more environmental agents. Additionally, studies initiated for questions other than environmental agents have proved valuable for research on environmental hazards. For example, the American Cancer Society's Cancer Prevention Study II (CPS II) has been a key source of evidence on air pollution exposure and all-cause and cause-specific mortality.[31,32] Originally established to investigate the causes of cancer, the original questionnaire data were supplemented by modeled estimates of exposure at the residential locations of the participants. Other cohort studies have been similarly complemented for investigating air pollution or other environmental exposures. As another example, the Strong Heart Study, the largest study of cardiovascular disease and its risk factors in American Indians, was initially funded to evaluate classical cardiovascular disease risk factors[33] but was subsequently expanded to assess the role of disproportionate metal exposure in the excess cardiovascular disease risk in American Indian communities.[34,35]

Study Designs

A broad array of study designs is used to address the effects of environmental agents on human health (Fig. 65-2 and Box 65-1). They can be broadly classified as population level or individual level, but in some multilevel designs, exposure may be classified at the population level, for example, by city, while covariate information is available at the individual level. Central to the design of studies in environmental epidemiology is establishing an exposure contrast or gradient, typically based around temporal or spatial patterns of exposure to an agent, although some interindividual differences in environmental exposures might be related to factors beyond geography or time, for example, dietary patterns, leisure time activities. The contrast may be on a short-term basis, for example, daily time-series studies of air pollution and mortality, or longer term, for example, declining levels of air pollution over several decades. By necessity, studies typically cover some specified period of time and cannot take a full life-course approach, given feasibility. With the follow-up of some birth cohorts being extended into adulthood, the potential for full life-course approaches should substantially increase in the coming decades.

Study designs may also have structure, at the simplest, individual level or population level. However, there may be additional structure incorporating levels that extend from individuals to neighborhoods, communities, states, and nations. Exposures at each of these levels affect health. Historically, population level designs had wide usage in early explorations of the environment and health, comparing, for example, health indicators in urban and nonurban areas and in more and less polluted locations. For example, when the rise of lung cancer was first identified, comparisons were made of lung cancer mortality in urban and rural areas in the United Kingdom.[36] The catastrophic consequences of the London Fog of 1952 were convincingly demonstrated by a plotting of mortality and air pollution levels over a several week period bracketing the days of extraordinarily high pollution.[37]

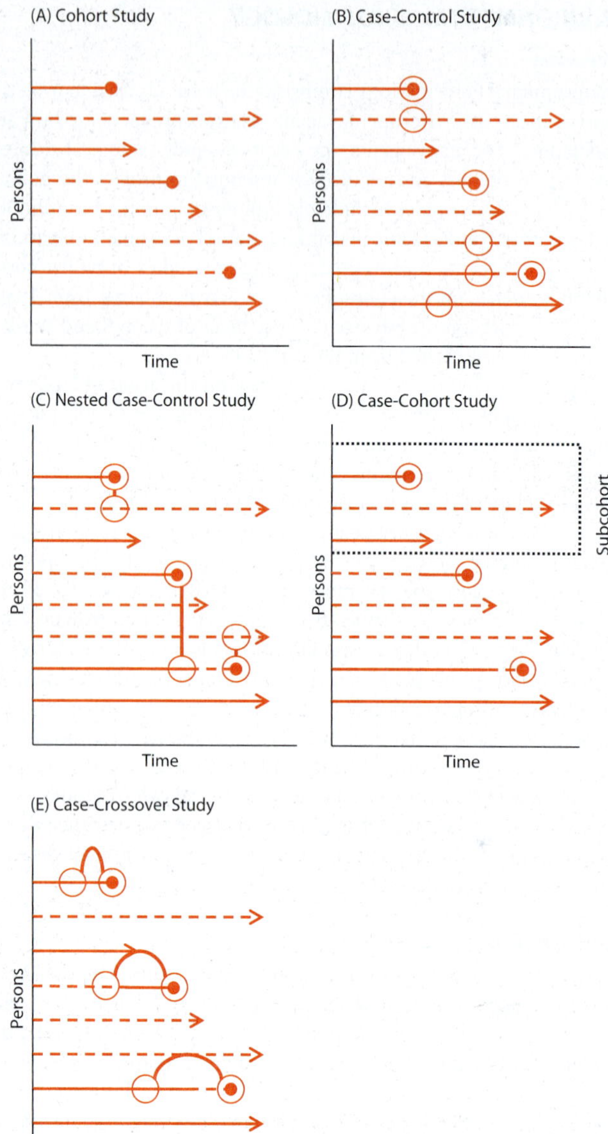

FIGURE 65-2. Schemas for basic epidemiologic designs. Note: Each figure shows the same hypothetical cohort of eight people. Solid line indicates time while exposed; dashed line indicates nonexposed time; solid circle indicates time at which outcome occurs, for example, death.

BOX 65.1 Study Designs Used to Address the Effects of Environmental Agents on Human Health

Population-Level Designs

- Ecological designs comparing patterns of exposure and disease over space and time at the population level
- Time-series designs assessing association of temporal variation in exposure with variation in disease occurrence
- Quasiexperimental designs addressing consequences of measures that change exposures

Multilevel Designs

- Studies involving multiple sites with differing exposures at the population-level and individual-level covariate information.

Individual-Level Designs

- Cross-sectional
- Case-control
- Cohort
  - Nested case-control
  - Case-cohort
- Case-crossover
- Randomized clinical trials

Figure 65-2A–E provides diagrams of the principal individual-level designs, including their foundation in the cohort design (Fig. 65-2A), which has the fundamental characteristic of following study participants over time and making observations concerning outcomes. The figures are based in a hypothetical cohort of eight persons followed over time with A–E—varying exposure for some. The figures show the various designs that could be used to assess association of exposure with risk for outcome. Cohorts are started at times that reflect feasibility, funding, public health exigencies, and other considerations. Exposures may have already taken place and may be continuing. The cross-sectional study or survey might be considered as a cohort study, that is, a population has been assembled, viewed at a single point of time without follow-up.

With regard to individual-level designs, surveys have long been a useful approach and a starting point for addressing health consequences of environmental agents. Some early surveys based exposure on the presence of a source or proximity to one or more sources, while contemporary surveys may use monitoring and models for exposure estimation.[38] Outcome assessment often involves a questionnaire, but may incorporate physiological assessment, for example, lung function testing with a spirometer, and collection of biological samples for measurement of exposure biomarkers, indicators of injury, and genomics. In the context of environmental epidemiology, the general limits of cross-sectional data collection remain: investigation of a prevalent population that may be affected by bias from loss of affected individuals and ambiguity as to causal directions underlying associations between exposures and outcomes.

The cohort design, generally used prospectively in addressing environmental exposures, has the advantage of supporting prospective collection of exposure to minimize measurement error and repeatedly assessing time-varying exposures (Fig. 65-2A). The cohort design also facilitates collection of information on potential confounding and modifying factors and on outcomes that may be time varying, for example, decline of lung function over time in a study of air pollution. The Harvard Six Cities Study of air pollution is exemplary.[39] This prospective cohort study, initiated in 1974, involved recruitment of schoolchildren and adults in six U.S. cities that were selected to cover a gradient of exposure to air pollution. Exposure was based on monitoring carried out at the city level, while information was collected on covariates, lung function, and respiratory symptoms and illnesses at the individual-level. A landmark paper published in 1993 found that mortality in the adults was associated with city of residence and level of exposure to airborne particulate matter.[39] There are many other landmark cohort studies, including diverse multiethnic populations,[40] and this design is essential for investigating the impact of adult exposures as well as prenatal and early-life exposures and later outcomes. There are barriers, including the challenges of recruiting and maintaining participation. The storage of biospecimens at baseline and over the follow-up also allows for analyzing exposures of interest when resources and technology make it possible, still preserving the advantages of the prospective design.

Some contemporary cohort studies have been based in administrative record systems, for example, the data for Medicare, which includes essentially all U.S. adults 65 years and above. Di et al. used this database to carry out a cohort study of air pollution exposure and mortality.[41] Exposure was estimated for zip code of residence using an artificial intelligence model incorporating multiple data streams. Similar approaches have been used in other countries, including use of census samples in Canada and various registries. There is an expectation that cohorts assembled from medical administrative data systems may be used to address environmental agents.

The case-control design has been primarily used to study environmental agents and noncommunicable diseases and related outcomes (Fig. 65-2B). Case-control studies involve sampling in a cohort by disease status, affected and unaffected (Fig. 65-2B). The presence of an underlying cohort is implicit, although the cohort may be ill defined, as with hospital-based case-control studies. Case-control studies may be conducted within defined populations, as with population-based case-control studies of cancer based in comprehensive cancer registries, for example, the population of a state represents the underlying cohort.[42] A case-control study may be nested within a specific cohort (Fig. 65-2C), most often as an efficient approach to conducting additional analyses for exposure assessment.[43]

The case-control design was the historical starting point for identifying the link between cigarette smoking and lung cancer risk. The early studies, initiated in the late 1940s, compared smoking histories in patients hospitalized for lung cancer with those of controls hospitalized for other diagnoses.[44–46] The design remains useful, if exposures can be estimated for the relevant timeframe. For example, a case-control study was carried out to identify risk factors for incident asthma in adults that addressed multiple environmental and occupational exposures.[47] The design has the advantage of supporting the assessment of multiple exposures, but the disadvantage of relying on the retrospective reconstruction of exposure. The temporal relationship between the exposure and the outcome is particularly challenging to interpret when exposure assessment relies on biomarkers that can be affected by the presence of the disease. An increasing challenge to the conduct of case-control studies is the identification of unbiased sources of cases from which appropriate controls can also be derived. This problem particularly affects case/control series recruited from medical care facilities.

The case-cohort design is used for efficiency (Fig. 65-2D); complete information is collected on a random sample of the full cohort (the subcohort) and outcomes determined on the full cohort with comparison of exposures in those having the outcome with those in the subcohort.[48] The case-cohort design has been used, for instance, to assess the role of baseline cumulative cadmium exposure with incident stroke and breast cancer.[49,50] Case-control studies may be nested within a cohort with cases representing those developing disease over follow-up and disease-free controls coming from those under follow-up having characteristics similar to the cases.[51] This design might be used, for example, to compare blood biomarkers of exposure in cases and controls; efficiency is gained and costs reduced by only making the measurements in a subset of the cohort. Many specific examples of nested case-control designs exist, for instance studies evaluating the prospective association of persistent organic pollutants (which require an expensive assay and quite large amount of blood) with incident diabetes.[52]

The case-crossover design is an individually matched approach to assessing risks of exposures that change relatively rapidly over time (Fig. 65-2E). It was originally proposed to assess triggers of myocardial infarction.[53] An exposure window is defined in relation to the occurrence of the event of interest, for example, a myocardial infarction; for the same individual, one or more control time-windows are also established, representing periods of risk for the same outcome during which the outcome did not occur. Because the design matches on the individual, confounding is implicitly controlled. Effect modification, however, can still play a role and requires assessment similar to other study designs. There are varying sampling methods to handle potential temporal confounding factors.[54]

For example, Peters and colleagues carried out a case-crossover study of traffic exposure and onset of acute myocardial infarction.[55] The study participants were in a registry of myocardial infarction victims in a city in Germany. Exposure was based on a detailed time-activity diary on the day of the event and the 4 prior days. The case periods were the one-hour periods in the six hours before the event while the control periods came from time 24–72 hours before the event. Exposure to traffic was associated with an almost threefold increase in risk for myocardial infarction.

Randomized controlled trials can be used to assess measures that will reduce the effects of exposures. Examples of randomized controlled trials relevant for environmental health include, for instance, air cleaning for indoor air pollutants,[56] lower-emission cookstoves and clean fuels to reduce household air pollution,[57] water arsenic mitigation,[58] metal chelating agents for cardiovascular disease prevention,[59,60] pest management interventions for asthma prevention and control,[61] and nutritional interventions to mitigate the health effects of environmental chemicals.[62,63]

Methodological Issues

The results of studies of environmental agents are subject to the same general limitations as other observational studies in human populations: measurement error, confounding, and selection bias. For the often high-stakes arenas where the findings of environmental epidemiology have impact, stakeholders may point to the limitations of epidemiological studies, often exaggerating the potential of well-known issues, for example, confounding, to produce misleading results. Such exaggeration dates to the early attacks of the tobacco industry on the findings linking smoking to lung cancer and it remains core to strategies for creating "doubt" about the findings of epidemiological studies.[64,65] Seasoned researchers anticipate such attacks and carefully consider potential limitations as studies are designed and data are collected and analyzed.

Exposure assessment is one of the most challenging elements in the design and conduct of an environmental epidemiology study. Many constraints around exposure assessment, including feasibility and costs, participant burden, and the complexities of obtaining biospecimens, exist. There may also be uncertainty about the relevant period(s) of exposure to the agent, for example, early life or cumulative across the lifespan, and exposures may change over time. For many environmental exposures, error in their measurement in the context of an epidemiological study is inherent. The consequences of measurement error depend on the nature of the error: random and introducing "noise," systematic and introducing bias either positive or negative in the effect estimated, or both.

Issues related to exposure measurement can often be anticipated when the exposure assessment strategy is planned and steps taken to minimize error through carefully designed protocols with sustained quality assurance. To gauge the degree of error, a validation study may be embedded in data collection, involving the collection of exposure data with the "gold standard" method in a sample of participants. Comparison of the results from the general exposure assessment strategy with those from the validation study provides an estimation of the degree of error. For example, in a study of lung function in 1172 coal miners with a total of 36,824 personal dust measures available, the mean difference in forced expiratory volume in the first second (FEV1) was -4.5 mL/mg/m^3 of exposure to respirable coal dust when all the personal dust measures were used (gold standard) in the analysis but only -3.6, -2.5, and -1.8 mL when 9, 6, and 3 dust samples were randomly selected per worker, respectively.[66]

Advances

There is an expectation that technology-driven advances in research methods will facilitate research on environmental agents. The emergence of exposomics promises to remedy some of the gaps in reconstructing longer-term and more comprehensive profiles of exposure and insights into susceptibility are anticipated from genomics.[67] Advances in exposure modeling and biomarkers support increasingly refined modeling of population and individual exposures. Use of administrative databases facilitates the development of large cohorts, although information may be lacking on key covariates and outcome assessment might be challenging for some endpoints (e.g., neurological endpoints).

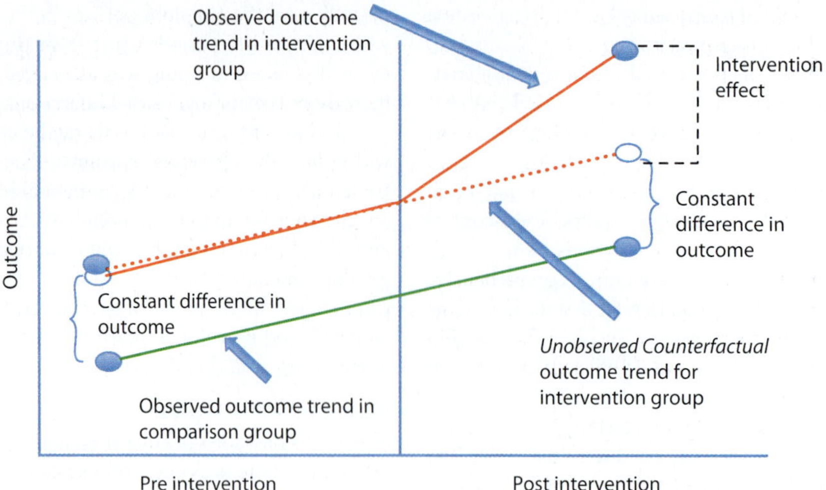

FIGURE 65-3. Difference-in-difference estimation, graphical explanation. (*Source:* Reproduced with permission from Difference-in-Difference Estimation. Columbia.edu. https://www.publichealth.columbia.edu/research/population-health-methods/difference-difference-estimation.) Reproduced with permission from Difference-in-Difference Estimation. Columbia.edu. https://www.publichealth.columbia.edu/research/population-health-methods/difference-difference-estimation. Accessed February 18, 2021.)

OCCUPATIONAL EPIDEMIOLOGY

Overview

Studies of environmental and occupational agents are overlapping and often address the same agents, albeit at higher levels in the occupational setting compared with the general population. Some aspects of occupational epidemiological studies are distinct, however, including the investigation of populations of workers who differ from the population at large in being sufficiently healthy to work, higher exposure concentrations in a defined environment but during shorter durations (e.g., 8 hours/day for 5 days/week), the possibility of documenting exposures through workplace records, and often limited availability of information on potential confounding factors particularly for mortality studies depending on the study design and resources. Historically, many workplaces had very high levels of exposure, for example, coal mines, and investigations were motivated by the occurrence of clinically evident disease, for example, severe, advanced black lung disease or coal workers' pneumoconiosis.[68] As a generalization, the field of occupational epidemiology has declined as industries have dropped units concerned with occupational health risks in their workers and funded fewer studies, in particular in places such as the United States and Europe. Internationally, however, numerous low and middle income countries continue to be affected by high exposure to numerous toxic chemicals in industries such as artisanal and low-scale gold mining,[69] e-waste recycling,[70] and exposure to agrochemicals and other toxic compounds in intensive farming.[71,72]

Study Designs

The study designs used in occupational epidemiology follow those listed in Box 65-1. In studying worker populations, surveys or cross-sectional studies are frequently carried out, for example, to assess lung function and respiratory health status. This design is feasible and useful to determine if adverse effects are occurring among workers. One mainstay of occupational epidemiology has been worker cohort studies, primarily directed at cause-specific mortality. Such studies have typically been carried out with retrospective timing, that is, as retrospective cohort studies, but prospective follow-up time can be added. Typically, mortality is compared with expectations based on the general population with the calculation of standardized mortality ratios (SMRs). Given that worker populations tend to be healthier than the general population, SMRs for all-cause mortality tend to be below unity as may other causes-of-death, for example, cardiovascular disease.[73,74] Studies based on internal comparisons, for example, within workers rather than comparing to external general populations, can facilitate comparisons,[75] although healthier workers can still be assigned the job tasks characterized by higher exposure levels to the agent of interest.[76] Analyses are also carried out to assess how SMRs vary with exposure, time since exposure, and time since the end of exposure.

Cohort studies may address endpoints other than mortality, including cancer incidence, changes in lung function, and other parameters. They are typically formed around specific exposure circumstances, such as the cohort of clean-up workers in the Gulf of Mexico, following the Deepwater Horizon disaster.[77] The Agricultural Health Study represents a unique longitudinal platform that involves agricultural workers and their spouses with enrollment of children now in progress.[78]

The consequences of occupational exposures may also be addressed in studies in the general population. Numerous population-based case-control studies of cancer have been carried out that explored associations of occupational agents with cancer risk. The National Cancer Institute developed a set of matrices to link jobs in particular industries to specific exposures, a so-called job-exposure matrix.[79] For example, in a case-control study of non-Hodgkin lymphoma in women from Connecticut, occupational exposure to chlorinated solvents and carbon tetrachloride, estimated based on a job-exposure-matrix, was higher among cases compared not non-cases.[80] Job exposure matrices have also been developed and widely used in countries with high quality occupational and industry nationwide records, allowing for large retrospective cohort studies by connecting the rich exposure data with mortality and medical records data.[81,82] Studies of lung function in general population cohorts have also addressed occupation and accelerated decline and risk for chronic obstructive pulmonary disease (COPD).[83]

Methodological Issues

While subject to the same general methodological issues as epidemiological studies in other areas, there are several considerations that have received specific attention with regard to occupational studies: most notably, the so-called "healthy worker effect."[84] This refers to the bias affecting studies of occupational cohorts through the selection of healthier people into cohorts of workers and the selective loss from those cohorts of those affected by a workplace exposure or those with health problems more generally. A consequence is the need to interpret associations in the context of potential bias from the healthy worker effect. For example, an SMR below one for all-cause mortality or for some specific causes of death such as cardiovascular disease can be expected in a worker population. It is an important bias when comparing workers to general populations but it also occurs when internal populations are used as referent, as job task assignment position changes are nonrandom with respect to the risk of disease.[76] Methods used to control for the healthy worker effect include the use of internal controls (partially successful strategy), account for time-since-hire and time-related work variables, lagging methods, adjustment for employment status and more advanced strategies.[85,86]

Advances

Studies of workers will be strengthened by some of the advances in epidemiology generally: the application of -omics technologies and particularly the exposome, and the application of advanced methods for the assessment of chemical mixtures. For many workplaces in the United States and other high-income countries, the agents that caused disease in the past are of lesser interest as exposures have declined or the industries have been moved to low- and middle-income countries. However, other stressors and job conditions are now of interest along with different types of outcomes, such as productivity and burnout syndrome.

NATURAL EXPERIMENTS

Overview

Changes in exposure levels over time affecting a specific population provide the opportunity to assess the impact of these changes on indicators of risk and disease burden. In interpreting the findings of observational studies of environmental exposures, there is an assumption that causal effects will occur "in reverse" when the exposure is reduced or eliminated. A reduction in exposure levels affecting a population is thus a potentially informative scenario, offering an opportunity to assess whether the reduction in exposure reduces exposure, risk, and disease burden. For instance, the rapid implementation of smoke-free legislation in multiple countries and states between 2005 and 2008 and substantial reductions in second-hand smoke exposure resulted in rapid reductions in hospital admissions for coronary heart disease[87,88] and asthma,[89] and of preterm births.[89] Biomonitoring of cotinine levels has shown a dramatic decline in secondhand smoke exposure in the United States.[90] These findings received substantial attention from the media and the medical/scientific community providing confirmatory evidence to decades of epidemiological research on the health effects of secondhand smoke exposure. When the change in exposure can be anticipated, for instance before and after the Beijing Olympic games, formal research studies can be prospectively planned and implemented.[91,92]

These studies are overall useful to evaluate the effectiveness of the implementation of policy and large-scale interventions/programs. With regard to air pollution, the term "accountability" research has been applied, responding to the questioning from policy-makers who seek documentation of the purported benefits of air pollution regulation.[93] In an initial report on the concept of accountability, a "chain of accountability" was proposed that moved from regulatory or other actions to reduction of emissions, changes in air quality, reduced exposure, and finally to risk for adverse health outcomes.[93]

Study Designs

A number of different designs can be implemented to leverage natural experiments and can be broadly defined as quasiexperiments.[94] Specific designs that apply particularly well in the context of a special circumstance that rapidly influences changes in environmental exposure levels include Difference in Difference and Regression Discontinuity (RD).[94-97] The Difference-in-Difference (DID) technique makes use of longitudinal data to estimate the effect of a specific intervention (e.g., policy enactment, program implementation, change in sources) comparing changes in outcomes over time between a population affected by the intervention and a population that is not (control group) (Fig. 65-3).[98,99] RD can be used when public health programs use a specific cut-off point on a continuous variable as the decision rule to assign treatment or program eligibility.[95,96] Thus, RD has been applied to studies assessing the effects of air quality alerts on human health,[100] the impact of sustained exposure to air pollution on life expectancy from programs that differentially affected air pollution exposure in China (Huai River policy),[101] and the impact of smoke-free legislation on birth outcomes,[102] for example.

Methodological Issues

Natural experiments and quasiexperiments are important tools when interventions cannot be randomized but they also involve important assumptions. For instance, DID relies on the exchangeability assumption, that is, absent treatment (intervention), the unobserved differences between treatment and control groups would have been the same over time.[98,99] Another assumption is that the allocation of the intervention is not determined by the outcome. DID studies provide intuitive interpretations and can estimate a causal effect using observational data if the assumptions are met. The requirement of baseline data and a nonintervention group can be a limitation if not available. The key assumption for RD methods are that (1) the decision rule and cutoff value of the variable used to assign the treatment are known, (2) the assignment variable is continuous near the cutoff value, and (3) potential outcomes with respect to the assignment variable are continuous at the threshold (i.e., lack of confounding around the threshold).[95,96] These RD assumptions can be tested with available data, an advantage of RD vs. other quasiexperimental designs.

Advances

The use of quasiexperimental designs in environmental epidemiology and environmental health at large is rapidly increasing. A search (carried out in December, 2019) in PubMed with the free text "quasiexperimental AND environmental health" resulted in 445 articles, including 78 in 2019, while before 2010 the number of publications was 10 or less per year. Given the urgent need to implement effective interventions to address the numerous environmental health problems affecting global populations, it is likely that quasiexperimental designs will continue to increase in the near future.

SUMMARY

The risks of environmental and occupational agents are addressed through a rich and complementary set of research approaches. New technologies benefit both toxicological and epidemiological approaches, and methods for exposure assessment have been strengthened by new -omics assays. Nonetheless, some long-standing challenges remain: the relevance of toxicological findings for risks to humans, and exposure estimation and handling potential confounding in epidemiological studies. Additionally, experience shows that studies with regulatory implications may come under intense scrutiny and that findings need to be robust to questioning about methods. Increasingly, research is addressing the consequences of interventions to reduce exposures through both randomized clinical trials and quasiexperimental designs.

References

1. Kreiss K, Gomaa A, Kullman G, Fedan K, Simoes EJ, Enright PL. Clinical bronchiolitis obliterans in workers at a microwave-popcorn plant. *N Engl J Med*. 2002;347(5):330–8.
2. Argos M, Kalra T, Pierce BL, et al. A prospective study of arsenic exposure from drinking water and incidence of skin lesions in Bangladesh. *Am J Epidemiol*. 2011;174(2):185–94.
3. Graber JM, Alexander C, Laumbach RJ, et al. Per and polyfluoroalkyl substances (PFAS) blood levels after contamination of a community water supply and comparison with 2013–2014 NHANES. *J Expo Sci Environ Epidemiol*. 2019;29(2):172–82.
4. Dominici F, Peng RD, Bell ML, et al. Fine particulate air pollution and hospital admission for cardiovascular and respiratory diseases. *JAMA*. 2006;295(10):1127–34.

5. USDHHS. *The health consequences of involuntary exposure to tobacco smoke. A report of the Surgeon General.* Atlanta, GA: U.S. Department of Health and Human Services, Centers for Disease Control and Prevention, Coordinating Center for Health Promotion, National Center for Chronic Disease Prevention and Health Promotion, Office on Smoking and Health; 2006.
6. National Research Council. *Critical Aspects of EPA's IRIS Assessment of Inorganic Arsenic: Interim Report.* Washington, DC: National Academies Press; 2013.
7. National Research Council, Committee on Toxicity Testing and Assessment of Environmental Agents, Board on Environmental Studies and Toxicology, Institute for Laboratory Animal Research, Division on Earth and Life Studies. *Toxicity Testing in the 21st Century: A Vision and a Strategy.* Washington, DC: National Academies Press; 2007.
8. European Chemicals Agency. Understanding REACH. 2019. https://echa.europa.eu/regulations/reach/understanding-reach. Accessed December 16, 2019.
9. U.S. Environmental Protection Agency. Risk Evaluations for Exisiting Chemicals under TSCA. *Assessing and Managing Chemicals under TSCA* 2019. https://www.epa.gov/assessing-and-managing-chemicals-under-tsca/risk-evaluations-existing-chemicals-under-tsca. Accessed December 30, 2019.
10. Linn WS, Avol EL, Shamoo DA, et al. A dose-response study of healthy, heavily exercising men exposed to ozone at concentrations near the ambient air quality standard. *Toxicol Ind Health.* 1986;2(1):99–112.
11. Frampton MW, Balmes J, Bromberg PA, et al. Multicenter ozone study in older subjects (MOSES): Part 1. Effects of exposure to low concentrations of ozone on respiratory and cardiovascular outcomes. *Res Rep Health Eff Inst.* 2017;(192, Pt 1):1–107.
12. Hatch GE, McKee J, Brown J, et al. Biomarkers of dose and effect of inhaled ozone in resting versus exercising human subjects: Comparison with resting rats. *Biomark Insights.* 2013;8:53–67.
13. Resnik DB, Portier C. Pesticide testing on human subjects: Weighing benefits and risks. *Environ Health Perspect.* 2005;113(7):813–7.
14. Cullen WR, Reimer KJ. Arsenic speciation in the environment. *Chem Rev.* 1989;89(4):713–64.
15. Institute of Medicine. *Veterans at Risk: The Health Effects of Mustard Gas and Lewisite.* Washington, DC: The National Academies Press; 1993.
16. Davies G. What is a humanized mouse? Remaking the species and spaces of translational medicine. *Body Soc.* 2012;18(3–4):126–55.
17. Walsh NC, Kenney LL, Jangalwe S, et al. Humanized mouse models of clinical disease. *Annu Rev Pathol.* 2017;12:187–215.
18. Bugel SM, Tanguay RL, Planchart A. Zebrafish: A marvel of high-throughput biology for 21(st) century toxicology. *Curr Environ Health Rep.* 2014;1(4):341–52.
19. Sant KE, Timme-Laragy AR. Zebrafish as a model for toxicological perturbation of yolk and nutrition in the early embryo. *Curr Environ Health Rep.* 2018;5(1):125–33.
20. Rodgers IS, Baetcke KP. Interpretation of male rat renal tubule tumors. *Environ Health Perspect.* 1993;101(Suppl 6):45–52.
21. National Toxicology Program. NTP Technical Report on the Toxicology and Carcinogenesis Studies in Hsd: Sprague Dawley SD Rats Exposed to Whole-Body Radio Frequency Radiation at Frequency (900 MHz) and Modulations (GSM and CDMA) Used by Cell Phones. Research Triangle, NC2018.
22. National Toxicology Program. NTP Technical Report on the Toxicology and Carcinogenesis Studies in B6C3F1/N Mice Exposed to Whole-Body Radio Frequency Radiation at a Frequency (1,900 MHz) and Modulations (GSM and CDMA) Used by Cell Phones. Research Triangle, NC2018.
23. National Toxicology Program. Cell Phone Radio Frequency Radiation. 2019. https://ntp.niehs.nih.gov/whatwestudy/topics/cellphones/index.html?utm_source=direct&utm_medium=prod&utm_campaign=ntp-golinks&utm_term=cellphone. Accessed December 30, 2019.
24. World Health Organization. Handbook: Good Laboratory Practice (GLP): Quality Practices for Regulated Non-clinical Research and Development. 2nd ed. Geneva, Switzerland: World Health Organization; 2009.
25. Park SE, Georgescu A, Huh D. Organoids-on-a-chip. *Science.* 2019;364(6444):960–5.
26. Truskey GA. Human microphysiological systems and organoids as in vitro models for toxicological studies. *Front Public Health.* 2018;6:185.
27. Organisation for Economic Co-Operation and Development. The Adverse Outcome Pathways development programme workplan. 2019. https://www.oecd.org/chemicalsafety/testing/projects-adverse-outcome-pathways.htm. Accessed December 30, 2019.
28. Kaufman JD, Adar SD, Barr RG, et al. Association between air pollution and coronary artery calcification within six metropolitan areas in the USA (the multi-ethnic study of atherosclerosis and air pollution): A longitudinal cohort study. *Lancet.* 2016;388(10045):696–704.
29. Lanphear BP, Hornung R, Khoury J, et al. Low-level environmental lead exposure and children's intellectual function: An international pooled analysis. *Environ Health Perspect.* 2005;113(7):894–9.
30. Moon KA, Oberoi S, Barchowsky A, et al. A dose-response meta-analysis of chronic arsenic exposure and incident cardiovascular disease. *Int J Epidemio.* 2018;46(6):1924–39.
31. Turner MC, Krewski D, Diver WR, et al. Ambient air pollution and cancer mortality in the cancer prevention study II. *Environ Health Perspect.* 2017;125(8):087013.
32. Eftim SE, Samet JM, Janes H, McDermott A, Dominici F. Fine particulate matter and mortality: A comparison of the six cities and American Cancer Society cohorts with a medicare cohort. *Epidemiology.* 2008;19(2):209–16.
33. Lee ET, Welty TK, Fabsitz R, et al. The strong heart Study. A study of cardiovascular disease in American Indians: design and methods. *Am J Epidemiol.* 1990;132(6):1141–55.
34. Moon KA, Guallar E, Umans JG, et al. Association between exposure to low to moderate arsenic levels and incident cardiovascular disease. A prospective cohort study. *Ann Intern Med.* 2013;159(10):649–59.
35. Tellez-Plaza M, Guallar E, Howard BV, Navas-Acien A. Cadmium and cardiovascular risk. *Epidemiology.* 2013;24(5):784–5.
36. Fairbairn AS, Reid DD. Air pollution and other local factors in respiratory disease. *Br J Prev Soc Med.* 1958;12(2):94–103.
37. Logan WP. Mortality in the London fog incident, 1952. *Lancet.* 1953;1(6755):336–8.
38. Prevention CfDCa. National Report on Human Exposure to Environmental Chemicals, Updated Tables, January 2019. 2017; Prevention of Childhood Lead Toxicity | From the American ... Accessed October 8, 2019.
39. Dockery DW, Pope CA, 3rd, Xu X, et al. An association between air pollution and mortality in six U.S. cities. *N Engl J Med.* 1993;329(24):1753–9.
40. Kaufman JD, Adar SD, Allen RW, et al. Prospective study of particulate air pollution exposures, subclinical atherosclerosis, and clinical cardiovascular disease: The multi-ethnic study of atherosclerosis and air pollution (MESA Air). *Am J Epidemiol.* 2012;176(9):825–37.
41. Di Q, Wang Y, Zanobetti A, et al. Air pollution and mortality in the medicare population. *N Engl J Med.* 2017;376(26):2513–22.
42. Humble CG, Samet JM. Smoking and lung cancer in New Mexico. *Am J Public Health.* 1986;76(11):1361.
43. Michaud DS, De Vivo I, Morris JS, Giovannucci E. Toenail selenium concentrations and bladder cancer risk in women and men. *Br J Cancer.* 2005;93(7):804–6.
44. Wynder EL, Graham EA. Tobacco smoking as a possible etiologic factor in bronchiogenic carcinoma; a study of 684 proved cases. *J Am Med Assoc.* 1950;143(4):329–36.
45. Levin ML, Goldstein H, Gerhardt PR. Cancer and tobacco smoking; a preliminary report. *J Am Med Assoc.* 1950;143(4):336–8.
46. Doll R, Hill AB. Smoking and carcinoma of the lung; preliminary report. *Br Med J.* 1950;2(4682):739–48.
47. Jaakkola JJK, Piipari R, Jaakkola MS. Occupation and asthma: A population-based incident case-control study. *Am J Epidemiol.* 2003;158(10):981–7.
48. Prentice RL. A case-cohort design for epidemiologic cohort studies and disease prevention trials. *Biometrika.* 1986;73(1):1–11.
49. Chen C, Xun P, Tsinovoi C, et al. Urinary cadmium concentration and the risk of ischemic stroke. *Neurology.* 2018;91(4):e382–91.
50. Adams SV, Shafer MM, Bonner MR, et al. Urinary cadmium and risk of invasive breast cancer in the women's health initiative. *Am J Epidemiol.* 2016;183(9):815–23.
51. Ernster VL. Nested case-control studies. *Prev Med.* 1994;23(5):587–90.
52. Wolf K, Bongaerts BWC, Schneider A, et al. Persistent organic pollutants and the incidence of type 2 diabetes in the CARLA and KORA cohort studies. *Environ Int.* 2019;129:221–8.
53. Mittleman MA, Maclure M, Robins JM. Control sampling strategies for case-crossover studies: An assessment of relative efficiency. *Am J Epidemiol.* 1995;142(1):91–8.
54. Levy D, Lumley T, Sheppard L, Kaufman J, Checkoway H. Referent selection in case-crossover analyses of acute health effects of air pollution. *Epidemiology.* 2001;12(2):186–92.

55. Peters A, von Klot S, Heier M, et al. Exposure to traffic and the onset of myocardial infarction. *N Engl J Med.* 2004;351(17):1721–30.
56. Peng RD, Butz AM, Hackstadt AJ, et al. Estimating the health benefit of reducing indoor air pollution in a randomized environmental intervention. *J R Stat Soc Ser A Stat Soc.* 2015;178(2):425–43.
57. Smith KR, McCracken JP, Weber MW, et al. Effect of reduction in household air pollution on childhood pneumonia in Guatemala (RESPIRE): A randomised controlled trial. *Lancet.* 2011;378(9804):1717–26.
58. Thomas ED, Gittelsohn J, Yracheta J, et al. The strong heart water study: Informing and designing a multi-level intervention to reduce arsenic exposure among private well users in Great Plains Indian Nations. *Sci Total Environ.* 2019;650(Pt 2):3120–33.
59. Lamas GA, Goertz C, Boineau R, et al. Effect of disodium EDTA chelation regimen on cardiovascular events in patients with previous myocardial infarction: The TACT randomized trial. *JAMA.* 2013;309(12):1241–50.
60. Lamas GA, Navas-Acien A, Mark DB, Lee KL. Heavy metals, cardiovascular disease, and the unexpected benefits of chelation therapy. *J Am Coll Cardiol.* 2016;67(20):2411–8.
61. Matsui EC, Perzanowski M, Peng RD, et al. Effect of an integrated pest management intervention on asthma symptoms among mouse-sensitized children and adolescents with asthma: A randomized clinical trial. *JAMA.* 2017;317(10):1027–36.
62. Gamble MV, Liu X, Slavkovich V, et al. Folic acid supplementation lowers blood arsenic. *Am J Clin Nutr.* 2007;86(4):1202–9.
63. Hernandez-Avila M, Gonzalez-Cossio T, Hernandez-Avila JE, et al. Dietary calcium supplements to lower blood lead levels in lactating women: A randomized placebo-controlled trial. *Epidemiology.* 2003;14(2):206–12.
64. Oreskes N, Conway EM. *Merchants of Doubt: How a Handful of Scientists Obscured the Truth on Issues from Tobacco Smoke to Global Warming.* New York: Bloomsbury Press; 2011.
65. Proctor R. *Golden Holocaust: Origins of the Cigarette Catastrophe and the Case for Abolition.* Berkeley, CA: University of California Press; 2012.
66. Heederik D, Attfield M. Characterization of dust exposure for the study of chronic occupational lung disease: A comparison of different exposure assessment strategies. *Am J Epidemiol.* 2000;151(10):982–90.
67. Wild CP. The exposome: From concept to utility. *Int J Epidemiol.* 2012;41(1):24–32.
68. Castranova V, Vallyathan V. Silicosis and coal workers' pneumoconiosis. *Environ Health Perspect.* 2000;108(suppl 4):675–84.
69. Veiga MM, Angeloci-Santos G, Meech JA. Review of barriers to reduce mercury use in artisanal gold mining. *Extract Ind Soc.* 2014;1(2):351–61.
70. Caravanos J, Clark E, Fuller R, Lambertson C. Assessing worker and environmental chemical exposure risks at an e-waste recycling and disposal site in Accra, Ghana. *J Health Pollut.* 2011;1(1):16–25.
71. Magauzi R, Mabaera B, Rusakaniko S, et al. Health effects of agrochemicals among farm workers in commercial farms of Kwekwe district, Zimbabwe. *Pan Afr Med J.* 2011;9:26.
72. Valcke M, Levasseur M-E, Soares da Silva A, Wesseling C. Pesticide exposures and chronic kidney disease of unknown etiology: An epidemiologic review. *Environ Health.* 2017;16(1):49.
73. Kirkeleit J, Riise T, Bjørge T, Christiani DC. The healthy worker effect in cancer incidence studies. *Am J Epidemiol.* 2013;177(11):1218–24.
74. Steenland K, Deddens J, Salvan A, Stayner L. Negative bias in exposure-response trends in occupational studies: Modeling the healthy worker survivor effect. *Am J Epidemiol.* 1996;143(2):202–10.
75. Hertz-Picciotto I, Arrighi HM, Hu SW. Does arsenic exposure increase the risk for circulatory disease? *Am J Epidemiol.* 2000;151(2):174–81.
76. Arrighi HM, Hertz-Picciotto I. The evolving concept of the healthy worker survivor effect. *Epidemiology.* 1994;5(2):189–96.
77. Kwok Richard K, Engel Lawrence S, Miller Aubrey K, et al. The GuLF STUDY: A prospective study of persons involved in the deepwater horizon oil spill response and clean-up. *Environ Health Perspect.* 2017;125(4):570–8.
78. Agricultural Health Study. 2019 Study Update. 2019. https://aghealth.nih.gov/news/2019.html. Accessed December 16, 2019.
79. National Cancer Institute, Division of Cancer Epidemiology & Genetics. Exposure Assessment Using Job Exposure Matrices. 2019. https://dceg.cancer.gov/research/how-we-study/exposure-assessment/job-exposure-matrices. Accessed December 16, 2019.
80. Wang R, Zhang Y, Lan Q, et al. Occupational exposure to solvents and risk of non-Hodgkin lymphoma in Connecticut women. *Am J Epidemiol.* 2009;169(2):176–85.
81. Navas-Acien A, Pollan M, Gustavsson P, Plato N. Occupation, exposure to chemicals and risk of gliomas and meningiomas in Sweden. *Am J Ind Med.* 2002;42(3):214–27.
82. Lope V, Perez-Gomez B, Aragones N, et al. Occupational exposure to chemicals and risk of thyroid cancer in Sweden. *Int Arch Occup Environ Health.* 2009;82(2):267–74.
83. Cullinan P. Occupation and chronic obstructive pulmonary disease (COPD). *Br Med Bull.* 2012;104(1):143–61.
84. McMichael AJ. Standardized mortality ratios and the "healthy worker effect": Scratching beneath the surface. *J Occup Med.* 1976;18(3):165–8.
85. Picciotto S, Hertz-Picciotto I. Commentary: Healthy worker survivor bias: A still-evolving concept. *Epidemiology.* 2015;26(2):213–15.
86. Buckley JP, Keil AP, McGrath LJ, Edwards JK. Evolving methods for inference in the presence of healthy worker survivor bias. *Epidemiology.* 2015;26(2):204–12.
87. Pell JP, Haw S, Cobbe S, et al. Smoke-free legislation and hospitalizations for acute coronary syndrome. *N Engl J Med.* 2008;359(5):482–91.
88. Jones MR, Barnoya J, Stranges S, Losonczy L, Navas-Acien A. Cardiovascular events following smoke-free legislations: An updated systematic review and meta-analysis. *Curr Environ Health Rep.* 2014;1(3):239–49.
89. Been JV, Nurmatov UB, Cox B, Nawrot TS, Van Schayck CP, Sheikh A. Effect of smoke-free legislation on perinatal and child health: A systematic review and meta-analysis. *Lancet.* 2014;383(9928):1549–60.
90. Centers for Disease Control and Prevention. Vital signs: Disparities in Nonsmokers' Exposure to Secondhand Smoke—United States, 1999–2012. *MMWR Morb Mortal Wkly Rep.* 2015;64(04):103–8. http://www.cdc.gov/mmwr/preview/mmwrhtml/mm6404a7.htm. Accessed July 29, 2016.
91. Rich DQ, Kipen HM, Huang W, et al. Association between changes in air pollution levels during the Beijing Olympics and biomarkers of inflammation and thrombosis in healthy young adults. *JAMA.* 2012;307(19):2068–78.
92. Rich DQ, Liu K, Zhang J, et al. Differences in birth weight associated with the 2008 Beijing Olympics air pollution reduction: Results from a natural experiment. *Environ Health Perspect.* 2015;123(9):880–7.
93. HEI Accountability Workgroup. *Assessing Health Impact of Air Quality Regulations: Concepts and Methods for Accountability Research. Communication 11.* Boston, MA: Health Effects Institute; 2003.
94. Morgenstern H, Thomas D. Principles of study design in environmental epidemiology. *Environ Health Perspect.* 1993;101 Suppl 4:23–38.
95. Moscoe E, Bor J, Barnighausen T. Regression discontinuity designs are underutilized in medicine, epidemiology, and public health: A review of current and best practice. *J Clin Epidemiol.* 2015;68(2):122–33.
96. Bor J, Moscoe E, Mutevedzi P, Newell ML, Barnighausen T. Regression discontinuity designs in epidemiology: Causal inference without randomized trials. *Epidemiology.* 2014;25(5):729–37.
97. Fletcher JM, Conley D. The challenge of causal inference in gene-environment interaction research: Leveraging research designs from the social sciences. *Am J Public Health.* 2013;103 Suppl 1:S42–5.
98. Columbia University Mailman School of Public Health. Difference-in-Difference Estimation. *Population Health Methods.* https://www.mailman.columbia.edu/research/population-health-methods/difference-difference-estimation. Accessed December 30, 2019.
99. Wing C, Simon K, Bello-Gomez RA. Designing difference in difference studies: Best practices for public health policy research. *Annu Rev Public Health.* 2018;39:453–69.
100. Chen H, Li Q, Kaufman JS, et al. Effect of air quality alerts on human health: A regression discontinuity analysis in Toronto, Canada. *Lancet Planet Health.* 2018;2(1):e19–26.
101. Chen Y, Ebenstein A, Greenstone M, Li H. Evidence on the impact of sustained exposure to air pollution on life expectancy from China's Huai River policy. *Proc Natl Acad Sci U S A.* 2013;110(32):12936–41.
102. Bakolis I, Kelly R, Fecht D, et al. Protective effects of smoke-free legislation on birth outcomes in England: A regression discontinuity design. *Epidemiology.* 2016;27(6):810–8.

CHAPTER

66

Participatory Research for Environmental Justice: Advancements in Community Science and Innovation

Christopher D. Heaney • Sacoby M. Wilson

INTRODUCTION

Low-income communities and communities of color living proximal to and at the fence line of legacy and ongoing hazards and industrial activities—including industrial food animal production (IFAP), fossil fuels-related industry, waste management, raw materials manufacturing, and goods movement—face a disproportionate burden of exposure to toxicants and other hazardous pollutants. Other large populations, primarily with low incomes and of color, also endure an inequitable burden of environmental exposures sustained because of where they are located. In urban areas, low-income residents and people of color typically live closer to industrial facilities, contaminated sites, and heavily trafficked roads than those who are white and with higher incomes.[1–7]

While the pollutants and their sources can be varied and complex, fence-line, and front-line communities and those living with higher levels of exposure to pollution share common concerns about whether and how such pollution is affecting their environment, and their health and well-being. They may look widely to find answers to their questions about risks they face and seek collaboration with researchers at agencies and in academia. Residents of these communities challenge environmental and public health scientists to conduct rigorous research that addresses the concerns that they identify as a result of their own grassroots observations about environmental conditions where they live, work, and play.[8–27] This chapter addresses the various types of community-engaged research that arise from partnerships between communities and researchers and where they fall along a continuum of community participation. Numerous academic researchers have engaged in participatory research that has been highly effective in enhancing the capacity and elevating the role of communities to become valid purveyors of new scientific knowledge that helps them to enhance health in their communities. Such findings from communities can advance environmental justice and strengthen the rationale for advancing community-engaged investigation.

New tools and approaches are also empowering communities to undertake their own investigations, often labeled as "citizen science." For example, low-cost monitors for air pollution can be used by community members to characterize pollutant concentrations at scales that are relevant to citizen concerns.

Throughout this chapter, we define community as an association of people, schools, religious and other organizations who share common interests, perspectives, and values to engage in joint action to reduce environmental exposure and health burdens. The U.S. Environmental Protection Agency (U.S. EPA) defines environmental justice as, "the fair treatment and meaningful involvement of all people regardless of race, color, national origin or income with respect to the development, implementation and enforcement of environmental laws, regulations, and policies."[28]

Herein, we aim to provide an overview of the principles and approaches that inform different incarnations of participatory research for environmental justice, demonstrate where they fall along a continuum, highlight a case example that demonstrates how the principles and approaches were applied to achieve community-driven policy change and actions to advance environmental justice, and close with an overview of best practices that can help to avoid threats to objectivity and validity that may arise when the disproportionately exposed communities meaningfully participate in every phase of the research process—from conception, design, measurement, interpretation, and environmental justice action.

PARTICIPATORY RESEARCH FOR ENVIRONMENTAL JUSTICE

Much participatory research related to the environment originates from concerns about inequitable exposures with unacceptable risks. Participatory research for environmental justice involves a combination of principles and approaches. Most successful examples of participatory research for environmental justice involve a sustained commitment of technical experts across multiple disciplines—for example, environmental health, toxicology, epidemiology, medicine, ecology, sociology, anthropology, social work, popular education, law, policy, civic engagement, and advocacy—collectively prioritizing the interests, norms, values, and organizing efforts of disproportionately exposed communities that seek reforms, solutions, and long-term positive impacts on self-determination, health, welfare, and quality of life (Fig. 66-1).[29–31] This approach requires a re-orientation of the norms, customs, values, and interests of traditional academic science to align with the norms, customs, values, and interests of communities who are most affected by historical and ongoing patterns of industrial pollution and who seek mitigation of exposures. Such alignment helps hone research questions around filling the most locally relevant knowledge gaps that once known and addressed, would advance community efforts to achieve structural change, environmental justice, and public health (Fig. 66-1).

Low-income communities and communities of color have emphasized the need to participate meaningfully and equitably when scientists are planning to conduct research such that its outputs and outcomes will improve understanding of how pollutants from diverse and often clustered industries affect their individual and community health and contribute to environmental health disparities.[9,14,25,27,29] Such participatory research encourages multidirectional communication on the part of environmental health scientists, biomedical researchers, and other technical experts to improve understanding of the community's concerns, which have been informed by cultural and contextual knowledge about environmental exposure and health burdens. It also encourages scientists to learn how modification of approaches used for more typical hypothesis-driven population-based

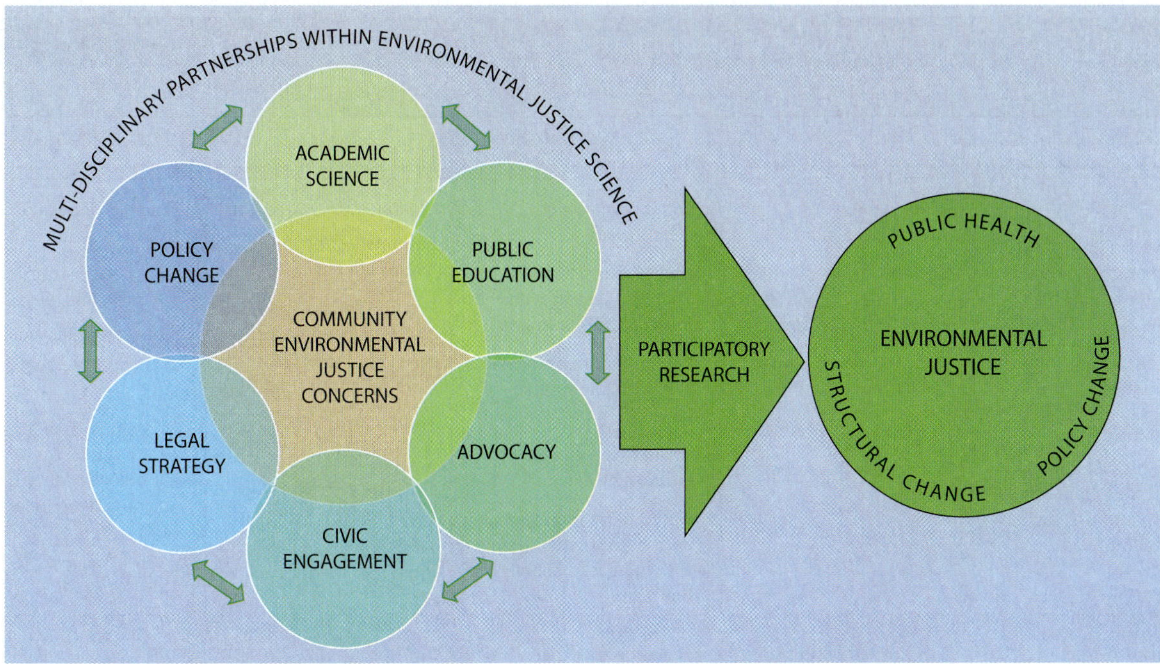

FIGURE 66-1. Conceptual framework showing how community environmental justice concerns drive technical partners' contributions across multiple disciplines to advance participatory research for structural and policy change, environmental justice, and public health.

and biomedical research can produce responsive, innovative, and impactful solutions to community-identified environmental health and well-being needs.[31] When done effectively, participatory research that addresses environmental justice concerns generates rigorous evidence to address community concerns and to counter industries' efforts to obfuscate and cast doubt about long-standing patterns of disproportionate exposure and health burdens within specific neighborhoods and populations.

Continuum of Participatory Research Principles and Approaches

In participatory research, one size does not fit all communities. Academic and community partners each possess different strengths, opportunities, and capacities, share different norms, values, and motivations, and face different pressures. Consequently, there is a range of different styles of participatory research, summarized by the Department of Health and Human Services (DHHS) as a community engagement continuum as presented in Fig. 66-2.[32] This concept of a continuum shows (from left to right) an increasing level of community involvement, impact, trust, and communication flow. Community engaged research is an umbrella term that encompasses a number of different forms of participatory research. The community engagement continuum shows that partnerships may vary from little interaction among communities and researchers to partnerships characterized by shared power, bidirectional communication, and trust.

We summarize several incarnations of participatory research in Fig. 66-3. These include community-based / placed research, community-based participatory research (CBPR), community-driven research (CDR), and community-owned and managed research (COMR). Our participatory research continuum shows (from left to right) increasing community participation, decision-making authority, power, and control over project leadership, budgeting, and accountability and reporting obligations. Definitions of each are provided below.

Community-Based/Placed Research

Community-based/placed research can involve little to no or some community input. Such research tends to involve an academic investigator prespecifying a research question designed to fill a scientific knowledge gap and that academic investigator needing to identify a community population within which to conduct a study. On the DHHS community engagement continuum, such a community-based/placed research project would fall to the left of, under "Outreach," or under "Consult" depending on the level of community input.[32] On one extreme, the process may involve a one-way flow of information and scientific inquiry directed by an academic principal investigator (PI) who seeks sufficient community input to carry out a prespecified research question. However, other forms of community-based/placed research can involve meaningful and iterative community input, by consulting community representatives or leaders or establishment of community advisory boards.

Community-Based Participatory Research

CBPR is defined by Israel et al. (2013)[33] as, "...a collaborative approach to research that equitably involves, for example, community members, organizational representatives, and researchers in all aspects of the research process. The partners contribute 'unique strengths and shared responsibilities'...to enhance understanding of a given phenomenon and the social and cultural dynamics of the community, and integrate the knowledge gained with action to improve the health and well-being of community members."

The core principles of CBPR further identified by Israel et al. (2018)[33] as, "1. Recognizing the community as a unit of identity; 2. Building on strengths and resources within the community; 3. Facilitating collaborative partnerships in all phases of the research; 4. Integrating knowledge and action for mutual benefit of all partners; 5. Promoting a co-learning and empowering process that attends to social inequalities; 6. Involving a cyclical and iterative process; 7. Addressing health from both positive and ecological perspectives; and 8. Disseminating findings and knowledge gained to all partners." Within Fig. 66-2, CBPR falls within the "Collaborate" and "Shared Leadership" sections of the continuum.

Community-Driven Research

CDR is characterized by shifting of power and decision-making authority away from academic investigators toward the community. Some forms—for example, the subsequent section on COMR—shift power entirely into the hands of community organizations to drive

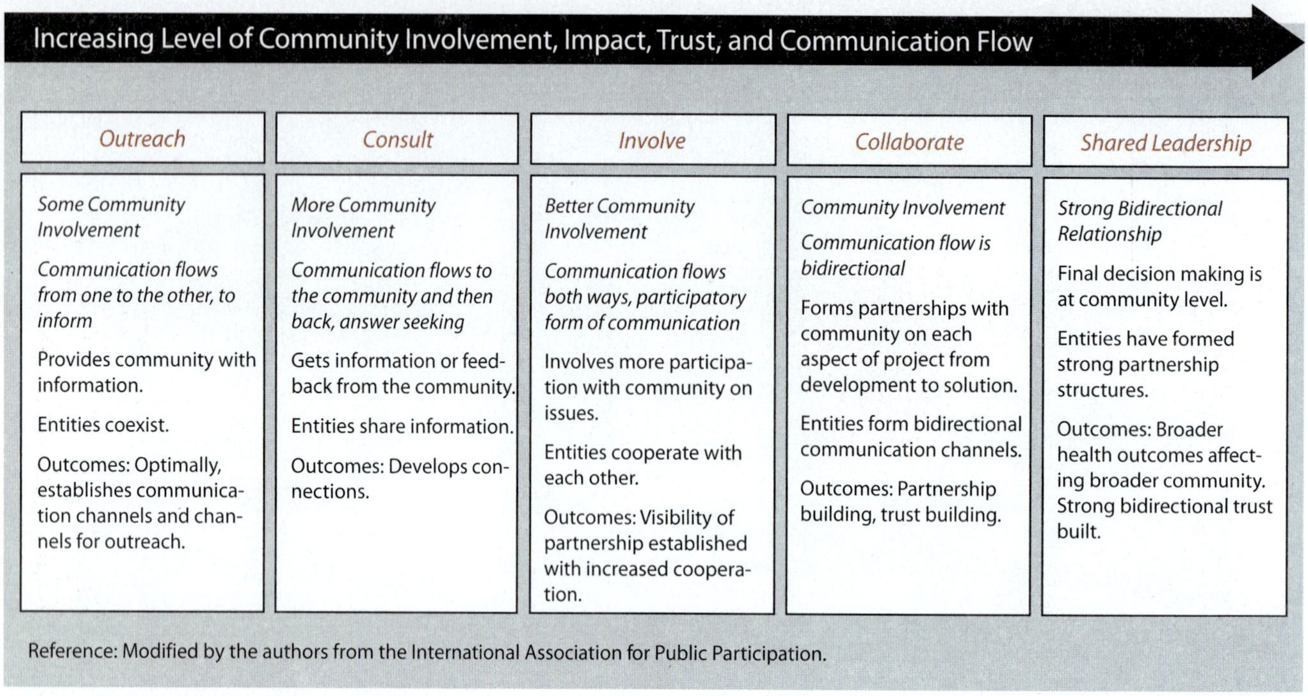

Increasing Level of Community Involvement, Impact, Trust, and Communication Flow

Outreach	*Consult*	*Involve*	*Collaborate*	*Shared Leadership*
Some Community Involvement *Communication flows from one to the other, to inform* Provides community with information. Entities coexist. Outcomes: Optimally, establishes communication channels and channels for outreach.	*More Community Involvement* *Communication flows to the community and then back, answer seeking* Gets information or feedback from the community. Entities share information. Outcomes: Develops connections.	*Better Community Involvement* *Communication flows both ways, participatory form of communication* Involves more participation with community on issues. Entities cooperate with each other. Outcomes: Visibility of partnership established with increased cooperation.	*Community Involvement* *Communication flow is bidirectional* Forms partnerships with community on each aspect of project from development to solution. Entities form bidirectional communication channels. Outcomes: Partnership building, trust building.	*Strong Bidirectional Relationship* Final decision making is at community level. Entities have formed strong partnership structures. Outcomes: Broader health outcomes affecting broader community. Strong bidirectional trust built.

Reference: Modified by the authors from the International Association for Public Participation.

FIGURE 66-2. Community-engagement continuum. (*Source:* From Principles of Community Engagement. 2011. Clinical and Translational Science Awards Consortium, Community Engagement Key Function Committee Task Force on the Principles of Community Engagement. 2011. Agency for Toxic Substances and Disease Registry, U.S. Centers for Disease Control and Prevention. https://www.atsdr.cdc.gov/communityengagement/pdf/PCE_Report_508_FINAL.pdf.)

all aspects of the research. Examples of CDR include the work of Dr. Steve Wing, who spent his life and career working in partnership with low-income communities and communities of color living at the fence line of diverse industries, including IFAP, municipal waste, and oil and gas production.[8,10–13,16,18,19,21,22,25,27,34–36]

Community-Owned and Managed Research

In response to some communities' exploitative and extractive experiences working with academic scientists purporting to conduct community-based research and CBPR, a new orientation of principles was created, called COMR.[37–40] COMR is farther along the CER continuum because it elevates the community to a higher level of power, management, and decision-making authority than CBPR. Within COMR, a community leader rather than an academic researcher serves as the PI of the project, the community decides which technical experts to hire and / or consult with, and research is conducted in ways that are aligned to advance their priorities for local, grassroots research. Principles of COMR will be further expanded upon in the Case Example below.

Community/Citizen Science

In its 2016 report NACEPT describes citizen science as a process in which: "the public participates voluntarily in the scientific process, addressing real-world problems in ways that may include formulating research questions, conducting scientific experiments, collecting and analyzing data, interpreting results, making new discoveries, developing technologies and applications, and solving complex problems."[41] Citizen science is a democratized extension of the participatory and community-engaged research principles and approaches described above that increase the public's access to science and scientific tools for measurement, inquiry, and applied action (Figs. 66-2 and 66-3). In terms of the continuum of participatory research and community-engagement (Figs. 66-2 and 66-3), citizen science has been described as a democratization of science, which may or may not involve partnerships or participation of professionally trained scientists or scientific institutions.[41] Community/citizen science can advance the field of participatory research for environmental justice in several ways. For example, advancements in low-cost sensors to measure air, water, and soil/sediment quality can support broader participation in science and greater access to locally relevant exposure data, at high-dimensional scales of observation. When integrated with mobile device crowd-sourcing apps such sensor networks can allow individuals and community groups to monitor pollution sources and track pollution levels in near-real time.[42] Some examples of the successful integration of these concepts include the Imperial County Community Air Monitoring Network,[43–47] the University of Southern California's Community Engagement and Outreach Core's work on low-cost air sensors, [48,49] and the Charleston Area Pollution Prevention Partnership led by the Low-Country Alliance for Model Communities.[50–52] Applying data science principles to such high-dimensional low-cost sensor and crowd sourcing data can reveal previously obscured evidence of disproportionate impacts at individual, household, neighborhood, and community scales along the fence-line and front-line of diverse hazards and industries.

PARTICIPATORY RESEARCH VIGNETTES

The following are questions to consider in approaching each vignette: (1) Where does each fall along the community engagement continuum? (2) Which participatory research principles are involved and how do they apply? and (3) How do they inform your conclusion about where the example falls along the community engagement continuum?

VIGNETTE 1

While attending a conference to learn more about health topic X, an executive director of a local community-based organization (CBO) meets a university professor with expertise relevant to the community's struggles to address health topic X. A week after the conference, the professor visits the community and meets with the executive director, CBO staff, and members of the community to learn more about the problem and discuss what the community sees as strategies to address health problem X. Several months go by until one day the executive director receives a call from the professor who says, "I have

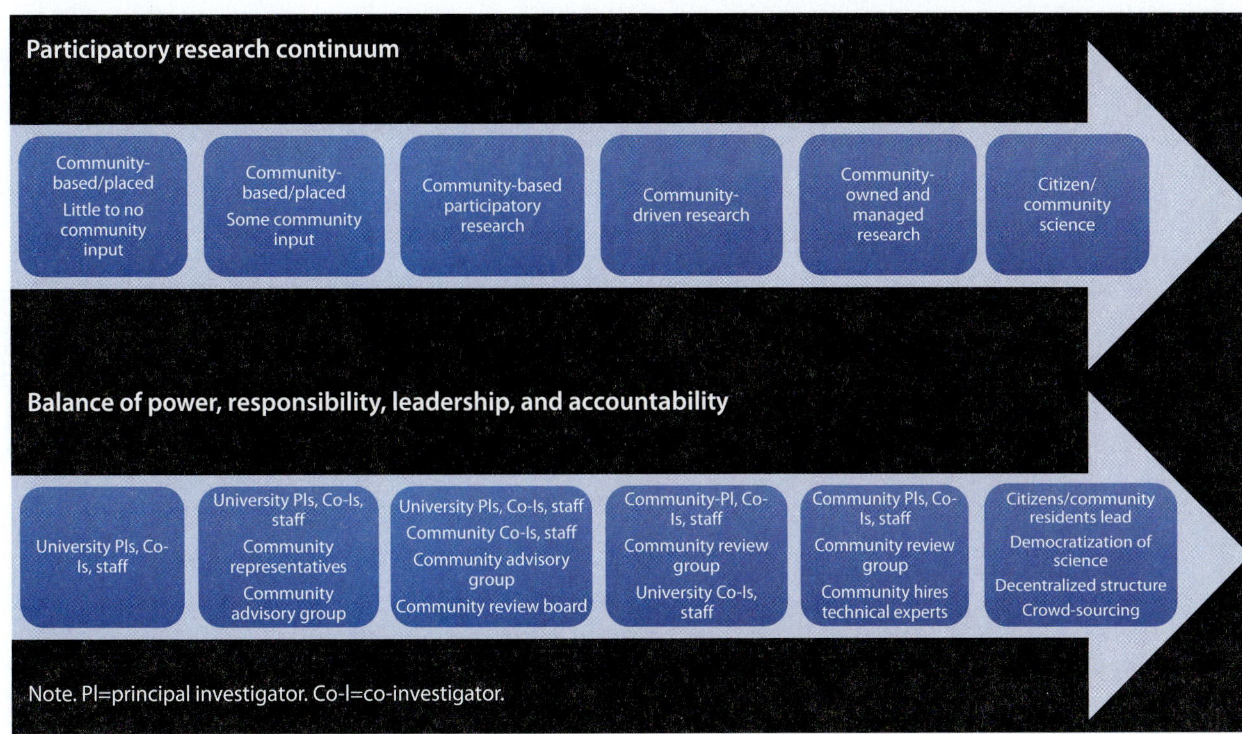

FIGURE 66-3. Participatory research continuum, showing (from left to right) increased community participation, decision-making authority, power, and control over research leadership, budgeting, reporting, dissemination, and policy mobilization actions.

wonderful news, our Center just received a $5 million grant to study the problem we discussed in your community related to health topic X. To get started with the grant we would like you to help us identify a community representative to work with us on the project. For the period of the project we will pay the community representative a full-time salary and benefits. We would also like to get more information about your experiences with health problem X since we last spoke."

VIGNETTE 2

A university research Center supports a community advisory group (CAG), consisting of one Center administrator and the leaders of several local CBOs. CAG members serve for distinct terms and some have served multiple terms since the establishment of the Center. CAG members are paid as part-time university contractors for the time they commit to CAG activities. CAG members are consulted regularly about research directions of the Center and are asked to review a diverse number of research proposals to internal and external funding agencies. All proposals that the CAG reviews have PIs and other investigators who are university faculty. Feedback provided by the CAG is used to make modifications to proposals before submission and the CAG is frequently listed as part of a proposal's "Approach" section as an example of how the PI will seek iterative community input and involvement in the research project. Several successful grants have been funded through this process and some have resulted in subcontracts to the CBOs of CAG members to assist with participant enrollment and data collection. For these subcontracts, the CBO retains the decision-making power to hire community research assistants and staff to work full time with benefits for the CBO for the period of the grant's subcontract.

VIGNETTE 3

A university professor has served on the board of directors of a local CBO for one term. Her research interests overlap with the mission and vision of the CBO and at a regular board meetings she shares a request for proposals (RFPs) for improving health outcomes in the area of their overlapping interests. The RFP does not require inclusion of a named community partner, but she proposes that they all work together and with affected community members to develop research questions, design a study, and submit a proposal. The board and executive director agree to write a letter of support to be included in the proposal. The university professor is listed as the PI and the executive director of the CBO is listed as a named Co-PI on the grant. The budget includes a subcontract to the CBO with salary support for the executive director, one full-time administrative staff position, two community research assistant staff positions, and 20% overhead. The grant is scored in the highest percentile but the team is notified that they need to cut 20% from the budget to be funded. The team gather to discuss how to respond. They achieve consensus to distribute the 20% cut evenly across the university and CBO-subcontract budgets and they are subsequently funded to start the research.

VIGNETTE 4

A CBO has a long history of working on health and social disparities problems in the local community. The CBO's executive director and board members all grew up in the affected community. Often the CBO has sought input and assistance from a number of technical experts and professionals at local universities, government agencies, law firms, and social services organizations. Over the years, the CBO and its community members have fostered trusting and mutually beneficial relationships with several of these professionals. One day the CBO receives an email through a listserv about a new government agency grants program that requires that funding for a proposed project go directly to the local CBO. The local CBO reaches out to several professionals with whom they have worked over the years and develop research questions, design a study, and submit a proposal. The executive director is the named PI of the grant and members of the board of directors are named as coinvestigators on the grant. Several technical experts and professionals are included on the grant as part-time paid consultants (without benefits) and others are listed as unpaid consultants who agree to implement specific technical aspects of the project. All listed technical experts and professionals write letters of support that are included in the proposal. The grant is funded and the CBO, as the leader of the team, starts the project, seeking input of team members as needed.

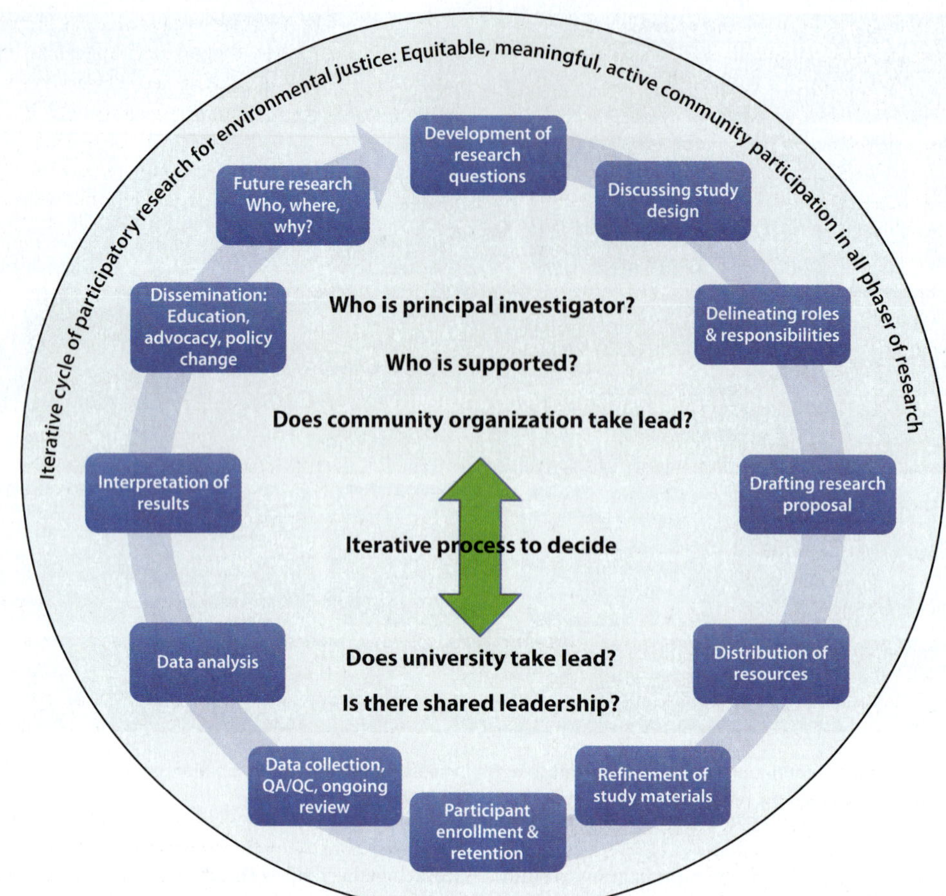

FIGURE 66-4. Participatory research for environmental justice science that involves cyclical iteration and equitable, meaningful, and active community participation in all phases of research.

Additional Discussion Questions after Reviewing Vignettes

Each of these vignettes raises important questions that need to be broached openly and equitably with community partners. Having reviewed the vignette, consider the following: What was missing from each scenario to determine whether it is an example of following best practices in participatory research? What happens after funding is obtained? How committed are academic partners to helping community partners sustain their operations after a grant? The long-term commitment of academics to partner with communities—often referred to as the "what next" after a funded grant period ends—is a critical determinant of the successful outcomes of participatory research. The sustainability or longevity of a partnership depends on the level of commitment of academics not only to the research, but also to nonresearch contributions to community efforts to build popular movements and educate the public to improve living and working conditions. This aspect of participatory projects can be one of the most challenging and time-consuming parts of the process. The degree of success is shaped in part by how academics and community partners: (a) work together to complete a project; (b) adapt to change—particularly changes in resources/funding; (c) disseminate findings, including interpret unexpected findings and remain faithful to/consistent with educational messaging about what the scientific evidence shows; and (d) maintain momentum for subsequent projects (both research and nonresearch).

CASE STUDY OF ENVIRONMENTAL INJUSTICE

Next, we present one case study that serves as an example of the application of COMR principles. This example provides additional context about a model that is farther along the continuum toward a higher level of community control and management of the participatory research process (see Figs. 66-2–66-4). COMR has led to successful advances and support of community efforts to achieve environmental justice.

The West End Revitalization Association (WERA) and Lack of Basic Amenities

Black residents in Mebane, North Carolina have been fighting against environmental racism for multiple decades. In 1994, residents of Mebane, North Carolina established the WERA to address the negative impacts of a proposed highway expansion.[37–40] The planned expansion of the 119 bypass would destroy several historic neighborhoods that are overwhelmingly African-American and in which most residents make less than $20,000 per year.[37–40] These neighborhoods were already differentially burdened by several environmental hazards including a sewage treatment plant, leaking underground storage tanks, brownfields, and a hazardous waste site.[37–40] In the case of the sewage treatment plant, sewer lines ran through one of the WERA neighborhoods, but residents were not connected to the lines even though they hosted the town's sewage treatment plant and were exposed to odorous compounds released from the facility on a daily basis.[37–40]

These neighborhoods were established after slavery and because of the racism that was part of the post-Reconstruction South and the Jim Crow South, development occurred that excluded these historic neighborhoods from basic amenities (e.g., publicly regulated sewer and water services, paved roads, good housing stock, and access to emergency services).[37–40] Some WERA neighborhoods are also under Mebane's extraterritorial jurisdiction, which gives the city land use decision-making authority without community input, even though they fall outside of Mebane's city limits.[37–40] Additionally, growth occurred that excluded these neighborhoods from being fully incorporated as part of the town. Since these neighborhoods are unincorporated, they do not have a town mayor or local council representative and consequently face further marginalization due to a lack of political power and voice in decision-making about zoning, planning, and community development activities.[37–40] This lack of power, representation, and voice in decision-making acts as a driver of environmental racism.

To address this environmental racism, WERA filed an administrative complaint.[37–40] In 1998, WERA and residents filed a complaint to the Civil Rights Office of the Federal Highway Administration (FHWA) as a result of racial harassment and intimidation by the North Carolina Department of Transportation (NCDOT).[37–40] In 1999, WERA also filed complaints under Title VI of the Civil Rights Act of 1964 and the Environmental Justice Executive Order 12898 at the U.S. Department of Justice, regarding plans for the 119 bypass that would destroy West End and White Level communities.[39,53] These complaints included details on noncompliance with public participation laws by governmental officials, inequities in zoning and planning, and differential impacts of the planned bypass on African-American and low-income neighborhoods in Mebane. WERA became the first CBO to submit an administrative complaint citing the lack of basic amenities as an environmental justice issue and act of environmental racism.[39,53]

After the complaints were filed, WERA members received Klan threats from local officials. Omega Wilson recalls the racial harassment[39]:

> On April 13, 1999, WERA and African-American residents spoke out when the North Carolina Secretary of Transportation came to Mebane to promote the 119 bypass, without a mitigation plan for low-income and minority homeowners in the path of the proposed highway. I made public comments for the record keepers regarding WERA's recent formal complaints at the United States Department of Justice. Mebane's mayor charged in the meeting room, screamed, and yelled at African American residents and frail senior citizens who opposed 119 bypass plans. A few days later, the Mebane city manager called me and stated: "I have six good friends and when I die and go to heaven you will be one of them." This is a Klan death threat that refers to six bullets in a pistol chamber for six "friends," used to intimidate people of color.

To achieve solutions to these environmental justice issues, WERA relied on relationships with local university researchers. These relationships failed to achieve resolution of the environmental justice concerns because the researchers were more focused on publications than on actually addressing and solving the community's issues. Moreover, communities were given no credit for or power over the findings that emerged from these studies.[38,39,53]

In response to the negative experience working with the researchers from the University of North Carolina, WERA developed the COMR framework, a community-driven citizen science framework.[38,39,53] COMR builds on the principles of CBPR by: (1) encouraging research partnerships with CBOs with the capacity to tackle an EJ issue; (2) requiring that CBOs be funded as PIs on a research issue; and (3) using research results to affect tangible change for communities.[38,39,53] By giving funding power to CBOs, COMR makes communities the principal decision-makers and experts in responding to environmental injustice concerns, with the ability to hire researchers as consultants and technical partners.[38,39,53] Furthermore, by using "science for compliance,"[37–40] COMR makes research actionable and focused on legal solutions under the Clean Air Act, Clean Water Act, Safe Drinking Water Act, Emergency Planning Community Right to Know Act (EPCRA), Superfund law, Civil Rights Act, housing laws, building codes, and public health statutes, a form of legal-based epidemiology.

In 2004, WERA pursued and received $100,000 in funding through EPA's Collaborative Problem-Solving (CPS) grant program, which makes CBOs that receive funding the project lead and primary grant recipient.[40] The CPS paradigm is meant to empower communities and build organizational capacity in a way more conventional funding initiative and community-university partnerships often fail to do.[40] Figure 66-2 illustrates the steps of the CPS model.

Under its CPS grant, WERA partnered with a new set of researchers from the University of North Carolina in the fields of environmental health, epidemiology, and regional planning including a core set of student researchers to study and address environmental health disparities associated with inequities in zoning, planning, and development and the lack of basic amenities.[37,38,40] WERA's research and management team designed projects in consultation with university researchers, who trained community members as citizen scientists to assess infrastructure and sample water from households on well water and households on public regulated water for fecal contamination.[37]

For instance, a survey was also developed for households to study indicators of septic system failure. Under this study, 48% of households reported issues with water quality, and 18% of households were found to have septic system failure. Of 94 water samples collected, 58 were tested for turbidity (i.e., cloudiness), which revealed higher levels of turbidity in water for private wells. Additionally, many private well samples tested positive for indicators of fecal contamination.[37] The results of this study showed a higher rate of septic system failure, and therefore a higher likelihood of exposure to fecal pollution, in households that rely on private drinking water wells, which are often found in lower income communities of color lacking access to publicly regulated and high-quality infrastructure.[37]

The results of COMR and the implementation of the CPS model allowed WERA to develop a quality assurance plan to monitor environmental issues and to advocate for improvements to local infrastructure by leveraging research findings.[37,38,40] WERA's CDR had a tremendous impact. It led to the first-time installation of sewer and water infrastructure for some residents, roads in these neighborhoods were paved for the first time, and the highway expansion project was delayed and eventually modified to preserve cultural assets including historic Black churches and cemeteries.

More recently, WERA has worked with state and federal officials, such as the head of the North Carolina Department of Environmental Quality (NCDEQ), through summits co hosted with the U.S. EPA and the North Carolina Environmental Justice Network (NCEJN) to advance an environmental justice agenda in the state of North Carolina. These events have provided a forum for impacted residents to engage with public officials and be part of the decision-making process on longstanding environmental justice concerns. WERA's efforts have contributed to the establishment of a new environmental justice commission in the state, which will provide recommendations on how state agencies can address environmental racism to the NCDEQ Director.

CONSIDERATIONS AND CHALLENGES IN CONDUCTING PARTICIPATORY RESEARCH FOR ENVIRONMENTAL JUSTICE

Low-income communities and communities of color with inequitable burdens of environmental exposures, whether from living at the fence-line adjacent to industry or from other place-based pollution sources, typically seek answers to causal research questions related to their concerns about whether disproportionate exposures have been occurring and what their impacts may be on their health. Examples of causal research questions are: "Is the water in my community safe to drink?," "Is the air in my community safe to breathe?," "What is an exposure study and how does it differ from a health study?," and "Does my community need a health study?"

As public health scientists endeavoring to develop participatory research that supports community struggles with questions of this nature, it is important to consider the following: What are public health scientists' roles, responsibilities, and capabilities to deliver answers to causal questions of community residents through a research study? How can they recognize, understand, and prepare in order to mitigate the range of potential biases and threats to objectivity and validity that can arise when communities participate meaningfully in the design and conduct of research? Although others have provided informative summaries of the trade-offs and concerns raised by these questions,[24,25,27,54–56] we outline five additional points on the topic of scientific objectivity and validity for public health scientists to consider as they absorb and begin to implement the principles and approaches of participatory research with communities.

Recognition of Academic Privilege

In order to build a foundation for effective participatory research to develop, it is critical for academics and technical experts to recognize the inherent *power and privilege* afforded by their positions within well-resourced scientific institutions whose scientific, technical, and administrative infrastructure and support are honed to respond to the priorities of hypercompetitive government, industry, and private foundation funders. Within this environment, academics cannot lose perspective about and must be sensitive to critical questions of equity raised by low-income communities and communities of color about why these resources, infrastructure, and support of academic institutions cannot similarly be leveraged to address their priorities and concerns of disproportionate exposure and adverse health effects. Pervasive pressures within academia to secure funding, publish, teach, perform academic service, and contribute to professional practice—which influence promotion, tenure, and job security—conflict with the time, effort, and relinquishment of power required for academics to build trust and develop long-term, sustainable participatory research partnerships with communities. Conflict can arise if these pressures influence the priorities of academic partners and they become introduced into the communications, decision-making, and power dynamics of a community participatory research partnership. Perspective must be maintained such that, regardless of the pressures, academics act to reverse the imbalance of privilege, power, and resources such that it can be leveraged to enhance the efforts of communities trying to reverse decades of structural environmental racism.[24,37,56] If scientists demonstrate awareness, sensitivity, and open communication about the inherent imbalances between the customs, norms, values, and structure of power and privilege within academia relative to fence-line communities, tension and conflict can be managed and mitigated—effective examples include Wing, 1998,[24] 2002,[25] and 2005,[56] and Scammell, 2019.[54]

Whose Agenda Drives the Questions That Are Prioritized?

A common critique of participatory research, particularly incarnations farther down the continuum toward involved, collaborative, and shared leadership (Fig. 66-2)—for example, CBPR, CDR, and COMR (Fig. 66-3)—is that the results and conclusions are inherently biased because the community residents most affected by an exposure or adverse health concern were prioritizing the questions to be asked, or even worse participating in data collection, analysis, and interpretation of results. Similar to the arguments of Wing, 1998[24] a critical examination is warranted as to who are the valid purveyors of new scientific knowledge? Participatory research challenges academic scientists to engage meaningfully with communities just as they would spend years cultivating relationships with government, industry, and private foundation funders, learn their customs, norms, values, and priorities, and position themselves to compete for an opportunity to produce valid and objective research responses to questions that address scientific knowledge gaps they have prioritized. If academics are willing to bring their considerable training, methodological expertise, skills, and technical infrastructure to bear for community rather than well-funded institutional interests why should the outputs and outcomes be any less valid or objective? Awareness of how the agendas of monied-institutions and funders shape the research questions that are prioritized versus those that do not can help counter industries' obfuscation of knowledge gaps about historical and ongoing patterns of exposure in specific places and among specific populations where few if any investigations may have been conducted—for example, fence-line communities seeking environmental justice. In these instances, a research question as simple as, "Is there evidence of exposure in my home, on my block, or in my neighborhood?" similar to a case report or case series can transform community understanding and mobilizing around mitigation efforts and solutions.

Transparency about Alignments and Conflicts of Interest

Once a researcher aligns around a research question that was prioritized through a participatory research approach with a community partner seeking to advance environmental justice, it is critical for to maintain transparency about how these relationships might be perceived as a conflict of interest given the shared goals, values, norms, and power structure that will drive decision-making about how the research will be conducted.[25] This applies the same, or a higher, standard to the management of relationships between an academic and a community partner as to an alignment, affiliation, relationship, or funding disclosure from government, industry, corporate, or foundation sponsors. Adherence to this high standard of transparency about alignments and conflicts of interest can require insistence depending on how broad scientific journals' policies are regarding when a declaration of a conflict of interest is required versus not. Given the history of industry and corporate efforts to hide alignments and funding relationships with academics[57]—some have involved claims of ghostwriting[58]—an adherence to the highest standards of transparency can put participatory research partnerships in a position of power by anticipating claims that community involvement in the research process could bias its outputs and outcomes.

Study Design and Methodology

"Absence of evidence is not evidence of absence"[59] is a well-recognized concept that has important implications for interpretation of scientific knowledge and transparency about null findings for clinical trials. This concept, popularized by, for example, Michaels, 2008,[60] serves as a powerful tool for polluting industries to limit public challenges to change their mode of operation by casting sufficient doubt given absence of evidence about disproportionate or adverse environmental exposure or health effects. This scenario creates challenges and opportunities within the context of participatory research for environmental justice. With no prior evidence for a specific home, block, or neighborhood often a pattern of exposure attributable to an industrial source of pollution can be captured through a case report or case series, where the research question is about whether there is indeed any evidence of exposure occurring in a given place at a given time. Similarly, a case series can be quite effective to reveal patterns of disease that may be related to industrial exposures.[61] The potential informativeness of these designs for community questions reverses a paradigm within the biomedical sciences that the highest weight of scientific evidence is achieved by employing a randomized controlled trial. This more pragmatic approach draws upon the weight of causal understanding achieved within ecological, geological, and other disciplines studying laws of nature that cannot employ randomization of exposure or treatment to advance knowledge. The repeated-measures panel study design and time-series designs represent powerful design strategies for community concerns that involve transient exposures and health outcomes. Within this design, the analysis of temporal relation between exposure and outcome measures allows each participant to serve as his / her own control, wherein the time-invariant characteristics of individual participants cannot confound the associations of interest. The design also eliminates common pitfalls of cross-sectional studies that aim to identify an elevated rate of exposure and/or disease in the partner community compare to some referent population.[62] The stochastic and transient nature of both exposure and outcome events mimics aspects of the quasiexperimental design which via exploitation of understanding of temporality has helped deliver causal evidence in support of community concerns related to the health effects of air pollution from industrial hog operations,[26,63] landfills,[9,14] and livestock-associated antimicrobial-resistant bacteria.[18,19,64] These provide examples of the methodological creativity that can be harnessed for studies that involve meaningful, active participation of community members most affected by exposure without compromising the rigor of the scientific conclusions.

Rationalization

As scientists committed to pursuit of participatory research with fence-line communities seeking environmental justice, the challenges to navigate the aforementioned academic pressures, high standards about what constitutes a conflict of interest, and goals to achieve methodological rigor in studies involving participation of communities most affected by exposure do not go away. This requires an understanding of how rationalization, as different decisions or situations are faced, may erode commitments to the foundational principles and approaches that can ensure that participatory research effectively advances community movements for environmental justice. This requires a deep level of awareness and self-criticism to avoid breakdowns in communication and power-sharing that can result from the persistent structure of academic incentives, rewards, and pressures.

CONCLUSIONS

Best Practices of Participatory Research for Environmental Justice

To achieve the right balance between community and academic power, responsibility, leadership and accountability most participatory research partnerships involve iterative, evolutionary processes with cyclical feedback loops that check and balance each partner's roles and responsibilities as the science unfolds from design, to implementation, interpretation, dissemination, and decisions about what research (if any) to pursue next (Fig. 66-4). This process can be time consuming, and may deter some academics whose career advancement goals and plans may conflict with the considerable investment of effort required to develop and build trust and mutual respect with communities and understanding about all stakeholders' roles, responsibilities, and priorities for decision-making. These trade-offs have produced diverse iterations of participatory research, which has been described using many terms that each reflect a different collection of principles and approaches along a continuum (Fig. 66-4).

Participatory research at its best seeks to advance cutting-edge and rigorous community science designed *with, by, and for* communities living at the fence line of diverse industries that are creating environmental injustice concerns. Among the principles highlighted in this chapter, those of open communication, trust, equity, power sharing, mutual accountability, and action, are critical to balance and tailor to achieve solutions within the context of each community-identified environmental injustice situation. The long-term goals of effective participatory research are to address these environmental injustice concerns, reduce and eliminate disproportionate and adverse exposure and disease burdens, and promote community self-determination, health, well-being, and quality of life. Realization of this goal requires a rebalancing of power, underpinned by community science, to compel those with the political connections and economic means to act in solidarity with fence-line environmental justice communities to mitigate the negative consequences of environmental hazards.

References

1. Mott L. The disproportionate impact of environmental health threats on children of color. *Environ Health Perspect.* 1995;103 Suppl 6:33–5.
2. Levy JI, Greco SL, Spengler JD. The importance of population susceptibility for air pollution risk assessment: A case study of power plants near Washington, DC. *Environ Health Perspect.* 2002;110(12):1253–60.
3. Morello-Frosch R, Pastor MJr, Porras C, Sadd J. Environmental justice and regional inequality in southern California: Implications for future research. *Environ Health Perspect.* 2002;110 Suppl 2:149–54.
4. Chakraborty J, Collins TW, Grineski SE, Montgomery MC, Hernandez M. Comparing disproportionate exposure to acute and chronic pollution risks: A case study in Houston, Texas. *Risk Anal.* 2014;34(11):2005–20.
5. Martenies SE, Milando CW, Williams GO, Batterman SA. Disease and health inequalities attributable to air pollutant exposure in Detroit, Michigan. *Int J Environ Res Public Health.* 2017;14(10):1243.
6. Ezeugoh RI, Puett R, Payne-Sturges D, Cruz-Cano R, Wilson SM. Air quality assessment of particulate matter near a concrete block plant and traffic in Bladensburg, Maryland. *Environ Justice.* 2020;13(3):75–85.
7. Shearston JA, Johnson AM, Domingo-Relloso A, et al. Opening a large delivery service warehouse in the South Bronx: Impacts on traffic, air pollution, and noise. *Int J Environ Res Public Health.* 2020;17(9):3208.
8. Avery RC, Wing S, Marshall SW, Schiffman SS. Odor from industrial hog farming operations and mucosal immune function in neighbors. *Arch Environ Health.* 2004;59(2):101–8.
9. Campbell RL, Caldwell D, Hopkins B, et al. Integrating research and community organizing to address water and sanitation concerns in a community bordering a landfill. *J Environ Health.* 2013;75(10):48–50.
10. Cole D, Todd L, Wing S. Concentrated swine feeding operations and public health: A review of occupational and community health effects. *Environ Health Perspect.* 2000;108(8):685–99.
11. Donham KJ, Wing S, Osterberg D, et al. Community health and socioeconomic issues surrounding concentrated animal feeding operations. *Environ Health Perspect.* 2007;115(2):317–20.
12. Guidry VT, Lowman A, Hall D, Baron D, Wing S. Challenges and benefits of conducting environmental justice research in a school setting. *New Solut.* 2014;24(2):153–70.
13. Heaney CD, Myers K, Wing S, Hall D, Baron D, Stewart JR. Source tracking swine fecal waste in surface water proximal to swine concentrated animal feeding operations. *Sci Total Environ.* 2015;511:676–83.
14. Heaney CD, Wing S, Campbell RL, et al. Relation between malodor, ambient hydrogen sulfide, and health in a community bordering a landfill. *Environ Res.* 2011;111(6):847–52.
15. Heaney CD, Wing S, Wilson SM, et al. Public infrastructure disparities and the microbiological and chemical safety of drinking and surface water supplies in a community bordering a landfill. *J Environ Health.* 2013;75(10):24–36.
16. Horton RA, Wing S, Marshall SW, Brownley KA. Malodor as a trigger of stress and negative mood in neighbors of industrial hog operations. *Am J Public Health.* 2009;99 Suppl 3:S610–5.
17. Lowman A, McDonald MA, Wing S, Muhammad N. Land application of treated sewage sludge: Community health and environmental justice. *Environ Health Perspect.* 2013;121(5):537–42.
18. Nadimpalli M, Rinsky JL, Wing S, et al. Persistence of livestock-associated antibiotic-resistant Staphylococcus aureus among industrial hog operation workers in North Carolina over 14 days. *Occup Environ Med.* 2015;72(2):90–9.
19. Pisanic N, Nadimpalli M, Rinsky JL, et al. Pig-2-Bac as a biomarker of occupational exposure to pigs and livestock-associated Staphylococcus aureus among industrial hog operation workers. *Environ Res.* 2015;143(Pt A):93–7.
20. Rinsky JL, Nadimpalli M, Wing S, et al. Livestock-associated methicillin and multidrug resistant Staphylococcus aureus is present among industrial, not antibiotic-free livestock operation workers in North Carolina. *PLoS One.* 2013;8(7):e67641.
21. Schinasi L, Horton RA, Guidry VT, Wing S, Marshall SW, Morland KB. Air pollution, lung function, and physical symptoms in communities near concentrated Swine feeding operations. *Epidemiology.* 2011;22(2):208–15.
22. Schinasi L, Horton RA, Wing S. Data completeness and quality in a community-based and participatory epidemiologic study. *Prog Community Health Partnersh.* 2009;3(2):179–90.
23. Wilson SM, Howell F, Wing S, Sobsey M. Environmental injustice and the Mississippi hog industry. *Environ Health Perspect.* 2002;110 Suppl 2:195–201.
24. Wing S. Whose epidemiology, whose health? *Int J Health Serv.* 1998;28(2):241–52.
25. Wing S. Social responsibility and research ethics in community-driven studies of industrialized hog production. *Environ Health Perspect.* 2002;110(5):437–44.
26. Wing S, Horton RA, Marshall SW, et al. Air pollution and odor in communities near industrial swine operations. *Environ Health Perspect.* 2008;116(10):1362–8.

27. Wing S, Horton RA, Muhammad N, Grant GR, Tajik M, Thu K. Integrating epidemiology, education, and organizing for environmental justice: Community health effects of industrial hog operations. *Am J Public Health.* 2008;98(8):1390–7.

28. USEPA. Learn about Environmental Justice. 2020. Accessed March 13, 2020.

29. Baron S, Sinclair R, Payne-Sturges D, et al. Partnerships for environmental and occupational justice: Contributions to research, capacity and public health. *Am J Public Health.* 2009;99 Suppl 3:S517–25.

30. O'Fallon LR, Dearry A. Commitment of the National Institute of Environmental Health Sciences to community-based participatory research for rural health. *Environ Health Perspect.* 2001;109 Suppl 3:469–73.

31. O'Fallon LR, Dearry A. Community-based participatory research as a tool to advance environmental health sciences. *Environ Health Perspect.* 2002;110 Suppl 2:155–9.

32. DHHS. *Principles of Community Engagement.* 2nd ed. Washington, DC: Department of Health and Human Services; 2011.

33. Israel BA, Eng E, Schulz AJ, Parker EA. *Methods for Community-Based Participatory Research for Health.* 2nd ed. San Francisco, CA: John Wiley & Sons; 2013.

34. Nachman KE, Lam J, Schinasi LH, Smith TC, Feingold BJ, Casey JA. O'Connor et al. systematic review regarding animal feeding operations and public health: Critical flaws may compromise conclusions. *Syst Rev.* 2017;6(1):179.

35. Schinasi L, Wing S, Augustino KL, et al. A case control study of environmental and occupational exposures associated with methicillin resistant Staphylococcus aureus nasal carriage in patients admitted to a rural tertiary care hospital in a high density swine region. *Environ Health.* 2014;13(1):54.

36. Schinasi L, Wing S, MacDonald PD, et al. Medical and household characteristics associated with methicillin resistant Staphylococcus aureus nasal carriage among patients admitted to a rural tertiary care hospital. *PLoS One.* 2013;8(8):e73595.

37. Heaney C, Wilson S, Wilson O, Cooper J, Bumpass N, Snipes M. Use of community-owned and -managed research to assess the vulnerability of water and sewer services in marginalized and underserved environmental justice communities. *J Environ Health.* 2011;74(1):8–17.

38. Heaney CD, Wilson SM, Wilson OR. The West End Revitalization Association's community-owned and -managed research model: Development, implementation, and action. *Prog Community Health Partnersh.* 2007;1(4):339–49.

39. Wilson OR, Bumpass NG, Wilson OM, Snipes MH. The West End Revitalization Association (WERA)'s right to basic amenities movement: Voice and language of ownership and management of public health solutions in Mebane, North Carolina. *Prog Community Health Partnersh.* 2008;2(3):237–43.

40. Wilson SM, Wilson OR, Heaney CD, Cooper J. Use of EPA collaborative problem-solving model to obtain environmental justice in North Carolina. *Prog Community Health Partnersh.* 2007;1(4):327–37.

41. NACEPT. Environmental Protection Belongs to the Public: A Vision for Citizen Science at EPA. USEPA; 2016.

42. https://smellmycity.org/. SmellMyCity. 2020. Accessed June 25, 2020.

43. English P, Amato H, Bejarano E, et al. Performance of a low-cost sensor community air monitoring network in Imperial County, CA. *Sensors (Basel).* 2020;20(11):3031.

44. Madrigal D, Claustro M, Wong M, Bejarano E, Olmedo L, English P. Developing youth environmental health literacy and civic leadership through community air monitoring in Imperial County, California. *Int J Environ Res Public Health.* 2020;17(5):1537.

45. Bi J, Stowell J, Seto EYW, et al. Contribution of low-cost sensor measurements to the prediction of PM2.5 levels: A case study in Imperial County, California, USA. *Environ Res.* 2020;180:108810.

46. Wong M, Bejarano E, Carvlin G, et al. Combining community engagement and scientific approaches in next-generation monitor siting: The case of the Imperial County community air network. *Int J Environ Res Public Health.* 2018;15(3):523.

47. English PB, Olmedo L, Bejarano E, et al. The Imperial County community air monitoring network: A model for community-based environmental monitoring for public health action. *Environ Health Perspect.* 2017;125(7):074501.

48. Collier-Oxandale A, Coffey E, Thorson J, Johnston J, Hannigan M. Comparing building and neighborhood-scale variability of CO(2) and O(3) to inform deployment considerations for low-cost sensor system use. *Sensors (Basel).* 2018;18(5):1349.

49. Clements AL, Griswold WG, Rs A, et al. Low-cost air quality monitoring tools: From research to practice (a workshop summary). *Sensors (Basel).* 2017;17(11):2478.

50. Burwell-Naney K, Wilson SM, Tarver SL, et al. Baseline air quality assessment of goods movement activities before the port of Charleston expansion: A community–university collaborative. *Environ Justice.* 2017;10(1):1–10.

51. Commodore A, Wilson SM, Muhammad O, Svendsen E, Pearce J. Community-based participatory research for the study of air pollution: A review of motivations, approaches, and outcomes. *Environ Monit Assess.* 2017;189(8):378.

52. Svendsen ER, Reynolds S, Ogunsakin OA, et al. Assessment of particulate matter levels in vulnerable communities in North Charleston, South Carolina prior to port expansion. *Environ Health Insights.* 2014;8:5–14.

53. Wilson O. Lack of basic amenities: Indicators of health disparities in low-income minority communities and tribal areas. *N C Med J.* 2011;72(2):145–8.

54. Scammell MK. Trust, conflict, and engagement in occupational health: North American epidemiologists conduct occupational study in communities affected by chronic kidney disease of unknown origin (CKDu). *Curr Environ Health Rep.* 2019;6(4):247–55.

55. Scammell MK, Howard GJ. Is a health study the answer for your community? A guide for making informed decisions. 2015. https://www.bu.edu/sph/files/2015/03/hsg_ch1_intro_1-26-16.pdf. Accessed March 13, 2020.

56. Wing S. Environmental justice, science, and public health. *Environ Health Perspect.* 2005;(special issue): 54–63.

57. Heath D. Meet the 'rented white coats' who defend toxic chemicals: How corporate-funded research is corrupting America's courts and regulatory agencies. 2016. https://www.publicintegrity.org/2016/02/08/19223/meet-rented-white-coats-who-defend-toxic-chemicals. Accessed March 13, 2020.

58. Pierson B. Plaintiffs in U.S. lawsuit say Monsanto ghostwrote Roundup studies. 2017. https://www.reuters.com/article/us-monsanto-cancer-lawsuit/plaintiffs-in-u-s-lawsuit-say-monsanto-ghostwrote-roundup-studies-idUSKBN16M01N

59. Altman DG, Bland JM. Absence of evidence is not evidence of absence. *BMJ.* 1995;311(7003):485.

60. Michaels D. *Doubt is their Product: How Industry's Assult on Science Threatens your Health.* Oxford: Oxford University Press; 2008.

61. Clapp RW, Ozonoff D. Environment and health: Vital intersection or contested territory? *Am J Law Med.* 2004;30(2-3):189–215.

62. Rothman KJ. A sobering start for the cluster busters' conference. *Am J Epidemiol.* 1990;132(1 Suppl):S6–13.

63. Wing S, Horton RA, Rose KM. Air pollution from industrial swine operations and blood pressure of neighboring residents. *Environ Health Perspect.* 2013;121(1):92–6.

64. Nadimpalli ML, Stewart JR, Pierce E, et al. Face mask use and persistence of livestock-associated Staphylococcus aureus nasal carriage among industrial hog operation workers and household contacts, USA. *Environ Health Perspect.* 2018;126(12):127005.

CHAPTER

67 Diseases Due to Physical Factors: Noise

Cristina Linares • Jesús de la Osa • Julio Díaz

INTRODUCTION

Noise is a physical atmospheric pollutant. Ambient noise is defined as all exterior sounds that are damaging or unwanted and originate from human activities, including noise from transportation (road, railway, and airplane traffic) and industrial activities.[1]

Noise pollution is a social and public health problem with important implications for quality of life, in particular for populations living in large urban areas, and there is growing evidence on long-term health effects including cardiovascular disease, neurocognitive effects in children, and other conditions. Multiple studies point to a significant association between urban noise and clinical cardiovascular outcomes such as acute myocardial infarction and stroke.[2–4] It is estimated that 3% of the burden of ischemic heart disease in large cities can be attributed to traffic noise.[5]

According to the Organization for Economic Cooperation and Development (OECD),[6] 130 million people are exposed to noise levels above the safety standards established by the World Health Organization (WHO)[7] and the U.S. Environmental Protection Agency (EPA) of 65 dB(A) during the day, and 55 dB(A) during the night. In 1974, the EPA estimated that nearly 100 million Americans lived in areas where the daily average noise levels exceeded those identified as being safe.[8] In 1991, it was estimated that environmental noise had increased by 10% in the decade of the 1980s.[9] In the 2000 United States Census, 30% of Americans complained of noise, and 11% found it to be bothersome. Among those who complained, noise was sufficiently bothersome to make nearly 40% want to change their place of residence.[10]

In the European Union (EU), 40% of the population is exposed to traffic noise levels over 55 dB(A), 20% exposed over 65 dB(A) during the day, and 30% exposed over 55 dB(A) at night.[11] Traffic noise is the most prevalent type of ambient noise and these exposure levels in the EU have an estimated burden of 61,000 disability adjusted life years (DALYs) and 1.6 million healthy life years lost,[12] making ambient noise the second most harmful environmental factor for health in the EU, behind air pollution. More specifically, in the countries of Western Europe 61,000 life years have been lost from ischemic heart disease, 45,000 due to cognitive problems in children, 900,000 due to sleep disorders, 22,000 due to tinnitus, and around 650,000 life years due to "discomfort."[13] In more recent exposure estimates, at least 100 million people in the European Union are affected by traffic noise.[14]

Hearing disorders and nonauditory health effects of noise have been studied for decades. In the United States and Europe, 26% of adults have a bilateral hearing disorder that impairs their ability to hear in noisy environments, and a further 2% have substantial unilateral hearing issues.[15] Age-adjusted prevalence of hearing disorders is similar in Asia.[16] In 2001, it was estimated that 12.5% of American children between the ages of 6–19 years had impaired hearing in one or both ears.[17] The nonauditory health effects of noise have been studied in trials with animals and in experimental human studies. The extrapolation of conclusions from such experiments to the findings of epidemiologic studies conducted under real-life conditions in populations exposed to ambient noise can be controversial, given the challenge of controlling individual and social factors: health conditions, lifestyles, individual sensitivity and adaptation, and the social representation of noise. However, the biological plausibility of these associations is solid, leading to consideration of noise as an inescapable public health problem that warrants residential- and community-level research.[18]

FROM AN OCCUPATIONAL TO A PUBLIC HEALTH PROBLEM

The health effects of ambient noise were first noted in people exposed to high levels in their work environments and research and control focused on auditory problems such as displacement of the hearing threshold, tinnitus, and hearing loss. Noise-induced hearing loss is the most common occupational disease in the United States: about 22 million U.S. workers are exposed to hazardous noise levels, and, annually, an estimated U.S. $242 million is spent on compensation for hearing loss disability.[19] In many countries, legislation recognizes deafness as an occupational disease produced by noise. In addition to auditory problems, less objective health problems including sleep disturbances, stress, and headaches, were also noticed. Then, occupational studies linked noise to chronic health outcomes, such as cardiovascular diseases and hormonal and metabolic responses.[20] Evidence shows that occupational noise exposure is related to unfavorable cardiovascular risk profiles including increased blood pressure, hyperglycemia, hyperlipidemia, and blood viscosity and coagulability of blood,[21] and increased risk of coronary artery disease, heart failure, and stroke.[22,23]

In the work environment, noise exposure is characterized by short periods and high sound intensity. Studies in general populations have shown that adverse health effects are related not only to high noise intensities during short intervals but also to lower noise intensities during longer intervals. Indeed, health outcomes previously related to noise in the work environment were also found in people exposed to ambient noise over a longer time period. The first studies in general populations were conducted in populations exposed to high noise exposure levels, such as those living close to airports. The health effects detected among the residents of these areas were similar to those found in the work environment. Later, studies included whole populations of city residents, with a particular interest in traffic-related noise. The concept of noise pollution shifted from being considered a work-related problem to being viewed today as a major environmental health problem affecting billions of people globally.[24]

BIOLOGICAL MECHANISMS INVOLVED IN THE EFFECTS OF NOISE ON HEALTH

Noise is processed as a stress factor at two levels: (a) psychological impact that begins with the arrival of the sound signal at the thalamic hearing structures and culminates with the excitation of the hypothalamus, and (b) an organic level that starts with the allostatic response from the hypothalamus and, in certain circumstances, ends with one or several adverse physiological effects.

In mammals, the primary mechanism that manages the physiological response to psychosocial stress is the hypothalamic-pituitary-adrenocortical axis (HPA) in coordination with the sympathetic-adrenal-medullary (SAM) system. The initial response to acute stress originates in the SAM axis with the release of catecholamines, while the HPA prolongs the physiological defensive response.[25] The hypothalamus activates the adrenal medullary and the sympathetic arm of the autonomic nervous system, starting SAM regulation with an increase in blood flow to the muscles, an increase in blood pressure and in heart rate and respiratory rate, along with a decrease in gastro intestinal activity. The hypothalamus then activates the adrenal cortex, which releases cortisol and other glucocorticoids. Among other activities, glucocorticoids are responsible for ensuring the flow of blood glucose to the brain and for elevating or stabilizing blood glucose levels, for mobilizing protein reserves, or regulating the immune system.

The physiological effects of catecholamines on the cardiovascular, respiratory, and metabolic systems are efficient when directly facing a physical short-term threat, but can be excessive in other situations, for instance, psychological or social threats, which affect people chronically and provoke continuous activation of the SAM axis (Fig. 67-1). Chronic catecholamine elevation has effects on development and can aggravate atherosclerosis, including increased blood coagulability. On the other hand, the chronic repressed response to acute stress results in the overactivation of the HPA axis and the overproduction of cortisol, which has been associated with an increase in insulin resistance, the accumulation of abdominal fat, and alterations in immune system function. High levels of cortisol can cause damage to the hippocampus and affect memory. Harm induced by excess cortisol can have far-reaching effects.

Environmental noise can be considered a psychosocial stress factor with organic effects equivalent to those triggered by other conventional physical, psychological, and social factors.[26] A situation of high stress can alter the balanced regulation of the adaptive response (allostasis) and cause organic damage and adverse effects on the cardiovascular, respiratory, metabolic, and immune systems.

Noise affects sleep, which inhibits several structures of the central nervous system. Consequently during sleep, the activity of the cortical connections is greatly reduced with the isolation from the outside world. During both sleep and wakefulness, the limbic system is on permanent alert, configuring the primary emotions that the hippocampus contributes to modeling through memory. During sleep, these unconscious emotions can cause autonomic awakenings and activate the hypothalamus, disturbing the REM phase by background noise, or the phases of deep sleep or slow wave sleep (SWS) by noise peaks.[27] If, during sleep, the sound signal is of such a nature and

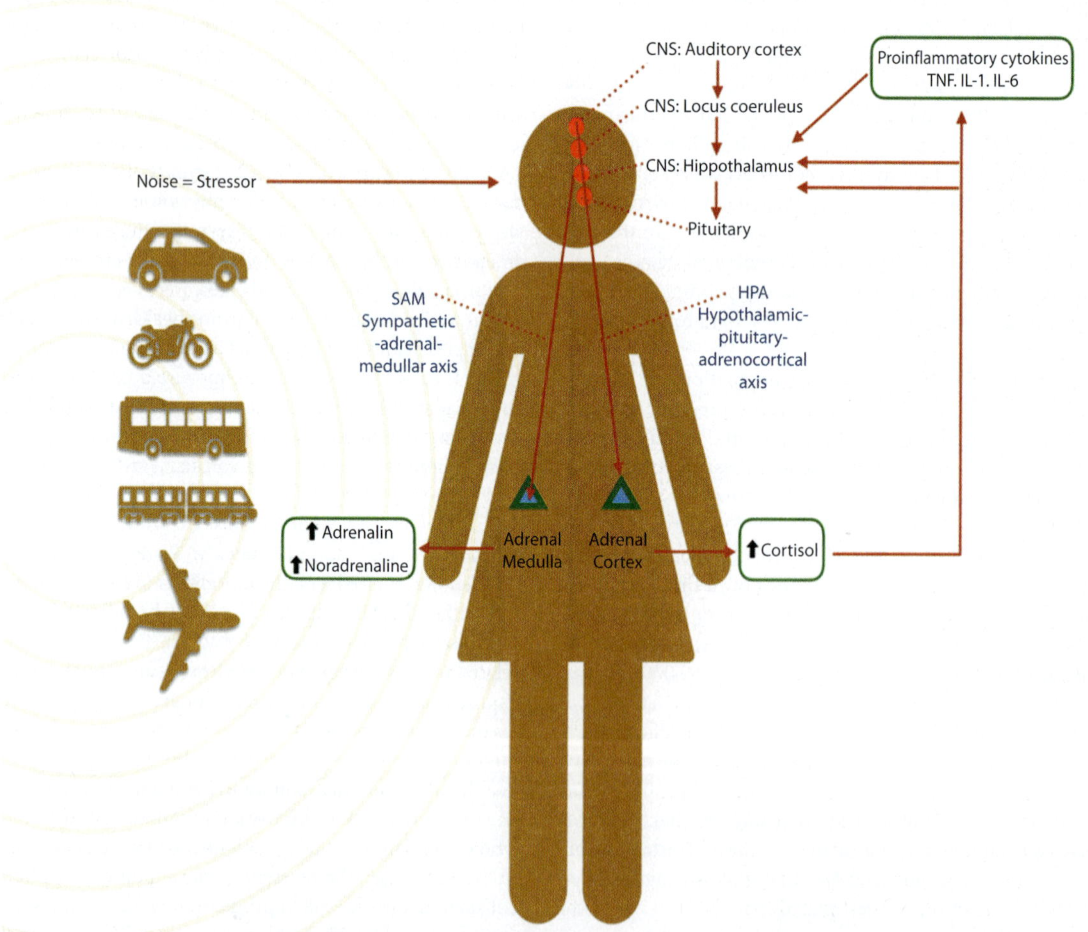

FIGURE 67-1. Roles of the sympathetic-adrenal-medullary (SAM) and hypothalamic-pituitary-adrenocortical (HPA) axes in the physiological response to acute psychic stress, from the activation of the central nervous system (CNS) to a warning or danger signal.

intensity that it activates the prefrontal cortex—generally by noise peaks—a cortical awakening occurs with SWS disturbance. The deep SWS promotes the repair of the acquired immune system, so that a lack of SWS prevents correct restitution, including adverse effects on the respiratory system and increased respiratory infections.[28]

SWS sleep also reduces systemic inflammation, and destabilization of atherosclerotic plaques, which disrupts cardiovascular health. In addition to affecting heart rate variability and raising blood pressure, SAM, and disproportionate HPA activity promotes the release of proinflammatory cytokines and systemic inflammation, which can increase oxidative stress, exacerbate endothelial dysfunction and aggravate atherosclerosis.[29–31] The excess of SAM activity inhibits the adhesion of lymphocytes to tissues and promotes blood coagulation. HPA activity decreases the number of lymphocytes, favors the accumulation of low-density lipoproteins in the arteries, and increases blood glucose levels.[32] Elderly people are more susceptible to the consequences of a marked decrease in SWS phases.[33] Allostatic overload has also been related to adverse respiratory outcomes through the inhibition of the innate immune system and increase of oxidative stress and connective tissue sclerosis.[34]

THE EFFECTS OF NOISE: AUDITORY AND NONAUDITORY EFFECTS

Adverse effects are changes in the morphology and physiology of an organism related to a maladjustment of its functional capacity, failure to compensate for additional stress, or increased susceptibility to the harmful effects of other environmental influences.[18] The adverse effects of noise include both alterations in the ear as well as in other organs and systems that are not directly related to the hearing process.[15]

Auditory Effects

Hearing loss. This occurs when an individual experiences an increase in the hearing threshold due to morphological and functional change in the inner cells of the cochlea that are connected to the auditory nerve. It is the most prevalent and irreversible occupational threat worldwide. Around 466 million people worldwide have disabling hearing loss, and 34 million of these are children. It is estimated that by 2050 over 900 million people will have disabling hearing loss. 1.1 billion young people (12–35 years) are at risk of hearing loss due to noise exposure in recreational settings.[35]

Cochlear recruitment. The theory of recruitment proposes that as the hair cells in the cochlea become ineffective, they "recruit" their (still working) neighbor hair cells to "hear" the frequency the damaged hair cell was supposed to hear. This phenomenon results in an abnormal perception of noise levels that is typically linked to hearing loss.

Tinnitus. This refers to sounds or noise effects generated by the inner ear. The condition can be permanent in the case of long exposures to occupational noise. It affects quality of life in different ways including sleep disruption, depression, and difficultly maintaining concentration. Tinnitus is responsible for 1.3% of healthy life-years lost each year in the EU due to exposure to ambient noise.[12]

Nonauditory Effects

Annoyance. Discomfort can be defined as a sense of displeasure associated with any factor or condition that an individual or group of people consider as the cause of adverse effects.[18] The first sign of discomfort is interference with verbal communication caused by noise, which results in fatigue, uncertainty, loss of confidence, erroneous interpretations, irritation, and other adverse effects that can result in stress. Other *annoyance* reactions include dissatisfaction, deception, nervousness, agitation, irritability, rage, desperation, anxiety, and aggressiveness. These responses are linked to a greater or lesser burden of psychological stress that can induce adverse physiological responses. The level of discomfort depends not only on the noise characteristics (source, level, low-frequency content), but also the characteristics of each person (sensitivity, capacity for stress management, current emotional situation, health status, feelings of defenselessness, or lack of control over the source of the noise, and fear of the noise). *Annoyance* is the most prevalent nonauditory effect of noise.[12]

Sleep disturbances. Sleep disturbances include difficulty falling asleep, waking up at night or sleep interruptions, and disturbances in the quality of sleep that affect the profundity of sleep or the proper succession of the phases of sleep. Physiological effects of disturbed sleep include increased blood pressure, increased heart rate frequency, cardia arrhythmia, vasoconstriction, and breathing changes. Effects that manifest during the day following disturbed sleep include fatigue, decline, clumsiness, low performance, and increased sensitivity to daily noise (with the associated sense of discomfort). Noise with Ln of 35 dB(A) or peaks over 50 dB(A) can prevent falling asleep and provoke nervous fatigue.[36] The adverse effects of nighttime noise depend on the level of background noise, maximum values, the number of noise events, and the difference between the noise level of those events and the background noise, in addition to certain noise characteristics such as tonal content and proportion of low frequencies.

Physiological stress. Exposure to noise induces stress, whether temporary or permanent, which manifests as increases in blood pressure, changes in heart rate, and vasoconstriction. These responses are mediated by the overactivation of the autonomic nervous system and endocrine system and, after prolonged exposure, can result in hypertension and cardiovascular diseases. These effects are greater for nighttime noise than daytime noise, possibly due to the difficulty in individual adaptation to nighttime noise in the absence of consciousness. Other effects related to continuous noise exposure include an increase in blood viscosity (coagulation factors) and increased lipids and glucose levels, which are established risk factors for atherosclerosis and diabetes. Studies in multiple countries support stress-induced by noise. For instance, a study in Japan[37] showed an association between traffic noise over 24 hours with certain psychological symptoms. Studies in Sweden[38] and Switzerland[39] related traffic noise to anxiety disorders and depressive symptoms. In a study in France, nighttime noise was associated to the consumption of anxiolytics.[40] In Germany, a study compared traffic noise in different locations with average noise over 24 hours, both above and below 55 dB(A), finding that traffic noise over 55 dB(A) increased the risk of depressive symptoms.[41]

Cognitive problems. Cognitive problems, including learning difficulties and low school performance, are especially relevant for children age 7–19 years.[42] The cognitive effects have been associated primarily with air traffic noise[43] and are the cause of 2.7% of healthy life years lost annually in the EU due to ambient noise exposure.[12]

Vestibular dysfunction. This condition includes symptoms like vertigo, nausea, and nystagmus. It is an understudied phenomenon and although evidence is limited, it may be caused by noise at low frequency in the audible and inaudible ranges. It has been associated with the growing installation of wind turbines in locations near urban centers, resulting in the so-called "air turbine syndrome."[44]

Cardiovascular effects and other health outcomes. The possible impact of noise on cardiovascular outcomes has been reported in multiple studies. The Stockholm conference on noise in 1988 concluded that noise is a risk factor for arterial hypertension. Intense noise between 95 and 105 dB(A) can provoke arterial vasoconstriction and blood pressure increase. The NAROMI study (*Noise burden and the risk of myocardial infarction*) found that chronic exposure to noise was associated with a small to moderate increase in the risk of acute myocardial infarction, both in men and women.[45] The association was not dose dependent. The HYENA study (*Hypertension and exposure to noise near airports)* was the first multicentric study to evaluate the effects of exposure to noise from airplanes and road traffic on blood pressure and heart disease.[46] There was a significant exposure–response relationships both for nighttime airplane noise and the average daily road traffic noise with hypertension. The LARES study (*Large analysis and reviews of European housing and health status)* reported that chronic discomfort due to traffic noise is associated with increased cardiovascular risk in adults 18–59 years. Generally, in the cited studies, the effects of noise pollution and air pollution were considered independently. Despite adjustment for air pollution, residual confounding is possible. Few studies have evaluated the potential interaction between air pollution and noise on cardiovascular outcomes.

THE SPECIAL CASE OF ROAD TRAFFIC NOISE EFFECTS ON HEALTH

Road traffic noise is the most relevant type of noise regarding the number of people exposed. Around 40% of the EU population is exposed to daytime levels of road traffic noise above 55 dB(A) and 20% to over 65 dB(A). At night, over 30% is exposed to levels above 55 dB(A) and suffers from sleep disturbances.[14] Traffic noise is generated primarily by the motor and by friction between the air and roadway. At speeds over 60 km/h, the noise from the friction of wheels with the ground is greater than the motor noise. In urban centers, motor noise is more important as the average speed of vehicles is under 60 km/h, except on large roads and when there is little traffic. At intersections regulated by traffic signals, noise levels are notable due to greater use of low gears. These levels can be estimated based on data related to the intensity of traffic, speed of automobiles, proportion of heavy vehicles, and the type of tread. In some cities, cultural factors can also influence noise levels. For example, the indiscriminate use of the horn can be an important source of urban noise related to road traffic, especially in Asian cities.[47]

Cardiovascular Diseases

Studies on exposure to road traffic noise and cardiovascular effects show an increase in the relative risk of ischemic heart disease when daytime traffic noise exceeds 65 dB(A) compared to lower levels.[48] Other studies support that people exposed to levels of traffic noise greater than or equal to 50 dB(A) have an increased risk of acute myocardial infarction compared to those exposed to levels under 50 dB(A). The associations remained even when excluding participants exposed to other sources of noise and those with hearing loss.[3] Noise-related interrupted sleep can also be a risk factor for acute myocardial infarction.[3] In addition to these observational epidemiologic studies, experimental studies have shown that exposure to ambient noise over 55 dB(A) can directly increase blood pressure levels in young people.[49]

The WHO 2018 Guide on Ambient Noise for the European Region, concluded that the quality of evidence for the positive relationship between long-term exposure to traffic noise and the incidence of ischemic heart disease is high.[14] Based on a meta-analysis, the relative risk for incident ischemic heart disease is 1.08 (95% CI: 1.01–1.15) for increases of 10 dB(A) in Lden (noise average for 24 hours), and the increased risk is continuous, starting at 50 dB(A).[23] Most of the studies included in the meta-analysis were conducted in Central and Northern Europe.[2,50] The relationship between traffic noise and ischemic heart disease mortality is also supported by a case-control study[3] and two prospective cohort studies.[51,52] While noise has been linked to hypertension, the quality of the evidence is low because most of the studies (N=26) were cross-sectional.[14]

In addition to these long-term health effects, short-term changes in traffic noise have also been related to hospital admissions for cardiovascular outcomes[53] and with cardiovascular mortality, including ischemic disease and stroke in those over age 65.[54] In this study, the estimated increase of cardiovascular mortality for 1 dB(A) in traffic noise was greater than for an increment of 10 mcg/m^3 of $PM_{2.5}$.

Respiratory Diseases

There are few studies on traffic noise and long-term respiratory outcomes and this health endpoint is not included in the above-mentioned 2018 WHO guide. Short-term exposure studies in Madrid showed an association with respiratory disease mortality in those over 65 years of age,[55] as well as with pneumonia and chronic obstructive pulmonary disease more specifically.[54] There is also a short-term association between noise levels in Madrid and hospital admissions due to respiratory causes in the general population.[53]

Metabolic Diseases

The 2018 WHO guide included three studies on the relationship between traffic noise and obesity. Since then, two cohort studies have evaluated the link between exposure to ambient noise and obesity development of obesity measures through the increase in abdominal perimeter.[56] In a cohort study in Switzerland, long-term exposure to transport-related noise, and traffic noise in particular, was related with obesity.[57]

The 2018, WHO guide indicated that the quality of evidence for the association between exposure to traffic noise and incidence of diabetes is moderate, based on a cohort study.[23] New cohort studies in Switzerland[58] and in Barcelona, Spain, shows that long-term exposure to noise is related to increased diabetes mortality.[59] Overall, the evidence for noise and metabolic diseases is limited by insufficient experimental evidence and the possibility of residual and unmeasured confounding.

Cognitive Development

According to the 2018 WHO guide, the quality of evidence was very low for the association between exposure to traffic noise and different dimensions of cognitive development in children (reading and oral comprehension, memory and attention, or performance at school), as few studies, all of them cross-sectional are available.[14]

Adverse Birth Outcomes

Few studies have evaluated the relationship between long-term traffic noise and birth weight[60,61] and premature birth.[62] The WHO classifies this evidence as of low quality.[14] In the city of Madrid, traffic noise was associated with acute adverse birth outcomes,[63–65] including fetal death.[66]

Annoyance

A systematic review carried out to support guidelines for Europe[67] found a quadratic association between levels of Lden and the percentage of discomfort reported. For values of Lden of 40 dB(A), the percentage of the population that experiences discomfort is around 9%. The threshold for 10% of the population suffering discomfort is 53.3 dB(A) of Lden.

Sleep

A systematic review of noise exposure and sleep outcomes included 44 studies for a qualitative review and 33 for a quantitative review.[68] The range of noise exposure reported in the studies reviewed was 37.5–77.5 dB Lnight (whole-night noise exposure metric, also called a noise night indicator). About 2% (95% CI: 0.90–3.15) of the population was characterized as highly sleep-disturbed at Lnight levels of 40 dB. The OR for the association between road traffic noise and the probability of being highly sleep-disturbed was 2.13 (95% CI: 1.82–2.48) per 10 dB increase in noise. Analyses for other sleep-related health outcomes provided supporting evidence on the overall relationship between road traffic noise and sleep disturbance. In general, the quality of evidence worldwide is moderate for the association between traffic noise and sleep indicators.

Figure 67-2 shows a summary of the studies conducted in Madrid on the short-term impact of noise on morbidity and mortality.

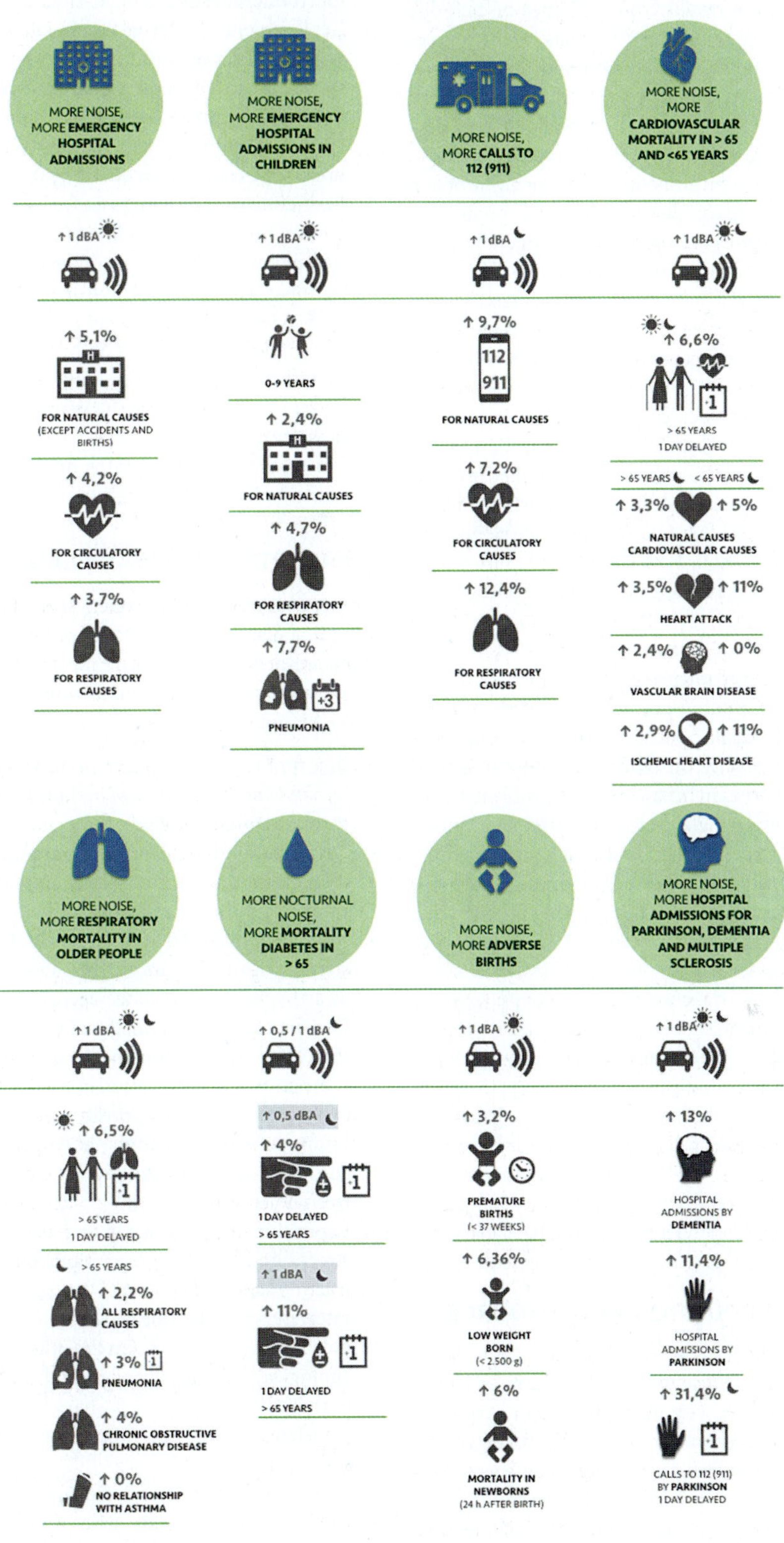

FIGURE 67-2. Summary of the studies conducted in Madrid on the short-term impact of noise on morbidity and mortality. (*Source:* Reproduced with permission from Recio A, Carmona R, Linares C, Ortiz C, Banegas JR, Díaz J. Efectos del ruido urbana sobre la salud: estudios de análisis de series temporales realizados en Madrid. Instituto de Salud Carlos III, Escuela Nacional de Sandidad: Madrid, 2016. Infograffia: Jesùs de la Osa, 2017, 2019. https://www.tiempo.com/ram/392902/entrevista-julio-diaz-cristina-linares/.)

MEASURES FOR MINIMIZING IMPACTS OF NOISE IN THE RESIDENTIAL ENVIRONMENT

Residential or community noise results from activities of daily life and excludes noise from occupational environments. Main sources include road, air, and train traffic, construction and service work, industrial activities, activities in public spaces (restaurants, bars, parks, and parking lots), and activities inside homes and offices (electronics, machines, musical instruments, animals, voices, parties). Noise pollution in residential environments is a growing problem related to urban and technological development and population growth. Existing control measures are limited and residential noise pollution will likely continue to affect coming generations.[18]

Urban noise due to industrial activity is characterized by the presence of low and high frequencies, tonal components, and sudden variations in intensity that are generated by increasingly powerful and sophisticated machines. Construction and maintenance projects, though temporary, lack measures of control for high-intensity sounds. Nocturnal services, such as trash collection, result in sudden elevations in the levels of nighttime noise that produce sleep disturbances. In some urban areas, there is a growing concern about noise of low frequency and modulating intensity from wind turbines. However, the principal source of community noise with a clear impact on public health is the noise caused by transportation. It is estimated that 50% of the population of the EU currently resides in problematic areas in terms of road, air, and train traffic.[69]

In terms of air traffic, the most intense noise is generated during take-offs, and certain types of motors produce high levels of tonal noise, which augments the disturbing effect of noise. The noise from train traffic depends on train velocity, the type of motor, train car, and train infrastructure. Closed curves in urban areas are problematic for road traffic noise, as they produce high levels of high-frequency noise due to squeaking wheels. Train stations are also a source of noise events: breaking and acceleration of trains, megaphones, and signals. In certain areas, high-speed trains constitute a growing problem due to their expanding presence and speeds over 250 km/h that emit noise similar in frequency and level to low-flying jet airplanes.

Noise control measures can be classified into two groups: (a) noise reduction measures related to the noise source and (b) measures involving planning and urban regulation. The first are linked to economic interests and the production system, and mostly they do not attempt to disrupt the unbridled use of motor vehicles, the main noise-generating machine in urban settings. They are, therefore, palliative measures that keep the urban landscape and the relationship of the individual with the environment unchanged. The second type of measures, on the other hand, aims to alter the urban physiognomy, adapting it to a healthy, habitable space where people recover the relational space usurped by machines.[18,70]

MEASURES FOR NOISE REDUCTION AT THE SOURCE

These measures are based on the transformation of vehicular technology and restrictive legislation of vehicle use. Road traffic noise comes mainly from the friction of the tires with the asphalt, engine combustion, expulsion of the gases derived from combustion, the friction of the chassis with the air (aerodynamic noise), and the horn. Noise reduction measures that address these mechanisms are described below. It should be noted, however, that some of these measures may be incompatible with others that aim to reduce air pollution; for example, the reduction of speed reduces noise but leads to an increase in traffic congestion and noise. These noise reduction measures should thus go hand in hand with measures related to better urban planning and regulation.

- Incorporation of silencers.
- Modernization of the automobile fleet. Modern vehicles are generally less noisy than old ones. In addition, they incorporate improvements such as automatic stopping of the engine when the car is stopped at a traffic light.
- Improvement of the quality of fuels. The type of fuel influences the combustion process and vibrations in the engine. The addition of lubricants such as cetane in diesel fuels reduces engine noise.
- Replacement of internal combustion engine vehicles with electric vehicles. This measure is certainly effective in cities, where the speed of cars on most traffic lanes is low and, therefore, engine noise predominates over noise due to friction with asphalt and air. If 12% of the current vehicles in the city of Paris were electric, noise levels could be reduced by 0.5 dB(A).[71]
- Reduction of speed limits on freeways close to residential places to control noise due to friction with the ground and air.
- Reduction of speed limits on urban roads, especially at night. For example, a car at 30 km/h instead of the typical 50 km/h generates 5 dB(A) less than equivalent noise level.
- Prohibition or awareness of the use of the horn for purposes other than those regulated, especially at night.
- Economic incentives to companies for the use of trucks with low noise emissions.
- More restrictive regulations on the maximum permissible noise emission levels for the car.

MEASURES FOR URBAN PLANNING AND REGULATION

These measures include reduction of traffic intensity and urban planning that discourages the use of private transport. They also contemplate antinoise infrastructure measures, particularly those related to green areas and plant structures in streets and facades. We outline some highlights here:

- Incorporation of aspects of healthy mobility into Sustainable Urban Mobility Plans that include the reduction of noise pollution through different tools.
- Design and urban planning that prioritizes modes of active mobility (commuting on foot and by bicycle) and silent public collective transport rather than private vehicles.
- More pedestrian-friendly streets in dense residential areas, so that streets with traffic are further away from people [moving traffic away by twice the distance decreases the noise levels by 3 dB(A)].
- Construction and extension of bicycle lane networks to encourage the use of nonpolluting means of transport.
- Limitation and pacification of road traffic in streets near homes by expanding residential priority areas.
- Limitations of road traffic and speed around hospitals, schools, and nursing homes to protect the most vulnerable population from noise, especially those over 65 years of age in these centers.
- Expansion of green areas and placement of plant structures in streets and facades. Vegetation, during the phenomena of diffraction and reflection of sound waves, promotes destructive interference and absorbs part of their energy transforming it into mechanical vibrations. On the other hand, vegetation exerts a psychological influence by altering the way people perceive and react to noise.[72,73]
- Construction of new homes with requirements for adequate soundproofing.
- Replacing the windows of old buildings with noise-proof windows.
- Construction of roads with noise-reducing surfaces (such as porous asphalt), especially on motorways close to residential environment, where the friction noise of the tires is greater due to the high speed of the vehicles. This measure must be complementary to a plan to maintain roads in optimum condition.

COMMUNICATION OF RISKS

In general, the population is unaware that noise pollution can affect health beyond causing discomfort. There is insufficient awareness among the population that exposure to noise, especially traffic, is a major health problem. This lack of awareness is related in part to media treatment. Media often focus on the auditory effects and the annoyance effects of leisure noise, or on the health effects of air pollution, rather than providing a more comprehensive perspective that also includes nonauditory effects. It gives less or no consideration to the source of the greatest population exposures, traffic noise. However, these aspects are being increasingly addressed, including interviews with researchers in the field. While knowledge, perception, and involvement of health professionals in the prevention and control of the health impacts of noise pollution are limited, training of health personnel on noise health effects and interventions is expanding, with a growing focus on the nonauditory health effects of noise and their public health impact. Some suggestions to improve communication of the health risks of noise pollution could be the following:

- Use the approach of Health in all Policies (HiAP). In this sense, the reduction of exposure to noise pollution, mainly traffic noise, but also from aircraft, railways, and leisure noise should be contemplated in all policies, strategies, plans, programs, and tools for territorial planning, urban planning, and healthcare planning.
- Messages should not alarm society but should reflect the total dimensions of the problem.
- When communicating information to the public, it should be transmitted in a way that is not overly technical and can be easily understood.
- A positive communication approach should be used. In addition to the negative impacts on health, we should also describe the health benefits of reducing exposure and the health assets of a quiet environment for health promotion, community health, and public health.
- The concrete practical measures that can be adopted to minimize the impact of noise on the health of the population, both at the citizen level and at the municipal, regional, or country level actions.
- Less noise is more health.

Health education and environmental education groups and professionals (scientists) can play a major role in developing prevention and control strategies for noise pollution. They can serve as mediators between technical groups and citizens. Their expertise in optimal communication skills for translation of the scientific evidence is a major asset.

References

1. Directive 2002/49/EC. Directive of the European Parliament and of the Council of 25 June 2002 relating to the assessment and management of environmental noise. *Off J Eur Comm.* 2002;L189:12–25.
2. Babisch W, Wölke G, Heinrich J, Straff W. Road traffic noise and hypertension--accounting for the location of rooms. *Environ Res.* 2014;133:380–7.
3. Selander J, Nilsson ME, Bluhm G, et al. Long-term exposure to road traffic noise and myocardial infarction. *Epidemiology.* 2009;20(2):272–9.
4. Sørensen M, Hvidberg M, Andersen ZJ, et al. Road traffic noise and stroke: A prospective cohort study. *Eur Heart J.* 2011;32:737–44.
5. Babisch W. Road traffic noise and cardiovascular risk. *Noise Health.* 2008;10(38):27–33.
6. OSE Informe de la Sostenibilidad en España. Observatorio de la Sostenibilidad en España. Madrid: MIMA, 2006.
7. WHO. World Health Organization. Guidelines for Community Noise. 2009.
8. EPA: Information on levels of environmental noise requisite to protect public health and welfare with an adequate margin of safety (EPA/ONAC Report 550/9-74-004). U.S. Environmental Protection Agency. Washington, DC, 1974.
9. Suter AH. Noise and its Effects. Administrative Conference of the United States, 1991.
10. U.S. Census Bureau, Housing and Economic Statistics Division. Available at: http://www.census.gov/hhes/www/housing/ahs/ahs99/tab28.html.
11. Hellmut T, Classens T, Khinr R, Kephalopoulos S, eds.Hellmut T, Classens T, Khinr R, Kephalopoulos S, eds. *World Health Regional Office for Europe and European Commission. Burden of Disease from Environmental Noise. Quantification of Healthy Life Years Lost in Europe.* Copenhagen: WHO Regional Publications; 2011.
12. WHO. World Health Regional Office for Europe. European Commission. Burden of disease from environmental noise. Quantification of healthy life years lost in Europe. Copenhagen. 2011.
13. Hänninen O, Knol AB, Jantunen M, et al. Environmental burden of disease in Europe: Assessing nine risk factors in six countries. *Environ Health Perspect.* 2014;122(5):439–46.
14. WHO, 2018. Environmental Noise Guidelines for the European Region. http://www.euro.who.int/en/publications/abstracts/environmental-noise-guidelines-for-the-european-region-2018.
15. Basner M, Babisch W, Davis A, et al. Auditory and non-auditory effects of noise on health. *Lancet.* 2014;383(9925):1325–32.
16. Fuente A, Hickson L. Noise-induced hearing loss in Asia. *Int J Audiol.* 2011;50(suppl):S3–10.
17. Niskar AS, Kieszak SM, Holmes AE, et al. Estimated prevalence of noise-induced hearing threshold shifts among children 6 to 19 years of age: The third national health and nutritional examination survey 1988–1994, United States. Pediatrics. 2001;108:40–3.
18. WHO. Guidelines for Community Noise. Geneva. 2000.
19. National Institute for Occupational Safety and Health (NIOSH); noise and hearing loss prevention. 2013.
20. Tomei G, Fioravanti M, Cerratti D, et al. Occupational exposure to noise and the cardiovascular system: A meta-analysis. *Sci Total Environ.* 2010;408:681–9.
21. Babisch W. The noise/stress concept, risk assessment and research needs. *Noise Health.* 2002;4:1–11.
22. van Kempen E, Casas M, Pershagen G, Foraster M. WHO environmental noise guidelines for the European Region: A systematic review on environmental noise and cardiovascular and metabolic effects: A summary. *Int J Environ Res Public Health.* 2018;15(2):pii: E379.
23. Tobías A, Linares C, Díaz J. El ruido de tráfico, un importante problema de salud pública en las grandes ciudades: De la pérdida de audición a causa de riesgo de muerte. Revista Actuarios. Edición de Otoño, 2013.
24. Aich P, Potter AA, Griebel PJ. Modern approaches to understanding stress and disease susceptibility: A review with special emphasis on respiratory disease. *Int J Gen Med.* 2009;2:19–32.
25. Prasher D. Is there evidence that environmental noise is immunotoxic? *Noise Health.* 2009;11(44):151–5.
26. Pirrera S, De Valck E, Cluydts R. Nocturnal road traffic noise: A review on its assessment and consequences on sleep and health. *Environ Int.* 2010;36(5):492–8.
27. Irwin MR. Sleep and infectious disease risk. *Sleep.* 2012;35(8):1025–6.
28. Yildirim I, Kilinc M, Okur E, et al. The effects of noise on hearing and oxidative stress in textile workers. *Ind Health.* 2007;45(6):743–9.
29. Schmidt FP, Basner M, Kröger G, et al. Effect of nighttime aircraft noise exposure on endothelial function and stress hormone release in healthy adults. *Eur Heart J.* 2013;34(45):3508–14a.
30. Hansson GK. Inflammation, atherosclerosis, and coronary artery disease. *N Engl J Med.* 2005;352(16):1685–95. Review.
31. Qureshi GM, Seehar GM, Zardari MK, Pirzado ZA, Abbasi SA. Study of blood ipids, cortisol and haemodynamic variations under stress in male adults. *J Ayub Med Coll Abbottabad.* 2009;21(1):158–61.
32. Recio A, Linares C, Banegas JR, Díaz J. Road traffic noise effects on cardiovascular, respiratory and metabolic health: An integrative model of biological mechanisms. *Environ Res.* 2016;146:359–70.
33. Santus P, Corsico A, Solidoro P, Braido F, Di Marco F, Scichilone N. Oxidative stress and respiratory system: Pharmacological and clinical reappraisal of N-acetylcysteine. *COPD.* 2014;11(6):705–17.
34. WHO, 2019. https://www.who.int/en/news-room/fact-sheets/detail/deafness-and-hearing-loss.
35. Ohrstrom E, Bjorkman M. Effects of noise disturbed-sleep: A laboratory study on habituation and subjective noise sensitivity. *J Sound Vibration.* 1998;122:277–90.
36. Yoshida T, Osada Y. Effects of road traffic noise on inhabitants of Tokyo. *J Sound Vibr.* 1997;205:517–22.
37. Persson R, Björk J, Ardö J, Albin M, Jakobsson K. Trait anxiety and modeled exposure as determinants of self-reported annoyance to sound, air pollution another environmental factors in the home. *Int Arch Occup Environ Health.* 2007;81(2):179–91.
38. Brand S, Heller P, Bicher AJ, et al. Patients with environment-related disorders: Comprehensive results of interdisciplinary diagnostics. *Int J Hyg Environ Health.* 2009;212:157–71.

39. Bocquier A, Cortaredona S, Boutin C, et al. Is exposure to night-time traffic noise a risk factor for purchase of anxiolytic–hypnotic medication? A cohort study. *Eur J Public Health.* 2014;24(2):298–303.
40. Münzel T, Sorensen M, Schmidt F, et al. The adverse effects of environmental noise exposure on oxidative stress and cardiovascular risk. *Antioxid Redox Signal.* 2018;28(9):873–908.
41. Orban E, McDonald K, Sutcliffe R, et al. Residential road traffic noise and high depressive symptoms after five years of follow-up: Results from the Heinz Nixdorf recall study. *Environ Health Perspect.* 2016;124(5):578–85.
42. Lopez AD, Mathers CD, Ezzati M, Jamison DT, Murray CJL. *Global Burden of Disease and Risk Factors.* Washington, DC and New York: The World Bank & Oxford University Press; 2006.
43. Stansfeld SA, Berglund B, Clark C, et al. Aircraft and road traffic noise and children's cognition and health: a cross-sectional study. *Lancet.* 2005;365:1942–9.
44. Harrison RV. On the biological plausibility of Wind Turbine syndrome. *Int J Environ Health Res.* 2015;25(5):463–8.
45. Willich SN, Wegscheider K, Stallmann M, Keial T. Noise burden and the risk of myocardial infarction. *Eur. Heart J.* 2012;27:276–82.
46. Jarup L. Babisch W, Houthuijs D, et al. Hypertension and exposure to noise near airports: The HYENA study. *Environ Health Perspect.* 2008;116:329–33.
47. Singh N, Davar SC. Noise pollution—Sources, effects and control. *J Hum Ecol.* 2004;16:181–7.
48. Argalášová-Sobotová L, Lekaviciute J, Jeram S, Sevcíková L, Jurkovicová J. Environmental noise and cardiovascular disease in adults: Research in Central, Eastern and South-Eastern Europe and Newly Independent States. *Noise Health.* 2013;15(62):22–31.
49. Lercher P, Botteldooren D, Widmann U, Uhrner U, Kammeringer E. Cardiovascular effects of environmental noise: Research in Austria. *Noise Health.* 2011;13(52):234–50.
50. Sørensen M, Hoffmann B, Hvidberg M, et al. Long-term exposure to traffic-related air pollution associated with blood pressure and self-reported hypertension in a Danish cohort. *Environ Health Perspect.* 2012;120(3):418–24.
51. Beelen R, Hoek G, Houthuijs D, et al. The joint association of air pollution and noise from road traffic with cardiovascular mortality in a cohort study. *Occup Environ Med.* 2009;66(4):243–50.
52. Gan WQ, Davies HW, Koehoorn M, Brauer M. Association of long-term exposure to community noise and traffic-related air pollution with coronary heart disease mortality. *Am J Epidemiol.* 2012;175(9):898–906.
53. Tobías A, Díaz J, Saez M, et al. Use of Poisson regression and Box-Jenkins models to evaluate the short-term effects of environmental noise levels on daily emergency admissions in Madrid, Spain. *Eur J Epidemiol.* 2001;17:765–71.
54. Recio A, Linares C, Banegas JR, Díaz J. Impact of road traffic noise on cause-specific mortality in Madrid (Spain). *Sci Total Environ.* 2017;590–1:171–3.
55. Tobías A, Recio A, Díaz J, Linares C. Does traffic noise influence respiratory mortality? *Eur Respir J.* 2014;44:797–9.
56. Pyko A, Eriksson C, Lind T, et al. Long-term exposure to transportation noise in relation to development of obesity—A cohort study. *Environ Health Perspect.* 2017;125(11):117005.
57. Foraster M, Künzli N, Aguilera I, et al. High blood pressure and long-term exposure to indoor noise and air pollution from road traffic. *Environ Health Perspect.* 2014;122(11):1193–200.
58. Eze IC, Foraster M, Schaffner E, et al. Long-term exposure to transportation noise and air pollution in relation to incident diabetes in the SAPALDIA study. *Int J Epidemiol.* 2017;46(4):1115–25.
59. Barceló MA, Varga D, Tobías A, Díaz J, Linares C, Sáez M. Long term effects of traffic noise on mortality in the city of Barcelona, 2004–2007. *Environ Res.* 2016;147:193–206.
60. Dadvand P, Ostro B, Figueras F, et al. Residential proximity to major roads and term low birth weight: The roles of air pollution, heat, noise, and road-adjacent trees. *Epidemiology.* 2014;25(4):518–25.
61. Hjortebjerg D, Andersen AM, Christensen JS, et al. Exposure to road traffic noise and behavioral problems in 7-year-old children: A cohort study. *Environ Health Perspect.* 2016;124(2):228–34.
62. Gehring U, Tamburic L, Sbihi H, Davies HW, Brauer M. Impact of noise and air pollution on pregnancy outcomes. *Epidemiology.* 2014;25(3):351–8.
63. Arroyo V, Díaz J, Ortíz C, Carmona R, Sáez M, Linares C. Short term effect of air pollution, noise and heat waves on preterm births in Madrid (Spain). *Environ Res.* 2016;145:162–8.
64. Arroyo V, Díaz J, Carmona R, Ortiz C, Linares C. Impact of air pollution and temperature on adverse birth outcomes: Madrid 2001–2009. *Environ Pollut.* 2016;218:1154–61. DOI: 10.106/j.envpol.2016.08.069.
65. Díaz J, Arroyo V, Carmona R, Ortiz C, Linares C. Effect of environmental factors on low weight in non-premature births: A time series analysis. *PLoS One.* 2016;11(10):e0164741. DOI:10.1371/journal.pone.0164741
66. Díaz J, Linares C. Traffic noise and adverse birth outcomes in Madrid: A time-series analysis. *Epidemiology.* 2016;27:e2–3. DOI: 10.1097/EDE.0000000000000406.
67. Guski R, Schreckenberg D, Schuemer R. WHO environmental noise guidelines for the European region: A systematic review on environmental noise and annoyance. *Int J Environ Res Public Health.* 2017 Dec 8;14(12):1539.
68. Basner M, McGuire S. WHO environmental noise guidelines for the European region: A systematic review on environmental noise and effects on sleep. *Int J Environ Res Public Health.* 2018;15(3):pii: E519.
69. EEA, 2019. Unequal exposure and unequal impacts: social vulnerability to air pollution, noise and extreme 122 temperatures in Europe, EEA Report No 22/2018, EEA, Copenhagen, Denmark.
70. Curran JH, Ward HD, Shum M, Davies HW. Reducing cardiovascular health impacts from traffic related noise and air pollution: Intervention strategies. *Environ Health Rev.* 2013;56(2):31–8.
71. Warburg N, Forell A, Guillon L, Teulón H, Canaguuier B. Elaboration selon Les Principes des ACV des Bilans Energetiques, des Emissions de Gaz es des autres impacts environmenteaux. Ademe (Agence de l'Environment et de la Maitrise de l'Energie). 2014.
72. Dzhambov AM, Dimitrova DD. Urban green spaces' effectiveness as a psychological buffer for the negative health impact of noise pollution: A systematic review. *Noise Health.* 2014 May–Jun;16(70):157–65.
73. Jang HS, Lee SC, Jeon JY, Kang J. Evaluation of road traffic noise abatement by vegetation treatment in a 1:10 urban scale model. *J Acoust Soc Am.* 2015 Dec;138(6):3884.

CHAPTER

68

Ionizing Radiation

Elizabeth Cahoon

Radiation is one of the most studied and best-characterized environmental exposures. Studies of the health effects of ionizing radiation have been motivated by the uses of radiation in medicine, science, and industry, as well as from the peaceful and military applications of atomic energy.[1] A main objective of these studies is to characterize risks of radiation exposure for the purpose of controlling these risks. An additional objective is to identify factors determining susceptibility to increased risk for cancer subsequent to radiation exposure.

Ionizing radiation causes chemical changes in cells and damage in DNA that may increase the risk of developing certain health conditions as an acute or late effect. Ionizing radiation can come from natural sources, such as radon, and manmade sources, such as medical imaging or therapeutic treatment. Nuclear power plant accidents and atomic weapon explosions have also led to releases of high levels of ionizing radiation. Thus, longitudinal studies of the atomic-bomb survivors in Hiroshima and Nagasaki have been a critical source of information on the consequences of radiation exposure. Being exposed to very high doses of ionizing radiation can cause damage to tissues and organs that becomes evident within a few days of exposure, while low to moderate doses can induce late effects on apparently undamaged tissues, such as cancer and cataracts. As one of the best-characterized environmental exposures, the extensive knowledge of the effects of ionizing radiation generated by both experimental and observational studies has led to numerous etiological insights and identified susceptible populations and windows of exposure. The research evidence has prompted policy and strategies for protection against radiation that have been influential in shaping measures for protection against other hazardous physical and chemical agents as well.

PHYSICAL PROPERTIES OF IONIZING RADIATION

Ionizing radiation is a type of high-energy radiation that has enough energy to remove an electron (negative particle) from an atom or molecule, causing it to become ionized. Ionizing radiations include (a) electromagnetic radiations of short-wavelength and high energy (e.g., x-rays and gamma rays) and (b) particulate radiations, which vary in mass and charge (e.g., electrons, protons, neutrons, alpha particles, and other atomic particles). Ionizing radiation, impinging on a living cell, collides randomly with atoms and molecules in its path, with some clustering at the ends of its track, giving rise to ions and free radicals and depositing enough localized energy to damage genes, chromosomes, or other vital macromolecules. The distribution of such events along the path of the radiation—that is, the *quality* or *linear energy transfer* (LET) of the radiation—varies with the energy and charge of the radiation, as well as the density of the absorbing medium.[2] Along the path of an alpha particle, for example, the collisions occur so close together that the radiation typically loses all of its energy in traversing only a few cells; beta particles, which consist of electrons, can penetrate up to 2 cm of soft tissue; whereas along the path of an x-ray the collisions are far enough apart so that the radiation may be able to traverse the entire body (Fig. 68-1).

Because the biological effects of ionizing radiation result from the deposition of energy in exposed cells, doses of ionizing radiation are customarily expressed in terms of energy deposition (Table 68-1). On traversing a given cell, a densely ionizing radiation (e.g., an alpha particle) is more likely than a sparsely ionizing radiation (e.g., an x-ray) to deposit enough energy in a critical site, such as a gene or chromosome, to injure the cell.[3–5] Hence an additional dose unit (the *equivalent dose)* is used in radiation protection to enable different types of radiation to be normalized in terms of their relative biological effectiveness (RBE). The equivalent dose (expressed in sievert [Sv]) is the dose in gray (Gy) multiplied by an appropriate weighting factor to adjust for differences in RBE; that is, 1 Sv of alpha radiation is that dose (in gray) of alpha radiation that is equivalent in biological effectiveness to 1 Gy of gamma rays (Table 68-1).

The uptake, distribution, and retention of an internally deposited radionuclide (one that enters the body, reaches one or more organs, and then decays) vary, depending on the physical and chemical properties of the element in question. Once deposited, the amount of radioactivity remaining in situ decreases with time as a result of both physical decay and biological removal. The physical half-lives, or times during which one-half of the atoms

Radionuclide	Radiation Type	Energy	Range in Tissue*
^{218}Po	Alpha (α)	6.1 MeV	0.052 mm[1]
^{63}Ni	Beta minus (β^-)	0.067 MeV (maximum)	0.072 mm[2] (maximum)
^{90}Y	Beta minus (β^-)	2.3 MeV (maximum)	11 mm[3] (maximum)
^{99m}Tc	Gamma (γ)	0.141 MeV	66 mm[4] (mean distance to collision)
^{40}K	Gamma (γ)	1.46 MeV	173 mm[5] (mean distance to collision)

*Decay data taken from LNHB recommended data, http://www.nucleide.org/DDEP_WG/DDEPdata.htm

1 CSDA (continuous slowing down approximation) range calculated in skeletal muscle ICRP using ASTAR, https://physics.nist.gov/PhysRefData/Star/Text/ASTAR-t.html

2 CSDA range calculated using spline interpolation of ESTAR data for soft tissue ICRP, https://physics.nist.gov/PhysRefData/Star/Text/ESTAR.html

3 CSDA range calculated using spline interpolation of ESTAR data for soft tissue ICRP, https://physics.nist.gov/PhysRefData/Star/Text/ESTAR.html

4 Mean free path calculated using mass attenuation coefficient for soft tissue ICRP interpolated from XCOM data, https://physics.nist.gov/PhysRefData/XrayMassCoef/ComTab/tissue.html

5 Mean free path calculated using mass attenuation coefficient for soft tissue ICRP interpolated from XCOM data, https://physics.nist.gov/PhysRefData/XrayMassCoef/ComTab/tissue.html

FIGURE 68-1. Differences among various types of ionizing radiation in penetrating power in tissue.[2] Notes: Range depictions are not to scale. Black dots represent points of ionization. Beta particles are emitted with a distribution of energy, while alpha and gamma are monoenergetic.

TABLE 68-1 UNITS OF RADIATION EXPSOURE

Quantity	Unit	Description
Absorbed dose	Gray (Gy)	Energy deposition in 1 kg of tissue without regard to type of radiation
Equivalent dose	Sievert (Sv)	Absorbed dose weighted for biological effectiveness of the radiation
Effective dose	Sievert (Sv)	Equivalent dose weighted for the sensitivity of the exposed organ
Collective effective dose	Sievert (Sv)	Effective dose applied to population
Radioactivity	Becquerel (Bq)	One atomic disintegration per second

Note: The units of measure listed are those of the International System, introduced in the 1970s to standardize usage throughout the world.[3] They have largely supplanted the earlier units; namely the rad (1 rad = 100 ergs/g = 0.01 Gy); the rem (1 rem = 0.01 Sv); and the curie (1 Ci = 3.7×10^{10} disintegrations per second = 3.7×10^{10} Bq).

TABLE 68-2 DOSE RANGES CONSIDERED IN EPIDEMIOLOGICAL STUDIES

Dose Level	Range of Absorbed Dose for Low LET-Radiation	Examples
Very low	Less than 10 mGy	Conventional radiology (excluding CT scans or fluoroscopy)
Low	10–100 mGy	Multiple whole-body CT scans
Moderate	100 mGy to 1 Gy	Clean-up workers following nuclear accident
High	Greater than 1 Gy	Dose following serious radiation accident or radiotherapy

Source: Modified from UNSCEAR 2012.

TABLE 68-3 PERCENT CONTRIBUTION OF VARIOUS SOURCES OF EXPOSURE

Background Radiation, Effective Dose per Individual = 3.1 mSv	Percent
Radon and thoron	73
Space radiation	11
Radionuclides in the body	9
Terrestrial radiation	7
Medical Radiation, Effective Dose per Individual = 3.0 mSv	
Computed tomography	49
Nuclear medicine	26
Interventional fluoroscopy	14
Conventional radiography and fluoroscopy	11
Other Sources, Effective Dose per Individual = 0.13 mSv[a]	

[a]Other sources include consumer products, industrial and occupational exposures contributed to less than 3% of total effective dose in 2006.
Source: NCRP2009.
Note: No update to whole report, just medical sources.

disintegrate, of the different radionuclides vary, from less than a second for some to billions of years for others.[2,6] Radionuclides with a short half-life, such as ^{131}I (8 days) decay more rapidly, emitting more of their total energy in a shorter period of time and potentially causing more biological damage over a given period. Biological half-lives, which reflect physical characteristics and biological processes, also vary, tending to be longer with radionuclides that localize in bone (e.g., radium, strontium, plutonium) than with those that are deposited predominantly in soft tissue (e.g., iodine, cesium, tritium).[4]

SOURCES AND LEVELS OF IONIZING RADIATION EXPOSURE

Sources of ionizing radiation have been broadly characterized as environmental, medical, and occupational. Occupational exposure can occur in both environmental (e.g., Chernobyl clean-up workers) and medical settings (e.g., radiologic technologists). Epidemiological studies characterize doses as low (<100 mGy), medium (100 mGy to <1 Gy), and high (1 Gy and higher) (Table 68-2). The general population is exposed to relatively low doses through background radiation and common diagnostic medical tests like CT scans, and nuclear industry workers are exposed to very low doses under normal working conditions. Higher doses may be received accidentally by certain groups of radiation workers and historically specific populations exposed to radiation from atomic bombs, nuclear fallout, and radiotherapy.

Environmental exposures to ionizing radiation include natural background and historical releases during from the atomic bombings in Japan and nuclear tests, and various nuclear accidents. The major sources of natural background radiation are (a) space radiation from solar particles and cosmic rays ; (b) terrestrial radiations, which emanate from the thorium, uranium, radium, and other radioactive constituents of the earth's crust; (c) internal radiation, which is emitted by the potassium-40, carbon-14, radium, and other radionuclides normally present in living cells; and (d) radon, thoron, and their daughter or progeny elements, which are inhaled in indoor air as shown in Table 68-3.[7] The dose from cosmic rays increases appreciably with increasing altitude, so that as few as five North America-Asia airplane trips can cause a passenger to exceed the recommended dose of 1 mSv per year.[8,9] Similarly, the dose from internally deposited radium may be higher by a factor of 2 or more in geographic regions where the earth's crust is rich in this element.[10] The doses to the bronchial epithelium from radon's decay products also may vary by an order of magnitude or more, depending on the concentration of radon in indoor air, which covers a wide range in homes reaching as high as levels in underground uranium mines.[7]

Radiation has been used in medicine for over a century, and undoubtedly has resulted in enormous advances in diagnosis and treatment of disease.[11] However, medical sources of ionizing radiation represent an increasingly greater proportion of ionizing radiation exposure in recent years, with an estimated doubling of effective dose from 3 to 6 mSv between 1980 and 2006 in the United States due largely to an increased administration of CT scans, nuclear medicine, and interventional fluoroscopy. The largest contributor is the use of CT scans in medical diagnosis (Table 68-3), which now represents nearly 50% of the effective dose to an individual living in the United States.[7] Changes in technology, campaigns for dose optimization, and changes in reimbursement appear to have reduced the annual nontherapeutic medical radiation dose to the U.S. population by 15–20% in 2016 when compared to 2006.[12]

Other sources of ionizing radiation include (a) consumer products such as cigarettes which expose pack-a-day smokers to additional annual effective doses ranging from 0.08 to 0.6 mSv from inhaled radionuclides in the smoke that deposit in the lungs, and radioactive minerals in building materials, phosphate fertilizers, and crushed rock; (b) radionuclides and radioactive fallout from nuclear weapons, nuclear accidents, and nuclear power generation; and (c) occupational radiation received by medical, aviation, and nuclear power workers who receive annual effective average doses of 1.1 mSv.[7]

Radiation accidents have been of heightened concern for workers and members of the public alike.[13,14] There have been five major nuclear accidents since nuclear power has been used to produce electricity. These include the 1957 accident at Windscale in the United Kingdom, the 1957 Mayak Production Association accident in Russia, the 1979 accident at Three Mile Island in the United States, the 1986 Chernobyl accident in Ukraine, and most recently, the 2011 accident at the Daiichi Nuclear Power Plant in Fukushima, Japan. These events resulted in the release of 1 PBq (petabecquerel, a standard international unit of radioactivity equal to 10^{15} becquerels), 740, 0006, 1760, and 120 PBq, respectively.[15–17] Prior to Chernobyl, there were over 280 nuclear reactor accidents reported across the world, resulting in the exposure of more than 1350 persons and 33 fatalities.[13] In the Chernobyl accident alone, enough radioactivity was released to require the evacuation of tens of thousands of people and farm animals from the surrounding area.[4,18,19] The large amounts of radioactive iodine that were released in the accident have since been implicated in an increase in the incidence of thyroid cancer in Belarus and the Ukraine.[20] More numerous than reactor accidents, although less catastrophic, are accidents involving medical and industrial sources.[19]

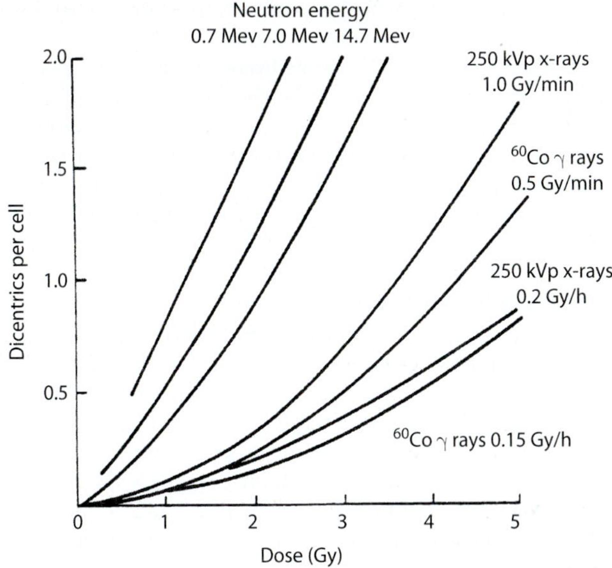

FIGURE 68-2. Frequency of dicentric chromosome aberrations in human lymphocytes in relation to dose, dose rate, and quality of irradiation in vitro. (*Source:* Adapted with permission from Lloyd DC, Purrott RJ. Chromosome aberration analysis in radiological protection dosimetry. *Radiat Protect Dosim*. 1981;1:19–28.[15])

RADIATION EFFECTS

Types of Effects

In radiation protection, it is customary to distinguish between effects for which there are dose thresholds and effects for which there may be no dose thresholds. The former—so-called *nonstochastic* (or *deterministic*) effects—include various tissue reactions that are elicited only by doses large enough to kill many cells in the affected organs.[21] The latter, by contrast—which include the mutagenic and carcinogenic effects of radiation—are viewed as *stochastic* (or *probabilistic*) phenomena of a type that may be produced by a subtle change within a single cell in an affected organ and which are therefore expected to increase in frequency as linear nonthreshold functions of the dose of radiation.[4,6,22–24]

Effects on Genes and Chromosomes

Any molecule in the cell may be damaged by ionizing radiation, but damage to a single gene, unless properly repaired, may permanently alter or kill the cell. Such damage may be caused by the radiation energy that is deposited within an affected cell itself, or it may be caused by the effects of radiation on one or more of its neighboring cells (the so-called "bystander effect").[25] A dose that is large enough to kill the average dividing cell (1–2 Sv) suffices to cause dozens of lesions in its DNA. Most such lesions tend to be reparable, depending on the effectiveness of the cell's repair processes, but residual or misrepaired damage, expressed in the form of mutations, appears to increase cancer risk as a linear-no threshold function of the dose in human somatic cells and the cells of other organisms. The frequency of such mutations approximates 10^{-5}–10^{-6} per locus per Sv, depending on the genetic locus and conditions of irradiation.[21,24]

Chromosomal aberrations also increase in frequency with the dose of ionizing radiation, approximating 0.1 aberrations per cell per Sv in the low-to-intermediate dose range (Fig. 68-2).[26] The dose-dependent increase in the frequency of such aberrations, which has been reported to be detectable in radiation workers and persons residing in areas of elevated natural background radiation levels, may be of use as a biological dosimeter or biomarker of radiation exposure in radiation accident victims.[27,28]

The yields of mutations and chromosome aberrations produced by a given dose of low-LET radiation are lower at low-dose rates than at high dose rates; but the weight of evidence suggests that there may be no threshold in the dose-response relationship for these effects.[22,24,29] Extensive studies of the children of the A-bomb survivors have been largely negative thus far, but the findings are not incompatible statistically with the results of experiments on laboratory animals, in which heritable mutagenic effects of radiation have been well documented.[22,24]

Cytotoxic and Mental Health Effects

As noted early in the twentieth century by Bergonie and Tribondeau, cells generally vary in radiosensitivity in proportion to their rate of proliferation and inversely in relation to their degree of differentiation. Cells of only few types (e.g., lymphocytes and oocytes) are radiosensitive in a nonproliferative state. The percentage of clonogenic human cells retaining the ability to proliferate decreases exponentially with increasing dose as higher doses kill more cells, acute exposure to 1–2 Sv typically sufficing to reduce the surviving population by 50%. In experiments, successive exposures tend to be less than fully additive in their cytotoxicity if they are sufficiently separated in time, owing to repair of radiation damage during the interim.[4,23,24]

Through cytotoxic effects on dividing cells, intensive irradiation can give rise to a wide variety of acute and chronic tissue reactions, depending on the tissue or organ irradiated, the dose, and the conditions of exposure.[4] In such reactions—exemplified by erythema, or redness, of the skin, depression of the blood count, impairment of fertility, and cataract of the lens—interference with normal cell replacement in the exposed area leads to hypoplasia, functional disturbances, and atrophy of the affected part. If enough stem cells remain viable to repopulate the tissue in question, regeneration may ensue within days or weeks; however, a second wave of degenerative changes may occur months or years later, as a result of residual damage and gradually progressive radiation-induced fibrosis, that is, scarring, of the exposed connective tissue and vasculature.[4,30] Depending on their anatomical location and severity, such changes can cause a dose-dependent decrease in the long-term survival of the affected individuals.[31,32]

A number of noncancer effects have been associated with increasing radiation dose in epidemiological studies, though with generally lower dose-response effects than observed for cancer. Among atomic bomb survivors who received low to moderate whole body external radiation, radiation-related risks were found for circulatory disease, including heart disease, stroke, and hypertension.[33] Risk of cataract among the atomic bomb survivors and occupationally exposed workers has also been established, with evidence of increased risk at lower dose levels than previously shown.[33,34] Noncancer thyroid diseases such as follicular adenoma and hypothyroidism have also been reported among childhood cancer survivors and residents of Ukraine and Belarus exposed to Chernobyl fallout.[35–39] Substantial mental health impacts have also been experienced by radiation exposed populations, particularly those affected by disasters, including cognitive impairment, depression, anxiety, social stigma, and lifestyle changes.[33]

Acute Radiation Syndrome

Intensive irradiation of the hemopoietic system, gastrointestinal tract, lungs, or brain can cause the *acute radiation syndrome.* This syndrome may take one of several forms, depending on the size and anatomical distribution of the dose (Table 68-4). In each of the forms, anorexia, nausea, and vomiting typically occur within minutes or hours after irradiation, to be followed by a symptom-free interval that lasts until the onset of the next phase of the illness. Acute radiation syndrome has occurred under extraordinary circumstances of accidents and major upsets, such as the Chernobyl reactor disaster.

Carcinogenic Effects

Cancers of various types have been observed to increase in frequency with the dose of ionizing radiation in atomic bomb survivors, nuclear industry workers, radiotherapy patients, early radiologists, radium dial painters, uranium and other radon-exposed underground miners, and other irradiated human populations.[4,22] With the exception of acute leukemia and thyroid cancer, the additional risk has generally not appeared until years or decades after irradiation, and despite important implications in identifying a molecular signature for radiation exposure, studies examining radiation sensitive cancers (e.g., sarcomas, thyroid cancer) have not yet identified signatures as being produced specifically by radiation, as opposed to some other cause.[16] The causal connection between such cancers and previous irradiation can, therefore, be inferred only from appropriate epidemiological analysis of the dose–response relationship interpreted in the context of deep understanding of how radiation affects cells and DNA in particular.[22–24]

The most extensive dose-response data available thus far have come from the study of the Japanese atomic bomb survivors, in whom the overall incidence of cancer has increased roughly in proportion with the radiation dose among females, while upward curvature

TABLE 68-4 MAJOR FORMS AND FEATURES OF THE ACUTE RADIATION SYNDROME

Time after Irradiation	*Cerebral Form (>50 Sv to Brain)*	*Gastrointestinal Form (10–20 Sv to Intestines)*	*Hemopoietic Form (2–10 Sv to Bone Marrow)*	*Pulmonary Form (>6 Sv to Lungs)*
First day	Nausea	Nausea	Nausea	Nausea
	Vomiting	Vomiting	Vomiting	Vomiting
	Diarrhea	Diarrhea	Diarrhea	
	Headache			
	Disorientation			
	Ataxia			
	Coma			
	Convulsions			
	Death			
Second week		Nausea		
		Vomiting		
		Diarrhea		
		Fever		
		Erythema		
		Prostration		
		Death		
Third–sixth weeks			Weakness	
			Fatigue	
			Anorexia	
			Fever	
			Hemorrhage	
			Epilation	
			Recovery or	
			Death	
Second–eighth months				Cough
				Dyspnea
				Fever
				Chest pain
				Respiratory failure

Source: Data from United Nations Scientific Committee on the Effects of Atomic Radiation (UNSCEAR). *Sources, Effects, and Risks of Ionizing Radiation, Report to the General Assembly, with Annexes.* New York: United Nations; 1988.[11]

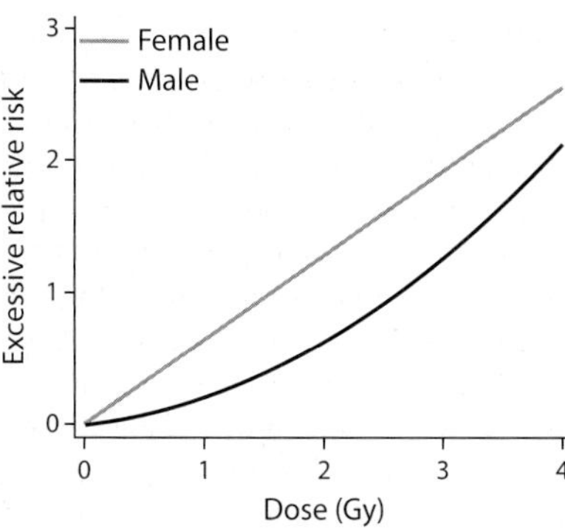

FIGURE 68-3. Excess relative risk of solid cancer for males and females in the Life Span Study of atomic bomb survivors at attained age 70 following exposure at age 30. Notes: Analyses of solid cancer use dose to the colon in Gray. The null value for the excess relative risk is zero. (*Source:* Modified from Grant EJ, et al. Solid cancer incidence among the life span study of atomic bomb survivors: 1958–2009. *Radiat Res.* 2017;187(5):513–37.)

TABLE 68-5 RELATIONSHIP OF IONIZING RADIATION TO CANCER RISKS AT 1 GY IN THE LIFE SPAN STUDY OF ATOMIC BOMB SURVIVORS*

Caused by Radiation	Cancer Sites
Yes	Bladder, breast, lung, leukemia (non-CLL), brain/CNS, ovary, thyroid, colon, esophagus, oral, stomach, liver, nonmelanoma skin, bone, soft tissue, pancreas, rectum
Possibly	Endometrial, CLL, multiple myeloma
Unclear	NHL, prostate, renal cell, cervix, gallbladder, melanoma

*For age at exposure at 30 and attained age at 70.
Sources: Preston 2007, HSU 2013, Modified from Thun.

in the dose–response relationship was noted for men (Fig. 68-3).[40] Considering the uncertainty in these findings, findings from the A-bomb survivors study, in agreement with other epidemiological studies, have largely demonstrated a linearity in the radiation dose–response relationship for all solid cancers, and many major cancer sites. The radiation-related risk of a disease is typically expressed as the excess relative risk per Gray (ERR/Gy), with zero representing the null of no association between radiation exposure and disease risk.

The magnitude of the dose-dependent increase varies, however, from one type of cancer to another, and not all organs appear to be radiation sensitive or there is insufficient data to draw a conclusion (Table 68-5).[41] The most extensive data available to date concerning dose-response relationships for individual types of cancer pertain to leukemia, cancer of the female breast, and cancer of the thyroid gland.

Leukemia. The frequencies of most major types of leukemia have been observed to increase with dose after exposure of the whole body or a major part of the hemopoietic system. In A-bomb survivors and other irradiated populations, the increases (except for chronic lymphocytic leukaemia) have appeared within 2–5 years after exposure; have been dose dependent, averaging approximately one to three cases per 10,000 persons per year per Sv to the bone marrow over the first 25 years after irradiation; and have persisted for 15 years or longer, depending on the type of leukemia, age at irradiation, and other variables.[22,24] A comparable excess has been reported in radiation workers, based on combined analyses of different occupational cohorts.[22,42,43] Risk of chronic lymphocytic leukemia has also been found to be associated with radiation exposure among Chernobyl clean-up workers.[44] While the data do not suffice to characterize the shape of the dose-incidence relationship precisely, they appear to be most consistent with a linear-quadratic function, that is, a curvilinear relationship without a threshold.[22,23]

Leukemia has also been observed to be increased in frequency in children who were x-irradiated prenatally through the abdominal radiographic examination of their mothers, the increase approximating 25 cases per 10,000 per Sv per year during the first 10 years of life.[22,24,43] Although no such increase was evident in prenatally exposed A-bomb survivors, the estimate is imprecise in view of the limited numbers of such survivors.[43] Irradiation of maternal or paternal germ cells also has been postulated to account for excesses of leukemia that have been observed in children subsequently conceived by some exposed individuals, but the weight of evidence argues against this hypothesis.[43]

Breast Cancer. The incidence of breast cancer has appeared to increase in proportion to the radiation dose in women surviving A-bomb irradiation, women given radiotherapy to the breast for acute postpartum mastitis, women fluoroscoped repeatedly in the treatment of pulmonary tuberculosis with artificial pneumothorax, a long-abandoned therapy, and women employed as radium dial painters.[4,22,45,46] In all four groups, the excess did not become evident until at least 5–10 years after irradiation, depending on age at the time of exposure, and it persisted for the duration of follow-up. The excess, averaged over all ages, has also been of similar magnitude in each group, in spite of marked differences among the groups in the rapidity with which the total doses of radiation were received, implying that successive small doses were highly additive in their cumulative carcinogenic effects.[4,22,46]

Susceptibility decreases markedly with increasing age at the time of irradiation, little excess being detectable in women exposed beyond the age of 40.[45,47,48] Following exposure during adolescence, moreover, the resulting cancers are similar in age distribution to those occurring in the general population, implying that the expression of the carcinogenic effects of radiation on the breast depends on the hormonal stimulation associated with sexual maturation.[47,48] The most recent study of breast cancer among A-bomb survivors found that radiation-related risk increased among women with earlier age at menarche and with radiation exposure during puberty.[45]

Thyroid Cancer. The thyroid gland is at particular risk because of the high rate of cell turnover. Dose-dependent excesses of thyroid cancer have been observed in A-bomb survivors, patients treated with x-rays for various benign conditions in childhood, Marshall Islanders and others exposed during childhood to radioactive fallout from nuclear weapons tests, and children exposed to radionuclides from the Chernobyl accident.[4,22] The cancers have consisted mainly of papillary carcinomas and have typically been preceded by a latent period of 10 years or longer, after which their frequency has remained elevated for the duration of follow-up, though risks do decline over time.[49] Children appear to be several times more susceptible to the induction of such tumors than adults, and females several times more susceptible than males.[4,22] The dose–incidence relationship after therapeutic x-irradiation of the neck in infancy has been observed to be consistent with a linear-no threshold function, corresponding to approximately four additional cancers per 10,000 persons per Sv per year, with an excess evident at doses as low as 65 mSv.[4,22,24]

Lung Cancer. Radiation dose-dependent excesses of lung cancer have been observed in A-bomb survivors, workers exposed to plutonium at the Mayak nuclear facility, radon-exposed miners, and people exposed to radon decay products in their homes.[50–52] Among atomic bomb survivors, smoking-associated excess relative risks were significantly larger for small-cell and squamous-cell carcinomas than for adenocarcinoma, while the excess relative risks of radiation were highest for small-cell carcinoma and adenocarcinoma.[53] In contrast to the radiation dose-response for most cancers in the atomic bomb survivors, increasing age at the time of exposure appears to be associated with increasing susceptibly for development of lung cancer.[50] Of continued interest is characterization of the joint effect of radiation with cigarette smoking, the leading cause of lung cancer worldwide. In the most recent study of atomic bomb survivors, the ERR/Gy for lung cancer was significantly higher for low-to-moderate smokers than for heavy smokers, with little evidence of any radiation-associated excess risk in heavy smokers.[50] An evaluation of studies of populations exposed to radon found evidence for a synergistic interaction between smoking and radon so that the number of cancers induced in ever-smokers by radon is greater than one would expect from the adding the number of cases from smoking alone and radon alone.[51] However, the degree of interaction is less than multiplicative, that is, that expected from the product of the risks of smoking and radon exposure separately.

Assessment of the Risks from Low-Level Exposure. This topic is of long-standing interest because of its relevance to radiation protection at the doses most commonly experienced. Although existing evidence does not suffice to characterize precisely the dose-incidence relationship for the carcinogenic effects of low-level radiation or to exclude the possibility that a threshold for such effects may exist in the millisievert dose range, the available epidemiologic and experimental data argue against the likelihood of such a threshold, in spite of evidence that cells have some capacity to adapt to low-level radiation.[4,22–24] Attempts to estimate the risks of radiation-induced cancers from low doses have, therefore, generally been based on the assumption that the overall incidence of cancer varies as a linear-nonthreshold function of the dose. Extrapolations based on the linear-nonthreshold model have yielded risk estimates for cancers of different organs (Table 68-6). These estimates imply that less than 3% of all cancers in the general population are attributable to natural background radiation, although a larger percentage—perhaps up to 10%—of lung cancers may be attributable to inhalation of indoor radon.

In radiation-exposed individuals with cancer, the issue of compensation arises in some circumstances: those exposed from testing of nuclear weapons, underground uranium miners, and others. In such individuals, some statutes base compensation around the extent to which radiation is estimated to have contributed to causation. The extent to which a cancer arising in a previously irradiated individual can be attributed to the radiation that he or she may have received cannot be determined with certainty; however, it may be assumed to increase with the radiation dose in question, all other things being equal.[54,55] On the basis of this assumption, one may arrive at a crude estimate of the probability of causation, given sufficient knowledge of the dose, when the dose was received, and the extent to which other causal factors also may have been involved.[54,55] Such estimates of probability of causation are used as a basis for compensation for certain radiation-exposed individuals and tools have been developed for that purpose.

TABLE 68-6 ESTIMATED LIFETIME RISKS OF CANCER ATTRIBUTABLE TO 0.1 SV (10 REM) LOW-DOSE-RATE IRRADIATION[*]

	Excess Cancer Deaths per 100,000	
Type or Site of Cancer	***(No.)***	***(%)[a]***
Colon	95	5
Lung	85	3
Bone marrow (leukemia)	50	10
Stomach	50	8
Breast	45	2
Urinary bladder	25	4
Esophagus	10	3
Liver	15	8
Gonads	15	3
Thyroid	5	5
Bone	3	3
Skin	2	2
Remainder	100	2
Total	500	2

[*]Modified from International Commission on Radiological Protection. Recommendations of the International Commission on Radiological Protection. ICRP Publication 60. Ann ICRP 21, No. 1–3. Oxford: Pergamon Press; 1991 and Puskin JS, Nelson CB. Estimates of radiological cancer risks. *Health Phys.* 1995;69:93–101.
[a]Percentage increase in spontaneous "background" risk expected for a nonirradiated population.

Effects of Prenatal Irradiation

Apart from the relatively high susceptibility of the unborn child to the carcinogenic effects of ionizing radiation, noted above, the embryo is also susceptible to tissue reaction effects and the teratogenic effects of radiation. Thus, although tissue reactions and teratonogenic effects are generally considered to be nonstochastic in nature, exposure to as little as 0.25 Sv during critical stages of organogenesis has sufficed to cause malformations of many types in laboratory animals,[56,57] and similar developmental disturbances have been reported to follow intensive prenatal irradiation in humans.[4,22,24,57] Noteworthy examples include a dose-dependent increase in the frequency of severe mental retardation and dose-dependent decreases in IQ and school performance scores in A-bomb survivors who were irradiated between the 8th and 15th weeks (and to a lesser extent the 16th and 25th weeks) after conception.[4,22,24,57] Furthermore, unlike mutagenic and carcinogenic effects, which are expressed in only a small percentage of exposed individuals, some disturbance of growth and development may be projected to affect all who are exposed at a susceptible stage to a dose that exceeds the relevant threshold. Thus, while only a small percentage of the individuals who were exposed prenatally to atomic bomb radiation at a critical stage in brain development (i.e., 8–26 weeks after conception) exhibited severe mental retardation, a larger percentage exhibited less marked decrements in intelligence and school performance, implying that there was a dose-dependent downward shift in the distribution of intelligence levels within the entire cohort.[19,24]

Adaptive Responses and Hormesis

A brief exposure to a small, "conditioning" dose of x-rays or gamma rays has been observed experimentally to elicit an adaptive response that enhances growth and survival, augments the immune response, and increases resistance to the cytotoxic, genetic, and carcinogenic effects of a subsequent, larger "test" dose of radiation.[4,19,23,24,58,59] The adaptive response to radiation resembles in many respects adaptive responses elicited by other toxicants,[59] and it may account in part for the decrease in the biological effectiveness of X-rays and gamma-rays that generally occurs as the dose rate is reduced. These features of the adaptive response have prompted some observers to postulate that the dose-response relationships for the genetic and carcinogenic effects of ionizing radiation are biphasic or "hormetic" in nature; that is, that it increases with the dose at moderate-to-high levels of exposure but decreases with the dose at low levels of exposure.[58] This hypothesis, far reaching in its implications for radiation protection, remains to be validated, however, and the weight of existing evidence argues against it.[23,24,29,60,61] The same arguments for hormesis have been raised around exposures to chemicals.

RADIATION PROTECTION

With the abandonment of the threshold dose-response hypothesis for the mutagenic and carcinogenic effects of radiation, the goal of minimizing the risks of such effects has become pre-eminent in radiation

TABLE 68-7 RECOMMENDED LIMITS OF EXPOSURE TO IONIZING RADIATION FOR RADIATION WORKERS AND MEMBERS OF THE PUBLIC*

Type of Exposure	*Maximum Permissible Dose (mSv)*
A. *Occupational Exposures*	
1. For protection against stochastic effects	
a. Annual effective dose	50
b. Cumulative effective dose	Age × 10
2. For protection against nonstochastic effects in individual organs	
a. Lens of the eye (annual effective dose)	150
b. All other organs (annual effective dose)	500
3. Planned special exposures (effective dose)[a]	100
4. Emergency exposure	—[b]
B. *Public Exposures*	
1. Continuous or frequent exposure (effective dose per year)	1
2. Infrequent exposure (effective dose per year)	5
3. Remedial action recommended if:	
a. Annual effective dose would exceed	5
b. Effective dose from radon would exceed	0.007 jhm^{-1}
C. *Education and Training Exposures*[c]	
1. Annual effective dose	1
2. Annual equivalent dose to lens of the eye, skin, extremities	50
D. *Exposure of the Embryo and Fetus*	
1. Total equivalent dose	5
2. Equivalent dose in any 1 month	0.5

[a]Sum of internal and external exposures, excluding medical irradiation.
[b]Effective dose in any one planned event; or cumulative effective dose in planned special exposures should not exceed 100 mSv (10 rem) over a working lifetime.
[c]Short-term exposure to more than 100 mSv (10 rem) is justified only in lifesaving emergency situations.
Source: From National Council on Radiation Protection and Measurements. Limitation of Exposure to Ionizing Radiation (NCRP) Report No. 116, Bethesda, MD: National Council on Radiation Protection and Measurements; 1993. *Including natural background radiation exclusive of that from internally deposited radionuclides.

protection. In pursuit of this goal, the following guidelines have been recommended for any activity involving exposure to ionizing radiation: (a) *justification*, that is, the activity should not be considered justifiable unless it produces a sufficient benefit to those who are exposed, or to society at large, to offset any harm it may cause; (b) *optimization*, that is, the dose and/or likelihood of exposure should be kept as low as is reasonably achievable (ALARA), all relevant economic and social factors considered; and (c) *dose limits*, that is, the likelihood of exposure and the resulting dose to any individual should be subject to control by operating limits.[6]

The dose limits that have been recommended (Table 68-7) are intended to restrict exposures sufficiently to completely prevent nonstochastic effects in any organ of the body, even in the most sensitive members of the population.[6] Although the limits are not expected to protect completely against the mutagenic and carcinogenic effects of radiation, since there may be no thresholds for such effects, the limits are judged to be low enough to prevent the risks of mutagenic and carcinogenic effects from reaching levels that are socially unacceptable.[6,62]

Implicit in the above guidelines are requirements that any facility dealing with ionizing radiation (a) be properly designed; (b) be carefully planned and its operating procedures be overseen, including dose calibration; (c) have in place a well-conceived radiation protection program; (d) ensure that its workers are adequately trained and supervised; and (e) maintain a well-developed and well-rehearsed emergency preparedness plan, to be able to respond promptly and effectively in the event of a malfunction, spill, or other type of radiation accident.[6,62]

Since the doses received from medical radiographic examinations and from indoor radon constitute the most important controllable sources of exposure to ionizing radiation for members of the general public, measures to limit these exposures are also called for.[6,62] Other potential sources of exposure against which protection is warranted are those posed by the millions of cubic feet of radioactive and mixed wastes (mine and mill tailings, spent nuclear fuel, waste from the decommissioning of nuclear power plants, dismantled industrial and medical radiation sources, radioactive pharmaceuticals and reagents, heavy metals, polyaromatic hydrocarbons, and other contaminants), which tax increasingly severely the existing storage capacities at numerous waste sites.[63,64]

SUMMARY

Ionizing radiation exposure from occupational, accidental, and medical sources continues to be of public health significance and regulatory concern. The health effects of ionizing radiation are widely diverse, ranging from rapidly fatal injuries to cancers, birth defects, cataracts, and cardiovascular disease detected months or decades following exposure. The nature, frequency, and severity of the effects depend on the type of the radiation in question, as well as on the dose and conditions of exposure and affected tissues/organs. For most effects, radiosensitivity varies with the rate of proliferation and inversely with the degree of differentiation of the exposed cells; as a result, the embryo and growing child are especially vulnerable to radiation injury. Although many types of effects require relatively high levels of exposure to detect with epidemiological studies, the genotoxic and carcinogenic effects of ionizing radiation appear to increase in frequency as linear-nonthreshold functions of the dose. To minimize the risks associated with ionizing radiation, therefore, exposures need to be limited accordingly. Many advancements have been made in understanding and mitigating health risk of radiation exposure. However, radiation will continue to be an exposure in human life and it is important to monitor changing sources of radiation exposure and their health effects.

References

1. Upton AC. Radiation carcinogenesis. *Current Oncology*. New York: Elsevier; 1986, p. xviii, 459.
2. Shapiro J. *Radiation Protection: A Guide for Scientists and Physicians*. 3rd ed., Cambridge, MA: Harvard University Press; 1972, p. xx, 339.
3. International Commission on Radiological Protection. 1990 *Recommendations of the International Commission on Radiological Protection: User's Edition*. Oxford; New York: Pergamon Press; 1992, p. vii, 83.
4. Mettler FA, Upton AC. *Medical Effects of Ionizing Radiation*. 2nd ed. Philadelphia: W.B. Saunders; 1995, p. xii, 430.
5. United Nations. *Scientific Committee on the Effects of Atomic Radiation. Sources and Effects of Ionizing Radiation: United Nations Scientific Committee on the Effects of Atomic Radiation: UNSCEAR 2008 Report to the General Assembly, with Scientific Annexes*. New York: United Nations; 2010.
6. International Commission on Radiological Protection. The 2007 Recommendations of the International Commission on Radiological Protection. ICRP publication 103. *Ann ICRP*. 2007; 37(2-4):1–332.
7. Schauer DA, Linton OW. NCRP report no. 160, ionizing radiation exposure of the population of the United States, medical exposure—Are we

doing less with more, and is there a role for health physicists? *Health Phys.* 2009;97(1):1–5.
8. Alvarez LE, Eastham SD, Barrett SR. Radiation dose to the global flying population. *J Radiol Prot.* 2016;36(1):93–103.
9. Lochard J, Bartlett DT, Rühm W, Yasuda H, Bottollier-Depois J-F, Authors on behalf of ICRP. ICRP Publication 132: Radiological protection from cosmic radiation in aviation. *Ann ICRP.* 2016;45(1):5–48.
10. UNSCEAR 2000. The United Nations Scientific Committee on the Effects of Atomic Radiation. *Health Phys.* 2000;79(3):314.
11. ICRP, Khong P-L, Ringertz H, et al. ICRP publication 121: Radiological protection in paediatric diagnostic and interventional radiology. *Ann ICRP.* 2013;42(2):1–63.
12. National Council on Radiation Protection and Measurements. Medical radiation exposure of patients in the United States. Report No. 184. 2019: Bethesda, MD.
13. Lushbaugh CC, Fry SA, Ricks RC. Medical and radiobiological basis of radiation accident management. *Br J Radiol.* 1987;60(720):1159–63.
14. Nenot JC. Overview of the radiological accidents in the world, updated December 1989. *Int J Radiat Biol.* 1990;57(6):1073–85.
15. Bouville A, Linet MS, Hatch M, Mabuchi K, Simon SL. Guidelines for exposure assessment in health risk studies following a nuclear reactor accident. *Environ Health Perspect.* 2014;122(1):1–5.
16. Thun MJ, Linet MS, Cerhan JR, Haiman CA, and Schottenfeld DThun MJ, Linet MS, Cerhan JR, Haiman CA, and Schottenfeld D, eds. *Schottenfeld and Fraumeni Cancer Epidemiology and Prevention.* 4th ed. New York: Oxford University Press; 2018, p. xix, 1308.
17. Akleyev AV, Krestinina LY, Degteva MO, Tolstykh EI. Consequences of the radiation accident at the Mayak production association in 1957 (the 'Kyshtym Accident'). *J Radiol Prot.* 2017;37(3):R19–42.
18. United Nations. *Scientific Committee on the Effects of Atomic Radiation. Sources, Effects and Risks of Ionizing Radiation: 1988 Report to the General Assembly, with Annexes.* New York: United Nations; 1988, p. v, 647.
19. United Nations. *Scientific Committee on the Effects of Atomic Radiation. Sources and Effects of Ionizing Radiation: United Nations Committee on the Effects of Atomic Radiation: UNSCEAR 1993 Report to the General Assembly, with Scientific Annexes.* New York: United Nations; 1993, p. 922.
20. Bouville A, Likhtarev IA, Kovgan LN, Minenko VF, Shinkarev SM, Drozdovitch VV. Radiation dosimetry for highly contaminated Belarusian, Russian and Ukrainian populations, and for less contaminated populations in Europe. *Health Phys.* 2007;93(5):487–501.
21. Fry RJ. Deterministic effects. *Health Phys.* 2001;80(4):338–43.
22. United Nations. *Scientific Committee on the Effects of Atomic Radiation. Sources and Effects of Ionizing Radiation: United Nations Scientific Committee on the Effects of Atomic Radiation: UNSCEAR 2000 Report to the General Assembly, with Scientific Annexes.* New York: United Nations; 2000.
23. Boice JDJr. The linear nonthreshold (LNT) model as used in radiation protection: An NCRP update. *Int J Radiat Biol.* 2017;93(10):1079–92.
24. National Research Council (U.S.). *Committee to Assess Health Risks from Exposure to Low Level of Ionizing Radiation. Health Risks from Exposure to Low Levels of Ionizing Radiation: BEIR VII Phase 2.* Washington, DC: National Academies Press; 2006, p. xvi, 406.
25. Mothersill C, Seymour C. Radiation-induced bystander effects: Past history and future directions. *Radiat Res.* 2001;155(6):759–67.
26. Lloyd DC, Purrott RJ, Dolphin GW. Chromosome aberration dosimetry using human lymphocytes in simulated partial body irradiation. *Phys Med Biol.* 1973;18(3):421–31.
27. Edwards AA. The use of chromosomal aberrations in human lymphocytes for biological dosimetry. *Radiat Res.* 1997;148(5 Suppl):S39–44.
28. International Atomic Energy Agency. Biological dosimetry: Chromosomal aberration analysis for dose assessment. Technological report no. 260. 1986: Vienna.
29. Vilenchik MM, Knudson AGJr. Inverse radiation dose-rate effects on somatic and germ-line mutations and DNA damage rates. *Proc Natl Acad Sci U S A.* 2000;97(10):5381–6.
30. Carnes BA, Gavrilova N, Grahn D. Pathology effects at radiation doses below those causing increased mortality. *Radiat Res.* 2002;158(2):187–94.
31. Preston DL, Shimizu Y, Pierce DA, Suyama A, Mabuchi K. Studies of mortality of atomic bomb survivors. Report 13: Solid cancer and noncancer disease mortality: 1950–1997. *Radiat Res.* 2003;160(4):381–407.
32. Carnes BA, Grahn D, Hoel D. Mortality of atomic bomb survivors predicted from laboratory animals. *Radiat Res.* 2003;160(2):159–67.
33. Cullings HM. Impact on the Japanese atomic bomb survivors of radiation received from the bombs. *Health Phys.* 2014;106(2):281–93.
34. Little MP, Kitahara CM, Cahoon EK, et al. Occupational radiation exposure and risk of cataract incidence in a cohort of US radiologic technologists. *Eur J Epidemiol.* 2018;33(12):1179–91.
35. Inskip PD, Veiga LHS, Brenner AV, et al. Hypothyroidism after radiation therapy for childhood cancer: A report from the childhood cancer survivor study. *Radiat Res.* 2018;190(2):117–32.
36. Ostroumova E, Brenner A, Oliynyk V, et al. Subclinical hypothyroidism after radioiodine exposure: Ukrainian-American cohort study of thyroid cancer and other thyroid diseases after the Chornobyl accident (1998–2000). *Environ Health Perspect.* 2009; 117(5): 745–50.
37. Ostroumova E, Rozhko A, Hatch M, et al. Measures of thyroid function among Belarusian children and adolescents exposed to iodine-131 from the accident at the Chernobyl nuclear plant. *Environ Health Perspect.* 2013;121(7):865–71.
38. Zablotska LB, Bogdanova TI, Ron E, et al. A cohort study of thyroid cancer and other thyroid diseases after the Chornobyl accident: Dose-response analysis of thyroid follicular adenomas detected during first screening in Ukraine (1998–2000). *Am J Epidemiol.* 2008;167(3): 305–12.
39. Zablotska LB, Nadyrov EA, Polyanskaya ON, et al. Risk of thyroid follicular adenoma among children and adolescents in Belarus exposed to iodine-131 after the Chornobyl accident. *Am J Epidemiol.* 2015;182(9):781–90.
40. Grant EJ, Brenner A, Sugiyama H, et al. Solid cancer incidence among the life span study of atomic bomb survivors: 1958–2009. *Radiat Res.* 2017;187(5):513–37.
41. Preston DL, Ron E, Tokuoka S, et al. Solid cancer incidence in atomic bomb survivors: 1958–1998. *Radiat Res.* 2007;168(1):1–64.
42. Cardis E, Gilbert ES, Carpenter L, et al. Effects of low doses and low dose rates of external ionizing radiation: Cancer mortality among nuclear industry workers in three countries. *Radiat Res.* 1995;142(2):117–32.
43. Wakeford R. The cancer epidemiology of radiation. *Oncogene.* 2004;23(38):6404–28.
44. Zablotska LB, Bazyka D, Lubin JH, et al. Radiation and the risk of chronic lymphocytic and other leukemias among chornobyl cleanup workers. *Environ Health Perspect.* 2013;121(1):59–65.
45. Brenner AV, Preston DL, Sakata R, et al. Incidence of breast cancer in the life span study of atomic bomb survivors: 1958–2009. *Radiat Res.* 2018;190(4):433–44.
46. Preston DL, Mattsson A, Holmberg E, Shore R, Hildreth NG, Boice JDJr. Radiation effects on breast cancer risk: A pooled analysis of eight cohorts. *Radiat Res.* 2002;158(2):220–35.
47. Mettler FA, Upton AC, Kelsey CA, Ashby RN, Rosenberg RD, Linver MN. Benefits versus risks from mammography: A critical reassessment. *Cancer.* 1996;77(5):903–9.
48. Land CE, Tokunaga M, Koyama K, et al. Incidence of female breast cancer among atomic bomb survivors, Hiroshima and Nagasaki, 1950–1990. *Radiat Res.* 2003;160(6):707–17.
49. Tronko M, Brenner AV, Bogdanova T, et al. Thyroid neoplasia risk is increased nearly 30 years after the Chernobyl accident. *Int J Cancer.* 2017;141(8):1585–8.
50. Cahoon EK, Preston DL, Pierce DA, et al. Lung, laryngeal and other respiratory cancer incidence among Japanese atomic bomb survivors: An updated analysis from 1958 through 2009. *Radiat Res.* 2017;187(5):538–48.
51. Douple EB, Samet JM. Health effects of exposure to radon (BEIR VI). *Radiat Res.* 2000; 2: 784–7.
52. Gilbert ES, Sokolnikov ME, Preston DL, et al. Lung cancer risks from plutonium: An updated analysis of data from the Mayak worker cohort. *Radiat Res.* 2013;179(3)332–42.
53. Egawa H, Furukawa K, Preston D, et al. Radiation and smoking effects on lung cancer incidence by histological types among atomic bomb survivors. *Radiat Res.* 2012;178(3):191–201.
54. Rall JE, Beebe GW, Hoel DG. Report of the National Institutes of Health Ad Hoc Working Group to Develop radio-epidemiological Tables. NIH Publication No. 85-2748. 1985: Washington, DC.
55. Wakeford R, Antell BA, Leigh WJ. A review of probability of causation and its use in a compensation scheme for nuclear industry workers in the United Kingdom. *Health Phys.* 1998;74(1):1–9.
56. United Nations. *Scientific Committee on the Effects of Atomic Radiation and United Nations. General Assembly. Ionizing Radiation: Sources and Biological Effects: 1982 Report to the General Assembly, with Annexes.* New York: United Nations; 1982, p. v, 773.
57. United Nations. *Scientific Committee on the Effects of Atomic Radiation and United Nations. General Assembly. Genetic and Somatic Effects of*

Ionizing Radiation: United Nations Scientific Committee on the Effects of Atomic Radiation: 1986 Report to the General Assembly, with Annexes. New York: United Nations; 1986, p. v, 366.

58. Calabrese EJ, Baldwin LA. Radiation hormesis: The demise of a legitimate hypothesis. *Hum Exp Toxicol.* 2000;19(1):76–84.
59. McBride WH, Chiang CS, Olson JL, et al. A sense of danger from radiation. *Radiat Res.* 2004;162(1):1–19.
60. Wojcik A, Shadley JD. The current status of the adaptive response to ionizing radiation in mammalian cells. *Hum Ecol Risk Assess.* 2000;6(2):281–300.
61. Upton AC. Radiation hormesis: Data and interpretations. *Crit Rev Toxicol.* 2001;31(4-5):681–95.
62. National Council on Radiation Protection and Measurements. Limitations of Exposure to Ionizing Radiation. Report No. 116. 1993: Bethesda, MD.
63. U.S. Department of Energy (USDOE). U.S. Department of energy Interim Mixed Waste Inventory Report: Waste Streams, Treatment Capacities, and Technologies. DOE/NBM 1100, G.P. Office, Editor. 1993: Washington, DC.
64. Bradley DJ, Frank CW, Mikerin Y. Nuclear contamination from weapons complexes in the former Soviet Union and the United States. *Phys Today.* 1996;49(4):40–5.

CHAPTER

69 Nonionizing Radiation

Elizabeth Cahoon

Exposure to nonionizing radiation is ubiquitous in everyday life, from both the natural environment and manmade sources. Ultraviolet radiation (UVR) from sunlight has been linked with skin cancer, the most common cancer in populations of European decent. Radiofrequency radiation is a common exposure in modern life, enabling the use of communication technologies such as AM/FM radio, television, Wi-Fi, and mobile phones. Even if some risks associated with certain types of nonionizing radiation are small, the ubiquity of the exposures could result in a large number of adverse health effects, loss of productivity, and direct and indirect costs. Estimating the magnitude of the health risks and understanding the underlying biological mechanisms of nonionizing radiation can support primary prevention programs and regulations aimed at reducing risks among highly exposed populations.

The electromagnetic spectrum is comprised of a range of all possible frequencies of electromagnetic radiation (Fig. 69-1). The term *nonionizing radiation* refers to several forms of electromagnetic radiation of wavelengths longer than those of ionizing radiation, where wavelengths represent the distance between the corresponding points of two consecutive waves. As wavelength lengthens, frequency (i.e., the number of waves that pass through a fixed point in a unit of time) decreases, and the energy level of electromagnetic radiation decreases.[1] In order of increasing wavelength, nonionizing radiation includes UVR, visible light, infrared radiation, microwave radiation, radiofrequency, low-frequency, extremely low-frequency, and static fields radiation (Fig. 69-1). The wavelength, frequency, and energy range for electromagnetic forces are shown in Table 69-1.

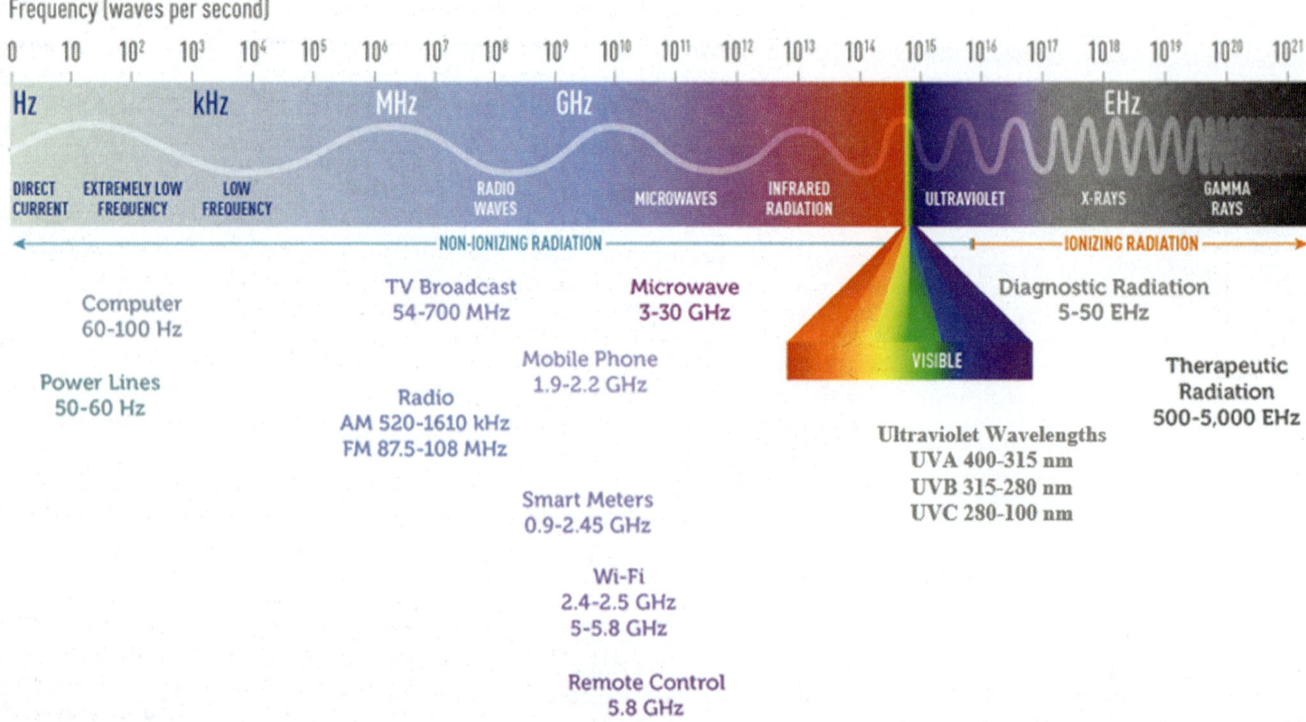

FIGURE 69-1. The electromagnetic spectrum. The electromagnetic spectrum represents all of the possible frequencies of electromagnetic energy. It ranges from extremely long wavelengths (extremely low-frequency exposures such as those from power lines) to extremely short wavelengths (x-rays and gamma rays) and includes both nonionizing and ionizing radiation. (*Source:* U.S. National Cancer Institute Electromagnetic Fields Fact Sheet Electromagnetic Fields and Cancer. Found at https://www.cancer.gov/about-cancer/causes-prevention/risk/radiation/electromagnetic-fields-fact-sheet.)

TABLE 69-1 ENERGY, FREQUENCY, AND WAVELENGTH RANGE FOR ELECTROMAGNETIC FORCES

Type of Radiation	Wavelength Range	Frequency Range	Energy Range
Ionizing (includes cosmic, gamma, and x-ray)	<100 nm	>3000 THz	>12.4 eV
Ultraviolet	100–400 nm	3000–750 THz	12.4–3.1 eV
UVC	100–280 nm	3000–1071 THz	12.4–4.4 eV
UVB	280–315 nm	1071–952 THz	4.4–3.9 eV
UVA	315–400 nm	952–750 THz	3.9–3.1 eV
Visible light	400–700 nm	750-429 THz	3.1–1.8 eV
Infrared	700 nm–1 mm	429 THz–300 GHz	1.8 eV–1.2 meV
Microwave	1 mm–1 m	300 GHz–300 MHz	1.2 meV–1.2 µeV
Radiofrequency	1 m–km	300 MHz–300 KHz	1.2 µeV–1.2 neV
Mobile phones		1.9–2.2 GHz	
AM radio		520–1610 kHz	
FM radio		87.5–108 MHz	
TV broadcast		54–700 MHz	
Low frequency	>90 km	<3000 Hz	0.012 neV
Extremely low frequency		3–300 Hz	
Power lines		50 Hz/60 Hz	
Static fields		0 Hz	

Source: Adapted from NIOSH Technical Report. Ionizing Radiation. Washington DC: NIOSH Publication No. 78–142; 1978.Abbreviations: nm = nanometer; m = meter; km = kilometer; Hz = Hertz; THz = terahertz; MHz = megahertz; KHz = kilohertz; eV = electron volt; meV = millielectron volt; µeV = microelectron volt; neV = nanoelectron volt.

The biological effect of radiation exposure depends on the type and duration of exposure and on the amount of energy absorbed by the tissue.[2] Although UV radiation penetrates through the body to a far lesser degree than ionizing radiation, UV radiation damages DNA, is responsible for the majority of skin cancers, and represents a major cause of eye disease, particularly cataracts.[3] The low- to mid-frequency electromagnetic radiations are also in the nonionizing radiation part of the electromagnetic spectrum, but in contrast to ionizing and UVR, are not known to cause direct damage to DNA, though several studies have shown they are able to increase the production of free radicals.[2]

ULTRAVIOLET RADIATION

Sources and Measurement

The sun is the major source of UVR. Radiation is emitted continuously from the sun with a range of wavelengths from 290 nanometers (nm) in the ultraviolet range to more than 2000 nm in the infrared range and maximum intensity at about 480 nm in the visible range. The UV spectrum spans wavelengths from 10 to 400 nm and is divided into far and extreme UV (10–120 nm), UVC (200–280 nm), UVB (280–320 nm), and UVA (320–400 nm).[4] The amount of UVR reaching the earth from the sun varies with season, time of day, latitude, altitude, and specific atmospheric conditions. The radiation from the sun is modified as it passes through the earth's atmosphere. Ozone, which is found in the upper atmosphere, that is, the stratosphere, absorbs the highest energy UVR. Approximately 95% of UVA and 5% of UVB penetrates the Earth's atmosphere, while nearly all of the shorter UVC wavelengths are filtered. The amount of solar UVR at the Earth's surface is greatest at midday and greater in summer than in winter. Window glass and light clothing efficiently filter out UVR, particularly in the UVB range.

Although sunlight is the main source of UVR for most of the population, some people are exposed to a nontrivial amount of UVR from artificial sources in cosmetic, medical, and occupational settings (Box 69-2). Artificial sources of UVR include, electric arc lights, welding arcs, and special ultraviolet lamps used in medical and industrial applications such as phototherapy, sterilization and disinfection, photocuring and hardening, and materials inspection.[5] Based on a 2014 systematic review and meta-analysis of 88 studies, for tanning beds used for cosmetic purposes the estimated prevalence rates for past-year exposure are 55% for university students, 19% for adolescents, and 34% for adults in Western countries.[6]

UVR is ubiquitous, making measurement of cumulative UV radiation exposure challenging in epidemiological studies. The UV Index, a standardized scale from 0 to 11+ (extreme UV) was developed to inform the public about UV protection. Environmental surrogates for personal UVR exposure used in epidemiological studies have include latitude, ground-based measurements (e.g., direct measurements with radiometers), and satellite-based measurements relying on information about an individual's residential history. Individual measures include self-reported time outdoors, occupation (Box 69-1), use of tanning beds, sunscreen, protective clothing, history of sunburns, polysulfone dosimeters, and measures of photoaging. These measures may be associated with exposure to UVR directly or personal susceptibility to skin cancer such as pigmentation. Some UV radiation measures reflect a combination of both environmental and individual-level factors such as history of sunburns.

Biological Mechanisms

Absorption of UVB photons by DNA causes direct DNA damage, which if not repaired can result in mutations to oncogenes and tumor suppressor genes, most frequently base substitutions of C by T at dipyrimidine sites, and also CC to TT tandem base substitutions.[7] These UV signature mutations are used to investigate whether UV radiation is a risk factor for a specific cancer. UV radiation of longer wavelengths, UVA, which is not absorbed by DNA, can induce DNA damage indirectly through the generation of reactive oxygen intermediates.[8] UVA has been found to induce mutations in the deeper basal layer of the epidermis, the location of the likely for skin cancers progenitor stem cells.[9] Exposure to UV radiation can also modulate the immune system both locally in the skin, and systemically at sites distant from the skin and location

BOX 69-1 Occupational Exposure to Ultraviolet Radiation

Outdoor construction workers
Agricultural and horticultural workers
Seamen and fisherman
Welders and glass blowers
Recreational workers (e.g., life guards and ski instructors)
Delivery persons
Policemen
Military personnel
Hospital and food irradiators (users of germicidal lamps for sterilization and disinfection)
Some scientific and medical workers (e.g., medical personnel administering phototherapy)
Workers in graphics, paper industry, and photocuring

Source: Adapted from International Commission on Non-Ionizing Radiation Protection. ICNIRP statement--Protection of workers against ultraviolet radiation. *Health Phys.* 2010;99(1):66-87. doi:10.1097/HP.0b013e3181d85908.

BOX 69-2 Occupational Exposure to Electromagnetic Fields

Radar workers (e.g., operators and repair of air traffic control, weather, military, marine, and speed control radars)
Electrical workers (e.g., electricians, electric power installers, power plant operators, telephone line installers and repairers, data processing repairers)
Machinists
Dental and medical device technicians (e.g., magnetic resonance imaging, cardiac monitors, ultrasounds, defibrillators, dentistry tools)
Broadcast equipment and photographic operators
Workers using computers
Train operators
Water and sewage treatment plant operators

Sources: Adapted from DHHS (NIOSH) Publication Number 96-129: EMFs In The Workplace. https://www.cdc.gov/niosh/docs/96-129/.html and Bowman JD et al., 2007.
https://www.who.int/peh-emf/publications/facts/fs226/en/.
**Bowman JD, Touchstone JA, Yost MG. A population-based job exposure matrix for power-frequency magnetic fields. J Occup Environ Hyg. 2007;4(9):715–28.Sources: Adapted from DHHS (NIOSH) Publication Number 96-129: EMFs In The Workplace. https://www.cdc.gov/niosh/docs/96-129/.html and Bowman JD et al., 2007.

of UV radiation exposure.[10] Immune responses to UV radiation involve both innate (i.e., nonspecific immunity that is naturally present and not due to prior sensitization to an antigen) and adaptive (i.e., acquired immunity that is activated by exposure to specific pathogens) immunity and have been linked to viral and bacterial infections, vaccination, carcinogenesis, and a number of autoimmune diseases.[11–13] Exposure to UV radiation also induces the production of vitamin D, an important hormone that controls calcium and phosphate metabolism and immune function.[14]

Carcinogenic Effects

Skin cancer is the most well-established adverse health effect of sun exposure, both through UV-induced DNA damage and the immunomodulatory effects of UV radiation.[11] Cutaneous malignant melanoma is responsible for the greatest number of skin cancer deaths worldwide and has been increasing over the last 30 years worldwide with differences observed between countries, by sex, and across different age groups.[15] Melanomas are more common among populations of northern European decent and in locations with higher ambient UV radiation. A number of inherited genes have also been found to be associated with increased melanoma risk including *CDKN2A*, which is common in familial melanoma, *MC1R* which regulates pigment, and *XP*, a mutation which hampers the repair of UV-induced DNA damage and is responsible for the condition xerodoma pigmentosum.[16,17] In 2012, an expert group from the International Agency for Research on Cancer (IARC), an intergovernmental agency part of the World Health Organization of the United Nations, concluded that there is sufficient evidence in humans that solar radiation causes cutaneous malignant melanoma.[4]

Skin cancers other than melanoma, notably keratinocyte carcinomas (basal and squamous cell carcinomas) have been consistently associated with measures of UV radiation. The majority of these lesions occurs on the sun-exposed sites of the head and neck and are much more common in areas of higher ambient UV radiation. While mortality is low in countries with adequate health care, the public health burden of these malignancies is considerable with total cases estimated to be over five million in 2012 and treatment, usually surgery, contributing to substantial health care expenditures.[18] Rare skin cancers such as Merkel cell carcinoma,[19] Kaposi sarcoma,[20] and sebaceous carcinoma[21] which occur disproportionately among individuals with severe immunosuppression (e.g., people infected with HIV or organ transplant recipients), have been recently associated with measures of ambient UV radiation.

UV radiation has also been suspected as a risk factor for a number of ocular tumors. The most common, uveal melanoma, located in the iris, ciliary body, or choroid of the eye has a mean age-adjusted incidence of 5.2 cases per million per year and a 5-year relative survival of 81% in the United States.[22] Uveal melanoma is more common in people with markers of a sun-sensitive phenotype such as those with light iris color, possibly because there is less protection from ultraviolet light with less melanin in the choroid and retinal pigment epithelium in blue or grey eyes.[23] However, epidemiological data do not consistently support UV radiation as a risk factor for uveal melanoma.[24] Less common ocular malignancies include ocular surface squamous neoplasia, which has been associated with increased time outdoors.[25] and conjunctival melanoma for which findings of UV mutational signature in tumor samples suggest a role for UVR.[26]

Noncarcinogenic Acute and Benign Ocular Effects

UVR exposure to the eye is associated with a number of acute and chronic benign ocular conditions resulting from damage to the cornea and lens. Accumulated UVR exposure to the cornea and conjunctiva may results in photokeratitis (e.g., ultraviolet keratitis), a painful eye condition lasting 6–24 hours also known as "snow blindness" or "welder's flash." Chronic UVR exposure has been associated with pterygium, triangular tissue growth on the cornea of the eye.[27] Cataract is the leading worldwide cause of blindness.[28] with cataract extraction representing the most common surgical procedure among Medicare beneficiaries in the United States.[29] A role for UVR in cataract development is supported by animal experiments conducted using high UVR doses,[30,31] biologic plausibility,[32,33] and some epidemiologic studies.[34–36]

Other Health Effects

The most common UV-induced skin disease is polymorphic light eruption (i.e., a rash caused by acquired photosensitivity), which occurs in approximately 18% of people of European ancestry.[37] UV-induced immune suppression has been found to play a role in reactivation and shedding of certain viruses, including herpes simplex virus and human papilloma virus.[12,13] Epidemiological studies have examined the association between UV radiation exposure and several autoimmune diseases including multiple sclerosis and type 1 diabetes mellitus. Evidence for reduced risk of multiple sclerosis with increasing ambient UV radiation comes from observations of reduced risk in populations living closer to the equator, particularly during early life, and animal studies showing the suppression of clinical symptoms in chronically UV-exposed mice.[13]

Ancient civilizations recognized that sunlight has a number of therapeutic properties.[38] UV radiation, through modulation of innate and adaptive immunity, has shown to be an effective treatment for cutaneous autoimmune disorders including psoriasis, atopic dermatitis, and vitiligo.[39,40] PUVA (psoralen and UVA) light therapy using psoralen to enhance the effect of UVA radiation has long been used to treat psoriasis, eczema, vitiligo, and cutaneous T-cell lymphoma. Photodynamic therapy is approved as a cancer treatment for certain sites by administering a photosensitising drug which is activated by UV radiation to kill nearby cancer cells.[41] Light therapy is also used in the treatment of sleep and mood disorders.[42]

Protection

Protective measures against the harmful effects of UVR include engineering controls, administrative controls, and personal protection.[5] Engineering controls involve the use of shading structures (e.g., solid or cloth roof structures, natural shade from trees) and protective equipment such as enclosures used to confine UV to a certain area. Administrative actions include educating and instructing of individuals who will be exposed, posting of notices, limiting access in the workplace, and regulating exposure time. Personal protection includes the use of sunscreens, appropriate clothing, sunglasses, and personal shields in occupationally exposed groups such as arc welders.

A number of community interventions and public health educational campaigns have been initiated to promote reduction in sun exposure in countries with high rates of skin cancer (e.g., Australia, New Zealand, the United Kingdom, the United States).[10,43–45] Much of the regulatory efforts aimed to reduce the skin cancer burden associated with UV radiation exposure is focused on indoor tanning devices and sunscreen formulations. Between 2003 and 2001, 11 countries enacted legislation to restrict access to indoor tanning.[46] Tanning salons were first restricted to adults only in France in 1997, banned for all ages in Brazil in 2009, Australia in 2015, and have been restricted to adults only by 42 U.S. states and the District of Columbia.[10,47] A primary concern in the formulation of sunscreens has been on providing broad-spectrum protection with filters against both UVB and UVA[48] since older formulations provided protection primarily from UVB-inducing sunburn.

ELECTRIC AND MAGNETIC FIELDS

Sources and Measurement

Electric and magnetic fields are produced by the movement of electrons, or current, through a wire and together are referred to as electromagnetic fields (EMFs). An electric field is produced by voltage, which is the pressure used to push charged electrons (current) through a wire and measured in volts per meter (V/m). Electric fields are produced even when a device is turned off but can be weakened by barriers such as walls. The flow of current through wires or electrical devices results in a magnetic field. As the current increases, the strength of a magnetic field, measured in microteslas (μT, or 10^{-6} T), also increases. Magnetic fields are produced when a device is turned on and current is flowing. In the case of power lines for which current is constantly flowing, magnetic fields are always present. However, the strength of a magnetic field decreases with increasing distance from its source. The units of measurement for radiofrequency radiation are watts per meter squared (W/m^2).

The two main categories of EMFs include (1) higher-frequency EMFs in the ionizing radiation part of the electromagnetic spectrum (**Chapter 69**) which can damage DNA directly and (2) low- to mid-frequency EMFs in the nonionizing radiation part of the electromagnetic spectrum, which are not known to directly damage DNA. Low- to mid-frequency EMFs include magnetic fields from electric power lines and appliances, radio waves, mobile phones, microwaves, infrared radiation, and visible light.

Whether there are health risks due to EMF exposure has been controversial for decades, largely because of the widespread penetration of mobile phones and the supporting infrastructure. Additionally, EMFs are emitted by many devices that are becoming ubiquitous in homes and offices.

Extremely Low-Frequency EMFs

EMFs in the 3–300 Hz frequency range are considered to be extremely low-frequency (ELF) EMFs. Transmission and distribution power lines (operating at 50–60 Hz) and electric appliances are the most common sources of ELF EMF exposures. The potential health effects of exposure to ELF EMFs remain controversial. No mechanism to explain how ELF EMFs can induce or promote cancer has been conclusively identified. In 2002, the IARC appointed a Working Group of experts to review all available evidence on static and extremely low frequency electric and magnetic fields.[49] This IARC Working Group classified ELF-EMFs as "possibly carcinogenic to humans," based on limited human evidence in for childhood leukemia seen at the highest power-frequency magnetic field levels. Pooled epidemiological studies have shown a less than twofold increase in risk for childhood leukemia for the highest exposed group, which represents approximately 3% of children.[50–52] No other cancers in children or adults have been associated with power-frequency magnetic field exposures. Static electric and magnetic fields and extremely low frequency electric fields were determined "not classifiable as to their carcinogenicity to humans."[49] A more recent report of the European Commission's Scientific Committee on Emerging and Newly Identified Health Risks concluded that, "new epidemiological studies are consistent with earlier findings of an increased risk of childhood leukemia with estimated daily average exposures above 0.3–0.4 μT."[53] However, "no mechanisms have been identified and no support is existing from experimental studies that could explain these findings, which, together with shortcomings of the epidemiological studies prevent a causal interpretation."

Radiofrequency Fields

Radiofrequency and microwave (RF/MW) radiation covers the 3 kHz–300 GHz frequency band of the electromagnetic spectrum. Sources of radiofrequency radiation include wireless telecommunication devices and equipment, including mobile phones, smart meters, and portable wireless devices, such as tablets and laptop computers.[54] Mobile phones operate in a frequency range of about 1.8–2.2 GHz in the United States.[49] The frequency spectrums associated with the wireless system vary with the protocol, for example, 3G or 5G. Other sources of radiofrequency radiation include radio and television signals, radar, satellite stations, magnetic resonance imaging, microwave ovens, television and computer screens, wireless local area networks, and mobile phone base stations. Exposures associated with electronic devices and base stations decrease with increasing distance from the source.

With over 5.1 billion subscribers worldwide by 2018, one of the most important public health concerns related to nonionizing radiation is the use of mobile phones.[55] Mobile phone use has been examined in relation to a broad range of health effects. Since the brain is the primary exposed organ, neurologic effects in children have been a focus of concern. Findings from studies examining memory, learning, and cognitive function have been inconsistent.[56–59] A consistent and major public health risk associated with mobile phone use is motor vehicle accidents caused by distracted driving.[60,61]

Over two decades ago, concern was raised about increased risk from brain cancer. Multiple epidemiological studies have been carried out, although there are challenging methodological issues and the technology has evolved over time. Several large epidemiological studies, conducted primarily in Europe, have examined the association between use of mobile phones and risk of benign and malignant brain tumors. The Interphone study was a multicenter large case-control study examining the risk of head and neck tumors using questionnaire data. Most of the analyses found no statistically significant increase in brain or central nervous system tumors related to mobile phone use.[55] However, an analysis among the Australian, Canadian, French, Israeli, and New Zealand components of the Interphone Study, there was a suggestion of an increased risk of glioma in long-term users with high exposures and, to a lesser extent for meningioma.[62] A large cohort study of 358,000 mobile phone subscribers set in Denmark found no significant increase in incidence of brain tumors with use of mobile phones.[63] In the Million Women Study, a large prospective cohort in the United Kingdom, self-reported long-term use of mobile phones was initially found to be associated with an increased risk of acoustic neuroma[64]; however, this association disappeared with updated follow-up.[65] A pooled analysis of two case-control studies in Sweden found a statistically significant increasing brain cancer risk for the cumulative hours of mobile phone use.[66] Analyses of brain cancer incidence trends in the United States and Europe during the time that mobile phone use increased considerably have not found evidence of increasing incidence over the relevant period.

In 1999, the Food and Drug Administration nominated mobile phone radiofrequency radiation exposures for study in experimental animal models by the U.S. National Toxicology Program (NTP). The NTP is an interagency program that coordinates toxicology research and testing across the U.S. Department of Health and Human Services. The NTP studied male and female rats and mice in a carefully designed 2-year experimental setting. A detailed description and peer-review summary of the research is available on the NTP website.[67] Briefly, animals were exposed to whole-body radiofrequency radiation in the range of 700–2700 mHz (i.e., 2G and 3G mobile phone frequencies) in highly specialized chambers. A small number of cancers of Schwann cells in the heart and noncancerous changes in the same tissues were observed for male rats, but not female rats, nor mice. Schwann cells in the hearts of rodents are similar to the type of cells that give rise to vestibular schwannomas (also known as acoustic neuromas), which some studies have suggested are increased in the heaviest mobile phone users. The NTP continues to study radiofrequency exposure in animal models to gain insight into the biological mechanisms of the findings.

An animal study carried out by the Ramazzini Institute reported an increase in heart schwannomas in male rats and nonmalignant Schwann cell growth in the hearts of male and female rats with the highest exposure levels.[68] However, details about the exposure methods and experimental conditions were missing, making the interpretation challenging.

In 2011, an IARC Working Group reviewed the evidence on radiofrequency EMF and concluded that this type of radiation is "possibly carcinogenic to humans (Group 2B)," based primarily on the epidemiological evidence on glioma and acoustic neuroma.[54] The animal bioassay results were not available at that time.

Protection

The International Commission on Non-Ionizing Radiation Protection and the Institute of Electrical and Electronics Engineers (IEEE) have set voluntary exposure limits based on acute exposures to EMF. For ELF, the standards seek to protect against shocks and burns, while for RF/MW radiation, they are designed to protect against thermal hazards. The United States does not have federally enforceable standards to regulate ambient exposures to any type of ELF EMFs or RF/MW radiation. There are two federal limits for specific products: one governing mobile phones and the other microwave ovens. The Federal Communications Commission has adopted the IEEE exposure limit for hand-held mobile phones: an SAR of 1.6 W/Kg averaged over 1 g of tissue. More than 30 years ago, the Food and Drug Administration adopted an emission standard of 1 mW/cm^2 at 5 cm from the door of a new microwave oven and 5 mW/cm^2 once it leaves the store.

References

1. Hall EJ, Giaccia AJ. *Radiobiology for the Radiologist*. 6th ed. Philadelphia: Lippincott Williams & Wilkins; 2006, p. ix, 546.
2. Saliev T, Begimbetova D, Masoud AR, Matkarimov B. Biological effects of non-ionizing electromagnetic fields: Two sides of a coin. *Prog Biophys Mol Biol*. 2019;141:25–36.
3. Lucas RM, McMichael AJ, Armstrong BK, Smith WT. Estimating the global disease burden due to ultraviolet radiation exposure. *Int J Epidemiol*. 2008;37(3):654–67.
4. IARC Working Group on the Evaluation of Carcinogenic Risks to Humans. Radiation. *IARC Monogr Eval Carcinog Risks Hum*. 2012;100(Pt D):303–7.
5. International Commission on Non-Ionizing Radiation Protection. ICNIRP statement—Protection of workers against ultraviolet radiation. *Health Phys*. 2010;99(1):66–87.
6. Wehner MR, Chren MM, Nameth D, et al. International prevalence of indoor tanning: A systematic review and meta-analysis. *JAMA Dermatol*. 2014;150(4):390–400.
7. Anna B, Blazej Z, Jacqueline G, Andrew CJ, Jeffrey R, Andezej S. Mechanism of UV-related carcinogenesis and its contribution to nevi/ melanoma. *Expert Rev Dermatol*. 2007;2(4):451–69.
8. Khan AQ, Travers JB, Kemp MG. Roles of UVA radiation and DNA damage responses in melanoma pathogenesis. *Environ Mol Mutagen*. 2018;59(5):438–60.
9. Halliday GM, Cadet J. It's all about position: The basal layer of human epidermis is particularly susceptible to different types of sunlight-induced DNA damage. *J Invest Dermatol*. 2012;132(2):265–7.
10. Thun MJ, Linet MS, Cerhan JR, Haiman C, Schottenfeld D.Thun MJ, Linet MS, Cerhan JR, Haiman C, Schottenfeld D. eds. *Schottenfeld and Fraumeni Cancer Epidemiology and Prevention*. 4th ed. New York: Oxford University Press; 2018, p. xix, 1308.
11. Hart PH, Norval M. Ultraviolet radiation-induced immunosuppression and its relevance for skin carcinogenesis. *Photochem Photobiol Sci*. 2018;17(12):1872–84.
12. Norval M. The effect of ultraviolet radiation on human viral infections. *Photochem Photobiol*. 2006;82(6):1495–504.
13. Norval M, Lucas RM, Cullen AP, et al. The human health effects of ozone depletion and interactions with climate change. Photochem Photobiol Sci. 2011;10(2):199–225.
14. Wacker M, Holick MF. Sunlight and vitamin D: A global perspective for health. *Dermatoendocrinol*. 2013;5(1):51–108.
15. Yang DD, Salciccioli JD, Marshall, Sheri A, Shalloub J. Trends in malignant melanoma mortality in 31 countries from 1985 to 2015. *Br J Dermatol*. 2020; 183(6):1056–64.
16. Tucker MA. Melanoma epidemiology. *Hematol Oncol Clin North Am*. 2009;23(3):383–95, vii.
17. Kraemer KH, DiGiovanna JJ. Xeroderma Pigmentosum. In: Adam MP, Ardinger HH, Pagon RA, et al., eds. *GeneReviews((R))*. Seattle, Washington: University of Washington; 1993.
18. Rogers HW, Weinstock MA, Fedman SR, Coldiron BM. Incidence estimate of nonmelanoma skin cancer (keratinocyte carcinomas) in the U.S. population, 2012. *JAMA Dermatol*. 2015;151(10):1081–6.
19. Clarke CA, Robbins HA, Tatalovich Z, et al. Risk of Merkel cell carcinoma after solid organ transplantation. *J Natl Cancer Inst*. 2015;107(2):dju382.
20. Cahoon EK, Engels EA, Freedman DM, Norval M, Pfeiffer RM. Ultraviolet radiation and Kaposi sarcoma incidence in a nationwide US cohort of HIV-infected men. *J Natl Cancer Inst*. 2017;109(5):djw267.
21. Sargen MR, Mai ZM, Engels EA, et al. Ambient ultraviolet radiation and sebaceous carcinoma incidence in the United States, 2000–2016. *JNCI Cancer Spectr*. 2020; 4(2):pkaa020.
22. Aronow ME, Topham AK, Singh AD. Uveal melanoma: 5-Year update on incidence, treatment, and survival (SEER 1973–2013). *Ocul Oncol Pathol*. 2018;4(3):145–51.
23. Kaliki S, Shields CL. Uveal melanoma: Relatively rare but deadly cancer. *Eye (Lond)*. 2017;31(2):241–57.
24. Shah CP, Weis E, Lajous M, Shields JA, Shields CL. Intermittent and chronic ultraviolet light exposure and uveal melanoma: A meta-analysis. *Ophthalmology*. 2005;112(9):1599–607.
25. Gichuhi S, Macharia E, Kabiru J, et al. Risk factors for ocular surface squamous neoplasia in Kenya: A case-control study. *Trop Med Int Health*. 2016;21(12):1522–30.
26. Swaminathan SS, Field MG, Sant D, et al. Molecular characteristics of conjunctival melanoma using whole-exome sequencing. *JAMA Ophthalmol*. 2017;135(12):1434–7.

27. Zhou WP, Zhu YF, Zhang B, Qiu WY, Yao YF. The role of ultraviolet radiation in the pathogenesis of pterygia (Review). *Mol Med Rep.* 2016;14(1):3–15.
28. Bourne RR, Stevens GA, White RA, et al. Causes of vision loss worldwide, 1990–2010: A systematic analysis. *Lancet Glob Health.* 2013;1(6):e339–49.
29. Schein OD, Cassard SD, Tielsch JM, Gower EW. Cataract surgery among Medicare beneficiaries. *Ophthalmic Epidemiol.* 2012;19(5):257–64.
30. Wu K, Shui YB, Kojima M, Murano H, Sasaki K, Hockwin O. Location and severity of UVB irradiation damage in the rat lens. *Jpn J Ophthalmol.* 1997;41(6):381–7.
31. Zigman S, Vaughan T. Near-ultraviolet light effects on the lenses and retinas of mice. *Invest Ophthalmol.* 1974;13(6):462–5.
32. Linetsky M, Raghavan CT, Johar K, et al. UVA light-excited kynurenines oxidize ascorbate and modify lens proteins through the formation of advanced glycation end products: Implications for human lens aging and cataract formation. *J Biol Chem.* 2014;289(24):17111–23.
33. Spector A. Oxidative stress-induced cataract: Mechanism of action. *FASEB J.* 1995;9(12):1173–82.
34. Delavar A, Freedman DM, Velazquez-Kronen R, et al. Ultraviolet radiation and incidence of cataracts in a nationwide US cohort. *Ophthalmic Epidemiol.* 2018;25(5–6):403–11.
35. West SK, Duncan DD, Munoz B, et al. Sunlight exposure and risk of lens opacities in a population-based study: The Salisbury Eye Evaluation project. *JAMA.* 1998;280(8):714–8.
36. Rosmini F, Stazi MA, Milton RC, Sperduto R D, Pasquini P, Maraini G. A dose-response effect between a sunlight index and age-related cataracts. Italian-American Cataract Study Group. *Ann Epidemiol.* 1994;4(4):266–70.
37. Rhodes LE, Bock M, Janssens SA, et al. Polymorphic light eruption occurs in 18% of Europeans and does not show higher prevalence with increasing latitude: multicenter survey of 6,895 individuals residing from the Mediterranean to Scandinavia. *J Invest Dermatol.* 2010;130(2):626–8.
38. Ackroyd R, Kelty C, Brown N, Reed M. The history of photodetection and photodynamic therapy. *Photochem Photobiol.* 2001;74(5):656–69.
39. Hart PH, Norval M, Byrne SN, Rhodes LE. Exposure to ultraviolet radiation in the modulation of human diseases. *Annu Rev Pathol.* 2019;14:55–81.
40. Singer S, Berneburg M. Phototherapy. *J Dtsch Dermatol Ges.* 2018;16(9):1120–9.
41. Dolmans DE, Fukumura D, Jain RK. Photodynamic therapy for cancer. *Nat Rev Cancer.* 2003;3(5):380–7.
42. Shirani A, St Louis EK. Illuminating rationale and uses for light therapy. *J Clin Sleep Med.* 2009;5(2):155–63.
43. Iannacone MR, Green AC. Towards skin cancer prevention and early detection: Evolution of skin cancer awareness campaigns in Australia. *Melanoma Manag.* 2014;1(1):75–84.
44. Tabbakh T, Volkov A,Wakefield M, Dobbinson S. Implementation of the SunSmart program and population sun protection behaviour in Melbourne, Australia: Results from cross-sectional summer surveys from 1987 to 2017. *PLoS Med.* 2019;16(10):e1002932.
45. Geller AC, Cantor M, Miller DR, et al. The Environmental Protection Agency's National SunWise School Program: Sun protection education in US schools (1999–2000). *J Am Acad Dermatol.* 2002;46(5):683–9.
46. Pawlak MT, Bui M, Amir M, Burkhardt DL, Chen AK, Dellavalle RP. Legislation restricting access to indoor tanning throughout the world. *Arch Dermatol.* 2012;148(9):1006–12.
47. Madigan LM, Lim HW. Tanning beds: Impact on health, and recent regulations. *Clin Dermatol.* 2016;34(5):640–8.
48. Mancuso JB, Maruthi R, Wang SQ, Lim HW. Sunscreens: An update. *Am J Clin Dermatol.* 2017;18(5):643–50.
49. Ahlbom A, Green A, Kheifets L, Savitz D, Swerdlow A, ICNIRP (International Commission for Non-Ionizing Radiation Protection) Standing Committee on Epidemiology. Epidemiology of health effects of radiofrequency exposure. *Environ Health Perspect.* 2004;112(17):1741–54.
50. Ahlbom A, Day N, Feychting M, et al. A pooled analysis of magnetic fields and childhood leukaemia. *Br J Cancer.* 2000;83(5):692–8.
51. Greenland S, Sheppard AR, Kaune WT, Poole C, Kelsh MA. A pooled analysis of magnetic fields, wire codes, and childhood leukemia. Childhood Leukemia-EMF Study Group. *Epidemiology.* 2000;11(6):624–34.
52. Kheifets L, Ahlbom A, Crespi CM, et al. Pooled analysis of recent studies on magnetic fields and childhood leukaemia. *Br J Cancer.* 2010;103(7):1128–35.
53. Scientific Committee on Emerging Newly Identified Health Risk. Opinion on potential health effects of exposure to electromagnetic fields. Bioelectromagnetics. 2015;36(6):480–4.
54. IARC, Non-Ionizing Radiation, Part 2: Radiofrequency Electromagnetic Fields. IARC Monographs on the Evaluation of Carcinogenic Risks to Humans, Volume 102. 1 ed. 2013: IARC Press.
55. GMSA. Global Data. 2020. https://www.gsmaintelligence.com/.
56. Zhang J, Sumich A, Wang GY. Acute effects of radiofrequency electromagnetic field emitted by mobile phone on brain function. *Bioelectromagnetics.* 2017;38(5):329–38.
57. Brzozek C, Benke KK, Zeleke BM, Abramson MJ, Benke G. Radiofrequency electromagnetic radiation and memory performance: Sources of uncertainty in epidemiological cohort studies. *Int J Environ Res Public Health.* 2018;15(4):592.
58. Foerster M, Thielens A, Joseph W, Eeftens M, Röösli M. A prospective cohort study of adolescents' memory performance and individual brain dose of microwave radiation from wireless communication. *Environ Health Perspect.* 2018;126(7):077007.
59. Guxens M, Vermeulen R, Steenkamer I, et al. Radiofrequency electromagnetic fields, screen time, and emotional and behavioural problems in 5-year-old children. *Int J Hyg Environ Health.* 2019;222(2):188–94.
60. Atchley P, Strayer DL. Small screen use and driving safety. *Pediatrics.* 2017;140(Suppl 2):S107–11.
61. Llerena LE, Aronow KV, Macleod J, et al. An evidence-based review: Distracted driver. *J Trauma Acute Care Surg.* 2015;78(1):147–52.
62. Cardis E, Armstrong BK, Bowman JD, et al. Risk of brain tumours in relation to estimated RF dose from mobile phones: Results from five Interphone countries. *Occup Environ Med.* 2011;68(9):631–40.
63. Frei P, Poulsen AH, Johansen C, Olsen JH, Steding-Jessen M, Schüz J. Use of mobile phones and risk of brain tumours: Update of Danish cohort study. *BMJ.* 2011;343:d6387.
64. Benson VS, Pirie K, Schüz J, et al. Mobile phone use and risk of brain neoplasms and other cancers: Prospective study. *Int J Epidemiol.* 2013;42(3):792–802.
65. Benson VS, Pirie K, Schüz J, Reeves GK, Beral V, Green J. Authors' response to: The case of acoustic neuroma: Comment on mobile phone use and risk of brain neoplasms and other cancers. *Int J Epidemiol.* 2014;43(1):275.
66. Hardell L, Carlberg M, Hansson K. Mild, pooled analysis of case-control studies on malignant brain tumours and the use of mobile and cordless phones including living and deceased subjects. *Int J Oncol.* 2011;38(5):1465–74.
67. NTP. Cell Phone Radio Frequency Radiation. 2018 [cited 2020 03/26/2020]. https://ntp.niehs.nih.gov/whatwestudy/topics/cellphones/index.html.
68. Falcioni L, Bua L, Tibaldi E, et al. Report of final results regarding brain and heart tumors in Sprague-Dawley rats exposed from prenatal life until natural death to mobile phone radiofrequency field representative of a 1.8GHz GSM base station environmental emission. *Environ Res.* 2018;165:496–503.

CHAPTER 70

Air Pollution

Jonathan M. Samet • Jim Zhang

INTRODUCTION

In 2020 as this chapter was written, the scientific evidence is certain: ambient air pollution, that is, contamination of outdoor air consequent to human activities, is a major, global cause of morbidity (ill health) and premature mortality (early death).[1] While the rise of ambient or outdoor air pollution is relatively recent in a historical context, air pollution has probably had adverse effects on human health throughout history. The use of fire for heating and cooking came with exposure to smoke outdoors and indoors, an exposure that persists today for the billions who use biomass fuels for cooking and heating. The rise of cities concentrated the emissions of pollutants from dwellings and industry and led to air pollution that received comment and was considered a danger to health. The problem of air pollution received attention centuries ago in London, polluted by widespread coal burning.[2] However, regulation was resisted even then.

The Industrial Revolution created new and powerful point sources of air pollution that were unregulated and placed throughout cities and other places where people lived and, with the twentieth century, continued industrialization and also electric power generation brought new point sources of pollution into areas adjacent to where people lived and worked. During the twentieth century, fossil fuel-powered vehicles became a ubiquitous and ever-increasing pollution source in higher income countries and created a new type of pollution—photochemical pollution, or "smog"—first recognized in the Los Angeles air basin in the 1940s.[3] The work of Haagen-Smidt identified the critical roles of sunlight, hydrocarbons, and nitrogen dioxides in the photochemical reactions that produced ozone and other oxidant species.[4] Now, ozone has become a ubiquitous pollutant globally as vehicle fleets have grown rapidly in cities around the world.[5]

In recent decades, air pollution has worsened across much of the world, driven by population growth, dense urbanization, and an explosive increase in vehicle numbers. The unprecedented growth of some urban areas into "megacities," such as Mexico City, São Paulo, London, Los Angeles, and Shanghai, has led to unrelenting and sometimes dangerously high air pollution from massive vehicle fleets and stagnant traffic and from polluting industries and coal-burning power plants. With population growth and urbanization, ever more megacities are anticipated; the current total of cities with a population over 10 million reached 33 in 2018 with a projected rise to 43 by 2030.[6]

While the problem of air pollution was noted centuries ago, the modern era of research on air pollution and health and evidence-driven air-quality regulation and management began at mid-twentieth century following a series of very high pollution episodes with disastrous health consequences in Europe and the United States.[7,8] The most dramatic was the London Fog of 1952, which caused thousands of deaths beyond expected based on the prior weeks and prompted some of the first studies of the health effects of air pollution (Fig. 70-1).[9] The levels of particulate matter (PM) air pollution reached during the 1952 Fog were approximately 100-fold greater than current air-quality standards for PM in the United States and Europe. In some cities in low- and middle-income countries, maximum PM concentrations still reach around 50% of the London Fog levels, raising concern that this disaster could be repeated.[10] In the United States, recognition of the public health consequences of air pollution also began at mid-twentieth century, driven by the rising problem of smog in southern California, episodes of visibly high pollution in major cities of the East Coast, such as New York City, and the 1948 air pollution episode in Donora, Pennsylvania, which caused 20 excess deaths and thousands of illnesses in a small town.[8,11]

The current era of air pollution research and control dates to these mid-century episodes, and regulations have been based around the stream of evidence on the adverse consequences of air pollution and the levels at which they occur. In the United States, the 1970 Clean Air Act and its subsequent Amendments directly acknowledge the critical role of evidence in driving regulation of major pollutants, the so-called "criteria" pollutants, where criteria refers to evidence in the Act.[12] The approach to understanding the health consequences of air pollution and strategies for control is broadly based and includes; characterization of pollutants in outdoor air as to their sources, concentrations, and chemical and physical properties; toxicological

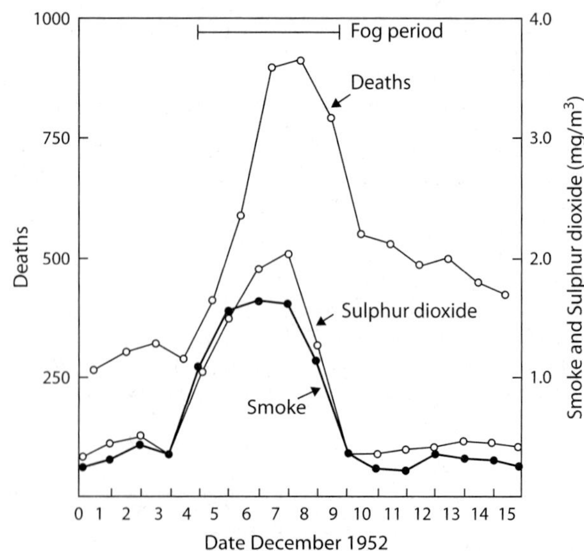

FIGURE 70-1. Deaths during the London Fog of 1952. (*Source:* Used with permission from Brimblecombe P. *The Big Smoke: A History of Air Pollution in London Since Medieval Times*. Routledge Kegan & Paul; 1987.

investigation on adverse effects caused by air pollutants and the underlying mechanisms of injury; and epidemiological studies of the health effects of air pollution in the real-world context. Application of these approaches has provided an increasingly strong and cohesive body of evidence that is the foundation for air-quality regulations worldwide.

There are a number of national and international groups that periodically assess the evidence on adverse effects of air pollution and provide guidance to the setting of standards and guidelines. In the United States, the Environmental Protection Agency (EPA) carries out reviews of the evidence as the basis for renewal of major air-quality standards (the National Ambient Air Quality Standards or NAAQS) on a 5-year cycle approximately.[13] Reviews are conducted by the United Kingdom, the European Commission and other nations. The World Health Organization (WHO) releases air-quality guidelines, which are currently being updated.[14] In reviewing the evidence, a judgment that the findings are strong enough to infer a causal relationship between a pollutant and an adverse outcome has great weight for regulation. The health risks associated with major air pollutants are reviewed below.

Evidence-driven regulations have had substantial impact on air quality in the United States and elsewhere, driving down levels of major pollutants (Fig. 70-2).[15] The success story in high-income countries, however, is not mirrored in many low- and middle-income countries where outdoor air pollution is a rising problem consequent to population growth, industrialization, and increasing numbers of vehicles. Many countries have given insufficient attention to air-quality management and regulation. As a result, the disease burden from ambient air pollution is substantial, sufficiently large for the World Health Organization Director, Tedros Ghebreyesus, to characterize air pollution as "the new tobacco." That comment reflects the attribution of 4.2 million premature deaths annually to outdoor air pollution.[1]

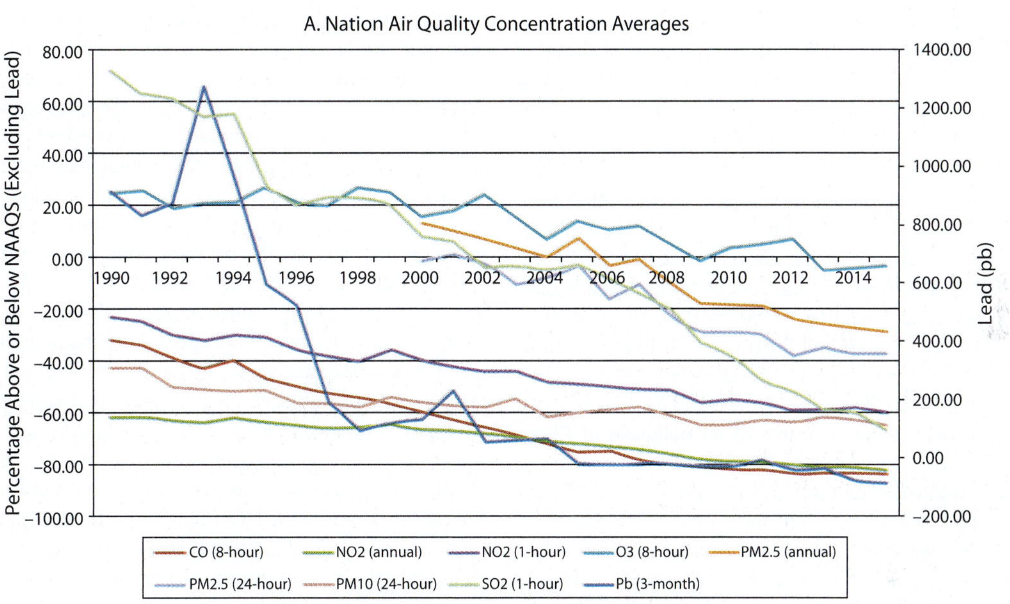

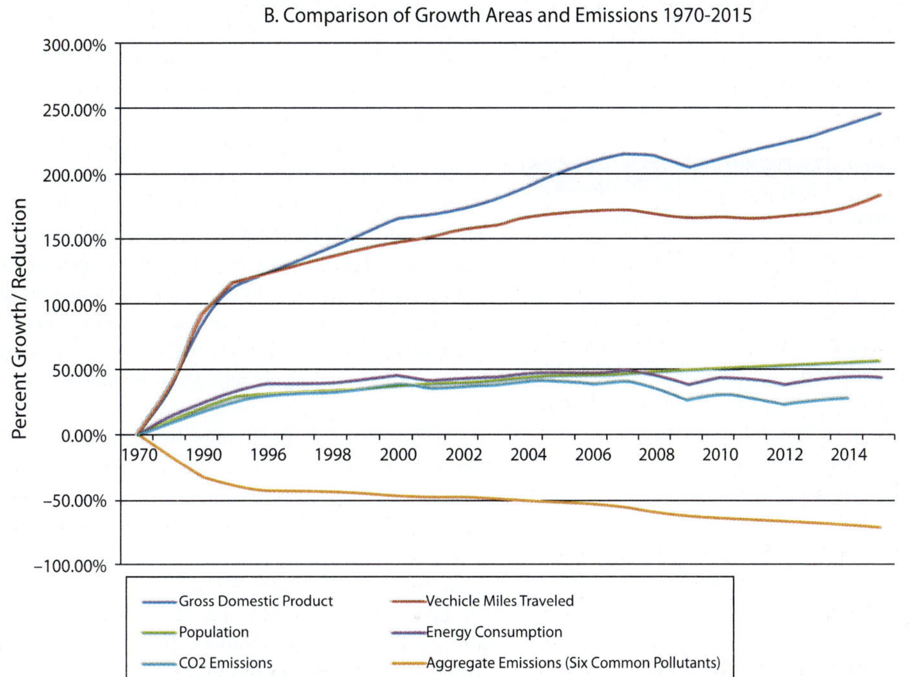

FIGURE 70-2. Changes in economic indicators, pollutant emissions, and concentrations of criteria pollutants over time. Note: Shown are changes in criteria pollutant concentrations from 1990 to 2015 (Panel A) and changes in economic growth indicators and emissions, 1970–2015 (Panel B). (*Source:* Drawn from EPA data[15] at https://gispub.epa.gov/air/trendsreport/2016/.)

This chapter covers the current state of knowledge on the adverse health effects of ambient air pollution and the associated disease burden. It emphasizes air pollution and its management in the United States, while considering the problem at the global level and the approaches being taken to address it. Ambient air pollution is closely linked to climate change, as the greenhouse gases emitted from combustion sources represent the bulk of the contributions to greenhouse gases globally. The literature on air pollution continues to expand and updated reviews can be found in the Integrated Science Assessments prepared approximately every 5 years by the EPA.

SOURCES AND TRANSPORT OF AIR POLLUTION

Air pollution may be defined as an atmospheric condition in which substances are present at elevated concentrations above their "normal" ambient levels and sufficient to exert adverse effects on humans, the ecosystem, and/or materials (e.g., buildings). There are numerous natural and anthropogenic sources (Table 70-1). Some natural events are well known to lead to air pollution, including volcanic eruptions (a source of SO_2, PM, and other pollutants), forest fires (a source of PM, CO, black carbon, and more), sea spray (a source of PM), and sand storms (a source of PM). Over human history, the earliest form of anthropogenic airborne emissions was wood smoke from biomass burning for cooking and warmth. Unfortunately, today nearly half of humanity still lives in conditions in which wood and other even more polluting biomass fuels, such as animal dung and crop residues, are used as a primary fuel for cooking and/or space heating.[16] Coal smoke contributed greatly to air pollution problems in the early days of the industrial revolution, leading to extremely high concentrations of PM and SO_2 in London and other cities in Europe, and in the United States. While coal ceased to be the major source of air pollution in western industrialized countries several decades ago, this same fossil fuel has been a major source of air pollution in China during the last three decades. Additionally, high use of other fossil fuels (mainly petroleum-derived fuels and natural gas) has resulted in urban air pollution around the globe and comprises a dominant contributor to the increasing emissions greenhouse gases.

The backbone supporting the modern lifestyle is the unprecedented demand for energy consumption that has largely been met by fossil fuels up to now. The combustion of fossil fuels for electricity generation or in motor vehicles occurs at high temperatures favorable for forming oxides of nitrogen (NO and NO_2) in addition to the ultimate combustion product of CO_2 (a greenhouse gas). Combustion also generates products of incomplete combustion in both the gaseous phase (e.g., CO and volatile organic compounds) and the solid phase—PM. During combustion, fuel impurities such as sulfur, mercury, and arsenic are also emitted as their oxidized products either as gas (e.g., SO_2) or as part of PM (e.g., sulfate, metal oxides). In contrast, biomass combustion, including tobacco smoking, does not generate a significant amount of oxides of nitrogen but does yield substantial amounts of products of incomplete combustion. When an individual combustion source (point source) is concerned, the emission is often called "smoke," representing a particulate and gaseous mixture. Smoke is typically visible when burning wood, coal, or tobacco; when starting or extinguishing kerosene (a petroleum-derived cooking or lighting fuel), candles, or incense; and during intentional or unintentional food cooking processes. When numerous point sources contribute to elevated concentrations of air pollutants, the affected area can experience a smog episode. The word smog, derived from the combination of the words smoke and fog, represents an atmospheric condition with substantially reduced visibility due to the elevated concentrations of PM and light-scattering or absorbing gases.[3] Through chemical reactions, the gaseous pollutants—sulfur dioxide and nitrogen dioxide—contribute sulfate and nitrate, respectively, to the mass of particles. Chemical reactions also drive the generation of myriad other toxic compounds, for example, carbonyl compounds, which include formaldehyde.

Historically, there have been two types of smog, namely sulfurous (sulfur-containing) smog and photochemical smog. Sulfurous smog is so named because the primary pollutants are SO_2 and soot particles emitted from burning coal (typically of high sulfur content) as observed in the early industrial age. It was also called London-type smog because it appeared frequently in London, United Kingdom, most infamously during the December 1952 episode.[7] The frequency and severity of sulfurous smogs depend on two major factors, source strength, and meteorology. Severe smog episodes occur mainly in winter months when coal combustion activity is at its peak (e.g., space heating using coal-fired fireplaces in London) and when atmospheric inversion is common, referring to an atmospheric condition when a layer of air above the ground is warmer than the air at the ground level. In cold winters during nighttime and nonsunny daytimes, the ground is colder than the air above, resulting in stagnation of pollutants released at the ground level as they are trapped and cannot move upward. This so-called radiation inversion, coupled with stagnant wind conditions, makes air movement very limited horizontally and vertically, essentially trapping air pollutants near the ground until the inversion condition ends.[17]

Photochemical smog was first recognized in Los Angeles, California, in the 1940s.[3] The primary pollutants leading to this type of smog are oxides of nitrogen (NO_x) and hydrocarbons or VOCs. In the presence of solar radiation, a series of photochemical chain reactions convert these primary pollutants (or precursor pollutants) into a complex mixture of secondary pollutants including ozone and aldehydes in the gas phase and nitrate, sulfate, and organic nitrates in the particulate phase. The presence of these primary and secondary pollutants at elevated levels reduces atmospheric visibility, making the atmospheric condition smoggy and irritating. Atmospheric inversion facilitates the development of photochemical smog episodes. Because photochemical reactions are stronger during hot and sunny summer days, it is a different type of inversion, namely, subsidence inversion that traps the constituents of the photochemical smog. A subsidence inversion develops when a high-pressure (warm) layer of air moves in atop colder air, thereby trapping the pollutants under the warm air. Long-range transport of precursor pollutants can be an important contributor to the photochemical smog observed in a particular locale. For example, certain VOCs emitted in Asia are responsible for some ozone measured in North America.

While sulfurous smog has diminished and photochemical pollution has risen in western industrialized countries for nearly half a century, both types of pollution now affect developing countries such

TABLE 70-1 MAJOR SOURCES OF AMBIENT AIR POLLUTION

Source Type	Primary Sources	Major Pollutants
Anthropogenic	Fuel combustion for utilities, industrial, and commercial	PM, CO, NO_x, VOCs, SO_2
	Industrial processes Solvent utilization On-road and off-road vehicles	PM, NO_x, VOCs, SO_2 VOCs, PM PM, CO, NO_x, VOCs, SO_2
	Fugitive dust from roads, construction, mining, and agriculture	PM
Natural	Forest fires Volcanic eruptions Lightning Dust and soil resuspension	PM, CO, VOCs, NO_x Sulfur, SO_2, PM NO_x PM
	See spray Biological actions (plant emissions, bacteria, fungal activities)	PM, sulfur VOCs, PM, sulfur, CO

Abbreviations: CO = carbon monoxide; NO_x = nitrogen oxides; O_3 = ozone, PM = particulate matter; VOCs = volatile organic compounds.

as China. In China, a third type of pollution has originated, namely Chinese haze, or *wu mai*, a complex mixture of air pollutants from a dynamic and growing set of sources.[18] This mixture includes PM (with a wide range of sizes) and gaseous pollutants (e.g., ozone, nitrogen dioxide, carbon monoxide, and sulfur dioxide). In addition to well-understood photochemical reactions, new chemistry has been discovered specific to the formation of Chinese haze.[19,20] Therefore, it is fair to say that Chinese haze is not only a combination of two historical types of smog, but it also has additional physiochemical characteristics reflecting the coexistence of many sources.

The pollutants released into or formed in the atmosphere, as described above, can enter indoor environments where people typically spend their majority of time. Additional indoor sources may further increase indoor levels and may even contribute to outdoor concentrations. Indoor sources include emissions from cooking/heating fuel combustion, cooking processes, tobacco smoking, bioeffluents from humans and pets, molds and fungi, VOCs from floor and wall coverings, synthetic paints, building products, furnishings, polishes/waxes, pesticides, etc. Health risks associated with indoor air pollutants emitted from cooking/heating, building products, and consumer products are typically addressed separately from health risks associated with ambient pollutants. However, interactions increasing risk to health have been found between indoor and outdoor pollutants.[21]

TABLE 70-2 SOURCES OF POLLUTION IN URBAN MICROENVIRONMENTS

Microenvironment	Sources	Pollutants
Home	Cooking, space heating, parked vehicles, hobbies, smoking, household products, pets, rodents, insects	PM, CO, NO_x, VOCs, allergens
Transportation environments	Vehicle and industrial emissions, road dust, background pollution, smoking	PM, including ultrafine PM, CO, NO_x, O_3, VOCs, aeroallergens, carcinogens
Streets	Vehicle emissions, road dust, background pollution	PM, including ultrafine PM, CO, NO_x, O_3, VOCs, carcinogens, lead
Work environments	Industrial processes, smoking, background pollution	PM, CO, VOCs, NO_x, carcinogens
Entertainment environments	Cooking and space heating, background pollution, smoking	PM, VOCs, carcinogens

Abbreviations: CO = carbon monoxide; NO_x = nitrogen oxides; O_3 = ozone; PM = particulate matter; VOCs = volatile organic compounds.

EXPOSURE TO AIR POLLUTION

General concepts of exposure are set out elsewhere in this volume. The concept of personal exposure is central to characterizing the risks of air pollution and formulating control strategies.[22] Exposure, defined as the contact of a person with the pollutant of concern, is calculated for air pollutants as the product of the concentration of the pollutant in the place(s) where time is spent with the time spent in that place or places. For example, a person working outdoors at a concentration of $PM_{2.5}$ of 100 µg per m^3 for 8 hours would have an exposure of 800 µg hr/m^3. Total personal exposure to an airborne pollutant reflects the concentrations in the various places where time is spent, weighted by the time spent in each. The microenvironmental model is useful for estimating personal exposure and for assessing the contributions of different environments to exposure; this concept defines total personal exposure as the sum of exposures received in the various microenvironments where time is spent. A microenvironment is defined as a place where time is spent that has a particular pollutant concentration profile during the time spent there; for example, a motor vehicle might represent a microenvironment during time spent commuting and a restaurant where a meal is eaten would be another.[22]

This model is useful for considering the numerous microenvironments relevant to estimating and controlling exposures to air pollution and associated risks to health. Table 70-2 lists some of these microenvironments along with pollution sources. Considered within the framework of the microenvironmental model, there are specific microenvironments of particular relevance to the health of urban and nonurban dwellers. The residence is particularly important regardless of urbanicity because most people spend the majority of time at home. For example, smoke and fumes from cooking and heating are prominent regardless of location as is tobacco smoke. In urban areas, the air contaminants in the home include those generated by indoor sources and the outdoor air pollutants penetrating indoors, including those pollutants generated by traffic and by nearby and more distant sources. The extent of penetration depends on the characteristics of the housing, including the exchange of indoor with outdoor air. The streets, which may have "hot spots" of air pollution generated by traffic or industrial sources, are another key and distinct microenvironment.

To date, most epidemiologic studies of ambient air pollution have used outdoor concentrations of air pollutants (e.g., $PM_{2.5}$ and ozone) as surrogates for population or individual exposures. This approach assumes that people's total exposure is proportional to outdoor concentrations and that the indoor source contribution to total exposure is either a constant or absent. This approach has been historically useful for regulatory purposes because a study can directly establish a relationship between risk for a health outcome and ambient pollutant levels that are subject to regulatory standards. In numerous time-series studies, exposure has been estimated as PM or other criteria pollutant concentrations measured at centrally located ambient monitoring stations. Exposure studies show that central site monitoring data cannot represent exposures of those who live closer to heavily trafficked roads or other local sources. Considerable effort, hence, has been made recently to use spatiotemporal models to estimate exposures at the residence level.[23,24] These models are often coupled with satellite data to estimate ambient concentrations at locations lacking a monitoring station.[25] These methods have proved adequate in large population studies, considering that influences from indoor sources and other personal sources may increase the random noise without causing significant differential measurement error.

However, in small-size cohort studies or panel studies, measuring personal exposure or considering indoor and personal sources becomes important and imperative. Personal exposure can be assessed either using direct personal monitoring or microenvironmental measurement methods. Recent advances in low-cost sensors for PM and gaseous pollutants make personal monitoring more feasible as these devices are small, lightweighted, and can be accurate when properly calibrated.[26] These sensors can also be used in various microenvironments to generate time-weighted average exposures as a proxy of total personal exposure. The microenvironmental approach has added value if a study is assessing health effects associated with specific microenvironments and sources specific to these microenviroments.

RESEARCH APPROACHES TO ASSESSING RISKS OF AIR POLLUTION

As with other environmental pollutants, the approaches to characterizing health risks draw on in vitro and in vivo toxicology, limited, brief, ethically allowable exposures of human volunteers to pollutants, and epidemiological studies. The approaches are complementary in providing information on mechanisms from the toxicological studies and on risks in populations from the epidemiological studies. Biomarkers bridge between these lines of investigation. In the past, toxicological studies often involved exposure of animals to a single pollutant, such as ozone, to isolate the pollutant's effect from those of other pollutants present in the air pollution mixture. For studying some pollutants, human volunteers have inhaled the pollutants in an exposure chamber over a short interval and their responses closely monitored. Additionally, pollutants are also studied in cell systems; these systems are likely to gain increasing prominence as new, sophisticated systems probe gene expression of different kinds of cells following exposure.[22]

The topic of research methods in environmental epidemiology is covered elsewhere. The full range of methods has been applied historically. Current research has used time-series methods, including the case-crossover design, to assess associations of daily mortality and morbidity counts with air pollution concentrations on a daily basis or averaged over several days. Over the last three decades, there has been a progression from considering data from single cities to large, pooled analyses, some at the national level; a 2019 publication described findings from 652 locations.[27] These time-series studies address short-term effects; cohort studies, which address longer-term effects, have also become a mainstay, facilitated by the development of modeling approaches that provide estimates on a sufficiently fine geographic scale, that is, zip code.

Longer-term effects have been primarily addressed in cohort studies. The Harvard Six-Cities Study, started in 1974, is a landmark.[28,29] The study population included children and adults in six cities across the United States, selected so as to provide a gradient of exposure to air pollution. Monitors were placed in each community and personal exposure assessments were done for some participants. Outcomes assessed including respiratory health and mortality. The study of adults, which included 8111 participants, provided some of the first evidence that air pollution increased mortality over the longer term. The Children's Health Study, carried out in Southern California, is another landmark. The study tracked lung growth and respiratory health in school children from communities having a range of pollution concentrations.[30,31] Exposure was initially estimated based on monitors placed in each community, later complemented by more dense monitoring to capture variation in exposure within communities. Now in progress for two decades, the study has shown that higher levels of air pollution slow lung growth and that reduction of pollution enhances it.[30,32]

More recent studies have had much larger numbers of participants. These large-scale studies have been facilitated by using national-level databases, which cover complete populations, for example, the Medicare data, and track vital status through record linkage. For example, in 2017, Di et al. reported a positive association between PM air pollution exposure and mortality in a dynamic Medicare cohort of approximately 65 million enrollees.[25] In addition, studies have been pooled to gain power and to facilitate exploration of heterogeneity of effects and its origins. For example, time-series studies were pooled from North America (Canada and the United States) and from Europe.[33] With these very large studies, adverse effects have been documented at ever lower exposures, some at concentrations below current National Ambient Air Quality Standards in the United States and the Air Quality Guidelines of the World Health Organization.[34] As air pollution levels declined with regulation, increasing emphasis was placed on understanding the quantitative risks of air pollution so that air-quality standards could be set that would be protective of public health. In other words, researchers did studies to understand how much risk changes as air pollution increases or decreases. Cohort studies have been informative in characterizing these risk relationships and large data sets have been particularly useful for exploring differing models for data analysis. In a line of research directed at "accountability," researchers have addressed the consequences of changes in policy, using a variety of quasiexperimental approaches.[35] For example, so-called "accountability studies" have addressed the aftermath of the coal-burning ban in Ireland and the congestion-charging scheme in London.

In interpreting the findings of epidemiological studies of air pollution, there are two commonly raised concerns: confounding and measurement error related to air pollution. Confounding, of course, is considered in the design and analysis of epidemiological studies generally. In studies of air pollution, it might arise because those individuals with higher exposures differ from those with lower exposures in such characteristics as socioeconomic status and correlates or tobacco smoking. A variety of strategies are used to consider potential confounding and the air pollution literature has proved robust to its influence. There is also a large literature on measurement error and its consequences and correction in investigating the health effects of air pollution.[36,37]

THE HEALTH EFFECTS OF AIR POLLUTION

Overview: Ambient air pollution comprises a complex and dynamic mixture of gaseous and particulate air pollutants that varies in physical and chemical characteristics over time and space. Table 70-3 provides a broad overview of major pollutants including sources, some major adverse health effects, and U.S. regulations and WHO guidelines. Combustion emissions, a dominant source of pollution, undergo physical and chemical changes following release. Airborne particles are the most widely used index of air pollution, as they reflect multiple sources, including primary and secondary particles from combustion processes. They are both primary, emitted directly, and secondary, formed from chemical transformations. Fresh PM emissions from motor vehicles are very small in size, in the ultrafine size range (smaller than 100 nm in diameter), but agglomerate quickly into larger particles. Thus, particles inhaled while driving on a freeway in traffic or walking on an urban sidewalk are in the ultrafine range, while particles present as a regional background or generated through mechanical processes (e.g., road dust resuspension and tire wear debris) are larger in size. Thus, particles inhaled while driving on a freeway in traffic or walking on an urban sidewalk are in the ultrafine range.

Although we are exposed to a dynamic mixture of inhaled pollutants across many different environments, the health effects of air pollution are largely considered in relationship to particular pollutants, both because of the complexity of understanding the toxicity of real-world pollution and because of regulatory frameworks that address particular source groups and specific pollutants. Consequently, many research studies are designed so as to disentangle the effects of mixture components, and some of the pollutants themselves comprise mixtures, for example, the particles comprising PM, which have countless physical properties and chemical components. Some studies have been directed at particular mixtures, most notably that from motor vehicles often referred to as traffic-related air pollution (TRAP).[38] The mixture of pollutants formed from vehicle emissions may have specific toxicity beyond that of well-studied individual components.

The array of health effects linked to ambient air pollution is broad and ever-growing (Table 70-3). The adverse effects causally linked to air pollution include excess mortality, as dramatic as the 10,000+ during the London Fog of 1952 to the far more subtle increases found in very large studies at current levels and in morbidity across a wide range of indicators. Adverse effects have been found for functioning and diseases of most organs and also for reproductive outcomes: increased risk for respiratory infections, exacerbation of asthma and chronic obstructive pulmonary disease (COPD—a disease involving destruction of the lung structure that is primarily attributable to cigarette smoking) and of cardiac (heart) heart events, contributions to development of major chronic diseases (coronary heart disease,

TABLE 70-3 MAJOR AMBIENT AIR POLLUTIONS: SOURCES, HEALTH EFFECTS, AND REGULATIONS[a]

	Source Types and Major Sources	Health Effects	Regulations and Guidelines
Lead	Primary Anthropogenic: Leaded fuel (phased out in some locations such as the United States), lead batteries, metal processing	Accumulates in organs and tissues. Learning disabilities, cancer, damage to the nervous system	*U.S. NAAQS:* Quarterly average: 1.5 μg/m^3 *WHO Guidelines:* Annual: 0.50 μg/m^3
Sulfur dioxide	Primary Anthropogenic: Combustion of fossil fuel (power plants), industrial boilers, household coal use, oil refineries Biogenic: Decomposition of organic matter, sea spray, volcanic eruptions	Lung impairment, respiratory symptoms. Precursor to PM. Contributes to acid precipitation	*U.S. NAAQS:* Annual arithmetic mean: 0.03 ppm (80 μg/m^3) 24-Hour average: 0.14 ppm (365 μg/m^3) *WHO Guidelines:* 10-Minute average: 500 μg/m^3 Annual: 20 μg/m^3
Carbon monoxide	Primary Anthropogenic: Combustion of fossil fuels (motor vehicles, boilers, furnaces) Biogenic: Forest fires	Interferes with delivery of oxygen. Fatigue, headache, neurological damage, dizziness	*U.S. NAAQS:* 1-Hour average: 35 ppm (40 mg/m^3) 8-Hour average: 9 ppm (10 mg/m^3) *WHO Guidelines:* 15-Minute average: 100 mg/m^3 30-Minute average: 60 mg/m^3 1-Hour average: 30 mg/m^3
Particulate matter[b]	Primary and secondary Anthropogenic: Burning of fossil fuel, wood burning, natural sources (e.g., pollen), conversion of precursors (NO_x, SO_x, VOCs) Biogenic: Dust storms, forest fires, dirt roads	Respiratory symptoms, decline in lung function, exacerbation of respiratory and cardiovascular disease (e.g., asthma), mortality	*U.S. NAAQS:* PM_{10} 24-Hour average 150 μg/m^3 $PM_{2.5}$ Annual arithmetic mean: 15 μg/m^3 24-Hour average: 35 μg/m^3 *WHO Guidelines:* PM_{10} Annual: 20 μg/m^3 24-Hour average: 50 μg/m^3 $PM_{2.5}$: Annual: 10 μg/m^3 24-Hour average: 25 μg/m^3
Nitrogen oxides	Primary and secondary Anthropogenic: Fossil fuel combustion (vehicles, electric utilities, industry), kerosene heaters Biogenic: Biological processes in soil, lightning	Decreased lung function, increased respiratory infectionPrecursor to ozone. Contributes to PM and acid precipitation	*U.S. NAAQS* for NO_2: Annual arithmetic mean: 0.053 ppm (100 μg/m^3) Related to compliance with NAAQS for ozone. *WHO Guidelines* for NO_2: 1-Hour average: 200 μg/m^3 Annual: 40 μg/m^3
Tropospheric ozone	Secondary Formed through chemical reactions of anthropogenic and biogenic precursors (VOCs and NO_x) in the presence of sunlight	Decreased lung function, increased respiratory symptoms, eye irritation, bronchoconstriction	*U.S. NAAQS:* 1-Hour average: 0.12 ppm (235 μg/m^3). Applies in limited areas. 8-Hour average: 0.075 ppm (147 μg/m^3) *WHO Guidelines:* 8-Hour average: 100 μg/m^3
"Toxic" pollutants ("Hazardous" pollutants) *(e.g., asbestos, mercury, dioxin, some VOCs)*	Primary and secondary Anthropogenic: Industrial processes, solvents, paint thinners, fuel	Cancer, reproductive effects, neurological damage, respiratory effects	EPA rules on emissions for more than 80 industrial source categories (e.g., dry cleaners, oil refineries, chemical plants) EPA and state rules on vehicle emissions
Volatile organic compounds (e.g., benzene, terpenes, toluene)	Primary and secondary Anthropogenic: Solvents, glues, smoking, fuel combustion Biogenic: Vegetation, forest fires	Range of effects, depending on the compound. Irritation of respiratory tract, nausea, cancer Precursor to ozone. Contributes to PM	EPA limits on emissions EPA toxic air pollutant rules Related to compliance with NAAQS for ozone
Biological pollutants (e.g., pollen, mold, mildew)	Primary Biogenic: Trees, grasses, ragweed, animals, debris Anthropogenic systems, such as central air conditioning, can create conditions that encourage production of biological pollutants	Allergic reactions, respiratory symptoms, fatigue, asthma	

[a]This table lists only a sample of the sources and health effects associated with each pollutant. Additionally, health effects may be the result of characteristics of the pollutant mixture rather than the independent effects of a pollutant. Additional legal requirements often apply, such as state regulations.

[b]Sources and effects of PM can differ by size.

Source: Used with permission from Bell ML, Samet JM. Air Pollution. In Frumkin H. (ed) *Environmental health*: From Local to Global. 2010;387-415. Figure 12.1.[84]

COPD, and cancer), and impaired lung growth and respiratory symptoms during childhood. Many additional adverse health outcomes are under study: autism and other neurodevelopmental disorders, various adverse reproductive outcomes, including prematurity and low birthweight, and more rapid "brain aging," for example.[39–41] Several general mechanisms are proposed as underlying these health effects, particularly oxidant stress, an excess of reactive molecules, and a heightened inflammatory state, given the oxidative nature of ambient air pollution. The increased risk for cancer causally linked to air pollution likely comes primarily from the presence of specific carcinogens, that is cancer-causing agents, in ambient air pollution, for example, polycyclic aromatic hydrocarbons, and inflammation; particles collected in outdoor air in hundreds of locations are mutagenic, that is, they can damage DNA.[42]

Particulate Matter: The literature on the health effects of particles is enormous, comprising many epidemiological and toxicological studies.[43] With regard to ambient air pollution, the risks of PM have assumed great prominence because particles are widely monitored and used as the principal indicator for estimating the burden of morbidity and premature mortality attributable to air pollution. Particles are a robust indicator of ambient air pollution because of their myriad sources and the contributions of sulfur and nitrogen oxides and organic compounds to secondary particle formation. Particles in outdoor air have numerous natural and manmade sources. The manmade sources are diverse and include power plants, industry, and motor vehicles, including diesel-powered vehicles that emit particles in the size range that penetrates into the lung. In areas where biomass fuels are used, the contributions of indoor combustion to outdoor air pollution may be substantial.

Particles in outdoor air span a wide range of sizes (Fig. 70-3) and are highly diverse in composition and physical characteristics, including size as indicated by aerodynamic diameter.[43] Thus, $PM_{2.5}$ includes those particles less than 2.5 μm in aerodynamic diameter, a size band that contains most manmade particles in outdoor air and also the particles of a size that can reach the smaller airways and air sacs of the lungs. The very small ultrafine particles less than 100 nm, which include freshly generated combustion particles, are another set of particles of concern. Much research has been done on characteristics of particles that determine toxicity. Hypotheses on determinants of particle toxicity have focused on acidity, transition metals like iron that can cause damaging injury, organic compounds, bioaerosols, and size and, as a further complication, different characteristics could be relevant to different health outcomes. However, in spite of extensive toxicological and epidemiological research, the evidence is not yet sufficiently definitive to link particular characteristics to toxicity. Making such linkages would be helpful for targeting control approaches. Typically, there are also larger, coarse mass particles that come from windblown dust, road traffic, and other sources.

There has been extensive epidemiological and toxicological investigation of the effects of particles on health since the air pollution disasters of mid-twentieth century. The toxicological studies have used approaches including exposing volunteers to generated particles or concentrated air particles, animal exposures, and diverse in vitro assays. This extensive body of evidence shows that particles are injurious and indicates mechanisms by which particles could cause adverse effects on the respiratory and cardiovascular systems. The epidemiological studies have grown in size and in the sophistication of their methodology. Recent studies involve large, national-level populations, like all people in the United States who are 65 years and older, and estimation of exposures at all household addresses using models that incorporate available monitoring data, satellite information, and land-use data, such as on roadways and manufacturing.[25,34] Both short-term and long-term adverse effects were found to be caused by PM. In the most recent completed review by the EPA, there was sufficient evidence to causally link $PM_{2.5}$ with adverse cardiovascular effects and mortality. There was also sufficient evidence to causally link long-term exposure to $PM_{2.5}$ with mortality.[43] The most recent epidemiological studies continue to find associations of $PM_{2.5}$ with increased risk for mortality, even at contemporary concentrations in the United States. In a study utilizing the Medicare data for persons 65 years of age and older, over 60 million people, Di and colleagues showed increased mortality at annual averages below 12 μg/m^3, the current annual standard for $PM_{2.5}$ in the United States.[25]

One analysis has suggested that reductions in particulate air pollution during the 1980s and 1990s have led to measurable improvements in life expectancy in the United States.[44] The researchers estimated that for each 10 μg/m^3 reduction in air pollution over this period the average gain in life expectancy was 0.61 years (about 7.3 months). The authors concluded that as much as 15% of the total life expectancy increase seen during this time in the United States was attributable to the air pollution reductions.

This strong evidence on the adverse health effects of PM has led to ever tighter ambient air-quality standards and improving air quality (Fig. 70-2). Nonetheless, adverse health effects are still observed and much of the world's population is exposed at high concentrations at which adverse effects are certain.

Ozone: Ozone is a specific gas that has been studied for hazard using toxicological approaches.[45,46] It is also used as the indicator for photochemical pollution, or "smog."[45] Smog has become a worldwide

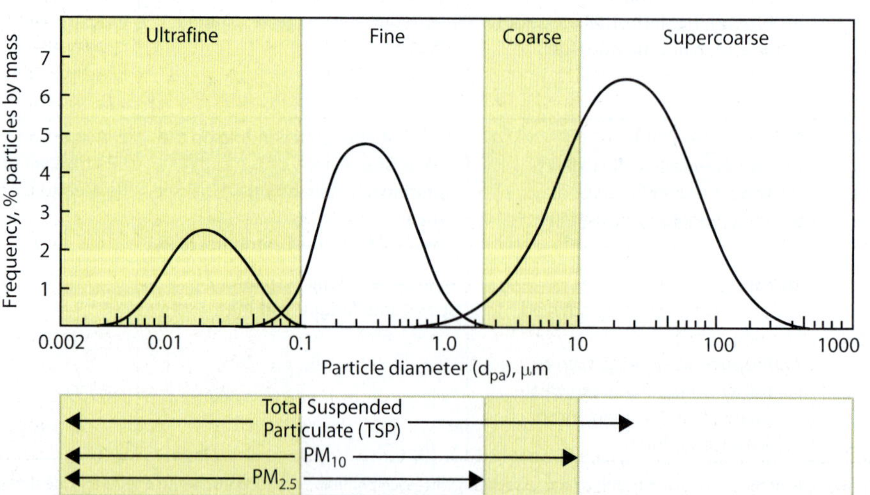

FIGURE 70-3. Ambient PM size distribution. (*Source*: Adapted from the EPA.[43])

problem as vehicle fleets have grown. The problem of tropospheric (ground-level) ozone pollution is distinct from the problem of depletion of the stratospheric (high-level) ozone layer.

Ozone, a highly reactive molecule, has been extensively investigated using toxicological approaches that have included exposures of human volunteers and short- and long-term exposures of animals.[47,48] The human studies have involved exposures of volunteers, generally young and healthy, to concentrations of ozone found in urban areas in the United States and elsewhere. Collectively, the studies show that exposures of up to 6–8 hours with intermittent exercise result in temporary drops in lung function and that some individuals have greater susceptibility to ozone. While the effects are transient, they are of sufficient magnitude in some people (loss of around 10% of function) to be considered adverse. In some of the studies, the lungs have been sampled and evidence of inflammation found by measuring concentrations of molecules that reflect the tissue's response. In experimental animals, sustained low-level exposure damages the small airways and leads to early changes of COPD; thus, there is concern about permanent structural alteration in ozone-exposed populations. In the human studies, asthmatics have not been shown to have increased susceptibility to ozone compared with nonasthmatics.

Epidemiological studies provide coherent evidence on short-term effects of ozone on respiratory health. There is also evidence from daily time-series studies (studies examining day-to-day variation in death counts in relationship to variation in pollution levels) that ozone increases risk for mortality.[49] There is inconsistent evidence for cardiovascular effects and a just-completed exposure study of older persons with cardiovascular disease did not find adverse effects.[50]

Reflecting the evidence on short-term effects on lung function, standards for ozone concentrations are directed at brief time spans (Table 70-3). Given the range of susceptibility of the population, it is likely that feasibly achieved standards will not protect the full population from adverse respiratory effects.

Nitrogen Oxides: Gaseous nitrogen oxides are produced by combustion processes and also contribute to the formation of aerosols. Nitrogen dioxide (NO_2), an oxidant gas, is the indicator that is generally monitored. The principal source of NO_2 in outdoor air is motor vehicle emissions and NO_2 is considered to be a useful indicator of TRAP in urban environments.[51] Power plants and industrial sources also contribute. The health effects of NO_2 emitted into outdoor air probably come mainly from the formation of secondary pollutants, including ozone and particles.[51] NO_2, along with hydrocarbons, is an essential precursor of ozone and the nitrogen oxides also form acidic nitrate particles.

Nitrogen dioxide itself has been studied in animal models and in clinical studies. It can reach the small airways and air sacs of the lung because of its low solubility. The toxicological evidence at high exposures has raised concern that NO_2 exposure can impair lung defenses against infectious agents like viruses and cause airway inflammation and thereby increase risk for respiratory infections.[52] Supporting epidemiological findings are problematic as population studies directed at NO_s are complicated by its role in the formation of ozone and its presence in the complex mixture of traffic-related pollutants. Nonetheless, several systematic reviews find associations between NO_2 and daily mortality and hospital admissions.[53,54] Human exposure studies have been performed to investigate the immediate effects of NO_2 on persons with asthma.[54] Nitrogen dioxide could plausibly increase airway responsiveness (the extent to which the airways constrict when irritated) by causing airway inflammation. The findings of the exposure studies have been inconsistent, but suggest that some people with asthma may be susceptible.[54]

Carbon Monoxide: Carbon monoxide (CO) is an invisible gas formed by incomplete combustion. It is a prominent indoor pollutant with sources including biomass fuel combustion and space heating with fossil fuels.[55] Carbon monoxide binds tightly to hemoglobin, thus reducing the oxygen-carrying capacity of the blood and the delivery of oxygen to the tissues. At high levels indoors, fatal CO poisoning may result. Outdoors, vehicle exhaust is the major source and concentrations are highly variable, reflecting vehicle density and traffic patterns. Urban locations with high traffic density, that is, "hot spots," tend to have the highest concentrations. Exposures to CO can be assessed by using the level of carboxyhemoglobin as a marker of exposure or by measuring the concentration of CO in the breath.

Because of the reduction of oxygen delivery, persons with cardiovascular disease are considered to be at greatest risk from CO exposure and research has focused on CO and adverse effects in this susceptible group.[55] The research has used the clinical study approach; volunteers with cardiovascular disease were exposed to levels of CO of interest and clinical measurements made, such as taking the electrocardiogram for indication of reduced oxygen delivery and its consequences. The evidence from such studies indicates that CO exposure leads to earlier indication of myocardial ischemia (inadequate oxygenation of the heart) following exposure compared with unexposed controls.[55] There is some coherent epidemiological evidence. There are other potential susceptible groups: fetuses, as well as persons with COPD, may also be harmed by CO, and normal persons may have reduced oxygen uptake during exercise at low levels of CO exposure.[55]

The exposure studies have provided robust evidence for standards for CO, which are based on brief time windows, reflective of the handling of CO in the body and its half-life. In higher-income countries, outdoor levels of CO have fallen greatly over recent decades as controls, particularly on motor vehicles, have greatly reduced emissions (see Fig. 70-2). Nonetheless, CO may be a concern in some high traffic locations and next to particular point sources. Less is known about CO exposure in middle- and low-income countries where ambient CO may be added to indoor exposure from biomass fuel combustion. In some countries, two-stroke motorcycles and other vehicles are a key source.

Sulfur Oxides: Sulfur oxides are generated by combustion of fuels containing sulfur, such as coal, petroleum-derived fuels such as gasoline, diesel, and heating oil, and by smelting operations.[56] The water-soluble gas, sulfur dioxide or SO_2, is the indicator that is generally monitored. However, other sulfur oxides are emitted and the sulfur oxides undergo transformation to form particulate sulfate compounds.[56] Scientific research has been directed primarily at SO_2, although epidemiological studies provide information on sulfur oxide exposure more generally.[56] Sulfur dioxide is a reactive gas that is effectively scrubbed or cleaned from inhaled air in the upper airway. With exercise and switch to oral breathing as ventilation increases, the inhaled dose of SO_2 increases and more reaches the lung.[56]

Much of the evidence that has driven regulation comes from human exposure studies that involve exposure of people with asthma and that show adverse effects without exposures to other pollutants. Asthmatics are particularly sensitive, with some asthmatics having more severe health responses at a particular concentration than others with asthma. With exercise and hyperventilation, some people with asthma respond with increased resistance of the lung to airflow with an associated drop in lung function and increased respiratory symptoms. Such effects have been demonstrated at concentrations that might be reached in the United States in high exposure situations and that may be common in some heavily industrialized countries. Epidemiological studies from Hong Kong examined the consequences of a major and rapid reduction in sulfur content in fuels.[57] The investigators found an associated substantial reduction in health effects (childhood respiratory disease and all age mortality outcomes). Over recent decades, sulfur dioxide concentrations have decreased substantially as use of high sulfur fuels has been reduced (Fig. 70-2).

Lead: Although lead in gasoline is now phased out in almost all nations, exposure to airborne continues from industrial activities, such as smelting, and sometimes results in dangerous exposures for children. Exposure to lead may occur through inhalation and also ingestion in food and water, routes of exposure that have become the most important in high-income countries.[58] A substantial body of epidemiological evidence links lead exposure of children to adverse neurodevelopmental effects, such as lowering the level of intelligence, and, as a result of that evidence, recommendations as to the acceptable level of lead for children have been lowered progressively.[58] Lead has also been linked to higher blood pressure and cardiovascular disease and to low bone mineral density and osteoporosis.[58] As the base of evidence has expanded, the blood concentrations of lead considered acceptable have dropped markedly.[59]

Toxic or Hazardous Air Pollutants: The term "toxic air pollutants" is a term used to a variety of primary and secondary pollutants that cause injury and increase risk for disease in the lungs and other organs. Under the Clean Air Act, as amended in 1990, 187 agents are classified as "hazardous."[60] Some are carcinogens, for example, benzene, while others are irritants, such as acrolein. These are to be regulated in a two-phase approach, first developing control technology, maximum achievable control technology, and then determining through risk assessment what residual risk remains.[61] To date, progress on the part of EPA has been limited with regard to this two-step progress. The toxic agents in outdoor air are not limited to these 187 agents, given the myriad sources contributing to outdoor air pollution and the potential for combustion to generate toxic species, even if they are short lived in the atmosphere.

TRAP: The mixture of pollutants coming from vehicle emissions has been investigated as a specific mixture, predominantly using epidemiological approaches. The hypothesis tested in these studies is whether there is an effect of the traffic mixture that exceeds that anticipated from the concentrations of the major pollutants, for example, PM and carbon monoxide. There is not a specific indicator of TRAP and hence such proxies as distance from major roadways and concentration of nitrogen dioxide, a primary engine exhaust pollutant, have been used as surrogates.[38] Evidence on the health consequences of TRAP shows multiple adverse consequences.[38]

THE DISEASE BURDEN FROM AMBIENT AIR POLLUTION

The estimation of disease burden as a means to quantify the importance of various risk factors has become a globally applied tool for policy purposes. Estimates are reported every 2 years by the Institute for Health Metrics and Evaluation. The estimates for air pollution, which cover household air pollution, ambient PM and ozone, have focused attention on the problem of air pollution, largely because of their magnitude. These estimates place air pollution among the leading causes of disease burden in the world, particularly if the burden from household air pollution is counted along with that from ambient air pollution.

These more recent global burden estimates are grounded in evermore sophisticated methodology for estimating burden: global models for estimation of the concentrations to which people are exposed and refined approaches for characterizing the concentration-response relationships for an increasing number of adverse health outcomes based on pooled analyses of cohort study data. However, the underlying concept of burden estimation dates to the 1953 seminal paper by Levin that described a method for calculating how much lung cancer in a population is attributable to cigarette smoking.[62] The calculation incorporates the prevalence of an exposure and the relative risk associated with that exposures. Comparison is made between the exposure distribution as it is and to a counterfactual distribution that represents the ideal in terms of avoidance of disease burden. Turning to the well-known example of cigarette smoking, the historical starting point for burden estimation, the implicit counterfactual is a smoking prevalence of zero, that is, there are no smokers.

For air pollution, the burden estimates are calculated by applying the concentration response relationships for the outcome of interest to the concentration distribution as estimated, making comparison to a "counterfactual" distribution of exposure concentrations that might be achieved. The air pollution concentration estimates are now estimated for all countries, using a combination of predictors that can be applied everywhere, even if actual monitoring data are unavailable, as for much of sub-Saharan Africa. These models draw on monitoring data as available, land-use information, satellite data, and other informative data sets. The counterfactual used in current estimates of burden represents the lower end of the distribution of exposure concentrations in the epidemiological studies of air pollution and mortality. The counterfactual value used by the Global Burden of Disease is well below typical values in urban areas.

Figure 70-4 illustrates the concept of the counterfactual based on the estimated global distribution, which shows that much of the population is exposed to $PM_{2.5}$ at concentrations above the WHO's annual guideline value of 10 μg/m^3. The assumed counterfactual shifts the population to the left and exposure is truncated at a value of approximately 4 μg/m^3. The enormous shift needed to meet the counterfactual range is evident, and for much of the population the counterfactual value is unachievable. Figure 70-4 highlights the distinction between attributable, that is, all exposures are below the counterfactual value, and achievable, that is, the extent to which exposures can be shifted to the left. This distinction needs be communicated in presenting disease burden estimates in policy contexts; the attributable burden represents the maximum benefit that would be achieved if the counterfactual could be met.

There is one further consideration related to using burden estimates in policy decisions: estimates of burden from different agents need to be compared with caution, given the differing bases on which counterfactual values are selected. The counterfactual value for $PM_{2.5}$ is derived from exposures in epidemiological studies of PM exposure and mortality, while prevalence of zero for smoking represents the target for tobacco control. Comparisons of attributable burdens mask differences in what is achievable.

Air Pollution Burden Estimates

The latest estimates confirm that air pollution is a leading cause of premature mortality around the world, ranking at the fourth position in 1990 and the fifth in 2017.[63] The total of deaths attributed to ambient air pollution globally in 2017 is 2.9 million distributed by cause as follows: IHD-977,000, lung cancer-265,000, COPD-633,000, and LRI-432,000.[64] There is substantial geographic variation globally (Fig. 70-4) with China and India together accounting for more than half of the attributable burden of premature mortality. From 1990 to 2017, estimates have increased in some countries, for example, India and China, as the population has grown and aged, and air pollution levels have risen. For ozone, the global mortality estimate is much smaller at 471,000, although this may be an underestimate, as this mortality estimate only considered ozone effects on respiratory death. Emerging evidence now shows that ozone can increase risk of cardiovascular mortality.[64]

The estimates of burden from air pollution have raised awareness of air pollution not only at the global level, but also at national, regional, and local levels. The policy implications of the estimates are evident, as they focus on public health problems that are the purview of national and local public health authorities. The comparison of the magnitude of the air pollution burden from air pollution to that from tobacco is attention getting, as the dangers of tobacco are well known.

APPROACHES TO AIR-QUALITY MANAGEMENT

Overview: Air-quality management has been based around setting standards for concentrations of air pollutants in ambient air and on source control, primarily using technology-based measures to reduce emissionsoi. For establishing standards, the starting point has been the foundation of evidence on the hazards posed by the air

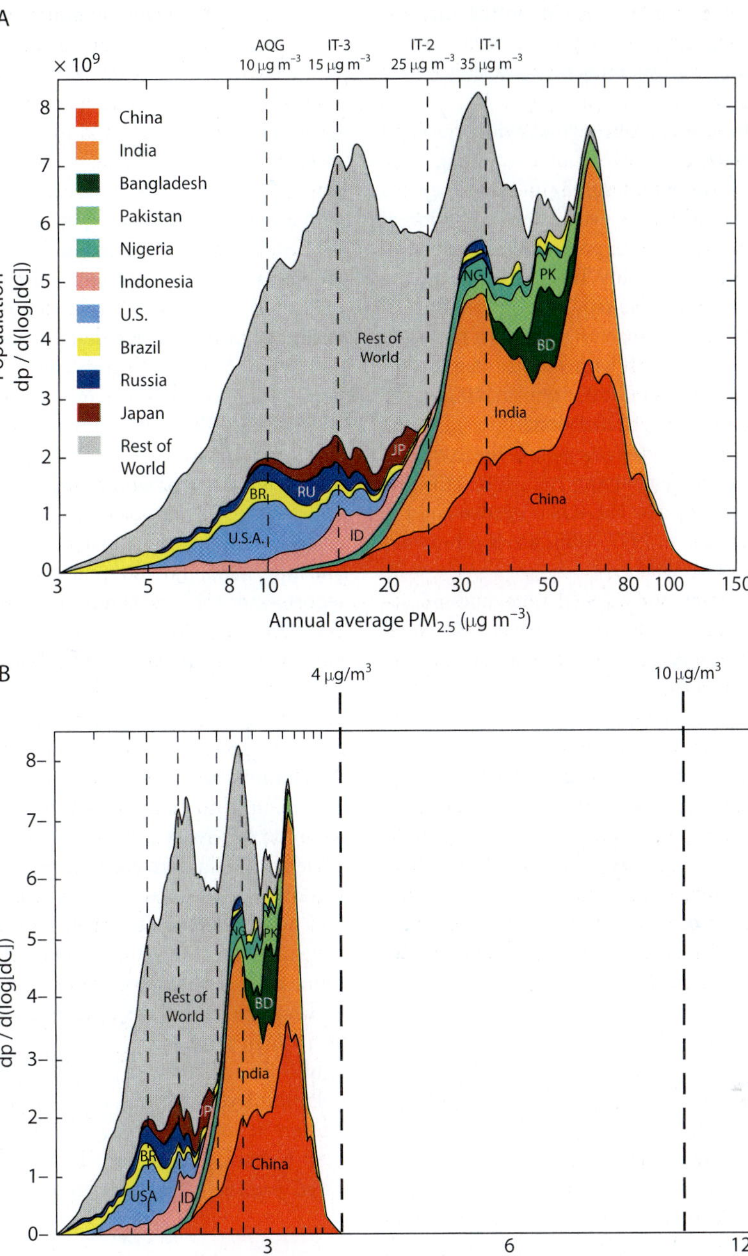

FIGURE 70-4. Global and regional distributions of population as a function of annual average ambient $PM_{2.5}$ concentration for the ten most populous countries in 2013 (A) and Distribution under Counterfactual Assumption (B). **A.** Global and regional distributions of population as a function of annual (2013) average ambient $PM_{2.5}$ concentration for the world's ten most populous countries. Plotted data reflect local smoothing of bin-width normalized distributions computed over 400 logarithmically spaced bins; equal-sized plotted areas would reflect equal populations. Dashed vertical lines indicate World Health Organization Interim Targets (IT) and the Air Quality Guideline (AQG). **B.** The attributable burden represents the maximum benefit that would be achieved if the counterfactual could be met. (*Source:* Adapted with permission from Brauer M, Freedman G, Frostad J, et al. Ambient Air Pollution Exposure Estimation for the Global Burden of Disease 2013. *Environ Sci Technol.* 2016;50(1):79-88.[82])

pollutant(s) of concern and how the risk associated with the hazard at current concentrations might be reduced through regulatory interventions. Intrinsically, setting air-quality standards or proposing guidelines involves judgment as to what constitutes an adverse health effect and as to what level of risk is acceptable.

U.S. Clean Air Act: In the United States, the Clean Air Act is the regulatory template for managing the major pollutants in ambient air.[60] Its major provisions include:

- Control of certain common, widespread pollutants using national air-quality standards, the National Ambient Air Quality Standards or NAAQS;
- Control of "hazardous air pollutants";
- Protection of visibility in national parks;
- Control of acid rain;
- Protection of the stratospheric ozone layer;
- Reduction of pollution that causes climate change;
- Operating permits;
- Enforcement; and
- Relation of the Act to State clean air laws.

The major outdoor air pollutants are regulated under Sections 108 and 109. These sections place a mandate for public health protection on the Administrator of the EPA by calling for NAAQS that "protect public health with an adequate margin of safety." The NAAQS apply to six major pollutants: PM (including PM_{10} and

$PM_{2.5}$ at the present), ozone, carbon monoxide, sulfur dioxide, nitrogen dioxide, and lead. For each pollutant, the standard supplies the indicator, for example, $PM_{2.5}$, the averaging time, the concentration, and the statistical form.

The standards are currently developed through an evidence-based process that begins with a comprehensive review of new findings over the 5 years since the previous evaluation; the resulting Integrated Science Assessment or ISA evaluates the strength of evidence for causation of adverse health effects, considers findings on exposure and mechanisms, and addresses welfare effects, such as visibility. The Risk and Exposure Analysis (REA) is generally the next in the sequence of translational steps. The REA uses risk assessment approaches to contrast the existing profiles of exposure and risk to health with various scenarios of change in the NAAQS. The goal is to support decision-making by the Administrator. The REA feeds into the final translational document, the Policy Analysis, With this foundation, and engagement of the Executive Branch through the Office of Management and Budget (OMB), the Administrator determines whether a new NAAQS is needed and the features of the NAAQS. For example, in 1997, Administrator Browner added $PM_{2.5}$ as an indicator for PM.

The NAAQS are regulatory limits and, as such, states and municipalities are required to meet them. With this regulatory structure, substantial progress have been made in the United States, and levels of the criteria pollutants have progressively declined, even as the economy has grown (Fig. 70-2).

World Health Organization (WHO) Guidelines: The WHO periodically releases Air Quality Guidelines that do not have direct regulatory impact, but provide a framework for implementation of air-quality standards for countries lacking infrastructure to set their own target values. These guidelines were last revised in 2006 and are currently (2020) being revised once more. The guidelines in effect at present cover the major pollutants and include not only guideline values but target values, as three tiers, recognizing that for many low- and middle-income countries the guidelines cannot be achieved on a short-term timeframe.

Personal Protective Measures

Conceptually, the risk to human health (e.g., increased risk for dying and for morbidity) attributable to air pollution can be represented as:

$$\text{Health risk} = \text{Exposure} \times \text{Toxicity}$$

That is, the risk to health reflects the magnitude of exposure to an agent and the toxicity of the agent with toxicity expressed as increased risk per unit exposure from the exposure–response relationship. For example, in an analysis of air pollution and daily mortality data collected from 652 cities in 24 countries or regions, on average, an increase of 10 $\mu g/m^3$ in 2-day moving average of $PM_{2.5}$ (representing the average exposure over the current and previous day), is associated with increases of 0.68%, 0.55%, and 0.74% in daily all-cause, cardiovascular, and respiratory mortality, respectively.[27] This equation with its two terms leads to two basic approaches to mitigate the health risk from air pollution: reduce exposure and reduce toxicity. As described earlier in this chapter, air pollution control regulations and polices have substantially reduced emissions of air pollutants, consequently resulting in lower ambient concentrations and exposures in North America and western Europe since regulations were implemented. Source controls may have also reduced the overall toxicity of the air pollution mixture, for example, by reducing sulfur and mercury emissions and eliminating lead in gasoline.

While protection of public health necessarily involves control of emission sources or their elimination (e.g., replacing fossil-fuel based electricity generation with wind or solar power), the public can take personal-level protective measures to reduce risk from air pollution.[65] While inhaling healthy air may be considered as a right,[66] residents in many places are continually exposed to high concentrations of air pollution, sometimes at peaks that are unquestionably dangerous and that necessitation protective measures. Warning systems are in place in some countries and cities to advise the population on the need for protective action. Such actions are particularly imperative for those who are susceptible, for example, the elderly and those with chronic heart and lung disease, and also at risk for very high exposures, for example, outdoor workers and women with the additional high exposure that comes with use of solid fuels for cooking.

Fundamental to implementing public health approaches based on individual action is communication with the public about high levels of air pollution and the associated risks and the actions that can be taken by individuals. For that purpose, the approach of reporting on the Pollution Standards Index (PSI) or Air Quality Index (AQI) has been developed and implemented in a number of countries. In the United States, the AQI values range from 0 to 500 with a value of 100 corresponding to the NAAQS for a particular pollutant.[67] The information is connected with color coding as a way to warn, that is, green indicates "good" air quality and higher levels are coded with hotter colors (red being the worst and orange being the second worst).[67] The information is communicated through such channels as weather reports and websites, empowering people (and the government) to take necessary actions as shown in Fig. 70-5. Some potential personal protective steps are described below.

Indoor air filtration. Indoor air cleaning devices have long been available, albeit with little evidence on their efficacy with regard to health protection. Now, however, there is increasing interest in their utility as air pollution levels are often at alert concentrations. For example, in Chinese cities over the last decade, it has become common to have red or orange alert days with an air-quality index value substantially exceeding the air-quality standards. At such times, schools are closed and people are advised to stay indoors. However, even with windows and doors closed, indoor $PM_{2.5}$ and NO_2 levels typically reach over 70% of outdoor levels, whereas highly reactive ozone can reach 20–30% of the outdoor levels.

Consequently, there is increasing interest in using air cleaning technology to reduce indoor air pollution concentrations, particularly as they are affected by outdoor pollution. In locations with high pollution levels, such as some mega-cities in China, there is rising interest in indoor air cleaning. For particles, the most commonly used technology has been high-efficiency particulate air (HEPA)-based particle filtration to remove $PM_{2.5}$ entering from outdoors.

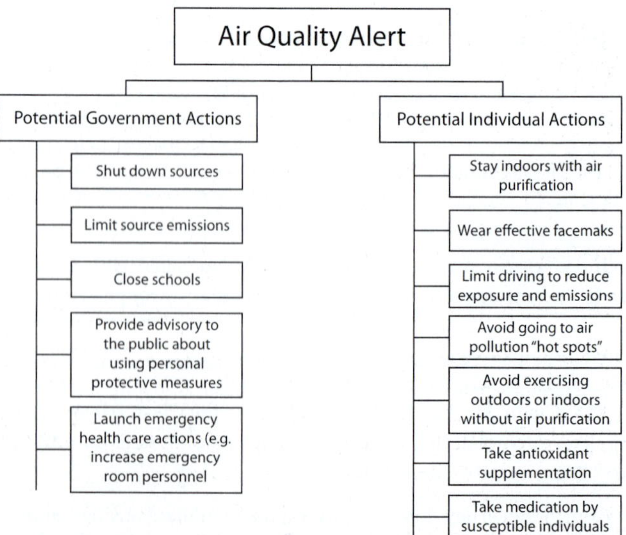

FIGURE 70-5. Potential responses to air-quality alerts at the governmental and the individual levels. (*Source:* Adapted from Samet, *Lancet Planet Health*. 2018;2:e6–7.[83])

This can be accomplished by adding HEPA filters within the HVAC system for mechanically vented buildings and by placing a portable air purifier containing a HEPA filter in a room. Studies conducted in western countries with low ambient $PM_{2.5}$ levels and in China all showed significant reductions in indoor $PM_{2.5}$ levels with indoor air HEPA filtration. The majority of these studies also showed improvements in health outcomes, although some of the outcomes are not directly related to a clinical benchmark, especially those biomarkers reflecting more of pathophysiologic changes than disease symptoms or organ function.[68]

Because HEPA filtration is relatively expensive due to high filter and maintenance costs as well as electricity consumption, other technologies have been used to remove $PM_{2.5}$. For example, electrostatic precipitation (ESP) is very efficient in removing particles with a cost substantially lower than HEPA filtration; and ESP devices have been used in large industrial facilities emitting particles. However, conventional ESP devices generate ozone as a byproduct. When ESP is used in occupied buildings, occupants will be exposed to ozone from this source and ozone reaction products.[69] Consequently, the United States has banned the sale of ESP for commercial and residential buildings. One recent study in participants who worked and lived in buildings equipped with an ESP and HEPA together in the HVAC system showed increased cardiovascular health risk compared to when the ESP was removed but the HEPA filtration remained operative.[70]

The most commonly used filters to remove gaseous pollutants have been filters impregnated with activated carbon. The HVAC system in some buildings contains an activated carbon filter, especially when odor is of concern in these buildings. Many commercial brands of portable air purifiers contain an activated carbon filter. These filters, when well-maintained or replaced before the adsorption capacity is saturated, have proven to remove certain volatile organic compounds (such as benzene, toluene, xylenes, and other nonpolar organics) efficiently. However, the removal efficiency of activated carbon filters for polar organics such as formaldehyde as well as for ozone and NO_2 is limited.[71,72] Research is recommended to develop more effective means to remove gaseous pollutants indoors.[73]

Facemasks. In some parts of the world, facemasks are commonly worn in public places. Typically, these masks are typically simple gauze or surgical masks. Although inexpensive and very common, they are not effective in providing protection against ambient air pollution. To achieve personal protection, a fitted N95 facemask is recommended for high-pollution days. The N95 facemask is capable of capturing $> 95\%$ of particles in inhaled air. This type of facemask is useful for people staying outdoors or indoors if effective indoor particle filtration is lacking. To be effective, it does require fitting and the N95 mask is not readily available for children. Furthermore, the mask may not be sufficiently comfortable, particularly in hot weather; it loads breathing; and it may not be culturally acceptable.

A few interventional studies have shown that wearing a facemask properly could lead to improved health outcomes.[68] However, these studies have a rigid study design requiring high compliance from study participants. In the real-world situation, people may not wear a facemask tightly over the full period when pollution levels are high. Whether efficacy, as documented in the clinical trials, will translate into effectiveness at the population level is unclear.

Dietary supplementation and therapeutic prevention. Exposure to air pollution increases oxidative stress and inflammation in the respiratory tract and systemically, leading to the hypothesis that antioxidants and inflammatory suppressants can reduce the risk of air pollution exposure.[74] The findings of a number of animal (rodent) studies confirm that using strong antioxidants such as N-acetyl cysteine (NAC), sulfide, ascorbate (vitamin C) or anti-inflammatory inhibitors (e.g., MitoTEMPO and VX765) can diminish injury from ozone.[75-77] Dietary interventional trials in humans showed that supplementation with antioxidants could alleviated respiratory effects of air pollution. For example, from October 1998 to April 2000 when photochemical pollution was severe in Mexico City, daily supplementation with a combination of vitamin C and vitamin E for 18 months significantly reduced the impact of ozone exposure on the small airways of Mexican children with moderate to severe asthma.[78] In a randomized, double-blinded, and placebo-controlled trial among 65 healthy college students living in Shanghai, dietary fish-oil supplementation of 2.5 g/day for 5 months (when average outdoor $PM_{2.5}$ concentration was 38 $\mu g/m^3$) resulted in significant improvements in biomarkers of systemic inflammation, blood coagulation, endothelial function, oxidative stress, antioxidant capacity, cardiometabolism, and neuroendocrine stress.[79] In a recent study, older people with COPD or free from cardiorespiratory diseases showed significantly worse lung function and cardiovascular function after walking in a street filled with traffic-related pollution. In contrast, older people with ischemic heart disease did not show these adverse effects following the same walk. The authors concluded that the routine medication use by the IHD patients helped to reduce the consequences of pollution exposure.[80]

Behavioral and lifestyle changes. For the long run, personal-level protective measures rely on a more health-oriented behavior and lifestyle. Personal protection is based on knowledge, awareness, and the capacity to take effective protective actions. With the constraints of feasibility, people can take steps to limit their exposure to traffic pollution, for example. They can also seek to reduce their contributions to pollution by using alternatives to personal motor vehicles. Such personal transportation choices may not only minimize their exposure to traffic pollution but also can minimize their contribution to traffic pollution. The availability of low-cost air pollution monitors allows communities and individuals to better understand the pollution to which they are exposed. Such sensors are now available at a cost as low as \$100.[81] Until recently, air-quality data were monitored at the central site monitoring stations set up for the regulatory purposes. These central site monitors cannot capture space heterogeneity in pollution levels, although the presence of air pollution "hotspots" (e.g., on or near a busy traffic road) is now well known. Governmental agencies and/or communities can add low-cost sensors in communities and neighborhoods to better inform community members' exposures. The monitoring data can be integrated to people's smartphones for instantaneous data access. Furthermore, the technology is becoming more readily available for individuals to wear an air pollution monitor. The data can guide people to make necessary activity changes to avoid high exposures. As personal health monitoring devices (e.g., wristbands capable of monitoring blood pressure, heart rate) are gaining popularity, integrating air pollution data into these wearable devices can also generate useful data for better understanding the risk of air pollution at the individual level.

SUMMARY

Ambient air pollution is a well-documented threat to global health that has worsened in some low- and middle-income countries, particularly in Asia. Because of expanding use of fossil fuels for manufacturing, vehicles, and power generation, the numbers of people worldwide exposed to risky levels of air pollution has increased progressively; some are exposed at levels historically associated with evident excess mortality and identification of risk-free levels of pollution has proved to be elusive. Ambient air pollution now affects large swathes of the world, as contaminated air crosses national boundaries and moves globally. Of course, greenhouse gases represent another form of global pollution that is linked to many of the same sources that contribute to ambient air pollution.

References

1. Cohen AJ, Brauer M, Burnett R, et al. Estimates and 25-year trends of the global burden of disease attributable to ambient air pollution: An analysis of data from the Global Burden of Diseases Study 2015. *Lancet.* 2017;389(10082):1907–18.
2. Corton C. *London Fog: The Biography.* 1st ed. Cambridge, MA: Belknap Press: An Imprint of Harvard University Press; 2015.
3. Jacobs C, Kelly WJ. *Smogtown. The Lung-Burning History of Pollution in Los Angeles.* New York: The Overlook Press, Peter Mayer Publishers, Inc.; 2008.
4. Haagen-Smit AJ. Chemistry and physiology of Los Angeles Smog. *Ind Eng Chem.* 1952;44(6):1342–6.
5. World Health Organization. Air pollution—Fact sheet. 2018. https://www.who.int/news-room/fact-sheets/detail/ambient-(outdoor)-air-quality-and-health. Accessed December 9, 2019.
6. United Nations, Department of Economic and Social Affairs, Population Division. *The World's Cities in 2018—Data Booklet.* 2018.
7. Brimblecombe P. *The Big Smoke: A History of Air Pollution in London Since Medieval Times.* 1st ed. London, UK: Routledge Kegan & Paul; 1987.
8. Davis D. *When Smoke Ran LIke Water: Tales of Environmental Deception and the Battle Against Pollution.* 1st ed. New York: Basic Books; 2002.
9. Logan WP. Mortality in the London fog incident, 1952. *Lancet.* 1953;1(6755):336–8.
10. AirNow. Homepage. https://www.airnow.gov/. Accessed December 30, 2019.
11. Jacobs ET, Burgess JL, Abbott MB. The Donora Smog revisited: 70 years after the event that inspired the Clean Air Act. *Am J Public Health.* 2018;108(S2):S85–8.
12. 42 U.S.C. Sect. 7401 *et seq.*—Clean Air Act (CAA). U.S. Environmental Protection Agency; 1990.
13. U.S. Environmental Protection Agency. Air Quality. 2016. https://www3.epa.gov/airquality/cleanair.html. Accessed December 19, 2019.
14. World Health Organization. *Air Quality Guidelines: Global Update 2005-Particulate Matter, Ozone, Nitrogen Dioxide and Sulfur Dioxide.* Copenhagen: World Health Organization; 2006.
15. U.S. Environmental Protection Agency. Our Nation's Air—Status and trends through 2015. 2016. https://gispub.epa.gov/air/trendsreport/2016/. Accessed September 9, 2016.
16. Stanaway JD, Afshin A, Gakidou E, et al. Global, regional, and national comparative risk assessment of 84 behavioural, environmental and occupational, and metabolic risks or clusters of risks for 195 countries and territories, 1990–2017: A systematic analysis for the Global Burden of Disease Study 2017. *Lancet.* 2018;392(10159):1923–94.
17. Godowitch J, Ching J, Clarke J. Evolution of the nocturnal inversion layer at an urban and nonurban location. *J Clim Appl Meteorol.* 1985;24(8):791–804.
18. Zhang JJ, Samet JM. Chinese haze versus Western smog: Lessons learned. *J Thorac Dis.* 2015;7(1):3–13.
19. An Z, Huang R-J, Zhang R, et al. Severe haze in northern China: A synergy of anthropogenic emissions and atmospheric processes. *Proc Natl Acad Sci U S A.* 2019;116(18):8657–66.
20. Cheng Y, Zheng G, Wei C, et al. Reactive nitrogen chemistry in aerosol water as a source of sulfate during haze events in China. *Sci Adv.* 2016;2(12):e1601530.
21. Leung DYC. Outdoor-indoor air pollution in urban environment: Challenges and opportunity. *Front Environ Sci.* 2015;2(69).
22 National Research Council. Committee on Human and Environmental Exposure Science in the 21st Century, Board on Environmental Studies and Toxicology, Division on Earth and Life Studies. *Exposure Science in the 21st Century : A Vision and a Strategy.* Washington, DC: National Academies Press; 2012.
23. van Donkelaar A, Martin RV, Brauer M, Boys BL. Use of satellite observations for long-term exposure assessment of global concentrations of fine particulate matter. *Environ Health Perspect.* 2015;123(2):135–43.
24. Di Q, Kloog I, Koutrakis P, Lyapustin A, Wang Y, Schwartz J. Assessing PM exposures with high spatio-temporal resolution across the continental United States. *Environ Sci Technol.* 2016;50(9):4712–21.
25. Di Q, Wang Y, Zanobetti A, et al. Air pollution and mortality in the medicare population. *N Engl J Med.* 2017;376(26):2513–22.
26. Collier-Oxandale A, Feenstra B, Papapostolou V, et al. Field and laboratory performance evaluations of 28 gas-phase air quality sensors by the AQ-SPEC program. *Atmos Environ.* 2020;220:117092.
27. Liu C, Chen R, Sera F, et al. Ambient particulate air pollution and daily mortality in 652 cities. *N Engl J Med.* 2019;381(8):705–15.
28. Dockery DW, Pope CA, 3rd, Xu X, et al. An association between air pollution and mortality in six U.S. cities. *N Engl J Med.* 1993;329(24):1753–9.
29. Ferris BG, Jr., Speizer FE, Spengler JD, et al. Effects of sulfur oxides and respirable particles on human health. Methodology and demography of populations in study. *Am Rev Respir Dis.* 1979;120(4):767–79.
30. Gauderman WJ, Urman R, Avol E, et al. Association of improved air quality with lung development in children. *N Engl J Med.* 2015;372(10):905–13.
31. Peters JM, Avol E, Navidi W, et al. A study of twelve Southern California communities with differing levels and types of air pollution. I. Prevalence of respiratory morbidity. *Am J Respir Crit Care Med.* 1999;159(3):760–7.
32. Gauderman WJ, Avol E, Gilliland F, et al. The effect of air pollution on lung development from 10 to 18 years of age. *N Engl J Med.* 2004;351(11):1057–67.
33. Katsouyanni K, Samet JM. *Air Pollution and Health: European and North American Approach (APHENA). Research Report 142.* Boston, MA: Health Effects Institute; 2009.
34. Pope CA, 3rd, Coleman N, Pond ZA, Burnett RT. Fine particulate air pollution and human mortality: 25+ Years of cohort studies. *Environ Res.* 2019;183:108924.
35. HEI Accountability Workgroup. *Assessing Health Impact of Air Quality Regulations: Concepts and Methods for Accountability Research. Communication 11.* Boston, MA: Health Effects Institute; 2003.
36. Zeger SL, Dominici F, Samet J. Harvesting-resistant estimates of air pollution effects on mortality. *Epidemiology.* 1999;10(2):171–5.
37. Krall JR, Chang HH, Sarnat SE, Peng RD, Waller LA. Current methods and challenges for epidemiological studies of the associations between chemical constituents of particulate matter and health. *Curr Environ Health Rep.* 2015;2(4):388–98.
38. Health Effects Institute. *Special Report 17: Traffic-Related Air Pollutions: A Critical Review of the Literature on Emissions, Exposure, and Health Effects.* Boston, MA: Health Effects Institute; 2010.
39. Lam J, Sutton P, Kalkbrenner A, et al. A systematic review and meta-analysis of multiple airborne pollutants and autism spectrum disorder. *PLoS One.* 2016;11(9):e0161851.
40. Li X, Huang S, Jiao A, et al. Association between ambient fine particulate matter and preterm birth or term low birth weight: An updated systematic review and meta-analysis. *Environ Pollut.* 2017;227:596–605.
41. Wilker EH, Preis SR, Beiser AS, et al. Long-term exposure to fine particulate matter, residential proximity to major roads and measures of brain structure. *Stroke.* 2015;46(5):1161–6.
42. IARC. *Outdoor Air Pollution.* Vol. 109. Lyon, France: International Agency for Research on Cancer; 2015.
43. U.S. EPA. *Final Report: Integrated Science Assessment for Particulate Matter.* Washington, DC: Agency USEP; 2009.
44. Pope CA3rd, Ezzati M, Dockery DW. Fine-particulate air pollution and life expectancy in the United States. *N Engl J Med.* 2009;360(4):376–86.
45. U.S. Environmental Protection Agency. Ozone Pollution and Your Patients' Health: What is Ozone? 2016. https://www.epa.gov/ozone-pollution-and-your-patients-health/what-ozone. Accessed December 10, 2019.
46. EPA US. *Final Report: Integrated Science Assessment of Ozone and Related Photochemical Oxidants.* Washington, DC: U.S. Environmental Protection Agency; 2013.
47. U.S. Environmental Protection Agency. Integrated Science Assessment for Ozone and Related Photochemical Oxidants. Research Triangle Park, NC2013. EPA/600/R-10/076F.
48. Frampton MW, Balmes J, Bromberg PA, et al. Multicenter ozone study in older subjects (MOSES): Part 1. Effects of exposure to low concentrations of ozone on respiratory and cardiovascular outcomes. *Res Rep Health Eff Inst.* 2017 Jun;(192, Pt 1):1–107;.
49. Bell ML, Dominici F, Samet JM. A meta-analysis of time-series studies of ozone and mortality with comparison to the national morbidity, mortality, and air pollution study. *Epidemiology.* 2005;16(4):436–45.
50. Zhang J, Wei Y, Fang Z. Ozone pollution: A major health hazard worldwide. *Front Immunol.* 2019;10:2518.
51. U.S. Environmental Protection Agency. *Integrated Science Assessment (ISA) For Oxides Of Nitrogen—Health Criteria (Final Report, 2016).* Washington, DC: U.S. EPA; 2016.
52. Agency for Toxic Substances and Disease Registry (ATSDR). ToxFAQs for Nitrogen Oxides. Atlanta, GA: Agency for Toxic Substances and Disease Registry; 2002.
53. Faustini A, Rapp R, Forastiere F. Nitrogen dioxide and mortality: Review and meta-analysis of long-term studies. *Eur Respir J.* 2014;44(3):744–53.
54. Achakulwisut P, Brauer M, Hystad P, Anenberg SC. Global, national, and urban burdens of paediatric asthma incidence attributable to ambient NO_2 pollution: Estimates from global datasets. *Lancet Planet Health.* 2019;3(4):e166–78.

55. U.S. Environmental Protection Agency. U.S. EPA. Integrated Science Assessment (ISA) For Carbon Monoxide (Final Report, Jan 2010). Washington, DC. 2010. EPA/600/R-09/019F.

56. U.S. Environmental Protection Agency. U.S. EPA. Integrated Science Assessment (ISA) For Sulfur Oxides—Health Criteria (Final). Washington, DC. 2017. EPA/600/R-17/451.

57. Hedley AJ, Wong CM, Thach TQ, Ma S, Lam TH, Anderson HR. Cardiorespiratory and all-cause mortality after restrictions on sulphur content of fuel in Hong Kong: An intervention study. *Lancet.* 2002;360(9346):1646–52.

58. U.S. Environmental Protection Agency. U.S. EPA. Integrated Science Assessment (ISA) For Lead (Final Report, Jul 2013). Washington, DC. 2013. EPA/600/R-10/075F.

59. Centers for Disease Control. Blood Lead Levels in Children. 2019. https://www.cdc.gov/nceh/lead/prevention/blood-lead-levels.htm. Accessed January 6, 2020.

60. U.S. Environmental Protection Agency. The Clean Air Act Amendments of 1990. 1990. https://www.epa.gov/laws-regulations/summary-clean-air-act. Accessed March 18, 2016.

61. U.S. Environmental Protection Agency. Controlling Hazardous Air Pollutants. 2017. https://www.epa.gov/haps/controlling-hazardous-air-pollutants. Accessed December 10, 2019.

62. Levin ML. The occurrence of lung cancer in man. *Acta Unio Int Contra Cancrum.* 1953;9(3):531–41.

63. Health Effects Institute. *State of Global Air 2019. Special Report.* Boston, MA: Health Effects Institute; 2019.

64. Institute for Health Metrics and Evaluation. Global Burden of Disease (GBD). 2017; http://www.healthdata.org/gbd. Accessed December 13, 2019.

65. Laumbach R, Meng Q, Kipen H. What can individuals do to reduce personal health risks from air pollution? *J Thorac Dis.* 2015;7(1):96–107.

66. Samet JM, Gruskin S. Air pollution, health, and human rights. *Lancet Respir Med.* 2015;3(2):98–100.

67. U.S. Environmental Protection Agency. The National Ambient Air Quality Standards for Particle Pollution: Revised Air Quality Standards for Particle Pollution and Updates to the Air Quality Index (AQI). 2012. https://www.epa.gov/sites/production/files/2016-04/documents/2012_aqi_factsheet.pdf. Accessed January 8, 2020.

68. Bard RL, Ijaz MK, Zhang JJ, et al. Interventions to reduce personal exposures to air pollution: A primer for health care providers. *Glob Heart.* 2019;14(1):47–60.

69. Xiang J, Weschler CJ, Mo J, Day D, Zhang J, Zhang Y. Ozone, electrostatic precipitators, and particle number concentrations: Correlations observed in a real office during working hours. *Environ Sci Technol.* 2016;50(18):10236–44.

70. Day DB, Xiang J, Mo J, et al. Combined use of an electrostatic precipitator and a high-efficiency particulate air filter in building ventilation systems: Effects on cardiorespiratory health indicators in healthy adults. *Indoor Air.* 2018;28(3):360–72.

71. Norris C, Fang L, Barkjohn KK, et al. Sources of volatile organic compounds in suburban homes in Shanghai, China, and the impact of air filtration on compound concentrations. *Chemosphere.* 2019;231:256–68.

72. Zhang X, Gao B, Creamer AE, Cao C, Li Y. Adsorption of VOCs onto engineered carbon materials: A review. *J Hazard Mater.* 2017;338:102–23.

73. Vikrant K, Cho M, Khan A, Kim K-H, Ahn W-S, Kwon EE. Adsorption properties of advanced functional materials against gaseous formaldehyde. *Environ Res.* 2019;178:108672.

74. Rich DQ, Kipen HM, Huang W, et al. Association between changes in air pollution levels during the Beijing Olympics and biomarkers of inflammation and thrombosis in healthy young adults. *JAMA.* 2012;307(19):2068–78.

75. Li F, Wiegman C, Seiffert JM, et al. Effects of N-acetylcysteine in ozone-induced chronic obstructive pulmonary disease model. *PLoS One.* 2013;8(11):e80782.

76. Li F, Zhang P, Zhang M, et al. Hydrogen sulfide prevents and partially reverses ozone-induced features of lung inflammation and emphysema in mice. *Am J Respir Cell Mol Bio.* 2016;55(1):72–81.

77. Li F, Xu M, Wang M, et al. Roles of mitochondrial ROS and NLRP3 inflammasome in multiple ozone-induced lung inflammation and emphysema. *Respir Res.* 2018;19(1):230.

78. Romieu I, Sienra-Monge JJ, Ramírez-Aguilar M, et al. Antioxidant supplementation and lung functions among children with asthma exposed to high levels of air pollutants. *Am J Respir Crit Care Med.* 2002;166(5):703–9.

79. Lin Z, Chen R, Jiang Y, et al. Cardiovascular benefits of fish-oil supplementation against fine particulate air pollution in China. *J Am Coll Cardiol.* 2019;73(16):2076–85.

80. Sinharay R, Gong J, Barratt B, et al. Respiratory and cardiovascular responses to walking down a traffic-polluted road compared with walking in a traffic-free area in participants aged 60 years and older with chronic lung or heart disease and age-matched healthy controls: A randomised, crossover study. *Lancet.* 2018;391(10118):339–49.

81. U.S. Environmental Protection Agency. Air Sensor Toolbox: What is EPA Doing? 2019. https://www.epa.gov/air-sensor-toolbox/air-sensor-toolbox-what-epa-doing. Accessed January 8, 2020.

82. Brauer M, Freedman G, Frostad J, et al. Ambient air pollution exposure estimation for the Global Burden of Disease 2013. *Environ Sci Technol.* 2016;50(1):79–88.

83. Samet JM. Do air quality alerts benefit public health? New evidence from Canada. *Lancet Planet Health.* 2018;2(1):e6–7.

84. Bell ML, Samet J. Air pollution. In: Frumkin H, ed.Frumkin H, ed. *Environmental Health: From Local to Global.* 2nd ed. San Francisco, CA: Jossey-Bass; 2010:387–415.

CHAPTER

71 Household Air Pollution in Low- and Middle-income Countries

Magdalena Fandiño-Del-Rio • Kirsten Koehler • Kristen Fedak • Jennifer Peel • William Checkley

INTRODUCTION

Household air pollution (HAP) is generated in resource-limited settings where people continue to depend on solid fuels including wood, dung, agricultural crop waste, and coal or kerosene, for their basic energy needs such as cooking and heating. The use of solid fuels results in inefficient combustion, which produce high levels of harmful air pollutants like particulate matter (PM), carbon monoxide (CO), and nitrogen oxides; carcinogenic organic compounds such as benzene, formaldehyde, and 1,3-butadiene; carcinogenic cyclic chemicals such as polycyclic aromatic hydrocarbons (PAHs); and, respiratory irritants such as phenols, cresols, acrolein, and acetaldehyde. Moreover, PM in HAP smoke contains compounds adsorbed to its surface including endotoxin, metals, and microbial components thought to play an important role in PM toxicity.[1-3] Thus, HAP is a complex mixture that varies widely in its characteristics.

It is estimated that three billion people worldwide use solid fuels for cooking.[4] While the proportion of households that rely on solid fuels for cooking has decreased in the last three decades (62%–33.7% between 1980 and 2016), the absolute number of people exposed to biomass fuel smoke has remained relatively stable due to population growth and rising lifespan.[5,6] Countries currently bearing the heaviest disease burdens from exposures to HAP include China, India, Pakistan, Bangladesh, Indonesia, Nigeria, Democratic Republic of Congo, Ethiopia, and Tanzania (Fig. 71-1). The greatest declines in percentages of the population using solid fuels have been documented in Asia, Southern Africa, and South America.[5] Despite improvements, the highest burden of exposure occurs in India and China with 560 million and 416 million exposed, respectively.[5] There has been little change in the proportion of the population using solid fuels in East, Central, and West sub-Saharan Africa. In particular, in Ethiopia, the Democratic Republic of the Congo, and Tanzania, where almost all of their populations are exposed to HAP.[5]

Current regulations for air pollutant concentrations are limited to ambient air quality and do not affect indoor air concentrations in the presence of HAP.[7] In an effort to address this concern, the World Health Organization (WHO) developed recommendations for several indoor air pollutants recognizing their importance regarding health impacts related to household fuel combustion.[8] Of these pollutants, PM and CO are the most commonly measured for indoor exposure quantification.[9,10] Typically, PM in the air covers a range of sizes and its aerodynamic properties determine how deeply it can penetrate and be deposited within the respiratory tract.[11] The composition of these particles depends on the combustion process and varies by fuel type, but most of the components include sulfate, nitrate, ammonium, black carbon (BC), and organic carbon in addition to various trace metals.[12] Particles larger than 10 micrometers in aerodynamic diameter (PM_{10}) are trapped in the nose and pharyngeal region. Fine particles, that consist of PM less than 2.5 micrometers in aerodynamic diameter ($PM_{2.5}$), are of particular importance due to their ability to penetrate to the bronchial and alveolar regions, initiate inflammatory cascades, and enter the pulmonary circulation.[13]

ASSESSMENT OF HOUSEHOLD AIR POLLUTION

The most common method to measure HAP is to use monitors in microenvironments such as the kitchen or living area. Stationary monitors, however, do not capture the movements of individuals and can result in biased exposure estimates compared to personal exposure assessment, which aims to estimate pollutant concentrations experienced by a person during normal daily activities. Measuring personal exposures directly reduces bias and increases the precision of estimates when quantifying the relationship of HAP with health risk in epidemiological studies.[9,14-16] However, personal exposure assessment can be challenging due to limitations in monitoring technology. Air pollution exposure assessment can be done through either integrated samples that collect information over a period of time and are returned to a laboratory for analysis, or continuous monitors that record concentrations as they are being measured and provide time-varying information. Monitors of either type can also be active (using a pump and a power source to collect air or pass it through a sensor) or passive (using a sensor that detects concentrations based on diffusion). Active monitors generally require a power source, are often heavy, noisy, and require frequent calibration.[17] as is often the case for PM sampling.

Personal sampling can be especially problematic when measuring PM, which generally requires the use of a personal sampling pump carried by people. Assessments of PM for HAP studies have been mostly done taking samples in fixed locations, such as the kitchen, and using an integrated sample collected gravimetrically.[9] Gravimetric integrated samples are active samples collected by pulling air through a filter using a pump for a known amount of time and with a known flow rate. These samples are precise, although they do not provide time-varying exposure information, instead giving a single time-weighted average exposure.[15,18] Nephelometric technology that is based on light scattering, can provide continuous measurements, but the measurements are subject to bias because of varying responses by different particle types and they can be very sensitive to temperature and relative humidity conditions.[19,20] Recently, smaller devices have been developed to be used as personal samplers and some incorporate simultaneous integrated gravimetric and continuous nephelometric technology.[16,21,22] Nevertheless, devices are generally not designed for remote low-income setting areas with lack of electricity or laboratory spaces for calibration and maintenance.[15] Moreover, there is a need for standardized indoor air pollution methods and for developing quality control on samples from urban low-income settings so as to increase the comparability between studies.[9]

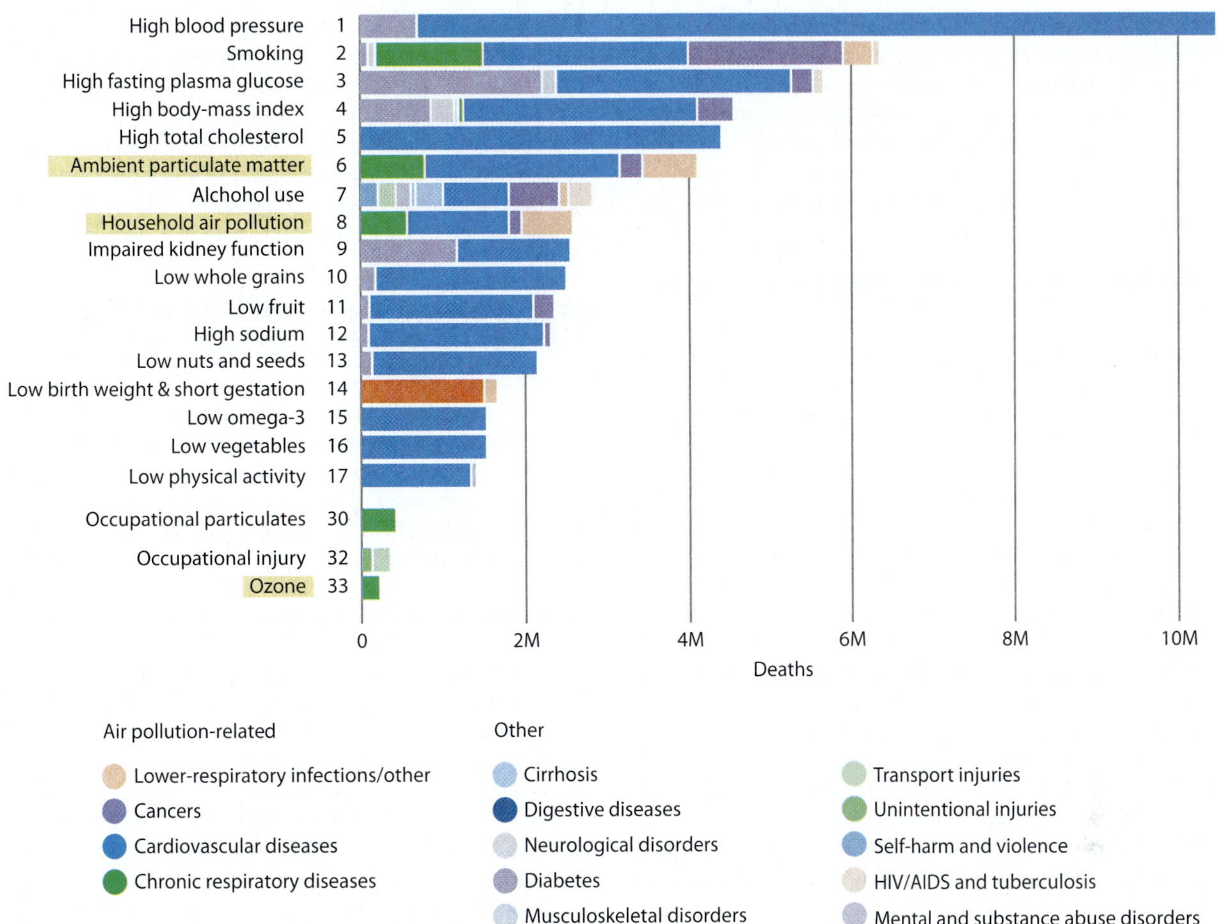

FIGURE 71-1. Global ranking of risk factors by total number of deaths from all causes for all ages and both sexes in 2016. (*Source:* Reproduced with Permission From Health Effects Institute. State of Global Air 2018. Special Report. Boston, MA: Health Effects Institute; 2018. https://www.stateofglobalair.org/report.[5])

Monitoring personal CO concentrations has generally been easer since it is commonly measured using electrochemical sensors or diffusion tubes that are small enough to be worn by study participants. Electrochemical sensors can also record personal exposure data continuously and can be powered using small batteries. Diffusion tubes are based on a color change and do not require power, although they are integrated samples and do not collect continuous data.[23,24] Some early studies measured CO as an indicator to estimate personal PM exposure.[25,26] Nevertheless, CO is not a consistent surrogate for $PM_{2.5}$ concentrations. Correlation between these two pollutants varies by site as well as many other factors that influence combustion characteristics and air exchange in a home or other structures.[27,28]

Biomarkers of exposure are also used to understand the effects of different exposure levels and health outcomes. The most common biomarkers of internal dose (the amount of pollutant entering the body) for HAP include urine PAHs, exhaled CO and carboxyhemoglobin.[20,24,29,30] Biomarkers of early biological effect such as inflammation, coagulation, oxidative stress and endothelial function are also being used given their relevance to documented disease endpoints related to ambient air pollution and also cigarette smoking.[31–36] Although biomarkers might provide accurate information on absorbed dose, very few metabolites have been assessed from HAP specifically and we lack information on risk linked to particular biomarkers that could to use as a reference to address indoor air pollution from biomass fuel use [15]. In addition, other sources of pollutants may also affect health given that biomass smoke is not the sole source of exposure to harmful indoor pollutants.

Little is known about the form of the dose-response curves of HAP with various health outcomes[37] and which components of PM play an important role in disease development. PM likely plays an important role since diminished immunotoxicity has been observed after removing the exposure.[38–40] PM is believed to affect the circulatory system through increased blood pressure, inflammation, enhanced coagulability, and increased blood viscosity.[41–44] While there is clear evidence of the toxicity of ambient air pollution and its consequent health effects,[13,45–48] the mechanisms by which HAP leads to the development of disease have not been fully explored.

When considering mitigation of the health effects of PM, there is particular interest in identifying components of PM responsible for triggering adverse health outcomes.[49] Recent reviews, mostly based on studies of traffic-related emissions, suggest that BC might play an important role in the relationship of PM with cardiovascular disease development.[49,50] BC is one of the main components of fine PM resulting from the incomplete combustion of carbonaceous materials. The total carbon content in fine particles reflects the organic fraction and the elemental fraction. The elemental fraction is often reported as elemental carbon (EC) or BC, used similarly in the literature, although measured differently. BC consists of EC with several organic and inorganic compounds absorbed on to its carbonaceous surface.[51–53] BC is defined as carbon content as measured by light absorption.[53]

Several literature reviews suggest that BC might have stronger association with cardiopulmonary outcomes than with PM mass or any other $PM_{2.5}$ species.[49,50,52,54,55] Studies that have looked at mortality, hospital admissions and emergency department visits, mostly on healthy adults and older susceptible populations, with both BC and PM from traffic-related exposures, suggest that the effect of BC was more robust than the effect of PM mass on outcomes.[49,50,52,54] In addition, the associations of cardiovascular and respiratory hospital admissions with ambient and traffic BC concentrations appear significantly greater than estimated effects of most other single PM elements in several studies involving adult populations.[55–61] In particular, the ultrafine fraction of particle emissions that contains BC coated with a mix of organic compounds, appears to be associated with oxidative stress and inflammation, as part of the pathways related to disease development.[47,52,54] Some recent studies are incorporating BC analysis in PM samples from biomass burning cookstoves.[62–64] There is a need to better understand the role of other relevant pollutants from biomass combustion and their relative toxicity.[15]

HOUSEHOLD AIR POLLUTION LEVELS FROM BIOMASS STOVES

Indoor air quality is not typically regulated by governments, even in high-income countries. The WHO has established guidelines for indoor environments and recommends $PM_{2.5}$ annual mean exposure to be less than 10 μg/m³ and a 24-hour mean less than 25 μg/m³. Nevertheless, existing evidence suggested that there is no safe level of $PM_{2.5}$ exposure.[65,66] The guidelines recommend that the mean CO concentrations levels not exceed 35 mg/m³ in one hour more than once a day, and the average should not exceed 7 mg/m³ in 24 hours. The WHO guidelines also suggest interim targets to promote progressive reductions for high pollution areas that are associated with risk reduction of acute and chronic health effects.[65] $PM_{2.5}$ interim targets are 35, 25, and 15 μg/m³ for annual mean concentrations and 75, 50, and 37.5 μg/m³ for the 24-hour means. Typical $PM_{2.5}$ concentrations for personal exposure of women in households that use biomass fuel can be more than seven times the most conservative interim daily guideline recommended by the WHO (35 μg/m³).

Several recent reviews have compiled data on HAP studies including the WHO database with information from more than 70 published studies in developing countries from households that use solid fuels. On average, 24-hour $PM_{2.5}$ concentrations indoors are around 980 μg/m³ (ranging from 200 to 3000 μg/m³).[9,18,67] Within the span of cooking events, levels of indoor air pollution can be as high as 30,000 μg/m³.[68] Typical CO concentrations (expressed as hourly averages) can be as high as 50 mg/m³ (ranging from 10 to 260 mg/m³) and 24-hour averages of kitchen concentrations are typically around 10 mg/m³ (ranging from 2 to 40 mg/m³).[9,18,68] Concentrations for personal exposures are on average around 250 μg/m³ (ranging from 50 to 1000 μg/m³) for $PM_{2.5}$ and 4 mg/m³ (ranging from 2 to 7 mg/m³) for CO.[9,18,68] Although annual averages have not been measured, given that household cooking activities take place daily, 24-hour concentrations are often considered estimates of annual averages for research and burden estimation.[68]

Several factors that influence combustion and home ventilation contribute to the high variability in indoor concentrations of air pollutants. For example, when comparing type of fuel, cooking practices that use animal dung as fuel produce much higher average concentrations compared to households that use wood. A model developed based on the WHO Global HAP database used 44 published studies in developing countries on households that use biomass, generated estimates of 24-hour $PM_{2.5}$ kitchen concentration and personal exposure measurements. Based on this model mean 24-hour $PM_{2.5}$ concentrations for traditional wood stoves were about 390 μg/m³ (95% CI 148–1039 μg/m³) in kitchens, 160 μg/m³ (95% CI 61–431 μg/m³) for personal exposure of an adult woman, and 140 μg/m³ (95% CI 53–375 μg/m³) for personal exposure of a child. In contrast, when using animal dung as fuel, mean exposures were about 960 μg/m³ (95% CI 359–2520 μg/m³) for kitchen concentrations, and 390 μg/m³ (95% CI 148–1047 μg/m³) and 340 μg/m³ (95% CI 129–911 μg/m³) for personal exposures in adult women and children, respectively.[67]

In addition to personal activity patterns and fuel type, there is a wide variability on the profiles on pollutant concentrations by site that will also depend on several factors such as cultural behaviors, cooking practices, seasonal patterns, and climate. Indeed, in some regions with hot climates biomass stoves are outdoors while they tend to be indoors in colder climates. Furthermore, variability in HAP concentrations is also expected within households from one day to the next.[15] Therefore, single, short-term exposure assessment may not adequately capture actual HAP exposures in a household.[18] Epidemiological studies assessing exposure in relation to health outcomes have used long-term repeated measurements and even develop models based on repeated samples and housing and community-level characteristics to predict longer-term exposure levels.[69,70]

EFFECTS OF HOUSEHOLD AIR POLLUTION ON CLIMATE AND AMBIENT AIR POLLUTION

HAP is a major contributor to outdoor air pollution.[8] It not only contributes to outdoor PM but also NOx emissions and volatile organic compounds from HAP that can contribute to ground-level formation of ozone. HAP accounts for 12% of ambient air pollution globally and contributes to almost 40% of $PM_{2.5}$ in regions such as sub-Saharan Africa.[71] In addition, BC, a major component of PM in HAP, is among the most important climate change pollutants after CO_2 and methane. HAP is estimated to contribute 25% of global emissions of BC. In particular, residential coal and biomass burning are estimated to contribute to more than 60% of BC emissions of Africa and Asia.[72] Biomass combustion also produces methane and N_2O, known greenhouse gases.

When comparing different alternatives to biomass-consuming stoves, use of LPG-fueled stoves has been shown to make a lower contribution to warming potential while a much greater contribution comes from charcoal and coal stove use.[73] In particular, when considering the scenario of providing LPG to replace traditional residential biomass use there is an estimated small but net overall reduction in greenhouse gas generation.[74] Expanding electrification to replace the use of solid fuels and using LPG stoves could have a negligible impact in greenhouse gas emissions, compared with continuing with the current fuel sources.[73] The consequences of switching traditional biomass stoves to electrical stoves alone has been estimated under several scenarios and assumptions. The net result ranges from potentially having a total reduction to having a very small impact increasing greenhouse gases by about 2–4%.[73]

EFFECTS OF HOUSEHOLD AIR POLLUTION ON HEALTH

HAP generated from biomass fuel combustion is currently identified as the eighth leading risk factor contributing to the global burden of disease (Fig. 71-2).[5,75] HAP exposure has been recognized as an important risk factor for the development of multiple diseases and other adverse effects: COPD, chronic bronchitis, lung cancer, childhood pneumonia and acute lower respiratory infections, hypertension, cardiovascular events, and lower birthweight.[76–78] HAP is not only a leading contributor to the global burden of disease but it has also been recognized among the largest environmental risk factors for preventable disease.[79–82] HAP from solid fuels was estimated to be responsible for 2.6 million premature deaths and 77.2 million disability-adjusted life-years (DALYs) lost in 2016.[75]

Burning of biomass fuels for cooking is an important risk factor for mortality in low and middle-income countries.[82] In particular, 60% of premature deaths from HAP in 2012 were attributed to women and children, who spend a considerable amount of their time near the combustion source and have the highest exposures to biomass fuel emissions.[83]

Exposure to HAP is a major risk factor for death and illness in children. In 2016, HAP was estimated to be responsible for 250,000 deaths in children under 5 years of age worldwide.[75,84] Almost 28% of total DALYs lost for children under 5 years are attributable to HAP.[5] Most of the burden for children comes from respiratory infections. Indeed, two meta-analyses have found that children were 3.52 times (95% CI 1.93–6.43) more likely to develop acute respiratory infections[85] and 2.51 times (95% CI 1.53–4.10) more likely to have an acute

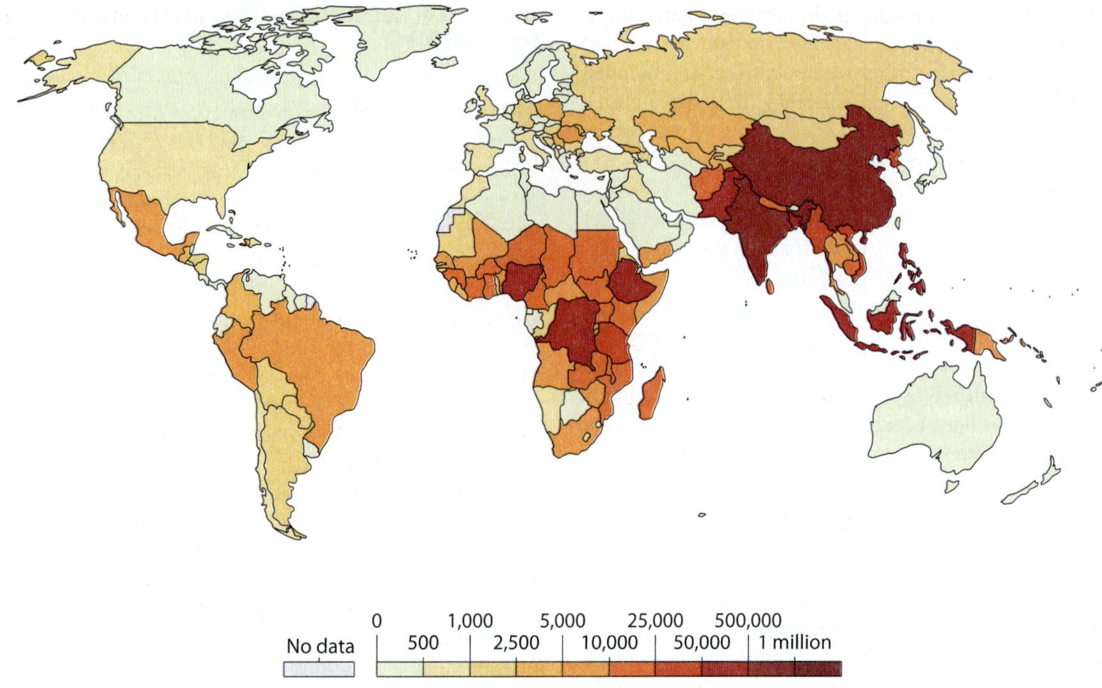

FIGURE 71-2. Number of deaths by country from HAP in 2016. (*Source:* From Global Burden of Disease Collaborative Network. Global Burden of Disease Study 2016 [GBD 2016] Results. Seattle, United States: Institute for Health Metrics and Evaluation [IHME]. 2017. http://ghdx.healthdata.org/gbd-results-tool.[150])

lower respiratory infection[86] when exposed to HAP than those without the exposure.

HAP exposure is also a strong contributor to poor health in adults, particularly among women who are the primary cooks. Several studies and meta-analyses have documented that HAP is associated with a higher prevalence of respiratory symptoms,[87,88] worse lung function and a higher prevalence of COPD,[87,89,90] higher blood pressure and hypertension,[42,91,92] a thicker carotid artery intima-media[93,94] and poorer pregnancy outcomes.[95] One meta-analysis of 18 studies found that use of solid fuels was associated with 2.80 greater odds (95% CI 1.85 to 4.00) of COPD and 2.32 greater odds of chronic bronchitis (95% CI 1.92–2.80).[98] In a subgroup analysis of studies that used spirometry for COPD, the use of solid fuels was associated with 2.96 greater odds (95% CI 2.01–4.37) of COPD. Another pooled analysis of population-based studies, involving 12,396 adults (aged 35–95 years) in 13 countries, found that those with HAP exposure had a 1.41 greater adjusted odds of having COPD (95% CI 1.18–1.68) than those without the exposure and estimated that 13.5% of COPD prevalence was attributable to HAP exposure.[101] In an analysis of data of premenopausal women (aged 15–49 years) from 12 Demographics and Health Surveys in ten countries, the investigators found that primary use of solid fuel was associated with a 0.58 mm Hg higher systolic blood pressure (95% CI 0.23–0.93 mm Hg) as compared to primary use of clean fuel.[103] Two studies found that adult participants exposed to HAP had a 0.03 mm (95% CI 0.01–0.06) greater adjusted carotid-intima media thickness and a higher prevalence of carotid plaques (OR = 2.6, 95% CI 1.1–6.0) in Peru and a 0.04 mm greater adjusted carotid intima media artery thickness (95% CI 0.01–0.09) in Nigeria when compared to those without the exposure.[104,105] A meta-analysis of 19 studies found that HAP exposure was associated with an average loss in birthweight of 86.3 grams (95% CI 55.5–117.4 grams), a 35% higher prevalence of low birthweight and 29% higher prevalence of stillbirth.[95,96] Another meta-analysis of five low birthweight studies and three stillbirth studies found that HAP exposure was associated with a higher prevalence of lower birthweight (OR = 1.38, 95% CI 1.25–1.52), a higher prevalence of lower stillbirth (OR = 1.51, 95% CI 1.23–1.85) and reduced mean birthweight (-95.6 grams, 95% CI -68.5 to -124.7 grams).[96]

However, many of these estimates were based on observational studies. In the sections below, we describe the effects of randomized controlled trials with cleaner cooking technologies or cleaner fuels on multiple health outcomes.

TYPES OF INTERVENTIONS TO REDUCE HOUSEHOLD AIR POLLUTION

Interventions to reduce the health burden of HAP generally fall into three broad areas: pollution source interventions, user behavior interventions, and living environment interventions.[97] The majority of cookstove users burn wood or charcoal in open-fire or rudimentary stoves,[6] resulting in uncontrolled, inefficient combustion that generates high pollutant emissions (e.g., ref. 98). Improved stoves can be designed to burn fuel more efficiently and deliver energy to the cooking task, thereby reducing emissions and exposures.[10] For example, design features can change combustion dynamics and alter the efficiency of the stove: insulated combustion chambers on a wood stove result in less energy lost as excess heat and more energy transferred to the cooking vessel or food, compared to an open-fire design.[99] This design can reduce the amount of fuel needed to complete a cooking task, which translates to less fuel use and less total pollutant generation. Other design features may not reduce emissions but change how the cook interacts with the stove during a cooking process, which can change exposures. Chimneys move the smoke emitted from the combustion away from the breathing zone of the cook and out of the house, reducing the pollutant concentrations in the cooking area and lowering personal exposures.[100] Stoves that are placed at waist height can reduce direct exposures by limiting the need for the cook to bend over close to the cooking; separation of cooking and living spaces can reduce exposures for noncook members of the household.[97] Integration of design features that do not serve a purpose in reducing stove emissions with other emissions-reducing design features may help encourage use of improved stoves over traditional stoves, for example, USB charging ports that enable cooking tasks to be combined with cellphone charging.[101]

Changes in fuel type can also impact pollution: pollutant composition can vary across fuel types, such as improved stoves over traditional stoves.[102,103] Combined with stove designs that are intended to maximize the thermal combustion efficiency for a specific fuel, interventions that target the replacement of a cooking system (stove/fuel combination) have the potential to reduce pollutant exposures and health burden.

Recent studies are also starting to evaluate the potential effect of stoves that use cleaner technologies such as the gas and in particular liquefied petroleum gas (LPG) stoves.[64,104–110] Laboratory-based testing shows that LPG stove use can reduce HAP enough to meet the WHO recommended guidelines.[8] As part of the HAP guidelines development, the WHO modeled emission rates and the potential impact of different technologies on indoor and personal exposure to air pollution. According to this model, 99% of homes could meet the WHO annual guideline Interim target-1 of 35 $\mu g/m^3$ for $PM_{2.5}$ with LPG stove use [8]. However, estimations based on laboratory data do not incorporate real social behaviors, cooking patterns, or other variables that affect actual reductions.

Few population-based studies have evaluated HAP from LPG stove use in low-income areas that traditionally use biomass as fuel for cooking.[9,104,106,111,112] Previous measurements show that kitchen $PM_{2.5}$ concentrations mostly range between 35 and 80 $\mu g/m^3$ in households that use clean fuels including gas.[8,111,112] Furthermore, according to recent estimates that model the potential impact of an LPG stove intervention in rural settings, personal exposure to $PM_{2.5}$ could decrease from 270 to 70 $\mu g/m^3$ due to potential continued use of traditional stove use.[113] When evaluating cleaner fuels, potential neighborhood contamination might also play an important role limiting reductions in HAP. Therefore, community-wide efforts should be incorporated in these types of interventions.[9] Evaluating the actual impact of the use of cleaner fuels in real settings is crucial to understand its potential impact on HAP and health.

Clean cooking transitions are often hindered by a variety of socioeconomic and cultural factors and lack of affordable access to stove and fuels. National policy can encourage the uptake and sustained use of clean cooking interventions. For example, government agencies in India, Guatemala, China, Cameroon, and Peru encourage the use of improved biomass and LPG stoves and offer incentives to reduce barriers to adoption, such as fuel subsidies to reduce costs, free or subsidized fuel delivery programs to ease access, and aid for startup costs such as free in-home gas connection installations.[114–117] China's government promoted improved stoves in rural households in the 1980s and 1990s, through public finance initiatives that improved coal access to rural households using biomass[118]; while successful, current knowledge suggests that coal use is not sufficiently improved, necessitating a second phase of governmental policy to promote clean stove adoption, the China Clean Stove Initiative collaboration with the World Bank.[119] In India, government initiatives to improve LPG access and encourage LPG use (including direct cash transfer programs, fuel subsidies, and campaigns to encourage high-income households to pass their subsidies to poorer families), have contributed to a rapid increase in LPG consumption.[120] However, use of cleaner fuels like LPG in India remains low, especially in rural areas, due to issues with affordability, accessibility, and awareness in poor communities.[120] Similarly, the government of Ghana has promoted LPG use through policy programs to encourage LPG production and distribution since 1989, such as offering free empty LPG canisters to the public, subsidizing the startup of LPG delivery services, building government LPG cylinder manufacturing facilities and refilling stations, and offering financial incentives for LPG distributors to travel to rural areas away from production centers; yet, LPG use country-wide remains less than 25%.[121]

IMPACT OF INTERVEZNTIONS ON HOUSEHOLD AIR POLLUTION

There is a large body of evidence demonstrating that in-home pollutant and personal exposure concentrations can differ across different stove and fuel types. A WHO review of 161 studies published through 2011 concluded that 24-hour average kitchen-area PM_{10} and $PM_{2.5}$ measurements in households using solid fuels (e.g., wood, charcoal) are consistently two to ten times above the WHO interim target guidelines limits for the annual average (the levels estimated to be associated with a 15% higher long-term mortality risk relative to the air quality guideline levels, set as 70 $\mu g/m^3$ for PM_{10} and 35 $\mu g/m^3$ for $PM_{2.5}$).[18] Comparatively, households using kerosene, gas or electric fuels for at least part of their energy needs were regularly at or below these limits. For example, the authors estimated pooled mean 24-hour kitchen concentrations (based on a subset of 46 studies with sufficient data for meta-analyses). In homes using solid fuel, the average concentration was 882 $\mu g/m^3$ (SD 971 $\mu g/m^3$) PM_{10} and 972 $\mu g/m^3$ (SD 876 $\mu g/m^3$) $PM_{2.5}$, versus 146 $\mu g/m^3$ (SD 94 $\mu g/m^3$) $PM_{2.5}$ for improved combustion cookstoves, and 148 $\mu g/m^3$ (SD 56 $\mu g/m^3$) PM_{10} and 66 $\mu g/m^3$ (SD 37 $\mu g/m^3$) $PM_{2.5}$ for gas, electric, or kerosene fuels. Concentrations of CO in kitchens were also elevated in homes using solid fuels in traditional stoves [8.60 ppm (SD 6.21 ppm) 24-hour average] compared to improved stoves (3.98 ppm, SD 4.14 ppm) and clean fuels (1.30 ppm, SD 0.60).[18]

Several other literature reviews and meta-analyses have summarized the effect of cookstove interventions on improving air-quality metrics.[9,122,123] For example, Quansah et al. (2017)[123] reviewed 55 studies and concluded that HAP interventions can reduce personal PM by 24%, kitchen PM by 18%, and kitchen CO by 3%. However, the authors noted high between-study variability due to a variety of intervention designs; further, most postintervention air pollutant concentrations were still above the WHO guidelines for air quality. Pope et al. (2017)[9] similarly concluded that improved stoves can result in large reductions in both kitchen/area $PM_{2.5}$ and CO concentrations and personal exposures. For example, they pooled data from 42 studies and estimated that advanced combustion stove interventions can reduce kitchen $PM_{2.5}$ by 29–50% (average 41%) compared to traditional solid fuel stoves; ethanol stoves can reduce result in even larger reductions of 64–94% (average 83%).[9] Thomas et al. (2015)[122] identified 36 studies published by April 2014 that reported on interventions to reduce HAP, primarily from improved stoves. The authors did not quantitatively summarize their findings but noted that while 29 of the 36 studies found reduced HAP with intervention, rarely did an intervention reduce HAP concentration to below WHO recommended limits.

IMPACTS OF HOUSEHOLD AIR POLLUTION INTERVENTIONS ON HEALTH OUTCOMES

The RESPIRE (Randomized Exposure Study of Pollution Indoors and Respiratory Effects) trial, conducted in Guatemala from 2002 to 2004, was the first randomized intervention trial aimed at reducing long-term cookstove-related air pollution exposures and subsequent health effects, primarily focused on clinical respiratory outcomes in young children. Participants were pregnant women or women with children < 4 months old. Half the enrolled households ($n = 269$) received a wood-burning plancha stove with a chimney while the other half ($n = 265$) maintained use of their traditional open wood fire. Results indicated a nonsignificant decrease in relative risk of physician-diagnosed pneumonia and significant decreases in relative risk of fieldworker-assessed pneumonia, physician-diagnosed severe pneumonia, and RSV-negative pneumonia, among children up to 18 months old who lived in intervention households compared to children in homes using traditional open fires.[124]

A decade after the RESPIRE trial, the Cooking and Pneumonia (CAPS) trial in Malawi[125] assessed the effect of an improved stove intervention on childhood pneumonia risk. The investigators used a gasifier stove, a technology intended to result in even greater exposure reductions compared to an open fire than the intervention of a chimney used in the RESPIRE trial. CAPS enrolled 10,750 children (8626 households) in a community-level cluster randomized design. Over 24 months of postintervention follow-up, researchers found no differences in pneumonia risk among children (<5 years old) who lived in homes using the intervention stove compared to children in homes using open fires (the control). However, overall adoption of the stove was low: by 12 months and through to 24 months postintervention, over 20% of the intervention group reported that they did not use the stove.

Impacts of cookstove interventions on adult respiratory health are unclear. In rural Mexico, a randomized control trial of 552 women found that those who received an improved stove intervention had a lower risk of reporting respiratory symptoms and lower lung function decline over a 1-year follow-up compared to women who continued to use open fires[126]; notably, adherence to the intervention was only 50%. However, in the RESPIRE trial, cross-sectional analysis of preintervention spirometry measurements among 319 women (all using open wood fires) indicated no association between FVC or FEV_1 and exhaled breath CO, an exposure biomarker.[127] Further, no associations were found between assignment of the intervention stove and FEV_1, FVC, or FEV_1/FVC at follow-up at 6, 12, or 18 months.[128] However, with exhaled CO in breath measured at the same time as spirometry was conducted, investigators observed a 35 mL decrease in FEV_1 (95% CI -61, -9 mL) for each one-unit increase in natural log transformed exhaled CO.[129] Among 120 women who had personal exposure measurements, those in the intervention group had lower personal 24-hour average $PM_{2.5}$ exposures (264 μg/m^3 versus 102 μg/m^3)[100]; however, exposure distributions between the control and intervention group overlapped,[124] likely resulting in measurement error in the categorical intent-to-treat analysis that would bias these results toward null.

Additional analyses conducted using data from the RESPIRE trial provide added insight into nonrespiratory health effects from cookstove air pollution, namely cardiovascular health and birth outcomes. Blood pressure measurements conducted on women indicated that the intervention was associated with lower systolic (-3.7 mm Hg, 95% CI -8.1, 0.60) and diastolic (-3.0 mm Hg, 95% CI -5.7, -0.4) pressure 1 year postintervention (average 293 days, range, 2–700 days).[100] Researchers also recorded birthweight of 174 newborns during the study period; weight was higher (89 grams; 95% CI -27, 204 grams) among infants born to mothers who had received the improved chimney stove during pregnancy compared to the mothers in the control group.[130]

The Ibadan Cookstoves and Low Birth Weight Study, conducted in Ibadan, Nigeria, between 2013 and 2015, has provided further insight into maternal blood pressure and birth outcomes. Researchers enrolled 324 pregnant women at < 18 weeks gestational age who used wood and/or kerosene as their primary cooking fuel from four community hospitals.[131–133] Half of the women were randomized into an intervention arm and received ethanol stoves and fuel supplies; follow-up was conducted six times during pregnancy. Researchers observed that diastolic blood pressure (DBP) was 2.8 mm Hg lower among women in the intervention arm at the last follow-up visit at approximately 38 weeks gestational age. However, they did not find differences in SBP throughout pregnancy or at final follow-up.[131] Birthweights were higher, average gestational age at delivery was higher, and there were less miscarriages and stillbirths in the ethanol arm compared to the control arm.[134] In a subset of 77 women who had both maternal blood collected at 34 weeks gestation and cord blood samples collected at delivery, levels of angiogenic factors placental growth factor and soluble fms-like tyrosine kinase 1 varied, but were not significantly different, between the groups.[132] Newborn length, placental weight to birth weight ratio, and infant head circumference were not different between the groups.[132] However, in an assessment on a subset of women (16 wood/kerosene users and 20 ethanol users), it was shown that various markers of chronic placental hypoxia (Hofbauer cells, syncytial knots, and chorionic vascular density and hypoxia-inducible factor) were increased significantly among wood/kerosene users compared to ethanol users.[133]

Additional experiments, while nonrandomized, provide further support for impacts of cookstove interventions on cardiovascular health. For example, Clark et al. (2011)[135] observed increases in systolic blood pressure with increased 48-hour indoor CO (1.78 mm Hg per 24 ppm increase in CO, 95% CI−1.25, 4.81) and 48-hour personal CO (1.89 mm Hg per 2 ppm increase in CO, 95% CI−0.48, 4.26) in a cross-sectional analysis of one-time measurements for 124 Nicaraguan women using traditional open-combustion wood stoves. No relationship was observed between blood pressure and 48-hour indoor $PM_{2.5}$. One year after intervention with a chimney stove among 74 of these women, Clark et al. (2013)[136] did not observe changes in systolic or diastolic blood pressure (SBP: -1.5 mm Hg 95% CI -4.9, 1.8; DBP: 0 mm Hg 95% CI -2.1, 2.1), despite marked reductions in 48-hour average kitchen $PM_{2.5}$ and CO measured among a subset of the women at follow-up ($PM_{2.5}$ average reduced from 1801 to 416 μg/m^3 in a sample of 25, CO reduced from 25.8 to 7.2 ppm in sample of 32). Subgroup analysis restricted to women greater than 40 years old, however, resulted in a 5.9 mm Hg reduction in systolic blood pressure (95% CI -11.3, -0.4). Notably, Clark et al. (2013)[136] found that about half of the participants still used their traditional stove. Alexander et al. (2015)[137] observed a 4.8% decrease in SBP (5.5 mm Hg, from 114.5 to 109.0 mm Hg) measured either during or immediately after cooking among 28 women in Bolivia, along with a 24-hour average kitchen $PM_{2.5}$ reduction from 240 to 48 μg/m^3 in a subset of 15 women, 1 year after an intervention that involved changing from indoor open-pit fires to better-insulated wood-burning stoves with chimneys. Stove adoption was around 90%, which may explain some of the difference in results between this work and that of Clark et al. More recently, an energy package intervention, comprised of a semigasifier cookstove, water heater, chimney, and supply of processed biomass fuel in rural China,[138] resulted in a decrease in air pollution exposures in both the treatment and control groups. This result is in part explained by participants in the control group unexpectedly switching to cleaner stoves (electric and gas) after baseline. Although significant differences comparing intervention and control groups were not observed, overall $PM_{2.5}$ and BC exposure reductions (range: +2% to −48% for $PM_{2.5}$; −49% to −69% for BC) resulted in small mean reductions in brachial and central blood pressure (−0.3 to −4.1 mm Hg).[138]

Although improved cookstoves have achieved important reductions in emissions, concentrations of indoor pollutants still remain significantly higher than the World Health Organization recommended levels,[9,139] and therefore show limited results in improving health.[10] For example, RESPIRE was unable to measure significant reductions in pneumonia occurrence despite reducing personal exposure to emissions by 50%.[26] Similarly, the cluster-randomized trial in Malawi did not find a reduction in child pneumonia with an improved biomass-burning stove intervention.[140] Previous exposure-response analyses have found that the greatest risk reductions occur with much lower exposure levels that are unlikely to be achieved with biomass and require interventions with cleaner fuels.[26,37,80] Thus, recent intervention efforts are shifting toward stoves that use cleaner fuels, such as LPG.[104–109]

ONGOING HOUSEHOLD AIR POLLUTION INTERVENTION TRIALS

Several additional randomized control trials that are currently underway or recently completed may help shed light on the respiratory and cardiovascular impacts of cookstove interventions; however, results related to longitudinal health impacts are not yet available for much of this work.[110,141–145] Ongoing trials focus primarily on LPG stove interventions,[64,110,145–147] considered by many researchers to be potentially the best available alternative to traditional biomass (in terms of reduced exposures). However, several ongoing trials consider interventions that potentially offer less emission reductions but may be more feasible long-term solutions. For example, improved rocket-elbow style or forced-draft wood stoves or biomass gasifiers that use a similar fuel source as traditional stoves and therefore require less of an infrastructure change.[141,142,146–149] Trends in the health outcomes studied in these interventions include a focus on biomarkers, such as inflammatory metabolites in urine and blood and health impacts of cookstove exposures on pregnant women, mothers, and young children, such as birth outcomes (e.g., birthweight, gestational age), gross motor development, childhood respiratory health (e.g., acute lower respiratory infection incidence), inflammatory biomarkers, blood pressure, and lung function.[64,142,146,147]

SUMMARY

Remarkably, one of the most common and potent sources of exposure to inhaled air pollutants, combustion of biomass fuels for cooking and heating, received little attention until three decades ago. The resulting research has provided insights into the nature of the exposure and the risks of HAP for children and adults. Many intervention studies have now been carried out and many are in progress, addressing ways to reduce exposures and disease burden. The findings to date indicate that exposures can be reduced, although generally not to levels that meet WHO guidelines for outdoor air. The burning of biomass fuels makes a substantial contribution to greenhouse gas emissions. Comprehensive approaches are needed to protect human health and planetary health.

References

1. Sussan TE, Ingole V, Kim J-H, et al. Source of biomass cooking fuel determines pulmonary response to household air pollution. *Am J Respir Cell Mol Biol.* 2014;50:538–48.
2. Edwards R, Karnani S, Fisher EM, et al. WHO | Indoor air quality guidelines: Household fuel combustion. Review 2: Emissions of Health-Damaging Pollutants from Household Stoves. World Health Organization; 2014. http://www.who.int/airpollution/guidelines/household-fuel-combustion/evidence/en/. Accessed 8 Jan 2019.
3. McDonald JD, White RK, Barr EB, Zielinska B, Chow JC, Grosjean E. Generation and characterization of hardwood smoke inhalation exposure atmospheres. *Aerosol Sci Technol.* 2006;40:573–84.
4. Yadama GN. *Fires, Fuel, and the Fate of 3 Billion: The State of the Energy Impoverished.* Oxford, New York: Oxford University Press; 2013.
5. Health Effects Institute. *State of Global Air 2018. Special Report.* Boston, MA: Health Effects Institute; 2018. https://www.stateofglobalair.org/report. Accessed 27 Sep 2018.
6. Bonjour S, Adair-Rohani H, Wolf J, et al. Solid fuel use for household cooking: Country and regional estimates for 1980–2010. *Environ Health Perspect.* 2013;121:784–90.
7. Avery CL, Mills KT, Williams R, et al. Estimating error in using ambient PM2.5 concentrations as proxies for personal exposures. *Epidemiol Camb Mass.* 2010;21:215–23.
8. World Health Organization. WHO indoor air quality guidelines: Household fuel combustion. World Health Organization; 2014. http://www.who.int/iris/handle/10665/141496. Accessed 23 Jan 2018.
9. Pope D, Bruce N, Dherani M, Jagoe K, Rehfuess E. Real-life effectiveness of 'improved' stoves and clean fuels in reducing PM2.5 and CO: Systematic review and meta-analysis. *Environ Int.* 2017;101 Supplement C:7–18.
10. Thomas E, Wickramasinghe K, Mendis S, Roberts N, Foster C. Improved stove interventions to reduce household air pollution in low and middle income countries: A descriptive systematic review. *BMC Public Health.* 2015;15:650.
11. Hinds WC. *Aerosol Technology: Properties, Behavior, and Measurement of Airborne Particles.* New York: John Wiley & Sons; 1999.
12. Wilson R, Spengler JD. *Particles in Our Air: Concentrations and Health Effects.* Cambridge, MA: Harvard School of Public Health; 1996.
13. Brook RD, Rajagopalan S, Pope C, et al. Particulate matter air pollution and cardiovascular disease: An update to the scientific statement from the American Heart Association. *Circulation.* 2010;121:2331–78.
14. Bruce N, Perez-Padilla R, Albalak R. Indoor air pollution in developing countries: A major environmental and public health challenge. *Bull World Health Organ.* 2000;78:1078–92.
15. Clark ML, Peel JL, Balakrishnan K, et al. Health and household air pollution from solid fuel use: The need for improved exposure assessment. *Environ Health Perspect.* 2013;121:1120–8.
16. Chartier R, Phillips M, Mosquin P, et al. A comparative study of human exposures to household air pollution from commonly used cookstoves in Sri Lanka. *Indoor Air.* 2017;27:147–59.
17. Watson AY, Bates RR, Kennedy D. *Assessment of Human Exposure to Air Pollution: Methods, Measurements, and Models.* Washington, DC: National Academies Press (US); 1988. https://www.ncbi.nlm.nih.gov/books/NBK218147/. Accessed 6 Mar 2019.
18. Balakrishnan K, Mehta S, Ghosh S, et al. WHO | Indoor air quality guidelines: Household fuel combustion. Review 5: Population levels of household air pollution and exposures. World Health Organization; 2014. http://www.who.int/airpollution/guidelines/household-fuel-combustion/evidence/en/. Accessed 8 Jan 2019.
19. Chakrabarti B, Fine PM, Delfino R, Sioutas C. Performance evaluation of the active-flow personal DataRAM PM2.5 mass monitor (Thermo Anderson pDR-1200) designed for continuous personal exposure measurements. *Atmos Environ.* 2004;38:3329–40.
20. Pollard SL, Williams DL, Breysse PN, et al. A cross-sectional study of determinants of indoor environmental exposures in households with and without chronic exposure to biomass fuel smoke. *Environ Health Glob Access Sci Source.* 2014;13:21.
21. Shi J, Chen F, Cai Y, et al. Validation of a light-scattering PM2.5 sensor monitor based on the long-term gravimetric measurements in field tests. *PLoS One.* 2017;12(11):e0185700.
22. Koehler KA, Peters TM. New methods for personal exposure monitoring for airborne particles. *Curr Environ Health Rep.* 2015;2:399–411.
23. Borghi F, Spinazzè A, Rovelli S, et al. Miniaturized monitors for assessment of exposure to air pollutants: A review. *Int J Environ Res Public Health.* 2017;14(8):909.
24. Balakrishnan K, Mehta S, Ghosh S, et al. WHO | Indoor air quality guidelines: Household fuel combustion. Review 5: Population levels of household air pollution and exposures. World Health Organization; 2014. http://www.who.int/airpollution/guidelines/household-fuel-combustion/evidence/en/. Accessed 8 Jan 2019.
25. Northcross A, Chowdhury Z, McCracken J, Canuz E, Smith KR. Estimating personal PM2.5 exposures using CO measurements in Guatemalan households cooking with wood fuel. *J Environ Monit JEM.* 2010;12:873–8.
26. Smith K, McCracken J, Weber M, et al. Effect of reduction in household air pollution on childhood pneumonia in Guatemala (RESPIRE): A randomised controlled trial. *Lancet.* 2011;378:1717–26.
27. Carter E, Norris C, Dionisio KL, et al. Assessing exposure to household air pollution: A systematic review and pooled analysis of carbon monoxide as a surrogate measure of particulate matter. *Environ Health Perspect.* 2017;125(7):076002.
28. Klasen EM, Wills B, Naithani N, et al. Low correlation between household carbon monoxide and particulate matter concentrations from biomass-related pollution in three resource-poor settings. *Environ Res.* 2015;142:424–31.
29. Torres-Dosal A, Pérez-Maldonado IN, Jasso-Pineda Y, Martínez Salinas RI, Alegría-Torres JA, Díaz-Barriga F. Indoor air pollution in a Mexican indigenous community: Evaluation of risk reduction program using biomarkers of exposure and effect. *Sci Total Environ.* 2008;390:362–8.
30. Lee A, Sanchez TR, Shahriar MH, Eunus M, Perzanowski M, Graziano J. A cross-sectional study of exhaled carbon monoxide as a biomarker of recent household air pollution exposure. *Environ Res.* 2015;143 Pt A:107–11.
31. Delfino RJ, Staimer N, Tjoa T, et al. Circulating biomarkers of inflammation, antioxidant activity, and platelet activation are associated with primary combustion aerosols in subjects with coronary artery disease. *Environ Health Perspect.* 2008;116:898–906.

32. Delfino RJ, Staimer N, Tjoa T, et al. Air pollution exposures and circulating biomarkers of effect in a susceptible population: Clues to potential causal component mixtures and mechanisms. *Environ Health Perspect.* 2009;117:1232–8.

33. Croft DP, Cameron SJ, Morrell CN, et al. Associations between ambient wood smoke and other particulate pollutants and biomarkers of systemic inflammation, coagulation and thrombosis in cardiac patients. *Environ Res.* 2017;154:352–61.

34. Rückerl R, Hampel R, Breitner S, et al. Associations between ambient air pollution and blood markers of inflammation and coagulation/fibrinolysis in susceptible populations. *Environ Int.* 2014;70:32–49.

35. Guarnieri MJ, Diaz JV, Basu C, et al. Effects of woodsmoke exposure on airway inflammation in rural Guatemalan women. *PLoS One.* 2014;9(3):e88455.

36. Olopade CO, Frank E, Bartlett E, et al. Effect of a clean stove intervention on inflammatory biomarkers in pregnant women in Ibadan, Nigeria: A randomized controlled study. *Environ Int.* 2017;98:181–90.

37. Burnett RT, Pope CA, Ezzati M, et al. An integrated risk function for estimating the global burden of disease attributable to ambient fine particulate matter exposure. *Environ Health Perspect.* 2014;122:397–403.

38. Thomas PT, Zelikoff JT. 17—Air pollutants: Modulators of pulmonary host resistance against infection. In: Holgate ST, Samet JM, Koren HS, Maynard RL, eds. *Air Pollution and Health.* London: Academic Press; 1999, pp. 357–79.

39. Lee A, Kinney P, Chillrud S, Jack D. A systematic review of innate immunomodulatory effects of household air pollution secondary to the burning of biomass fuels. *Ann Glob Health.* 2015;81:368–74.

40. Zelikoff JT, Chen LC, Cohen MD, Schlesinger RB. The toxicology of inhaled woodsmoke. *J Toxicol Environ Health Part B.* 2002;5:269–82.

41. Brook RD, Franklin B, Cascio W, et al. Air pollution and cardiovascular disease: A statement for healthcare professionals from the expert panel on population and prevention science of the American Heart Association. *Circulation.* 2004;109:2655–71.

42. Baumgartner J, Schauer JJ, Ezzati M, et al. Indoor air pollution and blood pressure in adult women living in rural China. *Environ Health Perspect.* 2011;119:1390–5.

43. Baumgartner J, Zhang Y, Schauer JJ, Ezzati M, Patz JA, Bautista LE. Household air pollution and children's blood pressure. *Epidemiology.* 2012;23:641–2.

44. Baumgartner J, Zhang Y, Schauer JJ, Huang W, Wang Y, Ezzati M. Highway proximity and black carbon from cookstoves as a risk factor for higher blood pressure in rural China. *Proc Natl Acad Sci U S A.* 2014;111: 13229–34.

45. Brook RD, Brook JR, Urch B, Vincent R, Rajagopalan S, Silverman F. Inhalation of fine particulate air pollution and ozone causes acute arterial vasoconstriction in healthy adults. *Circulation.* 2002;105:1534–6.

46. Rundell K, Hoffman J, Caviston R, Bulbulian R, Hollenbach A. Inhalation of ultrafine and fine particulate matter disrupts systemic vascular function. *Inhal Toxicol.* 2007;19:133–40.

47. Grahame TJ, Schlesinger RB. Cardiovascular health and particulate vehicular emissions: A critical evaluation of the evidence. *Air Qual Atmosphere Health.* 2010;3:3–27.

48. Mustafic H, Jabre P, Caussin C, et al. Main air pollutants and myocardial infarction: A systematic review and meta-analysis. *JAMA.* 2012;307:713–21.

49. Kelly FJ, Fussell JC. Size, source and chemical composition as determinants of toxicity attributable to ambient particulate matter. *Atmos Environ.* 2012;60 Supplement C:504–26.

50. World Health Organization. Health effects of black carbon (2012). 2012. http://www.euro.who.int/en/health-topics/environment-and-health/air-quality/publications/2012/health-effects-of-black-carbon-2012. Accessed 25 Sep 2017.

51. Cassee FR, Héroux M-E, Gerlofs-Nijland ME, Kelly FJ. Particulate matter beyond mass: Recent health evidence on the role of fractions, chemical constituents and sources of emission. *Inhal Toxicol.* 2013;25:802–12.

52. Grahame TJ, Klemm R, Schlesinger RB. Public health and components of particulate matter: The changing assessment of black carbon. *J Air Waste Manag Assoc.* 2014;64(6):620–60. http://www.tandfonline.com/doi/abs/10.1080/10962247.2014.912692. Accessed 25 Sep 2017.

53. Chow JC, Watson JG, Lowenthal DH, Antony Chen L-W, Motallebi N. PM2.5 source profiles for black and organic carbon emission inventories. *Atmos Environ.* 2011;45:5407–14.

54. Janssen NAH, Hoek G, Simic-Lawson M, et al. Black carbon as an additional indicator of the adverse health effects of airborne particles compared with PM10 and PM2.5. *Environ Health Perspect.* 2011;119:1691–9.

55. Achilleos S, Kioumourtzoglou M-A, Wu C-D, Schwartz JD, Koutrakis P, Papatheodorou SI. Acute effects of fine particulate matter constituents on mortality: A systematic review and meta-regression analysis. *Environ Int.* 2017;109:89–100.

56. Cakmak S, Dales RE, Gultekin T, et al. Components of particulate air pollution and emergency department visits in Chile. *Arch Environ Occup Health.* 2009;64:148–55.

57. Peng RD, Bell ML, Geyh AS, et al. Emergency admissions for cardiovascular and respiratory diseases and the chemical composition of fine particle air pollution. *Environ Health Perspect.* 2009;117:957–63.

58. Lipfert FW, Baty JD, Miller JP, Wyzga RE. PM2.5 constituents and related air quality variables as predictors of survival in a cohort of U.S. military veterans. *Inhal Toxicol.* 2006;18:645–57.

59. Ostro B, Feng W-Y, Broadwin R, Green S, Lipsett M. The effects of components of fine particulate air pollution on mortality in California: Results from CALFINE. *Environ Health Perspect.* 2007;115:13–9.

60. Cakmak S, Dales RE, Vida CB. Components of particulate air pollution and mortality in Chile. *Int J Occup Environ Health.* 2013;15:152–8.

61. Peng RD, Bell ML, Geyh AS, et al. Emergency admissions for cardiovascular and respiratory diseases and the chemical composition of fine particle air pollution. *Environ Health Perspect.* 2009;117:957–63.

62. Garland C, Delapena S, Prasad R, L'Orange C, Alexander D, Johnson M. Black carbon cookstove emissions: A field assessment of 19 stove/fuel combinations. *Atmos Environ.* 2017;169:140–9.

63. Downward GS, Hu W, Rothman N, et al. Outdoor, indoor, and personal black carbon exposure from cookstoves burning solid fuels. *Indoor Air.* 2016;26:784–95.

64. Household Air Pollution and Health: A Multi-country LPG Intervention Trial—Full Text View—ClinicalTrials.gov. https://clinicaltrials.gov/ct2/show/NCT02944682. Accessed 15 Feb 2019.

65. WHO | Air quality guidelines—Global update 2005. WHO. 2005. http://www.who.int/phe/health_topics/outdoorair/outdoorair_aqg/en/. Accessed 23 Jan 2018.

66. Raaschou-Nielsen O, Andersen ZJ, Beelen R, et al. Air pollution and lung cancer incidence in 17 European cohorts: Prospective analyses from the European Study of Cohorts for Air Pollution Effects (ESCAPE). *Lancet Oncol.* 2013;14:813–22.

67. Shupler M, Godwin W, Frostad J, Gustafson P, Arku RE, Brauer M. Global estimation of exposure to fine particulate matter (PM2.5) from household air pollution. *Environ Int.* 2018;120:354–63.

68. Rehfuess E, Bruce N, Smith K. Solid fuel use: Health effect. Nriagu JO, ed. *Encyclopedia of Environmental Health.* Burlington: Elsevier; 2011.

69. McCracken JP, Schwartz J, Bruce N, Mittleman M, Ryan LM, Smith KR. Combining individual- and group-level exposure information: Child carbon monoxide in the Guatemala woodstove randomized control trial. *Epidemiology.* 2009;20:127–36.

70. Dionisio KL, Howie SRC, Dominici F, et al. Household concentrations and exposure of children to particulate matter from biomass fuels in The Gambia. *Environ Sci Technol.* 2012;46:3519–27.

71. Chafe ZA, Brauer M, Klimont Z, et al. Household cooking with solid fuels contributes to ambient PM2.5 air pollution and the burden of disease. *Environ Health Perspect.* 2014;122:1314–20.

72. Bond TC, Doherty SJ, Fahey DW, et al. Bounding the role of black carbon in the climate system: A scientific assessment. *J Geophys Res Atmospheres.* 2013;118:5380–552.

73. Pachauri S, Ruijven BJ van, Nagai Y, et al. Pathways to achieve universal household access to modern energy by 2030. *Environ Res Lett.* 2013;8:024015.

74. Grieshop AP, Marshall JD, Kandlikar M. Health and climate benefits of cookstove replacement options. *Energy Policy.* 2011;39:7530–42.

75. Gakidou E, Afshin A, Abajobir AA, et al. Global, regional, and national comparative risk assessment of 84 behavioural, environmental and occupational, and metabolic risks or clusters of risks, 1990–2016: A systematic analysis for the Global Burden of Disease Study 2016. *Lancet.* 2017;390:1345–422.

76. Fullerton D, Bruce N, Gordon S. Indoor air pollution from biomass fuel smoke is a major health concern in the developing world. *Trans R Soc Trop Med Hyg.* 2008;102:843–51.

77. Miller KA, Siscovick DS, Sheppard L, et al. Long-term exposure to air pollution and incidence of cardiovascular events in women. *N Engl J Med.* 2007;356:447–58.

78. Gordon SB, Bruce NG, Grigg J, et al. Respiratory risks from household air pollution in low and middle income countries. *Lancet Respir Med.* 2014;2:823–60.

79. Bruce N, Perez-Padilla R, Albalak R. Indoor air pollution in developing countries: A major environmental and public health challenge. *Bull World Health Organ*. 2000;78:1078–92.

80. Smith KR, Bruce N, Balakrishnan K, et al. Millions dead: How do we know and what does it mean? Methods used in the comparative risk assessment of household air pollution. *Annu Rev Public Health*. 2014;35:185–206.

81. World Health Organization. *Global Health Risks: Mortality and Burden of Disease Attributable to Selected Major Risks*. Geneva: WHO Press; 2009. http://www.who.int/healthinfo/global_burden_disease/GlobalHealthRisks_report_full.pdf. Accessed 21 Jul 2016.

82. Cohen AJ, Brauer M, Burnett R, et al. Estimates and 25-year trends of the global burden of disease attributable to ambient air pollution: An analysis of data from the Global Burden of Diseases Study 2015. *Lancet Lond Engl*. 2017;389:1907–18.

83. World Health Organization. *Burning Opportunity: Clean Household Energy for Health, Sustainable Development, and Wellbeing of Women and Children*. Geneva: WHO Press; 2016. http://apps.who.int/iris/bitstream/10665/204717/1/9789241565233_eng.pdf.

84. Institute for Health Metrics and Evaluation (IHME). GBD Compare | IHME Viz Hub. 2015. http://vizhub.healthdata.org/gbd-compare. Accessed 7 Jan 2019.

85. Po JYT, FitzGerald JM, Carlsten C. Respiratory disease associated with solid biomass fuel exposure in rural women and children: Systematic review and meta-analysis. *Thorax*. 2011;66:232–9.

86. Misra P, Srivastava R, Krishnan A, Sreenivaas V, Pandav CS. Indoor air pollution-related acute lower respiratory infections and low birthweight: A systematic review. *J Trop Pediatr*. 2012;58:457–66.

87. Kurmi OP, Semple S, Simkhada P, Smith WCS, Ayres JG. COPD and chronic bronchitis risk of indoor air pollution from solid fuel: A systematic review and meta-analysis. *Thorax*. 2010;65:221–8.

88. Simkovich SM, Goodman D, Roa C, et al. The health and social implications of household air pollution and respiratory diseases. *NPJ Prim Care Respir Med*. 2019;29:12.

89. Jaganath D, Miranda JJ, Gilman RH, et al. Prevalence of chronic obstructive pulmonary disease and variation in risk factors across four geographically diverse resource-limited settings in Peru. *Respir Res*. 2015;16:40.

90. Siddharthan T, Grigsby MR, Goodman D, et al. Association between household air pollution exposure and chronic obstructive oulmonary disease outcomes in 13 low- and middle-income country settings. *Am J Respir Crit Care Med*. 2018;197:611–20.

91. Burroughs Peña M, Romero KM, Velazquez EJ, et al. Relationship between daily exposure to biomass fuel smoke and blood pressure in high-altitude Peru. *Hypertens Dallas Tex 1979*. 2015;65:1134–40.

92. Arku RE, Ezzati M, Baumgartner J, et al. Elevated blood pressure and household solid fuel use in premenopausal women: Analysis of 12 Demographic and Health Surveys (DHS) from 10 countries. *Environ Res*. 2018;160:499–505.

93. Painschab MS, Davila-Roman VG, Gilman RH, et al. Chronic exposure to biomass fuel is associated with increased carotid artery intima-media thickness and a higher prevalence of atherosclerotic plaque. *Heart Br Card Soc*. 2013;99:984–91.

94. Ofori SN, Fobil JN, Odia OJ. Household biomass fuel use, blood pressure and carotid intima media thickness; a cross sectional study of rural dwelling women in Southern Nigeria. *Environ Pollut Barking Essex 1987*. 2018;242 Pt A:390–7.

95. Amegah AK, Quansah R, Jaakkola JJK. Household air pollution from solid fuel use and risk of adverse pregnancy outcomes: A systematic review and meta-analysis of the empirical evidence. *PLoS One*. 2014;9(12):e113920.

96. Pope DP, Mishra V, Thompson L, et al. Risk of low birth weight and stillbirth associated with indoor air pollution from solid fuel use in developing countries. *Epidemiol Rev*. 2010;32:70–81.

97. Baumgartner J, Arku RE, Dickinson KL. Household energy solutions in low and middle income countries. In: Nriagu J, ed. *Encyclopedia of Environmental Health*, 2nd ed. Oxford: Elsevier; 2019, pp. 494–509.

98. Roden CA, Bond TC, Conway S, Osorto Pinel AB, MacCarty N, Still D. Laboratory and field investigations of particulate and carbon monoxide emissions from traditional and improved cookstoves. *Atmos Environ*. 2009;43:1170–81.

99. Sedighi M, Salarian H. A comprehensive review of technical aspects of biomass cookstoves. *Renew Sustain Energy Rev*. 2017;70:656–65.

100. McCracken JP, Smith KR, Díaz A, Mittleman MA, Schwartz J. Chimney stove intervention to reduce long-term wood smoke exposure lowers blood pressure among Guatemalan women. *Environ Health Perspect*. 2007;115:996–1001.

101. Wilson DL, Monga M, Saksena A, Kumar A, Gadgil A. Effects of USB port access on advanced cookstove adoption. *Dev Eng*. 2018;3:209–17.

102. Jetter J, Zhao Y, Smith KR, et al. Pollutant emissions and energy efficiency under controlled conditions for household biomass cookstoves and implications for metrics useful in setting international test standards. *Environ Sci Technol*. 2012;46:10827–34.

103. Shen G, Chen Y, Xue C, et al. Pollutant emissions from improved coal- and wood-fuelled cookstoves in rural households. *Environ Sci Technol*. 2015;49:6590–8.

104. Albalak R, Bruce N, McCracken JP, Smith KR, De Gallardo T. Indoor respirable particulate matter concentrations from an open fire, improved cookstove, and LPG/open fire combination in a rural Guatemalan community. *Environ Sci Technol*. 2001;35:2650–5.

105. Naeher LP, Leaderer BP, Smith KR. Particulate matter and carbon monoxide in Highland Guatemala: Indoor and outdoor levels from traditional and improved wood stoves and gas stoves. *Indoor Air*. 2000;10:200–5.

106. Begum BA, Paul SK, Dildar Hossain M, Biswas SK, Hopke PK. Indoor air pollution from particulate matter emissions in different households in rural areas of Bangladesh. *Build Environ*. 2009;44:898–903.

107. Nie P, Sousa-Poza A, Xue J. Fuel for life: Domestic cooking fuels and women's health in rural China. *Int J Environ Res Public Health*. 2016;13:810.

108. Anderman TL, DeFries RS, Wood SA, Remans R, Ahuja R, Ulla SE. Biogas cook stoves for healthy and sustainable diets? A case study in Southern India. *Nutr Environ Sustain*. 2015;2:28.

109. Sukhsohale ND, Narlawar UW, Phatak MS, Agrawal SB, Ughade SN. Effect of indoor air pollution during cooking on peak expiratory flow rate and its association with exposure index in rural women. *Indian J Physiol Pharmacol*. 2013;57:184–8.

110. Fandiño-Del-Rio M, Goodman D, Kephart JL, et al. Effects of a liquefied petroleum gas stove intervention on pollutant exposure and adult cardiopulmonary outcomes (CHAP): Study protocol for a randomized controlled trial. *Trials*. 2017;18(1):518.

111. Banerjee A, Mondal NK, Das D, Ray MR. Neutrophilic inflammatory response and oxidative stress in premenopausal women chronically exposed to indoor air pollution from biomass burning. *Inflammation*. 2012;35:671–83.

112. Dutta A, Ray MR, Banerjee A. Systemic inflammatory changes and increased oxidative stress in rural Indian women cooking with biomass fuels. *Toxicol Appl Pharmacol*. 2012;261:255–62.

113. Steenland K, Pillarisetti A, Kirby M, et al. Modeling the potential health benefits of lower household air pollution after a hypothetical liquified petroleum gas (LPG) cookstove intervention. *Environ Int*. 2018;111:71–9.

114. Troncoso K, Soares da Silva A. LPG fuel subsidies in Latin America and the use of solid fuels to cook. *Energy Policy*. 2017;107:188–96.

115. Pollard SL, Williams KN, O'Brien CJ, et al. An evaluation of the Fondo de Inclusión Social Energético program to promote access to liquefied petroleum gas in Peru. *Energy Sustain Dev*. 2018; 46:82–93.

116. Bruce N, de Cuevas RA, Cooper J, et al. The Government-led initiative for LPG scale-up in Cameroon: Programme development and initial evaluation. *Energy Sustain Dev*. 2018;46:103–110.

117. Calzada J, Sanz A. Universal access to clean cookstoves: Evaluation of a public program in Peru. *Energy Policy*. 2018;118 C:559–72.

118. Sinton JE, Smith KR, Peabody JW, et al. An assessment of programs to promote improved household stoves in China. *Energy Sustain Dev*. 2004;8:33–52.

119. Bank TW. China—Accelerating household access to clean cooking and heating. The World Bank; 2013. http://documents.worldbank.org/curated/en/401361468022441202/China-Accelerating-household-access-to-clean-cooking-and-heating. Accessed 29 Oct 2019.

120. Kumar P, Dhand A, Tabak RG, Brownson RC, Yadama GN. Adoption and sustained use of cleaner cooking fuels in rural India: A case control study protocol to understand household, network, and organizational drivers. *Arch Public Health Arch Belg Sante Publique*. 2017;75:70.

121. Asante KP, Afari-Asiedu S, Abdulai MA, et al. Ghana's rural liquefied petroleum gas program scale up: A case study. *Energy Sustain Dev*. 2018;46:94–102.

122. Thomas E, Wickramasinghe K, Mendis S, Roberts N, Foster C. Improved stove interventions to reduce household air pollution in low and middle

income countries: A descriptive systematic review. *BMC Public Health.* 2015;15:650.

123. Quansah R, Semple S, Ochieng CA, et al. Effectiveness of interventions to reduce household air pollution and/or improve health in homes using solid fuel in low-and-middle income countries: A systematic review and meta-analysis. *Environ Int.* 2017;103:73–90.
124. Smith KR, McCracken JP, Weber MW, et al. Effect of reduction in household air pollution on childhood pneumonia in Guatemala (RESPIRE): A randomised controlled trial. *Lancet.* 2011;378:1717–26.
125. Mortimer K, Ndamala CB, Naunje AW, et al. A cleaner burning biomass-fuelled cookstove intervention to prevent pneumonia in children under 5 years old in rural Malawi (the cooking and pneumonia study): A cluster randomised controlled trial. *Lancet.* 2017;389:167-75.
126. Romieu I, Riojas-Rodríguez H, Marrón-Mares A, Schilmann A, Perez-Padilla R, Masera O. Improved biomass stove intervention in rural Mexico: Impact on the respiratory health of women. *Am J Respir Crit Care Med.* 2009;180:649–56.
127. Díaz E, Bruce N, Pope D, et al. Lung function and symptoms among indigenous Mayan women exposed to high levels of indoor air pollution. *Int J Tuberc Lung Dis Off J Int Union Tuberc Lung Dis.* 2007;11:1372–9.
128. Smith-Sivertsen T, Díaz E, Pope D, et al. Effect of reducing indoor air pollution on women's respiratory symptoms and lung function: The RESPIRE Randomized Trial, Guatemala. *Am J Epidemiol.* 2009;170: 211–20.
129. Pope D, Diaz E, Smith-Sivertsen T, et al. Exposure to household air pollution from wood combustion and association with respiratory symptoms and lung function in nonsmoking women: Results from the RESPIRE trial, Guatemala. *Environ Health Perspect.* 2015;123:285–92.
130. Thompson LM, Bruce N, Eskenazi B, Diaz A, Pope D, Smith KR. Impact of reduced maternal exposures to wood smoke from an introduced chimney stove on newborn birth weight in rural Guatemala. *Environ Health Perspect.* 2011;119:1489–94.
131. Alexander D, Northcross A, Wilson N, et al. Randomized controlled ethanol cookstove intervention and blood pressure in pregnant Nigerian women. *Am J Respir Crit Care Med.* 2017;195:1629–39.
132. Dutta A, Brito K, Khramstova G, et al. Household air pollution and angiogenic factors in pregnant Nigerian women: A randomized controlled ethanol cookstove intervention. *Sci Total Environ.* 2017;599-600:2175–81.
133. Dutta A, Khramtsova G, Brito K, et al. Household air pollution and chronic hypoxia in the placenta of pregnant Nigerian women: A randomized controlled ethanol Cookstove intervention. *Sci Total Environ.* 2018;619–620:212–20.
134. Alexander DA, Northcross A, Karrison T, et al. Pregnancy outcomes and ethanol cook stove intervention: A randomized-controlled trial in Ibadan, Nigeria. *Environ Int.* 2018;111:152–63.
135. Clark ML, Bazemore H, Reynolds SJ, et al. A baseline evaluation of traditional cook stove smoke exposures and indicators of cardiovascular and respiratory health among Nicaraguan women. *Int J Occup Environ Health.* 2011;17:113–21.
136. Clark ML, Bachand AM, Heiderscheidt JM, et al. Impact of a cleaner-burning cookstove intervention on blood pressure in Nicaraguan women. *Indoor Air.* 2013;23:105–14.
137. Alexander D, Larson T, Bolton S, Vedal S. Systolic blood pressure changes in indigenous Bolivian women associated with an improved cookstove intervention. *Air Qual Atmosphere Health.* 2015;8:47–s53.
138. Clark SN, Schmidt AM, Carter EM, et al. Longitudinal evaluation of a household energy package on blood pressure, central hemodynamics, and arterial stiffness in China. *Environ Res.* 2019;177:108592.
139. Balmes J, Pope D, Dherani M, et al. WHO guidelines for indoor air quality: Household fuel combustion. Review 4: Health effects of household air pollution (HAP) exposure. 2014. http://www.who.int/indoorair/guidelines/hhfc/evidence/en/. Accessed 20 Jul 2016.
140. Mortimer K, Ndamala CB, Naunje AW, et al. A cleaner burning biomass-fuelled cookstove intervention to prevent pneumonia in children under 5 years old in rural Malawi (the cooking and pneumonia study): A cluster randomised controlled trial. *Lancet.* 2017;389(10065):167–75.
141. Dickinson KL, Kanyomse E, Piedrahita R, et al. Research on emissions, air quality, climate, and cooking technologies in Northern Ghana (REACCTING): Study rationale and protocol. *BMC Public Health.* 2015;15:126.
142. Thakur M, Boudewijns EA, Babu GR, et al. Low-smoke chulha in Indian slums: Study protocol for a randomised controlled trial. *BMC Public Health.* 2017;17:454.
143. Dickinson KL, Dalaba M, Brown ZS, et al. Prices, peers, and perceptions (P3): Study protocol for improved biomass cookstove project in northern Ghana. *BMC Public Health.* 2018;18:1209.
144. Patel S, Leavey A, Sheshadri A, et al. Associations between household air pollution and reduced lung function in women and children in rural southern India. *J Appl Toxicol JAT.* 2018;38:1405–15.
145. Carrión D, Dwommoh R, Tawiah T, et al. Enhancing LPG adoption in Ghana (ELAG): A factorial cluster-randomized controlled trial to Enhance LPG Adoption & Sustained use. *BMC Public Health.* 2018;18:689.
146. Tielsch JM, Katz J, Zeger SL, et al. Designs of two randomized, community-based trials to assess the impact of alternative cookstove installation on respiratory illness among young children and reproductive outcomes in rural Nepal. *BMC Public Health.* 2014;14:1271.
147. Jack DW, Asante KP, Wylie BJ, et al. Ghana randomized air pollution and health study (GRAPHS): Study protocol for a randomized controlled trial. *Trials.* 2015;16:420.
148. Jagger P, Das I. Implementation and scale-up of a biomass pellet and improved cookstove enterprise in Rwanda. *Energy Sustain Dev.* 2018;46:32–41.
149. Jagger P, Das I, Handa S, Nylander-French LA, Yeatts KB. Early adoption of an improved household energy system in urban Rwanda. *EcoHealth.* 2019;16:7–20.
150. Global Burden of Disease Collaborative Network. *Global Burden of Disease Study 2016 (GBD 2016) Results.* Seattle, United States: Institute for Health Metrics and Evaluation (IHME). 2017. http://ghdx.healthdata.org/gbd-results-tool. Accessed 18 Feb 2019.

CHAPTER

72

Water Pollution

Timothy J. Wade

INTRODUCTION

On July 28, 2010, the United Nations General Assembly adopted a resolution recognizing: "the right to safe and clean drinking water and sanitation as a human right that is essential for the full enjoyment of human life and all human rights."[1] Despite this international commitment, as of 2015 2.1 billion people lacked access to safe drinking water and 4.5 billion lacked access to safely managed sanitation worldwide.[2] An estimated 1.8 million deaths resulted from diseases related to water pollution in 2015, disproportionately affecting children under 5 years of age in lower-income countries.[3] Many of these deaths are preventable through access to safe and clean water for drinking and hygiene.[4] Although in most upper-income countries advances in drinking water and wastewater treatment over the past century have reduced the threat of diarrheal waterborne disease, new threats to the integrity and safety of water resources have emerged including treatment-resistant waterborne pathogens, persistent industrial and agricultural chemicals, a changing climate, and an aging water treatment and distribution infrastructure.

This chapter will discuss the main drivers and public health aspects of water pollution that result in human illness and mortality. The focus will be on diseases and other adverse health effects resulting from exposures via ingestion, inhalation, or absorption of water contaminated by pathogenic microorganisms (bacteria, viruses, protozoa) and chemicals. Vector-borne diseases associated with insect hosts, which may breed in water such as malaria, dengue, Zika, and yellow fever, will not be emphasized, nor will the ecological effects of water pollution or potential health effects resulting from exposures at treated water venues (pools, hot tubs, spas).

HISTORICAL PERSPECTIVE

Miasma Theory of Disease

Contaminated water has only been recognized as a cause of disease and illness for a little over 150 years. Before the mid-1800s, the "miasma" theory of disease prevailed which posited that bad air, unhealthy vapors and poisonous emanations from rotting carcasses or vegetation were responsible for most diseases and illnesses.[5] The miasma theory was first attributed to the Greek physician Hippocrates from the fourth or fifth century BCE,[5] and was used to explain many important diseases over the centuries including tuberculosis, plague, malaria, and cholera.[5] Miasma theory remained the prevalent disease theory for much of the nineteenth century.[6]

Ancient Sanskrit and Greek records indicate that treatments such as exposure to sunlight, filtering through charcoal and straining were used to improve water taste and clarity as early as 4000 BC. Alum was used in Egypt in 1500 BC to induce coagulation and help clarify water.[7] Aqueducts, established in ancient Rome and Assyria, helped to keep waste water separate from water used for drinking and bathing. Because water was not considered an important disease transmission route, these early water treatments were focused primarily on the aesthetic (clarity, taste, odor) qualities of water and not on disease prevention.

Cholera and John Snow

The earliest descriptions of cholera-like illnesses date back to approximately 500 BC in India[8] and were noted to primarily appear among those "living on the shores of big rivers."[9] In the early 1800s the first of seven global cholera pandemics began in India,[10] spreading through Russia and Europe by the 1830s.[11] Although now considered an archetypal waterborne disease, when cholera spread to England in the mid-1800s, most physicians, sanitarians, and scientists believed it was transmitted via poisoned air, reflecting their adherence to the miasma theory of disease,[6] and few believed it to be transmitted by water.[12] This emphasis on the miasma theory exacerbated cholera outbreaks, especially in the mid-1800s in London, as actions were taken that were counter to those that would have been taken to end waterborne transmission. Thus, in 1842 to reduce exposures to foul air, the sanitarian Edwin Chadwick advocated the drainage and disposal of all house and street refuse and cesspools into the Thames River, the source of drinking water for much of the population.[6,13] This resulted in a significant decline to the water quality of the river, and was followed by major cholera outbreaks in London between 1848 and 1854, killing over 15,000 people.[12] The London physician John Snow carefully mapped and analyzed cholera cases from this period and demonstrated that mortality due to cholera among customers of the Southwark and Vauxhall water company was six times higher than among customers of the Lambeth water company. He attributed this difference to the move by the Lambeth company of its source intake to a location upstream and above the pollution of the Thames whereas the Southwark company drew its water from the most polluted part of the river. A subsequent cholera outbreak occurred in 1854 in the Soho neighborhood of London in the vicinity of Broad Street, killing 500 within a month. By studying the geographic patterns of these deaths Snow identified significant clusters near the Broad Street pump. The water source for the Broad Street pump was later shown to be contaminated by a cesspool, the likely source of the cholera contamination. Snow then famously advocated for removal of the Broad Street pump handle to stem the outbreak. Despite Snow's careful and thorough evaluations, the waterborne theory of cholera transmission was not fully accepted until near the turn of the twentieth century. However, Snow's insights, together with the advancement of germ theory by Pasteur and Koch and the identification of the *Vibrio cholera* bacterium were a critical turning point in proving the waterborne transmission of cholera and the decline of the miasma theory of disease.

Water Treatment to Control Waterborne Disease

The acceptance of polluted water as an important vehicle for disease causation combined with advances in microbiology, engineering, public health and medicine, spurred the development of engineering and water treatment and management approaches to control waterborne diseases. In the late nineteenth century, waterborne diseases such as typhoid fever (caused by *Salmonella typhi*), dysentery and other diarrheal diseases (caused by a range of pathogens) as well as cholera, were often exacerbated by the growth of urban areas with community water systems but lacking appropriate waste management and treatment, resulting in contamination of drinking water sources.[14] Construction of a comprehensive sewage system that piped waste away from London's water source helped contain the persistent cholera epidemics of the mid-1800s. However, installation of sewage systems alone was often insufficient to prevent waterborne disease. When sewage was disposed directly to streams, lakes, and rivers that served as the drinking sources for urban centers, waterborne disease transmission could be exacerbated without any additional water treatment or disinfection. For example, exceptionally high typhoid fever death rates in Lowell and Lawrence, Massachusetts in the 1890s were attributed to sewage disposal of several upstream communities to the Merrimack River, the source of drinking water for these downstream communities.[14]

In response to these epidemics, municipal drinking water treatment began to be more widely implemented in the early 1900s. In 1903, Little Falls New Jersey implemented coagulation (using alum), sedimentation combined with filtration to treat water from the Passaic River. Chlorination was first used in to continuously treat drinking water in public drinking water systems in Jersey City, New Jersey in 1908. By 1941, 85% of drinking water supplies in the United States were chlorinated.[7] Municipal drinking water treatments and sewage systems (including increased chlorine disinfection of sewage), resulted in significant reductions in typhoid fever, cholera and dysentery (i.e., amoebic or bacillary dysentery caused by *Entamoeba histolytica* and *Shigella,* respectively) and other diarrheal diseases and virtually eliminated widespread outbreaks of these from diseases in the United States and Europe by the mid-1900s. There are numerous local examples of dramatic reductions of typhoid and other infectious waterborne diseases occurring immediately after the introduction of filtration, chlorination and effective municipal water management and treatment. For example, in 1854 in Chicago, 6% of the population died from cholera, and in 1891, the typhoid fever death rate was 173.8 per 100,000. Following effective source management and disinfection of drinking water (including chlorine disinfection and the reversal of the flow of the Chicago River so it no longer emptied into Lake Michigan, the drinking water source for the city), the typhoid fever mortality rate was reduced to 1.7 per 100,000 by 1917.[14] In 1900, the mortality rate attributable to typhoid in the United States was over 30 per 100,000 and by 1950 had decreased to less than 1 per 100,000 (Fig. 72-1).[15]

New Concerns

Despite the near elimination of large-scale outbreaks of waterborne infectious disease in upper income countries, with exponential population increases and the concentration of population to urban areas, municipal drinking water quality remained a public concern through the mid-twentieth century. Concerns included poor taste and bad odor as well as potential health effects from industrial and agricultural discharges and chlorination by products. Large rivers such as the Mississippi River received effluent from numerous sewage plants as well as runoff of chemicals from agriculture and industry adversely affecting water quality for downstream communities. In response to reports of poor taste, odor, and quality of drinking water, in 1964, the State of Louisiana requested that the federal government investigate the water quality in of the lower Mississippi River. The survey, completed in 1972, found that the river was contaminated with numerous industrial and agricultural compounds including cyanide, arsenic, mercury, lead, chromium, and over 50 organic compounds.[7] Many of these chemicals found their way into water supplies through factory discharges, street and farm field runoff, and leaking underground waste disposal areas. Chlorination of water sources, so effective in

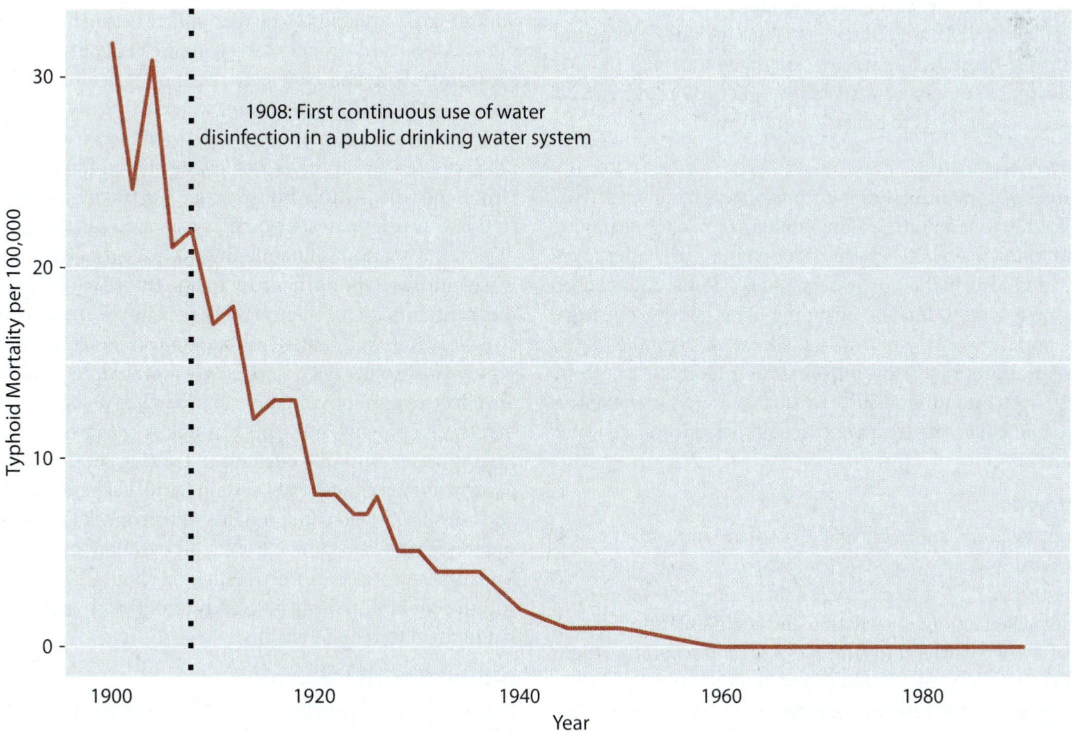

FIGURE 72-1. Reduction in mortality in the United States due to typhoid fever following treatment of public water supplies. (*Source:* Adapted from Armstrong GL, Conn LA, Pinner RW. Trends in infectious disease mortality in the United States during the 20th century. *J Am Med Assoc.* 1999;281(1):61–6.[157])

reducing the risk of microbial pathogens, also produced by products (disinfection by-products, DBPs) such as trihalomethanes (THMs), which were suspected to be harmful and possibly carcinogenic. An epidemiological analysis conducted in 1974 implicated an association between high rates of cancer mortality and drinking water obtained from the Mississippi River.[16] These concerns ultimately led to more systematic regulation of effluent discharges as part of the Federal Water Pollution Control Act (now known as the Clean Water Act) [17] and public drinking water supplies under the 1974 Safe Drinking Water Act. Similar European directives soon followed.[18]

Because large parts of the world still lack access to municipally treated drinking water or other sources of adequate and safe water, infectious waterborne diseases remain a major public health issue worldwide. However, modern treatment of water and sewage, in combination with source protection and management has been a major public health success, effectively eliminating the regular occurrence of major outbreaks of typhoid fever, cholera, and dysentery from countries with advanced drinking water infrastructure. In these areas, although acute outbreaks of infectious waterborne disease remain a threat that require careful management, there has been an increased focus on chemical contamination from pesticides, runoff, industrial waste, nutrients, DBPs (by-products that are formed as a result of chlorination and other treatment process) and treatment resistant waterborne pathogens (e.g., *Cryptosporidium* and norovirus).

WATER TREATMENT AND DISTRIBUTION

In addition to cholera, typhoid, and dysentery, raw and untreated water affected by sewage or fecal contamination can transmit a wide range of other infections from pathogenic bacteria, viruses, and protozoan parasites such as *Salmonella*, *Campylobacter*, enterovirus, rotavirus, norovirus, *Cryptosporidium* and *Giardia* which may occur in high densities in raw sewage.[19] Agricultural and industrial chemicals and heavy metals can also contaminate drinking water via sewage, runoff, industrial, and other discharges. Most urban areas in middle and upper income countries receive municipally treated and distributed water, designed to reduce or eliminate microbial pathogens and harmful chemicals from entering the water supply and endangering human health. Ensuring the safety of municipal drinking water usually involves a "multiple barrier" approach that includes protecting and preserving the quality of source water; water treatment; maintaining the quality of stored and distributed water; monitoring; and effective response capabilities to adverse conditions.[20]

Source Water Protection

Potential sources of contamination to source waters include agriculture, animal feeding operations, leaking underground storage tanks, industrial and municipal waste, storm water runoff, car washes, service stations, and individual homeowners and residents. Approaches to protect source waters include mapping and taking inventory of sources of pollution and runoff to the source of drinking water, managing them appropriately by implementing land use controls, reducing discharges into groundwater or surface water, maintaining septic systems and educating the public to help prevent source water contamination.[21]

Water Treatment

Source water protection cannot prevent all contaminants from entering water systems and some level of municipal water treatment is almost always necessary. The basic processes of municipal water treatment consist of: coagulation; flocculation and sedimentation (mixing and binding of small particles into large particles and separating them by gravity); filtration (granular or slow sand filter); and disinfection. Together, coagulation, flocculation, and filtration alone can reduce bacteria by two to three logs; viruses one to three logs, and protozoa (i.e., *Cryptosporidium*) two to three logs.[22] Disinfection following filtration is necessary to further reduce microbial contaminants to acceptable levels. Common disinfectants include chlorine, chloramine, ozone, and ultraviolet radiation. A secondary disinfection step is often included to maintain residual treatment through the distribution system and to reduce bacterial regrowth. There are numerous variations on these general processes depending on the nature and quality of the source water and specific contaminants of concern.[23] Bacteria are generally most susceptible to chlorination, followed by viruses and least susceptible are the protozoan pathogens *Cryptosporidium* and *Giardia*, which usually require filtration for effective removal. Reduction of potentially harmful chemicals in the source water is accomplished to a certain extent by coagulation, filtration, and chlorination but additional approaches such as granular activated carbon filtration, and ion exchange (i.e., removal of calcium ions to reduce water hardness) are effective in reducing certain chemicals. Membrane processes, such as reverse osmosis, ultrafiltration, microfiltration, and nanofiltration provide additional advanced treatment for both chemical and microbial contaminants, and in the case of reverse osmosis, for desalination of water. These techniques, although energy intensive, are highly effective at purifying water and are often employed to treat wastewater for potable or nonpotable reuse.[24]

Municipal and industrial sewage and sludge (produced from wastewater and drinking water treatment) also require treatment and management to ensure they are not a threat to human health and the environment and to protect surface water quality. Untreated domestic wastewater contains large numbers of microorganisms including potentially pathogenic bacteria, viruses, protozoa, and intestinal worms.[19] Modern wastewater treatment is designed to reduce organic material and biological oxygen demand, pathogens, nutrients, inorganic, and organic chemicals. It is generally comprised of three major steps. Primary treatment physically separates larger solids through screens and settling tanks. Secondary treatment consists of biological degradation and decomposition of remaining solids, organic material, removing nutrients (nitrogen, ammonia, phosphorus), and reduction of pathogens by biological degradation. Disinfection (chlorine, ozone, or ultraviolet radiation) is usually the last step of secondary treatment.[17] Tertiary or advanced treatment involves additional steps such as adsorption, membrane filtration, ion exchange, additional disinfection to further reduce organics, turbidity, nitrogen, phosphorus, and organics. Tertiary treated wastewater may be discharged to lake and rivers, or reuse in agriculture, watering of golf courses, or recharging of groundwater.

Water from private wells may be treated using a wide range of point of use (i.e., at the tap-or pitcher-based filter) or point of entry treatments (i.e., whole house water treatment systems) such as filtration, reverse osmosis, granular activated carbon, and disinfection depending on the contaminants of concern. Care must be taken to ensure the type of filter or treatment selected is appropriate for the contaminant of concern. For example, to effectively remove *Cryptosporidium* oocysts, reverse osmosis treatment or a filter with a 1-micron absolute pore size filter is required. Reverse osmosis filters are effective at removing most microbial as well as chemical contaminants by applying pressure through a semipermeable membrane. Boiling water is highly effective at treating most microbial contaminants, but may concentrate certain harmful chemicals such as arsenic and nitrate. Other contaminants commonly of concern for private water sources are chlorine and disinfection by products, arsenic, lead, and nitrate. In-home treatments should be certified to remove specific contaminants (e.g., NSF International) and must be properly maintained to remain effective.

Distribution and Storage

Following treatment, distribution, and storage of water can be a source of contamination and require additional management and treatment considerations. Biofilms (collection of organic and inorganic, living and dead material) may accumulate in piping and storage permitting potentially pathogenic microorganisms to persist and grow. Aging water infrastructure can result in breaks and leaks in the distribution system and low pressure that can allow intrusion of pathogens or other contaminants into the water supply. Older service pipes may also be constructed of lead, which can leach into drinking water systems especially when corrosion controls are not adequate. Inadequate corrosion control was the cause of recent widespread lead exposures in Washington DC in 2000 and more recently in Flint, Michigan in 2014.[25] Iron pipes, solders and fittings may leach iron, arsenic, lead, copper, and other metals into the water system.[26]

Main breaks and low-pressure events can allow pathogens and other contaminants into the distribution system, potentially causing significant adverse health effects. Distribution system breaks were likely the cause of a 1990 outbreak of *Escherichia coli* 0157:H7 in Cabool, Missouri that resulted in 243 cases of illness and four deaths. Because of high-quality source water, water treatment in this system did not include disinfection and the main breaks likely introduced sewage into the system.[20]

Contamination may also be introduced to the distribution system via cross-connections whereby the drinking water system is incorrectly connected to another (e.g., wastewater) source system. A cross-connection between the sewage system and the drinking water system during maintenance in Nokia, Finland in 2008 resulted in 450,000 liters of sewage entering the distribution system and 5000 cases of gastrointestinal illness due to *Campylobacter* and *Salmonella*.[26] Management measures to ensure distributed water quality include maintaining appropriate disinfection residual, leak detection and repair programs, routine water main flushing, and regular maintenance.[26]

Water systems may also be contaminated during storage prior to use and/or distribution. Several waterborne outbreaks of *Campylobacter* and *Salmonella* have been attributed to contamination of inadequately protected storage tanks and reservoirs by bird feces.[27–29] For example, bird contamination of storage tank in Gideon, Missouri in 1993 resulted in an outbreak of waterborne *Salmonella typhimurium* that affected more than 650 people and caused seven deaths.[27] Storage reservoirs should be designed to prevent microbial or chemical contamination of drinking water from environment pollutants or fecal contamination with regular maintenance to repair damage, gaps, and cracks.

Monitoring

Monitoring of source water, before, during, and after treatment and throughout the distribution and storage system is an integral part of ensuring a safe drinking water supply. An extensive discussion of monitoring is beyond the scope of this chapter but detailed discussions are available elsewhere.[30,31] Table 72-1 describes some commonly monitored parameters in water systems. These include turbidity, chlorine or disinfectant residual, and fecal contamination. The most commonly tested indicator for fecal contamination is coliform bacteria. Coliform (total or fecal) bacteria are generally not harmful themselves but are part of the normal bacterial flora of the intestinal tract of warm-blooded animals. Their presence in water systems is an indicator of fecal contamination and the possible presence of other, pathogenic microorganisms. *E. coli* is a coliform bacteria (most *E. coli* are generally harmless but there are notable pathogenic strains, e.g., *E. coli* 0157:H7), which is a more specific indicator of fecal contamination and may be used as a follow up or confirmatory test following a positive coliform result.

EXPOSURE ROUTES

A minimum of 50 liters of water per person per day is recommended to meet drinking and basic sanitation needs.[32] In the United States each person uses a total of about 100 liters daily for drinking, cooking, washing, bathing, and cleaning.[33] In addition to drinking and sanitation, recreation (swimming, boating) and occupation or subsistence (i.e., fishing, shellfish harvesting) may also result in contact with and/or ingestion of water. Pollution or contamination of waters used for these purposes can result in exposures to potentially harmful microorganisms, chemicals, or toxins.

The most common and direct exposure for most waterborne contaminants is ingestion. Estimates of the amount of drinking water consumed are used to calculate the potential total dose of a chemical or pathogen to exposed individuals for risk assessment. A commonly used conservative (i.e., high) estimate is 2 liters per day for adults and 1 liter per day for children under 10 years of age, which includes tap water in the form of juices and mixed beverages.[34,35] Estimates of daily water consumption by age group range from mean and 95th percentile values from 0.31 L/day to 1.3 L/day and from 0.86 L/day to 3.1 L/day, respectively, depending on the age group (highest in adults $>$ 20 years; lowest in children $<$ 1 year).[34] During swimming, it is estimated that children (under 18 years) swallow 1.2 L/hour and adults swallow 0.71 L/hour.[36,37]

Inhalation and dermal contact are also important routes of exposure to certain waterborne contaminants. For example, inhalation of aerosols and mists from showers, hot tubs and water sprays, is the primary transmission route for *Legionella*, which causes respiratory infection (Pontiac fever or the more severe form, Legionnaires' disease).[38] Nontuberculous mycobacteria (NTM), an opportunistic pathogen, are also transmitted via inhalation of aerosolized droplets (e.g., humidifiers, showers) among susceptible or vulnerable individuals.[39,40] *Vibrio vulnificus*, a naturally occurring bacterium in marine and brackish waters more commonly known as a foodborne pathogen, can also cause severe wound infections (often a necrotizing fasciitis) following contact with marine water. Those with chronic health conditions or compromised immune systems are particularly susceptible to *V. vulnificus* wound infections.[41–43] Aerosolized algal toxins may also be inhaled during recreation (swimming, jet-skiing, water skiing) or other activities causing respiratory irritation, resulting in upper and lower respiratory symptoms.[44,45] Dermal contact is also an important exposure route for some algal toxins (e.g., microcystin, lyngbyatoxin) that are associated with dermatitis and ear and eye irritation among swimmers, fishermen and those participating in water contact sports.[46] Inhalation and dermal exposures (e.g., showering, bathing, indoor swimming pools) to DBPs (e.g., THM, chloroform) are potentially important exposure routes.[47]

WATER SOURCES AND TYPES

Drinking Water

The World Health Organization classifies drinking water sources and supplies as "Improved," "Other Improved" and "Unimproved." Improved water sources are piped directly into a home or yard and confer the greatest protection from fecal and other contaminants. "Other improved" sources are more common in rural areas and are also likely to be protected from outside contamination. These include public taps or standpipes, tube wells or boreholes, protected dug wells, protected springs, and rainwater collection. "Unimproved" water supplies are usually not protected from outside contamination and include: Unprotected dug wells, unprotected springs, and surface water (river, dam, lake, pond, stream, canal, irrigation channels). These sources are highly susceptible to contamination, especially fecal contamination.[2] A meta-analysis of 319 studies worldwide found unimproved sources were nearly seven times more likely to be contaminated by indicators of fecal contamination (*E. coli* or fecal coliform) than other water sources.[48] As of 2015, the WHO estimated that 87% of the world's population used improved water sources with 54% using piped water into their residence and 33% using other improved sources. "At least basic" water sources are improved or other improved sources that can be collected within 30 minutes. Lack of access to an at least basic water source is most common in

TABLE 72-1 COMMONLY USED MEASURES OF WATER QUALITY

Parameter	Sampling Location	Description	Notes
Turbidity	Source water, treated water, distribution system	Measure of cloudiness of water	High turbidity may interfere with treatment. Some studies have associated high turbidity in treated water with increased risk for gastrointestinal illnesses
Heterotrophic bacteria count	Treated water, distribution system	Measure of culturable bacteria in water. Indicates microbial growth potential, increased biofilm	Not considered an indicator of adverse health effects. May indicate changes to source water or treatment
Coliform bacteria/*E. coli*/ enterococcus	Source water, distribution system, treated water, recreational waters	Markers of fecal contamination	Presence may indicate potential contamination with microbial pathogens
Total dissolved solids	Source water	Measure of combined inorganic and organic substances dissolved in water	Indicator of change in water quality and general water quality
Total organic carbon	Source water, treated water	Measure of organic matter in a sample	Nonspecific indicator of water quality
pH	Source water, distribution system, treated water	Measure of acidity/alkalinity of water	Low pH may cause corrosion, drinking water pH ranges between 6.5 and 8.5
Conductivity	Source water	Measure of ability of water to pass electric current	Indicator of changes in water quality and presence of dissolved solids
Total trihalomethanes	Treated water, distribution system	Disinfection by product formed between chlorine and organic matter	High levels in drinking water may be a health risk
Total chorine/residual chlorine	Treated water, distribution system	Disinfectant	Maintenance of some residual chlorine in distribution system may be desirable to reduce biofilm, microbial contamination
Algal toxins (microcystin, anatoxin-a, cylindrospermopsin)	Raw water, treated water, distribution system	Toxins produced by freshwater cyanobacteria	Potential health risk if found in treated water
Water hardness	Treated water, distribution system	Measure of naturally occurring mineral content (magnesium and calcium carbonate)	Hard water can form deposits and build un in plumbing and distribution systems

sub-Saharan Africa, followed by southern and south-eastern Asia (Fig. 72-2).[2]

Household or piped water used for drinking, cooking, washing, and bathing may be broadly classified as municipal water (processed, treated, and delivered to users) or private water (wells or springs for individual or small groups of households). *Groundwater* refers to water obtained from underground sources (i.e., springs, aquifers) and may have some natural protection from fecal contaminants and runoff associated pollution. Deep, protected wells may not require any additional treatment to be safe for drinking although regular monitoring and testing for fecal contamination (i.e., coliform bacteria) and chemical contaminants is recommended. *Surface water* includes water obtained from reservoirs, rivers, lakes, and streams and is more susceptible to fecal contamination as well as contamination from runoff, sewage, and industrial discharges. Surface water sources generally require a greater level of treatment (i.e., filtration, disinfection) to ensure safety from microbial and chemical contaminants. Shallow ground water sources that may be affected or influenced by surface water and may be considered *groundwater under influence of surface water* and regulatory bodies such as the U.S. EPA recommend treating this water as if it were surface water. These sources can be heavily contaminated during heavy rainfalls or floods, and inadequate management of these sources has resulted in several major outbreaks including the *E. coli* 0157:H7 outbreak in Walkerton, Canada (discussed later in this chapter).

Private water sources are usually wells or springs in countries with advanced water infrastructure. In the United States, an estimated 13 million households rely on private wells for drinking water.[49] Private wells often do not fall under the jurisdiction of environmental authorities and well owners are usually responsible for the safety of their water and should get their water tested regularly. Although wells may be at least partially protected from surface runoff and surface sewage discharges, they also can be susceptible to contamination from seepage of sewage from septic systems, leachate from underground storage tanks, groundwater movement from waste disposals, spills, nearby application of agricultural chemicals and fertilizers, or naturally occurring contaminants such as arsenic and fluoride.

Recreational and Occupational Water

Contact with water for recreational and occupational activities can also result in exposures to both naturally occurring and pollution-associated microbial pathogens and harmful contaminants. *Vibrio vulnificus,* discussed previously, is a potential risk for both recreators and fisherman in warm marine waters. Schistosomiasis, or bilharzia, is caused by infection with a trematode parasite of the genus *Shistosoma* that affects more than 230 million people worldwide mostly in sub-Saharan Africa, the Middle East, South America, and southeast Asia. Freshwater snails are the intermediate host and shed tens of thousands *Schistosoma* cercariae that can infect humans in contact with water by penetrating the skin. Long-term morbidity reflects anemia, malnutrition, and impaired childhood development due to continued inflammation caused by the infection.[50] Surface waters used for recreation are also commonly affected by fecal contamination from sewage discharge and runoff. Recreators themselves

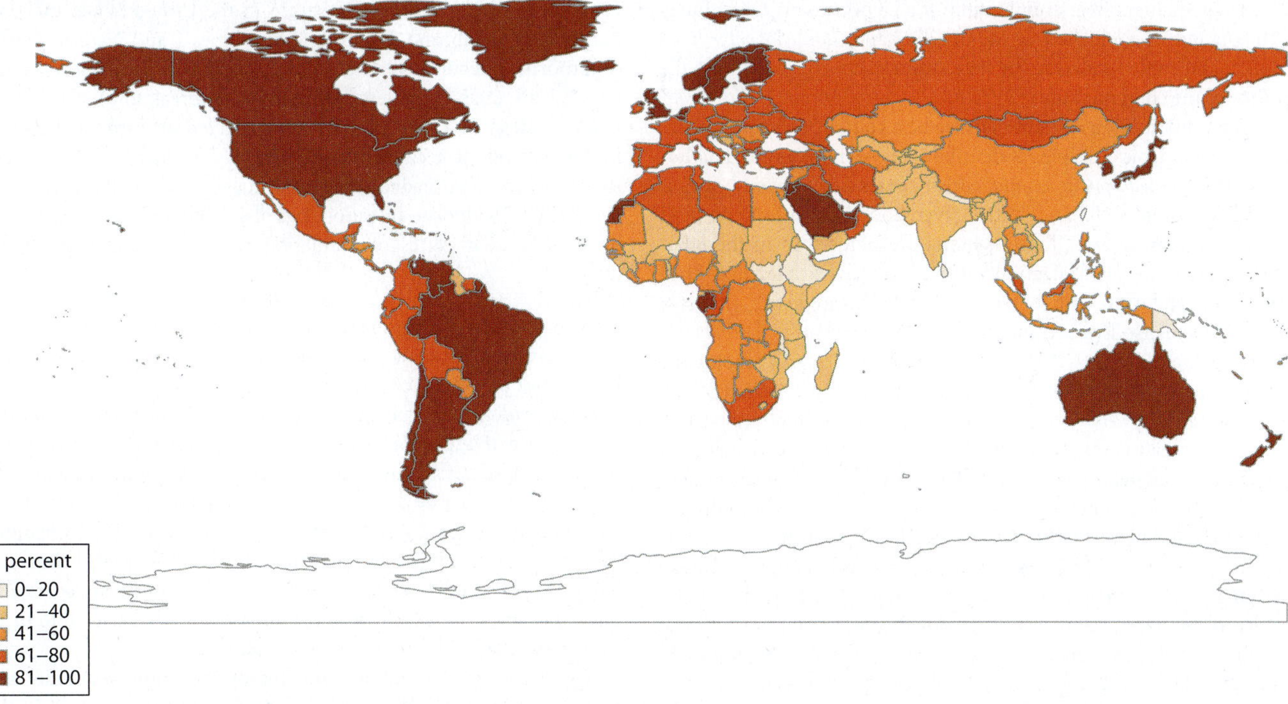

FIGURE 72-2. Percent of population with access to at least basic water source.* At least basic water sources are improved sources (piped water or protected wells) that require no more than 30-minute collection time. (*Source:* Adapted from World Health Organization, UNICEF. Progress on drinking water, sanitation and hygiene: 2017 update and SDG baselines. 2017.[2])

are also often a source of contamination, especially young children, as they may defecate in or near the water. Outbreaks in untreated recreational waters are most commonly attributed to norovirus, *E. coli* 0157:H7, *Shigella* and *Cryptosporidium*.[51] Epidemiological studies have also consistently demonstrated that the level of fecal contamination (measured by fecal indicator bacteria such as *Enterococcus*) is associated with self-reported gastrointestinal symptoms among swimmers.[52,53]

MAJOR WATERBORNE CONTAMINANTS

In lower income countries without adequate water and sewage infrastructure, a major source of water contamination is sewage and fecal contamination. Even in upper-income countries, lapses in treatment, aging water infrastructure, and severe climate events can result in fecal contamination of drinking water and other water sources. Other important sources of water contamination include industrial waste from factories, agriculture (nutrients, pesticides, animal waste), naturally occurring contaminants (arsenic, fluoride, radioactive substances, some microbial pathogens), disinfection by products, mining waste and by-products, and contaminants associated with water distribution or plumbing systems (lead, *Legionella,* NTM).

Pathogenic Micro-organisms

Pathogenic microorganisms (e.g., viruses, bacteria, protozoa, helminths) contaminate water sources most often through human fecal contamination (sewage, septic systems, runoff). Other sources include animal feces from agriculture or feeding operations, regrowth in distribution systems and storage systems, and free living/naturally occurring microorganisms. Many waterborne pathogens are also transmitted via other exposure routes, commonly food and person-to-person contact especially for pathogens transmitted via the fecal-oral route such as norovirus, *Shigella* and pathogenic *E. coli*. For these and wide range of other infections, waterborne transmission may make up a relatively small fraction of the total infections. Others, such as *Vibrio cholerae*, *Legionella*, and *Cryptosporidium* are predominantly waterborne.

Bacteria

Most bacterial waterborne pathogens are effectively treated by modern water treatment. Chlorination and other types of disinfection are particularly effective at killing or eliminating most harmful bacteria in water sources.[54] However, waterborne transmission and outbreaks still occur when treatment fails or is substandard, when water supplies are inadequate or when fecal contamination impacts surface water sources contacted by humans through occupation, recreation or daily living.

In 2000, an outbreak of bacterial waterborne pathogens *E. coli* 0157:H7 and *Campylobacter* in Walkerton, Ontario, Canada, illustrated how failures in source water protection, treatment, and oversight can result in serious and widespread disease transmission, even in upper-income countries with municipal water.[20] Heavy rains washed cattle manure from an adjacent farm into a shallow well that served as a drinking water source for the community. The well was inadequately chlorinated resulting in fecal contamination entering the water distribution system. Although fecal contamination was detected in well water samples by the water utility, no action was taken. In subsequent days, children were hospitalized with bloody diarrhea and increases in absenteeism were reported in the area schools. Ultimately over 2000 people were infected, 65 were hospitalized,

27 developed hemolytic uremic syndrome, a potentially fatal kidney ailment, and 7 people died. *E. coli* 0157:H7 and *Campylobacter* from human and cattle fecal samples were strain matched, confirming the source of the contamination.[20,55,56]

Water distribution systems can also be a source of bacterial infections. Two notable examples of distribution system-associated pathogens are *Legionella pneumophila,* which causes Legionnaires' disease as well as a milder illness, Pontiac fever, and NTM infections (e.g., *Mycobacterium avium*). These bacteria are ubiquitous in the environment but can cause infection when aerosolized and inhaled. They can persist and grow within "biofilms" that grow in distribution systems and can also live within amoeba that may protect the bacteria from harsh conditions.[57,58] In recent years, *Legionella* has become the primary cause of waterborne disease outbreaks in the United States, accounting for nearly 60% of drinking water associated outbreaks.[59] Infection is caused through inhalation of aerosolized droplets of water contaminated by *Legionella*. Major sources of *Legionella* infection are showers, cooling towers, whirlpools, fountains, humidifiers, and air conditioners. Outbreaks are common in hospitals and institutional settings.[38] Control of *Legionella* and NTM in distribution systems requires maintenance of appropriate disinfection residual levels in the distribution system, removal of nutrients to minimize biofilm formation and management of temperature to inhibit growth. For example, *Legionella* growth is inhibited above 50°C in hot water systems and below 25°C in cold water systems.[59,60]

Although human sources of fecal contamination are often viewed as the most risky to water sources, several bacterial pathogens such as *E. coli* 0157:H7, *Campylobacter* and nontyphoid *Salmonella* may also be transmitted by animal feces (i.e., zoonotic transmission). Leptospirosis is a strictly zoonotic disease transmitted via the urine of infected animals (rats, mice, cattle). Infection is caused by spirochete bacteria *Leptospira interrogans* and enters the body via cuts and abrasions or mucus membranes. Surface waters are susceptible to contamination with infected urine, especially after heavy rainfall or flooding, and contact with these waters is a risk factor for infection. Infection may be asymptomatic or cause a wide range of symptoms including fever, headache, jaundice, vomiting, diarrhea, and rash.[61] A second phase of illness can result in kidney or liver failure (Weil's disease) and pulmonary hemorrhage. An estimated 1.03 million cases and 58,900 deaths occur each year, predominantly in resource poor areas (South and Southeast Asia, Oceana, Latin America, Africa), making it among the leading zoonotic causes of morbidity worldwide.[62] Although rare in the continental United States, two cases were reported in 2016 following extensive flooding in south-central Louisiana.[63] The potential for increases in extreme weather events and flooding combined with population growth in urban areas with inadequate sanitation may further exacerbate morbidity and mortality due to leptospirosis.[62,64]

Viruses

Major viral causes of waterborne infection are summarized in Table 72-2. Notable waterborne viruses include hepatitis A and E, norovirus, rotavirus, enterovirus, and adenovirus. Waterborne transmission is usually associated with human sewage contamination.

Norovirus is an important waterborne pathogen and can be transmitted by drinking water and recreational water.[65] They are found in high densities in sewage, resistant to conventional water treatment, can survive in the environment, and have a low infectious dose. Norovirus is believed to be the most common cause of swimming associated-gastrointestinal illness.[66] A study at a beach in Puerto Rico contaminated by sewage found that 3.4% of those who immersed their head in water showed evidence of infection with Genogroup 1 or 2 norovirus based on increases in norovirus specific IgG response compared to only 0.4% who did not immerse their head.[67]

Numerous outbreaks of Hepatitis A and E have been caused by inadequately treated and fecally contaminated water. Hepatitis E genotype 3 is the predominant strain in the United States and predominantly foodborne. Hepatitis E genotypes 1 and 2 are primarily waterborne infections restricted to tropical and subtropical countries.[68] Naik et al. summarized a massive outbreak of Hepatitis E in Uttar Pradesh in 1991. The outbreak affected an estimated 79,091 individuals due to fecal contamination of the source water (Ganges River), which was inadequately chlorinated. [69] Hepatitis A, though primarily a foodborne infection, has also been associated with outbreaks caused by fecal contamination of drinking and recreational water.[70,71]

Parasitic Waterborne Pathogens

Protozoan and parasitic waterborne pathogens are listed in Table 72-2. Major pathogens of concern include *Acanthamoeba, Entamoeba, Cryptosporidium, Giardia*, and *Naegleria*. Other potential waterborne protozoan pathogens include *Toxoplasma gondii* and microsporidia. Amoebic dysentery caused by *Entamoeba histolytica* remains an important waterborne disease in areas with poor sanitary conditions and inadequate water treatment. Global public health campaigns have been successful in dramatically reducing and nearly eliminating guinea worm disease (Dracunculiasis) that can cause severe and disabling skin ulcers. Guinea worm disease is now restricted to three countries: Chad, Ethiopia, and South Sudan.[72]

Cryptosporidium oocysts are highly chlorine resistant and require 1-micron filtration for consistently effective removal. In the 1980s and 1990s, several drinking water associated outbreaks of *Cryptosporidium* sp. occurred in large cities with modern drinking water treatment.[73–75] In 1993 a massive drinking water associated outbreak of *Cryptosporidium parvum* may have affected up to 400,000 in Milwaukee, WI.[75] The outbreak was preceded by heavy rains that affected the quality of the water of Lake Michigan, the drinking water source, resulting in high levels of fecal contamination from both cattle and untreated sewage. This contamination resulted in exceptionally high turbidity in the source water that overwhelmed the filtration processes and leading to contamination of the water supply. Contamination of the water supply with *Cryptosporidium* likely lasted over a month and the community-wide outbreak was only discovered after antidiarrheal medications sold out of pharmacies and widespread absenteeism was reported by schools and hospital employees. These outbreaks drew significant attention to the quality of municipal drinking water supplies and resulted in more stringent criteria including source water monitoring for *Cryptosporidium*, strengthening of filtration requirements and covers on new finished water reservoirs.[76]

Naegleria fowleri is a free-living amoeba that naturally occurs in soil and warm freshwaters. Referred to in the press as the "brain eating amoeba," infection is extremely rare (0–8 infections per year; 142 cases between 1937 and 2014), but nearly always fatal (>97% fatality rate). Infection primarily affects healthy young males and occurs when amoebae are inhaled via the nasal cavity usually during swimming in freshwater lakes, ponds, reservoirs, rivers, or streams.[77] Although sensitive to chlorination, the amoeba can also contaminate drinking water systems and premise plumbing, possibly through cross-connections, pipe breaks, and pressure fluctuations. This pathogen has caused infection and death among Neti-pot users who used tap water for nasal irrigation.[78] Signs and symptoms of *Naegleria fowleri* infection are clinically similar to bacterial meningitis thereby lowering the chances of a correct initial diagnosis. A warming climate may increase the range of *Naegleria fowleri* and in recent years, cases have occurred as far north as Minnesota.[79]

Chemical Contaminants

Some of the major chemical contaminants affecting water supplies are shown in Table 72-3. Chemical contaminants may be naturally occurring, or may contaminate water from agricultural activities, industry, sewage, mining, pesticides, hazardous waste, or resulting

TABLE 72-2 MAJOR WATERBORNE MICROBIAL PATHOGENS

Contaminant	Source/Transmission	Health Effects	Notes
Bacteria			
Legionella pneumophila	Naturally occurring in soil and water. Infection occurs by inhalation of aerosolized bacteria. Common sources in water are distribution systems, cooling towers, showers, hot tubs.	Respiratory infection. Legionnaires' disease; Pontiac fever	Increase in outbreaks in recent years in the United States. Those with respiratory infection, smokers, lung disease or other chronic illnesses are more susceptible Legionnaires' disease.
Shigella sp.	Sewage, fecal contamination (human) of food or water. Transmitted via fecal-oral route.	Abdominal cramps, fever, watery diarrhea	Low infectious dose (10–100 bacteria). Numerous waterborne outbreaks have been documented. Not stable in water and susceptible to chlorination, presence reflects recent water contamination.
Campylobacter sp.	Sewage, fecal contamination (human, birds, cattle) of food or water. Usually transmitted via contact with animals (e.g., poultry) and their feces.	Gastroenteritis including abdominal pain, diarrhea, vomiting, chills, fever, Guillain Barre syndrome	Drinking water can be contaminated by fecal contamination of wild birds and cattle. Outbreaks in drinking water have occurred due to inadequate treatment and disinfection.
Salmonella sp. (nontyphoid)	Sewage, fecal contamination (human, birds other animals) of food or water. Spread via fecal-oral route and contact with animals and their feces.	Gastroenteritis including abdominal pain, diarrhea, fever, nausea	Waterborne outbreaks have occurred due to inadequately disinfected water supplies and fecal contamination of freshwater lakes.
Salmonella typhi/paratyphi	Sewage, fecal contamination (human) of food or water. Transmitted via fecal-oral route.	Infection causes typhoid fever. Symptoms include high fever, weakness, stomach pain, diarrhea.	Remains common in areas with inadequate water and sanitation infrastructure.
Escherichia coli(pathogenic strains)	Sewage, fecal contamination (human, cattle, livestock) of food or water. Transmitted via fecal-oral route.	Diarrhea, vomiting fever. Enterohaemorrhagic strains (0157:H7, 0111) can cause hemolytic uremic syndrome	Numerous documented outbreaks in inadequately treated and disinfected drinking water and fecally contaminated recreational water, often attributed to fecal releases from diaper age children.
Helicobacter pylori	Primary transmission route is believed to be person to person. but may be transmitted via fecal-oral route.	Gastric ulcers, gastric cancer, chronic gastritis. Most infections are asymptomatic	Water has not been confirmed as a source of transmission. Sensitive to chlorination but can survive in the environment and has been identified in surface waters and shallow groundwaters.
Leptospirosis(*Leptospira interrogans* and *Leptonoma sp.*)	Urine of infected animals (especially rodents). Can survive in water for days or weeks in water. Humans are infected when contact is made with contaminated surface waters.	Fever, headache, muscle pain, chills, abdominal pain, jaundice, vomiting, diarrhea, rash. May result in pulmonary bleeding and sequelae including depression, headaches, fatigue, joint pain, and renal failure (Weil disease)	Sensitive to disinfection, most waterborne outbreaks are associated with occupational or recreational contact with surface water or mud.
Mycobacteria (nontuberculous)	Inhalation, contact, and ingestion of contaminated water.	Pulmonary disease, skin/soft tissue disease. Most common in postmenopausal women and patients with underlying lung disease and AIDS	Naturally occurring in a variety of water and soil environments. Can grow or persist in biofilms of plumbing and distribution systems.
Vibrio cholerae	Ingestion of fecally contaminated water or food. Person to person route is an unlikely source of transmission.	Mild to severe watery diarrhea. Can cause death in up to 60% of untreated cases due to dehydration.	Cholera outbreaks continue to occur in many areas without adequate sanitation and water treatment. *V. cholera* occurs naturally occurring in water environments, the toxic strains are less common.
Vibrio (noncholerae)	Naturally occurring in marine, brackish and estuarine waters, Waterborne transmission occurs via recreational exposure or contact with flooded surface waters.	Wound infection, skin infection	Main agents are *Vibrio vulnificus and parahaemolyticus*. Primarily cause gastroenteritis due to foodborne infection, swimming, or wading can cause wound or skin infections.

(*Continued*)

TABLE 72-2 MAJOR WATERBORNE MICROBIAL PATHOGENS (*Continued*)

Contaminant	Source/Transmission	Health Effects	Notes
Viruses			
Norovirus (and human caliciviruses)	Sewage, fecal contamination (human).	Vomiting, diarrhea	Cause of drinking water and recreational water associated outbreaks. Relatively resistant to conventional water treatment, can survive in the environment.
Hepatitis A	Sewage, fecal contamination (human).	Fever, nausea, jaundice, liver damage. Asymptomatic infection is common.	Person-to-person spread most common route of transmission but strong evidence of waterborne transmission. Long incubation period (28–30 days). Relatively resistant to conventional water treatment.
Hepatitis E	Sewage, fecal contamination (human, swine), fecal-oral route.	Fever, fatigue, nausea, vomiting, jaundice, liver damage. Asymptomatic infection is common.	Present in raw and treated sewage. Contaminated water has been associated with large outbreaks. Relatively resistant to conventional water treatment. Swine are animal reservoirs.
Enterovirus	Sewage, fecal contamination (human).	Fever, runny nose, cough, rash, viral meningitis, myocarditis, hand-foot-and-mouth disease, acute flaccid paralysis. Asymptomatic infection is common.	Includes poliovirus, coxsackievirus. Occur in high numbers in sewage, raw water sources and treated drinking water and have been found in private wells. Water is not a common route of transmission.
Rotavirus	Sewage, fecal contamination (human).	Diarrhea, fever, abdominal pain	Water is not a common route of transmission but large waterborne outbreaks have been described.
Protozoa			
Entamoeba histolytica	Sewage, fecal contamination (human).	Dysentery, including diarrhea and cramping colitis. May infect liver, lungs and brain. Asymptomatic infection very common.	Cysts remain viable in aquatic environments for months. Relatively resistant to disinfection. Foodborne transmission is also common. More common in lower income countries.
Cryptosporidium sp.	Sewage, fecal contamination (human, cattle), fecal-oral route.	Watery diarrhea, fever, vomiting, nausea. Usually self-limiting in immune-competent individuals but can be life threatening in those with weakened immune systems	Role of drinking water and recreational water in transmission is well-established. Oocysts are extremely resistant to chlorination and can survive for months in the environment.
Giardia sp.	Sewage, fecal contamination (human, animal), fecal-oral route.	Diarrhea, cramps. In most cases self-limiting. Asymptomatic infection is common.	Person to person transmission is most common route, but waterborne transmission in drinking water and recreational water has been well established. Resistant to chlorination.
Toxoplasma gondii	Waterborne transmission may occur via contact or ingestion of water supplies contaminated by feces of infected cats. Cats are definitive host.	Usually asymptomatic in immune-competent hosts. May cause disseminated disease involving central nervous system, lungs, and neurological disorders. Infection during pregnancy can lead to stillbirth or fetal abnormality.	Foodborne transmission is most common route. Infrequently associated with waterborne transmission but associations with drinking water have been documented.
Acanthamoeba	Naturally occurring, widespread, and free living in aquatic environments. Also found in soil and dust.	Amoebic keratitis, affecting content lens wearers, causing eye pain, redness, blurred vision, and possible vision loss if untreated.	Amoebic keratitis has been associated with tap water used for washing contact lenses. May also be transmitted via swimming while wearing contact lenses.
Naegleria fowleri	Naturally occurring, widespread, and free living in aquatic environments and soil. Waterborne transmission occurs most commonly in warm, freshwater lakes and ponds through nasal inhalation.	Primary amoebic meningitis. Very rare but nearly always fatal.	Also transmitted via contaminated drinking water among Neti pot users.

(*Continued*)

TABLE 72-2 MAJOR WATERBORNE MICROBIAL PATHOGENS (Continued)

Contaminant	Source/Transmission	Health Effects	Notes
Microsporidia	Likely to occur in excreted feces, urine and respiratory excretions. Spores have been found in water sources.	Varies depending on site of infection. Intestinal infection results in chronic diarrhea.	Waterborne and foodborne transmission possible but not confirmed. An opportunistic infectious agent, occurs mainly in immunocompromised patients. Some now are classified as fungi.
Helminths			
Dracunculus medinensis ("Guinea worm")	Unfiltered, stagnant water containing small crustaceans infected with larvae	Swelling, fever, painful blisters about one year after infection. Blisters are immersed in water to relieve pain, releasing worm and larvae back into water	Now only occurs in Chad, Ethiopia and Sudan. Focus of global eradication effort.
Shistosoma sp.	Human schistosomes are found in tropical and subtropical fresh waters with freshwater snails. Transmission occurs through skin penetration by larvae.	Human schistosomes cause schistosomiasis, or bilharzia, which may result in allergic reaction, fever, chills, muscle pain. Chronic infection can cause liver fibrosis and renal failure.	Avian schistosomes, common in the United States and worldwide, cause cercarial dermatitis or "swimmer's itch."

TABLE 72-3 MAJOR WATERBORNE CHEMICAL CONTAMINANTS

Contaminant	Sources	Health Effects	Notes
Inorganic			
Lead	Corrosion of plumbing systems containing lead pipes or fittings.	Neurodevelopmental effects, cardiovascular effects, impaired renal function, hypertension, adverse reproductive outcomes. No level of exposure is considered safe, especially for children.	Infants and children are most sensitive to lead toxicity. Not a raw water contaminant.
Arsenic	Naturally occurring in soil and ground water. Waste product of mining and some industrial operations.	Cause of bladder, skin and lung cancer, skin lesions, and peripheral vascular disease. Also associated with of cardiovascular disease and diabetes.	Countries affected by high levels of arsenic in groundwater include: Argentina, Bangladesh, Chile, China, India, Mexico, Pakistan, United States.
Fluoride	Naturally occurring in earth's crust, rocks, soil, and ground water. Added to drinking water to provide protection against dental caries.	Low levels of exposure are highly effective in preventing dental caries (up to ~ 2 mg/L). High levels of exposure can cause dental and skeletal fluorosis.	High levels in water are found in parts of India, China, Central Africa and South America. Air, food, tea and other drinks may also significantly contribute to exposure.
Selenium	Naturally present in earth's crust, rocks, soil and ground and surface water. Discharge from petroleum refineries. Levels are usually less than 10 ppb in drinking water.	Hair or fingernail loss, numbness in fingers and toes, circulatory problems. May also be associated with respiratory, gastrointestinal and cardiovascular effects.	Essential nutrient for humans. Food is likely major exposure route. Health effects only likely to be observed well above 50 µg/L
Nitrate/nitrite	Runoff from agriculture, fertilizers, sewage. Wells in areas of intensive agriculture are particularly at risk of contamination	"Blue baby" syndrome (methaemoglobinaemia); thyroid effects. Some associations have been observed with gastric cancer and congenital malformations.	Food/diet is usually main source of exposure.
Chromium	Naturally occurring in rocks, soil, dust, and ground water. Used in industrial processes including production of dyes, wood preservation, chrome plating, discharges from cooling towers. Aqueous forms are chromium-6 and chromium-3	Inhaled chromium-6 is a cause of lung cancer. Oral ingestion of chromium-6 has been associated with stomach cancer.	Major contaminant of superfund sites in the United States.
Mercury	Naturally occurring in the environment; coal fired power plants; hazardous waste sites; dental amalgam fillings; fungicides; household products. Can impact water through erosion of natural deposits, industrial discharge, runoff from landfills or agriculture.	Nervous system effects, brain and kidney damage, nausea, diarrhea. Developing fetuses are particularly susceptible to nervous system effects.	Food is main source of exposure. Fish from contaminated waters are an important exposure in some areas.

(Continued)

TABLE 72-3 MAJOR WATERBORNE CHEMICAL CONTAMINANTS (*Continued*)

Contaminant	Sources	Health Effects	Notes
Cyanide	Gold mining, manufacturing, industrial chemical factories. May enter surface waters through runoff, spills or waste water discharges.	Highly acutely toxic. Shortness of breath, seizures, coma, and death. Thyroid toxicity.	Naturally found in some foods. Except following spills, usually occurs in levels too low in water to cause a health concern.
Copper	Corrosion of copper plumbing and fittings, erosion of natural deposits	Causes gastrointestinal symptoms at high exposures. Long-term exposures may cause liver or kidney damage.	Carriers of the gene for Wilson disease may be especially susceptible to adverse effects of waterborne copper exposure.
Cadmium	Wastewater; corrosion of plumbing; erosion of natural deposits; discharge from metal refineries; runoff from waste batteries and paints.	Kidney damage	Food is main source of exposure.
Organic			
Dioxane	Industrial chemical used as stabilizer in chlorinated solvents and as a solvent for resins, oils and waxes. Groundwater is susceptible to contamination.	Likely/possible human carcinogen, liver, kidney toxicity.	US EPA has not established a maximum contaminant level, but has established health advisory levels and states have developed guidelines levels.
Perchlorate	Used in rocket fuel, fireworks, fertilizers, and is also naturally occurring. Prevalent at hazardous waste sites. Can contaminate water supplies from environmental releases. Plumes in groundwater can be extensive.	Inhibits iodide uptake resulting in reduced production of thyroid hormone.	Difficult to remove by conventional water treatment. Prevalent in water supplies. Diet an important exposure route. Most humans have some exposure.
Polychlrorinated biphenyls (PCBs)	Highly persistent synthetic organic chemicals used as coolants, lubricants, lighting fixtures. No longer made in the United States. May be found in contaminated groundwater or surface water near hazardous waste sites.	Probable human carcinogen	Food, air, and soil are most important exposure routes.
Pesticides	Can impact ground or surface waters through agricultural and residential runoff, sewage, seepage, spills. Private wells in areas of intensive agriculture are at risk of contamination.	Range of potential health effects depending on the type of pesticide including nervous system effects, hormonal and endocrine effects, and cancer.	Examples of pesticides potentially impacting water sources include DDT, 2,4-D, atrazine, aldrin, lindane, methoxychlor, glypohsate
Per- and polyfluoroalkyl substances (PFAS)	Manufacturing of repellants and fire foam. Highly persistent and can impact surface or ground waters through industrial discharges.	Not well characterized, potentially associated with elevated cholesterol, thyroid function and immunological function.	EPA health advisory level of 70 ppt in drinking water for lifetime exposure.
Tri/Tetra chloroethylene (TCE/PCE)(chlorinated solvents)	Dry cleaning, textile processing, chemical manufacturing, can impact water sources as a result of improper disposal and leaching from landfills. Relatively frequently detected in groundwater.	PCE can have neurological effects and is a probable human carcinogen and causes liver and kidney cancer in animals. TCE known to cause kidney cancer and may cause liver cancer, lymphoma, adverse reproductive effects, and effects to the immune and endocrine systems.	Exposure also occurs in occupational settings. In the United States, between 9% and 34% of groundwater sources used for drinking water have some TCE.
Benzene	Chemical solvent used in production of plastics and synthetic fabrics. Found in crude oil, gasoline, and cigarette smoke. Introduced to water through industrial effluents, leaching from gas storage tanks and landfills and atmospheric deposition.	Human carcinogen, cause of leukemia	

(*Continued*)

TABLE 72-3 MAJOR WATERBORNE CHEMICAL CONTAMINANTS (*Continued*)

Contaminant	Sources	Health Effects	Notes
Vinyl chloride	Used in the manufacturing of if numerous products in building construction, automotive industry, in the rubber, paper and glass industries. Can migrate into groundwater from hazardous waste sites due to improper disposal or leakage, or spills.	Human carcinogen (multiple sites)	Rarely detected in surface waters due to high volatility. May also be formed as a degradation product of TCE/PCE.
Methyl tertiary butyl ether (MTBE)	Gasoline additive. Spills and leaking storage tanks can impact groundwater.	Although it can cause taste and odor problems MTBE is not known to cause health effects via drinking water exposure.	
Pharmaceuticals/ personal care products	Urban wastewater and discharges to surface waters.	Generally occur at low concentrations (parts-per-trillion), but effects of chronic exposures and exposures to breakdown products are not well characterized.	Antidepressants, antiviral drugs, antibiotics, fragrances.
Disinfection-by-products			
Trihalomethanes (THM)	By product of chlorination of raw water supplies containing organic matter.	Genotoxic, possible increased risk of bladder cancer and reproductive effects.	THMs include bromoform, bromodichloromethane, chloroform, dibromochloromethane
Haloacetic acids	By product of chlorination of raw water supplies containing organic matter.	Possible increased risk of gastric cancer.	
Halogenated acetonitriles (haloacetonitriles)	By product of chlorination or chloramination of raw water supplies containing organic matter.	Unknown/limited data. Animal toxicology studies suggest potential reproductive/ developmental toxicity.	
Bromate	By product of ozonation of raw water supplies containing bromide ion.	Possible human carcinogen	
Algal toxins			
Cyanobacteria/ cyanotoxins	Toxins are produced by cyanobacteria in freshwater. Blooms of cyanobacteria are influenced by increased nutrients (nitrogen and phosphorus) in waterbodies.	Microcystin is a liver toxin. Associated with dermal, respiratory, gastrointestinal symptoms. Can cause animal poisonings and death.	Examples include microcystin, cylindrospermopsin, anatoxin, saxitoxin.
Brevetoxin	Produced by marine dinoflagellates; associated with Florida red tides	Aerosol exposures from red tides can cause in respiratory symptoms, especially among asthmatics	Consumption of shellfish contaminated by brevetoxin can cause neurotoxic shellfish poisoning.
Radioactive substances			
Radon	Naturally occurring in groundwater sources. May be ingested or inhaled as radon is released from water to air.	Ingestion of water with radon increases risk stomach cancer; inhalation increases risk of lung cancer.	Those with private wells should get them tested. Does not affect surface waters. Most radon comes from soil underneath the home.
Uranium	Naturally occurring in mineral deposits, emissions from nuclear industry, mine tailings, coal combustion.	Kidney effects and kidney damage. Health effects of oral ingestion are generally due to the chemical and not radiation	Exposure through drinking water is generally very low, levels are generally < 1 ppb, though concentrations as high as 700 ppb have been observed

from water treatment or distribution.[80] Chemical contaminants may further be classified as inorganic (lead, arsenic), organic (pesticides, industrial compounds), disinfectants and DBPs, and algal toxins. There are many chemicals that can impact water sources and supplies but for many, human health effects are not well characterized. Some of the challenges in characterizing the health endpoints include low exposure levels, long-term exposure windows (i.e., for endpoints such as cancer), and lack of monitoring data.[81] For some chemicals found in water, the principal route may not be ingestion of water. For example, most exposure to nitrate and nitrite is through consumption of meat and vegetables and not drinking water,[82] thus complicating exposure assessment and characterization of the effects of waterborne nitrate exposures. Consequently, obtaining high-quality human or epidemiologic data linking chemicals in water directly to health effects is challenging, and health targets or regulatory limits are usually derived through extrapolation from high-dose animal studies.[81] The U.S. EPA regulates close to 80 chemicals in drinking water[30] and the World Health Organization provides guideline values for nearly 200 different chemicals.[31] These regulations do not include emerging contaminants such as pharmaceuticals, personal care products, and perfluorinated compounds for which limited information on occurrence and effects are currently available.

In this section, some of the globally important chemical contaminants are described. A more comprehensive overview can be found in the World Health Organization Guidelines for Drinking Water Quality (also supporting material)[31] and the U.S. Environmental Protection Agency's National Primary Drinking Water Standards (https://www.epa.gov/ground-water-and-drinking-water/national-primary-drinking-water-regulations).[30]

Inorganic Chemicals

Major inorganic chemical contaminants of water include lead, arsenic, nitrate, fluoride, and selenium. These contaminants may occur naturally or as a result of industrial or agricultural processes.

Mineral mining can produce large quantities of waste that include toxic chemicals such as cyanide, mercury, copper, arsenic, lead, cadmium, and sulfuric acid. These wastes can contaminate water sources that are used locally for drinking or fishing and adversely affect the ecological integrity of the region. Artisanal gold mining using mercury to dissolve and extract gold is practiced by about 13 million miners in 55 countries, including Brazil, Tanzania, Indonesia, and Vietnam, exposing mine workers to potentially hazardous levels of the neurotoxic metal and resulting in contamination of water resources. Following discharge to water, mercury then biomagnifies in the food chain, resulting in a health risk to indigenous populations relying on subsistence fishing.[80]

Waterborne arsenic is associated with significant morbidity and premature mortality around the world. It is a naturally occurring element distributed widely in soils, sediments, and groundwater. Arsenic also occurs in food, usually in its organic form, which is considerably less toxic, although rice contains substantial amounts of inorganic arsenic. Arsenic's toxic properties have been known since 370 BC and it has been used as a poison throughout history, and was even suspected in the poisoning death of Napoleon Bonaparte.[83] Symptoms of acute arsenic poisoning are similar to cholera, so poisonings often went undetected. Also used in cosmetics and medical treatments, its relationship to skin cancer was first described in 1888 following its use in treatments for psoriasis. Exposures to arsenic also cause characteristic skin lesions, depigmentation, and hyperkeratosis. Because it occurs naturally in groundwater, some populations have been exposed to excessively high arsenic as regions shifted to deep wells to avoid microbial contamination of shallower wells or surface water sources.

In the 1920s, Southwest Taiwan switched water sources from shallow wells and surface water to artesian well water, which was contaminated with extremely high levels of arsenic, up to 2000 μg/L (200 times current regulatory limits in the United States). Residents used this water for up to 60 years and in the mid-1900s, a severe peripheral arterial disease known as "blackfoot disease" was noted to be widespread in this region. By comparing nearby regions with similar population demographics that did not use the arsenic-affected wells, researchers determined that blackfoot disease was directly related to the arsenic contaminated water and cancer mortality rates among those exposed to arsenic were also significantly elevated. Bladder cancer mortality was over 11 times higher in this population and highly elevated rates of lung, kidney, skin, liver, and colon cancer mortality were also observed.[84] In Argentina and Chile, a switch to a drinking water source high in arsenic also resulted in a marked increase in bladder and lung cancer mortality.[85,86] Arsenic exposure through drinking water also been associated with cardiovascular disease[87–89] and diabetes.[90,91] Although there remains uncertainty regarding low exposure effects, both the World Health Organization and U.S. EPA threshold levels in water have a threshold level in water of 10 μg/L. This level was derived from the estimated excess cancer cases expected from exposures at this level ($\sim 1 \times 10^{-4}$), extrapolating from the Taiwan data, as well as taking into account the achievable levels of reduction for small systems.[30,31] In the state of New Jersey, the arsenic threshold level in water is 5 μg/L and in The Netherlands it is 1 μg/L, the lowest in the world. An estimated 140 million people across 50 countries are exposed to drinking water levels greater than 10 μg/L. Countries most affected include Bangladesh, China, Cambodia, India, Nepal, and Vietnam. Elevated levels of arsenic in drinking water have also been observed in Argentina, Bolivia, Chile, Mexico, and parts of the United States.[31]

Fluoride is a naturally occurring element that affects groundwater. At low levels (<1.5 mg/L) it is protective against dental caries and fluoridation of public water supplies has been shown to be an effective and safe preventative approach to reduce dental caries.[92] However, at higher levels of exposure fluoride can cause mild to severe and crippling dental and skeletal fluorosis. Dental fluorosis is characterized by staining and pitting of the teeth and damage to enamel. In skeletal fluorosis, fluoride accumulates in the bone, resulting in stiffness and pain in the joints and in severe cases, alterations to the bone structure, calcification of ligaments, and impairment of muscles and pain.[93] Exceptionally high levels up to 2800 mg/L may naturally occur in groundwater. Air, dental products, certain foods, and beverages (tea, wine) contribute additional fluoride exposure. High groundwater concentrations can be found in most parts of the world, but areas of India, Pakistan, West Africa, Thailand, China, Sri Lanka, and Southern Africa are especially affected. Endemic fluorosis is particularly problematic in India where 60–70 million are estimated to be at risk.[93]

Unlike arsenic and fluoride, most lead that occurs in drinking water is not a result of contamination of source water but from lead service connections and plumbing in buildings. Because it is a potent neurotoxicant, it is widely accepted that there is no safe level of lead exposure, particularly for children.[94] The U.S. EPA sets a public health regulatory goal for lead in water of zero, with a regulatory action limit of 15 μg/L. The removal of lead from major sources, such as gasoline, home paint, and consumer products has resulted in significant population declines in overall lead exposure.[95] However, lead piping and plumbing remain a source of lead exposure in drinking water, particularly in the presence of corrosive water.[96] Changes to water source, treatment, or distribution can trigger descaling of the pipes and the leaching of lead into water supplies as in Flint, Michigan in 2014 when the source water was changed from Lake Huron to the more corrosive Flint River without proper corrosion controls. This resulted in a marked increase in blood lead levels in children younger than 5 years in a community already impacted by high levels of lead exposure.[97]

In 1945, an Iowa physician linked two cases of methemoglobinemia ("blue baby syndrome") to infants fed bottled formula prepared with water from shallow wells with high levels of nitrate.[98] Nitrate (and nitrite) can contaminate drinking water most often from the application of fertilizer and manure and from human sewage or septic tanks, and animal waste. Wells located near intensive agriculture where nitrate from manure can seep into ground water are at particular risk of contamination. EPA's regulatory limit is 10 mg/L (parts per million) to protect against methemoglobinemia for public drinking water systems. Most cases of methemoglobinemia have occurred in infants fed bottled formula from ground water wells, which are not regulated or monitored.[99] However, there is some evidence that gastrointestinal infections may be a co factor or even an independent cause of infant methemoglobinemia.[100] Nitrates in water have been associated with other health effects including thyroid effects, gastric cancer, and adverse reproductive and developmental outcomes, although it has been difficult to confirm these associations since dietary nitrate and nitrite (root vegetables, cured meats, respectively) are usually the major source of exposure.[31]

Organic Chemicals

Organic chemicals including pesticides (e.g., herbicides, insecticides, fungicides), such as dichlorodiphenyltrichloroethane (DDT), lindane, glyphosate, atrazine, 2,4-dichlorophenoxyacetic acid (2,4-D), polychlorinated biphenyls (PCBs), and benzene contaminate water sources through agricultural and industrial discharge and runoff, runoff from gardens and lawns, and leaching of hazardous wastes sites and spills. Examples of organic chemicals that impact water sources are shown in Table 72-3. Although generally these chemicals are present in water sources at levels too low to result in acute health effects, some can persist and accumulate in the environment. DDT (banned in the United States in 1972, but still used in countries affected by malaria), PCBs (banned in the United States in 1978), aldrin, chlordane, and polycyclic aromatic hydrocarbons are known as persistent organic pollutants (POPs) because they do not readily degrade, can accumulate in the environment and magnify through food chains. Toxicology studies have found numerous potential adverse health effects from exposures to POPs including disruption of endocrine, immunological and reproductive systems, cancer, diabetes, and thyroid problems.[80] Although regulatory and health agencies provide criteria and guideline levels for many POPs in drinking water, diet is often a major exposure route to most POPs.[101]

Widespread pesticide use is associated with agricultural activities and those most at risk of exposure to pesticides via drinking water are those relying on private wells or other unmonitored/unregulated water sources in regions with intensive agriculture. Atrazine (herbicide used to control broadleaf weeds in corn, sugarcane and other crops) is one of the most common agricultural chemicals found in groundwater wells and surface waters, often co-occurring with nitrate in private wells. In Iowa, a state with intensive agriculture, atrazine or atrazine derivatives were found in 30% of private wells.[102] Atrazine is not commonly found in food, though soil contact and air are other potential exposure routes in addition to water. The human health effects of atrazine in humans are not well characterized, but toxicology studies indicate it can cause liver, kidney and heart damage in animals. Epidemiological studies have also noted associations between atrazine exposure and adverse reproductive outcomes.[103] Examples of other pesticides detected in water sources include metolachlor, cyanazine, trifluralin, and 2,4-D, diazinon and chlorpyrifos.[102]

Chlorinated solvents such as benzene, tetrachloroethylene (PCE), and trichloroethylene (TCE) are commonly used in a range of industries including dry cleaning, textile processing, and metal degreasing. These chemicals can cause numerous adverse health effects including cancer (e.g., leukemia, kidney cancer) and have caused localized contamination of ground water usually due to spills and improper disposal.

From 1953 to 1985, an estimated 500,000–1,000,000 military personnel, their families and other employees and residents of the Marine Corps Base Camp Lejeune in North Carolina were exposed to excessively high levels of chlorinated solvents (TCE, PCE, vinyl chloride, and benzene) in their drinking water.[104] Levels of these contaminants in ground water wells and the distribution system were often well above EPA's current regulatory criteria levels (in the early 1980s there were no drinking water regulations for these chemicals) with PCE measuring as high as 1580 μg/L in January 1985 (EPA's current regulatory criteria is 5 μg/L).[105] The suspected sources of contamination were an off-site dry cleaner and industrial and hazardous waste disposal and storage from the military base. The Centers for Disease Control and Prevention led detailed investigations of the exposures and potential health effects in the exposed population and found elevated risks for several cancers, including cancers of the kidney, rectum, prostate, lung, leukemias, and multiple myeloma as well as certain birth defects and preterm birth.[106] There was also some evidence for elevated risk of male breast cancer and Parkinson's disease.[107–109] Based on the epidemiological and toxicological evidence, the Department of Veteran's Affairs passed the "Diseases Associated With Exposure to Contaminants in the Water Supply at Camp Lejeune" rule in 2017. This rule provides VA medical benefits for those who served at Camp Lejeune for at least 30 days during this period, and who have been diagnosed with any of eight associated diseases (adult leukemia, aplastic anemia and other myelodysplastic syndromes, bladder cancer, kidney cancer, liver cancer, multiple myeloma non-Hodgkin's lymphoma, and Parkinson's disease) presumed to have been caused or exacerbated by exposure to the contaminated Camp Lejeune water.[110]

Disinfection By-products

DBPs are formed by chemical reactions between organic matter in water and the disinfectant used for treatment. The most common by-products are formed following disinfection with chlorine such as THMs (including chloroform) and haloacetic acids (HAAs).[111] There are an estimated over 700 different DBPs, only 11 of which are regulated by EPA.[112] Some have been shown to be genotoxic and carcinogenic in animals; animal studies have also demonstrated adverse reproductive effects. Epidemiological studies have demonstrated relatively small but statistically significant associations between total THMs and cancer, most notably bladder cancer, following long-term (~>40 years) exposures[111] and those with certain polymorphisms for genes involved in DBP metabolism may be at an increased risk.[113] Some epidemiological studies have also suggested associations between certain DBPs and risk for spontaneous abortion and infertility.[111] The EPA regulates total THMs and other DBPs for public water supplies to reduce these potential health risks; however, the risk from these by-products is likely outweighed by the benefits of pathogen inactivation. The WHO in their latest version of the Guidelines for Drinking Water Quality concluded that: "The use of chemical disinfectants in water treatment usually results in the formation of chemical by-products. However, the risks to health from these by-products are extremely small in comparison with the risks associated with inadequate disinfection, and it is important that disinfection efficacy not be compromised in attempting to control such by-products."[31] DBP formation can be minimized by reducing the level of organic material in the raw water, enhancing coagulation, or by alternating disinfectants (i.e., chloramination, ultraviolet radiation).

Algal Toxins

Algal toxins refer to a diverse array of toxic metabolites produced by marine and freshwater cyanobacteria ("blue-green algae") and algae. These include toxins such as microcystin and cylindrospermopsin produced by cyanobacteria, and brevetoxins and domoic acid produced by marine diatoms and dinoflagellates (the cause of "red tide"). Rapid growths of these algae result in visible blooms, known as "harmful algal blooms" or (HABs) and can be harmful to humans, animals, and ecosystems when enough toxins are produced. Not all algal blooms contain toxins, and algal toxins can also be present even in the absence of an obvious bloom or growth of algae. Algal blooms are caused by an abundance of nutrients in surface waters resulting from agricultural runoff, wastewater discharges, and land and resource management that facilitate eutrophication of surface waters. Exacerbating factors also include rising global temperatures and increasing atmospheric CO_2 concentrations.[114] Algal toxins have a diverse range of potential health effects, for example, cyanotoxins such as microcystin, cylindrospermopsin, and nodularin are hepatotoxins, whereas anatoxin is a neurotoxin. Short-term exposure may also cause irritation and gastrointestinal, respiratory, and dermal symptoms.[115] Freshwater cyanotoxins are known to poison and kill wildlife, livestock, and companion animals when the animals ingest surface water containing toxins.[116] Algal toxins also concentrate in shellfish and fish causing a range of adverse health effects, including paralytic shellfish poisoning (saxitoxin), gastrointestinal symptoms (domoic acid, ciguatoxin), and neurological symptoms (brevetoxin).[117]

The most common route of human exposure to algal toxins is through recreating on or near waters when blooms are present.[114] Exposure may be via ingestion, inhalation, or dermal contact. Freshwater outbreaks of dermatological, neurological, respiratory, and gastrointestinal symptoms attributable to algal blooms in recreational water have increased in recent years.[118] Persistent marine red-tide events can result in widespread fish kills, adversely impact recreation and tourism,[119] and are associated with increased asthma and respiratory symptoms.[45]

Although conventional water treatment is usually effective at removing both intact cyanobacterial cells and their toxins,[120] severe blooms or treatment failures can result in contamination of public drinking water supplies with algal toxins and the potential for severe human health effects. In 1996 in Brazil, contamination of a dialysis clinic's water supply with microcystin and cylindrospermopsin caused an outbreak of acute liver failure and 76 deaths.[115] In 2014, severe blooms in Lake Erie resulted in elevated levels of microcystin in the public drinking water supply for Toledo, Ohio, causing a "do not drink" advisory for over 400,000 people.[121] The frequency of harmful algal blooms is expected due to rise due to eutrophication of waterbodies, altered patterns of precipitation (i.e., more intense events that may increase runoff and extended drought that may lead to increased stagnation and reduced flow) and increasing global temperatures.[64]

Emerging Chemical Contaminants

Emerging chemical contaminants are those that have been observed in water sources or are believed to occur in water sources but the extent of their occurrence and/or their potential to harm human health or ecological integrity are not well understood. These chemicals are therefore not regulated or generally tested for in public water supplies. The U.S. EPA maintains a "candidate contaminant list" (CCL) which is "a list of contaminants that are currently not subject to any proposed or promulgated national primary drinking water regulations, but are known or anticipated to occur in public water systems" and may be considered for future regulation. The current list (CCL 4) contains 97 chemicals and these likely represent only a fraction of potential chemicals that can occur in water sources.[122] The identification of unregulated chemicals in drinking water sources is often alarming to the public as there is uncertainty about potential health effects even if they are found in low concentrations. Several examples of emerging chemical contaminants are discussed below.

Per- and Polyfluoroalkyl Substances (PFAS)

PFAS are a wide range of related compounds such as perfluorooctane sulfonate, perfluorooctanoic acid used in manufacturing of repellants, and in fire-fighting foam. The broad category of PFAS includes thousands of compounds. Although diet is likely the major source of human exposure,[81] water sources have become contaminated due to waste or discharges from industrial facilities where PFAS were produced or used to manufacture other products, or in locations where firefighting foam was used (e.g., oil refineries, or airfields).[123] "GenX" is a recently identified PFAS found in ground water wells and surface drinking water sources in North Carolina resulting from industrial discharge from a PFAS manufacturing facility to the Cape Fear River.[124] These chemicals are highly persistent in the environment and in the human body. Animal studies have identified reproductive, developmental, liver, kidney and immunological effects. Preliminary human studies indicate that PFAS may be associated with elevated cholesterol, impaired thyroid function, low infant birth weight, and impaired immunological function. EPA recently issued a health advisory for lifetime PFAS in water of 70 parts per trillion (0.07 μg/L).[125]

Perchlorate

Perchlorate is a naturally occurring anion that is used as an oxidizer in industrial products including missile fuel, matches, fireworks, signal flares, and in the manufacturing of fertilizers.[126] Perchlorate is highly stable in the environment and frequently detected in water, soil, and food, and most humans have some evidence of exposure over the course of their lifetimes.[126–128] Exposure occurs through diet, drinking water, and occupation (inhalation or ingestion). The major toxic effect of perchlorate is on thyroid metabolism, inhibiting iodide uptake leading to decreased secretion of thyroid hormone. Pregnant woman, fetuses, infants, and children may be particularly vulnerable to adverse health effects resulting from perchlorate's effects on thyroid metabolism.[127] Surveys across several countries have found that perchlorate is regularly detected in tapwater and public water systems. In the Republic of Korea and India, 80% of tapwater samples had detectable levels of perchlorate and in the United States 4.1% of public water systems surveyed had levels greater than 4 μg/L.[128] Guidelines and regulatory levels for perchlorate in water vary considerably, reflecting the uncertainty in its risk at low exposure as well as the contribution of water to overall exposure. The WHO guideline value for perchlorate is 70 μg/L in drinking water. Although EPA has not yet established formal regulatory criteria for perchlorate it has issued a health advisory level of 15 μg/L. Individual states have also issued lower regulations for perchlorate (California 6 μg/L and Massachusetts 2 μg/L).[129]

Pharmaceuticals and Personal-care Products

Pharmaceuticals, including over the counter or prescription medications for human or veterinary use, such as hormones, antibiotics, nonsteroidal anti-inflammatory drugs, and antidepressants; and personal-care products such as fragrances, preservatives, and sunscreen agents, have been detected at low concentrations (parts per trillion) in treated in and untreated water supplies and in surface waters.[130,131] Sewage discharge is the primary contributor as most conventional wastewater treatment methods are not designed to eliminate most pharmaceuticals and personal-care products (PPCPs). Swimming and direct disposal are other contributors of PPCPs in surface water. In a survey of source and treated drinking water at 25 treatment plants in the United States, commonly identified pharmaceuticals included: antidepressants bupropion (brand name: Wellbutrin), venlafaxine (brand name: Effexor), and lithium, found in 89%, 78%, and 60% of source water samples, respectively; the analgesic and anticonvulsant carbamazepine (78%); caffeine (67%); and the antibiotic sulfamethoxazole (56%). Steroidal estrogens were also frequently detected.[132] This study also found that drinking water treatment significantly reduced the concentration of PCPPs.[132] Theoretical health concerns include estrogenic effects and antimicrobial resistance in potentially pathogenic microorganisms. However, because levels of pharmaceuticals in water are several orders of magnitude below the minimum therapeutic dose, it is unlikely that exposure would result in adverse human health effects.[133] The effects of long-term exposures to mixtures of these chemicals are not known nor are the effects of exposure to the derivatives and degradation products of PCPPs.

Nanoparticles and Microplastics

Nanoparticles and microplastics are heterogenous materials, defined generally by their size. In recent years, there has been increased attention and concern with their potential impacts to the environment; however there are currently no regulations or criteria for these materials in drinking water.

Nanoparticles are particles between 1 and 100 nm in diameter and widely used in industry, research, and medicine. Examples of their use include adhesives, cosmetics, sunscreens, electronics, and biomedical engineering. Nanoparticles are also produced through diesel exhaust and combustion products.[134] Nanoparticles can enter water sources through wastewater treatment plant discharges, solid waste and landfills, direct discharges, accidental spills, and runoff.[134] They are highly persistent in the environment and most are unlikely to biodegrade. Some have been shown to be toxic to aquatic organisms and toxicological studies have found they can cause cell injury and induce oxidative stress, allergic reactions, and damage to liver and kidney function.[135] However, the potential for human exposures and health effects through drinking water are not well understood.[135]

Microplastics are plastics less than 5 mm in diameter that are either manufactured for use in cosmetics, facial cleansers, and abrasives, or produced as a result of degradation of larger plastic items. Microplastics can also enter water sources through wastewater treatment plant discharges, landfill leachate and sewage sludge as well as through physical/chemical degradation of plastic wastes and litter.[136,137] Aquatic organisms ingest microplastics and they can bioaccumulate in the food chain. Drinking water (also bottled water) may be a relevant exposure pathway, but human health effects and exposures through water exposures are not well characterized.

SUSCEPTIBLE AND VULNERABLE POPULATIONS

Depending on the type of waterborne contaminant and the nature of the exposure, certain individuals are at increased risk of adverse health effects. These individuals include those with weakened immune systems and certain chronic health conditions, children and infants, the elderly, and pregnant women.

Individuals with weakened immune systems due to AIDS, those taking immunosuppressive drugs due to cancer or organ transplant, or those with inherited immunodeficiencies, are at increased risk for severe illness resulting from waterborne infection. For example, *Cryptosporidium* was only recognized as an important cause of diarrhea in humans following 22 case reports in the late 1970s of severe protracted diarrhea among individuals with AIDS.[138] While infection with *Cryptosporidium* in immune competent individuals results in mild and self-limiting illness, among those with weakened immune system, infection can be severe and fatal.[139] Those with weakened immune systems are often advised to consider boiling or filtering their tap water to reduce their risk of becoming infected with *Cryptosporidium*. Those with weakened immune systems may also be at risk of infection with opportunistic waterborne pathogens such as *Legionella* and NTM as well as at increased risk for severe disease following infection with other waterborne pathogens, such as norovirus, *Toxoplasma gondii*, and microsporidia. Smoking, chronic respiratory and lung disease and organ transplantation are risk factors for development of severe Legionnaire's disease following infection with waterborne *Legionella*. [59]

Pregnant women and fetuses are also at increased risk of severe effects following infection with waterborne pathogens such as the parasite *Toxoplasma gondii*. Although most commonly associated with consumption of contaminated meat, soil, or contact with cat feces, outbreaks of *T. gondii* have been attributed to drinking water.[140] Infection with this parasite during pregnancy can result in congenital transmission to the infant causing miscarriage or stillbirth. Pregnant women may also be at increased risk of adverse hormonal effects resulting from exposures to organic chemicals in drinking water. Lead can cross the placenta and maternal lead exposure during pregnancy has been associated with reduced fetal growth and other adverse birth outcomes.[141] Exposures to high levels of other waterborne chemicals such as disinfection by products, arsenic, and nitrate during pregnancy may also increase the risk of adverse birth outcomes and pregnancy complications. Bottle-fed infants using formula made up with contaminated tap water are at risk of high exposure and adverse health effects due to contaminants such as nitrate and arsenic.

Young children are also at greater risk for certain waterborne infections due to lack of pre-existing immunity to some infections, poorer hygiene, and increased exposure. In areas lacking adequate water treatment and sanitation, waterborne infections are an important contributor to significant morbidity and mortality in children resulting from diarrheal diseases. Young males are at greatest risk for infection with *Naegleria fowleri* during recreation, resulting from activities that increase the likelihood of ingesting water through the nasal cavity (jumping, diving, etc.). Children younger than 10 years of age swallow more water during swimming and are at greater risk for developing gastrointestinal symptoms following exposures to fecally contaminated recreational waters, and are also presumed to be at increased risk of exposure to algal toxins during recreation.[77]

Because of their increased exposure and increased vulnerability due to higher ingestion of water per kilogram of body weight, higher absorption rates, poorer sanitation and hygiene and their developing and growing organ systems, children are also at increased risk for the adverse health effects of chemical waterborne contaminants. The neurotoxic effects of lead exposure in children are well documented[142] and in areas with high naturally occurring fluoride, children are at increased risk developing dental fluorosis.[143]

PUBLIC HEALTH SURVEILLANCE AND RESPONSE

Most countries with developed public health infrastructure maintain some type of routine surveillance and reporting system for waterborne diseases and outbreaks. In the United States, since 1971, the CDC and the U.S. EPA have conducted systematic surveillance for waterborne outbreaks through a national reporting system, relying on reporting from state and local health officials. Periodically (usually biennially) outbreaks are summarized in a report and classified according to strength of evidence, likely source, the nature of the deficiency and individuals impacted. The CDC defines a waterborne disease outbreak as: "an incident in which two or more epidemiologically linked persons experience a similar illness after exposure to the same water source and epidemiologic evidence implicates the water as the likely source of the illness." These systematic summaries are valuable to public health professionals and policy makers to document the impact of waterborne disease and have identified trends and emerging issues. For example, following implementation of the Surface Water Treatment Act in 1989, and subsequent revisions to the act, there was a notable decline in outbreaks in public drinking water systems relying on surface water sources[144] providing evidence of the effectiveness of these regulations in reducing waterborne disease. In addition, systematic analysis has documented a marked increase in outbreaks due to *Legionella* has in recent years.[59,144]

Public health surveillance and/or reports from clinicians can serve as actionable warnings of contamination of drinking water supplies. Alert identification and characterization of uncharacteristic clusters of waterborne infections or illnesses by clinicians or public health practitioners have often been important in identifying more widespread instances of waterborne disease. In Milwaukee, one of the first indications that drinking water was contaminated by *Cryptosporidium* was an increase in school absences and shortages of antidiarrheal medications.[145,146] In Flint, Michigan, physicians used routinely measured blood lead levels among infants to clearly document the impact of lead contaminated water on the community.[97] Consumer complaints regarding the taste, color, odor, and turbidity of their drinking water can also serve as indications of drinking water contamination and several outbreaks have been preceded by such complaints.[20] A few weeks after the drinking water source for the City of Flint was switched from Lake Huron to the Flint River, but before widespread lead contamination was found in drinking water, residents complained about the color, taste, and odor of their drinking water, and that the water was causing rashes.[147]

Clear communication and established relationships between water utilities and the clinical and public health community are critical to the timely investigation of water contamination events and mitigation of potential health impacts. Several waterborne outbreaks have been identified early as a result of clinicians identifying atypical clusters or spikes of predominantly waterborne infections with *Cryptosporidium* and *Giarida,* or gastroenteritis cases, and alerting the health and environmental authorities.[20] In contrast, poor communication and mistrust can delay the response and exacerbate the outbreak or contamination event. For example, response was critically delayed during the Walkerton outbreak (discussed earlier in this chapter) when operators of the water treatment plant failed to disclose contaminated sample results to public health authorities.[20]

The CDC's Agency for Toxic Substances and Disease Registry (ATSDR) responds to requests from federal, state, local governments, and community members to investigate waterborne and other environmental hazards. When environmental public health threats are identified, ATSDR collaborates with local communities and other state and federal agencies to investigate and characterize potential health risks and provide guidance to states and communities. In 2017, ATSDR conducted 49 investigations associated with waterborne contaminants across 20 states.[148] ATSDR also offers both accredited and nonaccredited continuing education courses in their "Case Studies in Environmental Medicine" series which include several courses related to waterborne contaminants, for example: Arsenic, lead, tetrachloroethylene, PFAS, and courses on taking an exposure history (https://www.atsdr.cdc.gov/emes/health_professionals/index.html).

EMERGING AND REIMERGING ISSUES

Global population increases and demographic shifts, changing weather and climate patterns, advancement of new technologies and industries bring new challenges to the management water resources. Several of these have been highlighted in other parts of this chapter (i.e., nanomaterials and microplastics). Other emerging and re-emerging issues include climate change and its impact to water quality and water treatment infrastructure, aging water treatment infrastructure, water reuse, water treatment for lower income countries, and potential impacts of unconventional natural gas extraction (i.e., hydraulic fracturing) to water sources.

Climate Change

Global climate change may alter weather and precipitation patterns that can impact water quality, quantity, and water treatment infrastructure. For example, climate change is anticipated to increase the frequency of heavy precipitation and other severe weather events (floods, hurricanes), which can damage water and sewage infrastructure and overwhelm water treatment processes resulting in lapses in treatment and discharges of untreated or partially treated sewage into surface waters. Increased frequency of severe precipitation events and flooding will also likely increase runoff and mobilization of nutrients, fecal contamination, and chemical contaminants from landfills and hazardous waste sites, resulting in the degradation of surface and ground water quality. Rising temperatures and increased nutrients in surface waters are anticipated to result in more frequent harmful algal blooms and may result in the expansion of naturally occurring waterborne pathogens such as noncholera *Vibrio*. Increasing air temperatures and drought may contribute to depletion of groundwater sources resulting in water scarcity. Sea-level rise poses a threat to the integrity and safety water and wastewater infrastructure, and may compromise groundwater quality by the intrusion of salt water into groundwater sources.[64]

Water Reuse

With increasing strain on water resources due to population growth, increased urbanization, and water scarcity,[149] the reuse of municipal wastewater has become increasingly important for sustainable water resource management. In Singapore, reused wastewater can meet up to 40% of total water demand.[149] Water reuse involves the use of highly treated wastewater (sewage) effluent (also called reclaimed water) for either potable or nonpotable purposes.[150] In practice, unplanned or "de facto" reuse of wastewater is a regular occurrence as sewage is discharged to rivers also used as drinking water sources for downstream communities. Common nonpotable uses of reclaimed water include irrigation of golf courses and parks and industrial cooling towers. Potable reuse may be indirect, where highly treated reclaimed water is discharged to existing surface or groundwater sources (i.e., recharging of groundwater aquifers), prior to drinking water treatment or direct, where reclaimed water is introduced into a drinking water supply without prior treatment or discharged to a water source without an environmental barrier. Wastewater treated for reuse is treated to a high degree with advanced treatment processes such as microfiltration, reverse osmosis, carbon filtration, and ultraviolet treatment. Despite the high quality of the treated water negative perceptions of "toilet to tap" presents challenges for water reuse gaining public acceptance, especially for direct potable reuse. Potable reuse systems require careful monitoring and management as treatment failures may result in widespread contamination of water supplies, especially in the case of direct potable reuse, but well-managed systems potable re-use systems have demonstrated the ability to consistently deliver high-quality water.[149,151]

Aging Water Infrastructure

In many areas, water infrastructure (pipes, treatment plants, reservoirs, storage systems) is over 40 years old and in the United States, 10% of water distribution pipes are over 80 years old.[152] Older pipes are more susceptible to breaks that can introduce contaminants to drinking water systems or discharge sewage into the environment. Older treatment plants may be more susceptible to failures and may lack sufficient capacity for high volumes resulting from an increased population sizes, or severe precipitation events and floods. Lead service lines were widely used in North America until as late as 1975 and in the United States an estimated 15–22 million people are served by full or partial lead service lines.[96] To reduce these vulnerabilities, significant investments are needed to replace and/or rehabilitate water infrastructure.

Household Water Treatment and Storage in Lower Income Countries

The World Health Organization estimates that 2 billion people rely on unimproved water sources or improved water sources that are fecally contaminated resulting in preventable morbidity and mortality due to waterborne disease.[4] Nonprofit organizations and public health agencies have tried to reduce this burden by encouraging point of use water treatments and safe storage. Examples include point of use ultrafiltration (i.e., LifeStraw), chemical disinfection (i.e., chlorine tablets), coagulation and flocculation, ultraviolet treatment, and solar disinfection.[153] While these treatments significantly improve microbiological quality, their ability to measurably reduce diarrheal disease has been more challenging. Several large-scale trials showed no reduction in diarrhea among those receiving improved water from household water treatments.[154] Possible explanations for these unexpected results include low adherence to the intervention, biases in self-reporting of illness, contamination of stored water after treatment, and exposures to pathogens from other sources (i.e., contaminated food and inadequate sanitation/hygiene). Interventions to reduce diarrheal disease may be more effective with the integration of improved sanitation, hygiene and nutrition as well as providing microbiologically safe household water.[154]

Unconventional Natural Gas Extraction

In recent years, there has been a rapid rise in unconventional natural gas and oil production through hydraulic fracturing, widely referred to as "fracking."[155] Potential effects to water resources resulting from hydraulic fracturing include increased use of water and contamination of surface waters and ground waters from well injection with fracturing fluid, wastewater disposal, or chemical spills. Hydraulic fracturing uses a large volume of water to produce fracturing fluids, approximately 1.5 million gallons per well, and typically uses freshwater sources from locally available ground water or surface water, potentially impacting availability of local water supplies.[156] Over 1500 different chemicals have been associated with the hydraulic fracturing process, most used in the production of hydraulic fracturing fluid. Chemical additives used in fracturing fluids include acids, biocides, friction reducers, corrosion inhibitors, foamers, and surfactants. The most commonly identified chemicals include hydrochloric acid, methanol, and hydrotreated light petroleum distillates and include known or probable human carcinogens such as ethanol and naphthalene. Other chemicals identified in fracturing fluid are associated with potential immune system effects, cardiotoxicity, neurotoxicity, liver and kidney toxicity, and reproductive and developmental toxicity. There are several documented cases where chemicals associated with nearby hydraulic fracturing activities including methanol, ethanol, naphthalene, 1,2,4-trimethylbenzene, diethylene glycol, and isopropanol have been identified in nearby ground water sources and private wells. Although direct human health effects resulting from exposure to water contaminated by hydraulic fracturing activities have not been confirmed, epidemiological studies have found associations between adverse birth outcomes including congenital heart defects and low birth weight and residential proximity to natural gas wells. Additional efforts and research are needed to better characterize environmental fate and transport of chemicals associated with hydrofracturing and their potential human health hazards.[156]

SUMMARY AND CONCLUSIONS

Modern water treatment and wastewater treatment and management have been among the most important public health achievements over the past 200 years, contributing to significant reductions in morbidity and mortality due to waterborne disease. Important challenges remain in ensuring safe water for lower income countries and areas that lack access to improved water sources. Climate change, aging water infrastructure, emerging infections, increased population growth and urbanization, and new industrial processes and materials will introduce new and future challenges for the continued access to safe water. Physicians and public health practitioners can play an important role in ensuring safe and healthy water by understanding local water quality concerns and their possible health effects, requesting laboratory tests for potential waterborne contaminants when warranted, early recognition and reporting of illness from waterborne exposures, and considering and recommending appropriate treatments or actions.

References

1. United Nations General Assembly. Resolution adopted by the General Assembly on 28 July 2010. The human right to water and sanitation. United Nations. *64/292*2010.
2. World Health Organization, UNICEF. Progress on drinking water, sanitation and hygiene: 2017 Update and SDG baselines. 2017.
3. Wang H, Naghavi M, Allen C, et al. Global, regional, and national life expectancy, all-cause mortality, and cause-specific mortality for 249 causes of death, 1980–2015: A systematic analysis for the Global Burden of Disease Study 2015. *Lancet.* 2016;388(10053):1459–544.
4. World Health Organization. *Preventing Diarrhoea through Better Water, Sanitation and Hygiene: Exposures and Impacts in Low-and-middle Income Countries.* Geneva, Switzerland: World Health Organization; 2014.
5. Last JM. Miasma theory. In: Breslow LBreslow L, ed. *Enycyclopedia of Public Health.* Vol. 3. New York: MacMillon Reference USA; 2002.
6. Halliday S. Death and miasma in Victorian London: An obstinate belief. *BMJ.* 2001;323(7327):1469.
7. US EPA. *25 Years of the Safe Drinking Water Act: History and Trends.* Washington, DC: Office of Water; December 1999.
8. Colwell RR. Global climate and infectious disease: The cholera paradigm. *Science.* 1996;274(5295):2025–31.
9. Pollitzer R. Cholera studies: 1. History of the disease. *Bull World Health Organ.* 1954;10(3):421.
10. Clemens JD, Nair GB, Ahmed T, Qadri F, Holmgren J. Cholera. 2017;(10101):1539–49.
11. Sack DA, Sack RB, Nair GB, Siddique AK. Cholera. *Lancet.* Jan 17 2004;363(9404):223–33.
12. Johnson S. *The Ghost Map: The Story of London's Most Terrifying Epidemic and How It Changed Science, Cities and the Modern World.* London, England: Penguin Books; 2006.
13. Chadwick E. *Report on the Sanitary Condition of the Labouring Population of Great Britain.* London: Clowes and Sons; 1843.
14. McGuire MJ. *The Chlorine Revolution: Water Disinfection and the Fight to Save Lives.* Denver, CO: American Water Works Association; 2013.
15. Armstrong GL, Conn LA, Pinner RW. Trends in infectious disease mortality in the United States during the 20th century. *JAMA.* 1999;281(1):61–6.
16. Page T, Harris RH, Epstein SS. Drinking water and cancer mortality in Louisiana. *Science.* Jul 2 1976;193(4247):55–7.
17. US EPA. *Primer for Municipal Wastewater Treatment Systems.* Washington, DC: US EPA; 2004.
18. European Environment Agency. *European Water Policies and Human Health.* Luxemborg: Publications Office of the European Union; 2016. 32/2016.
19. Gerba CP. Domestic wastes and waste treatment. In: Maier RM, Pepper IL, Gerba CPMaier RM, Pepper IL, Gerba CP, eds. *Environmental Microbiology.* San Diego: Academic Press; 2000, pp. 505–34.
20. Hrudey SE, Hrudey EJ. *Safe Drinking Water: Lessons from Recent Outbreaks in Affluent Nations.* London, UK: IWA Publishing; 2004.
21. US EPA. *Consider the Source: A Pocket Guide to Protecting Your Drinking Water.* 2002.
22. LeChevallier MW, Au K-K. *Water Treatment and Pathogen Control: Process Efficiency in Achieving Safe Drinking Water.* London, UK: IWA Publishing on behalf of the World Health Organization; 2004.
23. Stackelberg PE, Gibs J, Furlong ET, Meyer MT, Zaugg SD, Lippincott RL. Efficiency of conventional drinking-water-treatment processes in removal of pharmaceuticals and other organic compounds. *Sci Total Environ.* May 15 2007;377(2–3):255–72.
24. World Health Organization. *Guidelines for Drinking Water Quality-4th Edition: Annex 5 Treatment Methods and Performance.* Geneva: World Health Organization; 2017.
25. Pieper KJ, Tang M, Edwards MA. Flint water crisis caused by interrupted corrosion control: Investigating "ground zero" home. *Environ Sci Technol.* 2017;51(4):2007–14.
26. World Health Organization. *Water Safety in Distribution Systems.* Geneva, Switzerland: WHO; 2014. ISBN 978 92 4 154889 2.
27. Clark R, Geldreich E, Fox K, et al. A waterborne Salmonella typhimurium outbreak in Gideon, Missouri: Results from a field investigation. *Int J Environ Health Res.* 1996;6(3):187–93.
28. Palmer SR, Gully PR, White JM, et al. Water-borne outbreak of campylobacter gastroenteritis. *Lancet.* 1983;1(8319):287–90.
29. Sacks JJ, Lieb S, Baldy LM, et al. Epidemic campylobacteriosis associated with a community water supply. *Am J Public Health.* 1986;76(4):424–8.
30. US EPA. National Primary Drinking Water Regulations. Vol. 40 CFR 141 1998.
31. World Health Organization. *Guidelines for Drinking Water Quality-4th Edition.* Geneva: World Health Organization; 2017.
32. Gleick PH. Basic water requirements for human activities: Meeting basic needs. *Water Int.* 1996;21(2):83–92.
33. US Department of the Interior US Geological Survey. Water Questions & Answers: How much water does the average person use at home per day? 2016; https://water.usgs.gov/edu/qa-home-percapita.html. Accessed March 12, 2019.
34. US EPA. *Exposure Factors Handbook,* 2011 ed. Washington, DC: US Environmental Protection Agency; 2011.
35. World Health Organization. *Quantitative Microbial Risk Assessment: Application for Water Safety Management.* Geneva, Switzerland: WHO; 2016. ISBN 978 92 4 156537 0.
36. Dufour AP, Behymer TD, Cantu R, Magnuson M, Wymer LJ. Ingestion of swimming pool water by recreational swimmers. *J Water Health.* Jun 2017;15(3):429–37.
37. Dufour AP, Evans O, Behymer TD, Cantu R. Water ingestion during swimming activities in a pool: A pilot study. *J Water Health.* Dec 2006;4(4):425–30.
38. van Heijnsbergen E, Schalk JA, Euser SM, Brandsema PS, den Boer JW, de Roda Husman AM. Confirmed and potential sources of Legionella reviewed. *Environ Sci Technol.* 2015;49(8):4797–815.
39. Falkinham JO, 3rd. Environmental sources of nontuberculous mycobacteria. *Clin Chest Med.* Mar 2015;36(1):35–41.
40. Falkinham JO, 3rd. Current epidemiologic trends of the nontuberculous Mycobacteria (NTM). *Curr Environ Health Rep.* Jun 2016;3(2):161–7.
41. Baker-Austin C, Oliver JD. Rapidly developing and fatal Vibrio vulnificus wound infection. *IDCases.* 2016;6:13.
42. Klontz KC, Lieb S, Schreiber M, Janowski HT, Baldy LM, Gunn RA. Syndromes of Vibrio vulnificus infections: Clinical and epidemiologic features in Florida cases, 1981–1987. *Ann Intern Med.* 1988;109(4):318–23.

43. Oliver J. Wound infections caused by Vibrio vulnificus and other marine bacteria. *Epidemiol Infect.* 2005;133(3):383–91.
44. Backer LC, Manassaram-Baptiste D, LePrell R, Bolton B. Cyanobacteria and algae blooms: Review of health and environmental data from the Harmful Algal Bloom-Related Illness Surveillance System (HABISS) 2007–2011. *Toxins.* Mar 27 2015;7(4):1048–64.
45. Fleming LE, Kirkpatrick B, Backer LC, et al. Review of Florida red tide and human health effects. *Harmful Algae.* Jan 1 2011;10(2):224–33.
46. Codd GA, Bell SG, Kaya K, Ward CJ, Beattie KA, M JS. Cyanobacterial toxins, exposure routes and human health. *Eur J Phycol.* 1999;34(4):405–15.
47. Shimokura GH, Savitz DA, Symanski E. Assessment of water use for estimating exposure to tap water contaminants. *Environ Health Perspect.* 1998;106(2):55.
48. Bain R, Cronk R, Wright J, Yang H, Slaymaker T, Bartram J. Fecal contamination of drinking-water in low- and middle-income countries: A systematic review and meta-analysis. *PLoS Med.* May 2014;11(5):e1001644.
49. US EPA. Private Drinking Water Wells. 2018. https://www.epa.gov/privatewells. Accessed March 12, 2019.
50. Colley DG, Bustinduy AL, Secor WE, King CH. Human schistosomiasis. *Lancet.* 2014;383(9936):2253–64.
51. Graciaa DS, Cope JR, Roberts VA, et al. Outbreaks associated with untreated recreational water—United States, 2000–2014. *MMWR Morb Mortal Wkly Rep.* Jun 29 2018;67(25):701–6.
52. Wade TJ, Calderon RL, Sams E, et al. Rapidly measured indicators of recreational water quality are predictive of swimming-associated gastrointestinal illness. *Environ Health Perspect.* Jan 2006;114(1):24–8.
53. Wade TJ, Pai N, Eisenberg JN, Colford JM, Jr. Do U.S. Environmental Protection Agency water quality guidelines for recreational waters prevent gastrointestinal illness? A systematic review and meta-analysis. *Environ Health Perspect.* Jun 2003;111(8):1102–9.
54. Gerba CP. Drinking water treatment and distribution. In: Maier RM, Pepper IL, Gerba CPMaier RM, Pepper IL, Gerba CP, eds. *Environmental Microbiology.* San Diego: Academic Press; 2000, pp. 543–56.
55. Clark CG, Bryden L, Cuff WR, et al. Use of the oxford multilocus sequence typing protocol and sequencing of the flagellin short variable region to characterize isolates from a large outbreak of waterborne Campylobacter sp. strains in Walkerton, Ontario, Canada. *J Clin Microbiol.* May 2005;43(5):2080–91.
56. Clark CG, Bryden L, Cuff WR, et al. Use of the Oxford multilocus sequence typing protocol and sequencing of the flagellin short variable region to characterize isolates from a large outbreak of waterborne Campylobacter sp. strains in Walkerton, Ontario, Canada. *J Clin Microbiol.* 2005;43(5):2080–91.
57. Richards AM, Von Dwingelo JE, Price CT, Abu Kwaik Y. Cellular microbiology and molecular ecology of Legionella–amoeba interaction. *Virulence.* 2013;4(4):307–14.
58. Hilborn ED, Covert TC, Yakrus MA, et al. Persistence of nontuberculous mycobacteria in a drinking water system after addition of filtration treatment. *Appl Environ Microbiol.* 2006;72(9):5864–9.
59. Garrison LE, Kunz JM, Cooley LA, et al. Vital signs: Deficiencies in environmental control identified in outbreaks of Legionnaires' disease—North America, 2000–2014. *Am J Transplant.* 2016;16(10):3049–58.
60. Vaerewijck MJM, Huys G, Palomino JC, Swings J, Portaels F. Mycobacteria in drinking water distribution systems: Ecology and significance for human health. *FEMS Microbiol Rev.* 2005;29(5):911–34.
61. Bharti AR, Nally JE, Ricaldi JN, et al. Leptospirosis: A zoonotic disease of global importance. *Lancet Infect Dis.* 2003;3(12):757–71.
62. Costa F, Hagan JE, Calcagno J, et al. Global morbidity and mortality of leptospirosis: A systematic review. *PLoS Negl Trop Dis.* 2015;9(9):e0003898.
63. Frawley AA, Schafer I, Galloway R, Artus A, Ratard R. Notes from the field: Postflooding Leptospirosis-Louisiana, 2016. *MMWR Morb Mortal Wkly Rep.* 2017;66(42):1158–9.
64. USGCRP. *Impacts, Risks, and Adaptation in the United States: Fourth National Climate Assessment, Volume II.* Washington, DC: U.S. GLobal Change Research Program; 2018.
65. Craun GF, Brunkard JM, Yoder JS, et al. Causes of outbreaks associated with drinking water in the United States from 1971 to 2006. *Clin Microbiol Rev.* Jul 2010;23(3):507–28.
66. Soller JA, Bartrand T, Ashbolt NJ, Ravenscroft J, Wade TJ. Estimating the primary etiologic agents in recreational freshwaters impacted by human sources of faecal contamination. *Water Res.* 2010;44(16):4736–47 doi:4710.1016/j.watres.2010.4707.4064.
67. Wade TJ, Augustine SAJ, Griffin SM, et al. Asymptomatic norovirus infection associated with swimming at a tropical beach: A prospective cohort study. *PLoS One.* 2018;13(3):e0195056.
68. Dalton HR, Bendall R, Ijaz S, Banks M. Hepatitis E: An emerging infection in developed countries. *Lancet Infect Dis.* 2008;8(11):698–709.
69. Naik S, Aggarwal R, Salunke P, Mehrotra N. A large waterborne viral hepatitis E epidemic in Kanpur, India. *Bull World Health Organ.* 1992;70(5):597.
70. Bergeisen GH, Hinds MW, Skaggs JW. A waterborne outbreak of hepatitis A in Meade County, Kentucky. *Am J Public Health.* 1985;75(2):161–4.
71. Bryan JA, Lehmann JD, Setiady IF, Hatch MH. An outbreak of hepatitis-A associated with recreational lake water. *Am J Epidemiol.* 1974;99(2):145–54.
72. Hopkins DR. Progress toward global eradication of dracunculiasis—January 2015–June 2016. *MMWR Morb Mortal Wkly Rep.* 2016;65:1112–6.
73. Goldstein ST, Juranek DD, Ravenholt O, et al. Cryptosporidiosis: An outbreak associated with drinking water despite state-of-the-art water treatment. *Ann Intern Med.* 1996;124(5):459–68.
74. Hayes EB, Matte TD, O'Brien TR, et al. Large community outbreak of cryptosporidiosis due to contamination of a filtered public water supply. *N Engl J Med.* 1989;320(21):1372–6.
75. Mac Kenzie WR, Hoxie NJ, Proctor ME, et al. A massive outbreak in Milwaukee of cryptosporidium infection transmitted through the public water supply. *N Engl J Med.* 1994;331(3):161–7.
76. US EPA. National Primary Drinking Water Regulations: Long Term 2 Enhanced Surface Water Treatment Rule; Final Rule. Environmental Protection Agency, Vol. 40 CFR Parts 9, 141, and 142. Federal Register Vol. 71, No. 3, 2006.
77. Yoder J, Eddy B, Visvesvara G, Capewell L, Beach M. The epidemiology of primary amoebic meningoencephalitis in the USA, 1962–2008. *Epidemiol Infect.* 2010;138:968–75.
78. Yoder JS, Straif-Bourgeois S, Roy SL, et al. Primary amebic meningoencephalitis deaths associated with sinus irrigation using contaminated tap water. *Clin Infect Dis.* 2012;55(9):e79–85.
79. Kemble SK, Lynfield R, DeVries AS, et al. Fatal Naegleria fowleri infection acquired in Minnesota: Possible expanded range of a deadly thermophilic organism. *Clin Infect Dis.* 2012;54(6):805–9.
80. Schwarzenbach RP, Egli T, Hofstetter TB, Von Gunten U, Wehrli B. Global water pollution and human health. *Annu Rev Environ Res.* 2010;35:109–36.
81. Villanueva CM, Kogevinas M, Cordier S, et al. Assessing exposure and health consequences of chemicals in drinking water: Current state of knowledge and research needs. *Environ Health Perspect.* Mar 2014;122(3):213–21.
82. Levallois P, Ayotte P, Louchini R, et al. Sources of nitrate exposure in residents of rural areas in Quebec, Canada. *J Expo Sci Environ Epidemiol.* 2000;10(2):188.
83. Hughes MF, Beck BD, Chen Y, Lewis AS, Thomas DJ. Arsenic exposure and toxicology: a historical perspective. *Toxicological Sciences.* 2011;123(2):305–32.
84. Chen C-J, Chuang Y-C, Lin T-M, Wu H-Y. Malignant neoplasms among residents of a blackfoot disease-endemic area in Taiwan: High-arsenic artesian well water and cancers. *Cancer Res.* 1985;45(11 Part 2):5895–9.
85. Hopenhayn-Rich C, Biggs ML, Fuchs A, et al. Bladder cancer mortality associated with arsenic in drinking water in Argentina. *Epidemiology.* 1996;7(2):117–24.
86. Smith AH, Goycolea M, Haque R, Biggs ML. Marked increase in bladder and lung cancer mortality in a region of Northern Chile due to arsenic in drinking water. *Am J Epidemio.* 1998;147(7):660–9.
87. Chen Y, Graziano JH, Parvez F, et al. Arsenic exposure from drinking water and mortality from cardiovascular disease in Bangladesh: Prospective cohort study. *BMJ.* 2011;342:d2431.
88. Navas-Acien A, Sharrett AR, Silbergeld EK, et al. Arsenic exposure and cardiovascular disease: A systematic review of the epidemiologic evidence. *Am J Epidemiol.* 2005;162(11):1037–49.
89. Tseng C-H. Cardiovascular disease in arsenic-exposed subjects living in the arseniasis-hyperendemic areas in Taiwan. *Atherosclerosis.* 2008;199(1):12–18.
90. Lai M-S, Hsueh Y-M, Chen C-J, et al. Ingested inorganic arsenic and prevalence of diabetes mellitus. *Am J Epidemiol.* 1994;139(5):484–92.
91. Navas-Acien A, Silbergeld EK, Streeter RA, Clark JM, Burke TA, Guallar E. Arsenic exposure and type 2 diabetes: A systematic review of the experimental and epidemiologic evidence. *Environ Health Perspect.* 2005;114(5):641–8.
92. McDonagh MS, Whiting PF, Wilson PM, et al. Systematic review of water fluoridation. *BMJ.* 2000;321(7265):855–9.

93. Fawell J, Bailey K, Chilton J, Dahi E, Fewtrell L, Magara Y. *Fluoride in Drinking Water*. London, UK: IWA Publishing; 2006.
94. Bellinger DC. Lead contamination in Flint—An abject failure to protect public health. *N Engl J Med*. 2016;374(12):1101–3.
95. Pirkle JL, Brody DJ, Gunter EW, et al. The decline in blood lead levels in the United States: The National Health and Nutrition Examination Surveys (NHANES). *JAMA*. 1994;272(4):284–91.
96. Levallois P, Barn P, Valcke M, Gauvin D, Kosatsky T. Public health consequences of lead in drinking water. *Curr Environ Health Rep*. 2018;5(2):255–62.
97. Hanna-Attisha M, LaChance J, Sadler RC, Champney Schnepp A. Elevated blood lead levels in children associated with the Flint drinking water crisis: A spatial analysis of risk and public health response. *Am J Public Health*. 2016;106(2):283–90.
98. Comly HH. Cyanosis in infants caused by nitrates in well water. *JAMA*. 1945;129(2):112–6.
99. Knobeloch L, Salna B, Hogan A, Postle J, Anderson H. Blue babies and nitrate-contaminated well water. *Environ Health Perspect*. 2000;108(7):675.
100. Fewtrell L. Drinking-water nitrate, methemoglobinemia, and global burden of disease: A discussion. *Environ Health Perspect*. 2004;112(14):1371–4.
101. El-Shahawi M, Hamza A, Bashammakh A, Al-Saggaf W. An overview on the accumulation, distribution, transformations, toxicity and analytical methods for the monitoring of persistent organic pollutants. *Talanta*. 2010;80(5):1587–97.
102. Brender JD, Weyer PJ. Agricultural compounds in water and birth defects. *Curr Environ Health Rep*. 2016;3(2):144–52.
103. Agency for Toxic Substances and Disease Registry (ATSDR). *Toxicological Profile for Atrazine*. Atlanta, GA: US Department of Health and Human Services, Public Health Service; 2003.
104. Institute of Medicine. *Review of VA Clinical Guidance for the Health Conditions Identified by the Camp Lejeune Legislation*. Washington, DC: National Academies Press; 2015.
105. Maslia M, Aral M, Faye R, et al. Reconstructing historical exposures to volatile organic compound-contaminated drinking water at a US military base. *Water Qual Expo Health*. 2009;1(1):49–68.
106. Agency for Toxic Substances and Disease Registry (ATSDR). *ATSDR Assessment of the Evidence for the Drinking Water Contaminants at Camp Lejeune and Specific Cancers and Other Diseases*. Atlanta, GA: Department of Health and Human Services; 2017.
107. Bove FJ, Ruckart PZ, Maslia M, Larson TC. Evaluation of mortality among marines and navy personnel exposed to contaminated drinking water at USMC base Camp Lejeune: A retrospective cohort study. *Environ Health*. 2014;13(1):10.
108. Ruckart PZ, Bove FJ, Maslia M. Evaluation of exposure to contaminated drinking water and specific birth defects and childhood cancers at Marine Corps Base Camp Lejeune, North Carolina: A case-control study. *Environ Health*. 2013;12(1):104.
109. Ruckart PZ, Bove FJ, Maslia M. Evaluation of contaminated drinking water and preterm birth, small for gestational age, and birth weight at Marine Corps Base Camp Lejeune, North Carolina: A cross-sectional study. *Environ Health*. 2014;13(1):99.
110. Department of Veteran's Affairs. Diseases Associated With Exposure to Contaminants in the Water Supply at Camp Lejeune. 38 CFR Part 3 Vol. 82 FR 4173 2017:4173–85.
111. Villanueva CM, Cordier S, Font-Ribera L, Salas LA, Levallois P. Overview of disinfection by-products and associated health effects. *Curr Environ Health Rep*. 2015;2(1):107–15.
112. Richardson SD, Plewa MJ, Wagner ED, Schoeny R, DeMarini DM. Occurrence, genotoxicity, and carcinogenicity of regulated and emerging disinfection by-products in drinking water: A review and roadmap for research. *Mutat Res*. 2007;636(1–3):178–242.
113. Cantor KP, Villanueva CM, Silverman DT, et al. Polymorphisms in GSTT1, GSTZ1, and CYP2E1, disinfection by-products, and risk of bladder cancer in Spain. *Environ Health Perspect*. 2010;118(11):1545.
114. Otten TG, Paerl HW. Health effects of toxic cyanobacteria in US drinking and recreational waters: Our current understanding and proposed direction. *Curr Environ Health Rep*. 2015;2(1):75–84.
115. Carmichael WW, Azevedo S, An JS, et al. Human fatalities from cyanobacteria: Chemical and biological evidence for cyanotoxins. *Environ Health Perspect*. 2001;109(7):663.
116. Hilborn E, Beasley V. One health and cyanobacteria in freshwater systems: Animal illnesses and deaths are sentinel events for human health risks. *Toxins*. 2015;7(4):1374–95.
117. Visciano P, Schirone M, Berti M, Milandri A, Tofalo R, Suzzi G. Marine biotoxins: Occurrence, toxicity, regulatory limits and reference methods. *Front Microbiol*. 2016;7:1051.
118. Hilborn ED, Roberts VA, Backer L, et al. Algal bloom-associated disease outbreaks among users of freshwater lakes—United States, 2009–2010. *MMWR Morb Mortal Wkly Rep*. 2014;63(1):11–5.
119. Richlen ML, Morton SL, Jamali EA, Rajan A, Anderson DM. The catastrophic 2008–2009 red tide in the Arabian Gulf region, with observations on the identification and phylogeny of the fish-killing dinoflagellate Cochlodinium polykrikoides. *Harmful Algae*. 2010;9(2):163–72.
120. USEPA. *Water Treatment Optimization for Cyanotoxins*. Office of Water; October 2016. EPA 810-B-16-007.
121. Jetoo S, Grover VI, Krantzberg G. The Toledo drinking water advisory: Suggested application of the water safety planning approach. *Sustainability*. 2015;7(8):9787–808.
122. US EPA. Drinking Water Contaminant Candidate List 4-Final. Federal Register Vol. 81, FR 81099. Washington, DC; 2016, 81099–114.
123. Agency for Toxic Substances and Disease Registry (ATSDR). *Toxicological Profile for Perfluoroalkyls*. Atlanta, GA: US Department of Health and Human Services, Public Health Service; 2018.
124. Sun M, Arevalo E, Strynar M, et al. Legacy and emerging perfluoroalkyl substances are important drinking water contaminants in the Cape Fear River Watershed of North Carolina. *Environ Sci Technol Lett*. 2016;3(12):415–9.
125. US EPA. *Technical Fact Sheet-Perfluorooctain Sulfonate (PFOS) and Perfluorooctanoic Acid (PFOA)*. Washington, DC: Office of Land and Emergency Management; November 2017.
126. Agency for Toxic Substances and Disease Registry (ATSDR). *Toxicological Profile for Perchlorate*. Atlanta, GA: Department of Health and Human Services, Public Health Service; 2008.
127. Steinmaus CM. Perchlorate in water supplies: Sources, exposures, and health effects. *Curr Environ Health Rep*. 2016;3(2):136–43.
128. World Health Organization. *Perchlorate in Drinking-Water. Background Document for Development of WHO Guidelines for Drinking-Water Quality*. Geneva, Switzerland: World Health Organization; 2016.
129. EPA U. *Technical Fact Sheet-Perchlorate*. Washington, DC: Office of Solid Waste and Emergency Response; January 2014. EPA 505-F-14-003.
130. Glassmeyer ST, Furlong ET, Kolpin DW, et al. Nationwide reconnaissance of contaminants of emerging concern in source and treated drinking waters of the United States. *Sci Total Environ*. 2017;581:909–22.
131. Wang J, Wang S. Removal of pharmaceuticals and personal care products (PPCPs) from wastewater: A review. *J Environ Manage*. 2016;182:620–40.
132. Furlong ET, Batt AL, Glassmeyer ST, et al. Nationwide reconnaissance of contaminants of emerging concern in source and treated drinking waters of the United States: Pharmaceuticals. *Sci Total Environ*. 2017;579:1629–42.
133. Benson R, Conerly OD, Sander W, et al. Human health screening and public health significance of contaminants of emerging concern detected in public water supplies. *Sci Total Environ*. 2017;579:1643–8.
134. Klaine SJ, Alvarez PJ, Batley GE, et al. Nanomaterials in the environment: Behavior, fate, bioavailability, and effects. *Environ Toxicol Chem*. 2008;27(9):1825–51.
135. US EPA. *Technical Fact Sheet—Nanomaterials*. Washington, DC: Office of Land and Emergency Management; November 2017.
136. GESAMP. *Sources, Fate and Effects of Microplastics in the Marine Environment: Part Two of A Global Assessment*. London, UK: International Maritime Organization; 2016.
137. GESAMP. *Sources, Fate and Effects of Microplastics in the Marine Environment: Part One of A Global Assessment*. London, UK: International Maritime Organization; 2016.
138. CDC. Cryptosporidiosis: Assessment of chemotherapy of males with acquired immune deficiency syndrome (AIDS). *MMWR Morb Mortal Wkly Rep*. 1982;31(44):589.
139. Casemore D. Epidemiological aspects of human cryptosporidiosis. *Epidemiol Infect*. 1990;104:1–28.
140. Isaac-Renton J, Bowie WR, King A, et al. Detection of Toxoplasma gondii oocysts in drinking water. *Appl Environ Microbiol*. 1998;64(6):2278–80.
141. Landrigan PJ, Boffetta P, Apostoli P. The reproductive toxicity and carcinogenicity of lead: A critical review. *Am J Ind Med*. 2000;38(3):231–43.
142. Agency for Toxic Substances and Disease Registry (ATSDR). *Toxicological Profile for Lead*. Atlanta, GA: US Department of Health and Human Services, Public Health Service; 2007.
143. Rogan WJ, Brady MT. Drinking water from private wells and risks to children. *Pediatrics*. 2009;123(6):e1123–37.

144. Craun GF, Brunkard JM, Yoder JS, et al. Causes of outbreaks associated with drinking water in the United States from 1971 to 2006. *Clin Microbiol Rev*. Jul 2010;23(3):507–28.

145. Hrudey SE, Hrudey EJ. Published case studies of waterborne disease outbreaks evidence of a recurrent threat. *Water Environ Res*. 2007;79(3):233–45.

146. Mac Kenzie WR, Hoxie NJ, Proctor ME, et al. A massive outbreak in Milwaukee of cryptosporidium infection transmitted through the public water supply [published erratum appears in N Engl J Med 1994 Oct 13;331(15):1035] [see comments]. *N Engl J Med*. 1994;331(3):161–7.

147. Masten SJ, Davies SH, Mcelmurry SP. Flint water crisis: What happened and why? *J Am Water Works Assoc*. 2016;108(12):22–34.

148. Agency for Toxic Substances and Disease Registry. *2017 Annual Report: Investigating Environmental Hazards to Advance Community Health*. Centers for Disease Control and Prevention; 2017.

149. World Health Organization. *Potable Reuse: Guidance for Producing Safe Drinking Water*. Geneva, Switzerland: WHO; 2017.

150. National Research Council. *Water Reuse: Potential for Expanding the Nation's Water Supply Through Reuse of Municipal Wastewater*. Washington, DC: The National Academies Press; 2012.

151. National Research Council. *Water Reuse: Potential for Expanding the Nation's Water Supply Through Reuse of Municipal Wastewater*. Washington, DC: The National Academies Press; 2012.

152. US EPA. *Community Water System Survey*. Washington, DC: Office of Water; February 2009.

153. World Health Organization. *International Scheme to Evaluate Household Water Treatment Technologies Results of Round 1*. Geneva, Switzerland: WHO; 2016.

154. Clasen T. Household water treatment and safe storage to prevent diarrheal disease in developing countries. *Curr Environ Health Rep*. 2015;2(1):69–74.

155. Kondash A, Vengosh A. Water footprint of hydraulic fracturing. *Environ Sci Technol Lett*. 2015;2(10):276–80.

156. US EPA. *Hydraulic Fracturing for Oil and Gas: Impacts from the Hydraulic Fracturing Water Cycle on Drinking Water Resources in the United States*. Washington, DC: Office of Research and Development; 2016. EPA/600/R-16/236Fa.

157. Armstrong GL, Conn LA, Pinner RW. Trends in infectious disease mortality in the United States during the 20th century. *J Am Med Assoc*. 1999;281(1):61–6.

CHAPTER 73

Metals and Health: Science and Practice

Ana Navas-Acien • Maria Tellez-Plaza

INTRODUCTION

Humans are exposed to numerous metals and metalloids (referred to as metals for simplicity) that are ubiquitous in the environment, including the media of air, water, soil, and food. Many of these metals are toxic and have no essential function (e.g., arsenic, cadmium, lead). For most toxic metals, thresholds below which no risk occurs have not been identified and their distributions in human tissues tend to be right-skewed, indicating potentially high risk for some people. Other metals are essential (e.g., iron, selenium, zinc). Essential metals are needed for cellular function and optimal health, but they can also be toxic at higher exposure levels. Dose–response relationships in the form of a U shape are common for essential metals; that is, deficiency leads to excess risk as do higher doses. In human tissues, essential metal levels are often normally distributed as different metabolic and pharmacokinetic systems are in place to maintain adequate levels in the body.

Some metals are very common on the surface of the earth and have been part of the evolution of life on Earth since early on. This is true for essential metals, with the exception of some localized geographical areas where a certain metal might be rare. For instance, in some regions of China, selenium is rare, resulting in Kashin-Beck disease (a bone and cartilage disease) and Keshan disease (a form of congestive cardiomyopathy). For some elements, despite their toxicity, evolution facilitated the development of detoxification pathways. For instance, this is the case for arsenic, for which methylation converts highly toxic inorganic arsenic to dimethylated arsenic compounds that are less toxic and readily excreted through the urine, although some highly toxic intermediate compounds are formed during detoxification.

Some of the widespread metals, however, were deep in the ground and not present on the biosphere during evolution. This is the case of lead and cadmium, which have become ubiquitous in the surface of the earth only in recent geological times, due to anthropogenic activity. Lead was one of the first metals mined and smelted from rocks during prehistory (Box 73-1). Its use became widespread in the Roman era for water pipes and tools, and then again with the industrial revolution. These pre–twentieth-century exposures, however, were small compared to the massive exposures affecting most populations in most countries with the expansion of the automobile industry and use of lead-containing gasoline in the twentieth century, and in the United States with the production and marketing of lead-based paint. Automobiles used lead-acid batteries (each one containing 15–20 pounds of lead) and wheel balancing lead weights (still in use today), contributing to enormous amounts of lead being distributed in the environment. However, it was the addition of tetraethyl lead, as a gasoline antiknock agent, which contributed to massive airborne lead exposure affecting populations globally until being removed in the last decades of the twentieth century.

Cadmium was only discovered in the nineteenth century (as an impurity of zinc ores). Mining and production of cadmium exploded in the second-half of the twentieth century with the use of cadmium in numerous consumer products (e.g., nickel-cadmium batteries, pigments in jewelry, toys and plastic, stabilizers for plastic, ceramics and glassware, protective electroplating of metal surfaces, and others). Moreover, industrially produced fertilizer is high in cadmium because of the use of phosphate rock, which is naturally rich in cadmium. Cadmium contaminated soils and fertilizers are particularly worrisome, as cadmium is similar to zinc. Plants, in particular root vegetables and green leaf plants bioconcentrate cadmium from the soil in the belief it is zinc. This is the reason why cadmium levels are so high in tobacco leaves, in tobacco cigarettes, and ultimately in smokers. The lack of opportunity for animals and plants to adapt to toxic metals such as lead and cadmium during the evolution of life, their ability to form strong bonds with proteins in the body (these metals are cations and proteins are anions), and the resemblance of these metals to essential elements such as calcium and zinc likely explain our inadequate response to the adverse molecular and cellular effects of toxic metals that were rare in the biosphere before the Anthropocene such as lead, cadmium, mercury, and others.

In this chapter, we will review metals that are important for public health because of their ubiquitous exposure and contribution to health outcomes and the burden disease. Metals share characteristics but they are also distinct from each other in exposure sources, metabolism, mechanistic pathways, and health effects (e.g., see differences in health effects for different metals in Table 73-1). For the main metals, we will discuss the sources and routes of exposure, metabolism and pharmacokinetics, exposure assessment and biomonitoring, relevant mechanisms, summarize health effects, and potential interventions, including prevention, clinical and regulatory action, and policy. We will focus primarily on toxic metals (arsenic, lead, cadmium), cover some essential metals (selenium), and then discuss the importance of metal mixtures from an exposure, analytical, and health effects perspectives.

ARSENIC

Sources of Exposure

Humans may be exposed to different forms of arsenic, including inorganic (arsenite and arsenate) and organic [arsenobetaine, arsenosugars, dimethyl arsenic (DMA)] compounds. The sources of exposure, metabolism, and toxicity of inorganic and organic arsenic compounds differ substantially. Inorganic As is a potent toxic and carcinogenic metalloid found in water, soil, food, and air.[1] Known as a poison for centuries, it was widely used in medicine before the introduction of antibiotics. It is still used today as arsenic trioxide (inorganic compound) to treat acute promyelocytic leukemia and as melarsoprol (organic compound) to treat African trypanosomiasis

BOX 73-1 Lead Exposure Affecting Human Populations through Past and Recent Times[1–3]

- Evidence of intermittent, short-term lead exposure is present in 250k-year-old tooth samples from two Neanderthal children in Payre, France, an area with lead-rich ores nearby. No lead was found in tooth samples from a 100k-year-old Neanderthal child in Belgium. Lead exposure was rare before mining developed around 10,000 years ago.
- Lead was one of the first metals mined and smelted from rocks during prehistorical times. First known uses were in beads and statues, then pigments (first evidence 5000 years ago), and as a by-product of silver mining and refining.
- Lead was extensively mined during the Roman era for use in water pipes, tanks, cisterns, roofing, construction materials, cooking utensils, cosmetics, and pigments. Written reports of the health effects of lead are at least 2000 years old. Vitruvius, an architect, wrote that it is healthier to drink water from clay pipes than lead pipes.
- In the middle-ages and following centuries, lead was used for pottery, roofing, stained glass, alchemists' experiments, and in bullets following the invention of fire-arms in China.
- During the eighteenth and nineteenth centuries, industrial uses started, including lead paint, food cans, soldering, and sealed joints in water pipes. The lead-acid battery was invented in 1859 in France. Occupational lead poisoning became a major problem and measures to protect workers from acute lead poisoning and death were slowly introduced.
- During the twentieth century, the use of lead paint in the United States and the explosion of the automobile industry worldwide (lead-acid batteries, lead wheel weights, and tetraethyl lead use in gasoline), led to a massive increase in the use of lead. The health effects of lead in the general population, in particular long-term neurotoxicity affecting children was described and contributed to the banning of tetraethyl lead in gasoline.
- Twenty-first century: lead wheel weights and acid-lead batteries are still used today. Although they are recyclable, together with e-waste they remain a problem for many populations, especially in developing countries. Lead paints in toys, herbal products, cosmetics, water pipes, tobacco products, remain a problem in many countries including the United States.
- World lead production continues, rising from around 8 million tons in 2006 to almost 12 million tons in 2018.[11] China, Australia, Peru, the United States, and Mexico were the major global producers in 2019.[11]

(sleeping sickness). While occupational exposures to inorganic arsenic were common during the nineteenth and twentieth centuries, occupational arsenic exposure is rare today as arsenic mining and production have markedly declined in the last 50 years. The main source of exposure to inorganic arsenic, globally, is contaminated groundwater which affects populations worldwide (Fig. 73-1).[2,3] It is estimated that at least 140 million people, including 2 million people in the United States, are exposed to arsenic levels above the WHO and EPA arsenic standards for drinking water of 10 μg/L. Many more millions are exposed to water arsenic levels above 5 μg/L, which is the arsenic water standard in the states of New Jersey and New Hampshire, as well as Denmark. In the Western United States, the majority of the population is exposed to water arsenic levels above 1 μg/L, which is the water standard in The Netherlands.

In populations exposed to low levels of arsenic in water, diet is the major exposure source.[4,5] Contaminated soil and water, industrial contamination, and past use of As pesticides result in arsenic entering the food chain.[5–8] Rice is a major source of inorganic arsenic (iAs) and also of DMA (from cacodylic acid, an arsenic pesticide) as these arsenic compounds accumulate in the grain (Fig. 73-2).[9–14] U.S.-grown rice is particularly high in arsenic due to the past use of arsenic pesticides for cotton production and the transformation of cotton fields into rice fields. In U.S. populations, half cup of cooked rice is estimated to be equivalent to drinking 1 L of water at 10 μg/L, although this comparison does not account well for incomplete absorption of rice arsenic vs. complete absorption for water arsenic through the gastrointestinal tract.[15] Fruit juice, especially apple, pear, and grape concentrates, can have high levels of inorganic arsenic.[5,16] Poultry was a source of inorganic arsenic and other species before the ban of arsenic-based drugs in poultry in the United States (chicken in 2013, turkey in 2015).[17–20] In China and some other countries, arsenic-based drugs are still used today.[21] Foods that contain lower levels but are consumed in high quantities such as wheat and nonrice cereals can also contribute to arsenic exposure.[5] In the United States, rice and rice products contribute to 80.4%, 64.2%, and 41.7% of dietary As (excluding seafood) for Asian Americans, non-Mexican-American Hispanics, and non-Hispanic Whites, respectively; while cereals contribute to 1.8%, 9.0%, and 25.0%.[16] Seafood is generally low in inorganic arsenic but contains high levels of arsenobetaine, arsenosugars, and arsenolipids. These organic arsenicals are generally nontoxic but their presence complicate exposure assessment for inorganic arsenic.[22–24] Air pollution can also contribute to inorganic arsenic exposure, although airborne arsenic has been less studied compared to water arsenic.[25–27]

Exposure Sciences—Water Monitoring and Biomonitoring

Arsenic is an invisible poison—odorless, tasteless, and colorless. Measurement of arsenic in drinking water is thus needed to know if a community or household is affected by exposure to unacceptable levels. For monitoring and research purposes, measuring total arsenic in water—without speciation—is sufficient as both inorganic forms present in water (arsenite and arsenate) are toxic to humans, and although arsenite is more toxic, arsenate is reduced in the body to arsenite before methylation takes place (Fig. 73-3). Measuring arsenic species in water is useful to understand arsenic transport and mitigation options. For epidemiological research, measuring total water arsenic with sensitive methods [e.g., inductively coupled plasma mass spectrometry (ICPMS)] is sufficient. Laboratory methods are expensive, require advanced capabilities, and can be slow, especially if the number of samples is large. Semiquantitative colorimetric rapid testing can be useful in populations with high arsenic levels in the water (e.g., higher > 50 μg/L), where the test has high accuracy. Advantages of these rapid methods include their low cost and the immediate feedback to the household-members, allowing for rapid interventions.[28] Test sensitivity, however, can be low in populations where water arsenic levels are low (<50 μg/L, <10 μg/L). In the absence of interventions or change in water source, groundwater arsenic levels are generally stable so that one single water sample can reflect decades of exposure. Recent efforts to model the probability of groundwater arsenic above 10 μg/L in the United States[29] and globally[3,30] can help families and governmental organizations to test wells before authorizing them for water consumption in areas at high risk of elevated water arsenic.

Human studies have assessed arsenic exposure using environmental and indirect measures (drinking water, living in a high arsenic area, airborne arsenic levels, job titles), or arsenic biomarkers (urine, toenail, hair, blood). The use of environmental or indirect measures to assess exposure can result in substantial misclassification and is limited to settings where there is only one primary source of arsenic. Arsenic is primarily eliminated through the urine in three phases ranging from a few days to around a month. Urine arsenic thus serves as an integrated measure of recent and ongoing exposure

TABLE 73-1 MAIN SOURCES OF EXPOSURE, BIOTRANSFORMATION, AND HEALTH EFFECTS OF METALS AND METALLOIDS RELEVANT FOR HUMAN EXPOSURE

	As	Cd	Hg	Mn	Pb	Se
Sources of exposure	Water Rice	Smoking Food Air	Seafood (mHg) Air (iHg)	Food Welding	Old-paint Soil Water Smoking	Food Soil
Biotransformation	Yes	No	Yes	No	No	Yes
Elimination	Urine	No	mHg Bile iHg Urine	Bile	No	Urine
Health effects						
• Cancer	+++	+++	+		+	+
• CVD	+++	+++	+	+	+++	+
• Kidney	++	+++			+++	
• Respiratory	++	+++	++			
• Metabolic	+++	+	+		+	+++
• Neurocognitive	+	+	+++	+++	+++	
• Skin lesions	+++					+++
• Low birthweight	++	++		++	+	

Abbreviations: As = arsenic; Cd = cadmium; Hg = mercury; iHg = inorganic mercury; mHg = methylmercury; Mn = manganese; Pb = lead; Se = selenium.
+++: Strong evidence available in support of a relationship.
++: Moderate evidence available.
+: Some evidence available.
Blank: no evidence available.
The level of evidence (strong, moderate, some) is assigned based on the authors' interpretation of the epidemiological and experimental literature and agency evaluations [e.g., International Agency Research on Cancer (IARC) for cancer outcomes].

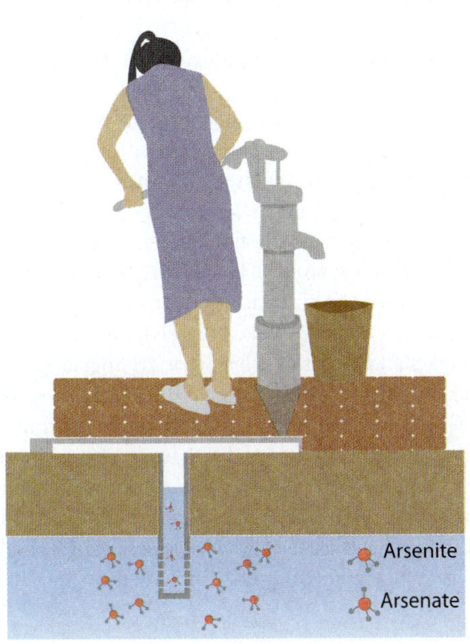

FIGURE 73-1. Inorganic arsenic species are common in groundwater globally. (*Source:* Used with Permission from Anne Bozac.)

and a marker of internal dose. Urine arsenic levels are the basis for exposure biomonitoring. Because collecting 24-hour urine samples is challenging, most research and biomonitoring studies collect spot urine samples. These samples require correction for urine dilution, either with the use of urine creatinine or specific gravity. In occupational settings, for instance, the Biological Exposure Index (BEI) for the sum of inorganic and methylated arsenic species is 35 μg/g creatinine. Several National Academy of Science reports on Arsenic in Drinking Water have concluded that urine arsenic is the biomarker of choice for epidemiologic studies.[31,32]

Many studies have used urine arsenic as a biomarker of exposure, and multiple studies have shown a good correlation between urine arsenic and arsenic in drinking water. For instance, a study of 96 people exposed to arsenic levels 8–620 μg/L in drinking water in Utah found a correlation coefficient of 0.66 between urine arsenic and arsenic in drinking water. In the same study, urine arsenic concentrations in samples collected over a 5-day period showed little short-term variation. In the Strong Heart Study (SHS), a study of American Indian adults primarily exposed to arsenic through drinking water, urine arsenic levels remained constant for a 10-year period from the late 1980s to the late 1990s, a period without regulatory policy or interventions. In the Health Effects of Arsenic Longitudinal Study (HEALS) in Bangladesh, the correlation between water and urinary arsenic in the year 2000 was also around 0.65. Water arsenic levels in Bangladesh have markedly declined in the last 20 years, resulting in a parallel decline in urinary arsenic levels in the population.

The half-life of arsenic in toenails is longer compared to that for urine. Each clipping represents several weeks of growth and is likely to reflect arsenic exposure, which occurred 3–12 months previously.[83] Toenail arsenic reflects mostly inorganic arsenic, which is bound to thiol groups as toenails grow. Arsenic in toenails can be measured using ICPMS, after digestion of the sample, or through nuclear activation analysis, which radiates but does not destroy the nails. The correlation coefficient for arsenic in toenail clippings taken 6 years apart was 0.54.[78] A limitation of toenail compared to urine arsenic is that analytical measurement error can be substantial, especially at low levels of arsenic exposure and when the toenail clippings are small. It also remains unclear how toenail growth rate affects metal levels, which factors influence toenail growth rates, including subclinical disease, and what are the best strategies to adjust for these sources of variation.

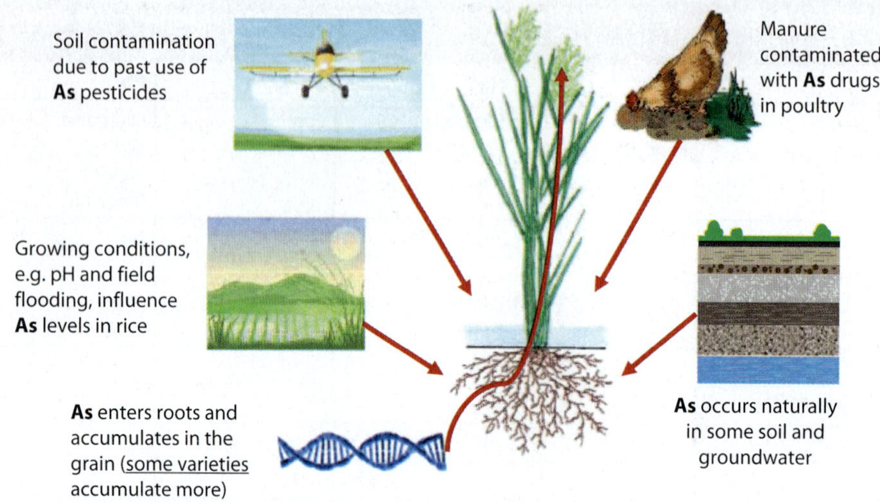
Soil contamination due to past use of As pesticides
Manure contaminated with As drugs in poultry
Growing conditions, e.g. pH and field flooding, influence As levels in rice
As enters roots and accumulates in the grain (some varieties accumulate more)
As occurs naturally in some soil and groundwater

FIGURE 73-2. Sources and reasons of arsenic (As) contamination and accumulation in rice.

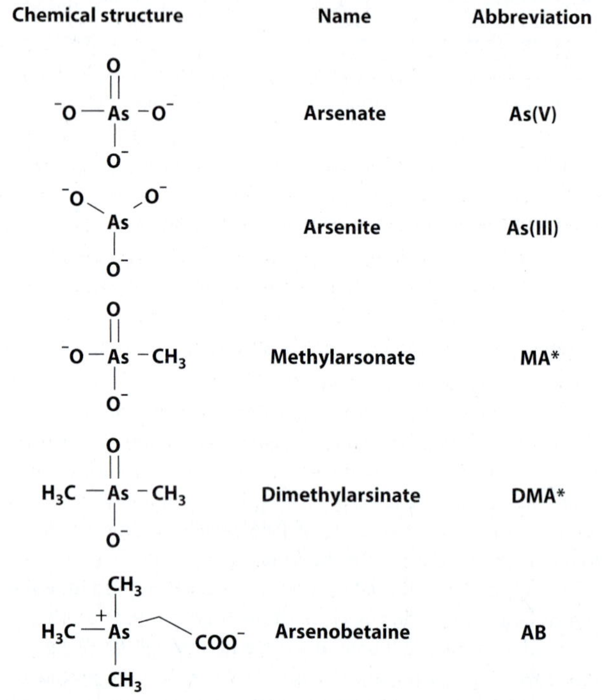

Chemical structure	Name	Abbreviation
$^-O-As(=O)(-O^-)-O^-$	Arsenate	As(V)
$^-O-As(-O^-)-O^-$	Arsenite	As(III)
$^-O-As(=O)(-O^-)-CH_3$	Methylarsonate	MA*
$H_3C-As(=O)(-O^-)-CH_3$	Dimethylarsinate	DMA*
$H_3C-As^+(CH_3)(CH_3)-CH_2-COO^-$	Arsenobetaine	AB

*MA and DMA are in +5 valence state. Methylarsonite [MA(III)] and dimethylarsinite [DMA(III)] are in +3 valence state and quickly revert to MA and DMA in urine

FIGURE 73-3. Chemical structure, name, and abbreviation of arsenic species relevant for human exposure.

Finally, an advantage of using urine arsenic compared to toenail or hair samples is the possibility to assess arsenic metabolism as reflected by arsenic species in urine samples. After exposure, inorganic arsenicals are metabolized into several compounds and cleared through urine. The main metabolic pathway of inorganic arsenic is methylation resulting in mono- (MMA) and dimethyl (DMA) arsenic compounds, which are excreted in the urine together with inorganic arsenic. Using S-adenosylmethionine (SAM) as the methyl donor, arsenic (3+) methyl transferase (AS3MT) is the main enzyme involved. Randomized clinical trials have demonstrated that supplementation with methyl donors, such as folate, increase arsenic methylation, facilitating its excretion through the urine and lowering blood arsenic levels. Heritability for the relative proportion of arsenic species in the urine is higher than 50% and Genetic variants in *AS3MT* have been related to variation in the profile of arsenic species in the urine in several genome-wide and candidate SNPs studies. There is also evidence of possible positive selection in Argentinean Indigenous communities exposed to arsenic for centuries, showing higher frequency for SNPs that are associated with a greater percentage of DMA in the urine. Overall, these data support that arsenic metabolism is genetically determined.

Measuring arsenic species in urine is particularly important in the presence of seafood intake. When seafood intake is low, the sum of inorganic arsenic species (arsenite and arsenate), MMA and DMA in urine reflects inorganic arsenic exposure (Fig. 73-4). Rice may also contain DMA in addition to inorganic arsenic, which is also excreted through urine. Seafood, including fish, shellfish, and seaweed are important sources of organic arsenicals (arsenobetaine, arsenosugars and arsenolipids); however, these species have low toxicity. Arsenobetaine (which can be simultaneously measured with inorganic arsenic, MMA and DMA), is rapidly cleared from the blood stream, excreted unchanged via the kidneys and contributes to total urine arsenic. In mouse models, iAs, MMA, and DMA, but not arsenobetaine, increased the size and number of atherosclerotic lesions. Seaweed, mollusks (e.g., scallops, mussels), and fatty fishes are rich in arsenosugars and/or arsenolipids that are metabolized to arsenic species such as DMA and dimethylated thiol As species. Therefore, in populations with moderate-high fish intake, the sum of iAs, MMA, and DMA in urine cannot be used as a biomarker of inorganic arsenic intake. To address this problem, methods such as adjusting for arsenobetaine and regressing inorganic arsenic, MMA and DMA on arsenobetaine and extracting the arsenobetaine-independent model residuals have been successfully implemented in epidemiologic studies.

Health Effects and Mechanisms

The median lethal dose of arsenic is estimated at 1–4 mg/kg. High nonlethal doses of arsenic can cause gastroenterological effects, shock, and neuritis.[42] Under chronic exposure levels (e.g., water arsenic > 10 μg/L), substantial human and experimental evidence support that arsenic adversely impacts numerous organs and systems in the body (Fig. 73-5). In 2004, the International Agency for Research on Cancer (IARC) classified inorganic arsenic in drinking water as a group 1 human carcinogen for lung, skin, kidney, and bladder cancer.[43,44] Human evidence supporting arsenic as a human carcinogen is more than 100 years old. Nonmelanoma skin cancer was the first type of cancer associated with arsenic. In 1973, the newly formed IARC concluded that arsenic was a skin carcinogen. Arsenic exposure has historically been associated with skin lesions in the palms and soles, a pathognomonic sign that has contributed to identifying outbreaks of arsenic exposure in Southwestern Taiwan, Northern Chile, Northern Argentina, and Mexico among other locations. In 2004, when the IARC classified inorganic arsenic as a lung carcinogen, the biological plausibility and coherence criteria were unclear despite the strong human evidence. At the time no animal model was capable of inducing cancer following arsenic exposure. In addition, it was unclear how a water contaminant could induce lung cancer. However, dose-response models comparing arsenic exposure through the air and water showed consistent findings and the evidence was strong even among women, most of them nonsmokers, chronically exposed to arsenic in drinking water in Taiwan and Chile. These data ultimately tilted the balance and water arsenic was classified as a lung carcinogen in 2004. The classification was further substantiated when the first animal model was published also in 2004.[33] While previous models had been unsuccessful, a transplacental model showed that inorganic arsenic exposure in pregnant mice produced a dose-dependent induction of tumors in the liver, adrenal, lung, and ovary in the offspring adults long after their arsenic exposure had ended. These scientific findings highlighted the importance of early-life vulnerability and long-lasting effects of arsenic exposure. These animal findings were further supported by human data from Northern Chile, where elevated risk of cancer mortality and lung disease following early-life exposure persisted decades after exposure had been reduced.[34–36]

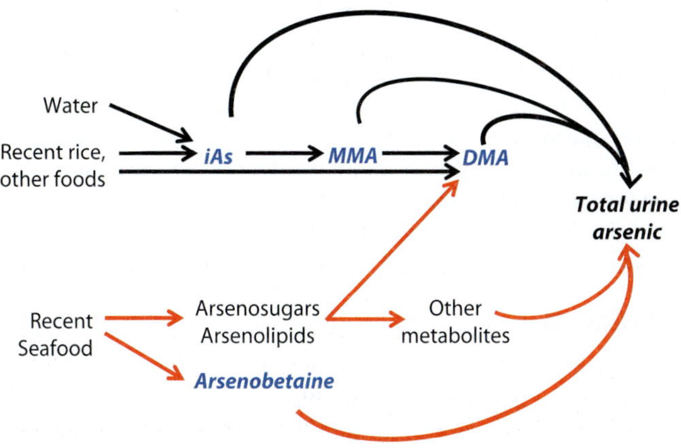

FIGURE 73-4. Arsenic exposure, metabolism, and urine biomarkers. Other sources of arsenic (occupational settings and air pollution) are not shown. Urine arsenic species commonly measured in epidemiologic studies are marked in blue. Red arrows reflect how adjusting for arsenobetaine and extracting model residuals can control the contribution of seafood arsenicals to DMA and total arsenic. (*Source:* Adapted with permission from Jones MR et al. Estimation of Inorganic Arsenic Exposure in populations with frequent seafood intake: evidence from MESA and NHANES. *AJE* 2016;184(8):590-602.)

Historical evidence indicates that arsenic plays a role in cardiovascular disease (CVD). Studies of populations in Taiwan,[37–39] Chile,[40] and Bangladesh[41,42] have consistently shown that high water As (>100 μg/L) constitutes a CVD risk factor. Occupational studies accounting for healthy worker effects[42] and experimental studies showing increased lesions covering the aortic intima among mice exposed to inorganic arsenic in drinking water (as low as 10 μg/L) compared to unexposed mice support these epidemiological findings. Cohort studies based on biomarkers in rural American Indian communities from Arizona, Oklahoma, and North and South Dakota (SHS)[11] and based on individual water As measures in White and Hispanic communities from rural Colorado [San Luis Valley Diabetes Study (SLVDS)][10] found higher risk of CVD, particularly coronary heart disease (CHD). In the SHS, the association of arsenic with incident CVD was attenuated after adjustment for hypertension and diabetes, which serve as mediators. In experimental and epidemiological studies, As at moderate to high levels has also been associated with subclinical outcomes including carotid intima media thickness,[43,44] plaque score,[45] and CVD risk factors such as hypertension,[46–48] diabetes,[49,50] and electrocardiographic abnormalities (prolonged QT interval),[51–53] although the findings are not entirely consistent.

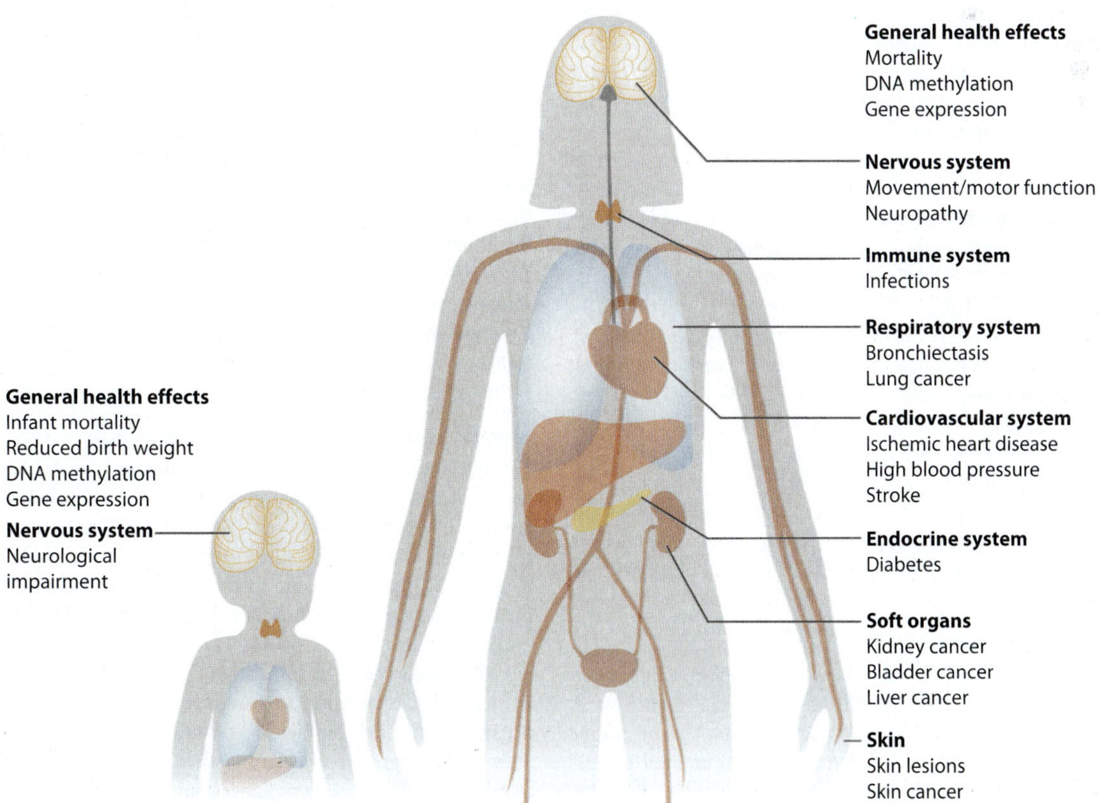

FIGURE 73-5. Health effects of arsenic exposure in children and adults. (Credit: Anne Bozack.)

Beyond cancer and cardiovascular disease, research studies in populations around the world have shown that arsenic also affects kidney function, immune function (resulting in a higher risk of infections including flu and pneumonia), respiratory diseases (restrictive lung disease patterns seem more common), and diabetes. For diabetes, the findings across studies have been inconsistent. One hypothesis, supported by animal studies and by recent epidemiological evidence is that early-life exposure rather than adult arsenic exposure contributes to metabolic reprograming and higher diabetes risk in adulthood. In children, arsenic exposure has been associated with increased reduced birth weight, infant mortality, and neurological impairment and lower IQ, appearing to affect in particular working memory[54] (Fig. 73-5).

The health effects of arsenic occur via numerous pathophysiological pathways, depending on exposure levels, genetic variants, arsenic metabolism, and nutritional status.[51,55] Elevated proinflammatory cytokines and markers of oxidative stress were detected in plasma, serum, and atherosclerotic lesions of arsenic-treated versus untreated mice.[56] In mouse models, arsenic interferes with macrophage function and induces upregulation of inflammatory signaling, enhanced oxidative stress, activation of nuclear factor-κB, and inhibition of NO availability.[57–63] Neovascularization, angiogenesis, and vessel remodeling have been shown even below the current water standard.[64–66] Relatively specific effects of arsenic exposure in animal experiments are cardiac electrophysiology changes, specifically QT prolongation, a risk factor for sudden cardiac death.[53,67,68] Prolonged QT-interval is also a common secondary effect of arsenic trioxide, a treatment for promyelocytic leukemia,[69–71] consistent with epidemiologic findings.[53] In recent years, support for the hypothesis that many of the toxic effects of arsenic may be mediated through epigenetic mechanisms, including DNA methylation (DNAm) continues to grow.[72–75] Epigenetic effects of arsenic exposure have been found in placenta and cord blood (with increased associations with pathways related to diabetes and metabolic disease) as well as in adult populations, although the specific signals have been inconsistent.[75,76]

Shape of the Dose Response

The shape of the dose response for low-moderate-high arsenic levels with cancer and noncancer health outcomes is uncertain but critical for risk assessment and regulatory purposes.[82] In the SHS, urine arsenic levels > 10 μg/g creatinine were associated with higher risk of CVD incidence and mortality.[11] Below 10 μg/g, however, the shape was inconsistent, showing a potential linear association for incident total CVD and stroke but a possible threshold for CHD. For all outcomes, the confidence intervals were consistent with multiple shapes. In a dose-response meta-analysis of prospective studies of arsenic and CVD, the pooled relative risks (95% CI) for a twofold increase in arsenic levels were 1.11 (1.05, 1.17) (number of studies $= 4$) and 1.16 (1.07, 1.26) ($n = 6$) for CHD incidence and mortality, respectively.[82] There was no evidence of nonlinearity using flexible splines, although a nonlinear dose response could not be discarded due to low power. Cardiovascular disease is probably the health outcome with more data available to assess the dose response. For cancer outcomes and for other outcomes, and even for CVD, the major limitation is the insufficient data below 10 μg/L. This gap is likely to be filled in incoming years, with new ongoing studies evaluating the health effects of low-level arsenic exposure in populations in the United States and other countries.

Public Health Implications

An update of the arsenic risks assessment by the EPA's Integrated Risk Information System (IRIS) is still ongoing, more than 8 years after the National Academy of Sciences (NAS) gathered a committee to guide the IRIS with this process.[32] A substantial amount of epidemiological and experimental evidence is available to conduct this risk assessment. Updating the risk assessment is important, as so far only cancer outcomes have been included. The 2013 NAS committee on inorganic arsenic recommended the EPA to give priority to the evaluation of CVD in addition to cancer and skin lesions.[32] Updating the risk assessment is needed for informing decisions regarding water arsenic standards, which are currently highly variable globally: the WHO and the U.S. EPA standards are both 10 μg/L while New Jersey and New Hampshire's standards are 5 μg/L (the lowest in the United States). Some of the controversies and delays with the arsenic risk assessment are related to the cost and challenges to reduce water arsenic levels below 10 μg/L, especially when the number of affected water systems is large, as in the Western United States. Regarding food arsenic, while the need to regulate As in food is agreed upon, the lack of data on health effects of dietary arsenic hinders regulation.[5,77,78] All current legislative actions for arsenic in food are nonbinding (e.g., As standards in juice and rice baby products are at different legislative stages). Efforts in Europe to regulate arsenic in food have also shown that they are very difficult to implement and enforce. From a clinical perspective, several strategies can be implemented, including the identification of individuals at risk of arsenic exposure because they use private wells for drinking, live in a community with high arsenic levels in the public water system, or rely on arsenic-rich diets (e.g., celiac disease patients, certain racial/ethnic groups).

CADMIUM

Sources of Exposure

Cadmium is a highly toxic metal widely distributed in the environment.[79,80] A by-product from mining, smelting and refining zinc, lead, and copper ores, its use has substantially increased in the last 100 years, particularly in nickel-cadmium batteries and in coatings and plastic stabilizers (Fig. 73-6). Cadmium is a widespread soil contaminant from industrial releases, fuel combustion, and the use of cadmium-containing phosphate fertilizers.[79,80] Soil contamination by cadmium is a major environmental health problem because leafy/root vegetables and grains bioconcentrate cadmium from soil, resulting in a major pathway for exposure to cadmium through diet and smoking.[81,82] Other dietary sources include shellfish and offal.[83,84] Ambient air can also contribute to cadmium exposure, particularly in urban areas and in the vicinity of industrial sources.[79,80] Asian countries are major producers of cadmium, resulting in higher cadmium concentrations in soils and foods produced from Asia and in several outbreaks of cadmium poisoning, for instance, the Itai-Itai disease outbreak in Japan and cadmium contamination in Thailand.[85,86] Belgium is also a country with historically high cadmium production and soil contamination. The Cadmibel, a study investigating the health effects of cadmium, recruited workers, and individuals living near cadmium-zinc smelters in four areas of Belgium.[87] This study found that cadmium levels in soil were related to distance to the smelters and correlated with concentrations in vegetables grown in those soils, with air and food representing major routes of exposure for the general population.[82,88,89]

Metabolism, Pharmacokinetics, and Biomonitoring

Human studies have evaluated cadmium exposure using environmental and indirect measures (airborne levels, job titles, living in contaminated areas) or biomarkers (blood, urine). Studies using indirect measures are problematic as there are multiple sources and routes for cadmium uptake in the body. Blood and urine cadmium provide integrated measures of exposure that are also informative of cumulative dose.

After absorption, cadmium binds to metallothionein forming a complex that is transferred primarily to the liver, kidney, and other organs. Cadmium's biological half-life in humans is very long (15–30 years), progressively accumulating with age in the kidney, liver, pancreas, and central nervous system.[79,80] In the kidney, the metallothionein-cadmium complex is filtered by the glomerulus and

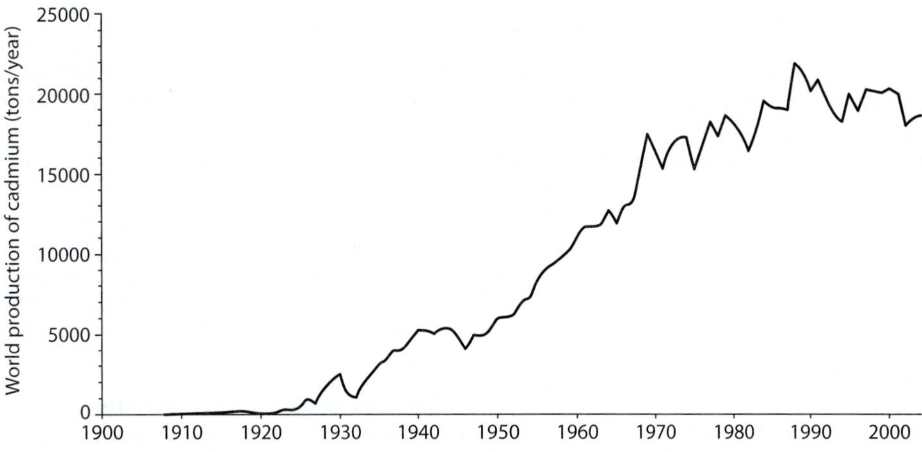

FIGURE 73-6. Cadmium production worldwide 1900–2000. The source is reference 80

then reabsorbed by the proximal tubule. The kidney cortex (tubular cells) contains more than half of the body burden of cadmium, with less than 0.01% of total body burden being excreted through urine every day.[79,90] Urine cadmium actually reflects long-term cumulative exposure and is widely used as a biomarker of lifetime exposure in biomonitoring and research studies. There are concerns, however, regarding the validity of urine as a biomarker of exposure when renal injury is present, and also with aging.[91] Urine cadmium accumulation in the renal cortex does not increase linearly with age and the increase appears to slow down at 50 years and older. Cadmium in blood is mainly found in red blood cells. The half-lives of cadmium in blood are 100 days for a fast component reflecting ongoing exposure and 7–16 years for a slow component reflecting internal body burden.[79,80] Both urine and blood cadmium are established biomarkers of cadmium internal dose.[79,80]

There are important differences in cadmium biomarker levels between men and women.[92] Women tend to have higher cadmium levels compared to men at equal levels of exposure. This sex effect is different compared to other metals, where levels tend to be higher in men because of higher exposure through occupation and lifestyles (e.g., lead, tungsten) or without clear differences in exposure levels by sex (e.g., arsenic). It is believed that higher cadmium internal dose among women at equal exposure levels than men is due to higher expression of iron transporters among women, as these transporters would also be used by cadmium.[93]

In the United States, data from NHANES between 1999 and 2016 show that the geometric mean (95% CI) of blood cadmium levels ranged from 0.41 (0.37–0.44) μg/L in 1999–2000 to 0.23 (0.22–0.25) μg/L in 2016.[94] A large fraction of the reduction in blood cadmium levels, but not all, could be explained by reductions in smoking prevalence.

Mechanisms of Toxicity

Cadmium is an established carcinogen and inhibits several DNA-repair mechanisms including base-excision and nucleotide-excision repair.[95] Cadmium is very similar to zinc in its properties and replaces zinc in key proteins and enzymes.[79,80] For instance, cadmium replaces zinc in zinc-finger structures in DNA-repair proteins. Other mechanisms relevant for cancer include conformational shifts of tumor suppressor protein p53, and down regulation of genes involved in DNA repair has been described.[95]

Cadmium can replace zinc in antioxidant enzymes that require or are enhanced by zinc such as paraoxonase 1, catalase, superoxide dismutase, and glutathione peroxidase.[79,80,96] Cadmium can deplete levels of glutathione, a major intracellular buffer for antioxidant defense, resulting in increased oxidative stress and reduce nitric oxide (NO) levels. Reduced NO levels can lead to increased oxidative damage, endothelial dysfunction, damage in the proximal tubule and atherosclerosis. Cadmium can also disrupt physiological responses to oxidative stress by competing with zinc for metallothioneins.[97,98] Metallothioneins are small cysteine-rich proteins that regulate homeostasis, storage, and transport of zinc needed for many antioxidant reactions. Metallothioneins are also effective free radical scavengers and could be even more effective than glutathione in quenching free radicals. Animal studies demonstrate that cadmium exposure, including chronic exposure at low levels, contributes to oxidative stress, inhibits antioxidant enzymes, and induces endothelial damage.[99,100]

Other potential mechanisms for cadmium toxicity include partial agonism for calcium channels, direct vasoconstrictor action, activation of the sympathetic nervous system, and endocrine disruption.[101,102] Because cadmium levels used in experimental models are generally much higher than exposures in general populations, the relevance of those mechanisms for human disease remains uncertain.

Health Effects

Cadmium is an established carcinogen for cancers of the lung and prostate, and possibly pancreatic cancer based on epidemiologic and experimental evidence.[95] Because cadmium has been described as an endocrine disruptor, and it is associated with prostate cancer, numerous studies have evaluated the potential association between cadmium and breast cancer, with inconsistent findings.[103,104]

In addition to cancer, cadmium is best known for its effects on bones, the kidney, and the vascular system.[79,80] Cadmium toxicity was discovered with Itai-itai disease, an outbreak that took place in Japan, affecting primarily menopausal women with microfractures, pain, and kidney disease.[105,106] In populations exposed to lower levels, such as the general U.S. population, cadmium has been associated with reduced grip strength and reduced walking speed in elderly populations.[107,108]

In the kidney, cadmium is known to induce tubular dysfunction. This effect of cadmium has been known for a long-time, and tubular biomarkers have been used as a sensitive marker for the health effects of cadmium by regulatory agencies. The implications of tubular dysfunction for chronic kidney disease, however, are not clear.

Regarding vascular disease, cadmium biomarkers (blood and urine) have been associated with CHD, stroke, and peripheral arterial disease. Studies from Europe, the United States, and Asia are available. In a recent meta-analysis, levels of cadmium biomarkers were associated with increased risk of clinical cardiovascular disease in a consistent manner across studies and with a monotonic dose response.[109] In analyses separated by sex, the association tends to be stronger and clearer for men, which could be related to the interpretation of the cadmium biomarkers among women.[110] The association between cadmium exposure and blood pressure endpoints has also been inconsistent.[111]

Public Health Implications

Studies in NHANES have shown that cadmium levels have declined in recent decades in the United States, in part due to declines in smoking.[94] Data from NHANES also support that the reduction in cadmium exposure in the United States has also contributed to a reduction in cardiovascular events.[112] Despite these positive changes, cadmium even at the low levels found today remains associated with adverse health outcomes in the general population and that additional interventions to reduce cadmium exposure through the diet, air pollution, and tobacco smoke are needed. Recently, it has also been proposed that intravenous chelation with edetate disodium, which is a nonspecific chelator of metal cations could also be beneficial to prevent some of the health effects of cadmium, in particular cardiovascular disease.[113] This is however, highly speculative (see more about chelation therapy for cardiovascular disease prevention in the lead section) as a large clinical trial is currently ongoing (trial to assess chelation therapy, TACT) and while chelation with edetate disodium increases cadmium in the urine in the few hours after starting the infusion (500% increase), no long-term changes in cadmium biomarkers were observed after repeated chelation, while for lead a reduction was observed with repeated chelation in a pilot study.[114]

LEAD

Sources of Exposure

Lead, together with arsenic, is probably the most studied metal. Lead remains ubiquitous in the environment in the twenty-first century despite the phase-out of leaded gasoline and lead-based paint during the 1970s–1990s (Box 73-1).[115,116] Current sources of lead exposure include old lead-containing paint, contaminated soil, tobacco products (conventional cigarettes and e-cigarettes), second-hand smoke, foods and drinks (including some baby formula), drinking water (water pipes), herbal remedies, toys, cosmetics, electronics, industrial emissions, and combustion sources. In the United States and in other countries, lead exposure disproportionately affects certain population subgroups, in particular poor urban communities and communities of color, resulting in environmental injustice.

Lead in the body is stored in bone. Bone lead levels of an average twentieth-century adult American were around 1000 times higher than those of preindustrial humans.[117] Because bone lead has a long-half life,[118] most people born before the 1990s still have a body lead burden that reflect past exposures to leaded gasoline and other sources. Internationally, lead remains a major concern in areas where e-waste recycling is common as well as in certain mining areas, such as Northern Nigeria.[119] Because of its widespread exposure and hazardous health effects (with no threshold), lead remains classified as one of the most dangerous chemicals of concern for humans by the Agency for Toxic Substances and Disease Registry (ATSDR)[120] and the World Health Organization (WHO).[121]

Metabolism and Pharmacokinetics

Following ingestion or inhalation, lead enters red blood cells, where it has a high affinity for δ-aminolevulinic acid dehydratase (ALAD), remaining there for the rest of the red cell's lifespan (average 120 days). When inhaled, lead absorption is practically 100%. Through ingestion, lead absorption depends on the type of food, metal transporters' expression in the gastrointestinal tract, and calcium body stores. Regular dairy product intake lowers lead absorption and people with high dairy product intake tend to have lower blood lead levels.[122] Because lead mimics calcium,[123,124] a large proportion of the absorbed lead is incorporated into bone tissue, where it binds to hydroxyapatite, the main bone mineral,[125] as well as to osteocalcin, a protein involved in bone mineralization.[126] In cortical bone (higher density bone, e.g., the tibia), the half-life of lead is 30 years or longer.[127,128] In trabecular bone (lower density bone, e.g., patella), the half-life of lead is about 5–10 years.[127,128] From the bone, lead is in recirculation with the blood serving as a continuous endogenous source of lead to other tissues. During periods of increased bone resorption (process through which the bone minerals are released and transferred to the blood, e.g., during menopause), lead levels in blood markedly increase. Endogenous lead exposure can thus occur for decades, many years after the main source of exposure has stopped. This persistence of lead in bone, and our inability to naturally eliminate it from the body, explains why so many individuals today are still affected by the excessive exposure to lead that occurred in the United States during the twentieth century. It also means that current exposures, for example, such as those in Flint, Michigan or Newark, New Jersey or those in urban communities still affected by lead paint and contaminated soil, could result in health effects that manifest many decades into the future.

Exposure Sciences—Biomonitoring

Lead exposure can be reliably assessed through several biomarkers of recent and long-term exposure, including whole blood, bone, and other specimens.[118] In blood, lead is predominantly bound to red blood cell proteins and whole blood has been the primary biomarker for the assessment of lead exposure for several decades.[118] Lead in blood has at least two compartments, one with a half-life of ~35 days and another with a half-life of decade(s).[118] As a consequence, blood lead reflects a combination of last month's and several years back exposures. Using repeated blood lead measures, the cumulative blood lead index (CBLI) can be calculated. The CBLI is an integrated, time-weighted average blood-lead level estimated as an area under the curve and is considered a biomarker of cumulative lead exposure. While repeated blood lead levels are considered the biomarker of choice to estimate total lead body burden, in populations with markedly lower current compared to past exposures (e.g., most adult populations in the United States today), a single blood lead can be a useful biomarker of long-term exposure.

More than 90% of the total lead burden is stored in bones. Lead turnover in bones is slow, and the half-life of lead in bones is decades, depending on the type of bone. Bone lead can be measured noninvasively using K-shell X-ray fluorescence (XRF). The measure of bone lead is taken through the surface of the skin during a period of 20 minutes or more. Although radiation levels are relatively low, radiation exposure is a concern during XRF measures. Multiple studies, especially in occupationally exposed populations but also in general populations, have shown that lead levels in the tibia, patella, and calcaneus correlate well with the CBLI, and that XRF bone lead measures could be considered a measure of cumulative lead exposure. A limitation, however, is measurement error, especially at the lower levels of bone lead that are relevant today for general populations.

Levels of lead in urine, hair, and toenails are not considered valid biomarkers of lead exposure and internal dose, as they do not generally correlate with actual exposure or with bone lead level, the generally used biomarker of internal dose. Indeed, urine is not a pathway for lead excretion. The exception is urine lead measured several hours after taking a chelating agent, either an intravenous agent such as edetate disodium (powerful but nonspecific chelator of lead and other cations), or an oral agent such as succimer (a specific lead chelator). In that situation, urine lead reflects lead that is unbound from the proteins in the body, bound to the chelating agent and eliminated through the urine (chelatable lead). It is well established that chelatable lead reflects internal dose and is an excellent biomarker of cumulative exposure. Because of the high past exposure in the United States, the level of lead in urine postchelation increases markedly. For instance, in a study of individuals from the general population without prior occupational lead exposure with coronary artery disease, lead increased by nearly 4000% after a single infusion of edetate disodium.[129]

Mechanisms of Toxicity

The lack of opportunity to adapt to lead during evolution, the ability of lead to form strong bonds with proteins, and the similarity of lead with zinc and particularly with calcium could explain the numerous adverse molecular and cellular effects of lead. Through protein binding and by replacing calcium and zinc in proteins and enzymes, lead alters important pathways for normal cell function including antioxidant defense mechanisms and internal signaling. Ultimately, dysfunction of these pathways results in clinical disease, accelerated aging, and premature mortality.

Lead increases oxidative stress through several mechanisms (Fig. 73-7). It can directly inactivate glutathione, a small peptide that serves as major buffer for antioxidant defense, through binding to thiol groups. Lead can also inactivate enzymes needed for glutathione synthesis (e.g., glutathione reductase, glutathione peroxidase, glutathione-S-transferase) and other antioxidant enzymes such as superoxide dismutase. The reduction in glutathione levels and the impairment of antioxidant enzymes reduces the ability of the cells to dispose of free radicals. These free radicals in turn increase lipid peroxidation and oxidative stress, and reduce NO levels. NO is a soluble gas synthesized by nitric oxide synthase, which has critical functions in the central nervous system and the endothelium (lining of the arteries).

Lead mimics calcium and binds to numerous proteins and enzymes that need calcium for their function, altering calcium-dependent internal signaling and interfering with cellular processes critical for normal cell functioning. Calmodulin, for instance, is a calcium-dependent protein that mediates neuronal communication, inflammation, apoptosis, and smooth muscle cell contraction and is also needed for the synthesis of NO. The binding of lead to calmodulin is one of the mechanisms explaining the neurocognitive effects of lead. By binding lead instead of calcium, the resulting impaired functioning of calmodulin could also explain the deleterious effects of lead on the cardiovascular system. Animal studies have shown that chronic lead exposures reduce NO availability, resulting in endothelial dysfunction and lead-induced hypertension in the absence of other risk factors. This reduction in NO could be mediated by improper functioning of calmodulin secondary to lead binding. It could also be due to an increase in NO degradation because of increased oxidative stress (as explained above). Impaired NO function is a major established mechanism for endothelial dysfunction, which leads to atherosclerosis and renal toxicity, and ultimately to premature death and disease.

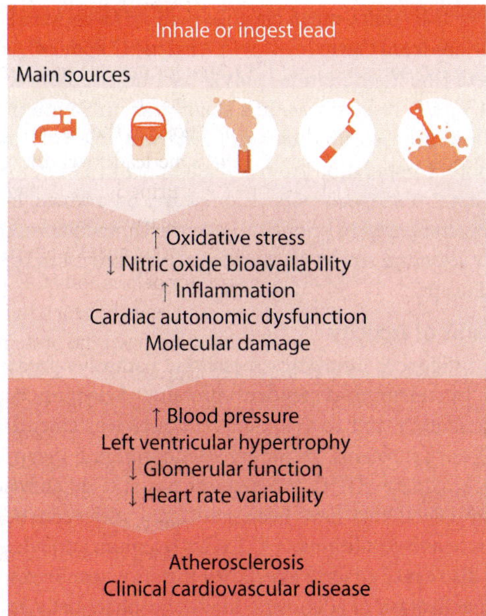

FIGURE 73-7. Lead as a risk factor for cardiovascular disease. (*Source:* Adapted with Permission from Lamas et al. *J Am Coll Cardiol.* 2016.)

Health Effects and Dose Response

Extensive research shows that even at levels considered low today (blood levels < 5 µg/dL), lead is toxic to the nervous system, cardiovascular system, kidney, immune system, red blood cells, and bones and teeth.[130–134] Lead, however, is not a clear carcinogen, distinguishing lead from arsenic and cadmium. Epidemiologic data indicate that the health effects of lead are supralinear (also called decelerating),[135] meaning that the estimated adverse health effects associated with a given increase in blood lead is greater at lower levels than at higher levels. This is well established for the effects of lead on intellectual function. In a pooled analysis of seven population-based cohort studies, the steepest declines in IQ were at blood lead levels < 10 µg/dL (3.9 IQ point decrement comparing a change in blood lead from 2.4 to 10 µg/dL), compared to 1.9 IQ decrements comparing a change in blood lead between 10 and < 20 µg/dL and 1.1 IQ decrement comparing a change in blood lead from 20 to 30 µg/dL.[133] In addition to the well-known effects of lead in impairing intellectual function early in life, increasing evidence also suggests that lead has adverse cognitive effects during aging, potentially contributing to the current dementia epidemic. Beyond cognition, other neurobehavioral effects of lead include aggressive behavior and violence, anxiety, and depression. Lead exposure during early life has been involved in violence and crime during adolescence, and declines in lead exposure have been related with declines in crime around 15–20 years later.[136]

Results of numerous studies indicate that lead is cardiotoxic.[130] The first papers documenting lead effects on the cardiovascular system were autopsy studies of workers affected by lead poisoning published in the nineteenth century.[137,138] These studies were ignored during most of the twentieth century; they were referenced again in the 1980s when the concerns about the cardiovascular effects of lead resurfaced and a number of prospective epidemiologic studies evaluated the association of lead exposure with cardiovascular disease.[139,140] In a recent meta-analysis of blood lead levels and fatal and nonfatal cardiovascular disease, which included 11 studies, the pooled relative risk comparing the highest to the lowest tertiles of lead was 1.43 (95% confidence interval 1.16, 1.76) for the 10 studies that included cardiovascular outcomes, 1.85 (1.27, 2.69) for the 8 studies that included CHD, and 1.63 (1.14, 2.34) for the 6 studies that included stroke (Fig. 73-8).[109] A formal dose-response analysis is not available for cardiovascular mortality. Data from NHANES, however, support a supralinear effect of lead on CVD risk, as the increased risks appear even stronger in populations exposed to lower lead levels

An additional body of evidence supporting the role of lead as a risk factor for cardiovascular disease comes from the TACT, a secondary prevention trial funded by the National Institutes of Health.[141] In TACT, repeated chelation with edetate disodium (EDTA), an agent that removes lead among other divalent cations from their internal body stores, led to lower risk for a composite cardiovascular outcome in people with a previous myocardial infarction as compared to repeated placebo infusions. The participants for TACT were recruited from the general population without any information on potential prior lead exposure. No data on lead biomarkers is available for this study, either at baseline or during the follow-up. All participants, however, were born before the 1980s and thus they have likely been exposed to high lead levels throughout their lifetime.

Public Health Implications

The public health and medical communities need to take an invigorated role to better protect the population from lead exposure and its health effects. It is not acceptable that so many children and adults, in the twenty-first century, remain exposed to lead levels that are above current standards, largely in part because of poor housing, old infrastructures, and insufficient public health programs and monitoring systems. Improving infrastructures and investing in communities is critical to prevent lead exposure from inadequately maintained public water systems and old housing. From the biomonitoring perspective,

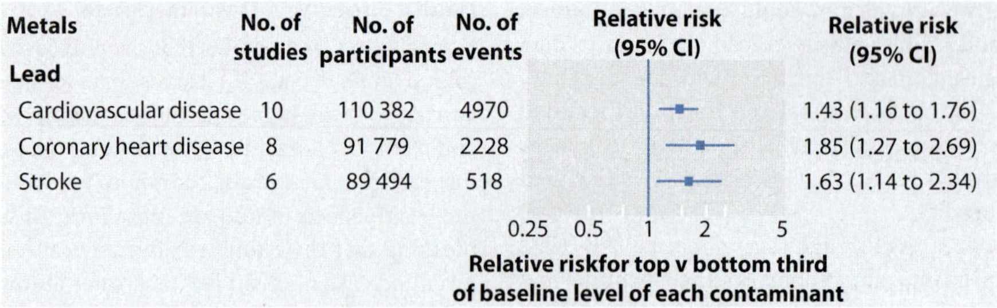

Metals	No. of studies	No. of participants	No. of events	Relative risk (95% CI)
Lead				
Cardiovascular disease	10	110 382	4970	1.43 (1.16 to 1.76)
Coronary heart disease	8	91 779	2228	1.85 (1.27 to 2.69)
Stroke	6	89 494	518	1.63 (1.14 to 2.34)

0.25 0.5 1 2 5

Relative riskfor top v bottom third of baseline level of each contaminant

FIGURE 73-8. Pooled relative risks and 95% confidence intervals (CI) for studies of blood lead levels and fatal and nonfatal clinical cardiovascular disease. (*Source:* Adapted with Permission from Chowdhury R, Ramond A, O'Keeffe LM, et al. Environmental toxic metal contaminants and risk of cardiovascular disease: systematic review and meta-analysis. BMJ (Clinical research ed). 2018;362:k3310.)

universal screening systems for children, in place in Maryland, rather than at risk programs as done in most states would be easier to implement and protect more children. Adults are currently not monitored for lead exposure. Medical organizations rarely consider the health effects of lead in adults. For instance, guidelines could indicate that when a child is diagnosed with elevated blood lead levels the whole family, including the parents should be evaluated. Workers, for instance, have been unprotected for decades as the current standard of the Occupational Safety and Health Administration remains at 40 ug/dL, when we know that the health effects in adults are present at levels well below 10 ug/dL. By focusing mostly on children, public health officials are neglecting numerous pockets of the population affected by lead exposure. Removing lead through chelation, which is approved by the Food and Drug Administration, is used rarely and generally only when blood lead levels are very high. The TACT trial, and potentially the ongoing replication trial TACT2, could further inform on the usefulness of lead chelation at the currently relevant levels of lead exposure in the U.S. population.

SELENIUM

Sources of Exposure

Selenium is an essential nutrient. It is a constituent of several selenoproteins needed for antioxidant enzyme activity, thyroid metabolism, and immune function. It is found in soil and water and enters the food chain through its incorporation into plants and aquatic organisms.[142] Food is the main source of selenium, with wide geographic variation across populations reflecting variability in soil selenium content. Foods that are generally rich in selenium, depending on soil content, include fruits, nuts, vegetables, wheat germ, fish, and meat.[143] Selenium soil levels are a major determinant of selenium intake across populations. Some parts of China have high selenium levels in soil resulting in selenosis (selenium intoxication) while other parts of China have low selenium levels resulting in selenium deficiency. Soils in the United States and the Americas in general are rich in selenium, while Europe tends to have lower selenium levels in soil. Selenium-containing supplements are another relevant source for the general population. In the United States, United Kingdom, and other Western countries, selenium supplement use has increased considerably in recent years, despite a lack of definitive evidence on the efficacy of supplementation for prevention of cancer and other chronic diseases.[144–147]

Metabolism

Selenium is a metalloid that enters the body generally through the gastrointestinal tract, most often from food and occasionally through drinking water. In food, selenium is generally found as selenomethionine, an amino acid containing selenium and incorporated into numerous proteins. In supplements, selenium generally comes as a form of selenomethionine. In water, selenium is generally found in inorganic forms, either as selenite or as selenate. After absorption, selenomethionine undergoes hepatic transsulfuration generating selenocystein and metabolically active selenium, which is incorporated into selenoproteins, including selenoprotein P, thioredoxin reductase, and other proteins.[148] In addition to this primary pathway, critical for the essential functions of selenium, a second pathway results in the production of selenosugars that are excreted in urine.[149,150] There seems to be substantial interindividual variability in selenium metabolism, although the implications for selenium function and health effects remain unclear.

The recommended dietary intake of selenium is 55 μg/day.[143,151–154] In selenium-replete populations, selenium intake above this level does not increase selenoprotein synthesis or activity, but rather increases plasma selenium concentrations as selenomethionine is incorporated nonspecifically into proteins[152] and also more selenium is excreted through the urine.

Exposure Assessment and Biomarkers

Plasma and serum selenium concentrations are well-established biomarkers of selenium levels, with a half-life of several days, and the most commonly used biomarkers to assess selenium status.[155] Other commonly used biomarkers of selenium include red blood cells, which have a half-life of around 2 months, and toenail selenium, which reflects several weeks of exposure taking place 6 months prior to sample selection. Urinary levels of selenium are not a commonly used biomarker as this pathway of selenium elimination is only relevant if selenium status is repleted.

In the United States, the median serum selenium level among participants in the Third National Health and Nutrition Examination Survey (NHANES III, 1988–94) was 124 μg/L, and most participants (99%) had serum selenium levels above ~100 μg/L, the level at which glutathione peroxidase is maximized.[152] In a nationally representative sample of British adults, mean plasma selenium levels were 86 μg/L.[156] In populations from Germany (Lipid Analytic Cologne (LIANCO)[157] and Finland (the Young Finns study),[158] serum selenium levels were 68 and 74.3 μg/L, respectively. In a small study in Southern Spain ($n = 84$),[159] the mean plasma selenium level was 76.6 μg/L, similar to that in another population from Valladolid ($n = 1445$), a Northern city in Spain.[160] European populations have, on average, lower selenium levels compared to populations in the United States, consistent with lower selenium soil levels and lower use of selenium supplementation in Europe.

Mechanisms of Toxicity

Selenium influences numerous metabolic pathways predominantly regulated by selenium-dependent proteins. Selenium acts as an anti-inflammatory and antioxidant micronutrient essential for the activity of selenoproteins, including selenoprotein P (Sepp) and glutathione peroxidase (GPx).[161] Selenium has anti-inflammatory and antioxidant effects that have been associated with reduction of risk for various health conditions.[162,163] Excess selenium and selenoprotein levels can also cause adverse effects, for instance, insulin resistance in mice by inactivation of adenosine monophosphate-activated protein kinase.[164] Selenium can also modulate the gut-barrier permeability and gut microbiota ecosystems.[165,166] Because of the dual role of selenium, as an essential but also toxic element, it is essential to study the effect of selenium intake at levels below and above selenoprotein saturation for better understanding of its role in the development of related disease.

GPx selenoproteins' activity correlates with blood selenium levels, especially in human populations with low selenium status.[167] In a population-based study,[160] the observed consistent associations of increasing plasma selenium concentrations with decreasing oxidized to reduced glutathione ratio (GSSG/GSH, a proxy for redox unbalance at the cellular level) and malondialdehyde (MDA, a proxy for oxidative stress at the lipid level) supports that selenium increases GPx-1 and 4 activity, respectively. Interestingly, the dose-response plateau for GSSG/GSH, but not for MDA, is consistent with a higher limiting point for the GPX-4 isoenzyme involved in MDA. Alternatively, 8-oxo-7,8-dihydroguanine (8-oxo-dG) is the product of DNA excision repair by multiple enzymes that have a complex regulation.[168] Plasma selenium concentrations above 110 μg/L was positively associated with 8-oxo-dG,[160] supporting that oxidative DNA damage, as measured by 8-oxo-dG, may partly mediate the associations of high selenium levels with adverse health outcomes, above selenoprotein saturation levels. Some experimental studies provide biological plausibility for a genotoxicity threshold for selenium.[169–173] Selenium excess could inhibit the expression and/or activity of enzymes involved in DNA repair (e.g., p53, BRCA1, and Gadd45),[169] which are related to cancer. In rodent models, high dietary intake of sodium selenite induced oxidative damage measured as 8-OH-dG levels in liver,[172] supporting that excessive selenium exposure may promote *in vivo* DNA oxidation. In canine models, a U-shaped dose response was observed between selenium status and prostatic DNA damage.[170]

Health Effects

Selenium can have health effects both at low and high levels of intake, often presenting with a U-shape dose response. Because of the antioxidant properties of selenium, there was interest in potential roles for dietary selenium and selenium supplements to prevent chronic diseases, including cancer and cardiovascular disease. However, the margin of safety for selenium is quite narrow, and consequently the selenium has become controversial as a strategy to prevent cancer and cardiovascular disease.[174] Plasma selenium levels above 95–120 μg/L have been associated with adverse health effects in observational studies and some clinical trials.[157,158,175–180] This finding has raised concern that high selenium concentrations may increase oxidative stress.

Meta-analyses of observational studies indicate an inverse association of selenium exposure at concentrations <100–125 μg/L with risk for several health outcomes including lung,[181,182] colorectal,[183] prostate cancers,[184] CHD,[185] and diabetes mellitus.[186] However, at higher serum selenium levels, recent observational studies from the United States, United Kingdom, Finland, and Germany reported positive associations with the prevalence of diabetes [13,52],[180,187,188] hypertension,[157,175] and dyslipemia.[158,176,189,190] In the United States, the associations between serum selenium levels and all-cancer and cancer mortality were nonlinear, with an inverse association at low selenium levels (<130 μg/L) and a modest increase in mortality at high selenium levels (>150 μg/L).[175] Data from the Nutritional Prevention of Cancer (NPC) trial support a significant protective effect of selenium supplementation on the overall incidence of prostate cancer only in participants with base line plasma selenium concentrations in the lowest two tertiles (<123.2 μg/L),[177] whereas in a recent analysis of the United States Selenium and Vitamin E Cancer Prevention Trial (SELECT), a selenium-replete study population, an increased risk of high-grade prostate cancer was observed among men who took selenium supplements for 5 years.[179] Substantial evidence also suggests that high selenium intake can increase the risk of type 2 diabetes, including evidence from cross-sectional and prospective cohort studies, some showing U-shape associations.[180,186,188,191,192] In a small randomized controlled trial in an elderly European population with low selenium status, the effect of selenium supplementation on changes in glycated hemoglobin followed a U-shaped dose-response curve.[193] Overall, while questions remain, it appears that excess selenium intake, above a relatively narrow safety margin compared to the level needed for essential functions, can increase risk for multiple diseases.

Public Health

Marketed selenium-containing supplements have become popular and easily accessible to consumers. A concern is that for populations with relatively high selenium intake through the diet (e.g., in the United States due to selenium rich soils), chronic selenium supplementation could increase the risk for several diseases due to selenium narrow safety margin. However, in some countries (e.g., the United Kingdom and parts of China), selenium intake might be relatively low and selenium supplementation might be appropriate, although additional trial data is needed. There is need to evaluate whether selenium standards for dietary and water intake, and other standards, should take into consideration the evidence pointing to the possibility that selenium-health effects are differential depending on the range of exposure levels.[194]

METAL MIXTURES

Monitoring, research, interventions, and policy generally deal with metals individually, trying to disentangle the health effects of one from another and the best strategies for exposure assessment and mitigation interventions for each metal, considered one at a time. This approach has proved useful, since, as discussed above, each metal has different properties and affects populations in different ways. In recent years, however, there is increasing awareness and interest in evaluating metals as a mixture rather than individually. Indeed, metal exposures do not occur in isolation and their health impact could depend on the presence of other metals in the mixture, including both toxic and essential metals. Intervention strategies might need to depend on what other metals are present, as removal methods might be different for one vs. multiple metals.

Advances in technology have facilitated mixture research, in particular the development of multielement analytical methods that measure metals simultaneously in the same sample (environmental or biological samples) with high specificity and sensitivity at very little additional cost for each metal added to the list of elements. The additional cost is related to the need for separate internal standards for each metal but the cost of sample collection, preparation, and processing is the same no matter the number of metals analyzed. The second factor greatly contributing to advancing metal mixtures research is the development of statistical methods for responding to different questions of interest such as identification of the toxic agent(s) in a mixture, pattern recognition, including patterns in exposure sources and tissue distribution, estimation of the overall effect of a mixture, and potential interactions among mixture members and patterns of metals. Progress in statistical methods for mixture analysis has been facilitated by an initiative from the National Institute of Environmental Health Sciences (NIEHS) called "Powering Research Innovative Methods for Mixtures in Epidemiology (PRIME)."[195] Some of the statistical methods that have been developed and used for studying metal health effects include Bayesian kernel machine regression,[196–198] principal component analysis (PCA),[199,200] exploratory factor analysis (EFA),[201,202] and weighted quantile sum (WQS),[203–205] among others.

Metal mixture analyses have been conducted both in epidemiological and in toxicological research. Examples of epidemiological studies include measuring the association of metal mixtures with intellectual function in adolescents in Bangladesh,[54,198] birthweight in a birth cohort from Belgium,[206] and CHD in adults in China[207] and Spain.[208] Examples of toxicological studies on metal mixtures include the investigation of metal mixtures and the development of hypertension[209] and cognitive deficits[210] in animal models, as well as in cell model systems.[210] While this area of research is still developing, some of the preliminary findings support that metals can be toxic to multiple organs and systems as a mixture; that individual metals can contribute more to the health effects associated with the mixture; that synergistic effects exist between metals as well as antagonistic effects (e.g., between toxic and essential metals); and that findings for metal mixtures are not necessarily generalizable across populations, possibly because the mixtures to which people are exposed differ among populations. Further improvements in analytical and statistical methods will advance research in this area, as the, as well as the application of the findings to practice and policy.

Overall, metals are a challenge to public health. Some are essential and deficiency can cause disease as may excess. Others are nonessential and toxic, particularly by mimicking essential metals. Exposures to toxic metals such as lead have been driven by economic considerations, even after hazards had been established. For naturally occurring metals, such as arsenic in groundwater, the need to drill deeper wells and to find new sources of water due to climate change and world over population, also drives exposures. Regulators have been challenged to establish safe levels of exposure for lead and arsenic, both having toxic effects at commonly experienced exposures. Remarkably, metals that were identified as posing a risk to health across the twentieth century remain as a threat to public health in the twenty-first century and the list of their adverse effects on health continues to lengthen. Health professionals, through the incorporation of environmental health knowledge into clinical and public health guidelines, and through the development of prevention and treatment interventions can contribute to the prevention of metal-related diseases.

References

1. Smith AH, Hopenhayn-Rich C, Bates MN, et al. Cancer risks from arsenic in drinking water. *Environ Health Perspect*. 1992;97:259–67.
2. Agency USEP. Fiscal year 2011 drinking water and ground water statistics. EPA 816-R-13-003. March 2013. 2013. http://water.epa.gov/scitech/datait/databases/drink/sdwisfed/howtoaccessdata.cfm. Accessed 11/18/2015, 2015.
3. Zheng Y. Global solutions to a silent poison. *Science*. 2020;368(6493):818–19.
4. Kurzius-Spencer M, Burgess JL, Harris RB, et al. Contribution of diet to aggregate arsenic exposures-an analysis across populations. *J Expo Sci Environ Epidemiol*. 2014;24(2):156–62.
5. Cubadda F, Jackson BP, Cottingham KL, Van Horne YO, Kurzius-Spencer M. Human exposure to dietary inorganic arsenic and other arsenic species: State of knowledge, gaps and uncertainties. *Sci Total Environ*. 2017;579:1228–39.
6. Nachman KE, Graham JP, Price LB, Silbergeld EK. Arsenic: A roadblock to potential animal waste management solutions. *Environ Health Perspect*. 2005;113(9):1123–4.
7. Navas-Acien A, Nachman KE. Public health responses to arsenic in rice and other foods. *JAMA Intern Med*. 2013;173(15):1395–6.
8. Yao L, Huang L, He Z, Zhou C, Lu W, Bai C. Delivery of roxarsone via chicken diet-->chicken-->chicken manure-->soil-->rice plant. *Sci Total Environ*. 2016;566-7:1152–8.
9. Meharg AA, Williams PN, Adomako E, et al. Geographical variation in total and inorganic arsenic content of polished (white) rice. *Environ Sci Technol*. 2009;43(5):1612–7.
10. Chen Y, Moore KL, Miller AJ, McGrath SP, Ma JF, Zhao F-J. The role of nodes in arsenic storage and distribution in rice. *J Exp Bot*. 2015;66(13):3717–24.
11. Carey A-M, Lombi E, Donner E, et al. A review of recent developments in the speciation and location of arsenic and selenium in rice grain. *Anal Bioanal Chem*. 2012;402(10):3275–86.
12. Robinson GR, Larkins P, Boughton CJ, Reed BW, Sibrell PL. Assessment of contamination from arsenical pesticide use on orchards in the Great Valley region, Virginia and West Virginia, USA. *J Environ Qual*. 2007;36(3):654–63.
13. Tariba B. Metals in wine—Impact on wine quality and health outcomes. *Biol Trace Elem Res*. 2011;144(1-3):143–56.
14. Hooper C, Shi X. Arsenic and lead in juice: Apple, citrus, and apple-base. *J Environ Health*. 2012;75(5):14.
15. Gilbert-Diamond D, Cottingham KL, Gruber JF, et al. Rice consumption contributes to arsenic exposure in US women. *Proc Natl Acad Sci U S A*. 2011;108(51):20656–60.
16. Xue J, Zartarian V, Wang SW, Liu SV, Georgopoulos P. Probabilistic modeling of dietary arsenic exposure and dose and evaluation with 2003–2004 NHANES data. *Environ Health Perspect*. 2010;118(3):345–50.
17. Nachman KE, Baron PA, Raber G, Francesconi KA, Navas-Acien A, Love DC. Inorganic arsenic, roxarsone and other arsenic species in chicken meat: A US-based market basket sample. *Environ Health Perspect*. 2013;121(7):818–24.
18. Nigra AE, Nachman KE, Love DC, Grau-Perez M, Navas-Acien A. Poultry consumption and arsenic exposure in the U.S. population. *Environ Health Perspect*. 2017;125:370–7.
19. Nachman KE, Love DC, Baron PA, et al. Nitarsone, inorganic arsenic, and other arsenic species in Turkey meat: Exposure and risk assessment based on a 2014 U.S. market basket sample. *Environ Health Perspect*. 2017;125(3):363–9.
20. Liu Q, Peng H, Lu X, Zuidhof MJ, Li XF, Le XC. Arsenic species in chicken breast: Temporal variations of metabolites, elimination kinetics, and residual concentrations. *Environ Health Perspect*. 2016;124(8):1174–81.
21. Zhao D, Wang J, Yin D, et al. Arsanilic acid contributes more to total arsenic than roxarsone in chicken meat from Chinese markets. *J Hazard Mater*. 2020;383:121178.
22. Taylor V, Goodale B, Raab A, et al. Human exposure to organic arsenic species from seafood. *Sci Total Environ*. 2017;580:266–82.
23. Francesconi KA, Edmonds JS. Arsenic and marine organisms. *AdvInorgChem*. 1996;44:147–89.
24. Francesconi KA, Kuehnelt D. Determination of arsenic species: A critical review of methods and applications, 2000–2003. *Analyst*. 2004;129(5):373–95.
25. Wai KM, Wu S, Li X, Jaffe DA, Perry KD. Global atmospheric transport and source-receptor relationships for arsenic. *Environ Sci Technol*. 2016;50(7):3714–20.
26. Wilson WE. The relationship between daily cardiovascular mortality and daily ambient concentrations of particulate pollutants (sulfur, arsenic, selenium, and mercury) and daily source contributions from coal power plants and smelters (individually, combined, and with interaction) in Phoenix, AZ, 1995–1998: A multipollutant approach to acute, time-series air pollution epidemiology: I. *J Air Waste Manag Assoc*. 2015;65(5):599–610.
27. Franklin M, Koutrakis P, Schwartz P. The role of particle composition on the association between PM2.5 and mortality. *Epidemiology*. 2008;19(5):680–9.
28. George CM, Zheng Y, Graziano JH, et al. Evaluation of an arsenic test kit for rapid well screening in Bangladesh. *Environ Sci Technol*. 2012;46(20):11213–9.
29. Ayotte JD, Medalie L, Qi SL, Backer LC, Nolan BT. Estimating the high-arsenic domestic-well population in the conterminous United States. *Environ Sci Technol*. 2017;51(21):12443–54.
30. Podgorski J, Berg M. Global threat of arsenic in groundwater. *Science*. 2020;368(6493):845–50.
31. National Research Council. *Arsenic in Drinking Water*. Washington, DC: National Academy Press; 1999.
32. National Research Council. Critical aspects of EPA's IRIS assessment of inorganic arsenic. In: *Interim Report*. Washington, DC: The National Academies; 2013.
33. Waalkes MP, Liu J, Ward JM, Diwan BA. Animal models for arsenic carcinogenesis: Inorganic arsenic is a transplacental carcinogen in mice. *Toxicol Appl Pharmacol*. 2004;198(3):377–84.
34. Roh T, Steinmaus C, Marshall G, Ferreccio C, Liaw J, Smith AH. Age at exposure to arsenic in water and mortality 30–40 years after exposure cessation. *Am J Epidemiol*. 2018;187(11):2297–305.
35. Steinmaus C, Ferreccio C, Acevedo J, et al. High risks of lung disease associated with early-life and moderate lifetime arsenic exposure in northern Chile. *Toxicol Appl Pharmacol*. 2016;313:10–5.
36. Smith AH, Marshall G, Roh T, Ferreccio C, Liaw J, Steinmaus C. Lung, bladder, and kidney cancer mortality 40 years after arsenic exposure reduction. *J Natl Cancer Inst*. 2018;110(3):241–9.
37. Chiou H-Y, Huang W-I, Su C-L, Chang S-F, Hsu Y-H, Chen C-J. Dose-response relationship between prevalence of cerebrovascular disease and ingested inorganic arsenic. *Stroke*. 1997;28(9):1717–23.
38. Tseng CH, Chong CK, Tseng CP, et al. Long-term arsenic exposure and ischemic heart disease in arseniasis-hyperendemic villages in Taiwan. *Toxicol Lett*. 2003;137(1–2):15–21.

39. Chen CJ, Chiou HY, Chiang MH, Lin LJ, Tai TY. Dose-response relationship between ischemic heart disease mortality and long-term arsenic exposure. *Arterioscler Thromb Vasc Biol*. 1996;16(4):504–10.

40. Yuan Y, Marshall G, Ferreccio C, et al. Acute myocardial infarction mortality in comparison with lung and bladder cancer mortality in arsenic-exposed region II of Chile from 1950 to 2000. *Am J Epidemiol*. 2007;166(12):1381–91.

41. Chen Y, Graziano JH, Parvez F, et al. Arsenic exposure from drinking water and mortality from cardiovascular disease in Bangladesh: Prospective cohort study. *BMJ*. 2011;342:d2431.

42. Sohel N, Persson LA, Rahman M, et al. Arsenic in drinking water and adult mortality: A population-based cohort study in rural Bangladesh. *Epidemiology*. 2009;20(6):824–30.

43. Osorio-Yanez C, Ayllon-Vergara JC, Aguilar-Madrid G, et al. Carotid intima-media thickness and plasma asymmetric dimethylarginine in Mexican children exposed to inorganic arsenic. *Environ Health Perspect*. 2013;121(9):1090–6.

44. Wang CH, Jeng JS, Yip PK, et al. Biological gradient between long-term arsenic exposure and carotid atherosclerosis. *Circulation*. 2002;105(15):1804–9.

45. Mateen FJ, Grau-Perez M, Pollak JS, Moon KA, Howard BV, Umans JG, Best LG, Francesconi KA, Goessler W, Crainiceanu C, Guallar E, Devereux RB, Roman MJ, Navas-Acien A. Chronic arsenic exposure and risk of carotid artery disease: The Strong Heart Study. *Environ Res*. 2017;157:127–34.

46. Abhyankar LN, Jones MR, Guallar E, Navas-Acien A. Arsenic exposure and hypertension: A systematic review. *Environ Health Perspect*. 2012;120(4):494–500.

47. Hall EM, Acevedo J, Lopez FG, et al. Hypertension among adults exposed to drinking water arsenic in Northern Chile. *Environ Res*. 2017;153:99–105.

48. Jiang J, Liu M, Parvez F, et al. Association between arsenic exposure from drinking water and longitudinal change in blood pressure among HEALS cohort participants. *Environ Health Perspect*. 2015;123(8):806–12.

49. Maull EA, Ahsan H, Edwards J, et al. Evaluation of the association between arsenic and diabetes: A National Toxicology Program workshop review. *Environ Health Perspect*. 2012;120(12):1658.

50. Kuo CC, Moon K, Thayer KA, Navas-Acien A. Environmental chemicals and type 2 diabetes: An updated systematic review of the epidemiologic evidence. *Curr Diab Rep*. 2013;13(6):831–49.

51. Wu F, Molinaro P, Chen Y. Arsenic exposure and subclinical endpoints of cardiovascular diseases. *Curr Environ Health Rep*. 2014;1(2):148–62.

52. Wang CH, Chen CL, Hsiao CK, et al. Arsenic-induced QT dispersion is associated with atherosclerotic diseases and predicts long-term cardiovascular mortality in subjects with previous exposure to arsenic: A 17-Year follow-up study. *Cardiovasc Toxicol*. 2010;10(1):17–26.

53. Mordukhovich I, Wright RO, Amarasiriwardena C, et al. Association between low-level environmental arsenic exposure and QT interval duration in a general population study. *Am J Epidemiol*. 2009;170(6):739–46.

54. Wasserman GA, Liu X, Parvez F, et al. A cross-sectional study of water arsenic exposure and intellectual function in adolescence in Araihazar, Bangladesh. *Environ Int*. 2018;118:304–13.

55. Cosselman KE, Navas-Acien A, Kaufman JD. Environmental factors in cardiovascular disease. *Nat Rev Cardiol*. 2015;12(11):627–42.

56. Srivastava S, Vladykovskaya EN, Haberzettl P, Sithu SD, D'Souza SE, States JC. Arsenic exacerbates atherosclerotic lesion formation and inflammation in ApoE-/- mice. *Toxicol Appl Pharmacol*. 2009;241(1):90–100.

57. Lemaire M, Negro Silva LF, Lemarie CA, et al. Arsenic exposure increases monocyte adhesion to the vascular endothelium, a pro-atherogenic mechanism. *PLoS One*. 2015;10(9):e0136592.

58. Lemaire M, Lemarie CA, Flores Molina M, Guilbert C, Lehoux S, Mann KK. Genetic deletion of LXRalpha prevents arsenic-enhanced atherosclerosis, but not arsenic-altered plaque composition. *Toxicol Sci*. 2014;142(2):477–88.

59. Padovani AM, Molina MF, Mann KK. Inhibition of liver x receptor/retinoid X receptor-mediated transcription contributes to the proatherogenic effects of arsenic in macrophages in vitro. *Arterioscler Thromb Vasc Biol*. 2010;30(6):1228–36.

60. Barchowsky A, Klei LR, Dudek EJ, Swartz HM, James PE. Stimulation of reactive oxygen, but not reactive nitrogen species, in vascular endothelial cells exposed to low levels of arsenite. *Free Radic Biol Med*. 1999;27(11–12):1405–12.

61. Barchowsky A, Dudek EJ, Treadwell MD, Wetterhahn KE. Arsenic induces oxidant stress and NF-kappa B activation in cultured aortic endothelial cells. *Free Radic Biol Med*. 1996;21(6):783–90.

62. Zhang C, Ferrari R, Beezhold K, et al. Arsenic promotes NF-kappab-mediated fibroblast dysfunction and matrix remodeling to impair muscle stem cell function. *Stem Cells*. 2016;34(3):732–42.

63. Wang L, Kou MC, Weng CY, Hu LW, Wang YJ, Wu MJ. Arsenic modulates heme oxygenase-1, interleukin-6, and vascular endothelial growth factor expression in endothelial cells: roles of ROS, NF-kappaB, and MAPK pathways. *Arch Toxicol*. 2012;86(6):879–96.

64. Soucy NV, Klei LR, Mayka DD, Barchowsky A. Signaling pathways for arsenic-stimulated vascular endothelial growth factor-a expression in primary vascular smooth muscle cells. *Chem Res Toxicol*. 2004;17(4):555–63.

65. Soucy NV, Mayka D, Klei LR, Nemec AA, Bauer JA, Barchowsky A. Neovascularization and angiogenic gene expression following chronic arsenic exposure in mice. *Cardiovasc Toxicol*. 2005;5(1):29–42.

66. States JC, Srivastava S, Chen Y, Barchowsky A. Arsenic and cardiovascular disease. *Toxicol Sci*. 2009;107(2):312–23.

67. Chen Y, Wu F, Parvez F, et al. Arsenic exposure from drinking water and QT-interval prolongation: Results from the health effects of arsenic longitudinal study. *Environ Health Perspect*. 2013;121(4):427–32.

68. Mumford JL, Wu KG, Xia YJ, et al. Chronic arsenic exposure and cardiac repolarization abnormalities with QT interval prolongation in a population-based study. *Environ Health Perspect*. 2007;115(5):690–4.

69. Siu C-W, Au W-Y, Yung C, et al. Effects of oral arsenic trioxide therapy on QT intervals in patients with acute promyelocytic leukemia: Implications for long-term cardiac safety. *Blood*. 2006;108(1):103–6.

70. Barbey JT, Pezzullo JC, Soignet SL. Effect of arsenic trioxide on QT interval in patients with advanced malignancies. *J Clin Oncol*. 2003;21(19):3609–15.

71. Ohnishi K, Yoshida H, Shigeno K, et al. Prolongation of the QT interval and ventricular tachycardia in patients treated with arsenic trioxide for acute promyelocytic leukemia. *Ann Intern Med*. 2000;133(11):881–5.

72. Koestler DC, Avissar-Whiting M, Houseman EA, Karagas MR, Marsit CJ. Differential DNA methylation in umbilical cord blood of infants exposed to low levels of arsenic in utero. *Environ Health Perspect*. 2013;121(8):971–7.

73. Reichard JF, Schnekenburger M, Puga A. Long term low-dose arsenic exposure induces loss of DNA methylation. *Biochem Biophys Res Commun*. 2007;352(1):188-92.

74. Bailey KA, Fry RC. Arsenic-associated changes to the epigenome: What are the functional consequences? *Curr Environ Health Rep*. 2014;1:22–34.

75. Argos M. Arsenic exposure and epigenetic alterations: Recent findings based on the illumina 450K DNA methylation array. *Curr Environ Health Rep*. 2015;2(2):137–44.

76. Bozack AK, Domingo-Relloso A, Haack K, et al. Locus-specific differential DNA methylation and urinary arsenic: An epigenome-wide association study in blood among adults with low-to-moderate arsenic exposure. *Environ Health Perspect*. 2020;128(6):67015.

77. Nachman KE, Ginsberg GL, Miller MD, Murray CJ, Nigra AE, Pendergrast CB. Mitigating dietary arsenic exposure: Current status in the United States and recommendations for an improved path forward. *Sci Total Environ*. 2017;581–2:221–36.

78. U.S. Food and Drug Administration. *Arsenic in Rice and Rice Products. Risk Assessment Report*. Center for Food Safety and Applied Nutrition, Food and Drug Administration, U.S. Department of Health and Human Services. March 2016.

79. Nordberg GF, Nogawa K, Nordberg M, Friberg LT. Cadmium. In: Nordberg GF, Fowler BA, Nordberg M, Friberg LT, eds.Nordberg GF, Fowler BA, Nordberg M, Friberg LT, eds. *Handbook on the Toxicology of Netals*. Vol. 3rd. Amsterdam: Elsevier; 2007, pp. 446–86.

80. U.S. Department of Health and Human Services. *Toxicological Profile for Cadmium*. Atlanta, GA: US Department of Health and Human Services; Public Health Service; 1999.

81. Lalor GC. Review of cadmium transfers from soil to humans and its health effects in the Jamaican environment. *Sci Total Environ*. 2008;400(1–3):162–72.

82. Staessen JA, Vyncke G, Lauwerys RR, et al. Transfer of cadmium from a sandy acidic soil to man: A population study. *Environ Res*. 1992;58(1):25–34.

83. Olmedo P, Grau-Perez M, Fretts A, et al. Dietary determinants of cadmium exposure in the strong heart family study. *Food Chem Toxicol*. 2017;100:239–46.

84. Choudhury H, Harvey T, Thayer WC, et al. Urinary cadmium elimination as a biomarker of exposure for evaluating a cadmium dietary exposure-biokinetics model. *J Toxicol Environ Health A*. 2001;63(5):321–50.

85. Satarug S, Swaddiwudhipong W, Ruangyuttikarn W, Nishijo M, Ruiz P. Modeling cadmium exposures in low- and high-exposure areas in Thailand. *Environ Health Perspect*. 2013;121(5):531–6.

86. Tsuchiya K. Causation of Ouch-Ouch disease (Itai-Itai Byo)—An introductory review. II. Epidemiology and evaluation. *Keio J Med.* 1969;18(4):195–211.

87. Lauwerys R, Bernard A, Buchet JP, et al. Does environmental exposure to cadmium represent a health risk? Conclusions from the Cadmibel study. *Acta ClinBelg.* 1991;46(4):219–25.

88. Hogervorst J, Plusquin M, Vangronsveld J, et al. House dust as possible route of environmental exposure to cadmium and lead in the adult general population. *Environ Res.* 2007;103(1):30–7.

89. Staessen JA, Buchet JP, Ginucchio G, et al. Public health implications of environmental exposure to cadmium and lead: An overview of epidemiological studies in Belgium. Working Groups. *J Cardiovasc Risk.* 1996;3(1):26–41.

90. Jarup L, Berglund M, Elinder CG, Nordberg G, Vahter M. Health effects of cadmium exposure—A review of the literature and a risk estimate. *Scand J Work Environ Health.* 1998;24 Suppl 1:1–51.

91. Vacchi-Suzzi C, Porucznik CA, Cox KJ, et al. Temporal variability of urinary cadmium in spot urine samples and first morning voids. *J Expo Sci Environ Epidemiol.* 2017;27(3):306–12.

92. Ali I, Engstrom A, Vahter M, et al. Associations between cadmium exposure and circulating levels of sex hormones in postmenopausal women. *Environ Res.* 2014;134:265–9.

93. Rentschler G, Kippler M, Axmon A, et al. Polymorphisms in iron homeostasis genes and urinary cadmium concentrations among nonsmoking women in Argentina and Bangladesh. *Environ Health Perspect.* 2013;121(4):467–72.

94. Tellez-Plaza M, Navas-Acien A, Caldwell KL, Menke A, Muntner P, Guallar E. Reduction in cadmium exposure in the United States population, 1988–2008: The contribution of declining smoking rates. *Environ Health Perspect.* 2012;120(2):204–9.

95. International Agency for Research on Cancer. Cadmium and Cadmium Compounds. https://monographs.iarc.fr/wp-content/uploads/2018/06/mono100C-8.pdf. 2018.

96. Nigam D, Shukla GS, Agarwal AK. Glutathione depletion and oxidative damage in mitochondria following exposure to cadmium in rat liver and kidney. *Toxicol Lett.* 1999;106(2–3):151–7.

97. Sone T, Koizumi S, Kimura M. Cadmium-induced synthesis of metallothioneins in human lymphocytes and monocytes. *Chem Biol Interact.* 1988;66(1–2):61–70.

98. Jin TY, Lu J, Nordberg M. Toxicokinetics and biochemistry of cadmium with special emphasis on the role of metallothionein. *Neurotoxicology.* 1998;19(4–5):529–35.

99. Almenara CC, Broseghini-Filho GB, Vescovi MV, et al. Chronic cadmium treatment promotes oxidative stress and endothelial damage in isolated rat aorta. *PLoS One.* 2013;8(7):e68418.

100. Domingo-Relloso A, Grau-Perez M, Galan-Chilet I, et al. Urinary metals and metal mixtures and oxidative stress biomarkers in an adult population from Spain: The Hortega study. *Environ Int.* 2019;123:171–80.

101. Sabir S, Akash MSH, Fiayyaz F, Saleem U, Mehmood MH, Rehman K. Role of cadmium and arsenic as endocrine disruptors in the metabolism of carbohydrates: Inserting the association into perspectives. *Biomed Pharmacother.* 2019;114:108802.

102. Roels HA, Lauwerys RR, Buchet JP, Bernard AM, Vos A, Oversteyns M. Health significance of cadmium induced renal dysfunction: a five year follow up. *BrJ IndMed.* 1989;46(11):755–64.

103. Liu R, Nelson DO, Hurley S, Hertz A, Reynolds P. Residential exposure to estrogen disrupting hazardous air pollutants and breast cancer risk: The California teachers study. *Epidemiology.* 2015;26(3):365–73.

104. Adams SV, Shafer MM, Bonner MR, et al. Urinary cadmium and risk of invasive breast cancer in the women's health initiative. *Am J Epidemiol.* 2016;183(9):815–23.

105. "Itai-itai byo" and other views on cadmium. *Food Cosmet Toxicol.* 1972;10(2):249–55.

106. Yasuda M, Miwa A, Kitagawa M. Morphometric studies of renal lesions in itai-itai disease—Chronic cadmium nephropathy. *Nephron.* 1995;69(1):14–9.

107. Garcia-Esquinas E, Carrasco-Rios M, Navas-Acien A, Ortola R, Rodriguez-Artalejo F. Cadmium exposure is associated with reduced grip strength in US adults. *Environ Res.* 2020;180:108819.

108. Kim J, Garcia-Esquinas E, Navas-Acien A, Choi YH. Blood and urine cadmium concentrations and walking speed in middle-aged and older U.S. adults. *Environ Pollut.* 2018;232:97–104.

109. Chowdhury R, Ramond A, O'Keeffe LM, et al. Environmental toxic metal contaminants and risk of cardiovascular disease: Systematic review and meta-analysis. *BMJ.* 2018;362:k3310.

110. Tellez-Plaza M, Jones MR, Dominguez-Lucas A, Guallar E, Navas-Acien A. Cadmium exposure and clinical cardiovascular disease: A systematic review. *Curr Atheroscler Rep.* 2013;15(10):356.

111. Tellez-Plaza M, Navas-Acien A, Crainiceanu CM, Guallar E. Cadmium exposure and hypertension in the 1999–2004 National Health and Nutrition Examination Survey (NHANES). *Environ Health Perspect.* 2008;116(1):51–6.

112. Ruiz-Hernandez A, Navas-Acien A, Pastor-Barriuso R, et al. Declining exposures to lead and cadmium contribute to explaining the reduction of cardiovascular mortality in the US population, 1988–2004. *Int J Epidemiol.* 2017;46(6):1903–12.

113. Ujueta F, Arenas IA, Diaz D, et al. Cadmium level and severity of peripheral artery disease in patients with coronary artery disease. *Eur J Prev Cardiol.* 2019;26(13):1456–8.

114. Alam ZH, Ujueta F, Arenas IA, Nigra AE, Navas-Acien A, Lamas GA. Urinary metal levels after repeated edetate disodium infusions: Preliminary findings. *Int J Environ Res Public Health.* 2020;17(13):4684.

115. Golding E. *A History of Technology and Environment: From Stone Tools to Ecological Crisis.* London and New York: Taylor and Francis; 2017.

116. Hanna-Attisha M, Lanphear B, Landrigan P. Lead poisoning in the 21st century: The silent epidemic continues. *Am J Public Health.* 2018;108(11):1430.

117. Patterson C, Ericson J, Manea-Krichten M, Shirahata H. Natural skeletal levels of lead in Homo sapiens sapiens uncontaminated by technological lead. *Sci Total Environ.* 1991;107:205–36.

118. Skerfving S, Bergdahl IA. CHAPTER 31—Lead. In: Nordberg GF, Fowler BA, Nordberg M, Friberg LT, eds.Nordberg GF, Fowler BA, Nordberg M, Friberg LT, eds. *Handbook on the Toxicology of Metals.* 3rd ed. Burlington: Academic Press; 2007, pp. 599–643.

119. CDC. Lead Poisoning Investigation in Northern Nigeria. *Centers for Disease Control and Prevention, National Center for Emerging and Zoonotic Infectious Diseases (NCEZID).* https://www.cdc.gov/onehealth/in-action/lead-poisoning.html#:~:text=Investigations%20of%20other%20villages%20in,of%20lead%20poisoning%20in%20history.

120. Agency for Toxic Substances and Disease Registry. ATSDR's Substance Priority List. 2019. https://www.atsdr.cdc.gov/spl/index.html.

121. WHO. World Health Organization. 2020.https://www.who.int/ipcs/assessment/public_health/chemicals_phc/en/.

122. de Almeida Lopes AC, Navas-Acien A, Zamoiski R, et al. Risk factors for lead exposure in adult population in southern Brazil. *J Toxicol Environ Health A.* 2015;78(2):92–108.

123. de Souza ID, de Andrade AS, Dalmolin RJS. Lead-interacting proteins and their implication in lead poisoning. *Crit Rev Toxicol.* 2018;48(5):375–86.

124. Kasten-Jolly J, Lawrence DA. The cationic (calcium and lead) and enzyme conundrum. *J Toxicol Environ Health B Crit Rev.* 2018;21(6–8):400–13.

125. Dowd TL, Rosen JF, Mints L, Gundberg CM. The effect of Pb(2+) on the structure and hydroxyapatite binding properties of osteocalcin. *Biochim Biophys Acta.* 2001;1535(2):153–63.

126. Dowd TL, Rosen JF, Gundberg CM, Gupta RK. The displacement of calcium from osteocalcin at submicromolar concentrations of free lead. *Biochim Biophys Acta.* 1994;1226(2):131–7.

127. Barbosa F, Jr., Tanus-Santos JE, Gerlach RF, Parsons PJ. A critical review of biomarkers used for monitoring human exposure to lead: Advantages, limitations, and future needs. *Environ Health Perspect.* 2005;113(12):1669–74.

128. Hu H, Shih R, Rothenberg S, Schwartz BS. The epidemiology of lead toxicity in adults: Measuring dose and consideration of other methodologic issues. *Environ Health Perspect.* 2007;115(3):455–62.

129. Arenas IA, Navas-Acien A, Ergui I, Lamas GA. Enhanced vasculotoxic metal excretion in post-myocardial infarction patients following a single edetate disodium-based infusion. *Environ Res.* 2017;158:443–9.

130. Navas-Acien A, Guallar E, Silbergeld EK, Rothenberg SJ. Lead exposure and cardiovascular disease—A systematic review. *Environ Health Perspect.* 2007;115(3):472–82.

131. NTP monograph on health effects of low-level lead. *NTP monogr.* 2012;(1):xiii, xv-148.

132. Dietert RR, Piepenbrink MS. Lead and immune function. *Crit Rev Toxicol.* 2006;36(4):359–85.

133. Lanphear BP, Hornung R, Khoury J, et al. Low-level environmental lead exposure and children's intellectual function: An international pooled analysis. *Environ Health Perspect.* 2005;113(7):894–9.

134. Moody EC, Coca SG, Sanders AP. Toxic metals and chronic kidney disease: A systematic review of recent literature. *Curr Environ Health Rep.* 2018;5(4):453–63.

135. Lanphear BP. Low-level toxicity of chemicals: No acceptable levels? *PLoS Biol.* 2017;15(12):e2003066.

136. Nevin R. Understanding international crime trends: The legacy of preschool lead exposure. *Environ Res.* 2007;104(3):315–36.

137. Lancéraux E. Nephrite et arthrite saturnine; coincidences de ces affections; parallèle ave la néphrite et l'arthrite goutteuses. *Transact Int Med Congr.* 1881;2:93–202.

138. Lorimer G. Saturnine gout, and its distinguishing marks. *Br Med J.* 1886;2(1334):163.

139. Pocock SJ, Shaper AG, Ashby D, Delves HT, Clayton BE. The relationship between blood lead, blood pressure, stroke, and heart attacks in middle-aged British men. *Environ Health Perspect.* 1988;78:23–30.

140. Kromhout D. Blood lead and coronary heart disease risk among elderly men in Zutphen, The Netherlands. *Environ Health Perspect.* 1988;78:43–6.

141. Lamas GA, Goertz C, Boineau R, et al. Effect of disodium EDTA chelation regimen on cardiovascular events in patients with previous myocardial infarction: The TACT randomized trial. *JAMA.* 2013;309(12):1241–50.

142. Weeks BS, Hanna MS, Cooperstein D. Dietary selenium and selenoprotein function. *Med Sci Monit.* 2012;18(8):RA127–32.

143. Rayman MP. Food-chain selenium and human health: Emphasis on intake. *Br J Nutr.* 2008;100(2):254–68.

144. Millen AE, Dodd KW, Subar AF. Use of vitamin, mineral, nonvitamin, and nonmineral supplements in the United States: The 1987, 1992, and 2000 National Health Interview Survey results. *J Am Dietetic Association.* 2004;104(6):942–50.

145. Rayman MP. Dietary selenium: Time to act. *BMJ.* 1997;314(7078):387–8.

146. Spina A, Guallar E, Rayman MP, Tigbe W, Kandala NB, Stranges S. Anthropometric indices and selenium status in British adults: The U.K. National Diet and Nutrition Survey. *Free Radic Biol Med.* 2013;65:1315–21.

147. Stranges S, Marshall JR, Natarajan R, et al. Effects of long-term selenium supplementation on the incidence of type 2 diabetes: A randomized trial. *Ann Intern Med.* 2007;147(4):217–23.

148. Burk RF, Norsworthy BK, Hill KE, Motley AK, Byrne DW. Effects of chemical form of selenium on plasma biomarkers in a high-dose human supplementation trial. *Cancer Epidemiol Biomarkers Prev.* 2006;15(4):804–10.

149. Kobayashi Y, Ogra Y, Ishiwata K, Takayama H, Aimi N, Suzuki KT. Selenosugars are key and urinary metabolites for selenium excretion within the required to low-toxic range. *Proc Natl Acad Sci U S A.* 2002;99(25):15932–6.

150. Kuehnelt D, Juresa D, Francesconi KA, Fakih M, Reid ME. Selenium metabolites in urine of cancer patients receiving L-selenomethionine at high doses. *Toxicol Appl Pharmacol.* 2007;220(2):211–5.

151. Burk RF. Selenium, an antioxidant nutrient. *Nutr Clin Care.* 2002; 5(2):75–9.

152. Monsen ER. Dietary reference intakes for the antioxidant nutrients: Vitamin C, vitamin E, selenium, and carotenoids. *J Am Diet Assoc.* 2000;100(6):637–40.

153. Papp LV, Lu J, Holmgren A, Khanna KK. From selenium to selenoproteins: Synthesis, identity, and their role in human health. *Antioxid Redox Signal.* 2007;9(7):775–806.

154. Rayman MP. The importance of selenium to human health. *Lancet.* 2000;356(9225):233–41.

155. Hogberg J, Alexander J. CHAPTER 38—Selenium. In: Nordberg GF, Fowler BA, Nordberg M, Friberg LT, eds.Nordberg GF, Fowler BA, Nordberg M, Friberg LT, eds. *Handbook on the Toxicology of Metals*, 3rd ed. Burlington: Academic Press; 2007, pp. 783–807.

156. Stranges S, Laclaustra M, Ji C, et al. Higher selenium status is associated with adverse blood lipid profile in British adults. *J Nutr.* 2010;140(1):81–7.

157. Berthold HK, Michalke B, Krone W, Guallar E, Gouni-Berthold I. Influence of serum selenium concentrations on hypertension: The lipid analytic cologne cross-sectional study. *J Hypertens.* 2012;30(7):1328–35.

158. Stranges S, Tabák AG, Guallar E, et al. Selenium status and blood lipids: The cardiovascular risk in Young Finns study. *J Intern Med.* 2011;270(5):469–77.

159. Millán Adame E, Florea D, Sáez Pérez L, et al. Deficient selenium status of a healthy adult Spanish population. *Nutr Hosp.* 2012;27(2):524–8.

160. Galan-Chilet I, Tellez-Plaza M, Guallar E, et al. Plasma selenium levels and oxidative stress biomarkers: A gene-environment interaction population-based study. *Free Radic Biol Med.* 2014;74:229–36.

161. Cominetti C, de Bortoli MC, Purgatto E, et al. Associations between glutathione peroxidase-1 Pro198Leu polymorphism, selenium status, and DNA damage levels in obese women after consumption of Brazil nuts. *Nutrition.* 2011;27(9):891–6.

162. Barakat G, Moustafa ME, Khalifeh I, Hodroj MH, Bikhazi A, Rizk S. Effects of exendin-4 and selenium on the expression of GLP-1R, IRS-1, and preproinsulin in the pancreas of diabetic rats. *J Physiol Biochem.* 2016;73(3):387–94.

163. Zou C, Qiu Q, Chen H, Dou L, Liang J. Hepatoprotective effects of selenium during diabetes in rats. *Hum Exp Toxicol.* 2016;35(2):114–23.

164. Chadani H, Usui S, Inoue O, et al. Endogenous selenoprotein P, a liver-derived secretory protein, mediates myocardial ischemia/reperfusion injury in mice. *Int J Mol Sci.* 2018;19(3):878.

165. Cani PD, Osto M, Geurts L, Everard A. Involvement of gut microbiota in the development of low-grade inflammation and type 2 diabetes associated with obesity. *Gut Microbes.* 2012;3(4):279–88.

166. Zhai Q, Xiao Y, Li P, et al. Varied doses and chemical forms of selenium supplementation differentially affect mouse intestinal physiology. *Food Funct.* 2019;10(9):5398–412.

167. Whanger PD, Beilstein MA, Thomson CD, Robinson MF, Howe M. Blood selenium and glutathione peroxidase activity of populations in New Zealand, Oregon, and South Dakota. *FASEB J.* 1988;2(14):2996–3002.

168. Il'yasova D, Scarbrough P, Spasojevic I. Urinary biomarkers of oxidative status. *Clin Chim Acta.* 2012;413(19–20):1446–53.

169. Bera S, De Rosa V, Rachidi W, Diamond AM. Does a role for selenium in DNA damage repair explain apparent controversies in its use in chemoprevention? *Mutagenesis.* 2013;28(2):127–34.

170. Chiang EC, Shen S, Kengeri SS, et al. Defining the optimal selenium dose for prostate cancer risk reduction: Insights from the U-shaped relationship between selenium status, DNA damage, and apoptosis. *Dose Response.* 2009;8(3):285–300.

171. Waters DJ, Shen S, Glickman LT, et al. Prostate cancer risk and DNA damage: Translational significance of selenium supplementation in a canine model. *Carcinogenesis.* 2005;26(7):1256–62.

172. Wycherly BJ, Moak MA, Christensen MJ. High dietary intake of sodium selenite induces oxidative DNA damage in rat liver. *Nutr Cancer.* 2004;48(1):78–83.

173. Zhang Q, Chen L, Guo K, et al. Effects of different selenium levels on gene expression of a subset of selenoproteins and antioxidative capacity in mice. *Biol Trace Elem Res.* 2013;154(2):255–61.

174. Vinceti M, Filippini T, Wise LA. Environmental selenium and human health: An update. *Curr Environ Health Rep.* 2018;5(4):464–85.

175. Bleys J, Navas-Acien A, Guallar E. Serum selenium levels and all-cause, cancer, and cardiovascular mortality among US adults. *Arch Intern Med.* 2008;168(4):404–10.

176. Bleys J, Navas-Acien A, Stranges S, Menke A, Miller ER 3rd, Guallar E. Serum selenium and serum lipids in US adults. *Am J Clin Nutr.* 2008;88(2):416–23.

177. Duffield-Lillico AJ, Dalkin BL, Reid ME, et al. Selenium supplementation, baseline plasma selenium status and incidence of prostate cancer: An analysis of the complete treatment period of the Nutritional Prevention of Cancer Trial. *BJU Int.* 2003;91(7):608–12.

178. Klein EA, Thompson IM Jr, Tangen CM, et al. Vitamin E and the risk of prostate cancer: The selenium and vitamin E cancer prevention trial (SELECT). *JAMA.* 2011;306(14):1549–56.

179. Kristal AR, Darke AK, Morris JS, et al. Baseline selenium status and effects of selenium and vitamin E supplementation on prostate cancer risk. *J Natl Cancer Inst.* 2014;106(3):djt456.

180. Laclaustra M, Navas-Acien A, Stranges S, Ordovas JM, Guallar E. Serum selenium concentrations and diabetes in U.S. adults: National Health and Nutrition Examination Survey (NHANES) 2003–2004. *Environ Health Perspect.* 2009;117(9):1409–13.

181. Fritz H, Kennedy D, Fergusson D, et al. Selenium and lung cancer: A systematic review and meta analysis. *PLoS One.* 2011;6(11):e26259.

182. Zhuo H, Smith AH, Steinmaus C. Selenium and lung cancer: A quantitative analysis of heterogeneity in the current epidemiological literature. *Cancer Epidemiol Biomarkers Prev.* 2004;13(5):771–8.

183. Jacobs ET, Jiang R, Alberts DS, et al. Selenium and colorectal adenoma: Results of a pooled analysis. *J Natl Cancer Inst.* 2004;96(22):1669–75.

184. Hurst R, Hooper L, Norat T, et al. Selenium and prostate cancer: Systematic review and meta-analysis. *Am J Clin Nutr.* 2012;96(1):111–22.

185. Flores-Mateo G, Navas-Acien A, Pastor-Barriuso R, Guallar E. Selenium and coronary heart disease: A meta-analysis. *Am J Clin Nutr.* 2006;84(4):762–73.

186. Bleys J, Navas-Acien A, Guallar E. Serum selenium and diabetes in U.S. adults. *Diabetes Care.* 2007;30(4):829–34.

187. Lei C, Niu X, Wei J, Zhu J, Zhu Y. Interaction of glutathione peroxidase-1 and selenium in endemic dilated cardiomyopathy. *Clin Chim Acta.* 2009;399(1–2):102–8.

188. Grau-Perez M, Navas-Acien A, Galan-Chilet I, et al. Arsenic exposure, diabetes-related genes and diabetes prevalence in a general population from Spain. *Environ Pollut*. 2018;235:948–55.

189. Galan-Chilet I, Guallar E, Martin-Escudero JC, et al. Do genes modify the association of selenium and lipid levels? *Antioxid Redox Signal*. 2015;22(15):1352–62.

190. Laclaustra M, Stranges S, Navas-Acien A, Ordovas JM, Guallar E. Serum selenium and serum lipids in US adults: National Health and Nutrition Examination Survey (NHANES) 2003–2004. *Atherosclerosis*. 2010;210(2):643–8.

191. Gao S, Jin Y, Hall KS, et al. Selenium level and cognitive function in rural elderly Chinese. *Am J Epidemiol*. 2007;165(8):955–65.

192. Stranges S, Galletti F, Farinaro E, et al. Associations of selenium status with cardiometabolic risk factors: An 8-year follow-up analysis of the Olivetti Heart study. *Atherosclerosis*. 2011;217(1):274–8.

193. Stranges S, Rayman MP, Winther KH, Guallar E, Cold S, Pastor-Barriuso R. Effect of selenium supplementation on changes in HbA1c: Results from a multiple-dose, randomized controlled trial. *Diabetes Obes Metab*. 2019;21(3):541–9.

194. Vinceti M, Filippini T, Cilloni S, et al. Health risk assessment of environmental selenium: Emerging evidence and challenges (Review). *Mol Med Rep*. 2017;15(5):3323–35.

195. NIEHS. Powering Research through Innovative Methods for Mixtures in Epidemiology (PRIME) Program. https://www.niehs.nih.gov/research/supported/exposure/mixtures/prime_program/index.cfm. Accessed November 7, 2018.

196. Coull BA, Bobb JF, Wellenius GA, et al. Part 1. Statistical learning methods for the effects of multiple air pollution constituents. *Res Rep Health Eff Inst*. 2015;(183 Pt 1–2):5–50.

197. Bobb JF, Valeri L, Claus Henn B, et al. Bayesian kernel machine regression for estimating the health effects of multi-pollutant mixtures. *Biostatistics*. 2015;16(3):493–508.

198. Valeri L, Mazumdar MM, Bobb JF, et al. The joint effect of prenatal exposure to metal mixtures on neurodevelopmental outcomes at 20–40 months of age: Evidence from rural Bangladesh. *Environ Health Perspect*. 2017;125(6):067015.

199. Pang Y, Peng RD, Jones MR, et al. Metal mixtures in urban and rural populations in the US: The multi-ethnic study of atherosclerosis and the strong heart study. *Environ Res*. 2016;147:356–64.

200. Sanchez TR, Slavkovich V, LoIacono N, et al. Urinary metals and metal mixtures in Bangladesh: Exploring environmental sources in the health effects of arsenic longitudinal study (HEALS). *Environ Int*. 2018;121 (Pt 1):852–60.

201. Caspersen IH, Thomsen C, Haug LS, et al. Patterns and dietary determinants of essential and toxic elements in blood measured in mid-pregnancy: The Norwegian Environmental Biobank. *Sci Total Environ*. 2019;671:299–308.

202. Han I, Whitworth KW, Zhang X, Afshar M, Berens PD, Symanski E. Characterization of urinary concentrations of heavy metals among socioeconomically disadvantaged black pregnant women. *Environ Monit Assess*. 2020;192(3):200.

203. Levin-Schwartz Y, Gennings C, Henn BC, et al. Multi-media biomarkers: Integrating information to improve lead exposure assessment. *Environ Res*. 2020;183:109148.

204. Levin-Schwartz Y, Gennings C, Schnaas L, et al. Time-varying associations between prenatal metal mixtures and rapid visual processing in children. *Environ Health*. 2019;18(1):92.

205. Moody EC, Colicino E, Wright RO, et al. Environmental exposure to metal mixtures and linear growth in healthy Ugandan children. *PLoS One*. 2020;15(5):e0233108.

206. Govarts E, Remy S, Bruckers L, et al. Combined effects of prenatal exposures to environmental chemicals on birth weight. *Int J Environ Res Public Health*. 2016;13(5):495.

207. Yuan Y, Xiao Y, Feng W, et al. Plasma metal concentrations and incident coronary heart disease in Chinese adults: The Dongfeng-Tongji cohort. *Environ Health Perspect*. 2017;125(10):107007.

208. Domingo-Relloso A, Grau-Perez M, Briongos-Figuero L, et al. The association of urine metals and metal mixtures with cardiovascular incidence in an adult population from Spain: The Hortega follow-up study. *Int J Epidemiol*. 2019;48(6):1839–49.

209. Wildemann TM, Siciliano SD, Weber LP. The mechanisms associated with the development of hypertension after exposure to lead, mercury species or their mixtures differs with the metal and the mixture ratio. *Toxicology*. 2016;339:1–8.

210. Jia Q, Zhang Y, Liu S, et al. Analysis of search strategies for evaluating low-dose heavy metal mixture induced cognitive deficits in rats: An early sensitive toxicological approach. *Ecotoxicol Environ Saf*. 2020;202:110900.

CHAPTER 74

Early-Life Environmental Exposures and Children's Health

Maria Foraster • Maribel Casas • Martine Vrijheid • Jordi Sunyer

INTRODUCTION

The seminal observation by Barker that low birth weight was linked to excess risk of cardiovascular disease (CVD) and mortality in adulthood[1] led to the concept of "developmental origins of health and disease" (DOHaD). The idea of "programming" during pregnancy development and risk for chronic diseases occurring late in life was first suggested by nutritional experiments inspired by the concept of early "imprinting" of behavior in birds that has been recognized for centuries.[2]

The programming stimulus exerts long-term effects when applied at a "critical" or "sensitive" period such as the prenatal period, when organs are forming and growing. The fact that in utero exposure to environmental factors may cause permanent injury is of particular interest. There are various examples of how development is very vulnerable in early life to various external stimuli.[3] In the late 1950s, the Japanese fishing town of Minamata suffered an epidemic of persistent mental retardation and spastic paresis in children. The children were born from unaffected pregnant mothers who ate seafood contaminated with methylmercury by a factory dumping effluent into Minamata Bay.[4] In France in the 1960s, alcohol dependence was found to be very common among the mothers of mentally retarded children at an institution. This finding contributed to identifying the fetal alcohol syndrome, which is characterized by chronic mental health and developmental disorders in the offspring of alcoholic mothers. Other historical examples of the importance of early-life windows of susceptibility include the long-term health effects in the offspring, including several cancers, caused by the widespread use of diethylstilbestrol, a synthetic nonsteroidal estrogen, during pregnancy between the 1940s and 1970s,[5] and the Dutch Hunger Winter Families Study (see Box). Studying the long-term structural and functional effects of environmental exposures during fetal and early life (i.e., during the entire childhood, but particularly during the first 2 years of life) is important, given the potential irreversible nature of these health effects and the critical opportunity for prevention during these periods.

In this chapter, we provide a general description of the evidence on early-life exposure to relevant environmental factors that can impact reproductive health, neurodevelopment, respiratory and immune health, growth, obesity, and cardiometabolic health in children (Table 74-1). In this context, "early life" refers to exposure during the prenatal period (fetal life) and postnatal period of childhood. In addition, the chapter covers exposure during adolescence, an important period for development too. This summary of the evidence is not a formal weight-of-evidence analysis. This summary is mainly based on epidemiological literature published between 2008 and 2018, including the review by Vrijheid et al. (2016)[6] and other existing reviews and relevant original manuscripts for chemical exposures and air pollution, noise and green spaces (Table 74-2).

We also aimed to provide a visual summary of the quality of the evidence (Table 74-3), to introduce the case of multiple exposures and the concept of "exposome," and to provide some illustrative historical cases.

BIOLOGICAL CONSIDERATIONS

Prenatal vulnerability to environmental hazards may involve all organ systems, but is probably most prominent in regard to the nervous system.[3] For example, experimentally reducing oxygen and nutrients to rabbits during the last third of gestation resulted in poorer neurobehavioral performance, an effect not seen in adults.[7] In children, lasting neurocognitive issues have been documented following *in utero* exposure to numerous neurotoxicants, for example, lead, methylmercury, and some persistent organic pollutants (POPs).[8] Other organ systems, such as the cardiovascular, the respiratory, the reproductive, and the immune systems are also known to be affected by early-life exposures. Early-life exposures can affect disease risks later in life after a substantial latency period, though evidence about persistence, tracking (i.e., the longitudinal course of increased risk), or recovery remains limited.

The protection the placenta provides to the fetus against maternal environmental hazards is incomplete.[3] For example, cotinine, a metabolite of nicotine, and polycyclic aromatic hydrocarbon (PAH) adducts are present in cord blood. The presence of these biomarkers suggests that tobacco smoke and air pollutants can effectively cross the placenta barrier. Moreover, environmental exposures during

TABLE 74-1 CHILDREN HEALTH OUTCOMES RELATED TO EARLY-LIFE[a] EXPOSURES TO CHEMICAL AND PHYSICAL FACTORS

Outcome Title	Outcomes
Reproductive outcomes	Birth weight, small for gestational age, preterm birth
Neurodevelopment	Cognitive development, intelligence quotient (IQ), behavioral disorders, autism, attention deficit hyperactivity disorder (ADHD)
Respiratory and immune health	Lung function, asthma, respiratory infections, antibody response, allergies
Children's growth and obesity	Change in growth patterns, weight gain, body mass index (BMI), waist circumference, body fat, overweight, obesity
Cardiometabolic outcomes	Fasting plasma lipids, insulin resistance, fasting glucose, blood pressure, type 1 and type 2 diabetes

[a]Prenatal period and postnatal period (basically childhood).

pregnancy that influence plasma viscosity, systemic low-grade inflammation, hormonal disruption, or epigenetics could impair placenta function leading to a disruption of the normal fetal development, for example, leading to cardiovascular or neurological fetal alterations.

Critical windows of susceptibility can be different for different environmental hazards and health outcomes depending on underlying mechanisms, embryological maturation, exposure pathways, and the intensity of exposure. Both the prenatal and postnatal periods are important and exposures during either can result in adverse effects depending on the environmental hazard. For instance, the mechanisms underlying the effects of air pollution on brain maturity are believed to be mediated through chronic stimulation of microglial cells and myelination.[3] The myelination process (which overlaps with the formation and function of synapses), starts around week 20 of gestation, reaches its peak around week 34, and continues actively during infancy. Consequently, the period starting from mid pregnancy to the first 2 years of life is the most vulnerable for environmental factors that affect the myelination process. While both prenatal and postnatal exposure are relevant, exposure to some environmental factors such as passive smoking or air pollutants such as lead could be more intense and direct for the child during the postnatal life.

TABLE 74-2 RELEVANT CHEMICAL AND PHYSICAL EXPOSURES DURING EARLY LIFE[a]

Exposure Title	Exposures
Outdoor air pollution	Nitrogen dioxide (NO_2), particulate matter (PM), ozone, sulfur dioxide (SO_2), carbon monoxide (CO), polycyclic aromatic hydrocarbons (PAHs)
Metals and metalloids	Arsenic (As), cadmium (Cd), lead (Pb), mercury (Hg)
Organochlorine compounds	Polychlorinated biphenyls (PCBs), dichlorodiphenyl-trichloroethane/dichloroethylene (DDT/DDE), hexachlorobenzene (HCB), dioxins
Perfluoroalkyl substances (PFAS)	Perfluorooctanesulfonate (PFOS) and perfluorooctanoate (PFOA)
Polybrominated diphenyl ethers (PBDEs)	Polybrominated diphenyl ethers
Phthalates	Phthalates
Bisphenol A	Bisphenol A
Transportation noise	Aircraft, railway, road traffic noise
Green spaces	Green spaces indicators

[a]Prenatal period and postnatal period (basically childhood).

REPRODUCTIVE OUTCOMES: FETAL GROWTH AND PRETERM BIRTH

Reproductive outcomes including fetal growth and preterm birth serve as sentinel events for detecting risks to humans. Fetal growth is commonly measured as continuous weight at birth and it can be categorized as low (<2500 g) and very low (<1500 g) birth weight in at term births, or as small for gestational age (birth weight lower than the 10th percentile of a suitable weight reference distribution specific to the sex and gestational age).[15] Gestational duration is measured as the time between the first day of the last menstrual period and birth and it is frequently used to derive the outcome of preterm birth (below 37 completed gestational weeks, Yes/No). Impaired fetal growth has been associated with poorer health in children and adverse health outcomes later in life (such as ischemic heart disease, metabolic syndrome, or chronic kidney disease in adults) and preterm birth is strongly associated with increased perinatal mortality and also long-term morbidity.[15] Environmental exposures during pregnancy have been associated with impaired fetal growth, such as with low birth weight or small for gestational age. The underlying mechanisms may involve low-grade inflammation, oxidative stress, and epigenetic changes during gestation affecting all organ systems and in particular the placenta and its function.

Outdoor Air Pollution

The main outdoor air pollutants studied in epidemiological studies of reproductive outcomes relate to traffic, generally, industrial sources, and specific pollutants including carbon monoxide (CO), nitrogen dioxide (NO_2), ozone (O_3), particulate matter (PM—including $PM_{2.5}$ and PM_{10}), PAHs, and sulfur dioxide (SO_2). In 2008,

TABLE 74-3 RELEVANT CHEMICAL AND PHYSICAL EXPOSURES DURING PRENATAL AND POSTNATAL PERIODS AND DEGREE OF EVIDENCE FOR THEIR ASSOCIATION WITH FUNCTIONAL AND CLINICAL CHILDREN HEALTH OUTCOMES AND QUALITY OF EVIDENCE*

	Fetal Growth and Preterm Birth	Neurodevelopment	Respiratory and Immune Health	Childhood Growth, Obesity, and Cardiometabolic Health
Outdoor air pollution	+++	++	+++	+
Metals and metalloids	++	+++	+	+
Organochlorine compounds	++ (+++ for PCBs)	+++	++	+ (++ for DDE)
Perfluoroalkyl substances	++	+	+	+ (++ for PFOA)
Polybrominated diphenyl ethers	+	++	0	0
Currently used pesticides	+	+++	+	0
Phthalates	+	+	+	+
Bisphenol A	+	+	+	+
Transportation noise	+	+	0	+
Green spaces	+	+	+	+

*Quality of evidence:
+++ = Strong evidence for an association based on consistent results from multiple studies and meta-analyses.
++ = Moderate evidence of an association based on multiple studies, but with some inconsistencies.
+ = Insufficient/inconsistent evidence. Evidence for an association based on only a few studies, or with substantial inconsistencies.
0 = No evidence or very few studies.
Abbreviations: PCBs = polychlorinated biphenyls; DDE = dichloroethylene; PFOA = perfluorooctanoate.
Note: At least two people rated the quality of the evidence reported in this table. The evidence summarized in this table is not a formal weight-of-evidence analyses.

BOX 74-1 The Dutch Hunger Winter Families Study

The winter of 1944–45 is known as the "Hunger Winter" in The Netherlands when Germans authorities blocked all food supplies in retaliation of a railway strike. Widespread starvation was more serious in the cities of the western Netherlands. The circumstances of the famine created a "natural experiment," since the Dutch population was well fed before and after that period. The cohort of famine-born infants followed until adulthood was used to study the *developmental origins of health and disease (DOHaD)*, also known as "Barker's hypothesis."[9] Individuals conceived during the famine period and exposed to an energy-poor fetal environment late during gestation had higher risk of obesity, glucose intolerance, and CVD compared to individuals conceived before the famine period.[10–12] A higher risk of schizophrenia in adulthood was also observed among individuals exposed to famine during prenatal life.[13] Epigenetic modifications that can shape the individual's phenotype through developmental plasticity have been postulated as one of the potential biological mechanisms for the long-term health consequences of early-life exposures.[14]

evidence for an effect of outdoor air pollution on preterm birth and fetal growth restriction was classified as limited[16] based on a small number of studies and inconsistent findings. Systematic reviews published in 2010 and 2011 concluded that the evidence was most consistent for the association between PM and fetal growth outcomes and between SO_2 and preterm birth.[17,18] Since then, a strong evidence base has emerged on the association between air pollution, especially CO, NO_2, PM_{10}, and $PM_{2.5}$, and greater risk of preterm birth and low birth weight as summarized in several systematic reviews with meta-analyses.[19–23] For example, odds ratios for low birth weight at term ranged from 1.03 per 10 μg/m³ of $PM_{2.5}$ in a meta-analysis of studies across the world[20] to 1.18 per 5 μg/m³ of $PM_{2.5}$ in a study pooling data from 14 longitudinal European birth cohorts.[21] A meta-analysis of Chinese studies observed pooled odds ratios for both low birth weight and preterm birth of 1.03 per interquartile range of $PM_{2.5}$.[23]

The consistent results from meta-analysis and pooled studies suggest there is strong evidence on the association between exposure to air pollutants and adverse reproductive outcomes.

Metals and Metalloids

An extensive nonsystematic review published in 2008[16] classified associations between lead and fetal growth and preterm birth as limited. Further studies found associations between prenatal exposure to lead with either no associations[24–26] or associations with adverse birth outcomes, for example,[27–31] For fetal growth, including birth weight, length, and preterm birth, multiple studies have found associations even at low levels of lead exposure (<10 g/dL maternal blood).[32–34]

Mercury exposure has been associated with birth weight[35–37] or with reduced fetal growth[38] in some studies. However, others have reported no association.[32,39–42]

Several studies have indicated associations between cadmium concentrations in maternal and cord blood with small-for-gestational-age and with reduced birth weight.[25,43–48]

A systematic review of 18 studies published in 2014 concluded that there was inconsistent evidence for an association between arsenic exposure and birth weight and preterm birth, mostly based on studies with small samples and conducted in populations exposed to high arsenic levels in contaminated drinking water.[49] However, a recent systematic review with meta-analysis[50] and further studies[51–55] support the association of arsenic (assessed either in water or in maternal tissues) with reduced birth weight. Regarding fetal growth, two recent studies observed an association between arsenic in maternal urine and fetal growth reductions.[56,57] In contrast, the evidence on the association between arsenic and preterm birth remains insufficient.[51]

In summary, the evidence for toxic metals/metalloids and increased risk for adverse reproductive outcomes is moderate to strong, based on the consistent findings with lead, the increasing evidence for arsenic, and the rather consistent results from the few studies available for cadmium and mercury.

Organochlorine Compounds

Organochlorine compounds (OCs) are POPs. POPs persist in the environment and bioaccumulate in animal fatty tissues, reaching the highest concentrations at the top of the food chain, such as in human beings. The Stockholm Convention (2001) has banned or restricted their production. Previous studies have concluded that there is sufficient evidence for an effect of high exposure to polychlorinated biphenyls (PCBs) levels on fetal growth.[16,58] There is strong evidence for the link between general population exposure levels to PCBs measured in maternal or cord blood and reductions in birth weight from two meta-analyses of 12 European birth cohort studies.[59,60] However, PCBs were not related to gestational age in one of them.[59] While most (but not all) the recent studies of biomarker concentrations of dioxins and organochlorine pesticides such as dichlorodiphenyl-trichloroethane (DDT), dichlorodiphenyl-dichloroethylene (DDE), and hexachlorobenzene (HCB) have observed associations between one of the organochlorine compounds studied and birth weight, there were inconsistencies between studies in the types of associated compounds or congeners, for example,[59,61–69] Therefore, the evidence for PCBs and reproductive outcomes was classified as strong and for the rest of POPs as moderate.

Perfluoroalkyl Substances (PFAS)

PFASs, which are also classified as POPs, are widely used for their water and oil repelling properties and found in products such as carpets, furniture, shampoo, shoes, clothes, nonstick cookware, and food packaging. They have also been used in fire-fighting foams, leading to contamination of water supplies. These compounds have extremely long half-lives in the environment and their fate and transport leads to various pathways for human exposure.

The most widely studied PFASs are perfluorooctanesulfonate (PFOS) and perfluorooctanoate (PFOA). Evidence for an association between PFOA and birth weight reduction is available from a meta-analysis of 9 studies of maternal plasma/serum concentration of PFOA[70] and a systematic review of 14 studies in utero PFOA exposure.[71] However, the later observed that associations in individual studies varied in magnitude and were not always statistically significant. The same review reported that PFOS exposure was associated with reduced birth weight in some studies, and with null associations in others.[71] Two other recent meta-analyses support associations with reduced birth weight both for PFOS and PFOA.[72,73] Interestingly, one of the meta-analysis[72] showed the challenges of PFAS exposure assessment, in other words, they observed that such associations remained but were partly explained by maternal glomerular filtration rates, that is, the kidney function of the mother. PFOS and PFOA are being substituted by other PFASs for which there is almost no information on possible toxicity. The findings from the different meta-analysis suggest that the evidence for PFAS and reproductive outcomes is currently moderate.

Polybrominated Diphenyl Ethers (PBDEs)

PBDEs, classified as POPs, are flame retardants commonly used to reduce flammability in many consumer products, including furniture, textiles, electronics, and building materials. A recent meta-analysis of seven studies reported an association between PBDE biomarker concentrations and reduced birth weight.[74] The study also observed indicative associations between different PBDE congeners and reduced birth weight. However, this was based only on three to four studies depending on the congener. Because of the limited number of studies, the evidence on PBDEs and reproductive outcomes was classified as "insufficient/inconsistent."

Currently Used Pesticides

Among the wide range of pesticides, the epidemiological literature mainly focuses on organophosphate pesticides and pyrethroids. Several studies have shown a negative impact on fetal growth of prenatal exposure to occupational pesticides,[75,76] to insecticides from nearby agricultural activity or household use,[77–79] and to organophosphate pesticides measured by biomarkers.[80–82] In contrast, a study of four cohorts[83] and a pilot study in Thailand[84] observed associations between biomarker levels of organophosphate pesticides and birth weight only in the subgroup with low detoxifying capacity with regard to the enzyme PON1 genotype or phenotype, respectively. There are very few studies on pyrethroid exposure and pregnancy outcomes and most of these report no association.[85] The evidence for the association between prenatal exposure to pesticides and preterm birth is limited to few studies, suggesting potential associations.[86–88] Overall, the evidence between currently used pesticides and reproductive outcomes was classified as "insufficient/inconsistent."

Phthalates

Phthalates are widely used in cosmetics, plastics, carpets, building materials, toys, and medical and cleaning products. In 2013, a systematic review of less than ten small ($N < 400$) studies reported inconsistent results, with associations between phthalates and both longer and shorter gestational duration, or reduced birth weight, or null associations.[89] A recent systematic review[90] and newer studies have added little further evidence, despite improved outcome assessment with detailed ultrasound fetal growth measurements compared with earlier studies: a study in China observed a link between phthalate exposure and preterm birth but not with fetal growth[91] and a Spanish study found no association between maternal phthalate urine concentrations and fetal growth parameters.[92] Two recent large studies identified associations with decreased birth weight either with one phthalate metabolite out of 16 organic pollutants[65] or with two phthalates out of seven in the entire sample and associations with the other five metabolites only in participant subgroups.[93] Such inconsistencies may be explained by the short biological half-lives of phthalates, which make them difficult to characterize and susceptible to exposure misclassification. In summary, because of the mixed findings, the evidence on phthalates and reproductive outcomes was classified as "insufficient/inconsistent."

Bisphenol A

BPA is produced in large quantities and used in the manufacture of plastic polymers, such as polycarbonate plastics and epoxy resins, for many consumer products. Systematic reviews of more than ten studies on BPA exposure in maternal urine and birth weight and preterm birth have reported inconsistencies between studies.[94,95] Two other studies indicated no association between prenatal BPA exposure and fetal growth.[92,96] A recent meta-analysis of eight studies did not find an association between prenatal exposure to BPA and birth weight, and alerted of the need of larger prospective studies to reach conclusions.[97] As indicated by this meta-analysis and the inconsistent findings, the evidence on BPA and reproductive outcomes was rated as "insufficient/inconsistent."

Transportation Noise

Exposure to noise is common, particularly with regard to road traffic noise, but few studies have evaluated its association with birth outcomes. A recent systematic review[98] of six studies for aircraft, five studies for road traffic, and three studies for railway noise observed low-quality evidence for an association with preterm birth or birth weight. Further studies have shown little evidence for an association between maternal exposure to road traffic noise and birth weight[99] and no association between total environmental noise and preterm birth.[100] Because of the limited number of studies, the evidence on transportation noise and reproductive outcomes was rated as "insufficient/inconsistent."

Green Spaces

Interest on the health effects of exposure to natural vegetation, generally evaluated as exposure to green spaces, has increased. Recent systematic reviews suggest that prenatal exposure to green spaces or urban green spaces may increase birth weight, although some studies found no associations with birth outcomes and the evidence is limited to few studies with comparable assessments.[101,102] Because of the limited number of comparable studies, the evidence on green spaces and reproductive outcomes was classified as "insufficient/inconsistent."

Summary of the Evidence

In general, the evidence is strong in support of an association of both outdoor air pollution and PCB exposure with measures of fetal growth; it is moderate for metals/metalloids and for PFOA and PFAS, and insufficient or inconsistent for phthalates, BPA, pesticides, noise, and green spaces.

NEURODEVELOPMENT

Brain development is the process of neuron maturation (proliferation, migration, differentiation, synaptogenesis, myelination, and apoptosis). This process continues from the embryonic period until late adolescence.[103] Exposure to environmental factors during this period may alter normal brain development and result in adverse effects on cognition, for example, reduction of global intelligence quotient (IQ) as the most studied outcome, and behavioral disorders including autism, autism spectrum disorder (ASD), attention deficit hyperactivity disorder (ADHD), and school failure or delinquent behavior.

Outdoor Air Pollution

The number of studies assessing the effects of air pollution on neurodevelopment has rapidly increased in the last decade.[104,105] Several systematic reviews have described fairly consistent evidence for an association of autism diagnosis with prenatal[106–108] and postnatal[108] exposure to air pollution. Another systematic review on autism

BOX 74-2 Maternal Smoking during Pregnancy and Offspring DNA Methylation

Maternal smoking during pregnancy, still frequent among gestating women in many countries, is a recognized risk factor for preterm birth, lower birth weight, and childhood diseases such as obesity, asthma, or neurobehavioral problems. However, the molecular mechanisms underlying this array of effects are poorly understood. The Pregnancy and Childhood Epigenetics (PACE) consortium investigated whether maternal smoking during pregnancy modified cord blood DNA methylation in a sample of nearly 7000 mother-child pairs.[6] Over 6000 CpG sites were differentially methylated at birth, and some of them were still affected in childhood. These CpGs were enriched in pathways critical to development and some had been described in blood of current smokers. A smaller study evaluated the association of maternal smoking with DNA methylation in the placenta, a key organ for fetal development. Fifty CpG sites were differentially methylated in relation to maternal smoking status during pregnancy. The top CpG sites, with around 20% hypomethylation in smokers, mapped to a locus that had previously been implicated in birth weight through genome-wide association studies. Interestingly, the signature of maternal smoking during pregnancy on the methylome was tissue specific, with not much overlap between cord blood and placenta.

concluded that the evidence was sufficient for pre- and postnatal exposure to $PM_{2.5}$, but inadequate for the rest of air pollutants.[103] Further studies suggest associations with postnatal exposure to $PM_{2.5}$ and also NO_2.[109,110] In contrast, a meta-analysis of European birth cohorts found no association between air pollution and autistic traits.[111]

A systematic review in 2015 reported that there was sufficient evidence for an association between both pre- and postnatal exposure to PAHs and decreased cognitive function (global IQ), but that evidence for an effect of other air pollutants on cognitive function (mainly global IQ) and on behavioral problems was inconsistent.[103] Further studies have shown mixed findings on the association between prenatal exposure to air pollution and cognitive function, for example,[112,113] and neurobehavioral problems.[114,115] Regarding postnatal exposure, further studies have observed that children attending schools with higher traffic-related air pollution had slower cognitive development over 1 year (in all measured cognitive functions).[116] Furthermore, air pollution exposure during commuting to schools was also associated with cognitive impairment.[117] Similarly, exposure to traffic-related pollution in these children was associated with more frequent behavioral problems.[118] It was also observed that only fine particles generated from traffic (not from other origins) were associated with impaired brain development.[119] Short-term exposures to traffic-related pollutants (the day before) were also associated with daily fluctuations in attention,[120] independently of longer-term exposure. Furthermore, a systematic review of 11 studies (6 in children, 4 in elderly, and 1 in rats) found associations between exposure to traffic-related pollutants and brain areas (white matter, cortical gray matter, and basal ganglia), which could be involved in the cognitive changes observed in epidemiological studies.[121]

The evidence is rather consistent for autism and for PAHs with neurodevelopment. There is increasing evidence for links between postnatal exposure to traffic-related air pollution and impaired neurodevelopment, including studies based on neuroimaging for outcome assessment. However, this new evidence is still based on few studies and few geographical areas and little is known about prenatal exposure. Therefore, the evidence for air pollution and neurodevelopment has been classified as moderate in strength.

Metals and Metalloids

Lead, methylmercury, and arsenic are recognized as developmental neurotoxicants.[8]

Findings for low-level exposure to prenatal methylmercury have been controversial, because of the different types of fish consumed in the studies of populations with high fish intake, and potential complex confounding due to beneficial effects of seafood intake. While cohort studies in the Faroe Islands with a high intake of whale meat have shown prenatal exposure to be related with a cognitive and neurophysiological impairment at age 14,[124] other cohort studies in high fish consumption communities such as the Seychelles Islands[125,126] and Spain,[127] have not shown these associations. These discrepancies may be due to the confounding effects of the essential fatty acids in fish, the main source of methylmercury that are beneficial for brain development.[124–127] Regarding neurobehavior, a meta-analysis on prenatal and postnatal mercury exposure and ADHD and autism found statistically significant associations for both outcomes, but the scope of evidence was limited.[128] Further studies have reported inconsistent results and suggest no association between prenatal exposure to mercury measured in blood and autism or neuropsychological impairment, provided women eat fish.[129,130]

The evidence for the neurotoxic effects of prenatal exposure to lead is heterogeneous as reviewed by Allen et al. (2015)[131] and it is difficult to disentangle the consequences of prenatal from postnatal exposure, for which there is more evidence. Recent studies for prenatal exposure have observed inconsistent results, reporting adverse neurobehavioral effects[132,133] or no effects,[134,135] or sex- or maternal-stress-dependent effects only.[136–138] Regarding postnatal exposure,

BOX 74-3 Prenatal Exposure to Air Pollution and Neurodevelopmental Effects—Is the Prenatal Period the Most Vulnerable Time Window for Air Pollution Effects on the Brain?

The human brain begins to develop very early in prenatal life and its maturation continues through adolescence and young adulthood. For some exposures such as mercury or organochlorine compounds, exposure during the prenatal period has shown larger effects than exposure occurring after birth. This is probably because during pregnancy, some brain processes are forming and growing and exposure to environmental hazards during that period may cause permanent brain injury. Is this similar for outdoor air pollution effects on the brain and if yes, what is the mechanism? Two recent studies showed that prenatal air pollution exposure exacerbates white matter lesions and reduces white matter volume, while exposure during childhood does not link to any structural alteration.[122,123] Placental dysfunction has been suggested as a potential mechanism by which air pollution may affect fetal brain development during pregnancy. Indeed, the placenta forms the barrier between the mother and the fetus and soot particles from polluted air have been recently shown to be able to reach the placenta via the bloodstream. The few available studies on placental function measured with Doppler ultrasound and air pollution did not measure the final impact on brain development. Studies evaluating placental function and its mediation role in the relationship between air pollution and brain development during pregnancy will advance understanding of the underlying mechanisms of air pollution effects on the brain.

meta-analyses have shown that children's blood lead concentrations, even those below 10 μg/dL, are inversely associated with cognitive function (IQ) following a nonlinear dose–response relationship.[139,140] A recent meta-analysis of 22 case-control studies corroborates the inverse association with IQ,[141] whereas another recent meta-analysis of seven studies observed associations with risk for ADHD.[142] Elevated early-life exposures to lead have been related to behavior disturbances and delinquency in adulthood.[143]

For cadmium, a systematic review found that there is suggestive evidence from ten recent studies for a detrimental effect of pre- and postnatal cadmium exposure on cognitive development, but that there is little evidence for an effect on ADHD and related symptoms.[144] Recent studies have also observed associations between pre- and postnatal cadmium exposure and cognitive development[145–147] or behavioral problems[145] but not with motor skills.[148] In turn, a recent cross-sectional study observed no association between postnatal exposure to cadmium and cognition in children aged 9–11 years.[149]

In a systematic review and meta-analysis on pre- and postnatal exposure to arsenic and manganese most studies reported significant adverse effects on neurodevelopment, and the meta-analysis results showed significant IQ decreases for exposures to both compounds; studies evaluating behavioral disorders were few (less than 5).[150] Recent studies have also observed associations between postnatal exposure to arsenic at different concentrations and cognitive development,[151,152] including an intervention study which observed improvements in working memory after reduction of arsenic in drinking water.[153] However, other studies found no association between arsenic exposure and cognitive development, neither in the postnatal[149,154] nor the prenatal periods,[155] although the latter was based on a small sample size ($n = 70$). Regarding neurobehavioral problems, two studies found associations with either prenatal[156] or postnatal exposure to arsenic,[157] whereas another found no association with ADHD and postnatal exposure.[152] A meta-analysis of three case-control studies and a cross-sectional study suggested an association between biomarker levels of manganese in children and ADHD.[158]

The evidence for the association of metals and metalloids with neurodevelopment was rated as "strong," because of the recognized neurodevelopmental effects of mercury and lead, and the recent evidence for other metals.

Organochlorine Compounds

In 2015, a systematic review updating the last 10 years of evidence found that prenatal or early postnatal exposure to PCBs was associated with adverse neurodevelopmental and behavioral outcomes in the entire sample or in boys, in around 13 out of 20 studies, whereas the rest reported null associations.[159] For DDE (12 studies), significant associations were particularly found for early infancy psychomotor development and for ADHD symptoms, whereas at school age no adverse associations were described.[159] Additionally, a recent pooled analysis of seven European birth cohorts did not report an association between pre- or postnatal exposure to PCB, DDE, and HCB and risk of ADHD in children aged 4–10 years.[160] According to several reviews, new concerns have arisen about the link between POPs, especially PCBs, and autism during the prenatal period[106] and the pre- and postnatal period,[108] but the number of studies is still small. Other POPs have been also linked to autism.[161–163] Because of the substantial evidence for PCBs based on a large systematic review and more recent evidence for other POPs, the evidence on their association with neurodevelopmental outcomes was rated as strong.

Perfluoroalkyl Substances

A recent narrative review concluded that most studies have evaluated prenatal and not postnatal exposure to PFAS in relation to neurodevelopment[164] and that the evidence is still inconclusive.[164,165] For PFOA, recent prospective analyses did not observe associations between PFOA and behavioral problems, ADHD and autism.[166–170] Therefore, the evidence on PFAS and neurodevelopment was rated as "insufficient/inconsistent."

Polybrominated Diphenyl Ethers

According to several reviews, there is growing concern for the effect of exposure to PBDEs on child behavior, cognition, and motor skills.[165,171] Despite the small number of studies, the majority found associations between prenatal or postnatal exposure to PBDE and adverse consequences for development. In additional studies, prenatal PBDE exposure has been associated with lower language and social development scores at 24 months,[172] and with lower IQ scores at age 5 years.[173] A recent systematic review concluded that there was sufficient evidence for an association between PBDE exposure and IQ ($n = 10$ studies) and limited evidence for ADHD ($n = 9$ studies), based on studies of moderate quality for both pre- and postnatal exposure.[174] The meta-analysis (four studies) reported a consistent association between PBDE exposure during gestation or at birth with IQ during childhood. There were not enough comparable studies on ADHD to perform a meta-analysis.[174] Because of the consistency in results, despite the limited number of studies, the evidence on PBDE and neurodevelopmental outcomes was classified as moderate.

Currently Used Pesticides

According to several systematic reviews, there is consistent evidence for an association between prenatal exposure to organophosphate pesticides and reduced IQ scores and other measures of mental and psychomotor development in children.[175,176] Further studies suggest that PON1gene polymorphisms may increase susceptibility to these effects.[176,177] Chlorpyrifos has previously been classified as a known developmental neurotoxicant[8] and prenatal exposure to chlorpyrifos has been related to alteration in brain morphology measured by structural magnetic resonance imaging.[82] The few studies on ADHD and autism are rather consistent in showing associations.[108,178–181] For postnatal organophosphate exposure there are fewer studies and results are inconsistent.[176] In turn, prenatal pyrethroid exposure has been related to adverse neurodevelopmental effects.[85] The greater consistency of associations with prenatal than postnatal exposure to organophosphates has been also reported in a subsequent summary of systematic reviews.[182] Because of the consistency of results, the evidence on the association between currently used pesticides and neurodevelopmental outcomes was classified as strong.

Phthalates

Different reviews of epidemiological studies have identified associations between phthalate exposure and adverse neurodevelopment outcomes in children,[89,183] mostly related to prenatal exposure, though with inconsistencies in the phthalate congeners studied, in the neurodevelopmental domains affected, and in the finding of sex-specific effects. A recent systematic review and meta-analysis of ten studies, reported associations between prenatal exposure to phthalates and reduced psychomotor development index (five studies) and between postnatal exposure to phthalates and reduced IQ (six studies) but not with other neurodevelopmental outcomes.[184] Findings regarding behavior and autism are inconsistent, for example, while a recent study reported associations between prenatal phthalate exposure and behavioral problems in 7- to 8-year-old children,[185] two other studies observed null associations with behavioral measures, and also with cognitive and psychomotor development[186] and ASDs.[187] A systematic review also reported inconsistent associations between pre- or postnatal exposure to phthalates and autism, based on few studies (five studies).[188] Based on the mixed findings, the evidence on phthalates and neurodevelopmental outcomes was classified as "insufficient/inconsistent."

Bisphenol A

A few reviews have suggested that BPA exposure is related to neurobehavioral problems in children[95,189] and behavioral problems,[190] though they were based on few studies. Inconsistencies remain regarding the direction of associations by sex and the affected neurobehavioral domains and time window of exposure (pre- or postnatal), for example.[191–193] Regarding cognitive development, some studies reported an association between prenatal BPA exposure and cognitive function[194,195] or with executive functions but not with intelligence in boys,[196] whereas others do not observe associations.[193,197,198] Based on the inconsistent findings, the evidence on BPA and neurodevelopmental outcomes was classified as "insufficient/inconsistent."

Transportation Noise

Studies have focused on postnatal exposure to noise. A recent systematic review reported that there was moderate-quality evidence for the association between long-term postnatal exposure to aircraft noise and cognitive impairment in terms of reading comprehension and long-term memory in school-age children. However, the authors concluded that, for other cognitive outcomes and transportation noise sources, more and better-quality studies were needed.[199] Another systematic review reported that evidence was of moderate quality for the association of exposure to road and railway noise with emotional conduct disorders in children and of low or moderate quality for the association of aircraft and road traffic noise, respectively, with hyperactivity.[200] Finally, another systematic review including two more recent studies until 2018 generally concluded that the evidence for an association between environmental noise and neurodevelopment and mental health in children is heterogeneous and limited to few studies but suggestive of associations.[201] Studies have also observed independent associations of air pollution and noise with neurobehavior in children.[118,199] Although there are reports of moderate evidence for some associations, there are few studies and inconsistencies for some others relationships. Therefore, the evidence for the association between transportation noise and neurodevelopmental outcomes was rated as "insufficient/inconsistent."

Green Spaces

Some studies have addressed whether access to green spaces affects neurodevelopment in children and they have focused on postnatal exposure to green spaces. One study observed beneficial associations between life-long exposure to green spaces from birth and inattention in children until age 7.[202] However, such exposure classification reflects both perinatal and postnatal exposure to green spaces and does not allow ruling out the impact of prenatal exposure. Studies on postnatal exposure have generally found beneficial associations of exposure to natural and/or green environments with cognition over the life-course, as reviewed recently[203] and with cognition and attention as observed in further studies.[202,204–206] Furthermore, a magnetic resonance study found that exposure to green space was positively associated with brain maturation.[207] Although initial findings have been consistent and were supported by one brain imaging study, there are still very few studies. Therefore, the evidence on green spaces and neurodevelopmental outcomes was rated as "insufficient/inconsistent"

Summary of the Evidence

An increasing number of environmental factors have been shown to have neurodevelopmental effects: there is strong evidence for organochlorine compounds, organophosphate pesticides and metals/metalloids, and moderate evidence for PBDEs, and air pollutants. Overall, the evidence is more limited for autism and behavioral problems.

RESPIRATORY AND IMMUNE HEALTH

The development of the lung and the immune system start *in utero* and continue throughout childhood.[212] Disruption of the developing respiratory and immune systems by environmental pollutants may lead to a reduced capacity to fight infection, a reduced lung function, and an increased risk to develop asthma and allergies.[213–216] In addition, lung function deficits that are established by school age may track into adult life and increase the risk of adult lung obstructive diseases.[217]

Outdoor Air Pollution

There is some evidence that prenatal exposure to air pollution is associated with reduced lung function development, for example,[218,219] The ESCAPE study, which combined data from multiple European birth cohorts, found associations between exposure to traffic-related air pollution at birth and pneumonia during early childhood[220] and between postnatal exposure to traffic-related air pollution, but not exposure at birth, and reduced lung function.[221] Other studies also indicate associations between postnatal exposure to air pollution and reduced lung function, for example,[222–224] A meta-analysis of 18 studies found associations between prenatal exposure to air pollution and risk of wheezing and asthma in children.[225] Different meta-analyses have consistently reported associations of postnatal exposure to air pollution with respiratory disease, that is, with risk of asthma,[226] asthma exacerbations,[227] pneumonia after short-term exposure,[228] and respiratory tract diseases (i.e., cough, wheezing, and lower tract respiratory diseases), being the latter association greater for traffic-related than nontraffic-related pollutants.[229] Because of the consistency in findings, the evidence on air pollution and respiratory health has been classified as strong.

Metals and Metalloids

There are very few studies on the link between exposure to heavy metals and the developing respiratory and immune systems.[230,231] A recent study found no association between maternal lead exposure and cord blood immune system biomarkers,[232] whereas two studies observed associations between postnatal blood lead levels and asthma in children.[233,234] Regarding exposure to mercury, no association was found between prenatal exposure to low mercury levels and immune system biomarkers.[235] For postnatal mercury exposure, the same study showed associations with one immune biomarker out of six (interleukin 10),[235] another study observed associations with asthma[236] and another one did not.[237] Regarding prenatal exposure to arsenic, a systematic review found only four studies,[238] which indicated associations with respiratory symptoms, respiratory infections, and/or pneumonia later on (7–17 years of age). A further study found associations between prenatal exposure to arsenic and lung function in children.[239] In contrast, the evidence is very limited for postnatal exposure to arsenic[238] with a recent study suggesting an association with airway inflammation in boys only.[239] Because of the few studies and inconsistencies, the evidence on metals and metalloids and respiratory and immune health was classified as "insufficient/inconsistent."

BOX 74-4 Duration of Breastfeeding and Better Intellectual Performance

Breast milk, which contains a large quantity of long-chain polyunsaturated fatty acids, has beneficial effects on offspring neurodevelopment, but it is also a source of exposure to POPs. Several cohort studies have shown that longer breastfeeding duration improves cognitive development in childhood. A study in two birth cohorts from high- and low-/middle-income countries showed that breastfeeding duration was associated with higher IQ in childhood. Results between breastfeeding and IQ were consistent in the different cultural settings where socioeconomic patterns in breastfeeding differ.[208] In contrast, breastfeeding was not consistently associated with blood pressure and body mass index (BMI) after comparing the confounding pattern of breastfeeding by socioeconomic status. These findings suggest that only the association of breastfeeding with intellectual performance is likely to be causal. Results from this cross-cohort comparison study were supported by a randomized trial where children fed on standard term formula had lower neurodevelopment scores at 2 years than those fed on donor breast milk.[209] Another cohort study showed that longer duration of breastfeeding was associated with better cognitive development and with fewer autistic traits in 5-year-old children.[210] Few studies have assessed whether the beneficial effects of breastfeeding persist until adulthood. A study in two independent samples and using two independent intelligence tests demonstrated that duration of breastfeeding was associated with higher IQ scores until young adulthood.[211]

Organochlorine Compounds

A large systematic review ($n = 41$ studies) classified evidence as limited (i.e., several good quality, independent, studies report an association, but with some inconsistencies) for the association between prenatal exposure to DDE, PCBs, and dioxins and risk of respiratory infections, and for postnatal exposure to PCBs and reduced immune response after vaccination in childhood.[216] Evidence was classified as inadequate for other organochlorine compounds and other outcomes.

A pooled-analysis of 4608 subjects from ten European birth cohort studies indicated that prenatal DDE exposure, but not PCB153, was associated with respiratory symptoms in young children.[240] A long-term follow-up study found that maternal concentrations of PCB118 and HCB were associated with increased risk of asthma medication use[241] and with increased airway obstruction[242] in offspring aged 20 years. Maternal occupational exposure to PCBs was also related to asthma, eczema/hay fever and ear infections in children.[243] In contrast, a few studies observed no association between prenatal biomarker concentrations of DDT and DDE with low tract respiratory infections in early childhood[244] and of PCB and DDE with asthma and eczema.[245] The role of the immune system remains unclear, no associations were observed between prenatal exposure to POPs and several immune biomarkers in recent studies,[232,246] except for interleukin 10.[246]

Regarding postnatal exposure, a recent study observed associations between children's DDE, PCB, and HCH serum concentrations and asthma in children.[247] They also reported associations between exposure to DDE, but not PCB, in indoor air and asthma,[248] whereas another study observed little evidence for an association between DDE and asthma.[249]

Because of the several associations with respiratory outcomes, the evidence for organochlorine compounds and respiratory health has been considered moderate.

Perfluoroalkyl Substances

There are indications for an association between PFASs and the developing immune system from studies showing that prenatal or postnatal exposure to PFAS may decrease antibody response to childhood vaccines and increase the risk of having low levels of the antibodies needed for long-term protection.[250–252] One study further identified associations between prenatal exposure to PFAS and lower levels of immune-related genes in cord blood.[253] Studies of other outcomes are inconsistent, with reports of increased, decreased and no risk of asthma, wheezing symptoms, and atopy in relation to prenatal or postnatal PFAS exposure.[216,245,254] Further studies have observed associations between prenatal exposure to PFAS and respiratory tract infections or lower levels of mumps and rubella antibodies but no link with asthma, lung function or allergies.[252,255] Recent studies observed associations between PFAS exposure and asthma, only in specific conditions, that is: A recent case-control study reported an association between postnatal exposure to PFAS and asthma in adolescents, which was stronger in children with higher hormone levels of estradiol and was attenuated with higher testosterone levels.[256] Results from the same population showed an association between PFAS and lung function but only among asthmatics.[257] Finally, another study observed associations between postnatal, not prenatal, PFAS exposure and asthma only in children without measles-mumps-rubella vaccination.[258] Because of the inconsistencies across studies, the evidence on PFAS and respiratory and immune health was rated as "insufficient/inconsistent."

Polybrominated Diphenyl Ethers

The three available studies evaluated the association of postnatal exposure to PBDEs in dust, indoor air or in children's serum with asthma and none observed an association.[247,248,259] Because of the very few studies, the evidence on PBDEs and respiratory and immune health was rated as "no evidence."

Currently Used Pesticides

The two studies on prenatal exposure to organophosphates have observed associations with respiratory symptoms at age 5 and 7 years[260] or inverse or no associations with immune biomarkers in newborns.[232] Prenatal but not postnatal exposure to pyrethroids has been also associated with cough, wheeze, and IgE in early childhood.[261] Furthermore, postnatal exposure to organophosphates has been associated with reduced lung function at age 7 years in a longitudinal study of an agricultural community,[262] but not with asthma in another study.[249] Because of the few studies, the evidence on currently used pesticides and respiratory and immune health was rated as "insufficient/inconsistent."

Phthalates

One prospective birth cohort study reported an association between prenatal exposure to one high molecular weight phthalate metabolite (monobenzyl phthalate: MBzP) and early onset eczema before age 2 years but not late onset eczema.[263] Three studies evaluating prenatal phthalate exposure have observed associations with risk of wheeze, asthma, and respiratory infections in children aged 5–11 years, but there were inconsistencies regarding the phthalate congeners.[264–266] Furthermore, a recent systematic review and meta-analysis reported an association between butylbenzyl phthalate (BBzP) exposure (out of six phthalates) and childhood asthma that was stronger in the prenatal than the postnatal period when assessed in urine metabolites (based on three and four studies, respectively). They also reported an association between postnatal exposure to di(2-ethylhexyl) phthalate (DEHP) and BBzP and childhood asthma when postnatal phthalates were assessed in dust (based on three studies).[267] A previous systematic review of similar studies (except one) had already reported the latter finding with asthma, and additionally observed a link with allergies.[268] Another study reported allergic sensitization in association with nondietary phthalate exposure in 3- to 5-year-old children.[269] Because of the few studies and the inconsistencies among them, the evidence on phthalates and respiratory and immune health was rated as "insufficient/inconsistent."

Bisphenol A

Few studies of sufficient quality have addressed the effects of BPA on respiratory health. The first evidence for a role of BPA in respiratory health (wheeze and asthma) of children emerged from two birth cohort studies from a systematic review in 2013.[95] A recent systematic review of cohort studies identified three studies showing an association between prenatal exposure to BPA and increased risk of childhood wheeze, whereas one study reported a reduced risk of wheeze.[270] Some of these studies also indicated that prenatal BPA exposure may lead to decreased lung function and chest infections in childhood.[264,271,272] The same systematic review reported that three out of four studies had observed an association between postnatal exposure to BPA and risk of childhood asthma/wheeze.[270] Further studies have observed either no association with respiratory and allergy health[273] or associations with allergic disease (i.e., eczema and wheeze) only in females.[274] Because of the few studies and the inconsistencies among them, the evidence on BPA and respiratory and immune health was rated as "insufficient/inconsistent."

Transportation Noise

It is hypothesized that noise could affect respiratory and/or immune health through different pathways,[275] but the little evidence available is for adults, for example.[276,277] There is no evidence on transportation noise and respiratory and immune health in children, therefore, this relationship was classified as "no evidence."

Green Spaces

A recent systematic review identified 11 studies. The meta-analysis reported null associations between green spaces and asthma (three studies) and allergic rhinitis (two studies). However, the assessment of the green spaces was very heterogeneous, which could have hampered the comparability of studies.[278] Because of the few comparable studies, the evidence for green spaces and respiratory and immune health was considered "insufficient/inconsistent."

Summary of the Evidence

Among all the environmental factors associated with respiratory and immune outcomes, there is only strong evidence for the association of air pollution and moderate for organochlorine compounds with respiratory health. The rest of environmental factors require further investigation.

CHILDHOOD GROWTH, OBESITY, AND CARDIOMETABOLIC HEALTH

The relatively recent "environmental obesogen" hypothesis is centered on the ability of chemicals that interfere with endocrine and metabolic systems to change growth patterns, and induce weight gain, obesity, and obesity-related diseases such as type 2 diabetes (T2D) and CVD.[279] Obesogens may perturb the neuroendocrine mechanisms involved in energy metabolism, appetite, adipogenesis, and glucose-insulin homeostasis.[279] Most epidemiologic studies have assessed generalized and central obesity in childhood using age- and sex-specific z-scores or percentile cutoffs for measured BMI and waist circumference, respectively, calculated based on national or international reference growth charts. Epidemiological studies have recently also started to evaluate cardiometabolic endpoints in childhood by including measures of fasting blood lipid concentrations (total cholesterol, high-density lipoprotein, triglycerides), insulin resistance and T2D (based on fasting blood insulin and glucose concentrations or medical records), and cardiovascular outcomes (mainly blood pressure).

Outdoor Air Pollutants

Few studies have evaluated the effects of exposure to air pollutants on childhood obesity and other metabolic outcomes. Recent studies have observed associations between prenatal exposure to air pollution and increases in childhood BMI,[280,281] but not associations with obesity[282] or decreases in infant growth, which might be mediated by impaired fetal growth or low birth weight.[283,284] Three studies have observed increased blood pressure levels in newborns or children in association with $PM_{2.5}$[285] or NO_2 (but not $PM_{2.5}$, PM_{10}, or ozone),[286] or $PM_{2.5}$ and black carbon[287]; though the latter reported decreased blood pressure levels in relation to ozone. Another study reported that living close to a major road at the time of delivery, but not the levels of black carbon or traffic density, were related to markers of cardiometabolic risk.[288]

Long-term postnatal exposure to air pollutants (PM_{10}, NO_2, SO_2, and O_3) was associated with increased risks for childhood obesity and hypertension in a large study ($N > 9000$) conducted in China[289] and NO_2 and $PM_{2.5}$, and several $PM_{2.5}$ constituents were associated with increased diastolic blood pressure in the Netherlands.[290,291] Higher concentrations of short-term PM_{10} and O_3 were also associated with increased blood pressure in China.[292] A recent study also observed associations between postnatal, but not prenatal, exposure to PAHs with childhood obesity.[293] In contrast, other studies observed either no association between postnatal exposure to air pollution and obesity[294] or reported delayed growth in infants with exposure to PM_{10}.[284] Several studies suggest an association between residential traffic density, roadway proximity, and/or traffic-related air pollution and rapid infant weight gain related to exposure at birth[295] and childhood obesity related to later postnatal exposure.[296–298] Regarding diabetes, a recent narrative systematic review suggested an association between air pollution and metabolic dysregulation and diabetes in children based on a summary of six studies performed between 2012 and 2017[299]; a further study also observed alterations in glucose levels in an adolescent population with overweight/obesity, though confounding for sociodemographical factors was not excluded.[300] Overall, there are still few studies and inconsistencies among them; therefore, the evidence on the association between early-life air pollution exposure and cardiometabolic outcomes in childhood and adulthood was rated as "insufficient/inconsistent."

Metals and Metalloids

Several studies have observed delayed (slower) growth or increased obesity in children prenatally or postnatally exposed to cadmium,[43,301–303] arsenic,[302,304,305] mercury,[306] and lead.[307–313] In other studies assessing postnatal exposure, mercury[314] and cadmium[313] were not associated with child growth; or lead or cadmium decreased obesity in children aged 6–19.[315]

Prenatal lead exposure has been associated with elevated blood pressure,[316–318] but not arsenic[317] or mercury.[319] In contrast, nonsignificant associations have been observed with blood pressure for postnatal exposure to lead,[317] mercury,[320] or cadmium.[321,322] For arsenic, postnatal exposure has been associated with blood pressure,[323] though others found no associations.[317,322] Postnatal arsenic exposure during childhood has been linked to greater carotid intima-media thickness,[324] and with lipid profile alterations in one[325] but not in another study.[324]

Because there are still few studies on the association of early-life exposure to metals and cardiometabolic outcomes during childhood and adulthood, the evidence was rated as "insufficient/inconsistent."

Organochlorine Compounds

The evidence for a relationship between prenatal exposure to organochlorine compounds and childhood obesity has been considered moderate in nonsystematic reviews.[326,327] Prenatal DDE exposure has been associated with accelerated weight gain in infancy, accelerated postnatal BMI trajectories, and risk of childhood obesity in several prospective studies[301,328–336] and with increased weight at age 12 but only in boys.[337] Only four recent studies found null or negative associations between prenatal DDE exposure and childhood growth and/or obesity.[338–341] In general, evidence for an association between childhood growth and obesity has been less consistent with prenatal PCB exposure[328,329,331,332,334,335,341] as well as with prenatal HCB and DDT exposure.[301,331–333,335,337,339,341,342] For postnatal exposure there is very little and inconsistent evidence. A study reported no association between DDE exposure during early infancy exposure and obesity in 5- to 9-year-old children.[340] A prospective study in Russian boys observed an association between peripubertal DDE and PCB exposure and delayed growth, instead of accelerated growth, between age 8 and 19 years; such findings were less consistent for HCB and HCH.[312] The effects of organochlorines on blood pressure have been rarely explored. One recent study reported no association between prenatal organochlorine exposures and child serum lipid concentrations in early childhood, but positive associations with blood pressure.[335] Because of the consistent prospective studies for DDE and growth and obesity, the evidence for DDE was rated as moderate. For the rest, it was rated as "insufficient/inconsistent" because of the yet few and inconsistent studies.

Perfluoroalkyl Substances

Some prospective studies evaluating prenatal PFASs exposure (mainly PFOS and PFOA) have reported positive associations between PFOS exposure and infant growth,[343] between PFOS and PFOA exposures and waist-to-height ratio at 5–9 years[344] and between PFOA and BMI and waist circumference in 20-year-old women but not in men.[345] However, other studies have found no association with child BMI and other obesity measures using cross-sectional,[346] retrospective,[347] and prospective[348] study designs. A recent systematic review of 10 prospective studies of PFOAs that included children older than 2 years of age reported associations with BMI (eight prenatal and two postnatal studies) and with overweight (seven prenatal and one postnatal studies).[349] Stratified meta-analysis for BMI showed associations for both the prenatal and postnatal periods.[349] Regarding cardiometabolic health, five recent studies for prenatal[350] and postnatal exposure to PFAS[346,351–353] have reported associations with elevated lipid concentrations in children[346,350] and in adolescents.[351–353] Furthermore, one cross-sectional study reported associations of postnatal exposure to PFNAS, but not other PFAS, with higher lipids and high systolic blood pressure in 48 obese children aged 8–12 years,[354] while another observed no relationship with blood pressure.[355] Some (but not all) previous studies[345,346] and a review[356] have further indicated a link with insulin resistance in relation to prenatal and postnatal PFAS exposure, whereas another one reported lower insulin resistance in adolescents.[353] Finally, a prospective study reported little evidence of an association between low-level prenatal exposure to PFAS and cardiometabolic risk in children.[357] Because of the consistent prospective studies for PFOA with BMI and overweight, the evidence for PFOA was rated as moderate. For the rest, it was rated as "insufficient/inconsistent" because of the yet few and inconsistent studies.

Polybrominated Diphenyl Ethers

There is little evidence on the potential association between PBDE exposure and childhood obesity. Studies on prenatal exposure to

PBDEs observed either increased BMI at 7 years in girls and decreased BMI in boys[358] or decreased BMI, waist circumference and percent body fat in children aged 1–8 years.[359] Another study observed no association between different PBDE congeners measured in colostrum and growth or weight measures in children.[336] Because of the few studies, the classification was "no evidence."

Currently Used Pesticides

Two studies on organophosphate pesticide exposure, defined by maternal employment in greenhouses, observed associations with childhood obesity[76] and with an interaction between PON1 enzyme genotypes and a range of cardiometabolic outcomes.[360] A recent review only identified two studies on blood pressure.[361] In a study of 84 children, only maternal greenhouse occupational exposure during pregnancy was associated with increased systolic blood pressure and a small decrease in BMI in children, but not prenatal paternal occupational exposure or postnatal urine concentrations in children.[362] A cross-sectional study ($n = 271$) observed that a decrease in the acetylcholinesterase activity (inhibited by common pesticides) was associated with lower systolic blood pressure in children living with flower workers, who were considered exposed to organophosphates, among others.[363] A 2018 review on diabetes only identified a preliminary case-control study on pesticides.[364] It observed an increased risk of diabetes type 1 linked to malathion measured in children's serum one month before diagnosis, but negative associations with profenofos and chlorpyrifosmethyl.[365] Because of the few studies by outcome, the classification was "no evidence."

Phthalates

In a 2013 review, six prospective studies indicated associations between phthalate metabolites and child anthropometry.[89] A recent nonsystematic review concluded that findings for prenatal exposure to phthalates in children are inconsistent, with reports of decreases and increases in BMI associated with different prenatal phthalate metabolites in boys or in girls.[366] Other studies report similar inconsistencies: either associations between one out of several phthalates and some adiposity markers both for prenatal and perinatal exposure,[367,368] or decreases in the adiposity markers,[369,370] or no effect at all,[371] or mixed results depending on the phthalate, outcome, and sex.[372–374] Besides, one study observed an association between prenatal exposure to phthalates and decreased blood pressure.[375] In relation to postnatal exposure to phthalates, the above-mentioned recent nonsystematic review indicated mixed findings for child growth and obesity, with five out of nine studies observing positive associations, whereas the rest reported either negative or no associations.[366] While several further studies have also observed increases between some phthalates and some adiposity markers and BMI[376–378] or delayed growth,[379] others have observed either increases or decreases depending on sex, phthalate and/or outcome.[369,370,380] The above-mentioned nonsystematic review also concluded that few studies had examined cardiometabolic outcomes, but they had consistently observed associations with postnatal exposure to phthalates.[366] Some studies have shown associations in children and adolescents in relation to increased blood pressure,[376,381] endothelial dysfunction and decreases in brachial artery distensibility,[382] insulin resistance,[382,383] or mixed results with the lipid profile.[376,382] Because of the inconsistencies in results, the evidence was rated as "insufficient/inconsistent."

Bisphenol A

A recent systematic review and meta-analysis of 33 studies on BPA exposure and cardiometabolic outcomes during childhood and adulthood found overall consistent positive cross-sectional associations between generalized (seven studies) and abdominal (five studies) obesity, CVD (five studies), and hypertension (three studies) and less consistent evidence from five prospective studies on obesity, CVD, and T2D.[384] Studies in children showed inconsistent results, which also depended on the time window of exposure (pre- or postnatal). Regarding prenatal exposure to BPA and child anthropometry, studies have observed either positive,[385–387] negative,[388] or no associations both in individual studies[96,369,374] and a review.[196] Other studies have observed a link between prenatal exposure to BPA and increases or decreases in anthropometric measures depending on sex[389] and associations with DNA methylation of an obesity promoter.[386] Regarding cardiometabolic outcomes, studies have reported associations between prenatal exposure to BPA and increases in blood pressure but decreases in pulse pressure[390] or null associations with blood pressure and lipid profile.[371,389]

Regarding postnatal exposure, studies have reported negative,[388] positive,[389,391,392] and also null associations[382] with child anthropometry, or positive associations either in boys[393] or girls.[369] One study observed associations between postnatal exposure to BPA and increases in blood pressure,[391] whereas others did not.[389] One study observed associations between postnatal exposure to BPA and oxidative stress and albuminuria but not with vascular function, BMI, or insulin resistance.[382] Recent studies have not observed associations with the lipid profile.[371,389,391]

Because of the still small number of studies and several inconsistencies in results, the evidence was rated as "insufficient/inconsistent."

Transportation Noise

Very few studies have examined the effect of environmental noise on children's growth. Two studies have evaluated and observed associations between prenatal exposure to road traffic noise and increased children's growth up to 7 or 8 years of age.[394,395] For postnatal exposure, Weyde et al. (2018) did not find any associations,[394] whereas Christensen et al. (2016) reported a suggestive association with increased overweight at age 7.[395] According to two recent systematic reviews and meta-analysis, the evidence for an association between postnatal exposure to road traffic noise and blood pressure in children is of very low quality,[396] inconsistent and based on very few studies (eight studies in total).[396,397] Most of these studies have evaluated road traffic noise. Kempen et al. (2018) only identified one study on postnatal exposure to aircraft noise, which found a positive but nonsignificant association with blood pressure in children.[396] There is no evidence for railway noise. Because of the few studies, the evidence was rated as "insufficient/inconsistent."

Green Spaces

The few studies available on the effects of green spaces on cardiometabolic health have focused on postnatal exposure and children anthropometry; they were mostly cross-sectional and used different greenness measurements. Some studies have reported associations between some of the greenness measurements and decreased overweight/obesity in children,[398–400] or suggested protective associations in boys but not in girls,[401] whereas others observed no association with obesity markers.[402,403] In turn, a recent study evaluated and observed a protective association between the time spent in green spaces and fasting blood glucose[404]; and also with impaired fasting blood glucose (fasting blood glucose $\geq$ 110 mg/dL) but only in relation to time spent in natural green spaces.[404] Because of the few studies, the evidence was rated as "insufficient/inconsistent."

Summary of the Evidence

Despite increasing concerns, there are still few studies and inconsistencies in findings for most environmental factors. Only the association of DDE and recently for PFOA with growth and/or obesity can be classified as "moderate" based on findings from prospective studies.

EXPOSOME

Pregnant women and children are not exposed to single chemicals, but to complex real-world mixtures. Traditionally, studies of the environmental influences on children's health and development have focused on one-to-one relationships between environmental exposures and health-related endpoints. Very recently, some studies have started studying effects of multiple chemicals, applying statistical techniques that may allow us to unravel some of the complex relationships between multiple exposures and health outcomes.[187,336,405–407] The exposome concept, encompassing the totality of lifetime environmental exposures, offers a useful framework for studying many exposures at the same time, avoiding the selective reporting of only the clearest associations.[408] This research is in its infancy with many outstanding challenges, but efforts are underway including in the field of pregnancy and child health.[409,410] One important challenge in associating the exposome with health outcomes is the simultaneous consideration of many correlated exposures.[411,412] In this context, methodological studies have established that statistical techniques are often limited in their ability to efficiently differentiate true predictors from correlated covariates and that false-positive findings are a concern.[413,414] First "exposome" studies in the area of child health have associated sets of around 100 exposures, from both chemical and physical exposure families, to child health outcomes. One such study based on six European cohorts as part of the HELIX (Human Early-Life Exposome) project, showed that, out of a large set of urban exposome factors measured during pregnancy, green space, and built environment characteristics were associated with birth weight.[415] Another study within HELIX showed that, out of over 100 exposures assessed, prenatal exposure to PFAS and postnatal exposure to phthalates, parabens, facility density, and house crowding were associated with child lung function.[416] These examples show that a systematic "exposome" approach to multiple exposures can avoid problems of selective reporting and publication bias (the cited work published all associations regardless of statistical significance) and, to some extent, confounding by coexposures by use of multiple exposure models. It also highlights challenges related to cross-sectional data, false-positive findings, confounding due to highly correlated exposures, differential measurement errors (i.e., different errors for different exposures), and absence of causal structure.

As an integral part of the exposome, internal, biological responses to environmental exposures can be measured at the molecular level using high-throughput omics techniques, which have great potential for broad and powerful characterization of complete sets of biological molecules; these include metabolomics, proteomics, transcriptomics, and epigenomics. Of particular interest is the identification of biological responses and pathways that respond to and interact with the exposures, leading to adverse health effects, that is, "early pathway perturbations." Such information may be used to improve biological plausibility of associations, to understand how different exposures may act on common pathways, and, ultimately, to predict environmental health-related disease. The early part of the life course is a particularly important period to study such early pathway perturbations: exposures during vulnerable periods may have pronounced effects at the molecular level but may remain clinically undetectable until adulthood. For example, first studies have identified DNA methylation markers related to specific early-life risk factors including smoking and air pollution.[6,417] Others have shown that chemical environmental contaminants (including arsenic, PCBs, tobacco smoke) have a detectable imprint on the metabolomic profiles of pregnant women.[418] In general, though, studies linking environmental exposure to omics have mainly been restricted to small studies on specific pollutants (e.g., phthalates).[419] In this area, larger and more systematic efforts are needed to understand the early biological responses to multiple environmental exposures, and to examine common mechanistic pathways by which different exposures may act to cause one or more health outcomes. Again, the exposome provides a useful framework to stimulate such efforts.

CONCLUSIONS

A relatively large body of evidence has investigated and provides support for the role of early-life exposures (pre- and/or postnatally), often at relatively low exposure levels, in offspring health outcomes. The level of evidence is strong for the association of air pollution and PCBs with fetal growth, the association of metals (particularly lead and methylmercury), organochlorine compounds, and organophosphate pesticides with neurotoxicity, and for the association of air pollution with respiratory outcomes (Table 74-3). There is moderate evidence for the association of PFAS with fetal growth, the association of lead, PCBs, and air pollution with ADHD and autism, the association of air pollution and PBDEs on cognitive development, the association of DDE and PCBs on respiratory and immune health, and the association of DDE and PFOA on childhood obesity (DDE). Such moderate evidence is recent and emerging for certain chemicals of recent concern such as PFAS and PBDEs. For other chemicals, particularly phthalates and BPA, the literature is sparse and characterized by large inconsistencies preventing solid conclusions. Besides, research is needed for their substitutes (e.g., bisphenol F and DINCH), which have similar structure and mechanisms of action. Due to common sharing of sources and routes of exposure (e.g., diet), these environmental exposures (and their measured congeners and metabolites) may be highly correlated, mainly within but also between the different chemical classes (e.g., PCBs, PBDEs, PFASs, and phthalates).[420] It is thus challenging to identify the chemicals, congeners, or metabolites that are responsible for certain effects. Pregnant women and children are not exposed to single chemicals, but to complex real-world mixtures. There is also increasing interest in understanding the early-life effects of noise and green spaces. For example, there is moderate evidence for the association of aircraft noise with reading comprehension and long-term memory and increasing evidence for the benefits of green spaces on cognitive development in children.

BOX 74-5 Measuring Biomarkers of Chemical Pollutants

In recent years, the use of exposure biomarkers has risen rapidly in the study of environmental contaminants and child health, often signifying a large improvement over other exposure assessments such as questionnaire-based ones or environmental measurements (e.g., pesticides). However, uncertainties also exist in the use of biomarkers. For example, for the nonpersistent chemicals (phthalates, BPA, currently used pesticides) it is difficult to characterize exposure since they have short biological half-lives and are eliminated from the body in a few hours or days. Studies measuring biomarkers in only one spot urine sample are thus prone to exposure misclassification, which is expected to cause attenuation bias in exposure-response functions, reducing our ability to detect true positive associations. Recent studies have shown that even when pooling many urine samples collected during an entire week, the variability of some of these compounds is still very high. Future studies assessing these compounds should consider a thoughtful sampling design based on many pooled urines. This contrasts sharply with the more persistent groups of chemicals (POPs, some metals) that have half-lives of years; here, one biomarker measurement can give a good estimate of long-term past exposure and more certainty in the epidemiological dose–response estimates. However, lack of understanding of physiological characteristics and pharmacokinetic issues still complicates the interpretation of biomonitoring data, even for the persistent chemicals. For example, urinary flowrate, glomerular filtration rate, and pregnancy weight gain may influence the concentrations of measured biomarkers. In addition, lipophilic POPs store in fat tissue and metabolic and physiological factors, including obesity itself, can influence the circulating concentrations of these chemicals in blood. For all these reasons, cross-sectional associations with biomarkers of both nonpersistent and persistent chemicals are subject to reverse causality.

However, the evidence is generally insufficient or inconsistent, due to few studies available with sufficient quality and/or with comparable assessments.

The childhood health endpoints included in this review may be important precursors of adult morbidity and mortality. The disease costs associated with these life-long consequences may be substantial: particulate air pollution (combined effects of ambient particles and household smoke) is the leading environmental contributor to the global burden of disease,[421,422] exposure to environmental noise has been ranked as the second greatest environmental contributor to the burden of disease in Europe, after air pollution,[423–426] and, together, air pollution and noise have been estimated to have a social cost of up to €1 trillion every year in the European Union, which is higher than that of smoking.[427] Exposure to endocrine disrupting chemicals has been estimated to cost the European Union $157 billion in total disease and dysfunction across the life-course,[428] and loss of IQ due to lead and mercury exposure has been estimated to cost the United States, respectively, $50 and $5 billion annually.[8]

Exposing the next generation to potential environmental hazards during early life, when the likely effects are irreversible and have long-term consequences for human health is a major issue for public health. Public health interventions have been shown to greatly reduce the burden of damage caused by environmental factors, such as for the case of early-life exposure to lead or second-hand smoking. However, it took decades to generate evidence that was considered sufficient to justify action given the need to provide "ideal evidence" and the resistance of economical forces. Moreover, for most of the current exposures of the hazards reviewed here, the risk assessment and management has been poorly conducted. The evaluation of the environmental hazards during early life and its potential management should be prioritized because of the vulnerably of the time period, the populations affected (i.e., children) and the likely long-term consequences on health.

Therefore, there is possibly need to apply the precautionary principle (take action on harmful issues without complete scientific certainty) and give social and legal institutions greater urgency to protect pregnancy and early life from environmental hazards. Because policy-makers may take decades to enact legislation, meanwhile parents may also need advice to understand the importance of avoiding or reducing early-life exposures to hazardous environmental factors such as, for example, prenatal exposure to lead or air pollution. This advice can be provided by acknowledgeable health actors for parents, such as the reproductive healthcare providers and pediatricians, as well as by other health professionals that act at community level and participate in health protection and promotion programs. For some cases, such as for smoking, mercury or lead, health professional societies have developed guidelines.

In conclusion, early life is a vulnerable period of exposure to environmental hazards for children's health and for long-term health consequences that requires special protection and public health interventions.

References

1. Barker DJP. The origins of the developmental origins theory. *J Intern Med.* 2007;261(5):412–7.
2. Lucas A. Role of nutritional programming in determining adult morbidity. *Arch Dis Child.* 1994;71(4):288–90.
3. Sunyer J, Dadvand P. Pre-natal brain development as a target for urban air pollution. *Basic Clin Pharmacol Toxicol.* 2019;125(Suppl 3):81–8.
4. Kondo K. Congenital Minamata disease: Warnings from Japan's experience. *J Child Neurol.* 2000;15(7):458–64.
5. Herbst AL, Ulfelder H, Poskanzer DC. Adenocarcinoma of the Vagina. *N Engl J Med.* 1971;284(16):878–81.
6. Joubert BR, Felix JF, Yousefi P, et al. DNA methylation in newborns and maternal smoking in pregnancy: Genome-wide consortium meta-analysis. *Am J Hum Genet.* 2016;98(4):680–96.
7. Illa M, Eixarch E, Muñoz-Moreno E, et al. Neurodevelopmental effects of undernutrition and placental underperfusion in fetal growth restriction rabbit models. *Fetal Diagn Ther.* 2017;42(3):189–97.
8. Grandjean P, Landrigan PJ. Neurobehavioural effects of developmental toxicity. *Lancet Neurol.* 2014;13(3):330–8.
9. Lumey LH, Stein AD, Kahn HS, et al. Cohort profile: The Dutch Hunger Winter families study. *Int J Epidemiol.* 2007;36(6):1196–204.
10. Roseboom TJ, van der Meulen JH, Osmond C, et al. Coronary heart disease after prenatal exposure to the Dutch famine, 1944–45. *Heart.* 2000;84(6):595–8.
11. Ravelli AC, van der Meulen JH, Osmond C, Barker DJ, Bleker OP. Obesity at the age of 50 y in men and women exposed to famine prenatally. *Am J Clin Nutr.* 1999;70(5):811–6.
12. Ravelli A, van der Meulen J, Michels R, et al. Glucose tolerance in adults after prenatal exposure to famine. *Lancet.* 1998;351(9097):173–7.
13. Susser E, Neugebauer R, Hoek HW, et al. Schizophrenia after prenatal famine. Further evidence. *Arch Gen Psychiatry.* 1996;53(1):25–31.
14. Tobi EW, Goeman JJ, Monajemi R, et al. DNA methylation signatures link prenatal famine exposure to growth and metabolism. *Nat Commun.* 2014;5(1):5592.
15. Slama R, Ballester F, Casas MC, et al. Epidemiologic tools to study the influence of environmental factors on fecundity and pregnancy-related outcomes. *Epidemiol Rev.* 2014;36(1):148–64.
16. Wigle DT, Arbuckle TE, Turner MC, et al. Epidemiologic evidence of relationships between reproductive and child health outcomes and environmental chemical contaminants. *J Toxicol Environ Health B Crit Rev.* 2008;11(5–6):373–517.
17. Bonzini M, Carugno M, Grillo P, Mensi C, Bertazzi PA, Pesatori AC. Impact of ambient air pollution on birth outcomes: Systematic review of the current evidences. *Med Lav.* 2010;101(5):341–63.
18. Shah PS, Balkhair T. Air pollution and birth outcomes: A systematic review. *Environ Int.* 2011;37(2):498–516.
19. Stieb DM, Chen L, Eshoul M, Judek S. Ambient air pollution, birth weight and preterm birth: A systematic review and meta-analysis. *Environ Res.* 2012;117:100–11.
20. Dadvand P, Parker J, Bell ML, et al. Maternal exposure to particulate air pollution and term birth weight: A multi-country evaluation of effect and heterogeneity. *Environ Health Perspect.* 2013;121(3):267–373.
21. Pedersen M, Giorgis-Allemand L, Bernard C, et al. Ambient air pollution and low birthweight: A European cohort study (ESCAPE). *Lancet Respir Med.* 2013;1(9):695–704.
22. Lai H-K, Tsang H, Wong C-M. Meta-analysis of adverse health effects due to air pollution in Chinese populations. *BMC Public Health.* 2013;13(1):360.
23. Li X, Huang S, Jiao A, et al. Association between ambient fine particulate matter and preterm birth or term low birth weight: An updated systematic review and meta-analysis. *Environ Pollut.* 2017;227:596–605.
24. Garcia-Esquinas E, Perez-Gomez B, Fernandez-Navarro P, et al. Lead, mercury and cadmium in umbilical cord blood and its association with parental epidemiological variables and birth factors. *BMC Public Health.* 2013;13:841.
25. Luo Y, McCullough LE, Tzeng J-Y, et al. Maternal blood cadmium, lead and arsenic levels, nutrient combinations, and offspring birthweight. *BMC Public Health.* 2017;17(1):354.
26. Tatsuta N, Kurokawa N, Nakai K, et al. Effects of intrauterine exposures to polychlorinated biphenyls, methylmercury, and lead on birth weight in Japanese male and female newborns. *Environ Health Prev Med.* 2017;22(1):39.
27. Li J, Wang H, Hao J-H, et al. Maternal serum lead level during pregnancy is positively correlated with risk of preterm birth in a Chinese population. *Environ Pollut.* 2017;227:484–9.
28. Rabito FA, Kocak M, Werthmann DW, Tylavsky FA, Palmer CD, Parsons PJ. Changes in low levels of lead over the course of pregnancy and the association with birth outcomes. *Reprod Toxicol.* 2014;50:138–44.
29. Rodosthenous RS, Burris HH, Svensson K, et al. Prenatal lead exposure and fetal growth: Smaller infants have heightened susceptibility. *Environ Int.* 2017;99:228–33.
30. Taylor CM, Golding J, Emond AM. Adverse effects of maternal lead levels on birth outcomes in the ALSPAC study: A prospective birth cohort study. *BJOG.* 2015;122(3):322–8.
31. Vigeh M, Yokoyama K, Seyedaghamiri Z, et al. Blood lead at currently acceptable levels may cause preterm labour. *Occup Environ Med.* 2011;68(3):231–4.

32. Gundacker C, Frohlich S, Graf-Rohrmeister K, et al. Perinatal lead and mercury exposure in Austria. *Sci Total Environ*. 2010;408(23):5744–9.
33. Zhu M, Fitzgerald EF, Gelberg KH, Lin S, Druschel CM. Maternal low-level lead exposure and fetal growth. *Environ Health Perspect*. 2010;118(10):1471–5.
34. Taylor CM, Tilling K, Golding J, Emond AM. Low level lead exposure and pregnancy outcomes in an observational birth cohort study: Dose-response relationships. *BMC Res Notes*. 2016;9:291.
35. Ramón R, Ballester F, Aguinagalde X, et al. Fish consumption during pregnancy, prenatal mercury exposure, and anthropometric measures at birth in a prospective mother-infant cohort study in Spain. *Am J Clin Nutr*. 2009;90(4):1047–55.
36. Vejrup K, Brantsæter AL, Knutsen HK, et al. Prenatal mercury exposure and infant birth weight in the Norwegian mother and child cohort study. *Public Health Nutr*. 2014;17(9):2071–80.
37. Kim B-M, Chen M-H, Chen P-C, et al. Path analysis of prenatal mercury levels and birth weights in Korean and Taiwanese birth cohorts. *Sci Total Environ*. 2017;605–6:1003–10.
38. Ballester F, Iniguez C, Murcia M, et al. Prenatal exposure to mercury and longitudinally assessed fetal growth: Relation and effect modifiers. *Environ Res*. 2018;160:97–106.
39. Drouillet-Pinard P, Huel G, Slama R, et al. Prenatal mercury contamination: Relationship with maternal seafood consumption during pregnancy and fetal growth in the 'EDEN mother–child' cohort. *Br J Nutr*. 2010;104(8):1096–100.
40. Ding G, Cui C, Chen L, et al. Prenatal low-level mercury exposure and neonatal anthropometry in rural northern China. *Chemosphere*. 2013;92(9):1085–9.
41. Miyashita C, Sasaki S, Ikeno T, et al. Effects of in utero exposure to polychlorinated biphenyls, methylmercury, and polyunsaturated fatty acids on birth size. *Sci Total Environ*. 2015;533:256–65.
42. Taylor CM, Golding J, Emond AM. Blood mercury levels and fish consumption in pregnancy: Risks and benefits for birth outcomes in a prospective observational birth cohort. *Int J Hyg Environ Health*. 2016;219(6):513–20.
43. Lin C-M, Doyle P, Wang D, Hwang Y-H, Chen P-C. Does prenatal cadmium exposure affect fetal and child growth? *Occup Environ Med*. 2011;68(9):641–6.
44. Menai M, Heude B, Slama R, et al. Association between maternal blood cadmium during pregnancy and birth weight and the risk of fetal growth restriction: The EDEN mother–child cohort study. *Reprod Toxicol*. 2012;34(4):622–7.
45. Kippler M, Tofail F, Gardner R, et al. Maternal cadmium exposure during pregnancy and size at birth: A prospective cohort study. *Environ Health Perspect*. 2012;120(2):284–9.
46. Sun H, Chen W, Wang D, Jin Y, Chen X, Xu Y. The effects of prenatal exposure to low-level cadmium, lead and selenium on birth outcomes. *Chemosphere*. 2014;108:33–9.
47. Johnston JE, Valentiner E, Maxson P, Miranda ML, Fry RC. Maternal cadmium levels during pregnancy associated with lower birth weight in infants in a North Carolina cohort. Chen A, editor. *PLoS One*. 2014;9(10):e109661.
48. Al-Saleh I, Al-Rouqi R, Obsum CA, et al. Interaction between cadmium (Cd), selenium (Se) and oxidative stress biomarkers in healthy mothers and its impact on birth anthropometric measures. *Int J Hyg Environ Health*. 2015;218(1):66–90.
49. Bloom MS, Surdu S, Neamtiu IA, Gurzau ES. Maternal arsenic exposure and birth outcomes: A comprehensive review of the epidemiologic literature focused on drinking water. *Int J Hyg Environ Health*. 2014;217(7):709–19.
50. Quansah R, Armah FA, Essumang DK, et al. Association of arsenic with adverse pregnancy outcomes/infant mortality: A systematic review and meta-analysis. *Environ Health Perspect*. 2015;123(5):412–21.
51. Milton AH, Hussain S, Akter S, Rahman M, Mouly TA, Mitchell K. A review of the effects of chronic arsenic exposure on adverse pregnancy outcomes. *Int J Environ Res Public Health*. 2017;14(6):556.
52. Rahman A, Granberg C, Persson L-A. Early life arsenic exposure, infant and child growth, and morbidity: A systematic review. *Arch Toxicol*. 2017;91(11):3459–67.
53. Rahman ML, Valeri L, Kile ML, et al. Investigating causal relation between prenatal arsenic exposure and birthweight: Are smaller infants more susceptible? *Environ Int*. 2017;108:32–40.
54. Liu H, Lu S, Zhang B, et al. Maternal arsenic exposure and birth outcomes: A birth cohort study in Wuhan, China. *Environ Pollut*. 2018;236: 817–23.
55. Liao K-W, Chang C-H, Tsai M-S, et al. Associations between urinary total arsenic levels, fetal development, and neonatal birth outcomes: A cohort study in Taiwan. *Sci Total Environ*. 2018;612:1373–9.
56. Davis MA, Higgins J, Li Z, et al. Preliminary analysis of in utero low-level arsenic exposure and fetal growth using biometric measurements extracted from fetal ultrasound reports. *Environ Health*. 2015;14(1):12.
57. Laine JE, Bailey KA, Rubio-Andrade M, et al. Maternal arsenic exposure, arsenic methylation efficiency, and birth outcomes in the Biomarkers of Exposure to ARsenic (BEAR) pregnancy cohort in Mexico. *Environ Health Perspect*. 2015;123(2):186–92.
58. Stillerman KP, Mattison DR, Giudice LC, Woodruff TJ. Environmental exposures and adverse pregnancy outcomes: A review of the science. *Reprod Sci*. 2008;15(7):631–50.
59. Govarts E, Nieuwenhuijsen M, Schoeters G, et al. Birth weight and prenatal exposure to polychlorinated biphenyls (PCBs) and dichlorodiphenyl-dichloroethylene (DDE): A meta-analysis within 12 European birth cohorts. *Environ Health Perspect*. 2012;120(2):162–70.
60. Casas M, Nieuwenhuijsen M, Martínez D, et al. Prenatal exposure to PCB-153, p,p′-DDE and birth outcomes in 9000 mother–child pairs: Exposure–response relationship and effect modifiers. *Environ Int*. 2015;74:23–31.
61. Basterrechea M, Lertxundi A, Iñiguez C, et al. Prenatal exposure to hexachlorobenzene (HCB) and reproductive effects in a multicentre birth cohort in spain. *Sci Total Environ*. 2014;466–7:770–6.
62. Guo H, Jin Y, Cheng Y, et al. Prenatal exposure to organochlorine pesticides and infant birth weight in China. *Chemosphere*. 2014;110:1–7.
63. Vafeiadi M, Vrijheid M, Fthenou E, et al. Persistent organic pollutants exposure during pregnancy, maternal gestational weight gain, and birth outcomes in the mother–child cohort in Crete, Greece (RHEA study). *Environ Int*. 2014;64:116–23.
64. Vafeiadi M, Agramunt S, Pedersen M, et al. In utero exposure to compounds with dioxin-like activity and birth outcomes. *Epidemiology*. 2014;25(2):215–24.
65. Lenters V, Portengen L, Rignell-Hydbom A, et al. Prenatal phthalate, perfluoroalkyl acid, and organochlorine exposures and term birth weight in three birth cohorts: Multi-pollutant models based on elastic net regression. *Environ Health Perspect*. 2016;124(3):365–72.
66. Arrebola JP, Cuellar M, Bonde JP, Gonzalez-Alzaga B, Mercado LA. Associations of maternal o,p'-DDT and p,p'-DDE levels with birth outcomes in a Bolivian cohort. *Environ Res*. 2016;151:469–77.
67. Woods MM, Lanphear BP, Braun JM, McCandless LC. Gestational exposure to endocrine disrupting chemicals in relation to infant birth weight: A Bayesian analysis of the HOME Study. *Environ Health*. 2017;16(1):115.
68. Callan AC, Hinwood AL, Heyworth J, Phi DT, Odland JO. Sex specific influence on the relationship between maternal exposures to persistent chemicals and birth outcomes. *Int J Hyg Environ Health*. 2016;219(8):734–41.
69. Valvi D, Oulhote Y, Weihe P, et al. Gestational diabetes and offspring birth size at elevated environmental pollutant exposures. *Environ Int*. 2017;107:205–15.
70. Johnson PI, Sutton P, Atchley DS, et al. The navigation guide—Evidence-based medicine meets environmental health: Systematic review of human evidence for PFOA effects on fetal growth. *Environ Health Perspect*. 2014;122(10):1028–39.
71. Bach CC, Bech BH, Brix N, Nohr EA, Bonde JPE, Henriksen TB. Perfluoroalkyl and polyfluoroalkyl substances and human fetal growth: A systematic review. *Crit Rev Toxicol*. 2015;45(1):53–67.
72. Verner M-A, Loccisano AE, Morken N-H, et al. Associations of perfluoroalkyl substances (PFAS) with lower birth weight: An evaluation of potential confounding by glomerular filtration rate using a physiologically based pharmacokinetic model (PBPK). *Environ Health Perspect*. 2015;123(12):1317–24.
73. Negri E, Metruccio F, Guercio V, et al. Exposure to PFOA and PFOS and fetal growth: A critical merging of toxicological and epidemiological data. *Crit Rev Toxicol*. 2017;47(6):489–515.
74. Zhao X, Peng S, Xiang Y, et al. Correlation between prenatal exposure to polybrominated diphenyl ethers (PBDEs) and infant birth outcomes: A meta-analysis and an experimental study. *Int J Environ Res Public Health*. 2017;14(3):268.
75. Sathyanarayana S, Basso O, Karr CJ, et al. Maternal pesticide use and birth weight in the agricultural health study. *J Agromedicine*. 2010;15(2):127–36.
76. Wohlfahrt-Veje C, Main KM, Schmidt IM, et al. Lower birth weight and increased body fat at school age in children prenatally exposed to modern pesticides: A prospective study. *Environ Health*. 2011;10(1):79.

77. Petit C, Chevrier C, Durand G, et al. Impact on fetal growth of prenatal exposure to pesticides due to agricultural activities: A prospective cohort study in Brittany, France. *Environ Health*. 2010;9(1):71.
78. Petit C, Blangiardo M, Richardson S, Coquet F, Chevrier C, Cordier S. Association of environmental insecticide exposure and fetal growth with a Bayesian model including multiple exposure sources: The PELAGIE mother-child cohort. *Am J Epidemiol*. 2012;175(11):1182–90.
79. Larsen AE, Gaines SD, Deschenes O. Agricultural pesticide use and adverse birth outcomes in the San Joaquin Valley of California. *Nat Commun*. 2017;8(1):302.
80. Wolff MS, Engel S, Berkowitz G, et al. Prenatal pesticide and PCB exposures and birth outcomes. *Pediatr Res*. 2007;61(2):243–50.
81. Harley KG, Huen K, Aguilar Schall R, et al. Association of organophosphate pesticide exposure and paraoxonase with birth outcome in Mexican-American women. Vitzthum VJ, editor. *PLoS One*. 2011;6(8):e23923.
82. Rauch SA, Braun JM, Barr DB, et al. Associations of prenatal exposure to organophosphate pesticide metabolites with gestational age and birth weight. *Environ Health Perspect*. 2012;120(7):1055–60.
83. Harley KG, Engel SM, Vedar MG, et al. Prenatal exposure to organophosphorous pesticides and fetal growth: Pooled results from four longitudinal birth cohort studies. *Environ Health Perspect*. 2016;124(7):1084–92.
84. Naksen W, Prapamontol T, Mangklabruks A, et al. Associations of maternal organophosphate pesticide exposure and PON1 activity with birth outcomes in SAWASDEE birth cohort, Thailand. *Environ Res*. 2015;142:288–96.
85. Saillenfait A-M, Ndiaye D, Sabaté J-P. Pyrethroids: Exposure and health effects—An update. *Int J Hyg Environ Health*. 2015;218(3):281–92.
86. Shaw GM, Yang W, Roberts EM, et al. Residential agricultural pesticide exposures and risks of spontaneous preterm birth. *Epidemiology*. 2018;29(1):8–21.
87. Winchester P, Proctor C, Ying J. County-level pesticide use and risk of shortened gestation and preterm birth. *Acta Paediatr*. 2016;105(3):e107–15.
88. Ferguson KK, O'Neill MS, Meeker JD. Environmental contaminant exposures and preterm birth: A comprehensive review. *J Toxicol Environ Health B Crit Rev*. 2013;16(2):69–113.
89. Braun JM, Sathyanarayana S, Hauser R. Phthalate exposure and children's health. *Curr Opin Pediatr*. 2013;25(2):247–54.
90. Zarean M, Keikha M, Poursafa P, Khalighinejad P, Amin M, Kelishadi R. A systematic review on the adverse health effects of di-2-ethylhexyl phthalate. *Environ Sci Pollut Res*. 2016;23(24):24642–93.
91. Huang Y, Li J, Garcia JM, Lin H, et al. Phthalate levels in cord blood are associated with preterm delivery and fetal growth parameters in Chinese women. Chen A, editor. *PLoS One*. 2014;9(2):e87430.
92. Casas M, Valvi D, Ballesteros-Gomez A, et al. Exposure to bisphenol A and phthalates during pregnancy and ultrasound measures of fetal growth in the INMA-Sabadell cohort. *Environ Health Perspect*. 2016;124(4):521–8.
93. Zhang Y-W, Gao H, Mao L-J, et al. Effects of the phthalate exposure during three gestation periods on birth weight and their gender differences: A birth cohort study in China. *Sci Total Environ*. 2018;613–4:1573–8.
94. Peretz J, Vrooman L, Ricke WA, et al. Bisphenol A and reproductive health: Update of experimental and human evidence, 2007–2013. *Environ Health Perspect*. 2014;122(8):775–86.
95. Rochester JR. Bisphenol A and human health: A review of the literature. *Reprod Toxicol*. 2013;42:132–55.
96. Philippat C, Botton J, Calafat AM, et al. Prenatal exposure to phenols and growth in boys. *Epidemiology*. 2014;25(5):625–35.
97. Hu C-Y, Li F-L, Hua X-G, Jiang W, Mao C, Zhang X-J. The association between prenatal bisphenol A exposure and birth weight: A meta-analysis. *Reprod Toxicol*. 2018;79:21–31.
98. Nieuwenhuijsen MJ, Ristovska G, Dadvand P. WHO environmental noise guidelines for the European region: A systematic review on environmental noise and adverse birth outcomes. *Int J Environ Res Public Health*. 2017;14(10):1252.
99. Smith RB, Fecht D, Gulliver J, Beevers SD, Dajnak D, Blangiardo M, et al. Impact of London's road traffic air and noise pollution on birth weight: Retrospective population based cohort study. *BMJ*. 2017 Dec;359:j5299.
100. Barba-Vasseur M, Bernard N, Pujol S, et al. Does low to moderate environmental exposure to noise and air pollution influence preterm delivery in medium-sized cities? *Int J Epidemiol*. 2017;46(6):2017–27.
101. Kondo M, Fluehr J, McKeon T, et al. Urban green space and its impact on human health. *Int J Environ Res Public Health*. 2018;15(3):445.
102. Banay RF, Bezold CP, James P, Hart JE, Laden F. Residential greenness: Current perspectives on its impact on maternal health and pregnancy outcomes. *Int J Womens Health*. 2017;9:133–44.
103. Suades-Gonzalez E, Gascon M, Guxens M, Sunyer J. Air pollution and neuropsychological development: A review of the latest evidence. *Endocrinology*. 2015;156(10):3473–82.
104. Block ML, Elder A, Auten RL, et al. The outdoor air pollution and brain health workshop. *Neurotoxicology*. 2012;33(5):972––84.
105. Levy RJ. Carbon monoxide pollution and neurodevelopment: A public health concern. *Neurotoxicol Teratol*. 2015;49:31–40.
106. Lyall K, Schmidt RJ, Hertz-Picciotto I. Maternal lifestyle and environmental risk factors for autism spectrum disorders. *Int J Epidemiol*. 2014;43(2):443–64.
107. Ornoy A, Weinstein-Fudim L, Ergaz Z. Prenatal factors associated with autism spectrum disorder (ASD). *Reprod Toxicol*. 2015;56:155–69.
108. Rossignol DA, Genuis SJ, Frye RE. Environmental toxicants and autism spectrum disorders: A systematic review. *Transl Psychiatry*. 2014;4(2):e360.
109. Flores-Pajot M-C, Ofner M, Do MT, Lavigne E, Villeneuve PJ. Childhood autism spectrum disorders and exposure to nitrogen dioxide, and particulate matter air pollution: A review and meta-analysis. *Environ Res*. 2016;151:763–76.
110. Raz R, Levine H, Pinto O, Broday DM, Yuval N, Weisskopf MG. Traffic-related air pollution and autism spectrum disorder: A population-based nested case-control study in Israel. *Am J Epidemiol*. 2018;187(4):717–25.
111. Guxens M, Ghassabian A, Gong T, et al. Air pollution exposure during pregnancy and childhood autistic traits in four European population-based cohort studies: The ESCAPE project. *Environ Health Perspect*. 2016;124(1):133–40.
112. Chiu Y-HM, Hsu H-HL, Coull BA, et al. Prenatal particulate air pollution and neurodevelopment in urban children: Examining sensitive windows and sex-specific associations. *Environ Int*. 2016;87:56–65.
113. Harris MH, Gold DR, Rifas-Shiman SL, et al. Prenatal and childhood traffic-related air pollution exposure and childhood executive function and behavior. *Neurotoxicol Teratol*. 2016;57:60–70.
114. Forns J, Sunyer J, Garcia-Esteban R, et al. Air pollution exposure during pregnancy and symptoms of attention deficit and hyperactivity disorder in children in Europe. *Epidemiology*. 2018;29(5):618–26.
115. Yorifuji T, Kashima S, Diez MH, Kado Y, Sanada S, Doi H. Prenatal exposure to outdoor air pollution and child behavioral problems at school age in Japan. *Environ Int*. 2017;99:192–8.
116. Sunyer J, Esnaola M, Alvarez-Pedrerol M, et al. Association between traffic-related air pollution in schools and cognitive development in primary school children: A prospective cohort study. Lanphear BP, editor. *PLoS Med*. 2015;12(3):e1001792.
117. Alvarez-Pedrerol M, Rivas I, Lopez-Vicente M, et al. Impact of commuting exposure to traffic-related air pollution on cognitive development in children walking to school. *Environ Pollut*. 2017;231(Pt 1):837–44.
118. Forns J, Dadvand P, Foraster M, et al. Traffic-related air pollution, noise at school, and behavioral problems in Barcelona schoolchildren: A cross-sectional study. *Environ Health Perspect*. 2016;124(4):529–35.
119. Basagaña X, Esnaola M, Rivas I, et al. Neurodevelopmental deceleration by urban fine particles from different emission sources: A longitudinal observational study. *Environ Health Perspect*. 2016;124(10):1630–6.
120. Sunyer J, Suades-Gonzalez E, Garcia-Esteban R, et al. Traffic-related air pollution and attention in primary school children: Short-term association. *Epidemiology*. 2017;28(2):181–9.
121. de Prado Bert P, Mercader EMH, Pujol J, Sunyer J, Mortamais M. The effects of air pollution on the brain: A review of studies interfacing environmental epidemiology and neuroimaging. *Curr Environ Health Rep*. 2018;5(3):351–64.
122. Peterson BS, Rauh VA, Bansal R, et al. Effects of prenatal exposure to air pollutants (polycyclic aromatic hydrocarbons) on the development of brain white matter, cognition, and behavior in later childhood. *JAMA Psychiatry*. 2015;72(6):531.
123. Guxens M, Lubczynska MJ, Muetzel RL, et al. Air pollution exposure during fetal life, brain morphology, and cognitive function in school-age children. *Biol Psychiatry*. 2018;84(4):295–303.
124. Debes F, Budtz-Jørgensen E, Weihe P, White RF, Grandjean P. Impact of prenatal methylmercury exposure on neurobehavioral function at age 14 years. *Neurotoxicol Teratol*. 2006;28(5):536–47.

125. van Wijngaarden E, Thurston SW, Myers GJ, et al. Prenatal methyl mercury exposure in relation to neurodevelopment and behavior at 19 years of age in the Seychelles child development study. *Neurotoxicol Teratol.* 2013;39:19–25.

126. Strain J, Yeates AJ, van Wijngaarden E, et al. Prenatal exposure to methyl mercury from fish consumption and polyunsaturated fatty acids: Associations with child development at 20 mo of age in an observational study in the Republic of Seychelles. *Am J Clin Nutr.* 2015;101(3):530–7.

127. Julvez J, Méndez M, Fernandez-Barres S, et al. Maternal consumption of seafood in pregnancy and child neuropsychological development: A longitudinal study based on a population with high consumption levels. *Am J Epidemiol.* 2016;183(3):169–82.

128. Yoshimasu K, Kiyohara C, Takemura S, Nakai K. A meta-analysis of the evidence on the impact of prenatal and early infancy exposures to mercury on autism and attention deficit/hyperactivity disorder in the childhood. *Neurotoxicology.* 2014;44:121–31.

129. Golding J, Rai D, Gregory S, et al. Prenatal mercury exposure and features of autism: A prospective population study. *Mol Autism.* 2018;9:30.

130. Llop S, Ballester F, Murcia M, et al. Prenatal exposure to mercury and neuropsychological development in young children: The role of fish consumption. *Int J Epidemiol.* 2017;46(3):827–38.

131. Allen KA. Is prenatal lead exposure a concern in infancy? What is the evidence? *Adv Neonatal Care.* 2015;15(6):416–20.

132. Tamayo Y Ortiz M, Tellez-Rojo MM, Trejo-Valdivia B, et al. Maternal stress modifies the effect of exposure to lead during pregnancy and 24-month old children's neurodevelopment. *Environ Int.* 2017;98:191–7.

133. Neugebauer J, Wittsiepe J, Kasper-Sonnenberg M, Schoneck N, Scholmerich A, Wilhelm M. The influence of low level pre- and perinatal exposure to PCDD/Fs, PCBs, and lead on attention performance and attention-related behavior among German school-aged children: Results from the Duisburg birth cohort study. *Int J Hyg Environ Health.* 2015;218(1):153–62.

134. Taylor CM, Kordas K, Golding J, Emond AM. Data relating to prenatal lead exposure and child IQ at 4 and 8 years old in the Avon Longitudinal Study of Parents and Children. *Neurotoxicology.* 2017;62:224–30.

135. Horton MK, Hsu L, Claus Henn B, et al. Dentine biomarkers of prenatal and early childhood exposure to manganese, zinc and lead and childhood behavior. *Environ Int.* 2018;121(Pt 1):148–58.

136. Joo H, Choi JH, Burm E, et al. Gender difference in the effects of lead exposure at different time windows on neurobehavioral development in 5-year-old children. *Sci Total Environ.* 2018;615:1086–92.

137. Singh G, Singh V, Sobolewski M, Cory-Slechta DA, Schneider JS. Sex-dependent effects of developmental lead exposure on the brain. *Front Genet.* 2018;9:89.

138. Zhou L, Xu J, Zhang J, et al. Prenatal maternal stress in relation to the effects of prenatal lead exposure on toddler cognitive development. *Neurotoxicology.* 2017;59:71–8.

139. Lanphear BP, Hornung R, Khoury J, et al. Low-level environmental lead exposure and children's intellectual function: An international pooled analysis. *Environ Health Perspect.* 2005;113(7):894–9.

140. Budtz-Jørgensen E, Bellinger D, Lanphear B, Grandjean P. An international pooled analysis for obtaining a benchmark dose for environmental lead exposure in children. *Risk Anal.* 2013;33(3):450–61.

141. Wu Y, Sun J, Wang M, Yu G, Yu L, Wang C. The relationship of children's intelligence quotient and blood lead and zinc levels: A meta-analysis and system review. *Biol Trace Elem Res.* 2018;182(2):185–95.

142. He J, Ning H, Huang R. Low blood lead levels and attention-deficit hyperactivity disorder in children: A systematic review and meta-analysis. *Environ Sci Pollut Res Int.* 2019;26(18):17875–84.

143. Beckwith TJ, Dietrich KN, Wright JP, Altaye M, Cecil KM. Reduced regional volumes associated with total psychopathy scores in an adult population with childhood lead exposure. *Neurotoxicology.* 2018;67:1–26.

144. Sanders AP, Claus Henn B, Wright RO. Perinatal and childhood exposure to cadmium, manganese, and metal mixtures and effects on cognition and behavior: A review of recent literature. *Curr Environ Health Rep.* 2015;2(3):284–94.

145. Gustin K, Tofail F, Vahter M, Kippler M. Cadmium exposure and cognitive abilities and behavior at 10years of age: A prospective cohort study. *Environ Int.* 2018;113:259–68.

146. Kippler M, Bottai M, Georgiou V, et al. Impact of prenatal exposure to cadmium on cognitive development at preschool age and the importance of selenium and iodine. *Eur J Epidemiol.* 2016;31(11):1123–34.

147. Wang Y, Chen L, Gao Y, et al. Effects of prenatal exposure to cadmium on neurodevelopment of infants in Shandong, China. *Environ Pollut.* 2016;211:67–73.

148. Taylor CM, Emond AM, Lingam R, Golding J. Prenatal lead, cadmium and mercury exposure and associations with motor skills at age 7 years in a UK observational birth cohort. *Environ Int.* 2018;117:40–7.

149. Pan S, Lin L, Zeng F, et al. Effects of lead, cadmium, arsenic, and mercury co-exposure on children's intelligence quotient in an industrialized area of southern China. *Environ Pollut.* 2018;235:47–54.

150. Rodríguez-Barranco M, Lacasaña M, Aguilar-Garduño C, et al. Association of arsenic, cadmium and manganese exposure with neurodevelopment and behavioural disorders in children: A systematic review and meta-analysis. *Sci Total Environ.* 2013;454–5:562–77.

151. Rodrigues EG, Bellinger DC, Valeri L, et al. Neurodevelopmental outcomes among 2- to 3-year-old children in Bangladesh with elevated blood lead and exposure to arsenic and manganese in drinking water. *Environ Health.* 2016;15:44.

152. Rodriguez-Barranco M, Gil F, Hernandez AF, et al. Postnatal arsenic exposure and attention impairment in school children. *Cortex.* 2016;74:370–82.

153. Wasserman GA, Liu X, Parvez F, et al. Child intelligence and reductions in water arsenic and manganese: A two-year follow-up study in Bangladesh. *Environ Health Perspect.* 2016;124(7):1114–20.

154. Desai G, Barg G, Queirolo EI, et al. A cross-sectional study of general cognitive abilities among Uruguayan school children with low-level arsenic exposure, potential effect modification by methylation capacity and dietary folate. *Environ Res.* 2018;164:124–31.

155. Parajuli RP, Umezaki M, Fujiwara T, Watanabe C. Association of cord blood levels of lead, arsenic, and zinc and home environment with children neurodevelopment at 36 months living in Chitwan Valley, Nepal. *PLoS One.* 2015;10(3):e0120992.

156. Wang B, Liu J, Liu B, Liu X, Yu X. Prenatal exposure to arsenic and neurobehavioral development of newborns in China. *Environ Int.* 2018;121(Pt 1):421–7.

157. Vibol S, Hashim JH, Sarmani S. Neurobehavioral effects of arsenic exposure among secondary school children in the Kandal Province, Cambodia. *Environ Res.* 2015;137:329–37.

158. Shih J-H, Zeng B-Y, Lin P-Y, et al. Association between peripheral manganese levels and attention-deficit/hyperactivity disorder: A preliminary meta-analysis. *Neuropsychiatr Dis Treat.* 2018;14:1831–42.

159. Berghuis SA, Bos AF, Sauer PJJ, Roze E. Developmental neurotoxicity of persistent organic pollutants: An update on childhood outcome. *Arch Toxicol.* 2015;89(5):687–709.

160. Forns J, Stigum H, Hoyer BB, et al. Prenatal and postnatal exposure to persistent organic pollutants and attention-deficit and hyperactivity disorder: A pooled analysis of seven European birth cohort studies. *Int J Epidemiol.* 2018;47(4):1082–97.

161. Brown AS, Cheslack-Postava K, Rantakokko P, et al. Association of maternal insecticide levels with autism in offspring from a national birth cohort. *Am J Psychiatry.* 2018;175(11):1094–101.

162. Guo Z, Xie HQ, Zhang P, et al. Dioxins as potential risk factors for autism spectrum disorder. *Environ Int.* 2018;121(Pt 1):906–15.

163. Lyall K, Croen LA, Sjodin A, et al. Polychlorinated biphenyl and organochlorine pesticide concentrations in maternal mid-pregnancy serum samples: Association with autism spectrum disorder and intellectual disability. *Environ Health Perspect.* 2017;125(3):474–80.

164. Liew Z, Goudarzi H, Oulhote Y. Developmental exposures to perfluoroalkyl substances (PFASs): An update of associated health outcomes. *Curr Environ Health Rep.* 2018;5(1):1–19.

165. Roth N, Wilks MF. Neurodevelopmental and neurobehavioural effects of polybrominated and perfluorinated chemicals: A systematic review of the epidemiological literature using a quality assessment scheme. *Toxicol Lett.* 2014;230(2):271–81.

166. Stein CR, Savitz DA, Bellinger DC. Perfluorooctanoate exposure in a highly exposed community and parent and teacher reports of behaviour in 6-12-year-old children. *Paediatr Perinat Epidemiol.* 2014;28(2): 146–56.

167. Strøm M, Hansen S, Olsen SF, et al. Persistent organic pollutants measured in maternal serum and offspring neurodevelopmental outcomes—A prospective study with long-term follow-up. *Environ Int.* 2014;68:41–8.

168. Lind DV, Priskorn L, Lassen TH, et al. Prenatal exposure to perfluoroalkyl substances and anogenital distance at 3 months of age as marker of endocrine disruption. *Reprod Toxicol.* 2016:S0890–6238(16): 30265–9.

169. Ode A, Källén K, Gustafsson P, et al. Fetal exposure to perfluorinated compounds and attention deficit hyperactivity disorder in childhood. Chen A, editor. *PLoS One.* 2014;9(4):e95891.

170. Liew Z, Ritz B, von Ehrenstein OS, et al. Attention deficit/hyperactivity disorder and childhood autism in association with prenatal exposure to perfluoroalkyl substances: A nested case-control study in the Danish national birth cohort. *Environ Health Perspect.* 2015;123(4):367–73.
171. Herbstman JB, Mall JK. Developmental exposure to polybrominated diphenyl ethers and neurodevelopment. *Curr Environ Health Rep.* 2014;1(2):101–12.
172. Ding G, Yu J, Cui C, et al. Association between prenatal exposure to polybrominated diphenyl ethers and young children's neurodevelopment in China. *Environ Res.* 2015;142:104–11.
173. Chen A, Yolton K, Rauch SA, et al. Prenatal polybrominated diphenyl ether exposures and neurodevelopment in U.S. children through 5 years of age: The HOME study. *Environ Health Perspect.* 2014;122(8):856–62.
174. Lam J, Lanphear BP, Bellinger D, et al. Developmental PBDE exposure and IQ/ADHD in childhood: A systematic review and meta-analysis. *Environ Health Perspect.* 2017;125(8):86001.
175. Muñoz-Quezada MT, Lucero BA, Barr DB, et al. Neurodevelopmental effects in children associated with exposure to organophosphate pesticides: A systematic review. *Neurotoxicology.* 2013;39:158–68.
176. González-Alzaga B, Lacasaña M, Aguilar-Garduño C, et al. A systematic review of neurodevelopmental effects of prenatal and postnatal organophosphate pesticide exposure. *Toxicol Lett.* 2014;230(2):104–21.
177. Eskenazi B, Kogut K, Huen K, et al. Organophosphate pesticide exposure, PON1, and neurodevelopment in school-age children from the CHAMACOS study. *Environ Res.* 2014;134:149–57.
178. Shelton JF, Geraghty EM, Tancredi DJ, et al. Neurodevelopmental disorders and prenatal residential proximity to agricultural pesticides: The CHARGE study. *Environ Health Perspect.* 2014;122(10):1103–9.
179. Fortenberry GZ, Meeker JD, Sánchez BN, et al. Urinary 3,5,6-trichloro-2-pyridinol (TCPY) in pregnant women from Mexico City: Distribution, temporal variability, and relationship with child attention and hyperactivity. *Int J Hyg Environ Health.* 2014;217(2–3):405–12.
180. Bouchard MF, Bellinger DC, Wright RO, Weisskopf MG. Attention-deficit/hyperactivity disorder and urinary metabolites of organophosphate pesticides. *Pediatrics.* 2010;125(6):e1270–7.
181. Marks AR, Harley K, Bradman A, et al. Organophosphate pesticide exposure and attention in young Mexican-American children: The CHAMACOS study. *Environ Health Perspect.* 2010;118(12):1768–74.
182. Hernandez AF, Gonzalez-Alzaga B, Lopez-Flores I, Lacasana M. Systematic reviews on neurodevelopmental and neurodegenerative disorders linked to pesticide exposure: Methodological features and impact on risk assessment. *Environ Int.* 2016;92–3:657–79.
183. Ejaredar M, Nyanza EC, Ten Eycke K, Dewey D. Phthalate exposure and childrens neurodevelopment: A systematic review. *Environ Res.* 2015;142:51–60.
184. Lee D-W, Kim M-S, Lim Y-H, Lee N, Hong Y-C. Prenatal and postnatal exposure to di-(2-ethylhexyl) phthalate and neurodevelopmental outcomes: A systematic review and meta-analysis. *Environ Res.* 2018v;167:558–66.
185. Lien Y-J, Ku H-Y, Su P-H, et al. Prenatal exposure to phthalate esters and behavioral syndromes in children at 8 years of age: Taiwan Maternal and Infant Cohort Study. *Environ Health Perspect.* 2015;123(1):95–100.
186. Gascon M, Valvi D, Forns J, et al. Prenatal exposure to phthalates and neuropsychological development during childhood. *Int J Hyg Environ Health.* 2015;218(6):550–8.
187. Braun JM, Kalkbrenner AE, Just AC, et al. Gestational exposure to endocrine-disrupting chemicals and reciprocal social, repetitive, and stereotypic behaviors in 4- and 5-year-old children: The HOME study. *Environ Health Perspect.* 2014;122(5):513–20.
188. Jeddi MZ, Janani L, Memari AH, Akhondzadeh S, Yunesian M. The role of phthalate esters in autism development: A systematic review. *Environ Res.* 2016;151:493–504.
189. Bellinger DC. Prenatal exposures to environmental chemicals and children's neurodevelopment: An update. *Saf Health Work.* 2013;4(1):1–11.
190. Ejaredar M, Lee Y, Roberts DJ, Sauve R, Dewey D. Bisphenol A exposure and children's behavior: A systematic review. *J Expo Sci Environ Epidemiol.* 2017;27(2):175–83.
191. Evans SF, Kobrosly RW, Barrett ES, et al. Prenatal bisphenol A exposure and maternally reported behavior in boys and girls. *Neurotoxicology.* 2014;45:91–9.
192. Mustieles V, Pérez-Lobato R, Olea N, Fernández MF. Bisphenol A: Human exposure and neurobehavior. *Neurotoxicology.* 2015;49:174–84.
193. Casas M, Forns J, Martínez D, et al. Exposure to bisphenol A during pregnancy and child neuropsychological development in the INMA-Sabadell cohort. *Environ Res.* 2015;142:671–9.
194. Braun JM, Kalkbrenner AE, Calafat AM, et al. Impact of early-life bisphenol A exposure on behavior and executive function in children. *Pediatrics.* 2011;128(5):873–82.
195. Hong S-B, Hong Y-C, Kim J-W, et al. Bisphenol A in relation to behavior and learning of school-age children. *J Child Psychol Psychiatry.* 2013;54(8):890–9.
196. Braun JM, Muckle G, Arbuckle T, et al. Associations of prenatal urinary bisphenol A concentrations with child behaviors and cognitive abilities. *Environ Health Perspect.* 2017;125(6):67008.
197. Minatoya M, Araki A, Nakajima S, et al. Cord blood BPA level and child neurodevelopment and behavioral problems: The Hokkaido study on environment and children's health. *Sci Total Environ.* 2017;607–8:351–6.
198. Stacy SL, Papandonatos GD, Calafat AM, et al. Early life bisphenol A exposure and neurobehavior at 8 years of age: Identifying windows of heightened vulnerability. *Environ Int.* 2017;107:258–65.
199. Clark C, Paunovic K. WHO environmental noise guidelines for the European region: A systematic review on environmental noise and cognition. *Int J Environ Res Public Health.* 2018;15(2):285.
200. Clark C, Paunovic K. WHO environmental noise guidelines for the European region: A systematic review on environmental noise and quality of life, wellbeing and mental health. *Int J Environ Res Public Health.* 2018;15(11):2400.
201. Zare Sakhvidi F, Zare Sakhvidi MJ, Mehrparvar AH, Dzhambov AM. Environmental noise exposure and neurodevelopmental and mental health problems in children: A systematic review. *Curr Environ Health Rep.* 2018;5(3):365–74.
202. Dadvand P, Tischer C, Estarlich M, et al. Lifelong residential exposure to green space and attention: A population-based prospective study. *Environ Health Perspect.* 2017;125(9):97016.
203. de Keijzer C, Gascon M, Nieuwenhuijsen MJ, Dadvand P. Long-term green space exposure and cognition across the life course: A systematic review. *Curr Environ Health Rep.* 2016;3(4):468–77.
204. Amicone G, Petruccelli I, De Dominicis S, et al. Green breaks: The restorative effect of the school environment's green areas on children's cognitive performance. *Front Psychol.* 2018;9:1579.
205. Cherrie MPC, Shortt NK, Mitchell RJ, et al. Green space and cognitive ageing: A retrospective life course analysis in the Lothian birth cohort 1936. *Soc Sci Med.* 2018;196:56–65.
206. Dadvand P, Nieuwenhuijsen MJ, Esnaola M, et al. Green spaces and cognitive development in primary schoolchildren. *Proc Natl Acad Sci U S A.* 2015;112(26):7937–42.
207. Dadvand P, Pujol J, Macià D, Martínez-Vilavella G, et al. The association between lifelong greenspace exposure and 3-dimensional brain magnetic resonance imaging in Barcelona schoolchildren. *Environ Health Perspect.* 2018;126(2):027012.
208. Brion M-JA, Lawlor DA, Matijasevich A, et al. What are the causal effects of breastfeeding on IQ, obesity and blood pressure? Evidence from comparing high-income with middle-income cohorts. *Int J Epidemiol.* 2011;40(3):670–80.
209. Lucas A, Morley R, Cole TJ, Gore SM. A randomised multicentre study of human milk versus formula and later development in preterm infants. *Arch Dis Child Fetal Neonatal Ed.* 1994;70(2):F141–6.
210. Boucher O, Julvez J, Guxens M, et al. Association between breastfeeding duration and cognitive development, autistic traits and ADHD symptoms: A multicenter study in Spain. *Pediatr Res.* 2017;81(3):434–42.
211. Mortensen EL. The association between duration of breastfeeding and adult intelligence. *JAMA.* 2002;287(18):2365.
212. Kajekar R. Environmental factors and developmental outcomes in the lung. *Pharmacol Ther.* 2007;114(2):129–45.
213. Luebke RW, Parks C, Luster MI. Suppression of immune function and susceptibility to infections in humans: Association of immune function with clinical disease. *J Immunotoxicol.* 2004;1(1):15–24.
214. Winans B, Humble MC, Lawrence BP. Environmental toxicants and the developing immune system: A missing link in the global battle against infectious disease? *Reprod Toxicol.* 2011;31(3):327–36.
215. Miller MD, Marty MA. Impact of environmental chemicals on lung development. *Environ Health Perspect.* 2010;118(8):1155–64.
216. Gascon M, Morales E, Sunyer J, Vrijheid M. Effects of persistent organic pollutants on the developing respiratory and immune systems: A systematic review. *Environ Int.* 2013;52:51–65.
217. Bui DS, Lodge CJ, Burgess JA, et al. Childhood predictors of lung function trajectories and future COPD risk: A prospective cohort study from the first to the sixth decade of life. *Lancet Respir Med.* 2018;6(7):535–44.
218. Jedrychowski WA, Perera FP, Maugeri U, et al. Effect of prenatal exposure to fine particulate matter on ventilatory lung function of

preschool children of non-smoking mothers. *Paediatr Perinat Epidemiol.* 2010;24(5):492–501.

219. Morales E, Garcia-Esteban R, Cruz OA de la, et al. Intrauterine and early postnatal exposure to outdoor air pollution and lung function at preschool age. *Thorax*. 2015;70(1):64–73.
220. MacIntyre EA, Gehring U, Mölter A, et al. Air pollution and respiratory infections during early childhood: An analysis of 10 European birth cohorts within the ESCAPE project. *Environ Health Perspect.* 2014;122(1):107–13.
221. Gehring U, Gruzieva O, Agius RM, et al. Air pollution exposure and lung function in children: The ESCAPE project. *Environ Health Perspect.* 2013;121(11–2):1357–64.
222. Schultz ES, Hallberg J, Bellander T, et al. Early-life exposure to traffic-related air pollution and lung function in adolescence. *Am J Respir Crit Care Med.* 2016;193(2):171–7.
223. Nordling E, Berglind N, Melén E, Emenius G, Hallberg J, Nyberg F, et al. Traffic-related air pollution and childhood respiratory symptoms, function and allergies. *Epidemiology.* 2008;19(3):401–8.
224. Mölter A, Agius RM, Vocht F de, et al. Long-term exposure to PM_{10} and NO_2 in association with lung volume and airway resistance in the MAAS birth cohort. *Environ Health Perspect.* 2013;121(10):1232.
225. Hehua Z, Qing C, Shanyan G, Qijun W, Yuhong Z. The impact of prenatal exposure to air pollution on childhood wheezing and asthma: A systematic review. *Environ Res.* 2017;159:519–30.
226. Khreis H, Kelly C, Tate J, Parslow R, Lucas K, Nieuwenhuijsen M. Exposure to traffic-related air pollution and risk of development of childhood asthma: A systematic review and meta-analysis. *Environ Int.* 2017;100:1–31.
227. Orellano P, Quaranta N, Reynoso J, Balbi B, Vasquez J. Effect of outdoor air pollution on asthma exacerbations in children and adults: Systematic review and multilevel meta-analysis. *PLoS One.* 2017;12(3):e0174050.
228. Nhung NTT, Amini H, Schindler C, et al. Short-term association between ambient air pollution and pneumonia in children: A systematic review and meta-analysis of time-series and case-crossover studies. *Environ Pollut.* 2017;230:1000–8.
229. Liu Q, Xu C, Ji G, et al. Effect of exposure to ambient $PM_{2.5}$ pollution on the risk of respiratory tract diseases: A meta-analysis of cohort studies. *J Biomed Res.* 2017;31(2):130–42.
230. Duramad P, Tager IB, Holland NT. Cytokines and other immunological biomarkers in children's environmental health studies. *Toxicol Lett.* 2007;172(1–2):48–59.
231. Cao J, Xu X, Hylkema MN, et al. Early-life exposure to widespread environmental toxicants and health risk: A focus on the immune and respiratory systems. *Ann Glob Health.* 2016;82(1):119–31.
232. Ashley-Martin J, Levy AR, Arbuckle TE, Platt RW, Marshall JS, Dodds L. Maternal exposure to metals and persistent pollutants and cord blood immune system biomarkers. *Environ Health.* 2015;14:52.
233. Wu K-G, Chang C-Y, Yen C-Y, Lai C-C. Associations between environmental heavy metal exposure and childhood asthma: A population-based study. *J Microbiol Immunol Infect.* 2019;52(2):352–62.
234. Wang I-J, Karmaus WJJ, Yang C-C. Lead exposure, IgE, and the risk of asthma in children. *J Expo Sci Environ Epidemiol.* 2017;27(5):478–83.
235. Hui LL, Chan MHM, Lam HS, et al. Impact of fetal and childhood mercury exposure on immune status in children. *Environ Res.* 2016;144(Pt A):66–72.
236. Kim K-N, Bae S, Park HY, Kwon H-J, Hong Y-C. Low-level mercury exposure and risk of asthma in school-age children. *Epidemiology.* 2015;26(5):733–9.
237. Heinrich J, Guo F, Trepka MJ. Brief report: Low-level mercury exposure and risk of asthma in school-age children. *Epidemiology.* 2017;28(1):116–8.
238. Sanchez TR, Perzanowski M, Graziano JH. Inorganic arsenic and respiratory health, from early life exposure to sex-specific effects: A systematic review. *Environ Res.* 2016;147:537–55.
239. Ahmed S, Akhtar E, Roy A, et al. Arsenic exposure alters lung function and airway inflammation in children: A cohort study in rural Bangladesh. *Environ Int.* 2017;101:108–16.
240. Gascon M, Sunyer J, Casas M, et al. Prenatal exposure to DDE and PCB 153 and respiratory health in early childhood: A meta-analysis. *Epidemiology.* 2014;25(4):544–53.
241. Hansen S, Strom M, Olsen SF, et al. Maternal concentrations of persistent organochlorine pollutants and the risk of asthma in offspring: Results from a prospective cohort with 20 years of follow-up. *Environ Health Perspect.* 2014;122(1):93–9.
242. Hansen S, Strom M, Olsen SF, et al. Prenatal exposure to persistent organic pollutants and offspring allergic sensitization and lung function at 20 years of age. *Clin Exp Allergy.* 2016;46(2):329–36.
243. Parker-Lalomio M, McCann K, Piorkowski J, Freels S, Persky VW. Prenatal exposure to polychlorinated biphenyls and asthma, eczema/hay fever, and frequent ear infections. *J Asthma.* 2018;55(10):1105–15.
244. Cupul-Uicab LA, Terrazas-Medina EA, Hernandez-Avila M, Longnecker MP. Prenatal exposure to p,p'-DDE and p,p'-DDT in relation to lower respiratory tract infections in boys from a highly exposed area of Mexico. *Environ Res.* 2014;132:19–23.
245. Smit LAM, Lenters V, Hoyer BB, et al. Prenatal exposure to environmental chemical contaminants and asthma and eczema in school-age children. *Allergy.* 2015;70(6):653–60.
246. Gascon M, Sunyer J, Martinez D, et al. Persistent organic pollutants and children's respiratory health: The role of cytokines and inflammatory biomarkers. *Environ Int.* 2014;69:133–40.
247. Meng G, Feng Y, Nie Z, et al. Internal exposure levels of typical POPs and their associations with childhood asthma in Shanghai, China. *Environ Res.* 2016;146:125–35.
248. Meng G, Nie Z, Feng Y, Wu X, Yin Y, Wang Y. Typical halogenated persistent organic pollutants in indoor dust and the associations with childhood asthma in Shanghai, China. *Environ Pollut.* 2016;211:389–98.
249. Perla ME, Rue T, Cheadle A, Krieger J, Karr CJ. Biomarkers of insecticide exposure and asthma in children: A national health and nutrition examination survey (NHANES) 1999–2008 analysis. *Arch Environ Occup Health.* 2015;70(6):309–22.
250. Grandjean P, Andersen EW, Budtz-Jørgensen E, et al. Serum vaccine antibody concentrations in children exposed to perfluorinated compounds. *JAMA.* 2012;307(4):391–7.
251. Granum B, Haug LS, Namork E, et al. Pre-natal exposure to perfluoroalkyl substances may be associated with altered vaccine antibody levels and immune-related health outcomes in early childhood. *J Immunotoxicol.* 2013;10(4):373–9.
252. Stein CR, McGovern KJ, Pajak AM, Maglione PJ, Wolff MS. Perfluoroalkyl and polyfluoroalkyl substances and indicators of immune function in children aged 12–19 y: National health and nutrition examination survey. *Pediatr Res.* 2016;79(2):348–57.
253. Pennings JLA, Jennen DGJ, Nygaard UC, et al. Cord blood gene expression supports that prenatal exposure to perfluoroalkyl substances causes depressed immune functionality in early childhood. *J Immunotoxicol.* 2016;13(2):173–80.
254. Okada E, Sasaki S, Kashino I, et al. Prenatal exposure to perfluoroalkyl acids and allergic diseases in early childhood. *Environ Int.* 2014;65:127–34.
255. Impinen A, Nygaard UC, Lodrup Carlsen KC, et al. Prenatal exposure to perfluoralkyl substances (PFASs) associated with respiratory tract infections but not allergy- and asthma-related health outcomes in childhood. *Environ Res.* 2018;160:518–23.
256. Zhou Y, Hu L-W, Qian ZM, et al. Interaction effects of polyfluoroalkyl substances and sex steroid hormones on asthma among children. *Sci Rep.* 2017;7(1):899.
257. Qin X-D, Qian ZM, Dharmage SC, et al. Association of perfluoroalkyl substances exposure with impaired lung function in children. *Environ Res.* 2017;155:15–21.
258. Timmermann CAG, Budtz-Jorgensen E, Jensen TK, et al. Association between perfluoroalkyl substance exposure and asthma and allergic disease in children as modified by MMR vaccination. *J Immunotoxicol.* 2017;14(1):39–49.
259. Canbaz D, van Velzen MJM, Hallner E, et al. Exposure to organophosphate and polybrominated diphenyl ether flame retardants via indoor dust and childhood asthma. *Indoor Air.* 2016;26(3):403–13.
260. Raanan R, Harley KG, Balmes JR, Bradman A, Lipsett M, Eskenazi B. Early-life exposure to organophosphate pesticides and pediatric respiratory symptoms in the CHAMACOS cohort. *Environ Health Perspect.* 2015;123(2):179–85.
261. Liu B, Jung KH, Horton MK, et al. Prenatal exposure to pesticide ingredient piperonyl butoxide and childhood cough in an urban cohort. *Environ Int.* 2012;48:156–61.
262. Raanan R, Balmes JR, Harley KG, et al. Decreased lung function in 7-year-old children with early-life organophosphate exposure. *Thorax.* 2016;71(2):148–53.
263. Just AC, Whyatt RM, Perzanowski MS, et al. Prenatal exposure to butylbenzyl phthalate and early eczema in an urban cohort. *Environ Health Perspect.* 2012;120(10):1475–80.

264. Gascon M, Casas M, Morales E, et al. Prenatal exposure to bisphenol A and phthalates and childhood respiratory tract infections and allergy. *J Allergy Clin Immunol.* 2015;135(2):370–8.

265. Whyatt RM, Perzanowski MS, Just AC, et al. Asthma in inner-city children at 5-11 years of age and prenatal exposure to phthalates: The Columbia Center for Children's Environmental Health Cohort. *Environ Health Perspect.* 2014;122(10):1141–6.

266. Ku HY, Su PH, Wen HJ, et al. Prenatal and postnatal exposure to phthalate esters and asthma: A 9-year follow-up study of a Taiwanese birth cohort. Chen Y-C, editor. *PLoS One.* 2015;10(4):e0123309.

267. Li M-C, Chen C-H, Guo YL. Phthalate esters and childhood asthma: A systematic review and congener-specific meta-analysis. *Environ Pollut.* 2017;229:655–60.

268. Jurewicz J, Hanke W. Exposure to phthalates: Reproductive outcome and children health. A review of epidemiological studies. *Int J Occup Med Environ Health.* 2011;24(2):115–41.

269. Bekö G, Callesen M, Weschler CJ, et al. Phthalate exposure through different pathways and allergic sensitization in preschool children with asthma, allergic rhinoconjunctivitis and atopic dermatitis. *Environ Res.* 2015;137:432–9.

270. Xie M-Y, Ni H, Zhao D-S, et al. Exposure to bisphenol A and the development of asthma: A systematic review of cohort studies. *Reprod Toxicol.* 2016;65:224–9.

271. Spanier AJ, Kahn RS, Kunselman AR, et al. Bisphenol A exposure and the development of wheeze and lung function in children through age 5 years. *JAMA Pediatr.* 2014;168(12):1131.

272. Spanier AJ, Fiorino EK, Trasande L. Bisphenol A exposure is associated with decreased lung function. *J Pediatr.* 2014;164(6):1403–8.e1.

273. Berger K, Eskenazi B, Balmes J, et al. Prenatal high molecular weight phthalates and bisphenol A, and childhood respiratory and allergic outcomes. *Pediatr Allergy Immunol.* 2019;30(1):36–46.

274. Zhou A, Chang H, Huo W, et al. Prenatal exposure to bisphenol A and risk of allergic diseases in early life. *Pediatr Res.* 2017;81(6):851–6.

275. Recio A, Linares C, Banegas JR, Díaz J. Road traffic noise effects on cardiovascular, respiratory, and metabolic health: An integrative model of biological mechanisms. *Environ Res.* 2016;146:359–70.

276. Eze IC, Foraster M, Schaffner E, et al. Transportation noise exposure, noise annoyance and respiratory health in adults: A repeated-measures study. *Environ Int.* 2018;121(Pt 1):741–50.

277. Recio A, Linares C, Banegas JR, Díaz J. The short-term association of road traffic noise with cardiovascular, respiratory, and diabetes-related mortality. *Environ Res.* 2016;150:383–90.

278. Lambert KA, Bowatte G, Tham R, et al. Residential greenness and allergic respiratory diseases in children and adolescents—A systematic review and meta-analysis. *Environ Res.* 2017;159:212–21.

279. Thayer KA, Heindel JJ, Bucher JR, Gallo MA. Role of environmental chemicals in diabetes and obesity: A national toxicology program workshop review. *Environ Health Perspect.* 2012;120(6):779–89.

280. Rundle A, Hoepner L, Hassoun A, et al. Association of childhood obesity with maternal exposure to ambient air polycyclic aromatic hydrocarbons during pregnancy. *Am J Epidemiol.* 2012;175(11):1163–72.

281. Michalaki E, Margetaki K, Roumeliotaki T, Vafeiadi M, Karachaliou M, Sarri K, et al. Air pollution during pregnancy and childhood obesity risk: Potential protective effect of diet. *Clin Nutr ESPEN.* 2018;24:187.

282. Frondelius K, Oudin A, Malmqvist E. Traffic-related air pollution and child BMI-A study of prenatal exposure to nitrogen oxides and body mass index in children at the age of four years in Malmo, Sweden. *Int J Environ Res Public Health.* 2018;15(10):2294.

283. Clemente DBP, Casas M, Janssen BG, et al. Prenatal ambient air pollution exposure, infant growth and placental mitochondrial DNA content in the INMA birth cohort. *Environ Res.* 2017;157:96–102.

284. Kim E, Park H, Park EA, et al. Particulate matter and early childhood body weight. *Environ Int.* 2016;94:591–9.

285. Zhang M, Mueller NT, Wang H, Hong X, Appel LJ, Wang X. Maternal exposure to ambient particulate matter $\leq$2.5 μm during pregnancy and the risk for high blood pressure in childhood. *Hypertension.* 2018;72(1):194–201.

286. Breton C V, Yao J, Millstein J, et al. Prenatal air pollution exposures, DNA methyl transferase genotypes, and associations with newborn LINE1 and Alu methylation and childhood blood pressure and carotid intima-media thickness in the children's health study. *Environ Health Perspect.* 2016;124(12):1905–12.

287. van Rossem L, Rifas-Shiman SL, Melly SJ, et al. Prenatal air pollution exposure and newborn blood pressure. *Environ Health Perspect.* 2015;123(4):353–9.

288. Fleisch AF, Luttmann-Gibson H, Perng W, et al. Prenatal and early life exposure to traffic pollution and cardiometabolic health in childhood. *Pediatr Obes.* 2017;12(1):48–57.

289. Dong G-H, Wang J, Zeng X-W, et al. Interactions between air pollution and obesity on blood pressure and hypertension in Chinese children. *Epidemiology.* 2015;26(5):740–7.

290. Bilenko N, Brunekreef B, Beelen R, et al. Associations between particulate matter composition and childhood blood pressure—The PIAMA study. *Environ Int.* 2015;84:1–6.

291. Bilenko N, van Rossem L, Brunekreef B, et al. Traffic-related air pollution and noise and children's blood pressure: results from the PIAMA birth cohort study. *Eur J Prev Cardiol.* 2015;22(1):4–12.

292. Zeng X-W, Qian ZM, Vaughn MG, et al. Positive association between short-term ambient air pollution exposure and children blood pressure in China—Result from the Seven Northeast Cities (SNEC) study. *Environ Pollut.* 2017;224:698–705.

293. Kim JS, Alderete TL, Chen Z, et al. Longitudinal associations of in utero and early life near-roadway air pollution with trajectories of childhood body mass index. *Environ Health.* 2018;17(1):64.

294. Fioravanti S, Cesaroni G, Badaloni C, Michelozzi P, Forastiere F, Porta D. Traffic-related air pollution and childhood obesity in an Italian birth cohort. *Environ Res.* 2018;160:479–86.

295. Fleisch AF, Rifas-Shiman SL, Koutrakis P, et al. Prenatal exposure to traffic pollution. *Epidemiology.* 2015;26(1):43–50.

296. Jerrett M, McConnell R, Wolch J, et al. Traffic-related air pollution and obesity formation in children: A longitudinal, multilevel analysis. *Environ Health.* 2014;13(1):49.

297. Jerrett M, McConnell R, Chang CCR, et al. Automobile traffic around the home and attained body mass index: A longitudinal cohort study of children aged 10–18 years. *Prev Med (Baltim).* 2010;50(Suppl 1):S50–8.

298. McConnell R, Shen E, Gilliland FD, et al. A longitudinal cohort study of body mass index and childhood exposure to secondhand tobacco smoke and air pollution: The southern California children's health study. *Environ Health Perspect.* 2015;123(4):360–6.

299. Alderete TL, Chen Z, Toledo-Corral CM, et al. Ambient and traffic-related air pollution exposures as novel risk factors for metabolic dysfunction and type 2 diabetes. *Curr Epidemiol Rep.* 2018;5(2):79–91.

300. Toledo-Corral CM, Alderete TL, et al. Effects of air pollution exposure on glucose metabolism in Los Angeles minority children. *Pediatr Obes.* 2018;13(1):54–62.

301. Delvaux I, Van Cauwenberghe J, Den Hond E, et al. Prenatal exposure to environmental contaminants and body composition at age 7–9 years. *Environ Res.* 2014;132:24–32.

302. Gardner RM, Kippler M, Tofail F, et al. Environmental exposure to metals and children's growth to age 5 years: A prospective cohort study. *Am J Epidemiol.* 2013;177(12):1356–67.

303. Chatzi L, Ierodiakonou D, Margetaki K, et al. Prenatal exposure to cadmium and child growth, obesity and cardiometabolic traits. *Am J Epidemiol.* 2019;188(1):141–50.

304. Saha KK, Engström A, Hamadani JD, Tofail F, Rasmussen KM, Vahter M. Pre- and postnatal arsenic exposure and body size to 2 years of age: A cohort study in rural Bangladesh. *Environ Health Perspect.* 2012;120(8):1208–14.

305. Su C-T, Lin H-C, Choy C-S, Huang Y-K, Huang S-R, Hsueh Y-M. The relationship between obesity, insulin and arsenic methylation capability in Taiwan adolescents. *Sci Total Environ.* 2012;414:152–8.

306. Kim B-M, Lee B-E, Hong Y-C, et al. Mercury levels in maternal and cord blood and attained weight through the 24 months of life. *Sci Total Environ.* 2011;410-1:26–33.

307. Afeiche M, Peterson KE, Sanchez BN, et al. Prenatal lead exposure and weight of 0- to 5-year-old children in Mexico city. *Environ Health Perspect.* 2011;119(10):1436–41.

308. Hong Y-C, Kulkarni SS, Lim Y-H, et al. Postnatal growth following prenatal lead exposure and calcium intake. *Pediatrics.* 2014;134(6):1151–9.

309. Scinicariello F, Buser MC, Mevissen M, Portier CJ. Blood lead level association with lower body weight in NHANES 1999–2006. *Toxicol Appl Pharmacol.* 2013;273(3):516–23.

310. Kim JH, Park Y, Kim SK, et al. Timing of an accelerated body mass increase in children exposed to lead in early life: A longitudinal study. *Sci Total Environ.* 2017;584–5:72–7.

311. Nye MD, King KE, Darrah TH, et al. Maternal blood lead concentrations, DNA methylation of MEG3 DMR regulating the DLK1/MEG3 imprinted domain and early growth in a multiethnic cohort. *Environ Epigenet.* 2016;2(1):dvv009.

312. Sergeyev O, Burns JS, Williams PL, et al. The association of peripubertal serum concentrations of organochlorine chemicals and blood lead with growth and pubertal development in a longitudinal cohort of boys: A review of published results from the Russian children's study. *Rev Environ Health*. 2017;32(1-2):83–92.
313. Zeng X, Xu X, Qin Q, Ye K, Wu W, Huo X. Heavy metal exposure has adverse effects on the growth and development of preschool children. *Environ Geochem Health*. 2019;41(1):309–21.
314. Chang JY, Park JS, Shin S, Yang HR, Moon JS, Ko JS. Mercury exposure in healthy Korean weaning-age infants: Association with growth, feeding and fish intake. *Int J Environ Res Public Health*. 2015;12(11):14669–89.
315. Shao W, Liu Q, He X, Liu H, Gu A, Jiang Z. Association between level of urinary trace heavy metals and obesity among children aged 6–19 years: NHANES 1999–2011. *Environ Sci Pollut Res Int*. 2017;24(12):11573–81.
316. Zhang A, Hu H, Sánchez BN, et al. Association between prenatal lead exposure and blood pressure in children. *Environ Health Perspect*. 2012;120(3):445–50.
317. Farzan SF, Howe CG, Chen Y, et al. Prenatal lead exposure and elevated blood pressure in children. *Environ Int*. 2018;121(Pt 2):1289–96.
318. Skroder H, Hawkesworth S, Moore SE, Wagatsuma Y, Kippler M, Vahter M. Prenatal lead exposure and childhood blood pressure and kidney function. *Environ Res*. 2016;151:628–34.
319. Gregory S, Iles-Caven Y, Hibbeln JR, Taylor CM, Golding J. Are prenatal mercury levels associated with subsequent blood pressure in childhood and adolescence? The Avon prebirth cohort study. *BMJ Open*. 2016;6(10):e012425.
320. Valera B, Muckle G, Poirier P, Jacobson SW, Jacobson JL, Dewailly E. Cardiac autonomic activity and blood pressure among Inuit children exposed to mercury. *Neurotoxicology*. 2012;33(5):1067–74.
321. Swaddiwudhipong W, Mahasakpan P, Jeekeeree W, et al. Renal and blood pressure effects from environmental cadmium exposure in Thai children. *Environ Res*. 2015;136:82–7.
322. Skroder H, Hawkesworth S, Kippler M, et al. Kidney function and blood pressure in preschool-aged children exposed to cadmium and arsenic—Potential alleviation by selenium. *Environ Res*. 2015;140:205–13.
323. Osorio-Yanez C, Ayllon-Vergara JC, Arreola-Mendoza L, et al. Blood pressure, left ventricular geometry, and systolic function in children exposed to inorganic arsenic. *Environ Health Perspect*. 2015;123(6): 629–35.
324. Osorio-Yáñez C, Ayllon-Vergara JC, Aguilar-Madrid G, et al. Carotid intima-media thickness and plasma asymmetric dimethylarginine in Mexican children exposed to inorganic arsenic. *Environ Health Perspect*. 2013;121(9):1090–6.
325. Kuo C-C, Su P-H, Sun C-W, Liu H-J, Chang C-L, Wang S-L. Early-life arsenic exposure promotes atherogenic lipid metabolism in adolescence: A 15-year birth cohort follow-up study in central Taiwan. *Environ Int*. 2018;118:97–105.
326. La Merrill M, Birnbaum LS. Childhood obesity and environmental chemicals. *Mt Sinai J Med*. 2011;78(1):22–48.
327. Tang-Péronard JL, Andersen HR, Jensen TK, Heitmann BL. Endocrine-disrupting chemicals and obesity development in humans: A review. *Obes Rev*. 2011;12(8):622–36.
328. Mendez MA, Garcia-Esteban R, Guxens M, et al. Prenatal organochlorine compound exposure, rapid weight gain, and overweight in infancy. *Environ Health Perspect*. 2011;119(2):272–8.
329. Iszatt N, Stigum H, Verner M-A, et al. Prenatal and postnatal exposure to persistent organic pollutants and infant growth: A pooled analysis of seven European birth cohorts. *Environ Health Perspect*. 2015;123(7):730–6.
330. Heggeseth B, Harley K, Warner M, Jewell N, Eskenazi B. Detecting associations between early-life DDT exposures and childhood growth patterns: A novel statistical approach. Pawluski J, editor. *PLoS One*. 2015;10(6):e0131443.
331. Valvi D, Mendez MA, Martinez D, et al. Prenatal concentrations of polychlorinated biphenyls, DDE, and DDT and overweight in children: A prospective birth cohort study. *Environ Health Perspect*. 2012;120(3):451–7.
332. Valvi D, Mendez MA, Garcia-Esteban R, et al. Prenatal exposure to persistent organic pollutants and rapid weight gain and overweight in infancy. *Obesity*. 2014;22(2):488–96.
333. Warner M, Wesselink A, Harley KG, Bradman A, Kogut K, Eskenazi B. Prenatal exposure to dichlorodiphenyltrichloroethane and obesity at 9 years of age in the CHAMACOS study cohort. *Am J Epidemiol*. 2014;179(11):1312–22.
334. Tang-Péronard JL, Heitmann BL, Andersen HR, et al. Association between prenatal polychlorinated biphenyl exposure and obesity development at ages 5 and 7 y: A prospective cohort study of 656 children from the Faroe Islands. *Am J Clin Nutr*. 2014;99(1):5–13.
335. Vafeiadi M, Georgiou V, Chalkiadaki G, et al. Association of prenatal exposure to persistent organic pollutants with obesity and cardiometabolic traits in early childhood: The Rhea mother-child cohort (Crete, Greece). *Environ Health Perspect*. 2015;123(10):1015–21.
336. Agay-Shay K, Martinez D, Valvi D, et al. Exposure to endocrine-disrupting chemicals during pregnancy and weight at 7 years of age: A multi-pollutant approach. *Environ Health Perspect*. 2015;123(10): 1030–7.
337. Warner M, Ye M, Harley K, Kogut K, Bradman A, Eskenazi B. Prenatal DDT exposure and child adiposity at age 12: The CHAMACOS study. *Environ Res*. 2017;159:606–12.
338. Garced S, Torres-Sánchez L, Cebrián ME, Claudio L, López-Carrillo L. Prenatal dichlorodiphenyldichloroethylene (DDE) exposure and child growth during the first year of life. *Environ Res*. 2012;113:58–62.
339. Cupul-Uicab LA, Klebanoff MA, Brock JW, Longnecker MP. Prenatal exposure to persistent organochlorines and childhood obesity in the US collaborative perinatal project. *Environ Health Perspect*. 2013;121(9):1103–9.
340. Høyer BB, Ramlau-Hansen CH, Henriksen TB, et al. Body mass index in young school-age children in relation to organochlorine compounds in early life: A prospective study. *Int J Obes*. 2014;38(7):919–25.
341. Lauritzen HB, Larose TL, Øien T, et al. Prenatal exposure to persistent organic pollutants and child overweight/obesity at 5-year follow-up: A prospective cohort study. *Environ Health*. 2018;17(1):9.
342. Coker E, Chevrier J, Rauch S, et al. Association between prenatal exposure to multiple insecticides and child body weight and body composition in the VHEMBE South African birth cohort. *Environ Int*. 2018;113:122–32.
343. Maisonet M, Terrell ML, McGeehin MA, et al. Maternal concentrations of polyfluoroalkyl compounds during pregnancy and fetal and postnatal growth in British girls. *Environ Health Perspect*. 2012;120(10):1432–7.
344. Høyer BB, Ramlau-Hansen CH, Vrijheid M, et al. Anthropometry in 5- to 9-year-old Greenlandic and Ukrainian children in relation to prenatal exposure to perfluorinated alkyl substances. *Environ Health Perspect*. 2015;123(8):841–6.
345. Halldorsson TI, Rytter D, Haug LS, et al. Prenatal exposure to perfluorooctanoate and risk of overweight at 20 years of age: A prospective cohort study. *Environ Health Perspect*. 2012;120(5):668–73.
346. Timmermann CAG, Rossing LI, Grøntved A, et al. Adiposity and glycemic control in children exposed to perfluorinated compounds. *J Clin Endocrinol Metab*. 2014;99(4):E608–14.
347. Barry V, Darrow LA, Klein M, Winquist A, Steenland K. Early life perfluorooctanoic acid (PFOA) exposure and overweight and obesity risk in adulthood in a community with elevated exposure. *Environ Res*. 2014;132:62–9.
348. Andersen CS, Fei C, Gamborg M, Nohr EA, Sorensen TIA, Olsen J. Prenatal exposures to perfluorinated chemicals and anthropometry at 7 years of age. *Am J Epidemiol*. 2013;178(6):921–7.
349. Liu P, Yang F, Wang Y, Yuan Z. Perfluorooctanoic acid (PFOA) exposure in early life increases risk of childhood adiposity: A meta-analysis of prospective cohort studies. *Int J Environ Res Public Health*. 2018;15(10):2070.
350. Maisonet M, Näyhä S, Lawlor DA, Marcus M. Prenatal exposures to perfluoroalkyl acids and serum lipids at ages 7 and 15 in females. *Environ Int*. 2015;82:49–60.
351. Geiger SD, Xiao J, Ducatman A, Frisbee S, Innes K, Shankar A. The association between PFOA, PFOS and serum lipid levels in adolescents. *Chemosphere*. 2014;98:78–83.
352. Zeng X-W, Qian Z, Emo B, et al. Association of polyfluoroalkyl chemical exposure with serum lipids in children. *Sci Total Environ*. 2015;512–3:364–70.
353. Koshy TT, Attina TM, Ghassabian A, et al. Serum perfluoroalkyl substances and cardiometabolic consequences in adolescents exposed to the World Trade Center disaster and a matched comparison group. *Environ Int*. 2017;109:128–35.
354. Khalil N, Ebert JR, Honda M, et al. Perfluoroalkyl substances, bone density, and cardio-metabolic risk factors in obese 8–12 year old children: A pilot study. *Environ Res*. 2018;160:314–21.
355. Geiger S, Shankar A, Xiao J. No association between perfluoroalkyl chemicals and hypertension in children. *Integr Blood Press Control*. 2014;7:1.
356. Taylor KW, Novak RF, Anderson HA, et al. Evaluation of the association between persistent organic pollutants (POPs) and diabetes in epidemi-

ological studies: A national toxicology program workshop review. *Environ Health Perspect.* 2013;121(7):774–83.

357. Manzano-Salgado CB, Casas M, Lopez-Espinosa M-J, et al. Prenatal exposure to perfluoroalkyl substances and cardiometabolic risk in children from the Spanish INMA birth cohort study. *Environ Health Perspect.* 2017;125(9):97018.
358. Erkin-Cakmak A, Harley KG, Chevrier J, et al. In utero and childhood polybrominated diphenyl ether exposures and body mass at age 7 years: The CHAMACOS study. *Environ Health Perspect.* 2015;123(6):636–42.
359. Vuong AM, Braun JM, Sjodin A, et al. Prenatal polybrominated diphenyl ether exposure and body mass index in children up to 8 years of age. *Environ Health Perspect.* 2016;124(12):1891–7.
360. Andersen HR, Wohlfahrt-Veje C, Dalgård C, et al. Paraoxonase 1 polymorphism and prenatal pesticide exposure associated with adverse cardiovascular risk profiles at school age. Amre D, editor. *PLoS One.* 2012;7(5):e36830.
361. Sanders AP, Saland JM, Wright RO, Satlin L. Perinatal and childhood exposure to environmental chemicals and blood pressure in children: A review of literature 2007–2017. *Pediatr Res.* 2018;84(2):165–80.
362. Harari R, Julvez J, Murata K, et al. Neurobehavioral deficits and increased blood pressure in school-age children prenatally exposed to pesticides. *Environ Health Perspect.* 2010;118(6):890–6.
363. Suarez-Lopez JR, Jacobs DR, Himes JH, Alexander BH, Alexander BH. Acetylcholinesterase activity, cohabitation with floricultural workers, and blood pressure in Ecuadorian children. *Environ Health Perspect.* 2013;121(5):619–24.
364. Howard SG. Exposure to environmental chemicals and type 1 diabetes: An update. *J Epidemiol Community Health.* 2019;73(6):483–8.
365. El Morsi DA, Rahman RHA, Abou-Arab AA. Pesticides residues in Egyptian diabetic children: A preliminary study. *J Clin Toxicol.* 2012;02(06):1–5.
366. Philips EM, Jaddoe VWV, Trasande L. Effects of early exposure to phthalates and bisphenols on cardiometabolic outcomes in pregnancy and childhood. *Reprod Toxicol.* 2017;68:105–18.
367. Kim JH, Park H, Lee J, et al. Association of diethylhexyl phthalate with obesity-related markers and body mass change from birth to 3 months of age. *J Epidemiol Community Health.* 2016;70(5):466–72.
368. Harley KG, Berger K, Rauch S, et al. Association of prenatal urinary phthalate metabolite concentrations and childhood BMI and obesity. *Pediatr Res.* 2017;82(3):405–15.
369. Yang TC, Peterson KE, Meeker JD, et al. Bisphenol A and phthalates in utero and in childhood: Association with child BMI z-score and adiposity. *Environ Res.* 2017;156:326–33.
370. Shoaff J, Papandonatos GD, Calafat AM, et al. Early-life phthalate exposure and adiposity at 8 years of age. *Environ Health Perspect.* 2017;125(9):97008.
371. Perng W, Watkins DJ, Cantoral A, et al. Exposure to phthalates is associated with lipid profile in peripubertal Mexican youth. *Environ Res.* 2017;154:311–7.
372. Botton J, Philippat C, Calafat AM, et al. Phthalate pregnancy exposure and male offspring growth from the intra-uterine period to five years of age. *Environ Res.* 2016;151:601–9.
373. Buckley JP, Engel SM, Braun JM, et al. Prenatal phthalate exposures and body mass index among 4- to 7-year-old children: A pooled analysis. *Epidemiology.* 2016;27(3):449–58.
374. Yang TC, Peterson KE, Meeker JD, et al. Exposure to bisphenol A and phthalates metabolites in the third trimester of pregnancy and BMI trajectories. *Pediatr Obes.* 2018;13(9):550–7.
375. Valvi D, Casas M, Romaguera D, et al. Prenatal phthalate exposure and childhood growth and blood pressure: Evidence from the Spanish INMA-Sabadell birth cohort study. *Environ Health Perspect.* 2015;123(10):1022–9.
376. Amin MM, Ebrahimpour K, Parastar S, et al. Association of urinary concentrations of phthalate metabolites with cardiometabolic risk factors and obesity in children and adolescents. *Chemosphere.* 2018;211:547–56.
377. Amin MM, Parastar S, Ebrahimpour K, et al. Association of urinary phthalate metabolites concentrations with body mass index and waist circumference. *Environ Sci Pollut Res Int.* 2018;25(11):11143–51.
378. Xia B, Zhu Q, Zhao Y, et al. Phthalate exposure and childhood overweight and obesity: Urinary metabolomic evidence. *Environ Int.* 2018;121(Pt 1):159–68.
379. Tsai Y-A, Lin C-L, Hou J-W, et al. Effects of high di(2-ethylhexyl) phthalate (DEHP) exposure due to tainted food intake on pre-pubertal growth characteristics in a Taiwanese population. *Environ Res.* 2016;149: 197–205.
380. Wu W, Wu P, Yang F, Sun D-L, Zhang D-X, Zhou Y-K. Association of phthalate exposure with anthropometric indices and blood pressure in first-grade children. *Environ Sci Pollut Res Int.* 2018;25(23):23125–34.
381. Trasande L, Sathyanarayana S, Spanier AJ, Trachtman H, Attina TM, Urbina EM. Urinary phthalates are associated with higher blood pressure in childhood. *J Pediatr.* 2013;163(3):747–53.e1.
382. Kataria A, Levine D, Wertenteil S, et al. Exposure to bisphenols and phthalates and association with oxidant stress, insulin resistance, and endothelial dysfunction in children. *Pediatr Res.* 2017;81(6):857–64.
383. Trasande L, Spanier AJ, Sathyanarayana S, Attina TM, Blustein J. Urinary phthalates and increased insulin resistance in adolescents. *Pediatrics.* 2013;132(3):e646–55.
384. Rancière F, Lyons JG, Loh VHY, et al. Bisphenol A and the risk of cardiometabolic disorders: A systematic review with meta-analysis of the epidemiological evidence. *Environ Health.* 2015;14(1):46.
385. Valvi D, Casas M, Mendez MA, et al. Prenatal bisphenol a urine concentrations and early rapid growth and overweight risk in the offspring. *Epidemiology.* 2013;24(6):791–9.
386. Junge KM, Leppert B, Jahreis S, et al. MEST mediates the impact of prenatal bisphenol A exposure on long-term body weight development. *Clin Epigenet.* 2018;10:58.
387. Hoepner LA, Whyatt RM, Widen EM, et al. Bisphenol A and adiposity in an inner-city birth cohort. *Environ Health Perspect.* 2016;124(10): 1644–50.
388. Harley KG, Schall RA, Chevrier J, et al. Prenatal and postnatal bisphenol A exposure and body mass index in childhood in the CHAMACOS cohort. *Environ Health Perspect.* 2013;121(4):514–20.
389. Vafeiadi M, Roumeliotaki T, Myridakis A, et al. Association of early life exposure to bisphenol A with obesity and cardiometabolic traits in childhood. *Environ Res.* 2016;146:379–87.
390. Bae S, Lim Y-H, Lee YA, Shin CH, Oh S-Y, Hong Y-C. Maternal urinary bisphenol A concentration during midterm pregnancy and children's blood pressure at age 4. *Hypertension.* 2017;69(2):367–74.
391. Amin MM, Ebrahim K, Hashemi M, et al. Association of exposure to bisphenol A with obesity and cardiometabolic risk factors in children and adolescents. *Int J Environ Health Res.* 2019;29(1):94–106.
392. Lee YM, Hong Y-C, Ha M, et al. Prenatal bisphenol-A exposure affects fetal length growth by maternal glutathione transferase polymorphisms, and neonatal exposure affects child volume growth by sex: From multiregional prospective birth cohort MOCEH study. *Sci Total Environ.* 2018;612:1433–41.
393. Wang Z, Liang H, Tu X, et al. Bisphenol A and pubertal height growth in school-aged children. *J Expo Sci Environ Epidemiol.* 2019;29(1):109–17.
394. Weyde KV, Krog NH, Oftedal B, et al. A longitudinal study of road traffic noise and body mass index trajectories from birth to 8 years. *Epidemiology.* 2018;29(5):729–38.
395. Christensen JS, Hjortebjerg D, Raaschou-Nielsen O, Ketzel M, Sorensen TIA, Sorensen M. Pregnancy and childhood exposure to residential traffic noise and overweight at 7 years of age. *Environ Int.* 2016;94:170–6.
396. van Kempen E, Casas M, Pershagen G, Foraster M. WHO environmental noise guidelines for the European region: A systematic review on environmental noise and cardiovascular and metabolic effects: A summary. *Int J Environ Res Public Health.* 2018;15(2):379.
397. Dzhambov AM, Dimitrova DD. Children's blood pressure and its association with road traffic noise exposure—A systematic review with meta-analysis. *Environ Res.* 2017;152:244–55.
398. Dadvand P, Villanueva CM, Font-Ribera L, et al. Risks and benefits of green spaces for children: A cross-sectional study of associations with sedentary behavior, obesity, asthma, and allergy. *Environ Health Perspect.* 2014;122(12):1329–35.
399. Lovasi GS, Schwartz-Soicher O, Quinn JW, et al. Neighborhood safety and green space as predictors of obesity among preschool children from low-income families in New York City. *Prev Med.* 2013;57(3):189–93.
400. Liu GC, Wilson JS, Qi R, Ying J. Green neighborhoods, food retail and childhood overweight: Differences by population density. *Am J Health Promot.* 2007;21(4_suppl):317–25.
401. Sanders T, Feng X, Fahey PP, Lonsdale C, Astell-Burt T. Green space and child weight status: Does outcome measurement matter? Evidence from an Australian longitudinal study. *J Obes.* 2015;2015:1–8.
402. Bloemsma LD, Wijga AH, Klompmaker JO, et al. The associations of air pollution, traffic noise and green space with overweight throughout childhood: The PIAMA birth cohort study. *Environ Res.* 2019;169:348–56.
403. Potestio ML, Patel AB, Powell CD, McNeil DA, Jacobson RD, McLaren L. Is there an association between spatial access to parks/green space

and childhood overweight/obesity in Calgary, Canada? *Int J Behav Nutr Phys Act.* 2009;6(1):77.

404. Dadvand P, Poursafa P, Heshmat R, et al. Use of green spaces and blood glucose in children; a population-based CASPIAN-V study. *Environ Pollut.* 2018;243(Pt B):1134–40.

405. Lenters V, Portengen L, Smit LAM, et al. Phthalates, perfluoroalkyl acids, metals and organochlorines and reproductive function: A multipollutant assessment in Greenlandic, Polish and Ukrainian men. *Occup Environ Med.* 2015;72(6):385–93.

406. Mogensen UB, Grandjean P, Heilmann C, Nielsen F, Weihe P, Budtz-Jørgensen E. Structural equation modeling of immunotoxicity associated with exposure to perfluorinated alkylates. *Environ Health.* 2015;14(1):47.

407. Zhang Y, Dong T, Hu W, et al. Association between exposure to a mixture of phenols, pesticides, and phthalates and obesity: Comparison of three statistical models. *Environ Int.* 2019;123:325–36.

408. Slama R, Vrijheid M. Some challenges of studies aiming to relate the exposome to human health. *Occup Environ Med.* 2015;72(6):383–4.

409. Maitre L, de Bont J, Casas M, et al. Human early life exposome (HELIX) study: A European population-based exposome cohort. *BMJ Open.* 2018;8(9):e021311.

410. Buck Louis GM, Yeung E, Sundaram R, Laughon SK, Zhang C. The exposome—Exciting opportunities for discoveries in reproductive and perinatal epidemiology. *Paediatr Perinat Epidemiol.* 2013;27(3):229–36.

411. Tamayo-Uria I, Maitre L, Thomsen C, et al. The early-life exposome: Description and patterns in six European countries. *Environ Int.* 2019;123:189–200.

412. Chung MK, Kannan K, Louis GM, Patel CJ. Toward capturing the exposome: exposure biomarker variability and coexposure patterns in the shared environment. *Environ Sci Technol.* 2018;52(15):8801–10.

413. Barrera-Gómez J, Agier L, Portengen L, et al. A systematic comparison of statistical methods to detect interactions in exposome-health associations. *Environ Health.* 2017;16(1):74.

414. Agier L, Portengen L, Chadeau-Hyam M, et al. A systematic comparison of linear regression-based statistical methods to assess exposome-health associations. *Environ Health Perspect.* 2016;124(12):1848–56.

415. Nieuwenhuijsen MJ, Agier L, Basagaña X, et al. Influence of the urban exposome on birth weight. *Environ Health Perspect.* 2019;127(4):47007.

416. Agier L, Basagaña X, Maitre L, et al. Early-life exposome and lung function in children in Europe: An analysis of data from the longitudinal, population-based HELIX cohort. *Lancet Planet Health.* 2019;3(2): e81–92.

417. Gruzieva O, Xu C-J, Breton CV, et al. Epigenome-wide meta-analysis of methylation in children related to prenatal NO_2 air pollution exposure. *Environ Health Perspect.* 2017;125(1):104–10.

418. Maitre L, Robinson O, Martinez D, et al. Urine metabolic signatures of multiple environmental pollutants in pregnant women: An exposome approach. *Environ Sci Technol.* 2018;52(22):13469–80.

419. Solomon O, Yousefi P, Huen K, et al. Prenatal phthalate exposure and altered patterns of DNA methylation in cord blood. *Environ Mol Mutagen.* 2017;58(6):398–410.

420. Robinson O, Basagaña X, Agier L, et al. The pregnancy exposome: Multiple environmental exposures in the INMA-Sabadell birth cohort. *Environ Sci Technol.* 2015;49(17):10632–41.

421. Cohen AJ, Brauer M, Burnett R, et al. Estimates and 25-year trends of the global burden of disease attributable to ambient air pollution: An analysis of data from the Global Burden of Diseases Study 2015. *Lancet.* 2017;389(10082):1907–18.

422. Stanaway JD, Afshin A, Gakidou E, et al. Global, regional, and national comparative risk assessment of 84 behavioural, environmental and occupational, and metabolic risks or clusters of risks for 195 countries and territories, 1990–2017: A systematic analysis for the Global Burden of Disease Study 2017. *Lancet.* 2018;392(10159):1923–94.

423. WHO Regional Office for Europe. *Environmental Noise Guidelines for the European Region (2018).* Copenhagen: World Health Organization; 2018 Oct.

424. WHO Regional Office for Europe, JRC. *WHO | Burden of Disease from Environmental Noise—Quantification of Healthy Life Years Lost in Europe [Internet].* Copenhagen: World Health Organization; 2011 [cited 2019 Jun 2]. Available at https://www.who.int/quantifying_ehimpacts/publications/e94888/en/.

425. Hänninen O, Knol AB, Jantunen M, et al. Environmental burden of disease in Europe: Assessing nine risk factors in six countries. *Environ Health Perspect.* 2014;122(5):439–46.

426. WHO. *World Health Organization—Burden of Disease from the Joint Effects of Household and Ambient Air Pollution for 2012 | Climate Clean Air Coalition [Internet].* Geneva, Switzerland: World Health Organization; 2014 [cited 2019 Jun 2]. Available at https://www.ccacoalition.org/es/resources/world-health-organization---burden-disease-joint-effects-household-and-ambient-air.

427. European Commission. *Links between Noise and Air Pollution and Socioeconomic Status [Internet].* Luxembourg: Publications Office of the EU; 2016 [cited 2019 Jun 2]. Available at https://publications.europa.eu/en/publication-detail/-/publication/1a3f0657-9a83-11e6-9bca-01aa75ed71a1.

428. Trasande L, Zoeller RT, Hass U, et al. Estimating burden and disease costs of exposure to endocrine-disrupting chemicals in the European Union. *J Clin Endocrinol Metab.* 2015;100(4):1245–55.

CHAPTER

75

Environmental Endocrine-disrupting Chemicals: Common Sources and Health Effects

Kathryn A. Crawford • Jessica R. Shoaff • Megan E. Romano

The environment around us has tremendous bearing on our health. Simply put, we need clean water to drink, unpolluted air to breathe, and healthy food to eat. We also need safe, comfortable neighborhoods, and homes to live in. Without access to these basic needs, human health quality suffers, increasing morbidity, and premature mortality among affected populations. The most vulnerable members of society often include children, pregnant women, the elderly, and people of minority or lower socioeconomic status. Although the field of environmental health is not often incorporated into training for medical practitioners, knowledge of the importance of environmental influences on health is critical for clinicians, particularly in preventative medicine, where patients have the opportunity to make lifestyle modifications in ways that reduce their exposure to environmental conditions causing harm. Public health practitioners working at levels ranging from local to national, and even global, monitor the environment and enforce regulations intended to protect public health. Clinicians together with public health practitioners and researchers can also play a major role in supporting policy development and regulations.

Environmental health is a broad, interdisciplinary field of public health, which draws on the collective expertise of epidemiologists, toxicologists, exposure scientists, risk assessors, chemists, biostatisticians, anthropologists, and sociologists, among others. Overall, the field serves to understand how exposures from our environment—air, water, food, neighborhood, indoor spaces—affect health. Much environmental heath attention is dedicated to understanding the effects of exposure to chemicals through various media, including the health risks associated with exposure and ways to reduce exposure. Why is there so much focus on chemical exposures? To begin, more than 80,000 chemicals are registered for use in the United States (U.S.) and serve as the basis for all industrial and manufacturing processes and commercial goods we have. As a result, chemicals are all around us, all the time, including in our air, water, food, neighborhoods, and personal spaces (e.g., homes, schools, workplaces, vehicles, and medical facilities). While some chemicals may pose little, if any, health risk to humans (or wildlife) as currently used, others pose considerable health threats, and many are untested for their toxicity. Chemicals can affect human health in many ways, including the ability to mimic endogenous molecules in the body, to disrupt cellular process and/or interfere with endocrine signaling, or to be teratogenic or carcinogenic. Since conditions to which a fetus or child are exposed can impact their health and, in turn, their children's health, the potential for environmental chemicals to adversely impact current and future generations is deeply concerning.

There are many sectors concerned with the risks of chemicals: the public itself, workers in the industries using chemicals, regulators, and public health practitioners. Clinicians may provide care for affected individuals, sometimes challenged to find the links between the presenting clinical picture and causal agents. Biomonitoring studies, such as the National Health and Nutrition Examination Survey (NHANES), show that chemical exposures are ubiquitous with large segments of the population having detectable levels of diverse chemicals in their bodies. For regulatory agencies and those concerned with population health, assessing the risks of the many agents to which we are exposed is challenging, albeit necessary for risk management.

The chemicals discussed in this chapter are known or suspected endocrine-disrupting chemicals, or exogenous chemicals that interfere with hormonal action or mechanisms within the body. These chemicals are broadly classified into two groups: persistent and nonpersistent compounds. Simply put, persistent chemicals are those not readily degrading in the environment, whereas, nonpersistent chemicals are those which are more susceptible to degradation processes and, thus, exist in the environment for less time. However, both persistent and nonpersistent chemicals are able to afflict harm on humans and wildlife, alike. Another common theme among many of the environmental chemicals described in this chapter is that of regrettable substitutions over time, or "the unwitting selection of an alternative that poses equal or higher risk" compared to the chemical being phased out.[1] Often more-persistent chemicals are replaced with nonpersistent ones, typically under the premise that nonpersistent chemicals will be less toxic. For example, when concerns were raised over the persistent polybrominated diphenyl ether flame retardants, they were phased out and replaced with nonpersistent OPFR, but relatively little is known regarding their toxicity to humans. A similar situation is unfolding for the persistent per- and polyfluoroalkyl substances (PFAS), which are being replaced with newer, less-persistent highly fluorinated compounds, yet the health effects of the replacement chemicals remain largely unknown. Frameworks, such as the Chemical Alternatives Assessment (CAA), have been created to assist relevant stakeholders in choosing safer chemical alternatives (Box 75-1), though suitable alternatives cannot always be identified through this process,[2–4] and the challenge of regrettable substitutions is one that will follow us into the future.

The following sections of this chapter outline the history, uses, and health concerns of several important groups of chemicals. The chapter begins with a description of the important differences between persistent and nonpersistent chemicals in terms of environmental fate and in the context of biomonitoring. Next, several classes of persistent chemicals are described. These include chlorinated chemicals, pesticides, fluorinated, and brominated chemicals (Table 75-1A). These are followed by the nonpersistent chemicals including, OPFRs, environmental phenols, and phthalates (Table 75-1B). Collectively, the chemicals described in this chapter reflect a wide spectrum of the chemical landscape encountered by

BOX 75-1 Chemical Alternatives Assessment

Chemical Alternatives Assessment

Establish Needs

- Industry, consumers, policy makers or other stakeholders determine that there is a need for a chemical alternatives assessment, often in response to recognition that a chemical may pose risks to human health or the environment.

Collect Info

- What previous work has been done to assess alternatives and are alternatives well characterized?
- Do the alternatives have a similar range of functional uses to the original chemical or will different alternatives need to be identified for varying uses?
- How do the structural, functional, and physical properties of alternatives compare to chemical in current use?
- What are the differences in the manufacturing processes and potential contaminants created by the alternative compared to the original chemical?

Stakeholder Feedback

- Chemical manufacturers, product manufacturers, retailers, end users, waste managers, government, nongovernment, and academic entities describe challenges and opportunities provided by the identified alternatives in order to describe the full scope of the implications of using proposed alternatives.

Hazard Assessment

- Select comparative hazard endpoints (e.g., carcinogenicity, bioaccumulation)
- Comprehensively review publicly available and confidential empirical data available through regulatory structures and identify data gaps.
- Apply criteria for safer chemical ingredients to transparently describe which alternatives are safer or less safe than current chemical.

Report Findings

- Information about alternatives and hazards assessments are communicated to decision makers.
- Reports focus on describing alternatives, typically without expressly identifying a favored alternative.

Apply Findings

- Stakeholders use information about alternatives, cost, performance, and other factors to make decisions about implementation of alternatives.

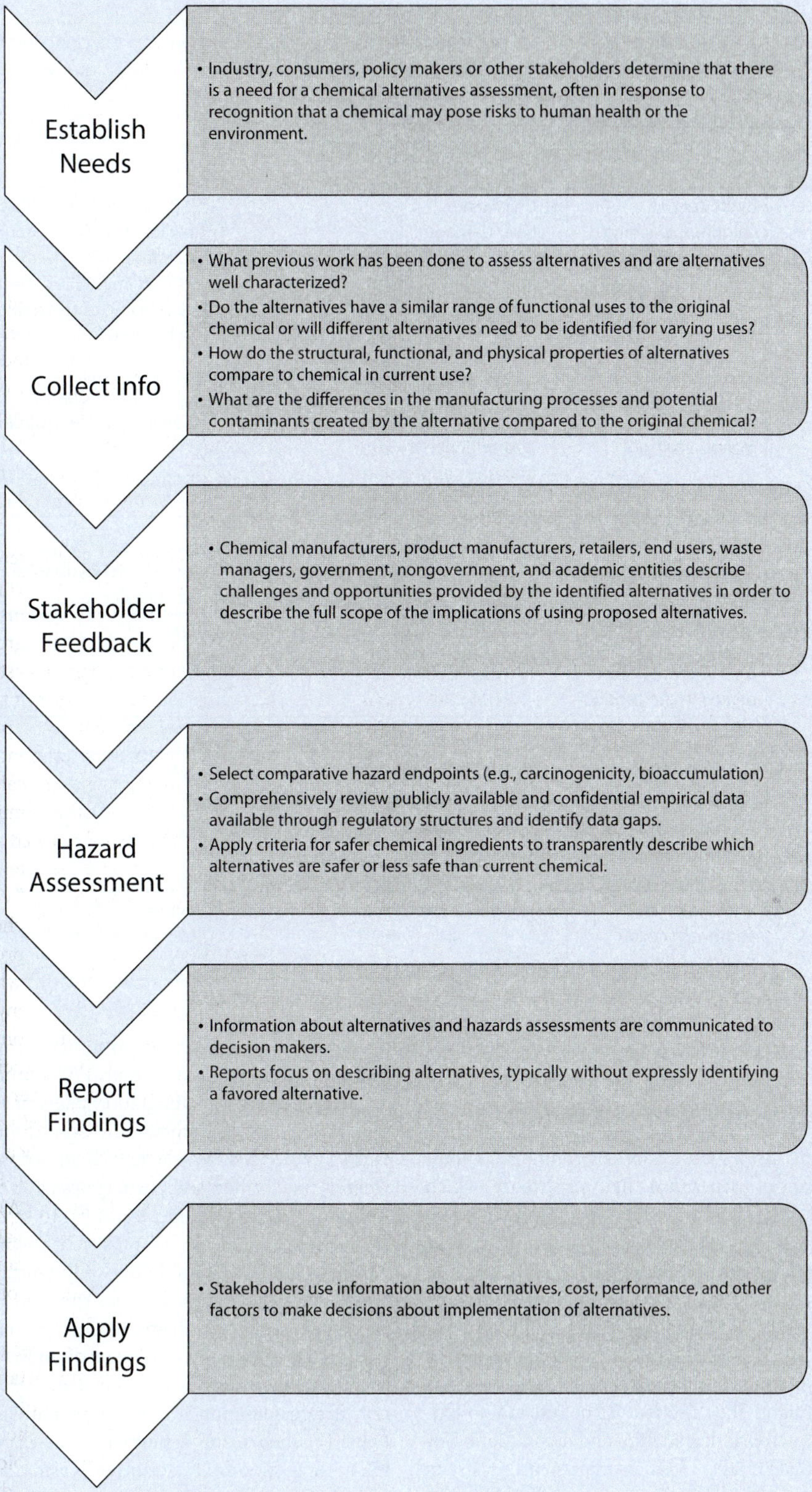

humans both historically and in contemporary daily life. The public health implications of these exposures close out the chapter. The focus of this chapter is on chemical exposures in the general population of developed countries. However, it is important to note that occupational exposures to chemicals tend to be greater than those sustained by the general population, and investigating the health effects of occupational exposures is often an important step in understanding the influence of chemical exposures on human health. Additionally, air pollution, metals, and nonchemical exposures, including exposures like noise (e.g., transportation), psychological stressors (e.g., neighborhood violence, poverty), radiation, and biological agents (e.g., foodborne or waterborne pathogens) are

TABLE 75-1A ORIGINAL USES, HUMAN HEALTH EFFECTS, AND CARCINOGENICITY OF PERSISTENT ORGANIC POLLUTANTS

Chemical Class or Name	Original Use	Main Noncancer Health Effects	IARC Classification for Carcinogenicity in Humans	Stockholm Convention Year
Chlorinated Chemicals				
Polychlorinated biphenyls (PCBs)	Heat and flame resistance; electrical equipment and electronics; paint additive; lubricant	• Skin conditions (chloracne, rashes) • Liver damage • Reproductive toxicity • Immune suppression • Impaired neurodevelopment • Endocrine disruption	Group 1: Carcinogenic to humans	2004
Polychlorinated dibenzo-p-dioxins (PCDDs)	Byproduct of chlorine-bleaching at paper mills, waste and drinking water treatment; trash incineration	• Chloracne • Liver damage • Reproductive toxicity • Immune suppression • Endocrine disruption • Altered glucose metabolism / Type II Diabetes	2,3,7,8-tetrachlorodibenzo-p-dioxin (TCDD) - Group 1: Carcinogenic to humans; Other PCDDs and PCDFs -Group 3: not classifiable as to carcinogenicity in humans	2004
Polychlorinated dibenzofurans (PCDFs)				
Diphenyltricholorethand (DDT)	Insecticide (agricultural and malaria control)	• Neurotoxicity • Impaired neurodevelopment • Reproductive toxicity • Immune suppression • Endocrine disruption	Group 2A: Probably Carcinogenic to Humans	2004
Fluorinated Chemicals				
Perfluorooctanoic acid (PFOA)	Nonstick coating on cookware or food packaging; water or stain resistant coating on clothing or carpet; personal care product	• Ulcerative colitis (PFOA) • Pregnancy-induced hypertension (PFOA) • High cholesterol • Thyroid disease	Group 2B: Possibly Carcinogenic to Humans	2019
Perfluorooctane sulfonic acid (PFOS)			NA	2009
Brominated Chemicals				
Polybrominated diphenyl ethers (PBDEs)	Flame retardant additive used in vehicles, aircrafts, textiles, plastics, polyurethane foam	• Thyroid hormone disruption • Impaired neurodevelopment	NA	2017
Tetrabromobisphenol A (TBBA)	Flame retardant additive in circuit boards, resins	• Thyroid hormone disruption	Group 2A: Probably Carcinogenic to Humans	NA

important in the field of environmental health, but are beyond the scope of this chapter and covered elsewhere.

PERSISTENT AND NONPERSISTENT CHEMICALS

One of the primary distinguishing features of environmental chemicals and a key determinant of their risk is their persistence, which relates to half-life in the body, recalcitrance in the environment, and bioaccumulation properties. The half-lives of compounds in various systems are key considerations for biomonitoring, exposure assessment, and risk assessment.[5] Persistent pollutants are those with long half-lives in the human body (months to years), that tend to bioaccumulate up the food chain. These compounds are often resistant to physical and chemical conditions such as heat, acidic or basic environments, and ultraviolet light. They also tend to be resistant to biological processes such as microbial degradation and detoxification by enzymes. Due to their recalcitrance, these chemicals can persist in the environment for prolonged periods of time (years, decades) and, in some cases are referred to as "forever" chemicals because they will likely exist for centuries. As such, persistent chemicals pose special challenges for environmental remediation and reduction of body burden once human exposure has occurred. In recognition of this complexity, the Stockholm Convention on Persistent Organic Pollutants, a United Nations treaty, aims to reduce the production, use, and release of 29 of the most harmful persistent organic pollutants (POPs). To protect humans and the environment from these toxic POPs, the European Union and more than 170 countries across the globe have created national implementation plans to reduce or eliminate POPs regulated under the Stockholm Convention from production, use, and waste streams.[6] While the U.S. signed the Stockholm Convention when it was formed and participates as an observer in meetings and technical working groups, it has yet to ratify the treaty.[7] In contrast to persistent chemicals, nonpersistent chemicals tend to have shorter half-lives (hours to days) in the body, typically do not bioaccumulate, are more easily degraded or destroyed in the environment, and are not regulated by the Stockholm Convention.

Because exposure assessment should reflect the etiologically relevant window of exposure, knowledge of chemical persistence is a critical consideration in environmental epidemiologic studies, particularly when using a biological matrix to quantify exposure. In many cases, blood (i.e., serum or plasma) is the matrix of choice for measurement of persistent chemicals. Sometimes fat or other alternative matrices will be preferred. Due to the episodic nature of exposure and short half-lives in the body, nonpersistent chemicals present some special challenges for exposure assessment. Biomonitoring of nonpersistent chemicals in humans is typically accomplished by measuring concentrations in urine.[5] However, the short half-lives of nonpersistent chemicals in the body often lead to greater within-person variability of individual exposure measurements. Conversely, levels

TABLE 75-1B PARENT COMPOUNDS, ORIGINAL USES, HUMAN HEALTH EFFECTS, CARCINOGENICITY, AND URINARY METABOLITES OF NONPERSISTENT POLLUTANTS

Parent Chemical	Original Use	Main Noncancer Health Effects	IARC Classification for Carcinogenicity in Humans	Urinary Metabolites
Pesticides				
Glyphosate	Herbicide	• Skin irritant • Respiratory toxicant • Suspected reproductive and neurotoxicity	Group 2A: Probably Carcinogenic to Humans	NA
Organophosphate flame retardants				
Tris(2-chloroethyl) phosphate (TCEP)	Flame retardant additives in textiles, electronics, and polyurethane foam	• Thyroid hormone disruption • Impaired neuro-development • Reproductive toxicity • Renal toxicity • Liver toxicity	Group 3: Not classifiable as to carcinogenicity in humans	Bis(2-chloroethyl) phosphate
Tributyl phosphate (TnBP)			NA	Dibutyl phosphate
Tris-(1,3-dichloro-2-propyl) phosphate (TDCP)				Bis-(1,3-dichloro-2-propyl) phosphate
Triphenyl phosphate (TPP)				Diphenyl phosphate
Tris-(1-chloro-2-propyl) phosphate (TCPP)				Bis-(1-chloro-2-propyl) phosphate
Tri-o-cresylphosphate (ToCP)				Di-o-cresylphosphate
Tri-p-cresylphosphate (TpCP)				Di-p-cresylphosphate
Environmental Phenols				
Bisphenol A	Synthetic estrogen; monomer in polycarbonate plastics and epoxy resins	• Reproductive toxicity • Thyroid hormone disruption • Cardiovascular disease • Obesity	NA	NA
Oxybenzone or Benzophenone-3	Ultraviolet light filter in personal care products	• Skin or photo allergy • Suspected developmental toxicant	Group 2B: Possibly Carcinogenic to Humans	NA
Triclosan	Antimicrobial in personal care products	• Allergies and asthma • Reproductive toxicant • Reduced birth size	NA	NA
Parabens	Preservatives/ antimicrobials in personal care products, pharmaceuticals and food	• Thyroid hormone disruption • Altered birth weight	NA	NA
Phthalates				
Diethyl phthalate (DEP)	Scent retainer in personal care products; excipient in pharmaceuticals	• Impaired neurodevelopment • Altered physical growth	NA	Monoethyl phthalate
Di-n-butyl phthalate (DBP or DnBP)	Scent retainer / plasticizer in personal care products; excipient in pharmaceuticals	• Impaired neurodevelopment • Decreased anogenital distance (males) • Delayed pubarche (females) • Altered birth size • Cardiometabolic disorders	NA	Mono-n-butyl phthalate
Benzylbutyl phthalate (BBzP)	Plasticizer in vinyl flooring, adhesives, food packaging	• Allergic diseases • Neurobehavioral effects	NA	Monobenzyl phthalate
Di(2-ethylhexyl) phthalate (DEHP)	Plasticizer in polyvinyl chloride plastics	• Allergic diseases • Neurobehavioral effects • Thyroid hormone disruption • Altered birth size and physical growth • Reproductive toxicity • Cardiometabolic disorders	Group 2B: Possibly Carcinogenic to Humans	Mono(2-ethylhexyl) phthalate; Mono(2-ethyl-5-hydroxyhexyl) phthalate; Mono(2-ethyl-5-oxohexyl) phthalate; Mono(2-ethyl-5-carboxypentyl) phthalate

of persistent chemicals tend to have lower within-person variability over time. Higher within-person variability leads to more exposure misclassification and necessitates the use of multiple urine samples for accurate exposure assessment.[8] Concentrations from a single urine sample, however, can sometimes successfully classify exposure over a period of weeks to months,[9] especially if exposure is constant over time. Exposure assessment of nonpersistent chemicals in environmental epidemiology studies relying on a single urine sample may lead to exposure misclassification. Therefore, an average concentration from multiple urine samples collected across the etiologically relevant period is often necessary to reflect the true exposure to nonpersistent chemicals. These challenges in the exposure assessment of nonpersistent chemicals may contribute to seemingly inconsistent results across studies geared toward investigating the health effects of nonpersistent chemicals.

POLYCHLORINATED BIPHENYLS, DIOXINS, AND FURANS

Polychlorinated biphenyls (PCBs), polychlorinated dibenzo-p-dioxins (PCDDs), and polychlorinated dibenzofurans (PCDFs) are three classes of chlorinated POPs with aromatic rings as central components of their chemical structures. PCBs encompass 209 individual compounds (congeners) comprised of two phenyl rings with a range of one to ten chlorines included in the chemical structure. The number and position of chlorine atoms determines the fate and transport of the congener in the environment, as well as its resistance to degradation and its toxicity. PCBs differ in terms of adverse health effect for humans and the environment, with higher chlorinated PCBs persisting longer in the environment.[10] PCBs are highly lipophilic and, when released into the environment, tend to sorb to organic material, where they may then be transported by sediment, soil, or dust via water and air. Historically, the volatility of PCBs was thought to be low, but more recent research shows that volatilization is an important route of PCB transport and human exposure (discussed below), particularly for congeners with fewer chlorines and, thus, lower molecular weight.[11,12] Due to their lipophilicity and resistance to microbial and enzymatic degradation, PCBs bioaccumulate in biota and biomagnify in the food chain. Therefore, top predators and humans tend to have higher concentrations of PCBs in their tissues than lower order organisms. A subset of PCBs are structurally similar to the synthetic, lipophilic, and also highly persistent, PCDDs and PCDFs.

Whereas PCBs consist of two connected biphenyl rings with no oxygen, PCDDs are comprised of two benzene rings joined by a middle ring containing oxygen. PCDDs incorporate two para position oxygen atoms in the middle ring, and PCDFs contain a single oxygen within the middle ring (Fig. 75-1). PCDDs and PCDFs are extremely toxic when chlorines are located in the 2, 3, 7, and 8 positions. For example, 2,3,7,8-tetrachlorodibenzo-p-dioxin (TCDD), often simply referred to as dioxin, is considered the most toxic dioxin congener and is defined as having the highest possible "Dioxin toxic equivalency factor" (TEF) of 1.0[13] (Table 75-2). PCDDs and PCDFs without chlorines in these positions are substantially less toxic with lower TEF. Some PCBs also have dioxin-like toxicity. For example 3,3′,4,4′,5-PentaCB (PCB-126) has a TEF of 0.1.[13]

PCBs were first produced for use in electrical products because low flammability characteristics and chemical properties made them desirable for use in electrical transformers and capacitors.[14] PCB use was expanded to include use in hydraulic fluids, building materials (e.g., caulking), microscope oil, paints, surface coatings, inks,

TABLE 75-2 PCDD, PCDF, AND PCB CONGENERS WITH TEF

PCDDs/PCDFs/PCBs	WHO TEF[a]
2,3,7,8-TetraCDD	1
1,2,3.7,8-PentaCDD	1
1,2,3,4,7,8-HexaCDD	0.1
1,2,3,6,7,8-HexaCDD	0.1
1,2,3,7,8,9-HexaCDD	0.1
1,2,3,4,6,7,8-HeptaCDD	0.01
OctaCDD	0.0001
2,3,7,8-TetraCDF	0.1
1,2,3,7,8-PentaCDF	0.05
2,3,4,7,8-PentaCDF	0.5
1,2,3,4,7,8-HexaCDF	0.1
1,2,3,6,7,8-HexaCDF	0.1
1,2,3,7,8,9-HexaCDF	0.1
2,3,4,6,7,8-HexaCDF	0.1
1,2,3,4,6,7,8-HeptaCDF	0.01
1,2,3,4,7,8,9-HeptaCDF	0.01
OctaCDF	0.0001
3,4,4′,5-TetraCB (#81)	0.0001
3,3′,4,4′-TetraCB (#77)	0.0001
3,3′,4,4′,5-PentaCB (#126)	0.1
3,3′,4,4′,5,5′-HexaCB (#169)	0.01
2,3,3′,4,4′-PentaCB (#105)	0.0001
2,3,4,4′,5-PentaCB (#114)	0.0005
2,3′,4,4′,5-PentaCB (#118)	0.0001
2′,3,4,4′,5-PentaCB (#123)	0.0001
2,3,3′,4,4′,5-HexaCB (#156)	0.0005
2,3,3′,4,4′,5′-HexaCB (#157)	0.0005
2,3′,4,4′,5,5′-HexaCB (#167)	0.00001
2,3,3′,4,4′,5,5′-HeptaCB (#189)	0.0001

[a]Data from the report of an expert meeting (1997) at the World Health Organization. *Source:* Van den Berg M, Birnbaum L, Bosveld ATC, et al. Toxic equivalency factors (TEFs) for PCBs, PCDDs, PCDFs for humans and wildlife. *Environ Health Perspect.* 1998;106:775–92.

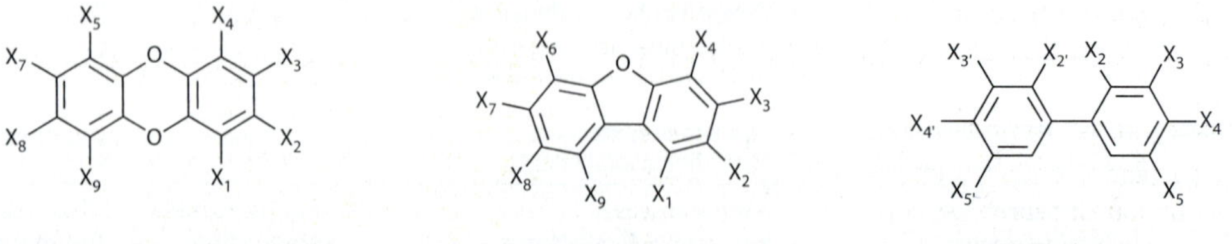

polychlorinated dibenzo-*p*-dioxins (PCDD) X_i = Cl or H

polychlorinated dibenzofurans (PCDF) X_j = Cl or H

polychlorinated biphenyls (PCB) X_k = Cl or H

FIGURE 75-1. General chemical structure of polychlorinated dibenzo-p-dioxins (PCDDs), polychlorinated dibenzofurans (PCDFs), and polychlorinated biphenyls (PCBs). (*Source:* Used with Permission from Sorg O. AhR signalling and dioxin toxicity. *Toxicology Letters.* 2013;230(2):225-233. doi:10.1016/j.toxlet.2013.10.039.)

adhesives, and in carbonless copy paper. The widespread use of PCBs in industrial process and building materials led to their ubiquity in the environment. The area surrounding some former industrial sites or industrial waste dumps may be contaminated due to poor waste handling and disposal. Additionally, indoor environments, notably schools, can have appreciable levels of PCBs in dust and air.[11] Unlike PCBs, PCDDs, and PCDFs are not manufactured as such, but are usually found as unwanted contaminants of other synthetic chemicals or as products of incineration of chlorinated organic compounds. Atmospheric transport is thus a major dispersal mechanism for PCDDs and PCDFs, with distribution depending upon vapor pressure and atmospheric temperature. Such dispersal results in deposition of these chemicals onto air, water, and soil. PCDDs and PCDFs are highly lipophilic, and as with PCBs, less-chlorinated congeners can be semivolatile. PCDDs and PCDFs resist most environmental degradation processes and can bioaccumulate.[15]

Exposure to Polychlorinated Biphenyls, Dioxins, and Furans. Because PCBs, PCDDs and PCDFs are ubiquitous in the environment, including in the food chain and indoor environments, human exposures to these compounds are common. In fact, measurable levels of these compounds are present in people around the globe. Furthermore, people are often exposed to mixtures of PCBs, PCDDs, and PCDFs. This co exposure complicates the assessment of the health consequences of exposure to individual chemicals among these related compounds.[16] Heterocyclic compounds, including some PCBs, PCDDs, PCDFs, often exert their toxicity through binding with the aryl hydrocarbon receptor.[17] Due to co-occurrence and potentially similar modes of toxicity across PCBs, PCDDs, and PCDFs, the dioxin toxic equivalency (TEQ) was developed to estimate the toxicity of the total mixture, and is determined by multiplying the measured level of each congener by the congener's TEF and then adding the products. The total dioxin toxicity of a mixture is the sum of the TEQs from the PCDDs, the PCDFs, and the dioxin-like PCBs. Intake of 1–6 pg/kg body weight (BW)/day of TEQ of dioxin-like chemicals (PCDDs, PCDFs, and PCBs) was characteristic of adult daily intake in the U.S. in the mid-1990s with intake primarily from food, especially meat, fish, and dairy products.[18]

Exposures to PCBs, PCDDs, and PCDFs are believed to be decreasing around the world, largely because PCBs were banned from manufacture and use in the late 1970s, and regulations have forced stricter limits on dioxin and furan emissions.[19] However, given the persistence of these chemicals and widespread environmental contamination, low-level exposure to the general population is likely to continue.

Health Effects of Polychlorinated Biphenyls, Dioxins, and Furans. Historic incidents of poisoning with cooking oil contaminated with PCBs, PCDFs, and PCDDs, and other chlorinated chemicals lead to clinical syndromes called Yusho and Yu-Cheng disease in 1968 and 1979, respectively.[20–22] Health effects of chlorinated chemicals include chloracne, hyperpigmentation, other skin abnormalities, swelling of the eyelids, and eye discharge.[21,22] Children exposed during gestation were at risk for low birth weight and exhibited dark skin pigmentation, pigmented nails, and abnormal dentition.[23–25] These children also experienced physical growth retardation and various other developmental effects.[26,27] Headache, joint swelling and pain, numbness of extremities, and irregular menstruation, were common among exposed adults.[28–30]

Some of the nondioxin-like PCBs have estrogenic properties that influence reproductive and endocrine systems, with PCB exposure associated with disruption of reproductive function, liver disease, thyroid, and immune system dysfunction.[31–33] Adverse developmental outcomes have been observed in North Carolina children born to women in the general population with higher levels of PCBs.[34,35] Striking and persistent long-term effects have been observed in children whose mothers were exposed to high levels of PCBs and PCDFs from the Taiwan Yu-Cheng rice oil poisoning outbreak.[36,37]

PCBs have been classified as "carcinogenic to humans" by the International Agency for Research on Cancer (IARC), because of evidence that they induce multiple types of cancers, such as liver, lung, and melanoma.[38] Occupational studies show that PCB exposure is associated with increased risk of death due to melanoma of the skin, lymphoma, brain, liver, and biliary tract cancers.[39–43] Furthermore, nonoccupational exposure has been associated with greater risk of non-Hodgkin's lymphoma[44–46] and testicular cancer.[47,48] TCDD is classified as "carcinogenic to humans" with experimental evidence in animals supporting its role as a multisite carcinogen acting through a mechanism involving the aryl hydrocarbon receptor.[49] A meta-analysis of 31 studies examining exposure to TCDD supports a positive exposure response relationship with increased cancer incidence and mortality regardless of cancer type.[50] Other PCDDs and all PCDFs are considered "not classifiable as to their carcinogenicity in humans," due primarily to inadequate animal and epidemiologic evidence for evaluation.[49] However, occupational exposure to PCDDs has been associated with greater risk of mortality from cancer,[51–53] suggesting that high levels of exposure to PCDDs may increase cancer risk.

PESTICIDES

Chemicals used to kill insects, vermin, weeds, or fungus are classified as pesticides. Only a brief overview is provided here, Persistent organochlorine pesticides [e.g., diphenyltricholorethand (DDT), hexachlorobenzene, hexachlorochyclohexane] are currently more commonly used in low-income countries, and often these countries purchase the chemicals from high- and middle-income countries where the chemicals have been banned for use.[54] Emerging concerns over glyphosate are worthy of note, as our understanding of its influence on the environment and human health are actively evolving. Because the herbicide glyphosate, n-(phosphonometyhl) glycine, is less persistent than other pesticides, such as the organochlorine pesticides, it has generally been assumed that glyphosate is less toxic than more-persistent herbicides.[55] However, global concern has increased over the 40 years during which glyphosate use has become increasingly common, raising questions about the health implications of chronic and low-level exposure to glyphosate and its breakdown product aminomethyl phosphonic acid.[55] In 2015, IARC classified glyphosate as "probably carcinogenic to humans," but the epidemiologic evidence has generally been mixed in terms of effects on both all cancers and site-specific cancers.[56] However, a meta-analysis of six studies supports an association of glyphosate exposure with non-Hodgkin Lymphoma.[57] Experimental evidence from rodent studies suggests that glyphosate exposure reduces male fertility[58,59] by causing abnormal sperm morphology and reduction in spermatids.[60] Epidemiologic studies have suggested that greater exposure to glyphosate may be associated with neurodevelopmental (e.g., autism)[61] or neurodegenerative conditions (e.g., Parkinson's disease),[62,63] and chronic kidney disease.[64] Additionally, it has been hypothesized that glyphosate is potentially involved in the proliferation of antibiotic resistant bacteria.[55] Due to the ubiquity of exposure and widespread applications of glyphosate, additional research is needed to clarify human toxicity and carcinogenicity of this herbicide, particularly to understand chronic low and ultralow levels of exposure.

PER- AND POLYFLUOROALKYL SUBSTANCES AND OTHER HIGHLY FLUORINATED CHEMICALS

PFAS are a class of more than 4000 individual synthetic compounds, collectively referred to as PFAS. The number of PFAS compounds continues to grow since organofluorine chemistry is an active area of research and development. PFAS are used in many consumer products and industrial applications, including firefighting foam, nonstick cookware, food packaging, outdoor clothing, carpets, leather products, ski and snowboard waxes, waterproof makeup (e.g., mascara), dental floss, and many more.[65] Because of the diversity of PFAS uses, which date back to the 1930s, PFAS are found ubiquitously in the environment and have received much attention and investigation over the past decade amid growing concern about their global distribution and potential toxicity to humans and wildlife. The following sections describe the evolution of use of PFAS in commerce, their environmental fate and transport, routes of human exposure, and their capacity to adversely impact health.

It should be noted that PFAS-related research is advancing quickly. While we have made every effort to report the most current science, the pace of certain areas of PFAS research, notably our understanding of their ability to adversely impact human health and information about emerging PFAS compounds, will almost certainly exceed the lifetime of this textbook. Readers are encouraged to review up-to-date information on government websites and within the scientific literature, particularly as more time passes since publication of this book. Additionally, the majority of PFAS-related research to date has focused on "legacy" PFAS (described in the following sections). By extension, much of the information presented here is most relevant to legacy PFAS compounds. Emerging, "replacement" compounds (also described below) have several key distinctions from legacy compounds so that caution is needed in extrapolating information known about legacy PFAS to the emerging PFAS chemicals.

History, Chemistry, and Use of Highly Fluorinated Chemicals. Per- and polyfluoroalkyls substances do not occur naturally in the environment. The earliest PFAS compound, polytetrafluoroethylene, was invented in the 1930s, followed shortly thereafter by, perfluorooctanoic acid (PFOA) and perfluorooctane sulfonic acid (PFOS), which were developed in the 1940s.[66] Per- and polyfluoroalkyl molecules are comprised of a carbon chain with fluorine atoms bound along the chain. The carbon-fluorine bond is one of the strongest, most stable bonds in organic chemistry, making PFAS highly durable in the environment (e.g., resistant to heat, acids, bases, oxidizing agents, microbial degradation, enzymatic transformation, photolysis) and hence classified as POPs.[65] Many PFAS also have a reactive moiety (e.g., sulfonic or carboxylic acid group) at one end of the carbon chain, affording them both lipophobic and lipophilic properties useful for surfactants, water- and stain-proof finishes, and nonstick coatings. The nomenclature used to name the more than 4000 PFAS compounds is complex, but generally categorizes compounds by their chemical properties. Importantly, PFAS can be categorized by the length of their carbon chain (e.g., C8 compounds have an eight-carbon chain), with six or more carbons colloquially referred to as "long-chain" PFAS compounds. The terms "perfluoro" and "polyfluoro" refer to whether a PFAS is either fully fluorinated ("perfluoro") or partially fluorinated ("polyfluoro"). PFAS may be further divided based on the reactive group attached to one end of the carbon chain (e.g., carboxylate, sulfonate, phosphonate/phosphinate). For example, perfluorooctane sulfonate (PFOS) has a fully fluorinated eight-carbon chain with a sulfonic acid reactive group at one end of the molecule. Additionally, PFAS can be classified chronologically. Legacy PFAS refer to compounds that were developed in the middle of the twentieth century and tend to be highly stable, longer-chain compounds [e.g., PFOA, PFOS, perfluorononanoic acid (PFNA), perfluorohexane sulfonic acid (PFHxS)]. Replacement PFAS, such as GenX chemicals and perfluorobutane sulfonic acid (PFBS) have shorter chains and have been developed and introduced into the global marketplace over the past two decades.[67]

The production and use of PFAS has risen since the 1950s; however, the specific application and frequency of use has varied for individual compounds over time. For example, PFOS was invented in the 1940s and was initially used in stain- and water-resistant products. Its use in firefighting foam emerged in the 1960s. The compound enjoyed widespread use until the mid-2000s, when its environmental persistence and adverse health effects were recognized. PFOS was added to Annex B of the Stockholm Convention on Persistent Organic Pollutants. In 2000, one of the largest PFAS produces, 3M Corporation, decided to voluntarily phase out PFOS (and PFOA) production, ending their use in 2002. In 2006, the U.S. Environmental Protection Agency (EPA) launched the PFOA Stewardship Program, which recommended that manufacturers cease production of long-chain PFAS. Major PFAS producers, including DuPont agree to do so over the following decade. However, the voluntary phase-outs of long-chain PFAS by major global producers ushered in the development of new, replacement PFAS compounds with shorter carbon chains, such as GenX in order to provide the array of industries that use PFAS with alternative compounds having similar beneficial properties when used in their products.

Environmental Fate and Transport and Human Exposure to Highly Fluorinated Chemicals. The extensive use of PFAS has led to their global distribution and PFAS are now ubiquitously found in the environment, including in water, sediment, soil, and biota. PFAS are also found in humans, including members of the general population. The global distribution of PFAS was first documented in a 2001 publication, which reported PFOS concentrations in fish, bird, and mammal tissue collected from around the world.[68] Since then, numerous studies have documented PFAS in environmental medium (e.g., surface and ground water, sediments) and human blood (whole, plasma and serum), and an increasing number of regulatory agencies have turned their attention toward PFAS due to both their ubiquity in consumer products, food, and water and concerns about their potential adverse health effects.[69,70]

The major sources of PFAS entering the environment include manufacturing and industrial sites, firefighting training facilities, landfills, and waste treatment operations (e.g., wastewater treatment plants or the application of biosolids to land).[65] From these sites, PFAS can sorb to dust or soil particles, dissolve into water or volatilize, after which they can be distributed by short- and long-range transport process, including atmospheric transport and deposition, and fresh water and oceanic circulation. PFAS are then detected in biota. In plants, PFAS may originate from atmospheric deposition onto surfaces (e.g., leaves) or by uptake from the soil, which has recently been shown to be an important source of PFAS in agricultural plants.[71] Animals are exposed to PFAS through a variety of pathways including ingestion, absorption, and inhalation and longer-chain PFAS in particular can bioaccumulate in tissues.

Like wildlife, humans are exposed to PFAS through ingestion, inhalation, and absorption. Pathways of human exposure to PFAS are an active area of scientific research as awareness of environmental contamination grows. These pathways have been recently reviewed.[72] Ingestion, particularly through diet and contaminated drinking water, is the primary route of human exposure. Important dietary sources include seafood, dairy, and foods stored or cooked in materials containing PFAS.[73] The unique combination of chemical properties of PFAS make their removal from water more challenging than other water contaminants typically eliminated by municipal or home water treatment systems. Reverse osmosis and granular activated carbon can be used to remove PFAS from water; however, safe disposal of used filters and carbon constitutes an unsolved problem. Efforts are ongoing in the U.S. and internationally to establish safe levels and enforceable standards for PFAS in food and drinking water. Overall, concentrations of PFAS in people have declined since regulatory measures were taken by world leaders in the early 2000s to reduce the manufacture and use of these compounds.[74] However, when human body burdens of individual PFAS compounds are considered, trends suggest that exposures to legacy compounds (e.g., PFOA, PFOS) have declined,[74,75] but concentrations of replacement PFAS compounds are increasing in the environment, suggesting that human exposure is also likely increasing.[76,77]

Health Effects of Highly Fluorinated Chemicals. The health effects of legacy PFAS (PFOA, PFOS, PFNA, and PFHxS) have been most extensively studied in humans. The most comprehensive evidence that PFAS can adversely impact human health comes from a longitudinal study conducted in a population of people living near the DuPont Washington Works, in West Virginia.[78] Manufacturing operations led to extensive contamination of groundwater with PFAS and, as a result, human exposure via drinking water. Based on this study and others, PFAS have been associated with high cholesterol, thyroid disorders, ulcerative colitis, kidney and testicular cancer, impaired neurodevelopment (learning and behavior) in infants and children, pregnancy-induced hypertension, immunotoxicity, and reduced fertility.[72,79–81] Investigations into the biological mechanisms underlying the roles that PFAS play in the disease development are ongoing. While toxicological studies play an important role in understanding disease development, there are differences between the disposition of PFAS within humans and rodents that complicate interpretation of the rodent assay results.

Recent discovery of emerging PFAS compounds, such as GenX and PFBS, in municipal drinking water and human tissue have raised concern over their toxicity.[67] Emerging PFAS tend to have shorter chains than legacy PFAS, making them potentially less likely to bioaccumulate and cause toxicity. Currently, studies on the human health effects of emerging PFAS are limited. Early toxicological studies in animals suggest that GenX exposure is associated with adverse effects on the liver, kidney, blood, immune system, and fetal development, and that GenX may also be carcinogenic.[82,83] Animal studies have also shown that PFBS exposure is associated with adverse health effects on the thyroid, kidney, reproductive organs, and fetal development, but there are insufficient data to evaluate carcinogenicity of newer highly fluorinated chemicals.[82,83] More research is warranted to identify safe alternatives to the legacy PFAS,[84] and caution in regards to limiting human exposure is prudent in the interim. Further, although the toxicological profiles of newer highly fluorinated compounds are less well understood than that of the legacy PFAS, the Madrid Statement, a consensus document signed by more than 200 scientists from 38 countries in 2015, supports stringent policy reform to reduce the threats to human health posed by highly fluorinated chemicals due to their potential persistence and toxicity.[85]

HALOGENATED AND ORGANOPHOSPHATE FLAME RETARDANTS

Given the risk of loss of property or life posed by fire, it is not surprising that efforts to prevent fires have existed for millennia and are multifaceted. Many naturally flame-resistant materials, such as brick, concrete, glass, and wool, have also been used throughout history to reduce the risk of loss by fire. Synthetic chemicals have also been developed for their flame-retardant properties.

Several key practices and policies have influenced continued use of flame retardants in consumer products from the 1970s, when PCBs were banned, through the present day. In the mid-1970s flame retardants were added to children's clothing with the goal of protecting children in the event of fire.[86] In 1975, the State of California adopted flammability standard Technical Bulletin 117 (TB117), which required that certain materials in consumer products be able to withstand a small open flame (e.g., a candle or cigarette) for at least 12 seconds.[87] The standard was designed to reduce risk and injury from fires associated with common in-home uses of fire, such as candles and cigarettes. TB117 specifically applies to upholstered furniture, including baby products polyurethane foams. Additionally, many electronics and electrical appliances contain flame retardants. In this chapter, we consider two classes of chemical flame: halogenated organic flame retardants and OPFRs.

Halogenated Organic Flame Retardants. Halogenated organic flame retardants are an important class of fire-retardant additives used in a wide array of consumer products. Brominated flame retardants (BFRs) are among the most widely used compounds in this class because they offer relatively low cost and high-efficiency fire resistance. More than 75 BFRs exist, however, five represent the majority of the entire class' production. Commercial mixtures of polybrominated diphenyl ethers (PBDEs) or biphenyl oxides have been used as additive or reactive components in a variety of polymers; these mixtures include, decabromodiphenyl ether (DBDE), octabromodiphenyl ether (OBDE), and pentabromodiphtnyl ether (PentaBDE), as well as Tetrabromobisphenol A (TBBPA) and hexabromocylododecane (HBCD).[88] The use of BFR compounds began in the 1950s. BFRs were added to materials to prevent fires by reducing their flammability through mechanisms such as reducing heat transfer, preventing ignition, and/or slowing fire growth. The use of these compounds in consumer products increased in scope in the 1970s, and has been used in electronics (e.g., televisions, computers, mobile phones), furniture, mattresses, carpet pads, insulation boards, and upholstered textiles. Due to the widespread use of these individual compounds and mixtures, BFRs are found ubiquitously around the globe.[89] Environmental fate and transport of BFRs have been studied extensively and BFRs have been identified in air, water, sediment, sewage sludge, and biota. These findings suggest their distribution occurs by short- and long-range transport mechanisms.[90] Additionally, much scientific research attention has been focused on understanding the toxic effects BFRs in wildlife and humans.

PBDEs were first commercially produced in the 1970s. A hallmark of PBDE chemistry is their recalcitrance to degradation in the environment. PBDEs have a biphenyl ring structure with 209 possible combinations of carbon-bromine bonds, each of which represents an individual compound, called a congener[89,91] (Fig. 75-2). The strength and stability of the carbon-bromine bonds serves as the basis for the ability of PBDEs to resist degradation. In addition to their persistence in the environment, PBDEs can also bioaccumulate in biota.[90] Monitoring data of PBDE concentrations in environmental medium show increases from the 1970s until the early 2000s, as use of these compounds increased. As these compounds were phased out of use and production throughout the early 2000s due to growing awareness of their toxicity to wildlife and humans, concentrations in environmental medium and biota have declined.[92,93] One exception to this pattern is Antarctica, where concentrations continue to increase.[92]

Humans are exposed to PBDEs through ingestion (diet), inhalation (primarily PBDEs sorbed to dust particles), and dermal absorption. The lower brominated congeners tend to be most well absorbed following ingestion and are most likely to bioaccumulate. PBDEs can induce Phase I and II liver enzymes, but are relatively poorly metabolized and slowly excreted. PBDEs accumulate in lipid-rich tissues in the body and their half-lives can exceed 2 years in humans. PBDEs have been detected in human tissue, blood, and breastmilk.[94,95] Scientific research has linked PBDEs to a range of adverse health effects. Toxicological studies in mice and rats have shown that PBDEs cause neurological, neurodevelopmental, reproductive, thyroid, immune, liver, pancreas, and teratogenic toxicity, with both epidemiologic and toxicologic studies suggesting that PBDEs are endocrine disrupting compounds.[88] The U.S. Environmental Protection Agency (EPA) and the National Toxicology Program (NTP) show evidence that some PBDEs (decaBDE and pentaBDE) are carcinogenic, but neither the International Agency for Research on Cancer nor the U.S. Department of Health and Human Services (DHHS) have classified

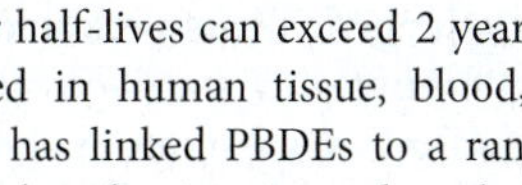

Br_m — O — Br_n

FIGURE 75-2. General chemical structure of polybrominated diphenyl ethers. (*Source:* https://commons.wikimedia.org/wiki/File:Polybrominated_diphenyl_ether.svg.)

PBDEs as carcinogenic.[96] At this time, evidence is strongest for PBDE-induced reduced thyroid hormone levels, impairment of neurodevelopment in children (particularly cognitive function, motor function, and behavior regulation), and endocrine disruption. Further information about the disposition of PBDEs in the body and their toxicity is available in a variety of formats, including government reports and primary literature.[88,97,98]

HBCDs have been less widely studied than PBDEs, however, their widespread use, persistence in the environment, and propensity for bioaccumulation, means that human exposures are common—likely via the same routes at PBDEs—and that HBCDs is long-lived within the body. Although fewer toxicological studies have investigated the effects of HBCD, those which have shown evidence of adverse impacts on a variety of organ systems, including neurodevelopmental,[99] the immune system,[100] and lipid and glucose homeostasis with high fat diet[101] among others. Like all BFRs, tetrabromobisphenol A (TBBPA) is used in a diverse set of products; however, it is particularly common in microelectronics (e.g., printed circuit boards) and resins. Although TBBPA also contains two phenyl rings, it is produced by the reaction of bisphenol A and bromine, resulting in a diphenylmethane structure that is distinct from the diphenyl structure of PBDEs. This feature distinguishes its commercial applications and disposition in the environment. Notably, TBBPA is more soluble in water than PBDEs. While human exposures to TBBPA can still occur via ingestion (primarily via diet), inhalation (sorbed to dust), and absorption, the half-life of TBBPA is shorter than other BFRs.[102] Nevertheless, TBBPA is still recognized as persistent and bioaccumulative. Toxicological studies in rodents show that TBBPA exposure is associated with changes in thyroid hormone levels, kidney toxicity, and impairment of adipose tissue physiology, as well as uterine tumors in females.[103–105]

Organophosphate Flame Retardants. As BFRs have largely been phased out amid concerns over toxicity, the use of less-persistent OPFRs has increased to meet flame resistant standards. OPFR refers to a class of phosphate ether compounds, which are flame resistant such that their addition to consumer products, helps manufacturers of an array of products (e.g., furniture foam, electronics) meet flammability standards. Currently, the most common and well-studied OPFRs include: tris(2-chloroethyl) phosphate (TCEP), tributyl phosphate (TnBP), tris(1,3-dichloro-2-propyl) phosphate (TDCP), triphenyl phosphate (TPP), tris(1-chloro-2-propyl) phosphate (TCPP), and tricresyl phosphate (TCP).[106] OPFRs have been in use and production since the 1940s. In response to a series of tragic deaths of children wearing clothing made from rayon and other highly flammable fabrics, the U.S. Flammable Fabrics Act of 1953 was passed, and then amended in 1967 to include other materials used in interior furnishings and clothing.[107] OPFRs were among the compounds used to comply with flammability standards of the time, though little was known about their disposition in the environment and effects on humans. From 1973 to 1978 children's clothing, notably sleepwear, was made from fabric treated with the OPFR, tris(2,3-dibromopropyl) phosphate.[86] Toxicological investigation showed that tris(2,3-dibromopropyl) phosphate was mutagenic,[108] and an epidemiologic study identified its metabolite in the urine of children who wore treated clothing, indicating dermal absorption. Shortly thereafter, tris(2,3-dibromopropyl) phosphate was removed from children's clothing.

The use of OPFRs in consumer products has been on the rise since the mid-2000s, when PBDEs were being phased out of use and production. Given the widespread use of OPFRs, human exposure is ubiquitous. In addition, given the structural similarity of modern OPFRs to earlier compounds, which have proven harmful to human health, it is not surprising that there is growing concern over human exposure to modern OFPRs. Humans are exposed to OPFRs through inhalation, ingestion, and dermal absorption. Inhalation and/or ingestion of dust to which OPFRs are sorbed are regarded as the primary route of exposure. OPFRs are rapidly metabolized by liver enzymes and excreted from the body, predominantly via urine (Table 75-1B). The half-lives of OPFRs in humans range from hours to days.[109–111] Regular detection of OPFR metabolites in urine samples collected from members of the general population of developed countries indicates that OPFRs are ubiquitous in the environment as they would otherwise be eliminated from the body quickly following exposure.

Toxicological and epidemiologic studies show that OPFRs are associated with an array of adverse health effects in animals. Since OPFRs are a diverse class of compounds with distinct chemical structures and biochemical properties, toxicity varies by compound. Broadly speaking, OPFRs have been associated with thyroid, neurodevelopmental, reproductive, kidney, liver, bladder, and adrenal toxicity. Toxicological studies also suggest that OPFRs may be carcinogenic, supporting associations of TCEP with kidney tumors, of TnBP with urinary bladder and liver tumors, and of TDCP with liver, kidneys, testes, and adrenal gland tumors,[112] and TDCP was listed as a carcinogen under California Proposition 65. More research is needed to understand the biological mechanisms underlying the toxicological effects that have been observed. Policies to remove OPFRs from consumer products are warranted given the weight of evidence showing many, if not all, members of the class can adversely affect health. Additionally, further consideration of flammability policy at state and federal scales to prevent repletion of another cycle of replacement flame retardant-turned environmental health villain.

ENVIRONMENTAL PHENOLS

Environmental phenols, including, bisphenol A (BPA) and its substitutes [bisphenol F (BPF) and bisphenol S (BPS)], benzophenones, triclosan, and parabens are nonpersistent phenolic compounds to which individuals living in industrialized countries are nearly ubiquitously exposed due to frequent use of these chemicals in consumer and personal-care products.[74] Environmental phenols cross the placenta and are detectable in the amniotic fluid of pregnant women.[113,114] Gestational exposure to environmental phenols presents special risks, because the developing fetus is particularly sensitive to endocrine-disrupting chemicals due to incompletely developed biologically protective mechanisms (e.g., detoxifying enzymes and DNA repair).[115]

Because environmental phenols are almost exclusively excreted in the urine, human exposure to environmental phenols is assessed by measuring urinary concentrations.[116–118] Blood levels are subject to exogenous contamination and tend to be considerably lower.[119] Although environmental phenols are nonpersistent chemicals with biological half-lives estimated to be < 24 hours, and thus do not persist in the body,[120–122] biomonitoring studies around the globe indicate nearly universal exposure to environmental phenols.[74,123–127] The short half-lives and episodic nature of dietary chemical exposures (e.g., BPA) result in more substantial within-person variability of urinary concentrations than chemical exposures from personal-care products (e.g., triclosan, parabens), which are used daily. Collectively, the environmental phenols represent a group of ubiquitous exposures with endocrine-disrupting properties, which may act through related biological mechanisms to cause adverse health outcomes.

Bisphenol A and Substitutes. BPA was synthesized in 1891. In the 1930s, it was considered for use as a potential synthetic estrogen, though diethylstilbestrol was ultimately adopted instead.[128] Beginning in the 1950s and continuing today, BPA is used as a monomer in polycarbonate plastics or epoxy resins, often used to line food and beverage cans despite its known estrogenic properties. Oral ingestion is the predominant exposure route since BPA can leach into food from packaging containers, and dermal absorption may be important for persons working with BPA-containing thermal receipts.[129,130] Leakage from dental amalgams that contain BPA is also a minor pathway of exposure.[131] As "BPA-free" products become increasingly prevalent, BPS and BPF are increasingly detected in urine samples of members of the general population of the United States (Fig. 75-3).[74,132] The toxicity of these BPA alternatives are less well understood, but early evidence suggest that BPF and BPS share similar or greater hormonal activity with BPA, indicating high potential that they possess similar endocrine-disrupting activity to BPA.[133] Epidemiologic research supports that adult exposure to BPA is associated with decreased fertility (e.g., reductions in ovarian reserve, in vitro fertilization success, miscarriage, sperm quality), disrupted hormones or hormonally mediated health outcomes (e.g., thyroid hormones, polycystic ovarian syndrome, type-2 diabetes), immunotoxicity, increased risk of cardiovascular disease (e.g., hypertension, cholesterol) and obesity, among others.[134] Gestational and early-life exposure to BPA has been associated with decreased birth weight and increased risk of childhood obesity and adverse neurodevelopmental/behavioral outcomes.[79,134,135]

Benzonphenone. Benzophenone-3 (BP-3), also known as oxybenzone, is an endocrine-disrupting chemical of emerging concern. Used as an ultraviolet light filter that is commonly incorporated into sunscreens, it is nearly ubiquitously present in the urine of individuals in the United States.[136] Dermal exposure to products containing BP-3 can sometimes cause a skin allergy or photo allergy.[137] BP-3 has been relatively understudied, but early evidence suggests that greater exposure to BP-3 is associated with sex-specific effects on birth weight (increased birth weight among male infants and decreased birth weight in females). Benzophenone has been classified by IARC as "possibly carcinogenic to humans."[138] An important consideration in the study of BP-3 is the potential for seasonal trends in exposure. BP-3 concentrations in urine of National Health and Nutrition Examination Survey (NHANES) participants are associated with sunscreen use[139] and peaks in urinary BP-3 concentrations during summer months has been observed in other populations as well.[140] Seasonal trends in exposure may prove to be an important consideration for other chemicals, such as triclosan and parabens (described below).

Triclosan. First introduced into commercial use in the 1960s, triclosan is an antimicrobial used in consumer and medical products. Though the U.S. Food and Drug Administration recently banned triclosan as an active ingredient in hand soap[141] and hand sanitizers,[142] dermal absorption may still occur due of its presence in other personal-care products such as antiperspirants or cosmetics.[143] Exposure through oral routes due to its use in toothpaste and mouthwashes is also common. However, triclosan has been removed from all human hygiene biocidal products in the European Union.[144] One important motivating factor in these bans were experimental studies indicating that environmentally relevant triclosan concentrations contributed to the development of bacterial resistance to antibiotics.[145] Epidemiologic evidence supports a role of triclosan exposure in the development of allergies and asthma, and adverse reproductive outcomes, including increased time to pregnancy.[144] Gestational exposure to triclosan has been associated with reduced size at birth, including reduced head circumference, suggesting a potential influence of triclosan on neurodevelopment; however, there is currently limited evidence in humans to support such associations.[79]

Parabens. Methyl-, ethyl-, propyl-, and butyl-parabens are esters of parahydroxybenzoic acid and are used as preservatives or antimicrobials in personal-care products, pharmaceuticals, food, and even water.[146,147] In the United States, women of reproductive age have higher urinary concentrations of parabens than men, likely due to greater use of personal-care products.[148] Use of these chemicals in personal-care products in the European Union is strictly regulated, and thus exposure is much less common. Parabens with longer alkyl side chains are more biologically active.[149] The paraben literature is somewhat inconsistent, but individual parabens have been associated with sperm DNA damage[150] and disruption of thyroid hormones (particularly among women).[151] Gestational exposure to parabens has been suggestively associated with birth weight.[152,153] In a study of maternal-son pairs from France, higher maternal urinary paraben levels were associated with greater birth weight,[127] and the positive association with methyl-paraben continued until 3 years of age.[154] However, the potential influence of parabens on childhood obesity is not presently well understood. Parabens have not been formally evaluated for carcinogenicity by IARC. Substantial controversy has surrounded the potential role of parabens in antiperspirants in the initiation and/or promotion of breast cancer, but some compelling evidence from experimental and epidemiologic studies suggests that caution may be warranted,[155–157] particularly when safer chemical alternatives and paraben-free formulations are available.

PHTHALATES

Phthalates are a class of nonpersistent synthetic chemicals that are diesters of phthalic acid (1,2-benzendicarboxylic acid). Phthalate diesters have a wide range of industrial uses and are frequently used as plasticizers to make polyvinyl chloride polymers softer or more flexible in a variety of products including: building materials, flooring, toys, medical devices, and food packaging/processing equipment. Phthalates are also used as fragrance retainers in a variety of personal-care products and cosmetics and as excipients in pharmaceuticals and dietary supplements.[117,158–160] Phthalate diesters are not chemically bound to products and are easily able to leach out. As such, there are multiple routes of phthalate exposure including ingestion (from contaminated food and pharmaceuticals/supplements), dermal contact, and inhalation.

After exposure, phthalate diesters are quickly metabolized into hydrolytic and/or oxidative monoester metabolites, conjugated to glucuronide or sulfate, and excreted in urine and feces.[159] Urine is the most common and reliable method for measuring phthalate metabolite concentrations (Table 75-1B). The pervasive use of phthalates has resulted in widespread exposure, and biomonitoring studies in the United States suggest that exposure to phthalates is nearly ubiquitous among members of general population.[74] However, the short half-lives of phthalates in the human body, combined with the frequent variability of an individual's exposure given typical alterations in diet and product use, create challenges for exposure assessment as a single biomarker measurement in urine may not accurately characterize a participant's typical exposure over time and could result in exposure misclassification. However, studies have shown that urinary concentrations of certain phthalate metabolites, particularly monoethyl phthalate, mono-n-butyl phthalate, mono-isobutyl phthalate,

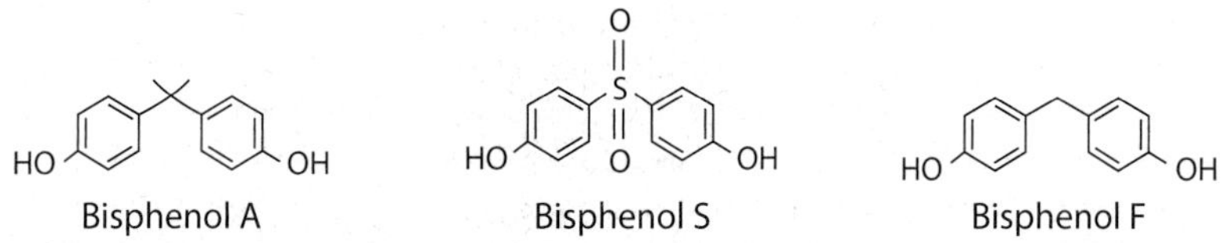

HO OH
Bisphenol A

O S O HO OH
Bisphenol S

HO OH
Bisphenol F

FIGURE 75-3. Chemical structures of bisphenol A, bisphenol S, and bisphenol F. (*Source:* Used with Permission from Eladak S, Grisin T, Moison D, et al. A new chapter in the bisphenol A story: Bisphenol S and bisphenol F are not safe alternatives to this compound. *Fertil Steril*. 2015;103(1):11–21.)

and monobenzyl phthalate, have fair to good correlation within individuals over time.[161-164]

Health Effects of Phthalates and Vulnerable Populations. Phthalates have well-documented antiandrogenic properties; they can not only mimic or inhibit hormones but can also alter target tissue response to hormonal signaling. Phthalates have been shown to interfere with the hypothalamic-pituitary-adrenal axis and thyroid axis, which are important for growth and development[165-168] and may also agonize or antagonize peroxisome proliferation activated receptors.[169]

While epidemiologic studies of the health effects of phthalate exposure have been mixed, with associations varying by phthalate metabolite, in general, phthalates been associated with a wide range of adverse health outcomes. Experimental evidence suggests that maternal-fetal transfer of phthalates occurs during gestation,[170] and phthalate monoester metabolites have been detected in amniotic fluid, umbilical cord blood, and meconium.[117,171,172] Exposure to phthalates during fetal development or early childhood may be particularly detrimental.

Increased maternal exposure to phthalates during gestation has been associated with alterations in birth outcomes (infant size and gestational duration), as well as alterations in anogenital distance and digit ratio (ratio of second digit to fourth digit), both of which are markers of fetal testosterone production.[159,173-176] Additionally, many studies have found adverse impacts of prenatal phthalate exposure on neurodevelopmental outcomes. Prospective epidemiologic studies have reported decreased cognition and increased behavioral problems [including anxiety, depression, autistic-like behaviors, internalizing and externalizing behaviors, aggressiveness, and attention deficit/hyperactivity disorder-like behaviors] in children born to mothers with higher urinary concentrations of select phthalate metabolites during pregnancy.[177-181] However, the direction and magnitude of these associations, as well as the implicated phthalates, have been inconsistent across studies. Many studies have reported sex-specific effects, indicating that the neurodevelopmental consequences of early-life phthalate exposure tend to be more detrimental in males.[182]

Collectively, the epidemiologic literature suggests that phthalate exposure may also impact somatic growth and obesity, pubertal development, reproductive health, thyroid hormones, allergies and asthma, respiratory heath, insulin resistance and diabetes risk, and cardiometabolic function.[159,173,174,183,184] Studies have also reported positive associations of di-*n*-butyl phthalate and diethyl phthalate exposure with breast cancer,[185,186] and IARC classifies diethylhexyl phthalate (DEHP) as a "possibly carcinogenic to humans."[138]

Phthalate Replacements. In recent years, some phthalates [e.g., di-2-ethylhexyl phthalate (DEHP) in children's toys] have been replaced by 1,2 cyclohexane dicarboxylic acid, diisononyl ester (DINCH).[187] While little is known about the potential human health effects of DINCH exposure, recent animal studies have reported that a metabolite of DINCH, cyclohexane-1,2-dicarboxylic acid monoisonyl ester (MHINCH), may interfere with the endocrine system,[188] and may alter female reproductive health in a similar manner to DEHP.[189]

PUBLIC HEALTH IMPLICATIONS OF ENVIRONMENTAL EXPOSURES: THE PAST, THE FUTURE, AND THE ROLE OF CLINICIANS

Clinicians, along with public health professionals, scientists, and policy makers play a central role in understanding environmental chemical exposures and conveying knowledge of associated health risks and modifiable lifestyle factors to the public so that individuals can take actions to reduce their chemical exposures. This chapter has summarized many of the most ubiquitous and widely studied chemicals and provides a broad overview of the associated health risks posed by these chemicals. The chapter also provides an overview of several areas of environmental health science that are emerging at this time.

As highlighted throughout the chapter, humans are exposed to a wide variety of environmental chemicals in their daily lives. Understanding the source(s) of exposure and their influence on both short- and long-term health is of critical public health importance. While much is known about some of these chemical exposures, particularly of legacy, persistent compounds, the field of environmental health is rapidly advancing. We are continuously learning about new chemicals that humans are exposed to and new health effects associated with previously known exposures. We are also constantly developing new analytical tools to better measure or estimate human exposures to chemicals in their environment. Another important recent advance in environmental health is the development of new statistical analysis and exposure assessment methodology to assist in moving away from the investigation of single exposures to more rigorous multipollutant models.[190] Studying complex mixtures provide insights into how chemical coexposures affect health and assists scientist in identifying the most relevant exposures. The clear delineation of potential exposure sources, as well as understanding of pharmacokinetics, being aware of possible synergism or antagonism across exposures, and being able to account for common biological mechanisms across chemicals is critically important in environmental health studies.[191]

Like the fields of epidemiology and toxicology, the field of risk assessment is beginning to move toward considering multiple types of environmental exposures. Presently, the U.S. EPA establishes health-based limits for human exposure to harmful chemicals (e.g., U.S. EPA Integrated Risk Information System oral reference doses or cancer slope factors), which can be interpreted as the maximum amount of a chemical that a person can be exposed to daily for their lifetime without experiencing an adverse health effect. Tools to conduct cumulative risk assessments, incorporating exposures to multiple chemical pollutants, as well as nonchemical stressors such as noise and social factors are being expanded and will hopefully catalyze improvements in risk minimization and environmental health policy in the future. Evaluating the "exposome," or the totality of all human environmental exposure from either the epidemiologic perspective or through a risk assessment framework remains an unattained ideal, though exposomic methods are rapidly improving.[192] Nevertheless, these efforts are providing insights into which environmental exposures are most detrimental to human health and how they can be intervened on by public health professionals and clinicians to reduce human exposures. Identifying the most critical exposures impacting the health of the general population can inform public health programs geared at reducing or eliminating the most harmful exposures at the population level and guide future policy reform that will improve population health and well-being.

The specific chemicals of concern for populations across the world will vary according to the regulatory landscape in individual countries. In the United States, the Toxics Substances Control Act (TSCA) was passed in 1976, providing the EPA with the authority to regulate chemicals that pose "unreasonable risk to health or to the environment," including many existing chemicals and those newly introduced into commerce.[193] In 2016, the Lautenberg Chemical Safety Act amended TSCA to require mandatory EPA evaluations of existing chemicals (beginning with chemicals most likely to cause risks), use of risk-based chemical assessments, increased transparency of chemical information to the public, and created consistent funding for EPA to enforce TSCA.[194] Many aspects of TSCA have proven challenging to implement, not the least of which is that the onus of demonstrating harm caused by chemicals falls to the EPA. By contrast, the European Union has adopted the precautionary principle, which indicates that "when an activity raises threats of harm to human health or the environment, precautionary measures should be taken even if some cause and effect relationships are not fully established scientifically."[195] As such, the European Commission's Registration, Evaluation, Authorisation, and Restriction of Chemicals (REACH) legislation, passed in 2007, requires manufacturers to provide safety data to support chemicals registered for use in the European Union.[196] Under REACH, the European Chemicals Agency (ECHA) identifies chemicals that pose "unacceptable hazards to human health and/or the environment" and has authority to restrict their use in commerce.[197] Quantification of disease burdens and economic costs associated with exposure to endocrine-disrupting chemicals suggests an advantage of the system employed by the EU. Human and animal studies were used to estimate the collective costs of 15 exposures (including PBDEs, phthalates, and bisphenol A, among others) based on their associations with several outcomes of interest (decrease in intelligence quotient points, attention deficit hyperactivity disorder, autism, obesity, diabetes, cryptorchidism, testicular cancer, male factor infertility, early cardiovascular mortality, leiomyomas, and endometriosis). Disease costs attributable to these exposures were estimated to be $340 billion [2.33% of gross domestic product (GDP)] in the U.S. versus $217 billion (1.28% of GDP in Europe).[198] China, Turkey, Japan, Taiwan, and South Korea have all adopted regulations similar to REACH.[196] Further implementation of the precautionary principle to preventing harmful exposures will likely benefit populations worldwide in terms of preventing adverse health outcomes associated with exposure to persistent and nonpersistent endocrine-disrupting chemicals.

Another important area of growth within the field of environmental health involves studying low and ultralow-level chronic exposures to environmental chemicals over the life course, including in sensitive subgroups within a population. New analytical methods have enabled increasingly low chemical detection limits in human biological samples, which has allowed scientists to begin to identify adverse health effects associated with lower levels of chemical exposures. This exposure scenario is highly relevant for the majority of the general population. As we consider the importance of chemical exposures on public health, we must keep in mind sensitive (e.g., pregnant women, children) and vulnerable (e.g., disadvantaged groups within society) populations, to whom low-level exposures may still pose a substantial threat. Further, we must remember that the effects of chemicals will vary by subpopulations. For instance, endocrine-disrupting chemicals may affect females and males differently. Thus, there is increasing focus on identifying sensitive subgroups within the population. Knowledge learned from studies evaluating low-level chronic exposures and their impacts on sensitive members of the general population will inform environmental health policy moving forward and is important for clinicians to be aware of in order to best treat and educate their patients.

In addition to environmental health policy and regulations, the importance of identifying modifiable risk factors for adverse health outcomes cannot be overstated. Modifiable risk factors can include lifestyle characteristics, behaviors, or comorbidities known to be risk factors for other disease, and are considered features of a person's life that they could alter to either reduce their exposure to environmental chemicals or the lessen the risk of developing associated adverse health effects. Clinicians play an important role in educating members of the general population about modifiable risk factors. For instance, a clinician could recommend testing water, for patients served by private wells, which are unregulated, installing a home water system if their drinking water is contaminated, or purchasing a flame retardant-free product when replacing their furniture. Similarly, a clinician could suggest eating organic fruits and vegetables and washing produce thoroughly to minimize pesticide residues, or choosing personal-care products that do not contain parabens, benzophenone, triclosan, PFAS, and phthalates. Nonprofit organizations such as the Silent Spring Institute and the Environmental Working Group publish useful guides for individuals and consumers looking to limit their exposures to the toxic chemicals in our environment.[199,200] Empowering individuals with knowledge and tools to reduce their exposure to chemicals of concern is an important public health priority. The largest public health gains will come when clinicians, scientists, and policy makers work together to inform and empower the general public.

References

1. Howard GJ. Chemical alternatives assessment: The case of flame retardants. *Chemosphere*. 2014;116:112–7.
2. Malloy TF, Zaunbrecher VM, Batteate CM, et al. Advancing alternative analysis: Integration of decision science. *Environ Health Perspect*. 2017;125(6):066001.
3. Jacobs MM, Malloy TF, Tickner JA, Edwards S. Alternatives assessment frameworks: Research needs for the informed substitution of hazardous chemicals. *Environ Health Perspect*. 2016;124(3):265–80.
4. Lavoie ET, Heine LG, Holder H, et al. Chemical alternatives assessment: Enabling substitution to safer chemicals. *Environ Sci Technol*. 2010;44(24):9244–9.
5. Calafat AM, Needham LL. Factors affecting the evaluation of biomonitoring data for human exposure assessment. *Int J Androl*. 2008;31(2): 139–43.
6. Stockholm Convention: Status of ratification. http://chm.pops.int/Countries/StatusofRatifications/PartiesandSignatoires/tabid/4500/Default.aspx. Accessed 29 October 2019.
7. U.S. State Department. Stockholm Conventiona on on Persistent Organic Pollutants 2019. https://www.state.gov/key-topics-office-of-environmental-quality-and-transboundary-issues/stockholm-convention-on-persistent-organic-pollutants/. Accessed 26 August 2019.
8. Johns LE, Cooper GS, Galizia A, Meeker JD. Exposure assessment issues in epidemiology studies of phthalates. *Environ Int*. 2015;85:27–39.
9. Teitelbaum SL, Britton JA, Calafat AM, et al. Temporal variability in urinary concentrations of phthalate metabolites, phytoestrogens and phenols among minority children in the United States. *Environ Res*. 2008;106(2):257–69.
10. Cogliano VJ. Assessing the cancer risk from environmental PCBs. *Environ Health Perspect*. 1998;106(6):317–23.
11. Marek RF, Thorne PS, Herkert NJ, Awad AM, Hornbuckle KC. Airborne PCBs and OH-PCBs inside and outside urban and rural U.S. schools. *Environ Sci Technol*. 2017;51(14):7853–60.
12. Martinez A, Hadnott BN, Awad AM, et al. Release of airborne polychlorinated biphenyls from New Bedford Harbor results in elevated concentrations in the surrounding air. *Environ Sci Technol Lett*. 2017;4(4):127–31.
13. Van den Berg M, Birnbaum L, Bosveld AT, et al. Toxic equivalency factors (TEFs) for PCBs, PCDDs, PCDFs for humans and wildlife. *Environ Health Perspect*. 1998;106(12):775–92.
14. Gilpin R, Wagel D, Solch J. Production, distribution and fate of polychlorinated dibenzo-p-dioxins, dibenzofurans and related organohalogens in the environment. In: Schecter A, Gasiewicz T, eds.Schecter A, Gasiewicz T, eds. *Dioxins and Health*. 2nd ed. Hoboken, NJ: Wiley-Interscience; 2003, pp. 55–87.
15. Institute of Medicine (US) Committee on the Implications of Dioxin in the Food Supply. Sources of dioxins and dioxin-like compounds in the environment. In: *Dioxins and Dioxin-like Compounds in the Food Supply: Strategies to Decrease Exposure*. Washington, DC: National Academies Press; 2003.
16. Braun JM, Gennings C, Hauser R, Webster TF. What can epidemiological studies tell us about the impact of chemical mixtures on human health? *Environ Health Perspect*. 2016;124(1):A6–9.
17. Martinez JM, Devito MJ, Birnbaum LS, Walker NJ. Toxicology of dioxins and dioxinlike compounds. In: Schecter A, Gasiewicz T, eds.Schecter A, Gasiewicz T, eds. *Dioxins and Health*. Hoboken, NJ: Wiley-Interscience; 2003, pp. 137–57.
18. Schecter A, Startin J, Wright C, et al. Congener-specific levels of dioxins and dibenzofurans in U.S. food and estimated daily dioxin toxic equivalent intake. *Environ Health Perspect*. 1994;102(11):962–6.
19. Hays SM, Aylward LL. Dioxin risks in perspective: Past, present, and future. *Regul Toxicol Pharmacol*. 2003;37(2):202–17.
20. Hsu C-C, Yu M-LM, Chen Y-CJ, Guo Y-LL, Rogan WJ. The Yu-Cheng rice oil poisoning incident. In: Schecter A, ed.Schecter A, ed. *Dioxins and Health*. Boston, MA: Springer US; 1994, pp. 661–84.

21. Masuda Y, Yoshimura H. Polychlorinated biphenyls and dibenzofurans in patients with yusho and their toxicological significance: A review. *Am J Ind Med.* 1984;5(1-2):31–44.
22. Masuda Y, Schecter A. The Yusho and Yucheng rice oil poisoning incidents. In: Schecter A, ed.Schecter A, ed. *Dioxins and Health: Including Other Persistent Organic Pollutants and Endocrine Disruptors.* 3rd ed. Hoboken, NJ: Wiley; 2012, pp. 521–51.
23. Rogan WJ. PCBs and cola-colored babies: Japan, 1968, and Taiwan, 1979. *Teratology.* 1982;26(3):259–61.
24. Rogan WJ, Miller RW. Prenatal exposure to polychlorinated biphenyls. *Lancet.* 1989;2(8673):1216.
25. Rogan WJ, Gladen BC, McKinney JD, et al. Neonatal effects of transplacental exposure to PCBs and DDE. *J Pediatr.* 1986;109(2):335–41.
26. Rogan WJ, Gladen BC, McKinney JD, et al. Polychlorinated biphenyls (PCBs) and dichlorodiphenyl dichloroethene (DDE) in human milk: Effects of maternal factors and previous lactation. *Am J Public Health.* 1986;76(2):172–7.
27. Rogan WJ, Gladen BC, McKinney JD, et al. Polychlorinated biphenyls (PCBs) and dichlorodiphenyl dichloroethene (DDE) in human milk: Effects on growth, morbidity, and duration of lactation. *Am J Public Health.* 1987;77(10):1294–7.
28. Yu ML, Guo YL, Hsu CC, Rogan WJ. Menstruation and reproduction in women with polychlorinated biphenyl (PCB) poisoning: Long-term follow-up interviews of the women from the Taiwan Yucheng cohort. *Int J Epidemiol.* 2000;29(4):672–7.
29. Guo YL, Yu ML, Hsu CC, Rogan WJ. Chloracne, goiter, arthritis, and anemia after polychlorinated biphenyl poisoning: 14-year follow-Up of the Taiwan Yucheng cohort. *Environ Health Perspect.* 1999;107(9):715–9.
30. Yu ML, Guo YL, Hsu CC, Rogan WJ. Increased mortality from chronic liver disease and cirrhosis 13 years after the Taiwan "yucheng" ("oil disease") incident. *Am J Ind Med.* 1997;31(2):172–5.
31. Crinnion WJ. Polychlorinated biphenyls: Persistent pollutants with immunological, neurological, and endocrinological consequences. *Altern Med Rev.* 2011;16(1):5–13.
32. Faroon O, Ruiz P. Polychlorinated biphenyls: New evidence from the last decade. *Toxicol Ind Health.* 2016;32(11):1825–47.
33. Longnecker M, Korrick S, Moysich K. Human health effects of polychlorinated biphenyls. In: Schecter A, Gasiewicz T, eds.Schecter A, Gasiewicz T, eds. *Dioxins and Health.* Hoboken, NJ: Wiley-Interscience; 2003, pp. 679–28.
34. Rogan WJ, Gladen BC. Study of human lactation for effects of environmental contaminants: The North Carolina breast milk and formula project and some other ideas. *Environ Health Perspect.* 1985;60:215–21.
35. Pan I-J, Daniels JL, Herring AH, et al. Lactational exposure to polychlorinated biphenyls, dichlorodiphenyltrichloroethane, and dichlorodiphenyldichloroethylene and infant growth: An analysis of the pregnancy, infection, and nutrition babies study. *Paediatr Perinat Epidemiol.* 2010;24(3):262–71.
36. Chen YC, Guo YL, Hsu CC, Rogan WJ. Cognitive development of Yu-Cheng ("oil disease") children prenatally exposed to heat-degraded PCBs. *JAMA.* 1992;268(22):3213–8.
37. Chen YC, Yu ML, Rogan WJ, Gladen BC, Hsu CC. A 6-year follow-up of behavior and activity disorders in the Taiwan Yu-cheng children. *Am J Public Health.* 1994;84(3):415–21.
38. IARC Working Group on the Evaluation of Carcinogenic Risk to Humans. Polychlorinated biphenyls and polybrominated biphenyls. In: *IARC Monographs on the Evaluation of Carcinogenic Risks to Humans, No. 107.* Lyon, France: International Agency for Research on Cancer; 2016.
39. Sinks T, Steele G, Smith AB, Watkins K, Shults RA. Mortality among workers exposed to polychlorinated biphenyls. *Am J Epidemiol.* 1992;136(4):389–98.
40. Loomis D, Browning SR, Schenck AP, Gregory E, Savitz DA. Cancer mortality among electric utility workers exposed to polychlorinated biphenyls. *Occup Environ Med.* 1997;54(10):720–8.
41. Yassi A, Tate R, Fish D. Cancer mortality in workers employed at a transformer manufacturing plant. *Am J Ind Med.* 1994;25(3):425–37.
42. Yassi A, Tate RB, Routledge M. Cancer incidence and mortality in workers employed at a transformer manufacturing plant: Update to a cohort study. *Am J Ind Med.* 2003;44(1):58–62.
43. Nicholson WJ, Landrigan PJ. Human health effects of polychlorinated biphenyls. In: Schecter A, ed.Schecter A, ed. *Dioxins and Health.* Boston, MA: Springer US; 1994, pp. 487–524.
44. Colt JS, Severson RK, Lubin J, et al. Organochlorines in carpet dust and non-Hodgkin lymphoma. *Epidemiology.* 2005;16(4):516–25.
45. Engel LS, Lan Q, Rothman N. Polychlorinated biphenyls and non-Hodgkin lymphoma. *Cancer Epidemiol Biomarkers Prev.* 2007;16(3):373–6.
46. Rothman N, Cantor KP, Blair A, et al. A nested case-control study of non-Hodgkin lymphoma and serum organochlorine residues. *Lancet.* 1997;350(9073):240–4.
47. Purdue MP, Engel LS, Langseth H, et al. Prediagnostic serum concentrations of organochlorine compounds and risk of testicular germ cell tumors. *Environ Health Perspect.* 2009;117(10):1514–9.
48. Hardell L, Van Bavel B, Lindström G, et al. Concentrations of polychlorinated biphenyls in blood and the risk for testicular cancer. *Int J Androl.* 2004;27(5):282–90.
49. IARC Working Group on the Evaluation of Carcinogenic Risk to Humans. Polychlorinated dibenzo-para-dioxins and polychlorinated dibenzofurans. In: *IARC Monographs on the Evaluation of Carcinogenic Risks to Humans, No. 69.* Lyon, France: International Agency for Research on Cancer; 2016.
50. Xu J, Ye Y, Huang F, et al. Association between dioxin and cancer incidence and mortality: A meta-analysis. *Sci Rep.* 2016;6:38012.
51. Manz A, Berger J, Dwyer JH, Flesch-Janys D, Nagel S, Waltsgott H. Cancer mortality among workers in chemical plant contaminated with dioxin. *Lancet.* 1991;338(8773):959–64.
52. Zober A, Messerer P, Huber P. Thirty-four-year mortality follow-up of BASF employees exposed to 2,3,7,8-TCDD after the 1953 accident. *Int Arch Occup Environ Health.* 1990;62(2):139–57.
53. Wang L, Weng S, Wen S, et al. Polychlorinated dibenzo-p-dioxins and dibenzofurans and their association with cancer mortality among workers in one automobile foundry factory. *Sci Total Environ.* 2013;443:104–11.
54. Jørs E, Neupane D, London L. Pesticide poisonings in low- and middle-income countries. *Environ Health Insights.* 2018;12:1178630217750876.
55. Van Bruggen AHC, He MM, Shin K, et al. Environmental and health effects of the herbicide glyphosate. *Sci Total Environ.* 2018;616–7: 255–68.
56. Mink PJ, Mandel JS, Sceurman BK, Lundin JI. Epidemiologic studies of glyphosate and cancer: A review. *Regul Toxicol Pharmacol.* 2012;63(3): 440–52.
57. Zhang L, Rana I, Shaffer RM, Taioli E, Sheppard L. Exposure to glyphosate-based herbicides and risk for non-Hodgkin lymphoma: A meta-analysis and supporting evidence. *Mutat Res.* 2019;781:186–206.
58. Abarikwu SO, Akiri OF, Durojaiye MA, Adenike A. Combined effects of repeated administration of Bretmont Wipeout (glyphosate) and Ultrazin (atrazine) on testosterone, oxidative stress and sperm quality of Wistar rats. *Toxicol Mech Methods.* 2015;25(1):70–80.
59. Dai P, Hu P, Tang J, Li Y, Li C. Effect of glyphosate on reproductive organs in male rat. *Acta Histochem.* 2016;118(5):519–26.
60. Nardi J, Moras PB, Koeppe C, Dallegrave E, Leal MB, Rossato-Grando LG. Prepubertal subchronic exposure to soy milk and glyphosate leads to endocrine disruption. *Food Chem Toxicol.* 2017;100:247–52.
61. von Ehrenstein OS, Ling C, Cui X, et al. Prenatal and infant exposure to ambient pesticides and autism spectrum disorder in children: Population based case-control study. *BMJ.* 2019;364:l962.
62. Caballero M, Amiri S, Denney JT, Monsivais P, Hystad P, Amram O. Estimated residential exposure to agricultural chemicals and premature mortality by Parkinson's disease in Washington state. *Int J Environ Res Public Health.* 2018;15(12):2885.
63. Eriguchi M, Iida K, Ikeda S, et al. Parkinsonism relating to intoxication with glyphosate. *Intern Med.* 2019;58(13):1935–8.
64. Jayasumana C, Gunatilake S, Senanayake P. Glyphosate, hard water and nephrotoxic metals: Are they the culprits behind the epidemic of chronic kidney disease of unknown etiology in Sri Lanka? *Int J Environ Res Public Health.* 2014;11(2):2125–47.
65. Buck RC, Franklin J, Berger U, et al. Perfluoroalkyl and polyfluoroalkyl substances in the environment: Terminology, classification, and origins. *Integr Environ Assess Manag.* 2011;7(4):513–41.
66. Interstate Technology Regulatory Council. Per- and Polyfluoroalkyl Substances (PFAS) Fact Sheets. n.d. 2020.
67. Gebbink WA, van Asseldonk L, van Leeuwen SPJ. Presence of emerging per- and polyfluoroalkyl substances (PFASs) in river and drinking water near a fluorochemical production plant in the Netherlands. *Environ Sci Technol.* 2017;51(19):11057–65.
68. Giesy JP, Kannan K. Global distribution of perfluorooctane sulfonate in wildlife. *Environ Sci Technol.* 2001;35(7):1339–42.
69. EFSA. Perfluoroctane sulfonate, perfluorooctanoic acid and their salts: Scientific opinion of the panel on contaminants in the food chain. *EFSA J.* 2008;653:1–131.
70. USEPA. Perfluorooctanoic Acid (PFOA) and Fluorinated Telomers. 2013. http://www.epa.gov/oppt/pfoa/, 2014.

71. Ghisi R, Vamerali T, Manzetti S. Accumulation of perfluorinated alkyl substances (PFAS) in agricultural plants: A review. *Environ Res.* 2019;169:326–41.

72. Sunderland EM, Hu XC, Dassuncao C, Tokranov AK, Wagner CC, Allen JG. A review of the pathways of human exposure to poly- and perfluoroalkyl substances (PFASs) and present understanding of health effects. *J Expo Sci Environ Epidemiol.* 2019;29(2):131–47.

73. Domingo JL, Nadal M. Per- and polyfluoroalkyl substances (PFASs) in food and human dietary intake: A review of the recent scientific literature. *J Agric Food Chem.* 2017;65(3):533–43.

74. Centers for Disease Control and Prevention. Fourth Report on Human Exposure to Environmental Chemicals, Updated Tables, January 2019. *CDC National Center for Environmental Health, Atlanta, GA, 30341.* 2019; 1.

75. Hurley S, Goldberg D, Wang M, et al. Time trends in per- and polyfluoroalkyl substances (PFASs) in California women: Declining serum levels, 2011–2015. *Environ Sci Technol.* 2018;52(1):277–87.

76. Hu XC, Tokranov AK, Liddie J, et al. Tap water contributions to plasma concentrations of Pply- and perfluoroalkyl substances (PFAS) in a nationwide prospective cohort of U.S. women. *Environ Health Perspect.* 2019;127(6):67006.

77. Sun M, Arevalo E, Strynar M, et al. Legacy and emerging perfluoroalkyl substances are important drinking water contaminants in the Cape Fear River watershed of North Carolina. *Environ Sci Technol Lett.* 2016;3(12):415–9.

78. Frisbee SJ, Brooks AP, Maher A, et al. The C8 health project: Design, methods, and participants. *Environ Health Perspect.* 2009;117(12):1873–82.

79. Braun JM. Early-life exposure to EDCs: Role in childhood obesity and neurodevelopment. *Nat Rev Endocrinol.* 2017;13(3):161–73.

80. Grandjean P, Andersen EW, Budtz-Jorgensen E, et al. Serum vaccine antibody concentrations in children exposed to perfluorinated compounds. *JAMA.* 2012;307(4):391–7.

81. Grandjean P, Heilmann C, Weihe P, et al. Estimated exposures to perfluorinated compounds in infancy predict attenuated vaccine antibody concentrations at age 5-years. *J Immunotoxicol.* 2017;14(1):188–95.

82. United States Environmental Protection Agency. *Fact Sheet: Draft Toxicity Assessments for GenX Chemicals and PFBS.* 2018.

83. Buck RC. Toxicology data for alternative "short-chain" fluorinated substances. In: DeWitt JC, ed.DeWitt JC, ed. *Toxicological Effects of Perfluoroalkyl and Polyfluoroalkyl Substances.* Cham: Springer International Publishing; 2015, pp. 451–77.

84. Birnbaum LS, Grandjean P. Alternatives to PFASs: Perspectives on the science. *Environ Health Perspect.* 2015;123(5):A104–5.

85. Blum A, Balan SA, Scheringer M, et al. The Madrid statement on poly- and perfluoroalkyl substances (PFASs). *Environ Health Perspect.* 2015;123(5):A107–11.

86. Blum A, Gold MD, Ames BN, et al. Children absorb tris-BP flame retardant from sleepwear: Urine contains the mutagenic metabolite, 2,3-dibromopropanol. *Science.* 1978;201(4360):1020–3.

87. State of California. *Technical Bulletin 117: Requirements, Test Procedure and Apparatus for Testing the Flame Retardance of Resilient Filling Materials Used in Upholstered Furniture.* State of California, 2000.

88. Birnbaum LS, Staskal DF. Brominated flame retardants: Cause for concern? *Environ Health Perspect.* 2004;112(1):9–17.

89. Rahman F, Langford KH, Scrimshaw MD, Lester JN. Polybrominated diphenyl ether (PBDE) flame retardants. *Sci Total Environ.* 2001;275(1–3):1–17.

90. Siddiqi MA, Laessig RH, Reed KD. Polybrominated diphenyl ethers (PBDEs): New pollutants-old diseases. *Clin Med Res.* 2003;1(4):281–90.

91. Siddique J, Lantos JD, VanderWeele TJ, Lauderdale DS. Screening tests during prenatal care: Does practice follow the evidence? *Matern Child Health J.* 2012;16(1):51–9.

92. Markham E, Brault EK, Khairy M, et al. Time trends of polybrominated diphenyl ethers (PBDEs) in Antarctic biota. *ACS Omega.* 2018;3(6):6595–4.

93. Zhou C, Pagano J, McGoldrick DJ, et al. Legacy polybrominated diphenyl ethers (PBDEs) trends in top predator fish of the Laurentian Great Lakes (GL) from 1979 to 2016: Will concentrations continue to decrease? *Environ Sci Technol.* 2019;53(12):6650–9.

94. Thomsen C, Haug LS, Stigum H, Frøshaug M, Broadwell SL, Becher G. Changes in concentrations of perfluorinated compounds, polybrominated diphenyl ethers, and polychlorinated biphenyls in Norwegian breast-milk during twelve months of lactation. *Environ Sci Technol.* 2010;44(24):9550–6.

95. Turyk ME, Anderson HA, Steenport D, Buelow C, Imm P, Knobeloch L. Longitudinal biomonitoring for polybrominated diphenyl ethers (PBDEs) in residents of the Great Lakes basin. *Chemosphere.* 2010;81(4):517–22.

96. United States Environmental Protection Agency. *Technical Fact Sheet—Polybrominated Diphenyl Ethers (PBDEs) (EPA 505-F-17-015).* Office of Land and Emergency Management (5106P); 2017.

97. ATSDR, U.S. Department of Health and Human Services, Public Health Service. *Toxicological Profile for Polybrominated Diphenyl Ethers (PBDEs).* U.S. Dept of Health and Human Services, Agency for Toxic Substances and Disease Registry; 2015.

98. Hudson-Hanley B, Irvin V, Flay B, MacDonald M, Kile ML. Prenatal PBDE exposure and neurodevelopment in children 7 years old or younger: A systematic review and meta-analysis. *Curr Epidemiol Rep.* 2018;5(1):46–59.

99. Pham-Lake C, Aronoff EB, Camp CR, Vester A, Peters SJ, Caudle WM. Impairment in the mesohippocampal dopamine circuit following exposure to the brominated flame retardant, HBCDD. *Environ Toxicol Pharmacol.* 2017;50:167–74.

100. Yasmin S, Whalen M. Flame retardants, hexabromocyclododecane (HCBD) and tetrabromobisphenol a (TBBPA), alter secretion of tumor necrosis factor alpha (TNFalpha) from human immune cells. *Arch Toxicol.* 2018;92(4):1483–94.

101. Yanagisawa R, Koike E, Win-Shwe TT, Yamamoto M, Takano H. Impaired lipid and glucose homeostasis in hexabromocyclododecane-exposed mice fed a high-fat diet. *Environ Health Perspect.* 2014;122(3):277–83.

102. Kodavanti Prs, Stoker TE, Fenton SE. Brominated flame retardants. In: Gupta R, ed.Gupta R, ed. *Reproductive and Developmental Toxicology.* 2nd ed. Hopkinsville, KY: Elsevier Academic Press; 2017, pp. 681–710.

103. Abou-Elwafa Abdallah M. Environmental occurrence, analysis and human exposure to the flame retardant tetrabromobisphenol-A (TBBP-A)—A review. *Environ Int.* 2016;94:235–50.

104. Kakutani H, Yuzuriha T, Akiyama E, Nakao T, Ohta S. Complex toxicity as disruption of adipocyte or osteoblast differentiation in human mesenchymal stem cells under the mixed condition of TBBPA and TCDD. *Toxicol Rep.* 2018;5:737–43.

105. Lai DY, Kacew S, Dekant W. Tetrabromobisphenol A (TBBPA): Possible modes of action of toxicity and carcinogenicity in rodents. *Food Chem Toxicol.* 2015;80:206–14.

106. ATSDR, U.S. Department of Health and Human Services, Public Health Service. *Toxicological Profile for Phosphate Ester Flame Retardants.* U.S. Dept of Health and Human Services, Agency for Toxic Substances and Disease Registry; 2012.

107. Bergman AB. Flammable Fabrics Act amendents of 1967. *Northwest Med.* 1967;66(7):627 passim.

108. Prival MJ, McCoy EC, Gutter B, Rosendranz HS. Tris(2,3-dibromopropyl) phosphate: Mutagenicity of a widely used flame retardant. *Science.* 1977;195(4273):76–8.

109. Nomeir AA, Kato S, Matthews HB. The metabolism and disposition of tris(1,3-dichloro-2-propyl) phosphate (Fyrol FR-2) in the rat. *Toxicol Appl Pharmacol.* 1981;57(3):401–13.

110. Chapman DE, Michener SR, Powis G. Metabolism of the flame retardant plasticizer tris(2-chloroethyl)phosphate by human and rat liver preparations. *Fundam Appl Toxicol.* 1991;17(2):215–24.

111. Burka LT, Sanders JM, Herr DW, Matthews HB. Metabolism of tris(2-chloroethyl) phosphate in rats and mice. *Drug Metab Dispos.* 1991;19(2):443–7.

112. ATSDR, U.S. Department of Health and Human Services, Public Health Service. *ToxFAQs™ for Phosphate Ester Flame Retardants.* U.S. Dept of Health and Human Services, Agency for Toxic Substances and Disease Registry; 2012.

113. Li LX, Chen L, Meng XZ, et al. Exposure levels of environmental endocrine disruptors in mother-newborn pairs in China and their placental transfer characteristics. *PLoS One.* 2013;8(5):e62526.

114. Philippat C, Wolff MS, Calafat AM, et al. Prenatal exposure to environmental phenols: Concentrations in amniotic fluid and variability in urinary concentrations during pregnancy. *Environ Health Perspect.* 2013;121(10):1225–31.

115. Newbold RR, Padilla-Banks E, Jefferson WN. Environmental estrogens and obesity. *Mol Cell Endocrinol.* 2009;304(1–2):84–89.

116. Calafat AM, Ye X, Wong LY, Reidy JA, Needham LL. Urinary concentrations of triclosan in the U.S. population: 2003–2004. *Environ Health Perspect.* 2008;116(3):303–7.

117. Silva MJ, Barr DB, Reidy JA, et al. Urinary levels of seven phthalate metabolites in the U.S. population from the National Health and Nutri-

tion Examination Survey (NHANES) 1999–2000. *Environ Health Perspect.* 2004;112(3):331–8.

118. Calafat AM, Ye X, Wong LY, Reidy JA, Needham LL. Exposure of the U.S. population to bisphenol A and 4-tertiary-octylphenol: 2003–2004. *Environ Health Perspect.* 2008;116(1):39–44.
119. Ye X, Zhou X, Hennings R, Kramer J, Calafat AM. Potential external contamination with bisphenol A and other ubiquitous organic environmental chemicals during biomonitoring analysis: An elusive laboratory challenge. *Environ Health Perspect.* 2013;121(3):283–6.
120. Sandborgh-Englund G, Adolfsson-Erici M, Odham G, Ekstrand J. Pharmacokinetics of triclosan following oral ingestion in humans. *J Toxicol Environ Health A.* 2006;69(20):1861–73.
121. Okereke CS, Abdel-Rhaman MS, Friedman MA. Disposition of benzophenone-3 after dermal administration in male rats. *Toxicol Lett.* 1994;73(2):113–22.
122. Volkel W, Colnot T, Csanady GA, Filser JG, Dekant W. Metabolism and kinetics of bisphenol A in humans at low doses following oral administration. *Chem Res Toxicol.* 2002;15(10):1281–7.
123. Meeker JD, Cantonwine D, Rivera-Gonzalez LO, et al. Distribution, variability and predictors of urinary concentrations of phenols and parabens among pregnant women in Puerto Rico. *Environ Sci Technol.* 2013;47(7):3439–47.
124. Bertelsen RJ, Longnecker MP, Lovik M, et al. Triclosan exposure and allergic sensitization in Norwegian children. *Allergy.* 2013;68(1):84–91.
125. Li X, Ying GG, Zhao JL, Chen ZF, Lai HJ, Su HC. 4-Nonylphenol, bisphenol-A and triclosan levels in human urine of children and students in China, and the effects of drinking these bottled materials on the levels. *Environ Int.* 2013;52:81–6.
126. Vandenberg LN, Chauhoud I, Heindel JJ, Padmanabhan V, Paumgartten FJ, Schoenfelder G. Urinary, circulating and tissue biomonitoring studies indicate widespread exposure to bisphenol A. *Environ Health Perspect.* 2010;118(8):1055–70.
127. Philippat C, Mortamais M, Chevrier C, et al. Exposure to phthalates and phenols during pregnancy and offspring size at birth. *Environ Health Perspect.* 2012;120(3):464–70.
128. Vogel SA. The politics of plastics: The making and unmaking of bisphenol a "safety." *Am J Public Health.* 2009;99(Suppl 3):S559–66.
129. Carwile JL, Ye X, Zhou X, Calafat AM, Michels KB. Canned soup consumption and urinary bisphenol A: A randomized crossover trial. *JAMA.* 2011;306(20):2218–20.
130. von Goetz N, Wormuth M, Scheringer M, Hungerbuhler K. Bisphenol A: How the most relevant exposure sources contribute to total consumer exposure. *Risk Anal.* 2010;30(3):473–87.
131. Löfroth M, Ghasemimehr M, Falk A, Vult von Steyern P. Bisphenol A in dental materials —Existence, leakage and biological effects. *Heliyon.* 2019;5(5):e01711.
132. Chen D, Kannan K, Tan H, et al. Bisphenol analogues other than BPA: Environmental occurrence, human exposure, and toxicity—A review. *Environ Sci Technol.* 2016;50(11):5438–53.
133. Rochester JR, Bolden AL. Bisphenol S and F: A systematic review and comparison of the hormonal activity of bisphenol A substitutes. *Environ Health Perspect.* 2015;123(7):643–50.
134. Rochester JR. Bisphenol A and human health: A review of the literature. *Reprod Toxicol.* 2013;42:132–55.
135. Braun JM, Hauser R. Bisphenol A and children's health. *Curr Opin Pediatr.* 2011;23(2):233–9.
136. Calafat AM, Wong L-Y, Ye X, Reidy JA, Needham LL. Concentrations of the sunscreen agent benzophenone-3 in residents of the United States: National Health and Nutrition Examination Survey 2003–2004. *Environ Health Perspect.* 2008;116(7):893–7.
137. Centers for Disease Control and Prevention. *Benzophenone-3.* Department of Health and Human Services; 2009.
138. IARC Working Group on the Evaluation of Carcinogenic Risk to Humans. Some chemicals present in industrial and consumer products, food and drinking-water. *IARC Monogr Eval Carcinog Risks Hum.* 2013;101:9–549.
139. Zamoiski RD, Cahoon EK, Michal Freedman D, Linet MS. Self-reported sunscreen use and urinary benzophenone-3 concentrations in the United States: NHANES 2003–2006 and 2009–2012. *Environ Res.* 2015;142:563–7.
140. Romano ME, Kalloo G, Etzel T, Braun JM. Re: Seasonal variation in exposure to endocrine-disrupting chemicals. *Epidemiology.* 2017;28(5):e42–3.
141. Food and Drug Administration HHS. Safety and effectiveness of consumer antiseptics; Topical antimicrobial drug products for over-the-counter human use (81 FR 42911). *Fed Regist.* 2016;81(126):42911–37.
142. Food and Drug Administration HHS. Safety and effectiveness of consumer antiseptics; Topical antimicrobial drug products for over-the-counter human use (81 FR 42911). *Fed Regist.* 2016;81(126):42911–37.
143. Dann AB, Hontela A. Triclosan: Environmental exposure, toxicity and mechanisms of action. *J Appl Toxicol.* 2011;31(4):285–311.
144. Weatherly LM, Gosse JA. Triclosan exposure, transformation, and human health effects. *J Toxicol Environ Health B Crit Rev.* 2017;20(8):447–69.
145. Schweizer HP. Triclosan: A widely used biocide and its link to antibiotics. *FEMS Microbiol Lett.* 2001;202(1):1–7.
146. Błędzka D, Gromadzińska J, Wąsowicz W. Parabens. From environmental studies to human health. *Environ Int.* 2014;67:27–42.
147. Guo Y, Kannan K. A survey of phthalates and parabens in personal care products from the United States and its implications for human exposure. *Environ Sci Technol.* 2013;47(24):14442–9.
148. Calafat AM, Ye X, Wong LY, Bishop AM, Needham LL. Urinary concentrations of four parabens in the U.S. population: NHANES 2005–2006. *Environ Health Perspect.* 2010;118(5):679–85.
149. Routledge EJ, Parker J, Odum J, Ashby J, Sumpter JP. Some alkyl hydroxy benzoate preservatives (parabens) are estrogenic. *Toxicol Appl Pharmacol.* 1998;153(1):12–9.
150. Meeker JD, Yang T, Ye X, Calafat AM, Hauser R. Urinary concentrations of parabens and serum hormone levels, semen quality parameters, and sperm DNA damage. *Environ Health Perspect.* 2011;119(2):252–7.
151. Koeppe ES, Ferguson KK, Colacino JA, Meeker JD. Relationship between urinary triclosan and paraben concentrations and serum thyroid measures in NHANES 2007–2008. *Sci Total Environ.* 2013;445–6:299–305.
152. Goodrich JM, Ingle ME, Domino SE, et al. First trimester maternal exposures to endocrine disrupting chemicals and metals and fetal size in the Michigan mother-infant pairs study. *J Dev Orig Health Dis.* 2019;10(4):447–58.
153. Messerlian C, Mustieles V, Minguez-Alarcon L, et al. Preconception and prenatal urinary concentrations of phenols and birth size of singleton infants born to mothers and fathers from the Environment and Reproductive Health (EARTH) study. *Environ Int.* 2018;114:60–8.
154. Philippat C, Botton J, Calafat AM, et al. Prenatal exposure to phenols and growth in boys. *Epidemiology.* 2014;25(5):625–35.
155. Harvey PW. Parabens, oestrogenicity, underarm cosmetics and breast cancer: A perspective on a hypothesis. *J Appl Toxicol.* 2003;23(5):285–8.
156. Konduracka E, Krzemieniecki K, Gajos G. Relationship between everyday use cosmetics and female breast cancer. *Pol Arch Med Wewn.* 2014;124(5):264–9.
157. Parada H, Jr., Gammon MD, Ettore HL, et al. Urinary concentrations of environmental phenols and their associations with breast cancer incidence and mortality following breast cancer. *Environ Int.* 2019;130:104890.
158. Koo HJ, Lee BM. Estimated exposure to phthalates in cosmetics and risk assessment. *J Toxicol Environ Health A.* 2004;67(23–24):1901–14.
159. Hauser R, Calafat AM. Phthalates and human health. *Occup Environ Med.* 2005;62(11):806–18.
160. Romano ME, O'Connell K, Du M, Rehm CD, Kantor ED. Use of dietary supplements in relation to urinary phthalate metabolite concentrations: Results from the National Health and Nutrition Examination Survey. *Environ Res.* 2018;172:437–43.
161. Adibi JJ, Whyatt RM, Williams PL, et al. Characterization of phthalate exposure among pregnant women assessed by repeat air and urine samples. *Environ Health Perspect.* 2008;116(4):467–73.
162. Ferguson KK, McElrath TF, Ko YA, Mukherjee B, Meeker JD. Variability in urinary phthalate metabolite levels across pregnancy and sensitive windows of exposure for the risk of preterm birth. *Environ Int.* 2014;70:118–24.
163. Watkins DJ, Eliot M, Sathyanarayana S, et al. Variability and predictors of urinary concentrations of phthalate metabolites during early childhood. *Environ Sci Technol.* 2014;48(15):8881–90.
164. Teitelbaum SL, Mervish N, Moshier EL, et al. Associations between phthalate metabolite urinary concentrations and body size measures in New York City children. *Environ Res.* 2012;112:186–93.
165. Boas M, Feldt-Rasmussen U, Main KM. Thyroid effects of endocrine disrupting chemicals. *Mol Cell Endocrinol.* 2012;355(2):240–8.
166. Howdeshell KL, Rider CV, Wilson VS, Gray LE Jr, Mechanisms of action of phthalate esters, individually and in combination, to induce abnormal reproductive development in male laboratory rats. *Environ Res.* 2008;108(2):168–76.
167. Ma X, Lian QQ, Dong Q, Ge RS. Environmental inhibitors of 11beta-hydroxysteroid dehydrogenase type 2. *Toxicology.* 2011;285(3):83–9.

168. Stout SA, Espel EV, Sandman CA, Glynn LM, Davis EP. Fetal programming of children's obesity risk. *Psychoneuroendocrinology*. 2015;53:29–39.

169. Casals-Casas C, Feige JN, Desvergne B. Interference of pollutants with PPARs: Endocrine disruption meets metabolism. *Int J Obes (Lond)*. 2008;32(Suppl 6):S53–61.

170. Singh AR, Lawrence WH, Autian J. Maternal-fetal transfer of 14C-di-2-ethylhexyl phthalate and 14C-diethyl phthalate in rats. *J Pharm Sci*. 1975;64(8):1347–50.

171. Latini G, De Felice C, Presta G, et al. Exposure to Di(2-ethylhexyl) phthalate in humans during pregnancy. A preliminary report. *Biol Neonate*. 2003;83(1):22–4.

172. Zhang YH, Chen BH, Zheng LX, Wu XY. [Study on the level of phthalates in human biological samples]. *Zhonghua Yu Fang Yi Xue Za Zhi*. 2003;37(6):429–34.

173. Benjamin S, Masai E, Kamimura N, Takahashi K, Anderson RC, Faisal PA. Phthalates impact human health: Epidemiological evidences and plausible mechanism of action. *J Hazard Mater*. 2017;340:360–83.

174. Braun JM, Sathyanarayana S, Hauser R. Phthalate exposure and children's health. *Curr Opin Pediatr*. 2013;25(2):247–54.

175. Radke EG, Braun JM, Meeker JD, Cooper GS. Phthalate exposure and male reproductive outcomes: A systematic review of the human epidemiological evidence. *Environ Int*. 2018;121(Pt 1):764–93.

176. Radke EG, Glenn BS, Braun JM, Cooper GS. Phthalate exposure and female reproductive and developmental outcomes: A systematic review of the human epidemiological evidence. *Environ Int*. 2019;130:104580.

177. Engel SM, Miodovnik A, Canfield RL, et al. Prenatal phthalate exposure is associated with childhood behavior and executive functioning. *Environ Health Perspect*. 2010;118(4):565–71.

178. Whyatt RM, Liu X, Rauh VA, et al. Maternal prenatal urinary phthalate metabolite concentrations and child mental, psychomotor, and behavioral development at 3 years of age. *Environ Health Perspect*. 2012;120(2): 290–5.

179. Lien YJ, Ku HY, Su PH, et al. Prenatal exposure to phthalate esters and behavioral syndromes in children at 8 years of age: Taiwan maternal and infant cohort study. *Environ Health Perspect*. 2015;123(1):95–100.

180. Kim JI, Hong YC, Shin CH, Lee YA, Lim YH, Kim BN. The effects of maternal and children phthalate exposure on the neurocognitive function of 6-year-old children. *Environ Res*. 2017;156:519–25.

181. Philippat C, Nakiwala D, Calafat AM, et al. Prenatal exposure to nonpersistent endocrine disruptors and behavior in boys at 3 and 5 Years. *Environ Health Perspect*. 2017;125(9):097014.

182. Ejaredar M, Nyanza EC, Ten Eycke K, Dewey D. Phthalate exposure and childrens neurodevelopment: A systematic review. *Environ Res*. 2015;142: 51–60.

183. Radke EG, Galizia A, Thayer KA, Cooper GS. Phthalate exposure and metabolic effects: A systematic review of the human epidemiological evidence. *Environ Int*. 2019;132:104768.

184. Engel SM, Villanger GD, Nethery RC, et al. Prenatal phthalates, maternal thyroid function, and risk of attention-deficit hyperactivity disorder in the Norwegian mother and child cohort. *Environ Health Perspect*. 2018;126(5):057004.

185. Ahern TP, Broe A, Lash TL, et al. Phthalate exposure and breast cancer incidence: A Danish nationwide cohort study. *J Clin Oncol*. 2019;37(21):1800–9.

186. Lopez-Carrillo L, Hernandez-Ramirez RU, Calafat AM, et al. Exposure to phthalates and breast cancer risk in northern Mexico. *Environ Health Perspect*. 2010;118(4):539–44.

187. Silva MJ, Jia T, Samandar E, Preau JL, Jr., Calafat AM. Environmental exposure to the plasticizer 1,2-cyclohexane dicarboxylic acid, diisononyl ester (DINCH) in U.S. adults (2000–2012). *Environ Res*. 2013;126:159–63.

188. Campioli E, Duong TB, Deschamps F, Papadopoulos V. Cyclohexane-1,2-dicarboxylic acid diisononyl ester and metabolite effects on rat epididymal stromal vascular fraction differentiation of adipose tissue. *Environ Res*. 2015;140:145–56.

189. Minguez-Alarcon L, Souter I, Chiu YH, et al. Urinary concentrations of cyclohexane-1,2-dicarboxylic acid monohydroxy isononyl ester, a metabolite of the non-phthalate plasticizer di(isononyl)cyclohexane-1,2-dicarboxylate (DINCH), and markers of ovarian response among women attending a fertility center. *Environ Res*. 2016;151:595–600.

190. Lazarevic N, Barnett AG, Sly PD, Knibbs LD. Statistical methodology in studies of prenatal exposure to mixtures of endocrine-disrupting chemicals: A review of existing approaches and new alternatives. *Environ Health Perspect*. 2019;127(2):26001.

191. Johns DO, Stanek LW, Walker K, et al. Practical advancement of multipollutant scientific and risk assessment approaches for ambient air pollution. *Environ Health Perspect*. 2012;120(9):1238–42.

192. DeBord DG, Carreón T, Lentz TJ, Middendorf PJ, Hoover MD, Schulte PA. Use of the "Exposome" in the practice of epidemiology: A primer on -omic technologies. *Am J Epidemiol*. 2016;184(4):302–14.

193. United States Environmental Protection Agency. Laws & Regulations: Summary of the Toxic Substances Control Act. https://www.epa.gov/laws-regulations/summary-toxic-substances-control-act. Accessed 29 October 2019.

194. United States Environmental Protection Agency. Assessing and Managing Chemicals under TSCA: The Frank R. Lautenberg Chemical Safety for the 21st Century Act. https://www.epa.gov/assessing-and-managing-chemicals-under-tsca/frank-r-lautenberg-chemical-safety-21st-century-act.

195. Hayes AW. The precautionary principle. *Arh Hig Rada Toksikol*. 2005;56(2):161–6.

196. Silbergeld EK, Mandrioli D, Cranor CF. Regulating chemicals: Law, science, and the unbearable burdens of regulation. *Annu Rev Public Health*. 2015;36:175–91.

197. Williams ES, Panko J, Paustenbach DJ. The European Union's REACH regulation: A review of its history and requirements. *Crit Rev Toxicol*. 2009;39(7):553–75.

198. Attina TM, Hauser R, Sathyanarayana S, et al. Exposure to endocrine-disrupting chemicals in the USA: A population-based disease burden and cost analysis. *Lancet Diabetes Endocrinol*. 2016;4(12):996–1003.

199. Silent Spring Institute. Detox Me app: Tips for healthier living.

200. Environmental Working Group. Environmental Working Group: Consumer Guides. https://www.ewg.org/consumer-guides. Accessed 29 October 2019.

CHAPTER 76

Work-related Asthma*

David N. Weissman • Paul K. Henneberger • Jean M. Cox-Ganser

INTRODUCTION

Work-related asthma (WRA) is an important topic in public health and preventive medicine. It is associated with a high population burden, affecting millions in the United States (U.S.) alone. It is also preventable through primary and secondary public health interventions. This chapter will provide a brief introduction to WRA, including pathophysiology, epidemiology, diagnosis, and prevention in individuals and populations.

Overview of Asthma

Asthma is a chronic relapsing, usually inflammatory disorder characterized by hyperreactive airways (increased responsiveness of the tracheobronchial tree to various stimuli) and episodic, reversible airways obstruction.[1,2] Recurring symptoms include wheeze, shortness of breath, chest tightness, and cough. Asthma is very common in the U.S. Based on estimates in 2017, 19 million adults currently had asthma for a prevalence of 7.7%, and lifetime prevalence was 13.4%.[3]

Work-Related Asthma

WRA includes both occupational asthma (OA) that is caused by exposures at work, and work-exacerbated asthma (WEA) in which pre-existing or concurrent asthma is worsened by exposures or conditions at work (Fig. 76-1).[4–7] OA is new-onset asthma or the recurrence of asthma that had been in remission (i.e., asymptomatic and not requiring asthma medications) attributable to either a sensitizer or an irritant in the work environment.[7,8]

Sensitizer-induced OA cases are typically categorized based on whether the causative agents are high-molecular weight (HMW) (i.e., > 10,000 Daltons) agents such as proteins, or low-molecular weight (LMW) (i.e., < 10,000 Daltons) agents such as reactive chemicals. Examples of common HMW agents include allergens from laboratory animals, insects, flour, enzymes, and natural rubber latex (NRL). Examples of common LMW agents include diisocyanates, colophony fluxes, solders, plicatic acid found in western red cedar wood dust, acrylates, and glutaraldehyde.[9] One of the more comprehensive and up-to-date online lists of OA agents is available from the Quebec provincial government.[10] A summary of this list of agents is shown in Table 76-1.

Sensitizer-induced OA characteristically presents after a latency period allowing for development of immune sensitization, airways inflammation, and clinically apparent asthma. HMW agents can frequently be demonstrated to be allergens that induce antigen-specific immunoglobulin E (IgE) responses. Thus, allergy skin tests or serological tests demonstrating specific IgE sensitization are often used to evaluate for specific causative agents. Some LMW agents can serve as haptens, inducing specific IgE responses after binding

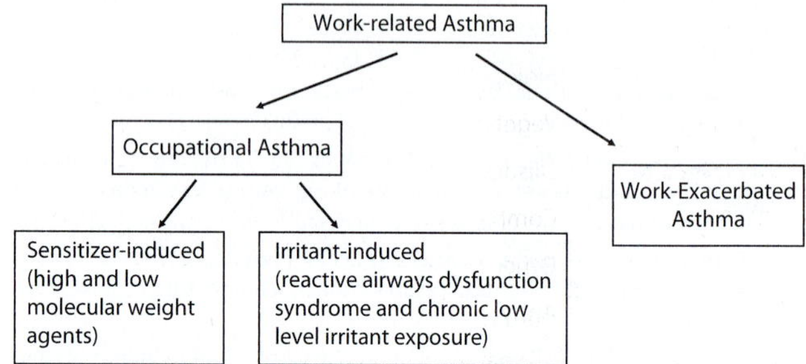

FIGURE 76-1. Relationship of work-related asthma, occupational asthma, and work-exacerbated asthma. See text for full description.

to larger molecules such as proteins. However, IgE sensitization does not always underlie sensitizer-induced OA, particularly OA induced by many LMW agents. In such cases, the immunologic mechanisms underlying OA remain unclear.[6,7]

The most widely accepted type of irritant-induced OA is reactive airways dysfunction syndrome (RADS), which is characterized by acute onset after a single high-level exposure to an irritant compound.[11] WRA cases might also be caused by long-term low-level irritant exposure at work, although evidence for this etiology is incomplete and remains a topic of investigation.[12]

WEA can occur in pre-existing or concurrent cases of asthma.[5] A pre-existing case experienced onset prior to entering a worksite of interest, which is a new job or changes in exposures or conditions at an existing job. A concurrent case of asthma had onset while in the worksite of interest but was not attributed to the suspected causes of exacerbation in that worksite. The exposures responsible for WEA are typically irritants but can also be allergens.[5,7,13] In addition to these agents, conditions in the workplace such as exercise or cold air can cause WEA.[7,13]

It is important to note that OA and WEA are not mutually exclusive. For example, an individual with OA attributed to a particular agent can subsequently develop WEA due to other workplace exposures or conditions. Some researchers make a distinction between WEA and work-aggravated asthma, with only the latter experiencing a permanent change in disease severity. However, most researchers and clinicians use these two terms interchangeably.[7]

PATHOPHYSIOLOGY OF WRA

A variety of pathogenic mechanisms associated with different biomarkers and phenotypes can lead to clinical asthma.[14–16] In 2019, the Global Initiative for Asthma (GINA) described phenotypes

*The findings and conclusions in this chapter are those of the authors and do not necessarily represent the views of the National Institute for Occupational Safety and Health.

TABLE 76-1 OCCUPATIONAL ASTHMA AGENTS COMPILED BY QUEBEC PROVINCIAL GOVERNMENT IN CANADA[10]

Molecular Weight	Category	Number of Agents	Examples of Agents
High molecular weight	Animal-derived antigens	27	Laboratory animal, cow dander
	Crustacea, seafoods, fish	23	Crab, prawn, salmon
	Arthropods	32	Locust, cricket, moth, butterfly
	Acarians	10	Grain mite
	Molds	12	*Aspergillus niger*, Alternaria
	Mushrooms	8	*Agaricus bisporus* (White mushroom)
	Algae	2	Chlorella
	Flours	7	Wheat, rye, and soya flour
	Pollens	12	Bell pepper, Chrysanthemum
	Plants	74	Grain dust, rice, herbal tea
	Plant-derived natural products	5	Soybean lecithin, pectin, latex
	Biologic enzymes	21	Bacillus subtilis, trypsin, papain
	Vegetable gums	5	Acacia, Tragacanth, Karaya
Low molecular weight	Diisocyanates	6	Toluene diisocyanate, diphenylmethane diisocyanate
	Combination of diisocyanates	3	TDI, MDI, HDI
	Other hardeners	3	Triglycidyl isocyanurate
	Anhydrides	11	Phthalic anhydride, trimellitic anhydride
	Aliphatic amines (ethyleneamines)	7	Ethylene diamine
	Aliphatic amines (ethanolamines)	4	Monoethanolamine
	Aliphatic amines (others)	1	3-(Dimethylamino)propylamine, 3-DMAPA
	Heterocyclic amines	3	Piperazine hydrochloride
	Aromatic amines	1	Paraphenylene diamine
	Quaternary amines	1	Benzalkonium chloride
	Mixture of amines	1	EPO 60
	Fluxes	5	Colophony
	Wood dust or bark	37	Western red cedar (*Thuja plicata*), Iroko (*Chlorophora excelsa*)
	Metals	16	Platinum, nickel sulfate, chromate
	Drugs	34	Cephalosporins, psyllium, spiramycin
	Reactive dye	11	Reactive dye, levafix brilliant yellow E36
	Biocides	11	Glutaraldehyde, chloramine T
	Fungicides	3	Tetrachloroisophthalonitrile, captafol
	Chemicals	30	Persulfate salts (ammonium, potassium, sodium), urea formaldehyde, azobisformamide
	Healthcare	11	Formaldehyde, methyl methacrylate, and cyanoacrylates
	Synthetic materials	3	Plexiglass
	Unidentified	10	(?) Aluminum

including allergic asthma, nonallergic asthma [including those with neutrophilic, eosinophilic, or few inflammatory cells (paucigranulocytic) in sputum], and adult (late)-onset asthma (which must be differentiated from OA).[1] Other phenotypes described were asthma with persistent airflow limitation, thought to be due to airway wall remodeling, and asthma with obesity, often with prominent respiratory symptoms and little eosinophilic airways inflammation. Asthma can also be more simply and broadly classified as eosinophilic or noneosinophilic based on evaluation of airways or peripheral blood.[14]

Whatever the underlying mechanism of airway inflammation or damage, airway narrowing and hyperreactivity are important final common pathways causing airflow obstruction and symptoms such as wheezing, chest tightness, and shortness of breath, often in response to environmental stimuli that would not affect a person without asthma.[17] This airway hyperreactivity likely underlies many cases of WEA. Reversible airway narrowing can result from excessive airway smooth muscle contraction (bronchoconstriction), airway edema (swelling), and mucus hypersecretion/plugging. Chronic disease can lead to airway narrowing that is not fully reversible because of structural changes such as wall thickening. This is called airway remodeling.

These characteristics of non-WRA also apply to WRA. As already noted, agents that cause OA can be broadly divided into HMW and LMW agents.[9,18] HMW agents frequently cause allergic OA via mechanisms identical to those causing nonoccupational allergic asthma. Briefly, exposure to a causative HMW agent induces an antigen-specific T-helper type 2 (Th2) T cell response which, in turn, promotes an antigen-specific B cell IgE response. Thus, the HMW agent is an allergen, or an antigen capable of inducing a specific IgE response. IgE circulates through blood to mediator-releasing cells throughout the body, including mast cells in the airways. Re-exposure by inhaling the HMW agent into the airway cross-links antigen-specific IgE on the surface of airway mast cells, resulting in release of mediators. These can trigger early asthmatic responses starting at about 15 minutes and resolving after about 3 hours by causing constriction of smooth muscle resulting in bronchoconstriction, increased vascular permeability resulting in airway edema, and mucus gland secretion, resulting in mucus plugging.[18,19] Release of chemotactic factors can also cause inflammatory late asthmatic responses starting about 3–4 hours later by recruiting inflammatory cells such as eosinophils from the circulation into the airway. Airway inflammation can damage the airway epithelium and is an important factor in development of airway hyperreactivity. Repeated, chronic airway inflammation can lead to airway remodeling.

An important clinical and diagnostic feature of allergic asthma caused by HMW agents is that systemic circulation of IgE can sensitize mast cells at other sites, such as in the nasal mucosa and skin, resulting in allergic manifestations at other sites such as allergic rhinitis, urticaria, or even anaphylaxis in response to the agent.

Some LMW agents, such as platinum, can also cause allergic OA.[20] It is thought that they are haptens, binding to larger molecules such as proteins and inducing IgE responses to the LMW agent-protein complex. However, for many LMW agents, specific IgE responses frequently cannot be demonstrated and the mechanism for causing OA is unclear. Based on features such as a latent period followed by symptoms induced by progressively lower levels of exposure, it is thought that immune sensitization plays an important role in OA induced by agents such as isocyanates and plicatic acid (found in western red cedar). In cases where specific IgE sensitization cannot be demonstrated, non-IgE immune mechanisms have been suspected. In the case of isocyanates, it has been argued that IgE sensitization may sometimes be missed due to technical challenges such as preparing the proper hapten-protein complex for immune testing.[21]

Differences in mechanisms underlying OA induced by HMW and LMW agents might underlie phenotypic differences described in a large international study.[22] OA caused by HMW agents was more associated with work-related rhinitis, work-related conjunctivitis, atopy (the tendency to develop IgE responses to allergens), early asthmatic reactions, and airflow limitation. OA caused by LMW agents was more associated with chest tightness at work, daily sputum, late asthmatic reactions, and severe asthma exacerbations.

The pathogenesis of OA induction in RADS and after chronic low-level irritant exposure remains unclear.[11,18] Chemical irritation or burn of the bronchial or bronchiolar mucosa likely plays a role, but it is not entirely clear how this insult progresses to chronic or even permanent OA. However, it has been suggested that activation of sensory nerves, epithelial cells, or cells of the innate immune system are likely to be important.[5]

Interaction between Upper and Lower Airway Disease, or United Airways Disease

It has been shown that people with asthma often have coexisting rhinitis and/or sinusitis and there is an increased risk of asthma in people with rhinitis. Accumulating evidence that the upper and lower airways have similar pathogenic allergic and inflammatory pathways led to a new term "allergic rhinobronchitis"[23] and a "united airways disease" concept.[24,25] In the 2016 revision of the "Allergic Rhinitis and Its Impact on Asthma (ARIA) Guidelines," it was noted that 15–38% of patients with allergic rhinitis have asthma, up to 85% of patients with asthma have allergic rhinitis, and that allergic rhinitis is a risk factor for asthma.[26] There is also some evidence that nonallergic rhinitis is a risk factor for asthma. In a longitudinal population-based study on asthma onset in over 6000 participants in the European Community Respiratory Health Surveys (ECRHS) I and II, both allergic and nonallergic rhinitis were risk factors for asthma onset.[27] Rhinosinusitis has also been considered part of the united airways disease continuum.[28,29]

Some studies have indicated the united airways disease theory is relevant to WRA. A 2018 review of the literature found some evidence that occupational rhinitis develops before OA in workers, especially when the etiologic agents were HMW allergens.[30] In a longitudinal study of employees in a large water-damaged office building that had indications of mold contamination, rhinosinusitus symptoms were a risk factor for the onset of asthma-like lower respiratory symptoms.[31] In a Belgian study of 363 patients referred for investigation of WRA symptoms, 105 were characterized as having WEA and 172 with OA. Both groups reported nasal symptoms at work, but these symptoms were less severe and less frequently preceded the developments of asthma symptoms in the WEA group as compared to the OA group.[32] Additional to the co-morbidity of rhinitis and asthma, there is evidence that occupational allergic rhinitis is associated with increased severity of OA as well as persistence of OA.[33] This body of work implies that removal from exposure with onset of rhinosinusitis symptoms may prevent the onset or lessen the severity of WRA, but more research is needed on this topic.

EPIDEMIOLOGY OF WRA

Burden of WRA

Frequency of WRA. WRA is the most common work-related respiratory disease in many industrialized countries. Specifically for OA, a recent statement of the American Thoracic Society (ATS) and European Respiratory Society (ERS) included results from nine longitudinal population-based studies that addressed the occupational burden of asthma.[4] The estimates of the population attributable fraction for the contribution to incident asthma ranged from 7% to 44%, with a pooled estimate of 16%. For WEA, an ATS committee summarized results from 12 studies conducted in general population or general healthcare settings.[5] The median estimate of WEA prevalence was 21.5%, with a range from 13% to 58%.

The frequency of OA cases and WEA cases can be similar, although the exact numbers vary by setting. For example, among 121 WRA cases identified in primary healthcare in Spain, OA ($n = 67$, 55%) was more common than WEA ($n = 54$, 45%).[34] At a tertiary care clinic in Toronto, Canada, the WRA cases diagnosed during 2008–15 were equally split between OA and WEA.[35] It is likely that a greater number of irritant agents and lower levels of exposure can exacerbate asthma than are responsible for asthma onset. In addition, WEA agents can include environmental conditions such as extreme cold and exercise that usually are not considered as causes of asthma.

Cost of WRA. Based on evidence from industrialized nations, WRA can involve a substantial cost. WRA cases frequently require more medical care than other individuals with asthma. For example, from the Behavioral Risk Factor Surveillance System (BRFSS) Asthma Call-back Survey conducted in the U.S. during 2006–08, WRA cases were more likely than other asthma cases to experience adverse outcomes such as very poorly controlled asthma and an asthma attack, as well as urgent care, an emergency department visit, and hospitalization for asthma.[36] These needs are associated with substantial costs. An economist estimated the total direct (i.e., medical) costs for WRA cases in the United States in 2007 were \$2.29 billion.[37] This economist also estimated indirect costs (e.g., lost earnings, fringe benefits, home production) for all occupational diseases but not specifically for WRA. However, knowing that nearly all WRA cases were nonfatal, and that the indirect costs for nonfatal diseases were about 2.87 times the corresponding direct costs (i.e., \$9.09/\$3.17), the indirect costs for WRA could be estimated as $2.87 \times \$2.29$ billion = \$6.57 billion.[37] Accordingly, total costs for WRA based on the sum of direct and indirect costs would be approximately $8.86 billion ($2.29 + $6.57) in 2007 prices.

A study conducted in the United Kingdom took a somewhat different approach to estimating both direct costs (e.g., for medical care, medications) and indirect costs (e.g., disability payments by the government, reduction in patient's income, cost of sickness absence for the employer) for OA cases identified in 2003.[38] The investigators estimated that the total lifetime cost per OA patient in 2004 prices was in the range of £70–£100 million, or about £3.4–£4.8 million each year for the lifetime of a patient. Most of these costs (97%) were divided almost equally between the patient and the government.

The burden of WRA for individual cases and society can also be measured in terms of employment status, job changes, loss of income, and reduced productivity. From a 2008 review of ten studies conducted in Western Europe, Canada, and the United States, the rate of prolonged unemployment for OA cases ranged from 14% to 69% (median 37.5%).[39] From the ATS Statement on WEA, unemployment is similarly frequent for this type of WRA case, with rates from 31% to 46% (median 43%) based on three estimates.[5] From the BRFSS Asthma Call-back Survey conducted during 2006–09, adults with any type of WRA were more likely to be currently unemployed or unable to work than asthma cases unrelated to work.[40] Many individuals with WRA change jobs or employers. The BRFSS Asthma Call-back Survey conducted during 2006–08 found that WRA cases were more likely to have changed or quit a job than other asthma cases.[41] The ATS Statement on WEA summarized results from five studies with rates of change in job or employer for both OA cases (range 33–94%, median 72%) and WEA cases (range 17–100%, median 54%).[5] Two of the studies had rates for OA and WEA that were about equal and the other three had higher rates for OA.

Adults with asthma tend to miss work (i.e., absenteeism) because of their disease. Based on data from the 2008 National Health Interview Survey (NHIS) conducted in the United States, employed adults with current asthma missed an estimated 14.2 million works days due to their asthma.[42] Among four studies that compared adults with WEA to adults with asthma unrelated to work, three of them reported that the frequency of lost workdays was similar for the two asthma groups, and in the fourth study the frequency was greater among WEA cases.[5] There is little published data about presenteeism (i.e., working while sick) and WRA. From a Canadian study conducted in 2010–12, WRA cases were less likely to have their symptoms controlled and more likely to have a productivity loss due to presenteeism (but not absenteeism) than cases that were not work related.[43]

Risk Factors for WRA

High-risk occupational exposures. A variety of workplace agents can cause or exacerbate asthma, numbering more than 300 in publications from the past 10 years.[44,45] OA cases are frequently categorized as being induced by either sensitizers or irritants, and/or by whether the causes are HMW or LMW agents. One of the more comprehensive and up-to-date online lists of OA agents is available from the Quebec provincial government.[10] The information is abstracted from publications (numbering over 500 by June 2019), and is organized either by whether the agents are HMW or LMW (with irritants in the LMW section), or by type of occupation. Table 76-1 summarizes the list by molecular weight and illustrates the variety of occupational agents that can contribute to the onset of asthma. Even discounting agents included in the final category of "Unidentified," the list includes 440 agents.

The online list maintained by Quebec is relatively inclusive, with various types of evidence to support the claim that the agents cause OA. In another effort, Xaver Baur and colleagues required evidence from more rigorous studies (i.e., excluding results from clinical studies, theoretical considerations, and clinical consensus) that agents and workplaces could cause OA.[9] The researchers abstracted relevant data from over 1300 publications about allergic and irritant causes of OA, evaluated the studies for potential biases and methodological quality, and rated the strength of the evidence for each cause. Even with the application of standards for quality of evidence, there was still a total of 137 different agents or workplaces judged as causing OA. The 137 causes included 66 that were only allergic, 59 that were only irritant, and 12 with both allergic and irritant qualities. No one has published a systematic evaluation of the causes of WEA similar to what Baur and colleagues did for OA.[9]

Another source of information about the agents responsible for WRA is provided by state-based surveillance activities in the United States, in which up to three putative agents could be assigned to each case. From the 4 years of 2009–12, this surveillance system identified 857 OA cases and 902 WEA cases with information about the type of agent.[46] The agent categories in Table 76-2 are ordered by decreasing frequency of OA cases. Both OA and WEA cases shared the same five most common agent categories: miscellaneous chemicals and materials, mineral and inorganic dusts, cleaning products, pyrolysis products, and indoor air pollutants. There were a few differences by specific agents within these categories. In particular, OA cases had a percentage at least 1.5 times that for WEA with the agent cigarette smoke (2.5% versus 1.2%) in the category pyrolysis products. In addition, WEA cases had percentages at least 1.5 times those for OA cases with perfumes, not otherwise specified (n.o.s) (5.8% versus 2.8%) in the category miscellaneous chemicals and materials, and floor wax (2.5% vs. 1.2%) in the category cleaning materials. Several categories less common than the top five had the same level of contrast between the two types of cases. Specifically, OA cases had higher percentages than WEA cases for the agents acids, bases, and oxidizing agents (5.3% vs. 3.0%); aldehydes and acetals (3.3% vs. 1.1%); halogens, inorganic (e.g., chlorine, chlorine dioxide) (2.1% vs. 1.3%); hydrocarbons, n.o.s. (e.g., cutting oils) (2.9% vs. 0.8%); isocyanates (3.6% vs. 0.6%); and polymers (1.8% vs. 0.7%). The reverse was true, with percentages higher for WEA versus OA cases, for ergonomics (e.g., exercise, stress) (7.4% vs. 1.2%) and physical factors (e.g., cold, heat, humidity) (3.2 vs. 1.8).

High-risk industries and occupations. It is of interest to understand in which industries and for what occupations WRA occurs most frequently. This information informs strategies for prevention on a work-force level as well as aiding clinicians in determining possible causes and triggers of a patient's asthma. Data on asthma for 21 states in the United States from the 2013 BRFSS survey were analyzed to describe the prevalence of asthma in relation to industry and occupation in adults employed during the 12 months prior to the interview.[47] For all states combined, the top industries for current asthma were: healthcare and social assistance (10.7%); education (9.1%); arts, entertainment, and recreation (9.0%); information (8.7%); and retail trade (8.7%). Lower down the ranking were: manufacturing (6.1%); mining, oil and gas (6.0%); and 5.9%. The five occupations with the highest current asthma prevalence for all states combined were: healthcare support (12.4%); community and social services (12.2%); personal care and service (12.1%); arts, design, entertainment, sports, and media (11.7%); and office and administrative support (10.2%). The occupation of education, training, and library was in the top five occupations for prevalence of current asthma in 11 of the 21 states, with the prevalence ranging from 7.0% in Florida to 18.6% in California.

An earlier publication used U.S. population-based data from the National Health and Nutrition Examination Survey (NHANES) 2001–04, to compare prevalence of current asthma by industry and occupation in working adults 20–59 years old.[48] The industries of mining (17.0%), health-related industries (12.5%), justice, public order—safety (9.7%), manufacturing—lumber (9.2%), and education services (9.0%) had the highest prevalences of asthma. The occupations of teachers (13.1%); health-related occupations (12.6%); technicians (9.2%), writers, artists, athletes, and entertainers (8.5%); and

TABLE 76-2 COMMON AGENTS FOR 857 OA CASES AND 902 WEA CASES AS DETERMINED BY STATE-BASED SURVEILLANCE PROGRAMS IN THE UNITED STATES, 2009–2012[46]

Agent Category[a]	OA		WEA	
	n	% of 857	*n*	% of 902
Miscellaneous chemicals and materials	203	23.7	206	22.8
Mineral and inorganic dusts	175	20.4	224	24.8
Cleaning products	184	21.5	184	20.4
Pyrolysis products	109	12.7	142	15.7
Indoor air pollutants	105	12.3	91	10.1
Mold	92	10.7	83	9.2
Plant/tree materials	67	7.8	59	6.5
Ergonomics (e.g., exercise, stress)[b]	10	1.2[b]	67	7.4[b]
Solvents, n.o.s. (e.g., paint, n.o.s.)	49	5.7	39	4.3
Animal/insect material	38	4.4	35	3.9
Acids, bases, and oxidizing agents[c]	45	5.3[c]	27	3.0[c]
Aliphatic and alicyclic hydrocarbons	28	3.3	24	2.7
Metals and metalloids	49	5.7	12	1.3
Physical factors (e.g., cold, heat, humidity)[b]	15	1.8[b]	29	3.2[b]
Aldehydes and acetals[c]	28	3.3[c]	10	1.1[c]
Halogens, inorganic (e.g., chlorine, chlorine dioxide)	18	2.1	12	1.3
Miscellaneous inorganic compounds	13	1.5	13	1.4
Hydrocarbons, n.o.s. (e.g., cutting oils)[c]	25	2.9[c]	7	0.8[c]
Isocyanates[c]	31	3.6[c]	5	0.6[c]
Polymers[c]	15	1.8[c]	6	0.7[c]

[a]Agent categories included if either OA or WEA had at least ten cases. The categories thus excluded were: microorganisms not including mold, ketones, alcohols, epoxy compounds, hydrocarbons, halogenated aliphatic hydrocarbons, aliphatic and alicyclic amines, glycol ethers, phenols and phenolic compounds, aromatic nitro and amino compounds, organophosphate and carbamate pesticides, aliphatic carboxylic acids and anhydrides, all other exposure categories, and hazard not on file.

[b]% WEA at least 1.5 × % OA.

[c]% OA at least 1.5 × % WEA.

Abbreviation: n.o.s. = not otherwise specified.

Data from NIOSH (National Institute for Occupational Safety and Health) 2019. Work-related asthma: Most frequently reported agents associated with work-related asthma cases by asthma classification, 2009–2012. File No. 2017-927. Originally accessed on NIOSH eWoRLD website, https://wwwn.cdc.gov/eworld/Grouping/Asthma/97#State-based, July 9, 2019. Currently available by request from WoRLD@CDC.gov.

management-related and clerical (7.9%) had the highest prevalence of current asthma. The study authors concluded that healthcare workers and teachers/educational services workers are at high risk for WRA and need more evaluation and control measures. This conclusion was supported by the findings in the previously discussed study.[47]

A study by the U.S. National Institute for Occupational Safety and Health (NIOSH) used data from the 2010 Occupational Health Supplement to the NHIS to examine the occupation held during the time that asthma symptoms first developed among adults with current asthma and who were employed in the past 12 months.[49] Current asthma was highest in the following currently held occupations: education, training, and library (10.3%); life, physical, and social science (10.1%); personal care and service (9.6%); healthcare support (9.1%); and healthcare practitioners and technical (8.8%). In comparison, using occupation when symptoms first developed indicated office and administrative support (13.3%); sales and related (9.4%); and management (8.5%); production (7.9%); and healthcare practitioners and technical (6.9%) as the highest risk occupations. The authors hypothesized the differences between these two lists of common occupations could indicate that workers may leave occupations where asthma develops or is worsened.

There have been a number of studies regarding asthma, industry, and occupation from countries other than the United States. In South Korea, data collected during 2004–09 by the Korea Work-Related Asthma Surveillance program indicated the highest risk industries for asthma incidence were: furniture and other instruments; manufacture of chemicals, rubber and plastics; vehicles and transport equipment; and manufacture of food and beverages.[50] The highest incidence for asthma was in the following occupations: craft and related trades workers; skilled agricultural, forestry and fishery workers; and plant workers, machine operators, and assemblers. The most frequent suspected agent was isocyanates (46.6% of cases). A study in New Zealand identified high-risk occupations for current asthma as: ever working as a printer, baker, sawmill laborer, metal processing plant operator, cleaner, teachers, and certain sales professionals.[51] These results show a different pattern to recent U.S. studies, in that crafts and trades and manufacturing occupations played a larger role in WRA in Korea and New Zealand. This could well be linked to the difference in the types of prevalent industries and differences in the nature of work between different regions. Data from patients at a Canadian tertiary care clinic were used to investigate changes over a 15-year period in high-risk industries and occupations for WRA.[35] While the manufacturing industry had the most cases in both time periods analyzed (2000–07 and 2008–15); the number of cases in the manufacturing industry (predominately due to isocyanate exposure) declined while cases in healthcare and education industries increased. This led the authors to conclude that cleaners and teachers should be a focus of intervention measures for WRA.

Emerging risk factors for WRA: Cleaning and disinfecting. Starting in the 1990s, various case reports[52–54] and published results from surveillance and epidemiologic studies[55–63] implicated workplace cleaning and disinfecting agents as increasingly common causes of the onset and exacerbation of asthma. Recent studies have documented the upward trend in the frequency of cleaning products as WRA agents. For example, among WRA cases identified in a tertiary care clinic in Toronto, Canada, the three most common causative agents for OA (in descending frequency) changed from isocyanates, flour and baking products, and construction/wood dusts in 2000–07 to cleaning products, isocyanates, and paint fumes in 2008–15.[35] From the same study, the top three agents for WEA went from isocyanates and airborne dusts, exhaust fumes, and construction dusts in the earlier time period to construction/wood dusts, cleaning products, and airborne dusts and scented products.[35] From 20 years (1991–2011) of surveillance for OA in the West Midlands, United Kingdom, there was a statistically significant increase in notifications for cleaning agents, and a decrease in notifications for several other agents.[64] Surveillance activities in France demonstrated that quaternary ammonium compounds used for cleaning and disinfecting were increasingly more common as a WRA agent during 2001–09.[56]

Institutions in the healthcare industry conduct cleaning and disinfecting in order to prevent infections, which means they pursue these activities with an intensity that is rare in most other industries. Consistent with these practices, the medical literature includes numerous reports about the association of asthma-related health outcomes with cleaning and disinfecting in healthcare. For example, among OA cases caused by cleaning products that were identified during 2000–16 by a surveillance program in the West Midlands, United Kingdom, the most frequently implicated industry was healthcare, which accounted for 55% of the cases.[65] Cleaning products were the most common putative agent for healthcare workers with WRA that were identified by state-based surveillance programs in the United States during 1993–97.[66] Findings from epidemiologic studies suggest that different types of cleaning products can contribute to WRA in healthcare. From a study of healthcare workers in France, current asthma was associated with using various cleaning products, including decalcifiers, ammonia, and sprays with moderate/high intensity.[67] From a study of healthcare workers in the U.S. state of Texas, posthire asthma was associated with surface cleaning products and instrument cleaning,[68] and WRA symptoms were associated with several products used for general purpose cleaning (i.e., bleach, cleaners/abrasives, cleaners for restrooms and toilets, detergents, and ammonia) and instrument cleaning/sterilization (i.e., glutaraldehyde/ortho-phthalaldehyde, chloramines, and ethylene oxide).[69] In the multinational ECRHS II study, asthma in hospital workers was associated with the use of ammonia and/or bleach at work.[70] From a large study of U.S. nurses who currently had asthma, a diminished control of asthma symptoms was associated with weekly use of disinfectants to clean instruments, weekly use of cleaning/disinfecting sprays, and several specific cleaning/disinfecting products (i.e., formaldehyde, glutaraldehyde, hypochlorite bleach, hydrogen peroxide, and enzymatic cleaners).[71]

Emerging risk factors for WRA: Indoor dampness and mold. Over the past 20 years, occupancy of damp indoor environments has increasingly been recognized as a risk factor for both asthma exacerbation and the onset of asthma (among a number of other respiratory conditions). Although the largest body of work exists on asthma in children in relation to damp and mold contaminated homes, there is substantial evidence that damp and mold contaminated working environments such as offices, healthcare facilities, and schools are important sources of exposures leading to asthma. In the United States, The Institute of Medicine of the National Academies published a report in 2004 that found sufficient evidence that exposure to damp indoor environments and mold led to exacerbation of asthma.[72] Then in 2009 the World Health Organization published a report that implicated both asthma exacerbation and asthma onset with exposure to dampness and mold.[73] This finding has been reinforced with updated reviews of the literature.[74,75] NIOSH in the United States has conducted a number of studies relating to dampness and mold and respiratory health, including asthma onset and exacerbation[76–80] and in 2012 published an Alert on Preventing Occupational Respiratory Disease from Exposures Caused by Dampness in Office Buildings, Schools, and Other Nonindustrial Buildings.[81]

Although the presence of dampness, water damage, visible signs of mold growth, and mold odor have consistently been associated with respiratory health outcomes including asthma development and exacerbation, there is much more research needed to elucidate the components of microbial exposures and other dampness-related exposures causing the health effects.[82–84] There has been some work that implicates water-loving (hydrophilic) fungi[85] and molds such as *Penicillium*, *Aspergillus*, *Cladosporium*, and *Alternaria* species.[86]

There is evidence in the literature that dampness and mold exposures can lead to both allergic (eosinophilic) and nonallergic (neutrophilic) asthma.[83,87] This has implications for clinical evaluation of possible WRA due to dampness and mold in that negative test results for allergic status or allergy to specific mold species does not rule out WRA.

Emerging risk factors for WRA: Psychosocial stress. Since the nineteen eighties, it has been increasingly recognized that psychological stress can affect the course and even the onset of asthma, although it has been a controversial issue and is still not clearly understood.[88–91]

Epidemiological studies have indicated that stress is associated with asthma prevalence, incidence, poor asthma control and a lower quality of life in both children and adults. A review on adult-onset asthma, (which often has a more severe course than childhood-onset asthma), concluded there is evidence for a number of contributing risk factors including stress, respiratory infections, environmental sensitizers, hormonal factors, and obesity.[92] In a Danish longitudinal cohort study on adults, perceived stress was positively associated with self-reported asthma incidence, asthma medication use, and first-time hospitalization for asthma.[89] Data from a large longitudinal study of the Finnish population indicated that participants with a score in the highest tertile for stressful life events that had occurred in the 5 years prior to the follow-up period had twice the risk of onset of new asthma during the 2-year follow-up.[93]

Recently, more attention has been paid to the role stress at work may play in asthma. As discussed by Loerbroks and colleagues,[94] there have been mixed findings with some studies finding no[95] or weak associations,[96,97] and others finding stronger associations. In a survey of 2903 workers in New Zealand, having a very or extremely stressful job as compared to a less stressful job was associated with being twice as likely to have current asthma.[98] Loerbroks and colleagues have studied work-related stress and asthma in German and Chinese populations, and found that work-related stress and job-insecurity is associated with asthma prevalence and incidence.[94,99–101] Although the literature implies that reducing work-stress should reduce the exacerbation or incidence of asthma, currently no intervention studies have been published.

There are a number of physiological responses to psychological stress that are important to asthma. It has been posited that psychological stress can increase airway inflammatory responses to asthma triggers in people with asthma.[102,103] Stress can lead to the release of hormones and neuropeptides that can influence the immune system response and may shift the immune response from a Th1 response to a Th2 allergic-type response.[91] Stress also can affect the sympathetic nervous system and lead to bronchorestriction.[104] Furthermore, recent findings suggest that stress can lead to changes in the expression of genes regulating these aforementioned physiological responses.[105] A review of human laboratory studies on the effects of acute psychological stress on physiological responses in people with asthma found that the type of stressor effected the response. Active stressors (those for which participants feel they can somewhat control and cope with) activate the sympathetic nervous system, may lead to a decrease in parasympathetic nervous system activity, but do not lead to bronchodilation. Active stressors also increase inflammation, and activate the hypothalamic-pituitary-adrenocortical axis, with increases in cortisol. Passive stressors (those over which the participant has no control and cannot use coping to resolve) activate the sympathetic nervous system with no changes in the parasympathetic nervous system but induce mild bronchoconstriction. The findings taken together suggest that active stressors could lead to asthma exacerbation hours after exposure due to increased immune activation while passive stressors can trigger immediate bronchorestriction.[106]

DIAGNOSIS OF WRA

Diagnosis of WRA is addressed in some detail in authoritative statements[7,107] and reviews.[108–111] Briefly, the first step in diagnosis of WRA is to make the diagnosis of asthma based on history, physical examination, and lung function testing to document variable expiratory airflow limitation.[1,2] It is important to confirm the diagnosis, because respiratory symptoms attributed to asthma often have another cause such as cardiac disease, COPD, vocal cord dysfunction, conditions causing large airways obstruction, and others.

Typical symptoms elicited in the medical history include wheeze, shortness of breath, cough, and chest tightness. It is important to ask about what triggers symptoms, frequency, and whether they interfere with ability to be active or cause nighttime awakenings. In an adult, it is important to ask if asthma has been a lifelong problem, if it occurred in childhood and has now recurred in adulthood, or if it is a new problem. If physical examination is performed between asthma attacks, it is likely to be normal. However, it is important to evaluate for chest findings such as wheeze and prolonged expiratory phase, signs of nonrespiratory allergic diseases such as rhinosinusitis and eczema, and signs of other conditions that might mimic asthma.

If asthma remains a diagnostic consideration, spirometry should be performed to assess for airway obstruction. If obstruction is present, an inhaled short-acting beta agonist bronchodilator should be administered, and spirometry repeated. Significant improvement documents the presence of variable airflow limitation. If spirometry is normal, as might be the case between asthma attacks, a bronchial challenge test can be performed to assess for airway hyperreactivity. This involves administering an inhaled agent that would not significantly affect spirometry findings in a healthy person in the doses used but could document variable airflow obstruction by causing a transient drop of 20% or more in the forced expiratory volume in one second (FEV_1) of a person with asthma. The agent most frequently used for this purpose in the U.S. is methacholine; the lower the dose of methacholine needed to drop the FEV_1 by 20%, the more severe the airways hyperreactivity.[112] Bronchial challenge with methacholine is highly sensitive for asthma and with only a few exceptions, a negative test essentially excludes asthma if symptoms were present within the previous few days. However, the test is not specific for asthma, since airway hyperreactivity also occurs in other diseases associated with airway inflammation or obstruction and is common among athletes, especially in winter sports.[112]

Additional tests can be useful in certain circumstances. For example, allergy skin tests or serological testing can help to confirm allergens contributing to asthma symptoms and exacerbations. Tests such as fractional concentration of exhaled nitric oxide (FENO) or measurements of eosinophils in sputum or blood can help to identify eosinophilic inflammation. Tests to identify comorbidities that might contribute to asthma symptoms, such as rhinosinusitis and gastroesophageal reflux disease are also often needed.

The possibility of WRA should be considered in all adults diagnosed with asthma.[7] Given that WEA is present in about 21.5% of adults with asthma, it is important to ask about workplace triggers for asthma even in those with long-standing asthma that preceded their line of work. Given that about 16% of adult asthma is attributable to work, it is important to question all adults with new-onset asthma about the possibility of OA. It is useful to ask if symptoms are worse at work and better on weekends and vacations. Information should also be sought about work and work exposures that might be associated with risk for OA. These might include HMW allergens like animal allergens in those working with animals and flour in bakers or LMW allergens like diisocyanates used in paints, glues, and insulating foams in a variety of occupations. It is important to ask about job duties, exposures, industry, use of protective devices and equipment, and whether coworkers have developed asthma. The patient should be able to obtain safety data sheets from the workplace that list hazardous agents used in the workplace. These should be obtained and reviewed. In addition, it is important to ask about acute irritant exposures that might cause RADS, and history of chronic irritant exposures. Even if the history is suggestive, additional evaluation should be undertaken to document the diagnosis of OA, since medical histories have high sensitivity but lower specificity,[107] and a diagnosis of OA can affect a patient's ability to work.

Ambulatory monitoring of peak expiratory flow rate (PEFR) or FEV_1 can be a useful, relatively noninvasive way to evaluate for the impact of work exposures on lung function. One common approach is for the patient to record peak flow four times a day over a period of 2 weeks at work and 2 weeks away from work.[7] Two weeks away from work can be difficult to arrange, but being away from work for a longer period of time allows for improvement in lung function that might not occur over just a weekend.[113] After obtaining data, software exists to help evaluate whether lung function variability is worse when working.[114] The sensitivity and specificity of PEFR monitoring for OA are reported to be 82% and 88%, respectively.[107] PEFR monitoring can be supplemented with measurement of nonspecific airway hyperreactivity at baseline and then after at least 2 weeks away from work to see if it improves.[7]

Another relatively noninvasive approach to assess for the relationship of asthma to work is to perform allergy skin testing or serological testing to determine if a patient demonstrates antigen-specific IgE-sensitization to an agent at work. Perhaps because of differing mechanisms of HMW and LMW asthma and technical challenges to measuring LMW agent-specific IgE, performance of serologic tests in identifying OA induced by HMW and LMW agents is quite different. For HMW agents, a systematic review found that sensitivity is 74% and specificity 71%. For LMW agents, sensitivity is 28% and specificity 89%.[115,116]

If other methods are not feasible or have not provided a clear diagnosis, specific inhalation challenge (SIC) testing can be performed.[7,107] One approach is to perform a workplace challenge by having the worker return to their job at the workplace or by having the worker reproduce job tasks in some other controlled setting with serial monitoring of lung function for early and late asthmatic reactions. Sputum eosinophil and FENO response to the challenge can also be measured. Another approach is to perform a controlled SIC in a laboratory. In this procedure, the patient breathes an atmosphere containing carefully controlled concentrations of the suspected work agent causing asthma and is carefully monitored. Usually, the patient is exposed to either air or a series of gradually increasing concentrations of the suspected causative agent on separate days. Serial spirometry is typically performed to detect early and late asthmatic responses. Sputum eosinophil and FENO responses are also monitored. SIC is often referred to as a gold standard for OA diagnosis, but it is expensive, time consuming, and not generally available. Also, diagnostic performance of SIC depends on using the correct agent in the correct doses, which may be difficult when the exact causative agent in a workplace is unstandardized or unknown.

PREVENTION AND TREATMENT OF WRA

Primary Prevention of WRA

Primary prevention of WRA asthma involves preventing the disease from ever occurring. Since exposures to airborne contaminants can be reduced or even eliminated in many workplaces, primary prevention is more likely for WRA than many other types of asthma that are caused by exposures in settings (e.g., the ambient environment) where exposure control is less certain. The ERS Task Force on the Management of Work-related Asthma systematically reviewed the available literature on prevention of WRA, evaluated the strength of the evidence, and published several recommendations. The preferred option for primary prevention is elimination of harmful exposures, and reduction of exposure is the second-best approach based on findings from studies of exposure–response relationships.[117] Evidence that respirators can prevent WRA is limited. Therefore, other approaches higher in the hierarchy of controls, notably elimination or reduction of exposure, should be used whenever possible instead of respirators. A low level of existing evidence suggests that skin exposure to certain chemicals (e.g., isocyanates) and perhaps some HMW protein allergens can increase the risk of OA. Minimizing skin exposure to asthma agents might contribute to primary prevention.

TABLE 76-3 PROTOCOLS TO FACILITATE SCREENING FOR WRA

Reference	Purpose(s) of Protocol	Items in Algorithm or System	Outcomes from Using Protocol
Bernstein 2017[126]	Provide clinical guidance to physicians for evaluating patients with lower respiratory symptoms at work and exposure to diisocyanates at work, with the goal of correctly diagnosing OA due to respiratory sensitization to these agents.	Applied in order: 1. History consistent with OA 2. Spirometry pre/postbronchodilator 3. Serial PEFR: 2 weeks at work, 2 weeks away from work 4. Methacholine inhalation test after 2 weeks at work	Depending on results, outcomes can include: 1. Continue work with diisocyanates 2. Continue work and monthly follow-up 3. Further testing 4. Removal from exposure 5. Referral to physician knowledgeable in occupational lung disease
Taghiakbari 2019[127]	Quantify individual probability of OA in a symptomatic worker who is exposed to HMW agents and still working one month prior to testing without using SIC. Algorithm is intended for use by physicians at secondary/tertiary centers, and/or have access to the objective tests.	Variables in regression model: • Age (≤40 years) • Rhinoconjunctivitis symptoms • Inhaled corticosteroid usage • Agent type: flour and associated agents • Sensitization to work-specific agents • NSBHR	Actions depend on probability of OA: • If low probability of OA: further evaluation with other tests, e.g., serial PEFR at and off work • If high probability of OA ◦ SIC if available ◦ If SIC not available: treatment, removal from exposure, and compensation claim (if an option). • Refer to specialist if cannot complete tests indicated.
Killorn 2015[129]	Assist primary-care providers when assessing for possible WRA in individuals with confirmed asthma.	Work-related asthma screening questionnaire (long version) [WRASQ(L)] has 14 items based on three concepts. • Job type and employment duration (3 items) ◦ Current occupation/industry ◦ Past occupation ◦ Current employment status • Relationship of asthma symptoms to work (8 items) Did asthma symptoms start under these circumstances? ◦ At work ◦ On day of spill or fire at work Do asthma symptoms worsen under these circumstances? ◦ At work ◦ First day back to work ◦ During work day ◦ At home after work ◦ Throughout work week Are chest symptoms different (less) under these circumstances? ◦ On days off work and/or holidays • Exposures at work and protection from exposure (3 items) ◦ Current exposures at work ◦ Past exposures at work ◦ Protective measures	Primary-care provider uses results from screening questionnaire to decide that patient does or does not need diagnostic work-up to confirm WRA. The primary-care provider can either conduct this work-up or refer the patient to a specialist.
Harber 2017[128]	Help primary-care clinicians recognize the possibility of WRA in working-age patients with asthma. It does not intend to be a complete diagnostic and management algorithm.	Primary-care providers use the clinical decision support system and document information in electronic health record (EHR).Sequential steps are applied to working age patients (i.e., >18 years old) who in past 2 years had either (a) onset of asthma, or (b) at least one ED visit or acute clinic/hospital visit for asthma (possible exacerbation of asthma).1a. Three screening questions about WR patterns of asthma symptoms: ◦ Started at work ◦ Worse at work ◦ Different (e.g., better) on days off work and/or holidays If "yes" to at least one question, then:1b. Confirm diagnosis of asthma with spirometry.If FEV1 < lower limit of normal and significant bronchodilator response, then:1c. Provide WRA information tools to clinician and patient, and have clinician document discussion with patient about their work and respiratory symptoms in EHR. The WRA tools should include three components: ◦ Checklist of high-risk exposures ◦ Educational materials on WRA ◦ Referral sources, including local specialists	Primary-care providers assess patients with asthma for possible WRA and refer suspected cases to specialists who have the expertise for diagnosing and managing WRA. Patients access information and resources to help them understand WRA and obtain the care they need.

Abbreviations: ED = emergency department; EHR = electronic health record; FEV1 = forced expiratory volume in one second; HMW = high molecular weight; NSBHR = nonspecific bronchial hyperreactivity; OA = occupational asthma; PEFR = peak expiratory flow rate; SIC = specific inhalation challenge; WR = work related; WRA = work-related asthma.

Research findings suggest the effectiveness of interventions to prevent asthma due to flour and fungal α-amylase in bakeries, diisocyanates, detergent enzymes, and the antigens in laboratory animal facilities. However, this evidence is less complete than what is available for the effectiveness of interventions that reduced the use of powdered NRL gloves in healthcare[117] as is described in the public health prevention case study below.

Public Health Prevention Case Study

Between 1987 and 1996, the use of NRL gloves increased more than tenfold among healthcare workers after CDC recommended glove use as part of universal precautions for the prevention of transmission of bloodborne pathogens such as hepatitis C virus and human immunodeficiency virus.[118] Together with this massive increase in use of NRL gloves came increased recognition of NRL allergy in healthcare workers, including NRL-induced OA, rhinitis, urticaria, and even life-threatening anaphylaxis.[119]

It was eventually recognized that an important source of NRL allergen exposure in healthcare workers was the cornstarch powder used on powdered gloves. Particles of glove powder became contaminated with allergenic NRL proteins during the manufacturing process and carried them aloft when aerosolized by activities like putting on and removing gloves. Using nonpowdered NRL gloves almost eliminated NRL allergen from the air.[120] A meta-analysis of relevant studies concluded that replacing protein-rich powdered NRL gloves with protein-poor nonpowdered NRL gloves or latex-free gloves had the effect of greatly reducing NRL aeroallergens, NRL sensitization, and NRL asthma in healthcare workers.[121] An especially persuasive study of the impact of this substitution on exposures was a longitudinal case crossover intervention, in which introducing low-protein, nonpowdered NRL gloves resulted in a tenfold decline in aeroallergen levels.[122]

To prevent NRL-induced WRA at the population level, Germany[123] and Belgium[124] banned the use of powdered NRL gloves. New cases of OA declined dramatically in parallel to declines in powdered NRL glove use. In the U.S., powdered NRL glove use also declined and the Food and Drug Administration formally banned powdered surgeons' and examination gloves, effective January 2017.[125]

Secondary Prevention of WRA

Secondary prevention of WRA involves early detection of WRA, when steps can be taken to prevent disease progression or even reverse it, with improvement in disease outcomes.

Approaches to medical screening for WRA. Early diagnosis and management of WRA contributes to better outcomes for patients and can help to prevent additional cases by alerting workers and management about potential problematic exposures in the workplace. Investigators have proposed protocols that support care providers in screening for WRA in those at risk, with the goal of reducing the time between the onset of WRA symptoms and diagnosis. Table 76-3 includes descriptions of four such protocols. They differ by the types of patients for whom they are intended, as defined by the likely WRA agent(s) and the patient's symptom status. In particular, one protocol was developed for screening diisocyanate-exposed workers who have symptoms at work,[126] another for symptomatic workers exposed to HMW agents,[127] and the other two for working-age individuals with asthma without specifications about type of agent or symptoms.[128,129] The two protocols that specify certain types of patients[126,127] include more tests (e.g., of serial PEFR, methacholine challenge to determine nonspecific bronchial hyperreactivity (NSBHR), and sensitization to workplace agents) than the other two protocols, which rely primarily on asking questions about topics such as job type, workplace exposures, and the relationship of symptoms to work.[128,129] The protocols with more specifications about patients and testing provide steps that could lead to a diagnosis of WRA, although also recommend referring patients to specialists when unable to perform specified tests. The primary intention of the other two protocols is to help primary care providers assess adults with asthma and decide whether to refer them to specialists who diagnose and manage WRA cases.

Outcome of exposure elimination or reduction. When cases of WRA are identified, an important issue in management is reduction in or removal from causative exposures. A Cochrane systematic review summarized evidence for whether eliminating or reducing workplace exposures are effective at treating OA.[130] The meta-analysis of results from several studies indicated that removal from exposure was superior to continued exposure, as indicated at follow-up by an increased likelihood of an absence of symptoms, improved FEV1 as a percent of a predicted value (FEV1%), and a decreased NSBHR. Removal was also superior to reduction of exposure as indicated by an increased likelihood of reporting absence of symptoms, but not by FEV1%, and data were not available to evaluate NSBH. When compared to continued exposure, reduction of exposure had an increased likelihood of reporting absence of symptoms, did not have better FEV1% findings, and data were unavailable to evaluate NSBH. Data from a pair of studies indicated that unemployment was more likely after removal from exposure than from reduction of exposure. In summary, removal from exposure had better health outcomes than reduction of exposure, but removal also had a greater risk of unemployment than reduction.

Tertiary Prevention of WRA

Tertiary prevention of WRA involves treatment of clinical disease. Other than acting to reduce or eliminate exposure, as already described, treatment of WRA asthma is essentially similar to treatment of non-OA. Detailed guidelines for asthma treatment are maintained by the Global Initiative for Asthma and are updated regularly.[1] Great advances have been made in recent years, particularly in treatment of severe asthma with monoclonal agents targeted to specific cytokines and cytokine receptors.[16] Impact of these newer agents on treatment of difficult WRA cases remains to be fully explored.

CONCLUSION

WRA is an important public health prevention issue. It includes OA, or asthma caused by work exposures, and WEA, or asthma exacerbated by work exposures. OA can be caused by immune sensitization after a latency by HMW and LMW agents. HMW agents are generally allergens inducing IgE sensitization. The mechanism of sensitization to many LMW agents remains less clear. OA can also be caused by single high-level irritant exposures or chronic exposures to lower levels of irritants. WRA is a common problem, affecting millions in the United States alone. It is important to consider the possibility of WRA in any working adult with asthma. WRA can be prevented by avoidance of causative exposures. In addition to primary prevention, there is an important role for secondary prevention of OA, since early detection and reduction or preferably elimination of exposure can alter the disease course and improve disease outcomes. The response to NRL allergy is an example of successfully addressing OA as a public health issue at the population level by removing a causative exposure.

References

1. GINA. Global strategy for asthma management and prevention. http://www.ginasthma.org: Global Initiative for Asthma; 2019.
2. NHLBI. Guidelines for the diagnosis and management of asthma. https://www.nhlbi.nih.gov/health-topics/guidelines-for-diagnosis-management-of-asthma: National Heart, Lung and Blood Institute; 2007.
3. CDC. *National Health Interview Survey*. Atlanta, GA: Department of Health and Human Services; 2017.
4. Blanc PD, Annesi-Maesano I, Balmes JR, et al. The occupational burden of nonmalignant respiratory diseases: An Official American Thoracic Society and European Respiratory Society Statement. *Am J Respir Crit Care Med*. 2019;199(11):1312–34.
5. Henneberger PK, Redlich CA, Callahan DB, et al. An Official American Thoracic Society statement: Work-exacerbated asthma. *Am J Respir Crit Care Med*. 2011;184(3):368–78.

6. Baur X, Sigsgaard T, Aasen TB, et al. Guidelines for the management of work-related asthma. *Eur Respir J*. 2012;39(3):529–45.
7. Tarlo SM, Balmes J, Balkissoon R, et al. Diagnosis and management of work-related asthma: American College of Chest Physicians consensus statement. *Chest*. 2008;134(3 Suppl):1S–41S.
8. NIOSH. WRA state reporting guidelines: Surveillance case definition for WRA. 2012. https://www.cdc.gov/niosh/topics/surveillance/ords/state-surveillance/reportingguidelines-wra.html. Accessed July 9, 2019.
9. Baur X. A compendium of causative agents of occupational asthma. *J Occup Med Toxicol*. 2013;8(1):15.
10. CNESST. Occupational Asthma. 2019. https://www.csst.qc.ca/en/prevention/reptox/occupational-asthma/Pages/occupational-asthma.aspx.
11. Brooks SM, Weiss MA, Bernstein IL. Reactive airways dysfunction syndrome (RADS). Persistent asthma syndrome after high level irritant exposures. *Chest*. 1985;88(3):376–84.
12. Dumas O, Le Moual N. Do chronic workplace irritant exposures cause asthma? *Curr Opin Allergy Clin Immunol*. 2016;16(2):75–85.
13. NIOSH. State-based Case Data—Work-related asthma: Most frequently reported agents associated with work-related asthma cases by state, 2009–2012. 2017. https://wwwn.cdc.gov/eworld/Grouping/Asthma/97#State-based Case Data. Accessed July 10, 2019.
14. Carr TF, Zeki AA, Kraft M. Eosinophilic and noneosinophilic asthma. *Am J Respir Crit Care Med*. 2018;197(1):22–37.
15. Quirce S, Sastre J. Occupational asthma: Clinical phenotypes, biomarkers, and management. *Curr Opin Pulm Med*. 2019;25(1):59–63.
16. Diamant Z, Vijverberg S, Alving K, et al. Towards clinically applicable biomarkers for asthma—An EAACI position paper. *Allergy*. 2019;74(10):1835–51.
17. GINA. *Global strategy for asthma management and prevention. Online appendix 2019*. http://www.ginasthma.com: Global Initiative for Asthma; 2019.
18. Cockcroft DW. Environmental causes of asthma. *Semin Respir Crit Care Med*. 2018;39(1):12–8.
19. O'Byrne P. Asthma pathogenesis and allergen-induced late responses. *J Allergy Clin Immunol*. 1998;102(5):S85–9.
20. Merget R, Schulte A, Gebler A, et al. Outcome of occupational asthma due to platinum salts after transferral to low-exposure areas. *Int Arch Occup Environ Health*. 1999;72(1):33–9.
21. Kimber I, Dearman RJ, Basketter DA. Diisocyanates, occupational asthma and IgE antibody: implications for hazard characterization. *J Appl Toxicol*. 2014;34(10):1073–7.
22. Vandenplas O, Godet J, Hurdubaea L, et al. Are high- and low-molecular-weight sensitizing agents associated with different clinical phenotypes of occupational asthma? *Allergy*. 2019;74(2):261–72.
23. Simons FE. Allergic rhinobronchitis: The asthma-allergic rhinitis link. *J Allergy Clin Immunol*. 1999;104(3 Pt 1):534–40.
24. Passalacqua G, Ciprandi G, Canonica GW. The nose-lung interaction in allergic rhinitis and asthma: United airways disease. *Curr Opin Allergy Clin Immunol*. 2001;1(1):7–13.
25. Passalacqua G, Ciprandi G, Canonica GW. United airways disease: Therapeutic aspects. *Thorax*. 2000;55(Suppl 2):S26–27.
26. Brozek JL, Bousquet J, Agache I, et al. Allergic rhinitis and its impact on asthma (ARIA) guidelines—2016 revision. *J Allergy Clin Immunol*. 2017;140(4):950–8.
27. Shaaban R, Zureik M, Soussan D, et al. Rhinitis and onset of asthma: A longitudinal population-based study. *Lancet*. 2008;372(9643):1049–57.
28. Feng CH, Miller MD, Simon RA. The united allergic airway: Connections between allergic rhinitis, asthma, and chronic sinusitis. *Am J Rhinol Allergy*. 2012;26(3):187–90.
29. Licari A, Caimmi S, Bosa L, Marseglia A, Marseglia GL, Caimmi D. Rhinosinusitis and asthma: A very long engagement. *Int J Immunopathol Pharmacol*. 2014;27(4):499–508.
30. Balogun RA, Siracusa A, Shusterman D. Occupational rhinitis and occupational asthma: Association or progression? *Am J Ind Med*. 2018;61(4):293–307.
31. Park JH, Kreiss K, Cox-Ganser JM. Rhinosinusitis and mold as risk factors for asthma symptoms in occupants of a water-damaged building. *Indoor Air*. 2012;22(5):396–404.
32. Vandenplas O, Van Brussel P, D'Alpaos V, Wattiez M, Jamart J, Thimpont J. Rhinitis in subjects with work-exacerbated asthma. *Respir Med*. 2010;104(4):497–503.
33. Moscato G, Pala G, Folletti I, Siracusa A, Quirce S. Occupational rhinitis affects occupational asthma severity. *J Occup Health*. 2016;58(3):310–13.
34. Vila-Rigat R, Panades Valls R, Hernandez Huet E, et al. Prevalence of work-related asthma and its impact in primary health care. *Arch Bronconeumol*. 2015;51(9):449–55.
35. Gotzev S, Lipszyc JC, Connor D, Tarlo SM. Trends in occupations and work sectors among patients with work-related asthma at a Canadian tertiary care clinic. *Chest*. 2016;150(4):811–8.
36. Knoeller GE, Mazurek JM, Moorman JE. Work-related asthma, financial barriers to asthma care, and adverse asthma outcomes: Asthma call-back survey, 37 states and District of Columbia, 2006 to 2008. *Med Care*. 2011;49(12):1097–104.
37. Leigh JP. Economic burden of occupational injury and illness in the United States. *Milbank Q*. 2011;89(4):728–72.
38. Ayres JG, Boyd R, Cowie H, Hurley JF. Costs of occupational asthma in the UK. *Thorax*. 2011;66(2):128–33.
39. Vandenplas O. Socioeconomic impact of work-related asthma. *Expert Rev Pharmacoecon Outcomes Res*. 2008;8(4):395–400.
40. White GE, Mazurek JM, Moorman JE. Work-related asthma and employment status—38 states and District of Columbia, 2006–2009. *J Asthma*. 2013;50(9):954–9.
41. Knoeller GE, Mazurek JM, Moorman JE. Characteristics associated with health care professional diagnosis of work-related asthma among individuals who describe their asthma as being caused or made worse by workplace exposures. *J Occup Environ Med*. 2012;54(4):485–90.
42. Moorman JE, Akinbami LJ, Bailey CM, et al. National surveillance of asthma: United States, 2001–2010. *Vital Health Stat*. 2012;(35):1-–58.
43. Wong A, Tavakoli H, Sadatsafavi M, Carlsten C, FitzGerald JM. Asthma control and productivity loss in those with work-related asthma: A population-based study. *J Asthma*. 2017;54(5):537–42.
44. Malo JL, Chan-Yeung M, Kennedy S. Occupational agents. In: Barnes PJ, Thomson NC, Drazen JM, Rennard SI, eds.Barnes PJ, Thomson NC, Drazen JM, Rennard SI, eds. *Asthma and COPD*. Oxford, UK: Academic Press; 2009, pp. 457–70.
45. Rosenman KD, Beckett WS. Web based listing of agents associated with new onset work-related asthma. *Respir Med*. 2015;109(5):625–31.
46. NIOSH. Work-related respiratory diseases: State-based case data. *eWORLD* 2019. https://wwwn.cdc.gov/eworld/Grouping/Asthma/97#State-based Case Data. Accessed July 9, 2019.
47. Dodd KE, Mazurek JM. Asthma among employed adults, by industry and occupation—21 States, 2013. *MMWR Morb Mortal Wkly Rep*. 2016;65(47):1325–31.
48. McHugh MK, Symanski E, Pompeii LA, Delclos GL. Prevalence of asthma by industry and occupation in the U.S. working population. *Am J Ind Med*. 2010;53(5):463–75.
49. Knoeller GE, Mazurek JM, Storey E. Occupation held at the time of asthma symptom development. *Am J Ind Med*. 2013;56(10):1165–73.
50. Kwon SC, Song J, Kim YK, Calvert GM. Work-related asthma in Korea—Findings from the Korea work-related asthma surveillance (KOWAS) program, 2004–2009. *Allergy Asthma Immunol Res*. 2015;7(1):51–9.
51. Eng A, A TM, Douwes J, et al. The New Zealand workforce survey II: Occupational risk factors for asthma. *Ann Occup Hyg*. 2010;54(2):154–64.
52. Burge PS, Richardson MN. Occupational asthma due to indirect exposure to lauryl dimethyl benzyl ammonium chloride used in a floor cleaner. *Thorax*. 1994;49(8):842–3.
53. Savonius B, Keskinen H, Tuppurainen M, Kanerva L. Occupational asthma caused by ethanolamines. *Allergy*. 1994;49(10):877–81.
54. Kujala VM, Reijula KE, Ruotsalainen EM, Heikkinen K. Occupational asthma due to chloramine-T solution. *Respir Med*. 1995;89(10):693–5.
55. Rosenman KD, Reilly MJ, Schill DP, et al. Cleaning products and work-related asthma. *J Occup Environ Med*. 2003;45(5):556–63.
56. Paris C, Ngatchou-Wandji J, Luc A, et al. Work-related asthma in France: Recent trends for the period 2001–2009. *Occup Environ Med*. 2012;69(6):391–7.
57. Kogevinas M, Anto JM, Sunyer J, Tobias A, Kromhout H, Burney P. Occupational asthma in Europe and other industrialised areas: A population-based study. European Community Respiratory Health Survey Study Group. *Lancet*. 1999;353(9166):1750–4.
58. Arif AA, Delclos GL, Whitehead LW, Tortolero SR, Lee ES. Occupational exposures associated with work-related asthma and work-related wheezing among U.S. workers. *Am J Ind Med*. 2003;44(4):368–76.
59. Zock JP, Kogevinas M, Sunyer J, et al. Asthma risk, cleaning activities and use of specific cleaning products among Spanish indoor cleaners. *Scand J Work Environ Health*. 2001;27(1):76–81.
60. Karjalainen A, Martikainen R, Karjalainen J, Klaukka T, Kurppa K. Excess incidence of asthma among Finnish cleaners employed in different industries. *Eur Respir J*. 2002;19(1):90–5.

61. Le Moual N, Kennedy SM, Kauffmann F. Occupational exposures and asthma in 14,000 adults from the general population. *Am J Epidemiol.* 2004;160(11):1108–16.
62. Medina-Ramon M, Zock JP, Kogevinas M, Sunyer J, Anto JM. Asthma symptoms in women employed in domestic cleaning: A community based study. *Thorax.* 2003;58(11):950–4.
63. Medina-Ramon M, Zock JP, Kogevinas M, et al. Asthma, chronic bronchitis, and exposure to irritant agents in occupational domestic cleaning: A nested case-control study. *Occup Environ Med.* 2005;62(9):598–606.
64. Walters GI, Kirkham A, McGrath EE, Moore VC, Robertson AS, Burge PS. Twenty years of SHIELD: Decreasing incidence of occupational asthma In the West Midlands, UK? *Occup Environ Med.* 2015;72(4):304–10.
65. Walters GI, Burge PS, Moore VC, Robertson AS. Cleaning agent occupational asthma in the West Midlands, UK: 2000–16. *Occup Med.* 2018;68(8):530–6.
66. Pechter E, Davis LK, Tumpowsky C, et al. Work-related asthma among health care workers: Surveillance data from California, Massachusetts, Michigan, and New Jersey, 1993–1997. *Am J Ind Med.* 2005;47(3): 265–75.
67. Dumas O, Donnay C, Heederik DJ, et al. Occupational exposure to cleaning products and asthma in hospital workers. *Occup Environ Med.* 2012;69(12):883–9.
68. Delclos GL, Gimeno D, Arif AA, et al. Occupational risk factors and asthma among health care professionals. *Am J Respir Crit Care Med.* 2007;175(7):667–75.
69. Arif AA, Delclos GL. Association between cleaning-related chemicals and work-related asthma and asthma symptoms among healthcare professionals. *Occup Environ Med.* 2012;69(1):35–40.
70. Mirabelli MC, Zock JP, Plana E, et al. Occupational risk factors for asthma among nurses and related healthcare professionals in an international study. *Occup Environ Med.* 2007;64(7):474–9.
71. Dumas O, Wiley AS, Quinot C, et al. Occupational exposure to disinfectants and asthma control in US nurses. *Eur Respir J.* 2017;50(4):1700237.
72. Institute of Medicine (US). *Damp Indoor Spaces and Health.* Washington, DC: National Academies Press; 2004.
73. WHO. *WHO Guidelines for Indoor Air Quality: Dampness and Mould.* Geneva: WHO; 2009.
74. Mendell MJ, Mirer AG, Cheung K, Tong M, Douwes J. Respiratory and allergic health effects of dampness, mold, and dampness-related agents: A review of the epidemiologic evidence. *Environ Health Perspect.* 2011;119(6):748-–56.
75. Caillaud D, Leynaert B, Keirsbulck M, et al. Indoor mould exposure, asthma and rhinitis: Findings from systematic reviews and recent longitudinal studies. *Eur Respir Rev.* 2018;27(148):170137.
76. Cox-Ganser JM, White SK, Jones R, et al. Respiratory morbidity in office workers in a water-damaged building. *Environ Health Perspect.* 2005;113(4):485–90.
77. Cox-Ganser JM, Rao CY, Park JH, Schumpert JC, Kreiss K. Asthma and respiratory symptoms in hospital workers related to dampness and biological contaminants. *Indoor Air.* 2009;19(4):280–90.
78. Park JH, Cox-Ganser J, Rao C, Kreiss K. Fungal and endotoxin measurements in dust associated with respiratory symptoms in a water-damaged office building. *Indoor Air.* 2006;16(3):192–203.
79. White SK, Cox-Ganser JM, Benaise LG, Kreiss K. Work-related peak flow and asthma symptoms in a damp building. *Occup Med.* 2013;63(4):287–90.
80. Kurth L, Virji MA, Storey E, et al. Current asthma and asthma-like symptoms among workers at a Veterans Administration Medical Center. *Int J Hyg Environ Health.* 2017;220(8):1325–32.
81. NIOSH MM, Cox-Ganser J, Kreiss K, Kanwal R, Sahakian N. NIOSH alert: Preventing occupational respiratory disease from exposures caused by dampness in office buildings, schools, and other non-industrial buildings. In: *National Institute for Occupational Safety and Health.* Department of Health and Human Services, DHHS (NIOSH); 2012.
82. Mendell MJ, Kumagai K. Observation-based metrics for residential dampness and mold with dose-response relationships to health: A review. *Indoor Air.* 2017;27(3):506–17.
83. Park JH, Cox-Ganser JM. Mold exposure and respiratory health in damp indoor environments. *Front biosci.* 2011;3:757–71.
84. National Academies of Sciences Engineering, and Medicine. *Microbiomes of the Built Environment: A Research Agenda for Indoor Microbiology, Human Health, and Buildings.* Washington, DC: The National Academies Press; 2017.
85. Park JH, Cox-Ganser JM, Kreiss K, White SK, Rao CY. Hydrophilic fungi and ergosterol associated with respiratory illness in a water-damaged building. *Environ health perspect.* 2008;116(1):45–50.
86. Sharpe RA, Bearman N, Thornton CR, Husk K, Osborne NJ. Indoor fungal diversity and asthma: A meta-analysis and systematic review of risk factors. *J Allergy Clin Immunol.* 2015;135(1):110–22.
87. Cox-Ganser JM. Indoor dampness and mould health effects—Ongoing questions on microbial exposures and allergic versus nonallergic mechanisms. *Clin Exp Allergy.* 2015;45(10):1478–82.
88. Rietveld S, Everaerd W, Creer TL. Stress-induced asthma: A review of research and potential mechanisms. *Clin Exp Allergy.* 2000;30(8):1058–66.
89. Rod NH, Kristensen TS, Lange P, Prescott E, Diderichsen F. Perceived stress and risk of adult-onset asthma and other atopic disorders: A longitudinal cohort study. *Allergy.* 2012;67(11):1408–14.
90. Wright RJ, Rodriguez M, Cohen S. Review of psychosocial stress and asthma: An integrated biopsychosocial approach. *Thorax.* 1998; 53(12):1066–74.
91. Yonas MA, Lange NE, Celedon JC. Psychosocial stress and asthma morbidity. *Curr Opin Allergy Clin Immunol.* 2012;12(2):202–210.
92. de Nijs SB, Venekamp LN, Bel EH. Adult-onset asthma: Is it really different? *Eur Resp Rev.* 2013;22(127):44–52.
93. Lietzen R, Virtanen P, Kivimaki M, Sillanmaki L, Vahtera J, Koskenvuo M. Stressful life events and the onset of asthma. *Eur Respir J.* 2011;37(6):1360–5.
94. Loerbroks A, Ding H, Han W, et al. Work stress, family stress and asthma: A cross-sectional study among women in China. *Int Arch Occup Environ Health.* 2017;90(4):349–56.
95. Renzaho AM, Houng B, Oldroyd J, Nicholson JM, D'Esposito F, Oldenburg B. Stressful life events and the onset of chronic diseases among Australian adults: Findings from a longitudinal survey. *Eur J Public Health.* 2014;24(1):57–62.
96. Heikkila K, Madsen IE, Nyberg ST, et al. Job strain and the risk of severe asthma exacerbations: A meta-analysis of individual-participant data from 100 000 European men and women. *Allergy.* 2014;69(6):775–83.
97. Runeson-Broberg R, Norback D. Work-related psychosocial stress as a risk factor for asthma, allergy, and respiratory infections in the Swedish workforce. *Psychol Rep.* 2014;114(2):377–89.
98. Eng A, Mannetje A, Pearce N, Douwes J. Work-related stress and asthma: Results from a workforce survey in New Zealand. *J Asthma.* 2011;48(8):783–9.
99. Loerbroks A, Bosch JA, Douwes J, Angerer P, Li J. Job insecurity is associated with adult asthma in Germany during Europe's recent economic crisis: A prospective cohort study. *J Epidemiol Community Health.* 2014;68(12):1196–9.
100. Loerbroks A, Gadinger MC, Bosch JA, Sturmer T, Amelang M. Work-related stress, inability to relax after work and risk of adult asthma: A population-based cohort study. *Allergy.* 2010;65(10):1298–305.
101. Loerbroks A, Herr RM, Li J, et al. The association of effort-reward imbalance and asthma: Findings from two cross-sectional studies. *Int Arch Occup Environ Health.* 2015;88(3):351–8.
102. Chen E, Miller GE. Stress and inflammation in exacerbations of asthma. *Brain Behav Immun.* 2007;21(8):993–9.
103. Haczku A, Panettieri RA, Jr. Social stress and asthma: The role of corticosteroid insensitivity. *J Allergy Clin Immunol.* 2010;125(3):550–8.
104. Wright RJ. Stress and atopic disorders. *J Allergy Clin Immunol.* 2005;116(6):1301–6.
105. Rosenberg SL, Miller GE, Brehm JM, Celedon JC. Stress and asthma: Novel insights on genetic, epigenetic, and immunologic mechanisms. *J Allergy Clin Immunol.* 2014;134(5):1009–15.
106. Plourde A, Lavoie KL, Raddatz C, Bacon SL. Effects of acute psychological stress induced in laboratory on physiological responses in asthma populations: A systematic review. *Respir Med.* 2017;127:21–32.
107. Aasen TB, Burge PS, Henneberger PK, Schlünssen V, Baur X. Diagnostic approach in cases with suspected work-related asthma. *J Occup Med Toxicol.* 2013;8(1):17.
108. Dao A, Bernstein DI. Occupational exposure and asthma. *Ann Allergy Asthma Immunol.* 2018;120(5):468–75.
109. Jares EJ, Baena-Cagnani CE, Gómez RM. Diagnosis of occupational asthma: An update. *Curr Allergy Asthma Rep.* 2012;12(3):221–31.
110. Pralong JA, Cartier A. Review of diagnostic challenges in occupational asthma. *Curr Allergy Asthma Rep.* 2017;17(1):1.
111. Trivedi V, Apala DR, Iyer VN. Occupational asthma: Diagnostic challenges and management dilemmas. *Curr Opin Pulm Med.* 2017;23(2):177–83.
112. Coates AL, Wanger J, Cockcroft DW, et al. ERS technical standard on bronchial challenge testing: General considerations and performance of methacholine challenge tests. *Eur Respir J.* 2017;49(5):1601526.

113. Moore VC, Jaakkola MS, Burge CB, et al. Do long periods off work in peak expiratory flow monitoring improve the sensitivity of occupational asthma diagnosis? *Occup Environ Med.* 2010;67(8):562–7.

114. Moore VC, Jaakkola MS, Burge CB, et al. A new diagnostic score for occupational asthma: The area between the curves (ABC score) of peak expiratory flow on days at and away from work. *Chest.* 2009;135(2):307–14.

115. Baur X, Akdis CA, Budnik LT, et al. Immunological methods for diagnosis and monitoring of IgE-mediated allergy caused by industrial sensitizing agents (IMExAllergy). *Allergy.* 2019;74(10):1885–97.

116. Lux H, Lenz K, Budnik LT, Baur X. Performance of specific immunoglobulin E tests for diagnosing occupational asthma: A systematic review and meta-analysis. *Occup Environ Med.* 2019;76(4):269–78.

117. Heederik D, Henneberger PK, Redlich CA. Primary prevention: Exposure reduction, skin exposure and respiratory protection. *Eur Respir Rev.* 2012;21(124):112–24.

118. Kellett PB. Latex allergy: A review. *J Emerg Nurs.* 1997;23(1):27–34; quiz 34-26.

119. Kelly KJ, Sussman G. Latex allergy: Where are we now and how did we get there? *J Allergy Clin Immunol Pract.* 2017;5(5):1212–6.

120. Tarlo SM, Sussman G, Contala A, Swanson MC. Control of airborne latex by use of powder-free latex gloves. *J Allergy Clin Immunol.* 1994;93(6):985–9.

121. LaMontagne AD, Radi S, Elder DS, Abramson MJ, Sim M. Primary prevention of latex related sensitisation and occupational asthma: A systematic review. *Occup Environ Med.* 2006;63(5):359–64.

122. Heilman DK, Jones RT, Swanson MC, Yunginger JW. A prospective, controlled study showing that rubber gloves are the major contributor to latex aeroallergen levels in the operating room. *J Allergy Clin Immunol.* 1996;98(2):325–30.

123. Allmers H, Schmengler J, Skudlik C. Primary prevention of natural rubber latex allergy in the German health care system through education and intervention. *J Allergy Clin Immunol.* 2002;110(2):318–23.

124. Vandenplas O, Larbanois A, Vanassche F, et al. Latex-induced occupational asthma: Time trend in incidence and relationship with hospital glove policies. *Allergy.* 2009;64(3):415–-20.

125. FDA. Banned devices: Powdered surgeon's gloves, powdered patient examination gloves, and absorbable powder for lubricating a surgeon's glove. *Fed Regist.* 2016;87(243):91722–31.

126. Bernstein DI. A Guide for the Primary Care Physician in Evaluating Diisocyanate Exposed Workers for Occupational Asthma. 2017.

127. Taghiakbari M, Pralong JA, Lemière C, et al. Novel clinical scores for occupational asthma due to exposure to high-molecular-weight agents. *Occup Environ Med.* 2019;76(7):495–501.

128. Harber P, Redlich CA, Hines S, Filios MS, Storey E. Recommendations for a clinical decision support system for work-related asthma in primary care settings. *J Occup Environ Med.* 2017;59(11):e231–5.

129. Killorn KR, Dostaler SM, Olajos-Clow J, et al. The development and test re-test reliability of a work-related asthma screening questionnaire. *J Asthma.* 2015;52(3):279–88.

130. De Groene GJ, Pal TM, Beach J, et al. Workplace interventions for treatment of occupational asthma: A Cochrane systematic review. *Occup Environ Med.* 2012;69(5):373–4.

CHAPTER

77 Infectious Diseases: Industrial Animal Operations

Meghan F. Davis

OVERVIEW

The raising of animals—for meat, for milk, for fiber, for draft—may be among the oldest of professions, dating back thousands of years to the domestication of animals.[1,2] Equally, anthropozoonotic infections, that is, those transmitted among humans and animals, are also among the first recorded diseases. For example, the Roman poet Virgil described transmission of anthrax from infected animals to humans via contact with wool: "The pelts of diseased animals were useless, and neither water or fire could cleanse the taint from their flesh...if anyone wore garments made from tainted wool, his limbs were soon attacked by inflamed papules and a foul exudate."[3] In the nineteenth century, anthrax was called "wool-sorters" disease, emphasizing the importance of the occupational routes of exposure.[4] Even today, anthrax remains a persistent, although rare, risk among a variety of professionals who work in agricultural or textile settings.[5] Public health success in the management of occupational anthrax may be due to several factors, in part to improved recognition and control of the disease at both the animal and the worker level, and in part to the reduction in the number of workers who handle animals and their products.

The number of farmers, in relation to the size of the world's population, has been on the decline, particularly in developed countries.[6] Driven by the Green Revolution in the 1930s, a movement that tackled the challenge of how to feed an exponentially growing world population, farm sizes have been increasing (see Fig. 77-1) but the number of farms—and in parallel, the number of people needed to work the farms—has been decreasing, particularly in more developed countries.[7] In the United States, the number of farmers, ranchers and agricultural managers is now less than 2% of the population, down from a peak in the 1900s when over 40% of the population were engaged in farming activities.[8] At the same time, global consumption of animal products has been on the rise.

The success of the agricultural sector to meet world demands for meat and other products stems in part from decades of industrialization and intensification. Industrial Food Animal Production (IFAP) is typified by the raising of a large number of animals on small plots of land.[9] These systems also typically use a variety of methods to ensure that animals are raised in a uniform manner to a target production size or weight—matched to an equally industrialized processing sector. Such methods include constraint of animal interactions, modification of genetic stock through selective breeding or newer methods of genetic manipulation, engineering of animal housing, use of animal waste management systems, and intervention with chemical agents, such as antimicrobial drugs and pesticides.[10] Unlike earlier agricultural systems where production was constrained by local resources such as water and nutrients, modern IFAP systems depend on resources that may be sourced globally.[10] For example, what we feed to animals may include grains and other commodities that are part of a global supply chain.[11]

Global movement of food-producing animals, animal feed, and related resources can contribute to emergence and spread of infectious agents that can impact both humans and animals, causing morbidity, mortality, and economic losses. For example, flexible feed totes (grain sacks) carrying soybeans or other products were implicated as a potential route for introduction of porcine epidemic virus that is believed to have entered the United States from Asia in 2013.[12] This virus devastated herds throughout the United States and led to severe economic losses for pork producers in 2013 and 2014.[13] Indeed, global supply chains and agricultural intensification can drive emergence of infectious diseases through a number of pathways, including encroachment of agricultural communities into areas that have not previously been developed, which may increase contact between wildlife and domestic animals.[14]

This chapter covers the intersection of animal production generally—and IFAP specifically—with infectious disease emergence and risk in an occupational and environmental health context. Specific examples and cases illustrate larger concepts of how IFAP systems can foster spread of infectious agents among animals and to humans using a One Health perspective, which is defined as the intersection of human health, animal health, and environmental health. Box 77-1

GLOBAL ONE HEALTH

The American Veterinary Medical Association (AVMA) defines One Health as "the collaborative effort of multiple disciplines—working locally, nationally, and globally—to attain optimal health for people, animals, and the environment."[15] Some have described it as the intersection of human health, animal health, and environmental health (Fig. 77-2). Given this framework, it is natural that a One Health approach is critical to understanding movement of infectious agents in IFAP systems, given the intensity of contact between human workers and animals via the confinement environments in which the animals are housed.

In a global health security framework, One Health is an approach or tool for response to threats—threats that often are in the form of outbreaks of endemic circulation of anthropozoonotic diseases.[16] It is a multisectoral approach that explicitly works to bring together stakeholders from diverse fields and backgrounds for problem solving. For example, the U.S. Centers for Disease Control (CDC) One Health Office developed a Zoonotic Disease Prioritization Tool, a voluntary and collaborative process to help organizations or institutions, such as the animal and human health agencies within a country, bring together key sectors to rank the zoonotic diseases of greatest threat to the health of their human and animal populations and identify strategies to prevent disease and respond to outbreaks.[17] Such activities are important to the Global Health Security Agenda (GHSA), a partnership of over 60 countries, international

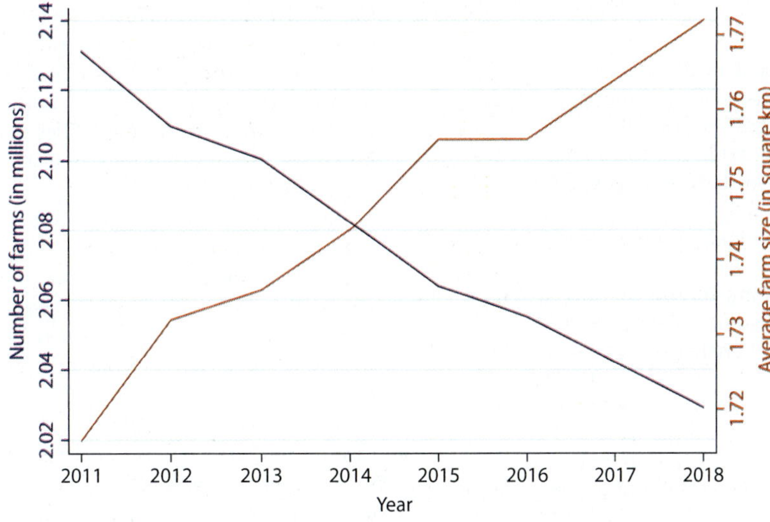

FIGURE 77-1. Number of farms compared to average farm size in the United States, 2011–18. (*Source:* Data from the USDA Farms and Land in Farms 2018 Summary. United States Department of Agriculture, April 2019. Report available from: https://downloads.usda.library.cornell.edu/usda-esmis/files/5712m6524/j098zk725/9z903749k/fnlo0419.pdf.)

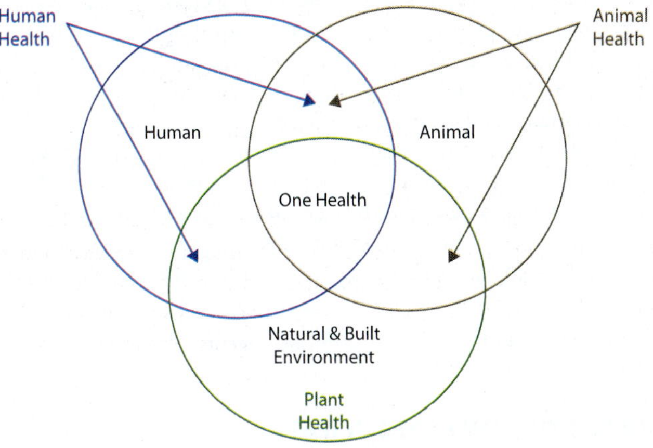

FIGURE 77-2. One Health is the intersection of human health, animal health, and environmental health domains. One Health motivates approaches to research, policy, and program development, and it includes consideration of the natural environment, including the health of plants and ecosystems, as well as consideration of the built environment, which encompasses all of the anthropogenic (human-made) inputs to our surroundings.

organizations, and nongovernmental organizations—advised by international groups such as the Food and Agriculture Organization (FAO), World Organization for Animal Health (OIE), and World Health Organization (WHO)—that work to secure the world from infectious disease threats. Livestock are particularly critical for GHSA activities since anthropozoonotic diseases that threaten food-producing animals not only can impact the health of the animals and farmers, but also can impact populations through food consumption, threaten food security, and result in economic losses. A One Health approach brings together stakeholders that include, not just disease experts, physicians, and veterinarians, but also other stakeholders that can include farmers, food industry professionals, economists, policy makers, and legal experts as needed for a complete local, country-level, or international response to an infectious disease threat.

INDUSTRIAL FOOD ANIMAL PRODUCTION (IFAP)

What we eat—and by extension how we grow or raise food, how we harvest and prepare it, and how we consume it—may differ from one country to the next, but the fact that we must eat is universal. Food production is foundational to societal stability; when a country faces a food shortage, the security of that country is threatened. This is true whether a country uses a traditional model of labor-intensive, small farms that might produce a diverse set of crops and/or animals or whether a country uses a modern industrialized model where each producer has a single, specialized output. What differs between the traditional, small-farm model and the modern industrialized model is the dependency the latter system has on a global network of trade.

The Green Revolution is a term coined by William Gaud in 1968 when he was Director of the U.S. Agency for International Development (USAID) to describe the specific transition in agriculture from traditional farming practices to more intensive systems, leading to dramatic growth in crop yields.[18] In particular, the Green Revolution is associated with the cultivation of specific genetic varieties in order to increase the yield of rice and wheat that occurred during the second half of the twentieth century.[18] One goal of the Green Revolution was to address concerns with how the world would feed an exponentially growing population. The challenge was that agriculture previously had been limited to local inputs of water and nutrients, and the solution was to de-couple production from the local ecology. This meant selective breeding and cultivation of just a few varieties chosen for their productivity rather than other traits (such as resistance to infectious diseases), use of fertilizers as a nutrient input, use of pesticides to reduce product waste or loss, and use of irrigation systems to supply water on a routine schedule. Because this transition required investment in agricultural research, inputs of modern fertilizers and pesticides, and engineering of water and other systems, the term Green Revolution has been applied to similar intensification that occurred shortly thereafter for other modes of crop and animal production.

Industrialization of food animal production began in the United States with the processing sector, where food animal products were subjected to increasing mechanization of the process to render whole animal or animal product (milk, eggs, or fiber) into the ultimate retail good that would be purchased by consumers, such as a package of chicken breasts or a gallon of 1% milk.[19] This meant substitution of machines to perform tasks previously performed by people, and process chains that were standardized from one plant to the next. In the United States, this next spread to the production sector, or farm. Instead of rotating different crops from 1 year to the next, farms increasingly employed monocropping techniques. Farms that once raised five different kinds of animals at low density where the animals lived off the productivity of the farm itself now raised only one kind of animal at high density under confinement. For example,

BOX 77-1 Definitions

Animal reservoir: A species of animal that can carry an infectious agent, where the infectious agent often does not cause severe disease in the animal reservoir itself.
Anthropozoonosis: A disease that can spread between humans and animals, typically in either direction (human to animal and animal to human).
Built environment: Anthropogenic (human-made) inputs to the environment.
Concentrated Animal Feeding Operation (CAFO): A term designated by the U.S. Environmental Protection Agency for the purposes of regulation of discharges of animal waste; the number of animals required for a production facility to be designated a large, medium, and small CAFOs is different for each species of animal.
Draft animal: Working animal that is used for transportation or hauling, which includes animals that pull a load, plow, or carriage.
Environmental reservoir: A location in the inanimate environment that can foster the survival of infectious agents outside of a host.
Fiber (or fiber) animal: Animal that is used primarily for the production of wool or pelts.
Fomite: Inanimate object that may harbor infectious disease agents and play a role in indirect transmission of those agents.
Industrial Food Animal Production (IFAP): The production of food animals at high density and under confinement conditions (N.B.: This term applies to food-animal production under high density and confinement, irrespective of whether the facility discharges animal waste and therefore meets the U.S. regulatory definition of a CAFO).
Meat animal: Animal that is used for the production of meat or related commodities, such as beef, chicken, pork, lamb, and goat.
Meat-and-bone meal (MBM): A feed commodity that consists of rendered products from other animals.
Milk animal: Animal that is used for the production of liquid milk or other dairy commodities, such as cheese.
Monocropping: An agricultural practice of specialization to grow just one variety of plant crop, such as corn, every year.
Natural environment: Portion of the environment that is not influenced by humans.
One Health: Multisectorial collaborative approach among stakeholders to advance knowledge at the intersection of human, animal, and environmental health, with a goal to optimize health in all sectors.
Vector: (1) An insect that may carry an infectious disease agent and be part of the lifecycle of that agent; (2) A living or nonliving object that is responsible for mechanical transmission of an infectious disease agent.
Zoonosis: A disease that spreads from animals to humans.

broiler poultry production in the United States is dominated by a single breed, the Cornish Cross, raised for 7 weeks in confinement on a facility where the median flock size is 160,000 birds.[10] Density alone can be a driver of infectious disease transmission, since each animal is in closer contact with its neighbors. This increase in animal density was enabled by bringing in feeds from off the farm, since the number of animals in modern IFAP systems typically exceeds the ability of the local ecology to provide sufficient nutrients for the animals. Increasingly, animals also are fed commodities, which are grains or by-products from other industries, and this can be on scales from local to global. For example, in California, dairy cows may be fed rations that contain almond hulls, a byproduct of the local almond industry. United States dairy cows also might be fed rendered products from other animals, termed meat-and-bone-meal (MBM). However, when MBM was implicated in the potential spread of bovine spongiform encephalopathy (BSE, or Mad Cow Disease) in the United Kingdom, the United States banned importation of MBM from Europe in 1997.[20] This highlights the potential for other globally traded grains and commodities to result in the introduction of infectious disease agents into countries or regions where the disease previously had not been detected.

As farms have changed, so has the management structure of the industry. The poultry and swine sectors in particular shifted from single-family operations to vertical integration. In this model, the company owns the animals, the processing facilities, and the product, and they often contract with "growers" to raise the animals to market weight. A consequence of this structure is that growers often must build their barns to the specifications of the company, and follow the company's requirements in terms of what the animals are fed. While this standardization likely has helped overcome certain challenges of animal health and productivity, it also has meant less diversity in production practices. If certain practices might drive spread of infectious disease, all the growers within a given integrator network are doing the same thing. This potential vulnerability extends to the kinds of animals being raised: if all the animals within a network come from the same breeder and genetic stock, then they all could be susceptible to a new infectious disease agent. Terrestrial species such as cattle, pigs, and poultry are not the only food-producing animals to be raised using this model; increasingly, the aquaculture sector has adopted similar strategies—including reliance on external inputs of feed, chemicals and drugs—to produce finfish and shellfish.[21]

What began in the United States has spread quickly throughout the world (see Fig. 77-3, a photograph of an industrial poultry operation on an island nation in the Caribbean). "Industrial food animal production is now the globalized model," writes Dr. Ellen Silbergeld in *Chickenizing Farms and Food.*[19] In countries that adopt the IFAP model, changes from traditional farms to confinement operations can happen rapidly, driven in part by international companies that do business around the world.

INFECTIOUS DISEASES IN IFAP

Infectious diseases are illnesses in people or animals that are caused by communicable agents that can be transmitted from person-to-person, from animal-to-animal, or among people and animals. These may be transmitted directly through contact or may be transmitted indirectly through the environment, a fomite, or an insect vector. The illness may be caused by the agent itself—such as a bacterium, virus, parasite, or prion (see Table 77-1)—or may be caused by a component of the agent or a substance produced by it. In the United States alone, the CDC estimates that there are over 3.6 million domestically acquired foodborne infections from the 31 most common pathogens that they include in surveillance efforts, including over 1 million infections due to nontyphoidal *Salmonella* species, over 900 thousand infections due to *Clostridium perfringens*, and over 800 thousand infections due to *Campylobacter* species.[22] Globally, the World Health Organization (WHO) estimates that, in 2010, there were 600 million foodborne infections with 420,000 deaths.[23]

Infection is not the only route by which infectious disease agents may cause disease. One example of a bacterial component that is associated with some diseases in people is endotoxin, which is the lipopolysaccharide coat of Gram-negative bacteria that can persist in the environment even after the bacteria die. Because endotoxin comes from Gram-negative bacteria, and because Gram-negative bacteria are found at high concentrations in fecal material, it is sometimes used as a marker of fecal contamination of the environment. Exposure to high concentrations of endotoxin, such as in closed barns or other IFAP confinement facilities, may elicit a fever and other inflammatory responses in people. However, not everyone exposed to high endotoxin concentrations will develop a fever.

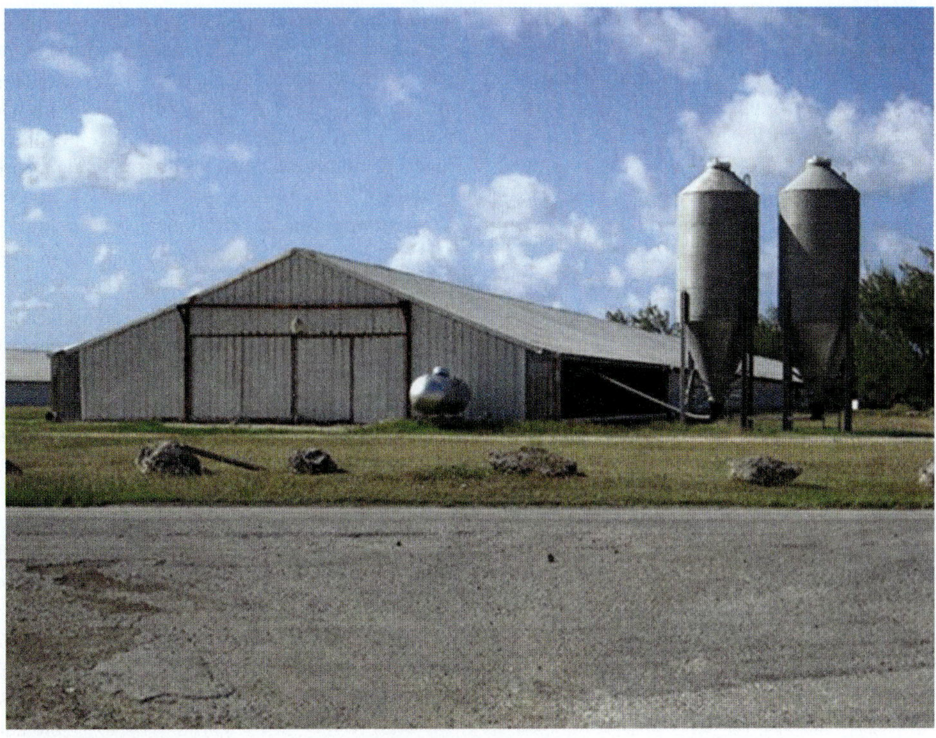

FIGURE 77-3. Industrial poultry facility in the Caribbean. (*Source:* Meghan F. Davis.)

TABLE 77-1 SELECTED INFECTIOUS AGENTS THAT MAY BE SPREAD AMONG PEOPLE AND ANIMALS IN THE CONTEXT OF IFAP

Infectious Agent	Disease in Animals	Disease in People	Control Strategies
Bacteria			
Campylobacter jejuni	Often asymptomatic	Gastrointestinal illness	Herd or flock eradication campaigns, good meat handling practices
E. coli O157:H7	Often asymptomatic	Gastrointestinal illness, hemolytic-uremic syndrome (HUS)	Good meat handling practices
Staphylococcus aureus	Often asymptomatic	Skin and soft-tissue infections; bloodstream infections	Hygiene practices
Viruses			
Influenza H1N1 "swine flu"	Respiratory and gastrointestinal illness	Respiratory and gastrointestinal illness	Vaccination of people, surveillance in animals
Nipah virus	Respiratory illness	Respiratory and neurologic illness	Animal culling
Parasites			
Cryptosporidium spp.	Gastrointestinal illness among younger populations (particularly dairy calves)	Gastrointestinal illness, particularly among younger, elderly or immunocompromised populations	Hygiene practices
Trichinella spp.	Often asymptomatic	Gastrointestinal illness	Confinement raising, rodent and wildlife control for animals
Prion diseases	Neurologic illness	Neurologic illness	Animal culling

There are many factors that determine whether or how exposure to an infectious agent can influence the kind of disease that may (or may not) manifest in the person or animal exposed (i.e., the host). The first is the infectious dose, which is the number of viable pathogens (e.g., virions, bacteria, parasites, etc.) needed to establish an infection. If a host is exposed to too few viable pathogens, these may be insufficient to overcome the host's innate immune response and other defenses and establish an infection. The number of pathogens needed to establish infection will vary from pathogen to pathogen, and may even vary within a species of pathogen according to strain. For example, the infectious dose for the bacterium *Escherichia coli* O157:H7 can be fewer than 100 organisms,[24] lower than for other strains of less pathogenic *E. coli*. In IFAP systems, animals are often housed in closed buildings, which (depending on the dynamics of the air ventilation system in the barn) could trap microorganisms, including pathogens, inside the building. This could mean that a worker is exposed to a higher number of pathogens while working inside the closed barn, and this could mean that the worker is more likely to get a dose that will be high enough to establish an infection.

Another key factor that determines whether exposure to an infectious agent will progress to infection is host susceptibility, which is a measure of whether the exposed person or animal has any innate or acquired resistance to the pathogen in question. An example of this is the limited livestock spread of the pandemic SARS-CoV-2 virus, which primarily impacted mink production in the Netherlands and the United States during 2020.[25] Experimental infection demonstrated that most livestock species, including pigs and chickens, are resistant to this novel coronavirus infection,[26] which is in contrast to the susceptibility of these same species for influenza viruses. Of note, SARS-CoV-2 primarily has been introduced to farms through infected workers,[25] suggesting that interventions to target people on the farm are critical for control efforts. One important way for a host to be resistant to a given pathogen is through prior exposure or vaccination. A person vaccinated against a disease is unlikely to be susceptible to the disease when exposed at a later time point. This is a point of potential intervention in IFAP systems, since some diseases that can transmit from animals to humans can be managed through vaccination of either or both the human workers and the animals—if such vaccines exist, if they are available to farmers or producers, and if they are cost effective to use. An example is the use of vaccination in cattle to prevent brucellosis, a zoonotic pathogen that causes disease in both humans and animals.[27] One challenge with the use of certain Brucella vaccines, such as *B. abortus* RB51, is the potential for workers who administer the vaccines to be exposed through accidental needlestick injury to the vaccine strain, and then to develop symptoms of brucellosis,[28] an occurrence suggesting that improvements to the safety and efficacy of such vaccines should be a research target.

In addition, the potential for exposure of a host to an infectious disease agent or its products (such as endotoxin) should be considered. When diseases are transmitted only through direct contact, it is possible that, even if there is an infected person or animal in a group, that the susceptible host in question may not come into direct contact with the infected one. In an IFAP system, where animals are housed under high density, they have high rates of direct contact with other animals, and so the chance to spread disease goes up. If the animals were housed under lower density, and with fewer other individuals, that chance of direct contact and disease spread would go down. This is one reason that many pathogens can spread quickly in an IFAP system, such that if any one animal is infected, often the pathogen spreads to infect many other members of the group. The more animals that are infected, the greater the chance that a worker will come into contact with an infected animal. However, for infectious agents to spread among animals within a facility, they first have to be introduced. Facilities closer to each other can experience this spread through wind, water, or wildlife conduits, such as via birds and rodents.[29,30] Some aquaculture facilities use sea cages or sea nets placed into the ocean or other large bodies of water, and these allows direct and indirect contact between farmed fish species and wild aquatic life. This can lead to introduction of infectious agents, such as sea lice (a parasite) in farmed salmon.[31] However, proximity is not required for spread among facilities. Networks of animal and product transport within companies and within the larger IFAP system can influence spread of infectious agents on a national or global scale.[32–35] In most cases, the spread occurs from new animals introduced to a facility, or via fomites and feed. However, the SARS-CoV-2 example demonstrates the importance of human personnel to expose animals for some infectious agents, as animal-to-animal spread on mink farms occurred after an infected worker introduced the coronavirus to the facility.[25]

When many animals are infected, when they shed the infectious agent into the environment, and when the infectious agent can survive in an environmental reservoir, then the environment itself can serve as a source of continued exposure to groups of animals and to people. The people exposed include workers, who may have direct contact with animals and the environment, and also people who might live in proximity to an IFAP facility. This is because infectious agents may be carried by wind or water off the facility and into surrounding communities. The use of ventilation fans on barns, with a goal to regulate the temperature inside the barn for animal health, and the spraying of manure, with a goal to provide nutrients to crop fields and manage the waste products of animal production, each may inadvertently spread infectious agents out of the barn and downwind of the facility.[36–39] Researchers have shown increased risk of certain zoonotic or potentially zoonotic pathogens, such as methicillin-resistant *Staphylococcus aureus* (MRSA), among people who live in close proximity to IFAP facilities or to fields where manure from these facilities is sprayed or spread.[40–42]

At the same time, estimating infectious disease risks to the population that are attributable directly to IFAP or IFAP practices is challenging, given the dynamic nature of infectious agents and given that transmission pathways can be bidirectional among the human, animal, and environmental domains. If IFAP workers apply chemicals, such as pesticides, that are not degraded quickly in the environment, then it is possible to measure the concentrations of the chemicals in the environment and in human samples, such as in blood or urine and expect to find some relationship between the concentration applied and the concentration that enters the worker's body. However, with infectious disease agents, the organism can replicate and can die, leading to fluctuations in the human, in the animal, and in the environment that may not reflect the original exposure. It is also possible for infectious agents to move in all directions, such that identifying which domain was the origin of the exposure (human, animal, or environment) often is not possible. In this complex system, uses of chemicals and pharmaceuticals, such as antimicrobial drugs, also can influence the population of bacteria in hosts or the environment and may drive emergence of or selection for drug-resistant strains.

CASE: ANTIMICROBIAL RESISTANCE

Antimicrobial drugs are critical to both human and veterinary medicine for the treatment of diseases. Shortly after mass production of the first antibiotic, penicillin, began in the early 1940s, uses of antimicrobial drugs became common in both humans and animals.[43] However, modern uses of antimicrobial drugs in treating animals globally may extend beyond therapeutic uses and encompass uses for prevention of disease and growth promotion, although the latter (uses for growth promotion or production) have been restricted in Europe and the United States.[7]

Microorganisms have the potential to have intrinsic or acquired traits that confer resistance to the effects of drugs, including antimicrobial drugs. Some bacteria are naturally resistant to certain antibiotics, such as *Pseudomonas aeruginosa* resistance to penicillin, and therefore physicians, veterinarians, pharmacists, clinical microbiologists, and other stakeholders take these known factors into account in the treatment of infections. The greater challenge is the potential for certain strains of microorganisms to acquire genes that confer resistance to one or more drugs to which that species of microorganism would typically be susceptible. This is what it typically meant by "drug-resistant" or "multidrug-resistant" strains. When a small number of resistant bacteria are present in a bacterial population, and the bacterial population is exposed to an antibiotic, then the resistant bacteria will tend to survive and the susceptible bacteria will tend to die. What happens over time is the resistant bacteria multiply, and then can outnumber the susceptible bacteria and dominate that bacterial population. When this occurs in the context of an infection, what clinicians observe is treatment failure, necessitating a switch to a different drug. This can mean more expensive and longer disease episodes, worse disease, and in some cases, fatal disease.

When bacteria exchange genes that confer resistance, this is termed horizontal gene transfer. This may occur through several mechanisms: conjugation (direct spread), transduction (spread via a

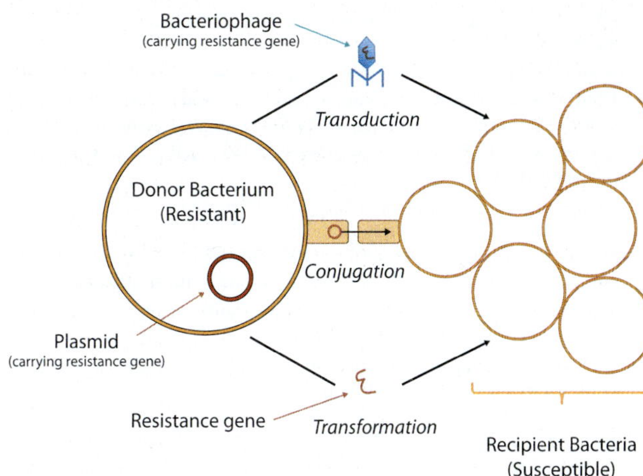

FIGURE 77-4. Mechanisms of bacterial horizontal gene transfer that may confer antimicrobial resistance to originally susceptible bacteria. Bacterial genes may be spread from a resistant bacterium to a susceptible bacterium multiple ways: (1) transduction involves movement of genes via bacteriophage viruses; (2) conjugation involves direct spread from one bacterium to another via conjugative pili, which allow direct cell-to-cell contact; and (3) transformation involves release of genetic material into the environment from the resistant bacterium, which may be taken up by another bacterium. (*Source:* Figure adapted from Furuya EY, Lowy FD. Antimicrobial-resistant bacteria in the community setting. *Nat Rev Microbiol.* 2006;4(1):36–45.)

virus), and transformation (spread via the environment), as depicted in Fig. 77-4. Sometimes, multiple genes that confer resistance to different antibiotics can be carried on a mobile genetic element, such as a plasmid, and transfer of that plasmid from one bacterium to another can confer resistance to multiple types of antibiotics at the same time. This means that if the population of bacteria where some member of the population carry plasmids of this type are exposed to even one of the antibiotics represented, the use of that single antibiotic can select for multidrug-resistant strains.

Researchers believe they have identified one case in the context of IFAP where genetic evidence suggests that this phenomenon has occurred and contributed to emergence of a particular strain of methicillin-resistant *Staphylococcus aureus* (MRSA) causing disease in people. In the early 2000s, a new strain of MRSA was identified in the Netherlands that was not typable by a conventional method for strain-typing: Pulsed-Field Gel Electrophoresis (PFGE).[44–47] This unusual strain was later categorized using a different strain-typing method, multilocus sequence typing (MLST), as Clonal Complex (CC) 398. Researchers identified that pig farmers and other people who had close contact with pigs were more likely than those without pig contact to carry CC398 or develop an infection with it.[44–47] As the number of cases of CC398 continued to rise, and CC398 was identified in pigs and people elsewhere in the world, researchers decided to perform whole genome sequencing to better understand how the global group of strains were related to each other.[48] They concluded that a progenitor strain of methicillin-susceptible *Staphylococcus aureus* (MSSA), present in humans, spread to livestock, and in the livestock population, the bacterial strain acquired the *mec*A gene for methicillin resistance, making the strain a MRSA.[48] Two other genes also were found to be associated with this new livestock strain: a gene that conferred resistance to the antibiotic drug tetracycline (*tet*M gene) and a gene that conferred resistance to zinc (*czr*C gene).[48] Since tetracycline is an antibiotic that can be used commonly in livestock production, and since zinc supplementation of feed also may be common, uses of tetracycline and zinc in IFAP pigs may have contributed to the emergence of CC398 MRSA.[49,50] More recent work in Denmark has identified that the structure of swine production in that country, where animals are raised on breeding farms and then shipped to farms where the animals are grown to harvest weight, contributed to the spread of CC398 in the animal population, which was associated with spread into the human population.[34,35]

How CC398 MRSA emerged and spread throughout the world is an interesting example of how global networks of trade, transport of animals and animal products, and human movement can play key roles in dissemination of infectious agents. This example also is important because it highlights the role of production practices—such as the uses of antimicrobial drugs and metal-based supplements—on selection for resistant pathogens. In this way, the structure of the swine industry and the IFAP practices employed with a goal to keep animals healthy may have inadvertently contributed to emergence and spread of a multidrug-resistant pathogen.

CONCLUSIONS

While this chapter has focused primarily on how intensification can drive spread of infectious disease agents and exposure to people, industrialization of food-animal production can have benefits to society and to food safety challenges. The food production chain and networks of trade are designed for reliable delivery of uniform animal products to consumers globally. On-farm food safety and other good management practices may target common pathogens that readily contaminate retail meat and other raw animal products. For example, a study in Argentina demonstrated that hogs raised outdoors were at greater risk than hogs raised in confinement for exposure to the parasite *Trichinella*, endemic to areas of that country.[51] The authors concluded that good management practices, which also included rodent control and prevention of hog contact with wildlife, on the IFAP facilities contributed to the low risk in those hogs.[51] Indeed, in the United States, where the vast majority of hogs are raised in confinement, rates of Trichinella are quite low, and most human cases are associated with consumption of pork products from home-reared hogs or wild boars.[52] Therefore, it is important to understand the interplay between the practices in IFAP that may contribute to infectious disease exposure for workers and the public, balanced with the practices that may mitigate human exposure to infectious agents throughout the food chain. This interplay may be different according to the infectious disease agent in question, and may be driven in part by local, state, national, or international factors, such as company policies to improve animal health (which could have additional economic benefits) and federal food safety regulations to safeguard consumers.

Various control strategies exist to reduce or eliminate human exposure to infectious disease agents in an IFAP context (see Table 77-1). For workers, the hierarchy of controls model is a guide to predict the success of intervention strategies. Under this model, strategies that focus on elimination of exposure through removal of the agent (disease eradication via animal culling, vaccination, biosecurity, or other methods) or through engineering controls, such as ventilation, to protect a worker from coming into contact with that agent, are assumed to be more successful than strategies that require people to adhere to certain behavioral practices, such as mask wearing or hand hygiene. For consumers, on-farm food safety practices and other strategies throughout the food chain may reduce or eliminate exposure. In the United States, producers, processors, transporters, and retailers follow the Hazard Analysis and Critical Control Points (HACCP) system, in which process controls are followed and monitored to improve food safety. An example of a critical control point is a target temperature and pressure for a certain period of time (pasteurization) that would be expected to kill bacteria in milk. Another key part of infection control relates to environmental contamination, and how practices may enhance or mitigate exposures in the soil or dust (surfaces), air, and water.

Infectious disease risks related to IFAP are dynamic and take place within a set of interconnected global industries. Over time, new infectious agents emerge, existing infectious agents change (e.g., through mutation or acquisition of resistance genes), and production practices may shift, sometimes driven by changes in global networks of trade. This underscores the importance of surveillance and other monitoring programs within the industry and in the public health sector to identify and respond to emerging and re-emerging threats to protect the health of workers, the community, and animals.

References

1. MacHugh DE, Larson G, Orlando L. Taming the past: Ancient DNA and the study of animal domestication. *Annu Rev Anim Biosci.* 2017;5:329–351.
2. Fuller DQ, Willcox G, Allaby RG. Cultivation and domestication had multiple origins: Arguments against the core area hypothesis for the origins of agriculture in the Near East. *World Archaeol.* 2011;43(4):628–52.
3. Sternbach G. The history of anthrax. *J Emerg Med.* 2003;24(4):463–7.
4. Plotkin SA, Brachman PS, Utell M, Bumford FH, Atchison MM. An epidemic of inhalation anthrax, the first in the twentieth century. I. Clinical features. *Am J Med.* 1960;29:992–1001.
5. Bales ME, Dannenberg AL, Brachman PS, Kaufmann AF, Klatsky PC, Ashford DA. Epidemiologic response to anthrax outbreaks: Field investigations, 1950–2001. *Emerg Infect Dis.* 2002;8(10):1163–74.
6. Roser M. Employment in Agriculture. 2018. Published online at OurWorldInData.org. Retrieved from: https://ourworldindata.org/employment-in-agriculture [Online Resource].
7. Davis MF, Rutkow L. Regulatory strategies to combat antimicrobial resistance of animal origin: Recommendations for a science-based approach. *Telj.* 2012;25:327–88.
8. Dimitri C, Effland A, Conklin N. The 20th Century Transformation of U.S. Agriculture and Farm Policy, Economic Information Bulletin No. (EIB-3). 2005, p. 17.
9. Silbergeld EK, Graham J, Price LB. Industrial food animal production, antimicrobial resistance, and human health. *Annu Rev Public Health.* 2008;29(1):151–69.
10. Davis MF, Price LB, Liu CM-H, Silbergeld EK. An ecological perspective on U.S. industrial poultry production: The role of anthropogenic ecosystems on the emergence of drug-resistant bacteria from agricultural environments. *Curr Opin Microbiol.* 2011;14(3):244–50.
11. FAO. World Mapping of Animal Feeding Systems in the Dairy Sector, 2014.
12. Scott A, McCluskey B, Brown-Reid M., et al. Porcine epidemic diarrhea virus introduction into the United States: Root cause investigation. *Prev Vet Med.* 2016;123:192–201.
13. Wang L, Byrum B, Zhang Y. New variant of porcine epidemic diarrhea virus, United States, 2014. *Emerg Infect Dis.* 2014;20(5):917–9.
14. Daszak P, Cunningham AA, Hyatt AD. Emerging infectious diseases of wildlife—Threats to biodiversity and human health. *Science.* 2000;287(5452):443–9.
15. AVMA. One health: A new professional imperative, American Veterinary Medical Association: One Health Initiative Task Force Final Report, 2008.
16. Mackenzie JS, Jeggo M, Daszak P, Richt JA., eds.Mackenzie JS, Jeggo M, Daszak P, Richt JA., eds. *One Health: The Human-Animal-Environment Interfaces in Emerging Infectious Diseases.* Berlin, Heidelberg: Springer Berlin Heidelberg; 2013.
17. nRist CL, Arriola CS, Rubin C. Prioritizing zoonoses: A proposed one health tool for collaborative decision-making. *PLoS One.* 2014;9(10): e109986–11.
18. International Food Policy Research Institute. Green Revolution: Curse or Blessing? 2002. Available at https://oregonstate.edu/instruct/css/330/three/Green.pdf.
19. Silbergeld EK. *Chickenizing Farms and Food: How Industrial Meat Production Endangers Workers, Animals and Consumers.* Baltimore, MD: Johns Hopkins University Press; 2016.
20. FDA. Bovine Spongiform Encephalopathy: Questions and Answers [website]. Food and Drug Administration, 2019. Downloaded 5/10/19. Available at https://www.fda.gov/vaccines-blood-biologics/safety-availability-biologics/bovine-spongiform-encephalopathy-bse-questions-and-answers.
21. Sapkota A, Sapkota AR, Kucharski M., et al. Aquaculture practices and potential human health risks: Current knowledge and future priorities. *Environ Int.* 2008;34(8):1215–26.
22. CDC. Estimated annual number of episodes of illnesses caused by 31 pathogens transmitted commonly by food, United States. *Centers for Disease Control and Prevention,* 2019. Report downloaded 5/10/2019. Available at https://www.cdc.gov/foodborneburden/pdfs/scallan-estimated-illnesses-foodborne-pathogens.pdf.
23. WHO. WHO estimates of the global burden of foodborne diseases: Foodborne disease burden epidemiology reference group 2007–2015. *World Health Organization.* Geneva: WHO Press; 2015. Available at https://apps.who.int/iris/bitstream/handle/10665/199350/9789241565165_eng.pdf?sequence=1.
24. Teunis PFM. Ogden ID, Strachan NJC. Hierarchical dose response of *E. coli* O157:H7 from human outbreaks incorporating heterogeneity in exposure. *Epidemiol Infect.* 2007;136(06):437–11.
25. Oude Munnink BB, Sikkema RS, Nieuwenhuijse DF., et al. Jumping back and forth: Anthropozoonotic and zoonotic transmission of SARS-CoV-2 on mink farms. *bioRxiv* 2020;277152.
26. Shi J, Wen Z, Zhong G., et al. Susceptibility of ferrets, cats, dogs, and other domesticated animals to SARS-coronavirus 2. *Science.* 2020;368(6494): 1016–20.
27. Khan M, Zahoor M. An overview of brucellosis in cattle and humans, and its serological and molecular diagnosis in control strategies. *Trop Med Infect Dis.* 2018;3(2):65–14.
28. CDC. Vaccination of cattle [website]. Centers for Disease Control and Prevention, 2018. Downloaded 11/1/2018. Available at https://www.cdc.gov/brucellosis/veterinarians/cattle.html.
29. van de Giessen AW, van Santen-Verheuvel MG, Hengeveld PD, Bosch T, Broens EM, Reusken, CBEM. Occurrence of methicillin-resistant *Staphylococcus aureus* in rats living on pig farms. *Prevent Vet Med.* 2009;91(2–4):270–73.
30. Vandegrift KJ, Sokolow SH, Daszak P, Kilpatrick AM. Ecology of avian influenza viruses in a changing world. *Ann N Y Acad Sci,* 2010;1195(1):113–28.
31. Tully O, Nolan D. A review of the population biology and host–parasite interactions of the sea louse Lepeophtheirus salmonis (Copepoda: Caligidae). *Parasitology.* 2002;124(7):165–82.
32. Leibler JH, Carone M, Silbergeld EK. Contribution of company affiliation and social contacts to risk estimates of between-farm transmission of avian influenza. *PLoS One.* 2010;5(3):e9888.
33. Mena I, Nelson MI, Quezada-Monroy F, et al. Origins of the 2009 H1N1 influenza pandemic in swine in Mexico. *Elife.* 2016;5:e16777.
34. Sieber RN, Skov RL, Nielsen J., et al. Drivers and dynamics of methicillin-resistant livestock-associated *Staphylococcus aureus* CC398 in pigs and humans in Denmark. *mBio.* 2018;9(6):e02142–18.
35. Smith T, Davis MF, Heaney CD. Pig movement and antimicrobial use drive transmission of livestock-associated *Staphylococcus aureus* CC398. *mBio.* 2018;9(6):e02459–18.
36. Burch TR, Spencer SK, Stokdyk JP., et al. Quantitative microbial risk assessment for spray irrigation of dairy manure based on an empirical fate and transport model. *Environ Health Perspect.* 2017;125(8):087009–11.
37. Ferguson DD, Smith TC, Hanson BM, Wardyn SE, Donham KJ. Detection of airborne methicillin-resistant *Staphylococcus aureus* inside and downwind of a swine building, and in animal feed: Potential occupational, animal health, and environmental implications. *J Agromedicine.* 2016;21(2):149–53.
38. Jahne MA, Rogers SW, Holsen TM, Grimberg SJ, Ramler IP. Emission and dispersion of bioaerosols from dairy manure application sites: Human health risk assessment. *Environ Sci Technol.* 2015;49(16):9842–9.
39. Sanz S, Olarte C, Martínez-Olarte R., et al. Airborne dissemination of *Escherichia coli* in a dairy cattle farm and its environment. *Int J Food Microbiol.* 2015;197(C):40–4.
40. Anker JCH, Koch A, Ethelberg S, Molbak K, Larsen J, Jepsen MR. Distance to pig farms as risk factor for community-onset livestock-associated MRSA CC398 infection in persons without known contact to pig farms—A nationwide study. *Zoonoses Public Health.* 2018;11(5):711–9.
41. Poulsen MN, Pollak J, Sills DL., et al. Residential proximity to high-density poultry operations associated with campylobacteriosis and infectious diarrhea. *Int J Hyg Environ Health.* 2018;221(2):323–33.
42. Casey JA, Curriero FC, Cosgrove SE, Nachman KE, Schwartz BS. High-density livestock operations, crop field application of manure, and risk of community-associated methicillin-resistant *Staphylococcus aureus* infection in Pennsylvania. *JAMA Intern Med.* 2013;173(21):1980–90.
43. Keyes K, Lee MD, Maurer JJ. Antibiotics: Mode of action, mechanisms of resistance, and transfer. In: Torrence ME, Isaacson RE, eds.Torrence ME, Isaacson RE, eds. *Microbial Food Safety in Animal Agriculture: Current Topics.* Ames, IA: Iowa State Press; 2003, pp. 45–56.
44. Armand-Lefevre L, Ruimy R, Andremont A. Clonal comparison of *Staphylococcus aureus* isolates from healthy pig farmers, human controls, and pigs. *Emerg Infect Dis.* 2005;11(5):711–4.

45. Voss A, Loeffen F, Bakker J, Klaassen C, Wulf M. Methicillin-resistant *Staphylococcus aureus* in pig farming. *Emerg Infect Dis.* 2005;11(12): 1965–6.

46. Huijsdens XW, van Dijke BJ, Spalburg E, et al. Community-acquired MRSA and pig-farming. *Ann Clin Microbiol Antimicrob.* 2006:5:26.

47. van Loo I, Huijsdens X, Tiemersma E, et al. Emergence of methicillin-resistant *Staphylococcus aureus* of animal origin in humans. *Emerg Infect Dis.* 2007;13(12):1834–9.

48. Price LB, Stegger M, Hasman H, et al. *Staphylococcus aureus* CC398: Host adaptation and emergence of methicillin resistance in livestock. *mBio.* 2012;3(1):e00305-11.

49. Aarestrup FM, Cavaco L, Hasman H. Decreased susceptibility to zinc chloride is associated with methicillin resistant *Staphylococcus aureus* CC398 in Danish swine. *Vet Microbiol.* 2010;142(3–4):455–7.

50. Cavaco LM, Hasman H, Aarestrup FM. Zinc resistance of *Staphylococcus aureus* of animal origin is strongly associated with methicillin resistance. *Vet Microbiol.* 2011;150(3–4):344–8.

51. Ribicich M, Gamble HR, Bolpe J., et al. Evaluation of the risk of transmission of Trichinella in pork production systems in Argentina. *Vet Parasitol.* 2009;159(3-4):350–3.

52. Wilson NO, Hall RL, Montgomery SP, Jones JL. Trichinellosis surveillance—United States, 2008–2012. *MMWR Morb Mortal Wkly Rep.* 2015;64(1):1–8.

CHAPTER

78

Managing Environmental and Occupational Risks

Jonathan M. Samet • Thomas A. Burke

INTRODUCTION

Risk refers to the likelihood that an untoward event will occur. Much environmental and occupational health research is directed at establishing whether an agent increases risk and by how much, laying the foundation for control. There are multiple evidence-based paths by which the risks posed by environmental and occupational agents are reduced and eliminated: regulatory actions directed at exposures, voluntary actions by those producing agents that pose a risk to the population and to workers, litigation directed at manufacturers and vendors of toxic agents, and protective measures taken by individuals and communities. Scientific evidence is central and often pivotal to motivating actions to reduce risk by providing: an indication as to the existence of a hazard; an understanding of the magnitude of the risk and how it varies with exposure or dose; and identifying points for interventions to reduce exposures and risks. Uncertainty, the complement to evidence, figures into decision-making as well. However, in actuality, numerous factors beyond scientific evidence and gaps in the evidence with attendant uncertainty drive actions related to policies on environmental and occupational agents (Fig. 78-1). These include stakeholder interests, the range extending from affected citizens and communities to the polluting parties. The power of political influence and of financial consequences of action need to be acknowledged, as does the impact of citizen's voices and nongovernmental organizations. A single figure cannot capture the multiple sectors and their interactions across the broad array of regulations and stakeholders that drive environmental and occupational health. This chapter provides a general introduction to the management of risk in these sectors.

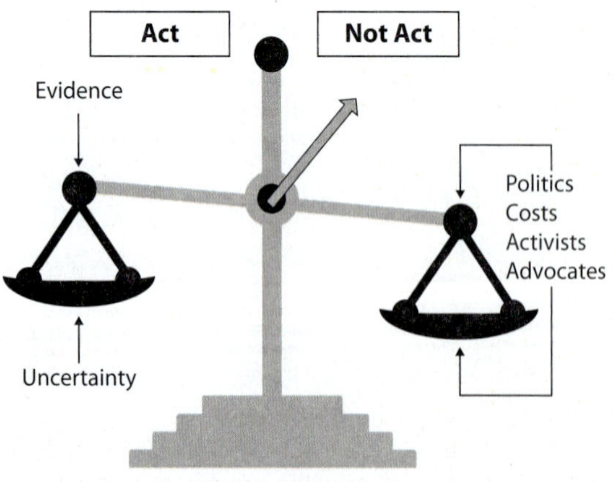

FIGURE 78-1. The weighing of evidence, uncertainty, and other factors in decision-making.

In the United States and globally, the regulation of exposures to environmental and occupational agents involves a patchwork of regulatory and nonregulatory approaches that have varied over time and differ to a substantial extent across nations. In the United States, there are enabling laws, for example, the Clean Air Act (Table 78-1), and agencies concerned with control of risks in specific domains: the Occupational Safety and Health Administration (OSHA), the Mine Safety and Health Administration (MSHA), the Environmental Protection Agency (EPA), the Food and Drug Administration (FDA), and others. There are international bodies that offer guidelines on exposure limits, for example, the World Health Organization (WHO) and the International Labour Organization (ILO), but none has direct regulatory authority within nations. Their recommendations may be adopted as the basis for national standards, however, as with the WHO Air Quality Guidelines.[1]

People's risk-increasing exposures come from sources that may be at least partially under their own control (e.g., tobacco use, ingestion of alcohol, and use of pesticides in the home) or that are not subject to their direct control (e.g., occupational carcinogens, asbestos in buildings, and pollution of ambient air). The latter exposures are the focus of regulation whereas the former are addressed by a blend of initiatives that range from education concerning risks to broader programs of control, as in the example of tobacco. Some societal activities are inevitably associated with exposure to injurious occupational and environmental agents so that harmful exposures cannot be completely eliminated. However, an overall goal of a broad array of regulatory and nonregulatory measures is to achieve acceptable levels of risk and to assure that individuals do not sustain exposures at levels known to cause adverse effects.

Consequently, principles are in use to guide the development of policies to control exposures to an acceptable level. These principles, considered below, have the general objective of achieving an acceptable level of risk and assuring safety to the extent possible. Lowrance classically defined safety as follows: "A thing is safe if its attendant risks are judged to be acceptable."[2] For public health protection, there are dual implications of this definition: information is needed on the risks associated with exposures, and principles are needed to judge the acceptability of the associated risk. Any principles used must reflect societal concerns and tolerance of risk, the necessity of using the materials or processes that lead to exposures, the feasibility of controls, and the potential costs of control measures as well. These costs need to be considered in the context of the damages from exposure: those of disease, disability and premature death, lost income, and other adverse consequences. Given this complex balancing, making judgments as to the acceptability of risk is not the domain of scientists or risk assessors, but lies with society at large. An extensive literature addresses risk perception and judgment as to the acceptability of different risks.[3]

TABLE 78-1 MAJOR ENVIRONMENTAL LAWS IN THE UNITED STATES

	Regulation	Year	Description
Clean Air Act (CAA)	42 U.S.C. §7401	1970, 1977, 1990	Authorizes the EPA to establish National Ambient Air Quality Standards (NAAQS) to protect public health and welfare from hazardous air pollutants. The law regulates air emissions from stationary and mobile sources.
Occupational Safety and Health Act (OSHA)	29 U.S. C. §651	1970	Ensure worker and workplace health safety by providing a place of employment free from recognized hazards such as exposure to toxic chemicals, excessive noise levels, mechanical dangers, heat or cold stress, or unsanitary conditions.
Clean Water Act (CWA)	33 U.S.C. §1251	1972	Establishes the fundamental structure for regulating discharges of pollutants into U.S. waters and quality standards for surface waters (e.g., pollution control programs such as setting wastewater standards for industry and permit programs to control discharges).
Safe Drinking Water Act (SDWA)	44 U.S.C. §300	1974, 1996	Protects the quality of drinking water—actually or potentially designed for drinking use, whether from above ground or underground sources. EPA establishes minimum standards to protect tap water and requires all owners or operators of public water systems to comply with health-related standards.
Toxic Substances Control Act (TSCA)	15 U.S.C. §2601	1976, 2016	Provides EPA authority to require reporting, recordkeeping and testing requirements, and restrictions relating to chemical substances and/or mixtures during production, importation, use, and disposal of chemicals. Chemicals include polychlorinated biphenyls (PCBs), asbestos, radon, and lead-based paint. Other substances like food, drugs, cosmetics, and pesticides are generally excluded.
Federal Insecticide, Rodenticide and Fungicide Act (FIFRA)	7 U.S.C. §136	1947, 1972, 1996	Governs the registration, distribution, sale and use of pesticides in the United States. All pesticides distributed or sold in the United States must be registered (and licensed) by EPA. According to the statute, a pesticide is any substance or mixture of substances intended for preventing, destroying, repelling, or mitigating any pest, or intended for use as a plant regulator, defoliant, or desiccant, or desiccant, or any nitrogen stabilizer.
National Environmental Policy Act (NEPA)	42 U.S.C. §4321	1969	Assures that all branches of government give proper consideration to the environment prior to commencing any major federal action that significantly affects the environment. The most notable NEPA requirements are the Environmental Assessments (EAs) and Environmental Impact Statements (EISs), which are assessments of the likelihood of impacts from alternative courses of action. Projects governed by this statue include airports, buildings, military complexes, highways, and parkland purchases.
Resource Conservation and Recovery Act (RCRA)	42 U.S.C. §6901	1979, 1986	Gives EPA the authority to control hazardous waste from the "cradle-to-grave." This involves the generation, transportation, treatment, storage, and disposal of hazardous waste. RCRA also sets a framework for the management of nonhazardous solid wastes by focusing on waste minimization and phasing out land disposal of hazardous waste.
Comprehensive Environmental Response, Compensation, and Liability Act (CERCLA or Superfund)	42 U.S.C. §9601	1980, 1986	Provides a Federal "Superfund" to clean up uncontrolled or abandoned hazardous-waste sites in addition to accidents, spills, and other emergency releases of pollutants and contaminants into the environment. EPA is authorized to implement the Act in all 50 states and U.S. territories. The identification, monitoring, and response activities in superfund sites are coordinated through the state environmental protection or waste management agencies.

Source: Samet JM, Burke TA. Deregulation and the assault on science and the environment. *Annu Rev Public Health.* 2020;41:1.

TOOLS FOR CHARACTERIZING RISK FOR DECISION-MAKING

Introduction

Central to management of dangers to human health and the environment posed by an environmental agent is the characterization of the risk: what is the source of the agent and how does exposure occur? What injuries and diseases does the agent cause and how do these risks vary with the level of exposure? How big is the problem and who is affected? Answers to these questions come from analysis of public health and surveillance data and research findings, and the integration of this information using tools that provide an informative synthesis.

Some of these tools have been in place for decades and refined over time based on experience. Some, for example, risk assessment, have become integral to statutes and agency practices.

As addressed in other chapters, information on environmental and occupational risks comes from complementary lines of investigation: toxicology—in vitro, that is, cell and molecular systems, and *in vivo*, that is, involving animals—epidemiology, and exposure sciences. Together, the findings of toxicological and epidemiological studies provide evidence on the existence of a risk or hazard; the variation of risk with the level of exposure or dose, and the scope of exposure. The resulting integration and synthesis of the evidence is the substrate for action.

Risk Assessment

Risk assessment is used in a variety of contexts and embedded in some laws and regulatory actions. The current general formalism of risk assessment was defined in a landmark 1983 report of the National Research Council, widely known as "the Red Book."[4] This pioneering report was initiated because of the increasing use of risk assessment across government agencies, but without any uniformity of approach. The general schema set out in the Red Book remains in use, although it has been refined over time through its application.

The Red Book described four interlocking elements in a risk assessment:

1. Hazard identification: Is a hazard posed by the exposure?
2. Exposure assessment: What is the distribution of the exposure?
3. Dose-response assessment: How does risk vary with exposure (or dose)?
4. Risk characterization: What is the extent of the risk to the population and what are the uncertainties in the characterization of risk?

The Red Book framework has been further elaborated through its application in practice and in subsequent reports from the National Academies of Science Engineering and Medicine. The 1994 report, *Science and Judgment in Risk Assessment*, elaborated on the need to characterize uncertainty and to fold that characterization into decision-making.[5] The 2009 report, *Science and Decisions. Advancing Risk Assessment* emphasized the critical need for formulating the risk assessment questions through early engagement of stakeholders to assure that the "right" questions were addressed.[6] This expanded formulation enfolds the original four elements from the Red Book into a stakeholder-engaged process (Fig. 78-2).

Various entities address the components of risk assessment, particularly the determination of whether a hazard exists and the assessment of the dose-response relationship. For carcinogens, for example, the International Agency for Research on Cancer (IARC) of the World Health Organization addresses the carcinogenicity of agents and exposures through a formal evidence-based review process.[7] The EPA's Integrated Risk Information System (IRIS) addresses whether cancer and noncancer hazards exist for agents and also characterizes exposure-response for both types of outcomes.[8] IRIS assessments are widely used for risk assessment and decision-making purposes.

A full risk assessment provides an informed picture of what is known and not known on a hazard in a form that will support decision-making and point to gaps that need to be addressed for better-informed decision-making. As risk assessment has evolved in the decades since the 1983 Red Book, the process helps to assure that the right questions will be targeted and critical points of uncertainty identified. Characterization of uncertainty in an informative fashion is key, as too much uncertainty may influence decision-making and also point to critical research gaps. There are abundant examples of the application of risk assessment: arsenic in drinking water, radon in indoor air, and air pollution from oil and gas extraction with hydraulic fracking, for example.

The lung cancer risk associated with radon in indoor air is exemplary, a problem that received widespread attention in the 1980s when radon testing was recommended by the government for most homes in the United States as the basis for determining whether some form of mitigation was needed. Controversy followed; the carcinogenicity of indoor radon was questioned although well established by studies of underground miners exposed to radon, and uncertainties were raised around the magnitude of the risk and the need for action,

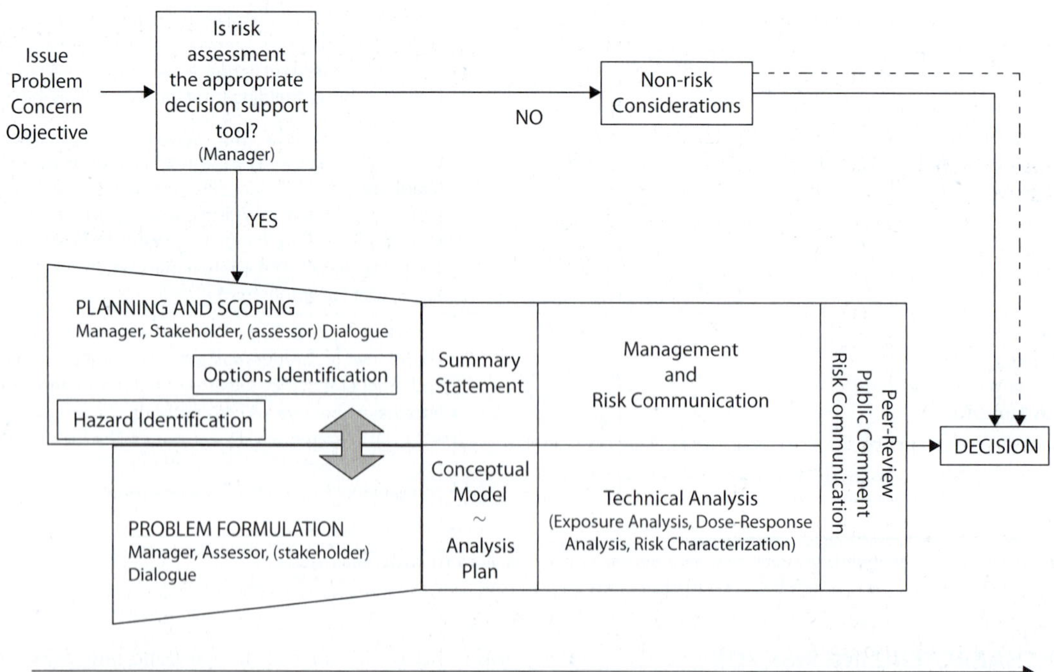

FIGURE 78-2. Schematic representation of the formative stages of risk-assessment design. Note: Dotted line in figure denotes that decisions informed by risk assessment will be influenced by nonrisk considerations. (*Source:* Used with permission from National Research Council 2009. Science and Decisions: *Advancing Risk Assessment*. Washington, DC: The National Academies Press. https://doi.org/10.17226/12209.)

particularly given the potential costs of implementing nationwide radon testing.[9] One of the most controversial issues was the shape of the dose-response curve and whether there was a threshold level of exposure below which there was not any risk. These issues were relevant to a policy of testing all homes and setting a guideline value for mitigation.

The most complete risk assessment for radon was carried out by the National Research Council's Biological Effects of Ionizing Radiation (BEIR) VI Committee.[10] By the 1990s, when the committee did its work, there was little question as to the carcinogenicity of radon, but risks at levels encountered in homes were not well characterized. At the time, epidemiological information on radon risks came primarily from cohort studies of underground miners exposed to radon; some case-control studies of lung cancer in the general population had been completed and some were in progress. The studies of underground miners uniformly documented excess lung cancer in comparison to expected numbers of cases and the excess was greater at higher cumulative exposures.

To provide more certain information on exposure-response, the committee analyzed data from 11 cohorts of radon-exposed underground miners and compared the results to meta-analytical estimates from the epidemiological studies of indoor radon and lung cancer. The committee also examined mechanisms by which the alpha particles released during the decay of radon progeny damaged cells and concluded on a mechanistic basis that there was no threshold. This conclusion was based on the dosimetry of the alpha particles released within the lung that damaged the cells lining the lung. The "hit" to these cells is invariant with the concentration since that energy reflects the energy from the decay of the progeny. The resulting epidemiologically based risk models were grounded in a well-supported linear no-threshold model from a mechanistic perspective that guided policy in the United States and elsewhere. Information on exposure was available from various surveys in which radon had been measured in homes. The committee used probabilistic approaches to describe the burden of radon-caused lung cancer and guided policy-makers on the distinction between the attributable burden of lung cancer from radon and how much that burden could be reduced with various mitigation strategies.

In terms of the elements of a risk assessment per the Red Book formulation, the BEIR VI Committee concluded that radon was causally associated with exposure to radon; derived several models for the relationship between radon progeny exposure and lung cancer risk; used population-based measurements to characterize the distribution of exposure to indoor radon; and used the dose–response model and the radon concentration distribution to characterize the lung cancer burden with consideration of uncertainty. The approach to characterizing uncertainty was both qualitative, that is, identifying the various contributors to uncertainty and providing expert judgment on their significance, and quantitative, that is, based on a probabilistic model that made assumptions about the range of uncertainty in key model parameters.

Cost-Benefit Analysis

Together, risk assessment and cost-benefit analysis bring a monetized, quantitative foundation to the control of environmental and occupational agents. A risk assessment can be qualitative, determining if a hazard exists, or quantitative, estimating the extent of the burden of disease caused by a particular agent. Cost-benefit analysis presents a comparison of two sets of costs: those estimated to arise from any disease and disability and premature death caused by the agent of concern and those associated with controlling exposures to the agent.[11,12] Estimation of "benefits" depends on being able to quantify disease rates and other harms addressed by a regulation or other action and the ability to assign costs to those conditions; consequently, risk assessment and cost-benefit analysis are very closely interrelated. In the United States, statutes have contained various standards, some of which have implicitly or explicitly required that agencies perform quantitative risk assessments as part of the process of controlling occupational and environmental carcinogens.

The costs of regulation may have major impacts on regulated industries. Regulatory impact analysis, including analysis of costs and benefits, has been required for evaluation of major rules (i.e., having > \$100 million impact) by Executive Order since the time of President Carter. The White House Office of Management and Budget (OMB) through its Office of Regulatory Impact Analysis (ORIA) have played a powerful role in the process of setting guidelines for such analyses and in the review of proposed major rules.[13]

Health Impact Assessment

Although less widely used than risk assessment, health impact assessment (HIA) takes a broader look at the consequences of an action for health. It is intended, as is risk assessment to be the basis for decision-making and brings a population health perspective. A 2011 report of the National Research Council defined HIA as:

> HIA is a systematic process that uses an array of data sources and analytic methods and considers input from stakeholders to determine the potential effects of a proposed policy, plan, program, or project on the health of a population and the distribution of those effects within the population. HIA provides recommendations on monitoring and managing those effects.[14]

Health Impact Assessment differs from conventional risk assessment, as previously discussed, by incorporating a holistic examination of the potential benefits and consequences of an action whether regulatory or nonregulatory. In its breadth and characterization of population impact and the distribution of population impact, a HIA goes beyond the Environmental Impact Statement (EIS) required in the United States under the National Environmental Policy Act (NEPA).[15] It can be applied in a wide range of decision-making processes extending beyond those specifically directed at environmental pollutants, for example, the construction of a new highway or of a new airport. Mueller et al. completed a systematic review of health impact assessments of active transport, that is, walking and cycling, identifying 30 studies.[16] Exemplifying the broad reach of the HIA approach; benefits came from physical activity and reduced air pollution, while risks were related to traffic incidents and the consequences of air pollution exposure during physical activities.

The 2011 report of the National Research Council identified six steps in the HIA process (Fig. 78-3), which begins with screening around a possible action and a determination as to whether a HIA is needed.[14] If undertaken, the full process ends with monitoring and evaluation of the consequences of actions taken by tracking appropriate health indicators. It ends with communication of findings to stakeholders and decision-makers and then tracking and evaluation to assess the impact of recommendations and decisions taken. The paradigm of HIA is versatile, potentially applicable to both local situations, for example, a specific pollution source, or to more generalized questions, as in the example of active transport.

PRINCIPLES FOR MANAGING RISK

Introduction

Risk management may be motivated by a variety of findings and carried out through a variety of routes, for example, regulatory and individual decision-making. Regardless of the risk management scenario, some principle for risk management will likely be invoked. These principles have come from precedent, regulatory mandates, public health guidance, legal decisions, and societal preferences and even individual behavior. In some situations, heterogeneous viewpoints may lead to differing approaches and opinions around the level of risk reduction to be achieved and the acceptability of residual risk after management. Below, some of the foundational principles are reviewed with coverage of some of those most widely applied or paradigm-setting.

As Low as Reasonably Achievable

The "as low as reasonably achievable" (ALARA) principle has largely been applied in relation to the risks of ionizing radiation, an exposure with consequences that gave rise to this approach. Historically, as understanding of the risks of radiation advanced through epidemiological studies of the Atomic Bomb Survivors and other exposed populations, risk for the stochastic outcomes, specifically cancer, was found to increase with dose and clear thresholds were not identified.[17] Additionally, early mechanistic work on radiation-caused mutations indicated that thresholds below which there was no risk might not be identified. Before the results of the epidemiological studies were reported, beginning in the 1950s and 1960s, limits for radiation exposure, tolerance limits, had been based primarily on identifying the radiation doses causing skin redness.[17,18]

With the emerging epidemiological evidence and growing mechanistic understanding, a new approach was needed for radiation protection for the rising numbers of workers exposed to radiation and the public, exposed through diagnostic radiation primarily. A shift was made from protecting individuals, as with the tolerance limits, to protecting populations. This principle was reflected in the standards proposed by the National Council on Radiation Protection and Measurements (NCRP) in the United States and the International Commission for Radiological Protection (ICRP); the former makes recommendations for the United States while the latter's have global reach. In the 1977 Publication 26, the ICRP[19] recommended that no procedure involving radiation exposure should be used unless beneficial and that all exposures should be in accordance with the ALARA principle, taking costs, and societal factors into consideration. Additionally, doses to individuals were not to exceed the limits of the ICRP.

The ALARA principle for guiding risk management acknowledges the necessity of radiation exposure to the population because of the benefits in several sectors, particularly diagnostic and therapeutic exposures. While the principle extends to worker protection, exposures to workers in the United States are regulated by the

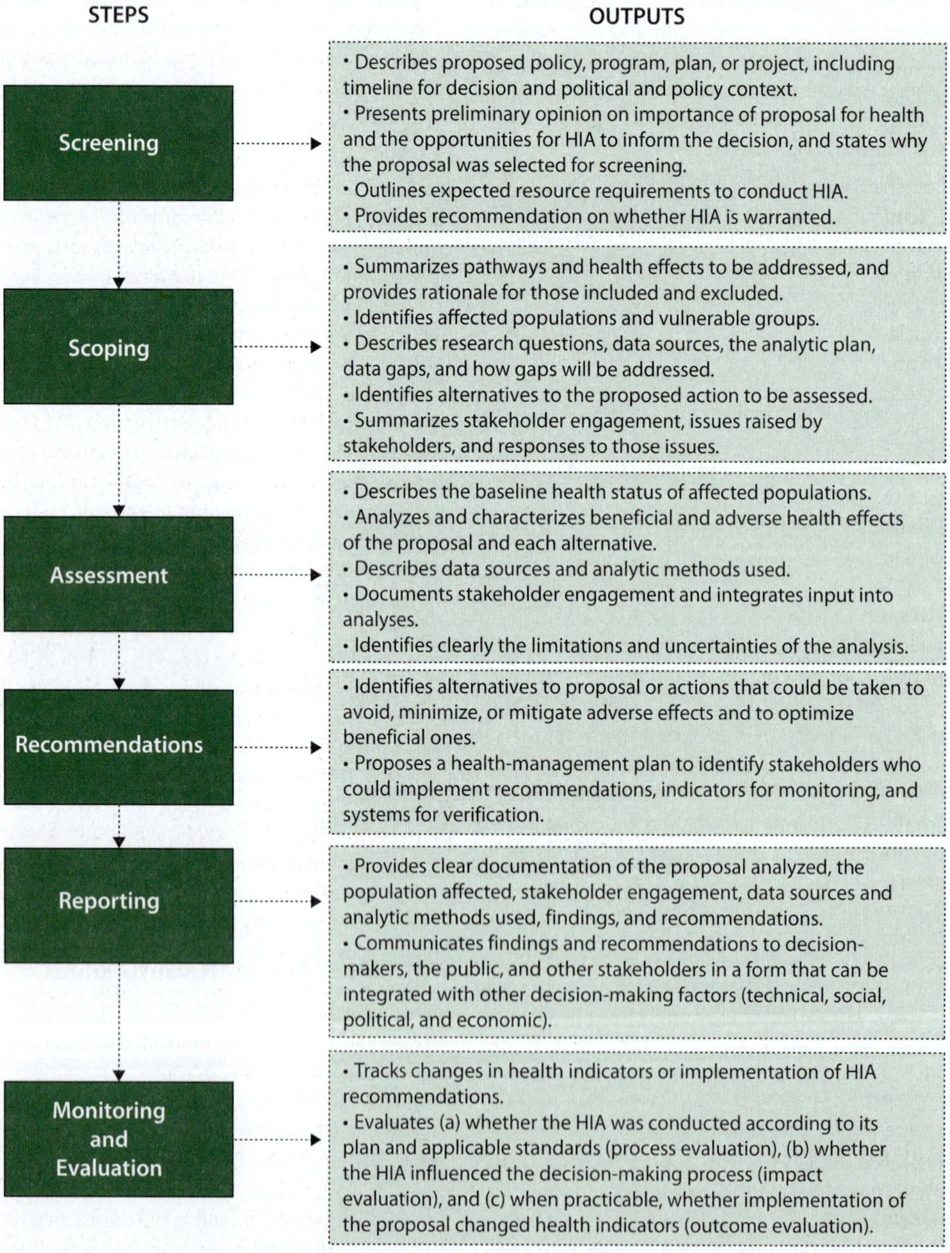

STEPS	OUTPUTS
Screening	• Describes proposed policy, program, plan, or project, including timeline for decision and political and policy context. • Presents preliminary opinion on importance of proposal for health and the opportunities for HIA to inform the decision, and states why the proposal was selected for screening. • Outlines expected resource requirements to conduct HIA. • Provides recommendation on whether HIA is warranted.
Scoping	• Summarizes pathways and health effects to be addressed, and provides rationale for those included and excluded. • Identifies affected populations and vulnerable groups. • Describes research questions, data sources, the analytic plan, data gaps, and how gaps will be addressed. • Identifies alternatives to the proposed action to be assessed. • Summarizes stakeholder engagement, issues raised by stakeholders, and responses to those issues.
Assessment	• Describes the baseline health status of affected populations. • Analyzes and characterizes beneficial and adverse health effects of the proposal and each alternative. • Describes data sources and analytic methods used. • Documents stakeholder engagement and integrates input into analyses. • Identifies clearly the limitations and uncertainties of the analysis.
Recommendations	• Identifies alternatives to proposal or actions that could be taken to avoid, minimize, or mitigate adverse effects and to optimize beneficial ones. • Proposes a health-management plan to identify stakeholders who could implement recommendations, indicators for monitoring, and systems for verification.
Reporting	• Provides clear documentation of the proposal analyzed, the population affected, stakeholder engagement, data sources and analytic methods used, findings, and recommendations. • Communicates findings and recommendations to decision-makers, the public, and other stakeholders in a form that can be integrated with other decision-making factors (technical, social, political, and economic).
Monitoring and Evaluation	• Tracks changes in health indicators or implementation of HIA recommendations. • Evaluates (a) whether the HIA was conducted according to its plan and applicable standards (process evaluation), (b) whether the HIA influenced the decision-making process (impact evaluation), and (c) when practicable, whether implementation of the proposal changed health indicators (outcome evaluation).

FIGURE 78-3. Framework for HIA, illustrating steps and outputs. (*Source:* Used with permission from National Research Council 2011. *Improving Health in the United States: The Role of Health Impact Assessment*. Washington, DC: The National Academies Press. https://doi.org/10.17226/13229.)

Occupational Safety and Health Administration (OSHA) generally and the Mine Safety and Health Administration (MSHA) for workers in underground mines. Inherently, ALARA aims to achieve the lowest possible dose to the population; under the assumption that radiation causes cancer at any dose, the risk to the population reflects the collective dose and guidelines or regulations based upon the ALARA embrace the principle of minimizing this dose.

Precautionary Principle

The precautionary principle calls for action when there is an indication of a potential threat of irreversible harm, even in the face of uncertainty as to the risks. This principle is frequently invoked when the consequences of an exposure are unknown or highly uncertain. The 1998 Wingspread Statement, the result of a meeting on the topic, offered four components for extending the principle:

1. "Taking action to reduce risk, even with uncertain evidence;
2. Giving the burden of proof of safety to those who are proposing something associated with risk;
3. Considering alternatives to the action that may have adverse consequences, and
4. Increasing the participation of the public in the decision-making process."[20]

To date, the precautionary principle has received more widespread discussion and consideration in Europe and it is embedded in risk management by the European Commission. It was also among the principles agreed to in the Rio Declaration.[21] In Europe, the European Union's REACH (Regulation, Evaluation, Authorization, and Restriction of Chemicals) regulation, which addresses the risks of chemicals, requires manufacturers to demonstrate that a compound can be used with safety, that is, without risk. Because of strong industry opposition, the precautionary principle has not yet been referenced in U.S. legislation but is frequently evoked in situations involving both known and unknown risks. Broader application of the precautionary principle has been proposed.[22–24]

"Bright Lines" for Risk

Risk assessment and projection methods permit the calculation of projected lifetime risks for disease, typically cancer, associated with various exposure scenarios. Such projections require assumptions concerning future disease and mortality trends, but nonetheless represent a useful tool for risk characterization. Such projections are offered in the following form: *exposure to substance x under these conditions increases lifetime risk for cancer (or other outcome) by 1 in a 1,000,000.* There is not an agreed to societal bright line for such incremental risk and by statute and practice there is variation across the EPA in its guidance.

For example, the 1996 Food Quality Protection Act incorporates a health-based standard of a "reasonable certainty of no harm" for all pesticides on all types of foods.[25] In hearings, but not in the statute, Congress stated the intent that, for a carcinogen, a 1 in 1,000,000 lifetime risk would be interpreted as meeting the standard of a reasonable certainty of no harm. Similarly, various statutes have required different targets for residual risk, that is, the risk persisting after regulation. For some exposures (e.g., for consumer products), this residual is not clearly stated by statute or by agency policies, whereas for others, the risk targets are clearly stated and have ranged between 10^{-4} and 10^{-6}.

The Benzene Decision and Material Impairment

A lasting precedent came from OSHA's attempt to regulate benzene based on increased risk for leukemia in benzene-exposed workers. In 1978, OSHA promulgated a standard for benzene, based on its risk as a cause of leukemia. The standard was challenged with the case reaching the Supreme Court.[26] In a momentous decision, the Court concluded that OSHA needed to demonstrate that "a significant risk of material health impairment exists" before it promulgates a health-and-safety standard for a toxic substance. The Court cited a substantive "significant risk" threshold requirement in the general language of the Occupational Safety and Health Act, specifically a statutory provision that regulatory standards must be "reasonably necessary or appropriate" to provide a safe place of employment.

The Supreme Court decision involved a complicated and divided interpretation of the OSHA Act.[27] The decision involved interpretation of what constituted a "significant risk"; the judges provided varying opinions of how such a level of risk might be defined. Issues related to the costs and benefits of the proposed benzene standard were considered in divergent ways by the Justices. The majority opinion required that OSHA demonstrate "that it is at least more likely than not that long-term exposure to 10 ppm of benzene presents a significant risk of material health impairment." The challenges to OSHA are clear: demonstrating a risk that is deemed "significant" on some basis and interpreting what constitutes "material health impairment." In response, OSHA carried out a risk assessment of the excess leukemia among workers in the United States that is caused by benzene.[28] In the agency's interpretation of the decision, the risk assessment was considered as responsive in its demonstration of "significant health risks." This decision still looms over standards for occupational exposures, specifically as to what levels of risk necessitate regulation.

The Clean Air Act, National Ambient Air Quality Standards, and Hazardous Air Pollutants

Under the Clean Air Act, the Administrator of the Environmental Protection Agency (EPA) sets evidence-based National Ambient Air Quality Standards (NAAQS) for major air pollutants. The Act places a strong mandate for public health protection on the Administrator; under Section 109 of the Clean Air Act, the Administrator sets "National primary ambient air quality standards, prescribed, under subsection (a) shall be ambient air quality standards the attainment and maintenance of which in the judgment of the Administrator, based on such criteria and allowing an adequate margin of safety, are requisite to protect the public health."[29] The underlying approach to risk management for the six indicator pollutants (currently, particulate matter, ozone, nitrogen dioxide, sulfur dioxide, carbon monoxide, and lead) is explicit and protective of public health.

The standard inherently posits that evidence will identify a threshold and that a margin of safety can be established by setting a standard below that threshold value. When the Clean Air Act was passed in 1970, there was a reasonable expectation that such thresholds might be identified. In actuality, however, thresholds have not been identified for the NAAQS pollutants and the most recent evidence generally indicates that risk persists below the current NAAQS for some pollutants, for example, particulate matter.[30] Since thresholds cannot be identified, the EPA has used a risk assessment approach to estimate risks under various scenarios of changes to the NAAQS, making comparison to the NAAQS in place.[31] This approach involves judgment by the Administrator as to the acceptability of the risk of adverse consequences and associated disease burden under various scenarios of changes to the NAAQS. Explicit criteria for guiding this judgment have not been made available.

One related issue for interpreting the evidence is what constitutes an adverse health effect of air pollution, given the broad spectrum of outcomes considered in the scientific literature. For some outcome measures, there is little question as to adversity: substantial life shortening from premature mortality, exacerbation of asthma leading to medical care, and heart attack, for example; for others, such as changes in biomarkers or transient drops in lung function, interpretation is more challenging. Guidance on this issue has been provided by the American Thoracic Society and the European Respiratory Society.[32]

Under Section 112, the EPA regulates hazardous air pollutants; a list of 189 targeted agents has been published based on the 1990 Amendments. The guiding language from the Act is: "The

Administrator shall establish any such standard at the level which in his judgement provides an ample margin of safety to protect the public health from such hazardous air pollutant."[33] A two-part strategy was called for, first using maximum available control technology (MACT) to reduce emissions from sources reach an "ample margin of safety," and in the second phase to address residual risk, if the ample margin of safety criterion had not been met. Implicitly, risk assessment is needed to estimate the level of residual risk so as to determine if an ample margin of safety has been achieved.

Goldstein[34] comments that the regulation of over 180 hazardous air pollutants under the 1990 Clean Air Act embodies elements of the precautionary principle. The Environmental Protection Agency does not have the burden of proof to demonstrate that environmental exposures to these pollutants were likely to produce adverse effects in order to impose maximal available control technology standards on industry. Broader application of the precautionary principle has been proposed.[22–24]

Environmental Justice

The distribution of environmental exposures harming health has long been shown to be heterogeneous, placing a higher burden of exposures on those with lower incomes, minority populations and other special groups. This inequitable burden reflects long-standing factors driving where people live, the quality of their dwellings, the siting of industry, proximity to crowded roadways, and more. In 1994, the Clinton Administration released Executive Order 12898, "Federal Actions to Address Environmental Justice in Minority Populations and Low-Income Populations."[35] This historic order called on all Federal agencies as follows: "…each Federal agency shall make achieving environmental justice part of its mission by identifying and addressing, as appropriate, disproportionately high and adverse human health or environmental effects of its programs, policies, and activities on minority populations and low-income populations…" Although variant orders have been released subsequently, EPA maintains the Office of Environmental Justice and reaffirmed its commitment to Environmental Justice in 2018.[36]

Many studies have described examples of populations affected by inequitable distributions of exposures. For example, a descriptive analysis of the Detroit metropolitan area documented greater exposure to air pollutants in census tracts with greater proportions of persons of color.[37] Multiple studies have documented that in the United States, communities with lower incomes have greater exposure to major air pollutants and higher rates of illness and mortality.[38] Health impact assessment has been proposed as a tool for characterizing the consequences of regulatory actions for specific groups within the population, beyond considering only population impact overall.[39] The World Health Organization's Health in All Policies are also intended to reduce health inequity by incorporating the reduction of health inequity in policies and actions across all sectors.[40] As a cross-cutting principle, environmental justice should underlie all actions to reduce environmental and occupational risks, as those with lower income and education and some minority populations are also more likely to work in more hazardous jobs with higher exposures to harmful agents.

LEGISLATIVE APPROACHES

Table 78-1 lists major U.S. statutes covering environmental and occupational exposures. The statutes cover media, for example, air and water, and substances, for example, toxic substances, fungicides and rodenticides, and exposure circumstances, for example, workers. All call for steps to reduce risk from environmental and occupational agents that are evidence-based. Across these laws, there is not uniformity in principles for moving from evidence to regulatory actions nor for determining what constitutes a significant level of risk and the extent to which risk should be reduced. For these long-standing laws, there is now a substantial body of precedent following from rule-making, litigation, and scientific and stakeholder input. Some are the enabling legislation for agencies, for example, the Occupational Safety and Health Act and the Occupational Safety and Health and the multiple statutes underlying the EPA.

Below the Federal level, state and local regulations and agencies are often central in environmental and occupational health. These are administered and reinforced by state and local agencies.

Nongovernmental Organizations

Nongovernmental organizations (NGOs) are often a powerful voice on environmental and occupational risk issues. They are varied in scope, for example, local or national and the range of topics considered, and also in their underlying purposes, principles and approaches. Some have substantial numbers of staff that include scientists with domain-specific expertise, along with policy analysts and attorneys: the National Resources Defense Council (NRDC) and the Environmental Defense Fund (EDF). These larger NGOs have the capability of bringing evidence-based perspectives to support their positions. They may focus on specific issues or general issues and their reach extends from global to local. Their mechanisms of action are extensive, possibly including: advocacy, public education, scientific research and reviews, testimony, and litigation. Thus, they can play multiple roles in the complexities of decision-making (Fig. 78-1).

CITIZEN ACTION

Citizen action can be a powerful force in shaping public opinion and driving political action for progress in addressing harmful environmental exposures.[41] The U.S. environmental movement is rooted in grassroots activism, local community members coming together to demand action to address risk to their health. Community activists at Love Canal concerned about impacts on their health from chemicals leaching from chemical dumping persisted in persisted in drawing national attention to uncontrolled hazardous waste sites and inaction by state and federal authorities.[42] Their protests were a catalyst for the passages of the "Superfund," the Comprehensive Environmental Response, Compensation, and Liability Act (CERCLA). Citizen action can now be mobilized through a variety of mechanisms including social media groups, and empowered by the findings of community-based participatory research and citizen science. For example, frustrated by city and state inaction to address drinking water contamination, residents of Flint Michigan partnered with a local medical doctor and university researchers to demonstrate high levels of lead in their water and elevated blood lead levels in children.[43]

Litigation

Litigation also drives risk management decisions and policies both in government and the private sector. Historically, lawsuits brought by citizen groups and advocacy organizations have shaped many national risk policies, from safe drinking water to workplace asbestos control. For example, recent major settlements for workers and communities exposed to per- and polyfluoroalkyl substances (PFAS) have led to the imposition of major financial penalties, discontinuance of use and manufacturing, exposure and medical monitoring and new legislation to develop risk management and remedial actions.[44] One settlement led to the implementation of a community-based research initiative, the C8 health project.[45]

Litigation and citizen action are sometimes intertwined with citizen groups turning to litigation to stop actions that may cause or are causing exposures. Individuals who have been harmed may also sue for compensation. For industries that threaten community environmental assets, for example, the water supply, litigation may be the most effective course for citizen groups and local governments. Of course, such litigation may be costly and resource intensive.

With regard to litigation in the domains of environmental and occupational health (workers' compensation is covered elsewhere), legal actions can be a powerful force and taken by multiple stakeholders. Myriad legal actions have been taken and it is the resulting case law that provides precedents for litigation. Some broad domains of litigation are set out below with selected examples.

With regard to litigation in the domains of environmental and occupational health, legal actions can be a powerful force and taken by multiple stakeholders (workers' compensation is covered elsewhere). Myriad legal actions have been taken and it is this case law that provides precedents for litigation. Some broad domains of litigation are set out below with selected examples.

- Tort litigation: A tort is a wrong and consequently tort litigation involves seeking compensation for the damages resulting to the defendant for the commission of the wrong. Litigation related to asbestos is a mass tort, that is, involving multiple injured parties.[46] Another major example of tort litigation is the settlements against the manufacturer of the broadly used weed-killer glyphosate awarding damages to plaintifs claiming their non-Hodgkins lymphoma is caused by exposure to the pesticide.[47]
- Enforcement: Environmental and occupational health law impose requirements for compliance on the regulated industries and facilities. Violations of these requirements are subject to enforcement actions by EPA and OSHA, in concert with the Department of Justice and the states. Enforcement actions can range from minor fines to major consent agreements to address violations and impose large financial penalties on the offending companies. The largest financial settlement in EPA history was the 2016 consent agreement with Volkswagen for alleged violations of the Clean Air Act.[48] Volkswagen was required to take mitigation efforts to reduce diesel emissions and paid a 1.45 billion dollar civil penalty.
- Litigation can also be initiated by stakeholders to block or spur actions by regulatory agencies. Twenty-four states sued EPA to block implementation of the Obama Clean Power Plan. Conversely, environmental groups often file suits against EPA to assure timely implementation of health-based regulations.

CONCLUSION

The concept of risk reduction underlies a broad, multilevel array of activities directed at environmental and occupational exposures. With a long trajectory of reducing risks from these exposures, there is a complicated web of regulations, agencies, organizations, and precedents for addressing them. This chapter provides a broad and high-level introduction to risk characterization and management. For many exposures, there are decades-long stories about efforts to manage them.

References

1. World Health Organization. *Air Quality Guidelines: Global Update 2005-Particulate Matter, Ozone, Nitrogen Dioxide and Sulfur Dioxide.* Copenhagen: World Health Organization; 2006.
2. Lowrance WW. *Of Acceptable Risk: Science and the Determination of Safety.* Los Altos, CA: William Kaufmann; 1976.
3. Council NR. *Improving Risk Communication: National Academies.* Washington, DC: The National Academies Press; 1989.
4. National Research Council. *Risk Assessment in the Federal Government: Managing the Process.* Washington, DC: National Academy Press; 1983.
5. National Research Council Committee on Risk Assessment of Hazardous Air Pollutants. *Science and Judgment in Risk Assessment.* Washington, DC: National Academy Press; 1994.
6. National Research Council. *Science and Decisions: Advancing Risk Assessment.* Washington, DC: National Academies Press; 2009, p. xviii, 403.
7. Samet JM, Chiu WA, Cogliano V., et al. The IARC monographs: Updated procedures for modern and transparent evidence synthesis in cancer hazard identification. *J Natl Cancer Inst.* 2019;112(1):30–7.
8. U.S. Environmental Protection Agency. EPA's Integrated Risk Information System (IRIS) Program. Progress Report and Report to Congress: Office of Research and Development, 2015.
9. Samet JM, Nero AV. Indoor radon and lung cancer. *N Engl J Med.* 1989;320(9):591–4.
10. National Research Council, *Committee on Health Risks of Exposure to Radon. Health Effects of Exposure to Radon: BEIR VI.* Washington, DC: National Academy Press; 1999.
11. Pearce D, Atkinson G, Mourato S. Cost-benefit analysis and the environment: Recent developments: Organisation for economic co-operation and development, 2006.
12. Pearce DW. *Cost-Benefit Analysis.* London: Macmillan International Higher Education; 2016.
13. Morrall J, Broughel J. The Role of Regulatory Impact Analysis in Federal Rulemaking. *Available at SSRN 2501096*, 2014.
14. National Research Council. *Improving Health in the United States: The Role of Health Impact Assessment.* Washington, DC: The National Academies Press; 2011.
15. National Environmental Policy Act of 1969. 42. United State of America, 1969.
16. Mueller N, Rojas-Rueda D, Cole-Hunter T, et al. Health impact assessment of active transportation: A systematic review. *Prev Med.* 2015;76:103–14.
17. Caufield C. *Multiple Exposures. Chronicles of the Radiation Age.* London, England: Stoddard Publishing, Ltd.; 1989.
18. Hendee WR, Edwards FM. ALARA and an integrated approach to radiation protection. *Semin Nucl Med.* 1986;16(2):142–50.
19. International Commission on Radiological Protection. Recommendations of the International Commission on radiological protection. *ICRP Publication 26 Ann ICRP.* 1977;1(3):87.
20. Wingspread statement on the precautionary principle. January 23–25, 1998; Racine, WI.
21. United Nations Conference on Environment Development. Rio declaration on environment and development. Geneva, Switzerland, 1992.
22. Kriebel D, Tickner J. Reenergizing public health through precaution. *Am J Public Health.* 2001;91(9):1351–5.
23. Kriebel D, Tickner J, Epstein P, et al. The precautionary principle in environmental science. *Environ Health Perspect.* 2001;109(9):871–6. [published Online First: 2001/10/24]
24. Tickner JA. Precautionary principle encourages policies that protect human health and the environment in the face of uncertain risks. *Public Health Rep.* 2002;117(6):493–7.
25. An Act to amend the Federal Insecticide, Fungicide, and Rodenticide Act and the Federal Food, Drug, and Cosmetic Act, and for other purposes. United States, 1996.
26. Industrial Union Department, AFL-CIO v. American Petroleum Institute, et al. Supreme Court of the United States, 1980.
27. Linet MS, Bailey PE. Benzene, leukemia, and the Supreme Court. *J Public Health Policy.* 1981;2(2):116–35.
28. White MC, Infante PF, Chu KC. A quantitative estimate of leukemia mortality associated with occupational exposure to benzene 3. *Risk Anal.* 1982;2(3):195–204.
29. U.S. Government Publishing Office. Title 42—THE PUBLIC HEALTH AND WELFARE, CHAPTER 85—AIR POLLUTION PREVENTION AND CONTROL, SUBCHAPTER I—PROGRAMS AND ACTIVITIES, Part A—Air Quality and Emission Limitations, Sec. 7409—National primary and secondary ambient air quality standards 2013 [Available at https://www.govinfo.gov/content/pkg/USCODE-2013-title42/html/USCODE-2013-title42-chap85-subchapI-partA-sec7409.htm. Accessed March 12, 2020.
30. Di Q, Wang Y, Zanobetti A., et al. Air pollution and mortality in the Medicare population. *N Engl J Med.* 2017;376(26):2513–22.
31. U.S. Environmental Protection Agency. Health Risk and Exposure Assessment for Ozone—Final Report. Resarch Triangle Park, North Carolina: Office of Air and Radiation. Office of Air Quality Planning and Standards. Health and Environmental Impacts Division. Risk and Benefits Group. 2014.
32. Thurston GD, Kipen H, Annesi-Maesano I, et al. A joint ERS/ATS policy statement: What constitutes an adverse health effect of air pollution? An analytical framework. *Eur Respir J.* 2017;49(1)
33. Ciaravella MW. Regulation of hazardous air pollutants under section 112 of the Clean Air Act Amendments of 1990. *Energy Law J.* 1994;15:485.
34. Goldstein BD. The precautionary principle also applies to public health actions. *Am J Public Health.* 2001;91(9):1358–61. [published Online First: 2001/08/31]
35. Federal Register. Executive Order 12898 of February 11, 1994—Federal actions to address environmental justice in minority populations and low-income populations, 1994.
36. Davis S. *Memorandum on EPA's Environmental Justice and Community Revitalization Priorities.* Washington, DC: EPA Office of Policy, U.S. Environmental Protection Agency; 2018.

37. Schulz AJ, Mentz GB, Sampson N., et al. Race and the distribution of social and physical environmental risk: A case example from the Detroit metropolitan area. *Du Bois Rev.* 2016;13(2):285–304.
38. Hajat A, Hsia C, O'Neill MS. Socioeconomic disparities and air pollution exposure: A global review. *Curr Environ Health Rep.* 2015;2(4):440–50.
39. Yuen TK, Payne-Sturges DC. Using health impact assessment to integrate environmental justice into federal environmental regulatory analysis. *New Solut.* 2013;23(3):439–66.
40. World Health Organization. Health in all policies: Helsinki statement. *Framework for Country Aaction*. Copenhagen: World Health Organization; 2014.
41. Korfmacher KS. *Bridging Silos: Collaborating for Environmental Health and Justice in Urban Communities*. Cambridge, MA: Mit Press; 2019.
42. Colten CE, Skinner PN. *The road to Love Canal: Managing Industrial Waste before EPA*. Austin, TX: University of Texas Press; 2010.
43. Hanna-Attisha M, LaChance J, Sadler RC., et al. Elevated blood lead levels in children associated with the Flint drinking water crisis: A spatial analysis of risk and public health response. *Am J Public Health.* 2016;106(2):283–90.
44. Leach. et al. v. E.I. Du Pont Nemours and Company: Circuit Court of Wood County, West Virginia, February 28, 2005, 608.
45. Frisbee SJ, Brooks JrAP, Maher A., et al. The C8 health project: Design, methods, and participants. *Environ Health Perspect.* 2009;117(12):1873–82.
46. Carroll SJ, Hensler DR, Gross J, et al. *Asbestos Litigation*. Santa Monica, CA: Rand Corporation; 2005.
47. Reuters. Monsanto Ordered to Pay $289 Million in Roundup Cancer Trial: The New York Times; 2018 [updated August 10, 2018. Available at https://www.nytimes.com/2018/08/10/business/monsanto-roundup-cancer-trial.html. Accessed March 27, 2019.
48. Cruden JC, Engel B, Cooney N., et al. Dieselgate: How the investigation, prosecution, and settlement of volkswagen's emissions cheating scandal illustrates the need for robust environmental enforcement. *Va Environ Law J.* 2018;36(2):118–84.

CHAPTER

79 Protecting Workers' Health, Safety, and Well-being

Gregory R. Wagner • Emily A. Spieler

RELATIONSHIP BETWEEN WORK AND HEALTH

People who are fully employed spend over one third of their lives at work, commuting to or from work, or engaged in other work-related activities. To a greater or lesser extent, work furnishes the material resources that enable people to address basic human needs, including housing, food, and access to health insurance. Work helps individuals flourish by providing a sense of purpose, meaning, and social support. And, when work provides adequate resources, it also enables people to address out-of-work responsibilities and pursue nonwork interests. On the other hand, employment and the work environment can pose serious threats to health and well-being by exposing workers to hazardous conditions that may result in physical injury, illness, disability or death, or to stressful, bullying or discriminatory environments that threaten psychological well-being. In private industry, work hazards account for at least 5200 injury-related deaths, almost 3 million serious injuries, and unnumbered deaths from occupational exposures annually.[1] By all measures, work is a significant determinant of health.

This chapter briefly explores selected U.S. laws and policies that are designed to protect people at work, assist them when they are injured, and ensure they are treated fairly. This encompasses not only direct regulation of hazards within workplaces, but also other legislation that is designed to promote worker—and therefore population—well-being.

Most of the relevant worker-protection legislation and policies were developed to address "standard" employment relationships in which individuals have an identified employer with defined responsibilities. While there has always been a range of work arrangements, the diversity of current forms of employment, often enabled by new technologies or creative profit seeking, have resulted in new threats to worker health and well-being and challenge the adequacy of current protections. Similarly, new technologies such as robotics, and workplace exposures to new substances such as manufactured nanoparticles, may themselves pose physical and psychological risks not adequately addressed by current standards and regulations. In the final section of this chapter, we touch briefly on these looming challenges.

PROTECTING WORKERS FROM WORKPLACE HAZARDS: LEGISLATION AND ITS ENFORCEMENT

Federal, state, and local government agencies have multiple opportunities to improve public health by regulating hazards and thereby reducing injury and disease from work. During the first half of the twentieth century, all states enacted some form of compensation program for workers injured on the job; these became known, collectively, as workers' compensation. Until the late 1960s, worker health and safety protection and workplace inspections were generally seen as functions of state government or were left to private market forces. The intensity of governmental oversight and the consequences of safety failures varied widely from state to state, and there were few laws providing any national harmonization.

While workplace hazards threaten public health, the motivation and possibility of government action to reduce these threats is based on a complex calculus involving an assessment of the extent to which a problem is widely recognized by the public; whether an available, politically acceptable solution is both technically and economically feasible; the balancing of stakeholder/constituent interests; and the trade-offs against other potential government actions. It was not until the late 1960s that these forces aligned to drive Congress to act.

The growing political activism of the United Mine Workers, health professionals, and others drew public attention to the unaddressed and usually uncompensated burden of Black Lung—a group of serious and fatal lung diseases afflicting coal miners. Then, in 1968, a fire and explosion at an underground coalmine in Farmington, West Virginia, and the subsequent failed efforts to rescue trapped miners, was covered nightly on national television—the first in-depth widespread TV coverage of an industrial disaster. Together these events set the stage for the development and passage of the first comprehensive national health and safety legislation, the Coal Mine Health and Safety Act of 1969 (Coal Act)[2] and the Occupational Safety and Health Act of 1970 (OSH Act).[3] After another mining disaster, the Coal Act was amended and extended by the Mine Safety and Health Act of 1977 (Mine Act)[4] to cover all miners and quarriers working in all underground and surface mines in the United States. The OSH Act and the Mine Act continue to provide the legal framework for protecting private sector workers in general industry and mining.

Occupational Safety and Health Act of 1970

Congress justified the passage of the OSH Act by noting that "personal injuries and illnesses arising out of work situations impose a substantial burden upon, and are a hindrance to, interstate commerce in terms of lost production, wage loss, medical expenses, and disability compensation payments."[3] The Act clarified that it is the responsibility of employers to create and maintain workplaces free of recognized hazards and to comply with mandatory health and safety standards. The OSH Act was intended to stimulate the development and implementation of new worksite programs to prevent harm, in addition to establishing legally enforceable standards mandating particular actions to control specific hazards and thus reduce risk. At the outset, the OSH Act authorized the conversion of a large number of existing voluntary standards into mandatory standards. These "interim" standards were then intended to be mandatory for private sector employers and legally enforced through inspections by a newly created federal agency, the Occupational Safety and Health Administration (OSHA). For unregulated, inadequately regulated, or newly recognized hazards, the OSH Act specified a process for establishing new standards. The OSH Act also gave OSHA the authority to collect data relevant to carrying out its responsibilities.

In addition, the OSH Act created the National Institute for Occupational Safety and Health (NIOSH) to conduct and support research regarding occupational health and safety hazards, including psychological hazards in the workplace, and approaches to address these hazards more effectively (e.g., through improved control technologies). Among other responsibilities, NIOSH was also charged with making recommendations to OSHA for new standards based on the best available science; the OSH Act instructed OSHA to respond meaningfully to these recommendations.

In tacit acknowledgement of a history of state involvement in occupational safety and health, the OSH Act encouraged coordination or, essentially, delegation of the administration of the Act to states, so long as the regulations and actions of the relevant state agencies provided a level of protection to workers in those states at least equivalent to that of workers covered by federal OSHA. When a state qualifies for this "state plan" status, federal OSHA does not conduct enforcement in that state, but instead attempts to monitor the state's compliance with the federal requirements.

For workers covered by either OSHA or the Mine Safety and Health Administration (MSHA), protections are supposed to be comprehensive. The vision guiding these agencies, as articulated in their legislative framework, is that no worker should suffer material impairment of health or death as a result of a lifetime of workplace exposures. In practice, however, legal, budgetary, and political constraints have limited the effectiveness of these agencies in fulfilling this vision.

In addition to its focus on improving the health and safety of workers directly, the OSH Act also mandated the creation of a separate national commission to investigate the status of existing state workers' compensation laws, while specifically noting that the Act was not intended to interfere with state control of these programs. The commission issued a scathing report in 1972 finding that "the protection furnished by workmen's [sic] compensation to American workers presently is, in general, inadequate and inequitable."[5] No federal legislation has ever been passed to address the inadequacies of these programs.

Federal Mine Safety and Health Act of 1977 (Mine Act)

The Mine Act and its subsequent amendments aim to protect the safety and health of all people who work in mines and quarries in the United States, including both underground and surface worksites. The Mine Act established the MSHA in the Department of Labor and gave the agency the responsibility to promulgate and enforce mandatory safety and health standards in order to reduce injuries, disease, and death resulting from workplace exposures. Mine operators retain the primary responsibility to prevent hazardous conditions and practices. NIOSH was also given specific responsibilities to conduct research and make recommendations. States are permitted to develop and enforce their own mine safety programs. Unlike under the OSH Act, these federal and state programs exist in parallel, and the federal government does not step back from enforcement in states that also have mine health and safety programs.

Congress justified and structured the Mine Act and the OSH Act to be similar in many ways, but the Mine Act provides higher levels of protections than the OSH Act in important ways:

- MSHA must inspect all underground mines in their entirety at least four times a year and inspect all surface mines in their entirety at least twice a year. In contrast, there is no minimum frequency of inspections of workplaces covered by the OSH Act, and most private worksites are rarely, if ever, inspected. OSHA inspectors generally perform limited inspections, sometimes restricted to a specific targeted problem.
- Both OSHA and MSHA inspectors can cite employers when they observe violations of mandatory safety or health standards (civil financial penalties may be imposed as a result of the citations); there is a legal process for employers to appeal these citations. However, mine operators must correct the problems for which they were cited even if they are appealing the citation, while employers in industries covered by the OSH Act can choose to delay making any workplace changes pending resolution of the appeal. This can be important: there are instances where workers have been killed by hazards cited by OSHA inspectors while the appeals process delayed mitigation of the hazard.
- MSHA inspectors who find conditions that they believe pose an imminent danger to the safety or health of miners working have the authority to shut down mining activities in that area until the problem is fixed. OSHA inspectors do not have this authority. Instead, under the OSH Act, Department of Labor lawyers must go to federal court for a judge-issued injunction in order to be able to shut down part of an operation in order to address an imminent hazard. This step has rarely been taken.
- Mine operators identified by MSHA as having a history of significant violations—known as a "Pattern of Violations"—must demonstrate their capability and commitment to maintain the mine without any serious violations or be shut down while violations are fixed. There is no comparably serious consequence for employers with a pattern of violating standards that are regulated by OSHA.
- MSHA is responsible for mandating and overseeing training for all miners. While OSHA standards may include mandated standard-specific training, there is no general training requirement for workers.
- MSHA, with the assistance of NIOSH, is responsible for overseeing a pulmonary health surveillance program for all coal miners and assuring that coal miners showing evidence of lung disease are informed of their right to work in a limited dust environment that is monitored frequently.[2,6]

Mandatory Health and Safety Standards

Promulgating mandatory workplace safety and health standards and enforcing the standards are critical functions of both MSHA and OSHA. The OSH Act and Mine Act established what was intended to be an efficient process to develop and enforce standards to address newly recognized hazards and to improve existing but inadequate regulations. Over time, however, a series of court decisions and administrative procedures constrained standard setting significantly. In fact, OSHA issued only 58 significant standards between 1981 and 2010, and the time frame from beginning the process to final publication of these standards averaged almost 8 years.[7] Since 2011, five additional significant standards were completed. Existing standards under these laws can be found in the Code of Federal Regulations.[8]

As a result of the limited setting of new standards, most workplace toxic exposures and new technologies are still not covered by specific standards. In fact, most of the existing exposure limits are contained in the interim standards, which were based on the initial conversion of voluntary industry standards to mandatory requirements in the first years following passage of the OSH Act. Although these are enforceable standards, they may be based on outdated science and set inadequately protective exposure limits. A clear example is the standard for lead exposure, based on an old standard of blood lead levels of 40 μg/dL, which was established in 1978 and has not been updated since then, despite substantial evidence on serious health effects at levels well below 10 μg/dL.[9,10] As a comparison, the CDC blood lead reference value for children was reduced to 5 μg/dL in 2012 to identify children at higher lead exposure levels and take action earlier to reduce the child's future lead exposure.[11]

An agency may decide to develop a new standard based on the knowledge and observations of agency staff including inspectors, in response to requests or formal petitions from stakeholders such as unions or employer associations, or in response to recommendations from NIOSH. Currently, by law and administrative practice, in order for a new standard that will regulate risks to be proposed, the agencies must use the best available science to (1) establish that exposed workers run a risk of significant injury, disease, or death that exceeds 1 case per 1000; (2) a technically and economically feasible approach to reduce the risk has been identified; (3) there is reason to believe that the implementation of the new standard will reduce the risk; and (4) less costly or constraining approaches to risk reduction have been evaluated thoroughly.

The requirement for a risk that exceeds one case per thousand is derived from a decision by the U.S. Supreme Court in 1980, generally known as the "Benzene Case."[12] In this case, the court interpreted the language of the OSH Act that requires a finding that there is a significant risk before a regulation can be issued. In the majority opinion, the court wrote, "Some risks are plainly acceptable and others are plainly unacceptable. If, for example, the odds are one in a billion that a person will die from cancer by taking a drink of chlorinated water, the risk clearly could not be considered significant. On the other hand, if the odds are one in a thousand that regular inhalation of gasoline vapors that are 2% benzene will be fatal, a reasonable person might well consider the risk significant and take appropriate steps to decrease of eliminate it." The agencies have taken this language to heart and will not issue a regulation unless this extent of risk can be demonstrated with strong scientific evidence.

The standard setting process involves ongoing public notice with many opportunities for members of the public to contribute knowledge and viewpoints along the way. Twice a year each agency publishes a listing of all new regulations that are in process or under consideration. At the early stages, the agency may issue a request for information so that anyone can weigh in on their view of the problem, experience in addressing it, and what if anything the agency should do to improve protections. After the agency drafts a potential regulation, the draft goes through legal and administrative review within the Department of Labor and then the Office of Management and Budget (part of the office of the President) to ensure that the proposal has been developed in a way that complies with the law and will not create an excessive burden on individuals or sectors. The proposed regulation is then published, and the Agency solicits further public comment (through written submission and sometimes public hearings) on all components of the proposal. Some stakeholders, particularly small businesses, have specific rights to be heard in OSHA's regulatory process. Independent scientists with new, relevant information are particularly valuable contributors to these processes.

After the public input, agency staff then collect and address all the new data or comments that have been provided and draft a revision of the rule that then goes through the entire review process again. Ultimately, after review and approval by both the Department of Labor and the Office of Management and Budget, a final standard is published with a date for enforcement set in the future to allow employers to prepare for compliance.

This window also provides for both Congressional and judicial review of the standard. For a limited period after publication of the final regulation, Congress has the authority to review (and revoke) new federal standards under the Congressional Review Act.[13] Congress can therefore make an independent political decision about the standard even if the agency met all of its legal and administrative responsibilities in the regulation development process. Once Congress reviews and rejects a regulation and the President approves that law, the agency is not allowed to work on substantially similar standards in the future. Prior to 2017, the *only* instance of Congress making use of this law was in 2001, when it rejected a final OSHA regulation intended to reduce risk of musculoskeletal injury, commonly known as the Ergonomics Rule.

Some regulations, known as *performance standards*, mandate specific limits (permissible exposure limits or PELs) to hazardous exposures and permit employers the flexibility to achieve those limits. Other standards, known as *specification standards*, are more prescriptive about the methods an employer must use to assure adequate protection. Comprehensive health standards may include specific requirements for a PEL, environmental monitoring, medical monitoring for exposed workers, recordkeeping, labeling, or sign posting to alert exposed workers to the hazards, training, and housekeeping (requiring specific approaches to workplace maintenance or clean-up). Some standards permit or require the use of personal protective equipment such as protective clothing or respirators in specific exposure situations. A few standards permit or mandate removal of workers from exposures if medical testing abnormalities exceed a defined threshold.

OSHA and MSHA standards reflect a commitment to what is known as a "hierarchy of controls," a common public health approach to population risk reduction. The most effective way to reduce risk from a specific hazard is to eliminate it from the workplace through process change or substitution of a less hazardous substance or process for the riskier one. When substitution is not possible, engineering controls such as enclosure or dilution and removal of hazards though effective ventilation may be effective. Administrative controls, for example, limiting the time a worker is exposed to hazardous exposures through scheduling, may provide supplementary protections. At the bottom of the hierarchy—the least protective approach—is the use of personal protective equipment such as respirators. As a rule, respiratory protection may be included in standards for emergency or other temporary situations. When permitted, respiratory protection requires the establishment of an overall program for respirator selection, fit testing (to make sure that the specific respirator will provide the necessary level of protection against the particular exposure), training (so the worker knows when and how to use the respirator), cleaning, maintenance, and appropriate replacement schedules.

In theory, OSHA and MSHA can establish a standard to mitigate risk from any exposures faced by workers under their jurisdictions. The regulatory process works best when there is a body of credible scientific evidence that shows a clear exposure–response relationship between a substance or condition in the workplace and the probability of death or serious injury as well as an existing set of controls that can limit exposures. In these cases, the agency can estimate the numbers of workers at risk, the probability of death, disability, or injury likely to occur at current exposure levels, and the benefits likely to accrue with reduction of exposure. Unfortunately, many common exposures, for example, the stresses caused by poor work organization, workplace bullying or violence, or irregular scheduling, are difficult to quantify in that fashion. Partly as a consequence, despite the data documenting adverse cardiovascular and mental health outcomes, there has been no regulatory approach to address workplace stress in the United States.

Enforcement

Mandatory standards define specific employer responsibilities. In addition, even in the absence of a specific regulation, the OSH Act imposes a general duty for employers furnish to each of their employees a workplace that is free from recognized hazards that are causing or likely to cause death or serious physical harm.

The implementation of the laws is based on the concept that employers, like most citizens, are law-abiding and will comply with the law. However, enforcement through on-site inspections is a critical component of the regulatory structure: Workplace inspections, or the threat of inspections, are intended to motivate compliance with both specific standards and with the general legal duty to maintain safe workplaces. There is evidence that inspections result in more compliance with health and safety requirements, and therefore safer workplaces.[14]

When OSHA inspectors show up at a workplace, the extent of their inspection may depend on the original stimulus for their visit.

For example, if the inspection is a result of a serious injury, the focus of the inspection is on the cause of that injury, although the inspection may be extended to hazards in plain sight. OSHA also has "special emphasis programs" under which inspections are limited to the substance or process that is the focus of the program. In general, OSHA inspectors rarely inspect the entire workplace (a "wall-to-wall" inspection); more often the inspection is limited. When there is not a specific standard, and the inspector relies on the general duty requirement, the inspector must determine that a significant hazard exists for which there is no specific standard and that the employer did not take reasonable steps to address the hazard using an existing feasible method for control.

As noted above, the powers of inspectors as well as the frequency of inspections—and the requirements during appeals—differ significantly between the Mine Act and the OSH Act. The Mine Act's stronger provisions reflect an historical commitment to the protection of people who work in this particularly dangerous industry. All mine sites are inspected at least annually, and multiple comprehensive annual inspections are a routine component of normal operations. In contrast, inspections are not required in the rest of private industry, and only a small number of employers covered by the OSH Act face inspections. As of 2020, federal and state-OSHA programs together employ approximately 2200 inspectors who conduct approximately 32,000 inspections annually to help safeguard approximately 130 million private sector nonmining workers in over 7 million workplaces. In fact, it would take more than 100 years for OSHA to reach every employer.[15]

The Roles of Other Federal and State Agencies

A number of other federal and state agencies have some responsibilities relevant to the health, safety, and well-being of workers. For example, the Federal Motor Carrier Safety Administration in the Department of Transportation limits hours of work for interstate truck drivers and the Federal Airline Administration limits working hours for flight personnel. The Federal Railroad Administration takes responsibility for the safety of railroad workers, and the Department of Energy is responsible for overseeing the health and safety of workers in nuclear facilities. Offshore drilling operations are the responsibility of the Bureau of Safety and Environmental Enforcement. The Environmental Protection Agency considers the toxic effects of the pesticides they review and approve, including the potential effects on both consumers and farm workers. In all of these cases, OSHA is preempted from authority over these workers or exposures. A number of mining states have agencies that oversee some parts of mine safety and miner training.

State OSHA plans have significant flexibility to extend the coverage of workers in their states, such as public employees, and can enact their own regulations to improve coverage for workers in private industry, so long at the regulations are at least as protective as those enforced by federal OSHA.

Localities as well as states have also passed ordinances protecting workers. For example, clean indoor air rules reduce tobacco smoke exposure to restaurant and bar employees. Contra Costa County, California, has a long standing "Industrial Safety Ordinance" applicable to chemical plants and refineries in that county. Some municipalities also consider safety records in the selection of contractors to perform public works projects.

Legal Protections for Workers who Face Retaliation after Raising Health and Safety Concerns

We rely on workers to report concerns about health and safety risks to their employers or to appropriate agencies. Logically, the health and safety laws include provisions against retaliation. Under these antiretaliation provisions, workers can file complaints raising concerns that discipline or discharge was due to the raising of these concerns. The Mine Act has the stronger provisions: if a miner can show that the claim is "not frivolous," then he is entitled to immediate reinstatement at work. Provisions under the OSH Act, the Mine Act, and many other laws provide that workers who can prove that their discipline was the result of raising concerns are entitled to recover damages, including pay that was lost and additional monetary damages. Under all of the laws, reinstatement to the job is also an option.

In addition to the specific provision under the OSH Act, OSHA is responsible for the investigation of more than 20 of these "whistleblower" laws.[16] MSHA investigates its own complaints.

NONREGULATORY APPROACHES TO WORKPLACE SAFETY

The Role of Federal Agencies: OSHA, MSHA, NIOSH

In addition to issuing and enforcing standards and regulations, OSHA and MSHA are actively engaged in producing and disseminating educational materials for both employers and workers about current hazards, how to address them, and how to comply with current regulations. In addition to performing workplace compliance inspections, agency staff makes consultative visits to help employers, particularly small businesses, understand how to recognize and then reduce or eliminate hazards commonly found in their industries.

OSHA also encourages the active development and implementation of safety and health management systems (also known as injury and illness prevention programs) to promote ongoing monitoring of both workplaces and the health of workers in order to anticipate, recognize, evaluate, and address hazardous conditions as they arise.[17] OSHA recognizes and rewards employers who implement health and safety management systems and are certified under the Voluntary Protection Programs (VPP). To attain certification, an employer must conduct a comprehensive, structured, self-audit that is then reviewed for accuracy by OSHA staff. As a rule, the injury and illness rates of certified employers are less than half that of others in their industry. A benefit of certification is avoidance of routine OSHA inspections, although inspections may still be conducted after a workplace death or in response to a worker complaint. OSHA offers a similar program, the Safety & Health Achievement Recognition Program (SHARP), aimed specifically at small employers.

NIOSH, a component of the Center for Disease Control and Prevention, also has legal responsibilities to contribute to nonregulatory approaches to workplace health and safety. NIOSH conducts original research and funds independent research on the causes of disease and injury from work and the means of preventing them, including the development and evaluation of new control technologies. NIOSH also produces guidelines based on their review of the scientific literature and communicates these to OSHA and MSHA and the general public.

In addition, in response to requests from employers, workers, or other government agencies, NIOSH may conduct workplace Health Hazard Evaluations (HHEs) to help identify and control hazards that are not regulated by specific standards. HHEs are often a vehicle for developing information on newly recognized hazards. One example was the NIOSH investigation of lung disease risk in popcorn manufacture.[18] NIOSH also conducts public health surveillance by collecting, analyzing, and communicating health, safety, and hazard data relevant to prevention by providing electronic access to data and issuing reports that are published in the technical and scientific literature.

The Role of Unions and Other Worker Organizations

Despite the efforts of the regulatory agencies, most workplaces are never inspected, and few workers call on regulatory agencies to intervene when they face risks at work. There are many reasons for this, but generally fear of retaliation—and skepticism that anything will get done—seem to underlie workers' reluctance to come forward. These concerns are reduced when workers belong to unions.

In fact, unionized workplaces have been shown to be safer than nonunion places of employment.[19] This is generally true for two reasons.

First, unions in workplaces have a range of rights that are not available to individual workers. For example, the employer must bargain with a union over safety and health issues when negotiating a contract. The terms of the contract may include requirements that the employer comply with the regulatory requirements, which then gives the union the power to enforce these provisions without waiting for a regulatory agency to show up. The specific terms covering health and safety can also be more protective than is required by law. In addition, unions can negotiate for broader ways in which to enforce safety requirements. For example, some unions, including the larger industrial unions, have been successful in negotiating clauses that establish safety committees that include union members, or give the union the right to bring in outside experts to review potential hazards, or establish more protective limits on exposures.[20]

Second, union contracts give individual workers protection from retaliation. Without a contract, private sector workers in the United States generally are considered to be "at-will" employees. This means that they can be discharged without cause, and that they have very few rights when an employer threatens them with retaliation. Nonunion workers often rely on laws against discrimination, but these laws are not directly applicable to many concerns that workers may raise. Union contracts, in contrast, provide for progressive discipline and require the employer to show "just cause" for disciplining or discharging an individual. Unions generally will be aggressive in enforcing these provisions.

However, only a small minority of workers have union protection. According to the Bureau of Labor Statistics, only 10.5% of the total United States workforce was unionized in 2018; the rate was higher for public sector employees (33.9%) than in the private sector (6.4%).[21] Public sector workers often also have additional protections through civil service and other laws. However, most private sector workers in dangerous occupations—including construction and mining—must rely on regulatory agencies to provide health and safety and other protections.

Public Health and Scientific Professional Organizations

Public health and scientific professionals and professional organizations also play critical roles in encouraging nonregulatory approaches to prevention of work-caused injuries and illnesses.

Organizations such as the American College of Occupational and Environmental Medicine, the American Occupational Health Nurses Association, The American Industrial Hygiene Association, the American Public Health Association, and the American Thoracic Society, among others, produce guidelines and official statements to promote and encourage recognition and reduction of risk from workplace risk. The Association of Governmental Industrial Hygienists (ACGIH), a private, nongovernmental organization, convenes committees to review scientific literature to arrive at recommendations for workplace limits to chemical exposures "Threshold Limit Values" (TLVs), sampling procedures, and other topics relevant to workplace protections. In fact, it was organizations like ACGIH that were responsible for development of the voluntary recommendations that because the interim OSHA standards. In addition, these organizations and their members respond to requests for information and requests for comments during the formal regulatory process and also have representatives sitting on advisory committees guiding and evaluating research and prevention priorities.

Internationally, the International Labour Organization (ILO) issues guidelines and recommendations that may drive improved worker protections. The International Organization for Standardization (ISO) develops and publishes many standards relevant to workplace safety. Many multinational companies adopt these standards companywide. The International Agency for Research on Cancer, a World Health Organization agency, reviews the scientific literature and classifies agents as to carcinogenicity. Their determinations are used both in the regulatory process and in OSHA's assessments of whether employers are following their general duty to maintain safe workplaces.

Summary

The regulatory and nonregulatory approaches to reducing health and safety risk from work, along with overall changes in industrial production and changes in employment patterns, have resulted in an overall reduction in deaths, serious injuries, and illnesses from work. For example, over the 30 years between 1989 and 2018, annual rates of reported lost-time injuries (including fatal injuries) per 100 full-time equivalent miners fell from 6.48 to 1.52, and fatalities per 100,000 FTE miners fell from 34.68 to 10.45. The reduction in fatalities in general industry also fell: Over the 20-year period from 1999 to 2018, the U.S. Bureau of Labor Statistics Census of Fatal Occupational Injuries show a drop from 6054 to 5200 fatalities annually, despite increases in the number of workers overall. Undoubtedly, some of this improvement may be attributed to changes in workplace technologies and types of jobs. However, public and private attention to workplace risks has been an important contributor to these improvements.

PROTECTING WORKERS WHO BECOME DISABLED AS A RESULT OF WORK: INCOME SUPPORT

Workers get injured at work despite the efforts of state and federal agencies, unions, and employers. Income and job protection for injured workers are part of the fabric of public health protection that is designed to safeguard the well-being of working people and their families. This section briefly summarizes the ways in which law and policy address the economic concerns of people who have been injured or sickened by their work.

For over a century, every state has had a workers' compensation system designed to provide healthcare and wage replacement benefits to workers whose injuries or illnesses arise out of their employment. All of these state programs provide weekly benefits for workers unable to work for a temporary period; healthcare coverage for the work-related injury or illness; some form of longer-term cash benefits for permanent disabilities; and, in the case of fatalities, burial expenses and benefits to surviving dependents. Weekly wage payments are based on the worker's earnings, but are generally capped, often at the state's average weekly wage. Temporary benefits are also generally limited by a defined number of weeks. Healthcare is provided without deductibles and co pays, but often with limitations regarding choice of providers. All of these programs are supported by payroll taxes paid by employers; in two states, employees also contribute directly to the cost of the program. In every state, the legislation provides benefits irrespective of fault; in return, workers gave up any right to sue their employers, even if the injury resulted from the employer's negligence or disregard for worker safety.

According to data maintained by the National Academy of Social Insurance, total benefit costs in these programs have been declining since about 1991, and the proportion of these benefits paid to medical care providers has risen in comparison to the amount paid directly to workers.[23] Much of the decline may be attributable to improved health and safety, as the decline in benefits tracks reasonably closely the data on injuries maintained by the U.S. Bureau of Labor Statistics. There are, however, other reasons that are contributing to the declines in paid benefits in these programs.

Large numbers of workers who are injured on the job never receive benefits. Some state statutes continue to exclude groups of workers including farmworkers and domestic employees. In addition, the barriers to filing and receiving benefits for eligible people are complex.[24] Workers may simply fail to file for benefits. This may be due to ignorance, or to reluctance to get involved in systems that have often been described as Kafkaesque, or to avoid the stigma that often follows beneficiaries of these programs, or to avoid retaliation by their employer. As a result, many eligible workers choose instead to make use of their general healthcare plans and employer's absence policies—and to bear any additional costs themselves.

It is not always easy for a worker to find a physician who will support a claim. Physicians play a critical role in these programs: without the support of a physician who can recognize and will certify that an injury or illness is arising out of work, the injured worker will not receive benefits. Unfortunately, because of billing limitations, complexity of reports, and delays in payment, many physicians are reluctant to participate in the programs.

At least in theory, both work-related injuries and illnesses are covered by these state programs. In fact, workers with occupationally related illnesses are rarely compensated. There are a host of reasons for this, including: ignorance on the part of workers and physicians; difficulty in proving that an individual's illness is work related if it is a disease that also appears in the general population; and long latency periods for some diseases, particularly cancers. Partly as a result, federal legislation has been passed to address a few specific diseases, most notably coal workers' pneumoconiosis.

State workers' compensation programs are often criticized by state business organizations, such as the Association of Manufacturers or the Chamber of Commerce. The success of probusiness advocacy in many states has resulted in recent changes in legislation that have erected barriers for collection of benefits. These changes include exclusions for conditions when the worker suffers from a preexisting condition that may have played a role in creating the disability. This means, for example, that in some states it is difficult for a worker with a preexisting lung condition to qualify for benefits when exposed to an acute respiratory hazard, or for someone with a preexisting but asymptomatic back condition to qualify for benefits after suffering a back injury at work. Other legislative changes have created procedural and evidentiary barriers to claims. It is difficult to tease apart the effects of this legislation from the effects of improved safety, but reductions in benefit availability appear to be a significant contributor.[25]

The state workers' compensation programs are supplemented by a variety of voluntary, state, and federal programs. Federal workers' compensation programs target specific subgroups of workers (e.g., federal employees, longshore and harbor workers, some radiation-exposed workers, workers exposed by the events of September 11, 2001) or specific diseases (e.g., black lung).

Public health research is critical to the compensation programs that provide benefits to workers with diseases. Epidemiologic studies of groups of workers or specific industries have been instrumental in the identification of excess disease risk in identified populations and the levels of exposure to hazardous substances that result in disability and death. The disease and exposure specific federal programs, in particular, would not have been created without this basis in scientific research. For example, findings of long-term systematic investigations of the hazards of radiation exposure were critical in the passage of the Radiation Exposure Compensation Act that provides benefits to workers in the nuclear industry sickened or killed by radiation exposure. Epidemiological findings were key to determining which workers would be eligible for compensation following the development of cancer or other covered diseases.

Workers who do not file or qualify for workers compensation may have access to benefits that do not require a showing that the disability was caused by work—and many workers with work-caused impairments do file for these other benefits. Several states have instituted mandatory temporary disability programs that provide some support to workers who are unable to work, irrespective of the cause of the disability. Employer-provided programs also provide income support through paid sick leave or paid disability leave, as well as general health insurance.

Workers with a sufficient history of participation in the U.S. labor market may qualify for a more general federal disability program, Social Security Disability Insurance (SSDI). SSDI requires that an individual prove total disability from all work. This can be proved by combining all impairments, including nonwork-related disabilities. For example, an individual with underlying heart disease or diabetes can combine these disabilities with those that may have occurred at work. In general, SSDI is the end of the road in terms of work participation, although the Social Security Administration has instituted various programs that try to encourage or force people out of the program.

In addition, while workers cannot bring lawsuits against their employers because of the exclusivity provisions of the workers' compensation laws, they may be able to supplement benefits they receive

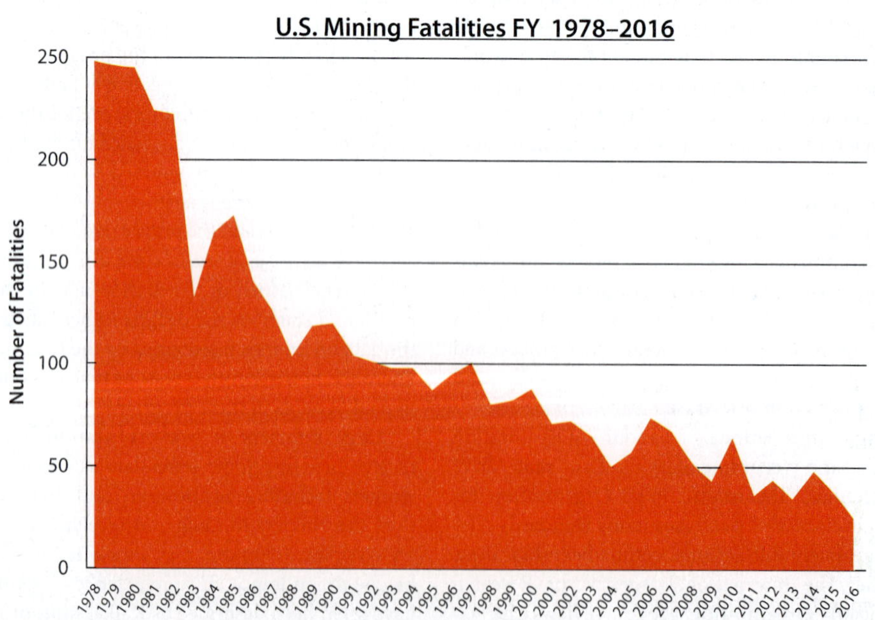

FIGURE 79-1. U.S. mining fatalities 1978–2016. (*Source:* Mine Safety and Health Administration.[22])

from these insurance programs by bringing lawsuits against the manufacturers of hazardous materials that are used in their workplaces. The public health consequences of this kind of litigation have sometimes been significant. For example, many of the legal cases involving asbestos exposure, requirements for ongoing medical monitoring, or compensation for disease have been brought by people who were exposed to asbestos at work. This litigation brought public attention to the extent of the asbestos problem and contributed to regulatory efforts, while also providing monetary benefits to the individuals involved. In another example, a lawsuit against the manufacturer of butter flavoring for popcorn, which resulted in a significant monetary victory for the worker, brought attention to the problem and added to the pressure on popcorn manufacturers to reduce or eliminate exposure to the flavoring.[26]

PROTECTING WORKERS AGAINST DISCRIMINATION AND HARASSMENT

In addition to income support and healthcare, workers with disabilities—whether caused by work or by other elements of life—often want to continue to work. It thus becomes important to establish an accommodation between the worker's need for continued work—and the accompanying income and sense of self-worth—and the employer's need for a productive, safe workforce. In the law, this is accomplished through laws that forbid discrimination on the basis of disability, including the federal Americans with Disabilities Act[27] and similar state laws.

This is one of a set of laws that forbid discrimination based on status, which also include prohibitions on discrimination based on race, age, sex, ethnicity, religion, national origin, and, in some states, sexual orientation. These laws attempt to address historical prejudice and exclusions in order to promote equality and well-being in the workplace. In general, individuals who bring claims must show they are members of the "protected class" and that an adverse action taken against them by their employer was linked to their membership in the class. Racial and sexual harassment are also addressed as a component of illegal discrimination.

Disability discrimination is somewhat more difficult to prove. The worker must show that she is disabled: that she has, or has a record of, or is regarded as having, a substantial impairment that significantly limits a major life activity such hearing, seeing, speaking, walking, breathing, performing manual tasks, caring for oneself, learning, or working. She then must show that she is capable of doing the job in question, with or without reasonable accommodation, that she was qualified to do the job, and that she was denied the opportunity to do the job due to the disability. Not surprisingly perhaps, these are all terms of art in the legal world.

As a matter of public health, the ability of individuals to access jobs is an important component of the well-being of the population. The bottom line of public policy that underlies these laws is that people with health impairments, or people who are members of groups who have faced historical prejudice and discrimination, should be assisted in overcoming barriers to full participation in the workforce. The U.S. Department of Labor Office of Disability Employment Policy provides resources for employers and for people with disabilities affecting their ability to work in order to encourage and improve employment possibilities. One of their funded projects, the Job Accommodation Network (JAN), has particular expertise in advising employers, workers and unions regarding how to accommodate an individual with disabilities in a workplace.[28]

PROTECTING WORKERS TO ENSURE MATERIAL WELL-BEING: FAIR WAGES, HOURS AND TIME ON AND OFF THE JOB

Employers have the responsibility to provide jobs and worksite free of recognized hazards. That is the purpose of the health and safety regulations discussed above. However, to be a "good job," work needs to contribute in positive ways to the well-being of individual workers—and thus to the health of the population as a whole. The need for adequate earnings, ability to take time off from work for leisure and to fulfil out-of-work responsibilities, and work reasonable hours are integral components to achieving this goal.

- Base earnings
For a century, the United States has mandated minimum wage levels, presumptively designed to keep workers out of poverty. As of January 2020, the federal minimum wage was \$7.25 per hour. Overtime is paid for hours over 40 hours per week. In most industries, there is no limit to the number of hours an employer can require an employee to work.

A change in the federal minimum wage requires Congressional action; it was last raised in 2009. Since it was first established in 1938 pursuant to the Fair Labor Standards Act,[29] Congress has never let it go unchanged for so long. When adjusted for inflation, researchers have estimated that its purchasing power declined over 17% over the ten subsequent years. In fact, in terms of purchasing power, the federal minimum wage reached its historical peak in 1968.[30] In reaction to the stagnation of the federal minimum wage, and in response to organizing by low wage workers and unions in a movement called "The Fight for Fifteen," more than half the states have now moved to increase the required minimum wage within the state.

This stagnation is not only in the minimum wage level. After adjusting for inflation, the average *hourly* wage in 2018 had about the same purchasing power it did in 1978. In fact, in real terms (adjusted for inflation) average *hourly* earnings peaked more than 45 years ago.[31]

The public health impact of declining purchasing power radiates out from work to families and communities. Individuals are forced to work more than one job—or to pick up a gig economy job such as driving for ride hailing companies (e.g., Uber or Lyft)—in order to earn sufficient income. Dual income households are more common. This creates greater need for adequate childcare and leave policies that allow families to care for children and aging parents. It also results in higher levels of stress and less time for sleep, recreation, or participation in community activities of all kinds. Thus, wage policies have broad implications for personal, family, and community health.

- Time off from work for family and medical reasons
A federal law, the Family and Medical Leave Act,[32] gives workers a job-protected right to take unpaid time off for specified medical and family reasons, including if they themselves are ill or to care for a newborn child or for a sick child or member of the immediate family. The qualifying illness must be serious; the FMLA does not allow workers to stay home due to a short-term illness that does not require medical treatment, such as the common cold. Time off is limited to 12 work weeks; the employer must have at least 50 employees; and the worker must have worked for the employer for at least 12 months.

Note that this leave is unpaid and does not provide protection for the millions of workers who are employed in smaller businesses. As of January 2020, there is no right in the United States to paid sick leave or to paid parental leave. This contrasts sharply with other developed countries, where this kind of social support is common.

A few states (including Arizona, California, Connecticut, Massachusetts, Michigan, Oregon, Vermont, New Jersey, and Maryland) and some cities have passed laws requiring at least some employers to provide paid sick leave to employees. However, as of January 2020, this is far from a universal legal protection.

The public health consequences of this are enormous. Workers with communicable diseases will come to work in order to be sure they will get paid. This puts not only their coworkers, but also the public at risk. Imagine, for example, the extent of risk that can be created by restaurant workers who feel they must go to work when sick in order to earn essential income and office workers who come to work with respiratory infections. Of course, many employers do provide paid sick leave voluntarily, but approximately 32% of the private sector workforce lacks paid sick leave.[33]

- Schedules and hours

Federal law in the United States guarantees that workers who are not administrative, professional, or managerial employees will be paid 150% of their regular hourly pay if they work more than forty hours per week. As with many laws, this provision is tricky to enforce. According to advocates for workers, many employees are paid salaries instead of hourly pay and misclassified as exempt from the overtime pay requirements.

Importantly, this overtime provision does not set any limit on the number of hours that an employee can be required to work. There are a few limited exceptions to this. For example, specific limits are set in federal law or regulations for children under 16, for airline pilots, and for interstate trucking and bus drivers. With the exception of the protection of children, these limits on hours are rooted in concern for the public at large and the dangers posed by excessive fatigue. The focus is not on the health and well-being of the worker him- or herself.

More recently, there has been a trend in some industries, particularly hospitality and retail, to move to "just-in-time" scheduling for workers. This type of scheduling is made possible by new technologies that can track business activities with great specificity. Workers may be required to be on-call for all hours that an establishment is open. A worker who goes to work may be sent home in the middle of a shift (and then possibly called back in) but will not be paid for hours off. Or, at the other end of the spectrum, workers may be required to work excessively long shifts. Schedules are often not posted in advance. This creates erratic pay—but it also means that workers are unable to plan for the needs of their families and communities. They are essentially "on-call" all the time but paid only when they appear at work. Obviously, this gives employers increased flexibility and reduced payroll costs, but at significant economic, social, and health consequences to the workers.

Again, there is no federal law that provides any protection against this random scheduling. There is a growing movement to persuade cities and states to adopt "fair workweek" laws that would require employers to post schedules in advance, offer compensation for on-call time, ban on-call scheduling entirely, or at least allow employees to make scheduling requests. As of 2019, some states (including New York, California, Washington, and Illinois) and cities (including Seattle and San Francisco) have passed some version of protective legislation regarding predictive scheduling in the affected industries.

The effect of unionization on all of these issues is profound: workers in unionized workplaces earn higher wages than the wages paid to nonunion workers in the same industry, have scheduling protections, and receive better benefits including long- and short-term disability plans, paid sick leave and vacation time, and richer health benefits.[34]

Notably, the failure of the federal government to act in these areas of pay and hours creates large disparities within the country. Moreover, recent wage growth, when local and state minimum wage increases are excluded, has been concentrated in the top 10% of wage earners.[35] Racial and gender disparities in wages persist. States that have moved to increase the minimum wage, create paid leave, and protect workers from the randomness of scheduling in the absence of adequate federal legislation contribute to deepening levels of inequality across the country.

The decline in unionization has also been linked to this growing income inequality. (See Fig. 79-2.)

The public health consequences of economic and social inequality are well covered elsewhere in this book. The role that work, and regulation of work, plays in this should not be underestimated.

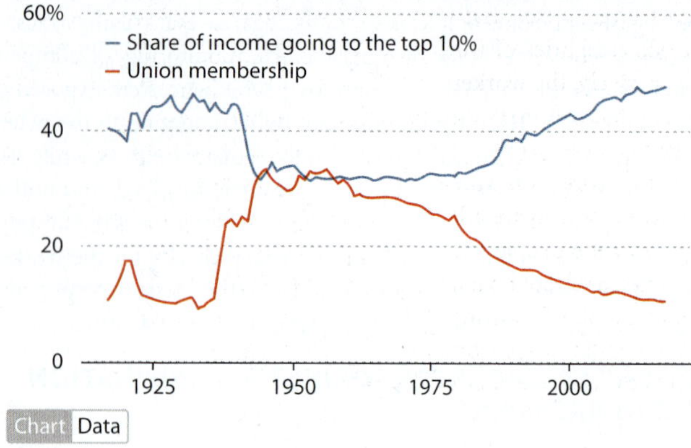

FIGURE 79-2. Union membership and share of income going to the top 10%, 1917–2017. As union membership declines, income inequality rises. (*Source:* Reproduced with Permission from Shierholz H. Working people have been thwarted in their efforts to bargain for better wages by attacks on unions Labor Day 2019.[35])

EMERGING CHALLENGES: NEW WAYS THAT TECHNOLOGY AND CONTRACTING IMPEDE OR ENHANCE WORKER WELL-BEING

It is impossible to leave the subject of the relationship between work and health without acknowledging the rapid changes that are occurring as this chapter is being written. Primarily three forces are transforming work for individuals and populations.

First, changing technology is affecting every type of work. These changes include new efficiencies and levels of autonomy for some workers, who can choose to work at home or in shared workplaces, and often at their chosen hours of work. This increase in autonomy can both increase well-being, but it may also increase social isolation. It is this same changing technology that has enabled the development of the "gig" economy: individuals who work on platforms, providing a variety of services, ranging from tiny tasks to driving for ride hailing companies such as Uber. The use of technology that has enabled the just-in-time scheduling increases business efficiency but has a deleterious effect on workers' lives.

These technologies also increase the ability of employers to monitor and control the work of many people, including those who work in warehouses or deliver goods. Where there was autonomy before—in choice of route, for example—there is now control that limits the ability of people to exercise judgment. The deskilling of jobs may increase productivity at the expense of job engagement and worker well-being.

Beyond the intervention of these technologies in existing jobs, it is also likely that artificial intelligence may change the nature of available jobs in the coming decades.

Second, new technologies create new workplace hazards that are, as yet, poorly understood. For example, nanotechnology has been embraced by many industries, from garment manufacture to cosmetics to military equipment. Knowledge about the health implications of exposure to nanoparticles is growing, but regulations are not yet under consideration. There is an attempt at coordination of research and information sharing across the federal government known as the National Nanotechnology Initiative.[36] Workers will continue to be exposed to these new hazards until reasonably conclusive research leads regulators to act.

Third, the nature of contracting among business organizations is changing dramatically. The idea of a single integrated firm that employs many types of workers is disintegrating. New arrangements often mean that in a single workplace, such as a hotel, the various categories of workers actually work for different employers. Alternatively, the workers in a factory may be employed by a "temp" agency that contracts with the primary business. Alternatively, a primary business may create franchises that it controls but which separate the workers from each other. These arrangements vary widely. The workers who are affected often have unclear supervision and do not know the people with whom they work; their ability to organize and exert collective voice is diminished; the possibility of adequate enforcement of existing employment laws, including health and safety regulation, is jeopardized; and their wages are depressed as a result of these contracting arrangements.[37,38]

CONCLUSION

The interactions between work, health, and well-being are diverse and complex. Nonetheless, in considering the need to protect workers, public health professionals often focus exclusively on hazards at work and the regulatory interventions designed to address these hazards. This approach is important, but inadequate. All aspects of work affect population health. To work without threats to safety and physical or mental health; the freedom to balance the demands of work with responsibilities to one's family, community, and self; and the opportunity to benefit both materially and socially from work are central to thriving individuals, families, and communities. The development, implementation, and evaluation of interventions that strengthen the benefits of work while better protecting the safety and health of workers are crucial public health functions.

References

1. Bureau of Labor Statistics Survey of Occupational Injuries and Illnesses, https://www.bls.gov/iif/soii-data.htm. 2019.
2. Federal Coal Mine Health and Safety Act of 1969, Public Law 91-173.
3. Occupational Safety and Health Act, Pub L. No. 91-596, Stat.1590, codified at 29 U.S.C. § 651 et seq.
4. Federal Mine Safety and Health Amendments Act of 1977, Public Law 91-173 as amended by Public Law 95-164, codified at 30 U.S.C. § 801 et seq.
5. Burton Jr JF. Letter of Transmittal, in The Report of the National Commission on State Workmen' s Compensation Laws. 1972, page 3.
6. https://www.cdc.gov/niosh/topics/cwhsp/.
7. US Government Accountability Office [GAO]. Multiple Challenges Lengthen OSHA's Standard Setting. GAO-12-330. April 2012.
8. Occupational Safety and Health Act Regulations, 29 C.F.R. Parts 1910–1928; Mine Act Regulations, 30 C.F.R. Parts 1–199.
9. U.S. Department of Labor. *1910.1025—Lead. Occupational Safety and Health Standards, Toxic and Hazardous Standards*. Washington, DC: Occupational Safety and Health Administration; 1978.
10. Schillaci WC. OSHA's 40-Year-Old Lead Standard Is Far Short of Protective. EHS Daily Advisor. July 18, 2018. Available at https://ehsdailyadvisor.blr.com/2018/07/oshas-40-year-old-lead-standard-far-short-protective/. Accessed February 5, 2020.
11. Centers for Disease Control. 2019. Available at https://www.cdc.gov/nceh/lead/prevention/blood-lead-levels.htm. Accessed January 6, 2020.
12. Industrial Union Department v. American Petroleum Institute (The Benzene Case), 448 U.S. 607. 1980.
13. Congressional Review Act, 5 U.S.C. § 801 et seq.
14. Levine DI, Toffel MW, Johnson MS. Randomized government safety inspections reduce worker injuries with no detectable job loss. *Science*. 2012;336(6083):907–11.
15. AFL-CIO. 2019. Death on the Job, The Toll of Neglect: A national and state-by-state profile of worker safety and health in the United States, 28 ed. https://aflcio.org/sites/default/files/2019-05/DOTJ2019Fnb_1.pdf.
16. https://www.whistleblowers.gov.
17. OSHA. Injury and Illness Prevention Programs White Paper. January 2012. Accessed at https://www.osha.gov/dsg/topics/safetyhealth/OSHAwhite-paper-january2012sm.pdf.
18. NIOSH HEALTH HAZARD EVALUATION REPORT HETA # 2000-0401-2991 Gilster-Mary Lee Corporation Jasper, Missouri, January 2006. Accessed at: https://www.cdc.gov/niosh/hhe/reports/pdfs/2000-0401-2991.pdf.
19. Morantz AD. *Coal Mine Safety: Do Unions Make a Difference?* February 2012. Accessed at https://law.utexas.edu/wp-content/uploads/sites/25/morantz-do-unions-make-a-difference.pdf.
20. Gray GR, Myers DW, Myers PS. Collective bargaining agreements: Safety and health provisions. *Mon Labor Rev*. 1998;13–35.
21. BLS, Union Members Summary. January 22, 2020. https://www.bls.gov/news.release/union2.nr0.htm.
22. Mine Safety and Health Administration.
23. Weiss E, Murphy G, Boden LI. Workers' Compensation Benefits, Costs, and Coverage—2017 Data, October 2019. Page 3 Figure 1.
24. Spieler EA, Burton Jr JF. The lack of correspondence between work-related disability and receipt of workers' compensation benefits. *Am J Ind Med*. 2012;55:487.
25. Guo X, Burton JFJr. Workers' compensation: Recent developments in moral hazard and benefit payments. *Ind Labor Relat Rev*. 2010;63:340–54.
26. Jury Gives Popcorn Worker $20M. CBS News; March 16, 2004. Available at https://www.cbsnews.com/news/jury-gives-popcorn-worker-20m/. Accessed February 5, 2020.
27. ADA Americans with Disabilities Act of 1990 (ADA), Pub. L. 101-336, July 26, 1990, 104 Stat. 327 codified at 42 USC § 12101 et seq.
28. https://askjan.org.
29. Fair Labor Standards Act, 29 U.S.C. § 201 et seq.
30. Cooper D. Congress has never let the federal minimum wage erode for this long, Economic Snapshot. June 17, 2019. https://www.epi.org/publication/congress-has-never-let-the-federal-minimum-wage-erode-for-this-long/.
31. DeSilver D. For most U.S. workers, real wages have barely budged in decades. August 7, 2018. https://www.pewresearch.org/fact-tank/2018/08/07/for-most-us-workers-real-wages-have-barely-budged-for-decades/.
32. FMLA, 29 USC § 2611 et seq.
33. BLS. 93 percent of managers and 46 percent of service workers had paid sick leave benefits in March 2017. August 02, 2017. https://www.bls.gov/opub/ted/2017/93-percent-of-managers-and-46-percent-of-service-workers-had-paid-sick-leave-benefits-in-march-2017.htm.
34. Long GI. Differences between union and nonunion compensation, 2001–2011. Monthly Labor Review. April 2013, pp. 16–23. https://www.bls.gov/opub/mlr/2013/04/art2full.pdf.
35. Shierholz H. Working people have been thwarted in their efforts to bargain for better wages by attacks on unions Labor Day. 2019. https://www.epi.org/publication/labor-day-2019-collective-bargaining/.
36. https://www.nano.gov/.
37. Weil D. *The Fissured Workplace: Why Work Became So Bad for So Many and What Can Be Done to Improve It*. Cambridge, MA: Harvard University Press; 2017.
38. Boden LI, Spieler EA, Wagner GR. The Changing Structure of Work: Implications for Workplace Health and Safety in the US. March 7, 2016. https://www.dol.gov/sites/dolgov/files/OASP/legacy/files/Future_of_work_the_implications_for_workplace_health_and_safety.pdf.

CHAPTER

80 Looking to the Future: Sustainability and Other Issues

John D. Spengler • Wendy M. Purcell

WHAT IS SUSTAINABILITY?

Sustainability is a goal for today and sustainable development an organizing **principle** that recognizes the interconnections between complex natural and social systems. Sustainability is a dialectical concept, like beauty and justice, and can be difficult to define, yet most will agree that it is an aspiration with **Sustainable Development** the means to deliver that end. The most widely accepted definition of sustainability is that determined by the World Commission on Environment and Development (WCED) published in 1987 in a report entitled **"Our Common Future"** by the **Brundtland Commission**; Gro Harlem Brundtland (Fig. 80-1), the former Prime Minister of Norway, led the Commission given her strong background in the sciences and public health. Her report strongly influenced the Earth Summit in Rio de Janeiro, Brazil, in 1992 and the 3rd United Nations (UN) Conference on Environment and Development in Johannesburg, South Africa, in 2002.

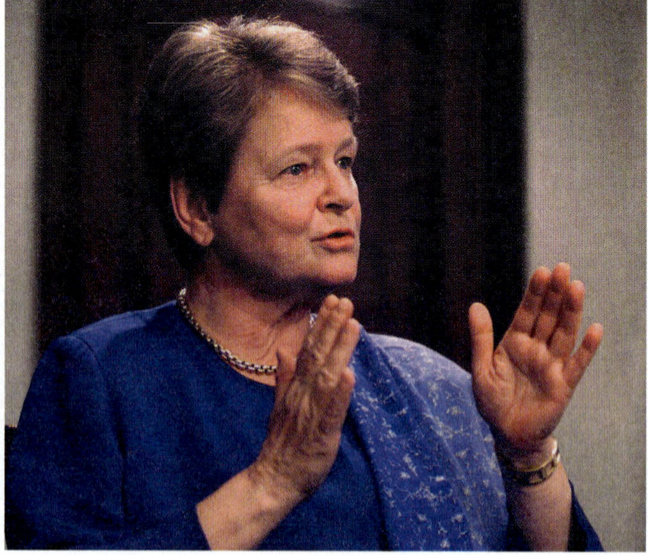

FIGURE 80-1. Gro Harlem Brundtland, MD was a Norwegian politician, who served three terms as Prime Minister of Norway and as Director-General of the World Health Organization from 1998 to 2003. She chaired the Brundtland Commission, which presented the Brundtland Report on sustainable development. (*Source*: B. Mathur JSG/Reuters/Alamy Stock Photo.)

> ***Sustainability is** ...development that meet the needs of the present without compromising the ability of future generations to meet their own needs.*[1]

Brundtland argued:

> *...the "environment" is where we live; and "development" is what we all do in attempting to improve our lot within that abode. The two are inseparable.*[1]

Sustainable development therefore deals with environmental issues as well as economic, social, and cultural matters. Given the increased demands being placed on societies and our planet, from increased urbanization, migration, and industrialization alongside the depletion of nonrenewable resources, concerted and global actions are required to create a more sustainable future. The UN, under General Secretary Javier Pérez de Cuéllar (1982–91), aimed to create a united international community with shared sustainability goals by identifying sustainability **problems** worldwide, raising awareness about them, and suggesting the implementation of **solutions**. The mission of the Brundtland Commission was to unite countries to pursue sustainable development together given it had long been recognized that the **tensions between economic growth and environmental resources** were exacerbating income disparities between developed and developing nations. Many poorer countries faced pressures from the extraction of resources that resulted in environmental degradation, while wealthier countries seem unwilling to arrest aggressive growth forecasts to reduce and/or remediate environmental damage. Sustainable development works as an organizing principle given it recognizes the interconnections between complex natural and social systems.

EARLY HISTORY

Indigenous Peoples

An intimacy with and reliance upon **nature and natural systems** for sustaining life has long shared behaviors and beliefs of many indigenous people. The northern plains along the front range of the Rockies Mountains in Montana were held in common among several Blackfeet family tribes, providing access to buffalo, natural plants and crops, and coordinating their seasonal migrations. The Swinomish, the Duwamish, the Suquamish and many other tribes of Salish people shared the fishing, clamming, and other natural resources of coastal British Columbia and Washington for many hundreds of years. Chief Seattle (c. 1786–June 7, 1866) (Fig. 80-2) was a Suquamish and Duwamish chief to whom many prophetic quotes about nature are attributed; his views in favor of ecological responsibility and respect of Native Americans' land rights resonate strongly today.

BOX 80-1 Definition of Sustainable Development

***Sustainable development** is the organizing principle for meeting human development goals while at the same time sustaining the ability of natural systems to provide the natural resources and ecosystem services upon which the economy and society depend. The desired result is a state of society where living conditions and resource use continue to meet human needs without undermining the integrity and stability of the natural system. Sustainable development can be classified as development that meets the needs of the present without compromising the ability of future generations.*[1]

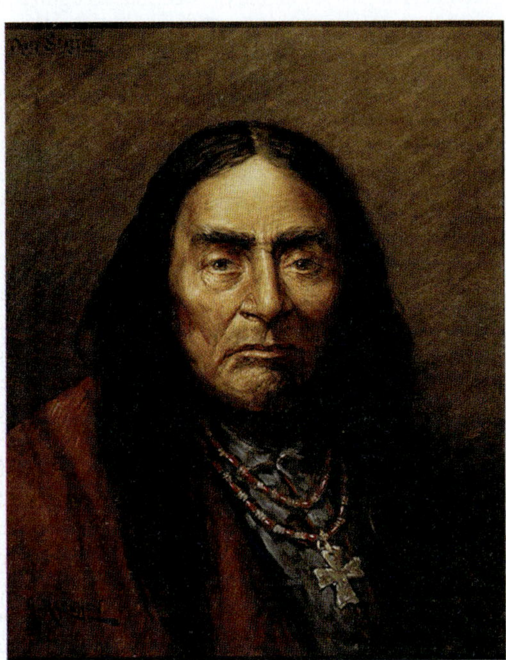

FIGURE 80-2. Chief Seattle. (*Source*: Volgi archive/Alamy Stock Photo.)

> *Will you teach your children what we have taught our children? That the earth is our mother? What befalls the earth befalls all the sons of the earth. This we know: the earth does not belong to man; man belongs to the earth. All things are connected like the blood that unites us all. Man did not weave the web of life; he is merely a strand in it. Whatever he does to the web, he does to himself.*[2]

In 2012, a statement by the Conference of Parties to the UN Framework Convention on Climate Change, the International Indigenous Peoples Forum on Climate Change (IIPFCC) acknowledged the importance of rethinking the value of some traditional practices.

> *...[W]e reiterate the need for recognition of our traditional knowledge, which we have sustainably used and practiced for generations; and the need to integrate such knowledge in global, national and sub-national efforts. This knowledge is our vital contribution to climate change adaptation and mitigation.*[3]

Many indigenous people have a sophisticated understanding of land and resource management. Fishing weirs, burning grasslands, using fish to enrich soil nutrients and developing complex irrigation systems were land management practice "discovered" by conquistadors, fur trappers, colonizers, and explorers of the "New World." In today's vernacular, indigenous peoples' traditional knowledge and management of their natural surroundings were a source of resilience for their tribes and communities. More examples of how indigenous people developed conservation practices to increase productivity of the natural resources they depended on for food, clothing and building materials can be found on the United Nations University site[4] However, not all indigenous peoples live in harmony with nature. Egregious self-aggrandizement, religious practices, climate change, and conflict have historically brought about the collapse of otherwise successful and sophisticated cultures. Capturing birds for their colorful plumage to enhance the symbolic importance of Hawaiian Royalty led to the extinction of some species; Easter Islanders on Rapa Nui are said to have experienced collapse of civilization after a century long drought, deforestation and conflict, and bustling cities in Tikal, in present-day Guatemala, were likely abandoned due to a combination of deforestation and drought. Today, we are seeing communities collapse, with places as diverse as Thailand's Koh Khai Islands, banning public access to three of its islands to reduce environmental degradation.

Rethinking Growth

The first few years of 1970s were marked by a growing environmental awareness and demands for strong governmental intervention to protect our atmosphere, water ways, oceans and land all showing signs of damage due to waste generated by economic activities. In the United States, the **Environmental Protection Agency** was established, and stronger Federal and State laws were enacted seeking to control and prevent air and water pollution and to remediate, restore and prevent further releases of toxic contaminants. In 1972, the Massachusetts Institute of Technology (MIT) published a report commissioned by the **Club of Rome**, a group founded in 1968 at Accademia dei Lincei in Rome, Italy, consisting of current and former heads of state, UN bureaucrats, high-level politicians and government officials, diplomats, scientists, economists, and business leaders from around the globe. The report, entitled "***Limits to Growth***"[5] was based on computer simulations of population and economic growth, and predicted that "business as usual" would deplete most natural resources over the twenty-first century, bringing to widespread public attention the idea that human activity was negatively impacting on planet Earth and we had to do something about it. While the Club of Rome has its critics, not least among academics who challenge the simplicity and assumptions of its models, the views of its founders, Aurelio Peccei, an Italian industrialist, and Alexander King, a Scottish scientist, are as true today as they were in the late 1960s.

> *Viewing the problems of mankind—environmental deterioration, poverty, endemic ill-health, urban blight, criminality—individually, in isolation or as "problems capable of being solved in their own terms," was doomed to failure. All are interrelated.*[5]

By the early 1980s many western European countries, the United States, Canada, and Japan were focused on addressing environmental problems associated with energy, transport, and industrial activities. However, many global environmental challenges had not been adequately addressed, such as manmade chemicals destroying the stratospheric ozone layer, acid rain, deforestation, and desertification along with mercury contamination of fish and many others threats to our shared natural environment.

GLOBALIZATION OF ENVIRONMENTAL CONCERNS

Earth Summit 1992

In 1992, the UN Conference on Environment and Development (UNCED), termed the "**Earth Summit**,"[6] drew delegates to Rio de Janeiro to participate in the world's first such gathering to explore the growing perils of environmental degradation. It was recognized that international cooperation and coordination was needed to address the challenges of sustainability on a global scale. Thus, began the truly multinational endeavor among UN member countries and numerous nongovernmental organizations (NGOs, civic, and corporate) that sought to alter patterns of human consumption, development and waste management that threatened both human well-being *and* the earth's ecosystems. The **Rio Earth Summit of 1992**[6] and the Brundtland Report of 1987[1] were transformational in their reach and impact offering a common and perhaps more acceptable lexicon for the Club of Rome's "limits to growth,"[5] Paul Ehrlich's "population bomb"[7] and Rachel Carson's "silent spring."[8] Framed as **Sustainable Development**, a way forward was being articulated to help shape policies, formulate consensus and raise social consciousness.

Global Reporting Initiative

The Global Reporting Initiative (GRI) is an NGO, its origin inspired by the Earth Summit. By 1998, GRI established a voluntary reporting framework for corporations that that included social, economic, and governance issues. It has been said of GRI, that its "guidance became a Sustainability Reporting Framework, with the Reporting Guidelines at its heart."[9] This remarkable effort sought to take the somewhat indefinite concept of sustainable development and translate it to measurable actions that corporations could pursue. GRI's consensus-driven efforts in establishing reporting guidelines and indicators to help companies document their social and environmental activities has been impactful. Many thousands of companies now publish an annual sustainability report, documenting progress across many sustainability domains, measuring consumption of energy, water, materials, and production of waste and identifying areas for action to drive efficiency and effectiveness and create value.

Many other NGOs have emerged in this social accountability space. They have developed reporting standards seeking to scrutinize, encourage, and activate governments, companies, and individuals to think and act more responsibly on a myriad of topics promoting social and environmental justice such as fair trade, child labor, work practices in the apparels industry, chemicals in personal care and cleaning products, sustainable practices in tourism and the like. It would be safe to say that a movement towards a more sustainable future was now well underway, although there is much more to do on developing metrics with high face validity.

First Attempt to Agree a Global Consensus to Curb Greenhouse Gases

The first Rio Earth Summit brought the world's focus to the problems of water scarcity, the negative impacts of energy, agriculture, transportation, and production of material goods. From this UN Summit emerged seminal actions, such as the **Climate Change Convention**[10] with its early agreements, known as the **Kyoto Protocol**,[11] where 41 countries and the European Union pledged to keep greenhouse gas (GHG) emissions at 5.2% below 1990 levels through the "commitment period" of 2008–12. Ratified in 2005, the Kyoto Protocol represented a significant international environmental treaty, albeit China and the United States as major polluters did not join. China as a "developing" country did not want to constrain its economic growth. While the US President, Bill Clinton, did sign up to the Kyoto Protocol at the end of his administration, his successor President George Bush decided the United States would not abide with it because the agreement did not impose as strict constraints on emissions in developing countries and concerns that compliance could harm the United States. It is widely understood that both China and the United States did not endorse the Kyoto Protocol given the influence of U.S. multinational energy companies.

Another important achievement of the Rio Summit was **Agenda 21**,[12] an important UN document that discloses the growing disparities between developed and developing economies. It calls for reforms of environmental protections and resource conversations and includes a blueprint for governments, businesses, communities and companies to make structural changes to improve access to education, technology, and financing. Agenda 21 was a prelude to the Millennium Development Goals,[13] followed by the Sustainable Development Goals.[14]

The United Nations Convention on Biological Diversity

The United Nations Convention on Biological Diversity (CBD)[15] is a multilateral treaty, introduced at the Rio Earth Summit 1992,[6] adopted in December 1993. All nations, except the United States, have ratified the CBD, which calls for conservation of biological diversity (or biodiversity), the sustainable use of nature, and an equitable sharing of benefits arising from genetic resources. The **Conference of the Parties** (COP)[16] to the Convention has come together on several occasions with responsibility for tracking progress and authoring amendments to the treaty. Departing from more traditional conservation efforts of primarily protecting species and habitats, members of the COP to the Conventions recognized human benefits provided by ecosystems. The CBD now asserts that utilizing natural systems, species, and genes needs to be done in a way and at a rate that preserves and enhances long-term biological diversity. However, the CBD is *not* working. Some 25 years after its adoption and 14 international meetings of the COP to the Convention, the UN issued a dire warning in 2019. In its report, the **"Intergovernmental Science-Policy Platform on Biodiversity and Ecosystem Services,"** the loss of species and natural habitat was said to be at a dangerous level and accelerating.[17]

Johannesburg Earth Summit 2002

The Rio Earth Summit 1992 also created the **Commission on Sustainable Development**,[18] tasked with following up on the first summit; the Earth Summit 2002 was held in Johannesburg, South Africa. Leaders from government, business, and NGOs agreed to the **Johannesburg Declaration**[19] that reinforced the aspirations of the Rio conference and provided important inflection points. Clearly, there was a need for better integration of sustainable development activities among several relevant UN agencies, programs, and funds. For the first time, on an international stage, there was discussion on the role of international financial institutions and multilateral development banks. Further, the voices of indigenous people were sought with an agreement *"not to carry out any activities on the lands of indigenous peoples that would cause environmental degradation or that would be culturally inappropriate."*[19] Delegates were confronted with the reality of reconciling "sustainable development" with extreme poverty and hunger worldwide,

BOX 80-2 Agenda 21 is a 350-page Document Divided into 40 Chapters, Grouping into Four Sections

- ***Section I: Social and Economic Dimensions*** *is directed toward combating poverty, especially in developing countries, changing consumption patterns, promoting health, achieving a more sustainable population, and sustainable settlement in decision making.*
- ***Section II: Conservation and Management of Resources for Development*** *includes atmospheric protection, combating deforestation, protecting fragile environments, conservation of biological diversity (biodiversity), control of pollution and the management of biotechnology, and radioactive wastes.*
- ***Section III: Strengthening the Role of Major Groups*** *includes the roles of children and youth, women, NGOs, local authorities, business and industry, and workers; and strengthening the role of indigenous peoples, their communities, and farmers.*
- ***Section IV: Means of Implementation*** *includes science, technology transfer, education, international institutions, and financial mechanisms.*[12]

with an important recognition that sustainability was far less relevant to about a third of the world's population. About 2 billion people experience disparities in health, housing, access to clean water and nutrition, sanitation, education, income and gender inequities, and the Johannesburg Declaration committed the almost 300 international participants to partnerships and initiatives to achieve the **Millennium Development Goals** (MGDs)[13]; these were elaborated 2 years earlier at the UN Millennium Summit and were to be achieved by 2015.

Rio+20: UN Conference on Sustainable Development, Rio 2012

In 2012, the UN Conference on Sustainable Development was also held in Rio and is commonly called **Rio+20** or the **Rio Earth Summit 2012**,[20] with officials representing 192 governments renewing their political commitment to sustainable development through the support of the nonbinding document "**The Future We Want**,"[21] which was an extension of Agenda 21.

World-thinking Begins to Pivot: Sustainable Development Goals and the Paris Agreement on Climate Change

Other outcomes of the 2012 Summit reflected a slow acceptance of the need to address some of the challenges hindering significant progress, recognizing the MDGs were not comprehensive and would likely not be achieved by 2015. There was discussion about replacing the MDGs with a suite of **Sustainable Development Goals** (SDGs; see Fig. 80-3)[22] accompanied by measurable targets and aimed at promoting sustainable development globally and including the environment. The use of gross domestic product (GDP: a monetary measure of the market value of all the final goods and services produced in a specific time period, often annually), as a measure of national wealth was challenged because it did not account for environmental and social factors. It was recognized that *"fundamental changes in the way societies consume and produce are indispensable for achieving global sustainable development"*[23] with **"environmental services"** and the economic value provided by nature, such as carbon sequestration and habitat protection, being considered.

The SDGs emerged from decades of work by countries and the UN, including the UN Department of Economic and Social Affairs, and can be traced back to Agenda 21[12] and the MDGs.[13] Formally initiated in 2013, when the UN General Assembly set up a 30-member Open Working Group to develop a proposal on the SDGs, the General Assembly began the negotiation process on the post-2015 development agenda in January 2015. When the **193-member countries of the United Nations adopted the SDGs**, it marked the first time the global community agreed on an actionable agenda with priorities, goals, and targets that include all countries and all citizens.

BOX 80-3 The Future We Want—Declaration of the UN Conference on Sustainable Development, Rio (2012)

Policy Document Topics: Policy instruments Sustainability transitions Resource efficiency and waste

The Future We Want is the declaration on sustainable development and a green economy adopted at the UN Conference on Sustainable Development in Rio on June 19, 2012. The Declaration includes broad sustainability objectives within themes of Poverty Eradication, Food Security and Sustainable Agriculture, Energy, Sustainable Transport, Sustainable Cities, Health and Population and Promoting Full and Productive Employment. It calls for the negotiation and adoption of internationally agreed Sustainable Development Goals by end 2014. It also calls for a UN resolution strengthening and consolidating UNEP both financially and institutionally so that it can better disseminate environmental information and provide capacity building for countries.[21]

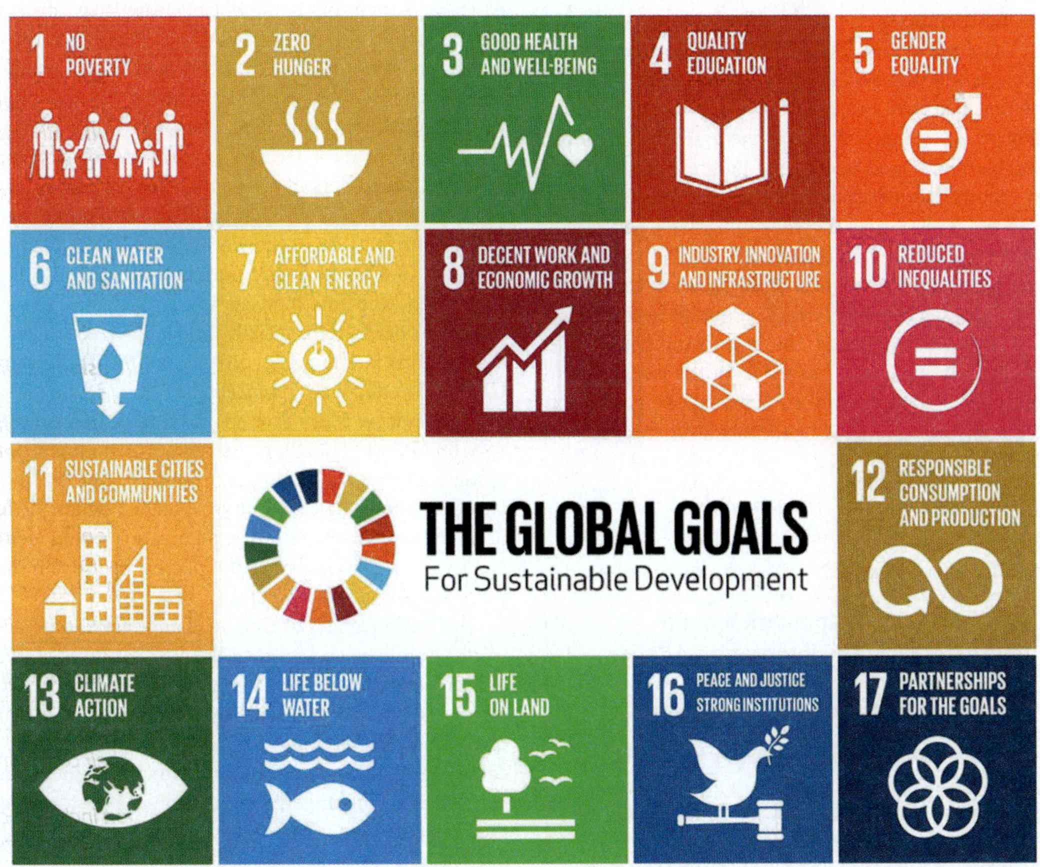
1 NO POVERTY
2 ZERO HUNGER
3 GOOD HEALTH AND WELL-BEING
4 QUALITY EDUCATION
5 GENDER EQUALITY
6 CLEAN WATER AND SANITATION
7 AFFORDABLE AND CLEAN ENERGY
8 DECENT WORK AND ECONOMIC GROWTH
9 INDUSTRY, INNOVATION AND INFRASTRUCTURE
10 REDUCED INEQUALITIES
11 SUSTAINABLE CITIES AND COMMUNITIES
THE GLOBAL GOALS
For Sustainable Development
12 RESPONSIBLE CONSUMPTION AND PRODUCTION
13 CLIMATE ACTION
14 LIFE BELOW WATER
15 LIFE ON LAND
16 PEACE AND JUSTICE STRONG INSTITUTIONS
17 PARTNERSHIPS FOR THE GOALS

FIGURE 80-3. The Sustainable Development Goals.[22]

The resulting **"Transforming our world: the 2030 Agenda for Sustainable Development"**[23] has **17 goals** at its core and provides a guide for global action on people, planet, prosperity, peace, and partnership. The near universal signings among country leaders of the SDGs and the Paris COP21 Climate Change[24] agreements in 2015 were significant in moving the issues of sustainability further up international, business, and public agendas.

With the SDGs, we have a **world strategy** that seeks to promote and improve the **health and well-being of the global population** in a concerted, coordinated, and accelerated manner. As a blueprint to achieve a better and more sustainable future for all, they seek to address the global challenges we face, including those related to poverty, inequality, climate, environmental degradation, prosperity, and peace and justice. The goals are **hyper-connected and interdependent** and call out the need for dynamic creativity and **radical collaboration** where no one is left. It is a **public health imperative** that we achieve each goal and underlying targets no later than 2030.

The annual **High-level Political Forum on Sustainable Development**[27] serves as the central UN platform for follow-up and review of the SDGs. The Division for Sustainable Development Goals (DSDG) in the UN Department of Economic and Social Affairs (UNDESA) provides substantive support and capacity-building for the SDGs and their related thematic issues including water, energy, climate, oceans, urbanization, transport, sciences and technology, the Global Sustainable Development Report (GSDR), partnerships and Small Island Developing States. DSDG plays a key role in the evaluation of UN system-wide implementation of the 2030 Agenda and on advocacy and outreach activities relating to the SDGs. In order to make the 2030 Agenda a reality, broad ownership of the SDGs must translate into a strong commitment by all stakeholders to implement the global goals; DSDG aims to help facilitate this engagement (see Fig. 80-4).

Annual SDG Progress Reports

In signing the SDGS, nations of the world acknowledge a collective responsibility to share prosperity. The 2030 Agenda for Sustainable Development pledges that the SDGs will be achieved by 2030 and progress toward that objective has been tracked since 2016 in the Annual SDGs Report. At the time of writing, the **2019 SDG Report**[28] is the latest available report and documents progress, highlighting those areas that require more attention. The **report** delivers a serious message, with sea levels rising, ocean acidification accelerating, and the past 4 years the warmest on record with 1 million plant and animal species at risk of extinction and land degradation continuing unchecked. Natural disasters, droughts, fires, excessive heat increase human suffering, particularly among the most vulnerable, with food supplies challenged and global hunger is on the rise. António Guterres, Secretary-General of the United Nations, offered the following perspective on the conditions of the world in the Forward section of the 2019 Report, stating that:

> *... progress is being made in some critical areas, and that some favorable trends are evident. Extreme poverty has declined considerably, the under-5 mortality rate fell by 49 per cent between 2000 and 2017, immunizations have saved millions of lives, and the vast majority of the world's population now has access to electricity. Countries are taking concrete actions to protect our planet: marine protected areas have doubled since 2010; countries are working concertedly to address illegal fishing; 186 parties have ratified the Paris Agreement on climate change, and almost all have communicated their first nationally determined contributions. About 150 countries have developed national policies to respond to the challenges of rapid urbanization, and 71 countries and the European Union now have more than 300 policies and instruments supporting sustainable consumption and production.*[28]

BOX 80-4 The Year 2015: A Landmark Year for Multilateralism and International Policy

- **Sendai Framework for Disaster Risk Reduction**, March 2015[25]
- **Addis Ababa Action Agenda on Financing for Development**, July 2015[26]
- **Transforming our world: The 2030 Agenda for Sustainable Development**, September 2015[23]
- **Paris Agreement on Climate Change**, December 2015[24]

Progress in meeting the **SDG goals is dependent on multisector engagement**. It is therefore encouraging that, along with national efforts, many academic institutions, businesses as well as international and local institutions across many sectors of private and civic society identify with the SDGs and are working toward their delivery in different ways. Given that agencies of national governments do not have the financial resources nor the regulatory reach to accomplish these ambitious goals alone, meeting and sustaining the SDGs will require fundamental restructuring of public and private institutions not least of which are financial markets. Of greatest concern now is the **deterioration of the natural environment**. The Stockholm Resilience Centre of Stockholm University offered an alternative way of displaying the SDGs, which is helpful to appreciating their interdependency and connectedness. Moving away from the typical graphic showing the SDGs as a series of blocks organized in rows, the revised graphic shows how the economy and society are nested into the biosphere which forms the basis of sustainable development. Positioning the earth's ecosystem as the foundation of all the other SDGs reflects the dynamic interdependency of the planet's natural systems with people and prosperity.[29]

Paris Agreement 2015

After a series of conferences mired in disagreements, the Conference of the Parties (COP)[16], referring to the countries that had signed up to the 1992 UN Framework Convention on Climate Change (UNFCC)[24], was held in Paris, France, in 2015. COP21[30] was negotiated by representatives of 196 state parties and adopted by consensus on 12 December 2015. As of November 2018, 195 UNFCCC members have signed the agreement, and 184 have become party to it. This global, but *nonbinding*, agreement seeks to limit the increase of the world's average temperature to no more than 2°C (3.6°F) above preindustrial levels, while at the same time striving to keep this increase to 1.5°C (2.7°F) above preindustrial levels in order to substantially reduce the risks and effects of climate change. This landmark accord, signed by all 196 signatories of the UNFCCC, effectively replaced the Kyoto Protocol. It mandated a progress review every 5 years and established a development fund of $100 billion by 2020, to be replenished annually, to help developing countries adopt nongreenhouse-gas-producing technologies. However, these goals are not yet matched by the pledges of individual countries which, even if implemented, would mean we could see 3°C by 2100—the last time the planet was this hot being 3 million years ago in the Pliocene era!

The consequences of climate change could dramatically alter our world, from sea-level rises to deadly heatwaves and killer floods as well as droughts. Climate migration is inevitable particularly of island nations. There will be climate refugees as well, as agriculture fails and conflicts over land and water arise. Marginalized people in low-income countries are more vulnerable to disruptions brought on by climate change. The underlying problem of how to reduce poverty and thus build resilience in low-income countries through a more productive agriculture and diversified economies without, in the process, exacerbating the global and local environmental burdens. Indeed,

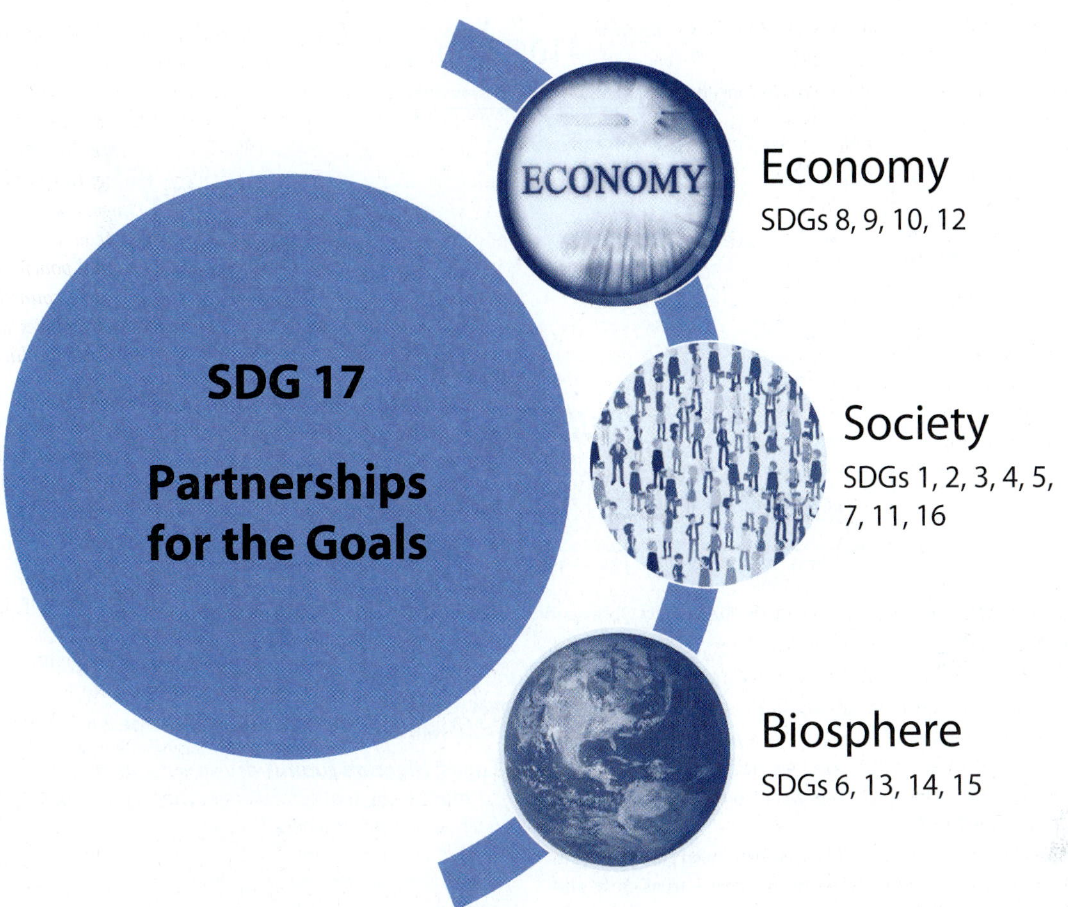

FIGURE 80-4. Schematic to show the earth's ecosystem as the foundation of all the other Sustainable Development Goals to illustrate the dynamic interdependency of the planet's natural systems with society and the economy.[29]

until recently, it appeared that neither high-income countries in the North nor low-income countries in the South were willing to give up economic development based on unfettered growth. The COP21 meeting in Paris in 2015 was in fact a remarkable departure from the traditional North-South divide, offering a viable way forward to address climate change and representing a concerted global recognition of climate as a shared human crisis.

WE ARE STILL IN TROUBLE!

The euphoria of the Paris Agreement has given way to a sober reality that the nations of the world are falling short on their pledged reductions in GHG. While many states and cities in the United States have confirmed their commitments to stay in the Paris Agreement, U.S. President Trump has pulled the United States out of the Agreement. The United States now stands apart from all the nations of the world having no federal commitment to reduce GHG.

The signs that we are losing ground on curbing the emission of atmospheric-warming gases are clear. When Charles Keeling[31] first began his pioneering measurements of background concentration of CO_2 at the remote NOAA observatory on Mona Loa, Big Island, Hawaii levels were about 250 ppm. These early records showed the season cycling in CO_2 concentrations and an upward trend of approximately 1 ppm per year. Currently, CO_2 levels are rising at an alarming rate of 3 ppm.[20] Global background levels of CO_2 measured at NOAA's Mona Loa observatory in a remote location on Hawaii's Big Island was 413.92 ppm in June 2019, which was 3ppm higher than a year earlier.

Population Growth and Urbanization

The world population in 2019 is 7.7 billion, nearly 2000 times what it was 12 millennia ago.[32] Historical demographers estimate the population grew very slowly, by just 0.04% annually, over the period 10,000 B.C. to the year 1700, reaching 1 billion around the year 1800. At the dawn of agriculture, about 8000 B.C., the population of the world was approximately 5 million. Over the 8000-year period up to 1 A.D. it grew to 200 million, with a growth rate of under 0.05% per year. After this time, it changed fundamentally with the industrial revolution: whereas it had taken all of human history until around 1800 for the world population to reach 1 billion, the second billion was achieved in only 130 years (1930), the third billion in 30 years (1960), the fourth billion in 15 years (1974), and the fifth billion in only 13 years (1987). During the twentieth century, the population grew from 1.65 billion to 6 billion and the median estimate for future growth sees the **world population reaching 8.6 billion in 2030**, 9.8 billion in 2050 and 11.2 billion by 2100 (assuming a continuing decrease in average fertility rate from 2.5 births per woman in 2010–15 to 2.2 in 2045–50 and to 2.0 in 2095–2100).[33]

Around 108 billion people have ever lived on our planet, meaning today's population makes up less than 10% of the total number of people ever born. **The global population growth rate** reached a peak in 1962 and 1963, with an annual growth rate of 2.2%. Since then, world population growth has been declining and the UN forecasts this will continue in the coming decades. In addition, yet, concerns around **overpopulation** abound as few countries can maintain their own welfare without technological and environmental intervention, with growing standards of living threaten our planetary ecosystem.

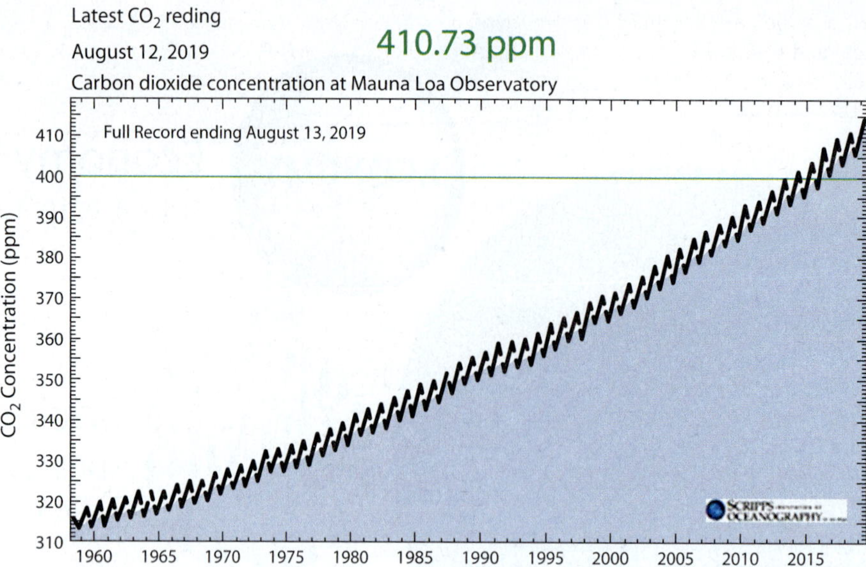

FIGURE 80-5. Carbon dioxide concentrations at the Mauna Loa Observatory.[31] (*Source*: Used with Permission from The Keeling Curve, Scripps Institution of Oceanography.https://keelingcurve.ucsd.edu/.)

With changes to climate, agricultural land and ocean food supplies are at risk; some call for population control policies, while others point to concerns over food waste noting we have enough resources to sustain over 10 billion people were we to steward our natural resources more sustainably.[34]

Urbanization is exacerbating strains on our natural systems, with some 55% of the world's population living in urban areas now and forecast to increase to 68% by 2050. This movement into cities will challenge quality of life across a range of domains as well as rural support systems. With India, China, and Nigeria together accounting for 35% of the projected growth of the world's urban population between 2018 and 2050, **the 100-million-person city**[33] is already predicted. Under an extreme scenario, where countries are unable to control fertility rates and urbanization continues apace, research has predicted that within 35 years more than 100 cities will have populations larger than 5.5 million people with the world's population centers shifting to Asia and Africa by the year 2100 and only 14 of the 101 largest cities in Europe or the Americas.

What happens to our cities over the next 30 years will determine the global environment and the quality of life of the world's projected 11 billion people. The UN notes[34] that much of humanity is young, fertile, and increasingly urban; for example, the median age of Nigeria is just 18, and under 20 across all Africa's 54 countries and the fertility rate of the continent's 500 million women is 4.4 births. Elsewhere, half of India's population is under age 25, and Latin America's average age is 29. The UN projects that the world's population will grow by nearly 3 billion people, equivalent to adding another China and India in the next 30 years, with 80–90% of people living in cities. Whether these cities are truly sustainable or are chaotic slums is an urgent issue for collective global action. Some suggest urbanization reduces humanity's environmental impact, while others fear cities will become ungovernable with conflict arising because of resource scarcity and ill health.

The United Nation's population forecasts show that countries experiencing the world's most rapid population growth over the coming decades will also be on the front line of climate change. The **Climate Vulnerability Index**[35] draws on datasets from bodies such as the World Bank and Intergovernmental Panel on Climate Change (IPCC) to determine the physical impacts of climate change on a given country and ranks 193 countries on their relative risk. Nine of out of the 10 most vulnerable countries are in sub-Saharan Africa, with total population predicted to double up to the year 2050; Europe and the United States are low risk with populations forecast to increase by 5% and 15%, respectively. This illustrates the **unequal distribution of climate change impacts** across developing and developed nations, and the difficulty of managing population growth in **climate-vulnerable environments** making it harder to reduce poverty levels. With the IPCC calling for a 45% cut in global emissions to have a chance of meeting the 1.5°C target, and just 11 years to go, it has been said that "winning slowly is the same as losing."[36]

BOX 80-5 Lagos, a 100-million-person city

Lagos, Nigeria's capital, *developed from a small coastal city surrounded by semirural villages that grew some 100-fold from under 200,000 people to some 20 million people in just two generation. Today, Lagos is one of the world's largest cities comprising wealthy neighborhoods alongside sprawling informal settlements or slums. Most people in the city are not connected to piped water or sanitation; traffic is dire and air quality poor. Forecast to become the world's largest metropolis, home to some 100 million people, the city boundary could stretch to hundreds of miles with accompanying negative environmental and quality of life effects.*[33]

Persistent Air Pollution

Air pollution has grown worse in both developed and developing countries given our global dependence on fossil fuels for electricity and transportation.[37] As the most significant contributor to climate-forcing GHG (CO_2 and methane), billions of people are exposed to harmful pollutants. While biomass fuels like wood, charcoal, peat, and dried animal dung bring warmth and can heat food for people it can also stunt their growth, harm their health and shorten their lives. Those living with the modern conveniences derived from "cleaner" fuels like electricity and gas cannot completely escape the hazards of air pollution. Besides localized exposure in homes and along roadways, emissions from combusting fossil fuels in factories generating electrical power can travel through the air for long distances. For example, pollution from coal burning in China drifts across Taiwan, Korea, and Japan and at times impacts the west coast of the United States and Canada. Illegal burning of forests in Sumatra and Indonesia to plant palm trees can poison the air in Malaysia and Singapore, while mercury from coal and other sources can enter our food chain and turn up in seafood dinners. The **Global Burden of**

Disease[38] attributes over 3.5 million deaths annually to bad air, with the worse impacts in India and China. Accounting for the attributable deaths from household use of dirty fuels there are an additional 4 million deaths annually. The UN World Health Organization (WHO) reports worldwide that ambient air pollution contributed to 7.6% of all deaths in 2016.

> *9 out of 10 people worldwide breathe polluted air, but more countries are acting.*[37]

Ecosystems in Peril

The UN Report "*Nature's Dangerous Decline 'Unprecedented'; Species Extinction Rates 'Accelerating,'*" provides the most comprehensive assessment of its kind noting some 1 million species are threatened with extinction.[39] The UN's latest report, May 2019, about humanity's impact on plant and animal species "Intergovernmental Science-Policy Platform on Biodiversity and Ecosystem Services"[17] estimates extinction rates are 100 times higher than ever before, predicting up to a million species becoming extinct in near decades, with negative impacts on seas, forests, agriculture, and humans. Calling on governments to shift subsidies and incentives away from polluting and extractive industries towards protecting and restoring natural systems, the report calls for a paradigm shift—a radical reorganizing of technological, economic, and social systems. There is therefore an urgent need for climate and resource risks to be better understood with new strategies required to put a value on natural and cultural assets as we move to a low carbon economy.

Mercury in the Environment

Mercury (Hg) is a dangerous neurotoxin that can disrupt brain function and harm the nervous system; it is especially threatening to pregnant women and young children. Hg in our food supply and in our bodies is an example of misuse of a public good: the atmosphere. Alkali and metal processing, incineration of coal, and medical and other waste, and mining of gold and mercury contribute greatly to mercury concentrations in some areas, but atmospheric deposition is the dominant source of mercury over most of the landscape.[40] Discharges of Hg from coal-fired power plants have long been recognized as the most important anthropogenic source of this bioaccumulating contaminant. Elemental Hg is methylated by bacteria and becomes biologically available in its organic form. Hg-contaminated fish in Nordic lakes far from the coal-burning power plants of Northern Europe were an early warning of the long distance transport of mercury.

Fortunately, there are useful guides available to help consumer select seafood containing less mercury, caught or raised in responsibly managed fisheries[41] along with the Monterey Aquarium Sea Watch recommendations.[42] Generally, smaller seafood such scallops and fish like sardines, contain less mercury than larger varieties like tuna and swordfish, which are higher up the food chain. While the UN Minamata Convention to reduce the global discharge of mercury was reversing levels of contamination in highly consumed species,[43] there is new evidence that heightens concern. The perverse coincidence of warmer waters in the Gulf of Maine and overfishing of feedstock is changing the levels of mercury in fish. In an article in *Nature*[44] researchers modelled how environmental factors, including increasing sea temperatures and overfishing, could affect levels of methylmercury in fish. The team found that while regulation of mercury emissions has successfully reduced methylmercury levels in fish, spiking temperatures are driving those levels back up and will play a major role in the methylmercury levels of marine life in the future.

Plastics

One word—plastics—"There's a great future in plastics,"[45] that iconic line from The Graduate (1967) takes on a new meaning as plastic pollution becomes widespread—with 94% of the Great Pacific Garbage Patch made up of plastic. Plastics have been at the center of the modern economy, with global production surging from 15 million metric tonnes in 1964 to 311 in 2014, projected to double to more than 600 in the next 20 years. Plastic packaging, especially the so-called single-use product, represents a quarter of the total volume of plastics and around 95% is lost to the economy each year but lives on in our environment for centuries. If plastics demand follows it current trajectory, global plastics waste volumes would increase from 260 million tons per year to nearly half a billion tons each year by 2030. The recent report[46] on "The New Plastics Economy: Rethinking the future of plastics" calls for the principles of the circular economy to be used to reshape the global plastic packaging flows and could drastically reduce negative externalities—valued by the United Nations at US$40 billion. Recycling plastics could also create a new business model, which has been estimated to represent a profit pool of U.S. $55 billion per year by 2020.[47]

Today, almost a third of all plastic packaging leaks into our oceans, with 8 million metric tons polluting our oceans each year. Plastic in our oceans matters. Plastic is a people problem, so we need to work upstream for impact and to save our oceans and humanity. The film "Albatross"[48] shows how beauty and grief can catalyze personal actions, leading to societal transformations. That is exactly what happened for Shaun Frankson, Co-Founder of The Plastic Bank[49] and his concept of "social plastic" through his work on plastic as currency. Empowering people to be social entrepreneurs, collecting ocean plastic and exchanging this for currency, and investing in their communities.

Microplastics, so-called because they are 5 mm in diameter or smaller, are everywhere, in the air we breathe, the food we eat, in our water and even our sewage coming from the disintegration of larger plastics into fragments.[50] Even if we stopped the production of all plastics today, we still have billions of tons to clean up worldwide. There is work underway to recycle ocean plastic, from Interface's[51] seminal work on creating carpets from ocean fishing nets to Prada's Re-nylon[52] project using regenerated nylon, called ECONYL made from ocean plastics and textile fiber waste, for its iconic bags. New technology, such as nanocoils[53] are also being trialed, a new hybrid material that generates free radicals that cause microplastics to break into tiny pieces that eventually become converted to CO_2 and water. The U.K. Government reported[54] single-use plastic bag sales in August 2019, noting that since the introduction in October 2015 of a mandatory small charge (equivalent to 6 cents U.S. currency) for bags by large retailers' distribution has fallen by 90%; the charge has raised just over $200M for charities since it began. Other nations, states, and cities however have implemented an outright ban on plastic bags, with the United Kingdom still distributing 1.1 billion bags in 2018–19.

A WAY FORWARD ON CLIMATE CHANGE SOLUTIONS

The Climate Agreement reached at the 2015 Paris Conference of the Parties[30] recognized the need to keep the earth's temperature from exceeding 2°C. The UN IPCC models[55] indicate that to accomplish this goal it would require keeping GHG below 500 ppm CO_2 equivalence (CO_2e); CO_2e accounts for the warming potential of other infrared-absorbing molecules in the atmosphere and considers the expected residence time for those molecules. Currently the global background levels of CO_2 are approaching 415 ppm (the CO_2e at the signing of the Paris Agreement was 485 CO_2e). Synthetic fluorinated hydrocarbons, long used as refrigerants, are potent GHG. While now less abundant, they can be released when equipment like air conditioners, chillers, and heat pumps is recharged. Alternative working fluids/gases could go a long way to controlling these GHG. Second to CO_2 from combustion of fuels (fossil and biomass) as an important contributor to the increasing in CO_2e is methane (CH_4), an invisible and odorless GHG. Natural gas consists largely of methane, which has a global warming potential

86 times greater than CO_2 in a 20-year period, tailing off to about 29 times the effect of CO_2 in a 100-year period on a molecule per molecule basis.[40]

With CO_2e concentrations, increasing between 2 and 4 ppm per year there is a growing gap between the actual emissions and what is required to meet the commitments of the Paris Agreement. The NGO **Climate Action Tracker**[56] monitors progress in reducing emissions at a global and a country level. Global emissions could be 20% higher in 2030 instead of 20% lower as required by the Paris Agreement. Many climate experts posit that more than a 50% reduction in GHG is necessary by 2030 to avoid a 1.5°C rise in global temperature. Delaying serious reductions puts people and planetary ecosystems in peril. The month of July 2019 was the hottest ever recorded, with heatwaves across Europe and by mid-summer ice melt on Greenland was at an all-time high. The calculated flow of ice melt into the North Atlantic for July was equivalent 90 million Olympic size swimming pools!

Previously, the long-term measurements and trends in global CO_2 concentrations were presented, but atmospheric levels of methane are also increasing. With the relative boom in **unconventional oil and gas development** (UOGD)[57] in the United States and elsewhere, commonly referred to as **hydrofracking**, wells can be drilled horizontally and then water, chemicals, and sand is injected under high pressure to "fracture" underground deposits of oil and gas.[58] Tens of thousands of wells have been drilled over the past decade and UOGD has made the United States a net exporter of energy. The abundance of natural gas has made coal-fired power plants economically uncompetitive, but there is growing concern that more methane is being released to the atmosphere from UOGD. Methane leaks can occur across all stages of operations from extraction, compression, transmission, to underground storage and from leaking pipes both inside and outside of homes, buildings, and factories of customers. The U.S. Environmental Protection Agency (EPA), other federal agencies, and companies maintain an emission inventory of CO_2e gases from onshore and offshore petroleum and natural gas production, transmission and storage.[57] To be clear the GHG from this energy sector include CO_2, methane, and nitrous oxide (N_2O); in CO_2e terms, CO_2 and N_2O each account for about one third. The concern is underreporting. There are hundreds of old well sites being used for underground storage which do not meet current technical standards for check values, casings and inspection/maintenance. The Aliso Canyon gas leak in Southern California in 2015/2016 was a tragic example of multiple failures with old natural gas storage facilities.[59]

There are other important sources of methane that can be attributed to personal choices about **food consumption**. According to the **Food and Agriculture Organization of the United Nations** (FAO)[60], agriculture is responsible for 18% of the total release of GHG worldwide that is, more than the whole transportation sector. Cattle raising is a significant factor for these GHG emissions. Ruminating animals like cows can release between 70 and 120 kilograms (kg) of methane per year; with some 1.5 billion cows in the world some 2 billion metric tons of CO_2e are released per year. Meeting the increasing demand for beef means that more tropical forests are cleared for grazing. Carbon sequestration is thus lost, and soil carbon released as more rain forests are cleared and burned. These ranching activities add another 2.8 billion metric tons of CO_2 emissions per year.

The table below indicates the CO_2 production in kg CO_2 equivalents per kg of meat depending on the animal; these values can be substantially reduced if animals are raised using sound environmental practices. Cattle-rearing uses 33% of the arable land used for food production while raising lambs, pigs, and chicken have a much smaller footprint.

REASONS TO BE (GUARDEDLY) OPTIMISTIC

Saving the earth from more serious effects of the existential threat of climate change requires a restructuring of energy generation to renewable sources, making the built environment far more energy efficient, electrification of transportation and changes to food systems. Relying on governments, corporations, and institutions for these transformations will not be enough. Financial and consumer markets need to value the services derived from nature and the damages being caused to earth's ecosystems and human infrastructure. The cost for inaction will greatly exceed the investments urgently needed now to reduce GHG and adapt to the significant changes already "built in" to decades of excessive warming stored in our ocean temperatures.

In their book "**Designing for Climate Solutions**,"[62] authors Harvey, Orvis, and Rissman claim there are ways to tackle climate change with the knowledge and technology that already exists. Distributive energy systems consisting of solar or wind generation and battery storage are commercially available, for example, with Tesla's Powerpack systems installed on the island of Ta'u in American Samoa in 2016.[63] Since then, internet firms Facebook and Microsoft have joined with investment firms to accelerate microgrid installations in parts of India, Indonesia, and East Africa—with an estimated addressable market of 212 million people. Integrated solar and battery systems have a role now in avoiding expensive generating capacity to meet peak demand and, as battery capacity improves, energy consumption can be shifted to take advantage of lower generating costs. Batteries will displace the need for auxiliary generators when severe weather disrupts service.

Global and national inventories of GHG identify that energy for powering industry, transportation, buildings and our cities along with industrial processes including agriculture account for ~95% of emissions and defining the contributions of anthropogenic sources of GHG is important. There are multiple strategies available to reduce or eliminate these emissions through market or regulatory mechanisms. Corporations, institutions, governments, consumers, insurance and financial markets need the proper economic signals, and legislative requirements to spur the transformations needed to combat climate change. Acting now *before* conditions get worse requires more than technological responses. Carbon-free electricity from hydro, wind, solar, and hydrogen with advanced battery storage is here now and disruptive companies like Tesla and Iberdrola are at the forefront of energy transformation.

While the power sector is changing, it will be a decade or more before most of the electricity supplied is with clean fuels. We therefore need to do more to reduce energy demand, for example, improving energy efficiency standards for consumer appliances, automobiles, homes, and buildings. While this is happening, we need to go further faster and some countries, states, and cities are exploring "net zero carbon building" requirements for new construction. However, most of what exists now will require energy to operate well into this twenty-first century such that efforts to retrofit with energy-efficient HVAC systems, lighting, insulation, windows, and cooler roofs are important. Greg Kats and Keith Glassbrook report "Delivering Urban Resilience"[64] make an economic case to cool cities with smart facades, white roofs, vegetation, and solar installations arguing that better choices of surfaces for cities are both cost-effective and essential for resilience in an increasingly warmer future.

The challenge ahead is to rapidly accelerate changes in markets and behaviors. Carbon pricing and/or carbon taxes have been put forward as ways to transform markets.[65] **Carbon pricing** starts with the premise that the use of fossil fuels and the release of GHGs are causing damage to the earth's ecosystem, agriculture, infrastructure, disruption to public services and commerce, and producing human suffering. For a free market to operate efficiently these external costs

BOX 80-6 Greenhouse gas and food

A Japanese study showed that producing 1 kg of beef leads to the emission of GHG with a global warming potential equivalent to 34.6 kg of CO_2 and releases fertilizing compounds equivalent to 340 grams of sulfur dioxide and 59 grams of phosphate and consumes 169 megajoules of energy. That is, a kg of beef is equivalent to the amount of CO_2 emitted by an average European car every 250 kilometers or enough energy to light a 100-watt bulb for nearly 20 days.[61]

BOX 80-7 1 kg Meat Produces CO_2e (kg)[47]

Beef 34.6
Lamb 17.4
Pork 6.35
Chicken 4.57
Source: Reference 61.

should be incorporated into what companies, governments, and consumers pay, being essentially an uncosted burden of unfettered shareholder capitalism. A **carbon tax** directly sets a price on carbon by defining a tax rate on GHGs or—more commonly—on the carbon content of fossil fuels. It is different from an **emission trading system** (ETS) in that the emission reduction outcome of a carbon tax is not predefined, but the carbon price is. An ETS, sometimes referred to as a **cap-and-trade system,** caps the total level of GHG emissions, and allows those industries with low emissions to sell their unused allowances to larger emitters. The trading establishes a market price for GHG emissions, while the cap helps ensure that the required emission reductions will take place in aggregate within a preallocated carbon budget.

By placing the financial burden on the polluter responsible for emitting the GHGs, carbon pricing sends an economic signal. As prices rise for commodities with higher carbon footprints, consumers should adjust their behaviors. For example, gasoline that is more expensive should mean an increase in ridership of public transit and purchases of more efficient cars and trucks. As electricity bills rise, if derived from coal and gas-fired generators, energy from renewable sources ought to be economically more viable. Polluters and consumers will then have to decide whether to stop paying higher prices. Alternatively, they can recalculate the return on investment (ROI) for energy conversation, fuel shifting, transportation, clean technologies, and industrial processes including carbon capture.

Carbon pricing schemes are now gaining momentum given leadership by the **World Bank**, with its overall environmental goal for carbon pricing to reduce, in the most flexible and least-cost way for society, dependency on fossil fuels. Its **Carbon Pricing Dashboard**[65] shows growing acceptance of financial mechanisms, covered 11 $GtCO_2e$, representing 20.1% of global GHG emissions in 2019. Encouragingly, some 40 countries and more than 20 cities, states, and provinces use carbon-pricing mechanisms, with more planning to implement them in the future. The **International Monetary Fund** also exercise responsible political and corporate leadership. At the **Carbon Pricing Leadership Coalition** (CPLC) Fourth Annual High-Level Assembly (HLA) (Spring 2018), efforts to organize a coalition of finance minister gained momentum. In February 2019, Finance Ministers from 19 countries met in Finland and signed the **Helsinki Principles** recognizing the seriousness of climate change and pledging to coordinate efforts.[66] This marked a significant shift in that governmental responsibilities, for climate change actions typically reside within environmental and/or health ministries. Realigning concerns for climate disruption to ministries of finance underscores how climate change represents an economic risk, as well as an opportunity, with infrastructure investments and taxing strategies that could be good fiscally while cutting carbon emissions. The World Bank estimates that responding to climate change could potentially require the investment of tens of trillion of dollars, yielding more than 50 million more jobs through 2030.[66]

While the February 2019 Helsinki meeting was a modest beginning, with just 19 nations represented, significant reductions in GHG *can* be accomplished if the top polluting countries commit. Of the approximately 50 gigatons of CO_2e currently emitted annually, just seven countries are responsible for more than half (China, USA, India, Indonesia, Russia, Brazil, and Japan). To build a worldwide consensus and make significant reductions, adding 13 more countries would account for nearly 80% of all global emissions; eight countries whose GHG emissions are 0.5–1 gigaton/year (Canada, Germany, Iran, Mexico, South Korai, Saudi Arabia, South Africa, and Australia) with five others in the top 20 GHG emitters at about 0.5 gigatons/year (United Kingdom, Nigeria, Argentina, Zambia, and Thailand). However, the re-emergence of nation states is a political reality promoted by more authoritarian leaders and populist political ideologies. This trend, if allowed to go unchallenged, may make it far more difficult to mobilize an international consensus to combat climate change. The adversarial, protectionist, and antiglobalism atmosphere disrupting the world's social order as we enter the 2020s, could not be happening at a worse time for our planet. Cooperation, at least among the 20 most polluting nations is desperately needed to reverse the trends in rising CO_2, methane, and other GHG. Concerted efforts to curb GHG emissions among the 20 named countries could change the course of human history in the twenty-first century. International agreements are needed to make financial mechanisms like carbon pricing and green fund investments effective. Without substantial progress in the next 10 years, it will be increasingly likely that technologies to remove CO_2 from stack gases and directly from the atmosphere will be needed. While "climate engineering" (see later) strategies are not popular now, if we are to avoid the devastating consequences of 3°C warming later in this century we may need to embrace them.

Carbon Capture and Storage

Carbon Capture and Storage (CCS) technology is not new but, given research and development efforts, is now becoming available at a price that makes it a viable proposition for industry.[67] CO_2 is highly concentrated in the discharge stacks of fossil fuel and biomass power stations, cement plants and other industrial facilities. Capture technology, by chemically absorbing CO_2 or by separation using membranes that allow the CO_2 molecule to pass through, could reduce emissions by 80–90%. The trapped gas can be deposited in underground storage sites or could be used in greenhouses to increase vegetation growth. As of 2019, there are 17 operating CCS projects in operation, mostly industrial facilities that are capturing 31.5Mt of CO_2 per year. Tax credits, carbon trading and carbon price will be necessary to accelerate CCS. The International Energy Agency (IEA)[68] calculates that CCS projects must capture 850 million tonnes of CO_2 by 2030 to meet the Paris commitments and estimates there will be a global market for CCS worth over $100B. CCS will provide investment opportunities as technology improves and applications expand, with projects already operating in many countries and for different types of facilities. The technology is getting better and offers significant health co benefits, from improved air quality, reduced air, and water pollution. As promising as CCS is, there are still technical challenges particularly with securing long-term stable storage. Further, not many electrical power plants are located where deep ocean or geological storage (abandoned oil and gas wells) would be feasible. There maybe technical solutions to overcome that limitation. CO_2 can be stored and degraded by algae or bacterium. Nature demonstrates long-term conversion and storage of carbon in limestone, a carbonate sedimentary rock. Ocean coral is composed of the skeletal remains of marine life that have capture carbon. For mineral storage, energy and catalyst are required to extract CO_2 and turn it into a stable form of carbonates. This technology is attractive because of it eliminates potential leaking from underground storage of compresses gas but currently comes with an energy penalty.[69]

Carbon Capture by Nature

Nature's ability to capture carbon is demonstrated in the Keeling CO_2 curves prepared from measurements make at NOAA's Mona Loa Observatory in Hawaii (Fig. 80-5).[31] During the growing season in the Northern Hemisphere (spring-summer), vegetation and algae incorporates vast amounts of carbon and global background CO_2 levels dip by a few ppm. Since most of the earth's land mass is above the equator, there is insufficient vegetation in the southern hemisphere to compensate for increased CO_2 emissions during the cooler months. Chapter 4 of the 2019 IPCC report[69] describes the complexities of land degradation and social need climate trade-offs. Agricultural soils have lost organic carbon content, deforestation, particularly of tropical forest (Amazon, Indonesia, Sumatra) for cattle and palm plantations result in important carbon sequestration loss and soil degradation. Even managed harvesting of old growth trees with replacement of new planning can be a net loss of carbon sequestration. Following years of reduced deforestation of the Amazon, it is on the rise again with trees covering an area the size of Yellowstone National Park cleared in 2017 to raise beef cattle. The report[69] suggests further land degradation can be avoided, reduced, or reversed by implementing sustainable land management, restoration, and rehabilitation practices as demonstrated on scales from small farms to large-scale recovery of watersheds and forest preserves. While well-managed forests systems can enhance carbon sinks and provide economic resources, replacing primary forest with new growth, managed forest comes at a price given carbon is released during logging and tilling and habitat disruption results in loss of biodiversity. If managed properly carbon storage in trees and long-lasting products made from wood can be an important climate mitigation strategy.

The restoration of forested land at a global scale could help capture atmospheric carbon and mitigate climate change. Thomas Crowther, a climate ecologist at the Swiss Federal Institute of Technology in Zurich coauthored an article published in *Science* on how planting a trillion trees could be done and the huge impact it could have on carbon capture.[70] The account states that "*...0.9 billion hectares is available for us to restore trees —and if we restored them and they grew to full mature forests, they would capture a major chunk of that excess carbon that is in the atmosphere and really help us in that fight against climate change*" Crowther and coauthors analyzed how much forest restoration potential across the globe was available outside existing forests and agricultural and urban land. Some 500 billion more trees could be grown on an additional 0.9 billion hectares, which could increase forested areas by more than 25%, and growing these forests to maturity would sequester more than 200 gigatonnes of additional carbon—equivalent to 4 years of current global emissions.

Direct Capture of CO_2 from the Air

With global levels of CO_2 exceeding 415 ppm, it might be too late for the countries of the world to get control of GHG sources to prevent more than a 2°C rise in global temperatures. Extracting CO_2 *directly* from the atmosphere is therefore attracting renewed attention, with a few enterprising companies showing that directly absorbing CO_2 from the air works. For example, Carbon Engineering,[71] a British Columbia, Canada firm has been working for nearly a decade on direct air capture technology using liquid potassium hydroxide flowed over grills across which a fan pulls air. Chemicals are then added, and the solution heated to create white pellets containing about 50% CO_2; further heating produces a highly concentrated CO_2, which can be combined with hydrogen extracted from water to make a clear, synthetic fuel like crude oil. Alternatively, the concentrated CO_2 or the pellets themselves can be stored. Closing the carbon loop by producing a valuable product that can be turned into products such as gasoline, diesel, and jet fuel is critical to the success of this innovative technology.[72] In 2017, the Swiss company Climeworks[73] set its goal to remove 1% of the atmospheric CO_2 by 2025 and opened the first commercial facility that can extract CO_2 from the atmosphere, using the concentrated CO_2 in a greenhouse operation close to the facility offering some optimism for our future. Scaled up, the recycled carbon could power vehicles, plants and be a substitute for petrochemicals without the additional use of fossil fuels. The concept of direct capture and conversion to a fuel does not however create a net reduction of CO_2 in the atmosphere.

Climate Engineering

Also known as "geoengineering," is the intentional large-scale intervention in the Earth's climate system to counter climate change.[74] It includes techniques to remove CO_2 from the atmosphere, and technologies to rapidly cool the Earth by reflecting solar energy back to space. Some proposed climate engineering technologies are highly controversial, spurring global debates about whether and under what conditions they should be considered, and reinforcing the pressing need for the United States and other nations to commit to aggressive reductions in heat-trapping emissions. Some CO_2 removal techniques (CDR), like reforestation, are well understood. Others entail using technologies to capture and sequester CO_2 that are in early research stages or currently are difficult to deploy at scale without high costs or substantial negative impacts on energy use, water, or land. Solar geoengineering, or "solar radiation management" (SRM) refers to technologies proposed to rapidly cool down Earth's temperature. Proposals include simulating the cooling effects of volcanic eruptions and enhancing the reflectivity of marine clouds. When volcanoes erupt, they spread into the atmosphere tiny light-colored aerosol particles that can reflect incoming energy from the sun in cloud-free air and dark particles can absorb it. A small fleet of aircraft, for example, could conceivably inject sulfate aerosols or other reflecting particles into the stratosphere and drive large-scale cooling. Marine cloud brightening proposals entail using sea salt to "seed" the formation of low-altitude clouds over the ocean, enhance their reflectivity, and extend their lifetimes. SRM technologies would however not limit some of the most serious impacts of rising CO_2 concentrations, including ocean acidification.

Capturing and removing CO_2 from the atmosphere (see above) could also be considered an example of climate engineering to mitigate the adverse effects of global warming. There are two main approaches to geoengineering: removing GHG or altering solar radiation, commonly done on smaller scales. The Kats and Glassbrook's "Delivering Urban Resilience"[64] provides a costs and benefits analysis of city-wide adoption of smart surfaces. Case studies of Washington DC, Philadelphia, and El Paso show possible benefits of billions of dollars over 40 years if these cities implement measures to cool buildings, streets, and parks. Benefits include improved health and livability, reduced urban inequality, and slowed global warming while strengthening the resiliency of these cities.[75] The challenge is how to bring climate engineering methods economically to a scale large enough to significantly reduce GHG and to cool extensive surfaces of the earth. Both the National

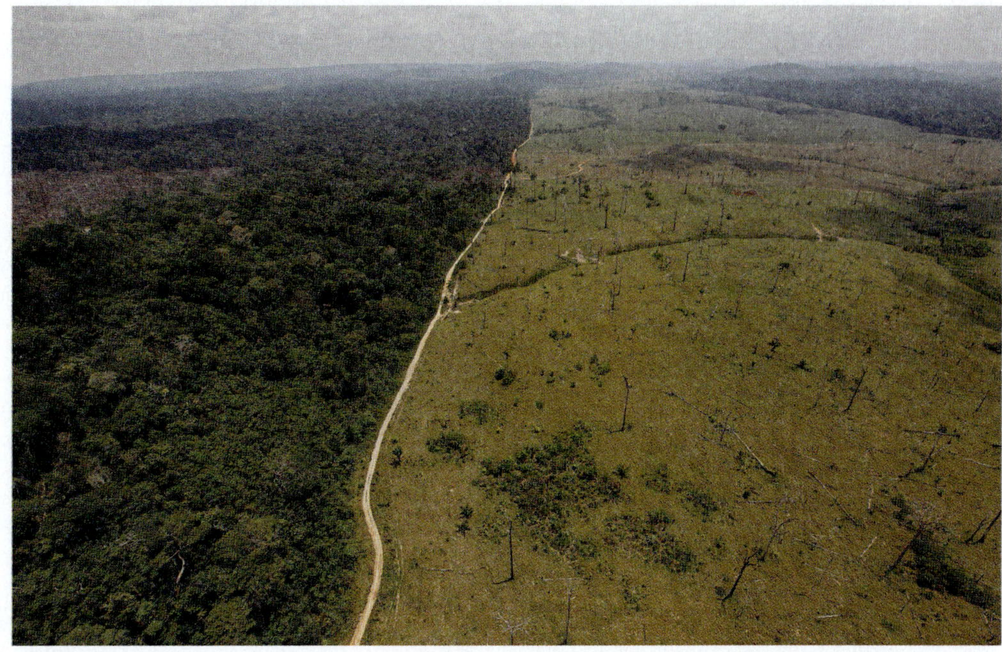

FIGURE 80-6. A deforested area near Novo Progresso in Brazil's northern state of Para. (*Source:* Andre Penner/AP Images.)

Academy of Science and the IPCC (5th Assessment Report) have assessed the feasibility and deliberated the benefits and risks for combating climate change with geoengineering approaches.[76] Climate engineering strategies for biological uptake of CO_2 are described in the IPCC 3rd Assessment Report.[77] One such method would be to "fertilize" specific areas of the ocean with iron to cause massive algae blooms, with the growing algae drawing carbon from the atmosphere, which would then remove the fixed carbon. Other examples of biological methods for removal that might be brought to scale include:

- Mixing biochar (i.e., in biomass-fired thermal power plants) into the soil to create terra preta;
- Bioenergy with carbon capture and storage to sequester carbon and simultaneously provide energy;
- Carbon air capture to remove CO_2 from ambient air; and
- Afforestation, reforestation, and forest restoration to absorb CO_2.

Reducing sunlight (ultraviolet, near infrared, and visible) absorbed in the atmosphere or at the surface, **Solar Radiation Management** (SRM)[76] techniques, can be achieved by deflecting sunlight away from the Earth, or by increasing the reflectivity (albedo) of the atmosphere or the Earth's surface. SRM approaches include:

- Protecting or expanding polar sea ice and glaciers, using pale-colored roofing materials;
- Marine cloud brightening, which would spray fine sea water to whiten clouds and thus increase cloud reflectivity;
- Creating reflective aerosols, such as stratospheric sulfate aerosols, specifically designed self-levitating aerosols or other substances; and
- Obstructing solar radiation with space-based mirrors, dust.

The **Union of Concerned Scientists**[78] offers an excellent explanation of climate engineering options, with precautionary discussions of unintended consequences. Calling for effective governance mechanisms to enable global society to consider the risks and potential benefits of these new technologies and make informed, they warn of "moral hazard" that investing in geoengineering may reduce our efforts to reduce net carbon emissions through proven and affordable means like renewable energy. They also raise issues relating to potential geopolitical conflict over "who decides" what the climate goals of deploying SRM would be. Forums like the **Carnegie Climate Geoengineering Governance Initiative** (C2G2), and the **Solar Radiation Management Governance Initiative** (SRMGI) consider the scientific and ethical implications of geoengineering.

Processes already occurring as part of the natural carbon, such as low-till agriculture, reforestation and afforestation, ocean iron fertilization, and land-and-ocean-based accelerated weathering, could amplify the rates of CO_2 removal.[75] Other CDR approaches, such as bioenergy with carbon capture and sequestration, direct air capture and sequestration, and traditional carbon capture and sequestration, seek to capture CO_2 from the atmosphere and dispose of it by pumping it underground at high pressure. Climate geoengineering has been viewed as a "last-ditch" response to climate change, but albedo modification—changing the fraction of incoming solar radiation that reaches the surface—is attracting attention.[76] However, a technology "fix" to modifying the Earth's albedo does not determine whether it should be done or what the consequences might be of such an action. Whatever portfolio of technologies are used, eliminating the CO_2 emissions from the global energy and transportation systems presents enormous technical, economic, and social challenges that will take decades of concerted effort to achieve.

SOME EXAMPLES OF SUSTAINABILITY SOLUTIONS

It is widely accepted that there is an urgent need for global collective action in support of delivery against the "wicked" challenges[79] reflected in Agenda 2030 the SDGs. The systemic transformational change needed will require new ways of working beyond simple incrementalism. This is a period of "punctuated equilibrium"[80] and will demand radical collaboration among public–private and plural organizations. Here we highlight a few examples of sustainability solutions that meet our criteria of **radical collaboration and systems thinking**, approaches we consider are urgently required to deliver against the SDGs. These examples highlight the importance of **local actions for global solutions** with delivery against the SDGs our shared purpose as humanity.

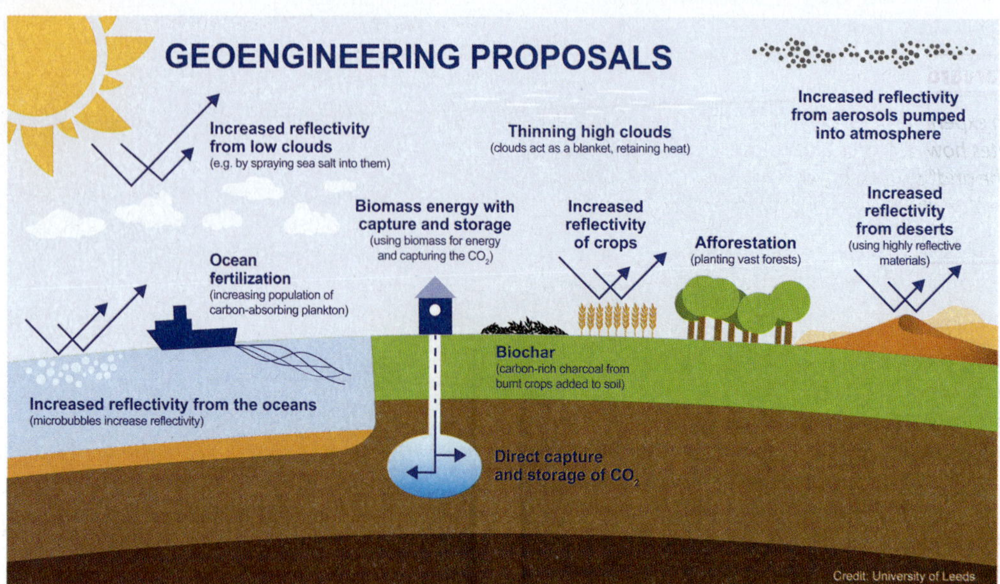

FIGURE 80-7. Approaches to climate engineering.[78] (*Source*: Reproduced with permission from University of Leeds.)

Communities of Opportunity

The work of Jonathon Rose Companies[81] relates to social housing and creating "communities of opportunity" that seek to attenuate the impact of adverse childhood experiences and promote well-being. By creating environmentally, socially, and economically responsible projects and plans Rose aims to equalize the landscape of opportunity for residents and improve the balance of human and nature. With a belief that every resident of every community deserves an equal opportunity to thrive, the team apply the transformative power of connected, integrative, well-designed, and thoughtfully planned places to help restore well-being. With buildings responsible for some one-third of GHG emissions, and transportation for another third, energy consumed by commuting by car can be as much as twice that of the building itself. Central to Jonathon Rose Companies mission as a sustainable, green real estate firm is its focus on greening the built environment by creating transit-oriented projects that are more healthful for tenants and residents. Energy-, water-, and waste-efficient development can help mitigate GHG and the effects of climate change. The goal for each project is to be a replicable model of environmental, social, and economic responsibility that contribute to the growing body of solutions to the challenges of inclusive twenty-first century cities.

> *The promise of a better life is too often constrained by ZIP code. Yet we know what it takes to more evenly distribute opportunity: affordable housing; meaningful work; accessible transportation; educational excellence; local health care; centers for arts and cultures, and community places of contemplation and compassion.*[81] Jonathan F.P. Rose

9 Foundations of Healthy Buildings

The nine foundations of a healthy building[82] is the result of multiactor dialogue and stakeholder engagement over many years, drawing upon academia as well as professionals in real estate, building owners, hospital administrators, facilities directors, and homeowners. Recognizing the opportunity for the public health community to translate research into actionable information for key decision-makers was the catalyst for the systems-approach adopted by Professor Joe Allen's group at Harvard.

> *The goal, to improve the lives of all people, in all buildings, everywhere, every day.*[82]

The nine Foundations apply universally to all building types, including homes, and represent the beginning of "Building Evidence for Health"—a collection of two-page curations of the scientific literature on key topics related to buildings and health. The group's research conducted at the Harvard T.H. Chan School of Public Health has already shown that substandard ventilation rates negatively impact cognitive function. For example, they used a real-life simulation tool to test the higher order cognitive function of office workers at the standard-specified minimum outdoor air ventilation rate of 20 cfm/person compared to 40 cfm/person and reported 26 participants shift upward from the 62nd to 70th percentile in terms of cognitive performance when compared to normative data of 70,000 people who had taken the cognitive tests in the past.[83] This change in performance is equivalent to a $6500 increase in salary per person per year, while the energy costs of achieving the same change in ventilation were less than $40 per person per year, and down to U.S.$1 per person per year when energy efficient systems are used. When combined with the comorbidity in terms of sick building symptoms and absenteeism, the benefits of higher ventilation rates far outweighed the costs in terms of energy by several orders of magnitude.

Citizen Participation for Sustainable Development in Ecuador

In the County of Pedro Moncayo, Ecuador, the Commonwealth of Decentralized Autonomous Rural Parishes of the North and Fundación Cimas del Ecuador (CIMAS), developed a demonstration project to implement at the local level national public policies aimed to improve sustainable human development.[85] Using a highly participatory planning process working at the grassroots-level, public, private, community, national, and international institutions (Rotary Clubs, United Nations Organizations, universities) worked together to defined needs and priority interventions, giving special attention to priority and vulnerable groups. Focusing on the reduction of poverty, undernutrition, and exposure to agrochemicals, the work led to community training in agroecology and programs for microlending and marketing aimed at small- and medium-production farmers. Research into child development underpins plans for a large nutritional supplementation intervention for children under 3 years of age, training for families in health and nutritional care for children and pregnant women.

BOX 80-8 Harvard House Zero

While built as an experimental research facility, Harvard's House Zero demonstrates how available technology can enable homes to operate "off the grid" and, with careful selection of materials, can provide a comfortable and toxic chemical free indoor environment.[84]

Universities Supporting Delivery of SDG Solutions

Universities and higher education institutions can play a critical role in developing new systemic and transformative solutions through multistakeholder collaboration. Given their primary role as knowledge producers, higher education can serve as a powerful means to help create a more sustainable future. They could offer "new platforms and new capacities that upgrade our mental and social operating system."[86] However, as organizations that have stood for many centuries in some cases, the ability of universities to deliver on the SDGs will demand that they too adapt to this new global agenda for change. Here, we need to be clear what we mean by "transformation"[79] and not endanger the independence, neutrality, and knowledge-driven community of practice represented by a university. The SDGs could become a powerful compass to guide transformation of universities, orienting both the university as an organization as well as its academic pursuits.

Many universities are already embracing the SDGs as a source of transformation, but are they acting fast enough and are the changes sufficiently deep given the pace and scale of change signaled by the SDGs across multiple domains? The established governance systems and processes may not be able to support organizational reform at scale, while also preserving those matters they were set up to manage such as quality and risk. Thus, we may need to develop a "second operating system devoted to the design and implementation of strategy, that uses an agile, network-like structure and a very different set of processes"[86] but complementing the traditional system. Purcell[87] described the senior management hierarchy of a university undergoing wholescale mission-led transformation as one operating system and the community of social networks as a second more agile system driving innovation. The main features of this second operating system, working in concert within established governance systems, are:

- A community convened around shared purpose[87];
- New functions at the center of the organization: integration; caring; facilitation; deep listening and conversation; curiosity, compassion, and courage[86];
- Holding environment to foster critical daily practices (hard conversations, accountability, information flow, etc.)[88];
- Promotion of self-management, wholeness, and evolutionary purpose[89,90];
- New governance and organization (from centralized to ecosystem)[86,87];
- Development of demonstration projects[91,92]; and
- A diverse community of legitimated and trustful members.[93,94]

Examples of university-led SDG projects abound and are showcased on an annual basis through the International Conference on Sustainable Development (http://ic-sd.org/).

Education for sustainable development (ESD) has become a principal educational subject, often embedded within a subject discipline but more typically featuring as stand-alone and offering cross-curricular courses that are not compulsory. With the world becoming increasingly globalized and interdependent, we expect ESD to feature more strongly in all programs of study and would support its mandatory inclusion to set up students for success in the twenty-first century and beyond. The United Nations Educational, Scientific and Cultural Organization (UNESCO)[95] defines ESD as that which "empowers people to change the way they think and work towards a sustainable future." So, while it should be a central part of formal education pathways, there is a need for us to upskill the adult population and recognize the important of ESD to lifelong learning and enabling equity of participation in the world of work and social justice.

We posit that ESD should not be limited to the teaching/learning domain of a university or college. Rather, it should feature across all domains and into research/innovation and community/service activities of higher educational institutions as well as its operations, strategy and governance.[92,94] Already, some leading universities are mapping their research portfolio against the SDGs while others are drawing upon the SDGs to promote inter- and transdisciplinary approaches to inquiry and knowledge exchange and transfer.[94] The theme of responsible and global citizenship has served to tie disparate strands of academic work together as has the concept of the university as a "living lab."[92] While we hear much of interdisciplinarity, this can sometimes be view as being antidisciplines and to be coterminus with shallow rather than deep learning. However, in practice ESD will support students to develop the requisite knowledge, skills, attitudes, and values in support of a sustainable future through the lens of their academic program whether it be a liberal arts pathway or a professional career-oriented one. We consider that ESD and the SDGs go hand in hand, and essential to a well-rounded public health education. Studies have shown that graduates expect to be involved in sustainability in some way during their career and believe the subject should be covered in their university course. Today's students and graduates are working out how to make a sustainable future happen.

Sustainable Impact Investing

It has been posited that the widely used "Return on Investment" tool is broken and is thus a key barrier to business planning for sustainability. While the idea of connecting actions to environmental and social impact is not new, measures and metrics of sustainability are becoming increasingly important in corporate environments. To inform stakeholders and consumers/clients through environmental, social, and governance (ESG) reporting, these measures also influence the wider investor community. Selecting and stewarding financial assets based on ESG measures is a growth area as investors want returns over the long term and thus to invest assets in sustainable companies. While the lack of standardized practices in the field, as compared to national and international codes and framework for financial accounting, currently do not allow a "like for like" comparison, there are some important advances in the field driven by science. Next-generation traceable indicators that seek to quantify external context and impact of investments and put this into a governance framework to guide decision-making are being developed. With growth in sustainable investment running way ahead of market growth rates worldwide, agencies like the Principles for Responsible Investment,[96] Sustainability Accounting Standards Board,[97] and Global Reporting Initiative[9] are all stepping into this space—and we predict there will be important future developments in scientifically assessing the impact of sustainable investment. Here we call for a more comprehensive approach to impact measurement by having the financial sector join with the scientific community.

Examples of metrics applied to the holding of a pension fund portfolio were recently reported[98] the development of intuitive, company-level metrics of value to sustainable investment decision-making and supported comparison across companies. The approach is to evaluate corporate products and services within broader environmental and human beneficiary settings. While the assumption is that a new basket of financial and impact metrics can be combined in a portfolio without adversely affecting financial returns, this has yet to be proven. However, we assert the cobenefits of sustainable transformation would result in the saving of trillions of dollars secured by mitigating climate change, water crises and loss of ecosystem services.

Circular Economy

There is a view that we can only square up to climate change by "going circular."[99] While there are lots of announcements heralding the latest news on transitioning to renewable energy, reducing emissions or water usage or banning single-use plastics, we need to go much further in embracing a circular economy. Unfettered growth is not sustainable, neither is the current position where the "real" cost of business—that is, pollution, health impacts and damage to ecosystems is not costed into products and services. The concept of the "circular economy" aims to eliminate waste and keep resources in use for as long as possible, with materials recovered and reused at the end of life. Circle Economy[100] produced a report of global circularity and reported that we are only 9% of the way there! Their advice was that we need to stop extracting, stop wasting, optimize what we already have, and recycle more and better." The Ellen Macarthur Foundation[101] forecasts in Europe alone some 500 billion euros in economic benefits. Dutch banking and financial services group ING highlight the fact that "externalities do not have a price."[102] given we do not have a global price on CO_2 emissions or water use. There are of course good-practice examples, from Cisco to Rolls-Royce, to Mud Jeans and Apple. Circularity Capital has already identified the circular economy as an opportunity for investors, which can drive behaviors by companies and consumers.

There are challenges, in terms of how we apply circular thinking to services as well as products, the lack of a common language and suitable metrics and measures. However, there are some easy wins from refilling and sharing to recycling packaging and food waste. In some ways, we are going back to bygone years with milk and other liquids being sold in glass bottles and firms like IKEA leasing furniture and offering upcycling and repair workshops. Proctor and Gamble's ocean plastic shampoo bottles is a public expression of its commitment to go to war on plastic, with the company coming a long way from the Greenpeace audit of Asian beaches. Its Ambition 2030[103] document pledges a 35% increase in water efficiency compared to 2010 and to source 10% of its water consumption from circular sources. While fast fashion has hit the headlines, there is work ongoing with, for example, the H&M Foundation[104] investing in recycling technologies with its stores selling regenerated nylon from fishing nets. There is so much more to do here—not least to quell consumer demand for "stuff" and the latest gadget or handbag. We generate some 45 million tonnes of electronic waste globally, worth an estimated $60 billion in material value, however only 20% is properly recycled.[105] Policy makers in the European Union will, from 2021, require products to consider disassembly and repair.[106] However, it is our considered view that companies are not moving fast enough on the circular economy, for example, fewer than 20% of packaging innovations were rolled out and household recycling remains constrained by lack of knowledge and limited local recycling services.

FORESIGHT ON CONTEMPORARY SUSTAINABILITY ISSUES

Here, we provide some further thoughts on **contemporary issues in sustainability**, from travel and tourism through to leadership and governance for sustainable development. We have also illustrated this section with some examples of **"sustainability solutions"** that meet our criteria of **radical collaboration** and **systems thinking**, approaches we consider are urgently required to deliver against the SDGs. These examples highlight the importance of local actions for global solutions and call upon policy makers to work in multiactor partnerships around the SDGs as a shared purpose and to disseminate their learning freely on an international stage.

Foresight—A New Era in Public Health

The twenty-first century heralds the promise and possibilities of a new era in public health seeking sustainability given challenges of demographics and globalization.[107] Inspired solutions, breakthrough research, and its translation alongside new generations of public health scholars and engaged lifelong education will enable us to tackle new frontiers in the field. Adopting a "cells to society" approach, public health is key to unlocking social and economic transformation necessary to deliver against the SDGs.

> *Public health transcends geography. Global problems, such as pandemics, threaten mankind as a whole, and if we have the change to solve them, we are all better off.*[108] Ronnie Chan

Powerful forces are, however, undermining efforts to protect and improve global health, necessitating changes in how we prevent, track, and respond to risks and disease outbreaks. Global demographic shifts, mounting environmental degradation and climate change, escalating humanitarian emergency, technology innovation, and a growing commitment to a universal right to healthcare are all driving change. The World Economic Forum's strategic intelligence efforts to map global transformations highlight key areas[109] for attention in global health from our aging global population, with some 2 billion people over 60 years by 2050, to increases in mental health conditions with costs rising to some $6 trillion by 2030 (from 2.5 trillion in 2010).[110]

Innovation in both digital technology and the biosciences is advancing at a furious pace, with analytics now a cornerstone of public health for individual and community benefit. New technologies will allow real-time data creations and insightful analyses driven by big data and mobile devices. Accelerating access to health interventions and health promotion will rebalance the dynamics between patient/client and healthcare/medical professionals with a shift from treating sickness to managing health. Evidence-based public health policy will adopt a more systems approach, drawing on the SDGs as a blueprint for how we sustain healthy people and healthy planet, working across industry and disciplinary boundaries. But becoming increasingly knowable to those who wish to know brings with it risk of new inequalities emerging in a so-called age of surveillance[111] with human experience translated into behavioral data channeled into prediction products with nudges toward outcomes—typically profit-based ones. This digital omnipresence brings with it new ways in which the individual can connect with their own data, for example, their liver function, and how they interact with others locally and globally with questions about who owns the data and who can "see" the data. Concerns already abound on how Amazon's "Alexa The Echo" is tuning into our lives, with people hired to transcribe our conversations and note our emotional states. Together with technology that seeks to discern how we feel as we engage with content, from microexpressions to voice and gestures, it has been contended that individual autonomy is being lost. Free will and determinism are venerable philosophical, scientific and theological notions of being "free," the question is will we remain free to choose when our reality is being actively curated? Will any "deviations" from what a society decides is "normal" be managed with dangers that a state or corporate actor could overthrow the very idea of what it means to be a person, challenging the construct of individuality.

Public health has been pursuing three key global ambitions: managing escalating costs, improving quality outcomes and expanding access.[112] The Lancet's Global Health Commission 2018 report on High quality health systems in the SDG era: time for a revolution[110] determined that high-quality health systems could save over 8 million lives each year in low-income and middle-income countries

(LMICs), of which 60% of the deaths from treatable conditions are due to poor quality with the remainder being the result of nonutilization of the health systems. High-quality health systems could prevent 2.5 million deaths from cardiovascular disease, 1 million newborn deaths, 900,000 deaths from tuberculosis, and half of all maternal deaths each year. Growing health needs and changing public expectations are demanding better health outcomes and greater social value from health systems.

> *...the human right to health is meaningless without good quality care because health systems cannot improve health without it. We propose that health systems be judged primarily on their impacts, including better health and its equitable distribution; on the confidence of people in their health system; and on their economic benefit, and processes of care, consisting of competent care and positive user experience.*[109]

In line with the SDGs goal 17 for partnerships, the Commission identified four values that define high-quality health in that they are for people, are equitable, resilient, and efficient.[109] The report examined health across the SDGs noting deficits in delivery at both individual and systems levels, with quality of care being worst in vulnerable groups, including the poor, the less educated, adolescents, those with stigmatized conditions, and those at the edges of health systems, such as people in prisons. Proposing **universal health coverage**, the report called on governments to establish a national quality guarantee for health services with appropriate measures in support of accountability and to inform improvements. The need for better metrics was noted, given that many of the outcomes that matter most to people are not measured. Given the complexity of health systems operating at multiple interconnected levels, foundational transformation of the system is required to meet the SDG targets and improve health system quality by 2030.

Initiatives to promote behavioral changes for healthier living are required given the chronic disease burden is expected to increase, largely due to aging populations in the developed world with people over 60 years forecast to double in number between 2010 and 2030. While most chronic diseases were present in affluent countries, with diets changing and a more sedentary lifestyle commonplace across the globe, we can expect deaths from chronic diseases to increase in low- and mid-income countries. A deeper understanding of our health status from mobile health technologies are empowering people to access information more easily with over 20,000 health apps making use of smart sensors and social media channels predicted to generate over 25,000 petabytes of healthcare data by 2020 (up from 50 petabytes in 2015). The next generation of sensor technology, cheaper, smaller, more efficient, will unbundle sensors from smart phones, embedding them in tattoos and adhesive bandages. The healthcare worker of the future may be a robot or, as we combine virtual- and augmented-reality may have a telescope 3-miles long! Robot dexterity revolves around building mechanical devices, such as robot hands, that can use AI to learn about environments as they encounter them and adapt to become more proficient. Dynamic interpersonal telemedicine, robotics, data analytics, and AI are changing how we sustain healthcare and wearable sensors will support a move from a passive recipient of healthcare to an active user pursuing health.

> *Empowering and trusting consumers with their own information could unleash huge efficiencies in healthcare.* Diego Miralles, MD, Head of Janssen Healthcare Innovation[113]

> *The whole idea of digital health reminds me that about 20 years ago we used to talk about e- commerce. We don't talk about e-commerce anymore; we just talk about commerce.*[114] Ashish Jha, Faculty Director of Harvard Global Health Institute

We are on the cusp of a vital new era in public health, one in which the focus is on a personal health manifesto based on prediction and prevention over simply addressing illness. Arising from a deepening understanding of our biology and the environment as well as social and cultural contexts, there is a growing trend towards personalization and health analytics. Given much of medicine involves heuristic, rules-based problem-solving based on symptoms and tests results, this is fertile ground for artificial intelligence (AI). Driven by AI and machine learning, real-time sensing and health apps will provide environmental data about what we are exposed to as we walk around, eat and work—from levels of benzene to exposure to UV rays. All the health data people generate will form a resourceful database of symptoms and behaviors. Using global databases as reference benchmarks, dynamic assessment of health and risk can help us to tailor interventions and risk-avoidance strategies to the individual within a community that is increasingly diverse.

> *Prevention as a new health worldview stems partly from sage advice of the past—an apple a day keeps the doctor away, wash your hands, and look both ways before crossing the street—and from public health pressures that understand that reckless individual behaviour leads to overall cost increases for all.*[112]

While spend on the biomedical sciences increases year-on-year, its translation into innovation and or drugs is declining. This translational gap, between basic science research funded largely from public funds and clinical development undertaken by business, needs to be addressed. This will require the creation of public–private–plural partnerships, in line with SDG goal 17, to advance a "lab-to-market" route. A focus on a new era of predictions, prevention, and personalized health is upon us and this will in turn require us to adopt a more balanced approach between reductionist science with a more integrated holistic systems approach to well-being. Shifting to a public health paradigm that embraces wellness is a major challenge, but the result will be in line with the SDGs with people living healthier and longer lives with purpose.

While unforeseen public health challenges can be vital in sparking innovation, many people still die due to preventable diseases and a vast discrepancy still exists between health outcomes in developed and developing countries, as well as extreme health disparities among communities within a nation state. Despite considerable health advances, over 6 million people die each year from malaria, HIV/AIDs, and TB with countless children dying from preventable conditions such as diarrhea. With one in five of the world's population living in extreme poverty, good public health and a focus on well-being is essential for economic development and delivery of the SDGs.

Foresight—Climate and Health

Climate change is an existential crisis and the single greatest threat to public health. Anthropogenic global warming has deleterious consequences on many aspects of our environment, including sea-level rises, heatwaves, droughts, invasive species migration, and wildfires. With 7 million people dying each year from diseases related to air pollution and numbers rising as extreme weather events lead to worsening chronic illnesses, increased infectious diseases spread by insects and decreased access to clean water and nutritious food. Yet, less than 2% of global change adaptation finance was allocated to health-related projects in the United States in 2016.[115] Despite evidence of mankind's negative impact on the planet, science is being challenged and the case against the climate crisis delays much-needed policy interventions. All sensible people can agree that climate change is real and that the consequences of not acting will be devastating. **Carbon justice is social justice.**

Tackling climate change is a significant global health opportunity, but we need to make it personal, actionable, and urgent. Science alone will not create the transformations necessary, and we need to engage the public and global decision makers to understand the health impacts of climate change. There is an obligation of governments, business and the public to act but the challenge is to make a global agenda personal. Community-led projects from hyperlocal initiatives where 40 million acres of private lawns were turned into edible landscapes[116] to rural electric co-operatives[117] can make a difference. Cities like Pittsburgh are reimagining themselves as technology-innovation hubs based on clean energy, global companies like Microsoft and Apple are moving into cities attracted by cheaper solar and wind energy. Climate change has wide-ranging consequences for many business sectors from agriculture to tourism, insurance to infrastructure all affected through linkages with socioeconomic and technological systems. For example, climate change could threaten food and resource security, which in turn can make poverty and conflict more likely in certain geographies. Meeting emission reduction targets requires investment in green technology, energy efficiency, and green finance. Despite lower costs for "clean" solutions, barriers to adoption include political positioning as well as switching costs and structural changes are urgently required.

When Greta Thunberg spoke in the fall of 2018, then a 15-year-old Swedish schoolgirl, she highlighted the impact of ecoanxiety on the young and drew the world's attention to climate change, putting pressure on politicians to act as she called for people to "...act like the house is on fire."[118] From a one-girl protest in front of the Swiss parliament, her climate activism ignited protests in Finland, the Netherlands, and Australia and other countries with the United Kingdom declaring "an environmental and climate emergency" on May 1, 2019.[119] University students across the world also started up campaigns to demand more climate-friendly organizations. Young people are worried about climate change and surveys show they rank it as the most important societal issue. However, the gap between their concern and lifestyle is no narrower than those of older age groups and in many cases is wider. This may reflect a pessimistic or even a fatalistic view of climate change, with young people feeling helpless as well as hopeless, and de-emphasizing the seriousness of the threat. Over a decade ago, sustainability scholar Richard Eckersley described "apocalyptic nihilism,"[103] where feelings of powerlessness take over and the person ceases to care and lives in the moment, and "apocalyptic fundamentalism," where people try to return to more certain times and adopt some extreme rules of what is good or bad. Those who adopt meaning-focused coping strategies, over emotion- or problem-focused ones, appear able to appreciate the seriousness of the climate problem and see positive trends, expressing trust in societal actors such as scientists, broadcasters, and some environmental organizations. Eckersley has now added "apocalyptic activism"[120] to describe constructive hope, the desire to create something new by facing challenges in a determined nonextremist way. Research shows that meaning-focused coping is associated with collective engagement and well-being. But there are those warning that we overestimate the ability of young adults to deal with uncertainty and complexity, such that feelings helplessness and hopelessness are increasing with concerns around growing mental health issues in young people.

There are real achievements in tackling climate change, for example, in breaking the link between growth and emissions through innovation in the power sector. Indeed, a recent poll in the United States found that 70% of respondents believed environmental protection is more important than growth.[121] There is, however, so much more to do at the level of the collective, for example, in Norway over half the new cars purchased in 2018 were electric while only 2% were in the United Kingdom. In addition, pollution is being "outsourced" with steel made in-country being counted toward emissions, but that manufactured overseas not being included. If we are to reduce global warming, it does not matter where the emissions take place! We saw this in Denmark, which adopted one of the most ambitious carbon reduction targets in the world at Kyoto in 1997, and went further in 2011 with a goal to phase out the use of all fossil fuels by 2050—but a recent report[122] highlighted the substantial increase in the carbon intensity of its important, all but wiping out any decarbonization benefits. Growth is not improving lives, for example, in the United States poverty rates are higher and real wages lower that in the 1970s, despite a doubling of GDP per capita; and Europe outperforms the United States on every social indicator, despite its GDP being 40% lower. It has been argued that we do not need more growth, rather we need an economy that focuses on good health, education, meaningful work and living wages—a new economy based on a **new world order**.

The hard part of transformation to address climate change lies ahead. Changing the ways, we heat, insulate, and cool our homes, taking petrol and diesel vehicles off the road, how we live, move and what we eat and use our land. This will not be done through business as usual and relies on communicating powerfully to change hearts and minds and turn knowing we need to do something into actions, with system change needed to facilitate individual change. From a framing of sacrifice and blame to a vision of hope and common endeavor, we need to demonstrate benefits in the present as well as for the future. A whole new infrastructure of change projects, supported by political and community leadership, is required with public health a clear reason to act and a key beneficiary of climate action.

Foresight—Pandemics

During the twenty-first century, global pandemics could cost in excess of $6 trillion, an expected loss of $60 billion per year and comparable to that of climate change, with the World Bank predicted a repeat of the 1918 flu pandemic could give rise to a 10% reduction in global GDP.[123] Global health crises do not respect national borders, cause devastation to human lives and livelihoods, and threaten global security and economic stability. Healthy nations tend to be more stable politically and are better economic partners such that global public health is a national security issue.

> *...epidemiologists say a fast-moving airborne pathogen could kill more than 30 million people in less than a year. There is a reasonable probability in the next 10 to 15 years.*[124] Bill Gates

> *No country can live to itself in disease prevention ... Failure of one is a failure of all.*[108] Wilbur Sawyer[125]

Foresight—Food: Hunger, Waste, and Diet

Many of us take for granted the easy access we enjoy to a variety of nutritious and safe food, while nearly a billion people still go hungry every day. Beyond nourishment, food is part of our culture, creating community and connecting us to one another and our planet. Food is a key lever to optimize human health and well-being as well as environmental sustainability and yet it currently poses a threat to both people and planet. Food is vulnerable to climate change, with the United Nations Food and Agricultural Organization estimating that 25% of fish stocks are overexploited today and 50% fully exploited.[126] An immense challenge facing humanity is to provide a growing world population with healthy diets from sustainable food systems, which relies upon ease of access to nutritious food. With nearly 40% of the world's ice-free surface used for crop and livestock productions, there is competition for land from cities as well as worrying levels of ecosystem decline and productivity with forecasts that we need to support a 60–120% increase in global crop demands by 2050. There are efficiency opportunities for food production, from precision agriculture to automated systems and food safety with big data and advanced analytics playing more important roles in the upstream steps of the value food chain.

Food hunger causes human misery and robs people of their dignity and ability to reach their potential. Some 160 million children under 5 years are malnourished and underweight, over 800 million people are chronically undernourished and hungry and 2 billion people suffer from nutrient deficiencies (hidden hunger). In 2012, the then secretary General of the United Nations, Ban Ki-Moon, issued a "Zero Hunger Challenge"[127] calling for a future where people enjoyed a fundamental right to food based on resilient and sustainable food systems. In some of our largest and most successful cities, like New York and Houston, people are hungry relying on charitable food banks and state aid. In London, England food poverty is real with teachers reporting most children in the city arrive at school without breakfast. Given issues in affluent areas, the situation in developing regions is challenging with the United Nations World Food Program (WFP; [128]) reaching 80 million people and distributing 2 million metric tons of food every year. Some 44 million people are driven into poverty by rising food prices, increasing 135% since the year 2000, with the poor spending a larger share of their income on food. Protests and riots in 48 countries were related to rising food prices.

Food waste is a sustainability issue, and accounts for one-third of the world's GHG emissions with the embodied CO_2 representing over 3 billion metric tons—more than twice the emission of all the vehicles in the United States. It is estimated that one third of all fruit and vegetables are wasted from farm to fork in North America and Oceania. Thomas Robert Mathus,[129] in his famous 1798 essay on population, predicted that the world's population growth would outrun the earth's food supply. Despite episodic and devastating famines, largely due to civil unrest over natural disasters, we have generally managed to feed most of the world's population. A report for the Millennium Institute in 2013[130] developed a range of scenarios concerning how food production could keep pace with a growing global population and concluded that even modest reductions in food waste could reduce the land needed as well as carbon emissions.

Our diet is changing such that the kinds of food we produce are becoming as important as the total amount of food. Dietary risk factors are among the most important contributors to the global burden of disease, with large numbers of premature deaths being due to inadequate consumption of vegetables, fruit, and nuts. Generally, diets with reduced animal product consumption, particularly from ruminants, are associated with reduced GHG emissions. More environmentally sustainable diets tend to be healthier than less sustainable diets, but not invariably so. The so-called "livestock revolution"[131] refers to our shift from a plant-based diet to one based on animal products, and growing demand for crop and pastureland could require an additional 90 million hectares of cropland. With a need to feed an estimated 9 billion people by 2050, requiring 70% more food than we consume now, and a growing middle class placing increased demands on food sources, governments are concerned about the sustainability of the food supply chain and food security. Beef, pork, and poultry production is increasing dramatically with consequent impact on land use and GHG (see earlier); to produce 1 kg of beef requires 6.5 kg of feed, compared to 2 kg and 1.2 kg for chicken and fish, respectively. Major proportions of the world's crops are being fed to animals (and are subject to conversion inefficiencies) or are used for biofuels, resulting in 41% of the calories available from global crop production being lost to the food system. Without changing crop mix, if food was exclusively grown for direct human consumption[132] enough extra calories would be available to feed an additional 4 billion people (more than the 2–3 billion people projected to be added to the world population in the coming decades).

Growing urbanization, with some 200,000 people moving each day into cities, also means we are losing our connection with nature, agriculture and the seasons with many people having little understanding of food sources and some children in urban settings unable to recognize simple vegetables in their original form. The recent Lancet Report "Food in the Anthropocene: the EAT–*Lancet* Commission on healthy diets from sustainable food systems"[133] called for the promotion of healthy, low environmental impact diets, noting the dietary shift towards high consumption of fats and oils, meats (particularly from ruminants), processed foods, and refined carbohydrates—including so-called empty calories—is a major contributor to the noncommunicable disease burden, and to GHG emissions, land use change, and agrochemical pollution. It also drew attention to innovative sources of nutrition, with over 1900 species of insects already part of the traditional diets of at least 2 billion people. Insects have substantial diversity in their nutritional value, but they can be a highly nutritious and a healthy food source with high fat, protein, vitamin, fiber, and mineral content. Insects have high feed conversion efficiencies, lower GHG emissions than conventional livestock, and usually require less land and are less likely to transmit zoonotic infections.

Given industrialization and concentration in the global food sector, publicly traded companies exercise significant control of food systems and food sovereignty. Despite having a small share of the global market the biggest supermarket corporations exercise influence on what vast swathes of the global population have access to eat given the food industry is largely responsible for food supplies. While global food production of calories has generally kept pace with population growth, many people consume either low-quality diets or too much food. Unhealthy diets pose a significant risk to morbidity and mortality, with adverse health effects associated with malnutrition, such as learning difficulties and stunted growth[133] or chronic noncommunicable diseases (NCDs)[110] related to overconsumption and obesity responsible for 72% of the world's 54.7 million deaths in 2016 (WHO).[134] Dietary changes from current diets toward healthier diets are likely to result in significant health benefits, with estimates of some 11 million adult deaths per year prevented. A radical transformation of the global food system is urgently needed given the substantial scientific evidence that links diet with human health and environmental sustainability; the data are strong enough to warrant urgent action.

Foresight—Business and the SDGs

Business is an engine for change and delivery of the SDGs will not happen without business being a key part of the solutions. Companies large and small, start-ups, and social enterprises can help deliver a more sustainable and inclusive future. While there are important questions around our current capitalist systems, business needs to place a greater emphasis on alleviating society's "miseries" and ensuring "blessings" are more evenly shared in order to maintain its legitimacy. Society is increasingly looking to business to embrace a wider sphere of responsibilities beyond the limits of their own operations and be proactive in developing solutions to tackle social and environmental challenges. In return, we are seeing a fundamental reassessment of the role business plays in society, moving beyond Corporate Social Responsibility (CSR) and ESG measures and placing its social compact as the core activity and purpose of business.

> *...the inherent vice of capitalism is the unequal sharing of blessings; the inherent virtue of socialism is the equal sharing of miseries.*[135] Winston Churchill

Navigating the tensions and opportunities of "sustainable growth," businesses are moving towards a more socially responsible model not as a point of differentiation but as the "new normal." The business case for sustainability has become much more powerful, although we see many organizations struggling to make the transition from current business models that focus on short-term profitability to address long-term challenges and long-term sustainability. Reinventing the business model for the future will require us to price in impact on people and planet and focus more on value creation across multiple stakeholder domains. In a world shaped by globalization and technological innovation, the underlying focus on markets and governments misses the critical third pillar of community in pursuing purpose-driven prosperity for all, a factor in the rise of populism. Reframing how we consider civil society and empower communities to restore the balance needed for sustainable development are key challenges. With community a safety net for when government fails, it can also serve to attenuate a key public health issue of loneliness as well as shaping market values and the concept of a just or fair profit.

Many businesses already recognize the need to drive transformational changes to align their purpose with the delivery of the SDGs and to harness new technologies and innovations to create value for society and the environment. Members of the Business and Sustainable Development Commission[136] argue that business has a unique opportunity, and responsibility, to find new sources of value creation that delivery for society.

> *It is incumbent on all of us to make the case for business to be at the heart of an open global economic system ... Business leaders need to strike out in new directions to embrace more sustainable and inclusive economic models.*[136]

Work by the Beacon Institute[137] found that "doing well by doing good" can enhance business performance by instilling strategic clarity, channeling innovation, providing a force for transformation and collaboration. However, the Cambridge Institute for Sustainability Leadership[138] calls for business to go beyond the sentiment of "do good" and sets out the conditions businesses need to meet to thrive from being relevant to the nature and scale of the challenges faced by the global economy and society to the agenda being holistic, authentic, owned across the organization and central to guiding strategy and actions.[139] Traditional leadership and governance frameworks and approaches do not yet acknowledge global challenges, nor do they equip leaders to navigate them. Connecting values, thinking and practice, new adaptive models are emerging that both challenge and complement traditional hierarchical management systems by creating new operating systems based on social networks and multiactor partnerships.[87,90,93]

> *Put simply, there is a need for businesses—and their leaders—to not only anticipate the future, but to shape the future we want. This is the leadership we need.*[139]

The past *was* a good predictor of the future, but no more and leaders need to re-invent strategy and governance for the world we live in today which is more turbulent and the future liable to be startlingly different. As the complexity of our physical and social systems increases, there is a premium on rapid prototyping and experimentation, so we learn quickly about what works. Moving beyond data into pattern recognition, leaders are finding new ways to delegate authority, learn from consumers and stakeholders in real-time and treat the organization and its supply chain as a team pursuing a shared purpose making "strategy a self-correcting series of intentional experiments."[140] Business must respond to the challenges humanity faces, recognizing that their permission to operate and make profits, comes only with the consent of society. Organizations need to anticipate change and position themselves appropriately, thinking at a systems level but acting entrepreneurially. Here, the SDGs as a global strategy can support leaders "zoom out" to develop strategic vision and then "zoom in" to action.

> *Plans are useless, but planning is everything.* Dwight D. Eisenhower[141]

Foresight—Sustainability Leadership and Governance

Leaders in the era of the SDGs need to be able to read the planet as well as the balance sheet, given their operational domain is largely outside the organization rather than within it. Now in the Fourth Industrial Revolution, characterized by unprecedented changes driven by new technologies and changing consumer behaviors, 21st leaders are prized for their ability to lead in situations characterized by so-called VUCA (volatility, uncertainty, complexity, ambiguity) conditions. With pervasive ambiguity a constant, leaders need to lead without certainty and embrace preparedness over predictions of the future with strategic agility a prized asset.

With the history of the twentieth century intimately linked with the human construct of "the firm" for creating money and meaning, in this new century leaders need to think differently and embrace the "edgeless" organization as it bumps up against issues of energy, water, security, public health, and so on as leaders are impacted by regulations and stakeholder activism. The construct of the hero leader, with leadership and the preserve of the few must be challenged as no individual leader can possibly possess either all the desirable capabilities nor all the necessary information.[87,139] Leadership in delivery of the SDGs requires a different set of attributes defined by the connections an organization has locally and with the rest of the world and how it enables human flourishing and purpose. Means to compete in the future will require a paradigm shift in leadership, focused on relational and trust capital as well as stakeholder engagement in a world where AI and machine learning challenge the very notion of an institution. Indeed, how do we develop policy and regulatory frameworks when organizations are no longer accountable for the decisions they make, with AI algorithms in widespread use.

Will the share price still be a primary metric of organizational value? Or, will we see more widespread engagement in a suite of measures that reflect the things the organization does? Going beyond optimizing shareholder return, outcomes measure already include benefits realized for employees and the community, but they are routinely not priced into company value. Given the complexity of delivery against the SDGs, partnerships among organizations in the public–private–plural sectors will reflect hybrid value chains and networked organizations that convene around shared purpose and value creation.

With high profile failures of institutional governance, a regular feature of press reports, from banks to churches, charities to retail stores and beyond, trust in organizations is weakening. There is an urgent need to strengthen decision-making and accountability, which will rely on greater thought diversity and hence driving inclusion and equity. Given the importance of goal 17 "partnerships for the goals," we need to promote cross-sector learning about governance and build governance literacy into public health as well as doing more to deepen the diversity of ideas to avoid the dangers of "groupthink" and increase public participation in governance. Drawing on different perspectives, experiences, and ideas is required for healthy governance, working across agencies to deliver against the SDGs and the health benefits and cobenefits arising. An activated citizenry is essential to effective governance, with means to encourage trust building in organizational settings urgently required.

While collective actions in the face of an emergency have typically relied on command-and-control techniques to effect change, this approach presumes we know the answers to the problem at hand; this is a closed-minded approach and can lead to stagnation. We need people to have the freedom and incentive to cocreate solutions, test them, fail and learn together calling for a more socially constructed inclusive leadership model[87,93,138] that has at its heart diversity of ideas. Governance for sustainability is a complex topic, and the rise of populist administration and growing nationalism movements are a clear and present danger to preserving the global environment.

Foresight—Travel and Tourism

The Travel and Tourism (T&T) sector is one of the world's largest and fastest growing economic sectors. It contributed nearly \$8.8 trillion to the global economy in 2018, representing 10.4% of all global economic activity, supporting one in ten jobs (319 million) worldwide and one in five new jobs, with 3.9% growth compared to the global economy at 3.2%.[142] The sector represents 27.2% of total service exports and fuels the economies of many nations, with domestic tourism representing 71.2% of total tourism spend, and business travel accounting for 21.5% and leisure travel 78.5%, with a high proportion of women in employment and a reliance on natural and cultural resources. With 1.4 billion international tourist arrivals in 2018, an additional 1 billion people are projected to join the global middle class by 2030. International travel is becoming more accessible and is predicted to grow by some 35%, with some 1.5 billion people travelling by 2030 and domestic tourism up to four times this figure.[142]

The health, social and environmental problems related to this mass T&T phenomenon are also growing. T&T is a public health issue, with matters as diverse as pandemics spread through travel to problems of water scarcity, environmental degradation, energy usage, waste and worker health and safety. Indeed, threats to public health are not only to the tourists but also to host communities and the tourists' home nations. In considering T&T and public health together, we can see how a community as a tourist destination could enhance and promote physical and mental health for both locals and tourists alike. Engagement with a well-being agenda is central to a public health strategy and could also form the basis for a well-being concept of tourism. Terms such as the "blue gym" and "green gym" are already common public health parlance, giving the community a reason for increased activity but also creating something of a unique selling point for tourist destinations. Indeed, the concept of well-being tourism is now a strategic priority for many destinations, dovetailing health, and well-being to sustaining the local economy.

Demographics, deforestation, deregulation, decentralization, privatization, and the fragmentation of power are among the global sustainability issues in the T&T sector. The infrastructure-supporting T&T impacts upon almost all other economic sectors, from food and farming, transportation, buildings, energy, and public health all straining natural resources. Travelers are not spread evenly around the world, with some 20 countries experiencing more international arrivals that the rest of the world combined with similar imbalances in cities and individual attractions. Overcrowding is already a global problem, with places as diverse as Thailand's Koh Khai Islands, which banned public access to three of its islands, Peru's Machu Picchu and Venice all experiencing negative side effects of the T&T they depend upon.[143] Restrictions on T&T are now commonplace, for example, Bruges has stopped advertising day trips, Dubrovnik has restricted cruises, and Rome has adopted measures to curb antisocial tourist behaviors. The U.K. Government's Environmental Audit Committee recently announced an inquiry into the environmental cost of tourism,[144] given that the number of visitors to the United Kingdom has grown to 40 million in 2018. Travelers use water, food, and energy and generate waste at higher rates than when at home, with a displaced negative burden experienced by some of our most fragile and/or poorest places on the planet. The International Sustainable Tourism Initiative (ISTI)[145] is advancing a science-based framework to monitor the cost of maintaining destinations and managing the future impact of climate change. Its report, published March 2019, focused on "The Invisible Burden of Tourism"[146] and revealed tourism's hidden costs that need to be accounted for to protect and manage ecosystems, cultural assets, and community life; this work was supported by ISTI's research in Tunisia.[147]

While many T&T companies have been integrating sustainable practices into their operations for years, performance and reporting across the sector is still in an early phase and remains largely confined to the corporate social responsibility agenda. Compared to other sectors, it does not feature strongly on indices like the Dow Jones Sustainability Index, FTSE4Good, CDP Climate Performance Leadership Index, or Newsweek Green Rankings. While there are many barriers to the mainstreaming of sustainability in business, such as consumer demand, policy failing to drive enough market incentives, the prevailing short termism of financial markets and so on, leading companies are widening their view beyond immediate operational impact and thinking about the broader systems in which they operate. The World Travel and Tourism council (WTTC)[142] supports private T&T businesses in their efforts to embrace sustainability and innovation to catalyze transformation of the sector in line with the SDGs. The WTTC is a not-for-profit membership organization representing the global T&T private sector, with over 170 Chief Executives, Chairs, and Presidents of the world's leading T&T companies from all geographies. WTTC has worked for some 30 years to raise awareness of, and practice in, T&T in pursuit of sustainable growth, seeking to accelerate sustainability in the sector, drawing upon the United Nations SDGs. WTTC has been undertaking research for over 25 years, working with universities and global consulting firms, to explore the economic impact of T&T in 185 countries. Advocating to world leaders and heads of state, WTTC uses empirical data to raise awareness of the sector. A key priority for WTTC relates to sustainable growth. In 2015, prior to the start of COP21 in Paris, WTTC published a report on "Connecting Global Climate Action"[148] in which it acknowledged that limited research has been undertaken to assess T&T's collective environmental footprint in line with delivery of the SDGs. The report stated that the next 20 years "will be characterized by the sector fully integrating climate change and related issues into business strategy, supporting the global transition to a low carbon economy, and strengthening resilience at a local level against climate risks." In 2018, WTTC made public commitments on behalf of its members to carbon reduction, agreeing on a common agenda for climate action in the sector with the UN Framework on Climate Change.[148] With climate change posing significant risks to some tourism destinations, in many of the most high-risk areas, tourism can provide opportunities for communities to build resilience to its impacts. It joined the fight against illegal wildlife trading in its Buenos Aires Declaration on Travel & Tourism and Illegal Wildlife Trade[150] setting out specific challenges the sector can take to address this challenge. WTTC also addresses destination stewardship, sustainability reporting, and issues relating to the future of work and advancing women's empowerment. It is now pursuing research to drive change in the sector by working with leaders to accelerate transformation toward stronger commitments and actions for sustainable development.

Key to unlocking the potential of T&T for sustainable growth is empowering leaders to reframe sustainability as a goal for today, integrating it within their core business strategy and decision-making architecture. Researchers have theorized about how organizations will change in line with delivery against the SDGs, describing how a move toward a more sustainable ethos presents a major challenge for leaders with tensions arising, for example, between strategic goals, cultural preferences, and individual and organizational drivers. The concept of "transformational leadership" relies upon systemic change, promoting sustainability through agile leadership and adaptive governance that position the SDGs as a strategic focus. Given the disruptive forces acting on organizations across a range of fronts, from technology to the sociopolitical agenda, together with interdependencies and the accelerating pace of change, the need to adapt relies upon innovation being a team effort within and across organizations. Indeed, the volume of ideas that deliver on sustainability and innovation in T&T require an understanding of natural capital, ecosystem services, and the ways in which the natural environment supports public health and well-being, demanding fundamental changes in global business practices and policy frameworks alongside consumer behaviors. Good practice sustainability innovation cases in the sector, highlighted by WTTC's "Tourism for Tomorrow" award winners and finalists[151] help identify enablers and barriers to reframing sustainability as a strategic imperative for the T&T sector.

Foresight—Nature and Mental Health, an Ecosystem Service

Evidence is amassing as to the connection between exposure to nature and good mental health. The rise of urbanization means that experiencing nature is no longer routine and becomes an activity we need to seek out—thus being dependent on having the resources to make this happen. A recent report[152] collated health insights on the impact of nature experience on cognitive functions, emotional well-being and other aspects of mental health. Actionable understanding of how human well-being is linked with the involvement in the natural environment allows us to explore the contribution living nature as "ecosystem services" can have on public health. Ecosystem services include diversity of organisms, ecosystems and their processes, water purification, provision of food, stabilization of climate, protection from flooding, and so on; the value of "services" offered and/or supported by nature are being explored in policy, finance and management domains. For example, the natural capital project's InVEST (Integrated Valuation of Ecosystems Services and Tradeoffs) models[153] are currently used in 183 countries; InVEST models are open source and are tested through a worldwide network and adapted through practice.

With mental illness on par with cardiovascular and circulatory diseases, in terms of the total global burden of disease, accounting for 35% of total years lived with a disability and 13% of disability-adjusted life-years, if nature can lessen this burden we could see a nature experience being a common public health intervention. Poor mental health can arise through a variety of factors from social to economic, psychological to physical, behavioral to environmental with genetic and epigenetic influences, with contextual factors influencing global levels of mental illness and health—such as the megatrends described earlier that include urbanization and the global move to living in cities. While we do not consider here the ways exposure to nature can be harmful, such as allergies, wildfires and attacks by pathogens and wildlife, these are all public health concerns. Our focus is to draw to the attention of future and current public health scientists the growing body of evidence in support of exposure to nature as a positive well-being event—framing nature as "psychological ecosystem services."

Laboratory and field studies, as well as cross-sectional and longitudinal research have found psychological well-being of a population can be linked to proximity to nature, whether that is green, in the form of land, trees and even domestic gardens/yards and/or blue as rivers, lakes, and seas.[153] What is only being unraveled through research is the causal link of nature and influence on long-terms mental health, albeit most studies are in the global North; exploring the global South and a diversity of sociocultural settings is required. To date, evidence supports an association between common types of nature experience and increased psychological well-being, a reduction of risk factors and burden of some types of mental illness and that opportunities for some types of nature experience are decreasing in quantity and quality for many people around the globe. Studies are now exploring the features of such exposure, in terms of type and qualities as well as time spent or "dose" and measuring effects. As an area for future studies in public health, ecosystem services are a ripe topic for concerted efforts.

Foresight—Sustaining Happiness and Loneliness as a Public Health Issue

Loneliness is increasingly recognized as a public health issue with social relationships critical to physical and mental well-being. The scholar John Cacioppa labeled loneliness as a "public health problem,"[154] and the problem is growing with some describing it as an epidemic. A 2018 survey from *The Economist* and the Kaiser Family Foundation (KFF; [155]), reported more than 22% of adults in the United States and 23% in the United Kingdom say they always or often feel lonely, lack companionship, or feel left out or isolated. Electing to spend time alone or chosen solitude are of course distinct from loneliness, which is held to be an affective state that results from a gap between the quality and quantity of relationships we think we have and what we want to have. Loneliness relates to a perceived deficiency in social relationships, is a subjective experience and an aversive one. Some have gone on to distinguish between social and emotional loneliness, the latter relating to an absence of emotional attachment,[156] others describe situational and chronic loneliness states. Overall, loneliness is a social construct, which can present psychologically in terms of feeling unwanted, worthless, hopeless, rejected, and depressed—with some 50% of people who are lonely reporting that they feel depressed. Whether loneliness is a cause of depression or depressed states associated with a loss of self-worth, which causes people to isolate themselves or become isolated by others is not clear.[157] Tools for depression screening, such as the Center for Epidemiological Studies Depression Scale[158] do however include items that ask people how lonely they feel.

The health consequences of loneliness have been equated to the negative impact of smoking 15 cigarettes daily. In 2018/19 nearly $7 billion in annual federal spending was attributable to social isolation among older adults, with poor social relationships associated with a 295 increase in the risk of coronary heart disease and a 32% rise in the risk of stroke with the public health impact of loneliness forecast to increase as the nation's population ages.[156] However, it would be wrong to view loneliness as an older person's condition. More young people are reporting feelings of being lonely; for example, in Japan, there are more than half a million people under 40 who have not left their house or interacted with anyone for at least 6 months. Tackling loneliness has largely been in the form of seeking to increase social networks, even though social isolation is not a precondition of loneliness. Indeed, a report from the "What Works Centre for Wellbeing" stated that there is no evidence that any of the existing loneliness interventions work.[159] The scourge of loneliness is a public health issue we shall hear more about in the future.

Are you happy? The World Happiness Report is a global happiness ranking[160] that offers an insight into the science of well-being and its connection with sustainability. A poll[161] among Americans revealed 30% were very happy, 55% were pretty happy and 15% not at all happy, with positive correlations to income/money, not having children and regular worship and age—with older people generally happier. Happiness is 50% genetics, 40% down to behaviors, choices, and attitudes and 20% down to external factors like beauty. Highlighting the importance of aligning values and purpose, meaningful work that ignites people emotionally and fits with a person's talents and strengths was a key part of being happy. The Kingdom of Bhutan first conceptualized and implemented "Gross National Happiness" in lieu of GDP to measure growth, development, and health; an idea that infused the world, and now a global pattern of thought.[162] In considering the question of "What are the supports of a good life?" the central premise of sustainability being that human value is the same everywhere. With inequality associated with reduced levels of happiness, even within in advantaged groups, the "Happiness Movement"[163] is a response to a perceived crisis of purpose and joy, especially among those under 35 years. Highlighting the importance of trust, mindfulness, gratitude, compassion, storytelling, self-reflection, meditation, spirituality, and empathy, the movement calls for a paradigm shift from GDP to happiness with a focus on human flourishing.

Global Happiness measured by: GDP per capita; social support; healthy life expectancy at birth; freedom to make life choices; generosity; perception of corruption[162]

Urbanization (see earlier) is interfering with traditional community practices of helping one another and seems to be making people unhappy. With widespread data collection eroding human agency, there is a call to track our purpose not our purchase! MIT's Center for

Bits and Atoms[164] has established a network of FabLabs, with a focus on sharing global knowledge for local fabrication with the consumer as creator; revisiting the practice of making, we are seeing communities making for self and others, developing microbusinesses as well as driving sustainable practice by avoiding transport of goods, etc.

Professor Kasisomayajula "Vish" Viswanath, Co-Director of Harvard's Lee Kum Sheung Center for Health & Happiness[165] highlights the importance of translating science to application, noting how long it takes for evidence to move into practice, for example, scurvy in the fifteenth century took some 500 years to move into prevention with research and development typically taking about 17 years to get to market. Can we yet promote policy and practice of happiness—is the evidence strong enough? First, we need to consider who is not at the table when we talk about migration, poverty, inclusion, and the SDGs and then move to cocreate solutions with scientific rigor and impact. While well-being and happiness are multidimensional states, the terms are used interchangeably, but are they the same? Health is still largely organized around body parts, not the person so how might we best include health measures in happiness measures, not least that happiness is sociocultural and relies upon context and place. For example, life expectancy in the United States is decreasing as a result of "diseases of despair."

Foresight—The Future of Work

Jobs remain the cornerstone of our economic and social lives, providing meaning and self-respect alongside income and a chance to make societal contributions.[166] These relationships are under strain as structural changes disrupt employment levels and occupational patterns, from the "gig economy" to the rise of women in work. While recent debates have focused on the risk of automation to the future of jobs, studies have tended to downplay the impact on job creation and influence of megatrends such as climate change, urbanization, increasing inequality, demographics, globalization, and political uncertainty. A false alarmism contributes to a culture of risk aversion and holds back technology adoption, innovation, and growth especially in countries like the United States which already face structural productivity problems. It has been predicted that around 10% of the workforce are in occupations likely to grow, with 20% in jobs likely to shrink typically low- and medium-skilled in nature.[167] Studies focus on a growing emphasis on interpersonal, higher-order cognitive and systems thinking skills with a premium on judgment and decision-making as well as fluency of ideas. Anticipating new occupations, education must be at the center of any long-term strategy for adjusting to structural change.

Either we are on the cusp of catastrophic job losses and economic misery for the masses, or new technologies will supercharge productivity, leading to a rise in living standards and an abundance of good quality jobs. We tend to fixate on just a handful of technologies—namely AI and robotics while paying little attention to less fashionable but powerful innovations like e-commerce platforms, the Internet of Things, distributed ledgers, cloud computing, and smartphones. We tend to focus on automation, as though this was the only way technology can shape the lives of workers, while machines are also changing recruitment practices, facilitating surveillance and monitoring, altering the nature of business models, and restructuring industries (with new technology often aiding market concentration). We too often dwell on what is theoretically possible while ignoring what is happening, focusing on breakthroughs in individual technologies like autonomous vehicles and personal voice assistants but paying less attention to whether these same innovations are adopted in the real world. We also we pay too little attention to the systemic effects of technology, such as how its adoption in one corner of the economy can affect the lives of workers in different sectors. For example, the phenomena of "recycled demand," whereby the deployment of technology in one industry leads to cost savings for consumers, which frees up cash to spur demand (and potentially job growth) in another part of the economy. What is however common in visioning the future of jobs and work, is the shifting balance of power placing consumers at the top of the food chain, securing concessions out of workers rather than employers.[175]

Greater connectivity and improvements in technology are enabling "intelligence" to be embedded into physical systems from cities to a human body. With peer-to-peer platforms, activities are open to decentralized production thereby muddying traditional definitions of ownership and employment. Globalization has impacted employment driving down wages and fueling worker migration, with efforts to frustrate these trends through tariffs and immigration policies. Exacerbated by ageing demographics, the global economy has passed an important threshold with the ratio of the nonworking age population greater than the working population and productivity challenges in many countries. With 68% world's population forecast to live in cities by 2050,[168] most of us will live *all* our lives in cities. This concentration illustrates the basic unevenness of economic development, with cities as magnets for high-value, knowledge-intensive business where physical proximity enables collaboration and pooling of resources. Indeed, innovation is often being designed into developments mixing work, with housing and recreation. While public health issues of diabetes and depression have been linked to aspects of the urban environment, there are movements to green cities and make them "smarter." However, challenges to affordable housing is increasing inequality with downstream issues related to access to education, employment, and healthcare. These concerns are showing up in political uncertainty, with the geopolitical landscape characterized by polarization of views and a rise in partisanship. With the SDGs demanding greater collaboration on a global scale, conflicts over policy are impeding delivery and increasing risks to humanity.

Breakthroughs in radical technologies with the potential to disrupt entire industries emerge on a regular basis. For example, Google's "DeepMind" drew attention to one of its health algorithms that could detect up to 50 eye conditions with the accuracy of a trained doctor[169] and the first 3D-printed concrete house was constructed in just 24 hours.[170] The positive impact on public health of such advanced technologies is obvious, as is the fact such advances will impact on jobs and work. Whether that impact is negative, with subsequent job losses and the health disbenefits of unemployment, and/or is positive with new, more intellectually stimulating work growing, with the health benefits associated with meaningful work are yet to be seen. Predicting the future is no easy task, and predictions around the number of jobs at risk range from 35% to just 5%.[167] Using scenario planning to help identify high-impact, highly uncertain drivers of change and then exploring the way these critical uncertainties could play out allow is to develop situations that include a broader range of factors. For example, how the Internet of Things and wearable devices might increase workplace monitoring, or how big data could create new disruptive platforms can be scenario planned and draw in issues like health of the global economy or involvement of unionized labor. This methodology was used[171] to determine four futures of work—the Big Tech Economy, the Precision Economy, the Exodus Economy and the Empathy Economy. While not complete depictions of the future, the scenarios serve to describe plausible outcomes in a vivid way so that people can engage practically with an emergent future. Looking at the brief description of the four futures, think about the public health issues emergent from each scenario.

- *Big Tech Economy* describes a world where technology had developed at pace with widespread automation. Self-driving vehicles, robots capable of complex tasks and human interactions are common in healthcare and other settings. Unemployment is rising and those in work typically do 20 hours a week. More leisure time, technological improvements in public services and lower costs mean people feel their living standards are good. Tech giants dominate, with the digital economy dominant.
- *Precision Economy* describes a world of hypersurveillance, where sensors are widespread, but technology has failed to deliver on

the hype. Workers are subject to new level of oversight and ratings, tracking data through wearables that drive on-demand labor strategies.

- *Exodus Economy* describes a world characterized by protracted economic slowdown, rising unemployment, and new austerity measures. Automation is limited by low investment in innovation, with a rise in the gig-economy and established companies closed. Resentment, activism, and a rise in alternative lifestyles abound.
- *Empathy Economy* describes a world of responsible stewardship, with breakthroughs in technology akin to the Big Tech Economy but where the public takes a more active role. Self-regulation by companies alongside more worker engagement see technology applied to augment human capabilities. There are improvements in living standards, with more investment in care and education.

Upskilling, reskilling, and lifelong learning are all needed to address the challenges embodied in considering the future of work. New safety nets, such as a universal living settlement providing a basic income for all, worker alliances and shared regulation may all emerge as parts of the necessary social reform arising from disruption in jobs and work.

CALL TO ACTION

> *World leaders sitting there, look up because the future generation is raising their voice.*[172] Matala Yousafzai speaking at the UN General Assembly 25th September 2015

There are many challenges ahead, but we are confident in your abilities to make a difference and be the change you want to see—a world where no one is left behind. As future and practicing public health professionals, you are our future, and we need you to step up now and promote sustainable development through the lens of public health.

While the SDGs are comprehensive and an agreed actionable agenda for the global community, it can be difficult to decide what to prioritize and where to target your efforts. Adopting a systems view can help us act in entrepreneurial ways to effect change, recognizing the centrality of the user voice in cocreating solutions with the community. Data and information can help us, with big data and real-time data capture helping us to pinpoint key areas where interventions can deliver maximum measurable benefits. Here, we must however caution on inherent biases in large datasets used to train artificial intelligent machine learning algorithms, ensuring that underrepresented groups are not further disadvantaged by context-blind data. Similarly, we need to call out for more robust governance mechanisms that support inclusive and equitable input to decision-making, and effective accountability mechanisms. Tackling the governance trap of democracy is important, given we expect our governments to act but they do not care about the issues enough to do so—here, collective action can drive accountability.

In science, we need a new social contract between scientists and society, working towards a deeper engagement with communication and policy. With behavior, we need to face up to "stealth denial," that is that the majority of those who understand the problem intellectually live as though they do not, and break "climate silence" moving away from whether it is happening or not to what we are going to doing about it. In technology, we need to invest in the future, moving towards renewables and deep carbonization with means to constrain extraction. Overall, we need to reframe sustainability as a goal for today, systemic in nature with a range of possible solutions.

There is a tangible need for a developmental concept that will allow the reconciliation of economic development with environmental protection. While there are different views on responsibility and accountability, for example, are local environmental problems the result of local developments or of a global economic system that forced low-income countries to exploit their environmental basis? Do environmental burdens result mainly from destructive economic growth-based development or from a lack of economic innovation and modernization? Would reconciling the economy and the environment require mainly technical solutions, using more resource-efficient technologies, or are social and structural changes needed that include political decision-making as well as changes in individual consumption patterns? Looking at the SDGs, they are interconnected and hyperdependent, as such we can look to work both upstream and downstream when seeking to codevelop solutions, recognizing that tackling, for example, education has cobenefits on maternal health, workforce equity, and so on while mitigating climate change has positive health and well-being impacts alongside economic benefits. Governments should be responsible for building a shared vision for sustainable development, but public–private–plural multiactor partnerships should also be held to account through regulatory and policy instruments as well as consumer and user behaviors. Challenges to delivering the SDGs are multifaceted but should be measured against the risk of not delivering on the goals—an existential threat to humanity.

There is so much more we could have included in this chapter; public health and sustainability are vast and all-encompassing subjects. We hope in curating a selection of materials provides some food for thought, but more importantly inspired you to act in delivering against the SDGs and pursue sustainable development. It has been said that we have around a decade to save the planet. We are more hopeful than that and are heartened by the concerted efforts of our students, universities, business, communities, cities, and national and global organizations coming together in common cause around a shared purpose. Our current global response is insufficient, with transformative changes needed to restore and protect nature for the public good. We need radical collaboration across private, public, and plural actors coming together in multiactor partnerships convened around the SDGs. While new advancements in science and technology help us wrestle with old challenges in new settings—a world where no one is left behind, our task is not "predicting the general shape of tomorrow's innovations," but instead, "figuring out what we will *do* with these technologies once we have them, and what they will do with *us* [italics original]."[173]

With compassion and justice for all, public health seeks to preserve human dignity and stop the loss of human potential and for that we need a healthy planet. It is time to act—it is time to lead. Over to you!

References

1. https://sustainabledevelopment.un.org/content/documents/5987our-common-future.pdf.
2. http://www.csun.edu/~vcpsy00h/seattle.htm.
3. https://i.unu.edu/media/tfm.unu.edu/publication/142/CCMLCIP-2012-Crn-3-Report-Final.pdf.
4. https://unu.edu/.
5. https://www.clubofrome.org/report/the-limits-to-growth/.
6. http://publications.gc.ca/Collection-R/LoPBdP/BP/bp317-e.htm.
7. Ehrlich P. *The Population Bomb*. New York: Ballantine Books; 1969.
8. Carson R. *Silent Spring*. Boston, MA: Houghton Mifflin Company; 1962.
9. https://www.globalreporting.org/Pages/default.aspx.
10. https://unfccc.int/.
11. https://unfccc.int/resource/docs/convkp/kpeng.pdf.
12. https://sustainabledevelopment.un.org/content/documents/Agenda21.pdf. https://www.dataplan.info/img_upload/7bdb1584e3b8a53d337518d988763f8d/agenda21-earth-summit-the-united-nations-programme-of-action-from-rio_1.pdf.
13. https://www.un.org/millenniumgoals/.
14. https://sustainabledevelopment.un.org/?menu=1300.
15. https://www.cbd.int/.
16. https://unfccc.int/process/bodies/supreme-bodies/conference-of-the-parties-cop.

17. https://www.ipbes.net/global-assessment-report-biodiversity-ecosystem-services.
18. https://sustainabledevelopment.un.org/csd.html.
19. https://earthsummit2002.org/.
20. https://sustainabledevelopment.un.org/rio20.
21. https://sustainabledevelopment.un.org/futurewewant.html.
22. https://sustainabledevelopment.un.org/?menu=1300.
23. https://sustainabledevelopment.un.org/post2015/transformingour world/publication.
24. https://sustainabledevelopment.un.org/frameworks/24agreement.
25. https://sustainabledevelopment.un.org/frameworks/sendaiframework.
26. https://sustainabledevelopment.un.org/frameworks/addisababaaction agenda.
27. https://sustainabledevelopment.un.org/hlpf.
28. https://unstats.un.org/sdgs/report/2019/The-Sustainable-Development-Goals-Report-2019.pdf.
29. https://www.stockholmresilience.org/research/research-news/2016-06-14-how-food-connects-all-the-sdgs.html.
30. http://www.cop21paris.org/.
31. https://scripps.ucsd.edu/programs/keelingcurve/.
32. https://population.un.org/wpp/.
33. Hoornweg D, Pope K. Population predictions for the world's largest cities in the 21st century. *Environ Urban*. 2016;29(1):195–216.
34. https://www.un.org/development/desa/en/news/population/world-urbanization-prospects.html.
35. https://www.maplecroft.com/risk-indices/climate-change-vulnerability-index/.
36. https://www.rollingstone.com/politics/politics-news/bill-mckibben-winning-slowly-is-the-same-as-losing-198205/.
37. https://www.who.int/news-room/detail/02-05-2018-9-out-of-10-people-worldwide-breathe-polluted-air-but-more-countries-are-taking-action.
38. http://www.healthdata.org/gbd.
39. https://www.un.org/sustainabledevelopment/blog/2019/05/nature-decline-unprecedented-report/.
40. https://www2.usgs.gov/themes/factsheet/146-00/.
41. https://www.nrdc.org/stories/smart-seafood-buying-guide.
42. https://www.seafoodwatch.org/.
43. http://www.mercuryconvention.org/.
44. https://www.nature.com/articles/s41586-019-1468-9?ftag=MSF0951a18.
45. https://www.quotes.net/mquote/114764.
46. https://www.ellenmacarthurfoundation.org/publications/the-new-plastics-economy-rethinking-the-future-of-plastics.
47. https://www.mckinsey.com/industries/chemicals/our-insights/how-plastics-waste-recycling-could-transform-the-chemical-industry.
48. http://www.albatrossthefilm.com/.
49. https://www.plasticbank.org/.
50. https://www.adventurescientists.org/microplastics.html.
51. https://www.interface.com/APAC/en-AU/about/mission/Net-Works-en_AU.
52. https://www.cnn.com/style/article/prada-nylon-sustainable-scli-intl/index.html.
53. https://www.cell.com/matter/fulltext/S2590-2385(19)30056-6.
54. https://www.theguardian.com/environment/2019/jul/31/shoppers-use-of-plastic-bags-in-england-continues-to-fall.
55. https://www.ipcc.ch/site/assets/uploads/2018/03/WG1AR5_Summary Volume_FINAL.pdf.
56. https://climateactiontracker.org/media/images/CAT-2030Emissions Gaps-2018.12.original.png.
57. https://www.epa.gov/uog.
58. https://www.epa.gov/ghgreporting/ghgrp-petroleum-and-natural-gas-systems.
59. https://en.wikipedia.org/wiki/Aliso_Canyon_gas_leak.
60. http://www.fao.org/home/en/.
61. Ogino A, Orito H, Shimada K, et al. Evaluating environmental impacts of the Japanese beef cow–calf system by the life cycle assessment method. *Anim Sci J*. 2007;78(4):424–32.
62. Harvey H, Orvis R, Rissman J. *Designing Climate Solutions: A Policy Guide for Low-Carbon Energy*. Washington, DC: Island Press; 2018.
63. https://www.theverge.com/2016/11/22/13712750/tesla-microgrid-tau-samoa.
64. https://www.staycoolsavecash.com/analysis/delivering-urban-resilience-full-report.
65. https://carbonpricingdashboard.worldbank.org/.
66. http://pubdocs.worldbank.org/en/646831555088732759/FM-Coalition-Brochure-final-v3.pdf.
67. https://www.mckinsey.com/business-functions/sustainability/our-insights/why-commercial-use-could-be-the-future-of-carbon-capture.
68. https://www.iea.org/.
69. https://www.ucsusa.org/global_warming/science_and_impacts/science/climate-engineering#bf-toc-1.
70. Bastin J-F, Finegold Y, Garcia C, et al. The global tree restoration potential. *Science*. 2019;365(6448):76–9.
71. https://carbonengineering.com/.
72. https://www.nap.edu/catalog/18805/climate-intervention-carbon-dioxide-removal-and-reliable-sequestration.
73. https://www.climeworks.com/.
74. https://web.archive.org/web/20120927031948/http://www.grida.no/publications/other/ipcc_tar/?src=%2FCLIMATE%2FIPCC_TAR%2Fwg3%2F176.htm.
75. https://www.nap.edu/catalog/18805/climate-intervention-carbon-dioxide-removal-and-reliable-sequestration.
76. https://www.nap.edu/catalog/18988/climate-intervention-reflecting-sunlight-to-cool-earth.
77. https://www.ipcc.ch/assessment-report/ar3/.
78. https://www.ucsusa.org/global_warming/science_and_impacts/science/climate-engineering.
79. Waddell. 2019. https://i2insights.org/2019/03/05/transformational-change/.
80. Schot J, Geels FW. Niches in evolutionary theories of technical change. *J Evol Econ*. 2007;17:605–22.
81. http://www.rosecompanies.com/development/.
82. https://9foundations.forhealth.org/9_Foundations_of_a_Healthy_Building.February_2017.pdf.
83. https://forhealth.org/globalbuildings/.
84. http://harvardcgbc.org/research/housezero/.
85. http://www.cimas.edu.ec/projects.html.
86. https://www.huffpost.com/entry/education-is-the-kindling-of-a-flame-how-to-reinvent_b_5a4ffec5e4b0ee59d41c0a9f.
87. Purcell WM. A conceptual framework of leadership and governance in sustaining entrepreneurial universities illustrated with case material from a retrospective review of a university's strategic transformation: The enterprise university. In Kliewe et al.,Kliewe et al., eds. *Developing Engaged and Entrepreneurial Universities*. Singapore: Springer; 2019.
88. Heifetz M, Linsky RA. *Leadership on the Line: Staying Alive through the Dangers of Leading*. Boston, MA: Harvard Business School Press; 2002.
89. Laloux F. *Reinventing Organizations: A Guide to Creating Organizations Inspired by the Next Stage of Human Consciousness*. Brussels, Belgium: Nelson Parker; 2014.
90. Purcell WM. Change management and metaphor in global higher education. In: *Critical Global Semiotics: Understanding Sustainable Transformational Citizenship*. London: Routledge Book;2019. https://www.routledge.com/Critical-Global-Semiotics-Understanding-Sustainable-Transformational-Citizenship/Ellis/p/book/9780367076986.
91. Purcell WM, Sharp L, Chahine T. New governance models for entrepreneurial universities: A conceptual framework. *Academic Proceedings of the 2017 University-Industry Engagement Conference: From Best Practice to Next Practice—Asia-Pacific Opportunities and Perspectives*. 2017; pp. 19–29.
92. Purcell WM, Hendriksen HA, Spengler J. Universities as the engine of transformational sustainability toward delivering the sustainable development goals: 'Living labs' for sustainability. *Int J Sustain High Educ*. 2019;20(8):1343–57.
93. Purcell W, Chahine T. Leadership and governance frameworks driving transformational change in an entrepreneurial UK university. *Leadersh Organ Dev J*. 2019;40(5):612–23.
94. Purcell WM. Universities as thought-leaders and collaborative partners in addressing local challenges. Global priorities educated solutions the

role of academia in advancing the sustainable development goals. A report on the program hosted by the international alliance of research universities during the annual conference of the international sustainable campus network, 12 June 2018 in KTH Royal Institute of technology, Stockholm. P18 track: Service for Society, 2018. http://www.iaruni.org/images/stories/Sustainability/IARU-SDG-Report-final-v4.pdf.

95. https://en.unesco.org/.
96. https://www.unprme.org/.
97. https://www.sasb.org/.
98. https://science.sciencemag.org/content/359/6375/523.
99. http://globalsustain.org/en/story/14557.
100. https://www.circularity-gap.world/.
101. https://www.ellenmacarthurfoundation.org/circular-economy/what-is-the-circular-economy.
102. http://www.ethicalcorp.com/rise-climate-emergency-we-have-turn-tap-waste.
103. https://www.pgsupplier.com/en-US/supplier-citizenship-blog/ambition-2030.
104. https://hmfoundation.com/.
105. https://www.weforum.org/agenda/2019/01/how-a-circular-approach-can-turn-e-waste-into-a-golden-opportunity/.
106. https://eeb.org/eu-governments-support-first-set-of-laws-for-more-repairable-products/.
107. https://intelligence.weforum.org/topics/a1Gb00000038pGiEAI?tab=–publications.
108. https://www.nytimes.com/2014/09/08/education/harvards-school-of-public-health-gets-350-million-from-the-morningside-foundation.html.
109. Kruk ME, Gage AD, Arsenault C, et al. High-quality health systems in the sustainable development goals era: Time for a revolution. *Lancet Glob Health*. 2018;6:e1196–252.
110. http://www3.weforum.org/docs/WEF_Harvard_HE_GlobalEconomicBurdenNonCommunicableDiseases_2011.pdf.
111. https://www.researchgate.net/publication/332288303_Digital_Inequalities_in_the_Age_of_Artificial_Intelligence_and_Big_Data.
112. Inayatullah S. Creating the prevention Prama Society. *The Health Advocate*. 2009;2:24–7. http://www.metafuture.org/library1/EmergingIssues/Creating-a-healthy-prama-society-Health-Advocate-2010.pdf.
113. https://www.manatt.com/insights/newsletters/health-update/10-megatrends-shaping-healthcare%E2%80%99s-next-1#Article1.
114. https://globalhealth.harvard.edu/people/ashish-jha.
115. https://www.wri.org/our-work/project/adaptation-finance-accountability-initiative.
116. https://civileats.com/>underline>2019/01>/underline>/14/edible-landscapes-are-un-lawning-america/.
117. https://www.ase.org/profile/national-rural-electric-cooperative-association.
118. https://www.euractiv.com/section/climate-environment/news/greta-thunberg-urges-meps-to-panic-like-the-house-is-on-fire/.
119. https://climateemergencydeclaration.org/united-kingdom-bipartisan-uk-parliament-declares-a-climate-emergency/.
120. https://www.researchgate.net/publication/281102433_Nihilism_fundamentalism_or_activism_Three_responses_to_fears_of_the_Apocalypse.
121. https://news.gallup.com/poll/23>underline>2007>/underline>/americans-want-government-more-environment.aspx.
122. https://wattsupwiththat.com/2019/05/09/decarbonisation-and-the-command-economy/.
123. https://www.worldbank.org/en/topic/pandemics.
124. https://www.securityconference.de/en/activities/munich-security-conference/munich-security-conference/msc-2017/speeches/speech-by-bill-gates/.
125. Wilbur Sawyer, Presidential Address, American Society of Tropical Medicine and Hygiene, 1944. https://www.astmh.org/ASTMH/media/Documents/Presidential%20Addresses/1944-Wilbur-A-Sawyer.pdf.
126. Whitmee S, Haines A, Beyrer C, et al. Safeguarding human health in the Anthropocene epoch: Report of the Rockefeller Foundation–Lancet Commission on Planetary Health. *Lancet*. 2015;386(10007):1973–2028.
127. https://www.un.org/zerohunger/.
128. https://www.wfp.org/.
129. https://oll.libertyfund.org/titles/malthus-an-essay-on-the-principle-of-population-1798-1st-ed.
130. https://docs.wixstatic.com/ugd/32519f_e622b238689e406895b54ec6af808a49.pdf.
131. http://www.fao.org/3/a-bp263e.pdf.
132. Cassidy ES, West PC, Gerber JS, Foley JA. Redefining agricultural yields: From tonnes to people nourished per hectare. *Environ Res Lett*. 2013;8(3):1–8.
133. https://www.thelancet.com/commissions/EAT.
134. https://www.who.int/nutrition/topics/sfa-tfa-public-consultation-4may2018/en/.
135. https://www.keepinspiring.me/winston-churchill-quotes/.
136. http://businesscommission.org/.
137. https://www.ey.com/Publication/vwLUAssets/ey-the-state-of-the-debate-on-purpose-in-business/$FILE/ey-the-state-of-the-debate-on-purpose-in-business.pdf.
138. https://www.cisl.cam.ac.uk/.
139. https://www.cisl.cam.ac.uk/resources/publication-pdfs/rewiring-leadership.pdf.
140. Stanford Social Innovation Review 'The Strategic Plan is Dead. Long Live Strategy'. https://ssir.org/articles/entry/the_strategic_plan_is_dead._long_live_strategy.
141. https://quoteinvestigator.com/2017/11/18/planning/.
142. https://www.wttc.org/.
143. https://www.news.com.au/travel/world-travel/asia/here-are-three-more-places-you-cant-visit-in-thailand-anymore/news-story/7329c8150749ee25d4234a3c3f178c30.
144. https://www.parliament.uk/business/committees/committees-a-z/commons-select/environmental-audit-committee/news-parliament-2017/sustainable-tourism-inquiry-launch-17-19/.
145. https://scholar.harvard.edu/sustainabletourism/home.
146. https://www.thetravelfoundation.org.uk/invisible-burden/.
147. https://scholar.harvard.edu/files/sustainabletourism/files/tunisia_tourism_and_a_changing_climate_final_report_final.pdf.
148. https://www.wttc.org/-/media/files/reports/policy-research/tt-2015--connecting-global-climate-action-a4-28pp-web.pdf?la=en.
149. https://unfccc.int/news/world-travel-tourism-industry-pledges-climate-neutrality.
150. https://www.wttc.org/-/media/files/summits/buenos-aires-2018/wttc-buenos-aires-declaration-with-signatures.pdf.
151. https://www.wttc.org/tourism-for-tomorrow-awards/.
152. https://advances.sciencemag.org/content/5/7/eaax0903.
153. https://www.ipbes.net/policy-support/tools-instruments/integrated-valuation-ecosystem-services-tradeoffs-invest.
154. https://www.nytimes.com/2016/09/06/health/lonliness-aging-health-effects.html.
155. https://www.kff.org/other/report/loneliness-and-social-isolation-in-the-united-states-the-united-kingdom-and-japan-an-international-survey/.
156. https://www.economist.com/international/2018/09/01/loneliness-is-a-serious-public-health-problem.
157. https://www.hrsa.gov/enews/past-issues/2019/january-17/loneliness-epidemic.
158. http://www.chcr.brown.edu/pcoc/cesdscale.pdf.
159. https://whatworkswellbeing.org/.
160. https://worldhappiness.report/ed/2019/.
161. https://theharrispoll.com/new-york-n-y-may-30-2013-has-the-pursuit-of-happiness-left-americans-unhappy-maybe-according-to-the-harris-polla-happiness-index-which-uses-a-series-of-questions-to-calculate-americans/.
162. https://ophi.org.uk/policy/national-policy/gross-national-happiness-index/.
163. https://www.livehappy.com/happiness-movement.
164. http://fab.cba.mit.edu/.
165. https://www.hsph.harvard.edu/health-happiness/.
166. https://www.thersa.org/discover/publications-and-articles/reports/field-guide-to-the-future-of-work-essay-collection.
167. http://www3.weforum.org/docs/WEF_Future_of_Jobs_2018.pdf.

168. https://www.un.org/development/desa/en/news/population/2018-revision-of-world-urbanization-prospects.html.
169. https://www.healthcaredive.com/news/deepminds-ai-detects-over-50-eye-diseases-with-94-accuracy-study-shows-1/530125/.
170. https://interestingengineering.com/this-10000-3d-printed-concrete-house-took-only-24-hours-to-build.
171. https://www.thersa.org/globalassets/pdfs/reports/rsa_four-futures-of-work.pdf.
172. https://news.un.org/en/story/2015/09/509752-malala-yousafzai-urges-world-leaders-un-promise-safe-quality-education-every.
173. Vallor S. *Technology and the Virtues: A Philosophical Guide to a World Worth Wanting*. New York: Oxford University Press; 2016.
174. https://global.oup.com/academic/product/technology-and-the-virtues-9780190498511?cc=us&lang=en&.
175. Rowson J, Corner A. The Seven Dimensions of Climate Change. *RSA Action and Research Centre*, 2015. https://www.thersa.org/discover/publications-and-articles/reports/the-seven-dimensions-of-climate-change-introducing-a-new-way-to-think-talk-and-act.

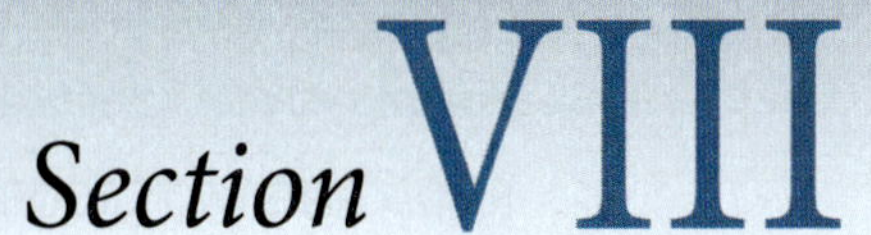

Section Editors
Ruth Lynfield, Timothy Jones, and Matthew L. Boulton

Communicable Diseases

CHAPTER

81

Agents of Infection and Principles of Transmission

Noreen A. Hynes • Diane Meyer

INTRODUCTION

Infectious diseases have posed significant threats to the public's health for millennia. Despite a change in global and domestic leading causes of morbidity and mortality with a shift to chronic diseases, infectious diseases continue to impose a high burden on individual and population health.[1] Therefore, public health practitioners must continue to attend to the prevention and control of infectious diseases. Common infectious diseases challenges in resource rich areas include influenza (which combined with pneumonia is the eighth leading cause of death in the United States), foodborne illnesses, health-care-associated infections, sexually transmitted diseases, hepatitis C, and human immunodeficiency virus (HIV) infections.[2] Although these same infectious diseases abound in lower resource countries, more traditional causes of infectious disease-associated morbidity and mortality prevail in these settings including tuberculosis (TB), malaria, soil-transmitted helminthic (STH) diseases, and diarrheal and acute respiratory infections (particularly in the under-5 age group). Adding to the complexity of the burden of infectious diseases is the identification of new infectious agents or the re-emergence of those in previously endemic areas. Demographic migrations among humans as well as animals, and the vectors and reservoirs of infectious agents, contribute to the introduction of new or the reintroduction of eliminated diseases as population threats where consideration of the classic epidemiological triad of determinants—the human host, the agent, and the human environment—comes into play.[3]

Selection and design of the optimal approach to prevent and control infectious diseases requires not only an understanding of the classic epidemiological triad but also the possible outcomes of the interactions of the host with a potentially infectious agent and the environment as it applies to both the host and the agent (Fig. 81-1). Although it is beyond the scope of this chapter to provide comprehensive information about every infectious agent, here we provide a general primer of infectious agents and their transmission to serve as a broad introduction to the subsequent communicable diseases chapters.

Terminology and definitions associated with infection and infectious diseases often reflect perspective, including the public, the clinician, the public health practitioner, the clinical laboratorian, the research scientist, the historian, or the lawyer. Here, we will use definitions used in the scientific domains, including public health, with the understanding that this lexicon is not standardized. Infectious agents encompass both microscopic and macroscopic organisms. An agent that gains access to and causes a response in the host resulting in an end-result termed infection. Importantly, not all exposures of a host to an infectious agent result in infection. This may be due to the presence of an inhospitable setting wherein the agent is seeking entry to a nonpermissive anatomic site, the host may lack the needed receptor for the agent, or the microenvironment of the host, such as pH, moisture content, or available nutrients, may ward off infection. If the result of the agent–host interaction causes both an infection and a disorder, then an infectious disease occurs; the etiological agent is a pathogen and its related processes define its pathogenesis.

An active disease state is only one of several outcomes following infection. The initial establishment of an ecological community on and within the human host, known as the human microbiota or normal flora, begins at birth. It consists primarily of bacterial species that create interactive states that do not harm the human host.[4] Mutualism exists when both the infecting agent and the host benefit from the interaction and when the interaction is longer term, it is referred to as, synergy. Commensalism occurs when the infecting organism is in a relationship wherein it derives nutrients or other benefits from the host without benefiting or harming the host. When an infectious agent—that is not part of the normal flora—is isolated from a nonsterile site of a human and there is no evidence of an adverse outcome, a state of colonization exists. Colonization may act as an immunizing event wherein the infection is asymptomatic or inapparent because the host's defenses have prevented multiplication of the infectious agent required to cause disease. Colonizing agents rarely go on to become invasive pathogens causing disease. The presence of antibodies reveals that prior infection has occurred.

PRINCIPLES OF TRANSMISSION

The triad of host, agent, and environment and their interactions are key to the transmission and occurrence of infectious disease as well as to designing appropriate prevention and control strategies. Each infectious agent falls into one of the following categories: infectious prions, viruses, bacteria (prokaryotes), fungi, protozoa, or multicellular organisms, such as worms (Table 81-1). The infectious diseases caused by these agents may be contagious or noncontagious in nature. The word contagious comes from the Latin *contagionem* meaning "to touch," originally with a sense of touch being something physically unclean. Historically, a contagious disease meant only those infections transmitted person-to-person through physical contact. The meaning now has expanded to include not only transmission to other people by physical contact with a person with an infection but also through casual contact with their secretions or objects touched by them (fomites) or via the airborne route. Noncontagious infectious diseases require a special mode of transmission to the host such as through a mosquito vector carrying the malaria parasite or a blood transfusion delivering human T-cell lymphoma virus. Contagious diseases (e.g., influenza) or noncontagious disease (e.g., dengue) can cause epidemics.

There are three important determinants to transmission of an infectious agent to a susceptible human host. First is the habitat or reservoir where the agent normally lives and multiplies; second is the route or mode of transmission to the host; and third is the portal

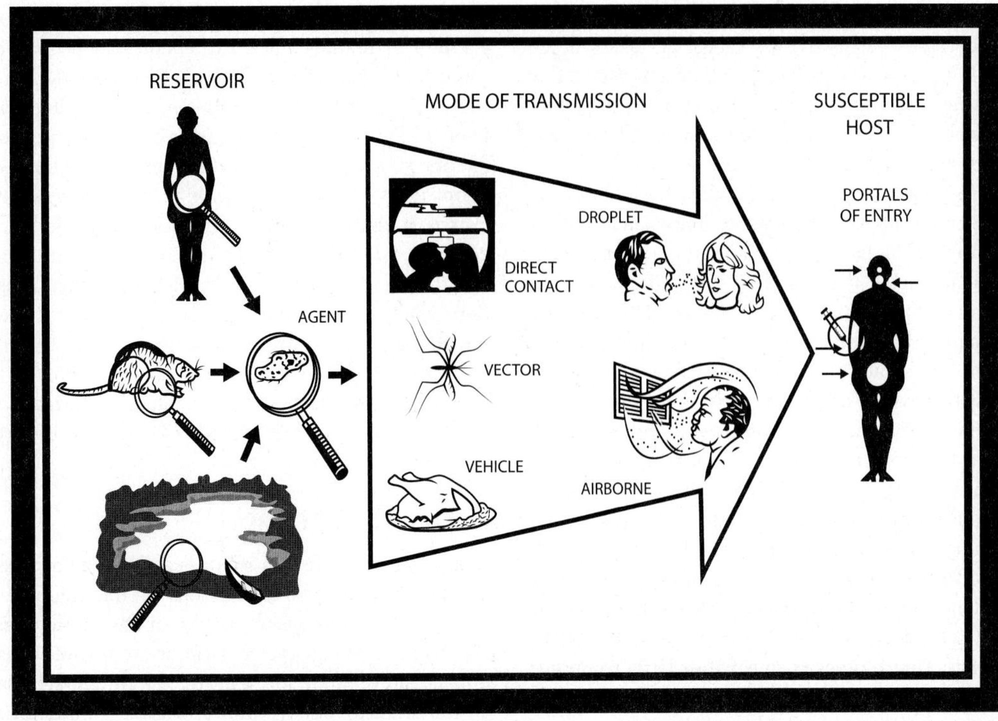

FIGURE 81-1. Chain of infection. (*Source:* Centers for Disease Control and Prevention. Principles of Epidemiology, 2nd ed. U.S. Department of Health and Human Services; 1992.)

TABLE 81-1 AGENTS OF INFECTION AND THEIR CHARACTERISTICS

Characteristic	Prions	Viruses	Bacteria	Fungi	Parasites[a]
Cell wall	No	No	Yes	Yes	+/-
Approximate diameter	0.02 nm	0.02–.3 μm	1–5 μm	3–10 μm (yeasts)	15–20 μm (trophozoites)[b]
Nucleic acids	No	Either DNA or RNA	Both DNA and RNA	Both DNA and RNA	Both DNA and RNA
Ribosomes	No	No	70s	80s	80s
Mitochondria	No	No	No	Yes	Yes
Cell wall containing peptidoglycan	No	No	Yes (Most)	No[c]	No
Chromosome number	None	None	Usually 1	More than 1	More than 1
Motility	No	No	No	No	Yes (most)
Replication	Unclear	Uses host mechanisms	Binary Fission, most acellularly[d]	Budding (yeasts) or mitosis (molds)	Reproduces self-using sexual life cycles

[a]Parasites include the protozoa and helminthes (worms).
[b]The lower limit of detection by the naked eye is ~ 40 μm; protozoa cannot be seen but proglottids of tapeworms and the egg of *Fasciola hepatica*, for example, can be seen.
[c]Fungal cells have a rigid cell wall due to the presence of chitin rather than peptidoglycan.
[d]Rickettsia and chlamydia require a living host cell for growth and replication.

of entry into the host (Fig. 81-1). The three reservoirs of infection—human, animal, and environmental—may or may not be mutually exclusive. For example, when humans are the only reservoir for infection, it may be possible to eradicate a pathogen and its associated disease. This occurred with the smallpox virus (Variola) and its associated disease, smallpox.[5] Other common infectious agents with only human reservoirs of infection include *Neisseria gonorrhoeae* (gonorrhea), measles virus, and Group A (beta hemolytic) streptococci. Human reservoirs may not show any signs of illness such as chronic carriers of *Salmonella enterica* serovar Typhi, the cause of typhoid fever. Animals or the environment may serve as an important reservoir of infection for other animals as well as humans. *Trichinella spiralis*, a roundworm infection found in carnivorous feral animals in the United Sates, such as polar bears and wild boar, causes trichinosis in human who consume inadequately cooked meat from such animals. Importantly, trichinosis is a zoonotic infection because humans are accidental or incidental hosts in the natural transmission and maintenance cycle of this infection. The dimorphic fungus *Blastomyces dermatitidis,* found in certain parts of North America, causes skin or lung disease; it lives in moist soil, particularly in wooded areas and its conidial form is inhaled in dust when an area with the agent is disturbed. Person-to-person or human-to-animal transmission does not occur following infection with this pathogen.

Each infectious agent may have one or more modes of transmission from its reservoir to the susceptible host; transmission can be either direct or indirect. An example of direct transmission is a hookworm infection contracted after direct contact with infected soil by a barefoot child living in the Mississippi delta area or the unvaccinated grandmother who develops pertussis after a large particle droplet[6] containing *Bordetella pertussis* is expelled from her grandchild that lands on her nasal mucosa. Indirect transmission of an infectious agent from its reservoir can occur in one of three ways: airborne, from inanimate objects, or animate ones, alternatively noted as the "three V's"—vapors, vehicles, and vectors. Understanding these modes of transmission is very important for designing and implementing control strategies. The "vapors" of the airborne route are very small particles (less than 5 μm in diameter) that flow through the air in a gas-like manner rather than in a trajectory seen with heavy droplets.[6] The best example of how this occurs is when an unvaccinated child develops measles traced to his attendance at a daycare center beginning one hour after a child with measles has gone home—because airborne particles stay suspended in air for a time.[7] Vehicles of indirect transmission include food, water, fomites (such as surgical instruments or towels), and biological products (such as blood products or transplanted organs). Consuming contaminated food and water causes many infectious diseases worldwide. In the United States, it is estimated that each year 31 major pathogens cause 9.4 million foodborne illnesses, over 50,000 hospitalizations, and over 1200 deaths.[8] Vectors include mosquitoes, ticks, fleas, and mites. Examples of vector-borne diseases include malaria (mosquitoes), Lyme disease (ticks), bubonic plague (fleas), and scrub typhus (mites). The vector-borne transmission route is the most complex among the three discussed because of the replication dynamics within the living vector, such as that seen with malaria.

The human host is also critical within the overall transmission model. Infection and infectious diseases require a susceptible host. There are several factors contributing to a host's susceptibility including genetic, immune, and nonspecific factors. Genetic factors may be important in increasing or decreasing risk for an infectious disease. Certain mutations are associated with "selective immunodeficiency," placing the host at increased risk of severe infectious disease outcomes. For example, the clinical outcomes following hepatitis B virus (HBV) infection are variable and only a small number develop chronic infection. A strong association between human leukocyte antigen (HLA) variants in the HLA class II region has been shown to protect against chronic infection in some Asian populations.[9] Specific immunity may also protect the human host as occurs following immunization or the transfer of material antibodies against pertussis to the fetus to protect the newborn in early months of life from possible life-threatening disease. Nonspecific factors that contribute to host susceptibility include disruption of host natural defenses such as immunosuppression due to drugs or disease. For example, persons with cirrhosis are at greatly increased risk of bacterial infections, such as urinary tract infections, when compared with persons without cirrhosis. Additionally, certain bacterial infections are more common and more severe in persons with cirrhosis including *Listeria, Campylobacter, Vibrio, and Yersinia* spp.[10]

In addition to the host, the reservoir, and the mode of transmission, other considerations in the design of prevention and control strategies including the natural progression of an infectious disease and its basic reproductive rate or number, abbreviated Ro (R-naught or R zero). There are four stages in the natural progression of an infectious disease. The incubation period is the time from exposure to the infectious agent or its elaborated toxin and the appearance of first clinical symptoms. When the symptoms are nonspecific, this is the prodromal period, followed by the specific illness period. The resolution of symptoms begins the convalescent period. Following this recovery period, and depending upon the infecting agent, the host may become a chronic carrier and as such may be a source of infection to others. Alternatively, following the recovery period of active infection, the host may continue to harbor latent infection that causes no ongoing harm to the host and is not transmissible to others or become a disease carrier. Finally, depending upon the infectious agent or toxin, the clinical expression may be local or systemic. The reproductive rate of an infection, often called the R naught (R_0), is the number of secondary infections in a susceptible population arising from a single person during his or her entire infectious period.[11] The factors contributing to R_0 include the average number of susceptible people who are in contact with an infectious person (factor c), the average probability, *p*, that transmission will take place during a given contact, and the average duration of infectiousness (*d*).[11] When R_0 is <1, the infection should die out whereas when R_0 is > 1, the infection will spread in the population.[11] In general, the greater the R_0, the harder it is to control an infectious disease epidemic. An effective public health intervention aimed at one or more of the three factors contributing to the reproductive rate should result in a decrease in the reproductive rate. See Chapter 82: "Epidemiology and Control of Infectious Diseases."

AGENTS OF INFECTION

The previous discussion examined the general principles of transmission. Here we provide a primer on the agents of infection. Many of these infectious agents will be discussed in greater detail in the chapters following, particularly in terms of their public health impact, prevention, and control. A full appreciation of the course of human history is incomplete without consideration of the causes and consequences of human disease, including infections, on the health, well-being, and success of populations.[12] Until the beginning of the twentieth century, infectious diseases posed the greatest disease threat to the health and well-being of the world's population. Although ischemic heart disease, stroke, and chronic obstructive pulmonary disease were the leading causes of death worldwide in 2016, lower respiratory tract infections, diarrheal diseases, and TB remain among the top ten causes.[13] Despite early inability to identify, isolate, and categorize infectious agents, we were able to ascribe names to their associated conditions and report on their impact on the outcome of armed conflicts (the plague),[14] colonization (smallpox—"the pox"),[15] crowding (TB),[16] and overall population health (cholera and trichinosis).[17,18] At times, there were demonstrated effective prevention strategies, often evidence based, on what we would now consider sound epidemiological methods, such as the identification of the source of the cholera epidemic in London's Soho district in 1849 by John Snow.[19]

Reliance on clinical observational skills in premodern times to today continues to be important in identifying disease in both individuals and populations when outbreaks occur. Laboratory diagnostics skills were later additions to the clinical and public health armamentarium, beginning with the invention of the compound light microscope in about 1595, followed by the creation of the simple one-lens microscope by Antoni van Leeuwenhoek,[20] which achieved twice the resolution of the earliest microscope. Macroscopic identification of worms predated the introduction of the light microscope that led to the rapid evolution of identification techniques for many bacteria.[21] Although the discovery of nonbacterial filterable infectious agents, termed viruses, occurred in the late 1800s, it was not until 1932 that the first human virus—yellow fever virus—was isolated from a human subject by Max Thieler.[22] The second half of the twentieth century and continuing into the current twenty-first century has seen exponential growth in our ability to identify and characterize infectious agents, identify possible pathological outcomes, understand the ways in which a potentially infectious agent can be transmitted and, at times, design more successful prevention and treatment strategies than previously existed.

Classification of Infectious Agents

As noted previously, infectious agents include prions, viruses, bacteria (prokaryotes), fungi, protozoa, and multicellular organisms, such as worms (helminths). Infectious prions and viruses are the smallest of the infectious agents and are incapable of independent replication and life and devoid of nucleic acids. A prion has a length of approximately 5–10 nanometers (10^{-9} m) whereas viruses range in size from 0.03 to 0.300 μm (10^{-6} m). Viruses are incapable of independent replication outside of a host cell. Complex, living agents have been traditionally stratified into three common subdivisions and two domains: the Archeae and the Bacteria, collectively called the Prokarya, and the Eukarya known as the Eurkaryotes.[23] The prokaryotes usually range from 0.2 to 2.0 μm. Notably, there is no substantive evidence to support that the Archeae are pathogenic[24] for humans and these will not be discussed further. The prokaryotes, characterized by the absence of true membrane-bound nuclei or organelles, reproduce by binary fission. Some bacteria are obligate intracellular organisms and are considered complete organisms within other organisms. The eukaryotes have true nuclei and division is by mitosis. There are several eukaryote subcategories including the protista (protozoa and algae), fungi (yeasts and molds), and helminths or worms (nematodes, cestodes, and trematodes).

Infectious Prions

Biologically distinct molecules involved in cellular processes were known in the eighteenth century, but had to await the next century for Jons Jakob Berzelius to assign the name protein.[25] A neurodegenerative condition, called sheep scrapie, was described in 1732 long before J.S. Griffith speculated, in 1967, that it was due to a protein rather than a slow virus or other microbe.[26,27] In the early 1920s, a human neurological condition of unknown etiology was described by Hans Gerhard Cruetzfeldt and Alfons Maria Jakob[25] and later named Creutzfeldt-Jakob disease (CJD). In 1959, William Hadlow reported on his observation of similar spongiform encephalopathies seen in both scrapie and kuru—a fatal neurodegenerative disease affecting a single language group in remote Papua New Guinea.[25] In the same year, Igor Klatzo reported the similarity in the histopathological features between scrapie and CJD. Although, CJD, kuru and other similar conditions subsequently were demonstrated to be transmissible, the specific etiologic agent was not defined until 1982 when Stanley Pruisner demonstrated the likely infectious nature of the proteins alone, that he named prions.[5]

The prion diseases, also known as transmissible spongiform encephalopathies (TSEs), constitute a family of rare, progressive neurodegenerative diseases, with specific types seen in humans and others in animals. Long incubation periods, with rapid progression following symptom onset to their fatal outcome are characteristic of the TSEs. Currently, there are five human-known prion diseases: kuru, CJD, variant Creutzfeldt-Jakob disease (vCJD), Gerstmann-Sträussler-Scheinker syndrome (GSS), and fatal familial insomnia (FFI). Among these human prion diseases CJD is the most commonly reported worldwide with an annual incidence of approximately one per million population. Most persons with CJD disease die within 1 year of symptom onset; these symptoms include rapid mental deterioration and myoclonus. About 85% of cases fall into the sporadic pattern of disease, with no recognizable transmission risk; 5–15% are classified as heritable to autosomal dominant inherited mutations in the prion protein gene (*PRNP* gene) causing heritable CJD, FFI, or GSS. A small of iatrogenic cases of CJD have occurred following contact within healthcare systems, including transmission following certain medical procedures such as blood transfusions, corneal transplants, and administration of human pituitary-derived growth hormone.[28–31] Their public health importance lies in preventing iatrogenic transmission.

So-called variant CJD (vCJD) was first described in 1995 in a sporadic case in the United Kingdom, with 22 additional cases identified the following year; all but one occurring in the United Kingdom.[32–34] It is not the same disease as the classic sporadic and heritable CJD forms described above; vCJD has different clinical and pathological characteristics. Notably, it has symptom onset at a younger age, with prominent sensory disturbances and psychiatric symptoms. In 1986, bovine spongiform encephalopathy (BSE) was discovered in cattle; it is believed to have evolved after consumption of offal from affected sheep.[35] Epidemiological data support bovine-to-human transmission as the human outbreak followed a change in processing of bovine offal that eliminated organic solvents (which inactivate PrP^{sc}) and the use of the offal in cattle feed. Exclusion of ruminant-derived proteins from animal and poultry feeds and a ban on consuming animals over the age of 30 months has dramatically decreased BSE and vCJD. Strict feed and animal import controls have been in place in the United States for many years. There have been only six BSE cases reported in U.S. cattle[36] and four cases of vCJD reported in the United States, all of whom had a likely identified exposure outside of the United States.[37]

These two diseases, BSE and vCJD, highlight the importance of "One Health" approaches in the prevention and control of disease, as six of every 10 infectious diseases in humans are spread from animals.[38] See Chapter 84: "One Health: A New Paradigm for Disease Prevention and Control." Historically, infectious prions have been transmitted though ritualistic cannibalism, causing the disease called kuru.[39] However, changes in cultural practices have led to only extremely rare cases reported today.

Viruses

Long before the isolation of the first human virus at the dawn of the twentieth century, many viral diseases caused unabated morbidity and mortality. Smallpox (Variola virus) and yellow fever (Flavivirus), for example, were responsible for millions of deaths each century and did not discriminate based upon societal wealth or status. Vaccination led to the eradication of smallpox and its virus, a uniquely human virus,[5] and elimination of yellow fever virus from many countries highlighting, the importance of this control strategy.

Historically, the first use of the word "virus" was in 1599, meaning poison, rather than a specific agent causing infection. By 1940, the definition of the word "virus" remained controversial and was often used to mean any transmissible agent, stratified by those that could be seen with a light microscope, also called microbes, and agents that could not be seen under a microscopic lens, called contagia.[40] In humans, the smallest virus causing infection, human parvovirus B19—its revised name is primate erythroparvovirus-1—is 20–26 nm in size;[41] the largest human virus, the smallpox virus, is 350 nm in its greatest dimension.

The first virus to be identified was a plant virus later known as tobacco mosaic virus, and was discovered when the extract taken from infected tobacco leaves was noted to still be infectious even after passage through a bacteria-impermeable filter, and only replicated in a host organism.[42] This was followed by the reporting of the first human virus identified—yellow fever virus—by Walter Reed when presenting a "preliminary note" on the subject at the American Public Health Association meeting, held in Indianapolis in October 1900, and immediately thereafter published in two journals.[43,44]

There are many known viruses of medical and public health importance among the nearly 5000 viruses known to exist today. In addition, new virus species continue to be identified.[41] A virus consists of a viral genome (made up of either DNA or RNA) packaged inside a protein coat known as the capsid. Some viruses also have a lipid bilayer, or envelope, that surrounds the capsid and is sensitive to environmental desiccation.[45] Virus entry into a target host cell is a multistep process that is dependent on specific receptors located on the host cell surface.[46] Once bound to the appropriate receptor, the virus enters the host cell's cytoplasm either through receptor-mediated endocytosis or through direct penetration of the cell's plasma membrane. Thereafter, the virus uses host-cell machinery for genome replication and protein production and processing. Successful replication within the host cell also requires that the newly produced progeny are able to avoid killing by the host, by evading its ability to kill infected cells.[47] Virus infection causes numerous cytopathic effects in host cells, including reduction in host-cell protein synthesis and various structural changes.[48,49]

Experts continue to struggle with the ideal classification system to use for viruses; classification may be by phenotypic characteristics such as nucleic acid type and morphology, type of disease they cause, how they replicate, or the host(s) they infect. One commonly used classification system stratifies viruses into different families according to whether or not they contain a lipid envelope, as well as by their nucleic acid type (DNA or RNA), structure (single or double stranded, linear or circular), and viral capsid symmetry (helical or icosahedral). Another schema used for virus classification is modes of transmission. Often, this is useful for medical and public health practitioners for designing prevention and control strategies. Together, these two classification approaches are critical for understanding the natural history, pathogenesis, diagnosis, treatment, prevention, and control of viral diseases. Several examples of important viruses using these schemata follow that make clear the difficulty in seeking a single taxonomy.

Rotavirus, a nonenveloped member of the family Reoviridae, is a double-stranded RNA virus. It is an enteric virus that is the most common cause of diarrhea-associated death in children less than 5 years of age, the vast majority in lower resource countries.[50] This fecal-orally transmitted virus requires only a small inoculum (approximately 100 colony-forming units) to infect the host; illness onset is within 48 hours and infectious virus is shed in the stool for 10 days or more. Development, licensure, and recommended use of rotavirus vaccine by the United States and the World Health Organization in 2006 and 2012, respectively, to prevent rotavirus morbidity and mortality has had measurable salutary effects.[51]

Respiratory syncytial virus (RSV), an enveloped member of the family Paramyxoviridae, is a linear negative sense RNA virus. It is a respiratory virus spread primarily by direct contact such as inoculation of ocular and nasopharyngeal mucous membranes after contact with virus-containing secretions or fomites. It is an important cause of illness and death in those under the age of 5 years and adults older than 65 years.[50] Infected persons are usually contagious for 3–8 days and the virus can persist on hard surfaces for many hours making RSV highly contagious, in general, and an important cause of health-care-associated and daycare infections. Targeted prevention strategies are key based upon the setting where transmission may occur or is occurring.

Influenza A viruses, enveloped members of the family Orthmyxoviridae, are RNA viruses with a segmented genome that allows high rates of genome segment reassortment among viruses co-infecting the same host cell. The modes of transmission and highest risk age groups are similar to RSV. However, the segmented genome can be associated, from time-to-time, with the evolution of combining animal and human RNA segments to produce a novel virus and a population pandemic with high mortality rates in all age groups. For example, influenza virus killed about 50 million people during the 1918–19 influenza pandemic.[52] The ever-changing antigenic nature of the virus necessitates reformulation and administration of a licensed vaccine annually prior to virus circulation, adding to the complexity of the prevention and control of this potentially deadly virus.[53]

The viral infections discussed above are associated with an acute viral infection during which time the host and the virus are in a constant state of disequilibrium. The host and the virus are constantly changing until the host's immune system clears the infection or the virus kills the host—no chronic infection occurs. However, interactions with some viruses lead to chronic infection wherein both the human host and the virus have evolved mechanisms to reach a metastable equilibrium. Under these conditions, the host's immune system downregulates to limit a continuous inflammatory response and dampen ongoing immunopathology.[54] Importantly, although at least 30 different viruses establish chronic infection following the inciting acute infection; the majority of these infections do not cause ongoing clinical disease.

Continuous viral replication, latency with reactivation, and invasion of the host's genome are the three strategies used by viruses to sustain chronic infection; one or more strategies may exist simultaneously.[54] Understanding the mode of virus transmission that leads to acute infection and the strategies in use to maintain chronic infection, assist in the design of public health prevention and control strategies. Examples of viruses that use continuous viral replication as a strategy include HIV, HBV, and hepatitis C virus (HCV). In the latency-reactivation strategy, virus replication with antigen expression ends after the acute infection in response to the host's immune system response. The virus then "hides" from the immune system. In their quiescent and hidden state, they are inaccessible to the host's immune clearance mechanisms. Importantly, these latent viruses must reactivate periodically to replicate and spread to new cells which is a strategy used by HIV. The Epstein-Barr virus (EBV) and some other herpes viruses also use this strategy of reactivation for replication. However, this approach may be thwarted in a process called abortive reactivation. This is common in EBV following acute infection in the immunocompetent host. The third strategy—invasion of the host's genome—is a long-standing strategy used by viruses. Vertically transmitted human endogenous retroviruses (ERVs) are normal components of the human genome and are remnants of germline infections eons ago by exogenous retroviruses. They appear to have a role in shaping the immune system and its responses[55]; therefore, they could be considered part of our normal metagenome, despite the relation of some ERVs to adverse disease states, including cancers and immune-mediated conditions. These ERVs are not currently amenable to prevention.

One important and preventable adverse outcome of some chronic virus infections is cancer. Hepatocellular carcinoma (HCC), the fifth most common cause of cancer worldwide,[56] usually presents after decades of chronic infection with HBV or HCV with a primary route of transmission via exposure to virus-containing blood or body fluids.[57] Hepatitis B is vaccine preventable and hepatitis C, accounting for one-third of all HCC cases in the United States,[58] can be treated and cured with antiviral agents. Human papillomavirus (HPV) may also cause cancer. There are over 170 serotypes of HPV. Some types may cause chronic infection and some have oncogenic potential, causing cancers of the cervix, penis, anus, or the head and neck. The sexual route of transmission is responsible for nearly all cases of cervical cancer, vulvar and vaginal cancer in women, most penile cancer in men and anal cancer cases in both sexes, and 25% of the head and neck cancers. A currently licensed vaccine directed at preventing nine serotypes of HPV, of which seven are directed at oncogenic strains causing invasive cervical cancer, could prevent 90% of invasive cervical cancer globally if administered to those between the ages of 11 and 45 years.[59–61] See Chapter 100: "Human Papillomavirus." Furthermore, chronic infection can lead to alterations in host-immune responsiveness that leads to increased risk of cancers when exposed to other viruses. This is exemplified by the range of cancers seen in HIV-infected persons that appear directly related to the immunosuppressive effect of HIV.[62] See Chapter 87: "The Epidemiology and Preventive of HIV and AIDS."

Bacteria

Bacteria are the oldest and most numerous independently replicating form of life. There are thousands of bacterial species, most of which are harmless or even beneficial to humans. For example, there are more than 2000 bacterial species making up the normal flora (also called the microbiome) on our skin and throughout the human gastrointestinal tract.[4] Importantly, there are fewer than 100 disease-causing pathogens known to infect humans;[63] disease expression is dependent on many factors including the need for a type and duration of exposure and the immune status of the human host. Certain bacterial diseases of antiquity are present today although their population burden is slowly decreasing. TB is an example of one such continuing disease.[64] The 2018 World Health Organization report of the top 10 causes of death in 2016 lists TB as the tenth leading cause.[65] The etiological agent, *Mycobacterium tuberculosis* complex (MTBC) is responsible for approximately 10 million new active cases of disease among adults and 1.3 million deaths globally, with one-third of the world population having a latent infection.[65] This burden of disease persists despite the existence of effective treatment since the 1940s. The global HIV epidemic has added to the challenges of prevention and control of TB.

Despite their primordial origins, our ability to characterize bacteria and their role in causing disease is relatively new. Antonie von Leeuwenhoek is credited with visualizing bacteria for the first time in 1677, which he called "animalcules."[20] However, he did not think of these entities as disease-causing agents. Proof that a bacterium could cause disease had to await Robert Koch and his postulates published in 1884.[66] In the same year, the Danish physician and scientist Hans Christian Gram published the results of the bacterial staining procedure that bears his name.[67] In the past, the Gram stain was one of the most important staining procedures in microbiology. Today, it retains a role as a rapid diagnostic screening tool. The staining procedure is useful for most medically important bacteria, capitalizing on differences in higher peptidoglycan (PG) and lower lipid content found in Gram-positive (purple-colored) bacteria compared with Gram-negative (pink-colored) bacteria lower PG content. Notably, approximately 100,000 bacteria/mL must be present in order to be able to visualize a single bacterium on a single oil immersion light microscopic field (100X). This highlights the low sensitivity of this staining methodology. Gram staining also led to subclassification of organisms based upon shape and arrangements including cocci in pairs, chains, clusters, coccobacilli, or rods. However, some bacteria cannot be seen by Gram stain and require other methods of identification including *Mycobacteria* species, *Treponema pallidum*, *Mycopslasma* spp., *Legionella* spp., *Chlamydia* spp. and rickettsia-like organisms.

Improved culture methodologies permitted further stratification into required growth conditions such as the need for oxygen, carbon dioxide, types of media, and supplements.

Furthermore, two decades before Gram introduced his stain, Johannes Fredrich Miescher took the first step into molecular biology by identifying "nuclein" in the nuclei of white blood cells[68] later named nucleic acids. Yet, even after publication of the first X-ray diffraction pattern of DNA in 1938, it took 15 years additional years before Watson and Crick determined the structure of this nucleic acid.[69,70] In rapid succession both DNA and/or RNA, the nucleic acids were found in all life forms. Sophisticated techniques in molecular biology have evolved such as cloning, polymerase chain reaction, microarrays, and matrix-assisted laser desorption/ionization-time of flight (MALDI-TOF).[71] Today, microbial taxonomy is focused on 16S ribosomal RNA (rRNA) relationships but they remain imprecise due to the cumbersome process of reclassifying an organism and should be considered *ad interim*.[72] For example, in the period 2012–15 there were 109 new bacterial species recovered from human clinical material along with revision of 28 bacterial taxa.[73]

Usual medical and public health laboratory practice has focused on microscopic morphology by Gram staining, colonial morphology on bacterial growth media, specific growth requirements and phenotypic (phonetic) test activity rather than evolutionary (cladistics) naming approaches, but the latter classification is gaining ground as diagnostic testing improves in sensitivity, specificity, and speed. Clinical medicine and public health practice tend to focus on using the bacterial genus and species designation to examine possible modes of transmission and disease outcomes, to guide treatment and prevention/control.

There is a wide spectrum of outcomes following infection with different bacteria or their elaborated toxins ranging from colonization to life-threatening illness. The particular outcome of infection is dependent upon characteristics of the host such as age or state of the immune system, the specific bacterium causing the infection, and the environmental setting responsible for the infection, including the agent's reservoir and mode of transmission to the host.

Importantly, our understanding of microbial interactions continues to expand. For example, bacteria and viruses are not mutually exclusive disease-causing agents. Human viruses may interact in direct manner with some bacteria or their products to gain an advantage when entering the human host to cause infection. Some viruses may interact indirectly with bacteria in a manner that may enhance the likelihood of bacterial colonization of the human host. The specter of untreatable bacterial diseases has grown as more bacteria, once treatable with several antimicrobial agents, grow resistant to this armamentarium. Most of these multidrug resistant organisms cause healthcare-associated infections and WHO has identified a list of priority organisms for research and development of new treatments for control of these infections.[74] For more information, see Chapter153:"Antibiotic Resistance and Stewardship."

Fungi

Fungi are eukaryotic, single-celled yeasts or multicellular molds, organisms that can cause disease in a number of hosts. Agostino Bassi first observed the infectious nature of fungi in an epidemic disease of silkworms in 1835.[75] Just a few years later, Gruby and Remak would discover the first human fungal infection, tinea favosa, a chronic fungal infection of the scalp.[75] There are an estimated 1.5–5 million fungal species on earth, and a few hundred of them are capable of causing human disease.[76] Most people will develop a superficial fungal infection at some time during their lifetimes and most are easily cured; they may present a public health challenge in the setting a rare outbreak.[77,78] However, certain invasive fungal diseases pose an important threat to public health including those which cause invasive opportunistic infections among immune-compromised persons, invasive bloodstream infections among hospitalized persons, and certain environmental fungi which can cause invasive human diseases in immune-competent hosts.

Superficial mycoses of the skin, nails, and hair are the most common type of human fungal infections, and affect a quarter of the world's population.[79] Superficial mycoses are caused primarily by keratinophilic dermatophytes, including the generas *Trichophton*, *Microsporum*, and *Epidermophyton*. *Trichophyton rubrum* is the most common dermatophyte in developed countries and causes chronic diseases such as athlete's foot (tinea pedis), jock itch (tinea cruris), and ringworm (tinea corporis). Dermatophyte infections are easily transmitted through contact with desquamated skin scales from an infected individual (i.e., through direct contact, contact with fomites). The scales contain dermatophyte spores, which attach to keratinocytes within the skin and subsequently germinate within 24 hours, leading to invasion of the fungus.[80]

Mucosal mycoses are common and include diseases such as thrush and vaginitis. *Candida* species are the most common cause of these mycoses and can be found in the human gastrointestinal tract, oral cavity, skin, and female genital tract.[77,81] Vulvovaginal candidiasis (VVC) is one of the most common genital tract mycoses, and occurs when a change in the vaginal environment leads to pathological effects of what is normally a commensal organism within the vagina. Approximately 70–75% of women will experience at least one episode of VVC during life.[82] The public health importance of this common condition is that it is associated with an increased risk of HIV acquisition and transmission.[83]

Invasive mycoses are much less common than superficial mycoses but are associated with much higher mortality rates. Globally, these infections kill at least 1.5 million people every year, although this is likely an underestimate due to misdiagnosis and/or lack of reporting requirements in most countries.[77] Most fungal-related deaths are attributed to species within the genera *Cryptococcus, Candida, Aspergillus,* and *Pneumocystis,* with mortality rates ranging from 20% to 95%, reflecting the underlying condition of the host and the availability to healthcare and treatment. While the human immune system has mechanisms to prevent mycoses, the increase of immunosuppressive drugs and infections has caused a dramatic rise in incidence of these invasive infections.[77]

Cryptococcus spp. are a common cause of invasive mycoses, usually due to *C. neoformans* infection. This group of infectious agents rarely causes disease in persons with healthy immune systems. It is a major cause of illness in persons with poorly controlled HIV infection with an estimated 220,000 cases of cryptococcal meningitis worldwide, most occurring in sub-Saharan Africa.[84] *C. albicans*, normally a human commensal organism, is the main cause of nosocomial invasive candidiasis worldwide, most detected as candidemia.[85] There has been a progressive shift to other *Candida* spp., often those resistant to the common antifungal treatments. Antimicrobial resistance across the spectrum of infectious diseases, not only fungal pathogens, is viewed a public health crisis.[86,87]

Protozoa

Protozoa are single-celled, microscopic, and eukaryotic organisms, with at least one membrane-bound nucleus; some are pathogenic for humans and some are free living. Protozoa diseases are important causes of morbidity and mortality, particularly in lower resource areas of the world. These infections are commonly classified by their mode of transmission. Intestinal protozoa are usually acquired through an oral-fecal route whereas those that are found in blood or tissue are transmitted by arthropod vector.

Protozoa were first described in 1681 by Dutch physician Antonie van Leeuwenhoek, who would later be known as the "father of protozoology."[88] However, more than two centuries passed before scientists began to suspect the parasite, initially described by van Leeuwenhoek, *Giardia duodenalis*, could cause diarrhea. Studies conducted during the World War I era would demonstrate that *Giardia* spp. cysts from infected soldiers could cause similar symptoms in laboratory animals and in 1954 scientists conclusively demonstrated the link between the parasite and diarrhea.[89] Many protozoa contain various organelles that are present in higher animals and some pathogenic protozoa contain specialized organelles that are involved in a variety of different processes and structures, such as those involved in locomotion.[90] Protozoa are classified into one of four groups based upon locomotion strategy—pseudopodia (the Sarcodina), flagella (the Mastigophora), cilia (the Cilophora), and motion limited to male gametes in the sexual phase (the Sporozoa).

Sarcodina, the largest group of protozoan organisms, are single cells that move and capture food by use of pseudopodia—temporary arm-like protrusions. *Entamoeba histolytica*, the cause of amoebic dysentery is a major pathogen in this group (Although a major infection found in low resource settings, it is increasingly found among returning travelers and immigrants from endemic areas and among men who have sex with men worldwide.[91]

The Mastigophora including *Giardia* spp., *Leishmania* spp., *Trypanosoma* spp., and *Trichomonas* spp. are flagellates. *Giardia* spp. is estimated to cause between 130 million and 250 million foodborne illnesses each year worldwide; no deaths but associated malabsorption can be associated with stunted grown in children.[92] *Leishmania* spp., vector-borne protozoa, cause 1–2 million new cases of cutaneous, mucocutaneous, and visceral disease, primarily in tropical areas.[93] Both *T. cruzi*, the cause of Chagas disease and *T. brucei*, the cause of human African trypanosomiasis, are vector-borne zoonotic diseases. (See Chapter 133: "Human African Trypanosomiasis"). Approximately 8 million people are infected with *T. cruzi* worldwide, with most living in Latin America; 240,000 U.S. residents are estimated to have chronic *T. cruzi* infection.[94] *Trichomonas vaginalis* causes trichomoniasis, the most common curable sexually transmitted disease. There are over 130 million incident cases annually and over 100 million prevalent cases.[95] The infection is common in both high and low resource countries, but prevalent cases are more common in low resource areas. Infection with *T. vaginalis* in women is associated with adverse reproductive outcomes, including preterm delivery and pelvic inflammatory disease. It is also thought to increase the risk for HIV acquisition, with one study attributing 6.2% of all HIV infections in women in the United States to *T. vaginalis* infection.

Among the Cilophora, *Balantidium coli* is the only ciliated protozoa known to be pathogenic in humans.[96] It is a zoonotic infection and acquired via the oral-fecal route from direct contact with pigs or contaminated water. It occurs in areas with poor access to clean water and lack of adequate sanitation.

The Sporozoa are a diverse group of protozoa causing important pathogenic infectious diseases including malaria, babesiosis, cryptosporidiosis, cylosporiasis, cystoiosporiasis, and toxoplasmosis. Malaria is the most important protozoan disease in terms of morbidity and mortality, with an estimated 216 million cases and 445,000 deaths in 2016 [97]. Malaria is a vector-borne disease transmitted by the *Anopheles* spp. mosquito and is caused primarily by protozoan species within the genus *Plasmodium*, including *P. falciparum, P. vivax, P. ovale, P. malariae,* and *P. knowlesi*. While *P. falciparum* and *P. vivax* are responsible for most human malaria infections, *P. falciparum* is known to cause the most severe complications, including cerebral malaria, pulmonary edema, renal failure, and severe anemia, and has the highest fatality rate of all the *Plasmodium* species.[98] Malaria can be prevented by the application of multiple prevention strategies both individual such as malaria chemoprophylactic agents and sleeping under bed nets, to community-wide strategies such as mosquito larvae destruction. Rapid diagnosis and treatment are also needed to control spread of malaria. Importantly, growing drug resistance has complicated treatment. Although the United States had successfully eradicated malaria by 1951,[99] imported cases by visitors, immigrants, and travelers returning from endemic areas continues to pose a public health challenge.[100]

Sporozoa intestinal protozoan parasites are also a major public health concern, causing an estimated 700 million to 1 billion illnesses each year.[92] These protozoan diseases are transmitted through person-to-person contact or through the consumption of contaminated food or water. *Crytosporidium* spp. cause one of the most common causes of diarrheal illness in low and middle-income countries, and is the leading cause of nationally notified recreational water–associated outbreaks and waterborne disease outbreaks in the United States.[101]

Helminths

Worms, or helminths, are multicellular invertebrate animals. Parasitic worms cause the most prevalent infections worldwide, with the greatest health impact noted in lower resource settings.[88] Helminths are not part of normal flora (microbiome) and do not colonize humans. This group includes multicellular organisms ranging in size from less than 1 cm to more than 10 meters in length. Adult worms are visible with the naked eye. These animals all have complex life cycles evolving from an ovum, through the juvenile larval stage(s), to adulthood. Importantly, most helminths cannot complete their lifecycle within the human host, with one or more preadult stage occurring in the environment, a vector, or an intermediate host.

Members of two groups of helminths are known to cause essentially all worm infections in humans—the round nematodes and the flat platyhelminths.[21] The *Nematoda* include round, elongated, bilaterally symmetrical worms, with a covering (the integument) consisting of a nonnucleated cuticle secreted by the underlying hypodermis, a body cavity, and a complete gastrointestinal tract. Those infecting humans are unisexual. The *Platyhelminthes*, are also bilaterally symmetrical but are flat giving them a tape-like or leaf-like shape. Like the roundworms, the flatworms that are infectious to humans are unisexual and fall into two classes: the *Trematoda* (flukes) and the *Cestoda* (tapeworms). A third group of helminths, the *Acanthocephala* (spiny-headed worms), incidentally infect humans after consumption of an arthropod intermediate host and will not be further discussed.[102]

Primitive man likely was aware of some infecting worms because often they were visible when seen in stool, for example. Greek and Roman physicians recognized large intestinal worms, including tapeworms and roundworms, and wrote about finding them in patient stools.[21] Over time the number of worms recognized expanded but with the maintenance of classification into the three groups previously noted—roundworms, tapeworms, and flukes.

The roundworms can reside in human blood, gastrointestinal tract, lymphatic system, or tissue depending upon the species. Due to the role of contaminated soil in the transmission of roundworms (*Ascaris lumbricoides*), hookworms (*Necator americanus* and *Ancylostoma duodenale*), whipworms (*Trichura trichicuris*), and threadworms (*Strongyloides stercoralis*), these agents are collectively called the STH. This group of roundworm infections is the most common cause of treatable infections worldwide. Most infections occur in low resource settings notable for poor sanitation; the worldwide prevalence is estimated to be greater than 1 billion infections.[103] Many people believed STH infections to be causally linked to poor health outcomes, poor school performance, and cognitive deficits leading to multiple clinical trials using repeated mass drug administration with effective medications in the hopes of having an impact on these adverse outcomes. However, a comprehensive review of all reported results of these clinical trials has failed to identify a salutary population effect.[104]

All human flatworms infections, except schistosomiasis, are foodborne. Some of the associated diseases include clonochiais, fascioliais, fasciolopsis, opisthorchiasis, and paragonamiasis. These foodborne illnesses are uncommon in the United States but when found are infections among travelers and immigrants from endemic areas. Schistosomiasis, a neglected tropical disease acquired when the skin is in contact with contaminated fresh water, is a major public health issue in many low resource areas, particularly sub-Saharan Africa. Most human infections are caused by *Schistosoma mansoni*, *S. haematobium*, and *S. japonicum*.

Among the tapeworms, *Taenia solium*, the pork tapeworm has the most significant medical and public health impact. On average, there are about 375,000 new infections each year and about 27,000 associated deaths from the foodborne parasitic disease. Cysticercosis is the parasitic infection of tissue by the larval cysts of *T. solium* that develop from ingested eggs or gravid proglottids found, for example, in food contaminated with human feces. These cysts can infect the brain, muscle and other tissue. Pigs are similarly infected from human fecal matter and consumption of poorly cooked pork containing cysticerci results in human tapeworm infection with subsequent shedding of eggs and egg-containing proglottids in stool. Unique among the tapeworms, *T. solium* is associated with neurocysticercosis (NCC), a known cause of epilepsy and other neurological sequelae. Brain lesions due to NCC are present in about 30% of persons with epilepsy in *T. solium* endemic areas where pork is consumed in locations characterized by poor sanitation and *poor pig management practices*. The *Echinococcus* spp. causes hydatid disease. *E. granulosis* and *E. multilocularis* causing cystic and alveolar disease, respectively, are associated with a lower global burden of disease than *T. solium* and fewer deaths. Cystic echinoccoccosis is found in many parts of the world including the western U.S. Multiple prevention and control strategies for these two cystic parasitic infections are needed as fewer than 50% of infections are transmitted by food.[92]

CONCLUSION

The prevention and control of communicable diseases requires an understanding of the interrelationships among the human host, the environment, and the infectious agent. The host may have factors that enhance or decrease risk of infection stemming from genetic, demographic, or immunological factors. Transmission of any of the categories of infectious agents outlined may be by one or more routes or only at a particular stage in its life cycle. The natural history of the infectious agent after initial infection provides important clues to possible prevention and control of the disease state. The environmental conditions may be permissive or hostile to agent transmission and/or host response. The remaining chapters in this section will further develop many of the concepts introduced here. It is prudent to keep in mind that newly emerging and reemerging infectious agents and environmental changes, including climate change, will continue to present public health challenges to the identification, prevention, and control of communicable diseases. Concurrent with these new challenges will be the growth of our knowledge about the human host that will assist in creating an optimal prevention and control toolbox.

References

1 CDC National Health Report: Leading Causes of Morbidity and Mortality and Associated Behavioral Risk and Protective Factors—United States, 2005–2013. https://www.cdc.gov/mmwr/preview/mmwrhtml/su6304a2.htm. Accessed August 27, 2018.

2 Heron M. Deaths: Leading causes for 2016. *Natl Vital Stat Rep.* 2018;67(6):1–77.

3 Morens DM, Fauci AS. Emerging infectious diseases: Threats to human health and global stability. *PLoS Pathog.* 2013;9(7):e1003467.

4 Ursell LK, Metcalf JL, Parfrey LW, Knight R. Defining the human microbiome. *Nutr Rev.* 2012;70(Suppl 1):S38–44.

5 Henderson DA. *Smallpox—The Death of a Disease: The Inside Story of Eradicating a Worldwide Killer.* Amherst, New York: Prometheus Books; 2009.

6 Stilianakis NI, Drossinos Y. Dynamics of infectious disease transmission by inhalable respiratory droplets. *J R Soc Interface.* 2010;7(50):1355–66.

7 Remington PL, Hall WN, Davis IH, Herald A, Gunn RA. Airborne transmission of measles in a physician's office. *JAMA.* 1985;253(11):1574–7.

8 Scallan E, Hoekstra RM, Angulo FJ, et al. Foodborne illness acquired in the United States—Major pathogens. *Emerg Infect Dis.* 2011;17(1):7–15.

9 Kamatani Y, Wattanapokayakit S, Ochi H, et al. A genome-wide association study identifies variants in the HLA-DP locus associated with chronic hepatitis B in Asians. *Nat Genet.* 2009;41(5):591–5. 8

10 Brann OS. Infectious complications of cirrhosis. *Curr Gastroenterol Rep.* 2001;3(4):285–92.

11 Anderson RM, May RM. *Infectious Diseases of Humans: Dynamics and Control.* Oxford, UK: Oxford University Press; 1992.

12 Brachman PS. Infectious diseases—Past, present, and future. *Int J Epidemiol.* 2003;32(5):684–6.

13 The top 10 causes of death. World Health Organization. http://www.who.int/news-room/fact-sheets/detail/the-top-10-causes-of-death. Accessed August 23, 2018.

14 Stenseth NC, Atshabar BB, Begon M, et al. Plague: Past, present, and future. *PLoS Med.* 2008;5(1):e3.

15 Pringle, H. How Europeans brought sickness to the New World. Science | AAAS. 04 June 2015. https://www.sciencemag.org/news/2015/06/how-europeans-brought-sickness-new-world. Published June 3, 2015. Accessed July 31, 2018.

16 Hargreaves JR, Boccia D, Evans CA, Adato M, Petticrew M, Porter JDH. The social determinants of tuberculosis: From evidence to action. *Am J Public Health.* 2011;101(4):654–62.

17 Tappero JW, Tauxe RV. Lessons learned during public health response to cholera epidemic in Haiti and the Dominican Republic. *Emerg Infect Dis.* 2011;17(11):2087–93.

18 Murrell KD, Pozio E. Worldwide occurrence and impact of human trichinellosis, 1986–2009. *Emerg Infect Dis.* 2011;17(12):2194–202.

19 Snow J. *On the Mode of Communication of Cholera.* London: John Churchill; 1849

20 Leeuwenhoek AV. Observations, communicated to the publisher by Mr. Antony van Leewenhoeck, in a Dutch letter of the 9th October. 1676. Here English'd: Concerning little animals by him observed in rain-well-sea- and snow water; as also in water wherein pepper had lain infused. *Phil Trans.* 1677;12(133):821–31.

21 Grove DI. *A History of Human Heminthology.* Wallingford, Oxon, UK: C.A.B International; 1990.

22 Frierson JG. The yellow fever vaccine: A history. *Yale J Biol Med.* 2010;83(2):77–85.

23 Ciccarelli FD, Doerks T, von Mering C, Creevey CJ, Snel B, Bork P. Toward automatic reconstruction of a highly resolved tree of life. *Science.* 2006;311(5765):1283–7.

24 Aminov RI. Role of archaea in human disease. *Front Cell Infect Microbiol.* 2013;3:42.

25 Zabel MD, Reid C. A brief history of prions. *Pathog Dis.* 2015;73(9):ftv087.

26 Griffith JS. Self-replication and scrapie. *Nature.* 1967;215(5105):1043–34.

27 Prusiner SB. Novel proteinaceous infectious particles cause scrapie. *Science.* 1982;216(4542):136–44.

28 Brandel J-P, Knight R. Chapter 11—Variant Creutzfeldt–Jakob disease. In: Pocchiari M, Manson J, eds. *Handbook of Clinical Neurology.* Vol. 153. Human Prion Diseases. New York: Elsevier; 2018, pp. 191–205.

29 Kobayashi A, Kitamoto T, Mizusawa H. Chapter 12—Iatrogenic Creutzfeldt–Jakob disease. In: Pocchiari M, Manson J, eds. *Handbook of Clinical Neurology.* Vol. 153. Human Prion Diseases. New York: Elsevier; 2018, pp. 207–18.

30 Heckmann JG, Lang CJG, Petruch F, et al. Transmission of Creutzfeldt-Jakob disease via a corneal transplant. *J Neurol Neurosurg Psychiatry.* 1997;63(3):388–90.

31 Deitz K, Raddatz G, Wallis J, et al. Blood transfusion and spread of variant Creutzfeldt-Jakob disease. *Emerg Infect Dis.* 2007; 13(1):89–96.

32 Britton TC, Al-Sarraj S, Shaw C, Campbell T, Collinge J. Sporadic Creutzfeldt-Jakob disease in a 16-year-old in the UK. *Lancet.* 1995; 346(8983):1155.

33 Bateman D, Hilton D, Love S, Zeidler M, Beck J, Collinge J. Sporadic Creutzfeldt-Jakob disease in a 18-year-old in the UK. *Lancet.* 1995;346(8983):1155–6.

34 Will RG, Ironside JW, Zeidler M, et al. A new variant of Creutzfeldt-Jakob disease in the UK. *Lancet.* 1996;347(9006):921–5.

35 Brown P, Bradley R. 1755 and all that: A historical primer of transmissible spongiform encephalopathy. *BMJ.* 1998;317(7174):1688–92.

36 BSE Cases Identified in the United States BSE (Bovine Spongiform Encephalopathy) | Prion Diseases | CDC. https://www.cdc.gov/prions/bse/case-us.html. Published October 2, 2018. Accessed August 29, 2018.

37 vCJD Cases Reported in the US | Variant Creutzfeldt-Jakob Disease, Classic (CJD) | Prion Disease | CDC. https://www.cdc.gov/prions/vcjd/vcjd-reported.html. Published October 2, 2018. Accessed August 29, 2018.

38 Asokan GV, Asokan V. Bradford Hill's criteria, emerging zoonoses, and One Health. *J Epidemiol Glob Health.* 2016;6(3):125–9.

39. Gajdusek DC, Zigas V. Degenerative disease of the central nervous system in New Guinea. *N Engl J Med.* 1957;257(20):974–8.

40 A virus by any other name. *Lancet.* 1940;236(6101):140–1.

41 Loeffelholz MJ, Fenwick BW. Taxonomic changes and additions for human and animal viruses, 2012 to 2015. *J Clin Microbiol.* 2017;55(1):48–52.

42 Harrison BD, Wilson TM. Milestones in the research on tobacco mosaic virus. *Philos Trans R Soc Lond B Biol Sci.* 1999;354(1383):521–9.

43 Reed W, Carroll J, Agramonte A, Lazear JW. The etiology of yellow fever—A preliminary note. *Public Health Pap Rep.* 1900;26:37–53.

44 Reed W, Carroll J, Agramonte A, Lazear JW. The etiology of yellow fever: A preliminary note. *Philadelphia Med J.* 1900;6:790–6.

45 Firquet S, Beaujard S, Lobert P-E, et al. Survival of enveloped and non-enveloped viruses on inanimate surfaces. *Microbes Environ.* 2015;30(2):140–4.

46 Boulant S, Stanifer M, Lozach P-Y. Dynamics of virus-receptor interactions in virus binding, signaling, and endocytosis. *Viruses.* 2015;7(6):2794–815.

47 Roulston A, Marcellus RC, Branton PE. Viruses and apoptosis. *Annu Rev Microbiol.* 1999;53:577–628.

48 Schneider RJ, Shenk T. Impact of virus infection on host cell protein synthesis. *Annu Rev Biochem.* 1987;56:317–32.

49 Tamm I. Cell injury with viruses. *Am J Pathol.* 1975;81(1):163–78.

50 GBD 2013 Mortality and Causes of Death Collaborators. Global, regional, and national age-sex specific all-cause and cause-specific mortality for 240 causes of death, 1990–2013: A systematic analysis for the Global Burden of Disease Study 2013. *Lancet.* 2015;385(9963):117–71.

51 Khabbaz RF, Moseley RR, Steiner RJ, Levitt AM, Bell BP. Challenges of infectious diseases in the USA. *Lancet.* 2014;384(9937):53–63.

52 Taubenberger JK, Morens DM. 1918 Influenza: The mother of all pandemics. *Emerg Infect Dis.* 2006;12(1):15–22.

53 Houser K, Subbarao K. Influenza vaccines: Challenges and solutions. *Cell Host Microbe.* 2015;17(3):295–300. doi:10.1016/j.chom.2015.02.012

54 Virgin HW, Wherry EJ, Ahmed R. Redefining chronic viral infection. *Cell.* 2009;138(1):30–50. doi:10.1016/j.cell.2009.06.036

55 Seifarth W, Frank O, Zeilfelder U, et al. Comprehensive analysis of human endogenous retrovirus transcriptional activity in human tissues with a retrovirus-specific microarray. *J Virol.* 2005;79(1):341–52.

56 Wong MCS, Jiang JY, Goggins WB, et al. International incidence and mortality trends of liver cancer: A global profile. *Sci Rep.* 2017;7:45846.

57 El-Serag HB. Epidemiology of viral hepatitis and hepatocellular carcinoma. *Gastroenterology.* 2012;142(6):1264–73.

58 Davila JA, Morgan RO, Shaib Y, McGlynn KA, El-Serag HB. Hepatitis C infection and the increasing incidence of hepatocellular carcinoma: A population-based study. *Gastroenterology.* 2004;127(5):1372–80.

59 Serrano B, Alemany L, Tous S, et al. Potential impact of a nine-valent vaccine in human papillomavirus related cervical disease. *Infect Agents Cancer.* 2012;7(1):38.

60 Use of 9-Valent Human Papillomavirus (HPV) Vaccine: Updated HPV Vaccination Recommendations of the Advisory Committee on Immunization Practices. https://www.cdc.gov/mmwr/preview/mmwrhtml/mm6411a3.htm. Accessed November 1, 2018.

61 Research C for BE and. Approved Products—Gardasil 9. https://www.fda.gov/biologicsbloodvaccines/vaccines/approvedproducts/ucm426445.htm. Accessed December 1, 2018.

62 Yarchoan R, Uldrick TS. HIV-associated cancers and related diseases. *N Engl J Med.* 2018;378(11):1029–41.

63 McFall-Ngai M. Adaptive immunity: Care for the community. *Nature.* 2007;445:153.

64 Witas HW, Donoghue HD, Kubiak D, Lewandowska M, Gładykowska-Rzeczycka JJ. Molecular studies on ancient M. tuberculosis and M. leprae: Methods of pathogen and host DNA analysis. *Eur J Clin Microbiol Infect Dis.* 2015;34(9):1733–49.

65 WHO | Global tuberculosis report 2018. WHO. http://www.who.int/tb/publications/global_report/en/. Accessed November 15, 2018.

66 Brock TD. *Milestones in Microbiology.* Englewood Cliffs, NJ: Prentice-Hall, Inc.; 1961. http://archive.org/details/MilestonesInMicrobiology. Accessed November 23, 2018.

67 Gram HCJ. Ueber die isolirte Farbung der Schizomyceten in Schitt- und Trockenpreparaten (Translation: The differential staining of Schixomycetes in tissue sections and in dried preparations published 1884 in Fortschritte der Medicin). In: *Milestones in Microbiology: 1556 to 1940.* Washington, DC: ASM Press; 1998.

68 Dahm R. Discovering DNA: Friedrich Miescher and the early years of nucleic acid research. *Hum Genet.* 2008;122(6):565–81.

69 Astbury WT, Bell FO. X-ray study of thymonucleic acid. *Nature.* 1938;141(3573):747–8.

70 Watson JD, Crick FHC. Molecular structure of nucleic acids: A structure for deoxyribose nucleic acid. *Nature.* 1953;171(4356):737–8.

71 Wolk D, Mitchell S, Patel R. Principles of molecular microbiology testing methods. *Infect Dis Clin North Am.* 2001;15(4):1157–204.

72 Yarza P, Yilmaz P, Pruesse E, et al. Uniting the classification of cultured and uncultured bacteria and archaea using 16S rRNA gene sequences. *Nat Rev Microbiol.* 2014;12(9):635–45.

73 Munson E, Carroll KC. What's in a name? New bacterial species and changes to taxonomic status from 2012 through 2015. *J Clin Microbiol.* 2017;55(1):24–42.

74 Tacconelli E, Carrara E, Savoldi A, et al. Discovery, research, and development of new antibiotics: The WHO priority list of antibiotic-resistant bacteria and tuberculosis. *Lancet Infect Dis.* 2018;18(3):318–27.

75 Espinel-Ingroff A. History of medical mycology in the United States. *Clin Microbiol Rev.* 1996;9(2):235–72.

76 Köhler JR, Casadevall A, Perfect J. The spectrum of fungi that infects humans. *Cold Spring Harb Perspect Med.* 2015;5(1):a019273.

77 Brown GD, Denning DW, Gow NAR, Levitz SM, Netea MG, White TC. Hidden killers: Human fungal infections. *Sci Transl Med.* 2012;4(165):165rv13.

78 Poisson DM, Rousseau D, Defo D, Estève E. Outbreak of tinea corporis gladiatorum, a fungal skin infection due to Trichophyton tonsurans, in a French high level judo team. *Eurosurveillance.* 2005;10(9):7–8.

79 Havlickova B, Czaika VA, Frederich M. Epidemiological trends in skin mycoses worldwide. *Mycoses.* 2008;51 Suppl 4:2–15.

80 Martinez-Rossi NM, Peres NTA, Rossi A. Pathogenesis of dermatophytosis: Sensing the host tissue. *Mycopathologia.* 2017;182(1):215–27.

81 Underhill DM, Iliev ID. The mycobiota: Interactions between commensal fungi and the host immune system. *Nat Rev Immunol.* 2014;14(6):405–16.

82 Sobel JD. Vulvovaginal candidosis. *Lancet.* 2007;369(9577):1961–71.

83 Johnson LF, Lewis DA. The effect of genital tract infections on Hiv-1 shedding in the genital tract: A systematic review and meta-analysis. *Sex Transm Dis.* 2008;35(11):946–59.

84 Rajasingham R, Smith RM, Park BJ, et al. Global burden of disease of HIV-associated cryptococcal meningitis: An updated analysis. *Lancet Infect Dis.* 2017;17(8):873–81.

85 Guinea J. Global trends in the distribution of Candida species causing candidemia. *Clin Microbiol Infect.* 2014;20 Suppl 6:5–10.

86 Ciorba V, Odone A, Veronesi L, Pasquarella C, Signorelli C. Antibiotic resistance as a major public health concern: Epidemiology and economic impact. *Ann Igiene.* 2015;27(3):562–79.

87 Toner E, Adalja A, Gronvall GK, Cicero A, Inglesby TV. Antimicrobial resistance is a global health emergency. *Health Secur.* 2015;13(3):153–5.

88 Cox FEG. History of human parasitology. *Clin Microbiol Rev.* 2002;15(4):595–612.

89 McCulloch R, Navarro M. The protozoan nucleus. *Mol Biochem Parasitol.* 2016;209(1–2):76–87.

90 Souza W de. Special organelles of some pathogenic protozoa. *Parasitol Res.* 2002;88(12):1013–25.

91 Shirley D-AT, Farr L, Watanabe K, Moonah S. A review of the global burden, new diagnostics, and current therapeutics for amebiasis. *Open Forum Infect Dis.* 2018;5(7):ofy161.

92 Torgerson PR, Devleesschauwer B, Praet N, et al. World Health Organization estimates of the global and regional disease burden of 11 foodborne parasitic diseases, 2010: A data synthesis. *PLoS Med.* 2015;12(12):e1001920.

93 Pigott DM, Bhatt S, Golding N, et al. Global distribution maps of the leishmaniases. *eLife.* 2014;3:1

94 Manne-Goehler J, Umeh CA, Montgomery SP, Wirtz VJ. Estimating the burden of Chagas disease in the United States. *PLoS Negl Trop Dis.* 2016;10(11):e0005033.

95 Newman L, Rowley J, Vander Hoorn S, et al. Global estimates of the prevalence and incidence of four curable sexually transmitted infections in 2012 based on systematic review and global reporting. *PLoS One.* 2015;10(12):e0143304.

96 Schuster FL, Ramirez-Avila L. Current world status of Balantidium coli. *Clin Microbiol Rev.* 2008;21(4):626–38.

97 Fact sheet about Malaria. World Health Organization. http://www.who.int/news-room/fact-sheets/detail/malaria. Accessed July 25, 2018.

98 Trampuz A, Jereb M, Muzlovic I, Prabhu RM. Clinical review: Severe malaria. *Crit Care.* 2003;7(4):315–23.

99 Williams LL. Malaria eradication in the United States. *Am J Public Health Nations Health.* 1963;53(1):17–21.

100 Dembele B, Yakubu A-A. Controlling imported malaria cases in the United States of America. *Math Biosci Eng.* 2017;14(1):95–109.

101 Adams DA. Summary of Notifiable Infectious Diseases and Conditions—United States, 2015. *MMWR Morb Mortal Wkly Rep.* 2017;64(53):1–143.

102 Berenji F, Fata A, Hosseininejad Z. A case of Moniliformis moniliformis (Acanthocephala) infection in Iran. *Korean J Parasitol.* 2007;45(2):145–8.

103 Jourdan PM, Lamberton PHL, Fenwick A, Addiss DG. Soil-transmitted helminth infections. *Lancet.* 2018;391(10117):252–65.

104 Tovey D, Littell JH, Grimshaw JM. The end of the wormwars? *Cochrane Database Syst Rev.* 2016;9:ED000116.

CHAPTER

82 Epidemiology and Control of Infectious Diseases

Sandra I. McCoy • Tomás J. Aragón • Arthur Reingold

INTRODUCTION

In this chapter, we review the epidemiologic concepts underlying the prevention and control of infectious diseases. While public health and medical professionals are familiar with the interventions commonly used to prevent or control infectious diseases, the underlying epidemiologic concepts that drive and guide these interventions may be less familiar. Although we focus on acute infectious diseases, these concepts are broadly applicable to communicable diseases, including chronic or neoplastic diseases caused by exogenous transmissible agents such as human immunodeficiency virus (HIV), hepatitis B and C viruses (HBV and HCV), human papilloma virus, and prions.

A better understanding of the core epidemiologic concepts can: (1) help researchers prioritize, design, and conduct studies to identify and optimize prevention and control interventions; (2) assist clinicians in understanding their role and how it directly and indirectly contributes to containment efforts; (3) aid field investigators in developing and using a systematic and comprehensive approach to hypothesis generation and testing when conducting outbreak investigations; (4) help responders design, implement, and evaluate interventions to control and prevent acute microbial threats (Box 82-1), as well as endemic infectious diseases; and (5) facilitate the design, testing, and evaluation of infectious disease emergency operations response plans by policy makers and planners.

Our primary focus is on infectious disease transmission mechanisms, transmission dynamics, and transmission containment. The design, implementation, and evaluation of strategies to control infectious diseases can be improved by using a systematic, integrated epidemiologic approach, especially for acute or novel microbial threats that require special public health actions (e.g., severe acute respiratory syndrome (SARS), human pandemic influenza, or bioterrorism). Furthermore, we stress the value and importance of understanding the epidemiologic control points that drive infectious disease transmission dynamics.

EPIDEMIOLOGIC CONCEPTS

Epidemiology is "[t]he study of the distribution and determinants of health related states and events in populations, and the application of this study to control health problems."[1] By health-related states or events, we mean the occurrence or condition of infection, disease, injury, disability, or death. Epidemiologic studies are designed to answer well-defined investigative questions while minimizing threats to valid inference (e.g., random and systematic error). Most medical and public health professionals are familiar with the epidemiologic approach to public health action. Infectious diseases differ in important ways from noninfectious diseases because of the mechanisms by which microbial agents are transmitted and the population dynamics of transmission and disease occurrence. To improve our conceptual understanding, we use a systematic, comprehensive, and integrated approach (Fig. 82-1). Specifically, we cover the following:

1. Transmission mechanisms
   a. Chain model of infectious diseases;
   b. Natural history of infection and infectiousness; and
   c. Convergence model of human-microbe interaction.
2. Transmission dynamics
   a. Reproductive number;
   b. Infection rate among susceptibles (i.e., susceptible individuals);
   c. Generation time; and
   d. The reproductive number and evolution of infectious agents.
3. Transmission containment
   a. Control points;
   b. Control strategies; and
   c. Control measures.

First, we review infectious disease transmission mechanisms. How are infections transmitted and why? Second, we review infectious disease transmission dynamics. At the population level, what mechanisms explain the transmission of microbial agents and the appearance of infectious cases? How do infectious cases interact with susceptible hosts? Third, we review transmission containment. From our study of transmission dynamics, we identify transmission control points for preventing and controlling infectious diseases. We then use these control points to guide the development of appropriate control measures. This process helps us to evaluate the success or failure of our control measures.

Transmission Mechanisms

Chain Model of Infectious Diseases

The Chain Model of infectious diseases contains the key components that must be "linked" in order for an infection to occur (Fig. 82-2). First, there is a susceptible host. Second, there is a microbial agent

BOX 82-1 Common Interventions to Prevent and Control Infectious Diseases

Control Measures
Alter risk factors
Prophylactic immunization
Postexposure management
Diagnosis and treatment
Infection control practices
Case finding and isolation
Contact tracing and quarantine
Environmental control measures
Identify and control infectious sources

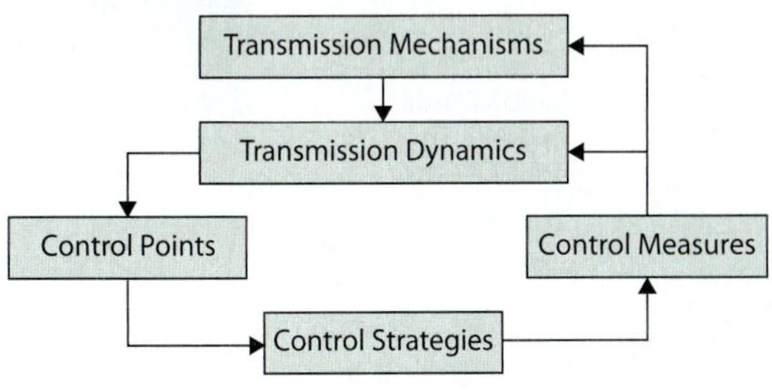

FIGURE 82-1. The relationship between infectious disease transmission mechanisms, transmission dynamics, and transmission containment (control points, control measures, and evaluation).

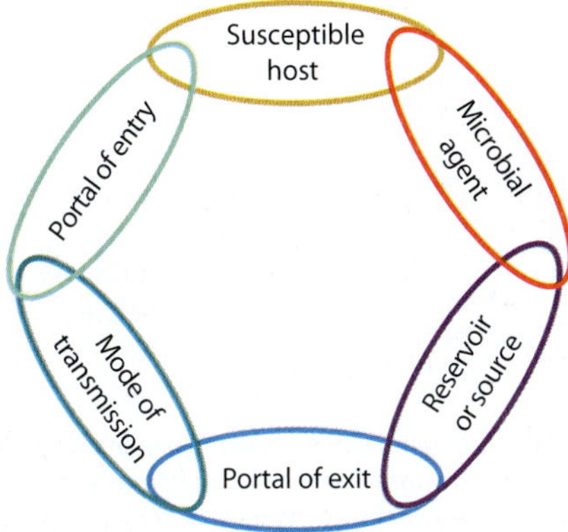

FIGURE 82-2. The chain model of infectious diseases.

capable of adhering, entering, infecting, and causing disease in the susceptible host. In its natural setting, the microbial agent multiplies and survives in a reservoir. The source is where the microbial agent resides at the time of transmission to the susceptible host. The reservoir can also be a source of infection. The portal of exit is the manner in which the agent exits the source. The mode of transmission is the mechanism by which the agent is transmitted from the source to the host (e.g., contact, droplet, airborne, etc.). In addition, the portal of entry is how the agent enters the susceptible host (e.g., respiratory tract, gastrointestinal tract, genitourinary tract, skin).

For example, enterohemorrhagic *Escherichia coli* (EHEC), most commonly *E. coli* O157:H7, elaborate Shiga toxins that can result in severe human disease, including hemorrhagic colitis and hemolytic uremic syndrome.[2] Cattle are the major reservoir for EHEC; up to 5% can be asymptomatic excretors of the organism. The source of infection for humans can be ingestion of contaminated foods or water, but also can be direct contact with colonized cattle or their environment or infected humans. The most commonly recognized mode of transmission to humans is ingestion of contaminated ground beef or produce.

Susceptible host. Human host susceptibility is a relative attribute and depends on the condition of host defenses. Host defenses consist of innate immunity and acquired immunity. Innate immunity consists of nonspecific mechanisms that do not require prior exposure to foreign agents in order to resist or fight invasion of the host by these foreign agents. The first lines of defense are intact skin and mucous membranes, and any breach in these can provide a portal of entry. Nonspecific inflammation and phagocytosis provide a second line of innate defense. The second type of host defense is acquired immunity, which can be active or passive. Acquired active immunity comprises host antibody or cellular immune defense mechanisms that target specific foreign agents based on prior exposure to this or antigenically similar agents or their components. Vaccination produces a form of active immunity. Acquired passive immunity is when a host receives preformed antibodies that were made in other hosts, such as the provision of immune globulin to people who have been exposed to rabies.

Microbial agent. Microbial agents or their products (e.g., toxins) can cause human disease. We focus on transmissible agents that are microbes or microbe-like and their toxins. Microbes are complex, reproducing microorganisms such as viruses, bacteria, parasites, and fungi. Prions are transmissible, self-propagating proteins that can cause disease (usually neurodegenerative diseases called spongiform encephalopathies). With respect to terminology, we refer generically to microbes (or microbial agents), a specific agent (e.g., *Clostridium botulinum*), or a microbial toxin (e.g., botulinum toxin). Although we are focusing on the transmission of microbial agents, diseases can also be caused by transmission of nonmicrobial agents, such as chemical toxicants.

Microbial reproduction can occur outside or inside the host. For example, staphylococcal food poisoning occurs when *Staphlococcus aureus* grows in food substrate and elaborates an enterotoxin. Ingestion of preformed enteroxin in food results in symptoms (nausea, vomiting, watery diarrhea) 1–6 hours after ingestion.[3] *S. aureus* can also grow inside a host, causing a local or systemic infection or causing systemic shock from the elaboration of toxin (e.g., toxic shock syndrome toxin). Host injury can occur directly from the invading microbe, from an inflammatory host immune response, or from organ hypoperfusion (septic shock).

Infection and transmission can be viewed as two sides of the same coin: infection is from the perspective of a susceptible host and transmission is from the perspective of an infectious host. Infection is acquisition of a microbe by a host[4] (Fig. 82-3) and infectivity describes the probability of infection, given exposure to a microbial agent. On the other hand, transmission describes the transfer of a microbe (infection) from an infectious source to a host. Transmission can occur within species (intraspecies), between species (interspecies), or between the environment and a species. Transmissibility is the probability of microbe transfer to a host, given contact (exposure). This is also called the *transmission probability*.

Infection can result in several possible states: elimination, commensalism, colonization, persistence, or disease.[5] Microbe elimination from the host can occur from physical factors, host flora interference, immune response, or medical therapy. Commensalism occurs when a microbe becomes part of the normal microbial flora. Commensals do not cause host damage unless there is impaired immunity or altered microbial flora. Infection can also result in colonization (i.e., microbial "carriage") whereby a microbe is recovered from a nonsterile site at which host damage may or may not be present but may not be clinically apparent. Colonization is transient and results in either microbe elimination, persistence, or host disease. Infection can result in microbial persistence when the microbe is not eliminated from the host and may or may not continue to cause host damage. Chronic hepatitis C infection and latent *Mycobacterium tuberculosis* infection are both examples of persistence.

Disease is a state of infection in which the host-microbe interaction results in sufficient host damage to cause clinical signs or symptoms and/or can be detectable by diagnostic tests.[5] Disease can occur quickly after infection or can develop from commensalism, colonization, or persistence states. The related term *pathogenicity* describes the probability of developing disease given infection. The term *virulence* describes the probability of severe disease, complication, or death, given disease and is a characteristic of the microbe. For example, *Neisseria meningitidis,* a causative agent of meningitis, colonizes the human oronasopharynx, resulting in a host immune response and eventual elimination. However, pathogenic strains can invade the bloodstream, causing meningococcemia, and the most

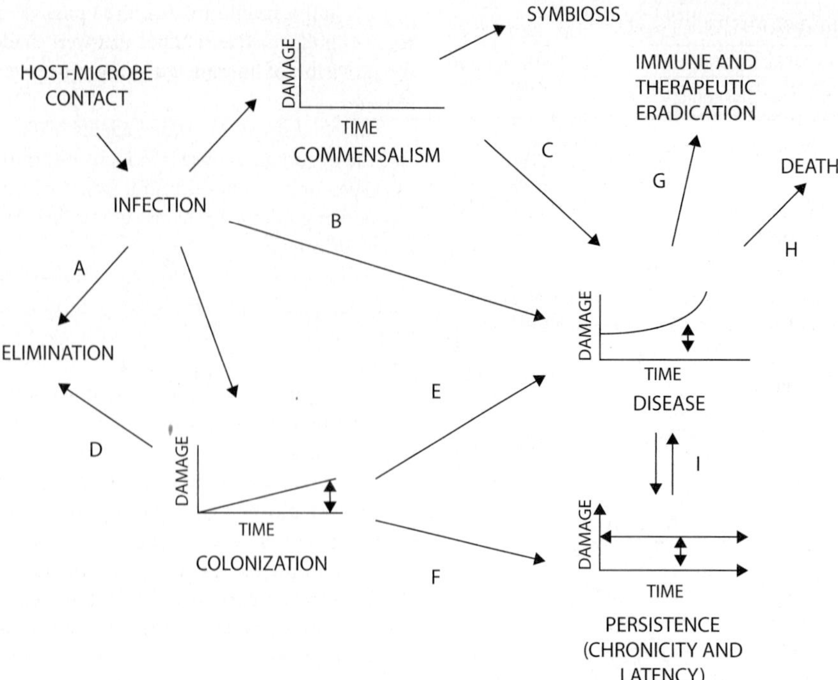

FIGURE 82-3. Damage-response framework of microbial pathogenesis: Infection (microbial acquisition by a host) leads to elimination, commensalism, colonization, persistence, or disease. The solid line represents host damage from host-microbe interaction. The dashed line represents the threshold at which the level or quality of host damage leads to persistence or disease. (*Source:* Adapted with Permission from Casadevall A, Pirofski L-A. Host-pathogen interactions:Basic concepts of microbial commensalism, colonization, infection, and disease, *Infect Immun*. 2000;68(12):6511–8.)

virulent strains cause severe meningococcal disease (meningitis or septic shock) and death.

Reservoir. Reservoirs for microbes can be either human, animal, or environmental. Generally, the reservoir contains nutritional substrate to support microbial growth. Bacteria that sporulate are an exception; for example, *Bacillus* and *Clostridium* species can survive extreme conditions as spores, and germinate into a vegetative form only when conditions are favorable. To control an infectious disease, we must know the primary reservoir(s). For some infectious diseases, humans are the only reservoir, examples being polio, hepatitis A (B and C), measles, mumps, rubella, varicella, and malaria. This feature was one of the factors that facilitated smallpox eradication, which is when the worldwide incidence of a specific agent is permanently reduced to zero as a result of deliberate efforts such that intervention measures are no longer needed.[6] Other necessary conditions for eradication include that the microbial agent is not part of the normal human flora, and that effective prevention measures exist (e.g., vaccination).

In contrast, the eradication of human infectious diseases is very unlikely when animals are the primary reservoir for the microbial agent. Examples of human infectious diseases for which animals are the primary reservoir include West Nile virus disease (West Nile virus in migratory birds transmitted via mosquito vectors), Lyme disease (*Borrelia burdorferi* in rodents and deer transmitted via tick vectors), enterohemorrhagic colitis (bloody diarrhea) and hemolytic-uremic syndrome (*E. coli* O157:H7 transmitted among cattle via ingestion), and cryptosporidiosis (*Cryptosporidium parvum* in calves). Human infectious diseases acquired from animals are called *zoonoses* or zoonotic infections. Several potential bioterrorism agents are zoonotic infections, including *Yersinia pestis* (plague), *Bacillus anthracis* (anthrax), *Francisella tularensis* (tularemia), and *Brucella* species (brucellosis). In general, these microbes are well adapted to survive in their animal reservoir and to being efficiently transmitted between animal hosts. However, when a zoonotic disease occurs in humans, the agent is often not adapted to the human host and sustained human-to-human transmission may not occur. We see this phenomenon with West Nile virus infection, bat and dog-variant rabies, and avian influenza virus—all of which cause human disease, but are then not transmitted efficiently from human to human.

Examples of human infectious diseases for which the environment is the reservoir for the agent include botulism (neurotoxin from *Clostridium botulinum* in soil), tetanus (neurotoxin from *Clostridium tetanus* in soil), legionellosis (*Legionella* species in water), *Mycobacterium avium* complex infections (*Mycobacterium avium* complex in soil and water), coccidioidomycosis (*Coccidioides immitis* in soil and dust), blastomycosis (*Blastomyces dermatitidis* in soil and dust), and aspergillosis (*Aspergillus* fungal species in the environment). Environmental microbes that are ubiquitous are often unavoidable, but many of these microbes are nonpathogenic in the face of a competent host immune system. However, in a severely immunocompromised host, these microbes can be deadly (e.g., *Pneumocystis jirovecii* pneumonia in people living with AIDS).

Source. The source is where the infectious agent survives or reproduces prior to transmission to a host. The source of infection is a primary focus in the investigation of an infectious disease outbreak, as controlling the source is often an effective strategy for intervention, even if the specific pathogen causing the outbreak is unknown. However, because the reservoir can serve as the source of infection, understanding microbe reservoirs is necessary to conduct a thorough investigation. Therefore, any reservoir is a potential source (human, animal, environment). A nonreservoir source can be almost anything; the only requirement is that the microbe must survive in or on the source until it is transmitted to the host. *Fomite* is a term to describe inanimate objects that can facilitate transmission, such as a door handle, mobile phone, or a contaminated toy at a day care center.[1]

In an outbreak investigation, if a known reservoir or one of the usual sources is not implicated as the source of the outbreak, then analytic studies may be necessary to identify an unsuspected or new source and redirect the investigation. For example, if an outbreak of gastrointestinal illness is suspected to be transmitted through food, investigators might first compare the frequency of consumption of various foods among ill individuals to population-based information about how often healthy individuals consume the same foods (e.g., a case-control study). Population-level data might be drawn from, for example, CDC's *Atlas of Exposures,* which summarizes food consumption patterns among healthy people in the 7 days before the interview.[7] More frequent consumption of a specific food, such as precut melon, among ill individuals might signal a possible exposure route. However, only hypotheses about potential exposures that are considered by investigators and either available in existing data or measurable can be tested in an analytic study. Therefore, if an analytic study does not identify a potential source, investigators may need to re-think their current hypotheses or consider new hypotheses. See Case Study (Box 82-2) for an example of identifying an unexpected route of nosocomial transmission of *Serratia marcescens* in the healthcare setting.[8]

Portal of exit. When a portal of exit exists, it describes how the infectious agent exits the source/reservoir. The portal of exit for an infectious human or animal is most commonly the respiratory, gastrointestinal or genitourinary tract, or a wound or ulcerative lesion on the skin or mucous membrane. Bloodborne pathogens exit the source through bleeding, phlebotomy, or sometimes genital secretions (e.g., HBV, HIV). When possible, covering portals of exit is a good control strategy; for example, covering one's mouth and nose when coughing or sneezing (i.e., "respiratory hygiene" and "cough etiquette"), or bandage dressing an oozing skin wound. However, the possibility of alternative portals of exit should always be considered in an acute outbreak setting. For example, during the SARS outbreaks, while the respiratory tract was quickly identified as a portal of exit, it was not appreciated that the gastrointestinal tract harbored a large viral load until a single SARS case with diarrhea produced a large outbreak.[9]

Mode of transmission. The mode of transmission is the mechanism by which the microbial agent is transported from the source to the susceptible host (Box 82-3). Multiple classification schemes have been proposed for systematizing similar transmission properties to facilitate comparison and to link appropriate control strategies. Here we present a common classification scheme that is aligned with the Centers for Disease Control and Prevention transmission-based precautions for infection control.[10] Nevertheless, students and professionals working in infectious disease epidemiology may encounter other systems.

Microbes can be transmitted from the source to the host by contact, respiratory droplets, airborne transmission, vehicle-borne, vector-borne, or vertical transmission routes. *Contact* transmission occurs from direct physical contact with a source (e.g., touching, kissing, sex) or indirect contact with a contaminated intermediate object (e.g., environmental surfaces or fomites). Transmission via *respiratory droplets* occurs when a susceptible host contacts large particles from secretions or those expelled during coughing or sneezing.

Transmission via *respiratory droplets* can be difficult to distinguish from *airborne transmission* and is therefore worthy of discussion. Transmission via respiratory droplets occurs via large droplets (>5 microns) and secretions generated from the respiratory tract during coughing, sneezing, or talking. These droplets can enter the eyes, nose, or mouth directly, or indirectly by self-inoculation with contaminated hands. Large respiratory droplets may be suspended briefly in the air but quickly settle to the ground and environmental surfaces less than 1 meter from the source; smaller droplets (6–10 microns) may be inhaled directly into the proximal respiratory tract of the host.[11]

In contrast, airborne transmission occurs when microbes are suspended in air on droplet nuclei (<5 microns) or dust, and can be transmitted over long distances and time intervals.[11] Suspended droplet nuclei can be inhaled deep into the lungs. Airborne transmission can be obligate, preferential, or opportunistic.[12] *Obligate* airborne transmission occurs with microbes (e.g., *Mycobacterium tuberculosis*) that, under natural conditions, can infect a host only when aerosols are inhaled deep into the lung. *Preferential* airborne transmission occurs with microbes that predominantly infect a host by deposition of droplet nuclei in distal airways but can also infect via other modes, such as droplet transmission. For example, measles virus is the most contagious human disease, a feature facilitated by its preferential airborne route of transmission. In some measles outbreaks, secondary cases never have direct contact with the index patients, as they only need to contact aerosols disbursed by the infectious case to become infected.[13] Measles has been transmitted through the air ventilation system at large stadium sporting events to susceptible individuals located far from infected cases.[14] However, measles can also infect via respiratory droplets in the case of close contact between infected and susceptible individuals.

Last, *opportunistic* airborne transmission occurs when a microbe infects a host predominantly by nonairborne modes but, under the right host or environmental conditions, can also infect via aerosolization. Opportunistic airborne transmission explains some of the "super spreading" events observed with the SARS outbreaks (for more on superspreading, a phenomenon whereby a minority of

BOX 82-2 Case Study. Postoperative *Serratia marcescens* Wound Infections Traced to an Out-of-Hospital Source [8]

"From 25 August to 28 September 1994, seven cardiovascular surgery patients at a California hospital acquired postoperative *Serratia marcescens* infections, and one died. To identify the outbreak source, a cohort study was done of all 55 adults who underwent cardiovascular surgery at the hospital during the outbreak. Specimens from the hospital environment and from hands of selected staff were cultured. *S. marcescens* isolates were compared using restriction-endonuclease analysis and pulsed-field gel electrophoresis. Several risk factors for *S. marcescens* infection were identified, but hospital and hand cultures were negative.

In October, a patient exposed to scrub nurse A (who wore artificial fingernails) and to another nurse—but not to other identified risk factors—became infected with the outbreak strain. Subsequent cultures from nurse A's home identified the strain in a jar of exfoliant cream. Removal of the cream ended the outbreak. *S. marcescens* does not normally colonize human skin, but artificial nails may have facilitated transmission via nurse A's hands."

Used with Permission Passaro DJ, Waring L, Armstrong R, et al. Postoperative Serratia marcescens wound infections traced to an out-of-hospital source. J Infect Dis. 1997;175(4):992-5

BOX 82-3 Chain Model of Infectious Diseases: Mode of Transmission

Modes of Transmission

1. Contact
   A. Direct contact (e.g., touching, kissing, sex)
   B. Indirect contact (e.g., intermediate object, fomites)
2. Respiratory droplets (i.e., large particles from secretions, coughing, sneezing)
3. Airborne (i.e., particles < 5 microns: droplet nuclei, dust)
4. Vehicle borne (e.g., ingestion of contaminated food or water, instrumentation, infusion/injection)
5. Vector borne (e.g., mechanical, biologic)
6. Vertical transmission (i.e., *in utero*, at birth, breastmilk)

infectious hosts produce a disproportionate amount of new infections, see below).[15,16]

The *vehicle-borne* transmission category includes ingestion of contaminated food or water (food and waterborne diseases), instrumentation (e.g., urinary catheter), injection (including injection drug use), and infusion (e.g., intravenous catheter). *Vector-borne* transmission can be biologic (vector feeding on the host) or mechanical (contaminated fly appendage contaminating a food item). Lastly, vertical transmission is transmission from mother to child before, during, or after birth. Transmission of HIV from mother-to-child via breast-feeding is considered a form of vertical transmission, but occurs via contaminated breast milk.

Some microbes can be transmitted via multiple modes. Shigellosis, an extremely infectious bacterial gastroenteritis of humans, is an example. *Shigella* is often described as being transmitted via the "fecal-oral" route. However, this description is insufficient to design control measures because it only summarizes the portals of exit and entry. More specifically, the modes of transmission include direct contact (person-to-person physical contact, including sexual), indirect contact (contaminated fomites), and vehicle-borne (ingestion of contaminated food or water). Therefore, understanding all the modes of transmission is necessary to implement preventive measures, to conduct an outbreak investigation, and to implement control measures during an outbreak.

Portal of entry. The portal of entry is where the infectious agent enters the host. Possible portals of entry include the following:

- Mucous membrane surfaces;
- Nose, mouth, oropharynx;
- Gastrointestinal tract;
- Genitourinary tract;
- Respiratory tract;
- Anorectum; and
- Cutaneous (or percutaneous) via skin or skin penetration.

Practical application. Understanding the chain model of infectious diseases is essential for implementing common sense infection control and worker safety measures. For example, agents transmitted primarily by large respiratory droplets and secretions include influenza virus, *Neisseria meningitidis* (meningococcal disease), *Yersinia pestis* (pneumonic plague), and *Variola* virus (smallpox). Large respiratory droplets fall out of the air, settling close to the source (usually within 3 feet). Therefore, common sense transmission control measures for these communicable agents include: covering the portal of exit (i.e., respiratory hygiene and cough etiquette); encouraging the susceptible host to use barrier methods to cover portals of entry (e.g., protective equipment such as face masks and goggles); handwashing (i.e., "hand hygiene"); and increasing awareness of hand contact with the face, mouth, nose, and eyes ("hand awareness"). Hand awareness may reduce self-inoculation from hands that have had contact with infectious patients or contaminated environmental surfaces.

Respiratory airborne agents transmitted by droplet nuclei include measles and varicella viruses and *Mycobacterium tuberculosis.* Droplet nuclei remain suspended in the air for longer periods of time and can travel over distances. Reducing the risk of airborne transmission requires diluting and/or filtering air. Air can be diluted by increasing ventilation (opening the windows), and it can be filtered by wearing a personal respirator. The common N-95 respirator is a snug-fitting facemask that filters air by the negative pressure generated by normal inspiration. To work properly, these respirators must be fitted and tested with the intended user. Better, albeit more expensive, protection can be obtained with a powered air-purifying respirator hood. Preventing the spread of droplet nuclei to distant areas in a given facility can be achieved by implementing engineering controls that might include a negative pressure room for the infectious patient and assuring that any potentially recirculated air undergoes high efficiency particulate air (HEPA) filtration or exposure to ultraviolet light. Hospital and community infection control practices are derived from these basic concepts.

Natural History of Infection and Infectiousness

To effectively interrupt transmission, we also need to understand the natural history of infection. This includes the concepts of infectiousness and disease, as well as how these time periods relate to each other. While clinicians focus on diagnosing and curing diseases and relieving symptoms, in public health we focus on understanding the dynamics of infection and infectiousness in order to prevent transmission (Fig. 82-4). The interval between when a susceptible person is infected until s/he develops symptoms is called the *incubation* period. Clinicians are familiar with the incubation period because it helps them narrow their differential diagnosis when the causative agent is unknown. Furthermore, in a "point source" outbreak when the times of disease exposure and onset are well documented, the incubation period can be used to generate hypotheses about the potential causative agent (and therefore source of the infection and potential control strategies). The interval between when a susceptible person becomes infected and s/he becomes infectious is called the *latent* period. The latent period is followed by the *infectious* period. The infectious period ends only when the host is no longer infectious, which typically means that the host has cleared the infection or has died.

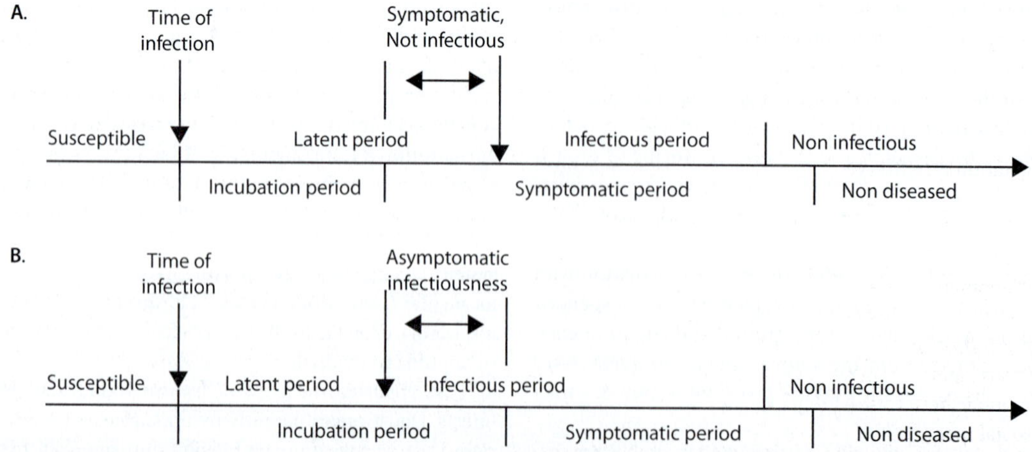

FIGURE 82-4. The natural history of infection and infectiousness. A: When the latent period is longer than the incubation period, an infected person develops symptoms before becoming infectious. B: When the latent period is shorter than the incubation period, the infected person becomes infectious before developing symptoms (asymptomatic infectiousness).

When these two intervals are considered together, they reveal both the natural history of infection as well as important insights about potential control strategies. For example, when the latent period is longer than the incubation period, an infected person develops symptoms before becoming infectious. However, when the latent period is shorter than the incubation period, the infected person becomes infectious before developing symptoms (asymptomatic infectiousness). In this way, this simple relationship can guide our understanding of transmission dynamics and can guide the public health response. Consider the following examples:

Asymptomatic infectiousness. Asymptomatic infectiousness is the important driver of several infectious diseases with a large public health impact. For example, HIV infection is transmitted by direct person-to-person contact via blood, genital fluids, or breast milk. In the absence of treatment, HIV-infected persons can be infectious for 10 years or more before developing symptoms of AIDS.[17] Hence, HIV-infected persons have the potential to infect many people (via sex or sharing injection drug use paraphernalia) for years before knowing they are infected. In the United States, nearly half of all new HIV infections are linked to the minority of persons living with HIV who are unaware of their infection.[18] Likewise, many HCV infected persons can be infectious decades before developing symptoms that lead to a diagnosis of chronic HCV infection.[19] Persons with hepatitis A, measles, and influenza infection are infectious about 1 week, 3–4 days, and 1–2 days before developing symptoms, respectively.[20] Identifying exposed contacts can be more difficult when the exposure occurred before the infectious source developed symptoms, especially if the exposure occurred years before.

In contrast, with smallpox (when it existed), the latent period was longer than the incubation period; therefore, patients developed symptoms (e.g., high fevers, muscle aches) before becoming infectious. In other words, there was little to no transmission by asymptomatic individuals. In fact, patients with smallpox were most infectious after the rash onset. This made detection and isolation of cases and contact tracing and vaccination an effective disease control strategy. Patients infected with the human SARS coronavirus were infectious after developing respiratory symptoms and were progressively more infectious as their disease worsened. Hence, most secondary infections occurred among healthcare workers and close household contacts caring for very ill persons. This also helped to explain why transmission of SARS in the community was not sustained.[21]

Convergence Model of Microbe-Human Interaction

In March, 2003, the "Convergence model of human-microbe interaction" (Fig. 82-5) was published by the Institute of Medicine (IOM), Committee on Emerging Microbial Threats to Health in the 21st Century.[22] This was a follow-up document to a landmark 1992 IOM report, which called for increasing vigilance against the threat that infectious diseases posed to national security.[23] The 2003 IOM report delineated the factors that can lead to the emergence and re-emergence of microbial threats to health, such as:

- Microbial adaptation and change;
- Human susceptibility to infection;
- Climate and weather;
- Changing ecosystems;
- Economic development and land use;
- Human demographics and behavior;
- Technology and industry;
- International travel and commerce;
- Breakdown of public health measures;
- Poverty and social inequality;
- War and famine;
- Lack of political will; and
- Intent to harm.

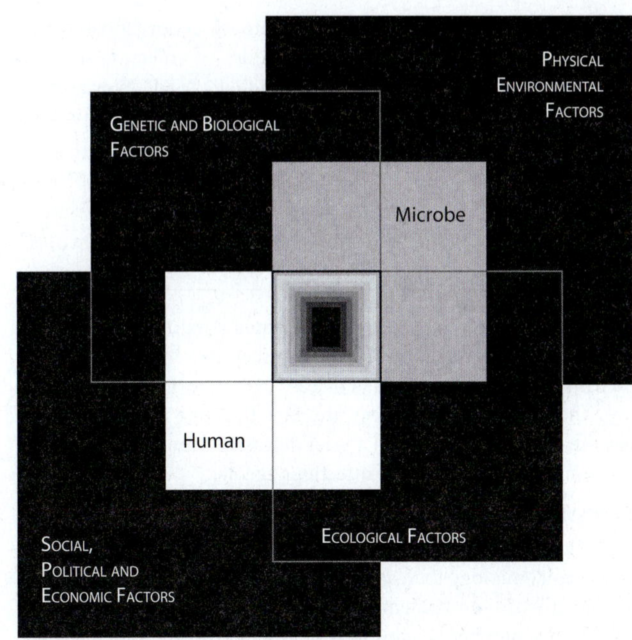

FIGURE 82-5. Convergence model of human–microbe interaction. At the center of the model is a box representing the convergence of factors leading to the emergence of an infectious disease. The interior of the box is a gradient flowing from white to black; the white outer edges represent what is known about the factors in emergence, and the black center represents the unknown (similar to the theoretical construct of the "black box" with its unknown constituents and means of operation). Interlocking with the center box are the two focal players in a microbial threat to health—the human and the microbe. The microbe–host interaction is influenced by the interlocking domains of the determinants of the emergence of infection: genetic and biological factors; physical environmental factors; ecological factors; and social, political, and economic factors. (Reproduced with Permission From Smolinski MS, Hamburg MA, Lederberg J, Institute of Medicine (U.S.). Committee on Emerging Microbial Threats to Health in the 21st Century. Washington, DC: National Academies Press; 2003.)

In addition to recognizing the challenges that each of the factors presents individually, the report posed that the *convergence* of these factors can create especially high-risk environments whereby infectious diseases may readily emerge or re-emerge. Specifically, the report describes the convergence model as follows:

> *The convergence of any number of factors can create an environment in which infectious diseases can emerge and become rooted in society. A model was developed to illustrate how the convergence of factors in four domains impacts the human-microbe interaction and results in infectious disease. The emergence and spread of microbial threats are driven by a complex set of factors, the convergence of which can lead to consequences of disease much greater than any single factor might suggest. Genetic and biological factors allow microbes to adapt and change, and can make humans more or less susceptible to infections. Changes in the physical environment can have impact on the ecology of vectors and animal reservoirs, the transmissibility of microbes, and the activities of humans that expose them to certain threats. Human behavior, both individual and collective, is perhaps the most complex factor in the emergence of disease. Emergence is especially complicated by social, political, and economic factors—including the development of megacities, the disruption of global ecosystems, the expansion of international travel and commerce, and poverty—which ensure that infectious diseases will continue to plague us. Today we also face the threats of intentionally introduced biological agents.*

Epidemiologists can think of this model as an updated version of the agent-host-environment model of infectious disease causation, also referred to as the "epidemiologic triad." However, the Convergence model offers an integrated approach that reminds us that causes can be complex, connected, and interdependent. The success or failure of our infectious disease prevention and control programs may depend on these factors, no matter how far upstream in the causal chain, and how they interact.

TRANSMISSION DYNAMICS

Transmission dynamics describe the population-level view of the consequences of interactions between susceptible and infected hosts and the accumulation of cases of disease over time. In this section, we cover the reproductive number, the infection rate among susceptibles, the generation time, and a brief discussion about the reproductive number and evolution of infectious agents.

The Basic Reproductive Number (R_0)

The basic reproductive number, R_0, is a central concept in infectious disease epidemiology that, along with the generation time, describes the rate at which an epidemic grows or recedes. To understand the reproductive number, it helps to adopt the perspective of a microbial agent that has infected and produced an infectious human case. In order for a communicable microbial agent to survive among humans, it must produce (directly or indirectly), on average, at least one other infectious human case. This "replacement rate" is the only way microbes can survive in a host population; otherwise, the microbe will die out. The basic reproductive number is defined as the average expected number of secondary infectious cases produced by one infectious host during his or her infectious period in a large population that is entirely susceptible (Fig. 82-6). It does not include new cases produced by secondary cases or cases that do not become infections. The interpretation is as follows: if $R_0 < 1$, the number of new cases will decline and eventually reach zero (i.e., epidemic burnout). If $R_0 \approx 1$, the production of new cases will assume a steady state. If $R_0 > 1$, the number of new cases will increase (growing epidemic).

R_0 helps to answer the following question: if an infectious case was introduced into a susceptible population with no control measures, what is the inherent potential for this case to cause an epidemic? More specifically, how many secondary infectious cases would be produced from a single infectious case, on average? In spite of the importance of R_0, it is difficult to measure empirically. This is because an important component in the definition of R_0 is the assumption that every host in the population is fully susceptible to the pathogen; there is no underlying partial or full immunity due to vaccination or genetic factors, for example. In reality, fully susceptible populations are rare and typically only occur when a pathogen is first introduced into a population (at time = 0). For example, during the SARS outbreak in 2003 the R_0 could be directly estimated from case counts and epidemiological data about contacts.[24] This is because it was hypothesized that nearly everyone in the population was susceptible to this new human coronavirus. These conditions were also likely met when HIV infection was introduced into San Francisco's gay male community in the late 1970s and early 1980s and when HCV spread among injection drug users before the availability of anti-HCV antibody testing.

The magnitude of R_0 at the start of an epidemic influences the epidemic pattern observed when an infectious disease is introduced into a population, whether that be in a closed or open population.[25] Consider a simple disease model whereby an infectious agent is introduced into a susceptible population and people are infected and then recover with immunity (e.g., measles, chicken pox). In epidemiological terms, this is often referred to as a "SIR model" (see Chapter 159: "Introduction to Infectious Disease Modeling") to indicate the successive states of susceptible, infected, and recovered. An agent following a SIR pattern with a high R_0 introduced into a susceptible

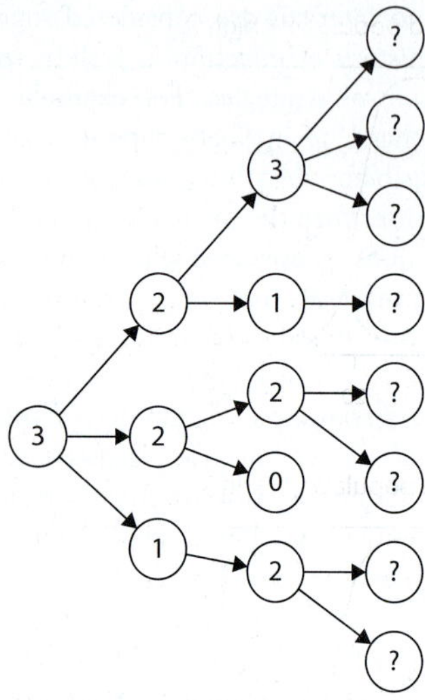

FIGURE 82-6. The reproductive number is the average number of secondary cases produced by infectious cases during their infectious periods. Each circle represents an infectious case, and the circle contains the number of secondary cases he or she produced. For example, the first case (at the far left) produced three secondary infectious cases, and so forth. Therefore, to calculate the average reproductive number, calculate the arithmetic average of the number of secondary cases: (3 + 2 + 2 + 1 + 3 + 1 + 2 + 0 + 2)/9 = 1.8.

closed population will produce an epidemic that eventually dies out once everyone has been infected. This is because the supply of susceptible hosts has been exhausted. In contrast, an agent with a high R_0 introduced into a susceptible open population, where there is replenishment of susceptible hosts through births, deaths, and/or immigration, will produce an epidemic followed by endemic persistence. In this scenario, the new supply of susceptibles produces a steady state whereby the incidence of new cases is constant. Figure 82-7 illustrates this general process.

The basic reproductive number can be defined quantitatively as follows:

$$R_0 = d\,c\,p \tag{1}$$

In Equation 1, from the perspective of an infectious host, d is the duration of infectiousness, the length of time that the host is infected and capable of infecting others, c is the contact rate with susceptible hosts, and p is the transmission probability—the conditional probability of infecting a susceptible host given that contact occurs.

Equation 1 is intuitive yet deceptively simple. By "infectious host," we are referring to an infectious human or animal case; however, it could also be, for example, an infectious mosquito or a contaminated blood product used for transfusion. In addition, for each microbial agent and infectious disease, "contact" and "transmission" need to be defined carefully. Contact is an exposure episode. For example, in the case of a woman living with HIV infection, contact might be defined as unprotected intercourse with another person. For a person living in an area where dengue is endemic, contact might be defined as the bite of an infected female *Aedes aegypti* mosquito. Transmission generally means sufficient transfer of the microbial agent to lead to an infection (pathological persistence in host, subclinical injury to host, or evidence of a host immune response). For example, transmission of hepatitis C virus can result in HCV infection (pathological persistence in blood), subclinical injury (liver inflammation with or without scarring), or presence of anti-HCV antibodies (evidence of a host immune response). Therefore, the operational definition of transmission varies, depending on the microbial agent and the outcomes under consideration.

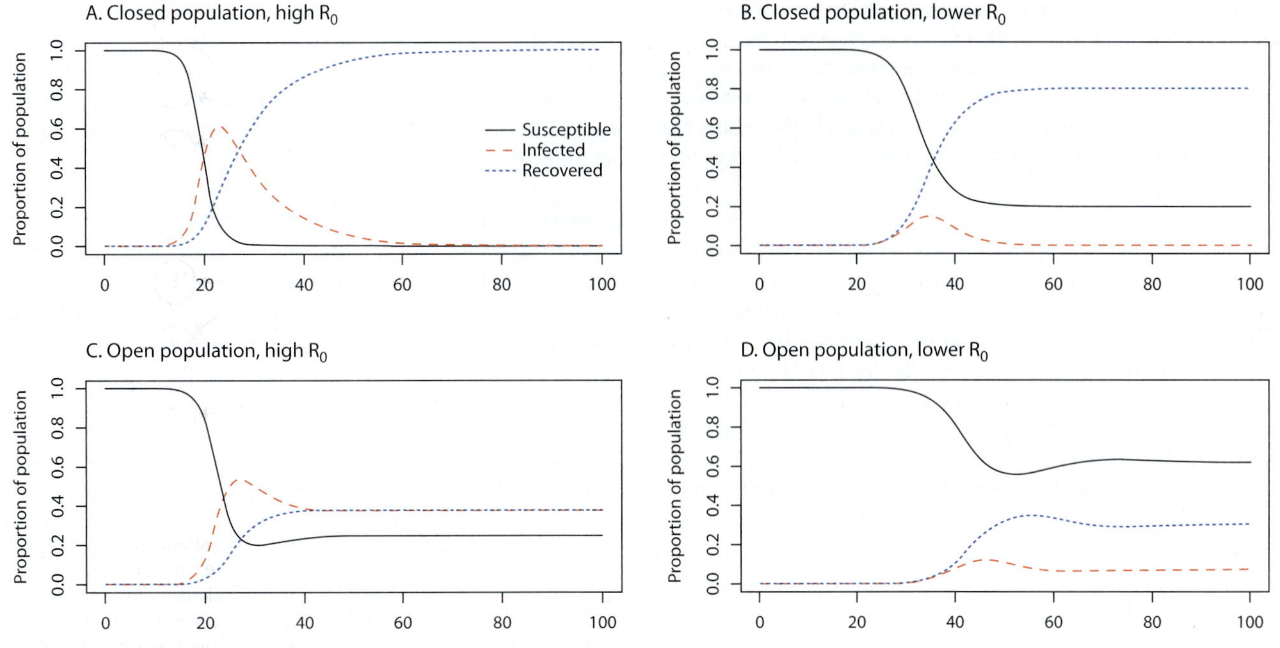

FIGURE 82-7. Simulated outbreak that follows a simple S-I-R pattern with microbes with high and low R_0 values in closed and open populations. The infected agent is introduced into a susceptible population whereby people become infected and then recover with immunity. Panel A: Epidemic in a closed population, high R_0. Everyone eventually is infected during the epidemic. Panel B: Epidemic in a closed population, lower R_0. The epidemic dies out before everyone is infected. Panel C: Epidemic in an open population, high R_0. Epidemic followed by epidemic persistence; the population reaches dynamic equilibrium and the infection does not die out due to replenishment of susceptible individuals. Panel D: Epidemic in an open population, lower R_0. Adapted with Permission from Halloran ER. Concepts of Transmission and Dynamics. In: Thomas JC, Weber DJ, editors. Epidemiologic Methods for the Study of Infectious Diseases, Oxford University Press, 2001

Understanding the transmission probability can be less intuitive, as it can vary widely even for the same pathogen. Consider sexual transmission of HIV infection. Exposure risks per sexual act range from extremely low for oral sex to 138 infections per 10,000 exposures for receptive anal intercourse.[26] The dual use of antiretroviral therapy (ART) for the HIV-infected partners and condoms can attenuate these risks by 99.2%,[26] underscoring the potential benefits of the global "Treat All" strategy to end the HIV epidemic.[27] In general, transmission probabilities depend on the microbe, the exposure conditions (e.g., airborne exposure, contact with respiratory droplets, use of personal protective equipment), and environmental conditions (e.g., temperature, humidity, airflow), as well as other cofactors. This might include the presence of an ulcerative sexually transmitted disease in the case of HIV or the presence or absence of a specific genetic cofactor that affects the efficiency of transmission.

Another familiar example of transmission probability is the secondary attack "rate" (correctly defined as a type of risk, but commonly referred to as a "rate"). It is a special case of the transmission probability and is defined as the proportion of susceptibles who become infected when exposed to an infectious person. Secondary attack rates are usually estimated for infections that can be transmitted through household contact, such as tuberculosis, measles, chicken pox, influenza, and viral gastroenteritis. Like R_0, the secondary attack rates are difficult to measure empirically. This is because the necessary conditions—an index infectious case being introduced into a susceptible population without control measures—rarely occurs except when a novel microbial agent is introduced and spreads before it has been identified.

The concept of superspreading further illustrates the complexity of measuring the transmission probability. Superspreading is a phenomenon observed for a variety of infectious diseases that refers to the minority of infectious hosts who are responsible for a disproportionate number of new infections relative to the average infected host.[28] For example, in the 2014–15 West Africa Ebola outbreak, although the reproductive number was approximately 2.4, modeling studies suggest that a minority of superspreaders played a key role in sustaining onward transmission of the epidemic and were responsible for approximately 61% of the total number of infections.[29] Superspreaders were also documented in the 2013 SARS outbreak. On average, it was estimated that a single infectious case of SARS infected about three secondary cases in a population that has not yet instituted control measures.[24] Nevertheless, a subset of cases each transmitted to more than ten healthcare workers, family and social contacts, or visitors to the healthcare facilities where the patients were hospitalized.[15] In this way, although R_0 provides important information about epidemic potential, it can obscure potentially relevant biological and epidemiologic phenomena.

Effective Reproductive Number (*R*)

The R_0 represents the inherent potential for an agent to cause an epidemic after the introduction of an infectious case into a completely susceptible population. However, in reality, populations are rarely completely susceptible, given heterogeneity in human susceptibility to infection and the presence of control measures such as vaccination. Thus, we can define the actual or effective reproductive number (R) as a function of the basic reproductive number (R_0) and the fraction of the population (x) that is susceptible upon the introduction (at time $= 0$) of the infectious case (Equation 2):

$$R = R_0 x \tag{2}$$

From Equation 2, there are at least two key insights. First, if $x = 1$, indicating a completely susceptible population, then $R = R_0$. Second, it is apparent from Equation 2 that an epidemic could eventually be ended ($R < 1$) by sufficiently reducing x because, on average, infectious cases would no longer produce at least one infectious case and subsequent generations of cases would be smaller (e.g., less than replacement rate). This might happen without intervention, for example if a fraction of the population was immune by virtue of their genetic profile or because of an effective control measure such as vaccination. In either case, as the fraction susceptible, x, falls below 100%, R eventually becomes less than 1. Therefore, decreasing the fraction of susceptibles is a strategy to achieve $R < 1$ and therefore slow or end an epidemic.

Herd Immunity Threshold

If vaccination is the control measure used to reduce population susceptibility to a pathogen, additional useful relationships emerge. The fraction of the population that is susceptible can be defined as $x = 1 - h\,f$, where f is the fraction of the population that has been vaccinated (vaccine coverage), and h is the fraction of those vaccinated who have complete protection (a type of vaccine efficacy). For a well-studied, vaccine-preventable disease, the basic reproductive number and vaccine efficacy are often known and we can estimate what fraction of the population would need to be vaccinated to bring $R < 1$ with simple algebra, $R = R_0(1 - h\,f) < 1$ becomes

$$f > 1 - (1 / R_0) / h, \qquad (3)$$

where f is the minimum vaccine coverage necessary to achieve $R < 1$. For example, R_0 was between 3 and 5 for smallpox. The smallpox vaccine had a pre-exposure vaccine efficacy of about 98%. Therefore, if smallpox were re introduced into the human population and spread naturally, then we would need to vaccinate at least 68% of the population if $R_0 \approx 3$, and at least 82% of the population if $R_0 \approx 5$, to get $R < 1$. This threshold of susceptibility, at which an epidemic will be prevented, is also known as the *herd immunity threshold* (Figs. 82-8 and 82-9).

Herd immunity was first described in 1923 as a population-level phenomenon related to, but distinct from, the immunity of individuals.[30] It refers to the protection of populations from infection through the presence and proximity of immune individuals.[31] In the 1970s, the theory of the herd immunity threshold was proposed, positing that the incidence of infection would decline if the proportion of a randomly mixing population who were immune exceeded $(R_0-1)/R_0$, or $1-1/R_0$.[32,33] One can see that these relationships are equivalent to Equation 3 if one assumes a perfect vaccine (i.e., $h = 1$). The herd immunity threshold is a useful, albeit overly simplified approach to determine the necessary level of coverage for a vaccine program to prevent epidemics. It also helps to explain interesting epidemic phenomena like epidemic cycling and "honeymoon periods," a time of very low incidence that immediately follows the introduction of a mass vaccination policy that approaches but fails to reach the herd immunity threshold.[34]

Displayed in Table 82-1 and Fig. 82-8 are various R_0 values and vaccine coverage thresholds (f) for selected vaccine-preventable diseases.[28] This information is useful in several ways. First, as described above, we can use R_0 to compare epidemic potential. Notice that the R_0 for smallpox is much smaller than the R_0 for, say, measles. These differences in R_0 are primarily explained by the transmission mechanisms. Smallpox was primarily transmitted by large respiratory droplets, and patients were not infectious until they developed a rash (that is, there was little to no asymptomatic infectiousness). In contrast, measles is spread by the airborne mode, and an infected person is infectious before the onset of the rash. As a result, measles is much more infectious than smallpox. Second, notice that some diseases have similar R_0 values despite different transmission mechanisms. SARS and HIV both have R_0 values in the 2–5 range. With a comparatively low-transmission probability, HIV's R_0 is largely driven by a long duration of infectiousness (d) that lasts years and sometimes decades. In contrast, patients with SARS are infectious for about 9 days on average[35] and may have a higher contact rate than HIV due to the mode of transmission (e.g., droplet transmission versus sexual transmission). The concept of *generation time*, introduced below, describes why epidemics caused by these pathogens with similar R_0 values occur on different time scales.

Also, notice from Fig. 82-8 that an effective control measure (in this case, vaccination) does not need to be applied to the whole susceptible population to be successful; it only needs to be implemented sufficiently to make $R < 1$, although in public health practice we strive to protect as many people as is feasible and affordable. Nevertheless, this is an important insight, as public health agencies are often operating in resource-constrained environments—even diseases with high R_0 values theoretically can, through effective control strategies, be contained.

Of course, there are important considerations when interpreting herd immunity thresholds that were recognized as early as 1971 in

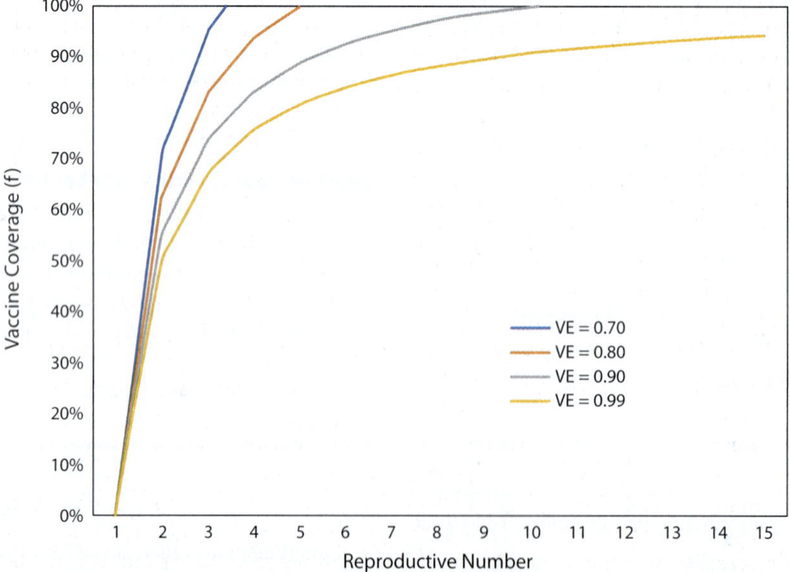

FIGURE 82-8. The vaccine coverage (f) required for an effective reproductive number less than one ($R < 1$) given the basic reproductive number (R_0) and vaccine effectiveness (h). For a highly effective vaccine or low R_0, only a proportion of the population needs to be vaccinated for R to fall below 1. This is a general property of interventions: they need to reach a sufficient proportion of the population to get $R < 1$ (100% vaccine coverage is shown on the figure with a dashed line).

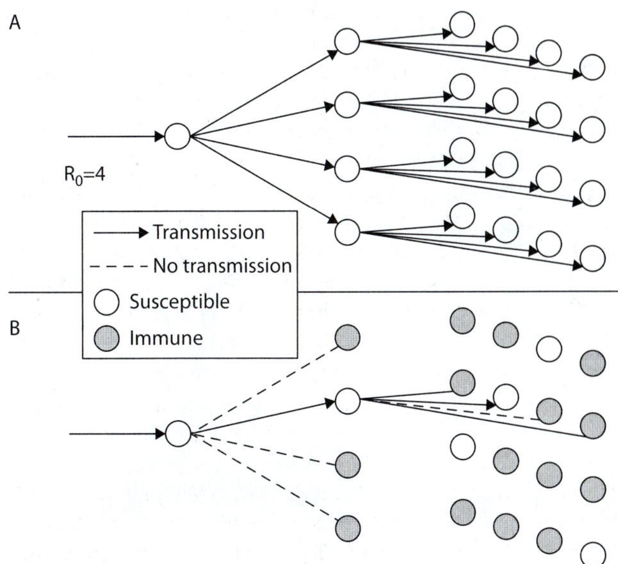

FIGURE 82-9. Diagram illustrating transmission of an infection with a basic reproduction number $R_0 = 4$. A: Transmission over three generations after introduction into a totally susceptible population (1 case would lead to 4 cases and then to 16 cases). B: Expected transmissions if $(R_0-1)/R_0 = 1-1/R_0 = 3/4$ of the population is immune. Under this circumstance, all but 1 of the contacts for each case is immune, and so each case leads to only 1 successful transmission of the infection. This implies constant incidence over time. If a greater proportion is immune, then incidence will decline. On this basis, $(R_0-1)/R_0$ is known as the "herd immunity threshold." (*Source*: Reproduced with Permission from From Fine P, Eames K, Heymann DL. "Herd immunity": a rough guide. *Clin Infect Dis.* 2011;52(7):911–6. © The Author 2011. Published by Oxford University Press on behalf of the Infectious Diseases Society of America. All rights reserved.)

TABLE 82-1 BASIC REPRODUCTIVE NUMBER FOR SELECTED VACCINE-PREVENTABLE DISEASES

Infection	Estimate	Confidence Interval or Range	Citation
Smallpox	4 (median)	3.84–5.20	Constantino
Influenza			Biggerstaff
-seasonal	1.28	1.19–1.37	--Ibid.
-1918 H1N1 pandemic	1.80 (median)	1.47–2.27	--Ibid.
-1957 H2N2 pandemic	1.65 (median)	1.53–1.70	--Ibid.
-1968 H3N2 pandemic	1.80 (median)	1.56–1.85	--Ibid.
-2009 H1N1 pandemic	1.46 (median)	1.30–1.70	--Ibid.
Diphtheria	7.2 (median)	4.7–14.8	Matsuyama
Zika virus	2.06		Gao
Ebola (West Africa, 2014)	see range	1.2–2.5	Van Kerkhove
Measles (pre-vaccine era)	11.1	6.1–27.0	Guerra
Polio virus	see range	5–6	Anderson
Pertussis	5.5	5.2.–5.9	Kretzschmar
SARS	4.6 (mean)	3.6–5.04	Gumel
HIV (100% assortative mixing and high sexual activity)	see range	4.18–6.69 (1991–96)5.43–36.75 (1997–2008)	Nsubuga

Sources: Costantino V, Kunasekaran MP, Chughtai AA, MacIntyre CR. How valid are assumptions about re-emerging smallpox? A systematic review of parameters used in smallpox mathematical models. *Mil Med.* 2018;183(7–8):e200–7. Biggerstaff M, Cauchemez S, Reed C, Gambhir M, Finelli L. Estimates of the reproduction number for seasonal, pandemic, and zoonotic influenza: A systematic review of the literature. *BMC Infect Dis.* 2014;14:480. Matsuyama R, Akhmetzhanov AR, Endo A, Lee H, Yamaguchi T, Tsuzuki S, Nishiura H. Uncertainty and sensitivity analysis of the basic reproduction number of diphtheria: A case study of a Rohingya refugee camp in Bangladesh, November–December 2017. *Peer J.* 2018;6:e4583. Gao D, Lou Y, He D, Porco TC, Kuang Y, Chowell G, Ruan S. Prevention and control of Zika as a mosquito-borne and sexually transmitted disease: A mathematical modeling analysis. *Sci Rep.* 2016;6:28070. Van Kerkhove MD, Bento AI, Mills HL, Ferguson NM, Donnelly CA. A review of epidemiological parameters from Ebola outbreaks to inform early public health decision-making. *Sci Data.* 2015;2:150019. Guerra FM, Bolotin S, Lim G, Heffernan J, Deeks SL, Li Y, Crowcroft NS. The basic reproduction number (R(0)) of measles: A systematic review. *Lancet Infect Dis.* 2017;17(12):e420–8. Anderson RM. Chapter 1. The impact of vaccination on the epidemiology of infectious diseases. In: *The Vaccine Book.* Academic Press; 2016. Kretzschmar M, Teunis PF, Pebody RG. Incidence and reproduction numbers of pertussis: Estimates from serological and social contact data in five European countries. *PLoS Med.* 2010 Jun 22;7(6):e1000291. Gumel AB, Ruan S, Day T, Watmough J, Brauer F, van den Driessche P, Gabrielson D, Bowman C, Alexander ME, Ardal S, Wu J, Sahai BM. Modelling strategies for controlling SARS outbreaks. *Proc Biol Sci.* 2004;271(1554):2223–32. Nsubuga RN, White RG, Mayanja BN, Shafer LA. Estimation of the HIV basic reproduction number in rural south west Uganda: 1991–2008. *PLoS One.* 2014;9(1):e83778.

a seminal paper by Fox et al.[36] The simple relationships presented above assume thorough and random mixing of members of the population, which is an unrealistic assumption in nearly all situations. Furthermore, although imperfect vaccination is represented by the parameter h, the impact of heterogeneous populations, nonrandom vaccination, and waning immunity are ignored. More complex dynamic models are needed to capture the impact of these real-world nuances. Regardless, the simple herd immunity thresholds presented above are useful ways to compare the epidemic potential of different pathogens and to consider how to define success for prevention programs.

Figure 82-10 displays a real-world example of these concepts—both R_0 and R.[37] On February 23, 2003, SARS was introduced into Toronto, Canada, and followed by two epidemic curves representing hospital outbreaks. In March, the early part of the first curve (number 1) rises rapidly and its slope approximates R_0: the average number of secondary cases when an index case was introduced into a completely susceptible population and without control measures. Once the outbreak was recognized and control measures were implemented, the epidemic curve peaked and returned to baseline approximately mid-to-late April. However, lulled by the disappearance of cases, infection control practices were relaxed and SARS was re-introduced in early May. Infection control measures were immediately reinstituted and we can see the subsequent "blunting of the curve" in late May. In this second curve, the initial slope was less steep and it approximates R. Therefore, in this completely susceptible population, the initial slope in the first curve measures R_0, the average number of secondary cases in the absence of control measures, and the initial slope in the second curve measures R, the average number of secondary cases in the presence of control measures.

Reproductive Number Over Time ($t > 0$)

So far, we have considered the reproductive number upon the introduction of an infectious case into a population. However, as an epidemic evolves over time ($t > 0$), the average number of secondary cases changes. This might be due, for example, to changing numbers of susceptibles in a closed population—as the epidemic continues, there will be fewer hosts to infect over time if they are not replaced by other susceptible hosts. It might also be due to a small number of hosts who are infected and infectious—pathogens with low R_0 values

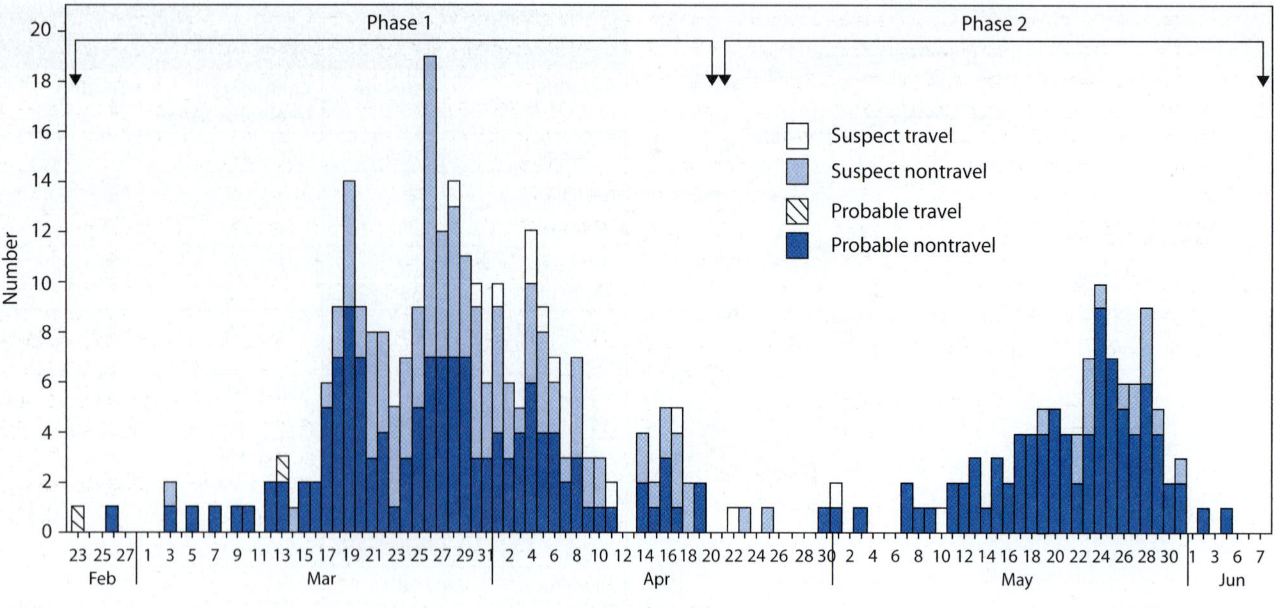

FIGURE 82-10. Number of reported cases of severe acute respiratory syndrome ($N = 361$), by classification and date of illness onset—Ontario, February 23–June 7, 2003. (*Source:* Morbidity and Mortality Weekly Report Vol. 52, No. 23 (June 13, 2003), pp. 547-550 (4 pages) Published by: Centers for Disease Control & Prevention (CDC).)

may not be able to sustain continual transmission because of low numbers of infected hosts and will therefore die out of the population. In both of these scenarios, the average number of secondary infections will continually decrease as the epidemic wanes and eventually burns out.

Consequently, we can define R as a function of time (t), or $R(t)$. For illustration of this phenomenon, we simulated a simple smallpox outbreak where an infectious case of smallpox was introduced into a closed population of 10,000 susceptible people under four different scenarios (Fig. 82-11). Curve A1 is the epidemic curve of prevalent smallpox cases in the absence of control measures. Curve B1 is the corresponding curve for the effective reproductive number, calculated from $R(t) = R_0x(t)$. R_0 drives the initial exponential increase in Curve A1. Even in the absence of control measures, the epidemic curve peaks and the number of prevalent cases declines. In a closed population, this happens because the supply of susceptible hosts is depleted [and $x(t)$ decreases]. This also happens with infections such as influenza, which move rapidly through open communities. Notice that the effective reproductive number changes with time (Curve B1). The effective reproductive number is a dynamic number and, in this case, eventually drops below 1, and the epidemic burns out. Even in the absence of control measures, the natural transmission dynamics of an epidemic may lead to extinction of the disease [$R(t) < 1$], particularly in a closed (or approximately closed) population. In Fig. 82-10, Curves A2, A3, and A4 are the epidemic smallpox curves in the presence of control interventions. Curves B2, B3, and B4 are the corresponding $R(t)$s. Notice that the effect of control measures is to shift and blunt the epidemic curve as $R(t) < 1$. This is ultimately our goal in communicable disease control as we want fewer cases, more time to respond, and, to drive $R < 1$ so that the epidemic burns out.

In general, as an epidemic spreads, susceptibles are infected and become infectious (known as "infectives"). Eventually, infectives are "removed" from the infectious state; they

- Become noninfectious and immune (e.g., measles, chicken pox);
- Become noninfectious and not immune (susceptible again, e.g., gonorrhea); or
- Die (typically a noninfectious state, although can also be temporarily infectious, as in the case of Ebola[38]).

For a closed population (no migration in or out) where infectives either die or become noninfectious with immunity, the number of susceptibles declines even in the absence of control measures. For an epidemic that moves rapidly through the population (e.g., a high R_0), the number of susceptibles also declines, even if the population is open. When the number of susceptibles declines the average number of secondary cases produced by infectious cases also declines with time. This explains the insight presented in the smallpox simulation above; the effective reproductive number [$R(t)$] changes over time, which has implications for the dynamics of the epidemic:

- If $R(t)$ persists above 1, the epidemic continues to grow.
- If $R(t)$ persists around 1, the infection becomes endemic.
- If $R(t)$ persists below 1, the infection becomes extinct.

In summary, when an infectious case is introduced into a population ($t = 0$), the basic reproductive number (R_0) represents the inherent epidemic potential when the population is completely susceptible and there are no control measures. This is somewhat of a theoretical measure as completely susceptible populations are typically rare. When a fraction x of the population is susceptible, the effective reproductive number (R) represents the actual epidemic potential where $R = R_0x$. Populations may not be fully susceptible if subpopulations have natural protection or control measures are in place (e.g., vaccination). If $R > 1$ at $t = 0$, an epidemic occurs; and $R(t)$ will continue to change as the epidemic evolves over time ($t > 0$). Consequently, using this framework, a logical goal of control measures is to (1) delay the outbreak peak, (2) decrease the magnitude of the outbreak peak, and (3) reduce the total number of infectious disease cases.[39]

Infection Rate Among Susceptibles

Understanding the reproductive number focused our attention on potential transmission control points, including the duration of infectiousness, contact rate, transmission probability, and fraction of the population that is susceptible. However, to complete the picture we must consider the transmission process from the perspective of a susceptible host. In epidemiology, the infection rate

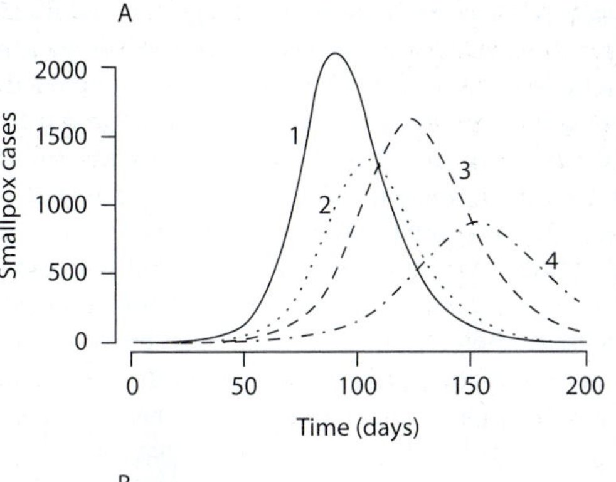

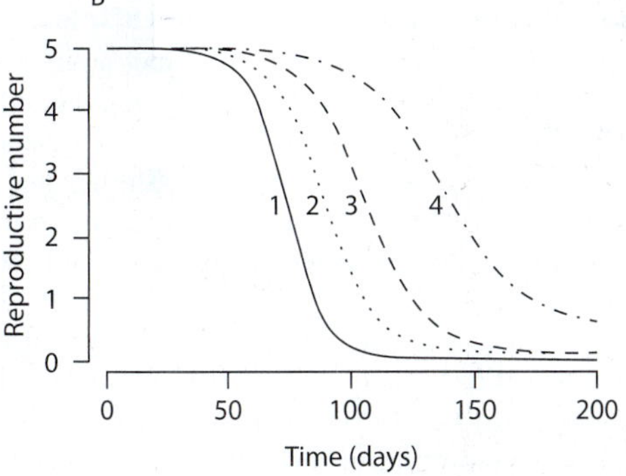

FIGURE 82-11. Simulated smallpox outbreak after introducing a single infectious case into a susceptible population of 10,000. Incubation period was 12 days, duration of infectiousness was 10 days, and $R_0 = 5$. Top curve (A) displays the prevalent cases, and bottom curve (B) displays the effective reproductive numbers. Curves A1 and B1 are without control measures. Curves A2 and B2 display the effect of vaccinating 70% of susceptible individuals. Curves A3 and B3 display the effect of case isolation, reducing the effective duration of infectiousness from 10 days to 7 days. Curves A4 and B4 display the effect of both control measures. Curves B2, B3, and B4 display the effective reproductive number (*R*).

among susceptibles, also known as *incidence*, is the number of new infections divided by the person-time at risk. It is a common and important epidemiologic measure of disease occurrence. However, we can also define incidence according to the drivers of infection (Equation 4):

$$I(t) = c\,p\,P(t), \tag{4}$$

where *c* is the contact rate (*c*) with potentially infectious sources, *p* is the transmission probability given contact with an infectious source, and *P*(*t*) is the probability that the potential source is infectious. This intuitive relationship introduces an important new parameter to consider—*P*(*t*), the probability the potential source is infectious. In this context, *P*(*t*) is usually approximated by estimating the *prevalence* of infectives.

Equation 4 is recognized as the fundamental "dependent happenings" relationship, a concept first described by Sir Ronald Ross more than 100 years ago,[40] in which the incidence of an infectious disease *depends* on the prevalence. This dependency, whereby the potential outcomes of an individual can depend on the status and treatment of other individuals in the population, means that interventions can have both direct and indirect effects.[41] For example, a vaccination program has *direct* benefit for the people receiving the vaccine. It also may have an *indirect* benefit for people living in communities where the vaccine program is implemented because they experience a lower *force of infection* due to the presence and proximity of immune individuals (e.g., herd immunity). However, indirect effects can also be harmful. For example, an effective vaccination program will typically increase the average age when people are first infected. Although there will be fewer cases overall than before the program, new infections will, on average, be among older individuals who may experience more severe manifestations of disease. Varicella (chickenpox) is an example of this phenomenon,[42] as is rubella, which is typically mild in infants and young children, but can cause devastating birth defects in the fetus (i.e., congenital rubella syndrome) when it occurs in a pregnant woman.

We now explore the parameters in Equation 4. Understanding the underlying components of incidence not only gives insights into the population level processes, but also helps us to develop and refine research questions, and to incorporate new research findings.

Contact Rate

Contact rates describe the rate of exposure episodes per unit time. They can describe, for example, the rate of bites from mosquitoes potentially infected with Dengue or Zika viruses, the rate of contact with students at a school with an ongoing influenza outbreak, or a sex worker's number of sex acts per week. Note that contact rates are assumed to be constant (unless explicitly modeled as time-varying rates) and typically apply to what is assumed to be a randomly mixing population. Note that this is a strong assumption: a randomly mixing population assumes that every person has an equal chance of contact with each other person and therefore an equal chance of being exposed to an infectious agent. Of course, most populations in the real world do not mix randomly. There may be subgroups of a population that preferentially interact, potentially constrained by boundaries defined by household, community, school, prisons, or other geographic or social structures.[25]

Several related concepts are worth mentioning here, although a detailed description is beyond the scope of this chapter. It is well known that individual preferences and social, cultural, and political influences shape the ways the individuals and populations interact and therefore spread infectious agents. In general, people "mix" with other people who are like them; this is also called *assortative* mixing (or, *homophily*). Depending on the specific context and the contact rates in these subpopulations, assortative mixing can amplify or inhibit the spread of infectious agents.

A second related concept is the structure of social and sexual networks and how it influences the spread of sexually transmitted infections. For example, *concurrency* is a network feature whereby sexual partnerships overlap and one partnership begins before another terminates, in contrast with "serial monogamy." Simulation studies have found that even small differences in concurrency can have dramatic effects on connectivity in sexual networks, and thereby the speed with which infection spreads and the number of people that can be infected.[43] Another interesting mixing pattern related to HIV transmission is *serosorting* and *seropositioning*. Serosorting is a decision process whereby people agree (or not) to engage in a sexual partnership based on HIV status, often with the goal of reducing the risk associated with condomless sex. Theoretically, a known HIV-negative person having condomless sex only with a known HIV-negative partner would be 100% effective at preventing HIV infection. The problem of course is that it is difficult for both participants to know with certainty each other's HIV serostatus. A systematic review of the effectiveness of serosorting among men who have sex with men and transgender people found that consistent condom use was a better harm reduction strategy than serosorting, but serosorting was better than no condom use.[44] A related concept is seropositioning, the practice of selectively engaging in insertive or receptive anal sex or selectively using condoms based on a partner's HIV status.

Probability a Source Is Infectious

The probability that a potential source is infectious, $P(t)$, describes the likelihood that a given contact is with an infected and infectious host. For example, Equation 4 suggests that if the prevalence is high, incidence may be high even in the presence of low contact rates and/or transmission probabilities. For example, the United States continues to experience alarming racial disparities in sexually transmitted diseases: in 2016, the rate of reported gonorrhea cases among Blacks (481.2 cases per 100,000 population) was 8.6 times the rate among Whites (55.7 cases per 100,000 population).[45] Although some have speculated that differences in individual level factors, like sexual behavior (e.g., contact rates), were the primary causes of health disparities, it is now widely recognized that differences in sexual network characteristics and the (higher) prevalence of infection $P(t)$ in those networks defined by high levels of homophily explain most of the disparities, along with other social factors, such as poverty, discrimination, and incarceration.[46] A reasonable first approximation of $P(t)$ is the prevalence of infected hosts circulating in the target community, which can be measured through community-based surveys or surveillance data. Of course, one must be cautious about when, if ever, it is appropriate to equate the prevalence of infection with the prevalence of *infectiousness*, as not all cases of a particular disease may be infectious.

The safety of the blood supply is an interesting illustration of the importance of monitoring and reducing $P(t)$. Blood banks prevent the transmission of bloodborne pathogens, such as HIV and HBV and HCV viruses, by donor deferral and screening blood to reduce the prevalence of contaminated blood units. The transmission probability (p)—the risk of infection after receiving a contaminated unit of blood,—is close to 1, and not amenable to postexposure interventions to reduce the risk. Reducing the contact rate (i.e., blood transfusions) has limited effectiveness because, for many patients, blood transfusions are medically indicated and life-saving. Hence, the most effective strategy to ensure the safety of the blood supply targets lowering the prevalence of contaminated units. The prevalence largely determines the per blood unit risk, and this risk has continued to decline as better methods for blood screening are developed and implemented.

Transmission Probability

The transmission probability (p) is the risk of infection given contact with an infectious source. The transmission probability is determined by:

- Susceptibility of the uninfected host;
- Infectiousness of the source; and
- Interruption of transmission (by physical, chemical, engineering, or environmental methods).

Consider the sexual transmission of HIV. For an HIV-uninfected person, an ulcerative sexually transmitted disease increases her or his susceptibility to HIV infection, whereas the use of pre-exposure prophylaxis decreases susceptibility. For HIV-infected persons, ART reduces their infectiousness by reducing the amount of HIV virus circulating in the blood and seminal/vaginal fluid viral load. People living with HIV who take ART as prescribed and who maintain an undetectable viral load, have effectively no risk of transmitting HIV to their HIV-negative sexual partners.[47] Finally, male and female condoms can interrupt HIV transmission via a physical barrier. Thus, the transmission probability can summarize the potential effect of multiple control strategies, if any, that share a common goal to block transmission, given contact between an infected and susceptible host.

Generation Time

Generation (or serial time) is the average time between the onset of symptoms in a given infectious individual and the onset of symptoms in individuals that person has infected. Communicable diseases with shorter generation times require more rapid detection and implementation of control measures as the outbreak will develop faster. For example, the generation time of influenza cases is about 3 days[48] and the reproductive number is less than 2.[49] Thus, in the absence of containment measures, the number of cases of epidemic influenza will approximately double about every 3 days. During human pandemic influenza, this leaves little time to identify, contact, and quarantine exposed persons. In contrast, the generation time of hepatitis A cases is measured in weeks, leaving more time to identify exposed persons and administer postexposure immune globulin or HAV vaccine. Thus, the reproductive number gives an indication of the magnitude of the potential outbreak, and the generation time is one indication of how fast control measures must be implemented.

The Reproductive Number and Evolution of Infectious Agents

In theory, from the perspective of an infectious agent, a "successful" pathogen would incite a long and highly infectious period in infected hosts corresponding to a high reproductive number and continual transmission of the agent in the population. The infected host would be infected and infectious but would not experience symptoms that would limit the number of potential contacts or otherwise inhibit transmission. Said in another way, in Equation 1 of R_0, duration (d) should be as long as possible for the pathogen to establish endemicity or to continually cause outbreaks. It would then follow that an agent associated with a very high mortality (measured as virulence or the case fatality proportion) is counterproductive in that it truncates the infectious period by prematurely killing the host and reducing d. There is therefore evolutionary pressure to develop a more benign relationship between the microbe and the host.[25]

Despite this logic, it is also possible that as virulence increases, the transmission probability (p) increases to counteract the decrease in d. For example, a respiratory pathogen like SARS may cause more coughing, sneezing, or other symptoms as virulence increases, which may increase the likelihood of transmission per contact as the disease worsens. In this way, there is evolutionary pressure to both increase and decrease virulence, and the way this balance plays out depends on the unique characteristics of each pathogen.

TRANSMISSION CONTAINMENT

Designing and implementing one or more interventions that can prevent or reduce transmission of infection involves three steps:

1. Identifying control points;
2. Deriving control strategies; and
3. Designing and implementing control measures.

Control Points

Given the equations presented in prior sections, it is possible to identify five transmission control points:

1. Contact rate (c);
2. Probability potential source is infectious (P);
3. Duration of infectiousness (d);
4. Transmission probability (p); and
5. Fraction of population that is susceptible (x).

The success or failure of a control measure is, ultimately explained by its impact on one or more of these five control points.

Control Strategies

Given these five transmission control points, it is possible to derive six control strategies that have the potential to reduce transmission or acquisition of infection. These control strategies are:

1. Reduce contact between those who are potentially infectious sources and possibly susceptible hosts;
2. Reduce the probability that potential sources of infection are infectious;

BOX 82-4 Examples of Control Measures Possibly Relevant to Control Strategies

Modes of Transmission

1. Reduce contact between those who are potentially infectious and possibly susceptible hosts
   A. Behavior change (infected, susceptible, or both)
   B. Isolation of cases
   C. Case finding and treatment or isolation
   D. Contact tracing and intervention (e.g., quarantine)
   E. Quarantine of exposed (individuals, households, communities)
   F. Sheltering (i.e., isolation of unexposed)
   G. Social distancing (e.g., school closures, travel restrictions)
2. Reduce probability that potential sources of infection are infectious
   A. Case finding and treatment or isolation
   B. Identification and control of infectious sources
   C. Vaccination
   D. Treatment of contacts (e.g., sexual partners)
3. Reduce susceptibility of susceptible hosts
   A. Vaccination (pre- and postexposure)
   B. Immune globulin (pre- and postexposure)
   C. Antimicrobial treatment (pre- and postexposure)
   D. Treatment of co-factors that facilitate transmission (e.g., ulcerative sexually transmitted infections)

Modes of Transmission

1. Reduce infectiousness of those who are infectious
   A. Treatment of cases
   B. Vaccination
2. Interrupt transmission between infectious sources and susceptible hosts
   A. Physical and chemical methods (e.g., masks, gloves, condoms, handwashing, hand sanitizers)
   B. Engineering controls (e.g., negative pressure rooms, UV lights, HEPA filters)
   C. Environmental controls (e.g., disinfection)
3. Reduce fraction of the population that is susceptible
   A. Vaccination
   B. Mass chemoprophylaxis

3. Reduce the susceptibility of susceptible hosts;
4. Reduce the infectiousness of those who are infectious;
5. Interrupt transmission between infectious sources and susceptible hosts; and
6. Reduce the fraction of the population that is susceptible.

These control strategies and the control measures that derive from them (see below) are best considered in the aggregate, rather than individually, and failure to do so can have unintended consequences. For example, a partially effective HIV vaccine given to an at-risk, susceptible population would reduce the fraction of the population that is susceptible to infection. However, if receipt of the vaccine is associated with a false sense of complete protection and a resultant increase in high-risk behavior (e.g., condomless sex), the overall effect could be to increase, rather than decrease transmission of HIV infection in the population. It is also important to point out that while some of these control strategies may be relevant only for infectious agents transmitted from person to person, others are also relevant for infectious agents transmitted via other routes (see below).

Control Measures

Given these six control strategies, it is possible to outline a number of control measures that, depending on the specific characteristics of the infectious agent and its transmission, may be effective in preventing or controlling an infectious disease. Examples of control measures that may be relevant to each of the six control strategies are listed in Box 82-4. It should be noted that a control measure (e.g., vaccination) may simultaneously contribute to more than one control strategy.

Multiple control measures are often necessary and appropriate in response to an infectious disease problem, although they typically constitute only a part of the overall public health and clinical response, which invariably requires multidimensional components. The need for and typical components of such a multidimensional response are illustrated by the diverse aspects of the optimal public health and medical response to an influenza pandemic (Box 82-5). At the same time, the specific control strategies and measures that are relevant in a given set of circumstances should flow from the concepts from the chain model of infectious diseases described above. For example, in the context of an influenza pandemic, isolation of cases and community mitigation measures are designed to reduce the contact rate between infectious and susceptible individuals, while treatment of cases may reduce the magnitude and duration of infectiousness.

It is also important to point out that many infectious disease agents can be transmitted via multiple routes, each of which may necessitate different control strategies and measures. For example, both HIV and HBV can be transmitted sexually, vertically from mother-to-infant, and via receipt of contaminated blood or blood products, and thus multiple control strategies and measures are required. Similarly, Shigella infections can be transmitted via ingestion of contaminated foods, contact with contaminated inanimate objects, sexually, and by direct contact, again requiring consideration of the use of diverse control strategies and measures to interrupt transmission.

SUMMARY

In this chapter, we have reviewed the epidemiologic concepts that are key to understanding the transmission and acquisition of infectious agents and that provide the basis for controlling or preventing infectious diseases at the individual and population level. While myriad infectious agents with diverse reservoirs, sources, and routes

BOX 82-5 Possible Components of a Public Health and Medical Response to Pandemic Influenza

Modes of Transmission

1. Surveillance and epidemiologic investigation
2. Laboratory testing
3. Transmission containment
   A. Community mitigation measures
      A. Isolation of cases at home
      B. Quarantine of exposed individuals at home
      C. Social distancing measures
         a. School closures, suspension of classes, or delays in school openings
         b. Cancellation of large public gatherings, events, etc.
         c. Travel restrictions (to and from affected areas)
         d. Modification of workplace practices and schedules
      D. Sheltering (isolation of unexposed individuals)
   B. Vaccine distribution and use
   C. Antiviral drug distribution and use, for treatment and prophylaxis
4. Provision of environmental and occupational health services
5. Infection control and promulgation of clinical guidelines in healthcare facilities
6. Provision of healthcare services, including mental health and surge capacity
7. Health communication to clinicians, healthcare facilities, the general public and the media

of transmission can cause infection and illness in humans (and animals), these epidemiologic concepts are broadly applicable, as well as highly useful in designing and prioritizing epidemiological, environmental, and laboratory studies of infectious disease and in developing, implementing, and assessing the impact of prevention and control activities, including emergency response plans.

References

1. Used with permission from Porta M, Last JM. *Dictionary of Epidemiology*. 5th ed. New York, NY: Oxford University Press; 2008.
2. Caprioli A, Morabito S, Brugere H, Oswald E. Enterohaemorrhagic *Escherichia coli*: Emerging issues on virulence and modes of transmission. *Vet Res*. 2005;36(3):289–311.
3. American Medical Association, American Nurses Association-American Nurses Foundation, Centers for Disease Control and Prevention, et al. Diagnosis and management of foodborne illnesses: A primer for physicians and other health care professionals. *MMWR Recomm Rep*. 2004;53(RR-4):1–33.
4. Pirofski LA, Casadevall A. The meaning of microbial exposure, infection, colonisation, and disease in clinical practice. *Lancet Infect Dis*. 2002;2(10):628–35.
5. Casadevall A, Pirofski LA. The damage-response framework of microbial pathogenesis. *Nat Rev Microbiol*. 2003;1(1):17–24.
6. Dowdle WR. The principles of disease elimination and eradication. *Bull World Health Organ*. 1998;76(Suppl 2):22–5.
7. Centers for Disease Control and Prevention (CDC). *Foodborne Active Surveillance Network (FoodNet) Population Survey Atlas of Exposures*. Atlanta, Georgia: U.S. Department of Health and Human Services; 2006–2007.
8. Passaro DJ, Waring L, Armstrong R, et al. Postoperative Serratia marcescens wound infections traced to an out-of-hospital source. *J Infect Dis*. 1997;175(4):992–5.
9. McKinney KR, Gong YY, Lewis TG. Environmental transmission of SARS at Amoy Gardens. *J Environ Health*. 2006;68(9):26–30; quiz 51-2.
10. Siegel JD, Rhinehart E, Jackson M, Chiarello L, Committee HICPA. *Guideline for Isolation Precautions: Preventing Transmission of Infectious Agents in Healthcare Settings*. Atlanta, Georgia: Centers for Disease Control and Prevention; 2007.
11. Kutter JS, Spronken MI, Fraaij PL, Fouchier RA, Herfst S. Transmission routes of respiratory viruses among humans. *Curr Opin Virol*. 2018;28:142–51.
12. Roy CJ, Milton DK. Airborne transmission of communicable infection—The elusive pathway. *N Engl J Med*. 2004;350(17):1710–2.
13. Bloch AB, Orenstein WA, Ewing WM, et al. Measles outbreak in a pediatric practice: Airborne transmission in an office setting. *Pediatrics*. 1985;75(4):676–83.
14. Ehresmann KR, Hedberg CW, Grimm MB, Norton CA, MacDonald KL, Osterholm MT. An outbreak of measles at an international sporting event with airborne transmission in a domed stadium. *J Infect Dis*. 1995;171(3):679–83.
15. Leo YS, Chen M, Heng BH, et al. Severe acute respiratory syndrome—Singapore, 2003. *MMWR Morb Mortal Wkly Rep*. 2003;52(18):405–11.
16. Yu IT, Li Y, Wong TW, et al. Evidence of airborne transmission of the severe acute respiratory syndrome virus. *N Engl J Med*. 2004;350(17):1731–9.
17. Pantaleo G, Graziosi C, Fauci AS. The immunopathogenesis of human immunodeficiency virus infection. *N Engl J Med*. 1993;328(5):327–35.
18. Hall HI, Holtgrave DR, Maulsby C. HIV transmission rates from persons living with HIV who are aware and unaware of their infection. *AIDS*. 2012;26(7):893–6.
19. Shepard CW, Finelli L, Alter MJ. Global epidemiology of hepatitis C virus infection. *Lancet Infect Dis*. 2005;5(9):558–67.
20. Heymann DL, ed. *Control of Communicable Diseases Manual*. 19th ed. Washington, DC: American Public Health Association; 2008.
21. Svoboda T, Henry B, Shulman L, et al. Public health measures to control the spread of the severe acute respiratory syndrome during the outbreak in Toronto. *N Engl J Med*. 2004;350(23):2352–61.
22. Smolinski MS, Hamburg MA, Lederberg J, Institute of Medicine (U.S.). *Committee on Emerging Microbial Threats to Health in the 21st Century. Microbial Threats to Health: Emergence, Detection, and Response [text]*. Washington, DC: National Academies Press; 2003. Available at http://www.nap.edu/catalog.php?record_id=10636 EBRARY. Restricted to UCB IP addresses. http://site.ebrary.com/lib/berkeley/Doc?id=10046909.
23. Institute of Medicine (U.S.) Committee on Emerging Microbial Threats to Health. In: Lederberg J, Shope RE, Oaks SC, eds. Emerging Infections: Microbial Threats to Health in the United States. Washington, DC: National Academy Press; 1992, p. xii, 294.
24. Lipsitch M, Cohen T, Cooper B, et al. Transmission dynamics and control of severe acute respiratory syndrome. *Science*. 2003;300(5627):1966–70.
25. Halloran ME. Concepts of transmission and dynamics. In: Thomas JC, Weber DJ, eds. *Epidemiologic Methods for the Study of Infectious Diseases*. New York: Oxford University Press; 2001.
26. Patel P, Borkowf CB, Brooks JT, Lasry A, Lansky A, Mermin J. Estimating per-act HIV transmission risk: A systematic review. *Aids*. 2014;28(10): 1509–19.
27. Joint United Nations Program on HIV/AIDS (UNAIDS). 90-90-90: An ambitious treatment target to help end the AIDS epidemic. Geneva, 2014.
28. Stein RA. Super-spreaders in infectious diseases. *Int J Infect Dis*. 2011;15(8): e510–3.
29. Lau MS, Dalziel BD, Funk S, et al. Spatial and temporal dynamics of superspreading events in the 2014–2015 West Africa Ebola epidemic. *Proc Natl Acad Sci U S A*. 2017;114(9):2337–42.
30. Topley WWC, Wilson GS. The spread of bacterial infection. The problem of herd immunity. *J Hyg (Lond)*. 1923;21:243–9.
31. Fine PE. Herd immunity: History, theory, practice. *Epidemiol Rev*. 1993;15(2):265–302.
32. Smith CE. Prospects for the control of infectious disease. *Proc R Soc Med*. 1970;63(11 Part 2):1181–90.
33. Dietz K. Transmission and control of arbovirus diseases. In: Ludwig D, Cooke KL, eds. *Epidemiology*. Philadelphia, PA: Society for Industrial and Applied Mathematics; 1975.
34. Scherer A, McLean A. Mathematical models of vaccination. *Br Med Bull*. 2002;62:187–99.
35. Cori A, Boelle PY, Thomas G, Leung GM, Valleron AJ. Temporal variability and social heterogeneity in disease transmission: The case of SARS in Hong Kong. *PLoS Comput Biol*. 2009;5(8):e1000471.
36. Fox JP, Elveback L, Scott W, Gatewood L, Ackerman E. Herd immunity: Basic concept and relevance to public health immunization practices. *Am J Epidemiol*. 1971;94(3):179–89.
37. Centers for Disease Control and Prevention. Update: Severe acute respiratory syndrome—Toronto, Canada, 2003. *MMWR Morb Mortal Wkly Rep*. 2003;52(23):547–50.
38. Prescott J, Bushmaker T, Fischer R, Miazgowicz K, Judson S, Munster VJ. Postmortem stability of Ebola virus. *Emerg Infect Dis*. 2015;21(5):856–9.
39. Homeland Security Council. *National Strategy for Pandemic Influenza: Implementation Plan*. Washington, DC: US Homeland Security Council; 2006.
40. Ross R. An application of the theory of probabilities to the study of a priori pathometry, Part 1. *Proc R Soc Series A*. 1916;92:204–30.
41. Halloran ME, Hudgens MG. Dependent happenings: A recent methodological review. *Curr Epidemiol Rep*. 2016;3(4):297–305.
42. Civen R, Lopez AS, Zhang J, et al. Varicella outbreak epidemiology in an active surveillance site, 1995–2005. *J Infect Dis*. 2008;197(Suppl 2): S114–9.
43. Morris M, Kretzschmar M. A micro-simulation study of the effect of concurrent partnerships on HIV spread in Uganda. *Math Popul Stud*. 2000;8:109–33.
44. Kennedy CE, Bernard LJ, Muessig KE, et al. Serosorting and HIV/STI infection among HIV-negative MSM and transgender people: A systematic review and meta-analysis to inform WHO guidelines. *J Sex Transm Dis*. 2013;2013:583627.
45. Centers for Disease Control and Prevention. *Sexually Transmitted Disease Surveillance 2016*. Atlanta, GA: U.S. Department of Health and Human Services; 2017.
46. Adimora AA, Schoenbach VJ. Social context, sexual networks, and racial disparities in rates of sexually transmitted infections. *J Infect Dis*. 2005;191 Suppl 1:S115–22.
47. Cohen MS, Chen YQ, McCauley M, et al. Prevention of HIV-1 infection with early antiretroviral therapy. *N Engl J Med*. 2011;365(6):493–505.
48. Cowling BJ, Fang VJ, Riley S, Malik Peiris JS, Leung GM. Estimation of the serial interval of influenza. *Epidemiology*. 2009;20(3):344–7.
49. Biggerstaff M, Cauchemez S, Reed C, Gambhir M, Finelli L. Estimates of the reproduction number for seasonal, pandemic, and zoonotic influenza: A systematic review of the literature. *BMC Infect Dis*. 2014;14:480.

CHAPTER

83 Principles of Disease Elimination and Eradication

Vincent L. Fenimore • Walter A. Orenstein

INTRODUCTION

Disease elimination and eradication have been the subject of infectious disease study for centuries.[1] Most public health attempts to fully eradicate communicable diseases in the past have proven unsuccessful across all global contexts.[2,3] Yet the lessons that were learned from these previous eradication endeavors paved the way for progress to be made with specific diseases. One of the highlights of public health history is the global eradication of smallpox. With this example at the forefront of more recent accomplishments, it has been more widely acknowledged that the global public health community is capable of eradicating other infectious diseases. This assumes, however, that the necessary conditions to eradicate diseases are met, including the establishment of biologic feasibility, economic feasibility, political will, and proof of principle in a large geographic area.[4,5]

In more recent years, global public health efforts have been focused on the eradication of polio.[6] It has been a longer than anticipated battle to eradicate transmission of polio virus, but transmission has been eliminated from four of the six World Health Organization (WHO) regions (the Americas, Europe, Western Pacific Region (including China), and Southeast Asia Region (including India)).[7,8] Guinea worm disease (Dracunculiasis) is also on the verge of eradication; the last human cases remain in the African countries of Chad and Ethiopia.[9,10] The International Task Force for Disease Eradication has determined the following global diseases have the potential to be eradicated: measles, mumps, rubella, lymphatic filariasis, cystocercosis, and yaws.[11]

DEFINING AND OPERATIONALIZING DISEASE ERADICATION AND ELIMINATION

A generally applied and recently advanced definition for *disease eradication* is "permanent reduction to zero of the worldwide incidence of infection caused by a specific agent as a result of deliberate efforts; intervention measures may be no longer needed."[4,5] There may be need to continue efforts to assure the infectious agent does not return. For example, once polio is declared eradicated, there may be a need to continue vaccinating to prevent a reintroduction into the human population (e.g., from a laboratory source that is not properly contained, see later discussion).

Disease elimination is defined as "the absence of a disease caused by a specific agent in a defined geographic area as a result of deliberate control efforts that must be continued in perpetuity to prevent re-emergence of disease.[1,4] Disease elimination (i.e., achieving zero incidence) is a necessary step toward the goal of global disease eradication.[4] The term "elimination" has also been used to define achievement of a disease control target in a sustained fashion. For example, neonatal tetanus elimination is defined as an annual incidence of $< 1/1000$ live births. However, because the microorganism still exists in a soil reservoir,[1] vaccination against tetanus should never stop.

Criteria to Identify Candidate Diseases for Eradication

To effectively eradicate a disease, global health experts generally agree that there are four major criteria that must be met: (1) biologic feasibility; (2) economic feasibility; (3) favorable sociopolitical conditions; and (4) proof of principle in a large geographic area.[4] Assessment and monitoring of these factors are essential to any eradication effort; indeed, if any of these criteria are not met, the viability of eradication may be quickly thwarted, especially in challenging field conditions.

Biologic Feasibility

The assessment of biologic feasibility of a specific disease agent for eradication depends on the fundamental properties of the agent and the disease it produces.[12] Most experts consider a key biologic criterion for a disease to be considered potentially eradicable is that humans are "essential" for maintaining the pathogen in nature.[4] If there is an animal or environmental reservoir, then the disease agent does not meet this criterion. Other components of biological feasibility include interventions that are effective to break the chains of transmission in humans (e.g., vaccines, water purification) and the ability to detect the infectious agent either through highly sensitive and specific clinical diagnosis (e.g., smallpox) or highly sensitive and specific laboratory diagnostic tools.[3,5]

Economic Feasibility

The economic resources that are needed and available must be carefully weighed and considered in terms of cost and benefits. Decisions on health resource management will vary in relation to other public health priorities and country health budgets.

Favorable Social and Political Conditions

Political and social will are integral to eradication efforts. Leadership support at all levels from local to national to global government bodies is essential for these endeavors. Strategic public health communication plays an important role in eliciting support for eradication. Often messages that focus on the benefit of disease eradication efforts to existing community health systems have been recognized as highly persuasive to those in government and leadership positions within community settings.[5] For disease eradication efforts to be feasible, epidemiologic response (including surveillance, monitoring, and assessment) must retain the ability to be nimble and responsive to broader conditions. Sociopolitical threats and challenges, such as security concerns within conflict areas, need early and ongoing identification and adjustments to unforeseen challenges must be made as eradication efforts are underway.[5] For example, ongoing conflict may require providing extra security for persons working in the eradication effort and/or efforts to get the warring parties to permit eradication efforts to be undertaken (such as truces that allow vaccinators to immunize target populations during particular times).

CHAPTER 83

Proof of Principle in a Large Geographic Area

Demonstration of operational feasibility in a large geographic area (i.e., elimination with a goal of zero indigenously acquired infections) is the fourth criterion (after humans essential for maintaining the organism in nature, effective interventions, and sensitive and specific tools for pathogen detection) for eradication feasibility. Proving operational feasibility can differ according to the pathogen. Operational feasibility can be particularly convincing, for example, if proven in areas with fragile health structures or high population districts.[13]

There are geographic and temporal aspects that must be accounted for in interpreting and applying these criteria. These issues have clear implications for strategic planning of resource allocation, community and environmental conditions, biologic factors, and other issues that affect how eradication and elimination efforts may be accomplished. The following cases highlight some differences with respect to the status of eradication and elimination efforts that have been undertaken in global settings.

Eradicated Diseases

Smallpox

The global eradication of smallpox, caused by the variola virus (*Orthopoxvirus* in the Poxviridae family), was certified and accepted by the World Health Assembly (WHA) in 1980 following absence of any cases of disease after the last naturally occurring case in Merca, Somalia in 1977 and two further cases in the United Kingdom in 1978 because of a break in laboratory containment.[14,15] The WHO Smallpox Eradication Program used surveillance and containment measures that led to the steady reduction of cases of the disease worldwide. WHO led the organization of visits to endemic countries for two or more years after the last smallpox case was recorded, to be confident that surveillance systems in place would have detected disease if present. The declaration by the WHA, in 1980 subsequently led to the discontinuation of routine smallpox vaccination, globally.[15] Smallpox is the only human disease to have been certified as eradicated.

The global gains of smallpox eradication have included greater health for citizens around the world and eliminated financial costs associated with control including costs associated with treating people with smallpox.[4] The success of the smallpox eradication program gave impetus to the consideration and search for other diseases for which to propose eradication efforts.[4]

The case of smallpox eradication illustrates the need for continuing evaluation of strategies, changing those strategies, when appropriate, and the importance of ongoing research to refine eradication strategies and to develop better tools. Efforts to eradicate smallpox began in 1959 when the 12th WHA approved a global smallpox eradication strategy.[15] Mass vaccination campaigns were undertaken worldwide, with mixed results. China eliminated smallpox, but progress lagged in Africa and South Asia. At that time, because the WHO was consumed with a very challenging global malaria eradication effort, it was less able to provide the necessary resources and support to battle the smallpox program.

Although there was skepticism around the feasibility of eradication as a concept, and frustration with the progress of the mass vaccination efforts, nonetheless, in 1966 the WHA decided to allocate more than two million dollars annually to support efforts to eradicate smallpox.[15] The campaign was composed of two parts. First, mass vaccination campaigns were held in countries using effective vaccines with the aim of reaching at least 80% of the population. Surveillance was always part of the strategy for eradication. It was critical to know who was getting smallpox, who were the major transmitters, where geographically the disease was endemic or epidemic, and whether cases were due to failure to vaccinate or vaccine failure. When the smallpox eradication campaign began, few countries had systematic immunization programs in place. Those who forged the smallpox campaign knew of the importance of management and a national surveillance system to ensure that vaccines reach as many inhabitants as possible. The second part of the eradication strategy, which proved to be vital to its ultimate success, was the use of surveillance and containment. Special programs were initiated to detect and isolate cases of smallpox disease, and to contain outbreaks.[15] Success was measured in lowered disease incidence, rather than just the number of vaccinations administered.

In the case of smallpox eradication, surveillance and containment proved to be a primary strategy to the success of the eradication efforts.[16] Surveillance and containment consisted of active community-based surveillance to detect cases of smallpox, isolating those cases to prevent further transmission, identifying the contacts of those cases who might be or have been exposed and vaccinating them, and then estimating who the contacts of the contacts might be to determine who the primary contacts might infect, should they come down with disease.[15] Once the secondary contacts were identified, they were also vaccinated. This often involved taking names and going back to vaccinate the contacts repeatedly until they accepted vaccination. A better understanding of the epidemiology of smallpox helped support the Surveillance and Containment approach. It was recognized that cases of smallpox were not generally contagious until rash appeared, that when cases were contagious, they often were not traveling around widely because they were very ill, with most travel to medical facilities, if it occurred, and that vaccine might be effective postexposure.[15] With a small program budget to utilize, and prevailing attitudes of skepticism around disease eradication, new and creative uses of underutilized personnel were put into action.[2] Community members around the world had valuable contributions to make in their own local environs. In addition, unlike the malaria eradication program, research initiatives were encouraged in the smallpox eradication effort. These research initiatives led to the development of new and improved vaccination techniques. Field studies revealed differences in the epidemiology of the disease than from those explained in current textbooks. These discoveries then led to changes in basic ground operations.

One factor leading to the success of the global smallpox eradication program was the introduction of improved vaccination techniques. In 1968, the bifurcated needle was introduced as an effective, easy-to-use means to vaccinate. A year later, bifurcated needles were being used by all countries. They were inexpensive, using only about one-fourth as much vaccine. In addition, the bifurcated needles were easy to use, and training was less arduous allowing workers who did not know how to use needles and syringes to vaccinate with the ability to vaccinate more people each day.[15]

Another significant advantage given to the smallpox eradication effort was the vaccine's favorable characteristic of heat-stability improving its efficiency in transport and storage.[2] Additionally, it was discovered during smallpox eradication research initiatives that the efficacy of the vaccine itself was much longer than originally thought, making the need for revaccination less critical.[2] Without the important benefits of research initiatives discovered during this time, smallpox may never have been eradicated.

Rinderpest Rinderpest is the only other disease besides smallpox to be globally eradicated.[17] The disease is caused by a virus (*Morbillivirus* in the Paramyxoviridae family) affecting cattle and other farming livestock and is transmitted through direct contact. Infected animals initially develop a fever. Sores appear in the mouth, and discharge is produced from the nose and eyes. Diarrhea and dehydration can lead to death, but the pathogenesis of the disease can vary, sometimes producing blindness without the gastrointestinal symptoms.[18] Historically, rinderpest pandemics killed huge numbers of cattle in the 1850s–1870s.[18] With the advent of steam transportation in Russia, infected cattle were moved by train to England creating epidemics of the disease.[19] Early efforts at eradication of rinderpest focused more on containment of the disease rather than an eradication plan. The highly effective Plowright tissue culture rinderpest vaccine (TCRV) enabled rinderpest eradication in Africa. Originally requiring a cold-chain for storage, researchers in the United States developed a thermostable form of the vaccine, which allowed for greater reach into hard to reach areas of the country.[20]

With the aid of the United Nations and the focused efforts of the countries within Southeast Asia, vaccine development and postwar peace enabled elimination of rinderpest from China in 1956.[21] India fought a longer battle to eliminate rinderpest. The National Project on Rinderpest Eradication (NPRE) in the 1980s helped to control the disease, but it took an epidemiologic approach and financial support from the European Commission to eliminate rinderpest from the remaining endemic area of the Indian peninsula.[21] While control measures were coordinated in Eastern Asia in collaboration with the United Nations Food and Agriculture Organization (FAO), Africa initiated the first coordinated effort to eradicate the disease throughout the continent. In 1960, the ambitious Joint Project 15 (JP15) was initiated with strong support from the United States to vaccinate all cattle of every age annually within Africa for three consecutive years.[18,19] After this initial effort, all countries would vaccinate their calves on an annual basis.[18] The plan proved quite effective, and by 1979, Sudan remained the only country in Africa reporting the disease. Unfortunately, satisfaction with these results led to a lack of surveillance and routine vaccine maintenance of young animals. A pandemic spread over sub-Saharan Africa in the 1980s. The FAO, European Commission (EC), and the African Union responded by initiating the Pan-African Rinderpest campaign. While the plan proved successful in many regions, in 1998, rinderpest still existed in Sudan, Somalia, and Kenya.[19]

A regional effort using the same methods was not going to eradicate the disease, so a new plan was implemented as the Global Rinderpest Eradication Campaign (GREP).[18,19] New strategies included identifying where rinderpest was in the world, and how the virus was continuing to be active.[19] Epidemiological studies provided the key to identifying the locations of the virus in Africa's pastoral areas and in dairy livestock transported from Asia.[18]

By the late 1990s, community-based Animal Health Workers (CAHW) in Africa were able to provide effective animal care and rinderpest vaccination to the remote effected areas within the continent. The last reported case of rinderpest was in Kenya in 2001.[19]

Diseases with Existing Eradication Targets and Programs

Polio

With large outbreaks of poliomyelitis occurring worldwide in the latter part of the nineteenth and early twentieth centuries, a search began that ultimately uncovered three polio virus serotypes. This knowledge, and the discovery that the polio virus could be grown in tissue led to the development of the polio vaccine.[22] Jonas Salk developed a vaccine in 1955 using formalin-inactivated polio virus (IPV), and Albert Sabin's oral polio virus vaccine (OPV) contains a mixture of three live attenuated serotypes of polio virus.[23] Polio, caused by polio virus in the Picornaviridae family, has not yet achieved global eradication status. Regional commissions have certified elimination of transmission of indigenous strains of wild polio viruses (WPVs) in the Americas, Europe, the Western Pacific, and Southeast Asia Regions. However, WPV continues to circulate in parts of Afghanistan and Pakistan, and while WPVs have not been detected in Nigeria since 2016, it is still considered endemic.[24,25] Access and security issues remain a challenge to the eradication program.[7] In addition, vaccine hesitancy is a current threat to the Global Polio Eradication Initiative (GPEI).[26]

In 1985, Rotary International, working with the Pan American Health Organization (PAHO) began a program to eventually eradicate polio globally by mass vaccination, ultimately contributing over $1.7 billion to the effort to date (https://my.rotary.org/en/document/rotary-and-polio accessed 2.13.18). Established in 1988, the GPEI is a public-private partnership that includes Rotary International, the World Health Organization, the U.S. Centers for Disease Control and Prevention, UNICEF, the Bill & Melinda Gates Foundation, and world governments. The GPEI has been an ongoing disease eradication effort from which we are continuing to derive lessons, which are of use not only to eventually eradicate polio but to future eradication efforts as well.[4,13] At the beginning of the eradication campaign, a basic strategy was laid out. The objective was to rid the world of WPV using OPV, and then discontinue use of OPV.[27] Prior to establishing the goal of polio eradication in 1988, mass immunization campaigns began in the former Soviet Union, followed by other countries around the world, including the United States in the 1960s. Controlling poliomyelitis in many developing countries has been a more recent phenomenon, as national vaccination programs became operational.[28] In addition, while overt cases are more easily detected, surveillance of "unseen" infections are more difficult to ascertain. Paralytic disease occurs in <1% of persons with primary infections. With smallpox, every infection was visible, and the period of contagiousness did not start until the patient was already ill, and hence less likely to travel. In contrast, because the clear majority of polio infections are subclinical or without paralysis, one cannot identify contacts exposed to the virus. Hence, mass campaigns were required to assure coverage of the whole population at risk of sustaining transmission. It is hoped that lessons learned from this massive effort will inform efficient strategy building in the fight against other diseases such as measles.

Although the use of OPV has contributed greatly to the eradication effort, the polio eradication endgame now requires the staged withdrawal of OPV. This is required, because in rare cases, the use of OPV can lead to vaccine-associated paralytic poliomyelitis (VAPP), in which the vaccine viruses gain the neurovirulence properties of WPVs, causing paralytic disease in vaccines or their close contacts. Polio viruses that cause VAPP do not cause outbreaks. On the other hand, vaccine viruses can develop into vaccine-derived polio viruses (VDPVs). There are two types of VDPVs. Persons with immune deficiencies, particularly B-cell deficiencies, can become chronically infected with immune-deficient vaccine-derived viruses (iVDPVs) including chronic shedding of those viruses. Of greater concern is circulating vaccine-derived polio viruses (cVDPVs).[29] These cVDPVs are derived through circulation of vaccine viruses among susceptible populations leading to mutations that reconfer both the neurovirulence and transmissibility properties of WPVs. Thus, cVDPVs can cause outbreaks of polio, similar to WPVs.[28] Therefore, true eradication of polio requires not only terminating transmission of the three serotypes of WPVs, but also discontinuing all use of OPV to prevent induction and transmission of cVDPVs. The first step was the removal of the type 2 component from the trivalent OPV to the bivalent (types 1 and 3) OPV[27] after WPV2 was certified as eradicated in 2015. This was accomplished during a 2-week period in April 2016. To combat the potential re-emergence of the polio type 2 virus by maintaining some population immunity against the type 2 polio virus, prior to the withdrawal of OPV, introduction of the inactivated polio vaccine (IPV), containing all three serotypes, was recommended for all OPV-using countries as part of their routine immunization programs.[27,30] These challenging intervention goals required stakeholders to implement new communication strategies to generate awareness and political will around these complex activities involved in the polio endgame.[31]

A predictive economic analysis of the GPEI indicates an extremely cost-effective program even with the more recent higher costs and longer delays to reach eradication that were unforeseen when the goal was formulated.[32] The net benefits are huge, and although poorer countries have high financial burdens with the effort, the analysis suggests their benefit is the greatest.[32]

In 2014, WHO introduced an accountability framework into its Polio Eradication program. An analysis of the framework revealed improvements in surveillance for acute flaccid paralysis (AFP) and staff performance.[33] Failure to detect WPV3 anywhere in the world since 2012 in Nigeria led to the certification that WPV3 has been eradicated in 2019. Therefore, all remaining WPV transmission is due to WPV1. The major challenge is terminating WPV1 in the remaining polio-endemic countries (Afghanistan, Pakistan, and Nigeria).[8]

Although the initiative to eradicate polio, began in 1988, most countries affected by polio did not begin their efforts until the mid-1990s. Along with financial problems, sociopolitical "buy-in" was a chief reason for delays in some areas.[4,13] Success of the polio elimination effort in the Americas was key to providing a feasibility model to other large countries that needed assurances that a huge polio eradication could be successful. Most countries were able to interrupt WPV within 2–3 years.[4,13] The countries that proved the exception to this rule and remain endemic, had challenges due to political crises or immunization fears which may provide lessons for future disease eradication initiatives.[34] With proven effective strategies to achieve eradication of polio in place, an obstacle that currently exists is the inability to implement these strategies in the three remaining polio-endemic countries.[28] Safety and security concerns of health workers are challenges that require innovative approaches.

A recent study of Muslim scholars in Pakistan revealed that security and vaccine management issues were the major barriers to polio immunization in Pakistan.[35] In addition, vaccine refusal, another factor affecting immunization rates, is developing in certain areas both in Europe and the United States. Muslim parents' vaccine hesitancy and refusal have been identified as a contributing factor in the increase of vaccine-preventable disease cases in Afghanistan, Malaysia, and Pakistan.[36] Additionally, immunization of hard to reach populations in the endemic countries is another challenge to overcome. Attempts to reach conflict-ridden areas with polio eradication efforts may require constant adaptation unique to each area. Local persons and major humanitarian outfits are willing and able to act on behalf of their children's futures. In addition, individuals are needed with special skills in conflict areas as well as the ability to build teams of workers to support eradication in conflict-ridden areas.

A further concern to the polio eradication endgame is the phasing out of financial support. With the polio virus still present in a few countries, and outbreaks of cVDPV, there remains a need for surveillance and vigilance as well as maintenance of high vaccine coverage.[25] Of additional concern is the fact that some countries are dependent upon polio funds for their other routine immunization and surveillance activities. With the phasing out of polio funding, there remains the question as to how countries will effectively continue these other important immunization efforts.

Sustained efforts are still needed to ensure polio eradication is achieved. Access and security issues remain with a need for solid-field operations. Surveillance, after all WPVs are certified as eradicated, will continue to be needed to monitor withdrawal of all Sabin polio viruses. Facility containment will help to complete the global certification of WPV eradication but will also be needed during the withdrawal of OPV, since laboratories may have vaccine viruses, which if released into the environment could lead to generation of cVDPVs.[7] Thus, containment of polio viruses in laboratories, which currently have known polio viruses or in laboratories which have specimens that could be potentially contaminated with polio viruses is critical to prevent reintroduction of viruses into the population posteradication with re-establishment of sustained transmission.

Guinea Worm

WHO's global plan of 2007 included a target for elimination of Guinea worm disease by 2015. Dracunculiasis (Guinea worm) has been certified as eliminated in 187 countries.[24] However, with continued cases in South Sudan, Chad, Ethiopia, and Mali, the timeframe for achieving the goal for eradication has been extended.[12] Increases in animal infections, security constraints, difficult to reach communities, and unsafe water are challenges that have slowed elimination progress.[9,10]

Dracunculiasis or Guinea worm disease is caused by a parasite passed to humans through contaminated drinking water. With the creation of the Guinea Worm Eradication Program (GWEP), cases of the disease have been reduced from 3.5 million in 20 countries in 1986 to 22 cases in just four countries in 2015. In 2016, 25 confirmed cases were reported in the three remaining endemic countries.[9] In Ethiopia, with its own national GWEP, and the support of other entities, the country reported just 3 human cases, 14 dog infections, and 2 baboon infections in 2016.[9] Remaining challenges to Guinea worm disease eradication in Ethiopia include refugee arrival, an increase in the number of animal infections, communities that are hard to reach, and a lack of safe water. Political instability in parts of South Sudan contributes to the challenges of eradicating Dracunculiasis.[34] Efforts to eradicate Guinea worm disease in this country include intervention strategies such as community behavioral change, improving surveillance systems, including cash awards for reporting Guinea worm disease and animal infections, case containment, and providing safe water.[9]

Diseases with Regional Elimination Goals (Achieving Zero Incidence)

Measles and Rubella

The WHA accepted the Global Vaccine Action Plan (GVAP) goal to eliminate measles caused by *Morbillivirus* in the family Paramyxoviridae, in four WHO regions by 2015 and in five regions by 2020.[37,38] One region (the Region of the Americas) has achieved measles elimination.[25] With a surge of recent measles cases in North America (due to importations from endemic areas) and Europe, efforts have been stalled. In fact, even though all six WHO regions have measles elimination targets and have established regional verification commissions (RVCs) to monitor measles and rubella elimination, none of them have achieved elimination as of 2018 except for the Americas. Five WHO regions have rubella elimination targets but only the Americas has achieved this target.[39] In Africa, regional immunization coverage has languished, and larger countries are experiencing outbreaks on an almost yearly basis.[40] In the South East Asian Region, challenges to measles and rubella elimination are primarily due to lower coverage rates and lack of surveillance resources in some areas.[40,41] Immunization services need greater reinforcement in specific, vulnerable geographic regions. An integrated plan for case-based surveillance for both measles and rubella is an integral component to achievement of elimination goals.[42] Outside of Europe, the failure to achieve high coverage is due in part to the weaknesses in the ongoing immunization systems.

Measles

After efforts to successfully eradicate smallpox, and progress made toward the eradication of polio disease around the world, the eradication of measles became a logical next target disease for consideration, as measles is still a major cause of child mortality.[43] Because of the success of measles vaccination efforts in the Americas including the United States, and globally, there is proof of principle that eradication is feasible. In 1994, the WHO Region of the Americas began an effort to eliminate measles by the year 2000. The strategy consisted of: (1) "catch-up" measles vaccination campaigns targeted to all children 9 months–14 years of age, regardless of prior vaccination status, to reduce susceptibility in that population;[11] (2) achieving high "keep-up" vaccination coverage with routine vaccination services; and (3) "follow-up" vaccination campaigns implemented when a susceptible birth cohort of children was estimated to accumulate, usually conducted about every 4 years. The calculation was based on estimates of 1 and 2 dose coverage in the population and estimates of the protective effect of each of the doses.[11]

Epidemiologic surveillance and laboratory confirmation, along with routine and "follow-up" immunizations campaigns have been necessary to prevent measles cases imported from other regions from re-establishing sustained indigenous transmission. In addition, there are high levels of political support in the Americas for laws to ensure funding as a line item in national budgets for immunization, and a "Revolving Fund" established by PAHO to facilitate vaccine procurement at good prices leading to widespread vaccine availability.[11] Additionally, PAHO and the WHO developed a regional action plan to standardize the process of documentation and verification of interruption of endemic measles (and rubella) virus transmission.[44] "Catch-up" campaigns, similar to those in the Americas, have also been implemented in other countries around the world to some success. Although the number of countries interrupting the transmission of measles virus has increased, particularly in the European, South-East Asia, and Western Pacific regions, global routine measles vaccine coverage stagnated at 85%, with only 41% of countries achieving a recommended target of approximately 95% for the first dose of measles vaccine.[25]

The greatest challenge to measles eradication is the very high immunity levels needed to interrupt transmission. The basic reproductive number (Ro) or rate for measles, a measure of contagiousness, is 12–18, meaning the average case of measles is capable of infecting 12–18 persons if all persons the case came in contact with were susceptible.[45] This means the herd immunity threshold is 92–94%. Measles is the most contagious of the vaccine-preventable diseases, but as demonstrated in the Americas, it can be eliminated. Other challenges to measles eradication include vaccine financing, supply issues, and safety concerns.[46–48] The introduction of new vaccines raises the cost of vaccination, and resources for measles eradication may need to compete for resources needed to introduce new vaccines.[46] One suggestion to strengthen measles elimination is to utilize lessons learned from the GPEI; this effort has existing assets, human resources, and infrastructure to refocus on the goal of measles elimination.[48] A transition from the numerous resources, created through the GPEI, to support measles and rubella elimination could be implemented. More funding would be required for global measles and rubella elimination as polio funding is eliminated. A Global Measles and Rubella Laboratory Network (GMRLN) operates currently to provide surveillance functions and data for quick response to outbreaks.[43] Although lessons learned from polio eradication can be efficiently modified to enhance measles and rubella elimination efforts, other challenges may require different tools with which to overcome those challenges.

An evaluation report of the GVAP was issued by the WHO Strategic Advisory Group of Experts on Immunization in 2017.[25] The GVAP was launched with an endorsement by the WHA in May 2012, with the aim of providing equitable access to immunizations for everyone. The assessment report while noting that the Region of the Americas eliminated measles, and seven additional countries in 2016 were verified free of measles, global routine measles vaccine coverage targets have not been met.[25]

Measles epidemiology plays a vital role in predicting patterns related to goals of elimination. When outbreak details are collected and analyzed, these sources of data become signposts along the way toward elimination.[49] Countries such as Egypt, which established goals for measles elimination, had to revise their goals when confronted with outbreaks (2005–2007). In response, a nation-wide immunization campaign targeted children, adolescents, and adults in 2008–2009. The two-phase campaign led to immunization rates of greater than 95%. Continuation of the recommended two-dose measles-rubella vaccine, surveillance strengthening, and the creation of congenital rubella syndrome (CRS) surveillance are suggested to help Egypt achieve measles and rubella elimination.[50] A recent midterm review report of the Measles and Rubella Initiative's Global Measles and Rubella Strategic Plan, 2012–2020, recommended greater country ownership and global political will to make progress toward elimination goals.[42]

Rubella

Rubella, caused by the *Rubivirus* belonging to the Togaviridae family, still affects people worldwide and infection during pregnancy (especially during the first trimester), can result in miscarriage, fetal death, stillbirth, and a collection of congenital birth defects known as congenital rubella syndrome (CRS).[11,51] Most cases are from low-income countries, where the vaccine has not been introduced or where coverage is poor. CRS in many infants could have been prevented if the rubella-containing vaccine (RCV) had been introduced into the country.[11] Like measles, rubella eradication is feasible given the fact that a vaccine currently exists, and the disease has no animal reservoir.[52] To achieve the 2020 rubella and CRS elimination goals established in the 2012–2020 GVAP, introduction of the vaccine, along with stronger surveillance of both rubella and CRS to measure progress is needed.[11] As was demonstrated in 2015 by the announcement of the interruption of rubella virus transmission in the Region of the Americas, introduction of RCV and wide-ranging immunization campaigns proved the feasibility of the elimination goals.[11]

Diseases with Control Targets

Tetanus

Elimination of maternal and neonatal tetanus is defined as "an incidence of <1 case of neonatal tetanus per 1000 live births per year in all districts or similar administrative units of a country."[53] The GVAP's objective for maternal and neonatal tetanus elimination established a 2015 global target of 40 priority countries. As of September 2017, elimination had yet to be achieved in 18 of those countries.[25] With the newer guidelines promoting tetanus containing vaccines as a component of routine maternal healthcare (i.e., Td immunization of pregnant women), the goal of elimination for pregnant women and infants may be within sight in the next decade with support of global obstetricians and allied health providers in North America, Australia, Europe, and other parts of the world. However, there remains a need for provider training on approaches to communication to increase vaccine acceptance and uptake.[54]

Hepatitis B and C

In May 2016, the WHA endorsed the Global Health Sector Strategy (GHSS) on viral hepatitis 2016–2021. Elimination of viral hepatitis as a public health threat by 2030 is defined as a 65% reduction in mortality and a 90% reduction in incidence compared with the 2015 baseline.[55,56] Incomplete data sources and outdated methods of surveillance related to hepatitis B virus (HBV) and hepatitis C virus (HCV) late outcomes, including cirrhosis and liver cancer, are one area of challenge identified.[57] In addition, awareness of HCV and access to healthcare have significant variance globally, thus creating wide differences in treatment eligibility and options.[58,59] People who inject drugs (PWID) have less access to healthcare and present a barrier to HCV elimination.[60,61]

Hepatitis B

Hepatitis B disease is a liver infection caused by HBV.[62] Acute HBV infection is treatable and does not always develop into chronic HBV infection, which can cause severe health problems over time. However, most people infected with HBV are unaware of their condition, because symptoms may be inapparent.[55] Infants and young children are at the greatest risk of developing chronic hepatitis when infected.[55] The highest prevalence of HBV infection is in the African and Western Pacific regions.[55] A major focus for hepatitis B elimination is widespread vaccination with vaccine, which is highly effective and leads to sustained long-term immunity.[63] For prevention of mother to child transmission of HBV, appropriate birth-dose HBV immunization is a primary intervention.

Hepatitis C

Hepatitis C disease is a liver infection caused by HCV.[64] A person may be infected for years before developing any symptoms of the disease. About 71 million people worldwide are living with chronic HCV infection.[55] The prevalence of HCV infection often is associated with unsafe medical injections or techniques. PWID also contribute to HCV epidemics around the globe.[55] The European and Eastern Mediterranean regions are more affected than other parts of the world with variation between and within countries. Recommendations for HCV prevention include guarantees that blood products are safe, safety around injection procedures, harm reduction services for PWID, and safe sex education.[65]

The WHA endorsed a global strategy to battle viral hepatitis in May 2016. The goal is to eliminate viral hepatitis worldwide by 2030. Although interventions are known and implemented to battle viral hepatitis globally, challenges exist including PWID who are unaware that they are infected with HCV.[61] Another major barrier to elimination is the fact that there are chronic asymptomatic carriers who are unaware of their infection, and continue to transmit infection for many years. Poor linkage to care and retention in treatment are challenges that currently exist.[60] Additionally, high prices for antiviral agents reduce the number of patients who can afford effective therapies.[59] Some countries have taken the lead on addressing and prioritizing this public health threat in their communities, but many others do not have national outfits dedicated to this issue, or as line items in their country's health priorities.

CONCLUSION

From global disease eradication efforts of the past, and the lessons that are being learned from current initiatives, disease eradication is a difficult undertaking. Diseases targeted for eradication must meet at least four biologic criteria including: (1) humans are essential for maintaining the pathogen in nature, (2) there must be a sensitive and specific diagnostic test to determine who is infected, (3) there is an effective intervention to terminate transmission, and (4) there is proof of principle in that disease transmission has been eliminated in large and diverse populations over a sustained period. Also, successful disease eradication programs require the highest levels of dedicated human resources along with willing financial support of donors. No one can predict with certainty how many resources will be needed to accomplish an eradication goal in advance, so there must be flexibility in getting additional resources beyond those initially projected, if needed.

Today, eradication efforts must take into consideration the political instability and insecurity of some regions in the world as challenges that must be overcome.[34] Bioterrorism is another factor that must be considered, especially in the case of polio eradication when routine immunization has stopped. Polio viruses have been synthesized in the laboratory and could be used to terrorize a population posteradication, particularly if vaccination has been stopped.[66]

Elimination Is Feasible for Specific Diseases

Feasibility of disease elimination initiatives requires meeting several criteria. First, biologic feasibility is necessary, which includes safe and effective interventions. Second, there must be enough public health infrastructure in place to manage the program along with an understanding of operational capacity. Third, there must be adequate funding available to support the necessary work involved. Last, feasibility requires prolonged political and societal will at all levels from local to national governments.[5]

One cannot predict all the trials that may present themselves when an initiative has begun. However, from past experiences in disease elimination and eradication, the role of continuing research programs remains a pivotal component of an initiative's success. Research services are necessary to identify persons who are not being immunized and the reasons why.[46] With the eradication of smallpox disease from the planet, the principles of disease eradication and elimination have become well established within the public health community. The necessary components of an effective disease eradication program can be utilized at the national level. Global plans for disease eradication can then proceed, given adequate central coordination. Sustained political and social will remain today at the forefront of challenges for success. Fortunately, disease eradication has a strong inherent appeal to people around the world for not only the economic benefits, but humanitarian benefits.[5]

ACKNOWLEDGMENT

We thank Stephen Cochi, MD, MPH for guidance, and for providing valuable comments on this chapter.

REFERENCES

1. Hopkins D. The allure of eradication. *Global Health Magazine*. 2009;3:14–17.
2. Henderson DA. Eradication: Lessons from the past. *Bull World Health Organ*. 1998;76(Suppl 2):17–21.
3. Dowdle WR. The principles of disease elimination and eradication. *Bull World Health Organ*. 1998;76(Suppl 2):22–25.
4. Cochi SL, Dowdle WR. *Disease Eradication in the 21st Century: Implications for Global Health*. Cambridge, MA.: MIT Press; 2011.
5. Dowdle WR, Cochi SL. The principles and feasibility of disease eradication. *Vaccine*. 2011;29(Suppl 4):D70–73.
6. Cochi SL, Hegg L, Kaur A, Pandak C, Jafari H. The global polio eradication initiative: Progress, lessons learned, and polio legacy transition planning. *Health Affairs*. 2016;35(2):277–83.
7. Bahl S, Bhatnagar P, Sutter RW, Roesel S, Zaffran M. Global polio eradication—Way ahead. *Indian J Pediatr*. 2018;85(2):124–31.
8. Kew OM, Cochi SL, Jafari HS, et al. Possible eradication of wild poliovirus type 3—Worldwide, 2012. *MMWR Morb Mortal Wkly Rep*. 2014;63(45):1031–3.
9. Beyene HB, Bekele A, Shifara A, et al. Elimination of Guinea worm disease in Ethiopia; current status of the disease's, eradication strategies and challenges to the end game. *Ethiop Med J*. 2017;55(Suppl 1):15–31.
10. WHO/Department of Control of Neglected Tropical Diseases. Dracunculiasis eradication: Global surveillance summary, 2017. *Wkly Epidemiol Rec*. 2018;93(21):305–20.
11. Meeting of the International Task Force for Disease Eradication, November 2015. *Wkly Epidemiol Rec*. 2016;91(6):61–71.
12. Galan-Puchades MT. WHO delays guinea-worm disease eradication to 2020: Are dogs the sole culprits? *Lancet Infect Dis*. 2017;17(11):1124–5.
13. Aylward R. *Lessons from the Late Stages of the Global Polio Eradication Initiative*. Cambridge, MA: MIT Press; 2011, pp. 13–23.
14. Deria A, Jezek Z, Markvart K, Carrasco P, Weisfeld J. The world's last endemic case of smallpox: Surveillance and containment measures. *Bull World Health Organ*. 1980;58(2):279–83.
15. Kennedy RB, Lane JM, Henderson DA, Poland GA. Smallpox and vaccinia. In: *Vaccines*. 6th ed. Washington, DC: Elsevier Inc.; 2012.
16. Heymann DL, Brilliant L. Surveillance in eradication and elimination of infectious diseases: A progression through the years. *Vaccine*. 2011;29(Suppl 4):D141–4.
17. Moutou F. The second eradication: Rinderpest. *Bull Soc Pathol Exot*. 2014;107(3):137–8.
18. Roeder P, Mariner J, Kock R. Rinderpest: The veterinary perspective on eradication. *Philos Trans R Soc Lond B Biol Sci*. 2013;368(1623): 20120139.
19. Roeder PL. Rinderpest: The end of cattle plague. *Prev Vet Med*. 2011;102(2):98–106.
20. Mariner JC, House JA, Mebus CA, et al. Rinderpest eradication: Appropriate technology and social innovations. *Science*. 2012; 337(6100):1309–12.
21. Roeder P, Rich K. *The Global Effort to Eradicate Rinderpest*. Vol. 923. Intl Food Policy Res Inst; 2009.
22. Sutter RW, Kew OM, Cochi SL, Aylward RB. Poliovirus vaccine—Live. In: *Plotkin's Vaccines*. Philadelphia, PA: Elsevier; 2018:866–917. e816.
23. Sabin AB. Oral poliovirus vaccine: History of its development and use and current challenge to eliminate poliomyelitis from the world. *J Infect Dis*. 1985;151(3):420–36.
24. Breman JG, Arita I. The certification of smallpox eradication and implications for guinea worm, poliomyelitis, and other diseases: Confirming and maintaining a negative. *Vaccine*. 2011;29(Suppl 4):D41–8.
25. Organization WH. *2017 Assessment Report of the Global Vaccine Action Plan Strategic Advisory Group of Experts on Immunization*. Geneva; 2017.

26. Taylor S, Khan M, Muhammad A, et al. Understanding vaccine hesitancy in polio eradication in northern Nigeria. *Vaccine*. 2017;35(47):6438–43.
27. Patel M, Cochi S. Addressing the challenges and opportunities of the polio endgame: Lessons for the future. *J Infect Dis*. 2017;216(suppl_1):S1–8.
28. Sutter RW, Kew OM, Cochi SL, Aylward RB. Poliovirus vaccine—Live. In: *Plotkin's Vaccines*. 7th ed. Philadelphia, PA: Elsevier; 2018:866–917. e816.
29. Zaffran M, McGovern M, Hossaini R, Martin R, Wenger J. The polio endgame: Securing a world free of all polioviruses. *Lancet*. 2018;391(10115):11–13.
30. Zipursky S, Vandelaer J, Brooks A, et al. Polio endgame: Lessons learned from the Immunization Systems Management Group. *J Infect Dis*. 2017;216(suppl_1):S9–14.
31. Menning L, Garg G, Pokharel D, et al. Communications, immunization, and polio vaccines: Lessons from a global perspective on generating political will, informing decision-making and planning, and engaging local support. *J Infect Dis*. 2017;216(suppl_1):S24–32.
32. Duintjer Tebbens RJ, Pallansch MA, Cochi SL, et al. Economic analysis of the global polio eradication initiative. *Vaccine*. 2010;29(2):334–43.
33. Kassahun A, Braka F, Gallagher K, Gebriel AW, Nsubuga P, M'Pele-Kilebou P. Introducing an accountability framework for polio eradication in Ethiopia: Results from the first year of implementation 2014–2015. *Pan Afr Med J*. 2017;27(Suppl 2):12.
34. Hopkins DR. Disease eradication. *N Engl J Med*. 2013;368(1):54–63.
35. Khan MU, Ahmad A, Salman S, et al. Muslim scholars' knowledge, attitudes and perceived barriers towards polio immunization in Pakistan. *J Relig Health*. 2017;56(2):635–48.
36. Ahmed A, Lee KS, Bukhsh A, et al. Outbreak of vaccine-preventable diseases in Muslim majority countries. *J Infect Public Health*. 2018;11(2):153–5.
37. Progress towards regional measles elimination—Worldwide, 2000–2016. *Wkly Epidemiol Rec*. 2017;92(43):649–59.
38. Peter M, Strebel MJP, Paul A, Gastanaduy, James L. Goodson. Measles vaccines. In: *Plotkin's Vaccines. 7th ed. Philadelphia, PA:* 2018:579–618.
39. O'Connor P, Jankovic D, Muscat M, et al. Measles and rubella elimination in the WHO Region for Europe: Progress and challenges. *Clin Microbiol Infect*. 2017;23(8):504–10.
40. Orenstein WA, Hinman A, Nkowane B, Olive JM, Reingold A. Measles and Rubella Global Strategic Plan 2012–2020 midterm review. *Vaccine*. 2018;36(Suppl 1):A1–34.
41. Orenstein WA, Cairns L, Hinman A, Nkowane B, Olive JM, Reingold AL. *Measles and Rubella Global Strategic Plan 2012-2020 Midterm Review*. World Health Organization.
42. Orenstein WA, Cairns L, Hinman A, Nkowane B, Olive JM, Reingold AL. Measles and Rubella Global Strategic Plan 2012–2020 midterm review report: Background and summary. *Vaccine*. 2018;36(Suppl 1):A35–42.
43. Goodson JL, Alexander JP, Linkins RW, Orenstein WA. Measles and rubella elimination: Learning from polio eradication and moving forward with a diagonal approach. *Expert Rev Vaccines*. 2017;16(12):1203–16.
44. Castillo-Solorzano C, Reef SE, Morice A, et al. Guidelines for the documentation and verification of measles, rubella, and congenital rubella syndrome elimination in the region of the Americas. *J Infect Dis*. 2011;204(Suppl 2):S683–9.
45. Fine PE, Mulholland K, Scott JA, Edmunds WJ. Community protection. In: *Plotkin's Vaccines*. 7th ed. Philadelphia, PA: Elsevier; 2018:1512–31. e1515.
46. Orenstein WA. The role of measles elimination in development of a national immunization program. *Pediatr Infect Dis J*. 2006;25(12):1093–101.
47. Patel MK, Gacic-Dobo M, Strebel PM, et al. Progress toward regional measles elimination—Worldwide, 2000–2015. *MMWR Morb Mortal Wkly Rep*. 2016;65(44):1228–33.
48. Cochi SL. Pivoting from polio eradication to measles and rubella elimination: A transition that makes sense both for children and immunization program improvement. *Pan Afr Med J*. 2017;27(Suppl 3):10.
49. Durrheim DN, Crowcroft NS, Strebel PM. Measles—The epidemiology of elimination. *Vaccine*. 2014;32(51):6880–3.
50. El Sayed N, Kandeel N, Barakat I, et al. Progress toward measles and rubella elimination in Egypt. *J Infect Dis*. 2011;204(Suppl 1):S318–24.
51. Reef SE, Plotkin SA. Rubella vaccines. In: *Plotkin's Vaccines*. Philadelphia, PA: Elsevier; 2018:970–1000. e1018.
52. Andrus JK, de Quadros CA, Solórzano CC, Periago MR, Henderson D. Measles and rubella eradication in the Americas. *Vaccine*. 2011;29: D91–6.
53. Global Vaccine Action Plan 2017 Secretariat Report. Available at http://www.who.int/immunization/global_vaccine_action_plan/gvap_2017_secretariat_report_mnt.pdf?ua=1. Accessed 5/2/18.
54. Frew PM, Randall LA, Malik F, et al. Clinician perspectives on strategies to improve patient maternal immunization acceptability in obstetrics and gynecology practice settings. *Hum Vaccin Immunother*. 2018;14(7):1548–57.
55. Global Hepatitis Report 2017. Geneva: World Health Organization; 2017.
56. Heffernan A, Barber E, Cook NA, et al. Aiming at the global elimination of viral hepatitis: Challenges along the care continuum. *Open Forum Infect Dis*. 2018;5(1):ofx252.
57. Duarte G, Williams CJ, Vasconcelos P, Nogueira P. Capacity to report on mortality attributable to chronic hepatitis B and C infections by member states: An exercise to monitor progress toward viral hepatitis elimination. *J Viral Hepat*. 2018;25(7):878–82.
58. Kershenobich D, Torre-Delgadillo A, Aguilar-Valenzuela LM. Heading toward the elimination of hepatitis C virus. *Rev Invest Clin*. 2018;70(1):29–31.
59. Par A, Par G. Three decades of the hepatitis C virus from the discovery to the potential global elimination: The success of translational researches. *Orv Hetil*. 2018;159(12):455–65.
60. Scott N, Doyle JS, Wilson DP, et al. Reaching hepatitis C virus elimination targets requires health system interventions to enhance the care cascade. *Int J Drug Policy*. 2017;47:107–16.
61. Taherkhani R, Farshadpour F. Global elimination of hepatitis C virus infection: Progresses and the remaining challenges. *World J Hepatol*. 2017;9(33):1239–52.
62. Available at https://www.cdc.gov/hepatitis/hbv/bfaq.htm#bFAQc01. Accessed June 30, 2018.
63. Van Damme P, Ward JW, Shouval D, Zanetti A. 25—Hepatitis B vaccines. In: Plotkin SA, Orenstein WA, Offit PA, Edwards KM, eds. *Plotkin's Vaccines*. 7th ed. Philadelphia, PA: Elsevier; 2018:342–74. e317.
64. Available at https://www.cdc.gov/hepatitis/hcv/cfaq.htm. Accessed June 30, 2018.
65. World Health Organization. Global health sector strategy on viral hepatitis 2016–2021; 2017.
66. Cello J, Paul AV, Wimmer E. Chemical synthesis of poliovirus cDNA: Generation of infectious virus in the absence of natural template. *Science*. 2002;297(5583):1016–18.

CHAPTER

84

One Health: A New Paradigm for Disease Prevention and Control

Lonnie J. King • Ruth Lynfield • Lisa Conti

INTRODUCTION

The world has become more complex. The convergence of people, animals, and the environment has created a new dynamic characterized by a profound and unprecedented interdependence in which the health of all three domains is inextricably linked. This is significant for public health and, especially, for infectious diseases. Over the last three decades, approximately 75% of new emerging human diseases have been zoonotic (diseases that are transmitted from or through animals to humans).[1] The human-animal interface is expanding, accelerating, and becoming more consequential. At the same time, we have permanently altered a significant portion of our ecosystems and have created a new ecological milieu that is changing the conditions of our human-animal interface, the conditions for microbial adaptation and the emergence and re-emergence of infectious diseases worldwide. Our challenge is to create and implement a transformational model based on a holistic and integrated approach that addresses our health threats with a new emphasis on prevention, and addresses problems closer to their origin, often within the animal and environmental domains. This approach is the essence of the One Health concept.

WHAT IS ONE HEALTH?

One Health can be defined as the collaborative effort of multiple disciplines—working locally, nationally, and globally to attain optimal health for people, other animals, and the environment.[2] The scope of One Health is impressive, broad, and growing. Much of the recent focus on One Health has been limited to emerging infectious diseases, yet the concept clearly embraces ecosystem health, social sciences, biodiversity, ecology, chronic diseases, and more. Although there may be other variations of the definition of One Health, there is broad consensus that a new framework for preventing diseases is essential for our future, rather than accepting the status quo which is a more reactive response.

Figure 84-1 is a simple Venn diagram depicting the three domains of One Health and their close inter-relationship. The size and influence of each domain is relative and variable depending on the events within each domain. Each domain, progressively and consistently, influences the health within the other spheres. The relationship among these domains is analogous to Newton's Third Law of Motion. Because of the intense interconnectivity of animal, human, and environmental risk factors, for almost every action in one domain, there is an equal and opposite reaction in the others.

ROOTS OF ONE HEALTH

The concept of One Health is not new and the idea can be traced to ancient history. Early societies learned that basic sanitation (clean water and removal of waste and vermin) was critical to the population's health. From Greek mythology, Apollo's son Asclepius was tasked by the gods to care for Greek mortals with his two daughters, Hygeia and Panacea. Hygeia championed the prevention of disease and the common-sense practices of sanitation as the basis of wellness (cleanliness is next to godliness), and Panacea-cured individuals who were already sick, one at a time. Communities remained healthier when they followed Hygeian principles, creating a healthy environment and preventing disease. Further, the ancient Greek physician, Hippocrates, recognized that the same "bad air" causing human illness would likely have similar negative health effects in animals.

Acceptance and support of One Health has waxed and waned over the centuries. However, nineteenth century advocates including Drs. Louis Pasteur, Robert Koch, and Edward Jenner, and their work conducted on rabies, anthrax, and tuberculosis exemplified the One Health approach of multidisciplinary collaboration. Drs. Rudolf Virchow and William Osler, medical and public health luminaries, also embraced the concept of One Health and encouraged cross-disciplinary efforts.[3] As human medicine became progressively more specialized, and scientific research more molecular and genomic, the concept of One Health seemed to lose focus and acceptance. Two influential veterinarians, Dr. Calvin Schwabe and Dr. James Steele were strong and persuasive advocates of One Health. Dr. Schwabe developed the term "One Medicine" and Dr. Steele introduced the concept of the veterinary medical officer category in public health to the Centers for Disease Control and Prevention (CDC).[4] Comparative medicine, the concept that human and veterinary medicine have similar issues and use similar approaches, became an accepted tenet in the biomedical community and viewed as mutually beneficial to human and animal health.[5]

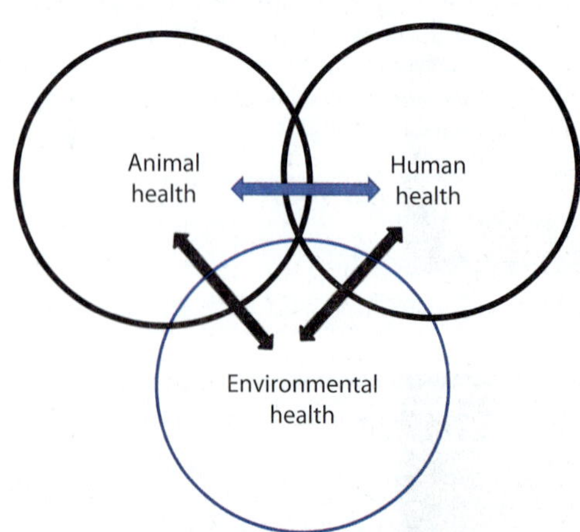

FIGURE 84-1. Dynamics of One Health domains; Newton's third law of motion: for every action, there is an equal and opposite reaction.

Our contemporary use and understanding of the term "One Health" originated from the Wildlife Conservation Society that adopted the phrase "One Health, One World" in 2004. Later the American Veterinary Medical Association (AVMA) passed a resolution in 2007, at the urging of both the Presidents of the AVMA and American Medical Association (AMA), adopting the term One Health in order to advance the collaboration of veterinary and human medicine. That same year, the AVMA formed the One Health Initiative Task Force which issued its report that formally defined the term and expanded on its principles and understanding. Today, the term One Health is gaining acceptance and recognition globally by health professionals, health organizations, and academic institutions.

The concept of One Health especially gained widespread interest over the last three decades, with the significant increase in emerging zoonoses, antimicrobial resistance, vector-borne, water-borne, and food-borne diseases. For example, during 2003, incursions of three zoonoses—West Nile virus, monkey pox, and severe acute respiratory syndrome (SARS), all occurred in the United States concurrently. None of these diseases had been reported previously in the Western Hemisphere. In addition, over the last few decades, notable zoonotic disease outbreaks and epidemics occurred along with a new appreciation of the impact of ecosystem changes on disease emergence. Diseases such as hantavirus, plague, new variant Creutzfeldt-Jakob disease, Nipah, Rift Valley fever, anthrax, Marburg, Ebola, Escherichia *coli* 0157:H7, Salmonella St. Paul, Q fever, avian influenza viruses (e.g., H_5N_1, H_7N_9), and numerous antimicrobial-resistant pathogens have created new challenges for public health. These significant global events give further credence and evidence that the human-animal-environmental interface is of growing significance to the health of all three domains.

THE PERFECT MICROBIAL STORM: EMERGING INFECTIOUS DISEASES

In a seminal publication, experts from the Institute of Medicine suggested that a group of factors have simultaneously been brought together to create a "Convergence model."[6] This model is a metaphor for a "perfect microbial storm" which stems from the book, *"The Perfect Storm,"* that describes a rare meteorological event in North American during 1991.[7] However, the perfect microbial storm (or epidemic) is hardly a rare event. Rather, such microbial events have become increasingly common. A group of factors have converged together resulting in a group of swirling forces or a "microbial storm" where the eye of the storm is the source of disease emergence and responsible for the global distribution of these new threats (Fig. 84-2). The factors and conditions that created perfect microbial storms are mostly anthropogenic and, today, microbes have abundant opportunities to establish new niches, cross species boundaries, travel globally, and establish new footholds in animals and in people. The interactions are complex and include social and ecologic systems. The factors converge and create a new, dynamic environment of entangled spatial and temporal webs.

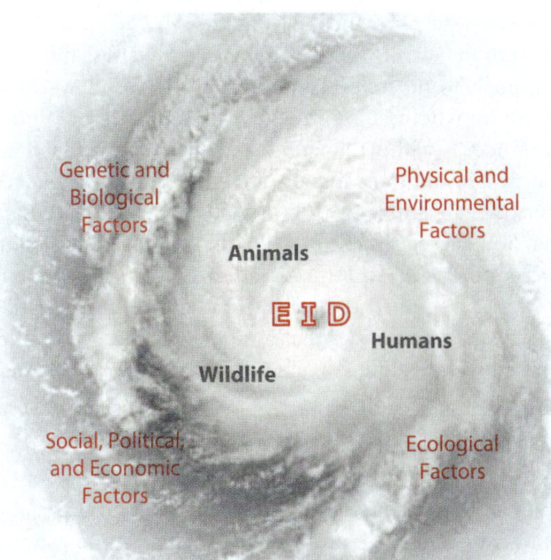

FIGURE 84-2. Convergence model of emerging infectious disease.

The most important of these convergence factors include:

- Microbial adaptation
- Global travel and transportation and commerce
- Host susceptibility
- Intent to do harm
- Climate and weather change
- Economic development and land use/changing ecosystems
- Human demographics and behavior
- Technology and industry
- A breakdown of both public and animal health infrastructures
- Poverty and social inequality
- War and famine

In a broad sense, the concept of convergence may be considered as both the "cause and cure" in addressing our contemporary challenges to health. Convergence factors have created conditions across the One Health domains that are largely responsible for new emerging and re-emerging diseases. In another sense, convergence of multiple disciplines, professions, collaborations, and thinking is essential to generate new innovations and interventions to tackle our vexing and difficult health issues of today.

EXPLORING THE DOMAINS OF ONE HEALTH

The Human Domain

Our human population has a global growth rate of 1.2% per year and is on a path of exponential growth. Today's global population is 7.6 billion and is expected to reach 8.6 billion by 2030, and 9.8 billion by 2050. At this rate, 10,000 people are added each hour, every day to the earth's human community.[8] There is also a significant demographic fault line between the population growth in countries with developing economies and that in developed countries. Approximately 90% of the world's population growth occurs in the former. The United Nations estimates that by 2030, five billion of the world's population of eight billion will be urban. Slums constitute a large part of today's urban reality. By 2020, a projected two billion people will live in slum settings with this population accounting for the fastest growing segment of the global population.[9] Slum inhabitants often have higher infant mortality, levels of food insecurity, undernutrition, and rates of infectious diseases. Most slums have inadequate public and animal health infrastructures, and lack the ability for both the rapid detection of an outbreak or generating an effective response. These limitations result in increased vulnerability to disease threats and, because of our remarkable interconnectedness, also create growing health threats globally. A One Health agenda that considers enhancements in the environment, sanitation, food access, socioeconomic status, reduced exposures to pests, and improved animal and public health services would improve slum conditions.

Currently, unprecedented human immigration and translocation to urban areas in developing countries and to wealthier countries are occurring, driven by economic and political circumstances and social instability. In low resource, densely populated areas, crowding and poor sanitation set the stage for easy spread of disease, including emerging and re-emerging infections. High rates of global travel and trade introduce new opportunities for infectious diseases to emerge in new areas. In addition to these occurrences, advances in medicine have resulted in large numbers of immunocompromised individuals who are especially susceptible to infections, including food- and water-borne illnesses.

The Animal Domain

Domestic Animal Issues in One Health

To meet the demands of a human population experiencing exponential growth, farmers will need to produce more food in the next 40 years than they did in the past 500 years. The Food and Agriculture Organization (FAO) of the United Nations estimates that food production must increase by 70% by 2050 to meet unprecedented demands of the projected 9.5 billion world population. In 2016, over 25 billion food animals (not counting aquaculture and wild fish) were produced, and 340 million metric tons of meat were consumed globally. The FAO projected that the demand for animal-produced protein will translate into the need to produce 50% more livestock and poultry over the next few decades as part of a 70% increase in food demand.[10] A new trend, urban agriculture, characterized by people moving from rural areas to urban settings who frequently bring livestock and poultry, is creating new city ecosystems and new zoonotic disease opportunities.[11]

Notably, one-third of the earth's crops is grown to feed livestock and poultry. The global food system will continue to shift to a more intensive, specialized, and integrated system, and expanded production systems will progressively move to the developing world. The higher consumption of protein from animal sources puts added pressure on natural resources and has serious environmental and health consequences, including on ecosystems, wildlife biodiversity, water resources, and greenhouse gas production.

Epidemics and pandemics within animal populations are evolving with greater frequency and significance. Porcine reproductive and respiratory syndrome (PRSS) and porcine epidemic diarrhea (PEDS), and highly pathogenic avian influenza are recent examples of global pandemics in hogs and poultry. Such diseases can substantially and quickly reduce food supplies and disrupt trade, thus indirectly impacting nutrition and human health. Food security is a global challenge and endemic and emerging livestock and poultry diseases are part of this challenge.

More intensive monoculture livestock production, especially poultry and hogs are at increased risk for massive pathogen amplification. Some pathogens (e.g., *Campylobacter and E. coli)* may be subclinical in production animals, yet pose a significant human food-borne disease concern. Antimicrobial-resistant food-borne pathogens exacerbate the situation. Conversely, livestock intensification may enhance biosecurity by better separating domestic and wild animals, improving animal health standards, and reducing species mixing. As the global human population increases, One Health models are critical for food animal production that simultaneously maximize the health of the involved humans (workers and consumers of food), animals, and local environment, and minimize the risks in all domains.

Companion animals (pets) are rapidly increasing globally. Over half the U.S. population closely share all facets of their lives with companion animals.[12] The lexicon change of "pet owners" to "pet parents" supports the importance of these animals to our everyday lives. The positive mental and physical aspects of companion animals are well documented. However, our shared exposures also allow for injury or disease transmission, which can be mitigated with proper hygiene and common-sense practices, even for immunocompromised people. Several million people in the United States experience animal (mostly dogs) bites each year, resulting in over 300,000 emergency room visits.[13] In addition to acute trauma, animal bites can result in envenomation, infection, and hypersensitivity reactions (e.g., following rodent and horse bites). Victims and animal owners may also suffer psychologically from the incident. In addition, companion animals that are bitten by other animals result in numerous veterinary visits. Rabies risk and management should be assessed in every animal bite situation in a human or pet.

Wildlife Issues in One Health

As food production facilities become more numerous, domestic animals and people frequently come in contact with wildlife, and wildlife habitats are being destroyed to accommodate more agriculture production, home and recreational sites for people. Emerging diseases are also responsible for deaths and population declines in wildlife. The fungus, *Batrachochytrium dendrobatidis*, resulted in dramatic reductions in global amphibian populations. At least 500 amphibian species have been infected across 54 countries and every continent. Another fungus, *Geomyces destructans* caused millions of bat deaths in Northeast and Midwest United States. These infections may have been introduced because of the pet trade (the former) or human movement (the latter).[14] Fungal infections caused some of the most severe die-offs and extinctions ever witnessed in wild species. Scientists believe that the world is in an era of unprecedented destruction, termed the Anthropocene Epoch, characterized by the loss of many wildlife species due to anthropogenic factors previously discussed, and especially alterations of our ecosystem.[15] One consequence of this phenomenon is the potential creation of a dilution factor enabling pathogens to pass more directly, and often more virulently, into human populations.[16]

One of the defining conditions of an emerging/re-emerging disease is pathogen shift to new hosts. At the domestic animal-wildlife interface, tuberculosis in wildlife is an example of this phenomenon. *Mycobacteria bovis* (*M. bovis* or bovine tuberculosis), the cause of tuberculosis primarily in cattle, is a very common infection in developing countries across the globe. The United States, as well as some other countries, successfully eradicated *M. bovis* from national cattle populations using the test and slaughter method. The U.S. Department of Agriculture reported that the prevalence of tuberculosis in U.S. cattle at the inception of the eradication program in 1917 was approximately 5% of all U.S. cattle.[17] Once the disease was eradicated from U.S. cattle, residual infections were found in white-tailed deer in several northeast counties of the lower peninsula of Michigan. Like many wild mammals, deer are highly susceptible to *M. bovis.* It was widely believed that deer were infected as a spill-over from cattle in the area prior to eradication, and maintained a low level of infection over time.[18] Experts further hypothesize that the spatial and temporal crowding of deer in winter months because of feeding and baiting practices (which increase the deer herd for hunters) was key to increased infection rates. Infection rates in white-tailed deer have persisted over the last two to three decades and the prevalence rate of white-tailed deer in the 5-county "hot spot" in this small area of Michigan is still in the 2–3% range.[18,19] This story has been repeated in other countries trying to finalize bovine tuberculosis eradication programs. However, different wildlife serve as both reservoir and spillover hosts. The European badger (*Meles meles*) has become a wildlife reservoir for *M. bovis* in England and Ireland, and the brushtail possum (*Trichosurus vulpecula*) is the wildlife reservoir in New Zealand. Eurasian wild boar in Portugal and Spain have relatively high infection rates and serve as the *M. bovis* wildlife host in that region of the world. These examples demonstrate the susceptibility of animals to tuberculosis and explain how spillover occurs back and forth from domestic animals and wildlife species. While the transmission occurs within the animal domain, the epidemiologic factors that enable the transmission are essentially anthropogenic. These factors include animal translocation, supplemental and artificial feeding, and encroachment on wildlife habitat. Transmission of *M. bovis* across the wildlife-domestic animal interface represents a serious obstacle to bovine tuberculosis eradication in a number of countries serving as a reminder that total eradication of any disease may be impossible if wildlife are infected, and serve as maintenance and spillover hosts.[19]

The Environmental Domain

Our environment continues to undergo dramatic changes, mostly to the detriment of our various ecosystems. The threat to the health of the environment is largely anthropogenic. While we are concerned about the sustainability of the environment itself, we also understand more clearly that diseases are often a result of environmental changes.

Today, environmental health focuses on the relationships between people, animals, plants, and the environment, ultimately preventing diseases of environmental origin. These diseases can be acute or chronic, and arise from exposures to:

- Infectious pathogens in food, water, animals (zoonoses), and/or vectors (e.g., mosquitoes, lice, fleas, mites, and ticks);
- Toxicants (e.g., pesticides, heavy metals, harmful algal blooms, carbon monoxide, and air-borne particulates);
- Excess radiation; or
- Lack of physical exercise (e.g., from a poorly built environment).

In developing countries, nearly 35% of mortality is attributed to environmental exposures in the home, work, and community.[20] Moreover, with socioeconomic growth comes demand for natural resources, including water, agricultural and residential land, minerals, lumber, and energy. Environmental changes alter both species composition and animal, vector, and human interactions. New opportunities are afforded for microbial transmission, for anthropogenic intoxications, and for diseases of sedentation.

Adversely altering our environment both directly and indirectly impacts long-term economics and community health. For example, sprawling communities centered on private transportation lead to issues such as traffic injury, air pollution-related asthma and hypertension, lack of exercise, and stress-related illness.[21] Automobiles are used for 80% of trips less than one mile in length in sprawling communities where few other travel options are available.[22] In the United States, dependence on automobiles, locating schools away from neighborhoods and the lack of attractive, accessible outdoor spaces contribute to physical inactivity. Veterinary health practitioners see a parallel rate of corpulence in companion animals. Moreover, failing to design communities in such a way as to promote neighborhood interaction reduces community resilience.

Community environments as well as indoor space design have a profound impact on health. When created with an eye toward accessibility and aesthetic attributes, built environments increase the likelihood of engaging in physical activity as well as "a sense of place" and the economic viability of a community.[23] Companion animals and wildlife are both impacted by changes in the built environment, and therefore may contribute to human health issues.

Alterations in temperature and precipitation patterns impact the habitats and growth of vectors such as mosquitoes and ticks, the replication rate of pathogens within vectors, and the vector-human bite rate. Malaria and dengue are expanding globally because of shifts in the geographic ranges of mosquito vectors associated with temperature and humidity change. Rift Valley fever has caused both animal and human epidemics in Africa after flooding rains have greatly increased the population of the vector mosquitoes. The last decade has ushered in increases in the incidence of tick-borne diseases such as Crimean Congo hemorrhagic fever, Lyme disease, and Rocky Mountain spotted fever. Leishmaniasis, a disease transmitted by sand flies, is also spreading.[24] The epidemiology of these diseases has altered, likely because of ecological changes.

The CDC recently reported that illnesses from mosquitoes, fleas, and ticks have more than tripled since 2004 in the United States, along with the discovery of nine vector-borne human diseases that were reported for the first time.[25] Although the majority of increased reported tick-borne diseases were Lyme disease, most experts agree that Lyme disease is still substantially under-reported. Lyme disease is the most widespread and frequently reported vector-borne disease in the earth's Northern Temperate Zone including North American, Europe, and Asia.[26] While this trend is well documented, it is often poorly understood. The conditions responsible for the unprecedented spread of Lyme disease comprise multiple, changing, and complex epidemiologic factors—a veritable One Health complex web. Focusing just on the deer, white-footed mice, *Ixodes* ticks, and pathogen (*Borrelia burgdorferi*) relationships may lead to an oversimplified ecologic model of infection. The true dynamic consists of the following factors: the diversity of other wildlife species; tick dynamics and biting habits; changing habitats and landscapes; changes in climate including rain, humidity, and temperatures; forest fragmentation; host range; access and abundance of food for wildlife; reservoir competence; differing genetic strains of the pathogen; and human behavior. Clearly, additional vector-borne disease studies and research are needed to understand and manage the One Health dynamics and offer new interventions to prevent Lyme infections.

Changing climate conditions, such as flooding or drought, increase the risk for infectious diseases to people, other animals, and plants. The classic example of a water-borne outbreak is cholera caused by *Vibrio cholera*. Typhoons that flood Bangladesh low lands produce a favorable environment for plankton growth, which enhance *Vibrio* growth. Crowded conditions, lack of toilets and lack of clean water amplify the risk for cholera. Excessive rainfall can also overwhelm sewage lines leading to contaminated water and spread of typhoid, other enteric pathogens, and leptospirosis. Water scarcity can increase risk for enteric disease due to limited options for clean water.

ENVIRONMENT, FOOD, AND AGRICULTURE

Like animals, plants suffer an array of diseases caused by bacteria, viruses, fungi, and other environmental stressors. Indeed, an example of an introduced vector-borne disease having a significant impact on plants is Citrus Greening (also known as Huang long bing, HLB, or yellow dragon disease). It is one of the most serious citrus diseases in the world, because once infected, the bacterium (*Candidatus Liberibacter*) attacks the plant vascular system. There is no cure for the disease, and most trees decline and die within a few years. In the United States, the vector Asian citrus psyllid (*Diaphorina citri*) preceded the causative bacterium, which was first identified in South Florida during 2005. By 2018, the disease spread throughout the state and resulted in an 80% reduction in citrus production. Integrated management programs make use of clean planting stock, ensuring timely removal of infected plants, and chemical and biological control of psyllid vectors. Antibiotics (tetracycline and streptomycin) have been approved to reduce the bacterial inoculum of infected trees.

Introduction of nonindigenous plants has the capacity to cause ecosystem changes that can enhance the risk of infectious diseases. For example, the spread of the Amur honeysuckle (*Lonicera maackii*) in Missouri, the United States increased the risk of exposure to ehrlichiosis. This occurred because the honeysuckle formed a dense monoculture with early and long-lasting leaves. White-tailed deer favored this habitat. Deer serve as the primary host for the lone star tick (*Amblyomma americanum*) and a reservoir for *Ehrlichia chaffeensis* and *Ehrlichia ewingii*. A study found that honeysuckle-invaded plots had a higher abundance of ticks and density of infected nymphs compared with native vegetation plots. Honeysuckle removal decreased deer activity and thus decreased the density of infected nymphs.[27]

Some pathogens' geographic range can expand even without vectors. For example, the fungus, *Cryptococcus gattii*, previously identified in Australia, has spread into Western Canada and Northwest United States. Sequencing studies suggest that the strain originated in tropical South America, spread to Australia, and from there to temperate British Columbia. In Australia, *C. gattii* has been recovered from eucalyptus trees. However, it has been isolated from indigenous trees such as the Douglas fir, coastal western hemlock, and cedar on Vancouver Island, British Columbia. *C. gattii* has infected people, domestic animals, marine mammals, and forests.[28]

Food production is dependent on weather, and changing conditions may favor undesirable plants, stress livestock, and provide other production challenges. Fortunately, plant production is benefitting from the innovative technology of "precision agriculture." Precision agriculture aims to optimize plant growth, and disease surveillance, diagnosis, and treatment. Three examples are as follows: by knowing the soil profile, nutrients are only applied to areas of need; infected or infested plants are identified with remote sensors quickly and "spot treated" rather than treating the entire acreage; and moisture sensors trip watering systems only when indicated. In this way, fertilizer, pesticides, and water are conserved targeting the plants' needs and eliminating potential run-off and water wastage.

Human health and nutrition are influenced by choice, access, quality, and relative costs of food. Plant and soil health is a global concern and key determinants to the future of food production, therefore, relevant to our health. However, the health of our food systems and environmental sustainability are often overlooked, and not fully appreciated as important features of One Health.

BACK TO THE FUTURE

Having just considered and reviewed the specifics and contexts of the One Health domains, the need for a more holistic and integrated strategy to address our contemporary health challenges is obvious, and biomedical concepts of the past, including One Health and One Medicine are once again relevant and pertinent to the future. The public health systems focus on prevention through population-based health promotion, services, and interventions. An important role of public health is to avert the onset and spread of diseases thus diminishing health threats to populations and communities. Some of these activities include preventing and addressing environmental contamination and pollution, contaminated food supply, and zoonotic diseases. The role and functions of public health are engaged in understanding the complex dynamics of the environmental, animal, and human health. The precepts of One Health are aligned well with these broad groups of determinants and their interactions. Today, One Health ideas and actions have enjoyed a resurgence. For the remainder of the twenty-first century, One Health is likely to be reconceptualized in contemporary heath management strategies. The CDC and World Health Organization (WHO) both have One Health offices to help integrate One Health into their thinking and actions. One Health is not intended to replace or diminish the importance and value of specific disciplines or specialties but rather, it emphasizes the need to share data across these fields to more effectively address and respond to risk threats. The One Health concept discussed and explored in the nineteenth and twentieth centuries has come full circle and has greater relevance to understanding and effectively addressing contemporary health threats than at any time other in our history. Until we address the underlying complexities of emerging diseases and work across discipline and professions, we are likely to continue to address each future epidemic or pandemic anew, forgetting lessons learned, and continue to act reactively.

WICKED PROBLEMS IN PUBLIC HEALTH: A NEED FOR NEW THINKING AND INNOVATIONS

In the world of business, the term "wicked problem" explains the complexities in which companies operate. Such problems cannot be resolved by gathering more data, redefining the problems, or just breaking them down into smaller components. They are wicked not because of their degree of difficulty, but rather because traditional processes and thinking cannot adequately resolve them. Wickedness is further based on the following criteria: the problems lack a single definition; do not have binary answers like yes or no; lack precedent; are entwined with other problems often outside the traditional realm; involve multiple stakeholders with different values; and a search for solutions never stops.[29]

The field of public health is increasingly faced with wicked and complex problems, such as obesity, addiction including the opioid crisis, and the spiraling costs of healthcare. Likewise, emerging and re-emerging diseases can be characterized as wicked, and One Health is an appropriate construct to better understand and successfully address such challenges. The key lesson learned in dealing with wicked problems is that conventional processes and interventions may no longer be effective and new, innovative, and systemic thinking is necessary to address many multifaceted contemporary disease threats. To comprehend the "wickedness" of our contemporary health challenges, further consideration is required for each of the One Health domains. Emerging zoonoses and antimicrobial resistance are further examples of wicked problems in human and animal health. A better understanding of these issues highlights the challenges of wicked problems and offer some direction into their resolution.

ZOONOTIC DISEASES

WHO recognizes over 200 zoonotic diseases involving agents including, bacteria, parasites, fungus, viruses, and novel agents such as prions.[30] A majority (61%) of known human pathogens have animal reservoirs, and nearly three quarters of emerging infections are zoonotic.[31] Zoonoses result in considerable human and animal disease burden globally, with millions of new cases annually. The ensuing economic impact is enormous. Communities suffer health service costs, lost wages, and animal production losses, as well as a multitude of indirect losses, including decreased trade and tourism. A study conducted by the International Livestock Research Institute (ILRI) concluded that zoonoses are major obstacles in pathways out of poverty for almost one billion poor livestock keepers worldwide. The study estimated that the top 13 zoonotic diseases were responsible for 2.4 billion human infections and 2.2 million deaths annually. In poor countries, these zoonoses may infect up to 1 out of every 7 livestock adding to a huge economic burden of these diseases.[32]

The pathogenic microorganisms causing zoonoses can be transmitted through vectors, via mucous membrane or transdermal contact, bites, scratches, or ingestion. Occasional iatrogenic intravenous or transplantation-associated transmissions occur. As discussed earlier, anthropogenic and natural environmental alterations influence the dynamics of disease transmission, and environmental factors impact the maintenance and distribution of zoonoses. Zoonotic pathogens can be encountered in shared air, food, water, soil, vectors, and wildlife. Pets and people typically live together in a home environment. People can be occupationally exposed to livestock. Animals can be sentinels for environmentally transmitted zoonoses. Alternatively, humans may be diagnosed first, providing an alert to the presence of a joint hazard.

Wildlife incorporated at the human-animal-environment interface have been associated with carrying and transmitting zoonotic diseases. Bats are special hosts for a variety of recently identified disease agents including Nipah, Ebola, and Marburg viruses. Consumption of "bush meat" has been associated with emerging infections such as human immunodeficiency virus, Ebola, and SARS. Influenza A viruses are also found across many animal species and can evolve, adapt, and move through avian and porcine hosts.

An example of an emerging infection that was a novel and widely spreading zoonosis is SARS. During 2003, the previously unrecognized SARS coronavirus caused a readily transmissible, atypical pneumonia in people. Small mammals, particularly the Himalayan palm civet, held in southern China food markets were thought to be the immediate source of the outbreak resulted in a massive culling campaign. Nevertheless, the SARS coronavirus quickly spread person-to-person to 29 countries in Asia, North America, South America, and Europe.[33] Losses due to SARS in East Asia and Canada were estimated U.S. $50 billion.[34] Horseshoe bats were identified as the likely natural virus reservoir.[35] SARS highlighted that a novel pathogen from a wildlife reservoir could threaten global health and global economies, and that responding to pandemic threats requires global cooperation across disciplines.

Another example of an emerging zoonotic virus is Nipah virus. The reservoir for Nipah virus is the Old World fruit bat (*Pteropus* spp.), which is found in many areas of Australia and Asia. Infected bats shed the virus in their saliva and urine. In 1998, a large outbreak of Nipah virus infection occurred in Malaysia and Singapore associated with 265 cases of encephalitis including 105 deaths in Malaysia, and another 11 cases and 1 death in Singapore.[36] Investigation revealed that fruit trees were planted next to pigsties (dual use agriculture) and attracted bats. The virus was transmitted to swine, likely from saliva on discarded fruit and/or direct exposure to bat excretions. The resulting infections in swine were often subclinical, or presented with respiratory and less commonly neurological disease. Infection spread among swine and transmission to humans occurred through exposure to the infected swine. Control measures included culling more than one million swine, and monitoring swine, restricting swine movement, and use of personal protective equipment.[37] Measures to prevent introduction and spread include removal of fruit trees from swine farms, utilizing wire screens to prevent bat-swine contact, and early identification and quarantine of affected farms. There have been no outbreaks of Nipah virus in Malaysia since 1999. In Bangladesh, Nipah virus infection was first detected in 2001, and multiple introductions of Nipah virus have occurred since that time. Interestingly, a higher proportion of severe respiratory disease occurred in human cases compared with infections in Malaysia. In Bangladesh, humans generally become infected through consumption of date sap that has been contaminated by bats licking the sap on the date palms. Person-to-person transmission has also occurred.[38] Putting "skirts" on the date palms to cover the sap-producing parts prevented bat-sap contact and has been suggested as a prevention measure.[39] A recent outbreak occurred in Kerala, India in 2018, encompassing 19 cases with 17 deaths. Most infections resulted from person-to-person transmission in healthcare facilities, including a fatality in a healthcare worker.[40]

The ease of genetic re-assortment, virulence, and pandemic potential of certain influenza A viruses heightened global concerns about novel zoonoses. Asymptomatic aquatic birds are considered reservoirs for most influenza A viruses, which can infect and cause devastating disease in poultry and occasionally other mammals, including people and dogs. Influenza A viruses are subtyped by two surface proteins, hemagglutinin (H) and neuraminidase (N). We are currently aware of 18 hemagglutinin subtypes, and 11 neuraminidase subtypes. Of the HN subtype combinations, all but H17N10 and H18N11 (bat subtypes) have been found in birds.[41]

In the largest U.S. poultry health disaster, over 50 million turkeys and chickens died or were depopulated due to a highly pathogenic avian influenza virus (HPAI H5N2) from December 2014 through June 2015. Issues related to premises biosecurity, mass euthanasia of poultry, and carcass disposal challenged responders. Although this virus did not cause human morbidity, approximately 12% of the U.S. egg layers and 8% of the U.S. meat turkeys died at a cost over one billion U.S. dollars during this outbreak.[42]

The intent to cause harm with bioterrorism agents is an unfortunate reality. CDC maintains a listing of priority bioterrorism agents and diseases. These are categorized as A, B, or C based on their likelihood of being easily transmitted, causing mass casualties, causing panic, and requiring enhanced preparedness actions.[43,44] Zoonotic pathogens comprise most of these select agents. Animals may become infected during an intentional release of an agent. Animals may also be infected naturally and serve as a reservoir for human infections such as tularemia. For more information on these diseases, please see Chap. 6.

With the existential threat of emerging pandemics naturally or intentionally instigated, new One Health surveillance systems, collaboration across health domains, and refocusing on more rapid interventions closer to the origin of these diseases, seem appropriate actions to ensure more effective prevention and control strategies. Effective methods of controlling zoonotic disease outbreaks require public investment of coordinated interventions, such as mass animal vaccination, public health education, feed bans, milk pasteurization, and "test and slaughter" operations.[43] Clearly, the challenges of intensive disease intervention are compounded in impoverished countries, including access to sufficient food and water, let alone access to human health and veterinary services. Undoubtedly, transdisciplinary collaboration and consideration of shared environments are requisite for zoonoses detection and, ultimately, management of environmental risks.

PREDICTABLE SURPRISES

The driving forces of convergence that have helped create our new era of emerging and re-emerging diseases are still firmly in place and the One Health domains are even more complex, active, and their interfaces more consequential. However, our health domains and their systems mostly remain "siloed" and narrowly focused, and epidemics usually come as a surprise. A predictable surprise is an event or set of events that take an individual or group by surprise, despite prior awareness of all the information necessary to anticipate the events and their consequences. There are, of course, true surprises that happen and are unpredictable. However, predictable surprises are different and occur when leaders or organizations unquestionably have all the data and insight needed to recognize the potential for, and even the inevitability of, a crisis but fail to respond with effective preventive action. Predictable surprises do not solve themselves, get worse over time, require investments in the short term, and benefits of the preventive actions are delayed or not recognized. The human tendency is often to maintain the status quo and avoid new actions especially if initial costs lead to uncertainty.[45] Although the exact location and timing of the next pandemic or the next antibiotic-resistant (AR) "superbug" may not be known today, the occurrence of the next complex epidemic is foreseeable and should not be a surprise. Understanding the One Health construct and being aware of the drivers and factors of disease emergence gives us evidence of the inevitability of ensuing disease catastrophes. However, we generally react to these occurrences as if they are a complete revelation—the response is re-invented, and we neither learn lessons of the past nor establish an integrated and holistic One Health strategy to better prepare for the inevitable.

Nearly all recent epidemics and pandemics have had a viral etiology and originated in animals. Thus, viral zoonoses are prime candidates for producing future pandemics. However, the diversity and potential pathogen emergence that create new risks of human disease are largely unknown but ultimately predictable. A U.S. Agency for International Development project, termed PREDICT, reported the discovery of over 1000 unique viruses from a pool of 74,000 samples from wildlife, livestock, and people located in Africa and Southeast Asia. The sampling was focused at the interface of humans and animals where there was potential for zoonotic pathogen spillover. Of these viruses, 820 were novel and 182 known, and all were either zoonotic or had zoonotic potential.[46] This seems to be just the tip of a global "viral iceberg." Modeling based on recent virus discovery data estimated that perhaps as many as 1.67 million yet undiscovered viral species exist in mammals and avian hosts. Further analyses suggest that possibly between 631,000 and 877,000 of these unknown viruses have zoonotic potential.[47] The twenty-first century mixing bowl of animals, animal products, and people contains the right ingredients to create pandemics along with the right conditions to accelerate spread and result in significant costs and consequences to our health.

In December 2019, the zoonotic coronavirus, SARS-CoronaVirus-2 (SARS-CoV-2) emerged marking the third zoonotic coronavirus to emerge in the twenty-first century and the one that has produced the most significant global health threat in the last century. Although the dissemination and impact of this pandemic was unusual, the emergence of yet another pathogen from an animal reservoir to humans certainly is not and qualifies as another "predictable surprise" in the world of infectious diseases. SARS-CoV-2 is just the latest example of why we need to embrace a One Health approach to better anticipate and understand such diseases, and improve our early detection and response and better manage these threats. Our extraordinary interconnectedness which continues to intensify and expand ensures that more "surprises" and similar disease events are guaranteed. (Chap. 86 discusses SARS-CoV-2 in detail.)

ANTIBIOTIC RESISTANCE

Another valuable One Health strategy area is combating antibiotic resistance. Antibiotics have had a major impact on human health, enabling whole fields of medicine such as intensive care, oncology, and transplant surgery. However, antibiotic use drives antibiotic resistance. Over the past 20 years, widespread recognition that decades of extensive (and often unnecessary) antibiotic use has resulted in multidrug-resistant infections that are challenging, and in some cases impossible to treat. Annually, over two million illnesses and 23,000 deaths in the United States are attributed to AR infections.[48] Urgent threats include *Clostridium difficile*, carbapenem-resistant Enterobacteriaceae, and AR *Neisseria gonorrhoeae*. Serious threats include AR *Campylobacter* and *Salmonella infections*, which can be acquired from food or animals. Recommendations and toolkits for antibiotic stewardship and surveillance systems across the continuum of human healthcare, including acute, long-term, and ambulatory care are available.[49]

Antibiotics are sold without oversight from clinicians in many parts of the world, particularly in developing countries where many cannot afford a doctor's evaluation. This led to overuse and misuse of antibiotics, and high selective pressure for the emergence of resistant organisms. AR infections are a challenging issue, where susceptibility testing for bacteria is limited and treatment options are scarce, expensive, and often toxic. Travel to receive healthcare in developing countries (medical tourism), although more affordable than some procedures in high resource countries, is associated with highly resistant infections such as the extensively drug resistant *E. coli* containing NDM (New Delhi Metallo-beta-lactamase) and KPC (*Klebsiella pneumoniae* carbapenamase) genes. Spread within healthcare settings and in the community has increased the prevalence of AR organisms.

Antibiotics are important in veterinary medicine and agriculture, and have been used to treat sick animals, for disease prevention, for growth promotion (low doses, long duration), and to control microbial plant diseases. After a 3-year voluntary period and beginning on January 1, 2017, the U.S. Food and Drug Administration (FDA) has acted to promote the judicious use of medically important drugs in food animals. This action was based on two guidances. One bans the use of medically important antibiotics to enhance growth or improve feed efficiency of food animals, and the second directs pharmaceutical companies to change the labels and claims on these products accordingly. Finally, the FDA expanded the scope of its existing Veterinary Feed Directive (VFD) by bringing the use of these antibiotics in feed and water under the oversight of licensed veterinarians for the prevention, control, and treatment of diseases.[50] Antibiotics used for growth promotion were banned in the European Union in 2006 but are still used in other parts of the world. In recent years, there has been an emphasis on antibiotic stewardship and infection prevention in veterinary medicine, including not only for agriculture (including food animals, aquaculture, and plants), but also for companion animals and horses. Animals and people can share AR organisms, through close contact and through contact with animal products, including handling meat.

Antibiotics can contaminate the natural environment and have been found in surface water, ground water, and soil.[51] Low-level antibiotic exposure can result in high-level resistance in microorganisms.[52] Up to 80% of antibiotics ingested by people and other animals are excreted through urine and feces, and waste flows (including agricultural run-off, manure, and wastewater), contain antibiotic residues and resistant bacteria.[53] Improperly disposed, unused antibiotics, and those used in aquaculture, crop agriculture, and pharmaceutical industries are other sources of antimicrobials in the environment. Highly resistant microorganisms have been found in water and sediment near discharges from industrial areas, urban areas, and aquaculture. Advances in wastewater treatment to effectively and efficiently remove antimicrobials and resistant bacteria are, therefore, needed. Determining the impact of this environmental contamination on health remains an important area of research.

Identifying and tracking the mcr-1 gene is a good example of the importance of a One Health approach. First identified in 2015 from a 2013 *E. coli* isolate of swine origin, the mcr-1 gene confers resistance to colistin, considered a "last-resort" antibiotic for Gram-negative bacteria.[54] This gene has subsequently been found in ten species of Enterobacteriaceae in numerous countries across five continents, on multiple plasmid types. It has been found in environmental isolates, and isolates from livestock, people, and companion animals.[55] Genetic analysis dates its emergence to mid-2000s in Chinese livestock, and it is hypothesized that global spread occurred through trade of food animals and meat. However, some spread may have occurred by colonized or infected humans.[56] Colistin had been used for livestock growth promotion in China (it was discontinued in April 2017, after the mcr-1 gene was identified). Mcr-1 producing *Klebsiella pneumoniae* has been reported in a healthcare setting, among children with leukemia.[57] Notably, a patient in Switzerland was found to have a mcr-1 containing isolate that also had a carbapenamase and other resistance genes: an extremely dangerous combination.[58] Antibiotic resistance and antibiotic stewardship are covered in detail in Chap. 153.

THE NEED FOR AN INTEGRATED ONE HEALTH SURVEILLANCE SYSTEM

Several excellent and successful models of One Health surveillance systems could be expanded or applied to different settings and systems. The FAO, World Organization for Animal Health (OIE), and WHO have established a "Global Early Warning System for Health Threats and Emerging Risks" at the Human-Animal-Ecosystems Interface (GLEWS). The GLEWS aim is for "a world capable of preventing, detecting, containing, eliminating, and responding to animal and public health risks attributable to zoonoses and animal diseases with an impact on food security, through multisectoral cooperation and strong partnerships."[59] Another surveillance system, ArboNet, is a U.S. example that monitors West Nile virus in birds, mosquito pools, and people. This system was useful in predicting future human infections based on infections in birds, horses, and mosquitoes, which all precede human exposures and infections.[60] A final example is the National Antimicrobial Resistance Monitoring System, which is supported by CDC, FDA, and U.S. Department of Agriculture, and tracks resistance in food-borne pathogens in humans, animals, and retail meats.[61]

ECONOMIC BENEFITS OF ONE HEALTH

The value proposition of One Health is based on the concept of optimizing investments to improve the efficiency and cost-effectiveness of public health strategies to maintain and improve human, animal, and ecosystem health. One Health emphasizes a proactive disease-prevention orientation by applying interventions "upstream," closer to the source of the problem, rather than a more reactive and disease-oriented approach focusing on addressing the disease after it has occurred. To fulfill its value proposition, One Health strategies must be more cost-effective and beneficial than the option of pursuing the status quo. Measuring the effectiveness of One Health can be difficult especially estimating savings from disease prevention results. However, much more is being done to establish relevant evaluations, such as by the International Network for Evaluation of One Health Activities. Like any new intervention, One Health must demonstrate added value to warrant its adoption and implementation.

Figure 84-3 quantitatively displays examples of the economic impacts of a few recent pandemics and the key sectors of the economy most impacted. The cost of these pandemics and others go well beyond the costs of medical expenses. Tourism, associated businesses, transportation, labor, education, and agricultural markets may also be negatively affected. The costs of response and recovery of pandemics including rebuilding communities, infrastructures, addressing environmental degradation, and loss of human capacity are additional costs. It is now estimated that future pandemics could cost an average of U.S. $60 billion for each event. The World Bank (2008) modeled the global economic impact of a serious influenza pandemic and, based on 2015 GDP, the economic impact would be approximately $6 trillion corresponding to a major global recession.[62] However, even with this reality and the knowledge that future outbreaks and possible pandemics are a certainty, investments in disease prevention and the mitigation of risks are still very limited. The World Bank estimates that an annual investment of between U.S. $1.9 and $3.4 billion annually to improve human and animal health systems and infrastructures would return upwards of U.S. $30 billion each year in avoided losses.[63] An additional financial benefit could be the gains expected to the agriculture sector through increases in productivity and expanding market access.

Figure 84-4 (World Bank Group: One Health: Operational Framework[63]) illustrates a temporal comparison of epidemic curves for zoonotic diseases. It demonstrates how early disease detection along with a rapid and effective response in animal populations can greatly limit subsequent infections, further amplification, and disease spread in human populations. In addition to reducing human morbidity and mortality, addressing zoonoses at the source in domestic animals or wildlife has a significant economic benefit to both animal and human populations but also to the broader society. Healthy animals can translate to healthier people. This has been proven in terms of advances in food safety and the successful campaigns to eliminate zoonoses like tuberculosis and brucellosis in livestock, which has been accomplished in the United States and other developed countries. Globally, WHO has estimated that there are 59,000 deaths annually due to rabies.[64] Canine rabies has been eradicated in the United States through ambitious and effective vaccination programs in dogs resulting in an immunologic barrier against human exposures. It is further estimated that the global burden of endemic canine rabies is approximately U.S. $8.6 billion annually based on postexposure prophylaxis, premature deaths, and loss of income.[65]

Given the scale of the financial consequences of emerging and re-emerging diseases, the case for disease prevention, early detection, and effective response using the One Health concept is both compelling and financially essential. A summary of the economic and biomedical benefits of One Health include:

- Avoiding morbidity and mortality in people, animals, and plants;
- Reducing the threat of zoonotic disease outbreaks, epidemics, and pandemics;
- Reducing and better controlling endemic zoonoses—the real beneficiaries are the poorest livestock keepers in the low-income countries;
- Protecting and in some cases correcting environmental insults and degradation;
- Enabling resource sharing and the added value of increased capacity and expertise;

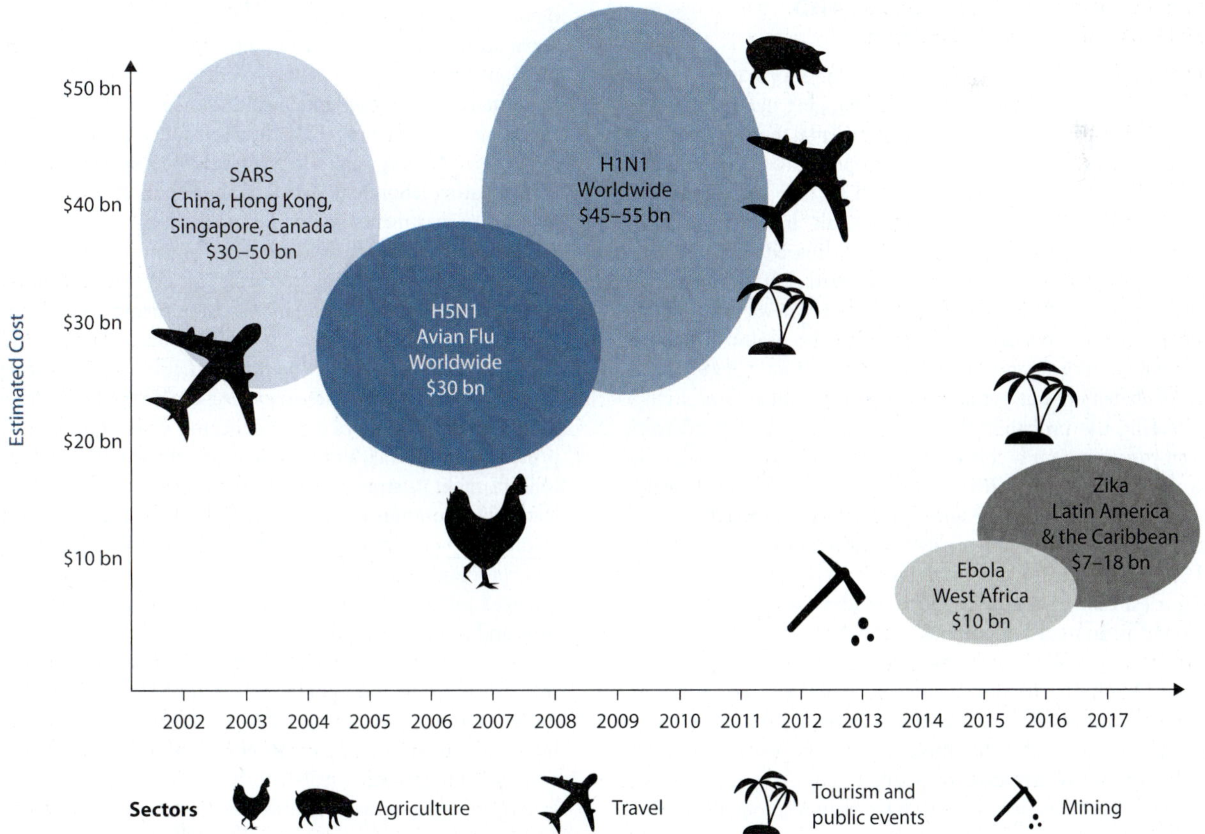

FIGURE 84-3. Examples of economic impacts of disease outbreaks; icons represent examples of highly affected sectors. (*Source:* Used with permission from the EcoHealthAlliance and World Bank Group.)

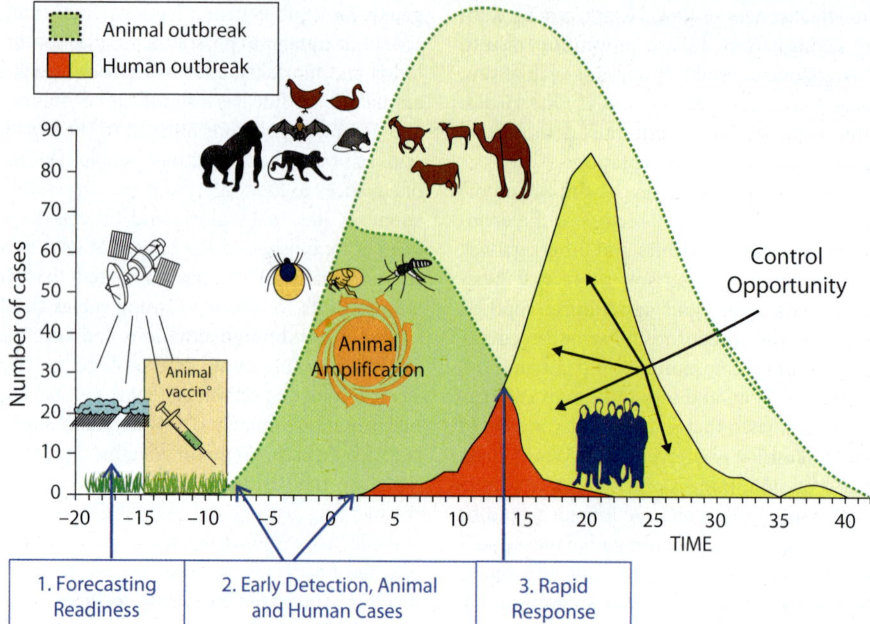

FIGURE 84-4. Stages, number of cases, and time-scale of emerging zoonotic disease outbreaks. (*Source:* Adapted from Karesh, W. B., Dobson, A., Lloyd-Smith, J. O., Lubroth, J., Dixon, M. A., Bennett, M., Aldrich, S., Harrington, T., Formenty, P., Loh, E. H., Machalaba, C. C., Thomas, M. J., and Heymann, D. L. (2012). Ecology of zoonoses: natural and unnatural histories. The Lancet 380(9857):1936–1945.)

- Improving animal health results in more efficient production, improved food safety and better food security for people;
- Protecting biodiversity and wildlife conservation; and
- Combating antimicrobial resistance and reducing the possible transfer of resistant organisms and genes from animals and the environment to human populations.

THE PATH FORWARD: DEVELOPING AND OPERATIONALIZING ONE HEALTH

This chapter has discussed the immensity of the contemporary challenges faced by public health due to the changing dynamics at the interface of human, animal, and environmental health domains. The world is now intricately connected geopolitically, economically, socially, culturally, and with shared health threats. Unprecedented population growth and movements of animals and people, and a remarkable global food system have created the ingredients necessary for perfect microbial storms, and an unparalleled global mixing bowl of convergent factors. The result of this reality is a new era of emerging and re-emerging diseases and threats to the health of people, other animals, and the environment. The driving forces demonstrate no signs of abatement but, rather, they are accelerating, intensifying, and increasing the probability of more epidemics and pandemics with even more profound consequences. One Health strategies are needed. This platform has real promise in reducing global health threats where the three domains of One Health are involved.

One Health strategies are consistent with, and included in, the Global Health Security Agenda (GHSA), a shared plan of 64-member countries, that envisions capacity building to prevent, detect, and respond to human and animal infectious disease threats. One of GHSA's recommendations pertains to zoonotic diseases that promote One Health approaches to policies, practices, and behaviors that could minimize the risk of zoonotic disease emergence and spread.[66] The agenda states that there needs to be a shared responsibility that cannot be achieved by a single action, organization, or sector. Future success depends upon collaboration among the health, security, environmental and agricultural sectors to advance a world safe and secure from infectious disease threats. The GHSA mission is synonymous with the goals and thinking of One Health. However, no agenda can be accomplished without effective actions. The path forward to operationalize One Health is built on existing and expanding disease prevention and response strategies that are relevant for complex and interconnected diseases and new actions critical to address today's wicked health challenges. A successful One Health action plan includes the following:

1. Base plans on scientific findings and rationale, evidence-based data, and a positive cost beneficial financial analysis.
2. Develop and implement One Health surveillance systems that are built on current human health surveillance systems, but expanded to animal and environmental health domains.
3. Invest in strengthening both human and animal health infrastructures and programs—there should be a special emphasis on consolidating laboratory data and sharing information across all domains. Investments should be made based on objective criteria that ensure proper prioritization of limited resources; such criteria should be derived from existing evaluation frameworks: International Health Regulations' Monitoring and Evaluation Framework; OIE's Performance of Veterinary Services and Gap Analysis; and the WHO-led Joint External Evaluation process.
4. Build further capacity and expertise—a new public health workforce needs to be trained and educated with knowledge of the principles of One Health and possess critical skills and abilities to implement its strategies. Critical competencies should include: leadership, communications, system thinking and working across traditional boundaries. The workforce should be highly diverse and represent experts in infectious diseases, behavior and social sciences, public policy, ecology, economics, environment, agriculture, and veterinary medicine.
5. Advance collaborative and integrative research and functionality–research funding and operations should be targeted to improve understanding of disease ecology, collaborative learning, and integration of knowledge and discovery. There should be a special emphasis on applied research to better identify and understand synergistic interventions and to develop and evaluate prevention and control strategies across One Health options.
6. Develop highly skilled and transdisciplinary One Health teams specialized in rapid response and control of emerging disease

situations and emergencies—such teams should be available on immediate notice and capable of working well within the human, animal, or environmental domains. Teams could be part of local, national, and international organizations. Teams need to be permanently funded and be embedded in national governance systems with strong leadership and authority to activate and support the teams, and ensure that members can work across boundaries and sectors.

7. Coordinate One Health actions with other efforts that help reduce poverty, improve the environment, and help advance social and other determinants of health. For example, programs and efforts focused on the global Sustainable Development Goals, Food Security programs, combating antimicrobial resistance, national preparedness and health security activities, and residual capacity from previous pandemic programs such as implemented for influenza, should be included to avoid duplication of effort and reduce excessive costs.
8. Create innovative financial strategies that are available for immediate use, and ensure long-term One Health capacity through programs of annual contributions. This could include public-private ventures, permanent funding from different sources emphasizing national security, or previous global commitments. For example, recent efforts of the World Bank and WHO to build a Pandemic Emergency Fund are laudable, but there also needs to be longer, sustainable financing strategies as well.
9. See with New Eyes—Marcel Proust once stated that "the real voyage of discovery consists not in seeing new landscapes, but in having new eyes." A One Health approach is seeing the world through the eyes and perspectives of others and suspend disbelief in favor of creating new options and possibilities. If wicked problems are characterized by defying old solutions, then seeing with new eyes is essential. One Health is a paradigm shift and overcoming the status quo and past organizational arrangements is difficult but essential to public health officials in the future.

CONCLUSION

A One Health approach is aligned well with the holistic perspective that practitioners in preventive medicine and public health employ. It builds upon the social determinants of health, defined by CDC as "conditions in the places where people live, learn, work and play affect a wide range of health risks and outcomes."[67] In understanding the root causes of health and diseases, particularly infectious diseases, it is essential that we understand the interplay of human activity, domesticated animals, wildlife, and the environment. Ecosystem health is key to public health. Global and local multidisciplinary partnerships and investments in local capacity to prevent, detect, and respond are crucial. We must invest in infrastructure, clean water, sanitation, agriculture, education, and public health systems. We need to anticipate and plan for unintended consequences of human activity. We must enhance our understanding of the factors that enable pathogens to move from spillover from another species to easy transmission among people. This includes understanding the distribution and activities of people, reservoir hosts, and vectors. Similarly, we must understand these factors in animals. Research into potential pathogens, effective methods of prevention and control, including nonpharmaceutical interventions, vaccine, and therapeutic development for humans and animals are important. Early warning systems through enhanced surveillance is crucial to provide control measures at the source of an outbreak. Public health leaders must understand the concepts of One Health and incorporate healthy ecology in their policies, plans, and practices. We have one world—let us keep it intact.

References

1. Taylor LH, Latham SM, Woolhouse ME. Risk factors for human disease emergence. *Philos Trans R Soc London B Biol Sci.* 2001;365:983–9.
2. King LJ, Anderson LR, Blackmore CG, et al. Executive Summary AVMA One Health Initiative Task Force Report. *J Am Vet Med Assoc.* 2008;233(2):259–61.
3. Kahn LH, Kaplan B, Monath TP, Steele JH. Teaching One Medicine, One Health. *Am J Med.* 2008;12(3):169–70.
4. Cowen P, Currier RW, Steele JH. A short history of One Health in the U.S. Veterinary Heritage. *Bull Am Vet History Soc.* 2016;29(1):1–15.
5. Mobasheri A. Comparative medicine in the 21st century: Where are we now and where do we go from here? *Front Vet Sci.* 2015;2(2):1–4.
6. Smolinski MS, Hamburg MA, Lederberg J. *Microbial Threats To Health: Emergence, Detection, and Response.* In: Smolinski MS, ed. Washington DC: National Academies Press; 2005, pp. 4–7.
7. Junger S. *The Perfect Storm.* New York, NY: WW Norton and Co; 1997.
8. United Nations. World Population Prospects. Available at https://esa.un.org/unpd/wpp. New York, NY, 2017.
9. Ezeh A, Mberu B, Haregu T. Slum health is not urban health. The Conversation. Publication (1-3), December 18, 2016. Available at https://theconversation.com/slum-health-is-not-urban-health-why-we-must-distinguish-between-the-two-69939. Boston, MA, 2016.
10. High Level Expert Forum. *How to Feed the World 2050: Global Agriculture Towards 2050.* Rome, Italy: FAO Bulletin; 2009:1–4.
11. National Public Radio. African cities test the limit of living with livestock. Available at http://www.npr.org/blogs/thesalt/2013/05/21/185763979/african-cities. New York, NY, 2013.
12. Chomel BB, Sun B. Zoonoses in the bedroom. *Emerg Infect Dis.* 2011;17(2):167–72.
13. Rabinowitz PM, Conti LA, Mainzer HM. *Public Health and Human-Animal Medicine: Human-Animal Medicine, Clinical Approaches to Zoonoses, Toxicants and Other Shared Health Risks.* In: Rabinowitz PM, Conti LA, eds. Maryland Heights, MO: Saunders Elsevier; 2010.
14. Fisher MC, Henk DA, Briggs CJ, et al. Emerging fungal threats to animal, plant and ecosystem health. *Nature.* 2012;484(7393):186–94.
15. Monastersky R. Anthropocene: The new human age. *Nature.* 2015;519:144–7.
16. Civitello DJ, Cohen J, Fatima H, et al. Biodiversity inhibits parasites: Broad evidence for the dilution effect. *Proc Natl Acad Sci USA.* 2015;112(28):8667–71.
17. Thoen C, Steele J, Kaneene J. *Zoonotic Tuberculosis: Mycobacterium bovis and Other Pathogenic Mycobacteria.* Hoboken, NJ: John Wily and Sons, Inc.; 2012, p. 235.
18. Okafor CC, Grooms DL, Bruning-Fann CS, Averill JJ, Kaneene JB. Descriptive epidemiology of Bovine Tuberculosis in Michigan (1975–2010): Lessons learned. *Veterinary Medicine International.* 2011;874924: 1–13. Available at https://www.hindawi.com/journals/vmi/2011/874924/.
19. Palmer MV, Thacker TC, Waters WR, Gortazar C, Corner LAL. *M. bovis*: A model pathogen at the interface of livestock, wildlife and humans. *Vet Med Int.* 2012:1–17. Article ID 236205. Available at http://dx.doi.org/10.1155/2012/236205.
20. World Health Organization. Environment and health in developing countries. Available at http://www.who.int/heli/risks/ehindevcoun/en/. Geneva, Switzerland, 2018.
21. Frumkin H. Urban sprawl and public health. *Public Health Rep.* 2002;117(3):201–17.
22. James P, Troped PJ, Hart JE, et al. Urban sprawl, physical activity, and body mass index: Nurses' health study and nurses' health study II. *Am J Public Health.* 2013;103(2):369–75.
23. Jackson RRJ, Dannenberg AL, Frumkin H. Health and the built environment: 10 years after. *Am J Public Health.* 2013;103(9):1542–4.
24. Carvalho BM, Rangel EF, Ready PD, Vale MM. Ecological niche modelling predicts southward expansion of *Lutzomyia (Nyssomyia) flaviscutellata* (Diptera: Psychodidae: Phlebotominae), vector of *Leishmania (Leishmania) amazonensis* in South America, under climate change. *PLOS One.* 2015;10(11):e0143282.
25. Centers for Disease Control and Prevention. Vital Signs: Trends in reporting vector-borne disease cases—U.S and Territories, 2004–2016. Available at https://www.cdc.gov/mmwr/volumes/67/wr/mm6717e1.htm. Atlanta, GA, 2018.

26. Ostfeld RS. *Lyme Disease*. New York, NY: Oxford University Press; 2011.
27. Allan BF, Dutra HP, Goessling LS, et al. Invasive honeysuckle eradication reduces tick-borne disease risk by altering host dynamics. *Proc Natl Acad Sci USA*. 2010;107(43):18523–7.
28. Chen SC, Meyer W, Sorrell TC. *Cryptococcus gattii* Infections. *Clin Microbiol Rev*. 2014;27(4):980–1024.
29. Camillus JC. Strategy as a Wicked Problem. *Harvard Business Review*. 2008;86(5):155–69.
30. World Health Organization. Zoonoses. Available at https://www.who.int/zoonoses/diseases/en. Geneva, Switzerland, 2016.
31. Jones KE, Patel NG, Levy MA, et al. Global trends in emerging infectious diseases. *Nature*. 2008;451(7181):990–3.
32. Grace D, Mutua F, Ochungo P, et al. Mapping of poverty and likely zoonoses hotspots. Report to the UK Dept. for International Development, Nairobi, Kenya. ILRI. Available at https://cgspace.cgiar.org/bitstream/handle/10568/21161/ZooMap_July2012_final.pdf. 2012.
33. Centers for Disease Control and Prevention. CDC SARS response timeline. Available at https://www.cdc.gov/about/history/sars/timeline.htm. Atlanta, 2018.
34. The World Bank. People, pathogens and our planet. Available at http://documents.worldbank.org/curated/en/214701468338937565/pdf/508330ESW0whit1410B01PUB. Washington DC, 2010.
35. Li W, Shi Z, Yu M, et al. Bats are natural reservoirs of SARS-like coronaviruses. *Science*. 2005;310(5748):676–9.
36. Chua KB, Bellini EJ, Roja PA, et al. Nipah virus: A recently emergent deadly paramyxovirus. *Science*. 2000;288(5470):1432–5.
37. Chua KB. Epidemiology, surveillance and control of Nipah virus infections in Malaysia. *Malaysian J Pathol*. 2010;32(2):69–73.
38. Gurley ES, Montgomery JM, Hossain MJ, et al. Person to person transmission of Nipah virus in a Bangladesh community. *Emerg Infect Dis*. 2007;13(7):1031–7.
39. Khan SU, Gurley ES, Hossain MJ, et al. A randomized controlled trial of interventions to impede date palm sap contamination by bats to prevent Nipah virus transmission in Bangladesh. *PLoS One*. 2012;7(8):e42689.
40. Arunkumar G, Abdulmajeed J, Aswathyraj S, et al. Outbreak of Nipah virus in Kerala, India, 2018. Abstract J4. The International Conference on Emerging Infectious Diseases. Available at https://custom.cvent.com/BA5667C9F30147A1BE057244E3AA6756/files/a394ab04ee224932a98e-4f5561ab962b.pdf. p. 191. Atlanta, GA, 2018.
41. Centers for Disease Control and Prevention. Transmission of influenza viruses from animals to people. Available at https://www.cdc.gov/flu/about/viruses/transmission.htm#subtypes. Atlanta, GA, 2017.
42. USDA. Highly pathogenic avian influenza response plan: The Red Book. Available at https://www.aphis.usda.gov/animal_health/emergency_management/downloads/hpai_response_plan.pdf. Riverdale, MD, 2017.
43. Keusch GT, Pappaioanou M, Gonzalez MC, Scott KA, Tsai P, eds. Sustaining global surveillance and response to emerging infectious diseases. National Research Council (US) Committee on Achieving Sustainable Global Capacity for Surveillance and Response to Emerging Diseases of Zoonotic Origin. Washington, DC: National Academies Press; 2009. Available at https://www.ncbi.nlm.nih.gov/pubmed/25009943.
44. Centers for Disease Control and Prevention. Bioterrorism Agents/Diseases. Available at https://emergency.cdc.gov/agent/agentlist-category.asp. Atlanta, GA, 2018.
45. Bazerman MH, Watkins MD. *Predictable Surprises*. Boston, MA: Harvard Business School Publishing Corporation; 2004:4–8.
46. United States Agency for International Development. USAID PREDICT Project: Semi-Annual Report. Available at https://www2vetmed.ucdavis.edu/ohi/local-resources/pdfs/SAR%202018%20Final. Washington, DC, 2018.
47. Carroll, D. Daszak P, Wolfe ND, et al. The global virome project. *Science*. 2018;359(6378):872–4.
48. Centers for Disease Control and Prevention. Available at https://www.cdc.gov/drugresistance/threat-report-2013/index.html. Atlanta, GA, 2013.
49. Centers for Disease Control and Prevention. Available at https://www.cdc.gov/antibiotic-use/index.html. Atlanta, GA, 2017.
50. US Food and Drug Administration. Available at https://www.fda.gov/animalveterinary/guidancecomplianceenforcement/guidanceforindustry/ucm216939.htm. Silver Spring, MD, 2018.
51. US Department of Interior. US Geological Survey. Available at https://toxics.usgs.gov/highlights/antibiotics_gw/. Reston, VA, 2018.
52. Wistrand-Yuen E, Knopp M, Hjort K, et al. Evolution of high-level resistance during low-level antibiotic exposure. *Nat Commun*. 2018;9(1):1599.
53. United Nations Environment Programme. Available at https://www.unenvironment.org/resources/frontiers-2017-emerging-issues-environmental-concern. Nairobi, Kenya, 2017.
54. Liu YY, Wang Y, Wash TR, et al. Emergence of plasmid-mediated colistin resistance mechanism MCR-1 in animals and human beings in China: A microbiological and molecular biological study. *Lancet Infect Dis*. 2016;16(2):161–68.
55. Zhang X, Doi Y, Huang X, et al. Possible transmission of mcr-1-harboring *Escherichia coli* between companion animals and human. *Emerging Infect Dis*. 2016;22(9):1679–81.
56. Wang R, van Dorp L, Shaw LP, et al. The global distribution and spread of the mobilized colistin resistance gene mcr-1. *Nat Commun*. 2018;9(1):1179.
57. Tian GB, Doi Y, Shen J, et al. MCR-1-producing *Klebsiella pneumoniae* outbreak in China. *Lancet Infect Dis*. 2017;17(6):577.
58. Poirel L, Kieffer N, Liassine N, Thanh D, Nordmann P. Plasmid-mediated carbapenem and colistin resistance in a clinical isolate of *Escherichia coli*. *Lancet Infect Dis*. 2016;16(3):282.
59. The Joint FAO–OIE–WHO global early warning system for health threats and emerging risks at the human–animal–ecosystems interface. Available at http://www.glews.net/. 2018.
60. Centers for Diseases Control and Prevention. Surveillance resources. Available at https://www.cdc.gov/westnile/resourcepages/SurResources.html. Atlanta, GA, 2015.
61. Centers for Disease Control and Prevention: Tracking trends in resistance. Available at https://www.cdc.gov/narms/index.html. Atlanta, GA, 2015.
62. World Bank Group. World Bank Report#122980-GLB: One Health: operational framework for strengthening human, animal, and environmental public health systems at their interface. Washington, DC, World Bank, Washington, DC. 2018.
63. World Bank Group. *Policy Brief: Investing in One Health*. Washington, DC: World Bank; 2018.
64. World Health Organization. Human Rabies: 2016 updates and call for data. *Wkly Epidemiology Rec*. 2017;92(7):77–88.
65. Hampson K, Coudeville L, Lembo T, et al., Estimating the global burden of endemic canine rabies. *PLoS Negl Trop Dis*. 2015;9(4):e0003709.
66. Global Health Security Agenda. Available at www.ghsagenda.org. 2018.
67. Centers for Disease Control and Prevention. Social determinants of health: Know what affects health. Available at https://www.cdc.gov/socialdeterminants/. Atlanta, GA, 2018.

CHAPTER

85 Emerging Microbial Threats to Health

Stephen M. Ostroff • James M. Hughes

INTRODUCTION

Our relationship to infectious pathogens is part of an evolutionary drama.

Joshua Lederberg

Nothing in the world of living things is permanently fixed.

Hans Zinsser

Despite great progress in the prevention and management of infectious diseases, microbial threats continue to evolve, proliferate, and result in human infection—the consequence of social and ecologic changes associated with a globalized society. The far-reaching effects of the 2003 outbreak of severe acute respiratory syndrome (SARS) highlight the ability of a previously unrecognized agent to appear unexpectedly, spread rapidly in the absence of diagnostics and effective disease prevention strategies, and cause widespread suffering as well as political, economic, and social turmoil. The emergence of SARS, a single example among many in recent years (Table 85-1), also illustrates the potential dangers of infectious agents and underscores the importance of preparedness for the unexpected. The 100th anniversary of the 1918 Spanish influenza pandemic is a reminder of the devastating impact of influenza and why concerns were raised when a new strain of influenza (H1N1) appeared in 2009. Previously known infectious diseases also continue to present new challenges. Some such as West Nile virus (WNV) infection and Zika virus have recently jumped to new continents, whereas others such as Ebola virus caused illness in urban centers of West Africa in numbers well beyond those that occurred previously. Many established diseases, such as malaria and tuberculosis, continue to exact a high burden, fueled in part by antimicrobial resistance.

In 1992, the Institute of Medicine (IOM) published a report[1] describing the increasing public health challenges posed by new, re-emerging, and drug-resistant infections and calling for improvements in the nation's public health infrastructure. The report identified six factors underlying infectious disease emergence (Box 85-1) and described their impact on diseases that had emerged in the United States in the previous two decades. In 2003, this report was updated[2] with expanded emphasis on the global impact of infectious disease threats and the international collaborative response needed to address them. In addition to the six underlying factors outlined in the first report, the new report cited seven other factors that contribute to the emergence of global microbial threats (Box 85-1). Combined, these 13 factors can be broadly categorized into four domains: genetic and biologic factors; physical environmental factors; ecologic factors; and social, political, and economic factors. These factors and their associated domains greatly affect the interaction of humans and microbes and can converge to produce an emerging global microbial threat.

This chapter describes recent emerging infectious diseases that present particular public health concerns, either because of the significance of their emergence or their continued or potential impact. The increasing problem of antimicrobial resistance—a major factor contributing to the impact of these diseases—is also discussed.

EMERGING ZOONOTIC INFECTIOUS DISEASES

Microbes that originate in animals and are transmitted to humans, either via direct transfer (zoonotic diseases) or through an intermediate vector (vector-borne diseases), are the source of a growing number of emerging infectious diseases.[3] Aided by a complex mix of social, technological, ecologic, and viral changes, zoonotic agents are increasingly crossing the barriers that once limited their geographic or host range and igniting the emergence, re-emergence, and spread of infectious diseases. Many of the new diseases that have appeared in recent years, as well as the established diseases that are increasing in incidence or expanding their range, are caused by zoonotic agents with wildlife reservoirs.[4,5] Wild mammals and birds provide a potentially rich pool of disease agents and hosts that can come into contact

TABLE 85-1 SELECTED INFECTIOUS DISEASE CHALLENGES, 1998–2017

Year	Disease (Location)
1998	Nipah virus encephalitis (Malaysia, Singapore)
1999	West Nile virus encephalitis (New York City)
2000	Rift Valley fever (Saudi Arabia, Yemen)
2001	Intentional Anthrax (USA)
2002	Vancomycin-resistant *Staphylococcus aureus* (USA)
2003	SARS (China); Monkeypox (USA)
2004	Influenza A (H5N1) (Southeast Asia)
2005	Chikungunya (Kenya, Indian Ocean Islands, India); Marburg (Angola)
2007	Zika virus (Micronesia)
2008	Lujo hemorrhagic fever (Southern Africa)
2009	Influenza A (H1N1) pandemic; *Candida auris* (Japan)
2011	Influenza A (H3N2)v (USA); *E. coli* O104:H4 (Germany)
2012	MERS (Saudi Arabia); Fungal meningitis (USA)
2013	Influenza A (H7N9) (China); Chikungunya (Caribbean)
2014	Ebola hemorrhagic fever (West Africa)
2015	Zika virus (Brazil)
2017	Monkeypox (Nigeria)

BOX 85-1 Factors Contributing to the Emergence of Infectious Diseases

Factors	Source
• Human demographics and behavior • Technology and industry • Economic development and land use • International travel and commerce • Microbial adaptation and change • Breakdown of public health measures	1992 Institute of medicine report
• Human susceptibility to infection • Climate and weather • Changing ecosystems • Poverty and social inequality • War and famine • Lack of political will	2003 Institute of medicine report

Sources: Adapted from *Institute of Medicine. Emerging Infections: Microbial Threats to Health in the United States*. Washington, DC: National Academy Press; 1992. *Institute of Medicine. Microbial Threats to Health: Emergence, Detection, and Response*. Washington, DC: National Academy Press; 2003.

with humans either naturally or, more likely, because of disruption or destabilization of their natural ecosystems.

Many emerging diseases result from transmission of infectious agents from animals to people. A literature review identified reports of 335 emerging disease events between 1940 and 2004.[6] Among these events, 60% involved transmission from animals to people, and 72% of those originated in wildlife.[6] Such events represent zoonotic spillover, defined as transmission of a pathogen from a vertebrate animal to a human which involves ecological, epidemiological, and behavioral determinants.[7,8] Of all mammals, bats harbor the highest proportion of potentially zoonotic viruses.[9] Geographic hotspots for zoonotic infectious diseases are areas of forested tropical regions experiencing land use changes (e.g., deforestation) and where wildlife diversity is high.[10] (See Chap. 84: One Health: A New Paradigm for Disease Prevention and Control.)

For example, hantavirus pulmonary syndrome was first recognized in the Four Corners area of the U.S. Southwest in 1993 when the deer mouse population increased rapidly due to climate-related food surpluses and the previously unrecognized virus spilled over into nearby human habitations. The mice were carrying an unrecognized subtype of hantavirus named Sin Nombre virus, which was transmitted to humans by direct contact with rodents or their excretions, or by inhalation of aerosolized infectious material (e.g., contaminated dust arising from disruption of rodent nests).[11,12] Sin Nombre virus is found in deer mice (*Peromyscus maniculatus*) in the western United States.[12] Spillover results in sporadic human illnesses and occasional outbreaks.

More recently, the highly lethal Nipah virus appeared after changes in agricultural practices and land use created first an emerging disease in livestock and then a health crisis in humans. The virus naturally infects *Pteropus* fruit bats, which are widely distributed in Asia and serve as the reservoir for the disease agent.[13] Nipah virus was discovered in Malaysia in 1998–1999 during an outbreak of encephalitis that killed 105 persons, most of whom had occupational exposure to ill pigs.[14–16] Changes from traditional to modern animal husbandry practices had increased the size and density of pig farms in the area, extending their reach into nearby orchards that harbored fruit bats whose natural habitats had been destroyed. Aerosolization of virus-containing bat droppings caused respiratory tract infection of the pigs, overcrowded conditions led to efficient pig-to-pig transmission, and close contact with ill animals led to infection in pig handlers that was manifested as encephalitis.[17] No person-to-person transmission was identified in this outbreak.

The virus has since caused multiple outbreaks in Bangladesh and India, causing a series of deadly outbreaks that appear to have resulted from direct contact with fruit contaminated with bat saliva.[14,18–20] Pigs have not played a role in the outbreaks in these countries. A large outbreak occurred in the Indian state of Kerala in April and May of 2018. In both the India and Bangladesh outbreaks, persons-to-person transmission has occurred, particularly involving household contacts and healthcare providers.[14]

Genetic analysis has shown Nipah virus to be closely related to Hendra virus, which was discovered in Australia as the cause of a fatal outbreak that killed 14 racehorses and two humans and also is maintained in pteropid fruit bats. The viruses constitute a new genus in the paramyxovirus family.[21]

International commerce, as well as changing human demographics, has provided opportunities for the amplification and spread of zoonotic microbes such as the monkeypox virus. Monkeypox occurs mainly in the rainforest areas of central and West Africa; disease is characterized by lesions that are similar to those seen in smallpox, which is caused by its orthopoxvirus relative variola.[22] In 2003, monkeypox appeared in prairie dogs and humans in the U.S. Midwest due to international trade in exotic pets.[23] The outbreak, which caused 47 documented human illnesses among persons exposed to ill prairie dogs that were sold or kept as pets, was traced to a shipment from Ghana of approximately 800 small mammals. A Gambian giant rat, three dormice, and two rope squirrels from the implicated shipment had laboratory evidence of monkeypox infection. After arrival in the United States, these imported animals were comingled with domestic prairie dogs, which proved to be a susceptible host for the virus and became infected. The outbreak was contained through a combination of healthcare infection control and contact tracing, identifying, and removing potentially infected animals, and a temporary ban on the capture, sale, and interstate shipment of prairie dogs. A ban on importation to the United States of rodents of African origin remains in place.

Monkeypox appears to be increasing in incidence in rainforest Africa.[24] The reason for this increase is likely multifactorial, and causes include waning immunity in persons previously vaccinated against smallpox (which is partially cross-protective for monkeypox), the increasing proportion of the population never vaccinated for smallpox, and increased opportunities for zoonotic transmission from rodent hosts.[25] One study in a health zone in the Democratic Republic of Congo (DRC) with active surveillance for monkeypox showed disease incidence increased from 0.72 cases per 10,000 persons in 1981–1986 to 14.42 cases per 10,000 persons in 2006–2007.[23] During that period the proportion of the population in that health zone ever vaccinated for smallpox decreased from 85% to 24%.[24] Large monkeypox outbreaks are now being recognized along with limited human-to-human transmission. A 2013 outbreak in the DRC involved 104 confirmed and suspected cases and a 2017 outbreak in Nigeria across 14 states involved 89 confirmed cases and many more suspected cases after no instances of this disease had been reported there in almost 40 years.[26–28]

The respiratory zoonosis SARS was first reported in late 2002 from the southern Chinese province of Guangdong.[29] It then dramatically spread to various parts of the world in February 2003, when several international travelers staying in a hotel in Hong Kong became infected after contact with an ill physician visiting from Guangdong.[30] These travelers returned home incubating the newly discovered SARS coronavirus (SARS-CoV), seeding multiple chains of transmission that, over the course of only 4 months, led to 8096 illnesses and 774 deaths in 29 locations around the world.[31,32] Retrospective analyses of banked respiratory and serologic specimens found no evidence of human infection before 2002. Studies in south China found potential zoonotic reservoirs for the virus in live wild animals such as civet cats sold for food in open markets and serologic evidence of human infections in workers in these markets.[33] Of note, no evidence of SARS-CoV was found in the same animal species in the wild in China. Subsequent studies suggested these animals were intermediate hosts, and that like other coronaviruses, the wildlife reservoir for SARS-CoV is bats.[34–36]

SARS is unique for several reasons. First, its sudden emergence and rapid spread caused worldwide panic along with economic, political, and transportation disruption on a scale that is fortunately not often seen with public health emergencies. Second, the virus could spread not only in zoonotic fashion, but also from person-to-person, especially through nosocomial "superspreading" events.[36,37] Third, its transmission dynamics, especially outside of healthcare settings, made control of the disease possible through the use of public health interventions like infection prevention in healthcare settings and community containment measures.[38] Since 2004, no SARS illnesses have been reported anywhere in the world despite ongoing surveillance. Whether the absence of reported disease means the virus is no longer in circulation is unknown. Recently, a closely related coronavirus (known as SADS-CoV) originating in bats from the same area of southern China as SARS-CoV was identified as the cause of a large outbreak of fatal swine acute diarrheal syndrome (SADS) in China that began in 2016.[39] Due to the global implications the re-emergence of SARS would have, it is only one of four diseases with mandatory notification to the World Health Organization (WHO) under the 2005 revisions of the International Health Regulations.[40]

Less than a decade after SARS appeared, in 2012 another previously unknown coronavirus-associated respiratory disease was identified, first in a Saudi Arabian patient with fatal illness and shortly afterwards in a Qatari patient hospitalized in London.[41,42] This new disease was named Middle East respiratory syndrome, or MERS, and the virus was designated MERS coronavirus (MERS-CoV). Retrospectively, a 13-person nosocomial outbreak that occurred in April 2012 in Jordan was determined to be caused by MERS and represented the earliest evidence of this infection in humans.[43]

Although SARS was rapidly contained in humans, this has not been the situation with MERS as cases have been continuously diagnosed since its initial detection. Through August 2018, a total of 2248 MERS cases have been reported, including 798 fatalities, for a case fatality ratio of 35%.[44] Mortality is more common in elderly patients, who often have underlying comorbidities.[41] Cases have been detected in 27 countries (Fig. 85-1), although 83% have been diagnosed in Saudi Arabia and an additional 7% in other Middle Eastern countries.[44] Illnesses elsewhere, including two cases in the United States, have been in persons who had recently been in the Middle East.[45] These include a 2015 outbreak in South Korea started by a traveler returning from the Middle East, which was characterized by superspreading events in hospitals that resulted in 185 illnesses and 38 (21%) deaths.[46] There has otherwise been limited secondary transmission outside of the Middle East. However, MERS in the Middle East has been characterized by household transmission and nosocomial outbreaks, where like SARS, large numbers of healthcare workers have been infected.[47] As infection control measures have improved in Middle Eastern countries, the incidence of MERS in healthcare workers has declined.[44]

Similar to SARS-CoV, MERS-CoV appears to be of bat origin although this link is not definitive.[48] However, there is extensive evidence that dromedary camels carry MERS-CoV and serve as the major reservoir for transmission to humans.[49] Serologic and virologic evidence indicates MERS-CoV-like viruses have been present in

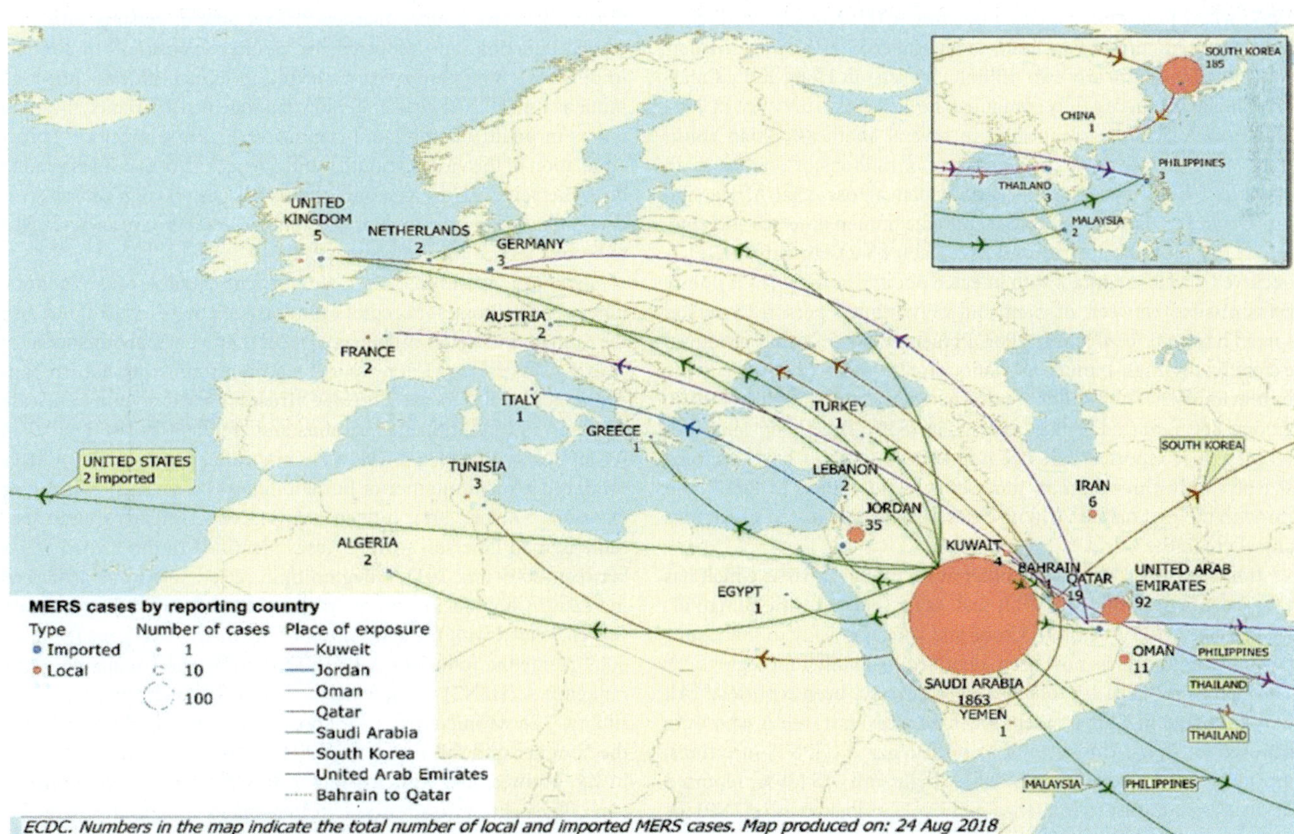

FIGURE 85-1. Distribution of cases of Middle East respiratory syndrome (MERS) by probable location of exposure 2013 through August 23, 2018. (*Source:* European CDC Rapid Risk Assessment, 22nd Update, August 29, 2018. https://ecdc.europa.eu/en/publications-data/rapid-risk-assessment-severe-respiratory-disease-associated-middle-east-11.)

dromedary camels for decades, including outside of the Middle East in Africa and Asia, despite no evidence of human illnesses prior to 2012.[50] Although this suggests the virus may have evolved to become pathogenic in humans, the reason for the recent emergence of MERS and why primary disease remains confined to exposure in the Middle East is unknown. Contact with camels is an epidemiologic risk factor for MERS-CoV infection, although many primary cases do not report recent camel exposure and the source of their infection is unclear.[41] At present, there is no specific therapeutic agent for MERS and no vaccine is available for humans or camels.

Scientists and public health officials worldwide remain concerned about the pandemic potential of avian influenza viruses, which are zoonotic agents with a wildlife reservoir.[51–53] Avian influenza is an infection of birds caused by type A strains of the influenza virus.[54] In birds, these viruses cause a wide spectrum of symptoms, ranging from mild illness to fatal disease. Migratory waterfowl, the natural reservoir of avian influenza viruses, are the most resistant to infection, whereas domestic poultry are particularly susceptible to highly pathogenic forms of avian influenza and develop rapidly fatal disease.[55] Direct or indirect contact of domestic flocks with wild migratory waterfowl has been implicated as an initiating event for poultry epidemics.[55]

In recent years, sporadic human infections with avian influenza viruses have raised concerns that currently circulating avian influenza viruses will adapt to humans through genetic mutation or reassortment with human influenza viruses and start a pandemic.[52] To date, human illnesses due to avian influenza have been caused by influenza A virus subtypes H5, H7, H9, and H10.[56,57] The two virus subtypes of greatest concern are influenza A (H5N1) and influenza A (H7N9), although small numbers of human illnesses have been caused by influenza A (H5N6), (H7N2), (H9N2), and (H10N8).[56,57]

Avian influenza viruses were first shown to cross the species barrier and cause human respiratory disease and death in Hong Kong in 1997, when highly pathogenic influenza A (H5N1) spread directly from infected chickens to humans and killed 6 of 18 infected persons.[58] Culling of nearly two million chickens in Hong Kong's markets and farms successfully contained the outbreak. However, in 2004 influenza A (H5N1) reappeared in several southeast Asian countries,[59] and despite mass culling of tens of millions of poultry in an effort to contain the virus, it spread widely across Asia, Africa, and Europe and to date has produced sporadic human illnesses and clusters in 16 countries in Africa and Asia (Table 85-2). Human illness has occurred via close contact with infected poultry, as the virus is poorly transmissible between humans and only limited person-to-person spread has been seen.[60] Since 2004, influenza A (H5N1) has produced exceptionally high human mortality despite most illness occurring in previously healthy children and young adults. Through July 2018, among 860 reported human cases, 454 (53%) have been fatal.[61] In recent years, reported cases of influenza A (H5N1) have declined sharply; only three human illnesses were identified in 2017, and through the first half of 2018 no cases have been reported in humans anywhere in the world.[56]

Influenza A (H7N9) is the other avian influenza virus which has raised pandemic concerns.[52,53] It first was associated with human illness in early 2013 in eastern China and spread quickly in that country; human illness has now been identified in 30 different regions.[56,62] Through August 2018, a total of 1567 cases have been reported.[63] All have occurred in China, except for three cases in travelers who were exposed in China. Similar to human influenza A (H5N1) infections, mortality from influenza A (H7N9) is high with 615 (39%) reported deaths.[63] In contrast to influenza A (H5N1), influenza A (H7N9) illness occurs in older persons (median age 57 years) who often have comorbidities.[56] Virtually all diagnosed cases of influenza A (H7N9) have been hospitalized with severe respiratory illness.[56] Human illness has occurred in seasonal waves, usually during the winter months.[62]

TABLE 85-2 CUMULATIVE NUMBER OF CASES OF HUMAN INFLUENZA H5N1—2003–2017

Country	Cumulative No. of Cases	Cumulative No. of Deaths (%)
Egypt	359	120 (33)
Indonesia	200	168 (84)
Vietnam	127	64 (50)
Cambodia	56	37 (66)
China	53	31 (58)
Thailand	25	17 (68)
Turkey	12	4 (33)
Azerbaijan	8	5 (63)
Bangladesh	8	1 (13)
Iraq	3	2 (67)
Pakistan	3	1 (33)
Laos	2	2 (100)
Canada	1	1 (100)
Djibouti	1	0 (0)
Myanmar	1	0 (0)
Nigeria	1	1 (100)
TOTAL	860	454 (53)

Source: WHO: http://www.who.int/influenza/human_animal_interface/2018_07_20_tableH5N1.pdf?ua=1.

Since seasonal influenza is also common in winter, laboratory confirmation of subtype is important.[62] Influenza A (H7N9) human infections have been epidemiologically linked to poultry exposure, especially in live poultry markets.[64] Over 90% of persons with confirmed infection have reported live poultry exposure.[56] In contrast to other avian influenza viruses linked to human illness, almost all influenza A (H7N9) viruses are low pathogenicity variants, meaning illness in poultry is mild and cannot serve as a sentinel to identify circulation of the virus in poultry and when control measures need to be implemented. However, once illness has been recognized, closure, depopulation, and cleaning of live poultry markets have been showed to be an effective control strategy.[65,66]

Influenza viruses that circulate in swine can also cause zoonotic illness. Swine possess receptors not only for these viruses, but also for human and avian influenza viruses, and can therefore serve as "mixing vessels" for viral reassortment into strains with human pandemic potential.[67] Swine influenza viruses that cause human disease are referred to as influenza variants and are identified with a "v." In recent years, influenza A (H1N1)v and influenza A (H1N2)v have produced a small number of human illnesses associated with swine exposure.[56] Before 2011, influenza A (H3N2)v similarly caused sporadic human illnesses, with 35 cases identified in the United States between 2005 and 2011.[68] Beginning in 2011, there was a marked increase in human infections in the United States.[69] This increase was correlated with the acquisition of the matrix (M) gene from the 2009 pandemic influenza A (H1N1) virus by the circulating swine influenza A (H3N2) virus, which was believed to enhance transmissibility.[70] These infections have mostly occurred in clusters during the summer and fall months among attendees at agricultural fairs in the Midwest and Mid-Atlantic states where swine were on display; illness has also occurred in persons exhibiting the swine.[71,72] Through 2017, 426 cases of influenza A (H3N2)v have been reported in 18 states, with the largest number linked to agricultural fairs in Indiana and Ohio (Fig. 85-2).[73] Symptoms caused by influenza A (H3N2)v have been similar to those seen with seasonal influenza,

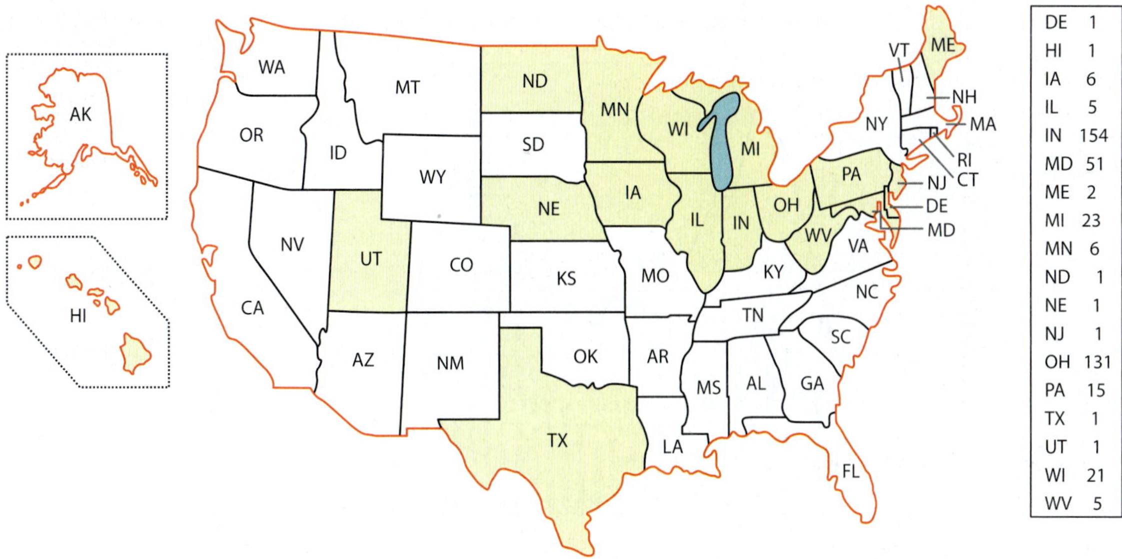

FIGURE 85-2. States with Influenza H3N2 variant infections, 2011–2017. (*Source:* CDC https://www.cdc.gov/flu/swineflu/h3n2v-case-count.htm.)

and only 26 hospitalizations and a single fatality in an individual with comorbidities have resulted.[73] Limited secondary human-to-human transmission has occurred, mostly in households, but has not been sustained.[69] Some swine exhibited at these agricultural fairs have had respiratory symptoms, but many others found to be infected have been asymptomatic.[74,75] Influenza H3N2 viruses isolated from swine at these fairs have shown high sequence homology to viruses isolated from humans.[75] In response to these clusters, public health officials have recommended a variety of measures to reduce the risk of zoonotic transmission at agricultural fairs, and have recommended that persons at high risk of influenza complications avoid exposure to pigs or swine barns at these fairs.[76]

There is no emerging infectious disease threat of greater concern to the global public health community than an influenza pandemic. The most dramatic demonstration of this threat occurred a century ago when the Spanish influenza H1N1 pandemic of 1918–1919 was estimated to have killed as many as 100 million persons worldwide.[77] That is why when in April 2009, two unrelated children near the Mexican border in California were separately diagnosed with an unusual influenza A (H1N1) virus, concerns were raised that the next pandemic could be emerging.[78] These concerns were based on several factors. First, there had not been an influenza pandemic since 1968, a period of over 40 years. Second, the virus that caused these two illnesses was a novel reassortant swine influenza virus that contained segments from a swine influenza H1N1 virus circulating in North American swine since the 1990s and segments from a Eurasian avian-like swine influenza virus.[79] Third, human illness due to swine influenza viruses usually occurs after contact with infected swine, as with the examples above. Yet neither child had a history of recent swine contact suggesting they had another means of exposure.[79]

Weeks before the two children became ill, Mexican health authorities noticed an increase in respiratory illness that resulted in 2155 cases of severe pneumonia and 100 deaths.[80] Among these deaths, 87% were in persons 5–59 years of age whereas typically only 17% of deaths from severe pneumonia in Mexico are in this age group. Upon learning of the novel influenza virus in California, nasopharyngeal specimens from patients who were part of the Mexican outbreak were examined for this virus and the identical novel influenza A (H1N1) virus (subsequently referred to as pandemic H1N1 virus, or pH1N1) was found in 29% of 8817 samples tested.[80] This confirmed the cause of the Mexican outbreak and the California findings showed it had already crossed international borders. Subsequent investigations determined that the Mexican outbreak began in February 2009 in an area of Veracruz State where swine farms were present.[81]

Other human illnesses caused by pH1N1 were quickly found in Texas, in universities, and among school students in New York City, some of whom had recent travel to Mexico.[79,82] Within weeks, pH1N1 had been detected in 41 U.S. states, 18% of whom had recently traveled to Mexico.[79] Within 8 weeks, a total of 48 countries had reported pH1N1 cases to WHO authorities, and by June 11, 2009, WHO declared that an influenza pandemic was underway.[83]

Initial reports indicated the Mexican pH1N1 outbreak was severe, but subsequent studies suggested that less severely ill patients had not been included in case counts and that the estimated mortality ratio in Mexico was 0.4%.[81] Studies examining the severity of illness associated with pH1N1 elsewhere found similar mortality ratios. Studies assessing the clinical features of pH1N1 illness found they were typical of those seen with nonpandemic seasonal influenza.[84] They also showed that pH1N1 disproportionately infected children and young adults and mostly spared the elderly, likely explaining the low mortality ratios.[85] The lack of illness in the elderly was hypothesized to result from residual immunity from exposure to influenza A (H1N1) viruses with antigenic similarities to pH1N1 that had circulated decades earlier before the 1957 Asian H2N2 influenza pandemic.[86]

As seen in previous pandemics, the 2009 pH1N1 pandemic occurred in waves (Fig. 85-3).[85,87] The initial wave dissipated in June of 2009 but was followed by a much larger wave that started in September 2009 and peaked a month later. During the pandemic period through April 2010, it was estimated that between 14% and 29% of the population (61 million persons, range estimates 43–89 million persons) in the United States was infected, although there were significant differences by age group.[88] A third of those infected were <18 years of age while only 10% were >65 years of age.[88] In one study of cases reported in the initial wave, 60% of all illnesses occurred in persons between the ages of 5 and 24 years.[85]

Mortality patterns showed that 87% of influenza-related deaths in the United States during the 2009 H1N1 pandemic occurred among persons <65 years whereas in typical influenza seasons 90% of influenza-related deaths occur in those above age 65 years.[88] This represented an 81% decrease in the risk of death from influenza over the course of the pandemic.[88] Data from outside the United States show the same pattern, with 80% of deaths globally in persons <65 years of age.[89] Two groups were found to be at especially high risk of severe illness and death during the pandemic. Pregnant women, especially

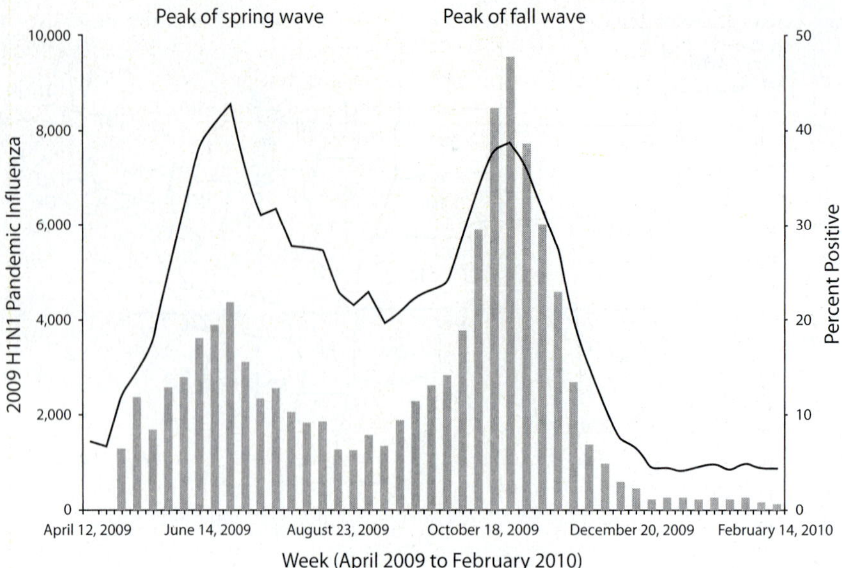

FIGURE 85-3. Waves of activity during the 2009 influenza A (H1N1) pandemic, by number of specimens tested and percent of specimens positive, United States, April 2009–February 2010. (*Source:* From Jhung MA et al. *Clin Infect Dis*. 2011;52 (Suppl 1):S13 -26.[85])

those in the third trimester, accounted for 5.7% of all deaths during the pandemic. Persons with morbid obesity (defined as a body mass index >40) were almost eight times more likely to die from influenza-related complications if hospitalized, compared to others who were hospitalized.[90,91] Impaired pulmonary function has been suggested as a cause in both risk groups.

Once the pandemic threat was identified, efforts were immediately launched to develop a monovalent pandemic vaccine, and mass-scale production occurred once studies showed the vaccine to be safe and immunogenic.[92] However, the first lots of vaccine were not available for administration until early October 2009, which was just weeks before the peak of the second wave. In the United States, the vaccine was purchased by the federal government and provided to the states for distribution and administration. Over a 3-month period, approximately 61 million doses of monovalent vaccine were administered.[93] Studies suggested vaccine efficacy for laboratory-confirmed disease was between 70% and 90%.[92] Although the vaccine became available too late to impact the trajectory of the second wave of disease, it helped to build herd immunity against the pandemic influenza virus. The pH1N1 virus displaced previously circulating influenza A (H1N1) viruses and its lineage has continued to circulate as the seasonal influenza A (H1N1) virus.[94]

Ebola virus was first identified in 1976, during the investigation of a large hemorrhagic fever outbreak in what was then Zaire, with high mortality and transmission to household contacts, healthcare workers, and funeral attendees. A number of outbreaks occurred over the next 40 plus years in Central and East African countries with high mortality. Index cases typically occurred in individuals working in forested areas as hunters or loggers with exposure to nonhuman primates. These primates were most likely infected by forest dwelling fruit bats, which are believed to be the reservoir for the virus.[95] The outbreaks were eventually controlled by international response teams working with local staff by utilizing surveillance, patient isolation, aggressive infection control efforts, contact tracing, and quarantine measures. However, countermeasure development efforts were not successful.

Beginning in 2014, an outbreak in West Africa that was centered in Guinea, Liberia, and Sierra Leone was recognized. The outbreak began in a remote area with a recent history of civil strife, porous national borders, extreme poverty, and limited healthcare capacity. Initial control efforts were not successful, and the outbreak spread to large urban centers for the first time, and to Senegal and Nigeria where aggressive surveillance and control efforts were successful in controlling the disease. By the time the outbreak was declared over in 2016, over 28,000 suspected, probable, and confirmed cases of Ebola virus disease and over 11,000 deaths had occurred. Many important lessons were learned regarding the broad clinical spectrum of the disease, the importance of compliance with rigorous infection control precautions in Ebola treatment centers, the role of sexual transmission by survivors, the importance of considering cultural factors in communication and community intervention, the role played by superspreaders, and the importance of conducting research while implementing outbreak control efforts.[96] As a result, a ring vaccination strategy with an unlicensed rVSV-ZEBOV vaccine introduced after approval for expanded access and compassionate use, was rapidly and safely implemented at scale.[97]

Four global commissions reviewed the global response to the West African epidemic and concluded that there was a need to strengthen national health systems, strengthen WHO emergency response capacity and coordination, enhance research and development programs, and provide sustainable and scalable financing to support these efforts.[98]

On May 8, 2018, an Ebola virus disease outbreak was declared in a remote rural area of Equateur Province by the Democratic Republic of the Congo (formerly Zaire), the ninth such outbreak in that country. The outbreak soon spread to Mbandaka, an urban center and transportation hub on the Congo River raising concern about regional cross-border spread. As in previous outbreaks, persons at greatest risk of infection were household contacts of cases, healthcare providers, and funeral attendees. An aggressive outbreak response involving international organizations and agencies in collaboration with local staff rapidly occurred and involved the use of a ring vaccination strategy for delivery of rVSV-ZEBOV vaccine beginning on May 21 in conjunction with a comprehensive control strategy.[99-102] One week after this outbreak ended, the tenth such outbreak was recognized in North Kivu Province in an area experiencing armed conflict, complicating control efforts, and highlighting the importance of political cooperation in the ability to control spread.

Plague is an ancient disease endemic in parts of many countries and capable of causing outbreaks with the potential for geographic spread. The disease was introduced into the continental United States by infected rats on board steamships in the late 1890s; the first documented autochthonous case occurred in the Chinatown section of San Francisco in March, 1900.[103] Plague is endemic in the western United States where sporadic cases occur each year; travel-associated cases occasionally occur in residents of eastern states.[104,105] Domestic pets, particularly cats which are highly susceptible to plague illness, are sometimes the source of human infection.[106]

Plague is also endemic in a number of countries in South America, Africa, and Asia. From 2004 to 2014, the Democratic Republic of the Congo reported 54% of the plague cases occurring worldwide. All cases occurred in Orientale Province where an endemic focus exists; two major outbreaks of pneumonic plague occurred in mining camps in the equatorial forest.[107]

The disease was introduced into Madagascar by steamships travelling from India at the end of the nineteenth century and infected the black rats in the country. Between 2010 and 2015, Madagascar accounted for three-quarters of the global burden of reported plague cases; most illness occurred in people living at 800 meters or more above sea level, where the endemic flea is found.[108] Madagascar recently experienced a large outbreak of pneumonic plague with more than 2200 confirmed, probable, and suspected reported cases and more than 200 deaths.[109] The index case in the outbreak was a 31-year-old man who became ill in late August, 2017 and took a bush taxi from the rural central highlands through the capital city to a city on the coast. He died in transit, after having exposed dozens of people who subsequently became ill.[110] A large international response was successful in controlling the outbreak, but efforts to strengthen the health system are required to address the problem and prevent a recurrence in the future.[109]

EMERGING VECTOR-BORNE INFECTIOUS DISEASES

Viruses that are spread by arthropod vectors have posed particular challenges, both in tropical areas where many previously controlled diseases have resurfaced and throughout the world as endemic diseases have appeared in new areas. There have been three examples of this phenomenon in the last 20 years marked by the sudden appearance in the Western Hemisphere of viral vector-borne diseases that have their origins in Africa.

The first of the vector-borne viruses to emerge in the Western Hemisphere is WNV. WNV is a mosquito-borne flavivirus that is maintained in a cycle primarily involving bird-feeding mosquitoes, with wild birds as the principal amplifying hosts.[111] It is occasionally transmitted by infected mosquitoes to humans and horses, in which disease may occur.[112] The virus was first isolated in the West Nile district of Uganda in 1937[113] but until 1999 was found only in Africa, southern and eastern Europe, western Asia, and western Russia, where it occasionally caused outbreaks of human and equine disease.[111] In 1999 it was identified as the cause of an epidemic of aseptic meningitis and encephalitis in New York City.[114,115] Genetic analysis of the New York City virus found, it was most closely related to a WNV identified 1 year earlier in Israel.[115] How the virus was introduced into North America is unknown, although speculation has focused on mosquitoes carried in cargo or an infected domesticated bird entered the country.[115] Once introduced into North America, the virus spread rapidly, likely through bird migratory routes, reaching the Pacific Coast by 2003 and as far south as Argentina by 2005.[116] Despite expanding throughout the Western Hemisphere, for unknown reasons epidemic disease has only occurred in the United States and Canada. In the United States, since its introduction in 1999, WNV disease has occurred annually in the summer and early fall months. Based on data reported through ArboNET, an electronic surveillance system used by the Centers for Disease Control and Prevention (CDC) and state and local health departments to track WNV infections, through 2017, 48,183 cases of WNV were reported, including 22,999 cases of severe neuroinvasive disease and 2163 deaths (4% of all reported cases) among U.S. residents.[117] The number of cases reported to ArboNET varies widely from year to year, from a low of 712 in 2011 to a high of 9862 in 2003.[117] The data show that through 2017, the highest annual incidence of disease has occurred in the high plains in the Midwest where *Culex tarsalis* mosquitoes predominate as the main transmission vector (Fig. 85-4). The virus has been identified in 65 mosquito species and 326 bird species.[116]

Numerous studies have demonstrated that 75–80% of WNV infections are asymptomatic, and the occurrence of symptomatic

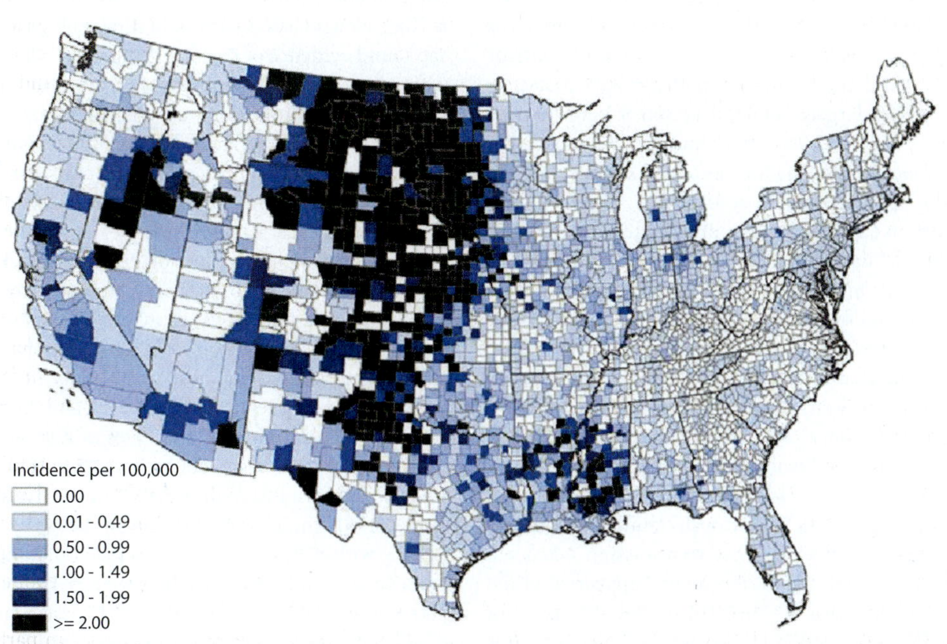

FIGURE 85-4. Average annual incidence of West Nile virus neuroinvasive disease reported to CDC by county, 1999–2017. (*Source:* https://www.cdc.gov/westnile/statsmaps/cumMapsData.html.)

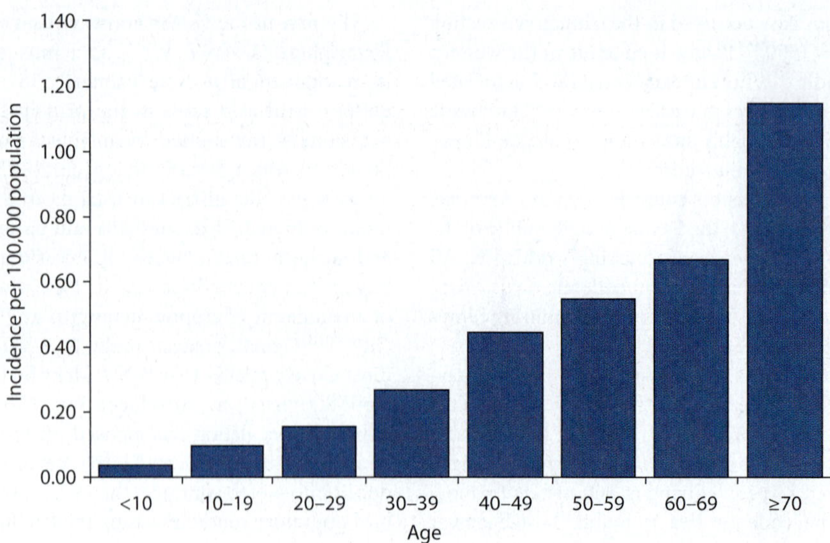

FIGURE 85-5. Average annual incidence of West Nile virus neuroinvasive disease reported to CDC by age group, 1999–2017. (*Source:* ArboNet. https://www.cdc.gov/westnile/statsmaps/cumMapsData.html.)

and severe disease and death rises with age (Fig. 85-5).[116,117] Therefore, the number of WNV infections in the United States is considerably higher than the number of ill individuals reported in ArboNET. Once large numbers of cases began to occur in the United States, previously unknown modes of transmission were identified, including through transfused blood and transplanted organs from asymptomatic donors, prompting screening of the blood supply to begin in 2003 which has resulted in the removal of >3000 infected units from the blood supply.[112] Intrauterine transmission and transmission through breast milk have also been seen.[112]

The second African-origin virus to emerge in the Americas is chikungunya (CHIKV) virus, which was first identified in Tanzania in 1952.[118] In rural Africa CHIKV has an enzootic sylvatic cycle involving nonhuman primates, but in other locations the virus cycles between humans and *Aedes* mosquitoes without an intermediate zoonotic host.[119] Therefore, CHIKV-infected travelers play an important role in the movement of the virus to new areas and increasing global air travel has likely contributed to its spread.[119] Until the beginning of the twenty-first century, CHIKV disease was largely confined to sub-Saharan Africa and southeast Asia.[120] But in 2004, a new lineage that was better adapted to *Aedes albopictus* mosquitoes emerged on the Kenyan coastline and then spread rapidly across the Indian Ocean islands to India, where in only a year beginning in late 2005 it caused >1.3 million illnesses.[120] In 2007, an infected traveler from India introduced the virus to Italy, resulting in 217 locally acquired cases of CHIKV. In 2014 a total of 11 cases occurred in southern France introduced by a traveler returning from Cameroon.[120,121]

Although travel-associated cases of CHIKV had been diagnosed in the Americas for many years, localized transmission did not result.[122] That changed in October 2013, when an outbreak of CHIKV infections was identified on the French side of the Caribbean island of St. Martin in persons with no history of travel.[123] The causative agent was an Asian lineage CHIKV previously found in southeast Asia and the Pacific Islands.[119] Once local transmission occurred, CHIKV moved rapidly through the Caribbean and appeared on the northern coast of South America.[119,124] In 2014, a total of 11 cases of locally acquired CHIKV occurred in Florida where *Aedes aegypti* is present but did not spread widely or persist.[125] Since its introduction to the Western Hemisphere, through 2017 more than 2.5 million suspected cases (with over 339,000 of these cases laboratory confirmed) of locally acquired CHIKV have been reported to the Pan American Health Organization from 43 countries in the Americas (Fig. 85-6).[126]

The third African virus to emerge in the Western Hemisphere is Zika virus, a flavivirus first detected in 1947 in a nonhuman primate in Uganda.[127] Zika was initially reported to have an enzootic cycle that only involved nonhuman primates and *Aedes* mosquitoes in Africa until a serosurvey conducted in Uganda in 1952 provided the first evidence of human infection.[128] As with CHIKV, Zika also has a nonzoonotic transmission cycle involving humans and *Aedes* mosquitoes.[129] In 1954, the first human illness due to Zika was confirmed in Nigeria.[130] However, over the next half century only 13 other human illnesses due to Zika had been recognized despite evidence that Zika virus continued to circulate in Africa and Asia.[131] In 2007, an outbreak of febrile rash illness with musculoskeletal symptoms and conjunctivitis occurred on the Micronesian island of Yap that was determined to be caused by the Asian lineage of Zika virus.[131] The outbreak consisted of 49 laboratory confirmed and 59 suspected cases of Zika, all associated with mild illness. A serosurvey performed on Yap found evidence of recent infection in 73% of island residents >3 years of age, only 19% of whom reported clinically compatible illness, suggesting most infections were asymptomatic.[131] In 2013, a larger outbreak due to Zika occurred in French Polynesia with an estimated 28,000 cases, representing 10% of the territory's population.[132] Outbreaks subsequently occurred elsewhere in the South Pacific.[129]

In March 2015, Zika virus appeared in the Americas when an outbreak was identified in northeastern Brazil.[133] Within months the outbreak spread to 14 Brazilian states and Colombia, and by January 2016, a total of 20 countries or territories in the Americas were reporting locally acquired Zika infections.[134] At the peak of the outbreak in early 2016, almost 40,000 suspected and confirmed cases of Zika were being reported (Fig. 85-7), and through the end of 2017, a total of 806,928 vector-borne cases of Zika virus (28% confirmed) had been reported by 48 countries and territories in the Americas; 46% of these cases were in Brazil.[135] In the United States during that time period, there were 231 locally acquired, vector-borne cases of Zika with 95% occurring in south Florida and the remainder in south Texas.[136] In Puerto Rico there were 37,139 locally acquired, vector-borne cases.[136] By the middle of 2017, cases of Zika had declined significantly throughout the Americas (Fig. 85-7).[137]

The upsurge of cases in the Americas led to the identification of both serious complications of Zika infection and previously unrecognized modes of transmission.[138,139] The most serious complication was

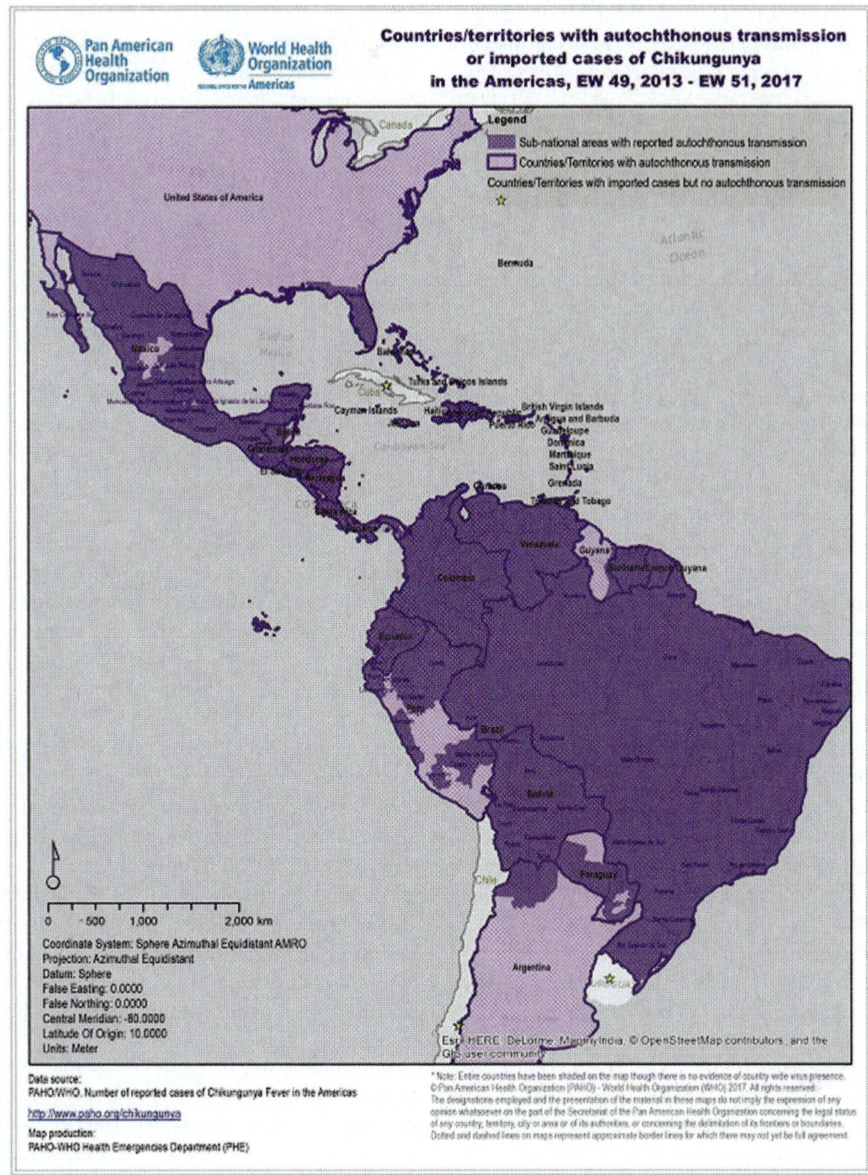

FIGURE 85-6. Countries/territories with autochthonous tranmission or imported cases of chikungunya in the Americas, EW 49, 2013 - EW 51, 2017.) *Source:* Used with Permission from © Pan American Health Organization (PAHO) – World Health organization (WHO) 2017. All rights reserved. Retrieved from https://www.paho.org/hq/images/stories/AD/HSD/IR/Viral_Diseases/Chikungunya/CHIKV-Data-Caribbean-2017-EW-51.jpg.

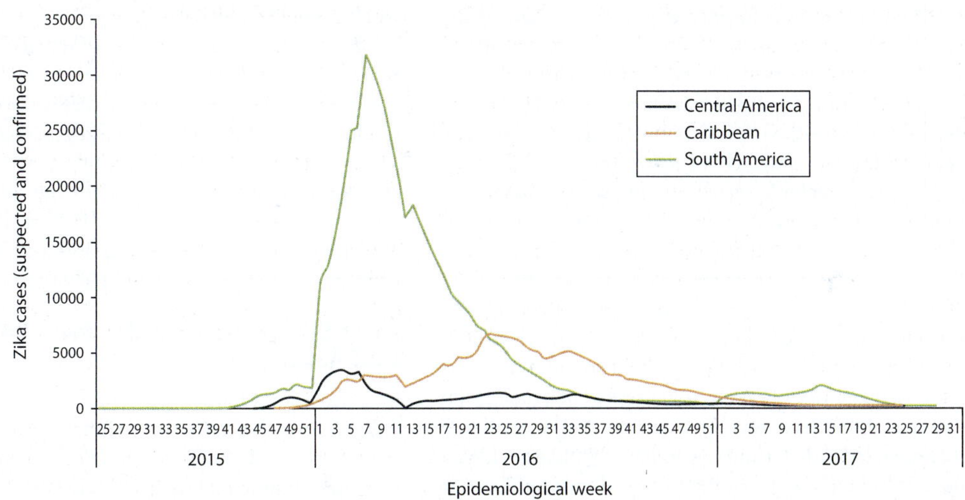

FIGURE 85-7. Reported suspected and confirmed cases of Zika virus reported to the Pan American Health Organization (PAHO) in three regions of the Americans, May 2015 to August 2017. (*Source:* Data provided by countries and territories of the Americas and reproduced by PAHO/WHO. Used with Permission. Retrieved from https://www.paho.org/hq/index.php?option=com_content&view=article&id=11599:regional-zika-epidemiological-update-americas&Itemid=41691&lang=en.)

the occurrence of microcephaly through transplacental transmission of the virus during pregnancy. This potential association was seen in Brazil in the autumn of 2015, and led to WHO declaring the Zika epidemic a public health emergency of international concern (PHEIC) under the 2005 revision of the International Health Regulations.[139,140] In Brazil alone, through mid-2017, a total of 2952 cases of microcephaly and other congenital malformations of the central nervous system were identified with 1023 of these cases having laboratory evidence of Zika infection.[141] Zika-associated cases of microcephaly were also identified in other affected countries and territories.

A second serious complication of Zika infection was Guillain-Barre syndrome (GBS), a complication that was also seen in the French Polynesia outbreak several years earlier.[129] In seven Latin American countries, rates of GBS rose between 2.0 and 9.8 times over baseline coincident with periods of high Zika activity.[142] While several instances of likely sexual transmission of Zika virus were reported prior to the onset of the epidemic in the Americas, this mode of transmission was confirmed among partners of infected travelers who had come to the United States from areas with vector-borne Zika transmission, and infectious virus has been identified in semen up to 69 days after symptom onset.[129,143] In the United States, 52 instances of sexual transmission have been identified.[136] Since many Zika infections are asymptomatic, concerns arose about the safety of the blood supply, and screening of the blood supply was initiated. In 2016 alone, a total of 38 presumptive viremic blood donors were identified in the United States (23 in Florida) along with 325 presumptive viremic blood donors in Puerto Rico.[136]

There are no licensed vaccines available for any of the three vector-borne viruses that were introduced into the Western Hemisphere in the last 20 years. However, given the significant public health impact of these diseases, especially Zika virus infection, efforts to develop vaccines are underway.[144]

Dengue viruses have become the most important human arboviral pathogens to emerge globally. Dengue is endemic in Africa, the tropical Americas, and parts of the Middle East, Asia, and the Western Pacific.[145] The frequency of dengue and its more severe complications, dengue hemorrhagic fever (DHF) and dengue shock syndrome (DSS), have increased dramatically since 1980.[145] Dengue is caused by four closely related flaviviruses transmitted by mosquitoes, primarily by domestic and peridomestic, day-biting *Aedes aegypti*. *Ae. albopictus* is also a competent vector. *Ae. aegypti* was historically found in Africa but spread through the world's tropical regions over the past two centuries through international commerce. A global pandemic of dengue began in Southeast Asia after World War II and has since intensified, with more frequent and progressively larger epidemics associated with severe disease.[146] The resurgence and spread of dengue and DHF have been most dramatic in Asia, Latin America, and the Caribbean including Puerto Rico and the U.S. Virgin Islands, where the uncontrolled growth of urban shanty towns with poor sanitation and unreliable water systems has led to the proliferation of the *Ae. aegypti* mosquito vector in open water pools.[146–148] Other contributing factors include climate change and population movements.

In the United States, outbreaks have occurred in south Texas in conjunction with outbreaks in northern Mexico in 1980, 1999, 2005, and 2013.[149] Outbreaks have also occurred in southern Florida including Key West, where autochthonous cases occurred in 2009 and 2010 followed by sporadic cases in additional counties in southern Florida in subsequent years.[150] A recently licensed dengue vaccine is currently approved, but has created a dilemma.[151] The vaccine is currently recommended only for those who have serologic evidence of prior dengue infection because of the observed increased risk of severe dengue in vaccines who have not had prior dengue infection.[152,153] The need for prevaccination screening may be a challenge for immunization programs managers to implement.

Yellow fever viruses are maintained in a sylvatic cycle involving nonhuman primates and mosquitoes in rain forest settings in South America and sub-Saharan Africa in which *Haemagogus* species of mosquitoes are involved. These viruses can also be transmitted to humans in an urban cycle in which *Ae. aegypti* mosquitoes play an important role. Reported cases have increased in recent years as a result of population growth, urbanization, globalization, and inadequate public health infrastructure.

Recent large outbreaks have occurred in Brazil,[154] Angola[155] with cross-border spread to the Democratic Republic of the Congo,[156] and Nigeria.[157] In Brazil, human cases have occurred near large urban centers posing the risk of urban transmission. Urban centers were affected in Angola. Control efforts included mass vaccination campaigns, highlighting the global shortage of yellow fever vaccine.[158,159]

These outbreaks illustrated the risk of infection in unvaccinated travelers from nonyellow fever countries,[160] the risk of cross-border spread (in addition to DRC, imported cases from Angola were identified in Kenya and China, the latter representing the alarming introduction of the virus into Asia).[161,162] Fortunately, no local transmission occurred in China.

In response to the issues raised by these outbreaks, WHO, UNICEF, and Gavi, the Vaccine Alliance, have launched the Eliminate Yellow Fever Epidemics (EYE) Strategy, which aims to eliminate yellow fever epidemics worldwide by 2026. The strategy includes developing the capacity to conduct preventive mass vaccination programs and the strengthening of routine immunization programs including yellow fever vaccine in endemic countries.[163,164]

Heartland virus, a member of the genus *Phlebovirus* in the Bunyavirus family, was initially described in 2012.[165] Cases have since been reported in men over the age of 50 years with a nonspecific febrile illness and history of a tick bite within 2 weeks prior to onset in most cases.[166–169] Illnesses have occurred in residents of Missouri, Oklahoma, Tennessee, and Arkansas between May and September. Two of nine reported cases have died, one of whom had widely disseminated infection with severe shock and multisystem organ failure.[170] The virus has been detected by PCR and culture in the lone star tick (*Amblyomma americanum*).[171] The reservoir has not been identified.

Bourbon virus, a member of the genus *Thogotovirus* in the Orthomyxovirus family, was first described in 2014 in a resident of Bourbon county in eastern Kansas.[172,173] The patient was a man over the age of 50 with a nonspecific febrile illness, a history of recent tick bites and removal of an engorged tick, and a diffuse maculopapular rash. His illness progressed to multisystem organ failure resulting in his death. A subsequent study detected the virus in adult males and nymphs of *A. americanum* collected in Bourbon county.[174] The reservoir has not been identified.

Oropouche virus, a member of the genus *Orthobunyavirus* in the Bunyavirus family, was first described in 1961 in Trinidad.[176] Large outbreaks and sporadic disease cases have since been reported in tropical areas of Brazil, Peru, and Panama.[178,179] The illness is characterized by fever, headache, myalgia, arthralgia, retro-orbital pain, photophobia, and skin rash.[175,177–180] The virus is transmitted by biting midges (*Culicoides paraensis*).[176,179–181] This midge can breed in piles of rotting banana plants and cacao husks; farmers exposed to these items appear to be at increased risk of infection.[180,181]

EMERGING FOOD-BORNE AND WATER-BORNE DISEASES

In a first-of-its-kind report released in 2015, the World Health Organization estimated the global burden of food-borne disease caused by 31 different food-borne agents that included bacteria, viruses, parasites, and toxins.[182] The WHO report found that an estimated 10% of the world's population experiences a food-borne illness every year, which translates to 600 million food-borne illnesses annually. Among those who became ill there were 420,000 deaths, with a third of the deaths occurring in children <5 years of age. Diarrhea was present in 91% (548 million) of food-borne illnesses episodes.

TABLE 85-3 AGENT SPECIFIC ILLNESS (600 MILLION) AND DEATHS (420,000)			
Agent	Illnesses (%)	Deaths (%)	CFR
Norovirus	124 m (21%)	35,000 (8%)	0.03%
Campylobacter	95 m (16%)	21,000 (5%)	0.02%
Enterotoxigenic *E. coli*	87 m (15%)	26,000 (6%)	0.03%
Nontyphi Salmonella	79 m (13%)	59,000 (14%)	0.07%
Protozoa	67 m (11%)	6,000 (1%)	<0.01%
Shigella	51 m (9%)	15,000 (4%)	0.03%
Enteropathogenic *E. coli*	24 m (4%)	37,000 (9%)	0.15%
Hepatitis A	14 m (2%)	28,000 (7%)	0.23%
Helminths	13 m (2%)	45,000 (11%)	0.35%
Salmonella typhi	12 m (2%)	52,000 (12%)	0.4%
Cholera	0.8 m (0.1%)	25,000 (6%)	3.3%
Aflatoxin	0.02 m	19,000 (5%)	86.4%

Source: WHO. *WHO Estimates of the Global Burden of Foodborne Diseases: Foodborne Disease Burden Epidemiology Reference Group 2007 -2015*. Geneva: WHO; 2015.[182]

Among the 31 agents, norovirus was the leading cause of illness causing 21% of all episodes, while nontyphoidal Salmonella caused the most deaths (14%) (Table 85-3).

In the WHO report, the vast majority of food-borne disease occurs in less-developed countries.[182] However, food-borne illness is also a significant problem in more developed settings. In the United States, CDC estimates that there are 48 million food-borne illnesses that result in 128,000 hospitalizations and 3000 deaths each year.[183,184] Among these 48 million illnesses, only 20% are estimated to be caused by known pathogens or toxins, suggesting there are agents of food-borne illness that have yet to be discovered.

To monitor the incidence of food-borne illness in the United States and assess trends, in 1996 CDC established FoodNet, which consists of 10 locations around the country with a combined population of almost 50 million persons that conduct active surveillance for infections caused by eight major food-borne pathogens.[185] In preliminary FoodNet data for 2017, there were 24,484 illnesses caused by these eight pathogens in the 10 surveillance locations, with *Salmonella* and *Campylobacter* infections having the highest incidence, at 19.0 and 16.2 cases per 100,000 population, respectively.[186] For six of the eight pathogens (*Cyclospora, Yersinia, Vibrio*, Shiga-toxin–producing *Escherichia coli* (STEC), *Listeria, and Campylobacter*) the incidence in 2017 was significantly higher than in the preceding 3-year time period (2014–2016).[186] Whether these results represent true increases in incidence or reflect changing diagnostic practices which include the increasing availability and use of culture-independent diagnostic tests (CIDTs) in clinical settings is unclear.[186]

Outbreaks of food-borne illness also provide insights into patterns of food-borne illness. They often are the first indications of emerging threats to the food supply. CDC recently summarized data on outbreaks that occurred in the United States over the 7-year period 2009–2015.[187] During this period, there were 5760 outbreaks reported by the states to CDC involving 100,939 illnesses and 145 deaths. Only 3% of these outbreaks were multistate, but these accounted for 11% of all illnesses and 54% of the deaths. For 1281 (22%) of the outbreaks, the cause of illness could be classified into a single food category. Among these outbreaks, 31% were due to meat products, 27% were due to seafood, and 26% were produce-associated. However, the seafood outbreaks involved considerably fewer cases on average than those involving meat and produce. Significant outbreaks that occurred during the 7-year period covered by the report include: listeriosis from cantaloupes that resulted in 33 deaths;[188] the first known outbreak of listeriosis associated with caramel apples;[189] *E. coli* O157:H7 from consumption of commercially packaged, ready-to-bake raw cookie dough,[190] and a massive egg-associated outbreak of *Salmonella enteritidis* involving 1519 cases that led to the recall of 550 million eggs.[191]

The epidemiology of food-borne illness continues to evolve as changes in food production, distribution, and consumption create opportunities for new pathogens to emerge, well-recognized pathogens to increase in prevalence or become associated with new food vehicles, and widespread outbreaks to occur.[192] Among the notable changes in the United States food system are increasing importation of foods in commodity categories such as seafood and produce; alterations in dietary patterns to promote consumer health and nutrition including increases in consumption of produce; and changing modes of food delivery such as online ordering of prepared foods and groceries.

The array of food-borne pathogens also changes and grows. Food-borne pathogens that have been added to the list include bacteria (*E. coli* O157:H7 and other STEC, *Listeria monocytogenes, Campylobacter jejuni, Yersinia enterocolitica*), parasites (*Cryptosporidium, Cyclospora*), and viruses (noroviruses). In addition, prions have been discovered to cause fatal neurodegenerative conditions (transmissible spongiform encephalopathies) in animals and humans. Many of these agents are zoonotic in origin.

First recognized as a human pathogen in 1982, *E. coli* O157:H7 has become a major cause of hemorrhagic colitis and hemolytic uremic syndrome.[193] In the United States, *E. coli* O157:H7 has been estimated to cause 63,000 food-borne illnesses annually and 20 deaths.[183] A zoonotic agent, *E. coli* O157:H7 colonizes the intestinal tract of agricultural animals, most often cattle,[194–196] and is transmitted to humans through fecally contaminated food, milk, or water and through direct animal contact. Food-borne transmission is estimated to account for 85% of *E. coli* O157:H7 illnesses and 65% of outbreaks.[197] Although most food-borne outbreaks due to *E. coli* O157:H7 in the United States were initially associated with consumption of undercooked ground beef,[198] the patterns of foods implicated in outbreaks is more diverse, with contaminated beef causing just over half of outbreaks followed by produce at 21%.[197] The two largest recent outbreaks in the United States have been due to leafy greens. A spinach associated outbreak in 2006 resulted in 199 illnesses and a romaine lettuce outbreak in 2018 resulted in 210 illnesses.[199,200]

The role of other STEC in causing food-borne illness is increasingly appreciated as surveillance and diagnostic assays improve.[201] The range of clinical manifestations varies widely for non-O157 STEC, but illness is generally milder and less likely to result in bloody diarrhea than illness seen with *E. coli* O157:H7.[202] Globally, STEC (including *E. coli* O157:H7) are estimated to annually cause more than 2.8 million acute infections; in the United States non-O157 STEC cause twice as much illness as *E. coli* O157:H7 with an estimated 113,000 illnesses occurring annually.[183,203] Serotypes associated with illness and outbreaks include *E. coli* O26, O45, O103, O104, O111, O121, and O145. A massive outbreak of *E. coli* O104:H4 infections occurred in Germany in 2011 that was caused by sprouts grown from fenugreek seeds imported from Egypt and resulted in 3816 illnesses, 845 instances of hemolytic uremic syndrome, and 54 deaths. Cases associated with this outbreak were also identified in 15 other countries.[204]

Increasing global trade in food, especially fresh fruits and vegetables, plays a significant role in the emergence of the coccidian parasite *Cyclospora cayetanensis* as an important food-borne pathogen.[205] *Cyclospora* was first definitively identified in the early 1990s in Peru, although diarrheal illnesses likely caused by this parasite were reported as early as the 1970s among residents and travelers in tropical locations and immunocompromised persons.[206] *C. cayetanensis* is found in tropical and subtropical locations worldwide. Humans are considered the host reservoir although person-to-person transmission does not occur, because after fecal excretion the parasite must mature in the environment for at least 7 days to become infectious.[207]

Transmission occurs via contaminated food or water. Between 1995 and 2000, *Cyclospora* was identified as the cause of repeated outbreaks of food-borne illness involving thousands of cases due to consumption of raspberries imported from Guatemala to the United States.[206,207] Other outbreaks in North America and Europe due to *Cyclospora* have been linked to imported basil, snow peas, cilantro, and bagged leafy greens.[206,207] Unsanitary conditions, including the use of water contaminated with the parasite in produce fields or poor worker hygienic practices, are thought to contribute to these outbreaks.[206] The number of cases identified in the United States has risen in recent years as surveillance has improved and diagnostic tests are more widely used.[208] More than 2000 nontravel associated cases were reported in the United States in 2018, which represents more nontravel associated cases than were identified during the preceding 17-year period.[209] That same year, two large outbreaks were identified in the United States. The first, involving 250 cases, was linked to vegetable trays containing broccoli, cauliflower, and carrots with ingredients of both domestic and international origin.[209] The second, involving 511 cases, occurred at a large fast-food chain and was due to bagged salad containing romaine lettuce and carrots that was potentially from domestic sources.[209] Investigations conducted in the United States in 2018 identified for the first time *Cyclospora* in domestically grown cilantro and romaine lettuce, demonstrating that this parasite is no longer only a problem in imported foods.[210]

Changes in agricultural practices are the basis for the recognition of a new class of food-borne pathogen, the prion. Although prion diseases in animals have long been recognized, the emergence in 1996 of a new variant form of Creutzfeld-Jakob disease (vCJD) brought these agents to international attention. The etiologic agent proved to be indistinguishable from that of bovine spongiform encephalopathy (BSE), a fatal neurodegenerative disease of cattle that caused a large-scale bovine epidemic in Great Britain beginning in 1986.[211] Cattle in Britain had presumably been exposed to the BSE agent since about 1982, when changes in the rendering process allowed contamination of cattle feed with infected tissues from previously slaughtered cows. Consumption of BSE-infected feed allowed the agent to recirculate within the cattle population and subsequently enter the human food chain via contaminated meat products.[211-213]

Since 1986, BSE has been confirmed in Japan, Israel, Canada, the United States, and more than 20 European countries;[214,215] most BSE cases outside of Britain have been traced to the importation of British cattle. BSE transmission to humans has led to more than 150 cases of invariably fatal vCJD, the vast majority occurring in Britain. Four cases of BSE have been reported in the United States; two appear to have been exposed in the United Kingdom and one in Saudi Arabia while the site of exposure of the fourth is uncertain.[216] Compared with the extent and speed of transmission of BSE in cattle, vCJD cases have increased very slowly. However, a likely long interval between exposure and development of symptoms raises concerns about the future appearance of additional cases as well as the risk of blood-borne transmission.[211,212,217]

Infections are also emerging through the water-borne route, i.e., from ingestion of contaminated drinking water or through immersion in contaminated water.[218] Increases in recreational water-associated outbreaks have also been reported, from both treated and fresh water sources.[219] The commonly recognized water-borne pathogens include several groups of enteric bacteria, protozoa, and viruses. For example, contaminated drinking water has been implicated in outbreaks of campylobacteriosis,[220] and *E. coli* O157:H7 has been transmitted via recreational water, well water, and contaminated municipal water.[197] In 1992, *Vibrio cholerae* O139, a novel strain, was first detected in South Asia and quickly spread to many regions of India and Bangladesh.[221] The most important parasitic protozoa associated with water-borne transmission are *Giardia lamblia* and chlorine-resistant *Cryptosporidium parvum*. The latter caused a municipal water outbreak of cryptosporidiosis that affected more than 400,000 people in Milwaukee, Wisconsin in 1993, and motivated authorities to reassess the adequacy of water-quality protections.[222] Although water-borne outbreaks of norovirus gastroenteritis are far less common than food-borne outbreaks, norovirus outbreaks have been associated with contaminated municipal water, well water, stream water, commercial ice, lake water, and swimming pool water.[223]

Cholera, an ancient disease, has emerged in Haiti following a natural disaster and in Yemen during armed conflict. Following a devastating earthquake in Haiti on January 12, 2010, a prolonged relief effort began.[224] On October 21, 2010, a cholera outbreak was confirmed by the Haitian National Public Health Laboratory.[225,226] An extensive epidemiologic and laboratory investigation provided evidence that the epidemic strain was closely related to Asian variant *V. cholerae* El Tor O1 strains previously isolated in Bangladesh in 2002 and 2008.[227] The outbreak began in a village downstream from a camp for the United Nations (UN) Stabilization Mission to Haiti, which had discharged sewage into a tributary of the Artibonite River. A contingent of soldiers from Nepal, where cholera is endemic, had recently arrived at the camp. Molecular genotyping indicated that the epidemic strain southern Asian type *V. cholerae* was introduced into Haiti as a result of population movement and human activity.[228] This strain is now endemic in Haiti. This experience highlights the importance and urgency of a comprehensive, integrated strategy for cholera prevention and control including use of cholera vaccine and improving access to safe water and adequate sanitation.[229-231]

A very large cholera epidemic that began in late 2016 has impacted Yemen in the setting of conflict, population displacement, destruction of healthcare facilities, and limited water supply and sanitation infrastructure.[232-234] The epidemic began during the dry season and exploded during the subsequent rainy season beginning in April 2017, becoming the largest cholera outbreak in modern times.[235] The epidemic strain is *V. cholerae* O1, serotype Ogawa. An international response involving WHO, the United Nations International Children's Fund (UNICEF), Medicins sans Frontieres, and the International Committee of the Red Cross among others, has succeeded in reducing the case-fatality rate to less than 1%,[235] a remarkable achievement given the devastating impact of the ongoing military conflict on healthcare facilities in the country.

Leptospirosis is a zoonotic disease with reservoirs in wild, peridomestic, and domestic animals. Leptospirosis outbreaks can occur following exposure to contaminated flood waters. [236,237] Outbreaks have involved adventure travelers,[238] multisport endurance race participants,[239] and triathalon participants[240] exposed to contaminated surface water. More recently, an outbreak in Puerto Rico following Hurricane Maria resulted in more than 50 cases and more than 20 deaths.[241]

ANTIMICROBIAL DRUG RESISTANCE

Adding to the health impact and challenges of emerging infections is the growing resistance of infectious agents to antimicrobial drugs.[242,243] Shortly after release of the IOM consensus report, *The Washington Post* published an article entitled "Running Out of Wonder Drugs."[244] This called attention to the continuing emergence of antibiotic resistance and raised concern about the possibility of a return to a preantibiotic era, because of the occurrence of serious bacterial infections caused by organisms resistant to all available antibiotics (sometimes referred to as superbugs), a concern that is very real today. Antibiotic resistance is an urgent, complex, multifaceted, local, national, and global challenge resulting in increased morbidity, mortality, and healthcare costs, threatening health security and the national and global economy, and challenging clinicians, veterinarians, microbiologists, infection preventionists, behavioral scientists, public health professionals, environmental scientists, and policy makers.

Not only are antimicrobial-resistant organisms increasing in number, but they are also expanding their geographic range, increasing the breadth of their resistance, and spreading from healthcare settings into the community.[242,245] Drug-resistant organisms include all major groups of disease-causing agents: bacteria such as staphylococci, enterococci, and gram-negative bacilli, which cause serious infections in hospitalized patients; bacteria that cause respiratory diseases such as pneumonia and tuberculosis; food-borne pathogens such as Salmonella and *Campylobacter*; sexually transmitted organisms such as *Neisseria gonorrhoeae*; strains of HIV and other viruses; *Candida* and other fungi; and protozoa such as *Plasmodium falciparum*.

In 2013, the CDC estimated that two million illnesses per year in the United States were caused by antibiotic-resistant organisms, resulting in eight million extra days of hospitalization, 23,000 deaths, and over $20 billion in direct healthcare costs.[246] An estimated 33,000 deaths per year in Europe are caused by antibiotic-resistant organisms.[247] The current worldwide estimate is 700,000 deaths per year with a projected increase to 10 million deaths per year by 2050 if current trends continue.[248] Antibiotic resistance has implications for public health, animal health, agriculture, and environmental health; resistance has the potential to compromise our ability to treat patients on chemotherapy for cancer, care for solid organ and bone marrow transplant patients, and to treat patients in critical care and trauma units and neonatal intensive care units (ICUs). In the United States, CDC has identified *Clostridioides difficile*, carbapenem-resistant *Enterobacteriaceae*, and multidrug-resistant (MDR) *N. gonorrhoeae* as top priority urgent threats to health.[246] Worldwide, WHO has identified carbapenem-resistant *Acinetobacter baumannii*, carbapenem-resistant *Pseudomonas aeruginosa*, and carbapenem-resistant, third-generation cephalosporin-resistant *Enterobacteriaceae* as top priority critical pathogens.[248] MDR and extensively drug-resistant (XDR) *Mycobacterium tuberculosis* and MDR *P. falciparum* are also of great concern.[249–251]

Why and how has this threat of antibiotic resistance emerged? The modern antibiotic era dates to the discovery of penicillin by Sir Alexander Fleming in 1928. However, it was not until 1940 that Howard Florey and Ernst Chain were able to purify the drug. Efforts to produce the drug, driven in part by the need for an effective treatment for injured soldiers with life-threatening infections during World War II, led to availability of small amounts of the drug by 1942. Its use resulted in dramatic responses in patients and a realization of the value of this wonder drug, leading Dr. Fleming to warn in 1945 of the potential for overuse and misuse of the agent to lead to resistance in bacteria-causing infections. Since numerous other antibiotics were developed in the late 1940s through the 1960s, the golden age of antibiotics, a sense of complacency developed as a result of the impression of the existence of a robust antibiotic development pipeline. However, the drug development pipeline withered in the 1970s and the early 1980s, with the last new class of antibiotics being introduced in the mid-1980s. The most important driver in the emergence of antibiotic resistance is microbial adaptation in response to selective pressures in the microbial environment (i.e., antibiotic pressure). Bacterial exposure to any antibiotic results in selective pressure, which is why judicious antibiotic use is emphasized by antibiotic stewardship efforts (the right drug in the right dose for the right diagnosis for the right duration).[252] In addition, many of the other factors in disease emergence contribute to the problem.

Staphylococcus aureus is one of the most common causes of hospital- and community-acquired infections.[253] Methicillin-resistant *S. aureus* (MRSA) strains were first recognized as a nosocomial pathogen in the United Kingdom in 1961, shortly after the introduction of methicillin. By 2000, approximately half of all nosocomial *S. aureus* isolates in the United States were methicillin-resistant.[254] Risk factors for healthcare-associated MRSA infection include recent hospitalization, residence in a long-term care facility, dialysis, and indwelling percutaneous medical devices and catheters. Since the late 1990s, MRSA infections have spread from the healthcare setting into the community, where outbreaks have occurred among persons with no prior hospital exposure.[255–257] Transmission has occurred by close physical contact in situations involving children in day care centers, children and adults on American Indian reservations, athletes, military personnel, inmates in correctional facilities, and men who have sex with men.[258–265] Available data suggest that community-associated strains are more likely than healthcare-derived isolates to carry virulence factors associated with pneumonia in children and skin and soft tissue infections in adults.[255]

A steadily increasing proportion of MRSA also shows low-level resistance to vancomycin, currently considered the treatment of last resort.[266] In 1996, the first appearance of intermediate resistance to vancomycin in *S. aureus* with minimum inhibitory concentrations (MICs) of 8 ug/mL was reported from Japan,[267] and additional cases were subsequently found in other countries.[268] By the end of 2004, 12 infections with vancomycin-intermediate *S. aureus* (VISA) had been confirmed in the United States. The first two confirmed clinical infections caused by *S. aureus* isolates with complete resistance to vancomycin (VRSA) occurred in the United States in 2002, both in outpatient settings.[269,270] These strains apparently acquired the resistance trait from vancomycin-resistant enterococci (VRE), which were first documented in 1986,[271] and are now endemic in many hospitals.[272] A third documented clinical isolate of VRSA from a U.S. patient was reported in 2004.[273] Through 2012, 13 cases have been identified in U.S. patients.[274,275]

C. difficile is the most common cause of healthcare-associated diarrhea and healthcare-associate infection in the United States.[276] The estimated annual cost is $4.8 billion.[277] A virulent toxigenic epidemic strain known as BI/NAP1/027 has been particularly problematic. The disease is a consequence of disruption of the intestinal microbiome as a consequence of antibiotic exposure. The overwhelming majority of cases are either healthcare facility–onset or community onset, healthcare facility–associated.[276,278] Less than 10% of cases have been classified as community-associated.[279] Transmission in healthcare facilities is associated with transient contamination of the hands of healthcare personnel and environmental contamination.[276] Infection control and antibiotic stewardship efforts are critical to reduce the risk of this infection.

Two recent dramatic examples of the rapid global spread of multidrug resistance due to newly recognized genetic mechanisms are particularly noteworthy. A report of the emergence of a new resistance mechanism mediated by an enzyme named New Delhi metal-lo-beta-lactamse-1 (NDM-1) in India, Pakistan, and the United Kingdom was published in 2010.[280] Strains of gram-negative bacteria expressing the gene for this enzyme were found on mobile genetic elements known as plasmids, which can contain multiple resistance genes and are transferable among bacteria. Bacteria producing this enzyme were resistant to nearly all available antibiotics with the exception of colistin and tigecycline—two old drugs that have been rarely used in recent years because of their toxicity. Infections caused by these multidrug-resistant organisms were initially recognized in individuals from the United Kingdom who had traveled to South Asia for medical treatment, became infected during their care, and required treatment for their infection following their return to the United Kingdom. Subsequent investigation revealed widespread environmental contamination by the NDM-1 gene in surface water and tap water samples collected in New Delhi.[281]

Reports of a second new genetic mechanism of resistance involved the emergence of plasmid-mediated colistin resistance mediated by the mcr-1 gene in organisms found in swine, poultry, and humans in China and multiple European countries.[282,283] Subsequent surveillance soon documented extensive global spread of this gene resulting in human infections for which few if any effective antibiotics are available.[283] Four additional variants (mcr-2—mcr-5) have been identified.[284] The first isolate of an organism containing the mcr-1 gene from a U.S. patient was reported in 2016.[285,286]

A recent report of a nosocomial outbreak caused by a hypervirulent, carbapenem-resistant, hypermucous *Klebsiella pneumoniae* ST 11 strain that had acquired a virulence plasmid has raised concern. The outbreak occurred in an ICU in Hangzhou, China and involved fatal pulmonary infections in five postoperative trauma patients on ventilators. All developed severe pneumonia, multiorgan system failure, or septic shock.[287] This outbreak highlights the need for ongoing surveillance and reporting of outbreaks caused by potentially emerging pathogens, especially those with novel resistance mechanisms.

Multidrug resistance has also expanded rapidly to other pathogens, fueled by antimicrobial use and misuse as well as economic decline and failing health infrastructures in many parts of the world.[242] Since the early 1990s, resistance of *Streptococcus pneumoniae* to penicillin and other antimicrobial agents has spread,[288,289] and an increasing trend of invasive pneumococci resistant to three or more drug classes threatens the treatment of pneumonia and ear infections, especially in children.[290,291] The frequency of fluoroquinolone-resistant *E. coli* has reached 70% in parts of Southeast Asia and China and nearly 10% in some industrialized countries, including the United States, and some strains of *E. coli* are resistant to as many as six drug classes.[242,243,292,293] Strains of *N. gonorrhoeae* have been widely resistant to both penicillin and tetracycline since the 1980s.[294] The appearance of fluoroquinolone-resistant strains severely limited therapeutic options for gonorrhea, the second most frequently reported communicable disease in the United States.[294,295] More recently, failures of dual therapy with ceftriaxone and azithromycin have been reported in the United Kingdom[296,297] and Australia.[298] Evidence supported acquisition during travel to Asia in all three cases, indicating that international dissemination is occurring.[299]

A recent report of an outbreak of typhoid fever caused by an XDR strain of *Salmonella enterica* serovar Typhi in Sindh, Pakistan affecting more than 300 people has raised considerable concern. The strain is resistant to all three first-line antibiotics for treatment of typhoid fever (chloramphenicol, ampicillin, and trimethoprim-sulfamethoxazole) as well as fluoroquinolones and third-generation cephalosporins.[300] Cases have occurred in returning travelers to the United States and the United Kingdom.[301]

In many countries, the failure to treat all patients properly has resulted in the emergence of *M. tuberculosis* strains that are resistant to increasing numbers of antituberculosis drugs and undermining disease-elimination efforts.[302,303] Of the estimated 300,000 new cases of drug-resistant tuberculosis occurring globally each year, 79% are resistant to three of the four first-line drugs.[304] *M. tuberculosis* strains resistant to at least isoniazid and rifampin (MDR-TB) are currently ten times more frequent in eastern Europe and central Asia than elsewhere in the world, although incomplete reporting precludes a true measure of the burden in all areas.[305] A WHO survey of 77 locations showed that, in 1999–2002, the prevalence of resistance to at least one antituberculosis drug ranged from none in some western European countries to 57% in Kazakhstan. In the United States, the incidence of drug resistance in new cases of tuberculosis is highest in foreign-born persons (1.2%).[306] The increased costs of treatment associated with the more expensive second-line drugs pose a major barrier to completion of treatment and increase the risk of progressive disease and death.[307] In 2016, 10.4 million people developed active tuberculosis, and 1.7 million died. WHO estimates that 490,000 had MDR-TB. About 6.2% of MDR-TB cases had extensively drug-resistant TB (XDR-TB) which does not respond to most second-line anti-TB drugs.[308] The MDR-TB burden is highest in India, China, and Russia; these three countries account for nearly 50% of global cases of MDR-TB.[308] An estimated one-third of global deaths due to AR are caused by MDR-TB.[309] The Sustainable Development Goals and the WHO End TB Strategy envision ending the TB pandemic by 2030. To do so will require sustained political will.[310]

Use of antibiotics in food animals also contributes to the emergence of resistance. Driven in large part by the use of antibiotics in livestock and poultry, antimicrobial resistance among food-borne bacterial pathogens is contributing to the health impact of food-borne infection.[288,311] For example, fluoroquinolone-resistant *Campylobacter* infections emerged in the United States in the early 1990s, coincident with the licensing of fluoroquinolones for treatment of respiratory disease in poultry. Similarly, the emergence of Salmonella strains resistant to cefriaxone is thought to be associated with the widespread use of third-generation cephalosporins in cattle.[288,311] Multidrug-resistant definitive phage type (DT) 104 strains of *Salmonella typhimurium* increased in prevalence from 0.6% in 1979–1980 to 34% in 1996, after spreading first among food animals.[288,290]

The use of antibiotics important in human medicine for production purposes (i.e., growth promotion and feed efficiency) in food animals has been a cause of concern for years.[312] Recent action by the U.S. Food and Drug Administration has eliminated the use of medically important antibiotics for production purposes in food animals in the United States effective in January 2017, and currently requires veterinary oversight of use of these drugs for prophylaxis and therapy in food animals.[312]

Environmental concerns relate to antibiotic residues and antibiotic-resistant organisms and genes in human and animal wastes (e.g., from healthcare settings and concentrated animal feeding operations), discharge of antibiotic residues from pharmaceutical manufacturing facilities, and use of large amounts of antibiotics in aquaculture.[313–317]

Globally, drug resistance has also become one of the greatest challenges to malaria control. Drug resistance has been associated with the spread of malaria to new areas, the re-emergence of malaria in previously affected locales, and the occurrence and spread of epidemics.[318] Resistance to chloroquine, the main affordable and available antimalarial treatment, is widespread in 80% of the 92 countries where malaria continues to be a major killer,[319] and resistance to newer antimalarial drugs is widespread and growing. The diminished efficacy of chloroquine represents a tremendous setback for malaria control, leading to a resurgence of malaria-related morbidity and mortality in Africa.[320] The ongoing outbreak of MDR *P. falciparum* malaria in South East Asia is a major concern.[250,251]

The multifaceted strategy needed to address this problem domestically and internationally includes strengthened surveillance of antimicrobial usage and resistance in humans and food animals at the local and national level, effective antimicrobial stewardship programs, strengthened infection control programs, improved sanitation and hygiene, strengthened healthcare systems and diagnostic laboratory capacity, development of rapid diagnostic tests for use at the point of care, reinvigoration of the drug development pipeline, development of alternative therapeutic approaches impacting the host or the pathogen, improving vaccine coverage to reduce the risk of infections requiring antibiotics, ensuring access to high-quality antibiotics, education of healthcare and animal health professionals and the public concerning principles of judicious antibiotic use, interdisciplinary research collaboration, public-private partnerships, and sustained political will.[321,322]

Effective implementation of this strategy requires a transdisciplinary approach as emphasized by the One Health concept, which emphasizes cooperation and collaboration at the interfaces between human health, animal health (both wildlife and domestic animals), and environmental health.[323,324] Other necessary components include timely feedback to prescribers regarding data on local resistance patterns and trends and data on their antibiotic usage. Other important areas include timely communication among healthcare professionals at the time of transfer to another facility regarding infection or colonization with drug-resistant organisms, educational approaches to empower patients to remind providers of the importance of hand hygiene and other prevention strategies, and empowering physicians and veterinarians to practice judicious antibiotic use, and ensuring communication with healthcare administrators and policymakers regarding the urgent need to develop and implement evidence-based policies. Last but not least, healthcare providers need to remain vigilant to ensure timely detection and reporting of the emergence or introduction of new drug-resistant strains. A recent report from a Joint Task Force convened by the Association of Public and Land Grant Universities and the American Association of Veterinary Medical Colleges issued a call to action to the veterinary community to use a One Health approach in addressing antibiotic resistance.[325]

The importance of a One Health approach in addressing these problems has been recognized by professional societies, national and international organizations, the animal agriculture and pharmaceutical industries, funding agencies, and civil society. These problems have recently been the focus of the President's Council of Advisors on Science and Technology,[326] the Presidential Advisory Council on Combating Antimicrobial Resistance,[327] the WHO World Health Assembly,[328] the Davos Declaration by the Pharmaceutical, Biotechnology, and Diagnostics Industries on Combating Antimicrobial Resistance,[329] the UN General Assembly High Level Meeting on Antimicrobial Resistance,[330] and a G20 Leaders' Meeting and Declaration.[331] All have emphasized the critical importance of investment in a One Health strategy to address these problems, which is also reflected in national action plans and the global strategy for confronting antibiotic resistance.[332,333]

EMERGING HEALTHCARE-ASSOCIATED INFECTIONS

Emerging infections can arise in healthcare settings for many reasons, including new or changing technologies, pharmacologic or nonpharmacologic interventions in complex healthcare systems; changing patient profiles, especially expanding populations of immunocompromised patients; microbial change and adaptation through mutations or development of antimicrobial resistance; changes in the healthcare industry and healthcare access; and even overseas travel for healthcare known as medical tourism. An extensive discussion of healthcare-associated infections is provided in Chap. 152 (Control of Infections in Institutions: Healthcare-Associated Infections). However, three recent examples of emerging infections in healthcare settings are noteworthy.

In 2012, a devastating iatrogenic outbreak of fungal meningitis and related fungal infections in otherwise normally sterile body sites occurred in the United States.[334,335] The outbreak was first recognized when several patients in Tennessee, who had been receiving epidural or paraspinal methylprednisolone injections for pain at the same clinic, were hospitalized with either fungal meningitis or meningitis of unknown etiology.[336] An investigation by the Tennessee Department of Health found that these patients had all been injected with compounded methylprednisolone from one of three separate lots produced by a compounding pharmacy in Massachusetts.[336] Further investigations showed that these three lots consisted of 17,675 vials that were distributed by the compounding pharmacy to 76 clinics in 23 states, and that as many as 13,534 patients had been administered methylprednisolone from the implicated lots and were at risk of infection.[335] Through systematic follow-up of these patients, a total of 753 cases of fungal meningitis, paraspinal abscess, and other related illnesses were identified in 20 states.[337] Among these cases, 64 (8.5%) were fatal and many survivors were left with chronic disability.[337]

Laboratory investigations identified the causative fungus as the brown-black soil mold *Exserohilum rostratum*. Prior to this outbreak, this organism was a rarely identified cause of human illness, having been reported <30 times as a cause of either localized posttraumatic infections or disseminated infections (only one of which involved the central nervous system) in immunocompromised hosts.[338] *E. rostratum* was cultured from unopened vials of methylprednisolone from the implicated lots, and the organism was found by whole genome sequencing to match fungal isolates obtained from patients.[335] Investigations at the compounding pharmacy found serious deficiencies in procedures and sterile practices, resulting in the recall of all of the products made in that facility, and its permanent closure. Other outbreaks due to contaminated compounded pharmaceuticals have occurred, and these and the 2012 fungal meningitis outbreak resulted in enhanced regulatory oversight of compounding pharmacies by the Food and Drug Administration.[335,339]

A second healthcare-associated fungal infection to recently emerge is *Candida auris*. This organism was first recognized as a human pathogen in 2009 when it was isolated from the ear of a patient in Japan, although it was retrospectively found to have caused illness in South Korea in 1996. Since its initial recognition, *C. auris* has been found to be the cause of infections and outbreaks in healthcare settings worldwide, including South Asia, the Middle East, Africa, South America, and most recently in Europe, North America, and Australia.[340,341] Investigations have shown that *C. auris* can be found colonizing patients and healthcare workers, and in the hospital environment, facilitating nosocomial transmission.[341] An outbreak occurring between 2015 and 2017 in Great Britain involved 70 patients who were either colonized or infected with *C. auris*, mostly in a neurological ICU, and that infection was associated with reusable skin-surface axillary temperature probes.[342] Despite implementing various infection control practices to control the outbreak, it was only terminated when these probes were removed from the hospital.

C. auris is MDR and can cause severe infections, including candidemia and meningitis, and is associated with high mortality.[340,342] Genetic analysis of *C. auris* isolates from around the world have identified four distinct clades (East Asian, South Asian, South American, and African).[343] A recent molecular investigation of 133 *C. auris* isolates collected in the United States between 2013, when the first cases were detected in the United States, and 2017 found all four clades present with regional clustering.[344] A number of these isolates were from patients who had either traveled to the United States for healthcare or obtained healthcare overseas, suggesting patient movement plays an important role in the spread of this organism to new locations.[344] Molecular analysis of the organism that caused the neurological ICU outbreak in Great Britain found it related to the South African clade, and it was thought to have been introduced to the hospital in 2013.[342] The reason *C. auris* has emerged is unclear, but infections caused by this organism appear to be a new phenomenon. Examination of collections of fungal isolates has not found evidence of the organism before 1996.[340] Potential explanations that have been advanced include changing patient demographics, empiric use of antifungals in ICUs, poor infection control, changing diagnostic and pathogen identification practice and international travel and medical tourism.[340,341]

A multinational outbreak of postcardiac surgery infections due to *Mycobacterium chimaera*, a slow-growing member of the *Mycobacterium avium* complex that was first described as a separate species in 2004, illustrates how the complex equipment used in hospital settings can precipitate an emerging healthcare-associated infection.[345,346] Most cases in this outbreak have involved prosthetic valve infections with disseminated disease, although locally invasive infections without dissemination have occurred in patients whose procedure did not involve an implanted device.[346] The common denominator among outbreak-associated patients with *M. chimaera* infections is that their procedure involved cardiopulmonary bypass where a heater-cooler device was used to chill and warm the patient.[347] The first clusters were recognized in Europe, followed by cases in the United States and Australia.[348–350] All *M. chimaera* isolates in these locations have been closely related by whole genome sequencing, indicating that this is a multisite, common-source outbreak.[351] Remarkably, investigations found that all involved healthcare facilities used heater-cooler units from the same manufacturer, and the outbreak strain of *M. chimaera* was found in water at the manufacturing plant and in heater-cooler units being shipped from the factory.[346,352,353] Studies have shown that while the heater-cooler unit is in use, contaminated water from the water tank can aerosolize and disseminate throughout the operating room via the unit's cooling fans, resulting in detection of *M. chimaera* in air samples and on settle plates.[353] *M. chimaera* infections can be indolent; so far cases have been identified up to 6 years postprocedure.[346] In some locations, after a case had been identified, systematic follow-up of patients who underwent procedures involving a heater-cooler unit have found other infected patients, including patients who were not yet symptomatic. Management of both presymptomatic and ill patients can be challenging.[346] As of 2017, more than 70 cases associated with this outbreak have been identified.[353] Because this organism has an incubation period of years, it is anticipated that cases associated with this outbreak will continue to be detected. Various risk mitigation strategies have been proposed to prevent the heater-cooler units from contaminating the operative field, if discontinuation of the units is not an option.[346]

STRATEGIES FOR ADDRESSING EMERGING INFECTIOUS DISEASES

Since earliest history, human populations have struggled against an evolving array of infectious diseases. However, the unprecedented succession of recent infectious disease emergencies—and the threat of more to come—brings new challenges that require novel solutions.[354,355] Unlike previous eras of infectious disease outbreaks, the scale is global and changes are occurring on many fronts, requiring the readiness of a coordinated international response.[1] The majority of emerging infections in recent years have resulted from cross-species transmission (spillover) of infectious agents from animals, especially wildlife, to people. In some cases, insect vectors have been involved. Examples, as discussed, include SARS, pandemic H1N1 influenza, Ebola virus disease, MERS, Chikungunya, and Zika. These agents are of particular concern as future pandemic and global security threats.[356]

Threats posed by influenza viruses (especially H7N9), the dissemination of MERS-CoV, and the possibility of yellow fever virus being introduced into large urban settings in South Asia where competent mosquito vectors exist, are concerns in 2018. In addition, recent experience with the rapid global spread of carbapenem-resistant bacterial strains producing New Delhi type 1 beta-lactamase enzymes and of strains containing the mcr-1 gene conferring resistance to colistin, are reminders of the threat posed by multidrug-resistant strains causing severe bacterial infections. The recent emergence and dissemination of the multidrug-resistant fungus *C. auris* is another such example. WHO has identified viral hemorrhagic fevers (Ebola, Marburg, CCHF, Rift Valley), SARS, MERS, Nipah, and Lassa viruses as severe outbreak threats.[355] WHO also added "Disease X" to this list in 2018, emphasizing the need to be prepared for the unexpected.[355]

The mainstay of infectious disease control continues to be public health surveillance and response systems that can rapidly detect unusual, unexpected, or unexplained disease patterns; track and exchange information on these occurrences in real time; manage a response effort that can quickly become global in scope; and contain transmission swiftly and decisively. The surveillance methods, investigational skills, diagnostic techniques, and physical resources needed to detect an unusual biologic event are similar, whether it is a seasonal influenza epidemic, a contaminated food in interstate commerce, or the intentional release of a deadly microorganism.

The next pandemic could begin at any moment, emphasizing the importance of sustained investments in health system strengthening and public health capacity building at the local, national, and global level. Alert healthcare providers have played critical roles in the initial recognition of many emerging diseases including AIDS, SARS, MERS, Ebola, and Zika.

In the United States, CDC works with state and local health departments and other agencies to detect and monitor microbial threats. Surveillance for notifiable diseases is conducted by state and local health departments, which receive reports from clinicians and laboratorians on the clinical front lines. To supplement routine public health surveillance functions, CDC funds and coordinates 10 Emerging Infections Program (EIP) sites in collaboration with state and local health departments, public health laboratories, and clinical and academic organizations and institutions (Fig. 85-8). These sites form a national network for population-based studies of emerging infectious diseases of public health importance.[357] CDC also supports sentinel networks in partnerships with specialists in infectious diseases,[358,359] emergency medicine,[360] and travel medicine[361] to track conditions that are likely to be seen by clinicians but that may be missed by traditional surveillance approaches. Much-needed collaborations with veterinary partners are improving the detection and monitoring of zoonotic agents.[362]

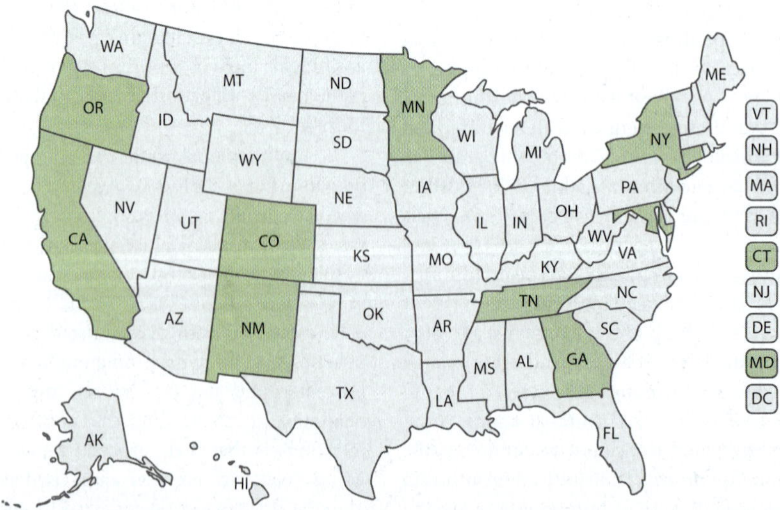

FIGURE 85-8. Emerging infections program sites, 2018. (*Source:* https://www.cdc.gov/ncezid/dpei/eip/eip-sites.html/.)

Control of food-borne illnesses provides added challenges due to the size and complexity of the food industry, the rapid changes that have occurred in its organization, products, and workforce, and the difficulty in tracking and monitoring these diseases. Prevention-based regulatory approaches that address the entire food supply chain are needed to ensure the safety of every food product "from farm to table."[363] Global food supplies and large distribution networks also demand strengthened capacity for disease surveillance and response to outbreaks that can quickly cross local, national, and international borders.[205] To address these needs, laboratory-based surveillance and molecular epidemiology tools have been developed to improve the understanding of the scope and source of food-borne outbreaks, and to direct investigative and research efforts. These include FoodNet, an active surveillance system designed to determine the frequency and severity of food-borne diseases in the United States, monitor trends, and determine the proportion of disease attributable to specific foods,[185,364] and PulseNET, a national molecular subtyping network for food-borne bacteria that facilitates rapid identification of and faster responses to outbreaks of food-borne disease.[365,366]

Internationally, the WHO coordinates these efforts through the Global Outbreak Alert and Response Network (GOARN), which was launched in 2000 as a mechanism for combating international disease outbreaks, ensuring the rapid deployment of technical assistance to affected areas, and contributing to long-term epidemic preparedness and capacity building.[367] The importance of such a network was demonstrated during the SARS epidemic and the 2018 Ebola outbreaks in the DRC, when WHO effectively coordinated disease surveillance, investigation, pathogen identification, laboratory diagnostics, and information dissemination.[368,369]

There has been progress in many countries in terms of coming into compliance with the International Health Regulations 2005, which entered into force in June 2007.[370,371] The Global Health Security Agenda (GHSA)[372] a partnership between WHO, the Food and Agriculture Organization (FAO), the World Organization for Animal Health (OIE), the European Union, and others, was launched in 2014 and currently includes more than 50 countries. It is focused on a vision of a world safe and secure from global health threats posed by infectious diseases. The recent experience with Ebola and Zika outbreaks have helped stimulate global efforts to strengthen national and global capacity to prevent, detect, and respond to global microbial threats in compliance with IHR 2005, but much more work needs to be done. In the United States, for example, an assessment of readiness conducted in 2017 revealed that half the states had achieved only two to five out of 10 public health preparedness indicators.[373] The GHSA includes 11 action packages in three categories (Prevent, Detect, and Respond); the Prevent category includes packages on antimicrobial resistance and zoonotic diseases.[372] Joint External Evaluations (JEEs) are one of the voluntary monitoring and evaluation instruments that provide a tool to assess progress and identify critical gaps in compliance with IHR 2005.[373,374] A JEE of the United States was conducted in May 2016. For the antimicrobial resistance and zoonotic diseases action packages, the evaluation concluded that "the United States might benefit from developing a more formal One Health strategy that encompasses federal, state, and local levels."[375] A score of three out of a possible five was obtained on antimicrobial stewardship activities and surveillance systems for priority zoonotic diseases, indicating that the capacity had been developed but not demonstrated.[375]

Increased security concerns since 2001 have placed a new focus on the importance of identifying unusual health events and responding rapidly to prevent large-scale devastation. A special strategic challenge is how to integrate bioterrorism preparedness into overall infectious disease preparedness in ways that are synergistic and cost-effective. One example of such "dual-use" capability is the Laboratory Response Network (LRN), a multilevel network of more than 120 laboratories that links U.S. public health agencies to advanced-capacity diagnostic facilities, and provides laboratory support during responses to naturally occurring as well as intentionally caused outbreaks.[376] Operational since 1999, the LRN builds on the nationwide system of public health and affiliated laboratories that conduct routine disease surveillance and are needed to combat the threat of emerging diseases.[377] Between 2001 and 2003, LRN member laboratories helped detect and monitor cases of SARS, WNV infection, and monkeypox, as well as intentionally caused anthrax.

New technologies are stimulating the development of other innovative public health tools that are invigorating disease surveillance and response systems. Internet-based information technologies are being used to improve national and international disease reporting, as well as facilitate emergency communications and the dissemination of public health information. Data from the Human Genome Project provide the foundation for public health genomics, a field that holds great promise for understanding the role of human genetic factors in susceptibility to disease, disease progression, and host responses to vaccines and other interventions.[378,379] As the genomic sequences of microbial pathogens become available, discoveries in microbial genetics are suggesting new methods and approaches for disease detection, control, and prevention.[380] Scientific advances are also facilitating the development of improved diagnostic techniques and new vaccines to prevent infection by emerging microbial agents such as dengue virus and H5N1 and H7N9 avian influenza viruses. Sophisticated geographic imaging systems (GIS) and remote sensing approaches are being used to monitor environmental changes that might influence disease emergence and transmission, and predict the occurrence of outbreaks.[17] Other novel technologies, although less sophisticated, nonetheless provide hope for the control of some persistent diseases. For example, the CDC Safe Water System uses point-of-use disinfection and safe water storage to prevent water-borne diseases in developing countries.[381,382] In rural Africa, insecticide-impregnated bednets have proven highly effective in reducing morbidity and mortality from malaria.[383–385]

The introduction of culture-independent diagnostic tests (CIDTs) into clinical medicine presents both challenges and opportunities.[386] These tests may be more rapid and more sensitive than culture-based tests. However, national infectious disease surveillance systems in the United States have been based for many years on isolation of organisms in clinical laboratories and performance of antibiotic susceptibility tests. Isolation of etiologic agents has enabled performance of molecular fingerprinting by pulsed field gel electrophoresis, which has been used in PulseNet for identification of many local, regional, national, and international food-borne disease outbreaks. CDC has launched an Advanced Molecular Detection effort[387] to help facilitate the transition of PulseNet and other outbreak investigation efforts to use of whole genome sequencing.[388,389] Efforts are in progress in collaboration with the Association of Public Health Laboratories and clinical and state public health laboratories to obtain bacterial isolates from CIDT-positive patient samples as a temporary measure during this transition period, while exploration of metagenomics and next-generation sequencing approaches and strengthening bioinformatics capacity are underway in an effort to eventually eliminate the need for bacterial isolates.[390]

Momentum has been building to address the antimicrobial resistance crisis. In the United States, the release of the President's Council of Science and Technology Advisors (PCAST) Report,[326] followed by President Barack Obama's Executive Order on Combating Antibiotic-Resistant Bacteria (CARB), and the White House National Strategy on CARB[391] in October 2014, set the stage. In March 2015, the White House issued the U.S. National Action Plan on CARB,[332] and President Obama established the Presidential Advisory Council on CARB.[327]

Internationally, the U.K. Government commissioned the Review on Antimicrobial Resistance led by Lord Jim O'Neill in July 2014.[309] The World Health Assembly passed a resolution on antimicrobial resistance in May, 2015, and the WHO issued a Global Action

Plan on Antimicrobial Resistance.[333] WHO launched the Global Antimicrobial Surveillance System (GLASS) in October 2015.[392]

In January 2016, the World Economic Forum adopted the Davos Declaration endorsed by pharmaceutical, biotechnology, and diagnostics companies representing those industries. In May 2016, the Review on Antimicrobial Resistance issued its final report and recommendations.[309] In addition, the World Health Assembly passed a resolution supporting the WHO Global Action Plan, the G7 declared antimicrobial resistance to be a national priority, and an Interagency Coordination Group chaired by the UN Deputy Secretary General and the WHO Director General was formed to provide guidance to political leaders on approaches needed to promote sustainable action on antimicrobial resistance. In July 2016, CARB-X, a public-private biopharmaceutical accelerator partnership, focused on accelerating antibacterial research on development of AMR countermeasures, was launched.[393] In September 2016, the Wellcome Trust published its Evidence for Action Report,[394] the G20 committed to reducing antimicrobial resistance, the UN High Level Meeting on AMR ratified the UN Declaration on a Global Effort on CARB,[330] the launch of a Global Antimicrobial Conservation Fund was proposed, nine organizations launched the Conscience of Antimicrobial Resistance Accountability,[395] and the World Bank published a report on Drug-Resistant Infections: A Threat to Our Economic Future.[396]

In January 2017, the FDA Guidance 213 and changes to the Veterinary Feed Directive took effect in the United States.[397] In February 2017, WHO published its Global Priority List of Antibiotic-Resistant Bacteria.[398] Consistent themes in these reports and documents were the urgency of the threat posed by AMR to public health, national and global security, and the stability of the global economy, and the need for a One Health approach across the human health, animal health, and environmental health sectors. The World Bank Group in collaboration with the EcoHealth Alliance, published a One Health operational framework for its work in countries around the world which includes highlighting the challenges posed by AMR.[399] National and international efforts to develop and implement antimicrobial resistance national action plans need ongoing support. In the second Tripartite country self-assessment survey in 2018, 93 of 154 responding countries reported completion of their national action plan, and 51 other countries indicated that they were in the process of developing a plan.[400]

Development of vaccines, therapeutic agents, and diagnostic tests for high priority threat agents is another priority, emphasizing the importance of increased research support for countermeasure development and improved epidemic predictive capacity. Efforts supported by the National Institutes of Health (NIH), the Biomedical Advanced Research and Development Authority (BARDA), and CARB-X are critical in the countermeasure development sphere. BARDA is focused on development of new antibiotics, and is working with NIH to foster development of rapid diagnostics for use at the point of care. The Coalition for Epidemic Preparedness Innovations (CEPI) has focused its initial vaccine countermeasure development efforts on Lassa, MERS, and Nipah viruses.[401,402]

As important as each of these strategies is, none can succeed in the long-term without the political will and actions to address the root causes of infectious diseases. As demonstrated by many of the examples cited above, infectious diseases do not exist in a social vacuum.[403] Ultimately, disease transmission may be affected less by the features of the etiologic agent than by factors such as poverty, overcrowding, poor nutrition, social inequities, inaccessibility of healthcare, workforce shortages, economic instability, and social and ecologic disturbances. In the midst of rapid global change, persistent health disparities, civil strife, armed conflict, and increasingly vulnerable populations add to the challenges. Governments need to supplement scientific and technologic breakthroughs with long-term policies and actions that recognize the complex social context of disease emergence, and that focus on underlying health, development, and sociopolitical determinants.

Promoting a transdisciplinary approach involving collaboration among the human, veterinary, and environmental health communities is particularly critical because of the threat of cross-species transmission (spillover). Such collaboration is central to One Health, EcoHealth, and Planetary Health approaches.[404] This is discussed extensively in chapter 84 (One Health: A New Paradigm for Disease Control and Prevention). Issues relevant to each discipline include vector-borne and zoonotic diseases, antimicrobial resistance, and food safety. Antimicrobial resistance has been described as a quintessential One Health issue,[405,406] while zoonotic diseases at the human–wild animal interface provide additional evidence for the utility of a One Health approach.[407] A recent review of membership in One Health networks concluded that environmental health was under-represented.[408,409] EcoHealth focuses on links between human health, animal health, and ecosystem status with emphasis on the impact of environmental degradation.[404] Planetary Health links health to climate change and migration.[410] Given the considerable common ground among these approaches, increasing communication and collaboration would likely represent value added in the future. The economic impacts of these threats provide further impetus for these three communities to increase dialogue and engagement with each other.

CONCLUSION

Microbes share our biosphere and possess the intrinsic genetic capacity to adapt, shift, and gain new hosts. Despite advances in science, technology, and medicine that have improved disease prevention and management, endemic and emerging infectious diseases continue to pose a threat to domestic and global health. The ever-increasing speed and volume of international travel, migration, and trade create additional opportunities for microbial spread. Increases in the world's most vulnerable populations and the prospect of a deliberate release of pathogenic microbes underscore the importance of expecting and being prepared to address the unexpected.

The best defense against these pathogens is a multifactorial solution characterized by international collaboration and communication; coordinated, well-prepared, and well-equipped public health systems; improved infrastructure and methods for detection and surveillance; effective preventive and therapeutic technologies; and strengthened response capacity. Establishment of an emergency preparedness fund in the United States is long overdue; such a fund is needed to ensure timely outbreak responses. There are numerous examples of the impact of delays in recognition of and response to emerging infection outbreaks leading to regional or global spread. Notable examples in recent years are SARS, MERS, Ebola, and Zika. Advocacy is critically important in making the case for the need for such a fund, the appropriate size of which is worthy of discussion and debate. Partnerships among clinicians, laboratorians, and local public health agencies,[411] as well as strengthened linkages between human health and veterinary organizations and professionals,[362] are also essential components of preparedness and response efforts. Above all, political commitment and adequate resources are needed to address the underlying social and economic factors that increase the vulnerability of human populations to pathogenic microbes. Sustained political will is vital to supporting these preparedness efforts. Therefore, ongoing public and policymaker education and dialogue are critically important.

References

1. Institute of Medicine. *Emerging Infections: Microbial Threats to Health in the United States*. Washington, DC: National Academy Press; 1992.
2. Institute of Medicine. *Microbial Threats to Health: Emergence, Detection, and Response*. Washington, DC: National Academies Press; 2003.
3. Taylor LH, Latham SM, Woolhouse ME. Risk factors for human disease emergence. *Philos Trans R Soc Lond B Biol Sci*. 2001;356(1411): 983–9.

4. Daszak P, Cunningham AA, Hyatt AD. Emerging infectious diseases of wildlife: Threats to biodiversity and human health. *Science.* 2000;287(5452):443–9.
5. Kruse H, Kirkemo AM, Handeland K. Wildlife as source of zoonotic infections. *Emerg Infect Dis.* 2004;10(12):2067–72.
6. Jones KE, Patel MG, Levy MA, et al. Global trends in emerging infectious diseases. *Nature.* 2008;451(7181):990–3.
7. Plowright RK, Parrish CR, McCallum H, et al. Pathways to zoonotic spillover. *Nat Rev Microbiol.* 2017;15(8):502–10.
8. Karesh WB, Dobson A, Lloyd-Smith WO, et al. Ecology of zoonoses: Natural and unnatural histories. *Lancet.* 2012;380(9857):1936–45.
9. Olival KJ, Husseini PR, Zambrana-Torrelio C, et al. Host and viral traits predict zoonotic spillover from mammals. *Nature.* 2017;546(7660):646–50.
10. Allen T, Murray KA, Zambrana-Torrelio C, et al. Global hotspots and correlates of emerging zoonotic diseases. *Nat Commun.* 2017;8(1):1124.
11. Ksiazek TG, Peters CJ, Rollin PE, et al. Identification of a new North American hantavirus that causes acute pulmonary insufficiency. *Am J Trop Med Hyg.* 1995;52(2):117–23.
12. Nichol ST, Spiropoulou CF, Morzunov S, et al. Genetic identification of a hantavirus associated with an outbreak of acute respiratory illness. *Science.* 1993;262(5135):914–7.
13. Yob JM, Field H, Rashdi AM, et al. Nipah virus infection in bats (order *Chiroptera*) in peninsular Malaysia. *Emerg Infect Dis.* 2001;7(3):439–41.
14. Ang BSP, Lim TCC, Wang L. Nipah virus infection. *J Clin Microbiol.* 2018;56(6):pii: eO1875-17.
15. Chua KB, Bellini WJ, Rota PA, et al. Nipah virus: A recently emergent deadly paramyxovirus. *Science.* 2000;288(5470):1432–5.
16. Chua KB. Nipah virus outbreak in Malaysia. *J Clin Virol.* 2003;26 (3):265–75.
17. Morens DM, Folkers GK, Fauci AS. The challenge of emerging and re-emerging infectious diseases. *Nature.* 2004;430(6996):242–9.
18. Cortes MC, Cauchemez S, Lefrancq N, et al. Characterization of the spatial and temporal distribution of Nipah virus spillover events in Bangladesh, 2007–2013. *J Infect Dis.* 2018;217(9):1390–4.
19. Donaldson H, Lucey D. Enhancing preparation for large Nipah outbreaks beyond Bangladesh: Preventing a tragedy like Ebola in West Africa. *Int J Infect Dis.* 2018;72:69–72.
20. Hsu VP, Hossain MJ, Parashar UD, et al. Nipah virus encephalitis reemergence, Bangladesh. *Emerg Infect Dis.* 2004;10(12):2082–7.
21. Nichol ST, Arikawa J, Kawaoka Y. Emerging viral diseases. *Proc Natl Acad Sci USA.* 2000;97(23):12411–2.
22. McCollum AM, Damon IK. Human monkeypox. *Clin Infect Dis.* 2014;58(2):260–7.
23. Reed KD, Melski JW, Graham MB, et al. The detection of monkeypox in humans in the Western Hemisphere. *N Engl J Med.* 2004;350(4):342–50.
24. Rimoin AW, Mulembakani PM, Johnston SC, et al. Major increase in human monkeypox incidence 30 years after smallpox vaccination campaigns cease in the Democratic Republic of Congo. *Proc Natl Acad Sci.* 2010;107(37):16262–7.
25. Kantele A, Chickering K, Vapalahti O, et al. Emerging diseases—The monkeypox epidemic in the Democratic Republic of the Congo. *Clin Microbiol Infect.* 2016;22:658–9.
26. Nolen LD, Osadebe L, Katomba J, et al. Extended human-to-human transmission during a monkeypox outbreak in the Democratic Republic of the Congo. *Emerg Infect Dis.* 2016;22(6):1014–21.
27. Durski KN, McCollum AM, Nakazawa Y, et al. Emergence of monkeypox—West and Central Africa, 1970–2017. *MMWR.* 2018;67(10):306–10.
28. Yinka-Ogunleye A, Aruna O, Ogoina D, et al. Reemergence of human monkeypox in Nigeria, 2017. *Emerg Infect Dis.* 2018;24(6):1149–51.
29. Wu W, Wang J, Liu P, et al. A hospital outbreak of severe acute respiratory syndrome in Guangzhou, China. *Chin Med J (Engl).* 2003; 116(6):811–8.
30. CDC. Update: Outbreak of Severe Acute Respiratory Syndrome—Worldwide, 2003. *MMWR.* 2003;52(12):241–8.
31. WHO. Summary of probable SARS cases with onset of illness from 1 November 2002 to 31 July 2003. December 31, 2003. Available at http://www.who.int/csr/sars/country/table2004_04_21/en/.
32. Hui DS, Chan PK. Severe acute respiratory syndrome and coronavirus. *Infect Dis Clin North Am.* 2010;24(3):619–38.
33. Guan Y, Zheng BJ, He YQ, et al. Isolation and characterization of viruses related to the SARS coronavirus from animals in southern China. *Science.* 2003;302(5643):276–8.
34. Balboni A, Battilani M, Prosperi S. The SARS-like coronaviruses: The role of bats and evolutionary relationships with SARS coronavirus. *New Microbiol.* 2012;35(1):1–16.
35. Hu B, Ge X, Wang LF, et al. Bat origin of human coronaviruses. *Virol J.* 2015;12:221.
36. de Wit E, van Doremalen N, Falzarano D, et al. SARS and MERS: Recent insights into emerging coronaviruses. *Nat Rev Microbiol.* 2016;14(8):523–34.
37. Wong G, Liu W, Liu Y, et al. MERS, SARS, and Ebola: The role of super-spreaders in infectious disease. *Cell Host Microbe.* 2015;18(4):398–401.
38. Anderson RM, Fraser C, Ghani AC, et al. Epidemiology, transmission dynamics, and control of SARS: The 2002–2003 epidemic. *Philos Trans R Soc Lond B Biol Sci.* 2004;359(1447):1091–105.
39. Zhou P, Fan H, Lan T, et al. Fatal swine acute diarrhoea syndrome caused by an HKU-2-related coronavirus of bat origin. *Nature.* 2018;556(7700):255–8.
40. WHO. International Health Regulations. 2005. 2nd ed. Available at http://apps.who.int/iris/bitstream/10665/43883/1/9789241580410_eng.pdf.
41. Arabi YM, Balkhy HH, Hayden FG, et al. Middle East respiratory syndrome. *N Engl J Med.* 2017;376(6):584–94.
42. Bermingham A, Chand MA, Brown CS, et al. Severe respiratory illness caused by a novel coronavirus, in a patient transferred to the United Kingdom from the Middle East, September 2012. *Euro Surveill.* 2012;17(40):20290.
43. Al-Abdallat MM, Payne DC, Alqaswari S, et al. Hospital-associated outbreak of Middle East respiratory syndrome coronavirus: A serologic, epidemiologic, and clinical description. *J Clin Infect Dis.* 2014;59(9):1225–33.
44. World Health Organization. MERS situation update. August 2018. Available at http://www.emro.who.int/pandemic-epidemic-diseases/mers-cov/mers-situation-update-august-2018.html.
45. Bialek SR, Allen D, Alvarado-Ramy F, et al. First confirmed cases of Middle East respiratory syndrome coronavirus (MERS-CoV) infection in the United States, updated information on the epidemiology of MERS-CoV infection, and guidance for the public, clinicians, and public health authorities—May 2014. *MMWR.* 2014;63(19):431–6.
46. Kim KH, Tandi TE, Choi JW, et al. Middle East respiratory syndrome coronavirus (MERS-CoV) outbreak in South Korea, 2015: Epidemiology, characteristics and public health implications. *J Hosp Infect.* 2017;95(2):207–13.
47. Al-Tawfiq JA, Auwaerter PG. Healthcare-associated infections: The hallmark of Middle East respiratory syndrome coronavirus with review of the literature. *J Hosp Infect.* 2019;101(1):20–29.
48. Mohd HA, Al-Tawfiq JA, Memish ZA. Middle East respiratory syndrome coronavirus (MERS-CoV) origin and animal reservoir. *Virol J.* 2016;13:87.
49. Wernery U, Lau SK, Woo PC. Middle East respiratory coronavirus (MERS) and dromedaries. *Vet J.* 2017;220(2):75–79.
50. Muller MA, Corman VM, Jones J, et al. MERS coronavirus neutralizing antibodies in camels. *Emerg Infect Dis.* 2014;20(12):2093–5.
51. Sutton TC. The pandemic threat of emerging H5 and H7 avian influenza viruses. *Viruses.* 2018;10(9):E461. doi:10.3390/v1009046.
52. Tanner WD, Toth DK, Gundlapalli AV. The pandemic potential of avian influenza A(H7N9) virus: A review. *Epidemiol Infect.* 2015;143(16): 3359–74.
53. Uyeki TM, Katz JM, Jernigan DB. Novel influenza A viruses and pandemic threats. *Lancet.* 2017;389(10085):2172–4.
54. Kaye D, Pringle CR. Avian influenza viruses and their implication for human health. *Clin Infect Dis.* 2005;40(1):108–12.
55. Alexander DJ. A review of avian influenza in different bird species. *Vet Microbiol.* 2000;74(1-2):3–13.
56. Hammond A, Fitzner J, Collins L, et al. Human cases of influenza at the human-animal interface, January 2015–April 2017. *Weekly Epidemiol Rec.* 2017:92(33):460–75.
57. Chen H, Yuan H, Gao R, et al. Clinical and epidemiological characteristics of a fatal case of avian influenza A H10N8 virus infection: A descriptive study. *Lancet.* 2014;383(9918):714–21.
58. Yuen KY, Chan PK, Peiris M, et al. Clinical features and rapid viral diagnosis of human disease associated with avian influenza A H5N1 virus. *Lancet.* 1998;351(9101):467–71.
59. deJong MD, Hien TT. Avian influenza A (H5N1). *J Clin Virol.* 2006; 35(1):2–13.
60. Fournie G, Hog E, Barnett T, et al. A systematic review and meta-analysis of practices exposing humans to avian influenza viruses, their prevalence, and rationale. *Am J Trop Med Hyg.* 2017;97(2):376–88.
61. World Health Organization. Cumulative number of confirmed human cases of avian influenza A(H5N1) reported to WHO. Available at http://www.who.int/influenza/human_animal_interface/H5N1_cumulative_table_archives/en/.

62. Wang X, Jiang H, Wu P, et al. Epidemiology of avian influenza A H7N9 virus in human beings across five epidemics in mainland China, 2013–17: An epidemiological study of laboratory-confirmed case series. *Lancet Infect Dis.* 2017;17(8):822–32.
63. World Health Organization. Human infection with avian influenza virus A(H7N9)—China: Update. Available at http://www.who.int/csr/don/05-september-2018-ah7n9-china/en/.
64. Liu B, Havers F, Chen E, et al. Risk factors for influenza A(H7N9) disease—China, 2013. *Clin Infect Dis.* 2013:59(6):787–94.
65. Wu P, Jiang H, Wu JT, et al. Poultry market closures and human infection with influenza A(H7N9) virus, China, 2013–14. *Emerg Infect Dis.* 2014;20(11):1891–4.
66. Yu H, Wu JT, Cowling BJ, et al. Effect of closure of live poultry markets on poultry-to-person transmission of avian influenza A H7N9 virus: An ecological study. *Lancet.* 2014;383(9916):541–8.
67. Ma W, Kahn RE, Richt JA. The pig as a mixing vessel for influenza viruses: Human and veterinary implications. *J Mol Genet Med.* 2009;3(1):158–66.
68. Shinde V, Bridges CB, Uyeki TM, et al. Triple-reassortant swine influenza A (H1) in humans in the United States, 2005–2009. *N Engl J Med.* 2009;360(25):2616–25.
69. Jhung MA, Epperson S, Biggerstaff M, et al. Outbreak of variant influenza A(H3N2) virus in the United States. *Clin Infect Dis.* 2013;57(12):1703–12.
70. Finelli L, Swerdlow DL. The emergence of influenza A (H3N2)v virus: What we learned from the first wave. *Clin Infect Dis.* 2013;57(Suppl 1):S1–3.
71. Greenbaum A, Quinn C, Bailer J, et al. Investigation of an outbreak of variant influenza A(H3N2) virus infection associated with an agricultural fair—Ohio, August 2012. *J Infect Dis.* 2015;212(10):1592–9.
72. Schicker RS, Rossow J, Eckel S, et al. Outbreak of influenza A(H3N2) variant virus infections among persons attending agricultural fairs housing infected swine—Michigan and Ohio, July–August 2016. *MMWR.* 2016;65(42):1157–60.
73. CDC. Case Count: Detected U.S. human infections with H3N2V by state since August 2011. Available at https://www.cdc.gov/flu/swineflu/h3n2v-case-count.htm.
74. Bowman AS, Nolting JM, Nelson SW, et al. Subclinical influenza A infections in pigs exhibited at agricultural fairs, Ohio, USA, 2009–2011. *Emerg Infect Dis.* 2012;18(12):1945–50.
75. Bowman AS, Walia RR, Nolting JM, et al. Influenza A(H3N2) virus in swine at agricultural fairs and transmission to humans, Michigan and Ohio, USA, 2016. *Emerg Infect Dis.* 2017;23(9):1551–5.
76. CDC. Issues for Fair Organizers to Consider When Planning Fairs. Available at https://www.cdc.gov/flu/swineflu/fairs-planning.htm.
77. Morens DM, Taubenberger JK. The mother of all pandemics is 100 years old (and going strong)! *Am J Public Health.* 2018;108(11):1449–54.
78. Neumann G, Noda T, Kawaoka Y. Emergence and pandemic potential of swine-origin H1N1 influenza virus. *Nature.* 2009;459(7249):931–9.
79. Novel Swine-Origin Influenza A (H1N1) Virus Investigation Team. Emergence of a novel swine-origin influenza A (H1N1) virus in humans. *N Engl J Med.* 2009;360(25):2605–15.
80. Chowell G, Bertozzi SM, Colchero MA, et al. Severe respiratory disease concurrent with the circulation of H1N1 influenza. *N Engl J Med.* 2009;361(7):674–9.
81. Fraser C, Donnelly CA, Cauchemez S, et al. Pandemic potential of a strain of influenza A (H1N1): Early findings. *Science.* 2009;324(5934):1557–61.
82. Jordan H, Mosquera M, Nair H, et al. Swine-origin influenza A (H1N1) virus infections in a school—New York City, April 2009. *MMWR.* 2009;58(dispatch)1:3.
83. World Health Organization. World now at the start of 2009 influenza pandemic. Available at http://www.who.int/mediacentre/news/statements/2009/h1n1_pandemic_phase6_20090611/en/.
84. Writing Committee of the WHO Consultation on Clinical Aspects of Pandemic (H1N1) 2009 Influenza. Clinical aspects of pandemic 209 influenza A (H1N1) virus infection. *N Engl J Med.* 2010;362(18):1708–19.
85. Reproduced with permission from Jhung MA, Swerdlow D, Olsen SJ, et al. Epidemiology of pandemic influenza A (H1N1) in the United States. *Clin Infect Dis.* 2011;52(Suppl 1):S13-26.
86. Broberg E, Nicoll A, Amato-Gauci A. Seroprevalence to influenza A (H1N1) 2009 virus—Where are we. *Clin Vacc Immunol.* 2011;18(8):1205–12.
87. Miller MA, Viboud C, Balinska M, et al. The signature features of influenza pandemics—Implications for policy. *New Engl J Med.* 2009;360(25):2595–8.
88. Shrestha SS, Swerdlow DL, Borse RH, et al. Estimating the burden of 2009 pandemic influenza A (H1N1) in the United States (April 2009–April 2010). *Clin Infect Dis.* 2011:52(Suppl 1):S75–82.
89. Dawood FS, Iuliano AD, Reed C, et al. Estimated global mortality associated with the first 12 months of 2009 pandemic influenza A H1N1 virus circulation: A modelling study. *Lancet Infect Dis.* 2012;12(9):687–95.
90. Mosby LG, Rasmussen SA, Jamieson DJ. 2009 pandemic influenza A (H1N1) in pregnancy: A systematic review of the literature. *Am J Obstet Gynecol.* 2011;205(1):10–18.
91. Morgan OW, Bramley A, Fowlkes A, et al. Morbid obesity as a risk factor for hospitalizations and deaths due to 2009 pandemic influenza A (H1N1) disease. *PLoS One.* 2010;5(3):e9694.
92. Yin JK, Khandaker G, Rashid H, et al. Immunogenicity and safety of pandemic influenza A (H1N1) 2009 vaccine: Systematic review and meta-analysis. *Influenza Other Respir Viruses.* 2011;5(5):299–305.
93. CDC. Interim results: Influenza A (H1N1) 2009 monovalent vaccination coverage—United States, October–December 2009. *MMWR.* 2010;59(2):44–8.
94. Garten R, Blanton L, Abd Elal AI, et al. Update: Influenza activity in the United States during the 2017–2018 season and composition of the 2018–2019 influenza vaccine. *MMWR.* 2018;67(22):634–42.
95. Rollin PE, Knust B, Nichol S. Ebola-Marburg viral diseases. In: Heymann DL, eds. *Control of Communicable Diseases Manual: An Official Report of the American Public Health Association.* Washington, DC: APHA Press, an imprint of the American Public Health Association; 2015, pp. 173–8.
96. Lau MS, Dalziel BD, Funk S, et al. Spatial and temporal dynamics of superspreading events in the 2015–2015 West Africa Ebola epidemic. *Proc Natl Acad Sci USA.* 2017;114(9):2337–42.
97. Gsell PS, Camacho A, Kucharski AJ, et al. Ring vaccination with rVSV-ZEBOV under expanded access in response to an outbreak of Ebola virus disease in Guinea, 2016: An operational and vaccine safety report. *Lancet Infect Dis.* 2017;17(12):1276–84.
98. Gostin LO, Tomori O, Wibulpolprasert S, et al. Towards a common secure future: Four global commissions in the wake of Ebola. *PLoS Med.* 2016;13(5):e1002042.
99. Green A. Ebola outbreak in the DR Congo: Lessons learned. *Lancet.* 2018;391(10135):2096.
100. Cohen J. Vaccine trial launched to stop Ebola. *Science.* 2018;360(6390):694–5.
101. The Ebola Outbreak Epidemiology Team. Outbreak of Ebola virus disease in the Democratic Republic of the Congo, April–May, 2018: An epidemiological study. *Lancet.* 2018;392(10143):213–21.
102. Nkengasong JN, Onyebujoh P. Response to Ebola virus disease outbreak in the Democratic Republic of the Congo. *Lancet.* 2018;391(10138):2395–8.
103. Kugeler KJ, Staples JE, Hinckley AF, et al. Epidemiology of human plague in the United States, 1900–2012. *Emerg Infect Dis.* 2015;21(1):16–22.
104. CDC. Plague—South Carolina. *MMWR.* 1983;32(32):417–8.
105. CDC. Imported plague—New York City, 2002. *MMWR.* 2003;52(31):725–8.
106. Kassem AM, Tengelson L, Atkins B, et al. Notes from the Field: Plauge in domestic cats-Idaho, 2016. *MMWR.* 2016;65(48):1378–9.
107. Abedi AA, Shako JC, Gaudart J, et al. Ecologic features of plague outbreak areas, Democratic Republic of the Congo, 2004–2014. 2018;24(2):210–20.
108. Burki T. Plague in Madagascar. *Lancet Infect Dis.* 2017;17(12):1241.
109. Bonds MH, Ouenzar MA, Garchitorena A, et al. Madagascar can build stronger health systems to fight plague and prevent the next epidemic. *PLoS Negl Trip Dis.* 2018;12(1):e0006131.
110. Mead PS. Plague in Madagascar—A tragic opportunity for improving public health. *N Engl J Med.* 2018;378(2):106–8.
111. Chancey C, Grinev A, Volkova E, et al. The global ecology and epidemiology of West Nile virus. *Biomed Res Int.* 2015;2015:376230.
112. Sejvar JJ. West Nile virus infection. *Microbiol Spectrum.* 2016;4(3):E|10-0021-2016.
113. Smithburn KC, Hughes TP, Burke AW, et al. A neurotropic virus isolated from the blood of a native of Uganda. *Am J Trop Med Hyg.* 1940;20:471–92.

114. Nash D, Mostashari F, Fine A, et al. The outbreak of West Nile virus infection in the New York city area in 1999. *N Engl J Med*. 2001;344(24):1807–14.
115. Roehrig JT. West Nile virus in the United States—a historical perspective. *Viruses*. 2013;5(12):3088–108.
116. Petersen LR, Brault AG, Nasci RS. West Nile virus: Review of the literature. *JAMA*. 2013;310(3):308–15.
117. CDC. West Nile virus statistics and maps. Available at https://www.cdc.gov/westnile/statsmaps/index.html.
118. Lumsden WH. An epidemic of virus disease in Southern Province, Tanganyika Territory, in 1952–53. II. General description and epidemiology. *Trans R Soc Trop Med Hyg*. 1955;49(1):33–57.
119. Morrison CR, Plante KS, Heise MT. Chikungunya virus: Current perspectives on a reemerging virus. *Microbiol Spectrum*. 2016;4(3): E|10-0017-2016.
120. Zeller H, Van Bortel W, Sudre B. Chikungunya: Its history in Africa and Asia and its spread to new regions in 2013–2014. *J Infect Dis*. 2016;214(Suppl 5):S436–40.
121. Rezza R, Nicolleti L, Angelini R, et al. Infection with chikungunya virus in Italy: An outbreak in a temperate region. *Lancet*. 2007;30 (9602):1840–6.
122. Gibney KB, Fischer M, Prince HE, et al. Chikungunya fever in the United States: A fifteen year review of cases. 2011;52(5):e121–6.
123. Khan K, Bogoch I, Brownstein JS, et al. Assessing the origin of and potential for international spread of chikungunya virus from the Caribbean. *PLoS Curr*. 2014;2014:6. pii: ecurrents.outbreaks.2134a0a7bf37fd8d388181539fea2da5.
124. Van Bortel W, Dorleans F, Rosine J, et al. Chikungunya outbreak in the Caribbean region, December 2013 to March 2014, and the significance for Europe. *Euro Surveill*. 2014;19(13):pii=20759.
125. Kendrick K, Stanek D, Blackmore C, et al. Notes from the field: Transmission of chikungunya virus in the continental United States—Florida, 2014. *MMWR*. 2014;63(48):1127.
126. Pan American Health Organization. Chikungunya. Available at https://www.paho.org/hq/index.php?option=com_topics&view=article&id=343&Itemid=40931&lang=en.
127. Dick GW, Kitchen SF, Haddow AJ. Zika virus I. Isolation and serological specificity. *Trans R Soc Trop Med Hyg*. 1952;46(5):509–20.
128. Dick GW. Zika virus II. Pathogenicity and physical properties. *Trans R Soc Trop Med Hyg*. 1952;46(5):521–34. ZV3.
129. Anderson KB, Thomas SJ, Endy TP. The emergence of Zika virus: A narrative review. *Ann Intern Med*. 2016;165(3):175–83.
130. Macnamara FN. Zika virus: A report on three cases of human infection during an epidemic of jaundice in Nigeria. *Trans R Soc Trop Med Hyg*. 1954;48(2):139–45.
131. Duffy MR, Chen TH, Hancock WT, et al. Zika virus outbreak on Yap Island, Federated States of Micronesia. *N Engl J Med*. 2009;360(24): 2536–43.
132. Aubry M, Teissier A, Huart M, et al. Zika virus seroprevalence, French Polynesia, 2014–2015. *Emerg Infect Dis*. 2017;23(4):669–72.
133. Zanluca C, Melo VC, Mosimann AL, et al. First report of autochthonous transmission of Zika virus in Brazil. *Mem Inst Oswaldo Cruz*. 2015;110(4):569–72.
134. Hennessey M, Fischer M, Staples JE. Zika virus spreads to new areas—Region of the Americas, May 2015—January 2016. *MMWR*. 2016;65(3):55–8.
135. Pan American Health Organization. Zika cumulative cases—4 January 2018. Available at https://www.paho.org/hq/index.php?option=com_content&view=article&id=12390:zika-cumulative-cases&Itemid=42090&lang=en.
136. CDC. Cumulative Zika virus disease case counts in the United States, 2015–2018. Available at https://www.cdc.gov/zika/reporting/case-counts.html.
137. Cohen J. Where has all the Zika gone? *Science*. 2017;357(6352):631–2.
138. Pierson TC, Diamond MS. The emergence of Zika virus and its new clinical syndromes. *Nature*. 2018;560(7720):573–81.
139. Saiz JC, Martin-Acebes MA, Bueno-Mari R, et al. Zika virus: What have we learnt since the start of the recent epidemic? *Front Microbiol*. 2017;8:1554.
140. Heymann DL, Hodgson A, Sell AA, et al. Zika virus and microcephaly: Why is this situation a PHEIC? *Lancet*. 2016;387(10020):719–21.
141. Pan American Health Organization. Zika-epidemiologic report. Brazil. Available at https://www.paho.org/hq/dmdocuments/2017/2017-phe-zika-situation-report-bra.pdf.
142. Dos Santos T, Rodriguez A, Almiron M, et al. Zika virus and the Guillain-Barre syndrome—Case series from seven countries. *N Engl J Med*. 2016;375(16):1598–1601.
143. Moreira J, Peixoto TM, Siqueira AM, et al. Sexually acquired Zika virus: A systematic review. *Clin Microbiol Infect*. 2017;23(5):296–305.
144. Abbink P, Stephenson KE, Barouch DH. Zika virus vaccines. *Nat Rev Microbiol*. 2018;16(10):594–600.
145. Gubler DJ. Epidemic dengue/dengue hemorrhagic fever as a public health, social and economic problem in the 21st century. *Trends Microbiol*. 2002;10(2):100–3.
146. Mackenzie JS, Gubler DG, Petersen LR. Emerging flaviviruses: The spread and resurgence of Japenese encephalitis, West Nile and dengue viruses. *Nat Med*. 2004;10(12 Suppl):S98–109.
147. Bhatt S, Gething PW, Brady OJ, et al. The global distribution and burden of dengue. *Nature*. 2013;496(7446):504–7.
148. Musso D, Rodriguez-Morales AJ, Levi JE, et al. Unexpected outbreaks of arboviral infections: Lessons learned from the Pacific and tropical America. *Lancet Infect Dis*. 2018;18(11):e355–61. pii: S1473-3099(18)30269-X.
149. Thomas DL, Santiago GA, Abeyta R, et al. Reemergence of dengue in southern Texas, 2013. *Emerg Infect Dis*. 2016;22(6):1002–7.
150. Rey JR. Dengue in Florida (USA). *Insects*. 2014;5(4):991–1000.
151. The Lancet Infectious Disease. The dengue vaccine dilemma. *Lancet Infect Dis*. 2018;18(2):123.
152. Sridhar S, Luedtke A, Langevin E, et al. Effect of dengue serostatus on dengue vaccine safety and efficacy. *N Engl J Med*. 2018;379(4):327–40.
153. WHO. Meeting of the Strategic Advisory Group of Experts on Immunization, April 2018—Conclusions and recommendations. *Wkly Epidemiol Rep*. 2018;93(23):329–44.
154. WHO. Yellow fever—Brazil. Emergencies preparedness, response (Disease Outbreak News) 2018. Available at http://www.who.int/csr/don/27-february-2018-yellow-fever-brazil/en.
155. Nishino K, Yactayo S, Garcia E, et al. Yellow fever urban outbreak in Angola and the risk of extension. *Wkly Epidemiol Rec*. 2016;91(14): 186–92.
156. Kraemer MUG, Faria NR, Reiner RCJr, et al. Spread of yellow fever outbreak in Angola and the Democratic Republic of the Congo 2015–2016: A modeling study. *Lancet Infect Dis*. 2017;17(3):330–8.
157. Muanya C, Atueyi U. Nigeria set to vaccinate 25m people against yellow fever, says WHO. The Guardian Nigeria. 2018.
158. Barrett AD. Yellow fever in Angola and beyond—The problem of vaccine supply and demand. *N Engl J Med*. 2016;375(4):301–3.
159. Lucey DR, Donaldson H. Yellow fever vaccine shortages in the United States and abroad: A critical issue. *Ann Intern Med*. 2017;167(9):664–5.
160. Hamer DH, Angelo K, Caumes E, et al. Fatal yellow fever in travelers to Brazil, 2018. *MMWR*. 2018;67(11):340–1.
161. Shrivastava S, Shrivastava P, Ramasamy J. Yellow fever outbreak in Angola: The potential global threat and the prevailing challenges in the control of the disease. *Ann Trop Med Public Health*. 2017;10(3):523–4.
162. Brent SE, Watts A, Cetron M, et al. International travel between global urban centres vulnerable to yellow fever transmission. *Bull World Health Org*. 2018;96(5):343–54B.
163. Anderson T. Stepping up local efforts to stop global spread of yellow fever. *Bull World Health Org*. 2018;96(6):374–5.
164. The Lancet. Yellow fever: A major threat to public health. *Lancet*. 2018;391(10119):402.
165. McMullen LK, Folk SM, Kelly AJ, et al. A new phlebovirus associated with severe febrile illness in Missouri. *N Engl J Med*. 2012;367(9): 834–41.
166. Muehlenbachs A, Fata CR, Lambert AJ, et al. Heartland virus-associated death in Tennessee. *Clin Infect Dis*. 2014;59(6):845–50.
167. Pastula DM, Turabelidze G, Yates KF, et al. Notes from the Field: Heartland virus disease—United States, 2012–2013. *MMWR*. 2014;63(12):270–1.
168. Oklahoma State Health Department. Oklahoma state health department confirms first case and death of Heartland virus, 2014. Available at https://www.ok.gov/health/Organization/Office_of_Communications/News_Releases/2014_News_Releases/Oklahoma_State_Health_Department_Confirms_First_Case_and_Death_of_Heartland_Virus.html.
169. Arkansas Department of Health. Case of Heartland virus found in Arkansas resident, 2017. Available at https://www.healthy.arkansas.gov/news/detail/case-of-heartland-virus-found-in-arkansas-resident.

170. Fill MA, Compton ML, McDonald EC, et al. Novel clinical and pathologic findings in a Heartland virus-associated death. *Clin Infect Dis.* 2017;64(4):510–2.

171. Savage HM, Godsey MSJr, Lambert A, et al. First detection of Heartland virus (Bunyaviridae: Phelbovirus) from field collected arthropods. *Am J Trop Med Hyg.* 2013;89(3):445–52.

172. Kansas Department of Health and Environment. KDHE and CDC investigate new virus—Bourbon virus is thought to be transmitted through mosquito or tick bites, 2014. Available at http://www.kdheks.gov/news/web_archives/2014/12222014.htm.

173. Kosoy OI, Lambert AJ, Hawkinson DJ, et al. Novel thogotovirus associated with febrile illness and death, United States. *Emerg Infect Dis.* 2015;21(5):760–4.

174. Savage HM, Burkhalter KL, Godsey MSJr, et al. Bourbon virus in field collected ticks, Missouri, USA. *Emerg Infect Dis.* 2017;23(12): 2017–22.

175. Mouraao MP, Bastos MS, Gimaqu JB, et al. Oropouche fever outbreak, Manaus, Brazil, 2007–2008. *Emerg Infect Dis.* 2009;15(12):2063–4.

176. Anderson CR, Spence L, Downs WG, et al. Oropouche virus: A new human disease agent from Trinidad, West Indies. *Am J Trop Med Hyg.* 1961;10:574–8.

177. Pinheiro FP, Travassos da Rosa AP, Travassos da Rosa JF, et al. Oropouche virus. I. A review of clinical, epidemiological, and ecological findings. *Am J Trop Med Hyg.* 1981;30(1):149–60.

178. Tesh RB. The emerging epidemiology of Venezuelan hemorrhagic fever and Oropouche fever in tropical South America. *Ann NY Acad Sci.* 1994;740:129–37.

179. Vasconcelos PH, Calisher CH. Emergence of human arboviral disease in the Americas, 2000–2016. *Vector Borne Zoonotic Dis.* 2016;16(5): 295–301.

180. Travassos da Rosa JF, de Sousa WM, Pinheiro FP, et al. Oropouche virus: Clinical, epidemiological, and molecular aspects of a neglected Orthobunyavirus. *Am J Trop Med Hyg.* 2017;96(5):1019–30.

181. Carpenter S, Groschup MH, Garros C, et al. Culicoides biting midges, arboviruses and public health in Europe. *Antiviral Res.* 2013;100(1): 102–13.

182. WHO. *WHO Estimates of the Global Burden of Foodborne Diseases: Foodborne Disease Burden Epidemiology Reference Group 2007-2015.* Geneva: WHO; 2015. Available at http://apps.who.int/iris/bitstream/handle/10665/199350/?sequence=1.

183. Scallan E, Hoekstra RM, Angulo FJ, et al. Foodborne illness acquired in the United States—Major pathogens. *Emerg Infect Dis.* 2011;17(1):7–15.

184. Scallan E, Griffin PM, Angulo FJ, et al. Foodborne illness acquired in the United States—Unspecified agents. *Emerg Infect Dis.* 2011;17(1):16–22.

185. Henao OL, Jones TF, Vugia DJ, et al. Foodborne disease active surveillance network—2 decades of achievements, 1996–2015. *Emerg Infect Dis.* 2015;21(9):1529–36.

186. Marder EP, Griffin PM, Cieslak PR, et al. Preliminary incidence and trends of infections with pathogens transmitted commonly through food—Foodborne Diseases Active Surveillance Network, 10 U.S. sites, 2006–2017. *MMWR.* 2018;67(11):324–8.

187. Dewey-Mattia D, Manikonda K, Hall AJ, et al. Surveillance for foodborne disease outbreaks—United States, 2009–2015. *MMWR Surveill Summ.* 2018;67(10):1–11.

188. McCollum JT, Cronquist AB, Silk BJ, et al. Multistate outbreak of listeriosis associated with cantaloupe. *N Engl J Med.* 2013;369(10):944–53.

189. Angelo KM, Conrad AR, Saupe A, et al. Multistate outbreak of *Listeria monocytogenes* infections linked to whole apples used in commercially produced, prepackaged caramel apples—United States, 2014–2015. *Epidemiol Infect.* 2017;145(5):848–56.

190. Neil KP, Biggerstaff G, MacDonald JK, et al. A novel vehicle for transmission of *Escherichia coli* O157:H7 to humans: Multistate outbreak of *E. coli* O157:H7 infections associated with consumption of ready-to-bake commercial prepackaged cookie dough—United States, 2009. *Clin Infect Dis.* 2012;54(4):511–8.

191. Kuehn BM. *Salmonella* cases traced to egg producers. *JAMA.* 2010;304(12):1316.

192. Tauxe RV. Emerging foodborne pathogens. *Int J Food Microbiol.* 2002;78(1-2):31–41.

193. Mead PS, Griffin PM. *Escherichia coli* O157:H7. *Lancet.* 1998;352 (9135):1207–12.

194. Lawson JM. Update on *Escherichia coli* O157:H7. *Curr Gastroenterol Rep.* 2004;6(4):297–301.

195. Orskov F, Orskov I, Villar JA. Cattle as reservoir of verotoxin-producing *Escherichia coli* O157:H7. *Lancet.* 1987;2(8553):276.

196. Faith NG, Shere JA, Brosch R, et al. Prevalence and clonal nature of *Escherichia coli* O157:H7 on dairy farms in Wisconsin. *Appl Environ Microbiol.* 1996;62(5):1519–25.

197. Heiman KE, Mody RK, Johnson SD, et al. *Escherichia coli* O157:H7 outbreaks in the United States, 2003–2012. *Emerg Infect Dis.* 2015;21(8):1293–1301.

198. Bell BP, Goldoft M, Griffin PM, et al. A multistate outbreak of *Escherichia coli* O157:H7-associated bloody diarrhea and hemolytic uremic syndrome from hamburgers. The Washington experience. *JAMA.* 1994;272(17):1349–53.

199. CDC. Multistate outbreak of *E. coli* O157:H7 infections linked to fresh spinach (final update). Available at https://www.cdc.gov/ecoli/2006/spinach-10-2006.html.

200. CDC. Multistate outbreak of *E. coli* O157:H7 infections linked to romaine lettuce (final update). Available at https://www.cdc.gov/ecoli/2018/o157h7-04-18/index.html.

201. Valilis E, Ramsey A, Sadiq S, et al. Non-O157 Shiga toxin-producing *Escherichia coli*—A poorly appreciated enteric pathogen: Systematic review. *Int J Infect Dis.* 2018;76:82–7.

202. Gould RH, Mody RK, Ong KL, et al. Increased recognition of non-O157 Shiga toxin-producing *Escherichia coli* infections in the United States during 2000–2010: Epidemiologic features and comparison with *E. coli* O157 infections. *Foodborne Pathog Dis.* 2013;10(5):453–60.

203. Majowicz SE, Scallan E, Jones-Bitton A, et al. Global incidence of Shiga toxin-producing *Escherichia coli* infections and deaths: A systematic review and knowledge synthesis. *Foodborne Pathog Dis.* 2014;11(6): 447–55.

204. Frank C, Werber D, Cramer JP, et al. Epidemic profile of Shiga-toxin-producing *Escherichia coli* O104:H4 outbreak in Germany. *N Engl J Med.* 2011;365(19):1771–80.

205. Dixon, BR. Parasitic illnesses associated with the consumption of fresh produce—an emerging issue in developed countries. *Curr Opinion Food Sci.* 2016;8:104–9.

206. Ortega YR, Sanchez R. Update on *Cyclospora cayatenensis*, a food-borne and waterborne parasite. *Clin Microbiol Rev.* 2010;23(1):218–34.

207. Herwaldt BL. *Cylcospora cayatenensis*: A review, focusing on the outbreaks of cyclosporiasis in the 1990s. *Clin Infect Dis.* 2000;31(4): 1040–57.

208. CDC. Parasites: Cyclosporiasis (Cyclospora Infection)—Outbreak investigations and updates. Available at https://www.cdc.gov/parasites/cyclosporiasis/outbreaks/index.html.

209. Casillas SM, Bennett C, Straily A. *Notes from the Field*: Multiple cyclosporiasis outbreaks—United States, 2018. *MMWR.* 2018;67(39):1101–2.

210. Food and Drug Administration. Statement from FDA Commissioner Scott Gottlieb, M.D., on the FDA's ongoing efforts to prevent foodborne outbreaks of *Cyclospora.* Available at https://www.fda.gov/NewsEvents/Newsroom/PressAnnouncements/ucm620867.htm.

211. Brown P, Will RG, Bradley R, et al. Bovine spongiform encephalopathy and variant Creutzfeldt-Jakob disease: Background, evolution, and current concerns. *Emerg Infect Dis.* 2001;7(1):6–16.

212. Donnelly CA. Bovine spongiform encephalopathy in the United States: An epidemiologist's view. *N Engl J Med.* 2004;350(6): 539–42.

213. Taylor DM, Woodgate SL. Bovine spongiform encephalopathy: The causal role of ruminant-derived protein in cattle diets. *Rev Sci Tech.* 1997;16(1):187–98.

214. Beisel CE, Morens DM. Variant Creutzfeldt-Jakob disease and the acquired and transmissible spongiform encephalopathies. *Clin Infect Dis.* 2004;38(5):697–704.

215. OIE-World Health Organisation for Animal Health. Bovine spongiform encephalopathy (BSE). Available at http://www.oie.int/doc/ged/D13944.PDF.

216. CDC. vCJD cases reported in the US. 2018. Available at https://www.cdc.gov/prions/vcjd-reported.html.

217. Belay ED, Schonberger LB. The public health impact of prion diseases. *Annu Rev Public Health.* 2005;26:191–212.

218. Perkins A, Trimmier M. Recreational waterborne illness: Recognition, treatment, and prevention. *Am Fam Physician.* 2017;95(9):554–60.

219. Hlavasa MC, Roberts VA, Kahler AM, et al. Outbreaks of illness associated with recreational water—United States, 2011–2012. *MMWR.* 2015;64(24):668–72.

220. CDC. Surveillance for waterborne disease outbreaks associated with drinking water and other nonrecreational water—United States, 2009–2010. *MMWR.* 2013;62(35):714–20.

221. Faruque SM, Sack DA, Sack RB, et al. Emergence and evolution of *Vibrio cholerae* O139. *Proc Natl Acad Sci USA.* 2003;100(3):1304–9.

222. MacKenzie WR, Hoxie NJ, Proctor ME, et al. A massive outbreak in Milwaukee of *Cryptosporidium* infection transmitted through the public water supply. *N Engl J Med*. 1994;331(3):161–7.

223. CDC. Norwalk-like viruses: Public health consequences and outbreak management. *MMWR*. 2001;50(RR-9):1–13.

224. Pape JW, Johnson WDJr, Fitzgerald DW. The earthquake in Haiti—Dispatch from Port-au-Prince. *N Engl J Med*. 2010;362(7):575–7.

225. CDC. Update: Cholera outbreak—Haiti, 2010. *MMWR*. 2010; 59(45):1473–9.

226. CDC. Update: Outbreak of cholera—Haiti, 2010. *MMWR*. 2010;59 (48):1586–90.

227. Chin CS, Sorenson J, Harris JB, et al. The origin of the Haitian cholera outbreak strain. *N Engl J Med*. 2011;364(1):33–42.

228. Eppinger M, Pearson T, Koenig SS, et al. Genomic epidemiology of the Haitian cholera outbreak: A single introduction followed by rapid, extensive, and continued spread characterized the onset of the epidemic. *MBio*. 2014;5(6):e01721.

229. Farmer P, Almazor CP, Bahnsen ET, et al. Meeting cholera's challenge to Haiti and the world: A joint statement on cholera prevention and cure. *PLoS Negl Trop Dis*. 2011;5(5):e1145.

230. Waldman RJ, Mintz ED, Papowitz HE. The cure for cholera—Improving access to safe water and sanitation. *N Engl J Med*. 2013;368(7):592–4.

231. WHO. Crisis-driven cholera resurgence switches focus to oral vaccine. *Bull World Health Org*. 2018;96(7):446–7.

232. The Lancet Infectious Disease. Cholera in Yemen: War, hunger, disease...and heroics. *Lancet Infect Dis*. 2017;17(8):781.

233. Devi S. Devastation in Yemen ongoing. *Lancet*. 2018;392(10142):110.

234. Qadri F, Islam T, Clemens JD. Cholera in Yemen—An old foe rearing its ugly head. *N Engl J Med*. 2017;377(21):2005–7.

235. Camacho A, Bouhenia M, Alyusfi R, et al. Cholera epidemic in Yemen, 2016–18: An analysis of surveillance data. *Lancet Glob Health*. 2018;6(6):e680–90.

236. Trevejo RT, Rigau-Perez JG, Ashford DA, et al. Epidemic leptospirosis associated with pulmonary hemorrhage—Nicaragua, 1995. *J Infect Dis*. 1998;178(5):1457–63.

237. Mohd Radi MF, Hashim JH, Jaafar MH, et al. Leptospirosis outbreak after the 2014 major flooding event in Kelantan, Malaysia: A spatial-temporal analysis. *Am J Trop Med Hyg*. 2018;98(5):1281–95.

238. CDC. Outbreak of leptospirosis among white-water rafters—Costa Rica, 1996. *MMWR*. 1997;46(25):577–9.

239. Sejvar J, Bancroft E, Winthrop K, et al. Leptospirosis in "Eco-challenge" athletes, Malaysian Borneo, 2000. *Emerg Infect Dis*. 2003;9(6):702–7.

240. Morgan J, Bornstein SL, Karpati AM, et al. Outbreak of leptospirosis among triathlon participants and community residents of Springfield, Illinois, 1998. *Clin Infect Dis*. 2002;34(12):1593–9.

241. Birnbaum E, Bacterial disease deaths in Puerto Rico hit 'epidemic' level after Hurricane Maria: Report. 2018. Available at http://thehill.com/homenews/news/395392-puerto-rico-saw-spike-in-deaths-from-bacterial-disease-after-hurricane-maria.

242. Levy SB, Marshall. Antibacterial resistance worldwide: Causes, challenges and responses. *Nat Med*. 2004;10(12 Suppl):S122–9.

243. Schmidt FR. The challenge of multidrug resistance: Actual strategies in the development of novel antibacterials. *Appl Microbiol Biotechnol*. 2004;63(4):335–43.

244. Boodman SG. Running out of wonder drugs. *The Washington Post*, March 16, 1993. Available at https://www.highbeam.com/doc/1P2-937206.html.

245. Marston HD, Dixon DM, Knisely JM, et al. Antimicrobial resistance. *JAMA*. 316(11):1193–204.

246. CDC. Antibiotics resistance threats in the United States, 2013. Available at https://www.cdc.gov/drugresistance/threat-report-2013/inndex.html.

247. Cassani A, Hogberg LD, Plachouras D, et al. Attributable deaths and disability-adjusted life-years caused by infections with antibiotic-resistant bacteria in the EU and the European Economic Area in 2015: A population-level modelling analysis. *Lancet Infect Dis*. 2019;19(1):56–66.

248. WHO. Global priority list of antibiotic-resistant bacteria to guide research, discovery, and development of new antibiotics. Geneva, Switzerland; 2007.

249. Shah NS, Auld SC, Brust JC, et al. Transmission of extensively drug-resistant tuberculosis in South Africa. *N Engl J Med*. 2017;376(3):243–53.

250. Amato R, Pearson RD, Almagro-Garcia J, et al. Origins of the current outbreak of mulitdrug-resistant malaria in southeast Asia: A retrospective genetic study. *Lancet Infect Dis*. 2018;18(3):337–45.

251. Menard D, Clain J, Ariey F. Multidrug-resistant *Plasmodium falciparum* malaria in the Greater Mekong subregion. *Lancet Infect Dis*. 2018;18(3):238–9.

252. Barlam TF, Cosgrove SE, Abbo LM, et al. Implementing an antibiotic stewardship program: Guidelines by the Infectious Diseases Society of America and the Society for Healthcare Epidemiology of America. *Clin Infect Dis*. 2016;62(10):51–77.

253. Que Y, Moreillon P. *Staphylococcus aureus* (including Staphylococcal Toxic Shock Syndrome). In: Bennett JE, Dolin R, Blaser MJ, eds. *Mandell, Douglas, and Bennett's Principals and Practice of Infectious Diseases*. Philadelphia, PA: Saunders; 2015.

254. Weinstein RA. Controlling antimicrobial resistance in hospitals: Infection control and use of antibiotics. *Emerg Infect Dis*. 2001;7(2):188–92.

255. Rybak MJ, LaPlante KL. Community-associated methicillin-resistant *Staphylococcus aureus*: A review. *Pharmacotherapy*. 2005;25(1):74–85.

256. Naimi TS, LeDell KH, Boxrud DJ, et al. Epidemiology and clonality of community-acquired methicillin-resistant *Staphylococcus aureus* in Minnesota, 1996–1998. *Clin Infect Dis*. 2001;33(7):990–6.

257. Baggett HC, Hennessy TW, Leman R, et al. An outbreak of community-onset methicillin-resistant *Staphylococcus aureus* skin infections in southwestern Alaska. *Infect Control Hosp Epidemiol*. 2003;24(6): 397–402.

258. CDC. Methicillin-resistant *Staphylococcus aureus* skin or soft tissue infections in a state prison—Mississippi, 2000. *MMWR*. 2000;50(42): 919–22.

259. CDC. Methicillin-resistant *Staphylococcus aureus* infections in correctional facilities—Georgia, California, and Texas, 2001–2003. *MMWR*. 2003;52(41):992–6.

260. Pan ES, Diep BA, Carleton HA, et al. Increasing prevalence of methicillin-resistant *Staphylococcus aureus* infection in California jails. *Clin Infect Dis*. 2003;37(10):1384–8.

261. Kazakova SV, Hageman JC, Matava M, et al. A clone of methicillin-resistant *Staphylococcus aureus* among professional football players. *N Engl J Med*. 2005;352(5):468–75.

262. Lindenmayer JM, Schoenfeld S, O'Grady R, et al. Methicillin-resistant *Staphylococcus aureus* in a high school wrestling team and the surrounding community. *Arch Intern Med*. 1998;158(8):895–9.

263. CDC. Methicillin-resistant *Staphylococcus aureus* infections among competitive sports participants—Colorado, Indiana, Pennsylvania, and Los Angeles County, 2000–2003. *MMWR*. 2003;52(33):793–5.

264. LeMar JE, Carr RB, Zinderman C, et al. Sentinel cases of community-acquired methicillin-resistant *Staphylococcus aureus* onboard a naval ship. *Mil Med*. 2003;168(2):135–8.

265. Zinderman CE, Connor B, Malakooti MA, et al. Community-acquired methicillin-resistant *Staphylococcus aureus* among military recruits. *Emerg Infect Dis*. 2004;10(5):941–4.

266. Fridkin SK. Vancomycin-intermediate and resistant *Staphylococcus aureus*: What the infectious disease specialist needs to know. *Clin Infect Dis*. 2001;32(1):108–15.

267. Hiramatsu K, Hanaki H, Ino T, et al. *Methicillin*-resistant *Staphylococcus aureus* clinical strain with reduced vancomycin susceptibility. *J Antimicrob Chemother*. 1997;40(1):135–6.

268. Hiramatsu K, Cui L, Kuroda M, et al. The emergence and evolution of methicillin-resistant Staphylococcus aureus. *Trends Microbiol*. 2001;9(10):486–93.

269. Weigel LM, Clewell DB, Gill SR, et al. Genetic analysis of a high-level vancomycin-resistant isolate of *Staphylococcus aureus*. *Science*. 2003;302(5650):1569–71.

270. Tenover FC, Weigel LM, Appelbaum PC, et al. Vancomycin-resistant *Staphylococcus aureus* isolate from a patient in Pennsylvania. *Antimicrob Agents Chemother*. 2004;48(1):275–80.

271. Leclercq R, Derlot E, Duval J, et al. Plasmid-mediated resistance to vancomycin and teicoplanin in *Enterococcus faecium*. *N Engl J Med*. 1988;319(3):157–61.

272. Chavers LS, Moser SA, Benjamin WH, et al. Vancomycin-resistant enterococci: 15 years and counting. *J Hosp Infect*. 2003;53(3):159–71.

273. CDC. Brief report: Vancomycin-resistant *Staphylococcus aureus*—New York, 2004. *MMWR*. 2004;53(15):322–3.

274. CDC. CDC reminds clinical laboratories and healthcare infection preventionists of their role in the search and containment of vancomycin-resistant *Staphylococcus aureus* (VRSA). 2014. Available at https://www.cdc.gov/hai/settings/lab/vrsa_lab_search_containment.html.

275. Limbago BM, Kallen AJ, Zhu W, et al. Report of the 13th vancomycin-resistant *Staphylococcus aureus* isolate from the United States. *J Clin Microbiol*. 2014;52(3):998–1002.

276. McDonald LC, Gerding DN, Johnson S, et al. Clinical practice guidelines for *Clostridium difficile* infection in adults and children: 2017 update by the Infectious Diseases Society of America (IDSA) and Society for Healthcare Epidemiology of America (SHEA). *Clin Infect Dis*. 2018:66(7):987–94.

277. The Lancet. A new approach to treating infection. *Lancet*. 2018;391 (10122):714.

278. Lessa FC, Mu Y, Winston LG, et al. Burden of *Clostridium difficile* infection in the United States. *N Engl J Med*. 2015;372(9):825–34.

279. Chitnis AS, Holzbauer SM, Belflower RM, et al. Epidemiology of community-associated *Clostridium difficile* infection, 2009 through 2011. *JAMA Intern Med*. 2013;173(14):1359–67.

280. Kumarasamy KK, Toleman MA, Walsh TR, et al. Emergence of a new antibiotic resistance mechanism in India, Pakistan, and the UK: A molecular, biological, and epidemiological study. *Lancet Infect Dis*. 2010;10(9):597–602.

281. Walsh TR, Weeks J, Livermore DM, et al. Dissemination of NDM-1 positive bacteria in the New Delhi environment and its implications for human health: An environmental point prevalence study. *Lancet Infect Dis*. 2011;11(5):355–62.

282. Liu YY, Wang Y, Walsh TR, et al. Emergence of plasmid-mediated colistin resistance mechanism MCR-1 in animals and human beings in China: A microbiological and biological study. *Lancet Infect Dis*. 2016;16(2):161–8.

283. Wang R, van Dorp L, Liam P, et al. The global distribution and spread of the mobilized colistin resistance gene mcr-1. *Nat Commun*. 2018; 9:1179.

284. Rebelo AR, Bortolaia V, Kjeldgaard JS, et al. Mulitplex PCR for detection of plasmid-mediated colistin resistance determinants, *mcr-1, mcr-2, mcr-3, mcr-4* and *mcr-5* for surveillance purposes. *Euro Surveill*. 2018;23(6):17–00672.

285. McGann P, Snesrud E, Maybank R, et al. *Escherichia coli* harboring *mcr-1* and $bla_{CTX\text{-}M}$ on a novel IncF plasmid: First report of *mcr-1* in the United States. *Antimicrob Agents Chemother*. 2016;60(7):4420–1.

286. Kline KE, Shover J, Kallen AJ, et al. Investigation of first identified *mcr-1* gene in an isolate from a U.S. patient—Pennsylvania, 2016. *MMWR*. 2016;65(36):977–8.

287. Gu D, Dong N, Zheng Z, et al. A fatal outbreak of ST11 carbapenem-resistant hypervirulent *Klebsiella pneumoniae* in a Chinese hospital: A molecular epidemiological study. *Lancet Infect Dis*. 2018;18(1):37–46.

288. Breiman RF, Butler JC, Tenover FC, et al. Emergence of drug-resistant pneumococcal infections in the United States. *JAMA*. 1994;271(23):1831–5.

289. Butler JC, Hofmann J, Cetron MS, et al. The continued emergence of drug-resistant *Streptococcus pneumoniae* in the United States: An update from the Centers for Disease Control and Prevention's Pneumococcal Sentinel Surveillance System. *J Infect Dis*. 1996;174(5):986–93.

290. Whitney CG, Farley MM, Halder J, et al. Increasing prevalence of multidrug-resistant *Streptococcus pneumoniae* in the United States. *N Engl J Med*. 2000;343(26):1917–24.

291. Schrag S, McGee L, Whitney CG, et al. Emergence of *Streptococcus pneumoniae* with very-high-level resistance to penicillin. *Antimicrob Agents Chemother*. 2004;48(8):3016–23.

292. Wang H, Dzink-Fox JL, Chen M, et al. Genetic characterization of highly fluoroquinolone-resistant clinical *Escherichia coli* strains from China: Role of *acrR* mutations. *Antimicrob Agents Chemother*. 2001;45(5):1515–21.

293. Karlowsky JA, Kelly LJ, Thornsberry C, et al. Trends in antimicrobial resistance among urinary tract infection isolates of *Escherichia coli* from female outpatients in the United States. *Antimicrob Agents Chemother*. 2002;46(8):2540–5.

294. Tapsall J & World Health Organization. Antimicrobial resistance in Neisseria gonorrhoeae. 2001, World Health Organization, Anti-Infective Drug Resistance and Containment Team: Geneva, Switzerland. Available at http://www.who.int/iris/handle/10665/66963.

295. CDC. Increases in fluoroquinolone-resistant Neisseria gonorrhoeae—Hawaii and California, 2001. *MMWR*. 2002;51(46):1041–4.

296. Fifer H, Natarajan U, Jones L, et al. Failure of dual antimicrobial therapy in treatment of gonorrhea. *N Engl J Med*. 2016;374(25):2504–6.

297. Public Health England. UK case of *Neisseria gonorrhoeae* with high-level resistance to azithromycin and resistance to ceftriaxone acquired abroad. 2018: PHE publications gateway number 2017893; HPR12(11).

298. Whiley DM, Jennison A, Pearson J, et al. Genetic characterization of *Neisseria gonorrhoeae* resistant to both ceftriaxone and azithromycin. *Lancet Infect Dis*. 2018;18(7):717–8.

299. Lahra MM, Martin I, Demczuk W, et al. Cooperative recognition of internationally disseminated ceftriaxone-resistant *Neisseria gonorrhoeae* strain. *Emerg Infect Dis*. 2018;24(4):735–40.

300. Klemm EJ, Shakoor S, Page AJ, et al. Emergence of an extensively drug-resistant *Salmonella enterica* serovar Typhi clone harboring a promiscuous plasmid encoding resistance to fluoroquinolones and third-generation cephalosporins. *Mbio*. 2018;9(1):e00105–18.

301. Cohen J. 'Frightening' drug-resistant strain of typhoid spreads in Pakistan. *Science*. 2018;361(6399):214.

302. Herbert N, Masham BS, Suttie BA, et al. Advancing political will to end the tuberculosis epidemic. *Lancet Infect Dis*. 2018;18(7):711–2.

303. Espinal MA, Laszlo A, Simonsen L, et al. Global trends in resistance to antituberculosis drugs. World Health Organization-International Union against Tuberculosis and Lung Disease Working Group on Anti-Tuberculosis Drug Resistance Surveillance. *N Engl J Med*. 2001;344(17): 1294–303.

304. WHO. Anti-tuberculosis Drug Resistance in the World. Third Global Report. The WHO/IUATLD Global Project on Anti-Tuberculosis Drug Resistance Surveillance, 1999–2002. 2004, World Health Organization: Geneva, Switzerland. apps.who.int/iris/handle/10665/43103.

305. WHO. Drug resistant tuberculosis: Levels are ten times higher in eastern Europe and central Asia. *Weekly Epidemiol Rep*. 2004;79(12):118–20.

306. CDC. Trends in tuberculosis—United States, 1998–2003. *MMWR*. 2004;53(10):209–14.

307. Bates I, Fenton C, Gruber J, et al. Vulnerability to malaria, tuberculosis, and HIV/AIDS infection and disease. Part II: Determinants operating at environmental and institutional level. *Lancet Infect Dis*. 2004;4(6):368–75.

308. WHO. Fact sheet on tuberculosis (updated January 2018). *Weekly Epidemiol Rep*. 2018;4-5:39–43.

309. O'Neill J. Tackling Drug-Resistant Infections Globally: Final Report and Recommendations. 2016. Available at https://amr-review.org/sites/default/files/160518_Final%20paper_with%20cover.pdf.

310. Herbert N, Sharma V, Masham BS, et al. Concrete action now: UN High-Level Meeting on Tuberculosis. *Lancet Infect Dis*. 2018;18(7):709–10.

311. Tauxe RV. Emerging foodborne pathogens. *Int J Food Microbiol*. 2002;78(1-2):31–41.

312. Lammie SL, Hughes JM. Antimicrobial resistance, food safety, and one health: The need for convergence. *Annu Rev Food Sci Technol*. 2016;7:287–312.

313. Lubbert C, Baars C, Dayakar A, et al. Environmental pollution with antimicrobial agents from bulk drug manufacturing industries in Hyderabad, South India, is associated with dissemination of extended-spectrum beta-lactamase and carbapenemase-producing pathogens. *Infection*. 2017;45(4):479–91.

314. Lancet Planetary Health. The natural environment an emergence of antimicrobial resistance. *Lancet Planet Health*. 2018;2(1):e1.

315. UNEP. Frontiers 2017: Emerging Issues of Environmental Concern. United Nations Environment Programme, Nairobi.

316. Cabello FC, Godfrey HP, Buschmann AH, et al. Aquaculture as yet another environmental gateway to the development and globalisation of antimicrobial resistance. *Lancet Infect Dis*. 2016;16(7):e127–33.

317. Luo Y, Yang F, Mathieu J, et al. Proliferation of multidrug-resistant New Delhi metallo-β-lactamase genes in municipal wastewater treatment plants in northern China. *Environ Science & Technol Letters*. 2014;1(1): 26–30.

318. Bloland PB. Drug resistance in malaria. 2001, World Health Organization, Anti-infective Drug Resistance Surveillance and Containment Team: Geneva, Switzerland. Available at http://www.who.int/drugresistance/publications/WHO_CDS_CSR_DRS_2001_4/en/.

319. WHO. Overcoming antimicrobial resistance. 2000. World Health Organization, Communicable Diseases Cluster: Geneva, Switzerland. Available at http://apps.who.int/iris/handle/10665/66672.

320. Wellems TE, Miller LH. Two worlds of malaria. *N Engl J Med*. 2003;349(16):1496–8.

321. Hughes JM. Preserving the lifesaving power of antimicrobial agents. *JAMA*. 2011;305(10):1027–8.

322. Hughes JM. Antimicrobial resistance: Current challenges and priorities. 2013, Infectious Disease News. Available at https://www.healio.com/infectious-disease/news/print/infectious-disease-news/%7B55565cc0-34ff-4979-b9f3-8865140a6c9d%7D/antimicrobial-resistance-current-challenges-and-priorities.

323. Kahn LH. *One Health and the Politics of Antimicrobial Resistance*. Baltimore, MD: Johns Hopkins University Press; 2016.

324. Atlas RM, Maloy S (eds). *One Health: People, Animals, and the Environment.* Washington, DC: ASM Press; 2014.

325. Addressing Antibiotic Resistance. A Report from the Joint APLU | AAVMC Task Force on Antibiotic Resistance in Production Agriculture. 2015. Available at http://aavmc.org/data/images/aplu_aavmc%20task%20force%20report%20final.pdf.

326. President's Council of Advisors on Science and Technology. Report to the President on Combating Antibiotic Resistant Bacteria. 2014: Washington, DC. Available at https://www.cdc.gov/drugresistance/pdf/report-to-the-president-on-combating-antibiotic-resistance.pdf.

327. Presidential Advisory Council on Combating Antibiotic-Resistant Bacteria. Initial Assessment of the National Action Plan for Combating Antibiotic Resistant Bacteria. 2016: Washington, DC. Available at https://www.hsdl.org/?abstract&did=805974.

328. Shallcross LJ, Davies SC. The World Health Assembly resolution on antimicrobial resistance. *J Antimicrob Chemother.* 2014;69(11):2883–5.

329. Declaration by the Pharmaceutical, Biotechnology and Diagnostics Industry on Combating Antimicrobial Resistance. 2016: Available at https://amr-review.org/industry-declaration.html.

330. United National High-Level Meeting on Antimicrobial Resistance. Draft political declaration of the high-level meeting of the General Assembly on antimicrobial resistance. 2016; New York NY. Available at https://digitallibrary.un.org/record/842813?ln=en.

331. G20 Health Ministers Germany 2017. Berlin Declaration of the G20 Health Ministers: Together Today for a Health Tomorrow, 2017. Available at https://www.bundesgesundheitsministerium.de/fileadmin/Dateien/3_Downloads/G/G20-Gesundheitsministertreffen/G20_Health_Ministers_Declaration_engl.pdf.

332. Task Force for Combating Antibiotic-Resistant Bacteria. National Action Plan for Combating Antibiotic-Resistant Bacteria. 2015. Available at https://www.cdc.gov/drugresistance/pdf/national_action_plan_for_combating_antibotic-resistant_bacteria.pdf.

333. WHO. Global Action Plan on Antimicrobial Resistance. 2015. Available at http://www.who.int/antimicrobial-resistance/global-action-plan/en/.

334. Smith RM, Schaefer MK, Kainer MA, et al. Fungal infections associated with contaminated methylprednisolone injections. *N Engl J Med.* 2013;369(17):1598–609.

335. Kauffman CA, Malani AN. Fungal infections associated with contaminated steroid injections. *Micriobiol Spectrum.* 2016;4(2): doi:10.1128/microbiolspec.EI10-0005-2015.

336. Kainer MA, Reagan DR, Nguyen DB, et al. Fungal infections associated with contaminated methylprednisolone in Tennessee. *N Engl J Med.* 2012;367(23): 2194–203.

337. CDC. Multistate outbreak of fungal meningitis and other infections. Available at https://www.cdc.gov/hai/outbreaks/meningitis.html.

338. Katragkou A, Pana ZD, Perlin DS, et al. *Exserohilum* infections: Review of 48 cases before the 2012 United States outbreak. *Med Mycol.* 2014;52(4):376–86.

339. Staes C, Jacobs J, Mayer J, et al. Description of outbreaks of health-care-associated infections related to compounding pharmacies, 2000–2012. *Am J Health Syst Pharm.* 2013;70(15):1301–12.

340. Chowdhary A, Sharma C, Meis JF. *Candida auris*: A rapidly emerging cause of hospital-acquired multidrug-resistant fungal infections globally. *PloS Pathog.* 2017;13(5):e1006290.

341. Meis JF, Chowdhary A. *Candida auris*: A global fungal public health threat. *Lancet Infect Dis.* 2018;18(10):doi:https//doi.org/10.1016/S1473-3099(18)30609-1.

342. Eyre DW, Sheppard AE, Madder H, et al. A *Candida auris* outbreak and its control in an intensive care setting. *N Engl J Med.* 2018;379(14): 1322–31.

343. Lockhart SR, Etienne KA, Vallabhaneni S. Simultaneous emergence of multidrug-resistant *Candida auris* on 3 continents confirmed by whole-genome sequencing and epidemiological analyses. *Clin Infect Dis.* 2017;64(2):134–40.

344. Chow NA, Gade L, Tsay SV, et al. Multiple introductions and subsequent transmission of multidrug-resistant *Candida auris* in the USA: A molecular epidemiological survey. *Lancet Infect Dis.* 2018;18(10): pii: S1473-3099(18)30597-8.

345. Tortoli E, Rindi L, Garcia MJ, et al. Proposal to elevate the genetic variant MAC-A, included in the *Mycobacterium avium* complex, to species rank as *Mycobacterium chimaera* sp. nov. *Int J Syst Evol Microbiol.* 2004:54 (Pt 4):1277–85.

346. Alexandre RM, Diekema DJ, Edmond MB. *Mycobacterium chimaera* infections associated with contaminated heater-cooler devices for cardiac surgery: Outbreak management. *Clin Infect Dis.* 2017;65(4):669–74.

347. Kohler P, Kuster SP, Bloemberg G, et al. Healthcare-associated prosthetic heart valve, aortic vascular graft, and disseminated *Mycobacterium chimaera* infections subsequent to open heart surgery. *Eur Heart J.* 2015:36(40):2745–53.

348. Sax H, Bloembert G, Hasse B, et al. Prolonged outbreak of *Mycobacterium chimaera* infection after open-chest heart surgery. *Clin Infect Dis.* 2015;61(1):67–75.

349. Lyman MM, Grigg C, Kinsey CB, et al. Invasive nontuberculous mycobacterial infections among cardiothoracic surgical patients exposed to heater-cooler devices. *Emerg Infect Dis.* 2017;23(5):796–805.

350. Robertson J, McClellan S, Donnan E, et al. Responding to *Mycobacterium chimaera* heater-cooler unit contamination: International and national intersectoral collaboration coordinated in the state of Queensland, Australia. *J Hosp Infect.* 2018;100(3):e77–84: pii: S0195-6701(18)30389-X.

351. van Ingen J, Kohl TA, Kranzer K, et al. Global outbreak of severe *Mycobacterium chimaera* disease after cardiac surgery: A molecular epidemiological study. *Lancet Infect Dis.* 2017;17(10):1033–41.

352. Haller S, Holler C, Jacobshagen A, et al. Contamination during production of heater-cooler units by *Mycobacterium chimaera* potential cause for invasive cardiovascular infections: Results of an outbreak investigation in Germany, April 2015 to February 2016. *Euro Surveill.* 2016;21(17): doi:10.2807/1560-7917.ES.2016.21.17.30215.

353. Sommerstein R, Schreiber PW, Diekema DJ, et al. *Mycobacterium chimaera* outbreak associated with heater-cooler devices: Piecing the puzzle together. *Infect Control Hosp Epidemiol.* 2017;38(1):103–8.

354. Stern AM, Markel H. International efforts to control infectious diseases, 1851 to the present. *JAMA.* 2004;292(12):1474–9.

355. WHO. 2018 Annual Review of Diseases Prioritized under the Research and Development Blueprint, Informal Consultation. 2018: Geneva, Switzerland. Available at http://www.who.int/blueprint/en/.

356. Sands P, Mundaca-Shah C, Dzau VJ. The neglected dimension of global security—A framework for countering infectious-disease crises. *N Engl J Med.* 2016;374(13):1281–7.

357. Pinner RW, Lynfield R, Hadler JL, et al. Cultivation of an adaptive network for surveillance and evaluation of emerging infections. *Emerg Infect Dis.* 2015;21(9):1499–509.

358. Pillai SK, Beekmann SE, Santibanez S, et al. The Infectious Diseases Society of America emerging infections network: Bridging the gap between clinical infectious diseases and public health. *Clin Infect Dis.* 2014;58(7):991–6.

359. Santibanez S, Polgreen PM, Beekmann SE, et al. Communication between infectious disease physicians and US state and local public health agencies: Strengths, challenges, and opportunities. *Public Health Rep.* 2016;131(5):666–70.

360. Santibanez S, Fischer LS, Krishnadasan, A, et al. *EMERGEncy* ID NET: Review of a 20-year multisite emergency department emerging infections research network. *Open Forum Infect Dis.* 2017;4(4):ofx218.

361. Leder K, Torresi J, Libman MD, et al. GeoSentinel surveillance of illness in returned travelers, 2007–2011. *Ann Intern Med.* 2013;158 (6):456–68.

362. King LJ, Marano N, Hughes JM. New partnerships between animal health services and public health agencies. *Rev Sci Tech.* 2004;23(2):717–25.

363. Acheson DW, Fiore AE. Preventing foodborne illness—What clinicians can do. *N Engl J Med.* 2004;350(5):437–40.

364. Allos BM, Moore MR, Griffin PM, et al. Surveillance for sporadic foodborne illness in the 21st century: The FoodNet perspective. *Clin Infect Dis.* 2004;38(Suppl 3):S115–20.

365. Swaminathan B, Barrett TJ, Hunter SM, et al. PulseNet: The molecular subtyping network for foodborne bacterial disease surveillance, United States. *Emerg Infect Dis.* 2001;7(3):382–9.

366. CDC. PulseNet: 20 years of making food safer to eat. 2016. Available at https://www.cdc.gov/pulsenet/anniversary/20-years.html.

367. Heymann DL, Rodier GR. WHO Operational Support Team to the Global Outbreak Alert and Response Network. *Lancet Infect Dis.* 2001;1(5):345–53.

368. Heymann DL. The international response to the outbreak of SARS in 2003. *Philos Trans R Soc Lond B Biol Sci.* 2004;359(1447):1127–9.

369. Heymann DL, Rodier G. Global surveillance, national surveillance, and SARS. *Emerg Infect Dis.* 2004;10(2):173–5.

370. Nuttall I. International Health Regulations (3005): Taking stock. *Bull World Health Org.* 2014;92(5):310.

371. Rodier G, Greenspan AL, Hughes JM, et al. Global public health security. *Emerg Infect Dis.* 2007;13(10):1447–52.

372. Global Health Security Agenda (GHSA). 2014. Available at https://www.ghsaagenda.org.

373. Trust for America's Health. Ready or Not? Protecting the Public's Health from Diseases, Disasters and Bioterrorism. 2017. Available at https://www.tfah.org/report-details/ready-or-not-1/.

374. WHO. Joint external evaluation in crisis countries—A perspective from the Eastern Mediterranean Region. *Weekly Epidemiol Rep.* 2018;93(25):357.

375. WHO. Joint external evaluation of IHR core capacities of the United States of America: Mission report, June 2016. 2017. Available at http://apps.who.int/iris/handle/10665/254701.

376. Morse SA, Kellogg RB, Perry S, et al. Detecting biothreat agents: The Laboratory Response Network. *ASM News.* 2003;69(9):433–7.

377. CDC. Facts about the Laboratory Response Network. 2018. Available at https://emergency.cdc.gov/lrn/factsheet.asp.

378. Rappuoli R. From Pasteur to genomics: Progress and challenges in infectious diseases. *Nat Med.* 2004;10(11):1177–85.

379. McNicholl JM, Promadej N. Insights into the role of host genetic and T-cell factors in resistance to HIV transmission from studies of highly HIV-exposed Thais. *Immunol Res.* 2004;29(1-3):161–74.

380. Robertson BH, Nicholson JK. New microbiology tools for public health and their implications. *Annu Rev Public Health.* 2005;26:281–302.

381. Quick RE, Venczel LV, Mintz ED, et al. Diarrhoea prevention in Bolivia through point-of-use water treatment and safe storage: A promising new strategy. *Epidemiol Infect.* 1999;122(1):83–90.

382. Quick RE, Kimura A, Thevos A, et al. Diarrhea prevention through household-level water disinfection and safe storage in Zambia. *Am J Trop Med Hyg.* 2002;66(5):584–9.

383. Lindblade KA, Eisele TP, Gimmig JE, et al. Sustainability of reductions in malaria transmission and infant mortality in western Kenya with us of insecticide-treated bednets: 4 to 6 years of follow-up. *JAMA.* 2004;291(21):2571–80.

384. ter Kuile FO, Terlouw DJ, Kariuki SK, et al. Impact of permethrin-treated bed nets on malaria, anemia, and growth in infants in an area of intense perennial malaria transmission in western Kenya. *Am J Trip Med Hyg.* 2003;68(4 Suppl):68–77.

385. Phillips-Howard PA, Nahlen BL, Kolczak MS, et al. Efficacy of permethrin-treated bed nets in the prevention of mortality in young children in an area of perennial malaria transmission in western Kenya. *Am J Trop Med Hyg.* 2003;68(4 Suppl):23–9.

386. Langley G, Besser J, Iwamoto M, et al. Effect of culture-independent diagnostic tests on future emerging infections program surveillance. *Emerg Infect Dis.* 2015;21(9):1582–8.

387. CDC. Advanced molecular detection (AMD). 2016. Available at https://www.cdc.gov/amd/.

388. den Bakker HC, Allard MW, Bopp D, et al. Rapid whole-genome sequencing for surveillance of *Salmonella* enterica serovar enteritidis. *Emerg Infect Dis.* 2014;20(8):1306–14.

389. Harris SR, Cole MJ, Spiteri G, et al. Public health surveillance of multidrug-resistant clones of *Neisseria gonorrhoeae* in Europe: A genomic survey. *Lancet Infect Dis.* 2018;18(7):758–68.

390. CDC. The future of PulseNet. 2016. Available at https://www.cdc.gov/pulsenet/next-generation.html.

391. President's Council of Advisors on Science and Technology. National Strategy for Combatting Antibiotic Resistant Bacteria. 2014. Available at https://obamawhitehouse.archives.gov/sites/default/files/docs/carb_national_strategy.pdf.

392. WHO. Global Antimicrobial Resistance Surveillance System (GLASS) Report, Early Implementation 2016–2017. 2018. Available at https://www.who.int/glass/resources/publications/early-implementation-report/en/.

393. Outterson K, Rex JH, Jinks T, et al. Accelerating global innovation to address antibacterial resistance: Introducing CARB-X. *Nat Rev Drug Discov.* 2016;15(9):589–90.

394. Wellcome Trust. Evidence for action on antimicrobial resistance. 2016. Available at https://wellcome.ac.uk/sites/default/files/evidence-for-action-on-antimicrobial-resistance-wellcome-sep16.pdf.

395. Gelbrand H. The UN, AMR, and CARA: The Conscience of Antimicrobial Resistance Accountability. 2016. https://cddep.org/blog/posts/un_amr_and_cara_conscience_antimicrobial_resistance_accountability/.

396. World Bank Group. Drug-Resistant Infections: A Threat to Our Economic Future. 2016. Available at http://www.worldbank.org/en/topic/health/publication/drug-resistant-infections-a-threat-to-our-economic-future.

397. Food and Drug Administration. Fact Sheet: Veterinary Feed Directive Final Rule and Next Steps. 2017. Available at https://www.fda.gov/animalveterinary/developmentapprovalprocess/ucm449019.htm.

398. WHO. Global priority list of antibiotic-resistant bacteria to guide research, discovery, and development of new antibiotics. 2017. Available at https://www.who.int/medicines/publications/global-priority-list-antibiotic-resistant-bacteria/en/.

399. World Bank Group. One Health: Operational framework for strengthening human, animal, and environmental public health systems at their interface. 2018. Available at http://documents.worldbank.org/curated/en/961101524657708673/pdf/122980-REVISED-PUBLIC-World-Bank-One-Health-Framework-2018.pdf.

400. WHO, Food and Agriculture Organization of the United Nations, World Organisation for Animal Health. Monitoring Global Progress on Addressing Antimicrobial Resistance (AMR). Analysis report of the second round of results of AMR country self-assessment survey. 2018. Available at http://www.who.int/antimicrobial-resistance/publications/Analysis-report-of-AMR-country-se/en/.

401. Rottingen JA, Gouglas D, Feinberg M, et al. New vaccines against epidemic infectious diseases. *N Engl J Med.* 2017;376(7):610–3.

402. Cheney C. CEPI, a year in: How can we get ready for the next pandemic. 2018. Available at https://www.devex.com/news/cepi-a-year-in-how-can-we-get-ready-for-the-next-pandemic-91987.

403. Singer M, Clair S. Syndemics and public health: Reconceptualizing disease in bio-social context. *Med Anthropol Q.* 2003;17(4):423–41.

404. Lerner H, Berg C. A comparison of three holistic approaches to health: One Health, EcoHealth, and Planetary Health. *Front Vet Sci.* 2017;4:163.

405. Robinson TP, Bu DP, Carrique-Mas J, et al. Antibiotic resistance is the quintessential One Health issue. *Trans R Soc Trop Med Hyg.* 2016;110(7):377–80.

406. Kahn LH. Antimicrobial resistance: A One Health perspective. *Trans R Soc Trop Med Hyg.* 2017;111(6):255–60.

407. Kelly TR, Karesh WB, Johnson CK, et al. One Health proof of concept: Bringing a transdisciplinary approach to surveillance in zoonotic viruses at the human-animal interface. *Prev Vet Med.* 2017;137(PtB):112–8.

408. Kahn MS, Rothman-Ostrow P, Spencer J, et al. The growth and strategic functioning of One Health networks: A systematic review. 2018;2(6):e264–73.

409. Essack SY. Environment: The neglected component of the One Health triad. *Lancet Planet Health.* 2018;2(6):e238–9.

410. Myers SS. Planetary health: Protecting human health on a rapidly changing planet. *Lancet.* 2018;390(10114):2860–8.

411. Gerberding JL, Hughes JM, Koplan JP. Bioterrorism preparedness and response: Clinicians and public health agencies as essential partners. *JAMA.* 2002;287(7):898–900.

CHAPTER

86 SARS CoV-2 and the COVID-19 Pandemic

Ryan E. Malosh • Hannah E. Segaloff • Arnold S. Monto

INTRODUCTION

In late 2019 a cluster of pneumonia cases of unknown cause was reported from the city of Wuhan, China in Hubei province. A novel coronavirus designated SARS-CoV-2 was determined to be the cause which subsequently spread world-wide causing the COVID-19 pandemic. The first wave of the pandemic, as of this writing, is still underway. As of the beginning of August, 2020, documented cases reported to the World Health Organization (WHO) have reached nearly 18 million globally with the largest number of cases in the United States and SARS-CoV-2 deaths are reported to be nearly 687,000 worldwide. The virus has spread to nearly all parts of the globe but the burden of disease has varied widely both within and among countries. Given that the pandemic is evolving on a daily basis, this chapter presents a snapshot of the situation which will change with the passage of time. Because of the novel nature of this virus, it is not possible to predict with any degree of certainty how the epidemiology of the pandemic will progress in countries around the world.

As SARS-CoV-2 emerged, many looked to recent examples of novel coronavirus emergence and influenza virus pandemics for guidance. The related coronavirus, SARS-CoV, for example, emerged in 2002, spread in 2003 to a small number of cities globally and then rapidly disappeared. There was no second wave associated with SARS-CoV and the virus did not cause a pandemic. Another novel coronavirus, MERS, has caused sporadic outbreaks but seems to be limited in terms of human-to-human transmission. In contrast, novel influenza viruses have caused four pandemics in the past 100 years, and have always produced several waves of disease before transitioning to seasonal viruses. While it is not possible to predict the path this virus will follow, most experts believe it will not simply disappear.

The most difficult related issue to predict is the speed with which vaccines and therapeutics for SARS CoV-2 might be developed. These will potentially play a key role in controlling the virus in the future, and it is only possible to discuss in general terms what their impact on the pandemic might be. Four other coronaviruses have been recognized in the population for years and they will be discussed as background to the three that have resulted in severe disease.

The Outbreak Begins

As with most pandemics, there is little certainty about the precise origins of the causative SARS-CoV-2. For reference, the precise locale where the 2009 pandemic influenza virus moved from swine to humans is not known, although it is generally acknowledged that the first outbreaks were detected in Mexico. Similarly, the SARS-CoV virus seems to have originated in bats but the host from which it moved to humans in Guangdong in 2002 is debated. The related SARS-CoV-2 virus appears also to have had a bat origin but how and exactly when it established human-to-human transmission is currently not settled. It appears that outbreaks of pneumonia of unexplained origin were occurring in Wuhan, China at the end of 2019 and thus the numerical designation of the disease (i.e., COVID-19). By the beginning of 2020, outbreaks in Wuhan had become widespread. There are different versions of the early timeline for COVID-19; the one proposed by WHO ostensibly represents a neutral source. On January 4, 2020, the WHO reported on social media that it had received reports of a cluster of pneumonia cases—with no deaths—in the city of Wuhan, Hubei Province, China. The next day, it published an advisory, entitled "Pneumonia of unknown cause-China" reporting 44 cases of pneumonia of which 11 were severely ill. It also stated that media reported a traditional food market was involved which had been closed on January 1 for decontamination. National authorities in China reported to WHO that close contacts of the pneumonia cases were being identified and followed and attempts to identify the etiologic agent were underway. The WHO statement also contained the following, "Based on the preliminary information from the Chinese investigation team, no evidence of significant human-to-human transmission and no healthcare worker infections have been reported." However, as additional information substantiating human-to-human transmission was reported, the WHO was prompted to publish guidelines on January 10 based on prior experience with SARS and MERS (both coronaviruses) and indicated the importance of protecting healthcare workers against coronavirus (CoV) transmission. On January 12, China shared the sequence of the causative coronavirus with the world, allowing development of diagnostic tests in various countries. Acknowledging questions about the official time line, the World Health Assembly held in May 2020 authorized an investigation into these early events to "review experience gained and lessons learned from the WHO-coordinated international health response to COVID-19."

The subsequent progression of events regarding the transmission of the novel coronavirus in China is well documented. An ominous early development was that on January 13 the first case outside China, in Thailand, was identified. This suggested that there were already sufficient numbers of cases, at least in the Wuhan area, to permit transmission outside of China through human-to-human transmission. The WHO, following the International Health Regulations (IHR) of 2005, formed an Emergency Committee on January 22 to advise the Director General (the first such committee was formed in 2009 to deal with the A(H1N1) influenza pandemic). The WHO Emergency Committee was unable to reach a consensus recommendation to declare a Public Health Emergency of International Concern at that point. On January 30, with limited reports of human-to-human transmission outside of China, the Emergency Committee activated the IHR by agreeing to make such a declaration. By that time, infection was documented in 18 countries outside of China. It was not until February 11 that the new disease was officially designated COVID-19 by WHO in consultation with other international organizations. The causative virus was named SARS-CoV-2, based on its relation to the virus which caused the coronavirus outbreaks (i.e., SARS) of 2002–2003. It should be noted that WHO did not officially refer to the global outbreak as a pandemic until March 11. The delay may be attributable to a lack of specific guidelines for making such a declaration which had previously been made in 2009 in response to the emergence of influenza A/H1N1pdm09.

The Pandemic Spreads Globally

The pandemic is still evolving globally and as such it is not possible to render a comprehensive picture of its epidemiology given variations in reporting from different areas of the world. The patterns of early dissemination are clear, with the initial epicenter in Wuhan, Hubei province, China. Spread to the remainder of China rapidly ensued and then to other countries before lock down measures were instituted by the government in Wuhan in an attempt to control transmission. As of February 1, there were over 4000 cases in China outside of Hubei province but only 152 in the remainder of the world based on WHO reported data. However, the virus spread rapidly and by February 29, there were over 6000 cases in 53 countries outside of China.

The earliest outbreaks beyond China occurred in Asia and varieties of interventions were implemented in response. When Hong Kong SAR, Taiwan, and Singapore had documented a small number of cases, each began to impose nonpharmaceutical interventions. Korea detected a major cluster of cases and instituted a large contact tracing program along with a number of nonpharmaceutical containment approaches. Japan was one the first countries to document within-country transmission, but did not initially commence with vigorous containment measures. The initial impact on control of the virus was encouraging although longer-term results were less uniform and reflected the difficulty early on in assessing interventions that did and did not work.

Spread Outside of Asia

Spread to Australia and New Zealand began early, with the first case documented in Australia on January 25. Social distancing measures were instituted in March, which proved successful in controlling transmission and keeping the number of deaths low. The pandemic progressed differently in Europe with the earliest epicenter of disease focused in the Lombardy region of Northern Italy. It is not clear at this time why this particular area in Europe was the first to be so severely affected. What is clear is that many cases were exported from Northern Italy to the remainder of Europe and North America.[1]

It is not apparent when the outbreak in Italy began, but it was first recognized early in February. Because of its severity and the high levels of associated mortality, it quickly transitioned into a national public health crisis. Among the other unusual features of the outbreak in Italy is that it was mainly confined to Lombardy and neighboring provinces. As of May 28, there were over 88,000 cases reported, while in Lazio, which includes Rome, the number cases as of that same date was under 8000. Nearly half of the 33,000 total deaths in Italy recorded on that date were in Lombardy itself.

As the pandemic progressed and evolved from March to April, new global epicenters of transmission arose in New York and London as densely and highly populated urban centers. In both cities the surge of cases created challenges for the healthcare system particularly in terms of shortages of personal protective equipment (PPE) for staff and ventilators for severely ill patients. As outbreaks in Europe began to wane and case counts in the United States plateaued, transmission began to increase in Central and South America, especially in Brazil. The delay in active transmission in Latin America occurred in spite of multiple earlier introductions including those from Spain to Ecuador. This highlights the difficulty in associating specific interventions with outbreak status since there has been a substantial degree of unpredictability why one country develops into a COVID-19 "hot spot" and another does not.

Outbreaks in the United States

Outside of New York City, the United States has experienced multiple major outbreaks that are unevenly distributed geographically and vary in their intensity epidemiologically. The first reported case in the United States was in Seattle, although it is now clear that disease introduction from China was already underway, particularly on the west coast, at the time the initial U.S. case was reported. The first recognized outbreak occurred in the Seattle, Washington area with the initial case's illness onset on January 15, 2020.[2] The outbreak did not begin to spread more rapidly until mid-February. At the time of this writing, viral sequence data cannot determine whether there was silent spread during the interval from mid-January to February or whether new introductions produced the surge in cases. There is a corresponding lack of viruses isolated from this period due to the lack of testing, which makes drawing conclusions about the early epidemiologic picture in the United States more difficult.[3]

In January and February, there were also early introductions into California but unlike the situation in Washington, these did not result in significant community transmission at that time. This may be due to early imposition of nonpharmaceutical interventions in California including stay-at-home orders, but other factors cannot be excluded. The first major U.S. epicenters of transmission developed during March 2020. New York City and its metropolitan area extending into New Jersey and Connecticut was the first region severely affected. Subsequently, New Orleans, Chicago, and Detroit also experienced substantial surges in cases and deaths straining healthcare systems. Other large cities, such as Boston and Washington DC, experienced early documented transmission, but did not experience the same expansion in cases, which came close to completely overwhelming hospital capacity in New York, Chicago, and Detroit. As of this writing, the New York outbreak remains the largest and best documented, with superspreading incidents in a suburban community to widespread infections, particularly in high population density areas inhabited mainly by minority residents. Stay-at-home recommendations were issued to control spread and were ultimately successful in reducing transmission in those states with higher infection frequency (Fig. 86-1). Others states that experienced less early transmission were also much less restrictive in instituting requirements on a variety of nonpharmaceutical interventions. In June, most states have become less restrictive in their policies and use of nonpharmaceutical interventions. This has resulted, in those places that lifted restrictions most rapidly such as Texas, Arizona, and Florida, in marked upsurges in cases. With modestly increased testing, it appears that young adults are driving the transmission and thus far death rates have not risen as dramatically, perhaps because of more compliant behavior in the elderly. In other regions, more modest lifting on restrictions has resulted in some increase in transmission. However, it is clear that virus transmission even at a reduced level is present universally and flair ups requiring control are to be expected. As of the beginning of August, 2020, while the United States has reported the greatest number of cases, other countries are experiencing surges in transmission, particularly Brazil and India. Because the number of cases is dependent on the amount of testing being carried out, deaths are also an important way to assess impact. While the United States still leads in mortality globally, other countries are closing the gap.

VIROLOGY

Phylogeny

The novel SARS-CoV-2 virus is a member of the *Coronaviradae* family of viruses and is the seventh coronavirus known to infect humans. Broadly, coronaviruses are enveloped, positive-sense single-stranded RNA viruses that infect humans and other animals. There are four genera: alpha, beta, gamma, and delta coronaviruses. Viruses from the alpha and beta genera primarily infect humans, while coronaviruses from the other genera infect birds. The four common human

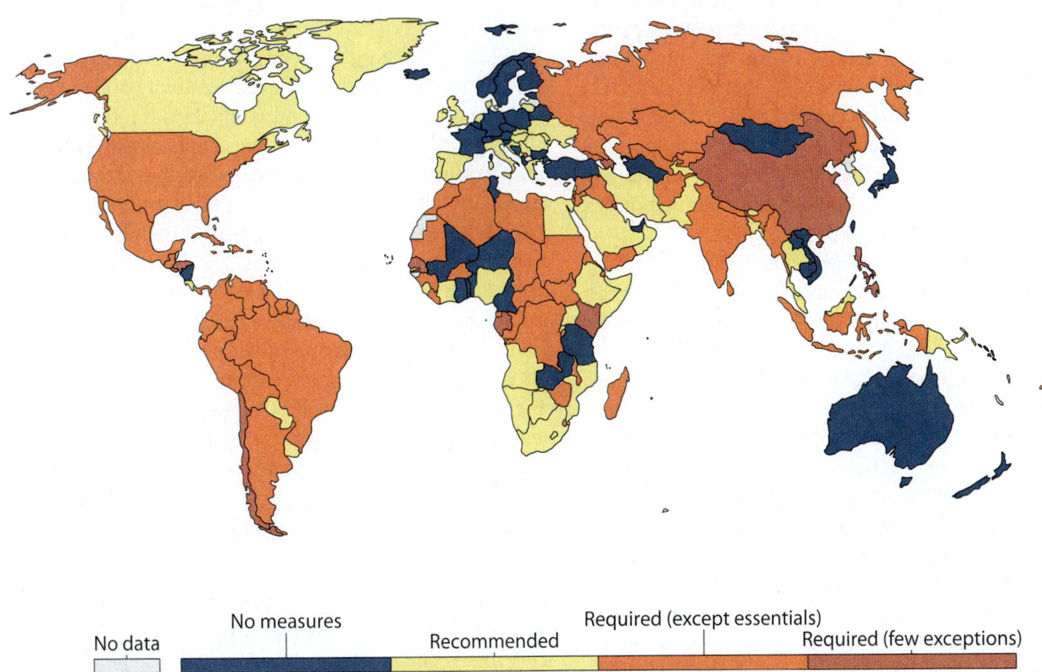

FIGURE 86-1. Stay-at-home requirements during COVID-19 pandemic, June 17, 2020. (*Source:* Hale, Webster, Petherick, Phillips, and Kira (2020). Oxford COVID-19 Government Response Tracker—Last Updated 17th June. OurWorldInData.org/coronavirus CC BY.)

coronaviruses (HCoV)—HKU1 (beta), OC43 (beta), 229E (alpha), and NL64 (alpha)—circulate seasonally in temperate regions and generally cause mild upper respiratory infections and infrequently more severe illnesses resulting in hospitalizations. In recent years two beta coronaviruses of animal origin have emerged that infect humans; severe acute respiratory syndrome (SARS) coronavirus appeared in 2002 and Middle East respiratory syndrome (MERS) coronavirus in 2012. Both of these novel viruses can cause severe illness in humans. Whole genome sequencing of the earliest identified COVID-19 cases indicated that SARS-CoV-2 is also a beta coronavirus, most closely related to SARS-CoV, with near 80% sequence homology compared to approximately 50% sequence homology between SARS-CoV-2 and MERS-CoV.[4]

SARS-CoV-2 shares many properties with SARS-CoV, including its manner of entry into the host cell through binding of angiotensin converting enzyme 2 (ACE2).[5] However, while the binding motif that directly interacts with ACE2 in SARS-CoV-2 is similar to that of SARS-CoV, the other regions of this receptor binding domain (RBD) have numerous amino acid substitutions, perhaps suggesting differences in some features of receptor binding and transmission.[4] Further research is needed to fully understand the virologic differences between SARS-CoV and SARS-CoV-2 and how these differences impact the clinical virology and severity of associated illness.

Origin

The potential origin of SARS-CoV-2 has been hotly debated in the early months of the pandemic. Both SARS-CoV and MERS-CoV emerged from viruses whose natural reservoir is bats through intermediate hosts; civets for SARS-CoV and certain camels for MERS-CoV. Whole genome sequencing of the first patients infected with SARS-CoV-2 indicates that while this virus is closely related to SARS-CoV, it is much more closely related to certain bat coronaviruses.

Certain unique features of SARS-CoV-2 may help point toward its origin. The RBD region is the most variable region in the coronavirus genome.[6] SARS-CoV-2 appears to have a RBD that gained efficient binding of human ACE2 through natural selection.[7,8] While SARS-CoV-2 is very closely related to certain bat coronaviruses, known bat coronaviruses have key mutations in RBD regions that suggest they would not efficiently bind human ACE2.[8,9] Some pangolin viruses have been identified that have similarities to SARS-CoV-2 in the entire RBD.[10]

The other key distinguishing feature of SARS-CoV-2 is a polybasic cleavage site in the spike protein, the exact function of this site is unknown.[11] However, other human coronaviruses do not contain this polybasic site. Currently, no animal coronavirus has been identified with this cleavage site. All closely related viruses described thus far have been missing key features of SARS-CoV-2, suggesting that the intermediate host, whether it be pangolin or another animal, is not yet known.

Media reports, and some politicians, have promoted hypotheses claiming that the SARS-CoV-2 could have been created in a laboratory at the Wuhan Institute of Virology, either as a laboratory construct or as a deliberately manipulated virus. These hypotheses are often based on nothing more than the proximity of the laboratory to the wet market linked to the first cluster of cases. Most scientists studying the origins of SARS-CoV-2 have vigorously refuted these hypotheses and maintained that scientific evidence points to a crossover event from a bat reservoir to humans, likely through an intermediate host.

TESTING

The first set of tests developed for detection of SARS-CoV-2 can largely be separated into two groups, polymerase chain reaction (PCR) tests for detecting current viral infection and serologic assays for detecting antibodies to SARS-CoV-2, indicating past infection. Widespread availability of both of groups of tests is important for understanding the epidemiology of SARS-CoV-2 and developing successful strategies for containing viral outbreaks.

PCR Testing—Creation and Availability

Controversies surrounding testing for SARS-CoV-2 persisted during the first part of the pandemic. As the virus emerged from Wuhan China, the genetic sequence was quickly characterized and released, leading to the creation of a variety of PCR tests, with protocols published from multiple countries in January. The German protocol was endorsed by the WHO and was used to make kits that were delivered to low- and middle-income countries (LMIC) that requested aid. Encouragingly this pandemic has been marked by extreme speed in identifying, sequencing, and isolating the etiologic agent and creating a diagnostic test but conversely has also been marred by limitations in the global supply chain and errors in test production.

In the United States in particular, quickly making and distributing sufficient tests has been challenging. The early PCR kit created by the U.S. CDC targeted three sequences in SARS-CoV-2. These kits were distributed on February 2 to states. However, reports suggested contamination issues in early test manufacturing that resulted in false positives.[12] Days after the kits were sent to state health departments and public health labs, testing was halted. Due to FDA regulations, neither WHO-approved kits nor kits developed from private companies could be rapidly deployed. Eventually, after weeks of extremely limited testing, states were allowed to continue testing with CDC kits without using the problematic third target. Still, testing availability remained limited. Private companies and hospitals were moving to develop their own tests, but the approval process was slowed by the necessity of receiving an emergency use authorization (EUA) from the FDA. It was not until mid-March that any commercial test received an EUA, though the FDA eventually changed regulations to speed up the approval process considerably. However, the result was that less than a thousand COVID-19 PCR tests were performed in the United Sates per day until early March and it was not until the end of March that daily testing levels reached into the tens of thousands. The impact of this delayed rollout of testing is difficult to assess, but it is clear that it adversely affected the ability of the United States to monitor and contain the virus.

This lack of test kits was not only an issue in the United States, but also persisted across many other countries. As the pandemic spread across Europe many countries found themselves limited to testing only the most severe clinical cases due to lack of supplies. Inadequate testing capacity made it impossible to fully implement a COVID-19 control strategy that relied on tracing case contacts, as identifying a high percentage of cases was difficult. Test kits were not the only supplies with limited availability as viral media, RNA extraction kits, and swabs were all marked by restricted accessibility which greatly impacted testing capacity globally. These shortages and delays in building testing capacity appeared to have a considerable negative effect on the ability to control outbreaks of SARS-CoV-2, as countries were overwhelmed with cases by the time testing resources were more fully developed and secured. Difficulties were not uniform across countries; some, such as Korea were able to develop and use testing early to control spread.

Virologic Tests—Utility and Limitations

There are a variety of PCR-based testing strategies available throughout the world, including rapid point of care tests, more traditional PCR tests, and antigen tests.

Traditionally, appropriate patient samples for PCR detection of respiratory viruses include nasopharyngeal (NP), oropharyngeal, and mid-turbinate swabs and bronchiolar lavage (BAL) specimens. Early in the pandemic it was recognized that NP swabs and other traditional collection techniques involved high levels of contact with trained medical personnel, requiring use of full personal protective equipment, and also often had aerosol-generating potential. As a result, alternative specimens, such as saliva, were evaluated for reliable virus detection. The ability to detect SARS-CoV-2 from saliva has increased the opportunity to expand PCR testing to include specimens collected in the home. In the United States, home saliva collection was approved in early May by the FDA. Expansion of this type of testing should allow for more convenient ways to test for SARS-CoV-2 while reducing discomfort and potential contact with ill patients.

While PCR testing has good reliability, there have been some concerns about the impact of reduced sensitivity of results from a single specimen on clinical care and public health interventions. The sensitivity of PCR varies both by the sample quality and the time from onset to sample collection. Some research has shown that viral load is highest just after symptom onset and that a substantial proportion of patients tested either before they are symptomatic or late in their disease course may be false negatives.[13] Additionally, while SARS-CoV-2 seems to replicate in high concentration in the nasopharynx, BAL specimens may be more sensitive than NP swabs in patients with profound pneumonia. False-negative specimens can disrupt control of the virus if hospital infection control policy or public health quarantine policy is based solely off PCR positive results. On the other hand, some recovered patients may be PCR-positive for long periods but with evidence that this late presence of RNA is not correlated with the presence of replicating virus. This has created some confusion concerning when an individual becomes noninfectious post-illness.

Serology

Serologic tests, or blood tests that detect antibodies to SARS-CoV-2, are used to determine whether a person has previously contracted COVID-19. These tests are useful for practical public health response and research. Unlike PCR, a positive result does not indicate that a person is currently infected with SARS-CoV-2.

A few strategies using serological data to better characterize the epidemiology of COVID-19 are large-scale geographic studies, smaller community-level studies, and studies in special populations such as schools or healthcare workers. The large geographic studies generally focus on widely available data in an area, such as a survey of blood donors or other types of blood specimens stored in biorepositories. These surveys generally serve to improve our understanding of the level of infection in a large geographic area or population catchment that may have experienced a major COVID-19 outbreak. However, using blood banked from donation or from other medical care can bias results of the studies, as these individuals may not be representative of the community or population as a whole.

Community-based serology surveys are generally smaller than geographical surveys and aim to include a representative sample of individuals in the community, hopefully reducing some of the biases that affect large geographical surveys. The intent is to extend the results of these seroprevalence studies to other similar communities. Studies of special populations help inform the seroprevalence in specific groups, such as healthcare workers or long-term care facility residents. This permits development of a more comprehensive profile of the burden of COVID-19 in a given special population, although those results may not extend to other populations.

After the delayed and gradual launch of PCR tests in the United States, the FDA reduced many of the regulatory hurdles associated with making a new diagnostic test obtainable on the market by use of Emergency Use Authorizations. Unfortunately, this allowed numerous serological tests with suboptimal reliability to inundate the marketplace. The FDA has since added additional guidelines to the approval process and many of the poorly functioning tests are no longer commercially available. Even when using reliable serological tests, interpretation of results can be difficult. If the prevalence of previous SARS-CoV-2 infection is low, then a large percentage of people who are seropositive for SARS-CoV-2, potentially more than 50% of the positives, may be false positives. For this reason, and others, such as the possibility of reinfection, use of serological testing as an "immunology passport" to allow people to travel or return to work will likely not be a successful containment strategy.

CLINICAL CHARACTERISTICS

Common clinical symptoms of COVID-19 include fever, cough, fatigue, and anorexia. Many persons with COVID-19 also exhibit shortness of breath, change in amount of or presence of sputum, and myalgia.[14–16] Not all symptoms are present with illness onset but may develop over the course of disease. Less-frequently–reported symptoms include gastrointestinal upset such as diarrhea or nausea and sore throat, headache, confusion, or rhinorrhea.[17] Loss of taste (i.e., ageusia) and/or smell (i.e., anosmia) have also occasionally been reported as uniquely predictive symptoms of COVID-19.[18]

COVID-19 is characterized by a remarkable variability in symptom severity. Many infected individuals, potentially over one-third, do not show any symptoms, while others have only mild symptoms A minority of infected individuals require supplemental oxygen, invasive mechanical ventilation, or have other serious complications.[19,20] Importantly, testing availability initially limited the characterization of the full range of clinical symptoms as virtually all states limited diagnostic testing to patients presenting to the hospital with characteristic symptoms who typically had more serious disease.

Complications

Many individuals who have severe cases of COVID-19 report mild symptoms for the first week of illness and then rapidly progress to experience severe shortness of breath and dyspnea. Other severe complications of COVID-19 include pneumonia, acute respiratory distress syndrome (ARDS), sepsis, acute kidney injury, and cardiomyopathy.[18] Some patients with more severe illness present with or develop extremely high D-dimer levels, indicating hypercoagulability. This state of hypercoagulability is associated with stroke and other clotting complications and may correlate with higher probability of COVID-19 mortality.[21,22] A distinguishing feature of severe COVID-19 is the prolonged disease course. Some individuals remain on ventilators for weeks and may require a tracheostomy if they cannot be successfully weaned off mechanical ventilatory assistance. Other individuals are re-readmitted to the hospital after continuing to experience lasting effects infection following recovery from acute infection. At this time, the longer-term clinical effects of COVID-19 have not been fully characterized but there are emerging reports of continuing pulmonary, cardiovascular, and neurologic abnormalities.

The majority of COVID-19 infections are asymptomatic or mild, consisting of typical respiratory symptoms much like a common cold and are self-limited in nature. However, hospitalization and mortality rates for this virus are higher than that seen with typical seasonal influenza. Extensive study has been dedicated to estimating the case fatality ratio and infection fatality ratio for COVID-19. These estimates have been difficult to establish and, since are dependent on recognition of infection and availability of appropriate therapy, have varied. While there is no definitive consensus about these metrics at this time, it is clear that pandemic COVID-19 is a much more serious infection than seasonal influenza.[23] A better comparator might be historic influenza pandemics; for example, in the pandemic of 1918, many have estimated the global mortality to have been 50 million.

Risk Factors for Severe Disease

Most other respiratory viruses, including influenza, have a "U-shaped" curve regarding the age with younger children and older adults the most likely to experience illness and clinical complications. In contrast, COVID-19 illness and more severe disease are rare in children, and exceedingly rare in young children. Risk for severe COVID-19 complications increases with increasing age, with those 65 years and older at the highest risk. Other risk factors associated with severe illness include preexisting comorbid conditions. While the data on specific conditions is not completely clear, it appears that chronic lung disease, heart disease, immunocompromising conditions, diabetes, liver disease, and severe obesity are risk factors for severe illness.[24]

Severe Complications Among Children

While children rarely show severe symptoms of illness, some children have exhibited an inflammatory condition following COVID-19 infection typically in the most highly impacted areas of the world. This condition, termed multisystem inflammatory syndrome in children (MIS-C), is rare. While it has not been definitively shown that this condition is directly related to COVID-19, it has appeared in areas of the world with higher levels of SARS-CoV-2 transmission, and the majority of children who have MIS-C either had known COVID-19 infection or tested positive for antibodies to SARS-CoV-2.[25] This condition has also been linked temporally to the peak of viral transmission and appears to primarily occur in children who previously had an asymptomatic or mild COVID-19 infection and is characterized by fever, severe abdominal pain, and rash. This syndrome exhibits some similarities clinically to both Kawasaki's disease and Toxic Shock Syndrome and can be life threatening, leading to cardiac and kidney damage.[26] MIS-C may originate with a hyperimmune response to infection as it is characterized by a cytokine storm and hyperinflammation. Unlike Kawasaki's disease, which mostly impacts children under 5 years of age, the mean age of children with MIS-C is approximately 10 years of age.[27] Older children and young adults have also been identified with the syndrome, which is currently being further defined as is appropriate therapy for its treatment.

EPIDEMIOLOGY

Transmission

Transmission of SARS-CoV-2 is possible via multiple routes. As with other coronaviruses, evidence from the earliest documented outbreaks suggested that respiratory droplets were the most efficient means of transmission. Subsequent studies in various settings also suggested the potential for aerosol transmission as a secondary form of transmission. In particular, laboratory studies documented the potential for recovery of viral RNA from aerosolized particles. One outbreak investigation in a restaurant in Guangzhou, China found that poor ventilation likely contributed to a probable aerosol transmission.[28]

A consistent finding throughout the early phases of the pandemic suggest that transmission is most likely to occur in indoor, congregate settings with poor ventilation. Evidence supporting this setting as the most efficient for transmission include high secondary infection risks among household contacts and in prisons, long-term care facilities (e.g. nursing homes), and food processing plants.

The basic reproductive number (R_0), or the average number of new infections from single infectious person in a completely susceptible population, is a key parameter describing the transmissibility of a novel pathogen. Early in the initial outbreak of SARS-CoV-2 in China R_0 was estimated to be between 2 and 3. Subsequent estimates have varied by location. In Italy the R_0 estimate was 2.4–3.1. In South Korea, the initial estimate was approximately 1.5. R_0 is a population-level average measure of transmissibility and cannot capture potentially important heterogeneity in infectiousness and is specific to a population based on factors such as the age structure and control measures.

Asymptomatic and Presymptomatic Transmission

Some studies have suggested that transmission is possible prior to the onset of symptoms.[29–31] One early study from Germany purported to show evidence of asymptomatic transmission,[32] but follow-up investigations found that some of these cases subsequently developed symptoms.[33] A number of studies followed that also described transmission before the onset of symptoms.[30] These studies frequently did not include long-term follow-up of index cases to determine if the transmission even was truly asymptomatic or presymptomatic.

Superspreading Events

Heterogeneity in the number of secondary infections from a single index case (reproductive number) has been documented for a number of infectious diseases, including previous novel coronaviruses that cause SARS and MERS.[34] Superspreader events are transmission occurrences where one infectious individual infects multiple, sometimes dozens of susceptible individuals.[35] Multiple studies have suggested that so-called superspreader events contribute substantially to transmission of SARS-CoV-2.[35,36] In one cluster from a choir practice in Washington State, 32 confirmed and 20 probable infections were linked to a single symptomatic index case.[37]

Cases

Through the end of May 2020 nearly 6 million cases of COVID-19 have been confirmed worldwide. The United States is the country with the most cases, with 1.7 million confirmed through the end of May. There is substantial heterogeneity in the number of cases and the proportion of cases per 100,000 population by location. In the United States, cases are disproportionately Black, even with incomplete reporting of race/ethnicity data by states.

Rates of severe disease and mortality have thus far been difficult to estimate with precision due to issues related to availability of testing, asymptomatic infection, and variation by population.

Hospitalization

In the United States, CDC adapted the FLUSurvNet network, a population-based surveillance network of laboratory-confirmed influenza hospitalizations, to estimate rates of hospitalization for COVID-19. The newly named COVID-19-Associated Hospitalization Surveillance Network (COVID-NET) uses the same population-based surveillance for laboratory-confirmed COVID-19-associated hospitalizations.

Hospitalization rates differ by age, race/ethnicity, and underlying comorbidities.[20] Through the end of May the cumulative hospitalization rate by age group is listed in Table 86-1. Hospitalization rates increase with increasing age group, and also increase linearly within age groups.[20] One retrospective cohort study conducted from March to April 11, 2020 in New Orleans, Louisiana found that 40% of those with laboratory-confirmed infection were hospitalized, and that hospitalized patients were predominantly (77%) Black. Black race, socioeconomic status, and higher Charlson comorbidity index were all associated with increased odds of hospitalization in this population.[38] Among 5700 COVID-19 hospitalizations in New York City, the most prevalent comorbid conditions were hypertension, obesity, and diabetes.

Mortality

Typical measures of mortality include the case fatality rate (CFR) and the infection fatality rate (IFR). The CFR is calculated as the number of deaths among symptomatic cases of disease. The IFR is the number of deaths among all those infected, regardless of whether they develop symptoms. Both parameters are extremely sensitive to the denominator. During the early phases of any outbreak, and especially with the COVID-19 pandemic, these denominators have been notoriously difficult to estimate. Case-finding and contact-tracing methods can improve estimates of each of these denominators but have been done in relatively limited settings. In addition, these measures are highly contextual, varying based on the age-structure, control measures, and the underlying prevalence of comorbidities of the population in which they are estimated. IFR has been particularly difficult to estimate as most cases are identified when they present for care, due to limited testing capacity.

The Diamond Princess cruise ship and similar settings where all members of a population are tested for infection can give a clear denominator for both the CFR and IFR. In the case of the Diamond Princess, 3711 individuals were quarantined and repeatedly tested for SARS-CoV-2 infection. Out of these, 705 developed symptomatic disease and 7 individuals died, leading to a CFR of 1%.[23] In other settings, the CFR has been highly variable. One study estimated that the CFR ranged from 0.1% in Austria to 5.0% in the United Kingdom, prior to each country instituting a lockdown.[39]

TABLE 86-1 HOSPITALIZATION RATE PER 10,000 PERSONS COVID-NET AS OF MAY 25, 2020

Age Group	Cumulative Rate per 100,000 Persons
Overall	67.9
0–4 years	3.5
5–17 years	1.7
18–49 years	37.2
18–29 years	17.8
30–39 years	36.8
40–49 years	62.8
50–64 years	105.9
65+ years	214.4
65–74 years	156.6
75–84 years	258.3
85+ years	396.4

MATHEMATICAL MODELING

During the COVID-19 pandemic mathematical modeling of disease dynamics has played a large role in predicting the impact of the disease as it spread to new locations. Some of the most influential models have guided governmental policies. A wide variety of approaches has been used to attempt to better understand and predict the future epidemiology of the pandemic. While all models are limited by the extent and quality of the available data used, the best approaches acknowledge these limitations and are transparent about assumptions made and appropriate use of a given model. With an unprecedented number of modeling studies presented to the public in the popular press, or appearing on preprint servers and in peer-reviewed journals, making determinations about the quality and predictive value of this surfeit of models has become progressively more difficult. As a result, calls for open science practices including publishing source code, model parameterizations, and providing detailed documentation are increasingly important.[40]

Forecasting Hospitalizations and Deaths

The focus of many models has been forecasting the number of hospitalizations and deaths due to COVID-19. Initially, one of the most relied upon models was developed by the Institute for Health Metrics and Evaluation (IHME) at the University of Washington.[41] This model represents a hybrid between forecasting and curve-fitting techniques, which also provide frequently updated predictions as to when cases and deaths would peak in each U.S. state. However, the model was notoriously inaccurate on several occasions. Other groups developing influential models that have found wider use include researchers at Imperial College, Harvard University, and the Johns Hopkins Infectious Disease Dynamics Lab.

These models were frequently used to guide government policy around public health interventions and control measures. But often the uncertainty inherent in these types of modes was lost in translation from modeling groups to policy makers. As a result, in April and May there was a substantial backlash and criticism of any model that was deemed to produce incorrect predictions of disease burden. Some prominent researchers decried the lack of quality data and suggested that model inferences were deeply flawed, resulting in stricter lockdown policies than were necessary. Proponents of modeling approaches argued that while data were not perfect, there was enough evidence to act decisively to save more lives.

Modeling Interventions

Another group of models was used to demonstrate the relative effectiveness of various interventions. Rather than attempting to predict a specific number of cases, hospitalizations, or deaths at a future point in time, these models instead start with clear assumptions about virus transmission parameters and model the effect of an intervention or group of interventions.

A prime example is the model developed by Kissler et al.[42] to examine transmission dynamics and ICU capacity with and without use of intermittent widespread social distancing. These researchers determined that in the absence of seasonal patterns of transmission there would be several peaks and troughs of cases that would require social distancing for at least 2 years to keep the number of ICU cases below hospital capacity. The authors determined that the key to effective social distancing was when to institute these measure (and went not to) which would necessitate intense public health surveillance and extensive use of contact tracing. Additional models were used to examine the potential effect of universal masking policies[43] and school closures,[44,45] among other possible interventions.

NONPHARMACEUTICAL INTERVENTIONS

Given an immunologically naïve population without any preexisting immunity to COVID-19, and the lack of effective treatments or vaccines, nonpharmaceutical interventions (NPIs) were adopted as the primary public health intervention(s) to reduce the burden of infection and disease. Specific NPIs discussed here include quarantine and isolation through contact tracing, wide-scale social distancing, school closures, use of face masks and hand hygiene, banning of public gatherings, and implementation of travel restrictions. These measures were undertaken to varying degrees between and within countries, and generally were correlated with both the number of cases and the number of deaths, as hot spots of transmission generally put more restrictions in place. As the pandemic spread globally, variation in the specific NPI measures utilized decreased suggesting that a common set of interventions was increasingly used by many countries.[46]

The effectiveness of many of these NPIs was originally tested during the SARS outbreaks in 2002–2003 with a virtual shut down of a number of cities in Asia. More recently, concerns about the pandemic potential of avian influenza A/H5N1-generated studies on social distancing and other nonpharmaceutical interventions. However, aside from those measures implemented solely at the individual level, most of the above NPI, when fully applied, have a potentially negative effect on normal economic activity. As a result, there is often a lack of political will in many cities, states, and countries to sustain these interventions over long periods of time. Indeed, the approaches developed when avian influenza was the primary concern assumed that the full measures used to "flatten the curve" would be time-limited and only used until vaccines were available. That was thought to be a period of months, as development of specific influenza vaccines is a relatively predictable process involving strain replacement in an existing vaccine. Without a licensed human coronavirus vaccine, however, the timeline for vaccine development is substantially longer, with the most optimistic estimates ranging from 12 to 18 months (i.e., availability sometime in 2021).

Quarantine and Isolation Through Contact Tracing

One of the primary NPI used to control the COVID-19 pandemic has been isolation of cases and quarantine of contacts. Quarantine is the separation and monitoring of exposed but non-ill individuals, while isolation is the separation of individuals who are already clinically symptomatic with disease. Contact tracing can be used to identify both cases and their contacts who can subsequently isolate and/or quarantine to disrupt chains of transmission.

Some countries successfully contained COVID-19 outbreaks with extensive testing, contract tracing, and use of strict quarantine/isolation protocols. The primary examples of these measures leading to successful control of the virus are New Zealand, Hong Kong, and Singapore. Many of the areas that successfully employed these measures had previous experience with SARS or other respiratory viruses with pandemic potential, and therefore understood the importance of disrupting community transmission early in the course of the pandemic. Some studies in locations that successfully contained the first wave of their outbreak reported a reduction in time from exposure to isolation or quarantine of up to 2 days.[47] Countries who were able to control their outbreaks with these interventions were those who introduced widespread testing and contact tracing before experiencing exponential growth of cases that can render these measures ineffective or simply impossible to continue from a resource perspective.

Wide-Scale Social Distancing

Social, or physical, distancing has also been used to prevent and control the spread of SARS-CoV-2. The goal of social distancing is to reduce the contact rate between susceptible and infectious individuals in the population, by limiting interactions between all people. In the context of the COVID-19 pandemic, recommended social distancing practices generally include staying at least 6 feet or 2 meters away from others, not gathering in groups, and avoiding crowded venues. Additional measures include limiting the use of public transportation, working from home (telework), school or child care closures, and using contactless delivery services to obtain food and other essential goods. Novel methods for tracking adherence to social distancing measures include the use of cellphone geolocation data usually aggregated to the county level.

China set the precedent for community-wide shutdowns early in the outbreak in Wuhan. The Lombardy region in Italy similarly employed strong restrictions on the movement of its citizens as the outbreak began to overwhelm the health system in Northern Italy. In the United States, there was not any type of governmentally recommended nation-wide policy on use of stay-at-home measures. Rather, the federal government deferred to such decisions to the state or local level. The first region to implement strict stay-at-home orders and other NPI measures was the San Francisco Bay Area in March. California was also the first state to institute a state-wide stay-at-home order, on March 19. Almost all states eventually issued some form of a stay-at-home order by the beginning of April. Similarly, many countries throughout the world issued similar mandates specifying that people only leave their homes to obtain essential goods and services as the disease spread worldwide through April. One notable exception was Sweden, which never issued a governmental requirement or even a recommendation to stay at home. The unstated goal was to reach herd immunity and to spot the infection without using vaccine or other pharmaceutical interventions. However, based on antibody testing, the country is far from that point and mortality is much higher than in several Nordic countries that used NPIs for various periods.

Social distancing measures, however, cannot be adopted by all populations with comparable ease or equally. So-called essential workers (i.e., workers required to continue reporting to work despite potential health risks) like grocery store clerks and healthcare personnel are not able to work from home.

School Closures

Similarly, school closures were eventually ordered by a majority of countries. Through the end of February very few countries had closed schools, but by the end of March nearly all countries had required such closures at all administrative levels. Most schools remained closed through April at which point over 90% of all enrolled school-aged children globally were affected by closures at the national, regional, or local level.[48] Several European countries began to relax school closures throughout May. Sweden is a notable example of a country which never instituted a nation-wide closure and they instead remained open with no major changes to class size, lunch, or recess policies. South Korea, Singapore, and Israel all opened schools as the initial stages of their outbreak declined and subsequently experienced outbreaks among children and/or teachers, and in some cases resulting in schools closing down again.

Face Masks and Hand Hygiene

Some of the earliest recommendations for NPIs to prevent COVID-19 included improving hand hygiene practices in the form of more frequent handwashing. Previously, hand hygiene interventions have shown little effectiveness in preventing respiratory illnesses. Nevertheless, as a relatively low-cost and easy intervention it was widely recommended by public health authorities.

The use of face masks had been controversial. In an effort to conserve resources for healthcare workers, public health authorities like WHO and CDC originally declared face masks ineffective at protecting healthy individuals and recommended face mask use only for sick individuals. Previous research, however, has shown some effectiveness of face masks against influenza-like illness in healthy individuals. When evidence emerged suggesting the possibility of presymptomatic or asymptomatic transmission of SARS-CoV-2, these leading public health agencies adjusted their recommendations accordingly. Subsequent modeling studies showed that meaningful reductions in transmission could be achieved through universal masking. Also supporting this recommendations has been the value of surgical face masks in interrupting nosocomial transmission.

Travel Restrictions

Importation of cases was of special concern early in the outbreak. As a result, almost all countries instituted some level of travel restrictions. New Zealand, for example, first implemented a quarantine period for all persons entering the country in mid-March but by March 19, 2020, as the pandemic became more severe, the country banned international travelers altogether from entering the country. Similar outright travel restrictions or required quarantine for visitors were enacted throughout the Asia-Pacific including Hong Kong, Taiwan, Vietnam, and South Korea. Some other countries, such as the United States, originally instituted travel bans among travelers originating from only highly affected areas. By the end of April, most countries had closed their borders completely to all international travel.

VACCINE

Many media, governmental, and academic commentators have proposed that society cannot return to prepandemic normalcy until an effective vaccine is available and extensively administered with a goal of achieving herd immunity (i.e., a sufficiently large proportion of the population is immune providing indirect protection to those who are not). Vaccine testing in humans is just underway making it difficult or impossible to predict with any degree of certainty the population effect from using a newly developed vaccine. Vaccine development has been accelerated with governmental assistance in many countries accompanied by an unprecedented push to rapidly move production forward. Licensure is typically only granted after there has been some demonstration of vaccine safety and effectiveness through clinical trials. The purpose of this accelerated timeframe is to generate sufficient quantities of vaccine ready for distribution virtually simultaneous with licensure by the appropriate regulatory authority.

The principal vaccine candidates receiving governmental assistance for development of all use novel technologies, mainly involving platforms not previously employed for approved human vaccines. There are, however, precedents for work on coronavirus vaccines as during and immediately after the SARS-CoV outbreaks some vaccine development did occur. While much of that original work on SARS-CoV was terminated prior to identifying a viable vaccine candidate, it was replaced by research on a MERS vaccine which has continued to the present day. This is of the regular reappearance of MERS in the Middle East and the perception, that is, represents an ongoing disease threat. The research into a vaccine for MERS has clear relevance for insights it may provide into development of a SARS-CoV-2 vaccine.

The major focus in SARS-CoV vaccine development was directed to developing neutralizing antibodies to the S or spike protein, the same portion of the virus targeted by the current SARS-CoV-2 vaccine candidates. Methods to achieve this have been varied. Traditional approaches have included virus growth in substrates and inactivation, production of viral subunits, or even development of live-attenuated variants by creating deletions in the viral genome. Other less traditional research was directed at development of recombinant vaccines in which vectors such as vaccinia virus Ankara (MVA) were engineered to encode the full length S protein. There was also research into DNA vaccines which at the time were being evaluated for a number of diseases.

The MERS vaccines under development were intended not only for humans but also for camels, the major zoonotic host of that virus. The human candidate vaccines, similar to the SARS-CoV vaccines, include the following approaches: viral vectored, DNA, subunit, nanoparticle, inactivated-whole viral, and live-attenuated. While other components of the virus were present in some of the vaccines, the S protein was present in all candidates, given the likely association between the presence of antibodies and protection from disease.

Vaccines in development for SARS-CoV-2 have largely used the same platforms as both the SARS-CoV and MERS-CoV vaccine candidates. As mentioned, some research groups were actively developing MERS vaccines and, as such, they have simply updated the viral components to those of the novel coronavirus. A large number of countries and companies globally are working on these vaccines which include whole virus and subunit vaccines. However, lead candidates, which are now in advanced stages of development, use the recombinant-vectored approach. The University of Oxford, in partnership with AstraZeneca, is in late stage trials with a vaccine using a nonreplicating chimpanzee adenovirus as the vector. Similarly, Janssen Pharmaceutical Companies is in earlier stage development using an adenovirus 26 vector. Further, a nanoparticle vaccine produced by Novavax with a stable perfusion viral protein in both an adjuvanted and unadjuvanted formulations is also in development. One of the more novel vaccine approaches being used is the mRNA vaccine developed by the NIH Vaccine Research Center in conjunction with Moderna. This represents a new technology which is attractive because of its relatively rapid production with stabilization of the mRNA accomplished by encapsulation in lipid nanoparticles (LNPs) for delivery. Other mRNA vaccines are also in various stages of development, led by one being evaluated by Pfizer.

When vaccines utilizing new technologies are introduced, there is heightened concern about the potential for adverse events. For that reason, regulatory authorities generally require that such vaccines be administered to much larger numbers in clinical trials than would typically be necessary to demonstrate efficacy. However, low-frequency adverse events can occur when a new vaccine is approved and used in larger numbers of individuals who often express greater social, ethnic, racial, and health status heterogeneity than is present in clinical trials. In addition, careful evaluation of the safety of coronavirus vaccines in the context of previous exposure to infection is warranted. Specifically, some people may develop antibodies to SARS-CoV-2 following the first wave(s) of the pandemic. Moreover, many individuals may have preexisting antibodies to the common coronaviruses, which may cross react with vaccine-induced SARS-CoV-2 antibodies. In some animal challenge studies with SARS-CoV-1, investigators have reported antibody-dependent enhancement (ADE). The question as to whether this should be a concern going forward has been reviewed in detail.[49,50]

It has been generally proposed that an effective SARS-CoV-2 vaccine will be used to achieve herd immunity. This concept, described elsewhere, suggests that production of population-level antibody exceeding a level predetermined by transmission models and often based on the R_0 will result in interruption of community transmission of infection through both direct and indirect mechanisms. Protection would be conferred by antibodies resulting from infection supplemented by that produced through vaccination. Currently, the seroprevalence of antibody in the population, even in COVID-19 epicenters, is relatively low, in affected New York groups under 20% suggesting a necessary role for vaccination to achieve herd immunity.

It is unclear whether achieving herd immunity is realistic given many years of experience with influenza for which little evidence exists that vaccination can significantly interrupt transmission even at vaccination rates of 60% or higher in some population subgroups. Important considerations in achieving herd immunity will be vaccine effectiveness as well as potential reductions in transmissibility in the event of vaccine failure. The initial goal may be prevention or reduction of illness severity in those at highest risk of infection or disease. Potential target groups would likely be healthcare or other essential workers in the former case and older adults and those with underlying comorbidities in the latter.

THERAPEUTICS

During the emergence of SARS-CoV there was no known antiviral with demonstrated treatment effectiveness. Because the SARS-CoV outbreak was limited in scope and duration, there were few clues about other treatment approaches beyond the apparent lack of usefulness of corticosteroids when administered early and in high doses. Similarly, there were no effective antiviral treatments for MERS-CoV infections.

A number of treatment options have been proposed, although many are without any clear demonstration of efficacy. Some proposed therapies are antiviral drugs while other proposed therapeutics aim to manage one or more of the specific effects of infection. There have numerous preliminary reports on potential therapeutics, often providing conflicting conclusions. One of the primary issues is the complexity of the clinical manifestations of COVID-19, as described above. In addition, the lengthy duration of the illness from infection to symptom onset and resolution has meant that studies with short-term follow-up are not applicable or appropriate. All of these factors suggest that a single therapeutic intervention may only be sufficient to address a limited or very specific significant clinical issue and combination therapies may be needed.

One antiviral, remdesivir, is being evaluated, along with other potential therapeutics.[51] Remdesivir is a nucleotide analogue prodrug that interferes with viral replication. It was originally developed as a drug, which might work against Ebola in the 2014 outbreak. It was not found to be effective against that virus, but on screening was found to have activity against coronaviruses. Studies by NIAID indicated that it had a clinical benefit when given early in treatment of rhesus macaques challenged with SARS-CoV-2.[52] Clinical trials are being carried out using different designs both by NIAID and Gilead, the company promoting the drug. The first published study[53] demonstrated a significant reduction in time of illness in a controlled trial. More than 25% of those treated were on invasive mechanical ventilation and the mean duration of illness before randomization was 9 days. The latter factor was of interest, since it indicated that there was an effect even with use later in the course of illness. Further studies following this preliminary report are underway and the drug is being studied for inhaled rather than intravenous use. Alternative modes of administration might make the drug available for use in postexposure prophylaxis as it would not require hospitalization to be administered.

There have not been positive results as yet for immunotherapy. Many of the initial studies are based on blood donated by individuals who have recovered from infection making it too early to draw definitive conclusions. However, it is possible to conjecture that many of the later manifestations of illness occur at a time when antibody is already developing. There is, of course, speculation that there might be some role for immunopathogenesis in the course of the disease, but studies have not found any safety concerns with the use of antibody therapy.

Many of the other drugs being used are intended to modify the cytokine storm or other over reactions of the immune system. One drug, which is being studied in conjunction with remdesivir, is tocilizumab,[54] approved for treatment of rheumatoid arthritis. There are preliminary reports of success in using this drug. A surprise finding is the report of significant reduction in 28-day mortality using a 10-day course of treatment with dexamethasone, a readily available and inexpensive medication, in patients with severe illness.[55] This study, which requires further confirmation, is in contrast to observations that patients with high levels of cortisol are at particular risk.

Research on potential treatment modalities for SARS-CoV-2 is very much in flux and drugs that have shown promise in the laboratory, and sometimes in animal models, such as hydroxychloroquine, have not had comparable success in human studies. Discovering effective treatments to improve clinical outcomes for those with severe disease is critical to addressing future surges in infection and disease and reducing the related burden of morbidity and mortality.

SPECIAL POPULATIONS

Throughout the pandemic, certain populations have garnered special interest either through their vulnerabilities to severe disease or high rates of SARS-CoV-2 infection. The populations described here include healthcare workers (HCWs), individuals living in institutional settings such as nursing homes, long-term care facilities or prisons, those working in large factories such as meat-packing plants, and persons belonging to racial/ethnic minority groups.

HCWs

Since the emergence of COVID-19 in China, there has been intense concern about the potential for mass infection of HCWs. This in part resulted from lessons learned in the SARS epidemic of 2003 during which large numbers of HCWs became infected and nosocomial infections drove much of the epidemic worldwide.[56] HCWs were generally at much greater risk for nosocomial transmission than non-healthcare workers, making SARS an occupational hazard in some cases.[57] Much of this transmission was related to a lack of or incorrect use of personal protective equipment such as surgical masks, gowns, and N95 respirators.[58]

At the beginning of the SARS-CoV-2 outbreak, there were initial reports from Hubei Provence of numerous HCW infections. However, the WHO Joint Mission to China found that while there were specific instances of nosocomial infection during the outbreak, it did not appear to be a major impetus for transmission overall as it was during the SARS outbreak.[59] In addition, the majority of HCW infections appeared to occur in the early phase of the outbreak in China, mostly in Wuhan, suggesting that supply and personnel limitations increase the probability transmission in the hospital setting. This was evident with the rapid rise of cases in Northern Italy, when HCW infection was a significant issue. In Lombardy, HCWs represented a significant proportion of those infected, with reports that near 10% of cases in that region at the end of March were HCW.[60] This region experienced a rapid rise in cases accompanied by overcrowding in hospitals and lack of adequate PPE.

The major factor associated with infection of HCWs in hospitals or other clinical settings is lack of access to PPE. In facilities with appropriate controls related to HCW contact with patients and proper use of PPE, transmission from the latter to the former appears to be minimal. However, limited access to PPE has been a dominant feature of this pandemic in the United States and elsewhere. In the United States, production of N95s was not accelerated early part of the pandemic leading to dramatic shortages as cases increased rapidly. Many of the N95s secured for use by health systems in the United States were from other countries and often did not meet safety standards of the United

States, potentially putting HCW at heightened risk. Guidance as to when HCW should use surgical masks and when they require N95s has not always been clear, likely due to both the shortages of supplies and the unknown contribution of small aerosol transmission of COVID-19 in healthcare settings. At this time, the CDC recommends that N95 respirators or other similar respirators be used for HCWs in a room with COVID-19 patients and when involved in potentially aerosol generating or surgical procedures on such patients. Only a surgical mask with added eye protection is recommended in settings when there is the possibility of moderate to substantial community transmission.[61] These recommendations are frequently updated and are different in different jurisdictions. Infections in HCWs are especially tragic since they provide care to the ill and as such greater levels of infection can limit their ability to treat all patients with in need with COVID-19 and otherwise. Therefore, protecting healthcare professionals is of paramount importance to any successful strategy for control the pandemic.

Efforts have been made to quantify the number and proportion of HCW infected thus far in the outbreak. It is expected that this will vary widely by city and setting, and will depend on both the intensity of the outbreak in the area of interest as well as a given healthcare setting's infection control practices and policies. It is clear that with proper practices, the threat can be reduced markedly. Moving forward, more systematic serology-surveys testing HCWs can assist with estimating this number in different hospitals and healthcare systems particularly among those HCW treating or in direct contact with COVID-19 patients. Recent reports have also suggested that many infections in HCWs have really been community acquired.

Nursing Homes, Long-Term Care Facilities, and Skilled Nursing Facilities

Nursing homes, long-term care facilities (LTCFs), and skilled nursing facilities (SNFs) have been severely impacted by the COVID-19 outbreak. The older age group which is subject to multiple comorbidities and living in close proximity in these settings renders them especially prone to COVID-19 transmission and outbreaks. In some U.S. states, nursing home outbreaks have caused upwards of 40% of total infections and 25% of total deaths. One of the first identified SNF outbreaks in the United States occurred in King County, Washington in which over 60% of residents became infected and over 25% of infected residents died.[30] This illustrates the potential devastation possible in a population of elderly individuals, often with multiple comorbid conditions that place them at greater risk of serious disease, living in an institutional setting that fostering extensive close personal contact. This phenomenon is not specific to the United States and the WHO has reported that through April, half of deaths from COVID-19 in Europe occurred in LTCFs such as nursing homes.

In an attempt to intervene and control these outbreaks, several measures have been taken in the United States and in other countries. Many LTCFs have banned visitors to help reduce introduction of COVID-19. Others have introduced regular and more systematic testing of residents and staff to identify infected individuals before they can transmit the virus. Finally, the CDC recommends universal masking of patients and staff in LTCF to help reduce spread.[62]

Prisons

Another institutional setting that has been an important source for COVID-19 transmission and cases is prisons. These settings are often overcrowded, and involve a large population of individuals sharing spaces and resources making it difficult or impossible to socially distance. In the United States, where there are more inmates per capita than in most of Europe, outbreak in prisons has contributed significantly to total case counts. Notably, testing has not been extensively undertaken in most prisons, although Ohio reported results from universal testing and found that two-thirds of prisoners had tested positive for COVID-19. Many human rights advocacy groups have proposed release of some nonviolent inmates to reduce jail and prison crowding which has been done in some states. Most countries have not widely tested prisoners, though outbreaks have been reported in China and across Europe in that setting. Prisons may prove to be an important location for outbreaks in Latin America, where many countries have exceptionally overcrowded prison populations.

Factories and Meat-Packing Plants

More densely congregated work environments are well suited to spread of COVID-19. One such occupational setting, meat-packing plants, has been a hotspot for COVD-19 transmission in the United States. A large proportion of all cases in Utah were associated with meat-packing plant outbreaks. Because a large number of outbreaks across the country have occurred in this setting, many meat-packing plants have temporarily closed down for restructuring and cleaning in an attempt to reduce transmission risk which was anticipated to lead to potential meat shortages nationwide. To avoid this hypothetical shortage an executive order was signed obligating meat-packing plants to remain open and workers to report to the plants. In order to mitigate risks, the CDC published guidance to improve physical distancing in plants, enhance hand hygiene, cleaning and disinfection, and to encourage plants to mandate that sick employees stay at home.[63]

Racial/Ethnic Minority Groups

In the United States and in other countries, such as the United Kingdom, the COVID-19 pandemic has disproportionally affected nonwhite minority groups, particularly those who are Black or of African descent and, in parts of the United States, Latinx and Native American populations as well. Initially, the discussion of this phenomenon focused on whether this reflected genetic differences, but, as observations rapidly accumulated, it became clear that a number of other factors, namely racism and other forms of discrimination, are involved. These factors may contribute to increased likelihood of infection or poor outcome in those infected or both. Increased exposure to COVID-19 may be associated with crowded housing conditions, increasing the probability of transmission. Multigenerational households increase the likelihood of vulnerable older individuals being exposed. Occupational factors are also involved with some racial and ethnic minorities in urban areas more likely to be employed as part of the essential workforce. Many of these jobs are less likely to have access to remote work or paid sick leave, putting employees in contact with many potentially infected persons. This includes work in healthcare, often in roles where protective equipment is not routinely used. Finally, there is often reduced availability of prompt and appropriate medical care, which is a chronic issue in some areas. The U.S. CDC has a specific website titled, Health Equity Considerations and Racial and Ethnic Minority Groups, which provides additional relevant information at the following link: https://www.cdc.gov/coronavirus/2019-ncov/community/health-equity/race-ethnicity.html.

CONCLUSION

As the first cases of COVID-19 emerged in the United States, Dr. Nancy Messonnier at the CDC issued a prescient and dire warning, stating in a news conference, "Disruption to everyday life might be severe." Several months into the COVID-19 pandemic, there is still much that we do not understand about this virus, its epidemiology and the clinical course of disease with which it is associated. At the time of this writing, people across the globe are living vastly different lives than preceding the pandemic with many working from home, their children are out of school and day care, and often barred from engaging in commonplace activities like eating at a restaurant, watching a movie, or getting a haircut. The profound disruptions to everyday life have been severe and reveal the overwhelming enduring capacity for an infectious disease to alter life for people in every corner of the globe.

It remains almost impossible to predict how long the COVID-19 pandemic will continue. The question of whether there will be any seasonality to COVID-19 transmission is hard to predict. The common human coronaviruses mainly occur in the winter in temperate settings, but all indications point to efficient transmission of this virus at high temperatures as well. Whether this lack of seasonality is mainly due to a lack of immunity in the global population may become more evident with the passage of time. Another major unknown is when (and if) a vaccine will be available, and how effective and durable the immunity produced by vaccination will be. This has given rise to questions about the ability of vaccination to produce high enough levels of population immunity to interrupt transmission. Combination use of a vaccine with therapeutics should theoretically make a return to near prepandemic status possible. The COVID-19 pandemic may eventually be recognized as an event unprecedented in recent human history. The 1918 influenza epidemic produced far more deaths than COVID-19 has, but it did not maintain its lethality indefinitely. How COVID-19 will behave in the future virologically, epidemiologically, and clinically, we simply do not know at this time.

What is clear is that despite high transmissibility, the SARS-CoV-2 virus does not seem to be spreading sufficiently fast to produce population or herd immunity following the first waves. Thus, modification of that spread will need to be attained by other means. Currently, much effort is focused on reducing contact rates to control transmission, bolstering hospital capacity, and, when possible, opening up the economy to ease the financial burden of the pandemic. Open science and global partnerships are being used both to improve reporting and analysis of surveillance data and in the development of an effective vaccine and therapeutics. What has, at times, been a disheartening display of the prioritization of politics over policy has also been marked by the world's collective effort to "flatten the curve" and save lives.

The coming months and years will determine whether efforts to control SARS-CoV-2 and develop effective treatment options are sufficient and successful. As we look to the immediate future, with the prospect of cocirculation of SARS-CoV-2 with influenza and other respiratory viruses, the need for continued effort and engagement against this virus globally is as urgent as ever. Only time will tell whether we heed the call.

References

1. Italy: Coronavirus cases by region. Statista. Accessed June 23, 2020. Available at https://www.statista.com/statistics/1099375/coronavirus-cases-by-region-in-italy/.
2. Holshue ML, DeBolt C, Lindquist S, et al. First case of 2019 novel coronavirus in the United States. *N Engl J Med.* 2020;382(10):929–36.
3. Worobey M, Pekar J, Larsen BB, et al. The emergence of SARS-CoV-2 in Europe and the US. *bioRxiv.* Published online May 23, 2020:2020.05.21.109322.
4. Lu R, Zhao X, Li J, et al. Genomic characterisation and epidemiology of 2019 novel coronavirus: Implications for virus origins and receptor binding. *Lancet.* 2020;395(10224):565–74.
5. Zhou P, Yang X-L, Wang X-G, et al. A pneumonia outbreak associated with a new coronavirus of probable bat origin. *Nature.* 2020;579(7798):270–3.
6. Wu F, Zhao S, Yu B, et al. A new coronavirus associated with human respiratory disease in China. *Nature.* 2020;579(7798):265–9.
7. Tang X, Wu C, Li X, et al. On the origin and continuing evolution of SARS-CoV-2. *Natl Sci Rev.* Published online 2020 Mar 3.
8. Andersen KG, Rambaut A, Lipkin WI, Holmes EC, Garry RF. The proximal origin of SARS-CoV-2. *Nat Med.* 2020;26(4):450–2.
9. Xu X, Chen P, Wang J, et al. Evolution of the novel coronavirus from the ongoing Wuhan outbreak and modeling of its spike protein for risk of human transmission. *Sci China Life Sci.* 2020;63(3):457–60.
10. Lau SKP, Luk HKH, Wong ACP, et al. Early release—Possible bat origin of severe acute respiratory syndrome coronavirus 2. *Emerg Infect Dis.* 2020;26(7):1542–7.
11. Hoffmann M, Kleine-Weber H, Pöhlmann S. A multibasic cleavage site in the spike protein of SARS-CoV-2 is essential for infection of human lung cells. *Mol Cell.* 2020;78(4):779–84.e5.
12. Willman D. Contamination at CDC lab delayed rollout of coronavirus tests. *The Washington Post.* Accessed June 22, 2020. https://www.washingtonpost.com/investigations/contamination-at-cdc-lab-delayed-rollout-of-coronavirus-tests/2020/04/18/fd7d3824-7139-11ea-aa80-c2470c6b2034_story.html.
13. He X, Lau EHY, Wu P, et al. Temporal dynamics in viral shedding and transmissibility of COVID-19. *Nat Med.* 2020;26(5):672–5.
14. Xu X-W, Wu X-X, Jiang X-G, et al. Clinical findings in a group of patients infected with the 2019 novel coronavirus (SARS-Cov-2) outside of Wuhan, China: Retrospective case series. *BMJ.* 2020;368:m606.
15. Huang C, Wang Y, Li X, et al. Clinical features of patients infected with 2019 novel coronavirus in Wuhan, China. *The Lancet.* 2020;395(10223):497–506.
16. Chen N, Zhou M, Dong X, et al. Epidemiological and clinical characteristics of 99 cases of 2019 novel coronavirus pneumonia in Wuhan, China: A descriptive study. *The Lancet.* 2020;395(10223):507–13.
17. Pan L, Mu M, Yang P, et al. Clinical characteristics of COVID-19 patients with digestive symptoms in Hubei, China: A descriptive, cross-sectional, multicenter study. *Am J Gastroenterol.* 2020;115(5):766–73.
18. CDC. Interim Clinical Guidance for Management of Patients with Confirmed Coronavirus Disease (COVID-19). Centers for Disease Control and Prevention. Published February 11, 2020. Accessed June 17, 2020. Available at https://www.cdc.gov/coronavirus/2019-ncov/hcp/clinical-guidance-management-patients.html.
19. Gandhi M, Yokoe DS, Havlir DV. Asymptomatic transmission, the Achilles' Heel of current strategies to control Covid-19. *N Engl J Med.* 2020;382(22):2158–60.
20. Epidemiological Characteristics of COVID-19: A Systemic Review and Meta-Analysis—Abstract—Europe PMC. Accessed June 17, 2020. Available at https://europepmc.org/article/ppr/ppr139410.
21. Oxley TJ, Mocco J, Majidi S, et al. Large-vessel stroke as a presenting feature of Covid-19 in the young. *N Engl J Med.* 2020;382(20):e60.
22. Magro C, Mulvey JJ, Berlin D, et al. Complement associated microvascular injury and thrombosis in the pathogenesis of severe COVID-19 infection: A report of five cases. *Transl Res.* 2020;220:1-13.
23. Russell TW, Hellewell J, Jarvis CI, et al. Estimating the infection and case fatality ratio for coronavirus disease (COVID-19) using age-adjusted data from the outbreak on the Diamond Princess cruise ship, February 2020. *Eurosurveillance.* 2020;25(12):2000256.
24. CDC. People Who are at Higher Risk for Severe Illness. Centers for Disease Control and Prevention. Published February 11, 2020. Accessed June 17, 2020. Available at https://www.cdc.gov/coronavirus/2019-ncov/need-extra-precautions/people-at-higher-risk.html.
25. Chiotos K, Bassiri H, Behrens EM, et al. Multisystem inflammatory syndrome in children during the coronavirus 2019 pandemic: A case series. *J Pediatr Infect Dis Soc.* 2020;9(3):393–8.
26. Greene AG, Saleh M, Roseman E, Sinert R. Toxic shock-like syndrome and COVID-19: A case report of multisystem inflammatory syndrome in children (MIS-C). *Am J Emerg Med.* 2020;S0735-6757(20):30492–7.
27. Zahra B, Mathilde M, Fanny B, et al. Acute heart failure in multisystem inflammatory syndrome in children (MIS-C) in the context of global SARS-CoV-2 pandemic. *Circulation.* 2020;142(5):429–36.
28. Li Y, Qian H, Hang J, et al. Evidence for probable aerosol transmission of SARS-CoV-2 in a poorly ventilated restaurant. *medRxiv.* Published online April 22, 2020:2020.04.16.20067728.
29. Bai Y, Yao L, Wei T, et al. Presumed asymptomatic carrier transmission of COVID-19. *JAMA.* 2020;323(14):1406–7.
30. Arons MM, Hatfield KM, Reddy SC, et al. Presymptomatic SARS-CoV-2 infections and transmission in a skilled nursing facility. *N Engl J Med.* 2020;382(22):2081–90.
31. Cheng H-Y, Jian S-W, Liu D-P, Ng T-C, Huang W-T, Lin H-H. Contact tracing assessment of COVID-19 transmission dynamics in Taiwan and risk at different exposure periods before and after symptom onset. *JAMA Intern Med.* 2020;180(9):1156–63.
32. Rothe C, Schunk M, Sothmann P, et al. Transmission of 2019-nCoV infection from an asymptomatic contact in Germany. *N Engl J Med.* 2020;382(10):970–1.
33. Böhmer MM, Buchholz U, Corman VM, et al. Investigation of a COVID-19 outbreak in Germany resulting from a single travel-associated primary case: A case series. *Lancet Infect Dis.* 2020;20(8):920–8.
34. Wong G, Liu W, Liu Y, Zhou B, Bi Y, Gao GF. MERS, SARS, and Ebola: The role of super-spreaders in infectious disease. *Cell Host Microbe.* 2015;18(4):398–401.

35. Frieden TR, Lee CT. Identifying and interrupting superspreading events—Implications for control of severe acute respiratory syndrome coronavirus 2. *Emerg Infect Dis.* 2020;26:1059–66.
36. Liu Y, Eggo RM, Kucharski AJ. Secondary attack rate and superspreading events for SARS-CoV-2. *The Lancet.* 2020;395(10227):e47.
37. Hamner L. High SARS-CoV-2 attack rate following exposure at a choir practice—Skagit County, Washington, March 2020. *MMWR Morb Mortal Wkly Rep.* 2020;69.
38. Price-Haywood EG, Burton J, Fort D, Seoane L. Hospitalization and mortality among black patients and white patients with Covid-19. *N Engl J Med.* 2020;382:2534-43.
39. Rajgor DD, Lee MH, Archuleta S, Bagdasarian N, Quek SC. The many estimates of the COVID-19 case fatality rate. *Lancet Infect Dis.* 2020;20(7):776–7.
40. Dyal JW. COVID-19 among workers in meat and poultry processing facilities—19 States, April 2020. *MMWR Morb Mortal Wkly Rep.* 2020;69.
41. Barton CM, Alberti M, Ames D, et al. Call for transparency of COVID-19 models. *Science.* 2020;368(6490):482–3.
42. IHME | COVID-19 Projections. Institute for Health Metrics and Evaluation. Accessed June 24, 2020. Available at https://covid19.healthdata.org/.
43. Kissler SM, Tedijanto C, Goldstein E, Grad YH, Lipsitch M. Projecting the transmission dynamics of SARS-CoV-2 through the postpandemic period. *Science.* 2020;368(6493):860–8.
44. Stutt ROJH, Retkute R, Bradley M, Gilligan CA, Colvin J. A modelling framework to assess the likely effectiveness of facemasks in combination with 'lock-down' in managing the COVID-19 pandemic. *Proc R Soc Math Phys Eng Sci.* 2020;476(2238):20200376.
45. Bayham J, Fenichel EP. Impact of school closures for COVID-19 on the US health-care workforce and net mortality: A modelling study. *Lancet Public Health.* 2020;5(5):e271–8.
46. Hale T, Angrist N, Kira B, Petherick A, Phillips T, Webster S. "Variation in Government Responses to COVID-19" Version 6.0 Blavatnik School of Government Working Paper. Published online May 25, 2020. Available at www.bsg.ox.ac.uk/covidtracker.
47. Bi Q, Wu Y, Mei S, et al. Epidemiology and transmission of COVID-19 in 391 cases and 1286 of their close contacts in Shenzhen, China: A retrospective cohort study. *Lancet Infect Dis.* 2020;20(8):911–9.
48. https://plus.google.com/+UNESCO. Education: From disruption to recovery. UNESCO. Published March 4, 2020. Accessed June 23, 2020. Available at https://en.unesco.org/covid19/educationresponse.
49. Jiang S, He Y, Liu S. SARS vaccine development. *Emerg Infect Dis.* 2005;11(7):1016–20.
50. Yong CY, Ong HK, Yeap SK, Ho KL, Tan WS. Recent advances in the vaccine development against Middle East respiratory syndrome-coronavirus. *Front Microbiol.* 2019;10:1781.
51. Eastman RT, Roth JS, Brimacombe KR, et al. Remdesivir: A review of its discovery and development leading to emergency use authorization for treatment of COVID-19. *ACS Cent Sci.* 2020;6(5):672–83.
52. Williamson BN, Feldmann F, Schwarz B, et al. Clinical benefit of remdesivir in rhesus macaques infected with SARS-CoV-2. *Nature.* 2020;585(7824):273–6.
53. Beigel JH, Tomashek KM, Dodd LE, et al. Remdesivir for the treatment of Covid-19—Final report. *N Engl J Med.* 2020;383(19):1813–26. Online ahead of print.
54. Kewan T, Covut F, Al–Jaghbeer MJ, Rose L, Gopalakrishna KV, Akbik B. Tocilizumab for treatment of patients with severe COVID-19: A retrospective cohort study. *EClinicalMedicine.* 2020;24:100418.
55. Horby P, Lim WS, Emberson J, et al. Effect of dexamethasone in hospitalized patients with COVID-19: Preliminary report. *N Engl J Med.* 2020. Published online June 22, 2020:2020.06.22.20137273.
56. Mackenzie JS, Drury P, Ellis A, et al. The Who Response to SARS and Preparations for the Future. Washington, DC: National Academies Press; 2004. Accessed June 7, 2020. Available at https://www.ncbi.nlm.nih.gov/books/NBK92476/.
57. Lee N, Sung JJY. Nosocomial transmission of SARS. *Curr Infect Dis Rep.* 2003;5(6):473–6.
58. WHO | SARS (Severe Acute Respiratory Syndrome). WHO. Accessed June 7, 2020. Available at https://www.who.int/ith/diseases/sars/en/.
59. who-china-joint-mission-on-covid-19-final-report.pdf. Accessed June 7, 2020. Available at https://www.who.int/docs/default-source/coronaviruse/who-china-joint-mission-on-covid-19-final-report.pdf.
60. Paterlini M. On the front lines of coronavirus: The Italian response to covid-19. *BMJ.* 2020;368:m1065.
61. CDC. Coronavirus Disease 2019 (COVID-19). Centers for Disease Control and Prevention. Published February 11, 2020. Accessed June 10, 2020. Available at https://www.cdc.gov/coronavirus/2019-ncov/hcp/infection-control-recommendations.html.
62. Interim Infection Prevention and Control Recommendations for Healthcare Personnel During the Coronavirus Disease 2019 (COVID-19) Pandemic. Published July 15, 2020.
63. CDC. Coronavirus Disease 2019 (COVID-19) Preparing for COVID-19 in Nursing Homes. Centers for Disease Control and Prevention. Published February 11, 2020. Accessed June 10, 2020. Available at https://www.cdc.gov/coronavirus/2019-ncov/hcp/long-term-care.html.

CHAPTER

87

The Epidemiology and Prevention of HIV and AIDS

Jeb Jones • Colleen Kelley • Patrick S. Sullivan • James W. Curran

INTRODUCTION

Human immunodeficiency virus (HIV) infection and the immune impairments it can lead to (acquired immune deficiency syndrome or AIDS) continue to be leading causes of morbidity and mortality globally. As of 2015, AIDS continues to be a top-ten cause of death among many low-income countries,[1] and HIV infection continues to be a major public health problem worldwide, particularly among certain risk groups. Significant advancements have been made in our understanding of HIV prevention and treatment in recent years; however, the HIV/AIDS epidemic continues to present numerous unique behavioral, medical, and societal challenges that have made control of the epidemic difficult.

HISTORY AND ORIGIN

The June 5, 1981 issue of the Centers for Disease Control and Prevention's (CDC's) *Morbidity and Mortality Weekly Report* included a description of five cases of *Pneumocystis carinii* pneumonia (PCP) among previously healthy men who have sex with men in Los Angeles, California.[2] These would become the first reports of AIDS. HIV was identified as the cause of AIDS in 1983.[3,4] In the United States, incidence and prevalence of HIV and AIDS have been disproportionately high among men who have sex with men (MSM) since the beginning of the epidemic.[5] Other groups have also experienced greater risk compared to the general population including injection drug users[6,7] and, initially, persons with hemophilia and other blood transfusion recipients.[8] The clustering of the epidemic among marginalized and minority populations, along with early fears and misunderstanding of how HIV is transmitted, has led to persistent stigma associated with HIV infection. Stigma continues to exacerbate disparities in HIV prevention and treatment outcomes.[9]

In addition to stigma, several other factors specific to HIV/AIDS led to the rapid propagation of the epidemic. Because of the long incubation period from HIV infection until the onset of AIDS, HIV was able to circulate extensively before the clinical manifestations of AIDS led to its recognition as a public health problem. Factors that increased the spread of HIV included increases in the numbers of sexual partners and sexually transmitted diseases among substantial numbers of men who have sex with men, high rates of injection drug use with sharing of contaminated needles and syringes, and the utilization of clotting factor concentrates made from unheated plasma pooled from thousands of donors to treat hemophilia. These factors represented amplification systems that, in combination with the long incubation period for AIDS, allowed extensive transmission of HIV to occur even before the first clinical cases were discovered. The first antiretroviral drug (zidovudine) to treat HIV infection was not available until 1987,[10] by which time the epidemic was widespread. Highly active antiretroviral therapy (HAART), which involves treating HIV-infected patients with a combination of antiretroviral drugs, became common practice for management of HIV in 1996.[11,12] A cure continues to remain elusive.

Two strains of HIV have been identified: HIV-1 and HIV-2. HIV-1 is the predominant circulating strain of HIV. HIV-2 is less efficiently transmitted and less pathogenic; however, it can still lead to AIDS.[13] Retrospective studies have identified the earliest known case of HIV-1 to have been in a patient in Kinshasa, Zaire in 1959. The first known HIV-2 infection in humans has been traced to the 1960s.[14] However, molecular analysis methods have been used to demonstrate that HIV-1 and HIV-2 were originally transmitted to humans from nonhuman primates in the 1930s.[15]

ETIOLOGIC AGENT AND NATURAL HISTORY

In 1983 and 1984, researchers at the Institut Pasteur (Paris) and the National Cancer Institute isolated a retrovirus, subsequently named HIV, and demonstrated it to be the etiologic agent of AIDS.[4,16–19] In 1985, a genetic variant of the AIDS virus was isolated and subsequently named HIV-2.[14,20] HIV-1 has great genetic diversity, and is divided in to groups thought to represent independent zoonotic transmission events of simian immunodeficiency virus into humans.[21] These are classified as group M (main), O (outlier), N (non-M, non-O), and P (proposed new group) HIV-1 viruses, with almost all of the globally transmitted strains being from group M.[21] Group M is composed of eleven distinct subtypes and several additional recombinant forms, with predominantly subtype B in North America and Western Europe; subtypes B and F in South America; subtype C in Southern Africa; subtypes A and D in East Africa; recombinant subtype A/G in West Africa; subtype B and recombinant subtype A/E in Asia; and a great diversity of subtypes found in Central Africa, where HIV-1 is believed to have first been introduced in humans.

HIV can enter the body parenterally or by mucosal transmission through the distal gastrointestinal tract or the genitourinary tract. HIV infects local cells such as macrophages, dendritic cells, and/or CD4+ T cells, which are the primary target for HIV, and replicates locally in the tissues after mucosal transmission for a few days before it becomes a systemic infection. Within about 7–10 days after infection, HIV nucleic acids are detectable in blood, and antibodies to HIV are detectable as early as 2–6 weeks following infection, although delayed HIV seroconversion can occur. HIV preferentially infects CD4 T-helper lymphocytes (so-named by the receptor molecule on their surface that identifies them), white blood cells that are critical to human immune function, through a complex mechanism whereby a glycoprotein (gp 120) of the HIV viral envelope binds strongly to the surface of the CD4 lymphocytes and a few other cell types.[22,23]

HIV is an RNA virus, which replicates by a process known as reverse transcription. HIV RNA is initially transcribed into DNA of the host cell which is then transcribed into RNA, which in turn is then copied multiple times, turning the cell into a virtual "factory" for producing multiple HIV viral particles. These particles are then released from the CD4 lymphocyte into the bloodstream, destroying the host cell in the process. When these particles invade many new CD4 cells, the life cycle of HIV is complete.[24] This direct cellular destruction, in addition to CD4+ T cell bystander destruction, results in the characteristic decrease in CD4 cell and total lymphocyte counts causing a progressive immunodeficiency. When the immune compromise is severe enough (typically defined as a CD4 count of less than 200 cells/uL), an HIV-infected person becomes more susceptible to potentially life-threatening "opportunistic" infections and diseases. Although the immune system is extraordinarily resilient and regenerative, HIV reproduces at a rate of 10 billion new virions per day,[25] and the immune system eventually succumbs in almost all HIV-infected individuals unless effective antiretroviral therapy (ART) is initiated.

In addition to maintaining productive infection in CD4+ T cells, HIV DNA integrates into the host genome where it can remain latent (i.e., persistence but no production of new virion progeny) for the life of the cell. Only a minority of CD4+ T cells harbor integrated HIV DNA; however, it is estimated that the time for natural elimination of all latently infected cells exceeds an individual's lifespan. The totality of infected cells in the blood and body tissues that contain integrated HIV DNA is referred to as the HIV reservoir and current antiretroviral therapies do not eliminate the reservoir. Elimination or reduction in size of this HIV reservoir in people on effective ART could lead to HIV cure, and is an area of active, ongoing research.[26–28]

MODES OF TRANSMISSION AND DISTRIBUTION OF INFECTION

HIV has been recovered from peripheral blood, semen, vaginal secretions, breast milk, other body fluids, and numerous anatomical sites.[29,30] There are three main modes of transmission: sexual transmission through rectal, vaginal, and (rarely) oral contact; parenteral transmission through injection, transfusion, or accidental exposure to infected blood or its components; and perinatal transmission from infected mothers to their infants either before, during, or after childbirth. Epidemiologic observations and controlled studies have confirmed these routes of transmission in homosexual and bisexual men,[31] heterosexual men and women,[32] injecting drug users,[33] and infants.[34] Previously documented risks to persons with hemophilia[35–37] and transfusion recipients[8] have been remarkably well controlled by educating donors, testing all donations of blood and plasma for HIV-1 and HIV-2 antibody, HIV-1 antigen, HIV RNA, and by developing safe clotting factor concentrates.[38,39] A systematic review conducted in 2014 estimated the risk of HIV transmission per exposure among multiple routes. The highest risk route was blood transfusion with a risk of 9250 per 10,000 exposures followed by mother-to-child transmission (2260 per 10,000 exposures), receptive anal intercourse (138 per 10,000 exposures), needle-sharing injection drug use (63 per 10,000 exposures), percutaneous needle stick (23 per 10,000 exposures), insertive anal intercourse (11 per 10,000 exposures), receptive penile-vaginal intercourse (8 per 10,000 exposures), and insertive penile-vaginal intercourse (4 per 10,000 exposures).[40] Risks associated with insertive and receptive oral sex are assumed to be nonzero but were too small to be estimated.

Healthcare and laboratory workers have been infected through occupational exposure to blood or specimens from HIV-infected patients. Using data from 23 studies, the estimated risk of HIV seroconversion following percutaneous exposure to HIV-infected blood was estimated to be approximately 0.3%[41]; risk following mucous-membrane exposure has been estimated to be approximately 0.09%.[42] Reports of seroconversion and HIV infection following skin exposure to HIV-infected blood indicate that these can occur, but the risk is much lower than following parenteral exposures. The United States Public Health Service (USPHS) has published guidelines for standard practices to avoid infection when exposed to blood and other bodily fluids.[43] USPHS Guidelines recommend following Standard Precautions[44] in all healthcare settings, including home healthcare settings when indicated. Postexposure prophylaxis (PEP) with antiretroviral medications should be initiated within 72 hours of a suspected exposure and should be continued for 4 weeks. Exposures indicated for PEP include percutaneous, mucous membrane, or nonintact skin exposure to potentially infectious bodily fluids. The PEP regimen should consist of a combination of three antiretroviral medications. HIV testing should be conducted at the time that PEP is initiated and again at 6 weeks, 12 weeks, and 6 months following exposure. Guidelines allow for follow-up HIV testing to conclude after 4 months if a fourth-generation combination HIV Ag/Ab test is used. Nonoccupational PEP (nPEP) is recommended for individuals with potential HIV exposure with a substantial risk of transmission via sexual, injection drug use, or other exposures outside of an occupational setting.[45] Timing of initiation, duration of treatment, and recommended medication regimens are similar regardless of exposure type (i.e., occupational or nonoccupational).

There is no evidence that HIV is spread by air, water, food, casual contact, or insect vectors. If such modes of transmission did exist, the epidemiology of HIV and AIDS would be much different, with clusters occurring in schools, nursing homes, and households. Only a small fraction of the reported cases do not fall readily into a characteristic patient group. Extensive follow-up of household contacts of both adults and children with AIDS has failed to demonstrate evidence of HIV transmission via shared living space, kitchens, or bathrooms or through casual contact.[46]

SURVEILLANCE OF HIV AND AIDS

History of HIV/AIDS Surveillance. Before the etiologic agent was known, AIDS was initially defined as the occurrence of a severe opportunistic illness in a person without a previously known cause of immunodeficiency; the most frequently reported illnesses in the United States were *Pneumocystis carinii* pneumonia and Kaposi's sarcoma.[47,48] Identification of HIV as the cause of AIDS and growing knowledge of the disease's epidemiology and clinical presentations led to the expansion of the United States. AIDS surveillance case definition, in 1987, to include HIV testing and such conditions as HIV encephalopathy and wasting syndrome, and in 1993 to include tuberculosis, invasive bacterial pneumonia, invasive cervical cancer, and severe immunodeficiency as measured by a CD4 cell count less than 200 cells/uL.[49,50] Currently, the most frequently reported AIDS condition is a CD4 count less than 200 cells/uL, responsible for the majority of newly reported AIDS diagnoses in the United States. Because the natural history and distribution of time from infection to development of opportunistic infections was known through cohort studies, AIDS incidence was used initially to estimate historical HIV incidence. However, the addition of CD4 count criteria to the AIDS case definition and the efficacy of HAART eliminated the ability to estimate HIV incidence through the reporting of AIDS cases. Subsequently, the HIV incidence in the United States was estimated using a number of imprecise methods to be approximately 40,000 cases per year between 1992 and 2000.[51]

In 1996, when the use of HAART became widespread in the United States, the interval between HIV infection and the development of severe HIV-related disease was greatly increased and trends in AIDS cases became much less useful in modeling trends in HIV transmission. This made it critical to monitor the number of persons reported with HIV as well as with AIDS.[52] National surveillance systems for HIV/AIDS were consequently expanded to include monitoring of new HIV diagnoses, HIV incidence, behaviors that put people at high risk for HIV, and HIV-related morbidity and mortality. In the United States, a National Behavioral Surveillance System was established to monitor behaviors that place individuals at high risk for

HIV infection[53]; this surveillance system uses serial cross-sectional surveys in high-risk populations including MSM, injection drug users, and heterosexuals at high risk for HIV infection throughout the United States.

HIV/AIDS Surveillance in the United States. Reliable, population-level estimates of HIV incidence are not available due to frequent delays between HIV infection and diagnosis. Thus, HIV surveillance data are reported as diagnoses, not incident infections. HIV surveillance in the United States is conducted at the state level and states submit de-identified surveillance data to the CDC for national surveillance reports. Surveillance practices were inconsistent at the state level in the early years of the epidemic. However, by 2008, all 50 states, the District of Columbia, and six dependent areas had fully implemented confidential name-based surveillance of HIV diagnoses. This consistency in surveillance practices and reporting allows for more reliable observations of trends in HIV diagnosis rates in the United States. As of 2014, CDC has classified HIV diagnoses into four categories—stages 0–3—and an additional "unknown" category for those diagnoses that cannot be classified. Stage 0 represents recent infections; stage 1 are infections with no AIDS-defining opportunistic illnesses (OI), CD4 count of $\geq$ 500 cells/uL or CD4 percentage of total leukocytes $\geq$ 29%; stage 2 also have no AIDS-defining OI but reduced CD4 count (200–499 cells/uL) or CD4 percentage (14–28%); and stage 3 is characterized by AIDS-defining OI, CD4 count $<$ 200 cells/uL or CD4 percentage of total leukocytes $<$ 14%.[54]

HIV and stage 3 (AIDS) diagnoses in 2016, cumulative AIDS diagnoses through 2016, and deaths among persons diagnosed with AIDS through 2015 are presented in Table 87-1. Despite progress that has been made in reducing the HIV epidemic in the United States key racial and behavioral groups continue to experience a disproportionate burden of HIV infection. In 2016, 44% (N = 17,528) of new diagnoses occurred among black/African American individuals despite the fact that they comprise approximately 13% of the population in the United States.[55] In the same year, two-thirds (N = 26,570) occurred among MSM; an additional 1201 (3%) occurred among MSM who also inject drugs. MSM have been estimated to comprise approximately 2% of the adult population, or 4% of adult men, in the United States.[56]

Despite the high number of AIDS deaths that have occurred since the epidemic began, progress in ART has led to a steady decline in the rate of AIDS deaths. Figure 87-1 depicts AIDS diagnoses, prevalence, and deaths from 1985 through 2015. Sharp decreases in the number of diagnoses and deaths occurred following the development and implementation of successful ART in the mid-1990s. As with HIV infection in general, prevalence continues to rise reflecting the successful treatment and longer lifespan of individuals living with an AIDS diagnosis. Similar disparities to those observed among HIV diagnoses are reflected in cumulative AIDS diagnoses and deaths. Of the 1,232,346 cumulative AIDS diagnoses through 2016, 508,711 (41%) occurred among black/African American individuals and 599,230 (49%) occurred among MSM. Similarly, of the 692,789 cumulative AIDS deaths through 2015, 285,744 (41%) were among black/African American individuals and 325,330 (47%) were among MSM.

The prevalence of HIV infection among children age 13 years and younger has declined significantly due to advances in the prevention of mother-to-child transmission of HIV. An early study demonstrating the successful prevention of mother-to-child transmission was the Pediatric AIDS Clinical Trial 076 Study, which demonstrated 67.5% reduction in the risk of HIV transmission among mothers and infants treated with zidovudine.[57] The CDC recommends testing all pregnant women for HIV.[58] Maternal use of ARV during pregnancy and delivering ART to the newborn, elective cesarean section, and avoidance of breastfeeding can reduce the risk of mother to child transmission to less than 1%.[59–61] In 2015, fewer than 0.4% of HIV diagnoses occurred among individuals age 13 and younger.

In addition to providing current estimates of the populations recently diagnosed and those living with HIV and death rates from AIDS, surveillance is also useful in understanding trends in behavioral risk factors and treatment uptake and adherence. As described above, CDC conducts behavioral surveillance via the National HIV Behavioral Surveillance System (NHBS) to better characterize HIV risk among three subgroups: MSM, people who inject drugs (PWIDs), and high-risk heterosexual men and women. Each risk group is surveyed every 3 years. NHBS data have been useful in understanding, for example, current rates of HIV testing among PWID,[62] changes in condom use among MSM,[63] and the occurrence of anal sex among high-risk heterosexual men and women.[64] CDC also conducts surveillance of people living with HIV via the Medical Monitoring Project (MMP).[65] MMP has increased our understanding of the behavioral and clinical characteristics of people living with HIV in the United States, such as rates of viral suppression among persons in care[66] and rates of hypertension among persons living with HIV.[67]

Global Surveillance. Globally, the United Nations Joint Programme on AIDS (UNAIDS) and the World Health Organization issue annual updated HIV/AIDS surveillance estimates. There were an estimated 36,100,000 people living with HIV globally in 2016 with an estimated 1,800,000 new HIV diagnoses (Table 87-2). Complete HIV surveillance is resource-intensive and is not feasible in all countries. In many low- to middle-income countries, counts of new HIV diagnoses are approximated based on prevalence estimates obtained from antenatal clinics. The characteristics of the HIV epidemic vary globally. In contrast to the concentrated epidemic among specific subgroups in the United States, many countries, particularly in Africa, continue to have generalized epidemics. Approximately 19.4 million people are living with HIV in eastern and southern Africa. The countries with the highest prevalence of HIV among adults age 15–49 in 2016 were Swaziland (27.2%), Lesotho (25.0%), and Botswana (21.9%).[68] Although deaths from AIDS have been declining globally, from 2010 to 2016 the number of AIDS-related deaths increased in the Middle East, North Africa, Eastern Europe, and Central Asia.[69] Injection drug use is an important factor in the HIV epidemic in high-income countries in Eastern Europe; however, these countries also tend to report low or no HIV infections among MSM, indicating that there might be some misclassification of mode of transmission.[70]

Recent developments in HIV prevention and treatment have improved control of the HIV epidemic. Pre-exposure prophylaxis (PrEP),[71] PEP,[72] voluntary medical male circumcision,[73–75] HIV treatment as prevention (TaSP),[76] consistent condom use,[77,78] and needle and syringe exchange[79] have all been shown to be effective methods of reducing HIV incidence. UNAIDS member countries have adopted the 90-90-90 targets, which aim to have 90% of people living with HIV to be aware of their infection, 90% of those who are aware to be on ART, and 90% of those on ART to be virally suppressed. Scaled-up surveillance and monitoring efforts will be necessary to evaluate national, regional, and global progress towards the 90-90-90 targets in terms of awareness of infection, treatment coverage, and viral suppression.

TREATMENT OF HIV IN THE ERA OF HIGHLY ACTIVE ANTIRETROVIRAL THERAPY

Before the era of combination ART, approximately 50–70% of HIV-infected adults developed AIDS within 10 years of HIV infection. The introduction of zidovudine (ZDV or AZT) in the United States in 1987 ushered in the era of ART. As additional anti-HIV drugs were introduced, HIV-infected patients were treated with monotherapy through about 1993 and subsequently the concurrent use of two antiretrovirals ("dual therapy") became common from 1993 to 1996. However, due in part to its rapid replication rate, HIV exhibits a remarkable rate of mutation and became largely resistant to both mono- and dual therapy. However, when the use of three concurrent

TABLE 87-1 DIAGNOSES OF HIV, AIDS, AND CUMULATIVE DEATHS AMONG INDIVIDUALS EVER DIAGNOSED WITH AIDS, 2016

	HIV Diagnoses	AIDS Diagnoses	Cumulative AIDS Diagnoses	Cumulative AIDS Deaths (Through 2015)[a]
Total	39,782	18,160	1,232,346	692,789
age				
<13	122	38	9,573	4,968
13–14	23	12	1,478	296
15–19	1,652	209	9,298	1,313
20–24	6,776	1,252	53,874	10,077
25–29	7,964	2,426	145,223	47,563
30–39	9,943	4,692	475,322	232,157
40–49	6,490	4,201	351,523	223,040
50–59	4,882	3,664	137,208	116,633
60+	1,930	1,666	48,847	56,742
Race/Ethnicity				
American Indian/Alaska Native	243	102	3,580	1,988
Asian	977	335	10,067	3,542
Black/African American	17,528	8,501	508,711	285,744
Hispanic/Latino	9,766	4,111	231,473	106,644
Native Hawaiian/Pacific Islander	48	15	837	369
White	10,345	4,442	439,998	279,807
Multiple races	875	654	37,588	14,647
Men				
All men	32,131	13,851	971,120	561,296
MSM	26,570	10,075	599,230	325,330
IDU	1,285	952	185,414	134,466
MSM/IDU	1,201	751	87,872	53,521
Heterosexual	3,037	1,992	86,911	38,727
Perinatal	--	--	--	463
Other	38	80	11,694	8,789
Women				
All women	7,529	4,271	251,653	126,525
IDU	939	728	91,021	59,438
Heterosexual	6,541	3,434	154,584	62,839
Perinatal	--	--	--	592
Other	49	109	6,048	3,655
Region				
Northeast	6,309	3,088	354,229	213,084
Midwest	5,068	2,359	132,116	73,965
South	20,588	9,584	501,523	272,756
West	7,817	3,129	244,478	132,984

[a]Deaths among individuals ever diagnosed with AIDS.

agents ("triple therapy," or combination "ART") began in 1996, highly successful therapy for HIV became commonplace in high-income countries. Although cure of HIV infection remains an active area of research, replication of the virus can now be held in check and immune function can effectively be preserved with long-term ART. Today, a young HIV-infected person who initiates ART prior to advanced immunosuppression can aspire to a near-normal life expectancy.[80–82]

Historically, clinical decisions regarding when to initiate ART in HIV-infected persons were based on laboratory measurements of the patient's immune status (CD4 lymphocyte count) and on the concentration of HIV in the patient's blood ("HIV viral load"). Department of Health and Human Services (DHHS) guidelines recommend that ART be initiated for all HIV-infected persons regardless of CD4 count or viral load to reduce morbidity and mortality associated with HIV infection,[83] but also to prevent HIV transmission as those who maintain durable viral suppression with ART do not transmit HIV to sexual partners.[84,85] The more than 20 licensed antiretroviral medications in the United States as of 2018 fall into five general categories—nucleoside/nucleotide reverse transcriptase inhibitors (NRTIs), nonnucleoside reverse transcriptase inhibitors (NNRTIs), protease inhibitors, entry inhibitors, and integrase inhibitors.

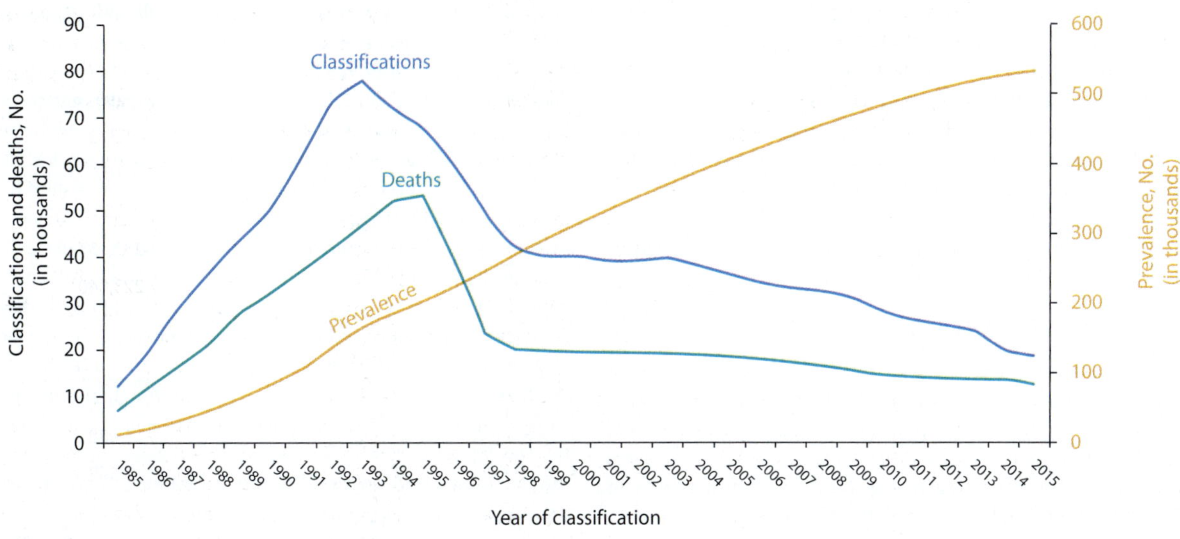

FIGURE 87-1. Stage 3 (AIDS) classifications deaths, and persons living with diagnosed HIV infection ever classified as stage 3 (AIDS) 1985–2015—United States and six dependent areas. Centers for Disease Control and Prevention. https://www.cdc.gov/hiv/pdf/library/slidesets/cdc-hiv-infection-trends-stage3-2016.pdf

TABLE 87-2 GLOBAL SURVEILLANCE OF HIV/AIDS, 2016

	New HIV Diagnoses	Living with HIV	Deaths from AIDS
Asia and the Pacific	270,000	5,100,000	170,000
Caribbean	18,000	310,000	9,400
East and Southern Africa	790,000	19,400,000	420,000
Eastern Europe and Central Asia	190,000	1,600,000	40,000
Latin America	97,000	1,800,000	36,000
Middle East and North Africa	18,000	230,000	11,000
West and Central Africa	370,000	6,100,000	310,000
Western and Central Europe and North America	73,000	2,100,000	18,000
Total	1,800,000	36,100,000	36,700,000

Source: aidsinfo.unaids.org.

Current guidelines recommend initiation of an integrase inhibitor in combination with two NRTIs for most treatment naïve HIV-infected adults; however, multiple alternative regimens are available and chosen based in individual patient characteristics and needs.[83] In addition, the use of prophylactic oral antibiotics such as trimethoprim-sulfamethoxazole to prevent opportunistic infections such as pneumocystis pneumonia are recommended for patients whose CD4 lymphocyte counts are less than 200 cells/uL.[86] The impact of ART in countries where it has been widely available has been almost as dramatic as was the dawn of the antibiotic era following World War II, with steep declines in the incidence of AIDS and deaths among HIV-infected persons.[87-89] It is critical that HIV-infected individuals remain engaged in clinical care over their lifetime to ensure durable viral suppression and to monitor for long-term complications of aging with HIV infection.

Despite the successes of ART, important challenges remain. Since infection with HIV is lifelong, patients beginning on ART need to take these pills daily indefinitely because therapy suppresses viral replication but does not eradicate HIV from the host. HIV is unique among viruses in that it can integrate into the host genome and lay dormant (latent) for an individual's lifetime, even in the setting of effective ART. Once ART is stopped, the virus reactivates from latency and the disease progresses. Eradication from the host, or "HIV cure," has been definitively achieved to date in only one individual after he received two bone marrow transplants for leukemia with CD4 cells harboring a mutation in the CCR5 coreceptor for HIV entry rendering them resistant to infection.[90,91] While bone marrow transplantation is too invasive to consider for all HIV positive patients, multiple other mechanisms for HIV cure are under investigation including initiating ART at the earliest time points after HIV infection and latency reversing agents.[92]

In addition to the need for lifelong therapy to suppress viral replication, patients must adhere very closely to the prescribed regimens. All regimens currently require daily dosing, because missing multiple doses can allow the virus to mutate and become resistant to antiretroviral drugs, which will then necessitate changing to potentially more complex, toxic, and/or expensive regimens. ART treatment interruptions have also been associated with increased morbidity and mortality and should be avoided.[93] New, long-acting ART regimens that might obviate the need for daily dosing and hopefully improve adherence for those who struggle with daily dosing are currently under investigation.[94] Finally, it must be noted that critical inequities remain in achievement of durable viral suppression with ART both in the United States and globally. In the United States, blacks are less likely to achieve viral suppression with ART than whites[95] due to a myriad of contributing social determinant of health[96] and, globally, universal access to antiretroviral drugs remains challenging.[88]

Several important global initiatives began to address disparities in global access to ART in the early 2000s. The World Health Organization launched the "3 by 5" initiative with the goal of treating 3 million persons with HAART by 2005. WHO promulgated the first guidelines for scaling up ART in resource-limited settings in 2003. A "Global Fund" was established in 2002 to finance international efforts to address AIDS, tuberculosis, and malaria in the developing world. In 2003, The United States government committed significant resources to expanding ART in the developing world through the President's Emergency Plan for AIDS Relief that established initial 5-year goals to provide treatment to 2 million persons and to prevent 7 million HIV infections in 15 designated countries. Over time, these programs sustained important advances in delivery of ART in resource-limited settings. In 2014, UNAIDS released the ambitious 90-90-90 treatment targets to help end the AIDS epidemic: By 2020, 90% of all people living with HIV will know their status; 90% of all people with diagnosed HIV infection will received sustained ART; and 90% of people receiving ART will have viral suppression.[97] As of mid-2017, UNAIDS reported that more than 20 million of the approximately 37 million people living with HIV infection worldwide were receiving ART.[98]

PREVENTION AND CONTROL

At the end of 2015, approximately 1.1 million people in the United States were living with HIV. An estimated 15% of these were unaware of their infection[99] and approximately 40,000 new cases are diagnosed annually.[100] There have been substantial decreases in HIV incidence since early in the epidemic, largely due to increased awareness and understanding of HIV and advances in the effectiveness and number of HIV prevention interventions.[101,102]

HIV Testing. HIV testing and counseling has long been the cornerstone of HIV prevention and control. Since 2006, CDC has recommended routine opt-out HIV testing for patients of age 13–64 years in primary care settings, with repeat screening occurring at least annually among high-risk populations.[103] The United States Preventive Services Task Force (USPSTF) recommends HIV screening for all adolescents and adults age 15–65 and all pregnant women.[104] Once an individual is aware of their HIV status, they tend to take steps to reduce the risk of transmitting the virus to others. Indeed the majority of new HIV infections are estimated to originate from persons who are unaware they are living with HIV, despite the fact that they comprise a minority of people living with HIV.[105] A variety of testing options are now available. Traditionally, individuals learned their HIV status during an individual testing and counseling session in a physician's office or through an HIV prevention community-based organization. Recently, however, the additional value of couples testing together has been recognized. Originally developed as a HIV prevention intervention in Africa,[106] couples voluntary counseling and testing (CVCT) highlights the importance of couples making decisions together about HIV risk reduction, and when necessary, HIV treatment for one or both members of the couple. CVCT has been shown to be safe, acceptable, and effective as a HIV testing method and prevention tool in the United States[107–110] and has been adopted by the CDC as an evidence-based intervention.[111] Finally, home-based testing kits are now available which increase the convenience and ease of HIV testing; such kits have been found to be broadly acceptable.[112,113] These kits allow users to receive their results at home within a few minutes or mail the test to a lab for next-day results.

HIV tests are not able to detect the presence of HIV immediately after infection. Instead, there is a "window period" during which an individual is infected but tests will return a negative result. The period immediately following infection is characterized by high viremia[114] resulting in a high probability of onward transmission, so prolonged window periods are problematic from the perspective of HIV control. The window period for the first HIV antibody tests was approximately 3 months. Later, third- and fourth-generation tests were developed that significantly reduced the window period. Third-generation tests expanded the classes of immunoglobulins that are detected, and are capable of detecting antibodies that develop earlier in infection than previous tests, leading to a window period of approximately 20–25 days. Fourth-generation tests have reduced the window period to approximately 2 weeks. Nevertheless, the window period persists, limiting our ability to detect the most recent infections, and sometimes requiring more than one test after possible exposure.

Barriers to HIV testing have been reduced. The Internet has made it easier for people to find testing locations, and the advent of home testing has made HIV testing more convenient. As mentioned previously, individuals can test and obtain their results at home using rapid HIV testing or collect a blood sample at home to send to a lab for testing.[115] In a sample of men who have sex with men, both methods were deemed acceptable, with 72% of men reporting that would be likely or extremely likely to use an at-home rapid HIV test,[112] and distribution of at-home HIV test kits increases HIV testing frequency for MSM.[116]

Behavioral Prevention Methods. Correct and consistent condom use continues to be the primary behavioral method to prevent transmission of HIV and other sexually transmitted diseases. Consistent condom use among MSM reduces the risk of HIV from anal sex by about 70%[117]; condoms have been estimated to be approximately 80% effective in preventing HIV among heterosexuals.[77] However, rates of condomless sex remain high. According to NHBS surveys, condomless vaginal sex was reported by 91.7% of high-risk heterosexual women and 87.9% of high-risk heterosexual men[118]; condomless anal sex was reported by 65.4% of MSM.[119] A review of behavior change interventions for MSM found generally small effect sizes and nonsignificant results across studies.[120]

Biomedical Prevention. Huge advancements have been made in the development of biomedical HIV prevention interventions. Historically, when an individual entered HIV treatment their CD4 count and viral load were monitored until one or both measures fell below threshold values (e.g., CD4 count < 350 cells/uL), at which point they would initiate ART. Evidence now indicates that earlier initiation into treatment of someone living with HIV is effective in reducing HIV risk for partners. A randomized controlled trial of early initiation of HIV therapy demonstrated a 96% reduction in HIV risk for the partners of participants who initiated therapy at HIV diagnosis instead of waiting; a strategy known as TasP.[76] A Consensus Statement signed by a multinational collection of governmental and nongovernmental organizations supports the conclusion that the risk of transmission from people living with HIV who have had an undetectable viral load for at least 6 months is negligible. Current Department of Health and Human Services guidelines recommend that all persons diagnosed with HIV initiate ART regardless of CD4 count.[83]

Antiretroviral drugs have been also been found to prevent HIV infection when taken by individuals at risk of HIV; this strategy is known as PrEP. Currently one drug, Truvada (200 mg emtricitabine/300 mg tenofovir disoproxil fumarate) is approved for use as PrEP in the United States via daily dosing. A trial conducted among MSM and transgender women found 44% protection against HIV infection.[71] However, among participants with detectable drug in their system, the protection from HIV was 92%. PrEP has also been found to be effective in some heterosexual populations. A 75% reduction of HIV risk was observed in the Partners PrEP trial conducted in Kenya and Uganda among serodiscordant couples[121] and a 62.5% reduction in HIV risk was observed in a trial conducted in Botswana.[122] Other trials have not demonstrated efficacy, potentially due to poor compliance.[122] Uptake of PrEP has been slow in the 6 years since its licensure.[123]

Prevention of Mother-to-Child Transmission. Effective methods are available to virtually eliminate the risk of transmission of HIV from mother to child. The CDC recommends HIV testing of all pregnant women and antiretroviral treatment initiation for all pregnant women living with HIV.[103] Mothers who receive HAART for at least 4 weeks reduce the risk of transmission to less than 1%.[124] Caesarean section deliveries reduce the risk of transmission of HIV to the infant compared to vaginal deliveries[125,126]; however, there are no differences in HIV risk for caesarean compared to vaginal birth if the mother is on HAART.[124] Infants who test positive for HIV can be provided antiretroviral PEP to prevent HIV infection.[103] HIV is present in breastmilk,[127] so mothers should continue on therapy (as is recommended for all persons living with HIV) while breastfeeding or use formula for feeding. Official recommendations regarding breastfeeding by mothers living with HIV differ. In the United States, CDC[128] and the American Academy of Pediatrics[129] recommend the exclusive use of infant formula, regardless of ART status, for mothers living with HIV because this is the only guaranteed method to completely prevent HIV transmission from mother to child via feeding. However, the World Health Organization recommends breastfeeding exclusively for the first 6 months of life for all children, with continued breastfeeding up to at least the first birthday, and ART therapy to prevent mother-to-child HIV transmission.[130]

Blood Transfusions. The risk of HIV due to blood transfusions has been virtually eliminated in the United States. Screening of donated blood was implemented in the 1990s and the risk of HIV due to blood transfusions is now less than 1 per 2 million transfusions.[131] Globally, some countries still do not screen donated blood and access to safe blood there remains a challenge.[132]

Mobile and Internet-based Interventions. The vast expansion in the availability of the Internet and Internet-connected mobile devices has broadened the landscape of HIV prevention interventions, as well as expanding the availability of sexual partners. Numerous mobile-based interventions have been developed or are being tested to increase uptake of HIV prevention services and promote behavior change.[133–135] Geolocation services in mobile apps can make it easier for individuals to find geographically convenient HIV testing locations. The CDC maintains databases of HIV test site locations and PrEP providers that can facilitate locating testing and care providers. Multiple mobile apps developed based on theories of behavior change are currently in development to increase access. Common features include information about HIV and HIV prevention methods, HIV testing and PrEP provider locators, guidance on developing a plan to test for HIV, reminders to prompt the user to test for HIV on a given schedule, and telemedicine components for services like PrEP navigation or counseling to accompany rapid at-home HIV testing. This is an approach that is economical to bring to scale and has the potential to dramatically broaden the landscape of HIV prevention.

HIV PREVENTION RESEARCH ISSUES

There have been vast improvements in HIV prevention and HIV-related outcomes since the beginning of the epidemic. Several behavioral and biomedical prevention options are now available including HIV testing, voluntary male circumcision, methods to prevent mother to child transmission of HIV, TaSP, needle and syringe exchange, and PrEP. Despite the remarkable gains in HIV prevention and treatment research, a number of areas of research remain to further our understanding of individual, group, and community-level HIV prevention methods and to improve treatment regimens. Broadly, HIV prevention methods can be grouped into behavioral and biomedical domains.

A number of advancements have been made in biomedical HIV prevention, with the most notable being TasP and the efficacy of PrEP.[71,121,136] However, more research is needed to explore additional options for PrEP including other antiretroviral drugs,[137] dosing regimens,[138] and modes of administration.[139,140] As of May 2018, a combination of emtricitabine and tenofovir disoproxil fumarate is approved for use as oral PrEP in individuals age 15 and older. CDC publishes recommendations with indications for PrEP among PWID, MSM, and heterosexual men and women.[141] PrEP is most effective with regular dosing,[136] so adherence is an important component of PrEP. Uptake, adherence, and persistence (continued use of PrEP over an extended period of time) have been suboptimal in the first years of PrEP availability. Continued research to identify barriers to PrEP therapy will be necessary to realize the full potential of this HIV-prevention method. Other biomedical prevention options, including vaginal and rectal microbicides, are currently under study.[142] Microbicides have the potential to provide a prevention method that does not require frequent pill-taking as with PrEP. Microbicides could provide women with additional control over their sexual health in comparison with condoms, use of which must be negotiated with sexual partners, but trial results have not been encouraging to date.[143,144]

An effective HIV vaccine has thus far proven elusive. Of six vaccine efficacy trials,[145–150] only one has demonstrated any efficacy for preventing HIV.[145] Primary analyses in the RV144 trial,[145] conducted among a primarily heterosexual population in Thailand, did not demonstrate statistically significant efficacy. However, a modified intention-to-treat analysis excluding participants who were found to have been living with HIV at baseline showed that the vaccine had moderate, statistically significant efficacy of 31.2%. Results of the RV144 trial have been used to further develop a vaccine regimen that is currently being tested in the HIV Vaccine Trials Network 702 study,[151] with results expected in 2020. Another active trial, HVTN 705,[152] is investigating a mosaic-based vaccine strategy. The mosaic vaccine is intended to be broadly effective against a wide variety of HIV strains, a potentially promising strategy given the global diversity of HIV strains. Earlier trials of the mosaic vaccine have demonstrated promising results in monkeys.[153]

The Internet and mobile technology have altered the landscape of HIV prevention. These technologies have made it much easier to access at-risk, marginalized, and traditionally hidden populations[154,155] such as MSM, transgender populations, and injection drug users. Internet- and mobile-based interventions are also much more cost effective to bring to scale[156] because of the low marginal costs associated with reaching additional populations. These types of interventions can take many forms including informational websites, inclusion of HIV prevention information in existing social and sexual networking websites and mobile apps, and standalone mobile apps with integrated HIV prevention resources. Thus, these interventions vary from passively providing information to actively engaging users, for example, to create a plan to be tested for HIV. Continued research will be needed to identify the most effective methods for delivering HIV prevention information and interventions online and via mobile devices. Researchers must also continue to adapt to ever-changing technical capabilities to ensure that interventions will be acceptable to their target populations.

Mathematical modeling is another growing area of research that has utility in assessing the expected outcomes associated with different HIV prevention programs and to explore research questions that are difficult or impossible to answer using empirical research methods. In particular, agent-based models (ABM) are a relatively new type of model that allows the creation of virtual populations. Characteristics of the population such as formation of sexual partnerships, sexual behavior, and disease transmission can be modeled based on estimates from empirical studies. Using ABM, these virtual populations can be used to conduct virtual experiments to answer questions about treatment effectiveness under particular conditions and to assess the potential effects of, for example, increasing coverage levels of existing interventions. Such models have been used to estimate the expected declines in HIV incidence under different levels of PrEP coverage,[157] to examine synergistic effects of combination prevention packages,[120] and to examine the expected impact of universal ART for serodiscordant couples,[158] among other applications.

Finally, a growing area of research within public health that has implications for each of the areas discussed above is implementation science. Biomedical and behavioral HIV prevention methods are only useful to the extent they can be scaled up and implemented broadly among at-risk communities. Implementation science is the study of how evidence-based interventions can be effectively extended into real-world public health and medical practice.[159] For example, PrEP must be implemented among communities that have been traditionally marginalized and who might face stigma in healthcare settings. These individuals require long-term monitoring, HIV/STI testing, and behavioral counseling for risk reduction and adherence support.[160] Increasingly, funding agencies and scientists are recognizing the need for implementation science to form the bridge between evidence and practice.

SUMMARY

Incredible progress in our ability to prevent and treat HIV/AIDS has been made since the beginning of the epidemic. Thanks to advocacy, multisectoral leadership,[161] and advances in HIV prevention research, we have the ability with existing methods to nearly eliminate HIV transmissions due to blood transfusions and mother-to-child transmission, especially in middle- to upper-income countries. Highly effective methods to prevent HIV transmission due to sexual exposures and injection drug use, such as needle and syringe exchange, drug treatment, and PrEP, have the potential to drastically curtail the epidemic. This progress has led governmental and nongovernmental institutions to begin to advocate for an AIDS-free generation. However, significant challenges remain. Access to HIV prevention and treatment services is not universal. Stigma and cost continue to be substantial barriers to the healthcare system generally, and to HIV prevention and treatment resources specifically, among many of the marginalized populations at greatest risk of HIV. Continued efforts are needed to reduce barriers to access and to bring effective interventions to scale so that all individuals at risk will be able to benefit from them. At the same time, biomedical research into additional methods of PrEP (e.g., different formulations and/or modes of delivery) and, eventually, a safe and effective vaccine or curative therapy must continue to meet the goal of bringing the HIV/AIDS epidemic to an end.

References

1. World Health Organization. WHO | The Top 10 Causes of Death. 2018. http://www.who.int/mediacentre/factsheets/fs310/en/index1.html. Accessed May 23, 2018.
2. Centers for Disease Control. Pneumocystis pneumonia—Los Angeles. *MMWR Morb Mortal Wkly Rep.* 1981;30(21):250–2.
3. Barre-Sinoussi F, Chermann JC, Rey F, et al. Isolation of a T-lymphotropic retrovirus from a patient at risk for acquired immune deficiency syndrome (AIDS). *Science.* 1983;220(4599):868–71.
4. Popovic M, Sarngadharan MG, Read E, Gallo RC. Detection, isolation, and continuous production of cytopathic retroviruses (HTLV-III) from patients with AIDS and pre-AIDS. *Science.* 1984;224(4648):497–500.
5. Jaffe HW, Valdiserri RO, De Cock KM. The reemerging HIV/AIDS epidemic in men who have sex with men. *JAMA.* 2007;298(20):2412–14.
6. Masur H, Michelis MA, Greene JB, et al. An outbreak of community-acquired Pneumocystis carinii pneumonia: Initial manifestation of cellular immune dysfunction. *N Engl J Med.* 1981;305(24):1431–8.
7. Masur H, Michelis MA, Wormser GP, et al. Opportunistic infection in previously healthy women. Initial manifestations of a community-acquired cellular immunodeficiency. *Ann Intern Med.* 1982;97(4):533–9.
8. Curran JW, Lawrence DN, Jaffe H, et al. Acquired immunodeficiency syndrome (AIDS) associated with transfusions. *N Engl J Med.* 1984;310(2):69–75.
9. Mahajan AP, Sayles JN, Patel VA, et al. Stigma in the HIV/AIDS epidemic: A review of the literature and recommendations for the way forward. *AIDS.* 2008;22(Suppl 2):S67–79.
10. Yarchoan R, Mitsuya H, Broder S. AIDS therapies. *Sci Am.* 1988;259(4): 110–9.
11. Hammer SM, Squires KE, Hughes MD, et al. A controlled trial of two nucleoside analogues plus indinavir in persons with human immunodeficiency virus infection and CD4 cell counts of 200 per cubic millimeter or less. AIDS Clinical Trials Group 320 Study Team. *N Engl J Med.* 1997;337(11):725–33.
12. Gulick RM, Mellors JW, Havlir D, et al. Treatment with indinavir, zidovudine, and lamivudine in adults with human immunodeficiency virus infection and prior antiretroviral therapy. *N Engl J Med.* 1997;337(11):734–9.
13. Nyamweya S, Hegedus A, Jaye A, Rowland-Jones S, Flanagan KL, Macallan DC. Comparing HIV-1 and HIV-2 infection: Lessons for viral immunopathogenesis. *Rev Med Virol.* 2013;23(4):221–40.
14. Barin F, M'Boup S, Denis F, et al. Serological evidence for virus related to simian T-lymphotropic retrovirus III in residents of west Africa. *Lancet.* 1985;2(8469–70):1387–9.
15. Hillis DM. AIDS. Origins of HIV. *Science.* 2000;288(5472):1757–9.
16. Barre-Sinoussi F, Chermann JC, Rey F, et al. Isolation of a T-lymphotropic retrovirus from a patient at risk for acquired immune deficiency syndrome (AIDS). 1983. *Rev Invest Clin.* 2004;56(2):126–9.
17. Gallo RC, Salahuddin SZ, Popovic M, et al. Frequent detection and isolation of cytopathic retroviruses (HTLV-III) from patients with AIDS and at risk for AIDS. *Science.* 1984;224(4648):500–3.
18. Schupbach J, Popovic M, Gilden RV, Gonda MA, Sarngadharan MG, Gallo RC. Serological analysis of a subgroup of human T-lymphotropic retroviruses (HTLV-III) associated with AIDS. *Science.* 1984;224(4648):503–5.
19. Sarngadharan MG, Popovic M, Bruch L, Schupbach J, Gallo RC. Antibodies reactive with human T-lymphotropic retroviruses (HTLV-III) in the serum of patients with AIDS. *Science.* 1984;224(4648):506–8.
20. Clavel F, Guetard D, Brun-Vezinet F, et al. Isolation of a new human retrovirus from West African patients with AIDS. *Science.* 1986;233(4761):343–6.
21. Peeters M, Jung M, Ayouba A. The origin and molecular epidemiology of HIV. *Expert Rev Anti Infect Ther.* 2013;11(9):885–96.
22. Shaw GM, Hunter E. HIV transmission. *Cold Spring Harb Perspect Med.* 2012;2(11):a006965.
23. Pope M, Haase AT.Transmission, acute HIV-1 infection and the quest for strategies to prevent infection. *Nat Med.* 2003;9(7):847–52.
24. Iwasa J. Science of HIV. http://scienceofhiv.org/wp/. Accessed June 28, 2018.
25. Ho DD, Neumann AU, Perelson AS, Chen W, Leonard JM, Markowitz M. Rapid turnover of plasma virions and CD4 lymphocytes in HIV-1 infection. *Nature.* 1995;373(6510):123–6.
26. Chun TW, Carruth L, Finzi D, et al. Quantification of latent tissue reservoirs and total body viral load in HIV-1 infection. *Nature.* 1997;387(6629):183–8.
27. Estes JD, Kityo C, Ssali F, et al. Defining total-body AIDS-virus burden with implications for curative strategies. *Nat Med.* 2017;23(11):1271–6.
28. Henrich TJ, Deeks SG, Pillai SK. Measuring the size of the latent human immunodeficiency virus reservoir: The present and future of evaluating eradication strategies. *J Infect Dis.* 2017;215(suppl 3):S134–41.
29. Ho DD, Schooley RT, Rota TR, et al. HTLV-III in the semen and blood of a healthy homosexual man. *Science.* 1984;226(4673):451–3.
30. Zagury D, Bernard J, Leibowitch J, et al. HTLV-III in cells cultured from semen of two patients with AIDS. *Science.* 1984;226(4673):449–51.
31. Auerbach DM, Darrow WW, Jaffe HW, Curran JW. Cluster of cases of the acquired immune deficiency syndrome. Patients linked by sexual contact. *Am J Med.* 1984;76(3):487–92.
32. Peterman TA, Stoneburner RL, Allen JR, Jaffe HW, Curran JW. Risk of human immunodeficiency virus transmission from heterosexual adults with transfusion-associated infections. *JAMA.* 1988;259(1):55–8.
33. Guinan ME, Thomas PA, Pinsky PF, et al. Heterosexual and homosexual patients with the acquired immunodeficiency syndrome. A comparison of surveillance, interview, and laboratory data. *Ann Intern Med.* 1984;100(2):213–8.
34. Ammann AJ, Cowan MJ, Wara DW, et al. Acquired immunodeficiency in an infant: Possible transmission by means of blood products. *Lancet.* 1983;1(8331):956–8.
35 Centers for Disease Control. Pneumocystis carinii pneumonia among persons with hemophilia A. *MMWR Morb Mortal Wkly Rep.* 1982;31(27):365–7.
36. Stehr-Green JK, Holman RC, Jason JM, Evatt BL. Hemophilia-associated AIDS in the United States, 1981 to September 1987. *Am J Public Health.* 1988;78(4):439–42.
37. Goedert JJ, Kessler CM, Aledort LM, et al. A prospective study of human immunodeficiency virus type 1 infection and the development of AIDS in subjects with hemophilia. *N Engl J Med.* 1989;321(17):1141–8.
38. Ward JW, Holmberg SD, Allen JR, et al. Transmission of human immunodeficiency virus (HIV) by blood transfusions screened as negative for HIV antibody. *N Engl J Med.* 1988;318(8):473–8.
39 Centers for Disease Control. U.S. Public Health Service guidelines for testing and counseling blood and plasma donors for human immunodeficiency virus type 1 antigen. *MMWR Morb Mortal Wkly Rep.* 1996;45(Rr-2):1–9.

40. Patel P, Borkowf CB, Brooks JT, Lasry A, Lansky A, Mermin J. Estimating per-act HIV transmission risk: A systematic review. *AIDS.* 2014;28(10):1509–19.
41. Bell DM. Occupational risk of human immunodeficiency virus infection in healthcare workers: An overview. *Am J Med.* 1997;102(5b):9–15.
42. Ippolito G, Puro V, De Carli G. The risk of occupational human immunodeficiency virus infection in health care workers. Italian Multicenter Study. The Italian Study Group on Occupational Risk of HIV infection. *Arch Intern Med.* 1993;153(12):1451–8.
43. Kuhar DT, Henderson DK, Struble KA, et al. Updated US Public Health Service guidelines for the management of occupational exposures to human immunodeficiency virus and recommendations for postexposure prophylaxis. *Infect Control Hosp Epidemiol.* 2013;34(9):875–92.
44. Siegel JD, Rhinehart E, Jackson M, Chiarello L. 2007 Guideline for isolation precautions: Preventing transmission of infectious agents in health care settings. *Am J Infect Control.* 2007;35(10):S65–164.
45. Centers for Disease Control and Prevention. Announcement. Updated Guidelines for Antiretroviral Postexposure Prophylaxis after Sexual, Injection Drug Use, or Other Nonoccupational Exposure to HIV—United States, 2016. *MMWR Morb Mortal Wkly Rep.* 2016;65:458.
46. Friedland G, Kahl P, Saltzman B, et al. Additional evidence for lack of transmission of HIV infection by close interpersonal (casual) contact. *AIDS.* 1990;4(7):639–44.
47. Centers for Disease Control. Epidemiologic aspects of the current outbreak of Kaposi's sarcoma and opportunistic infections. *N Engl J Med.* 1982;306(4):248–52.
48. Centers for Disease Control. Kaposi's sarcoma and Pneumocystis pneumonia among homosexual men—New York City and California. *MMWR Morb Mortal Wkly Rep.* 1981;30(25):305–8.
49. Centers for Disease Control. 1993 revised classification system for HIV infection and expanded surveillance case definition for AIDS among adolescents and adults. *MMWR Recomm Rep.* 1992;41(Rr-17):1–19.
50. Centers for Disease Control. Revision of the CDC surveillance case definition for acquired immunodeficiency syndrome. Council of State and Territorial Epidemiologists; AIDS Program, Center for Infectious Diseases. *MMWR Suppl.* 1987;36(1):1s–15s.
51. Karon JM, Fleming PL, Steketee RW, De Cock KM. HIV in the United States at the turn of the century: An epidemic in transition. *Am J Public Health.* 2001;91(7):1060–8.
52. Centers for Disease Control. Guidelines for national human immunodeficiency virus case surveillance, including monitoring for human immunodeficiency virus infection and acquired immunodeficiency syndrome. *MMWR Recomm Rep.* 1999;48(Rr-13):1–27, 29–31.
53. Gallagher KM, Sullivan PS, Lansky A, Onorato IM. Behavioral surveillance among people at risk for HIV infection in the U.S.: The National HIV Behavioral Surveillance System. *Public Health Rep.* 2007;122(Suppl 1): 32–8.
54. Centers for Disease Control and Prevention. HIV Surveillance Report, 2016; Vol. 28. 2017. http://www.cdc.gov/hiv/library/reports/hiv-surveillance.html. Accessed March 2018.
55. United States Census Bureau. QuickFacts: United States. 2016. https://www.census.gov/quickfacts/fact/table/US/PST045216. Accessed June 8, 2018.
56. Purcell DW, Johnson CH, Lansky A, et al. Estimating the population size of men who have sex with men in the United States to obtain HIV and syphilis rates. *Open AIDS J.* 2012;6:98–107.
57. Connor EM, Sperling RS, Gelber R, et al. Reduction of maternal-infant transmission of human immunodeficiency virus type 1 with zidovudine treatment. Pediatric AIDS Clinical Trials Group Protocol 076 Study Group. *N Engl J Med.* 1994;331(18):1173–80.
58. Centers for Disease Control and Prevention. Revised recommendations for HIV testing of adults, adolescents, and pregnant women in health-care settings. *MMWR Recomm Rep.* 2006;55(RR-14):1–17; quiz CE11-14.
59. Nesheim S, Harris LF, Lampe M. Elimination of perinatal HIV infection in the USA and other high-income countries: Achievements and challenges. *Curr Opin HIV AIDS.* 2013;8(5):447–56.
60. Sollai S, Noguera-Julian A, Galli L, et al. Strategies for the prevention of mother to child transmission in Western countries: An update. *Pediatr Infect Dis J.* 2015;34(5 Suppl 1):S14–30.
61. Townsend CL, Byrne L, Cortina-Borja M, et al. Earlier initiation of ART and further decline in mother-to-child HIV transmission rates, 2000–2011. *AIDS.* 2014;28(7):1049–57.
62. Cooley LA, Wejnert C, Spiller MW, Broz D, Paz-Bailey G. Low HIV testing among persons who inject drugs-National HIV Behavioral Surveillance, 20 U.S. cities, 2012. *Drug Alcohol Depend.* 2016;165:270–4.
63. Paz-Bailey G, Mendoza M, Finlayson T, et al. Trends in condom use among men who have sex with men in the United States: The role of antiretroviral therapy and sero-adaptive strategies. *AIDS.* 2016;30(12):1985–90.
64. Hess KL, DiNenno E, Sionean C, Ivy W, Paz-Bailey G. Prevalence and correlates of heterosexual anal intercourse among men and women, 20 U.S. cities. *AIDS Behav.* 2016;20(12):2966–75.
65. McNaghten AD, Wolfe MI, Onorato I, et al. Improving the representativeness of behavioral and clinical surveillance for persons with HIV in the United States: The rationale for developing a population-based approach. *PLoS One.* 2007;2(6):e550.
66. Wohl AR, Benbow N, Tejero J, et al. Antiretroviral prescription and viral suppression in a representative sample of HIV-infected persons in care in 4 large metropolitan areas of the United States, Medical Monitoring Project, 2011–2013. *J Acquir Immune Defic Syndr.* 2017;76(2):158–70.
67. Olaiya O, Weiser J, Zhou W, Patel P, Bradley H. Hypertension among persons living with HIV in medical care in the United States-Medical Monitoring Project, 2013–2014. *Open Forum Infect Dis.* 2018;5(3):ofy028.
68. UN AIDS. AIDSinfo. 2014. http://www.unaids.org/en/dataanalysis/datatools/aidsinfo/. Accessed March 12, 2018.
69. UNAIDS. Fact Sheet—World AIDS Day 2017. 2017. http://www.unaids.org/sites/default/files/media_asset/UNAIDS_FactSheet_en.pdf. Accessed March 12, 2018.
70. Sullivan PS, Jones JS, Baral SD. The global north: HIV epidemiology in high-income countries. *Curr Opin HIV AIDS.* 2014;9(2):199–205.
71. Grant RM, Lama JR, Anderson PL, et al. Preexposure chemoprophylaxis for HIV prevention in men who have sex with men. *N Engl J Med.* 2010;363(27):2587–99.
72. Smith DK, Grohskopf LA, Black RJ, et al. Antiretroviral postexposure prophylaxis after sexual, injection-drug use, or other nonoccupational exposure to HIV in the United States: Recommendations from the U.S. Department of Health and Human Services. *MMWR Recomm Rep.* 2005;54(Rr-2):1–20.
73. Auvert B, Taljaard D, Lagarde E, Sobngwi-Tambekou J, Sitta R, Puren A. Randomized, controlled intervention trial of male circumcision for reduction of HIV infection risk: The ANRS 1265 Trial. *PLoS Med.* 2005;2(11):e298.
74. Bailey RC, Moses S, Parker CB, et al. Male circumcision for HIV prevention in young men in Kisumu, Kenya: A randomised controlled trial. *Lancet.* 2007;369(9562):643–56.
75. Gray RH, Kigozi G, Serwadda D, et al. Male circumcision for HIV prevention in men in Rakai, Uganda: A randomised trial. *Lancet.* 2007;369(9562):657–66.
76. Cohen MS, Chen YQ, McCauley M, et al. Prevention of HIV-1 infection with early antiretroviral therapy. *N Engl J Med.* 2011;365(6):493–505.
77. Weller S, Davis K. Condom effectiveness in reducing heterosexual HIV transmission. *Cochrane Database Syst Rev.* 2002(1):Cd003255.
78. Holmes KK, Levine R, Weaver M. Effectiveness of condoms in preventing sexually transmitted infections. *Bull. World Health Organ.* 2004;82(6):454–61.
79. Wilson DP, Donald B, Shattock AJ, Wilson D, Fraser-Hurt N. The cost-effectiveness of harm reduction. *Int J Drug Policy.* 2015;26(Suppl 1):S5–11.
80. Mills EJ, Bakanda C, Birungi J, et al. Life expectancy of persons receiving combination antiretroviral therapy in low-income countries: A cohort analysis from Uganda. *Ann Intern Med.* 2011;155(4):209–16.
81. Teeraananchai S, Kerr SJ, Amin J, Ruxrungtham K, Law MG. Life expectancy of HIV-positive people after starting combination antiretroviral therapy: A meta-analysis. *HIV Med.* 2017;18(4):256–66.
82. The Antiretroviral Therapy Cohort Collaboration. Life expectancy of individuals on combination antiretroviral therapy in high-income countries: A collaborative analysis of 14 cohort studies. *Lancet.* 2008;372(9635):293–9.
83. Panel on Antiretroviral Guidelines for Adults and Adolescents. Guidelines on the use of Antiretroviral Agents in Adults and Adolescents Living with HIV.
84. Cohen MS, Chen YQ, McCauley M, et al. Antiretroviral therapy for the prevention of HIV-1 transmission. *N Engl J Med.* 2016;375(9):830–9.
85. Rodger AJ, Cambiano V, Bruun T, et al. Sexual activity without condoms and risk of HIV transmission in serodifferent couples when the HIV-positive partner is using suppressive antiretroviral therapy. *JAMA.* 2016;316(2):171–81.
86. Masur H, Brooks JT, Benson CA, Holmes KK, Pau AK, Kaplan JE. Prevention and treatment of opportunistic infections in HIV-infected adults and adolescents: Updated guidelines from the Centers for Disease Control and Prevention, National Institutes of Health, and HIV Medicine Association of the Infectious Diseases Society of America. *Clin Infect Dis.* 2014;58(9):1308–11.

87. Palella FJJr, Baker RK, Moorman AC, et al. Mortality in the highly active antiretroviral therapy era: Changing causes of death and disease in the HIV outpatient study. *J Acquir Immune Defic Syndr.* 2006;43(1):27–34.

88. World Health Organization. WHO | HIV/AIDS. 2018. http://www.who.int/gho/hiv/en/. Accessed June 29, 2018.

89. Palella FJ, Jr., Delaney KM, Moorman AC, et al. Declining morbidity and mortality among patients with advanced human immunodeficiency virus infection. HIV Outpatient Study Investigators. *N Engl J Med.* 1998;338(13):853–60.

90. Hutter G, Nowak D, Mossner M, et al. Long-term control of HIV by CCR5 Delta32/Delta32 stem-cell transplantation. *N Engl J Med.* 2009;360(7):692–8.

91. Brown TR. I am the Berlin patient: A personal reflection. *AIDS Res Hum Retroviruses.* 2015;31(1):2–3.

92. Deeks SG, Lewin SR, Ross AL, et al. International AIDS Society global scientific strategy: Towards an HIV cure 2016. *Nat Med.* 2016;22(8):839–50.

93. El-Sadr WM, Lundgren J, Neaton JD, et al. CD4+ count-guided interruption of antiretroviral treatment. *N Engl J Med.* 2006;355(22):2283–96.

94. Margolis DA, Gonzalez-Garcia J, Stellbrink HJ, et al. Long-acting intramuscular cabotegravir and rilpivirine in adults with HIV-1 infection (LATTE-2): 96-Week results of a randomised, open-label, phase 2b, non-inferiority trial. *Lancet.* 2017;390(10101):1499–510.

95. Crepaz N, Dong X, Wang X, Hernandez AL, Hall HI. Racial and ethnic disparities in sustained viral suppression and transmission risk potential among persons receiving HIV care—United States, 2014. *MMWR Morb Mortal Wkly Rep.* 2018;67(4):113–8.

96. Dasgupta S, Oster AM, Li J, Hall HI. Disparities in consistent retention in HIV care—11 States and the district of Columbia, 2011–2013. *MMWR Morb Mortal Wkly Rep.* 2016;65(4):77–82.

97. UNAIDS. 90-90-90: An ambitious treatment target to help end the AIDS epidemic. 2014. http://www.unaids.org/en/resources/documents/2017/90-90-90.

98. UNAIDS. UNAIDS. 2018. http://www.unaids.org/. Accessed June 29, 2018.

99. Centers for Disease Control and Prevention. HIV Basic Statistics. 2017. https://www.cdc.gov/hiv/basics/statistics.html. Accessed March 16, 2018.

100. Centers for Disease Control and Prevention. HIV Surveillance Report, 2015; Vol. 27. November 2016. https://www.cdc.gov/hiv/pdf/library/reports/surveillance/cdc-hiv-surveillance-report-2015-vol-27.pdf.

101. Hall HI, Ruiguang S, Rhodes P, et al. Estimation of HIV incidence in the United States. *JAMA.* 2008;300(5):520–9.

102. Hall HI, Song R, Tang T, et al. HIV trends in the United States: Diagnoses and estimated incidence. *JMIR Public Health Surveill.* 2017;3(1):e8.

103. Branson BM, Handsfield HH, Lampe MA, et al. Revised recommendations for HIV testing of adults, adolescents, and pregnant women in health-care settings. *MMWR Recomm Rep.* 2006;55(Rr-14):1–17; quiz CE11-14.

104. Moyer VA. Screening for HIV: U.S. Preventive Services Task Force recommendation statement. *Ann Intern Med.* 2013;159(1):51–60.

105. Marks G, Crepaz N, Janssen RS. Estimating sexual transmission of HIV from persons aware and unaware that they are infected with the virus in the USA. *AIDS.* 2006;20(10):1447–50.

106. Allen S, Tice J, Van de Perre P, et al. Effect of serotesting with counselling on condom use and seroconversion among HIV discordant couples in Africa. *BMJ.* 1992;304(6842):1605–9.

107. Sullivan PS, Stephenson R, Grazter B, et al. Adaptation of the African couples HIV testing and counseling model for men who have sex with men in the United States: An application of the ADAPT-ITT framework. *Springerplus.* 2014;3:249.

108. Sullivan PS, Wall KM, O'Hara B, et al. The prevalence of undiagnosed HIV serodiscordance among male couples presenting for HIV testing. *Arch Sex Behav.* 2014;43(1):173–80.

109. Sullivan PS, White D, Rosenberg ES, et al. Safety and acceptability of couples HIV testing and counseling for US men who have sex with men: A randomized prevention study. *J Int Assoc Provid AIDS Care.* 2014;13(2):135–44.

110. Wagenaar BH, Christiansen-Lindquist L, Khosropour C, et al. Willingness of US men who have sex with men (MSM) to participate in couples HIV voluntary counseling and testing (CVCT). *PLoS One.* 2012;7(8):e42953.

111. Centers for Disease Control and Prevention. Testing Together. 2017. https://effectiveinterventions.cdc.gov/en/HighImpactPrevention/PublicHealthStrategies/testing-together. Accessed March 14, 2018.

112. Sharma A, Stephenson RB, White D, Sullivan PS. Acceptability and intended usage preferences for six HIV testing options among internet-using men who have sex with men. *Springerplus.* 2014;3:109.

113. Kalibala S, Tun W, Cherutich P, Nganga A, Oweya E, Oluoch P. Factors associated with acceptability of HIV self-testing among health care workers in Kenya. *AIDS Behav.* 2014;18 Suppl 4:S405–14.

114. Robb ML, Ananworanich J. Lessons from acute HIV infection. *Curr Opin HIV AIDS.* 2016;11(6):555–60.

115. UNAIDS. WHO, UNAIDS Statement on HIV Testing Services: New Opportunities and Ongoing Challenges. Geneva, Switzerland; 2017.

116. Macgowan R, Chavez P, Borkowf C, Sullivan P, Mermin J. The impact of HIV self-testing among internet-recruited men who have sex with men, eSTAMP, 2015–2016. *International AIDS Conference.* Durban, South Africa, 2017.

117. Smith DK, Herbst JH, Zhang X, Rose CE. Condom effectiveness for HIV prevention by consistency of use among men who have sex with men (MSM) in the U.S. *J Acquir Immune Defic Syndr.* 2015;68(3):337–44.

118. Centers for Disease Control and Prevention. HIV Infection, Risk, Prevention, and Testing Behaviors among Heterosexuals at Increased Risk of HIV Infection—National HIV Behavioral Surveillance, 20 U.S. Cities, 2013. HIV Surveillance Special Report 13. 2015. http://www.cdc.gov/hiv/library/reports/surveillance/#panel2. Accessed March 14, 2018.

119. Centers for Disease Control and Prevention. HIV Infection Risk, Prevention, and Testing Behaviors among Men Who Have Sex With Men—National HIV Behavioral Surveillance, 20 U.S. Cities, 2014. HIV Surveillance Special Report 15. 2016. http://www.cdc.gov/hiv/library/reports/surveillance/#panel2. Accessed March 14, 2018.

120. Sullivan PS, Carballo-Diéguez A, Coates T, et al. Successes and challenges of HIV prevention in men who have sex with men. *Lancet.* 2012;380(9839):388–99.

121. Baeten JM, Donnell D, Ndase P, et al. Antiretroviral prophylaxis for HIV prevention in heterosexual men and women. *N Engl J Med.* 2012;367(5):399–410.

122. Thigpen MC, Kebaabetswe PM, Paxton LA, et al. Antiretroviral preexposure prophylaxis for heterosexual HIV transmission in Botswana. *N Engl J Med.* 2012;367(5):423–34.

123. Sullivan PS, Giler RM, Mouhanna F, et al. Trends in use of oral emtricitabine/tenofovir disoproxil fumarate for pre-exposure prophylaxis against HIV infections, United States, 2012–2017. *Ann Epidemiol.* 2018;28(12):833–40.

124. Forbes JC, Alimenti AM, Singer J, et al. A national review of vertical HIV transmission. *AIDS.* 2012;26(6):757–63.

125. Andiman W, Bryson Y, de Martino M, et al. The mode of delivery and the risk of vertical transmission of human immunodeficiency virus type 1—A meta-analysis of 15 prospective cohort studies. *N Engl J Med.* 1999;340(13):977–87.

126. European Mode of Delivery Collaboration. Elective caesarean-section versus vaginal delivery in prevention of vertical HIV-1 transmission: A randomised clinical trial. *Lancet.* 1999;353(9158):1035–9.

127. Miotti PG, Taha TE, Kumwenda NI, et al. HIV transmission through breastfeeding: A study in Malawi. *JAMA.* 1999;282(8):744–9.

128. Centers for Disease Control and Prevention. Breastfeeding. 2018. https://www.cdc.gov/breastfeeding/breastfeeding-special-circumstances/maternal-or-infant-illnesses/hiv.html. Accessed July 9, 2018.

129. Committee on Pediatric AIDS. Infant feeding and transmission of human immunodeficiency virus in the United States. *Pediatrics.* 2013;131(2):391–6.

130. World Health Organization. Infant feeding for the prevention of mother-to-child transmission of HIV. 2018. http://www.who.int/elena/titles/hiv_infant_feeding/en/. Accessed July 9, 2018.

131. National Heart L, and Blood Institute. Blood Transfusion—What Are the Risks of a Blood Transfusion? https://www.nhlbi.nih.gov/node/3593. Accessed March 16, 2018.

132. World Health Organization. Global Database on Blood Safety Report. 2011. http://www.who.int/bloodsafety/global_database/GDBS_Summary_Report_2011.pdf. Accessed March 16, 2018.

133. Sullivan PS, Jones J, Kishore N, Stephenson R. The roles of technology in primary HIV prevention for men who have sex with men. *Curr HIV/AIDS Rep.* 2015;12(4):481–8.

134. Muessig KE, Pike EC, Legrand S, Hightow-Weidman LB. Mobile phone applications for the care and prevention of HIV and other sexually transmitted diseases: A review. *J Med Internet Res.* 2013;15(1):e1.

135. Forrest JI, Wiens M, Kanters S, Nsanzimana S, Lester RT, Mills EJ. Mobile health applications for HIV prevention and care in Africa. *Curr Opin HIV AIDS.* 2015;10(6):464–71.

136. Grant RM, Anderson PL, McMahan V, et al. Uptake of pre-exposure prophylaxis, sexual practices, and HIV incidence in men and transgender women who have sex with men: A cohort study. *Lancet. Infect Dis.* 2014;14(9):820–9.

137. Fox J, Tiraboschi JM, Herrera C, et al. Brief report: Pharmacokinetic/pharmacodynamic investigation of single-dose oral maraviroc in the context of HIV-1 pre-exposure prophylaxis. *J Acquir Immune Defic Syndr.* 2016;73(3):252–7.

138. Anderson PL, Garcia-Lerma JG, Heneine W. Nondaily preexposure prophylaxis for HIV prevention. *Curr Opin HIV AIDS.* 2016;11(1):94–101.

139. Landovitz RJ, Kofron R, McCauley M. The promise and pitfalls of long-acting injectable agents for HIV prevention. *Curr Opin HIV AIDS.* 2016;11(1):122–8.

140. Abdool Karim Q, Abdool Karim SS, Frohlich JA, et al. Effectiveness and safety of tenofovir gel, an antiretroviral microbicide, for the prevention of HIV infection in women. *Science.* 2010;329(5996):1168–74.

141. Centers for Disease Control and Prevention. US Public Health Service: Preexposure prophylaxis for the prevention of HIV infection in the United States—2017 Update: A clinical practice guideline. 2018.

142. Abdool Karim SS, Baxter C. Microbicides for prevention of HIV infection: Clinical efficacy trials. *Curr Top Microbiol Immunol.* 2014;383:97–115.

143. Marrazzo JM, Ramjee G, Richardson BA, et al. Tenofovir-based preexposure prophylaxis for HIV infection among African women. *N Engl J Med.* 2015;372(6):509–18.

144. Baeten JM, Palanee-Phillips T, Brown ER, et al. Use of a vaginal ring containing dapivirine for HIV-1 prevention in women. *N Engl J Med.* 2016;375(22):2121–32.

145. Rerks-Ngarm S, Pitisuttithum P, Nitayaphan S, et al. Vaccination with ALVAC and AIDSVAX to prevent HIV-1 infection in Thailand. *N Engl J Med.* 2009;361(23):2209–20.

146. Buchbinder SP, Mehrotra DV, Duerr A, et al. Efficacy assessment of a cell-mediated immunity HIV-1 vaccine (the Step Study): A double-blind, randomised, placebo-controlled, test-of-concept trial. *Lancet.* 2008;372(9653):1881–93.

147. Pitisuttithum P, Gilbert P, Gurwith M, et al. Randomized, double-blind, placebo-controlled efficacy trial of a bivalent recombinant glycoprotein 120 HIV-1 vaccine among injection drug users in Bangkok, Thailand. *J Infect Dis.* 2006;194(12):1661–71.

148. Flynn NM, Forthal DN, Harro CD, Judson FN, Mayer KH, Para MF. Placebo-controlled phase 3 trial of a recombinant glycoprotein 120 vaccine to prevent HIV-1 infection. *J Infect Dis.* 2005;191(5):654–65.

149. Gray GE, Allen M, Moodie Z, et al. Safety and efficacy of the HVTN 503/Phambili study of a clade-B-based HIV-1 vaccine in South Africa: A double-blind, randomised, placebo-controlled test-of-concept phase 2b study. *Lancet Infect Dis.* 2011;11(7):507–15.

150. Hammer SM, Sobieszczyk ME, Janes H, et al. Efficacy trial of a DNA/rAd5 HIV-1 preventive vaccine. *N Engl J Med.* 2013;369(22):2083–92.

151. ClinicalTrials.gov. Pivotal Phase 2b/3 ALVAC/Bivalent gp120/MF59 HIV Vaccine Prevention Safety and Efficacy Study in South Africa (HVTN702). https://clinicaltrials.gov/ct2/show/NCT02968849. Accessed 5/21/2018, 2018.

152. ClinicalTrials.gov. A Study to Assess the Efficacy of a Heterologous Prime/Boost Vaccine Regimen of Ad26.Mos4.HIV and Aluminum Phosphate-Adjuvanted Clade C gp140 in Preventing Human Immunodeficiency Virus (HIV) -1 Infection in Women in Sub-Saharan Africa. https://clinicaltrials.gov/ct2/show/NCT03060629.

153. Barouch DH, Stephenson KE, Borducchi EN, et al. Protective efficacy of a global HIV-1 mosaic vaccine against heterologous SHIV challenges in rhesus monkeys. *Cell.* 2013;155(3):531–9.

154. Shrestha R, Huedo-Medina TB, Altice FL, Krishnan A, Copenhaver M. Examining the acceptability of mHealth technology in HIV prevention among high-risk drug users in treatment. *AIDS Behav.* 2017;21(11):3100–10.

155. Grov C, Bux DJr, Parsons JT, Morgenstern J. Recruiting hard-to-reach drug-using men who have sex with men into an intervention study: Lessons learned and implications for applied research. *Subst Use Misuse.* 2009;44(13):1855–71.

156. Iribarren SJ, Cato K, Falzon L, Stone PW. What is the economic evidence for mHealth? A systematic review of economic evaluations of mHealth solutions. *PLoS One.* 2017;12(2):e0170581.

157. Jenness SM, Goodreau SM, Rosenberg E, et al. Impact of the Centers for Disease Control's HIV preexposure prophylaxis guidelines for men who have sex with men in the United States. *J Infect Dis.* 2016;214(12):1800–7.

158. Roberts ST, Khanna AS, Barnabas RV, et al. Estimating the impact of universal antiretroviral therapy for HIV serodiscordant couples through home HIV testing: Insights from mathematical models. *J Int AIDS Soc.* 2016;19(1):20864.

159. Odeny TA, Padian N, Doherty MC, et al. Definitions of implementation science in HIV/AIDS. *Lancet. HIV.* 2015;2(5):e178–80.

160. Underhill K, Operario D, Skeer M, Mimiaga M, Mayer K. Packaging PrEP to prevent HIV: An integrated framework to plan for pre-exposure prophylaxis implementation in clinical practice. *J Acquir Immune Defic Syndr.* 2010;55(1):8–13.

161. Killen J, Harrington M, Fauci AS. MSM, AIDS research activism, and HAART. *Lancet.* 2012;380(9839):314–6.

CHAPTER

88 Tuberculosis

Douglas B. Hornick

Tuberculosis (TB) has been an affliction of humankind since before recorded history. TB inspired the writer John Bunyan to aptly describe this deadly and mysterious disease in 1660 as "the captain of all these men of death that came against him to take him away, was the consumption for it was that brought him down to the grave."[1] As with classic works of literature, tuberculosis endures. In spite of the heralded medicinal cures developed in the 1940s and 1950s, tuberculosis still devastates populations throughout the world. Aspects of the pathogenesis of this disease still remain shrouded in mystery. Even more disturbing, *Mycobacterium tuberculosis*, the etiologic agent of TB, has become increasingly resistant to antimycobacterial medications and travels with, and has been especially virulent among those suffering from acquired immunodeficiency syndrome (AIDS). These trends keep tuberculosis at the forefront among the deadly infections of humankind.

THE MICROBIOLOGY OF *M. TUBERCULOSIS*

M. tuberculosis is classified within a group nearly genetically identical organisms and is thus referred to as the *M. tuberculosis* complex. The members of the *M. tuberculosis* complex include *Mycobacterium bovis*, and several uncommon and very rare human pathogens: *M. pinnipedii*, *M. microti*, *M. cannettii*, *M. orygis*, *M. caprae*, and *M. africanum*.[2] *M. tuberculosis* and *M. bovis* along with *Mycobacterium leprae* cause communicable disease, which set these species apart from the more than 170 other species of *Mycobacteria*, which are generally found within the environment and referred to as nontuberculous mycobacteria (NTM). In contrast, *M. tuberculosis* is not found within the environment.[3]

M. tuberculosis organisms exhibit a bacillary morphology and produce an impervious waxy cell wall. The cell wall, composed mostly of a beta-hydroxy fatty acid, mycolic acid, excludes most antimicrobial agents and is resistant to alkali and acid. The latter property is taken advantage of by the acid-fast stains (e.g., Ziehl-Neelsen, Kinyoun, fluorochrome). *M. tuberculosis* organisms can be killed relatively easily by ultraviolet (UV) light at 254-nm wavelength, sunlight, heat, and specific disinfectants such as tricresol and phenol. Modern molecular techniques applied to *M. tuberculosis*, have resulted in sequencing and annotation of entire genome, comprising about 4000 genes.[4] Currently, whole genome sequencing (WGS) has evolved into a powerful automated tool within the contemporary clinical microbiology laboratory, which provides a comprehensive method for *M. tuberculosis* identification and importantly concurrent detection of mutations that predict resistance to first- and second-line antimycobacterial drugs.[5]

Mycobacteria divide every 18–24 hours compared to every 1–2 hours for most other bacterial pathogens. Mycobacteria have traditionally been cultured on egg-potato–based solid media, Lowenstein-Jensen (L-J) slants, or Middlebrook 7H10 or 7H11 agar-based solid media. Following a 3- to 4-week incubation, an array of biochemical tests and additional growth on artificial media have been necessary traditionally to distinguish *M. tuberculosis* from the other multiple species of mycobacteria.[6] Final identification by these nearly outdated methods introduce a 6- to 8-week delay in diagnosis. More about how modern laboratory techniques that shorten the time to identification will be described later.

Antimycobacterial Resistance. Mutations producing resistance to the first-line medications such as isoniazid (INH) and rifampin occur spontaneously. Genetic data have shown that at least two mechanisms account for INH resistance: deletion of *katG*, the gene encoding for catalase or mutation in *inhA*, a gene involved in the synthesis of mycolic acid.[7,8] Rifampin resistance results from mutations within the *ropB* gene which encodes for β subunit of RNA polymerase.[9]

The probability of spontaneous resistance is estimated at 10^{-6} for isoniazid and 10^{-8} for rifampin, and the probabilities for resistance to the other first-line medications fall within the same range.[10] The occurrence of these mutations is an unlinked phenomenon, so the probability that a single organism will be resistant to both INH and rifampin is the product of the probability of each mutation or 10^{-14}. The estimated burden of organisms in a patient varies as follows: 10^3 bacteria for a latent infection, 10^4–10^5 bacteria per gram of tissue for noncavitary pulmonary disease, and 10^9–10^{11} organisms per gram of tissue for cavitary pulmonary disease. The use of INH alone in a patient with latent TB infection is not believed to risk selection of resistant strains. The use of INH alone in a patient with cavitary pulmonary disease, however, allows spontaneously resistant strains to grow selectively. Resistance to multiple medications can develop with time if other antimycobacterial medications are added sequentially. Resistance that develops in this fashion is defined as acquired (or secondary) drug resistance.

Drug resistance that is discovered in an isolate from a patient who has not previously received antituberculous medications is called primary drug resistance. Primary resistance is usually found in patients who have been infected by transmission from another individual with drug-resistant TB. *M. tuberculosis* isolates that exhibit simultaneous resistance to at least INH and rifampin are referred to as multidrug-resistant tuberculosis (MDRTB).[11,12] The rationale for this specific definition is that treatment outcomes are compromised significantly when the two most potent first-line medications, INH and rifampin, are ineffective. The new millennium brought an even more ominous strain, the extensively drug-resistant tuberculosis (XDRTB).[13] These organisms are MDRTB strains exhibiting second-line drug resistance as follows: any within the fluoroquinolone class, plus one or more of the three second-line injectables (amikacin, capreomycin, or kanamycin).[14]

PATHOGENESIS AND TRANSMISSION OF *M. TUBERCULOSIS*

M. tuberculosis infects the human host following inhalation of small infectious particles called droplet nuclei.[15,16] At least three possible consequences result if the organisms are not killed and cleared immediately: progressive development of active infection (primary TB), latent tuberculosis infection (LTBI) that persists throughout the life of the host, or active infection that emerges many months or years after the initial infection (reactivation TB).

Infectious droplet nuclei measure approximately 1–5 μm in diameter, which allows them to deposit in the terminal bronchioles and alveoli of the host. Theoretically, they may contain as few as one viable organism. The bacteria may multiply briefly at the site of deposition but eventually are ingested by pulmonary macrophages. Following phagocytosis, *M. tuberculosis* inhibits phagolysosomal fusion, allowing the organism to survive and multiply intracellularly within lysosomes.[17]

The infected macrophages then initiate the cellular immune response that in most individuals eventually contains the infection. During this initial phase of infection and multiplication, the inflammatory response can be of sufficient intensity to cause a localized pneumonitis. In general, the host is asymptomatic or minimally symptomatic. During this phase, also, the organisms are carried into the regional lymphatics, then into the hilar and mediastinal lymph nodes.[18] Lymphohematogenous dissemination occurs with deposition of the bacteria at multiple extrapulmonary sites, where further multiplication can continue. During dissemination, specific cell-mediated immunity matures and further multiplication and dissemination of the organism is halted in the majority of healthy individuals. Subsequently the infection remains contained or latent.[19] The immune response produces granulomas known as tubercles with characteristic caseous necrosis seen microscopically within the lung, mediastinal lymph nodes and other tissues. When the cell-mediated immune response is overwhelmed (approximately 5% of all infected individuals) rapidly progressive infection or primary TB results. Human immunodeficiency virus (HIV)-infected patients, due to impaired cellular immunity, are much more likely compared to normal hosts, to develop primary TB after exposure.

Reactivation TB (approximately 5% of all infected individuals) results when previously contained organisms begin uncontrolled proliferation. This may occur in the nonimmunosuppressed host within approximately 2 years of the initial infection, accounting for roughly half of the cases of reactivation TB. The other cases arise randomly after 2 years through the remaining years of life, in some spontaneously and in others when cell-mediated immunity becomes compromised.

The cell-mediated immune response takes approximately 4–8 weeks to mature in the naive host,[20] and it can be detected in the human host by either the Tuberculin Skin Test (TST) response or a positive blood test called the interferon-gamma release assay (IGRA). Both tests measure the intensity of T-cell response to either tuberculin, a purified protein derivative of *M. tuberculosis* culture extract *in vivo* in the case of TST, or to very select and specific *M. tuberculosis* derived antigens *in vitro*, in the case of the IGRA.[21]

Factors listed in Box 88-1 consist of disease states that weaken cell-mediated immunity and situations that reflect an increased burden of latent organisms and greater potential to transition into active tuberculosis.[22,23] The relative risk of progression approximates tenfold among untreated HIV, substantially higher compared to the rest on the list. By comparison immunosuppressant agents such as chronic steroids and tumor necrosis factor inhibitor therapies (e.g., infliximab, etanercept) increase the risk of reactivation TB by 2–3 fold.[23] Smoking, poorly controlled diabetes and other medical conditions listed range between 1.5- and 2-fold.[23]

Transmission of Tuberculosis. Transmission of tuberculosis to other human hosts is strictly via airborne droplet nuclei. *M. tuberculosis* within secretions or droplet nuclei that have deposited on a surface loses the potential for infection. Patients with pulmonary or laryngeal TB produce infectious droplet nuclei.[24,25] Those with extrapulmonary tuberculosis do not, unless the site of TB infection is manipulated in such a way that an aerosol is generated (e.g., wound irrigation, autopsy). The data from the Centers for Disease Control and Prevention (CDC) show that approximately 21–23% of individuals in close contact to patients with infectious tuberculosis become infected. Most of these are LTBIs. Recent data reported from nine United States (US) and Canada health departments indicates that 4% of close contacts develop active tuberculosis and that most of the cases, 75%, are diagnosed within the first 3 months of the index case diagnosis.[26] Transmission of infection to another human host is generally a function of the concentration of infectious droplet nuclei, duration of contact with the infectious case, and the susceptibility of the host exposed.

BOX 88-1 Risk Factors for Developing Active Disease from Latent Tb Infection

HIV (especially when CD4 < 200 mm^3)
One or more of the following medical conditions:
Persons who inject drugs (including those that are HIV negative)
Tobacco abuse
Poorly controlled diabetes
Silicosis
Renal failure and those on chronic hemodialysis
Immunosuppressive therapy:
Steroids ($>$15 mg/day for $>$ 1 month)
Tumor necrosis factor-α inhibitor treatment
Chemotherapy
Solid organ and stem cell transplant
Hematologic malignancy (e.g., leukemia, Hodgkin's disease)
Head and neck malignancy
Chronic malabsorption syndrome or body weight 10% below ideal
Intestinal bypass or gastrectomy
Close contact to person(s) with active pulmonary TB
TB infection documented in the previous 2 years
Chest x-ray showing healed prior pulmonary TB, untreated
History of active TB in the past, but treatment incomplete or inadequate

Classic experiments attempting to quantify TB transmission and identifying key factors in droplet nuclei concentration were done in the late 1950s and early 1960s by Riley and investigators in the Baltimore City veterans hospital.[16] In these studies, air from a room containing patients with active pulmonary tuberculosis was diverted to either a UV light chamber and then a control group of guinea pigs, or directly past a test group of guinea pigs. By monitoring the rate of guinea pig infections and the volume of air circulated over the study period, the average concentration of infectious units was calculated at approximately 1 per 15,000–20,000 cubic feet of air. If an adult person ventilates approximately 18 cubic feet of air per hour, the probability of infection for an hour of exposure would be approximately 1 in 800–1000, which is comparable to risk data from other studies examining nosocomial tuberculosis transmission. The guinea pig investigations also demonstrated significant variation in the concentration of infectious units or droplet nuclei.[27] The variation depended upon clinical characteristics of TB in the source patient (e.g., cavitary vs. noncavitary lung disease). In addition, transmission dropped rapidly after the source patient was started on antimycobacterial treatment.

Factors effecting transmission can be related to the source case, the environment, the recipient host, and/or the organism. Most source cases with active pulmonary disease produce droplet nuclei within aerosols produced by coughing, sneezing, or speaking. The behavior of the infectious patient also affects the concentration of droplet nuclei released. When a patient with active pulmonary disease cooperates by covering their nose and mouth when coughing or sneezing, or by wearing an ordinary surgical mask, the large droplets with the potential to form infectious droplet nuclei are captured and inactivated.[24] The effect as a physical barrier rather than the filtration properties are what is important with such techniques. Also, the large number of organisms in the sputum from patients with cavitary disease and more precisely, a shorter time-to-detection in culture (less than 9 days),[28] increases the probability of infection among contacts. A study from Finland even suggested that the probability of active tuberculosis was also higher among contacts of patients who produced sputum smears that contained a high number of organisms.[29] At the other end of the spectrum, patients who produce a low concentration of organisms in sputum, those who are smear-negative, but culture-positive, are the least likely to transmit infection, yet transmission does occur at low levels.[30]

Environmental factors also affect the concentration of droplet nuclei in the air.[24] The volume of air common to the source and the recipient host is one such factor. The smaller the room, the more concentrated the droplet nuclei. The amount of outside air ventilated into a room is another factor, since fresh air will dilute the number of droplet nuclei. Modern buildings are engineered for air recirculation. The closed heating and air-conditioning systems increase the concentration of droplet nuclei since not much outside air is introduced into such a system. Engineering controls that reduce contamination include passage of recirculated air across a UV light source or across high-efficiency particulate air (HEPA) filters.

Duration of exposure and immune status of the recipient host (also referred to as a close contact) of an infectious case also affect the probability of transmission. The longer the duration of exposure, the greater the probability the close contact will inhale a critical number of droplet nuclei and exceed the threshold for infection. Naive hosts who are immunosuppressed or at the extremes of age (under 5 or over 65 years) are more likely to become infected when they are in close contact with a patient with a positive sputum smear. In contrast, close contacts who have been infected previously, demonstrable by a positive TST, are unlikely to be reinfected as long immune and health status are intact.[31,32] However, reinfection has been documented for nonimmunosuppressed individuals where TB prevalence is high.[33]

Tuberculosis strain-specific transmissibility was supported by older studies from New York City using DNA fingerprinting methodology to precisely track the *M. tuberculosis* isolates, but subsequent studies examining transmissibility and other virulence characteristics have been inconsistent. The data suggest that variation in host vulnerability determinants obscure the influence of specific strain virulence characteristics.[34,35]

CLINICAL ASPECTS OF TUBERCULOSIS

Active TB must be suspected in specific clinical settings. The confirmation of active TB relies on the acquisition of sputum, body fluid, or infected tissue, followed by identification of the organism.[21] The recent decade has been marked by the development of faster and more reliable diagnostic tests.

Characteristics of Patients with Tuberculosis. The majority of primary infections (approximately 90%) result in healing and granuloma formation. The organism then becomes dormant and the infection remains latent. Individuals with LTBI are completely asymptomatic and are detected only by a positive TST or IGRA. These individuals cannot transmit tuberculosis to others and represent the most prevalent form of tuberculosis.

Active tuberculosis in the nonimmunocompromised adults is frequently infectious because it presents as a pulmonary infection in 85% of the cases. Symptoms are insidious in onset and develop over several weeks or months. The typical pulmonary symptoms are a productive cough of small or scant amounts of a nonpurulent sputum, hemoptysis, and vague chest discomfort. Patients also have systemic symptoms such as chills, night sweats, fever, easy fatigue, loss of appetite, and weight loss. A physical examination of adults with active pulmonary tuberculosis usually contributes little to the diagnosis of tuberculosis. Active tuberculosis manifests differently in children compared to adults. Neonates and infants more often present with miliary TB or meningitis. Pulmonary or nodal involvement is more frequent in children over age 5, but difficult to diagnose because nonspecific symptoms, plus few organism cause intense inflammation, making them noncontagious but affecting the yield of diagnostic tests negatively.[36]

Adults with active tuberculosis and HIV or AIDS coinfection, present differently than nonimmunosuppressed patients. Atypical chest findings or extrapulmonary disease is far more common in HIV-infected hosts. Extrapulmonary disease can occur in up to 70% of patients.[37] The probability of an atypical presentation increases as the CD4+ T-cell count falls. Sputum samples, IGRA and TST also are less reliable adjuncts to diagnosis. The reaction to the TST is often blunted and as many as 40% of HIV patients with active TB will not react to the TST.[38] One study showed that 100% of AIDS patients with CD4+ T-cell counts below 100 and active TB had a negative TST.[39] IGRAs also show reduced sensitivity among HIV patients.[40] Furthermore, histologic samples from patients infected with TB may not demonstrate a mature granuloma. In general, specific diagnosis of tuberculosis in patients with AIDS often requires a high index of suspicion, a comprehensive search for site of infection, and biopsy to demonstrate and identify the organisms in the tissue site.

Sputum Examination. The standard sputum acid-fast smear is less sensitive and not specific compared to culture for detecting *M. tuberculosis*. To detect organisms in a sputum smear, the concentration needs to exceed approximately 10,000 organisms/mL.[41,42] Only 50–80% of patients with active pulmonary TB will have a positive acid-fast smear. Acid-fast smears also cannot distinguish *M. tuberculosis* from acid-fast staining NTM.

Currently molecular diagnostics, which either rely on nucleic acid probes or WGS, extend information provided by sputum specimens, but also can be applied to *M. tuberculosis* isolated in culture, if sputum specimen insufficient. Nucleic acid amplification (NAA) techniques have developed into rapid (1- to 2-day turnaround), commercially available, uncomplicated lab procedures that improve the specificity and sensitivity of *M. tuberculosis* identification. They also add drug resistance data. Two commercial NAA kits have been advocated by the World Health Organization (WHO): the Xpert MTB/RIF (Cepheid, Sunnyvale, Ca) cartridge-based system and the Hain Line Probe assay (Hain Lifescience, Inc, Nehren, Germany). These NAA assays amplify short, specific RNA or DNA sequences followed by hybridization with probes designed to detect *M. tuberculosis* and the most frequent resistance conferring mutations (see Molecular Detection of Drug Resistance). The Xpert MTB/RIF Ultra, a recent modification, provides enhanced detection of organisms within specimens that are smear negative, but also extra pulmonary specimens such as spinal fluid.[43] Because of these advanced techniques, the diagnostic value of the sputum specimen has been augmented substantially: improved sensitivity, immediate *M. tuberculosis* confirmation with very high specificity, and preliminary drug susceptibility information.[44]

Culture of Clinical Specimens. Refinements in culture techniques have cut the time for growth and identification down to approximately 1–3 weeks. Culture-based identification and drug susceptibility testing remains the gold standard and is referred to as phenotypic testing, distinguishing it from molecular techniques which are also widely used. Conventional culture can detect as few as 10 organisms/mL, making it a very sensitive tool for detecting tuberculosis.[45] Although solid media culture back-up is often done concurrently, most clinical laboratories rely on a commercial system consisting of selective liquid media, Middlebrook 7H12, and a fluorescence, pressure or other detector system to sense growth. Liquid media culture methods are faster compared to solid media, with a median time of 15 versus 26 days, but are more often compromised by contaminant overgrowth.[21] Once the threshold growth index is achieved, *M. tuberculosis* complex confirmation follows within 1 day in most clinical labs, using nucleic acid hybridization with a RNA or DNA probe. Phenotypic assessment of antibiotic susceptibility for the first-line medications have been adapted to the rapid culture process so that notification of resistant isolates can be made after an additional 4–13 days.

Molecular Detection of Drug Susceptibility. The phenotypic assessment of drug resistance has become routinely supplemented by genotypic-based diagnostic testing that detect mutations associated with drug resistance either by WGS, DNA sequencing, or amplifying target mutations using PCR, followed by a specific probe. The two commercially available probe-based systems for identifying *M. tuberculosis* were mentioned above. The standard Xpert MTB/RIF assay detects rifampin resistance as a surrogate for MDRTB with sensitivity and specificity that exceed 95%, probing for specific mutations within the *rpoB* gene.[46] The Hain Line Probe Assay (LPA) detects mutations conferring resistance to both isoniazid and rifampin with similar sensitivity and specificity on culture isolates.[47] Recently an upgraded cartridge for the Xpert MTB/RIF system and an extension of the Hain LPA (MTBDR*sl*) have been developed and tested, and both show high sensitivity and specificity for detecting mutations in *gyrA* and *rrs* genes, which correlate with resistance to key second-line medications: fluoroquinolones and aminoglycosides (i.e., amikacin, kanamycin).[47,48] Although powerful, these probe-based assays come with drawbacks. Both of the following are examples of clinically misleading results that occur uncommonly: missense and silent mutations creating a false negative result, or in cases of TB relapse or new active infection in someone with previous active disease, the assays are sensitive enough to detect residual DNA or RNA fragments from the prior infectious isolate, creating a false positive result.[49,50] DNA sequencing assays (i.e., pyrosequencing, Sanger) in contrast provide mutation data that are not subject to those limitations and provides accurate predictions of resistance.[5] Although DNA sequencing for detection of resistance remains categorized as an investigational technique, it is readily available in the US with 2- to 4-day turnaround, through state public health laboratories in connection with the laboratory for Molecular Detection of Drug Resistance (MDDR) supported by the CDC. The process can be performed on sputum, culture specimens, or isolates. DNA sequencing provides robust data about genetic polymorphisms, which when coupled with clinical outcome metadata, improve predictions about resistance, such that the sensitivity and specificity approaches that of phenotypic susceptibility results for first-line drugs.[51] For second line and new drugs, the data provide useful information for planning initial therapy, but discrepancies remain between sequencing data and conventional drug susceptibility results. With time and more research one can anticipate those will be reconciled, making it possible to confidently select a specific drug regimen at the time of diagnosis which avoids amplifying drug resistance and transmission of drug resistant isolates.[52]

Chest Radiography. The chest x-ray in active pulmonary tuberculosis typically demonstrates infiltrates within the apical and/or posterior segments, and often the infiltrates contain variably sized cavities. In patients with disseminated TB, the chest x-ray as well as the CT, often demonstrates a miliary pattern with countless uniformly 1–3 mm nodules diffusely distributed throughout all lung fields and pleural surfaces.[53] The name stems from the visual resemblance to millet seeds. In immunocompromised and particularly HIV patients, the chest x-ray may be normal or exhibit only hilar or mediastinal adenopathy or infiltrates in any lung zone. Cavities within infiltrates are uncommon.

The Tuberculin Skin Test. The Mantoux or standard TST requires intradermal injection of 5 tuberculin units. The test identifies persons who have been infected by *M. tuberculosis* and have developed the specific cellular immune response. Infected individuals will develop induration at the site of injection at 48–72 hours. The diameter of induration is measured to determine whether the test is positive or negative. The classification of a positive Mantoux tuberculin skin test depends upon the pretest probability that the person was infected with *M. tuberculosis*.[22]

False-positive reactions can arise from subclinical infection by other similar organisms such as NTM, which express antigens that cross-react with *M. tuberculosis*. False-positive results have the greatest impact in populations with a low incidence of tuberculosis. For persons living in regions of low tuberculosis incidence, such as those in rural parts of the United States, a high threshold, 15 mm of induration, minimizes the possibility of a false-positive test misidentifying someone as having tuberculosis. The 5 mm threshold is established for those persons with a high probability of being infected and who may exhibit an attenuated cellular immune response. HIV-infected persons, close contacts of an active case of tuberculosis, and individuals with a chest x-ray compatible with old or healed tuberculosis lesions are those in which the smaller reaction is still considered positive. The standard cut point of 10 mm of induration effectively identifies all other patient populations where the incidence of TB is significant. These groups include foreign-born persons (Africa, Asia, Pacific Islands, Eastern Europe, and Central and South America), medically underserved and low-income populations, persons who inject drugs (PWID), residents of long-term care facilities, and individuals with medical conditions (other than HIV) known to increase the risk of TB (Box 88-1).

The *booster phenomenon* should be taken into consideration when performing serial screening (i.e., annually, semiannually). An insignificant skin test reaction may be exhibited by a person who was infected in the distant past, because the cellular immune response to *M. tuberculosis* wanes with time. Within a week, however, a boosted reaction can be seen upon placing a second TST. The first TST induces a recall of the immune response so that the second test should be classified as a true-positive result. The boosted response can last up to a year, so that it potentially can be confused with a TST conversion. Therefore two tests separated by 1–2 weeks, or *two-step* testing, is recommended for screening populations that contain a significant number of persons infected in the distant past (e.g., at a long-term care facility).[20,24]

TB vaccination [bacillus Calmette-Guérin (BCG)] is used in many parts of the world and may confound the interpretation of the TST reaction when screening foreign-born populations for tuberculosis infections. Prior BCG vaccination can induce a TST reaction ranging from 0 to 19 mm of induration. A larger reaction cannot be used reliably to differentiate those also infected with *M. tuberculosis*.[54] In the absence of performing an IGRA, most agree that a significant skin test reaction indicates latent TB infection in an individual from a high TB prevalence area regardless of whether they were previously vaccinated with BCG.[22,55]

Interferon-Gamma Release Assay. As with the TST, the IGRA tests for tuberculosis specific cell-mediated immunity, but does so *in vitro*, measuring interferon-γ release from T lymphocytes stimulated by two to three antigens specific for *M. tuberculosis*. T lymphocytes from individuals with prior infection compared to naïve individuals produce high levels of interferon-γ.[21] An IGRA, as with the TST, does not distinguish active from latent TB infection. Since an IGRA also can be negative because of transient energy that occurs early in active TB, it should be reserved for diagnosis of latent TB.[56] IGRA specificity exceeds 95%, and cross reaction with BCG and many NTM does not occur, but for a few rarely occurring exceptions: *M. kansasii*, *M. marinum*, *M. szulgai*, and *M. flavescens*.[57,58] The IGRA can be used instead of the TST for detecting LTBI and it is recommended over the TST for testing people who have had prior BCG vaccine.[21] In the

US, two commercial tests are available. The QuantiFERON-TB (QFT; Cellestis LTD, Carnegie, Australia), an enzyme-linked immunosorbent assay (ELISA), was first approved by the US Food and Drug Administration in 2005 and the QFT-Plus is the most recent update released in 2017. The T-SPOT.TB, an enzyme-linked immunospot (ELISPOT) assay, was approved in 2008.

The IGRA in contrast to the TST shows improved specificity, no booster effect, and results after only one visit. However, the IGRA costs more than a TST and other limitations include the requirement for fresh lymphocytes (i.e., impacted by blood acquisition inconsistency, transport delay, environmental factors), and laboratory personnel trained in specialized techniques.[57,58] The IGRA has also turned out to be a problematic replacement for the TST in testing healthcare providers serially because of an annual 5–8% false conversion rate, which is six to nine times higher than serial testing by TST.[59,60] These shortcomings have been enough to slow more extensive transition to the IGRA in place of the TST.

Genotyping M. tuberculosis Isolates. Advancing molecular biology technology introduced genotyping strains originally to enhance epidemiologic research.[61,62] Currently, molecular epidemiology characterizing genetic differences and similarities between TB strains is used routinely for verifying false positive cultures and understanding more precisely the transmission dynamics within outbreaks. In the United States, the National TB Genotyping Service (NTGS) has the capacity for genotyping all isolates from culture positive cases and relies on two techniques: spacer oligonucleotide typing (spoligotyping) and 24-locus variable-number tandem repeat mycobacterial interspersed repetitive units analysis (MIRU-VNTR).[63] Although powerful, these techniques can be limited by genotype clustering unrelated by transmission when a genotype is common within a region or population. WGS along with analysis of sequential accumulation of single nucleotide polymorphisms can provide higher molecular resolution to reveal chains of transmission. For example, the MIRU-VNTR and social network analysis of isolates from 32 patients in a Canadian TB outbreak classified it as an identical genotype cluster, but combining social network data with WGS analysis revealed two distinct TB transmission networks rather than a single outbreak.[64]

Reporting a Verified Case of Tuberculosis. Every active tuberculosis case and associated epidemiologic data must be reported to state or local health departments in the United States. State health departments, report data on confirmed cases to CDC as part of ongoing public health surveillance. Specific criteria have been established to generate a valid report of a verified case of tuberculosis (RVCT). Case definition for an RVCT relies on laboratory and clinical criteria. The laboratory criteria for diagnosis of *M. tuberculosis* require any of the following: isolation by culture from a clinical specimen, or demonstration by NAA test or acid-fast bacilli on smear when a culture has not or cannot be obtained. In the absence of laboratory data, a valid case must meet the following clinical criteria: (a) a positive TST or IGRA, (b) signs and symptoms compatible with active TB (e.g., clinical evidence of active disease, changing chest x-ray), (c) treatment with two or more antituberculous medications, and (d) completed diagnostic evaluation.[65]

TREATMENT OF TUBERCULOSIS

Treatment of tuberculosis requires distinguishing patients with active TB from those with a LTBI. The current approach to treatment of active TB reflects the emphasis on ensuring adherence to treatment to head off the development of secondary resistance. The updated recommendations for LTBI screening and treatment focuses on patients most likely infected and/or at higher risk for developing active TB. In the United States, detailed diagnosis and treatment guidelines for adults, pregnant women, HIV-infected individuals, and children can be found at the tuberculosis website managed by the CDC[66] and in consensus documents, which are regularly updated and provide ratings for the quality of evidence supporting recommendations.[21,67,68] In the United States, when more complex treatment questions arise, contact with clinicians expert in TB management is facilitated through the state public health departments.

Treatment of Active Tuberculosis. The basic principles of therapy are to provide a safe, cost-effective medication regimen in the shortest period of time. Multiple drugs are used in the initiation phase of treatment to rapidly reduce the number of viable organisms. In addition, steps are taken to ensure adherence to treatment.

To treat pulmonary and most forms of extrapulmonary tuberculosis in nonimmunosuppressed patients as well as those co-infected with HIV, four first-line medications are used during the first 8 weeks and referred to as the Intensive Phase of treatment: isoniazid, rifampin, pyrazinamide, and ethambutol. The Continuation Phase follows during which isoniazid and rifampin are given for an additional 18 weeks. This four-medication regimen has been shown to be highly effective. CDC data for the US indicate that 95% of patients treated by this regimen will receive at least two drugs to which the infecting organism is susceptible. In addition, patients who default before completing this regimen are more likely to be cured than those receiving fewer medications at the onset.[68]

The duration of airborne infection isolation (AII) for a patient who has started on treatment may be variably interpreted by practitioners. It is known from the guinea pig studies cited earlier that once treatment is started, the risk of transmission of infection rapidly diminishes, and by approximately 2 weeks of effective treatment, the risk approaches zero.[27] The sputum smear and culture from patients on therapy, however, may remain positive well beyond 2 weeks. For example, in a study that achieved a 98.4% cure rate, the median time to culture negativity was 4.6 weeks, and 25% of the patients had sputum samples still culture positive at 8 weeks.[69] The persistently positive sputum raises concern for continued contagion. Practical recommendations for certifying an outpatient at low risk for contagion are as follows: documented adherence to recommended multidrug TB therapy for 2–3 weeks, low risk for MDRTB and evidence for clinical improvement (e.g., less cough, reduced organism load in sputum smear). More conservative recommendations are suggested for patients within a healthcare setting. One would require the above criteria, but rather than release isolation upon demonstration of reduced organism load on sputum smear, continue AII until three consecutive sputum samples (8–24 hours apart and at least one early morning sample) are negative for acid-fast bacilli.[70]

Most patients with active tuberculosis are not severely ill, and treatment can be initiated safely in the outpatient setting. Temporary hospitalization for isolation of an active pulmonary case may be necessary while treatment is initiated, if household members include highly susceptible contacts such as HIV-positive individuals or children less than 5 years of age. Miliary tuberculosis and tuberculous meningitis are examples of serious extrapulmonary TB that require inpatient management. Enforcement of adherence for a patient who has been repeatedly nonadherent with treatment as an outpatient is another reason to use the inpatient setting for treatment.

INH-resistant bacteria can be treated successfully with the four-medication regimen noted above.[69,71] MDRTB strains, however, pose a more complicated treatment problem. The treatment is generally extended much longer than 6 months. At least three medications to which the organism is susceptible need to be provided. Second-line medications are required, which are less effective generally and carry a higher side effect and intolerance profile.

Treatment Adherence Issues for Patients with Active TB. Adherence to therapy is essential for successful outcome and to prevent the development of resistance. Nonadherence to tuberculosis therapy occurs commonly with self-administered regimens. Approximately 25% of patients with active tuberculosis fail to complete the 6-month standard regimen by 12 months. In homeless and substance-abusing patients, the number approaches 90%.[72] In addition, the ability of physicians to predict nonadherence is generally poor.[73] A study in a tuberculosis clinic showed that only 68% of all patients nonadherent to therapy were identified.

Physicians can improve upon their ability to anticipate nonadherence through continuing education that teaches them the most reliable predictors. A history of poor adherence to therapy, for example, has been shown to be among the best predictors. Other predictive factors include homelessness, substance abuse, mental health issues, and lack of family and social support.[74] Cultural factors also influence adherence to tuberculosis therapy. For example, within certain ethnic groups, persons with active TB risk rejection by their family.

The current approach to tuberculosis treatment incorporates supervised or directly observed therapy (DOT) to improve patient adherence. The advantages of DOT have been proven in multiple studies. A prospective study in Tarrant County, Texas, demonstrated that DOT, compared to standard self-administered therapy, decreased relapse rates and decreased incidence of drug-resistant strains of *M. tuberculosis*.[75] In New York City, prior to introducing a DOT program, a dismal 35% of the patients returned for follow-up appointments, with an overall 11% adherence to therapy. After a DOT program was introduced, 88% of patients were adherent to treatment and all sterilized their sputum. Relapses became rare and only in those with primary drug resistance.[76] Data such as these support recommendations that DOT be the core management strategy for all patients with active pulmonary tuberculosis.[68]

Treatment of Latent Tuberculosis Infection. Approximately 5–10% of patients with LTBI progress to active TB in their lifetime. US evidence-based consensus guidelines recommend using the IGRA or TB skin testing for screening individuals at risk for developing active TB and in populations in whom active TB is prevalent.[21,67] These individuals form the reservoir from which new cases of active TB arise. Treatment reduces the rate of active TB cases within these populations. Isoniazid self-administered daily for 6–9 months is 65–80% effective in treating a nonimmunosuppressed individual with LTBI.[22,77] Recent data indicate that shorter, self-administered rifampicin-based regimens may be provided with similar efficacy and less hepatotoxicity: Rifampin daily for 4 months or rifapentine plus isoniazid once a week for 12 weeks (doses).[78,79] When considering LTBI treatment for TB case contacts where resistance is known, one would treat isoniazid monoresistance with rifampin daily for 4 months and treat rifampin monoresistance with isoniazid daily for 9 months. In treating contacts of an MDRTB infected case, uncertainty remains, but data suggest treating for 6–12 months with at least two drugs to which the isolate was susceptible especially if one includes quinolones.[80,81] Treatment for LTBI in an HIV patient not only reduces the risk of developing active TB (i.e., 4.7–1.6 cases per 100 patient-years),[82] but also reduces TB transmission with in the population.[83]

The targeted testing paradigm focuses public health efforts on those who benefit from treatment and reduces waste of valuable resources on groups at low or no risk for reactivation TB. The highest priority group targeted for TST or IGRA screening are the following: HIV patients, patients whose HIV status is unknown but suspected, PWID who are HIV negative, close contacts of a newly diagnosed person with tuberculosis, persons exhibiting recent tuberculosis skin test conversion from negative to positive (less than 2 years), persons with old fibrotic lesion on chest x-ray consistent with prior pulmonary TB, and persons with certain non-HIV medical conditions that are known to increase the risk for developing active tuberculosis (Box 88-1).[80] A review of published data quantified more precisely lifetime risk for reactivation TB among persons with a positive TST. Individuals with either HIV infection or evidence of old healed TB on chest x-ray were the highest risk populations, each more than 20%. Population groups within a 10–20% lifetime risk included the following: those recently infected (less than 2 years), those receiving tumor necrosis factor antagonist treatment and under 35 years old with a TST > 15 mm, and those under 5 years old and demonstrating a TST > 5 mm.[84]

Also targeted for TST or IGRA screening and treatment are individuals in whom TB is more prevalent: immigrants to the United States from high TB prevalence countries, medically underserved individuals, residents of long-term care facilities, and staff of schools, correctional, health, and child-care facilities.[80]

When considering treatment, one must balance the risk of treatment against that of developing TB disease. Estimates for the risk of hepatitis from INH treatment vary between 0.1% and 0.15%, which is lower than earlier data indicated.[80] A US public health department 7-year study involving 11,141 patients receiving INH in which nurses performed monthly symptom surveys and intervention revealed only 11 cases of clinical hepatitis, one of which required hospitalization and none resulted in death.[85] In general, the risk of INH hepatotoxicity increases in the following clinical situations: age over age 60, pre-existing liver disease, pregnancy plus early postpartum period, and heavy alcohol consumption.[80] Rifamycin-based regimens provide noninferior alternative with less hepatotoxicity, higher rates of hypersensitivity reactions, but overall lower rates of adverse effects.[79,86]

Efficacy of the BCG Vaccine and Novel Vaccine Development. An *M. bovis* strain was continuously subcultured by Calmette and Guérin from 1908 to 1922 to produce the live attenuated strain named for them, bacillus Calmette-Guérin (BCG). BCG has been used as the basis for the live attenuated vaccine against tuberculosis since 1922. BCG vaccine remains the best available TB vaccine today and is used in many parts of the world.

Assessment of efficacy of the BCG vaccine has been clouded by multiple variables, which include the variability of BCG strains from which vaccines have been prepared, method and route of administration, characteristics of populations studied, and endpoints selected. Two meta-analyses of best studies dating back to 1950 indicate that the vaccine's efficacy is more than 80% in preventing TB meningitis and miliary TB in children.[87,88] These meta-analyses were unable to unravel the disparate data regarding prevention of pulmonary TB in adults. It is likely that the BCG vaccine does not prevent infection in adults, but likely decreases the probability of active TB.[89] Modest additional reductions have been reported by boosting the BCG vaccine effect using a vaccine containing *M. tuberculosis* proteins plus adjuvant.[90]

The CDC continues to recommend that the current BCG vaccine be used rarely because of the questions surrounding its efficacy, the issues relative to TST interpretation, and the overall risk for TB exposure in the United States remains low. Infants and young children at high risk for repeated TB exposure are the main indication for BCG vaccine use in the United States.[55]

The development of new effective vaccines promises to more rapidly reduce the global burden of TB and contain MDRTB. Vaccine development remains an international focus and priority for the WHO, which has compiled a consensus document describing the preferred product characteristics. Besides boosting the BCG vaccine effect for prevention of TB infection as mentioned above, the vaccine pipeline includes testing candidate vaccines that make use of viral vectors to deliver mycobacterial antigens, whole cell component vaccines, and vaccines with adjuvanted proteins. The new strategies target prevention of infection as well as supplementing therapy to prevent progression to active disease, shorten the course of treatment, and decrease risk of recurrence.[91]

EPIDEMIOLOGY OF TUBERCULOSIS

Crowded conditions, poverty, and host susceptibility facilitate the spread of this disease within populations. These situations have evolved over the past millennium and over the past two decades affecting the trends in TB incidence in the United States, the rest of the world, and specific subpopulations.

Tuberculosis Trends through History. Evidence for tuberculosis in ancient civilizations has come from the remains of ancient Egyptians, early Hindu writings referring to a disease called consumption, and ancient Greek medical literature referring to tuberculosis as phthisis. Also, documentation comes from granulomata found in a 1000-year-old pre-Columbian Peruvian mummy containing DNA compatible with *M. tuberculosis* by NAA studies,[92] as well as spinal and psoas abscesses, and a lung granuloma containing acid-fast staining bacilli found in another Peruvian mummy dated to 700 A.D.[93]

Initial theories logically speculated that *M. bovis* may have been the evolutionary precursor of *M. tuberculosis*.[94] *M. bovis* was known to be endemic within bovine and other animal populations before humans evolved. After humans evolved and particularly once cattle were herded and in close contact with humans, *M. bovis* could have been transmitted from animals causing the most ancient forms of human tuberculosis. However, phylogenic analysis of genomic deletions in the DNA from *M. tuberculosis* complex strains indicates that *M. tuberculosis* and *M. bovis* evolved separately within human and bovine ancestors long before cattle and humans were in close contact through domestication.[95,96]

Tuberculosis became widespread after 1600 A.D. with the onset of the Industrial Revolution in Europe.[94,97] Crowded conditions, poor sanitation, and poor nutrition were all features of rapidly expanding cities. Conditions were ideal for transmission of tuberculosis and it became epidemic. At its peak, 100% of western European urban dwellers may have been infected and the mortality rate was extremely high.[94] Tuberculosis struck predominantly the young people. Those that survived to reproductive age are believed to have had a selective advantage. After several generations, a degree of natural immunity and a greater prevalence of chronic infection developed. The higher prevalence of chronic infection, however, facilitated transmission of infection. TB naturally followed the Europeans to the Americas, where the immunologically naive Native Americans were extremely susceptible to tuberculosis upon first exposure. The same can be said for the peoples in the interior of Africa, where the disease arrived with western culture around 1910. Similar transmission to naive populations occurred in New Guinea in 1950 and in the deep Amazon region of South America in the 1970s.[98]

During the twentieth century before the development of effective antituberculosis medications in 1945, TB mortality in the United States and Europe continuously declined, probably in part because of the continued development of natural immunity. In the United States from 1900 to 1945, the number of new cases dropped from 194 to 40 per 100,000.[99] Improved socioeconomic conditions (including decreased crowding) and public health interventions are other factors that likely contributed to the decline in incidence.[97] The public health interventions for finding active cases included the widespread use of fluorography, skin testing, and chest x-ray for patients with a positive TST. The patients with active disease were removed from society and placed into sanitaria, which helped break the transmission cycle. Sanitaria-focused care was the state-of-the-art for tuberculosis management prior to the development of effective antimycobacterial medications. In the sanitaria, patients received rest and fresh air therapy supplemented by surgical lung collapse and resection. Mortality remained as high as 50%.

Widespread use of effective drug treatment finally reduced TB mortality to nearly zero in the United States during the 1950s through the early 1980s. The decline in incidence of TB disease continued over the same period, but the rate of decline did not change or accelerate. The most plausible explanation is that socioeconomic conditions and public health measures produced the predominant effect on TB incidence, while treatment improvements affected mortality rates. It is disconcerting to realize that in many parts of the world over the last two decades, the incidence of tuberculosis has risen and antituberculosis drugs are becoming less effective.

Recent Tuberculosis Trends within the United States. In 1984, the incidence of new cases of tuberculosis had declined to 9.4 per 100,000 and mortality was low at 0.7 per 100,000. Federal funding for TB control declined concurrently, while different public health needs moved to the forefront, diverting money away from TB programs. City and state governments downgraded their TB control and treatment supervision programs. Nearly simultaneously, there was an unanticipated upswing in TB incidence from 1985 to 1992. Incidence peaked at 10.5 cases per 100,000 population producing 51,700 excess new cases of tuberculosis.[38,100] Other factors contributing to the resurgence in tuberculosis, besides the failure of public health system, included the exponential growth in the AIDS epidemic, the development of drug-resistant strains of tuberculosis, the influx of immigrants from countries with high TB prevalence, the increase in homelessness in urban centers, and the increase in PWID.

The combination of AIDS and drug-resistant TB made treatment and control of infections more difficult and allowed for more prolonged transmission of infection. The greatest upswing in cases were in geographically restricted, congested urban centers such as New York City, Miami, and San Francisco, where AIDS and drug-resistant tuberculosis were most prevalent.[101] The drug resistance problem in particular was a by-product of the failing public health system (e.g., poor case management, poor patient compliance with treatment) and the importation of drug-resistant *M. tuberculosis* with immigrants.

By 1993, the infusion of money from the US government for TB control programs had increased substantially and was targeted to the urban centers where the most significant outbreaks were occurring. The incidence of new cases has slowly trended downward since. In 2017, the incidence of new cases was down to 2.8 per 100,000.[102] Although the annual TB rate continued a steady decrease, the proportion of cases accounted for by foreign-born individuals increased steadily (see section: TB in Foreign-Born Immigrants). The small fraction of US-born cases were concentrated among the homeless (61%), those in long-term care facilities (45%), and incarcerated persons (40%).[102] The national policy on screening and treating LTBI remains focused on the high-risk immigrants, homeless, and those within congregate settings.[67]

HIV and Tuberculosis in the United States. HIV impairs cell-mediated immunity and the host's ability to resist tuberculous infection. In addition, TB accelerates the progression to AIDS, other opportunistic infections and death.[103,104] The resurgence of TB in the United States during 1986–92 was closely interwoven with the HIV epidemic.[105,106] This was supported by the following findings: approximately 57% of the excess cases of tuberculosis were attributable to HIV coinfection,[107] the AIDS epidemic and the resurgence of TB followed similar time courses, persons in the 25- to 44-year-old age group exhibited the highest increase in TB and included the majority of AIDS cases,[108,109] and the geographic distribution of the two epidemics correlated closely on state-by-state analyses as well as by specific urban TB clinics (e.g., New York City, Newark, and Miami). These found a prevalence of HIV among the TB cases, approximately 30%, and up to 58%.[108]

Other facts about TB and HIV coinfection came to light during the 1986–92 resurgence. In contrast to non-HIV, new TB cases more likely represented recent infection.[82] Many persons within populations with a high incidence of HIV were independently at high risk for exposure to tuberculosis.[106,110] Many HIV-positive individuals living in urban areas were more likely to be exposed to others with active TB. In addition, AIDS patients with active tuberculosis acquired a new infection exogenously, which was uncommon in the non-HIV host. By studying the RFLP patterns of *M. tuberculosis* isolates from patients with AIDS, investigators found that among active tuberculosis cases who responded poorly to tuberculosis treatment,[111] or that relapsed during or after successful completion of therapy, a significant proportion were caused by a new *M. tuberculosis* strain. Thus, infectious TB patients who also have AIDS not only require isolation for public health reasons, but also for protection from others with active TB.

In the past data about the HIV status of TB patients in the US remained incomplete as a result of concerns about confidentiality, reluctance to report HIV status to TB surveillance program staff and varying interpretation of state and local laws.[112] In the current era, those no longer create barriers. In 2017, HIV status was reported for 86.3% of TB cases in the United States and 5.6% were HIV coinfected.[102]

Effective antiretroviral therapy, essentially restoring normal immune function, contributed to improved outcomes for TB in HIV patients over the last two decades. Restoration of the immune function simultaneous with active TB infection, however, may cause the immune reconstitution inflammatory syndrome (IRIS). These patients, due to revitalization of their immune system, will develop high fevers, adenopathy, and advancing pulmonary infiltrates as a result of a marked increase in the inflammation within existing TB lesions.[113] Besides this confusing and paradoxic treatment response, managing antiretroviral along with TB therapy remains complex due to many factors including prophylactic prednisone administration to diminish IRIS, malabsorption of TB drugs,[114] acquired rifampin resistance,[115] antiretroviral and TB drug interactions, and high rates of adverse effects and intolerances. Despite the complexities, the benefits of successful treatment of HIV and TB in the United States have been realized. However, the burden of HIV and TB coinfection remains substantial in developing countries of the world (see Global Tuberculosis below).

US Data for Drug-Resistant Tuberculosis (including MDR- and XDRTB). The threat of drug-resistant tuberculosis arose during the 1990s. Most concerning was the emergence of MDRTB isolates. Treatment of such patients relied on selecting a regimen based on resistance surveillance data, prior treatment history, drug susceptibility data of the isolate (often not available), and the use of second-line medications (aminoglycosides, fluoroquinolones, ethionamide, cycloserine, and para-aminosalicyclic acid), which generally were less effective, costlier, and more toxic. Compounding the difficulties has been the emergence of XDRTB cases that impose greater management complexity than MDRTB.

The theoretical explanations for how drug resistance develops (see earlier text) have been borne out in epidemiologic data. Patients with cavitary pulmonary TB are fourfold more likely to exhibit resistant isolates compared to those with noncavitary disease. In addition, among *M. tuberculosis* isolates from patients who relapse after previous treatment, resistance is demonstrated 4.7 times more frequently compared to those with no history of prior treatment. The combination of cavitary disease and prior treatment produce a risk of resistance that is additive.[116] Errors in prescribing treatment are a too frequent reason for development of drug resistance.[117] Inappropriate use of monotherapy for active TB, failure to provide an adequate medication regimen at time of TB diagnosis, failure to ensure adherence to treatment, and not recognizing and treating medication failure all account for the typical prescribing errors. Patient errors such as taking partial doses or only some of the drugs prescribed also contribute significantly when treatment occurs without supervision.[118]

The peak concentrations of drug-resistant cases were found in New York City and in urban populations in California in 1991. The CDC national survey revealed that single drug resistance was at 14.2%, two or more drug resistance was at 6%, and MDRTB was found in 3.5% of all cases surveyed.[119] The New York City region accounted for 63% of the MDRTB cases, while only 1% of the other counties surveyed reported MDRTB. The New York City TB Control Bureau reported in 1991 that 26% of *M. tuberculosis* isolates exhibited resistance to INH and 19% exhibited multidrug resistance.[120] Subsequent intensive efforts to ensure appropriate treatment, adherence, and effective isolation of infectious TB cases, led to reduced rates of resistant *M. tuberculosis* strains.[121] Yet in New York City, reports of outbreaks of cases infected by a particularly resistant MDRTB, strain W (resistant to INH, rifampin, ethambutol, streptomycin, and several second-line drugs) persisted throughout the 1990s.[122,123] By 2004, however, US rates for MDRTB had come down to approximately 1%, remaining stable since, accounting for less than 100 cases, 92% attributable to foreign-born immigrants.[102,112] One XDRTB case was reported in 2016.[102] Management of MDR- and XDRTB cases remain difficult, complex, and cost approximately 8- and 25-fold, respectively, that of a nondrug resistant TB patient, making intensive containment an ongoing focus.[124]

Global Tuberculosis. Since 1997, the WHO has been annually updating and publishing worldwide tuberculosis surveillance data and marking the magnitude of the problem as well as the uncertainty in the data, the large financial resources needed to follow-through with the newest strategies for worldwide TB control, and where small incremental gains have been made.[125] Approximately 25% of the world's population is infected with tuberculosis (1.7 billion persons with LTBI). Since about 2005 global incidence of new TB cases has been falling slowly, approximately 2% annually. All six WHO designated regions (Africa, Americas, Eastern Mediterranean, Europe, Southeast Asian, and Western Pacific) showed falling case rates in 2017. The number of new tuberculosis cases in that year was estimated to be 10 million, of which 1.3 million died.[125] The 30 WHO designated high TB burden countries (HBC) account for 87% of global TB cases. Two-thirds of the cases can be found in eight countries (order high to low): India, China, Indonesia, Philippines, Pakistan, Nigeria, Bangladesh, and South Africa. The rates for the Philippines and South Africa exceed 500 per 100,000, while most of the other HBC range between 150 and 400. The gap between the officially reported cases and the estimate is 3.6 million, which represents under diagnosis (inadequate diagnostic tools or patient access) and underreporting and 80% can be found in India, Indonesia, and Nigeria. Deaths from tuberculosis among HIV-negative cases globally have fallen by nearly 30% since 2000. Countries among the HBC showing the fastest declines from 2013 to 2017 include: Russian Federation, Ethiopia, Sierra Leone, Kenya, and Viet Nam.[125] Analogous to Western Europe during the Industrial Revolution, those under the age of 50 years, the most productive fraction of the population, are hit hardest.[126]

HIV infection complicates treatment and control of tuberculosis globally. The impact of AIDS and HIV on TB makes it a major driver by increasing risks of acquisition and progression to active TB and death from TB. HIV remains most prevalent in the same populations in whom tuberculosis prevalence is the greatest. Antiretroviral therapy reduces the risk of TB and distribution of therapy is becoming more widespread through joint initiatives like the FIND.TREAT.ALL.#ENDTB partnership, which since 2018 aims to close the financial gaps, while combining forces with the WHO, the Stop TB partnership and the Global Fund to Fight AIDS, tuberculosis, and malaria.[127] In 2017 the WHO estimated 0.9 million TB/HIV cases and 72% occurred in Africa and mostly affected young adults and children. There were 300,000 TB deaths among HIV-positive cases, which have continued to fall and since 2015 have fallen by 20%.[125]

Managing drug-resistant tuberculosis also remains an important barrier to controlling TB worldwide. Drug resistance prevalence correlates indirectly with available resources and the quality of tuberculosis control practices.[128] Overall global prevalence for MDRTB remains difficult to measure due to inconsistent reporting, but 2017 estimates ranged between 483,000 and 639,000 cases resistant to rifampin, 82% were MDRTB, and account for 3.5% of new and 18% of previously treated tuberculosis cases. India, China, and the Russian Federation contribute about half of the MDRTB cases. Between 6.2% and 11% of the MDRTB cases classify as XDRTB.[125] The persistence of XDRTB remains concerning since rates of death or therapeutic failure exceed 50% outstripping poor outcomes recorded for MDRTB cases.[13]

The WHO in 1993 initially declared that tuberculosis is a global health emergency. Strategies for control were developed and were published in 1994.[129] This document established the following two main targets for tuberculosis control: to cure 85% of newly detected smear-positive tuberculosis cases, and to find at least 70% of existing cases by the year 2000. In 2005, the WHO continued to report shortfalls: the goal for 85% treatment success was at 82% based on selected cohort of 1.7 million patients diagnosed in 2003 and the goal for case detection was only at 60%. The WHO established Global Plan to Stop TB in 2005 and a key element in the control programs emphasized the administration of the standard short-course regimen with a very strong effort toward supervised treatment (referred to as DOTS—directly observed treatment, short course), adequate drug supplies, and effective program management and evaluation. Further enhancements included an expanded scope of interventions in regions of high HIV prevalence, the development of the DOTS-Plus, which extended treatment for MDRTB in regions of high prevalence. Financial constraints within the WHO and the HBC stood as the major obstacle to widely instituting these well-intentioned programs.[130] Since 2015, WHO recognized that TB is a nation development challenge in addition to public health concern and rolled out the End TB program. Adopting Sustainable Development Goals, a strategy adaptable to diverse country settings, WHO aims to reduce the incidence of TB by 80%, deaths from TB by 90%, and eliminate the costs for TB affected families, all by 2030. The End TB Strategy sets four key principals: government stewardship and accountability with monitoring and evaluation; strong coalition with civil society organizations and communities; protection and promotion of human rights, ethics, and equity; and adaptation of the strategy and targets at country level, with global collaboration.[131] In 2018, although $6.9 billion (double that of 2005 dollars) went to the low- and middle-income countries accounting for 97% of TB cases, but at least $10.4 billion is required annually to reach the End TB milestones 2025 and 2030. Insufficient funding continues to undermine the well-structured and intentioned WHO strategies.[125]

Tuberculosis in Foreign-Born Immigrants to the United States. Given the high prevalence of tuberculosis globally, it is not surprising that foreign-born immigrants generate a substantial fraction of the new cases within the United States. The rate of TB cases due to foreign-born is 15 times that of US-born persons, which is 1.0/100,000 per year. The highest TB rate is reported among Asian immigrants at 27/100,000 per year. The proportion of US cases comprised by the foreign-born population increased steadily from 22% to 70% over the period from 1986 to 2017. The top five countries: Mexico (19%), Philippines (12%), India (9%), Vietnam (8%), and China (6%), account for nearly half of the tuberculosis cases among new immigrants.[102,132] Tuberculosis rates for these countries are many times greater than the US rate, ranging from 22 (Mexico) to 554/100,000 per year (Philippines).[125] Most of the foreign-born cases of active tuberculosis (55%) are diagnosed during the first 5 years in the United States, and most often arises from activation of a prior infection.[133] Also, progression from latent to active tuberculosis among these immigrants has been reported to be 100–200 times the US rate.[134] Another potential contributor to the tuberculosis rate, which is difficult to measure, are the millions of nonimmigrant, foreign arrivals per year that are in the United States as tourists, visiting family members, business visitors, and students. Many of these people do not receive any sort of screening for tuberculosis before they arrive.[135] California, Florida, New York, and Texas are the states where the largest numbers of immigrants arrive and settle, and also report more than half of the total TB cases in the United States.[102]

Drug resistance remains a more significant problem than HIV coinfection within the foreign-born population. In 2016, 1 XDRTB and 97 MDRTB cases were reported in the United States and 92% were among foreign-born persons.[102]

Nosocomial Transmission of Tuberculosis. The major causes of tuberculosis transmission within hospitals are from those cases where it is not suspected, the diagnosis is delayed, or the respiratory isolation procedure breaks down.[136,137]

The following unusual example of extrapulmonary tuberculosis aptly illustrates these aspects of nosocomial transmission.[138] A deep thigh abscess, not suspected to be tuberculous, was surgically debrided in an Arkansas hospital, then irrigated daily for approximately 2 weeks using a Water Pik-type device. Eventually, of the 70 healthcare workers (HCWs) either directly exposed to or working on the same hallway as this patient, 63% became infected and 14% developed active tuberculosis between 9 and 12 weeks after the exposure. The high rate of transmission resulted from the combined effect of the following factors: (a) unsuspected, high concentration of *M. tuberculosis* in the abscess tissues; (b) unrecognized generation of aerosol densely contaminated with *M. tuberculosis* because of wound irrigation (perhaps further facilitated by the high intensity of the water stream produced by the irrigating device); and (c) unanticipated positive air pressure in the patient's room so that the contaminated air circulated outside the room and up and down the hallways.

Medical students, pathologists, and assistants working in an autopsy room exhibit a higher risk for tuberculosis infection and active disease.[139,140] The autopsy suite stands out as one of the hospital sites where the heaviest exposure to tuberculosis may occur for several reasons. An aerosol with a high density of bacteria will likely be generated when cutting infected lung or bone with a knife or oscillating saw. Recent data show that the concentration can be as high as 1 infectious unit per 3.5 cubic feet of air,[141] a far more dense concentration when one considers that on a tuberculosis ward the concentration measures approximately 1 infectious unit per 24,000 cubic feet of air.[16] Also, autopsy workers, especially within areas such as South Africa where HIV and TB prevalence is high, are more frequently exposed to patients unsuspected of having tuberculosis antemortem and abide great risk if adequate respiratory protection is neglected.[142]

The extensive MDRTB outbreaks that occurred during the late 1980s in eight hospitals and an upstate New York state prison displayed overlapping chains of transmission and illustrated unfortunate, but common characteristics of nosocomial transmission.[11,12,143–145] Delayed diagnosis, delay in effective treatment, lack of effective isolation procedures, and a high proportion of patients with severe AIDS (CD4+ lymphocytes less than 100/mL) were all common features. Advanced AIDS altered the clinical picture of active TB and contributed significantly to the delayed diagnosis. The laboratory confirmation of *M. tuberculosis* was also delayed for several of the following reasons: TB went unsuspected, so confirmation tests were not done; acid-fast bacilli present on smears of clinical specimens were assumed to be *M. avium* complex instead of *M. tuberculosis*; and the mean time between specimen collection and identification of *M. tuberculosis* was 6 weeks. The realization that the *M. tuberculosis* strain isolated was resistant was further delayed because the task of susceptibility testing required at least an additional 6 weeks. All of these factors together resulted in extended opportunities for transmission of MDRTB in the hospitals, outpatient clinics, and among the prisoners. Approximately 300 individuals developed active MDRTB and most were coinfected by HIV. A high attack rate, short incubation time, and rapid progression to active disease and death were among the most striking characteristics and were a function of the high prevalence of patients with AIDS and MDRTB. The mortality rate in most of the hospitals approached 100%, with a median time from diagnosis to death of 4 weeks. Over 150 HCWs were directly exposed and 27% became infected. Seventeen of these developed active MDRTB, eight were co-infected with HIV, and four of those persons died from MDRTB. Three others died, one of whom may also have been immunosuppressed as a result of a malignancy.

Both the irrigated tuberculous abscess and the extensive MDRTB outbreak in upstate New York demonstrated clear and dramatic evidence for overlapping chains of nosocomial transmission and the danger to healthcare workers and patients when active cases go unsuspected. The upstate New York outbreak in particular, provided the motivation behind subsequent government efforts to tighten isolation procedures for healthcare facilities (discussed below).

Guidelines for Protection of Healthcare Workers. The resurgence of tuberculosis, and in particular the lessons learned from the MDRTB outbreaks reviewed above, drove the process for re-evaluating the 1990 CDC guidelines for tuberculosis containment in the hospital environment.[146,147] These efforts culminated in detailed, broad guidelines published by the CDC and the National Institute for Occupational Safety and Health (NIOSH) at the end of 1994 and introduced the three-tier control hierarchy within hospitals: administrative controls, environmental controls, and respiratory protection.[148] The changes in the update to these guidelines in 2005 were not driven by dramatic tuberculosis outbreaks in the years after 1994. Rather, the latest guidelines recognized that the risk for healthcare associated tuberculosis transmission has decreased, that healthcare practices have changed since 1994, and that better scientific data regarding transmission and control could be applied.[149] The three-tier control hierarchy continued with the latest iteration. Among the biggest changes were that the guidelines included much more practical and detailed information, and encompassed the entire healthcare arena, beyond hospitals, including chronic-care facilities, outpatient settings, laboratories, and nontraditional settings.

The administrative control portion of the plan assigns the responsibility for developing, installing, and maintaining TB infection control, as well as identifying how it should be coordinated with the public health department. The administrative controls also include a detailed local risk assessment worksheet and annual reassessment plan. Based on local risk assessment the rate and intensity for screening, training, and educating HCW for and about tuberculosis can be established. A consensus document[149] and the CDC tuberculosis website[150] describe how for screening HCWs, IGRAs may be substituted for TST, and provide updated recommendations for initial and serial screening of HCWs. A recent consensus paper compiled by the National TB Controllers Association in conjunction with the CDC recommends no routine annual TB screening in the absence of ongoing exposure or transmission.[151]

Environmental controls portion of the guidelines serve to control the source of infection by reducing the concentration of droplet nuclei within the patient's room, adjacent rooms, and hallway. Expanded information includes detailed specific information about designing negative pressure *AII* rooms, room air circulation, cleaning air by use of HEPA filtration (minimum efficiency 99.97% for particles > 0.3 μm diameter), and UV germicidal irradiation.[149]

The respiratory protection measures described in the current guidelines spell out the details for use of the N95 disposable respirator, fit testing, user training, and includes how to train patients in proper respiratory hygiene and cough techniques.[149]

Appropriate respiratory protection historically has been a contentious issue particularly around the proper respirator and the issue of fit-testing healthcare workers.[147] In 1992, NIOSH took the stance that the risk to HCWs had to be completely eliminated and therefore all who were at risk for exposure to TB patients should wear HEPA-filtered, powered, personal respirators, and participate in a mandatory respirator fit-testing program. These recommendations were put forward even though there were no specific data to support the necessity of such a sweeping upgrade from the standard surgical masks. Subsequent revision of the guidelines released a year later in the *Federal Register* by NIOSH recommended HEPA-filtered disposable particulate respiratory protection and fit-testing, yet adequate data to support this recommendation were still not available. After reviewing the extensive public criticism (comprising 2700 responses) to those revised guidelines, the CDC and NIOSH agreed to accept the use of disposable personal particulate respirators that met the less-stringent specifications of 95% efficiency at filtering 1-μm particles (N95 classification). Fit-testing was still recommended to ensure that the appropriate-size mask works properly in at least 90% of individuals at risk for exposure.[148] The Occupational Safety and Health Administration (OSHA) were left to develop and enforce regulations. Initially hospitals were required to conform to the 1987 OSHA Respiratory Protection Standard, which required initial fit-testing but not annual testing. In 1998 OSHA revised the Respiratory Protection Standard (29 CFR 110.134) to require initial and annual fit-testing but excluded TB until December 30, 2003. Subsequently, the threat of OSHA enforcement has driven the maintenance of the Respiratory Protection Standard for tuberculosis.

Several classic studies have demonstrated that administrative and environmental portions of infection control plans most successfully arrest nosocomial transmission. For example, a study by Wenger et al.[152] demonstrated that strict implementation of the least stringent 1990 CDC tuberculosis control guidelines substantially reduced transmission of MDRTB to HCWs and among HIV-positive inpatients. However, multiple factors were tested simultaneously, making it difficult to determine which component of the infection control practices was most essential. Blumberg et al.[153] evaluated a broad upgrade of administrative controls, engineering controls, and respiratory protection. The administrative controls specifically were an expanded isolation policy mandating discharge from isolation only after three sputa were acid-fast bacilli smear negative, an expanded infection control department, increased HCW education, and more frequent TST screening of workers at risk for TB exposure. The engineering controls included simply introducing negative-pressure ventilation via a window fan installation in isolation rooms so that air was vented directly to the outdoors. For respiratory protection, the hospital switched to a disposable personal particulate respirator from the standard surgical mask. The result of these changes was a significant reduction in nosocomial transmission. Maloney et al.[146] demonstrated that the combination of early isolation and treatment of patients with tuberculosis, the use of techniques which more rapidly identify *M. tuberculosis* in specimens, configuration of isolation rooms with negative-pressure ventilation, and provision of molded surgical masks for HCWs greatly reduced transmission within the hospital studied. Taken together these studies confirm that stricter adherence to standard infection control measures greatly reduce nosocomial transmission of tuberculosis, but do not provide data to evaluate the impact of individual control measures. Subsequent surveys of hospital TB control plans instituted in the 1990s show that TST conversion rates fell or remained low more as a result of administrative and environmental controls than respiratory protection.[154–157] These results and the lack of data for added protection produced by expensive high-filtration respirators and fit-testing continues to fuel debate.

Tuberculosis in Correctional Institutions. Globally, prisons represent a considerable incubator for tuberculosis as more than 10 million persons are incarcerated.[125] In the United States as a result of criminalization of illicit drug use, the number of people incarcerated increased from about 500,000 in 1980 to more than 2 million in 2004, and currently comprises 1% of the adult population, the highest rate in the world.[158,159] People at high risk for tuberculosis are more prevalent within prison populations: those who were homeless, within low income, racial/ethnic groups, those with HIV infection as well as PWID.[159,160]

Worldwide, the average incidence of tuberculosis has been estimated at 23 times that of the general population, plus the prevalence of MDRTB is much higher.[161,162] Chronic overcrowding, inadequate ventilation, delays in diagnosis, lack of access to effective treatment, and inability to isolate active cases make correctional institutions around the world as well as within the United States, ideal for transmission of tuberculosis among inmates, plus to the correctional workers. Further, evidence indicates that prisoners released into the communities extend transmission.[159] Recidivism is high and the transitions in and out of prison interrupts LTBI and active TB treatment, which exacerbates drug-resistant TB as well as disease transmission.[160]

The high rate of HIV coinfection is a particularly potent multiplier that is not fully appreciated because studies of tuberculosis and coinfection with HIV among prison populations remain scarce. The data that are available indicate that problems, which promote the spread of TB exist. They include segregation of HIV prisoners from the rest of the population, ART inconsistently provided despite the UN's Mandela Rules requiring prisoner healthcare be equal to community standards, and in some US prisons, Hispanic prisoners may be tested for HIV and TB less frequently than white prisoners.[159,160]

All of these factors taken together contribute to the excessive rate of tuberculosis among individuals housed in correctional institutions. The magnitude remains to be fully determined. This may enable more comprehensive treatment and control.

Tuberculosis in Persons Who Inject Drugs. PWID have a higher incidence of tuberculosis than does the general population in areas of the United States where tuberculosis is prevalent.[163] Higher rates of HIV coinfection within the PWID population increase the risk of a tuberculosis infection and the development of active disease in this population. The data are somewhat conflicting regarding whether drug use in absence of coinfection with HIV is an independent risk factor for tuberculosis.[164,165] Data suggest that non-HIV–infected PWID may exhibit lower levels of cellular immunity, and the TST has been reported as less reliable in this population.[166]

Other risk factors for tuberculosis are prevalent among populations of PWID. PWID as well as those who abuse alcohol have a poor record adherence to tuberculosis therapy.[167] They frequent similar locales, so they are more likely to transmit to others within the cohort. They are a mobile population that is difficult to retain in tuberculosis treatment programs. Thus, they are also at higher risk for acquired drug resistance because they may elope before completing therapy or take therapy on an irregular basis.

Tuberculosis in the Elderly. Analogous to that in the foreign-born population, the majority of tuberculosis cases in the elderly population are a result of activation of a prior infection, and only approximately 10–20% of active cases are due to primary infection.[168,169] Into the 1930s, approximately 80% of the US population was infected by tuberculosis once they reached the age of 30. In a study from 1987, of 43,000 nursing home residents from Arkansas, it was found that the rate of positive TST was 13.2%.[170]

Pulmonary infection occurs in 75% of active cases in the elderly in contrast to 85% of a younger cohort.[168] A higher proportion of elderly patients present with disseminated tuberculosis, tuberculous meningitis, and skeletal tuberculosis. Signs can be nonspecific and the TST (or IGRA) may be nonreactive.[171] Active tuberculosis in the elderly has a greater probability of going undiagnosed for an extended period of time, with the increased risk of transmission to other individuals.

Transmission of Tuberculosis during Airline Flights. The risk of *M. tuberculosis* transmission to other passengers during airline flight is not greater than in any other confined spaces. Several studies have shown that passengers with documented cavitary pulmonary disease did not infect other passengers.[172,173] These data may have been confounded by the fact that the investigations were initiated many weeks to months following the flight, which limited successful contact tracing and the effectiveness of the tuberculosis skin test to detect conversions.

Airplane ambient air is relatively sterile.[174,175] The fresh air is compressed and passed through the jet engines, where it is heated to 250°C and then cooled at high pressures (450 pounds per square inch). Since the 1980s, however, airplanes have not used 100% fresh air circulation. About 50% of the air is recirculated. The air is introduced as vertical laminar sheets from the top of the cabin to the floor and is recirculated every 3–4 minutes. This is more frequent than the standard of 5–12 minutes that is seen in offices and homes. In newer airplanes, the recirculated air passes across a HEPA filtration unit. Investigators have shown that the usual bacteria contamination of airplane air is less than 100 colony-forming units (CFUs) per 160 L, which is significantly less than the approximately 1000 CFUs per 160 L found in city buses, shopping malls, or even airline terminals. These data suggest that transmission risk may be lower within airplanes.

The CDC identifies three critical factors necessary to increase the probability that others may be infected during flight.[172,176] Clear-cut evidence of infectiousness at the time of the flight (e.g., cavitary disease, laryngeal TB, evidence of household transmission prior to flight), prolonged flight time (probably exceeding 8 hours), and proximity to the active case (risk is measurable within 15 rows of the active case).

BOVINE TUBERCULOSIS

M. bovis, the species from which the BCG vaccine is derived, is a member of *M. tuberculosis* complex, and like *M. tuberculosis* causes communicable disease. *M. bovis* causes primary and reactivation infection, as well as both pulmonary and extrapulmonary disease. Bovine tuberculosis is clinically and radiologically indistinguishable from cases caused by *M. tuberculosis*, and the standard AFB smear, culture identification, and molecular testing (i.e., Gene Xpert) cannot distinguish *M. bovis* from *M. tuberculosis*.[177] DNA from *M. bovis* is almost 100% homologous to DNA from *M. tuberculosis*. Distinguishing one from the other requires the capacity to combine genomic data with biochemical testing, which is available only in specialized laboratories such as the NTGS laboratory in the United States.[63] However, *M. bovis* isolates almost always demonstrate monoresistance to pyrazinamide, which should raise suspicion for *M. bovis* rather than *M. tuberculosis* infection.[178]

Bovine tuberculosis commonly results from livestock (usually a cow)-to-human transmission. *M. bovis* remains endemic in beef and dairy cattle herds in many regions of Mexico, and Central America, for example. Cervical adenitis due to *M. bovis* occurs more often in children and usually results from the ingestion of unpasteurized milk from contaminated cows. In general, a higher proportion of extrapulmonary infections are found among bovine tuberculosis cases due to ingestion of unpasteurized dairy products. Besides animal to human, human-to-human aerosol transmission occurs also.[177] In 2017, the WHO estimated there were 142,000 new cases and 12,500 deaths due to *M. bovis*.[125] These data likely underestimate the true number since the areas where bovine tuberculosis should be more common lack sufficient molecular and laboratory technology, even susceptibility testing to detect pyrazinamide monoresistance. When efforts to segregate out *M. bovis* are made, such as in Mexico City from 2000 to 2014, 19% of pulmonary and 26% of all isolates were found to be *M. bovis* among 1100 tuberculosis isolates.[179] Southern California may have a higher prevalence due to its geographic proximity and immigration from Mexico. In an older US study, up to 3% of the tuberculosis respiratory isolates in San Diego were reported to be *M. bovis*, and most were from Hispanic adult immigrants.[180] A recent California registry report showed that the problem likely persists, as new bovine tuberculosis cases in 2003 had increased from 3.4% to 5.4% by 2011.[181]

The prognosis for bovine tuberculosis is worse than that for tuberculosis. In Mexico, the mortality has been reported as high as 31%.[182] In the United States, the mortality for *M. bovis* is 9% compared to 5%

for tuberculosis.[183] There are few data to guide treatment and most cases receive isoniazid, rifampin, and ethambutol daily for 2 months, followed by isoniazid and rifampin daily for an additional 7 months.

The problem of bovine tuberculosis can be substantially reduced globally by finding and removing infected cows from the contaminated herds and pasteurizing the milk.

CONCLUSION

Tuberculosis remains a notorious airborne contagious disease, caused by *M. tuberculosis* and primarily produces an insidious, subacute lung infection in humans. Although curable, its more resistant modern iteration persists worldwide and coinfection with HIV facilitates continuing spread. TB still reigns globally as the leading cause of death by infectious disease. Optimistic projections for reducing incidence and mortality 90% or more worldwide by 2035 could be achieved by concerted effort and redoubled resources. Whether the long acknowledged "Captain of the Men of Death" surrenders remains to be seen.

References

1. Dubos R, Dubos J. *The White Plague: Tuberculosis, Man and Society*. New Brunswick, NJ: Rutgers University Press; 1952.
2. Wlodarska M, Johnston JC, Gardy JL, Tang P. A microbiological revolution meets an ancient disease: Improving the management of tuberculosis with genomics. *Clin Microbiol Rev*. 2015;28(2):523–39.
3. Comas I, Coscolla M, Luo T, et al. Out-of-Africa migration and Neolithic coexpansion of *Mycobacterium tuberculosis* with modern humans. *Nat Genet*. 2013;45(10):1176–82.
4. Cole STBR, Parkhill J, Garnier T, et al. Deciphering the biology of *Mycobacterium tuberculosis* from the complete genome sequence. *Nature*. 1998;393(6685):537–44.
5. Papaventsis D, Casali N, Kontsevaya I, Drobniewski F, Cirillo DM, Nikolayevskyy V. Whole genome sequencing of *Mycobacterium tuberculosis* for detection of drug resistance: A systematic review. *Clin Microbiol Infect*. 2017;23(2):61–8.
6. Wayne L, Kubica L. *Genus Mycobacterium*. Vol. 2. Baltimore: Wlliams & Wilkins; 1986.
7. Zhang Y, Heym B, Allen B, Young D, Cole S. The catalase-peroxidase gene and isoniazid resistance of *Mycobacterium tuberculosis*. *Nature*. 1992;358(6387):591–3.
8. Telenti A. Genetics of drug resistant tuberculosis. *Thorax*. 1998;53(9): 793–7.
9. Telenti A, Imboden P, Marchesi F, et al. Detection of rifampicin-resistance mutations in *Mycobacterium tuberculosis*. *Lancet*. 1993;341(8846):647–50.
10. Iseman MD, Madsen LA. Drug-resistant tuberculosis. *Clin Chest Med*. 1989;10(3):341–53.
11. Pearson ML, Jereb JA, Frieden TR, et al. Nosocomial transmission of multidrug-resistant *Mycobacterium tuberculosis*. A risk to patients and health care workers. *Ann Intern Med*. 1992;117(3):191–6.
12. Beck-Sague C, Dooley SW, Hutton MD, et al. Hospital outbreak of multidrug-resistant *Mycobacterium tuberculosis* infections. Factors in transmission to staff and HIV-infected patients. *JAMA*. 1992;268(10):1280–6.
13. Center for Disease Control. Emergence of *Mycobacterium tuberculosis* with extensive resistance to second-line drugs—Worldwide, 2000–2004. *MMWR Morb Mortal Wkly Rep*. 2006;55(11):301–5.
14. Cegielski P, Nunn P, Kurbatova EV, et al. Challenges and controversies in defining totally drug-resistant tuberculosis. *Emerg Infect Dis*. 2012;18(11):e2.
15. Wells W, Ratcliffe H, Crumb C. On the mechanics of droplet nucleii infection. *Am J Hyg*. 1948;47:11–28.
16. Riley R, Mills C, Nyka W, et al. Aerial dissemination of pulmonary tuberculosis. A two year study of contagion in a tuberculsis ward. *Am J Hyg*. 1959;70:185–96.
17. Schlesinger L. *The Role of Mononuclear Phagocytes in Tuberculosis*. New York: Marcel Dekker; 1997.
18. Harmsen AG, Muggenburg BA, Snipes MB, Bice DE. The role of macrophages in particle translocation from lungs to lymph nodes. *Science*. 1985;230(4731):1277–80.
19. Cooper AM, Flynn JL. The protective immune response to *Mycobacterium tuberculosis*. *Curr Opin Immunol*. 1995;7(4):512–6.
20. Menzies D. Interpretation of repeated tuberculin tests. Boosting, conversion, and reversion. *Am J Respir Crit Care Med*. 1999;159(1):15–21.
21. Lewinsohn DM, Leonard MK, LoBue PA, et al. Official American Thoracic Society/Infectious Diseases Society of America/Centers for Disease Control and Prevention Clinical Practice Guidelines: Diagnosis of tuberculosis in adults and children. *Clin Infect Dis*. 2017;64(2):e1–33.
22. Bass JB, Jr., Farer LS, Hopewell PC, et al. Treatment of tuberculosis and tuberculosis infection in adults and children. American Thoracic Society and The Centers for Disease Control and Prevention. *Am J Respir Crit Care Med*. 1994;149(5):1359–74.
23. Horsburgh CR Jr, Rubin EJ. Clinical practice. Latent tuberculosis infection in the United States. *N Engl J Med*. 2011;364(15):1441–8.
24. American Thoracic Society, Centers for Disease Control and Prevention. Control of tuberculosis in the United States. *Am Rev Respir Dis*. 1992;146(6):1623–33.
25. Braden CR. Infectiousness of a university student with laryngeal and cavitary tuberculosis. Investigative team. *Clin Infect Dis*. 1995;21(3):565–70.
26. Reichler MR, Khan A, Sterling TR, et al. Risk and timing of tuberculosis among close contacts of persons with infectious tuberculosis. *J Infect Dis*. 2018;218(6):1000–8.
27. Riley RL, Mills CC, O'Grady F, Sultan LU, Wittstadt F, Shivpuri DN. Infectiousness of air from a tuberculosis ward. Ultraviolet irradiation of infected air: Comparative infectiousness of different patients. *Am Rev Respir Dis*. 1962;85:511–25.
28. O'Shea MK, Koh GC, Munang M, Smith G, Banerjee A, Dedicoat M. Time-to-detection in culture predicts risk of *Mycobacterium tuberculosis* transmission: A cohort study. *Clin Infect Dis*. 2014;59(2):177–85.
29. Liippo KK, Kulmala K, Tala EO. Focusing tuberculosis contact tracing by smear grading of index cases. *Am Rev Respir Dis*. 1993;148(1):235–6.
30. Grzybowski S, Barnett GD, Styblo K. Contacts of cases of active pulmonary tuberculosis. *Bull Int Union Tuberc*. 1975;50(1):90–106.
31. Stead WW. Management of health care workers after inadvertent exposure to tuberculosis: A guide for the use of preventive therapy. *Ann Intern Med*. 1995;122(12):906–12.
32. Bandera A, Gori A, Catozzi L, et al. Molecular epidemiology study of exogenous reinfection in an area with a low incidence of tuberculosis. *J Clin Microbiol*. 2001;39(6):2213–8.
33. van Rie A, Warren R, Richardson M, et al. Exogenous reinfection as a cause of recurrent tuberculosis after curative treatment. *N Engl J Med*. 1999;341:1174–9.
34. Driver CR, Macaraig M, McElroy PD, et al. Which patients' factors predict the rate of growth of *Mycobacterium tuberculosis* clusters in an urban community? *Am J Epidemiol*. 2006;164(1):21–31.
35. Warner DF, Koch A, Mizrahi V. Diversity and disease pathogenesis in *Mycobacterium tuberculosis*. *Trends Microbiol*. 2015;23(1):14–21.
36. Cruz AT, Starke JR. Clinical manifestations of tuberculosis in children. *Paediatr Respir Rev*. 2007;8(2):107–17.
37. Chaisson RE, Slutkin G. Tuberculosis and human immunodeficiency virus infection. *J Infect Dis*. 1989;159(1):96–100.
38. Centers for Disease Control and Prevention. Tuberculosis morbidity—United States, 1992. *MMWR*. 1993;42(36):696–7, 703–4.
39. Jones BE, Young SM, Antoniskis D, Davidson PT, Kramer F, Barnes PF. Relationship of the manifestations of tuberculosis to CD4 cell counts in patients with human immunodeficiency virus infection. *Am Rev Respir Dis*. 1993;148(5):1292–7.
40. Cattamanchi A, Smith R, Steingart KR, et al. Interferon-gamma release assays for the diagnosis of latent tuberculosis infection in HIV-infected individuals: A systematic review and meta-analysis. *J Acquir Immune Defic Syndr*. 2011;56(3):230–8.
41. Yeager H Jr, Lacy J, Smith LR, LeMaistre CA. Quantitative studies of mycobacterial populations in sputum and saliva. *Am Rev Respir Dis*. 1967;95(6):998–1004.
42. Hobby GL, Holman AP, Iseman MD, Jones JM. Enumeration of tubercle bacilli in sputum of patients with pulmonary tuberculosis. *Antimicrob Agents Chemother*. 1973;4(2):94–104.
43. Chakravorty S, Simmons AM, Rowneki M, et al. The new Xpert MTB/RIF ultra: Improving detection of *Mycobacterium tuberculosis* and resistance to rifampin in an assay suitable for point-of-care testing. *mBio*. 2017;8(4):e00812–17.
44. Koch A, Cox H, Mizrahi V. Drug-resistant tuberculosis: Challenges and opportunities for diagnosis and treatment. *Curr Opin Pharmacol*. 2018;42:7–15.
45. Morgan MA, Horstmeier CD, DeYoung DR, Roberts GD. Comparison of a radiometric method (BACTEC) and conventional culture media for recovery of mycobacteria from smear-negative specimens. *J Clin Microbiol*. 1983;18(2):384–8.

46. Steingart KR, Schiller I, Horne DJ, Pai M, Boehme CC, Dendukuri N. Xpert(R) MTB/RIF assay for pulmonary tuberculosis and rifampicin resistance in adults. *Cochrane Database Syst Rev.* 2014;(1):CD009593.
47. Tomasicchio M, Theron G, Pietersen E, et al. The diagnostic accuracy of the MTBDRplus and MTBDRsl assays for drug-resistant TB detection when performed on sputum and culture isolates. *Sci Rep.* 2016;6:17850.
48. Xie YL, Chakravorty S, Armstrong DT, et al. Evaluation of a rapid molecular drug-susceptibility test for tuberculosis. *N Engl J Med.* 2017;377(11):1043–54.
49. Sanchez-Padilla E, Merker M, Beckert P, et al. Detection of drug-resistant tuberculosis by Xpert MTB/RIF in Swaziland. *N Engl J Med.* 2015;372(12):1181–2.
50. Friedrich SO, Rachow A, Saathoff E, et al. Assessment of the sensitivity and specificity of Xpert MTB/RIF assay as an early sputum biomarker of response to tuberculosis treatment. *Lancet Respir Med.* 2013;1(6): 462–70.
51. Consortium CR, the GP, Allix-Beguec C, et al. Prediction of susceptibility to first-line tuberculosis drugs by DNA sequencing. *N Engl J Med.* 2018;379(15):1403–15.
52. Cox H, Mizrahi V. The coming of age of drug-susceptibility testing for tuberculosis. *N Engl J Med.* 2018;379(15):1474–5.
53. Mu XD, Wang GF. Images in clinical medicine. Miliary tuberculosis. *N Engl J Med.* 2010;363(11):1059.
54. American Thoracic Society—CDC. The tuberculin skin test. *Am Rev Respir Dis.* 1981;124:356–63.
55. Centers for Disease Control and Prevention. The role of BCG vaccine in the prevention and control of tuberculosis in the United States. A joint statement by the Advisory Council for the Elimination of Tuberculosis and the Advisory Committee on Immunization Practices. *MMWR Recomm Rep.* 1996;45(RR-4):1–18.
56. Metcalfe JZ, Everett CK, Steingart KR, et al. Interferon-gamma release assays for active pulmonary tuberculosis diagnosis in adults in low- and middle-income countries: Systematic review and meta-analysis. *J Infect Dis.* 2011;204(Suppl 4):S1120–9.
57. Pai M, Zwerling A, Menzies D. Systematic review: T-cell-based assays for the diagnosis of latent tuberculosis infection: An update. *Ann Intern Med.* 2008;149(3):177–84.
58. Menzies D, Pai M, Comstock G. Meta-analysis: New tests for the diagnosis of latent tuberculosis infection: Areas of uncertainty and recommendations for research. *Ann Intern Med.* 2007;146(5):340–54.
59. Zwerling A, Pai M, Michael JS, Christopher DJ. Serial testing using interferon-gamma release assays in nursing students in India. *Eur Respir J.* 2014;44(1):257–60.
60. Dorman SE, Belknap R, Graviss EA, et al. Interferon-gamma release assays and tuberculin skin testing for diagnosis of latent tuberculosis infection in healthcare workers in the United States. *Am J Respir Crit Care Med.* 2014;189(1):77–87.
61. Small PM, Hopewell PC, Singh SP, et al. The epidemiology of tuberculosis in San Francisco. A population-based study using conventional and molecular methods. *N Engl J Med.* 1994;330(24):1703–9.
62. Alland D, Kalkut GE, Moss AR, et al. Transmission of tuberculosis in New York City. An analysis by DNA fingerprinting and conventional epidemiologic methods. *N Engl J Med.* 1994;330(24):1710–6.
63. (CDC) Centers for Disease Control and Prevention. Prioritizing Tuberculosis Genotype Clusters for Further Investigation and Public Health Action. US Department of Health and Human Services. Atlanta, GA; 2017.
64. Gardy JL, Johnston JC, Ho Sui SJ, et al. Whole-genome sequencing and social-network analysis of a tuberculosis outbreak. *N Engl J Med.* 2011;364(8):730–9.
65. Centers for Disease Control and Prevention. Report of verified case of tuberculosis (RVCT) instruction manual. Services USDoHaH. Atlanta, GA; 2009.
66. https://www.cdc.gov/tb/topic/treatment/default.htm. Accessed June 7, 2019.
67. Kahwati LC, Feltner C, Halpern M, et al. Primary care screening and treatment for latent tuberculosis infection in adults: Evidence report and systematic review for the US Preventive Services Task Force. *JAMA.* 2016;316(9):970–83.
68. Nahid P, Dorman SE, Alipanah N, et al. Official American Thoracic Society/Centers for Disease Control and Prevention/Infectious Diseases Society of America Clinical Practice Guidelines: Treatment of drug-susceptible tuberculosis. *Clin Infect Dis.* 2016;63(7):e147–95.
69. Cohn DL, Catlin BJ, Peterson KL, Judson FN, Sbarbaro JA. A 62-dose, 6-month therapy for pulmonary and extrapulmonary tuberculosis. A twice-weekly, directly observed, and cost-effective regimen. *Ann Intern Med.* 1990;112(6):407–15.
70. Centers for Disease Control and Prevention. Controlling tuberculosis in the United States: recommendations from the American Thoracic Society, CDC, and the Infectious Diseases Society of America. *MMWR.* 2005;54(RR-12):1–81.
71. Combs DL, O'Brien RJ, Geiter LJ. USPHS tuberculosis short-course chemotherapy trial 21: Effectiveness, toxicity, and acceptability. The report of final results. *Ann Intern Med.* 1990;112(6):397–406.
72. Brudney K, Dobkin J. Resurgent tuberculosis in New York City. Human immunodeficiency virus, homelessness, and the decline of tuberculosis control programs. *Am Rev Respir Dis.* 1991;144(4):745–9.
73. Sbarbaro JA. Tuberculosis in the 1990s. Epidemiology and therapeutic challenge. *Chest.* 1995;108(Suppl 2):58S–62S.
74. Sumartojo E. When tuberculosis treatment fails. A social behavioral account of patient adherence. *Am Rev Respir Dis.* 1993;147(5):1311–20.
75. Weis SE, Slocum PC, Blais FX, et al. The effect of directly observed therapy on the rates of drug resistance and relapse in tuberculosis. *N Engl J Med.* 1994;330(17):1179–84.
76. Schluger N, Ciotoli C, Cohen D, Johnson H, Rom WN. Comprehensive tuberculosis control for patients at high risk for noncompliance. *Am J Respir Crit Care Med.* 1995;151(5):1486–90.
77. Ferebee SH, Mount FW. Tuberculosis morbidity in a controlled trial of the prophylactic use of isoniazid among household contacts. *Am Rev Respir Dis.* 1962;85:490–510.
78. Sterling TR, Villarino ME, Borisov AS, et al. Three months of rifapentine and isoniazid for latent tuberculosis infection. *N Engl J Med.* 2011;365(23):2155–66.
79. Menzies D, Adjobimey M, Ruslami R, et al. Four months of rifampin or nine months of isoniazid for latent tuberculosis in adults. *N Engl J Med.* 2018;379(5):440–53.
80. American Thoracic Society, Centers for Disease Control and Prevention. Targeted tuberculin testing and treatment of latent tuberculosis infection. *Am J Respir Crit Care Med.* 2000;161(4):S221–47.
81. Marks SM, Mase SR, Morris SB. Systematic review, meta-analysis, and cost-effectiveness of treatment of latent tuberculosis to reduce progression to multidrug-resistant tuberculosis. *Clin Infect Dis.* 2017;64(12):1670–77.
82. Markowitz N, Hansen NI, Hopewell PC, et al. Incidence of tuberculosis in the United States among HIV-infected persons. The pulmonary complications of HIV infection study group. *Ann Intern Med.* 1997;126(2):123–32.
83. Foster S, Godfrey-Faussett P, Porter J. Modelling the economic benefits of tuberculosis preventive therapy for people with HIV: The example of Zambia. *AIDS.* 1997;11(7):919–25.
84. Horsburgh C. Priorities for the treatment of latent tuberculosis infection in the United States. *N Engl J Med.* 2004;350(20):2060–7.
85. Nolan CMGS, Buskin SE.. Hepatotoxicity associated with isoniazid preventive therapy: A 7-year survey from a public health tuberculosis clinic. *JAMA.* 1999;281(11):1014–18.
86. Stagg HR, Zenner D, Harris RJ, Munoz L, Lipman MC, Abubakar I. Treatment of latent tuberculosis infection: A network meta-analysis. *Ann Intern Med.* 2014;161(6):419–28.
87. Colditz GA, Brewer TF, Berkey CS, et al. Efficacy of BCG vaccine in the prevention of tuberculosis. Meta-analysis of the published literature. *JAMA.* 1994;271(9):698–702.
88. Rodrigues LC, Diwan VK, Wheeler JG. Protective effect of BCG against tuberculous meningitis and miliary tuberculosis: A meta-analysis. *Int J Epidemiol.* 1993;22(6):1154–8.
89. Aronson NE SM, Comstock GW, Howard RS, Moulton LH, Rhoades ER, Harrison LH. Long-term efficacy of BCG vaccine in American Indians and Alaska Natives. A 60-year follow-up study. *JAMA.* 2004;291(17):2086–91.
90. Van Der Meeren O, Hatherill M, Nduba V, et al. Phase 2b controlled trial of M72/AS01E vaccine to prevent tuberculosis. *N Engl J Med.* 2018;379(17):1621–34.
91. https://www.who.int/immunization/research/development/tuberculosis/en/. Accessed June 6, 2019.
92. Salo WL, Aufderheide AC, Buikstra J, Holcomb TA. Identification of *Mycobacterium tuberculosis* DNA in a pre-Columbian Peruvian mummy. *Proc Natl Acad Sci U S A.* 1994;91(6):2091–4.
93. Allison M, Medoza P, Pezziea A. Documentation of a case of tuberculosis in pre-Columbian Peruvian America. *Am Rev Respir Dis.* 1972;107:985–91.
94. Bates JH, Stead WW. The history of tuberculosis as a global epidemic. *Med Clin North Am.* 1993;77(6):1205–17.

95. Mostowy SCD, Brinkman J, Aranaz A, Behr MA.. Genomic deletions suggest a phylogeny for the *Mycobacterium tuberculosis* complex. *J Infect Dis*. 2002;186(1):74–80.
96. Brosch RGS, Marmiesse M, Brodin P,et al. A new evolutionary scenario for the *Mycobacterium tuberculosis* complex. *Proc Natl Acad Sci U S A*. 2002;99(6):3684–9.
97. Blower SM, McLean AR, Porco TC, et al. The intrinsic transmission dynamics of tuberculosis epidemics. *Nat Med*. 1995;1(8):815–21.
98. Black FL. Infectious diseases in primitive societies. *Science*. 1975;187(4176):515–18.
99. Pinner M. *Pulmonary Tuberculosis in the Adult: Its Fundamental Aspects*. Springfield, IL: Charles C Thomas; 1945.
100. Centers for Disease Control and Prevention. Expanded tuberculosis surveillance and tuberculosis morbidity—United States, 1993. *MMWR*. 1994;43(20):361–6.
101. Jereb JA, Kelly GD, Dooley SW Jr, Cauthen GM, Snider DE Jr. Tuberculosis morbidity in the United States: Final data, 1990. *MMWR CDC Surveill Summ*. 1991;40(3):23–7.
102. Stewart RJ, Tsang CA, Pratt RH, Price SF, Langer AJ. Tuberculosis—United States, 2017. *MMWR Morb Mortal Wkly Rep*. 2018;67(11): 317–23.
103. Munsiff SS, Alpert PL, Gourevitch MN, Chang CJ, Klein RS. A prospective study of tuberculosis and HIV disease progression. *J Acquir Immune Defic Syndr Hum Retrovirol*. 1998;19(4):361–6.
104. Lopez-Gatell H, Cole SR, Hessol NA, et al. Effect of tuberculosis on the survival of women infected with human immunodeficiency virus. *Am J Epidemiol*. 2007;165(10):1134–42.
105. Daley CL, Small PM, Schecter GF, et al. An outbreak of tuberculosis with accelerated progression among persons infected with the human immunodeficiency virus. An analysis using restriction-fragment-length polymorphisms. *N Engl J Med*. 1992;326(4):231–5.
106. Selwyn PA, Hartel D, Lewis VA, et al. A prospective study of the risk of tuberculosis among intravenous drug users with human immunodeficiency virus infection. *N Engl J Med*. 1989;320(9):545–50.
107. Bloom BR, Murray CJ. Tuberculosis: Commentary on a reemergent killer. *Science*. 1992;257(5073):1055–64.
108. Centers for Disease Control and Prevention. HIV/AIDS Surveillance Report 1992. 1993.
109. Cantwell MF, Snider DE Jr, Cauthen GM, Onorato IM. Epidemiology of tuberculosis in the United States, 1985 through 1992. *JAMA*. 1994;272(7):535–9.
110. Markowitz N, Hansen NI, Wilcosky TC, et al. Tuberculin and anergy testing in HIV-seropositive and HIV-seronegative persons. Pulmonary complications of HIV infection study group. *Ann Intern Med*. 1993;119(3):185–93.
111. Small PM, Shafer RW, Hopewell PC, et al. Exogenous reinfection with multidrug-resistant *Mycobacterium tuberculosis* in patients with advanced HIV infection. *N Engl J Med*. 1993;328(16):1137–44.
112. Centers for Disease Control and Prevention. Reported tuberculosis in the United States. US Department of Health and Human Services; 2004.
113. French MAPP, Stone SF. Immune restoration disease after antiretroviral therapy. *AIDS*. 2004;18(12):1615–27.
114. Peloquin CA, MacPhee AA, Berning SE. Malabsorption of antimycobacterial medications. *N Engl J Med*. 1993;329(15):1122–3.
115. Sandman LSN, Davidow AL, Bonk S. Risk factors for rifampin-monoresistant tuberculosis: A case-control study. *Am J Respir Crit Care Med*. 1999;159(2):468–72.
116. Ben-Dov I, Mason GR. Drug-resistant tuberculosis in a southern California hospital. Trends from 1969 to 1984. *Am Rev Respir Dis*. 1987;135(6):1307–10.
117. Mahmoudi A, Iseman MD. Pitfalls in the care of patients with tuberculosis. Common errors and their association with the acquisition of drug resistance. *JAMA*. 1993;270(1):65–8.
118. Kopanoff DE, Snider DE Jr, Johnson M. Recurrent tuberculosis: Why do patients develop disease again? A United States Public Health Service cooperative survey. *Am J Public Health*. 1988;78(1):30–3.
119. Bloch AB, Cauthen GM, Onorato IM, et al. Nationwide survey of drug-resistant tuberculosis in the United States. *JAMA*. 1994;271(9):665–71.
120. Frieden TR, Sterling T, Pablos-Mendez A, Kilburn JO, Cauthen GM, Dooley SW. The emergence of drug-resistant tuberculosis in New York City. *N Engl J Med*. 1993;328(8):521–6.
121. Frieden TR, Fujiwara PI, Washko RM, Hamburg MA. Tuberculosis in New York City—Turning the tide. *N Engl J Med*. 1995;333(4):229–33.
122. Frieden TRSL, Maw KL, Fujiwara PI, Crawford JT, Nivin B, Sharp V, Hewlett D Jr, Brudney K, Alland D, Kreisworth BN. A multi-institutional outbreak of highly drug-resistant tuberculosis: Epidemiology and clinical outcomes. *JAMA*. 1996;276(15):1229–35.
123. Agerton TBVS, Blinkhorn RJ, Shilkret KL, Reves R, Schluter WW, Gore B, Pozsik CJ, Plikaytis BB, Woodley C, Onorato IM. Spread of strain W, a highly drug-resistant strain of *Mycobacterium tuberculosis*, across the United States. *Clin Infect Dis*. 1999;29(1):85–92.
124. Marks SM, Flood J, Seaworth B, et al. Treatment practices, outcomes, and costs of multidrug-resistant and extensively drug-resistant tuberculosis, United States, 2005–2007. *Emerg Infect Dis*. 2014;20(5):812–21.
125. World Health Organization. Global Tuberculosis Report 2018. World Health Organization. https://www.who.int/tb/publications/global_report/en/. Published 2018. Accessed January 9, 2019.
126. Maher D, Raviglione M. Global epidemiology of tuberculosis. *Clin Chest Med*. 2005;26(2):167–82.
127. https://www.who.int/tb/joint-initiative/en/. Accessed January 20, 2019.
128. Zignol M, Dean AS, Falzon D, et al. Twenty years of global surveillance of antituberculosis-drug resistance. *N Engl J Med*. 2016;375(11):1081–9.
129. World Health Organization. WHO Tuberculosis Programme: Framework for Effective Tuberculosis Control. Geneva: World Health Organization. 1994;94(179): p.13.
130. World Health Organization. *Global Tuberculosis Control: Surveillance, Planning, Financing: WHO Report 2006*. Geneva: World Health Organization; March 2006.
131. https://www.who.int/tb/strategy/en/. Accessed January 18, 2019.
132. McKenna MT, McCray E, Onorato I. The epidemiology of tuberculosis among foreign-born persons in the United States, 1986 to 1993. *N Engl J Med*. 1995;332(16):1071–6.
133. Zuber PLMM, Binkin NJ, Onorato IM, Castro KG. Long-term risk of tuberculosis among foreign-born persons in the United States. *JAMA*. 1997;278(4):304–7.
134. Styblo K. Overview and epidemiologic assessment of the current global tuberculosis situation with an emphasis on control in developing countries. *Rev Infect Dis*. 1989;11(Suppl 2):S339–46.
135. Raviglione MC, Snider DE Jr, Kochi A. Global epidemiology of tuberculosis. Morbidity and mortality of a worldwide epidemic. *JAMA*. 1995;273(3):220–6.
136. Kantor HS, Poblete R, Pusateri SL. Nosocomial transmission of tuberculosis from unsuspected disease. *Am J Med*. 1988;84(5):833–8.
137. Schwartzman K, Loo V, Pasztor J, Menzies D. Tuberculosis infection among health care workers in Montreal. *Am J Respir Crit Care Med*. 1996;154(4 Pt 1):1006–12.
138. Hutton MD, Stead WW, Cauthen GM, Bloch AB, Ewing WM. Nosocomial transmission of tuberculosis associated with a draining abscess. *J Infect Dis*. 1990;161(2):286–95.
139. Morris L. Tuberculosis as an occupational hazard during medical training. *Am Rev Tuberculosis*. 1946;54:140–57.
140. Reid D. Incidence of tuberculosis among workers in medical laboratories. *Br Med J*. 1957;2:10–4.
141. Templeton GL, Illing LA, Young L, Cave D, Stead WW, Bates JH. The risk for transmission of *Mycobacterium tuberculosis* at the bedside and during autopsy. *Ann Intern Med*. 1995;122(12):922–5.
142. Bates M, Mudenda V, Shibemba A, et al. Burden of tuberculosis at post mortem in inpatients at a tertiary referral centre in sub-Saharan Africa: A prospective descriptive autopsy study. *Lancet Infect Dis*. 2015;15(5):544–51.
143. Centers for Disease Control and Prevention. Transmission of Multidrug-resistant tuberculosis among HIV-infected persons—Florida and New York, 1988–1991. *MMWR*. 1991;40(34):585–91.
144. Edlin BR, Tokars JI, Grieco MH, et al. An outbreak of multidrug-resistant tuberculosis among hospitalized patients with the acquired immunodeficiency syndrome. *N Engl J Med*. 1992;326(23):1514–21.
145. Valway SE, Richards SB, Kovacovich J, Greifinger RB, Crawford JT, Dooley SW. Outbreak of multi-drug-resistant tuberculosis in a New York State prison, 1991. *Am J Epidemiol*. 1994;140(2):113–22.
146. Maloney SA, Pearson ML, Gordon MT, Del Castillo R, Boyle JF, Jarvis WR. Efficacy of control measures in preventing nosocomial transmission of multidrug-resistant tuberculosis to patients and health care workers. *Ann Intern Med*. 1995;122(2):90–5.
147. Jarvis WR, Bolyard EA, Bozzi CJ, et al. Respirators, recommendations, and regulations: The controversy surrounding protection of health care workers from tuberculosis. *Ann Intern Med*. 1995;122(2):142–6.

148. Centers for Disease Control and Prevention. Guidelines for preventing the transmission of *Mycobacterium tuberculosis* in health-care facilities, 1994. *MMWR Recomm Rep.* 1994;43(RR-13):1–132.

149. Centers for Disease Control and Prevention. Guidelines for preventing the transmission of *Mycobacterium tuberculosis* in health-care settings, 2005. *MMWR Morb Mortal Wkly Rep.* 2005;54(RR-17):1–140.

150. https://www.cdc.gov/tb/topic/testing/healthcareworkers.htm. Accessed June 9, 2019.

151. Sosa LE, Njie GJ, Lobato MN, et al. Tuberculosis screening, testing, and treatment of U.S. health care personnel: Recommendations from the National Tuberculosis Controllers Association and CDC, 2019. *MMWR Morb Mortal Wkly Rep.* 2019;68(19):439–43.

152. Wenger PN, Otten J, Breeden A, Orfas D, Beck-Sague CM, Jarvis WR. Control of nosocomial transmission of multidrug-resistant *Mycobacterium tuberculosis* among healthcare workers and HIV-infected patients. *Lancet.* 1995;345(8944):235–40.

153. Blumberg HM, Watkins DL, Berschling JD, et al. Preventing the nosocomial transmission of tuberculosis. *Ann Intern Med.* 1995;122(9):658–63.

154. Bangsberg DRCK, Moss A, Dobkin JF, McGregor C, Neu HC. Reduction in tuberculin skin-test conversions among medical house staff associated with improved tuberculosis infection control practices. *Infect Control Hosp Epidemiol.* 1997;18(8):566–70.

155. Fella PRP, Hale M, Squires K, Sepkowitz K. Dramatic decrease in tuberculin skin test conversion rate among employees at a hospital in New York City. *Am J Infect Control.* 1995;23(6):1995.

156. Jernigan JAAK, Anglim AM, Byers KE, Farr BM. *Mycobacterium tuberculosis* transmission rates in a sanatorium: Implications for new preventive guidelines. *Am J Infect Control.* 1994;22(6):329–33.

157. Fridkin SKML, Bolyard E, Jarvis WR. SHEA-CDC TB survey, Part II: Efficacy of TB infection control programs at member hospitals, 1992. Society for Healthcare Epidemiology of America. *Infect Control Hosp Epidemiol.* 1995;16(3):135–40.

158. The number of adults in the correctional population has been increasing. U.S. Department of Justice, Office of Justice Programs; 2004. http://www.ojp.usdoj.gov/bjs/glance/corr2.htm. Accessed January 2006.

159. Dolan K, Wirtz AL, Moazen B, et al. Global burden of HIV, viral hepatitis, and tuberculosis in prisoners and detainees. *Lancet.* 2016;388(10049):1089–102.

160. Edge CL, King EJ, Dolan K, McKee M. Prisoners co-infected with tuberculosis and HIV: A systematic review. *J Int AIDS Soc.* 2016;19(1):20960.

161. Baussano I, Williams BG, Nunn P, Beggiato M, Fedeli U, Scano F. Tuberculosis incidence in prisons: A systematic review. *PLoS Med.* 2010;7(12):e1000381.

162. Ndeffo-Mbah ML, Vigliotti VS, Skrip LA, Dolan K, Galvani AP. Dynamic models of infectious disease transmission in prisons and the general population. *Epidemiol Rev.* 2018;40(1):40–57.

163. Perlman DC, Salomon N, Perkins MP, Yancovitz S, Paone D, Des Jarlais DC. Tuberculosis in drug users. *Clin Infect Dis.* 1995;21(5):1253–64.

164. Reichman LB, Felton CP, Edsall JR. Drug dependence, a possible new risk factor for tuberculosis disease. *Arch Intern Med.* 1979;139(3):337–9.

165. Friedman LN, Sullivan GM, Bevilaqua RP, Loscos R. Tuberculosis screening in alcoholics and drug addicts. *Am Rev Respir Dis.* 1987;136(5):1188–92.

166. Graham NM, Nelson KE, Solomon L, et al. Prevalence of tuberculin positivity and skin test anergy in HIV-1-seropositive and -seronegative intravenous drug users. *JAMA.* 1992;267(3):369–73.

167. Nazar-Stewart V, Nolan CM. Results of a directly observed intermittent isoniazid preventive therapy program in a shelter for homeless men. *Am Rev Respir Dis.* 1992;146(1):57–60.

168. Stead WW, Dutt AK. Tuberculosis in elderly persons. *Annu Rev Med.* 1991;42:267–76.

169. Stead WW, Lofgren JP, Warren E, Thomas C. Tuberculosis as an endemic and nosocomial infection among the elderly in nursing homes. *N Engl J Med.* 1985;312(23):1483–7.

170. Stead WW, To T. The significance of the tuberculin skin test in elderly persons. *Ann Intern Med.* 1987;107(6):837–42.

171. Battershill JH. Cutaneous testing in the elderly patient with tuberculosis. *Chest.* 1980;77(2):188–9.

172. Centers for Disease Control and Prevention. Exposure of passengers and flight crew to *Mycobaterium tuberculosis* on commercial aircraft, 1992–1995. *MMWR.* 1995;44(08):137–40.

173. McFarland JW, Hickman C, Osterholm M, MacDonald KL. Exposure to *Mycobacterium tuberculosis* during air travel. *Lancet.* 1993;342(8863):112–3.

174. Wick RL Jr, Irvine LA. The microbiological composition of airliner cabin air. *Aviat Space Environ Med.* 1995;66(3):220–4.

175. Wenzel RP. Airline travel and infection. *N Engl J Med.* 1996;334(15):981–2.

176. Kenyon TA, Valway SE, Ihle WW, Onorato IM, Castro KG. Transmission of multidrug-resistant *Mycobacterium tuberculosis* during a long airplane flight. *N Engl J Med.* 1996;334(15):933–8.

177. Scott C, Cavanaugh JS, Pratt R, Silk BJ, LoBue P, Moonan PK. Human tuberculosis caused by *Mycobacterium bovis* in the United States, 2006–2013. *Clin Infect Dis.* 2016;63(5):594–601.

178. Hlavsa MC, Moonan PK, Cowan LS, et al. Human tuberculosis due to *Mycobacterium bovis* in the United States, 1995–2005. *Clin Infect Dis.* 2008;47(2):168–75.

179. Bobadilla-del Valle M, Torres-Gonzalez P, Cervera-Hernandez ME, et al. Trends of *Mycobacterium bovis* isolation and first-line anti-tuberculosis drug susceptibility profile: A fifteen-year laboratory-based surveillance. *PLoS Negl Trop Dis.* 2015;9(9):e0004124.

180. Dankner WM, Waecker NJ, Essey MA, Moser K, Thompson M, Davis CE. *Mycobacterium bovis* infections in San Diego: A clinicoepidemiologic study of 73 patients and a historical review of a forgotten pathogen. *Medicine (Baltimore).* 1993;72(1):11–37.

181. Gallivan M, Shah N, Flood J. Epidemiology of human *Mycobacterium bovis* disease, California, USA, 2003–2011. *Emerg Infect Dis.* 2015;21(3):435–43.

182. Portillo-Gomez L, Sosa-Iglesias EG. Molecular identification of *Mycobacterium bovis* and the importance of zoonotic tuberculosis in Mexican patients. *Int J Tuberc Lung Dis.* 2011;15(10):1409–14.

183. Scott C, Cavanaugh JS, Silk BJ, et al. Comparison of Sputum-culture conversion for *Mycobacterium bovis* and *M. tuberculosis*. *Emerg Infect Dis.* 2017;23(3):456–62.

CHAPTER 89

Malaria

S. Patrick Kachur

INTRODUCTION

Malaria is an ancient disease that continues to exact a toll on human health and livelihood. In 2017, the World Health Organization (WHO) estimates that malaria was responsible for 219,000,000 [uncertainty interval: 203–262 million] clinical cases and 435,000 deaths worldwide.[1] While potentially disabling or fatal, it is also largely preventable and treatable. Malaria remains an important health concern both in those countries where it is transmitted regularly as well as in those that experience imported cases or that may be susceptible to reintroduction. An extremely complex condition, malaria manifests differently in different individuals and different parts of the world depending on a range of considerations: parasite species, insect vectors, antimalarial and insecticide susceptibility, climate and environmental conditions, health systems factors, and the genetic composition, acquired immunity, and behavior of the human population. Children, pregnant women, and nonimmune visitors to malarious areas are at greatest risk of severe or fatal infections. Multiple public health interventions can combat malaria by targeting the parasite, vector, environment, and human host. No one intervention is completely effective. The optimal combination of intervention strategies should carefully consider local context. In recent years, substantial progress toward reducing the global burden of malaria has been achieved through committed efforts of endemic countries and their development partners. An international effort to eradicate malaria in the mid-twentieth century was suspended in 1969 after mixed progress. Since 2001, global attention and commitment have revitalized enthusiasm and encouraged reinvigorated calls to eliminate this ancient public health menace. Continued progress demands sustained attention to proven interventions and investments in promising new tools.

BURDEN AND DISTRIBUTION

Malaria is a mosquito-borne illness caused by a protozoan parasite. Thirty-six percent of the global population lives in areas where there is risk of malaria transmission.[2] Each year, more than 200 million clinical cases of malaria and 400,000 malaria deaths occur, making it one of the most prevalent infectious diseases. Malaria can be a devastating disease with high morbidity and mortality, demanding a rapid and comprehensive response. In other settings, it can be a more pernicious public health threat. In many malarious areas of the world, especially sub-Saharan Africa, malaria is ranked among the most frequent causes of morbidity and mortality among children and is often the leading identifiable cause. WHO estimates that more than 60% of the deaths attributed to malaria each year occur in African children.[1] Estimates of global burden are necessary because few of the most intensely malaria-endemic countries can report accurate health data. There have been recent calls to improve the quality of reported morbidity and mortality data. Advances in diagnostic and information technology are rapidly making this feasible. In addition to its morbidity and mortality burden, the economic effects of malaria infection can be tremendous. These include direct costs for treatment and prevention, as well as indirect costs such as lost productivity from morbidity and mortality, time spent seeking treatment and diversion of household resources. This heavy toll can hinder economic and community development. Global malaria partners have estimated that aggressively reducing the malaria burden over the next two decades could avert 3 billion illnesses, save 10 million lives and generate trillions of dollars in additional economic output. At US$ 5–8 per case averted, currently recommended malaria interventions are highly cost effective and malaria prevention and treatment could produce a return on investment of as much as US$ 40 for each dollar spent.[2,3] This represents one of the best global health investments available, exceeded only by childhood immunization.

Malaria transmission occurs primarily in tropical and subtropical regions in sub-Saharan Africa, Central and South America, the Caribbean island of Hispaniola, the Middle East, the Indian subcontinent, Southeast Asia, and Oceania. The global distribution of malaria transmission in 2017 is shown in Fig. 89-1. In areas where malaria occurs, however, there is considerable variation in the intensity of transmission and risk of malaria infection, illness, and death. Highland (>1500 meters above sea level) and arid (<1000 mm of rainfall per year) areas typically have little to no ongoing transmission, although they may be prone to epidemic malaria when parasitemic individuals provide a source of infection and conditions are favorable to mosquito and parasite development. The greatest burden of malaria affects remote rural locations where resources to prevent and treat it may be most constrained. Although urban areas have typically been at lower risk, explosive, unplanned population growth has contributed to the growing problem of urban malaria. In addition, vectors that thrive in urban and periurban settings may be particularly difficult to control with tools that have been developed for rural settings.

AGENT AND LIFE CYCLE

Human malaria is caused by one or more of four species of intracellular protozoan parasite. *Plasmodium falciparum*, *P. vivax*, *P. ovale*, and *P. malariae* differ in their geographic distribution, microscopic appearance, clinical features (periodicity of fever, potential for severe or complicated disease, and tendency for relapse or recrudescence), and immunogenic potential. Humans are, almost exclusively, the natural intermediate host for all four. *P. falciparum* and *P. vivax* account for the overwhelming majority of cases. *P. falciparum* is the most common by far and accounts for more than 99% of the malaria burden in Africa. Falciparum malaria may represent the most serious public health threat because of its tendency to produce severe and fatal infections and the global distribution of drug-resistant parasite

Countries with indigenous cases in 2000 and their status by 2017 Countries with zero indigenous cases over at least the past 3 consecutive years are considered to be malaria free. All countries in the WHO European Region reported zero inidigenous cases in 2016 and again in 2017. In 2017, both China and El Salvador reportes zero indigenous cases. *Source: WHO database.*

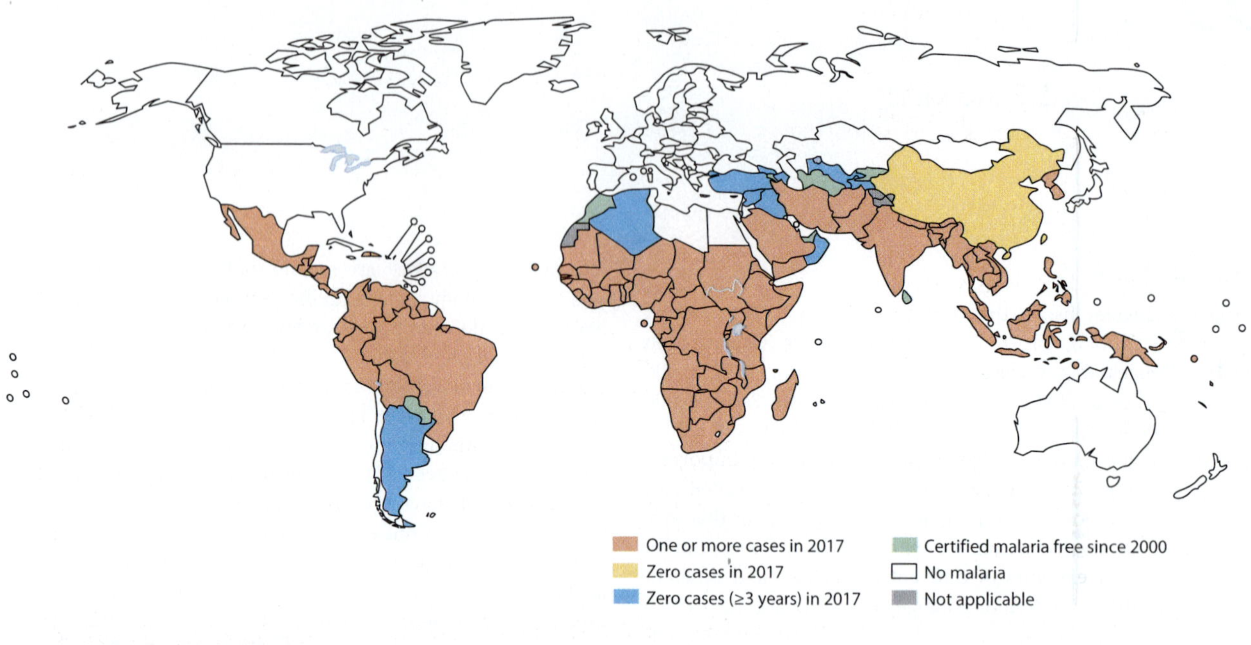

WHO:World Health Organization.

FIGURE 89-1. Global distribution of malaria in 2017.[1] (*Source:* Reprinted with permission of the World Health Organization.)

strains. However, *P. vivax* accounts for 40–75% of malaria cases outside of Africa.[1] Vivax malaria should not be underestimated as a cause of morbidity and mortality and a particular challenge for public health programs given its ability to relapse months or years after initial infection. *P. ovale* and *P. malariae* malaria occur far less frequently but are distributed widely. Like vivax malaria their relapsing and recrudescing potential is an important consideration for prevention and treatment. In recent years, simian malaria parasites, particularly *P. knowlesi* and *P. cynomolgi*, have also been recognized as infecting humans in nature and could represent an additional source of biological complexity for malaria programs, particularly in Asia. At present, it is unclear whether human-to-mosquito-to-human transmission of these parasites can occur without the natural intermediate nonhuman primate host.[4]

Routes of Transmission. Malaria is nearly always transmitted by the bite of an infective female *Anopheles* sp. mosquito. Mosquito-borne cases can be classified as indigenous, imported, or introduced. An **indigenous** case is one contracted locally with no evidence of importation and no direct link to transmission from an imported case. A malaria infection or clinical illness acquired outside the geographic area where it is diagnosed is an **imported** case. An **introduced** case is one contracted locally, with strong epidemiological evidence linking it directly to a known imported case (first-generation local transmission). Although far less common than mosquito-borne transmission, malaria infection can be passed directly from person to person under certain circumstances. **Congenital** malaria refers specifically to infection passed from mother to infant *in utero* or during delivery. An **induced** case occurs when infection occurs via blood transfusion or other form of parenteral inoculation (needle stick, solid organ transplantation, malariotherapy, and controlled human malaria infection) of the parasite.[5] Finally, when a route of transmission cannot be established, even after careful investigation, a case may be classified as **cryptic** malaria.

Life Cycle. Although there are important differences between the infecting species, malaria parasites share a common life cycle, as illustrated in Fig. 89-2.[6] Human infection typically begins when an infective mosquito injects *Plasmodium* sp. sporozoites during a blood meal. The sporozoites circulate in the blood stream only briefly before arriving at the liver and infecting parenchymal cells. They undergo asexual reproduction (exoerythrocytic schizogony) producing hepatic schizonts. In 6–14 days, these schizonts mature and rupture releasing numerous free merozoites into the blood stream. Merozoites then infect individual red blood cells (RBCs) where they develop as trophozoites and undergo a second phase of asexual reproduction (erythrocytic schizogony). Once mature, erythrocytic schizonts rupture releasing still more free merozoites into the blood stream, and another round of RBC infection, development, multiplication, and maturation. Clinical symptoms such as fever are associated with the rupture of erythrocytic schizonts and usually manifest after several erythrocytic cycles. The classical presentation of periodic fever occurs when cycles of erythrocytic schizogony are synchronized. Malaria parasites can continue to proliferate in the RBCs until (a) immune responses limit or eliminate infection, (b) effective antimalarial drugs kill off all the erythrocytic parasites, or (c) the host patient dies from the infection.

Some blood-stage parasites develop along a different pathway and result in the sexual forms—male and female gametocytes. Gametocytes can circulate and mature without contributing to illness symptoms (and unaffected by many antimalarial drugs) until they are ingested by a mosquito during a subsequent blood meal. Sexual reproduction occurs in the mosquito midgut. The fertilized zygote quickly transforms into an amoeboid ookinete which penetrates the

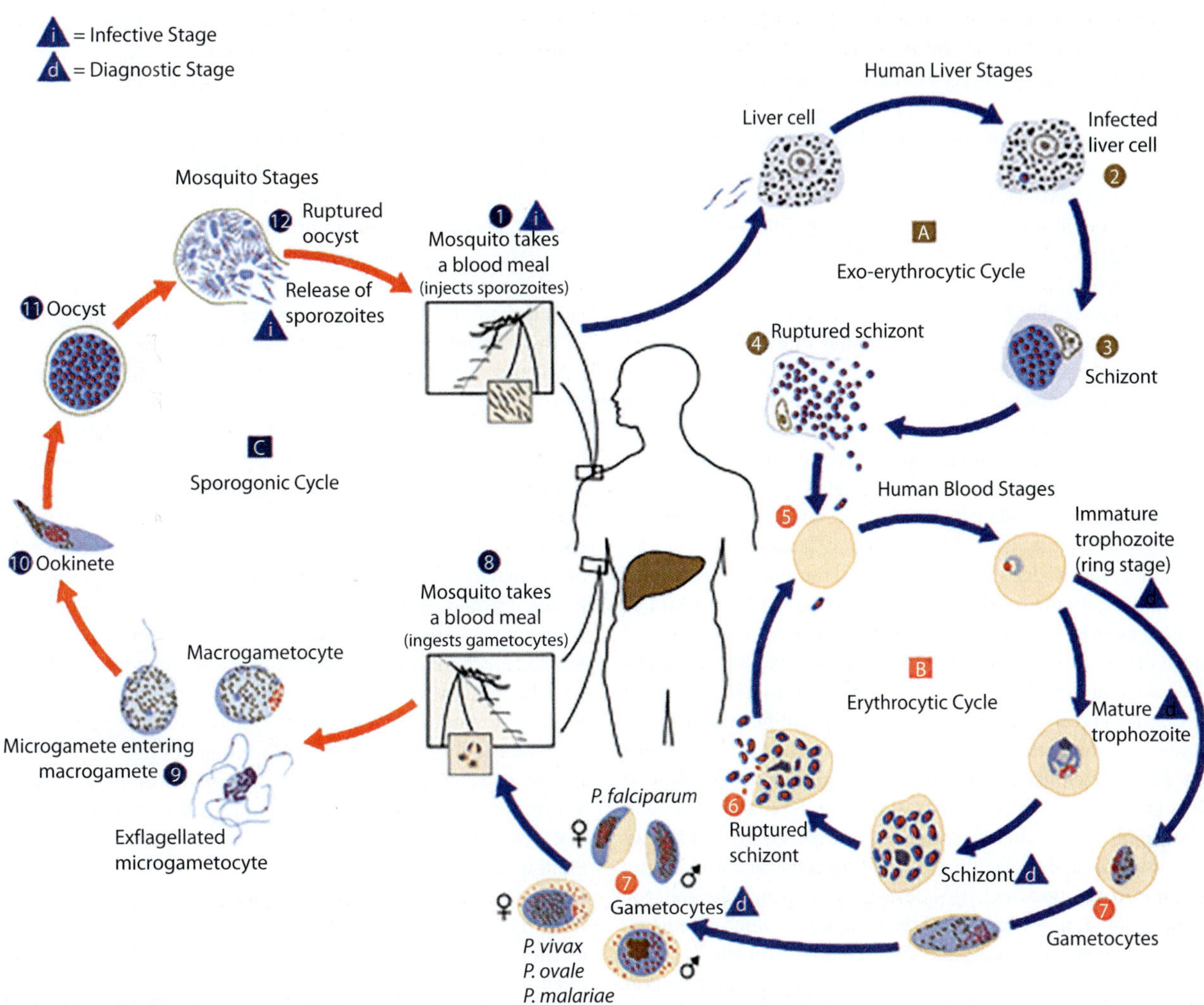

FIGURE 89-2. Life cycle of human malaria parasites.[6]

midgut wall and forms an oocyst. After maturing for several days or weeks, the oocyst ruptures, releasing sporozoites which migrate to the salivary glands. The life cycle is complete and starts anew when the infective mosquito bites another human and injects sporozoites. As the definitive host, the mosquito is essential to the development of the malaria parasite as well as its transmission. The sporogonic cycle—the period of time between ingesting mature gametocytes and becoming infective to humans—varies among the different species of malaria parasites and anopheline vectors and is affected by ambient environmental conditions as well.

The timing of various stages in the life cycle and the number of merozoites produced from each hepatic or erythrocytic schizont differ among the four human malaria parasite species. Additionally, *P. vivax* and *P. ovale* sporozoites can establish a dormant form (hypnozoite) that persists in the liver for months or years, before replicating and causing periodic relapses of parasitemia and illness. Hypnozoites arise only from mosquito-borne infections and are not present following induced or congenital transmission. While *P. falciparum* and *P. malariae* do not form hypnozoites, blood stream infection with these parasites can persist at subpatent levels not associated with clinical symptoms. This very low-level parasitemia can result in recrudescent patent infection and clinical disease later. Except in partially immune persons, *P. falciparum* rarely results in patent or clinical recrudescence more than several weeks following initial infection. However, recrudescent *P. malariae* infection or illness can manifest decades later.

HISTORICAL PERSPECTIVE

More than 150 named species of *Plasmodium* parasites infect a range of vertebrate animals, including closely related nonhuman primates. For decades, it was widely accepted that falciparum malaria parasites evolved alongside humans over millions of years and that vivax malaria arose more recently as humans expanded into Asia and came into close contact with Old World monkeys and the morphologically similar appearing malaria parasites that infect them. However, more recent evidence based on comparative population and genomic studies of naturally occurring malaria parasites in wild populations of great apes strongly suggests that both *P. falciparum* and *P. vivax* transitioned to humans far more recently. Human *P. falciparum* appears to be traceable to a single cross-species transmission event from a gorilla parasite as recently as 10,000 years ago. *P. vivax* malaria most likely evolved from a parasite that infected humans, chimpanzees, and gorillas, alike—also in Africa. But vivax malaria has since been largely driven from the continent by the selection and spread of the Duffy-negative blood group. More information about the origins of *P. ovale* and *P. malariae* may also arise from these studies.[7] Even with this recently revised evolutionary perspective, malaria has been part of the human experience longer than written language. Human activity, particularly settled agriculture, almost certainly facilitated a transformative expansion of both the human and malaria parasite populations. Over this time, malaria has exerted influence on human evolution, selecting for protective blood group (Duffy) and other surface markers, hemoglobin variants (hemoglobins S and C, alpha-thalassemia), and metabolic diversity (G6PD deficiency), as well as a growing number of recognized genes involved in infection and immunity.[8]

Malaria expanded out of Africa with human migration, finding suitable vectors in parts of Europe and Asia. Parasite antigens and genetic sequences have been identified in paleopathologic examination of human remains dating from as far back as 3000 years ago and through the European Renaissance[9]—most notably those of Egypt's King Tutankhamun[10] and several of the Florentine Medici family.[11] In addition, malaria-like illnesses are described in ancient writings from Mesopotamia, India, China, Greece, and Rome. Chinese writings from as far back as 300 years BCE describe the botanical "qinghaosu" or sweet wormwood (*Artemesia annua*) as an effective fever treatment. Some Sanskrit texts associated malarial fever with biting insects. And many Roman writers attributed the disease to the foul atmosphere around swampy areas—giving rise to the name "malaria," for "bad air." For thousands of years malaria influenced patterns of human migration, settlement, civilization, and decline.[12]

It is unlikely that malaria parasites survived the long human migration traversing extreme northern Asia and across the Bering Straits. The Americas may have been malaria-free prior to the arrival of European explorers, colonists, and their African slaves.[13] By the eighteenth century, however, malaria was widespread throughout tropical Latin America and the Caribbean, and had spread far into temperate regions in North and South America. Early in the seventeenth century, Jesuit missionaries learned from indigenous peoples how to use "Peruvian bark" as an effective treatment for fever and eventually brought samples of *Cinchona* sp. back to Europe. By 1820, Pelletier and Caventou isolated the quinine alkaloid from the bark and identified it as the active ingredient. This development opened the door for mass cultivation and production of the compound which ultimately became centered in Indonesia under Dutch colonial control.[14]

Malaria parasites were first observed microscopically in the blood of a febrile soldier by Charles Alphonse Laveran in 1880, who recognized multiple life-cycle stages and attributed the cause of illness to these forms in a series of patients. His observations were confirmed by Camillo Golgi who specifically associated the onset of cyclic fevers with the rupture of blood schizonts and clearly recognized at least two forms of the disease based on the periodicity of cyclic fevers. While studying avian parasites, Ronald Ross discovered pigment-containing cells in mosquitoes that had fed on malaria-infected blood in 1897. Gionvanni Battista Grassi and colleagues confirmed that human malaria parasites could also be transmitted in the same way and specifically identified *Anopheles maculipennis* as a vector of human disease.[12] Ross and Laveran were each recognized with the Nobel Prize in Physiology or Medicine for their contributions to the understanding of malaria. Julius Warner-Juaregg found that deliberately inducing high fevers could be effective at reversing severe psychiatric conditions including "generalized paralysis." After some initial success using various agents to induce fever, he turned to direct inoculation with malaria-infected blood. Malariotherapy—a form of controlled human infection with malaria—actually became a standard treatment for tertiary syphilis in the first half of the twentieth century,[15] and Warner-Juaregg's discovery earned him a Nobel Prize in 1927. Although the erythrocytic stages of the parasite life cycle associated with illness were characterized, it was not until the 1940s that the liver stage parasites were identified.[13]

Accompanying this scientific understanding of the cause and transmission of malaria, the twentieth century also saw the systematic development and deployment of tools to combat it. Mosquito control and personal protection were essential to the completion of the Panama Canal and became a priority for limiting the impact of malaria and other illnesses elsewhere. In many parts of Europe and North America, civil engineering and land use improvements contributed both to disease control and economic development. Although first isolated in 1874, DDT (dichlorodiphenyltrichloroethane) was discovered to have strong insecticidal properties by Paul Hermann Müller in 1939 (earning a Nobel Prize in 1948), and quickly became used for control of typhus, malaria, yellow fever, and insect pests.[16] Large quantities of quinine were essential to European colonial and military enterprises. The search for an alternative to quinine became a strategic priority in World War II, particularly after large scale plantations came under Japanese control. In 1934, Hans Andersag had isolated the compound resorchin, later known as chloroquine. But it was not until after the war that the importance of this compound as an antimalarial treatment was widely recognized and chloroquine became the mainstay of malaria treatment for generations.[17]

Equipped with synthetic insecticides and antimalarial drugs, public health efforts to control and eliminate malaria locally could be undertaken in earnest. In the decade following the war, many of the tools and approaches currently used to diagnose, treat, prevent, and control malaria had been established, and a deeper understanding of the malaria life-cycle-permitted mathematical modeling that suggested it would be possible to interrupt transmission.[18] In the United States, a concerted national effort to eliminate malaria in the southern states where it persisted resulted in the creation of the Centers for Disease Control and Prevention. Accurate diagnostic and surveillance information permitted the targeted and strategic deployment of strategies including flood control, housing improvement, larviciding, indoor residual spraying (IRS), and mass use of antimalarial drugs, which contributed—along with unplanned economic development and population migration—to eliminating transmission by 1951.[19] Similar successes occurred in parts of southern Europe and the Soviet Union, Venezuela, and island nations like Ceylon and Mauritius.[20] In 1955 the World Health Organization adopted a resolution to eradicate malaria. The efforts led to certification of 25 countries and territories as malaria-free by 1987.[21] However, even from the start, it was recognized that eradication depended on the continued efficacy of key tools like chloroquine and DDT. The opportune window to achieve lasting impact would close when resistant parasites and mosquitoes appeared and spread. And they inevitably did. A lack of alternatives and the inflexibility of the paradigm, coupled with flagging international support and dissipating financial and political commitment finally led the international community to suspend its drive for eradication in 1969. A revised global malaria strategy evolved, emphasizing control over elimination, and remained the paradigm until recently. While the twentieth-century eradication effort had enduring impact in places—especially where transmission was exclusively seasonal or relatively low—it achieved little in others, and malaria resurged after the attention waned.[12]

In addition, the mid-century "global" malaria eradication effort never fully took hold across the highest burden settings. Some of the leading voices in the eradication movement at the time, like Paul Russell and George MacDonald, recognized that the available tools would be inadequate in the face of the highly efficient vectors, weak public health infrastructure, and logistical challenges that prevailed across sub-Saharan Africa.[20] Beyond settings where European economic interests prompted larval control or mass quinine administration, little organized malaria control had been implemented in Africa prior to 1945. The broad introduction of chloroquine and focal use of DDT probably contributed to reducing the overall burden of malaria on the continent between 1945 and 1949. Even after the eradication agenda was suspended and progress reversed elsewhere, malaria prevalence slowly declined in Africa between 1960 and 1984. It then reverted to its historically high levels by 2004 as chloroquine resistance intensified and spread. In the years since, expansion of insecticide treated nets and highly efficacious antimalarial treatments have been credited with an unprecedented reduction in malaria risk across

Africa, and it is likely this impact has been boosted by longer-term cyclical changes.[22] As many as 7 million lives have been saved, but this remarkable progress is fragile and may have stalled by 2015.[1]

CLINICAL FEATURES AND PATHOPHYSIOLOGY

Patients with malaria illness can present with a wide range of symptoms and a broad spectrum of severity depending on factors such as the infecting species and level of acquired immunity in the host. In general, partial immunity to malaria is effectively acquired and maintained only after repeated exposure. Individuals who survive multiple malaria infections can tolerate the presence of malaria parasites in their blood with a minimum of symptoms. In areas where malaria transmission is intense, the first exposure often occurs very early in childhood. After many subsequent infections the likelihood of severe illness or death lessens, although infection and illness may still occur. This protection wanes when individuals are no longer exposed to repeated infection, and it can be disrupted by pregnancy, nutritional status, and other conditions including HIV/AIDS.

Clinical Presentation. Symptomatic malaria most commonly manifests as a febrile illness and may appear mild at first. Typical symptoms among nonimmune individuals with malaria include fever, chills, myalgias and arthralgias, headache, diarrhea, vomiting, and other nonspecific complaints. Respiratory symptoms are common in children in high transmission areas. Splenomegaly, anemia, thrombocytopenia, pulmonary or renal dysfunction, and neurological signs can also be present. When synchronous infections (occurring when large numbers of intraerythrocytic schizonts rupture at once) develop, each of the four human malarias can cause a characteristic pattern of periodic fever. Paroxysms of *P. vivax* and *P. ovale* have been described as recurring every 48 hours, while those of *P. malariae* have been characterized by a 72-hour cycle. *P. falciparum* can feature a daily, 48-hour, or irregular periodicity. These classically described presentations with predictably recurring fever and chill cycles can be highly variable and may not occur at all, especially shortly after the onset of illness, when individuals have access to antipyretic or antimalarial medications, or when partial immunity has developed.

Signs and symptoms of malaria can be greatly modified by the patient's immune status; malaria infections among partially immune individuals can range from asymptomatic to severe. Presentation may be atypical or subtle, especially among infants or young children with immature immune systems. Because the manifestations of uncomplicated malaria illness can be so protean and nonspecific, it is a common practice to suspect malaria in all patients with fever living or traveling in endemic areas. Until recently, it was routine in many high burden areas to treat all febrile illness cases for malaria—especially among young children and pregnant women who are at greatest risk for severe or fatal illness. The availability of affordable point-of-care diagnostic testing is transforming this practice. Since 2010, diagnostic confirmation of malaria has been recommended for all demographic groups in all transmission settings and has become a global standard of care.[23] Malaria illness case definitions generally require the presence of clinical symptoms (almost always fever) and laboratory evidence of parasite infection.

Severe or Complicated Malaria. Uncomplicated malaria can progress to severe disease or death within hours. The potential for severe and complicated illness is particularly ominous in patients with high levels of parasitemia and without partial immunity from prior infections. *P. falciparum* is the species most commonly associated with severe and fatal illness and the diagnostic criteria for severe malaria appear in Table 89-1.[24] Organ system failure and death are far less common among nonfalciparum infections—but severe and fatal episodes can occur, especially when there is underlying illness, malnutrition, or coinfection with falciparum malaria. Aside from the risk of splenic rupture in the presence of overwhelming parasitemia, the full range of severe and complicated illness associated with nonfalciparum malaria has long gone underappreciated, but recent evidence, especially for *P. vivax*[25] and *P. knowlesi*[26] confirms that these conditions should not be regarded as universally benign.

TABLE 89-1 FEATURES OF SEVERE MALARIA[24]

- *Impaired consciousness:* A Glasgow coma score < 11 in adults or a Blantyre coma score < 3 in children
- *Prostration: Generalized weakness so that the person is unable to sit, stand, or walk without assistance*
- *Multiple convulsions:* More than two episodes within 24 hours
- *Acidosis:* A base deficit of > 8 mEq/L or, if not available, a plasma bicarbonate level of < 15 mmol/L or venous plasma lactate ≥ 5 mmol/L. Severe acidosis manifests clinically as respiratory distress (rapid, deep, labored breathing)
- *Hypoglycemia: Blood or plasma glucose < 2.2 mmol/L (<40 mg/dL)*
- *Severe malarial anemia:* Hemoglobin concentration ≤ 5 g/dL or a hematocrit of $\leq 15\%$ in children < 12 years of age (<7 g/dL and $< 20\%$, respectively, in adults) with a parasite count $> 10,000/\mu$L
- *Renal impairment:* Plasma or serum creatinine > 265 μmol/L (3 mg/dL) or blood urea > 20 mmol/L
- *Jaundice:* Plasma or serum bilirubin > 50 μmol/L (3 mg/dL) with a parasite count $> 100,000/$ μL
- *Pulmonary edema: Radiologically confirmed or oxygen saturation $< 92\%$ on room air with a respiratory rate > 30/minute, often with chest indrawing and crepitations on auscultation*
- *Significant bleeding:* Including recurrent or prolonged bleeding from the nose, gums, or venipuncture sites; hematemesis or melena
- *Shock:* Compensated shock is defined as capillary refill ≥ 3 seconds or temperature gradient on leg (mid to proximal limb), but no hypotension. Decompensated shock is defined as systolic blood pressure < 70 mm Hg in children or < 80 mm Hg in adults, with evidence of impaired perfusion (cool peripheries or prolonged capillary refill).
- *Hyperparasitemia: P. falciparum* parasitsemia $> 10\%$.

Note: For epidemiological purposes, **severe falciparum malaria** is defined as one or more of the following, occurring in the absence of an identified alternative cause and in the presence of *P. falciparum* asexual parasitemia.

Neurological manifestations are the best known severe malaria presentation in infants, children, and nonimmune adults. Malaria with central nervous system (CNS) involvement can present as fever with subtle mental status changes, and can progress to coma and death rapidly unless aggressively treated. The initial neurological symptoms are often drowsiness, confusion, failure to eat or drink, or repeated convulsions. Cerebral malaria refers to *P. falciparum* malaria with impaired consciousness (Glasgow coma scale < 11, Blantyre coma scale < 3) persisting for more than 30 minutes.[27] Cerebral malaria is almost universally fatal if not treated promptly. Impaired consciousness, metabolic acidosis, and respiratory compromise are particularly grave clinical features associated with higher rates of fatal outcome. In carefully conducted contemporary clinical trials, case fatality ranged from $<10\%$ to $>20\%$, despite state-of-the-art treatment.[28,29] Other acute complications denoting severe disease include renal failure, metabolic acidosis, jaundice, hemolytic anemia, splenic rupture, hypoglycemia, coagulopathy, shock, and pulmonary edema with acute respiratory distress. In patients who survive severe or complicated malaria, long-term sequelae can include permanent cognitive and CNS deficits, or lasting impairment of kidney or liver function.

Not all severe manifestations of malaria present acutely. Persistent, repeated, or inadequately treated infections can cause chronic anemia, especially among infants and young children, or populations with underlying nutritional deficiency. Malaria-related anemia can become severe enough to require transfusion and is an important, often underappreciated, cause of malaria-related severe morbidity and mortality.[30] The rate of development and severity of anemia are affected by the duration of parasitemia and complexity of infection.[31]

Malaria prevention and treatment in high burden areas can have an important role in ameliorating the effects of childhood anemia. Persistent falciparum malaria infection due to repeated and inadequately treated infection can also result in hyperreactive malarial splenomegaly, which is only reversible by adequate antimalarial treatment and removing the risk of reinfection.[32]

In addition, falciparum and vivax malaria can have devastating effects during pregnancy. In nonimmune women, acute malaria during pregnancy can be more likely to progress to severe or complicated illness than malaria in women who are not pregnant, carrying a high risk of poor maternal and fetal outcomes if not treated promptly and adequately. Among partially immune women in endemic areas, however, malaria infection can persist for weeks or months without producing overt clinical illness. Parasites may sequester in the placenta in large numbers, even if they are not visible in peripheral blood films. This placental infection is an important cause of maternal and fetal anemia, intrauterine growth retardation, fetal loss, and low birthweight—the single greatest risk factor for neonatal and infant mortality. In high transmission settings, malaria is most concerning during a woman's first and second pregnancies, although placental infection can occur in all pregnancies, and certain conditions, such as HIV infection, can reduce the protective effect of multigravidity.[33]

Host Factors. As noted, partial immunity acquired through repeated malaria infection can affect the prevalence of malaria infection as well as the clinical presentation and course of an individual illness. Population or community level of immunity to malaria is highest in areas where malaria transmission is most intense. In rural sub-Saharan Africa, where a majority of malaria-associated deaths occur, malaria illness is most common and the highest mortality is seen in children under 5 years of age. In such settings the burden of illness and death shifts to young children and severe malaria manifests more frequently as malaria associated anemia than cerebral disease. Where transmission intensity is lower, community-level immunity develops later, if at all, and illness is seen across all age groups, while cerebral disease and other acute complications are more likely than severe malaria-related anemia.[34] Any condition that disrupts the immune response can affect malaria. In particular, HIV-infected individuals are at higher risk of patent malaria infection and clinical illness. Some HIV care and treatment strategies, however, can afford a measure of protection—such as suppression of opportunistic infections with trimethoprim/sulfamethoxazole. Other host considerations that affect the distribution and clinical impact of malaria infection in humans include biological as well as social and behavioral factors.

Heritable genetic traits can influence host's susceptibility to malaria infections and their likelihood of progressing to severe or fatal malaria. Perhaps the best recognized group of host factors associated with malaria are the hemoglobinopathies. Hemoglobin S, in its homozygous state, causes sickle cell disease, which is universally fatal in childhood without medical intervention. Although both persons with sickle cell disease and heterozygous carriers of the sickle trait can become infected and clinically ill from malaria, heterozygous individuals are afforded 80–95% protection from severe or complicated *P. falciparum*. The high prevalence of falciparum malaria in Africa has perpetuated the Hb S gene. Other hemoglobinopathies, including hemoglobins C and E, the thalassemias, and persistence of fetal hemoglobin have also been associated with some level of protection from severe or complicated malaria. *P. vivax* merozoites invade RBCs by recognizing the Duffy antigen on the surface. Persons who are genetically Duffy-negative, therefore, are less able to sustain vivax infections. As noted, the prevalence of Duffy-negative individuals played an important role in the evolution of vivax malaria and its spread in human populations outside of Africa. Hereditary ovalocytosis, glucose-6-phosphate dehydrogenase deficiency, and human leukocyte antigens of the major histocompatibility complex—have also been associated with mediating the clinical presentation of malaria infection in various settings.[8]

The interaction between malaria and nutritional status is complex and incompletely understood. Some nutritional states may exacerbate the severity of malaria illness, while others appear protective. Data are not always consistent across different studies and settings.[35,36] Earlier studies suggested that iron deficiency may protect some children against malaria infection, and iron supplementation was even linked to increased risk of death. More recent evidence, however, suggests that iron supplements are a valuable intervention for reducing both anemia and clinical malaria,[37] potentially improving child survival and development—and that supplements should not be withheld from children who could benefit as long as regular malaria surveillance, prevention, diagnosis, and treatment services are available. Social and behavioral factors including use of preventive measures, housing construction, education, relative poverty, and ethnomedical beliefs and practices can all affect the risk of infection or influence the clinical presentation and risk of progression to severe disease or fatal outcomes. Among these, the recognition of febrile illness and the household and individual responses that shape access to malaria diagnosis and effective treatment are amenable to malaria treatment and control efforts.

Pathophysiology. The incubation period from infective mosquito bite to onset of symptoms can range from 9 to 30 days, or longer, depending on the species of parasite, host immune status, complexity of infection, and use of drugs with antimalarial activity. The clinical symptoms associated with malaria are caused by a complex interplay between the parasite and the host immune response. Symptoms are associated exclusively with asexual erythrocytic stage parasites; exoerythrocytic forms (sporozoites, exoerythrocytic schizonts, and hypnozoites) and gametocytes do not cause symptoms or pathology. In general, higher levels of parasitemia are associated with clinical symptoms, especially in partially immune populations, and with severe and complicated illness. Larger infecting doses have been associated with shorter prepatent periods. The size of the infecting dose does not appear to correlate consistently with severity of infection, level of parasitemia, number of paroxysms, or likelihood of complications. However, there is evidence that complex infections with greater genetic and antigenic diversity are more likely to elicit symptomatic or severe illness.

Falciparum malaria is more likely than other forms to result in severe or fatal illness based on several features of the parasite. First, exoerythrocytic and erythrocytic schizonts of *P. falciparum* release larger numbers of merozoites when they rupture, resulting in a more rapid rate of increasing parasitemia. *P. falciparum* is also able to infect both mature RBCs and some of their precursor stages. In contrast *P. vivax* and *P. ovale*, which are less commonly associated with complicated illness, selectively infect immature RBCs and reticulocytes. Finally, erythrocytes infected with *P. falciparum* adhere to the vascular endothelium of postcapillary venules or form rosettes *in vitro*; factors that appear to mediate this property—adherence factors—have been characterized and associated with severe or complicated malaria manifestations.[38]

The host response to malaria parasitemia includes both humoral and cellular immune processes and contributes substantially to disease pathogenesis. Several specific mediators have been implicated both for uncomplicated illness and severe disease. Malaria fever appears to arise from cytokines released by host mononuclear cells in response to the rupture of erythrocytic schizonts and release of free merozoites. Tumor necrosis factor alpha has been detected at elevated levels in patients during malarial fever episodes and immediately preceding paroxysms of *P. vivax* infection. Other cytokines that may contribute to febrile episodes include interferon-gamma and interleukins. The occurrence of severe and complicated illness remains unpredictable and incompletely understood. However, it appears that both parasite and host immunologic processes play important roles in each of the major complications. Cerebral malaria is associated with sequestration of infected RBCs in the deep capillaries of the brain where these infected cells demonstrate sludging in the microvasculature, poor deformability, and cytoadherence which contribute to impaired perfusion. The presence of large numbers of sequestered parasites induces further cytokine production and high levels of several of these have been linked to hypoglycemia, hyperparasitemia, and anemia. The coma in cerebral malaria is often mediated through metabolic encephalopathy, resulting in abnormal neurotransmitter synthesis, release, and binding. Cytokine-induced production of nitric oxide is also associated with coma and CNS manifestations. Renal failure from acute tubular necrosis may involve both parasite and host response processes. Malaria-related anemia results from direct effects—destruction of infected RBCs and their removal by the spleen—as well as inhibition of erythropoiesis, autoantibodies to RBC antigens, and immune-mediated removal of uninfected RBCs.[38,39]

DIAGNOSIS AND TREATMENT

Diagnostic Approaches. Malaria should be considered in the differential diagnosis of any patient living in or traveling from endemic areas, as well as those who may have received blood products, tissues, or organs from persons who have been to such areas. Fever alone is unreliably specific, but it can be a sensitive marker for suspected malaria illness. As noted, presumptive clinical diagnosis was once widely recommended in highly endemic settings where laboratory confirmation was unavailable. Attempts to improve the specificity of clinical diagnosis for malaria by considering other signs and symptoms in addition to fever or history of fever have not led to satisfying alternative syndromic algorithms. In some African countries, presumptive treatment of febrile illness with antimalarial drugs had been the only tool for malaria control or prevention and probably averted countless severe illness episodes and deaths, for decades.[22] It is also likely that it led to overuse of antimalarial drugs, may have contributed to poor adherence to complete treatment and selection for drug resistant parasites, and discouraged clinicians from considering other potentially treatable causes of fever.[40] Since 2010, it is recommended that clinical suspicion of malaria be confirmed by laboratory evidence of active blood stage infection.[23] A definitive diagnosis can be made by several approaches including light microscopy, rapid antigen tests, and nucleic acid detection.

Direct microscopic examination of intracellular parasites on stained blood films has long been the standard for definitive diagnosis. Blood slide microscopy has been supplanted as the most common tool for diagnostic confirmation, but it still remains a valuable tool. A skilled microscopist can distinguish the circulating forms of the various species of human malaria, identify mixed infections, quantify the parasite density and burden of infection, and discriminate between clinically important asexual parasites and transmissible gametocyte forms. This can be critical for guiding treatment choice and assessing its efficacy. While several different stains can be used, Giemsa generally gives the best results. Slide collection, staining and reading can be time consuming and microscopists must be trained and supervised carefully to ensure consistent reliability. Even when performed as recommended, microscopic diagnosis does have important limitations. In partially immune persons, asymptomatic parasitemia may be detected which can be of limited clinical significance and may mask another cause of illness. Conversely, particularly in nonimmune persons, symptoms may develop before there are detectable levels of circulating parasites. For this reason, several blood slide examinations are usually required to exclude the diagnosis of malaria. High-quality microscopy services are often not available in remote rural settings where most malaria cases occur, and where they are, microscopists' performance can vary markedly. Logistic, technical and human resource demands often limit malaria microscopy to hospital or referral level health facilities in many endemic country settings.

More recently, rapid diagnostic tests (RDTs) developed for point-of-care settings have transformed malaria diagnosis, precisely where microscopy is most difficult. A number of lateral flow immunochromatographic test platforms and products are now available. The most commonly used ones detect the histidine-rich protein 2 (HRP2), produced by *P. falciparum* parasites. Other diagnostic targets of malaria RDTs include parasite enzymes like aldolase or lactate dehydrogenase—which may be pan-specific across all malaria species or specific to vivax or falciparum parasites. Some products incorporate more than one antigen in a multichannel format. In general, HRP2-based RDTs perform as well as expert microscopy for identifying *P. falciparum* infections associated with clinical illness. RDTs are not useful as a test of cure, since the HRP2 antigen persists for weeks after treatment. Most do not detect very low-density infections that are usually asymptomatic. RDTs targeting other antigens and nonfalciparum parasites are generally less sensitive than *P. falciparum*-specific ones, but improvements are rapidly being made. The scalability and affordability of malaria RDTs—particularly HRP2-based ones—has made it possible to recommend universal parasitological diagnosis as a standard practice for malaria case management everywhere. The exact function of HRP2 is not known, but it does not appear to be essential. Some *P. falciparum* parasites produce large quantities, and others, none at all. Evidence from the Americas, South Asia, and parts of Africa is accumulating to confirm that parasites with genetic deletions, producing no detectable HRP2 (or HRP3), will be undetectable by RDTs with that exclusive target. These can be sufficiently prevalent in some areas, that alternative test kits or microscopy should be recommended to optimize detection of infection and guard against selection of deleted parasite populations. Guidelines for how to monitor the prevalence of HRP deletions and when to rely on alternative diagnostic approaches have been developed.[41] It is likely that RDTs will continue to improve in coming years, incorporating new diagnostic targets and approaches that may extend their utility beyond diagnosing illness, to tracking and helping eliminate transmission.[42]

Nucleic acid detection techniques—including polymerase chain reaction (PCR)—continue to gain prominence as a valuable malaria research tool. Specific primers have been identified for each of the malaria parasite species infecting humans. Some targets can even distinguish the infectious stages. While currently not operationalized for routine clinical diagnosis of malaria illness, an important use of this new technology is in detecting mixed infections or differentiating between infecting species at reference laboratories when microscopic examination is inconclusive. Characterizing parasites at the start of treatment and at the time of recurrent parasitemia is an essential step in recommended therapeutic efficacy studies for antimalarial drug resistance. In addition, specific molecular markers have been associated with phenotypic resistance to chloroquine, amodiaquine, antifolates, lumefantrine, piperaquine, mefloquine, atovaquone, and the artemisinin derivatives. It is impractical to fully characterize the antimalarial drug-resistance potential as part of treatment decisions, but tracking these markers has been informative in understanding the evolution and spread of drug-resistant parasites.[27] PCR techniques can also be valuable for tracing molecular epidemiology in investigations of malaria clusters or epidemics and as a research tool.

Techniques also exist for detecting antimalaria antibodies in serum specimens. Specific serological markers have been identified for each of the species of malaria affecting humans as well as for markers expressed by parasites at different stages of the life cycle. Positive studies do not distinguish current from past infection. Serology is not useful for diagnosing acute infection because detectable levels of antimalarial antibodies do not appear until weeks into infection and may persist long after clinically significant parasitemia has resolved. However, in particular settings, such as screening blood donors in the epidemiological investigation of a potential transfusion-induced case of malaria, serologic studies have been an appropriate and valuable tool for some time. More recently technological refinements have made it practical and more affordable to screen samples for multiple serologic markers efficiently in multiplex platforms. At a population level, serologic conversion rates and the age distribution of antibodies marking recent and remote infection, can provide evidence of how transmission is evolving and may contribute to malaria elimination efforts in years to come.[43]

Treatment Modalities. There are a limited number of drugs that can be used to treat or prevent malaria, but the drug development pipeline is more robust now than in recent decades, in part because of specific attention to research and development efforts. Currently available antimalarial drug classes and compounds are listed below along with information about their activity. Not all are efficacious, practical, appropriate, or recommended to use in every given situation or regulatory environment. The selection of preferred treatment options by national programs—as well as the specific regimen suited to an individual patient—must consider multiple factors. Local and national treatment guidelines should be based on evidence of clinical efficacy, and treatment of imported malaria should consider the evidence from the countries where infection was acquired. In addition, individual considerations including age, infecting species, clinical features, pregnancy and breastfeeding status, concomitant medical conditions, drug allergies, prior antimalarial drug use, and other medications, are important to guide decisions about how to treat malaria in each specific patient. Treatment recommendations for patients diagnosed with malaria in the United States are available from the Centers for Disease Control and Prevention (CDC) at www.cdc.gov/malaria/diagnosis_treatment/treatment.html; assistance obtaining diagnosis and treatment is also available through the CDC Malaria Hotline (770-488-7788) from 9:00 am to 5:00 pm Eastern Time. After hours or on weekends and holidays, call the CDC Emergency Operation Center at 770-488-7100.

Most of the drugs commonly used to treat malaria are **blood schizonticides**, active against the asexual intraerythrocytic stages of the parasites that are associated with clinical symptoms. Common drug classes and key compounds with this property include:

- Arylamino alcohols: quinine, quinidine, mefloquine, lumefantrine;
- 4-aminoquinolines: chloroquine, amodiaquine, piperaquine, pyronaridine, naphthoquine;
- Artemisinins and synthetic peroxides: artesunate, artemether, dihydroartemisinsin;
- Antifolates: sulfadoxine, sulfalene, dapsone, pyrimethamine, proguanil, trimethoprim;
- Electron transport inhibitors: atovaquone; and
- Other antibiotics: tetracyclines, quinolones, rifampicin, azithromycin, chloramphenicol, clindamycin.

Treatment of the erythrocytic stages alone can be curative for *P. falciparum* and *P. malariae* infection. To achieve a radical cure, naturally transmitted *P. vivax* and *P. ovale* infections also require treatment of liver stage parasites with an active **tissue schizonticide** or **hypnozoiticide**. The 8-aminoquinoline drugs, primaquine and tafenoquine, are the only approved compounds with this activity. Some antimalarial treatments also affect the production of gametocytes and influence the likelihood of ongoing transmission. Both the artemisinins and 8-aminoquinolines have activity as **gametocytocides** in addition to their value in treating acute illness.[17]

Antimalarial Drug-Resistance Concerns. In the past, sequential monotherapies were used extensively until drug resistance limited their effectiveness. Chloroquine resistance arose independently in *P. falciparum* parasites in Southeast Asia and South America. It eventually spread from Asia to Africa and became well established there in the 1980s and 1990s. Because of resistance, chloroquine became substantially compromised as a treatment option nearly everywhere *P. falciparum* occurred—with notable exceptions in Central America, the Caribbean, and Middle East. As the clinical importance of chloroquine resistance was recognized, few alternatives were available. Antifolate drugs, particularly sulfadoxine-pyrimethamine (SP), were recommended in some places, but resistance developed shortly after widespread use in Southeast Asia and South America as well. In Africa, conflicting clinical advice and sparse evidence, longstanding trust in chloroquine, and the lack of an affordable locally available alternative, contributed to it remaining the foundation of malaria control programs long after it failed to cure more than half the infections in many areas. The result was an insidious loss of life. Children might have appeared to be improving at first but were left vulnerable by repeated bouts of incompletely treated illness. By the time more than the first few countries in East and Southern Africa abandoned chloroquine for SP, resistance to antifolate drugs had already reached saturation. SP on its own or in combination with amodiaquine remains a valuable drug for some chemoprevention interventions in pregnant women after their first trimester, as well as in infants and young children, in some settings—even where it has been abandoned for treatment of clinical illness.

The drive to replace quinine during World War II had yielded promising leads that U.S. military interests pursued again beginning in 1963, leading to the development and release of mefloquine.[44] Similarly, by the early 1970s, Chinese investigators, having isolated the active ingredient from *A. annua* and began producing artemisinin derivatives.[17] Youyou Tu was recognized with the Nobel Prize in Physiology or Medicine in 2015 for her contribution to the latter. Both alternatives were promising but each had its limitations. A major advance was realized in the mid-1990s when they were applied in combination for treatment of *P. falciparum* malaria along the Thai-Cambodian border. Not only did the combination successfully cure most infections that were resistant to multiple other drugs, the combination remained efficacious for decades in a setting where one drug after another—chloroquine, SP, SP plus mefloquine, and mefloquine monotherapy—had failed. By 2001 WHO recommended artemisinin-based combination therapies (ACTs) for falciparum malaria, and resources to procure them became available through the Global Fund to Fight AIDS, Tuberculosis and Malaria. As ACTs have largely replaced failing monotherapies, they have without question contributed to substantial progress in reducing malaria-related morbidity and mortality. But they have not proven invincible. Resistance to many of the partner drugs and to artemisinin derivatives themselves is a challenge in the countries of the Greater Mekong subregion. Well-founded concerns about the limited number of treatment options remaining in parts of the region and the risk of resistant parasites spreading beyond this setting demand coordinated action to eliminate malaria where transmission persists in these countries.

Treatment of Uncomplicated Falciparum Malaria. Nonsevere illness caused by *P. falciparum* alone can usually be treated with a single course of an oral ACT. ACTs specifically include partner drugs with a mechanism of action distinct from the artemisinin component, and frequently one with a longer half-life. Coformulated fixed-dose combination drugs are generally recommended over coadministration of separate tablets. The specific regimen depends on antimalarial drug resistance patterns and local regulatory approvals, as well as individual patient characteristics. Recommended options currently include fixed dose combinations of: artemether/lumefantrine, artesunate/amodiaquine, artesunate/mefloquine, dihydroartemisinin/piperaquine, and, occasionally, the co-administration of SP plus artesunate. Some potential partner drugs, like SP and amodiaquine, should be avoided where they must be reserved for chemoprevention indications, particularly in sub-Saharan Africa. WHO specifically discourages monotherapy formulations of artemisinin derivatives, and their partner drugs—amodiaquine, mefloquine, and SP—recommending they be withdrawn wherever they are recommended as part of a first-line ACT.[27] All recommended ACTs include at least 3 days treatment with the artemisinin component. Patients with uncomplicated falciparum malaria who are in care and treatment for HIV coinfection may avoid combinations with SP (if they also receive trimethoprim/sulfamethoxazole) or amodiaquine (if they are taking efavirenz or zidovudine). In settings where ACTs are unavailable or in patients for which they are unsuitable (first trimester of pregnancy) alternative treatments for uncomplicated *P. falciparum* can include quinine or quinidine with another drug like clindamycin or a tetracycline. Under conditions of close observation, *P. falciparum* infections acquired in areas where the threat of drug resistance is known to be minimal, can be successfully treated with chloroquine, mefloquine, atovaquone/proguanil, or quinine combination treatments.

Treatment of Uncomplicated Nonfalciparum Malaria. Chloroquine remains active against most nonfalciparum malaria infections. But *P. vivax* resistance has reached a high level across New Guinea and elsewhere in the Western Pacific; lower levels of resistance occur in Southeast Asia and South America.[27] Isolated chloroquine resistance in *P. malariae* has also been reported.[45] If the infecting malaria species is not known or uncertain, and in cases of mixed species infection, it is always recommended that uncomplicated malaria be treated with an ACT as for *P. falciparum*. In most areas, adults and children with uncomplicated illness from *P. vivax*, *P. ovale*, *P. malariae*, or *P. knowlesi* can be treated equally well with chloroquine or an ACT. Chloroquine or quinine is recommended for women in the first trimester of pregnancy. If there is any question of chloroquine resistance, nonfalciparum malaria can be treated with an ACT or quinine. Patients with *P. vivax* or *P. ovale* should be tested for G6PD deficiency as part of the initial evaluation (or as early as feasible) in order to guide the use of 8-aminoquinolines for radical cure. Both primaquine and tafenoquine are effective for this indication but should be avoided in patients with insufficient G6PD activity, pregnant women, infants < 6 months old, and women breastfeeding infants < 6 months old, or older infants who are not known to have adequate G6PD activity. Some individuals with certain levels of diminished G6PD activity can be treated with an adjusted dose of primaquine. Women who are pregnant or breast feeding may benefit from weekly chloroquine until delivery or breastfeeding is completed.

Treatment of Severe Malaria. Malaria is a life-threatening condition and requires immediate intervention whenever signs or symptoms of severe disease are present. Parenteral artesunate is the recognized drug of choice for all adults and children with severe malaria—including infants, pregnant women, and lactating mothers. Parenteral therapy should be continued for a minimum of 24 hours or until the patient can tolerate oral medication. At that point they should receive a complete 3-day treatment course of a recommended ACT, regardless of the duration of parenteral artesunate prior to that point. Dose adjustments are necessary for children under 20 kg. If parenteral artesunate is not available, artemether is the preferred alternative. Despite evidence that artesunate is clinically superior and safer, quinine and quinidine remain widely used for severe malaria, especially where no other parenteral antimalarial drug has received regulatory approval or is available.[24] Since April 2019, CDC has moved to make IV artesunate available for the management of severe malaria in the United States and it can be obtained upon consultation with subject matter experts through the CDC Malaria Hotline (at 770-488-7788 from 9:00 am to 5:00 pm Eastern Time and through the CDC Emergency Operation Center at 770-488-7100 at other times). There is some evidence that prereferral treatment, initiated with intramuscular or rectal artemisinin drugs, can improve survival of young children with severe disease in settings where definitive referral care is accessible.[46] This practice has yet to be widely adopted. Definitive treatment of severe malaria frequently also requires additional supportive and critical care treatment of the end-organ syndromes, and coinfection even after malaria parasitemia may be cleared; respiratory and hemodynamic support, fluid and electrolyte replacement, blood transfusion, and hemodialysis can all be life-saving where available. Some common and recommended treatment practices can precipitate or predispose to some manifestations of severe disease. Once recommended, exchange transfusion to rapidly reduce high-density malaria parasitemia may pose more risk than benefit,[47] particularly as rapidly acting artemisinin treatment becomes more widely used.[48] Aggressive intravenous fluid resuscitation to address shock can be associated with additional iatrogenic risk of death in children with severe infections including malaria.[49] Incomplete or insufficiently efficacious antimalarial treatment can contribute to prolonged infection, anemia, and risk of death after discharge.[50] Even life-saving artemisinin-treatment of high-density malaria infection can be associated with a late onset hemolytic anemia.[51] For these reasons, patients with severe malaria should always be managed in an inpatient setting with careful follow-up.

PREVENTION AND CONTROL

Since 2001, a revitalized commitment to fighting malaria—through the efforts of endemic countries and their development partners, global advocacy including the Roll Back Malaria Partnership, and coordinated procurement via the Global Fund to Fight AIDS, Tuberculosis, and Malaria—has mobilized as much U.S.$3 billion per year for prevention and control.[1] While still barely half of the projected need, this level of funding has made unprecedented progress possible.[2,3] Contemporary malaria efforts aim to reduce morbidity and mortality, through a combination of multiple interventions that affect the transmission cycle at several points. As none of these is completely effective on its own, and resources are generally insufficient to implement all the strategies everywhere at once, public health officials need to make informed decisions about when and where to apply the options available to them. The effectiveness of different malaria tools, and the optimal timing and mix of intervention strategies can depend heavily on local conditions. At a minimum, good access to proven vector control and high-quality diagnosis and treatment of malaria illness are essential for all populations at risk.[52] The prevailing global strategy is presented in Fig. 89-3 and emphasizes three pillars: universal access to effective vector control and case management, accelerating transmission reduction, and real-time case-based surveillance. These rest on supporting elements that specifically address shortcomings of the previous eradication experience: strengthening innovation and research as

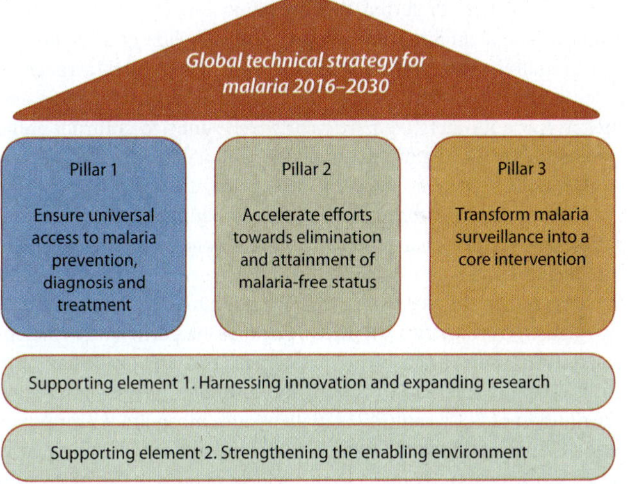

FIGURE 89-3. Global technical strategy for malaria 2015–30, featuring pillars, and supportive strategies.[2] (*Source:* Reprinted with permission of the World Health Organization.)

well as the political and health system environment.[2] While many of the effective strategies used today derive from approaches that were successful in past decades, there have been several key advances and economies of scale that have unlocked their potential to reach millions. In addition, new tools that could overcome technical limitations or affect the transmission cycle in different ways are poised for deployment or in development.

Vector Control. Even before the malaria life cycle was understood, humans had devised approaches for avoiding insect pests. Applied with an awareness of the biology and behavior of malaria vectors, interventions aimed at reducing contact between people and mosquitoes can be highly effective. Generally, these approaches target vector species either in their developmental stages or as adults. Environmental measures, such as preferentially locating housing or settlements, controlling flooding, and otherwise eliminating breeding sites where the aquatic stages of the malaria vector mosquitoes develop can reduce human-mosquito contact and malaria infection. These measures were important historically, but are not applicable everywhere.[53] Each mosquito species that transmits malaria has adapted to a specific environmental niche. In situations where breeding sites are well characterized and semipermanent but not amenable to elimination, they can be treated with chemical or biological agents to kill or arrest the development of juvenile mosquito life-cycle stages.[54] Chemical larvicides currently recommended for mosquito control include those of the benzoylurea, juvenile hormone mimic, organophosphate, and spinosyn classes; recommended biological larvicides are limited to bacterial strains of *Bacillus thuringiensis israelensis* and *B. sphaericus*.[55] Stocking rivers and ponds with fish that feed on mosquito larvae has been promoted as a malaria control tool in some settings, but evidence of its effectiveness is not clear.[56] Larval source reduction and larviciding contribute to malaria and vector control in many settings, and can potentially be effective against mosquitoes wherever they bite or rest. But they are not well suited to settings where important vector species exploit numerous small and temporary breeding sites, as is the case in much of Africa and South Asia.[53]

Killing, repelling, or avoiding adult mosquitoes is the most common vector-control approach currently applied for malaria prevention. Personal protective measures such as clothing and repellants are routinely recommended for malaria prevention among nonimmune travelers. But the impact of these personal protection measures on malaria at a population level is undocumented and constrained by the feasibility of large numbers of people using them consistently and correctly for an indefinite period of time.[57] Differences in the behavior of adult mosquitoes can have a marked effect on their capacity to transmit malaria and may suggest which control strategies may be more effective. Preferred time of biting can vary from daylight hours to late at night. Some vectors prefer to bite or rest indoors and predominantly feed on human blood. Others seek a range of potential blood meal sources or rest wherever they find shade and shelter. Mosquito nets are particularly well suited to anthropophilic (preferentially feeding on humans) and indoor-biting vectors. When treated with a durable chemical insecticide, they can be a highly effective malaria control tool, which acts by killing adult mosquitoes and providing personal protection to the persons resting beneath. Insecticide-treated mosquito nets (ITNs) have been credited with the largest part of the twenty-first century malaria control gains, especially in rural Africa where *An. gambiae*—a particularly efficient malaria vector—exhibits biting preferences that are ideally suited to an intervention deployed indoors and at night.[58] Community-wide distribution of ITNs can substantially reduce mosquito vector populations, malaria transmission, and morbidity and mortality in nearly every transmission setting.[59] When widely deployed, the protection they provide may even extend to individuals and households without nets, so long as enough of their neighbors are using them. Through the efforts of endemic countries and their global partners, billions of ITNs have been deployed across endemic communities since 2001. Until recently, synthetic pyrethroids were the only class of insecticide approved for use on ITNs—making this tool vulnerable to insecticide resistance against these compounds. Newer ITNs incorporate additional insecticides, chemical synergists, and combinations of active ingredients; evidence on their relative effectiveness is being developed. In addition, applying insecticide to curtains, hammocks, bed linens, clothing, and building materials have all been explored as future tools for specific settings.[60]

IRS—the application of durable insecticide to the interior walls of houses—is another form of vector control that acts by killing adult vectors, particularly after they have taken a blood meal. IRS can be effective against vectors that bite and rest indoors and does not require being deployed nightly through individual behavior like ITNs. IRS and ITNs can have very comparable efficacy for malaria outcomes.[61] In some settings, however, the logistic complexity and cost of repeated application of IRS have constrained its deployment to relatively limited geographic settings and risk populations.[53] During the twentieth-century eradication era, DDT was deployed widely for IRS and undoubtedly contributed to the interruption of transmission in temperate areas and decreased burden in others. The use of DDT fell out of favor in the latter decades, both because of the development of insecticide resistance and because of the recognition of the potentially damaging environmental impact of persistent organic pesticides.[16] Malaria control is one of the few indications where careful application of DDT can outweigh its environmental risk, especially when resistance to other classes of insecticide is a concern. Other formulations currently recommended—and more commonly deployed—for IRS include active ingredients in the carbamate, neonicotinoid, organophosphate, and synthetic pyrethroid classes.[55] Like ITNs, the next-generation IRS products will incorporate new active ingredients, other insecticide classes, chemical synergists, insecticide combinations, and technologies that enhance durability.[60]

Deploying chemical insecticides on a large scale—such as through universal coverage of ITNs or expanded use of IRS—exposes populations of insect vectors to active compounds and requires careful planning. Basic entomological surveillance to characterize local mosquito populations and the suitability of specific interventions should occur as part of planning and be continued throughout the application and expected duration of action. Most of the insecticides employed in public health programs may also be used for agricultural and household pest control. Selective pressure from insecticide use inevitably favors the emergence and intensification of insecticide resistance. Integrated vector management strategies that can mitigate the impact of resistance should be a priority, especially when the options are limited. This is especially true for pyrethroid insecticides used on ITNs. There is evidence of pyrethroid resistance from many areas where ITN use is high, and it has the potential to undermine this critically important tool.[62] Deploying pyrethroids for IRS in the same areas can intensify selection and risks compromising a successful ITN strategy. However, IRS with other chemical classes may be particularly useful for disrupting insecticide resistance through strategies like rotational, mosaic, or combined application. To date, much of the practical experience has been limited to rotating active compounds in IRS only after documented resistance has arisen locally, but the growing awareness of this concern may spark more proactive deployment. In addition, research and development into new active ingredients for both IRS and ITNs, as well as nonchemical vector control alternatives, is urgently needed.[63]

Vector control options suitable for mosquitoes that bite outdoors or throughout the day, and those that feed on a range of nonhuman hosts are more limited and potentially less favorable as public health strategies. In some settings, use of IRS and ITNs has preferentially eliminated anthropophilic indoor biters, leaving more challenging adversaries behind to carry on transmission. Indoor and outdoor space-spraying has seldom been shown effective against malaria,[64] but is often invoked in mosquito-abatement and pest-control programs. Applying insecticides to livestock or through outdoor spraying, positioning attractants and traps, and deploying spatial repellants may have an impact in some settings and are the focus of ongoing research and development. Genetically modifying mosquitoes to reduce their numbers or to replace effective transmitters with populations refractory to malaria may also result in new approaches to malaria control. Likewise, viral, fungal, and bacterial symbionts of mosquitoes may eventually be developed specifically to alter or deter development of mosquito stage parasites. Basic research along these lines may result in new paradigms for vector control in the years to come.[60]

Malaria Case Management. Diagnosis and treatment of malaria cases remains the cornerstone of malaria prevention and control in most endemic areas. Prompt case management of uncomplicated malaria can prevent severe and complicated illness and avert deaths. It can also contribute to controlling transmission by reducing the prevalence and duration of infection and the infectiousness of humans to mosquitoes. As noted above, providing malaria treatment on the basis of clinical fever alone was widely practiced in highly endemic areas for decades. This almost certainly mitigated some of the devastating impact of malaria. As point of care diagnostic technologies improved it has become possible to recommend their universal application as a first step in malaria case management. Targeting malaria treatment to individuals with demonstrated infection has the potential to reduce costs, contain overuse of antimalarial drugs, avoid side effects from unnecessary treatments, enhance compliance, and encourage detection of nonmalarial illnesses. Along with antimalarial combination treatments, it may even contribute to slowing the emergence and selection of drug resistant parasites. Despite relatively large investments in diagnostic and treatment commodities, the overall coverage of malaria case management has been disappointing in many high burden countries.[1] Efforts to expand malaria case management through community health workers,[65] market subsidies, and engagement of private and retail sector providers[66] can improve coverage, but these seldom operate at scale. Unlike vector-control efforts for malaria, which are often conducted in campaign style, quality case management largely depends on functional health systems that must operate without interruption, even in remote and under-resourced settings. Infusion of malaria-specific diagnostic and treatment commodities only addresses a small part of the complex environment of health-seeking and delivery.[67] In addition, the consistent use of malaria diagnostic testing as the basis of malaria case management still requires attention. In 2017 national malaria programs distributed 245 million RDT kits and reported a test positivity between 40% and 50%. At the same time, they distributed 206 million doses of ACTs, suggesting that at least 30% of first line treatments were provided to persons who either tested negative or did not receive a diagnostic test.[1]

In addition, it is uncertain to what extent clearing circulating infections in symptomatic individuals with blood schizonticidal drugs alone can impact malaria transmission in many settings.[68] Some of the drugs commonly used to treat malaria in prior decades may have enhanced gametocytogenesis and transmissibility.[69] Artemisinin derivatives, even when used in combination therapies, have activity against immature gametocytes, and may contribute more to transmission reduction than conventional monotherapies, but this effect is incomplete.[70] Co-administering a single low dose of primaquine as part of routine malaria case management has been recommended more recently as a safe, affordable, and effective adjunct treatment that can reliably reduce onward transmission, without the risk of inducing hemolysis from undetected G6PD deficiency.[71] To date, relatively few malaria programs have implemented this strategy. This single low dose will not be active against liver-stage parasites. Radical cure for vivax and ovale malaria, as described earlier, requires a higher total dose of an 8-aminoquinoline, which will also be sufficient to eliminate gametocytes.

Surveillance and Response. As noted, planning, operating, and evaluating malaria programs requires accurate and reliable surveillance data. WHO's Global Technical Strategy for Malaria, 2016–30 specifically calls for transforming malaria surveillance into a core intervention, alongside vector control and case management.[2] Nearly all countries convey aggregate annual numbers of malaria cases and deaths recorded in their national health information systems as part of the process of compiling the World Malaria Report. Many also use this information to estimate their malaria program needs. In decades past, many of these reports were based solely on clinical cases and data had been notably incomplete, inaccurate, and untimely. In many high burden countries, control programs and WHO are still forced to estimate the realistic burden. With the wide acceptance of diagnostic confirmation and advances in information and communication technology, it is becoming increasingly possible to improve the quality of malaria surveillance, eliminate delays, and develop a more real-time picture of where and when malaria cases are presenting for treatment. Most surveillance depends on passive case detection—reporting only those cases that come to health facilities for diagnosis and treatment.[72] The ability to detect and report cases that occur at community outlets and private providers is limited, and the large portion of malaria infections that do not cause illness are missed altogether. In addition, most deaths from malaria go unrecorded outside of health facilities. Even so, improving surveillance based on passively detected cases alone, can go a long way toward providing information that will help malaria programs anticipate and target their efforts.

As countries approach elimination, surveillance becomes even more critical. When the disease burden is low enough, it becomes possible for local health officials to investigate each individual case to explore the likelihood that it was imported or transmitted locally, and to ensure adequate treatment and coverage with preventive interventions. This is an important step along the way toward being able to be internationally certified as malaria free. Individual case investigations can also present an opportunity to search for additional malaria illnesses or infections by testing individuals in the same or nearby households. The exact perimeter around each case that such reactive case detection should target will depend on local epidemiology, ecology, and geography, as well as the available personnel and resources. In some settings, untargeted active case detection activities such as mass testing and treatment (or mass screening and treatment) may help to identify and treat individuals infected with malaria before they develop clinical illness or as a way to limit the likelihood that they will contribute to local malaria transmission. Screen and treat strategies have been proposed for evaluating malaria infection prevalence and treating groups such as pregnant women or returning travelers in different settings. In general, the limit of detection for currently available point of care tests is not sufficient to detect all individuals who may contribute to malaria transmission or be at risk of future illness. But new tools with enhanced sensitivity may become practical and should be evaluated for the added role they might be able to play in accelerating progress toward elimination.[72,73]

In addition to surveillance for malaria cases and infections, coverage and use of malaria interventions are commonly assessed through periodic population surveys. Malaria programs in nearly all settings should also collect data on the continued utility of their key intervention tools, and this requires specific attention and capability. Antimalarial drug efficacy can be monitored through regular therapeutic efficacy studies conducted at sentinel sites to ensure that recommended and alternative treatment regimens are active against the malaria infections commonly seen. Molecular markers have been identified for some of the key classes of antimalarial drugs, but the most useful information comes from enrolling patients with documented malaria parasitemia and following them closely for several weeks to ensure that infection has been completely cleared and does not recrudesce.[27] In areas where malaria transmission is so infrequent that these *in vivo* follow-up studies are impractical, monitoring the frequency of established molecular markers and day 7 cure rate can be useful. Entomological surveillance is also important to characterize the prevalent malaria vector species and their susceptibility to insecticides used in vector control strategies.[72] The appearance of *P. falciparum* parasites that fail to produce HRP-2 should also prompt control program managers and their partners to be alert for diagnostic failures when relying on RDTs that depend on detecting this antigen.[41]

Chemoprevention. Malaria case management is based on treating infections that cause symptoms and can be detected on a laboratory test. But in many transmission settings, this represents only a small fraction of the individuals carrying parasites—including those who could eventually develop illness or transmit the infection to others. Antimalarial drugs can play an important role in reducing the burden of malaria in particular risk groups. Applied strategically, they offer promise as potential tools to reduce transmission and accelerate progress toward elimination. The most widely recommended chemoprevention strategy is antimalarial chemoprophylaxis for nonimmune travelers visiting endemic areas. The choice of drugs for prophylaxis must be made on an individual basis. Travelers and their providers should consider the intended travel destination(s), potential for antimalarial drug resistance, type of exposure and accommodation, timing and duration of travel, and the traveler's age, drug allergies, other medications and medical history. In the United States, the Centers for Disease Control and Prevention (CDC) issues recommendations on what drugs can be used for prevention of malaria in travelers at www.cdc.gov/malaria/travelers/index.html along with guidance for selecting the best option. One important consideration is adherence, as some drugs must be taken daily and others are dosed once a week. In general, antimalarial chemoprophylaxis should be initiated before travel (from as few as 1 or 2 days to as much as a week) and continued from 1 to 4 weeks after leaving a malarious area. Many of the drugs commonly used for chemoprophylaxis act primarily as blood schizonticides. Even when used appropriately they cannot prevent primary infection or the establishment of liver-stage hypnozoites. For travelers returning from an area where *P. vivax* or *P. ovale* infection risk is high—particularly after an extended stay—a complete course of antirelapse therapy is recommended as well. Failure to take a recommended chemoprophylaxis drug or to complete its full course is among the most common avoidable factors contributing to imported malaria.[74]

Chemoprophylaxis can also reduce the impact of malaria among high-risk populations in endemic country settings as well. Suppressive doses of antimalarial drugs can reduce illness and mortality and improve cognitive performance in children as well as improve birth outcomes among pregnant women in clinical trial and project settings in rural Africa. Unfortunately, the intervention can be difficult to sustain indefinitely and stopping it was associated with rebound mortality.[75] Strategies that aimed to deliver low doses of antimalarial drugs through treated salt produced less clear evidence of impact[76] and may have contributed to the selection and intensification of antimalarial drug resistance. By the mid-1990s a new strategy had evolved—providing complete treatment doses of antimalarial drugs to risk groups at determined intervals. Intermittent preventive treatment (IPT) replaced chemoprophylaxis as a recommended strategy for pregnant women and children in high transmission settings.[77,78] IPT strategies are effective by eliminating chronic persistent parasitemia that may be subclinical but contributes to anemia and vulnerability and by providing a window of protection from subsequent blood-stage infections. SP, delivered at intervals of at least 1 month, is recommended for IPT in pregnancy (IPTp). This intervention remains effective at reducing placental malaria, anemia, and low birth weight, even in settings where SP is no longer useful as a monotherapy treatment for malaria illness. Recent studies with a range of alternative antimalarial drugs have yet to identify one that is as effective as SP for IPTp.[79] SP is highly affordable and simple to deliver and a majority of women attend facility-based antenatal care in nearly every setting where IPTp is recommended. Even so, although 35 million women could benefit from IPTp each year, as of 2017 only one country, Zambia, reported providing three or more doses to more than 50% of eligible women. Challenges with health systems and suboptimal timing of antenatal visits have made it difficult to achieve high coverage with at least three doses of IPTp.[1]

IPT strategies have also been elaborated for infants and children under 5 years. In very high transmission settings of sub-Saharan Africa, providing IPT at scheduled immunization visits during infancy (IPTi) can contribute to reducing clinical illness episodes and anemia associated with repeated and chronic parasitemia. Large-scale intervention trials failed to provide conclusive evidence of an impact on mortality.[80] IPTi with at least three doses of SP has been recommended by WHO since 2010, at least for settings where the antimalarial drug resistance profile is favorable. Despite some early success with subnational implementation, as of 2017, no malaria endemic country reported having implemented a national policy for IPTi.[1] In stark contrast, another IPT strategy for children 3–59 months old has rapidly been adopted in areas of highly seasonal malaria transmission in Sahelian West Africa. Seasonal malaria chemoprevention (SMC) involves delivering full treatment with SP plus amodiaquine at monthly intervals to children in settings where the majority of malaria cases are reported in a predictable 3- to 4-month period each year. Under such conditions, SMC can reduce the incidence of malaria illness and severe malaria by nearly a third in children who receive the recommended doses and may also reduce all-cause mortality to a more modest degree.[81] WHO began recommending SMC in 2015 and within just 3 years nearly half of the 30 million children eligible across 12 countries had received at least one dose.[1] Unlike IPTp and IPTi, SMC is usually delivered in stand-alone campaigns by health workers who provide the service door-to-door.

Mass drug administration is an untargeted form of chemoprevention that involves providing a complete treatment course of an effective antimalarial regimen to whole populations without assessing whether individuals are infected at the time. MDA was invoked in some late twentieth-century malaria efforts and is a common strategy in campaigns focused on eliminating neglected tropical diseases. The evidence for MDA as a malaria intervention is somewhat mixed. It can definitely reduce the immediate prevalence of malaria infection and the onset of clinical illness, but that effect is usually short-lived.[82] MDA for malaria may be useful for reducing the malaria burden in extreme settings of complex emergencies when the health system that ordinarily provides malaria case management is severely disrupted. It was used to this end in the 2014–15 Ebola crisis.[83,84] By temporarily clearing asymptomatic and potentially undetectable malaria parasitemia, there is growing interest in the potential of MDA as a tool for disrupting malaria transmission and accelerating progress toward elimination. There is less objective evidence of its effectiveness for this indication, but evaluation studies are currently planned or underway which may be informative. Whether used for burden reduction or as part of an elimination effort, high population coverage with MDA is key.[85] Door-to-door delivery strategies, mop up visits, and repeated rounds can be useful strategies for reaching as many potential beneficiaries as possible.

In order to avoid contributing to selection of resistant parasites, it is generally not recommended that MDA be undertaken with the same regimen used for treatment of malaria illness. To have an optimum impact on transmission, an ideal MDA regimen would be simple to dose and have a relatively long half-life, extending the period of protection. In addition to drugs that clear blood-stage parasites, the gametocytocidal properties of artemisinin drugs and 8-aminoquinolines are particularly attractive as adjunct MDA candidates for their transmission blocking potential. Endectocides are veterinary antiparasitic drugs active both against endoparasites and ectoparasites. Ivermectin has been widely used in humans for MDA against onchocerciasis and lymphatic filariasis and will kill mosquitoes that feed on individuals who have recently taken it. This observation has sparked an interest in exploring the use of ivermectin or related drugs as part of malaria case management[86] or malaria-specific MDA—either delivered to human populations, livestock,[87] or both. Preliminary studies are promising, and show the impact is highly dependent on dosage and timing. In addition, the pathway toward developing a promising adjunct transmission blocking or vector control tool based on a pharmacological intervention may not be straightforward.[88]

Malaria Vaccines. The search for an effective vaccine against malaria has been an area of active research and development work for decades. Scores of candidate vaccine antigens and constructs have been proposed and evaluated in laboratory and preclinical settings—often with disappointing results. RTS,S, a pre-erythrocytic *P. falciparum* malaria vaccine, has been shown to prevent malaria illness in African children, been granted a favorable opinion by the European Medicines Agency, and deployed in large scale pilot evaluation projects in Ghana, Kenya, and Malawi. Its efficacy against clinical illness and severe malaria in children was modest, but the clinical trials showed that it could make a substantial contribution to reducing malaria, especially in highly endemic settings where vector control and case management were optimized.[89] The large-scale evaluation is planned to explore the safety and feasibility of delivering this multidose vaccine as well as its potential impact on child survival. The late-stage clinical trials of RTS,S did not evaluate the potential impact on transmission that might be possible if it were administered to all age groups or in a fractionated dosing regimen, and these outcomes are also being evaluated independently. Several other pre-erythrocytic vaccines are also being evaluated. In particular, a whole parasite vaccine composed of irradiated (PfSPZ) or genetically attenuated *P. falciparum* sporozoites shows promise in infection challenge and early field studies.[90,91] Next-generation malaria vaccines are likely to address multiple targets across multiple life-cycle stages. Specific vaccines for placental malaria and *P. vivax* or *P. ovale* are also in development. Vaccines that have the potential to interrupt transmission, particularly if they do not provide individual protection from infection or illness as well, could also prove useful for malaria elimination and control efforts, but may require careful regulatory and policy considerations.[60]

Malaria Elimination and Prevention of Reestablishment. Since 2007 there is a renewed call for elimination and even eradication[92]—embraced widely as the ultimate goal of malaria efforts collectively.[73] Dozens of countries and territories have elaborated plans for reaching malaria-free status in the medium-term.[93] A global framework document lays out the general approach, illustrated in Fig. 89-4.[73] Recapitulating the Global Technical Strategy, it emphasizes the importance of optimizing access to vector control, case management, and surveillance as core interventions for all transmission settings. As the total burden of malaria cases declines, individual case and focus investigations can be initiated and other interventions may be more targeted. In addition, specific transmission reduction efforts focused on population-level parasite clearance, such as MDA or potential new tools can be introduced to accelerate the progress toward elimination. The programmatic goal is to be able to investigate and contain each individual case and document when local transmission has been interrupted or re-established. Once a country has achieved zero indigenous malaria cases for 3 consecutive years, it can request certification of malaria-free status.

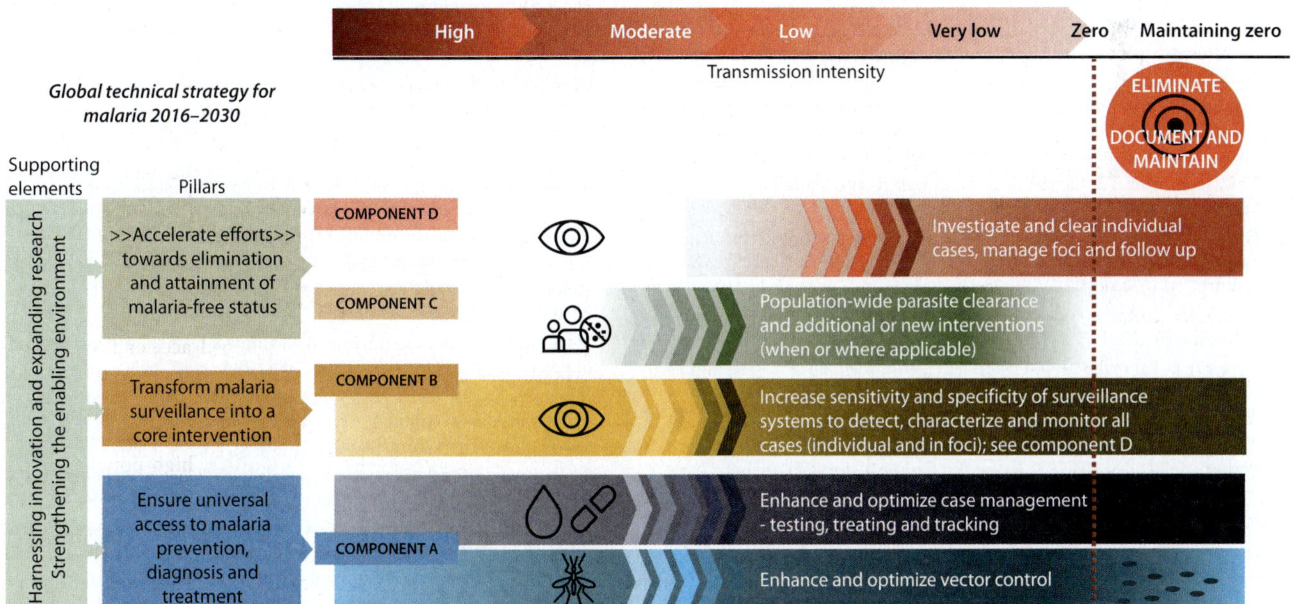

Illustrative intervention package
The package of intervention strategies can be adapted for different geographical areas in a country. The choice of interventions should be based on transmission intensity (from "high" to " very low" to zero and maintaining zero) and also on operational capacity and system readiness. The diagram should be seen as illustrative rather than prescriptive, as the onset and duration of interventions will depend on local circumstances. The shading in the boxes showing components indicates the enhancements and quality required as programmes progress towards elimination, with darker colours indicating more intense actions and shading from light to dark indicating enhancement of the quality and scale or focus of the work.
High
Moderate
Low
Very low
Zero
Maintaining zero
Transmission intensity
Global technical strategy for malaria 2016–2030
ELIMINATE
DOCUMENT AND MAINTAIN
Supporting elements
Pillars
Harnessing innovation and expanding research
Strengthening the enabling environment
>>Accelerate efforts>> towards elimination and attainment of malaria-free status
Transform malaria surveillance into a core intervention
Ensure universal access to malaria prevention, diagnosis and treatment
COMPONENT D
COMPONENT C
COMPONENT B
COMPONENT A
Investigate and clear individual cases, manage foci and follow up
Population-wide parasite clearance and additional or new interventions (when or where applicable)
Increase sensitivity and specificity of surveillance systems to detect, characterize and monitor all cases (individual and in foci); see component D
Enhance and optimize case management - testing, treating and tracking
Enhance and optimize vector control
*Acceleration – as represented by arrow bars (>>>>>) here – relates to time-limited efforts made across all components in order to (1) achieve universal/optimal coverage in malaria prevention and case management (Component A), and increase sensitivity and specificity of surveillance systems so they are able to detect, characterize and monitor all malaria cases and foci (Component B); and (2) bring malaria transmission to sufficiently low levels (with or without population-wide parasite clearance and other strategies, Component C as an option) where remaining cases can be investigated/cleared and foci can be managed and followed up (Component D).

FIGURE 89-4. Elements of the global framework for malaria elimination.[73] (*Source:* Reprinted with permission of the World Health Organization.)

CONCLUSION

Malaria, with its attendant burden of illness, disability, and mortality, remains one of the most challenging global health threats despite being preventable and treatable. In recent decades, the efforts of endemic countries and their global partners have resulted in delivery of billions of ITNs, diagnostic tests and treatment drugs. This massive expansion of access to proven interventions has met with unprecedented progress and rekindled the promise that malaria can be eliminated as a public health problem. Yet familiar challenges threaten to slow or reverse hard-won gains. Incremental improvements in surveillance, prevention, diagnosis, and treatment technologies are encouraging. Potentially transformative new tools and paradigms may already be taking shape. Better understanding and application of basic and implementation science is likely to produce others in coming years. The boldest ambitions will certainly require, as well, a stronger emphasis on complex health systems factors, better engagement across numerous sectors of human activity and development, and more sustained global financial and political commitment—than attended the mid-twentieth-century eradication project. Even so, the opportunities for maintaining and expanding recent successes in combatting malaria and mitigating its public health impact have never been better.

References

1. World Health Organization. *World Malaria Report, 2018*. Geneva: World Health Organization; 2018.
2. World Health Organization. *Global Technical Strategy for Malaria, 2016–2030*. Geneva: World Health Organization; 2015.
3. Roll Back Malaria Partnership Secretariat. *Action and Investment to defeat Malaria, 2016–2030. For a Malaria-Free World*. Geneva: World Health Organization; 2015.
4. Imwong M, Madmanee W, Suwannasin K, et al. Asymptomatic natural human infections with the simian malaria parasites *Plasmodium cynomolgi* and *Plasmodium knowlesi*. *J Infect Dis.* 2019;219(5):695–702.
5. World Health Organization. *WHO Malaria Terminology*. Geneva: World Health Organization; 2016.
6. DPDx—Laboratory Identification of Parasites of Public Health Concern. https://www.cdc.gov/dpdx/malaria/index.html.
7. Loy DE, Liu W, Li Y, et al. Out of Africa: Origins and evolution of the human malaria parasites *Plasmodium falciparum* and *Plasmodium vivax*. *Int J Parasitol.* 2017;47:87–97.
8. Kwiatkowski DP. How malaria has affected the human genome and what human genetics can teach us about malaria. *Am J Hum Genet.* 2005;77:171–92.
9. Bianucci R, Araujo A, Pusch CM, Nerlich AG. The identification of malaria in paleopathology—An in-depth assessment of the strategies to detect malaria in ancient remains. *Acta Trop.* 2015;152:176–80.
10. Hawass Z, Gad YZ, Ismail S, et al. Ancestry and pathology in King Tutankhamun's family. *JAMA.* 2010;303:638–47.
11. Fornaciari G, Giuffra V, Bianucci R. Identification of pathogens in ancient skeletal series: The malaria of the Medici Grand Dukes (Florence, XVI century). *Med Secoli.* 2010;22(1–3):261–72.
12. Najera JA. Malaria control: Achievements, problems and strategies. *Parassitologia.* 2001;43(1–2):1–89.
13. Arrow KJ, Panosian C, Gelband H. Committee on the Economics of Antimalarial Drugs: Saving lives, buying time. In: *Economics of Malaria Drugs in an Age of Resistance*. Washington, DC: Institute of Medicine; 2004.
14. Permin H, Norn S, Kruse E, Kruse PR. On the history of Cinchona bark in the treatment of Malaria. *Dan Medicinhist Arbog.* 2016;44:9–30.
15. Wagner-Jauregg J. The history of the malaria treatment of general paralysis. 1946. *Am J Psychiatry.* 1994;151:231–5.
16. Roberts D, Tren R, Bate R, Zambone J. *The Excellent Powder: DDT's Political and Scientific History*. Indianapolis: Dog Ear Publishing; 2010.
17. Schlitzer M. Malaria chemotherapeutics part I: History of antimalarial drug development, currently used therapeutics, and drugs in clinical development. *ChemMedChem.* 2007;2(7):944–86.
18. Macdonald G. Theory of the eradication of malaria. *Bull World Health Organ.* 1956;15(3–5):369–87.
19. Humpheys M. *Malaria: Poverty, Race and Public Health in the United States*. Baltimore: Johns Hopkins University Press; 2001.
20. Packard RM. *The Making of a Tropical Disease: A Short History of Malaria*. Baltimore: Johns Hopikins University Press; 2007.
21. World Health Organization. *World Malaria Report, 2009*. Geneva: World Health Organization; 2009.
22. Snow RW, Sartorius B, Kyalo D, et al. The prevalence of *Plasmodium falciparum* in sub-Saharan Africa since 1900. *Nature.* 2017;550(7677):515–8.
23. World Health Organization. *Universal Access to Malaria Diagnostic Testing: An Operational Manual*. Geneva: World Health Organization; 2011.
24. World Health Organization. Severe malaria. *Trop Med Int Health.* 2014;19(Suppl 1):7–131.
25. Price RN, Douglas NM, Anstey NM. New developments in *Plasmodium vivax* malaria: Severe disease and the rise of chloroquine resistance. *Curr Opin Infect Dis.* 2009;22(5):430–5.
26. Barber BE, William T, Grigg MJ, et al. A prospective comparative study of knowlesi, falciparum, and vivax malaria in Sabah, Malaysia: High proportion with severe disease from *Plasmodium knowlesi* and *Plasmodium vivax* but no mortality with early referral and artesunate therapy. *Clin Infect Dis.* 2013;56(3):383–97.
27. World Health Organization. *Guidelines for the Treatment of Malaria*, 3rd ed. Geneva: World Health Organization; 2015.
28. Dondorp A, Nosten F, Stepniewska K, Day N, White N, South East Asian Quinine Artesunate Malaria Trial Group. Artesunate versus quinine for treatment of severe falciparum malaria: A randomised trial. *Lancet.* 2005;366(9487):717–25.
29. Dondorp AM, Fanello CI, Hendriksen IC, et al. Artesunate versus quinine in the treatment of severe falciparum malaria in African children (AQUAMAT): An open-label, randomised trial. *Lancet.* 2010;376(9753):1647–57.
30. Bloland PB, Boriga DA, Ruebush TK, et al. Longitudinal cohort study of the epidemiology of malaria infections in an area of intense malaria transmission II. Descriptive epidemiology of malaria infection and disease among children. *Am J Trop Med Hyg.* 1999;60(4):641–8.
31. McElroy PD, ter Kuile FO, Lal AA, et al. Effect of *Plasmodium falciparum* parasitemia density on hemoglobin concentrations among full-term, normal birth weight children in western Kenya, IV. The Asembo Bay Cohort Project. *Am J Trop Med Hyg.* 2000;62(4):504–12.
32. Bisoffi Z, Leoni S, Angheben A, et al. Chronic malaria and hyper-reactive malarial splenomegaly: A retrospective study on the largest series observed in a non-endemic country. *Malar J.* 2016;15:230.
33. Rogerson SJ, Desai M, Mayor A, Sicuri E, Taylor SM, van Eijk AM. Burden, pathology, and costs of malaria in pregnancy: New developments for an old problem. *Lancet Infect Dis.* 2018;18(4):e107–18.
34. Snow RW, Omumbo JA, Lowe B, et al. Relation between severe malaria morbidity in children and level of *Plasmodium falciparum* transmission in Africa. *Lancet.* 1997;349(9066):1650–4.
35. Oldenburg CE, Guerin PJ, Berthe F, Grais RF, Isanaka S. Malaria and nutritional status among children with severe acute malnutrition in Niger: A prospective cohort study. *Clin Infect Dis.* 2018;67(7):1027–34.
36. Wilson AL, Bradley J, Kandeh B, et al. Is chronic malnutrition associated with an increase in malaria incidence? A cohort study in children aged under 5 years in rural Gambia. *Parasit Vectors.* 2018;11(1):451.
37. Neuberger A, Okebe J, Yahav D, Paul M. Oral iron supplements for children in malaria-endemic areas. *Cochrane Database Syst Rev.* 2016;2(2):CD006589.
38. Mackintosh CL, Beeson JG, Marsh K. Clinical features and pathogenesis of severe malaria. *Trends Parasitol.* 2004;20(12):597–603.
39. Marsh K, English M, Crawley J, Peshu N. The pathogenesis of severe malaria in African children. *Ann Trop Med Parasitol.* 1996;90(4):395–402.
40. Njama-Meya D, Clark TD, Nzarubara B, Staedke S, Kamya MR, Dorsey G. Treatment of malaria restricted to laboratory-confirmed cases: A prospective cohort study in Ugandan children. *Malar J.* 2007;6(1):7.
41. World Health Organization. *Protocol for Estimating the Prevalence of pfhrp2/pfhrp3 Gene Deletions among Symptomatic Falciparum Patients with False-Negative RDT Results*. Geneva: World Health Organization; 2018.
42. Slater HC, Ross A, Ouedraogo AL, et al. Assessing the impact of next-generation rapid diagnostic tests on *Plasmodium falciparum* malaria elimination strategies. *Nature.* 2015;528(7580):S94–101.
43. Simmons RA, Mboera L, Miranda ML, et al. A longitudinal cohort study of malaria exposure and changing serostatus in a malaria endemic area of rural Tanzania. *Malar J.* 2017;16(1):309.
44. Masterson KM. *The Malaria Project: the US Government's Secret Mission to Find a Miracle Cure*. New York: New American Library; 2014.

45. Maguire JD, Sumawinata IW, Masbar S, et al. Chloroquine-resistant *Plasmodium malariae* in south Sumatra, Indonesia. *Lancet.* 2002;360(9326):58–60.
46. Siribie M, Ajayi IO, Nsungwa-Sabiiti J, et al. Compliance with referral advice after treatment with prereferral rectal artesunate: A study in 3 sub-Saharan African countries. *Clin Infect Dis.* 2016;63(Suppl 5):S283–9.
47. Tan KR, Wiegand RE, Arguin PM. Exchange transfusion for severe malaria: Evidence base and literature review. *Clin Infect Dis.* 2013;57(7):923–8.
48. Calvo-Cano A, Gomez-Junyent J, Lozano M, et al. The role of red blood cell exchange for severe imported malaria in the artesunate era: A retrospective cohort study in a referral centre. *Malar J.* 2016;15:216.
49. Maitland K, Kiguli S, Opoka RO, et al. Mortality after fluid bolus in African children with severe infection. *N Engl J Med.* 2011;364(26):2483–95.
50. Zucker JR, Lackritz EM, Ruebush TK2nd, et al. Childhood mortality during and after hospitalization in western Kenya: Effect of malaria treatment regimens. *Am J Trop Med Hyg.* 1996;55(6):655–60.
51. Centers for Disease Control and Prevention. Published reports of delayed hemolytic anemia after treatment with artesunate for severe malaria—worldwide, 2010–2012. *MMWR Morb Mortal Wkly Rep.* 2013;62(1): 5–8.
52. Walker PG, Griffin JT, Ferguson NM, Ghani AC. Estimating the most efficient allocation of interventions to achieve reductions in *Plasmodium falciparum* malaria burden and transmission in Africa: A modelling study. *Lancet Glob Health.* 2016;4(7):e474–84.
53. Lobo NF, Achee NL, Grieco J, Collins FH. Modern vector control. In: Wirth DF, Alonso PL, eds. *Malaria: Biology in the Era of Eradication.* Cold Spring Harbor: Cold Spring Harbor Laboratory Press; 2017, pp. 69–86.
54. Tusting LS, Thwing J, Sinclair D, et al. Mosquito larval source management for controlling malaria. *Cochrane Database Syst Rev.* 2013;(8):CD008923.
55. World Health Organization. *Pesticides and Their Application for the Control of Vectors and Pests of Public Health Importance*, 6th ed. Geneva: World Health Organization Pesticide Evaluation Scheme; 2006.
56. Walshe DP, Garner P, Adeel AA, Pyke GH, Burkot TR. Larvivorous fish for preventing malaria transmission. *Cochrane Database Syst Rev.* 2017;12(12):CD008090.
57. Maia MF, Kliner M, Richardson M, Lengeler C, Moore SJ. Mosquito repellents for malaria prevention. *Cochrane Database Syst Rev.* 2018;2(2):CD011595.
58. Bhatt S, Weiss DJ, Cameron E, et al. The effect of malaria control on *Plasmodium falciparum* in Africa between 2000 and 2015. *Nature.* 2015;526(7572):207–11.
59. Pryce J, Richardson M, Lengeler C. Insecticide-treated nets for preventing malaria. *Cochrane Database Syst Rev.* 2018;11(11):CD000363.
60. malERA Refresh Consultative Panel on Tools for Malaria Elimination. malERA: An updated research agenda for diagnostics, drugs, vaccines, and vector control in malaria elimination and eradication. *PLoS Med.* 2017;14(11):e1002455.
61. Pluess B, Tanser FC, Lengeler C, Sharp BL. Indoor residual spraying for preventing malaria. *Cochrane Database Syst Rev.* 2010;2010(4):CD006657.
62. Kleinschmidt I, Bradley J, Knox TB, et al. Implications of insecticide resistance for malaria vector control with long-lasting insecticidal nets: A WHO-coordinated, prospective, international, observational cohort study. *Lancet Infect Dis.* 2018;18(6):640–9.
63. malERA Refresh Consultative Panel on Insecticide and Drug Resistance. malERA: An updated research agenda for insecticide and drug resistance in malaria elimination and eradication. *PLoS Med.* 2017;14(11):e1002450.
64. Pryce J, Choi L, Richardson M, Malone D. Insecticide space spraying for preventing malaria transmission. *Cochrane Database Syst Rev.* 2018;11(11):CD012689.
65. Hazel E, Bryce J, The Iip-Jhu iCCM Evaluation Working Group. On bathwater, babies, and designing programs for impact: Evaluations of the integrated community case management strategy in Burkina Faso, Ethiopia, and Malawi. *Am J Trop Med Hyg.* 2016;94(3):568–70.
66. Tougher S, Mann AG, Group AC, et al. Improving access to malaria medicine through private-sector subsidies in seven African countries. *Health Aff (Millwood).* 2014;33(9):1576–85.
67. malERA Refresh Consultative Panel on Health Systems and Policy Research. malERA: An updated research agenda for health systems and policy research in malaria elimination and eradication. *PLoS Med.* 2017;14(11):e1002454.
68. Ghani AC. Can improving access to care help to eliminate malaria? *Lancet.* 2018;391(10133):1870–1.
69. Abdul-Ghani R, Beier JC. Strategic use of antimalarial drugs that block falciparum malaria parasite transmission to mosquitoes to achieve local malaria elimination. *Parasitol Res.* 2014;113(10):3535–46.
70. Okell LC, Drakeley CJ, Ghani AC, Bousema T, Sutherland CJ. Reduction of transmission from malaria patients by artemisinin combination therapies: A pooled analysis of six randomized trials. *Malar J.* 2008;7:125.
71. Taylor WR, Naw HK, Maitland K, et al. Single low-dose primaquine for blocking transmission of *Plasmodium falciparum* malaria—A proposed model-derived age-based regimen for sub-Saharan Africa. *BMC Med.* 2018;16(1):11.
72. World Health Organization. *Malaria Surveillance, Monitoring & Evaluation: A Reference Manual.* Geneva: World Health Organization; 2018.
73. World Health Organization. *A Framework for Malaria Elimination.* Geneva: World Health Organization; 2017.
74. Mace KE, Arguin PM, Tan KR. Malaria surveillance—United States, 2015. *MMWR Surveill Summ.* 2018;67(7):1–28.
75. Greenwood BM, David PH, Otoo-Forbes LN, et al. Mortality and morbidity from malaria after stopping malaria chemoprophylaxis. *Trans R Soc Trop Med Hyg.* 1995;89(6):629–33.
76. Clyde DF. Suppression of malaria in Tanzania with the use of medicated salt. *Bull World Health Organ.* 1966;35(6):962–8.
77. Athuman M, Kabanywanyi AM, Rohwer AC. Intermittent preventive antimalarial treatment for children with anaemia. *Cochrane Database Syst Rev.* 2015;1(1):CD010767.
78. Radeva-Petrova D, Kayentao K, ter Kuile FO, Sinclair D, Garner P. Drugs for preventing malaria in pregnant women in endemic areas: Any drug regimen versus placebo or no treatment. *Cochrane Database Syst Rev.* 2014;2014(10):CD000169.
79. Muanda FT, Chaabane S, Boukhris T, et al. Antimalarial drugs for preventing malaria during pregnancy and the risk of low birth weight: A systematic review and meta-analysis of randomized and quasi-randomized trials. *BMC Med.* 2015;13:193.
80. Schellenberg JR, Maokola W, Shirima K, et al. Cluster-randomized study of intermittent preventive treatment for malaria in infants (IPTi) in southern Tanzania: Evaluation of impact on survival. *Malar J.* 2011;10:387.
81. Meremikwu MM, Donegan S, Sinclair D, Esu E, Oringanje C. Intermittent preventive treatment for malaria in children living in areas with seasonal transmission. *Cochrane Database Syst Rev.* 2012;2012(2):CD003756.
82. Poirot E, Skarbinski J, Sinclair D, Kachur SP, Slutsker L, Hwang J. Mass drug administration for malaria. *Cochrane Database Syst Rev.* 2013;2013(12):CD008846.
83. Aregawi M, Smith SJ, Sillah-Kanu M, et al. Impact of the mass drug administration for malaria in response to the Ebola outbreak in Sierra Leone. *Malar J.* 2016;15:480.
84. Kuehne A, Tiffany A, Lasry E, et al. Impact and lessons learned from mass drug administrations of malaria chemoprevention during the Ebola outbreak in Monrovia, Liberia, 2014. *PLoS One.* 2016;11(8):e0161311.
85. Newby G, Hwang J, Koita K, et al. Review of mass drug administration for malaria and its operational challenges. *Am J Trop Med Hyg.* 2015;93(1):125–34.
86. Ouedraogo AL, Bastiaens GJ, Tiono AB, et al. Efficacy and safety of the mosquitocidal drug ivermectin to prevent malaria transmission after treatment: A double-blind, randomized, clinical trial. *Clin Infect Dis.* 2015;60(3):357–65.
87. Pooda HS, Rayaisse JB, Hien DF, et al. Administration of ivermectin to peridomestic cattle: a promising approach to target the residual transmission of human malaria. *Malar J.* 2015;13(Suppl 1):496.
88. Chaccour C, Rabinovich NR. Ivermectin to reduce malaria transmission II. Considerations regarding clinical development pathway. *Malar J.* 2017;16(1):166.
89. RTS,S Clinical Trials Partnership, Agnandji ST, Lell B, et al. A phase 3 trial of RTS,S/AS01 malaria vaccine in African infants. *N Engl J Med.* 2012;367(24):2284–95.
90. Jongo SA, Shekalaghe SA, Church LWP, et al. Safety, immunogenicity, and protective efficacy against controlled human malaria infection of *Plasmodium falciparum* sporozoite vaccine in Tanzanian adults. *Am J Trop Med Hyg.* 2018;99(2):338–49.
91. Seder RA, Chang LJ, Enama ME, et al. Protection against malaria by intravenous immunization with a nonreplicating sporozoite vaccine. *Science.* 2013;341(6152):1359–65.
92. Edge L. Benefiting from the Gates' billions. Where next for malaria? *Lancet Infect Dis.* 2008;8(5):269.
93. World Health Organization. *Update on the e-2020 Initiative of 21 Malaria-Eliminating Countries.* Geneva: World Health Organization; 2018.

CHAPTER

90

Vaccine Preventable Diseases

Vaccine Innovation and Development

Charlene M.C. Rodrigues • Lori Kestenbaum Handy • Barton F. Haynes • Stanley A. Plotkin

GENERAL

Vaccine manufacture began in humble academic laboratories such as that of Louis Pasteur in the Rue d'Ulm in Paris[1] or on the cow farms in which vaccinia was produced.[2] The results of vaccine application hardly needs emphasis, and numerous data testify to the impact of vaccination with regard to disease incidence, mortality, and economics.[3-8] However, by the beginning of the twentieth century, it was obvious that a large number of doses was needed and that standardization was necessary. At first this was accomplished in government laboratories but soon the scale of effort exceeded the personnel and facilities, and also the possibility of profit became evident, so that manufacture passed to pharmaceutical laboratories. These were concentrated in Europe and the United States. After the Second World War, when the number of routine vaccines increased, lawsuits against vaccine manufacturers began to increase sharply. The result was the withdrawal of some manufacturers from the vaccine field, and the contraction of the industry to four major players: GlaxoSmithKline, Merck, Pfizer, and Sanofi.

The development of the Vaccine Compensation System in 1986 rescued vaccine manufacturing, in that the United States government paid those who claimed damage from vaccination, often without proof of an association. This allowed commercial manufacturers immunity from most lawsuits, and brought new players into the field. Thus, organizations that have succeeded or are seeking to develop vaccines for the American market now include Janssen, Takeda, Astellas, and Dynavax, among others. In addition, the growing economies in other countries allowed for the growth of many companies that were producing vaccines for domestic markets, but which had aspirations for selling in foreign markets. These include notably, Serum Institute of India, Bharat, Biological E, Butantan, Indonesia, Sinovac, Chengdu, and Commonwealth Serum Laboratories. Thus, the vaccine industry is once again strong and fertile.

However, problems remain. The cost of vaccine development to the point of registration, has mounted considerably. There have been variable estimates, but half a billion dollars for development of a new vaccine appears to be a reasonable one.[9] Nevertheless, the cost of the Sanofi developed vaccine against dengue exceeded 1 billion dollars, and it appears that Dengvaxia will not give return on investment because of unanticipated safety problems.[10] The length of time for vaccine development from the end of preclinical research to licensure has also become elongated, 11 years being about average. In addition, most projects end in failure.[11]

These difficulties have been inhibitory to vaccine development in two ways. First, it inhibits companies from investing in vaccines with small markets or markets predominantly in developing countries. Second, the research and development costs are not afforded by most companies in the developing world, although that is beginning to change for the better. A consequence of the difficulties has been the birth of the Coalition for Epidemic Preparedness (CEPI), an organization funded by multiple countries and charitable organizations specifically to develop vaccines for emerging (usually tropical) diseases.[12-14] Ideally, CEPI would develop a vaccine before the disease has a high incidence in order to prevent epidemics. However, CEPI already has a considerable task to develop vaccines against already prevalent diseases like Lassa fever, Nipah, and Chikungunya.

Once vaccines have been developed the question arises as to who will pay for the number of doses necessary for control of the disease. Fortunately, there are at least three organizations that support purchase of vaccines for poor countries: GAVI, the Gates Foundation, and PATH. Without those organizations the world would be in bad shape, since many countries cannot afford to buy vaccines on the open market. Yet, the cost of vaccines is still an inhibitory factor to vaccination. An example from our experience may serve: the Palestinian territories are unable to buy vaccines at standard prices. A private foundation, the Rostropovich-Vishnevskaya Foundation has supported the introduction of pneumococcal and rotavirus vaccines based on prices negotiated with the manufacturers that are almost as low as GAVI prices.[15] Arrangements such as this, together with those mentioned above, are allowing vaccination of at least 80% of the world's children, but there is much that remains to be done.

UNSOLVED PROBLEMS IN VACCINE DEVELOPMENT

By and large current vaccines were developed by attenuation or inactivation of replicating agents, with the aim that on injection or oral administration they will induce a protective antibody response. The only exceptions have been vaccines against zoster, which protect against the reactivation of varicella virus through reactivation of cellular immune responses, and against tuberculosis, where the correlate of protection is unknown but is also thought to be a cellular immune response.[16] As the current disease targets of vaccine development have more complex strategies of disease causation, vaccine development must also solve more immunologic difficulties. Thus, vaccinologists are looking toward the future and the use of new technologies.[17-19]

For example, a problem that vexes vaccination against both pertussis and mumps is loss of immune memory.[20,21] With regard to pertussis, immunity in school children and adolescents is rapidly lost after booster doses of vaccines containing only protective antigens (acellular vaccines) without whole cells of *Bordetella pertussis*. The immunological basis of this problem is known: acellular vaccines evoke Th2 responses without the Th1 and Th17 responses that the older whole cell vaccine evoked.[22,23] The lack of IL-17 permits persistence of the organism in the throat and increasing susceptibility with time to expression of virulence factors by the organism. The most obvious approach to solving this problem is the addition of an adjuvant to pertussis vaccines that evokes stronger responses.

However, changing later in life the Th2 orientation given in infancy to a Th1 orientation has not yet been achieved. An attenuated *Bordetella pertussis* under current development, is the best candidate and might be successful.[24]

A vaccine against the human immunodeficiency virus (HIV) has long been a goal, but has been frustrating.[25,26] Most efforts have been directed towards eliciting neutralizing antibodies directed against the V3 loop, the CD4 binding site, or the gp41. Now it appears that non-neutralizing antibodies against the V1/V2 loop may play a major role in protection, as shown in the vaccine trial conducted in Thailand.[27] Trials in Africa are now in motion and will tell us if antibodies can be protective. Another lead toward prevention is the ability of SIV proteins carried by rhesus cytomegalovirus (CMV) to evoke HLA-e cytotoxicity that is able to abort SIV infections.[28]

Whereas rotavirus vaccination has been spectacularly successful in the United States and Europe, efficacy has been much less in developing countries due to interference with replication of the vaccine viruses.[29] Although transplacental maternal antibodies, breast milk antibodies, and simultaneous oral polio vaccine may decrease efficacy, the main problem seems to be the effect of the microbiome.[30,31] It is not yet clear which organisms in the intestine are responsible for interference with viral replication, but current studies should clarify matters.

There are many unsolved general problems for vaccinology. Certainly, generation of long immune memory is one, as mentioned for pertussis and mumps, but it applies to most inactivated vaccines, including the old standbys of tetanus and diphtheria.[32,33] Even Natural Killer (NK) cells can develop memory.[34] Adjuvants that strongly stimulate innate immunity, perhaps through Toll-like receptors, are helpful in prolonging immunity.[35] Identification of broadly protective epitopes is another issue, particularly for influenza and HIV vaccines.[36,37] The answer seems to lie in structural biology analysis of where epitopes are hidden or masked by glycan groups.

The identification of correlates of protection is another important area. As we learn more about them, we realize that they may be mechanistic or nonmechanistic, and that they are often much more complex than we first thought.[38–40] The discovery that NK cells may have memory has been an eye opener, and it is obvious that B cell, T cell, and NK functions may all be important. Moreover, it is clear that antibody has many different functions, not only neutralization. For example, antibody-dependent cellular cytotoxic antibodies have been shown to be a correlate of protection in the case of HIV,[41] and antibody-dependent cellular phagocytosis to be important in protection against CMV.[42] Fc receptor functions may be important for broad protection against influenza.[43] Moreover, correlates of protection may replace each other: in other words, in the absence of antibody, cellular response may protect, and in the absence of cellular responses, high antibody levels may protect. It is hoped that systems biology will identify gene functions that could serve as correlates of protection.

Vaccination at both the beginning and end of life presents special problems. Infants lack lymph nodes containing T follicular helper (Tfh) cells, and therefore require multiple injections to mount good immune responses. Fortunately, that situation seems to change at 1–2 years of age.[44] On the other hand, the elderly have reduced ability to respond with either arm of the immune system, but may make aberrant responses. After age 50 it is clear that T cell immunity is not good: after all T stands for thymus, which atrophies with age.[45,46]

Another important difficulty is to find other routes of immunization besides intramuscular or subcutaneous. Of course, there are vaccines given orally, but they are agents that replicate in the gastrointestinal tract. The problem is that the GI tract is constructed so as not to respond to antigens in the lumen that do not invade cells. Perhaps sublingual administration is a way around this problem.[47] More basic is the difficulty in producing prolonged mucosal responses, which tend to fade with time.[48] That being said, the use of vectors carrying vaccine antigens which can replicate in the gastrointestinal tract, requires more exploration.

Perhaps the solution to these problems lies in the so-called "omics."[49] These include genomics to identify conserved protective antigens; transcriptomics to identify proteins produced at different stages of infection; proteomics to analyze those proteins; antigenomics to identify host responses to those proteins; and adversomics to identify people genetically likely to have reactions to vaccines. Systems serology may also identify protective mechanisms.[50] These analytic methods might allow us to create synthetic vaccines from scratch, which could make them safer and more immunogenic.

In addition, we need to learn more about the influence of the microbiome on vaccine responses. That influence has already become evident with regard to the success or failure of rotavirus vaccine in developing countries.[51] Although there is an impact of maternal antibodies and interference with other oral vaccines on rotavirus immunization, the main factor seems to be the microbial flora of the intestine, and the future lies in changing the microbiome or giving vaccine early in life before the establishment of the microbiome.[52]

THE VACCINE INDUSTRY

There are numerous companies throughout the world that sell vaccines. However, only some of those actually make the vaccines they sell, and only a small number of manufacturers are engaged in vaccine research and development. Over the years their number has shrunk because of the sophistication and cost required for modern vaccinology. In the latter group are the four major European and American manufacturers: Glaxo SmithKline, Merck, Pfizer, and Sanofi (Box 90-1). Of lesser size but still important in vaccine development in developed countries are Astellas (Japan), CSL (Australia), Johnson & Johnson (U.S. and Netherlands), and Takeda (Japan). Indian companies, including the Serum Institute, Bharat and Biological E are rapidly ramping up their development departments. Butantan is important in Brazil and there are numerous Chinese manufacturers, including Sinovac and Chengdu (Box 90-2).

The problems are similar for all the manufacturers, although to a variable degree: cost, time, and regulatory barriers. At least in the United States and Europe, the cost of development for a new vaccine varies between $500 million and over $1 billion.[9] The interval between initial research and a licensed vaccine is variable but is generally over 15 years.[11] So far, no manufacturer outside developed

BOX 90-1 The "Big Four" Vaccine Manufacturers

GlaxoSmithKline
Merck
Pfizer-Wyeth
Sanofi Pasteur

BOX 90-2 Vaccine Manufacturers with Smaller Market Share or Limited Range

Johnson & Johnson	Avant
MedImmune-AstraZeneca	Bharat
Serum Institute of India	Bioport
	Emergent
	ID Biomedical
	Solvay
	Statens Serum Inst.
	Takeda

countries has succeeded in obtaining a license from the U.S. Food and Drug Administration (FDA) or the European Medicines Agency.

Thus, the future must hold solutions that will allow developing world manufacturers to supply their citizens with the vaccines of the future. Either they will have to upgrade their manufacturing facilities and controls or buy technology from the developed world manufacturers. We believe that eventually they will improve their standards to allow development and manufacture to occur locally, particularly as many diseases have markets only in parts of the world that have no interest for the major manufacturers.

SELECTED PROBLEMS IN VACCINE DEVELOPMENT

Maternal Vaccination: Optimizing Vaccination Strategies

Immunizations are most effective when given to an individual prior to entering the period of highest risk for acquiring the infection. Currently, the infant vaccination schedule is initiated at quite a young age (2 months in the United States, 6 weeks in many low- and middle-income countries). Even so, this leaves infants at risk for the period before they have completed their primary series, which is between 14 weeks in low-income countries and 6 months of age throughout the rest of the world. For this reason, administering vaccines to pregnant women to provide passive immunity would optimize the protection that can be offered. Currently in the United States, pregnant women are recommended to receive inactivated influenza and a combined tetanus-diphtheria-acellular pertussis (Tdap) vaccine.[53]

To support expansion of a maternal vaccination platform, understanding response to vaccination during the gestational period is critical. Pregnancy has been considered an immunosuppressed state, though recent data from animal models demonstrate that the immune system is dynamic throughout gestation, with changing levels of hormones.[54] The majority of studies measuring antibody response to vaccination while pregnant have been conducted related to inactivated influenza vaccine, though response to yellow fever vaccine and pertussis vaccine have also been conducted. Studies of influenza vaccination and yellow fever vaccine have inconclusive results by measurement of antibody alone, with some evidence supporting lower immunogenicity of influenza vaccine or yellow fever vaccine in pregnant women compared to nonpregnant women, while others demonstrate equivalent response.[55–58] Due to the changes in hormone levels throughout pregnancy, timing may also impact immunogenicity, with evidence for pertussis vaccination to be most effective at 27–30 weeks.[59]

Effectiveness data, however, demonstrate clear benefit for pregnant women and their infants. Randomized controlled trials have been relatively small, but epidemiologic studies of 250,000 women in the United States demonstrated an 83% reduction in hospitalizations with laboratory confirmed influenza in vaccinated women.[60] An analysis of multiple randomized controlled trials of infants born to mothers receiving influenza vaccine, demonstrated approximately 20% reduction in severe pneumonia in young infants, while a retrospective study of a cohort of infants in the United States estimated effectiveness at 25%.[61,62] Vaccine effectiveness for infants of pertussis vaccination during pregnancy in the United Kingdom was found to be 91% (CI 84–95%).[63]

Transfer of maternal IgG must be done efficiently to protect the neonate until the infant is old enough to receive vaccination.[64] Pertussis vaccination is an excellent example of this phenomenon. A vaccination trial of pregnant women with Tdap resulted in high concentrations of pertussis antibodies in the first 2 months of life.[65] Additional factors may impact IgG transfer, such as co infections in the mother and her nutritional state, though infections of concern such as malaria and HIV, require further study for conclusive results.[66] With the demonstrated capabilities of the maternal platform, there has been increased attention to creating vaccines for maternal vaccination for both respiratory syncytial virus (RSV) and group B streptococcus (GBS). Because of concerns about induction of disease-enhancing immune responses, maternal vaccination circumvents this issue as maternal antibodies are transferred without the aberrant vaccine-associated response. As adult women have already had significant exposures to RSV, they have minimal risk for having enhanced RSV disease themselves.[67–69]

Current public health measures aimed at reducing neonatal GBS infections focus on reducing burden of GBS present by use of intrapartum antibiotics. While this has definitely reduced early-onset disease, it has not impacted late-onset disease and GBS remains a leading cause of neonatal infection.[70] A maternal GBS vaccine would be most effective for reducing the burden of late onset GBS invasive disease. Research has focused on development of a GBS vaccine since the 1990s. Worldwide, disease is caused by a number of serotypes (Ia, Ib, II, III, and V) and a maternal vaccine would need to address all of these serotypes. Recently, a trivalent GBS polysaccharide-protein conjugate vaccine was studied, but likely will not be further tested. Additional candidate vaccines are described below. Trials are challenged by lack of a correlate of disease, which is needed, due to the relatively low rate of outcomes.[71]

While maternal vaccination for influenza, pertussis, GBS, and RSV have been extensively studied, an additional barrier to effectiveness at the population level is increasing acceptance of a maternal vaccination platform. Currently, only 53.6% of pregnant women receive influenza vaccine, and 50% receive Tdap.[72,73] As the science of maternal vaccination needs to move forward, the acceptability of the practice also needs to advance for this to be effective. For maternal immunization to be effective, a program requires strong provider "buy in" for immunization including office champions and appropriate reimbursement. Logistical challenges, such as having a nurse available to provide the vaccine, need to be overcome. Optimal timing of vaccination needs to be determined. IgG transfer occurs robustly during the third trimester, and is dependent on maternal levels of IgG. Timing of vaccination of the mother must therefore occur to maximize maternal IgG levels during the third trimester.[74] Current literature indicates that second trimester vaccination for pertussis maximizes antibody transfer, while ideal timing of vaccination for influenza is unclear.[75–77] Effective communication is needed to increase acceptance of maternal vaccination to protect infants.[78]

Consideration should include not only the benefits to infants born to mothers vaccinated during pregnancy, but also the protection provided to the mother from diseases known to be more severe in pregnant women, namely, influenza. During pregnancy, women have varied immune responses and are more susceptible to influenza due to altered cell-mediated immunity.[79] The only other vaccinations considered for use during pregnancy for maternal protection are those related to maternal exposures, such as yellow fever and anthrax. In the event of an exposure, the risks and benefits need to be weighed, to determine the value of maternal vaccination.

Concerns have been raised that maternal antibodies, both due to prior infections in a mother as well as vaccination, can interfere with an infant's own vaccine response.[44,80] Immune responses in infants after their 2-, 4-, and 6-month DTaP vaccines were lower in those infants born to vaccinated mothers, but by the time of their 12- to 18-month booster, antibody levels in infants born to either vaccinated or unvaccinated mothers were equivalent. Additional studies have had conflicting results which are challenging to interpret, as the definite correlate for protection by pertussis immunization remains unknown.[44] Widespread use of maternal vaccination will require further study on the impact on clinical effectiveness of the primary vaccination series.[81]

The regulatory challenges of bringing new vaccines to market is even more pronounced when trying to develop vaccines effective in the neonate. Pregnant women at this time are generally excluded from prelicensure clinical trials of vaccines.[82] A significant amount of safety data are therefore collected postlicensure, when a pregnant woman is vaccinated prior to recognizing she is pregnant. Data through safety registries are therefore the best mechanism for understanding safety in pregnant women. However, to truly determine the effectiveness of utilizing the maternal platform to protect neonates, regulations will need to be changed to include pregnant women in trials.[83] Despite these challenges, the current evidence supporting maternal immunization indicates that more widespread vaccination would likely reduce vaccine-preventable diseases in neonates.[84]

SELECTED PROBLEMS IN VACCINE DEVELOPMENT

Cytomegalovirus: A Complex Pathogenesis

Pathogen Description

The human CMV is ubiquitous and the cause of many different clinical manifestations. Most prominently, CMV is the most prevalent cause of congenital malformation, and the most common infectious complications of both solid organ and hematogenous stem cell transplantation.[85–87] CMV is also suspected to play a role, though still poorly defined, in immunosenescence, glioblastoma, and atherosclerosis.[88–90] Thus, this virus, which ultimately infects the vast majority of the world's population, deserves considerable study and the development of prophylactic measures. Antiviral drugs to treat or prevent CMV infection are available and used both in infants and transplant recipients, but will not be discussed in this chapter.[91]

Epidemiology

CMV is excreted in pharyngeal secretions, including saliva, and in urine.[92,93] Toddlers are thought to be the principal sources of infection,[94] although CMV may be transmitted between adults via the same secretions and perhaps also through sexual intercourse. In developed countries, approximately 50% of women of child-bearing age have been previously infected and are seropositive, whereas in developing countries almost all adults have been previously infected.[95] However, seropositive individuals may be chronically excreting the virus and congenital infections take place even where seropositivity is almost 100%.[96]

Nevertheless, multiple facts argue for the possibility of prevention of CMV infection by vaccination. In seropositive pregnant women it has been demonstrated that infection can still occur, particularly in settings where there are multiple exposures from children.[96–99] However, whereas CMV infection in seronegative women during early pregnancy results in 30–40% affected infants, similar infection in seropositive women results in a much lower percentage, variously estimated as 3–10%.[100,101] Thus, prior CMV infection does confer protection against fetalinjury.

Challenges in Vaccine Development

Unfortunately, the correlates of protection afforded by natural infection or vaccination are not well established. However, it is reasonably clear that they revolve around three viral antigens: the gB surface glycoprotein, the gH/gL/UL128/UL130/UL131 surface pentamer, and the pp65 tegument protein.[102–104] Antibodies to the gB glycoprotein were shown to protect women against natural acquisition of CMV and to prevent solid organ transplant recipients from CMV carried in the transplanted organ.[105–107] Interestingly, the protective antibodies to gB were non-neutralizing and possibly functioning to phagocytose virus,[108] but in any case gB would be an essential part of a vaccine if its efficacy can be augmented by adjuvantation or other means. Moreover, the protective functions of gB relate to CD4+ T cell responses, as well as B cell responses.[103,109,110]

The pp65 tegument protein is certainly not the only CMV inducer of CD8+ T cells, but together with the nonstructural immediate-early proteins is the most likely to generate cellular immunity.[87,111,112] It has been possible to present pp65 to the immune system by several means, resulting in cellular responses that protected against reactivation of CMV. However, whereas those responses appear critical to protection against reactivation of the virus in hematogenous stem cell recipients, it is not certain that they are necessary to protect pregnant women against acquisition.

The pentamer protein complex is key to a complete vaccine. Most of the neutralizing antibodies in naturally seropositive individuals are directed against the pentamer and those antibodies are responsible for prevention of entry into epithelial cells, in contrast to gB antibodies, which only prevent entry into fibroblasts.[113,114] Thus, current efforts to develop vaccines against congenital infection usually, though not always, focus on the pentamer as a key component.

Development of candidate vaccines against CMV began as long ago as the 1970s, but was slowed by a general lack of appreciation concerning the importance of congenital infection.[115–117] However, in 2001 the National Academy of Medicine (then the Institute of Medicine) issued a report on vaccines that ranked a CMV vaccine among the highest priority for development, citing the evidence for frequent causation of congenital abnormalities in infants infected during pregnancy.[118] This report caused vaccine companies to reassess CMV as a target, and eventually vaccine development projects were launched by GSK, Merck, Pfizer, and Sanofi, in addition to numerous biotechnology firms and academic laboratories. The result is a profusion of candidate vaccines, among which many have progressed to clinical testing. Table 90-1 lists these many candidates.

As stated above, the candidate vaccines turn on the presentation of gB, pentamer, and pp65; the former two antigens in order to prevent congenital infection, whereas the latter antigen is needed for CD8+ T cell control, particularly in hematogenous stem cell transplant recipients. The approaches that should stimulate responses to all three antigens are the replication defective virus of Merck and the purified dense bodies of Serum Institute of India.[119,120] Attenuated viruses, such as the reassortants of attenuated and low-passage CMV strains produced by MedImmune, do not express the pentamer.[121] The pentamer has been synthesized by GSK, Humabs, and Redbiotech. City of Hope uses peptides from the pentamer.[113,122] Many organizations have produced gB by inserting the gene in viral vectors, including the Queensland Institute, GSK, Hookipa, City of Hope, Sanofi, and Yale University.[111,123–126] DNA plasmids have been created by Astellas

TABLE 90-1 CMV VACCINES IN DEVELOPMENT

Type of vaccine	Developer
Attenuated strain (Towne)	Wistar Inst./Med Coll VA
Recombinants with wild virus (Towne-Toledo)	Medimmune
Replication-defective virus	Merck
Vectored:	
Canary Pox	Sanofi
MVA	City of Hope
Adeno	Queensland Inst.
LCMV	Hookipa
VSV	Yale
Recombinant gB glycoprotein with adjuvant	Sanofi Pasteur, GSK
Soluble Pentamers	Redbiotech, GSK, Humabs
DNA plasmids	Astellas, Inovio
Self-replicating RNA	Moderna
Peptides	City of Hope
Dense bodies	Vaccine Project Management (Germany) and Serum Inst. India
Virus-like particles	Variations Bio

and Invovio that express gB,[88,95] and Moderna has used mRNA for the same purpose.[127]

At the time of writing, a limited number of vaccine candidates have progressed to clinical trials, including attenuated strains, reassortant attenuated strains, subunit gB, alphavirus-vectored replicons, canarypox vector, the replication-defective virus, the gB virus-like particle vaccine of Variations Bio, and the DNA gB/pp65 vaccine of Astellas. The City of Hope is testing MVA vectored CMV antigens and peptide antigens in the hope of preventing CMV disease after transplantation.[105–107,111,116,119–121,123,128]

Thus, there is a profusion of vaccine candidates, but none so far has been tested for efficacy in prevention of congenital infection. Some efficacy was shown in clinical trials of the Sanofi gB vaccine to prevent acquisition of CMV by seronegative women,[105,106] and considerable efficacy was shown by the same vaccine in the prevention of CMV disease after solid organ transplantation.[107] However, a successful vaccine for congenital CMV infection must show either high efficacy in prevention of acquisition by women, or high efficacy in preventing maternal infection from passing to the fetus. A successful vaccine for transplant patients should induce gB antibody and CD8+ T cells to prevent reactivation of CMV in the presence of immunosuppression.

However, even if the goal of vaccine prevention is difficult to reach, efforts must continue because of the worldwide importance of congenital CMV infection and its contribution to morbidity after transplantation.[96,129–131] With regard to congenital infection in naturally seropositive women, the immediate goal is to define whether it occurs by chance due to high exposure, or if a deficiency of acquired immune functions is responsible. In the latter case, a vaccine could restore protection against transplacental passage of the virus.

Even if it is not possible to prevent congenital infection in the developing country situation where exposure to CMV is constant, a vaccine for seronegative women in developed countries where exposure is occasional, would still be worthwhile on condition that such a vaccine would provide a reasonable duration of protection during the child-bearing years. If a vaccine could prevent or reduce viral excretion, vaccination of toddlers could be contemplated to interrupt circulation and reduce exposure of their mothers to CMV.

Understanding Host Immunity

Inasmuch as it is clear that natural immunity is imperfect, a key question is whether immune responses to a vaccine can prevent CMV infection during later exposure. It is known that proteins produced by the US2-11 genes act to inhibit HLA-mediated responses, and perhaps immunization against those proteins might help.[132] However, only vaccines containing full length genomes could do that.

There are a number of unanswered questions about vaccine prevention, including whether or not cellular immune responses are needed to prevent maternal-fetal transmission, whether boosting antibody responses could prevent infection in seropositives, and whether a vaccine could protect women throughout their child-bearing years.[42,95,108]

To demonstrate efficacy of a CMV vaccine several courses can be envisaged. Artificial challenge of volunteers with a low-passage virus, which was done in the past, could demonstrate resistance.[133] However, more acceptable would be to show protection of women whose children are in day care, where they are likely to acquire CMV and to thereby expose their mothers. Considering that infants are the most likely source of infection, it has been suggested that they should be the target of vaccination in order to protect their mothers.[10] Nevertheless, the FDA has indicated that it would prefer a study in which vaccinated women are followed through subsequent pregnancies, with demonstration that their newborns are uninfected by CMV.[134]

Demonstration of efficacy in transplant patients should be relatively simple. However, one must distinguish between solid organ transplant recipients, in whom the problem is CMV contained in the transplanted organ, and hematogenous stem cell transplant recipients, in whom reactivation of a prior CMV infection under immunosuppression is the risk.[107,120] In both cases, the endpoints would be lowered viral load, less use of antivirals, and most important, less rejection of the graft.

Thus, the probable first targets for CMV vaccination would be preadolescent girls in association with other vaccines given at that age, seronegative women of child-bearing age, transplant recipients, and perhaps all infants, to reduce viral circulation.[42,95,108]

SELECTED PROBLEMS IN VACCINE DEVELOPMENT

Dengue Vaccines: Understanding the Correlates of Protection

Pathogen Description and Epidemiology

Dengue virus is a single-stranded RNA virus, from the Flavivirus family. The flaviviruses are transmitted via arthropod vectors. There are four serotypes of dengue viruses that are antigenically distinct, namely DENV-1, DENV-2, DENV-3, and DENV-4. Infection with dengue virus requires the vector, genus *Aedes* mosquitoes, to be present to transmit the disease, most commonly *A. aegypti* and *A. albopictus*. Regions that have endemic dengue disease include tropical and subtropical areas of Asia, the Pacific, Americas, Caribbean, and Africa, in particular urban and semiurban areas. In some areas of Asia and South America, severe dengue is a major cause of morbidity and mortality amongst children.[135] In these regions, most people are seropositive, reflecting the degree of exposure and infection. Infection confers long-term immunity with serotype-specific antibodies, but only short-lived immunity to other serotypes.[136,137] As this cross-protection wanes, the individual is then more at risk of severe dengue following a future infection with a different serotype to the original infection. Outside of endemic regions, dengue virus is now being seen in more temperate regions including southern Europe. Dengue virus is transmitted to humans following a bite from *Aedes* mosquitoes, with an incubation period of 4–10 days.

Clinical Disease

Patients who acquire dengue virus may be asymptomatic. In 2009, the World Health Organization (WHO) classification for disease severity categorized into dengue without warning signs, dengue with warning signs, and severe dengue, in an attempt to stratify management responses.[138] Patients presenting with fever and two of nausea/vomiting, rash, myalgia/arthralgia, leukopenia, and a positive tourniquet test were considered to have dengue without warning signs. Warning signs that require further medical evaluation and intervention include; abdominal pain, persistent vomiting, extracellular fluid accumulation, mucosal bleeding, lethargy, hepatomegaly of > 2 cm or hematological changes including increasing hematocrit with decreasing platelet count. Severe dengue includes the presence of plasma leak with shock or respiratory distress secondary to pulmonary edema, severe hemorrhage, or other organ involvement. Management is largely supportive of fluid, metabolic and blood product requirements and with timely and appropriate management mortality can be controlled at $< 1\%$.[139] The major concern with dengue infection occurs the second time a person is infected with a different serotype to the first infection. For reasons that remain unclear, there is a heightened immune response on reinfection with a different serotype. This is of particular concern in children and the elderly who have higher mortality rates from severe dengue (also known as dengue hemorrhagic fever or dengue shock syndrome).

Prior Vaccine Development

There were no licensed vaccines for dengue fever until 2015, so prior to this measures to reduce dengue disease were focused on vector control. One reason for the lack of vaccine development was the poor understanding of the immune response to dengue fever and immune enhancement observed with secondary infection. In 2015, the first dengue vaccine CYD-TDV was licensed for use in endemic regions. It is a live, attenuated, tetravalent vaccine containing recombinant chimeric virus premembrane (prM) and envelope (E) proteins from all four serotypes. These are all inserted into the 17D yellow fever vaccine backbone, with the aim on inducing antibodies to all serotypes.

Challenges with Vaccines on the Market or Vaccines in Development

The CYD-TDV vaccine was highly anticipated for the prevention of a disease that has been considered neglected in many regions of the world. With increasing rates of dengue disease due to factors such as population growth, climate change, globalization, and travel, a vaccine would not only reduce morbidity and mortality, but also the strain it placed on developing healthcare settings. The aim had been to develop a vaccine that induced equal immunity to all four serotypes in order to prevent the immune enhancement seen with heterotypic reinfection. Large clinical trials took place in South America and Asia with overall efficacy reported as 56.5–60.8%.[140,141] However, the efficacy varied between serotypes, with 74.9% efficacy against serotype 3 and 76.6% efficacy against serotype 4. Lowest efficacy was observed against serotype 2 (39.6%) and serotype 1 (50.2%). Many reasons have been suggested for this apparent variability in host responses to different serotypes which include serotype-specific differences in the dose of antigen required to induce a protective response, variable antibody titers required to confer protection against clinical disease, and the different pathogenesis of serotype 2 virus which precipitously infect monocytes and poorly replicates, potentially lessening the functional role of antibodies. There have been observations that HLA type may be involved in determining the degree of and breadth of CD8 T cell responses, independent of antibody production.[142]

Further, structural changes that occur during vaccine development and administration, may affect the epitopes presented to the immune system and their responses to them. The chimeric E protein contained in the vaccine may take on a different conformational shape than the naturally occurring protein. Further studies of the antigens' physical arrangements, identified that dimers of E protein were found to be tightly packed on the viral surface at 28°C when cultured in mosquito cells.[143] When the virus was exposed to temperatures above 34°C (human body temperature is generally exceeds 36°C), irreversible changes in this arrangement occurred, with spaces opening up and exposing viral membrane.[144,145] E protein plays an important role in during the entry of the virus into host cells, and antibodies to the E protein can interfere with this process, so it is important to understand the inadvertent alterations to key antigenic epitopes.

There remains no accepted correlate of protection for measuring the immunogenicity to CYD-TDV. During clinical trials, serotype-specific neutralizing antibodies were measured and noted to be higher in seropositive individuals compared to seronegative individuals at the point of vaccination. However, the relationship between titers of this neutralizing antibody and protection against clinical disease is still under evaluation. As mentioned earlier, T cell responses are also likely to be important in protection to dengue virus, but the mechanism remains unclear and there is no clear marker which can be defined and measured. Thus, primary endpoints in efficacy trials were virologically confirmed dengue infection. CYD-TDV was licensed for use in endemic regions only and in individuals aged 9 years and older, due to safety concerns in children aged 2–5 years. There was an increased rate of hospitalization with dengue illness, in the 2- to 5-year-old group, during the first- and second-year post dose 1 of the vaccine. The proposed explanations include the fact that a higher proportion of this age group is likely to be seronegative, and in these individuals, the vaccine may be acting like a first episode of natural infection, thereby priming them for immune enhancement at the next infection. As young children, they are also more likely to suffer from severe illness compared to older children and adults. It remains to be seen how effective the first dengue vaccine is, which because of the safety issues is recommended only in previously infected individuals. The safety concerns identified through clinical trials, highlight the importance of understanding the natural immunity to a disease in order to determine meaningful correlates of protection.

SELECTED PROBLEMS IN VACCINE DEVELOPMENT

Human Immunodeficiency Virus

Pathogen Description and Epidemiology

In 2017, there were 1.8 million new HIV infections, 37 million people globally living with HIV, and 15 million of those did not have access to antiretroviral therapy (www.unaids.org). Thus, while treatment of HIV infection can prevent the development of AIDS and death, development of an efficacious AIDS vaccine remains a major global priority to combine with other preventive and therapeutic modalities to end the AIDS epidemic.[146] While HIV, a lentivirus, was discovered in 1983[147] and shown to be the cause of AIDS in 1984,[148] no efficacious vaccine has been approved to prevent HIV infection. The reasons the HIV vaccine has been so difficult to develop are multifactorial and include HIV diversity, the ability of HIV to integrate into the host genome, decoration of the HIV envelope with dense glycans and host control of induction of protective neutralizing antibodies.[149] There are three types of potentially protective immune responses to HIV, (1) difficult-to-induce broadly neutralizing antibodies (bnAbs) that can neutralize diverse transmitted founder (TF) HIV strains,[150] (2) easy-to-induce antibodies that do not neutralize TF viruses but do recognize envelope epitopes on the surface of HIV-infected CD4 T cells (nonneutralizing antibodies, NNAbs),[40] and (3) CD8+ T cell responses that eliminate HIV-infected T cells.[151]

Induction of bnAbs by an HIV vaccine would be the most desirable outcome for HIV vaccine development.[149] While bnAbs occur in up to 50% of HIV-infected individuals over time, they have not been induced in humans with current investigational vaccines. The roadblocks to bnAb induction are control of some bnAb induction and expansion by host immune tolerance mechanisms,[152] the need for extensive somatic mutations for bnAb maturation,[149] and the requirement for multiple antibody insertions and deletions for acquisition of the ability to neutralize HIV.[153] The sites on the HIV envelope on virions are well guarded by glycans such that the shape and type of antibodies that can recognize bnAb Env epitopes can be both restricted and unusual.[154] For example, bnAbs have either long HCDR3 regions required to reach between glycans but this trait also predisposes the B cells with such B cell receptors to be vulnerable to immune tolerance controls.[155] Other classes of bnAbs that bind to the CD4 binding site all utilized the same or similar immunoglobulin heavy-chain variable genes.[150,154] Virtually all bnAbs isolated from HIV-infected individuals have unusually high levels of somatic mutations, a trait thought to reflect the tortuous and disfavored status of bnAbs.[149] Finally, bnAbs require very improbable mutations[156] or insertions or deletions[154] to achieve neutralizing status, thus further preventing bnAb affinity maturation.

Antibodies that do not bind to the native trimer and do not neutralize virions, can bind to the surface of HIV-infected cells and mediate antibody-dependent cellular cytotoxicity or other Fc receptor-mediated anti-HIV activities.[40] Indeed, these types of antibody effector mechanisms were the correlates of decreased transmission risk in the only HIV efficacy trial that showed any protection, the ALVAC/AIDSVAX B/E RV144 trial in Thailand.[157,158] However, these types of antibodies are not as potent nor broad as bnAbs.

Finally, CD8+ cytotoxic T lymphocytes (CTL) can kill HIV-infected CD4 T cells but frequently escape MHC class-1a-mediated HIV peptide recognition.[159] Recently however, a vaccine delivered by rhesus cytomegalovirus (rhCMV) has protected 50% of macaques from persistent simian immunodeficiency virus (SIV) infection by inducing CD8+ CTL that kill SIV-infected CD4+ T cells by nonclassical HLA-E peptide recognition.[151]

Prior Vaccine Development: HIV Vaccine or Neutralizing Antibody Administration Efficacy Trials

Table 90-2 outlines HIV vaccine or bnAb administration efficacy trials that are completed or ongoing. Trials testing either dual gp120s in alum and antibody induction (Vax003, Vax004)[160,161] or adenovirus type 5 for CD8 T cell induction (HVTN 502, HVTN 503)[162,163] showed no efficacy, and both the latter adenovirus type 5 trials showed enhanced infection with the vaccine, likely by activating CD4 cells by the vaccine, thus promoting infection. Addition of DNA prime to recombinant adenovirus type 5 with multiclade Envs likewise showed no vaccine efficacy (HVTN 505).[164]

The only HIV vaccine trial to date to show any efficacy was the ALVAC/AIDSVAX B/E gp120 trial that showed an estimated 60% efficacy at 12 months that declined rapidly to 31.2% vaccine efficacy at 42 months.[157,165] An immune correlates analysis of the RV144 trial demonstrated that antibodies against the second variable (V2) region of gp120 envelope were the prime correlate of decreased transmission risk.[158] The ongoing HVTN 702 HIV vaccine efficacy trial hopes to improve on RV144 by incorporating a more potent adjuvant (MF59 for Alum) and using two clade C Envs, one of which is a TF Env (1086C).[166] A second ongoing vaccine efficacy trial for the induction of nonneutralizing antibodies is HVTN 705 that tests an adenovirus 26 vector with a gp140 envelope boost.[167,168]

While bnAbs are protective against simian/human chimeric immunodeficiency viruses (SHIVs) in passive administration trials in rhesus macaques, bnAb protective efficacy in humans is not known. If bnAbs are protective, the serum bnAb level that can prevent infection is also not known. VRC01 is one of the most potent bnAbs isolated and it binds to the Env CD4 binding site.[169] The two antibody mediated prevention (AMP) studies, one in South Africa (HVTN 703/HPTN 081) and one in the United States (HVTN 704/HPTN 085), infuse the VRC01 bnAb intravenously to determine VRC01 efficacy in HIV prevention, and if protective, determine the protective serum level[170] (Table 90-2). The hope is that bnAb administration will be protective and prevent HIV infection, and provide a guide for the level of bnAb that must be induced by vaccination in future vaccine efficacy trials targeted to inducing bnAbs.

New HIV Vaccine Concepts: Obtaining the Right Functional Response

The newer HIV vaccine concepts are targeted to inducing HIV bnAbs that will be broadly protective or that can eradicate the first round of HIV infection. Table 90-3 lists some of the newer HIV vaccine concepts that are currently either in clinical trials or are in preclinical studies. Key concepts for bnAb induction that derived from the realization that bnAb B cell lineages are disfavored and negatively controlled at multiple steps by host tolerance mechanisms, are the need for targeting the naïve B cell receptors of bnAbs,[171,172] and the need for sequential immunization for bnAb induction.[154,171,173] Thus, many Env forms have been isolated or designed that can bind and activate bnAb B cell precursors or induce autologous neutralizing antibodies.[172,174–180] Currently, a candidate for expression of a near-native trimer is a stabilized trimer that is also moving into clinical trials.[177]

Studies of antibody virus co-evolution from the time of acute HIV infection to the time of bnAb development, have taught that bnAbs only develop when HIV Env undergoes extraordinary mutations, demonstrating that sequential Env immunogens after germline targeting will be required for full bnAb development.[173] From such co-evolution studies are several sequential Env regimens, the first of which (EnvSeq-1) that is comprised of 4 Envs sequentially isolated between the time of infection with a TF virus and the development of bnAbs. This is currently being investigated in the HVTN 115 Phase 1 trial.[173,176]

If germline targeting and sequential Env immunizations are insufficient for inducing full bnAb B cell lineage development, then additional strategies to enhance germinal center B cell and Tfh responses may be needed.[149,181] Concepts currently being tested are the use of

TABLE 90-2 HIV VACCINE OR NEUTRALIZING ANTIBODY ADMINISTRATION EFFICACY TRIALS

Trial	Vaccine	Goal	Status
Vax004	Bivalent clade B gp120s in Alum	Induce protective antibodies in US and Europe vaccines	Completed: No efficacy
VAX003	Bivalent CRF_01AE/B gp120s in Alum	Induce protective antibodies in Thailand and vaccines	Completed: No efficacy
HVTN 502 (Step)	Adenovirus type 5 clade B	Induce protective T cell responses in United States vacinees	Completed: No efficacy; increased infection in vaccines
HVTN503 (Phambili)	Adenovirus type 5 clade B gag/pol/nef	Induce protective T cell responses in South African vaccines	Completed: No efficacy; increased infection in male vaccines
RV144	ALVAC-AE vCP1521) with gag/pro/env; Bivalent clade CRF_01AE A244/B MN gp120s in Alum	Induce protective antibody and T cell responses in Thailand vaccines	Completed: Estimated 31.2% vaccine efficacy at 42 months; 60% efficacy at 12 months
HVTN505	DNAs with clade B gag/pol/nef: DNAs with clade A, B and C Envs: Adenovirus type 5 with gag/pol and clades A, B and C Envs	Induce protective T or B cell responses in United States vaccines	Completed: No efficacy
HVTN702	ALVAC-C vCP2438 with gag/pro/env; Bivalent clade C TV-1/C 1086 gp120s in MF59	Induce protective T or B cell responses in South Africa; Improve on RV144 efficacy.	Ongoing
HVTN 703/HPTN 081 (The Antibody Mediated Prevention [AMP] Study)	Recombinant VRC01 neutralizing antibody	Infuse neutralizing antibody VRC01 every 8 weeks to determine efficacy in preventing HIV infection, and determine the protective serum level in Sub Saharan Africa	Ongoing
HVTN 704/HPTN 085 (The Antibody Mediated Prevention [AMP] Study)	Recombinant VRC01 neutralizing antibody	Infuse neutralizing antibody VRC01 every 8weeks to determine efficacy in preventing HIV infection, and determine the protective serum level in the United States	Ongoing
HVTN 705	Ad26.Mos4.HIV; clade C gp140 Env	Induce protective T or B cell responses in South Africa; Improve on RV144 efficacy	Ongoing

TABLE 90-3 STATUS OF NEW EXPERIMENTAL HIV VACCINE CONCEPTS

Concept	Experimental Vaccine Examples	Goal	Status
Induce Broadly Reactive Neutralizing Antibodies (bnAbs)			
Envelope immunogens to target the germline (GL) B cell receptors (BCRs) of bnAbs	eOD8 env, CH505 Transmitted/founder Env, 426c Env for CD4 binding site bnAb GLs; membrane proximal external region peptide-liposome; multiple Env candidates for V3- or V1V2-glycan bnAbs	Initiate bnAb B cell lineages and expand and precursor pool of B cells capable of expanding protective neutralizing bnAb precursors	First clinical trials to start in 2019
Sequential envelope immunogens designed to select for rare or disfavored stages of bnAb B cell lineage development	CH505 sequential Envs (EnvSeq-1) comprised of 4-valent gp 120s identified in an individual who made broadly reactive CD4bs bnAbs after HIV infection.	Initiate CD4 binding site bnAb B cell lineages, expand precursors and drive bnAb B cell lineage to completion	HVTN 115 trial ongoing; multiple sequential Env designs in development
Transiently modify host immunoregulatory controls of antibody responses	Checkpoint inhibitors or modifiers of T regulatory or NK cell regulatory activity used with vaccination	Transiently and safely inhibit host negative immunoeregulatory activities in responding immune sites to allow otherwise disfavored bnAbs to be made	In preclinical studies
Induce Protective Non-Neutralizing Antibodies (NNAbs)			
Multimeric natural Env mixture	Broaden protective NNAb induction; Improve on RV144 and on any efficacy seen in HVTN 702 or HVTN 705 ongoing trials	Improve NNAb diversity and therefore efficacy by increasing the number of epitopes targeted by NNAbs	In preclinical studies
Multimeric centralized Env mixture	Broaden protective NNAb induction; Improve on RV144 and on any efficacy seen in HVTN 702 or HVTN 705 ongoing trials	Improve NNAb diversity and therefore efficacy by increasing the number of epitopes targeted by NNAbs	In preclinical studies
Vector or DNA prime, Env boost strategies	Protective NNAb induction; Improve on RV144 and on any efficacy seen in HVTN 702 or HVTN 705 ongoing trials	Improve vaccine efficacy by inducing potent protective T and B cell responses	In preclinical studies
Induce Protective T Cell Responses			
Modified Cytomegalovirus (CMV) vector	Human ortholog to rhesus CMV that protects 50% after SIV challenge	To determine if a modified human CMV vector can protect from HIV infection by CD8+ T cell recognition of HLA-E/peptide complexes	In preclinical studies

immune checkpoint inhibitors, or modifiers of cellular regulatory cells that dampen the germinal center response, such as NK cells. In this regard, it has recently been demonstrated that those HIV-infected individuals that make bnAbs have elevated Tfh,[182,183] decreased T regulatory cells,[183] high frequency of autoantibodies,[183] and dysfunctional NK cells with decreased capacity to kill target cells.[184] A current hypothesis is that in HIV-infected individuals that make bnAbs, normal NK regulation of germinal center B cells or Tfh cells is defective, allowing bnAbs to be made.[184] Thus, a number of new strategies are being developed to facilitate the Env germinal center response for bnAb development.

In contrast to difficult to induce bnAbs, NNAbs are easily induced but are less potent and less broad. New concepts for induction of NNAbs include the use of multimeric Env mixtures (either centralized or wild-type Envs) to boost ALVAC-Env primes in order to broaden coverage of Env diversity by NNAbs. In this regard, a multivalent wild-type Env mixture protected rhesus macaques at 67% per exposure rate from mucosal SHIV challenge.[185] Several preclinical studies in rhesus macaques have used additional various vector/protein combinations for prime and boost, each with the goal to induce optimal potency and diversity of coverage of NNAbs, and these vector/protein combinations are in advanced preclinical evaluation.[186–189]

As noted, HVTN 502, HVTN 503 and HVTN 505 vaccine efficacy trials that were each designed to induce HLA class 1a (HLA-A, -B, or -C-restricted CD8+ CTL) responses all showed no vaccine efficacy (Table 90-2). A new attenuated CMV vaccine for rhesus macaques has eliminated SIV in 50% of vaccinated monkeys and the effect is mediated by nonclassical HLA-E presentation of SIV peptides to CD8+ T cells.[190,191] Preclinical work is ongoing to determine if this strategy can be broadened to more than 50% of vaccinated monkeys and if it can be translated to an attenuated human CMV vector (Table 90-3).

Thus, HIV vaccine development has progressed rapidly during the last 10 years and demonstrated the roadblocks preventing a successful vaccine. The current HIV vaccine efficacy trials coupled with the ongoing and planned clinical trials of new concepts are very promising and should lead to the eventual development of a successful vaccine.

SELECTED PROBLEMS IN VACCINE DEVELOPMENT

Influenza Vaccines: Adapting to Pathogen Variation

Pathogen Description

The influenza viruses are categorized into four groups A–D based on antigenic similarity.[159] Influenza viruses can be isolated from a range of human and animal hosts. Influenza A viruses are found most commonly in their natural hosts, aquatic birds, but some antigenic variants have been identified in pigs, whales, horses, seals, bats, and humans.[36] Human disease can be caused by types A, B, and C, with pandemics associated with type A and epidemic or seasonal outbreaks with types A and B. Influenza D viruses infect cattle and are not known to cause infection in humans. Influenza is a single-stranded RNA virus, with the central RNA surrounded by an M protein layer with glycoproteins inserted and the surface exposed. It is these glycoproteins, namely hemagglutinin (HA) and neuraminidase (NA) that act as antigens during host infection and have been exploited as vaccine antigens; there are 18 HA subtypes (H1–H18) and 11 NA subtypes

(N1–N11).[36] In the pathogenic process, HA is an attachment protein, which binds to sialic acid on human cells. NA breaks down sialic acid thereby promoting the dissemination of new virus particles from the infected host cell. The virus is transmitted by respiratory droplet spread or contact with contaminated surfaces and infects the upper respiratory tract. The incubation period is 1–4 days, and importantly viral shedding can persist for much longer after infection in young children (~13 days) compared to adults (6–8 days).

Clinical Disease and Epidemiology

Influenza infections occur in temperate regions during the winter months, with distinct HA variants responsible for the disease depending on the circulating virus. Severity of seasonal influenza also depends on the circulating variants. Increasingly, influenza infections in the tropics are being recognized and investigated. All age groups can become infected, with 250,000–500,000 people succumbing to infection worldwide annually.[192] More severe illness with increased morbidity and mortality affects high-risk groups, including: the very young (<2 years), > 65 year olds, and those with pre-existing co-morbidities such as asthma, diabetes, chronic heart or lung conditions, or the immunocompromised. Clinical features in adults are well-recognized as coryza, dry cough, fever, myalgia, malaise, pharyngitis, and headaches. In young infants or neonates, poor feeding, irritability, and apnea may also occur. Complications can occur, more readily in those at high risk, involving the respiratory system with otitis media, sinusitis, secondary bacterial pneumonia; the neurological system with encephalitis, Reye's syndrome, Guillain-Barre syndrome, transverse myelitis; and the cardiovascular system with myocarditis.

Prior Vaccine Development

The phenomenon of antigenic drift and antigenic shift are responsible for the lack of persistent immunity to influenza in humans and the concern about pandemics, respectively. Antigenic drift describes the accumulation of minor genetic changes in HA, and less frequently in NA. Point mutations in the genome result in sufficient changes in the protein structure that evade recognition by neutralizing antibodies produced by previous exposure, infection, or vaccination. Antigenic drift is a continuous process, which explains why the influenza vaccine antigens need frequent updating. Antigenic shift is much less frequent, but describes the emergence of a novel combination of influenza A HA or NA antigenic variants occurring in a human population which is immune and therefore highly susceptible. Four major pandemics occurred in the last hundred years: 1918 H1N1 (Spanish flu), 1957 H2N2 (Asian flu), 1968 H3N2 (Hong Kong flu), and 2009 H1N1 (Swine flu).

There are two types of vaccine available against seasonal influenza; inactivated vaccines and live attenuated influenza vaccines (LAIV). Vaccines are redesigned annually to account for the changes to circulating virus in that period due to antigenic drift. The vaccine antigens are from the HA glycoprotein, and each year, the WHO selects the optimal epitopes to include based on the circulating strains.[193] Inactivated vaccines are available for all age groups in the United States and are especially recommended for vulnerable groups. The live vaccine is licensed for 2–49 years olds, excluding pregnant women. However, because of poor replication and effectiveness the LAIV was not recommended in 2017, but recently reinstated for 2018.

Challenges with Vaccines on the Market or Vaccines in Development

Antigenic drift and antigenic shift produce two different challenges in optimizing influenza vaccine formulation. To address antigenic drift, at present, WHO annually predicts the antigenic variants based on known circulating strains, to prepare vaccines for the next influenza season. The resulting efficacy of the seasonal influenza vaccine is therefore dependent on age, degree of similarity between the vaccine strain and circulating strain, and type of vaccine used.[194] Estimates of vaccine efficacy taking into account these variables identified that the overall efficacy was 65% to any strain, with efficacy higher against type A than type B nonmatching strains. The LAIV was observed to be more efficacious in children compared to adults, with the converse true of the inactivated vaccine. Both vaccines showed similar efficacy against nonmatching strains.[194]

Vaccines traditionally contained only three variants, two from influenza A and one from influenza B. However, more recent attempts to improve efficacy include the inclusion of an additional B variant, or increasing the overall HA dose. The current approaches, however, still rely on using variable parts of the influenza viral proteins, with the risk of mismatch to the seasonal strain, and unknown efficacy against emerging pandemic strains. The search for influenza antigens that are universally present between subtypes of influenza A, has identified some potential vaccine targets.[195–197] The development and trials of vaccines using highly conserved influenza epitopes formulated as virus-like particles have shown encouraging results. By using antigens based on the conserved matrix protein 2 ectodomain and the hemaglutinin stalk, cross-reactive antibodies were generated that protected naive mice against infection.[198] Further stimulation of the cellular responses was seen to intranasal vaccination of mice with a vaccine containing multiple conserved ectodomains of matrix protein 2.[199]

Alternative strategies for optimizing influenza vaccines include modifying the adjuvants in order to produce broader and longer-lasting protection. MF59 has been developed and included in influenza vaccines with the aim of improving antigen presenting cell recruitment and activation, $CD4^+$ T lymphocytes, and optimizing the antibody binding sites. The increasing use of MF59-adjuvanted vaccines is providing more evidence of their safety and tolerability, as well as their improved immunogenicity in both young children and the elderly, compared to nonadjuvanted inactivated vaccines.[200,201] Other adjuvants under investigation include Toll-like receptor stimulating adjuvants such as adjuvant family AS01, used in licensed malaria and herpes zoster vaccines, and flagellin.

To address the concerns about the speed of development of effective vaccines in the setting of an influenza pandemic, different methodologies could be considered. Newly developing vaccine platforms incorporating DNA or RNA encoding the required antigen, offer the prospect of rapid, cell-free vaccine development in response to an emerging pathogenic strain. These vaccines are in the early stages of development but self-amplifying RNA vaccine against H7N9 was immunogenic in mice models.[202] Despite the challenges of influenza's highly variable nature, there are a number of technologies that appear to be leading influenza vaccine development in new directions.

SELECTED PROBLEMS IN VACCINE DEVELOPMENT

Pertussis Vaccines: Short Effector Memory

Pathogen Description

Bordetella pertussis is a fastidious gram-negative bacterium. It specifically infects humans, making animal models of disease challenging. Infection with *B. pertussis* causes a prolonged illness, commonly called whooping cough and comprising three clinical stages. The catarrhal stage is characterized by mild upper respiratory tract symptoms such as cough and rhinorrhea. Following this, the illness progresses to the paroxysmal stage, during which patients have a characteristic inspiratory "whoop," potentially followed by vomiting. Over weeks to months, symptoms slowly wane in the convalescent stage. Duration of illness ranges 6–10 weeks. Disease is most severe in infants due to gagging and gasping, and infants can experience apnea and bradycardia. Pneumonia is not uncommon; seizures, acute encephalopathy, and permanent brain damage can occur. In older teens and adults, complications include sleep disturbance, incontinence, rib fractures, and pneumonia. Typically, complications increase with age in adults. In the most vulnerable populations, disease can be fatal.

Epidemiology

B. pertussis is transmitted person to person via aerosolized droplets. Susceptible hosts with close exposures are highly likely to develop disease. Individuals are most contagious during the catarrhal stage, and the first 2 weeks after onset of cough. Approximately 16 million cases of pertussis occur worldwide, with close to 200,000 deaths.[203] Since introduction of vaccines in the 1940s, incidence of disease has dramatically declined, particularly in developed countries with high vaccine coverage. Infants, unvaccinated populations, and individuals, who have remote history of vaccination but immunity that has waned, remain at risk for disease.

Vaccine Development

Because this organism has humans as the only host, is highly contagious, and has organism components that can be vaccine targets, it was a clear candidate for vaccine development. Certain components of the organism are known to contribute to its pathogenicity, include pertussis toxin (PT), filamentous hemagglutinin (FHA), pertactin (PRN), agglutinin which is fimbriae-associated (FIM), adenylate cyclase toxin, and tracheal toxin.[204] Several of these molecules are critical for attachment to respiratory epithelium, while others impair leukocyte function and cause local damage of epithelial tissue. Vaccines to protect children from pertussis were first developed in the early twentieth century. Initially, all vaccines were derived from the whole cell (wP), with either inactivated or alum adjuvants. A number of manufacturers produced the vaccine, and whole cell vaccines overall proved efficacy of approximately 78%.[205] By the end of the twentieth century, concerns were raised about reactions to wP vaccines, including high fevers and potential correlation with seizure. Acellular vaccines were developed (aP). Acellular vaccines differed in composition between manufacturers, with varied antigen content of PT, FHA, PRN, and FIM. Multicomponent pertussis antigen vaccines are likely superior in efficacy to those containing one or two antigens, but concentration of antigens also influences efficacy.[206] While aP vaccines are less reactogenic, most experts agree that good wP vaccines are superior in efficacy to any aP vaccine.

As acellular vaccines were better tolerated, they were adopted first in Japan in the 1980s, followed by the United States and Europe in the 1990s. At this time, the available aP vaccines are safe, and provide protection worldwide to prevent widespread disease from *Bordetella pertussis*. Worldwide, approximately 86% of the population has completed a three-dose series, but pertussis remains the most prevalent vaccine-preventable illness.[207]

Challenges: Waning Immunity

Sporadic outbreaks have led to questions about the ability of the aP vaccine to support long-term protection. In a meta-analysis of studies including both three- and five-dose series of DTaP, McGirr, and Fisman found predictable waning of immunity after series completion, and concluded that the odds of pertussis disease increases by 1.33 times (95% CI 1.23–1.43) for every year after receipt of DTaP.[208] This was also apparent in an outbreak in California in 2010, confirming that unvaccinated infants were at highest risk of disease, but identifying that 66% of cases in fully vaccinated children were in the 7- to 10-year-old age group who had received only aP.[209] Additional studies support this epidemiology indicating that primary vaccination with acellular vaccines does not confer long-term protection, both due to waning effectiveness after a primary series, but also with less response to aP boosters.[209–211] The immunologic response induced by aP versus wP vaccines is largely responsible for waning immunity. There are known differences in the immune system response to aP versus wP vaccines, though even countries utilizing wP vaccines still have had pockets of disease.[212] Research has elucidated that the immune response to aP vaccines leads to less optimal priming of the immune system than either wP vaccines or natural infection, which in turn limits long-term protection and our ability to boost the initial response.[213] Both natural infection and wP vaccination have a higher proportion of response by Th1 and Th17 cells compared to immunization with aP vaccines, which induce stronger Th2 responses.[214] Additionally, in a baboon model of infection, aP vaccines reduce incidence of disease, but do not prevent colonization, which can then lead to ongoing transmission in the population.[215] The differential T cell response may contribute to this colonization, which in turn can contribute to ongoing transmission in populations despite use of vaccine. Studies of small cohorts of children have indicated that humans may asymptomatically carry the organism leading to ongoing spread to unvaccinated individuals.[216] Other concerns have been raised related to studying the epidemiology of pertussis vaccine effectiveness including evolution of the organism, changes in testing practices, improved surveillance by public health authorities, and changes in vaccination rates in select populations. However, these are insufficient to explain the resurgence of disease and force the examination of vaccine design.[217]

New Approaches

As the aP vaccines can boost existing response, albeit for a brief period, one approach to improve effectiveness is to alter the childhood vaccination schedule to reduce waning immunity.[218] Use of "cocooning," that is, vaccinating individuals who are in contact with the most vulnerable population (infants) has been suggested, but is challenging to carry out on a large scale. This, combined with vaccination during pregnancy to support transmission of antibody as discussed, will reduce morbidity and mortality from *B. pertussis*.[219,252] At present, acceptability of returning to wP is likely to be low. Long term, the current aP vaccines will need to be improved by either changing adjuvants or adding antigens to increase long-term protection and decrease colonization. Alternate adjuvants have been proposed, including ASO4, CpG oligonucleotides, or TLR-2 agonists.[214] New pertussis vaccines in preclinical development include wP with low endotoxin content, outer membrane vesicles, new formulations of aP with additional antigens, and a live attenuated vaccine.[220] Of these, live attenuated nasal BPZE1, which is a genetically modified pertussis derivative, is the most promising.[221,222] Of course, with any of these alternatives, regulatory approval, ethically sound trials in populations where an effective vaccine is available, and measuring an appropriate correlate of protection present challenges in bringing a new vaccine to market.

SELECTED PROBLEMS IN VACCINE DEVELOPMENT

Rotavirus Vaccines: Variation between Different Populations

Pathogen Description

Rotaviruses are part of the Reoviridae family and the 100 nm viral particle consists of a three-layer capsid surrounding double stranded RNA, encoding six structural (VP1–4, VP6, VP7) and six nonstructural proteins (NSP1–6).[223] Rotavirus are categorized into seven groups (A–G) based on antigenic and genotypic homology of the VP6 protein. Only group A, B, and C rotaviruses are known to cause human disease, with group A further classified by the VP7 (G-type) and VP4 (P-type) proteins which are on the outer layer of the capsid and induce potent neutralizing antibodies, relevant for diagnostics and vaccine development.[223] Worldwide there is a predominance of the prevalence of G types (G1–4 and G9) and P types (P4, P6, and P8).[224] However, despite nonlinkage of the genes for these, they tend to occur in discrete combinations, with five types occurring in over 90% of circulating rotaviruses: P8,G1, P4,G2, P8,G3, P8,G4, and P8,G9.[224] This has profound implications for targeting disease-causing strains in combinatorial vaccines. Rotavirus is transmitted by faeco-oral spread from an infected individual. The incubation period is 1–3 days.

Clinical Disease and Epidemiology

Rotavirus is the most important cause of gastroenteritis and dehydration in children globally. Severe and symptomatic infection is most common in children from 3 months to 24 months old. The impact of this infection is highly dependent on socioeconomic status and global region. In developing countries, there is elevated morbidity and mortality from the consequences of rotavirus infection, mainly through dehydration and shock that follow profuse vomiting and diarrhea. Improved healthcare provision, access to clean water, and oral rehydration solutions (ORS) have dramatically improved the outcomes for many children with gastroenteritis caused by rotavirus and other pathogens, but it remains problematic. In industrialized settings, the burden of disease causes high morbidity, resulting in mild/moderate gastroenteritis illness, transmission to other family members, time off school and work and the societal costs that this entails. In temperate regions, rotavirus infection peaks in winter whereas in tropical regions, disease can occur all year round, but peaks in cooler or drier seasons. Rotavirus infects the proximal small intestine with the resulting reduction in absorptive function of the enterocytes and production of enterotoxin. Clinical presentation is with abrupt fever, profuse vomiting, diarrhea or both, leading to varying degrees of dehydration, depending on the oral intake. The disease is self-limiting in most children, though they often transmit the virus to caregivers during the illness. Major morbidity and mortality arise from the consequences of dehydration, including metabolic acidosis and electrolyte disturbances, particularly in regions with poor hygiene and access to healthcare facilities.

Prior Vaccine Development

The study of natural infection with rotavirus led to the observations that these children developed adaptive immunity preventing reinfection.[225–227] On this basis, oral live vaccines were developed against rotavirus strains and this remains the principle on which current vaccines work. The first generation of rotavirus vaccines contained a single, attenuated animal strain. These were superceded by reassortant vaccines, exploiting the virus' propensity to reassort genetic material. These vaccines contain an animal backbone with human VP7 and VP4 genes introduced.[228] At the time of writing, the most widely used rotavirus vaccines worldwide were the monovalent human G1 vaccine (Rotarix®, containing G1, P8) and the pentavalent human-bovine reassortant vaccine (Rotateq®, containing G1, G2, G3, G4, P8).

Challenges with Vaccines in Development

The safety of oral, live rotavirus vaccines has been demonstrated as part of their development. However, vaccine efficacy remains highly variable among different regions of the world. In industrialized settings there has been a dramatic reduction in rotavirus infection following introduction of Rotarix®. Emergency department visits and hospitalization in the United Kingdom fell by 48% and 53%, respectively, in particular in the vaccinated age groups (infants) through direct protection, but also in older children and adults, through herd immunity, an effect observed in the US and western Europe examples.[229–231] In Rwanda, introduction of Rotateq® into the immunization program, with high vaccine uptake of 88%, reduced hospital admission of under 5 years olds by 48–49%.[232] However, in developing regions, there has been a much lower efficacy for rotavirus vaccines when compared to industrialized countries. Randomized controlled trials of the pentavalent vaccine RotaTeq®, vaccine efficacy was reported at 98% in eleven developed countries after the first season.[233] Vaccine efficacy was reported in Kenya, Ghana and Mali at 64% and in Bangladesh and Vietnam at 51% for the same period.[234,235] This has significant implications as there is a clear inverse relationship between vaccine efficacy and childhood mortality.[236] There have been a number of proposed reasons for the reduced efficacy of oral vaccines including: higher titers of maternally derived transplacental antibody, interaction with components of human breast milk in regions where breastfeeding rates are higher, micronutrient deficiencies including zinc and vitamin A, and comorbidities in the infant such as HIV or helminth infection. However, there has also been experimental evidence to support the theory that the different gut microbiota may be, at least in part, implicated. The gut microbiota is still poorly understood, in particular the changes throughout infancy and childhood, and its interactions with the host immune system. Germ-free mice have extensively been used to explore the interplay with immune system maturation. Both infection and antibiotic use can lead to perturbations in the diversity and extent of bacterial species found in the gut. Following disturbance of the mouse gut microbiota with antimicrobials, there was a reduction in the susceptibility to infection with poliovirus and reduced infection with rotavirus.[237] Thus, depleting the resident microbiota, may limit the ability of the virus to replicate and limit the infectious load. Further, immunological response measured by serum and fecal IgA titers suggested that the magnitude and duration of antibodies was higher after pretreatment with the oral antibiotics neomycin and ampicillin.[238] Probiotics have been studied in this regard, as an alternative way of manipulating the gut flora. A Finnish study showed a significant increase in seroconversion following supplementation with lactobacillus (LGG), similar to results in a larger study in India, where children were supplemented with LGG and zinc.[239] However, overall seroconversion rates were much lower in India compared to Finland (27.4–39.4% seroconversion in nonsupplemented and supplemented children in India compared to 74% and 93%, respectively, in Finland). Analysis of the microbiome of human fecal samples from the Ghanaian vaccine responders and nonresponders from the RotaTeq® RCTs, found that Ghanaian responders were more similar to healthy age-matched Dutch children, than to the Ghanaian nonresponders.[240]

There is likely a complex interplay between all the predisposing factors and the ensuing response to rotavirus vaccines, but as more is understood about the interaction between the host microbiome and immune system, it is likely that we will be able to optimize the response to oral live vaccines against not only rotavirus, but other important diseases including poliovirus and cholera.

SELECTED PROBLEMS IN VACCINE DEVELOPMENT

RSV Vaccines

Advances in Structural Biology

Pathogen Description RSV belongs to the Paramyxoviridae virus family, and Pneumovirininae subfamily, along with human metapneumovirus. The RSV structure consists of a single-stranded negative-sense RNA, encoding eleven proteins. The genome is enclosed in a helical nucleocapsid and is encapsulated in a lipid bilayer obtained from the host cell membrane. Surface glycoproteins, glycosylated attachment (G) and fusion (F) proteins are important virulence factors, as well as targets for neutralizing antibodies.[241] Viral entry into host cells is mediated by the F protein which facilitates fusion to target host epithelial cells. Viral entry into the upper respiratory tract is followed by spread into and around the lower respiratory tract between epithelial cells through syncitia, a further function of the F protein when observed using human cell lines. RSV can be broadly categorized into two subgroups, A and B, based on reactivity to polyclonal sera.[242,243] Both subgroups can circulate and cause disease in the same geotemporal setting, but there is genetic diversity between them.[244] However, the F protein showed 50% homology between the two subgroups and demonstrates little antigenic drift, thereby is relatively stable through time, in comparison to other respiratory viruses such as influenza. RSV is transmitted by droplet spread and can survive on surfaces for 4–7 hours. The incubation period is 3–5 days.

Clinical Disease and Epidemiology RSV infection causes bronchiolitis or viral pneumonia, predominantly in infants, the immunocompromised and elderly. RSV disease occurs worldwide and there is marked seasonal variation in the incidence of RSV infections. The disease peaks in the winter months, in temperate climates, with maximal hospital admissions with RSV disease during this period. Clinical disease manifests as coryza followed by cough, wheeze, crepitations, and respiratory distress. For the majority of infants, RSV infection is a self-limiting illness, with symptoms worsening for the first 5 days and then improving. A residual postbronchiolitic cough can be problematic for some weeks after infection, but no long-term consequences are recognized following mild/moderate bronchiolitis. Almost all children will be infected with RSV in their first winter. There is major morbidity and resulting hospital admission, with admission estimated at 2–3% in the United Kingdom and the United States.[245] In severe RSV infection, ensuing respiratory failure will follow initial symptoms in premature or very young infants or immunocompromised hosts in the absence of ventilatory support, in 2–5% of those admitted. Further, secondary bacterial infection is a recognized complication of RSV infection. There is no antiviral treatment licensed for use in bronchiolitis, and management is largely supportive of oxygen, ventilatory, and feeding requirements. Hence, there is a major need for a vaccine to prevent this disease, which is ubiquitous to infants facing their first winter, with minimal protective immunity. The health and economic implications of reduced hospital admission, morbidity and mortality, and parental leave are clear.

PRIOR VACCINE DEVELOPMENT

Prevention of RSV infection has been a research priority for decades, with the first formalin-inactivated RSV (FI-RSV) vaccine developed in the 1960s by Pfizer Laboratories Inc. The Bernett strain was passaged in human and monkey kidney cell cultures, and inactivated using formalin treatment.[246] This Fi-RSV vaccine antigenic component was the F protein. In subsequent clinical trials in the United States from 1965 to 1966, it was observed that the vaccine offered no protection against disease, with vaccinees having higher rates and more severe disease than unvaccinated controls.[246,247] This enhanced RSV disease, was likely due to the alterations to the RSV F protein during the formalin-inactivation process, which produced imbalanced immune responses and skewed Th2 responses. Since this time, there have been no new RSV vaccines implemented and great caution amongst scientists to introduce an infant vaccine. Instead alternative vaccine strategies have been considered to deliver safe and efficacious protection. At present, the only means of RSV disease prevention is through passive immunization with monoclonal antibodies such as palivizumab, administered to certain high-risk young children throughout the winter season.

CHALLENGES WITH VACCINES IN DEVELOPMENT

A further challenge is the observation that natural immunity to RSV infection is incomplete and not persistent, resulting in reinfection. There was also concern following the FI-RSV vaccine trials, that the presence of antibodies may have been involved in the pathogenesis of disease, an assertion consistent with the increased rates of disease in infants under 6 months old, who had maternally derived antibodies. However, passive immunity with monoclonal antibodies such as palivizumab, has been highly successful in preventing severe RSV disease and has been the only means of protection for the increasing number of premature and immunocompromised children in the last decade.[187] This monoclonal antibody is directed at the F protein, and this remains the target antigen of choice for vaccine development, for this reason as well as its biological role in host cell entry and genetic conservation.[248] The main challenge for RSV antigen development has been to optimize the conformational state of the F protein, whose metastable prefusion F (pre-F) epitopes have a far greater neutralizing activity than the stable postfusion F (post-F), when tested with human sera.[249] In order to stabilize this pre-F structure, an in depth understanding of the protein structure and conformational changes on fusion, have been required. Insights in structural biology, allowing atomic-level analyses have helped to understand these structures and make further progress toward generating stable and effective antigens.[250] In 2013, monoclonal antibodies (D25, 5C4, and AM22) were used to target pre-F specific epitopes.[251] The crystal structure of these interactions were visualized and it was possible to identify novel antigenic sites. These antigenic sites were not present on the post-F structure due to the conformational changes associated with host cell entry. The subsequent challenge was to stabilize this structure for use as a vaccine antigen. This was achieved by inserting cysteine residues which formed disulfide bonds and cavity filling mutations. The resultant stable pre-F structure, termed pre-F DS-Cav1 was used to immunize mice and macaques, and induced potent neutralizing antibodies to both subgroups of RSV.[251] The efficacy of pre-F RSV vaccines is under investigation, but there is much anticipation that there may be a real possibility of reducing the morbidity and mortality from the disease.

Vaccine strategy and deployment has been a sensitive issue in RSV vaccine development, due to the safety lessons learned from the past. Alternative strategies including vaccination of pregnant women have shown great efficacy in protection of infants for diseases such as pertussis, which also affects young infants.[252] Clinical trials are in progress to assess safety and efficacy of RSV vaccines in pregnant women. Other strategies include vaccinating older children to induce direct protection and reduce transmission, and vaccination of at risk groups who at present receive passive immunization with palivizumab including; premature infants, chronic lung or heart disease, immunocompromised, and if deemed efficacious, the elderly with co-morbidities.

Due to technological advances we are now able to harness the potential of these molecular approaches, to discover and design better vaccine antigens modified and integrated according to information derived from the analysis of the B cell repertoire. These advances will drive vaccinology to make more effective and innovative vaccine designs, but history will continue to remind us of the rigorous safety testing required beyond the laboratory.

SELECTED PROBLEMS IN VACCINE DEVELOPMENT

Streptococcus, Group B

Pathogen Description

GBS is the leading cause of invasive bacterial infection in neonates and young infants, with disease manifestations including bacteremia, meningitis, sepsis, pneumonia, osteomyelitis, cellulitis, and adenitis.[253] In pregnant women, GBS can cause endometritis and chorioamnionitis, as well as urinary tract infections. GBS is an aerobic gram-positive organism. There are 10 serotypes (Ia, Ib, II–IX) identified by different capsular polysaccharides, though five types (Ia, Ib, II, III, and V) cause the majority of disease.[254] Virulence factors include these capsular polysaccharides, as well as β-hemolysin, C proteins, and pilus-like proteins.[255–258] Antibodies to these proteins lead to protection from clinical disease.

Clinical Disease and Epidemiology

The immune system of a neonate is particularly ineffective in forming antibodies against polysaccharides, leaving this population at risk of invasive disease due to GBS.[259] Infections occur in neonates throughout the first 3 months of life, with early-onset disease categorized as infection in the first week. Most infants with early-onset disease will become ill within the first 12 hours of life, consistent with the pathogenesis of transmission from the exposure during labor and delivery. Infections at day 7 or later are considered late-onset disease and are mainly due to bacteremia or meningitis. Mortality associated with these infections is approximately 4–6%, and morbidity includes neurologic sequelae from meningitis, as well as disabilities associated with severe illness so early in life.[260] At times, GBS can infect adults with medical co morbidities including diabetes, liver disease, or malignancies. The organism can be treated with penicillin, with only a few isolates identified with resistance of unclear clinical significance.[261]

Colonization of the maternal vaginal or rectal area with GBS is a major risk factor for neonatal disease. Approximately 30% of pregnant women are colonized.[253] In the absence of an effective vaccine, intrapartum antibiotic prophylaxis (IAP) with penicillin or ampicillin during labor and delivery, has been utilized to reduce neonatal disease. In the United States, IAP has been utilized since 1996. While at first a number of different criteria were identified to determine which pregnant women warranted prophylaxis, screening all pregnant women by culture has been recommended by the U.S. Centers for Disease Control and Prevention since 2002.[262] It is critical to note that IAP has only reduced early-onset GBS disease without impacting the incidence of late-onset disease. Prior to the introduction of IAP, the rate of early-onset disease was 1.8 per 1000 live births; that is now 0.26/1000 live births (Fig. 90-1).[262a] Reassuringly, since beginning IAP, penicillin nonsusceptible GBS have rarely been identified, but concerns have been raised that exposure of the population to penicillin for prophylactic measures can lead to resistance in other bacteria such as *Escherichia coli*.[263]

Vaccine Development

Since the 1970s, investigators have acknowledged that GBS-specific antibodies in a pregnant woman that can be transmitted to the neonate are critical in reducing the incidence of disease in the neonate.[264] Development of a polysaccharide vaccine for pregnant women would allow for transfer of antibody to the unborn infant. As discussed earlier, while transfer of antibodies begins around 17-week gestation, it is most robust after 33 weeks.[265] Vaccines for types Ia, II, and III were developed but did not lead to predictable immunogenicity, with concern that adults were not sufficiently primed.[266] However, infants born to responders of vaccination did have protective antibodies in their sera until 3 months of age.[267]

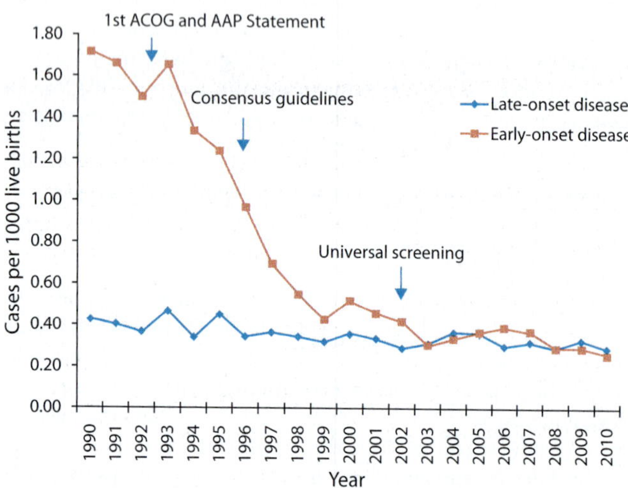

FIGURE 90-1. Incidence of invasive early- and late-onset group B streptococcal disease, Active Bacterial Core surveillance, United States, 1990–2010. (*Source:* Used, with permission, from Schrag SJ, Verani JR. Intrapartum antibiotic prophylaxis for the prevention of perinatal group B streptococcal disease: Experience in the United States and implications for a potential group B streptococcal vaccine. *Vaccine.* 2013;31 Suppl 4:D20–6.)

Current Challenges: Determining Breadth of Protection

In the 1990s, serotype V emerged in the United States, accounting for 23% of maternal cases and 14% of neonatal cases.[268] With the recognition that five serotypes need to be included in an effective vaccine, conjugate vaccines for all five serotypes have been developed and tested.[269–272] These were all well tolerated without serious adverse events. Conjugation appeared to have improved immunogenicity compared to earlier polysaccharide vaccines, but also demonstrated a dose-dependent response particularly in those individuals with low levels of antibody prior to vaccination.[272] While polysaccharide vaccines require T-cell independent B-cell activation, glycoconjugate vaccines can induce both B- and T-cell memory. The result is a more robust IgG response from class-switching.[273]

Efforts are ongoing to develop an effective conjugate vaccine, summarized in Table 90-4. A bivalent vaccine with types II and III conjugated to tetanus toxoid demonstrated an immune response not statistically different from those demonstrated by monovalent vaccines.[274] A candidate trivalent (Ia, Ib, III-CRM$_{197}$) vaccine was in development and was demonstrated to be safe and immunogenic, but further development was stopped in 2015.[275] Alternate targets for vaccine development include surface-expressed proteins. In 2002, whole genome sequencing of GBS was completed leading to more comprehensive identification of pathogenic proteins. C proteins, C5a peptidase, rib protein, GBS immunogenic bacterial adhesion (*bibA*), and surface immunogenic protein have all been explored. One vaccine in trials is based on fusion of AlphaC and Rib protein, which could protect against up to 95% of isolates.[276] Clearly, a pentavalent vaccine or vaccine against a universal GBS protein is the goal, but as pharmaceutical companies continue to change targets, we will need many more years to demonstrate immunogenicity, safety, and efficacy.

Licensure of a GBS vaccine would require a candidate vaccine to be manufactured and studied with a pharmaceutical company in a phase 3 trial. This would include vaccination of pregnant women to demonstrate true efficacy, or an appropriate immune correlate of protection. Invasive GBS disease in an infant is likely to be a relevant primary efficacy endpoint. As summarized by Kobayashi et al., there is an inverse relationship between a pregnant woman's serotype-specific IgG levels and disease risk in her infant,[277] though without standardized assays this is not likely to be an appropriate measure for licensure.

At the public health level, vaccination is clearly beneficial. In a model predicting the benefits of vaccination versus continued use of IAP, immunization was superior. Immunization of pregnant women early in the third trimester can prevent 4% of preterm births, 61–67%

TABLE 90-4 GROUP B STREPTOCOCCUS VACCINES IN DEVELOPMENT. DEVELOPMENT STATUS OF CURRENT VACCINE CANDIDATE (ADAPTED FROM 329)

Developer	Candidate name/identifier	Preclinical	Phase I	Phase II	POC	Phase III
NIH	Tetanus toxoid-CPS conjugates: monovalent (multiple studies), bivalent (one study); CRM$_{197}$-CPS conjugate: monovalent (one study)	X	X	X	X (trial in pregnant women)	
Novartis/GSK	CRM$_{197}$-CPS conjugate: monovalent (multiple), trivalent (several)	X	X	X	X (trial in pregnant women)	
Minervax	N-terminal domains of the Rib ad AlphaC surface proteins	X	X			
Novartis/GSK	Pilus proteins	X				
Various academic groups	Other protein(s) and/or protein-GPS conjugates	X				

of early-onset disease, and 70–72% of late-onset disease. The reduction of maternal and late-onset disease simply cannot be achieved by IAP. Alternatively, if immunity were long-lasting, vaccination could be provided to adolescent females to reduce maternal disease and infections in the preterm population.[278–280]

Control of Emerging Diseases

The increase in travel between the developed and the developing world, plus the increased movement of insect and other vectors of microbes, has increased the number of infections that grow from an isolated focus into worldwide epidemics. The cases in point include Ebola, Chikungunya, and Zika viruses, all originating in Africa but ultimately becoming problems in multiple continents.[281–283] Unfortunately, these emerging diseases do not furnish attractive markets for major manufacturers as they occur particularly in poor populations.

The Ebola outbreak in West Africa was a "wakeup call" to the world that vaccine development would need to change. In fact, as is often the case, scientists had anticipated the need for an Ebola vaccine and had developed candidate vaccines that seemed efficacious in experimental animals, but they had not gone further because of lack of funds and facilities. Although considerable vaccine development had taken place before the West African outbreak,[284] the outbreak was almost over before the first candidate vaccine could be tested in an efficacy trial.[285] The case of Zika was more typical in that no vaccine development had taken place before it became notorious.[283]

Accordingly, in 2015 a proposal was published suggesting the establishment of an international fund and organization to develop usable vaccines.[12,285,286] It was the right time for this proposal, since it was evident that there was no existing mechanism to accomplish that goal and even now there is still no licensed Ebola vaccine, despite evidence for efficacy. An organization came into being, called the Coalition for Epidemic Preparedness and Innovation, headquartered in London and Oslo. Funds were forthcoming from a number of governments and charitable foundations. A list of target diseases was constructed, as indicated in Table 90-5. Proposals have been solicited for candidate vaccines against Lassa fever, MERS, and Nipah viruses, as well as innovative platforms for rapid vaccine development, such as DNA and mRNA technology. The first grants have been made based on the criteria in Table 90-6. In addition to providing vaccines for immediate use, the idea is to create stockpiles so that in an emergency there will be immediate access to vaccines.[13]

As its first targets CEPI has chosen Lass, Nipah, and MERS. Grants have been awarded to multiple vaccine developers for these agents in order to have products within several years.

TABLE 90-5 PRIORITY PATHOGEN LISTS

WHO List of Priority Pathogens	FVR
Filovirus diseases (Ebola, Marburg)	Filovirus disease (Ebola, Marburg)
Rift Valley Fever	Rift Valley Fever
Coronaviruses (SARS, MERS)	Coronaviruses (SARS, MERS)
Lassa	Lassa
Chikungunya	Chikungunya
Zika	Zika
Severe Fever with Thrombocytopenia Syndrome	Paratyphoid A (Salmonella enterical)
New Disease	Hepatitis E
	Enterovirus 71, 68, Coxsackievirus
	West Nile
	Plague

New Approaches to Vaccine Development

The old paradigms of chemical inactivation and selection of nonpathogenic mutants are disappearing, while new methods to develop vaccines are flourishing, as listed in Box 90-3. We will discuss those new methods by giving examples of their use.

In the category of "live" vaccines, we will give examples of reassortment, codon deoptimization, micro RNA insertion, and replicating vectors. Reassortment led to the pentavalent rotavirus vaccine, which combines the RNA segments that code for internal antigens of a bovine rotavirus strain that is attenuated for humans, with the RNA segments for the vp4 and vp7 surface proteins that induce protective antibodies.[287]

Codon deoptimization clearly has an impact on virulence. That strategy was used to further attenuate arenaviruses by codon changes for the viral glycoprotein, and may be useful for development of a vaccine against Lassa fever. The insertion of a particular micro RNA associated with influenza virus nucleoprotein has an attenuating effect on the virus.[288]

The use of vectors to present vaccine antigens is a burgeoning field. In some cases the viral vector itself is replicating, producing more of the protein coded for by the inserted gene, whereas in other cases the vector is incapable of replicating but nevertheless produces the vaccine protein *in vivo*. Examples include the use of poxviruses, adenoviruses, vesicular stomatitis virus, or lymphocytic choriomeningitis

TABLE 90-6 MOST IMPORTANT CRITERIA

Criteria	Comment to interpretation
Protection in a relevant animal model	Protection in mice also scored but rated lower than protection in models closer to humans.
Evidence for a correlate of protection	Preferably inferred from date in humans, but also counted if inferred from animal or natural history data.
A viable platform for vaccine manufacture exists	Preferably more than one. If the proposed vaccine was accomplished by an important technological advance in vaccinology that could be applied to other vaccines its score was increased.

BOX 90-3 New Strategies for Vaccine Development

Attenuated vaccines

- Reverse genetics, temperature-sensitive mutations, and reassortment.
- Viral recombinants and deletion mutants.
- Codon deoptimization.
- Control of replication fidelity.
- MicroRNA insertion.
- Replicating vectors that contain genes from pathogens.
- Gene delivery by invasive bacteria.

Inactivated vaccines

- DNA plasmids and DNA shuffling.
- Reverse vaccinology.
- Antigen identification by transcriptomics and proteomics.
- Development of fusion proteins.
- Development of new adjuvants (including cytokines).
- Induction of innate immunity.

Source: Used, with permission, from Plotkin SA, Plotkin SL. *Nat Rev Microbiol.* 2011;9(12):889–93, Box 90-2.

viruses as vectors for HIV, Ebola, and Lassa fever antigens.[289–292] A problem with this strategy is immunity to the vector, but certain vectors, for example, canarypox and lymphocytic choriomeningitis do not seem to induce immune responses against themselves when used as vectors. The MVA vaccinia mutant is another frequently used vector.[293]

With regard to inactivated vaccines, new strategies also abound. Reverse vaccinology has become a familiar term. This boils down to sequencing the genome of a pathogen of interest, and then placing bits of the DNA or RNA translated to DNA in bacteria capable of synthesizing the coded proteins r. Those proteins are collected from the supernatants of the cultivated bacteria and used to immunize mice. The sera from the inoculated mice are then tested for their ability to neutralize the organism. Those proteins that produce protective responses are further investigated for use in vaccines. In addition, systems vaccinology promises to reveal immune responses associated with efficacy that can be targeted.[294]

Considerable interest is now being directed at nucleic acid vaccines, based either on DNA plasmids or mRNA segments. The former require relatively large doses and delivery by electroporation in order to generate important immune responses, but are particularly adept at inducing T cell responses. The latter are promising to produce good immune responses if their stability can be assured. There are already veterinary vaccines based on DNA plasmids[295] and the mRNA strategy is being explored for rapid immunization against influenza and HIV.[296]

Nevertheless, despite the availability of these new strategies, several vaccine targets remain difficult, among them universal influenza, RSV, and HIV. A universal influenza vaccine will necessitate the use of antigens other than the head of the hemagglutinin. Those antigens include neuraminidase, nucleoprotein, the M2e ion exchange protein, and the stalk of the hemagglutinin.[297–300] Although moderate efficacy has been achieved with the current influenza vaccines,[194] improvements can be made through the use of cell culture-derived vaccines,[301] epitope optimization,[302] increasing HA dose,[70] the addition of neuraminidase[303] stronger adjuvants,[304] and the search for better correlates of immunity than HA titers.[305–308] Success with RSV appears to depend on creating a fusion protein of the virus in its prefusion form.[249] Progress toward an effective HIV vaccine is focused on using multiple parts of the viral glycoprotein to induce multiple immune responses, including neutralization, antibody-dependent cellular cytotoxicity, and atypical CD8+ T cells.[309,310] In addition, efficacy may depend on so-called prime-boost regimens, in which the prime is a nucleic acid vaccine or a vector producing HIV proteins and the boost is the viral glycoprotein.[311]

Two other problem vaccines include dengue and CMV. In the case of dengue there is the problem that antibodies may be neutralizing and protective against one of the four serotypes immediately after vaccination, but heterotypic antibody against another serotype may wane after vaccination, leaving antibody that enhances entry into macrophages and causes hemorrhagic disease.[312] This phenomenon has already been problematic for one candidate vaccine.[313–315] In the case of CMV, immunity is not absolute and large challenge doses may overwhelm nominal immunity, even that induced by natural infection.[316] However, progress is being made to provide substantial protection against CMV through vaccination.[42]

Optimizing Breadth of Vaccin e Coverage—Genomics and Protein-based Vaccines

For most of the established vaccines in global use, the antigens selected for inclusion in the vaccine are present almost universally across the disease-causing bacterial population. For example, diphtheria and tetanus toxoid vaccines, are based on antigens ubiquitous to disease-causing *Corynebacterium diptheriae* and *Clostridium tetani*. Similarly, with the polysaccharide capsular vaccines used to prevent *Haemophilus influenzae* type b (Hib), *Streptococcus pneumoniae* (pneumococcus), and *Neisseria meningitidis* (meningococcus), the polysaccharide is a key virulence factor and depending on capsular types included in the vaccine, any organism possessing the respective capsules should be prevented from causing disease in an immunocompetent host. However, as the vaccine field faces challenges with optimizing existing vaccines or developing ones for new diseases, proteins are increasingly being studied as vaccine antigens.

Reverse vaccinology provided an antigen discovery method that enabled proteins to be identified using *in silico* techniques to assess cellular location and potential B and T cell epitopes.[317] These proteins were then generated *in vitro* and recombinant antigens were tested using mouse models to establish their immunogenic potential. However, proteins are subject to peptide sequence variation, through genetic mutations or recombination. When selecting proteins to use, properties such as cellular location, function, degree of conservation as well as the presence in other species need to be considered. An example of such vaccines are protein-based meningococcal vaccines, which were developed during the start of the twenty-first century to address the lack of serogroup B capsular vaccines. The B capsule shared structural similarity to human neural tissue and elicited poor immunogenicity in early studies. Capsular group B vaccine development was abandoned due to concerns regarding autoimmunity. Alternative, subcapsular proteins were identified and are the basis of the two licensed capsular group B meningococcal protein vaccines. The 4CMenB vaccine contains four major components namely: factor-H binding protein (fHbp), *Neisseria* heparin binding antigen (NHBA), *Neisseria* adhesin A (NadA), and Porin A (porA) all inserted into the outer membrane vesicle (OMV) vaccine MenNZB™.[318] The recombinant lipoprotein rLP2086 vaccine contains two different variants of the fHBP recombinant protein.[319] Although these proteins are found on the surface of most meningococci (except NadA), there is considerable meningococcal diversity which impacts potential efficacy. As we start introducing these multivalent protein-based vaccines, the breadth of coverage of such vaccines becomes appreciably more difficult to estimate than traditional vaccines. Outer membrane proteins are inherently more variable than periplasmic or cytoplasmic proteins, due to the influence of host immune selection, particularly as *N. meningitidis* exists in the normal nasopharyngeal microbiota, and is an organism with a solely human reservoir. Due to the rarity of invasive meningococcal disease, the accepted correlate of protection for meningococcal vaccines is the serum bactericidal activity (SBA) assay, which measures immunogenicity, that is, the ability of antibodies produced against all meningococcal vaccines to kill meningococci through complement-mediated pathways. Using this assay, meningococci with the same protein variants as contained in the vaccine were tested using postvaccination sera. For 4CMenB, 93–100% of infant vaccinees demonstrated acceptable titers in the SBA assays when strains matched the vaccine variants (peptide variants fHbp 1, NadA 8, PorA 7.2,4).[320] However, titers against nonvaccine strains were much lower for some variants and absent for others. Therefore it follows, that for this vaccine to remain effective, the vaccine needs to match strains, and therefore antigenic variants, that are circulating in the geographic region where it is being implemented or the antibodies generated need to show a degree of cross-protection. For rLP2086, the immunogenicity was also tested using SBA assays in subjects aged 10–18 years, and showed protective titers against four heterologous strains in 78.8–90.2%.[321]

In order to assess strain coverage, prior to licensure of the protein-based meningococcal vaccines, new laboratory assays were developed to determine strain coverage in view of these concerns. For 4CMenB vaccines, the Meningococcal Antigen Typing System (MATS) was developed.[322] For rLP2086, the Meningococcal Antigen Surface Expression (MEASURE) was developed.[323] Both assays aim to determine the protein variants and expression of representative isolates from regions of interest and then correlate this to bactericidal killing. Both assays are relatively complex, and can only be performed in specialist laboratories. These assays are also costly and labor intensive, so large-scale analysis is not feasible. Additionally, it is important to use contemporaneous strain collections, due to the secular changes in bacterial populations or clonal complexes, as defined by multilocus sequence typing.[324] As whole genome sequencing of microbial genomes becomes increasingly affordable, genomic analysis allows high-throughput and scalable methods of surveying bacterial population structure. By studying carriage or disease collections of meningococcal genomes, it is possible to identify the vaccine antigenic variants. One such study of meningococcal disease genomes identified low incidence of the vaccine variants in the United Kingdom prior to implementation of the 4CMenB vaccine into the infant immunization schedule.[325] However, cross-protective immune responses to similar, but not necessarily identical, vaccine antigens are also important, for which there were limited data at the time of writing, beyond the antigens identified using the MATS assay. The MATS assay estimated 66% coverage of meningococcal isolates from epidemiological year 2014/15, prior to national vaccine implementation.[326] Over this same period genomic estimates were 60.8% and a genotype-phenotype model estimated 66%.[327]

The true impact of the vaccine on infant meningococcal B disease is awaited, but vaccine efficacy estimated 10 months after implementation were 82.9% (95% confidence interval 24–94%).[328] If efficacy continues to be high, then the estimation of coverage needs to consider the antigens included in the outer membrane vesicle, which contains hundreds of proteins and lipo-oligosaccharide. These are not measured formally, beyond the identification of PorA, and there is suggestion for early studies of OMV vaccines, that these may be acting as minor antigens with a cumulative or synergistic effect.

The capsular group B meningococcal vaccines exemplify how novel approaches to vaccine development can raise further challenges that need to be addressed to aid in vaccine licensure, implementation, and ongoing surveillance. It is imperative that the postimplementation surveillance is as rigorous as the vaccine development, to ensure we are providing efficacious vaccines despite dynamic disease epidemiology. Collaboration between industry, academia, and public health are invaluable in allowing this to happen in a transparent way.

References

1. Bazin H. *Vaccination: A History: From Lady Montagu to Genetic Engineering*. Montrouge, France: John Libbey Eurotext; 2011, pp. 407–54.
2. Bailey I. Edward Jenner: Benefactor to mankind. *Proc R Coll Physicians Edinb*. 1997;27(1):5–15.
3. van Wijhe M, McDonald SA, de Melker HE, Postma MJ, Wallinga J. Effect of vaccination programmes on mortality burden among children and young adults in the Netherlands during the 20th century: A historical analysis. *Lancet Infect Dis*. 2016;16(5):592–8.
4. Orenstein WA, Ahmed R. Simply put: Vaccination saves lives. *Proc Natl Acad Sci U S A*. 2017;114(16):4031–3.
5. Saadatian-Elahi M, Horstick O, Breiman RF, et al. Beyond efficacy: The full public health impact of vaccines. *Vaccine*. 2016;34(9):1139–47.
6. Jit M, Hutubessy R, Png ME, et al. The broader economic impact of vaccination: Reviewing and appraising the strength of evidence. *BMC Med*. 2015;13:209.
7. Gessner BD, Kaslow D, Louis J, et al. Estimating the full public health value of vaccination. *Vaccine*. 2017;35(46):6255–63.
8. Doherty M, Buchy P, Standaert B, Giaquinto C, Prado-Cohrs D. Vaccine impact: Benefits for human health. *Vaccine*. 2016;34(52):6707–14.
9. Waye A, Jacobs P, Schryvers AB. Vaccine development costs: A review. *Expert Rev Vaccines*. 2013;12(12):1495–501.
10. Aguiar M, Stollenwerk N. Dengvaxia efficacy dependency on serostatus: A closer look at more recent data. *Clin Infect Dis*. 2018;66(4):641–2.
11. Pronker ES, Weenen TC, Commandeur H, Claassen EH, Osterhaus AD. Risk in vaccine research and development quantified. *PLoS One*. 2013;8(3):e57755.
12. Plotkin SA, Mahmoud AA, Farrar J. Establishing a global vaccine-development fund. *N Engl J Med*. 2015;373(4):297–300.
13. Rottingen JA, Gouglas D, Feinberg M, et al. New vaccines against epidemic infectious diseases. *N Engl J Med*. 2017;376(7):610–3.
14. Plotkin SA. Vaccines for epidemic infections and the role of CEPI. *Hum Vaccines Immunother*. 2017;13(12):2755–62.
15. Rennert WP, Hindiyeh M, Abu-Awwad FM, Marzouqa H, Ramlawi A. Introducing rotavirus vaccine to the Palestinian territories: The role of public-private partnerships. *J Public Health*. 2019;41(1):e78–83.
16. Plotkin SA. Correlates of protection induced by vaccination. *Clin Vaccine Immunol*. 2010;17(7):1055–65.
17. Rappuoli R, Bottomley MJ, D'Oro U, Finco O, De Gregorio E. Reverse vaccinology 2.0: Human immunology instructs vaccine antigen design. *J Exp Med*. 2016;213(4):469–81.
18. Mentzer AJ, O'Connor D, Pollard AJ, Hill AV. Searching for the human genetic factors standing in the way of universally effective vaccines. *Philos Trans R Soc Lond B Biol Sci*. 2015;370(1671):20140341.
19. Poland GA, Whitaker JA, Poland CM, Ovsyannikova IG, Kennedy RB. Vaccinology in the third millennium: Scientific and social challenges. *Curr Opin Virol*. 2016;17:116–25.
20. Burdin N, Handy LK, Plotkin SA. What is wrong with pertussis vaccine immunity? The problem of waning effectiveness of pertussis vaccines. *Cold Spring Harb Perspect Biol*. 2017;9(12):a029454.
21. Plotkin SA. Mumps: A pain in the neck. *J Pediatr Infect Dis Soc*. 2018;7(2):91–2.
22. Pinto MV, Merkel TJ. Pertussis disease and transmission and host responses: Insights from the baboon model of pertussis. *J Infect*. 2017;74 Suppl 1:S114–9.
23. Diavatopoulos DA, Edwards KM. What is wrong with pertussis vaccine immunity? Why immunological memory to pertussis is failing. *Cold Spring Harb Perspect Biol*. 2017;9(12):a029553.
24. Locht C. Live pertussis vaccines: Will they protect against carriage and spread of pertussis? *Clin Microbiol Infect*. 2016;22 Suppl 5:S96–102.
25. Kwong PD, Mascola JR. HIV-1 vaccines based on antibody identification, B cell ontogeny, and epitope structure. *Immunity*. 2018;48(5):855–71.
26. Williams LD, Ofek G, Schatzle S, et al. Potent and broad HIV-neutralizing antibodies in memory B cells and plasma. *Sci Immunol*. 2017;2(7):eaal2200.
27. Corey L, Gilbert PB, Tomaras GD, Haynes BF, Pantaleo G, Fauci AS. Immune correlates of vaccine protection against HIV-1 acquisition. *Sci Transl Med*. 2015;7(310):310rv317.
28. McMichael AJ, Picker LJ. Unusual antigen presentation offers new insight into HIV vaccine design. *Curr Opin Immunol*. 2017;46:75–81.
29. Burnett E, Jonesteller CL, Tate JE, Yen C, Parashar UD. Global impact of rotavirus vaccination on childhood hospitalizations and mortality from diarrhea. *J Infect Dis*. 2017;215(11):1666–72.
30. Magwira CA, Taylor MB. Composition of gut microbiota and its influence on the immunogenicity of oral rotavirus vaccines. *Vaccine*. 2018;36(24):3427–33.
31. Desselberger U. Differences of rotavirus vaccine effectiveness by country: Likely causes and contributing factors. *Pathogens*. 2017;6(4):65.
32. Crotty S, Ahmed R. Immunological memory in humans. *Semin Immunol*. 2004;16(3):197–203.
33. Hale JS, Ahmed R. Memory T follicular helper CD4 T cells. *Front Immunol*. 2015;6:16.
34. Geary CD, Sun JC. Memory responses of natural killer cells. *Semin Immunol*. 2017;31:11–9.
35. Topfer E, Boraschi D, Italiani P. Innate immune memory: The latest frontier of adjuvanticity. *J Immunol Res*. 2015;2015:478408.
36. Wu NC, Wilson IA. A perspective on the structural and functional constraints for immune evasion: Insights from influenza virus. *J Mol Biol*. 2017;429(17):2694–709.
37. Andrabi R, Bhiman JN, Burton DR. Strategies for a multi-stage neutralizing antibody-based HIV vaccine. *Curr Opin Immunol*. 2018;53:143–51.
38. Plotkin SA, Gilbert PB. Nomenclature for immune correlates of protection after vaccination. *Clin Infect Dis*. 2012;54(11):1615–7.
39. Plotkin SA. Complex correlates of protection after vaccination. *Clin Infect Dis*. 2013;56(10):1458–65.
40. Tomaras GD, Plotkin SA. Complex immune correlates of protection in HIV-1 vaccine efficacy trials. *Immunol Rev*. 2017;275(1):245–61.
41. Karnasuta C, Paris RM, Cox JH, et al. Antibody-dependent cell-mediated cytotoxic responses in participants enrolled in a phase I/II ALVAC-HIV/AIDSVAX B/E prime-boost HIV-1 vaccine trial in Thailand. *Vaccine*. 2005;23(19):2522–9.

42. Permar SR, Schleiss MR, Plotkin SA. Advancing our understanding of protective maternal immunity as a guide for development of vaccines to reduce congenital cytomegalovirus infections. *J Virol.* 2018;92(7):e00030-18.
43. Jegaskanda S. The potential role of Fc-receptor functions in the development of a universal influenza vaccine. *Vaccines.* 2018;6(2):27.
44. Voysey M, Kelly DF, Fanshawe TR, et al. The influence of maternally derived antibody and infant age at vaccination on infant vaccine responses: An individual participant meta-analysis. *JAMA Pediatr.* 2017;171(7):637–46.
45. Swain SL, Kugler-Umana O, Kuang Y, Zhang W. The properties of the unique age-associated B cell subset reveal a shift in strategy of immune response with age. *Cell Immunol.* 2017;321:52–60.
46. McElhaney JE, Kuchel GA, Zhou X, Swain SL, Haynes L. T-cell immunity to influenza in older adults: A pathophysiological framework for development of more effective vaccines. *Front Immunol.* 2016;7:41.
47. Bekri S, Bourdely P, Luci C, et al. Sublingual priming with a HIV gp41-based subunit vaccine elicits mucosal antibodies and persistent B memory responses in non-human primates. *Front Immunol.* 2017;8:63.
48. Xiao Y, Daniell H. Long-term evaluation of mucosal and systemic immunity and protection conferred by different polio booster vaccines. *Vaccine.* 2017;35(40):5418–25.
49. Poland GA, Kennedy RB, McKinney BA, et al. Vaccinomics, adversomics, and the immune response network theory: Individualized vaccinology in the 21st century. *Semin Immunol.* 2013;25(2):89–103.
50. Poland GA, Ovsyannikova IG, Kennedy RB. Personalized vaccinology: A review. *Vaccine.* 2018;36(36):5350–7.
51. Lazarus RP, John J, Shanmugasundaram E, et al. The effect of probiotics and zinc supplementation on the immune response to oral rotavirus vaccine: A randomized, factorial design, placebo-controlled study among Indian infants. *Vaccine.* 2018;36(2):273–9.
52. Zimmermann P, Curtis N. The influence of probiotics on vaccine responses—A systematic review. *Vaccine.* 2018;36(2):207–13.
53. Omer SB. Maternal immunization. *N Engl J Med.* 2017;376(25):2497.
54. Kourtis AP, Read JS, Jamieson DJ. Pregnancy and infection. *N Engl J Med.* 2014;370(23):2211–8.
55. Suzano CE, Amaral E, Sato HK, Papaiordanou PM. Campinas group on yellow fever immunization during P. The effects of yellow fever immunization (17DD) inadvertently used in early pregnancy during a mass campaign in Brazil. *Vaccine.* 2006;24(9):1421–6.
56. Schlaudecker EP, McNeal MM, Dodd CN, Ranz JB, Steinhoff MC. Pregnancy modifies the antibody response to trivalent influenza immunization. *J Infect Dis.* 2012;206(11):1670–3.
57. Christian LM, Porter K, Karlsson E, Schultz-Cherry S, Iams JD. Serum proinflammatory cytokine responses to influenza virus vaccine among women during pregnancy versus non-pregnancy. *Am J Reprod Immunol.* 2013;70(1):45–53.
58. Nasidi A, Monath TP, Vandenberg J, et al. Yellow fever vaccination and pregnancy: A four-year prospective study. *Trans R Soc Trop Med Hyg.* 1993;87(3):337–9.
59. Abu Raya B, Bamberger E, Almog M, Peri R, Srugo I, Kessel A. Immunization of pregnant women against pertussis: The effect of timing on antibody avidity. *Vaccine.* 2015;33(16):1948–52.
60. Regan AK, Klerk N, Moore HC, Omer SB, Shellam G, Effler PV. Effectiveness of seasonal trivalent influenza vaccination against hospital-attended acute respiratory infections in pregnant women: A retrospective cohort study. *Vaccine.* 2016;34(32):3649–56.
61. Omer SB, Clark DR, Aqil AR, et al. Maternal influenza immunization and prevention of severe clinical pneumonia in young infants: Analysis of randomized controlled trials conducted in Nepal, Mali and South Africa. *Pediatr Infect Dis J.* 2018;37(5):436–40.
62. Regan AK, de Klerk N, Moore HC, Omer SB, Shellam G, Effler PV. Effect of maternal influenza vaccination on hospitalization for respiratory infections in newborns: A retrospective cohort study. *Pediatr Infect Dis J.* 2016;35(10):1097–103.
63. Amirthalingam G, Andrews N, Campbell H, et al. Effectiveness of maternal pertussis vaccination in England: An observational study. *Lancet.* 2014;384(9953):1521–8.
64. Marchant A, Sadarangani M, Garand M, et al. Maternal immunisation: Collaborating with mother nature. *Lancet Infect Dis.* 2017;17(7):e197–208.
65. Munoz FM, Bond NH, Maccato M, et al. Safety and immunogenicity of tetanus diphtheria and acellular pertussis (Tdap) immunization during pregnancy in mothers and infants: A randomized clinical trial. *JAMA.* 2014;311(17):1760–9.
66. Cumberland P, Shulman CE, Maple PA, et al. Maternal HIV infection and placental malaria reduce transplacental antibody transfer and tetanus antibody levels in newborns in Kenya. *J Infect Dis.* 2007;196(4):550–7.
67. Glenn GM, Smith G, Fries L, et al. Safety and immunogenicity of a Sf9 insect cell-derived respiratory syncytial virus fusion protein nanoparticle vaccine. *Vaccine.* 2013;31(3):524–32.
68. Glenn GM, Fries LF, Thomas DN, et al. A randomized, blinded, controlled, dose-ranging study of a respiratory syncytial virus recombinant fusion (F) nanoparticle vaccine in healthy women of childbearing age. *J Infect Dis.* 2016;213(3):411–22.
69. The IMpact-RSV Study Group. Palivizumab, a humanized respiratory syncytial virus monoclonal antibody, reduces hospitalization from respiratory syncytial virus infection in high-risk infants. *Pediatrics.* 1998;102(3):531–7.
70. Edmond KM, Kortsalioudaki C, Scott S, et al. Group B streptococcal disease in infants aged younger than 3 months: Systematic review and meta-analysis. *Lancet.* 2012;379(9815):547–56.
71. Dzanibe S, Madhi SA. Systematic review of the clinical development of group B streptococcus serotype-specific capsular polysaccharide-based vaccines. *Expert Rev Vaccines.* 2018:17(7):635–51.
72. Kerr S, Van Bennekom CM, Liang JL, Mitchell AA. Tdap vaccination coverage during pregnancy—Selected sites, United States, 2006–2015. *MMWR Morb Mortal Wkly Rep.* 2017;66(41):1105–8.
73. Ding H, Black CL, Ball S, et al. Influenza vaccination coverage among pregnant women—United States, 2016–17 influenza season. *MMWR Morb Mortal Wkly Rep.* 2017;66(38):1016–22.
74. Saji F, Samejima Y, Kamiura S, Koyama M. Dynamics of immunoglobulins at the feto-maternal interface. *Rev Reprod.* 1999;4(2):81–9.
75. Eberhardt CS, Blanchard-Rohner G, Lemaitre B, et al. Maternal immunization earlier in pregnancy maximizes antibody transfer and expected infant seropositivity against pertussis. *Clin Infect Dis.* 2016;62(7):829–36.
76. Lumbreras Areta M, Eberhardt CS, Siegrist CA, Martinez de Tejada B. Antenatal vaccination to decrease pertussis in infants: Safety, effectiveness, timing, and implementation. *J Matern Fetal Neonatal Med.* 2019;32(9):1541–6.
77. Katz J, Englund JA, Steinhoff MC, et al. Impact of timing of influenza vaccination in pregnancy on transplacental antibody transfer, influenza incidence, and birth outcomes: A randomized trial in rural Nepal. *Clin Infect Dis.* 2018;67(3):334–40.
78. Frew PM, Randall LA, Malik F, et al. Clinician perspectives on strategies to improve patient maternal immunization acceptability in obstetrics and gynecology practice settings. *Hum Vaccin Immunother.* 2018;14(7):1548–57.
79. Grohskopf LA, Sokolow LZ, Broder KR, et al. Prevention and control of seasonal influenza with vaccines: Recommendations of the Advisory Committee on Immunization Practices—United States, 2017–18 influenza season. *Am J Transplant.* 2017;17(11):2970–82.
80. Hardy-Fairbanks AJ, Pan SJ, Decker MD, et al. Immune responses in infants whose mothers received Tdap vaccine during pregnancy. *Pediatr Infect Dis J.* 2013;32(11):1257–60.
81. Madhi SA, Nunes MC. Experience and challenges on influenza and pertussis vaccination in pregnant women. *Hum Vaccin Immunother.* 2018;14(9):2183–8.
82. Chamberlain AT, Lavery JV, White A, Omer SB. Ethics of maternal vaccination. *Science.* 2017;358(6362):452–3.
83. Beigi RH, Omer SB, Thompson KM. Key steps forward for maternal immunization: Policy making in action. *Vaccine.* 2018;36(12):1521–3.
84. Vojtek I, Dieussaert I, Doherty TM, et al. Maternal immunization: Where are we now and how to move forward? *Ann Med.* 2018;50(3):193–208.
85. Kenneson A, Cannon MJ. Review and meta-analysis of the epidemiology of congenital cytomegalovirus (CMV) infection. *Rev Med Virol.* 2007;17(4):253–76.
86. Camargo JF, Komanduri KV. Emerging concepts in cytomegalovirus infection following hematopoietic stem cell transplantation. *Hematol Oncol Stem Cell Ther.* 2017;10(4):233–8.
87. Ljungman P, Boeckh M, Hirsch HH, et al. Definitions of cytomegalovirus infection and disease in transplant patients for use in clinical trials. *Clin Infect Dis.* 2017;64(1):87–91.
88. Sansoni P, Vescovini R, Fagnoni FF, et al. New advances in CMV and immunosenescence. *Exp Gerontol.* 2014;55:54–62.
89. Joseph GP, McDermott R, Baryshnikova MA, Cobbs CS, Ulasov IV. Cytomegalovirus as an oncomodulatory agent in the progression of glioma. *Cancer Lett.* 2017;384:79–85.

90. Tracy RP, Doyle MF, Olson NC, et al. T-helper type 1 bias in healthy people is associated with cytomegalovirus serology and atherosclerosis: The Multi-Ethnic Study of Atherosclerosis. *J Am Heart Assoc.* 2013;2(3):e000117.

91. Kimberlin DW, Jester PM, Sanchez PJ, et al. Valganciclovir for symptomatic congenital cytomegalovirus disease. *N Engl J Med.* 2015;372(10):933–43.

92. Balcarek KB, Warren W, Smith RJ, Lyon MD, Pass RF. Neonatal screening for congenital cytomegalovirus infection by detection of virus in saliva. *J Infect Dis.* 1993;167(6):1433–6.

93. Boppana SB, Ross SA, Shimamura M, et al. Saliva polymerase-chain-reaction assay for cytomegalovirus screening in newborns. *N Engl J Med.* 2011;364(22):2111–8.

94. Griffiths P, Plotkin S, Mocarski E, et al. Desirability and feasibility of a vaccine against cytomegalovirus. *Vaccine.* 2013;31 Suppl 2:B197–203.

95. Plotkin SA, Boppana SB. Vaccination against the human cytomegalovirus. *Vaccine.* 2019;37(50):7437–42.

96. Yamamoto AY, Mussi-Pinhata MM, Isaac Mde L, et al. Congenital cytomegalovirus infection as a cause of sensorineural hearing loss in a highly immune population. *Pediatr Infect Dis J.* 2011;30(12):1043–6.

97. Fowler KB, Pass RF. Sexually transmitted diseases in mothers of neonates with congenital cytomegalovirus infection. *J Infect Dis.* 1991;164(2):259–64.

98. Leruez-Ville M, Magny JF, Couderc S, et al. Risk factors for congenital cytomegalovirus infection following primary and nonprimary maternal infection: A prospective neonatal screening study using polymerase chain reaction in saliva. *Clin Infect Dis.* 2017;65(3):398–404.

99. Wang C, Zhang X, Bialek S, Cannon MJ. Attribution of congenital cytomegalovirus infection to primary versus non-primary maternal infection. *Clin Infect Dis.* 2011;52(2):e11–3.

100. Schopfer K, Lauber E, Krech U. Congenital cytomegalovirus infection in newborn infants of mothers infected before pregnancy. *Arch Dis Child.* 1978;53(7):536–9.

101. Sohn YM, Park KI, Lee C, Han DG, Lee WY. Congenital cytomegalovirus infection in Korean population with very high prevalence of maternal immunity. *J Korean Med Sci.* 1992;7(1):47–51.

102. Schleiss MR, Permar SR, Plotkin SA. Progress toward development of a vaccine against congenital cytomegalovirus infection. *Clin Vaccine Immunol.* 2017;24(12):e00268-17.

103. Lilleri D, Fornara C, Furione M, Zavattoni M, Revello MG, Gerna G. Development of human cytomegalovirus-specific T cell immunity during primary infection of pregnant women and its correlation with virus transmission to the fetus. *J Infect Dis.* 2007;195(7):1062–70.

104. Lilleri D, Gerna G. Maternal immune correlates of protection from human cytomegalovirus transmission to the fetus after primary infection in pregnancy. *Rev Med Virol.* 2017;27(2).

105. Pass RF, Zhang C, Evans A, et al. Vaccine prevention of maternal cytomegalovirus infection. *N Engl J Med.* 2009;360(12):1191–9.

106. Bernstein DI, Munoz FM, Callahan ST, et al. Safety and efficacy of a cytomegalovirus glycoprotein B (gB) vaccine in adolescent girls: A randomized clinical trial. *Vaccine.* 2016;34(3):313–9.

107. Griffiths PD, Stanton A, McCarrell E, et al. Cytomegalovirus glycoprotein-B vaccine with MF59 adjuvant in transplant recipients: A phase 2 randomised placebo-controlled trial. *Lancet.* 2011;377(9773):1256–63.

108. Baraniak I, Kropff B, McLean GR, et al. Epitope-specific humoral responses to human cytomegalovirus glycoprotein-B vaccine with MF59: Anti-AD2 levels correlate with protection from viremia. *J Infect Dis.* 2018;217(12):1907–17.

109. Revello MG, Lilleri D, Zavattoni M, et al. Lymphoproliferative response in primary human cytomegalovirus (HCMV) infection is delayed in HCMV transmitter mothers. *J Infect Dis.* 2006;193(2):269–76.

110. Fornara C, Cassaniti I, Zavattoni M, et al. Human cytomegalovirus-specific memory CD4+ T-cell response and its correlation with virus transmission to the fetus in pregnant women with primary infection. *Clin Infect Dis.* 2017;65(10):1659–65.

111. Berencsi K, Gyulai Z, Gonczol E, et al. A canarypox vector-expressing cytomegalovirus (CMV) phosphoprotein 65 induces long-lasting cytotoxic T cell responses in human CMV-seronegative subjects. *J Infect Dis.* 2001;183(8):1171–9.

112. Cayatte C, Schneider-Ohrum K, Wang Z, et al. Cytomegalovirus vaccine strain towne-derived dense bodies induce broad cellular immune responses and neutralizing antibodies that prevent infection of fibroblasts and epithelial cells. *J Virol.* 2013;87(20):11107–20.

113. Wang D, Shenk T. Human cytomegalovirus virion protein complex required for epithelial and endothelial cell tropism. *Proc Natl Acad Sci U S A.* 2005;102(50):18153–8.

114. Ha S, Li F, Troutman MC, et al. Neutralization of diverse human cytomegalovirus strains conferred by antibodies targeting viral gH/gL/pUL128-131 pentameric complex. *J Virol.* 2017;91(7):e02033-16.

115. Elek SD, Stern H. Development of a vaccine against mental retardation caused by cytomegalovirus infection in utero. *Lancet.* 1974;1(7845):1–5.

116. Plotkin SA, Furukawa T, Zygraich N, Huygelen C. Candidate cytomegalovirus strain for human vaccination. *Infect Immun.* 1975;12(3):521–7.

117. Plotkin SA, Higgins R, Kurtz JB, et al. Multicenter trial of towne strain attenuated virus vaccine in seronegative renal transplant recipients. *Transplantation.* 1994;58(11):1176–8.

118. Institute of Medicine Committee to Study Priorities for Vaccine Development. The national academies collection: Reports funded by National Institutes of Health. In: Stratton KR, Durch JS, Lawrence RS, eds. *Vaccines for the 21st Century: A Tool for Decisionmaking.* Washington, DC: National Academies Press; 2000.

119. Fu TM, An Z, Wang D. Progress on pursuit of human cytomegalovirus vaccines for prevention of congenital infection and disease. *Vaccine.* 2014;32(22):2525–33.

120. Wloch MK, Smith LR, Boutsaboualoy S, et al. Safety and immunogenicity of a bivalent cytomegalovirus DNA vaccine in healthy adult subjects. *J Infect Dis.* 2008;197(12):1634–42.

121. Adler SP, Manganello AM, Lee R, et al. A phase 1 study of 4 live, recombinant human cytomegalovirus towne/toledo chimera vaccines in cytomegalovirus-seronegative men. *J Infect Dis.* 2016;214(9):1341–8.

122. Nakamura R, La Rosa C, Longmate J, et al. Viraemia, immunogenicity, and survival outcomes of cytomegalovirus chimeric epitope vaccine supplemented with PF03512676 (CMVPepVax) in allogeneic haemopoietic stem-cell transplantation: Randomised phase 1b trial. *Lancet Haematol.* 2016;3(2):e87–98.

123. La Rosa C, Longmate J, Martinez J, et al. MVA vaccine encoding CMV antigens safely induces durable expansion of CMV-specific T cells in healthy adults. *Blood.* 2017;129(1):114–25.

124. Flatz L, Hegazy AN, Bergthaler A, et al. Development of replication-defective lymphocytic choriomeningitis virus vectors for the induction of potent CD8+ T cell immunity. *Nat Med.* 2010;16(3):339–45.

125. Zhong J, Khanna R. Delineating the role of CD4+ T cells in the activation of human cytomegalovirus-specific immune responses following immunization with Ad-gBCMVpoly vaccine: Implications for vaccination of immunocompromised individuals. *J Gen Virol.* 2010;91(Pt 12):2994–3001.

126. Wilson SR, Wilson JH, Buonocore L, Palin A, Rose JK, Reuter JD. Intranasal immunization with recombinant vesicular stomatitis virus expressing murine cytomegalovirus glycoprotein B induces humoral and cellular immunity. *Comp Med.* 2008;58(2):129–39.

127. Geall AJ, Verma A, Otten GR, et al. Nonviral delivery of self-amplifying RNA vaccines. *Proc Natl Acad Sci U S A.* 2012;109(36):14604–9.

128. Kirchmeier M, Fluckiger AC, Soare C, et al. Enveloped virus-like particle expression of human cytomegalovirus glycoprotein B antigen induces antibodies with potent and broad neutralizing activity. *Clin Vaccine Immunol.* 2014;21(2):174–80.

129. Lanzieri TM, Dollard SC, Bialek SR, Grosse SD. Systematic review of the birth prevalence of congenital cytomegalovirus infection in developing countries. *Int J Infect Dis.* 2014;22:44–8.

130. Manicklal S, Emery VC, Lazzarotto T, Boppana SB, Gupta RK. The "silent" global burden of congenital cytomegalovirus. *Clin Microbiol Rev.* 2013;26(1):86–102.

131. Dar L, Namdeo D, Kumar P, et al. Congenital cytomegalovirus infection and permanent hearing loss in rural North Indian children. *Pediatr Infect Dis J.* 2017;36(7):670–3.

132. Hansen SG, Powers CJ, Richards R, et al. Evasion of CD8+ T cells is critical for superinfection by cytomegalovirus. *Science.* 2010;328(5974):102–6.

133. Starr SE, Friedman HM, Plotkin SA. The status of cytomegalovirus vaccine. *Rev Infect Dis.* 1991;13 Suppl 11:S964–5.

134. Krause PR, Bialek SR, Boppana SB, et al. Priorities for CMV vaccine development. *Vaccine.* 2013;32(1):4–10.

135. Murray NE, Quam MB, Wilder-Smith A. Epidemiology of dengue: Past, present and future prospects. *Clin Epidemiol.* 2013;5:299–309.

136. Rodrigo WWSI, Block OKT, Lane C, et al. Dengue virus neutralization is modulated by IgG antibody subclass and Fcγ receptor subtype. *Virology.* 2009;394(2):175–82.

137. Wu RSL, Chan KR, Tan HC, Chow A, Allen JC, Ooi EE. Neutralization of dengue virus in the presence of Fc receptor-mediated phagocytosis distinguishes serotype-specific from cross-neutralizing antibodies. *Antiviral Res.* 2012;96(3):340–3.

138. Dengue: Guidelines for Diagnosis, Treatment, Prevention and Control. 2009; *New Edition.*
139. Gibbons RV, Vaughn DW. Dengue: An escalating problem. *BMJ.* 2002;324(7353):1563–6.
140. Capeding MR, Tran NH, Hadinegoro SRS, et al. Clinical efficacy and safety of a novel tetravalent dengue vaccine in healthy children in Asia: A phase 3, randomised, observer-masked, placebo-controlled trial. *Lancet.* 2014;384(9951):1358–65.
141. Villar L, Dayan GH, Arredondo-García JL, et al. Efficacy of a tetravalent dengue vaccine in children in Latin America. *N Engl J Med.* 2015;372(2):113–23.
142. de Alwis R, Bangs DJ, Angelo MA, et al. Immunodominant dengue virus-specific CD8+T cell responses are associated with a memory PD-1+ phenotype. *J Virol.* 2016;90(9):4771–9.
143. Rey FA. Dengue virus: Two hosts, two structures. *Nature.* 2013;497(7450):443–4.
144. Zhang X, Sheng J, Plevka P, Kuhn RJ, Diamond MS, Rossmann MG. Dengue structure differs at the temperatures of its human and mosquito hosts. *Proc Natl Acad Sci U S A.* 2013;110(17):6795–9.
145. Fibriansah G, Ng TS, Kostyuchenko VA, et al. Structural changes in dengue virus when exposed to a temperature of 37 degrees C. *J Virol.* 2013;87(13):7585–92.
146. Eisinger RW, Fauci AS. Ending the HIV/AIDS pandemic. *Emerg Infect Dis.* 2018;24(3):413–6.
147. Barre-Sinoussi F, Chermann JC, Rey F, et al. Isolation of a T-lymphotropic retrovirus from a patient at risk for acquired immune deficiency syndrome (AIDS). *Science.* 1983;220(4599):868–71.
148. Schupbach J, Popovic M, Gilden RV, Gonda MA, Sarngadharan MG, Gallo RC. Serological analysis of a subgroup of human T-lymphotropic retroviruses (HTLV-III) associated with AIDS. *Science.* 1984;224(4648):503–5.
149. Haynes BF, Shaw GM, Korber B, et al. HIV-host interactions: Implications for vaccine design. *Cell Host Microbe.* 2016;19(3):292–303.
150. McCoy LE, Burton DR. Identification and specificity of broadly neutralizing antibodies against HIV. *Immunol Rev.* 2017;275(1):11–20.
151. McMichael AJ, Picker LJ. Unusual antigen presentation offers new insight into HIV vaccine design. *Curr Opin Immunol.* 2017;46:75–81.
152. Haynes BF, Verkoczy L. AIDS/HIV. Host controls of HIV neutralizing antibodies. *Science.* 2014;344(6184):588–9.
153. Kepler TB, Liao HX, Alam SM, et al. Immunoglobulin gene insertions and deletions in the affinity maturation of HIV-1 broadly reactive neutralizing antibodies. *Cell Host Microbe.* 2014;16(3):304–13.
154. Mascola JR, Haynes BF. HIV-1 neutralizing antibodies: Understanding nature's pathways. *Immunol Rev.* 2013;254(1):225–44.
155. Meffre E, Milili M, Blanco-Betancourt C, Antunes H, Nussenzweig MC, Schiff C. Immunoglobulin heavy chain expression shapes the B cell receptor repertoire in human B cell development. *J Clin Invest.* 2001;108(6):879–86.
156. Wiehe K, Bradley T, Meyerhoff RR, et al. Functional relevance of improbable antibody mutations for HIV broadly neutralizing antibody development. *Cell Host Microbe.* 2018;23(6):759–65 e756.
157. Robb ML, Rerks-Ngarm S, Nitayaphan S, et al. Risk behaviour and time as covariates for efficacy of the HIV vaccine regimen ALVAC-HIV (vCP1521) and AIDSVAX B/E: A post-hoc analysis of the Thai phase 3 efficacy trial RV 144. *Lancet Infect Dis.* 2012;12(7):531–7.
158. Haynes BF, Gilbert PB, McElrath MJ, et al. Immune-correlates analysis of an HIV-1 vaccine efficacy trial. *N Engl J Med.* 2012;366(14):1275–86.
159. Goonetilleke N, Liu MK, Salazar-Gonzalez JF, et al. The first T cell response to transmitted/founder virus contributes to the control of acute viremia in HIV-1 infection. *J Exp Med.* 2009;206(6):1253–72.
160. Gilbert PB, Peterson ML, Follmann D, et al. Correlation between immunologic responses to a recombinant glycoprotein 120 vaccine and incidence of HIV-1 infection in a phase 3 HIV-1 preventive vaccine trial. *J Infect Dis.* 2005;191(5):666–77.
161. Flynn NM, Forthal DN, Harro CD, et al. Placebo-controlled phase 3 trial of a recombinant glycoprotein 120 vaccine to prevent HIV-1 infection. *J Infect Dis.* 2005;191(5):654–65.
162. Buchbinder SP, Mehrotra DV, Duerr A, et al. Efficacy assessment of a cell-mediated immunity HIV-1 vaccine (the Step Study): A double-blind, randomised, placebo-controlled, test-of-concept trial. *Lancet.* 2008;372(9653):1881–93.
163. Duerr A, Huang Y, Buchbinder S, et al. Extended follow-up confirms early vaccine-enhanced risk of HIV acquisition and demonstrates waning effect over time among participants in a randomized trial of recombinant adenovirus HIV vaccine (Step Study). *J Infect Dis.* 2012;206(2):258–66.
164. Hammer SM, Sobieszczyk ME, Janes H, et al. Efficacy trial of a DNA/rAd5 HIV-1 preventive vaccine. *N Engl J Med.* 2013;369(22):2083–92.
165. Rerks-Ngarm S, Pitisuttithum P, Nitayaphan S, et al. Vaccination with ALVAC and AIDSVAX to prevent HIV-1 infection in Thailand. *N Engl J Med.* 2009;361(23):2209–20.
166. Wen Y, Trinh HV, Linton CE, et al. Generation and characterization of a bivalent protein boost for future clinical trials: HIV-1 subtypes CR01_AE and B gp120 antigens with a potent adjuvant. *PLoS One.* 2018;13(4):e0194266.
167. Barouch DH, Tomaka FL, Wegmann F, et al. Evaluation of a mosaic HIV-1 vaccine in a multicentre, randomised, double-blind, placebo-controlled, phase 1/2a clinical trial (APPROACH) and in rhesus monkeys (NHP 13-19). *Lancet.* 2018;392(10143):232–43.
168. Baden LR, Walsh SR, Seaman MS, et al. First-in-human randomized, controlled trial of mosaic HIV-1 immunogens delivered via a modified vaccinia ankara vector. *J Infect Dis.* 2018;218(4):633–44.
169. Zhou T, Georgiev I, Wu X, et al. Structural basis for broad and potent neutralization of HIV-1 by antibody VRC01. *Science.* 2010;329(5993):811–7.
170. Gilbert PB, Juraska M, deCamp AC, et al. Basis and statistical design of the passive HIV-1 antibody mediated prevention (AMP) test-of-concept efficacy trials. *Stat Commun Infect Dis.* 2017;9(1):20160001.
171. Haynes BF, Kelsoe G, Harrison SC, Kepler TB. B-cell-lineage immunogen design in vaccine development with HIV-1 as a case study. *Nat Biotechnol.* 2012;30(5):423–33.
172. Stamatatos L, Pancera M, McGuire AT. Germline-targeting immunogens. *Immunol Rev.* 2017;275(1):203–16.
173. Liao HX, Lynch R, Zhou T, et al. Co-evolution of a broadly neutralizing HIV-1 antibody and founder virus. *Nature.* 2013;496(7446):469–76.
174. Jardine JG, Kulp DW, Havenar-Daughton C, et al. HIV-1 broadly neutralizing antibody precursor B cells revealed by germline-targeting immunogen. *Science.* 2016;351(6280):1458–63.
175. Zhang R, Verkoczy L, Wiehe K, et al. Initiation of immune tolerance-controlled HIV gp41 neutralizing B cell lineages. *Sci Transl Med.* 2016;8(336):336ra362.
176. Williams WB, Zhang J, Jiang C, et al. Initiation of HIV neutralizing B cell lineages with sequential envelope immunizations. *Nat Commun.* 2017;8(1):1732.
177. Sanders RW, van Gils MJ, Derking R, et al. HIV-1 vaccines. HIV-1 neutralizing antibodies induced by native-like envelope trimers. *Science.* 2015;349(6244):aac4223.
178. Pauthner M, Havenar-Daughton C, Sok D, et al. Elicitation of robust tier 2 neutralizing antibody responses in nonhuman primates by HIV envelope trimer immunization using optimized approaches. *Immunity.* 2017;46(6):1073–88 e1076.
179. Voss JE, Andrabi R, McCoy LE, et al. Elicitation of neutralizing antibodies targeting the V2 apex of the HIV envelope trimer in a wild-type animal model. *Cell Rep.* 2017;21(1):222–35.
180. Saunders KO, Verkoczy LK, Jiang C, et al. Vaccine induction of heterologous tier 2 HIV-1 neutralizing antibodies in animal models. *Cell Rep.* 2017;21(13):3681–90.
181. Kelsoe G, Haynes BF. Host controls of HIV broadly neutralizing antibody development. *Immunol Rev.* 2017;275(1):79–88.
182. Locci M, Havenar-Daughton C, Landais E, et al. Human circulating PD-1+ CXCR3-CXCR5+ memory Tfh cells are highly functional and correlate with broadly neutralizing HIV antibody responses. *Immunity.* 2013;39(4):758–69.
183. Moody MA, Pedroza-Pacheco I, Vandergrift NA, et al. Immune perturbations in HIV-1-infected individuals who make broadly neutralizing antibodies. *Sci Immunol.* 2016;1(1):aag0851.
184. Bradley T, Peppa D, Pedroza-Pacheco I, et al. RAB11FIP5 expression and altered natural killer cell function are associated with induction of HIV broadly neutralizing antibody responses. *Cell.* 2018;175(2):387–99.e17.
185. Bradley T, Pollara J, Santra S, et al. Pentavalent HIV-1 vaccine protects against simian-human immunodeficiency virus challenge. *Nat Commun.* 2017;8:15711.
186. Vaccari M, Gordon SN, Fourati S, et al. Adjuvant-dependent innate and adaptive immune signatures of risk of SIVmac251 acquisition. *Nat Med.* 2016;22(7):762–70.
187. Vaccari M, Fourati S, Gordon SN, et al. HIV vaccine candidate activation of hypoxia and the inflammasome in CD14(+) monocytes is associated with a decreased risk of SIVmac251 acquisition. *Nat Med.* 2018;24(6):847–56.

188. Buchbinder SP, Grunenberg NA, Sanchez BJ, et al. Immunogenicity of a novel Clade B HIV-1 vaccine combination: Results of phase 1 randomized placebo controlled trial of an HIV-1 GM-CSF-expressing DNA prime with a modified vaccinia Ankara vaccine boost in healthy HIV-1 uninfected adults. *PLoS One.* 2017;12(7):e0179597.

189. Goepfert PA, Elizaga ML, Sato A, et al. Phase 1 safety and immunogenicity testing of DNA and recombinant modified vaccinia Ankara vaccines expressing HIV-1 virus-like particles. *J Infect Dis.* 2011;203(5):610–9.

190. Hansen SG, Wu HL, Burwitz BJ, et al. Broadly targeted CD8(+) T cell responses restricted by major histocompatibility complex E. *Science.* 2016;351(6274):714–20.

191. Hause BM, Ducatez M, Collin EA, et al. Isolation of a novel swine influenza virus from Oklahoma in 2011 which is distantly related to human influenza C viruses. *PLoS Pathog.* 2013;9(2):e1003176.

192. Palache A. Seasonal influenza vaccine provision in 157 countries (2004–2009) and the potential influence of national public health policies. *Vaccine.* 2011;29(51):9459–66.

193. Gerdil C. The annual production cycle for influenza vaccine. *Vaccine.* 2003;21(16):1776–9.

194. DiazGranados CA, Denis M, Plotkin S. Seasonal influenza vaccine efficacy and its determinants in children and non-elderly adults: A systematic review with meta-analyses of controlled trials. *Vaccine.* 2012;31(1):49–57.

195. Steel J, Lowen AC, Wang TT, et al. Influenza virus vaccine based on the conserved hemagglutinin stalk domain. *mBio.* 2010;1(1):e00018-10.

196. Gao X, Wang W, Li Y, et al. Enhanced influenza VLP vaccines comprising matrix-2 ectodomain and nucleoprotein epitopes protects mice from lethal challenge. *Antiviral Res.* 2013;98(1):4–11.

197. Ekiert DC, Friesen RH, Bhabha G, et al. A highly conserved neutralizing epitope on group 2 influenza A viruses. *Science.* 2011;333(6044):843–50.

198. Ramirez A, Morris S, Maucourant S, et al. A virus-like particle vaccine candidate for influenza A virus based on multiple conserved antigens presented on hepatitis B tandem core particles. *Vaccine.* 2018;36(6):873–80.

199. Lee YT, Ko EJ, Lee Y, et al. Intranasal vaccination with M2e5x virus-like particles induces humoral and cellular immune responses conferring cross-protection against heterosubtypic influenza viruses. *PLoS One.* 2018;13(1):e0190868.

200. Zedda L, Forleo-Neto E, Vertruyen A, et al. Dissecting the immune response to MF59-adjuvanted and nonadjuvanted seasonal influenza vaccines in children less than three years of age. *Pediatr Infect Dis J.* 2015;34(1):73–8.

201. Nakaya HI, Clutterbuck E, Kazmin D, et al. Systems biology of immunity to MF59-adjuvanted versus nonadjuvanted trivalent seasonal influenza vaccines in early childhood. *Proc Natl Acad Sci U S A.* 2016;113(7):1853–8.

202. Hekele A, Bertholet S, Archer J, et al. Rapidly produced SAM((R)) vaccine against H7N9 influenza is immunogenic in mice. *Emerg Microbes Infect.* 2013;2(8):e52.

203. WHO. Immunization, Vaccines and Biologicals: Pertussis. 2011. http://www.who.int/immunization/topics/pertussis/en/. Accessed August 1, 2018.

204. Kerr JR, Matthews RC. Bordetella pertussis infection: Pathogenesis, diagnosis, management, and the role of protective immunity. *Eur J Clin Microbiol Infect Dis.* 2000;19(2):77–88.

205. Jefferson T, Rudin M, DiPietrantonj C. Systematic review of the effects of pertussis vaccines in children. *Vaccine.* 2003;21(17-18):2003–14.

206. Zhang L, Prietsch SO, Axelsson I, Halperin SA. Acellular vaccines for preventing whooping cough in children. *Cochrane Database Syst Rev.* 2014(9):CD001478.

207. Feldstein LR, Mariat S, Gacic-Dobo M, Diallo MS, Conklin LM, Wallace AS. Global routine vaccination coverage, 2016. *MMWR Morb Mortal Wkly Rep.* 2017;66(45):1252–5.

208. McGirr A, Fisman DN. Duration of pertussis immunity after DTaP immunization: A meta-analysis. *Pediatrics.* 2015;135(2):331–43.

209. Winter K, Harriman K, Zipprich J, et al. California pertussis epidemic, 2010. *J Pediatr.* 2012;161(6):1091–6.

210. Acosta AM, DeBolt C, Tasslimi A, et al. Tdap vaccine effectiveness in adolescents during the 2012 Washington State pertussis epidemic. *Pediatrics.* 2015;135(6):981–9.

211. Koepke R, Eickhoff JC, Ayele RA, et al. Estimating the effectiveness of tetanus-diphtheria-acellular pertussis vaccine (Tdap) for preventing pertussis: Evidence of rapidly waning immunity and difference in effectiveness by Tdap brand. *J Infect Dis.* 2014;210(6):942–53.

212. Tan T, Dalby T, Forsyth K, et al. Pertussis across the globe: Recent epidemiologic trends from 2000 to 2013. *Pediatr Infect Dis J.* 2015;34(9):e222–32.

213. Bolotin S, Harvill ET, Crowcroft NS. What to do about pertussis vaccines? Linking what we know about pertussis vaccine effectiveness, immunology and disease transmission to create a better vaccine. *Pathog Dis.* 2015;73(8):ftv057.

214. Allen AC, Mills KH. Improved pertussis vaccines based on adjuvants that induce cell-mediated immunity. *Expert Rev Vaccines.* 2014;13(10):1253–64.

215. Warfel JM, Zimmerman LI, Merkel TJ. Acellular pertussis vaccines protect against disease but fail to prevent infection and transmission in a nonhuman primate model. *Proc Natl Acad Sci U S A.* 2014;111(2):787–92.

216. Matthias J, Pritchard PS, Martin SW, et al. Sustained transmission of pertussis in vaccinated, 1–5-year-old children in a preschool, Florida, USA. *Emerg Infect Dis.* 2016;22(2):242–6.

217. Cherry JD. Why do pertussis vaccines fail? *Pediatrics.* 2012;129(5):968–70.

218. Sharma SK, Pichichero ME. Functional deficits of pertussis-specific CD4+ T cells in infants compared to adults following DTaP vaccination. *Clin Exp Immunol.* 2012;169(3):281–91.

219. Plotkin SA. Pertussis: Pertussis control strategies and the options for improving current vaccines. *Expert Rev Vaccines.* 2014;13(9):1071–2.

220. Locht C. Will we have new pertussis vaccines? *Vaccine.* 2018;36(36):5460–9.

221. Locht C. Pertussis: Where did we go wrong and what can we do about it? *J Infect.* 2016;72 Suppl:S34–40.

222. Debrie AS, Coutte L, Raze D, et al. Construction and evaluation of Bordetella pertussis live attenuated vaccine strain BPZE1 producing Fim3. *Vaccine.* 2018;36(11):1345–52.

223. Desselberger U. Rotaviruses. *Virus Res.* 2014;190:75–96.

224. Santos N, Hoshino Y. Global distribution of rotavirus serotypes/genotypes and its implication for the development and implementation of an effective rotavirus vaccine. *Rev Med Virol.* 2005;15(1):29–56.

225. Bishop RF, Barnes GL, Cipriani E, Lund JS. Clinical immunity after neonatal rotavirus infection. A prospective longitudinal study in young children. *N Engl J Med.* 1983;309(2):72–6.

226. Fischer TK, Valentiner-Branth P, Steinsland H, et al. Protective immunity after natural rotavirus infection: A community cohort study of newborn children in Guinea-Bissau, west Africa. *J Infect Dis.* 2002;186(5):593–7.

227. Velazquez FR, Matson DO, Calva JJ, et al. Rotavirus infections in infants as protection against subsequent infections. *N Engl J Med.* 1996;335(14):1022–8.

228. Jiang V, Jiang B, Tate J, Parashar UD, Patel MM. Performance of rotavirus vaccines in developed and developing countries. *Hum Vaccin.* 2010;6(7):532–42.

229. Marlow R, Muir P, Vipond B, Lyttle M, Trotter C, Finn A. Assessing the impacts of the first year of rotavirus vaccination in the United Kingdom. *Euro Surveill.* 2015;20(48):30077.

230. Rha B, Tate JE, Payne DC, et al. Effectiveness and impact of rotavirus vaccines in the United States—2006-2012. *Expert Rev Vaccines.* 2014;13(3):365–76.

231. Giaquinto C, Dominiak-Felden G, Van Damme P, et al. Summary of effectiveness and impact of rotavirus vaccination with the oral pentavalent rotavirus vaccine: A systematic review of the experience in industrialized countries. *Hum Vaccin.* 2011;7(7):734–48.

232. Ngabo F, Tate JE, Gatera M, et al. Effect of pentavalent rotavirus vaccine introduction on hospital admissions for diarrhoea and rotavirus in children in Rwanda: A time-series analysis. *Lancet Glob Health.* 2016;4(2):e129–36.

233. Vesikari T, Matson DO, Dennehy P, et al. Safety and efficacy of a pentavalent human-bovine (WC3) reassortant rotavirus vaccine. *N Engl J Med.* 2006;354(1):23–33.

234. Armah GE, Sow SO, Breiman RF, et al. Efficacy of pentavalent rotavirus vaccine against severe rotavirus gastroenteritis in infants in developing countries in sub-Saharan Africa: A randomised, double-blind, placebo-controlled trial. *Lancet.* 2010;376(9741):606–14.

235. Zaman K, Dang DA, Victor JC, et al. Efficacy of pentavalent rotavirus vaccine against severe rotavirus gastroenteritis in infants in developing countries in Asia: A randomised, double-blind, placebo-controlled trial. *Lancet.* 2010;376(9741):615–23.

236. World Health Organisation. Rotavirus vaccines: An update. *Wkly Epidemiol Rec.* 2009;84:553–40.

237. Kuss SK, Best GT, Etheredge CA, et al. Intestinal microbiota promote enteric virus replication and systemic pathogenesis. *Science.* 2011;334(6053):249–52.

238. Uchiyama R, Chassaing B, Zhang B, Gewirtz AT. Antibiotic treatment suppresses rotavirus infection and enhances specific humoral immunity. *J Infect Dis.* 2014;210(2):171–82.

239. Isolauri E, Joensuu J, Suomalainen H, Luomala M, Vesikari T. Improved immunogenicity of oral D x RRV reassortant rotavirus vaccine by *Lactobacillus casei* GG. *Vaccine.* 1995;13(3):310-312.

240. Harris VC, Armah G, Fuentes S, et al. Significant correlation between the infant gut microbiome and rotavirus vaccine response in rural Ghana. *J Infect Dis.* 2017;215(1):34–41.

241. Zhao X, Singh M, Malashkevich VN, Kim PS. Structural characterization of the human respiratory syncytial virus fusion protein core. *Proc Natl Acad Sci U S A.* 2000;97(26):14172–7.

242. Anderson LJ, Hierholzer JC, Tsou C, et al. Antigenic characterization of respiratory syncytial virus strains with monoclonal antibodies. *J Infect Dis.* 1985;151(4):626–33.

243. Mufson MA, Orvell C, Rafnar B, Norrby E. Two distinct subtypes of human respiratory syncytial virus. *J Gen Virol.* 1985;66 (Pt 10):2111–24.

244. Peret TC, Hall CB, Schnabel KC, Golub JA, Anderson LJ. Circulation patterns of genetically distinct group A and B strains of human respiratory syncytial virus in a community. *J Gen Virol.* 1998;79 (Pt 9):2221–9.

245. Drysdale SB, Sande CJ, Green CA, Pollard AJ. RSV vaccine use—The missing data. *Expert Rev Vaccines.* 2016;15(2):149–52.

246. Kim HW, Canchola JG, Brandt CD, et al. Respiratory syncytial virus disease in infants despite prior administration of antigenic inactivated vaccine. *Am J Epidemiol.* 1969;89(4):422–34.

247. Kapikian AZ, Mitchell RH, Chanock RM, Shvedoff RA, Stewart CE. An epidemiologic study of altered clinical reactivity to respiratory syncytial (RS) virus infection in children previously vaccinated with an inactivated RS virus vaccine. *Am J Epidemiol.* 1969;89(4):405–21.

248. Beeler JA, van Wyke Coelingh K. Neutralization epitopes of the F glycoprotein of respiratory syncytial virus: Effect of mutation upon fusion function. *J Virol.* 1989;63(7):2941–50.

249. Graham BS, Modjarrad K, McLellan JS. Novel antigens for RSV vaccines. *Curr Opin Immunol.* 2015;35:30–8.

250. McLellan JS, Chen M, Joyce MG, et al. Structure-based design of a fusion glycoprotein vaccine for respiratory syncytial virus. *Science.* 2013;342(6158):592–8.

251. McLellan JS, Chen M, Leung S, et al. Structure of RSV fusion glycoprotein trimer bound to a prefusion-specific neutralizing antibody. *Science.* 2013;340(6136):1113–7.

252. Gkentzi D, Katsakiori P, Marangos M, et al. Maternal vaccination against pertussis: A systematic review of the recent literature. *Arch Dis Child Fetal Neonatal Ed.* 2017;102(5):F456–63.

253. Verani JR, McGee L, Schrag SJ. Division of bacterial diseases NCfI, respiratory diseases CfDC, prevention. Prevention of perinatal group B streptococcal disease—Revised guidelines from CDC, 2010. *MMWR Recomm Rep.* 2010;59(RR-10):1–36.

254. Harrison LH, Elliott JA, Dwyer DM, et al. Serotype distribution of invasive group B streptococcal isolates in Maryland: Implications for vaccine formulation. Maryland Emerging Infections Program. *J Infect Dis.* 1998;177(4):998–1002.

255. Buccato S, Maione D, Rinaudo CD, et al. Use of *Lactococcus lactis* expressing pili from group B Streptococcus as a broad-coverage vaccine against streptococcal disease. *J Infect Dis.* 2006;194(3):331–40.

256. Lauer P, Rinaudo CD, Soriani M, et al. Genome analysis reveals pili in Group B Streptococcus. *Science.* 2005;309(5731):105.

257. Rosini R, Rinaudo CD, Soriani M, et al. Identification of novel genomic islands coding for antigenic pilus-like structures in *Streptococcus agalactiae. Mol Microbiol.* 2006;61(1):126–41.

258. Maisey HC, Hensler M, Nizet V, Doran KS. Group B streptococcal pilus proteins contribute to adherence to and invasion of brain microvascular endothelial cells. *J Bacteriol.* 2007;189(4):1464–7.

259. Siegrist CA, Aspinall R. B-cell responses to vaccination at the extremes of age. *Nat Rev Immunol.* 2009;9(3):185–94.

260. Schuchat A. Epidemiology of group B streptococcal disease in the United States: Shifting paradigms. *Clin Microbiol Rev.* 1998;11(3):497–513.

261. Kimura K, Suzuki S, Wachino J, et al. First molecular characterization of group B streptococci with reduced penicillin susceptibility. *Antimicrob Agents Chemother.* 2008;52(8):2890–7.

262. Schrag SJ, Zell ER, Lynfield R, et al. A population-based comparison of strategies to prevent early-onset group B streptococcal disease in neonates. *N Engl J Med.* 2002;347(4):233–9.

262a. Schrag SJ, Verani JR. Intrapartum antibiotic prophylaxis for the prevention of perinatal group B streptococcal disease: Experience in the United States and implications for a potential group B streptococcal vaccine. *Vaccine.* 2013;31 Suppl 4:D20–6.

263. Metcalf BJ, Chochua S, Gertz RE Jr, et al. Short-read whole genome sequencing for determination of antimicrobial resistance mechanisms and capsular serotypes of current invasive *Streptococcus agalactiae* recovered in the USA. *Clin Microbiol Infect.* 2017;23(8):574.e7–14.

264. Rentz AC, Samore MH, Stoddard GJ, Faix RG, Byington CL. Risk factors associated with ampicillin-resistant infection in newborns in the era of group B streptococcal prophylaxis. *Arch Pediatr Adolesc Med.* 2004;158(6):556–60.

265. Baker CJ, Kasper DL. Correlation of maternal antibody deficiency with susceptibility to neonatal group B streptococcal infection. *N Engl J Med.* 1976;294(14):753–6.

266. Edwards MS, Rench MA, Baker CJ. Relevance of age at diagnosis to prevention of late-onset group B streptococcal disease by maternal immunization. *Pediatr Infect Dis J.* 2015;34(5):538–9.

267. Baker CJ, Kasper DL. Group B streptococcal vaccines. *Rev Infect Dis.* 1985;7(4):458–67.

268. Baker CJ, Rench MA, Edwards MS, Carpenter RJ, Hays BM, Kasper DL. Immunization of pregnant women with a polysaccharide vaccine of group B streptococcus. *N Engl J Med.* 1988;319(18):1180–5.

269. Zaleznik DF, Rench MA, Hillier S, et al. Invasive disease due to group B Streptococcus in pregnant women and neonates from diverse population groups. *Clin Infect Dis.* 2000;30(2):276–81.

270. Baker CJ, Paoletti LC, Rench MA, et al. Use of capsular polysaccharide-tetanus toxoid conjugate vaccine for type II group B Streptococcus in healthy women. *J Infect dis.* 2000;182(4):1129–38.

271. Baker CJ, Paoletti LC, Wessels MR, et al. Safety and immunogenicity of capsular polysaccharide-tetanus toxoid conjugate vaccines for group B streptococcal types Ia and Ib. *J Infect Dis.* 1999;179(1):142–50.

272. Baker CJ, Edwards MS. Group B streptococcal conjugate vaccines. *Arch Dis Child.* 2003;88(5):375–8.

273. Paoletti LC, Rench MA, Kasper DL, Molrine D, Ambrosino D, Baker CJ. Effects of alum adjuvant or a booster dose on immunogenicity during clinical trials of group B streptococcal type III conjugate vaccines. *Infect Immun.* 2001;69(11):6696–701.

274. Chen VL, Avci FY, Kasper DL. A maternal vaccine against group B Streptococcus: Past, present, and future. *Vaccine.* 2013;31 Suppl 4:D13–9.

275. Baker CJ, Rench MA, Fernandez M, Paoletti LC, Kasper DL, Edwards MS. Safety and immunogenicity of a bivalent group B streptococcal conjugate vaccine for serotypes II and III. *J Infect Dis.* 2003;188(1):66–73.

276. Madhi SA, Koen A, Cutland CL, et al. Antibody kinetics and response to routine vaccinations in infants born to women who received an investigational trivalent group B Streptococcus polysaccharide CRM197-conjugate vaccine during pregnancy. *Clin Infect Dis.* 2017;65(11):1897–904.

277. Lin SM, Zhi Y, Ahn KB, Lim S, Seo HS. Status of group B streptococcal vaccine development. *Clin Exp Vaccine Res.* 2018;7(1):76–81.

278. Kobayashi M, Vekemans J, Baker CJ, Ratner AJ, Le Doare K, Schrag SJ. Group B Streptococcus vaccine development: Present status and future considerations, with emphasis on perspectives for low and middle income countries. *F1000Res.* 2016;5:2355.

279. Kristeva M, Tillman C, Goordeen A. Immunization against group B *Streptococci* vs. intrapartum antibiotic prophylaxis in peripartum pregnant women and their neonates: A review. *Cureus.* 2017;9(10):e1775.

280. Johnson K, Posner SF, Biermann J, et al. Recommendations to improve preconception health and health care—United States. A report of the CDC/ATSDR Preconception Care Work Group and the Select Panel on Preconception Care. *MMWR Recomm Rep.* 2006;55(RR-6):1–23.

281. Prescott JB, Marzi A, Safronetz D, Robertson SJ, Feldmann H, Best SM. Immunobiology of Ebola and Lassa virus infections. *Nat Rev Immunol.* 2017;17(3):195–207.

282. Weaver SC, Lecuit M. Chikungunya virus and the global spread of a mosquito-borne disease. *N Engl J Med.* 2015;372(13):1231–9.

283. Depoux A, Philibert A, Rabier S, Philippe HJ, Fontanet A, Flahault A. A multi-faceted pandemic: A review of the state of knowledge on the Zika virus. *Public Health Rev.* 2018;39:10.

284. Fausther-Bovendo H, Mulangu S, Sullivan NJ. Ebolavirus vaccines for humans and apes. *Curr Opin Virol.* 2012;2(3):324–9.

285. Suder E, Furuyama W, Feldmann H, Marzi A, de Wit E. The vesicular stomatitis virus-based Ebola virus vaccine: From concept to clinical trials. *Hum Vaccin Immunother.* 2018;14(9):2107–13.

286. Kieny MP, Rottingen JA, Farrar J. The need for global R&D coordination for infectious diseases with epidemic potential. *Lancet.* 2016;388(10043):460–1.

287. Clark HF, Offit PA, Ellis RW, et al. The development of multivalent bovine rotavirus (strain WC3) reassortant vaccine for infants. *J Infect Dis.* 1996;174 Suppl 1:S73–80.

288. Waring BM, Sjaastad LE, Fiege JK, et al. MicroRNA-based attenuation of influenza virus across susceptible hosts. *J Virol.* 2018;92(2):e01741-17.

289. Humphreys IR, Sebastian S. Novel viral vectors in infectious diseases. *Immunology.* 2018;153(1):1–9.

290. Geisbert TW, Feldmann H. Recombinant vesicular stomatitis virus-based vaccines against Ebola and Marburg virus infections. *J Infect Dis.* 2011;204 Suppl 3:S1075–81.

291. Ring S, Flatz L. Generation of lymphocytic choriomeningitis virus based vaccine vectors. *Methods Mol Biol.* 2016;1404:351–64.

292. Keele BF, Li W, Borducchi EN, et al. Adenovirus prime, Env protein boost vaccine protects against neutralization-resistant SIVsmE660 variants in rhesus monkeys. *Nat Commun.* 2017;8:15740.

293. Shen X, Basu R, Sawant S, et al. HIV-1 gp120 and modified vaccinia virus ankara (MVA) gp140 boost immunogens increase immunogenicity of a DNA/MVA HIV-1 vaccine. *J Virol.* 2017;91(24):e01077-17.

294. Amenyogbe N, Levy O, Kollmann TR. Systems vaccinology: A promise for the young and the poor. *Philos Trans R Soc Lond B Biol Sci.* 2015;370(1671):20140340.

295. Kudchodkar SB, Choi H, Reuschel EL, et al. Rapid response to an emerging infectious disease—Lessons learned from development of a synthetic DNA vaccine targeting Zika virus. *Microbes Infect.* 2018;20(11–12):676–84.

296. Pardi N, Hogan MJ, Naradikian MS, et al. Nucleoside-modified mRNA vaccines induce potent T follicular helper and germinal center B cell responses. *J Exp Med.* 2018;215(6):1571–88.

297. Krammer F, Fouchier RAM, Eichelberger MC, et al. NAction! How can neuraminidase-based immunity contribute to better influenza virus vaccines? *mBio.* 2018;9(2):e02332-17.

298. Nachbagauer R, Palese P. Development of next generation hemagglutinin-based broadly protective influenza virus vaccines. *Curr Opin Immunol.* 2018;53:51–7.

299. Cox F, Juraszek, J., Stoop, E., Goudsmit, J. Universal influenza vaccine design: Directing the antibody repertoire. *Future Virol.* 2016;11(6):451–67.

300. Clemens EB, van de Sandt C, Wong SS, Wakim LM, Valkenburg SA. Harnessing the power of T cells: The promising hope for a universal influenza vaccine. *Vaccines.* 2018;6(2):18.

301. Perez-Rubio A, Eiros Bouza JM. Cell culture-derived flu vaccine: Present and future. *Hum Vaccin Immunother.* 2018;14(8):1874–82.

302. Allen JD, Owino SO, Carter DM, et al. Broadened immunity and protective responses with emulsion-adjuvanted H5 COBRA-VLP vaccines. *Vaccine.* 2017;35(38):5209–16.

303. Eichelberger MC, Morens DM, Taubenberger JK. Neuraminidase as an influenza vaccine antigen: A low hanging fruit, ready for picking to improve vaccine effectiveness. *Curr Opin Immunol.* 2018;53:38–44.

304. Domnich A, Arata L, Amicizia D, Puig-Barbera J, Gasparini R, Panatto D. Effectiveness of MF59-adjuvanted seasonal influenza vaccine in the elderly: A systematic review and meta-analysis. *Vaccine.* 2017;35(4):513–20.

305. Vanderven HA, Jegaskanda S, Wines BD, et al. Antibody-dependent cellular cytotoxicity responses to seasonal influenza vaccination in older adults. *J Infect Dis.* 2017;217(1):12–23.

306. de Vries RD, Nieuwkoop NJ, Pronk M, et al. Influenza virus-specific antibody dependent cellular cytoxicity induced by vaccination or natural infection. *Vaccine.* 2017;35(2):238–47.

307. Wilkinson TM, Li CK, Chui CS, et al. Preexisting influenza-specific CD4+ T cells correlate with disease protection against influenza challenge in humans. *Nat Med.* 2012;18(2):274–80.

308. Sridhar S, Begom S, Bermingham A, et al. Cellular immune correlates of protection against symptomatic pandemic influenza. *Nat Med.* 2013;19(10):1305–12.

309. Haynes BF, Burton DR. Developing an HIV vaccine. *Science.* 2017;355(6330):1129–30.

310. Montefiori DC, Roederer M, Morris L, Seaman MS. Neutralization tiers of HIV-1. *Curr Opin HIV AIDS.* 2018;13(2):128–36.

311. Saunders KO, Santra S, Parks R, et al. Immunogenicity of NYVAC prime-protein boost human immunodeficiency virus type 1 envelope vaccination and simian-human immunodeficiency virus challenge of nonhuman primates. *J Virol.* 2018;92(8):e02035-17.

312. Katzelnick LC, Gresh L, Halloran ME, et al. Antibody-dependent enhancement of severe dengue disease in humans. *Science.* 2017; 358(6365):929–32.

313. Halstead SB. Dengvaxia sensitizes seronegatives to vaccine enhanced disease regardless of age. *Vaccine.* 2017;35(47):6355–8.

314. Godoi IP, Lemos LL, de Araujo VE, Bonoto BC, Godman B, Guerra Junior AA. CYD-TDV dengue vaccine: Systematic review and meta-analysis of efficacy, immunogenicity and safety. *J Comp Eff Res.* 2017;6(2):165–80.

315. Whitehead SS, Subbarao K. Which dengue vaccine approach is the most promising, and should we be concerned about enhanced disease after vaccination? The risks of incomplete immunity to dengue virus revealed by vaccination. *Cold Spring Harb Perspect Biol.* 2018;10(6):a028811.

316. Plotkin SA, Starr SE, Friedman HM, Gonczol E, Weibel RE. Protective effects of Towne cytomegalovirus vaccine against low-passage cytomegalovirus administered as a challenge. *J Infect Dis.* 1989;159(5):860–5.

317. Sette A, Rappuoli R. Reverse vaccinology: Developing vaccines in the era of genomics. *Immunity.* 2010;33(4):530–41.

318. Serruto D, Bottomley MJ, Ram S, Giuliani MM, Rappuoli R. The new multicomponent vaccine against meningococcal serogroup B, 4CMenB: Immunological, functional and structural characterization of the antigens. *Vaccine.* 2012;30 Suppl 2:B87–97.

319. Jiang HQ, Hoiseth SK, Harris SL, et al. Broad vaccine coverage predicted for a bivalent recombinant factor H binding protein based vaccine to prevent serogroup B meningococcal disease. *Vaccine.* 2010;28(37):6086–93.

320. Findlow J, Borrow R, Snape MD, et al. Multicenter, open-label, randomized phase II controlled trial of an investigational recombinant Meningococcal serogroup B vaccine with and without outer membrane vesicles, administered in infancy. *Clin Infect Dis.* 2010;51(10):1127–37.

321. Shirley M, Taha MK. MenB-FHbp Meningococcal group B vaccine (Trumenba(R)): A review in active immunization in individuals aged >/= 10 years. *Drugs.* 2018;78(2):257–68.

322. Donnelly J, Medini D, Boccadifuoco G, et al. Qualitative and quantitative assessment of meningococcal antigens to evaluate the potential strain coverage of protein-based vaccines. *Proc Natl Acad Sci U S A.* 2010;107(45):19490–5.

323. Donald RG, Hawkins JC, Hao L, et al. Meningococcal serogroup B vaccines: Estimating breadth of coverage. *Hum Vaccin Immunother.* 2017;13(2):255–65.

324. Maiden MC, Bygraves JA, Feil E, et al. Multilocus sequence typing: A portable approach to the identification of clones within populations of pathogenic microorganisms. *Proc Natl Acad Sci U S A.* 1998;95(6):3140–5.

325. Rodrigues CMC, Lucidarme J, Borrow R, et al. Genomic surveillance of 4CMenB vaccine antigenic variants among disease-causing Neisseria meningitidis isolates, United Kingdom, 2010–2016. *Emerg Infect Dis.* 2018;24(4):673–82.

326. Parikh SR, Newbold L, Slater S, et al. Meningococcal serogroup B strain coverage of the multicomponent 4CMenB vaccine with corresponding regional distribution and clinical characteristics in England, Wales, and Northern Ireland, 2007–08 and 2014–15: A qualitative and quantitative assessment. *Lancet Infect Dis.* 2017;17(7):754–62.

327. Brehony C, Rodrigues CMC, Borrow R, et al. Distribution of Bexsero(R) Antigen Sequence Types (BASTs) in invasive meningococcal disease isolates: Implications for immunisation. *Vaccine.* 2016;34(39):4690–7.

328. Parikh SR, Andrews NJ, Beebeejaun K, et al. Effectiveness and impact of a reduced infant schedule of 4CMenB vaccine against group B meningococcal disease in England: A national observational cohort study. *Lancet.* 2016;388(10061):2775–82.

CHAPTER

91 Vaccine Decision-making and Vaccine Hesitancy

Abram L. Wagner • Leah C. Pinckney • Brian J. Zikmund-Fisher

HISTORICAL CONTEXT

Negative attitudes toward vaccination are not a recent phenomenon. Medical and political leaders have had to respond to these attitudes for hundreds of years. The precursor to smallpox vaccination, variolation with smallpox inocula, was introduced from the Ottoman Empire into the United Kingdom by Lady Mary Montague in the first quarter of the eighteenth century.[1] Within Europe and the New World, it quickly faced religious and philosophical objections suggesting variolation countered God's will in determining who was sick and who was healthy. Pamphlets produced by political and religious leaders, such as Cotton Mather, were important in countering negative sentiments and popularizing the spread of variolation in the American colonies.[2]

The physician Edward Jenner developed the first vaccine in 1796, using a cowpox inoculum to protect against smallpox. Although this vaccination did not have the serious adverse effects associated with the smallpox inoculum,[2] it was almost immediately followed by the establishment of antivaccination societies and misgivings about the vaccine. Figure 91-1 displays an exaggerated belief that the vaccine would turn vaccinees into cows. Many antivaccine advocates still relied on arguments grounded in religious and personal liberty.[3] However, the U.S. Supreme Court affirmed in *Jacobson vs. Massachusetts* in 1905 that "upon the principle of self-defense, of paramount necessity, a community has the right to protect itself against an epidemic of disease which threatens the safety of its members."[3] The era of the government instituting vaccine mandates had begun.

The development of vaccines against diphtheria, tetanus, and pertussis (DTP) in the 1920s and 1930s[4,5] and against polio in the 1950s, were seen as further milestones in the medical world. The roll out of these vaccines, however, was not entirely without incident. In one major vaccine production problem—the Cutter Incident of 1955—eight lots of polio vaccine were improperly inactivated, resulting in the paralysis of 196 individuals and 10 deaths.[6] At the time, this incident did little to dampen enthusiasm for the vaccine. Many parents had seen polio first-hand or read extensive news about polio,[7] and their concern about contracting the disease was greater than concerns about the safety of the vaccine.

By the time parents in high-income countries were making vaccination decisions for their children in the 1990s, they were already one or two generations removed from the most widespread lived experiences of vaccine-preventable disease. It was in this environment, in which people largely lacked first-hand experience with vaccine-preventable diseases, that Andrew Wakefield published a report in *The Lancet* linking measles-mumps-rubella (MMR) vaccination with neurodevelopmental issues, and, by implication, autism.[8] Although problems with the report were immediately discovered, coauthors were slow to distance themselves from the published manuscript, and it was only retracted by *The Lancet* in 2010.[9] This article has done lasting damage. MMR vaccination coverage in the United Kingdom dipped from close to 90% in 1996 to under 80% in the early 2001, which corresponded to trends in rising concerns about vaccine safety.[10]

While concerns about vaccination have existed for centuries, only recently has the concept of vaccine hesitancy been defined. According to the World Health Organization's (WHO) Strategic Advisory Group of Experts on Immunization (SAGE) Vaccine Hesitancy Working Group's 2011 definition: "Vaccine hesitancy refers to delay in acceptance or refusal of vaccines despite availability of vaccination services. Vaccine hesitancy is complex and context specific, varying across time, place, and vaccines. It is influenced by factors such as complacency, convenience and confidence."[11] Later researchers have expanded the psychological dimensions of vaccine hesitancy to include the following[12]:

- Confidence (attitudes);
- Complacency (perceived vulnerability toward changes in health status);
- Constraints (self-control);
- Calculation (disposition toward deliberation); and
- Collective responsibilities (preference for communal vs. individualistic actions).

Vaccine hesitancy explicitly excludes other drivers of vaccine uptake[13]:

- Access (availability of vaccination providers);
- Affordability (time and financial costs associated with vaccination);
- Awareness (knowledge of a vaccine); and
- Activation (e.g., receiving SMS reminders to go to a vaccination appointment).

In this chapter, we will discuss aspects of vaccine hesitancy and vaccine decision-making, which are relevant to clinicians. We describe vaccine hesitancy, along with the applicability of health behavior models, psychological decision-making, and stated preference methods to the world of vaccination. Subsequently, we cite specific examples related to pediatric vaccinations, human papillomavirus (HPV) vaccine, influenza vaccines, and pandemic vaccines. The novel coronavirus disease (COVID-19) pandemic in particular will likely have a lasting impact on vaccination programs and attitudes toward vaccines. Several groups of individuals have specific vaccine requirements, notably pregnant women, the elderly, and healthcare workers. These three groups are touched upon separately. Next, we address special considerations or time points when vaccine decision-making encounters particular challenges. These include: when first introducing a vaccine, how concerns may differ across countries, and the role of religion on vaccination. We conclude by bringing up several techniques to improve vaccination coverage, such

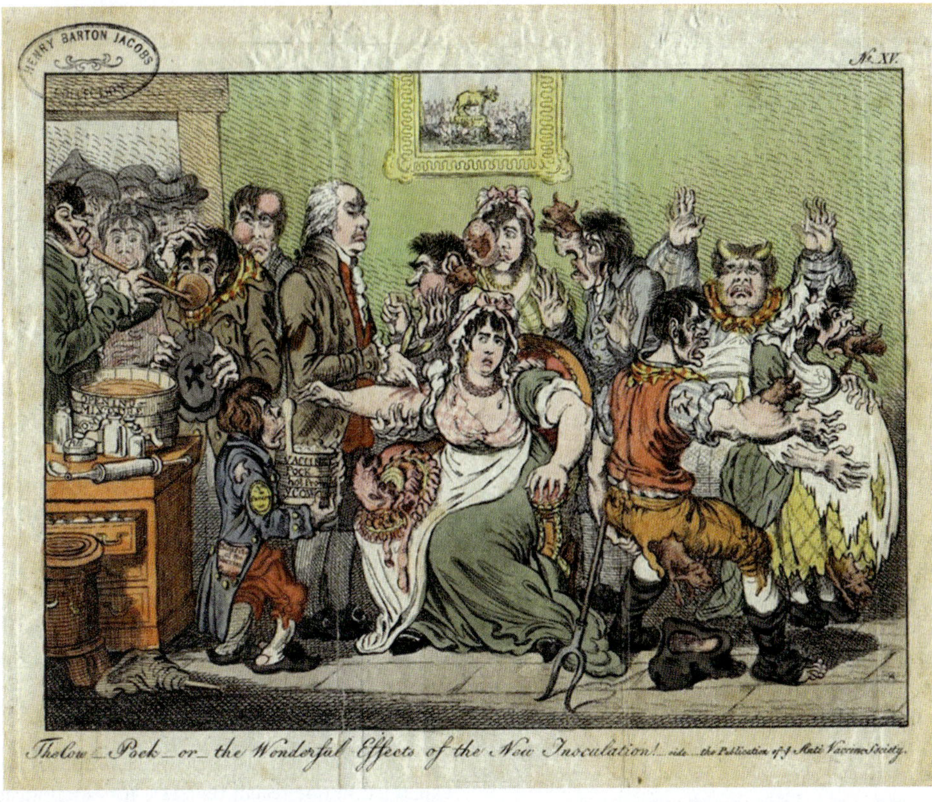

FIGURE 91-1. James Gillray. 1802. The Cow Pock or the Wonderful Effects of the New Inoculation. (*Source:* Library of Congress Prints and Photographs Division [LC-DIG-ds-14062].)

as instituting mandatory vaccination programs, nudges, negotiating with parents, excluding vaccine-hesitant parents from clinical practices, and developing effective narratives to frame vaccination.

TYPES OF VACCINE HESITANCY

The WHO definition for vaccine hesitancy presupposes a continuum from full acceptance of vaccines and administered on time to refusal of all vaccines.[14] Various researchers have attempted to develop categorization schemes that could be useful for different purposes, ranging from determining how much parents may be willing to negotiate on following the pediatric immunization schedule[15] to identifying what groups of parents hold intractable beliefs and which ones are open to changes.[16]

For example, Forbes et al. have classified individuals into five different groups based on degree of vaccine hesitancy.[17] According to this approach, there are "unquestioning acceptors" and "cautious acceptors," the latter of whom vaccinate despite some concerns, and then there are three distinct groups of vaccine hesitant parents: the "hesitant," "late or selective vaccinators," and "refusers." The hesitant generally vaccinate but have substantial concerns, which can be ameliorated by healthcare providers. Late or selective vaccinators have high levels of vaccine knowledge, leading them to have large concerns about the scheduling of vaccines or certain vaccine doses. Refusers, on the other hand, tend to have lower levels of vaccine knowledge and refuse to vaccinate based on religious, cultural, or philosophical principles.

In another, qualitative study,[18] individuals were grouped into six categories: those following the national recommended vaccination schedule, those following the Dr. Sears schedule[19] for delaying or withholding certain vaccines, parents more generally interested in limiting co-administered vaccines during each office visit, individuals selectively delaying or withholding certain vaccines distinct from the Dr. Sears schedule, those making visit-by-visit decisions, and at the extreme, those refusing all vaccines.

Many multi-item vaccine hesitancy measurements are available, including a 10-item vaccine hesitancy scale developed by the WHO SAGE Working Group on Vaccine Hesitancy,[20] and an 18-item Parent Attitudes About Childhood Vaccines survey (PACV).[21] These scales may attempt to measure vaccine hesitancy comprehensively or across several different domains. For instance, PACV encompasses three domains: behavior, safety and efficacy, and general attitudes.

It is important to also recognize that vaccine hesitancy is not static and can change based on an individual's experiences. Mothers are often most unsure about vaccination during pregnancy,[22] and a cohort study of young mothers in Washington state found that vaccine hesitancy significantly decreased between the child's birth and 24 months.[23] A study of parents sampled in the community and in hospitals found that parents whose children were hospitalized were more sensitive to safety issues and to their child's immune system than parents in the community.[24] Parents of children with autism spectrum disorder (AS) will be less likely to vaccinate younger siblings without ASD,[25] most likely because of the de-bunked belief that vaccination may be causally related to ASD.[26]

The distribution of vaccine hesitancy—including "refuser," "hesitant," or "visit-by-visit" groups can also vary across demographic groups. Within high-income countries, vaccine hesitancy is thought to be more common in more affluent groups that are more highly educated or have a higher income,[27] leading to lower vaccine uptake in more affluent communities.[28] This relationship is unclear in low- and middle-income countries.[29–31]

APPLICATION OF HEALTH BEHAVIOR MODELS TO VACCINATION

Vaccine-related communications include both providers' brief interactions with parent/patients who are making vaccine decisions and broader clinic- or community-level interventions. Regardless of communication type, however, vaccination providers should focus on honing a message that is both audience-appropriate and that addresses key concepts from relevant health behavior or behavioral change models, such as the Health Belief Model, the Theory of Planned Behavior, and the Social Cognitive Theory.[32] These models are particularly suited to helping develop population-level interventions on how to encourage vaccination using a motivational and persuasive message.

The Health Belief Model is one of the earliest and most used health behavior models,[33] and its constructs include perceived susceptibility (which aligns somewhat to the mathematical concept of perceived likelihood), perceived severity of disease, perceived benefits of health actions, and barriers that may inhibit a recommended health action.[34] Communications that clearly address perceptions of disease susceptibility and severity and/or benefits of vaccination can therefore be particularly valuable. Across studies, the Health Belief Model encourages vaccine providers to emphasize vaccine safety and benefits accruing from vaccination.[35,36]

Two other theories that are relevant to vaccination attitudes are the Theory of Planned Behavior[37,38] and the Social Cognitive Theory.[39] The Theory of Planned Behavior, previously known as the Theory of Reasoned Action, focuses on intention, and intention is theorized to be predicted by three sets of constructs: (1) behavioral beliefs and attitudes toward the behavior, (2) social and subjective norms, and (3) control beliefs and perceived behavioral control.[32,40] The Social Cognitive Theory, previously known as the Social Learning Theory, emphasizes the social nature of learning. At its basis, the theory includes the concept of reciprocal determinism, whereby an individual's experiences, environment/social context, and behavior are all interrelated.[32]

The Theory of Planned Behavior and Social Cognitive Theory include norms. Normative beliefs, or social norms, refer to the standard codes of behaviors within a specified group or community. Subjective norms (i.e., what an individual believes others thinks the individual should be doing) are typically thought to be influenced by these social norms.[32] The significance of norms in research related to vaccination would imply that physicians could increase parent/patients' willingness to get vaccinated by discussing the number of individuals in their practice or in the community who get vaccinated.

Beliefs about these norms have parallels to herd immunity. Vaccinated individuals not only protect themselves but also others around them, including those not age eligible or otherwise contraindicated for vaccination. Studies in China[30] and Ethiopia[41] have shown that a large proportion of parents will express agreement with a statement that vaccines can protect others in the community. Similarly, a study in the United States found that parents were willing to pay more for vaccines to increase vaccination coverage and attain herd immunity,[42] suggesting that framing the community benefits of vaccination can be helpful for promoting uptake in certain circumstances.

It is important to acknowledge, however, that there are limitations to these behavioral change models. In one systematic review, various constructs from behavioral change models—knowledge, attitudes, and beliefs—were all related to vaccine uptake,[43] but interventions aimed at educating individuals directly about these attitudes or beliefs had limited utility in increasing vaccine uptake.[44] Recent research has focused on how vaccination decision-making can be colored by irrational beliefs, experiences that the individual has had, and mental models. Behavioral change models offer a good explanation for the association between proposed factors and vaccination outcomes on an observational or cross-sectional level, but their predictive power is more variable in longitudinal or experimental settings.

DECISION PSYCHOLOGY PERSPECTIVES

An alternate approach to communicating with vaccine hesitant individuals derives from decision psychology. This approach assumes that individuals (patients or parents) make autonomous decisions that are influenced by risk perceptions, risk tolerance, experiences, and mental models. At the heart of this perspective on risk is a recognition that all people simultaneously *think* about risk in cognitive and analytical ways and *feel* a sense of risk or safety that is derived from unconscious associations, lived experience, and emotional responses.[45] When thinking and feeling align, behavior is motivated.[46] In the context of vaccination, however, analysis and feelings often conflict. For example, parents can be aware of statistics that vaccine side effects are rare, but they can also simultaneously have unconscious negative emotions derived, for example, from seeing their child's reaction to being injected with a vaccine or not understanding how exposing their healthy child to something derived from a virus could not cause them harm. The "risk-as-feelings" framework suggests that in these cases, feelings often win.[45]

Decision psychology can also explain how best to consider risks in population-level policies versus when talking with an individual patient. For policies, the rarity of adverse events is important, and a small chance of adverse effects is acceptable given the large beneficial output. However, at the patient level, the chance of adverse effects is often thought of in terms of possibility that "it might happen to my kid" rather than probability.[47] After all, there is only one outcome: either the patient gets the adverse effect or not. Healthcare providers need to recognize that parents and patients may give significant consideration to even very rare adverse events and acknowledge the feelings that that prospect may evoke.

Risk Perceptions

The formation of risk perceptions differs across individuals, as explained in one recent review.[48] For example, more numerate individuals are more likely to value and use "more relevant" numerical information.[49] As might be expected given the Health Belief Model, a meta-analysis of risk perception and vaccination found that vaccination behavior was highly related to perceptions of risk likelihood, susceptibility, and severity.[50] Because both infectious diseases and vaccine-related adverse events are rare in most societies, however, presenting these risks in terms of absolute probabilities (e.g., an overall percent) can reinforce thoughts that the risk is a small amount. Alternate presentations (e.g., relative risk) amplify peoples risk perceptions upward and may be relevant for highly persuasive messaging, but their use raises ethical concerns regarding manipulation.[47]

Longitudinally, increased risk perceptions can influence vaccine uptake by creating a sense of motivation to reduce future risk. However, vaccine uptake can also impact risk perceptions through a risk reappraisal process.[51] For example, a study of Lyme disease vaccination in the United States found that individuals with higher initial risk perceptions of Lyme disease were more likely to get vaccinated. After vaccination, however, they had reduced perceptions of risk.[51]

The fact that risk perceptions can evolve postvaccination is important because the change in risk perceptions after vaccination might theoretically create space for novel, unhealthy behaviors,[52] and such beliefs might therefore lead people to be less willing to vaccinate. This problem is epitomized by the introduction of the HPV vaccine, at which time many parents—particularly those socially conservative[53]—raised the concern that adolescents vaccinated against HPV would change their behaviors and become more sexually disinhibited.[54] It is important to note, however, that a systematic review of 21 articles has found no evidence that HPV vaccination has, in fact, contributed to disinhibitions and higher likelihoods of unsafe behaviors.[55]

Risk Tolerance

It may sometimes seem that those who manifest degrees of vaccine hesitancy are intolerant of any degree of vaccine-related risk. However, most research in this area has shown some tolerance for vaccine-related risks. In a population of highly educated mothers in Ontario, Canada, 25% would accept a 1 in 1 million chance of a severe side effect.[56]

Focusing on likelihood statistics presumes that parents and patients will change as the likelihood of a negative outcome changes. After all, purely rational people, as defined by Expected Utility Theory, should vary their preferences proportionately to changes in the probabilities of the relevant events (risks).[57]

Extensive evidence demonstrates, however, that people's reactions to likelihood information do not adhere to rational models. First, people pay much more attention to a risk new to them, no matter how small, than they do to a change in the likelihood of a risk (e.g., an increase of a risk from 10% to 12%).[58] Furthermore, people pay even less attention to changes in likelihood for events, which are affect-heavy.[59] For example, participants in one study were willing to pay similar amounts of money for widely varying chances to kiss their favorite celebrity, an affect-rich outcome.[59]

Because vaccine-preventable diseases and vaccination are both highly emotional outcomes, people focus more on the possibility of something like an adverse reaction happening instead of its quantitative probability.[58] Some parents state that they will not accept any vaccine with any possible risk (13.7% in one study from Ontario).[56] Parents and patients thinking this way may use wording such as, they know the adverse event "might happen, might not" or "It could happen to me."[47] People's emotional investment in the outcome—potentially seeing their child have an adverse reaction after deciding to obtain a vaccination—decreases their sensitivity to changes in the probability that this adverse reaction would actually occur.

Furthermore, the emotional component of people's reactions implies that how vaccine-related risks are framed can change people's level of concern. In one study examining trade-offs between vaccine safety and effectiveness, a large majority (82%) preferred a 95% effective vaccine where 1% developed a fever compared to an 80% effective vaccine where 0.5% developed a fever.[60] However, when the side effect was changed to a febrile seizure (0.2% chance for 95% effective vaccine, 0.1% chance for 80% effective vaccine), only 55% preferred the more effective vaccine. Thus, people appeared more concerned with safety when the highlighted side effect evoked stronger emotions even though it was less likely. Individuals' perceptions of risk probability were heavily colored by their emotional response to that risk.[61]

The key implication of people's insensitivity to vaccine-related probabilities is that communications that simply throw risk statistics at patients and parents are unlikely to change beliefs. Because emotion-rich risks will be considered regardless of their likelihood, communications must both clarify the relative likelihood of different events and acknowledge the feelings people have about the possibility of those outcomes, no matter how unlikely they are.

Another key finding of decision psychology is that people use emotions as a common currency to allow them to integrate perceptions of varied risks and benefits. The implications of this "affect heuristic" is that people tend to believe that there must be an inverse relationship between risk and benefit, even though risk and benefit are usually positively correlated in the real world.[62] In other words, people tend to feel that something with high benefits must not be very risky, and vice versa. In an empirical study, this inverse relationship is heightened under high-pressure situations.[63]

The affect heuristic is important for understanding how perceptions of vaccination risk are intimately linked to perceptions of vaccine benefit. When people perceive diseases as highly threatening and hence vaccine-based protection to be valuable, they will tend to perceive those vaccines as less risky. By contrast, vaccines that are perceived to convey little to no practical benefit are likely to be seen as more risky even if the absolute level of risk is unchanged.

Experiences

Perhaps the most important lesson of decision-making research for discussions of vaccination is the recognition that for most individuals, risk perceptions—and by extension medical decision-making—is a function of individual's experience with disease, and not merely the analytical knowledge they obtain about the disease. Relevant experiences include individual behaviors—engaging in risky behaviors results in higher risk perceptions[64]—as well as the experience of having a family member diagnosed with a disease.[65] Experiential learning can also occur through exposure to stories or media about other individuals' experiences.[66]

It is critical to note, however, that people's experiential learning involves both cases (situations where people get diseases or vaccine-related events) and noncases (situations where people know they were at risk yet nothing happens). This is part of the reason why the effect of disease experience likely varies across time. For example, acceptance of the polio vaccine was higher in the 1950s,[67] when polio outbreaks commonly occurred at communal swimming pools and summer camps.[7] News reports at the time focused on imagery and stories of individuals affected by the disease.[68] The polio vaccine trials, which included 1.8 million children,[6] were widely reported on, with most families being highly willing to participate given their own understanding of the polio disease.[7]

In the late 1900s and early 2000s, however, the majority of parents had no first hand experience with most vaccine-preventable diseases. This fact is plausibly related to a decrease in the acceptability of the polio vaccine.[69] A qualitative study of parents who pursue an alternative vaccination schedule found that many did not have personal experience and perceived risk of disease to be low.[18] The relationship between time and experience with vaccine-preventable disease raises the hypothesis that grandparents could be useful groups to discuss disease and the importance of vaccination with parents who are making vaccination decisions. However, there is little empirical research on this point,[70] and its value may become moot with the passing of the older generations that have more experience with specific vaccine-preventable diseases.

The effect of disease experience could also explain some diversity in the acceptance of vaccines across countries.[71] This separation in experience could also be a reason for why healthcare providers and the general population approach vaccines differently. Healthcare providers may be more likely to have seen severe and serious cases of vaccine-preventable disease than members of the general population.

Although experience with vaccine-preventable disease is often thought to lead to increased acceptance of the vaccine, the relationship could be inverted in some circumstances. For some diseases, like chickenpox, the clinical presentation in childhood is perceived to be less severe, and so parents who have had chickenpox may think vaccination unnecessary, thereby increasing the risk of more severe presentations in adult patients.[72] A similar pattern could be seen with influenza,[73] especially since many individuals conflate influenza with the common cold or disease from other respiratory viruses.[74]

Outbreaks represent an opportunity for healthcare providers and public health professionals to reacquaint the public with a vaccine-preventable disease in order to increase individuals' experiences (even if only through media) with the disease. Compared to before the 2014–15 outbreak of measles around Disneyland in California, adults surveyed afterward had higher perceptions of vaccine safety and effectiveness,[75] which is consistent with the affect heuristic. Furthermore, an ongoing outbreak of measles in Washington state resulted in one traditionally vaccine hesitant community to increase compliance in state-mandated vaccinations for kindergarteners from 56% to 74%.[76]

More generally, the COVID-19 pandemic globally impacted people's perceptions of infectious disease risks. While part of the pandemic's effect stems from how it made infectious diseases salient again, personal experience likely moderates the impact of this event both on perceptions of coronavirus-specific vaccines and on attitudes regarding vaccines in general. The more that individuals have direct or indirect experience with COVID-19-related harm (e.g., by being infected themselves or by observing the effects of family, friends, or close others becoming infected), the more risk perceptions shift toward disease concern. Per the affect heuristic discussed above, this effect not only increases perceived benefits of vaccination but also likely decreases potential concerns about vaccine-related risks. Experience with COVID-19 might generalize to perceptions of other infectious diseases (e.g., by making concrete how easily infections spread and their potential severity), but it is as of yet unclear how much COVID-19 experiences will have global effects on vaccine hesitancy.

Yet, at the same time, it is also possible that experiences with an individual disease can increase vaccine hesitancy. Over the course of the 2009 H1N1 pandemic in France, there was a substantial increase in the number of vaccine hesitant individuals.[77] This decrease in vaccine confidence could plausibly be tied to individuals perceiving H1N1 influenza as not severe because they did not experience this disease themselves. Similarly, with regards to COVID-19, the more that individuals are exposed to coronavirus disease statistics, warning messages, and stay-at-home orders but do not see or experience actual harms themselves, the less concerned they become about the disease and the less tolerant they become of other factors, such as physical distancing measures and potential risks of a newly developed coronavirus vaccine. Put simply, being alarmed without experiencing actual threat or harm tends to reduce people's perceptions of the risk in question. These lowered risk perceptions and this lack of experience could then be projected onto other vaccines.

Mental Models

Another important line of decision-related research has concerned the mental models that people hold about different risks and why they occur. Mental models explain how individuals develop thoughts about a concept, in particular how are various components thought to be causally related. Understanding the public's mental models about risks can help to clarify patterns of health-related beliefs in individuals.[78] For example, with infectious diseases, researchers using a mental models approach can include individuals' understanding of disease transmission and can identify how individuals think the disease can be prevented.[79] The ideas that influenza vaccines cause influenza or that mercury in vaccines causes autism are also examples of mental model components. These mental models can have wide-ranging impacts, including a decision in the United States to remove thimerosal from also all vaccines by 2001.[80]

Another key mental model component of people's mental models related to vaccination is the idea of whether, and under what circumstances, vaccines can cause disease. This idea is biologically relevant in certain cases, such as the difference between the oral polio vaccine (OPV), which can result in vaccine-associated paralytic polio (VAPP), and the inactivated polio vaccine (IPV), which cannot. Similarly, parents may be confused by reports that a possible measles case turned out to be a vaccine-induced rash if they lack an understanding of the difference between a live and an inactive attenuated virus.

Another application of mental models toward vaccination decision-making examines the simplicity versus complexity of people's concepts of vaccines and diseases. For example, one study revealed that parents tended to have a simplified understanding of vaccination and were therefore highly susceptible to misinformation from antivaccine sources.[81] Yet, complexity of model is not always better. When examining sources of vaccination information, this same study found that, while a CDC website displayed a very simple provaccine message, sources from antivaccine activists addressed all the issues raised in the CDC source and additionally provided narrative explanations of other phenomena, such as the benefits of having a preventable disease over obtaining a vaccine.[81] From an antivaccine perspective, the fact that the CDC source presented an oversimplified perspective may contribute to perceptions that provaccination sources are not "telling the whole story."

Gist Messages vs. Detailed Messages

Healthcare providers do not need to and do not have the time to provide parent/patients with all information about vaccines. Fortunately, according to Fuzzy Trace Theory, people rely on a general, bottom-line gist of information more so than precise verbatim details when making decisions.[82] Individuals can process verbatim information into gist-level understanding through mental models, although communications emphasizing a gist-level information to begin with is both easier and more effective. For example, a study of news articles shared after the 2016 measles outbreak at Disneyland in California found that articles expressing a bottom-line gist were more often shared than those emphasizing statistics.[83] One study of verbatim versus gist information found that gist messages led to individuals having higher risk perceptions but greater levels of using protective health behaviors, whereas verbatim messages increased risk perceptions but also increased risky behaviors.[64]

EXAMPLES OF VACCINE DECISION-MAKING

Routine Pediatric Immunizations

Vaccine-hesitant parents are not a homogeneous group. Instead, this group tends to express a variety of views and have mental models that incorporate various misconceptions about vaccine-related risks. Understanding these models may be of value in guiding conversations about routine pediatric immunizations.

One common mental model component of late or selective vaccinators is a belief that certain vaccines may overload the child's immune system, especially in terms of the currently recommended vaccination schedules. The natural implication of this model is an expectation that certain vaccines should not be given at certain times and that the program should overall be spaced out. As one qualitative study discovered, parents were not able to explain why vaccine antigens would overly burden their child's immune system, but these beliefs still impacted the scheduling of their child's vaccine doses.[18] Other observed mental model beliefs include that some vaccines may cause various allergies, chronic diseases, or autoimmune diseases. Empirical research has shown no evidence of such a relationship.[84] Parents also may want to selectively choose which vaccines to skip, based on their perceptions of disease severity or on their concerns with a specific vaccine. In one study in the United States, 24% of parents expressed interest in skipping certain vaccines, and the most commonly cited vaccines were influenza (33%), varicella (27%), and HPV (27%).[85]

The structure of vaccination schedules can amplify patient and parental concerns about perceived risks of vaccine administration. The increase in vaccines administered in countries' Expanded Program on Immunization (EPI) mean that vaccines must (1) be coadministered during one office visit, (2) be combined into a single vial, or (3) be administered at separate office visits, adding to parents' time costs in obtaining the full regimen of vaccinations. A systematic review of parental attitudes toward combination vaccines has detailed many of these beliefs. For instance, parents may be concerned about overloading their child's immune system through multiple antigens present in combination vaccines, but they were also concerned about infecting their child with multiple shots in one visit.[86] One qualitative study examined these tensions between coadministered and combination vaccines in depth: some parents preferred seeing their child receive fewer injections, but for those concerned about antigen amount, combination or coadministered vaccines were perceived as equally bad.[18] Engaging to determine what exactly they are concerned about may therefore help guide conversations in productive ways.

Beliefs about vaccines are heavily influenced by other beliefs, such as trust in Western vs alternative science. For example, qualitative interviews with Australian parents who refused some vaccine found that many preferred to use complementary and alternative medicine (CAM) for a financial reason—they believed CAM practitioners were less corrupted by Big Pharma, and for a scientific belief—they believed it was more "natural" than Western medicine and vaccination.[87] A study of vaccination preferences in France found that individuals who regularly used alternative medicine had substantially reduced preferences for vaccination in general compared to those who did not regularly use alternative medicine.[88]

Parental Relationship with Vaccination Provider

Having a strong, positive relationship with a healthcare provider can help parents change antivaccination thoughts.[89] Obtaining information from physicians, as opposed to from other parents or from the internet leads to parents being less concerned about the vaccine schedule, according to studies in the United States[90] and in China.[31] This association could be thought to be causal. If a parent has trust in the "system," a strong recommendation for vaccination from a provider can strongly predict their own vaccination behaviors.[91] Different groups of individuals may be more predisposed to be trusting of health authorities. In one survey of vaccine attitudes in the United States, Hispanic parents were more likely than others to follow doctor recommendations while still reporting a high degree of concern over vaccine side effects.[92]

Yet, many vaccine-hesitant parents are not trusting of the government as a source of information and prefer to receive information indirectly from the media or other nonofficial sources.[93] Vaccine-hesitant parents trust anecdotal evidence and unofficial sources rather than the established medical system.[93,94] Parents who seek exemptions for vaccinations, for example, tend to have lower trust in the medical establishment and more confidence in their own decision-making.[95] Additionally, the relationship between provider recommendations and vaccine hesitancy is not always clear, because parents who are strongly vaccine hesitant may choose a healthcare provider who is more accommodating of their beliefs.[96]

In short, providers with vaccine-hesitant parents will need to be mindful that they are both an individual who can build personal relationships and a representative of the health system. Some parents or patients may value providers being a source of reliable, vetted information, but others will trust a provider that is willing to "work with them" more than one who "toes the line."

Human Papillomavirus Vaccine

Adolescent vaccines, which include diphtheria-tetanus-pertussis boosters and the HPV vaccine, have been more recently introduced into countries' immunization schedule.[97] Parents' concerns about these adolescent vaccines can differ from what they believe about pediatric vaccines.

Attitudes about the HPV vaccine appear particularly shaped by parents' experiences and perceptions of benefits. Mothers in one qualitative study were excited about the potential for the HPV vaccine to reduce burdensome and affect-heavy cervical cancer screenings (an action that is not recommended).[98] Studies from England[99] and China[100] have shown that mothers with a family history of cancer were more likely to accept the vaccine for their daughters. Vaccination providers should be aware of the impact of leveraging these experiences and findings of benefit when discussing HPV vaccination with parents and adolescents. As rates of HPV-related cancers are demonstrated to decrease in countries such as Australia with longer HPV vaccination histories, sharing that information with parents may be of particular value.

Although other vaccines for sexually transmitted diseases, notably hepatitis B, had previously been on the market prior to the HPV vaccine, the sexually transmitted nature of HPV was more salient in the framing of the initial roll-out of the vaccine in the United States.[101–103] This resulted in providers, parents, and adolescents having conversations during office visits that are framed about gender and sexual activity more than cancer screening. Parents have remained concerned about the HPV vaccine's impact on their child's sexual behaviors,[104] and uptake remains low in the United States—37% for girls and 13% for boys in 2014.[105] Programs that have attempted to promote HPV vaccination since its introduction in the United States have met with mixed success.[106] In contrast, the hepatitis B vaccine—which protects against an infection largely spread through injection drug use or sexual intercourse—has not had such pushback from the public. This is likely due to the fact that it was marketed as vaccine that protects against the development of chronic infection in young infants.[107]

The influence of the sexual activity-based nature of HPV risk has had slightly less impact on parents' decisions over time. Between 2010 and 2016, the number of parents in the United States citing their child's lack of sexual activity as a reason for refusing the HPV vaccine was cut by about half.[54] However, even hesitant parents are not necessarily categorically opposed to an STD vaccine. In one discrete choice experiment, parents placed more value on a vaccine that protected against warts in addition to cervical cancer than one that only protected against cervical cancer.[108]

More recently, introduction of HPV vaccine into low- and middle-income countries has focused on it being a cervical cancer vaccine for girls.[97] Ethicists in Bangladesh, where the vaccine was rolled out as a cervical cancer vaccine, raised the concern that this discussion excludes the contribution of males to the spread of HPV and may lead to young women being less concerned about cervical cancer and getting regular cervical cancer screening.[109] Healthcare workers throughout the world should be prepared to discuss gender issues and sexual activity when promoting the HPV vaccine.

Using Nudges and Overcoming Barriers to HPV Vaccination

For the HPV vaccine, physicians can increase vaccination coverage by using nudges, which are different ways that physicians can alter their discussion with parents so that vaccination is presented as the default option.[110,111] Nudges can smooth over barriers, such as the time barrier of setting up multiple office visits to discuss an issue, and can leverage social norms to create a presumption of action by implying most individuals in the community are receiving a vaccine. For example, in appointments with parents and adolescents, presumptively offering the HPV vaccine puts less cognitive burden on the parent or adolescent to decide whether they should give the vaccine while allowing them the choice to refuse it.

Beyond nudges, it is well known that lubricating the healthcare system so that it is as easy as possible for individuals to get vaccinated is important. For instance, a systematic review from 2000 found that issuing reminders and recalls about vaccine appointments to parent-clients, offering vaccinations in Women, Infant, Child (WIC) settings and home visits, and having standing order for vaccination are all effective in improving vaccination coverage.[112]

Offering vaccinations like HPV at school can also be extremely beneficial. One systematic review found that school-based interventions (e.g., offering the vaccine at schools) was effective in increasing uptake, and much more effective than informational or behavioral interventions.[44] As one example, in South Africa, the HPV vaccine was rolled out within schools. Vaccination uptake reached 86.6% at the end of the campaign even with misinformation being spread through social media.[113]

Governmental support for the HPV vaccine is key. The HPV vaccination in Japan was recommended for use in 2013, but this governmental recommendation was suspended later in the year due to reports of adverse events following immunization. HPV vaccination coverage has dropped precipitously, to under 1%, and doctors remain unwilling to recommend the vaccine without an official government endorsement.[114] A contrasting example is the introduction of HPV vaccine into Australia.[115] The school-aged cohort has maintained a vaccination coverage of around 70% within Australia.[116]

Another issue of contention is whether adolescents should be able to consent to vaccinations even if their parents are "antivaccine."[117,118]

Most adolescents and college students' healthcare decisions are heavily influenced by parents. In the United States, this link is due to the fact that these individuals are relying on their parents for medical insurance.[119] Parents may be influenced by their child's wishes, but this is often in the context of the adolescent not wanting to get vaccinated.[120] Fifteen states in the United States have allowed adolescents to consent with various payment mechanisms in place (e.g., with charges being billed to Medicaid).[121] Medical doctors should be encouraged to discuss vaccination options with adolescents, even if the doctors know the parents are antivaccine.[119]

Influenza Vaccine

The World Health Organization does not issue a blanket recommendation for countries to include influenza vaccines on their immunization schedule, although they do recommend pregnant women, children, the elderly, individuals with chronic disease, and healthcare workers be prioritized for vaccination programs.[122] In contrast to other vaccines, influenza requires an annual vaccination while having widely varying effectiveness depending on the match between the vaccine and predominant circulating strain of virus.

Experiences surrounding influenza and influenza vaccination are key for understanding vaccine-decision making. In general, young adults, including college students, are apt to think they are not at risk for disease,[123] and many view influenza as a minor illness.[85] Even among older adults, many individuals have had first- or second-hand experiences with influenza or various respiratory illnesses thought of as influenza[74] that were not severe, and these experiences tend to influence perceptions of vaccine benefit. As a result, influenza is commonly thought of as a vaccine that healthy individuals could reasonably skip.[85] Another challenging effect of experience is when individuals experience respiratory illness after getting vaccinated. The incongruity between the protective action (vaccination) and their experience (getting sick) may lead these individuals to have a mental model that suggests that the vaccine itself caused the illness or that the vaccine is not actually effective at preventing illness.[124] Accordingly, in one study in four middle-income countries, perceived vaccine safety was the most important attitude related to intent to receive an influenza vaccine.[125] And parents who see their child have an adverse event or who worry about vaccine side effects are less likely to re-vaccinate their child against influenza in subsequent seasons.[126]

In line with the regular nature of the vaccine, having a previous seasonal influenza vaccination has been shown to be strongly predictive of vaccination in the current influenza season across many different risk groups—healthcare providers, individuals with chronic diseases, children, the elderly, and the general public.[127] Although this pattern could speak to some individuals being more health-oriented, it suggests that repeated experience with getting vaccinated generally is associated with positive attitudes toward vaccination.

Because influenza vaccine must be annually readministered, promoting vaccination is difficult and may need to incorporate diverse strategies. One proposal—to vaccinate children at schools—was explored in a qualitative study based out of Alberta, Canada, where parents discussed program advantages, like convenience, but were worried that they would lose the ability to make decisions for their children.[128] Offering parents choices in the type of influenza vaccine their child receives could promote uptake of the vaccine. Multiple influenza vaccines are available, although any individual practice may have a limited selection. Currently, trivalent and quadrivalent vaccines are on the market, along with nasal sprays and injected vaccines. Studies of parents[129] and children[130] have shown that nasal sprays are preferred to injected vaccines when all other attributes (e.g., safety and effectiveness) are held equal. Targeted reminders from the state health department or from vaccination providers, particularly to high-risk groups, can also improve influenza vaccination rates.[131]

Optimizing the timing of influenza vaccination is difficult because influenza is a seasonal disease with a variable start date, and because vaccination requires 2 weeks to mount an immune response. One study has suggested that waiting until late November (in a northern hemisphere country) to vaccinate individuals would prevent more cases from contracting disease.[132] This has raised the concern that doctors should not vaccinate individuals against influenza "too early."[133] Doctors should vaccinate against influenza in accordance with the epidemiology of disease within their own region. In addition, although purposefully scheduling vaccinations for patients early is not optimal, it could be useful for physicians to vaccinate patients who are at the office early in the season, if the doctor believes the patient may not return for a follow-up visit. Additionally, instilling in an individual an experience of vaccination can also bear dividends for the future as vaccination becomes regularized.

Pandemic Vaccines

Pandemics typically manifest as a new disease (e.g., COVID-19), when the possibility of disease arises in a population. Perceived risks of disease and serious outcomes decline over time as the public habituates to the disease, and intention to engage in preventive behaviors like vaccination also decreases over time. These trends have been seen in recent outbreaks, including for the 2009 H1N1 outbreak in the United States,[134] an Ebola exposure at a U.S. university,[135] and the COVID-19 pandemic during early- to mid-2020.[136] Thus, the early period of a pandemic (which is likely measured in weeks, not months) is a unique situation where fear of disease is high and experience with the vaccine is low. In such contexts, vaccination is often relatively accepted. However, a vaccine may not be available until the tail end of a pandemic,[137,138] or after the population has become more habituated to the disease.

Certain populations may be prioritized or targeted for vaccination during a pandemic.[139] Interventions would have to address concerns that targeted individuals and the larger population have about the pandemic and the vaccine, and, at the very basis, stressing vaccination as a way to protect high-risk individuals will be important.[140,141] How this information is displayed becomes very important, especially has individuals can have a highly emotional response to a pandemic. One study, comparing the length of messages, found that shorter messages which emphasized several key points (anyone is at risk of disease, vaccine is safe and effective) were most effective in increasing intent to vaccinate.[142] Concern about the disease is a particularly salient point, because some pandemics may receive more notice in the news than others. A study of pregnant women found that women who worried about Zika were much more likely to want to receive a vaccine.[143] Lastly, if people have more confidence in vaccines in general, they will be more accepting of an individual vaccine. For example, a study in Indonesia found more positive attitudes toward vaccine safety and efficacy in general were associated with acceptance of a Zika vaccine.[144]

Because pandemic vaccines may be rapidly deployed after development, parent/patients may have concerns about the vaccine's safety record. These concerns came to the forefront during the development of a COVID-19 vaccine and have arisen in response to past vaccination events. For instance, during its rollout in Philippines, one dengue vaccine was found in some circumstances to prime vaccinees for a severe reaction to future infection.[145] After the media publicized these vaccine safety issues, there was a precipitous drop in vaccine confidence in Philippines, from 93% in 2015 before the incident to 32% in 2018.[146] Predictably, subsequent vaccine uptake decreased and incidence of vaccine-preventable diseases increased.[147]

On the whole, studies have found pandemic vaccines to be safe,[148,149] and modern-day vaccine development techniques are recognized as safe.[150] However, members of the general population have little understanding of the vaccine development process.[150] Focusing on patients' risk perceptions of the pandemic disease can be helpful to encourage vaccination early on in the pandemic cycle. Given long development times for vaccines, however, this approach may be limited for vaccines introduced later on.

In summary, public health officials, medical doctors, and other vaccination providers should be aware that pandemics can be an opportunity to reinforce positive attitudes toward vaccines. At the same time, they can also be a time when vaccination rates decrease—either because individuals are hesitant to go out in public and visit a doctor[151] or because individuals' perceptions of the pandemic vaccine can affect their attitudes about vaccines in general.

VACCINATION PROGRAMS IN SPECIFIC POPULATIONS

Vaccines for Pregnant Women

Throughout the world, coverage of vaccines during pregnancy is low,[152] and pregnant women are selective in which vaccines they choose to receive. For instance, in one study in Australia, 85% of pregnant women had received a pertussis booster, whereas only 37% had received an influenza vaccine.[153] Many of these women cite a lack of recommendation from an OB/GYN. Some vaccines are contraindicated during pregnancy, like the MMR and varicella vaccines,[154] and so vaccination providers should take care to frame their recommendations on the available evidence.[155] Mothers who had received a seasonal vaccine in the previous year were more likely to have gotten an additional dose while pregnant.[153] Another study looking at pandemic influenza vaccination during pregnancy found very low levels of uptake in the United Kingdom, but uptake was related to increased maternal age and having a previous delivery.[156] This last study's findings indicate that accumulated experience—from previous children and other life events—can dispose a mother toward vaccination.

Interventions to increase maternal uptake of vaccines have shown mixed results.[157] However, it is notable that increasing the convenience of vaccination (letting community health workers in the antenatal period vaccinate, using automated reminders, and increasing provider awareness of vaccines) in observational studies has been shown to be effective at increasing uptake of the pertussis vaccine during pregnancy.[157]

Because pregnant women tend to be particularly concerned about protecting their baby, framing the vaccination decision in terms of benefits to the child (vs. the parent) is a promising strategy to increase motivation to vaccinate. Ensuring that family members beyond the mother are protected against vaccine-preventable diseases, particularly pertussis, is known as "cocooning" and could potentially prevent transmission of disease to young infants.[158,159] This strategy may be relevant to all family members, not just the mother, especially when messages highlight how vaccination can protect others. Increasing awareness of vaccination among family members and making the vaccine available in pediatric offices can promote vaccine uptake among these family members.[159]

Vaccines for the Elderly

Across different countries, various vaccines for older adults are available, including influenza vaccines, shingles vaccines, and pneumococcal vaccines. However, lack of awareness and convenience in getting these vaccines is a huge issue in their relatively low uptake.[152,160,161] For example, in the United States, shingles vaccination coverage in older adults is estimated at 31.8% in 2017,[162] and influenza vaccination coverage was 67% in 2014–15, and pneumococcal vaccination coverage was less than 60% in 2013.[152] In the Netherlands, coverage of shingles, influenza, and pneumococcal vaccination in older adults was separately estimated to be 49.5%, 42.2%, and 58.1%.[163]

As with vaccines in other age groups, vaccination uptake in older adults is related to constructs from health behavior theories (including perceptions of severity, susceptibility, and side effects) as well as risk perceptions and attitudes toward vaccination in general.[161] One discrete choice experiment from the Netherlands revealed that seriousness of disease (risk of mortality), susceptibility of disease, and vaccine effectiveness were all important factors that affected vaccine preference.[163]

As with other age groups, personal experiences may affect willingness to get vaccinated among older adults. Shingles provides a strong example. A study in South Korea found that knowing someone with singles was the second most commonly mentioned reason for having interest in the vaccine, after concern about the severity of disease.[160] This association between history and vaccination has also been seen with influenza and pneumonia.[161]

However, there are limits to how personal experiences can affect vaccine uptake. The influenza and pneumococcal vaccine protect against respiratory illnesses, which may have a wide range of etiologies. As a result, individuals may not know what specifically caused a bout of pneumonia or influenza-like illness. A qualitative study of older adults in Michigan found that these individuals did think that influenza and pneumonia could be serious, especially for elderly adults, but they balanced their past experiences with these diseases with their perceptions that they have gotten an illness after receiving a vaccine.[164]

Some adults receive care from multiple specialist doctors and less care from primary-care providers who vaccinate.[152] Having a regular general practitioner is predictive of vaccination.[165] Broadening where individuals can get vaccinated (e.g., pharmacies, at specialists' offices) would increase the convenience of vaccination and decreasing the burden of older adults having to make decision about vaccine and seek out a vaccination provider.

Another challenge with vaccination of older adults is that many vaccines for this age group are newer—so they may be perceived to be less effective or not as safe,[164] and some vaccines are less effective in older adults than younger adults.[166] In their communication with older adult patients, doctors can acknowledge these issues if they are raised by patients, while stressing the benefits of vaccination and the experiences the doctors have had in vaccinating other adults (social norms) and preventing serious disease.

Vaccines for Healthcare Workers

Vaccination is particularly important for healthcare providers given their propensity to come into contact with infectious or susceptible patients. This potential for exposure, and healthcare workers' relatively high science and health literacy would seem to predispose them to having an extremely high uptake of vaccines. Although vaccination coverage is generally higher among healthcare workers compared to the general population,[33] there are still many who do not vaccinate. In China, for example, only 60% of healthcare workers had received the complete series of hepatitis B vaccination.[167] Vaccination coverage may also vary across provider groups. During the 2009 H1N1 outbreak in Minnesota, 85% of physicians, but only 62% of nurses were vaccinated against the pandemic influenza virus.[168]

Although healthcare workers are often thought of as vaccine champions, some may be vaccine skeptic themselves, choosing not to receive certain vaccines, or encouraging patients to not vaccinate.[169,170] For influenza vaccination, they may have similar misconceptions or beliefs as the general population, such as believing influenza vaccine can cause influenza or that the risk of acquiring influenza is low.[171] Similar to members of the general population, healthcare providers may have vague anxieties about vaccinations.[172] More often, though, suboptimal vaccination coverage among healthcare providers is due to inertia or difficulties in obtaining vaccination. Increasing ease of vaccination and providing the vaccine for free can significantly increase healthcare worker's uptake of vaccines.[167]

Vaccination against influenza and other vaccines for workers in hospitals and other medical settings is becoming more common and may be mandatory in some locations. Compared to those facilities without mandates, healthcare facilities with influenza mandates have 11% greater coverage of influenza vaccine.[173] Many healthcare workers dislike the idea of mandatory vaccination, even if they realize the benefits of preventing disease spread to patients.[174] Acceptance of mandatory vaccination may vary across healthcare provider groups. In one study, it was higher among physicians than nurses.[168] Relying on social norms (e.g., publicizing vaccination rates by department) for vaccination could be one way to promote vaccination among healthcare workers.

Interventions to increase acceptance of influenza and other vaccinations among healthcare workers can rely on health behavior theories and decision psychology. A systematic review of pandemic influenza vaccination among healthcare workers found that many studies used the Health Belief Model constructs as a framework for studying attitudes toward vaccination, and that major concerns about this vaccination were vaccine safety (related to rapid development following the 2009 pandemic), conflicting messages from mass media, and receiving negative cues, like political figures refusing vaccination.[175] Vaccination coverage is higher among those providers who believe in an ethical or professional obligation to get vaccinated or to follow public health recommendations.[168] Healthcare providers may be more accepting of vaccination if the stories surrounding vaccination rely on gist-based messages instead of statistics.[171] Interventions can also take advantage of social norms due to the fact that large numbers of healthcare providers are already vaccinated. Messages that include information on how many individuals are vaccinated, along with their personal experiences getting vaccinated, would be one step in this direction.

Beyond protecting themselves against disease, vaccination providers can use this personal experience with vaccination when discussing vaccination with patients. One study of healthcare workers who had and who had not received a pandemic influenza vaccine found those who had received the vaccine often talked about this experience with patients. In contrast, healthcare workers who had not received the vaccine viewed their patients' decisions as relying on official recommendations, not their own.[176]

SPECIAL CONSIDERATIONS

Introduction of New Vaccines

The introduction of vaccines into the existing vaccination schedule can be considered problematic to many parents,[177] who may already be concerned with "overwhelming" the immune system of their child through coadministering multiple doses of vaccines during one office visit, or increasing the number of vaccines given to a young infant.[31,178] As a result, a substantial proportion of the population (11% in one Dutch study)[177] would not want any future additions to the vaccine schedule.

The period around the introduction of a new vaccine into the private market or the government-funded EPI is a sensitive time.[179] Most parents will reasonably be asking why the change or additional vaccine is necessary. Messaging at this time should address both prevalent questions about the need for the vaccine and potential concerns regarding its safety.[180] For example, parents are more willing to accept new vaccines for severe or fatal diseases,[181] so messaging can emphasize serious complications caused by the disease in question. Individuals may be more willing to get vaccinated when they first learn about a disease (when the *possibility* of illness becomes first apparent),[134] and so a logistically smooth introduction of the vaccine, where individuals have easy access to vaccination points, becomes very important. As noted above, messaging to increase perceptions of vaccine benefit may also have beneficial impacts on perceptions of a newly required vaccine's safety. Regardless, communicators should recognize that parents are likely asking themselves why they should put their child at risk from this vaccine that is new to them when contemplating a new requirement.

This contextualization of the vaccine can include not only information on disease severity and susceptibility but also social norms and experiences. These can be particularly important when receiving a vaccine may carry with it negative associations. As previously mentioned, the early association of HPV with sexual behavior or cancer prevention was very apparent in the United States,[101–103] and has resulted in long-term concerns about the vaccine[106] and low uptake[105]. A better strategy for physicians developing messaging for the HPV vaccine and other, future vaccines for sexually transmitted disease would be to humanize cases of the disease by talking with cases with serious complications (pelvic inflammatory disease, various cancers, arthritis, etc.).

Modifying Vaccines or Vaccine Schedule

Vaccines have been pulled from the market in the past due to safety concerns. For example, a killed measles vaccine on the market in the United States between 1963 and 1967 resulted in a hypersensitivity to subsequent exposure to measles virus.[182] The first rotavirus vaccine in the United States, available between 1998 and 1999, was associated with some cases of intussusception (i.e., bowel telescoping), with much negative news reporting.[183] These examples may influence vaccine decision-making in some, but it is important to note the speed at which they were able to be removed from the market.

Clinicians should acknowledge when safety scares are occurring in order to be able to engage patients about their concerns. However, it is unclear if vaccine safety scares will influence parents' perceptions not just of the affected vaccine but also of other vaccines. For instance, a 2010 vaccine safety incident related to influenza in Australia did not apparently affect parents' perceptions of other vaccines.[184] However, a substantive drop in measles vaccination coverage in the Philippines (from 88% in 2014 to 55% in 2018) was attributed to a highly visible political battle over the roll-out of a novel dengue vaccine, which was found to have severe side effects in certain circumstances.[185]

There have been other examples of the U.S.-modifying vaccine composition in response to political or public concerns, but again it remains unclear whether these changes actually resulted in changes in public perceptions of safety. Between 1997 and 2000, the United States switched from using the OPV to the injected, IPV, over concerns about VAPP.[186] A gradual global effort on this front started in 2016.[187] Somewhat similarly, Japan switched from a whole cell pertussis (DTwP) to acellular pertussis (DTaP) vaccine in 1981,[188] followed by other countries like the United States in 1996,[189] because DTaP is less reactogenic and was initially thought to have similar levels of effectiveness as DTwP.[188] More recently, lower levels of effectiveness of DTaP have led to outbreaks of pertussis and have changed vaccine policy in other ways—in introducing acellular pertussis antigens to a tetanus-diphtheria booster.[190] Loss of vaccine effectiveness could lower popular confidence in the vaccine. Another example of vaccine changes is the removal of thimerosal from most vaccines—starting in 1992 in Denmark and Sweden—over concerns that it might be related to autism or other neurodevelopmental issues. Subsequent studies in the United States, Canada, and Europe have found no relationship between amount of thimerosal exposure, or removal of thimerosal from vaccines, and autism rates.[178]

Vaccine Decision-Making Globally

Global, widespread use of vaccines has dramatically reduced childhood mortality and morbidity, but antivaccine and antiscience movements could threaten further progress.[191] Although most scientific literature about vaccine decision making has focused on high-income countries in North America and Europe, the literature from low- and middle-income countries (LMICs) shows similar patterns about how decisions are made, although specific concerns about vaccines may vary. There have been few studies that have systematically looked at vaccine attitudes across different countries. One study, using data from 67 countries, found substantial differences among countries. European countries were least confident about vaccine safety, and higher education appeared somewhat related to increased confidence in vaccine effectiveness but less confidence in vaccine safety.[192]

It is difficult, however, to make sweeping statements about the geographical distribution of vaccine confidence. For instance, Azerbaijan and Iran—two contiguous countries at a similar per capita income level—are among the least and most confident about vaccines, respectively.[192] The heterogeneity found across countries makes it difficult to group generalize concerns into those mainly affecting high-income countries, and those more relevant to LMICs.[27]

Especially in LMIC settings, it is important to recognize that undervaccination can result from not only vaccine hesitancy but also other reasons, such as vaccination provider readiness or community access to vaccinations.[193] One systematic review found that individuals who had refused or delayed vaccines in LMICs held beliefs that vaccines were harmful and were distrustful of the vaccination program.[194] Across countries, delayed vaccination from both lack of access and lack of confidence in vaccination is higher among families with greater numbers of children and in those with lower maternal education and lower socioeconomic status.[195] The distribution of these characteristics (trust in vaccination program, family, and mother's socioeconomic status) certainly varies across countries. Vaccination providers should be aware of the socioeconomic circumstances affecting vaccine uptake, either through access issues or vaccine hesitancy, in their local area.

Improving vaccine confidence across global settings will likely require the use of many different components involving leaders, social mobilization, and employing dialogue-based interventions.[196] These interventions can be adapted to local circumstances and should be cognizant of how subpopulations within a country may view vaccines differently, and that the proportion of the overall population who belong to these subpopulations differs country to country.

It is also important to consider that individuals in any country can look up information about vaccines sourced from other countries. This can result in confusion if there are differing policies across the globe, which is notable especially for influenza vaccination.[197] Since country-specific websites about influenza vaccination are accessible across the globe, individuals placing content about vaccines online can look at how global organizations like the World Health Organization frame the vaccine and can explicitly contextualize any vaccination recommendations to their specific country.

Religion

Globally, no major religious group objects to vaccination in principle.[198] However, vaccination providers should be aware of some religious dimensions to vaccine hesitancy, in particular the use of aborted fetal tissue and some Muslim groups' interpretations about substances in vaccines as not halal. Additionally, for many individuals stressing religious objections, religious and philosophical ideals overlap, and the connection between religious beliefs and vaccination attitudes is difficult to disentangle. Religious objections to vaccinations are often vague and related to purity, in that the vaccine is purported to have impure properties, have an impure mode of administration, or result in the vaccine becoming impure.[199]

There are region- and country-specific characteristics of religion and vaccination. A global survey found that Catholics were among the groups most associated with positive vaccine sentiment, whereas religious groups in the Western Pacific region were most likely to report that vaccines were incompatible with their religion.[192] In Israel, Jewish parents were more hesitant than Muslim parents.[200] In the United States, many states offer a religious exemption toward vaccines.[201] Religious exemptions are particularly common among traditionalist Christian denominations, like the Amish and Mennonites.[202]

Islam raises some questions about vaccines, as vaccines may include porcine ingredients in their production processes. Consumption of pork is not halal, but many Muslim groups do not consider vaccination as "consumption" in the technical sense.[198] Prior to 2018, Muslim councils in Europe and Malaysia had issued fatwas indicating that vaccination was permissible, even as some ingredients were not halal.[203] In 2018, regional and national Muslim religious bodies in Indonesia issued fatwas describing the measles vaccine as not halal.[204] The bodies did not prohibit vaccination, but measles vaccination coverage dropped to 68% in the aftermath. Measles coverage in Aceh province, a more religiously conservative area, was just 8%.[204] Creating vaccines and medicinal drugs that adhere to halal standards is one possible solution,[205] but doing so is not logistically feasible in the short term.

Some individuals may also object to certain vaccines because of concerns that the vaccines contain tissue from aborted fetuses. In particular, this stance has been associated with some Catholic groups, although other denominations and religions may have similar beliefs. Vaccines relevant to this concern include the rubella vaccine in the United States, which was isolated from an infected fetus,[206] as well as rubella single-antigen vaccines, measles-mumps-rubella vaccines, chickenpox vaccines, and hepatitis A vaccines, which are grown in cell lines extracted from voluntarily aborted fetuses.[198,207] The Catholic Church has issued statements allowing for the use of these vaccines.[198] Globally there are some alternatives to these vaccines in use or in development, including a rubella vaccine grown in rabbit tissue and a hepatitis vaccine grown in monkey tissue,[198] but their availability is limited.

TECHNIQUES TO IMPROVE VACCINATION COVERAGE

Researchers have only recently started to develop an evidence base for changing antivaccine beliefs. Suggestions include using presumptive and not participatory discussions with parent/patients (nudges), engaging with parent/patients about their beliefs and risk perceptions, reframing their values, and developing stories about experiences.[208] Physicians will do best if they can have families develop a routine for getting vaccinated.[209]

Given the fact discussed above that vaccine hesitancy represents a spectrum of views, it is important for healthcare providers not to divide parent/patients into those who do vaccinate and those who do not. Many parents who do adhere to the typical vaccination schedule still may have concerns about adverse events, possible links between vaccination and autism, and the safety of newer vaccines.[92] Some vaccine-hesitant parent/patients may be amenable to receiving vaccines, whereas it is difficult to change the beliefs of individuals heavily antivaccine.[16]

Mandatory Vaccination

Mandatory vaccination is one policy mechanism to increase vaccination coverage. Mandatory vaccination policies exist in a continuum across countries or even within countries: some countries offer opt outs without penalty, others allow for personal/philosophical, or religious waivers, but some countries impose serious financial penalties or social/educational restrictions on those not vaccinated.[210] Political jurisdictions seeking to implement mandatory vaccination policies will have to consider the legal justification, vaccine doses involved, penalties and incentives, enforcement, and evaluation.[210] Among 62 countries which were identified in one study to have mandatory vaccine policies, only 7 (11%) had no fault vaccine injury compensation schemes.[211] However, injury compensation policies are important in settings with strict mandatory policies and may encourage more parents to support the vaccination program.

The long-term effectiveness of changes to vaccine mandates may be limited. Research across U.S. states shows that removing a philosophical waiver (but keeping a religious waiver) results in substantial movement of families into seeking a religious waiver instead.[212] There is some evidence in California that absence of both religious and philosophical waivers has increased the use of medical exemptions,[213] possibly from parents seeking exemptions from pliable physicians.[202]

However, overall the absence of nonmedical exemptions is associated with greater diphtheria-pertussis-tetanus vaccine uptake and lower pertussis incidence rate.[214] Removing philosophical and religious waivers is probably much more effective than increasing the difficulty or amount of administrative hoops than a family needs to go through to request an exemption. Connecticut, Michigan, Alaska, and Oregon instituted such administrative changes between 2012 and 2016, but within a couple years of implementation had again seen a rise in the number of individuals seeking a nonmedical exemption.[212] Within the United States, a higher rate of nonmedical exemptions does lead to decreased vaccination coverage.[215]

Vaccine concerns brought up by parents requesting personal exemptions to vaccination reveal several topics that clinicians should be prepared to discuss with vaccine-hesitant parents. In one cross-sectional study of parents in Utah, the most common reasons for seeking a vaccine exemption included higher perceived risk of vaccine adverse events compared to risk of disease, belief in link between vaccination and autism, and concerns about vaccine ingredients.[216]

Vaccination providers should also be aware of the sociodemographic context of families seeking vaccination waivers. Vaccination waivers are more common in private schools than public schools—and are particularly high in Waldorf schools.[202] In California, areas that were rural, had more white people, and had more college-educated individuals, were more likely to request waivers to vaccination.[217]

Dismissing or Negotiating with Vaccine-Hesitant Parents

Physicians and other vaccination providers encountering vaccine-hesitant families face difficult choices. Should they dismiss families who refuse (some/all) vaccines?[218] Should they be open to negotiating a reduced or delayed "alternative" schedule?[219] The American Academy of Pediatrics issued guidance that physicians should not dismiss families that are refusing vaccines for their children (statement released in 2005[220] and reaffirmed in 2012[221]). Instead, the American Academy of Pediatrics recommends physicians to engage with parents in targeted discussions.[222] Regardless, 21% of pediatricians and 4% of family physicians in the United States reported dismissing families who refused vaccines.[223]

Alternative schedules refer to immunization schedules different from ones recommended by a National Immunization Technical Advisory Group, like the Advisory Committee on Immunization Practices. Robert Sears, for example, has proposed an alternative schedule which delays many vaccines and which is popular with many vaccine-hesitant families.[19] Another physician created an alternate schedule, which limits coadministrations but adds in more office visits to keep children relatively up-to-date.[15]

Physicians' choice to use alternative schedules or dismiss families that refuse vaccines is ultimately their own decision based their preferences for keeping vaccine hesitant parents in their practice. In qualitative and quantitative studies of parents following alternative vaccination schedules, many expressed annoyance at the lack of choices, and that they preferred doctors being able to have a conversation about the pros and cons of vaccination with the parents.[18,85] When encountering families that are refusing or hesitant about vaccines, physicians should be available to have a discussion, should be aware of presumptive discussion tactics, and should be able to frame their discussions in a evidence-based way.

Nudges and Presumptive Vaccination

Nudges are one way to alter the "choice architecture" by providing parent/patients with a default choice.[110,111] Nudges are a presumptive form of discussion, where physicians use phrases like "Today your teenager will get a Tdap and HPV vaccine" instead of a participatory approach, where a doctor in a similar appointment would ask, "Do you want to vaccinate your teenager against Tdap and HPV today?" Although the change in language is simple, these formats can have real impacts on vaccination uptake: doctors initiating conversation with parents about HPV vaccination in a presumptive way had 17.5 times higher odds of vaccinating the teenager compared to doctors starting with a participatory approach.[224]

One concern is that nudges are ethically problematic.[225] In the pursuit of encouraging individuals to get vaccinated—a worthy goal of any government—can public health be manipulative, or how can public health treat parent/patients as autonomous individuals and promote good decisions? Vaccination nudges are a way for doctors to present vaccination as the default choice without encouraging parent/patients to think deeply about the vaccination choice.[225]

At the same time, the overall structure of physician-patient conversation can influence vaccination uptake. Parents more satisfied with their provider's communication with them were more likely to get the HPV vaccine,[226] and providers who spent more time talking with parents about the HPV vaccine were also more likely to successfully vaccinate.[227] Therefore, nudges can be a start to discussions during an office visit, but healthcare providers encountering vaccine hesitant parents should be available for longer discussions.

Framing of Vaccinations

Discussions about vaccines with parent/patients should rely on health behavior theories and decision psychology. Presenting information about the benefits of vaccination is important, as increasing benefit perceptions are linked with decreasing risk perceptions according to the affect heuristic.[63] However, the government and public health authorities often overemphasize specific facts, statistics, and details in vaccine education, whereas vaccine recipients may be more persuaded by heuristics, experiences, and a "risks as feelings" approach.[228]

Physicians' discussions with parent/patients can take the form of a variety of narratives. The ability of narratives to influence vaccination is limited, but narratives vary widely in content.[229] The limited effectiveness seen in previous studies may be due to mismatched narrative types or incorrectly written narratives. For example, in the United States, Nyhan et al. developed a five-arm experiment to improve attitudes toward the MMR vaccine.[230] Controls were compared to parents randomized into the groups that received the following messages: (1) information correcting common misconceptions, (2) risks of measles, (3) a dramatic narrative, or (4) visuals about risks. No intervention increased parental intent to vaccinate a future child.

In contrast, Shourie et al. did find in a cluster randomized controlled trial that a web-based MMR decision aid or an MMR leaflet were both associated with parents having reduced concerns in their decision-making and both resulted in increased vaccine uptake.[231] And a study, which randomized individuals into those talking with cases of vaccine-preventable disease and those who did not, found that exposure to a case changed vaccine-hesitant individuals into being much more provaccine.[232] These two studies indicate that vaccine attitudes can change—even when simple decision aids are used, and especially when individuals develop a personal connection with a case and learn more about their experiences.

Ultimately, physicians can rely on personal anecdotes and decision psychology—for example, vaccinating their own family members, talking about their experiences with cases, and emphasizing the benefits and social norms of vaccination. These discussions often take a lot of time[233] but are ultimately worth it if a child ends up getting vaccinated.

Use of Social Media

Social media represents an opportunity to spread positive messages about vaccines, although historically it is has been more effectively manipulated by antivaccine forces. Vaccine-related topics that are highly relevant on social media can also inform the content of discussions that doctors have with parent/patients.[234] Social media is characterized by user participation, openness, and network effects. These characteristics lead to increased power of personal narratives, using multiple sources for informed decision-making, and social norms.[66] Personal narratives, and other stories involving categorical gist, are more likely to be shared than statistics-heavy stories on Twitter[83] and Youtube[235].

Social media users also need to be cognizant of how they frame provaccine messages. Provaccine activists can also frame social media posts in terms of reinforcing positive views or countering negative views.[236] This latter point can be particularly salient because correcting health information on social media platforms can limit misperceptions,[237] but other research has shown that online debates strengthened polarization of vaccination beliefs.[238]

CONCLUSIONS

Attitudes toward vaccinations have been described by some as a pendulum swinging, in which the public at certain points views vaccines particularly favorable (especially if this is in line with their lived experiences with vaccine-preventable disease) and at other points is more fixated on vaccine adverse events—whether these are causally related to the immunization event or not. Vaccination was popularized in Western Europe and the United States because of people like Lady Mary Montague, who understood that many infectious diseases were a preventable scourge. Policymakers and vaccination providers who are able to grasp how experiences—personal, family, friend, or media-mediated—with vaccine-preventable disease and vaccine safety are different in different areas and at different times will be better able to develop policies and advocate for vaccination across diverse groups of individuals.[239] Healthcare providers play a key role in advocating for vaccines and in correcting the mental model misconceptions and omissions related to vaccines that affect the beliefs that parents and patients hold.

References

1. Marcuse EK. Reflections on US immunization challenges: Lady Montague, where are you? *Pediatrics*. 2011;128(6):1192–4.
2. Riedel S. Edward Jenner and the history of smallpox and vaccination. *Baylor Univ Med Cent Proc*. 2017;18(1):21–5.
3. Parmet WE, Goodman RA, Farber A. Individual rights versus the public's health—100 Years after Jacobson v. Massachusetts. *N Engl J Med*. 2005;352(7):652–4.
4. Parkman PD. Combined and simultaneously administered vaccines: A brief history. *Ann New York Acad Sci*. 1995;754(1):1–9.
5. Fitzpatrick MC, Wenzel NS, Scarpino SV, et al. Cost-effectiveness of next-generation vaccines: The case of pertussis. *Vaccine*. 2016;34(29):3405–11.
6. Furesz J. Developments in the production and quality control of poliovirus vaccines—Historical perspectives. *Biologicals*. 2006;34(2):87–90.
7. Lambert SM, Markel H. Making history. *Arch Pediatr Adolesc Med*. 2000;154(May):512–7.
8. Saint-Victor DS, Omer SB. Vaccine refusal and the endgame: Walking the last mile first. *Phil Trans R Soc B*. 2013;368:20120148.
9. Eggertson L. Lancet retracts 12-year-old article linking autism to MMR vaccines. *CMAJ*. 2010;182(4):199–200.
10. Smith A, Yarwood J, Salisbury DM. Tracking mothers' attitudes to MMR immunisation 1996–2006. *Vaccine*. 2007;25(20):3996–4002.
11. The Strategic Advisory Group of Experts (SAGE). Report of the SAGE working group on vaccine hesitancy. http://www.who.int/immunization/sage/meetings/2014/october/SAGE_working_group_revised_report_vaccine_hesitancy.pdf. Published 2014. Accessed June 14, 2018.
12. Betsch C, Schmid P, Heinemeier D, Korn L, Holtmann C, Böhm R. Beyond confidence: Development of a measure assessing the 5C psychological antecedents of vaccination. Angelillo IF, ed. *PLoS One*. 2018;13(12):e0208601.
13. Thomson A, Robinson K, Vallée-Tourangeau G. The 5As: A practical taxonomy for the determinants of vaccine uptake. *Vaccine*. 2016;34(8):1018–24.
14. The Strategic Advisory Group of Experts (SAGE). Report of the SAGE working group on vaccine hesitancy. http://www.who.int/immunization/sage/meetings/2014/october/SAGE_working_group_revised_report_vaccine_hesitancy.pdf. Published 2014. Accessed June 14, 2018.
15. Block SL. Taking a 'PASS' on alternative immunization schedules. *Pediatr Ann*. 2013;42(10):399–406.
16. Leask J. Target the fence-sitters. *Nature*. 2011;473:443–5.
17. Forbes TA, McMinn A, Crawford N, Leask J, Danchin M. Vaccination uptake by vaccine-hesitant parents attending a specialist immunization clinic in Australia. *Hum Vaccines Immunother*. 2015;11(12):2895–903.
18. Saada A, Lieu TA, Morain SR, Zikmund-Fisher BJ, Wittenberg E. Parents' choices and rationales for alternative vaccination schedules: A qualitative study. *Clin Pediatr (Phila)*. 2015;54(3):236–43.
19. Offit PA, Moser CA. The problem with Dr Bob's alternative vaccine schedule. *Pediatrics*. 2009;123(1):e164–9.
20. Larson HJ, Jarrett C, Schulz W, et al. Measuring vaccine hesitancy: The development of a survey tool. *Vaccine*. 2015;33:4165–75.
21. Opel DJ, Taylor JA, Zhou C, Catz S, Myaing M, Mangione-Smith R. The relationship between parent attitudes about childhood vaccines survey scores and future child immunization status: A validation study. *JAMA Pediatr*. 2013;167(11):1065–71.
22. Corben P, Leask J. Vaccination hesitancy in the antenatal period: A cross-sectional survey. *BMC Public Health*. 2018;18(1):1–14.
23. Henrikson NB, Anderson ML, Opel DJ, Dunn J, Marcuse EK, Grossman DC. Longitudinal trends in vaccine hesitancy in a cohort of mothers surveyed in Washington State, 2013–2015. *Public Health Rep*. 2017;132(4):451–4.
24. Costa-Pinto JC, Willaby HW, Leask J, et al. Parental immunisation needs and attitudes survey in paediatric hospital clinics and community maternal and child health centres in Melbourne, Australia. *J Paediatr Child Health*. 2018;54(5):522–9.
25. Zerbo O, Modaressi S, Goddard K, et al. Vaccination patterns in children after autism spectrum disorder diagnosis and in their younger siblings. *JAMA Pediatr*. 2018;94612(5):469–75.
26. Cooper LZ, Larson HJ, Katz SL. Protecting public trust in immunization. *Pediatrics*. 2008;122(1):149–53.
27. Larson HJ, Jarrett C, Eckersberger E, Smith DMD, Paterson P. Understanding vaccine hesitancy around vaccines and vaccination from a global perspective: A systematic review of published literature, 2007–2012. *Vaccine*. 2014;32(19):2150–9.
28. Hegde ST, Wagner AL, Clarke PJ, Potter RC, Swanson RG, Boulton ML. Neighborhood influence on diphtheria-tetanus-pertussis booster vaccination. *Public Health*. 2019;167:41–9.
29. Domek GJ, O'Leary ST, Bull S, et al. Measuring vaccine hesitancy: Field testing the WHO SAGE Working Group on Vaccine Hesitancy survey tool in Guatemala. *Vaccine*. 2018;35:5273–81.
30. Ren J, Wagner AL, Zheng A, et al. The demographics of vaccine hesitancy in Shanghai, China. *PLoS One*. 2018;13(12):e0209117.
31. Wagner AL, Boulton ML, Sun X, et al. Parents' concerns about vaccine scheduling in Shanghai, China. *Vaccine*. 2017;35(34):4362–7.
32. LaMorte WW. Behavioral Change Models.
33. Bish A, Yardley L, Nicoll A, Michie S. Factors associated with uptake of vaccination against pandemic influenza: A systematic review. *Vaccine*. 2011;29(38):6472–84.
34. Strecher VJ, Becker MH, Rosenstock IM. Social learning theory and the health belief model. *Heal Educ Behav*. 1988;15(2):175.
35. Wagner AL, Boulton ML, Sun X, et al. Perceptions of measles, pneumonia, and meningitis vaccines among caregivers in Shanghai, China, and the health belief model: A cross-sectional study. *BMC Pediatr*. 2017;17(1):143.
36. Smith PJ, Humiston SG, Marcuse EK, et al. Parental delay or refusal of vaccine doses, childhood vaccination coverage at 24 months of age, and the health belief model. *Public Health Rep*. 2011;126:135–46.
37. Agarwal V. A/H1N1 vaccine intentions in college students: An application of the theory of planned behavior. *J Am Coll Heal*. 2014;62(6):416–24.
38. Harmsen IA, Lambooij MS, Ruiter RAC, et al. Psychosocial determinants of parents' intention to vaccinate their newborn child against hepatitis B. *Vaccine*. 2012;30(32):4771–7.
39. Priest HM, Knowlden AP, Sharma M. Social cognitive theory predictors of human papillomavirus vaccination intentions of college men at a southeastern university. *Int Q Community Health Educ*. 2015;35(4):371–85.
40. Ajzen I. The theory of planned behavior. *Organ Behav Hum Decis Process*. 1991;50:179–211.
41. Masters NB, Tefera YA, Wagner AL, Boulton ML. Vaccine hesitancy among caregivers and association with childhood vaccination timeliness in Addis Ababa, Ethiopia. *Hum Vaccin Immunother*. 2018;14(10):2340–7.

42. Gidengil C, Lieu TA, Payne K, Rusinak D, Messonnier M, Prosser LA. Parental and societal values for the risks and benefits of childhood combination vaccines. *Vaccine.* 2012;30(23):3445–52.
43. Wilson L, Rubens-Augustson T, Murphy M, et al. Barriers to immunization among newcomers: A systematic review. *Vaccine.* 2018;36(8):1055–62.
44. Walling EB, Benzoni N, Dornfeld J, et al. Interventions to improve HPV vaccine uptake: A systematic review. *Pediatrics.* 2016;138(1):e20153863.
45. Slovic P, Finucane ML, Peters E, MacGregor DG. Risk as analysis and risk as feelings. *Risk Anal.* 2004;24(2):311–22.
46. Loewenstein GF, Hsee CK, Weber EU, Welch N. Risk as feelings. *Psychol Bull.* 2001;127(2):267–86.
47. Zikmund-Fisher BJ. The right tool is what they need, not what we have. *Med Care Res Rev.* 2013;70(1_suppl):37S–49S.
48. Ferrer RA, Klein WMP. Risk perceptions and health behavior. *Curr Opin Psychol.* 2015;5:85–9.
49. Peters E, Västfjäll D, Slovic P, Mertz CK, Mazzocco K, Dickert S. Numeracy and decision making. *Psychol Sci.* 2006;17(5):407–13.
50. Brewer NT, Chapman GB, Gibbons FX, Gerrard M, McCaul KD, Weinstein ND. Meta-analysis of the relationship between risk perception and health behavior: The example of vaccination. *Heal Psychol.* 2007;26(2):136–45.
51. Brewer NT, Weinstein ND, Cuite CL, Herrington JE. Risk perceptions and their relation to risk behavior. *Ann Behav Med.* 2004;27(2):125–30.
52. Brewer NT, Cuite CL, Herrington JE, Weinstein ND. Risk compensation and vaccination: Can getting vaccinated cause people to engage in risky behaviors? *Ann Behav Med.* 2007;34(1):95–9.
53. Schuler CL, Reiter PL, Smith JS, Brewer NT. Human papillomavirus vaccine and behavioural disinhibition. *Sex Transm Infect.* 2011;87(4):349–53.
54. Beavis A, Krakow M, Levinson K, Rositch AF. Reasons for lack of HPV vaccine initiation in NIS-Teen over time: Shifting the focus from gender and sexuality to necessity and safety. *J Adolesc Heal.* 2018;63(5):652–6.
55. Madhivanan P, Pierre-Victor D, Mukherjee S, et al. Human papillomavirus vaccination and sexual disinhibition in females: A systematic review. *Am J Prev Med.* 2016;51(3):373–83.
56. Freeman TR, Bass MJ. Determinants of maternal tolerance of vaccine-related risks. *Fam Pract.* 1992;9(1):36–41.
57. Caplin A, Leahy J. Psychological expected utility theory and anticipatory feelings. *Q J Econ.* 2001;(February):55–79.
58. Kahneman D, Tversky A. Prospect theory: An analysis of decision under risk. *Econometrica.* 1979;47(2):263–91.
59. Hsee CK, Rottenstreich Y. Money, kisses, and electric shocks: On the affective psychology of risk. *Psychol Sci.* 2001;12(3):185–90.
60. Zikmund-Fisher BJ, Wittenberg E, Lieu TA. Parental weighting of seizure risks vs. fever risks in vaccination tradeoff decisions. *Vaccine.* 2016;34(50):6123–5.
61. Zikmund-Fisher BJ, Fagerlin A, Ubel PA. Risky feelings: Why a 6% risk of cancer does not always feel like 6%. *Patient Educ Couns.* 2010;81(SUPPL. 1): S87–93.
62. Slovic P, Peters E. Risk perception and affect. *Curr Dir Psychol Sci.* 2006;15(6):322–25.
63. Alhakami A, Finucane ML, Johnson SM, Slovic P. The affect heuristic in judgments of risks and benefits. *J Behav Decis Mak.* 2000;13(1):1–17.
64. Mills B, Reyna VF, Estrada S. Explaining contradictory relations between risk perception and risk taking. *Psychol Sci.* 2008;19(5):429–33.
65. Chen LS, Kaphingst KA. Risk perceptions and family history of lung cancer: Differences by smoking status. *Public Health Genomics.* 2011;14(1):26–34.
66. Witteman HO, Zikmund-Fisher BJ. The defining characteristics of Web 2.0 and their potential influence in the online vaccination debate. *Vaccine.* 2012;30(25):3734–40.
67. Glasser MA. Attitudes and reactions of the public to health programs. *Am J Public Heal Nations Heal.* 1958;48(2):141–6.
68. Cunningham RM, Boom JA. Telling stories of vaccine-preventable diseases: Why it works. *South Dakota Med.* 2013;Special Ed:21–6.
69. Sturm LA, Mays RM, Zimet GD. Parental beliefs and decision making about child and adolescent immunization: From polio to sexually transmitted infections. *J Dev Behav Pediatr.* 2005;26(6):441–52.
70. Karthigesu SP, Chisholm JS, Coall DA. Do grandparents influence parents' decision to vaccinate their children? A systematic review. *Vaccine.* 2018;36(49):7456–62.
71. Nichter M. Vaccinations in the third world: A consideration of community demand. *Soc Sci Med.* 1995;41(5):617–32.
72. Taylor JA. Parental attitudes toward varicella vaccination. *Arch Pediatr Adolesc Med.* 2013;154(3):302–6.
73. Ward L, Draper J. A review of the factors involved in older people's decision making with regard to influenza vaccination: A literature review. *J Clin Nurs.* 2008;17(1):5–16.
74. Baer R, Weller S, Pachter L, et al. Cross-cultural perspectives on the common cold: Data from five populations. *Hum Organ.* 1999;58(3):251–60.
75. Cacciatore MA, Nowak GJ, Evans NJ. It's complicated: The 2014–2015 U.S. measles outbreak and parents' vaccination beliefs, confidence, and intentions. *Risk Anal.* 2018;38(10):2178–92.
76. Ho S. Vaccinations rise on Vashon Island, challenging its reputation as anti-vax 'poster child.' The Associated Press. https://www.seattletimes.com/life/lifestyle/vaccine-rates-rise-on-vashon-island-challenging-its-reputation-as-anti-vaccine-poster-child/. Published 2019. Accessed May 21, 2019.
77. Peretti-Watel P, Verger P, Raude J, et al. Dramatic change in public attitudes towards vaccination during the 2009 influenza A(H1N1) pandemic in France. *Eurosurveillance.* 2013;18(44):1–8.
78. Morgan MG, Fischhoff B, Bostrom A, Atman CJ. Mental models. In: *Risk Communication: A Mental Models Approach.* Cambridge, United Kingdom: Cambridge University Press; 2002, pp. 63–83.
79. Southwell BG, Ray SE, Vazquez NN, Ligorria T, Kelly BJ. A mental models approach to assessing public understanding of Zika virus, Guatemala. *Emerg Infect Dis.* 2018;24(5):938–9.
80. Wessel L. Vaccine myths. *Science.* 2017;356(6336):368–72.
81. Downs JS, de Bruin WB, Fischhoff B. Parents' vaccination comprehension and decisions. *Vaccine.* 2008;26(12):1595–607.
82. Reyna VF. A theory of medical decision making and health: Fuzzy trace theory. *Med Decis Mak.* 2008;28(6):850–65.
83. Broniatowski DA, Hilyard KM, Dredze M. Effective vaccine communication during the Disneyland measles outbreak. *Vaccine.* 2016;34(28):3225–8.
84. Offit PA, Hackett CJ. Addressing parents' concerns: Do vaccines cause allergic or autoimmune diseases? *Pediatrics.* 2003;111(3):653–9.
85. Lieu TA, Zikmund-Fisher BJ, Chou C, Ray GT, Wittenberg E. Parents' perspectives on how to improve the childhood vaccination process. *Clin Pediatr (Phila).* 2017;56(3):238–46.
86. Hulsey E, Bland T. Immune overload: Parental attitudes toward combination and single antigen vaccines. *Vaccine.* 2015;33(22):2546–50.
87. Attwell K, Ward PR, Meyer SB, Rokkas PJ, Leask J. "Do-it-yourself": Vaccine rejection and complementary and alternative medicine (CAM). *Soc Sci Med.* 2018;196(May 2017):106–14.
88. Seanehia J, Treibich C, Holmberg C, et al. Quantifying population preferences around vaccination against severe but rare diseases: A conjoint analysis among French university students, 2016. *Vaccine.* 2017;35(20):2676–84.
89. Gust DA, Darling N, Kennedy A, Schwartz B. Parents with doubts about vaccines: Which vaccines and reasons why. *Pediatrics.* 2008;122(4):718–25.
90. Wheeler M, Buttenheim AM. Parental vaccine concerns, information source, and choice of alternative immunization schedules. *Hum Vaccines Immunother.* 2013;9(8):1782–9.
91. Smith PJ, Kennedy AM, Wooten K, Gust DA, Pickering LK. Association between health care providers' influence on parents who have concerns about vaccine safety and vaccination coverage. *Pediatrics.* 2006;118(5):e1287–92.
92. Freed GL, Clark SJ, Butchart AT, Singer DC, Davis MM. Parental vaccine safety concerns in 2009. *Pediatrics.* 2010;125(4):654–9.
93. Brown KF, Kroll JS, Hudson MJ, et al. Factors underlying parental decisions about combination childhood vaccinations including MMR: A systematic review. *Vaccine.* 2010;28(26):4235–48.
94. Eller NM, Henrikson NB, Opel DJ. Vaccine information sources and parental trust in their child's health care provider. *Heal Educ Behav.* 2019;46(3):445–53.
95. Salmon DA, Moulton LH, Omer SB, DeHart MP, Stokley S, Halsey NA. Factors associated with refusal of childhood vaccines among parents of school-aged children. *Arch Pediatr Adolesc Med.* 2005;159(5):470.
96. Karlamangla S. S.F. city attorney investigates doctor for excusing kids from mandatory vaccines. *Los Angeles Times.* https://www.latimes.com/local/california/la-me-vaccines-herrera-stoller-exemption-20190508-story.html. Published 2019. Accessed May 10, 2019.
97. Gallagher KE, LaMontagne DS, Watson-Jones D. Status of HPV vaccine introduction and barriers to country uptake. *Vaccine.* 2018;36(32):4761–7.

98. Waller J, Marlow LAV, Wardle J. Mothers' attitudes towards preventing cervical cancer through human papillomavirus vaccination: A qualitative study. *Cancer Epidemiol Biomarkers Prev*. 2006;15(7):1257–61.

99. Marlow LAV, Waller J, Wardle J. Parental attitudes to pre-pubertal HPV vaccination. *Vaccine*. 2007;25(11):1945–52.

100. Han YF, Zhuang YN, Li Y, Fang Y. Analysis of mothers' acceptance of HPV vaccination of adolescent girls in Xiamen. *Chinese J Prev Med*. 2018;52:38–42.

101. Velan B, Yadgar Y. On the implications of desexualizing vaccines against sexually transmitted diseases: Health policy challenges in a multicultural society. *Isr J Health Policy Res*. 2017;6(1):30.

102. Clark A. Should HPV vaccination be mandatory? *CBS News*. http://www.cbsnews.com/news/should-hpv-vaccine-be-mandatory/. Published 2007. Accessed March 27, 2017.

103. Clark A. Controversy Swirls around HPV Vaccine. *CBS News*. http://www.cbsnews.com/news/controversy-swirls-around-hpv-vaccine/. Published 2007. Accessed March 27, 2017.

104. Brewer NT, Fazekas KI. Predictors of HPV vaccine acceptability: A theory-informed, systematic review. *Prev Med*. 2007;45(2–3):107–14.

105. Lancet T. HPV vaccination: A decade on. *Lancet*. 2016;388(10043):438.

106. Walling EB, Benzoni N, Dornfeld J, et al. Interventions to improve HPV vaccine uptake: A systematic review. *Pediatrics*. 2016;138(1):e20153863.

107. Hardt K, Bonanni P, King S, et al. Vaccine strategies: Optimising outcomes. *Vaccine*. 2016;34(52):6691–9.

108. Brown DS, Johnson FR, Poulos C, Messonnier ML. Mothers' preferences and willingness to pay for vaccinating daughters against human papillomavirus. *Vaccine*. 2010;28(7):1702–8.

109. Salwa M, Abdullah Al-Munim T. Ethical issues related to human papillomavirus vaccination programs: An example from Bangladesh. *BMC Med Ethics*. 2018;19(S1):39.

110. Attwell K, Smith DT. Hearts, minds, nudges and shoves: (How) can we mobilise communities for vaccination in a marketised society? *Vaccine*. 2017;36(44):6506–8.

111. Thaler RH, Sunstein CR. *Nudge: Improving Decisions about Health, Wealth, and Happiness*. New Haven, CT: Yale University Press; 2008.

112. Briss PA, Rodewald LE, Hinman AR, et al. Reviews of evidence regarding coverage in children, adolescents, and adults. *Am J Prev Med*. 2000;18(1):97–140.

113. Delany-Moretlwe S, Kelley KF, James S, et al. Human papillomavirus vaccine introduction in South Africa: Implementation lessons from an evaluation of the national school-based vaccination campaign. *Glob Heal Sci Pract*. 2018;6(3):425–38.

114. Katsuta T, Moser CA, Offit PA, Feemster KA. Japanese physicians' attitudes and intentions regarding human papillomavirus vaccine compared with other adolescent vaccines. *Papillomavirus Res*. 2019;7:193–200.

115. Shefer A, Markowitz L, Deeks S, et al. Early experience with human papillomavirus vaccine introduction in the United States, Canada and Australia. *Vaccine*. 2008;26(SUPPL. 10):68–75.

116. Garland SM, Skinner SR, Brotherton JML. Adolescent and young adult HPV vaccination in Australia: Achievements and challenges. *Prev Med*. 2011;53(SUPPL. 1):S29–35.

117. World Health Organization. Considerations regarding consent in vaccinating children and adolescents between 6 and 17 years old. https://www.who.int/immunization/programmes_systems/policies_strategies/consent_note_en.pdf. Published 2014. Accessed May 13, 2019.

118. Silverman RD, Opel DJ, Omer SB. Vaccination over parental objection—Should adolescents be allowed to consent to receiving vaccines? *N Engl J Med*. 2019;381(2):104–6.

119. Ragan KR, Bednarczyk RA, Butler SM, Omer SB. Missed opportunities for catch-up human papillomavirus vaccination among university undergraduates: Identifying health decision-making behaviors and uptake barriers. *Vaccine*. 2018;36(2):331–41.

120. Gowda C, Schaffer SE, Dombkowski KJ, Dempsey AF. Understanding attitudes toward adolescent vaccination and the decision-making dynamic among adolescents, parents and providers. *BMC Public Health*. 2012;12(1):1.

121. Iannelli V. How Can I Get Vaccinated If My Parents Are Anti-Vaccine? Vaxopedia. 2018.

122. World Health Organization. Vaccines against influenza WHO position paper—November 2012. *Wkly Epidemiol Rec*. 2012;47(87):461–76.

123. Ramsey MA, Marczinski CA. College students' perceptions of H1N1 flu risk and attitudes toward vaccination. *Vaccine*. 2011;29(44):7599–601.

124. Nyhan B, Reifler J. Does correcting myths about the flu vaccine work? An experimental evaluation of the effects of corrective information. *Vaccine*. 2015;33(3):459–64.

125. Wagner AL, Gordon A, Tallo VL, et al. Intent to obtain pediatric influenza vaccine among mothers in four middle income countries. *Vaccine*. 2020;38(27):4325–35.

126. Smith LE, Amlôt R, Weinman J, Yiend J, Rubin GJ. Why do parents not re-vaccinate their child for influenza? A prospective cohort study. *Vaccine*. 2020;38(27):4230–5.

127. Schmid P, Rauber D, Betsch C, Lidolt G, Denker ML. Barriers of influenza vaccination intention and behavior—A systematic review of influenza vaccine hesitancy, 2005–2016. Cowling BJ, ed. *PLoS One*. 2017;12(1):e0170550.

128. Lind C, Russell ML, MacDonald J, Collins R, Frank CJ, Davis AE. School-based influenza vaccination: Parents' perspectives. *PLoS One*. 2014;9(3):e93490.

129. Flood EM, Ryan KJ, Rousculp MD, et al. Parent preferences for pediatric influenza vaccine attributes. *Clin Pediatr (Phila)*. 2011;50(4):338–47.

130. Flood EM, Ryan KJ, Rousculp MD, et al. A survey of children's preferences for influenza vaccine attributes. *Vaccine*. 2011;29(26):4334–40.

131. Dombkowski KJ, Cowan AE, Potter RC, Dong S, Kolasa M, Clark SJ. Statewide pandemic influenza vaccination reminders for children with chronic conditions. *Am J Public Health*. 2014;104(1):39–45.

132. Ray GT, Lewis N, Klein NP, et al. Intraseason waning of influenza vaccine effectiveness. *Clin Infect Dis*. 2018;68:1623–30.

133. Rambhia KJ, Rambhia MT. Early bird gets the flu: What should be done about waning intraseasonal immunity against seasonal influenza? *Clin Infect Dis*. 2019;68(7):1235–40.

134. Gidengil CA, Parker AM, Zikmund-Fisher BJ. Trends in risk perceptions and vaccination intentions: A longitudinal study of the first year of the H1N1 pandemic. *Am J Public Health*. 2012;102(4):672–9.

135. Shook E, Curtis A, Curtis J, et al. Assessing the geographic context of risk perception and behavioral response to potential Ebola exposure. *Int J Environ Res Public Health*. 2019;16:831.

136. McFadden SM, Malik AA, Aguolu OG, Willebrand KS, Omer SB. Perceptions of the adult US population regarding the novel coronavirus outbreak. *PLoS One*. 2020;15(4):e0231808.

137. Lurie N, Saville M, Hatchett R, Halton J. Developing COVID-19 vaccines at pandemic speed. *N Engl J Med*. 2020;382(21):1969–73.

138. Poland GA. Tortoises, hares, and vaccines: A cautionary note for SARS-CoV-2 vaccine development. *Vaccine*. 2020;38(27):4219–20.

139. Xiao Y, Moghadas SM. The impact of ethnicity and geographical location of residence on the 2009 influenza H1N1 pandemic vaccination. *Epidemiol Infect*. 2015;143(4):757–65.

140. Crowley KA, Myers R, Riley HEM, Morse SS, Brandt-Rauf P, Gershon RRM. Using participatory action research to identify strategies to improve pandemic vaccination. *Disaster Med Public Health Prep*. 2013;7(4):424–30.

141. Poland GA, Kennedy RB, Ovsyannikova IG, Palacios R, Ho PL, Kalil J. Development of vaccines against Zika virus. *Lancet Infect Dis*. 2018;18(7):e211–9.

142. Godinho CA, Yardley L, Marcu A, Mowbray F, Beard E, Michie S. Increasing the intent to receive a pandemic influenza vaccination: Testing the impact of theory-based messages. *Prev Med*. 2016;89:104–11.

143. Fraiz LD, de Roche A, Mauro C, et al. U.S. pregnant women's knowledge and attitudes about behavioral strategies and vaccines to prevent Zika acquisition. *Vaccine*. 2018;36(1):165–9.

144. Harapan H, Mudatsir M, Yufika A, et al. Community acceptance and willingness-to-pay for a hypothetical Zika vaccine: A cross-sectional study in Indonesia. *Vaccine*. 2019;37(11):1398–406.

145. Meissner HC. Complexity in assessing the benefit vs risk of vaccines: Experience with rotavirus and dengue virus vaccines. *JAMA*. 2019;322(19):1861–2.

146. Larson HJ, Hartigan-Go K, de Figueiredo A. Vaccine confidence plummets in the Philippines following dengue vaccine scare: why it matters to pandemic preparedness. *Hum Vaccin Immunother*. 2019;15(3):625–7.

147. The Lancet Infectious Diseases. Infectious disease crisis in the Philippines. *Lancet Infect Dis*. 2019;19(12):1265.

148. Håberg SE, Aaberg KM, Surén P, et al. Epilepsy in children after pandemic influenza vaccination. *Pediatrics*. 2018;141(3):e20170752.

149. Pasternak B, Svanström H, Mølgaard-Nielsen D, et al. Vaccination against pandemic A/H1N1 2009 influenza in pregnancy and risk of fetal death: Cohort study in Denmark. *BMJ*. 2012;344(7857):1–13.

150. Poland GA, Jacobson RM, Ovsyannikova IG. Trends affecting the future of vaccine development and delivery: The role of demographics, regulatory science, the anti-vaccine movement, and vaccinomics. *Vaccine.* 2009;27(25-26):3240–4.
151. Bramer CA, Kimmins LM, Swanson R, et al. Decline in child vaccination coverage during the COVID-19 pandemic—Michigan Care Improvement Registry, May 2016–May 2020. *MMWR Morb Mortal Wkly Rep.* 2020;69(20):630–1.
152. Doherty M, Schmidt-Ott R, Santos JI, et al. Vaccination of special populations: Protecting the vulnerable. *Vaccine.* 2016;34(52):6681–90.
153. Van Buynder PG, Van Buynder JL, Menton L, Thompson G, Sun J. Antigen specific vaccine hesitancy in pregnancy. *Vaccine.* 2019;37(21):2814–20.
154. Sur DK, Wallis DH, O'Connell TX. Vaccinations in pregnancy. *Am Fam Physician.* 2003;68(2):299–304.
155. Nasser R, Rakedzon S, Dickstein Y, et al. Are all vaccines safe for the pregnant traveller? A systematic review and meta-analysis. *J Travel Med.* 2020;27(2):1–16.
156. Sammon CJ, McGrogan A, Snowball J, de Vries CS. Pandemic influenza vaccination during pregnancy. *Hum Vaccin Immunother.* 2013;9(4):917–23.
157. Mohammed H, McMillan M, Roberts CT, Marshall HS. A systematic review of interventions to improve uptake of pertussis vaccination in pregnancy. Borrow R, ed. *PLoS One.* 2019;14(3):e0214538.
158. Visser O, Kraan J, Akkermans R, et al. Assessing determinants of the intention to accept a pertussis cocooning vaccination: A survey among Dutch parents. *Vaccine.* 2016;34(39):4744–51.
159. Lessin HR, Edwards KM. Immunizing parents and other close family contacts in the pediatric office setting. *Pediatrics.* 2012;129(1):e247–53.
160. Roh NK, Park YM, Kang H, et al. Awareness, knowledge, and vaccine acceptability of herpes zoster in Korea: A multicenter survey of 607 patients. *Ann Dermatol.* 2015;27(5):531–8.
161. Eilers R, Krabbe PFM, de Melker HE. Factors affecting the uptake of vaccination by the elderly in Western society. *Prev Med (Baltim).* 2014;69:224–34.
162. Lu PJ, O'Halloran A, Williams WW, Harpaz R. National and state-specific shingles vaccination among adults aged ≥60 years. *Am J Prev Med.* 2017;52(3):362–72.
163. Eilers R, de Melker HE, Veldwijk J, Krabbe PFM. Vaccine preferences and acceptance of older adults. *Vaccine.* 2017;35(21):2823–30.
164. Kaljee LM, Kilgore P, Prentiss T, et al. "You need to be an advocate for yourself": Factors associated with decision-making regarding influenza and pneumococcal vaccine use among US older adults from within a large metropolitan health system. *Hum Vaccines Immunother.* 2017;13(1):206–12.
165. Ang LW, Cutter J, James L, Goh KT. Factors associated with influenza vaccine uptake in older adults living in the community in Singapore. *Epidemiol Infect.* 2017;145(4):775–86.
166. de Gomensoro E, Del Giudice G, Doherty TM. Challenges in adult vaccination. *Ann Med.* 2018;50(3):181–92.
167. Yuan Q, Wang F, Zheng H, et al. Hepatitis B vaccination coverage among health care workers in China. *PLoS One.* 2019;14(5):e0216598.
168. Henriksen Hellyer JM, DeVries AS, Jenkins SM, et al. Attitudes toward and uptake of H1N1 vaccine among health care workers during the 2009 H1N1 pandemic. *PLoS One.* 2011;6(12):e29478.
169. Suryadevara M, Handel A, Bonville CA, Cibula DA, Domachowske JB. Pediatric provider vaccine hesitancy: An under-recognized obstacle to immunizing children. *Vaccine.* 2015;33(48):6629–34.
170. Paterson P, Meurice F, Stanberry LR, Glismann S, Rosenthal SL, Larson HJ. Vaccine hesitancy and healthcare providers. *Vaccine.* 2016;34(52):6700–6.
171. Sundaram N, Duckett K, Yung CF, et al. "I wouldn't really believe statistics"—Challenges with influenza vaccine acceptance among healthcare workers in Singapore. *Vaccine.* 2018;36(15):1996–2004.
172. Manca T. "One of the greatest medical success stories:" Physicians and nurses' small stories about vaccine knowledge and anxieties. *Soc Sci Med.* 2018;196(April 2017):182–9.
173. Lindley MC, Mu Y, Hoss A, et al. Association of state laws with influenza vaccination of hospital personnel. *Am J Prev Med.* 2019;56(6):e177–83.
174. Chor JSY, Pada SK, Stephenson I, et al. Seasonal influenza vaccination predicts pandemic H1N1 vaccination uptake among healthcare workers in three countries. *Vaccine.* 2011;29(43):7364–9.
175. Prematunge C, Corace K, McCarthy A, Nair RC, Pugsley R, Garber G. Factors influencing pandemic influenza vaccination of healthcare workers—A systematic review. *Vaccine.* 2012;30(32):4733–43.
176. Marcu A, Rubinstein H, Michie S, Yardley L. Accounting for personal and professional choices for pandemic influenza vaccination amongst English healthcare workers. *Vaccine.* 2015;33(19):2267–72.
177. Hak E, Schönbeck Y, De Melker H, Van Essen GA, Sanders EAM. Negative attitude of highly educated parents and health care workers towards future vaccinations in the Dutch childhood vaccination program. *Vaccine.* 2005;23(24):3103–7.
178. Chatterjee A. The controversy that will not go away: Vaccines and autism. In: *Vaccinophobia and Vaccine Controversies of the 21st Century.* New York: Springer New York; 2013, pp. 181–211.
179. Chen X-X, Wagner AL, Zheng X-B, et al. Hepatitis E vaccine in China: Public health professional perspectives on vaccine promotion and strategies for control. *Vaccine.* 2019;37(43):6566–72.
180. Ren H, Wagner AL, Xie J-Y, et al. How do experts and nonexperts want to promote vaccines? Hepatitis E vaccine as example. *Heal Serv Insights.* 2019;12:117863291989727.
181. Bakhache P, Rodrigo C, Davie S, et al. Health care providers' and parents' attitudes toward administration of new infant vaccines—A multinational survey. *Eur J Pediatr.* 2013;172(4):485–92.
182. Centers for Disease Control and Prevention. Measles. In: Hamborsky J, Kroger A, Wolfe SHamborsky J, Kroger A, Wolfe S, eds. *Epidemiology and Prevention of Vaccine-Preventable Diseases.* 13th ed. Washington, DC: Public Health Foundation; 2015, pp. 209–30.
183. Danovaro-Holliday MC, Wood AL, LeBaron CW. Rotavirus vaccine and the news media, 1987–2001. *JAMA.* 2002;287(11):1455–62.
184. King C, Leask J. The impact of a vaccine scare on parental views, trust and information needs: A qualitative study in Sydney, Australia. *BMC Public Health.* 2017;17(1):1–10.
185. Dyer O. Philippines measles outbreak is deadliest yet as vaccine scepticism spurs disease comeback. *BMJ.* 2019;739(February):l739.
186. Alexander LN, Seward JF, Santibanez TA, et al. Vaccine policy changes and epidemiology of poliomyelitis in the United States. *J Am Med Assoc.* 2004;292(14):1696–701.
187. Jiang B, Patel M, Glass RI. Polio endgame: Lessons for the global rotavirus vaccination program. *Vaccine.* 2019;37(23):3040–9.
188. Sato Y, Sato H. Development of acellular pertussis vaccines. *Biologicals.* 1999;27(2):61–9.
189. Tanaka M, Vitek CR, Pascual FB, Bisgard KM, Tate JE, Murphy T V. Trends in pertussis among infants in the United States, 1980–1999. *JAMA.* 2003;290(22):2968–75.
190. Guiso N, Liese J, Plotkin S. The global pertussis initiative: Meeting report from the fourth regional roundtable meeting, France, April 14–15, 2010—Commentary. *Hum Vaccin.* 2011;7(4):481–8.
191. Hotez PJ. Science tikkun: A framework embracing the right of access to innovation and translational medicine on a global scale. Dutra WO, ed. *PLoS Negl Trop Dis.* 2019;13(6):e0007117.
192. Larson HJ, de Figueiredo A, Xiahong Z, et al. The State of Vaccine Confidence 2016: Global insights through a 67-country survey. *EBioMedicine.* 2016;12:295–301.
193. Phillips DE, Dieleman JL, Lim SS, Shearer J. Determinants of effective vaccine coverage in low and middle-income countries: A systematic review and interpretive synthesis. *BMC Health Serv Res.* 2017;17(1):681.
194. Cobos Munoz D, Monzon Llamas L, Bosch-Capblanch X. Exposing concerns about vaccination in low- and middle-income countries: A systematic review. *Int J Public Health.* 2015;60(7):767–80.
195. Tauil M de C, Sato APS, Waldman EA. Factors associated with incomplete or delayed vaccination across countries: A systematic review. *Vaccine.* 2016;34(24):2635–43.
196. Jarrett C, Wilson R, O'Leary M, Eckersberger E, Larson HJ. Strategies for addressing vaccine hesitancy—A systematic review. *Vaccine.* 2015;33(October 2014):4180–90.
197. Ohlrogge AW, Suggs LS. Flu vaccination communication in Europe: What does the government communicate and how? *Vaccine.* 2018;36(44):6512–9.
198. Pelčić G, Karačić S, Mikirtichan GL, et al. Religious exception for vaccination or religious excuses for avoiding vaccination. *Croat Med J.* 2016;57(5):516–21.
199. Antommaria AH, Prows CA. Content analysis of requests for religious exemptions from a mandatory influenza vaccination program for healthcare personnel. *J Med Ethics.* 2018;44:389–91.
200. Gesser-Edelsburg A, Walter N, Shir-Raz Y, Sassoni Bar-Lev O, Rosenblat S. The behind-the-scenes activity of parental decision-making discourse regarding childhood vaccination. *Am J Infect Control.* 2017;45(3):267–71.

201. Seither R, Calhoun K, Street EJ, et al. Vaccination coverage for selected vaccines, exemption rates, and provisional enrollment among children in Kindergarten—United States, 2016–17 school year. *MMWR Morb Mortal Wkly Rep*. 2017;66(40):1073–80.

202. Bednarczyk RA, King AR, Lahijani A, Omer SB. Current landscape of nonmedical vaccination exemptions in the United States: Impact of policy changes. *Expert Rev Vaccines*. 2019;18(2):175–90.

203. Ahmed A, Lee KS, Bukhsh A, et al. Outbreak of vaccine-preventable diseases in Muslim majority countries. *J Infect Public Health*. 2018;11:153–5.

204. Rochmyaningsih D. Indonesian 'vaccine fatwa' sends measles immunization rates plummeting. *Science*. 2018.

205. Norazmi MN, Lim LS. Halal pharmaceutical industry: Opportunities and challenges. *Trends Pharmacol Sci*. 2015;36(8):496–7.

206. CDC. Rubella virus. In: *Epidemiology and Prevention of Vaccine-Preventable Diseases*. Washington, DC: Public Health Foundation Pubns; 2012, pp. 275–90.

207. Moffatt K, McNally C. Vaccine refusal: Perspectives from pediatrics. In: Chatterjee AChatterjee A, ed. *Vaccinophobia and Vaccine Controversies of the 21st Century*. New York: Springer New York; 2013, pp. 97–118.

208. Haelle TS. Why parents fear vaccines. In: *22nd Annual Conference on Vaccinology Research*. Baltimore, MD: National Foundation for Infectious Diseases; 2019.

209. Sobo EJ, Huhn A, Sannwald A, Thurman L. Information curation among vaccine cautious parents: Web 2.0, Pinterest thinking, and pediatric vaccination choice. *Med Anthropol Cross Cult Stud Heal Illn*. 2016;35(6):529–46.

210. MacDonald NE, Harmon S, Dube E, et al. Mandatory infant and childhood immunization: Rationales, issues and knowledge gaps. *Vaccine*. 2018;36(39):5811–8.

211. Attwell K, Drislane S, Leask J. Mandatory vaccination and no fault vaccine injury compensation schemes: An identification of country-level policies. *Vaccine*. 2019;37(21):2843–8.

212. Garnier R. Policy changes in vaccine exemptions in the United States may shape herd immunity. In: *22nd Annual Conference on Vaccinology Research*. Baltimore, MD: National Foundation for Infectious Diseases; 2019.

213. Delamater PL, Pingali SC, Buttenheim AM, Salmon DA, Klein NP, Omer SB. Elimination of nonmedical immunization exemptions in California and school-entry vaccine status. *Pediatrics*. 2019;143(6):e20183301.

214. Yang YT, Debold V. A longitudinal analysis of the effect of nonmedical exemption law and vaccine uptake on vaccine-targeted disease rates. *Am J Public Health*. 2014;104(2):371–7.

215. Olive JK, Hotez PJ, Damania A, Nolan MS. The state of the antivaccine movement in the United States: A focused examination of nonmedical exemptions in states and counties. *PLoS Med*. 2018;15(6):e1002578.

216. Luthy KE, Beckstrand RL, Meyers CJH. Common perceptions of parents requesting personal exemption from vaccination. *J Sch Nurs*. 2013;29(2): 95–103.

217. Richards JL, Wagenaar BH, Van Otterloo J, et al. Nonmedical exemptions to immunization requirements in California: A 16-year longitudinal analysis of trends and associated community factors. *Vaccine*. 2013;31(29):3009–13.

218. Navin MC. The ethics of vaccination nudges in pediatric practice. *HEC Forum*. 2017;29(1):43–57.

219. Smith MJ. Alternative schedules: Why not? In: Chatterjee AChatterjee A, ed. *Vaccinophobia and Vaccine Controversies of the 21st Century*. New York: Springer New York; 2013, pp. 307–20.

220. Diekema DS, American Academy of Pediatrics Committee on Bioethics. Responding to parental refusals of immunization of children. *Pediatrics*. 2005;115(5):1428–31.

221. American Academy of Pediatrics. Reaffirmation: Responding to parents who refuse immunization for their children. *Pediatrics*. 2013;131(5):e1696.

222. Edwards KM, Hackell JM, Committee on Infectious Diseases, Committee on Practice and Ambulatory Medicine. Countering vaccine hesitancy. *Pediatrics*. 2016;138(3):e20162146.

223. O'Leary ST, Allison MA, Fisher A, et al. Characteristics of physicians who dismiss families for refusing vaccines. *Pediatrics*. 2015;136(6):1103–11.

224. Opel DJ, Heritage J, Taylor JA, et al. The architecture of provider-parent vaccine discussions at health supervision visits. *Pediatrics*. 2013;132(6):1037–46.

225. Navin MC. The ethics of vaccination nudges in pediatric practice. *HEC Forum*. 2017;29:43–57.

226. Kornides ML, Fontenot HB, McRee AL, Panozzo CA, Gilkey MB. Associations between parents' satisfaction with provider communication and HPV vaccination behaviors. *Vaccine*. 2018;36(19):2637–42.

227. Smith PJ, Stokley S, Bednarczyk RA, Orenstein WA, Omer SB. HPV vaccination coverage of teen girls: The influence of health care providers. *Vaccine*. 2016;34(13):1604–10.

228. Poland CM, Poland GA. Vaccine education spectrum disorder: The importance of incorporating psychological and cognitive models into vaccine education. *Vaccine*. 2011;29(37):6145–8.

229. Shaffer VA, Zikmund-Fisher BJ. All stories are not alike: A purpose-, content-, and valence-based taxonomy of patient narratives in decision aids. *Med Decis Mak*. 2012;33(1):4–13.

230. Nyhan B, Reifler J, Richey S, Freed GL. Effective messages in vaccine promotion: A randomized trial. *Pediatrics*. 2014;133(4):e835–42.

231. Shourie S, Jackson C, Cheater FM, et al. A cluster randomised controlled trial of a web based decision aid to support parents' decisions about their child's measles mumps and rubella (MMR) vaccination. *Vaccine*. 2013;31(50):6003–10.

232. Johnson DK, Mello EJ, Walker TD, Hood SJ, Jensen JL, Poole BD. Combating vaccine hesitancy with vaccine-preventable disease familiarization: An interview and curriculum intervention for college students. *Vaccines (Basel)*. 2019;7:39.

233. Saitoh A, Saitoh A, Sato I, Shinozaki T, Kamiya H, Nagata S. Improved parental attitudes and beliefs through stepwise perinatal vaccination education. *Hum Vaccines Immunother*. 2017;13(11):2639–45.

234. Lama Y, Hu D, Jamison A, Quinn SC, Broniatowski DA. Characterizing trends in HPV vaccine discourse on Reddit (2007–2015). *JMIR Public Heal Surveill*. 2019;5(1):e12480.

235. Yiannakoulias N, Slavik C, Chase M. Expressions of pro- and anti-vaccine sentiment on YouTube. *Vaccine*. 2019;37(15):2057–64.

236. Vanderslott S. Exploring the meaning of pro-vaccine activism across two countries. *Soc Sci Med*. 2019;222:59–66.

237. Bode L, Vraga EK. See something, say something: Correction of global health misinformation on social media. *Health Commun*. 2018;33(9):1131–40.

238. Meyer SB, Violette R, Aggarwal R, Simeoni M, MacDougall H, Waite N. Vaccine hesitancy and Web 2.0: Exploring how attitudes and beliefs about influenza vaccination are exchanged in online threaded user comments. *Vaccine*. 2019;37(13):1769–74.

239. Leask J, Willaby HW, Kaufman J. The big picture in addressing vaccine hesitancy. *Hum Vaccines Immunother*. 2014;10(9):2600–2.

CHAPTER

92 Measles

Matthew L. Boulton • Abram L. Wagner

HISTORY

Measles is considered perhaps the most infectious disease known to humans, possibly equaled only by pertussis in its communicability.[1,2] Measles was described and differentiated from smallpox by the Persian physician Al-Razi in the tenth century,[3] but was not recognized as a viral disease until 1911, with the virus first successfully cultured in tissue in the late 1930s.[4] In the prevaccine era, virtually every child became infected with measles. With increasing development and availability of vaccines in the 1960s, the incidence of disease decreased dramatically.[5] Measles-containing vaccines were among the very first vaccines to be incorporated into the World Health Organization's (WHO) Expanded Program on Immunization (EPI)—those recommended vaccines that every country should publicly promote and fund.[6] The United States was able to achieve measles elimination (i.e., complete control of any endemic chain of transmission to < 12 months), in 1997.[7] Today, all regions of the WHO have established target dates for measles elimination.[8,9] However, recent years have seen striking increases in the number of measles cases, even in countries with historically robust immunization programs.[10] Measles remains a sentinel disease whose emergence within a country may represent a failure of the government to provide timely vaccinations to all residents or an increase in vaccine hesitancy, a growing concern following the now-discredited study reporting a link between measles vaccination and autism.

CLINICAL PRESENTATION

Measles can be transmitted both through direct contact with large respiratory droplets and through indirect contact with measles virus in aerosolized droplet nuclei. Transmission of measles after the virus has been suspended in the air for over 2 hours has been documented.[11,12] Infectiousness is extremely high, with 75–90% of susceptible household contacts developing disease.[13]

Measles has an incubation period of roughly 8–12 days before developing a characteristic viral prodrome initially consisting of high fever and malaise followed shortly thereafter by onset of cough, coryza, and conjunctivitis (the three Cs). Approximately 2–4 days after the viral prodrome, a distinctive erythematous, maculopapular rash appears consisting of lesions 3–8 mm in dimension, which spreads centrifugally starting on the face, before spreading to the trunk and extremities with the rash sometimes becoming confluent, especially on the face. Koplik's spots, small blue-white enanthem in the mouth, are pathognomonic for measles, but are typically only seen 2 days before and after the onset of rash. Only about 62.5% of cases will develop Koplik's spots.[14] The patient's temperature peaks 1–3 days following rash with fever as high as 104 degrees, with gradual fading of the rash about 3–7 days after onset in order of its appearance on the patient's body. Measles typically resolves 10–14 days after symptom onset.[13]

Complications and death are not uncommon after measles infection. In the United States, prevalent complications include diarrhea (8%), otitis media (7%), and pneumonia (6%).[13,15] The rate of complications, including morbidity and mortality, is higher in some countries, possibly mediated by crowding, malnutrition, and vitamin A deficiency. Crowding, and having a prolonged household exposure to a primary case, can result in a secondary case having a higher inoculum after exposure, and subsequently more serious disease. Malnourished children may have impaired immune systems, resulting in higher case fatalities, although measles also contributes to malnutrition through an increased metabolic demands and decreases in food intake. Children with vitamin A deficiency more frequently have pneumonia or diarrhea after measles.[13]

Infection with the measles virus can also lead to neurological complications. Measles encephalitis occurs 4–7 days after onset of rash (range 1–15 days) in approximately 1 out of every 1000 cases of measles.[13,16] Approximately 15% of patients with measles encephalitis die, and one-third will have permanent neurologic sequelae. Subacute sclerosing panencephalitis (SSPE) is a degenerative neurological condition that arises on average 4–10 years after initial infection with measles.[17] The estimated incidence of SSPE varies from 1 to 22 per 100,000 measles cases,[18,19] with incidence likely higher for individuals infected during infancy.[18] SSPE is characterized by an insidious onset and progressively severe personality changes, myoclonic seizures, and motor impairment. It almost invariably results in death.

Other clinical presentations of measles of note include modified measles and atypical measles. Modified measles is a milder clinical presentation of measles, characterized by a prolonged incubation period up to 20 days, a mild viral prodrome, and sparse rash, among individuals with passive immunity to measles—either through maternal antibodies in young infants or patients who received measles immune globulin. Atypical measles is a more severe presentation of measles, characterized by high fever, pneumonia, and edema of the extremities, among individuals who received the killed measles vaccine in the United States between 1963 and 1967.[20]

Measles is a serious disease. In the United States, the reported case fatality ratio is 1–3 deaths per 1000 cases.[13] However, in some settings it has been higher. For example, during an outbreak of measles in a religious community in Philadelphia opposed to medical interventions, 6 individuals died out of 486 cases.[21] The case fatality ratio may be higher in developing countries, and frequently ranges between 50 and 100 deaths per 1000 cases.[22]

There has been increased recognition that morbidity from measles extends beyond an acute presentation of illness. For example, measles early in life leads to children with significantly lower weight.[23,24] Additionally, individuals infected with measles can become immunosuppressed. Long-term immunological sequelae lasting 2–3 years can predispose individuals who have recovered from measles to more frequently acquire other infectious diseases. Thus, measles vaccination provides a benefit in preventing not only measles disease but also all-cause infectious disease.[25]

There are no specific treatments for measles and clinical care is supportive. Because vitamin A deficiency impacts recovery and potentiates complications, the WHO recommends treating all acute cases with vitamin A.[6] Secondary bacterial infections, which may lead to pneumonia or other complications, often require specific antibiotic therapy.[12,26]

VIRUS

Measles is caused by a single-stranded RNA virus in the genus *Morbillivirus* and the family *Paramyxoviridae*. Measles is a human disease and there are no known animal reservoirs. The Paramyxoviruses include pathogens that are important causes of respiratory disease in children including infantile bronchiolitis, croup, and pneumonia (i.e., parainfluenza and respiratory syncytial viruses) in addition to the causative agent of mumps. Three membrane proteins play critical roles in measles pathogenesis: hemagglutinin protein (H) attaches to cell surfaces, the fusion protein (F) allows for cell-to-cell spread, and the matrix protein (M) generates intact viral particles.[27] Immunity to measles is attributable to antibodies against the H protein,[28] and there is only one antigenic type of measles virus.

Because of clinical similarities between measles and other febrile rash-based illnesses, like rubella, varicella, Exanthem subitum, and Erythema infectiosum,[29] laboratory confirmation of suspected measles cases is an essential component of measles diagnostics and surveillance. Laboratory studies of measles are coordinated through the Global Measles Laboratory Network, which includes 506 subnational laboratories, 180 national laboratories, 14 regional reference laboratories, and 3 global specialized laboratories.[30] Measles virus can be cultured from respiratory secretions, urine, or serum. These tests take more time than other methods, and are more sensitive to shipping methods and specimen collection. However, reverse transcriptase polymerase chain reaction (RT-PCR) can allow for determination of the viral genotype, which is important for tracking chains of transmission.[31] A total of 24 different genotypes of measles virus have been identified based on the nucleoprotein (N) nucleotide sequence, although not all genotypes are actively circulating.[32,33] These genotypes show a varied regional distribution and can be used to monitor the geographical source of disease: for example, D4 is common in western Europe, D6 in eastern Europe, H1 in China, D4 in western and south Asia, B3 in north Africa, and D2 in southern Africa.[32]

Laboratory confirmation relies on enzyme linked immunosorbent assays (ELISA) to measure measles antibodies from serum samples. Infection with wild-type measles or live virus vaccine induces production of immunoglobulin M (IgM) antibodies within 72 hours. IgM antibodies decline within 2 months after onset of disease, and are evidence of recent infection. IgG antibodies appear shortly after rash onset, and appear to last a lifetime (Fig. 92-1). A fourfold rise in IgG titer across 10 days is indicative of recent infection.[34] Besides ELISA kits, plaque reduction neutralization assays can provide a quantitative measure of antibodies' ability to prevent pathogenesis of measles disease, and therefore represent the gold standard. Serological tests cannot distinguish between wild-type infection and live measles virus vaccination. Moreover, no standardized tests for cellular immunity to measles are currently available.

In most clinical settings, serum samples collected from venipuncture are used to supply specimens for antibody testing. Additionally, studies testing the prevalence of antibodies in a population, that is, seroprevalence surveys, are important for identifying demographic groups and geographical settings that are at high risk for measles outbreaks,[35] particularly because vaccination records are limited in many locations. For these epidemiological studies, venipuncture may be overly labor intensive and could be a disincentive to enroll in the study for some participants. Other methods to collect specimens, such as through oral fluid samples or dried blood spots (DBS) may be preferable. Results from a study in Bangladesh found that oral fluid samples were 60.2% sensitive and 75.7% specific for measles antibodies as compared to a serum gold standard.[36] A published study from the United States found that measles IgG tests from oral fluid were 97% sensitive and 100% specific compared to a serum gold standard.[37] A study of DBS in Australia found that they were 90.2% sensitive and 98.8% specific for measles, compared to serum samples.[38]

PASSIVE IMMUNIZATION

If mothers have been previously infected with measles or vaccinated with the measles vaccine, they can impart measles antibodies to their fetus in the third trimester of pregnancy, through an active transport process, whereby the antibody titers in the infant will typically be about twice as high compared to titers in the mother.[39] Historically, it was thought that protective levels of maternal antibodies would persist in infants up to 1 year, and was the primary justification for initiating measles vaccination at 12 months of age in the United States. However, recent research has found rapidly declining protective levels of maternal antibodies in infants, which may not be present beyond

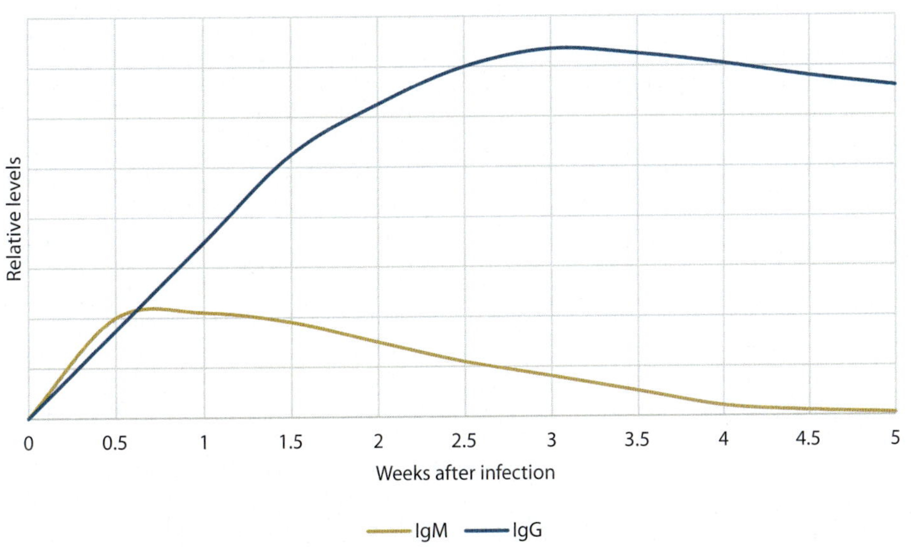

FIGURE 92-1. Immune response in acute measles infection. (*Source:* Adapted from World Health Organization. *Manual for the Laboratory Diagnosis of Measles and Rubella Virus Infection*, 2nd ed. Geneva, Switzerland: World Health Organization; 2007.[34])

3 months of age.[40,41] These declines in infant antibodies could be due, in part, to a large contingent of mothers who have been vaccinated (which results in lower antibody titers than natural infections)—often only once, or who may not have been vaccinated or had disease, but who were protected due to herd immunity.

Passive immunity can also be induced by administering homologous pooled human antibody (i.e., immune globulin) which is produced by combining the IgG antibody fraction from thousands of adult donors and contains antibody to measles among other antigens. Immune globulin can be given to individuals exposed to contacts of a measles case within 6 days of exposure, and is especially indicated for susceptible household contacts, immunocompromised individuals, pregnant women, and infants < 1 year, who are too young to be vaccinated.[42]

ACTIVE IMMUNIZATION

The first two measles vaccines were licensed in the United States in 1963. One was a live-attenuated virus using the Edmonston strain, and the other was a killed vaccine. The live-vaccine had a high rate of adverse reactions, and the killed vaccine could result in atypical measles. The killed vaccine was withdrawn from the market in the United States in 1967.[43] The Edmonston strain was further attenuated and additional live-attenuated vaccines were developed and licensed in 1965 (based on the Schwarz strain) and 1968 (based on the Moraten strain). Most vaccine strains derive from the original Edmonston strain, but the CAM-70 strain (used in Asia), Shanghai (or Hu)-191 (used in China), and Leningrad-4 (used in Russia) strains were all derived from unique wild-type isolates.[33]

The recommended age for initial measles vaccination varies across countries and is based primarily on local epidemiological, logistical, and financial considerations. A review of field studies on vaccine effectiveness found it to be 77.0% if administered at 9–11 months and 92.0% if administered at ≥ 12 months.[44] In settings with endemic transmission of disease where infants may comprise a disproportionately high number of measles cases, vaccinating at earlier ages, such as 9 or even 8 months, may be epidemiologically and clinically warranted.

A small proportion of individuals do not respond to the first dose of measles vaccine. In response to outbreaks of measles in the late 1980s, the U.S. Advisory Committee on Immunization Practices (ACIP) and the Committee on Infectious Diseases of the American Academy of Pediatrics both recommended in 1989 that all children receive a second dose of measles-containing vaccine.[45,46] Given the high infectiousness of measles disease and the less-than-perfect effectiveness of the measles vaccine, two doses of the vaccine are considered necessary to limit spread and control measles in a population.

Common adverse reactions to measles vaccine include fever and rash. Fever is estimated to occur in 5–11% of vaccinees, and rash in 12–20%.[47] In rare cases measles vaccination can also result in a clinical presentation indistinguishable from natural disease.[48]

A number of different formulations of measles-containing vaccines are used globally. In most high-income countries, measles is combined with rubella and mumps into a single measles-mumps-rubella (MMR) vaccine. Low- and middle-income countries may use a measles monovalent vaccine or combine it with a rubella as a measles-rubella combined vaccine (MR). A measles-mumps-rubella-varicella combined vaccine (MMRV) is also available, but it is noted for relatively high reactogenicity. For example, in a randomized clinical trial in the United States, adverse events were higher after an MMRV vaccine (rash, 5.9%; fever, 27.7%) than after separate administration of MMR and varicella (rash, 1.9%; fever, 18.7%), although immunogenicity was comparable between the different clinical arms.[49]

More serious adverse reactions to measles vaccines have been documented only in specific circumstances. For example, a study of the efficacy of high-titer vaccines in children in Senegal found that the risk of mortality was 1.80 times higher for a high-titer Edmonston vaccine (95% CI: 1.18, 2.74) and 1.51 times higher for a high-titer Schwartz vaccine (95% CI: 0.97, 2.34), compared to a standard low-titer Schwarz vaccine.[50] The female to male mortality ratio was 1.84 (95% CI: 1.19, 2.84).[51] This high-titer vaccine was recommended by the WHO in 1989, but was withdrawn in 1992 after these results came to light in efficacy trials.

No epidemiological study has shown a relationship between the administration of measles vaccine and autism. This hypothesis was popularized by Andrew Wakefield, a now discredited doctor who published an article based on a very small and methodologically weak study in the Lancet in 1998 purporting a link between MMRV and developmental disorder.[52] Subsequent large-scale and much more rigorous studies have found no association between measles vaccination and autism. For example, in a retrospective cohort study of all children born in Denmark from 1991 to 1998 ($n = 537{,}303$), the risk of autism was 0.92 times as high in vaccinated children compared to unvaccinated children (95% CI: 0.68, 1.24). Wakefield was later accused of falsifying data and deriving financial benefit from proposing the measles-autism link. All but one of his coauthors withdrew their co-authorship, Lancet retracted the paper, and Wakefield lost his medical license in the United Kingdom as a result of a formal investigation into his research.[53]

RECOMMENDATIONS FOR CONTROL

Measles is a highly infectious disease. The basic reproductive number (R_0), a measure of the average number of secondary cases, varies by setting, but the median value from one review of surveillance data was 13.2.[54] Theoretically, this means that the herd immunity threshold is around 95%, in that this proportion of the population needs to be immune to measles (either through vaccination or natural infection) in order to prevent further transmission of disease. In practice, calculating population-level immunity on a broad geographical scale has little practical value because pockets of susceptible individuals will almost invariably be present and may be more likely to mix with each other than vaccinated individuals.[55] For example, an analysis of schools in King and Snohomish counties, Washington State, in 2011–12 found that 86 schools had vaccination exemption rates $>$ 10%, and these schools were clustered.[56] And in April and May 2017, an outbreak of measles occurred in the Somali American population, whose vaccination coverage had been declining for several years after being targeted by messaging from antivaccine groups.[57]

Many parents express vaccine hesitancy—ranging from complete distrust in and refusal for all vaccines to a desire to space out vaccine administration (see chapter on Vaccine Decision-Making and Vaccine Hesitancy). The American Academy of Pediatrics (AAP) has reported that 75% of pediatricians in 2006 and 87% of pediatricians in 2013 had encountered parents who have refused a vaccine.[58] Many educational materials (including refuting antivaccine claims, showing parents images of or narratives about sick children) appear to have little effect on parents' desire to get a vaccine.[59] Executing a presumptive delivery strategy (i.e., "nudging"), where the doctor confidently inform parents about which vaccines their child should be receiving, is an ethically sound intervention to increase parents' adherence to the recommended vaccination schedule.[60] The AAP suggests dismissing parents who do not vaccinate only as a last resort.[58] Temporary dismissal of susceptible students (i.e., school exclusion) may be necessary to limit the spread of infectious diseases to children who are medically ineligible for vaccination; measles outbreaks in the past have been tied to exposure in clinical settings.[61]

Measles vaccination is indicated for all children. Contraindications to vaccination include individuals with immunosuppression and individuals with allergies to vaccine components (although the risk of serious reaction in those with egg allergies is extremely low, and therefore the vaccine should be administered to egg-allergic children).[15] Due to the possibility of outbreaks occurring even in countries where measles has been eliminated, unvaccinated adults should also be immunized. As of 2008, 192 out of 193 countries had adopted a two-dose vaccination strategy.[6] In the United States, individuals can be vaccinated as early as 6 months in an outbreak setting although must then be revaccinated at the standard recommended age of 12 months, which would count as the first dose in the two-dose schedule. In the United States and many other countries, measles is a mandatory vaccine, and required for school entry. In the United States, states require two doses prior to school entry, although almost all states allow for nonmedical waivers (philosophical, religious) with varying degrees of ease in obtaining them. The relative administrative ease with which one can obtain a waiver has been linked to the incidence of vaccine-preventable diseases, and it is recommended on a policy-level to limit the use of waivers in order to control measles.[62]

In countries that have already eliminated measles, contact tracing is expensive but necessary to seek out individuals who have been exposed and are at higher risk of acquiring disease. In a 2008 outbreak, contact tracing cost $10,376 per case.[61] In travel settings, contact tracing is particularly important due to the potential for reintroducing measles into regions where it has already been eliminated. Current guidelines from the CDC for potential exposures occurring during international flights are to contact any individual within two rows of either side of a laboratory-confirmed case, along with any infant and flight crew in the same cabin.[63]

Supplementary Immunization Activities

Supplementary immunization activities (SIAs) have been frequently used as a component of measles control strategies and are a mechanism to provide individuals with vaccines outside of routine immunization services. There are several varieties of SIAs. "Catch-up" SIAs target a broad age range of children; "follow-up" campaigns which target children born since the previous SIA; "mop-up" campaigns aimed at children in geographically remote regions or who were employed during the previous campaign; and "speed-up" campaigns which target adolescents and adults.[64,65] Typically, most SIAs target all individuals, regardless of previous vaccination status. This is necessary to vaccinate individuals with a second dose of measles vaccine, but could also lead to substantial vaccine wastage or vaccination fatigue, if parents are obtaining ≥ 3 doses of measles vaccine for their children.

Previously, SIAs have been found to lead to large reductions in measles incidence in the following year. Two studies examining provincial- and national-level SIAs in China found that the incidence of disease bounced back to pre-SIA levels after a few years.[66,67] This could be due to the follow-up, mop-up, or speed-up campaigns not being strategically implemented after an initial catch-up campaign, or it could be due to routine immunization services not adequately capturing populations migrating between provinces.

Another criticism of SIAs is that they take funding and focus away from a broad spectrum of communicable diseases and wellness programs (which can be packaged together at public immunization clinics) and instead focus vertically on a specific disease. This means healthcare workers may not be vaccinating children against other conditions during a measles vaccine-specific SIA. Interviews with officials in health departments in some low- and middle-income countries have revealed concerns that measles SIAs can undermine local decisions on resource allocation.[68] One study in Zambia did show SIAs to be cost effective, and even cost saving, but it assumed SIAs were able to reach children not previously vaccinated.[69] Considering all these challenges, SIAs are most valuable when targeting individuals not typically serviced through routine immunization programs, like children in remote regions or adults. For example, speed-up campaigns targeting adults in many Central and South American countries may have contributed to the early elimination of measles in the region.[64]

CHANGING EPIDEMIOLOGY OF MEASLES

The introduction of measles vaccines has had a dramatic impact on morbidity and mortality from measles. For example, in the United States, there has been a > 99% decline in cases and deaths, comparing annual averages before and after vaccination was introduced.[5] In certain situations, that is, a small limited population with low immigration and high access to vaccination programs, this decline can be quite rapid. For instance, a 12-year program using two doses of measles-containing vaccine limited outbreaks of measles in Finland to imported cases.[70]

Introduction of a measles vaccine has also led to a decrease in the rate of complications from measles disease. After introduction of a vaccine, noticeable declines in SSPE have occurred, after accounting for a 7-year lag because of the incubation period. For example, compared to a multiyear period of high measles incidence and low vaccination coverage, a later period of low measles incidence and high vaccination coverage had 0.04 times the rate of SSPE in the United States and 0.07 times the rate of SSPE in the Netherlands.[17]

As incidence of measles decreases, several challenges arise in realizing further declines in disease occurrence.[71] (1) Low incidence of disease for several years can build up a substantial population of susceptible individuals, who can then rapidly spread disease after it has been apparently controlled. (2) The age at infection increases so that it more frequently occurs in adolescents and adults, who are less likely to participate in immunization programs, especially in low- and middle-income countries. In addition, (3) sources of infection are different from in the pre-elimination era. The experiences controlling measles in Tianjin, China, a city with high coverage of measles-containing vaccines, reflect these issues. Years of low measles incidence (2008–09 and 2011–13) were followed by years of high measles incidence, and the average age of measles cases shifted upward—with young adults 20–39 years comprising a growing proportion in the overall number of cases.[72]

Several studies have documented how measles has spread among families who intentionally do not vaccinate their children. In high-income countries, it is often highly educated populations who express negative attitudes toward vaccinations and have lower vaccination coverage.[73] In an outbreak of measles in California in 2008, an intentionally unvaccinated child was infected during a trip to Switzerland, and led to an outbreak of 11 additional cases in unvaccinated children, 1 hospitalized infant too young for vaccination, and a total of 839 exposed persons.[61] In another outbreak associated with attendance at Disney theme parks in 2014–15, among 110 cases from California, 49 were unvaccinated—of these 12 (24%) were too young to be vaccinated, 28 (67%) were intentionally unvaccinated.[74]

Elimination and Eradication

Elimination is the reduction of endemic transmission of disease within a specific geographical region, with endemic transmission defined as a continued chain of infection over a 1-year span. Eradication is the global elimination of disease—currently smallpox is the only human pathogen to be eradicated (see Chapter 83: Principles of Disease Elimination and Eradication).[71]

The difficulties in eliminating measles are exemplified by the experience with controlling measles in the Americas. The United States was one of the first countries to declare measles elimination in 1997.[75] However, the United States has recently had large outbreaks of disease, including 1282 cases in 2019, of which 73% were linked to outbreaks in New York.[76] The American region of the WHO was the first to declare elimination throughout the region in 2002. Brazil had previously eliminated measles in 2001, however, starting in December 2013 and lasting 20 months, 1052 confirmed cases with the same genotype (D8) were identified in Ceará, Brazil.[77] After intensive measles control efforts, Brazil, and the entire Americas region, was re-certified as having eliminated measles in 2016. No other regional office of the WHO has been certified to have eliminated measles, but several other countries have been able to eliminate measles, including Australia in 2014,[78] and Bhutan and the Maldives in 2017.[79]

All WHO regions have agreed to eliminate measles by 2020.[8,9] Large outbreaks of measles in the 2010s in Europe cast doubt as to whether this goal is feasible, even in high-income countries. In 2015, there were still 25,283 cases in Europe, and all countries had below 95% immunity against measles.[80] High-income countries that are more than one generation beyond measles infection as the status quo face a populace, which is vaccine hesitant.[58] At the same time, developing countries may lack the resources to provide regular routine immunization services. Along with the WHO, several organizations, notably the GAVI Alliance, funded in part through the Bill and Melinda Gates Foundation, and the Measles & Rubella Initiative are providing support to countries to provide robust immunization services, and pushing them to take cost-effective steps toward sustainably financing these important services.

Several features are common to countries approaching the measles elimination end game.[71] Measles becomes more common in infants (below the age of vaccination) and young and middle-aged adults, often who grew up in an era of noncomprehensive one-dose vaccination programs. The future of measles control includes robust routine immunization programs, SIAs that target individuals not commonly serviced by these routine programs (such as adults and migrants), combined with educational efforts to increase individuals trust in measles vaccination.

References

1. Wallinga J, Teunis P, Kretzschmar M. Reconstruction of measles dynamics in a vaccinated population. *Vaccine*. 2003;21(19–20):2643–50.
2. Kretzschmar M, Teunis PFM, Pebody RG. Incidence and reproduction numbers of pertussis: Estimates from serological and social contact data in five European countries. *PLoS Med*. 2010;7(6):e1000291.
3. Ligon BL. Biography: Rhazes: His career and his writings. *Semin Pediatr Infect Dis*. 2001;12(3):266–72.
4. Babbott FL, Gordon JE. Modern measles. *Am J Med Sci*. 1954;228(3):334–61.
5. Roush SW, Murphy TV. Historical comparisons of morbidity and mortality for vaccine-preventable diseases in the United States. *JAMA*. 2007;298(18):2155–63. doi:10.1001/jama.298.18.2155.
6. World Health Organization. Measles vaccines: WHO position paper. *Wkly Epidemiol Rec*. 2009;84(35):349–60.
7. Katz SL, Hinman AR. Summary and conclusions: Measles elimination meeting, 16–17 March 2000. Orenstein WA, Samuel KL, Hinman AR. eds. *J Infect Dis*. 2004;189(Suppl 1):S43–7.
8. World Health Organization. *Global Measles and Rubella Strategic Plan 2012–2020*. Geneva, Switzerland: World Health Organization; 2012.
9. Thapa A, Khanal S, Sharapov U, et al. Progress toward measles elimination—South-East Asia region, 2003–2013. *MMWR Morb Mortal Wkly Rep*. 2015; 64(22):613–7.
10. Cottrell S, Roberts RJ. Measles outbreak in Europe. *BMJ*. 2011;342: d3724.
11. DeJong JG, Winkler KC. Survival of measles virus in air. *Nature*. 1964;201: 1054–5.
12. Bloch AB, Orenstein WA, Ewing WM, et al. Measles outbreak in a pediatric practice: Airborne transmission in an office setting. *Pediatrics*. 1985;75(4): 676–83.
13. Perry RT, Halsey NA. The clinical significance of measles. *J Infect Dis*. 2004;189(Suppl 1):S4–16.
14. Zenner D, Nacul L. Predictive power of Koplik's spots for the diagnosis of measles. *J Infect Dev Ctries*. 2012;6(3):271–5.
15. CDC. Measles virus. In: *Epidemiology and Prevention of Vaccine-Preventable Diseases*. Washington, DC: Public Health Foundation; 2012, pp. 173–92.
16. Bloch AB, Orenstein WA, Wassilak SG, et al. Epidemiology of measles and its complications. In: Gruenberg E, Lewis C, Goldston SEGruenberg E, Lewis C, Goldston SE, eds. *Vaccinating Against Brain Syndromes: The Campaign Against Measles and Rubella*. New York: Oxford University Press; 1986, pp. 5–20.
17. Campbell H, Andrews N, Brown KE, Miller E. Review of the effect of measles vaccination on the epidemiology of SSPE. *Int J Epidemiol*. 2007;36(6): 1334–48.
18. Miller C, Andrews N, Rush M, Munro H, Jin L, Miller E. The epidemiology of subacute sclerosing panencephalitis in England and Wales 1990–2002. *Arch Dis Child*. 2004;89(12):1145–8.
19. Bellini WJ, Rota JS, Lowe LE, et al. Subacute sclerosing panencephalitis: More cases of this fatal disease are prevented by measles immunization than was previously recognized. *J Infect Dis*. 2005;192(10):1686–93.
20. Fulginiti VA, Eller JJ, Downie AW, Kempe CH. Altered reactivity to measles virus. *JAMA*. 1967;202(12):1075–80.
21. Rodgers DV, Gindler JS, Atkinson WiL, Markowitz LE. High attack rates and case fatality during a measles outbreak in groups with religious exemption to vaccination. *Pediatr Infect Dis J*. 1993;12:288–92.
22. Aaby P. Malnutrition and overcrowding/intensive exposure in severe measles infection: Review of community studies. *Clin Infect Dis*. 1988;10(2): 478–91.
23. Vargas PA, Bernardi FDC, Alves VAF, et al. Uncommon histopathological findings in fatal measles infection: Pancreatitis, sialoadenitis and thyroiditis. *Histopathology*. 2000;37(2):141–6.
24. Halsey NA, Boulos R, Mode F, et al. Response to measles vaccine in Haitian infants 6 to 12 months old. *N Engl J Med*. 1985;313(9):544–9.
25. Mina M, Metcalf C, de Swart RL, Osterhous A, Grenfell B. Long-term measles-induced immunomodulation increases overall childhood infectious disease mortality. *Science*. 2015;348(6235):694–700.
26. Barkin RM. Measles mortality. *Am J Dis Child*. 1975;129(3):307.
27. Griffin DE. Measles virus. In: Knipe DM, Howley PMKnipe DM, Howley PM, eds. *Field's Virology*. Philadelphia: Lippincott-Williams Wilkins; 2001, pp. 1401–41.
28. de Swart RL, Yüksel S, Osterhaus ADME. Relative contributions of measles virus hemagglutinin- and fusion protein-specific serum antibodies to virus neutralization. *J Virol*. 2005;79(17):11547–51.
29. Kang JH. Febrile illness with skin rashes. *Infect Chemother*. 2015;47(3): 155–66.
30. Xu W, Zhang Y, Wang H, et al. Global and national laboratory networks support high quality surveillance for measles and rubella. *Int Health*. 2017;9(3):184–9.
31. Rota JS, Heath JL, Rota PA, et al. Molecular epidemiology of measles virus: Identification of pathways of transmission and implications for measles elimination. *J Infect Dis*. 1996;173(1):32–7.
32. World Health Organization. New genotype of measles virus and update on global distribution of measles genotypes. *Wkly Epidemiol Rec*. 2005;80:341–52.
33. Strebel PM, Papania MJ, Fiebelkorn AP, Halsey NA. Measles vaccine. In: Plotkin SA, Orenstein WA, Offit PA, eds.Plotkin SA, Orenstein WA, Offit PA, eds. *Vaccines*. 6th ed. Philadelphia: Elsevier; 2013, pp. 352–87.
34. World Health Organization. *Manual for the Laboratory Diagnosis of Measles and Rubella Virus Infection*, 2nd ed. Geneva, Switzerland: World Health Organization; 2007.
35. Thompson KM, Odahowski CL. Systematic review of measles and rubella serology studies. *Risk Anal*. 2016;36(7):1459–86.
36. Hayford KT, Al-Emran HM, Moss WJ, Shomik MS, Bishai D, Levine OS. Validation of an anti-measles virus-specific IgG assay with oral fluid samples for immunization surveillance in Bangladesh. *J Virol Methods*. 2013;193(2):512–8.
37. Thieme T, Piacentini S, Davidson S, Steingart K. Determination of measles, mumps, and rubella immunization status using oral fluid samples. *JAMA*. 1994;272(3):219–21.
38. Riddell MA, Leydon JA, Catton MG, Kelly HA. Detection of measles virus-specific immunoglobulin M in dried venous blood samples by using a commercial enzyme immunoassay. *J Clin Microbiol*. 2002;40(1):5–9.
39. Leuridan E, Van Damme P. Passive transmission and persistence of naturally acquired or vaccine-induced maternal antibodies against measles in newborns. *Vaccine*. 2007;25(34):6296–304.
40. Gans HA, Maldonado YA. Loss of passively acquired maternal antibodies in highly vaccinated populations: An emerging need to define the ontogeny of infant immune responses. *J Infect Dis*. 2013;208(1):1–3.
41. Boulton ML, Wang X, Wagner AL, et al. Measles antibodies in mother-infant dyads in Tianjin, China. *J Infect Dis*. 2017;216(9):1122–9.
42. American Academy of Pediatrics. In: Pickering LKPickering LK, ed. *Red Book 2000*. Elk Grove Village, IL: American Academy of Pediatrics; 2000.
43. Centers for Disease Control and Prevention. Measles. In: Hamborsky J, Kroger A, Wolfe SEHamborsky J, Kroger A, Wolfe SE, eds. *Epidemiology and Prevention of Vaccine-Preventable Diseases*, 13th ed. Washington, DC: Public Health Foundation; 2015, pp. 209–30.
44. Uzicanin A, Zimmerman L. Field effectiveness of live attenuated measles-containing vaccines: A review of published literature. *J Infect Dis*. 2011; 204(Suppl 1):S133–48.

45. Plotkin SA, Daum RS, Giebink GS, et al. Measles: Reassessment of the current immunization policy. *Pediatrics*. 1989;84:1110–3.
46. Centers for Disease Control and Prevention (CDC). Measles prevention: Recommendations of the Advisory Committee for Immunization Practices (ACIP). *MMWR Morb Mortal Wkly Rep*. 1989;38(S-9):1–18.
47. Lerman SJ, Bollinger M, Brunken JM. Clinical and serologic evaluation of measles, mumps, and rubella (HPV-77:DE-5 and RA27/3) virus vaccines, singly and in combination. *Pediatrics*. 1981;68(1):18–22.
48. Berggren KL, Tharp M, Boyer KM. Vaccine-associated "wild-type" measles. *Pediatr Dermatol*. 2005;22(2):130–2.
49. Shinefield H, Black S, Digilio L, et al. Evaluation of a quadrivalent measles, mumps, rubella and varicella vaccine in healthy children. *Pediatr Infect Dis J*. 2005;24(8):665–9.
50. Garenne M, Leroy O, Beau JP, Sene I. Child mortality after high-titre measles vaccines: Prospective study in Senegal. *Lancet*. 1991;338(8772): 903–7.
51. Aaby P, Jensen H, Samb B, et al. Differences in female-male mortality after high-titre measles vaccine and association with subsequent vaccination with diphtheria-tetanus-pertussis and inactivated poliovirus: Reanalysis of West African studies. *Lancet*. 2003;361(9376):2183–8.
52. Eggertson L. Lancet retracts 12-year-old article linking autism to MMR vaccines. *CMAJ*. 2010;182(4):199–200.
53. Knopf A. MMR vs. autism: A false choice. *Brown Univ Child Adolesc Behav Lett*. 2015;31(S4):1–2.
54. Guerra FM, Bolotin S, Lim G, et al. The basic reproduction number (R0) of measles: A systematic review. *Lancet Infect Dis*. 2017;17(12):e420–8.
55. Fine P, Eames K, Heymann DL. "Herd immunity": A rough guide. *Clin Infect Dis*. 2011;52(7):911–6.
56. Balk G. Vaccine exemptions exceed 10% at dozens of Seattle-area schools. *Seattle Times*.
57. Hall V, Banerjee E, Kenyon C, et al. Measles outbreak—Minnesota April–May 2017. *MMWR Morb Mortal Wkly Rep*. 2017;66(27):713–7.
58. Edwards KM, Hackell JM, The Committee on Infectious Diseases, The Committee on Practice and Ambulatory Medicine. Countering vaccine hesitancy. *Pediatrics*. 2016;138(3):e20162146.
59. Nyhan B, Reifler J, Richey S, Freed GL. Effective messages in vaccine promotion: A randomized trial. *Pediatrics*. 2014;133:e835–42.
60. Navin MC. The ethics of vaccination nudges in pediatric practice. *HEC Forum*. 2017;29:43–57.
61. Sugerman DE, Barskey AE, Delea MG, et al. Measles outbreak in a highly vaccinated population, San Diego, 2008: Role of the intentionally undervaccinated. *Pediatrics*. 2010;125(4):747–55.
62. Omer SB, Salmon DA, Orenstein WA, et al. Vaccine refusal, mandatory immunization, and the risks of vaccine-preventable diseases. *N Engl J Med*. 2009;360(19):1981–8.
63. Beard F, Franklin L, Donohue S, et al. Contact tracing of in-flight measles exposures: Lessons from an outbreak investigation and case series, Australia, 2010. *Western Pac Surveill Response J*. 2011;2(3):25–33.
64. Castillo-Solorzano C, Marsigli C, Danovaro-Holliday MC, Ruiz-Matus C, Tambini G, Andrus JK. Measles and rubella elimination initiatives in the Americas:Lessonslearnedandbestpractices.*JInfectDis*.2011;204(Suppl.1): 279–83.
65. Aaby P. Measles infection. In: Schenck-Gustafsson K, DeCola P, Pfaff D, Pisetsky DSchenck-Gustafsson K, DeCola P, Pfaff D, Pisetsky D, eds. *Handbook of Clinical Gender Medicine*. Basel: Karger; 2012, pp. 405–13.
66. Ma C, An Z, Hao L, et al. Progress toward measles elimination in the People's Republic of China, 2000–2009. *J Infect Dis*. 2011;204:S447–54.
67. Wagner AL, Zhang Y, Mukherjee B, Ding Y, Wells E, Boulton ML. The impact of supplementary immunization activities on the epidemiology of measles in Tianjin, China. *Int J Infect Dis*. 2016;45:103–8.
68. Hanvoravongchai P, Mounier-Jack S, Oliveira Cruz V, et al. Impact of measles elimination activities on immunization services and health systems: Findings from six countries. *J Infect Dis*. 2011;204(Suppl 1):S82–9.
69. Dayan GH, Cairns L, Sangrujee N, Mtonga A, Nguyen V, Strebel P. Cost-effectiveness of three different vaccination strategies against measles in Zambian children. *Vaccine*. 2004;22(3–4):475–84.
70. Peltola H, Heinonen OP, Valle M, et al. The elimination of indigenous measles, mumps, and rubella from Finland by a 12-year, two-dose vaccination program. *N Engl J Med*. 1994;331(21):1397–402.
71. Klepac P, Metcalf CJE, McLean AR, Hampson K. Towards the endgame and beyond: Complexities and challenges for the elimination of infectious diseases. *Phil Trans R Soc Lond B Biol Sci*. 2013;368(1623):20120137.
72. Wang X, Boulton ML, Montgomery JP, et al. The epidemiology of measles in Tianjin, China, 2005–2014. *Vaccine*. 2015;33(46):6186–91.
73. Hak E, Schönbeck Y, De Melker H, Van Essen GA, Sanders EAM. Negative attitude of highly educated parents and health care workers towards future vaccinations in the Dutch childhood vaccination program. *Vaccine*. 2005;23(24):3103–7.
74. Zipprich J, Winter K, Hacker J, Xia D, Watt J, Harriman K. Measles outbreak—California, December 2014–February 2015. *MMWR Morb Mortal Wkly Rep*. 2015;64(6):153–4.
75. Centers for Disease Control and Prevention. Measles—United States, 1997. *MMWR Morb Mortal Wkly Rep*. 1998;47(14):273–6.
76. Centers for Disease Control and Prevention. Measles (Rubeola) Measles Cases and Outbreaks. https://www.cdc.gov/measles/cases-outbreaks.html. Published 2020. Accessed July 8, 2020.
77. Rocha D, Lemos Q, Ramirez A, et al. Measles epidemic in Brazil in the post-elimination period : Coordinated response and containment strategies. *Vaccine*. 2017;35(13):1721–8.
78. Gidding HF, Martin NV, Stambos V, Tran T, Dey A. Verification of measles elimination in Australia: Application of World Health Organization regional guidelines. *J Epidemiol Glob Health*. 2016;6(3):197–209.
79. World Health Organization: Regional Office for South-East Asia. Bhutan, Maldives eliminate measles. SEAR/PR/1651. http://www.searo.who.int/mediacentre/releases/2017/1651/en/. Published 2017. Accessed August 11, 2017.
80. Plans-Rubió P. Why does measles persist in Europe ? *Eur J Clin Microbiol Infect Dis*. 2017;36(10):1899–906.

CHAPTER

93

Mumps*

Mariel A. Marlow

Mumps disease was described in the literature as early as fifth century BC by Hippocrates. The etiologic agent was identified as a virus in 1934 by Johnson and Goodpasture who demonstrated transmission to rhesus monkeys[1]; propagation of the virus ultimately led to the development of vaccines by the late 1960s.[2] Mumps vaccine has resulted in dramatic decreases in the incidence and associated morbidity in the United States and in other countries that have introduced the vaccine in their routine childhood immunization programs. However, starting in the mid-2000s, mumps epidemics have occurred in countries with high mumps vaccination coverage, with the majority of cases occurring among persons who previously received two doses of mumps vaccine.[3–7] Still, incidence remains much higher in countries where there is no routine vaccination for mumps.[8]

CLINICAL DESCRIPTION

Mumps is an acute viral infection that typically presents as parotitis or other salivary gland swelling, and may be proceeded by a prodrome characterized by fever, headache, malaise, myalgias, anorexia, and fatigue.[9] Infection may be asymptomatic in approximately 15–24% of unvaccinated persons.[10–12] The frequency of subclinical or asymptomatic infection in vaccinated persons is unknown, but mumps symptoms are usually milder among vaccinated persons.[13–19]

Uncomplicated mumps illness typically resolves within 10 days. Mumps reinfection or recurrent mumps (parotid swelling resolves on one side and then weeks to months later occurs on the other side) can occur.[20–24]

COMPLICATIONS

Complications associated with mumps infection are usually more severe in adults than children,[12,19] and are less common in vaccinated persons.[13–19] Orchitis is the most frequently reported complication and occurs in about 30% of unvaccinated and 6% of vaccinated postpubertal men.[16,18] About half of patients with mumps orchitis develop testicular atrophy of the affected testicles.[25,26] While orchitis and testicular atrophy from mumps can cause oligospermia, azoospermia, asthenospermia, no studies have documented cases of or assessed risk for sterility. Oophoritis and mastitis have been reported to occur in 7–30% of unvaccinated postpubertal women during outbreaks,[10,11,16,18] and in < 1% of vaccinated postpubertal women with mumps in population-based studies.[16,27,28] Sensorineural deafness associated with mumps infection can occur in up to 4% of unvaccinated patients and may result in permanent hearing loss.[29,30] Pancreatitis occurs in up to 4% of unvaccinated patients and is usually mild.[12] Hearing loss and pancreatitis occur in < 1% of vaccinated mumps patients.[4,13,16,19,27,31,32]

Aseptic meningitis is the most common CNS complication and is typically mild or subclinical.[26] In studies involving vaccinated and unvaccinated cases, clinically apparent meningitis and encephalitis occurred in ≤ 1% of mumps cases.[4,13,16,19,27,32] Nephritis, myocarditis, and other sequelae, including paralysis, seizures, cranial nerve palsies, and hydrocephalus, in mumps patients have also been reported. Mumps infection during pregnancy has not been associated with congenital malformations[33] but first-trimester infections may result in spontaneous abortion.[34] Death from mumps is very rare.

ETIOLOGIC AGENT AND TRANSMISSION

Mumps is caused by a ribonucleic acid virus in the family *Paramyxoviridae*. Humans are the only known natural reservoir. Mumps virus is transmitted through direct contact with saliva or respiratory droplets of an infected person. Transmission among populations with high vaccination coverage usually involves intense close contact behaviors, such as sharing drinks, dancing, playing sports, or prolonged or frequent contact. The incubation period averages 16–18 days after exposure to the virus but can range from 12 to 25 days.[9] A person is considered infectious from 2 days before until 5 days after onset of parotitis or other salivary gland swelling,[35] but virus has been detected in patients' saliva as early as 7 days before and until 9 days after onset.[36,37] Mumps virus has been isolated from urine[38] and seminal fluids[39] up to 14 days after onset of parotitis. Mumps virus is the only infectious agent known to cause epidemic parotitis.

DIAGNOSIS AND LABORATORY TESTING

Acute mumps infection is confirmed by virus detection by real-time reverse transcriptase polymerase chain reaction (RT-qPCR) or viral isolation in specimens collected from the parotid duct (Stensen's duct), saliva, urine, or cerebral spinal fluid. Serologic testing for presence of IgM antibodies, IgG seroconversion, or a fourfold rise in IgG antibody titer can also aid in mumps diagnosis, but are not confirmatory. Other etiologic agents that cause parotitis may cause false-positive serologic results. Vaccinated persons may have transient or undetectable IgM response and IgG titers may already be positive or elevated at the initial blood draw.

Proper buccal swab collection includes massaging the parotid for 30 seconds prior to buccal specimen collection. Timing of specimen collection is important for both RT-qPCR and serological tests. The proportion of buccal swab samples with positive results by RT-qPCR decreases as the interval between onset and specimen collection increases. The optimal timing for buccal swab collection is ≤ 3 days after symptom onset. Urine samples may not be RT-qPCR positive for mumps virus until > 4 days. IgM antibodies may be detectable

*Note: The findings and conclusions in this chapter are those of the author and do not necessarily represent the official position of the Centers for Disease Control and Prevention.

within the first few days of illness, but usually peak at 7 days following onset of illness, and remain elevated for several weeks to months.[40]

Persons in the United States are considered to have presumptive immunity to mumps if they (a) have documented evidence of age-appropriate vaccination, (b) have laboratory evidence of immunity, (c) have laboratory confirmation of disease, or (d) were born before 1957.

IMMUNIZATION

An inactivated mumps virus vaccine was developed in 1946 but did not provide lasting protection and was withdrawn.[2] Since then, several mumps vaccine strains have been developed and used in vaccines throughout the world. In 1967, the Jeryl Lynn strain of live attenuated vaccine was licensed and has been the only mumps vaccine strain used in the United States.[41] In addition to the Jeryl Lynn strain, the RIT 4385 strain, the Leningrad-3 strain, and the Leningrad-Zagreb strain are the most widely used. Two strains, Rubini and Urabe AM 9, were widely distributed globally but are no longer available. The immunogenicity, efficacy, and adverse events associated with different vaccine strains can vary substantially.

The World Health Organization (WHO) reports that 122 member countries include mumps in their routine vaccination program.[42] Most countries that include mumps vaccine as part of their routine immunization program recommend two doses of mumps vaccine for children. The trivalent measles, mumps, and rubella (MMR) vaccine formulation is the most commonly used formulation for the mumps vaccine. In the United States, the first dose of MMR vaccine (or measles, mumps, rubella and varicella vaccine) is recommended at 12–15 months of age and the second dose at 4–6 years. Two doses of MMR vaccine are recommended for school-aged children, students in high-school and educational facilities, healthcare workers born in and after 1957, and international travellers.[43]

Vaccination provides persistent antibodies against mumps. Currently available mumps vaccines induce seroconversion in more than 90% of vaccine recipients, but mumps antibodies decline overtime.[44] The protective efficacy of vaccines in controlled clinical trials with short duration of follow-up (up to 20 months) was observed to be approximately 95%,[45–47] Vaccine effectiveness of mumps vaccines in field studies has been lower. The median vaccine effectiveness is estimated to be 80% (range: 49–92%) for one dose and 88% (range: 32–95%) for two doses of Jeryl Lynn mumps vaccine.[3,9,44] The level of mumps antibodies that would indicate a person is protected against mumps remains unknown.

For the Jeryl Lynn strain vaccine, the most common adverse reactions to vaccination are parotitis and low-grade fever; parotitis occurs in < 1% of vaccine recipients.[43] For all mumps vaccines, postvaccine aseptic meningitis does occur, but is rare, generally mild to moderate, and resolves within a week. The rates of reported aseptic meningitis after mumps vaccination were the lowest with the Jeryl Lynn strain (<1 per 100,000 doses).[44]

Postexposure MMR vaccination does not prevent or alter the clinical severity of mumps. However, vaccination of persons who were exposed may protect against subsequent infection in the event that the intial exposure did not cause infection. The vaccine does not increase the severity of disease when administered following exposure. Passive immunization with either immune globulin or mumps immune globulin has not been shown to be effective for postexposure prophylaxis or for the prevention of complications. Maternal antibody crosses the placenta and provides protection to infants against clinical mumps.[44]

Contraindications to MMR vaccination include pregnancy, history of anaphylactic reactions to neomycin, history of severe allergic reaction to any component of the vaccine, and immunosuppression. Persons with human immunodeficiency virus (HIV) infection who are not severely immunosuppressed may receive MMR vaccine.[43]

OUTBREAK CONTROL

While mumps is usually a mild illness, mumps outbreaks cause major disruption to the community where they occur, as well as a notable burden on public health resources. Despite being a vaccine preventable disease, mumps outbreak response can be challenging since mumps can occur in fully vaccinated individuals, has a long incubation period, aspymtomatic persons may transmit the virus, and there is no postexposure prophylaxis to prevent disease in those already exposed and infected.

Standard mumps outbreak response measures include isolation of patients during their infectious period (until 5 days after parotitis onset), educating people in the outbreak setting on mumps symptoms and transmission, and catch-up vaccination or vaccination of persons at increased risk for mumps.[9] Public health officials may also exclude people who do not have presumptive immunity[*] from the outbreak setting.[9]

During mumps outbreaks in populations with high two-MMR dose coverage, a third dose of MMR vaccine is recommended for groups of people who public health authorities determine are at increased risk for acquiring mumps.[3] People in the group at increased risk who have unknown vaccination status, one dose of MMR vaccine, or have other evidence of presumptive immunity may also be recommended to receive a dose of MMR vaccine. In three studies, incremental vaccine effectiveness of the third versus the second MMR dose has been shown to range from 61% to 88%; one estimate was statistically significant (78%, 95% confidence interval = 61–88%).[48–50] The duration of protection from a third dose of MMR vaccine is unknown; immunological studies have shown the increase in antibodies following receipt of a third dose might not persist longer than 1 year after vaccination.[51] For this, a third dose of MMR vaccine is recommended only for individual protection during outbreaks and not for routine vaccination.

OCCURRENCE

Mumps occurs worldwide. Since mumps is not a reportable disease in most countries, global mumps incidence is unknown. Countries that report mumps cases to the World Health Organization reported an average of ~ 500,000 mumps cases annually since 1999.[8] In countries that do not have routine mumps vaccination, mumps epidemics typically occur every 2–5 years[52] and most infections occur during childhood. In the United States, prior to the introduction of vaccine, mumps was a universal childhood disease, with most children affected by age 14 years.[43] During this time, mumps accounted for approximately 10% of reported aseptic meningitis cases[53] and 36% of reported encephalitis cases.[54] Mumps continues to be a significant cause of hearing impairment in regions with low vaccination coverage.[55]

Following vaccine introduction in 1967 in the United States, the annual number of mumps cases reported decreased from more than 100,000 cases to less than 300 cases during 2001–04, a reduction of greater than 99% (Fig. 93-1).[17]

In 2006, the first large postvaccine era mumps epidemic occurred among college-age adults in the United States.[56] Mumps epidemics subsequently occurred in 2009–10[49,57] and 2016–17.[3] While most cases during these epidemics occurred among college students or close-knit communities, such as the Orthodox Jewish community in New York[14] or the Marshallese community in Arkansas,[58] outbreaks in 2016–17 varied widely in size and included many different settings. From January 2016 to June 2017, U.S. health departments reported 150 outbreaks (9200 cases) that occurred in universities, schools, athletics teams and facilities, church groups, workplaces, large parties or events, households, among other settings, with a median outbreak size of 10 cases (IQR: 4–26 cases).[3] Over 70% of cases in these outbreaks had received two doses of MMR vaccine before developing mumps.

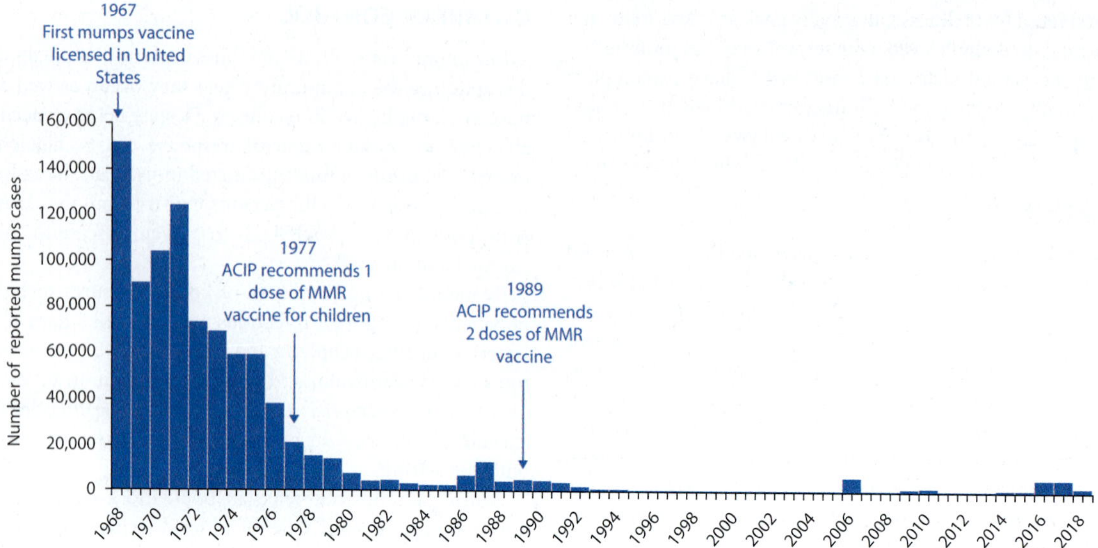

FIGURE 93-1. Reported mumps cases—United States, 1968–2018. ACIP, Advisory Committee on Immunization Practices; MMR, measles, mumps, rubella. (*Source:* Adapted from National Notifiable Diseases Surveillance System.)

The reemergence of mumps among highly vaccinated populations is believed to be due to waning immunity overtime, absence of natural boosting from exposure to wild-type virus during periods of low disease incidence, an average two-dose vaccine effectiveness of 88%, introduction of the virus into close contact settings that facilitate transmission, and antigenic differences between circulating wild-type virus strains and the vaccine virus strains.[59–61] Several studies have documented the increased risk of mumps with longer time since last vaccination.[48,62,63] However, waning of immunity does not explain the typically focal distribution of outbreaks, that about a third of recent mumps cases in the United States are ≤ 18 years of age, and that the oldest vaccinated cohorts are not always the most affected. Mumps virus circulating in the United States has predominantly been one genotype (genotype G) since the first resurgence in 2006.[64] All sera from vaccinated children neutralized diverse mumps virus strains; however, significantly lower neutralizing antibody response to genotype G virus strain compared with vaccine virus strain (genotype A)[59,65,66] support that antigenic variation plays a role in reduced vaccine-induced protection against currently circulating mumps virus. While two doses of the current mumps vaccines appears to be sufficient for mumps control in the general population, a new vaccine that has a better and more long lasting response against circulating mumps virus strains may be needed to prevent mumps epidemics.[67]

References

1. Johnson CD, Goodpasture EW. An investigation of the etiology of mumps. *J Exp Med.* 1934;59(1):1–19.
2. Habel K. Preparation of mumps vaccines and immunization of monkeys against experimental mumps infection. *Public Health Rep.* 1946;61(46):1655–64.
3. Marin M, Marlow M, Moore KL, Patel M. Recommendation of the Advisory Committee on Immunization Practices for use of a third dose of mumps virus-containing vaccine in persons at increased risk for mumps during an outbreak. *MMWR Morb Mortal Wkly Rep.* 2018;67(1):33–8.
4. Sane J, Gouma S, Koopmans M, et al. Epidemic of mumps among vaccinated persons, the Netherlands, 2009–2012. *Emerg Infect Dis.* 2014;20(4):643–8.
5. Willocks LJ, Guerendiain D, Austin HI, et al. An outbreak of mumps with genetic strain variation in a highly vaccinated student population in Scotland. *Epidemiol Infect.* 2017;145(15):3219–25.
6. Westphal DW, Eastwood A, Levy A, et al. A protracted mumps outbreak in Western Australia despite high vaccine coverage: A population-based surveillance study. *Lancet Infect Dis.* 2019;19(2):177–84.
7. Vygen S, Fischer A, Meurice L, et al. Waning immunity against mumps in vaccinated young adults, France 2013. *Euro Surveill.* 2016;21(10):30156.
8. World Health Organization. Mumps reported cases. 2018. http://apps.who.int/immunization_monitoring/globalsummary/timeseries/tsincidencemumps.html. Accessed April 16, 2019.
9. Clemmons N, Hickman C, Lee A, Marin M, Patel M. Mumps. In. *CDC Manual for the Surveillance of Vaccine-Preventable Diseases.* Atlanta, GA: US Department of Health and Human Services, CDC; 2018.
10. Philip RN, Reinhard KR, Lackman DB. Observations on a mumps epidemic in a virgin population. *Am J Hyg.* 1959;69(2):91–111.
11. Reed D, Brown G, Merrick R, Sever J, Feltz E. A mumps epidemic on St. George Island, Alaska. *JAMA.* 1967;199(13):113–7.
12. Falk WA, Buchan K, Dow M, et al. The epidemiology of mumps in southern Alberta 1980–1982. *Am J Epidemiol.* 1989;130(4):736–49.
13. Yung CF, Andrews N, Bukasa A, Brown KE, Ramsay M. Mumps complications and effects of mumps vaccination, England and Wales, 2002–2006. *Emerg Infect Dis.* 2011;17(4):661–7;quiz 766.
14. Barskey AE, Schulte C, Rosen JB, et al. Mumps outbreak in Orthodox Jewish communities in the United States. *N Engl J Med.* 2012;367(18):1704–13.
15. Zamir CS, Schroeder H, Shoob H, Abramson N, Zentner G. Characteristics of a large mumps outbreak: Clinical severity, complications and association with vaccination status of mumps outbreak cases. *Hum Vaccin Immunother.* 2015;11(6):1413–7.
16. Orlikova H, Maly M, Lexova P, et al. Protective effect of vaccination against mumps complications, Czech Republic, 2007–2012. *BMC Public Health.* 2016;16(1):293.
17. Gouma S, Hahne SJ, Gijselaar DB, Koopmans MP, van Binnendijk RS. Severity of mumps disease is related to MMR vaccination status and viral shedding. *Vaccine.* 2016;34(16):1868–73.
18. Havlickova M, Limberkova R, Smiskova D, et al. Mumps in the Czech Republic in 2013: Clinical characteristics, mumps virus genotyping, and epidemiological links. *Cent Eur J Public Health.* 2016;24(1):22–8.
19. Ma R, Lu L, Zhou T, Pan J, Chen M, Pang X. Mumps disease in Beijing in the era of two-dose vaccination policy, 2005–2016. *Vaccine.* 2018;36(19):2589–95.
20. Biedel CW. Recurrent mumps parotitis following natural infection and immunization. *Am J Dis Child.* 1978;132(7):678–80.
21. Crowley B, Afzal MA. Mumps virus reinfection—Clinical findings and serological vagaries. *Commun Dis Public Health.* 2002;5(4):311–3.
22. Yoshida N, Fujino M, Miyata A, et al. Mumps virus reinfection is not a rare event confirmed by reverse transcription loop-mediated isothermal amplification. *J Med Virol.* 2008;80(3):517–23.
23. Terada K, Hagihara K, Oishi T, et al. Cellular and humoral immunity after vaccination or natural infection of mumps. *Pediatr Int.* 2017;59(8):885–90.
24. Gut JP, Lablache C, Behr S, Kirn A. Symptomatic mumps virus reinfections. *J Med Virol.* 1995;45(1):17–23.
25. Masarani M, Wazait H, Dinneen M. Mumps orchitis. *J R Soc Med.* 2006;99(11):573–5.

26. Rubin S, Eckhaus M, Rennick LJ, Bamford CG, Duprex WP. Molecular biology, pathogenesis and pathology of mumps virus. *J Pathol.* 2015;235(2): 242–52.
27. Dayan GH, Quinlisk MP, Parker AA, et al. Recent resurgence of mumps in the United States. *N Engl J Med.* 2008;358(15):1580–9.
28. Donahue M, Schneider A, Ukegbu U, et al. Notes from the field: Complications of mumps during a university outbreak among students who had received 2 doses of measles-mumps-rubella vaccine—Iowa, July 2015–May 2016. *MMWR Morb Mortal Wkly Rep.* 2017;66(14):390–1.
29. Vuori M, Lahikainen EA, Peltonen T. Perceptive deafness in connection with mumps. A study of 298 servicemen suffering from mumps. *Acta Otolaryngol.* 1962;55:231–6.
30. Everberg G. Deafness following mumps. *Acta Otolaryngol.* 1957;48(5–6): 397–403.
31. Takla A, Bohmer MM, Klinc C, et al. Outbreak-related mumps vaccine effectiveness among a cohort of children and of young adults in Germany 2011. *Hum Vaccin Immunother.* 2014;10(1):140–5.
32. Takla A, Wichmann O, Klinc C, Hautmann W, Rieck T, Koch J. Mumps epidemiology in Germany 2007–11. *Euro Surveill.* 2013;18(33):20557.
33. Siegel M. Congenital malformations following chickenpox, measles, mumps, and hepatitis. Results of a cohort study. *JAMA.* 1973;226(13): 1521–4.
34. Siegel M, Fuerst HT, Peress NS. Comparative fetal mortality in maternal virus diseases. A prospective study on rubella, measles, mumps, chicken pox and hepatitis. *N Engl J Med.* 1966;274(14):768–71.
35. Centers for Disease Control and Prevention. Updated recommendations for isolation of persons with mumps. *MMWR Morb Mortal Wkly Rep.* 2008;57(40):1103–5.
36. Ennis FA, Jackson D. Isolation of virus during the incubation period of mumps infection. *J Pediatr.* 1968;72(4):536–7.
37. Nunn A, Masud S, Krajden M, Naus M, Jassem AN. Diagnostic yield of laboratory methods and value of viral genotyping during an outbreak of mumps in a partially vaccinated population in British Columbia, Canada. *J Clin Microbiol.* 2018;56(5):e01954-17.
38. Utz JP, Szwed CF, Kasel JA. Clinical and laboratory studies of mumps. II. Detection and duration of excretion of virus in urine. *Proc Soc Exp Biol Med.* 1958;99(1):259–61.
39. Jalal H, Bahadur G, Knowles W, Jin L, Brink N. Mumps epididymo-orchitis with prolonged detection of virus in semen and the development of anti-sperm antibodies. *J Med Virol.* 2004;73(1):147–50.
40. Rota JS, Rosen JB, Doll MK, et al. Comparison of the sensitivity of laboratory diagnostic methods from a well-characterized outbreak of mumps in New York city in 2009. *Clin Vaccine Immunol.* 2013;20(3):391–6.
41. Hilleman MR, Buynak EB, Weibel RE, Stokes JJr. Live, attenuated mumps-virus vaccine. *N Engl J Med.* 1968;278(5):227–32.
42. World Health Organization. Immunization coverage. 2018. http://www.who.int/mediacentre/factsheets/fs378/en/. Accessed 29 November 2018.
43. McLean HQ, Fiebelkorn AP, Temte JL, Wallace GS, Centers for Disease Control and Prevention. Prevention of measles, rubella, congenital rubella syndrome, and mumps, 2013: Summary recommendations of the Advisory Committee on Immunization Practices (ACIP). *MMWR Recomm Rep.* 2013;62(RR-04):1–34.
44. McLean HQ, Hickman CJ, Seward JF. *The Immunological Basis for Immunization Series, Module 16: Mumps.* Geneva: World Health Organization; 2010.
45. Hilleman MR, Weibel RE, Buynak EB, Stokes Jr. J, Whitman Jr. JE. Live attenuated mumps-virus vaccine. IV. Protective efficacy as measured in a field evaluation. *N Engl J Med.* 1967;276(5):252–8.
46. Weibel RE, Stokes J Jr., Buynak EB, Whitman JE Jr., Hilleman MR. Live attenuated mumps-virus vaccine. 3. Clinical and serologic aspects in a field evaluation. *N Engl J Med.* 1967;276(5):245–51.
47. Sugg WC, Finger JA, Levine RH, Pagano JS. Field evaluation of live virus mumps vaccine. *J Pediatr.* 1968;72(4):461–6.
48. Cardemil CV, Dahl RM, James L, et al. Effectiveness of a third dose of MMR vaccine for mumps outbreak control. *N Engl J Med.* 2017;377(10):947–56.
49. Nelson GE, Aguon A, Valencia E, et al. Epidemiology of a mumps outbreak in a highly vaccinated island population and use of a third dose of measles-mumps-rubella vaccine for outbreak control—Guam 2009 to 2010. *Pediatr Infect Dis J.* 2013;32(4):374–80.
50. Ogbuanu IU, Kutty PK, Hudson JM, et al. Impact of a third dose of measles-mumps-rubella vaccine on a mumps outbreak. *Pediatrics.* 2012;130(6): e1567–74.
51. Latner DR, Parker Fiebelkorn A, McGrew M, et al. Mumps virus nucleoprotein and hemagglutinin-specific antibody response following a third dose of measles mumps rubella vaccine. *Open Forum Infect Dis.* 2017;4(4):ofx263.
52. Galazka AM, Robertson SE, Kraigher A. Mumps and mumps vaccine: A global review. *Bull World Health Organ.* 1999;77(1):3–14.
53. Litman N, Baum SG. Mumps virus. In: Mandell GL, Bennett JE, Dolin R, eds Mandell GL, Bennett JE, Dolin R, eds. *Mandell, Douglas, and Bennett's Principles and Practice of Infectious Diseases.* Philadelphia, PA: Churchill Livingstone Elsiever; 2010, pp. 2201–6.
54. Centers for Disease Control. *Mumps Surveillance: January 1972–June 1974.* Atlanta, GA: U.S. Department of Health, Education, and Welfare, Public Health Service; 1974.
55. Olusanya BO, Neumann KJ, Saunders JE. The global burden of disabling hearing impairment: A call to action. *Bull World Health Organ.* 2014;92:367–73.
56. Centers for Disease Control and Prevention. Update: Multistate outbreak of mumps—United States, January 1–May 2, 2006. *MMWR Morb Mortal Wkly Rep.* 2006;55(20):559–63.
57. Centers for Disease Control and Prevention. Update: Mumps outbreak—New York and New Jersey, June 2009–January 2010. *MMWR Morb Mortal Wkly Rep.* 2010;59(5):125–9.
58. Fields VS, Safi H, Waters C, et al. Mumps in a highly vaccinated Marshallese community in Arkansas, USA: An outbreak report. *Lancet Infect Dis.* 2019;19(2):185–92.
59. Rubin SA, Qi L, Audet SA, et al. Antibody induced by immunization with the Jeryl Lynn mumps vaccine strain effectively neutralizes a heterologous wild-type mumps virus associated with a large outbreak. *J Infect Dis.* 2008;198(4):508–15.
60. Gouma S, Vermeire T, Van Gucht S, et al. Differences in antigenic sites and other functional regions between genotype A and G mumps virus surface proteins. *Sci Rep.* 2018;8(1):13337.
61. Vermeire T, Barbezange C, Francart A, et al. Sera from different age cohorts in Belgium show limited cross-neutralization between the mumps vaccine and outbreak strains. *Clin Microbiol Infect.* 2019;25(7):907.e1–6.
62. Cortese MM, Jordan HT, Curns AT, et al. Mumps vaccine performance among university students during a mumps outbreak. *Clin Infect Dis.* 2008;46(8):1172–80.
63. Castilla J, Garcia Cenoz M, Arriazu M, et al. Effectiveness of Jeryl Lynn-containing vaccine in Spanish children. *Vaccine.* 2009;27(15):2089–93.
64. McNall RJ. In:2019.
65. Rubin S, Mauldin J, Chumakov K, Vanderzanden J, Iskow R, Carbone K. Serological and phylogenetic evidence of monotypic immune responses to different mumps virus strains. *Vaccine.* 2006;24(14):2662–8.
66. Hickman C, Mohammed A, Sowers S, et al. Humoral and cellular immune responses to mumps in young adults immunized with MMR vaccine. Paper presented at: Clinical Virology Symposium; May 6–9, 2018; West Palm Beach, FL.
67. Plotkin SA. Mumps: A pain in the neck. *J Pediatr Infect Dis Soc.* 2018;7(2): 91–2.

CHAPTER

94

Rubella

Jennifer K. Knapp • Susan E. Reef

In 1941, an epidemic of congenital cataracts in Australia was observed in the wake of a large outbreak of rubella.[1] Until then, Rubella was considered a mild and self-limited illness. However, it assumed new importance when the association with congenital cataracts demonstrated its ability to induce congenital malformations in infants born to susceptible women who acquired rubella during pregnancy. In the following years, a broad spectrum of congenital malformations associated with congenital infection and Congenital Rubella Syndrome (CRS) were described.[2–4] The subsequent success in developing and licensing an effective vaccine to prevent rubella in 1969 remains a major public health achievement. Until recently, however, the use of rubella-containing vaccine has occurred mainly in developed countries. According to the World Health Organization (WHO) only 99 (51%) countries/territories were using rubella vaccine in their national immunization programs in 2000,[5] but by February 2019, 168 (87%) countries reported using rubella-containing vaccine in their national programs.[6]

ETIOLOGICAL AGENT, IMMUNOLOGY, AND DIAGNOSIS

Rubella disease (also known as German measles or 3-day measles) is caused by an RNA virus of the Togavirus family. This family also includes Eastern and Western Equine Encephalitis viruses. Rubella virus is highly communicable, though less so than measles or varicella viruses, and humans are the only known reservoir. It is transmitted by the respiratory route, and infection usually occurs as a result of droplet spread through nasopharyngeal secretions of infected persons.

Primary rubella infection induces lifelong immunity. Rarely, reinfections with rubella virus have occurred in persons with natural or vaccine-induced immunity, but they are usually asymptomatic and recognized only by serological testing.[7] Reinfections in pregnant women pose minimal risk to the unborn fetus.[7–9]

Clinical diagnosis of rubella disease is unreliable without laboratory confirmation because rubella infection is frequently asymptomatic or presents as a mild illness with a nonspecific rash. A history of exposure to rubella can be helpful in the absence of the full complement of clinical signs and symptoms. Serologic testing is the simplest means of confirming rubella infection. Both antirubella immunoglobulin M (IgM) and immunoglobulin G (IgG) antibodies appear shortly after the onset of rash. IgM antibodies generally do not persist more than 8–12 weeks after rash onset, while IgG antibodies usually persist for the lifetime of the patient. Rubella virus is present in a variety of clinical specimens from infected persons. However, some intrinsic characteristics make detection of rubella virus more challenging than detection of measles virus, which causes a similar febrile rash illness. Rubella infection usually results in a lower-titer viremia, making it more challenging to grow virus in cell culture. Rubella virus has a higher G-C content in its RNA than measles, thus making it more difficult to detect by reverse transcriptase-polymerase chain reaction (RT-PCR).[10]

Approximately 84% of neonates with congenital rubella infection have detectable rubella virus, and virus can be found in most bodily fluids, including pharyngeal secretions, cerebrospinal fluid, tears, and urine.[4] Some infants with congenital rubella infection shed virus for more than a year.[4,11] Antirubella IgM antibodies are present at birth, and more than half of infected infants have detectable antibody at 6 months of age. Because IgM antibody normally does not cross the placenta, the presence of rubella-specific IgM antibody in cord blood is evidence of congenital infection. Paired IgG serology can also be used for diagnosis in infants, particularly after 6 months of age. When rubella-specific IgG titers are sustained or increasing across two specimens obtained a month apart, congenital infection is suggested, since the half-life of maternal antibodies in infants is 1 month.

CLINICAL CHARACTERISTICS

Postnatal Infection. Rubella is an acute, mild disease in children and young adults. The first symptoms occur after an incubation period ranging from 14 to 21 days. Adolescents and adults may exhibit a 1- to 5-day prodrome of low-grade fever, headache, malaise, anorexia, mild conjunctivitis, coryza, sore throat, and lymphadenopathy. These manifestations rapidly subside after the first day of the rash. The contagious period may begin as early as 7 days before onset of rash and may persist up to 7 days after rash onset.

While asymptomatic infections are common (up to 50% of infections occur without rash[12]), the cardinal manifestation of symptomatic infection is a nonspecific maculopapular rash lasting 3 days or less (hence the term "3-day measles"). The rash appears first on the face and then spreads downward rapidly to the neck, arms, trunk, and extremities; it can be pruritic. Associated with the rash is generalized lymphadenopathy, particularly of the postauricular, suboccipital, and posterior cervical lymph nodes. Rashes similar to those observed with rubella infection have been described in *echovirus, coxackievirus, and parvovirus* (fifth disease) infections and with mild measles; however, these infections are not commonly associated with postauricular or suboccipital adenopathy.

COMPLICATIONS OF POSTNATAL INFECTION

Complications of postnatal rubella infections are generally rare in children but are more common among adults. Arthralgia and arthritis are common among women, who have reported rates as high as 70%. Joint involvement usually occurs after the rash fades and typically lasts 5–10 days. Rare complications include optic neuritis, thrombocytopenic purpura, and myocarditis. Postinfectious encephalitis of short duration may occur 1–6 days after the appearance of rash; its incidence rate is estimated at 1 in 1600[13] to 1 in 6000 cases.[14]

Prenatal Infection. Primary rubella infection of a susceptible woman during pregnancy, whether clinical or asymptomatic, carries a significant risk of fetal infection. Fetal infection can result in the greatest morbidity and mortality associated with rubella infection, including spontaneous abortion, stillbirth, or CRS, a constellation of birth defects affecting heart, vision, and/or hearing. The gestational age of the fetus at the time of primary rubella infection of the mother is the main factor determining the risk of adverse consequences of fetal infection. The risk of CRS in the first 10 weeks of pregnancy may be as high as 90%, but the risk decreases sharply after the 11th week and is absent after the 20th week of gestation.[15]

Fetal rubella infection often results in a disseminated and chronic infection that may persist throughout fetal life and for many months after birth. Disrupted organogenesis and hypoplastic organ development lead to the characteristic structural defects of CRS; common manifestations are listed in Box 94-1. Up to 50–70% of infants infected *in utero* may appear normal at birth,[3] but numerous manifestations have delayed detection or onset.[2,16] Among infants born with congenital rubella infection, the most common delayed diagnosis is hearing impairment/deafness; other delayed diagnoses include learning and speech development and behavioral and psychiatric disorders. Autism has been reported to occur at a rate of 7.4%.[2,17] More than 20% of children with CRS also experience late-onset manifestations including endocrinopathies such as diabetes mellitus, thyroiditis with hypothyroidism or hyperthyroidism, and Addison's disease.[16]

Even as rubella infection results in significant morbidity due to CRS, there is also high mortality among CRS cases ranging from 13% to 41%.[4,18–22] Mortality is common among infants with congenital heart defects at 37–38%,[19,22] and particularly among infants with patent ductus arteriosus with pulmonary hypertension at 56%.[22] If these conditions resolve naturally or with treatment then the likelihood of survival also increases. Other manifestations associated with mortality include hepatosplenomegaly (46%)[22] and thrombocytopenic purpura (35%).[4,22]

BOX 94-1 Manifestations of Congenital Rubella Infection

- ***Spontaneous abortions***
- ***Stillbirths***
- ***Bone lesions***
- ***Cardiac defects***
  Patent ductus arteriosus
  Pulmonary stenosis and coarctation
- ***Neurologic***
  Encephalitis
  Mental retardation
  Microcephaly
  Progressive panencephalitis
  Spastic quadriparesis
- ***Hearing impairment (deafness)***
- ***Endocrinopathies***
  Thyroid disorders (hypothyroidism, hyperthyroidism)
  Addison's disease
  Diabetes mellitus
  Precocious puberty
  Growth hormone deficiency
- ***Eye defects***
  Cataracts
  Glaucoma
  Microphthalmos
  Retinopathy
- ***Genitourinary defects***
- ***Hematologic disorders***
  Anemia
  Thrombocytopenia
  Immunodeficiencies
- ***Hepatitis***
- ***Interstitial pneumonitis***
- ***Psychiatric disorders***

RUBELLA VACCINES

In 1969, three live-attenuated rubella vaccines were licensed for use in the United States: the HPV-77 DE-5 strain, prepared in duck embryo cell culture; the HPV-77 DK-12 strain, prepared in dog kidney cell culture; and the Cendehill strain, prepared in rabbit kidney cell culture. In 1979, the RA 27/3 strain, which is prepared in human diploid cells, was licensed as a combination vaccine with measles and mumps combined as MMR, and all previous strains were discontinued. In the United States, rubella vaccine is exclusively administered in a combination MMR vaccine or as MMR with varicella as MMRV. In at least 95% of vaccinees, all four of the rubella vaccine strains induce antibodies that persist for more than 15 years.[23–25] While there is some evidence of waning rubella antibody titers, half-life estimates exceed the average human lifespan,[26] suggesting immunity is durable and lifelong. In countries with robust vaccination programs, outbreaks of rubella have occurred in adolescents[21,27,28] and adults[29,30] but few cases have been observed among persons with documented prior vaccination.

Rubella-specific side effects were characterized in single-antigen vaccine trials. Side effects include low-grade fever, rash, and lymphadenopathy.[31–34] The rubella vaccine currently used in the United States (RA 27/3) also is associated with a 14% (95% confidence interval 13–15%) prevalence of joint pain in adult females.[35] Such side effects are less common than with natural infection, but vaccinated women are still more frequently and more severely affected than either vaccinated men or children. Among vaccinated children, as many as 2% of have reported arthralgia, but reports of arthritis have been rare. In contrast, 8% of susceptible women who were vaccinated have reported acute arthritis.[33,35] These side effects usually do not disrupt daily activities and generally do not persist.

In 1991, the Institute of Medicine (now the National Academy of Medicine) reviewed evidence about persistent or chronic arthropathy as a result of rubella vaccination and concluded: "Evidence is consistent with a causal relation between the currently used rubella vaccine strain (RA 27/3) and chronic arthritis in adult women, although the evidence is limited in scope and confined to reports from one institution."[35] One study then evaluated persistent arthropathy among women with acute arthropathy or arthritis; among the small proportion with acute arthropathy, chronic manifestation was documented in 72% of vaccinees and 75% of the women in the placebo arm, a difference that was not statistically different.[36] Other studies have re-affirmed those findings, suggesting that postvaccination arthropathy is generally rare and is not causally related to administration of RA 27/3 strain rubella vaccines.[37,38]

Transient peripheral neuritis complaints, such as paresthesia and pain in the arms and legs, have also occurred very rarely.[35,36] These rare reactions usually occur only in susceptible vaccinees; persons already immune to rubella by previous vaccination or natural infection are not at increased risk of local or systemic reactions following rubella vaccine receipt.

Although use of rubella vaccine is contraindicated in pregnant women or women planning pregnancy within 4 weeks, the risk of CRS following administration of the vaccine to unknowingly pregnant women has been evaluated. Data were reviewed for 2478 live births to 2931 susceptible women who were inadvertently vaccinated while pregnant or who became pregnant within 3 months of vaccination.[14,39] None of these live-births resulted in an infant with CRS, but 3.3% had congenital rubella infection as detected by IgM. A maximal theoretical risk of CRS estimated at 0.2% could not be ruled out[39]; however, this was substantially less than the more than 20% risk for CRS associated with maternal infection during the first 20 weeks of pregnancy.

Similar to other live-attenuated viral vaccines, reasonable practices for avoiding vaccination of pregnant women should include (a) asking women if they are pregnant, (b) excluding those who say they are pregnant from vaccination, and (c) explaining the theoretical risks to women of childbearing age before vaccinating.

In addition to pregnancy, contraindications for rubella vaccine include immunodeficiency or a compromised immune system resulting from disease or treatment, since there is a theoretical possibility of potentiated vaccine virus replication. Other contraindications to vaccination are recent administration of immune globulin (IG) and severe febrile illness.

IMMUNIZATION STRATEGIES

Since licensure of live attenuated rubella virus vaccines in 1969, efforts to control rubella in the United States have focused on interrupting rubella transmission by vaccinating all preschool and elementary schoolchildren. It was hypothesized that decreased transmission of rubella virus would indirectly protect susceptible pregnant women by decreasing the risk of exposure. This strategy substantially reduced the incidence of both rubella and CRS in the United States. In the mid-1970s, however, it was recognized that there was still susceptibility in persons over 15 years old, who had not been eligible for vaccination as children.[40] Consequently, in 1978, the Advisory Committee on Immunization Practices (ACIP) expanded vaccination recommendations to susceptible postpubertal females and high-risk groups such as military recruits and university students.

An alternate vaccination strategy was implemented in certain other countries to protect females directly and prevent congenital rubella. Immunization was recommended for girls aged 11–14 years and for susceptible adult women of child-bearing age. While fewer congenital infections occurred, there was evidence of continuing susceptibility in unvaccinated women and in men who were neither eligible for vaccination nor naturally exposed, resulting in recurring epidemics among adolescent and young adult men and women.[40,41] Since 2013, vaccination of girls and adolescent women is no longer the primary rubella vaccination strategy in any country; however, there is still a risk of rubella outbreaks among susceptible males in those countries that implemented the alternate strategy.[29]

In the United States, vaccination against rubella is recommended for all susceptible persons 12 months of age and older without a contraindication. Persons should be considered susceptible to rubella unless they have (a) documentation of immunization with rubella virus-containing vaccine at age $\geq$ 12 months, (b) laboratory evidence of immunity, (c) laboratory evidence of disease, or (d) birth before 1957.[9]

Postexposure prophylaxis for rubella with IG has not been shown to reliably prevent infection or viremia but may modify or suppress symptoms.[3,42] Further, infants with CRS have been born to women given IG before or shortly after exposure.[43] Therefore, the routine use of IG for postexposure prophylaxis of rubella in early pregnancy is not recommended unless termination of the pregnancy would not be considered.

OCCURRENCE

In temperate climates, rubella is endemic year-round with a regular seasonal peak during springtime. Before the advent of rubella vaccination, major epidemics of rubella tended to occur in the United States at 6- to 9-year intervals. The last major U.S. epidemic of rubella occurred during 1964–65, and resulted in an estimated 12,500,000 cases of rubella, 20,000 cases of CRS, and 11,250 fetal losses (because of death or therapeutic abortion).

The incidence of rubella in the United States began to decrease in 1969 with the licensure and use of live attenuated rubella vaccines. Initially, vaccines were administered to children from 1 to 12 years of age. By 1977, rubella incidence had diminished across all age groups, including adults, with the greatest decreases among persons less than 15 years of age.[40] During the 1970s and 1980s, there were record low numbers of cases but two outbreaks occurred: the first occurred in 1977–78 among adolescents and young adults who had not been targeted for immunization; the second, in 1989–91, among unvaccinated adults in group settings (e.g., colleges, workplaces, prisons) and in religious communities that did not accept vaccination.[44] The latter outbreak resulted in 66 (56%) of 117 CRS cases reported in the 1990s. In the mid-1990s, a notable change occurred in the distribution of most rubella cases, from non-Hispanic children to Hispanic adults.[45] In 2000, the proportion of rubella case-patients who had been born outside the United States was 77% (404 of 533),[45] indicating that infections were occurring primarily in people who received childhood vaccinations outside the United States and might not have been vaccinated against rubella.

In 2001, endemic rubella virus transmission was interrupted in the United States. Thereafter, cases among the foreign born decreased to 58% (33 of 57) of the sporadic cases that occurred during 2004–11,[46] indicating that infections detected in the United States among unvaccinated persons are now mostly independent of country of birth. However, the proportion of cases where infection was acquired overseas increased to 40%.[46] During 2002–18, a median of seven (range, 1–18) rubella cases were reported annually in the United States, and a median of 1 CRS case was reported per year with a maximum of five in 2017.[47] Since elimination of endemic rubella virus transmission in the United States, 18 CRS cases have been identified. All but one case were clearly the result of importations; the origin of infection was countries in the African Region for nine (50%) cases, the Eastern Mediterranean Region for seven (39%) cases, and the Southeast Asian Region for one (5%) case. Importations continue, but fluctuate with global disease trends and travel patterns.

ABSENCE OF RUBELLA IN THE UNITED STATES

The intent of the United States immunization program has always been to interrupt indigenous rubella virus transmission. In 1989, a goal to eliminated indigenous rubella and CRS was included in the "Healthy People 2000" objectives.[44] Interruption of indigenous transmission is defined as the absence of a continuous domestically acquired chain of transmission of rubella virus for $\geq$ 12 months in any defined geographic area.[45] When interruption has been sustained for 36 months, elimination can then be verified. The United States convened an expert panel in October 2004 to evaluate progress toward the elimination goal. The panel examined data from 1998 to 2004 that showed that fewer than 25 reported rubella cases had occurred annually since 2001(Fig. 94-1), documented vaccination coverage among school-age children was $\geq$ 95%, population immunity was more than 91%, surveillance was sensitive enough to detect outbreaks of two or more cases, and virus genotypes detected in cases in the United States originated in other parts of the world. Based on these available data, panel members concluded unanimously that rubella was no longer endemic in the United States.[45] In 2011, verification of rubella elimination in the World Health Organization (WHO) Region of the Americas required that U.S. data be reviewed again, and the evidence supported the maintenance of elimination of endemic rubella virus transmission in the United States.[46]

WORLDWIDE CONTROL AND ELIMINATION OF RUBELLA

In 1997, all countries in the WHO Region of the Americas adopted an initiative for accelerated rubella control,[48] and in 2003, they set a goal for rubella elimination by 2010 which accelerated rubella

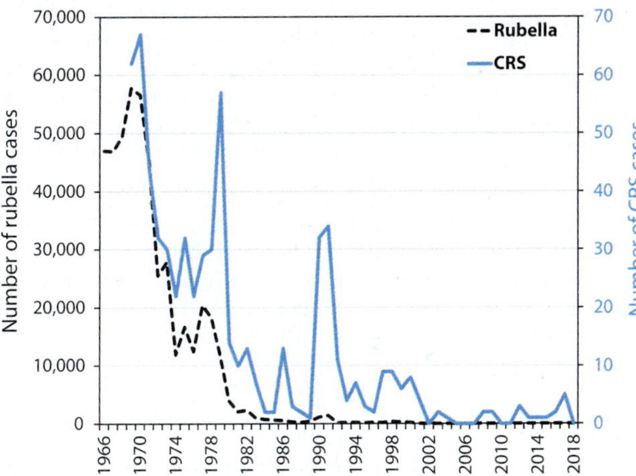

FIGURE 94-1. Reported number of rubella and CRS—United States, 1966–18.* This curve shows the decline in rubella and CRS from 1966 when rubella became reportable. On the X axis is the years and the left Y axis shows the number of rubella cases and the second Y shows the number of CRS cases.*2018 data is provisional.

vaccine introduction and control strategies in these 35 nations/territories.[49] The Americas was verified for rubella elimination in 2015.[50]

Two other WHO regions also have rubella elimination goals while a third has a control goal, but rubella continues to be endemic in many parts of the world. Since only 87% of countries provide routine vaccination against rubella, there is an ongoing risk of virus importation into the United States by people infected in other countries. Vigilance is necessary on three fronts to prevent the re-establishment of endemic rubella virus transmission and the occurrence of CRS in the United States: maintaining high vaccination rates among children; assuring immunity among women of childbearing age, including those women born outside the United States; and continuing to conduct surveillance for both rubella and CRS.

Note: The findings and conclusions in this chapter are those of the authors and do not necessarily represent the views of the Centers for Disease Control and Prevention.

References

1. Gregg NM. Congenital cataract following German measles in the mother. *Trans Ophthalmol Soc Aust.* 1942;3:35–45.
2. Giles JP, Cooper LZ, Krugman S. The rubella syndrome. *J Pediatr.* 1965;66:434–7.
3. Schiff GM, Sutherland JM, Light IJ, Bloom JE. Studies on congenital rubella. Preliminary results on the frequency and significance of presence of rubella virus in the newborn and the effect of gamma-globulin in preventing congenital rubella. *Am J Dis Child.* 1965;110(4):441–3.
4. Cooper LZ, Krugman S. Clinical manifestations of postnatal and congenital rubella. *Arch Ophthalmol.* 1967;77(4):434–9.
5. Grant GB, Reef SE, Patel M, Knapp JK, Dabbagh A. Progress in rubella and congenital rubella syndrome control and elimination—Worldwide, 2000–2016. *MMWR Morb Mortal Wkly Rep.* 2017;66(45):1256–60.
6. World Health Organization: Vaccine introduction slides. [ppt]. 2019. https://www.who.int/immunization/monitoring_surveillance/VaccineIntroStatus.pptx?ua=1. Geneva, 2019.
7. Skendzel LP. Rubella immunity. Defining the level of protective antibody. *Am J Clin Pathol.* 1996;106(2):170–4.
8. Miller E. Rubella reinfection. *Arch Dis Child.* 1990;65(8):820–1.
9. McLean HQ, Fiebelkorn AP, Temte JL, Wallace GS, Centers for Disease Control and Prevention. Prevention of measles, rubella, congenital rubella syndrome, and mumps, 2013: Summary recommendations of the Advisory Committee on Immunization Practices (ACIP). *MMWR Recomm Rep.* 2013;62(RR-04):1–34.
10. Hubschen JM, Bork SM, Brown KE, et al. Challenges of measles and rubella laboratory diagnostic in the era of elimination. *Clin Microbiol Infect.* 2017;23(8):511–5.
11. Sugishita Y, Akiba T, Sumitomo M, et al. Shedding of rubella virus among infants with congenital rubella syndrome born in Tokyo, Japan, 2013–2014. *Jpn J Infect Dis.* 2016;69(5):418–23.
12. Yusof AB, Selvanesan S, Norizah I, et al. Rubella outbreak amongst residential students in a military vocational school of Malaysia. *Med J Malaysia.* 2006;61(3):296–301.
13. Moriuchi H, Yamasaki S, Mori K, Sakai M, Tsuji Y. A rubella epidemic in Sasebo, Japan in 1987, with various complications. *Acta Paediatr Jpn.* 1990;32(1):67–75.
14. Plotkin SA, Reef SE. In: Plotkin SA, Offit PA, Orenstein WA, Edwards KMPlotkin SA, Offit PA, Orenstein WA, Edwards KM, eds. *Rubella Vaccines, in Plotkin's Vaccines,* 7th ed., Philadelphia, PA: Elsevier; 2018, pp. 918–42.
15. Miller E, Cradock-Watson JE, Pollock TM. Consequences of confirmed maternal rubella at successive stages of pregnancy. *Lancet.* 1982;2(8302):781–4.
16. Sever JL, South MA, Shaver KA. Delayed manifestations of congenital rubella. *Rev Infect Dis.* 1985;7(Suppl 1):S164–9.
17. Chess S, Fernandez P, Korn S. Behavioral consequences of congenital rubella. *J Pediatr.* 1978;93(4):699–703.
18. Forrest JM, Burgess M, Donovan T. A resurgence of congenital rubella in Australia? *Commun Dis Intell Q Rep.* 2003;27(4):533–6.
19. Al-Awaidy ST, Allison RD. Early clinical manifestations of congenital rubella syndrome in Oman, 1980–2015. *Int J Vaccines Res.* 2016;3(3):23–30.
20. Motaze NV, Manamela J, Smit S, et al. Congenital rubella syndrome surveillance in South Africa using a sentinel site approach: A cross-sectional study. *Clin Infect Dis.* 2019;68(10):1658–64.
21. Lazar M, Abernathy E, Chen MH, et al. Epidemiological and molecular investigation of a rubella outbreak, Romania, 2011 to 2012. *Euro Surveill.* 2016;21(38):30345.
22. Toizumi M, Motomura H, Vo HM, et al. Mortality associated with pulmonary hypertension in congenital rubella syndrome. *Pediatrics.* 2014;134(2):e519–26.
23. Chu SY, Bernier RH, Stewart JA, et al. Rubella antibody persistence after immunization. Sixteen-year follow-up in the Hawaiian Islands. *JAMA.* 1988;259(21):3133–6.
24. Davidkin I, Peltola H, Leinikki P, Valle M. Duration of rubella immunity induced by two-dose measles, mumps and rubella (MMR) vaccination. A 15-year follow-up in Finland. *Vaccine.* 2000;18(27):3106–12.
25. Just M, Just V, Berger R, Burkhardt F, Schilt U. Duration of immunity after rubella vaccination: A long-term study in Switzerland. *Rev Infect Dis.* 1985;7(Suppl 1):S91–4.
26. Amanna IJ, Carlson NE, Slifka MK. Duration of humoral immunity to common viral and vaccine antigens. *N Engl J Med.* 2007;357(19):1903–15.
27. Hukic M, Hubschen JM, Seremet M, et al. An outbreak of rubella in the Federation of Bosnia and Herzegovina between December 2009 and May 2010 indicates failure to vaccinate during wartime (1992–1995). *Epidemiol Infect.* 2012;140(3):447–53.
28. Chang C, Ma H, Liang W, et al. Rubella outbreak and outbreak management in a school setting, China, 2014. *Hum Vaccin Immunother.* 2017;13(4):772–5.
29. Sugishita Y, Shimatani N, Katow S, Takahashi T, Hori N. Epidemiological characteristics of rubella and congenital rubella syndrome in the 2012–2013 epidemics in Tokyo, Japan. *Jpn J Infect Dis.* 2015;68(2):159–65.
30. D'Agaro P, Dal Molin G, Zamparo E, et al. Epidemiological and molecular assessment of a rubella outbreak in North-Eastern Italy. *J Med Virol.* 2010;82(11):1976–82.
31. Kehrer AF, Isacson P. A comparative field evaluation of three live, attenuated rubella virus vaccines. *Am J Public Health.* 1971;61(1):152–6.
32. Lipman RP, Bethel MB, Wooten JH, Levine RH, Pagano JS. Attenuated rubella vaccine (HPV-77): Evaluation in a large controlled trial. *Am J Public Health.* 1971;61(7):1392–402.
33. Weibel RE, Stokes Jr. J, Buynak EB, Hilleman MR. Influence of age on clinical response to HPV-77 duck rubella vaccine. *JAMA.* 1972;222(7):805–7.
34. Balfour Jr. HH, Balfour CL, Edelman CK, Rierson PA. Evaluation of Wistar RA27/3 rubella virus vaccine in children. *Am J Dis Child.* 1976;130(10):1089–91.
35 Institute of Medicine (US) Committee to Review the Adverse Consequences of Pertussis and Rubella Vaccines. In: Howson CP, Howe CJ, Fineberg HVHowson CP, Howe CJ, Fineberg HV, eds. *Adverse Effects of Pertussis and Rubella Vaccines: A Report of the Committee to Review the Adverse Consequences of Pertussis and Rubella Vaccines.* Washington, DC: National Academies Press; 1991, pp. 187–205.

36. Tingle AJ, Mitchell LA, Grace M, et al. Randomised double-blind placebo-controlled study on adverse effects of rubella immunisation in seronegative women. *Lancet*. 1997;349(9061):1277–81.
37. Slater PE, Ben-Zvi T, Fogel A, Ehrenfeld M, Ever-Hadani S. Absence of an association between rubella vaccination and arthritis in underimmune postpartum women. *Vaccine*. 1995;13(16):1529–32.
38. Ray P, Black S, Shinefield H, et al. Risk of chronic arthropathy among women after rubella vaccination. *JAMA*. 1997;278(7):551–6.
39. Castillo-Solorzano C, Reef SE, Morice A, et al. Rubella vaccination of unknowingly pregnant women during mass campaigns for rubella and congenital rubella syndrome elimination, the Americas 2001–2008. *J Infect Dis*. 2011;204(Suppl 2):S713–7.
40. Hinman AR, Bart KJ, Orenstein WA, Preblud SR. Rational strategy for rubella vaccination. *Lancet*. 1983;1(8314–5):39–40.
41. Vyse AJ, Gay NJ, White JM, et al. Evolution of surveillance of measles, mumps, and rubella in England and Wales: Providing the platform for evidence-based vaccination policy. *Epidemiol Rev*. 2002;24(2):125–36.
42. Young MK, Cripps AW, Nimmo GR, van Driel ML. Post-exposure passive immunisation for preventing rubella and congenital rubella syndrome. *Cochrane Database Syst Rev*. 2015;(9):CD010586.
43. Butler NR, Dudgeon JA, Hayes K, Peckham CS, Wybar K. Persistence of rubella antibody with and without embryopathy. A follow-up study of children exposed to maternal rubella. *Br Med J*. 1965;2(5469):1027–9.
44. Reef SE, Cochi SL. The evidence for the elimination of rubella and congenital rubella syndrome in the United States: A public health achievement. *Clin Infect Dis*. 2006;43(Suppl 3):S123–5.
45. Reef SE, Redd SB, Abernathy E, Zimmerman L, Icenogle JP. The epidemiological profile of rubella and congenital rubella syndrome in the United States, 1998–2004: The evidence for absence of endemic transmission. *Clin Infect Dis*. 2006;43(Suppl 3):S126–32.
46. Papania MJ, Wallace GS, Rota PA, et al. Elimination of endemic measles, rubella, and congenital rubella syndrome from the Western hemisphere: The US experience. *JAMA Pediatr*. 2014;168(2):148–55.
47. CDC Division of Health Informatics and Surveillance: National Notifiable Diseases Surveillance System, 2016–2017 annual tables of infectious disease data. https://wonder.cdc.gov/nndss/nndss_annual_tables_menu.asp. Atlanta, GA, 2018. Accessed March 18, 2019.
48. Hinman AR, Hersh BS, de Quadros CA. Rational use of rubella vaccine for prevention of congenital rubella syndrome in the Americas. *Rev Panam Salud Publica*. 1998;4(3):156–60.
49. New goal for vaccination programs in the Region of the Americas: To eliminate rubella and congenital rubella syndrome. 2003. *Rev Panam Salud Publica*. 2003;14(5):359–63.
50. Kirby T. Rubella is eliminated from the Americas. *Lancet Infect Dis*. 2015;15(7):768–9.

CHAPTER

95 Diphtheria*

Anna M. Acosta • Tejpratap S. P. Tiwari

At the beginning of the twentieth century, respiratory diphtheria was a major cause of childhood disease and death worldwide, but widespread use of safe and efficacious diphtheria toxoid-containing vaccines (DTCV) in industrialized nations starting in the 1940s reduced disease incidence significantly by the 1980s. However, diphtheria re-emerged as a public health threat in the 1990s, when a massive diphtheria epidemic occurred in the newly independent states of the former Soviet Union, with over 157,000 cases and 5000 deaths reported.[1] Since 2010, multiple large diphtheria outbreaks been reported globally, including in Indonesia,[2] Laos,[3] Thailand,[4] Haiti,[5] Venezuela,[5] South Africa,[6] India,[7] Bangladesh,[8] and Yemen.[9] Recent outbreaks illustrate the potential for this vaccine-preventable disease to spread following decades of successful control, particularly in countries with economic decline and civil unrest, population displacement, and collapse of public health infrastructure accompanied by decreased delivery of childhood vaccination programs. In addition to causing outbreaks, diphtheria is endemic in under- and unvaccinated populations and in countries where childhood DTCV coverage is persistently below 80%.[10,11] Maintaining high levels of vaccination in both children and adults is critical to provide both individual protection and population immunity.

ETIOLOGICAL AGENT, TRANSMISSION, PATHOGENESIS, AND DIAGNOSIS

Diphtheria is a potentially life-threatening disease caused by toxin-producing strains of *Corynebacterium diphtheriae*. The organism is a gram-positive, nonmotile, nonencapsulated, nonsporulating rod-shaped bacillus that was first described as the etiologic agent of diphtheria in 1884. Some *C. diphtheria* strains can produce diphtheria toxin, a very potent exotoxin; strains becomes toxigenic when lysogenized by beta-(β) corynebacteriophages that harbor *tox*, the structural gene for diphtheria toxin.[12] There are four biotypes of *C. diphtheria*: gravis, mitis, intermedius, and belfanti. All *C. diphtheria* biotypes can become toxigenic and cause disease with similar pathogenicity and severity. In addition, two other zoonotic *Corynebacterium* species, *C. ulcerans* and *C. pseudotuberculosis*, can be lysogenized by β-corynebacteriophages and cause toxin-mediated illness in humans with a similar clinical presentation to that of toxigenic *C. diphtheriae*.[13,14] Although possible, person-to-person transmission of these two zoonotic species has not been established.[14,15]

The reservoir for *C. diphtheriae* is humans, although toxigenic organisms have been occasionally recovered from other animals, including infected horses and dogs.[16–18] Transmission of *C. diphtheriae* generally occurs by droplet spread from respiratory sites of either infected persons or carriers. Transmission can also occur through direct contact with discharge from infected skin lesions. Environmental contamination with *C. diphtheriae* has been documented; however, transmission via contaminated fomites is presumed to be rare.[19,20]

The most common anatomic sites for infection are the mucosal lining of the respiratory tract (i.e., nares, nasopharynx, tonsils, or larynx), and the skin. Rarely, other mucosal sites, such as the conjunctiva, ear, and genitalia are affected. In susceptible persons, diphtheria toxin binds to a wide range of cells, blocks protein synthesis, and causes cell damage and cell death, leading to severe tissue inflammation and necrosis. An ensuing fibrinous exudate with trapped necrotic epithelial debris, blood cells, and bacteria rapidly organizes into a thick grayish, leather-like pseudomembrane. As local inflammation worsens and the pseudomembrane expands, diphtheria toxin may be absorbed and disseminated in the blood stream. Diphtheria toxin has a predilection for causing inflammation of cardiac, neural, and renal tissues.

Specific diagnosis of diphtheria depends on the recovery of toxigenic *C. diphtheriae* from specimens obtained from the nares or throat, or from cutaneous or other lesions. Specimens are more likely to be culture-positive if obtained before the patient receives antibiotic treatment. Clinical specimens should be placed in a transport medium (e.g., Amies transport media) and immediately shipped to the testing laboratory. If a long delay is anticipated from specimen collection to laboratory processing and culturing (e.g., when transport from remote locations is required), specimens should be transported in silica gel. Isolation of organisms is enhanced by using selective tellurite-containing medium for culture. Identification of *C. diphtheriae* and its biotypes is made from colony morphology (black colonies with a surrounding halo) and from biochemical tests.[21] The Elek test is an in vitro immunoprecipitation (immunodiffusion) test that confirms toxin production and is considered a confirmatory test.[22] Diphtheria polymerase chain reaction (PCR) tests for *tox*, the gene coding for the A and B fragments of diphtheria toxin.[23,24] Because PCR cannot confirm production of toxin protein, as the Elek test does, it is considered a supplementary test, and is most useful in settings when antibiotic treatment was initiated prior to specimen collection.

Laboratory capacity for diphtheria testing and confirmation varies by country, with many low- and middle-income countries having little or no capacity for culture and PCR testing for *C. diphtheriae*. Certain tests, such as genomic sequencing, PCR assays that can simultaneously determine presence of the diphtheria *tox* gene and distinguish *C. diphtheriae* from *C. ulcerans* and *C. pseudotuberculosis*, or molecular assays that can subtype *C. diphtheriae* strains, can aid in epidemiologic investigations. However, these tools are only available at very few reference or research laboratories.

*The findings and conclusions in this chapter are those of the authors and do not necessarily represent the official position of the Centers for Disease Control and Prevention.

CLINICAL CHARACTERISTICS

After an incubation period of 2–5 days (range 1–10 days), respiratory diphtheria caused by toxigenic strains of *C. diphtheriae* develops insidiously over 1–2 days.[25] Anatomic sites of respiratory diphtheria include the mucous membranes of the nose, pharynx, tonsils, larynx, or trachea, with the pharynx the most common site. Patients with respiratory diphtheria frequently present with sore throat, difficulty swallowing, and low-grade fever. On clinical examination, the throat may show only mild erythema with localized tenacious exudate in the early stage, or a pseudomembrane that initially begins as a localized patch in the posterior pharynx or over the tonsil(s). The pseudomembrane is firmly adherent to the underlying mucosa, and erythema is usually present around the edges. Attempts at removal usually result in profuse bleeding. The pseudomembrane may expand and cover the soft and hard palates and the posterior portion of the pharynx. Palatal paralysis is often present. Patients with severe disease have marked submandibular soft tissue edema in the anterior portion of the neck. Together with accompanying cervical lymphadenopathy, this results in the characteristic "bullneck" appearance.

Laryngeal diphtheria is an uncommon but severe form of respiratory diphtheria.[26] It is usually preceded by pharyngotonsillar disease that later extends into the tracheobronchial tree. Symptoms include hoarseness and a croupy cough that may be clinically indistinguishable from viral croup or epiglottitis. Nasal diphtheria generally is the mildest, but very contagious form of respiratory diphtheria and typically presents as a cold-like illness with accompanying blood-tinged discharge.[26] The pseudomembrane is usually localized on the nasal septum or turbinates of one side of the nose and may occasionally extend into the pharynx.

Cutaneous infection with toxigenic *C. diphtheriae* is more common in tropical areas, where diphtheritic cutaneous infections may occur in association with poor hygiene.[27,28] Cutaneous infections can be primary or secondary. Primary infection is uncommon, presenting as a small nodule that breaks down to form an ulcer with a base covered by a dirty-looking pseudomembrane, surrounded by an erythematous margin. Secondary *C. diphtheriae* infection occurs as a coinfection with other bacteria, typically in preexisting skin ulcers or sores from insect bites. The lesions can sometimes be confused with impetigo, or eczema. Cutaneous diphtheria infection rarely progresses to systemic disease.

Occasionally, pharyngitis caused by other infectious agents (e.g., group A *Streptococcus*, Ebstein Bar vrus, Arcanobacter, adenoviruses, herpes simplex viruses, *Candida albicans*) and noninfectious exposures (e.g., prolonged steroid use, chemotherapy) can present with pseudomembranes or exudate, resembling *C. diphtheriae* infection.

Disease caused by nontoxigenic strains of *C. diphtheriae* is being increasingly recognized. Manifestations of infection can range from mild to moderate respiratory disease, cutaneous infection, septic arthritis, and systemic disease, including endocarditis and bacteremia.[29–33]

COMPLICATIONS

Major causes of diphtheria-associated death include airway obstruction by the pseudomembrane and toxin-mediated myocarditis. Airway obstruction can result from direct extension or sudden detachment and aspiration of the pseudomembrane into the larynx and the bronchial tree, or external compression of the airway by neck swelling. Diphtheria toxin may be absorbed into the blood stream and preferentially affects the heart, nerves, and kidneys. Myocarditis usually begins in the second through the sixth week of clinical illness.[34,35] Earlier onset (i.e., during the first week of illness) is associated with higher mortality, and cardiac abnormalities can persist as long-term sequelae.[35] Cranial or peripheral polyneuropathy, primarily involving motor loss, usually develops 1–8 weeks or longer after disease onset.[36] However, paralysis of the soft palate can be present at disease onset. Loss of visual accommodation, diplopia, nasal-sounding voice, and difficulty in swallowing are the most frequent manifestations of cranial nerve involvement.[37,38] Complete recovery of neurologic impairment is the rule in patients who survive. Other complications include renal failure, thrombocytopenia, disseminated intravascular coagulation and shock, and death. Although data are limited, diphtheria case fatality in the prevaccine era is thought to have been substantial. A 2015 study of a diphtheria outbreak in South Africa reported 27% case fatality, even with diphtheria antitoxin treatment.[6]

OCCURRENCE

Occurrence of diphtheria in the United States has fallen dramatically, from 147,000 cases in 1920 to an annual average of < 1 reported cases from 1996 through 2018 (CDC, unpublished data). Fourteen cases were reported in the United States from 1996 through 2018; there was one associated death, and greater than 85% (12/14) of cases were among persons aged 15 years or older. Although diphtheria has been nearly eliminated in the United States and other countries with high vaccination coverage, it remains endemic in some areas and large outbreaks continue to occur.

From 1990 to 1998, more than 157,000 diphtheria cases and 5000 associated deaths, primarily among adults, were reported in the Newly Independent States (NIS) of the former Soviet Union.[1] Increased susceptibility in the adult population, likely due to low booster vaccine coverage and decreased natural exposure to disease, was a major factor in the diphtheria epidemic in the NIS, where diphtheria incidence had been reduced to very low levels since the early 1960s.[10] Other contributory factors for the resurgence included decreased childhood immunization rates due to vaccine hesitancy among the general population and physicians, increased population movement, vaccine shortages, and socioeconomic hardships.[10] Effective control of the NIS epidemic was accomplished by organizing mass DTCV vaccination campaigns to raise childhood and adult DTCV vaccination coverage.[1]

In low- and middle-income countries (LMIC), a steady decrease in diphtheria occurred after the establishment of the World Health Organization (WHO) Expanded Programme on Immunization in 1974. Global childhood vaccination coverage rates with three doses of DTCV increased from 20% in 1980 to 86% in 2018.[39] Correspondingly, global diphtheria cases reported to WHO declined by >80%, from ~ 97,200 cases in 1980 to ~ 16,600 in 2018.[39] However, diphtheria has recently re-emerged in countries with persistently low infant DTCV vaccination coverage, DTCV vaccine shortage, prolonged civil unrest and breakdown in public health infrastructure, and with population displacement. Between 2010 and 2018, large laboratory-confirmed outbreaks occurred in Haiti, Venezuela, Indonesia, Laos, Thailand, South Africa, Yemen, and camps for Forcibly Displaced Myanmar Nationals in Bangladesh. From 2011 to 2016, countries of the South East Asia regions of WHO contributed from 56% to 99% of all cases reported globally.[40]

Prior to the introduction of universal immunization programs, diphtheria in LMIC was predominantly reported in very young children. The lower incidence among adults was attributed to immunity acquired through high rates of skin infections with *C. diphtheriae* in early childhood, followed by recurrent boosting of immunity through environmental exposures. Outbreaks of diphtheria that occur in countries with effective childhood immunization programs in place for at least 5–10 years typically show a shift in the affected age groups to older children and young adults.[11] In the absence of natural environmental boosting, routine booster doses are needed to maintain protective immunity in these age groups.

TREATMENT

The mainstay of treatment of respiratory diphtheria is antitoxin, which neutralizes free, circulating toxin. Treatment should not be delayed pending laboratory confirmation, as increasing delay between onset of illness and treatment correlate with higher rates of complications and death.[41] The dose of antitoxin ranges between 20,000 and 100,000 units and depends on the interval since onset of the illness, site of infection, and severity of disease. All commercially available diphtheria antitoxin products are produced from serum obtained from hyperimmunized horses. Equine antitoxin can produce severe reactions and rarely fatal anaphylaxis in previously sensitized individuals; sensitivity testing prior to administering diphtheria antitoxin is recommended.

Currently, there is a global shortage of diphtheria antitoxin due to reduced manufacturing of the product.[42] In the United States, no licensed diphtheria antitoxin product is available. However, diphtheria antitoxin product can be made available on a case-by-case basis through the Centers for Disease Control and Prevention (CDC) under a Food and Drug Administration (FDA)-approved Investigational New Drug protocol to treat suspected diphtheria cases.[43] Alternatives to equine diphtheria antitoxin for diphtheria treatment, such as diphtheria monoclonal antibodies, are currently being clinically evaluated.[44]

In addition to diphtheria antitoxin treatment, a 2-week course of penicillin or erythromycin is used to eliminate the organism and prevent transmission.[25] Though some countries have used azithromycin in recent outbreaks, this drug and other macrolides have not been clinically validated in studies. As disease may not confer immune protection, patients should receive a primary series of DTCV if previously unvaccinated, or booster doses if not up to date.

MANAGEMENT OF CLOSE CONTACTS OF PATIENTS WITH SUSPECTED DISEASE

Paired nasal and throat swabs for diphtheria culture should be obtained from all close contacts, including household contacts, and sent to the laboratory for testing as early as possible. After specimen collection, prophylactic antibiotic therapy with a 7- to 10-day course of oral erythromycin (40–50 mg/kg, maximum 2 g/day) is recommended for all persons exposed to diphtheria, regardless of vaccination status.[25] If follow-up or compliance with an oral antibiotic cannot be assured, a single dose of intramuscular benzathine penicillin (600,000 units for persons less than 6 years old and 1.2 million units for persons 6 years and older) can be given instead. A booster dose with an age-appropriate DTCV should be given if more than 5 years have elapsed since completion of a five-dose childhood series or since the last booster dose. A primary immunization series with an age-appropriate DTCV should be started in previously unvaccinated contacts.

PREVENTION AND CONTROL

Vaccination is highly protective against diphtheria. In 1918, New York City initiated an immunization program for children using a mixture of antitoxin and toxin and the results provided the first large-scale demonstration that such a program could decrease diphtheria incidence and mortality. In 1923, Ramon demonstrated the safety and immunogenicity of diphtheria toxoid (formalin-inactivated diphtheria toxin). Subsequent improvement in efficacy with alum-precipitated diphtheria toxoid was demonstrated by 1931.

Vaccination provides individual protection against diphtheria by inducing circulating antibodies to diphtheria toxin, which limit the extent of local invasion of the organism and neutralize unbound absorbed toxin. A three-dose series of DTCV is highly immunogenic in all age groups and significantly reduces both the risk of diphtheria and the severity of the illness.[40] While vaccination with DTCV does not prevent colonization or infection with either nontoxigenic or toxigenic organisms, $\geq$ 80% population coverage with DTCV appears to have decreased diphtheria transmission in the United States and in other countries. Because vaccine-induced antibody levels wane over time in the absence of the natural environmental boosting that is present with ongoing low-level disease circulation, booster doses of diphtheria toxoid are required to maintain protective immunity. Duration of immunity is at least 10 years from the last booster dose, but depends on multiple factors, including vaccine schedule and antigenic content of the primary vaccine series.

For children below 7 years of age, diphtheria toxoid is available in combination with tetanus toxoid and pertussis vaccine (whole cell or acellular), or as a diphtheria toxoid and tetanus toxoid only combination vaccine (DT); the antigenic content of these preparations ranges from 6.7 to 15 limit of flocculation (Lf) units. Because the frequency and severity of local reactions increase with increasing age, a diphtheria toxoid and tetanus toxoid combination vaccine (Td) with lower diphtheria toxoid content ($\leq$2) Lf is formulated for use in older children and adults.[45]

For diphtheria prevention, the WHO recommends a three-dose primary series of DTCV, with the first dose administered as early as 6 weeks of age and the third dose completed by 6 months of age if possible, with a minimum interval of 4 weeks between doses. Booster doses with age-appropriate formulations of DTCV are recommended at 12–23 months of age, 4–7 years of age, and 9–15 years of age.[40] Vaccination schedules and strategies vary by country and depend on country immunization service capacity and local epidemiological pattern of diphtheria. While few countries recommend routine boosters for older children and adults, global coverage with a three-dose DTCV primary series exceeded 85% in 2018.[39]

In the United States, the Advisory Committee on Immunization Practices recommends three doses of a diphtheria toxoid, tetanus toxoid, and acellular pertussis (DTaP) vaccine at 4- to 8-week intervals beginning at 2 months of age. A fourth dose is recommended at 15–18 months and may be administered as early as 12 months of age provided that 6 months elapsed since the third dose and that the child is unlikely to return at the recommended age. A fifth dose is administered at 4–6 years of age. An adolescent booster dose with a tetanus toxoid, reduced diphtheria toxoid, and acellular pertussis vaccine (Tdap) is recommended at age 11–12 years.[45] To ensure continued protection against diphtheria, a booster dose of either Td or Tdap should be administered every 10 years throughout life.[46] Unimmunized individuals 7 years of age or older should receive a series of three tetanus toxoid and diphtheria toxoid–containing vaccines, including at least 1 Tdap dose.[46]

CONCLUSION

Routine diphtheria vaccination has been highly successful in reducing the once devastating burden of disease. However, recent large diphtheria outbreaks in the Americas, Southeast Asia, and Africa highlight the importance of maintaining high levels of vaccination coverage in both children and adults, in order to provide both individual protection and population immunity.

References

1. Dittmann S, Wharton M, Vitek C, et al. Successful control of epidemic diphtheria in the states of the Former Union of Soviet Socialist Republics: Lessons learned. *J Infect Dis*. 2000;181 Suppl 1:S10–22.
2. Hughes GJ, Mikhail AF, Husada D, et al. Seroprevalence and determinants of immunity to diphtheria for children living in two districts of contrasting incidence during an outbreak in East Java, Indonesia. *Pediatr Infect Dis J*. 2015;34(11):1152–6.
3. Sein C, Tiwari T, Macneil A, et al. Diphtheria outbreak in Lao People's Democratic Republic, 2012–2013. *Vaccine*. 2016;34(36):4321–6.
4. Wanlapakorn N, Yoocharoen P, Tharmaphornpilas P, Theamboonlers A, Poovorawan Y. Diphtheria outbreak in Thailand, 2012; seroprevalence of diphtheria antibodies among Thai adults and its implications for immunization programs. *Southeast Asian J Trop Med Public Health*. 2014;45(5): 1132–41.
5. Pan American Health Organization and World Health Organization. Epidemiological Update: Diphtheria. 2020. http://www.paho.org/hq/index.php?option=com_docman&task=doc_view&Itemid=270&gid=44497&lang=en. 2020.

6. Mahomed S, Archary M, Mutevedzi P, et al. An isolated outbreak of diphtheria in South Africa, 2015. *Epidemiol Infect*. 2017;145(10):2100–8.
7. Murhekar M. Epidemiology of Diphtheria in India, 1996–2016: Implications for prevention and control. *Am J Trop Med Hyg*. 2017;97(2):313–8.
8. Finger F, Funk S, White K, Siddiqui MR, Edmunds WJ, Kucharski AJ. Real-time analysis of the diphtheria outbreak in forcibly displaced Myanmar nationals in Bangladesh. *BMC Med*. 2019;17(1):58.
9. Dureab F, Al-Sakkaf M, Ismail O, et al. Diphtheria outbreak in Yemen: The impact of conflict on a fragile health system. *Confl Health*. 2019;13:19.
10. Galazka A. Implications of the diphtheria epidemic in the Former Soviet Union for immunization programs. *J Infect Dis*. 2000;181 Suppl 1:S244–8.
11. Galazka A. The changing epidemiology of diphtheria in the vaccine era. *J Infect Dis*. 2000;181 Suppl 1:S2–9.
12. Holmes RK, Barksdale L. Genetic analysis of tox+ and tox- bacteriophages of Corynebacterium diphtheriae. *J Virol*. 1969;3(6):586–98.
13. Peel MM, Palmer GG, Stacpoole AM, Kerr TG. Human lymphadenitis due to Corynebacterium pseudotuberculosis: Report of ten cases from Australia and review. *Clin Infect Dis*. 1997;24(2):185–91.
14. Hacker E, Antunes CA, Mattos-Guaraldi AL, Burkovski A, Tauch A. Corynebacterium ulcerans, an emerging human pathogen. *Future Microbiol*. 2016;11:1191–208.
15. Konrad R, Hormansdorfer S, Sing A. Possible human-to-human transmission of toxigenic Corynebacterium ulcerans. *Clin Microbiol Infect*. 2015; 21(8):768–71.
16. Leggett BA, De Zoysa A, Abbott YE, Leonard N, Markey B, Efstratiou A. Toxigenic Corynebacterium diphtheriae isolated from a wound in a horse. *Vet Rec*. 2010;166(21):656–7.
17. Henricson B, Segarra M, Garvin J, et al. Toxigenic Corynebacterium diphtheriae associated with an equine wound infection. *J Vet Diagn Invest*. 2000;12(3):253–7.
18. Kraszewska A, Anusz Z. [Appearance in domestic animals of Corynebacterium diphtheriae and other Corynebacterium strains pathogenic for man]. *Przegl Epidemiol*. 1979;33(2):269–76.
19. Belsey MA. Isolation of Corynebacterium diphtheriae in the environment of skin carriers. *Am J Epidemiol*. 1970;91(3):294–9.
20. Larsson P, Brinkhoff B, Larsson L. Corynebacterium diphtheriae in the environment of carriers and patients. *J Hosp Infect*. 1987;10(3):282–6.
21. Efstratiou A, Maple PAC. *Manual for the Laboratory Diagnosis of Diphtheria*. Copenhagen: World Health Organization, Expanded Programme on Immunization in the European Region; 1994.
22. Engler KH, Glushkevich T, Mazurova IK, George RC, Efstratiou A. A modified Elek test for detection of toxigenic corynebacteria in the diagnostic laboratory. *J Clin Microbiol*. 1997;35(2):495–8.
23. Nakao H, Popovic T. Development of a direct PCR assay for detection of the diphtheria toxin gene. *J Clin Microbiol*. 1997;35(7):1651–5.
24. Mothershed EA, Cassiday PK, Pierson K, Mayer LW, Popovic T. Development of a real-time fluorescence PCR assay for rapid detection of the diphtheria toxin gene. *J Clin Microbiol*. 2002;40(12):4713–9.
25. AAP Committee on Infectious Diseases. *Red Book (2018): Report of the Committee on Infectious Diseases*. Elk Grove Village, IL: American Academy of Pediatrics; 2018.
26. Hadfield TL, McEvoy P, Polotsky Y, Tzinserling VA, Yakovlev AA. The pathology of diphtheria. *J Infect Dis*. 2000;181 Suppl 1:S116–20.
27. Quick ML, Sutter RW, Kobaidze K, et al. Risk factors for diphtheria: A prospective case-control study in the Republic of Georgia, 1995–1996. *J Infect Dis*. 2000;181 Suppl 1:S121–9.
28. Murakami H, Phuong NM, Thang HV, Chau NV, Giao PN, Tho ND. Endemic diphtheria in Ho Chi Minh City; Viet Nam: A matched case-control study to identify risk factors of incidence. *Vaccine*. 2010;28(51):8141–6.
29. Fricchione MJ, Deyro HJ, Jensen CY, Hoffman JF, Singh K, Logan LK. Non-toxigenic Penicillin and Cephalosporin-resistant Corynebacterium diphtheriae endocarditis in a child: A case report and review of the literature. *J Pediatric Infect Dis Soc*. 2014;3(3):251–4.
30. Muttaiyah S, Best EJ, Freeman JT, Taylor SL, Morris AJ, Roberts SA. Corynebacterium diphtheriae endocarditis: A case series and review of the treatment approach. *Int J Infect Dis*. 2011;15(9):e584–8.
31. Damade R, Pouchot J, Delacroix I, Boussougant Y, Vinceneux P. Septic arthritis due to Corynebacterium diphtheriae. *Clin Infect Dis*. 1993;16(3): 446–7.
32. Dewinter LM, Bernard KA, Romney MG. Human clinical isolates of Corynebacterium diphtheriae and Corynebacterium ulcerans collected in Canada from 1999 to 2003 but not fitting reporting criteria for cases of diphtheria. *J Clin Microbiol*. 2005;43(7):3447–9.
33. Wagner KS, White JM, Neal S, et al. Screening for Corynebacterium diphtheriae and Corynebacterium ulcerans in patients with upper respiratory tract infections 2007–2008: A multicentre European study. *Clin Microbiol Infect*. 2011;17(4):519–25.
34. Boyer NH, Weinstein L. Diphtheritic myocarditis. *N Engl J Med*. 1948;239(24): 913–9.
35. Lumio JT, Groundstroem KW, Melnick OB, Huhtala H, Rakhmanova AG. Electrocardiographic abnormalities in patients with diphtheria: A prospective study. *Am J Med*. 2004;116(2):78–83.
36. Dyck PJTP, McDonald WI, Kocen R. Diphtheritic neuropathy. In: Dyck PJTP, ed. *Peripheral Neuropathy*. Vol. 2. Philadelphia: WB Saunders; 1991, pp 1412–7.
37. Piradov MA, Pirogov VN, Popova LM, Avdunina IA. Diphtheritic polyneuropathy: Clinical analysis of severe forms. *Arch Neurol*. 2001;58(9): 1438–42.
38. Prasad PL, Rai PL. Prospective study of diphtheria for neurological complications. *J Pediatr Neurosci*. 2018;13(3):313–6.
39. World Health Organization. WHO vaccine-preventable disease monitoring system, 2019 global summary. 2019. http://www.who.int/immunization/monitoring_surveillance/data/gs_gloprofile.pdf?ua=1. Accessed June 14, 2019.
40. World Health Organization. Diphtheria vaccine: WHO position paper—August 2017. *Wkly Epidemiol Rec*. 2017;31(90):417–36. https://apps.who.int/iris/bitstream/handle/10665/258681/WER9231.pdf?sequence=1. Accessed August 1, 2019.
41. Naiditch MJ, Bower AG. Diphtheria; a study of 1,433 cases observed during a ten-year period at the Los Angeles County Hospital. *Am J Med*. 1954;17(2):229–45.
42. Kupferschmidt K. Life-saving diphtheria drug is running out. *Science*. 2017;355(6321):118–9.
43. Centers for Disease Control and Prevention. Expanded Access Investigational New Drug (IND) Application Protocol: Use of Diphtheria Antitoxin (DAT) for Suspected Diphtheria Cases. 2019. https://www.cdc.gov/diphtheria/downloads/protocol.pdf. 2019.
44. Smith HL, Saia G, Lobikin M, Tiwari T, Cheng SC, Molrine DC. Characterization of serum anti-diphtheria antibody activity following administration of equine anti-toxin for suspected diphtheria. *Hum Vaccin Immunother*. 2017;13(11):2738–41.
45. Liang JL, Tiwari T, Moro P, et al. Prevention of pertussis, tetanus, and diphtheria with vaccines in the United States: Recommendations of the Advisory Committee on Immunization Practices (ACIP). *MMWR Recomm Rep*. 2018;67(2):1–44.
46. Havers FP, Moro PL, Hunter P, Hariri S, Bernstein H. Use of tetanus toxoid, reduced diphtheria toxoid, and acellular pertussis vaccines: Updated recommendations of the Advisory Committee on Immunization Practices—United States, 2019. *MMWR Morb Mortal Wkly Rep*. 2020;69(3):77–83.

CHAPTER

96

Tetanus

Tejpratap S. P. Tiwari • Amy E. Blain

INTRODUCTION

Tetanus is a noncommunicable, toxin-mediated disease caused by *Clostridium tetani,* an organism that is ubiquitous in the environment. The disease is characterized by muscle rigidity and spasms, and medical treatment requires hospitalization and costly intensive care management. The case-fatality rate remains high (>10%), even among patients treated in modern care facilities. In developed countries, the disease has become uncommon following the implementation of universal childhood vaccination programs using safe and effective tetanus toxoid-containing vaccines (TTCVs); however, tetanus remains a public health problem in developing countries.

Etiological Agent, Pathogenesis, and Diagnosis

The causative agent, *C. tetani,* is an anaerobic, gram-positive rod that exists in both vegetative and sporulated forms. The vegetative form of *C. tetani* is sensitive to heat and does not survive in the presence of oxygen. Tetanus spores are ubiquitous in the environment and are found in soil, dust, animal and human feces, and on human skin. Spores can survive in the environment for years and are resistant to dry environments, most household disinfectants, ethanol, phenol, and hydrogen peroxide, and can survive boiling for 20 minutes, but are destroyed by autoclaving at 121°C and 103 kPa (15 psi).[1]

Spores enter the body through skin abrasions or breaches. Tetanus can occur in association with a number of acute and chronic conditions and exposures, including puncture wounds, compound fractures, abrasions, avulsions, burns, crush injuries, animal bites or scratches, surgery, injections, dental and ear infections, chronic skin ulceration, abscesses, gangrene, abortions, childbirth, and infections of the umbilical stump. Puncture and deep wounds, especially those associated with devitalized tissue, are more prone to tetanus infection than superficial abrasions. However, skin breaches may be trivial and not recalled in 7–21% of cases.[1]

After entry into the body, the spores vegetate and multiply under anaerobic conditions such as occur in necrotic tissue, purulent accumulations, and deep puncture wounds. The bacilli produce two known powerful exotoxins—tetanolysin and tetanospasmin. While the role of tetanolysin is not well understood, it may promote tissue necrosis and bacterial proliferation at the injury site. Tetanospasmin is one of the most potent neurotoxins, and the minimum human lethal dose is estimated to be 2.5 ng/kg of body weight.[2] Tetanospasmin travels along nerves toward the central nervous system by retrograde intra-axonal transport, binds to gangliosides at the neuromuscular junction, and proceeds to the ventral horns of the spinal cord or motor horns of the cranial nerves. The toxin blocks the release of neurotransmitter substances such as γ-aminobutyric acid (GABA) and glycine and increases unopposed motor activity that results in spasms or convulsions that are characteristic of generalized tetanus.[3] Similarly, disinhibition of autonomic nerve fibers can cause cardiovascular instability. The toxin does not cross the blood-brain barrier.

The diagnosis of tetanus depends on symptoms and clinical signs rather than laboratory confirmation. Isolation of *C. tetani* from infected wounds is neither sensitive nor specific for tetanus diagnosis. Tetanus bacilli are infrequently recovered from contaminated wounds and may be isolated from persons who do not have the disease. Serum collected before administration of tetanus immune globulin (TIG) can demonstrate susceptibility to the disease if antitetanus antibody levels are below 0.01 IU/mL as measured by an *in vivo* neutralization assay[4]; however, a higher level in the protective range does not rule out the diagnosis. A clinical test, the "spatula test," may be useful for diagnosis. Touching the posterior wall of the pharynx with a soft instrument or spatula causes reflex spasm and clenching of the jaw. This "spatula test" has high specificity (100%) and sensitivity (94%).[5]

Clinical Characteristics

The incubation period for nonneonatal tetanus ranges from 2 days to 21 days or longer, with a median interval of 7 days. Clinical manifestation depends on the quantity of tetanospasmin produced, and severity of symptoms is inversely related to incubation period.[6] The disease is characterized by skeletal muscle spasms, rigidity, and autonomic disorders. Four clinical forms of tetanus are described: generalized, localized, neonatal, and cephalic.

Generalized tetanus, resulting from systemic dissemination of toxin, is the most common form. The earliest sign of tetanus is difficulty in opening of the mouth as a result of spasm of the jaw muscles or trismus, commonly known as "lockjaw." Spasm of the facial muscles leads to a grimacing facial expression or risus sardonicus (sardonic smile) that is characterized by clenching of the jaw, laterally drawn lips and widening of the mouth, raised eyebrows, tight closure of the eyelids, and wrinkling of the forehead. Severe generalized spasm may give rise to a characteristic backward arching of the back known as opisthotonos that is characterized by retraction of the neck muscles, spasm of the erector spinae muscles of the back, thorax, and abdomen, flexion of the elbows and knees, dorsiflexion of the feet, and hyperextension of the toes. External stimuli such as light, sound or movements can aggravate spasms and should be minimized during care. With severe disease, tonic seizure-like activity may also occur. Instability of the autonomic nervous system is a relatively common complication. Spasms may be powerful enough to cause vertebral injury. Recovery from the acute episode of tetanus may require several weeks and can be complicated by conditions associated with generalized debility and poor nutrition, such as pneumonia, embolism, fecal impaction, and decubitus ulcers. In general, the risk of death is related to the quality of supportive care provided, but is higher among infants, the elderly, and unvaccinated persons.[6]

Localized tetanus develops when the toxin diffuses locally to the nerves supplying adjacent muscles. It is an uncommon form of tetanus characterized by stiffness and rigidity around the site of injury due to muscle spasm. Localized tetanus usually resolves without sequelae but can progress to generalized tetanus.

Tetanus neonatorum is a form of generalized tetanus occurring in newborn infants 28 days old or less, but symptoms commonly manifest at 7 days of life (range, 3–14 days). Neonatal tetanus is characterized by increasing irritability and difficulty feeding. Signs of neonatal tetanus are similar to tetanus in older age groups. The World Health Organization (WHO) definition of neonatal tetanus is "an illness occurring in a child who has the normal ability to suck and cry in the first 2 days of life but who loses this ability between days 3 and 28 of life and becomes rigid and has spasms." Case-fatality rates vary, ranging from 10% in modern hospital facilities to 100% in settings without intensive care units.[7]

Cephalic tetanus is a rare manifestation of the disease that is generally associated with localized lesions of the head or face. In contrast to the other forms of tetanus, cephalic tetanus is associated with atonic cranial nerve palsies.

Occurrence

Tetanus is rare in industrialized countries; however, despite the availability of an effective vaccine, the disease continues to be a burden, particularly in developing countries, with over 15,000 cases reported globally in 2018.[8] In the United States, case reporting began in the late 1940s, with an annual incidence of 4 per million population and a case-fatality rate of 91%. Tetanus-associated mortality declined at a relatively constant rate from the mid-1900s to 2000s.[9] By 2017, the average annual incidence declined to 0.1 per million with a case-fatality rate of 6.1%.

A total of 264 cases and 19 deaths from tetanus were reported from 2009 to 2017. Sixty four percent of cases were in persons 20–64 years of age, and 23% cases were in persons 65 years of age or older; the remaining 13% were in persons younger than 20 years, including three cases of neonatal tetanus. All tetanus-related deaths occurred among patients > 55 years of age (CDC, unpublished data). Acute trauma accounted for 72% of 233 United States cases of non-neonatal tetanus between 2001 and 2008. No wound could be recalled in over 9% of cases; 64% of these cases were in people who inject drugs (PWID).[10]

Diabetes and intravenous drug use are independent risk factors for tetanus. From 2009 through 2017, persons with diabetes accounted for 12% of all reported tetanus cases and 26% of all tetanus deaths. PWID accounted for 8% of cases from 2009 through 2017 (CDC, unpublished data).

Immunization status is inversely correlated with risk for disease and mortality from tetanus. Among the 264 cases from 2009 to 2017, complete vaccination status was known for 72 (27%) and only 18 (25%) were in persons who received three or more doses of TTCV (CDC, unpublished data). Tetanus fatalities among patients who have received at least three tetanus toxoid doses are very rare.

Neonatal tetanus occurs during the month following delivery, usually as the result of *C. tetani* infection of the umbilical stump of a child born to a mother who did not possess sufficient antibodies to provide passive protection by transplacental antibody transfer. Contamination of the umbilical stump occurs most often following deliveries not attended by trained personnel, especially when clean birthing surfaces and equipment for cutting the umbilical cord and dressing the cord stump are unavailable. In 1988, WHO estimated 787,000 neonatal tetanus deaths (6.5 per 1000 live births) worldwide. The estimated number of deaths declined by 96% to approximately 30,848 in 2017.[11]

Prevention and Treatment

Because the quantity of toxin sufficient to cause disease is generally insufficient to induce an immune response, tetanus infection does not confer immunity.

Pre-exposure Vaccination. Pre-exposure active immunization with TTCVs offers the best and most efficient method of preventing tetanus.[7] The results of active immunization of U.S. Army personnel during World War II demonstrated the effectiveness of the toxoid. Only 12 cases occurred among 2.73 million wounded or injured personnel (4.4 per million) compared with 70 cases among 0.52 million wounded or injured during World War I (134 per million).[12]

Vaccination-acquired immunity wanes over time. Nationally representative data from 1988 to 1994 showed decreasing tetanus seroprotection (defined as minimum antibody concentration of 0.15 IU/mL) with increasing age.[13] The lower prevalence of seroprotection in older age groups likely reflected a combination of a lower likelihood of having completed a primary series of TTCV (birth before initiation of routine childhood immunization with tetanus toxoid), noncompliance with recommended decennial tetanus toxoid booster doses, and waning immunity with time since last dose. Overall, 17% more men than women had protective levels of antibody to tetanus, likely due to immunization received as part of military service or employment, or in conjunction with wound care.

For protection against tetanus, WHO recommends that an individual receive six doses (three primary plus three booster doses) of TTCV. The three-dose primary series should begin as early as 6 weeks of age. Subsequent doses should be given with a minimum interval of 4 weeks between doses. The three booster doses should preferably be given one each during the second year of life (12–23 months), at 4–7 years, and at 9–15 years of age. Ideally, there should be at least 4 years between booster doses.[7]

In the United States, the Advisory Committee on Immunization Practices recommends three doses of a diphtheria toxoid, tetanus toxoid, and acellular pertussis (DTaP) vaccine at 4- to 8-week intervals beginning at 2 months of age. A fourth dose is recommended at 15–18 months of age but may be administered as early as 12 months of age provided that 6 months have elapsed since the third dose and that the child is unlikely to return at the recommended age. A fifth dose should be administered at 4–6 years of age. An adolescent booster dose with Tdap is recommended at 11–12 years of age and a booster dose with Td is recommended every 10 years thereafter throughout adulthood.[14]

Mild local reactions such as pain, erythema and mild swelling at the injection site are relatively common following receipt of tetanus toxoid. Severe systemic reactions are very rare. In patients with a history of possible anaphylactic reaction to tetanus toxoid, skin testing with appropriately diluted toxoid should be performed before a decision is made to discontinue further tetanus toxoid vaccination.[6,15] Severe local swelling following tetanus toxoid (Arthus reaction) is rare and usually occurs in those who have received multiple doses of tetanus booster and have high preexisting antitoxin levels.[15–17] Neurologic reactions after tetanus toxoid are rare but can occur. In a 1994 review, the U.S. Institute of Medicine (now the National Academy of Medicine) concluded that a causal link exists between tetanus toxoid and brachial plexus neuropathy, but that insufficient evidence exists to assign causality to the observed association between tetanus toxoid and Guillain-Barré syndrome.[18] A subsequent study failed to find an association between tetanus toxoid and Guillain-Barré syndrome.[19]

Treatment

Treatment of tetanus includes appropriate wound care and antimicrobial therapy to help eliminate the organism and thereby prevent further toxin elaboration. Tetanus immunoglobulin (TIG) should also be given, in a single intramuscular dose to neutralize unbound tetanus toxin. Although the optimum therapeutic dose of TIG has not been established, studies suggest that a dose of 500 units is as effective as higher doses ranging from 3000 to 6000 units.[20,21] Treatment to control muscle spasm and autonomic dysfunction is critical. In addition, intensive supportive care and maintaining patent airway are essential to patient survival. Because tetanus disease does not induce immunity to tetanus, all persons with tetanus should complete a primary series or receive a booster dose of a TTCV, as indicated.[14]

Wound Management. The management of wounds includes adequate wound cleaning and debridement and evaluation of immunization status.[14] The need for vaccination with a TTCV (active immunization) with or without TIG (passive immunization) depends on both the condition of the wound and the patient's vaccination history (Table 96-1). Patients with unknown or uncertain previous

TABLE 96-1 GUIDE TO TETANUS PROPHYLAXIS IN ROUTINE WOUND MANAGEMENT[14]

	Clean, Minor Wound		All Other Wounds[a]	
Number of adsorbed tetanus toxoid-containing vaccine doses	DTaP, Tdap, or Td[c]	TIG	DTaP, Tdap or Td[c]	TIG[b]
Unknown or < 3	Yes	No[d]	Yes	Yes
≥3	No	No	No[e]	No

Abbreviations: DTaP = diphtheria and tetanus toxoids and acellular pertussis vaccine; Tdap = tetanus toxoid, reduced diphtheria toxoid, and acellular; pertussis; Td = tetanus and diphtheria toxoids; TIG = tetanus immune globulin.

[a]Such as, but not limited to, wounds contaminated with dirt, feces, soil, and saliva; puncture wounds; avulsions; and wounds resulting from missiles, crushing, burns, and frostbite.

[b]Persons with HIV infection or severe immunodeficiency who have contaminated wounds should also receive TIG, regardless of their history of tetanus immunization.

[c]DTaP is recommended for children aged < 7 years. Tdap is preferred to Td for persons aged ≥ 11 years who have not previously received Tdap. Persons aged ≥ 7 years who are not fully immunized against pertussis, tetanus, or diphtheria should receive one dose of Tdap for wound management and as part of the catch-up series.

[d]Yes, if ≥ 10 years since the last tetanus toxoid-containing vaccine dose.

[e]Yes, if ≥ 5 years since the last tetanus toxoid-containing vaccine dose.

immunization histories should be considered to have received no previous tetanus toxoid.[14]

When passive tetanus prophylaxis is indicated, 250 units of TIG should be given intramuscularly. TTCV and TIG can be given simultaneously but should be administered at separate sites. Protection conferred by TIG can be expected to last about 4 weeks. The use of equine antitoxin has serious disadvantages compared with the use of the human product, including short-lived protection, risk of serum sickness, and occasional anaphylaxis. Since TIG of human origin has become widely available, there is little rationale for the use of equine antitoxin for postexposure prophylaxis and treatment, except in countries where human TIG is not available.

Maternal and Neonatal Tetanus Elimination

In 1989, the World Health Assembly adopted a goal of global elimination of neonatal tetanus, defined as less than one neonatal tetanus case per 1000 live births at the district level.[22,23] In 1999, this goal was reaffirmed and extended to the elimination of maternal tetanus as well.[24] In 2000, 59 countries were at risk for maternal and neonatal tetanus and, while progress continues to be made, as of early 2019, 13 countries had still not achieved elimination of maternal and neonatal tetanus.

The key strategies for maternal and neonatal tetanus elimination are achievement and maintenance of high TTCV vaccination coverage levels among women of childbearing age in high-risk areas and promotion of clean delivery and cord care practices. Active immunization of unimmunized pregnant women with two doses of appropriately timed TTCV prevents maternal and neonatal tetanus for that pregnancy; additional doses can be given with each subsequent pregnancy or at intervals of 1 year or more. The five TTCV doses recommended by WHO for previously unimmunized women of childbearing age are likely to provide protection throughout reproductive life.[25,26] The rarity of neonatal tetanus in developed countries is a consequence of the high proportion of institutional births attended by trained personnel, clean delivery practices, and the high proportion of mothers adequately vaccinated against tetanus.

SUMMARY

Tetanus is a serious disease that is almost completely preventable through immunization. As there is no natural immunity, all persons should receive an age-appropriate primary series of TTCV vaccine followed by recommended booster doses to maintain protective immunity throughout life. Healthcare providers should use every patient encounter to evaluate tetanus vaccination status and administer vaccine if indicated.

References

1. Bleck TP. Tetanus: Pathophysiology, management, and prophylaxis. *Dis Mon.* 1991;37(9):545–603.
2. Gill DM. Bacterial toxins: A table of lethal amounts. *Microbiol Rev.* 1982;46(1): 86–94.
3. Rossetto O, Scorzeto M, Megighian A, Montecucco C. Tetanus neurotoxin. *Toxicon.* 2013;66:59–63.
4. World Health Organization. Tetanus vaccines: WHO position paper, February 2017—Recommendations. *Vaccine.* 2018;36(25):3573–5.
5. Apte NM, Karnad DR. Short report: The spatula test: A simple bedside test to diagnose tetanus. *Am J Trop Med Hyg.* 1995;53(4):386–7.
6. Roper MRWS, Tiwari TSP, Orenstein WA. Tetanus toxoid. In: Plotkin SA, Orenstein WA, Offit P, eds. *Vaccines,* 6th ed. Philadelphia: Saunders; 2013, pp. 447–92.
7. WHO. Tetanus vaccines: WHO position paper—February 2017. *Wkly Epidemiol Rec.* 2017;92(6):53–76.
8. World Health Organization. Immunization, Vaccines and Biologicals. Tetanus. https://www.who.int/immunization/monitoring_surveillance/burden/vpd/surveillance_type/passive/tetanus_coverage_2018.jpg?ua=1. Accessed on July 1, 2019.
9. Pascual FB, McGinley EL, Zanardi LR, Cortese MM, Murphy TV. Tetanus surveillance—United States, 1998–2000. *MMWR Surveill Summ.* 2003;52(3):1–8.
10. Tiwari T, Thomas C, Clark T. Tetanus surveillance—United States, 2001–2008. *MMWR Morb Mortal Wkly Rep.* 2011;60(12):365–9.
11. World Health Organization. Immunization, Vaccines and Biologicals. Maternal and Neonatal Tetanus Elimination (MNTE). https://www.who.int/immunization/diseases/MNTE_initiative/en/. Accessed on July 1, 2019.
12. Long AP, Sartwell PE. Tetanus in the United States Army in World War II. *Bull U S Army Med Dep.* 1947;7(4):371–85.
13. McQuillan GM, Kruszon-Moran D, Deforest A, Chu SY, Wharton M. Serologic immunity to diphtheria and tetanus in the United States. *Ann Intern Med.* 2002;136(9):660–6.
14. Liang JL, Tiwari T, Moro P, et al. Prevention of pertussis, tetanus, and diphtheria with vaccines in the United States: Recommendations of the Advisory Committee on Immunization Practices (ACIP). *MMWR Recomm Rep.* 2018;67(2):1–44.
15. Jacobs RL, Lowe RS, Lanier BQ. Adverse reactions to tetanus toxoid. *JAMA.* 1982;247(1):40–2.
16. Edsall G, Elliott MW, Peebles TC, Eldred MC. Excessive use of tetanus toxoid boosters. *JAMA.* 1967;202(1):17–9.
17. White WG, Barnes GM, Barker E, Gall D, Knight P, Griffith AH, et al. Reactions to tetanus toxoid. *J Hyg (Lond).* 1973;71(2):283–97.
18. Institute of Medicine Vaccine Safety Committee. Diphtheria and tetanus toxoids. Adverse events associated with childhood vaccines: Evidence bearing on causality. In: Sratton Kr , Howe CJ, Johnston RB, eds. *Research Strategies for Assessing Adverse Effects Associated with Vaccines.* Washington, DC: National Academy Press; 1994, pp. 67–117.
19. Tuttle J, Chen RT, Rantala H, Cherry JD, Rhodes PH, Hadler S. The risk of Guillain-Barre syndrome after tetanus-toxoid-containing vaccines in adults and children in the United States. *Am J Public Health.* 1997;87(12):2045–8.
20. Blake PA, Feldman RA, Buchanan TM, Brooks GF, Bennett JV. Serologic therapy of tetanus in the United States, 1965–1971. *JAMA.* 1976;235(1):42–4.
21. Brauner JS, Vieira SR, Bleck TP. Changes in severe accidental tetanus mortality in the ICU during two decades in Brazil. *Intensive Care Med.* 2002;28(7):930–5.
22. Vandelaer J, Birmingham M, Gasse F, Kurian M, Shaw C, Garnier S. Tetanus in developing countries: An update on the maternal and neonatal tetanus elimination initiative. *Vaccine.* 2003;21(24):3442–5.
23. World Health Organization. *Handbook of Resolutions and Decisions of the World Health Assembly and the Executive Board (1985–1992).* Vol III. 3rd ed. Resolution 42.32. Geneva: World Health Organization; 1993, p. 102.
24. World Health Organization, *UNICEF, UNFPA. Maternal and Neonatal Tetanus Elimination by 2005. Strategies for Achieving and Maintaining Elimination.* Geneva: World Health Organization, UNICEF, UNFPA; 2000 (WHO/V&B/02.09).
25. World Health Organization. *Expanded Program on Immunization. Immunization Policy.* Geneva: World Health Organization; 1996 (WHO/EPI/Gen/95.03 Rev.1).
26. World Health Organization. *The Immunological Bases for Immunization Series. Module 3. Tetanus.* Geneva: World Health Organization; 1993 (WHO/ EPI/Gen/93.13).

CHAPTER

97

Pertussis*

Tami H. Skoff • Lucia C. Pawloski • Anna Acosta

Pertussis is a highly communicable, vaccine-preventable, respiratory illness caused by the bacterium *Bordetella pertussis*. It is typically characterized by paroxysms of severe coughing that can last for many weeks and are often associated with inspiratory whooping and posttussive vomiting. In the prevaccine era, pertussis was a significant cause of morbidity and mortality among infants and children in the United States.[1] With introduction of pertussis vaccines in the 1940s, the number of reported cases declined substantially; however, in more recent years, a resurgence of disease has been observed (Fig. 97-1).[1-4]

EPIDEMIOLOGY

Pertussis is an endemic disease worldwide. The disease is cyclic in nature, with epidemic cycles typically occurring every 2–5 years. While differences in surveillance methodology, vaccination schedules, and diagnostic capacity make accurate estimates of disease burden across countries challenging, data from a recent modeling study suggest that more than 24 million new pertussis cases occurred globally among children less than 5 years of age in 2014, and caused an estimated 160,700 deaths.[5]

Before pertussis vaccine introduction in the United States in the late 1940s, an average of 200,000 cases and 4000 pertussis-related deaths were reported each year.[1] However, following the introduction of pertussis vaccines, a > 99% reduction in reported pertussis was observed, highlighting the success of the vaccination program. Although reported cases reached a nadir of approximately 1000 cases in 1976, case counts have gradually increased since the late 1980s (Fig. 97-1). A recent analysis of U.S. national surveillance data showed that the average annual incidence of pertussis increased significantly between 2000 and 2016, with notable cyclicity in disease, ranging from a low of 2.7/100,000 in 2001, to a high of 15.4/100,000 in 2012.[4] Numerous factors are thought to be contributing to this observed increase, including changes in diagnostic testing and reporting, increased provider recognition, and molecular changes in the *B. pertussis* organism.[6,7] However, recent data support waning of vaccine-induced immunity as an important cause of the increase in the United States as well as in other countries that have transitioned from whole cell to acellular pertussis vaccine formulations.[8-12]

In the United States, the incidence of pertussis is highest in infants too young to have received adequate vaccination (i.e., at least three doses), although incidence among school-aged children and adolescents has been increasing (Fig. 97-2). Evaluation of U.S. national surveillance data revealed an increase in disease among 7–10 years olds during the late 2000s and then later among adolescents, groups thought to be well-protected by pertussis vaccines. Increases in reported disease in these age groups coincided with the aging of the first acellular-primed birth cohorts in the United States.[4]

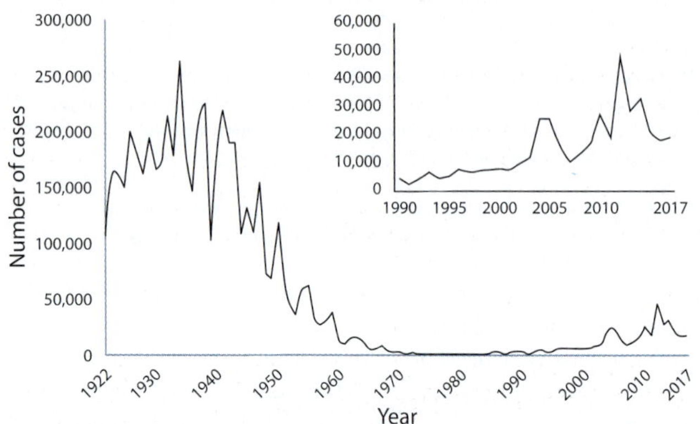

FIGURE 97-1. Nationally reported pertussis cases in the United States: 1922–17. (*Source:* Based on CDC, National Notifiable Diseases Surveillance System and 1922–49, passive reports to the Public Health Service.)

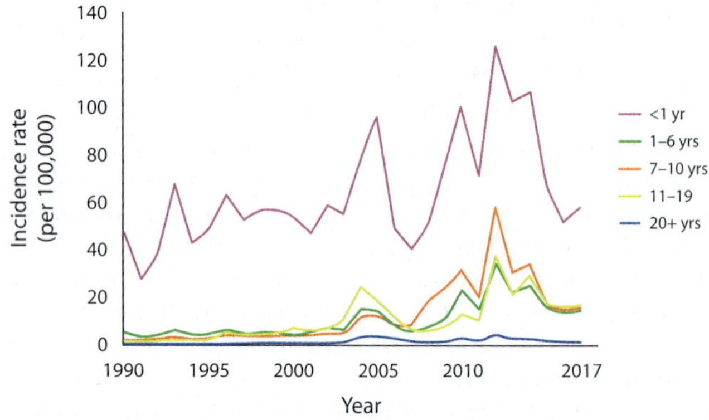

FIGURE 97-2. Nationally reported U.S. pertussis incidence, by age group: 1990–17. (*Source:* Based on CDC, National Notifiable Diseases Surveillance System.)

TRANSMISSION

Humans are the only known reservoir for *B. pertussis*. Pertussis is spread from person to person by large respiratory droplets generated by an infected person, or by direct contact with secretions from the respiratory tract. Pertussis is highly contagious, with secondary attack rates in unimmunized susceptible household contacts as high as 90%.[13] The incubation period of pertussis is usually 7–10 days (range 4–21 days).[14] A person is considered infectious from the onset

*The findings and conclusions in this chapter are those of the authors and do not necessarily represent the official position of the Centers for Disease Control and Prevention.

of symptoms (during the catarrhal stage) through the first 3 weeks of paroxysmal cough or until 5 days after the start of effective antimicrobial treatment.

Etiological Agent and Pathogenesis

Pertussis is caused by the gram-negative coccobacillus, *Bordetella pertussis*. A slow growing and fastidious microorganism, *B. pertussis* was first isolated by Bordet and Gengou in 1906. It is aerobic, nonmotile, and capable of hemolysis.

While the mechanism of pathogenesis is not completely defined, *B. pertussis* is known to infect the respiratory tract by attaching to ciliated epithelial cells along the throat and lungs. Pertussis is a toxin-mediated disease, utilizing a wide range of virulence factors, such as pertussis toxin (PT), along with cell-surface adherence proteins, including filamentous hemagglutinin, fimbriae 2 and 3, and pertactin, that play critical roles during infection and disease. Historic histopathologic reports of severe, fatal cases of pertussis in infants inform most of the current knowledge of disease pathogenesis, including observed leukocytosis, lymphocytosis, and pulmonary hypertension.[15] Pathological specimens from these infants demonstrated necrotizing bronchiolitis and intra-alveolar hemorrhage. The recent development of the baboon model has provided valuable insight into pathogenesis in nonfatal cases, indicating that infection causes severe inflammation localized to the lungs.[16]

CLINICAL CHARACTERISTICS

The clinical course of a classic pertussis infection can be divided into three distinct phases: *catarrhal*, *paroxysmal*, and *convalescent*.[13] The onset of illness is insidious, and during the first 1–2 weeks of illness, known as the *catarrhal* phase, coryza may be accompanied by shallow, nonproductive coughing. During the next phase, the *paroxysmal* phase, coughing progressively becomes more severe and paroxysmal in nature (i.e., repeated violent coughs without intervening respirations). The typical clinical feature of pertussis now manifests: paroxysmal coughing followed by an inspiratory whoop or vomiting.[13] After a few weeks of paroxysmal coughing, the disease peaks in severity and begins to subside. The *convalescent* phase, characterized by diminished but continuing cough, is protracted, and can last for months.

Classic pertussis symptoms can occur in persons at any age; however, disease presentation can vary with age, history of previous vaccination or exposure, and intervention with antibiotics. Mild or atypical pertussis (without severe paroxysms or whooping) can occur in individuals who have a level of protection from vaccination or previous natural exposure that has waned, or who have received antibiotics at an early point in the course of illness.[17–21] Infants aged $\leq$ 12 months, especially those aged $<$ 2 months, are at highest risk for severe disease; the clinical presentation may include apnea, cyanosis, or bradycardia with relatively minimal cough, and pertussis may not be initially suspected.[22–26]

Other causes of illnesses with a similar presentation to pertussis include *B. parapertussis*, *B. holmesii*, and *B. bronchiseptica*. Infections caused by *B. parapertussis and B. holmesii* are generally milder than pertussis[27–29] and the duration of infection may be shorter. *B. bronchiseptica* commonly causes respiratory infections in dogs and other animals, but can also be transmitted to humans, especially those who are immunocompromised.[30]

COMPLICATIONS

Major complications from pertussis, including hypoxia, pneumonia, pulmonary hypertension, seizures, encephalopathy, and death, are most commonly observed in young, unimmunized infants, especially in the early months of life.[26,31,32] Of the 53,226 pertussis cases reported between 2000 and 2017 in U.S. infants $<$ 12 months of age, 37.9% resulted in hospitalization, and 37.7% were in infants $<$ 2 months of age [unpublished data, National Notifiable Diseases Surveillance system (NNDSS)].[33] Of those ill infants with information on complications available, 10.5% had radiographed-confirmed pneumonia, 50.7% had apnea, 0.9% had seizures, and 0.3% had encephalopathy. Younger infants were more likely to be hospitalized than older infants: 63.8% infants $<$ 4 months of age were hospitalized, compared to 20.1% of infants 4–11 months of age.[33]

In developed countries, deaths from pertussis are almost always in infants, with the majority occurring in infants too young to have received three doses of a pertussis-containing vaccine.[23,24,34] Of the 307 pertussis deaths reported in the United States between 2000 and 2017, 270 (88%) were in infants aged $<$ 12 months, and 264 (86%) were in infants aged $<$ 4 months (unpublished data, NNDSS).[33] A recent study examining risk factors for pertussis infant death found that infants with fatal disease had significantly lower birth weight, younger gestational age, younger age at time of cough onset, and higher peak white blood cell and lymphocyte counts, compared to infants with nonfatal disease.[35] Infants with fatal disease were also more likely to have developed pulmonary hypertension, seizures, encephalitis, and pneumonia.

Adolescents and adults can also develop complications from pertussis, although data are limited because the disease may go unrecognized in these populations. Based on a recent analysis of pertussis cases reported between 2011 and 2015 in several sites across the United States, 0.5% of adolescents aged 11–18 years and 3.5% of adults aged $\geq$ 19 years with reported pertussis were hospitalized as a result of their pertussis infection. The most common complications reported among hospitalized adolescents and adults included pneumonia, new onset seizures, and encephalopathy.[36] However, little is known about the potential long-term sequelae of pertussis infections in these age groups.

TREATMENT AND CHEMOPROPHYLAXIS

Pertussis symptoms may be attenuated and communicability decreased when effective antimicrobial therapy is started during the *catarrhal* stage. However, after this time frame, initiation of antimicrobial therapy has no clear effect on the course of illness, and antibiotics would no longer be required to prevent transmission.[37] Patients who are treated with an effective course of antibiotics are no longer considered infectious after 5 days of treatment; untreated patients are considered infectious until 21 or more days after cough onset.[37] The preferred antimicrobial agents for treatment and prophylaxis of pertussis are macrolide antibiotics: azithromycin, erythromycin, or clarithromycin. Erythromycin was for a long time the drug of choice for treatment of pertussis, however, azithromycin is now more commonly administered to treat pertussis, because it has reduced gastrointestinal side effects and a simpler dosing regimen.[38–40] Trimethoprim-sulfamethoxazole is an alternative for patients who cannot tolerate macrolides.[13] In selecting an antibiotic for treatment, providers should consider the potential for adverse events: macrolide use has been associated with infantile hypertrophic pyloric stenosis, as well as with cardiac arrhythmias in certain populations.[13,41–45] In some situations, the benefit of treating disease may outweigh the risk of associated adverse events.

In the United States, the objective of postexposure chemoprophylaxis is to prevent death and serious complications in those who were exposed to a pertussis case. In the current setting of ongoing community transmission and rising pertussis incidence, widespread use of chemoprophylaxis may not be an effective strategy to control pertussis. Therefore, current chemoprophylaxis recommendations target the following groups: household contacts, contacts at high risk for developing severe disease (infants $<$ 12 months of age, pregnant women in the third trimester), contacts with pre-existing health conditions that may be exacerbated by a pertussis infection (e.g., but not limited to, immunocompromised people and those with moderate to severe medically treated asthma), or contacts who themselves have close contact with either infants, pregnant women, or individuals with pre-existing health conditions at risk of severe illness or complications.[46]

ANTIMICROBIAL RESISTANCE

The first known case of pertussis caused by a strain of *B. pertussis* resistant to high concentrations of erythromycin was reported in the United States in 1994; the isolate was sensitive to trimethoprim-sulfamethoxazole and the infected infant responded well to this therapy.[47] While other erythromycin-resistant isolates have been reported only very rarely in this country, China has observed a higher prevalence of macrolide resistance.[48–52] Therefore, outside of surveillance activities, susceptibility testing is recommended only when there is therapeutic failure.

IMMUNIZATION

Immunization is the most effective method for the prevention and control of pertussis. The first generation of pertussis vaccines were developed and tested in the 1940s and consisted of whole-cell preparations of *B. pertussis* combined with diphtheria and tetanus toxoids (DTP). These vaccines have been used worldwide since the 1950s and have substantially reduced pertussis morbidity and mortality. However, concerns about the safety of whole-cell pertussis vaccines led to the development of less reactogenic acellular vaccines containing purified antigenic components of *B. pertussis* combined with diphtheria and tetanus toxoids (DTaP); the composition and quantities of antigens vary by vaccine type and manufacturer. Acellular pertussis vaccines were licensed in the United States in 1991 for use as the fourth and fifth doses of the childhood pertussis vaccination series; they were additionally approved and recommended for use in the infant three-dose primary series in 1997.[53] Currently, no whole-cell pertussis vaccine formulations are licensed for use in the United States but these formulations are still used widely around the world, especially in low- and middle-income countries.

Eight different acellular pertussis vaccines were evaluated and compared with four whole-cell vaccines in controlled trials in the 1990s for safety and efficacy when administered to infants.[54–58] The protective efficacy of the acellular vaccines against moderately severe disease ranged from 59% to 85% while vaccine efficacy for the four whole-cell vaccines ranged from 36% to 98%; one lot of whole-cell pertussis vaccine, manufactured and distributed in the United States, had unexpectedly low vaccine efficacy when used as a three-dose series in studies conducted in Sweden and Italy. In these trials, all the acellular vaccines evaluated were associated with fewer local (pain, redness, and swelling at the site of injection) and systemic (fever and fussiness) adverse reactions than whole-cell vaccines.

The efficacy of immunization with whole-cell pertussis vaccines for preventing classical pertussis was good initially but waned over several years.[59,60] While follow-up studies of children in the acellular vaccine efficacy trials did not detect reductions in efficacy for up to 6 years,[61,62] more recent postlicensure studies of DTaP found that protection wanes more quickly than whole-cell vaccines.[8,10,63] In a large case-control study conducted by Misegades et al., DTaP vaccines were approximately 98% effective within 1 year of receiving the fifth dose but effectiveness dropped to 70% by 5 years postvaccination.[8] This documented waning of immunity correlates well with the epidemiology of reported disease in the United States, and the emergence of disease among cohorts recently vaccinated with acellular vaccines.[4]

Although pertussis vaccines are less immunogenic in younger infants compared with older infants, it is recommended that immunization begin at 6–8 weeks of age because young infants are at highest risk for severe pertussis-related morbidity and mortality. Three or more doses of DTP or DTaP vaccine are required to reliably confer protection; a single dose of the childhood vaccine has been shown to protect against infant death, hospitalization, and pneumonia.[31] In the United States, five doses of DTaP vaccine are recommended: three primary doses at 2, 4, and 6 months of age, a booster dose in the second year of life (15–18 months) and a second booster dose at school entry (4–6 years).[53]

Because neither pertussis vaccines nor natural infection confer lifelong protection against disease, two tetanus toxoid, reduced diphtheria toxoid, and acellular pertussis vaccines (Tdap) were licensed and recommended for use in the United States in 2005 as a single booster dose to provide protection to adolescents and adults.[53] Well-defined correlates of protection are lacking for pertussis; therefore, the efficacy of the Tdap vaccine components was inferred based on serologic bridging to DTaP vaccine efficacy data, with efficacy ranging from 79% to 89%.[57,64] Postlicensure vaccine effectiveness evaluations among adolescents have estimated Tdap effectiveness between 63% and 78%.[9,29,65,66] Similar to DTaP, significant waning of vaccine-induced immunity has also been observed following Tdap vaccination, with a significant reduction in vaccine effectiveness by 2–4 years postvaccination.[9,67,68] Neither prelicensure safety data nor routine postlicensure monitoring have identified any safety concerns associated with Tdap.[69,70]

While the main goal of Tdap vaccination was to directly protect adolescents and adults from pertussis, targeted Tdap vaccination of infant caregivers and household contacts was recommended at the time of Tdap introduction to provide indirect protection to young infants, a strategy known as cocooning. However, the cocooning strategy has encountered substantial logistical hurdles, such as difficulty achieving high vaccine uptake among cocoon members, making widespread implementation challenging. Furthermore, the effectiveness of the strategy remains inconclusive.[71–74]

In an effort to reduce the burden of pertussis in infants, the United States introduced maternal Tdap immunization during pregnancy in 2011 as a way to provide direct protection to young infants through the passive transfer of maternal antibodies; because maternal antipertussis antibodies are short lived, the recommendation was expanded in 2012 to include a dose during *each* pregnancy.[75] Although the United States was the first country to introduce the strategy, numerous countries now recommend Tdap immunization during pregnancy, with most recommending vaccination during every pregnancy. Immunization during pregnancy has been shown to be safe and highly effective among young infants, with vaccine effectiveness estimates ranging from 69% to 93%.[76–81]

Laboratory Diagnosis

Laboratory confirmation of pertussis can be difficult. A complementary, multitest algorithm that includes culture, polymerase chain reaction (PCR), and serology should be considered, as each individual test has its strengths and limitations. A patient's age, prior vaccination, antimicrobial therapy, and the timing of specimen collection in relation to cough onset all greatly affect test performance and need to be considered when deciding which assay(s) to use. When interpreting test results, a patient's clinical presentation should also be considered.

Isolation of *B. pertussis* by bacterial culture remains the gold standard for diagnosing pertussis. It is highly specific, but has very poor sensitivity (most sensitive for infants, unvaccinated children, and patients with $<$ 2 weeks of cough) and test performance is affected by antibiotics. Culture specimens are obtained either by nasopharyngeal (NP) aspiration or swabbing.[82] Sterile, flocked polyester, rayon or nylon swabs can be used for both bacterial isolation and PCR. Agar media that use horse blood, like Bordet-Gengou or Regan-Lowe, should be used, ideally with the selective antimicrobial agent, cephalexin, to suppress the overgrowth of normal flora. Bacilli appear as small, pearly colonies. Though *B. pertussis* colonies may appear after 3 days, plates should be incubated for up to 10 days at 37°C with high humidity and observed daily.

Compared with culture, PCR testing is more rapid, can be more sensitive, is less affected by antibiotic administration, and can be used up to 4 weeks postcough onset, as the bacterium does not need to be viable for testing. The most common PCR target, insertion sequence IS*481*, is present in *B. pertussis* with at least 238 copies, making it a very highly sensitive target that can also be prone to false-positivity by contamination. IS*481* is also found in other *Bordetella* species, making it a less specific target. Ideally, PCR should include additional targets that are specific for *B. pertussis*, *B. parapertussis*, and *B. holmesii*.[83,84]

A reference-calibrated anti-PT IgG titer in a single serum sample taken 2–12 weeks after cough onset can be used to diagnose pertussis.[85–88] Serology can be particularly useful in adolescents and adults, who often present to medical care later in the course of their cough illness when it is too late to be diagnosed by culture or PCR, and in suspected respiratory outbreaks for retrospective confirmation of *B. pertussis*. Because recent vaccination can confound anti-PT IgG diagnostic interpretation, many countries have implemented various waiting periods for serologic testing following vaccination.[85–87,89]

While direct fluorescence antibody (DFA) staining of mucous smears from NP swabs has also been used for laboratory diagnosis, rates of false-positive and false-negative results can be high and DFA is no longer recommended for the diagnosis of pertussis.[85–88]

Molecular Epidemiology

There are multiple molecular typing methods for *B. pertussis*, such as pulsed-field gel electrophoresis (PFGE), that characterize isolates by genomic fragment sizes, and nucleotide sequence-based typing schemes, such as multilocus sequence typing (MLST) and multiple locus variable-number tandem repeat analysis (MLVA). While circulating strains display a wider range of MLVA types than MLST, single, monomorphic MLST and MLVA profiles have become predominant in the United States since the introduction of vaccination.[90,91] This is in contrast to PFGE, for which five to six types typically predominate at any given time.[91,92] Whole genome sequencing has helped improve sequence typing by substantially increasing the number of sequence targets to be analyzed, thereby providing more discriminatory power.[93] Furthermore, it has revealed a vast extent of complex chromosomal restructuring that the bacterium has undergone over time, largely negating the original consensus that *B. pertussis* evolution was relatively static.[94,95]

Analysis of genomes of current, circulating isolates in several countries has revealed many differences, both at the sequence and structural level, between modern strains and the historic reference strains that informed current vaccine formulations. This suggests that part of the current resurgence and waning of immunity may be due to vaccine-induced pathogen adaptation. Part of the bacterial evolution includes the loss of pertactin, one of the primary immunogens included in the acellular pertussis vaccine, observed in most countries that employ the acellular vaccine.[96,97] Analysis has shown that this phenomenon is likely vaccine driven,[98] but clinical presentation and vaccine efficacy appear unaffected.[99] To date, only a handful of isolates have lost the production of other vaccine immunogens.[100–102]

SUMMARY

Although pertussis can occur in persons of all ages, infants are at greatest risk for severe pertussis-related morbidity and mortality. Despite the dramatic decline in disease following the introduction of pertussis vaccines, numerous countries have been experiencing a pertussis resurgence in recent years. While the reasons for the resurgence are likely multifactorial, waning of immunity from current pertussis vaccines appears to be an important factor. However, even in the setting of waning immunity, vaccination continues to be the single most important way to protect against pertussis, and new strategies, such as maternal immunization during pregnancy, are highly effective at preventing disease in the most vulnerable age groups.

References

1. CDC. Annual summary 1979: Reported morbidity and mortality in the United States. *MMWR*. 1980;28(54):12–7.
2. Farizo KM, Cochi SL, Zell ER, Brink EW, Wassilak SG, Patriarca PA. Epidemiological features of pertussis in the United States, 1980–1989. *Clin Infect Dis*. 1992;14(3):708–19.
3. Guris D, Strebel PM, Bardenheier B, et al. Changing epidemiology of pertussis in the United States: Increasing reported incidence among adolescents and adults, 1990–1996. *Clin Infect Dis*. 1999;28(6):1230–7.
4. Skoff TH, Hadler S, Hariri S. The epidemiology of nationally reported pertussis in the United States, 2000–2016. *Clin Infect Dis*. 2019;68(10): 1634–40.
5. Yeung KHT, Duclos P, Nelson EAS, Hutubessy RCW. An update of the global burden of pertussis in children younger than 5 years: A modelling study. *Lancet Infect Dis*. 2017;17(9):974–80.
6. Clark T. Changing pertussis epidemiology: Everything old is new again. *J Infect Dis*. 2014;209(7):978–81.
7. Tan T, Dalby T, Forsyth K, et al. Pertussis across the globe: Recent epidemiologic trends from 2000 to 2013. *Pediatr Infect Dis J*. 2015;34(9):e222–32.
8. Misegades L, Winter K, Harriman K, et al. Association of childhood pertussis with receipt of 5 doses of pertussis vaccine by time since last vaccine dose, California, 2010. *JAMA*. 2012;308(20):2126–32.
9. Acosta AM, DeBolt C, Tasslimi A, et al. Tdap vaccine effectiveness in adolescents during the 2012 Washington State pertussis epidemic. *Pediatrics*. 2015;135(6):981–9.
10. Tartof S, Lewis M, Kenyon C, et al. Waning immunity to pertussis following 5 doses of DTaP. *Pediatrics*. 2013;131(4):e1047–52.
11. Liko J, Robison SG, Cieslak PR. Priming with whole-cell versus acellular pertussis vaccine. *N Engl J Med*. 2013;368(6):581–2.
12. Sheridan SL, Frith K, Snelling TL, Grimwood K, McIntyre PB, Lambert SB. Waning vaccine immunity in teenagers primed with whole cell and acellular pertussis vaccine: Recent epidemiology. *Expert Rev Vaccines*. 2014;13(9): 1081–106.
13. American Academy of Pediatrics. Pertussis (whooping cough). In: Kimberlin DW, Brady MT, Jackson MA, Long SS, eds. *Red Book: 2018 Report of the Committee on Infectious Diseases*. 31st ed. Itasca, IL: American Academy of Pediatrics; 2018, pp. 620–34.
14. Fine PE. Herd immunity: History, theory, practice. *Epidemiol Rev*. 1993;15(2):265–302.
15. Paddock CD, Sanden GN, Cherry JD, et al. Pathology and pathogenesis of fatal *Bordetella pertussis* infection in infants. *Clin Infect Dis*. 2008;47(3):328–38.
16. Zimmerman L, Papin J, Warfel J, Wolf R, Kosanke S, Merkel T. Histopathology of *Bordetella pertussis* in the Baboon Model. *Infect Immun*. 2018;86(11):e00511-8.
17. Bortolussi R, Miller B, Ledwith M, Halperin S. Clinical course of pertussis in immunized children. *Pediatr Infect Dis J*. 1995;14(10):870–4.
18. Heininger U, Klich K, Stehr K, Cherry JD. Clinical findings in *Bordetella pertussis* infections: Results of a prospective multicenter surveillance study. *Pediatrics*. 1997;100(6):e10.
19. Barlow RS, Reynolds LE, Cieslak PR, Sullivan AD. Vaccinated children and adolescents with pertussis infections experience reduced illness severity and duration, Oregon, 2010–2012. *Clin Infect Dis*. 2014;58(11):1523–9.
20. McNamara L, Skoff T, Faulkner A, et al. Reduced severity of pertussis in persons with age-appropriate pertussis vaccination—United States, 2010–2012. *Clin Infect Dis*. 2017;65(5):811–8.
21. Tozzi A, Ravà L, Ciofi degli Atti ML, Salmaso S. Clinical presentation of pertussis in unvaccinated and vaccinated children in the first six years of life. *Pediatrics*. 2003;112(5):1069–75.
22. Christie CD, Baltimore RS. Pertussis in neonates. *Am J Dis Child*. 1989; 143(10):1199–202.
23. Vitek CR, Pascual FB, Baughman AL, Murphy TV. Increase in deaths from pertussis among young infants in the United States in the 1990s. *Pediatr Infect Dis J*. 2003;22(7):628–34.
24. Crowcroft NS, Booy R, Harrison T, et al. Severe and unrecognised: Pertussis in UK infants. *Arch Dis Child*. 2003;88(9):802–6.
25. O'Riordan A, Cleary J, Cunney R, Nicholson AJ. Pertussis in young infants: Clinical presentation, course and prevention. *Ir Med J*. 2014;107(7):217–9.
26. Marshall H, Clarke M, Rasiah K, et al. Predictors of disease severity in children hospitalized for pertussis during an epidemic. *Pediatr Infect Dis J*. 2015;34(4):339–45.
27. Koepke R, Bartholomew M, Eickhoff J, et al. Widespread *Bordetella parapertussis* infections-Wisconsin, 2011–2012: Clinical and epidemiologic

features and antibiotic use for treatment and prevention. *Clin Infect Dis.* 2015;61(9):1421–31.

28. Pittet L, Emonet S, Schrenzel J, Siegrist C-A, Posfay Barbe K. *Bordetella holmesii*: An under-recognised Bordetella species. *Lancet Infect Dis.* 2014;14(6):510–9.
29. Rodgers L, Martin S, Cohn A, et al. Epidemiologic and laboratory features of a large outbreak of pertussis-like illnesses associated with cocirculating *Bordetella holmesii* and *Bordetella pertussis*—Ohio, 2010–2011. *Clin Infect Dis.* 2013;56(3):322–31.
30. Mattoo S, Cherry JD. Molecular pathogenesis, epidemiology, and clinical manifestations of respiratory infections due to *Bordetella pertussis* and other Bordetella subspecies. *Clin Microbiol Rev.* 2005;18(2):326–82.
31. Tiwari TSP, Baughman AL, Clark TA. First pertussis vaccine dose and prevention of infant mortality. *Pediatrics.* 2015;135(6):990–9.
32. Cherry J, Wendorf K, Bregman B, et al. An observational study of severe pertussis in 100 infants ≤120 days of age. *Pediatr Infect Dis J.* 2018;37(3):202–5.
33. Bozio C, Skoff T, Pondo T, Liang J. Epidemiology and trends of pertussis among infants: United States, 2000–2015. *Open Forum Infect Dis.* 2017;4(Suppl_1):S5.
34. Tanaka M, Vitek CR, Pascual FB, Bisgard KM, Tate JE, Murphy TV. Trends in pertussis among infants in the United States, 1980–1999. *JAMA.* 2003;290(22):2968–75.
35. Winter K, Zipprich J, Harriman K, et al. Risk factors associated with infant deaths from pertussis: A case-control study. *Clin Infect Dis.* 2015;61(7): 1099–106.
36. Mbayei SA, Faulkner A, Miner C, et al. Severe pertussis infections in the United States, 2011–2015. *Clin Infect Dis.* 2019;69(2):218–26.
37. CDC. Pertussis (whooping cough): Treatment. https://www.cdc.gov/pertussis/clinical/treatment.html. Accessed July 2, 2019.
38. Langley J, Halperin S, Boucher F, Smith B. Azithromycin is as effective as and better tolerated than erythromycin estolate for the treatment of pertussis. *Pediatrics.* 2004;114(1):e96–101.
39. Lebel MH, Mehra S. Efficacy and safety of clarithromycin versus erythromycin for the treatment of pertussis: A prospective, randomized, single blind trial. *Pediatr Infect Dis J.* 2001;20(12):1149–54.
40. Tiwari T, Murphy T, Moran J. Recommended antimicrobial agents for the treatment and postexposure prophylaxis of pertussis 2005 CDC guidelines. *Morb Mortal Wkly Rep.* 2005;54(RR-14):1–16.
41. Honein MA, Paulozzi LJ, Himelright IM, et al. Infantile hypertrophic pyloric stenosis after pertussis prophylaxis with erythromcyin: A case review and cohort study. *Lancet.* 1999;354(9196):2101–5.
42. Mahon BE, Rosenman MB, Kleiman MB. Maternal and infant use of erythromycin and other macrolide antibiotics as risk factors for infantile hypertrophic pyloric stenosis. *J Pediatr.* 2001;139(3):380–4.
43. Eberly M, Eide M, Thompson J, Nylund C. Azithromycin in early infancy and pyloric stenosis. *Pediatrics.* 2015;135(3):483–8.
44. Ray W, Murray K, Hall K, Arbogast P, Stein CM. Azithromycin and the risk of cardiovascular death. *N Engl J Med.* 2012;366(20):1881–90.
45. Albert R, Schuller J. Macrolide antibiotics and the risk of cardiac arrhythmias. *Am J Respir Crit Care Med.* 2014;189(10):1173–80.
46. CDC. Postexposure antimicrobial prophylaxis: Information for health professionals. https://www.cdc.gov/pertussis/outbreaks/pep.html. Accessed 07/02/2019.
47. Lewis K, Saubolle MA, Tenover FC, Rudinsky MF, Barbour SD, Cherry JD. Pertussis caused by an erythromycin-resistant strain of *Bordetella pertussis*. *Pediatr Infect Dis J.* 1995;14(5):388–91.
48. Bartkus JM, Juni BA, Ehresmann K, et al. Identification of a mutation associated with erythromycin resistance in *Bordetella pertussis*: Implications for surveillance of antimicrobial resistance. *J Clin Microbiol.* 2003;41(3):1167–72.
49. Wilson KE, Cassiday PK, Popovic T, Sanden GN. *Bordetella pertussis* isolates with a heterogeneous phenotype for erythromycin resistance. *J Clin Microbiol.* 2002;40(8):2942–4.
50. Hill BC, Baker CN, Tenover FC. A simplified method for testing *Bordetella pertussis* for resistance to erythromycin and other antimicrobial agents. *J Clin Microbiol.* 2000;38(3):1151–5.
51. Fu P, Wang C, Tian H, Kang Z, Zeng M. *Bordetella pertussis* infection in infants and young children in Shanghai, China, 2016–2017: Clinical features, genotype variations of antigenic genes and macrolides resistance. *Pediatr Infect Dis J.* 2019;38(4):370–6.
52. Wang Z, Cui Z, Li Y, et al. High prevalence of erythromycin-resistant *Bordetella pertussis* in Xi'an, China. *Clin Microbiol Infect.* 2014;20(11): O825–30.
53. Liang J, Tiwari T, Moro P, et al. Prevention of pertussis, tetanus, and diphtheria with vaccines in the United States: Recommendations of the Advisory Committee on Immunization Practices (ACIP). *MMWR Recomm Rep.* 2018;67(2):1–44.
54. Gustafsson L, Hallander HO, Olin P, Reizenstein E, Storsaeter J. A controlled trial of a two-component acellular, a five-component acellular, and a whole-cell pertussis vaccine. *N Engl J Med.* 1996;334(6):349–55.
55. Stehr K, Cherry JD, Heininger U, et al. A comparative efficacy trial in Germany in infants who received either the Lederle/Takeda acellular pertussis component DTP (DTaP) vaccine, the Lederle whole-cell component DTP vaccine, or DT vaccine. *Pediatrics.* 1998;101(1 Pt 1):1–11.
56. CDC. Pertussis vaccination: Use of acellular pertussis vaccines among infants and young children. Recommendations of the Advisory Committee on Immunization Practices (ACIP). *MMWR.* 1997;46(RR-7):1–25.
57. Schmitt HJ, von Konig CH, Neiss A, et al. Efficacy of acellular pertussis vaccine in early childhood after household exposure. *JAMA.* 1996;275(1): 37–41.
58. Trollfors B, Taranger J, Lagergård T, et al. A placebo-controlled trial of a pertussis-toxoid vaccine. *N Engl J Med.* 1995;333(16):1045–50.
59. Fine PE, Clarkson JA. Reflections on the efficacy of pertussis vaccines. *Rev Infect Dis.* 1987;9(5):866–83.
60. Jenkinson D. Duration of effectiveness of pertussis vaccine: Evidence from a 10 year community study. *Br Med J.* 1988;296:612–4.
61. Salmaso S, Mastrantonio P, Tozzi AE, et al. Sustained efficacy during the first 6 years of life of 3-component acellular pertussis vaccines administered in infancy: The Italian experience. *Pediatrics.* 2001;108(5):e81.
62. Lugauer S, Heininger U, Cherry JD, Stehr K. Long-term clinical effectiveness of an acellular pertussis component vaccine and a whole cell pertussis component vaccine. *EurJ Pediatr.* 2002;161(3):142–6.
63. Klein NP, Bartlett J, Rowhani-Rahbar A, Fireman B, Baxter R. Waning protection after fifth dose of acellular pertussis vaccine in children. *N Engl J Med.* 2012;367(11):1012–9.
64. Gustafsson L, Hallander HO, Olin P, Reizenstein E, Storsaeter J. A controlled trial of a two-component acellular, a five-component acellular, and a whole-cell pertussis vaccine. *N Engl J Med.* 1996;334(6):349–55.
65. Rank C, Quinn HE, McIntyre PB. Pertussis vaccine effectiveness after mass immunization of high school students in Australia. *Pediatr Infect Dis J.* 2009;28(2):152–3.
66. Wei SC, Tatti K, Cushing K, et al. Effectiveness of adolescent and adult tetanus, reduced-dose diphtheria, and acellular pertussis vaccine against pertussis. *Clin Infect Dis.* 2010;51(3):315–21.
67. Klein N, Bartlett J, Fireman B, Baxter R. Waning Tdap effectiveness in adolescents. *Pediatrics.* 2016;137(3):e20153326.
68. Koepke R, Eickhoff J, Ayele R, et al. Estimating the effectiveness of tetanus-diphtheria-acellular pertussis vaccine (Tdap) for preventing pertussis: Evidence of rapidly waning immunity and difference in effectiveness by Tdap brand. *J Infect Dis.* 2014;210(6):942–53.
69. Yih WK, Nordin J, Kulldorff M, et al. An assessment of the safety of adolescent and adult tetanus-diphtheria-acellular pertussis (Tdap) vaccine, using active surveillance for adverse events in the Vaccine Safety Datalink. *Vaccine.* 2009;27(32):4257–62.
70. Chang S, O'Connor P, Slade B, Woo E. U.S. Postlicensure safety surveillance for adolescent and adult tetanus, diphtheria and acellular pertussis vaccines: 2005–2007. *Vaccine.* 2013;31(10):1447–52.
71. Quinn HE, Snelling TL, Habig A, Chiu C, Spokes PJ, McIntyre PB. Parental Tdap boosters and infant pertussis: A case-control study. *Pediatrics.* 2014;134(4):713–20.
72. Carcione D, Regan AK, Tracey L, et al. The impact of parental postpartum pertussis vaccination on infection in infants: A population-based study of cocooning in Western Australia. *Vaccine.* 2015;33(42):5654–61.
73. Castagnini LA, Healy CM, Rench MA, Wootton SH, Munoz FM, Baker CJ. Impact of maternal postpartum tetanus and diphtheria toxoids and acellular pertussis immunization on infant pertussis infection. *Clin Infect Dis.* 2012;54(1):78–84.
74. Healy CM, Rench MA, Wootton SH, Castagnini LA. Evaluation of the impact of a pertussis cocooning program on infant pertussis infection. *Pediatr Infect Dis J.* 2015;34(1):22–6.
75. Centers for Disease Control and Prevention (CDC). Updated recommendations for use of tetanus toxoid, reduced diphtheria toxoid, and acellular pertussis vaccine (Tdap) in pregnant women—Advisory Committee on Immunization Practices (ACIP), 2012. *MMWR Morb Mortal Wkly Rep.* 2013;62(7):131–5.
76. Skoff TH, Blain AE, Watt J, et al. Impact of the US maternal tetanus, diphtheria, and acellular pertussis vaccination program on preventing

pertussis in infants <2 months of age: A case-control evaluation. *Clin Infect Dis.* 2017;65(12):1977–83.

77. Dabrera G, Amirthalingam G, Andrews N, et al. A case-control study to estimate the effectiveness of maternal pertussis vaccination in protecting newborn infants in England and Wales, 2012–2013. *Clin Infect Dis.* 2015;60(3):333–7.
78. Winter K, Nickell S, Powell M, Harriman K. Effectiveness of prenatal versus postpartum tetanus, diphtheria, and acellular pertussis vaccination in preventing infant pertussis. *Clin Infect Dis.* 2017;64(1):3–8.
79. Saul N, Wang K, Bag S, et al. Effectiveness of maternal pertussis vaccination in preventing infection and disease in infants: The NSW Public Health Network case-control study. *Vaccine.* 2018;36(14):1887–92.
80. Baxter R, Bartlett J, Fireman B, Lewis E, Klein NP. Effectiveness of vaccination during pregnancy to prevent infant pertussis. *Pediatrics.* 2017;139(5): e20164091.
81. McMillan M, Clarke M, Parrella A, Fell D, Amirthalingam G, Marshall H. Safety of tetanus, diphtheria, and pertussis vaccination during pregnancy: A systematic review. *Obstet Gynecol.* 2017;129(3):560–73.
82. CDC. Pertussis (whooping cough): Specimen collection. https://www.cdc.gov/pertussis/clinical/diagnostic-testing/specimen-collection.html. Accessed July 15, 2019.
83. Templeton K, Scheltinga S, van der Zee A, et al. Evaluation of real-time PCR for detection of and discrimination between *Bordetella pertussis*, *Bordetella parapertussis*, and *Bordetella holmesii* for clinical diagnosis. *J Clin Microbiol.* 2003;41(9):4121–6.
84. Tatti K, Sparks K, Boney K, Tondella M. Novel multitarget real-time PCR assay for rapid detection of Bordetella species in clinical specimens. *J Clin Microbiol.* 2011;49(12):4059–66.
85. Guiso N, Berbers G, Fry NK, He Q, Riffelmann M, von König CHW. What to do and what not to do in serological diagnosis of pertussis: Recommendations from EU reference laboratories. *Eur J Clin Microbiol Infect Dis.* 2011;30(3):307–12.
86. van der Zee A, Schellekens JFP, Mooi F. Laboratory diagnosis of pertussis. *Clin Microbiol Rev.* 2015;28(4):1005–26.
87. World Health Organization. Vaccine-preventable diseases surveillance standards: Pertussis. Accessed July 15, 2019.
88. CDC. Manual for the surveillance of vaccine-preventable diseases: Pertussis. https://www.cdc.gov/vaccines/pubs/surv-manual/chpt10-pertussis.html. Accessed July 15, 2019.
89. Pawloski L, Kirkland K, Baughman A, et al. Does tetanus-diphtheria-acellular pertussis vaccination interfere with serodiagnosis of pertussis infection? *Clin Vaccine Immunol.* 2012;19(6):875–80.
90. Schmidtke A, Boney K, Martin S, Skoff T, Tondella ML, Tatti K. Population diversity among *Bordetella pertussis* isolates, United States, 1935–2009. *Emerg Infect Dis.* 2012;18(8):1248–55.
91. van Gent M, Heuvelman CJ, van der Heide HG, et al. Analysis of *Bordetella pertussis* clinical isolates circulating in European countries during the period 1998–2012. *Eur J Clin Microbiol Infect Dis.* 2015;34(4):821–30.
92. Cassiday P, Skoff T, Jawahir S, Tondella ML. Changes in predominance of pulsed-field gel electrophoresis profiles of *Bordetella pertussis* isolates, United States, 2000–2012. *Emerg Infect Dis.* 2016;22(3):442–8.
93. Bouchez V, Guglielmini J, Dazas M, et al. Genomic sequencing of *Bordetella pertussis* for epidemiology and global surveillance of whooping cough. *Emerg Infect Dis.* 2018;24(6):988–94.
94. Bowden K, Weigand M, Peng Y, et al. Genome structural diversity among 31 *Bordetella pertussis* isolates from two recent U.S. whooping cough statewide epidemics. *mSphere.* 2016;1(3):e00036-16.
95. Weigand M, Peng Y, Loparev V, et al. The history of *Bordetella pertussis* genome evolution includes structural rearrangement. *J Bacteriol.* 2017;199(8):e00806-16.
96. Hegerle N, Paris AS, Brun D, et al. Evolution of French *Bordetella pertussis* and *Bordetella parapertussis* isolates: Increase of Bordetellae not expressing pertactin. *Clin Microbiol Infect.* 2012;18(9):E340–6.
97. Pawloski LC, Queenan AM, Cassiday PK, et al. Prevalence and molecular characterization of pertactin-deficient *Bordetella pertussis* in the United States. *Clin Vaccine Immunol.* 2014;21(2):119–25.
98. Martin S, Pawloski L, Williams M, et al. Pertactin-negative *Bordetella pertussis* strains: Evidence for a possible selective advantage. *Clin Infect Dis.* 2015;60(2):223–7.
99. Breakwell L, Kelso P, Finley C, et al. Pertussis vaccine effectiveness in the setting of pertactin-deficient pertussis. *Pediatrics.* 2016;137(5):e20153973.
100. Bouchez V, Hegerle N, Strati F, Njamkepo E, Guiso N. New data on vaccine antigen deficient *Bordetella pertussis* isolates. *Vaccines.* 2015;3(3):751–70.
101. Williams M, Sen K, Weigand M, et al. *Bordetella pertussis* strain lacking pertactin and pertussis toxin. *Emerg Infect Dis.* 2016;22(2):319–22.
102. Weigand M, Pawloski L, Peng Y, et al. Screening and genomic characterization of filamentous hemagglutinin-deficient *Bordetella pertussis*. *Infect Immun.* 2018;86(4):e00869-17.

CHAPTER

98 Poliomyelitis*

Roland W. Sutter • Stephen L. Cochi

Poliomyelitis, or infantile paralysis, is an acute contagious disease characterized by fever, flaccid paralysis, and muscle atrophy as a result of the destruction of motor neurons in the spinal cord and less commonly the brain stem. Three serotypes of poliovirus cause infections that result in severity ranging from inapparent illness to acute flaccid paralysis (AFP) and death. Paralysis may resolve or lead to permanent disability and deformity. Decades after the acute episode, new paralysis or progressive weakness may appear.[1] This clinical entity is referred to as postpolio syndrome. Poliomyelitis probably has afflicted mankind for thousands of years, as manifested by an Egyptian stele originating from the eighteenth dynasty (dating from 1403 to 1365 BC) that depicts a priest with a typical leg deformity. However, only in 1789 was the disease first described. Epidemic poliomyelitis emerged as a public health problem in the United States and Northern Europe in the late nineteenth and early twentieth centuries, with tens of thousands of cases reported annually. Improved hygiene and sanitation delayed poliovirus exposure to older children and young adults that were at higher risk for severe paralytic disease ("central polio dogma"). Effective vaccines, developed in the 1950s and 1960s, rapidly eliminated poliomyelitis in industrialized countries as a public health problem, but not in the developing world.[2] To remedy this, the World Health Assembly, the governing body of the World Health Organization, resolved in 1988 to eradicate poliomyelitis globally by the year 2000.[3] Although this target has not yet been reached, substantial progress has been made, and achievement of eradication remains feasible. The last wild poliovirus type 2 was detected in 1999, the last wild poliovirus type 3 in 2012, and wild poliovirus 1 circulation appears to be restricted to parts of Afghanistan and Pakistan with 22–33 paralytic cases per year during 2017–18. However, a resurgence of cases in 2019 led to major increases in case count, with over 176 paralytic cases (data as of June 2, 2019).

ETIOLOGY

In 1908, Landsteiner and Popper demonstrated that poliomyelitis was caused by a virus ("filterable agent"). Polioviruses caused paralytic disease in monkeys by intraperitoneal inoculation of spinal cord materials from a patient with fatal poliomyelitis. In 1931, Burnet and Macnamara established that more than one virus strain can cause poliomyelitis, and that immunity to one strain was not protective against the other strain (i.e., no heterotypic immunity). A typing effort by the Committee on Typing of the National Infantile Paralysis Society in 1951 determined that there were only three serotypes of polioviruses, designated as poliovirus types 1, 2, and 3.[4] The closely related but antigenically distinct viruses are part of the Enterovirus genus and belong to the family Picornaviruses.[5] In the early 1940s, it was shown that the infectious agent was present usually in the stools of patients with symptomatic disease and their symptom-free contacts. In 1949, Enders, Weller, and Robbins successfully propagated poliovirus for the first time in human embryonic nonnervous tissue, and documented virus growth directly in cell cultures (i.e., "cytopathogenic effect"). This method eliminated the need for *in vivo* methods (e.g., monkeys) to confirm virus replication.[6] Together, these breakthroughs were critical to pave the way for efficient virus growth needed for the eventual production of vaccines.

PATHOGENESIS

After ingestion into the oral cavity, polioviruses replicate initially in the oropharyngeal mucosa (tonsils) and the Peyer's patches in the ileum after gaining access into cells using the human poliovirus receptor.[7] Viremia may ensue and central nervous system (CNS) infection may follow; in the latter instance, the virus specifically targets the motor neurons of the spinal cord and occasionally the brain stem. Viral replication in the motor neurons results in cell destruction and flaccid paralysis of the muscles they innervate. Death is usually a result of bulbar involvement with respiratory paralysis.

Infection with polioviruses may result in a spectrum of clinical outcomes. The vast majority of infected persons remain asymptomatic, or experience a mild illness characterized by fever, malaise, headache with nausea, vomiting, constipation, diarrhea, and sore throat. Infections with limited CNS involvement may cause illness with fever and evidence of meningeal irritation—stiff neck and back and elevated protein and leukocyte levels in the spinal fluid—followed by complete recovery. This syndrome is clinically identical to aseptic meningitis caused by other viral agents such as mumps virus, echovirus, and coxsackie viruses. Finally, approximately 1:100–1:1000 infected persons may experience the typical paralytic consequences of poliovirus infection. The differences in attack rates may be due to variations in neurovirulence among the three serotypes, with type 1 being the most neurovirulent viral serotype.

After an interval of 30–40 years, many persons (25–40%) who contracted paralytic poliomyelitis in their childhood may experience muscle pain and exacerbation of existing weakness, or may develop new weakness or paralysis. This condition is referred to as postpolio syndrome. To date, this syndrome has only been described in persons infected during the era of wild poliovirus circulation. Factors that enhance the risk of post-polio syndrome include: (a) increasing

*Note: The findings and conclusions in this chapter are those of the authors and do not necessarily represent the views of the Centers for Disease Control and Prevention.

length of time since acute poliovirus infection; (b) presence of permanent residual impairment after recovery from the acute illness; and (c) female gender. The pathogenesis of postpolio syndrome is thought to involve late attrition of oversized motor units that developed during the recovery process of paralytic poliomyelitis.[1]

EPIDEMIOLOGY

Following development and widespread use of effective poliovirus vaccines, first inactivated poliovirus vaccine (the "Salk vaccine") and then live attenuated oral poliovirus vaccine (the "Sabin vaccine"), in the United States and other industrialized countries, paralytic poliomyelitis was largely eliminated as a public health concern.[8] The same success had yet to be achieved in much of the developing world; therefore, in 1988, the World Health Assembly resolved to eradicate poliomyelitis globally by 2000[3] (see Global Poliomyelitis Eradication Initiative). In 1988, an estimated 350,000 cases of poliomyelitis occurred worldwide, and in many countries paralytic disease due to poliomyelitis was the single most important contributor to permanent disability.[2,9,10] The vast majority of the cases emanated from tropical and subtropical regions, where crowding, poor sanitation, and inadequate hygiene facilitate transmission of polioviruses and other enteric pathogens.

Humans (and some nonhuman primates) are the only known reservoir of poliovirus infection and excrete the agent in pharyngeal secretions and feces. The incubation period is most commonly 7–24 days, with a range of 3–36 days. Patients can be infectious before symptoms develop; virus is subsequently excreted in pharyngeal secretions for a few days and in the stool for several weeks. Transmission occurs via the fecal-oral route, particularly in settings where sanitation and personal hygiene are poor, and via the oral-oral route in settings with good hygiene. Male gender is a risk factor for paralytic outcomes. In developing countries, poliomyelitis primarily afflicts infants less than 2 years of age, while in industrialized countries members of groups objecting to vaccination are at highest risk for poliomyelitis.

During the past several years, considerable information has been obtained on the epidemiologic features of poliovirus transmission using molecular techniques.[11] In contrast to influenza viruses, which tend to spread globally on an annual basis, most polioviruses appear to circulate within relatively limited geographic areas, with occasional instances of spread to adjacent countries and infrequently across continents. The more widespread use of genomic sequencing in recent years has provided an effective tool to monitor the circulation of poliovirus genotypes, to document the spread of poliovirus from endemic areas to nonendemic areas, and to substantiate the gradual elimination of different lineages of poliovirus genotypes in polio-endemic areas. Recombinant mouse cell lines cloned with the human poliovirus receptor gene will facilitate the isolation of poliovirus because these cell lines are relatively resistant to supporting other enterovirus growth. The use of these cell lines and/or application of polymerase chain reaction facilitates detection of wild virus in sewage, water, and increasingly environmental samples as an additional means of surveillance at the national, regional, and global levels as global eradication of poliomyelitis approaches. The progress in sequencing over the past few decades has created a new "molecular epidemiology" discipline that provides high-level resolution on virus transmission, length of circulation and origin (wild or Sabin), and tracking of geographic spread of polioviruses over time.[11]

PREVENTION AND CONTROL

Vaccine Development and Use After Enders' successful propagation of poliovirus in human nonembryonic nonnervous tissue culture, Salk used this method to prepare inactivated poliovirus vaccine (IPV), which, after the largest field trial, until that time in 1954, conducted by Thomas Francis, was shown to be highly effective in preventing paralytic disease.[12] Sabin and others soon developed live attenuated strains of the three poliovirus types, which were ultimately incorporated into an orally administered, trivalent poliovirus vaccine (OPV). Because of ease of administration of OPV and improved effectiveness in preventing gut infection with wild polioviruses, Sabin's vaccine largely supplanted IPV for use in the United States and most of the world beginning in the early 1960s.

The apparent elimination of indigenous spread of wild-poliovirus infections in the United States since 1979 is due to the high coverage with effective poliovirus vaccines. After licensure of IPV in 1955, more than 450 million doses were administered to children and adults during the next 5 years. During this period, the incidence of poliomyelitis declined precipitously from 18 cases per 100,000 total population to less than 2 cases per 100,000. After licensure of OPV in 1961, the incidence of poliomyelitis declined rapidly in the United States and most other industrialized nations, as well as in some developing countries that have achieved high levels of coverage with three or more doses of OPV.[2]

Immunization, first with IPV, then OPV, eliminated the indigenous wild poliovirus genotypes in the United States in the 1960s. Subsequently, only three outbreaks of poliomyelitis occurred in the 1970s; all of these outbreaks were presumed to be due to imported virus. The only forms of poliomyelitis reported in the United States from 1979 to 1997 were the 8–10 cases annually of vaccine-associated paralytic poliomyelitis (VAPP).[13] In addition, during this period on average one poliomyelitis case classified as imported was reported each year. Changes in vaccination policy first decreased, and then eliminated VAPP in the United States after 1999.[8]

Current U.S. Polio Vaccination Policy Vaccination policies are adjusted periodically to take advantage of new products or scientific findings. From 1955 to 1961, IPV was the sole vaccine available for poliomyelitis prevention. Starting in 1961, first monovalent OPVs, and since 1963, trivalent OPV were recommended for routine immunization in the United States. From 1997 to 1999, a sequential schedule of IPV followed by OPV was used.[14] Since 2000, poliomyelitis prevention in the United States relies exclusively on IPV.[15]

The recent changes in polio-prevention policies were prompted by what in the mid-1990s became an unacceptable risk of VAPP following OPV use, especially since polio had been eliminated in the entire Western Hemisphere by 1991, and the Americas had been certified as free of indigenous wild poliovirus transmission by an international commission in 1994.

A primary series of IPV consists of three doses, administered at 2, 4, and 6–18 months, followed by a booster dose at age 4–6 years just before school entry.[15] One dose of IPV vaccine should be given to previously immunized adults who may be at increased risk of exposure to wild poliovirus (e.g., travelers to polio-endemic areas).

Consequences of OPV Use While the United States has relied since 2000 on the exclusive use of IPV for polio prevention, more than 150 countries used OPV exclusively for routine immunization and campaigns until the withdrawal of Sabin type 2 in 2016.[16] The use of OPV until 2016 was associated with VAPP (approximately 250–500 cases each year worldwide), and the emergence of vaccine-derived polioviruses (VDPVs), including circulating vaccine-derived polioviruses (cVDPVs) and immunodeficient vaccine-derived polioviruses (iVDPVs). Since the withdrawal of Sabin type 2 from OPV in 2016, the VAPP burden has decreased considerably.

cVDPVs, first described in an outbreak in Hispaniola in 2000–2001, have acquired the neurovirulent and transmission characteristics of wild polioviruses, and caused occasional outbreaks in the pretype 2 withdrawal era, but after the withdrawal of type 2 are causing outbreaks in many countries in sub-Saharan Africa, and more recently in Asia (China, Philippines, and Pakistan).[17] cVDPVs typically have more than 1% sequence diversity in the VP1 region of the genome from the parental Sabin strains (except for type 2 with

0.6% diversity) and often show evidence of recombination with other nonpolio enteroviruses. In the trivalent OPV era, extensive control efforts relying on massive use of OPV have rapidly controlled these outbreaks.

The World Health Organization (WHO) maintains a registry of cases that have excreted polioviruses for more than 6 months. As of 2019, 125 cases of iVDPVs accumulated over almost 60 years of observation are included in the registry. All individuals are immunodeficient (with disorders either affecting the B-cell system alone or together with T-cell defects), and a shift from upper- to middle-income countries was observed in the past decade. At least one individual in a high-income country has documented evidence of poliovirus excretion for more than 30 years.[18] Analysis of cases from the registry identified two patterns. While most long-term carriers stop virus excretion spontaneously or expire within a 1- to 3-year period, rarely replication and excretion of virus may continue for a much longer period, usually associated with common-variable immunodeficiency syndrome.[19] Since these patients are also at risk to develop paralytic disease and could be a source of reseeding communities with poliovirus in the future, the clearing of chronic infection and the development of effective antiviral drugs is a high priority.[20]

Global Poliomyelitis Eradication Initiative (GPEI) In 1988, the World Health Assembly adopted the goal of global polio eradication by the year 2000.[3] The initiative relies on OPV and the following strategies to accomplish the eradication target: (a) achievement and maintenance of high routine vaccination coverage levels among children with at least three doses of OPV; (b) development of sensitive systems of epidemiologic and laboratory surveillance, including the use of standard case definitions (i.e., AFP surveillance); (c) administration of supplementary doses of OPV to preschool-aged children (generally age < 5 years) during National Immunization Days (NIDs) to rapidly interrupt poliovirus transmission; and (d) "mopping-up" vaccination campaigns—localized campaigns targeted at high-risk areas where poliovirus is most likely to persist at low levels.

An extraordinary program of work, and an impressive coalition of core partners consisting of Rotary International, UNICEF, WHO, CDC, the Bill and Melinda Gates Foundations, and more recently Gavi, the Vaccine Alliance, are committed to the eradication of polio. The program of work focuses on surveillance for AFP with stool specimens collected from each case of AFP for virologic investigation in one of the 145 WHO-accredited polio network laboratories, and on support for planning, execution, and evaluation of mass vaccination campaigns. Currently, more than 10,000 staff are employed by WHO in the polio-endemic or recently endemic countries.

These efforts have had marked impact on the incidence of reported poliomyelitis cases, which has declined by more than 99.99% (from an estimated 350,000 cases in 1988 to 33 reported cases in 2018) (Fig. 98-1). During this period, the number of polio-endemic countries decreased from 125 to 3 (Afghanistan, Pakistan, and Nigeria). Four WHO regions, comprising $> 80\%$ of the world's population, including the Region of the Americas in 1991, the Western Pacific Region in 2000, the European Region in 2001, and the Region of South East Asia in 2014 are certified as polio-free by regional certification commissions. In addition, two poliovirus serotypes have already been eradicated; wild poliovirus type 2 and wild poliovirus type 3 were certified eradicated in 2015 and 2019, respectively, by the Global Certification Commission.[21]

Although substantial progress toward a polio-free world has been achieved,[9,22] by 2019 two countries continued to have ongoing transmission of poliovirus—Afghanistan and Pakistan. Nigeria, the last polio-endemic country in the African Region has not reported wild poliovirus type 1 cases since September 2016, and may have eliminated the last reservoirs of this virus. However, further review and careful assessment will be needed before the Region can be declared free of all wild poliovirus.

In 2018, a total of 33 AFP associated with wild poliovirus type 1 isolation were detected in Afghanistan and Pakistan. Unfortunately, a relative resurgence in wild poliovirus type 1 cases occurred in 2019, with 176 cases reported (data as of June 2, 2020). The reasons for the resurgence and ongoing transmission of wild poliovirus type 1 in these countries are twofold: (1) access constraints, often due to internal strife and (2) insufficient program quality. Access, at least

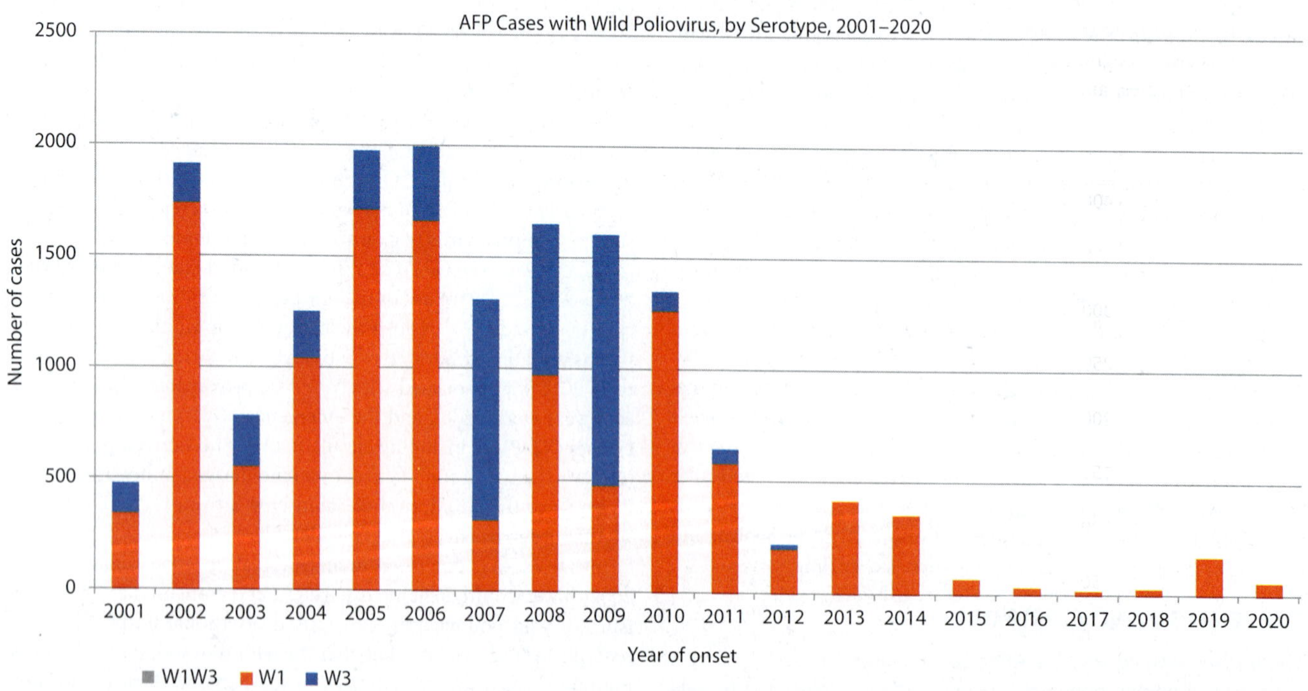

FIGURE 98-1. Wild poliovirus cases, by serotype, 2001–20.

temporarily, is mandatory both to implement the polio-eradication strategies, especially the supplemental immunization activities (SIAs), the monitoring of such activities, and to perform highly sensitive surveillance. In areas where access is assured the program needs to reach as high a proportion of the targeted children (usually those < 5 years of age). While access negotiations are often complex, in some countries local time-limited solutions are often feasible. However, to interrupt the final poliovirus transmission chains, coverage with poliovirus vaccine needs to be high, likely more than 90%. The most intractable access challenges present in Southern Afghanistan, North-Eastern Nigeria (parts of Borno), and South Somalia where large populations are living in insurgency-controlled areas. The key question is whether these populations are sufficiently large to support ongoing transmission. The quality of SIAs is carefully monitored by national and international partnership. However, despite incremental improvements in SIAs vaccination coverage over the past decades, the population immunity is not sufficiently high, or is too heterogeneous with pockets of low population immunity, to stop transmission. In Northern India, just before interruption of transmission in 2011, the seroprevalence reached > 98% in infants 6–7 months of age (usually the lowest level because of decay of passively acquired maternally derived antibody and the increase in actively induced immunity from poliovirus vaccine).[23] Thus, further sustained efforts are required in gaining access, especially in Afghanistan, and improving the quality of program efforts, both in Afghanistan and Pakistan.

The arsenal of poliovirus vaccines has greatly expanded since 2005, first with monovalent oral poliovirus vaccines type 1 (mOPV1) being rapidly developed and used massively in SIAs to interrupt transmission. Monovalent type 3 (mOPV3) and monovalent type 2 (mOPV2) followed rapidly. These monovalent vaccines are substantially more immunogenic than the corresponding Sabin serotype contained in the trivalent OPV and allow a highly targeted approach to improve the population immunity (and induce type-specific mucosal immunity). In 2009, bivalent (types 1 and 3) OPV (bOPV) was licensed and by-and-large replaced mOPVs in SIAs, and since 2016 in routine EPI vaccination schedules. bOPV is nearly as efficient as the mOPVs in inducing immunity to types 1 and 3, primarily because it has eliminated the interference of Sabin type 2. Since 2016, all countries also have included at least one dose of IPV in routine immunization schedules to mitigate the risks of poliovirus type 2 circulation. The program is also recognizing the need for genetically more stable oral poliovirus vaccines, and is in the late stages of developing a novel OPV2 vaccine.[24] This vaccine may become available in 2020 for outbreak response.

Although the goal of eradication is an ambitious one, the global poliomyelitis eradication initiative has demonstrated the feasibility of this goal in all but two countries that report wild poliovirus type 1, and it remains for mankind to demonstrate the will and tenacity to see this initiative to a successful conclusion.

Policy Development for the Post-OPV Era Progress in polio eradication suggests that the program is now dealing with two distinct challenges: (1) ongoing massive efforts to eradicate wild poliovirus type 1 in Afghanistan and Pakistan; and (2) the control of large number of cVDPV2 outbreaks after the withdrawal of Sabin type 2 from OPV in 2016 (Fig. 98-2).

The program is addressing these challenges in parallel following the blueprint contained in the detailed Strategic Plan 2013–18 (extended to 2019).[25] The plan addresses eradication, routine immunization, and sequential Sabin strain withdrawal (starting with poliovirus type 2), containment and transition. The plan was implemented and resulted in the largest withdrawal of vaccine in history. All 150 OPV-using countries changed from trivalent to bivalent OPV each individually in a 2-week period in April 2016. The plan called for the introduction of at least a single dose of inactivated poliovirus vaccine (IPV), primarily for risk mitigation purposes to ensure that a base immunity against type 2 poliovirus would be maintained that could be boosted rapidly in case of a reintroduction of epidemic or endemic spread of poliovirus type 2. More than 120 countries intended to introduce IPV for routine vaccination since 2011.

Although the withdrawal of Sabin type 2 for bivalent OPV was meticulously planned and implemented, with only a few countries experiencing emergence of circulating vaccine-derived type 2 poliovirus (cVDPV2), probably originating from a dose of trivalent OPV administered before the switch, a number of countries have experienced new outbreaks that were seeded after the switch, and either could be attributed to left-over trivalent OPV stocks or the control efforts themselves (Fig. 98-3). To control these outbreaks of cVDPV2 very large-scale immunization rounds with mOPV2 are needed. mOPV2 is the vaccine-of-choice because it induces robust mucosal immunity, a feat that IPV cannot achieve. The polio eradication program has entered a new era where the global birth cohorts grow up without mucosal immunity to poliovirus type 2. Thus, the risk of further spread of cVDPV2 and large-scale outbreaks is a new challenge that the program needs to address.

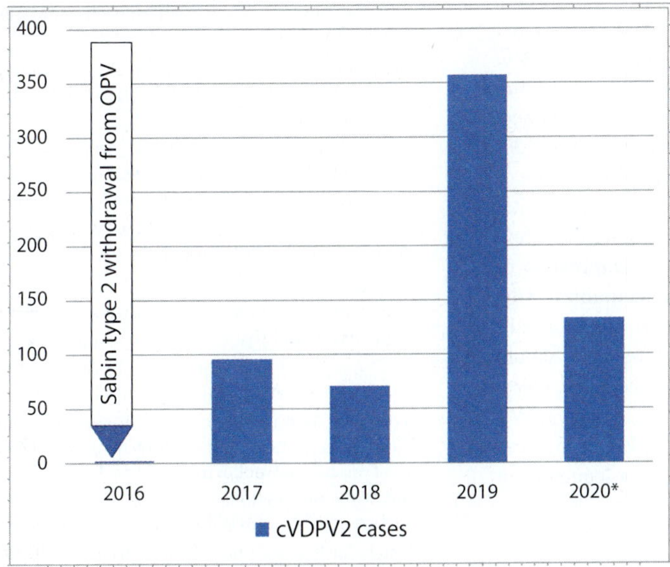

*Data as of 09 Jun 2020

FIGURE 98-2. Circulating vaccine-derived poliovirus type 2, 2016–20.

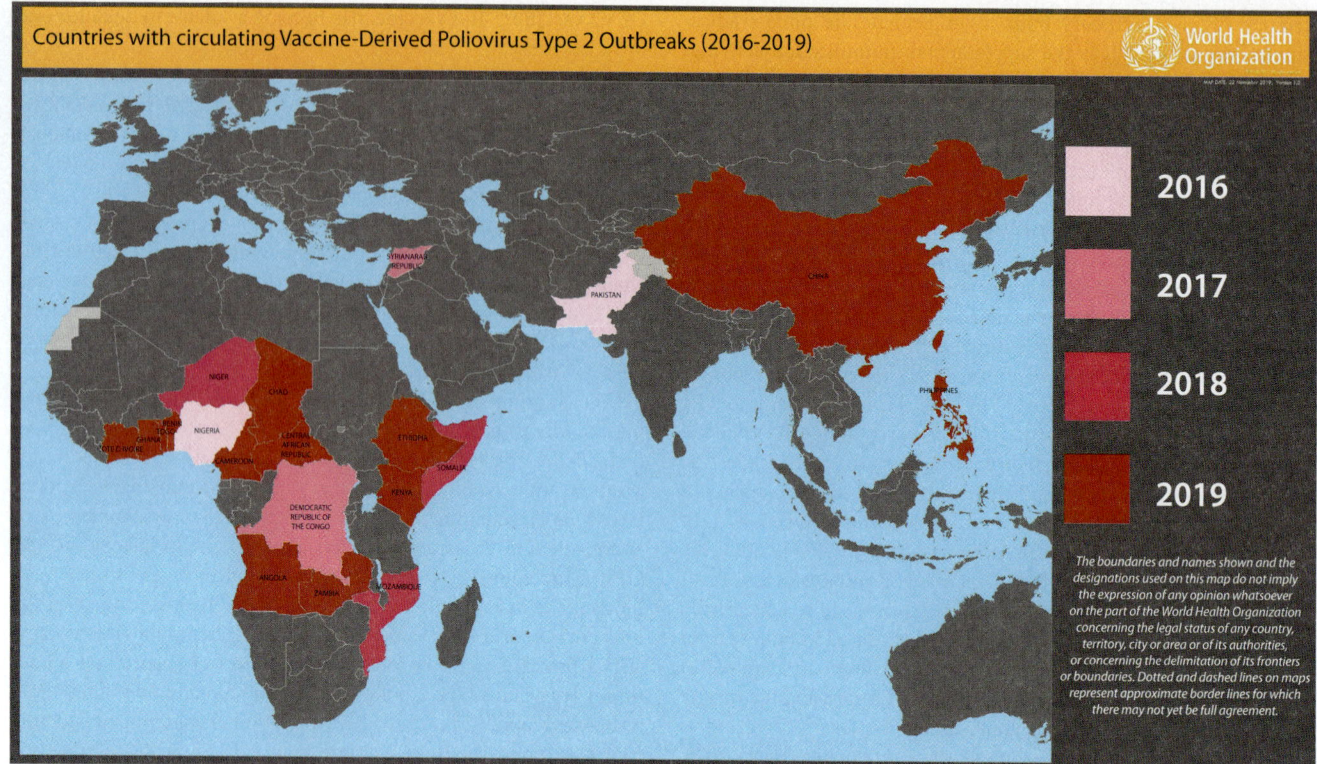
Countries with circulating Vaccine-Derived Poliovirus Type 2 Outbreaks (2016-2019)
World Health Organization
2016
2017
2018
2019
NIGER
NIGERIA
CHAD
CAMEROON
ETHIOPIA
SOMALIA
KENYA
DEMOCRATIC REPUBLIC OF THE CONGO
ANGOLA
ZAMBIA
MOZAMBIQUE
PAKISTAN
CHINA
The boundaries and names shown and the designations used on this map do not imply the expression of any opinion whatsoever on the part of the World Health Organization concerning the legal status of any country, territory, city or area or of its authorities, or concerning the delimitation of its frontiers or boundaries. Dotted and dashed lines on maps represent approximate border lines for which there may not yet be full agreement.

FIGURE 98-3. Countries with circulating vaccine-derived poliovirus type 2, 2016–20. (*Source*: Used with Permission from World Health Organisation, Geneva, Switzerland, 2020.)

Highlighted above, vaccine-derived polioviruses (VDPVs) can establish endemic or epidemic transmission, making continued use of OPV incompatible with polio eradication. Continued use of OPV after interruption of wild poliovirus transmission can generate paralytic disease due to: (a) cases of vaccine-associated paralytic poliomyelitis (VAPP), (b) outbreaks due to circulating vaccine-derived polioviruses (cVDPVs), and (c) long-term excretion of vaccine-derived poliovirus among individuals with primary immunodeficiency disorders (iVDPVs). In addition, there is a risk of paralytic cases due to wild polioviruses from: unintentional release from a contained facility (laboratory or manufacturing site) or intentional release due to an act of bioterrorism or biological warfare. These risk estimates have been quantified, and the evolution of these risks over time estimated.

An extensive program of work has been established for ensuring that the risks of facility release (from poliovirus vaccine manufacturers and diagnostic and research laboratories) of poliovirus can be minimized. This program is based on conducting inventories of poliovirus, followed by the "detect, transfer, or destroy policy," and then the designation by national competent authorities of polio-essential facilities. The latter must be certified by national authorities (i.e., national containment authority) with review and concurrence of the international authorities.

Planning for OPV cessation is focusing on managing the future risks of paralytic disease due to polioviruses. Total elimination of these risks is not feasible. Effective containment should minimize the risks of reintroduction of any poliovirus strains from laboratories or vaccine production sites. Continuing sensitive surveillance should detect the circulation of polioviruses. A coordinated OPV cessation strategy should minimize the risks of emergence of cVDPVs, and the availability of sufficient quantities of stockpile vaccines and the related response capacity should minimize the consequences of poliovirus introduction in a community.

References

1. Ramlow J, Alexander M, LaPorte R, Kaufman C, Kuller L. Epidemiology of post-polio syndrome. *Am J Epidemiol.* 1992;136:769–86.
2. Sutter RW, Kew OM, Cochi SL, Aylward BA. Poliovirus vaccine-live. In: Plotkin SA, Orenstein WA, eds . *Vaccines.* Vol. 49. 7th ed. Philadelphia, PA: Elsevier Inc.; 2018, pp. 866–916.
3. World Health Assembly. *Global Eradication of Poliomyelitis by the Year 2000. Resolutions of the 41st World Health Assembly.* Geneva, Switzerland: World Health Organization; 1988: Resolution WHA 41.28.
4. Paul JR. *A History of Poliomyelitis.* New Haven, CT: Yale University Press; 1971.
5. Evans AS, ed. *Viral Infections of Humans: Epidemiology and Control.* 3rd ed. New York: Plenum Medical Book Company; 1991.
6. Enders JF, Weller TH, Robbins FC. Cultivation of the Lansing strains of poliomyelitis virus in cultures of various human embryonic tissue. *Science.* 1949;109:85–7.
7. Mendelsohn CL, Wimmer E, Racaniello VR. Cellular receptor for poliovirus: Molecular cloning, nucleotide sequence, and expression of a new member of the immunoglobulin superfamily. *Cell.* 1989;56:855–65.
8. Alexander LN, Seward JF, Santibanez TA, et al. Vaccine policy changes and epidemiology of poliomyelitis in the United States. *JAMA.* 2004;292:1696–701.
9. Greene SA, Ahmed J, Datta SD, et al. Progress toward polio eradication—Worldwide, January 2017–March 2019. *MMWR Morb Mortal Wkly Rep.* 2019;68:458–62.
10. Lambert ML, François I, Salort C, Slypen V, Bertrand F, Tonglet R. Household survey of locomotor disability caused by poliomyelitis and landmines in Afghanistan. *BMJ.* 1997;315:1424–5.
11. Burns CC, Diop OM, Sutter RW, Kew OM. Vaccine-derived polioviruses. *J Infect Dis.* 2014;210(Suppl 1):S283–93.
12. Francis T, Napier JA, Voight RB, et al. *Evaluation of the 1954 Field Trial of Poliomyelitis Vaccine.* Ann Arbor, Michigan: Edward Brothers, Inc.; 1957.
13. Strebel PM, Sutter RW, Cochi SL, et al. Epidemiology of poliomyelitis in the United States one decade after the last reported case of indigenous wild virus-associated disease. *Clin Infect Dis.* 1992;14:568–79.
14. Centers for Disease Control and Prevention. Poliomyelitis prevention in the United States: Introduction of a sequential vaccination schedule of inactivated poliovirus vaccine followed by oral poliovirus vaccine. Recommendations of the Advisory Committee on Immunization Practices (ACIP). *MMWR Recomm Rep.* 1997;46(RR-3):1–25.
15. Centers for Disease Control and Prevention. Updated recommendations of the ACIP regarding routine poliovirus vaccination. *Morb Mortal Wkly Rep.* 2009;58:829–30.

16. Gonzalez AR, Farrell M, Menning L et al. Implementing the synchronized global switch from trivalent to bivalent oral polio vaccines—Lessons learned from the global perspective. *J Infect Dis*. 2017;216 (Suppl 1):S183–92.
17. Jorba J, Diop OM, Iber J, et al. Update on vaccine-derived poliovirus outbreaks—Worldwide, January 2018–June 2019. *MMWR Morb Mortal Wkly Rep*. 2019;15;68(45):1024–8.
18. MacLennan C, Dunn G, Huissoon AP, et al. Failure to clear persistent vaccine-derived neurovirulent poliovirus infection in an immunodeficient man. *Lancet*. 2004;363:1509–13.
19. Macklin G, Liao Y, Takane M, et al. Prolonged excretion of poliovirus among individuals with primary immunodeficiency disorder: An analysis of the World Health Organization Registry. *Front Immunol*. 2017;8:1103.
20. Collett MS, Hincks JR, Benschop K, et al. Antiviral activity of pocapavir in a randomized, blinded, placebo-controlled human oral poliovirus vaccine challenge model. *J Infect Dis*. 2017;215:335–43.
21. Global Commission for the Certification of Poliomyelitis Eradication. *14th Meeting of the Global Commission for the Certification of Poliomyelitis Eradication. Bali, Indonesia, 20–21 September 2015. Summary of Findings, Decisions and Recommendations*. Geneva: World Health Organization; 2015. http://polioeradication.org/wp-content/uploads/2016/07/1Report.pdf. Accessed November 19, 2019.
22. Mach O, Tangermann RH, Wassilak SG, Singh S, Sutter RW. Outbreaks of paralytic poliomyelitis during 1996–2012: The changing epidemiology of a disease in the final stages of eradication. *J Infect Dis*. 2014;210 (Suppl 1):S275–82.
23. Patriarca PA, Linkins RW, Sutter RW, Orenstein WA. Optimal schedule for the administration of oral poliovirus vaccine. In: Kurstak E, ed. *Measles and Poliomyelitis. Vaccines, Immunization, and Control*. Vol. 24. Wien: Springer Verlag; 1993, pp. 303–13.
24. Van Damme P, De Coster I, Bandyopadhyay AS, et al. The safety and immunogenicity of two novel live attenuated monovalent (serotype 2) oral poliovirus vaccines in healthy adults: A double-blind, single-centre phase 1 study. *Lancet*. 2019;394(10193):148–58.
25. Global Polio Eradication Initiative. *Polio Eradication & Endgame Strategic Plan 2013–2018*. Geneva: Wolrd Health Organization; 2013 (WHO/POLIO/13.02).

CHAPTER 99 Varicella*

Mona Marin

PUBLIC HEALTH SIGNIFICANCE

Varicella (chickenpox) is a highly contagious infectious disease caused by the varicella-zoster virus (VZV). Varicella is the primary infection caused by VZV, which, like other herpes viruses maintains latency in the human body and can reactivate to result in the secondary or reactivated form of disease known as herpes zoster or shingles. In temperate climates without a routine vaccination program, varicella is a common, highly communicable, childhood illness characterized by fever and a generalized pruritic vesicular exanthem. In the United States, prior to the availability of a varicella vaccine, this disease affected essentially everyone during their lifetime, with more than 95% of adults demonstrating antibodies to VZV by age 20–29 years.[1,2] In tropical climates, varicella may be acquired at older ages with more infections and a higher susceptibility in adults. Varicella may result in serious consequences both in healthy persons and those at higher risk for severe disease including newborn infants, immunocompromised persons, pregnant women, and adults.[3–6] Severe complications of varicella include sepsis, pneumonia, encephalitis, coagulation defects, shock, and death.[5–9] In the United States before the vaccine era, annually varicella was responsible for an average of 11,000–13,500 hospitalizations and 100–150 deaths.[7,8,10–12] Substantial burden of school absenteeism, costs of parental leave, and medical costs were associated with childhood varicella with net benefit to cost estimates for a routine childhood vaccination program.[13,14]

A live, attenuated, varicella vaccine (VARIVAX) was licensed for use in the United States in 1995. A combination measles, mumps, rubella, and varicella vaccine (MMRV, ProQuad) was licensed in 2005. Recommendations for routine use of varicella vaccine among children at 12–18 months of age, older susceptible children, and priority adult groups including healthcare workers were established in 1996 and further expanded in 1999.[15] Widespread use of varicella vaccine has resulted in substantial decline in varicella morbidity, mortality, and related healthcare expenditures. Despite the success of an initial one-dose childhood varicella vaccination program, one-dose vaccine effectiveness of approximately 85% has not been sufficient to prevent varicella outbreaks, which, although less common than in the prevaccine era, have continued to occur in highly vaccinated populations. In 2007, the varicella vaccination policy in the United States was changed to include a routine second dose of varicella vaccine for children.[15] Additional declines in incidence and occurrence of outbreaks have occurred since the second dose implementation.[16–18]

ETIOLOGIC AGENT AND TRANSMISSION

The varicella-zoster virus is a DNA virus of the herpes family (Herpesviridae). Humans are the only natural host. Although the etiological agent responsible for varicella and herpes zoster was not identified and named until the 1950s, herpes zoster was described in the early medical literature. Varicella, however, was frequently confused with another "pox" illness, smallpox (variola), until the end of the nineteenth century. In the early 1900s, the association between varicella and herpes zoster was suggested when von Bokay reported on the occurrence of varicella following cases of herpes zoster in two families, and this was confirmed experimentally in 1925 by demonstrating that inoculation of vesicular fluid from persons with herpes zoster led to varicella in susceptible volunteers. In 1943, herpes zoster was first suggested to be reactivation of a latent agent that had been originally acquired during varicella. Weller, in 1953, confirmed that varicella and herpes zoster have a common etiology by isolating and propagating the etiological agent from both diseases *in vitro*. He and colleagues then demonstrated that the viruses were morphologically and serologically identical, and the agent was named varicella-zoster virus in 1958.[19]

Varicella is highly contagious, with secondary attack rates in susceptible household contacts ranging from 65% to 100%.[20–23] Transmission occurs from person-to-person primarily via the respiratory route by inhalation of aerosols from vesicular fluid of skin lesions of varicella or herpes zoster; the virus can also spread by direct contact with the vesicular fluid of skin lesions and possibly infected respiratory tract secretions. The path of entry of the virus is the upper respiratory tract. The incubation period for varicella ranges from 10 to 21 days, most commonly 14–16 days. This period may be prolonged (usually for up to 28 days) in recipients of Varicella-Zoster Immune Globulin (VZIG).[15,24] A person with varicella is considered infectious from 1 to 2 days before the rash appears until all of the lesions have crusted, usually 5–7 days after onset of rash.

IMMUNE RESPONSE

VZV induces both humoral and cell-mediated immune responses. Cell-mediated immunity (CMI) to VZV is believed to be particularly important in providing long-term protection against varicella and preventing recurrences of varicella after reexposure, and in maintaining the latent state of the virus in dorsal root ganglia to prevent symptomatic reactivation as herpes zoster. Life-long immunity usually occurs following one episode of varicella. Reexposure to wild-type varicella frequently results in reinfection that boosts immunity without causing clinical illness or detectable viremia. However, rarely, recurrence of varicella has been reported in immunocompetent individuals with documented VZV immunity.[25,26] Although population-based studies suggest that symptomatic second infections of varicella may occur more frequently than anticipated, cases reported in these studies were not laboratory-confirmed.[27]

* The findings and conclusions in this chapter are those of the author and do not necessarily represent the views of the Centers for Disease Control and Prevention.

DIAGNOSIS AND LABORATORY TESTING

Laboratory tests are available to (a) confirm diagnosis of varicella, (b) assess immune status, and (c) genotype VZV strains. Diagnosis of varicella is usually made on clinical grounds, based on rash characteristics and on epidemiologic features, such as contact with other varicella patients. However, for severe or for mild vaccinated cases (i.e., with few lesions, mostly or all maculopapular) laboratory confirmation is needed. Polymerase chain reaction (PCR) is the preferred test for laboratory confirmation of acute varicella. Serologic tests are useful for identifying the immune status of individuals whose history of varicella is negative or uncertain. Viral genotyping is used to distinguish wild-type VZV from the vaccine strain (Oka) and assessing wild-type strains circulating.[28]

PCR. PCR allows rapid amplification of specific sequences of viral DNA and provides results fast (within hours). Recommended clinical samples for PCR testing are vesicular fluid, scabs, or scrapings from maculopapular lesions. In addition, respiratory secretions, cerebrospinal fluid (CSF), autopsy specimens, and buccal smear can be used.

PCR and restriction fragment length polymorphism analysis can be used to differentiate between vaccine strains and wild-type strains.[29] These are useful tools to identify vaccine-associated adverse events and differentiate vaccine-associated rash from disease that occurs among vaccinated persons (breakthrough disease).

Serology. Serological tests are available to measure IgG and IgM antibodies against VZV. Testing for IgM antibody may not be useful clinically since available methods lack sensitivity and specificity. A capture assay is the preferred method for IgM testing to decrease false positive results that may occur in the presence of high IgG levels but it is not available commercially.[30] Many tests have been used to detect IgG antibody to VZV.[31] Rising IgG antibody levels from paired acute and convalescent sera taken 2–3 weeks apart is evidence of acute infection with VZV. Single IgG assays are used to screen or verify an individual's immune status. With automation of testing equipment and high-volume testing in the laboratory setting, the enzyme-linked immunosorbent assay (ELISA) test using whole-cell VZV has replaced both latex agglutination (LA) and fluorescent antibody to membrane antigen (FAMA) as the most common serological test available. In unvaccinated persons, the presence of antibody detectable by one of these assays may be considered evidence of past infection with VZV and hence evidence of immunity. In addition, in unvaccinated persons, reported history of disease was highly predictive of serological immunity and likely continues to be for adults. However, a study conducted after 7–8 years of varicella vaccine use in the United States indicates that positive predictive value of disease history in children may not be high.[32] Therefore, laboratory testing or epidemiological link to typical cases at the time of infection are recommended to be sought to assess evidence of immunity.

Levels of antibody following vaccination are usually lower than those following natural varicella infection and may not be detected by commercially available whole-cell ELISA tests. A highly sensitive gpELISA test, using purified viral glycoproteins as antigens, was developed for testing of immunogenicity in vaccine clinical trials but is not commercially available at the present time.[33] This test, as well as fluorescent antibody to membrane antigen (FAMA), are considered gold standards for testing immunity in vaccinees.[31]

Other Virologic Tests. The most commonly available and widely used test is the direct immunofluorescent antibody (DFA) test which is rapid (results are available in several hours) and highly specific, however, it is only about 60% as sensitive as PCR. The DFA test uses immunofluorescence procedures to label polyclonal or monoclonal antibodies, which bind to VZV antigens to allow the rapid identification of VZV proteins in cells from the base of skin lesions. Direct and indirect immunofluorescence methods may detect VZV infected cells in tissue sections of lung, liver, brain, and other organs in patients with disseminated primary or recurrent VZV infection. Crusts from lesions are not suitable for use with DFA.

Cultures for VZV, though confirming unequivocally the diagnosis of VZV infection, require a minimum of 2 days, more frequently at least 5 days, to detect infectious virus in cell culture and are less sensitive compared with PCR because the virus is very labile outside cells. Although in clinical cases of varicella, VZV is difficult to isolate from sites other than skin lesions, VZV has been cultured from clinical specimens such as autopsy samples or CSF, and rarely from throat, pharyngeal, and conjunctival specimens. Viable VZV cannot be recovered from crusted lesions.

CLINICAL CHARACTERISTICS

Varicella is generally a mild disease in children and most people recover without serious complications. The disease presents with a characteristic rash often accompanied by fever. In older children and adults the exanthem is preceded by a short (1–3 days) prodromal period (fever, malaise, irritability); younger children may have no prodrome. Systemic symptoms also are milder in children than in adults. Fever [~38–390°C (100–1020°F)] is present during the peak of rash evolution and disappears by the time all the vesicles have either dried or crusted over. Infection usually produces a typical clinical illness; clinically inapparent or asymptomatic primary infection is estimated to occur in no more than 5% of susceptible children.[34]

The characteristic rash is pruritic, appears in successive crops and quickly (24 hours) evolves from macules to papules to clear, fluid-filled vesicles approximately 2–4 mm in diameter. Early in the illness all stages of the rash coexist. The vesicles are initially surrounded by an erythematous base, which fades during the process of crusting. Vesicles sequentially become purulent and dry and crust over. The crust, which is not infectious, may remain intact from 1 to 3 weeks. The rash is distributed centrally with more lesions occurring on the face, scalp, and trunk than on the extremities; in a typical presentation ~250–300 vesicles are present. Lesions are not confined to the skin and can develop on any mucosal surface including inside the mouth and vagina. They can also develop on the cornea[35] and tympanic membranes. Patients with altered immunity may develop new lesions for an extended period.

Approximately 20% of one-dose vaccinated persons may develop varicella if exposed to VZV. Persons who received two doses of vaccine are less likely to develop disease than those who received one dose.[15] Varicella that occurs *more than* 42 days after vaccination is known as "breakthrough" disease. Breakthrough varicella is substantially less severe, with shorter duration of illness and with approximately 80% of the patients developing less than 50 lesions.[36,37] Fever may not be present, and most or all lesions may be of pruritic maculopapular type, rather than vesicular. Therefore, it is easy to miss breakthrough varicella or misclassify it (e.g., insect bites, enteroviral infection). However, vaccinated patients who develop breakthrough disease are infectious. Patients with breakthrough varicella with > 50 lesions are as infectious as unvaccinated patients[23] whereas vaccinated patients with < 50 lesions are one-third as infectious as unvaccinated patients.

COMPLICATIONS

Varicella may be followed by complications. The risk of complications is higher among immunocompromised persons, neonates, adolescents, and adults than among children.[5,7,8,10,11,38] Severe disease and deaths do occur in previously healthy individuals. Serious complications include secondary bacterial infections, pneumonia, postinfectious encephalitis, cerebellar ataxia, Reye's syndrome, and death.[5,39–41] Rarer complications include nephritis, arthritis, Guillain-Barré syndrome, stroke, thrombocytopenia, and clinical hepatitis. Though clinical hepatitis occurs rarely, evidence of subclinical hepatitis is frequent.[30]

Complications from varicella vary by age. In healthy children with varicella, secondary bacterial infections of skin lesions, usually due to *Staphylococcus* or *Streptococcus*, are the most common complications requiring hospitalization.[10,11,40] Reports of life-threatening or lethal invasive group A beta-hemolytic streptococcus infections include cellulitis, necrotizing fasciitis, septic arthritis, osteomyelitis, septicemia, and toxic shock syndrome. Neurologic complications are the second most common indication for hospitalization for healthy children with varicella. Central nervous system (CNS) complications, meningoencephalitis, and cerebellar ataxia are more frequent in children younger than 5 years and in adults aged 20 years and older.[4] Among unvaccinated children, varicella-associated encephalitis is estimated to occur in 1 case per 50,000 reported varicella cases,[4] and cerebellar ataxia in approximately 1 per 4000 cases.[38] Reye's syndrome has become a rare complication following the marked decline in use of salicylates among children with varicella.[42]

A higher rate of complications occurs in adults where systemic involvement is more prominent. Primary varicella pneumonia is the most common, life-threatening complication in adults.[40] Estimates of the frequency of pneumonia complicating varicella in healthy adults have varied widely from 0.3% to 50% with wide ranges also in fatality from pneumonia of 9% to 50%.[43–46] Hemorrhagic complications occur more commonly in adults than in healthy children and include thrombocytopenia associated with bleeding into skin lesions, petechiae, purpura, hematuria, and gastrointestinal hemorrhage. This may proceed to disseminated intravascular coagulopathy, shock, and death. Some, but not all, studies have suggested that pregnant women have a higher risk of complications than do nonpregnant adults of childbearing age.[47] However, these data are predominantly from case reports and case series from referral hospitals.

Varicella has been identified as an underlying cause of death every year in the United States. Septic and CNS complications, pneumonia, and hemorrhagic conditions are the most common causes of death following varicella disease.[6–8] Overall varicella case-fatality rate is highest among infants, adults, and persons with immunocompromising conditions, and lowest among children 1–9 years of age.[7] In the United States, during the prevaccine years of 1970–94, the varicella mortality rate was 0.4 deaths per million population. Most varicella deaths occurred among previously healthy individuals; during 1990–94, 89% and 75% of child and adult deaths, respectively, occurred among individuals without severe underlying conditions.[7]

In immunocompromised patients, all expressions of the infection may be markedly enhanced.[3,30,48] In such patients, atypical severe presentations of varicella may be difficult to distinguish from disseminated herpes zoster. Severe varicella and serious complications with multiorgan system involvement have been described in many situations associated with an immunocompromised state including leukemia and other cancers, HIV/AIDS, disorders of the immune system and immunosuppression secondary to use of steroids or cancer chemotherapeutic drugs.[49,50] Numerous studies suggest that an impaired cellular immune state is the major contributing factor.

Neonatal Varicella. Prior to the advent of antiviral therapy, as many as 30% of infected infants whose mothers had a varicella rash within 5 days before delivery died of the disease. The risk of serious illness is highest when maternal onset of varicella is from 5 days before delivery to 2 days afterward since the baby acquires VZV via a viremia but does not acquire passive immunity transplacentally. Disease earlier in pregnancy is associated with the passage of protective maternal antibody to the fetus.[51]

Congenital (Fetal) Varicella Syndrome. Maternal infection within the first 26 weeks of gestation can lead to congenital varicella syndrome, a constellation of congenital defects including hypoplasia of an extremity, cicatricial skin scarring, localized muscular atrophy, encephalitis, microcephaly, cortical atrophy, ocular abnormalities, mental retardation, and low birth weight. This syndrome has been estimated to occur in about 0.4% of infections that occur from weeks 0 to 12 and 2.0% of infections that occur from weeks 13 to 20; the latest infection reported in pregnancy that resulted in congenital varicella syndrome is 25 1/2 weeks.[52,53] Gestational varicella is also associated with an increased risk of zoster occurring at an early age especially within the first year of life.[51]

TREATMENT

Antiviral drugs are available for treatment of varicella. Acyclovir is a synthetic nucleoside analog that inhibits replication of human herpes viruses including VZV; it is available in both oral and intravenous forms and is most effective when administered within 24 hours of rash onset.[15,54] Oral acyclovir is not recommended routinely for the treatment of uncomplicated varicella in healthy children, but is recommended for treatment of primary varicella among certain groups at increased risk of severe disease or its complications. This includes people older than 12 years of age, people with chronic cutaneous or pulmonary disorders, people receiving long-term salicylate therapy, and people receiving short intermittent or aerosolized courses of corticosteroids.[54] Valacyclovir and famciclovir can also be used. These drugs are highly active against VZV by the same mechanism as acyclovir and are better absorbed by the oral route. Since oral acyclovir is poorly absorbed, IV acyclovir is recommended for the treatment of severe primary varicella and/or serious complications of varicella in healthy or immunocompromised individuals and for recurrent zoster in immunocompromised persons. VZV resistance to acyclovir has not proven to be a problem in immunocompetent hosts. In immunocompromised hosts, acyclovir-resistant VZV infections have been reported and may become an increasing problem with the use of prolonged acyclovir therapy for patients with chronic or recurrent herpes zoster infections. For such patients, the best alternative therapy is foscarnet.[55,56]

EPIDEMIOLOGY

In temperate climates, in the absence of vaccination, varicella is a disease of childhood with 80–90% cases occurring before 10 years of age.[2,20,57,58] In the United States, during the 1980s, the highest annual incidence rate was described in 5- to 9-year-old children followed by the 1–4 age group[2,57,58]; by early adulthood, 95% of the population was immune to varicella; among persons more than 30 years of age, varicella seroprevalence was > 99%.[1] This pattern was also described in many European countries.[59,60]

Varicella has been less commonly a childhood disease in the tropics, with more frequent disease occurring among adults. The reasons for this difference in the age-specific incidence of varicella in tropical compared with temperate climates are unclear but may include differences in population size, population density, crowding, and higher ambient temperatures or humidity resulting in decreased transmission in the tropics.

The routine varicella vaccination program implemented in the United States in 1996 resulted in rapid increases in vaccination coverage and dramatic declines in varicella morbidity and mortality. One-dose vaccination coverage among children 19–35 years of age increased from 27% in 1997 to 90–91% during 2007–17.[61] During the one-dose vaccination program (1996–06) overall, incidence declined 80–90%; the median age of infection has increased however, the incidence has declined in all age groups.[62] Varicella-related hospitalizations and deaths declined by 88% from prevaccine years through 2002 and 2006, respectively, with 92–95% decline among persons age < 20 years, representing the cohort who had received routine vaccination.[63,64] Although the varicella vaccination program resulted in substantial declines in cases, hospitalizations, and deaths due to varicella, outbreaks continued to be reported among both unvaccinated and vaccinated school children, including in highly vaccinated school populations.[65–67] These outbreaks prompted a recommendation in

2007 for a routine second dose of varicella vaccine for children.[15] Additional declines in disease burden have occurred during the two-dose era: incidence declined 98% during 1990–2016, hospitalizations declined 93% in 2012 versus the prevaccine period, and deaths declined 96% during 2012–16 compared with 1990–94.[16,68,69] Varicella outbreaks have also declined in size (i.e., number of cases) and duration.[17,18] Each year, more than 3.5 million cases of varicella, 9000 hospitalizations, and 100 deaths are prevented by varicella vaccination in the United States.

PREVENTION AND CONTROL

Active Immunization. Varicella is a vaccine-preventable disease. Several varicella vaccines are licensed; all contain live attenuated VZV and all, except for the vaccine used in South Korea, are based on the Oka strain of VZV isolated in Japan. Varicella vaccines are available as monovalent and combination MMRV vaccine. Although varicella vaccines have worldwide availability, they are recommended for routine use only in a small number of primarily developed countries. As of 2018, 18% of countries have introduced a routine varicella vaccination program and an additional 6% have varicella vaccination programs for risk groups only.[70] In 1996, the United States became the first country to introduce varicella vaccine into its routine childhood immunization program. The formulation licensed for use in the United States (VARIVAX) contains more than 1350 plaque forming units (PFU) (~1.13 log10) of Oka/Merck VZV in each 0.5 mL dose. In the MMRV combination vaccine (ProQuad), the varicella dose has been increased to 3.99 log10 PFU to obtain comparable immunogenicity provided by VARIVAX. Varicella vaccine is administered subcutaneously (0.5 mL dose).

In the United States, monovalent varicella vaccine is approved for use in healthy persons aged 12 months and older and MMRV is approved for children 12 months through 12 years of age. The Advisory Committee on Immunization Practice (ACIP) and the American Academy of Pediatrics (AAP) recommend that all children receive a first dose of varicella vaccine at 12–15 months of age and a second dose at 4–6 years of age.[15,54] Catch-up two-dose vaccination is recommended for persons who are older than 6 years of age and do not have evidence of immunity. Evidence of immunity includes: (1) age appropriate vaccination one dose for preschool-aged children 12 months or older and two doses for school-aged children, adolescents, and adults), (2) laboratory evidence of immunity or laboratory confirmation of disease, (3) birth in the United States before 1980, (4) diagnosis or verification of a history of varicella by a healthcare provider, and (5) diagnosis or verification of a history of herpes zoster by a healthcare provider.[15,54] The minimum interval between doses is 3 months for persons through 12 years of age and 4 weeks for persons 13 years of age or older. In outbreak settings, a second dose of vaccine is recommended for persons who have received one dose of vaccine to prevent further spread. ACIP recommends assessment of pregnant women for varicella immunity and postpartum vaccination of susceptible women. HIV-infected children with age-specific CD4+T lymphocyte percentages of $\geq$ 15% and adolescents and adults with CD4+T lymphocyte counts > 200 cells/μL should be considered for vaccinations with two doses of varicella vaccine (only monovalent vaccine can be used for HIV+ persons).

Vaccine Immunogenicity and Effectiveness. Approximately 73–86% of children vaccinated in clinical trials have achieved titers 5 gpELISA units and more (level considered to be associated with protection against disease[71,72]) 4–6 weeks after a single dose vaccination.[73,74] The proportion of subjects with antibody titers 5 gpELISA units and more was significantly higher 6 weeks after the second dose compared with the first dose (99.6% vs. 85.7%) and remained high at the end of the 9-year follow-up, although the difference between the two regimens did not persist (97% vs. 95%).[74]

The humoral immunity has been shown to persist for more than 20 years in a study in Japan and for up to 10 years in studies in the United States in 93–100% of child vaccinees.[74–77] However, other studies found that 25–31% of adult vaccinees who seroconverted lost detectable antibodies (FAMA) at intervals ranging from 1 to 11 years after vaccination and that 9–21% of vaccinees developed breakthrough disease.[78–80] CMI persisted in 87–94% vaccinated children and adults for 5–6 years following vaccination.[77,81,82]

Clinical trials prior to licensure demonstrated vaccine efficacies for one dose of vaccine ranging from 70% to 100% depending on the age at vaccination, dosage, number of doses given, type of exposure (household or community), length of follow-up, and outcome of disease studied, that is, level of severity of disease. In the randomized clinical trial of one versus two doses of varicella vaccine administered three months apart, the estimated vaccine efficacy of one versus two doses for a 10-year observation period was 94.4% and 98.3%, respectively ($p < 0.001$).[74]

Since licensure, effectiveness of varicella vaccine under field conditions has been assessed in childcare, school, and household and community settings using a variety of methods. Effectiveness has frequently been estimated against varicella and against moderate and/or severe varicella. Outbreak investigations have assessed effectiveness against clinically defined varicella. The majority of these investigations in the United States have found one-dose vaccine effectiveness for prevention of varicella in the range most commonly described in prelicensure trials (70%–90%) with some lower estimates < 50% (20% and 44%) and some higher (100%) estimates.[83] A meta-analysis that included 58 vaccine effectiveness estimates for one dose and 34 for two doses, found a pooled vaccine effectiveness of 81% [95% confidence interval (CI): 78–84%] for one dose and 92% (95% CI: 88–95%) for two doses.[84] Most of the studies were conducted within the first decade after vaccination.

Post-licensure studies that have assessed vaccine performance in preventing moderate and severe varicella have consistently demonstrated extremely high effectiveness against these outcome measures. Definitions for disease severity have varied between studies from using a defined scale of illness that includes number of skin lesions, fever, complications, and investigator assessment of illness severity to using the number of skin lesions and reported complications or hospitalizations. Irrespective of definition differences, one-dose varicella vaccine has been 90% and more effective in preventing moderate or severe disease, pooled vaccine effectiveness was 98% (95% CI: 97–99%).[84] When effectiveness against severe disease was measured separately, 24 estimates reported 100% with one study reporting 86% (for prevention of varicella-related hospitalizations).

Several studies, including those conducted during outbreak investigations identified younger age at vaccination (varying between less than 14 and 19 months of age), time since vaccination ($\geq$3 years or $\geq$ 5 years), asthma, or eczema as potential risk factors for vaccine failure but the majority have not included sample sizes sufficient for independent assessment.[83,84] However, to date, no factor has been clearly established as a risk factor for developing breakthrough disease. Only one cohort study controlled simultaneously for the effect of multiple risk factors and found that the use of oral steroids within the last 3 months of varicella vaccine, age at vaccination (<15 months) and administration MMR within 28 days of varicella vaccination were risk factors for breakthrough varicella disease.[85] Another study found that the effectiveness of vaccine in the first year after vaccination was substantially lower (73%) among children vaccinated at age less than 15 months; however, the difference between children vaccinated at age less than 15 months and at 15 months and more did not persist in the 7 subsequent years.[86] A multivariate logistic regression analysis of U.S. surveillance data revealed that the annual rate of breakthrough varicella significantly increased with the time since vaccination and that varicella was twice as likely to be moderate/severe (defined as > 50 skin lesions) in those who developed disease > 5 years after vaccination compared with those who became ill < 5 years after vaccination.[87] Further studies are needed to confirm this finding. To date, no increases in rate of complications, hospitalizations, or deaths have been reported with time since vaccination in countries with a one-dose program. A longitudinal study of a cohort of more than 7500 children and adolescents found a major reduction in varicella incidence and hospitalization in the 15 years after the introduction of varicella vaccine, with no evidence of a shift in the burden of varicella to older age groups.[88] Persistence of immunity in the absence of exposure to the wild virus and natural boosting of immunity needs to continue to be monitored.

Vaccine Safety. The vaccine is well tolerated in healthy individuals. Local pain and/or redness at the injection site, fever, and generalized varicella-like rash may occur. From prelicensure clinical trials, the reported incidence of rash at the injection site post vaccination was approximately 3–4% among children, adolescents, and adults following the first dose. For generalized rash, these rates are 4% for children and 6% for adolescents and adults, respectively. The median number of lesions was low—two at the injection site and five for generalized rash.[15] Fever was reported in a higher proportion after the first dose of MMRV compared with the first dose of MMR vaccine and varicella vaccine administered as separate injections at the same visit (22% vs. 15%) in young children.[89] The vaccine virus is capable of reactivating to cause HZ.[90,91] Postlicensure data indicated that the risk for HZ among vaccinated children is 80% less than among unvaccinated children.[92] Other rarely reported adverse events include pharyngitis, cellulitis, hepatic pathology, pneumonia, erythema multiforme and Stevens-Johnson Syndrome (SJS), arthropathy, thrombocytopenia, anaphylaxis, and aplastic anemia.[93,94] They all accounted for reporting rates lower than 1 case per 100,000 doses sold. Neurological adverse events accounted for a reporting rate of 3.8 per 100,000 doses sold and included neuropathy, convulsion, ataxia, encephalopathy, and meningitis.[95]

Postlicensure data suggest that the risk of transmission of varicella vaccine virus from healthy persons is very low; in particular, in the absence of rash in the vaccinee. Through 2018, and with > 140 million doses of varicella vaccine distributed in the United States alone, only 13 cases of transmission of the varicella vaccine virus from 11 immunocompetent vaccine recipients have been reported, 6 had a varicella-like rash and 5 had HZ.[96] Secondary cases have typically been mild.

MMRV is associated with a slightly higher risk for febrile seizures compared with MMR and varicella vaccine as separate injections, one additional febrile seizure is expected to occur per 2300–2600 young children vaccinated with a first doses of MMRV compared with a first dose of MMR plus varicella vaccine.[97]

Contraindications and Precautions. Contraindications and precautions to vaccination include pregnancy (women should avoid pregnancy for 1 month after receiving a dose of varicella vaccine), allergy to vaccine components (vaccine contains neomycin, but does not contain egg protein or preservatives), recent administration of blood, plasma or immune globulin, altered immunity including malignant conditions, and conditions that require steroid therapy (>2 mg/kg/day or a total of 20 mg/day of prednisone or its equivalent). The vaccine is not recommended for persons with cellular immunodeficiencies but can be administered to persons with impaired humoral immunity. VARIVAX is contraindicated for HIV-infected children with age-specific CD4+ T-lymphocyte of less than 15%.[15] A pregnancy registry established to monitor outcomes of pregnant women inadvertently vaccinated 3 months before or at any time during pregnancy did not detect any cases with abnormal features suggestive of congenital varicella syndrome or increased prevalence of other birth defects.[98,99]

Postexposure Vaccination. One dose of varicella vaccine administered within 3 days of exposure to a person with rash is at least 90% effective in preventing varicella. If administered within 5 days of exposure vaccine is approximately 70% effective in preventing disease and 100% effective in modifying it.[100] Therefore, vaccination is recommended within 3–5 days of exposure; however, vaccination after this interval is still recommended given that the vaccine will provide protection against future exposures for those whose current exposure might not result in efficient transmission.[15]

Passive Immunization. VZIG (available product in the United States is Varizig) is recommended for postexposure prophylaxis in susceptible persons at high risk for developing severe disease who have been exposed to VZV. Varizig has been shown to be effective in reducing the severity of varicella when given up to 10 days after exposure.[101] It should, however, be given as soon as possible after exposure. The decision to administer Varizig to a person exposed to varicella is based on whether (a) the person is susceptible, (b) the exposure is likely to result in infection, and (c) the patient is at greater risk for complications than the general population. Identified high-risk groups include newborn infants whose mothers developed varicella around the time of delivery (from 5 days before to 2 days after delivery), immunocompromised persons including those on immunosuppressive medications and steroids, pregnant women without evidence of immunity, hospitalized premature infants born at 28 weeks or longer gestation whose mothers have no history of varicella and/or antibodies to VZV, and hospitalized premature infants born at less than 28 weeks gestation or who weigh 1000 g or less at birth regardless of the mother's history of varicella.[15] The recommended dose is one vial (125 U) per 10 kg body weight and up to a maximum of 625 U/person given by intramuscular injection.

Isolation Guidelines. Isolation of individuals with varicella until all lesions have crusted is a routine outbreak control measure. Quarantine is recommended for exposed susceptible individuals who may be in contact with persons at high risk of serious complications, for example, healthcare workers and families of immunocompromised persons. Such isolation is required for the duration of the period of communicability, that is, from the eighth until the twenty-first day postexposure or until the twenty-eighth day if the exposed individual receives Varizig.

FUTURE PUBLIC HEALTH NEEDS

More than 20 years of experience with the varicella vaccination program in the Unites States show that varicella vaccine is safe and effective in preventing varicella-related morbidity and mortality. The varicella vaccination program has been tremendously successful in reducing morbidity and mortality (90% or more). Therefore, wider use of vaccine through its integration into routine childhood vaccination programs is beneficial in other countries where this disease is an important public health and socioeconomic problem. One dose varicella vaccine is approximately 80–85% effective in preventing any disease and close to 100% in preventing severe disease. Therefore, if the country focus is to reduce mortality and severe morbidity from varicella, a one-dose schedule could be implemented into routine immunization. Two doses induce higher effectiveness (~92%) and are needed in countries where the programmatic goal is, in addition to decreasing mortality and severe morbidity, to further reduce the number of cases and outbreaks which might continue to occur with a one-dose schedule. Long-term duration of protections for both one and two doses of varicella vaccine, especially in the absence of exposure to the wild virus and natural boosting of immunity needs to continue to be monitored. An additional benefit of varicella vaccination is the reduction of the risk for herpes zoster documented among children. Continued monitoring is needed to assess whether this reduced herpes zoster risk is maintained as varicella vaccinated persons age and reach the age at higher risk for herpes zoster (50 years and older).

Surveillance is critical to establish and monitor impact of vaccination programs. However, varicella surveillance in many countries, is a challenge as the number of varicella cases remains high and varicella in vaccinated persons is mostly a mild disease and difficult to diagnose. In addition to increasing completeness of reporting, surveillance will benefit greatly from reduction in varicella incidence and wide availability of diagnostic tests. Countries with varicella vaccination programs in place need to continue to monitor the changing epidemiology of both varicella and herpes zoster.

References

1. Kilgore PE, Kruszon-Moran D, Seward JF, et al. Varicella in Americans from NHANES III: Implications for control through routine immunization. *J Med Virol*. 2003;70(Suppl 1):S111–8.
2. Wharton M. The epidemiology of varicella-zoster virus infections. *Infect Dis Clin North Am*. 1996;10(3):571–81.
3. Feldman S, Hughes WT, Daniel CB. Varicella in children with cancer: Seventy-seven cases. *Pediatrics*. 1975;56(3):388–97.
4. Preblud SR. Age-specific risks of varicella complications. *Pediatrics*. 1981; 68(1):14–7.
5. Preblud SR. Varicella: Complications and costs. *Pediatrics*. 1986;78(4 Pt 2): 728–35.
6. Preblud SR, Orenstein WA, Bart KJ. Varicella: Clinical manifestations, epidemiology and health impact in children. *Pediatr Infect Dis*. 1984; 3(6):505–9.
7. Meyer PA, Seward JF, Jumaan AO, Wharton M. Varicella mortality: Trends before vaccine licensure in the United States, 1970–1994. *J Infect Dis*. 2000;182(2):383–90.
8. Nguyen HQ, Jumaan AO, Seward JF. Decline in mortality due to varicella after implementation of varicella vaccination in the United States. *N Engl J Med*. 2005;352(5):450–8.
9. Weller TH. Varicella: Historical perspective and clinical overview. *J Infect Dis*. 1996;174(Suppl 3):S306–9.
10. Davis MM, Patel MS, Gebremariam A. Decline in varicella-related hospitalizations and expenditures for children and adults after introduction of varicella vaccine in the United States. *Pediatrics*. 2004;114(3):786–92.
11. Galil K, Brown C, Lin F, Seward J. Hospitalizations for varicella in the United States, 1988 to 1999. *Pediatr Infect Dis J*. 2002;21(10):931–5.
12. Ratner AJ. Varicella-related hospitalizations in the vaccine era. *Pediatr Infect Dis J*. 2002;21(10):927–31.
13. Lieu TA, Cochi SL, Black SB, et al. Cost-effectiveness of a routine varicella vaccination program for US children. *JAMA*. 1994;271(5):375–81.
14. Zhou F, Ortega-Sanchez IR, Guris D, Shefer A, Lieu T, Seward JF. An economic analysis of the universal varicella vaccination program in the United States. *J Infect Dis*. 2008;197(Suppl 2):S156–64.
15. Marin M, Guris D, Chaves SS, Schmid S, Seward JF. Prevention of varicella: Recommendations of the Advisory Committee on Immunization Practices (ACIP). *MMWR Recomm Rep*. 2007;56(RR-4):1–40.
16. Lopez AS, Zhang J, Marin M. Epidemiology of varicella during the 2-dose varicella vaccination program—United States, 2005–2014. *MMWR Morb Mortal Wkly Rep*. 2016;65(34):902–5.
17. Leung J, Lopez AS, Blostein J, et al. Impact of the US two-dose varicella vaccination program on the epidemiology of varicella outbreaks: Data from nine states, 2005–2012. *Pediatr Infect Dis J*. 2015;34(10):1105–9.
18. Lopez AS, LaClair B, Buttery V, et al. Varicella outbreak surveillance in schools in sentinel jurisdictions, 2012–2015. *J Pediatr Infect Dis Soc*. 2019;8(2):122–7.
19. Weller TH, Witton HM, Bell EJ. The etiologic agents of varicella and herpes zoster; isolation, propagation, and cultural characteristics *in vitro*. *J Exp Med*. 1958;108(6):843–68.
20. Hope Simpson RE. Infectiousness of communicable diseases in the household (measles, chickenpox, and mumps). *Lancet*. 1952;2(6734):549–54.
21. Ross AH. Modification of chicken pox in family contacts by administration of gamma globulin. *N Engl J Med*. 1962;267:369–76.
22. Asano Y, Nakayama H, Yazaki T, Kato R, Hirose S. Protection against varicella in family contacts by immediate inoculation with live varicella vaccine. *Pediatrics*. 1977;59(1):3–7.
23. Seward JF, Zhang JX, Maupin TJ, Mascola L, Jumaan AO. Contagiousness of varicella in vaccinated cases: A household contact study. *JAMA*. 2004;292(6):704–8.
24. Hanngren K, Falksveden L, Grandien M, Lidin-Janson G. Zoster immunoglobulin in varicella prophylaxis. A study among high-risk patients. *Scand J Infect Dis*. 1983;15(4):327–34.
25. Gershon AA, Steinberg SP, Gelb L. Clinical reinfection with varicella-zoster virus. *J Infect Dis*. 1984;149(2):137–42.
26. Junker AK, Angus E, Thomas EE. Recurrent varicella-zoster virus infections in apparently immunocompetent children. *Pediatr Infect Dis J*. 1991;10(8):569–75.
27. Hall S, Maupin T, Seward J, et al. Second varicella infections: Are they more common than previously thought? *Pediatrics*. 2002;109(6): 1068–73.
28. Jensen NJRP, Tseng HF, Quinlivan M, et al. Revisiting the genotyping scheme for varicella-zoster viruses based on whole-genome comparisons. *J Gen Virol*. 2017;98(6):1434–8.
29. LaRussa P, Lungu O, Hardy I, Gershon A, Steinberg SP, Silverstein S. Restriction fragment length polymorphism of polymerase chain reaction products from vaccine and wild-type varicella-zoster virus isolates. *J Virol*. 1992;66(2):1016–20.
30. Arvin AM. Varicella-zoster virus. *Clin Microbiol Rev*. 1996;9(3):361–81.
31. Krah DL. Assays for antibodies to varicella-zoster virus. *Infect Dis Clin North Am*. 1996;10(3):507–27.
32. Perella D, Fiks AG, Jumaan A, et al. Validity of reported varicella history as a marker for varicella zoster virus immunity among unvaccinated children, adolescents, and young adults in the post-vaccine licensure era. *Pediatrics*. 2009;123(5):e820–8.
33. Wasmuth EH, Miller WJ. Sensitive enzyme-linked immunosorbent assay for antibody to varicella-zoster virus using purified VZV glycoprotein antigen. *J Med Virol*. 1990;32(3):189–93.
34. Gordon JE. Chickenpox: An epidemiological review. *Am J Med Sci*. 1962;244: 362–89.
35. Pavan-Lanston D. Ophthalmic zoster. In: Arvin AM, Gershon AA, eds. *Varicella-Zoster Virus, Virology and Clinical Management*. Cambridge, UK: Cambridge University Press; 2000, pp. 276–98.
36. Chaves SS, Zhang J, Civen R, et al. Varicella disease among vaccinated persons: Clinical and epidemiological characteristics, 1997–2005. *J Infect Dis*. 2008;197(Suppl 2):S127–31.
37. Bernstein HH, Rothstein EP, Watson BM, et al. Clinical survey of natural varicella compared with breakthrough varicella after immunization with live attenuated Oka/Merck varicella vaccine. *Pediatrics*. 1993;92(6):833–7.
38. Guess HA, Broughton DD, Melton LJ3rd, Kurland LT. Population-based studies of varicella complications. *Pediatrics*. 1986;78(4 Pt 2):723–7.
39. Aebi C, Ahmed A, Ramilo O. Bacterial complications of primary varicella in children. *Clin Infect Dis*. 1996;23(4):698–705.
40. Choo PW, Donahue JG, Manson JE, Platt R. The epidemiology of varicella and its complications. *J Infect Dis*. 1995;172(3):706–12.
41. Jackson MA, Burry VF, Olson LC. Complications of varicella requiring hospitalization in previously healthy children. *Pediatr Infect Dis J*. 1992;11(6): 441–5.
42. Remington PL, Rowley D, McGee H, Hall WN, Monto AS. Decreasing trends in Reye syndrome and aspirin use in Michigan, 1979 to 1984. *Pediatrics*. 1986;77(1):93–8.
43. Krugman S, Goodrich CH, Ward R. Primary varicella pneumonia. *N Engl J Med*. 1957;257(18):843–8.
44. Nilsson A, Ortqvist A. Severe varicella pneumonia in adults in Stockholm County 1980–1989. *Scand J Infect Dis*. 1996;28(2):121–3.
45. Gogos CA, Bassaris HP, Vagenakis AG. Varicella pneumonia in adults. A review of pulmonary manifestations, risk factors and treatment. *Respiration*. 1992;59(6):339–43.
46. Feldman S. Varicella-zoster virus pneumonitis. *Chest*. 1994;106(1 Suppl): 22S–7.
47. Gnann JWJr. Varicella-zoster virus: Prevention through vaccination. *Clin Obstet Gynecol*. 2012;55(2):560–70.
48. LaRussa P. Clinical manifestations of varicella. In: Arvin AM, Gershon AA, eds. *Varicella-Zoster Virus: Virology and Clinical Management*. Cambridge, England: Cambridge University Press; 2000, pp. 206–19.
49. Dowell SF, Bresee JS. Severe varicella associated with steroid use. *Pediatrics*. 1993;92(2):223–8.
50. Reiches NA, Jones JF. Steroids and varicella. *Pediatrics*. 1993;92(2):288–9.
51. Brunell PA. Fetal and neonatal varicella-zoster infections. *Semin Perinatol*. 1983;7(1):47–56.
52. Salzman MB, Sood SK. Congenital anomalies resulting from maternal varicella at 25 1/2 weeks of gestation. *Pediatr Infect Dis J*. 1992;11(6): 504–5.
53. Enders G, Miller E, Cradock-Watson J, Bolley I, Ridehalgh M. Consequences of varicella and herpes zoster in pregnancy: Prospective study of 1739 cases. *Lancet*. 1994;343(8912):1548–51.
54. American Academy of Pediatrics. Varicella-zoster infections. In: Kimberlin DW, Brady MT, Jackson MA, Long SS, eds. *Red Book: 2018 Report of the Committee on Infectious Diseases*. 31st ed. Itasca, IL: American Academy of Pediatrics; 2018, pp. 869–83.
55. Enright AM, Prober C. Antiviral therapy in children with varicella zoster virus and herpes simplex virus infections. *Herpes*. 2003;10(2):32–7.

56. Whitley RJ. Treatment of varicella. In: *Varicella-Zoster Virus, Virology and Clinical Management.* Cambridge, UK: Cambridge University Press; 2000, pp. 385–95.
57. Finger R, Hughes JP, Meade BJ, Pelletier AR, Palmer CT. Age-specific incidence of chickenpox. *Public Health Rep.* 1994;109(6):750–5.
58. Seward JF, Watson BM, Peterson CL, et al. Varicella disease after introduction of varicella vaccine in the United States, 1995–2000. *JAMA.* 2002;287(5):606–11.
59. Nardone A, de Ory F, Carton M, et al. The comparative sero-epidemiology of varicella zoster virus in 11 countries in the European region. *Vaccine.* 2007;25(45):7866–72.
60. Boelle PY, Hanslik T. Varicella in non-immune persons: Incidence, hospitalization and mortality rates. *Epidemiol Infect.* 2002;129(3):599–606.
61. Hill HA, Elam-Evans LD, Yankey D, Singleton JA, Kang Y. Vaccination coverage among children aged 19–35 Months—United States, 2017. *MMWR Morb Mortal Wkly Rep.* 2018;67(40):1123–28.
62. Bialek SR, Perella D, Zhang J, et al. Impact of a routine two-dose varicella vaccination program on varicella epidemiology. *Pediatrics.* 2013;132(5): e1134–40.
63. Lopez AS, Zhang J, Brown C, Bialek S. Varicella-related hospitalizations in the United States, 2000–2006: The 1-dose varicella vaccination era. *Pediatrics.* 2011;127(2):238–45.
64. Marin M, Zhang JX, Seward JF. Near elimination of varicella deaths in the US after implementation of the vaccination program. *Pediatrics.* 2011;128(2):214–20.
65. Lopez AS, Guris D, Zimmerman L, et al. One dose of varicella vaccine does not prevent school outbreaks: Is it time for a second dose? *Pediatrics.* 2006;117(6):e1070–7.
66. Gould PL, Leung J, Scott C, et al. An outbreak of varicella in elementary school children with two-dose varicella vaccine recipients—Arkansas, 2006. *Pediatr Infect Dis J.* 2009;28(8):678–81.
67. Tugwell BD, Lee LE, Gillette H, Lorber EM, Hedberg K, Cieslak PR. Chickenpox outbreak in a highly vaccinated school population. *Pediatrics.* 2004;113(3 Pt 1):455–9.
68. Leung J, Bialek SR, Marin M. Trends in varicella mortality in the United States: Data from vital statistics and the national surveillance system. *Hum Vaccin Immunother.* 2015;11(3):662–8.
69. Leung J, Harpaz R. Impact of the maturing varicella vaccination program on varicella and related outcomes in the United States: 1994–2012. *J Pediatr Infect Dis Soc.* 2016;5(4):395–402.
70. World Health Organization. WHO vaccine-preventable diseases: Monitoring system. 2017 global summary [cited 2018 Mar 13]. http://apps.who.int/immunization_monitoring/globalsummary.
71. Chan IS, Li S, Matthews H, et al. Use of statistical models for evaluating antibody response as a correlate of protection against varicella. *Stat Med.* 2002;21(22):3411–30.
72. Li S, Chan IS, Matthews H, et al. Inverse relationship between six week postvaccination varicella antibody response to vaccine and likelihood of long term breakthrough infection. *Pediatr Infect Dis J.* 2002;21(4):337–42.
73. White CJ, Kuter BJ, Ngai A, et al. Modified cases of chickenpox after varicella vaccination: Correlation of protection with antibody response. *Pediatr Infect Dis J.* 1992;11(1):19–23.
74. Kuter B, Matthews H, Shinefield H, et al. Ten year follow-up of healthy children who received one or two injections of varicella vaccine. *Pediatr Infect Dis J.* 2004;23(2):132–7.
75. Asano Y, Suga S, Yoshikawa T, et al. Experience and reason: Twenty-year follow-up of protective immunity of the Oka strain live varicella vaccine. *Pediatrics.* 1994;94(4 Pt 1):524–6.
76. Kuter BJ, Weibel RE, Guess HA, et al. Oka/Merck varicella vaccine in healthy children: Final report of a 2-year efficacy study and 7-year follow-up studies. *Vaccine.* 1991;9(9):643–7.
77. Watson B, Gupta R, Randall T, Starr S. Persistence of cell-mediated and humoral immune responses in healthy children immunized with live attenuated varicella vaccine. *J Infect Dis.* 1994;169(1):197–9.
78. Ampofo K, Saiman L, LaRussa P, Steinberg S, Annunziato P, Gershon A. Persistence of immunity to live attenuated varicella vaccine in healthy adults. *Clin Infect Dis.* 2002;34(6):774–9.
79. Gershon AA, Steinberg SP, LaRussa P, Ferrara A, Hammerschlag M, Gelb L. Immunization of healthy adults with live attenuated varicella vaccine. *J Infect Dis.* 1988;158(1):132–7.
80. Saiman L, LaRussa P, Steinberg SP, et al. Persistence of immunity to varicella-zoster virus after vaccination of healthcare workers. *Infect Control Hosp Epidemiol.* 2001;22(5):279–83.
81. Nader S, Bergen R, Sharp M, Arvin AM. Age-related differences in cell-mediated immunity to varicella-zoster virus among children and adults immunized with live attenuated varicella vaccine. *J Infect Dis.* 1995;171(1):13–7.
82. Zerboni L, Nader S, Aoki K, Arvin AM. Analysis of the persistence of humoral and cellular immunity in children and adults immunized with varicella vaccine. *J Infect Dis.* 1998;177(6):1701–4.
83. Seward JF, Marin M, Vazquez M. Varicella vaccine effectiveness in the US vaccination program: A review. *J Infect Dis.* 2008;197(Suppl 2): S82–9.
84. Marin M, Marti M, Kambhampati A, Jeram SM, Seward JF. Global varicella vaccine effectiveness: A meta-analysis. *Pediatrics.* 2016;137(3): e20153741.
85. Verstraeten T, Jumaan AO, Mullooly JP, et al. A retrospective cohort study of the association of varicella vaccine failure with asthma, steroid use, age at vaccination, and measles-mumps-rubella vaccination. *Pediatrics.* 2003;112(2):e98–103.
86. Vazquez M, LaRussa PS, Gershon AA, et al. Effectiveness over time of varicella vaccine. *JAMA.* 2004;291(7):851–5.
87. Chaves SS, Gargiullo P, Zhang JX, et al. Loss of vaccine-induced immunity to varicella over time. *N Engl J Med.* 2007;356(11):1121–9.
88. Baxter R, Tran TN, Ray P, et al. Impact of vaccination on the epidemiology of varicella: 1995–2009. *Pediatrics.* 2014;134(1):24–30.
89. Kuter BJ, Brown ML, Hartzel J, et al. Safety and immunogenicity of a combination measles, mumps, rubella and varicella vaccine (ProQuad). *Hum Vaccin.* 2006;2(5):205–14.
90. Sharrar RG, LaRussa P, Galea SA, et al. The postmarketing safety profile of varicella vaccine. *Vaccine.* 2000;19(7–8):916–23.
91. Weinmann S, Chun C, Schmid DS, et al. Incidence and clinical characteristics of herpes zoster among children in the varicella vaccine era, 2005–2009. *J Infect Dis.* 2013;208(11):1859–68.
92. Weinmann S, Naleway AL, Koppolu P, et al. Incidence of herpes zoster among children: 2003–2014. *Pediatrics.* 2019;144(1):e20182917.
93. Chaves SS, Haber P, Walton K, et al. Safety of varicella vaccine after licensure in the United States: Experience from reports to the vaccine adverse event reporting system, 1995–2005. *J Infectious Dis.* 2008;197(Suppl 2): S170–7.
94. Galea SA, Sweet A, Beninger P, et al. The safety profile of varicella vaccine: A 10-year review. *J Infect Dis.* 2008;197(Suppl 2):S165–9.
95. Wise RP, Salive ME, Braun MM, et al. Postlicensure safety surveillance for varicella vaccine. *JAMA.* 2000;284(10):1271–9.
96. Marin M, Leung J, Gershon AA. Transmission of vaccine-strain varicella-zoster virus: A systematic review. *Pediatrics.* 2019;144(3):e20191305.
97. Marin M, Broder KR, Temte JL, Snider DE, Seward JF. Use of combination measles, mumps, rubella, and varicella vaccine: Recommendations of the Advisory Committee on Immunization Practices (ACIP). *MMWR Recomm Rep.* 2010;59(RR-3):1–12.
98. Marin M, Willis ED, Marko A, et al. Closure of varicella-zoster virus-containing vaccines pregnancy registry—United States, 2013. *MMWR Morb Mortal Wkly Rep.* 2014;63(33):732–3.
99. Wilson E, Goss MA, Marin M, et al. Varicella vaccine exposure during pregnancy: Data from 10 years of the pregnancy registry. *J Infect Dis.* 2008;197(Suppl 2):S178–84.
100. Macartney K, McIntyre P. Vaccines for post-exposure prophylaxis against varicella (chickenpox) in children and adults. *Cochrane Database Syst Rev.* 2008;(3):CD001833.
101. Levin MJ, Duchon JM, Swamy GK, Gershon AA. Varicella zoster immune globulin (VARIZIG) administration up to 10 days after varicella exposure in pregnant women, immunocompromised participants, and infants: Varicella outcomes and safety results from a large, open-label, expanded-access program. *PLoS One.* 2019;14(7):e0217749.

CHAPTER

100 Human Papillomavirus

Julia W. Gargano • Lauri E. Markowitz

Advances in virology during the 1970s established the existence of multiple distinct types of human papillomavirus (HPV). These virologic discoveries, when combined with epidemiologic studies, and the recognition that viral DNA can be integrated into the host genome, enabled the eventual identification of the causal role of specific HPV types in cervical cancers and later other cancers, as well as anogenital warts and recurrent respiratory papillomatosis (RRP).[1,2] These advances and the identification of HPV types 16 and 18 in the majority of cervical cancers, as well as in precancers, later led to the development of prophylactic HPV vaccines; this work was recognized with a portion of the 2008 Nobel Prize in Physiology or Medicine for Harald zur Hausen.[1,3]

Genital HPV infection is the most common sexually transmitted infection worldwide[4,5] Studies have shown that HPV is prevalent in all regions of the world, with an average prevalence of 11% in females with normal cervical cytology, a correlation between prevalence in females and males, and variation by geographic region.[4] An estimated 4.5% of all cancers worldwide, 630,000 cancers annually, are attributable to HPV.[6] In the United States, an estimated 14 million persons are newly infected every year, resulting in an estimated U.S.$1.7 (U.S.$0.8–U.S.$2.9) billion in direct medical costs.[7] HPV infections are commonly acquired soon after initiation of sexual activity.[8,9] Although the vast majority of HPV infections cause no symptoms and are self-limited, persistent HPV infection can cause cervical cancer as well as other anogenital cancers in women, penile cancer in men, and oropharyngeal and anal cancers in men and women[6,10] HPV is also the cause of anogenital warts and RRP.[11]

NOMENCLATURE AND CLASSIFICATION

HPVs are in the family *Papillomaviridae.*[12] All are double-stranded DNA viruses, with a small (8 kb) circular genome, share a common organization, and encode two late (L) and several early (E) proteins. HPVs have two capsid proteins, L1 and L2. L1 is the major capsid protein. The L1 capsid proteins can self-assemble to form virus-like particles (VLPs), with type-specific conformational epitopes; these are the basis of currently available prophylactic vaccines.[13] The early proteins are responsible for viral DNA replication and transcriptional regulation (E1 and E2), virus assembly and virion release (E4), and transformation (E5, E6, and E7).[12,14] Not all early genes are present in all HPV types; E6 and E7 are the primary oncoproteins in oncogenic HPV types.[12,15]

More than 200 HPV types have been identified.[12,15,16] These are classified into five genera (evolutionary groups) based on the degree of L1 sequence homology[12,15]: alpha, beta, gamma, mu, and nu. All five genera include cutaneous types, and the alpha genus also includes all mucosal types.[15] Within genera, species are denoted with numbers (e.g., alpha-1, alpha-2, beta-3, gamma-10). HPV types were numbered in order of discovery, therefore the type numbers bear no relation to the genus and species designation. Types differ by at least 10% in L1.[12] Future changes to the nomenclature system for HPV are under consideration.[12]

Many HPV types preferentially infect nonmucosal skin surfaces. Most of these cutaneous HPV types are in the beta and gamma genera. They can be transmitted through direct and indirect contact and can cause common skin warts. Some epidemiologic evidence has linked squamous cell carcinoma of the skin and its precursor lesion, actinic keratosis, with nontype-specific HPV infection; however, it is not yet known whether this is a causal association. If there is a causal association, it is possibly a complex one that also includes ultraviolet damage, immunosuppression, or genetics as cofactors.[17]

Approximately 40 types, all in the alpha genus, preferentially infect the genital mucosa.[15,16,18] These genital HPV types are categorized according to their epidemiologic association with cervical cancer.[17] The International Agency for Research on Cancer (IARC), has classified 12 HPV types (16, 18, 31, 33, 35, 39, 45, 51, 52, 56, 58, and 59) as human carcinogens based on their association with cervical cancer. These are typically referred to as high-risk (HR), or oncogenic, HPV types. Additionally, several other types in the alpha genus have limited evidence linking them to cervical cancer, including one type classified as probably carcinogenic (HPV 68) and seven types classified as possibly carcinogenic (HPV 26, 53, 66, 67, 70, 73, and 82).[17] High-risk HPV types can cause low-grade cervical cell abnormalities, and high-grade cervical cell abnormalities that are precursors to cancer.[2,17,19] Nearly all cervical cancers are attributable to high-risk HPV types,[20] and approximately 70% of cervical cancer cases worldwide are caused by two types: 16 and 18.[21] HPV 16 infection is also responsible for most cases of other HPV-attributable anogenital cancers such as cancers of the vulva, vagina, penis, and anus, as well as cancers arising in some oropharynx subsites.[17] Nonhigh-risk HPV types, also sometimes called low-risk types, can cause anogenital warts, benign or low-grade cervical cell changes, and RRP.[11] Nonhigh-risk HPV types 6 and 11 cause 90% of anogenital warts and nearly all RRP.

PATHOGENESIS AND NATURAL HISTORY

The HPV life cycle consists of a sequence of several distinct phases that allow the viruses to be sustained in the population.[12,14] Infection is initiated when viral episomes infect the basal layer of the epithelium, which is exposed through microabrasions, or at the squamocolumnar junction. Infection is established as low copy number episome in basal and parabasal layers. Viral DNA is amplified as the infected cells migrate toward the epithelial surface. The DNA is subsequently packaged into infectious virions, and is shed through desquamation.

While HPV is a common infection, most HPV infections are transient and do not cause disease. Over 90% of incident HPV infections, including those with high-risk types, clear or become undetectable within 2 years; clearance usually occurs in the first 6 months after infection.[22–24] Persistent infection with high-risk HPV is the most important risk factor for HPV-attributable diseases including cancer precursors and invasive cancer.[22,23,25–27] Although persistent infection with high-risk HPV types is considered necessary for cervical cancer development, it is not sufficient because the vast majority of women with high-risk HPV infection do not develop cancer.[22,28,29] The risk for persistence and progression to cancer varies by both HPV type and host factors.[30] For instance, HPV 16 is more likely to persist and progress to cancer than other high-risk HPV types.[31–33] Usually, decades elapse between incident HPV infection and development of cervical cancer, but more rapid progression can occur.[34] Some aspects of the natural history of HPV are not well understood, including latent infections and redetection and the role and duration of naturally acquired immunity after HPV infection.[35,36]

EPIDEMIOLOGY OF HPV INFECTIONS

Prevalence and Incidence

Because HPV cannot be cultured directly from patient specimens, epidemiologic studies to estimate prevalence and incidence of HPV infections are based on molecular testing, most commonly assays that detect HPV DNA.[12] Incidence and prevalence of genital (cervical or vaginal) HPV infection in women are highest in young women aged $<$ 25 years, coinciding with high incidence following sexual debut.[9,37] Studies in female university students found that the cumulative incidence of HPV infection within 1 year of initiating sex with their first male partner was 28.5%.[38] Another study found that the 3-year cumulative incidence in college women was 43%.[29] Incidence and prevalence are lower in successively older age groups after the early 20s, although a second smaller prevalence peak in middle age has been observed in some, but not all, regions of the world.[9,38] In the United States, as part of the nationally representative National Health and Nutrition Examination Surveys (NHANES), the prevalence of genital HPV has been monitored since 2003 using self-collected vaginal swabs in girls and women aged 14–59 years.[39] Data from NHANES have been used to define demographic characteristics and behaviors associated with HPV prevalence and to monitor declines in HPV prevalence after introduction of the United States vaccination program in 2006, In NHANES, as well as in many studies worldwide, the total number of lifetime sex partners is the most important determinant of HPV prevalence.[39–41]

Genital HPV prevalence in males follows a somewhat different pattern than that observed in females. Following the initial peak in prevalence soon after initiation of sexual activity, similar to that seen in females, prevalence is not much lower in in older age groups.[8,40,42,43] While the reasons for this sex difference are not known with certainty, possible explanations include a higher number of sex partners throughout the life course for males[44] and/or differences in type specific immunity after clearance of infection, both of which would contribute to higher incidence in older age groups among males.[45,46] In the United States, prevalence of HPV DNA in male genital (penile) swabs has been monitored in NHANES since 2013. As with females, the lifetime number of sex partners is the most important determinant of HPV prevalence.[40]

Overall, among all sexually experienced persons aged 14–59 years in the U.S. population, the estimated prevalence of any HPV detected at genital sites was slightly higher in males than in females (45.8% in males vs. 40.1% in females); a similar difference was observed for HR-HPV prevalence (25.7% in males, 20.7% in females).[40] However, the overall prevalence estimates obscured age-specific prevalence differences by sex. Generally, HPV prevalence was higher in females in the younger age groups and higher in males in their 40s and 50s.

Epidemiologic studies have provided some insight into risk factors for anal HPV infection. In women, concurrent HPV infections with the same type can often be detected at the anus and cervix, which suggests a shared exposure or autoinoculation from one site to the other, with the cervix suggested as a viral reservoir; the total number of lifetime sex partners is a more important determinant of anal HPV infection than experience with anal intercourse.[47,48] In men, cohort studies have identified a higher incidence of anal HPV infections in men who have sex with men (MSM) than in men who have sex with women (MSW).[49]

Oral HPV prevalence, at 6.9% in the general population, is much lower than genital or anal HPV prevalence.[50] Oral HPV prevalence is higher in men than in women overall (10.1% vs. 3.6%) and in all age groups.[50] The higher incidence and prevalence of oral HPV among males compared with females is not explained by differences in number of lifetime sex partners or oral sex partners.[51,52] Similar to genital HPV infections, the vast majority of oral HPV infections become undetectable and do not progress to cancer.

Antibody responses to HPV infection differ by sex; females are more likely to seroconvert from a natural HPV infection than males.[45,46,53] This may be the result of tissue differences at site of initial HPV infection, as seroconversion may be more likely following exposure at mucosal sites with nonkeratinized epithelium (e.g., cervix) than keratinized epithelium (e.g., penis).[45,46] Prior to vaccine introduction, seroprevalence in populations can be used as a measure of lifetime exposure to specific HPV types among females, although it underestimates exposure as not all females develop antibody after infection; it is a poor measure of exposure among males.[54,55]

Transmission

Mucosal HPV types are mainly transmitted through skin-to-skin sexual contact, including through vaginal, anal, or oral sex, or through other close genital contact.[56–60] Some studies suggest that deep kissing can also transmit oral HPV infections.[61,62] Transmission has been hypothesized via shared sex toys or hands, but more recent research suggests that hand to genital transmission is unlikely.[56,63] Autoinoculation from one body site to another (e.g., from genitals to mouth) is believed to occur. Vertical transmission of HPV from a mother to her infant, most likely at the time of delivery, is believed to be the main route of transmission for juvenile onset RRP.[11,64]

High-risk Populations

Several population groups are known to have higher risk of acquiring an HPV infection, and/or have a higher risk of disease following infection. In general, immunocompromised persons are less likely to clear HPV infections and more likely to develop anogenital warts, cervical precancer and cancers, and other HPV-associated diseases. Individuals who have had solid organ transplants have higher risk of HPV-associated cancers than the general population, likely attributable to immunosuppressive medications.[65] Individuals with HIV infection are more likely to have persistent HPV infection and to be infected with multiple HPV types simultaneously, and are less likely to clear their HPV infection. The risk of invasive cancer is several times higher in HIV-infected persons with HPV.[66–69] Other groups, including MSM, are considered high-risk for infection because they have a higher risk of HPV exposure, through sexual behavior and sexual networks having a higher prevalence of infection.[70] In a systematic review that included studies evaluating prevalence in MSM and MSW, HPV16 prevalence was significantly higher in MSM than MSW, among those HIV-negative (14% vs. 3%) and HIV-positive (30% vs. 11%).[70] Anal cancer rates are much higher in MSM, especially among MSM living with HIV/AIDS.[66]

HPV-ASSOCIATED DISEASES

Diseases Caused by Oncogenic HPV Types

Oncogenic HPV can cause cervical, vulvar, and vaginal cancers in women, penile cancer in men, and oropharyngeal and anal cancers in women and men. Worldwide oncogenic HPV causes an estimated 630,000 cancers annually, including 570,000 cancers in women and 60,000 cancers in men.[6] The most common HPV-attributable cancers

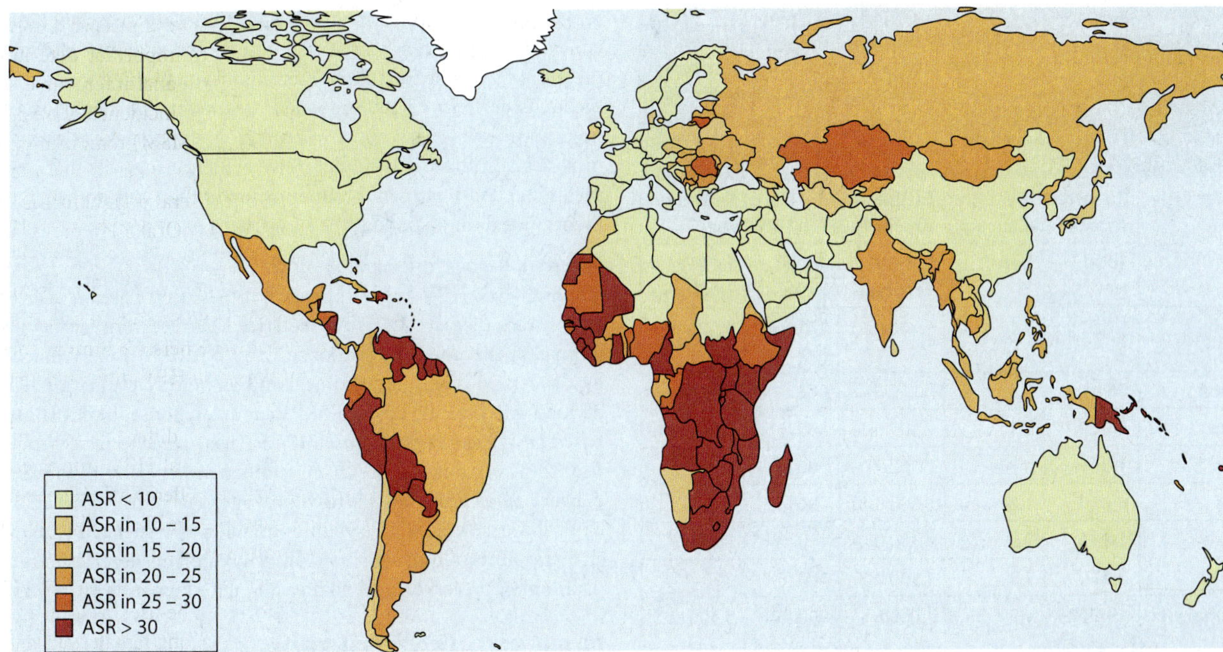

FIGURE 100-1. Age-standardized (world) incidence rates (per 100,000) of cervical cancer cases attributable to HPV in 2012. It is available on page 2 of this pdf: 23-Cervix-uteri-fact-sheet.pdf (iarc.fr). ASR = age-standardized rate. (*Source*: Used with permission from de Martel C, Plummer M, Vignat J, Franceschi S. Worldwide burden of cancer attributable to HPV by site, country and HPV type. *Int J Cancer*. 2017;141(4):664–670. doi:10.1002/ijc.30716.)

in males are of the oropharynx (24,000/year), anus (17,000/year), and penis (13,000/year). The most common HPV-attributable cancers in females are of the uterine cervix (530,000/year), anus (18,000/year), and vagina (12,000/year).

Global Distribution of HPV-attributable Neoplasia

Among the cancers attributable to HPV infection, invasive cervical cancer has historically been considered the most important worldwide, with about 570,000 new cases and 311,000 deaths in 2018.[71] The geographic distribution of HPV-attributable cancers varies by anatomic site, with cervical cancer concentrated in sub-Saharan Africa, some Latin American countries, and other areas lacking cervical cancer screening infrastructure and/or a high burden of HIV infection (Fig. 100-1). Deaths from cervical cancer predominantly occur in low-income countries that lack sufficient cervical cancer screening programs; as many of these deaths occur in relatively young women, deaths from cervical cancer are particularly consequential for their families and communities.[6] By contrast, oropharyngeal cancers are concentrated in higher-income countries; noncervical anogenital HPV-associated cancers more evenly distributed worldwide. While cervical cancer remains the most important HPV-attributable cancer in women, oropharyngeal cancer has surpassed cervical cancer as the highest-incidence HPV-attributable cancer in the United States, and the majority of the oropharyngeal cancer burden is in men.[72]

HPV-type Attribution

Data on the attribution of HPV in various HPV-associated cancers has been reported through tissue typing studies. The largest study to date, an international effort including paraffin-embedded specimens from 38 countries, identified HPV in 85% of specimens. Of cervical cancers with any HPV detected, HPV types 16 and 18 were identified in 71%, and HPV types 31, 33, 35, 45, 52, and 58 were identified in a further 20%.[21] In the United States, the HPV-type distribution in HPV-associated cancers was determined through a special typing study using tissues obtained from cases diagnosed prior to vaccine introduction. HPV was detected in about 90% of cervical cancers, 90% of anal cancers, 75% of vaginal cancers, 70% of oropharyngeal cancers, 70% of vulvar cancers, and 60% of penile cancers.[73]

Epidemiology of HPV-associated Cancers in the United States

For the United States, estimates of HPV-attributable cancers are made by applying the HPV type distribution measured in special typing studies to incidence data for HPV-associated cancers from cancer registries.[73–75] For the years 2012–16, an estimated 43,999 cancers were reported annually at HPV-associated anatomic sites; Of these, 32,100 were cancers attributable to an HPV type targeted by the 9-valent HPV vaccine (9vHPV), and 2700 were attributable to other HPV types (Table 100-1).[75] Cancer rates vary by anatomic site and sex. In recent years, the highest rate observed was for oropharyngeal cancer in males, at 8.5 per 100,000. This was higher than the cervical cancer rate (7.2) or oropharyngeal cancer rate in females (1.7). Rates of anal squamous cell carcinoma were higher among females (2.3) than males. There are differences in rates of some cancers by race; for example, non-Hispanic black and Hispanic females have the highest incidence of cervical cancer and white males have the highest incidence of oropharyngeal cancer.[74]

The age at cancer diagnosis varies by anatomic site and sex.[74,76] The median age at diagnosis of cervical cancer is 49 years. Other HPV-associated cancers in women are diagnosed later: 62 years for anus and oropharynx, 66 years for vulva, and 67 years for vagina. In men, the median age at diagnosis for anal cancer is 59 years, for oropharyngeal cancer is 61 years, and for penile cancer is 69 years.

Diseases Caused by Nononcogenic HPV Types

Anogenital Warts

Almost all anogenital warts are caused by nononcogenic HPV types 6 or 11.[77,78] Anogenital warts typically develop approximately 2–3 months after HPV infection, but can appear much later. Anogenital warts should be assessed by a clinician; they are usually diagnosed by visual inspection, although biopsy may be helpful in some cases. Untreated, anogenital warts can resolve spontaneously (20–30%), remain unchanged, or increase in size or number. Because warts might spontaneously resolve, an acceptable approach for some persons is to forego treatment and monitor for spontaneous resolution within 1 year. Unfortunately, anogenital warts commonly recur within 3 months, whether clearance occurs spontaneously or following treatment.[79]

Detailed treatment guidelines for anogenital warts have been published.[80] The main aim of treatment is removal of the wart

TABLE 100-1 AVERAGE ANNUAL NUMBER AND RATE OF HUMAN PAPILLOMAVIRUS (HPV)-ASSOCIATED CANCERS AND ESTIMATED PERCENTAGE AND ANNUAL NUMBER OF CANCERS ATTRIBUTABLE TO HPV, BY HPV TYPE, CANCER TYPE, AND SEX—UNITED STATES,* 2012–16[74]

Cancer Type	Reported HPV-Associated Cancers[a]		Estimated No.[b] (%) of Cancers Attributable to HPV Types		
	Total No.[c]	Rate[d]	9vHPV-Targeted	Other HPV	HPV-Negative
Cervix	**12,015**	7.2	9,700 (81)	1,200 (10)	1,100 (9)
Vagina	**862**	0.4	600 (73)	0 (2)	300 (25)
Vulva	**4,009**	2.1	2,500 (63)	300 (6)	1,200 (31)
Penis	**1,303**	0.8	700 (57)	100 (6)	500 (37)
Anus	**6,810**	1.8	6,000 (88)	200 (3)	600 (9)
Female	**4,539**	2.3	4,100 (90)	100 (2)	300 (8)
Male	**2,270**	1.3	1,900 (83)	100 (6)	300 (11)
Oropharynx	**19,000**	4.9	12,600 (66)	900 (5)	5,500 (29)
Female	**3,460**	1.7	2,100 (60)	100 (3)	1,300 (37)
Male	**15,540**	8.5	10,500 (68)	800 (5)	4,200 (28)
Total	**43,999**	**12.2**	**32,100 (73)**	**2,700 (6)**	**9,200 (21)**
Female	**24,886**	**13.7**	**19,000 (76)**	**1,700 (7)**	**4,200 (17)**
Male	**19,113**	**10.6**	**13,100 (69)**	**1,000 (5)**	**5,000 (26)**

*Compiled from population-based cancer registries that participate in the CDC National Program of Cancer Registries, and/or the National Cancer Institute's Surveillance, Epidemiology, and End Results Program and meet the criteria for high data quality for all years during 2012–2016, covering 100% of the U.S. population. This information is in the original source, here: https://www.cdc.gov/mmwr/volumes/68/wr/mm6833a3.htm (Table 100-1).

[a]HPV-associated cancers were defined as invasive cancers at anatomic sites with cell types in which HPV DNA frequently is found. All cancers were histologically confirmed. Cervical cancers (ICD-O-3 site codes C53.0–C53.9) are limited to carcinomas (ICD-O-3 histology codes 8010–8671, 8940–8941). Vaginal (ICD-O-3 site code C52.9), vulvar (ICD-O-3 site codes C51.0–C51.9), penile (ICD-O-3 site codes C60.0–60.9), anal (ICD-O-3 site codes C20.9, C21.0–C21.9) and oropharyngeal (ICD-O-3 site codes C01.9, C02.4, C02.8, C05.1, C05.2, C09.0, C09.1, C09.8, C09.9, C10.0, C10.1, C10.2, C10.3, C10.4, C10.8, C10.9, C14.0, C14.2, and C14.8) cancer sites are limited to squamous cell carcinomas (ICD-O-3 histology codes 8050–8084, 8120–8131).

[b]HPV-attributable cancers are cancers that are probably caused by HPV (https://academic.oup.com/jnci/article/107/6/djv086/872092external icon). Estimates for attributable fraction were based on studies that used population-based data from cancer tissue studies to estimate the percentage of those cancers probably caused by HPV. The estimated number of cancers attributable to HPV was calculated by multiplying the number of reported HPV-associated cancer cases by the percentage of each cancer type attributable to HPV. The total of HPV-attributable cancers is the sum of cancers attributable to types included in the 9vHPV and cancers attributable to other HPV types (e.g. 32,100 + 2,700 = 34,800). Estimated counts were rounded to the nearest 100 (counts <100 are not displayed) and might not sum to total because of rounding. "9vHPV-targeted" types include oncogenic HPV types 16, 18, 31, 33, 45, 52, and 58. "Other HPV" includes other oncogenic HPV types. "HPV-negative" cancers are those that occur at anatomic sites in which HPV-associated cancers are often found, but HPV DNA was not detected.

[c]The total reported count is the annual count averaged over the 5-year period and might not sum to total because of rounding.

[d]Rates are per 100,000 persons; age-adjusted to the 2000 U.S. standard population.

and relief of symptoms, such as pain and pruritis, if present. Wart removal can relieve cosmetic concerns related to the appearance of warts and resulting psychosocial distress. In most patients, treatment results in resolution of the wart(s). Whether therapies for anogenital warts reduce infectivity and likelihood of future transmission remains unknown. Treatment of anogenital warts may be guided by considerations such as wart size, number, and anatomic site; patient preference; cost of treatment; convenience; adverse effects; and clinician experience. Recommended treatment regimens for external anogenital warts can be classified as either patient-applied or provider-administered. No definitive evidence suggests that any one recommended treatment is superior to another, and no single treatment is ideal for all patients or all warts.

Recurrent Respiratory Papillomatosis

Nonhigh-risk HPV types (primarily types 6 or 11) can also cause RRP, a rare disease that is characterized by recurrent warts or papillomas in the upper respiratory tract.[11,64] RRP is usually diagnosed by a specialist based upon clinical and pathologic evaluation. RRP is divided into juvenile onset (JORRP) and adult onset (AORRP) forms based on age at symptom onset. JORRP is believed to result from vertical transmission of HPV from mother to her baby at the time of delivery. Age of diagnosis is usually at age younger than 5 years.[81] The clinical course of JORRP is highly variable and associated with extensive morbidity, requiring a median of 4.3 annual surgeries to remove papillomas, preserve vocal quality, and maintain an open airway.[81]

PREVENTION AND CONTROL

Primary Prevention of HPV Infection

Highly effective HPV vaccines are available for primary prevention of vaccine targeted HPV types (see Primary prevention through HPV vaccination). Other primary prevention measures have been less effective. Because HPV infections are sexually transmitted, general measures recommended for prevention of other sexually transmitted infections may be helpful for reducing transmission of HPV. These measures include abstinence, monogamy or limiting number of sex partners, and consistent use of condoms and dental dams. Because HPV can infect areas that are not covered by condoms, condoms are not completely effective at preventing sexual transmission.[82] In randomized controlled trials, circumcision decreased the prevalence of HPV infection among circumcised males and their females partners,[83,84]

No treatment is required or available for asymptomatic HPV infections; instead, treatment is directed at the HPV-associated conditions.[80] Molecular HPV testing for a subset of oncogenic HPV types is performed clinically as part of cervical cancer screening and management of abnormal screening tests in certain age groups.[85–87] Unlike many sexually transmitted infections, there are no recommendations for partner notification following awareness of an HPV infection (such as an infection identified through cancer screening).[80] There are no other clinical indications for HPV testing, including no clinical HPV testing recommended for males. While assays have been developed for HPV typing of a broader array of HPV types than those included in clinical HPV tests, these are for research use only and have not been validated against clinical outcomes.[88] Additionally, serologic tests are available for research use but are not used clinically evaluations. HPV cannot be detected through culture methods.

Early Detection of Cancer

Cervical Cancer Screening

Persistent HPV infections can result in precancerous cervical lesions; some of these lesions progress to invasive cervical cancer. With regular cervical cancer screening and appropriate follow-up, most cervical cancer precursors can be identified and treated to prevent progression to invasive disease. In the United States, cervical cancer incidence and mortality rates have decreased approximately 57% and 60% respectively since 1975.[89] These decreases are mainly attributable to increased use of cytology screening [i.e., Papanicolaou (Pap) smears] and effective treatment of precancerous lesions.[87,90,91] Cervical cancer screening strategies have evolved from cytology-based screening alone, to incorporation of molecular HPV testing. Some countries particularly those with high HPV vaccine coverage, are moving to HPV testing alone, and no longer offer cytology-based screening.[92] In low-resource settings, screen-and-treat strategies have been employed, in which women are screened using visual inspection with acetic acid (VIA), and acetowhite areas are treated with cryotherapy or thermocoagulation.[93,94] In many high-resource settings, including the United States, precancerous cervical lesions and invasive cancers are diagnosed based on the histology of tissues obtained with biopsy or excision, and these specimens guide further treatment decisions.[85,95] Guidelines for management of and treatment aim to balance cancer prevention with minimization of reproductive and other harms from overtreatment.[85]

Recommendations for cervical cancer screening in the United States are based on systematic reviews of evidence and are largely consistent across the major medical organizations, including American Cancer Society (ACS), American College of Obstetricians and Gynecologists (ACOG), and the United States Preventive Services Task Force (USPSTF).[80,86,87,96–98] Current recommendations for women in the United States include routine cervical screening starting at age 21 years and through age 65 years. Conventional or liquid-based cytologic tests (i.e., Pap tests) are recommended every 3 years from ages 21–29 years. During age 30–65 years, women should either receive a Pap test every 3 years, a Pap test plus HPV test (co-test) every 5 years, or HPV test alone every 5 years. Because of the high negative predictive value of HPV tests, women with normal results for HPV or for both HPV and Pap tests do not need to be screened again for 5 years. Cervical screening recommendations do not currently differ for unvaccinated women and those who have received HPV vaccination. ACS, ACOG, and USPSTF concur that no Pap testing is recommended before age 21 years, and that women with a history of negative tests can cease screening after age 65. ACOG issued interim recommendations for primary HPV screening in 2015, following FDA approval of a test for this use. The USPSTF now includes primary HPV screening every 5 years as an additional screening option on women at least 30 years of age.[87]

Although cervical precancers are asymptomatic, those identified through screening are an important aspect of preventable disease attributable to HPV infections. Approximately 200,000 cervical precancers are diagnosed annually in the United States.[99,100] Treatment for cervical precancers may be associated with subsequent risk of preterm birth, and management guidelines have a goal of minimizing unnecessary treatment for precancers that may resolve spontaneously, particularly those in young women.[101,102]

Early Detection of Other HPV-associated Cancers

Aside from those for cervical cancer, there are no recommendations or organized screening programs for other HPV-associated cancers. Although pathogenesis and natural history of HPV-associated cancers at other anatomic sites may be analogous to the pathogenesis of cervical cancer, there are a number of gaps in the evidence base that preclude recommendations for screening. For some HPV-associated cancers, there are fundamental biological challenges with early detection, and for others, methods of detecting precancers exist, but evidence for safety and effectiveness of screening and treatment to prevent cancer is lacking.

Like cervical cancers, anal cancers arise from the squamocolumnar junction. Anal intraepithelial neoplasia is a precancerous lesion similar to cervical intraepithelial neoplasia (CIN). Cytology screening, similar to the Pap test for cervical cancer, can be performed to detect abnormal anal cells. Some specialized clinics conduct high-resolution anoscopy (HRA) to identify precancerous anal lesions in MSM.[80] Data regarding anal cancer screening were reviewed in development of the 2015 CDC Sexually Transmitted Diseases Treatment Guidelines; the available data were deemed insufficient to recommend screening with anal cytology in people living with HIV, MSM without HIV, or the general population.[103] The American Society for Colposcopy and Cervical Pathology (ASCCP) has reviewed evidence regarding screening for anal cancer in women, and made recommendations for screening for several groups at higher risk for anal cancer, such as HIV-infected women, women with organ transplants or certain autoimmune conditions, and women with lower genital tract cancers or high-grade lesions.[48] Recommended screening methods include asking patients about anal cancer symptoms and performing digital anorectal examinations (DARE); HIV-infected women could be considered for screening using anal cytology and HRA-directed biopsies. Data from an ongoing trial of anal cancer screening (NCT02135419) may provide data to inform future development anal cancer screening recommendations.

Precancerous lesions of the penis and vulva can sometimes be identified through skin lesions or symptoms, such as pruritis. Vulvar and vaginal precancers can also be identified during colposcopy exams indicated by cervical cancer screening results. No specific recommendations exist for screening for these lesions, however.[104]

No precancerous lesion for oropharyngeal cancer has been identified, likely because the site of the lesion is inaccessible.[105] Oral HPV testing has no prognostic value for cancer risk.[106] Neoplasias of the oropharynx are typically diagnosed as invasive cancers, often at advanced stages.[105]

Treatment of Cervical and Other HPV-associated Cancers

For invasive cervical and other HPV-associated cancers, treatment options include surgery, radiation therapy, and chemotherapy, alone or in combination depending on stage of disease. The survival rate 5 years after diagnosis of cervical cancer varies depending upon the stage of cervical cancer, ranging from 93% among those diagnosed at the earliest invasive state to only about 15% of those diagnosed at the latest stages.[107]

Primary Prevention through HPV Vaccination

Three HPV vaccines are licensed in the United States: a quadrivalent vaccine (4vHPV; Gardasil, Merck and Co, Inc.), a bivalent vaccine (2vHPV; Cervarix, GlaxoSmithKline), and a 9-valent vaccine (Table 100-2) (9vHPV; Gardisil 9, Merck and Co, Inc.).[108] All three vaccines are composed of VLPs prepared from recombinant L1 capsid protein of the targeted HPV types and are not live vaccines. Availability of 9vHPV, 4vHPV, and 2vHPV varies internationally; different countries use different vaccines in their national programs.

2vHPV is directed against two oncogenic types (HPV 16 and 18). 4vHPV is directed against two oncogenic types (HPV 16 and 18) and two nononcogenic types (HPV 6 and 11). 9vHPV is directed against all 4vHPV types plus five additional oncogenic types (HPV 31, 33, 45, 52, and 58). The vaccines are prophylactic and have no therapeutic effect on HPV-attributable disease, nor on risk of progression to disease in persons already infected with vaccine-type HPV at the time of vaccination.

Recommendations for Use of HPV Vaccines

Following regulatory approval (licensure), National Immunization Technical Advisory Groups develop recommendations for use in individual countries. Recommendations for use, and funding for public health vaccination programs, may vary substantially from country to country, depending on disease burden, health economic analyses, funding availability, disease reduction goals, overall vaccination program characteristics, acceptability, and other values.

After HPV vaccine was licensed in 2006, the United States, Australia, Canada, and some European countries were the first to introduce it into national vaccination programs.[110] Initially, cost prevented vaccine introductions into middle-income and low-income countries. Additional challenges to HPV vaccine introductions included targeting the adolescent age group and competing health priorities. Starting in 2011, tiered pricing of vaccines and lower vaccine prices obtained through the Pan American Health Organization's Revolving Fund allowed vaccine introductions in middle-income

TABLE 100-2 CHARACTERISTICS OF THE THREE LICENSED HUMAN PAPILLOMAVIRUS (HPV) VACCINES, UNITED STATES

Characteristic	Bivalent (2vHPV)[a]	Quadrivalent (4vHPV)[b]	9-valent (9vHPV)[c]
Brand name	Cervarix	Gardasil	Gardasil 9
VLPs	16, 18	6, 11, 16, 18	6, 11, 16, 18, 31, 33, 45, 52, 58
Manufacturer	GlaxoSmithKline	Merck and Co., Inc.	Merck and Co., Inc.
First FDA licensure	2009	2006	2014
Manufacturing	*Trichoplusia ni* insect cell-line infected with L1 encoding recombinant baculovirus	*Saccharomyces cerevisiae* (Baker's yeast), expressing L1	*Saccharomyces cerevisiae* (Baker's yeast), expressing L1
Adjuvant	500 μg aluminum hydroxide50 μg 3-O-desacyl-4' monophosphoryl lipid A	225 μg amorphous aluminum hydroxyphosphate sulfate	500 μg amorphous aluminum hydroxyphosphate sulfate
Volume per dose	0.5 mL	0.5 mL	0.5 mL
Administration	Intramuscular	Intramuscular	Intramuscular

Abbreviation: L1 = the HPV major capsid protein; VLPs = virus-like particles.
[a]Only licensed for use in females in the United States. Package insert available at http://www.fda.gov/downloads/BiologicsBloodVaccines/Vaccines/ApprovedProducts/UCM186981.pdf.
[b]Package insert available at http://www.fda.gov/downloads/BiologicsBloodVaccines/Vaccines/ApprovedProducts/UCM111263.pdf.
[c]Package insert available at http://www.fda.gov/downloads/BiologicsBloodVaccines/Vaccines/ApprovedProducts/UCM426457.pdf.
Source: Adapted from ref. 109.

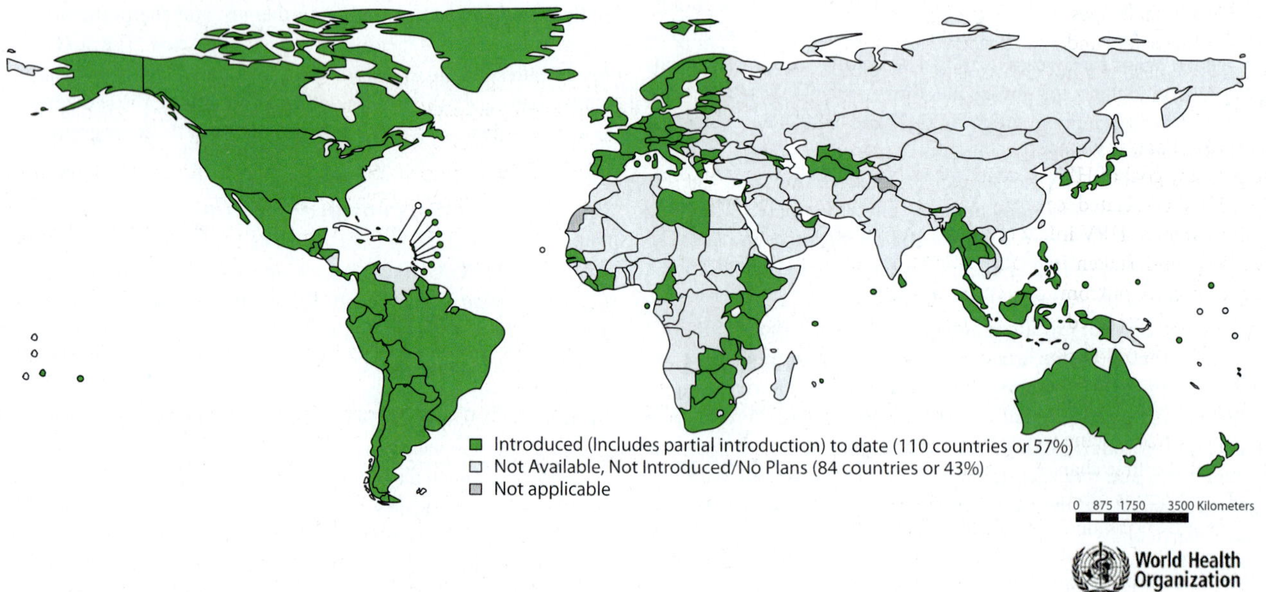

FIGURE 100-2. Countries with HPV vaccine in the national immunization program 2020. (*Source:* Used with permission WHO/IVB Database, as of 15 May 2018 URL: https://www.who.int/docs/default-source/documents/immunization/data/vaccine-intro-status.pdf?sfvrsn=bb2857ec_2 (slide 5).)

countries in the Americas. Funding of the HPV vaccine by the Gavi starting in 2012 (with vaccine costs of less than U.S.$5 per dose) and donation programs made possible HPV demonstration projects in some low-income countries.[111] As of 2020, use of HPV vaccine had expanded to 110 countries worldwide (Fig. 100-2).[112] Although all HPV vaccination programs target young adolescent girls, target age groups, inclusion of males, and catch-up vaccination recommendations differ between countries. In 2009, WHO recommended a three-dose schedule targeting just one birth cohort between the ages of 9 and 13 years.[113] In 2014, WHO revised recommendations to a two-dose schedule for girls who start the vaccination schedule before age 15 years. Vaccination policies have evolved owing to the availability of additional data from clinical trials and new regulatory approvals. The first countries to include boys and young men in their national HPV immunization programs were the United States in 2011, and Australia in 2013.[110,114] Other countries subsequently included males in their programs, but most still target only girls.

In the United States, national recommendations for use of HPV vaccines are developed by the Advisory Committee on Immunization Practice (ACIP) and harmonized with other professional organizations.[10,109,115,116] ACIP recommends routine HPV vaccination for U.S. girls and boys at age 11 or 12 years. Vaccination can be given starting at age 9 years. ACIP also recommends vaccination through age 26 years for anyone who was not adequately vaccinated previously.[117] During 2006–2016, a three-dose vaccination schedule was recommended. In October 2016, ACIP voted to recommend a two-dose schedule for persons initiating vaccination at age 9–14 years.[116] The second dose should be administered 6–12 months after the first dose

(0, 6–12 month schedule). For persons initiating vaccination on or after their 15th birthday, the recommended immunization schedule is three doses of HPV vaccine. The second dose should be administered 1–2 months after the first dose, and the third dose should be administered 6 months after the first dose (0, 1–2, 6 month schedule). For age-eligible persons with immunocompromising conditions that might reduce cell-mediated or humoral immunity a three-dose schedule is recommended.

HPV Vaccination Programs

HPV vaccination has been delivered through school-based programs in some countries and through primary care providers or health facilities in others. In the United States, HPV vaccine is mainly provided through primary care providers, at the same age that some other vaccines are recommended, age 11 or 12 years. At least one dose coverage has increased gradually in the United States, reaching 70% among 13- to 17-year-old females and 66% among males in 2018.[118] There are ongoing national and local efforts to increase coverage, including work with multiple partners and stakeholders to provide education to providers so that strong recommendations can be made for vaccination.[119] In general, countries with school-based vaccination have achieved higher coverage.[120] Rwanda, the first country in Africa to introduce HPV vaccination, achieved > 90% coverage in the first year of the program through school-based vaccination[121] Antivaccine groups have been active in many countries. A few countries have experienced challenges with their programs due to concerns about HPV vaccine safety and misinformation promulgated by antivaccine groups,[122–125] despite a now robust body of evidence about HPV vaccine safety.[126,127]

Evidence of Vaccine Impact

The primary goal of HPV vaccination is to prevent cervical cancers, other HPV-associated cancers, and genital warts associated with vaccine-targeted HPV infections. Vaccine impact monitoring efforts have been undertaken in many countries, and evidence of vaccine impact on early outcomes (prevalence of HPV infections, anogenital warts) and intermediate outcomes (cervical precancers) has been observed in many high-income countries.[128] Few data are available on vaccine impact from low- and middle-income countries (LMIC), as vaccine impact monitoring efforts are resource-intensive and many LMIC prioritize vaccine provision over monitoring efforts.

One of the first changes that can be observed after introduction of HPV vaccine is a reduced prevalence of vaccine-type HPV DNA from genital swabs or other relatively noninvasive specimen in the general population. Within 4 years of vaccine introduction, a pooled analysis of multiple studies showed a 70% decline in the prevalence of HPV 16/18 in 13- to 19-year-old girls (10 studies), a 37% decline in 20- to 24-year-old women (11 studies), and a nonsignificant 14% decline in 25- to 29-year-old women (6 studies).[128] Within 5–8 years of vaccine introduction, the declines were greater: 83% in 13–19 years olds (six studies), 66% in 20–24 years olds (eight studies), and 37% (and statistically significant, five studies) in 25–29 years olds; most women in this latter age group had not been vaccinated, suggesting the role of herd protection.[128] Few countries evaluated HPV prevalence among males during the time that only females were vaccinated routinely. In Australia, which started vaccinating girls only with 4vHPV and achieved high coverage quickly, the prevalence of vaccine types in unvaccinated males declined within a few years of the start of the female vaccination program, before male vaccination was recommended in that country.[130] National data from the United States on HPV prevalence in males suggests herd impact from vaccination of females in the youngest age groups.[41] Scotland achieved high coverage with 2vHPV administered at ages 12–13 years, and documented marked declines in the prevalence of HPV types 16 and 18 within 7 years after vaccination, as well as declines in HPV types 31, 33, and 45, demonstrating cross-protection.[143]

In countries with vaccination programs that include a vaccine that targets HPV types 6 and 11, another outcome that can provide an early measure of vaccine impact is anogenital warts, because warts usually develop soon after exposure to HPV. In the published pooled analyses, within 4 years of 4vHPV vaccine introduction, anogenital wart diagnoses declined 40% in females aged 15–19 years, 24% in females aged 20–24 years, and 11% in females aged 25–29 years.[128,129] Within 8 years of 4vHPV introduction, anogenital wart diagnoses had declined further: 67% in females aged 15–19 years, 54% in females aged 20–24 years, and 31% in females aged 25–29 years. Several studies also evaluated changes in anogenital warts in females aged 30–39 years (who were not targeted by any vaccination program), and no significant declines were observed. However, males in some age groups also experienced declines in anogenital wart diagnoses during the time of female-only vaccination, indicating herd protection. In 5–8 years after 4vHPV female-only vaccination programs, anogenital wart diagnoses in males declined 48% in boys aged 15–19 years and 32% in males 20- to 24-aged years. Subgroup analyses showed that much stronger herd effects in countries where vaccination coverage was high (>=50%) or multicohort vaccination was done, than in countries with lower coverage or single-cohort vaccination. Australia achieved high coverage with 4vHPV quickly, and was among the first countries to observe herd protection in unvaccinated males for this outcome.[131]

Cervical precancers have also been monitored for vaccine impact, as the most important proxy for cervical cancer prevention potential. The impact on precancers was expected to be observed somewhat later than impact on prevalence and anogenital warts because of the time it takes for precancers to develop after vaccination and for these asymptomatic lesions to be detected through cervical cancer screening. Nevertheless, declines in cervical precancers have already been observed during the vaccine era. Within 5–8 years after vaccine introductions, pooled analyses identified a 51% decrease in diagnoses of cervical intraepithelial neoplasia grade 2 or worse (CIN2+) in girls aged 15–19 years, and a 31% decrease in women aged 20–24 years, among those screened for cervical cancer.[128] However, analyses have also shown increases in CIN2+ in age groups 25–29 years and 30–39 years during the vaccine era; reasons for these increases are not known with certainty, but may reflect continuing increases in incidence in unvaccinated populations that began prior to vaccination programs, and changes in screening recommendations, particularly increased use of more sensitive HPV testing over cytology alone. Changes in screening practices during the vaccine era must be taken into account when interpreting changes in cervical disease incidence; one common approach has been to use the number of screened women, rather than the number of women in the population, as the denominator in incidence calculations.[128,132–134]

Ultimately, cancer registries will provide a source of information on vaccine impact on HPV-associated cancers. Because cervical cancer is diagnosed at younger ages than other HPV-associated cancers, on average, vaccine impact should be observed for cervical cancers first. In the United States, data on HPV-associated cancers are collected by the National Program on Cancer Registries (NPCR) and Surveillance, Epidemiology, and End Results (SEER) population-based cancer registries which together collect data on cancers diagnosed in 100% of the U.S. population.[72,73] Data from these registries have been used to assess the prevaccine burden of HPV-associated cancers and will be the basis for monitoring relevant cancers postvaccine introduction. However, the full impact of HPV vaccination on preventing invasive cancers is not expected until several decades after widespread adoption of the vaccine. Many high-income countries have robust cancer registries; in middle- and low-income countries, cancer registration is less complete.[135] Due to the extensive resources needed to establish and maintain strong cancer registries, and the many years between HPV infection and diagnosis of invasive cancer, strengthening cancer registries in low-income countries may not be a feasible vaccine impact monitoring strategy.

Future of HPV Vaccination

The introduction of HPV vaccination programs has had a substantial impact in just over a decade of use, but work remains to realize the full potential of HPV vaccines. Continuing efforts to improve vaccination coverage in countries that have introduced the vaccine and to mitigate the negative impacts of unsubstantiated safety concerns will be important for continuing to increase vaccine impact.[127,136–139] Further introductions of HPV vaccine in low-income countries are needed to maximize the global benefits and equity of HPV vaccine.[111] Introductions have been slowed in recent years by a global imbalance in supply and demand. Efforts are underway to optimize vaccination schedules, including evaluation of one-dose schedules, which could greatly simplify vaccination programs.[140] Further L1 VLP vacines are in development, which could increase global HPV vaccine supply (World Health Organization. Global Market Study. See https://www.who.int/immunization/programmes_systems/procurement/mi4a/platform/module2/WHO_HPV_market_study_public_summary_Dec2019.pdf), and research is ongoing into other HPV vaccines including vaccines based on the L2 capsid protein, which might impact a broader range of HPV types.[141] The recognition that HPV vaccines are highly effective has generated enthusiasm about the possibility of eliminating of cervical cancer as a global public health concern.[128,142]

References

1. zur Hausen H. Papillomaviruses in the causation of human cancers—A brief historical account. *Virology*. 2009;384:260–5.
2. Munoz N, Bosch FX, de Sanjose S, et al. Epidemiologic classification of human papillomavirus types associated with cervical cancer. *N Engl J Med*. 2003;348:518–27.
3. NobelPrize.org. Harald zur Hausen—Facts. https://www.nobelprize.org/prizes/medicine/2008/hausen/facts/. Accessed August 12, 2019.
4. Forman D, de Martel C, Lacey CJ, et al. Global burden of human papillomavirus and related diseases. *Vaccine*. 2012;30(Suppl 5):F12–23.
5. Satterwhite CL, Torrone E, Meites E, et al. Sexually transmitted infections among US women and men: Prevalence and incidence estimates, 2008. *Sex Transm Dis*. 2013;40:187–93.
6. de Martel C, Plummer M, Vignat J, Franceschi S. Worldwide burden of cancer attributable to HPV by site, country and HPV type. *Int J Cancer*. 2017;141:664–70.
7. Owusu-Edusei K Jr, Chesson HW, Gift TL, et al. The estimated direct medical cost of selected sexually transmitted infections in the United States, 2008. *Sex Transm Dis*. 2013;40:197–201.
8. Smith JS, Gilbert PA, Melendy A, Rana RK, Pimenta JM. Age-specific prevalence of human papillomavirus infection in males: A global review. *J Adolesc Health*. 2011;48:540–52.
9. Smith JS, Melendy A, Rana RK, Pimenta JM. Age-specific prevalence of infection with human papillomavirus in females: A global review. *J Adolesc Health*. 2008;43:S5–25, S.e1–41.
10. Markowitz LE, Dunne EF, Saraiya M, et al. Human papillomavirus vaccination: Recommendations of the Advisory Committee on Immunization Practices (ACIP). *MMWR Recomm Rep*. 2014;63:1–30.
11. Lacey CJ, Lowndes CM, Shah KV. Chapter 4: Burden and management of non-cancerous HPV-related conditions: HPV-6/11 disease. *Vaccine*. 2006;24(Suppl 3):S3/35–41.
12. Burd EM. Human papillomavirus laboratory testing: The changing paradigm. *Clin Microbiol Rev*. 2016;29:291–319.
13. Schiller JT, Lowy DR. Understanding and learning from the success of prophylactic human papillomavirus vaccines. *Nat Rev Microbiol*. 2012;10:681–92.
14. Middleton K, Peh W, Southern S, et al. Organization of human papillomavirus productive cycle during neoplastic progression provides a basis for selection of diagnostic markers. *J Virol*. 2003;77:10186–201.
15. Doorbar J, Quint W, Banks L, et al. The biology and life-cycle of human papillomaviruses. *Vaccine*. 2012;30(Suppl 5):F55–70.
16. International Human Papillomavirus (HPV) Reference Center. Reference Clones, 2017. Available at: https://www.hpvcenter.se/human_reference_clones/.
17. IARC Working Group on the Evaluation of Carcinogenic Risks to Humans. Biological agents. Volume 100 B: A review of human carcinogens. *IARC Monogr Eval Carcinog Risks Hum*. 2012;100(Pt B):1–441.
18. de Villiers EM. Cross-roads in the classification of papillomaviruses. *Virology*. 2013;445:2–10.
19. Combes JD, Guan P, Franceschi S, Clifford GM. Judging the carcinogenicity of rare human papillomavirus types. *Int J Cancer*. 2015;136:740–2.
20. Walboomers JM, Jacobs MV, Manos MM, et al. Human papillomavirus is a necessary cause of invasive cervical cancer worldwide. *J Pathol*. 1999;189:12–9.
21. de Sanjose S, Quint WG, Alemany L, et al. Human papillomavirus genotype attribution in invasive cervical cancer: A retrospective cross-sectional worldwide study. *Lancet Oncol*. 2010;11:1048–56.
22. Molano M, Van den Brule A, Plummer M, et al. Determinants of clearance of human papillomavirus infections in Colombian women with normal cytology: A population-based, 5-year follow-up study. *Am J Epidemiol*. 2003;158:486–94.
23. Ho GY, Burk RD, Klein S, et al. Persistent genital human papillomavirus infection as a risk factor for persistent cervical dysplasia. *J Natl Cancer Inst*. 1995;87:1365–71.
24. Franco EL, Villa LL, Sobrinho JP, et al. Epidemiology of acquisition and clearance of cervical human papillomavirus infection in women from a high-risk area for cervical cancer. *J Infect Dis*. 1999;180:1415–23.
25. Schlecht NF, Platt RW, Duarte-Franco E, et al. Human papillomavirus infection and time to progression and regression of cervical intraepithelial neoplasia. *J Natl Cancer Inst*. 2003;95:1336–43.
26. Schiffman M, Kjaer SK. Chapter 2: Natural history of anogenital human papillomavirus infection and neoplasia. *J Natl Cancer Inst Monogr*. 2003;(31):14–9.
27. Hildesheim A, Schiffman MH, Gravitt PE, et al. Persistence of type-specific human papillomavirus infection among cytologically normal women. *J Infect Dis*. 1994;169:235–40.
28. Franco EL, Duarte-Franco E, Ferenczy A. Cervical cancer: Epidemiology, prevention and the role of human papillomavirus infection. *CMAJ*. 2001;164:1017–25.
29. Ho GY, Bierman R, Beardsley L, Chang CJ, Burk RD. Natural history of cervicovaginal papillomavirus infection in young women. *N Engl J Med*. 1998;338:423–8.
30. Wheeler CM, Hunt WC, Schiffman M, Castle PE. Human papillomavirus genotypes and the cumulative 2-year risk of cervical precancer. *J Infect Dis*. 2006;194:1291–9.
31. Moscicki AB, Schiffman M, Kjaer S, Villa LL. Chapter 5: Updating the natural history of HPV and anogenital cancer. *Vaccine*. 2006;24(Suppl 3):S3/42–51.
32. Wheeler CM, Skinner SR, Del Rosario-Raymundo MR, et al. Efficacy, safety, and immunogenicity of the human papillomavirus 16/18 AS04-adjuvanted vaccine in women older than 25 years: 7-Year follow-up of the phase 3, double-blind, randomised controlled VIVIANE study. *Lancet Infect Dis*. 2016;16:1154–68.
33. Monsonego J, Cox JT, Behrens C, et al. Prevalence of high-risk human papilloma virus genotypes and associated risk of cervical precancerous lesions in a large U.S. screening population: Data from the ATHENA trial. *Gynecol Oncol*. 2015;137:47–54.
34. Hildesheim A, Hadjimichael O, Schwartz PE, et al. Risk factors for rapid-onset cervical cancer. *Am J Obstet Gynecol*. 1999;180:571–7.
35. Beachler DC, Jenkins G, Safaeian M, Kreimer AR, Wentzensen N. Natural acquired immunity against subsequent genital human papillomavirus infection: A systematic review and meta-analysis. *J Infect Dis*. 2016;213:1444–54.
36. Gravitt PE, Winer RL. Natural history of HPV infection across the lifespan: Role of viral latency. *Viruses*. 2017;9(10):267.
37. Muñoz N, Méndez F, Posso H, et al. Incidence, duration, and determinants of cervical human papillomavirus infection in a cohort of Colombian women with normal cytological results. J Infect Dis. 2004;190:2077-2087.
38. Winer RL, Feng Q, Hughes JP, O'Reilly S, Kiviat NB, Koutsky LA. Risk of female human papillomavirus acquisition associated with first male sex partner. *J Infect Dis*. 2008;197:279–82.
39. Hariri S, Unger ER, Sternberg M, et al. Prevalence of genital human papillomavirus among females in the United States, the National Health And Nutrition Examination Survey, 2003–2006. *J Infect Dis*. 2011;204:566–73.
40. Lewis RM, Markowitz LE, Gargano JW, Steinau M, Unger ER. Prevalence of genital human papillomavirus among sexually experienced males and females aged 14–59 Years, United States, 2013–2014. *J Infect Dis*. 2018;217:869–77.

41. Vaccarella S, Franceschi S, Herrero R, et al. Sexual behavior, condom use, and human papillomavirus: Pooled analysis of the IARC human papillomavirus prevalence surveys. *Cancer Epidemiol Biomarkers Prev.* 2006;15:326–33.
42. Gargano JW, Unger ER, Liu G, Steinau M, Meites E, Dunne E, Markowitz LE. Prevalence of genital human papillomavirus in males, United States, 2013–2014. *J Infect Dis.* 2017;215(7):1070–9.
43. Giuliano AR, Lu B, Nielson CM, et al. Age-specific prevalence, incidence, and duration of human papillomavirus infections in a cohort of 290 US men. *J Infect Dis.* 2008;198:827–35.
44. Giuliano AR, Lee JH, Fulp W, et al. Incidence and clearance of genital human papillomavirus infection in men (HIM): A cohort study. *Lancet.* 2011;377:932–40.
45. Edelstein ZR, Carter JJ, Garg R, et al. Serum antibody response following genital α9 human papillomavirus infection in young men. *J Infect Dis.* 2011;204:209–16.
46. Giuliano AR, Nyitray AG, Kreimer AR, et al. EUROGIN 2014 roadmap: Differences in human papillomavirus infection natural history, transmission and human papillomavirus-related cancer incidence by gender and anatomic site of infection. *Int J Cancer.* 2015;136:2752–60.
47. Lin C, Slama J, Gonzalez P, et al. Cervical determinants of anal HPV infection and high-grade anal lesions in women: A collaborative pooled analysis. *Lancet Infect Dis.* 2019;19:880–91.
48. Moscicki AB, Darragh TM, Berry-Lawhorn JM, et al. Screening for anal cancer in women. *J Low Genit Tract Dis.* 2015;19:S27–42.
49. Nyitray AG, Carvalho da Silva RJ, Baggio ML, et al. Six-month incidence, persistence, and factors associated with persistence of anal human papillomavirus in men: The HPV in men study. *J Infect Dis.* 2011;204:1711–22.
50. Gillison ML, Broutian T, Pickard RK, et al. Prevalence of oral HPV infection in the United States, 2009–2010. *JAMA.* 2012;307:693–703.
51. Chaturvedi AK, Graubard BI, Broutian T, et al. NHANES 2009–2012 findings: Association of sexual behaviors with higher prevalence of oral oncogenic human papillomavirus infections in U.S. men. *Cancer Res.* 2015;75:2468–77.
52. D'Souza G, Wentz A, Kluz N, et al. Sex differences in risk factors and natural history of oral human papillomavirus infection. *J Infect Dis.* 2016;213:1893–6.
53. Carter JJ, Koutsky LA, Hughes JP, et al. Comparison of human papillomavirus types 16, 18, and 6 capsid antibody responses following incident infection. *J Infect Dis.* 2000;181:1911–9.
54. Jit M, Vyse A, Borrow R, Pebody R, Soldan K, Miller E. Prevalence of human papillomavirus antibodies in young female subjects in England. *Br J Cancer.* 2007;97:989–91.
55. Markowitz LE, Sternberg M, Dunne EF, McQuillan G, Unger ER. Seroprevalence of human papillomavirus types 6, 11, 16, and 18 in the United States: National Health and Nutrition Examination Survey 2003–2004. *J Infect Dis.* 2009;200:1059–67.
56. Malagon T, Louvanto K, Wissing M, et al. Hand-to-genital and genital-to-genital transmission of human papillomaviruses between male and female sexual partners (HITCH): A prospective cohort study. *Lancet Infect Dis.* 2019;19:317–26.
57. Marrazzo JM, Koutsky LA, Stine KL, et al. Genital human papillomavirus infection in women who have sex with women. *J Infect Dis.* 1998;178:1604–9.
58. Moscicki AB, Schiffman M, Burchell A, et al. Updating the natural history of human papillomavirus and anogenital cancers. *Vaccine.* 2012;30(Suppl 5):F24–33.
59. Shew ML, Weaver B, Tu W, Tong Y, Fortenberry JD, Brown DR. High frequency of human papillomavirus detection in the vagina before first vaginal intercourse among females enrolled in a longitudinal cohort study. *J Infect Dis.* 2013;207:1012–5.
60. Winer RL, Lee SK, Hughes JP, Adam DE, Kiviat NB, Koutsky LA. Genital human papillomavirus infection: Incidence and risk factors in a cohort of female university students. *Am J Epidemiol.* 2003;157:218–26.
61. D'Souza G, Agrawal Y, Halpern J, Bodison S, Gillison ML. Oral sexual behaviors associated with prevalent oral human papillomavirus infection. *J Infect Dis.* 2009;199:1263–9.
62. Fu TC, Hughes JP, Feng Q, et al. Epidemiology of human papillomavirus detected in the oral cavity and fingernails of mid-adult women. *Sex Transm Dis.* 2015;42:677–85.
63. Anderson TA, Schick V, Herbenick D, Dodge B, Fortenberry JD. A study of human papillomavirus on vaginally inserted sex toys, before and after cleaning, among women who have sex with women and men. *Sex Transm Infect.* 2014;90:529–31.
64. Derkay CS, Bluher AE. Recurrent respiratory papillomatosis: Update 2018. *Curr Opin Otolaryngol Head Neck Surg.* 2018;26:421–5.
65. Chin-Hong PV, Reid GE. Human papillomavirus infection in solid organ transplant recipients: Guidelines from the American Society of Transplantation Infectious Diseases Community of Practice. *Clin Transplant.* 2019;33(9):e13590.
66. Machalek DA, Poynten M, Jin F, et al. Anal human papillomavirus infection and associated neoplastic lesions in men who have sex with men: A systematic review and meta-analysis. *Lancet Oncol.* 2012;13:487–500.
67. Schim van der Loeff MF, Mooij SH, Richel O, de Vries HJ, Prins JM. HPV and anal cancer in HIV-infected individuals: A review. *Current HIV/AIDS reports.* 2014;11:250–62.
68. Shiels MS, Pfeiffer RM, Gail MH, et al. Cancer burden in the HIV-infected population in the United States. *J Natl Cancer Inst.* 2011;103:753–62.
69. Shiels MS, Pfeiffer RM, Hall HI, et al. Proportions of Kaposi sarcoma, selected non-Hodgkin lymphomas, and cervical cancer in the United States occurring in persons with AIDS, 1980–2007. *JAMA.* 2011;305:1450–9.
70. Marra E, Lin C, Clifford GM. Type-specific anal human papillomavirus prevalence among men, according to sexual preference and HIV status: A systematic literature review and meta-analysis. *J Infect Dis.* 2019;219:590–8.
71. International Agency for Research on Cancer. Cervix Uteri. http://gco.iarc.fr/today/data/factsheets/cancers/23-Cervix-uteri-fact-sheet.pdf.
72. Van Dyne EA, Henley SJ, Saraiya M, Thomas CC, Markowitz LE, Benard VB. Trends in human papillomavirus-associated cancers—United States, 1999–2015. *MMWR Morb Mortal Wkly Rep.* 2018;67:918–24.
73. Saraiya M, Unger ER, Thompson TD, et al. US assessment of HPV types in cancers: Implications for current and 9-valent HPV vaccines. *J Natl Cancer Inst.* 2015;107:djv086.
74. Viens LJ, Henley SJ, Watson M, et al. Human papillomavirus-associated cancers—United States, 2008–2012. *MMWR Morb Mortal Wkly Rep.* 2016;65:661–6.
75. Senkomago VHS, Thomas CC, Mix JM, Markowitz LE, Saraiya M. Human papillomavirus–attributable cancers—United States, 2012–2016. *MMWR Morb Mortal Wkly Rep.* 2019;68:724–8.
76. Centers for Disease Control and Prevention. HPV-Associated Cancer Diagnosis by Age. https://www.cdc.gov/cancer/hpv/statistics/age.htm. Accessed August 14, 2019.
77. Garland SM, Steben M, Sings HL, et al. Natural history of genital warts: Analysis of the placebo arm of 2 randomized phase III trials of a quadrivalent human papillomavirus (types 6, 11, 16, and 18) vaccine. *J Infect Dis.* 2009;199:805–14.
78. Winer RL, Kiviat NB, Hughes JP, et al. Development and duration of human papillomavirus lesions, after initial infection. *J Infect Dis.* 2005;191:731–8.
79. Chuang TY, Perry HO, Kurland LT, Ilstrup DM. Condyloma acuminatum in Rochester, Minn, 1950–1978. II. Anaplasias and unfavorable outcomes. *Arch Dermatol.* 1984;120:476–83.
80. Workowski KA, Bolan GA, Centers for Disease Control and Prevention. Sexually transmitted diseases treatment guidelines, 2015. *MMWR Recomm Rep.* 2015;64:1–137.
81. Reeves WC, Ruparelia SS, Swanson KI, Derkay CS, Marcus A, Unger ER. National registry for juvenile-onset recurrent respiratory papillomatosis. *Arch Otolaryngol Head Neck Surg.* 2003;129:976–82.
82. Winer RL, Hughes JP, Feng Q, et al. Condom use and the risk of genital human papillomavirus infection in young women. *N Engl J Med.* 2006;354:2645–54.
83. Gray RH, Serwadda D, Kong X, et al. Male circumcision decreases acquisition and increases clearance of high-risk human papillomavirus in HIV-negative men: A randomized trial in Rakai, Uganda. *J Infect Dis.* 2010;201:1455–62.
84. Tobian AA, Kacker S, Quinn TC. Male circumcision: A globally relevant but under-utilized method for the prevention of HIV and other sexually transmitted infections. *Annu Rev Med.* 2014;65:293–306.
85 Massad LS, Einstein MH, Huh WK, et al. 2012 updated consensus guidelines for the management of abnormal cervical cancer screening tests and cancer precursors. *J Low Genit Tract Dis.* 2013;17:S1–27.
86. Saslow D, Solomon D, Lawson HW, et al. American Cancer Society, American Society for Colposcopy and Cervical Pathology, and American Society for Clinical Pathology screening guidelines for the prevention and early detection of cervical cancer. *CA Cancer J Clin.* 2012;62:147–72.
87. Curry SJ, Krist AH, Owens DK, et al. Screening for cervical cancer: US Preventive Services Task Force recommendation statement. *JAMA.* 2018;320:674–86.
88. Schiller JT, Lowy DR. Immunogenicity testing in human papillomavirus virus-like-particle vaccine trials. *J Infect Dis.* 2009;200:166–71.
89. Howlader N NA, Krapcho M, Miller D, Brest A, Yu M, Ruhl J, Tatalovich Z, Mariotto A, Lewis DR, Chen HS, Feuer EJ, Cronin KA, eds. *SEER*

Cancer Statistics Review, 1975–2016. Bethesda, MD: National Cancer Institute; 2018.

90. Benard VB, Thomas CC, King J, Massetti GM, Doria-Rose VP, Saraiya M. Vital signs: Cervical cancer incidence, mortality, and screening—United States, 2007–2012. *MMWR Morb Mortal Wkly Rep*. 2014;63:1004–9.
91. Lippman SM, Hawk ET. Cancer prevention: From 1727 to milestones of the past 100 years. *Cancer Res*. 2009;69:5269–84.
92. Machalek DA, Roberts JM, Garland SM, et al. Routine cervical screening by primary HPV testing: Early findings in the renewed National Cervical Screening Program. *Med J Aust*. 2019;211:113–9.
93. WHO Guidelines Approved by the Guidelines Review Committee. *WHO Guidelines for Screening and Treatment of Precancerous Lesions for Cervical Cancer Prevention*. Geneva: World Health Organization; 2013.
94. Viviano M, Kenfack B, Catarino R, et al. Feasibility of thermocoagulation in a screen-and-treat approach for the treatment of cervical precancerous lesions in sub-Saharan Africa. *BMC Womens Health*. 2017;17:2.
95. Jeronimo J, Castle PE, Temin S, et al. Secondary prevention of cervical cancer: ASCO resource-stratified clinical practice guideline. *J Glob Oncol*. 2017;3:635–57.
96. Committee on Practice B-G. ACOG practice bulletin number 131: Screening for cervical cancer. *Obstet Gynecol*. 2012;120:1222–38.
97. Moyer VA, Force USPST. Screening for cervical cancer: U.S. Preventive Services Task Force recommendation statement. *Ann Intern Med*. 2012;156:880–91, W312.
98. Huh WK, Ault KA, Chelmow D, et al. Use of primary high-risk human papillomavirus testing for cervical cancer screening: interim clinical guidance. *Gynecologic oncology*. 2015;136:178–82.
99. Henk HJ, Insinga RP, Singhal PK, Darkow T. Incidence and costs of cervical intraepithelial neoplasia in a US commercially insured population. *J Low Genit Tract Dis*. 2010;14:29–36.
100. McClung NM, Gargano JW, Park IU, et al. Estimated number of cases of high-grade cervical lesions diagnosed among women—United States, 2008 and 2016. *MMWR Morb Mortal Wkly Rep*. 2019;68:337–43.
101. Bjorge T, Skare GB, Bjorge L, Trope A, Lonnberg S. Adverse pregnancy outcomes after treatment for cervical intraepithelial neoplasia. *Obstet Gynecol*. 2016;128:1265–73.
102. Kyrgiou M, Mitra A, Paraskevaidis E. Fertility and early pregnancy outcomes following conservative treatment for cervical intraepithelial neoplasia and early cervical cancer. *JAMA Oncol*. 2016;2:1496–8.
103. Park IU, Introcaso C, Dunne EF. Human papillomavirus and genital warts: A review of the evidence for the 2015 Centers for Disease Control and Prevention sexually transmitted diseases treatment guidelines. *Clin Infect Dis*. 2015;61(Suppl 8):S849–55.
104. Smith RA, Andrews KS, Brooks D, et al. Cancer screening in the United States, 2019: A review of current American Cancer Society guidelines and current issues in cancer screening. *CA Cancer J Clin*. 2019;69:184–210.
105. Taberna M, Mena M, Pavon MA, Alemany L, Gillison ML, Mesia R. Human papillomavirus-related oropharyngeal cancer. *Ann Oncol*. 2017;28:2386–98.
106. Lingen MW, Tampi MP, Urquhart O, et al. Adjuncts for the evaluation of potentially malignant disorders in the oral cavity: Diagnostic test accuracy systematic review and meta-analysis—A report of the American Dental Association. *J Am Dent Assoc*. 2017;148:797–813.e52.
107. American Cancer Society. Survival Rates for Cervical Cancer, by Stage. https://www.cancer.org/cancer/cervical-cancer/detection-diagnosis-staging/survival.html.
108. Food and Drug Administration. Vaccines Licensed for Use in the United States. http://www.fda.gov/BiologicsBloodVaccines/Vaccines/ApprovedProducts/ucm093833.htm. Accessed January 30, 2017.
109. Petrosky E, Bocchini JA, Hariri S, et al. Use of 9-valent human papillomavirus (HPV) vaccine: Updated HPV vaccination recommendations of the advisory committee on immunization practices. *MMWR Morb Mortal Wkly Rep*. 2015;64:300–4.
110. Markowitz LE, Tsu V, Deeks SL, et al. Human papillomavirus vaccine introduction—The first five years. *Vaccine*. 2012;30(Suppl 5):F139–48.
111. Gavi. More than 30 million girls to be immunised with HPV vaccines by 2020 with GAVI support. https://www.gavi.org/library/news/press-releases/2012/more-than-30-million-girls-immunised-with-hpv-by-2020/. Accessed August 14, 2019.
112. World Health Organization. Immunizations, Vaccines, and Biologicals: Monitoring and Surveillance. https://view.officeapps.live.com/op/view.aspx?src=https%3A%2F%2Fwww.who.int%2Fimmunization%2Fmonitoring_surveillance%2FVaccineIntroStatus.pptx.
113. World Health Organization. Human papillomavirus vaccines: WHO position paper. *Biologicals*. 2009;37:338–44.
114. Australian Government Department of Health. Human papillomavirus (HPV). http://www.health.gov.au/internet/immunise/publishing.nsf/Content/immunise-HPV Accessed December 18, 2014.
115. Markowitz LE, Dunne EF, Saraiya M, et al. Quadrivalent human papillomavirus vaccine: Recommendations of the Advisory Committee on Immunization Practices (ACIP). *MMWR Recomm Rep*. 2007;56:1–24.
116. Meites E, Kempe A, Markowitz LE. Use of a 2-dose schedule for human papillomavirus vaccination—Updated recommendations of the Advisory Committee on Immunization Practices. *MMWR Morb Mortal Wkly Rep*. 2016;65:1405–8.
117. Meites E, Szilagyi PG, Chesson HW, Unger ER, Romero JR, Markowitz LE. Human papillomavirus vaccination for adults: Updated recommendations of the Advisory Committee on Immunization Practices. *MMWR Morb Mortal Wkly Rep*. 2019;68:698–702.
118. Walker TY, Elam-Evans LD, Yankey D, Markowitz LE, Williams CL, Fredua BSJ, Stokley S. National, regional, state, and selected local area vaccination coverage among adolescents aged 13–17 years—United States, 2018. *MMWR Morb Mortal Wkly Rep*. 2019;68:718–23.
119. Gilkey MB, Calo WA, Moss JL, Shah PD, Marciniak MW, Brewer NT. Provider communication and HPV vaccination: The impact of recommendation quality. *Vaccine*. 2016;34:1187–92.
120. Brotherton JML, Bloem PN. Population-based HPV vaccination programmes are safe and effective: 2017 Update and the impetus for achieving better global coverage. *Best Pract Res Clin Obstet Gynaecol*. 2018;47:42–58.
121. Binagwaho A, Wagner CM, Gatera M, Karema C, Nutt CT, Ngabo F. Achieving high coverage in Rwanda's national human papillomavirus vaccination programme. *Bull World Health Organ*. 2012;90:623–8.
122. Hanley SJ, Yoshioka E, Ito Y, Kishi R. HPV vaccination crisis in Japan. *Lancet*. 2015;385:2571.
123. Okuhara T, Ishikawa H, Okada M, Kato M, Kiuchi T. Newspaper coverage before and after the HPV vaccination crisis began in Japan: A text mining analysis. *BMC Public Health*. 2019;19:770.
124. Suppli CH, Hansen ND, Rasmussen M, Valentiner-Branth P, Krause TG, Molbak K. Decline in HPV-vaccination uptake in Denmark—The association between HPV-related media coverage and HPV-vaccination. *BMC Public Health*. 2018;18:1360.
125. World Health Organization. Denmark campaign rebuilds confidence in HPV vaccination program. https://www.who.int/features/2018/hpv-vaccination-denmark/en/. Accessed August 14, 2019.
126. Gee J, Weinbaum C, Sukumaran L, Markowitz LE. Quadrivalent HPV vaccine safety review and safety monitoring plans for nine-valent HPV vaccine in the United States. *Hum Vaccin Immunother*. 2016;12:1406–17.
127. World Health Organization. Safety Update of HPV Vaccines. https://www.who.int/vaccine_safety/committee/topics/hpv/June_2017/en/. Accessed August 14, 2019.
128. Drolet M, Benard E, Perez N, Brisson M. Population-level impact and herd effects following the introduction of human papillomavirus vaccination programmes: Updated systematic review and meta-analysis. *Lancet*. 2019;394:497–509.
129. Drolet M, Benard E, Boily MC, et al. Population-level impact and herd effects following human papillomavirus vaccination programmes: A systematic review and meta-analysis. *Lancet Infect Dis*. 2015;15:565–80.
130. Chow EPF, Machalek DA, Tabrizi SN, et al. Quadrivalent vaccine-targeted human papillomavirus genotypes in heterosexual men after the Australian female human papillomavirus vaccination programme: A retrospective observational study. *Lancet Infect Dis*. 2017;17:68–77.
131. Chow EP, Fairley CK. Assortative sexual mixing among heterosexuals in Australia: Implications for herd protection in males from a female human papillomavirus vaccination program. *Sex Health*. 2016. Online ahead of print.
132. Benard VB, Castle PE, Jenison SA, et al. Population-based incidence rates of cervical intraepithelial neoplasia in the human papillomavirus vaccine era. *JAMA Oncol*. 2017;3(6):833–7.
133. Flagg EW, Torrone EA, Weinstock H. Ecological association of human papillomavirus vaccination with cervical dysplasia prevalence in the United States, 2007–2014. *Am J Public Health*. 2016;106:2211–8.
134. Gargano JW, Park IU, Griffin MR, et al. Trends in high-grade cervical lesions and cervical cancer screening in five states—United States, 2008–2015. *Clin Infect Dis*. 2019;68(8):1282–91.
135. Znaor A, Eser S, Anton-Culver H, et al. Cancer surveillance in northern Africa, and central and western Asia: Challenges and strategies in support of developing cancer registries. *Lancet Oncol*. 2018;19:e85–92.
136. Gallagher KE, Howard N, Kabakama S, et al. Human papillomavirus (HPV) vaccine coverage achievements in low and middle-income countries 2007–2016. *Papillomavirus Res*. 2017;4:72–8.

137. Gilkey MB, Parks MJ, Margolis MA, McRee AL, Terk JV. Implementing Evidence-Based Strategies to Improve HPV Vaccine Delivery. *Pediatrics*. 2019;144:e20182500.

138. Lu PJ, Yankey D, Fredua B, et al. Association of Provider Recommendation and Human Papillomavirus Vaccination Initiation among Male Adolescents Aged 13–17 Years-United States. *J Pediatr*. 2019;206:33–41.e1.

139. Smulian EA, Mitchell KR, Stokley S. Interventions to increase HPV vaccination coverage: A systematic review. *Hum Vaccin Immunother*. 2016;12:1566–88.

140. Kreimer AR, Herrero R, Sampson JN, et al. Evidence for single-dose protection by the bivalent HPV vaccine—Review of the Costa Rica HPV vaccine trial and future research studies. *Vaccine*. 2018;36:4774–82.

141. Schiller JT, Muller M. Next generation prophylactic human papillomavirus vaccines. *Lancet Oncol*. 2015;16:e217–25.

142. Canfell K. Towards the global elimination of cervical cancer. *Papillomavirus Res*. 2019;8:100170.

143. Kavanagh K, Pollock KG, Cuschieri K, et al. Changes in the prevalence of human papillomavirus following a national bivalent human papillomavirus vaccination programme in Scotland: a 7-year cross-sectional study. *Lancet Infect Dis*. 2017;17:1293–1302.

CHAPTER

101 Hepatitis B

Aaron M. Harris

ETIOLOGIC AGENT

Hepatitis B virus (HBV) is a member of the family Hepadnaviridae, the members of which replicate in the liver and cause hepatic dysfunction. The only natural host for HBV appears to be humans, but the Hepadnaviridae family also includes viruses that infect woodchucks, ducks, ground squirrels, and herons.

HBV has a small (3.2 kilobase) genome with a circular DNA that is partially double stranded and a retroviral replication strategy with an RNA intermediate. The genome codes for a surface glycoprotein, nucleocapsid protein, DNA polymerase, and the X protein, a small transcriptional transactivator that influences the transcription of HBV genes.[1,2]

The complete HBV virion (Dane particle) is 42 nm in diameter and is composed of an outer lipoprotein coat containing the hepatitis B surface antigen (HBsAg) and a 27-nm nucleocapsid core, the hepatitis B core antigen (HBcAg). In addition to being a component of lipoprotein coat of the virus, HBsAg circulates independently in the blood as 22-nm spheres and tubules. HBsAg is antigenically heterogeneous, with a common antigen, *a*, and two pairs of mutually exclusive antigens, *d* and *y*, and *w* and *r*, resulting in four possible subtypes: adw, adr, ayw, and ayr.[3,4] Antibodies to the *a* antigen confer immunity to all the subtypes. Although no clinical differences have been identified between subtypes, there are distinct geographic distributions, which have been useful in epidemiologic studies.[5] A third hepatitis B antigen, the *e* antigen (HBeAg) is a soluble protein that is not part of the virus particle, but can be detected in the serum of patients with acute HBV infection, and in patients with chronic HBV infection who have high virus titers.

HBV has a higher frequency of mutations than other DNA viruses due to its replication via an RNA intermediate, using a reverse transcriptase that seems to lack a proofreading function.[4] The clinical significance of these mutations is not well established, but may include increased virulence, decreased host response to therapy, and viral replication in the presence of protective levels of antibody to HBsAg after vaccination or hepatitis B immune globulin (HBIG) administration.[6,7]

HBV has been shown to retain infectivity in serum for at least 1 month when stored at either room temperature or frozen. HBV is also stable on environmental surfaces for 7 days or longer; thus, indirect inoculation of HBV can occur through inanimate objects.[8,15] Infectivity is destroyed at 90°C after 1 hour.[9]

CLINICAL ILLNESS, PATHOGENESIS, AND IMMUNE RESPONSE

HBV infection can be asymptomatic, cause acute self-limited hepatitis, or result in fulminant hepatitis and death. Persons infected with HBV also may develop chronic infection, which can lead to chronic liver disease and death from cirrhosis or hepatocellular carcinoma (HCC).

The incubation period for acute infection is an average of 90 days (range: 60–150 days) after exposure to HBV.[8] The age that HBV infection is acquired is the main factor determining clinical expression of disease. Fewer than 10% of children under 5 years of age who become infected have initial clinical signs or symptoms of disease (i.e., acute hepatitis B) compared with 30–50% of older children and adults.[10] In persons who develop symptomatic infection, the clinical onset of hepatitis B is usually insidious, with malaise, weakness, and anorexia being the most common findings. In 5–10% of patients, a serum sickness-like syndrome may develop during the prodromal phase that is characterized by arthralgias or arthritis, rash, and angioedema.[4] In 10–30% of patients with acute hepatitis B, myalgias, and arthralgias have been described without jaundice or other clinical signs of hepatitis; in one-third of these patients, a maculopapular rash appears with joint symptoms.[4,11] In patients with icteric hepatitis (30% or more of infected adults), jaundice usually develops within 1–2 weeks after onset of illness; dark urine and clay-colored stools may appear 1–5 days before onset of clinical jaundice.[4,12] Liver enzyme elevations usually occur prior to the onset of jaundice. HBV infection is also associated with extrahepatitic disease such as vasculitis and membranoproliferative glomerulonephritis.[12] Clinical signs and symptoms of acute hepatitis B usually resolve within 1–3 months.

Since the mid-1990s, the incidence of acute HBV infection in the United States has declined significantly. National surveillance data indicate that the incidence decreased from 11.5 per 100,000 population in 1985 to 1.0 per 100,000 in 2018 (https://www.cdc.gov/hepatitis/hbv/hbvfaq.htm#overview). Incidence is estimated to be about six times the reported number of cases after adjustment for underreporting of cases and asymptomatic infections. In 2018, an estimated 21,600 (12,300–52,800) people were newly infected (https://www.cdc.gov/hepatitis/hbv/hbvfaq.htm#overview). However, from 2014 to 2018, there was an increase in the rate of acute hepatitis B cases in some geographic areas, likely due to injection drug use (IDU).[13] Fulminant liver failure occurs in approximately 0.5–1% of infected adults, but rarely in infected infants or children.

The risk of developing chronic HBV infection (persistence of HBsAg for longer than 6 months) varies inversely with age: approximately 90% of infants infected during the first year of life, 25–50% of children infected between 1 year and 5 years of age, and 5% of adults develop chronic infection.[10] Among individuals in whom HBV infection persists, both HBsAg and anti-HBc remain detectable, usually indefinitely (Fig. 101-1). During the early stage of chronic HBV infection, HBeAg is present and indicates a high level of viral replication and infectivity. Each year approximately 10% of persons with chronic HBV infection will lose HBeAg and up to 1% per year may naturally lose HBsAg.[14] Persons with chronic HBV infection are at risk of chronic liver disease (i.e., chronic active hepatitis, cirrhosis) and HCC. Prospective studies have shown that 25% of persons

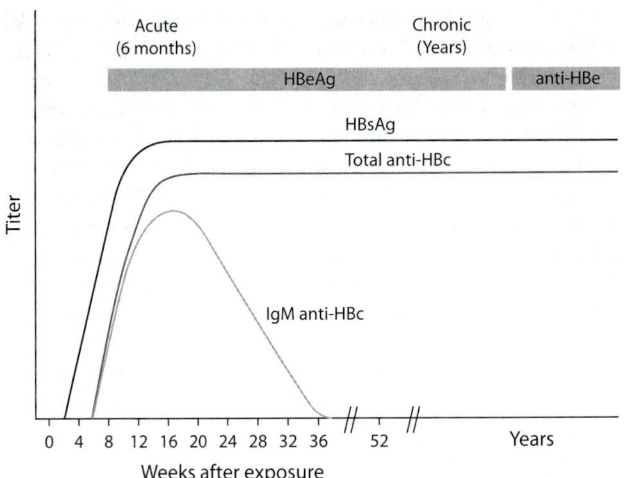

FIGURE 101-1. Serologic course for progression to chronic hepatitis B virus infection. Anti-HBc, antibody to hepatitis B core antigen; anti-HBe, antibody to hepatitis early antigen; HBeAg, hepatitis B early antigen; HBsAg, hepatitis B surface antigen; IgM anti-HBc, antibody of the immunoglobulin M subclass to hepatitis B core antigen. (*Source:* CDC Website, https://www.cdc.gov/hepatitis/resources/healthprofessionaltools.htm.)

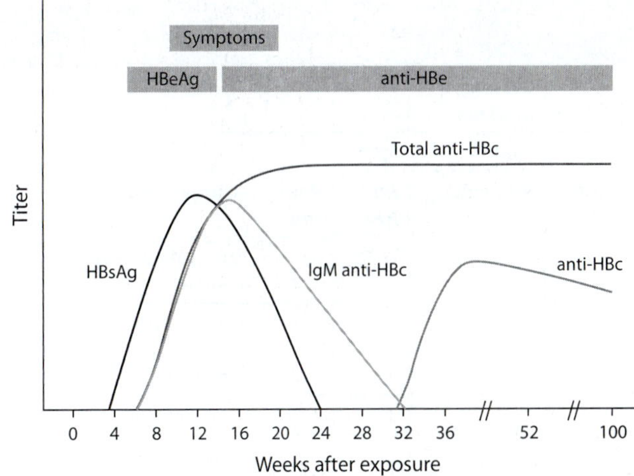

FIGURE 101-2. Serologic course for acute hepatitis B virus infection, with recovery. Anti-HBc, antibody to hepatitis B core antigen; anti-HBe, antibody to hepatitis early antigen; anti-HBs, antibody to hepatitis B surface antigen; HBeAg, hepatitis early antigen; HBsAg, hepatitis B surface antigen; IgM anti-HBc, antibody of the immunoglobulin M subclass to hepatitis B core antigen. (*Source:* CDC Website, https://www.cdc.gov/hepatitis/resources/healthprofessionaltools.htm.)

who acquired chronic HBV infection as infants or young children will die as adults (average age 45 years) from HBV-related cirrhosis or HCC.[15,16] Among persons who acquire chronic HBV infection as adults, it is estimated that 15% will die from HBV-related chronic liver disease at an average age of 55 years.[16]

HBV is transmitted via percutaneous or mucosal exposure to infected blood and various body fluids, as well as through saliva, menstrual, vaginal, and seminal fluids and requires hepatocytes for replication. Access occurs through direct percutaneous inoculation, breaks in the skin that allow inapparent inoculation, or passage through mucous membranes. Although HBsAg has been detected in tissues other than the liver, there is little evidence to suggest sustained replication at these sites.[17,18] The number of hepatocytes affected during the acute phase of replication is variable and can reach almost 100%.[19] During persistent infection, approximately 10% of hepatocytes remain infected.[19]

There is strong evidence that the hepatocellular injury that occurs during HBV infection is immune mediated, rather than due to a direct cytopathic effect of HBV.[4,8] Cell-mediated injury is targeted at hepatocytes through a combination of human leukocyte antigen (HLA) molecules and HBV antigens.[20] The precise mechanism(s) that lead to viral persistence are unknown, but may include the induction of immune tolerance by HBeAg. Integration of HBV DNA does occur during chronic infection, which may be important for the development of HCC.

During acute infection, HBsAg may become detectable 1–2 months prior to the onset of clinical symptoms and is soon followed by the appearance of IgM anti-HBc (Fig. 101-2). In late convalescence, there is a transition period (window phase) when the levels of HBsAg decline and the levels of antibody to HBsAg (anti-HBs) increase. As these markers reach equivalency, neither may be detectable because they form immune complexes; however, both total anti-HBc and IgM anti-HBc remain detectable. For infections that resolve, HBsAg disappears from circulation and the virus-neutralizing anti-HBs become detectable, along with total anti-HBc. Although HBV-specific humoral and cellular immunity is maintained for life, this immunity is not sterilizing. Trace amounts of HBV DNA persist and remain intermittently detectable in blood and liver using sensitive diagnostic techniques.[8] These trace amounts of HBV appear to continuously activate and maintain HBV-specific immune responses, which control and limit HBV replication.

DIAGNOSIS

Serologic tests are available commercially for a number of antigens and antibodies associated with HBV infection, including HBsAg, anti-HBs, total [immunoglobulin (Ig) G and IgM] antibody to HBcAg (total anti-HBc), IgM anti-HBc, HBeAg, and anti-HBe (Table 101-1). In addition, there are NAATs to detect HBV DNA. Although HBsAg, IgM anti-HBc, total anti-HBc, and HBeAg can all be detected in serum or plasma as early as 1–2 months after exposure to HBV, IgM anti-HBc is the only reliable marker of acute infection, as the other three can also be detected in persons with chronic HBV infection. IgM anti-HBc usually becomes undetectable within 6–9 months after acute infection, and HBsAg and HBeAg are usually cleared within 6 months following illness onset in those who recover from the acute infection. Anti-HBs and anti-HBe develop during the convalescent phase, with anti-HBs acting as a protective antibody that neutralizes the virus. Presence of anti-HBs following acute infection indicates recovery and immunity from reinfection. Anti-HBs can also be detected in persons who have received hepatitis B vaccine, and transiently in persons who have received HBIG.

In persons who develop chronic HBV infection, HBsAg and total anti-HBc remain detectable, generally for life (Fig. 101-1). Although all persons with detectable HBsAg should be considered infectious, the presence of HBeAg and HBV DNA, which are variably present in chronically infected persons, correlates with higher titers of HBV and greater infectivity.

EPIDEMIOLOGY

Routes of Transmission. HBV is transmitted by either percutaneous or mucosal exposure to infected blood or blood-derived body fluids. The virus is found in highest concentrations in blood and serous exudates (as high as 108–109 virions/mL); 1–2 log lower concentrations are found in various body secretions, including saliva, semen, and vaginal fluid.[12] The most probable mechanisms of person-to-person transmission involve inapparent percutaneous or permucosal contact with infectious body fluids such as exudates from dermatologic lesions, breaks in the skin, or mucous membranes with blood or serous secretions. HBV may also spread because of contact with saliva through bites or other breaks in the skin, as a consequence of the premastication of food, and through contact with virus from inanimate objects such as shared towels, toothbrushes, or reuse of

TABLE 101-1 INTERPRETATION OF SEROLOGIC TEST RESULTS FOR HEPATITIS B VIRUS INFECTION

	Serologic Markers			
	Total	*IgM*[c]		
HBsAg[a]	*Anti-HBc*[b]	*Anti-HBc*	*Anti-HBs*[d]	**Interpretation**
−	−	−	−	Susceptible; never infected
+	−	−	−	Early acute infection; transient (21 days) after vaccination
+	+	+	−	Acute infection
−	+	+	−	Acute resolving infection
−	+	−	+	Past infection; recovered and immune
+	+	−	−	Chronic infection
−	+	−	−	Past infection; "low-level" chronic infection[e]; or passive transfer to infant born to HBsAg-positive mother
−	−	−	+	Immune if titer is ≥10 mIU/mL[f] when tested 1–2 months following the full vaccination series[g]

[a]Hepatitis B surface antigen; repeat reactive should be confirmed with a licensed neutralizing confirmatory test; all HBsAg-positive persons are potentially infectious.
[b]Antibody to hepatitis B core antigen.
[c]Immunoglobulin M.
[d]Antibody to hepatitis B surface antigen.
[e]Persons positive for anti-HBc alone are unlikely to be infectious except under unusual circumstances involving direct percutaneous exposure to large quantities of blood (e.g., blood transfusion).
[f]Milli-international units per milliliter.
[g]A titer of 10 mIU/mL or higher obtained 1–2 months after the completion of the vaccine series is considered protective; without repeated exposure to HBV, titres will naturally decline over time, but immunity is likely maintained despite a decline below this level.

needles.[21,22] HBV remains infectious for at least 7 days outside the body and can be found in titers of 102–103 virions/mL on objects, even in the absence of visible blood.[23,24] The primary routes of transmission are perinatal, nonsexual person-to-person exposures, sexual contact, and percutaneous exposure to blood (e.g., IDU, unsafe injections in medical settings). HBV is not transmitted by air, food, or water.

Perinatal Transmission. Perinatal HBV transmission is one of the most efficient modes of infection. Most perinatal HBV infections occur among infants of pregnant women with chronic HBV infection. Pregnant women with acute hepatitis B in the first and second trimester rarely transmit HBV to the fetus or neonate.[25] However, the risk of transmission from pregnant women who acquire infection during the third trimester is approximately 60%.[26] Perinatal transmission occurs most often at the time of birth, with in utero transmission rarely accounting for infections transmitted from mother to infant. Although HBV can be detected in breast milk, there is no evidence that HBV is transmitted by breast-feeding.[27] The primary determinant of infection is a high concentration of maternal HBV DNA.[28] Without postexposure immunization, 70–90% of infants born to HBeAg-positive mothers will become infected by 6 months of age; about 90% of these children will remain chronically infected.[29,30] In addition, up to 20% of HBeAg negative mothers have moderately high levels of HBV DNA and may infect their newborns during the perinatal period.[30]

Nonsexual Person-to-Person Transmission. Nonsexual person-to-person HBV transmission during early childhood accounts for a high proportion of HBV infections worldwide.[4] Most early childhood transmission occurs in households of persons with chronic infection, and widespread HBsAg contamination of surfaces has been demonstrated in homes of persons with chronic infection.[23] Approximately 30% of children living in a household with an HBsAg-positive person become infected, and infants born to HBsAg-positive mothers and not infected at birth remain at high risk of infection during the first 5 years of life.[31] Transmission has rarely occurred in child day-care centers, but has not been identified between children in school settings.[22]

Before integration of hepatitis B vaccine into the infant immunization schedule in the United States, an estimated 16,000 children less than 10 years of age were infected annually with HBV beyond the postnatal period.[32] Although these infections represented only 5–10% of all HBV infections in the United States, it is estimated that 18% of persons with chronic HBV infection acquired their infection postnatally during early childhood, before implementation of perinatal hepatitis B immunization programs and routine infant hepatitis B immunization.[33] In some populations, childhood transmission was more important than perinatal transmission as a cause of chronic HBV infection before hepatitis B immunization was widely implemented. For example, in studies conducted among U.S.-born children of Southeast Asian refugees during the 1980s, approximately 60% of chronic infections in young children were among those born to HBsAg-negative mothers.[34–36]

Sexual Transmission. HBV in semen and vaginal secretions provides the means for efficient transmission by sexual contact, which is one of the most frequent routes of transmission among adults.[8,37] The most common sexual-risk factors for acute infection among heterosexual adults include having more than one sex partner in the 6-week to 6-month period prior to infection or having sex with a known infected person during this time period.[4,37] Among prevalent cases of HBV infection (presence of any HBV marker), the most common risk factors among heterosexuals include increased number of sex partners, history of sexually transmitted disease, and a history of sex with an infected partner.[8] Men who have sex with men (MSM) are one of the groups at highest risk for sexual transmission of HBV, with infection associated with receptive anal intercourse, increased numbers of sex partners, and numbers of years of sexual activity.[8]

Percutaneous Transmission. HBV is efficiently transmitted by percutaneous exposures, which predominantly occur in healthcare settings or among IDUrs. The risk of HBV infection is approximately 30–60% from needlestick exposures to HBsAg-positive, HBeAg-positive blood, and approximately 10–30% from needlestick exposures to HBsAg-positive, and HBeAg-negative blood.[38,39] By comparison, the risks of hepatitis C virus and human immunodeficiency virus transmission from percutaneous exposures are approximately 2% and 0.2%, respectively.[40,41]

Patient-to-patient transmission of HBV from percutaneous exposures has been identified in a variety of healthcare settings, including chronic hemodialysis centers, inpatient services, outpatient clinics, and long-term care facilities.[8,42] In most cases, transmission resulted from noncompliance with aseptic techniques for administering injections and recommended infection control practices designed to prevent cross-contamination of medical equipment and devices.

Although HBV infection was recognized as a frequent occupational hazard among persons who worked in laboratories or were exposed to blood while caring for patients, hepatitis B vaccination of healthcare workers and implementation of standard precautions has made HBV infection a rare event in these populations in countries where prevention measures have been implemented.[43,44] Chronically infected healthcare workers performing invasive procedures may, on rare occasions, transmit infection. Risk factors associated with these infections have been high levels of HBV DNA in the healthcare worker and the blind palpation of suture needles.[45] While an increased frequency of exposure to blood or body fluids occurs in a number of other occupations (e.g., policemen, firefighters, correctional officers), increased rates of HBV have not been identified that are attributable to occupational exposures.[46]

The primary nonmedical source of percutaneous HBV exposures is through injection of illicit drugs, which is a common mode of HBV transmission in many countries. The prevalence of chronic HBV infrection among injection drug users is an estimated 12%.[47] In the United States, the incidence of HBV has increased 114% among persons reporting IDU.[13]

Worldwide Patterns of Transmission. The endemicity of HBV infection varies greatly throughout the world (Fig. 101-3).[48] Endemicity is considered high in those areas where the prevalence of chronic infection is 8% or more and where 60–90% of the populations have serologic evidence of previous infection. In these areas, infection during the perinatal period and early childhood accounts for high rates of chronic infection and its sequelae. In most developed countries, the prevalence of HBV infection is low, with rates of HBsAg positivity being less than 1%, and the overall infection rate 5–7%.[48] For example, the prevalence of chronic HBV infection in the United States is approximately 0.28%, and approximately 4% of the general population has serologic evidence of HBV infection.[49,50] In these low-endemic areas, most infections occur among young adults, and high-risk sexual activity and injecting drug use account for most cases of newly acquired hepatitis B.[13,37] Historically, within some areas of low endemicity, the prevalence of infection has varied widely. For example, within North America, Native Alaskan populations have had a high endemicity of HBV infection, and first-generation immigrant populations from high endemic areas (e.g., Asia, Africa, Middle East, former Soviet Union) have continued to have high rates of HBV transmission.[34–36,51] In those parts of the world with an intermediate endemicity of HBV infection, transmission in all age groups maintains the level of chronic infection.

Worldwide, nosocomial transmission of HBV from inadequate sterilization of medical and dental instruments and unsafe injection practices continues to be a significant problem in developing countries and may cause as many as 8–16 million HBV infections each year.[52–56] In most developed countries, nosocomial transmission of HBV from inadequately sterilized medical instruments or reuse of injection equipment has not been a significant problem. However, occasional outbreaks continue to occur from the contamination of multiple dose vials, the reuse of disposable needles and syringes, and inadequately sterilized medical devices.[57–59] These outbreaks usually represent lapses in infection control practices.

Direct transmission via blood or blood products has been eliminated in those countries that routinely screen donors for HBsAg and require viral inactivation of clotting factor concentrates.[8] However, blood transfusion is a major source of HBV transmission in countries where the blood supply is not screened for HBsAg.

Epidemiology in the United States. With the implementation of a comprehensive immunization strategy to eliminate hepatitis B in the United States since 1991, the incidence of hepatitis B has declined dramatically, particularly among younger age groups covered by the recommendation for routine childhood immunization.[60] Since 1990, the incidence of acute hepatitis B declined from 8.5 to 1.0 per 100,000 population, with the lowest incidence among persons aged 0–19 years (less than 0.1 per 100,000), although the highest among those aged 40–49 years (2.6 per 100,000).[60] In 2018, the incidence for males (1.3 per 100,000) was approximately 1.5 times higher than that for females (0.8 per 100,000).[60]

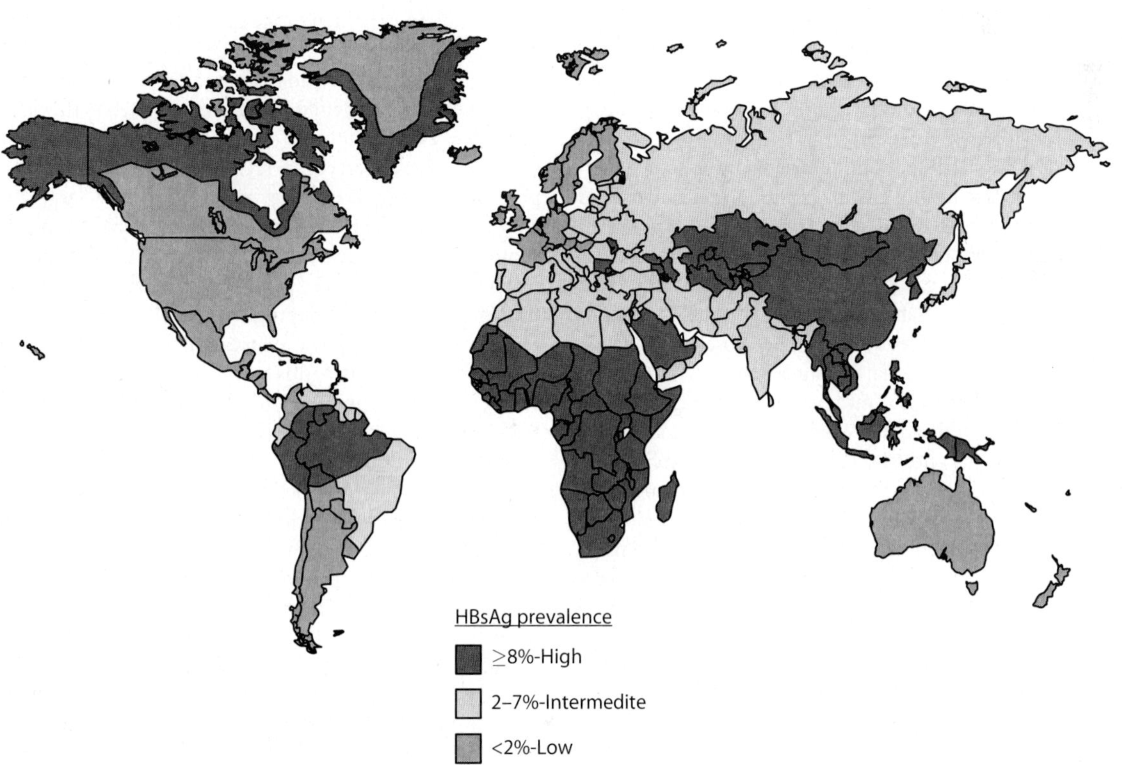

FIGURE 101-3. Geographic distribution of chronic hepatitis B virus infection. (*Source:* CDC Website, https://www.cdc.gov/hepatitis/resources/healthprofessionaltools.htm.)

In addition to declines by age, racial disparities in hepatitis B incidence have narrowed. The reduction of the disparity between Asian/Pacific Islanders and other children is consistent with recent observations noting a decline in seroprevalence of HBV infection and successful implementation of routine hepatitis B vaccination among Asians who have recently immigrated to the United States. Rates of hepatitis B have been declining among all racial and ethnic groups, and rates are now highest among non-Hispanic Whites (1.0 per 100,000) in 2018, which may be due to the opioid epidemic.[13,60]

While the proportion of reported acute hepatitis B cases reporting risk factors has been declining, the proportion of persons reporting IDUas a risk factor has increased from 15% in 2005 to 30% in 2018. Outbreaks among injection drug users continue to be reported.[61]

Among other U.S.-reported cases of acute hepatitis B in 2018 for which information on exposures during the incubation period was determined, receiving hemodialysis or a blood transfusion, both of which were previously major sources of infection, accounted for less than 0.5% of cases each.[60] This is likely a result of the vaccination of dialysis patients, improvements in infection control, and the required screening of donated blood for markers of HBV infection. Similarly, the percentage of cases attributable to occupational exposure to blood is approximately 0.5%, following widespread hepatitis B vaccination of healthcare workers.

PREVENTION AND CONTROL

The goals of hepatitis B prevention programs is the prevention of acute hepatitis B, reduction of chronic HBV infection, and mitigation of HBV-related chronic liver disease. Hepatitis B immunization is the most effective prevention measure. In addition, HBV infection can be prevented by screening blood, plasma, organ, tissue, and semen donors; virus inactivation of plasma-derived products; risk-reduction counseling and service; and implementation and maintenance of infection control practices.[8]

Two products are available to prevent HBV infection, hepatitis B vaccine, and HBIG. Hepatitis B vaccines are composed of HBsAg adsorbed to either an aluminum or cytidine-phsphate-guanosine oligodeoxynucleotide (1018) adjuvant. Both plasma-derived and recombinant vaccines are available worldwide, although only recombinant vaccines are used in the United States. HBIG is prepared from plasma containing high concentrations of anti-HBs. It provides short-term (i.e., 3–6 months) protection and is recommended in certain postexposure settings.[62]

Hepatitis B vaccines are highly immunogenic, with seroconversion rates of at least 95% in healthy infants, children, adolescents, and adults.[62] Seroprotection to HBV infection is defined as an anti-HBs response of 10 milli-International Units per milliliter (mIU/mL) or more 1–2 months after the vaccination series. There is long-term protection against hepatitis B after vaccination despite the loss of detectable levels of anti-HBs over time; booster doses are not recommended for persons with normal immune status.[62–64] Due to the high immunogenicity of hepatitis B vaccines, postvaccination testing to detect anti-HBs is not indicated after routine vaccination, except for the following groups: (a) healthcare personnel and public safety workers, (b) hemodialysis patients and others who might require outpatient hemodialysis (e.g., predialysis, peritoneal dialysis, and home dialysis), (c) HIV-infected persons or other immunocompromised persons (e.g., hematopoietic stem-cell transplant recipients or persons receiving chemotherapy), (d) sex partners of HBsAg-positive persons, and (e) infants born whose mother's HBsAg status remains unknown (e.g., when a parent or person with lawful custody safely surrenders an infant confidentially shortly after birth infants safely surrendered at or shortly after birth).

More than three decades of experience have shown that hepatitis B vaccination is a safe and cost-effective means to prevent HBV infection and its acute and chronic consequences.[62,65–67] The effectiveness of routine infant hepatitis B immunization in significantly reducing or eliminating the prevalence of chronic HBV infection has been demonstrated in many countries. In general, studies conducted in high HBV-endemic areas have demonstrated the elimination of chronic HBV among children after introduction of the vaccine.[68–71] The greatest impact has been achieved in countries that have attained high vaccine coverage among infants, and where a birth dose of vaccine was administered. In Alaska, where high vaccine coverage among infants has been achieved and all infants receive a birth dose of vaccine, HBV transmission among children has been eliminated.[68]

Since 1992, the World Health Organization has called for all countries to add hepatitis B vaccine into their national childhood immunization services, and substantial progress has been made in implementing this recommendation.[72] By 2017, 188 countries worldwide had introduced the hepatitis B vaccine.[73] In addition to routine infant vaccination, WHO recommends considering administration of a dose at birth to prevent perinatal HBV transmission, particularly in countries where a high proportion of chronic HBV infections is acquired perinatally (e.g., East and Southeast Asia, Pacific Islands). As of 2017, 105 countries have introduced hepatitis B birth dose.[73]

In the United States, a comprehensive immunization strategy has been recommended to prevent HBV-related chronic liver disease in all age groups, and to ultimately eliminate HBV transmission. Components of this strategy are: (a) prevention of perinatal HBV infection through routine screening of all pregnant women for HBsAg and appropriate immunoprophylaxis of infants born to HBsAg-positive women, (b) universal vaccination of infants beginning at birth, (c) routine vaccination of all adolescents who have not previously been vaccinated, and (d) vaccination of adults at high risk of infection, who have not been previously vaccinated.[62]

To date, most of these components have been widely implemented. Hepatitis B vaccine has been successfully integrated into the childhood vaccine schedule, and infant vaccine coverage levels are now equivalent to those of other vaccines in the childhood schedule. As of 2016, more than 90.5% of 19- to 35-month-old children had been fully immunized with three doses of hepatitis B vaccine, and 91.4% of 13–17 year olds have been fully immunized.[74] Part of this success can be attributed to the established infrastructure for vaccine delivery to children, which ensures high coverage levels. Because hepatitis B vaccine provides long-term protection against chronic HBV infection, these children will be protected as they move through adolescence and adulthood.

High HBsAg screening rates have also been achieved among pregnant women. Currently, every state and large metropolitan area receives federal funding to support perinatal hepatitis B prevention programs. An analysis of commercially insured pregnant women indicated more than 82% of pregnancies receive HBsAg testing.[75] Timely immunoprophylaxis and completion of the ACIP-recommended three-dose hepatitis B vaccine series is the corner stone of perinatal hepatitis B prevention. Hepatitis B vaccine or HBIG given alone are 75% and 71% effective in preventing perinatal HBV transmission, respectively; their combined efficacy is 94%.[62] In addition, the mother's HBV DNA level (viral titer) or HBeAg status determines the risk of mother to child transmission; the risk is considered higher with viral titers (HBV DNA) >200,000 IU/mL and/or HBeAg-positive status.[62,76] However, only about 50% of new births to HBsAg-positive women are identified for case management for ensuring completion of postexposure immunoprophylaxis.[77] For women without prenatal care, the need for proper management, including HBsAg testing of the mother at the time of admission for delivery and administration of the first dose of hepatitis B vaccine to the infant within 12 hours of birth is underscored by the higher prevalence of HBsAg seropositivity in this group compared to women who are screened prenatally.[78] However, studies have found that infants born to mothers with unknown HBsAg status at the time of delivery often do not receive a birth dose.[79,80] In addition, errors in maternal HBsAg testing and omissions in test reporting have resulted in failure to administer postexposure immunoprophylaxis to infants born to HBsAg-positive mothers.[81] Pregnant women who test HBsAg positive should also receive HBV DNA testing.[62] Antiviral therapy (i.e., lamivudine, telbivudine, and tenofovir) has been studied as an intervention to reduce perinatal HBV transmission among pregnant women with high HBV DNA levels (e.g., average HBV DNA levels >200,000 IU/mL).[82,83] Maternal antiviral therapy started at 28- to 32-week gestation, as an adjunct to hepatitis B vaccine and HBIG administered to the infant shortly after deliver, has been associated with significantly reduced rates of perinatal transmission.[82,83] Since lamivudine and telbivudine is limited by viral resistance and mutations, and tenofovir is not, tenofovir is the preferred antiviral agent.[76] Clinical guidelines recommend antiviral therapy to reduce perinatal HBV transmission when maternal HBV DNA is >200,000 IU/mL.[76] At 3 months postpartum, antiviral therapy may be stopped unless there is another clinical indication to continue antiviral therapy in the mother.[76] In addition, postvaccination serologic testing for anti-HBs and HBsAg should be performed after completion of the vaccine series at age 9–12 months, or 1–2 months after the final dose in the series.[62]

The greatest remaining challenge for hepatitis B prevention in the United States is suboptimal testing and vaccination of high-risk adults. It is estimated that fewer than half of foreign-born adults, MSM, and patients receiving chemotherapy receive HBV testing.[84–86] Regular assessment of liver enzymes and HBV DNA levels is critical for evaluation of disease progression and treatment eligibility. Eight therapeutic agents have been approved by the Food and Drug Administration (FDA) for treatment of chronic hepatitis B: alpha-interferon, pegylated interferon, telbivudine, lamivudine, adefovir, entecavir, tenofovir alafenamide, and tenofovir dipovoxil fumarate.[76] The aims of treatment are to achieve sustained suppression of HBV replication and remission of liver diseases. Fewer than 50% of persons living with chronic HBV infection are being monitored for disease progression, and only 15% of treatment eligible persons are receiving treatment.[76,87]

Vaccination coverage (>3 doses) is about 25% among all adults aged 19 years or older, and is approximately 45% among high-risk adults.[88,89] The vaccination coverage among specific risk groups include 21% for foreign-born adults residing in the United States, 27% among adults with chronic liver conditions, and 65% among healthcare workers.[88]

As a best practice, clinicians should perform HBV testing with HBsAg, total antibody to HBcAg, and anti-HBs among adults at risk for HBV infection; and vaccination among those who test negative to all three seromarkers.[90] Various strategies have been implemented in clinical and community settings to increase hepatitis B vaccination, screening, and linkage to care, and these include: partnerships with community organizations and local health centers, use of culturally and linguistically competent patient navigators, and utilization of the electronic health record.[90–92] Increased HBV testing in high-risk populations is the first step in the care cascade to identify persons with chronic HBV infection, and vaccination and linkage to care are effective at reducing HBV-associated mortality and achieving the national elimination goals.[93]

References

1. Tiollais P, Charnay P, Vyas GN. Biology of hepatitis B virus. *Science*. 1981;213:406.
2. Rossner MT. Review: Hepatitis B virus X gene product: A promiscuous transcriptional activator. *J Med Virol*. 1992;36(2):101–17.
3. Benenson AS, Chin J, eds. Viral hepatitis B. In: *Control of Communicable Diseases Manual*. 16th ed. Washington, DC: American Public Health Association; 1995, pp. 221–7.
4. Mast E, Mahoney F, Kane M, et al. Hepatitis B vaccine. In: Plotkin SA, Orenstein WA, eds. *Vaccines*. Philadelphia: WB Saunders; 2004, pp. 299–337.
5. Brown JL, Carman WF, Thomas HC. The clinical significance of molecular variation within the hepatitis B virus genome. *Hepatology*. 1992;15:144.
6. Hunt CM, McGill JM, Allen MI, et al. Clinic relevance of hepatitis B viral mutations. *Hepatology*. 2000;31(5):1037–44.
7. Zuckerman AJ. Effect of hepatitis B virus mutants on efficacy of vaccination. *Lancet*. 2000;355(9213):1382–4.
8. Seto W-K, Lo Y-R, Pawlotsky J-M, Yuen M-F. Chronic hepatitis B virus infection. *Lancet*. 2018;392(10161):2313–24.
9. Kobayashi H, Tsuzuki M, Koshimuzu K, et al. Susceptibility of hepatitis B virus to disinfection or heat. *J Clin Micro*. 1984;20(2):214.
10. McMahon BJ, Alward WL, Hall DB, et al. Acute hepatitis B virus infection: Relation of age to the clinical expression of disease and subsequent development of the carrier state. *J Infect Dis*. 1985;151(4):599–603.
11. Dienstag JL. Immunogenesis of extrahepatic manifestations of hepatitis. *Springer Semin Immunopathol*. 1982;3(4):461–72.
12. Margolis HS, Alter MJ, Hadler SC. Viral hepatitis. In: Evans AS, Kaslow RA, eds. *Viral Infections of Humans: Epidemiology and Control*. 4th ed. New York: Plenum Medical Book Co.; 1997, pp. 363–418.
13. Harris AM, Iqbal K, Schillie S, et al. Increases in acute hepatitis B virus infections—Kentucky, Tennessee, and West Virginia, 2006–2013. *MMWR*. 2016;65(3):47–50.
14. Zhou K, Contag C, Whitaker E, Terrault N. Spontaneous loss of surface antigen among adults living with chronic hepatitis B virus infection: A systematic review and pooled meta-analyses. *Lancet Gastroenterol Hepatol*. 2019;4(3):227–38.
15. Beasley RP, Hwang L-Y. Overview on the epidemiology of hepatocellular carcinoma. In: Hollinger FB, Lemon SM, Margolis HS, eds. *Viral Hepatitis and Liver Disease*. Baltimore: Williams and Wilkins; 1991, pp. 532–5.
16. McMahon BJ. The natural history of chronic hepatitis B virus infection. *Hepatology*. 2009;49(Suppl 5):S45–55.
17. Korba BE, Gowans EJ, Wells FV, et al. Systemic distribution of woodchuck hepatitis virus in the tissues of experimentally infected woodchucks. *Virology*. 1988;165(1):172–81.
18. Halpern MS, England JM, Deery DT, et al. Viral nucleic acid synthesis and antigen accumulation in pancreas and kidney of Peking ducks infected with duck hepatitis B virus. *Proc Natl Acad Sci U S A*. 1983;80(15):4865–9.
19. Asabe S, Wieland SF, Chattopadhyay PK, Roederer M, Engle RE, Purcell RH, Chisari FV. The size of the viral inoculum contributes to the outcome of hepatitis B virus infection. *J Virology*. 2009;83(19):9652–62.
20. Penna A, Chisari FV, Bertoletti A, et al. Cytotoxic T lymphocytes recognize an HLA-A2-restricted epitope within the hepatitis B virus nucleocapsid antigen. *J Exp Med*. 1991;174(6):1565–70.
21. Scott RM, Snitbhan R. Bancroft WH, et al. Experimental transmission of hepatitis B virus by semen and saliva. *J Infect Dis*. 1980;142(1):67–71.
22. Williams I, Smith MG, Sinha D, et al. Hepatitis B virus transmission in an elementary school setting. *JAMA*. 1997;278(24):2167–9.
23. Bond WW, Favero MS, Peterson NJ, et al. Survival of hepatitis B virus after drying and storage for one week. *Lancet*. 1981;1(8219):550–1.
24. Petersen NJ, Barrett DH, Bond WH, et al. HBsAg in saliva, impetigenous lesions and the environment in two remote Alaskan villages. *Appl Environ Microbiol*. 1976;32(4):572–4.
25. Tong MJ, Thursby M, Rakela J, et al. Studies of the maternal-infant transmission of the viruses which cause acute hepatitis. *Gastroenterology*. 1981;80(5 Pt 1):999–1004.
26. Levy M, Koren G. Hepatitis B vaccine in pregnancy: Maternal and fetal safety. *Am J Perinatol*. 1991;8(3):227–32.
27. Beasley RP, Stevens CE, Shiao IS, et al. Evidence against breast-feeding as a mechanism for vertical transmission of hepatitis B. *Lancet*. 1975;2(7938):740–1.
28. Stevens CE, Neurath RA, Beasley RP, et al. HBeAg and anti-HBe detection by radioimmunoassay: Correlation of verticle transmission of hepatitis B virus in Taiwan. *J Med Virol*. 1979;3(3):237–41.
29. Xu ZY, Liu CB, Francis DP, et al. Prevention of perinatal acquisition of hepatitis B virus carriage using vaccine: Preliminary report of a randomized double-blind placebo-controlled and comparative trial. *Pediatrics*. 1985;76(5):713–8.
30. Lee SD, Lo KJ, Wu JC, et al. Prevention of maternal-infant hepatitis B transmission by immunization: The role of serum hepatitis B virus DNA. *Hepatology*. 1986;6(3):369–73.

31. Beasley RP, Hwang LY. Postnatal infectivity of hepatitis B surface antigen-carrier mothers. *J Infect Dis.* 1983;147(2):185–90.
32. Armstrong GL, Mast EE, Wojczynski M, et al. Childhood hepatitis B virus infections in the United States before hepatitis B immunization. *Pediatrics.* 2001;108(5):1123–8.
33. Margolis HS, Coleman PJ, Brown RE, et al. Prevention of hepatitis B virus transmission by immunization: An economic analysis of current recommendations. *JAMA.* 1995;274(15):1201–8.
34. Hurie MB, Mast EE, Davis JP. Horizontal transmission of hepatitis B virus infection to United States-born children of Hmong refugees. *Pediatrics.* 1992;89(2):269–73.
35. Mahoney FJ, Lawrence M, Scott K, et al. Continuing risk for hepatitis B virus transmission among children born in the United States to Southeast Asian children in Louisiana. *Pediatrics.* 1995;95(6):1113–6.
36. Franks AL, Berg CJ, Kane MA, et al. Hepatitis B infection among children born in the United States to Southeast Asian refugees. *New Engl J Med.* 1989;321(19):1301–5.
37. Goldstein ST, Alter MJ, Williams IT, et al. Incidence and risk factors for acute hepatitis B in the United States, 1982–1998: Implications for vaccination programs. *J Infect Dis.* 2002;185(6):713–9.
38. Seeff LB, Wright EC, Zimmerman HJ, et al. Type B hepatitis after needle-stick exposure: Prevention with hepatitis B immune globulin: Final report of the Veterans Administration Cooperative Study. *Ann Intern Med.* 1978;88(3):285–93.
39. Grady GF, Lee VA, Prince AM, et al. Hepatitis B immune globulin for accidental exposures among medical personnel: Final report of a multi-center controlled trial. *J Infect Dis.* 1978;138(5):625–38.
40. Gerberding JL. Management of occupational exposures to blood-borne viruses. *N Engl J Med.* 1995;332(7):444–51.
41. Centers for Disease Control and Prevention. Recommendations for prevention and control of hepatitis C virus (HCV) infection and HCV-related chronic disease. *MMWR.* 1998;47(RR-19):1–39.
42. Centers for Disease Control and Prevention. Outbreaks of hepatitis B virus infection among hemodialysis patients--California, Nebraska, and Texas, 1994. *MMWR.* 1996;45(14):285–9.
43. Hadler SC, Doto IL, Maynard JE, et al. Occupational risk of hepatitis B infection in hospital workers. *Infect Control.* 1985;6(1):24–31.
44. Shapiro CN. Occupational risk of infection with hepatitis B and hepatitis C viruses. *Surg Clin North Am.* 1995;75(6):1047–56.
45. Harpaz R, Von Seidlein L, Averhoff FM, et al. Transmission of hepatitis B virus to multiple patients from a surgeon without evidence of inadequate infection control. *New Eng J Med.* 1996;334(9):549–54.
46. Woodruff BA, Moyer LA, O'Rourke KM, et al. Blood exposure and risk of hepatitis B virus infection in firefighters. *J Occup Med.* 1993;35:1048–54.
47. Nelson PK, Mathers BM, Cowie B, et al. Global epidemiology of hepatitis B and hepatitis C in people who inject drugs: Results of systematic reviews. *Lancet.* 2011;378(9791):571–83.
48. Polaris Observatory Collaborators. Global prevalence, treatment, and prevention of hepatitis B virus infection in 2016: A modelling study. *Lancet Gastroenterol Hepatol.* 2018;3(6):383–403.
49. Patel EU, Thio CL, Boon D, Thomas DL, Tobian AAR. Prevalence of hepatitis B and hepatitis D virus infections in the United States, 2011–2016. *Clin Infect Dis.* 2019;69(4):709–12.
50. Roberts H, Kruszon-Moran D, Ly KN, et al. Prevalence of chronic hepatitis B virus (HBV) infection in U.S. households: National Health and Nutrition Examination Survey (NHANES), 1988–2012. *Hepatology.* 2016;63(2):388–97.
51. Schreeder MT, Bender TR, McMahon BJ, et al. Prevalence of hepatitis B in selected Alaskan Eskimo villages. *Amer J Epidemiol.* 1983;118(4):543–9.
52. Hutin YJ, Harpaz R, Drobenuic J, et al. Injections given in healthcare settings as a major source of acute hepatitis B in Moldova. *Int J Epidemiol.* 1999;27(4):782–6.
53. World Health Organization. Global database on blood safety: Summary report 1998–1999. www.who.int/bct/.
54. Hutin Y, Stilwell B, Hauri AM, et al. Transmission of blood-borne pathogens through unsafe injections and proposed approach for the Safe Injection Global Network. In: Margolis HS, Alter MJ, Liang TJ, et al., eds. *Viral Hepatitis and Liver Disease.* London: International Medical Press; 2002, pp. 219–27.
55. Hutin YJF, Chen RT. Injection safety: A global challenge. *Bull World Health Organ.* 1999;77(10):787–8.
56. Kane A, Lloyd J, Zaffran M, et al. Transmission of hepatitis B, hepatitis C, and human immunodeficiency viruses through unsafe injections in the developing world: Model-based regional estimates. *Bull World Health Organ.* 1999;77(10):801–7.
57. Polish LB, Shapiro CN, Bauer F, et al. Nosocomial transmission of hepatitis B virus associated with a spring-loaded fingerstick device. *New Eng J Med.* 1992;326(11):721–5.
58. Centers for Disease Control and Prevention. Transmission of hepatitis B and C viruses in outpatient settings--New York, Oklahoma, and Nebraska, 2000–2002. *MMWR.* 2003;52(38):901–6.
59. Centers for Disease Control and Prevention. Transmission of hepatitis B virus among persons undergoing glucose monitoring in long-term care facilities: Mississippi, North Carolina, and Los Angeles County, California, 2003–2004. *MMWR.* 2005;54(09):220–3.
60. Centers for Disease Control and Prevention. Viral Hepatitis Surveillance, United States. https://www.cdc.gov/hepatitis/statistics/SurveillanceRpts.htm.
61. Comer M, Matthias J, Nicholson G, Asher A, Holmberg S, Wilson C. Notes from the field: Increase in acute hepatitis B infections--Pasco County, Florida, 2011–2016. *MMWR Morb Mortal Wkly Rep.* 2018;67(7):230–1.
62. Schillie S, Vellozzi C, Reingold A, et al. Prevention of hepatitis B virus infection in the United States: Recommendations of the Advisory Committee on Immunization Practices. *MMWR Recomm Rep.* 2018;67(1):1–31.
63. Simons BC, Spradling PR, Bruden DJ, et al. A longitudinal hepatitis B vaccine cohort demonstrates long-lasting hepatitis B virus (HBV) cellular immunity despite loss of antibody against HBV surface antigen. *J Infect Dis.* 2016;214(2):273–80.
64. Williams IT, Goldstein ST, Tufa J, et al. Long-term antibody response to hepatitis B vaccination beginning at birth and to subsequent booster vaccination. *Pediatr Infect Dis J.* 2003;22(2):157–63.
65. Fan L, Owusu-Edusei Jr. K, Schillie SF, Murphy TV. Cost-effectiveness of active-passive prophylaxis and antiviral prophylaxis during pregnancy to prevent perinatal hepatitis B virus infection. *Hepatology.* 2016;63(5):1471–80.
66. Barbosa C, Smith EA, Hoerger TJ, et al. Cost-effectiveness analysis of the national perinatal hepatitis B prevention program. *Pediatrics.* 2014;133(2):243–53.
67. Hoerger TJ, Bradley C, Schillie SF, Reilly M, Murphy TV. Cost-effectiveness of ensuring hepatitis B protection for previously vaccinated healthcare personnel. *Infect Control Hosp Epidemiol.* 2014;35(7):845–54.
68. McMahon BJ, Bulkow LR, Singleton RJ, et al. Elimination of hepatocellular carcinoma and acute hepatitis B in children 25 years after a hepatitis B newborn and catch-up immunization program. *Hepatology.* 2011;54(3):801–7.
69. Cui Y, Jia J. Update on epidemiology of hepatitis B and C in China. *J Gastroenterol Hepatol.* 2013;28(Suppl 1):7–10.
70. Cui F, Shen L, Li L, et al. Prevention of chronic hepatitis B after 3 decades of escalating vaccination policy, China. *Emerg Infect Dis.* 2017;23(5):765–72.
71. Fan R, Yin X, Liu Z, Liu Z, Lau G, Hou J. A hepatitis B-free generation in China: From dream to reality. *Lancet Infect Dis.* 2016;16(10):1103–5.
72. Cooke GS, Andrieux-Meyer I, Applegate TL, et al. Accelerating the elimination of viral hepatitis: A Lancet Gastroenterology & Hepatology Commission [published correction appears in Lancet Gastroenterol Hepatol. 2019 May;4(5):e4]. *Lancet Gastroenterol Hepatol.* 2019;4(2):135–84.
73. WHO/UNICEF coverage estimates 2017 revision, July 2018, and WHO database as at 06 July 2018. Immunization Vaccines and Biologicals, (IVB), World Health Organization. 194 WHO Member States. Date of slide: 15 July 2018.
74. Hill HA, Elam-Evans LD, Yankey D, Singleton JA, Kang Y. Vaccination coverage among children aged 19–35 months—United States, 2016. *MMWR Morb Mortal Wkly Rep.* 2017;66(43):1171–7.
75. Harris AM, Isenhour C, Schillie S, Vellozzi C. Hepatitis B virus testing and care among pregnant women using commercial claims data, United States, 2011–2014. *Infect Dis Obstet Gynecol.* 2018;2018:4107329.
76. Terrault NA, Lok ASF, McMahon BJ, et al. Update on prevention, diagnosis, and treatment of chronic hepatitis B: AASLD 2018 hepatitis B guidance. *Hepatology.* 2018;67(4):1560–99.
77. Ko SC, Fan L, Smith EA, Fenlon N, Koneru AK, Murphy TV. Estimated annual perinatal hepatitis B virus infections in the United States, 2000–2009. *J Pediatric Infect Dis Soc.* 2016;5(2):114–21.
78. Silverman NS, Darby MJ, Ronkin SL, et al. Hepatitis B prevalence in an unregistered prenatal population: Implications for neonatal therapy. *JAMA.* 1991;266(20):2852–5.

79. Biroscak BJ, Fiore AE, Fasano N, et al. Impact of the thimerisol controversy on hepatitis B vaccine coverage of infants born to women of unknown hepatitis B surface antigen status in Michigan. *Pediatrics.* 2003;111(6 Pt 1):e645–9.
80. Thomas AR, Fiore AE, Corwith HL, et al. Hepatitis B vaccine coverage among infants born to women without prenatal screening for hepatitis B virus infection: Effects of the joint statement on thimerosal in vaccines. *Pediatr Infect Dis J.* 2004;23(4):313–8.
81. Centers for Disease Control and Prevention. Impact of the 1999 AAP/USPHS joint statement on thimerosal in vaccines on infant hepatitis B vaccination practices. *MMWR.* 2001;50(6):94–7.
82. Pan CQ, Duan Z, Dai E, et al. Tenofovir to prevent hepatitis B transmission in mothers with high viral load. *N Engl J Med.* 2016;374(24):2324–34.
83. Jourdain G, Ngo-Giang-Huong N, Harrison L, et al. Tenofovir versus placebo to prevent perinatal transmission of hepatitis B. *N Engl J Med.* 2018;378(10):911–23.
84. Vijayadeva V, Spradling PR, Moorman AC, et al. Hepatitis B virus infection testing and prevalence among Asian and Pacific Islanders. *Am J Manag Care.* 2014;20(4):e98–104.
85. Hechter RC, Jacobsen SJ, Luo Y, et al. Hepatitis B testing and vaccination among adults with sexually transmitted infections in a large managed care organization. *Clin Infect Dis.* 2014;58(12):1739–45.
86. Hwang JP, Somerfield MR, Alston-Johnson DE, et al. Hepatitis B virus screening for patients with cancer before therapy: American Society of Clinical Oncology provisional clinical opinion update. *J Clin Oncol.* 2015;33(19):2212–20.
87. Cohen C, Holmberg SD, McMahon BJ, et al. Is chronic hepatitis B being undertreated in the United States?. *J Viral Hepat.* 2011;18(6):377–83.
88. Williams WW, Lu PJ, O'Halloran A, et al. Surveillance of vaccination coverage among adult populations—United States, 2015. *MMWR Surveill Summ.* 2017;66(11):1–28.
89. Centers for Disease Control and Prevention (CDC). Hepatitis B vaccination coverage among adults—United States, 2004. *MMWR Morb Mortal Wkly Rep.* 2006;55(18):509–11.
90. Abara WE, Qaseem A, Schillie S, McMahon BJ, Harris AM; High Value Care Task Force of the American College of Physicians and the Centers for Disease Control and Prevention. Hepatitis B vaccination, screening, and linkage to care: Best practice advice from the American College of Physicians and the Centers for Disease Control and Prevention. *Ann Intern Med.* 2017;167(11):794–804.
91. Chak E, Taefi A, Li CS, et al. Electronic medical alerts increase screening for chronic hepatitis B: A randomized, double-blind, controlled trial. *Cancer Epidemiol Biomarkers Prev.* 2018;27(11):1352–7.
92. Harris AM, Link-Gelles R, Kim K, et al. Community-based services to improve testing and linkage to care among non-U.S.-born persons with chronic hepatitis B virus infection—Three U.S. programs, October 2014–September 2017. *MMWR Morb Mortal Wkly Rep.* 2018;67(19):541–6.
93. National Academies of Sciences, Engineering Medicine. A national strategy for the elimination of hepatitis B and C: Phase two report. 2017. https://www.nap.edu/catalog/24731/a-national-strategy-for-the-elimination-of-hepatitis-b-and-c.

CHAPTER 102

Hepatitis A

Martha P. Montgomery • Mark Weng • Michael A. Purdy • Megan G. Hofmeister

INTRODUCTION

Reports of illness resembling hepatitis A virus (HAV) infection were described in Greek writings from the fourth century BC.[1] Once referred to as epidemic jaundice, catarrhal jaundice, and infectious hepatitis, hepatitis A outbreaks have been well documented since the eighteenth century.[1] In 1973, hepatitis A viral particles were visualized for the first time using electron microscopy and were identified as the etiologic agent of hepatitis A.[2,3] These findings led to the development of diagnostic tests that could differentiate acute from past HAV infection, the propagation of HAV in cell culture, and the development and licensure of hepatitis A vaccines. HAV spreads primarily by the fecal-oral route, either by direct contact with an infected individual or through consumption of contaminated food or water. In 2015, the World Health Organization estimated that 1.4 million hepatitis A cases occur globally each year.[4]

ETIOLOGIC AGENT

HAV is a 27 nm, spherical, nonenveloped virus with an icosahedral capsid configuration, and is a member of the *Hepatovirus A* species in the genus *Hepatovirus* and the family *Picornaviridae*.[5,6] The HAV genome is composed of a single-stranded, positive sense RNA molecule whose organization and replication scheme are similar to poliovirus and other members of the family *Picornaviridae*. Unlike other picornaviruses, HAV does not commandeer the host replication machinery but coexists with the host by using codons rarely used by the host. HAV infects primates and replicates predominantly in the liver where it infects hepatocytes. HAV can also infect epithelial cells in the small intestine. The virus hijacks host cellular membranes to cloak itself from host immune response and is excreted as naked virions in feces and into the blood stream as enveloped virions.[7]

Antibody binding studies indicate there is only a single HAV serotype. HAV isolates from diverse geographic areas are recognized by polyclonal antibody generated against capsid proteins (anti-HAV) and by neutralizing monoclonal antibodies to human HAV. Although HAV has little phenotypic diversity, enough genetic diversity exists in the capsid region to define six genotypes and allow for studies of molecular relatedness.[8] Genotypes I–III infect humans while genotypes IV–VI infect simians.

Compared to other picornaviruses, HAV is more resistant to inactivation by heating, to pH less than 3, to drying at ambient temperature, and to low concentrations of free chlorine or hypochlorite.[9,10] HAV is also resistant to freezing and remains infectious in feces or on environmental surfaces for several weeks.[11,12] HAV can be inactivated by many common disinfecting chemicals, including hypochlorite (bleach) and quaternary ammonium formulations containing 23% HCl, found in many toilet bowl cleaners.[13] HAV is only partially inactivated by pasteurization (60°C for 1 hour) but is completely inactivated in food by heating to temperatures higher than 85°C (>185°F) for at least 1 minute.[13] HAV grows poorly in cell culture where it requires a very long adaptation period (up to 1 month), rarely produces a cytopathic effect, and rapidly becomes attenuated.[9,10]

CLINICAL ILLNESS, PATHOGENESIS, AND IMMUNE RESPONSE

HAV infection can cause both acute disease and asymptomatic infection but does not cause chronic infection.[14] Manifestations of HAV infection include fecal shedding of virus, viremia, age-dependent expression of clinical illness (e.g., jaundice), and the occasional occurrence of fulminant liver failure. HAV infections among children under 6 years of age are usually (70%) asymptomatic.[15] If symptomatic, they generally have mild, nonspecific symptoms that include malaise, nausea, vomiting, diarrhea, fever, and dark urine. Jaundice is uncommon in children; less than 5% of children aged less than 3 years and about 10% of children aged 4–6 years are icteric.[16] Among adolescents and adults infected with HAV, the majority have classic signs or symptoms (e.g., fever, malaise, nausea, vomiting, loss of appetite, abdominal pain, and dark urine), with jaundice occurring in more than 70% of patients.[17,18]

Fulminant hepatitis A is uncommon. Before hepatitis A vaccine was licensed, an estimated 100 people died as a result of acute liver failure due to hepatitis A each year in the United States.[19] Host factors reported to be associated with an increased risk of fulminant hepatitis include older age and underlying chronic liver disease.[20–24] In the postvaccination era, hospitalization rates have increased as incident infection has shifted to older populations with more severe disease.[25] Among nationally reported hepatitis A cases with available information on hospitalization status, 67% were hospitalized in 2017.[26] The overall case-fatality rate for hepatitis A is less than 1% but increases to 1.8% among adults aged > 50 years.[19]

Although HAV infection does not cause chronic liver disease or persistent infection, up to 20% of symptomatic cases may have prolonged or relapsing disease lasting up to 6 months.[27] In addition, a cholestatic form of hepatitis A has been reported in which patients experience persistent jaundice, usually accompanied by itching.[28] Other atypical clinical manifestations are rare and may include immunologic, neurologic, hematologic, or renal manifestations.[24]

The pathogenic events that occur during the course of infection have been determined from experimental infections in chimpanzees and naturally acquired infections in humans (Fig. 102-1). The incubation period ranges from 15 to 50 days after exposure, with a median of 28 days.[9,10] Virus is found in hepatocytes throughout the course of infection and is excreted in bile. Viral shedding declines rapidly after jaundice appears in adults, although shedding may be prolonged in infected infants and children.[29–32] Using polymerase chain reaction (PCR) techniques, HAV RNA has been detected in stools of infected newborns for up to 6 months after infection and from 1 to 3 months

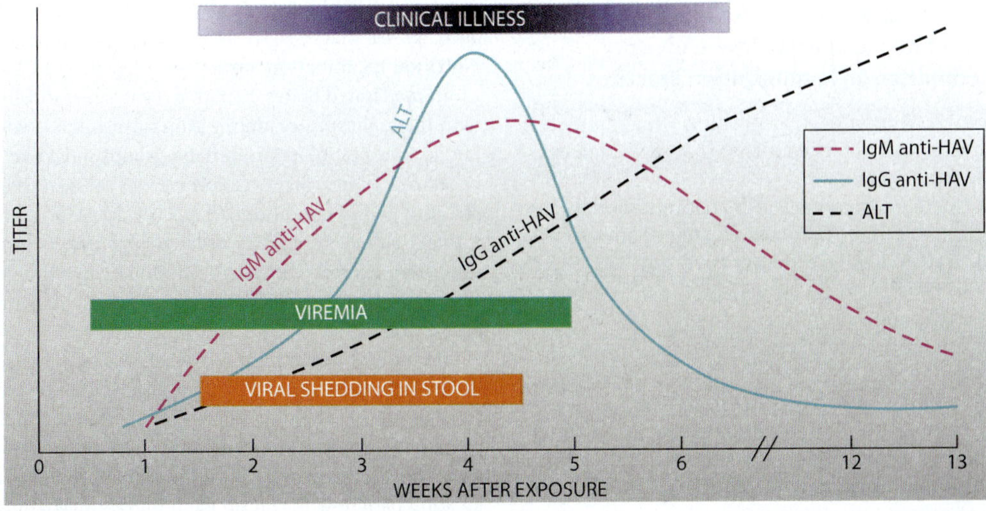

FIGURE 102-1. Events during hepatitis A virus infection. HAV, hepatitis A virus; ALT, alanine aminotransferase; IgM, antibody of the immunoglobulin M subclass to HAV; IgG, antibody of the immunoglobulin G subclass to HAV. (*Source:* CDC Website, https://www.cdc.gov/hepatitis/resources/professionals/training/serology/training.htm.)

after clinical illness in older children and adults.[31,33] Chronic HAV shedding does not occur, but virus has been detected in feces during relapsing illness.[34] Data from epidemiologic studies suggest that peak infectivity occurs during the 2 weeks before symptom onset to 1 week after jaundice appears.[35]

Available data suggest the pathogenesis of liver injury is immune-mediated rather than due to direct cytotoxicity and probably involves cell-mediated immune responses.[36] Although liver damage occurs at the same time that circulating antibodies become detectable, studies have failed to show that the pathologic process is antibody dependent. A specific immunoglobulin M (IgM) antibody response to HAV capsid proteins develops prior to the onset of clinical illness, which is accompanied by a nonspecific rise in the concentration of serum IgM.[9,10] Neutralizing IgG antibodies are usually detectable shortly after the onset of clinical illness and persist to provide lifelong immunity.[37–39]

DIAGNOSIS

Because hepatitis A is clinically indistinguishable from other forms of acute viral hepatitis, diagnosis requires the detection of either serologic markers of infection or HAV RNA. IgM anti-HAV, a serologic marker of acute illness, is present in > 99% of patients within 1 week of symptom onset, usually peaks within 1 month of illness, and declines to undetectable levels within 6 months after infection (Fig. 102-1).[32,40–42] IgG anti-HAV is produced either in response to natural infection or after immunization with hepatitis A vaccine and persists for life.[37–39] Some commercially available immunoassays detect total anti-HAV (IgM and IgG) and therefore require supplemental testing for IgM anti-HAV to distinguish acute HAV infection from past infection or previous immunization.

HAV RNA in feces, blood, cell culture, or environmental samples can be detected using PCR methodologies.[43] Detection of HAV RNA can be qualitative or quantitative, and nucleic acid sequencing can be performed on PCR products to compare genetic relatedness of isolates. However, detection of HAV RNA by PCR does not necessarily correlate with infectivity. HAV antigen can be detected in feces, cell culture, and some environmental specimens by enzyme immunoassay.[9] Currently, antigen detection is based on a research laboratory-based assay.[44] Growth in cell culture requires a long period of adaptation and changes the genetic makeup of the virus.

Biochemical evidence of hepatitis includes elevated levels of serum bilirubin and serum hepatic enzymes, including alanine aminotransferase (ALT), aspartate aminotransferase (AST), alkaline phosphatase, and gamma-glutamyltranspeptidase. Elevations in AST and ALT may occur a week or more prior to symptom onset. Serum bilirubin and ALT levels usually return to normal by 2–3 months after illness onset.

EPIDEMIOLOGY

Routes of Transmission. Person-to-person transmission by the fecal-oral route is the predominant mode of HAV transmission, both in the United States and throughout the world. In addition, because HAV can remain infectious in the environment, common-source outbreaks and sporadic cases can occur from exposure to fecal-contaminated food or water.

Bloodborne exposure is a rare route of HAV transmission, which can result from transfusion of blood or blood derivatives from a donor during the viremic phase of their infection. Outbreaks of post-transfusion hepatitis A have occurred in neonatal intensive care units with silent transmission to hospital staff and parents from infants infected by whole-blood or packed-cell transfusions.[31] Clotting factor concentrates (factor VIII, factor IX) prepared from plasma have also been implicated in the transmission of HAV, and one study indicated that people routinely receiving clotting factors prepared from plasma might be at increased risk of HAV infection.[45,46] Vertical intrauterine transmission from an infected mother and transmission from organ transplantation are also rare modes of HAV transmission.[47,48]

Worldwide Patterns of Disease. Hepatitis A is an important cause of illness throughout the world, and there are several patterns of endemicity of infection. Endemicity of HAV infection is closely related to hygiene, water, and sanitation.[49] In areas of high endemicity, represented by low-income countries (e.g., parts of sub-Saharan Africa and South Asia), socioeconomic and environmental conditions facilitate easy transmission of HAV, which is transmitted person-to-person through the fecal-oral route.[50] In these areas, almost all adults have been infected, usually as children before 10 years of age.[51]

In middle-income countries (e.g., parts of East and Southeast Asia, Eastern and Central Europe, Latin America, the Middle East, and North Africa), improved sanitation and access to clean drinking water have significantly reduced the endemic rate of HAV infection.[51] In such areas, a significant decrease in the prevalence of HAV infection has occurred among young children. However, HAV infection continues to occur among older children and young adults, and a paradoxical increase in the incidence of hepatitis A may occur

BOX 102-1 Recommendations for Routine Pre-exposure Use of Hepatitis a Vaccine—Advisory Committee on Immunization Practices

All children at age 12–23 months
Persons traveling to or working in countries that have high or intermediate HAV endemicity
Persons who anticipate close contact with an international adoptee from a country of high or intermediate endemicity during the first 60 days following arrival of the adoptee in the United States
Men who have sex with men
Users of injection and noninjection drugs
Persons with chronic liver disease
Persons with clotting factor disorders
Persons who work with HAV-infected primates or with HAV in a research laboratory setting
Persons experiencing homelessness
Anyone wishing to obtain immunity

Sources: CDC. Prevention of hepatitis A through active or passive immunization: Recommendations of the Advisory Committee on Immunization Practices. *MMWR Recomm Rep* 2006;55(No. RR-7).
CDC. Updated recommendations from the Advisory Committee on Immunization Practices (ACIP) for use of hepatitis A vaccine in close contacts of newly arriving international adoptees. *MMWR Morb Mortal Wkly Rep.* 2009;58:1006–7.
Nelson NP, Link-Gelles R, Hofmeister MG, et al. Update: Recommendations of the Advisory Committee on Immunization Practices for use of hepatitis a vaccine for postexposure prophylaxis and for preexposure prophylaxis for international travel. *MMWR Morb Mortal Wkly Rep.* 2018;67:1216–20.
Doshani M, Weng M, Moore KL, Romero JR, Nelson NP. Recommendations of the Advisory Committee on Immunization Practices for use of hepatitis A vaccine for persons experiencing homelessness. MMWR Morb Mortal Wkly Rep. 2019;68(6):153–6.

because of the greater likelihood of symptomatic infection in older age groups. In addition, as long as HAV is present in the population or the environment, including food sources, the potential remains for epidemics to occur. Shifts in infection patterns were observed in 1988 in Shanghai, China, when over 300,000 young adults became ill when shellfish contaminated with HAV were sold in the marketplace and subsequently prepared at temperatures that did not kill the virus.[52]

Low endemic rates of HAV infection are found in the United States, Canada, Western Europe, Australia, and other developed countries. There is an increased risk of hepatitis A among people from these countries traveling or working in countries with a high or intermediate endemicity of infection, and risk of infection increases with the length of stay in the country.[53]

Epidemiology in the United States. Transmission of HAV in the United States has been greatly reduced since the hepatitis A vaccine was first licensed by the U.S. Food and Drug Administration in 1995 and was first recommended by the Advisory Committee on Immunization Practices (ACIP) for use in individuals at least 2 years of age in 1996.[19,54,55] In 2014, the overall reported hepatitis A rate was the lowest yet recorded (0.4 per 100,000). During 2016–18, large increases were observed primarily due to outbreaks among people who use drugs and people experiencing homelessness.[56,57]

Hepatitis A rates among all age groups in the United States today are substantially lower than in 1995. In 2016, the lowest rates occurred among children aged 0–9 years (0.1 cases per 100,000 population); whereas adults aged 20–39 years had the highest rates (0.9 cases per 100,000 population).[55] This is similar to anti-HAV prevalence, which was highest in children aged 2–11 years (60%) and lowest in adults aged 40–49 years (16%) as measured in the National Health and Nutrition Examination Survey during 2007–12.[58]

In the United States, hepatitis A rates historically differed by race, with the highest rates among American Indians/Alaskan Natives.[20,54] Higher rates of infection in these groups most likely reflected differences in the risk for infection related to socioeconomic levels and resulting living conditions (e.g., crowding). Rates among American Indians, which were greater than 60 per 100,000 prior to 1995, however, have decreased dramatically following widespread vaccination in this group and since 2002 have been approximately the same as in other races.[55,59]

Because young children are more likely to have asymptomatic or unrecognized infections, they played an important role in HAV transmission in the prevaccine era.[20] Serologic studies demonstrated in the prevaccine era that an asymptomatic child with serologic evidence of recent HAV infection was often present in the household of an adult patient who had no identified source of infection.[60] Since the adoption of universal childhood vaccination recommendations, the rate of acute HAV infection among young children has been very low (0.1 cases/100,000), and the role of children in HAV transmission has declined.[55]

Since the adoption of universal childhood vaccination in the United States, common risk factors for hepatitis A during nonoutbreak years include international travel and sexual or household contact with a person known to have hepatitis A. Other risk factors include use of injection or noninjection drugs, being a man who reports having sex with men, exposure during a common-source outbreak, and association with a child care center. Frequently a specific risk factor cannot be identified.

In both low and high endemic populations, HAV infection behaves like most other acute infectious diseases, producing periodic epidemics as the pool of susceptible individuals increases. In the United States, cyclic increases in the incidence of hepatitis A have occurred approximately every 10–15 years, with the last nationwide increase in the prevaccine era in 1995.[54,61]

Most U.S. cases of hepatitis A result from person-to-person transmission during community-wide outbreaks.[20,62,63] During outbreaks in the prevaccine era, increases of hepatitis A were observed across all ages and racial and ethnic groups, although some risk factors [men who have sex with men (MSM) and injection drug use] were reported more frequently than in nonoutbreak years.[63] More recently, community-wide outbreaks have occurred predominantly among adults who report specific risk factors including MSM, drug use, or homelessness.[56,64]

Periodic outbreaks of hepatitis A have occurred among MSM and among people who use injection or noninjection drugs.[56,65–69] Although these two populations have been included in ACIP vaccine recommendations since 1996, vaccine uptake has been low in many areas.[56,69–71] In 2019, homelessness was recognized as an independent risk factor for HAV infection and for severe outcomes, and this population has been included in ACIP hepatitis A vaccine recommendations.[64,72,73]

Common source outbreaks due to contaminated food continue to occur. Implicated foods are generally eaten raw and have been contaminated during growing, harvest, final processing, or preparation.[9,74] Shellfish-associated outbreaks have been due to eating raw or partially cooked oysters, clams, scallops, or mussels harvested from contaminated waters.[9,75,76] Fruits or vegetables contaminated during harvest or packing and eaten raw (e.g., lettuce, green onions, strawberries, raspberries, pomegranate arils) have accounted for a number of hepatitis A outbreaks, including a large outbreak (>700 people infected) at a single restaurant, associated with imported green onions.[9,77–81] No hepatitis A outbreaks transmitted through contaminated public water systems have been reported in the United States in the last several decades. Water treatment processes and dilution within public water systems appear to be sufficient to render HAV noninfectious.[74] Hepatitis A has previously been reported among people using small private or community wells or swimming pools, and contamination by adjacent septic systems has been implicated as the source.[9,74]

PREVENTION AND CONTROL

Active immunization is the primary means for preventing HAV infection. Currently licensed hepatitis A vaccines are well tolerated, highly immunogenic, and produce long-term immunity. The hepatitis A vaccines licensed in the United States are produced from cell-culture–adapted virus that is formalin inactivated and adsorbed on an alum adjuvant.[82–84] Two single-antigen vaccines are currently licensed in the United States for use in people 12 months of age and older.[65] A third combination vaccine containing both HAV and hepatitis B virus antigens is licensed for use in people aged 18 years or older.[65] The single-antigen vaccines have been shown to be highly immunogenic in children, adolescents, and adults using a two-dose vaccination schedule.[20,65] In controlled clinical trials, preexposure vaccination with inactivated hepatitis A vaccine has been shown to be more than 95% effective in preventing HAV transmission.[85,86] With completion of the two-dose childhood vaccine series, hepatitis A vaccine is observed to provide protective levels of anti-HAV for at least 20 years.[87,88] Furthermore, detectable antibodies are estimated to persist for over 40 years and could be lifelong based on mathematical modeling and anti-HAV kinetic studies.[89,90]

In the United States, recommendations for the use of hepatitis A vaccine are directed at the prevention and control of community-wide outbreaks of disease, the protection of individuals in groups at high risk of HAV infection, and the protection of people who experience significantly increased morbidity or mortality from HAV infection.[44,65] Since 1996, ACIP has introduced hepatitis A vaccination recommendations incrementally in the United States, initially in states with high rates of hepatitis A. Beginning in 2006, all children aged 12–23 months were recommended to be routinely vaccinated with consideration of catch-up vaccination. Dramatic declines in hepatitis A cases occurred nationally after vaccine introduction.[91]

People traveling or working in countries with high or intermediate endemicity of HAV infection should be vaccinated prior to departure.[65] For most healthy people, one dose of single-antigen hepatitis A vaccine administered any time before departure can provide adequate protection.[92] According to current ACIP recommendations, hepatitis A vaccine should be administered to infants aged 6–11 months traveling outside the United States when protection against hepatitis A is recommended.[92]

Occupational risk of HAV infection has been evaluated for certain occupations. Studies conducted among U.S. workers exposed to raw sewage do not indicate a significantly increased risk for HAV infection; therefore, occupational exposure to raw sewage is not a recommended indication for vaccination.[65,93] Similarly, hepatitis A vaccine is not routinely recommended for healthcare personnel in the United States because healthcare personnel do not have increased prevalence of HAV infection and healthcare-associated outbreaks are rare.[92] Routine vaccination of food handlers is not recommended because their profession does not put them at higher risk for infection.[65,74]

When vaccinating people in groups at high risk of HAV infection, some will already have been infected with HAV. Vaccinating a person who is immune because of prior infection does not increase the risk of adverse events.[65] In populations expected to have high prevalence of previous HAV infection, prevaccination testing may be considered to reduce costs by not vaccinating people who are already immune. Decisions to test should be based on: (1) the expected prevalence of immunity, (2) the cost of vaccination compared with the cost of serologic testing (including the cost of an additional visit), and (3) the likelihood that testing will not interfere with initiation of vaccination.[65] Postvaccination testing is not warranted, as vaccine response rate is high.

When HAV exposure occurs, postexposure prophylaxis can prevent illness if administered within 2 weeks after exposure. Two options for postexposure prophylaxis include vaccination or immune globulin (IG). In most instances, hepatitis A vaccine for postexposure prophylaxis is preferred to IG, as the vaccine induces active immunity and has longer duration of protection.[92] Vaccine is also comparatively easier to administer, more acceptable, and more readily available. Hepatitis A vaccine and IG are considered safe for pregnant women and are recommended for pregnant women who have a specific risk for hepatitis A.[94,95]

Although hepatitis A vaccine is preferred in most situations, passive immunization with IG is also available as a preventive measure and provides short-term protection from HAV infection. IG is preferred to vaccination for postexposure prophylaxis in infants aged < 12 months, infant travelers aged 6–11 months, and in people for whom vaccine is contraindicated. IG and hepatitis A vaccine should be administered simultaneously in different anatomic sites for people aged ≥ 12 months who are immunocompromised or have chronic liver disease and who have not previously completed the two-dose hepatitis A vaccination series and need postexposure prophylaxis. Lastly, IG may be administered in addition to hepatitis A vaccine to people aged > 40 years for postexposure prophylaxis, depending on the provider's risk assessment. The updated dose of IG for postexposure prophylaxis is 0.1 mL/kg.[96] Preparations of human IG that contain anti-HAV are more than 85% effective in preventing symptomatic HAV infection if given before or within 2 weeks of exposure.[65,97] After administration of IG, at least 3 months must pass before MMR and varicella vaccines can be given.[96,98,99]

Postexposure prophylaxis should be administered as soon as possible, but no more than 2 weeks after the last exposure, to unvaccinated household and sexual contacts of individuals with hepatitis A, to people who have shared illicit drugs with a person with hepatitis A, and to children and staff exposed in child care or certain other institutional settings.[65] Postexposure prophylaxis should not be routinely given when a single case occurs in schools, offices, other professional settings, or hospital settings. Rather, attention should be given to standard precautions, including good hand hygiene.

Most food handlers with HAV infection do not transmit HAV to exposed consumers or restaurant patrons.[100–102] If a food handler is diagnosed with hepatitis A, postexposure prophylaxis should be administered to other unvaccinated food handlers at the same establishment. Because common-source transmission to patrons is unlikely, postexposure prophylaxis administration to patrons is usually not recommended but can be considered if (a) during the time when the food handler was likely to be infectious, the food handler both directly handled uncooked foods or foods after cooking and had diarrhea or poor hygienic practices; and (b) patrons can be identified and offered postexposure prophylaxis within 2 weeks after the exposure. In situations where repeated HAV exposures might have occurred such as institutional cafeterias, postexposure prophylaxis may be considered.[92]

Other prevention and control measures include attention to good personal hygiene and environmental sanitation, which can serve as useful adjuncts to vaccination. Complete inactivation of HAV in food requires heating to 85°C (>185°F) for at least 1 minute, or disinfection with a 1:100 dilution of household bleach in water or cleaning solutions containing quaternary ammonium and/or HCl.[13] Although vaccination coupled with improved sanitation and socioeconomic conditions in the United States have led to the decline in disease incidence, further progress toward prevention and reduction of HAV disease transmission will require strategies aimed at an emerging cohort of susceptible adults.[91]

References

1. Cockayne EA. Catarrhal jaundice, sporadic and epidemic, and its relation to acute yellow atrophy of the liver. *QJM*. 1912;6(1):1–29.
2. Feinstone SM, Kapikian AZ, Purceli RH. Hepatitis A: Detection by immune electron microscopy of a viruslike antigen associated with acute illness. *Science*. 1973;182(4116):1026–8.
3. Gravelle CR, Hornbeck CL, Maynard JE, Schable CA, Cook EH, Bradley DW. Hepatitis A: Report of a common-source outbreak with recovery of a possible etiologic agent. II. Laboratory studies. *J Infect Dis*. 1975;131(2):167–71.
4. World Health Organization. Immunization, vaccines and biologicals: Hepatitis A. https://www.who.int/immunization/diseases/hepatitisA/en/.
5. Drexler JF, Corman VM, Lukashev AN, et al. Evolutionary origins of hepatitis A virus in small mammals. *Proc Natl Acad Sci U S A*. 2015;112(49):15190–5.
6. Zell R, Delwart E, Gorbalenya AE, et al. ICTV virus taxonomy profile: Picornaviridae. *J Gen Virol*. 2017;98(10):2421–2.
7. Feng Z, Hensley L, McKnight KL, et al. A pathogenic picornavirus acquires an envelope by hijacking cellular membranes. *Nature*. 2013;496(7445):367–71.
8. Vaughan G, Rossi LMG, Forbi JC, et al. Hepatitis A virus: Host interactions, molecular epidemiology and evolution. *Infect Genet Evol*. 2014;21:227–43.
9. Hui YH, Sattar SA, Murrell KD, Nip W-K, Stanfield PS, eds. *Foodborne Disease Handbook*. Boca Raton: CRC Press; 2001.
10. Lemon SM. Type A viral hepatitis. New developments in an old disease. *N Engl J Med*. 1985;313(17):1059–67.
11. Butot S, Putallaz T, Sanchez G. Effects of sanitation, freezing and frozen storage on enteric viruses in berries and herbs. *Int J Food Microbiol*. 2008;126(1–2):30–5.
12. Sattar SA, Jason T, Bidawid S, Farber J. Foodborne spread of hepatitis A: Recent studies on virus survival, transfer and inactivation. *Can J Infect Dis*. 2000;11(3):159–63.
13. Favero MS, Bond WW. In: *Viral Hepatitis*. Thomas HC, Lemon SM, Zuckerman AJ, eds Malden, MA: Blackwell Pub; 2005, Ch. 53, pp. 804–14.
14. Stapleton JT. Host immune response to hepatitis A virus. *J Infect Dis*. 1995;171(Suppl 1):S9–14.
15. Hadler SC, Webster HM, Erben JJ, Swanson JE, Maynard JE. Hepatitis A in day-care centers. A community-wide assessment. *N Engl J Med*. 1980;302(22):1222–7.
16. Gingrich GA, Hadler SC, Elder HA, Ash KO. Serologic investigation of an outbreak of hepatitis A in a rural day-care center. *Am J Public Health*. 1983;73(10):1190–3.
17. Lednar WM, Lemon SM, Kirkpatrick JW, Redfield RR, Fields ML, Kelley PW. Frequency of illness associated with epidemic hepatitis A virus infections in adults. *Am J Epidemiol*. 1985;122(2):226–33.
18. Tong MJ, el-Farra NS, Grew MI. Clinical manifestations of hepatitis A: Recent experience in a community teaching hospital. *J Infect Dis*. 1995;171(Suppl 1):S15–8.
19. Shapiro CN, Bell BP, Margolis HS, Centers for Disease Control and Prevention. Prevention of hepatitis A through active or passive immunization: Recommendations of the Advisory Committee on Immunization Practices (ACIP). *MMWR Recomm Rep*. 1996;45:1–30.
20. Bell BP, Wasley A, Shapiro CN, Margolis HS, Advisory Committee on Immunization Practices. Prevention of hepatitis A through active or passive immunization: Recommendations of the Advisory Committee on Immunization Practices (ACIP). *MMWR Recomm Rep*. 1999;48(RR-12):1–37.
21. Akriviadis EA, Redeker AG. Fulminant hepatitis A in intravenous drug users with chronic liver disease. *Ann Intern Med*. 1989;110(10):838–9.
22. Vento S, Garofano T, Renzini C, et al. Fulminant hepatitis associated with hepatitis A virus superinfection in patients with chronic hepatitis C. *N Engl J Med*. 1998;338(5):286–90.
23. Keeffe EB. Is hepatitis A more severe in patients with chronic hepatitis B and other chronic liver diseases? *Am J Gastroenterol*. 1995;90(2):201–5.
24. Willner IR, Uhl MD, Howard SC, Williams EQ, Riely CA, Waters B. Serious hepatitis A: An analysis of patients hospitalized during an urban epidemic in the United States. *Ann Intern Med*. 1998;128(2):111–4.
25. Ly KN, Klevens RM. Trends in disease and complications of hepatitis A virus infection in the United States, 1999–2011: A new concern for adults. *J Infect Dis*. 2015;212(2):176–82.
26. Centers for Disease Control and Prevention. Surveillance for Viral Hepatitis—United States, 2017. 2019.
27. Glikson M, Galun E, Oren R, Tur-Kaspa R, Shouval D. Relapsing hepatitis A. Review of 14 cases and literature survey. *Medicine*. 1992;71(1):14–23.
28. Gordon SC, Reddy KR, Schiff L, Schiff ER. Prolonged intrahepatic cholestasis secondary to acute hepatitis A. *Ann Intern Med*. 1984;101(5):635–7.
29. Carl M, Kantor RJ, Webster HM, Fields HA, Maynard JE. Excretion of hepatitis A virus in the stools of hospitalized hepatitis patients. *J Med Virol*. 1982;9(2):125–9.
30. Tassopoulos NC, Papaevangelou GJ, Ticehurst JR, Purcell RH. Fecal excretion of Greek strains of hepatitis A virus in patients with hepatitis A and in experimentally infected chimpanzees. *J Infect Dis*. 1986;154(2):231–7.
31. Rosenblum LS, Villarino ME, Nainan OV, et al. Hepatitis A outbreak in a neonatal intensive care unit: Risk factors for transmission and evidence of prolonged viral excretion among preterm infants. *J Infect Dis*. 1991;164(3):476–82.
32. Bower WA, Nainan OV, Han X, Margolis HS. Duration of viremia in hepatitis A virus infection. *J Infect Dis*. 2000;182(1):12–7.
33. Yotsuyanagi H, Koike K, Yasuda K, et al. Prolonged fecal excretion of hepatitis A virus in adult patients with hepatitis A as determined by polymerase chain reaction. *Hepatology*. 1996;24(1):10–3.
34. Sjogren MH, Tanno H, Fay O, et al. Hepatitis A virus in stool during clinical relapse. *Ann Intern Med*. 1987;106(6):221–6.
35. Krugman S, Ward R, Giles JP, Bodansky O, Jacobs AM. Infectious hepatitis: Detection of virus during the incubation period and in clinically inapparent infection. *N Engl J Med*. 1959;261:729–34.
36. Vallbracht A, Fleischer B. Immune pathogenesis of hepatitis A. *Arch Virol*. 1992;4(Suppl 4):3–4.
37. Decker RH, Overby LR, Ling CM, Frösner G, Deinhardt F, Boggs J. Serologic studies of transmission of hepatitis A in humans. *J Infect Dis*. 1979;139(1):74–82.
38. Lemon SM, Binn LN. Serum neutralizing antibody response to hepatitis A virus. *J Infect Dis*. 1983;148(6):1033–9.
39. Locarnini SA, Ferris AA, Lehmann NI, Gust ID. The antibody response following hepatitis A infection. *Intervirology*. 1977;8(5):309–18.
40. Liaw YF, Yang CY, Chu CM, Huang MJ. Appearance and persistence of hepatitis A IgM antibody in acute clinical hepatitis A observed in an outbreak. *Infection*. 1986;14(4):156–8.
41. Lemon SM. Type A viral hepatitis: Epidemiology, diagnosis, and prevention. *Clin Chem*. 1997;43(8 Pt 2):1494–9.
42. Lee HK, Kim K-A, Lee JS, Kim N-H, Bae WK, Song TJ. Window period of anti-hepatitis A virus immunoglobulin M antibodies in diagnosing acute hepatitis A. *Eur J Gastroenterol Hepatol*. 2013;25(6):665–8.
43. Nainan OV, Xia G, Vaughan G, Margolis HS. Diagnosis of hepatitis a virus infection: A molecular approach. *Clin Microbiol Rev*. 2006;19(1):63–79.
44. Averhoff FM, Khudyakov Y, Nelson NP. In: Plotkin SA, Orenstein WA, Offit PA, Edwards KM, eds. *Plotkin's Vaccines*. 7th ed. New York: Elsevier; 2018, pp. 319–41.e315.
45. Centers for Disease Control and Prevention. Hepatitis A among persons with hemophilia who received clotting factor concentrate—United States, September–December 1995. *MMWR Morb Mortal Wkly Rep*. 1996;45(2):29–32.
46. Mah MW, Royce RA, Rathouz PJ, et al. Prevalence of hepatitis A antibodies in hemophiliacs: Preliminary results from the Southeastern Delta Hepatitis Study. *Vox Sang*. 1994;67(Suppl 1):21–2; discussion 23.
47. Watson JC, Fleming DW, Borella AJ, Olcott ES, Conrad RE, Baron RC. Vertical transmission of hepatitis A resulting in an outbreak in a neonatal intensive care unit. *J Infect Dis*. 1993;167(3):567–71.
48. Foster MA, Weil LM, Jin S, et al. Transmission of hepatitis A virus through combined liver-small intestine-pancreas transplantation. *Emerg Infect Dis*. 2017;23(4):590–6.
49. Wasley A, Fiore A, Bell BP. Hepatitis A in the era of vaccination. *Epidemiol Rev*. 2006;28:101–11.
50. Jacobsen KH. Globalization and the changing epidemiology of hepatitis A virus. *Cold Spring Harb Perspect Med*. 2018;8(10):a031716.
51. Jacobsen KH, Wiersma ST. Hepatitis A virus seroprevalence by age and world region, 1990 and 2005. *Vaccine*. 2010;28(41):6653–7.
52. Halliday ML, Kang LY, Zhou TK, et al. An epidemic of hepatitis A attributable to the ingestion of raw clams in Shanghai, China. *J Infect Dis*. 1991;164(5):852–9.
53. Steffen, R. Kane MA, Shapiro CN, Billo N, Schoellhorn KJ, van Damme P. Epidemiology and prevention of hepatitis A in travelers. *JAMA*. 1994;272(11):885–9.
54. Wasley A, Miller JT, Finelli L, Centers for Disease Control and Prevention. Surveillance for acute viral hepatitis—United States, 2005. *MMWR CDC Surveill Summ*. 2007;56:1–24.

55. Centers for Disease Control and Prevention. Surveillance for Viral Hepatitis—United States, 2016. 2017.
56. Foster M, Ramachandran S, Myatt K, et al. Hepatitis A virus outbreaks associated with drug use and homelessness—California, Kentucky, Michigan, and Utah, 2017. *MMWR Morb Mortal Wkly Rep.* 2018;67(43):1208–10.
57. Foster MA, Hofmeister MG, Kupronis BA, et al. Increase in Hepatitis A virus infections—United States, 2013–2018. *MMWR Morb Mortal Wkly Rep.* 2019;68(18):413–5.
58. Klevens RM, Denniston MM, Jiles-Chapman RB, Murphy TV. Decreasing immunity to hepatitis A virus infection among US adults: Findings from the National Health and Nutrition Examination Survey (NHANES), 1999–2012. *Vaccine.* 2015;33(46):6192–8.
59. Bialek SR, Thoroughman DA, Hu D, et al. Hepatitis A incidence and hepatitis a vaccination among American Indians and Alaska Natives, 1990–2001. *Am J Public Health.* 2004;94(6):996–1001.
60. Staes CJ, Schlenker TL, Risk I, et al. Sources of infection among persons with acute hepatitis A and no identified risk factors during a sustained community-wide outbreak. *Pediatrics.* 2000;106(4):E54.
61. Shapiro CN, Coleman PJ, McQuillan GM, Alter MJ, Margolis HS. Epidemiology of hepatitis A: Seroepidemiology and risk groups in the USA. *Vaccine.* 1992;10(Suppl 1):S59–62.
62. Shaw FE, Sudman JH, Smith SM, et al. A Community-wide epidemic of hepatitis A in Ohio. *Am J Epidemiol.* 1986;123(6):1057–65.
63. Bell BP, Shapiro CN, Alter MJ, et al. The diverse patterns of hepatitis A epidemiology in the United States-implications for vaccination strategies. *J Infect Dis.* 1998;178(6):1579–84.
64. Wooten DA. Forgotten but not gone: Learning from the hepatitis A outbreak and public health response in San Diego. *Top Antivir Med.* 2019;26(4):117–21.
65. Fiore AE, Wasley A, Bell BP, Advisory Committee on Immunization Practices. Prevention of hepatitis A through active or passive immunization: Recommendations of the Advisory Committee on Immunization Practices (ACIP). *MMWR Recomm Rep.* 2006;55(RR-7):1–23.
66. Corey L, Holmes KK. Sexual transmission of hepatitis A in homosexual men: Incidence and mechanism. *N Engl J Med.* 1980;302(8):435–8.
67. Cotter SM, Sansom S, Long T, et al. Outbreak of hepatitis A among men who have sex with men: Implications for hepatitis A vaccination strategies. *J Infect Dis.* 2003;187(8):1235–40.
68. Hutin YJ, Sabin KM, Hutwagner LC, et al. Multiple modes of hepatitis A virus transmission among methamphetamine users. *Am J Epidemiol.* 2000;152(2):186–92.
69. Latash J, Dorsinville M, Rosso PD, et al. Notes from the field: Increase in reported hepatitis A infections among men who have sex with men—New York City, January–August 2017. *MMWR Morb Mortal Wkly Rep.* 2017;66(37):999–1000.
70. Williams WW, Lu P-J, O'Halloran A, et al. Surveillance of vaccination coverage among adult populations—United States, 2015. *MMWR Surveill Summ.* 2017;66(11):1–28.
71. Campbell JV, Garfein RS, Thiede H, et al. Convenience is the key to hepatitis A and B vaccination uptake among young adult injection drug users. *Drug Alcohol Depend.* 2007;91(Suppl 1):S64–72.
72. Doshani M, Weng M, Moore KL, Romero JR, Nelson NP. Recommendations of the Advisory Committee on Immunization Practices for use of hepatitis A vaccine for persons experiencing homelessness. *MMWR Morb Mortal Wkly Rep.* 2019;68(6):153–6.
73. Kim DK, Hunter P. Advisory Committee on Immunization Practices recommended immunization schedule for adults aged 19 years or older—United States, 2019. *MMWR Morb Mortal Wkly Rep.* 2019;68(5):115–8.
74. Fiore AE. Hepatitis A transmitted by food. *Clin Infect Dis.* 2004; 38(5):705–15.
75. Desenclos JC, Klontz KC, Wilder MH, Nainan OV, Margolis HS, Gunn RA. A multistate outbreak of hepatitis A caused by the consumption of raw oysters. *Am J Public Health.* 1991;81(10):1268–72.
76. Viray MA, Hofmeister MG, Johnston DI, et al. Public health investigation and response to a hepatitis A outbreak from imported scallops consumed raw-Hawaii, 2016. *Epidemiol Infect.* 2018;1–8.
77. Rosenblum LS, Mirkin IR, Allen DT, Safford S, Hadler SC. A multifocal outbreak of hepatitis A traced to commercially distributed lettuce. *Am J Public Health.* 1990;80(9):1075–9.
78. Niu MT, Polish LB, Robertson BH, et al. Multistate outbreak of hepatitis A associated with frozen strawberries. *J Infect Dis.* 1992;166(3):518–24.
79. Dentinger CM, Bower WA, Nainan OV, et al. An outbreak of hepatitis A associated with green onions. *J Infect Dis* 2001;183(8):1273–6.
80. Centers for Disease Control and Prevention. Hepatitis A outbreak associated with green onions at a restaurant—Monaca, Pennsylvania, 2003. *MMWR. Morb Mortal Wkly Rep.* 2003;52(47):1155–7.
81. Collier MG, Khudyakov YE, Selvage D, et al. Outbreak of hepatitis A in the USA associated with frozen pomegranate arils imported from Turkey: An epidemiological case study. *Lancet Infect Dis.* 2014;14(10):976–81.
82. Siegl G, Lemon SM. Recent advances in hepatitis A vaccine development. *Virus Res.* 1990;17(2):75–92.
83. Armstrong ME, Giesa PA, Davide JP, et al. Development of the formalin-inactivated hepatitis A vaccine, VAQTA from the live attenuated virus strain CR326F. *J Hepatol.* 1993;18(Suppl 2):S20–6.
84. Peetermans J. Production, quality control and characterization of an inactivated hepatitis A vaccine. *Vaccine.* 1992;10(Suppl 1):S99–101.
85. Innis BL, Snitbhan R, Kunasol P, et al. Protection against hepatitis A by an inactivated vaccine. *JAMA.* 1994;271(17):1328–34.
86. Werzberger A, Mensch B, Kuter B, et al. A controlled trial of a formalin-inactivated hepatitis A vaccine in healthy children. *N Engl J Med.* 1992;327(7):453–7.
87. Plumb ID, Bulkow LR, Bruce MG, et al. Persistence of antibody to Hepatitis A virus 20 years after receipt of Hepatitis A vaccine in Alaska. *J Viral Hepat.* 2017;24(7):608–12.
88. Mosites E, Gounder P, Snowball M, et al. Hepatitis A vaccine immune response 22 years after vaccination. *J Med Virol.* 2018;90:1418–22.
89. Theeten H, Van Herck K, Van Der Meeren O, et al. Long-term antibody persistence after vaccination with a 2-dose Havrix™ (inactivated hepatitis A vaccine): 20 Years of observed data, and long-term model-based predictions. *Vaccine.* 2015;33(42):5723–7.
90. Hens N, Habteab Ghebretinsae A, Hardt K, Van Damme P, Van Herck K. Model based estimates of long-term persistence of inactivated hepatitis A vaccine-induced antibodies in adults. *Vaccine.* 2014;32(13):1507–13.
91. Murphy TV, Denniston MM, Hill HA, et al. Progress toward eliminating hepatitis A disease in the United States. *MMWR Suppl.* 2016;65(1):29–41.
92. Nelson NP, Link-Gelles R, Hofmeister MG, et al. Update: Recommendations of the Advisory Committee on Immunization Practices for use of hepatitis A vaccine for postexposure prophylaxis and for preexposure prophylaxis for international travel. *MMWR. Morb Mortal Wkly Rep.* 2018;67(43):1216–20.
93. Venczel L, Brown S, Frumkin H, Simmonds-Diaz J, Deitchman S, Bell BP. Prevalence of hepatitis A virus infection among sewage workers in Georgia. *Am J Ind Med.* 2003;43(2):172–8.
94. Moro PL, Museru OI, Niu M, Lewis P, Broder K. Reports to the Vaccine Adverse Event Reporting System after hepatitis A and hepatitis AB vaccines in pregnant women. *Am J Obstet Gynecol.* 2014;210(6):561.e1-6.
95. Kim DK, Hunter P. Recommended adult immunization schedule, United States, 2019. *Ann Intern Med.* 2019;170(3):182–92.
96. Nelson NP. Updated dosing instructions for immune globulin (Human) GamaSTAN S/D for hepatitis A virus prophylaxis. *MMWR. Morb Mortal Wkly Rep.* 2017;66(36):959–60.
97. Winokur PL, Stapleton JT. Immunoglobulin prophylaxis for hepatitis A. *Clin Infect Dis.* 1992;14(2):580–6.
98. Kroger AT, Sumaya CV, Pickering LK, Atkinson WL. General recommendations on immunization: Recommendations of the Advisory Committee on Immunization Practices (ACIP). *MMWR. Recomm Rep.* 2006;55:1–48.
99. McLean HQ, Fiebelkorn AP, Temte JL, Wallace GS. Prevention of measles, rubella, congenital rubella syndrome, and mumps, 2013: Summary recommendations of the Advisory Committee on Immunization Practices (ACIP). *MMWR. Recomm Rep.* 2013;62(RR-4):1–34.
100. Sharapov UM, Kentenyants K, Groeger J, Roberts H, Holmberg SD, Collier MG. Hepatitis A infections among food handlers in the United States, 1993–2011. *Public Health Rep.* 2016;131(1):26–9.
101. Morey RJ, Collier MG, Nelson NP. The financial burden of public health responses to hepatitis A cases among food handlers, 2012–2014. *Public Health Rep.* 2017;132(4):443–7.
102. Ridpath A, Reddy V, Layton M, et al. Hepatitis A cases among food handlers: A local health department response—New York City, 2013. *J Public Health Manag Pract.* 2017;23(6):571–6.

CHAPTER

103 *Haemophilus influenzae* Infections*

Sara E. Oliver • Fernanda C. Lessa

Haemophilus influenzae was proposed by Pfeiffer in 1892 as the etiologic agent of influenza because of its recovery from the respiratory tracts of persons with that disease. It was later identified as a major bacterial cause of pneumonia and meningitis in children and immunocompromised or chronically ill adults. *H. influenzae* type b (Hib) was the most common cause of bacterial meningitis and invasive bacterial disease in children in the United States before the introduction of Hib polysaccharide-protein conjugate vaccines in the late 1980s. Routine infant immunization against Hib has led to the near elimination of Hib disease in the United States.[1,2] Of the 194 WHO member countries, 192 (99%) have introduced conjugate Hib vaccine, which contributed to substantial declines in Hib deaths globally.[3–5] The success of the Hib conjugate vaccines has paved the way for a new generation of vaccines against the other major bacterial diseases of children, *Streptococcus pneumoniae* and *Neisseria meningitidis*. However, in the post-Hib vaccine era, increases in nonserotype b *H. influenzae* infections, particularly *H. influenzae* serotype a (Hia) and nontypeable *H. influenzae*, have occurred in some countries, including Canada and the United States.[2,6]

BACTERIOLOGY

H. influenzae is a nonmotile, gram-negative bacterium with varied form, appearing as cocci to small rods in clinical specimens. It can be difficult to stain and may be confused with gram-positive diplococci in spinal fluid. *In vitro* culture requires the use of specialized media supplemented with essential growth factors (hemin or "factor X" and nicotinamide adenine dinucleotide or "factor V") and a carbon dioxide rich atmosphere.

H. influenzae are classified into six capsular serotypes (designated a, b, c, d, e, and f) that were first identified by Pittman in 1931. There are also unencapsulated strains that are referred to as "nontypeable." In clinical or reference laboratories, serotyping can be performed using slide agglutination serotyping (SAST), which takes advantage of type-specific agglutination of organisms by antisera. Although used since the 1930s, this technique requires subjective interpretation, and cross-reactivity can result in misclassification.[7] DNA-based methods, such as the polymerase chain reaction (PCR) and whole genome sequencing (WGS), can also be used to determine capsular genotypes. Real-time PCR is highly sensitive and specific for distinguishing *H. influenzae* capsular genotypes. Both real-time PCR and WGS have shown good agreement with SAST in determining *H. influenzae* capsule types.[8]

Antibiotic resistance among isolates is widespread, but prevalence varies geographically. *H. influenzae* strains may acquire resistance to common beta-lactam antibiotics, such as penicillin and ampicillin, via plasmids containing genes for beta lactamase. Approximately one-third of U.S. invasive isolates are β-lactamase positive.[9,10] In two global assessments, 16–17% of isolates from the respiratory tract were β-lactamase positive, ranging from 2% in Italy to 65% in South Korea.[11,12] In addition, β-lactamase-negative ampicillin-resistant (BLNAR) strains have been detected. While BLNAR strains are rare overall,[12,13] nearly 40% of *H. influenzae* strains in one study in Japan were BLNAR positive.[14] Continued monitoring of antimicrobial susceptibilities of *H. influenzae* is important to inform clinical treatment guidelines.

CLINICAL CHARACTERISTICS AND PATHOPHYSIOLOGY

Meningitis is the most severe, life-threatening illness caused by *H. influenzae*. Prior to routine immunization, Hib was the leading cause of bacterial meningitis among young children in the United States. Peak incidence occurred in infants 6–8 months of age, and case-fatality was approximately 3–5%,[15] which is lower compared to low- and middle-income countries, where case-fatality rates for Hib meningitis were $\geq$ 10%.[16] Among adults with Hib infection, meningitis was less common than other invasive syndromes, including pneumonia or bacteremia. In the vaccine era, nontypeable (unencapsulated) strains account for over 70% of invasive *H. influenzae* disease in the United States, with bacteremic pneumonia being the principal clinical presentation.[2] Invasive Hia has similar clinical presentations to Hib disease, with meningitis primarily noted in children.[17] Epiglottitis, a potentially severe inflammation and edema of the epiglottis and surrounding soft tissue due to *H. influenzae,* is now uncommon among children.

H. influenzae colonizes the respiratory tract; organisms enter the bloodstream of susceptible hosts and disseminate throughout the tissues. Bacteria may cross the blood-brain barrier and seed the central nervous system to cause meningitis. Epiglottitis and pneumonia may result from infection of soft tissue by organisms colonizing the respiratory tract. *H. influenzae* evades the host immune system by inhibition of mucosal cilia and proteolytic cleavage of secretory IgA antibody. Capsular polysaccharides play a role in blocking complement-mediated phagocytosis. Immunocompromised hosts, such as people with asplenia or human immunodeficiency virus (HIV) infection, may be more vulnerable to infection. Chronic smoke exposure or preceding viral infections may increase susceptibility by disrupting respiratory clearance of the organism.[18]

In the United States, nontypeable *H. influenzae* and *S. pneumoniae* remain the two most common causes of acute otitis media. Following the introduction of pneumococcal conjugate vaccine for infants in

*Note: The findings and conclusions in this chapter are those of the authors and do not necessarily represent the official position of the Centers for Disease Control and Prevention.

2000, nontypeable *H. influenzae* has been identified as the etiology in an increased proportion of otitis media cases.[19,20] Otitis media is the most common reason for pediatric outpatient visits and is the leading indication for antimicrobial use in the United States, resulting in > 10,000,000 annual antibiotic prescriptions.[21,22]

TREATMENT

Initial empiric treatment for infections caused by *H. influenzae* involves utilizing available antibiotics that cover the most likely bacterial pathogens. In the United States, practice guidelines for empiric antibiotic treatment of bacterial meningitis and pneumonia are based on patient age and predisposing conditions.[23,24] Once *H. influenzae* has been identified as the etiologic agent, a third-generation cephalosporin, such as ceftriaxone and cefotaxime, is recommended for targeted treatment of severe infections, particularly due to the current prevalence of ampicillin-resistance.[25] For noninvasive infections that could be caused by *H. influenzae*, such as otitis media, current treatment guidelines reflect efforts to avoid the unnecessary use of antibiotics.[21,22] Individual clinical decisions to treat with antibiotics reflect a patient's age, severity of illness, and underlying medical conditions.

IMMUNITY

In 1933, Fothergill and Wright described a nadir in serum bactericidal activity in children from age 3 months to 2 years, the age range at which *H. influenzae* meningitis incidence among children peaks.[26] Protective immunity against *H. influenzae* is mediated by maternal antibodies or antibodies naturally acquired as a result of nasopharyngeal carriage or infection with the organism. Protection from *H. influenzae* type b disease is associated with antibodies against a capsular polysaccharide, polyribosyl-ribitol-phosphate (PRP).[27] Pioneers in vaccinology realized that stimulation of anti-PRP antibody in infants could protect against Hib disease.[27]

The first Hib vaccine was made from purified PRP polysaccharide and was variably effective. A large efficacy study in Finland demonstrated protection for children who received vaccine at 18 months or older, but poor immunogenicity in younger children.[28] The immune response to polysaccharide vaccine administered in infancy had no evidence of long-term immunity.[29] The polysaccharide vaccine was licensed in the United States in 1985 for children 18 months and older, and postlicensure studies showed inconsistent results, with substantial variations in estimates of vaccine efficacy.[30] The limitations of the polysaccharide vaccine were overcome by a new generation of Hib vaccines. Investigators found that PRP polysaccharide could be coupled with protein antigens that stimulated interaction with T-lymphocytes, so called T-cell–dependent antigens, such as tetanus and diphtheria toxoids.[31] The ability of the PRP-protein conjugate to induce T-cell–dependent immunity improved antibody response in infancy and primed the immune system for subsequent doses.[32]

All currently available Hib vaccines contain PRP polysaccharide conjugated to one of a number of protein antigens, including tetanus toxoid derivatives and the major outer membrane protein from *N. meningitidis*. The choice of carrier protein influences the immunogenicity of the PRP polysaccharide, with PRP conjugated to the *N. meningitidis* outer membrane protein stimulating higher levels of antibody after the first dose compared to other conjugate vaccines, which require two or three doses to produce protective levels of antibody.[33] A booster dose of Hib vaccine is recommended after 12 months of age to sustain protective antibody levels throughout childhood.[34]

TRANSMISSION

H. influenzae causes disease only in humans, and the human nasopharynx is its natural reservoir. Unencapsulated organisms predominate in the nasopharynx and can be isolated frequently from asymptomatic children. The prevalence of nasopharyngeal colonization increases from infancy through early childhood; approximately 50–60% of children 4–6 years of age can be colonized with nontypable *H. influenzae*.[35,36] Hib carriage was uncommon even before the introduction of conjugate vaccines, identified in just 3–5% of children < 5 years of age in high-income settings[37] and 10–18% of children of that age in low-income settings.[38,39] Higher prevalence of Hib carriage has been reported in association with clusters of invasive infections in childcare centers and, in some studies, from populations with high rates of invasive disease.[37]

Asymptomatic carriers are the major source of transmission; most patients with invasive *H. influenzae* disease have not had contact with a person who had invasive disease.[37] *H. influenzae* is spread via contact with respiratory droplets or secretions. However, clusters of invasive Hib cases may occur even in the absence of a high prevalence of nasopharyngeal carriage.[40]

OCCURRENCE

High-income Countries. In the United States, the incidence of invasive Hib disease among children < 5 years of age dropped from more than 50 cases per 100,000 children in the prevaccine era to less than 1 case per 100,000 within 10 years of vaccine introduction.[2,41] The average annual incidence of invasive Hib disease among children < 5 years of age has been well below the United States' Healthy People 2020 goal (<0.27/100,000) since 2000.[34]

In the prevaccine era, American Indian, Alaska Native, and Australian Aboriginal populations experienced high rates of Hib disease, with the highest occurrence in infants < 1 year of age.[16,42] Rates among American Indian and Alaska Native children have declined substantially, but remain higher than those in the general U.S. population.[43,44] Historically, higher incidence of Hib disease among black children compared to white children in the United States has largely disappeared.[2] Children with HIV infection, sickle-cell disease, or disorders of immunoglobulin synthesis are at increased risk of *H. influenzae* disease.

Although Hib disease has been nearly eliminated in the postvaccine era, invasive disease caused by non-b *H. influenzae* has been increasingly reported in the United States (see Fig. 103-1). The largest burden of invasive *H. influenzae* occurs in people at the extremes of ages, with the highest incidence among the youngest (<1 year of age) and oldest (≥80 years of age) individuals.[2] Nontypeable *H. influenzae* is the most common cause of invasive *H. influenzae* disease and is also associated with the highest case fatality (16.1%). Across 12 European countries, nontypeable *H. influenzae* caused 78% of all invasive *H. influenzae* cases from 2007 to 2014, and incidence of *H. influenzae* disease increased among persons < 1 month and ≥ 20 years of age during this period.[45] Additionally, nontypeable *H.*

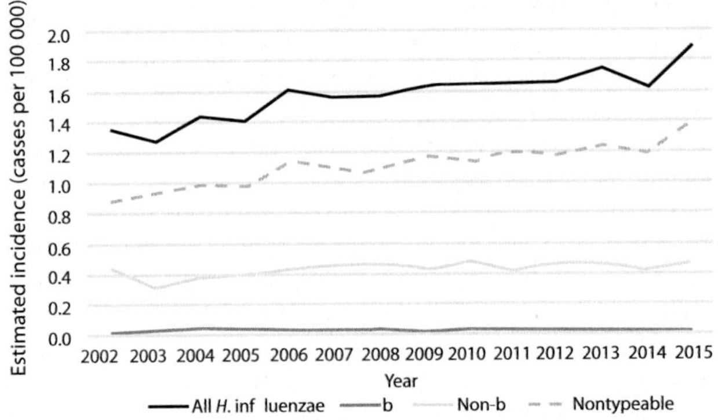

FIGURE 103-1. Trends in estimated incidence of invasive *Haemophilus influenzae* disease, by serotype—United States, 2002–15. (*Source:* From Soeters H, Blain A, Pondo T, et al. Current epidemiology and trends in invasive *Haemophilus influenzae* disease—United States, 2009–2015. *Clin Infect Dis.* 2018:67(6):881–9.)

influenzae has been noted as an emerging pathogen among pregnant women and neonates (infants <1 month of age). In the United Kingdom, the incidence of invasive nontypeable *H. influenzae* disease was 17 times higher among pregnant women, compared to nonpregnant women[46] and 28 times higher among preterm neonates, compared to term neonates.[47] *H. influenzae* infection in all but two of the cases in pregnant women resulted in the end of the pregnancy, either through miscarriage, stillbirth, or birth of the infant at the time of infection.[47] Additional surveillance capturing pregnancy status and pregnancy outcome for women of reproductive age can provide further information on this emerging clinical picture.

The incidence of invasive *H. influenzae* serotype a (Hia) disease has increased in North American countries. Among the general U.S. population, invasive Hia disease incidence was nearly 150% higher in 2009–15, compared to 2002–08, with the largest increases seen in children <1 year of age.[2] Similar to Hib, indigenous children in North America are at increased risk for invasive Hia disease compared to other races. In Alaska, the incidence of Hia among Alaska Native children <5 years of age was 36 times higher than that among non-Native children from 2002 to 2011.[48] In areas of Northern Canada, where most Indigenous Canadian people live, the incidence of Hia among children has been reported to be as high as 200–400 cases per 100,000 persons.[49,50] However, the incidence of Hia across 12 European countries remains low.[45] The incidence of invasive Hia disease in other regions of the world is not well characterized because serotyping of isolates is not routinely performed or only distinguishes between Hib and non-Hib disease. No Hia vaccine is currently available, and cross-protection against Hia disease is not expected from Hib vaccines. However, a conjugate Hia vaccine is currently under development.[51,52] The development of an effective Hia vaccine could prevent substantial morbidity and mortality, particularly among indigenous populations.

Low and Middle-income Countries

After the World Health Organization recommended Hib vaccination worldwide in 2006,[53] and with financial support from Gavi, the Vaccine Alliance, Hib vaccine has been introduced into national immunization programs in most countries.[3,54] By 2015, all countries except China and Thailand had introduced Hib vaccine into their infant immunization programs.[3] An increase in the number of countries using Hib vaccine, from 60 countries in 2000 to 192 countries in 2015, has been associated with a decline of approximately 1.2 million Hib deaths globally.[5] Despite great success with Hib vaccine introduction, 30–40% of children <5 years of age remain unvaccinated.[55] Hib continues to be an important cause of morbidity and mortality among young children in low- and middle-income countries, and the most prevalent serotype causing *H. influenzae* meningitis in Africa.[56-60] Recent estimates suggest that Hib was responsible for over 900,000 cases of pneumonia and 31,000 cases of meningitis in 2015.[5] Of an estimated 29,800 annual deaths due to Hib in 2015, 82% occur in Africa and Southeast Asia. The countries with the largest number of Hib deaths were India, Nigeria, China, and South Sudan. Southeast Asia was the region with the highest Hib mortality rate per 100,000 children <5 years of age (range 6–13).[5]

Globally, pneumonia is the most common manifestation of invasive Hib disease.[5] Hib pneumonia is three to four times more common than Hib meningitis, and case-fatality ranges from 5% to 10%.[5] Studies in Chile and the Gambia showed that as many as 20% of severe, x-ray confirmed cases of pneumonia in children <2 years of age were prevented by Hib conjugate vaccine,[61,62] and that five times more cases of Hib pneumonia were prevented as cases of Hib meningitis. In contrast, a community-randomized trial in Indonesia found no reduction of severe pneumonia in children who received Hib vaccine but identified a large burden of Hib meningitis preventable through vaccination.[63] Sustaining high coverage of Hib vaccine will be critical to further declines in Hib disease globally.

PREVENTION

Immunization is the most effective means of preventing Hib disease. Hib vaccines were the first protein-polysaccharide conjugate vaccines against bacterial infections, and they have proven to be extremely safe and efficacious. These conjugate vaccines are immunogenic in early infancy, eliciting protective antibodies in young children at highest risk of invasive disease. Most Hib conjugate vaccines require three doses in the first 6 months of life to achieve protective levels of antibody. Countries vary in their schedules for administration of Hib vaccine and the inclusion of a booster dose. In the United States, Hib vaccinations are recommended at 2, 4, and 6 months of age, with a booster dose in the second year of life.[34] The vaccine is usually administered at the same time as other vaccines in the routine childhood immunization series, most commonly diphtheria-tetanus-pertussis and hepatitis B. For some high-risk populations, specific Hib conjugates may be recommended for different doses of the vaccination schedule. For example, the Hib conjugate vaccine containing the *N. meningitidis* outer membrane protein (PRP-OMP) has been recommended for primary immunization in American Indian and Alaska Native communities that experience high rates of disease in early infancy.[34] Different from the United States and other high-income countries, many low- and middle-income countries introduced Hib vaccine without a booster dose.[53]

Globally, undervaccination or failure to vaccinate accounts for a substantial percentage of the remaining invasive Hib disease among children.[2,55] Undervaccination also contributes to continued circulation of Hib, as increased disease transmission has been reported in communities with low vaccination coverage.[64]

Hib conjugate vaccines elicit "herd immunity" by preventing nasopharyngeal carriage of Hib and decreasing transmission.[37] In the United States, Hib conjugate vaccines were first licensed for use in children 18 months of age and older. Before these vaccines were licensed for use in infants, rates in infants had already started to fall as a result of herd effects achieved by vaccinating older children.[65] The magnitude of the herd effects of Hib conjugate vaccine was unexpected when the vaccine was introduced.

In the Hib vaccine era in the United States, chemoprophylaxis is recommended to interrupt transmission for household contacts of cases in specific circumstances when unimmunized young children are present. Rifampin eliminates carriage of *H. influenzae* and is given to protect children at increased risk of invasive disease.[66] These include immunocompromised children (regardless of immunization status), household contacts less than 4 years of age who are not fully vaccinated, and household contacts less than 12 months of age who have not completed the primary Hib series. If there are no at-risk children present, chemoprophylaxis is not recommended. Chemoprophylaxis is also recommended for preschool and child care center contacts when two or more cases of Hib invasive disease have occurred within 60 days.

The success of Hib conjugate vaccines has led the way for introduction of other protein-polysaccharide vaccines against common bacterial infections, including *Streptococcus pneumoniae* and *Neisseria meningitidis*. The pitfalls encountered with Hib vaccine introduction in lower income countries have served as lessons for the introduction of newer vaccines such as pneumococcal and meningococcal conjugate vaccines. With coordinated international effort, it is hoped that the delay between the introduction of these life-saving vaccines in high-income countries and their ensuing availability in lower income countries can be minimized. The Hib conjugate vaccine represents a public health triumph, although the goal of eliminating Hib disease among all the world's children may require more years to be achieved. A challenge for the future will be to improve surveillance globally to evaluate if declines in Hib disease and deaths are being sustained, and to monitor for serotype replacement with non-b *H. influenzae*.

References

1. Centers for Disease Control and Prevention. Progress toward elimination of *Haemophilus influenzae* type b invasive disease among infants and children—United States, 1998–2000. *MMWR Morb Mortal Wkly Rep.* 2002;51(11):234–7.
2. Soeters H, Blain A, Pondo T, et al. Current epidemiology and trends in invasive *Haemophilus influenzae* disease—United States, 2009–2015. *Clin Infect Dis.* 2018;67(6):881–9.
3. View-hub report: Global Vaccine Introduction and Implementation (https://www.jhsph.edu/ivac/wp-content/uploads/2019/08/VIEW-hub_Report_Jun2019.pdf). Accessed August 27, 2019.
4. Wenger JD, DiFabio J, Landaverde JM, et al. Introduction of Hib conjugate vaccines in the non-industrialized world: Experience in four "newly adopting" countries. *Vaccine.* 1999;18(7–8):736–42.
5. Wahl B, O'Brien K, Greenbaum A, et al. Burden of *Streptococcus pneumoniae* and *Haemophilus influenzae* type b disease in children in the era of conjugate vaccines: Global, regional and national estimates for 2000–2015. *Lancet Glob Health.* 2018;6(7):e744–57.
6. Brown VM, Madden S, Kelly L, et al. Invasive *Haemophilus influenzae* disease caused by non-type b strains in Northwestern Ontario, Canada, 2002–2008. *Clin Infect Dis.* 2009;49(8):1240–3.
7. LaClaire LL, Tondella ML, Beall DS, et al. Identification of *Haemophilus influenzae* serotypes by standard slide agglutination serotyping and PCR-based capsule typing. *J Clin Microbiol.* 2003;41(1):393–6.
8. Potts CC, Topaz N, Rodriguez-Rivera LD, et al. Genomic characterization of *Haemophilus influenzae*: A focus on the capsule locus. *BMC Genomics.* 2019;20(1):733.
9. Doern GV, Brueggemann AB, Pierce G, et al. Antibiotic resistance among clinical isolates of *Haemophilus influenzae* in the United States in 1994 and 1995 and detection of beta-lactamase-positive strains resistant to amoxicillin-clavulanate: Results of a national multicenter surveillance study. *Antimicrob Agents Chemother.* 1997;41(2):292–7.
10. Triden L, Glennen A, Juni B, Lynfield R. Invasive *Haemophilus influenzae* disease and antibiotic susceptibility of invasive isolates in Minneosta, 2002–2005. *Infect Dis Clin Pract.* 2007;15:373–6.
11. Jacobs MR, Felmingham D, Appelbaum PC, et al. The Alexander project 1998–2000: Susceptibility of pathogens isolated from community-acquired respiratory tract infection to commonly used antimicrobial agents. *J Antimicrob Chemother.* 2003;52(2):229–46.
12. Hoban D, Felmingham D. The PROTEKT surveillance study: Antimicrobial susceptibility of *Haemophilus influenzae* and *Moraxella catarrhalis* from community-acquired respiratory tract infections. *J Antimicrob Chemother.* 2002;50(Supp 2):49–59.
13. Karlowsky JAZ, Critchley IA, Blosser-Middleton RS, et al. Antimicrobial surveillance of *Haemophilus influenzae* in the United States during 2000–2001 leads to detection of clonal dissemination of a β-lactamase-negative and ampicillin-resistant strain. *J Clin Microbiol.* 2002;40(3):1063–6.
14. Hasegawa K, Yamamoto K, Chiba N, et al. Diversity of ampicillin-resistance genes in *Haemophilus influenzae* in Japan and the United States. *Microb Drug Resist.* 2003;9(1):39–46.
15. Wenger JD, Hightower AW, Facklam RR, et al. Bacterial meningitis in the United States, 1986: Report of a multistate surveillance study. The Bacterial Meningitis Study Group. *J Infect Dis.* 1990;162(6):1316–23.
16. Bennett J, Platonov A, Slack MP, et al. *Haemophilus influenzae Type b (Hib) Meningitis in the Pre-Vaccine Era: A Global Review of Incidence, Age Distributions, and Case-Fatality Rates.* Geneva: WHO; 2002:92.
17. Plumb ID, Lecy KD, Singleton R, et al. Invasive *Haemophilus influenzae* serotype a infection in children: Clinical description of an emerging pathogen—Alaska, 2002–2014. *Pediatr Infect Dis J.* 2018;37(4):298–303.
18. Wilson R, Read R, Cole P. Interaction of *Haemophilus influenzae* with mucus, cilia, and respiratory epithelium. *J Infect Dis.* 1992;165(Suppl 1):S100–2.
19. Van Dyke MK, Pirçon JY, Cohen R, et al. Etiology of acute otitis media in children less than 5 years of age: A pooled analysis of 10 similarly designed observational studies. *Pediatr Infect Dis J.* 2017;36(3):274–81.
20. Kaur R, Morris M, Pichichero ME. Epidemiology of acute otitis media in the postpneumococcal conjugate vaccine era. *Pediatrics.* 2017;140(3):e20170181.
21. Siddiq S, Grainger J. The diagnosis and management of acute otitis media: American Academy of Pediatrics Guidelines 2013. *Arch Dis Child Educ Pract Ed.* 2015;100(4):193–7.
22. Lieberthal AS, Carroll AE, Chonmaitree T, et al. The diagnosis and management of acute otitis media. *Pediatrics.* 2013;131(3):e964–99. www.pediatrics.org/cgi/content/full/131/3/e964.
23. Tunkel AR, Hartman BJ, Kaplan SL, et al. Practice guidelines for the management of bacterial meningitis. *Clin Infect Dis.* 2004;39(9):1267–84.
24. Metlay JP, Waterer GW, Long AC et al. Diagnosis and treatment of adults with community-acquired pneumonia. An official clinical practice guideline of the American Thoracic Society and Infectious Diseases Society of America. *Am J Respir Crit Care Med.* 2019;200(7):e45–67.
25. Brouwer MC, Tunkel AR, van de Beek D. Epidemiology, diagnosis and antimicrobial treatment of acute bacterial meningitis. *Clin Microb Rev.* 2010;23(3):467–92.
26. Fothergill L, Wright J. Influenzal meningitis: The relation of age incidence to the bactericidal power of blood against the causal organism. *J Immunol.* 1933;24(4):273–84.
27. Robbins JB, Schneerson R, Argaman M, et al. *Haemophilus influenzae* type b: Disease and immunity in humans. *Ann Intern Med.* 1973;78(2):259–69.
28. Peltola H, Kayhty H, Sivonen A, et al. *Haemophilus influenzae* type b capsular polysaccharide vaccine in children: A double-blind field study of 100,000 vaccinees 3 months to 5 years of age in Finland. *Pediatrics.* 1977;60(5):730–7.
29. Kelly DF, Moxon ER, Pollard AJ. *Haemophilus influenzae* type b conjugate vaccines. *Immunology.* 2004;113(2):163–74.
30. Ward JI, Broome CV, Harrison LH, Shinefield HR, Black SB. *Haemophilus influenzae* type b vaccines: Lessons for the future. *Pediatrics.* 1988;81(6):886–93.
31. Schneerson R, Robbins JB, Wang Z, et al. Characterization of serum *Haemophilus influenzae* type b and Pneumococcus type 6A antibodies elicited by polysaccharide-protein conjugates in adult volunteers. In: Robbins JB, Schneerson R, Klein D, Sadoff J, Hardegree MC, eds. *Bacterial Vaccines.* New York: Praeger Publishers; 1987:425–37.
32. Eskola J, Kayhty H, Takala AK. A randomized, prospective field trial of a conjugate vaccine in the protection of infants and young children against invasive *Haemophilus influenzae* type b disease. *N Engl J Med.* 1990;323(20):1381–7.
33. Santosham M, Wolff M, Reid R, et al. The efficacy in Navajo infants of a conjugate vaccine consisting of *Haemophilus influenzae* type b polysaccharide and *Neisseria meningitidis* outer-membrane protein complex. *N Engl J Med.* 1991;324(25):1767–72.
34. Briere EC, Rubin L, Moro P, et al. Prevention and control of *Haemophilus influenzae* type b disease: Recommendations of the Advisory Committee on Immunization Practices (ACIP). *MMWR Recomm Rep.* 2014;63(RR-01):1–14.
35. St Geme JW 3rd. The pathogenesis of nontypable *Haemophilus influenzae* otitis media. *Vaccine.* 2000;19(Suppl 1):S41–50.
36. Howard AJ, Dunkin KT, Millar GW. Nasopharyngeal carriage and antibiotic resistance of *Haemophilus influenzae* in healthy children. *Epidemiol Infect.* 1988;100(2):193–203.
37. Barbour ML. Conjugate vaccines and the carriage of *Haemophilus influenzae* type b. *Emerg Infect Dis.* 1996;2(3):176–82.
38. Adegbola RA, Secka O, Lahai G et al. Elimination of *Haemophilus influenzae* type b (Hib) disease from The Gambia after the introduction of routine immunization with a Hib conjugate vaccine: A prospective study. *Lancet.* 2005;366(9480):144–50.
39. Bijlmer HA, Evans NL, Campbell H et al. Carriage of *Haemophilus influenzae* in healthy Gambian children. *Trans R Soc Trop Med Hyg.* 1989;83(6):831–5.
40. McVernon J, Morgan P, Mallaghan C, et al. Outbreak of *Haemophilus influenzae* type b disease among fully vaccinated children in a day-care center. *Pediatr Infect Dis J.* 2004;23(1):38–41.
41. Broome C. Epidemiology of *Haemophilus influenzae* type b infections in the United States. *Pediatr Infect Dis J.* 1987;6:779–82.
42. Bijlmer HA. Worldwide epidemiology of *Haemophilus influenzae* meningitis; industrialized vs non-industralized countries. *Vaccine.* 1991;9(suppl):S5.
43. Singleton R, Bulkow LR, Levine OS, et al. Experience with the prevention of invasive *Haemophilus influenzae* type b disease by vaccination in Alaska: The impact of persistent oropharyngeal carriage. *J Pediatr.* 2000;137(3):313–20.
44. Millar EV, O'Brien KL, Levine OS, et al. Toward elimination of *Haemophilus influenzae* type b carriage and disease among high-risk American Indian children. *Am J Public Health.* 2000;90(10):1550–4.
45. Whittaker R, Economopoulou A, Gomes Dias J. Epidemiology of invasive *Haemophilus influenzae* disease, Europe, 2007–2014. *Emerg Infect Dis.* 2017;23(3):396–404.
46. Collins S, Ramsay M, Slack MPE. Risk of invasive *Haemophilus influenzae* infection during pregnancy and association with adverse fetal outcomes. *JAMA.* 2014;311(11):1125–32.

47. Collins S, Litt DJ, Flynn S. Neonatal invasive *Haemophilus influenzae* disease in England and Wales: Epidemiology, clinical characteristics and outcome. *Clin Infect Dis.* 2015;60(12):1786–92.
48. Bruce MG, Zulz T, DeByle C. *Haemophilus influenzae* serotype a invasive disease, Alaska, USA, 1983–2011. *Emerg Infect Dis.* 2013;19(6):932–7.
49. McConnell A, Tab B, Scheifele D, et al. Invasive infectious caused by serotypes in twelve Candian IMPACT centers, 1996–2001. *Pediatr Infect Dis J.* 2007;26:1025–31.
50. Tsang RSW, Li YA, Mullen A. Laboratory characterization of invasive *Haemophilus influenzae* isolates from Nunavut, Canada, 2000–2012. *Int J Circumpolar Health.* 2016;75(1):29798. doi:10.3402/ijch.v75.29798.
51. Cox AD, Barreto L, Ulanova M, Bruce MG, Tsang RSW. Developing a vaccine for *Haemophilus influenzae* serotype a: Proceedings of a workshop. *Can Commun Dis Rep.* 2017;43(5):89–95.
52. Cox AD, Williams D, Cairns C. Investigating the candidacy of a capsular polysaccharide-based glycoconjugate as a vaccine to combat *Haemophilus influenzae* type a disease: A solution for an unmet public health need. *Vaccine.* 2017;35(45):6129–39.
53. World Health Organization. The WHO position paper on *Haemophilus influenzae* type b conjugate vaccines. *Wkly Epidemiol Rec.* 2006;81(47):445–52.
54. The Global Alliance for Vaccines and Immunization *Haemophilus influenzae* type b vaccine support. https://www.gavi.org/support/nvs/hib/ Accessed August 27, 2019.
55. World Health Organization. WHO-UNICEF estimates of Hib3 coverage. https://apps.who.int/immunization_monitoring/globalsummary/timeseries/tswucoveragehib3.html. Accessed August 27, 2019.
56. Howie SRC, Oluwalana C, Secka O, et al. The effectiveness of conjugate *Haemophilus influenzae* type b vaccine in the Gambia 14 years after introduction. *Clin Infect Dis.* 2013;57(11):1527–34.
57. Von Gottberg A, de Gouveia L, Madhi SA, et al. Respiratory and meningeal disease surveillance in South Africa: Impact of conjugate *Haemophilus influenzae* type b (Hib) vaccine introduction in South Africa. *Bull World Health Organ.* 2006;84(10):811–8.
58. Hammitt LL, Crane RJ, Karani A, et al. Effect of *Haemophilus influenzae* type b vaccination without a booster dose on invasive *H. influenzae* type b disease, nasopharyngeal carriage, and population immunity in Kilifi, Kenya: A 15-year regional surveillance study. *Lancet Glob Health.* 2016;4(3):e185–94.
59. Mwenda JM, Soda E, Weldegebriel G, et al. Pediatric bacterial meningitis surveillance in the World Health Organization African Region using the invasive bacterial vaccine—Preventable Disease Surveillance Network, 2011–2016. *Clin Infect Dis.* 2019;69(Suppl 2):S49–57.
60. Mackenzie GA, Ikumapayi UN, Scott S, et al. Increased disease due to *Haemophilus influenzae* type b: Population-based surveillance in eastern Gambia, 2008–2013. *Pediatr Infect Dis J.* 2015;34(5):e107–12.
61. Mulholland K, Smith PG, Broome CV, et al. A randomized trial of a *Haemophilus influenzae* type b conjugate vaccine in a developing country for the prevention of pneumonia—Ethical considerations. *Int J Tuberc Lung Dis.* 1999;3(9):749–55.
62. Levine OS, Lagos R, Munoz A, et al. Defining the burden of pneumonia in children preventable by vaccination against *Haemophilus influenzae* type b. *Pediatr Infect Dis J.* 1999;18(12):1060–4.
63. Gessner BD, Sutanto A, Linehan M, et al. Incidences of vaccine-preventable *Haemophilus influenzae* type b pneumonia and meningitis in Indonesian children: Hamlet-randomised vaccine-probe trial. *Lancet.* 2005;365(9453):43–52.
64. Fry AM, Lurie P, Gidley M, et al. *Haemophilus influenzae* type b disease among Amish children in Pennsylvania: Reasons for persistent disease. *Pediatrics.* 2001;108(4):E60.
65. Adams WG, Deaver KA, Cochi SL, et al. Decline of childhood *Haemophilus influenzae* type b (Hib) disease in the Hib vaccine era. *JAMA.* 1993;269(2):221–6.
66. American Academy of Pediatrics. Haemophilus influenzae infections. In: Kimberlin DW, Brady MT, Jackson MA., eds. *Red Book: Report of the Committee on Infectious Diseases.* 31st ed. Elk Grove Village, IL: American Academy of Pediatrics; 2018:367–75.

CHAPTER

104

Meningococcal Disease*

Sarah Mbaeyi

Meningococcal disease, due to the bacterium *Neisseria meningitidis* (meningococcus), is a serious cause of bacterial meningitis and sepsis globally. The high mortality and epidemic potential of meningococcal disease have led to extensive prevention and control efforts.

BACTERIOLOGY

N. meningitidis is an aerobic, gram-negative bacterium that is closely related to other *Neisseria* species including *N. gonorrhoeae* and commensal organisms such as *N. lactamica*. The outer membrane proteins and polysaccharide capsule are important virulence factors that help the bacterium attach to the naso- and oropharyngeal epithelium and evade phagocytosis and complement-mediated lysis.[1] *N. meningitidis* is classified into 12 serogroups based on characteristics of the polysaccharide capsule, with serogroups A, B, C, W, X, and Y the most common causes of meningococcal disease worldwide.[2]

EPIDEMIOLOGY

Meningococcal disease occurs globally, though the incidence and serogroup distribution varies by region. Average annual incidence in recent years has ranged from <0.10 cases per 100,000 population in parts of Latin America and Asia to 7.5 cases per 100,000 population in areas of the meningitis belt of sub-Saharan Africa.[3,4] In the United States, incidence has steadily declined since the late 1990s, with an incidence of 0.11 cases per 100,000 population in 2017.[5] In many regions of the world, incidence of meningococcal disease is highest in infants and young children, followed by a peak in incidence in adolescents, who have the highest rates of asymptomatic oropharyngeal carriage, and thus are thought to be the primary sources of transmission to other groups.[6,7] Globally, serogroup B and C cause a significant burden of invasive disease, though in recent years several regions have experienced rapid expansion of a serogroup W clone.[2,8] Serogroup A was historically the primary cause of the high rates of endemic meningococcal disease and large-scale epidemics in sub-Saharan Africa.[9] A variety of meningococcal vaccination strategies have been implemented globally, further influencing the epidemiology of disease in vaccinated areas over time.[10]

Outbreaks of meningococcal disease can occur in community settings or may affect persons in organization-based settings, such as schools, universities, childcare facilities, or healthcare facilities. Outbreaks are relatively uncommon in the United States, accounting for approximately 5% of all cases.[11] In recent years, several serogroup B meningococcal disease outbreaks at universities and serogroup C outbreaks among men who have sex with men have been reported in the United States.[11,12] In other areas of the world, outbreaks are a significant cause of morbidity and mortality. In the "meningitis belt" of sub-Saharan Africa, periodic large-scale epidemics occur every 5–10 years, with incidence rates as high as 1000 cases per 100,000 population.[9] Following introduction of a serogroup A meningococcal conjugate vaccine starting in 2010, large serogroup A epidemics were eliminated in this region, though several large outbreaks due to serogroups C and W have been reported, along with increased incidence of serogroup X.[4,13–17]

Certain persons are at increased risk for meningococcal disease due to underlying medical conditions, including complement deficiency (e.g., C3, C5-9, properdin, Factor D, or Factor H deficiencies), use of a type of medication called a complement inhibitor [e.g., eculizumab (Soliris®), ravulizumab (Ultomiris®)], functional or anatomic asplenia, and human immunodeficiency virus (HIV) infection.[18–22] Additionally, microbiologists who routinely handle isolates of *N. meningitidis*, travelers to areas where meningococcal disease is endemic or hyperendemic (such as the meningitis belt of sub-Saharan Africa), and persons identified as part of the population at risk during an outbreak, are at increased risk of exposure, and thus acquisition, of *N. meningitidis* infection. Additionally, college freshmen living in residence halls and military recruits have an increased incidence of meningococcal disease, likely due in part to crowded living conditions, which has been identified as a risk factor for meningococcal disease.[23,24] Additional risk factors include antecedent viral infection and exposure to active or passive smoking.[25,26]

TRANSMISSION

N. meningitidis is found only in humans and is spread by respiratory droplets. The organism can be transmitted from asymptomatic carriers or patients with *meningococcal disease*. Oropharyngeal carriage of meningococci is common, affecting approximately 10% of the population at any given time, though prevalence can vary depending on the population, season, age, and living conditions, and typically persists for several weeks to months.[27] Rates of meningococcal carriage vary with age, with the highest carriage rates among adolescents and young adults.[6] In most persons, carriage is harmless and serves as an immunizing process in which antibodies against *N. meningitidis* are developed.[28] However, in a small proportion of carriers, the bacteria penetrate the mucosal epithelium and enter the bloodstream, resulting in invasive disease. Secondary cases most commonly occur in closed, crowded conditions in which extensive close contact occurs, such as in households or childcare centers.[29,30] Risk of disease among close contacts is highest in the first few days after symptom onset in the index patient.

*Disclaimer: The findings and conclusions in this chapter are those of the author and do not necessarily represent the official position of the U.S. Centers for Disease Control and Prevention.

CLINICAL CHARACTERISTICS

Meningococcal disease primarily presents as meningitis and/or meningococcemia (septicemia), though other manifestations of invasive infection, such as bacteremic pneumonia, arthritis, or pericarditis, are reported.[31] Additionally, noninvasive infections, such as urethritis and conjunctivitis, can occur.[31] The incubation period for invasive meningococcal disease is usually less than 4 days, but can range from 1 to 10 days after exposure. Early symptoms of invasive meningococcal disease are often nonspecific and resemble flulike or other self-limiting illnesses, with subsequent rapid progression of symptom severity and appearance of classic meningococcal disease symptoms occurring late in the illness course.[31,32] Symptoms of meningitis include fever, headache, nuchal rigidity, photophobia, nausea, and vomiting. In infants, meningitis may present with irritability, poor feeding, bulging fontanelle, and without stiff neck. Meningococcemia is associated with fever, malaise, cold hands and feet, leg and other body pain, vomiting, diarrhea, and in later stages, presence of a maculopapular, petechial or purpuric rash. Meningococcemia may lead to multiorgan failure, disseminated intravascular coagulation, and acute adrenal hemorrhage (Waterhouse-Friderichsen syndrome), which is detected on autopsy. Overall, 10–15% of persons with meningococcal disease die despite appropriate medical treatment, with higher death rates in persons with meningococcemia compared to those with meningitis, and increasing death rates in older patients. Among survivors, 10–20% experience long-term sequelae, such as hearing loss, neurologic disability, limb scarring, or amputations.[31]

DIAGNOSIS

While meningococcal disease may be suspected based on clinical signs and symptoms, laboratory confirmation is necessary to distinguish *N. meningitidis* from other causes of bacterial meningitis or sepsis.[33] Identification of gram-negative diplococci is useful for presumptive meningococcal disease diagnosis, but is not confirmatory. Diagnosis of meningococcal disease is made through isolation of *N. meningitidis* or detection of *N. meningitidis*-specific nucleic acid using a validated polymerase chain reaction assay in a specimen obtained from a normally sterile body site, such as the blood or cerebrospinal fluid. Whole genome sequencing allows further characterization of *N. meningitidis and can help determine relatedness of meningococcal strains, which is often useful during a suspected outbreak of meningococcal disease.*[34]

TREATMENT

Several antimicrobial agents are active against *N. meningitidis.*[35] Empiric treatment for suspected meningococcal disease should include ceftriaxone or cefotaxime. Some treatment guidelines recommend that antimicrobial therapy may be switched to penicillin upon confirmation of *N. meningitidis* and after completion of antimicrobial susceptibility testing. Resistance to cephalosporins and penicillin remains rare in the United States. However, several countries have reported increases in rates of intermediate resistance to penicillin, though the clinical significance of this remains unclear. Patients are considered infectious until 24 hours after initiation of appropriate antimicrobial therapy.

CHEMOPROPHYLAXIS

Antimicrobial chemoprophylaxis among close contacts of meningococcal disease patients is recommended to prevent secondary spread. Close contacts include household members, day-care center contacts, and anyone directly exposed to the patient's oral secretions (e.g., through kissing, mouth-to-mouth resuscitation, endotracheal intubation, or endotracheal tube management).[36] Because the risk of secondary disease among close contacts is highest during the first few days after the onset of disease in the index patient, chemoprophylaxis should be administered as soon as possible and is of limited use if administered more than 14 days after exposure. Neither vaccination status nor oropharyngeal carriage status are used to determine whether chemoprophylaxis is indicated. Antibiotic options for chemoprophylaxis include ciprofloxacin, rifampin, and ceftriaxone.[35] Azithromycin may be considered for chemoprophylaxis in areas with fluoroquinolone-resistant strains of *N. meningitidis.*

VACCINATION

Vaccination is the primary means of meningococcal disease prevention. Globally, an increasing number of countries have introduced vaccines against serogroups A, B, C, W, and/or Y; no licensed vaccines against serogroup X currently exist. Vaccine recommendations vary by country, based on factors such as incidence, age groups or other populations at increased risk, and serogroup distribution.[10,37]

For prevention of serogroups A, C, W, and Y, polysaccharide vaccines have been available since the 1960s to protect against one or more serogroups.[38] However, they have several disadvantages compared to conjugate vaccines, such as poor immunogenicity in young children, shorter duration of protection, poor response to a booster dose, hyporesponsiveness to repeat doses, and no impact on oropharyngeal carriage of *N. meningitidis.* Thus, conjugate vaccines have largely replaced polysaccharide vaccines, except in a few countries that use them for routine immunization and in outbreak response in sub-Saharan Africa.[10]

Conjugate meningococcal vaccines have been available since the late 1990s: monovalent serogroup C vaccine, followed by multivalent formulations against serogroups A, C, W, and Y, and a monovalent serogroup A vaccine.[10] Since introduction in a variety of settings, meningococcal conjugate vaccines have been shown to be safe and effective for the prevention of meningococcal disease. Following implementation of serogroup C vaccination in several countries in Europe through routine infant immunization and catch-up vaccination of children and adolescents, marked declines were observed in rates of serogroup C meningococcal disease and carriage, with induction of herd protection in unvaccinated cohorts.[39,40] However, as a result of increases in incidence of serogroup W disease in recent years, several countries have now replaced MenC vaccine with MenACWY and/or introduced MenACWY vaccination of adolescents and/or infants.[8] Since 2005, all adolescents aged 11–18 years in the United States are recommended to receive MenACWY vaccination, with the first dose at age 11–12 years and a booster dose at age 16 years.[41] Vaccine effectiveness of a single MenACWY (Menactra®, Sanofi Pasteur) dose among U.S. adolescents is estimated at 69% (95% confidence intervals: 51–80%) overall, with waning observed in the 3 to <8 years following vaccination.[42] Assessing population impact of MenACWY vaccination has been difficult, given low incidence and declining rates prior to vaccine introduction in the United States and very recent introduction of the vaccine among adolescents in other countries; however, evidence to-date suggests an impact of vaccination on incidence rates among adolescents.[43] In sub-Saharan Africa, a serogroup A meningococcal conjugate vaccine has been progressively introduced since 2010, and has been introduced in 22 countries to-date. In the first 5 years since vaccine introduction in nine countries, the incidence of serogroup A declined by over 99%.[17] Additionally, evaluations have demonstrated the vaccine's impact on reducing oropharyngeal carriage and generation of herd immunity in unvaccinated populations.[44]

As a result of similarities of the serogroup B polysaccharide capsule with human neural cell adhesion molecules, development of either a polysaccharide or conjugate serogroup B meningococcal vaccine is not possible. Thus, recombinant serogroup B meningococcal (MenB) vaccines have recently been developed using different subcapsular proteins. A multicomponent vaccine (MenB-4C, Bexsero®, GlaxoSmithKline) with three recombinant proteins [neisserial-heparin binding antigen (NHBA), *Neisseria* adhesion A (NadA), and factor H binding protein (FHbp)], along with Porin A (PorA) from an outer membrane vesicle, was first licensed in Europe in 2013 and has been introduced into the routine infant immunization program in the United Kingdom and several other countries.[45] Early data suggest that the vaccine is 70% (95% confidence intervals: 1–89%) effective up to 2 years following completion of an infant series (at 2, 4, and 12 months).[46] MenB-4C, as well as a second MenB vaccine containing two FHbp subvariants (MenB-FHbp, Trumenba®, Pfizer), have also been recently licensed in the United States and may be administered to adolescents aged 16–23 years based on shared clinical decision-making.[47]

In addition to routine vaccination, several countries recommend meningococcal vaccination for persons at increased risk for meningococcal disease. In the United States, persons with certain underlying medical conditions (complement component deficiency, complement inhibitor use, functional or anatomic asplenia) and microbiologists routinely exposed to *N. meningitidis* isolates are recommended to receive both MenACWY and MenB vaccines.[41,48] MenACWY alone is recommended for travelers to the meningitis belt of sub-Saharan Africa, persons with HIV, college freshmen living in residence halls, and military recruits.[41] Vaccination with either MenACWY or MenB is recommended for persons at increased risk during an outbreak, depending on the causative serogroup.[41,48]

Vaccination has led to major advancements in the control of meningococcal disease globally. In addition, because the subcapsular proteins in the current MenB vaccines are also found in other serogroups as well as other *Neisseria* species, additional evaluations are currently ongoing to assess the potential for broader benefits of MenB vaccines, including protection against gonorrhea infections.[49,50] In addition, meningococcal vaccines are currently in development that protect against five serogroups: a serogroup A, C, W, X, and Y vaccine for use in sub-Saharan Africa as well as a serogroup A, B, C, W, and Y vaccine that combines the existing MenACWY and MenB vaccines.[51,52] With the ever-evolving epidemiology of meningococcal disease, rapid diagnosis and treatment, strong surveillance systems, and meningococcal vaccination will continue to be important for the prevention and control of meningococcal disease globally.

References

1. Rouphael NG, Stephens DS. Neisseria meningitidis: Biology, microbiology, and epidemiology. *Methods Mol Biol.* 2012;799:1–20.
2. Peterson ME, Li Y, Bita A, et al. Meningococcal serogroups and surveillance: A systematic review and survey. *J Glob Health.* 2019;9(1):010409.
3. Acevedo R, Bai X, Borrow R, et al. The Global Meningococcal Initiative meeting on prevention of meningococcal disease worldwide: Epidemiology, surveillance, hypervirulent strains, antibiotic resistance and high-risk populations. *Expert Rev Vaccines.* 2019;18(1):15–30.
4. Soeters HM, Diallo AO, Bicaba B, et al. Bacterial meningitis epidemiology in 5 countries in the meningitis belt of sub-Saharan Africa, MenAfriNet, 2015–2017. *J Infect Dis.* 2019;220(Suppl 4):S165–74.
5. Centers for Disease Control and Prevention. Enhanced Meningococcal Disease Surveillance Reports, 2015–2017. https://www.cdc.gov/meningococcal/surveillance/index.html#enhanced-reports. 2019.
6. Christensen H, May M, Bowen L, Hickman M, Trotter CL. Meningococcal carriage by age: A systematic review and meta-analysis. *Lancet Infect Dis.* 2010;10(12):853–61.
7. Jafri RZ, Ali A, Messonnier NE, et al. Global epidemiology of invasive meningococcal disease. *Popul Health Metr.* 2013;11(1):17.
8. Booy R, Gentile A, Nissen M, Whelan J, Abitbol V. Recent changes in the epidemiology of Neisseria meningitidis serogroup W across the world, current vaccination policy choices and possible future strategies. *Hum Vaccin Immunother.* 2019;15(2):470–80.
9. Greenwood B. Manson lecture. Meningococcal meningitis in Africa. *Trans R Soc Trop Med Hyg.* 1999;93(4):341–53.
10. Ali A, Jafri RZ, Messonnier N, et al. Global practices of meningococcal vaccine use and impact on invasive disease. *Pathog Glob Health.* 2014;108(1):11–20.
11. Mbaeyi SA, Blain A, Whaley MJ, Wang X, Cohn AC, MacNeil JR. Epidemiology of meningococcal disease outbreaks in the United States, 2009–2013. *Clin Infect Dis.* 2019;68(4):580–5.
12. Soeters HM, McNamara LA, Blain AE, et al. University-based outbreaks of meningococcal disease caused by serogroup B, United States, 2013–2018. *Emerg Infect Dis.* 2019;25(3):434–40.
13. Lingani C, Bergeron-Caron C, Stuart JM, et al. Meningococcal meningitis surveillance in the African meningitis belt, 2004–2013. *Clin Infect Dis.* 2015;61(Suppl 5):S410–5.
14. MacNeil JR, Medah I, Koussoube D, et al. Neisseria meningitidis serogroup W, Burkina Faso, 2012. *Emerg Infect Dis.* 2014;20(3):394–9.
15. Nnadi C, Oladejo J, Yennan S, et al. Large outbreak of Neisseria meningitidis serogroup C—Nigeria, December 2016–June 2017. *MMWR Morb Mortal Wkly Rep.* 2017;66(49):1352–6.
16. Sidikou F, Zaneidou M, Alkassoum I, et al. Emergence of epidemic Neisseria meningitidis serogroup C in Niger, 2015: An analysis of national surveillance data. *Lancet Infect Dis.* 2016;16(11):1288–94.
17. Trotter CL, Lingani C, Fernandez K, et al. Impact of MenAfriVac in nine countries of the African meningitis belt, 2010–15: An analysis of surveillance data. *Lancet Infect Dis.* 2017;17(8):867–72.
18. Densen P. Complement deficiencies and meningococcal disease. *Clin Exp Immunol.* 1991;86(Suppl 1):57–62.
19. Francke EL, Neu HC. Postsplenectomy infection. *Surg Clin North Am.* 1981;61(1):135–55.
20. Harris CM, Wu HM, Li J, et al. Meningococcal disease in patients with human immunodeficiency virus infection: A review of cases reported through active surveillance in the United States, 2000–2008. *Open Forum Infect Dis.* 2016;3(4):ofw226.
21. McNamara LA, Topaz N, Wang X, Hariri S, Fox L, MacNeil JR. High risk for invasive meningococcal disease among patients receiving eculizumab (Soliris) despite receipt of meningococcal vaccine. *MMWR Morb Mortal Wkly Rep.* 2017;66(27):734–7.
22. Miller L, Arakaki L, Ramautar A, et al. Elevated risk for invasive meningococcal disease among persons with HIV. *Ann Intern Med.* 2014;160(1):30–7.
23. Bruce MG, Rosenstein NE, Capparella JM, Shutt KA, Perkins BA, Collins M. Risk factors for meningococcal disease in college students. *JAMA.* 2001;286(6):688–93.
24. Stuart JM, Cartwright KA, Dawson JA, Rickard J, Noah ND. Risk factors for meningococcal disease: A case control study in south west England. *Community Med.* 1988;10(2):139–46.
25. Cartwright KA, Jones DM, Smith AJ, Stuart JM, Kaczmarski EB, Palmer SR. Influenza A and meningococcal disease. *Lancet.* 1991;338(8766):554–7.
26. Fischer M, Hedberg K, Cardosi P, et al. Tobacco smoke as a risk factor for meningococcal disease. *Pediatr Infect Dis J.* 1997;16(10):979–83.
27. Yazdankhah SP, Caugant DA. Neisseria meningitidis: An overview of the carriage state. *J Med Microbiol.* 2004;53(Pt 9):821–32.
28. Kremastinou J, Tzanakaki G, Pagalis A, Theodondou M, Weir DM, Blackwell CC. Detection of IgG and IgM to meningococcal outer membrane proteins in relation to carriage of Neisseria meningitidis or Neisseria lactamica. *FEMS Immunol Med Microbiol.* 1999;24(1):73–8.
29. De Wals P, Hertoghe L, Borlee-Grimee I, et al. Meningococcal disease in Belgium. Secondary attack rate among household, day-care nursery and pre-elementary school contacts. *J Infect.* 1981;3(Suppl 1):53–61.
30. Munford RS, Taunay Ade E, de Morais JS, Fraser DW, Feldman RA. Spread of meningococcal infection within households. *Lancet.* 1974;1(7869):1275–8.
31. Pace D, Pollard AJ. Meningococcal disease: Clinical presentation and sequelae. *Vaccine.* 2012;30(Suppl 2):B3–9.
32. Thompson MJ, Ninis N, Perera R, et al. Clinical recognition of meningococcal disease in children and adolescents. *Lancet.* 2006;367(9508):397–403.
33. Roush SB B, McGee L, Cassiday P, et al. Chapter 22: Laboratory support for surveillance of vaccine-preventable diseases. Manual for the Surveillance of Vaccine-Preventable Diseases. Atlanta, GA: Centers for Disease Control and Prevention, 2013. https://www.cdc.gov/vaccines/pubs/surv-manual/chpt22-lab-support.html.
34. Centers for Disease Control and Prevention. Guidance for the evaluation and public health management of suspected outbreaks of meningococcal disease. https://www.cdc.gov/meningococcal/downloads/meningococcal-outbreak-guidance.pdf. Accessed November 29, 2017.
35. American Academy of Pediatrics. Haemophilus influenzae infections. In: Kimberlin DW, Brady MT, Jackson MA., eds. *Red Book: Report of the Committee on Infectious Diseases.* 31st ed. Elk Grove Village, IL: American Academy of Pediatrics; 2018.
36. MacNeil J, Patton M. Chapter 8: Meningococcal disease. *Manual for the Surveillance of Vaccine-Preventable Diseases.* Atlanta, GA: Centers for Disease Control and Prevention; 2013. https://www.cdc.gov/vaccines/pubs/surv-manual/chpt08-mening.html.

37. Borrow R, Alarcon P, Carlos J, et al. The Global Meningococcal Initiative: Global epidemiology, the impact of vaccines on meningococcal disease and the importance of herd protection. *Expert Rev Vaccines.* 2017;16(4):313–28.
38. Gotschlich EC, Goldschneider I, Artenstein MS. Human immunity to the meningococcus. V. The effect of immunization with meningococcal group C polysaccharide on the carrier state. *J Exp Med.* 1969;129(6):1385–95.
39. Maiden MC, Ibarz-Pavon AB, Urwin R, et al. Impact of meningococcal serogroup C conjugate vaccines on carriage and herd immunity. *J Infect Dis.* 2008;197(5):737–43.
40. Trotter CL, Andrews NJ, Kaczmarski EB, Miller E, Ramsay ME. Effectiveness of meningococcal serogroup C conjugate vaccine 4 years after introduction. *Lancet.* 2004;364(9431):365–7.
41. Cohn AC, MacNeil JR, Clark TA, et al. Prevention and control of meningococcal disease: Recommendations of the Advisory Committee on Immunization Practices (ACIP). *MMWR Recomm Rep.* 2013;62(RR-2):1–28.
42. Cohn AC, MacNeil JR, Harrison LH, et al. Effectiveness and duration of protection of one dose of a meningococcal conjugate vaccine. *Pediatrics.* 2017;139(2):e20162193.
43. MacNeil JR, Blain AE, Wang X, Cohn AC. Current epidemiology and trends in meningococcal disease-United States, 1996–2015. *Clin Infect Dis.* 2018;66(8):1276–81.
44. Kristiansen PA, Diomande F, Ba AK, et al. Impact of the serogroup A meningococcal conjugate vaccine, MenAfriVac, on carriage and herd immunity. *Clin Infect Dis.* 2013;56(3):354–63.
45. European Medicines Agency. Summary of the European public assessment report (EPAR) for Bexsero. https://www.ema.europa.eu/en/medicines/human/EPAR/bexsero. Access June 8, 2019.
46. Joint Committee on Vaccination and Immunisation. Minute of the meeting on 03 October 2018: Meningococcal Epidemiology. London, UK. https://app.box.com/s/iddfb4ppwkmtjusir2tc/file/349905639306. 2018.
47. MacNeil JR, Rubin L, Folaranmi T, Ortega-Sanchez IR, Patel M, Martin SW. Use of serogroup B meningococcal vaccines in adolescents and young adults: Recommendations of the Advisory Committee on Immunization Practices, 2015. *MMWR Morb Mortal Wkly Rep.* 2015;64(41):1171–6.
48. Folaranmi T, Rubin L, Martin SW, Patel M, MacNeil JR, Centers for Disease Control and prevention. Use of serogroup B meningococcal vaccines in persons aged >/=10 years at increased risk for serogroup B meningococcal disease: Recommendations of the Advisory Committee on Immunization Practices, 2015. *MMWR Morb Mortal Wkly Rep.* 2015;64(22):608–12.
49. Ladhani SN, Giuliani MM, Biolchi A, et al. Effectiveness of meningococcal B vaccine against endemic hypervirulent Neisseria meningitidis W Strain, England. *Emerg Infect Dis.* 2016;22(2):309–11.
50. Petousis-Harris H, Paynter J, Morgan J, et al. Effectiveness of a group B outer membrane vesicle meningococcal vaccine against gonorrhoea in New Zealand: A retrospective case-control study. *Lancet.* 2017;390(10102):1603–10.
51. Block SL, Szenborn L, Daly W, et al. A comparative evaluation of two investigational meningococcal ABCWY vaccine formulations: Results of a phase 2 randomized, controlled trial. *Vaccine.* 2015;33(21):2500–10.
52. Chen WH, Neuzil KM, Boyce CR, et al. Safety and immunogenicity of a pentavalent meningococcal conjugate vaccine containing serogroups A, C, Y, W, and X in healthy adults: A phase 1, single-centre, double-blind, randomised, controlled study. *Lancet Infect Dis.* 2018;18(10):1088–96.

CHAPTER

105 Influenza

Hannah E. Segaloff • Mark A. Katz

Influenza is an acute respiratory illness caused by influenza A, B, and C viruses.[1–3] Influenza A and B cause annual or near annual epidemics of febrile respiratory illness throughout the world.[4] In temperate climates, influenza epidemics follow a typical pattern, peaking annually during colder months.[1] In regions with tropical or subtropical climates, influenza epidemics have more variable seasonality often associated with the rainy season and influenza can circulate for longer periods annually.[4–6] In addition to annual epidemics, new influenza A subtypes can emerge during epidemic and nonepidemic periods among humans and cause a worldwide outbreak, known as a pandemic, leading to larger than usual numbers of severe disease, deaths, and societal disruption.[3]

Although most cases of influenza are self-limited, influenza may cause more severe illness, hospitalization, and death, particularly among young children, elderly individuals, people with underlying medical conditions, pregnant women, and people with morbid obesity.[7] The public health impact of influenza is considerable; every year influenza causes an increase in absenteeism in schools and the workplace, patient visits to physicians, hospitalizations, and deaths.[8,9] Influenza-related visits can overwhelm hospitals, clinics, and emergency rooms during the influenza season.[10]

Vaccination remains the most effective means of prevention of influenza illness. However, vaccine effectiveness is generally only moderate and varies by influenza type, subtype, and season.[11] Vaccination coverage for influenza is relatively low throughout much of the world, and influenza remains a largely uncontrolled disease.[12,13] Eradication of influenza is unlikely because influenza A viruses circulate among several animal species, especially wild aquatic birds, which form the primary reservoir for all influenza A virus subtypes.

HISTORY

Influenza viruses that infect humans were first identified in 1933, but outbreaks of rapidly spreading febrile respiratory diseases consistent with influenza have been documented as early as the twelfth century. The term "influenza" was first used in the fourteenth century, when Buonissequi described an epidemic as the "grande influenza."[14] The Italian word for "influence" was used as a collective term for various causes of widespread epidemics. Cold weather, or "influenza di freddo," was considered a causal factor for many years.[15]

The first clearly described pandemic consistent with influenza occurred in 1580. Pandemics have appeared periodically since then with four pandemics occurring in the twentieth century.[16–18] The first of those, the 1918 Pandemic, which is sometimes referred to as the "Spanish flu," is estimated to have caused at least 50 million deaths worldwide, including nearly 700,000 in the United States.[18,19] Deaths occurred mainly among healthy 20- to 40-year-olds, in contrast to the usual pattern in interpandemic influenza seasons, in which most deaths occur among the elderly.[20] In the era of HIV and AIDS, it is often forgotten that influenza caused the most deadly pandemic in recorded history.

During the twentieth century, a series of important discoveries led to the modern understanding of the influenza virus and to the first use of influenza vaccines. The first influenza virus isolated was a type A virus cultured from ferrets in 1933 by Smith et al.[21] In 1936, Burnet showed that the virus could be grown in embryonated chicken's eggs. This discovery facilitated the study of viral characteristics and the development of inactivated vaccines.[14] Influenza B was first isolated in 1940 by Francis.[15] Hirst's discovery of the hemagglutination protein on the virus' surface in 1941 led to better characterization of these viruses and improved detection of antibodies to influenza. In the 1940s, the U.S. military developed the first inactivated vaccines for influenza, which were used to vaccinate U.S. soldiers toward the end of World War II.[22] Public health control measures related to influenza, including the widespread use of inactivated vaccines, began in the 1950s. In 1952, the World Health Organization established the Global Influenza Surveillance Network. The network, still currently operating, was renamed the Global Influenza Surveillance and Response System in 2011.[23] Since the 1957 pandemic, targeted vaccination of selected segments of the population, especially those considered at risk for serious complications, has been the basis for reducing the health impact of influenza.[24] Influenza antiviral agents for therapy and chemoprophylaxis first became available in the United States in 1966.[14]

ETIOLOGIC AGENT

Influenza is a medium-sized virus (80–120 nm) of the family Orthomyxoviridae. The virus consists of single-stranded segments of negative sense ribonucleic acid (RNA) enclosed in a helical protein shell, or nucleocapsid. The virus is covered by a lipid envelope with protruding surface proteins consisting of hemagglutinin (HA) and neuraminidase (NA). Influenza viruses are classified on the basis of their ribonucleoprotein into four distinct types, A, B, C, and D, of which only types A, B, and C are known to cause illness in humans.[3] Influenza types A and B cause widespread seasonal epidemics in humans.[3,25] Influenza C viruses are generally associated with a mild, upper respiratory illness, but these viruses have been identified in cases of severe influenza and in outbreak scenarios as well.[26,27] Influenza A viruses have been isolated from many species, including humans, horses, dogs, cats, swine, seals, ferrets, mink, whales, tigers, and avian species. Wild aquatic birds serve as the natural reservoir for all known influenza A viruses. Influenza B and C viruses mainly cause human infections, but there have been documented infections of influenza B virus in seals, and influenza C virus in pigs and dogs.[28–30]

Influenza A viruses are subtyped based on their surface proteins, HA, and NA. The HA and NA surface proteins are highly antigenic and are the target for the humoral immune response to influenza virus infection. HA is named for its ability to cause agglutination of erythrocytes (hemagglutination) in vitro. The virus binds to host cell receptors using an attachment site that is located on the HA protein. NA functions as an enzyme that cleaves neuraminic acid from mucoproteins, allowing newly formed viruses to be released from the host cell surface.

Currently, 18 HA and 11 NA subtypes are known to exist. Most of these subtypes were found in viruses isolated from birds, but the most recently identified HA subtypes, H17 and H18, were found in viruses isolated from bats.[31,32] By contrast, only three HA subtypes (H1, H2, and H3) and two NA subtypes (N1 and N2) are known to have circulated widely among humans.[33] H2 viruses have not been in circulation since 1968.

The nomenclature for influenza virus strains includes the virus type, geographical origin, laboratory reference number, and year of isolation. For example, the first type B strain isolated by a laboratory in Oregon in 1965 would be designated B/Oregon/1/65. Among influenza A viruses, a description of the HA and NA subtypes follows the strain designation, for example: A/Mississippi/1/85 (H3N2).

ANTIGENIC VARIATION

Antigenic Drift

Because the antigenicity of the virus changes frequently through antigenic drift, levels of immunity among human populations vary from year to year.[34] In antigenic drift, point mutations in the viral RNA genomes of both influenza A and B viruses can result in immunologically significant alterations to HA and NA. Drift results in more frequent antigenic changes of influenza A viruses than in influenza B viruses.[1] Predominant antigenic variants often circulate for a few years before being supplanted by a new predominant influenza strain.

Antigenic Shift

Antigenic shift occurs only among influenza A viruses. It reflects a more radical change in the virus, and requires by definition the emergence of a novel HA or a combination of both a novel HA and NA in a virus that causes human infection. Antigenic shift can occur when influenza A viruses of two different subtypes simultaneously infect the same host, leading to "reassortment," or the exchange of viral RNA segments in the host's cells, which results in a hybrid virus containing genes from both subtypes. Pigs have been considered effective hosts or "mixing vessels" for reassortment, because they contain receptors for both avian and human viruses. A coinfection of human and avian influenza A viruses in pigs or other animals, can create a new "reassorted" virus that contains genetic material from both parental viruses. If such an emergent virus were able to infect people and spread easily from person-to-person in an immunologically naïve population, an influenza pandemic could result. This mechanism likely created the viruses that were responsible for the pandemics of 1957 (H2N2), 1968 (H3N2), and 2009 (H1N1).[35–37] The exact mechanism of the emergence of the 1918 (H1N1) pandemic virus is not known.

Another way that circulating influenza in humans can undergo large-scale changes involves the direct transmission of influenza virus from avian or other animal species to humans with subsequent adaptation by mutation to the new human host.[38] Direct human infections with avian influenza viruses A(H5N1),[39] A(H7N9),[39] A(H7N7),[40] A(H9N2),[39] and A(H6N1)[41] have occurred in the past few decades. While these infections are typically associated with high case-fatality rates, human-to-human transmission of these avian viruses has been rare.

EPIDEMIOLOGY

Seasonality

Patterns of influenza epidemics vary by climate and region. In temperate climate zones in the northern and southern hemispheres, seasonal epidemics of influenza usually begin in the late fall to winter months and peak in mid to late winter.[42,43] However, sporadic cases and institutional outbreaks can occur in any season.[44] In tropical regions, influenza activity is more variable. In some tropical and subtropical countries, there are predictable annual peaks, often coinciding with the rainy season; in other countries, semiannual or year-round transmission of influenza occurs.[6,43] Annual epidemics generally last between 6 and 12 weeks, though duration varies based on location, climate, season, and influenza subtype.[4]

The beginning, peak, duration, and health impact of individual influenza seasons vary considerably from year to year.[45] The pattern of influenza epidemics reflects several factors: the extent of the antigenic variation; virulence and transmissibility of the virus; the extent of immunity in the population; the specific population groups that are affected; and seasonal factors that remain poorly understood.[45]

Two influenza A virus subtypes, A(H1N1)pdm09 and A(H3N2); and two influenza B virus lineages, B/Victoria and B/Yamagata currently circulate in humans worldwide. The predominant influenza virus in circulation may vary temporally and geographically in any given year.[46]

Burden

Influenza virus can cause mild symptomatic infection, illness requiring ambulatory medical visits, hospitalizations, and deaths. In addition, the economic impact of influenza due to healthcare utilization and missed workdays is considerable.[47,48] During influenza seasons, 10–20% of the U.S. population may become infected by influenza. Attack rates may be higher or lower in certain communities or age groups.[1,45,49,50] During seasonal epidemics, influenza cases often appear first among school-age children, who generally have relatively high attack rates.[51] However, the burden of serious disease remains greatest among the elderly, the very young, and individuals with underlying medical conditions.[52,53]

Understanding the overall disease burden of influenza—how many illnesses, doctor's visits, hospitalizations, and deaths occur due to influenza annually, and their associated costs, is critical for producing effective influenza prevention and control programs. However, estimating the global burden of influenza is particularly difficult due to the lack of detailed surveillance data among many countries around the world. Annual influenza epidemics vary in severity from year to year. In the United States, in recent years, the Centers for Disease Control and Prevention (CDC) began calculating estimates of the influenza burden annually (Fig. 105-1). From the 2010–11 to 2017–18 influenza seasons, the CDC estimated that annually there were between 9,300,000 (2011–12) and 49,000,000 (2017–18) symptomatic influenza illnesses, 4,300,000–23,000,000 medically attended influenza illnesses, 140,000–960,000 hospitalizations, and 12,000–79,000 deaths.[51]

Many low- to middle-income countries have recently published country-specific burden estimates from previous influenza seasons, most commonly focused on influenza-related hospitalizations and deaths.[54–62] A recent study that included data from low, middle, and high-income countries estimated that between 291,243 and 645,832 influenza-associated respiratory deaths occur annually depending on season severity[53] (Fig. 105-2).

Pandemics

Influenza pandemics occur when a novel influenza A virus subtype emerges and spreads among populations. Pandemics are usually associated with significant worldwide increases in morbidity and mortality. Four pandemics were documented in the last century: the "Spanish flu" of 1918, associated with influenza A(H1N1) viruses[63]; the "Asian flu" of 1957 [influenza A(H2N2)], "Hong Kong flu" of 1968 [influenza A(H3N2)], and the 2009 influenza A(H1N1) pandemic.

The ability of pandemic influenza to spread rapidly was well documented in 1957. The Asian influenza pandemic of 1957 began in

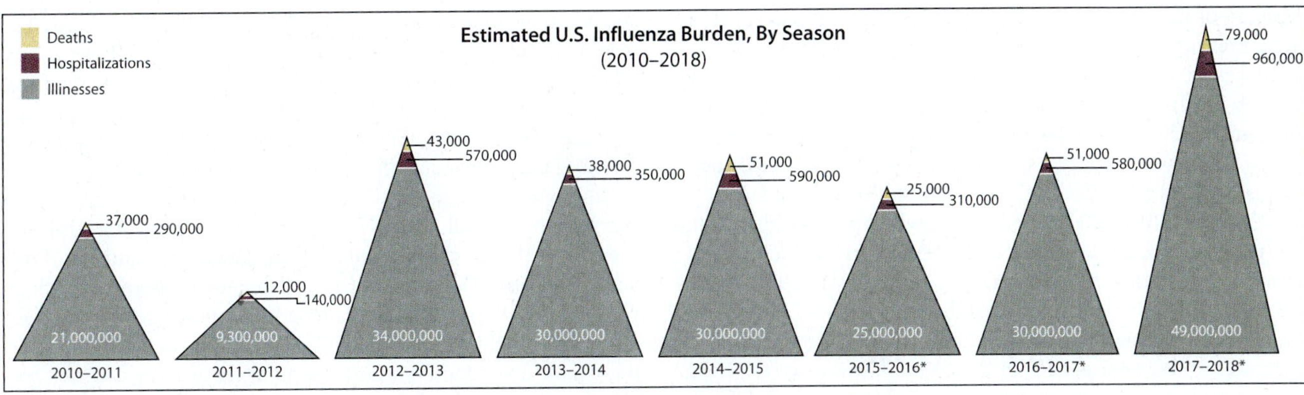

FIGURE 105-1. Influenza burden by season and level of disease severity in the United States, 2010–18. (*Source:* Modified from Centers for Disease Control and Prevention. Disease Burden of Influenza. https://www.cdc.gov/flu/about/burden/index.html. October 5, 2020.

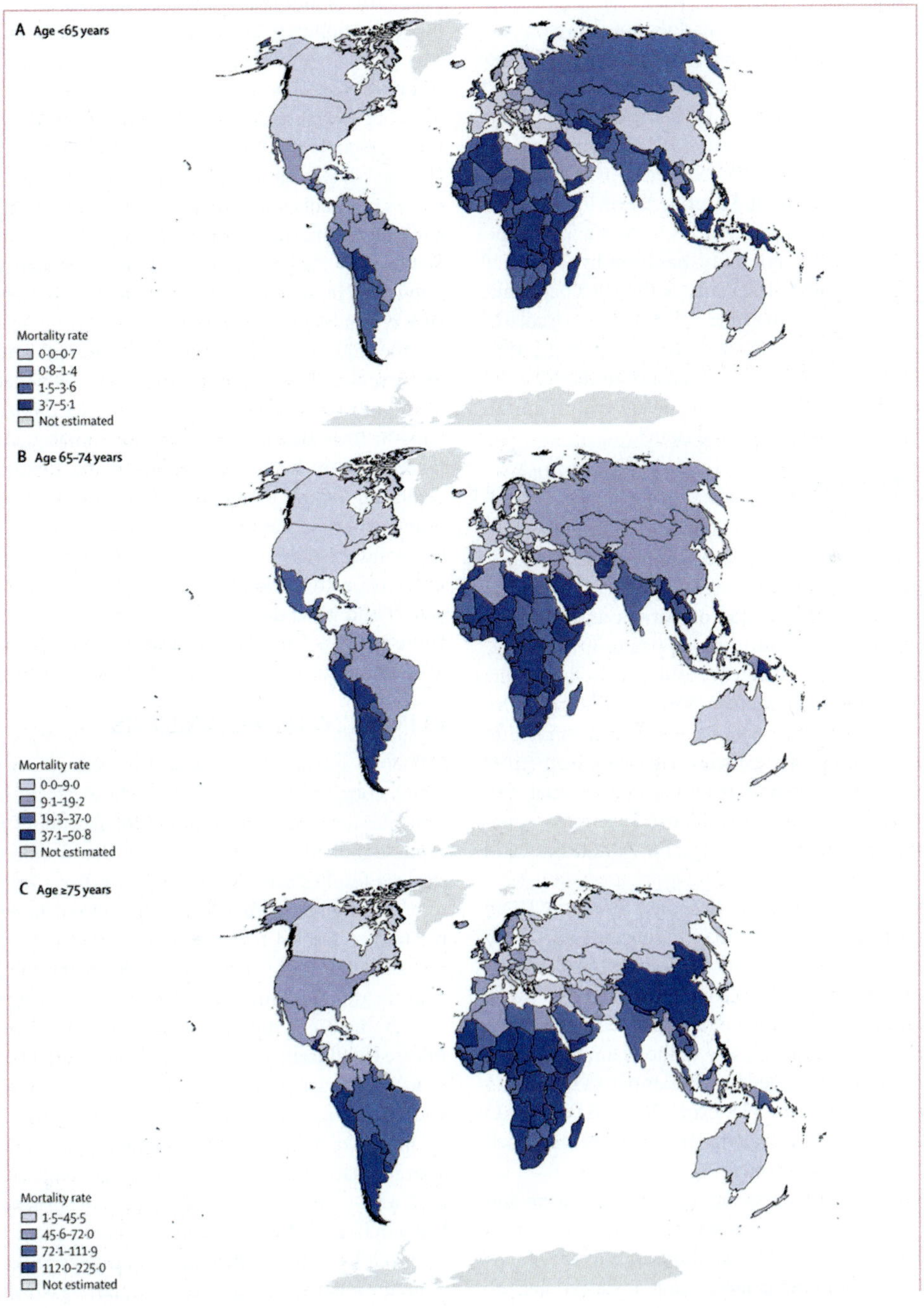

FIGURE 105-2. Estimated country-specific and age-specific global influenza-associated respiratory mortality rates. (*Source:* Used with Permission from Iuliano AD, Roguski KM, Chang HH, et al. Estimates of global seasonal influenza-associated respiratory mortality: A modelling study. Lancet. 2018;391(10127):1285–1300

February of that year in southern China. By April, it had spread to Hong Kong and Singapore. In May, the causative agent, an influenza A(H2N2) virus, was isolated in Japan.[35] The virus spread rapidly through the South Pacific, Southeast Asia, and the Middle East by June, and into Europe and North America by midsummer. By the end of 1957, the new subtype had spread worldwide. In the United States, the pandemic of 1957 resulted in an estimated 70,000 deaths.[35]

The morbidity, mortality, and epidemiology associated with the four pandemics of the last century varied considerably. The A(H1N1) virus that caused the 1918 pandemic was extremely virulent.[64] Deaths were especially prevalent among healthy young adults, a group that has relatively low morbidity and mortality from seasonal influenza.[64] In contrast to the 1918 pandemic, the 2009 influenza A(H1N1) pandemic was associated with less morbidity and mortality.[65] Like the 1918 pandemic, the beginning of the 2009 pandemic was characterized by an increase in severity among young adults.[66] However, mortality and hospitalization rates remained relatively low, and the pandemic was ultimately classified as one of "moderate" severity by the World Health Organization (WHO).[35]

Pandemic influenza, while a global threat, does not always impact individuals across the world uniformly. The 1968 influenza pandemic was characterized by the rapid spread of a new influenza A(H3N2) virus through Asia, Europe, and North America.[67] While mortality rates in North America during the first wave (1968–69 influenza season) were similar to those described in the 1957 pandemic, mortality levels were comparatively low in Asia and Europe.[67] Previous population-wide exposure to similar influenza viruses in Asia and Europe, which may have conferred partial immunity, has been hypothesized as an explanation for the variability in severity of the 1968 pandemic by region. The 1968 pandemic virus had a HA that had not circulated in humans before, but the NA was similar to the NA from the 1957 virus. It has been hypothesized that recent exposure to the N2 from the H2N2 virus that emerged in 1957 led to the relatively low mortality in Europe and Asia during the 1968–69 season.[68]

INFLUENZA SURVEILLANCE

Although influenza A and B viruses circulate virtually every winter in temperate zones of the Northern and Southern hemispheres, surveillance for influenza remains challenging. Clinical testing for influenza occurs infrequently in both the outpatient and inpatient settings, leading to missed cases and underreporting in discharge summaries and death certificates—sources routinely used to conduct surveillance. In the late twentieth century, formal influenza virologic and epidemiologic surveillance systems were mostly limited to high-income countries in temperate climates. However, in the past two decades new seasonal and year-round national and regional platforms for laboratory-based influenza surveillance have been established throughout Asia, Eastern Europe, Africa, the Middle East, and Latin America.[5,69–72]

The Global Influenza Surveillance and Response System (GISRS) is a platform for global influenza surveillance coordinated by the WHO. As of 2019, the GISRS network included 144 National Influenza Centers (NICs) in 114 WHO Member States. The Network includes sites that collect both epidemiologic and virologic data. Network laboratories test approximately one million clinical samples per year.[23,73] Virologic data are uploaded by laboratories to FluNet, an electronic database and data-sharing platform supported by WHO that was established in 1997.[23] Epidemiologic data are uploaded through FluID, another WHO platform.[74]

Data from GISRS are used to assess the start, end, duration and severity of influenza seasons each year, and the type and subtype of circulating viruses each season. In addition, thousands of specimens are analyzed at WHO collaborating centers using advanced genetic and antigenic techniques and antiviral susceptibility testing.[23] These data help inform the composition of the influenza vaccine each season and aid in the understanding of influenza virus evolution.[75] Another mission of the network is to identify novel influenza pathogens and other respiratory viruses[73]; during the last century NICs identified novel pandemic viruses in 1957 (Singapore) and 1968 (Hong Kong). In the last two decades, GISRS laboratories have identified and characterized many avian influenza viruses in humans in animals.[23,73]

Components of regional and national surveillance systems can vary. In the United States, the Centers for Disease Control and Prevention (CDC) collects and analyzes data from a number of different sources. U.S.-based WHO collaborating laboratories, along with National Respiratory and Enteric Virus Surveillance System laboratories, which include both clinical and public health laboratories throughout the country, report the numbers of types and subtypes of influenza A viruses detected throughout the year.[76] In addition, in order to compare how closely currently circulating influenza viruses match vaccine strains that were included in the influenza vaccine of a given year, and to monitor for changes in circulating influenza viruses, CDC antigenically characterizes approximately 2000 influenza viruses annually. CDC laboratories also test influenza viruses for susceptibility to antiviral medications.[77] CDC oversees outpatient surveillance for influenza-like illness through the US Outpatient Influenza-like Illness Surveillance Network (ILINet), conducts surveillance for laboratory-confirmed influenza-associated hospitalizations through the Influenza Hospitalization Surveillance Network (FluSurv-NET), and collects data on influenza-associated deaths in children. Finally, on a weekly basis, mortality attributed to influenza and pneumonia are reported through the National Center for Health Statistics Mortality Reporting System, and state and territorial epidemiologists report on the geographic distribution and spread of influenza within their jurisdiction.[78]

The 2009 pandemic exposed potential areas for improvement in current influenza surveillance systems. Since the pandemic, the WHO has invested heavily in improving influenza surveillance systems in low- and middle-income countries, as only 54% of WHO member states had functional influenza surveillance systems at the beginning of the pandemic.[79] The WHO has also certified a large number of new national influenza centers. As a result, more member states are now able to detect novel viruses and monitor domestic influenza activity. Similarly, the CDC has increased its capacity to collect and genetically test viruses from laboratories throughout the United States. The CDC has also developed risk assessment tools to understand the potential impact of a novel virus.[80]

CLINICAL CHARACTERISTICS

Influenza spreads from person-to-person when an infected individual coughs or sneezes and produces virus-laden droplets.[81] Most transmission occurs from direct interaction of the mucosa of a susceptible individual with the virus-laden droplets although transmission via fomites can also occur. Most direct transmission is believed to be through large droplets, although recent evidence suggests that the role of aerosol transmission is more important than previously recognized.[82,83] The incubation period for the virus is 1–4 days.[84] Viral shedding in infected individuals can occur from approximately one day before symptoms begin through 5 days after illness onset. Infected children, in particular young infants, can shed influenza virus for longer periods. In severely immunocompromised people, viral shedding can occur for weeks to months.[85–88]

Influenza infection can cause illnesses that range in severity, from asymptomatic infection, to mild uncomplicated illness, to severe illness with complications that can result in hospitalization or death. Uncomplicated primary influenza illness often begins abruptly with fever, chills, fatigue, headache, myalgias, decreased appetite, and a nonproductive cough. In children, gastrointestinal symptoms, including diarrhea, may also occur.[89] Fever usually ranges from 38°C to 40°C but may be higher. In some elderly people, fever may be absent.[90] In infants, influenza may present as a sepsis-like illness, and in children, high fevers due to influenza can be associated with febrile seizures.[91,92] Influenza illness usually resolves within 1 week, but cough and malaise can persist for several weeks.[93]

Complications

Complications from influenza infection include sinusitis, otitis media, pneumonia, inflammation of the heart (myocarditis), brain (encephalitis), or muscle (myositis, rhabdomyolysis) tissues, exacerbation of underlying chronic diseases and multiorgan failure.[94,95] While complications can be mild to moderate, they can also result in hospitalization and death.

The risk of complications from influenza, which may lead to hospitalization, is elevated among people 65 years and older, children younger than 5 and especially children younger than 2 years of age, pregnant women, and residents of nursing homes or long-term-care facilities.[96–100] In addition, some evidence suggests that in the United States, American Indians, and Alaska Natives may be at higher risk for influenza complications than other Americans.[101] Individuals of any age with underlying chronic medical conditions, including asthma, neurological or neurodevelopmental conditions, chronic lung diseases, blood disorders, heart disease, kidney or liver disease, endocrine disorders, blood disorders, individuals with morbid obesity, or immunocompromised individuals, are at increased risk of influenza complications.[102] Influenza infection can also exacerbate underlying chronic cardiopulmonary diseases, such as asthma, chronic obstructive pulmonary disease, and congestive heart failure, and has been shown to increase the risk of myocardial infarction.[95,103–108] Individuals aged 75 or older have the high rates of excess mortality due to influenza.[109]

Influenza infection can lead to the development of secondary bacterial pneumonia, which is associated with increased morbidity and mortality.[110] Common etiologic agents associated with bacterial coinfection include *Streptococcus pneumoniae*, *Haemophilus influenzae*, and *Staphylococcus aureus*.[111] Uncommonly, influenza infection can cause primary viral pneumonia, which can also cause severe illness during seasonal influenza outbreaks.[112]

Reye's syndrome, which is characterized by acute encephalopathy and fatty degeneration of the liver,[20] has been reported mainly in children with influenza infection who were previously treated with salicylates, most commonly aspirin, for controlling fever.[113,114] Since the 1980s the incidence of Reye's syndrome has decreased dramatically in the United States following warnings regarding the use of aspirin to treat children.[115]

Influenza infection can also lead to neurological complications, although these are rare. Cases of influenza-associated acute encephalopathy (IAE) have been reported since the 1990s, primarily in Japanese children,[116,117] but also in adults and in countries other than Japan.[118–120] The incidence of IAE has been reported to be approximately 1 per every 1 million Japanese citizen; rates are higher in children than adults.[121,122] A recent survey in Japan found that 37% of individuals with IAE did not fully recover and 7% died.[116,117,121] Mortality rates are higher in adults than in children.[122] Additional neurological complications, such as encephalitis, transverse myelitis, and Guillain-Barré syndrome (GBS), have been reported in association with influenza, but a causal relationship remains unclear.[1] Influenza infection has been associated with myocarditis, a complication reported during the pandemics of 1918, 1957, and 2009, and in the context of seasonal influenza infections.[123–125]

Immune Response and Immunity

The immune response to influenza infection is a complex process involving the innate and adaptive immune systems. After infection with influenza, the innate immune system is the body's first line of defense. Cellular immune responses consisting of proinflammatory cytokines and type I interferons can disrupt influenza pathogenesis by halting protein synthesis in host cells.[126] Systemic symptoms of influenza illness, such as fever and myalgia, are thought to be mediated primarily by innate immune responses elicited by viral infection of the respiratory tract.[127,128] Interleukins and cytokine levels increase with increasing viral load and tend to peak around day 3 of influenza infection. Extreme increases in specific interleukins and cytokines has been associated with severe disease in patients with influenza infection, suggesting that influenza disease pathology is linked to the innate immune response.[129]

Activation of the adaptive immune response is necessary for viral clearance of influenza. During the innate immune response to influenza dendritic cells are activated by type I interferons leading to enhancement of CD4+ and CD8+ T cell activity, both of which contribute to an effective adaptive immune response against influenza. CD8+ T cells mature into cytotoxic T cells and help eliminate influenza-infected epithelial cells in the respiratory tract.[130] CD4+ T cells contribute to the maturation of B cells and production of influenza-specific antibodies. Development of antibodies, primarily to the HA protein, but also to the NA protein, is the most important protective immune response to influenza virus infection or vaccination.[131] Most people infected with influenza develop specific antibodies within 2 weeks.

DIAGNOSIS

While diagnosis of influenza is often made on clinical grounds alone during periods of widespread influenza activity, laboratory confirmation of influenza can aid in clinical management when the incidence of influenza is low. When influenza is circulating within the community, the combined symptoms of fever and cough suggest a significantly increased likelihood of influenza.[132,133]

A number of laboratory tests for influenza are available: viral tissue cell culture, rapid cell culture, reverse transcriptase polymerase chain reaction (RT-PCR), immunofluorescence (direct and indirect), rapid diagnostic tests, and rapid molecular assays. Serologic testing, while used in research studies, is not recommended for clinical testing.[134] Various specimens can be used for testing, including throat swabs, nasopharyngeal swabs and aspirates, nasal swabs, nasal washes, and sputum. The appropriate specimens depend on the test employed. RT-PCR, a molecular method used to detect viral RNA, is considered the gold standard for laboratory diagnosis of influenza because of its high sensitivity and specificity. It can provide information on virus type, influenza A virus subtype, and influenza B virus lineage type.[135] Rapid detection assays which detect viral antigen have lower sensitivity and specificity compared to viral culture but offer the advantage of fast results (<30 minutes).[136] Rapid tests, along with RT-PCR, are commonly used in clinical settings. Newer rapid tests that use PCR rather than viral antigen detection are becoming more common and combine the sensitivity and specificity of RT-PCR with the speed afforded by rapid antigen tests.[137] The use of rapid influenza diagnostic testing in emergency rooms and other clinical settings has been shown to reduce further ancillary testing, and to reduce antibiotic use, although the latter finding has been variable.[138–140]

PREVENTION AND TREATMENT

The antigenic variability of influenza, combined with its rapid spread, short incubation period, and limited vaccine coverage in many populations, complicate efforts to control it. Influenza vaccination is the most effective approach to disease prevention. Antiviral medications are used for treatment and chemoprophylaxis of influenza. Beyond vaccination and antiviral treatment, nonpharmaceutical interventions can be used to reduce the risk of infection and slow the spread of influenza.

Nonpharmaceutical Interventions for the Control of Influenza Outbreaks

A number of nonpharmaceutical interventions have been shown to reduce the risk of influenza infection and the spread of the virus. These include actions that can be undertaken at the individual level as well as broader institution- and population-level policies. Evidence from observational and modelling studies suggests that staying home from school or work when sick, washing hands regularly, and covering one's mouth and nose when sneezing or coughing can reduce the spread of influenza in a household and in the community.[141–144] On the community level, policies that promote social distancing when sick, such as flexible attendance at school and sick leave from work, can also help reduce spread. In addition, cleaning commonly touched surfaces at home, at schools, in workplaces and in common community gathering places can help mitigate transmission.[145–147]

Nonpharmaceutical interventions can be especially critical to mitigate virus spread during a pandemic. In the past, pandemic vaccines have not been available until after the peak of the pandemic has passed. For this reason, individual and community interventions are likely to be the main methods of influenza prevention in the beginning of a pandemic.[148]

Influenza Vaccines

Global recommendations for the antigenic composition of the influenza vaccine are made twice a year based on antigenic and genetic characterization of viruses from both the Northern and Southern hemispheres. In the Northern Hemisphere, vaccine strains are selected between January and March, most often in February, to allow for adequate production time prior to the start of the next influenza season. Each year a representative virus from each influenza A subtype and one influenza B lineage is selected for inclusion in the trivalent vaccine. A representative virus from the other influenza B lineage is also included in the quadrivalent vaccine.[149]

In the United States, the CDC recommends that people receive influenza vaccine by October, a month that usually precedes the beginning of the influenza season in the United States. However, because the immune protection from influenza vaccines, and thus the effectiveness of the vaccine, can wane over time,[150] and the timing of the influenza season can change from year to year, identifying the optimal time for vaccination remains a challenge.[151–153] The U.S. CDC recommends that unvaccinated individuals should receive influenza vaccine throughout the influenza season, because influenza season may persist well into the spring.[154]

A number of different kinds of influenza vaccines are currently available worldwide, including inactivated, live attenuated, recombinant, and cell-based vaccines.[155] Inactivated influenza vaccines are the most widely used, and consist of subvirion preparations, which retain the immunogenic properties of the viral proteins but are associated with fewer adverse reactions.[156–160]

In the United States, three classes of influenza vaccine are currently available: inactivated (i.e., killed virus) influenza vaccine, live attenuated influenza vaccine (LAIV), and a recombinant vaccine that contains a recombinant HA. Details on the available vaccines for the 2018–19 influenza seasons are in Table 105-1. Inactivated influenza vaccine, the most commonly used vaccine, is approved for healthy people and people with chronic medical conditions aged at least 6 months. The recombinant vaccine is approved for adults aged $\geq$ 18. Currently LAIV is approved only for healthy individuals aged 2–49 years. Because LAIV is a live vaccine, it is contraindicated in certain populations, such as immunocompromised persons and pregnant women. All vaccine types should be used with caution in individuals who have had Gullian-Barré syndrome in the past 6 weeks or who have had an allergic reaction following prior influenza vaccination.[7]

Influenza viruses for most inactivated vaccines and all live attenuated vaccine are initially grown in embryonic hens' eggs. One type of inactivated influenza vaccine, the Flucelvax Quadrivalent vaccine,

TABLE 105-1 INFLUENZA VACCINES—UNITED STATES, 2019–20 INFLUENZA SEASON

Trade Name (Manufacturer)	Presentation	Age Indication	HA (IIVs and RIV4) or Virus Count (LAIV4) for Each Vaccine Virus (Per Dose)
IIV4—Standard dose—Egg based[†]			
Afluria Quadrivalent (Seqirus)	0.25-mL PFS[§] 0.5-mL PFS[§] 5.0-mL MDV[§]	6 through 35 mos ≥3 yrs ≥6 mos (needle/syringe);18 through 64 yrs (jet injector)	7.5 µg/0.25 mL[§];15 µg/0.5 mL[§]
Fluarix Quadrivalent (GlaxoSmithKline)	0.5-mL PFS	≥6 mos	15 µg/0.5 mL
FluLaval Quadrivalent (GlaxoSmithKline)	0.5-mL PFS 5.0-mL MDV	≥6 mos ≥6 mos	15 µg/0.5 mL
Fluzone Quadrivalent (Sanofi Pasteur)	0.25-mL PFS[**] 0.5-mL PFS[**] 0.5-mL SDV[**] 5.0-mL MDV[**]	6 through 35 mos ≥6 mos ≥6 mos ≥6 mos	7.5 µg/0.25 mL[**]; 15 µg/0.5 mL[**]
IIV4—Standard dose—Cell culture based (ccIIV4)			
Flucelvax Quadrivalent (Seqirus)	0.5-mL PFS 5.0-mL MDV	≥4 yrs ≥4 yrs	15 µg/0.5 mL
IIV3—High dose—Egg based[†] (HD-IIV3)			
Fluzone High-Dose (Sanofi Pasteur)	0.5-mL PFS	≥65 yrs	60 µg/0.5 mL
IIV3—Standard dose—Egg based[†] with MF59 adjuvant (aIIV3)			
Fluad (Seqirus)	0.5-mL PFS	≥65 yrs	15 µg/0.5 mL
RIV4—Recombinant HA			
Flublok Quadrivalent (Sanofi Pasteur)	0.5-mL PFS	≥18 yrs	45 µg/0.5 mL
LAIV4—Egg based[†]			
FluMist Quadrivalent (AstraZeneca)	0.2-mL prefilled single-use intranasal sprayer	2 through 49 yrs	$10^{6.5-7.5}$ fluorescent focus units/0.2 mL

[†]Persons with a history of egg allergy may receive any licensed, recommended influenza vaccine that is otherwise appropriate for their age and health status. Those who report having had reactions to egg involving symptoms other than urticaria (e.g., angioedema or swelling, respiratory distress, lightheadedness, or recurrent emesis) or who required epinephrine or another emergency medical intervention should be vaccinated in an inpatient or outpatient medical setting (including, but not necessarily limited to, hospitals, clinics, health departments, and physician offices). Vaccine administration should be supervised by a health care provider who is able to recognize and manage severe allergic reactions.

[§] The dose volume for Afluria Quadrivalent is 0.25 mL for children aged 6 through 35 months and 0.5 mL for persons aged ≥3 years. [¶] Intramuscularly-administered influenza vaccines should be given by needle and syringe only, with the exception of the MDV presentation of Afluria Quadrivalent, which may alternatively be given by the PharmaJet Stratis jet injector for persons aged 18 through 64 years only. For adults and older children, the recommended site for IM influenza vaccination is the deltoid muscle. The preferred site for infants and young children is the anterolateral aspect of the thigh. Additional guidance regarding site selection and needle length for intramuscular administration is available in the ACIP General Best Practice Guidelines for Immunization (https://www.cdc.gov/vaccines/hcp/acip-recs/general-recs/downloads/general-recs.pdf pdf icon). [**] Fluzone Quadrivalent may be given to children aged 6 through 35 months as either 0.25 mL per dose or 0.5 mL per dose. No preference is expressed for one or the other dose volume for this age group. Persons aged ≥3 years should receive the 0.5-mL dose volume. Also from the same source (footnotes from Grohskopf et al, 2019)

Source: Grohskopf LA, Alyanak E, Broder KR, Walter EB, Fry AM, Jernigan DB. Prevention and control of seasonal influenza with vaccines: Recommendations of the Advisory Committee on Immunization Practices—United States, 2019–20 influenza season. *MMWR Recomm Rep.* 2019;68(No. RR-3):1–21.

is propagated in mammalian cells rather than in eggs. Recombinant influenza vaccines are "egg-free" vaccines. These vaccines are produced by inserting the hemagglutinin gene from an influenza vaccine virus into cultured cells to make many copies of the hemagglutinin protein that are purified to be used in the vaccine.[161] In the United States, inactivated vaccine and recombinant vaccine are currently only approved for intramuscular administration. In contrast, LAIV is administered intranasally. Currently, inactivated vaccines are available as either trivalent vaccines, containing contemporary circulating strains of influenza A(H1N1), influenza A(H3N2), and one influenza B virus lineage, or quadrivalent vaccines, containing one virus from each influenza A subtype and one of each influenza B virus lineage. Recombinant vaccine and LAIV are only currently available as quadrivalent vaccines.

Two types of inactivated influenza vaccines, the high-dose vaccine and the adjuvanted vaccine, were designed to produce an improved immune response compared to traditional influenza vaccines. Both vaccines are licensed in the United States for individuals aged 65 years and older, an age group that tends to have a lower immune response after vaccination.[162,163] The high-dose vaccine contains four times the antigen of the standard dose. Results from randomized trials indicate that it is more effective at preventing influenza in older adults than the standard-dose vaccine.[164,165] The adjuvanted vaccine contains an adjuvant designed to produce a stronger immune response compared to vaccines that only include antigen. In clinical trials, the adjuvanted vaccine has demonstrated increased immunogenicity compared to the standard-dose vaccine in the elderly.[166–168] In addition, an observational study also showed increased effectiveness of the adjuvanted vaccine compared to the standard-dose vaccine.[169] The adjuvanted vaccine is available in many countries throughout the world, including most of Europe. As of 2019, the high-dose vaccine was only licensed in the United States, Brazil, Canada, and Australia, but it was approved for use in the 2019–20 influenza season in the United Kingdom.[170]

In addition to injectable influenza vaccines, an intradermal inactivated vaccine is currently available in multiple countries throughout the world. This vaccine has a much smaller needle than other inactivated vaccines and the antigen is delivered into the skin rather than the intramuscularly. Clinical trials have found that the intradermal vaccination elicits similar or superior immune response compared to conventional intramuscular vaccinations.[171–173] This vaccine was not available in the United States during the 2018–19 season but had been available previously. Details pertaining to the composition and availability of common vaccine types are listed in Table 105-1.

Efficacy and Effectiveness of Influenza Vaccine

The efficacy and effectiveness of influenza vaccine depends on a number of factors, including the type of vaccine, host factors such as the age and immunocompetence of the vaccine recipient, the influenza type and subtype in circulation, and the degree of similarity between the viruses in the vaccine and those in circulation in a certain year.[11,174] Due to the rapid evolution of influenza, particularly due to frequent changes in HA, vaccination must be given each season to ensure protection. It is hypothesized that natural infection may provide broader immune protection compared to vaccination, but even those infected with influenza in a season maybe be at risk for infection with a different type or subtype.

Studies of influenza vaccine effectiveness have generally found moderate and highly variable effectiveness. A 2016 systemic review and meta-analysis found that inactivated vaccines had a effectiveness of 33% (confidence interval 26–39%) against influenza A(H3N2), 61% (confidence interval 29–85%) against influenza A(H1N1) pdm09, and 54% (confidence interval 46–61%) against influenza B pooled across the period from 2004 to 2005 influenza season through the 2014–15 season in all groups. Studies in this review reported vaccine effectiveness from -66% to 93%, reflecting the wide variability in vaccine effectiveness by season, subtype, and age.[11] In recent years, vaccines have been less effective against influenza A(H3N2) viruses, particularly in years when the H3N2 virus strain contained in the vaccine did not match the circulating virus strain antigenically.[11] Even when the vaccine does not prevent influenza illness, the vaccine may reduce the severity of influenza illness.[175,176]

Randomized studies using a variety of outcome measures (seroconversion, culture-confirmed influenza, clinically diagnosed disease) have shown inactivated vaccine to be effective in preventing infection in children and the elderly.[177] Although some studies have found inactivated vaccine can decrease influenza-related complications in children, such as otitis media, by as much as 30%, other studies have not shown such an effect.[178,179] Inactivated vaccine was also found to prevent hospitalizations by 28–65% and death from all causes by 27–30% in the elderly.[180]

Studies in the past decade have evaluated the effectiveness of more recently approved influenza vaccines such as LAIV (approved by the FDA in 2007), cell-based influenza vaccine (approved in 2012), recombinant influenza vaccine (approved in 2013), high-dose vaccine (approved in 2014), and influenza vaccine with adjuvant (approved in 2015).

In the 2014–15 season, based on available evidence from randomized trials showing that LAIV was more effective than inactivated vaccine in children,[181–184] the Advisory Committee on Immunization Practice (ACIP) recommended that LAIV be used preferentially to inactivated vaccine in children aged 2–8 years old. However, studies from the 2013 to 2014 and 2015 to 2016 influenza seasons in the United States found that LAIV was not effective at preventing influenza A(H1N1pdm09) in children.[185,186] For this reason, the ACIP removed the preferential recommendation in the 2016–17 season and recommended that LAIV not be used in the 2017–18 influenza season.[187,188] Interestingly, during the same time period studies of LAIV outside the United States showed continued effectiveness.[189,190] After reformulation of LAIV by the manufacturer, it was again recommended, though not preferentially, for use in the 2018–19 influenza season in the United States.[191]

Despite the limitations of current influenza vaccines, national and international organizations recommend that individuals receive influenza vaccine annually, and influenza vaccine has been shown to reduce morbidity and mortality every year. From the 2010–11 to the 2015–16 season, U.S. CDC estimated that the influenza vaccine prevented 1.6–6.7 million illness, 793,000–3.1 million medical visits, and 39,000–86,700 hospitalizations each season in the United States,[9] and during the 2017–18 season the U.S. CDC estimated that the influenza vaccine prevented 7.1 million illnesses, 3.7 million medical visits, 109,000 hospitalizations, and 8000 deaths.[192]

Influenza vaccination has been shown to reduce healthcare costs and productivity losses associated with influenza infection. Studies in people aged 65 years or older have found that inactivated influenza vaccine reduced both direct and indirect medical costs. A recent literature review of cost-effectiveness studies of influenza vaccine found that influenza vaccine was cost-effective among children, pregnant women, and high-risk adults and to a limited degree, working age healthy adults.[193–195]

Vaccine Adverse Effects

The most frequent side effect associated with inactivated influenza vaccine is soreness at the vaccination site, which usually lasts less than 2 days.[177] Fever, malaise, and myalgia do not occur more often among inactivated influenza vaccine recipients than controls.[196–199] Acute allergic reactions, including anaphylaxis, can occur infrequently after administration of inactivated influenza vaccine in people who have anaphylactic reactions to eggs or documented immunoglobulin E (IgE)-mediated hypersensitivity to eggs. Protocols have been created to allow administration of influenza vaccine that is grown in eggs to persons with egg allergies.[200–202]

Influenza vaccine has rarely been associated with more severe events. The 1976–77 swine influenza vaccine was associated with 1 additional case of GBS per 100,000 persons vaccinated above the background rate of GBS.[203] From 1978 to 1988, no increased incidence of GBS was reported with influenza vaccine, but evaluation of the 1992–93 and 1993–94 influenza seasons found slightly more than one additional case of GBS per million persons vaccinated with inactivated influenza.[204–206] The estimated risk for vaccine-related GBS is substantially less than the risk of severe influenza in people at high risk, and the potential benefits of influenza vaccination in preventing serious complications and death in this group outweigh the possible risk for developing vaccine-associated GBS.[177] After the pandemic influenza A(H1N1) vaccination campaign in 2009, multiple countries in Europe noticed an increase in narcolepsy. In 2011, epidemiological links between Pandemrix, a vaccine specifically used to protect against the pandemic influenza subtype in 2009, and narcolepsy were found in Finland and several other European countries.[207,208] A meta-analysis of available literature found that the risk of narcolepsy in the next year was 5–14 times higher in children and two to seven times higher in adults who were vaccinated with Pandemrix compared to those who did not receive this vaccine.[209]

Randomized, placebo-controlled safety trials have not shown an association between LAIV and adverse events such as pneumonia or CNS complications compared to placebo in healthy persons aged 5–49 years.[177] In studies involving children and adults, LAIV recipients reported runny nose, nasal congestion, and headache more often than placebo recipients.[177] Trials examining the safety of newer vaccines, such as the recombinant, cell-based, high-dose, and adjuvanted vaccines, have not shown an increased risk of serious adverse events associated with these vaccines compared to standard-dose inactivated influenza vaccines. In studies of adjuvanted and high-dose vaccines, participants reported increases in some mild to moderate side effects, such as discomfort around the injection site.[168,210] Studies that compared the recombinant or cell-based vaccines found no increase in mild or moderate side effects in participants who received these newer vaccines compared to those who received the inactivated influenza vaccine.[211,212]

Thimerosal is a mercury-containing preservative used in some inactive influenza vaccines to prevent bacterial contamination. In 2001, a committee was convened by the Institute of Medicine (now the National Academy of Medicine) of the National Academy of Sciences to examine whether the use of thimerosal-containing vaccines was associated with neurodevelopmental disorders. The committee concluded that the evidence was "inadequate to accept or reject a causal relationship" between thimerosal exposures from childhood vaccines and neurodevelopmental disorders.[213] Nonetheless, efforts have been made in the United States to reduce the amount of thimerosal in inactivated influenza vaccine, and preservative-free formulations of inactivated vaccine are available.[213–215]

Current Vaccination Recommendations

Influenza vaccine recommendations vary throughout the world. The WHO recommends annual vaccination for high-risk groups, which include pregnant women, young children 6–59 months of age, adults with specific chronic illnesses, persons aged 65 years or older, and healthcare workers.[216] In 2014, 115/194 (59%) WHO member states reported having a national influenza immunization policy.[217] The countries with national policies were disproportionately high income and upper middle income, and tended to have a National Immunization Technical Advisory Committee in place. Among all countries with national influenza immunization, target groups for vaccination included healthcare workers (47%), adults with chronic medical conditions (46%), elderly individuals (45%), pregnant women (42%), and young children (28%).[217]

In the United States, the ACIP serves as the federal advisory committee that develops written recommendations, subject to approval by the director of the CDC, that provide guidance for the administration of FDA-licensed vaccines to children, adolescents, and adults in the United States. The ACIP is composed of 15 experts in immunization-related fields who have been selected by the secretary of the U.S. Department of Health and Human Services.[218] In order to make its recommendations, the ACIP reviews available scientific data, including disease morbidity and mortality in the general U.S. population and in specific risk groups, vaccine safety and efficacy, cost-effectiveness, and other relevant available information.[218] ACIP makes annual recommendations for influenza prevention and control in the United States. Currently, the ACIP recommends that all individuals aged 6 months and older receive the influenza vaccine annually in the United States, and puts particular emphasis on vaccination in persons who are at high risk for influenza-related complications.[7]

Vaccine Coverage

In the United States, influenza vaccine use has increased considerably since the early 1990s, in part because of a Medicare program authorizing federal reimbursement for influenza vaccination of the elderly that began in 1993.[219] However, use of influenza vaccine among ACIP target groups continues to be highly variable. Between 1989 and 1999, influenza vaccination levels in persons older than 65 years rose from 33% to 66%.[220] Results of a national cross-sectional survey showed an average vaccination rate of 70% among respondents aged 65 years and older for the 2002 influenza season; coverage in this population was estimated to be approximately 67% in the 2010–11 season.[221] Recent vaccination campaigns have focused on target groups such as healthcare workers. Many hospitals and other health facilities in the United States now require mandatory vaccination. In the 2018–19 influenza season approximately 78% of healthcare workers were estimated to have been vaccinated.[222]

Global vaccine coverage is highly variable and difficult to estimate in certain countries and regions. A 2015 manuscript examined vaccine doses distributed globally from 2004 to 2013. They found that doses distributed increased 87% from 2004 through 2013, but with the vast majority of this increase occurring between 2004 and 2008. Doses distributed also varied widely be WHO region, with a large majority of the doses being distributed in the Americas. Dose distribution by region per 1000 population is illustrated in Fig. 105-3.

Looking Forward—Universal Influenza Vaccines

Current influenza vaccines have numerous limitations.[223] First, the influenza vaccine must be updated each season, both because the circulating influenza viruses change frequently and because immunity conferred by the vaccine wanes over time.[151] The necessity of annual production and receipt of influenza vaccine increases costs and decreases influenza vaccination coverage. Due to the difficult process involved in vaccine production, it can take up to 6 months to prepare the seasonal influenza vaccine for production.[148] This limitation is especially important in the case of a pandemic; a vaccine made with current technologies may not be available for distribution until well into the pandemic. In addition, viruses included in the vaccine each season do not always match the circulating influenza viruses. When the viruses included in the vaccine do not match the circulating influenza viruses, the vaccine is considered "mismatched" to circulating influenza viruses, and likely confers minimal or no protection.

In order to address these limitations, there has been a recent global push to produce a universal influenza vaccine that could provide broad and durable protection against a variety of influenza viruses, including potential pandemic viruses. In 2018, the National Institute of Allergy and Infectious Diseases (NIAID) of the NIH in the United States released a strategic plan that outlined key research areas that would need to be prioritized in order to develop a universal influenza vaccine.[224] Currently, a number of universal vaccines are in both phase III and phase II clinical trials, but no vaccine is near licensure.

Antiviral Medications

Antiviral medications can be used for early treatment and chemoprophylaxis of influenza. Multiple classes of antiviral medications are licensed for use in multiple countries; as of 2019 these included amantadines, NA inhibitors, endonuclease inhibitors, membrane fusion inhibitors, and RNA-dependent RNA polymerase inhibitors.[3] The amantadines, amantadine and rimantadine, are not currently

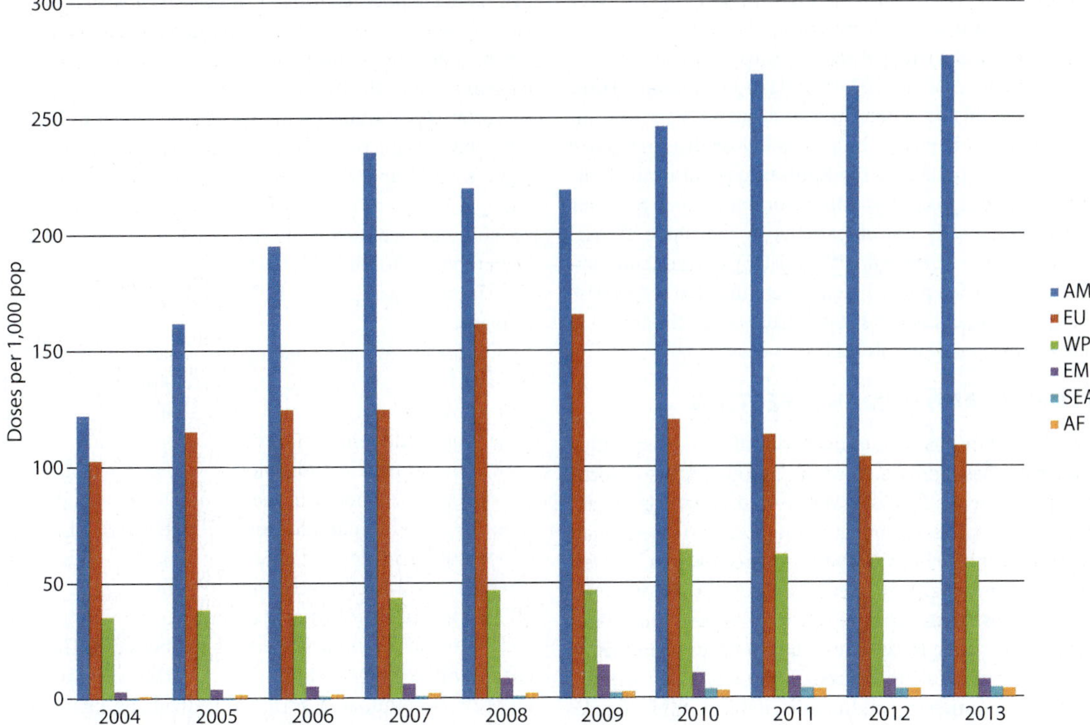

FIGURE 105-3. Seasonal influenza vaccine doses distributed per 1000 population by WHO region. (*Source:* Used with Permission from Palache A et al. Seasonal influenza vaccine dose distribution in 195 countries (2004–2013): little progress in estimated global vaccination coverage. *Vaccine* 2015;33(42): 5598–5605)

recommended for use due to widespread resistance in circulating influenza viruses. RNA polymerase inhibitors, such as favipiravir, and membrane fusion inhibitors, such as Arbidol, are not commonly used. Medications that fall into these categories are only licensed in a few countries and are not licensed in the United States.

In the United States, three types of NA inhibitors and one endonuclease inhibitor are approved for use. The three NA inhibitors include oseltamivir, an oral medication that is licensed in many countries, zanamivir, an inhaled powder that is also widely licensed, and peramivir, which is used intravenously and is only available in South Korea, China, Japan, and the United States.[225] Lanamivir is a NA inhibitor that is only licensed in Japan.[226] Baloxavir is an endonuclease inhibitor that was approved by the FDA in the United States in 2018. It works against both influenza A and B and is taken orally.[227]

All influenza antiviral agents were licensed on the basis of results from randomized control trials that demonstrated the effectiveness of the medications for treating uncomplicated influenza. When administered within 2 days of illness onset, all four antiviral agents recommended in the United States have been shown to reduce the duration of uncomplicated influenza illness by approximately 1 day.[227–229] A pooled analysis of 10 randomized, double-blind, placebo-controlled trial found that oseltamivir significantly reduced lower respiratory tract complications, particularly bronchitis, by 55% among influenza-infected adults and adolescents (from 10.3% in untreated patients to 4.6% in treated patients).[230] A similar meta-analysis in children that included data from five clinical trials found that oseltamivir reduced the duration of illness by 17.6 hours, was more effective in children with asthma, and also reduced otitis media.[231] Data on the effectiveness of antiviral medications in the treatment of more serious outcomes are limited, and mostly reflect results from observational studies with oseltamivir. In three observational studies of individuals who were either hospitalized or admitted to the intensive care unit with influenza, administration of oseltamivir up to 5 days after onset significantly reduced odds of death or severe illness.[232–234] Most studies have shown that oseltamivir is more effective the sooner it is taken after illness onset, and that it is most effective when taken within 48 hours of illness onset.

In the United States, the CDC recommends that all individuals with confirmed or suspected influenza who are hospitalized or at high risk for severe influenza complications be treated with oselatamivir as soon as possible after illness onset. In addition, the CDC states that treatment of individuals with uncomplicated suspected or confirmed influenza within 48 hours of illness onset can be considered based on clinical judgement.[235]

Antiviral medications can be used for chemoprophylaxis against influenza, especially to prevent outbreaks in institutional settings. Among NA inhibitors, oseltamivir and zanamivir are approved for prophylaxis. One study of oseltamivir prophylaxis in a nursing home showed a 92% reduction in influenza illness among nursing home residents.[236] Two randomized control trials measuring the efficacy of prophylactic zanamivir in preventing symptomatic influenza among community-dwelling healthy adults in households found that zanamivir was between 67% and 82% effective at preventing symptomatic illness.[237,238]

Each antiviral medication has its unique side effects, drug interactions, and drug resistance profile. Among the NA inhibitors, zanamivir, which is inhaled orally, may exacerbate respiratory problems in patients with underlying airway disease. Oseltamivir was associated with nausea and vomiting in clinical trials; the side effects may be reduced if the medication is taken with food.[2] Peramivir may be associated with diarrhea.[239] In a phase III clinical trial, baloxavir did not have increased side effects compared to placebo or oseltamivir.[227]

Prior to the 2007 influenza season, resistance to oseltamivir in circulating influenza viruses was quite rare (<1%). However, during the 2007–08 season a mutation in circulating A(H1N1) seasonal influenza viruses led widespread resistance to oseltamivir.[240,241] The seasonal influenza A(H1N1) virus stopped circulating after the emergence of the A(H1N1)pdm09 virus, which was susceptible to oseltamivir. Since the pandemic, circulating influenza viruses have mostly remained susceptible to NA inhibitors. However, in 2011 a cluster of A(H1N1)pdm09 viruses resistant to oseltamivir with the same mutation found in resistant 2007–08 A(H1N1) seasonal viruses was detected.[242] While this mutation did not occur in high levels in A(H1N1)pdm09 viruses, it raised the possibility of the emergence of resistance. Data from published randomized control trials, indicate that resistance to baloxavir is more common than resistant NA-inhibitors; approximately 2% of patients in the phase II trial treated with baloxavir were infected with resistant viruses, and 10% of baloxivir recipients in the phase III trial were infected with resistant viruses.[227] The fitness of these resistant viruses (e.g., the ability of these viruses to survive and replicate) is less understood.

AVIAN INFLUENZA AND HUMAN INFECTION

Since 1997, human infections by a number of different avian influenza A viruses have been documented in Europe, Africa, North America, and, most extensively, Asia. While wild aquatic birds are thought to be the primary reservoir for influenza A viruses, avian influenza A viruses have also been isolated from horses, pigs, whales, seals, cats, and tigers and pigs.[17]

Influenza A viruses occur naturally in wild aquatic birds and are very contagious to other birds. The majority of avian influenza viruses are "low pathogenic avian influenza" viruses. Birds infected with these viruses are either asymptomatic or have mild disease. Highly pathogenic avian influenza, while less common, is equally contagious to other birds and can cause serious illness or death among water fowl. If domesticated birds come into contact with infected water fowl, they can become infected and spread the virus to other birds and to humans handlers. To date, human infections with avian influenza viruses have occurred sporadically and have not spread from person to person. However, avian influenza infection can cause severe disease and death in humans.[243] If a highly pathogenic strain were to infect humans and become easily transmissible from person-to-person, it could lead to a pandemic with potentially devastating health effects. For this reason, a variety of surveillance systems exist to detect influenza illness in wild and domesticated birds. These surveillance systems, run by the WHO and the U.S. CDC, routinely monitor influenza viruses in birds to detect changes or potential risks. The WHO states that any human infection with an avian influenza virus should reported to the WHO.[244]

In recent decades, outbreaks of avian influenza A H5, H6, H7, H9, and H10 viruses in humans have occurred. The majority of human avian influenza cases have been due to highly pathogenic H5N1 and low pathogenic H7N9.[243] The first human cases of highly pathogenic avian influenza were identified in 1997, when an outbreak of highly pathogenic avian influenza A(H5N1) occurred in poultry and spread to humans in Hong Kong.[245] Eighteen people were infected, six of whom died. Nearly all of the infected individuals had been exposed to live poultry. Further spread of disease was probably curbed by the prompt culling of approximately 1.5 million chickens in Hong Kong.[245(p1)]

Since the influenza A(H5N1) re-emerged in 2003, periodic outbreaks of high pathogenic avian influenza A(H5N1) have occurred in poultry, primarily in East Asia but also in Central and South Asia, in a variety of European countries, North Africa, and the Middle East.[245(p1)] H5N1 is now considered endemic in poultry in 6 countries in Asia and North Africa. In order to control the spread of avian influenza during outbreaks of H5N1 in poultry, millions of birds have been culled. From December 2003 through April 2017, 859 human cases of influenza A(H5N1) from 16 countries were reported to the WHO, of whom approximately 50% died.[244(p1)] Most cases have been detected in Asia, though one case was detected in in a Canadian traveler returning from China in 2014.[243] Human-to-human transmission has been documented rarely, primarily between family members with very close contact, but concern remains that the H5N1 virus could adapt to the human host and acquire the ability to conduct sustained transmission in the human population.[246–248]

A variety of other highly pathogenic avian influenza A H5 subtypes have been reported in poultry in increasing frequency since 2012. In 2016 and 2017, cases of H5N8 were detected in birds across Europe, as well as in Asia and Africa.[249] In addition, as of July 2019, 23 laboratory-confirmed human cases of A(H5N6), all in China, had been reported to the WHO; seven of the 23 cases resulted in deaths.[250] No H5 cases aside from H5N1 and H5N6 have been detected in humans.

Outbreaks of highly pathogenic Asian influenza H7 viruses have occurred in poultry in Europe, North America, and South America, and a low pathogenic Asian lineage of H7N9 virus has circulated widely in poultry in China since 2013. Sporadic human infections with low and high pathogenic H7 viruses have occurred in a number of countries, mostly in Asia. From 2013 through 2017, the WHO reported 1565 human infections with H7N9, of which approximately 40% resulted in death.[251] The vast majority of cases resulted from direct exposure to infected poultry; however, a small number of H7N9 cases have occurred via human-to-human transmission.[252,253]

The most common risk factor for human infection avian influenza A viruses appears to be direct contact with infected live or dead birds or contaminated surfaces. Individuals involved in slaughtering or preparing poultry for consumption are at increased risk for avian influenza infection.[17,106] There is no evidence that transmission can occur through consumption of cooked poultry or eggs, but consumption of raw poultry blood has been linked to some cases of H5N1.[254,255] Avian influenza A infection in humans can cause a wide range of symptoms, from mild self-limited influenza-like illness (i.e., fever, cough, sore throat, and myalgia) to severe disease involving rapid progression to life-threatening complications and death.[256–258] Frequently, influenza H5N1 and H7N9 infections in humans cause severe complications such as pneumonia, respiratory failure, multiorgan failure, and sepsis. Gastrointestinal symptoms such as diarrhea and vomiting have also been reported, more commonly with H5N1 than with other types of avian influenza. Conjunctivitis has been reported as a symptoms of influenza A(H7).[256]

Research on the effectiveness of antiviral treatment in cases of avian influenza infection is limited. One study using global registry data found that oseltamivir given within 6–8 days of illness onset reduced mortality in patients with influenza A(H5N1) infection.[259] Oseltamivir, peramivir, and zanamivir have all been used to treat influenza A(H7N9) infection but their effectiveness has not been determined. Most H5N1 and H7N9 influenza viruses tested have been susceptible to NA inhibitors but resistant to admantadines, and therefore amantadines are not recommended for the treatment of H5N1 in humans.[260]

CONCLUSION

Influenza is a common respiratory illness that causes severe disease and death throughout the world every year. Prevention and control of influenza continues to be a global challenge. In recent years, epidemiologic and laboratory surveillance efforts have expanded globally, tracking seasonal influenza activity, potential pandemic viruses, and avian influenza circulation. Numerous influenza vaccines and antiviral drugs are now available, which have variable effectiveness in reducing different influenza-associated outcomes. Continued global efforts to monitor influenza epidemiology, disease burden and virus circulation are essential in order to identify and mitigate potential drifted or pandemic influenza viruses. In addition, continued investment to improve vaccines and therapeutics is critical to reduce the global burden of influenza.

References

1. Harper S, Klimov A, Uyeki T, Fukuda K. Influenza. *Clin Lab Med.* 2002;22:863–82.
2. Call SA, Vollenweider MA, Hornung CA, Simel DL, McKinney WP. Does this patient have influenza? *JAMA.* 2005;293(8):987–97.
3. Paules C, Subbarao K. Influenza. *Lancet.* 2017;390(10095):697–708.
4. Li Y, Reeves RM, Wang X, et al. Global patterns in monthly activity of influenza virus, respiratory syncytial virus, parainfluenza virus, and metapneumovirus: A systematic analysis. *Lancet Glob Health.* 2019;7(8):e1031–45.
5. Hirve S, Newman LP, Paget J, et al. Influenza seasonality in the tropics and subtropics—When to vaccinate? *PLoS One.* 2016;11(4):e0153003.
6. Moura FE. Influenza in the tropics. *Curr Opin Infect Dis.* 2010;23(5): 415–20.
7. Grohskopf LA, Sokolow LZ, Broder KR, Walter EB, Fry AM, Jernigan DB. Prevention and control of seasonal influenza with vaccines: Recommendations of the Advisory Committee on Immunization Practices—United States, 2018–19 influenza season. *MMWR Recomm Rep.* 2018;67(03):1–20.
8. Petrie JG, Cheng C, Malosh RE, et al. Illness severity and work productivity loss among working adults with medically attended acute respiratory illnesses: US Influenza Vaccine Effectiveness Network 2012–2013. *Clin Infect Dis.* 2016;62(4):448–55.
9. Rolfes MA, Foppa IM, Garg S, et al. Annual estimates of the burden of seasonal influenza in the United States: A tool for strengthening influenza surveillance and preparedness. *Influenza Other Respir Viruses.* 2018;12(1):132–7.
10. Glaser CA, Gilliam S, Thompson WW, et al. Medical care capacity for influenza outbreaks, Los Angeles. *Emerg Infect Dis.* 2002;8(6):569–74.
11. Belongia EA, Simpson MD, King JP, et al. Variable influenza vaccine effectiveness by subtype: A systematic review and meta-analysis of test-negative design studies. *Lancet Infect Dis.* 2016;16(8):942–51.
12. Jorgensen P, Mereckiene J, Cotter S, Johansen K, Tsolova S, Brown C. How close are countries of the WHO European Region to achieving the goal of vaccinating 75% of key risk groups against influenza? Results from national surveys on seasonal influenza vaccination programmes, 2008/2009 to 2014/2015. *Vaccine.* 2018;36(4):442–52.
13. Palache A, Abelin A, Hollingsworth R, et al. Survey of distribution of seasonal influenza vaccine doses in 201 countries (2004–2015): The 2003 World Health Assembly resolution on seasonal influenza vaccination coverage and the 2009 influenza pandemic have had very little impact on improving influenza control and pandemic preparedness. *Vaccine.* 2017;35(36):4681–6.
14. Doebbeling B. Influenza. In: *Public Health and Preventative Medicine.* New York: McGraw-Hill; 1998.
15. Noble G. Epidemiological and clinical aspects of influenza. In: Beare AS, ed. *Basic and Applied Influenza Research.* Boca Raton, Florida: CRC Press; 1982, pp. 2–50.
16. Doebbeling B. Influenza. In: *Public Health and Preventative Medicine.* New York: McGraw-Hill; 1998.
17. Cox NJ, Subbarao K. Global epidemiology of influenza: Past and present. *Annu Rev Med.* 2000;51(1):407–21.
18. Taubenberger JK, Morens DM. Influenza: The once and future pandemic. *Public Health Rep Wash DC 1974.* 2010;125 Suppl 3:16–26.
19. Reid AH. The origin of the 1918 pandemic influenza virus: A continuing enigma. *J Gen Virol.* 2003;84(9):2285–92.
20. Nobel G. Epidemiological and clinical aspects of influenza. In: *Basic and Applied Influenza Research.* Boca Raton Florida: CRC Press; 1982, pp. 12–50.
21. Smith W, Andrewes CH, Laidlaw PP. A virus obtained from influenza patients. *Lancet.* 1933;2:66–8.
22. Ratto-Kim S, Yoon I-K, Paris RM, Excler J-L, Kim JH, O'Connell RJ. The US Military commitment to vaccine development: A century of successes and challenges. *Front Immunol.* 2018;9:1397.
23. Ziegler T, Mamahit A, Cox NJ. 65 years of influenza surveillance by a World Health Organization-coordinated global network. *Influenza Other Respir Viruses.* 2018;12(5):558–65.
24. Uyeki TM, Fowler RA, Fischer WA. Gaps in the clinical management of influenza: A century since the 1918 pandemic. *JAMA.* 2018;320(8):755–6.
25. Nicholson K, Wood J, Zambon M. Influenza. *Lancet.* 2003;363(9397): 1733–45.
26. Katagiri S, Ohizumi A, Homma M. An outbreak of type C influenza in a children's home. *J Infect Dis.* 1983;148(1):51–6.
27. Thielen BK, Friedlander H, Bistodeau S, et al. Detection of influenza C viruses among outpatients and patients hospitalized for severe acute respiratory infection, Minnesota, 2013–2016. *Clin Infect Dis.* 2017;66(7):1092–8.
28. Bodewes R, Morick D, de Mutsert G, et al. Recurring influenza B virus infections in seals. *Emerg Infect Dis.* 2013;19(3):511–2.
29. Ohwada K, Kitame F, Homma M. Experimental infections of dogs with type C influenza virus. *Microbiol Immunol.* 1986;30(5):451–60.
30. Yuanji (Kuo Yuanchi) G, Fengen J, Ping W, Min W, Jiming (Chu Chinming) Z. Isolation of influenza C virus from pigs and experimental infection of pigs with influenza C virus. *J Gen Virol.* 1983;64(1):177–82.
31. Mehle A. Unusual influenza A viruses in bats. *Viruses.* 2014;6(9):3438–49.
32. Tong S, Li Y, Rivailler P, et al. A distinct lineage of influenza A virus from bats. *Proc Natl Acad Sci U S A.* 2012;109(11):4269–74.
33. Byrd-Leotis L, Cummings RD, Steinhauer DA. The interplay between the host receptor and influenza virus hemagglutinin and neuraminidase. *Int J Mol Sci.* 2017;18(7):1541.
34. Murphy B, Webster RG. Orthomyxoviruses. In: Fields B, Knipe D, Howley P, eds. *Fields Virology*, 3rd ed. Philadelphia: Lippincott-Raven; 1996, pp. 1397–445.
35. Monto AS, Webster RG. Influenza pandemics: History and lessons learned. In: Webster RG, Monto AS, Braciale TJ, Lamb RA, eds. *Textbook of Influenza.* West Sussex, UK: John Wiley & Sons, Ltd; 2013, pp. 20–33.
36. Kawaoka Y, Krauss S, Webster RG. Avian-to-human transmission of the PB1 gene of influenza A viruses in the 1957 and 1968 pandemics. *J Virol.* 1989;63(11):4603–8.
37. Mena I, Nelson MI, Quezada-Monroy F, et al. Origins of the 2009 H1N1 influenza pandemic in swine in Mexico. *Elife.* 2016;5:e16777.
38. Schrauwen EJ, Fouchier RA. Host adaptation and transmission of influenza A viruses in mammals. *Emerg Microbes Infect.* 2014;3(1):1–10.
39. Hammond A, Fitzner J, Collins L, Kun Ong S, Vandemaele K. *Human Cases of Influenza at the Human-Animal Interface, January 2015–April 2017.* Geneva: WHO; 2017. https://apps.who.int/iris/bitstream/handle/10665/258731/WER9233.pdf;jsessionid=85A4635BB47BDFBCA7FF206522B1C77D?sequence=1. Accessed February 24, 2019.
40. WHO. World Health Organization Influenza at the Human-Animal Interface. Geneva; 2013.
41. Yuan J, Zhang L, Kan X, et al. Origin and molecular characteristics of a Novel 2013 Avian Influenza A(H6N1) virus causing human infection in Taiwan. *Clin Infect Dis.* 2013;57(9):1367–8.
42. Finkelman BS, Viboud C, Koelle K, Ferrari MJ, Bharti N, Grenfell BT. Global patterns in seasonal activity of influenza A/H3N2, A/H1N1, and B from 1997 to 2005: Viral coexistence and latitudinal gradients. Myer L, ed. *PLoS One.* 2007;2(12):e1296.
43. Tamerius JD, Shaman J, Alonso WJ, et al. Environmental predictors of seasonal influenza epidemics across temperate and tropical climates. Riley S, ed. *PLoS Pathog.* 2013;9(3):e1003194.
44. Kohn MA, Farley TA, Sundin D, Tapia R, McFarland LM, Arden NH. Three summertime outbreaks of influenza type A. *J Infect Dis.* 1995;172(1):246–9.
45. Fukuda K, Levandowski RA, Bridges CB, Cox NJ. Inactivated influenza vaccines. In: Plotkin SA, Orenstein WA, eds. *Vaccines.* Philadelphia PA: Elsevier Inc.; 1994, pp. 339–70.
46. Bedford T, Riley S, Barr IG, et al. Global circulation patterns of seasonal influenza viruses vary with antigenic drift. *Nature.* 2015;523(7559):217–20.
47. Keech M, Scott AJ, Ryan PJ. The impact of influenza and influenza-like illness on productivity and healthcare resource utilization in a working population. *Occup Med Oxf Engl.* 1998;48(2):85–90.
48. Thorrington D, Balasegaram S, Cleary P, Hay C, Eames K. Social and economic impacts of school influenza outbreaks in England: Survey of caregivers. *J Sch Health.* 2017;87(3):209–16.
49. Chunara R, Goldstein E, Patterson-Lomba O, Brownstein JS. Estimating influenza attack rates in the United States using a participatory cohort. *Sci Rep.* 2015;5(1):9540.
50. Somes MP, Turner RM, Dwyer LJ, Newall AT. Estimating the annual attack rate of seasonal influenza among unvaccinated individuals: A systematic review and meta-analysis. *Vaccine.* 2018;36(23):3199–207.
51. Centers for Disease Control and Prevention. Disease Burden of Influenza. February 2019. https://www.cdc.gov/flu/about/burden/index.html. Accessed February 23, 2019.
52. Nair H, Brooks WA, Katz M, et al. Global burden of respiratory infections due to seasonal influenza in young children: A systematic review and meta-analysis. *Lancet Lond Engl.* 2011;378(9807):1917–30.

53. Iuliano AD, Roguski KM, Chang HH, et al. Estimates of global seasonal influenza-associated respiratory mortality: A modelling study. *Lancet.* 2018;391(10127):1285–300.
54. Dawa JA, Chaves SS, Nyawanda B, et al. National burden of hospitalized and non-hospitalized influenza-associated severe acute respiratory illness in Kenya, 2012–2014. *Influenza Other Respir Viruses.* 2018;12(1):30–7.
55. Nyamusore J, Rukelibuga J, Mutagoma M, et al. The national burden of influenza-associated severe acute respiratory illness hospitalization in Rwanda, 2012–2014. *Influenza Other Respir Viruses.* 2018;12(1):38–45.
56. Theo A, Tempia S, Cohen AL, et al. The national burden of influenza-associated severe acute respiratory illness hospitalization in Zambia, 2011–2014. *Influenza Other Respir Viruses.* 2018;12(1):46–53.
57. Ahmed M, Aleem MA, Roguski K, et al. Estimates of seasonal influenza-associated mortality in Bangladesh, 2010–2012. *Influenza Other Respir Viruses.* 2018;12(1):65–71.
58. Narayan VV, Iuliano AD, Roguski K, et al. Evaluation of data sources and approaches for estimation of influenza-associated mortality in India. *Influenza Other Respir Viruses.* 2018;12(1):72–80.
59. Susilarini NK, Haryanto E, Praptiningsih CY, et al. Estimated incidence of influenza-associated severe acute respiratory infections in Indonesia, 2013–2016. *Influenza Other Respir Viruses.* 2018;12(1):81–7.
60. Stewart RJ, Ly S, Sar B, et al. Using a hospital admission survey to estimate the burden of influenza-associated severe acute respiratory infection in one province of Cambodia—Methods used and lessons learned. *Influenza Other Respir Viruses.* 2018;12(1):104–12.
61. Sotomayor V, Fasce RA, Vergara N, Fuente FD, la Loayza S, Palekar R. Estimating the burden of influenza-associated hospitalizations and deaths in Chile during 2012–2014. *Influenza Other Respir Viruses.* 2018;12(1):138–45.
62. Abdel-Hady DM, Balushi RMA, Abri BAA, et al. Estimating the burden of influenza-associated hospitalization and deaths in Oman (2012–2015). *Influenza Other Respir Viruses.* 2018;12(1):146–52.
63. Chowell G, Echevarría-Zuno S, Viboud C, et al. Characterizing the epidemiology of the 2009 influenza A/H1N1 pandemic in Mexico. Peiris JSM, ed. *PLoS Med.* 2011;8(5):e1000436.
64. Johnson NPAS, Mueller J. Updating the accounts: Global mortality of the 1918–1920 "Spanish" influenza pandemic. *Bull Hist Med.* 2002;76(1):105–15.
65. WHO. Pandemic (H1N1) 2009—Update 94. https://www.who.int/csr/don/2010_04_01/en/. Accessed August 9, 2019.
66. Jain S, Kamimoto L, Bramley AM, et al. Hospitalized patients with 2009 H1N1 influenza in the United States, April–June 2009. *N Engl J Med.* 2009;361(20):1935–44.
67. Cockburn WC, Delon PJ, Ferreira W. Origin and progress of the 1968–69 Hong Kong influenza epidemic. *Bull World Health Organ.* 1969;41(3-5):343–8.
68. Viboud C, Grais RF, Lafont BAP, Miller MA, Simonsen L. Multinational impact of the 1968 Hong Kong influenza pandemic: Evidence for a smoldering pandemic. *J Infect Dis.* 2005;192(2):233–48.
69. Caini S, Séblain CE-G, Ciblak MA, Paget J. Epidemiology of seasonal influenza in the Middle East and North Africa regions, 2010–2016: Circulating influenza A and B viruses and spatial timing of epidemics. *Influenza Other Respir Viruses.* 2018;12(3):344–52.
70. Cowling BJ, Caini S, Chotpitayasunondh T, et al. Influenza in the Asia-Pacific region: Findings and recommendations from the Global Influenza Initiative. *Vaccine.* 2017;35(6):856–64.
71. Katz MA, Schoub BD, Heraud JM, Breiman RF, Njenga MK, Widdowson MA. Influenza in Africa: Uncovering the epidemiology of a long-overlooked disease. *J Infect Dis.* 2012;206(suppl_1):S1–4.
72. Rakocevic B, Grgurevic A, Trajkovic G, et al. Severe acute respiratory infection surveillance in Montenegro, 2014–2017. *Curr Med Res Opin.* 2018;34(8):1513–7.
73. Monto AS. Reflections on the Global Influenza Surveillance and Response System (GISRS) at 65 years: An expanding framework for influenza detection, prevention and control. *Influenza Other Respir Viruses.* 2018;12(1):10–2.
74. WHO. FluID—A global influenza epidemiological data sharing platform. WHO. http://www.who.int/influenza/surveillance_monitoring/fluid/en/. Accessed July 31, 2019.
75. WHO. National Influenza Centres. https://www.who.int/influenza/gisrs_laboratory/national_influenza_centres/en/. Published 2019. Accessed February 24, 2019.
76. Xu X. Update: Influenza activity in the United States during the 2018–19 season and composition of the 2019–20 influenza vaccine. *MMWR Morb Mortal Wkly Rep.* 2019;68(24):544–51.
77. CDC. Antigenic Characterization. https://www.cdc.gov/flu/about/professionals/antigenic.htm. Published March 26, 2019. Accessed July 31, 2019.
78. Blanton L, Dugan VG, Abd Elal AI, et al. Update: Influenza activity—United States, September 30, 2018–February 2, 2019. *MMWR Morb Mortal Wkly Rep.* 2019;68(6):125–34.
79. Briand S, Mounts A, Chamberland M. Challenges of global surveillance during an influenza pandemic. *Public Health.* 2011;125(5):247–56.
80. CDC. Summary of Progress since 2009. Pandemic Influenza (Flu). https://www.cdc.gov/flu/pandemic-resources/h1n1-summary.htm. Published June 7, 2019. Accessed August 7, 2019.
81. Murphy B, Webster R. Orthomyxoviruses. In: Fields B, Knipe D, Howley P, eds. *Fields Virology.* New York: Raven Press; 1996, pp. 1397–445.
82. Cowling BJ, Ip DKM, Fang VJ, et al. Aerosol transmission is an important mode of influenza A virus spread. *Nat Commun.* 2013;4(1):1935.
83. Smieszek T, Lazzari G, Salathé M. Assessing the dynamics and control of droplet- and aerosol-transmitted influenza using an indoor positioning system. *Sci Rep.* 2020;9:2185. https://www.nature.com/articles/s41598-019-38825-y. Accessed August 22, 2019.
84. Lessler J, Reich NG, Brookmeyer R, Perl TM, Nelson KE, Cummings DAT. Incubation periods of acute respiratory viral infections: A systematic review. *Lancet Infect Dis.* 2009;9(5):291–300.
85. Frank AL, Taber LH, Wells CR, Wells JM, Glezen WP, Paredes A. Patterns of shedding of myxoviruses and paramyxoviruses in children. *J Infect Dis.* 1981;144(5):433–41.
86. Klimov AI, Rocha E, Hayden FG, Shult PA, Roumillat LF, Cox NJ. Prolonged shedding of amantadine-resistant influenza A viruses by immunodeficient patients: Detection by polymerase chain reaction-restriction analysis. *J Infect Dis.* 1995;172(5):1352–5.
87. Englund JA, Champlin RE, Wyde PR, et al. Common emergence of amantadine- and rimantadine-resistant influenza A viruses in symptomatic immunocompromised adults. *Clin Infect Dis.* 1998;26(6):1418–24.
88. Boivin G, Goyette N, Bernatchez H. Prolonged excretion of amantadine-resistant influenza A virus quasi species after cessation of antiviral therapy in an immunocompromised patient. *Clin Infect Dis.* 2002;34(5):e23–5.
89. Dilantika C, Sedyaningsih ER, Kasper MR, et al. Influenza virus infection among pediatric patients reporting diarrhea and influenza-like illness. *BMC Infect Dis.* 2010;10:3.
90. Gravenstein S, Ambrozaitis A, Schilling M, et al. Surveillance for respiratory illness in long-term care settings: Detection of illness using a prospective research technique. *J Am Med Dir Assoc.* 2000;1(3):122–8.
91. Chiu SS, Tse CYC, Lau YL, Peiris M. Influenza A infection is an important cause of febrile seizures. *Pediatrics.* 2001;108(4):e63.
92. Chiu SS, Catherine, Tse YC, Lau YL, Peiris M, Dphil F. Influenza A infection is an important cause of febrile seizures. *Pediatrics.* 2001;108(4):1–7.
93. Kelnk H, Garten W. Matrosovich M. pathogenesis. In: Webster RG, Monto AS, Braciale TJ, Lamb RA, eds. *Textbook of Influenza.* 2nd ed. Oxford, UK: John Wiley & Sons, Ltd; 2013, pp. 157–75.
94. CDC. Flu Symptoms & Complications. Centers for Disease Control and Prevention. https://www.cdc.gov/flu/symptoms/symptoms.htm. Published April 26, 2019. Accessed August 1, 2019.
95. Kwong JC, Schwartz KL, Campitelli MA, et al. Acute myocardial infarction after laboratory-confirmed influenza infection. *N Engl J Med.* 2018;378(4):345–53.
96. Poehling KA, Edwards KM, Weinberg GA, et al. The underrecognized burden of influenza in young children. *N Engl J Med.* 2006;355(1):31–40.
97. O'Brien MA, Uyeki TM, Shay DK, et al. Incidence of outpatient visits and hospitalizations related to influenza in infants and young children. *Pediatrics.* 2004;113(3):585–93.
98. Centers for Disease Control and Prevention (CDC). Maternal and infant outcomes among severely ill pregnant and postpartum women with 2009 pandemic influenza A (H1N1)—United States, April 2009–August 2010. *MMWR Morb Mortal Wkly Rep.* 2011;60(35):1193–6.
99. Hartert TV, Neuzil KM, Shintani AK, et al. Maternal morbidity and perinatal outcomes among pregnant women with respiratory hospitalizations during influenza season. *Am J Obstet Gynecol.* 2003;189(6):1705–12.
100. Pop-Vicas A, Gravenstein S. Influenza in the elderly—A mini-review. *Gerontology.* 2010;25(5):397–404.
101. La Ruche G, Tarantola A, Barboza P, et al. The 2009 pandemic H1N1 influenza and indigenous populations of the Americas and the Pacific. *Euro Surveill.* 2009;14(42):19366.
102. Fiore A, Fry A, Shay D, Gubareva L, Bresee J, Uyeki T. Antiviral agents for the treatment and chemoprophylaxis of influenza recommenda-

tions of the Advisory Committee on Immunization Practices (ACIP). *MMWR*. 2011;60(1):1–25.

103. Gordon A, Reingold A. The burden of influenza: A complex problem. *Curr Epidemiol Rep*. 2018;5(1):1–9.
104. Corrales-Medina VF, Alvarez KN, Weissfeld LA, et al. Association between hospitalization for pneumonia and subsequent risk of cardiovascular disease. *JAMA*. 2015;313(3):264.
105. Johnston SL, Pattemore PK, Sanderson G, et al. Community study of role of viral infections in exacerbations of asthma in 9–11 year old children. *BMJ*. 1995;310(6989):1225–9.
106. Nicholson KG, Kent J, Ireland DC. Respiratory viruses and exacerbations of asthma in adults. *BMJ*. 1993;307(6910):982–6.
107. Warren-Gash C, Smeeth L, Hayward AC. Influenza as a trigger for acute myocardial infarction or death from cardiovascular disease: A systematic review. *Lancet Infect Dis*. 2009;9(10):601–10.
108. Wedzicha JA. Role of viruses in exacerbations of chronic obstructive pulmonary disease. *Proc Am Thorac Soc*. 2004;1(2):115–20.
109. Thompson WW, Shay DK, Weintraub E, et al. Mortality associated with influenza and respiratory syncytial virus in the United States. *JAMA*. 2003;289(2):179–86.
110. Rothberg MB, Haessler SD, Brown RB. Complications of viral influenza. *Am J Med*. 2008;121(4):258–64.
111. Morris DE, Cleary DW, Clarke SC. Secondary bacterial infections associated with influenza pandemics. *Front Microbiol*. 2017;8:1041.
112. Rello J, Pop-Vicas A. Clinical review: Primary influenza viral pneumonia. *Crit Care*. 2009;13(6):235.
113. Corey L, Rubin RJ, Hattwick MA, Noble GR, Cassidy E. A nationwide outbreak of Reye's Syndrome. Its epidemiologic relationship of influenza B. *Am J Med*. 1976;61(5):615–25.
114. Hurwitz ES, Nelson DB, Davis C, Morens D, Schonberger LB. National surveillance for Reye syndrome: A five-year review. *Pediatrics*. 1982;70(6):895–900.
115. Belay ED, Bresee JS, Holman RC, Khan AS, Shahriari A, Schonberger LB. Reye's syndrome in the United States from 1981 through 1997. *N Engl J Med*. 1999;340(18):1377–82.
116. Morishima T, Togashi T, Yokota S, et al. Encephalitis and encephalopathy associated with an influenza epidemic in Japan. *Clin Infect Dis*. 2002;35(5):512–7.
117. Togashi T, Matsuzono Y, Narita M, Morishima T. Influenza-associated acute encephalopathy in Japanese children in 1994–2002. *Virus Res*. 2004;103(1–2):75–8.
118. Welk A, Schmeh I, Knuf M, et al. Acute encephalopathy in children associated with influenza A: A retrospective case series. *Klin Pädiatr.* 2016;228(05):280–1.
119. Meijer WJ, Linn FHH, Wensing AMJ, et al. Acute influenza virus-associated encephalitis and encephalopathy in adults: a challenging diagnosis. *JMM Case Rep*. 2016;3(6):e005076.
120. Ochi N, Takahashi K, Yamane H, Takigawa N. Acute necrotizing encephalopathy in an adult with influenza A infection. *Ther Clin Risk Manag*. 2018;14:753–6.
121. Morita A, Ishihara M, Kamei S, et al. Nationwide survey of influenza-associated acute encephalopathy in Japanese adults. *J Neurol Sci*. 2019;399:101–7.
122. Okuno H, Yahata Y, Tanaka-Taya K, et al. Characteristics and outcomes of influenza-associated encephalopathy cases among children and adults in Japan, 2010–2015. *Clin Infect Dis*. 2018;66(12):1831–7.
123. Ukimura A, Satomi H, Ooi Y, Kanzaki Y. Myocarditis associated with influenza A H1N1pdm2009. *Influenza Res Treat*. 2012;2012:351979.
124. Aykac K, Ozsurekci Y, Kahyaoglu P, et al. Myocarditis associated with influenza infection in five children. *J Infect Public Health*. 2018;11(5):698–701.
125. Rezkalla SH, Kloner RA. Influenza-related viral myocarditis. *WMJ*. 2010;109(4):209–13.
126. Kreijtz JHCM, Fouchier RAM, Rimmelzwaan GF. Immune responses to influenza virus infection. *Virus Res*. 2011;162(1):19–30.
127. Hayden FG, Fritz R, Lobo MC, Alvord W, Strober W, Straus SE. Local and systemic cytokine responses during experimental human influenza A virus infection. Relation to symptom formation and host defense. *J Clin Invest*. 1998;101(3):643–9.
128. Webster RG, Marie R, Thomas Chair F, Monto AS, et al. Innate immunity. In: Webster RG, Monto AS, Braciale TJ, Lamb RA, eds. *Textbook of Influenza*. Oxford, UK: John Wiley & Sons, Ltd; 2013.
129. Lee N, Chan PK, Wong CK, et al. Viral clearance and inflammatory response patterns in adults hospitalized for pandemic 2009 influenza A(H1N1) virus pneumonia. *Antivir Ther*. 2011;16(2):237–47.
130. Hufford MM, Kim TS, Sun J, Braciale TJ. The effector T cell response to influenza infection. *Curr Top Microbiol Immunol*. 2015;386: 423–55.
131. Baumgarth N, Carroll M, Gonzalez S. Antibody-mediated immunity. In: Webster RG, Monto AS, Braciale TJ, Lamb RA, eds. *Textbook of Influenza*. Oxford, UK: John Wiley & Sons, Ltd; 2013.
132. Monto AS, Gravenstein S, Elliott M, Colopy M, Schweinle J. Clinical signs and symptoms predicting influenza infection. *Arch Intern Med*. 2000;160(21):3243–7.
133. Dugas AF, Hsieh Y-H, Lovecchio F, et al. Derivation and validation of a clinical decision guideline for influenza testing in four U.S. Emergency Departments. *Clin Infect Dis*. 2020;70(1):49–58.
134. CDC. Influenza Virus Testing Methods. https://www.cdc.gov/flu/professionals/diagnosis/table-testing-methods.htm. Published April 17, 2019. Accessed August 1, 2019.
135. Stockton J, Ellis JS, Saville M, Clewley JP, Zambon MC. Multiplex PCR for typing and subtyping influenza and respiratory syncytial viruses. *J Clin Microbiol*. 1998;36(10):2990–5.
136. Uyeki TM, Fukuda K, Cox NJ. Influenza surveillance with rapid diagnostic tests. *Clin Infect Dis*. 2002;34(10):1422.
137. Chu HY, Englund JA, Huang D, et al. Impact of rapid influenza PCR testing on hospitalization and antiviral use: A retrospective cohort study: Impact of Rapid Flu PCR Testing on clinical outcomes. *J Med Virol*. 2015;87(12):2021–6.
138. Nesher L, Tsaban G, Dreiher J, et al. The impact of incorporating early rapid influenza diagnosis on hospital occupancy and hospital acquired influenza. *Infect Control Hosp Epidemiol*. 2019;40(8):897–903.
139. Lee JJ, Verbakel JY, Goyder CR, et al. The clinical utility of point-of-care tests for influenza in ambulatory care: A systematic review and meta-analysis. *Clin Infect Dis*. 2019;69(1):24–33.
140. Blaschke AJ, Heyrend C, Byington CL, et al. Molecular analysis improves pathogen identification and epidemiologic study of pediatric parapneumonic empyema. *Pediatr Infect Dis J*. 2011;30(4):289.
141. Godoy P, Castilla J, Delgado-Rodríguez M, et al. Effectiveness of hand hygiene and provision of information in preventing influenza cases requiring hospitalization. *Prev Med*. 2012;54(6):434–9.
142. Mizumoto K, Yamamoto T, Nishiura H. Contact behaviour of children and parental employment behaviour during school closures against the pandemic influenza A (H1N1-2009) in Japan. *J Int Med Res*. 2013;41(3):716–24.
143. Nasrullah M, Breiding MJ, Smith W, et al. Response to 2009 pandemic influenza A H1N1 among public schools of Georgia, United States—Fall 2009. *Int J Infect Dis*. 2012;16(5):e382–90.
144. Kumar S, Grefenstette JJ, Galloway D, Albert SM, Burke DS. Policies to reduce influenza in the workplace: Impact assessments using an agent-based model. *Am J Public Health*. 2013;103(8):1406–11.
145. Thomas Y, Vogel G, Wunderli W, et al. Survival of influenza virus on banknotes. *Appl Environ Microbiol*. 2008;74(10):3002–7.
146. Simmerman JM, Suntarattiwong P, Levy J, et al. Influenza virus contamination of common household surfaces during the 2009 influenza A (H1N1) pandemic in Bangkok, Thailand: Implications for contact transmission. *Clin Infect Dis*. 2010;51(9):1053–61.
147. Weber TP, Stilianakis NI. Inactivation of influenza A viruses in the environment and modes of transmission: A critical review. *J Infect*. 2008;57(5):361–73.
148. WHO. Pandemic influenza vaccine manufacturing process and timeline. WHO. https://www.who.int/csr/disease/swineflu/notes/h1n1_vaccine_20090806/en/. Accessed August 31, 2019.
149. Hampson A, Barr I, Cox N, et al. Improving the selection and development of influenza vaccine viruses—Report of a WHO informal consultation on improving influenza vaccine virus selection, Hong Kong SAR, China, 18–20 November 2015. *Vaccine*. 2017;35(8): 1104–9.
150. Young B, Sadarangani S, Haur SY, et al. Semiannual versus annual influenza vaccination in older adults in the tropics: An observer-blind, active-comparator–controlled, randomized superiority trial. *Clin Infect Dis*. 2019;69(1):121–9.
151. Ferdinands JM, Fry AM, Reynolds S, et al. Intraseason waning of influenza vaccine protection: Evidence from the US Influenza Vaccine Effectiveness Network, 2011–12 through 2014–15. *Clin Infect Dis*. 2016;64(5):ciw816.
152. Radin JM, Hawksworth AW, Myers CA, Ricketts MN, Hansen EA, Brice GT. Influenza vaccine effectiveness: Maintained protection throughout the duration of influenza seasons 2010–2011 through 2013–2014. *Vaccine*. 2016;34(33):3907–12.

153. Kissling E, Nunes B, Robertson C, et al. I-MOVE multicentre case–control study 2010/11 to 2014/15: Is there within-season waning of influenza type/subtype vaccine effectiveness with increasing time since vaccination? *Euro Surveill.* 2016;21(16):30201.

154. CDC. Everyone 6 months of age and older should get a flu vaccine. Centers for Disease Control and Prevention. https://www.cdc.gov/flu/prevent/vaccinations.htm. Published August 31, 2018. Accessed August 5, 2019.

155. CDC. Influenza vaccines—United States, 2018–19 influenza season. https://www.cdc.gov/flu/professionals/vaccines.htm. Published April 26, 2019. Accessed August 4, 2019.

156. Cate TR, Couch RB, Kasel JA, Six HR. Clinical trials of monovalent influenza A/New Jersey/76 virus vaccines in adults: Reactogenicity, antibody response, and antibody persistence. *J Infect Dis.* 1977;136(Supplement 3):S450–5.

157. Cate TR, Couch RB, Parker D, Baxter B. Reactogenicity, immunogenicity, and antibody persistence in adults given inactivated influenza virus vaccines—1978. *Rev Infect Dis.* 1983;5(4):737–47.

158. Wright PF, Cherry JD, Foy HM, et al. Antigenicity and reactogenicity of influenza A/USSR/77 virus vaccine in children—A multicentered evaluation of dosage and safety. *Rev Infect Dis.* 1983;5(4):758–64.

159. Wright PF, Thompson J, Vaughn WK, Folland DS, Sell SHW, Karzon DT. Trials of influenza A/New Jersey/76 virus vaccine in normal children: An overview of age-related antigenicity and reactogenicity. *J Infect Dis.* 1977;136(Supplement 3):S731–41.

160. Quinnan GV, Schooley R, Dolin R, Ennis FA, Gross P, Gwaltney JM. Serologic responses and systemic reactions in adults after vaccination with monovalent A/USSR/77 and trivalent A/USSR/77, A/Texas/77, B/Hong Kong/72 influenza vaccines. *Rev Infect Dis.* 1983;5(4):748–57.

161. CDC. How Influenza (Flu) Vaccines are Made. https://www.cdc.gov/flu/prevent/how-fluvaccine-made.htm. Published July 10, 2019. Accessed August 4, 2019.

162. CDC. Fluzone High-Dose Seasonal Influenza Vaccine. https://www.cdc.gov/flu/prevent/qa_fluzone.htm. Published April 18, 2019. Accessed August 5, 2019.

163. CDC. Flu Vaccine with Adjuvant. https://www.cdc.gov/flu/prevent/adjuvant.htm. Published April 18, 2019. Accessed August 5, 2019.

164. DiazGranados CA, Dunning AJ, Kimmel M, et al. Efficacy of high-dose versus standard-dose influenza vaccine in older adults. *N Engl J Med.* 2014;371(7):635–45.

165. Gravenstein S, Davidson HE, Taljaard M, et al. Comparative effectiveness of high-dose versus standard-dose influenza vaccination on numbers of US nursing home residents admitted to hospital: A cluster-randomised trial. *Lancet Respir Med.* 2017;5(9):738–46.

166. De Donato S, Granoff D, Minutello M, et al. Safety and immunogenicity of MF59-adjuvanted influenza vaccine in the elderly. *Vaccine.* 1999;17(23):3094–101.

167. Podda A. The adjuvanted influenza vaccines with novel adjuvants: Experience with the MF59-adjuvanted vaccine. *Vaccine.* 2001;19(17):2673–80.

168. Tsai TF. Fluad®-MF59®-adjuvanted influenza vaccine in older adults. *Infect Chemother.* 2013;45(2):159–74.

169. Van Buynder PG, Konrad S, Van Buynder JL, et al. The comparative effectiveness of adjuvanted and unadjuvanted trivalent inactivated influenza vaccine (TIV) in the elderly. *Vaccine.* 2013;31(51):6122–8.

170. Pasteur S. Sanofi UK marketing authorisation granted for Sanofi Pasteur's Trivalent Influenza Vaccine (Split Virion, Inactivated) High Dose ▼(TIV High Dose). *GlobeNewswire News Room.* http://www.globenewswire.com/news-release/2019/01/21/1703026/0/en/Sanofi-UK-marketing-authorisation-granted-for-Sanofi-Pasteur-s-Trivalent-Influenza-Vaccine-Split-Virion-Inactivated-High-Dose-TIV-High-Dose.html. Published January 21, 2019. Accessed August 5, 2019.

171. Holland D, Booy R, De Looze F, et al. Intradermal influenza vaccine administered using a new microinjection system produces superior immunogenicity in elderly adults: A randomized controlled trial. *J Infect Dis.* 2008;198(5):650–8.

172. Arnou R, Icardi G, De Decker M, et al. Intradermal influenza vaccine for older adults: A randomized controlled multicenter phase III study. *Vaccine.* 2009;27(52):7304–12.

173. Van Damme P, Oosterhuis-Kafeja F, Van der Wielen M, Almagor Y, Sharon O, Levin Y. Safety and efficacy of a novel microneedle device for dose sparing intradermal influenza vaccination in healthy adults. *Vaccine.* 2009;27(3):454–9.

174. CDC. Immunogenicity, Efficacy, and Effectiveness of Influenza Vaccines. https://www.cdc.gov/flu/professionals/acip/2018-2019/background/immunogenicity.htm. Published April 17, 2019. Accessed August 5, 2019.

175. Thompson MG, Pierse N, Sue Huang Q, et al. Influenza vaccine effectiveness in preventing influenza-associated intensive care admissions and attenuating severe disease among adults in New Zealand 2012–2015. *Vaccine.* 2018;36(39):5916–25.

176. Arriola CS, Anderson EJ, Baumbach J, et al. Does influenza vaccination modify influenza severity? Data on older adults hospitalized with influenza during the 2012–2013 season in the United States. *J Infect Dis.* 2015;212(8):1200–8.

177. Harper SA, Fukuda K, Uyeki TM, Cox NJ, Bridges CB, Centers for Disease Control and Prevention (CDC) Advisory Committee on Immunization Practices (ACIP). Prevention and control of influenza: Recommendations of the Advisory Committee on Immunization Practices (ACIP). *MMWR Recomm.* 2004;53(RR-6):1–40.

178. Hoberman A, Greenberg DP, Paradise JL, et al. Effectiveness of inactivated influenza vaccine in preventing acute otitis media in young children: A randomized controlled trial. *JAMA.* 2003;290(12):1608–16.

179. Clements DA, Langdon L, Bland C, Walter E. Influenza A vaccine decreases the incidence of otitis media in 6- to 30-month-old children in day care. *Arch Pediatr Adolesc Med.* 1995;149(10):1113–7.

180. Gross PA, Hermogenes AW, Sacks HS, Lau J, Levandowski RA. The efficacy of influenza vaccine in elderly persons. A meta-analysis and review of the literature. *Ann Intern Med.* 1995;123(7):518–27.

181. Rhorer J, Ambrose CS, Dickinson S, et al. Efficacy of live attenuated influenza vaccine in children: A meta-analysis of nine randomized clinical trials. *Vaccine.* 2009;27(7):1101–10.

182. Belshe RB, Edwards KM, Vesikari T, et al. Live attenuated versus inactivated influenza vaccine in infants and young children. *N Engl J Med.* 2007;356(7):685–96.

183. Ashkenazi S, Vertruyen A, Arístegui J, et al. Superior relative efficacy of live attenuated influenza vaccine compared with inactivated influenza vaccine in young children with recurrent respiratory tract infections. *Pediatr Infect Dis J.* 2006;25(10):870–9.

184. Fleming DM, Crovari P, Wahn U, et al. Comparison of the efficacy and safety of live attenuated cold-adapted influenza vaccine, trivalent, with trivalent inactivated influenza virus vaccine in children and adolescents with asthma. *Pediatr Infect Dis J.* 2006;25(10):860–9.

185. Gaglani M, Pruszynski J, Murthy K, et al. Influenza vaccine effectiveness against 2009 pandemic influenza A(H1N1) virus differed by vaccine type during 2013–2014 in the United States. *J Infect Dis.* 2016;213(10):1546–56.

186. Jackson ML, Chung JR, Jackson LA, et al. Influenza vaccine effectiveness in the United States during the 2015–2016 season. *N Engl J Med.* 2017;377(6):534–43.

187. Grohskopf LA. Prevention and control of seasonal influenza with vaccines. *MMWR Recomm Rep.* 2016;65:1–54.

188. Grohskopf LA, Sokolow LZ, Broder KR, et al. Prevention and control of seasonal influenza with vaccines: Recommendations of the Advisory Committee on Immunization Practices—United States, 2017–18 influenza season. *MMWR Recomm Rep.* 2017;66(2):1–20.

189. Pebody R, Warburton F, Ellis J, et al. Effectiveness of seasonal influenza vaccine for adults and children in preventing laboratory-confirmed influenza in primary care in the United Kingdom: 2015/16 End-of-season results. *Euro Surveill.* 2016;21(38):30348.

190. Pebody R, Sile B, Warburton F, et al. Live attenuated influenza vaccine effectiveness against hospitalisation due to laboratory-confirmed influenza in children two to six years of age in England in the 2015/16 season. *Euro Surveill.* 2017;22(4):30450.

191. Grohskopf LA. Update: ACIP recommendations for the use of quadrivalent live attenuated influenza vaccine (LAIV4)—United States, 2018–19 influenza season. *MMWR Morb Mortal Wkly Rep.* 2018;67:643–5.

192. Rolfes MA, Flannery B, Chung J, et al. Effects of influenza vaccination in the United States during the 2017–2018 influenza season. *Clin Infect Dis.* 2019;69(11):1845–53.

193. Ting EEK, Sander B, Ungar WJ. Systematic review of the cost-effectiveness of influenza immunization programs. *Vaccine.* 2017;35(15):1828–43.

194. Wood SC, Nguyen VH, Schmidt C. Economic evaluations of influenza vaccination in healthy working-age adults. Employer and society perspective. *PharmacoEconomics.* 2000;18(2):173–83.

195. Postma MJ, Baltussen RM, Heijnen ML, de Berg LT, Jager JC. Pharmacoeconomics of influenza vaccination in the elderly: Reviewing the available evidence. *Drugs Aging.* 2000;17(3):217–27.

196. Bridges CB, Thompson WW, Meltzer MI, et al. Effectiveness and cost-benefit of influenza vaccination of healthy working adults: A randomized controlled trial. *JAMA.* 2000;284(13):1655–63.

197. Govaert TM, Dinant GJ, Aretz K, Masurel N, Sprenger MJ, Knottnerus JA. Adverse reactions to influenza vaccine in elderly people: Randomised double blind placebo controlled trial. *BMJ.* 1993;307(6910):988–90.

198. Margolis KL, Nichol KL, Poland GA, Pluhar RE. Frequency of adverse reactions to influenza vaccine in the elderly. A randomized, placebo-controlled trial. *JAMA.* 1990;264(9):1139–41.

199. Nichol KL, Margolis KL, Lind A, et al. Side effects associated with influenza vaccination in healthy working adults. A randomized, placebo-controlled trial. *Arch Intern Med.* 1996;156(14):1546–50.

200. James JM, Zeiger RS, Lester MR, et al. Safe administration of influenza vaccine to patients with egg allergy. *J Pediatr.* 1998;133(5):624–8.

201. Murphy KR, Strunk RC. Safe administration of influenza vaccine in asthmatic children hypersensitive to egg proteins. *J Pediatr.* 1985;106(6):931–3.

202. Zeiger RS. Current issues with influenza vaccination in egg allergy. *J Allergy Clin Immunol.* 2002;110(6):834–40.

203. Schonberger LB, Bregman DJ, Sullivan-Bolyai JZ, et al. Guillain-Barre syndrome following vaccination in the National Influenza Immunization Program, United States, 1976–1977. *Am J Epidemiol.* 1979;110(2):105–23.

204. Kaplan JE, Katona P, Hurwitz ES, Schonberger LB. Guillain-Barré syndrome in the United States, 1979–1980 and 1980–1981. Lack of an association with influenza vaccination. *JAMA.* 1982;248(6):698–700.

205. Hurwitz ES, Schonberger LB, Nelson DB, Holman RC. Guillain-Barré syndrome and the 1978–1979 influenza vaccine. *N Engl J Med.* 1981;304(26):1557–61.

206. Lasky T, Terracciano GJ, Magder L, et al. The Guillain-Barré syndrome and the 1992–1993 and 1993–1994 influenza vaccines. *N Engl J Med.* 1998;339(25):1797–802.

207. Miller E, Andrews N, Stellitano L, et al. Risk of narcolepsy in children and young people receiving AS03 adjuvanted pandemic A/H1N1 2009 influenza vaccine: Retrospective analysis. *BMJ.* 2013;346:f794.

208. Nohynek H, Jokinen J, Partinen M, et al. AS03 adjuvanted AH1N1 vaccine associated with an abrupt increase in the incidence of childhood narcolepsy in Finland. *PLoS One.* 2012;7(3):e33536.

209. Sarkanen TO, Alakuijala APE, Dauvilliers YA, Partinen MM. Incidence of narcolepsy after H1N1 influenza and vaccinations: Systematic review and meta-analysis. *Sleep Med Rev.* 2018;38:177–86.

210. Falsey AR, Treanor JJ, Tornieporth N, Capellan J, Gorse GJ. Randomized, double-blind controlled phase 3 trial comparing the immunogenicity of high-dose and standard-dose influenza vaccine in adults 65 years of age and older. *J Infect Dis.* 2009;200(2):172–80.

211. CDC. Cell-Based Flu Vaccines. https://www.cdc.gov/flu/prevent/cell-based.htm. Published April 18, 2019. Accessed August 6, 2019.

212. Cox MMJ, Izikson R, Post P, Dunkle L. Safety, efficacy, and immunogenicity of Flublok in the prevention of seasonal influenza in adults. *Ther Adv Vaccines.* 2015;3(4):97–108.

213. Institute of Medicine (US) Immunization Safety Review Committee, Stratton K, Gable A, McCormick M. *Thimerosal-Containing Vaccines and Neurodevelopmental Disorders.* Washington, DC: National Academies Press; 2001. https://www.ncbi.nlm.nih.gov/books/NBK223724/. Accessed May 12, 2019.

214. Centers for Disease Control and Prevention. Recommendations regarding the use of vaccines that contain thimerosal as a preservative. *Morb Mortal Wkly Rep.* 1999;48(43):996–8.

215. Pichichero ME, Cernichiari E, Lopreiato J, Treanor J. Mercury concentrations and metabolism in infants receiving vaccines containing thiomersal: A descriptive study. *Lancet.* 2002;360(9347):1737–41.

216. World Health Organization. Vaccine Position Paper. https://www.who.int/wer/2012/wer8747.pdf?ua=1. Accessed August 6, 2019.

217. Ortiz JR, Perut M, Dumolard L, et al. A global review of national influenza immunization policies: Analysis of the 2014 WHO/UNICEF Joint Reporting Form on immunization. *Vaccine.* 2016;34(45):5400–5.

218. Smith JC. Immunization policy development in the United States: The role of the Advisory Committee on Immunization Practices. *Ann Intern Med.* 2009;150(1):45.

219. Fedson DS, Hirota Y, Shin HK, et al. Influenza vaccination in 22 developed countries: An update to 1995. *Vaccine.* 1997;15(14):1506–11.

220. Bridges CB, Fukuda K, Uyeki TM, Cox NJ, Singleton JA, Centers for Disease Control and Prevention, Advisory Committee on Immunization Practices. Prevention and control of influenza. Recommendations of the Advisory Committee on Immunization Practices (ACIP). *MMWR Recomm Rep.* 2002;51(RR-3):1–31.

221. Centers for Disease Control and Prevention (CDC). Influenza and pneumococcal vaccination coverage among persons aged > or =65 years and persons aged 18–64 years with diabetes or asthma—United States, 2003. *MMWR Morb Mortal Wkly Rep.* 2004;53(43):1007–12.

222. CDC. Influenza Vaccination Information for Health Care Workers. https://www.cdc.gov/flu/professionals/healthcareworkers.htm. Published April 25, 2019. Accessed August 6, 2019.

223. Paules CI, Sullivan SG, Subbarao K, Fauci AS. Chasing seasonal influenza—The need for a universal influenza vaccine. *N Engl J Med.* 2018;378(1):7–9.

224. Erbelding EJ, Post DJ, Stemmy EJ, et al. A universal influenza vaccine: The strategic plan for the National Institute of Allergy and Infectious Diseases. *J Infect Dis.* 2018;218(3):347–54.

225. Ison MG. Optimizing antiviral therapy for influenza: Understanding the evidence. *Expert Rev Anti Infect Ther.* 2015;13(4):417–25.

226. Ison MG. Clinical use of approved influenza antivirals: Therapy and prophylaxis. *Influenza Other Respir Viruses.* 2013;7(s1):7–13.

227. Hayden FG, Sugaya N, Hirotsu N, et al. Baloxavir marboxil for uncomplicated influenza in adults and adolescents. *N Engl J Med.* 2018;379(10):913–23.

228. Moscona A. Neuraminidase inhibitors for influenza. *N Engl J Med.* 2005;353(13):1363–73.

229. Nakamura S, Miyazaki T, Izumikawa K, et al. Efficacy and safety of intravenous peramivir compared with oseltamivir in high-risk patients infected with influenza A and B viruses: A multicenter randomized controlled study. *Open Forum Infect Dis.* 2017;4(3):ofx129.

230. Kaiser L, Wat C, Mills T, Mahoney P, Ward P, Hayden F. Impact of oseltamivir treatment on influenza-related lower respiratory tract complications and hospitalizations. *Arch Intern Med.* 2003;163(14):1667–72.

231. Malosh RE, Martin ET, Heikkinen T, Brooks WA, Whitley RJ, Monto AS. Efficacy and safety of oseltamivir in children: Systematic review and individual patient data meta-analysis of randomized controlled trials. *Clin Infect Dis.* 2018;66(10):1492–500.

232. Muthuri SG, Venkatesan S, Myles PR, et al. Effectiveness of neuraminidase inhibitors in reducing mortality in patients admitted to hospital with influenza A H1N1pdm09 virus infection: A meta-analysis of individual participant data. *Lancet Respir Med.* 2014;2(5):395–404.

233. Louie JK, Yang S, Acosta M, et al. Treatment with neuraminidase inhibitors for critically ill patients with influenza A (H1N1)pdm09. *Clin Infect Dis.* 2012;55(9):1198–204.

234. Yu H, Feng Z, Uyeki TM, et al. Risk factors for severe illness with 2009 pandemic influenza A (H1N1) virus infection in China. *Clin Infect Dis.* 2011;52(4):457–65.

235. Uyeki TM, Bernstein HH, Bradley JS, et al. Clinical practice guidelines by the Infectious Diseases Society of America: 2018 Update on diagnosis, treatment, chemoprophylaxis, and institutional outbreak management of seasonal influenza. *Clin Infect Dis.* 2019;68(6):e1–47.

236. Peters PH, Gravenstein S, Norwood P, et al. Long-term use of oseltamivir for the prophylaxis of influenza in a vaccinated frail older population. *J Am Geriatr Soc.* 2001;49(8):1025–31.

237. Monto AS, Pichichero ME, Blanckenberg SJ, et al. Zanamivir prophylaxis: An effective strategy for the prevention of influenza types A and B within households. *J Infect Dis.* 2002;186(11):1582–8.

238. Monto AS, Robinson DP, Herlocher ML, Hinson JM, Elliott MJ, Crisp A. Zanamivir in the prevention of influenza among healthy adults: A randomized controlled trial. *JAMA.* 1999;282(1):31–5.

239. CDC. What You Should Know About Flu Antiviral Drugs. https://www.cdc.gov/flu/treatment/whatyoushould.htm. Published April 22, 2019. Accessed August 7, 2019.

240. Meijer A, Lackenby A, Hungnes O, et al. Oseltamivir-resistant influenza virus A (H1N1), Europe, 2007–08 season. *Emerg Infect Dis.* 2009;15(4):552–60.

241. Dharan NJ, Gubareva LV, Meyer JJ, et al. Infections with oseltamivir-resistant influenza A(H1N1) virus in the United States. *JAMA.* 2009;301(10):1034–41.

242. Hurt AC, Hardie K, Wilson NJ, et al. Community transmission of oseltamivir-resistant A(H1N1)pdm09 influenza. *N Engl J Med.* 2011;365(26):2541–2.

243. CDC. Avian Influenza A Virus Infections in Humans. https://www.cdc.gov/flu/avianflu/avian-in-humans.htm. Published April 18, 2017. Accessed August 9, 2019.

244. WHO. Cumulative number of confirmed human cases of avian influenza A(H5N1) reported to WHO. http://www.who.int/influenza/human_animal_interface/H5N1_cumulative_table_archives/en/. Accessed August 9, 2019.

245. H5N1_avian_influenza_update20141204.pdf. https://www.who.int/influenza/human_animal_interface/H5N1_avian_influenza_update20141204.pdf?ua=1. Accessed August 9, 2019.

246. Katz JM, Lim W, Bridges CB, et al. Antibody response in individuals infected with avian influenza A (H5N1) viruses and detection of anti-H5 antibody among household and social contacts. *J Infect Dis.* 1999;180(6):1763–70.

247. Ungchusak K, Auewarakul P, Dowell SF, et al. Probable person-to-person transmission of avian influenza A (H5N1). *N Engl J Med.* 2005;352(4):333–40.

248. Kandun IN, Wibisono H, Sedyaningsih ER, et al. Three Indonesian clusters of H5N1 virus infection in 2005. *N Engl J Med.* 2006;355(21):2186–94.

249. Napp S, Majó N, Sánchez-Gónzalez R, Vergara-Alert J. Emergence and spread of highly pathogenic avian influenza A(H5N8) in Europe in 2016–2017. *Transbound Emerg Dis.* 2018;65(5):1217–26.

250. ai-20190719.pdf. https://www.who.int/docs/default-source/wpro--documents/emergency/surveillance/avian-influenza/ai-20190719.pdf?sfvrsn=30d65594_28. Accessed August 9, 2019.

251. WHO. Weekly Epidemiological Record, 18 August 2017, vol. 92, 33 (pp. 453–76). http://www.who.int/wer/2017/wer9233/en/. Accessed August 9, 2019.

252. Chen H, Liu S, Liu J, et al. Nosocomial co-transmission of avian influenza A(H7N9) and A(H1N1)pdm09 viruses between 2 patients with hematologic disorders. *Emerg Infect Dis.* 2016;22(4):598–607.

253. Fang C-F, Ma M-J, Zhan B-D, et al. Nosocomial transmission of avian influenza A (H7N9) virus in China: Epidemiological investigation. *BMJ.* 2015;351:h5765.

254. WHO. Avian influenza: Food safety issues. http://www.who.int/foodsafety/areas_work/zoonose/avian/en/. Accessed August 9, 2019.

255. Harder TC, Buda S, Hengel H, Beer M, Mettenleiter TC. Poultry food products—A source of avian influenza virus transmission to humans? *Clin Microbiol Infect.* 2016;22(2):141–6.

256. Tweed SA, Skowronski DM, David ST, et al. Human illness from avian Influenza H7N3, British Columbia. *Emerg Infect Dis.* 2004;10(12):2196–9.

257. Yuen K, Chan P, Peiris M, et al. Clinical features and rapid viral diagnosis of human disease associated with avian influenza A H5N1 virus. *Lancet.* 1998;351(9101):467–71.

258. Apisarnthanarak A, Kitphati R, Thongphubeth K, et al. Atypical avian influenza (H5N1). *Emerg Infect Dis.* 2004;10(7):1321–4.

259. Adisasmito W, Chan PKS, Lee N, et al. Effectiveness of antiviral treatment in human influenza A(H5N1) infections: Analysis of a Global Patient Registry. *J Infect Dis.* 2010;202(8):1154–60.

260. CDC. Interim Guidance on the Use of Antiviral Medications for Treatment of Human Infections with Novel Influenza A Viruses Associated with Severe Human Disease. Avian Influenza (Flu). https://www.cdc.gov/flu/avianflu/novel-av-treatment-guidance.htm. Published December 26, 2018. Accessed August 9, 2019.

CHAPTER 106

Pneumococcal Infections

Abram L. Wagner • Matthew L. Boulton

HISTORY

Streptococcus pneumoniae (i.e., pneumococcus) was independently isolated in American and French laboratories in the early 1880s.[1,2] It was one of the first bacteria to be observed using Gram stain, and advances in microscopic techniques allowed it to become established as a cause of pneumonia, meningitis, and otitis media by the end of the nineteenth century.[1] During the 1918 Flu Pandemic, secondary bacterial infections—predominantly pneumococcal, contributed to a high infectious disease-related mortality rate.[3]

Pneumococcus was one of the earliest pathogens for which attempts were made to develop a vaccine. Clinical trials among mineworkers in South Africa in the 1910s found whole-cell, killed vaccines to have limited and transient efficacy.[4] Widespread distribution of vaccines did not begin until after the development of a pneumococcal polysaccharide vaccine (PPSV) targeting 14 serotypes (licensed in 1977) and later 23 serotypes (licensed in 1983).[4] In 1981, the U.S. Advisory Committee on Immunization Practices (ACIP) recommended all adults $\geq$ 65 years to be vaccinated with PPSV14, and this was updated to PPSV23 in 1984.[5] Polysaccharide vaccines do not induce a substantial antibody response in infants, however, and they elicit only a short term immunity.[6] A more immunogenic pediatric vaccine formulation was licensed in 2000, in the form of the 7-valent pneumococcal conjugate vaccine (PCV), which was expanded to a 13-valent form, licensed in 2010.[7,8] PCV is notable for being one of the most expensive vaccines currently available at over $150 per dose, although many studies have shown it cost-effective.[9,10] The World Health Organization (WHO) recommended inclusion of PCV in every country's immunization schedule—the Expanded Program on Immunization, in 2012.[11] The widespread introduction of pneumococcal vaccines has led to a rapid decline in pneumococcal pneumonia and invasive pneumococcal disease (i.e., meningitis and bacteremia),[12] but there remain theoretical concerns about serotype replacement.

BACTERIOLOGY

There are 97 known serotypes of pneumococcus, which can be classified according to what is commonly known as the Danish system.[13] Pneumococcal serotypes, or strains, are typically differentiated based on the polysaccharide capsule surrounding the bacterium, the role of which is to help the bacteria avoid the immune system and prevent phagocytosis.[14,15] However, nonencapsulated strains exist and can also cause disease, particularly in cases of conjunctivitis with 80% of pneumococcal infections involving nonencapsulated strains and in cases of otitis media with 8% nonencapsulated.[16] Immunity to pneumococcus is serotype-specific, although related serotypes (termed "serogroups") may provide some cross protection, particularly for serogroup 6.[17] Understanding the serotype distribution within a population has been an important area of research both to identify which serotypes should be targeted by vaccines and to evaluate the cost-effectiveness and success of public immunization programs.

The distribution of pneumococcal serotypes varies by age, geographical location, time, site of infection, and in their propensity to result in asymptomatic colonization versus invasive disease. Seven serotypes (in descending order: 14, 6B, 19F, 18C, 23F, 4, and 9V) were found in 78% of pneumococcal cases of meningitis, bacteremia, and otitis media among children < 6 years in the United States between 1978 and 1994, which was a time period preceding pediatric pneumococcal vaccination.[18] In contrast, adults contend with a greater diversity of strains; the ten most common serotypes isolated from blood and cerebrospinal fluid (CSF) between 1978 and 1992 in U.S. adults were 4, 14, 23F, 9V, 12F, 6B, 3, 8, 1, and 9N, which collectively comprised 65% of all invasive pneumococcal infections.[19]

Globally the six most common serotypes among cases of invasive disease have been, in order from highest to lowest, 14, 6B, 1, 23F, 5, and 19F. Serotypes 1 and 5, in particular, are more common in low- and middle-income countries in Africa, Asia, and Latin America, whereas serotype 18C is more frequently found in high-income countries. However, there exists substantial variability among countries in a given region with regard to the pneumococcal serotype distribution and occurrence.[20]

Serotype strains could also vary based on the location of sampling (nasopharynx vs. other site) or based on whether the case represents invasive versus noninvasive disease. Only 20–30 serotypes regularly cause invasive disease.[13] For example, in a study of children in China which compared samples taken from cases of noninvasive to invasive disease, serotypes 19A, 14, and 5 were more commonly found in invasive cases.[21]

PNEUMOCOCCAL COLONIZATION

Pneumococcal disease follows asymptomatic nasopharyngeal colonization, or carriage. It is likely that most individuals afflicted with pneumococcal infection will have been colonized at one point in their lifetime, and carriage is especially common in infants and young children. Among studies of children < 2 years of age examined in one review,[15] carriage ranged from 2% to 86%, with a median value between 34% and 40%. A study of children in Finland found that nasopharyngeal carriage increased from 9% at 2 months to 43% at 24 months.[22] Another study in the United Kingdom found that carriage decreased at older ages in children, from 52% for children 0–2 years to 21% for children 5–17 years.[23] Because of their high potential rate of carriage of pneumococcus, children are thought to be the principle disseminators of pneumococcal colonization, and therefore disease, within a community. Pneumococcal carriage is particularly elevated in crowded settings, including daycare centers.[24]

The nasopharynx can be colonized by various other bacteria, including *Moraxella cattarrhalis*, *Haemophilus influenzae*, *Neisseria meningitides* (meningococcus), and *Staphylococcus aureus*, and other α-hemolytic streptococci.[15] Various synergistic and antagonistic relationships exist between these bacteria.[15] For example, growth of pneumococcus increases in the presence of meningococcus,[25] whereas pneumococcus is impeded by the presence of α-hemolytic streptococci[26] and viridans streptococci.[27] Pneumococcus can impede the growth of *S. aureus*, and this competitive inhibition explains some of the age-related patterns of pneumococcal and *S. aureus* carriage—with the former being more common in young children, and the latter more frequently found in older children and young adolescents.[28,29] Viral-bacterial interactions are also common, as exemplified by the influenza-pneumococcus superinfection during the 1918 flu pandemic,[3,30] and viral infection could promote secondary bacterial infections through a variety of mechanisms, including disrupting the epithelial layer of the respiratory tract mucosa, upregulating adhesion proteins, and impairing immune system functioning.[30]

A broad range of disease can occur if pneumococcal colonization persists. A local, mucosal immune response can clear colonization while also preventing recolonization.[15] In contrast, disease can result if the pathogen is able to infect other areas of the respiratory tract. As for pathogen-specific factors that can potentiate disease, some polysaccharide capsules may be more virulent (especially with a thicker layer), although phase variation could result in genetically identical colonies expressing different phenotypes with one being more predisposed to asymptomatic colonization and another to survival in the bloodstream.[31]

PNEUMOCOCCAL DISEASE

Symptomatic pneumococcal disease results after disruption has occurred in the commensal relationship between host and bacteria. As bacteria invade areas beyond the nasopharynx, including the middle-ear space or the terminal airways, infection can eventually cause otitis media or more severe illness like pneumonia. More serious invasive complications such as bacteremia occur following pneumonia in most cases, although, less often, the bacteria can spread directly from the nasopharynx into the bloodstream as a form of occult bacteremia.[32] Mortality from invasive pneumococcal disease can be high; in a cohort study in Denmark between 1997 and 2007, 30-day mortality was 17% following bacteremia and 22% following meningitis.[33] Mortality from pneumonia accompanied by invasive disease was found to be 12% across nine geographic regions of North America[34] and 15.1% in Spain.[35] Although pneumococcal carriage is highest in young children, mortality for invasive disease is lowest in young children, and greatest in older adults.[34]

Invasive pneumococcal disease has been a national notifiable disease in the United States since 2010. For surveillance purposes, a confirmed case of invasive disease requires that pneumococcus be isolated from a normally sterile body site (e.g., blood, CSF, or joint, pleural, or pericardial fluid). The 2010 case definition mentions acute otitis media, pneumonia, bacteremia, or meningitis as possible clinical syndrome, but only bacteremia or meningitis are mentioned in the 2017 updated case definition,[36] as acute otitis media and pneumonia often occur in the absence of bacteria in sterile body sites.

Severe community-acquired pneumonia (CAP) is defined as pneumonia acquired in the community that requires admission to an intensive-care unit. The Infectious Disease Society of America and American Thoracic Society have issued a strong recommendation for admission to an ICU for patients with either of two major criteria; the need for mechanical ventilation and/or a clinical presentation of septic shock requiring vasopressor therapy, as shown in Box 106-1, in addition to a moderate recommendation for ICU admission for patients if they fulfill three of the minor criteria.[37]

Several distinct epidemiological patterns have emerged with pneumococcal disease. Prior to the introduction of pneumococcal vaccination programs, Australian aboriginals, Native Alaskans, and Native American groups in the United States, experienced some of the world's highest incidence of invasive pneumococcal disease.[38] Certain socioeconomic factors, including exposure to smoke among smokers but also from secondhand exposure and from indoor cooking—has been associated with a higher risk for developing invasive pneumococcal disease.[38]

BOX 106-1 Criteria for Severe Community-acquired Pneumonia[37]

Major criteria
Invasive mechanical ventilation
Septic shock with the need for vasopressors
Minor criteria
Respiratory rate > 30 breaths/min
PaO_2/FiO_2 ratio < 250
Multilobar infiltrates
Confusion/disorientation
Uremia (BUN level > 20 mg/dL)
Leukopenia (WBC count < 4000 cells/mm^3)
Thrombocytopenia (platelet count < 1000,000 cells/mm^3)
Hypothermia (core temperature < 36°C)
Hypotension requiring aggressive fluid resuscitation

Reproduce with Permission from Mandell LA, Wunderink RG, Anzueto A, et al. Infectious Diseases Society of America / American Thoracic Society Consensus Guidelines on the Management of Community-Acquired Pneumonia in Adults. Clin. Infect. Dis. 2007;44:S27-72.

Pneumococcal infections are also a theoretical and practical concern for individuals with certain medical conditions, especially those affecting immune response. Immune deficiencies (like agammaglobulinemia, IgG subclass deficiency, multiple myeloma, chronic lymphocytic leukemia, lymphoma, and defective complement) lead to impaired availability of opsonizing antibody and diminished effectiveness of phagocytosis. Individuals with untreated HIV infection are ten times more likely to acquire pneumococcal pneumonia and 100 times more likely to incur pneumococcal bacteremia than the general population.[39] Functional or anatomic splenectomy also increases the risk of pneumococcal infection through impaired clearance of pneumococcal bacteremia. In many areas of the world, individuals with sickle cell disease are the group that mostly commonly experiences this risk, and consequently are an important target for prevention programs, including prophylactic use of antibiotics and priority uptake of pneumococcal vaccines.

DIAGNOSIS

Several diagnostic methods for pneumococcus are available, although their accuracy and usage varies. The historical gold standard for pneumococcal diagnosis has been isolation and culture of the pneumococcal bacterium. For noninvasive pneumonia, this typically requires a sputum sample. Unfortunately, this technique has significant drawbacks: collecting an acceptable sputum sample can be difficult, and the accuracy of Gram stains is low—with a sensitivity of 60% and specificity of 80%[40] with substantial variations between operators.[41] For invasive cases, current CDC guidelines indicate that confirmed cases require isolation and culture of pneumococcus from normally sterile body sites; culture independent diagnostic tests, such as polymerase chain reaction (PCR)-based testing or rapid urinary antigen tests, currently can only provide supportive information.[36] For clinical purposes, the current consensus guidelines from the Infectious Diseases Society of America and the American Thoracic Society state that patients with severe CAP (see Box 106-1) should have both blood samples and expectorated sputum samples cultured, along with urinary antigen tests performed for pneumococcus and *Legionella pneumophila*.[37]

A rapid urine antigen test for pneumococcus was licensed by the Food and Drug Administration in 1999, and was used by 65%

of physicians who were members of the Infectious Disease Society of America in a survey in the United States in 2013.[42] This test uses an immunochromatographic membrane technique to detect the C-polysaccharide antigen of pneumococcus. Its sensitivity is 80% and specificity 97%.[43,44]

The gold standard for pneumococcal serotyping is considered to be the Quellung reaction. In this laboratory test, a cultured sample of pneumococcus is exposed to agglutinizing anticapsular antibodies, and the capsule will appear "swollen" under microscopic investigation. By sequentially testing the sample with different serotype-specific antibodies, experienced investigators can determine which serotype is present. The latex agglutination procedure is similar, except the antibodies are passively attached to latex materials. Latex agglutination is simpler and less expensive than the Quellung reaction.[45] Finally, PCR-based methods are also available. Real-time PCR is more sensitive than multiplex-sequential PCR.[46] Although epidemiologically interesting as certain serotypes are associated with greater mortality,[33] serotyping pneumococcus has less direct utility for clinical decision-making.

TREATMENT AND SUSCEPTIBILITY TESTING

Treatment of acute otitis media does not need to include antibiotics for children over 2 years with a mild presentation of illness. Amoxicillin is often the first choice for patients without a penicillin allergy.[47] Amoxicillin can also be used for mild and moderate pneumococcal pneumonia.[48,49]

Due to widespread antibiotic resistance, initial treatment for invasive pneumococcal disease generally begins with a broad-spectrum antibiotic,[50] such as cephalosporin and often vancomycin, until results of antibiotic sensitivity testing can guide the clinician with regard to the preferred class of antibiotics to use.

Limiting the spread of antibiotic resistance is an important component to any clinical treatment regimen and public health surveillance program. One of the first known instances of antibiotic resistance was in pneumococcus, which demonstrated resistance to Optochin in one patient in 1916.[51] Resistance to penicillin was first identified in 1943, but did not become commonplace until after 1965.[52] The problem of antibiotic resistance in pneumococcus was recognized as a global phenomenon soon after, with resistant strains isolated in Papua New Guinea, Australia, and South Africa.[53] In the United States, the Active Bacterial Core (ABC) Surveillance in the Emerging Infections Program Network monitors antibiotic resistance patterns across ten states in the United States.[54]

Inappropriate use of antibiotics can undoubtedly influence the incidence of resistance. There is a general supposition that antibiotics are overprescribed, especially in low- and middle-income countries. For example, a study of drug prescriptions in ten provinces of western China found that 48.53% were for antibiotics—much higher than would be expected given healthcare usage and incidence of bacterial diseases.[55] In the United States, a study of antibiotic prescriptions undertaken by the Centers for Disease Control and Prevention found that almost one-third of prescriptions were unnecessary.[56] Beyond prescribing antibiotics in circumstances where they are not clinically indicated, physicians may be prescribing a regimen for an inappropriate duration, treating the patient longer than is necessary. Early studies on efficacy of antibiotics for pneumococcal pneumonia used 2–4 days of antibiotics, and findings from a randomized control trial find similar efficacy in treating patients for 3 versus 8 days. Empirical evidence points to prolonged courses of antibiotic therapy as contributing to antibiotic resistance, even while many sources of educational marketing encourage patients to take a full course of antibiotics to prevent antibiotic resistance.[57]

There has been some evidence that the introduction of pediatric vaccines into a population decreases the prevalence of antibiotic resistance within pneumococcal isolates found in the community,[58] likely because decreases in the incidence of disease—particularly in infants and young children—leads to decreases of antibiotic use in those populations, combined with reductions as fewer antibiotic-resistant strains are spread to family members. Along with antibiotic prescription patterns, vaccine use could explain how antibiotic resistance differs across regions of the world. For example, around 25% of pneumococcal isolates in the United States from invasive disease are nonsusceptible to penicillin,[54] compared to 44.8% in China.[21] Guidelines on susceptibility cut-offs changed in 2008, after the National Committee for Clinical Laboratory concluded that pneumococcal infections were responding to penicillin when in vitro studies would have suggested otherwise.[59]

IMMUNIZATION

All pneumococcal vaccine formulations currently on the market are based on immunity to the polysaccharide capsules of the bacteria, and therefore immunity is serotype specific. The first polysaccharide vaccines (PPSV) targeted 14 serotypes (in 1979) and 23 serotypes (licensed in 1983).[4] In the United States, PPSV was initially only recommended for adults $\geq$ 65 years, but in 1997, the Advisory Committee on Immunization Practices issued a recommendation for children $>$ 2 years with certain medical conditions to be vaccinated (see Table 106-1).[60] There are a number of deficiencies associated with PPSV. It is not immunogenic in children $<$ 2 years—who have a high prevalence of carriage and are epidemiologically important as an age group which spreads infection. Additionally, the vaccine has limited duration of effectiveness, and might induce hyporesponsiveness, that is, lower antibody response on subsequent re challenge with pneumococcal antigens.[60]

Conjugation—the covalent attachment of a poor antigen (i.e., a polysaccharide) to a strongly immunogenic antigen (i.e., a protein)—is a newer technology that has improved polysaccharide vaccines. It was first used for *Haemophilus influenzae* type b vaccines, which were licensed for use in the United States in 1987.[61] PCVs were developed in the 1990s, with the polysaccharides conjugated to an outer membrane protein from *H. influenzae*, from the diphtheria toxoid, or from the tetanus toxoid. The 7-valent PCV was licensed in 2000. Subsequently, higher-valence vaccines have been developed: a PCV-13 was licensed in the United States in 2010, and a PCV-15 is currently under development.[7,8,62] The World Health Organization (WHO) recommended PCV to be included on every country's immunization schedule—the Expanded Program on Immunization, in 2012.[11] Although measuring efficacy and effectiveness is difficult for a vaccine protecting against an infection with multifarious clinical presentations, and for which isolation is difficult, all indications point to a highly effective vaccine. Studies in healthy children have found efficacy against invasive disease from vaccine serotypes to be 97% and effectiveness at preventing invasive disease caused by vaccine serotypes to be between 91% and 96%, although effectiveness is potentially lower (91%) in children with comorbid medical conditions.[63]

TABLE 106-1 MEDICAL CONDITIONS THAT ARE INDICATIONS FOR PNEUMOCOCCAL VACCINATION[60]

Risk Group	Condition
Immunocompetent children	Chronic heart disease,chronic lung disease,diabetes mellitus,cerebrospinal fluid leaks,cochlear implant
Children with functional or anatomic asplenia	Sickle cell disease,other hemoglobinopathies,congenital or acquired asplenia,splenic dysfunction
Children with immunocompromising conditions	HIV infection,chronic renal failure and nephrotic syndrome,treatment with immunosuppressive drugs or radiation therapy,congenital immunodeficiency

Current Vaccine Recommendations

The U.S. ACIP and the WHO recommend all children to be vaccinated against pneumococcus with a conjugate vaccine. Per manufacturer's instructions, followed by ACIP, the number of doses required depends on the age at first vaccine administration: four doses (three primary + one booster) if first vaccinated when the child was < 6 months; three doses (two primary + one booster) if first vaccinated 7–11 months; two primary doses if vaccinated 12–23 months, and 1 primary dose if vaccinated 24–59 months.[60] The WHO recommends that countries choose between two schedules comprising three doses each: two primary + one booster, or three primary doses. A study in the United Kingdom comparing infants given a 3 + 1 schedule versus 2 + 1 schedule found no differences in antibody titer.[64] Further studies of the effectiveness of different pediatric schedules are ongoing.[65]

PCV has a similar schedule to many other pediatric vaccines, such as diphtheria-tetanus-pertussis, hepatitis B, and polio, for which all have receipt of the primary series recommended within the first year and a booster shot after a set interval. Coadministering these vaccines during the same office visit has been shown to be a safe and efficient mechanism to ensure infants are vaccinated with recommended doses as early as possible (for a three-dose primary series: either 6, 10, and 14 weeks, or 2, 4, and 6 months[66]). However, coadministration of certain vaccinations, like the PCV and influenza vaccine,[67] may result in a slight increase in the risk of adverse events like febrile seizures compared to nonconcomitant administration, but this small increase in risk is thought to be negligible compared to the potential benefit of providing early protection to a child against a full range of infectious diseases. Among adults, a randomized clinical trial found somewhat lower serotype-specific titers when PCV-13 was coadministered with a trivalent influenza vaccine.[68] However, these differences were not judged to be significant enough to recommend separately administering vaccines.

Children with certain chronic diseases (see Table 106-1) should also receive PPSV after completing the complete PCV series. These children are also to be prioritized for receiving PCV during vaccine shortages.

According to the U.S. ACIP, adults ≥ s65 are recommended to be vaccinated with both vaccines: preferably with PCV first and then PPSV, but PCV can also be administered after PPSV.[69]

Future Use of Pneumococcal Vaccines

Pneumonia can be associated with many different types of pathogens, but pneumococcal infection is the predominant bacterial cause of pneumonia-related deaths.[70] Because of the historical associations between pneumonia and pneumococcus, the pneumococcal vaccine is often marketed as the "pneumonia vaccine." This may be an inadequate and ineffective marketing strategy. First, vaccinated individuals who later come down with (nonpneumococcal) pneumonia may become distrustful of the pneumococcal vaccine's effectiveness or vaccines generally. Additionally, even if most pneumococcal deaths are due to pneumonia, pneumococcal infections also result in more meningitis deaths than *Haemophilus influenzae* type b or meningococcal infections. Because individuals may be more attuned to performing health behaviors based on severity of the event (e.g., perceiving meningitis as more severe than pneumonia) than probability of the event (e.g., pneumonia is more common than meningitis),[71] healthcare providers can emphasize that pneumococcal vaccines protect against meningitis.

Harkening back to the earliest pneumococcal vaccines, the formulation of future vaccines may try to induce broad protection against many, if not all, serotypes, by focusing on targets beyond the polysaccharides. For instance, cell-surface proteins (choline-binding proteins and lipoproteins) are one promising target.[32]

CHANGING EPIDEMIOLOGY OF PNEUMOCOCCAL DISEASE

Pneumococcal disease is highly prevalent and morbid. Each year there are approximately 2.6 million episodes of severe pneumococcal pneumonia globally.[72] Estimates from various modeling studies suggest that 36% (95% CI: 27%, 40%) of all-cause pneumonia deaths in children < 5 years are attributable to pneumococcus, and 18.3% (95% CI: 15.6%, 21.6%) of all deaths in children are attributable to pneumococcal infection.[73] Due to limited global uptake of PCV in the first decade of the 2000s, there was little change in absolute morbidity patterns in all ages between 1990 and 2010: deaths from pneumococcal pneumonia and meningitis, respectively, were 858,000 and 125,000 in 1990 (983,000 total) and 827,000 and 118,000 in 2010 (946,000 total).[70]

Countries, which have introduced PCV as a recommended vaccine on their EPI schedule, have seen substantial decreases in morbidity from pneumococcal disease, both directly among ages targeted by the vaccine program and indirectly in other age groups. For instance, a study from the United States modeling differences between observed incidence of disease and expected incidence in the absence of the PCV-13 introduction, incidence of disease declined 45% (95% CI: −50% to −40%) among children < 5 years, but it also declined 33% (95% CI: −45%, −18%) among children 5–17 years and 12% (95% CI: −20%, −5%) among adults 18–49 years.[74] In a meta-analysis of 172 studies from 34 countries that reported on the direct and indirect effects of PCV introduction, the overall incidence of vaccine-covered pneumococcal disease was 0.79 times as high (95% CI: 0.75, 0.81) for each year after vaccine introduction. Children < 5 years—the targeted vaccination group—experienced the greatest decline [risk ratio (RR): 0.62, 95% CI: 0.55, 0.70], but all age groups experienced substantial declines, including adults ≥ 65 years (RR: 0.77, 95% CI: 0.75, 0.80).[75] That herd immunity extends to groups not typically covered by the vaccine is indicative of the role infants play in spreading disease within the population.

Serotype replacement is a theoretical concern, which refers to nonvaccine serotypes increasing in incidence after introduction of the vaccine. Such a scenario would attenuate the benefit of PCVs in preventing all pneumococcal disease. It could be expected that serotype replacement is more likely applicable to pneumococcal carriage than pneumococcal disease, because a wider distribution of serotypes are commonly found in the nasopharynx as asymptomatic infections compared to invasive infections.[63] Some initial studies in limited geographical areas have found evidence of serotype replacement; for instance studies have found increases in nonvaccine-type disease in Utah,[76] and among Native Alaskans in Alaska.[77] A model from a meta-analysis of effectiveness studies estimates a nonsignificant yearly increase in incidence of nonvaccine-type disease of 1.18 times (95% CI: 0.96, 1.41) among adults 19–64 years, but significantly greater (RR: 1.18, 95% CI: 1.12, 1.25) for adults ≥ 65 years. In aggregate among all age groups, however, the incidence of invasive pneumococcal disease for all vaccine and nonvaccine serotypes is estimated to decrease after vaccine introduction.[75] The possibility of serotype replacement could be minimized in the future by using higher-valent vaccines or polysaccharide-independent vaccines.

References

1. Watson DA, Musher DM, Jacobson JW, et al. A brief history of the pneumococcus in biomedical research : A panoply of scientific discovery. *Clin Infect Dis*. 1993;17(5):913–24.
2. Austrian R. A brief history of pneumococcal vaccines. *Drugs Aging*. 1999;15(Suppl 1):1–10.
3. Morens DM, Taubenberger JK, Fauci AS. Predominant role of bacterial pneumonia as a cause of death in pandemic influenza : Implications for pandemic influenza preparedness. *J Infect Dis*. 2008;198(7):962–70.
4. Grabenstein JD, Klugman KP. A century of pneumococcal vaccination research in humans. *Clin Microbiol Infect*. 2012;18(Suppl 5):15–24.
5. Centers for Disease Control and Prevention. Recommendations of the Immunization Practices Advisory Committee (ACIP) update: Pneumococcal polysaccharide vaccine usage—United States. *MMWR Morb Mortal Wkly Rep*. 1984;33(20):273–6, 281.
6. Goldblatt D. Conjugate vaccines. *Clin Exp Immunol*. 2000;119(1):1–3.

7. Advisory Committee on Immunization Practices. Preventing pneumococcal disease among infants and young children. *MMWR Morb Mortal Wkly Rep.* 2000;49(RR-9):1–35.
8. Centers for Disease Control and Prevention (CDC). Licensure of a 13-valent pneumococcal conjugate vaccine (PCV13) and recommendations for use among children—Advisory Committee on Immunization Practices (ACIP), 2010. *MMWR Morb Mortal Wkly Rep.* 2010;59(9):258–61.
9. Levine OS, Knoll MD, Jones A, et al. Global status of Haemophilus influenzae type b and pneumococcal conjugate vaccines: Evidence, policies, and introductions. *Curr Opin Infect Dis.* 2010;23(3):236–41.
10. Maurer KA, Chen H-F, Wagner AL, et al. Cost-effectiveness analysis of pneumococcal vaccination for infants in China. *Vaccine.* 2016;34(50):6343–9.
11. World Health Organization. Pneumococcal vaccines: WHO position paper—2012. *Wkly Epidemiol Rec.* 2012;87(14):129–44.
12. National Center for Immunization and Respiratory Diseases. Pneumococcal disease: Types of infection [Internet]. Centers Disease Control and Prevention. 2017. https://www.cdc.gov/pneumococcal/about/infection-types.html.
13. Geno KA, Gilbert GL, Song Y, et al. Pneumococcal capsules and their types: Past, present, and future. *Clin Microbiol Rev.* 2015;28(3):871–99.
14. Kim JO, Romero-steiner S, Sørensen UBS, et al. Relationship between cell surface carbohydrates and intrastrain variation on opsonophagocytosis of *Streptococcus pneumoniae*. *Infect Immun.* 1999;67(5):2327–33.
15. Bogaert D, De Groot R, Hermans PWM. *Streptococcus pneumoniae* colonisation: The key to pneumococcal disease. *Lancet Infect Dis.* 2004;4(3): 144–54.
16. Keller LE, Robinson DA, McDaniel LS. Nonencapsulated *Streptococcus pneumoniae*: Emergence and pathogenesis. *mBio.* 2016;7(2):e01792–15.
17. Kim HW, Lee S, Kim K. Serotype 6B from a pneumococcal polysaccharide vaccine induces cross-functional antibody responses in adults to serotypes 6A, 6C, and 6D. *Medicine (Baltimore).* 2016;95(37):e4854.
18. Butler JC, Breiman RF, Lipman HB, et al. Serotype distribution of *Streptococcus pneumoniae* infections among preschool children in the United States, 1978–1994: Implications for development of a conjugate vaccine. *J Infect Dis.* 1995;171(4):885–9.
19. Butler JC, Breiman RF, CJ F, et al. Pneumococcal polysaccharide vaccine efficacy. *JAMA.* 1993;270(15):1826–31.
20. Johnson HL, Deloria-Knoll M, Levine OS, et al. Systematic evaluation of serotypes causing invasive pneumococcal disease among children under five: The pneumococcal global serotype project. *PLoS Med.* 2010;7(10):e1000348.
21. Liu Y, Wang H, Chen M, et al. Serotype distribution and antimicrobial resistance patterns of *Streptococcus pneumoniae* isolated from children in China younger than 5 years. *Diagn Microbiol Infect Dis.* 2008;61(3):256–63.
22. Syrjanen RK, Kilpi TM, Kaijalainen TH, et al. Nasopharyngeal carriage of *Streptococcus pneumoniae* in Finnish children younger than 2 years old. *J Infect Dis.* 2001;184(4):451–9.
23. Hussain M, Melegaro A, Pebody RG, et al. A longitudinal household study of *Streptococcus pneumoniae* nasopharyngeal carriage in a UK setting. *Epidemiol Infect.* 2005;133(5):891–8.
24. Huang SS, Finkelstein JA, Lipsitch M. Modeling community- and individual-level effects of child-care center attendance on pneumococcal carriage. *Clin Infect Dis.* 2005;40(9):1215–22.
25. Pericone CD, Overweg K, Hermans PWM, Weiser JN. Inhibitory and bactericidal effects of hydrogen peroxide production by *Streptococcus pneumoniae* on other inhabitants of the upper respiratory tract. *Infect Immun.* 2000;68(7):3990–7.
26. Ghaffar F, Friedland IR, McCracken GH. Dynamics of nasopharyngeal colonization by *Streptococcus pneumoniae*. *Pediatr Infect Dis J.* 1999;18(7): 638–46.
27. Ghaffar F, Muniz LS, Katz K, et al. Effects of large dosages of amoxicillin/clavulanate or azithromycin on nasopharyngeal carriage of *Streptococcus pneumoniae, Haemophilus influenzae*, nonpneumococcal α-hemolytic streptococci, and *Staphylococcus aureus* in children with acute otitis media. *Clin Infect Dis.* 2002;34(10):1301–9.
28. Regev-Yochay G, Dagan R, Raz M, et al. Is nasopharyngeal carriage of *Streptococcus pneumoniae* protective against carriage of *Staphylococcus aureus*? *43rd ICAAC.* Chicago, IL; 2003, p. G-2048.
29. Bogaert D, Koppen S, Boelens H, et al. Epidemiology and determinants of nasopharyngeal carriage of bacterial pathogens in healthy Dutch children. *21st Annual Meeting of the European Society for Paediatric Infectious Diseases*, Giardini Naxos; 2003.
30. Bosch AATM, Biesbroek G, Trzcinski K, et al. Viral and bacterial interactions in the upper respiratory tract. *PLoS Pathog.* 2013;9(1):e1003057.
31. Simell B, Auranen K, Käyhty H, et al. The fundamental link between pneumococcal carriage and disease. *Expert Rev Vaccines.* 2012;11(7):841–55.
32. Kadioglu A, Weiser JN, Paton JC, et al. The role of *Streptococcus pneumoniae* virulence factors in host respiratory colonization and disease. *Nat Rev Microbiol.* 2008;6(4):288–301.
33. Harboe ZB, Thomsen RW, Riis A, et al. Pneumococcal serotypes and mortality following invasive pneumococcal disease: A population-based cohort study. *PLoS Med.* 2009;6(5):e1000081.
34. Feikin DR, Schuchat A, Kolczak M, et al. Mortality from invasive pneumococcal pneumonia in the era of antibiotic resistance, 1995–1997. *Am J Public Health.* 2000;90(2):223–9.
35. Aspa J, Rajas O, Huertas MC, et al. Impact of initial antibiotic choice on mortality from *Pneumococcal pneumonia*. *Eur Respir J.* 2006;27(5):1010–9.
36. Centers for Disease Control and Prevention. Invasive pneumococcal disease (IPD) (*Streptococcus pneumoniae*) [Internet]. 2017 [cited August 4, 2017]. https://wwwn.cdc.gov/nndss/conditions/invasive-pneumococcal-disease/.
37. Mandell LA, Wunderink RG, Anzueto A, et al. Infectious Diseases Society of America/American Thoracic Society consensus guidelines on the management of community-acquired pneumonia in adults. *Clin Infect Dis.* 2007;44(Suppl 2):S27–72.
38. Greenwood B. The epidemiology of pneumococcal infection in children in the developing world. *Philos Trans R Soc Lond B Biol Sci.* 1999; 354(1384):777–85.
39. Janoff EN, Breiman RF, Daley CL, et al. Pneumococcal disease during HIV infection. *Ann Intern Med.* 1992;117(4):314–24.
40. Bartlett JG, Breiman RF, Mandell LA, et al. Community-acquired pneumonia in adults: Guidelines for management. *Clin Infect Dis.* 1998;26(4): 811–38.
41. Fine MJ, Orloff JJ, Rihs JD, et al. Evaluation of housestaff physicians' preparation and interpretation of sputum gram stains for community-acquired pneumonia. *J Gen Intern Med.* 1991;6(3):189–98.
42. Harris AM, Beekmann SE, Polgreen PM, et al. Rapid urine antigen testing for *Streptococcus pneumoniae* in adults with community-acquired pneumonia: Clinical use and barriers. *Diagn Microbiol Infect Dis.* 2014;79(4): 454–7.
43. Pesola GR. The urinary antigen test for *Pneumococcal pneumonia*. *Chest.* 2001;119(1):9–11.
44. Domínguez J, Galí N, Blanco S, et al. Detection of *Streptococcus pneumoniae* antigen by a rapid immunochromatographic assay in urine samples. *Chest.* 2001;119(1):243–9.
45. Porter BD, Ortika BD, Satzke C. Capsular serotyping of *Streptococcus pneumoniae* by latex agglutination. *J Vis Exp.* 2014;91:e51747.
46. Azzari C, Moriondo M, Indolfi G, et al. Realtime PCR is more sensitive than multiplex PCR for diagnosis and serotyping in children with culture negative pneumococcal invasive disease. *PLoS One.* 2010;5(2):e9282.
47. Harmes KM, Blackwood RA, Burrows HL, et al. Otitis media: Diagnosis and treatment. *Am Fam Physician.* 2013;88(7):435–40.
48. Pallares R. Treatment of pneumococcal pneumonia. *Semin Respir Infect.* 1999;14(3):276–84.
49. Teepe J, Little P, Elshof N, et al. Amoxicillin for clinically unsuspected pneumonia in primary care: Subgroup analysis. *Eur Respir J.* 2016;47(1): 327–30.
50. Centers for Disease Control and Prevention (CDC). Pneumococcal disease | Diagnosis and treatment [Internet]. 2017 [cited July 9, 2020]. http://www.cdc.gov/pneumococcal/about/diagnosis-treatment.html.
51. Moore HF, Chesney AM. A study of ethylhydrocuprein (optochin) in the treatment of acute lobar pneumonia. *Arch Intern Med.* 1917;XIX(4): 611–82.
52. Kislak JW, Razavi LMB, Daly AK, et al. Susceptibility of pneumococci to nine antibiotics. *Am J Med Sci.* 1965;250(3):261–8.
53. Venkatesan P, Innes JA. Antibiotic resistance in common acute respiratory pathogens. *Thorax.* 1995;50(5):481–3.
54. Schuchat A, Hilger T, Zell E, et al. Active bacterial core surveillance of the emerging infections program network. *Emerg Infect Dis.* 2001;7(1): 92–9.
55. Dong L, Yan H, Wang D. Antibiotic prescribing patterns in village health clinics across 10 provinces of Western China. *J Antimicrob Chemother.* 2008;62(2):410–5.
56. Fleming-Dutra KE, Hersh AL, Shapiro DJ, et al. Prevalence of inappropriate antibiotic prescriptions among US ambulatory care visits, 2010–2011. *JAMA.* 2016;315(17):1864–73.

57. Rice LB. The Maxwell Finland lecture: For the duration—Rational antibiotic administration in an era of antimicrobial resistance and *Clostridium difficile*. *Clin Infect Dis*. 2008;46(4):491–6.
58. Whitney CG, Klugman KP. Vaccines as tools against resistance: The example of pneumococcal conjugate vaccine. *Semin Pediatr Infect Dis*. 2004;15(2):86–93.
59. Weinstein MP, Klugman KP, Jones RN. Rationale for revised penicillin susceptibility breakpoints versus *Streptococcus pneumoniae:* Coping with antimicrobial susceptibility in an era of resistance. *Clin Infect Dis*. 2009;48(11):1596–600.
60. Advisory Committee on Immunization Practices. Prevention of pneumococcal disease among infants and children—Use of 13-valent pneumococcal conjugate vaccine and 23-valent pneumococcal polysaccharide vaccine. *MMWR Morb Mortal Wkly Rep*. 2010;59(RR-11):1–18.
61. CDC. *Haemophilus influenzae. Epidemiology and Prevention of Vaccine-Preventable Diseases*. 12th ed. Washington, DC: Public Health Foundation; 2012, pp. 87–100.
62. Ginsburg AS, Alderson MR. New conjugate vaccines for the prevention of pneumococcal disease in developing countries. *Drugs Today (Barc)*. 2011;47(3):207–14.
63. Trotter CL, McVernon J, Ramsay ME, et al. Optimising the use of conjugate vaccines to prevent disease caused by *Haemophilus influenzae* type b, *Neisseria meningitidis* and *Streptococcus pneumoniae*. *Vaccine*. 2008;26(35):4434–45.
64. Goldblatt D, Southern J, Ashton L, et al. Immunogenicity and boosting after a reduced number of doses of a pneumococcal conjugate vaccine in infants and toddlers. *Pediatr Infect Dis J*. 2006;25(4):312–9.
65. Temple B, Toan NT, Uyen DY, et al. Evaluation of different infant vaccination schedules incorporating pneumococcal vaccination (The Vietnam Pneumococcal Project): Protocol of a randomised controlled trial. *BMJ Open*. 2018;8(6):e019795.
66. World Health Organization. *Introduction of Pneumococcal Vaccine PCV10, Two Dose Presentation: A Handbook for District and Health Facility Staff World Health Organization*. Geneva: World Health Organization; 2013.
67. Tse A, Tseng HF, Greene SK, et al. Signal identification and evaluation for risk of febrile seizures in children following trivalent inactivated influenza vaccine in the Vaccine Safety Datalink Project, 2010–2011. *Vaccine*. 2012;30(11):2024–31.
68. Schwarz TF, Flamaing J, Rümke HC, et al. A randomized, double-blind trial to evaluate immunogenicity and safety of 13-valent pneumococcal conjugate vaccine given concomitantly with trivalent influenza vaccine in adults aged ≥ 65 years. *Vaccine*. 2011;29(32):5195–202.
69. Tomczyk S, Bennett NM, Stoecker C, et al. Use of 13-valent pneumococcal conjugate vaccine and 23-valent pneumococcal polysaccharide vaccine among adults aged ≥ 65 years: Recommendations of the Advisory Committee on Immunization Practices (ACIP). *MMWR Morb Mortal Wkly Rep*. 2014;63(37):822–5.
70. Lozano R, Naghavi M, Foreman K, et al. Global and regional mortality from 235 causes of death for 20 age groups in 1990 and 2010: A systematic analysis for the Global Burden of Disease Study 2010. *Lancet*. 2012;380(9859):2095–128.
71. Wagner ALAL, Boulton MLML, Sun X, et al. Perceptions of measles, pneumonia, and meningitis vaccines among caregivers in Shanghai, China, and the Health Belief Model: A cross-sectional study. *BMC Pediatr*. 2017;17(1):143.
72. Fischer Walker CL, Rudan I, Liu L, et al. Global burden of childhood pneumonia and diarrhoea. *Lancet*. 2013;381(9875):1405–16.
73. Izadnegahdar R, Cohen AL, Klugman KP, et al. Childhood pneumonia in developing countries. *Lancet Respir Med*. 2013;1(7):574–84.
74. Moore MR, Link-Gelles R, Schaffner W, et al. Effect of use of 13-valent pneumococcal conjugate vaccine in children on invasive pneumococcal disease in children and adults in the USA: Analysis of multisite, population-based surveillance. *Lancet Infect Dis*. 2015;15(3):301–9.
75. Shiri T, Datta S, Madan J, et al. Indirect effects of childhood pneumococcal conjugate vaccination on invasive pneumococcal disease: A systematic review and meta-analysis. *Lancet Glob Health*. 2017;5(1): e51–9.
76. Byington CL, Samore MH, Stoddard GJ, et al. Temporal trends of invasive disease due to *Streptococcus pneumoniae* among children in the intermountain west: Emergence of nonvaccine serogroups. *Clin Infect Dis*. 2005;41(1):21–9.
77. Singleton RJ, Hennessy TW, Bulkow LR, et al. Invasive pneumococcal disease caused by nonvaccine serotypes among Alaska native children with high levels of 7-valent pneumococcal conjugate vaccine coverage. *JAMA*. 2007;297(16):1784–92.

CHAPTER 107 Introduction to Food Safety

Kari Irvin

INTRODUCTION

Each year, the average American consumes about 2000 pounds (1 ton) of food.[1] These foods are sourced both domestically and globally. About 19% of food is imported, including approximately 97% of fish and shellfish, 50% of fresh fruits, and 20% of fresh vegetables.[2] Foods are distributed to Americans through over 1 million restaurants, 40,000 grocery stores, and numerous other points of sale.[3,4] Most foods in the United States make their way to consumers through a supply chain that includes producers, processors, distributors, and points of sale. Along this complicated pathway from farm to fork, consumers expect high quality and safe food. Food served, packed, prepared, or grown under conditions that allow for contamination by pathogenic bacteria, viruses, parasites, or other adulterants result in 48 million people sickened by foodborne illness each year.[5] Foodborne illness costs the United States between $152 billion and $1.4 trillion annually.[6]

A safe food supply is necessary to combat the public health burden generated by foodborne illnesses. The goal of this chapter is to understand what food safety is, how it is accomplished, and what challenges exist in implementation.

WHAT IS FOOD SAFETY?

Food safety is the scientific discipline of preventing food from becoming a vehicle for health threat, risk, or injury. Food is vulnerable to contamination along the entire supply chain. At each point from farm to fork, special considerations need to be considered to protect food from those vulnerabilities. Growers, manufacturers, distributers, and end users all play a role in food safety, albeit the roles vary. It is important to consider how the approach to food safety may change along the supply chain.

Growers/Suppliers. In addition to meeting the demands of operating a profitable business, growers and suppliers have food-safety responsibilities that are regulated across different levels of government. The size and scope of the operation often determines the degree and type of government regulation.

Food safety at the grower/supplier level is paramount given that food and animals in farming environments are exposed to many potential environmental conditions that could lead to contamination or cross-contamination. In addition, point source contamination on a farm could lead to adulteration of additional products that are comingled further along the supply chain. Farms responsible for producing fruits and vegetables are challenged with balancing successful harvests with the risk involved in supplying food to consumers absent a kill step to control microbial contamination. For example, analysis of foodborne illness attribution data from 1998 to 2008 determined that 46% of all foodborne illnesses were a result of exposure to contaminated produce.[10]

Considerations need to be made about how food or animals used for food are grown or raised in a way that limits risk of contamination with a foodborne pathogen or adulterant. Growers and suppliers need to consider issues such as:

- The type of soil or fertilizer used, and whether it contains animal by-products that could lead to contamination of food;
- The type of water used to irrigate fields, how the water is applied, and the potential for the water to be contaminated;
- The type of food and water consumed by animals intended for slaughter;
- The potential hazards that exist when food is harvested; and
- Training staff and employees to avoid contaminating food.

Food-safety agencies provide many educational materials to growers and suppliers. For fruits and vegetables, the United States Department of Agriculture (USDA) and the Food and Drug Administration (FDA) have developed a voluntary list of practices noted as Good Agricultural Practices (GAPs) and Good Handling Practices (GHPs). These science-based practices help government and industry work together to ensure farms utilize safe practices preharvest and postharvest.[7]

Manufacturers. Monitoring food safety in the manufacturing environment is an important public health protection initiative. Whether ingredients come into a manufacturing firm already contaminated or a food becomes contaminated during the process, food manufacturers can prevent food-safety issues by identifying and controlling hazards.

Food manufacturers are responsible for maintaining equipment and facilities to process safe and wholesome food. In the United States, food manufactures are required to produce food using the minimum requirements outlined by the good manufacturing practices (GMPs) published in Title 21 of the Code of Federal Regulations Part 110.[8] These practices lay out a framework for safe manufacturing, including:

- Requirements for cleaning/sanitizing facilities, food contact surfaces, and equipment;
- Pest control;
- Worker hygiene (hand-washing, waste management, etc.);
- Control of raw ingredients used in processed food;
- Training for employees on a variety of food-safety topics;
- Documentation of policies and processes to ensure food safety; and
- Maintaining records of control measures (cleaning, temperatures, etc.), training activities, and ingredient and product storage/distribution.

Failure of food manufacturers to follow GMPs may have severe consequences for both the business and their customers. In 2017, soy nut butter from one manufacturing firm sickened 32 people, 12 of whom required hospitalization. The root cause of the contamination event was not identified, but inspections conducted at the manufacturing firm identified problems with rodent and insect control, equipment cleanliness and operation, and worker hygiene practices.[41] The FDA suspended the registration of the firm, preventing food from leaving the facility for sale or distribution.

Distributors. Food moves into and across the United States utilizing planes, trains, boats, and trucks to move it to locations of purchase by consumers. As food moves through this complicated distribution system, it is important that the product be stored and maintained at temperatures that keep the food safe. If refrigerated food is not kept at a suitable temperature, not only can the quality of the food be impacted, but also more importantly it may facilitate propagation of pathogens.

Distributors of food are charged with storing foods in locations that are free from insects, rodents, and other pests. Warehouses should be well maintained, with dry food kept from high moisture settings. Distributors are also responsible for maintaining documentation on where food came from and where it is going. These records are important to help identify the supply chain of food that may be contaminated and needs to be removed, or recalled, from the market.

Service Industry. Retail establishments such as restaurants and grocery stores present several major food-safety risk factors related to employee and preparation practices, including:

- Improper holding temperatures;
- Inadequate cooking;
- Contaminated equipment;
- Food from unsafe sources; and
- Poor personal hygiene.[9]

In the United States, the FDA Food Code is one of the most widely used food-safety documents in the country because it helps lay out suggested regulations for restaurants, retailers, and other food service locations. It is a comprehensive "model that assists food control jurisdictions at all levels of government by providing them with a scientifically sound technical and legal basis for regulating the retail and food service segment of the industry (e.g., restaurants, grocery stores, and institutions such as nursing homes)."[9]

Local, state, tribal, and federal regulators use the Food Code to develop or update food-safety rules within their jurisdictions that are consistent with national food regulatory policy. The document outlines scientifically sound and legally justifiable regulations established by government bodies with jurisdictional authority over the retail segment.

The content of the Food Code covers the following areas: management and personnel; food; equipment, utensils and linens; water, plumbing, and waste; physical facilities; poisonous or toxic materials; and compliance and enforcement. Each area contains definitions and specific instructions to help establish a common understanding of food-safety problems and solutions across industry and government. For example, the Food Code provides detailed information about cooking temperatures and times for poultry, meat, seafood, and other commodities. It also contains detailed information on how to clean specific equipment, and how to store equipment used for cleaning safely. The Food Code is updated every 2 years as industry and government officials provide proposed updates and changes to the content.

Deviations from practices and procedures that are in place to control hazards increase the risk for a food-safety incident. For example, norovirus is a leading cause of foodborne outbreaks in the United States. Food can become contaminated with norovirus when it is handled by an ill person that has not washed their hands or when aerosolized particles from infectious vomit or stool are introduced into food or food preparation surfaces. Poor personal hygiene practices or lack of proper equipment cleaning in the restaurant setting can allow for the transmission of the virus to customers.[42]

Consumer Responsibility. Once food makes it way to the consumer, additional food-safety practices are important. While consumers should expect that the food they purchase from the supply chain is safe, contamination events can go undetected, creating hazards for consumers. Consumers are encouraged to follow four basic steps for food safety in their homes:

- Keep hands, cooking utensils, and countertops clean;
- Keep raw foods (meat, poultry, seafood, and eggs) away from other foods;
- Heat food to safe temperatures
  - Beef, Pork, Lamb 145°F,
  - Fish 145°F,
  - Ground Beef, Pork, Lamb 160°F,
  - Turkey, Chicken, Duck 165°F; and
- Keep food appropriately refrigerated.[11]

In addition, the FDA recommends individuals with an increased risk of foodborne illness (e.g., pregnant women, elderly, or immunocompromised individuals) avoid high-risk foods (Table 107-1).[12]

OVERSIGHT OF FOOD SAFETY

With millions of food establishments throughout the United States, government authorities must work together across jurisdictions to assist with the education and enforcement of food-safety regulations. In general, local, state, tribal, and federal agencies share this responsibility, but doing so requires effective information sharing.

Government. In the United States, local and state governments began regulating food safety in the mid-1800s. Federal regulations were instituted in 1906, when the Pure Food and Drugs Acts and Federal Meat Inspection Act of 1906 were passed by Congress. These acts paved the way for the creation of subsequent laws, which authorized the U.S. FDA and the United States Food Safety and Inspection Service (FSIS) to oversee the safety of meat, poultry, food, drugs, and cosmetics.[13]

HACCP. Hazard Analysis Critical Control Point (HACCP) is a management system in which food safety is addressed through the analysis and control of biological, chemical, and physical hazards along the food supply chain. HACCP plans are scientifically based

TABLE 107-1. FOODS TO AVOID FOR VULNERABLE CONSUMERS BY FOOD GROUP

Meat and Poultry	Seafood and Shellfish	Eggs	Dairy	Vegetables and Fruit
Raw or undercooked meat and poultry	Raw and undercooked seafood and shellfish	Raw and undercooked eggs	Raw milk	Unwashed fresh vegetables
Unheated deli-style meats, hot dogs, and sausage	Deli-made seafood salad	Batters and dressings containing raw eggs	Products made with raw milk (yogurt)	Unpasteurized vegetable and fruit juices
Deli made chicken salad, ham salad, etc.	Refrigerated smoked seafood		Soft cheeses made with unpasteurized milk (feta, brie, queso fresco, etc.)	Raw sprouts
Unpasteurized, refrigerated pâtés or meat spreads				

and well-researched strategies to combat food-safety issues along the supply chain. Assessing the hazards within a facility and establishing control points protects consumers, product integrity, and promotes a culture of food safety within an organization. The development of a HACCP plan is a widely accepted strategy to promote food safety across all jurisdictions responsible for keeping food safe.

Hazards are identified from raw material production, procurement, and handling, to manufacturing, distribution, and consumption of the finished product. Firms along the supply chain are asked to utilize seven guiding principles when establishing a HACCP plan of their own: conducting a hazard analysis; identify critical control points; establish critical limits; monitor procedures; implement corrective actions; verify procedures; and record and document plans and outcomes.[20]

A **hazard analysis** is defined as the process of collecting and evaluating information on hazards associated with the food under consideration to decide which are significant.[20] A comprehensive hazard analysis should consider ingredients, raw materials, flow of food through the facility, storage, distribution, and even final preparation and use by the consumer. A **critical control point (CCP)** is defined as a step at which control can be applied and is essential to prevent or eliminate a food-safety hazard or reduce it to an acceptable level. **Critical limits** are values used to determine whether food is safe or unsafe at the CCP. Critical limits may be based upon factors such as: temperature, time, physical dimensions, humidity, moisture level, water activity (aw), pH, titratable acidity, salt concentration, available chlorine, viscosity, preservatives, or sensory information such as aroma and visual appearance.[20]

Once critical limits are established for the critical control points, **monitoring procedures** should be assigned. Monitoring is a planned sequence of observations or measurements to assess whether a CCP is under control and to produce an accurate record for future use in verification.[20] A firm's HACCP plan will contain **corrective actions** that address what a firm will do with product if a critical control point failure has occurred. Implementation of corrective action strategies, such as destroying product if control failures occur, can be difficult decisions for firms to make due to lost profit margins and fulfillment deadlines, but they represent necessary public health protections. **Verification** of the plan determines the validity of the HACCP plan and that the system is operating per the plan.[20] The HACCP system is evaluated to confirm that changes or updates are not necessary. HACCP plans should be well **documented** and widely available within firm.

Food Safety Modernization Act. In 2011, the U.S. Congress signed into law the Food Safety Modernization Act (FSMA). This bill focuses on not only reacting to food-safety failures, but also preventing failures before they cause harm. FSMA has granted FDA a mandate to require science-based preventive controls across the food supply chain.

By 2018, the FDA has finalized seven rules in the implementation of FSMA. These rules focus on:

- Produce safety;
- Sanitary transportation;
- Preventive controls for human food and animal feed;
- Foreign supplier verification;
- Accredited third-party certification; and
- Protection of food from intentional adulteration

While each of these rules is complicated, the underlying theme of each is to ensure those responsible for regulating, growing, processing, distributing, or preparing food are implementing plans to prevent food contamination events.[21]

In addition to mandating preventive control strategies, FSMA also grants US FDA the authority to respond urgently to failures in the food supply chain. Specifically, FSMA allows U.S. FDA to issue mandatory recalls if a company fails to voluntarily recall contaminated food from the market place. FSMA also grants U.S. FDA the authority to suspend the registration of a facility if it determines that the food poses a reasonable probability of serious adverse health consequences or death. A facility that is under suspension is prohibited from distributing food.

Finally, FSMA charges U.S. FDA with building an integrated food-safety system, by collaborating with local, state, federal, and international governments. These collaborations allow U.S. FDA to fund state partners and leverage resources in visiting and inspecting the numerous food facilities across the United States. FSMA also directs U.S. FDA to train international government partners on U.S. food-safety requirements.

Federal Meat Inspection Act. The Federal Meat Inspection Act (FMIA) was enacted by the U.S. Congress in 1906 to prevent contaminated meat from reaching consumers. Meat products that fall under the Act include cattle, sheep, goats, pigs, and equines. Some historians maintain that the FMIA was passed based on the well-known novel "The Jungle" n by Upton Sinclair, which highlighted the unsanitary conditions in the Chicago meat packing industry.[22] FMIA requires the mandatory inspection of livestock before slaughter, mandatory post-mortem inspection of every carcass, and sets explicit sanitary standards for slaughterhouses. The Act also authorized USDA to conduct ongoing monitoring and inspection of the meat packing industry.

Enforcement of FMIA has evolved over the years to address emerging public health threats (such as *E. coli* O157:H7) and address improvements in inspection strategies (such as HACCP). Today, USDA's FSIS conducts inspections at over 6000 slaughter and food processing establishments.

Poultry Products Inspection Act. After World War II, consumption of poultry products skyrocketed, requiring the need for regulation of the industry. In 1957, the U.S. Congress established the Poultry Products Inspection Act (PPIA) to protect consumers from adulterated poultry products by ensuring sanitary conditions at establishments conducting poultry processing. The Act mandates USDA FSIS to inspect all domesticated birds when slaughtered and further processed as food for consumers. The act defines "domesticated birds" as chickens, turkeys, geese, ducks, and other birds used for food (such as ostrich).

Industry. Balancing consumer demands with regulatory oversight while maintaining viability can be challenging for industry. Firms that supply, manufacture, or transport similar commodities are often subject to the same regulations. Industry associations take a leadership role in promoting comprehensive food-safety initiatives, educating their members on the need to prioritize food safety, training members on relevant food-safety content, and conducting research on topics pertaining to their member base. For example, the Grocery Manufacturers Association (GMA) represents approximately 250 food, beverage, and consumer product companies and "helps its members produce safe products through a strong and ongoing commitment to scientific research, testing and evaluation."[14]

Industry is dramatically impacted by failures in the food-safety system. In 2006, the U.S. leafy green industry lost millions of dollars after an *E. coli* O157:H7 outbreak caused by contaminated spinach sickened 199 people and killed 3.[15] While the outbreak was caused by one supplier, for a time many consumers avoided spinach from all suppliers. In 2014, an outbreak of *Listeria monocytogenes* in caramel apples caused 35 illnesses and 7 deaths. The source was traced back to a single U.S. apple supplier[16] but its market effect reached the international apple trade community and many U.S. apple suppliers that were not part of the outbreak.

Consumer Groups. Consumer groups are instrumental in advocating for safe foods. These groups engage government and industry to understand how each entity is working toward ensuring a safe food supply. They play a key role in advocating for changes and improvements in the food-safety system.

Consumer groups are integral in identifying new food trends, which may lead to the detection of food hazards not previously considered. They educate citizens on food-safety hazards and provide resources to consumers about foodborne illnesses and ways to protect themselves. For example, the Partnership for Food Safety Education develops and promotes education programs for teachers and parents to reduce foodborne illness risk for consumers.[17] STOP Foodborne Illness is an example of nonprofit group initiated by victims and their families to raise awareness about foodborne pathogens, advocate for stricter regulations, and assist families personally impacted by foodborne illness.[18]

Academia. Effective food-safety activities are driven by sound scientific evidence. Scientific research can feed directly into the development of new policies and regulations, as well as processes and practices adopted by industry. For example, after the aforementioned *Listeria monocytogenes* outbreak in caramel apples, researchers at the University of Wisconsin-Madison identified that insertion of the stick and storage of the caramel coated apples at room temperature allowed *Listeria monocytogenes* to grow to levels capable of causing illness.[19] This research led to recommendations for caramel apple manufacturers and retailers to refrigerate the product rather than shipping and selling them at room temperature.[38]

GLOBAL FOOD-SAFETY ASSURANCE MEASURES

Improvements in the food distribution system have allowed consumers access to foods from around the world. In the United States, consumer demand for year-round fresh produce and products that must be sourced internationally have led to advancements in how industry fulfills these demands.

Codex Alimentarius. U.S. government officials work closely with the World Health Organization (WHO) and the Food and Agriculture Organization (FAO) of the United Nations. The WHO has offices in over 150 countries and works within the United Nations' (UN) system to promote public health. The FAO works in over 130 countries to promote food safety and security. In 1963, WHO and FAO created the Codex Alimentarius Commission, which establishes international food standards, guidelines, and codes of practice that contribute to the safety, quality, and fairness of international food trade.[23]

Codex standards are not intended to replace the food-safety laws of individual countries. Rather, the standards serve to establish common definitions and requirements, creating harmonization of food-safety practices to facilitate international trade. A governing body's choice to comply or not may have significant impacts on the country's ability to offer food into international trade. The World Trade Organization (WTO) designates the Codex Alimentarius as the reference standard for establishing sanitary measures to protect public health.

The Codex Alimentarius includes provisions covering food hygiene, food additives, residues of pesticides and veterinary drugs, contaminants, labelling and presentation, methods of analysis and sampling, and import and export inspection and certification. Codex also sets the maximum residue limits for nearly 200 different pesticides.

ISO 22000. The International Organization for Standardization (ISO) is a private, nongovernment, international organization responsible for bringing together international experts to provide support and solutions to global challenges. ISO addresses issues of quality, safety, and efficiency of many products, services, and systems. The standards established by ISO are keys facilitators in international trade.

ISO 22000 specifies the requirements for a food-safety management system that combines the generally recognized key elements of interactive communication, system management, prerequisite programs, and HAACP principles to ensure food safety along the food chain, up to the point of final consumption.[24]

Each requirement specified by ISO 22000 encourages industry to create standards for effective supplier audits. ISO 22000 builds on the principles of the HAACP system to ensure that food-safety issues are managed in a consistent way. The identified hazards and controls require an appropriate system in place to manage those elements along the supply chain. ISO 22000 also identifies prerequisite programs, such as pest control programs or personnel hygiene programs that must be put into place to create a safe food-processing environment.

Together, Codex and ISO 22000 allow governments and food suppliers across the world to speak a similar food-safety language. With billions of tons of food being distributed globally each year, food-safety expectations are not bound by international borders.

CHALLENGES WITH ADDRESSING FOOD-SAFETY ISSUES

Novel Foods. As Americans become better educated on the importance of healthy eating habits, trends in novel uses for ingredients can introduce new food-safety hazards. For example, in 2013, 94 persons from the United States and Canada were sickened with multiple Salmonella serotypes from consuming a powder produced by sprouting, drying, and grinding chia seeds.[25] Sprouts have been implicated in 33 outbreaks from 1998 to 2010.[26] The FDA issued sprout guidance in 1999, recommending that seeds undergo a chlorine treatment prior to sprouting, but in this case, the treatment interfered with product quality, and the final product had no critical control point.

Antimicrobial Resistance. Foodborne pathogens resistant to antibiotics are an emerging public health concern. *Salmonella* and *Campylobacter*, two of the many bacteria commonly transmitted through food, cause an estimated 410,000 antibiotic-resistant infections in the United States each year.[27]

Animals raised for food on farms are often fed antibiotics to prevent the spread of disease across flocks and herds, and to prevent contamination of food with pathogenic bacteria. Bacteria that survive these treatments are resistant to the antibiotics and may end up in the food supply. The WHO has published guidelines recommending reductions in the overall use of medically important antimicrobials in food-producing animals, including complete restriction of use of antimicrobials for growth promotion and for disease prevention.[28]

Food Allergens. Food allergies affect approximately 4–6% of children living in the United States.[29] Most food allergies reported by individuals involve eight types of food: milk, eggs, peanuts, tree nuts, fish, shellfish, soy, and wheat.[30] Symptoms can range from mild tingling of the tongue to severe anaphylactic shock and death. The number of individuals reporting food allergies is increasing, creating a need for accurate food labeling with detailed allergen information and increasing the demand for foods free of allergens. In the United States, the Food Allergen Labeling and Consumer Protection Act (FALCPA) of 2004 requires that food labels declare the presence of any of the eight major food allergens. FALCPA covers all products regulated by the U.S. FDA, but not the USDA. Nonetheless, many producers voluntarily comply with FALCPA in order to protect consumers.

Centralization of Food Production. Safety breakdowns in a large supply chain can have devastating impacts on a broad consumer base. In 2015, a *Salmonella* Poona outbreak linked to cucumbers sickened 907 people, resulting in 204 hospitalizations and 6 deaths. People from 40 different states were impacted.[31] The source of contamination was traced to a large farming operation in Baja, Mexico. Investigations of the grower did not identify a root cause for contamination, but multiple food-safety failures were found. Concerns with wastewater management, equipment design in the washing area, and storage of packing material indicated that food supplied by the grower were prepared, packed, and held under unsanitary conditions. Food-safety failures at one supplier led to one of the largest outbreaks of salmonellosis in U.S. history.

Climate Change. Changes in the environment due to global warming will have a substantial impact on the food industry. Weather-related events have been associated with more than 90% of all disasters worldwide in the past 20 years.[32] The food-safety sector will need to consider the potential impact rising temperatures and sea levels will have on how products are grown, manufactured, and transported. In addition, the natural disasters intensified by climate change will require the food industry to be prepared to conduct hazard analysis postdisaster. In 2017, Hurricanes Harvey, Irma, and Maria caused substantial damage to Texas, Florida, Puerto Rico, and the United States Virgin Islands. Flooding and power outages left food vulnerable to contamination. These extreme weather events may lead to contamination of soil, agricultural lands, water and food, and animal feed with pathogens, chemicals, and other hazardous substances, originating from sewage, agriculture, and industrial settings.[33]

As climate change intensifies, the food-safety sector will need to be prepared to address the ongoing challenge of keep food safe under evolving climatic conditions.

Globalization. Harmonization of food-safety regulations and improved trade agreement standards open markets to food from a wide variety of sources. The United States imports food from all over the world, ranging in commodities from fresh produce to frozen seafood. The sourcing of ingredients from this global market requires constant evaluation of food-safety systems along the supply chain. The removal of contaminated food from a global market presents a challenging logistical concern, especially for shelf-stable commodities that can last years in consumer's homes. To address this challenge, the WHO and FAO jointly manage the International Food Safety Authorities Network (INFOSAN). INFOSAN provides a forum for international members to manage food-safety risks, ensure rapid sharing of information during food-safety emergencies, and potentially stop the spread of contaminated food from one country to another.[34]

Country of origin labeling on products has also been helpful, but as product traceability systems through the supply chain improve, more detailed information may be available to consumers. For example, some packaged produce items like fresh berries maintain the same coding throughout the supply chain, allowing a consumer to plug in the code and determine the specific farm the berries were sourced.

In the United States, the FSMA rule on the Foreign Supplier Verification Programs (FSVP) for Importers of Food for Humans and Animals requires that importers perform certain risk-based activities to verify that food imported into the United States has been produced in a manner that meets applicable U.S. safety standards.

CHANGING THE CULTURE OF FOOD SAFETY

What Is a Food-Safety Culture? For growers, suppliers, manufacturers, distributors, and points of service along the supply chain, awareness about ongoing and potential food-safety risks, regulations, and challenges are just the first step in keeping foods safe for consumption. A food-safety culture requires going one step beyond awareness and creates an environment where each responsible entity along the food supply chain understands the underlying reasons behind each process in place to protect food. When employees understand the reasoning behind fundamental food-safety concepts commitment to those practices are likely to improve.

Consumers should also create a culture of food safety in their day-to-day lives. Consumers should know and understand the risk of food they eat, especially high-risk options. Food should be prepared in the home per instructions, cooking temperatures should be followed, cutting boards and counter tops should be cleaned, and hands should be washed. While consumers should expect safe food is supplied to them, taking extra precautions at home can further prevent foodborne illness.

Reactive Approach. Unfortunately, the importance of many food-safety practices is sometimes appreciated only after experiencing the consequences of a failure. In 1993, a historically renowned foodborne illness outbreak occurred when undercooked hamburgers from Jack in the Box restaurants sickened 732 people with *E. coli* O157:H7.[35] Subsequently, Jack in the Box has developed an awarded and highly regarded food-safety system.[36] In addition to changes in the business, federal food-safety regulations were modified in response to this outbreak. For example, the USDA initiated research into establishing a Pathogen Reduction Program in federally inspected meat-processing facilities.[39]

Preventive Approach. New food-safety regulations, such as FSMA require food-safety professionals to work to prevent contamination and illness before they happen. In addition to better preparing industry, FSMA is changing the way regulators look to identify food-safety issues. FSMA mandates a series of risk-based preventive controls, rather than a reactive regulatory strategy. This strategy will allow industry and regulators to start thinking about hazards along the supply chain that could lead to an outbreak and put controls in place to prevent those hazards.[40]

Influencing Management. New regulations and the barrage of foodborne outbreaks making national headlines have emphasized the importance of food safety within the leadership teams of many companies responsible for serving and supplying food. In 2008–09, products containing peanut butter supplied by Peanut Corporation of America (PCA) sickened 714 people in 46 states. Nine people died and more than half of those sickened were under the age of 16.[37] PCA owner Stewart Parnell, and other company leadership were convicted on criminal charges and sentenced to prison.

CONCLUSIONS

U.S. consumers eat almost 1 billion meals each day. Approximately 11% of jobs in the United States are within the food and agriculture sector. Collaboration among government, industry, consumer groups, and academia is essential in advancing food-safety policy and effectively preventing or reducing the burden of foodborne illness.

References

1. U.S. Department of Agriculture, Agricultural Research Service, Beltsville Human Nutrition Research Center, Food Surveys Research Group (Beltsville, MD) and U.S. Department of Health and Human Services, Centers for Disease Control and Prevention, National Center for Health Statistics (Hyattsville, MD). *What We Eat in America, NHANES 2007-2010 Type of File: Average daily intake of food by food source and demographic characteristics*. 2014.
2. US Department of Agriculture. Import share of consumption. 2016. [cited August 12, 2016]. http://www.ers.usda.gov/topics/international-markets-trade/us-agricultural-trade/import-share-of-consumption.aspx
3. http://www.restaurant.org/News-Research/Research/Facts-at-a-Glance.
4. Nielsen TDLinx. Progressive Grocer's 85th Annual Report of teh Grocery Industry, 2018; pp. 30–1.
5. Scallan E, Hoekstra RM, Angulo FJ, et al. Foodborne illness acquired in the United States—Major pathogens. *Emerg Infect Dis*. 2011;17(1):7–15.
6. Scharff RL. Health related costs from foodborne illness in the United States. Produce Safety Project. 2010. http://www.pewtrusts.org/~/media/legacy/uploadedfiles/phg/content_level_pages/reports/pspscharff20v9pdf.pdf.
7. U.S. Food and Drug Administration, Center for Food Safety and Applied Nutrition. Guidance for Industry—Guide to Minimize Microbial Food Safety Hazards for Fresh Fruits and Vegetables. 1998.
8. Current Good Manufacturing Practice in Manufacturing, Packing, or Holding Human Food. 21 C.F.R. § 110 2017.
9. U.S. Department of Health and Human Services. Public Health Service. U.S. Food and Drug Administration. Food Code. 2017.
10. Painter JA, Hoekstra RM, Ayers T, et al. Attribution of foodborne illnesses, hospitalizations, and deaths to food commodities by using outbreak data, United States, 1998–2008. *Emerg Infect Dis*. 2013;19(3):407–15.
11. U.S. Department of Agriculture, Food Safety and Inspection Service. Basics for Handling Food Safely. 2013.
12. U.S. Food and Drug Administration. Food Safety: It's Especially Important for At-Risk Groups. 2017.
13. U.S. Food and Drug Administration. *National Integrated Food Safety System (IFSS) Program and Initiatives*. 2017. https://www.fda.gov/ForFederalStateandLocalOfficials/ProgramsInitiatives/default.htm.
14. Grocery Manufacturers Association. *About GMA*. https://www.gmaonline.org/about/. Cited 2018.

15. U.S. Centers for Disease Control and Prevention. *Multistate Outbreak of E. coli O157:H7 Infections Linked to Fresh Spinach (Final Update)*. 2006. https://www.cdc.gov/ecoli/2006/spinach-10-2006.html.
16. Angelo KM, Conrad AR, Saupe A, Dragoo H, et al. Multistate outbreak of Listeria monocytogenes infections linked to whole apples used in commercially produced, prepackaged caramel apples: United States, 2014–2015. *Epidemiol Infect*. 2017;145(5):848–56.
17. Partnership for Food Safety and Education. *Partnership and History*. Cited 2018. http://www.fightbac.org/about-us/partnership-history/
18. Stop Foodborne Illness. *What We* Do. Cited 2018. http://www.stopfoodborneillness.org/about-us/get-to-know-us/
19. Glass KA, Golden MC, Wanless BJ, Bedale W, Czuprynski C. Growth of Listeria monocytogenes within a caramel-coated apple microenvironment. *mBio*. 2015;6(5):e01232-15.
20. U.S. Food and Drug Administration. *HACCP Principles and Application Guidelines*. 2017. https://www.fda.gov/Food/GuidanceRegulation/HACCP/ucm2006801.htm.
21. U.S. Food and Drug Administration. *Background on the FDA Food Safety Modernization Act (FSMA)*. 2018. https://www.fda.gov/Food/GuidanceRegulation/FSMA/ucm239907.htm.
22. U.S. Department of Agriculture, Food Safety and Inspection Service. *FSIS History*. 2018. https://www.fsis.usda.gov/wps/portal/informational/aboutfsis/history.
23. World Health Organization, Food and Agriculture Organization of the United Nations. *Codex Alimentarius: International Food Standards. About Codex Alimentarius*. Cited 2018. http://www.fao.org/fao-who-codexalimentarius/about-codex/en/.
24. International Organization for Standardization. Food safety management systems—Requirements for any organization in the food chain. (ISO/DIS Standard No. 22000:2005). 2009.
25. Harvey RR, Heiman Marshall KE, et al. International outbreak of multiple Salmonella serotype infections linked to sprouted chia seed powder—USA and Canada, 2013–2014. *Epidemiol Infect*. 2017;145(8):1535–44.
26. Dechet AM, Herman KM, Chen Parker C, et al. Outbreaks caused by sprouts, United States, 1998–2010: Lessons learned and solutions needed. *Foodborne Pathog Dis*. 2014;11(8):635–44.
27. U.S Centers for Disease Control and Prevention. *Antibiotic Resistance Threats in the United States, 2013*. Atlanta, GA: U.S. Department of Health and Human Services, CDC; 2013, p. 7, 36–7.
28. Aidara-Kane A, Angulo FJ, Conly JM, et al. World Health Organization (WHO) guidelines on use of medically important antimicrobials in food-producing animals. *Antimicrob Resist Infect Control*. 2018;7:7.
29. Branum AM, Lukacs SL. Food allergy among U.S. children: Trends in prevalence and hospitalizations. *NCHS Data Brief*. 2008;10:1–8.
30. Sicherer SH. Food allergy. *Lancet*. 2002;360(9334):701–10.
31. U.S. Food and Drug Administration. *FDA investigated multistate outbreak of Salmonella Poona linked to cucumbers*. 2016. https://www.fda.gov/Food/RecallsOutbreaksEmergencies/Outbreaks/ucm461317.htm.
32. Watts N, Amann M, Ayet-Karlsson S, et al. The Lancet Countdown on health and climate change: From 25 years of inaction to a global transformation for public health. *Lancet*. 2018;391(10120):581–630.
33. Tirado MC, Clarke R, Jaykus LA, McQuatters-Gollop A, Frank JM. Climate change and food safety: A review. *Food Res Int*. 2010;43(7):1745–65.
34. World Health Organization. *International food safety authorities network (INFOSAN)*. Cited 2018. http://www.who.int/foodsafety/areas_work/infosan/en/
35. U.S. Centers for Disease Control and Prevention. Update: Multistate outbreak of *Escherichia coli* O157:H7 infections from hamburgers—Western United States, 1992–1993. *MMWR Morb Mortal Wkly Rep*. 1993;42(14):258–63.
36. Benedict J. *Poisoned*. Buena Vista, VA: Inspire Books; 2011.
37. U.S. Centers for Disease Control and Prevention. *Multistate outbreak of Salmonella Typhimurium infections linked to peanut butter, 2008–2009 (final update)*. 2009. https://www.cdc.gov/salmonella/2009/peanut-butter-2008-2009.html.
38. Jackson K, Iwamoto M, Swerdlow D. Pregnancy-associated listeriosis. *Epidemiol Infect*. 2010;138(10):1503–9.
39. Crowe SJ, Bottichio L, Shade LN, et al. Shiga toxin producing *E. coli* infections associated with flour. *N Engl J Med*. 2017; 377:2036–43.
40. Firestone MJ, Hoelzer K, Hedberg C, Conroy CA, Guzewich JJ. Leveraging current opportunities to communicate lessons learned from root cause analysis to prevent foodborne illness outbreaks. *Food Prot Trends*. 2018;38(2):134–8.
41. U.S. Food and Drug Administration. *FDA Suspends Food Facility Registration of Dixie Dew Products, Inc*. 2017. https://www.fda.gov/Food/RecallsOutbreaksEmergencies/SafetyAlertsAdvisories/ucm549734.htm.
42. U.S. Centers for Disease Control and Prevention. *Norovirus and working with food*. 2016. https://www.cdc.gov/norovirus/food-handlers/work-with-food.html.

CHAPTER

108 Acute Diarrheal Illness—An Overview

Martyn Kirk

INTRODUCTION

Acute diarrhea results in substantial morbidity and mortality. Globally, there were an estimated 6.3 billion episodes of diarrheal disease in 2017.[1] Among children less than 5 years of age, the incidence is approximately three episodes per person per year, while among older children and adults it is less than one episode per person per year.[2] Diarrheal disease is a key cause of childhood mortality. In 2017, the Global Burden of Disease study—a global collaborative effort to understand the burden and causes of morbidity from all causes—estimated that diarrheal diseases resulted in 1.6 million deaths globally, with 533,000 occurring among children less than 5 years old.[3] These resulted in 41.4 million Disability Adjusted Life Years (DALY's) lost, which equates to years of life lost due to ill health, disability, or death.[4] Infectious diarrhea is also important for its propensity to spread globally via infected humans and animals and contaminated foods. In countries of all levels of development, there are regular outbreaks of diarrheal disease requiring intervention that are tailored to the pathogen and nature of spread.

This chapter summarizes the major causes of acute diarrhea, the agents responsible, how they are transmitted, and the main public health interventions.

DIARRHEA AND ITS CAUSES

Diarrhea is a common symptom of gastrointestinal infection and is commonly defined as "≥3 or more loose stools in a 24-hour period."[5] The syndrome of acute diarrhea is caused by a range of pathogens that vary in their characteristics of infectiousness, clinical manifestations, and transmission. These pathogens result in different symptoms and duration of illness. For example, norovirus—one of the most common causes of gastroenteritis globally—results in the majority of infected persons experiencing diarrhea less than 48 hours in duration. In fact, many persons infected with norovirus do not even experience diarrhea, but may experience nausea and vomiting alone. In contrast, people infected with bacterial pathogens, such as Shiga-toxin-producing *Escherichia coli* may experience bloody diarrhea that can progress to serious sequelae including hemolytic uremic syndrome (Table 108-1).

In addition to acute illness, many diarrheal agents result in acute injury or chronic sequelae that can have significant consequences. For instance, approximately 3–6% of persons presenting with diarrhea due to Shiga-toxin-producing *E. coli* (STEC) infection progress to hemolytic uremic syndrome as a result of toxin damage to blood and blood vessels. Similarly, *Salmonella*, *Campylobacter*, and *Yersinia* infections can result in postinfectious reactive arthritis that may last for several months. Some agents that are spread predominantly from person-to-person or from contact with contaminated surfaces, such as *Clostridium Difficile* or norovirus present a particular problem for healthcare facilities and long-term care facilities, as they result in protracted serious outbreaks affecting administrative functioning.

The predominant agents and their effects vary for the level of country development. This is largely due to differences in hygiene and sanitation and among children—nutrient intake. Children in low- and middle-income countries (LMIC) are at higher risk of stunting and malnutrition when subclinically infected with various bacterial and parasitic enteric infections, including those from *Shigella*, *Campylobacter*, *E. coli*, and *Giardia*.[6] Reducing exposure to enteric pathogens in children may reduce global rates of stunting.

MICROBIOLOGICAL TESTING

Despite the commonness of acute diarrheal illness, many of the main microbiological causes of diarrhea are poorly understood. Traditional microbiological methods of culture and microscopy of fecal specimens are only able to identify the causes of approximately 20–30% of all cases of diarrhea, depending on the tests carried out. Culture-based methods of detection are insensitive even for common pathogens, such as *Campylobacter* and *Salmonella*. There are two main reasons for the difficulty of detecting pathogens. First, due to delays in presenting with symptoms, people who are ill often collect specimens after the peak of their diarrheal infection when shedding of infective organisms is lower. Second, the tests used to diagnose diarrheal infections are insensitive. For many agents, such as STEC, special laboratory media, and culture conditions are required that are not universally used on all stools submitted for testing. This can result in differences in reported disease rates within and across countries that may be the result of laboratory testing practices.[7]

In the last decade, there has been a revolution in diagnosis of enteric infections through the use of polymerase chain reaction-based panels detecting multiple agents at the same time. These culture-independent diagnostic tests have shone a light on the main causes of diarrhea and reignited interest in others. These tests are usually far more sensitive than traditional tests, resulting in identification of pathogens in 40–60% of stool specimens depending on the patient population and test characteristics.[8] These kits have the advantage of being rapid with results available in hours rather than the days needed to culture and identify an organism. Clinically, they assist with early identification of an expanded range of pathogens and improve antibiotic stewardship by reducing reliance on unnecessary antibiotics.[8,9]

Efforts to understand the causes of diarrheal disease in children using these newer diagnostic tests have resulted in vastly improved estimates of incidence by etiological agents. The Global Enteric Microbial Study (GEMS) was a multicenter case control study in children investigating etiological agents of diarrhea.[10] The GEMS study revealed when laboratories used traditional culture-based methods many enteric pathogens were significantly underestimated as a cause of diarrheal disease, particularly for *Shigella*, adenoviruses,

TABLE 108-1 LISTS THE MAIN AGENTS, INFECTIOUSNESS, MAIN MANIFESTATIONS AND PREDOMINANT MODE OF TRANSMISSION

Pathogen	Incubation Period	Duration of Illness	Main Manifestations	Predominant Mode of Transmission
Bacillus cereus	1–6 hours (emetic toxin) 6–24 hours (diarrheal toxin)	24 hours	Rapid onset of vomiting and diarrhea depending on toxin	Foodborne intoxication
Campylobacter sp.	2–10 days	2–10 days	Diarrhea, fever, abdominal cramps, vomiting	Foodborne and zoonotic
Clostridium perfringens	6–24 hours	24 hours	Diarrhea, abdominal pain	Foodborne intoxication
Clostridium difficile	2–3 days	1–5 weeks	Diarrhea, abdominal cramps, fever, nausea	Person-to-person and environmental
Cryptosporidium sp.	2–10 days	1–2 weeks	Watery diarrhea, abdominal pain, nausea, vomiting	Person-to-person, waterborne, and zoonotic
Enterotoxigenic *Escherichia coli* (ETEC)	6–48 hours	1–14 days	Diarrhea, fever, loss of appetite, abdominal pain	Foodborne
Enteropathogenic *E. coli* (EPEC)	1–2 days	1–2 weeks	Diarrhea, abdominal pain, nausea, fever	Person-to-person, foodborne, waterborne
Enterohaemmorrhagic (Shiga-toxin producing) *E. coli*	1–10 days	1–2 weeks	Bloody diarrhea, abdominal cramps	Person-to-person, foodborne, zoonotic
Giardia sp.	1–3 weeks	1–4 weeks	Diarrhea, bloating, abdominal cramps	Person-to-person, waterborne, zoonotic
Norovirus	12–48 hours	1–3 days	Nausea, vomiting, diarrhea	Person-to-person, waterborne, foodborne
Rotavirus	1–2 days	3–8 days	Watery diarrhea, vomiting, fever, abdominal pain	Person-to-person, waterborne
Salmonella enterica	12–72 hours	1–7 days	Diarrhea, fever, nausea, abdominal cramps	Foodborne, zoonotic, person-to-person, waterborne
Shigella sp.	1–2 days	5–7 days	Diarrhea (sometimes bloody), fever, abdominal pain	Person-to-person, waterborne, foodborne
Staphylococcus aureus intoxication	30 minutes–8 hours	1 day	Nausea, vomiting, diarrhea	Foodborne
Yersinia sp.	4–7 days	1–3 weeks	Diarrhea, abdominal pain, fever	Foodborne, zoonotic
Vibrio cholerae (cholera)	1–5 days	1–10 days	Watery diarrhea, vomiting, dehydration	Waterborne, person-to-person, foodborne

E. coli, and *Campylobacter*. The study was able to identify an etiological cause for 89.3% of diarrheal episodes using molecular methods compared to 51.5% using culture-based methods.[11]

There are two major challenges for public health agencies where pathology laboratories start to use these methods as routine testing for diarrhea: identification of questionable pathogens and lack of cultures for molecular subtyping. In many of the multiplex panels used for testing, there are agents included that are not considered a cause of disease in feeding studies or laboratory-based case control studies. These organisms include *Aeromonas* sp., *Blastocystis hominis*, and *Dientamoeba fragilis*. This can lead to clinicians attributing patient's illness to these agents where there is little evidence for them as a cause of diarrhea, and the treatments may be questionable and ineffective. The second challenge for health departments is subtyping enteric agents to identify relatedness of strains for surveillance and outbreak investigation.[12] For many typing tests, such as serotyping or whole genome sequencing (WGS), there is a requirement for a reference laboratory to receive and use a pure culture to extract DNA. Rapid test kits do not generate pure cultures and the pathology laboratories are often reluctant to culture positive samples.

SOURCES OF INFECTION

The source of diarrheal disease varies by pathogen and setting. Most enteric agents are transmissible through a variety of modes of transmission, although many are fecal-oral spread. It is difficult to identify the source of infection for an individual patient's diarrhea due to variable incubation periods of different pathogens and multicausal nature of such symptoms. However, estimates of etiologies can be made at a population level, either through epidemiological studies, investigation of outbreaks, or expert opinion. Understanding the modes of transmission is important for identifying appropriate means of intervening to prevent disease (Fig. 108-1).

The primary sources of infection for diarrheal diseases include contact with infected persons, animals or contaminated environments, and consumption of contaminated foods and waters. The proportion of infections transmitted by these main sources varies depending on the infectiousness of the agent, ability of the pathogen to survive, development of immunity, and sociocultural factors. For example, norovirus has a very low infectious dose, with only several viral particles required to cause infection, which results in easy transmission from one infected person to another, either through direct contact with body fluids or touching contaminated surfaces. This means that the predominant mode of transmission for norovirus is person-to-person infection, although it can cause very large foodborne outbreaks when food becomes contaminated during production, processing, or point of service setting.[13]

In LMIC where the greatest burden of diarrheal disease occurs, the main mode of transmission is poor sanitation and hygiene as demonstrated by many epidemiological studies.[14,15] In 2017, GBD 2017 collaborators estimated that diarrhea from unsafe water sources resulted

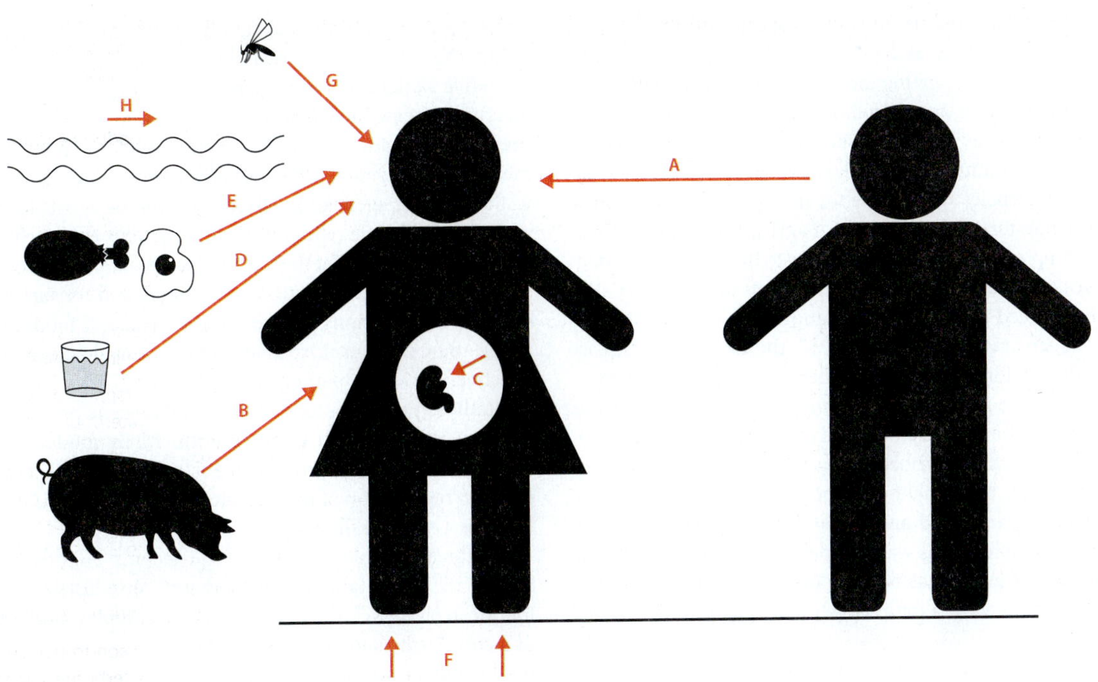

FIGURE 108-1. The main sources of infection for enteric agents.)

in 1.2 million deaths and 64 million DALYs.[16] The World Health Organization (WHO) has estimated the main sources of many enteric infections using expert elicitation at a global level.[17] In this structured estimation process, 78 experts were asked to estimate based on their investigative experience what the main sources were at the global and regional levels, along with their level of certainty. For many pathogens, the foodborne route was more important in high-income subregions than in LMIC regions of the world. For example, experts estimated that 73% of *Campylobacter* infections were foodborne in high-income American countries, compared to 57% in African countries. For foodborne transmission, experts also estimated the contribution of different foods for certain pathogens, which is important for agents like *Salmonella* and *Campylobacter* that may be transmitted largely through consumption of poultry-based foods.[18]

PUBLIC HEALTH SURVEILLANCE AND OUTBREAK INVESTIGATION

Surveillance for acute diarrheal illness is important for public health due to the preventable nature of many illnesses. In high-income countries, surveillance for acute diarrheal illness relies on additional tests on organisms detected in stool specimens, while in LMIC surveillance often relies on reporting of specific diarrheal syndromes, such as acute watery diarrhea, from clinics or hospitals. Increases in laboratory-based diagnoses or reports of syndromic diarrhea may mean that there is an emerging source of infection in the population that requires public health action. It is impossible to know the nature of transmission and potential interventions from surveillance data without investigation of cases and collation of risk factor information to determine the etiology and cause.

In high-income countries, surveillance of diarrheal diseases is based on microbiology laboratories and clinicians reporting cases of specific infections, such as those caused by *Salmonella*, *Campylobacter*, and STEC, to the local and state health departments. The health department will capture these in databases and regularly analyze data to identify signals indicating changes in the epidemiology or increases at local or larger geographic areas that might signify an outbreak. For many pathogens, specialized or reference laboratories will further characterize strains of enteric agents using phenotypic (e.g., antimicrobial susceptibility tests), or genotypic tests, such as WGS. These typing tests can identify whether pathogens infecting different people are related and potentially indicating an outbreak or common source.

With increasing use of WGS, rapid sharing of sequence data can improve detection of multicountry spread of infectious diarrhea from contaminated food or infected persons. Multistate and country spread of infectious agents is reasonably common, particularly for foodborne infections. High-income countries have established routine systems to subtype or sequence all enteric pathogens reported to central reference laboratories. The PulseNet system in the United States and Canada has proven extremely successful at surveillance of enteric infections for identification of widely distributed outbreaks.[19] PulseNet was originally based on pulsed field gel electrophoresis of enteric bacteria, but is in the process of transitioning to WGS that has allowed comparison with sequences from isolates obtained from foods and uploaded to the Food and Drug Administration's GenomeTrackr database.

Public Health England was one of the earliest agencies to conduct countrywide laboratory-based surveillance for enteric infections using only WGS, which started in 2014.[20] This results in detection of outbreaks that continue over a longer period of time or are more geographically dispersed. In addition, as WGS data are often shared in public domain databases it is possible for researchers to conduct comparative genomic analysis to explore trends, origins, and emergence of strains. This newer type of analysis of surveillance data for *Shigella* has demonstrated new insights into international spread of drug-resistant strains among high-risk populations, such as men who have sex with men.[21]

A key public health action arising from surveillance of diarrhea and enteric pathogens is investigation of outbreaks. An outbreak is defined as the occurrence of disease at higher levels than normal. This may be indicated by clustering of cases of diarrhea in a village, or among friends who have shared a meal. The nature and focus of these investigations vary from country-to-country specifically with regards to capacity of microbiology and public health services. In LMIC, there is less focus on investigating individual cases and smaller outbreaks and more emphasis on controlling epidemic diseases that persist in poor sanitation environments, such as cholera and typhoid.

In high-income countries, outbreak investigation is often a partnership between agencies responsible for infectious disease control, public health laboratories, departments of agriculture, and food regulators. This complex situation has arisen due to the difficulty of identifying sources of infection from epidemiological or laboratory data alone. There is a need to include information on traceback of foods or animals as a stream of evidence. In 2015, the Centers for Disease Control and Prevention and U.S. health departments investigated an outbreak of 50 people infected with *S. enterica* serotype Paratyphi C biovar Java that was linked to eating sushi containing tuna. The identification of frozen tuna relied heavily on food-safety investigations and was traced back to a single supplier of tuna originating from Indonesia, which was recalled and removed from public sale.[22] An animal-related example of this was the identification of an outbreak multidrug resistant *Campylobacter* infection affecting 118 persons in 18 states that was linked to a national pet store chain in the United States.[23]

There are several reasons why it is important to investigate outbreaks of enteric infection, including to:

- Remove a contaminated food products or infected animals from the marketplace,
- Identify food and agricultural production system failures to prevent future disease,
- Introduce regulatory measures to stop further outbreaks from occurring,
- Treat contacts of persistent infections, such as typhoid, to prevent further infections, and
- Provide training opportunities for field staff, such as epidemiologists, microbiologists and agricultural and food-safety specialists.

Importantly, as diarrheal diseases are multicausal, there is often no way to tell how infections are being transmitted without a robust investigation to identify the source.

CONTROL MEASURES

Control of diarrheal diseases relies on a range of strategies depending on the main sources of infection. There are many different means of controlling infectious diarrhea, most of which focus on improvements in hygiene and sanitation. Water, sanitation, and hygiene interventions are the key control measure in LMIC, which is shown by the difference in the types of infections and the health outcomes occurring in these countries compared to high-income countries.[24] GBD collaborators estimated that between 2007 and 2017 improvements in water, sanitation and handwashing resulted in a 31.6% reduction in age-standardized deaths and 36% reduction in DALYs lost.[16] These interventions rely on improving access to safe water supplies, toilets, disposal of wastewater, and adequate soap and water to wash hands properly.

Vaccines for humans and animals also play a role in controlling infectious diarrhea. Many countries have introduced human vaccines for rotavirus, which is a common cause of childhood mortality and morbidity. Where it has been introduced as a routine vaccine for children, this has resulted in spectacular declines in reduction in incidence and deaths among all age groups. Most other enteric agents do not have efficacious vaccines for population use, although there are vaccines in development for norovirus and other agents. Effective vaccines against typhoid and cholera are commonly used for travelers. Vaccines against *Salmonella* are routinely used in food production animals to control spread through the food chain. For foodborne and zoonotic agents, there is significant potential for new vaccines to reduce the burden of disease in human populations.

While sanitation and hygiene improvements are key to reducing diarrheal disease incidence, there is a need for the global health community to prioritize food-safety interventions in LMIC.[25] The control measures to prevent foodborne disease are elaborate and complex due to the multiple agencies involved. Controlling agents like *Salmonella* and *Campylobacter* relies on taking a systems approach where there are adequate controls at the food producer, suppliers, processors, food service industry (restaurants and caterers), and consumers. The most effective interventions reduce the prevalence of foodborne bacteria at the source on farm, so that interventions downstream are more effective. For other pathogens, such as norovirus, the focus should be on those preparing food taking good hygiene precautions and not working while ill with gastroenteritis. Many foodborne pathogens are easily killed by appropriate cooking. However, there has been a growing recognition of fresh produce and other raw and ready-to-eat foods as a cause of illness.[26]

Outbreak investigations in high-income countries have highlighted the important role of food service industries in preventing foodborne illness.[27] The main causes are complex, but largely consist of factors such as inadequate cooking, inadequate washing of hands, food handlers working while ill, unsanitary food cooking and preparation environments, and poor-quality ingredients. In many countries, food-safety agencies have implemented regulatory controls based on a systems approach to food production, such as Hazard Analysis and Critical Control Points (HAACP). These food-safety systems rely on food businesses analyzing processes and identifying points where contamination entry could occur and implementing adequate monitoring and controls.

CONCLUSIONS

Infectious diarrhea is a global concern causing significant morbidity and mortality. While the burden of infection has improved dramatically in recent decades, the pathogens causing diarrhea are still a persistent problem even in industrialized countries. There are many different modes of transmission for diarrhea, making control complex. Changing diagnostic tests and technologies for characterizing infecting strains are providing novel insights into transmission and sources. There is a need to deploy these on a wider scale and introduce new control measures for diarrheal disease in both high and LMIC.

References

1 GBD 2017 Disease and Injury Incidence and Prevalence Collaborators. Global, regional, and national incidence, prevalence, and years lived with disability for 354 diseases and injuries for 195 countries and territories, 1990–2017: A systematic analysis for the Global Burden of Disease Study 2017. *Lancet.* 2018;392(10159):1789–858.

2. Fischer Walker CL, Sack D, Black RE. Etiology of diarrhea in older children, adolescents and adults: A systematic review. *PLoS Negl Trop Dis.* 2010;4(8):e768.

3 GBD 2017 Causes of Death Collaborators. Global, regional, and national age-sex-specific mortality for 282 causes of death in 195 countries and territories, 1980–2017: A systematic analysis for the Global Burden of Disease Study 2017. *Lancet.* 2018;392(10159):1736–88.

4 GBD 2017 DALYs and HALE Collaborators. Global, regional, and national disability-adjusted life-years (DALYs) for 359 diseases and injuries and healthy life expectancy (HALE) for 195 countries and territories, 1990–2017: A systematic analysis for the Global Burden of Disease Study 2017. *Lancet.* 2018;392(10159):1859–922.

5 Majowicz SE, Hall G, Scallan E, et al. A common, symptom-based case definition for gastroenteritis. *Epidemiol Infect.* 2008;136(7):886–94.

6 Rogawski ET, Liu J, Platts-Mills JA, et al. Use of quantitative molecular diagnostic methods to investigate the effect of enteropathogen infections on linear growth in children in low-resource settings: Longitudinal analysis of results from the MAL-ED cohort study. *Lancet Glob Health.* 2018;6(12):e1319–e28.

7 Vally H, Hall G, Scallan E, Kirk MD, Angulo FJ. Higher rate of culture-confirmed Campylobacter infections in Australia than in the USA: Is this due to differences in healthcare-seeking behaviour or stool culture frequency? *Epidemiol Infect*. 2009;137(12):1751–8.

8 Piralla A, Lunghi G, Ardissino G, et al. FilmArray GI panel performance for the diagnosis of acute gastroenteritis or hemorragic diarrhea. *BMC Microbiol*. 2017;17(1):111.

9 Beal SG, Tremblay EE, Toffel S, Velez L, Rand KH. A Gastrointestinal PCR Panel improves clinical management and lowers health care costs. *J Clin Microbiol*. 2018;56(1):e01457–17.

10 Levine MM, Kotloff KL, Nataro JP, Muhsen K. The Global Enteric Multicenter Study (GEMS): Impetus, rationale, and genesis. *Clin Infect Dis*. 2012;55 Suppl 4:S215–24.

11 Liu J, Platts-Mills JA, Juma J, et al. Use of quantitative molecular diagnostic methods to identify causes of diarrhoea in children: A reanalysis of the GEMS case-control study. *Lancet*. 2016;388(10051):1291–301.

12 Shea S, Kubota KA, Maguire H, et al. Clinical microbiology laboratories' adoption of culture-independent diagnostic tests is a threat to foodborne-disease surveillance in the United States. *J Clin Microbiol*. 2017;55(1):10–9.

13 de Graaf M, van Beek J, Koopmans MP. Human norovirus transmission and evolution in a changing world. *Nat Rev Microbiol*. 2016;14(7):421–33.

14 Wolf J, Hunter PR, Freeman MC, et al. Impact of drinking water, sanitation and handwashing with soap on childhood diarrhoeal disease: Updated meta-analysis and meta-regression. *Trop Med Int Health*. 2018;23(5):508–25.

15 Baker KK, O'Reilly CE, Levine MM, et al. Sanitation and hygiene-specific risk factors for moderate-to-severe diarrhea in young children in the Global Enteric Multicenter Study, 2007–2011: Case-control study. *PLoS Med*. 2016;13(5):e1002010.

16 GBD 2017 Risk Factor Collaborators. Global, regional, and national comparative risk assessment of 84 behavioural, environmental and occupational, and metabolic risks or clusters of risks for 195 countries and territories, 1990–2017: A systematic analysis for the Global Burden of Disease Study 2017. *Lancet*. 2018;392(10159):1923–94.

17 Hald T, Aspinall W, Devleesschauwer B, et al. World Health Organization estimates of the relative contributions of food to the burden of disease due to selected foodborne hazards: A structured expert elicitation. *PLoS One*. 2016;11(1):e0145839.

18 Hoffmann S, Devleesschauwer B, Aspinall W, et al. Attribution of global foodborne disease to specific foods: Findings from a World Health Organization structured expert elicitation. *PLoS One*. 2017;12(9):e0183641.

19 Scharff RL, Besser J, Sharp DJ, Jones TF, Peter GS, Hedberg CW. An economic evaluation of PulseNet: A Network for Foodborne Disease Surveillance. *Am J Prev Med*. 2016;50(5 Suppl 1):S66–73.

20 Mook P, Gardiner D, Verlander NQ, et al. Operational burden of implementing Salmonella Enteritidis and Typhimurium cluster detection using whole genome sequencing surveillance data in England: A retrospective assessment. *Epidemiol Infect*. 2018;146(11):1452-60.

21 Baker KS, Dallman TJ, Ashton PM, et al. Intercontinental dissemination of azithromycin-resistant shigellosis through sexual transmission: A cross-sectional study. *Lancet Infect Dis*. 2015;15(8):913–21.

22 Hassan R, Tecle S, Adcock B, et al. Multistate outbreak of Salmonella Paratyphi B variant L(+) tartrate(+) and Salmonella Weltevreden infections linked to imported frozen raw tuna: USA, March–July 2015. *Epidemiol Infect*. 2018;146(11):1461–7.

23 Montgomery MP, Robertson S, Koski L, et al. Multidrug-resistant Campylobacter jejuni uutbreak linked to puppy exposure—United States, 2016–2018. *MMWR Morb Mortal Wkly Rep*. 2018;67(37):1032–5.

24 GBD 2016 DALYs and HALE Collaborators. Estimates of global, regional, and national morbidity, mortality, and aetiologies of diarrhoeal diseases: A systematic analysis for the Global Burden of Disease Study 2015. *Lancet Infect Dis*. 2017;17(9):909–48.

25 Kirk MD, Angulo FJ, Havelaar AH, Black RE. Diarrhoeal disease in children due to contaminated food. *Bull World Health Organ*. 2017;95(3):233–4.

26 Callejon RM, Rodriguez-Naranjo MI, Ubeda C, Hornedo-Ortega R, Garcia-Parrilla MC, Troncoso AM. Reported foodborne outbreaks due to fresh produce in the United States and European Union: Trends and causes. *Foodborne Pathog Dis*. 2015;12(1):32–8.

27 Gould LH, Rosenblum I, Nicholas D, Phan Q, Jones TF. Contributing factors in restaurant-associated foodborne disease outbreaks, FoodNet sites, 2006 and 2007. *J Food Prot*. 2013;76(11):1824–8.

CHAPTER

109 Campylobacter

Craig W. Hedberg

CAMPYLOBACTER

Campylobacter spp. are the most common bacterial etiology of diarrhea in the United States, causing more than 1,300,000 acute illnesses with 80% attributed to foodborne transmission.[1] The clinical significance of these illnesses is compounded by the occasional occurrence of Guillain-Barre syndrome (GBS), the most common cause of acute flaccid paralysis worldwide.[2] Globally, *Campylobacter* spp. cause an estimated 96 million foodborne illnesses and 21,000 deaths.[3] As a result of GBS, *Campylobacter* spp. accounts for the most years lived with disability among diarrheal disease agents.[3] In the United States an estimated 17% of confirmed infections result in hospitalization with a 0.1% death rate.[1] *C. jejuni* causes approximately 86% of human infections with 10% caused by *C. coli*.[4] Both *Campylobacter* species are carried by a variety of food animals and domestic pets. Despite their prominence as causes of foodborne illness, confirmed foodborne outbreaks caused by *Campylobacter* spp. are remarkably uncommon.[5] Less than 1% of *Campylobacter* cases reported to the Foodborne Diseases Active Surveillance Network (FoodNet) from 1996 to 2018 were associated with outbreaks.[6] Outbreak detection among reported *Campylobacter* cases has been limited, in part, due to the lack of routine subtype characterization of isolates needed to identify clusters of likely related cases, and by the lack of routine interviewing of cases to identify potential common exposures. However, the bigger reason appears to be the characteristics of *Campylobacter* spp. that limit amplification of contamination in common exposure settings linked to foodborne outbreaks.

Microbiology

Campylobacter spp. are motile, nonspore forming, Gram-negative rods with a distinctive curved morphology.[7] They share growth characteristics that distinguish them from other foodborne pathogens, such as *Salmonella* spp., in epidemiologically important ways. *Campylobacter* spp. are microaerophilic. Their growth may be inhibited at atmospheric oxygen concentrations, which limits their growth in ambient environments, such as kitchens.[7] This also limits their survival in clinical samples during transport and culture by clinical laboratories. *C. jejuni* are thermophilic with growth temperature ranges from 37°C to 42°C, reflecting the body temperatures of their primary reservoir hosts.[8] They do not grow at temperatures below 30°C.[9] This also prevents amplification in most ambient environments. They are sensitive to drying, heating, freezing, common disinfectants, and low pH environments.[7,9] Under conditions of stress they may enter a viable but nonculturable state that permits survival under unfavorable conditions.[8] The role of these cells in transmission of foodborne illness is unknown. Because *Campylobacter* spp. are limited in their ability to survive and grow in the environment, they pose a food safety threat primarily from direct contamination of raw or ready-to-eat foods.

C. jejuni possess several virulence and stress response factors associated with motility, chemotaxis, adhesion, invasion, multidrug resistance, and survival.[8] These include specific antimicrobial resistance determinants and a multidrug efflux pump that promotes resistance to bile salts, heavy metals, and a broad range of other antimicrobial agents.[8] The proportion of human *C. jejuni* isolates submitted to the National Antimicrobial Resistance Monitoring System (NARMS) that were resistant to two or more classes of antibiotics increased from 13.1% in 2006 to 25.3% in 2015.[4] with resistance to ciprofloxacin increasing from 19.6% to 25.3%. Importantly, the proportion of human *C. jejuni* isolates resistant to both a macrolide and a quinolone remains low, ranging from 0.7% in 2006 to 2.1% in 2015.[4] Rates of antimicrobial resistance among *C. coli* tend to be somewhat higher, with 39% exhibiting resistance to two or more classes of antimicrobial agents in 2015, including 39.8% resistant to ciprofloxacin and 8.5% resistant to both a macrolide and a quinolone.[4]

Strains of *C. jejuni* that exhibit enhanced aerotolerance have been found to cluster among clonal complexes, or clades, that are frequently associated with human illness.[10] These strains have also been found to be highly prevalent in raw chicken samples at retail.[10] More recently, *C. jejuni* strains exhibiting tolerance to multiple stress conditions associated with food-production environments, including aerotolerance, disinfectant exposure, freeze-thaw cycles, heat treatment, and osmotic stress have been identified in clades associated with human illness.[11] It is not clear whether these represent emerging traits within *C. jejuni*, or whether they reflect the emergence of new tools that can be used to explore these characteristics.

Of particular importance from a public health perspective are a polysaccharide capsule and lip-oligosaccharides (LOS) on the surface of *C. jejuni* cells that facilitate host cell adhesion, invasion and evasion of the host immune system.[8] Capsular genotypes and sialylated LOS have been associated with the occurrence of GBS.[12] Molecular similarity between ganglioside-like epitopes in these structures and on human nerve cells elicits autoantibodies in some hosts that attack peripheral nerves.[13]

Diagnosis and Treatment

Campylobacteriosis is characterized by diarrhea, fever, and abdominal cramps.[7] The illness is usually self-limited, but symptoms may persist for a week or longer. Diarrhea may be accompanied by blood in the stool. The constellation of acute symptoms and 2–5 day incubation period are similar to other enteric bacterial agents, such as *Salmonella* and *Shigella*. Cases of reactive arthritis and irritable bowel syndrome have been associated with *Campylobacter* infections.[14] Approximately one in every 2000 cases of *Campylobacter* results in GBS.[2]

The nonspecific nature of the symptoms requires laboratory testing to establish a diagnosis and guide decisions on antimicrobial treatment. Stool culture for *C. jejuni* requires special conditions, which may limit the sensitivity of culture compared to other enteric bacteria.[7] Stool may be inoculated directly onto selective media to limit growth of competing organisms, or into an enrichment broth to increase recovery. Cultures are incubated for 48–72 hours under microaerophilic conditions at 42°C.[7] However, in recent years clinical laboratories have been moving away from stool culture in favor of culture-independent diagnostic tests (CIDT). DNA-based syndrome panels that can provide test results for multiple agents in a matter of hours are now in widespread use by clinical laboratories.[15] Although these tests provide rapid diagnostic information, they do not isolate an organism for antimicrobial resistance testing or further molecular characterization by whole genome sequencing (WGS). In 2018, 45% of *Campylobacter* cases reported to FoodNET were diagnosed by DNA-based syndrome panels.[15] A reflex culture was attempted for 64% of *Campylobacter*-positive CIDT results and 59% of these samples yielded a *Campylobacter* isolate. Thus 28% of *Campylobacter* cases were diagnosed solely by CIDT.

Most *Campylobacter* illnesses are self-limited, can be managed with oral rehydration therapy, and do not require antimicrobial treatment. However, persons with illnesses that last for several days, are accompanied by fever or blood in the stool, or that occur following international travel are more likely to seek medical care.[16] The availability of rapid CIDT that can distinguish *Campylobacter* from *Salmonella* or other enteric infections may increase the likelihood that antimicrobial treatment would be prescribed.

Azithromycin is recommended as a first choice for antimicrobial treatment of *Campylobacter*, with ciprofloxacin as an alternative.[16] Increasing rates of resistance to ciprofloxacin warrant use of antimicrobial susceptibility testing of clinical isolates. Antimicrobial resistance may also be inferred from results of WGS. However, increased use of CIDT may limit the availability of isolates for antimicrobial susceptibility testing or WGS. Current antimicrobial sensitivity data compiled through public health surveillance may be useful to guide treatment options.[16]

Occurrence

The incidence of *Campylobacter* illnesses in the United States has been systematically tracked by FoodNET since 1996.[6] The incidence of illness over this time period has been 14.4 cases per 100,000 population. Overall, 15% of cases were hospitalized and < 1% died. A history of international travel was reported by 11% of cases.[6]

From 2001 to 2010, rates of *Campylobacter* illnesses were consistently under 14 cases per 100,000.[6] Since 2012, analysis of trends related to *Campylobacter* has been complicated by the increasing use of CIDT. Adjusting for the use of CIDT, CDC estimated that *Campylobacter* incidence rates remained stable through 2015.[17] However, when including cases diagnosed by CIDT, the incidence rate of *Campylobacter* illnesses reported by FoodNET in 2018 was 19.6 cases per 100,000. This represented a 12% increase over the mean incidence rate reported for 2015–17.[17]

Less than 1% of cases reported to FoodNET were associated with outbreaks.[6] From 2009 to 2017, 552 outbreaks involving *Campylobacter* infections were reported to the CDC National Outbreak Reporting System (NORS).[5] The median size of outbreaks was four cases, with a range from 2 to 628 cases. Outbreaks associated with food or waterborne transmission tended to be somewhat larger, involving a median of six and seven cases, respectively. The absence of routine, molecular subtype-based surveillance for *Campylobacter* means that most outbreaks are identified as local clusters of cases associated with common exposure settings. The likelihood of detecting and investigating these outbreaks varies considerably by state. For example, five states accounted for 43% of all *Campylobacter* outbreaks reported to NORS from 2009 to 2017.[5] Only six multistate outbreaks were reported during this time frame.

Modes of Transmission

Based on results of a FoodNET case-control study of sporadic *Campylobacter* illnesses, approximately 80% of *Campylobacter* infections are attributed to foodborne transmission, with approximately 11% related to animal contact, 6% related to environmental exposures and 3% due to untreated surface water.[1] A meta-analysis of case-control studies of sporadic *Campylobacter* infections confirmed the significance of food, direct contact with farm animals and pets, water and environmental exposures, but could not determine what proportion of cases were attributable to these sources.[18] More directly, NORS has collected reports of outbreaks by all modes of transmission since 2009.[5] Among outbreaks where the primary mode of transmission could be determined, 69% were attributed to food, 12% were attributed to animal contact, 5% were attributed to water, and 1% were attributed to environmental exposures other than food or water.

Overall, 13% of *Campylobacter* outbreaks reported to NORS were attributed to person-to-person transmission. However, the size and settings of these outbreaks limit our ability to draw firm conclusions regarding the results of the investigations. More than half of these outbreaks involved only two or three cases, about one-third occurred in nursing homes or childcare settings, and several involved multiple pathogens. Thus, person-to-person transmission of *Campylobacter* appears to be very uncommon.

Recent studies have demonstrated increased occupational risk of *Campylobacter* infections among farmers and workers in chicken slaughter plants.[19,20] Although animal contact at fairs and petting zoos have been implicated in numerous outbreaks of shigatoxin-producing *E. coli* and *Salmonella*, relatively few outbreaks of *Campylobacter* infections have been linked to these same settings.[21] The role of pets in the transmission of *Campylobacter* was demonstrated by a multistate outbreak involving 118 cases from 18 states, with illnesses occurring over a 2-year time period.[22] Cases ranged from < 1 to 85 years, and 24% of cases for whom information was available were hospitalized. Outbreak-associated isolates were shown to be highly related by WGS, within three different clades, and all were resistant to azithromycin, ciprofloxacin, and multiple other antimicrobials. Interviews with cases revealed that almost all had contact with a puppy in the week before onset of illness. The vast majority of puppies were from a single chain of pet stores, although six different pet store chains were involved in the outbreak. Among a sample of puppies evaluated, 95% had been given one or more courses of antibiotics at the pet store. *Campylobacter* strains isolated from pet store puppies were closely related to human isolates by WGS. A complex distribution chain involving multiple breeders, transportation companies, and distributors provided various points at which puppies from one breeder may have commingled with puppies from other breeders to spread infection.[22]

The vast majority of reported foodborne outbreaks for which a food vehicle could be identified have been associated with consumption of animal products that were consumed without sufficient heat treatment to kill *Campylobacter*.[5] Of 176 *Campylobacter* outbreaks with a food vehicle reported to NORS from 2009 to 2017, 84 (48%) were associated with unpasteurized dairy products. Of 34 outbreaks associated with chicken, 26 (76%) were associated with chicken liver. Eight (33%) of 24 outbreaks in which multiple food items were implicated also included chicken, of which three included chicken liver. Four outbreaks were associated with duck livers or foie gras. Two of five beef associated outbreaks identified consumption of raw beef and two others identified beef liver. Six outbreaks were associated with oysters or raw clams. One outbreak was attributed to unpasteurized apple cider.[5] This pattern of outbreaks associated with raw or undercooked foods was confirmed by contributing factors identified in outbreak investigations.[23] Among 38 confirmed *Campylobacter* outbreaks with contributing factors identified from 2014 to 2016, 15 (39%) were attributed to consumptions of raw foods intended to be consumed raw and 14 (37%) were attributed to consumption of raw foods intended to be eaten after cooking. In 15 (39%) outbreaks, inadequate cooking was identified as a contributing factor.[23]

The lack of *Campylobacter* transmission by ill food handlers is notable. Among published foodborne outbreaks, there is only one with credible evidence implicating transmission from an ill food handler.[24] The food handler in that outbreak was reported to have had profuse diarrhea and made numerous trips to the bathroom while refilling serving dishes.[24]

Prevention and Control

Prevention of *Campylobacter* infections requires a combination of actions, from modifying individual behaviors to enhancing regulatory actions that reduce contamination of raw agricultural commodities and control transmission within the pet industry. Risks associated with consumption of unpasteurized milk and dairy products are well known and widely publicized. Commercial distribution of unpasteurized milk is prohibited in many states, although many also allow sales to individuals at the farm.[25] However, consumer demand for raw milk has led to internet sales and novel arrangements such as "cow shares," where urban residents can buy partial ownership in a cow and thereby obtain raw milk from their "own" cow. Legal and political battles have surrounded many of these novel arrangements.[25] It may be less obvious to consumers that pate made from chicken livers is undercooked. In this regard, consumers need clear information about the product and regulators need to work with industry to reduce the level of contamination in the raw materials.

Data on foodborne outbreaks reported to NORS is being used by the Interagency Food Safety Analytics Collaborative (IFSAC) to improve source attribution for *Campylobacter* infections, and to guide regulatory prevention measures.[26] Excluding outbreaks associated with dairy products, 47.5% of *Campylobacter* cases were attributed to chicken in 2016.[26] Over 80% of nondairy illnesses were attributed to chicken, seafood, turkey, other meat and poultry, and vegetable row crops. These data support efforts by USDA's Food Safety Inspection Service (FSIS) to focus on working with industry to reduce *Campylobacter* contamination of the poultry and meat supply. As part of a Healthy People 2020 initiative, FSIS established a target of a 25% reduction in human illnesses by the year 2020. Results of their Pathogen Reduction/HACCP verification testing program demonstrated a reduction in *Campylobacter* contamination of young chicken from 9.3% of samples in 2011 to 6.0% of samples in 2014.[27] Reduction of source contamination needs to be accompanied by appropriate food handling practices at the point of food preparation and service. The FDA Model Food Code provides guidance on proper cooking and safe handling procedures for restaurants to avoid cross-contamination of ready-to-eat foods.[28] Consumer education also needs to continue to emphasize safe handling and proper cooking of poultry and meat products.[29]

References

1. Scallan E, Hoekstra RM, Angulo FJ, et al. Foodborne illness acquired in the United States—Major pathogens. *Emerg Infect Dis.* 2011;17(1):7–15.
2. Halpin AL, Gu W, Wise ME, Sejvar JJ, Hoekstra RM, Mahon BE. Post-Campylobacter Guillain Barré syndrome in the USA: Secondary analysis of surveillance data collected during the 2009–2010 novel Influenza A (H1N1) vaccination campaign. *Epidemiol Infect.* 2018;146(13):1740–5.
3. Havelaar AH, Kirk MD, Torgerson PR, et al. World Health Organization global estimates and regional comparisons of the burden of foodborne disease in 2010. *PLoS Med.* 2015;12(12):e1001923.
4. Food and Drug Administration. The National Antimicrobial Resistance Monitoring System: NARMS integrated report, 2015. https://www.fda.gov/animal-veterinary/national-antimicrobial-resistance-monitoring-system/2015-narms-integrated-report. Laurel, MD, 2017.
5. Centers for Disease Control and Prevention. National Outbreak Reporting System. https://wwwn.cdc.gov/norsdashboard/. Atlanta, GA, 2019.
6. Centers for Disease Control and Prevention. FoodNet Fast. https://www.cdc.gov/foodnetfast/. Atlanta, GA, 2019.
7. Food and Drug Administration. Campylobacter jejuni. In: *Bad Bug Book, Foodborne Pathogenic Microorganisms and Natural Toxins.* 2nd ed. College Park, MD: Center for Food Safety and Applied Nutrition (CFSAN); 2012, pp.14–17.
8. Bolton DJ. Campylobacter *virulence* and survival factors. *Food Microbiol.* 2015;48:99–108.
9. Nachamkin I. Campylobacter jejuni. In: Doyle MP, Beuchat LR, Montville TJ, eds. *Food Microbioloy: Fundamentals and Frontiers*, 2nd ed. Washington, DC: ASM Press; 2001, pp. 179–92.
10. Oh E, McMullen L, Jeon B. High prevalence of hyper-aerotolerant *Campylobacter jejuni* in retail poultry with potential implication in human infection. *Front Microbiol.* 2015;6:1263.
11. Oh E, Chui L, Bae J, et al. Frequent implication of multistress-tolerant Campylobacter jejuni in human infections. *Emerg Infect Dis.* 2018;24(6):1037–44.
12. Heikema AP, Islam Z, Horst-Kreft D, et al. *Campylobacter jejuni* capsular genotypes are related to Guillain-Barré syndrome. *Clin Microbiol Infect.* 2015;21(9):852.
13. Nachamkin I, Allos BM, Ho T. Campylobacter species and Guillain-Barré syndrome. *Clin Microbiol Rev.* 1998;11(3):555–67.
14. Batz MB, Henke E, Kowalcyk B. Long-term consequences of foodborne infections. *Infect Dis Clin North Am.* 2013;27(3):599–616.
15. Tack DM, Marder EP, Griffin PM, et al. Preliminary incidence and trends of infections with pathogens transmitted commonly through food—Foodborne Diseases Active Surveillance Network, 10 U.S. sites, 2015–2018. *MMWR Morb Mortal Wkly Rep.* 2019;68:369–73.
16. Shane AL, Mody RK, Crump JA, et al. 2017 Infectious Diseases Society of America Clinical Practice guidelines for the diagnosis and management of infectious diarrhea. *Clin Infect Dis.* 2017;65 (12):e45–80.
17. Gu W, Dutta V, Patrick M, et al. Statistical adjustment of culture-independent diagnostic tests for trend analysis in the Foodborne Diseases Active Surveillance Network (FoodNet), USA. *Int J Epidemiol.* 2018;47(5):1613–22.
18. Domingues AR, Pires SM, Halasa T, Hald T. Source attribution of human campylobacteriosis using a meta-analysis of case-control studies of sporadic infections. *Epidemiol Infect.* 2012;140(6):970–81.
19. Su C, Stover DT, Buss BF, Carlson AV, Luckhaupt SE. Occupational animal exposure among persons with campylobacteriosis and cryptosporidiosis —Nebraska, 2005–2015. *MMWR Morb Mortal Wkly Rep.* 2017;66:955–8.
20. Su C, de Perio MA, Fagan K, et al. Occupational distribution of campylobacteriosis and ssalmonellosis cases—Maryland, Ohio, and Virginia, 2014. *MMWR Morb Mortal Wkly Rep.* 2017;66:850–3.
21. Conrad CC, Stanford K, Narvaez-Bravo C, Callaway T, McAllister T. Farm fairs and petting zoos: A review of animal contact as a source of zoonotic enteric disease. *Foodborne Pathog Dis.* 2017;14(2):59–73.
22. Montgomery MP, Robertson S, Koski L, et al. Multidrug-resistant *Campylobacter jejuni* outbreak linked to puppy exposure—United States, 2016–2018. *MMWR Morb Mortal Wkly Rep.* 2018;67:1032–5.
23. Centers for Disease Control and Prevention (CDC). Surveillance for foodborne disease outbreaks, United States, 2016, annual report. https://www.cdc.gov/fdoss/pdf/2016_FoodBorneOutbreaks_508.pdf. Atlanta, GA, 2018.
24. Olsen SJ, Hansen GR, Bartlett L, et al. An outbreak of *Campylobacter jejuni* infections associated with food handler contamination: The use of pulsed-field gel electrophoresis. *J Infect Dis.* 2001;183(1):164–7.
25. David SD. Raw milk and the first amendment: Implications for public health policy and practice. *Public Health Rep.* 2014;129(5):455–7.
26. Interagency Food Safety Analytics Collaboration. Foodborne illness source attribution estimates for 2016 for Salmonella, *Escherichia coli* O157, Listeria monocytogenes, and Campylobacter using multi-year outbreak surveillance data, United States. https://www.cdc.gov/foodsafety/ifsac/pdf/P19-2016-report-TriAgency-508.pdf. Atlanta, GA and Washington, DC, 2018.
27. Food Safety and Inspection Service. FSIS progress report on Salmonella and Campylobacter testing of raw meat and poultry products, 1998–2014. https://www.fsis.usda.gov/wps/portal/fsis/topics/data-collection-and-reports/microbiology/annual-progress-report. Washington, DC, 2015.
28. Food and Drug Administration. Food Code, 2017. Recommendations of the United States Public Health Service, Food and Drug Administration. https://www.fda.gov/Food/GuidanceRegulation/RetailFoodProtection/FoodCode/ucm595139.htm. College Park, MD, 2018.
29. Centers for Disease Control and Prevention. Four steps (clean, separate, cook, chill) to food safety. https://www.cdc.gov/foodsafety/keep-food-safe.html. Atlanta, GA, 2019.

CHAPTER

111

Salmonella Infections (Nontyphoidal)

Jessica M. Healy • Robert V. Tauxe • Beau B. Bruce

INTRODUCTION

Salmonellosis is the general term for infection caused by bacteria in the genus *Salmonella*, excluding *Salmonella* Typhi and three other typhoidal bioserotypes (i.e., Paratyphi A, Paratyphi B tartrate-negative, and Paratyphi C) that cause typhoid or enteric fever. Salmonellosis is a common gastrointestinal infection in the United States and around the world. Each year, an estimated 1.22 million *Salmonella* infections occur in the United States, and approximately 150 foodborne outbreaks of salmonellosis are investigated and reported by public health officials[1,2] (Fig. 111-1). Large and severe outbreaks of salmonellosis have driven major advances in public health surveillance and prevention, such as routine serotyping of clinical isolates in public health laboratories to determine major strains responsible for illness and to detect outbreaks.[3] The many types of *Salmonella* have become adapted to number of different host animals, particularly reptiles, amphibians, birds, and a variety of mammals, in which they usually cause little observed illness. Part of the adaptation includes strategies to reach the next generation of hosts by silently contaminating fertile eggs or mammalian milk. Humans can encounter the bacteria in their food supply, in water or other environmental sources, and through direct contact with animals carrying it.

Most illnesses caused by nontyphoidal *Salmonella* are characterized by diarrhea, sometimes bloody, along with fever, abdominal cramps, and vomiting, which can last for several days to a week, and usually resolves without antibiotic treatment. Symptoms typically begin 24–48 hours after ingesting the bacteria, as early as 8 hours and as late as 92 hours, and sometimes longer.[4] Some infections can lead to bloodstream invasion with a clinical picture more like that of typhoid fever, with high fever, sometimes complicated by sepsis, shock, organ failure, and death; in these patients, antibiotic treatment can be lifesaving. These invasive infections more commonly occur in persons with deficient immunity due to malignancy, medical treatment, diabetes, hemoglobinopathy, or HIV infection; recurrent *Salmonella* bacteremia is a defining condition for AIDS. Some serotypes, including Typhimurium and Enteritidis, are opportunistically invasive, and are particularly likely to cause bacteremia in persons with AIDS.[5] Other serotypes, such as Dublin, Choleraesuis, and Heidelberg are more likely to be invasive even in the normal host.[6] The likelihood of bacteremia depends on the dose ingested; persons with normal immunity may develop bacteremia following an overwhelming dose. In young infants, febrile bacteremia is not an uncommon outcome. *Salmonella* can also spread from the GI tract to distant parts of the body, leading to focal infections such as osteomyelitis, meningitis, and urinary tract infections. There is little apparent lasting immunity following natural infection, and humans infected with one strain remain susceptible to infection with others.

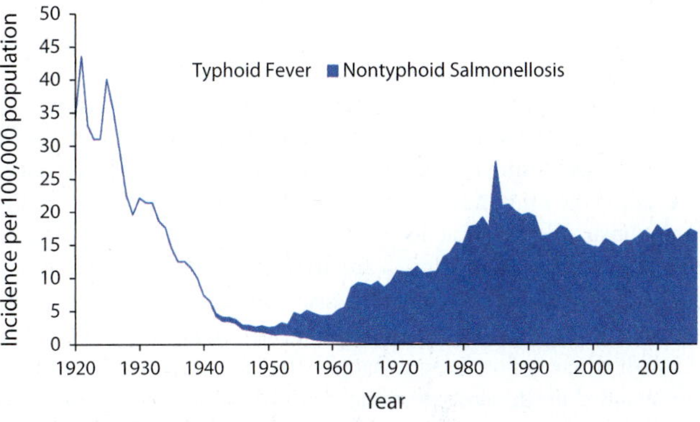

FIGURE 111-1. Reported combined incidence of typhoid fever and nontyphoidal salmonellosis (confirmed and suspected) in the United States from 1920 to 2015.

DIAGNOSIS

Salmonellosis is diagnosed based on clinical presentation and laboratory testing of a patient's specimen. For nontyphoidal *Salmonella* infection, isolation of organisms from a culture is the mainstay of clinical diagnostic testing. Approximately 90% of isolates are obtained from routine stool culture; isolates also come from other sites, including blood, urine, and abscesses. Recently, diagnostic laboratories have begun to incorporate culture-independent diagnostic testing (CIDT) of stool samples into their routine testing practices. These tests detect the pathogen's genetic material via methods such as real-time polymerase chain reaction. Diagnosis using CIDT produces rapid results, but culturing for and testing bacterial isolates remains necessary for determining antimicrobial susceptibility, serotyping, and for the molecular subtyping that is critical for public health surveillance, including the detection of widespread outbreaks. For these reasons, specimens that are positive by CIDT should be cultured for *Salmonella* ("reflex culture").[7] Serological diagnostic testing is not advised due to cross-reactivity with other genera of *Enterobacteriaceae.*

TREATMENT

In most cases of *Salmonella* gastroenteritis, symptoms resolve within 5–7 days with symptomatic treatment and oral rehydration therapy.[8] Antibiotic treatment is not recommended in these cases because it may prolong bacterial shedding and will disrupt the microbiome.[8,9] Antibiotic therapy should, however, be considered for patients with severe symptoms (e.g., high fever and severe diarrhea), with extraintestinal infection, or who are at increased risk for invasive disease, such as infants, persons over 65 years old, and the immunosuppressed. When antibiotic therapy is indicated, treatment is empiric until susceptibility testing is completed. Fluoroquinolones, such as ciprofloxacin, are considered first-line treatment in adults, and ceftriaxone is used for children. Approximately 2% of isolates tested by the National Antimicrobial Resistance Monitoring System (NARMS) exhibited nonsusceptibility to the fluoroquinolone ciprofloxacin, and 3% of isolates were resistant to ceftriaxone.[10]

MICROBIOLOGICAL CHARACTERISTICS

Salmonella spp. are Gram-negative bacilli of the genus *Salmonella* and the family *Enterobacteriaceae,* which includes other common pathogens such as *Escherichia coli and Shigella.* There are two species of *Salmonella*: *enterica* and *bongori;* the latter is an extremely rare cause of human illness and found largely in reptiles. *S. enterica* is subdivided into six subspecies, within which about 2500 serotypes have been identified. Serotypes are distinguished by the O antigens of the cell surface lipopolysaccharide and the H antigens of the flagellar protein filaments. Most serotypes can alternately express two different flagella, so they have two phenotypes, or phases, for the H antigen. This is unique to *Salmonella* among bacteria, and may relate to evading the immune response, or to attachment or motility in different hosts or environments.[11,12] Serotypes with only one flagella, or phase, are termed monophasic, and some serotypes, termed nonmotile, lack any H antigen. O and H antigens are identified through antisera agglutination assays, and the responsible genes can be identified through whole genome sequencing.[13] The type of O and H antigens are included in the serotype name, denoted by various numbers and letters according to the Kauffman-White scheme[14]:

> Subspecies Roman numeral O antigens: Phase 1 H antigen: Phase 2 H antigen

For example, *S. enterica* subspecies II with type 47 O antigen, type b phase 1 H antigen, and types 1 and 5 phase 2 H antigen could be written as II 47:b:1,5. Serotypes belonging to subspecies I, or S. *enterica subsp. enterica*, are the only serotypes to have proper names.*

Due to regular use of antibiotics in agriculture and medicine, antimicrobial resistance has emerged in numerous serotypes. Multiple antibiotic resistance gene clusters that confer multi drug resistance (e.g., *Salmonella* Genomic Island 1 and 2) have been identified and many are transferable via plasmids to other bacteria.[15]

PUBLIC HEALTH BURDEN

The estimated 1.22 million acute gastrointestinal illnesses caused by nontyphoidal *Salmonella* infections in the United States each year include mild infections that were not laboratory-confirmed (Fig. 111-2). The Centers for Disease Control and Prevention (CDC) receives approximately 47,000 reports of laboratory-confirmed nontyphoidal *Salmonella* infection each year.[16] Among these illnesses, an estimated 27% led to hospitalization, and 0.5% to death.[1] Reported cases can be associated with an outbreak or occur in individuals without a known connection, referred to as sporadic cases. About 6% of all reported salmonellosis cases are associated with a known outbreak.[17]

The five most common serotypes (Enteritidis, Typhimurium, Newport, Javiana, and I 4,[5],12:I:-) account for about half of all reported laboratory-confirmed cases (Table 111-1). They have similar seasonal patterns, peaking in late summer,[18] and trends over several years show that Typhimurium is decreasing whereas the other four are increasing (Fig. 111-3).[17,19] Four of these serotypes also show

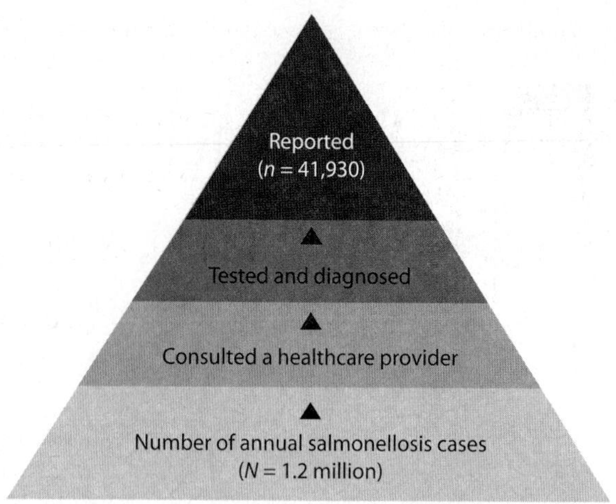

FIGURE 111-2. Surveillance pyramid for salmonellosis cases occurring in the United States. An estimated 1.2 million cases occur each year, yet only a proportion of these consult a healthcare provider about their illness, and further only a proportion of these cases will be tested and diagnosed, and, finally, a proportion of these cases are reported.[1] Data from Scallan E, Hoekstra RM, Angulo FJ, et al. Foodborne illness acquired in the United States—major pathogens. *Emerg Infect Dis.* 2011;17(1):7–15.

TABLE 111-1 THE 20 MOST COMMON SEROTYPES REPORTED TO THE LABORATORY-BASED ENTERIC DISEASE SURVEILLANCE SYSTEM DURING 2016, UNITED STATES[16]

Serotype	Number Reported	Percent	Incidence (per 100,000)
Enteritidis	7,830	16.8	2.44
Newsport	4,728	10.1	1.47
Typhimurium	4,581	9.8	1.43
Javiana	2,719	5.8	0.85
I 4,[5],12:i:-	2,179	4.7	0.68
Infantis	1,281	2.7	0.40
Muenchen	1,216	2.6	0.38
Montevideo	1,018	2.2	0.32
Braenderup	1,001	2.1	0.31
Thompson	792	1.7	0.25
Saintpaul	778	1.7	0.24
Heidelberg	754	1.6	0.23
Oranienburg	692	1.5	0.22
Mississippi	536	1.1	0.17
Typhi	423	0.9	0.13
Bareilly	412	0.9	0.13
Berta	369	0.8	0.11
Agona	362	0.8	0.11
Paratyphi B var. L(+) tartrate+	343	0.7	0.11
Anatum	257	0.6	0.08

*The nomenclature of *Salmonella* has evolved over time. Each of the thousands of serotypes was once described as a separate species, with a full Linnaean italicized name, thus: *Salmonella* typhimurium. After genetic studies indicated that almost all strains causing human infections are part of a single species, now called *Salmonella enterica*, the serotype is indicated either by a name or by an antigenic formula; neither is italicized. Thus, *Salmonella enterica* serotype Typhimurium is often shortened to *Salmonella* Typhimurium or, after introducing the genus name, to serotype Typhimurium.

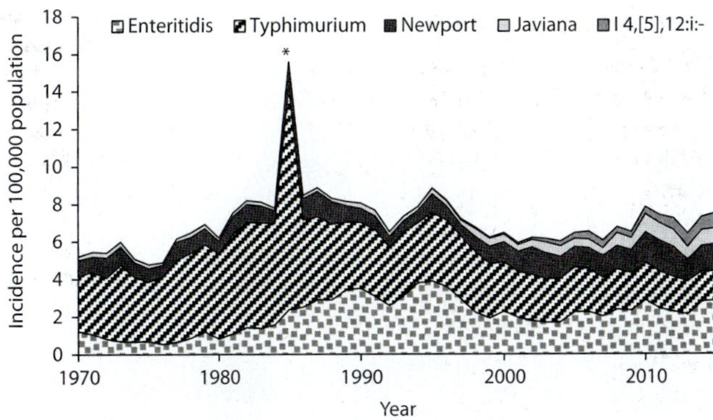

FIGURE 111-3. Incidence of culture confirmed salmonellosis cases reported to laboratory-based enteric disease surveillance system by year for the five most common serotypes, United States, 1970–2015.[16] *In 1985 a multistate outbreak of *Salmonella* Typhimurium in milk occurred, and accounted for over 16,000 cases.[52]

little variation in their regional distribution and have been associated with widely distributed food vehicles such as poultry, eggs, and pork, whereas Javiana is most commonly reported in the Southeastern region of the United States, where it has been associated with contact with amphibians and the presence of wetlands, indicating a possible ecological niche.[20,21]

The population groups most likely to have salmonellosis are similar across the serotypes. Risk is highest among children under the age of 5 and adults 70 and older. Risk of infection may increase after a course of antibiotics, which can alter the gut flora.[22] The proportion hospitalized is highest in the older population.[23] Serious outcomes, such as septicemia and death, are most common among young children, older adults, and those with compromised immune responses.

SURVEILLANCE

National *Salmonella* surveillance data are collected through multiple systems, which capture different information. Reports of diagnosed cases at the local level (city, county, state, or territory) are often investigated and are compiled to estimate the incidence and changes over time. Cases are detected when a patient's specimen yields *Salmonella* by culture or is positive by CIDT. The diagnosed case is reported to the local public health department, and if possible, an isolate or, in the case of diagnosis by CIDT without a reflex culture, a patient specimen is forwarded to the public health department laboratory. State public health laboratories culture the specimen if necessary, and perform confirmatory testing, serotyping, and additional characterization such as whole genome sequencing. Case reports are compiled by the National Notifiable Diseases Surveillance System (NNDSS), a passive system that includes both laboratory-confirmed and probable salmonellosis cases, but that does not capture serotype or subtyping data.[24] Because some cases may not be reported in passive surveillance, an enhanced network, CDC's Foodborne Diseases Active Surveillance Network (FoodNet), supports ten representative sentinel sites to seek and gather reports of all laboratory-confirmed salmonellosis cases.[25]

Public health laboratory-based surveillance, based on serotype and additional subtyping, has been vital since the 1960s to help find widespread outbreaks and track them to their sources. The Laboratory-based Enteric Disease Surveillance system, LEDS, and its predecessor systems have gathered and summarized serotype results since the 1960s.[3] Beginning in 1996, state and large city public health laboratories have participated in the national network for molecular subtyping, known as PulseNet. PulseNet also includes federal food safety agency laboratories, and has been the key to finding and stopping many widespread and large outbreaks of salmonellosis and other enteric bacterial infections.[26] In 2018, PulseNet began switching to the more advanced whole genome sequencing methodology, which promises to provide even greater resolution than the previous method used—pulsed-field gel electrophoresis.[27] In addition, also beginning in 1996, state public health laboratories have referred a subset of 1 in 20 *Salmonella* case isolates to be tested against a standard panel of antibiotics to monitor trends in antibiotic resistance as part of the National Antimicrobial Resistance Monitoring System for Enteric bacteria (NARMS).[28] As part of NARMS, *Salmonella* isolates from retail food samples and food animals are collected by the Food and Drug Administration (FDA) and U.S. Department of Agriculture (USDA), Food Safety and Inspection Service (FSIS), to help track trends and sources of antimicrobial resistance in *Salmonella* and other enteric bacteria.

In addition to surveillance for individual cases, the National Outbreak Reporting System (NORS) collects and compiles information from state and local health departments on enteric disease outbreaks along with the multistate outbreak investigations coordinated by the CDC.[29] This includes salmonellosis and outbreaks caused by other pathogens, and includes reports of outbreaks due to foodborne, waterborne, animal contact, and person-to-person transmission.

TRANSMISSION

Salmonella can be transmitted through contaminated food or water, through contact with animals or their environment, or, less often, from one person to another. *Salmonella* is commonly found in the intestinal tract of mammals, birds, amphibians, and reptiles, and is also found in the environment. *Salmonella* can multiply in many moist environments, and can persist in a dry environment for years.[30] Consequently, salmonellosis has been linked to an extremely broad range of transmission modes and vehicles.

A serotype's common transmission routes can be identified using exposure data from outbreak investigations in which multiple individuals report the same exposure source. Exposures among sporadic cases can also be used to identify transmission routes through case-control studies. In the United States, approximately 81% of *Salmonella* outbreaks with an identified source that occurred from 2009 to 2014 were attributed to contaminated food, followed by 11% from animal contact, 8% person-to-person, and fewer than 1% from water or the environment.[29] Case-control studies have identified travel and consumption of chicken as the highest risk exposures in cases of sporadic illness compared with all other exposures, including contaminated water and animal contact.[31]

Food

The majority of salmonellosis cases are thought to be caused by foodborne transmission. Based on U.S. foodborne outbreak surveillance data from 1998 to 2013, the most common food sources were "seeded vegetables" (e.g., tomatoes and cucumbers), eggs, chicken, pork, beef, and fruit (Fig. 111-4).[32] Some serotypes are commonly associated with one food item (e.g., *S.* Enteritidis and eggs) and others may be associated with several food items.[33]

Contamination of animal-derived foods can occur during slaughter, production, processing, or any time when food comes into contact with fecal matter. Meat can become contaminated by transfer of feces from intestines, hides, or feathers during the slaughter process. Milk can be contaminated by feces or inapparent udder infections in cows. Eggs can harbor *Salmonella* internally as a result of transovarian (vertical) transmission as the egg forms inside the hen or be contaminated on the shell as they are laid. Produce can be contaminated during cultivation from manure used as fertilizer or contributed by wild animals and birds. Water used for irrigation, pesticide applications, or washing and cooling steps can introduce and spread

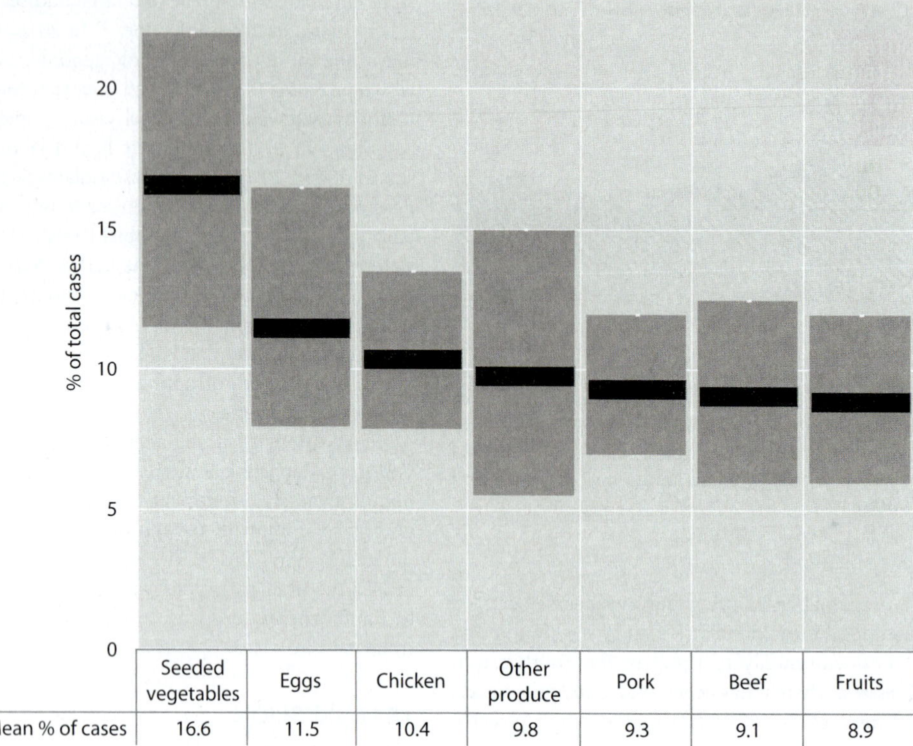

FIGURE 111-4. Top food categories identified as the source of salmonellosis outbreaks in 2013 in the United States, and the associated estimated percentage (black bar; 90% credible interval dark gray bar) of salmonellosis cases attributed to each food category. These top categories account for 75.4% of all outbreak-associated salmonellosis cases in 2013.[32] Data from Interagency *Food Safety Analytics Collaboration. Foodborne Illness Source Attribution Estimates for 2013 for Salmonella, Escherichia coli O157, Listeria monocytogenes, and Campylobacter Using Multi-Year Outbreak Surveillance Data, United States*. GA and D.C.: Available from: https://www.cdc.gov/foodsafety/pdfs/IFSAC-2013FoodborneillnessSourceEstimates-508.pdf.

contamination. Processed foods like precooked roast beef, pasteurized milk, and peanut butter can be contaminated if processing or postprocessing sanitation is inadequate. Food prepared by someone working with raw meat or poultry can be cross-contaminated with meat juices, and food prepared by someone who has *Salmonella* in the feces can be directly contaminated. Human illness results when contaminated foods are consumed raw or lightly cooked, or when cooked foods are recontaminated after cooking.

Water

Waterborne outbreaks of salmonellosis are extremely rare. A large waterborne outbreak occurred after an untreated municipal water system was contaminated, possibly by birds in water towers.[34] It is also possible that sporadic cases of salmonellosis result from ingesting untreated, improperly treated, or contaminated water, though such occurrences have not been well documented.[31]

Zoonotic

Salmonella infection can result from occupational, recreational, or household contact with animals. Household pets such as dogs, cats, and birds have transmitted *Salmonella* to humans, and recently, backyard poultry have caused recurrent large outbreaks.[35] Reptiles and amphibians including turtles, iguanas, frogs, and bearded dragons have also caused outbreaks and numerous sporadic cases. In fact, in the early 1970s, until their sale was banned, approximately 14% of salmonellosis cases in the United States were attributed to small pet turtles.[36] Severe outcomes, such as meningitis and soft-tissue abscesses, have more frequently been linked to reptiles than to food, specifically in young children.[37] Animals may shed the bacteria in their feces whether or not they are symptomatic, and can contaminate the environment, leading to indirect transmission. Animals may become infected through contaminated feed or their environment.

Person-to-Person

Salmonella can be transmitted person-to-person via direct contact with infected feces or through contact with contaminated surfaces. This risk is likely highest among household members of or those who care for persons in diapers (i.e., children and incontinent adults). Persons with salmonellosis may contaminate food they prepare, or transmit the infection to an infant or high-risk patient; therefore, many jurisdictions exclude food handlers, patient caregivers, and childcare workers while they are ill with salmonellosis. The period of greatest communicability lasts for the duration of diarrhea. Some patients experience relapsing bouts of diarrhea.[9] Approximately 45% of children under the age of 5 and up to 6% of patients over 5 years old shed the bacteria three months after symptoms begin, depending on the serotype.[38]

SPECIAL SETTINGS

Salmonellosis outbreaks are typically associated with consumption of a contaminated food product; the settings in which clusters of persons were exposed to the pathogen are commonly facilities where many people are served the same food item at approximately the same time or restaurants using the same food source. The type of facility can dictate if further transmission to secondary cases is likely to occur, and which control measures are most effective.

Restaurants

Approximately 48% of *Salmonella* foodborne outbreaks with an identified setting that occurred in 2009–16 were the result of an exposure in a restaurant (Table 111-2).[29] During an investigation of a suspected outbreak, finding one restaurant or chain of restaurants where multiple cases reported eating can be an important lead in finding the source of contamination. For instance, in 2014 multiple people infected with serotype Newport had eaten at seven restaurants, six of which received cucumbers from the same distributor. The distributor received cucumbers from several produce brokers, and each of the brokers identified the same single farm, leading investigators to believe the source of contamination was on the farm.[39] In another instance, an unusual strain of *Salmonella* Enteritidis had caused a series of restaurant outbreaks, but was controlled after it was shown

TABLE 111-2 COMMON SETTINGS* OF SALMONELLA OUTBREAKS, THE CORRESPONDING NUMBER OF OUTBREAKS, RELATIVE FREQUENCY OF SETTING, AND MEDIAN NUMBER OF ILLNESSES, 2009–2014, UNITED STATES[29]

Setting	Number of Outbreaks	% of Outbreaks	Median Number Ill
Restaurant/Caterer	305	50.0	9.0
Private home	171	28.0	8.0
School/Camp/Daycare	59	9.6	4.0
Healthcare/Correctional	44	7.2	6.0
Grocery store	19	3.1	8.0
Fair/Festival	14	2.3	12.5

*Does not include outbreaks in which no setting was identified/reported, the setting was unknown, or when multiple settings were reported ($n = 547$).

that all the affected restaurants, but not others in the same area, got their eggs from the same source farm.[40]

Careful interviews of cases based on the menus, determination of the ingredients in each item, and kitchen inspections can all contribute to the investigation; testing food handlers for the pathogen may identify some infected, likely because they were exposed to the implicated food themselves. In some instances, improper hygiene among food handlers or cross contamination in the kitchen may be why contamination occurred in the kitchen, but more frequently, the food items were contaminated at some point between the farm and delivery to the restaurant. Recalls of food items associated with case clusters or outbreaks are shared with the food-service industry, and it is expected that these items will then be disposed of to prevent further transmission, and that customers who were served will be informed of the possible exposure and advised to seek medical care if symptoms arise.

Institutional

Settings where many people gather with close or lengthy contact, often eating the same foods and sharing bathrooms, can pose a risk for *Salmonella* transmission. This is especially a concern when the population is already at higher risk for salmonellosis and for severe outcomes from it (e.g., the elderly and the immunocompromised). These types of settings can include nursing homes, hospitals, daycare centers, and correctional facilities (Table 111-2). Settings such as military bases and children's camps can pose a risk for transmission for the same reasons, but the populations in these settings are not likely to be in high-risk groups. Secondary cases can occur when an ill individual spreads the pathogen to others by contaminating surfaces and through unhygienic behaviors. From 2009 to 2014, CDC received reports of 84 outbreaks in institutional settings, and 52 of these outbreaks were attributed to person-to-person transmission.

PREVENTION

There is no human vaccine for salmonellosis. Understanding pathways of transmission well enough to prevent transmission has been critical to reducing the risk of infection. Specific measures and technologies have controlled some salmonellosis risk, but the overall infection rate has not declined in recent years, so additional prevention measures are warranted.[41] Foodborne salmonellosis can be prevented with measures taken from the farm through food processing to the final kitchen, or farm-to-table. Measures taken on the farm can reduce the likelihood that food animals are themselves infected, and reduce the risk that fresh produce is contaminated from animal waste. In slaughter plants, careful attention to sanitation and specific measures that reduce the microbial load on meat and poultry are important to prevention. In food processing, principles of good manufacturing, and hazard control should be standard. In the final kitchen, the basic principles of food safety apply, and are the last food-safety step. Throughout the food chain, a culture of food safety can encourage all participants to recognize the role that they play in keeping foods safe.

It often takes multiple prevention efforts to make a food safe and keep it safe. Grade A pasteurized milk, for example, represents the product of a series of prevention measures. To qualify as grade A, milk must be produced by healthy cows that are milked in dairy parlors that meet strict standards of hygiene, and the milk must be tested for white blood cells, an indicator of infection in the cows' udders. Only grade A milk is pasteurized, to specific combinations of time and temperature required to kill even the hardiest pathogens. Finally, the pasteurized milk is transported and delivered in sealed containers held under constant refrigeration. However, outbreaks and illnesses can occur when a step in this basic preventive system is bypassed.[42]

On the farm, animals may be infected with *Salmonella*, and are sometimes made ill themselves. The prevention and control of *Salmonella* on the farm requires "good agricultural practices" or GAPS, such as providing uncontaminated drinking water, maintaining sanitation, isolating ill animals, and vaccinating them against specific strains. Animals ill with invasive infections can contaminate the food supply and need to be excluded from it.[43] Rodents can harbor *Salmonella* of many types, and rodent control is an important prevention strategy.

At processing, food animals often carry *Salmonella* in their intestines and on their skins when they arrive at a slaughter plant. Until the late 1990s, most slaughter inspection was focused on finding and excluding animals with visible illness. A new strategy based on Hazard Analysis—Critical Control Point (HACCP) was then introduced by the USDA's FSIS to reduce invisible microbial contamination of meat and poultry. HACCP applies safety engineering to food safety. Likely sources of contamination of the food product are identified, and specific steps are taken at key points to reduce that likelihood. HACCP is often combined with systematic product sampling to verify that the pathogen reduction measures are working.

Preventing contamination on the farm and during processing is important for fresh fruits and vegetables that may be eaten without further cooking.[44] On produce farms, GAPs can reduce the likelihood of contamination by avoiding fecally tainted irrigation water, not using uncomposted manure as fertilizer, and by keeping wild animals out of the fields. Washing and chilling produce can be problematic, as wash water can be readily contaminated unless levels of chlorine in the wash tanks are carefully maintained. Even water temperature is important, as some fruits and vegetables coming warm from the field and plunged in to cold water will rapidly draw water into their interiors, along with any contaminants in the water.[45] New produce safety regulations developed by the Food and Drug Administration under the Food Safety Modernization Act of 2011 (FSMA) are now being implemented, and are likely to improve produce safety and decrease the frequency of produce-related outbreaks.

Eggs have been a particularly frequent source of salmonellosis. Two mechanisms of contamination lead to two especially important prevention strategies. The first is external contamination, as the egg is laid and comes in contact with the hen's feces. Following outbreaks of egg-associated salmonellosis in the 1960s, systematic procedures for washing, disinfecting, and inspecting eggs were mandated.[3] The result of these mandated changes is the grade A egg, and such outbreaks are now rare, though they still can occur when application is slipshod. The second mechanism is transovarial internal contamination, when *Salmonella* present around the hen's ovarian tissues contaminate the yolk as it forms, resulting in a normal-looking but contaminated egg. If the egg is fertile, the chick that hatches from it grows up to lay infected eggs herself. If the egg is eaten, then *Salmonella* can infect the hapless consumer who likes eggs with runny yolks or foods made with raw eggs. Serotypes that can spread by this means (Enteritidis, and to a lesser degree Typhimurium and Heidelberg) caused numerous outbreaks in the 1980s and the 1990s related to grade A eggs. Prevention of these infections depends on measures that reduce infection in the laying flocks, on testing those flocks for those *Salmonella* strains, and diverting eggs from flocks with *Salmonella* to further processing. Eggs can be pasteurized in bulk or in the shell; using pasteurized eggs is a major safety measure in high-risk locations such as nursing homes and hospitals. Refrigerating eggs during transport, sale, and storage keeps *Salmonella* inside an egg from growing, and educating chefs and the public on the hazard of raw egg dishes can reduce risk.

A variety of processed foods caused outbreaks after breaks in sanitation introduced *Salmonella*; fruit juices, peanut butter, and imported spices are just a few of the foods that have repeatedly been sources of outbreaks. Fruit juice can be pasteurized, and HACCP principles apply to these foods as well as to meat and poultry.[46] Pathogen contamination can also be reduced by technologies such as high-pressure processing, radio-frequency heating of dry foods, and irradiation. The new Preventive Controls Rule and Imported Foods Rule promulgated by the FDA after FSMA may reduce the frequency of these contamination events.

In the kitchen, prevention starts with the basic rules of food safety, including refrigeration of perishable meat, poultry, eggs, and milk, thorough cooking of meat, poultry, and eggs, preventing cross contamination by keeping raw foods of animal origin well separated from fresh produce, holding hot foods hot and cold foods cold, and careful attention to hand hygiene. A food service manager trained in the principles of food safety can reduce the risk of outbreaks in a commercial kitchen. Restaurant inspections by the health department can help make sure the facility is clean, properly equipped, and that the kitchen staff are properly trained.

Routine disinfection of drinking and swimming water eliminates the risk of waterborne transmission, as *Salmonella* is inactivated by even low levels of chlorine.

Pets can carry *Salmonella* into the home, particularly reptiles, amphibians, and birds. After the popular small pet turtle was estimated to account for 14% of all salmonellosis in the United States, particularly affecting small children, the sale of these turtles was banned. This measure reduced illnesses from these attractive but dangerous pets substantially, and remains in place today.[47] However, outbreaks traced to illegally sold turtles show that the risk is still present.[48] Exotic reptiles are also likely to harbor salmonella, though are not as likely to be given to small children to play with; avoiding them as pets in households with small children, and careful handwashing after contact can help prevent reptile-associated salmonellosis.[49] The growing popularity of backyard chickens has brought the farmyard to many suburbs, and caused many cases of salmonellosis.[50] A multitiered prevention strategy includes hatchery hygiene to prevent chicks from being colonized, sanitation in the stores where chicks are sold, and educating the new chicken owner on how to avoid getting *Salmonella*.[50]

Humans themselves can on occasion serve as sources of salmonellosis. It is prudent to exclude persons ill with *Salmonella* infections from working in high risk settings such as hospitals, nursing homes, restaurants, and day-care centers. However, the risk of transmission from the asymptomatic shedder is low, and does not justify routine periodic stool cultures of food handlers or healthcare providers.[51] The spread of salmonellosis from ill salmonellosis patients in hospitals can be prevented with routine enteric precautions, such as strict handwashing, and other basic tenets of infection control, as well as attention to food-safety efforts in the kitchen.

FURTHER RESOURCES

CDC information on salmonellosis: https://www.cdc.gov/salmonella/index.html

WHO and Institut Pasteur antigenic formulae guidelines: https://www.pasteur.fr/sites/default/files/veng_0.pdf

CDC Atlas of *Salmonella* serotypes: https://www.cdc.gov/salmonella/pdf/salmonella-atlas-508c.pdf

References

1. Scallan E, Hoekstra RM, Angulo FJ, et al. Foodborne illness acquired in the United States—Major pathogens. *Emerg Infect Dis.* 2011;17(1):7–15.
2. Centers for Disease Control and Prevention. *Surveillance for foodborne disease outbreaks, United States, 2015: Annual Report.* https://www.cdc.gov/foodsafety/pdfs/2015FoodBorneOutbreaks_508.pdf.
3. Centers for Disease Control and Prevention. Proceedings of the National Conference on Salmonellosis. Atlanta, GA, 1964.
4. Brooks JT, Matyas BT, Fontana J, et al. An outbreak of *Salmonella* serotype Typhimurium infections with an unusually long incubation period. *Foodborne Pathog Dis.* 2012;9(3):245–8.
5. Levine WC, Buehler JW, Bean NH, et al. Epidemiology of nontyphoidal *Salmonella* bacteremia during the human immunodeficiency virus epidemic. *J Infect Dis.* 1991;164(1):81–7.
6. Jones TF, Ingram LA, Cieslak PR, et al. Salmonellosis outcomes differ substantially by serotype. *J Infect Dis.* 2008;198(1):109–14.
7. Shane AL, Mody RK, Crump JA, et al. 2017 Infectious Diseases Society of America Clinical Practice Guidelines for the diagnosis and management of infectious diarrhea. *Clin Infect Dis.* 2017;65(12):e45–80.
8. Onwuezobe IA, Oshun PO, Odigwe CC. Antimicrobials for treating symptomatic non-typhoidal *Salmonella* infection. *Cochrane Database Syst Rev.* 2012;11:Cd001167.
9. Marzel A, Desai PT, Goren A, et al. Persistent infections by nontyphoidal *Salmonella* in humans: Epidemiology and genetics. *Clin Infect Dis.* 2016;62(7):879–86.
10. Medalla F, Gu W, Mahon BE, et al. Estimated incidence of antimicrobial drug-resistant nontyphoidal *Salmonella* infections, United States, 2004–2012. *Emerg Infect Dis.* 2016;23(1):29–37.
11. Silverman M, Zieg J, Hilmen M, et al. Phase variation in *Salmonella*: Genetic analysis of a recombinational switch. *Proc Natl Acad Sci U S A.* 1979;76(1):391–5.
12. McQuiston JR, Fields PI, Tauxe RV, et al. Do *Salmonella* carry spare tyres? *Trends Microbiol.* 2008;16(4):142–8.
13. Zhang S, Yin Y, Jones MB, et al. *Salmonella* serotype determination utilizing high-throughput genome sequencing data. *J Clin Microbiol.* 2015;53(5):1685–92.
14. Grimont PAD, Weill FX. *Antigenic formulae of the Salmonella serovars, 2007.* https://www.pasteur.fr/sites/default/files/veng_0.pdf.
15. Michael GB, Schwarz S. Antimicrobial resistance in zoonotic nontyphoidal *Salmonella*: an alarming trend? *Clin Microbiol Infect.* 2016;22(12):968–74.
16. Centers for Disease Control and Prevention. *Salmonella Annual Report, 2016.* https://www.cdc.gov/nationalsurveillance/pdfs/2016-Salmonella-report-508.pdf.
17. Centers for Disease Control and Prevention. FoodNet Fast. 2017 [cited 2018 May 10, 2018]. https://wwwn.cdc.gov/foodnetfast/.
18. Boore AL, Hoekstra RM, Iwamoto M, et al. *Salmonella enterica* infections in the United States and assessment of coefficients of variation: A novel approach to identify epidemiologic characteristics of individual serotypes, 1996–2011. *PLoS One.* 2015;10(12):e0145416.
19. Powell MR, Crim SM, Hoekstra RM, et al. Temporal patterns in principal *Salmonella* serotypes in the USA; 1996–2014. *Epidemiol Infect.* 2018;146(4):437–41.
20. Huang JY, Patrick ME, Manners J, et al. Association between wetland presence and incidence of *Salmonella enterica* serotype Javiana infections in selected US sites, 2005–2011. *Epidemiol Infect.* 2017;145(14):2991–7.
21. Srikantiah P, Lay JC, Hand S, et al. *Salmonella enterica* serotype Javiana infections associated with amphibian contact, Mississippi, 2001. *Epidemiol Infect.* 2004;132(2):273–81.
22. Gradel KO, Dethlefsen C, Ejlertsen T, et al. Increased prescription rate of antibiotics prior to non-typhoid *Salmonella* infections: A one-year nested case-control study. *Scand J Infect Dis.* 2008;40(8):635–41.
23. Centers for Disease Control and Prevention. *FoodNet 2015 Surveillance Report.* https://www.cdc.gov/foodnet/pdfs/FoodNet-Annual-Report-2015-508c.pdf.

24. Council for State and Territorial Epidemiologists. *Public Health Reporting and National Notification for Salmonellosis.* http://c.ymcdn.com/sites/www.cste.org/resource/resmgr/PS/11-ID-08.pdf.
25. Centers for Disease Control and Prevention. *Salmonella Surveillance Overview.* Atlanta, Georgia. https://www.cdc.gov/nationalsurveillance/pdfs/NationalSalmSurveillOverview_508.pdf.
26. Tauxe RV. Molecular subtyping and the transformation of public health. *Foodborne Pathog Dis.* 2006;3(1):4–8.
27. Jackso n BR, Tarr C, Strain E, et al. Implementation of nationwide real-time whole-genome sequencing to enhance listeriosis outbreak detection and investigation. *Clin Infect Dis.* 2016;63(3):380–6.
28. Karp BE, Tate H, Plumblee JR, et al. National Antimicrobial Resistance Monitoring System: Two decades of advancing public health through integrated surveillance of antimicrobial resistance. *Foodborne Pathog Dis.* 2017;14(10):545–57.
29. Centers for Disease Control and Prevention. National Outbreak Reporting System Dashboard. 2017 [cited 2018 May 8, 2018]. https://wwwn.cdc.gov/norsdashboard/.
30. Burgess CM, Gianotti A, Gruzdev N, et al. The response of foodborne pathogens to osmotic and desiccation stresses in the food chain. *Int J Food Microbiol.* 2016;221:37–53.
31. Domingues AR, Pires SM, Halasa T, et al. Source attribution of human salmonellosis using a meta-analysis of case-control studies of sporadic infections. *Epidemiol Infect.* 2012;140(6):959–69.
32. Interagency Food Safety Analytics Collaboration. *Foodborne Illness Source Attribution Estimates for 2013 for Salmonella, Escherichia coli O157, Listeria monocytogenes, and Campylobacter Using Multi-Year Outbreak Surveillance Data, United States.* GA and D.C. https://www.cdc.gov/foodsafety/pdfs/IFSAC-2013FoodborneillnessSourceEstimates-508.pdf.
33. Jackson BR, Griffin PM, Cole D, et al. Outbreak-associated *Salmonella enterica* serotypes and food commodities, United States, 1998–2008. *Emerg Infect Dis.* 2013;19(8):1239–44.
34. Angulo FJ, Tippen S, Sharp DJ, et al. A community waterborne outbreak of salmonellosis and the effectiveness of a boil water order. *Am J Public Health.* 1997;87(4):580–4.
35. Basler C, Nguyen T-A, Anderson TC, et al. Outbreaks of human salmonella infections associated with live poultry, United States, 1990–2014. *Emerg Infect Dis.* 2016;22(10):1705–11.
36. Lamm SH, Taylor JA, Gangarosa EJ, et al. Turtle-associated salmonellosis I. An estimation of the magnitude of the problem in the United States, 1970–1971. *Am J Epidemiol.* 1972;95(6):511–7.
37. Hoelzer K, Moreno Switt AI, Wiedmann M. Animal contact as a source of human non-typhoidal salmonellosis. *Vet Res.* 2011;42:34.
38. Buchwald DS, Blaser MJ. A review of human salmonellosis: II. Duration of excretion following infection with nontyphi Salmonella. *Rev Infect Dis.* 1984;6(3):345–56.
39. Angelo KM, Chu A, Anand M, et al. Outbreak of *Salmonella* Newport infections linked to cucumbers—United States, 2014. *MMWR Morb Mortal Wkly Rep.* 2015;64(6):144–7.
40. Sobel J, Hirshfeld AB, McTigue K, et al. The pandemic of *Salmonella enteritidis* phage type 4 reaches Utah: A complex investigation confirms the need for continuing rigorous control measures. *Epidemiol Infect.* 2000;125(1):1–8.
41. Marder EP, Cieslak PR, Cronquist AB, et al. Incidence and trends of infections with pathogens transmitted commonly through food and the effect of increasing use of culture-independent diagnostic tests on surveillance—Foodborne Diseases Active Surveillance Network, 10 U.S. Sites, 2013–2016. *MMWR Morb Mortal Wkly Rep.* 2017;66:397–403.
42. Langer AJ, Ayers T, Grass J, et al. Nonpasteurized dairy products, disease outbreaks, and state laws—United States, 1993–2006. *Emerg Infect Dis.* 2012;18(3):385–91.
43. Su LH, Wu TL, Chiu CH. Decline of *Salmonella enterica* serotype Choleraesuis infections, Taiwan. *Emerg Infect Dis.* 2014;20(4):715–6.
44. Lynch MF, Tauxe RV, Hedberg CW. The growing burden of foodborne outbreaks due to contaminated fresh produce: Risks and opportunities. *Epidemiol Infect.* 2009;137(3):307–15.
45. Penteado AL, Eblen BS, Miller AJ. Evidence of *Salmonella* internalization into fresh mangos during simulated postharvest insect disinfestation procedures. *J Food Prot.* 2004;67(1):181–4.
46. Vojdani JD, Beuchat LR, Tauxe RV. Juice-associated outbreaks of human illness in the United States, 1995 through 2005. *J Food Prot.* 2008;71(2):356–64.
47. Cohen ML, Potter M, Pollard R, et al. Turtle-associated salmonellosis in the United States. Effect of Public Health Action, 1970 to 1976. *JAMA.* 1980;243(12):1247–9.
48. Bosch S, Tauxe RV, Behravesh CB. Turtle-associated salmonellosis, United States, 2006–2014. *Emerg Infect Dis.* 2016;22(7):1149–55.
49. Friedman CR, Torigian C, Shillam PJ, et al. An outbreak of salmonellosis among children attending a reptile exhibit at a zoo. *J Pediatr.* 1998;132(5):802–7.
50. Behravesh CB, Brinson D, Hopkins BA, et al. Backyard poultry flocks and salmonellosis: A recurring, yet preventable public health challenge. *Clin Infect Dis.* 2014;58(10):1432–8.
51. Tauxe RV, Hassan LF, Findeisen KO, et al. Salmonellosis in nurses: Lack of transmission to patients. *J Infect Dis.* 1988;157(2):370–3.
52. Ryan CA, Nickels MK, Hargrett-Bean NT, et al. Massive outbreak of antimicrobial-resistant salmonellosis traced to pasteurized milk. *JAMA.* 1987;258(22):3269–74.

CHAPTER

112 Cholera*

Rupa Narra • Maryann Turnsek • William Davis • Eric Mintz

Cholera is an acute infection of the small intestine caused by fecal-oral transmission of the toxigenic bacterium *Vibrio cholerae* serogroup O1 or O139. In individual patients, cholera presents with the sudden onset of profuse watery diarrhea that can rapidly lead to dehydration and death. In epidemic form, cholera can spread rapidly through entire countries, filling hospitals, cholera treatment centers, and cemeteries. Despite our knowledge of cholera epidemiology, microbiology, and its clinical management, and our success in protecting populations in many countries from epidemic cholera, it remains a major public health concern in Africa, Asia, and the Americas, where populations with limited access to safe drinking water and sanitation continue to suffer cholera illnesses, hospitalizations, and deaths.

Today, cholera is at a crossroads. The current and seventh cholera pandemic, which began in 1961, has lasted far longer and spread further than any of its six predecessors. Climate change, population growth, and armed conflict all have the potential to increase the risk for epidemic cholera. However, recent developments in cholera vaccination, low-cost technologies for improved access to water, sanitation, and hygiene, and the growing capacity to collect, analyze, and map data, could enable us to rapidly reduce that risk. In 2018, the World Health Assembly endorsed "Ending Cholera—A Global Roadmap to 2030," an ambitious initiative to reduce cholera deaths by 90% and to end cholera as a public health threat in 20 countries by 2030.[1] If it succeeds, the end of the seventh cholera pandemic, and perhaps of cholera as a public health threat worldwide, could be within reach.

AGENT AND DIAGNOSIS

Vibrio cholerae is a curved, motile, aerobic Gram-negative bacterium classified principally by serogroup based on the somatic O antigen.[2] It survives as a free-living environmental microorganism in brackish surface waters. Although over 200 serogroups exist, only toxigenic *V. cholerae* serogroups O1 and O139 cause widespread epidemic and pandemic disease. Strains of *V. cholerae* O1 and O139 that do not produce cholera toxin may be isolated from persons with sporadic cases of acute watery diarrhea, but have not caused large epidemics.[2] *V. cholerae* serogroup O1 is classified into two biotypes—classical and El Tor; the biotypes are further classified by serotype—Inaba, Ogawa and, rarely, Hikojima.

Isolation and identification of *V. cholerae* serogroup O1 or O139 from stool or rectal swabs is necessary for the confirmation of cholera.[3] Fecal specimens should be collected from clinically suspect patients prior to treatment with antibiotics, preferably within 4 days after the onset of illness. Specimens can be transported to a reference laboratory at ambient temperature and should be preserved in Cary-Blair transport media if they cannot be processed within 2 hours after collection.[4] In field conditions, use of filter paper as a transport medium for stool specimens is an acceptable alternative to Cary-Blair and can be as effective for the recovery and diagnosis of cholera.[5,6] Traditionally, culture-based tests have been the gold standard method of identification. Specimens are directly plated onto a selective media such as thiosulfate citrate, bile salts, sucrose agar and incubated overnight. Growth suspicious for *V. cholerae*—shiny, yellow colonies with a slightly raised center, 2–4 mm in diameter—are subcultured to nonselective growth media, such as heart infusion agar or Mueller Hinton agar, and incubated overnight before performing the confirmatory slide agglutination test with polyvalent O1 and O139 antisera. Pre-enrichment in alkaline peptone water will increase the number of organisms present in the specimen and is the recommended first step for isolation in specimens from convalescent patients and asymptomatic carriers.[7] Molecular tests, such as polymerase chain reaction (PCR), have gained acceptance as an alternative to culture for identification and characterization of *V. cholerae* O1 and O139.[8–11] Confirmed *V. cholerae* O1 or O139 isolates should be tested by PCR for cholera toxin gene sequences (*ctxAB*), since this is invariably present in epidemigenic strains.[6,12] Commercially available rapid diagnostic tests are a useful surveillance tool but do not replace stool culture or PCR to confirm cholera due to variation in their performance.[13]

HISTORY

The first known appearance of the Sanskrit word for cholera is in the Sushruta Samhita, estimated to be written in 500–400 BC. Soon afterward, a cholera-like illness was described in Athens by Hippocrates. Descriptions of diarrhea epidemics in India in the late fifteenth century suggest that the Bengal region of India and Bangladesh was a continuous endemic region for cholera.[14,15]

The worldwide spread of cholera began in 1817, and by 1823 the first pandemic of cholera had spread from the Ganges River delta to much of Asia and Africa. Five periods of pandemic spread occurred before 1900: from 1817 to 1823; from 1826 to 1837; from 1846 to 1862; from 1864 to 1875; and from 1887 to 1896. John Snow's observations on the waterborne transmission of cholera were from the third and fourth pandemics, and Robert Koch accurately described the cholera bacillus during the fifth pandemic. During these early pandemics, thousands of people were sickened in affected countries, with reported case fatality rates (CFRs) often approaching 50%.

The sixth pandemic (1902–23) also involved severe epidemics, especially in Asia, but outbreaks in Africa and Europe were more limited than in previous pandemics, and the Western Hemisphere

*The findings and conclusions in this chapter are those of the authors and do not necessarily represent the official position of the Centers for Disease Control and Prevention.

was not involved. The sixth pandemic and the second pandemic are known to be caused by the classical biotype of *V. cholerae*; presumably, other pandemics before 1900 were as well.[16] This biotype decreased in frequency of isolation in the 1960s and has largely disappeared except in Bangladesh, where it reemerged in epidemic form in 1982.[17]

The seventh pandemic, which is generally considered to have started in 1961, is ongoing and shows no signs of slowing down, with genetic evidence of three independent, but temporally overlapping waves of transmission.[18] The causative agent of this pandemic was first isolated in 1905 by Gotchlich from pilgrims returning from Mecca at the El Tor quarantine camp in Egypt. Although this organism was initially considered nonpathogenic, outbreaks of severe disease between 1937 and 1958 confirmed its ability to cause epidemics.[19] An outbreak caused by *V. cholerae* biotype El Tor in Sulawesi in 1961 was the beginning of the seventh pandemic. From there it quickly spread to Java, Sarawak, Borneo, the Philippines, and most of Southeast Asia; in 1962, the El Tor biotype of *Vibrio cholerae* was recognized by WHO as a cause of cholera. Between 1963 and 1969, this organism continued its spread across the Asian mainland, eventually replacing classical *V. cholerae*. In 1970, the pandemic continued its westward progression through the Middle East and the Soviet Union, resulting in major outbreaks in Spain, Portugal, and Italy. From 1970 to the present, nearly all countries in sub-Saharan Africa have been affected by cholera outbreaks, and with few exceptions, it is the region with the highest cholera burden reported to WHO each year.[20]

North America had no indigenous cases of cholera in the twentieth century until a single case was detected in Texas in 1973. Five years later, a case investigation in Louisiana ultimately detected infection in 11 persons.[21] In this outbreak, *V. cholerae* O1, biotype El Tor, serotype Inaba was recovered from sewage and canal water and from crabs, which were implicated as the vehicle of infection. In 1981, cholera was found in two residents of the Gulf Coast of Texas and another 16 persons on an oil rig in the gulf near Texas. Investigations of these outbreaks determined that they were due to the same unique strain of *V. cholerae* that apparently persisted in the environment.[22] This observation and other evidence have led to the conclusion that cholera is indigenous to the Gulf Coast area of the United States, where the organism has a persistent environmental reservoir. In 1983, a U.S. tourist apparently became infected with *V. cholerae* while visiting the Caribbean coast of Mexico and developed cholera after returning home. The strain causing this infection was the same as the U.S. Gulf Coast strains, and subsequent cases have supported the hypothesis that the environmental reservoir also runs south around the Gulf of Mexico.[23] It appears that Australia also has a similar environmental reservoir, in this case freshwater rivers instead of brackish water of the Gulf estuaries, resulting in a small number of cases and small outbreaks.

Latin America was spared from cholera epidemics in the twentieth century until January 1991, when cholera appeared in Peru.[24,25] The outbreak, which began in several cities along the Pacific coast, subsequently spread throughout Peru, and to 14 other countries within the year. By the end of 1992, over 745,000 cholera cases and 6300 cholera deaths had been reported from 21 countries in North, Central, and South America. The source of the initial contamination is unknown, but subsequent transmission was shown to be related to both water and foods.[24,26,27] The epidemic never reached the Caribbean, and ended soon after the turn of the century, with regional CFRs never exceeding 1%.[28,29] Interestingly, the investments in improved access to safe water and sanitation spurred by epidemic cholera, led to documented improvements in infant mortality and decreases in other waterborne and foodborne diseases in certain countries.[30–32]

All known cholera pandemics have been due to *V. cholerae* serogroup O1, although other toxigenic serogroups, such as O75 and O141 have caused sporadic cases of cholera-like illness.[33,34] In October 1992, cases of cholera associated with a *V. cholerae* strain that did not agglutinate with O1 antisera were reported from Madras, India, and subsequently other cities in southern and eastern India and Bangladesh.[35] This strain, ultimately designated serogroup O139, caused epidemic disease throughout Bangladesh, with cases in Malaysia, Nepal, Pakistan, China, and Thailand. Imported cases were documented in the United States and the United Kingdom.[36] Although cases of cholera in Asia due to *V. cholerae* serogroup O1 are now far more common, *V. cholerae* serogroup O139 persists as a cause of sporadic cases in Bangladesh. Molecular analysis has clearly demonstrated that serotype O139 arose from the O1 El Tor strain that caused the seventh pandemic. Unlike *V. cholerae* O1, *V. cholerae* serogroup O139 strains are encapsulated, and therefore immunologically distinct; neither naturally acquired nor vaccine-derived antibodies against *V. cholerae* O1 provide protection against infection with *V. cholerae* O139. Regardless of genetic origins, the emergence of epidemic cholera caused by serogroup O139 has demonstrated the potential for newly emerging serogroups of *V. cholerae* to cause deadly waterborne epidemics.

The El Tor biotype strain responsible for the seventh pandemic produces a slightly different toxin than the classical strain, and causes a higher proportion of asymptomatic infections, and a lower proportion of severe cholera infections.[37–39] More recently, genetic rearrangements have led to the emergence of El Tor variant strains, which have phenotypical features of the original El Tor strain, but have the genes to secrete the classical-type enterotoxin. As a result, the spectrum of illness attributable to the seventh cholera pandemic has shifted from a relatively low proportion of severe illness during the first four decades, to a mixed picture with relatively greater proportions of severe illness caused by variant El Tor strains, as has been reported in Bangladesh, sub-Saharan Africa, and Haiti.[40–42] Although most people infected with cholera are asymptomatic, they still shed vibrios in stool while infected, adding to the transmission burden.[43]

EPIDEMIOLOGY

Despite advances in access to safe water and waste disposal, improvements in clinical case management, and new cholera vaccines, the global burden of cholera remains high. From 1990 to 2017, the number of cholera cases and deaths reported annually to WHO has ranged from 74,000 to 1,227,000 cases, with the greatest variation attributable to epidemic surges associated with the introduction of cholera to Peru in 1991 and to Haiti in 2010–11 and to a surge exceeding 1 million reported cholera cases in war-torn Yemen in 2017 (Figs. 112-1 and 112-2a).[44–48] Reported cholera deaths over the same period have ranged from 1304 to 19,302 per year, with a global CFR between 0.5% and 4.4% (Figs. 12-1 and 112-2b). Because many cholera cases and deaths do not present to healthcare facilities, and are therefore not captured by passive surveillance systems, and because political and economic concerns may favor underreporting, estimates of cholera burden by public health researchers exceed those reported to WHO several-fold.[49,50] The most commonly cited estimates, which are based on incidence rates and CFRs from population-based studies, and on estimates of the population without access to sanitation, are that 2.86 million (1.3–4.0 million) cholera cases, including 95,000 (21,000–143,000) cholera deaths, occurred each year from 2008 to 2012.[51] Sub-Saharan Africa has consistently reported the largest proportion of cholera cases and deaths each year, except during 1991–93 and 2010–13 when epidemics in cholera naïve populations in Latin America and the Caribbean (respectively) were predominant, and during the epidemic surge in Yemen in 2017 (Fig. 112-2a and b). The cholera case-fatality ratio has also been consistently higher in sub-Saharan Africa than in other regions. Although it has gradually decreased, in 2016, it was 2.5%, compared with 1.1% in the Americas and 1.0% in Asia.[52] More recently, large outbreaks of cholera in Afghanistan, Iraq, and Yemen suggest that cholera has established a firm foothold in the Middle East.[26,46,53]

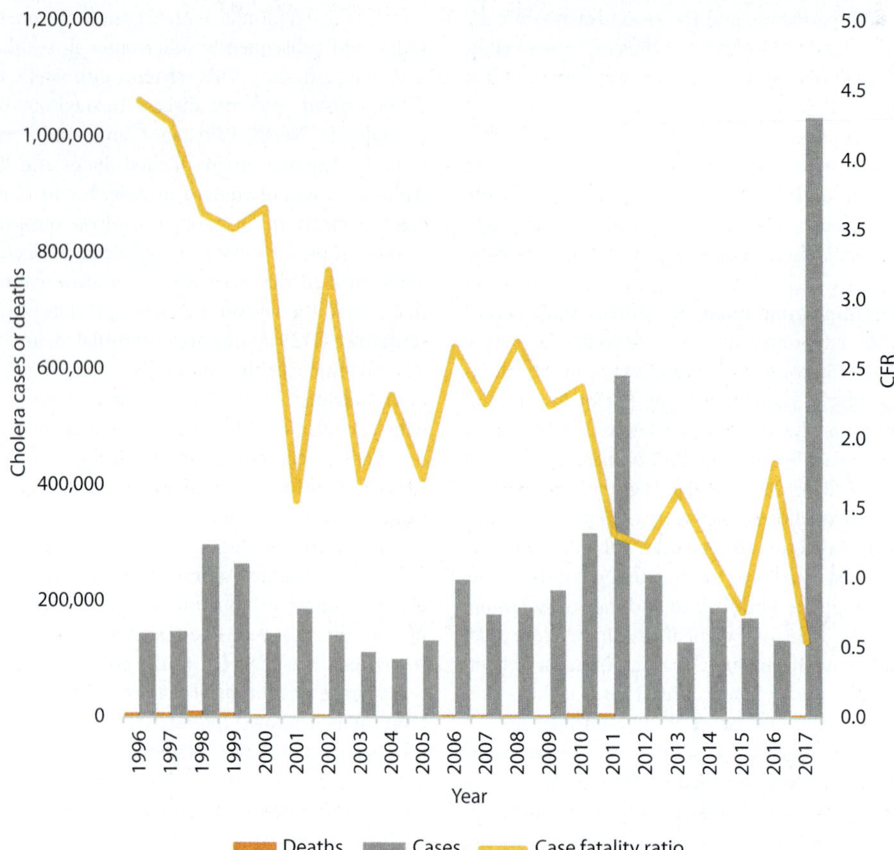

FIGURE 112-1. Global cholera cases, deaths and CFR by year, 1996–2017.

Although sporadic cholera cases may arise from consumption of raw or inadequately cooked seafood contaminated by free-living toxigenic *Vibrio cholerae* O1, infected persons spread cholera epidemics primarily through fecal contamination of drinking water, and occasionally food.[54] A recent review and meta-analysis of the role of water, sanitation, and hygiene exposures in 51 case-control studies found several factors significantly associated with case status: use of an unimproved water source, contact with surface water, unsafe water transport and storage, untreated drinking water, open defecation, unimproved sanitation, shared sanitation, and poor hand hygiene.[55] Several recent studies found that household contacts of cholera patients had high risk of infection, which could occur through contaminated fomites, food, or drinking water.[56–58] Another study found that proximity to a case's home increased risk of cholera in neighbors.[59]

Infection with certain strains of *Vibrio cholerae*, including the recently described El Tor variant, increases the likelihood of severe disease, as does a larger inoculum of *Vibrio cholerae* ingested.[60,61] Host factors, such as achlorhydria or blood group O also increase the risk of severe illness.[62] Risk factors for cholera mortality have been studied in outbreaks in rural and urban settings, but can be challenging to investigate due to underreporting and limitations in surveillance.[49–51] People at the extremes of age, and those with certain comorbidities, are more susceptible to the effects of dehydration.[63] However, limited access to healthcare, poor health-seeking behavior, and inadequate rehydration are the salient preventable risk factors for cholera deaths.[64–67] Despite these challenges, simple strategies such as improving access to oral rehydration are proven to lower mortality rates from cholera and other dehydrating diarrheal diseases.[30]

The World Health Organization defines a cholera-endemic area as an area where confirmed locally acquired cholera cases have been detected in 3 of the previous 5 years with evidence of local transmission.[53,68] Epidemic cholera can occur in endemic and nonendemic areas when more cases of cholera occur than expected over a particular period.[69] Besides the presence of toxigenic *V. cholerae* O1 or O139, the primary determinant of cholera outbreaks and endemicity is a failure to protect drinking water, food, and the environment from fecal contamination. Many other factors influence cholera risk, including environmental and meteorological conditions, population density, mobility, and immunity, and social customs, such as those associated with burials.[70] A core component of The Global Roadmap to 2030 is the identification of cholera hotspots for intensive prevention and preparedness efforts. A 2017 paper suggests three key types of hotspots: "burden hotspots," where disease prevalence or incidence is high; "risk hotspots," where transmission efficacy or risk of disease acquisition and amplification is high; and "emergence hotspots," where there is increased likelihood of disease emergence.[71] Identifying these hotspots is critical to cost-effective cholera prevention and control. Initial efforts have relied on historical cholera data, enhanced by more granular mapping of GIS data on cholera cases, population density, and drinking water and sanitation services.[72] Improvements in environmental models that predict conditions where *V. cholerae* thrive, the use of migration and cell phone data to predict areas with high transmission risk, and more accurate estimates of cases and fatalities through improved surveillance will enable more timely disease control measures and more accurate hotspot identification.[73–76]

ECOLOGY OF DISEASE

The association between cholera outbreaks and environmental drivers has been recognized for decades.[77] *V. cholerae* are free-living organisms commonly found in brackish waters in close conjunction with zooplankton, shellfish, and other flora and fauna.[78–80] Conditions of temperature and salinity that promote growth of these organisms may also

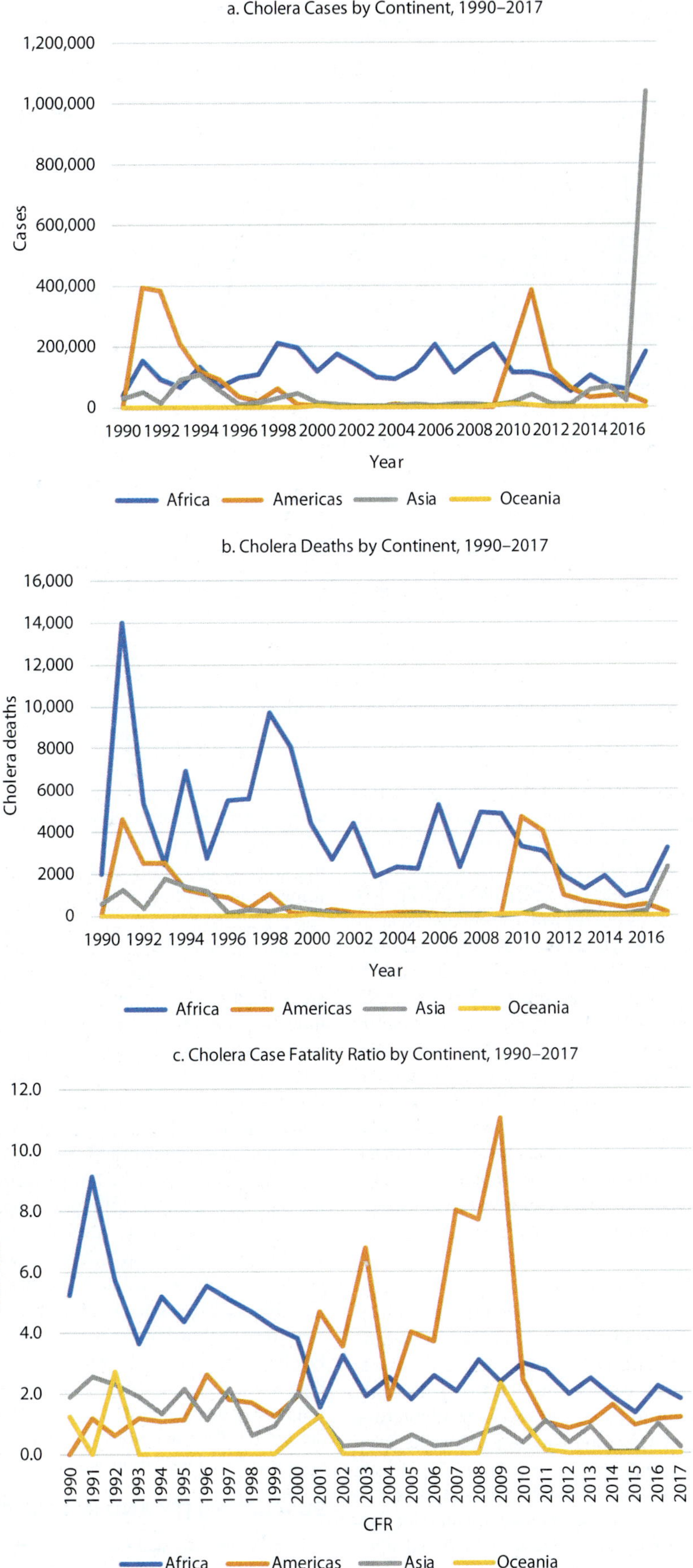

FIGURE 112-2. **A.** Cholera cases by continent, 1990–2017. **B.** Cholera deaths by continent, 1990–2017. **C.** Cholera case fatality ratio by continent, 1990–2017.

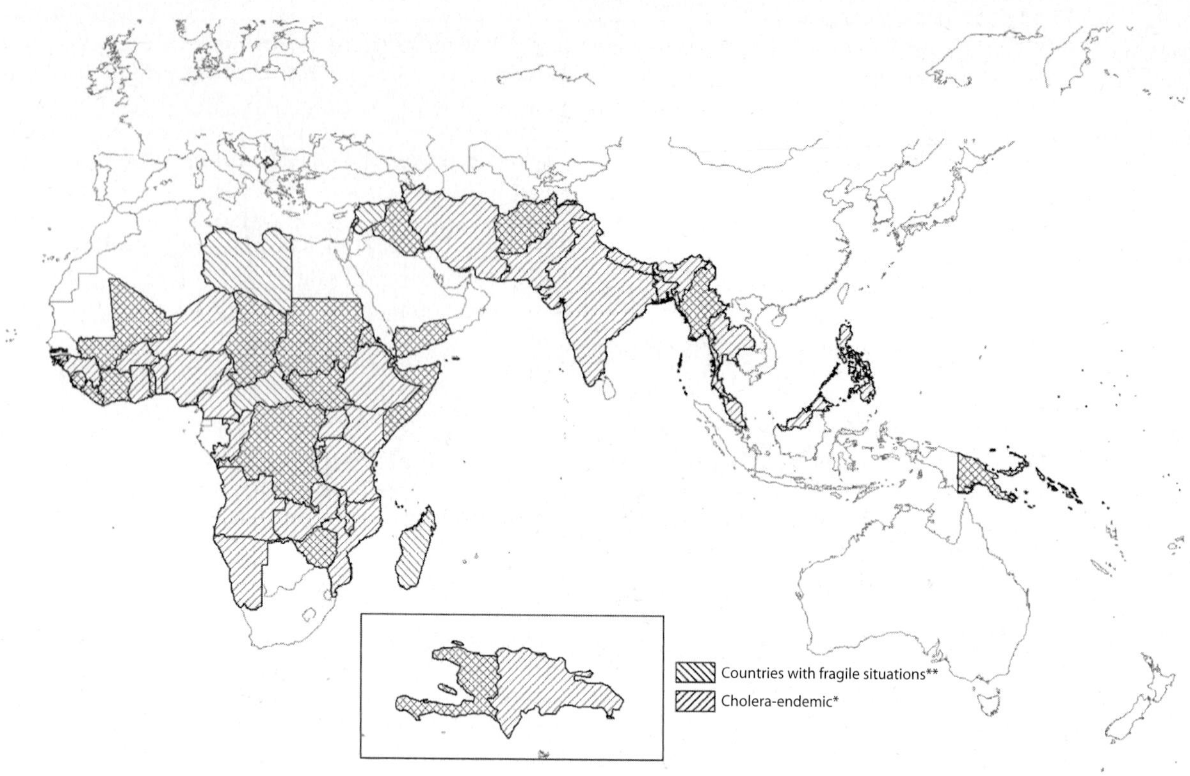

FIGURE 112-3. Cholera-endemic countries and fragile situations, 2018. (*Source:* Used, with permission, from Davis W, Narra R, Mintz ED. Cholera. *Curr Epidemiol Rep*. 2018;5:303–15, Fig 112-3.)

promote growth of *V. cholerae*. These conditions, and algal blooms and other proxy indicators, are measurable by satellite imagery and may help predict cholera outbreak risk in vulnerable nearby populations.[81,82] The El Niño Southern Oscillation (ENSO), a periodic warming of a section of the Pacific Ocean, was associated with cholera outbreaks in Bangladesh and Peru, though its effects are modified by local climate and other variables, complicating accurate outbreak prediction.[83–85] ENSO also affects inland temperature and rainfall.[46,81,86–89] A study of cholera incidence in Africa over a 15-year period found decreases in Madagascar and parts of Western, Central, and Southern Africa, and increases in Eastern Africa during El Niño. Several papers have noted a relationship between cholera incidence and rainfall.[46,81,86–88,90] Proposed pathways include fecal contamination of drinking water sources due to excessive precipitation and flooding; increased use of unsafe water sources due to reduced rainfall and drought; and the effects on other factors related to *Vibrio* survival and growth in water sources, including zooplankton, bacteriophage, and iron content.[91–93]

TRANSMISSION DYNAMICS

In recent years, cholera outbreaks have occurred in the capital cities of Benin, Ghana, Guinea, Guinea Bissau, Haiti, Ivory Coast, Kenya, Sierra Leone, Tanzania, Togo, Uganda, Zambia, and Zimbabwe, whereas cholera is considered endemic in Dhaka, Bangladesh and Kolkata, India. According to data from the Joint Monitoring Programme (JMP), improved sanitation coverage decreased from 2010 to 2015 among urban populations in 36 (67%) of 54 African countries, a net increase of 24 million city-dwellers without access.[94,95] Crowded urban environments with poor sanitation conditions in Europe and the United States were frequent foci of cholera epidemics in the nineteenth century; similar unsanitary conditions prevail in parts of many cities today.[62,96–98]

A recent paper examined associations between high cholera burden and socioeconomic characteristics in districts in India. Districts with higher rates of literacy, mobile phone ownership, and households using tap water from a treated source had lower risk of reporting cholera, and districts with higher proportions of households using latrines without a slab or using open drainage for sanitation had higher risk.[99]

Cholera may persist in states with weak governments that place low priority on healthcare, and in conflict areas where interventions are difficult to implement. Conflict can damage water and sanitation infrastructure directly, as in Yemen, and it weakens economies and health systems, which can limit people from accessing healthcare, safe drinking water, or proper sanitation and hygiene facilities.[100–102] Conflict can also limit the potential for outside support from NGOs, UN agencies, or bilateral donors. The World Bank's list of fragile situations includes countries and territories with ongoing conflict or risk of conflict, and those with low performance on indicators of governance.[103] The proportion of the population without access to safe drinking water is twice as large in fragile states as it is in nonfragile states, and the proportion who lack basic sanitation is fourfold greater.[104] Of the 34 countries on the World Bank list of fragile situations for FY 2018, 22 have endemic cholera and 3 more share a border with countries identified by GTFCC as cholera endemic (Fig. 112-3).[103,105] Fragile states that border states with endemic cholera are at higher than average risk for cholera, and need prevention, detection, and response protocols. Most countries with endemic cholera share a border with at least one other country with endemic cholera, making cross-border coordination essential.

SUSCEPTIBILITY AND IMMUNITY

Several biological factors have been shown to modify the incidence and severity of disease following exposure to *V. cholerae*. Susceptibility to *V. cholerae* infection depends on innate host factors including age, blood type, nutritional factors and gastric acidity, and adaptive immune responses produced by previous infection or vaccination.[37,62,106,107] Furthermore, severity of disease depends on dose of *V. cholerae* ingested, virulence of the agent and underlying medical problems of the host.[62,108]

It has long been noted that patients with achlorhydria (postgastrectomy or from autoimmune disease) were severely affected with cholera and acquired the disease more frequently than normal hosts. More recently severity of cholera has been linked to *H. pylori* infection with the likely mechanism being the development of hypochlorhydria secondary to chronic atrophic gastritis of the acid-secreting gastric portion of the stomach.[108] For reasons that remain unclear, the risk of developing severe cholera is much greater in patients with blood group O.[109,110]

Cholera infection provides at least 3 years of protection against subsequent symptomatic disease, particularly by a homologous strain.[111] Immune protection is more pronounced and longer lasting after symptomatic infection by classical biotype organisms compared to El Tor organisms.[111] Additionally, Inaba serotype evokes stronger protection than the Ogawa serotype.[111] Furthermore, infection with O1 serogroup strains provides no protection against O139 infection, and vice versa.[112]

Lower socioeconomic groups have a higher incidence of cholera for a variety of reasons: (a) occupational exposures (e.g., boatmen in several areas have a high incidence of cholera, probably because they often drink raw river water, eat seafood, and lack proper sanitation or handwashing facilities); (b) unsanitary conditions in low-income housing areas, primarily reflected in inadequate sewage disposal and contaminated water sources; and (c) high population density in low-income areas, increasing the risk of introduction of *V. cholerae* and possibly enhancing transmission of the organism after it has been introduced.[113] Once illness occurs, the poor may be more likely to encounter barriers to care and be at greater risk of mortality.

CLINICAL PRESENTATION

The clinical spectrum of cholera is broad, ranging from asymptomatic infection, to mild or moderate symptoms, to a massive outpouring of watery diarrhea that can lead to hypotensive shock and death within hours if left untreated.[114,115] Asymptomatic cases may represent approximately half of all cholera cases in endemic settings.[62,107] The incubation period for cholera is 12 hours–5 days and it typically presents as an abrupt onset of watery, painless diarrhea, often profuse, and described as "rice-water" stools. Vomiting often accompanies the diarrhea in the early stages of illness, but fever is uncommon unless there is coinfection. Toxigenic *V. cholerae* serogroups O1 and O139 produce cholera toxin which disrupts normal absorption and secretion of fluid when it attaches to the intestinal cells.[116–120]

In severe cases, the loss of diarrheal stool can be extreme and rapidly reach 1 L/hr. In addition to diarrhea and vomiting, patients may experience lightheadedness, anxiety, thirst, and abdominal and muscle cramps. On exam, patients may present with dry mucous membranes, sunken eyes, a rapid, but weak pulse, decreased skin turgor and decreased urine output. The initial clinical assessment of a cholera patient should focus on determining the level of dehydration; the recognition of hypovolemic shock is critical, and survival is dependent on immediate treatment. In those who survive the acute phase, the disease usually subsides spontaneously in 2–7 days. Shedding of bacteria, however, may continue in symptomatic and asymptomatic patients for days, and rarely for weeks after recovery.[43]

Specific considerations are important when caring for special populations, such as children, pregnant patients, and patients with human immunodeficiency virus (HIV). Compared to adults with cholera, children are at a higher risk of hypoglycemia which can lead to lethargy, coma, seizures, and death.[121] Children with cholera are also more susceptible to hypokalemia due to greater potassium loss in the stool.[122,123] Pregnant mothers in their third trimester with vomiting and severe dehydration were found to have higher rates of fetal death.[124] Additionally, due to increased circulating plasma volume, assessment of dehydration can be challenging in pregnant patients. Patients with HIV suffer CD4+ T-cell deficiency in the intestine resulting in a decrease in secretory IgA production.[125] Secretory IgA neutralizes cholera toxin and prevents *Vibrios* from attaching to the intestinal cells.[126] As a result, it is presumed that patients with HIV would have an impaired immune response to *V. cholerae*. Findings from a study in cholera-endemic Mozambique suggested HIV infection was associated with an increased risk for cholera, although this has not been consistently reported.[127]

TREATMENT

Timely rehydration with the proper combination of fluids and electrolytes is the cornerstone of cholera treatment and is essential to save lives. Prompt and effective treatment can reduce cholera mortality rates from $> 50\%$ to less than 1%.[128] If a patient is able to drink, treatment should begin at home with oral rehydration solution (ORS) while seeking medical care. ORS is a prepared by mixing a sachet of prepackaged electrolytes with 1 liter of safe drinking water. ORS is usually sufficient to treat the majority of symptomatic cholera patients. Intravenous therapy with Ringer's Lactate is recommended for patients with severe dehydration and for those who cannot drink sufficient ORS due to vomiting or profuse fluid losses. Failure to identify patients with severe dehydration, which can occur quickly, results in delayed treatment and underhydration that can lead to hypovolemic shock and death. Underhydration is a frequent error in therapy in centers without experience in the treatment of cholera.[129]

If possible, patients should be weighed at treatment centers. Rehydration fluids and volumes depend on the level of dehydration, body weight, and ongoing losses. Frequent reassessment of dehydration status is critical, and patients should be encouraged to begin drinking ORS as soon as possible. Among other important electrolytes, ORS contains glucose, which activates an alternative mechanism for absorption of sodium from the intestine, and potassium, which is important to replace, especially in children. Oral therapy at home, or in community-based oral rehydration points, is important, because in many areas where cholera occurs, access to medical care for intravenous rehydration may be difficult. Patients with progressive dehydration despite oral rehydration must be referred to treatment centers or units that can provide intravenous rehydration. Educational campaigns should motivate populations to seek care in health centers and to start taking ORS at home as soon as possible during this process.

Antibiotics can decrease the duration of diarrhea, volume of stool, and duration of *V. cholerae* carriage when used in conjunction with rehydration therapy in severely ill patients.[130–133] Current guidance from the Global Task Force on Cholera Control (GTFCC) recommends a single dose of doxycycline for all patients, including pregnant women and children.[134] However, due to emerging antimicrobial resistance in *V. cholerae*, antimicrobial sensitivity testing is essential in guiding treatment.[134–137] Zinc supplementation also reduces fluid losses and duration of cholera in children.[138] Zinc dosage is age dependent and should be administered over 10–14 days in children with cholera.[138]

PREVENTION

During the late nineteenth and early twentieth centuries, the "sanitary revolution" helped lead to the elimination of cholera from Europe and North America by improving municipal water and sanitation infrastructure.[139] More recently, improved access to safe drinking water, safe collection and disposal of fecal waste, and hygiene promotion helped dramatically reduce the transmission of cholera, other enteric diseases, and infant and child mortality in Central and South America, leading to the end of the Latin American pandemic in the early 2000s.[31,32,140]

Timely disease surveillance is critical for detecting and containing cholera outbreaks. Surveillance should include the registration of cases of acute watery diarrhea in individuals < 5 years old and those ≥ 5 years old, and stool culture or PCR for the identification and isolation of *Vibrio cholerae* O1 or O139 in those patients who meet the definition for a suspected cholera case (acute watery diarrhea with severe dehydration or death in a person ≥ 5 years old).[141] Isolates of *V. cholerae* should be serotyped and tested for susceptibility to antimicrobial agents. Sudden increases in acute watery diarrhea in adults should prompt the expanded testing of samples; samples from areas where microbiologic testing is not available should be preserved and transported in Cary Blair media to appropriate regional and national diagnostic centers. Cholera outbreaks require significant logistic activity, and disease control and treatment will be optimized only when notification has allowed for the early reinforcement of healthcare systems and an increased awareness of the disease among the public and healthcare providers.

When a cholera outbreak has been confirmed, mass media messages can have an important role in limiting its spread and lethality. The population must be made aware of the potential severity of disease and the importance of seeking treatment with ORS or IV fluids at a health center or hospital. Education about the importance of drinking only treated water and eating only food that has been safely prepared and stored is essential.[64–67]

An effective public health response requires rapid and coordinated mobilization of national and local governments, international agencies, nongovernmental organizations, along with resources to meet the logistical needs of responding to an outbreak that can rapidly overwhelm health systems. Training or retraining healthcare providers will help improve case management. Often, affected areas will require additional healthcare staff and treatment structures, which can be co-located with existing healthcare facilities, or set-up as standalone cholera treatment centers. Treatment supplies need to be monitored carefully, as deaths can result from shortages of critical items, such as IV fluids, catheters, or tubing.

Although antimicrobial treatment is recommended for patients with severe dehydration, or moderate dehydration that is worsening despite IV rehydration. However, antibiotic chemoprophylaxis of cholera case contacts is rarely advisable.[136] Often, by the time antibiotics can be delivered to contacts of a case, targeted individuals have either already acquired or have little chance of acquiring the infection. Exceptions to this include chemoprophylaxis of institutionalized populations, such as individuals in prisons or boarding schools, who may be rapidly accessible following the identification of an index case.[142] Mass chemoprophylaxis of whole communities is never indicated and is discouraged, as it promotes the development of drug resistance and wastes resources.[135,137]

Disinfection of households by spraying them with chlorine is a popular intervention that has not been proven effective in decreasing cholera transmission. It can stigmatize a family, damage the home, and waste considerable resources and time. Instead, these resources should be focused on procurement of safe water through chlorination, ORS for early home treatment and improving hygiene.[143]

Oral cholera vaccines (OCVs) can be a useful complementary tool when used together with timely and appropriate case management, improved access to safe water and sanitation, and hygiene promotion.[144] OCV campaigns should never disrupt other crucial cholera control measures, and can be considered in (i) endemic settings targeting high-risk groups; (ii) epidemic settings either as a preemptive or reactive strategy; or (iii) during humanitarian emergencies when the risk of cholera is high.[68,145] Three OCVs are prequalified by the World Health Organization: Dukoral® (SBL Vaccines), Shanchol® (Shanta Biotec), and Euvichol® (Eubiologics). Dukoral is monovalent and contains only *V. cholerae* serogroup O1 with the recombinant B subunit of cholera toxin. It requires a buffer and is licensed for children ≥ 2 years old. Shanchol and Euvichol are bivalent and contain both O1 and O139 *V. cholerae* without the toxin subunit; they do not require buffer and are licensed for children ≥ 1 year old [148]. All three vaccines are licensed as a two-dose regimen with doses ideally given between 2 and 6 weeks apart. OCVs have been found safe in pregnant women.[146–148] Shanchol has demonstrated protection for 5 years among adults and children ≥ 5 years old, but protective effectiveness in children < 5 years old is not as high and does not last as long.[149–153] Recent studies have shown that single-dose regimens can be useful in special circumstances and provide short-term effectiveness for approximately 6 months.[144,151–153]

The global OCV stockpile was established by Gavi and other partners in 2013 to ensure rapid access to cholera vaccine in endemic and emergency settings.[144] Gavi has recently renewed its commitment through 2025, and the number of doses available in the stockpile is expected to increase as current manufacturers scale-up their production capacity. The stockpile has empowered governments and NGOs to be able to take rapid action to prevent, or combat cholera outbreaks. As a result, some countries that did not previously declare cholera outbreaks, or report cholera cases to WHO, have begun to do so. In addition, over a dozen countries have begun developing multisectoral National Cholera Plans aligned with the "Global Roadmap to 2030," and a few countries have already begun to implement these plans. Many obstacles will have to be overcome to obtain the resources necessary for implementation of these plans, but to the extent that populations living in cholera hotspots receive improved drinking water, sanitation, and hygiene, the return on these investments is expected to be high. As happened in the United States and Europe during the late nineteenth century and early twentieth centuries, infant and child mortality is expected to decrease dramatically—not just because of fewer cholera deaths, but also because of fewer deaths due to other enteric infections that are transmitted through the same routes as cholera. By 2030, we will know if early adopters have validated the promise of this approach.

References

1. The Global Task Force on Cholera Control. Ending Cholera A Global Roadmap to 2030. WHO. 2018. http://www.who.int/cholera/publications/global-roadmap/en. Accessed May 23, 2018.
2. Abbott S, Janda J, Farmer J. Vibrio and related organisms. In: *Manual of Clinical Microbiology*. Vol. 1. Washington, DC: ASM Press; 2011:666–76.
3. Centers for Disease Control. *Vibrio Cholerae Infection, Diagnosis and Detection*. http://www.cdc.gov/cholera/diagnosis.html.
4. Centers for Disease Control and Prevention. Chapter 2: Collection and transport of fecal specimens. In: Laboratory Methods for the Diagnosis of Epidemic Dysentery and Cholera. Atlanta, GA: Centers for Disease Control and Prevention; 1999. https://www.cdc.gov/cholera/pdf/Laboratory-Methods-for-the-Diagnosis-of-Epidemic-Dysentery-and-Cholera.pdf.
5. Page A-L, Alberti KP, Guenole A, et al. Use of filter paper as a transport medium for laboratory diagnosis of cholera under field conditions. *J Clin Microbiol.* 2011;49(8):3021–3.
6. Keddy KH, Sooka A, Parsons MB, Njanpop-Lafourcade B-M, Fitchet K, Smith AM. Diagnosis of *Vibrio cholerae* O1 infection in Africa. *J Infect Dis.* 2013;208(Suppl 1):S23–31.
7. Centers for Disease Control and Prevention. Chapter 6: Isolation and identification of *Vibrio cholerae* serogroups 01 and 0139. In: Laboratory Methods for the Diagnosis of Epidemic Dysentery and Cholera. Atlanta, GA: Centers for Disease Control and Prevention; 1999. https://www.cdc.gov/cholera/pdf/Laboratory-Methods-for-the-Diagnosis-of-Epidemic-Dysentery-and-Cholera.pdf.
8. Global Task Force on Cholera Control. *Interim Technical Note, Introduction of DNA-Based Identification and Typing Methods to Public Health Practitioners for Epidemiological Investigation of Cholera Outbreaks*; 2017. https://www.who.int/cholera/task_force/GTFCC-Laboratory-support-public-health-surveillance.pdf.
9. Tarr CL, Patel JS, Puhr ND, Sowers EG, Bopp CA, Strockbine NA. Identification of Vibrio isolates by a multiplex PCR assay and rpoB sequence determination. *J Clin Microbiol.* 2007;45(1):134–40.

10. Nandi B, Nandy RK, Mukhopadhyay S, Nair GB, Shimada T, Ghose AC. Rapid method for species-specific identification of *Vibrio cholerae* using primers targeted to the gene of outer membrane protein OmpW. *J Clin Microbiol.* 2000;38(11):4145–51.
11. Keasler SP, Hall RH. Detecting and biotyping *Vibrio cholerae* O1 with multiplex polymerase chain reaction. *Lancet.* 1993;341(8861):1661.
12. Fields PI, Popovic T, Wachsmuth K, Olsvik O. Use of polymerase chain reaction for detection of toxigenic *Vibrio cholerae* O1 strains from the Latin American cholera epidemic. *J Clin Microbiol.* 1992;30(8):2118–21.
13. Global Task Force on Cholera Control. *Interim Technical Note, The Use of Cholera Rapid Diagnostic Tests.* 2016. https://www.who.int/cholera/task_force/Interim-guidance-cholera-RDT.pdf.
14. Kousoulis AA. Etymology of cholera. *Emerg Infect Dis.* 2012;18(3):540.
15. Pollitzer R. Cholera Monograph No. 43. World Health Organisation. 1959, p. 1019.
16. Devault AM, Golding GB, Waglechner N, et al. Second-pandemic strain of *Vibrio cholerae* from the Philadelphia cholera outbreak of 1849. *N Engl J Med.* 2014;370(4):334–40.
17. Samadi AR, Huq MI, Shahid N, et al. Classical *Vibrio cholerae* biotype displaces El Tor in Bangladesh. *Lancet.* 1983;1(8328):805–7.
18. Weill F-X, Domman D, Njamkepo E, et al. Genomic history of the seventh pandemic of cholera in Africa. *Science.* 2017;358(6364):785–9.
19. Glass R. Epidemiology of cholera. In: *Cholera.* New York: Plenum Medical Books; 1992:129–54.
20. WHO. Cholera, 2015. *Wkly Epidemiol Rec.* 2016;91(38):432–40.
21. Blake PA, Allegra DT, Snyder JD, et al. Cholera—A possible endemic focus in the United States. *N Engl J Med.* 1980;302(6):305–9.
22. Shandera WX, Hafkin B, Martin DL, et al. Persistence of cholera in the United States. *Am J Trop Med Hyg.* 1983;32(4):812–7.
23. Blake PA, Wachsmuth K, Davis BR, Bopp CA, Chaiken BP, Lee JV. Toxigenic *Vibrio cholerae* O1 strain from Mexico identical to United States isolates. *Lancet.* 1983;2(8355):912.
24. Swerdlow DL, Mintz ED, Rodriguez M, et al. Waterborne transmission of epidemic cholera in Trujillo, Peru: Lessons for a continent at risk. *Lancet.* 1992;340(8810):28–33.
25. Wachsmuth I, Blake P, Olsvik O. *Vibrio Cholerae and Cholera.* Washington, DC: ASM Press; 1994.
26. Ries AA, Vugia DJ, Beingolea L, et al. Cholera in Piura, Peru: A modern urban epidemic. *J Infect Dis.* 1992;166(6):1429–33.
27. Tauxe RV, Mintz ED, Quick RE. Epidemic cholera in the new world: Translating field epidemiology into new prevention strategies. *Emerg Infect Dis.* 1995;1(4):141–6.
28. Cholera situation in the Americas, 1996. *Epidemiol Bull.* 1997;18(1):5–10.
29. WHO. Cholera, 2009. *Wkly Epidemiol Rec.* 2010;31:293–308.
30. Gutierrez G, Tapia-Conyer R, Guiscafre H, Reyes H, Martinez H, Kumate J. Impact of oral rehydration and selected public health interventions on reduction of mortality from childhood diarrhoeal diseases in Mexico. *Bull World Health Organ.* 1996;74(2):189–97.
31. Sepulveda J, Valdespino JL, Garcia-Garcia L. Cholera in Mexico: The paradoxical benefits of the last pandemic. *Int J Infect Dis.* 2006;10(1):4–13.
32. Marco C, Delgado I, Vargas C, Munoz X, Bhutta ZA, Ferreccio C. Typhoid fever in Chile 1969–2012: Analysis of an epidemic and its control. *Am J Trop Med Hyg.* 2018;99(Suppl 3):26–33.
33. Tobin-D'Angelo M, Smith AR, Bulens SN, et al. Severe diarrhea caused by cholera toxin-producing *Vibrio cholerae* serogroup O75 infections acquired in the southeastern United States. *Clin Infect Dis.* 2008;47(8):1035–40.
34. Crump JA, Bopp CA, Greene KD, et al. Toxigenic *Vibrio cholerae* serogroup O141-associated cholera-like diarrhea and bloodstream infection in the United States. *J Infect Dis.* 2003;187(5):866–8.
35. Faruque SM, Sack DA, Sack RB, Colwell RR, Takeda Y, Nair GB. Emergence and evolution of *Vibrio cholerae* O139. *Proc Natl Acad Sci U S A.* 2003;100(3):1304–9.
36. Boyce TG, Mintz ED, Greene KD, et al. *Vibrio cholerae* O139 Bengal infections among tourists to Southeast Asia: An intercontinental foodborne outbreak. *J Infect Dis.* 1995;172(5):1401–4.
37. Bart KJ, Huq Z, Khan M, Mosley WH. Seroepidemiologic studies during a simultaneous epidemic of infection with El Tor Ogawa and classical Inaba *Vibrio cholerae. J Infect Dis.* 1970;121(Suppl):17–24.
38. Woodward WE, Mosley WH, McCormack WM. The spectrum of cholera in rural East Pakistan. I. Correlation of bacteriologic and serologic results. *J Infect Dis.* 1970;121(Suppl):10–6.
39. Gangarosa E, Mosley W. *Epidemiology and Surveillance of Cholera.* Philadelphia, PA: WB Saunders Co; 1974.
40. Siddique AK, Nair GB, Alam M, et al. El Tor cholera with severe disease: A new threat to Asia and beyond. *Epidemiol Infect.* 2010;138(3):347–52.
41. Safa A, Sultana J, Dac Cam P, Mwansa JC, Kong RYC. *Vibrio cholerae* O1 hybrid El Tor strains, Asia and Africa. *Emerg Infect Dis.* 2008;14(6):987–8.
42. Chin C-S, Sorenson J, Harris JB, et al. The origin of the Haitian cholera outbreak strain. *N Engl J Med.* 2011;364(1):33–42.
43. Weil AA, Begum Y, Chowdhury F, et al. Bacterial shedding in household contacts of cholera patients in Dhaka, Bangladesh. *Am J Trop Med Hyg.* 2014;91(4):738–42.
44. Barzilay EJ, Schaad N, Magloire R, et al. Cholera surveillance during the Haiti epidemic—The first 2 years. *N Engl J Med.* 2013;368(7):599–609.
45. WHO. Global Health Observatory data repository: Cholera. http://apps.who.int/gho/data/node.main.174?lang=en. Published 2017.
46. Camacho A, Bouhenia M, Alyusfi R, et al. Cholera epidemic in Yemen, 2016–18: An analysis of surveillance data. *Lancet Glob Health.* 2018;6(6):e680–90.
47. Al-Mandhari A, Musani A, Abubakar A, Malik M. Cholera in Yemen: Concerns remain over recent spike but control efforts show promise (Editorial). *East Mediterr Health J.* 2018;24(10):971–2.
48. Weill F-X, Domman D, Njamkepo E, et al. Genomic insights into the 2016–2017 cholera epidemic in Yemen. *Nature.* 2019;565(7738):230–3.
49. Shikanga O-T, Mutonga D, Abade M, et al. High mortality in a cholera outbreak in western Kenya after post-election violence in 2008. *Am J Trop Med Hyg.* 2009;81(6):1085–90.
50. McCrickard LS, Massay AE, Narra R, et al. Cholera mortality during urban epidemic, Dar es Salaam, Tanzania, August 16, 2015–January 16, 20161. *Emerg Infect Dis.* 2017;23(Suppl 1):S154–7.
51. Ali M, Nelson AR, Lopez AL, Sack DA. Updated global burden of cholera in endemic countries. Remais JV, ed. *PLoS Negl Trop Dis.* 2015;9(6):e0003832.
52. WHO. Cholera, 2016. *Wkly Epidemiol Rec.* 2017;92(36):521–36.
53. WHO. Meeting of the Strategic Advisory Group of Experts on Immunization, April 2017—conclusions and recommendations. *Wkly Epidemiol Rec.* 2017;92(22):301–20.
54. Estrada-García T, Mintz ED. Cholera: Foodborne transmission and its prevention. *Eur J Epidemiol.* 1996;12(5):461–9.
55. Wolfe M, Kaur M, Yates T, Woodlin M, Lantagne D. A systematic review and meta-analysis of the association between water, sanitation, and hygiene exposures and cholera in case-control studies. *Am J Trop Med Hyg.* 2018;99(2):534–45.
56. Sugimoto JD, Koepke AA, Kenah EE, et al. Household Transmission of *Vibrio cholerae* in Bangladesh. *PLoS Negl Trop Dis.* 2014;8(11):e3314.
57. Burrowes V, Perin J, Monira S, et al. Risk factors for household transmission of *Vibrio cholerae* in Dhaka, Bangladesh (CHoBI7 Trial). *Am J Trop Med Hyg.* 2017;96(6):1382–7.
58. Weil AA, Khan AI, Chowdhury F, et al. Clinical outcomes in household contacts of patients with cholera in Bangladesh. *Clin Infect Dis.* 2009;49(10):1473–9.
59. Debes AK, Ali M, Azman AS, Yunus M, Sack DA. Cholera cases cluster in time and space in Matlab, Bangladesh: Implications for targeted preventive interventions. *Int J Epidemiol.* 2016;45(6):2134–9.
60. Jackson BR, Talkington DF, Pruckler JM, et al. Seroepidemiologic survey of epidemic cholera in Haiti to assess spectrum of illness and risk factors for severe disease. *Am J Trop Med Hyg.* 2013;89(4):654–64.
61. Watson AP, Armstrong AQ, White GH, Thran BH. Health-based ingestion exposure guidelines for *Vibrio cholerae*: Technical basis for water reuse applications. *Sci Total Environ.* 2018;613–4:379–87.
62. Clemens JD, Nair GB, Ahmed T, Qadri F, Holmgren J. Cholera. *Lancet.* 2017;390(10101):1539–49.
63. Gunnlaugsson G, Angulo FJ, Einarsdottir J, Passa A, Tauxe RV. Epidemic cholera in Guinea-Bissau: The challenge of preventing deaths in rural West Africa. *Int J Infect Dis.* 2000;4(1):8–13.
64. Tauxe RV, Holmberg SD, Dodin A, Wells JV, Blake PA. Epidemic cholera in Mali: High mortality and multiple routes of transmission in a famine area. *Epidemiol Infect.* 1988;100(2):279–89.
65. Quick RE, Vargas R, Moreno D, et al. Epidemic cholera in the Amazon: The challenge of preventing death. *Am J Trop Med Hyg.* 1993;48(5):597–602.
66. Routh JA, Loharikar A, Fouche M-DB, et al. Rapid assessment of cholera-related deaths, Artibonite Department, Haiti, 2010. *Emerg Infect Dis.* 2011;17(11):2139–42.

67. Morof D, Cookson ST, Laver S, et al. Community mortality from cholera: Urban and rural districts in Zimbabwe. *Am J Trop Med Hyg.* 2013;88(4):645–50.

68. WHO. Cholera vaccines: WHO position paper—August 2017. 2017. http://apps.who.int/iris/bitstream/handle/10665/258763/WER9234.pdf?sequence=1.

69. WHO. *Outbreak Surveillance and Response in Humanitarian Emergencies. WHO Guidelines for EWARN Implementation.* Geneva: WHO; 2012. https://apps.who.int/iris/bitstream/handle/10665/70812/WHO_HSE_GAR_DCE_2012_1_eng.pdf;jsessionid=5E7EC43AE157C40A7C8F63C676B6196C?sequence=1.

70. McAteer JB, Danda S, Nhende T, et al. Notes from the field: Outbreak of *Vibrio cholerae* associated with attending a funeral—Chegutu District, Zimbabwe, 2018. *MMWR Morb Mortal Wkly Rep.* 2018;67(19):560–1.

71. McKay HS, Lessler J, Moore SM, Azman AS. What is a hotspot anyway? *Am J Trop Med Hyg.* 2017;96(6):1270–3.

72. Lessler J, Moore SM, Luquero FJ, et al. Mapping the burden of cholera in sub-Saharan Africa and implications for control: An analysis of data across geographical scales. *Lancet Lond Engl.* 2018;391(10133):1908–15.

73. Moore SM, Azman AS, Zaitchik BF, et al. El Niño and the shifting geography of cholera in Africa. *Proc Natl Acad Sci U S A.* 2017;114(17):4436–41.

74. Finger F, Genolet T, Mari L, et al. Mobile phone data highlights the role of mass gatherings in the spreading of cholera outbreaks. *Proc Natl Acad Sci U S A.* 2016;113(23):6421–6.

75. Bengtsson L, Gaudart J, Lu X, et al. Using mobile phone data to predict the spatial spread of cholera. *Sci Rep.* 2015;5(1):8923.

76. Mintz ED, Tauxe RV. Cholera in Africa: A closer look and a time for action. *J Infect Dis.* 2013;208(Suppl 1):S4–7.

77. Colwell RR. Global climate and infectious disease: The cholera paradigm. *Science.* 1996;274(5295):2025–31.

78. Huq A, West PA, Small EB, Huq MI, Colwell Rita R.. Influence of water temperature, salinity, and pH on survival and growth of toxigenic *Vibrio cholerae* serovar O1 associated with live copepods in laboratory microcosms. *Appl Environ Microbiol.* 1984;48(2):420–4.

79. Kaneko T, Colwell RR. Ecology of *Vibrio parahaemolyticus* in Chesapeake Bay. *J Bacteriol.* 1973;113(1):24–32.

80. Oliver JD, Warner RA, Cleland DR. Distribution of *Vibrio vulnificus* and other lactose-fermenting vibrios in the marine environment. *Appl Environ Microbiol.* 1983;45(3):985–98.

81. Jutla A, Aldaach H, Billian H, Akanda A, Huq A, Colwell R. Satellite based assessment of hydroclimatic conditions related to cholera in Zimbabwe. Schumann GJ-P, ed. *PLoS One.* 2015;10(9):e0137828.

82. Chretien J-P, Anyamba A, Small J, et al. Global climate anomalies and potential infectious disease risks: 2014–2015. *PLoS Curr.* 2015;7.

83. Cash BA, Rodó X, Emch M, Yunus M, Faruque ASG, Pascual M. Cholera and shigellosis: Different epidemiology but similar responses to climate variability. *PLoS One.* 2014;9(9):e107223.

84. Martinez PP, Reiner RC, Cash BA, et al. Cholera forecast for Dhaka, Bangladesh, with the 2015–2016 El Niño: Lessons learned. *PLoS One.* 2017;12(3):e0172355.

85. Ramírez IJ, Grady SC. El Niño, climate, and cholera Associations in Piura, Peru, 1991–2001: A wavelet analysis. *EcoHealth.* 2016;13(1):83–99.

86. Munyuli MT, Kavuvu JM, Mulinganya G, Bwinja GM. The potential financial costs of climate change on health of urban and rural citizens: A case study of *Vibrio cholerae* infections at Bukavu town, South Kivu Province, eastern Democratic Republic of Congo. *Iran J Public Health.* 2013;42(7):707.

87. Leckebusch GC, Abdussalam AF. Climate and socioeconomic influences on interannual variability of cholera in Nigeria. *Health Place.* 2015;34:107–17.

88. Stoltzfus JD, Carter JY, Akpinar-Elci M, et al. Interaction between climatic, environmental, and demographic factors on cholera outbreaks in Kenya. *Infect Dis Poverty.* 2014;3(1):37.

89. Rebaudet S, Sudre B, Faucher B, Piarroux R. Environmental determinants of cholera outbreaks in inland Africa: A systematic review of main transmission foci and propagation routes. *J Infect Dis.* 2013;208 (Suppl 1):S46–54.

90. Constantin de Magny G, Thiaw W, Kumar V, et al. Cholera outbreak in Senegal in 2005: Was climate a factor? *PLoS One.* 2012;7(8):e44577.

91. Ruiz-Moreno D, Pascual M, Bouma M, Dobson A, Cash B. Cholera seasonality in Madras (1901–1940): Dual role for rainfall in endemic and epidemic regions. *EcoHealth.* 2007;4(1):52–62.

92. Hashizume M, Faruque ASG, Wagatsuma Y, Hayashi T, Armstrong B. Cholera in Bangladesh: Climatic components of seasonal variation. *Epidemiology.* 2010;21(5):706–10.

93. Rieckmann A, Tamason CC, Gurley ES, Rod NH, Jensen PKM. Exploring droughts and floods and their association with cholera outbreaks in sub-Saharan Africa: A register-based ecological study from 1990 to 2010. *Am J Trop Med Hyg.* 2018;98(5):1269–74.

94. UNPOP. World Urbanization Prospects—Population Division—United Nations. https://esa.un.org/unpd/wup/. Published 2017. Accessed May 24, 2018.

95. JMP. WHO/UNICEF JMP data. https://washdata.org/data. Published 2018. Accessed May 24, 2018.

96. Sack DA, Sack RB, Nair GB, Siddique AK. Cholera. *Lancet Lond Engl.* 2004;363(9404):223–33.

97. Snow J. *Mode of Communication of Cholera.* London: John Churchill; 1855.

98. Johnson S. The Ghost Map : *The Story of London's Most Terrifying Epidemic—and How It Changed Science, Cities, and the Modern World.* New York: Riverhead Books; 2007.

99. Ali M, Gupta SS, Arora N, et al. Identification of burden hotspots and risk factors for cholera in India: An observational study. *PLoS One.* 2017;12(8):e0183100.

100. Almosawa S, Hubbard B, Griggs T. 'It's a Slow Death': The World's Worst Humanitarian Crisis. *The New York Times.* https://www.nytimes.com/interactive/2017/08/23/world/middleeast/yemen-cholera-humanitarian-crisis.html, https://www.nytimes.com/interactive/2017/08/23/world/middleeast/yemen-cholera-humanitarian-crisis.html. Published August 23, 2017. Accessed May 24, 2018.

101. Bruckner C, Checchi F. Detection of infectious disease outbreaks in twenty-two fragile states, 2000–2010: A systematic review. *Confl Health.* 2011;5(1):13.

102. Beyrer C, Villar JC, Suwanvanichkij V, Singh S, Baral SD, Mills EJ. Neglected diseases, civil conflicts, and the right to health. *Lancet.* 2007;370(9587):619–27.

103. World Bank. Harmonized List of Fragile Situations. World Bank. http://www.worldbank.org/en/topic/fragilityconflictviolence/brief/harmonized-list-of-fragile-situations. Published 2018. Accessed May 24, 2018.

104. JMP. *Progress on Drinking Water, Sanitation and Hygiene.* UNICEF, WHO Joint Monitoring Project; 2017. http://www.who.int/mediacentre/news/releases/2017/launch-version-report-jmp-water-sanitation-hygiene.pdf.

105. Global Task Force on Cholera Control. Personal communication. May 2018.

106. Harris JB, LaRocque RC, Chowdhury F, et al. Susceptibility to *Vibrio cholerae* infection in a cohort of household contacts of patients with cholera in Bangladesh. *PLoS Negl Trop Dis.* 2008;2(4):e221.

107. Nelson EJ, Harris JB, Morris JGJ, Calderwood SB, Camilli A. Cholera transmission: The host, pathogen and bacteriophage dynamic. *Nat Rev Microbiol.* 2009;7(10):693–702.

108. Leon-Barua R, Recavarren-Arce S, Chinga-Alayo E, et al. Helicobacter pylori-associated chronic atrophic gastritis involving the gastric body and severe disease by *Vibrio cholerae. Trans R Soc Trop Med Hyg.* 2006;100(6):567–72.

109. Swerdlow DL, Mintz ED, Rodriguez M, et al. Severe life-threatening cholera associated with blood group O in Peru: Implications for the Latin American epidemic. *J Infect Dis.* 1994;170(2):468–72.

110. Glass RI, Holmgren J, Haley CE, et al. Predisposition for cholera of individuals with O blood group. Possible evolutionary significance. *Am J Epidemiol.* 1985;121(6):791–6.

111. Ali M, Emch M, Park JK, Yunus M, Clemens J. Natural cholera infection-derived immunity in an endemic setting. *J Infect Dis.* 2011;204(6):912–8.

112. Qadri F, Wenneras C, Albert MJ, et al. Comparison of immune responses in patients infected with *Vibrio cholerae* O139 and O1. *Infect Immun.* 1997;65(9):3571–6.

113. Grandesso F, Rafael F, Chipeta S, et al. Oral cholera vaccination in hard-to-reach communities, Lake Chilwa, Malawi. *Bull World Health Organ.* 2018;96(12):817–25.

114. Tariq M, Memon M, Jafferani A, et al. Massive fluid requirements and an unusual BUN/creatinine ratio for pre-renal failure in patients with cholera. *PLoS One.* 2009;4(10):e7552.

115. Pollitzer R. Cholera studies. IX. Symptomatology, diagnosis, prognosis, and treatment. *Bull World Health Organ.* 1957;16(2):295–430.

116. DE SN. Enterotoxicity of bacteria-free culture-filtrate of Vibrio cholerae. *Nature.* 1959;183(4674):1533–4.
117. Banwell JG, Pierce NF, Mitra RC, et al. Intestinal fluid and electrolyte transport in human cholera. *J Clin Invest.* 1970;49(1):183–95.
118. Lonnroth I, Holmgren J. Subunit structure of cholera toxin. *J Gen Microbiol.* 1973;76(2):417–27.
119. Holmgren J, Lonnroth I, Svennerholm L. Tissue receptor for cholera exotoxin: Postulated structure from studies with GM1 ganglioside and related glycolipids. *Infect Immun.* 1973;8(2):208–14.
120. Ganguly NK, Kaur T. Mechanism of action of cholera toxin and other toxins. *Indian J Med Res.* 1996;104:28–37.
121. Hirschhorn N, Lindenbaum J, Greenough WB3rd, Alam SM. Hypoglycemia in children with acute diarrhoea. *Lancet.* 1966;2(7455):128–32.
122. Griffith LS, Fresh JW, Watten RH, Villaroman MP. Electrolyte replacement in paediatric cholera. *Lancet.* 1967;1(7501):1197–9.
123. Molla AM, Rahman M, Sarker SA, Sack DA, Molla A. Stool electrolyte content and purging rates in diarrhea caused by rotavirus, enterotoxigenic *E. coli*, and *V. cholerae* in children. *J Pediatr.* 1981;98(5):835–8.
124. Schillberg E, Ariti C, Bryson L, et al. Factors related to fetal death in pregnant women with cholera, Haiti, 2011–2014. *Emerg Infect Dis.* 2016;22(1):124–7.
125. McGhee JR, Mestecky J, Elson CO, Kiyono H. Regulation of IgA synthesis and immune response by T cells and interleukins. *J Clin Immunol.* 1989;9(3):175–99.
126. Murthy AK, Chaganty BKR, Troutman T, et al. Mannose-containing oligosaccharides of non-specific human secretory immunoglobulin A mediate inhibition of *Vibrio cholerae* biofilm formation. *PLoS One.* 2011;6(2):e16847.
127. von Seidlein L, Wang X-Y, Macuamule A, et al. Is HIV infection associated with an increased risk for cholera? Findings from a case-control study in Mozambique. *Trop Med Int Health.* 2008;13(5):683–8.
128. Lindenbaum J, Greenough WB, Islam MR. Antibiotic therapy of cholera in children. *Bull World Health Organ.* 1967;37(4):529–38.
129. Siddique AK, Salam A, Islam MS, et al. Why treatment centres failed to prevent cholera deaths among Rwandan refugees in Goma, Zaire. *Lancet.* 1995;345(8946):359–61.
130. Greenough WB3rd, Gordon RSJ, Rosenberg IS, Davies BI, Benenson AS. Tetracycline in the treatment of cholera. *Lancet Lond Engl.* 1964;1(7329):355–7.
131. Rahaman MM, Majid MA, AKMJ A, Islam MR. Effects of doxycycline in actively purging cholera patients: A double-blind clinical trial. *Antimicrob Agents Chemother.* 1976;10(4):610–2.
132. Kaushik JS, Gupta P, Faridi MM, Das S. Single dose azithromycin versus ciprofloxacin for cholera in children: A randomized controlled trial. *Indian Pediatr.* 2010;47(4):309–15.
133. Roy SK, Islam A, Ali R, et al. A randomized clinical trial to compare the efficacy of erythromycin, ampicillin and tetracycline for the treatment of cholera in children. *Trans R Soc Trop Med Hyg.* 1998;92(4):460–2.
134. Global Task Force on Cholera Control. *Technical Note: Use of Antibiotics for the Treatment of Cholera.* 2018. https://www.who.int/cholera/task_force/use-of-antibiotics-for-the-treatment-of-cholera.pdf?ua=1.
135. Weber JT, Mintz ED, Canizares R, et al. Epidemic cholera in Ecuador: Multidrug-resistance and transmission by water and seafood. *Epidemiol Infect.* 1994;112(1):1–11.
136. Reveiz L, Chapman E, Ramon-Pardo P, et al. Chemoprophylaxis in contacts of patients with cholera: Systematic review and meta-analysis. von Seidlein L, ed. *PLoS One.* 2011;6(11):e27060.
137. Towner KJ, Pearson NJ, Mhalu FS, O'Grady F. Resistance to antimicrobial agents of *Vibrio cholerae* El Tor strains isolated during the fourth cholera epidemic in the United Republic of Tanzania. *Bull World Health Organ.* 1980;58(5):747–51.
138. Roy SK, Hossain MJ, Khatun W, et al. Zinc supplementation in children with cholera in Bangladesh: Randomised controlled trial. *BMJ.* 2008;336(7638):266–8.
139. Cutler D, Miller G. The role of public health improvements in health advances: The twentieth-century United States. *Demography.* 2005;42(1):1–22.
140. Alcayaga S, Alcayaga J, Gassibe P. Changes in the morbidity profile of certain enteric infections after the cholera epidemic. *Rev Chile Infect.* 1993;1:5–10.
141. Global Task Force on Cholera Control. *Interim Guidance Document on Cholera Surveillance.* 2017. https://www.who.int/cholera/task_force/GTFCC-Guidance-cholera-surveillance.pdf?ua=1.
142. UNICEF. UNICEF Cholera Toolkit. 2017. https://www.unicef.org/cholera/index_71222.html.
143. UNICEF, CDC, MSF. Draft document for a position paper against chlorine spraying at households of cholera patients. 2011. https://www.unicef.org/cholera/Chapter_9_community/Haiti-POs_paper_against_chlorine_HH_spraying_cholera.docx.
144. Desai SN, Pezzoli L, Alberti KP, et al. Achievements and challenges for the use of killed oral cholera vaccines in the global stockpile era. *Hum Vaccines Immunother.* 2017;13(3):579–87.
145. WHO. Deployments from the oral cholera vaccine stockpile, 2013–2017-Déploiements à partir du stock de vaccins anticholériques oraux (VCO), 2013-2017. *Wkly Epidemiol Rec.* 2017;92(32):437–42.
146. Khan AI, Ali M, Chowdhury F, et al. Safety of the oral cholera vaccine in pregnancy: Retrospective findings from a subgroup following mass vaccination campaign in Dhaka, Bangladesh. *Vaccine.* 2017;35(11):1538–43.
147. Hashim R, Khatib AM, Enwere G, et al. Safety of the recombinant cholera toxin B subunit, killed whole-cell (rBS-WC) oral cholera vaccine in pregnancy. *PLoS Negl Trop Dis.* 2012;6(7):e1743.
148. Grout L, Martinez-Pino I, Ciglenecki I, et al. Pregnancy outcomes after a mass vaccination campaign with an oral cholera vaccine in Guinea: A retrospective cohort study. *PLoS Negl Trop Dis.* 2015;9(12):e0004274.
149. Bhattacharya SK, Sur D, Ali M, et al. 5 year efficacy of a bivalent killed whole-cell oral cholera vaccine in Kolkata, India: A cluster-randomised, double-blind, placebo-controlled trial. *Lancet Infect Dis.* 2013;13(12):1050–6.
150. Ivers LC, Hilaire IJ, Teng JE, et al. Effectiveness of reactive oral cholera vaccination in rural Haiti: A case-control study and bias-indicator analysis. *Lancet Glob Health.* 2015;3(3):e162–8.
151. Azman AS, Parker LA, Rumunu J, et al. Effectiveness of one dose of oral cholera vaccine in response to an outbreak: A case-cohort study. *Lancet Glob Health.* 2016;4(11):e856–63.
152. Qadri F, Wierzba TF, Ali M, et al. Efficacy of a single-dose, inactivated oral cholera vaccine in Bangladesh. *N Engl J Med.* 2016;374(18):1723–32.
153. Qadri F, Ali M, Lynch J, et al. Efficacy of a single-dose regimen of inactivated whole-cell oral cholera vaccine: Results from 2 years of follow-up of a randomised trial. *Lancet Infect Dis.* 2018;18(6):666–74.

CHAPTER

113

Escherichia coli, Diarrheagenic

Jennifer C. Hunter • Alison Winstead • Nancy A. Strockbine • Patricia M. Griffin

Escherichia coli are Gram-negative bacteria that are part of the normal intestinal flora of humans and animals. Most strains do not cause illness in healthy persons, but some have virulence attributes that enable them to cause disease. Pathogenic *E. coli* are categorized into pathotypes based on virulence genes that reflect distinctive aspects of their pathogenesis. Several pathotypes are associated with diarrhea, including enteropathogenic *E. coli* (EPEC), enterotoxigenic *E. coli* (ETEC), enteroinvasive *E. coli* (EIEC), Shiga toxin-producing *E. coli* (STEC),[1] and enteroaggregative *E. coli* (EAEC). Other pathotypes cause urinary tract infections, bloodstream infections, and meningitis. The relative importance of diarrheagenic pathotypes in the burden of disease globally and regionally has been difficult to assess because routine diagnostic methods for their detection are not readily available. Prevalence estimates for the different pathotypes largely come from studies that have used a variety of laboratory-developed tests.[1] As syndromic-focused assays that target a broad range of diarrheal pathogens are adopted, our estimates for the global and regional burden of disease attributable to these pathotypes should improve.

E. coli are also characterized by serotype, which is defined by a combination of up to four surface antigens (O, K, H, and F). The two commonly used surface antigens for serotyping diarrheagenic *E. coli* are the O antigen (repeating oligosaccharides of the lipopolysaccharide molecule) and the H antigen (flagellin of the flagellum). Historically, O:H serotyping has been useful for subtyping strains and predicting a strain's pathotype, because a relatively strong correlation exists between specific serotypes and combinations of virulence genes. Predicting pathotype is more reliably done by determining virulence gene content. Serotyping, however, still provides valuable context for understanding a strain's pathogenesis and relating historical with current findings. Because virulence genes are commonly on mobile genetic elements (e.g., bacteriophages, plasmids, and pathogenicity islands), *E. coli* often have virulence factors associated with more than one pathotype. The continuous movement of virulence genes within *E. coli* leads to the emergence of new strains capable of causing disease with clinical features reflective of new combinations of genes. An example is the O104:H4 strain that caused a large outbreak of bloody diarrhea in Germany in 2011; it produced Shiga toxin and, unlike other STEC, had adherence properties typical of EAEC.[2]

ENTEROPATHOGENIC *ESCHERICHIA COLI*

EPEC was the first pathotype widely recognized as a cause of diarrheal illness. In the 1940s, bacteria later classified as EPEC were linked to "infantile summer diarrhea." Investigations of outbreaks in newborn nurseries in industrialized countries, many with high fatality rates, implicated EPEC.[3,4] Although outbreaks in nurseries are now almost never reported from industrialized countries, EPEC continue to be an important cause of diarrheal illness in developing countries.[5]

Pathogenesis. EPEC produce an attaching and effacing (A/E) lesion; they do not produce Shiga toxins. Adherence to enterocytes in the small bowel is facilitated by production of intimin, a protein encoded by the *eae* gene. EPEC also produce the protein Tir, which is translocated into the enterocyte; Tir then acts as a receptor for intimin. The interaction of intimin and Tir and the cytoskeletal changes they induce result in intimate adherence of EPEC to the enterocyte and the formation of the characteristic A/E pedestal lesion.[6–8] EPEC are classified as "typical" or "atypical" based on the presence of the EPEC adherence factor (EAF) plasmid, which carries the genes that encode the bundle-forming pili (BFP). Typical EPEC (tEPEC) carry the EAF plasmid and cause diarrheal illness; atypical EPEC (aEPEC) do not have the EAF plasmid and their role as pathogens is unclear.[9]

Clinical characteristics. The diarrhea is watery, and illness ranges in severity from mild to severe; some patients develop persistent diarrhea. Fever and vomiting have been reported in fewer than half of cases. Among adult volunteers, diarrhea occurred, on average, 7–16 hours after inoculation and lasted fewer than 2 days.[10] However, multiple outbreak investigations indicate a longer duration of illness for infants. Among infants with moderate-to-severe diarrhea, a study published in 2013 found that those with tEPEC infection had a higher risk of dying than those without tEPEC.[5]

Epidemiology. Although EPEC are frequently detected in children younger than 5 years in countries with a low sociodemographic index, their contribution to the burden of diarrheal disease is unclear.[5,11–13] Codetection with other enteric pathogens is common, and EPEC are frequently detected in asymptomatic persons, which makes the interpretation of results challenging. The World Health Organization estimates that EPEC cause over 81 million illnesses and nearly 122,000 deaths globally each year.[14] The Global Enteric Multicenter Study (GEMS) reported attributable fractions of 0.3–3.4% for EPEC among medically attended children with moderate-to-severe diarrhea.[5]

Diagnosis. Identifying which *E. coli* with EPEC virulence properties are pathogens is a challenge. Laboratories now use genotypic tests, such as polymerase chain reaction (PCR) assays, that target the three major characteristics: *eae* gene, EAF plasmid, and lack of Shiga toxin genes. Clinicians should be aware that many asymptomatic persons harbor *E. coli* that test positive for the *eae* gene or the EAF plasmid in the gut, so identification of EPEC in a patient with diarrhea does not

[1] STEC are also called verotoxigenic *E. coli* (VTEC), and the term enterohemorrhagic *E. coli* is sometimes used to specify STEC strains capable of causing human illness, especially bloody diarrhea and hemolytic uremic syndrome (HUS).

confirm that EPEC is the etiology of illness. Diagnostic testing is not recommended for most cases of uncomplicated travelers' diarrhea.[15] Research laboratories can also use phenotypic testing, requiring the use of cell culture and fluorescence microscopy.

Treatment. Replacement of water and electrolytes by the oral or parenteral route is the only treatment usually required. Antimicrobial therapy should be considered for moderate-to-severe diarrhea if EPEC is thought to be a possible cause, for example, in a traveler who returned the week before illness began from an area with a lower sociodemographic index. Because antimicrobial resistance is common in EPEC,[16] selection of an agent would ideally be tailored to local resistance patterns. In resource-limited settings, nutritional rehabilitation, including supplementation with zinc and vitamin A, should be considered for children.

Prevention and control. Similar to other diarrheagenic *E. coli*, transmission is by the fecal-oral route, and the primary vehicles are thought to be contaminated water and food. Humans are the major reservoir for tEPEC,[17] whereas aEPEC have been isolated in animals traditionally kept as pets and those used for food production.[9]

Avoiding possibly unsafe water, undercooked foods, and perishable foods left at room temperature for more than 2 hours can help prevent illness. Fruits that are eaten peeled should be peeled by the person who eats them. Drinking water may be disinfected by boiling or by adding 1/8 teaspoon (or eight drops) of regular, unscented, liquid household bleach to a gallon of water at least 30 minutes before drinking. Beverages made with boiled water and served steaming hot (such as tea and coffee) are generally safe to drink. When served in unopened, factory-sealed cans or bottles, carbonated beverages, commercially prepared fruit drinks, water, alcoholic beverages, and pasteurized drinks can generally be considered safe (https://wwwnc.cdc.gov/travel/yellowbook/2018/the-pre-travel-consultation/food-water-precautions).[18]

Antimicrobial prophylaxis is not recommended for routine use in travelers to areas with high risk of disease transmission. When antimicrobial prophylaxis is indicated, rifaximin should be considered.[19] Probiotics, which are composed of live bacteria such as *Lactobacillus*, have not been shown to prevent travelers' diarrhea.[20]

ENTEROTOXIGENIC *ESCHERICHIA COLI*

In the late 1960s, investigators recognized that some *E. coli* strains that cause diarrhea in many animals and in humans produce enterotoxins. Research in the following decade led to the recognition that these organisms are a major cause of diarrhea in countries with a low sociodemographic index and an important etiology of travelers' diarrhea.

Pathogenesis. ETEC produce two plasmid-encoded enterotoxins, one heat-labile (LT) and the other heat-stable (ST). The heat-labile toxin is structurally similar to cholera toxin; it stimulates adenylate cyclase, resulting in loss of fluid and electrolytes from the intestine. The heat-stable toxin acts in a similar way through stimulation of guanylate cyclase.[21] In recent studies, ETEC that produce ST (with or without LT) have been associated with more severe disease than ETEC that produce only LT.[5,22] The relative frequency with which ETEC produce either or both toxins varies in different regions of the world. Strains producing both toxins appear to be largely restricted to a small number of serotypes. The ability to produce only one toxin or the other seems to occur in a broader range of serotypes. Colonization factors, also plasmid-encoded, appear to be essential for ETEC to establish itself in the small intestine and are the primary target of vaccine development.[23,24]

Clinical characteristics. The diarrhea, which is nonbloody, ranges from mild to dehydrating, similar to cholera; it lasts 1–7 days. Most patients have vomiting but fewer than 20% have fever.

Epidemiology. ETEC are a commonly identified etiology of travelers' diarrhea and a major cause of illness in countries with a low socioeconomic index.[25] The World Health Organization estimates that ETEC cause over 240 million illnesses and nearly 74,000 deaths globally each year.[14] The Global Enteric Multicenter Study (GEMS) identified ETEC as one of four major pathogens contributing to moderate-to-severe diarrhea in children younger than 5 years at selected sites.[5]

Diagnosis. ETEC can be identified by PCR assays, with most commercially available assays targeting the presence of the heat-stable human and porcine (STh and Stp) or heat-labile (LT) toxins. However, most clinical laboratories do not test for ETEC. Diagnostic testing is not recommended for most cases of uncomplicated travelers' diarrhea.[15]

Treatment. Replacement of water and electrolytes by the oral or parenteral route is the only treatment usually required. Antimicrobial therapy should be considered for moderate-to-severe diarrhea if ETEC is thought to be the likely cause, for example, in a traveler who returned the week before illness began from an area with a lower sociodemographic index. First-line therapy for children is azithromycin; either azithromycin or ciprofloxacin can be used for adults. Nutritional rehabilitation, including supplementation with zinc and vitamin A, should also be considered for malnourished children.

Prevention and control. Transmission is by the fecal-oral route, and the primary vehicles are thought to be contaminated water and food. Foodborne outbreaks have been reported, although rarely, in the United States[26] and other countries.[27–29] Contaminated water supplies have been identified as sources in domestic and international settings.[30–32]

Prevention measures are the same as for enteropathogenic *E. coli*.

ENTEROINVASIVE *ESCHERICHIA COLI*

The first EIEC was reported in 1947 as "paracolon bacillus," later identified as *E. coli* O124. During the 1950s and 1960s, EIEC strains, initially classified as *Shigella* species, were implicated as a cause of dysentery. In 1971, a U.S. outbreak of EIEC O124:B17 infections transmitted by imported French cheese affected 387 persons.[33] More recently, outbreaks affecting over 100 persons have been reported in Italy and the United Kingdom.[34,35] However, EIEC infections are most common in developing countries.

EIEC shares many features with *Shigella* species, including a virulence plasmid that facilitates invasion of the intestinal mucosa. Illness is usually characterized by watery diarrhea. Less commonly, EIEC infection can present with bloody stools and fever, similar to shigellosis and other enteric infections.[36] The invasion plasmid antigen H gene sequence, *ipaH*, which is used to detect *Shigella*, is also found in EIEC,[37] and many investigators consider EIEC and *Shigella* to be genetically the same species.[38] Uncertainty in identification makes it difficult to estimate disease burden.

SHIGA TOXIN-PRODUCING *ESCHERICHIA COLI*

STEC were first recognized as a cause of human disease after two outbreaks of illness in 1982 characterized by severe abdominal cramps, grossly bloody diarrhea, and little or no fever were associated with *E. coli* O157:H7.[39] STEC are defined by the presence of a gene for Shiga toxin in, or demonstrated production of Shiga toxin by, an *E. coli*.

Pathogenesis. All STEC produce one or both Shiga toxins (Stx1 and Stx2) that are highly similar to the toxin produced by *Shigella dysenteriae* type 1. These toxins are thought to travel through the blood, perhaps in blood cell-derived microvesicles, and bind to epithelial and endothelial cells, particularly in the kidney and central nervous system.[40] Toxin-mediated renal endothelial cell injury and subsequent host response can result in life-threatening hemolytic uremic syndrome (HUS) characterized by hemolytic anemia, thrombocytopenia, and acute renal dysfunction. HUS is more commonly associated with STEC strains that produce only Stx2 than those that produce both toxins or only Stx1.[41–44] Certain Stx2 subtypes (e.g.,

Stx2a) have been more strongly linked to HUS than others. STEC adhere to enterocytes; most use a type of intimin, encoded by *eae*, and produce an A/E lesion by a mechanism similar to EPEC. The increasing use of whole genome sequencing of isolates from ill persons as part of routine public health surveillance has the potential to advance our understanding of STEC virulence.[45–48]

Clinical characteristics. STEC cause nonbloody diarrhea, bloody diarrhea, and HUS. The incubation period for STEC O157 has been best studied; it is 3–4 days (range, 1–10 days). Progression from watery to bloody diarrhea occurs in most patients with diagnosed STEC O157 infection, usually on the second or third day of illness; it occurs in about half of those with diagnosed non-O157 STEC infection.[49,50] Most patients have abdominal pain, about one-third have fever, and vomiting occurs in some. The most severe manifestation is HUS, which is typically diagnosed a week after onset of illness, often after diarrhea has resolved.[51] Many patients with HUS have neurologic abnormalities. Approximately 15% of young children and a much smaller proportion of adults with laboratory-confirmed STEC O157 diarrhea develop HUS; only about 1% of patients with non-O157 STEC infection develop HUS. Half of patients with STEC-associated HUS require dialysis and 3–5% die. In a study of adults aged 60 years and older with STEC O157 infection, 33% with HUS died compared with 2% without.[52] STEC O157 is the major cause of diarrhea-associated HUS. Limited data suggest a mild increase in the risk of hypertension and reduced kidney function among persons with moderate or severe STEC O157 gastroenteritis.[53] Hypertension or long-term renal insufficiency occur in 25% of patients who survive diarrhea-associated HUS; these outcomes are more common among patients who had severe acute illness.[54] Other sequelae occur rarely, such as chronic neurologic deficits, diabetes mellitus, pancreatic insufficiency, and gastrointestinal complications.[55]

Epidemiology. In the United States, an estimated 265,000 STEC infections occur each year, most are not laboratory confirmed. Whereas infections caused by STEC O157 (approximately 40% of infections) have decreased in the past 10 years, the number of recognized non-O157 infections has increased, likely due to increasing use of culture-independent diagnostic tests.[56] In the United States, the most common serogroups isolated from people are (in descending order) O157, O26, O103, O111, O121, O45, and O145. The most common serogroups for which 50% or more of human isolates produce only Stx2 are O157, O121, and O145. In several European countries, a strain of STEC O26 has emerged that, unlike most STEC O26, produces Stx2; it has become an important cause of HUS.[57–60]

In outbreaks, STEC have been most frequently transmitted by ground beef and vegetable row crops (e.g., leafy vegetables),[61] but have also been linked to unchlorinated water, unpasteurized juice and milk, other raw fruits and vegetables, flour, and other vehicles. Person-to-person transmission is common in homes and has been the mode in outbreaks among children in day care centers, elderly adults in nursing homes, and in institutions for the mentally disabled.

Diagnosis. The Infectious Diseases Society of America (IDSA) clinical practice guidelines recommend that stool testing be performed when diarrhea is accompanied by fever, bloody or mucoid stools, severe abdominal cramping or tenderness, or signs of sepsis. A stool specimen should be tested for STEC O157 by culture on selective media and for non-O157 STEC by an assay that detects Shiga toxin or the genes that encode them.[15] All specimens with positive CIDT results should be cultured, either by the clinical laboratory or by arrangement with a public health laboratory, to obtain isolates for public health surveillance and response.[62] All confirmed and presumptive O157 STEC isolates and Shiga toxin-positive broths should be sent to a public health laboratory for isolation and characterization of the *E. coli*, including pulsed-field gel electrophoresis or whole genome sequencing, which is critical for outbreak detection.

Treatment. Primary treatment should focus on ensuring hydration to decrease the risk of oligoanuric renal failure. Antimicrobial therapy is not recommended.

Prevention and control. Because the primary reservoir for STEC O157 is cattle, prevention includes control measures in farming, cattle raising, slaughtering, and processing, as well as thoroughly cooking beef and pasteurizing milk. Fecal matter from animals can contaminate streams and the environment, leading to contamination of crops. Therefore, washing vegetables, chlorinating water, and pasteurizing juice can also prevent infections. Other STEC are widely spread among animal populations including cattle, and STEC O157 can also be found in other animals; control measures for all STEC are similar. The low infectious dose facilitates spread in child-care centers and among children who touch objects in petting zoos, so hygienic practices to reduce environment contamination and person-to-person spread can limit infections. Prompt epidemiologic investigation and implementation of control measures, such as excluding sick children from child-care centers, can limit the scope of outbreaks. A 10-year analysis of surveillance data in central Ireland found the median clearance time for STEC among children under age 6 is approximately 40 days; the predominant strains—O157 (41%) and O26 (44%)—did not have significantly different clearance times.[63] Vaccination of cattle against type III secretion proteins (e.g., Tir) decreases the percentage of animals shedding the bacteria, the bacterial load in positive animals, and the duration of shedding, so it might decrease the risk of human disease.[64]

Novel Strains

STEC strains associated with severe disease continue to be recognized, including those with virulence factors of other *E. coli* pathotypes. An example is the O104:H4 strain that caused an outbreak in Germany in 2011; it produced Stx2 and had adherence properties typical of EAEC.[65] In France, a virulent strain of STEC O80:H2 was identified in 2005 and is now recognized as an important cause of pediatric HUS there. This strain carries genes encoding Stx2 and intimin as well as genes characteristic of the pS88 plasmid associated with extraintestinal virulence.[2]

ENTEROAGGREGATIVE *ESCHERICHIA COLI*

EAEC have a "stacked brick" pattern of adherence to tissue culture cells and glass slides. It is not known how EAEC cause illness, although multiple virulence factors have been proposed. The extent of intestinal inflammation present is dependent on a proinflammatory flagellin.[66] These bacteria have been variably associated with acute[67–69] and persistent diarrhea[70,71] in children in developing countries. EAEC have also been implicated as an important cause of diarrhea in persons living with AIDS[72] and travelers.[73,74] However, in recent case-control studies among children younger than 5 years at selected sites in developing countries, EAEC was frequently found in a similar percentage of those with and without diarrhea.[5,22] A statistically significant attributable fraction of diarrheal illness was reported at only one site in one age group.[5,11]

The typical illness is characterized by watery or mucoid diarrhea with or without fever and vomiting.[70] Grossly bloody stools have been reported.[75] Like EPEC, the diagnosis of pathogenic EAEC is challenging. EAEC is known to cause asymptomatic colonization as well as diarrheal disease, and discrimination between the organisms by laboratory testing is difficult. PCR assays often identify EAEC by targeting genes such as *aggR* and *aat4*. However, nondiarrheagenic strains have also been found to possess *aggR*, and some *aggR*-negative strains have been associated with diarrhea.[76] Clinicians should interpret PCR assays carefully as identification of EAEC in a patient may not indicate that EAEC is the etiology of the illness.

Control measures, as for other forms of *E. coli*-associated diarrhea, consist of limiting fecal-oral transmission. Following safe food handling practices and avoiding fecally contaminated water can help prevent illness.

OTHER ENTEROVIRULENT *E. COLI*

Diffusely adherent *E. coli* (DAEC) is so named for its adherence pattern in cell culture. The clinical relevance of DAEC is well described for urinary tract infections, but their role in diarrhea is not well understood.[77,78] Cytolethal distending toxin-producing *E. coli* have been described,[79] but the presence of the toxin in many serotypes and pathotypes (predominantly EPEC)[80] makes it hard to delineate the epidemiology and public health importance of strains producing this toxin. It seems likely that new pathotypes of *E. coli* will continue to be described.

References

1. Kirk MD, Pires SM, Black RE, et al. World Health Organization estimates of the global and regional disease burden of 22 foodborne bacterial, protozoal, and viral diseases, 2010: A data synthesis. *PLoS Med.* 2015;12(12):e1001921.
2. Frank C, Werber D, Cramer JP, et al. Epidemic profile of Shiga-toxin–producing *Escherichia coli* O104: H4 outbreak in Germany. *N Engl J Med.* 2011;365(19):1771–80.
3. Kauffmann F, Dupont A. Escherichia strains from infantile epidemic gastroenteritis. *Acta Pathol.* 1950;27:552–64.
4. Wu S, Peng R. Studies on an outbreak of neonatal diarrhea caused by EPEC 0127:H6 with plasmid analysis restriction analysis and outer membrane protein determination. *Acta Paediatr.* 1992;81:217–21.
5. Kotloff KL, Nataro JP, Blackwelder WC, et al. Burden and aetiology of diarrhoeal disease in infants and young children in developing countries (the Global Enteric Multicenter Study, GEMS): A prospective, case-control study. *Lancet.* 2013;382(9888):209–22.
6. Hu J, Torres AG. Enteropathogenic *Escherichia coli*: Foe or innocent bystander? *Clin Microbiol Infect.* 2015;21(8):729–34.
7. Guttman JA, Li Y, Wickham ME, et al. Attaching and effacing pathogen-induced tight junction disruption in vivo. *Cell Microbiol.* 2006;8(4):634–45.
8. Frankel G, Phillips AD, Rosenshine I, Dougan G, Kaper JB, Knutton S. Enteropathogenic and enterohaemorrhagic *Escherichia coli*: More subversive elements. *Mol Microbiol.* 1998;30:911–21.
9. Hernandes RT, Elias WP, Vieira MAM, Gomes TAT. An overview of atypical enteropathogenic *Escherichia coli. FEMS Microbiol Lett.* 2009;297(2):137–49.
10. Levine M, Nalin D, Hornick R, et al. *Escherichia coli* strains that cause diarrhea but do not produce heat-labile or heat-stable enterotoxins and are non-invasive. *Lancet.* 1978;311(8074):1119–22.
11. Liu J, Platts-Mills JA, Juma J, et al. Use of quantitative molecular diagnostic methods to identify causes of diarrhoea in children: A reanalysis of the GEMS case-control study. *Lancet.* 2016;388(10051):1291–301.
12. Lanata CF, Fischer-Walker CL, Olascoaga AC, et al. Global causes of diarrheal disease mortality in children <5 years of age: A systematic review. *PLoS One.* 2013;8(9):e72788.
13. Donnenberg MS, Kaper JB. Enteropathogenic *Escherichia coli. Infect Immun.* 1992;60(10):3953–61.
14. World Health Organization. The World Health Organization estimates of the global burden of Foodborne Diseases: FERG Project Report. http://www.who.int/foodsafety/areas_work/foodborne-diseases/ferg/en/. 2015.
15. Shane AL, Mody RK, Crump JA, et al. 2017 Infectious Diseases Society of America clinical practice guidelines for the diagnosis and management of infectious diarrhea. *Clin Infect Dis.* 2017;65(12):e45–80.
16. Malvi S, Appannanavar S, Mohan B, et al. Comparative analysis of virulence determinants, antibiotic susceptibility patterns and serogrouping of atypical enteropathogenic Escherichia coli versus typical enteropathogenic *E. coli* in India. *J Med Microbiol.* 2015;64(10):1208–15.
17. Trabulsi LR, Keller R, Gomes TAT. 10.321/eid0805.Typical and atypical enteropathogenic *Escherichia coli. Emerg Infect Dis.* 2002;8(5):508–13.
18. Centers for Disease Control and Prevention. *CDC Health Information for International Travel 2016.* New York: Oxford University Press; 2016.
19. Riddle MS, Connor BA, Beeching NJ, et al. Guidelines for the prevention and treatment of travelers' diarrhea: A graded expert panel report. *J Travel Med.* 2017;24(Suppl 1):S63–80.
20. Sazawal S, Hiremath G, Dhingra U, et al. Efficacy of probiotics in prevention of acute diarrhoea: A meta-analysis of masked, randomized, placebo-controlled trials. *Lancet Infect Dis.* 2006;6(6):374–82.
21. Richards KL, Douglas SD. Pathophysiological effects of Vibrio cholerae and enterotoxigenic *Escherichia coli* and their exotoxins on eucaryotic cells. *Microbiol Rev.* 1978;42(3):592–613.
22. Platts-Mills JA, Babji S, Bodhidatta L, et al. Pathogen-specific burdens of community diarrhoea in developing countries: A multisite birth cohort study (MAL-ED). *Lancet Glob Health.* 2015;3 (9):e564–75.
23. McKenzie R, Bourgeois AL, Engstrom F, et al. Comparative safety and immunogenicity of two attenuated enterotoxigenic *Escherichia coli* vaccine strains in healthy adults. *Infect Immun.* 2006;74(2):994–1000.
24. Qadri F, Ahmed T, Ahmed F, et al. Safety and immunogenicity of an oral, inactivated enterotoxigenic *Escherichia coli* plus cholera toxin B subunit vaccine in Bangladeshi children 18–36 months of age. *Vaccine.* 2003;21(19–20):2394–403.
25. Lääveri T, Vilkman K, Pakkanen S, et al. Despite antibiotic treatment of travellers' diarrhoea, pathogens are found in stools from half of travellers at return. *Travel Med Infect Dis.* 2018;23:49–55.
26. Qadri F, Das SK, Faruque AS, et al. Prevalence of toxin types and colonization factors in enterotoxigenic *Escherichia coli* isolated during a 2-year period from diarrhea patients in Bangladesh. *J Clin Microbiol.* 2000;38:27–31.
27. Dalton CB, Mintz ED, Wells JG, Bopp CA, Tauxe RV. Outbreaks of enterotoxigenic Escherichia coli infection in American adults: A clinical and epidemiologic profile. *Epidemiol Infect.* 1999;123:9–16.
28. MacDonald E, Møller KE, Wester AL, et al. *Epidemiol Infect.* 2015;143(3):486–93.
29. Ethelberg S, Lisby M, Bottiger B, et al. Outbreaks of gastroenteritis linked to lettuce, Denmark, January 2010. *Euro Surveill.* 2010;15(6):19484.
30. Rosenberg ML, Koplan JP, Wachsmuth IK, et al. Epidemic diarrhea at Crater Lake from enterotoxigenic *Escherichia coli.* A large waterborne outbreak. *Ann Intern Med.* 1977;86(6):714–8.
31. Sack RB, Hirschhorn N, Brownlee I, Cash RA, Woodward WE, Sack DA. Enterotoxigenic *Escherichia coli*-associated diarrheal disease in Apache children. *N Engl J Med.* 1975;292(20):1041–5.
32. Ryder RW, Sack DA, Kapikian AZ, et al. Enterotoxigenic *Escherichia coli* and Reovirus-like agent in rural Bangladesh. *Lancet.* 1976;1(7961):659–63.
33. Marier R, Wells JG, Swanson RC, et al. An outbreak of enteropathogenic *Escherichia coli*: Foodborne disease traced to imported French cheese. *Lancet.* 1973;302(7842):1376–8.
34. Escher M, Scavia G, Morabito S, et al. A severe foodborne outbreak of diarrhoea linked to a canteen in Italy caused by enteroinvasive Escherichia coli, an uncommon agent. *Epidemiol Infect.* 2014;142:2559–66.
35. Newitt S, MacGregor V, Robbins V, et al. Two linked enteroinvasive *Escherichia coli* outbreaks, Nottingham, UK, June 2014. *Emerg Infect Dis.* 2016;22:1178–84.
36. Nataro JP, Kaper JB. Diarrheagenic *Escherichia coli. Clin Microbiol Rev.* 1998;11(1):142–201.
37. Aranda KRS, Fagundes-Neto U, Scaletsky ICA. Evaluation of multiplex PCRs for diagnosis of infection with diarrheagenic *Escherichia coli* and *Shigella* spp. *J Clin Microbiol.* 2004;42(12):5849–53.
38. Pettengill EA, Pettengill JB, Binet R. Phylogenetic analyses of *Shigella* and enteroinvasive *Escherichia coli* for the identification of molecular epidemiological markers: Whole-genome comparative analysis does not support distinct genera designation. *Front Microbiol.* 2015;6:1573.
39. Riley LW, Remis RS, Helgerson SD, et al. Hemorrhagic colitis associated with a rare *Escherichia coli* serotype. *N Engl J Med.* 1983;308(12):681–5.
40. Ståhl AL, Arvidsson I, Johansson KE, et al. A novel mechanism of bacterial toxin transfer within host blood cell-derived microvesicles. *PLoS Pathog.* 2015;11(2):e1004619.
41. Messens W, Bolton D, Frankel G, et al. Defining pathogenic verocytotoxin-producing *Escherichia coli* (VTEC) from cases of human infection in the European Union, 2007–2010. *Epidemiol Infect.* 2015;143(8):1652–61.
42. Ardissino G, Salardi S, Colombo E, et al. Epidemiology of haemolytic uremic syndrome in children. Data from the North Italian HUS network. *Eur J Pediatr.* 2016;175(4):465–73.
43. Brandal LT, Wester AL, Lange H, et al. Shiga toxin-producing *Escherichia coli* infections in Norway, 1992–2012: Characterization of isolates and identification of risk factors for haemolytic uremic syndrome. *BMC Infect Dis.* 2015;15(1):324.
44. Naseer U, Løbersli I, Hindrum M, Bruvik T, Brandal LT. Virulence factors of Shiga toxin-producing *Escherichia coli* and the risk of developing haemolytic uraemic syndrome in Norway, 1992–2013. *Eur J Clin Microbiol Infect Dis.* 2017;36(9):1613–20.
45. Dallman TJ, Byrne L, Launders N, Glen K, Grant KA, Jenkins C. The utility and public health implications of PCR and whole genome

sequencing for the detection and investigation of an outbreak of Shiga toxin-producing Escherichia coli serogroup O26:H11. *Epidemiol Infect.* 2015;143(8):1672–80.

46. Griffin PM, Tauxe RV. The epidemiology of infections caused by *Escherichia coli* O157:H7, other enterohemorrhagic *E. coli*, and the associated hemolytic uremic syndrome. *Epidemiol Rev.* 1991;13:60–98.
47. Thomas A, Chart H, Cheasty T, et al. Vero cytotoxin-producing *Escherichia coli*, particularly serogroup O157, associated with human infections in the United Kingdom: 1989–1991. *Epidemiol Infect.* 1993;110(3):591–600.
48. Thomas A, Cheasty T, Frost JA, et al. Vero cytotoxin-producing *Escherichia coli*, particularly serogroup O157, associated with human infections in England and Wales: 1992–1994. *Epidemiol Infect.* 1996;117(1):1–10.
49. Gould LH, Mody RK, Ong KL, et al. Increased recognition of non-O157 Shiga toxin-producing *Escherichia coli* infections in the United States during 2000–2010: Epidemiologic features and comparison with *E. coli* O157 infections. *Foodborne Pathog Dis.* 2013;10(5):453–60.
50. Ostroff SM, Kobayashi JM, Lewis JH. Infections with *Escherichia coli* 0157:H7 in Washington State: The first year of statewide disease surveillance. *JAMA.* 1989;262(3):355–9.
51. Tarr PI, Gordon CA, Chandler WL. Shiga-toxin-producing *Escherichia coli* and haemolytic uraemic syndrome. *Lancet.* 2005;365(9464):1073–86.
52. Gould LH, Demma L, Jones TF, et al. Hemolytic uremic syndrome and death in persons with *Escherichia coli* O157:H7 infection, foodborne diseases active surveillance network sites, 2000–2006. *Clin Infect Dis.* 2009;49(10):1480–5.
53. Garg AX, Moist L, Matsell D, et al. Risk of hypertension and reduced kidney function after acute gastroenteritis from bacteria-contaminated drinking water. *CMAJ.* 2005;173(3):261–8.
54. Garg AX, Suri RS, Barrowman N, et al. Long-term renal prognosis of diarrhea-associated hemolytic uremic syndrome: A systematic review, meta-analysis, and meta-regression. *JAMA.* 2003;290(10):1360–70.
55. Rosales A, Hofer J, Zimmerhackl LB, et al. Need for long-term follow-up in enterohemorrhagic *Escherichia coli*-associated hemolytic uremic syndrome due to late-emerging sequelae. *Clin Infect Dis.* 2012;54(10):1413–21.
56. Marder EP, Griffin PM, Cieslak PR, et al. Preliminary incidence and trends of infections with pathogens transmitted commonly through food—Foodborne Diseases Active Surveillance Network, 10 US Sites, 2006–2017. *Morb Mortal Wkly Rep.* 2018;67(11):324.
57. Tozzi AE, Caprioli A, Minelli F, et al. Shiga toxin-producing *Escherichia coli* infections associated with hemolytic uremic syndrome, Italy, 1988–2000. *Emerg Infect Dis.* 2003;9(1):106.
58. Scavia G, Gianviti A, Labriola V, et al. A case of haemolytic uraemic syndrome (HUS) revealed an outbreak of Shiga toxin-2-producing *Escherichia coli* O26:H11 infection in a nursery, with long-lasting shedders and person-to-person transmission, Italy 2015. *J Med Microbiol.* 2018;67(6):775–82.
59. Usein CR, Ciontea AS, Militaru CM, et al. Molecular characterisation of human Shiga toxin-producing *Escherichia coli* O26 strains: Results of an outbreak investigation, Romania, February to August 2016. *Euro Surveill.* 2017;22(47).
60. Bielaszewska M, Mellmann A, Bletz S, et al. Enterohemorrhagic *Escherichia coli* O26:H11/H−: A new virulent clone emerges in Europe. *Clin Infect Dis.* 2013;56(10):1373–81.
61. Interagency Food Safety Analytics Collaboration. Foodborne illness source attribution estimates for 2013 for Salmonella, *Escherichia coli* O157, Listeria monocytogenes, and Campylobacter using multi-year outbreak surveillance data, United States. Atlanta, Georgia and Washington, DC: U.S. Department of Health and Human Services, CDC, FDA, USDA/FSIS; 2018. https://www.cdc.gov/foodsafety/pdfs/IFSAC-2013FoodborneillnessSourceEstimates-508.pdf. 2017 December. Accessed on May 28, 2018.
62. Gould LH, Bopp C, Strockbine N, et al. Recommendations for diagnosis of Shiga toxin–producing *Escherichia coli* infections by clinical laboratories. *Morb Mortal Wkly Rep.* 2009;58(12):1–4.
63. Collins A, Fallon UB, Cosgrove M, Meagher G, Shuileabhan CN. A 10-year analysis of VTEC microbiological clearance times, in the under-six population of the Midlands, Ireland. *Epidemiol Infect.* 2017;145(8):1577–83.
64. Potter AA, Klashinsky S, Li Y, et al. Decreased shedding of *Escherichia coli* O157:H7 by cattle following vaccination with type III secreted proteins. *Vaccine.* 2004;22(3–4):362–9.
65. Soysal N, Mariani-Kurkdjian P, Smail Y, et al. Enterohemorrhagic *Escherichia coli* hybrid pathotype O80:H2 as a new therapeutic challenge. *Emerg Infect Dis.* 2016;22(9):1604.
66. Steiner TS, Nataro JP, Poteet-Smith CE, et al. Enteroaggregative *Escherichia coli* expresses a novel flagellin that causes IL-8 release from intestinal epithelial cells. *J Clin Invest.* 2000;105(12):1769–77.
67. Albert MJ, Faruque SM, Faruque AS, et al. Controlled study of *Escherichia coli* diarrheal infections in Bangladeshi children. *J Clin Microbiol.* 1995;33(4):973–7.
68. Salmanzadeh-Ahrabi S, Habibi E, Jaafari F, et al. Molecular epidemiology of *Escherichia coli* diarrhoea in children in Tehran. *Ann Trop Paediatr.* 2005;25(1):35–9.
69. Orlandi PP, Magalhaes GF, Matos NB, et al. Etiology of diarrheal infections in children of Porto Velho (Rondonia, Western Amazon region, Brazil). *Braz J Med Biol Res.* 2006;39(4):507–17.
70. Bhan MK, Raj P, Levine MM, et al. Enteroaggregative *Escherichia coli* associated with persistent diarrhea in a cohort of rural children in India. *J Infect Dis.* 1989;159(6):1061–4.
71. Bhan MK, Bhandari N, Sazawal S, et al. Descriptive epidemiology of persistent diarrhoea among young children in rural northern India. *Bull World Health Organ.* 1989;67(3):281–8.
72. Wanke CA, Mayer H, Weber R, et al. Enteroaggregative *Escherichia coli* as a potential cause of diarrheal disease in adults infected with human immunodeficiency virus. *J Infect Dis.* 1998;178(1):185–90.
73. Adachi JA, Jiang ZD, Mathewson JJ, et al. Enteroaggregative *Escherichia coli* as a major etiologic agent in traveler's diarrhea in three regions of the world. *Clin Infect Dis.* 2001;32(12):1706–9.
74. Adachi JA, Ericsson CD, Jiang ZD, et al. Natural history of enteroaggregative and enterotoxigenic *Escherichia coli* infection among U.S. travelers to Guadalajara, Mexico. *J Infect Dis.* 2002;185(11):1681–3.
75. Cravioto A, Tello A, Navarro A, et al. Association of *Escherichia coli* HEp-2 adherence patterns with type and duration of diarrhoea. *Lancet.* 1991;337(8736):262–4.
76. Nüesch-Inderbinen MT, Hofer E, Hächler H, Beutin L, Stephan R. Characteristics of enteroaggregative *Escherichia coli* isolated from healthy carriers and from patients with diarrhoea. *J Med Microbiol.* 2013;62(12):1828–34.
77. Kaper JB, Nataro JP, Mobley HL. Pathogenic *Escherichia coli*. *Nat Rev Microbiol.* 2004;2(2):123.
78. Servin AL. Pathogenesis of human diffusely adhering *Escherichia coli* expressing Afa/Dr adhesins (Afa/Dr DAEC): Current insights and future challenges. *Clin Microbiol Rev.* 2014;27(4):823–69.
79. Johnson WM, Lior H. A new heat-labile cytolethal distending toxin (CLDT) produced by *Escherichia coli* isolates from clinical material. *Microb Pathog.* 1988;4(2):103–13.
80. Ansaruzzaman M, Albert MJ, Nahar S, et al. Clonal groups of enteropathogenic *Escherichia coli* isolated in case-control studies of diarrhoea in Bangladesh. *J Med Microbiol.* 2000;49(2):177–85.

CHAPTER 114

Shigellosis

Katie Fullerton • Beth E. Karp • Grace D. Appiah • Nancy A. Strockbine

Worldwide, shigellosis is estimated to cause more than 188 million cases of diarrhea each year, including about 500,000 cases in the United States.[1,2] "Bacillary dysentery," a term used to describe a diarrheal illness with fever, abdominal pain, and blood and pus (leukocytes) in the stool, is often used to refer to shigellosis in lower income countries. Transmission of *Shigella* spp. is most likely when there is crowding and hygiene and sanitation are insufficient. Shigellosis is predominantly caused by *S. sonnei* in industrialized countries, whereas *S. flexneri* prevails in lower income countries; there is evidence that *S. sonnei* is increasing in industrializing regions in Asia, Latin America, and the Middle East.[3] Infections caused by *S. boydii* and *S. dysenteriae* are uncommon globally but can make up a substantial proportion of *Shigella* spp. isolated in sub-Saharan Africa and South Asia.

In the United States, outbreaks and sporadic disease typically occur among young children in childcare centers,[4–7] international travelers,[8–11] men who have sex with men (MSM),[12–22] persons with weakened immune systems,[23] and those in small social groups such as traditionally observant Jewish communities.[24–27] Antibiotic resistance among *Shigella* is a serious and growing worldwide problem that is limiting options for effective treatment. The Centers for Disease Control and Prevention (CDC) has categorized drug-resistant *Shigella* as a serious threat to public health, and the World Health Organization (WHO) has included fluoroquinolone-resistant *Shigella* on its global priority list of antibiotic-resistant pathogens.[28,29]

BACTERIOLOGY

The Shigella species are a fairly homogeneous group of Gram-negative, facultatively anaerobic, nonmotile, nonlactose-fermenting bacilli classified in the family *Enterobacteriaceae*. The genus *Shigella* has 4 species or subgroups (A, B, C, and D) and 43 serotypes. Subgroups A, B, C, and D have historically been treated as species: subgroup A is referred to as *S. dysenteriae*; subgroup B as *S. flexneri;* subgroup C as *S. boydii*, and subgroup D as *S. sonnei*. Subgroups and serotypes are differentiated from each other by biochemical characteristics (e.g., ability to ferment D-mannitol) and antigenic properties. The most recently recognized serotype belongs to subgroup C.[30–32]

Shigella species are becoming increasingly resistant to first-line treatment agents, including ciprofloxacin and azithromycin, and, in some areas, cephalosporins.[33–40] The mechanisms underlying these resistance phenotypes in *Shigella* include mobile genetic elements with resistance genes [e.g., plasmids with *mph(A)* and CTX-M genes conferring resistance to azithromycin and cephalosporins, respectively], and chromosomal mutations (e.g., *gyrA* and *parC* mutations conferring fluoroquinolone resistance).[33,34,41–45] Both clonal expansion of resistant strains and horizontal transfer of resistance determinants have contributed to the spread of clinically important resistance.[43,46] Genetic studies suggest that fluoroquinolone resistance in *Shigella sonnei* has been largely driven by the expansion of a clone that emerged and spread in South Asia before disseminating intercontinentally to Europe, America, and other areas.[33,46] In contrast, the genes conferring azithromycin resistance among *Shigella* are carried on conjugative plasmids and are multiphyletic; the genes are strongly associated with sublineages found in MSM.[41–43]

Shigella with plasmid-mediated quinolone resistance (PMQR) mechanisms have been reported in several countries and now have emerged in the United States. Isolates with PMQR usually have elevated ciprofloxacin minimum inhibitory concentrations (MICs), but are considered ciprofloxacin susceptible according to current clinical breakpoints; the clinical impact of such elevations in fluoroquinolone MICs is not known.[104] Although azithromycin epidemiological cutoff values for *Shigella* have been published,[113] clinical breakpoints are not available to help guide treatment. Additionally, clinical laboratories should be aware that a dual-zone phenomenon seen with disk diffusion and Etest® (bioMérieux, St. Louis, MO) methods for *Shigella sonnei* can make interpretation difficult.[114]

TRANSMISSION

The primary reservoir for *Shigella* organisms is humans, although Shigella species occasionally infect other primates. The infective dose can be as low as ten organisms.[32,47,48] The primary mode of transmission is direct or indirect fecal-oral transmission from a symptomatic patient or asymptomatic carrier. Transmission can occur via contaminated objects and food or water; houseflies can also be vectors in settings with environmental fecal contamination.[7,49–52] However, *Shigella* is most often transmitted person-to-person, including through sexual contact. Many outbreaks of multidrug-resistant *Shigella* have occurred in recent years among MSM.[16,20,53,54] Childcare center-associated outbreaks are common and often difficult to control.[7,55–57] Secondary attack rates are high in homes of preschool children with shigellosis.[58–60] *Shigella* infections can also be transmitted by contaminated food,[61–63] ill food handlers,[64–66] and contaminated water used for drinking or recreational purposes.[67–72] Other groups with an increased risk of shigellosis include persons in situations where personal hygiene is difficult to maintain such as those in custodial institutions or the homeless[54,73,74]; and social groups with large households containing many children such as traditionally observant Jews.[24–27]

OCCURRENCE

In the United States, shigellosis is a nationally notifiable disease (required to be reported to state health departments, which then send the data to CDC).[75] In 2016, the incidence of confirmed and probable cases shigellosis reported in the United States was 6.5 cases per 100,000 population.[75,76] As in previous years, the highest rates occurred among children aged 1–14 years. In the United States, shigellosis does not demonstrate marked seasonality, likely reflecting the contribution of year-round person-to-person transmission.[75] Preliminary data for 2017 from the CDC's Foodborne Diseases Active Surveillance Network shows that the incidence of laboratory-diagnosed *Shigella* infections was 4.3 cases per 100,000 population in ten sentinel U.S. sites.[77]

Globally, most shigellosis occurs in children 1–4 years old living in lower income countries; the Global Enteric Multicenter Study (GEMS) found *Shigella* to be the most common cause of acute moderate-to-severe diarrhea in children aged 24–59 months living in sub-Saharan Africa and south Asia. *Shigella* was the second leading cause of diarrhea in children aged 12–23 months.[78–80]

CLINICAL CHARACTERISTICS

The usual incubation period is 1–3 days, but may range from 12 to 96 hours and up to 1 week for *S. dysenteriae* type 1 (Sd1).[32] In normal hosts, *Shigella* gastroenteritis is usually self-limited with symptoms generally lasting less than a week if untreated. Shigellosis is characterized by watery, bloody, or mucoid diarrhea, fever, stomach cramps, and nausea. Shigellosis often begins with fever, headache, malaise, and vomiting followed by abdominal pain and watery diarrhea without blood.[81,82] At this stage, the diarrhea is difficult to distinguish from that caused by other agents; abdominal pain may mimic appendicitis or, in young infants, intussusception and necrotizing enterocolitis.[39] Following invasion of the colonic mucosa, stools often become bloody, mucoid, and scant. Large bowel microabscesses and ulcers may form, and the patient may suffer from urgency and tenesmus. Infection with *S. sonnei* typically causes milder illness than infection with the other *Shigella* species; illness associated with *S. dysenteriae* type 1 is often severe. *Shigella* of any species can cause severe illness among people with compromised immune systems. Intestinal complications, including obstruction, rectal prolapse, toxic megacolon, and colonic perforation,[82] occur most commonly with *S. dysenteriae* type 1. Prolonged carriage is uncommon in healthy people, but carriage for more than 1 year has been reported.[83]

Complications include postinfectious arthritis, bloodstream infection, seizure, and hemolytic-uremic syndrome. Postinfectious arthritis, also known as reactive arthritis, is an immune-mediated syndrome of joint pain, eye irritation, and painful urination after an infection. It occurs in approximately 2% of persons infected with *Shigella flexneri*. Few cases have been reported in association with *S. sonnei* or *S. dysenteriae* infection. The syndrome can last for months or years, and can lead to chronic arthritis. Postinfectious arthritis is caused by a reaction to infection that happens more often in those who have HLA B27.[82,84–91] *Shigella* bloodstream infections are rare; they are most common among patients with weakened immune systems, such as those with HIV, cancer, or severe malnutrition.[82,92,93] Generalized seizures have been reported occasionally among young children with shigellosis, and usually resolve without treatment. Children who experience seizures while infected with *Shigella* typically have a high fever or abnormal blood electrolytes, but it is not well understood why the seizures occur.[39,94–98] In patients with shigellosis, hemolytic-uremic syndrome is infrequently associated with Shiga toxin-producing *Shigella*, almost exclusively *Shigella dysenteriae*.[99]

DIAGNOSIS AND TREATMENT

Culture has been the mainstay for diagnosis although rapid, culture-independent diagnostic tests (CIDT) are increasingly being used for diagnosis.[77,100–103] Specimens with CIDT-positive results should be cultured to obtain isolates for antimicrobial susceptibility testing and essential public health surveillance activities, such as subtyping, detecting outbreaks, and determining routes of transmission.[100,104] Many *Shigella* organisms are present in the intestinal mucus or feces during the first several days of the illness. If direct inoculation of culture media is not possible, fecal material or rectal swabs should be placed in Cary-Blair transport medium. The organism can be isolated from commonly used enteric media; however, so-called "*Salmonella-Shigella*" agar is actually inhibitory to some *Shigellae*. Commercially available antisera can be used for grouping and typing.[105]

Shigellosis is generally a self-limited infection. Supportive care and correcting fluid and electrolyte losses is the mainstay of treatment.[82] Antimicrobial treatment is not required for mild infections, but it is recommended for patients with severe disease or immunosuppressive conditions.[79,102] Early treatment with antibiotics can slightly shorten the duration of symptoms and excretion of *Shigella*.[34,106] Due to widespread resistance, ampicillin and trimethoprim-sulfamethoxazole are no longer recommended for empiric treatment.[34,82,107,108] Ciprofloxacin, azithromycin, and ceftriaxone are now considered first-line agents for empiric treatment.[39,82,108] Because resistance to these agents is common in some areas and emerging in others, antibiograms from the area where the patient likely acquired the infection should guide treatment until susceptibility results are available.[34,39,104,109] In the United States and Canada, resistance to ciprofloxacin and reduced susceptibility to azithromycin have been increasing among *Shigella*. Persons at increased risk for infection with drug-resistant *Shigella* include international travelers, HIV-infected persons, and MSM.[10,13–16,20,53,54,110–112]

PREVENTION AND CONTROL

The best defense against shigellosis is thorough handwashing, strict adherence to standard food and water safety precautions, minimizing fecal-oral exposures during sexual contact, and avoiding sexual activity with people who have diarrhea or who recently recovered from shigellosis (as *Shigella* may be present in stool for several weeks). Alcohol-based hand sanitizers can be a useful adjunct to washing hands with soap and water or when soap and water are not available.[106] Once begun, outbreaks of shigellosis are difficult to contro.[25,55] Interrupting the fecal-oral transmission cycle is the key objective, and handwashing with soap and running water is the most effective intervention.[56,115] In childcare settings, children who recently recovered from shigellosis can be grouped together in one room to reduce spread of *Shigella* to children who are not sick. Adults who recently recovered from shigellosis can be moved to jobs that are less likely to spread infection (e.g., administrative work instead of food preparation), depending on local health regulations; an increased focus on hygiene is usually needed to control outbreaks in childcare facilities.[116,117] Use of antimicrobial agents to control outbreaks may be ineffective, particularly among MSM, due to the emergence of multidrug-resistant strains.[16,53] Efforts to develop *Shigella* vaccines are ongoing, but have been complicated by the large number of antigenically distinct serotypes.[39,118,119]

References

1. Scallan E, Hoekstra RM, Angulo FJ, et al. Foodborne illness acquired in the United States—Major pathogens. *Emerg Infect Dis*. 2011;17(1):7–15.
2. Pires SM, Fischer-Walker CL, Lanata CF, et al. Aetiology-specific estimates of the global and regional incidence and mortality of diarrhoeal diseases commonly transmitted through food. *PLoS One*. 2015;10(12):e0142927.
3. Thompson CN, Duy PT, Baker S. The rising dominance of *Shigella sonnei*: An intercontinental shift in the etiology of bacillary dysentery. *PLoS Negl Trop Dis*. 2015;9(6):e0003708.
4. Scallan E, Mahon BE, Hoekstra RM, Griffin PM. Estimates of illnesses, hospitalizations and deaths caused by major bacterial enteric pathogens in young children in the United States. *Pediatr Infect Dis J*. 2013;32(3):217–21.
5. Haley CC, Ong KL, Hedberg K, et al. Risk factors for sporadic shigellosis, FoodNet 2005. *Foodborne Pathog Dis*. 2010;7(7):741–7.
6. Adams DA, Thomas KR, Jajosky RA, et al. Summary of notifiable infectious diseases and conditions—United States, 2015. *MMWR Morb Mortal Wkly Rep*. 2017;64(53):1–143.
7. Wikswo ME, Kambhampati A, Shioda K, et al. Outbreaks of acute gastroenteritis transmitted by person-to-person contact, environmental contamination, and unknown modes of transmission—United States, 2009–2013. *MMWR Surveill Summ*. 2015;64(12):1–16.

8. Kantele A. As far as travelers' risk of acquiring resistant intestinal microbes is considered, no antibiotics (absorbable or nonabsorbable) are safe. *Clin Infect Dis.* 2015;60(12):1872–3.
9. Kendall ME, Crim S, Fullerton K, et al. Travel-associated enteric infections diagnosed after return to the United States, Foodborne Diseases Active Surveillance Network (FoodNet), 2004–2009. *Clin Infect Dis.* 2012;54(Suppl 5):S480–7.
10. Bowen A, Hurd J, Hoover C, et al. Importation and domestic transmission of *Shigella sonnei* resistant to ciprofloxacin—United States, May 2014–February 2015. *MMWR Morb Mortal Wkly Rep.* 2015;64(12):318–20.
11. Gray MD, Lampel KA, Strockbine NA, Fernandez RE, Melton-Celsa AR, Maurelli AT. Clinical isolates of Shiga toxin 1a-producing *Shigella flexneri* with an epidemiological link to recent travel to Hispaniola. *Emerg Infect Dis.* 2014;20(10):1669–77.
12. Aragon TJ, Vugia DJ, Shallow S, et al. Case-control study of shigellosis in San Francisco: The role of sexual transmission and HIV infection. *Clin Infect Dis.* 2007;44(3):327–34.
13. Gaudreau C, Ratnayake R, Pilon PA, Gagnon S, Roger M, Lévesque S. Ciprofloxacin-resistant *Shigella sonnei* among men who have sex with men, Canada, 2010. *Emerg Infect Dis.* 2011;17(9):1747–50.
14. Gaudreau C, Pilon PA, Cornut G, Marchand-Senecal X, Bekal S. *Shigella flexneri* with Ciprofloxacin resistance and reduced azithromycin susceptibility, Canada, 2015. *Emerg Infect Dis.* 2016;22(11):2016–8.
15. Gaudreau C, Barkati S, Leduc J-M, Pilon PA, Favreau J, Bekal S. Shigella spp. with reduced azithromycin susceptibility, Quebec, Canada, 2012–2013. *Emerg Infect Dis.* 2014;20(5):854–6.
16. Heiman KE, Karlsson M, Grass J, et al. Notes from the field: Shigella with decreased susceptibility to azithromycin among men who have sex with men—United States, 2002–2013. *MMWR Morb Mortal Wkly Rep.* 2014;63(6):132–3.
17. Morgan O, Crook P, Cheasty T, et al. *Shigella sonnei* outbreak among homosexual men, London. *Emerg Infect Dis.* 2006;12(9):1458–60.
18. Okame M, Adachi E, Sato H, et al. *Shigella sonnei* outbreak among men who have sex with men in Tokyo. *Jpn J Infect Dis.* 2012;65(3):277–8.
19. Centers for Disease Control and Prevention (CDC). Shigella flexneri serotype 3 infections among men who have sex with men—Chicago, Illinois, 2003–2004. *MMWR Morb Mortal Wkly Rep.* 2005;54(33):820–2.
20. Bowen A, Eikmeier D, Talley P, et al. Notes from the field: Outbreaks of *Shigella sonnei* infection with decreased susceptibility to azithromycin among men who have sex with men—Chicago and Metropolitan Minneapolis-St. Paul, 2014. *MMWR Morb Mortal Wkly Rep.* 2015;64(21):597–8.
21. Borg ML, Modi A, Tostmann A, et al. Ongoing outbreak of *Shigella flexneri* serotype 3a in men who have sex with men in England and Wales, data from 2009–2011. *Euro Surveill.* 2012;17(13):20137.
22. Simms I, Field N, Jenkins C, et al. Intensified shigellosis epidemic associated with sexual transmission in men who have sex with men—*Shigella flexneri* and *S. sonnei* in England, 2004 to end of February 2015. *Euro Surveill.* 2015;20(15):16.
23. Hoffmann C, Sahly H, Jessen A, et al. High rates of quinolone-resistant strains of *Shigella sonnei* in HIV-infected MSM. *Infection.* 2013;41(5):999–1003.
24. De Schrijver K, Bertrand S, Garitano IG, Van den Branden D, Van Schaeren J. Outbreak of *Shigella sonnei* infections in the Orthodox Jewish community of Antwerp, Belgium, April to August 2008. *Euro Surveill.* 2011;16(14):19838.
25. Garrett V, Bornschlegel K, Lange D, et al. A recurring outbreak of *Shigella sonnei* among traditionally observant Jewish children in New York City: The risks of daycare and household transmission. *Epidemiol Infect.* 2006;134(6):1231–6.
26. Sobel J, Cameron DN, Ismail J, et al. A prolonged outbreak of *Shigella sonnei* infections in traditionally observant Jewish communities in North America caused by a molecularly distinct bacterial subtype. *J Infect Dis.* 1998;177(5):1405–9.
27. Baker KS, Dallman TJ, Behar A, et al. Travel- and community-based transmission of multidrug-resistant *Shigella sonnei* lineage among International Orthodox Jewish Communities. *Emerg Infect Dis.* 2016;22(9):1545–53.
28. World Health Organization (WHO). Global priority list of antibiotic-resistant bacteria to guide research, discovery, and development of new antibiotics. 2017 [cited 2018 5/8/2018]. http://www.who.int/medicines/publications/global-priority-list-antibiotic-resistant-bacteria/en/.
29. Centers for Disease Control and Prevention (CDC). Antibiotic Resistance Threats in the United States, 2013. 2013 [cited 2018 5/8/2018]. https://www.cdc.gov/drugresistance/threat-report-2013/.
30. Ewing WH, Reavis RW, Davis BR. Provisional Shigella serotypes. *Can J Microbiol.* 1958;4(2):89–107.
31. Centers for Disease Control and Prevention (CDC). National Shigella Surveillance, 2014. 11/21/2017 [cited 2018 5/8/2018]. https://www.cdc.gov/nationalsurveillance/shigella-surveillance.html.
32. Bowen A. In: Heymann DL, ed. *Shigellosis, in Control of Communicable Diseases Manual.* Washington, DC: American Public Health Association; 2015.
33. The HC, Baker S. Out of Asia: The independent rise and global spread of fluoroquinolone-resistant Shigella. *Microb Genom.* 2018;4(4):e000171.
34. Klontz KC, Singh N. Treatment of drug-resistant Shigella infections. *Expert Rev Antiinfect Ther.* 2015;13(1):69–80.
35. Baker KS, Dallman TJ, Ashton PM, et al. Intercontinental dissemination of azithromycin-resistant shigellosis through sexual transmission: A cross-sectional study. *Lancet Infect Dis.* 2015;15(8):913–21.
36. Centers for Disease Control and Prevention (CDC). CDC HAN 00379: Ciprofloxacin- and Azithromycin-Nonsusceptible Shigellosis in the United States, 2015. [cited 2018 5/8/2018]. https://emergency.cdc.gov/han/han00379.asp.
37. Gu B, Cao Y, Pan S, et al. Comparison of the prevalence and changing resistance to nalidixic acid and ciprofloxacin of Shigella between Europe-America and Asia-Africa from 1998 to 2009. *Int J Antimicrob Agents.* 2012;40(1):9–17.
38. Gu B, Zhou M, Ke X, et al. Comparison of resistance to third-generation cephalosporins in Shigella between Europe-America and Asia-Africa from 1998 to 2012. *Epidemiol Infect.* 2015;143(13):2687–99.
39. Kotloff KL, Riddle MS, Platts-Mills JA, Pavlinac P, Zaidi AKM. Shigellosis. *Lancet.* 2018;391(10122):801–12.
40. Chang Z, Zhang J, Ran L, et al. The changing epidemiology of bacillary dysentery and characteristics of antimicrobial resistance of Shigella isolated in China from 2004–2014. *BMC Infect Dis.* 2016;16(1):685.
41. Darton TC, Tuyen HT, The HC, et al. Azithromycin resistance in Shigella spp. in Southeast Asia. *Antimicrob Agents Chemother.* 2018;62(4):e01748-17.
42. Baker KS, Dallman TJ, Ashton PM, et al. Intercontinental dissemination of azithromycin-resistant shigellosis through sexual transmission: A cross-sectional study. *Lancet Infect Dis.* 2015;15(8):913–21.
43. Baker KS, Dallman TJ, Field N, et al. Horizontal antimicrobial resistance transfer drives epidemics of multiple Shigella species. *Nat Commun.* 2018;9(1):1462.
44. Zhang CL, Liu Q-Z, Wang J, Chu X, Shen L-M, Guo Y-Y. Epidemic and virulence characteristic of Shigella spp. with extended-spectrum cephalosporin resistance in Xiaoshan District, Hangzhou, China. *BMC Infect Dis.* 2014;14:260.
45. Nuesch-Inderbinen M, Heini N, Zurfluh K, Althaus D, Hächler H, Stephan R. Shigella antimicrobial drug resistance mechanisms, 2004–2014. *Emerg Infect Dis.* 2016;22(6):1083–5.
46. The HC, Rabba MA, Thanh DP, et al. South Asia as a reservoir for the global spread of ciprofloxacin-resistant *Shigella sonnei*: A cross-sectional study. *PLoS Med.* 2016;13(8):e1002055.
47. Ross AI. The role of the symptomless excreter in the spread of Sonne dysentery. *Mon Bull Minist Health Public Health Lab Serv.* 1957;16:174–9.
48. DuPont HL, Levine MM, Hornick RB, Formal SB. Inoculum size in shigellosis and implications for expected mode of transmission. *J Infect Dis.* 1989;159(6):1126–8.
49. Tuttle J, Ries AA, Chimba RM, Perera CU, Bean NH, Griffin PM. Antimicrobial-resistant epidemic *Shigella dysenteriae* type 1 in Zambia: Modes of transmission. *J Infect Dis.* 1995;171(2):371–5.
50. George CM, Ahmed S, Talukder KA, et al. Shigella infections in household contacts of pediatric shigellosis patients in rural Bangladesh. *Emerg Infect Dis.* 2015;21(11):2006–13.
51. Cohen D, Green M, Block C, Slepon R, Ambar R, Wasserman SS, Levine MM. Reduction of transmission of shigellosis by control of houseflies (*Musca domestica*). *Lancet.* 1991;337(8748):993–7.
52. Levine OS, Levine MM. Houseflies (*Musca domestica*) as mechanical vectors of shigellosis. *Rev Infect Dis.* 1991;13(4):688–96.
53. Bowen A, Grass J, Bicknese A, Campbell D, Hurd J, Kirkcaldy RD. Elevated risk for antimicrobial drug-resistant Shigella infection among men who have sex with men, United States, 2011–2015. *Emerg Infect Dis.* 2016;22(9):1613–6.
54. Hines JZ, Pinsent T, Rees K, et al. Notes from the field: Shigellosis outbreak among men who have sex with men and homeless persons—Oregon, 2015–2016. *MMWR Morb Mortal Wkly Rep.* 2016;65(31):812–3.

55. Arvelo W, Hinkel CJ, Nguyen TA, et al. Transmission risk factors and treatment of pediatric shigellosis during a large daycare center-associated outbreak of multidrug resistant *Shigella sonnei*: Implications for the management of shigellosis outbreaks among children. *Pediatr Infect Dis J.* 2009;28(11):976–80.
56. Mohle-Boetani JC, Stapleton M, Finger R, et al. Communitywide shigellosis: Control of an outbreak and risk factors in child day-care centers. *Am J Public Health.* 1995;85(6):812–6.
57. Litwin CM, Leonard RB, Carroll KC, Drummond WK, Pavia AT. Characterization of endemic strains of *Shigella sonnei* by use of plasmid DNA analysis and pulsed-field gel electrophoresis to detect patterns of transmission. *J Infect Dis.* 1997;175(4):864–70.
58. Painter JE, Walker AT, Pytell J, et al. Notes from the field: Outbreak of diarrheal illness caused by *Shigella flexneri*—American Samoa, May–June 2014. *MMWR Morb Mortal Wkly Rep.* 2015;64(1):30.
59. Shane AL, Tucker NA, Crump JA, Mintz ED, Painter JA. Sharing Shigella: Risk factors for a multicommunity outbreak of shigellosis. *Arch Pediatr Adolesc Med.* 2003;157(6):601–3.
60. Wilson R, Feldman RA, Davis J, LaVenture M. Family illness associated with Shigella infection: The interrelationship of age of the index patient and the age of household members in acquisition of illness. *J Infect Dis.* 1981;143(1):130–2.
61. Naimi TS, Wicklund JH, Olsen SJ, et al. Concurrent outbreaks of *Shigella sonnei* and enterotoxigenic *Escherichia coli* infections associated with parsley: Implications for surveillance and control of foodborne illness. *J Food Prot.* 2003;66(4):535–41.
62. Kapperud G, Rorvik LM, Hasseltvedt V, et al. Outbreak of *Shigella sonnei* infection traced to imported iceberg lettuce. *J Clin Microbiol.* 1995;33(3):609–14.
63. Guzman-Herrador B, Vold L, Comelli H, et al. Outbreak of *Shigella sonnei* infection in Norway linked to consumption of fresh basil, October 2011. *Euro Surveill.* 2011;16(44):20007.
64. Lee LA, Ostroff SM, McGee HB, et al. An outbreak of shigellosis at an outdoor music festival. *Am J Epidemiol.* 1991;133(6):608–15.
65. Kimura AC, Johnson K, Palumbo MS, et al. Multistate shigellosis outbreak and commercially prepared food, United States. *Emerg Infect Dis.* 2004;10(6):1147–9.
66. Hedberg CW, Levine WC, White KE, et al. An international foodborne outbreak of shigellosis associated with a commercial airline. *JAMA.* 1992;268(22):3208–12.
67. He F, Han K, Liu L, et al. Shigellosis outbreak associated with contaminated well water in a rural elementary school: Sichuan Province, China, June 7–16, 2009. *PLoS One.* 2012;7(10):e47239.
68. Beer KD, Gargano JW, Roberts VA, et al. Surveillance for waterborne disease outbreaks associated with drinking water—United States, 2011–2012. *MMWR Morb Mortal Wkly Rep.* 2015;64(31):842–8.
69. Hlavsa MC, Roberts VA, Kahler AM, et al. Outbreaks of illness associated with recreational water—United States, 2011–2012. *MMWR Morb Mortal Wkly Rep.* 2015;64(24):668–72.
70. Bancroft JE, Keifer SB, Keene WE. Shigellosis from an interactive fountain: Implications for regulation. *J Environ Health.* 2010;73(4):16–20.
71. Keene WE, McAnulty JM, Hoesly FC, et al. A swimming-associated outbreak of hemorrhagic colitis caused by *Escherichia coli* O157:H7 and *Shigella sonnei*. *N Engl J Med.* 1994;331(9):579–84.
72. Centers for Disease Control and Prevention (CDC). *Shigella sonnei* outbreak associated with contaminated drinking water—Island Park, Idaho, August 1995. *MMWR Morb Mortal Wkly Rep.* 1996;45(11):229–31.
73. DuPont HL, Gangarosa EJ, Reller LB, et al. Shigellosis in custodial institutions. *Am J Epidemiol.* 1970;92(3):172–9.
74. Hines JZ, Jagger MA, Jeanne TL, et al. Heavy precipitation as a risk factor for shigellosis among homeless persons during an outbreak—Oregon, 2015–2016. *J Infect.* 2018;76(3):280–5.
75. Centers for Disease Control and Prevention (CDC). CDC WONDER (Wide-ranging Online Data for Epidemiologic Research)—National Notifiable Infectious Diseases and Conditions: United States. [cited 2018 5/9/2018]. https://wonder.cdc.gov/nndss/nndss_annual_tables_menu.asp.
76. Centers for Disease Control and Prevention (CDC). National Notifiable Disease Surveillance System (NNDSS): Shigellosis (Shigella spp.) 2012 Case Defintion. 2012 [cited 2018 5/30/2018]. https://wwwn.cdc.gov/nndss/conditions/shigellosis/case-definition/2012/.
77. Marder EP, Griffin PM, Cieslak PR, et al. Preliminary incidence and trends of infections with pathogens transmitted commonly through food—Foodborne Diseases Active Surveillance Network, 10 U.S. sites, 2006–2017. *MMWR Morb Mortal Wkly Rep.* 2018;67(11):324–8.
78. Liu J, Platts-Mills JA, Juma J, et al. Use of quantitative molecular diagnostic methods to identify causes of diarrhoea in children: A reanalysis of the GEMS case-control study. *Lancet.* 2016;388(10051):1291–301.
79. Kotloff KL. The burden and etiology of diarrheal illness in developing countries. *Pediatr Clin North Am.* 2017;64(4):799–814.
80. Kotloff KL, Nataro JP, Blackwelder WC, et al. Burden and aetiology of diarrhoeal disease in infants and young children in developing countries (the Global Enteric Multicenter Study, GEMS): A prospective, case-control study. *Lancet.* 2013;382(9888):209–22.
81. DuPont HL, Hornick RB, Dawkins AT, Snyder MJ, Formal SB. The response of man to virulent *Shigella flexneri* 2a. *J Infect Dis.* 1969;119(3):296–9.
82. Committee on Infectious Diseases; American Academy of Pediatrics; Kimberlin DW, et al. Shigella infections. In: Kimberlin D, et al, eds. *Red Book: 2018–2021 Report of the Committee on Infectious Diseases.* 31st ed. Washington, DC: American Academy of Pediatrics; 2018:723–7.
83. Levine MM, DuPont HL, Khodabandelou M, Hornick RB. Long-term Shigella-carrier state. *N Engl J Med.* 1973;288(22):1169–71.
84. Finch M, Rodey G, Lawrence D, Blake P. Epidemic Reiter's syndrome following an outbreak of shigellosis. *Eur J Epidemiol.* 1986;2(1):26–30.
85. Simon DG, Kaslow RA, Rosenbaum J, Kaye RL, Calin A. Reiter's syndrome following epidemic shigellosis. *J Rheumatol.* 1981;8(6):969–73.
86. Noer HR. An "experimental" epidemic of Reiter's syndrome. *JAMA.* 1966;198(7):693–8.
87. van Bohemen CG, Lionarons RJ, van Bodegom P, et al. Susceptibility and HLA-B27 in post-dysenteric arthropathies. *Immunology.* 1985;56(2):377–9.
88. Lauhio A, Lähdevirta J, Janes R, Kontiainen S, Repo H. Reactive arthritis associated with *Shigella sonnei* infection. *Arthritis Rheum.* 1988;31(9):1190–3.
89. Chen M, Delpech V, O'Sullivan B, Donovan B. *Shigella sonnei*: Another cause of sexually acquired reactive arthritis. *Int J STD AIDS.* 2002;13(2):135–6.
90. Mazumder RN, Salam MA, Ali M, Bhattacharya MK. Reactive arthritis associated with Shigella dysenteriae type 1 infection. *J Diarrhoeal Dis Res.* 1997;15(1):21–4.
91. Hannu T, Mattila L, Siitonen A, Leirisalo-Repo M. Reactive arthritis attributable to Shigella infection: A clinical and epidemiological nationwide study. *Ann Rheum Dis.* 2005;64(4):594–8.
92. Morduchowicz G, Huminer D, Siegman-Igra Y, Drucker M, Block CS, Pitlik SD. Shigella bacteremia in adults. A report of five cases and review of the literature. *Arch Intern Med.* 1987;147(11):2034–7.
93. Appannanavar SB, Goyal K, Garg R, Ray P, Rathi M, Taneja N. Shigellemia in a post renal transplant patient: A case report and literature review. *J Infect Dev Ctries.* 2014;8(2):237–9.
94. Galanakis E, Tzoufi M, Charisi M, Levidiotou S, Papadopoulou ZL. Rate of seizures in children with shigellosis. *Acta Paediatr.* 2002;91(1):101–2.
95. Khan WA, Dhar U, Salam MA, Griffiths JK, Rand W, Bennish ML. Central nervous system manifestations of childhood shigellosis: Prevalence, risk factors, and outcome. *Pediatrics.* 1999;103(2):E18.
96. Lahat E, Katz Y, Bistritzer T, Eshel G, Aladjem M. Recurrent seizures in children with Shigella-associated convulsions. *Ann Neurol.* 1990;28(3):393–5.
97. Goldberg EM, Balamuth F, Desrochers CR, Mittal MK. Seizure and altered mental status in a 12-year-old child with *Shigella sonnei* gastroenteritis. *Pediatr Emerg Care.* 2011;27(2):135–7.
98. Shamsizadeh A, Nikfar R, Bavarsadian E. Neurological manifestations of shigellosis in children in southwestern Iran. *Pediatr Int.* 2012;54(1):127–30.
99. Butler T. Haemolytic uraemic syndrome during shigellosis. *Trans R Soc Trop Med Hyg.* 2012;106(7):395–9.
100. Huang JY, Henao OL, Griffin PM, et al. Infection with pathogens transmitted commonly through food and the effect of increasing use of culture-independent diagnostic tests on surveillance—Foodborne Diseases Active Surveillance Network, 10 U.S. sites, 2012–2015. *MMWR Morb Mortal Wkly Rep.* 2016;65(14):368–71.
101. Atkinson R, Maguire H, Gerner-Smidt P. A challenge and an opportunity to improve patient management and public health surveillance for food-borne infections through culture-independent diagnostics. *J Clin Microbiol.* 2013;51(8):2479–82.
102. Cronquist AB, Mody RK, Atkinson R, et al. Impacts of culture-independent diagnostic practices on public health surveillance for bacterial enteric pathogens. *Clin Infect Dis.* 2012;54(Suppl 5):S432–9.

103. Jones TF, Gerner-Smidt P. Nonculture diagnostic tests for enteric diseases. *Emerg Infect Dis*. 2012;18(3):513–4.

104. Centers for Disease Control and Prevention (CDC). CDC HAN 00401: CDC Recommendations for Diagnosing and Managing Shigella Strains with Possible Reduced Susceptibility to Ciprofloxacin. 2017 [cited 2018 5/9/2018]. https://emergency.cdc.gov/han/han00401.asp.

105. World Health Organization. *Laboratory Methods for the Diagnosis of Epidemic Dysentery and Cholera*. Atlanta, GA: Centers for Disease Control and Prevention (CDC); 1999.

106. Bowen A. Shigellosis. In: *Yellow Book*. Atlanta, GA: Centers for Disease Control and Prevention (CDC); 2018.

107. Allen GP, Harris KA. In vitro resistance selection in *Shigella flexneri* by azithromycin, ceftriaxone, ciprofloxacin, levofloxacin, and moxifloxacin. *Antimicrob Agents Chemother*. 2017;61(7):e00086-17.

108. Shane AL, Mody RK, Crump JA, et al. 2017 Infectious Diseases Society of America (IDSA) clinical practice guidelines for the diagnosis and management of infectious diarrhea. *Clin Infect Dis*. 2017;65(12):1963–73.

109. Lane CR, Sutton B, Valcanis M, et al. Travel destinations and sexual behavior as indicators of antibiotic resistant Shigella strains—Victoria, Australia. *Clin Infect Dis*. 2016;62(6):722–9.

110. Murray K, Reddy K, Kornblum JS, et al. Increasing antibiotic resistance in Shigella spp. from infected New York City residents, New York, USA. *Emerg Infect Dis*. 2017;23(2):332–5.

111. Centers for Disease Control and Prevention (CDC). NARMS NOW: Human Data. 2018 [cited 2018 5/9/2018]. https://wwwn.cdc.gov/narmsnow/.

112. Kim JS, Kim JJ, Kim SJ, et al. Outbreak of ciprofloxacin-resistant *Shigella sonnei* associated with travel to Vietnam, Republic of Korea. *Emerg Infect Dis*. 2015;21(7):1247–50.

113. Clinical and Laboratory Standards Institute (CLSI). In: Weinstein MP, ed. CLSI supplement M100. *Performance Standards for Antimicrobial Susceptibility Testing*. 28th ed. Wayne, PA: Clinical and Laboratory Standards Institute; 2018.

114. Jain SK, Gupta A, Glanz B, Dick J, Siberry GK. Antimicrobial-resistant *Shigella sonnei*: Limited antimicrobial treatment options for children and challenges of interpreting in vitro azithromycin susceptibility. *Pediatr Infect Dis J*. 2005;24(6):494–7.

115. Khan MU. Interruption of shigellosis by hand washing. *Trans R Soc Trop Med Hyg*. 1982;76(2):164–8.

116. Centers for Disease Control and Prevention (CDC). Shigella-Shigellosis: Information for Childcare Facilities. 2018 [cited 2018 5/9/2018]. https://www.cdc.gov/shigella/information-for-childcare-facilities.html.

117. Centers for Disease Control and Prevention (CDC). Shigella-Shigellosis: Intensified control measures for shigellosis outbreaks in a childcare setting. 2018 [cited 2018 5/9/2018]. https://www.cdc.gov/shigella/intensified-control-measures.html.

118. Chen WH, Kotloff KL. Shigella vaccine development: Finding the path of least resistance. *Clin Vaccine Immunol*. 2016;23(12):904–7.

119. Kotloff KL, Platts-Mills JA, Nasrin D, Roose A, Blackwelder WC, Levine MM. Global burden of diarrheal diseases among children in developing countries: Incidence, etiology, and insights from new molecular diagnostic techniques. *Vaccine*. 2017;35(49 Pt A):6783–9.

CHAPTER

115 A Multidisciplinary Approach for the Control and Prevention of Legionellosis[1]

Brian H. Raphael • Claressa E. Lucas • Cynthia G. Whitney

INTRODUCTION

Legionnaires' disease is a unique bacterial pneumonia that is transmitted to individuals from environmental water sources contaminated with *Legionella* spp. The disease can be associated with both complex building water systems (e.g., in hospitals, institutions, long-term care facilities, hotels) and with community settings. Outbreaks involving community-associated Legionnaires' disease cases can escalate rapidly and gain significant attention. In other situations, cases of Legionnaires' disease may continue within buildings for extended periods of time before an outbreak is detected.

When an outbreak is detected, a multidisciplinary approach involving epidemiology, laboratory science, and environmental health can be key to identifying and controlling the source of an outbreak. In settings with complex water systems, the expertise of environmental health specialists can be useful to understanding parts of the system that may be at risk for *Legionella* growth. In many outbreaks, source attribution can involve analysis of both epidemiological data and molecular subtyping of *Legionella* strains in the laboratory. Primary prevention efforts, such as the development and review of water management plans, also require a multidisciplinary approach. Communication specialists can be particularly helpful in designing public health messages on Legionnaires' disease prevention and providing complex messaging on the progress of public health investigations during outbreaks.

MICROBIOLOGY

Legionella spp. are Gram-negative aerobic rods with fastidious growth requirements. Approximately 60 species of *Legionella* are currently recognized.[1] At least one-third of these species have been associated with disease.[2] *L. pneumophila* causes the vast majority (~90%) of disease, although *L. longbeachae* is a major cause of illness in Australia and New Zealand.[3] While *L. pneumophila* is commonly found in aquatic sources, *L. longbeachae* has been found in potting soils.[4] Nearly all species of *Legionella* require cysteine for growth and the use of specialized media such as buffered charcoal yeast extract (BCYE) is one of the most commonly used media for cultivation of these organisms. Supplementation of BCYE with various antimicrobial agents helps to reduce competing microorganisms present in samples that can hinder isolation of *Legionella* spp.[5]

At least 15 serogroups of *L. pneumophila* have been reported; however, *L. pneumophila* serogroup 1 causes more than 80% of Legionnaires' disease cases in the United States.[4,6] Serogroup 1 strains can be further characterized using panels of monoclonal antibodies.[7,8] Monoclonal antibody 2 (MAb2), also called 3/1 when part of the Dresden panel, recognizes a component of the lipopolysaccharide and strains reacting with this reagent have been shown to contain the gene *lag-1*.[9] Interestingly, MAb2 strains are more commonly isolated from cases of sporadic disease and recovered during outbreak investigations.[10] Although it remains unclear if *lag-1* provides a selective advantage for isolates causing human disease, it is possible that strains expressing this gene are capable of surviving inhospitable environmental niches or able to evade immune responses.

Clinical disease due to non-*Legionella pneumophila* spp. is most frequently attributed to *L. bozemanii*, *L. dumoffii*, *L. longbeachae*, and *L. micdadei*.[3,11–13] Other species are detected in clinical specimens only rarely (in some cases only associated with a single report) and are often associated with transplant patients, those undergoing treatment for various cancers, and those with other significant immune system deficiencies.

ECOLOGY AND PATHOGENESIS OF *LEGIONELLA*

Legionellae are extremely common residents of natural freshwater environments worldwide and, depending upon the conditions, can be associated with complex human-made water systems. Yet, legionellae have also been detected in marine and groundwater sources as well as all phases of the sewage treatment process, including treated effluent. Nonaquatic sources of legionellae include native soils, potting soils and compost, and garden soils. In industrial settings, a mix of aquatic milieus have been identified as potential sources of disease-causing legionellae, with the most frequent association being liquid used to cool machine processes. However, the habitats where legionellae are able to persist and thrive seem to be limited only by the imagination of the researchers looking for them since the bacteria have also been detected in such unlikely places as windshield wiper fluid, bracts of rainforest epiphytic plants, and acid mine drainage.[14]

In most parts of the world, especially North America, Europe, and Asia, the species *L. pneumophila* predominates in both natural and human-made aquatic environments.[15–20] In Australasia, the species *L. longbeachae* is predominant in terrestrial environments like compost and garden soils.[21] Some studies suggest that human activities may affect the relative distribution of *Legionella* species in both the natural and built environment.[16,20,22,23] A recent large-scale metagenomic study detected wide distribution but low abundance of the bacterial order containing *Legionella*, even in habitats previously thought inimical to their survival, such as marine Antarctica.[24] In this study, temperature was identified as a major determinant of *Legionella* species distribution and prevalence, but more research is needed to identify and define the contributions of local conditions to *Legionella* persistence in a given environment.

Where *L. pneumophila* represents the most abundant species in the environment, the most clinically relevant subtypes often display

[1]The findings and conclusions in this chapter are those of the authors and do not necessarily represent the official position of the Centers for Disease Control and Prevention.

limited geographical distribution and low relative abundance. For instance, *L. pneumophila* serogroup 1 sequence type (ST) 47 is the most frequent cause of Legionnaires' disease in France, The Netherlands, and Belgium but not in other parts of Europe, indicating an extremely narrow geographic distribution. Yet, this subtype of *L. pneumophila* is also rarely recovered from either the built or natural environment during routine sampling in the absence of cases of disease in countries where it is clinically relevant.[25] Taken together, these observations suggest that while ST47 may be widely distributed in these countries, it is typically found in very low abundance in either the natural or built environment. Thus, more study is needed to better define the distribution and prevalence of clinically relevant strains.

Legionellae are parasites of free-living protozoa with an extremely broad host range that can also include fungi, slime molds, and even some lower order worms and insects.[26] Although the bacteria may be found as free-living cells in the environment, amplification of the bacteria only occurs intracellularly.[24] Legionellae are able to evade fusion of the phagosome with lysosomes and subvert the host's cellular machinery for their own purposes, interacting closely with the endoplasmic reticulum.[27] The bacteria replicate within the cytoplasm of the host cell until they are released back into the extracellular environment. Legionellae exhibit numerous forms during this lifecycle.[28,29] Similar molecular mechanisms that help *Legionella* survive within amoebae and protozoa are also important for the ability of this organism to invade and grow within alveolar macrophages in the human lung.[30]

This facultative intracellular lifestyle may provide a partial explanation for the extremely wide distribution of *Legionella* species worldwide yet low abundance of clinically relevant subtypes in a given habitat. As generalists, legionellae are able to invade multiple hosts in diverse environments using a conserved, but extremely broad, repertoire of bacterial effectors.[26] This allows the bacteria to spread extensively throughout natural and built environments, wherever a suitable host for intracellular replication can be found. However, evolutionary biology experiments using multiple passages of *L. pneumophila* through either macrophages or amoebae have demonstrated the accumulation of point mutations in both effectors and transcription control sequences that are believed to tailor effector utilization for the current host. As legionellae parasitize similar hosts successively in an environment with a predominant protozoan host class, the bacteria accumulate mutations and induce production of effectors that make them more "fit" for the most abundant hosts. Such host specialization often comes with a cost for *Legionella* that narrows their host range or otherwise make them less generally fit for the environment. Accordingly, the currently prevailing theory is that legionellae are only accidental pathogens, which confuse human alveolar macrophages for their natural protozoan host. However, protozoan host types that bear functional similarity to human alveolar macrophages would individually be rare in the natural or built environment, leading to only low abundance of "human adapted" *Legionella*. Thus, selective pressure that favors the most clinically relevant subtypes of legionellae would be low, resulting in "human adapted" strains in lower abundance than generally "environmentally adapted" ones.[31] Similarly, Australian researchers link the prevalence of the species *L. longbeachae* in that island continent's composts to the unique protozoa associated with their novel, archaic flora.[21]

The majority of the interactions between legionellae and their protozoan hosts take place not in the free-flowing liquid environment as planktonic cells, but within biofilms.[32] Biofilms are complex structures that form on any wet surface. Biofilms are composed of a variety of microorganisms that include not only bacteria and protozoa, but also viruses, fungi, and sometimes even lower order multicellular organisms such as nematodes. Mature biofilms may behave in a manner similar to multicellular organisms, with stratified segregation of constituent microorganisms, excreted polysaccharide infrastructure, and organized distribution of nutrients through internal fluid channels. Biofilm development is a complex process whose stages roughly correlate to attachment, colonization, and maturation. Legionellae are thought to participate in all stages of this process, with conditions such as stagnation, nutrient availability, substrate material, and temperature being the most relevant determinants of *Legionella* colonization and persistence within biofilms.[33] Where legionellae have colonized established biofilms, they may infect successive protozoan hosts and can be physically protected from harsh environmental conditions including attempts at chemical disinfection or thermal eradication.[22,32]

CLINICAL ASPECTS OF LEGIONELLOSIS

Legionellosis

There are two clinical forms of legionellosis—Legionnaires' disease and Pontiac fever. Legionnaires' disease is characterized by the presence of pneumonia, which can be severe. In the United States, approximately 40% of patients with Legionnaires' disease required admission to the intensive-care unit in an active surveillance study conducted between 2011 and 2013.[34] In this study, the case fatality rate for Legionnaires' disease was 9%. Patients typically report cough, shortness of breath, fever, muscle aches, and headaches. Other symptoms such as diarrhea, nausea, and confusion may occur. Although the incubation period for Legionnaires' disease is typically 2–10 days, symptom onset may take as long as 2 weeks after exposure. An incubation period of up to 19 days has been reported.[35]

Pontiac fever generally presents with fever and muscle aches but without pneumonia. It is a milder illness compared to Legionnaires' disease, and symptom onset may occur within 24–72 hours after exposure to the bacterium. During outbreaks, it is sometimes possible to identify cases of Pontiac fever in persons who report similar environmental exposures to those reported by Legionnaires' disease patients.[36–38] The pathogenesis of Pontiac fever is poorly understood. Patients with Pontiac fever may develop antibodies against *Legionella* spp. and in some cases, patients may excrete antigen in the urine.[38,39] It remains unclear if Pontiac fever results from infection with *Legionella* spp. or represents a host reaction to the inhalation of the organism or a component of the organism.

Diagnostic Testing

The most commonly used diagnostic test for Legionnaires' disease is the urinary antigen test (UAT). The UAT detects *L. pneumophila* serogroup 1 antigen secreted in the urine. The test is highly sensitive and specific.[4] Antigen is detectable within a few days of symptom onset and infrequently may remain detectable for weeks. It is important to note that the UAT is intended for diagnosis of Legionnaires' disease in patients with pneumonia and it is unclear how a positive result should be interpreted in an asymptomatic individual.

Although culture of lower respiratory tract secretions (e.g., sputum, bronchoalveolar lavage fluid, etc.) is considered the "gold standard" for diagnosis of this disease, a lack of appropriate specimens and the technically challenging microbiological identification of the organism remain major hurdles. Culture allows for identification of any serogroup of *L. pneumophila* or *Legionella* spp. Extended incubation of specimens (up to 14 days) may be required for isolation of some *Legionella* spp. Moreover, recovering an isolate allows for further molecular subtyping, which can help in source attribution studies. Development of subtyping methods that could be performed directly from specimens is ongoing. Although infrequently used, serological methods (showing a fourfold antibody titer increase between acute and convalescent sera) and direct fluorescent antibody testing of respiratory secretions have been historically used in diagnostic testing.

In recent years, PCR has emerged as an important diagnostic assay. While PCR requires a lower respiratory tract specimen, it offers the ability to provide a result rapidly. In some cases, a positive PCR result can be obtained even when culture is negative (e.g., due to initiation of antibiotic treatment). Some laboratory-developed PCR tests offer the ability to detect multiple markers such as those for *Legionella* spp., *L. pneumophila*, and *L. pneumophila* serogroup 1.[40,41] As a result, PCR offers the ability to detect cases of Legionnaires' disease that may be missed by the UAT alone.

ENVIRONMENTAL SOURCES

Sources and Transmission

Legionella spp. are commonly found in aquatic environments. In a metagenomic study of watersheds in British Columbia, Canada, *Legionella* spp. were found in low abundance (<2% of bacterial taxa) throughout the year and in various land use settings.[16] However, transmission of the organism to humans occurs when *Legionella* spp. enter human-made water systems in which a variety of conditions may be suitable for amplification and ongoing growth of the organism (Fig. 115-1). *Legionella* may adhere to biofilms and survive within resident amoebae. Moreover, water conditions such as elevated temperature (e.g., in hot water systems), lack of a disinfectant residual, and extended water stagnation time may also result in organism growth. In experimental plumbing systems, lower water heater set points and low tap usage (compared to recirculating systems) were associated with increased *L. pneumophila* growth.[42] Moreover, such experimental setups have also revealed an association between the abundance of the amoebal host, *Vermamoeba vermiformis,* and *L. pneumophila*.[42,43]

Various devices can serve to aerosolize the bacteria in water droplets, which can be inhaled by susceptible hosts. Devices disseminating nonpotable water include pools, spas, cooling towers, and decorative fountains. Notably, cooling towers have been implicated in the transmission of *Legionella* across several kilometers.[44] Devices that can aerosolize potable water sources include showers, tubs, and sink faucets.

Sampling and Laboratory Testing

During outbreak investigations, environmental sampling is important for helping to confirm an environmental source of *Legionella* causing disease. When isolates are available, it is possible to compare environmental and clinical isolates to help establish genetic links confirming the identification of a suspected source. Selecting appropriate sites to sample involves identifying locations of possible exposure (often based on case interviews). During investigations of specific buildings, extensive sampling may also be conducted to characterize a building water system (including central locations within hot water systems as well as proximal and distal sites). A 1-liter sample volume is preferred, and sodium thiosulfate should be added to neutralize any residual disinfectant. In some cases, swabs of sink faucets and showers (with aerators and/or shower heads removed) can help detect localized formation of biofilm where *Legionella* may reside. Samples should be processed within 72 hours of collection by a laboratory familiar with environmental testing for *Legionella*. The abundance of *Legionella* in water samples can vary widely. In general, potable water samples (which are expected to contain a low abundance of *Legionella*) are concentrated using membrane filtration and aliquots of the concentrate is plated to selective BCYE media, while nonpotable sources are plated directly without the concentration step.[5]

CDC operates the Environmental *Legionella* Isolation Techniques Evaluation (ELITE) program, which allows external laboratories to evaluate their ability to isolate (i.e., grow and identify) *Legionella* from a water sample using a culture method. Details about laboratories participating in this program can be found on the CDC website.[45] More recently, laboratories have begun using more rapid methods such as PCR to detect *Legionella* DNA present in environmental samples.[15,41,46] As environmental samples may contain substances which can interfere with PCR, the use of a PCR inhibition control is advised.

EPIDEMIOLOGY

Epidemiology of Legionellosis

The burden of Legionnaires' disease is increasing in the United States. From 2000 to 2017, the rate of Legionnaires' disease reported to CDC increased from about 0.4 to 1.9 cases per 100,000 population, including persons of all ages (Fig. 115-2).[47] The increase in disease rates is striking, but not well understood, and is likely multifactorial. Most cases of Legionnaires' disease are diagnosed using UAT, and some have speculated that availability of antigen tests may have improved over time; at the same time, the increase in outbreaks and related publicity has raised awareness of Legionnaires' disease, which could have resulted in more use of specific diagnostic tests such as urinary antigen or culture. The U.S. population is aging, and persons with underlying conditions or advanced age that put them at higher risk for Legionnaires' disease are an increasing proportion of the population. Given the annual peak of Legionnaires' disease occurs in months with the warmest weather, the changing climate with increasingly warm temperatures and greater rainfall in some areas may be providing a better environment for *Legionella* growth.[48] In addition, aging buildings found in many cities mean that plumbing systems can have poor water flow or "dead legs," in particular in areas that have undergone renovation or drops in water use. Stagnation in water systems has been linked to *Legionella* growth.[49]

The epidemiology of Legionnaires' disease is similar in some ways to pneumonia caused by other pathogens. For example, the risk of Legionnaires' disease increases with increasing age among adults and is more common in smokers and those with chronic lung disease; persons with immunocompromising conditions are at very high risk and can have disease caused by the typically less invasive non-*pneumophila* strains such as *L. micdadei*.[50] In contrast to other types of pneumonia, Legionnaires' disease is much more common among

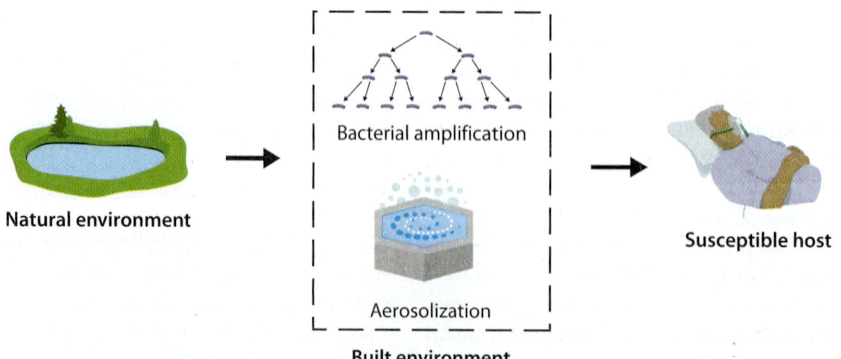

FIGURE 115-1. Schematic of the ecology of *Legionella* and its transmission. *Legionella* are present in natural water systems. Within the built environment (e.g., buildings, cooling towers, spas, or fountains), conditions may permit *Legionella* to amplify in number and be dispersed by aerosol generating devices. Inhalation of these bacteria containing aerosols by a susceptible individual can result in transmission of Legionnaires' disease.

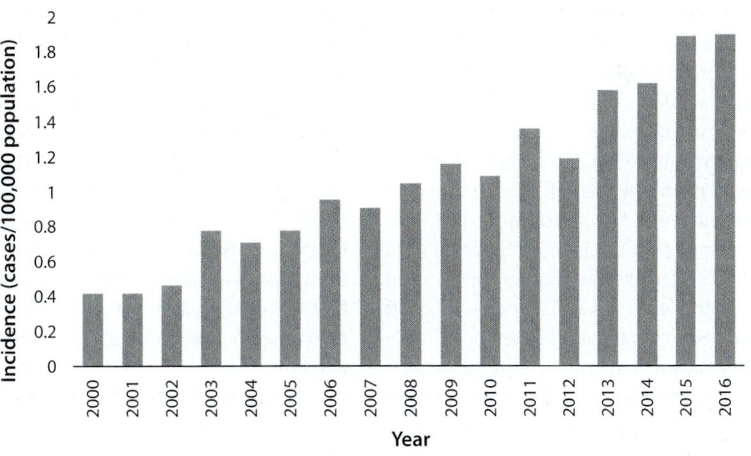

FIGURE 115-2. Incidence (cases/100,000 population) of Legionnaires' disease in the United States by year, 2000–16. Cases are from reports collected through the National Notifiable Disease Reporting System. (*Source:* Data from Centers for Disease Control and Prevention. Legionella (Legionnaires' Disease and Pontiac Fever). https://www.cdc.gov/legionella/qa-media.html.)

men than women and is rarely diagnosed in children, other than in those with immune compromising medical conditions.[51] In addition, the peak incidence of Legionnaires' disease occurs in warmer summer and early fall months rather than in the colder months of the "respiratory season."[51,52] Legionnaires' disease cases and outbreaks can occur in winter months, especially outbreaks linked to potable water systems or among travelers to warm climates. Rates of disease differ with geography; in the United States, Legionnaires' disease is most common in the northeast states.[52] Studies from urban areas suggest that incidence is higher among areas with more persons living in poverty.[53] In Australia and New Zealand, where *Legionella longbeachae* is a common cause of Legionnaires' disease, exposure to potting soil has been linked to disease.[54] Other common exposures among persons with Legionnaires' disease are recent travel, found in about 10–15%,[47] and hospitalization or other types of healthcare visits, found in up to 20%.[55] The vast majority of reported cases in the United States are not linked to a known outbreak.

Because young or healthy persons are at lower risk for developing Legionnaires' disease and water systems may only intermittently shed live *Legionella* bacteria, attack rates (i.e., the number of persons who become ill among those exposed) in Legionnaires' disease outbreaks are typically low; even in outbreaks in long-term care facilities, usually fewer than 20% of residents will develop Legionnaires' disease.[56] The epidemiology of Pontiac fever is quite different from that of Legionnaires' disease; attack rates can be $>$ 50% among those exposed in some settings and young and healthy persons are often among those affected.[57]

Tracking Legionellosis

Cases of Legionnaires' disease or Pontiac fever are required to be reported to state or local health authorities, who will then conduct an investigation, the extent of which depends on the situation and resources. The first step in any investigation is confirming whether the patient's illness meets accepted clinical and laboratory definitions of Legionnaires' disease or Pontiac fever (https://www.cdc.gov/legionella/health-depts/surv-reporting/case-definitions.html).[47] To be classified as a confirmed case, a patient's illness should be compatible with Legionnaires' disease (i.e., pneumonia) or Pontiac fever and a specific laboratory test should indicate *Legionella* infection; accepted tests include culture of respiratory secretions, *Legionella* urinary antigen testing, or paired serology for *L. pneumophila* serogroup 1. At the time of the last case definition update (2009), positive tests using other laboratory methods such as PCR were considered as contributing to meeting the "suspected" case definition. Most legionellosis outbreaks are detected through investigations conducted by local or state health department staff before notification forms are sent to CDC.

At the national level, CDC uses three different reporting systems to track different aspects of legionellosis.[47] Case reports from all states and territories are reported through the National Notifiable Diseases Surveillance System (NNDSS). NNDSS reports include basic information on all patients who meet the case definitions for Legionnaires' disease or Pontiac fever. NNDSS reports are reviewed periodically and used to track total cases in the United States, but data gathered through NNDSS are not usually timely or detailed enough for outbreak detection or investigation. A second system, the Supplemental Legionnaires' Disease Surveillance System (SLDSS), includes additional information on individual cases such as the tests used for diagnosis and exposures that may have led to *Legionella* infection. As of 2015, about half of all reported Legionnaires' disease cases through NNDSS included supplemental information in SLDSS.[55]

Importantly, the SLDSS platform allows for rapid reporting of travel-related cases—Legionnaires' disease occurring in persons who may have been exposed to *Legionella* while traveling or staying away from home. CDC staff use the reported information on travel exposures to link cases in persons who had the same exposure (e.g., hotel X in state A) and to ensure that U.S. health departments are notified of cases occurring in travelers to their areas. CDC staff also exchange information on travel-related Legionnaires' disease cases with public health officials in other countries. The European Centre for Disease Prevention and Control (eCDC) operates a similar system for rapid tracking of travel-related cases of Legionnaires' disease as part of the European Legionnaires' disease Surveillance Network.[58]

The third U.S. surveillance system is the National Outbreak Reporting System (NORS). NORS collects information on a range of outbreaks detected and investigated by health departments, including outbreaks caused by *Legionella* other waterborne pathogens. A total of 42 drinking-water-associated outbreaks reported to CDC in 2012–13 accounted for 1006 cases of disease and 13 deaths.[59] *Legionella* was responsible for 24 (57%) of these outbreaks and all 13 (100%) of the deaths. While the actual number of clusters occurring annually in the United States is unknown, CDC staff provided technical input on $>$ 100 Legionnaires' disease investigations in 2017 (CDC unpublished data). More information on U.S. surveillance systems, methods, and forms can be found at www.cdc.gov/legionella.

CONTROL

Outbreak Detection and Investigation

Most outbreaks are detected by local health departments or by astute clinicians or infection control professionals who notice links between cases or an uptick in the number of cases over baseline. Nonetheless, a diagnosis of Legionnaires' disease is unusual enough that two or more cases occurring among persons with the same exposure in a short amount of time is not likely to be a chance occurrence. Therefore, any links identified between persons with Legionnaires' disease, such as more than one case occurring in residents of a particular apartment building, neighborhood, work place, or long-term care facility, suggests a common environmental exposure. CDC's *Legionella* Program recommends that state or local public health officials conduct an investigation of environmental sources that could transmit *Legionella* when two or more cases are detected within a 12-month period with links to a particular building.[47] When two or more cases are reported among travelers on a cruise ship that docks in a U.S. port, CDC staff work with the U.S. Vessel Sanitation Program and cruise line officials to investigate and conduct any needed remediation of water systems.[60]

In the 10–14 days before illness onset, most people are exposed to several different sources of water that could, if contaminated with *Legionella*, spread Legionnaires' disease. Therefore, finding the likely source for individual cases of Legionnaires' disease can be difficult, and environmental sampling is not routinely conducted for investigating single cases. The exception is for situations in which a patient with Legionnaires' disease has only been in one location, such as a prison, long-term care facility, or hospital for the entire 10–14 days before illness onset. In these situations, CDC recommends conducting an investigation after even a single case, as the water source that led to the person's illness must be in or very near the facility.[47]

Legionnaires' disease cases that occur in persons who are or were recently hospitalized, live in long-term care facilities, or have other types of healthcare exposures warrant special attention. Such healthcare-associated Legionnaires' disease cases result in death in about one of every four episodes, more often than among persons who developed Legionnaires' disease after an exposure in the community.[55] In addition, persons in healthcare facilities often have pre-existing illnesses or are receiving immune-suppressing treatments that place them at high risk for developing Legionnaires' disease if exposed to water containing the organism. Therefore, CDC recommends performing an investigation after a single case in someone who was in the healthcare facility for the entire 10–14 days before illness onset (definite healthcare-associated Legionnaires' disease), or two cases of Legionnaires' disease in a 12-month period among persons who were in a facility for only part of the 10–14 days before symptom onset (possible healthcare-associated Legionnaires' disease).[47]

Outbreaks that occur among persons in a larger community pose significant challenges to investigate. Identifying links between cases by area and time of exposure can be difficult for outdoor exposures, such as those from cooling towers or fountains that have not been properly maintained. Susceptible persons can be exposed in a variety of locations. In most urban settings, the locations of cooling towers are unknown, as most cities do not require cooling towers to be registered. New analytic methods and software are being employed for investigating space and time links between cases in urban locations with many possible water exposures. SaTScan™ (https://www.satscan.org) is one such tool that has been used successfully to identify Legionnaires' disease outbreaks in New York City.[61] For outbreaks with larger numbers of cases, public health investigators can use mapping programs to outline areas in which sources that can aerosolize water should be identified and tested for *Legionella*. Information and forms to help with outbreak investigations are available on the CDC website.[47]

Conducting Environmental Assessments

Performing an environmental assessment should be one of the first activities conducted on-site during the investigation of a building associated with cases of Legionnaires' disease. The environmental assessment identifies all sources of possible water exposure at a building and records current operating parameters so that potentially hazardous conditions can be recognized. Performing an environmental assessment can greatly help to direct environmental sampling activities to ensure that a comprehensive sampling strategy is achieved. An environmental assessment should also help to identify locations where control measures can be applied to ameliorate hazardous conditions in building water systems. CDC provides an online environmental assessment form[62] to help conduct these procedures.

The environmental assessment describes the building characteristics such as use (i.e., healthcare, travel, residential, etc.), size, age, and typical occupancy. Buildings that are older than a decade and include at least 10 stories are more likely colonized by legionellae.[63] Healthcare facilities used to house or treat people with weakened immunity, underlying disease, or advanced age may host a population that is at greater risk for Legionnaires' disease and may generate more specific questions about exposure to medical devices and ice machines.

The environmental assessment should also describe the flow of water through a building such as presented in CDC toolkit entitled "Developing a Water Management Program to Reduce *Legionella* Growth and Spread in Buildings: A Practical Guide to Implementing Industry Standards."[64] Specific attention should be directed to cooling towers and whirlpool spas, which are most frequently associated with explosive clusters of disease.[65,66] It should be noted that intermittent disinfection of devices, especially cooling towers, has been linked to several outbreaks.[56,65] Finally, the environmental assessment should describe external factors that could contribute to *Legionella* colonization of a building such as construction and water main breaks.

Source Attribution

Analysis of exposures among persons with Legionnaires' disease or Pontiac fever often points to one or a limited number of likely environmental sources from which they were infected. Sampling of these environmental sources to look for the presence of *Legionella* is a next step in an outbreak investigation. A comprehensive sampling plan based on the analysis of exposures and a thorough environmental assessment may involve different types of samples (e.g., bulk water and swabs) and various locations within a building (e.g., proximal and distal sites of a hot water system). In outbreak settings, healthcare providers should be encouraged to collect lower respiratory track specimens from patients with pneumonia in order to obtain isolates that can be compared to isolates from environmental specimens. Generally, the goal of source attribution studies is to use genetic relationships among isolates to help confirm the identification of a specific environmental source(s) of an outbreak. Genetic comparison of clinical and environmental isolates is especially helpful when the source of outbreak cannot be determined from other data (such as the analysis of patient exposures) and provides further confirmation of the environmental source.

Several methods have been applied to compare clinical and environmental isolates collected during outbreak investigations, including pulsed-field gel electrophoresis (PFGE), sequence-based typing (SBT), and whole genome sequencing (WGS). Using SBT, investigators amplify and sequence seven "housekeeping" genes.[67,68] Differences in the nucleotide sequences of these alleles are cataloged and a resulting allele profile yields a ST. This method is supported by an international database containing isolate information such as geographical location and sources.[69] A 10-year (1982–2012) retrospective study of *L. pneumophila* serogroup 1 isolates in the CDC culture collection revealed that ST1 was the most frequent type associated with sporadic clinical cases and environmental sources.[70] The top five types associated with outbreak investigations were ST1, ST35, ST36, ST37, and ST222.

More recently, WGS has shown effectiveness for resolving strains collected during outbreak investigations. Isolates collected during a large outbreak occurring in New York City during the summer of 2015 and analyzed using single nucleotide polymorphisms not only confirmed a specific cooling tower as the source of the outbreak but also revealed the presence of an endemic strain of *L. pneumophila* which had been associated with previous cases of disease occurring in the same regions over several years.[65] In a study of clinical and environmental isolates collected from investigations occurring across New York State, whole genome multilocus sequence typing (wgMLST) demonstrated improved resolution among isolates compared to PFGE or SBT.[71] wgMLST is a useful method for public health investigations because allele profiles based on thousands of genes are catalogued using a centralized database allowing for standardized genome sequence analysis across jurisdictions. It is possible that more routine genomic analysis of *L. pneumophila* isolates using a wgMLST approach could supplement surveillance activities for this disease. For instance, a cluster of highly related isolates recovered from travelers to the same location but residing in different jurisdictions could alert public health officials to investigate a potential travel-associated event.

Culture-independent methods for subtyping strains of *Legionella* spp. directly within clinical specimens and environmental sources are developing rapidly. These methods have the benefit of bypassing the lengthy time-to-result for culture. A recent report using deep sequencing of the 16S rRNA gene on sputa specimens from pneumonia patients revealed that *Legionella* could be detected in specimens for which culture failed to recover isolates.[72] Interestingly, this study also found that *Legionella* presence was associated with other respiratory pathogens as well as aquatic bacteria. For environmental samples, it is critical to ascertain if the recovered DNA is associated with viable bacteria that pose a risk for human transmission.

PREVENTION

Almost all outbreaks of Legionnaires' disease or Pontiac fever can be linked to lapses in or a lack of water management programs. Such programs are designed to decrease the risk of *Legionella* growth and spread. A retrospective review of outbreaks from 2000 to 2014 found that over half identified a maintenance deficiency that could have led to *Legionella* growth in the system.[73] In two-thirds of the outbreaks, a water management program was missing or inadequate; human errors or equipment failures were also common programs. In one-third of outbreak reports reviewed, problems were noted outside the building that could have contributed to low disinfectant levels, such as water main breaks that introduced dirt into a building's water system. In short, the report suggests that nearly all Legionnaires' disease outbreaks are preventable with careful water management programs.

Water Management Programs

The goal of water management programs is to reduce the risk of Legionnaires' disease associated with building water systems. Several industrial societies and government agencies have provided guidance for this process.[63,64,74] A multidisciplinary team should be established with members who have the knowledge and skills to understand the operations of building water systems, ecology of legionellae as it relates to the built environment, and the authority to oversee operations including purchases, personnel, and contracts. The team should describe the building water system, identify areas where *Legionella* can grow and spread, determine where control measures should be applied (e.g., flushing program to ensure water movement), and identify corrective actions to restore control to a system that has exceeded established limits. Confirmation that the program has been implemented and is effective is an important part of the plan. Testing for *Legionella* may be one way to confirm that a water management program is effective. However, some authorities suggest that more emphasis should be placed on managing appropriate control measures and protecting high-risk population groups. This may be especially applicable in healthcare settings where disease caused by other waterborne microorganisms is of greater concern than legionellae and active surveillance of all cases of pneumonia is possible.[75,76] Finally, the program must document and communicate activities. Additional details on developing water management plans can be found at: https://www.cdc.gov/legionella/wmp/index.html.

Water management programs should undergo a thorough review at least annually to assess the data and address the root causes of any recurring issues. A successful water management program should evolve over time as more data are generated. For example, in a study that detailed the implementation and optimization of a water management program for a campus healthcare facility, the authors noted the need for additional control in pressure tanks and automatic faucets.[77]

The Role of Testing and Regulations to Prevent Legionnaires' Disease

Experts on Legionnaires' disease do not agree on an amount of *Legionella* in a water system that is safe for human exposure. Whether a water system containing *Legionella* poses a risk can depend on several factors, including the concentration of *Legionella* in the system, whether the *Legionella* strains are one of the types most likely to cause disease, the amount of aerosols produced by the systems' showers, faucets, cooling towers or other devices, and the susceptibility of those exposed to the aerosols. For example, some buildings could have *Legionella* in the water system but pose little risk because either exposures to water aerosols are minimal or people using the building are generally healthy, such as office buildings in which generally healthy people work. In other settings, such as hospitals, even minimal exposures to *Legionella* in water aerosols could pose a serious risk to patients undergoing treatment who may be immune compromised.

Many water management programs may not include routine testing of water for *Legionella*. In some settings, such as in hospitals with seriously ill patients, the water management team should consider routine testing as part of their activities where *Legionella* testing can be a means to validate that water management measures are controlling *Legionella* growth in the building's water systems.[63] If a water management team finds *Legionella* during routine environmental sampling, CDC suggests exploring possible reasons for the growth.[47] Note that complete eradication of *Legionella* may not be possible for some large, complex water systems. Active surveillance for *Legionella* infections among those with healthcare-associated pneumonia can also help monitor whether *Legionella* growth is adequately controlled in healthcare facility water systems.

In the United States, few states or municipalities have legislation or regulations regarding control of *Legionella* in building water systems. In 2005, the city of Garland, Texas, implemented a citywide *Legionella* ordinance that required those operating multifamily residences to conduct routine testing of any cooling towers serving the buildings; an evaluation conducted 10 years later suggested that the ordinance resulted in a drop in the number of cooling towers testing positive over time.[78] In response to an outbreak in 2015 that resulted in 138 cases of Legionnaires' disease and 16 deaths, New York City enacted regulations that called for registration of all cooling towers and annual certification with evidence of proper maintenance.[79] The State of New York followed in 2016 with similar rules for cooling towers and included additional mandates for hospitals and other healthcare facilities to have water management programs, conduct annual environmental assessments, and perform routine water sampling for *Legionella*.[80] Whether these requirements for registration and maintenance of cooling towers results in fewer cases of Legionnaires' disease is currently being evaluated.

While no U.S. regulations address Legionnaires' disease prevention generally, the U.S. Centers for Medicaid and Medicare Services (CMS) added an element on prevention to their certification checklist for healthcare facilities in 2017.[81] CMS now requires that Medicare-certified hospitals and long-term care facilities have water management policies and procedures in place that are designed to reduce the risk of growth and spread of *Legionella* and other opportunistic pathogens in building water systems; the programs should adhere to the American Society of Heating, Refrigerating and Air-Conditioning Engineers (ASHRAE) industry standard.[63]

SUMMARY

A multifactorial process involving increases in susceptible populations, aging infrastructure, and improved recognition likely contributes to an increasing trend in Legionnaires' disease incidence. Control and prevention of Legionnaires' disease requires a multifaceted approach. A critical component of this approach involves primary prevention efforts aimed at implementing water maintenance programs in high-risk buildings. Investment in the investigation of Legionnaires' disease cases, promotion of water management programs in buildings as risk for growth and transmission of *Legionella*, and research into the ecology, detection, and control of *Legionella* spp. remains the key to decreasing the incidence of this disease.

ACKNOWLEDGMENTS

We thank Laura Cooley (CDC) for critical review of the manuscript.

References

1. List of prokaryotic names with standing in nomenclature. http://www.bacterio.net/legionella.html. Accessed October 29, 2018.
2. Muder RR, Yu VL. Infection due to *Legionella* species other than *L. pneumophila*. *Clin Infect Dis.* 2002;35(8):990–8.
3. Yu VL, Plouffe JF, Pastoris MC, et al. Distribution of *Legionella* species and serogroups isolated by culture in patients with sporadic community-acquired legionellosis: An international collaborative survey. *J Infect Dis.* 2002;186(1):127–8.
4. Mercante JW, Winchell JM. Current and emerging *Legionella* diagnostics for laboratory and outbreak investigations. *Clin Microbiol Rev.* 2015;28(1): 95–133.
5. Kozak NA, Lucas CE, Winchell JM. Identification of *Legionella* in the environment. *Methods Mol Biol.* 2013;954:3–25.
6. Gomez-Valero L, Rusniok C, Buchrieser C. *Legionella pneumophila*: Population genetics, phylogeny and genomics. *Infect Genet Evol.* 2009;9: 727–39.
7. Joly JR, McKinney RM, Tobin JO, et al. Development of a standardized subgrouping scheme for *Legionella pneumophila* serogroup 1 using monoclonal antibodies. *J Clin Microbiol.* 1986;23:768–71.
8. Helbig JH, Kurtz JB, Pastoris MC, et al. Antigenic lipopolysaccharide components of *Legionella pneumophila* recognized by monoclonal antibodies: Possibilities and limitations for division of the species into serogroups. *J Clin Microbiol.* 1997;35:2841–5.
9. Zou CH, Knirel YA, Helbig JH, et al. Molecular cloning and characterization of a locus responsible for O acetylation of the O polysaccharide of *Legionella pneumophila* serogroup 1 lipopolysaccharide. *J Bacteriol.* 1999;181(13):4137–41.
10. Kozak NA, Benson RF, Brown E, et al. Distribution of *lag-1* alleles and sequence-based types among *Legionella pneumophila* serogroup 1 clinical and environmental isolates in the United States. *J Clin Microbiol.* 2009;47: 2525–35.
11. Amodeo MR, Murdoch DR, Pithie AD. Legionnaires' disease caused by *Legionella longbeachae* and *Legionella pneumophila*: Comparison of clinical features, host-related risk factors, and outcomes. *Clin Microbiol Infect.* 2010;16:1405–7.
12. Fang GD, Yu VL, Vickers RM. Disease due to the Legionellaceae (other than *Legionella pneumophila*). Historical, microbiological, clinical, and epidemiological review. *Medicine.* 1989;68:116–32.
13. Reingold AL, Thomason BM, Brake BJ, et al. *Legionella pneumonia* in the United States: The distribution of serogroups and species causing human illness. *J Infect Dis.* 1984;149:819.
14. van Heijnsbergen E, Schalk JA, Euser SM, et al. Confirmed and potential sources of *Legionella* reviewed. *Environ Sci Technol.* 2015;49:4797–815.
15. Llewellyn AC, Lucas DE, Roberts SE, et al. Distribution of *Legionella* and bacterial community composition among regionally diverse US cooling towers. *PLoS One.* 2017;12(12):e0189937.
16. Peabody MA, Caravas JA, Morrison SS, et al. Characterization of *Legionella* species from watersheds in British Columbia, Canada. *mSphere.* 2017;2: e00246-17.
17. Zhang L, Li Y, Wang X, et al. High prevalence and genetic polymorphisms of *Legionella* in natural and man-made aquatic environments in Wenzhou, China. *Int J Environ Res Public Health.* 2017;14(3):222–35.
18. Kanatani JI, Isobe J, Norimoto S, et al. Prevalence of *Legionella* species isolated from shower water in public bath facilities in Toyama Prefecture, Japan. *J Infect Chemother.* 2017;23(5):265–70.
19. Steege L, Moore G. The presence and prevalence of *Legionella* spp. in collected rainwater and its aerosolisation during common gardening activities. *Perspect Public Health.* 2018;138(5):254–60.
20. Parthuisot N, West NJ, Lebaron P, et al. High diversity and abundance of *Legionella* spp. in a pristine river and impact of seasonal and anthropogenic effects. *Appl Environ Microbiol.* 2010;76(24):8201–10.
21. Whiley H, Bentham R. *Legionella longbeachae* and legionellosis. *Emerg Infect Dis.* 2011;17(4):579–83.
22. Whiley H, Bentham R, Brown MH. *Legionella* persistence in manufactured water systems: Pasteurization potentially selecting for thermal tolerance. *Front Microbiol.* 2017;8:1330.
23. Huan SW, Hsu BM, Ma PH, Chien KT. *Legionella* prevalence in wastewater treatment plants of Taiwan. *Water Sci Tecnol.* 2009;60(5):1303–10.
24. Graells T, Ishak H, Larsson M, et al. The all-intracellular order Legionellales is unexpectedly diverse, globally distributed and lowly abundant. *FEMS Microbiol Ecol.* 2018;94(12):fiy185. doi: 10.1093/femsle/fiy185.
25. Euser SM, Brion JP, Brandsema P, et al. *Legionella* prevention in the Netherlands: An evaluation using genotype distribution. *Eur J Clin Microbiol Infect Dis.* 2013;32(8):1017–22.
26. Boamah DK, Zhou G, Ensminger AW et al. From many hosts, one accidental pathogen: The diverse protozoan hosts of *Legionella*. *Front Cell Infect Microbiol.* 2017;7:477.
27. Sherwood RD, Roy CR. Autophagy evasion and endoplasmic reticulum subversion: The yin and yang of *Legionella* intracellular infection. Ann *Rev Microbiol.* 2016;70:413–33.
28. Robertson P, Abdelhady H, Garduno RA, et al. The many forms of a pleomorphic bacterial pathogen—The developmental network of *Legionella pneumophila*. *Front Microbiol.* 2014;5:670.
29. Oliva G, Sahr T, Buchrieser C. The life cycle of *L. pneumophila*: Cellular differentiation is linked to virulence and metabolism. *Front Cell Infect Microbiol.* 2018;8:3.
30. Newton HJ, Ang DK, van Driel IR, et al. Molecular pathogenesis of infections caused by *Legionella pneumophila*. *Clin Microbiol Rev.* 2010;23(2): 274–98.
31. Ensminger AW. *Legionella pneumophila*, armed to the hilt: Justifying the largest arsenal of effectors in the bacterial world. *Curr Opin Microbiol.* 2016;29:74–80.
32. Abdel-Nour M, Duncan C, Low DE, et al. Biofilms: The stronghold of *Legionella pneumophila*. *Int J Mol Sci.* 2013;14(11):21660–75.
33. Wang H, Masters S, Edwards MA, et al. Effect of disinfectant, water age, and pipe materials on bacterial and eukaryotic community structure in drinking water biofilm. *Env Sci Technol.* 2014;48(3):1426–35.
34. Centers for Disease Control and Prevention. Active bacterial core surveillance for legionellosis—United States, 2011–2013. *Morb Mortal Wkly Rep.* 2015;64:1190–3.
35. Den Boer JW, Yzerman EPF, Schellekens J, et al. A large outbreak of Legionnaires' disease at a Flower Show, the Netherlands, 1999. *Emerg Infect Dis.* 2002;8(1):37–43.
36. Ambrose J, Hampton LM, Fleming-Dutra KE, et al. Large outbreak of Legionnaires' disease and Pontiac fever at a military base. *Epidemiol Infect.* 2014;142(11):2336–46.
37. Ward M, Boland M, Nicolay N, et al. A cluster of Legionnaires' disease and associated Pontiac fever morbidity in office workers, Dublin, June–July 2008. *J Environ Public Health.* 2010;2010:463926.
38. Burnsed LJ, Hicks LA, Smithee LMK, et al. A large travel-associated outbreak of legionellosis among hotel guests: Utility of the urine antigen assay in confirming Pontiac fever. *Clin Infect Dis.* 2007;44(2):222–8.
39. Edelstein PH. Urine antigen tests positive for Pontiac fever: Implications for diagnosis and pathogenesis. *Clin Infect Dis.* 2007;44(2):229–31.
40. Benitez AJ, Winchell JM. Clinical application of a multiplex real-time PCR assay for simultaneous detection of *Legionella* species, *Legionella pneumophila*, and *Legionella pneumophila* serogroup 1. *J Clin Microbiol.* 2013;51(1): 348–51.
41. Nazarian EJ, Bopp DJ, Saylors A, et al. Design and implementation of a protocol for the detection of *Legionella* in clinical and environmental samples. *Diagn Microbiol Infect Dis.* 2008;62(2):125–32.
42. Rhoads WJ, Ji P, Pruden A, et al. Water heater temperature set point and water use patterns influence *Legionella pneumophila* and associated microorganisms at the tap. *Microbiome.* 2015;3:67.
43. Ji P, Rhoads WJ, Edwards MA, et al. Impact of water heater temperature setting and water use frequency on the building plumbing microbiome. *ISME J.* 2017;11(6):1318–30.
44. Nguyen TM, Ilef D, Jarraud S, et al. A community-wide outbreak of Legionnaires disease linked to industrial cooling towers—How far can contaminated aerosols spread? *J Infect Dis.* 2006;193(1):102–11.

45. Centers for Disease Control and Prevention. Environmental Legionella Isolation Techniques Evaluation Program. https://www.cdc.gov/legionella/labs/elite.html. Updated September 28, 2017. Accessed October 29, 2018.

46. Benowitz I, Fitzhenry R, Boyd C, et al. Rapid identification of a cooling tower-associated Legionnaires' disease outbreak supported by polymerase chain reaction testing of environmental samples, New York City, 2014–2015. *J Environ Health.* 2018;80(8):8–12.

47. Centers for Disease Control and Prevention. Legionella (Legionnaires' Disease and Pontiac Fever). https://www.cdc.gov/legionella. Updated April 30, 2018. Accessed August 20, 2018.

48. Simmering JE, Polgreen LA, Hornick DB, et al. Weather-dependent risk for Legionnaires' disease, United States. *Emerg Infect Dis.* 2017;23(11):1843–51.

49. Völker S, Schreiber C, Kistemann T. Modelling characteristics to predict *Legionella* contamination risk—Surveillance of drinking water plumbing systems and identification of risk areas. *Int J Hyg Environ Health.* 2016;219(1):101–9.

50. Sivagnanam S, Podczervinski S, Butler-Wu SM, et al. Legionnaires' disease in transplant recipients: A 15-year retrospective study in a tertiary referral center. *Transpl Infect Dis.* 2017;19(5).

51. Neil K, Berkelman R. Increasing incidence of legionellosis in the United States, 1990–2005: Changing epidemiologic trends. *Clin Infect Dis.* 2008;47:591–9.

52. Centers for Disease Control and Prevention. Legionellosis—United States, 2000–2009. *Morb Mortal Wkly Rep.* 2011;60:1083–6.

53. Farnham A, Alleyne L, Cimini D, et al. Legionnaires' disease incidence and risk factors, New York, New York, USA, 2002–2011. *Emerg Infect Dis.* 2014;20(11):1795–802.

54. Kenagy E, Priest PC, Cameron CM, et al. Risk factors for *Legionella longbeachae* Legionnaires' disease, New Zealand. *Emerg Infect Dis.* 2017;23(7):1148–54.

55. Soda EA, Barskey AE, Shah PP, et al. Vital signs: Health care-associated Legionnaires' disease surveillance data from 20 states and a large metropolitan area—United States, 2015. *Morb Mortal Wkly Rep.* 2017;66:584–9.

56. Quinn C, Demirjian A, Lucas C, et al. Legionnaires' disease outbreak at a long-term care facility caused by a cooling tower using an automated disinfection system—Ohio, 2013. *J Environ Health.* 2015;78(5):8–13.

57. Leoni E, Catalani F, Marini S, et al. Legionellosis associated with recreational waters: A systematic review of cases and outbreaks in swimming pools, spa pools, and similar environments. *Int J Environ Res Public Health.* 2018;15(8):1612.

58. European Legionnaires' Disease Surveillance Network (ELDSNet), European Centre for Disease Prevention and Control. https://ecdc.europa.eu/en/about-us/partnerships-and-networks/disease-and-laboratory-networks/eldsnet. Accessed October 29, 2018.

59. Benedict KM, Reses H, Vigar M, et al. Surveillance for waterborne disease outbreaks associated with drinking water—United States, 2013–2014. *Morb Mortal Wkly Rep.* 2017;66:1216–21.

60. Centers for Disease Control and Prevention. Vessel Sanitation Program. https://www.cdc.gov/nceh/vsp/default.htm Updated June 20, 2018. Accessed August 31, 2018.

61. Greene SK, Peterson ER, Kapell D, et al. Daily reportable disease spatiotemporal cluster detection, New York City, New York, USA, 2014–2015. *Emerg Infect Dis.* 2016;22(10):1808–12.

62. Centers for Disease Control and Prevention. *Legionella* Environmental Assessment Form. https://www.cdc.gov/legionella/downloads/legionella-environmental-assessment.pdf. Accessed October 29, 2018.

63. ASHRAE. Legionellosis: Risk management for building water systems. *ANSI/ASHRAE Standard 188–2015.* Atlanta, GA: ASHRAE; 2015. http://www.mesc.org/downloads/v/PCTI/ASHRAE%20188%20-%202015%20FINAL.pdf. Accessed October 29, 2018.

64. Centers for Disease Control and Prevention. Developing a Water Management Program to Reduce *Legionella* Growth & Spread in Buildings. https://www.cdc.gov/legionella/downloads/toolkit.pdf. Accessed October 29, 2018.

65. Lapierre P, Nazarian E, Zhu Y, et al. Legionnaires' disease outbreak caused by endemic strain of *Legionella pneumophila*, New York, New York, USA, 2015. *Emerg Infect Dis.* 2017;23(11):1784–91.

66. Campese C, Roche D, Clément C, et al. Cluster of Legionnaires' disease associated with a public whirlpool spa, France, April–May 2010. *Euro Surveill.* 2010;15(26):pii:19602.

67. Gaia V, Fry NK, Afshar B, et al. Consensus sequence-based scheme for epidemiological typing of clinical and environmental isolates of *Legionella pneumophila. J Clin Microbiol.* 2005;43:2047–52.

68. Ratzow S, Gaia V, Helbig JH, et al. Addition of *neuA*, the gene encoding N-acylneuraminate cytidylyl transferase, increases the discriminatory ability of the consensus sequence-based scheme for typing *Legionella pneumophila* serogroup 1 strains. *J Clin Microbiol.* 2007;45:1965–8.

69. European Working Group for Legionella Infections. *Legionella pneumophila* sequence based typing. http://bioinformatics.phe.org.uk/legionella/legionella_sbt/php/sbt_homepage.php.

70. Kozak-Muiznieks NA, Lucas CE, Brown E, et al. Prevalence of sequence types among clinical and environmental isolates of *Legionella pneumophila* serogroup 1 in the United States from 1982 to 2012. *J Clin Microbiol.* 2014;52(1):201.

71. Raphael BH, Baker DJ, Nazarian E, et al. Genomic resolution of outbreak-associated *Legionella pneumophila* aerogroup 1 isolates from New York State. *Appl Environ Microbiol.* 2016;82(12):3582–90.

72. Mizrahi H, Peretz A, Lesnik R, et al. Comparison of sputum microbiome of legionellosis-associated patients and other pneumonia patients: indications for polybacterial infections. *Sci Rep.* 2017;7:40114.

73. Garrison LE, Kunz JM, Cooley LA, et al. Vital Signs: deficiencies in environmental control identified in outbreaks of Legionnaires' disease—North America, 2000–2014. *Morb Mortal Wkly Rep* 2016;65:576–84.

74. World Health Organization. Legionella *and the Prevention of Legionellosis.* Geneva, Switzerland: WHO; 2007.

75. Whiley H. Legionella risk management and control in potable water systems: Argument for the abolishment of routine testing. *Int J Environ Res Public Health.* 2016;14(1):pii: E12.

76. Gamage SD, Ambrose M, Kralovic SM, et al. Water safety and *Legionella* in health care: Priorities, policy, and practice. *Infect Dis Clin North Am.* 2016;30(3):689–712.

77. Krageschmidt DA, Kubly AF, Browning MS, et al. A comprehensive water management program for multicampus healthcare facilities. *Infect Control Hosp Epidemiol.* 2014;35(5):556–63.

78. Whitney EA, Blake S, Berkelman RL. Implementation of a *Legionella* ordinance for multifamily housing, Garland, Texas. *J Public Health Manag Pract.* 2017;23(6):601–7.

79. City of New York. NYC Health: Cooling tower registration and maintenance. https://www1.nyc.gov/site/doh/business/permits-and-licenses/cooling-towers.page. Accessed August 20, 2018.

80. New York State. New York codes, rules and regulations. Volume A (Title 10): Part 4—protection against *Legionella*. https://regs.health.ny.gov/content/part-4-protection-against-legionella. Accessed August 20, 2018.

81. Center for Clinical Standards and Quality/Survey and Certification Group, Centers for Medicaid and Medicare Services. Requirement to reduce Legionella risk in healthcare facility water systems to prevent cases and outbreaks of Legionnaires' disease. S&C 17-30-*Hospitals/CAHs/NHs* REVISED 06.09.2017. https://www.cms.gov/Medicare/Provider-Enrollment-and-Certification/SurveyCertificationGenInfo/Downloads/Survey-and-Cert-Letter-17-30.pdf. Accessed September 1, 2018.

CHAPTER

116 Giardiasis*

Katharine M. Benedict • Jonathan S. Yoder • Mohsin Ali

Giardiasis is caused by the protozoan parasite *Giardia duodenalis* (formerly called *G. lamblia* or *G. intestinalis*). This anaerobic flagellate protozoan is found on surfaces or in soil, food, or water that has been contaminated by feces from humans or animals hosting the parasite. The disease has substantial global burden; for 2010, the World Health Organization estimated that there were 183.8 million cases worldwide (95% uncertainty interval, 130.0–262.8 million).[1] Annually, more than 1 million cases occur in the United States.[2]

LIFE CYCLE

Giardia has two stages in its life cycle—cyst and trophozoite—and is transmitted by the fecal–oral route. While both cysts and trophozoites can be found in the feces, only cysts cause disease transmission, partly because their outer shell allows them to survive for weeks to several months in the environment and makes them moderately chlorine tolerant.[3] These properties, combined with a low infectious dose, make *Giardia* ideally suited for transmission through ingestion of contaminated water.[4,5] However, transmission also occurs through contact with feces (e.g., through caring for an infected person), eating contaminated food, or contact with contaminated surfaces.[4–9]

Infection typically begins with cyst ingestion from contaminated water, food, or fomites (e.g., hands). In the small intestine, excystation releases trophozoites, with each cyst producing two trophozoites.[4–6] Trophozoites multiply by longitudinal binary fission, remaining in the lumen of the proximal small intestine where they can be free or attached to the mucosa by a ventral sucking disk. Encystation occurs as the parasites transit toward the colon. The cyst is the stage found most commonly in nondiarrheal feces.

CLINICAL MANIFESTATIONS

While *Giardia* infections can be asymptomatic,[10] patients with giardiasis classically present with gradual onset of two to five loose stools per day and gradually increasing fatigue.[11,12] Stools are often described as foul-smelling, greasy, and tend to float. Other symptoms include nausea, anorexia, abdominal cramps, bloating, flatulence, and dehydration, whereas fever, vomiting, pruritus, hives, and swelling of the eye and joints are more uncommon.[11–14] Weight loss may occur over time, and giardiasis is also associated with fat, lactose, vitamin A, and vitamin B12 malabsorption.[11,12,15,16]

Giardiasis has an incubation period of 1–2 weeks and generally resolves within 2–4 weeks.[5,12] However, chronic sequelae have also been recognized, including reactive arthritis[17,18] and irritable bowel syndrome[6,19]; in children, in particular, severe giardiasis may cause growth stunting, developmental delay, failure to thrive, and malnutrition.[20–24]

EPIDEMIOLOGY AND RISK FACTORS

Giardia is the most common intestinal parasite of humans identified in the United States,[25,26] and a common cause of outbreaks associated with untreated surface and groundwater.[27–29] Annually, an estimated 1.2 million cases of giardiasis occur in the United States,[2] costing U.S.$34 million in hospitalizations.[30]

Transmission occurs indirectly through the consumption of fecally contaminated water or food and directly through person-to-person transmission and animal-to-person transmission. Most reported giardiasis outbreaks have been associated with waterborne transmission.[27] Drinking untreated water from lakes and rivers, swimming, having contact with some animal species, and sexual activity involving fecal contact might increase risk for giardiasis (Box 116-1).[7,31,32] *Giardia* infection rates have been known to rise in late summer and children are more commonly infected.[25] Giardiasis is often diagnosed in international travelers and among internationally adopted children.[32–34]

Giardia cysts are infectious when passed in the stool or shortly afterward, making person-to-person transmission possible in the absence of frequent hand washing. While animals such as cats, dogs, cattle, deer, and beavers can host *Giardia*, their role in infecting humans or contaminating the environment with human-pathogenic *Giardia* is unclear.[35–38] The risk of humans acquiring *Giardia* infection from dogs or cats is small.[39,40] The exact type of *Giardia* that is pathogenic to humans is usually not the same type that is pathogenic in dogs and cats[37,41,42] (Table 116-1). *Giardia duodenalis* can be subdivided based on molecular analysis into what are known as different genetic assemblages (A, B, C, D, E, F, G, and H). Some of these assemblages can be classified even further into subtypes (e.g., A-I, A-II, A-III, A-IV). Each assemblage is capable of infecting certain species, and some assemblages are more commonly seen than others.[36,39,42]

In the United States, *Giardia* has been reported since 1992 and became a nationally notifiable disease in 2002.[43] Federal, state, and local public health agencies can use giardiasis surveillance data to better understand the epidemiology of giardiasis in the United States, design efforts to prevent the spread of disease, and establish research priorities.

*The findings and conclusions in this report are those of the authors and do not necessarily represent the official position of the Centers for Disease Control and Prevention.

BOX 116-1 Persons at Greatest Risk for *Giardia* Infection

While anyone may become infected with *Giardia*, those at greatest risk are:

- Travelers to countries where giardiasis is common;
- People in childcare settings;
- Those who are in close contact with someone who has the disease;
- People who swallow contaminated drinking water;
- Backpackers or campers who drink untreated water from springs, lakes, or rivers (i.e., surface water);
- People who have contact with infected animals or animal environments contaminated with feces; and
- People who have contact with feces during sexual activity.

TABLE 116-1 MOLECULAR CHARACTERIZATION OF *GIARDIA DUODENALIS*

Assemblages	Species Commonly Infected
A-I	Humans and animals (cats, dogs, livestock, deer, muskrats, beavers, voles, guinea pigs, ferrets, nonhuman primates, birds, marsupials)
A-II	Humans; nonhuman primates (more common than A-I)
A-III, A-IV	Exclusively animals
B	Humans and animals (livestock, chinchillas, beavers, marmosets, rodents, marsupials, nonhuman primates, cats, dogs, birds)
C and D	Dogs, wild canids
E	Alpacas, cattle, goats, pigs, sheep
F	Cats
G	Rats
H	Pinnipeds

DIAGNOSIS

Giardia cysts or trophozoites are not consistently seen in the stools of infected patients. Diagnostic sensitivity can be increased by examining up to three stool specimens over several days.[44] New molecular enteric panel assays generally include *Giardia* as a target pathogen. Diagnostic techniques include microscopy with direct fluorescent antibody testing (DFA; considered the gold standard), rapid immunochromatographic cartridge assays, enzyme immunoassay (EIA) kits, microscopy with trichrome staining, and molecular assays. Only enhanced molecular testing [i.e., polymerase chain reaction (PCR)] can be used to identify the *Giardia* assemblage; the assemblage cannot be determined based on morphology alone.[44,45] Retesting is only recommended if symptoms persist after treatment (see Treatment section).

TREATMENT

Several drugs can be used to treat giardiasis, including metronidazole, tinidazole, and nitazoxanide.[46] Alternatives include paromomycin, quinacrine, and furazolidone.[46,47] Treatment is often empiric in patients with the appropriate history and typical symptoms since making a definitive diagnosis is difficult. The effectiveness of drug regimens depends on several factors, including medical history, nutritional status, and condition of the immune system.[48–50] Dehydration due to diarrhea can be particular risk among pregnant women and can be life threatening for infants. Thus, rehydration is especially important for these groups.

When dealing with possible cases of *Giardia* clinical treatment failure and before switching therapies, consider the following algorithm:

1. Determine if the patient is still infected. Test 3 stool samples every other day by antigen testing or microscopy.
2. Consider reinfection through the environment (i.e., home, daycare) or household members, rather than treatment failure.
3. Consider inadequate dosing or duration of treatment. Confirm that the patient took the entire course of medication as prescribed.
4. If *Giardia* is confirmed by positive stool test, reinfection and inadequate dosing have been ruled out, and the patient remains symptomatic, retreat. Combination therapy can be safe, effective, and a useful alternative in the case of treatment failure.[51] Wait at least 2 weeks after the last dose of anti-*Giardia* medication is taken and re-exam stool specimens as outlined in Step One for the presence of *Giardia*.
5. If *Giardia* is not found after three stool exams, *and* if a parasite concentration method is used to process the stool specimen before the exam, one can be roughly 95% confident that the patient is no longer infected.

PREVENTION AND CONTROL

Prevention messages to share with those at risk of giardiasis:

Safe water, appropriate sanitation, and hand washing are the most important measures to avoid giardiasis. Avoid drinking and recreational water that may be contaminated. If the safety of drinking water is in doubt (e.g., during travel to a location with poor sanitation or lack of water treatment systems), do one of the following:

- Drink commercially bottled water from an unopened factory-sealed container.
- Disinfect tap water by heating it to a rolling boil for 1 minute.
- Use a filter that has been certified for cyst and oocyst reduction.

Avoid swallowing water while swimming in pools, hot tubs, interactive fountains, lakes, rivers, springs, ponds, streams, or the ocean or drinking untreated water from lakes, rivers, springs, ponds, streams, or shallow wells.

Wash hands frequently with soap and clean, running water for at least 20 seconds; rub your hands together to make a lather and be sure to scrub the backs of your hands, between your fingers, and under your nails. Specific times when washing hands is especially important are:

- Before, during, and after preparing food;
- Before eating food;
- Before and after caring for someone who is sick;
- After using the toilet, changing diapers or cleaning up a child who has used the toilet; and
- After touching an animal, animal waste, or animal environments.

Prevent contact and contamination with feces during sex:

- Use a barrier during oral–anal sex.
- Wash hands right after handling a condom used during anal sex and after touching the anus or rectal area.

For additional prevention guidance, visit the CDC *Giardia* website: https://www.cdc.gov/parasites/giardia.

References

1. Kirk MD, Pires SM, Black RE, et al. World Health Organization estimates of the global and regional disease burden of 22 foodborne bacterial, protozoal, and viral diseases, 2010: A data synthesis. *PLoS Med.* 2015;12(12):e1001921.
2. Scallan E, Hoekstra RM, Angulo FJ, et al. Foodborne illness acquired in the United States—Major pathogens. *Emerg Infect Dis.* 2011;17(1):7–15.
3. Jarroll EL, Bingham AK, Meyer EA. Effect of chlorine on Giardia lamblia cyst viability. *Appl Environ Microbiol.* 1981;41(2):483–7.

4. Leggett HC, Cornwallis CK, West SA. Mechanisms of pathogenesis, infective dose and virulence in human parasites. *PLoS Pathog.* 2012;8(2):e1002512.
5. Ortega YR, Adam RD. Giardia: Overview and update. *Clin Infect Dis.* 1997;25(3):545–9; quiz 550.
6. Einarsson E, Ma'ayeh S, Svard SG. An up-date on Giardia and giardiasis. *Curr Opin Microbiol.* 2016;34:47–52.
7. Escobedo AA, Almirall P, Alfonso M, Cimerman S, Chacin-Bonilla L. Sexual transmission of giardiasis: A neglected route of spread? *Acta Trop.* 2014;132:106–11.
8. Keystone JS, Krajden S, Warren MR. Person-to-person transmission of Giardia lamblia in day-care nurseries. *Can Med Assoc J.* 1978;119(3):241–2, 247–8.
9. Rose JB, Slifko TR. Giardia, Cryptosporidium, and Cyclospora and their impact on foods: A review. *J Food Prot.* 1999;62(9):1059–70.
10. Huang DB, White AC. An updated review on Cryptosporidium and Giardia. *Gastroenterol Clin North Am.* 2006;35(2):291–314, viii.
11. Gardner TB, Hill DR. Treatment of giardiasis. *Clin Microbiol Rev.* 2001;14(1):114–28.
12. Robertson LJ, Hanevik K, Escobedo AA, Morch K, Langeland N. Giardiasis—Why do the symptoms sometimes never stop? *Trends Parasitol.* 2010;26(2):75–82.
13. Farthing MJ. Giardiasis. *Gastroenterol Clin North Am.* 1996;25(3):493–515.
14. Wolfe MS. Giardiasis. *Clin Microbiol Rev.* 1992;5(1):93–100.
15. Notis WM. Giardiasis and vitamin B 12 malabsorption. *Gastroenterology.* 1972;63(6):1085.
16. Solomons NW. Giardiasis: Nutritional implications. *Rev Infect Dis.* 1982;4(4):859–69.
17. Halliez MC, Buret AG. Extra-intestinal and long term consequences of Giardia duodenalis infections. *World J Gastroenterol.* 2013;19(47):8974–85.
18. Painter JE, Collier SA, Gargano JW. Association between Giardia and arthritis or joint pain in a large health insurance cohort: Could it be reactive arthritis? *Epidemiol Infect.* 2017;145(3):471–7.
19. Nakao JH, Collier SA, Gargano JW.Giardiasis and subsequent irritable bowel syndrome: A longitudinal cohort study using health insurance data. *J Infect Dis.* 2017;215(5):798–805.
20. Berkman DS, Lescano AG, Gilman RH, Lopez SL, Black MM. Effects of stunting, diarrhoeal disease, and parasitic infection during infancy on cognition in late childhood: A follow-up study. *Lancet.* 2002;359(9306):564–71.
21. Botero-Garces JH, Garcia-Montoya GM, Grisales-Patino D, Aguirre-Acevedo DC, Alvarez-Uribe MC. Giardia intestinalis and nutritional status in children participating in the complementary nutrition program, Antioquia, Colombia, May to October 2006. *Rev Inst Med Trop Sao Paulo.* 2009;51(3):155–62.
22. Farthing MJ, Mata L, Urrutia JJ, Kronmal RA. Natural history of Giardia infection of infants and children in rural Guatemala and its impact on physical growth. *Am J Clin Nutr.* 1986;43(3):395–405.
23. Newman RD, Moore SR, Lima AA, Nataro JP, Guerrant RL, Sears CL. A longitudinal study of Giardia lamblia infection in north-east Brazilian children. *Trop Med Int Health.* 2001;6(8):624–34.
24. Sullivan PB, Marsh MN, Phillips MB, et al. Prevalence and treatment of giardiasis in chronic diarrhoea and malnutrition. *Arch Dis Child.* 1991;66(3):304–6.
25. Painter JE, Gargano JW, Collier SA, Yoder JS, Centers for Disease Control and Prevention. Giardiasis surveillance—United States, 2011–2012. *MMWR Suppl.* 2015;64(3):15–25.
26. Schnell K, Collier S, Derado G, Yoder J, Gargano JW. Giardiasis in the United States—An epidemiologic and geospatial analysis of county-level drinking water and sanitation data, 1993–2010. *J Water Health.* 2016;14(2):267–79.
27. Adam EA, Yoder JS, Gould LH, Hlavsa MC, Gargano JW. Giardiasis outbreaks in the United States, 1971–2011. *Epidemiol Infect.* 2016;144(13):2790–801.
28. Craun GF, Brunkard JM, Yoder JS, et al. Causes of outbreaks associated with drinking water in the United States from 1971 to 2006. *Clin Microbiol Rev.* 2010;23(3):507–28.
29. Wallender EK, Ailes EC, Yoder JS, Roberts VA, Brunkard JM. Contributing factors to disease outbreaks associated with untreated groundwater. *Groundwater.* 2014;52(6):886–97.
30. Collier SA, Stockman LJ, Hicks LA, Garrison LE, Zhou FJ, Beach MJ. Direct healthcare costs of selected diseases primarily or partially transmitted by water. *Epidemiol Infect.* 2012;140(11):2003–13.
31. Reses HE, Gargano JW, Liang JL, et al. Risk factors for sporadic Giardia infection in the USA: A case-control study in Colorado and Minnesota. *Epidemiol Infect.* 2018;146(9):1071–8.
32. Swirski AL, Pearl DL, Peregrine AS, Pintar K. A comparison of exposure to risk factors for giardiasis in non-travellers, domestic travellers and international travellers in a Canadian community, 2006–2012. *Epidemiol Infect.* 2016;144(5):980–99.
33. Connor BA. Chronic diarrhea in travelers. *Curr Infect Dis Rep.* 2013;15(3):203–10.
34. Staat MA. Infectious disease issues in internationally adopted children. *Pediatr Infect Dis J.* 2002;21(3):257–8.
35. Cacciò SM. Giardiasis: A zoonotic infection or not? In: *Zoonoses-Infections Affecting Humans and Animals: Focus on Public Health Aspects.* New York: Springer; 2015, pp. 821–48.
36. Feng Y, Xiao L. Zoonotic potential and molecular epidemiology of Giardia species and giardiasis. *Clin Microbiol Rev.* 2011;24(1):110–40.
37. Pijnacker R, Mughini-Gras L, Heusinkveld M, Roelfsema J, van Pelt W, Kortbeek T. Different risk factors for infection with Giardia lamblia assemblages A and B in children attending day-care centres. *Eur J Clin Microbiol Infect Dis.* 2016;35(12):2005–13.
38. Tsui CK, Miller R, Uyaguari-Diaz M, et al. Beaver fever: Whole-genome characterization of waterborne outbreak and sporadic isolates to study the zoonotic transmission of giardiasis. *mSphere.* 2018;3(2):e00090-18.
39. Ballweber LR, Xiao L, Bowman DD, Kahn G, Cama VA. Giardiasis in dogs and cats: Update on epidemiology and public health significance. *Trends Parasitol.* 2010;26(4):180–9.
40. Patton S. *Overview of Giardiasis.* United States: Merck; 2013.
41. Mohamed AS, Levine M, Camp JW Jr., et al. Temporal patterns of human and canine Giardia infection in the United States: 2003–2009. *Prev Vet Med.* 2014;113(2):249–56.
42. Xiao L, Fayer R. Molecular characterisation of species and genotypes of Cryptosporidium and Giardia and assessment of zoonotic transmission. *Int J Parasitol.* 2008;38(11):1239–55.
43. CDC. National Notifiable Diseases Surveillance System (NNDSS): Giardiasis. https://wwwn.cdc.gov/nndss/conditions/giardiasis/.
44. Garcia LS, Arrowood M, Kokoskin E, et al. Laboratory diagnosis of parasites from the gastrointestinal tract. *Clin Microbiol Rev.* 2018;31(1):e00025-17.
45. Soares R, Tasca T. Giardiasis: An update review on sensitivity and specificity of methods for laboratorial diagnosis. *J Microbiol Methods.* 2016;129:98–102.
46. The Medical Letter, Inc. Drugs for parasitic infections. *Med Lett.* 2013;11(Suppl)(143):e1–31.
47. Escobedo AA, Cimerman S. Giardiasis: A pharmacotherapy review. *Expert Opin Pharmacother.* 2007;8(12):1885–902.
48. Muller J, Ley S, Felger I, Hemphill A, Muller N. Identification of differentially expressed genes in a Giardia lamblia WB C6 clone resistant to nitazoxanide and metronidazole. *J Antimicrob Chemother.* 2008;62(1):72–82.
49. Solaymani-Mohammadi S, Genkinger JM, Loffredo CA, Singer SM. A meta-analysis of the effectiveness of albendazole compared with metronidazole as treatments for infections with Giardia duodenalis. *PLoS Negl Trop Dis.* 2010;4(5):e682.
50. Upcroft JA, Upcroft P. Drug resistance and Giardia. *Parasitol Today.* 1993;9(5):187–90.
51. Escobedo AA, Lalle M, Hrastnik NI, et al. Combination therapy in the management of giardiasis: What laboratory and clinical studies tell us, so far. *Acta Tropica.* 2016;162:196–205.

CHAPTER 117

Amebiasis

Jennifer R. Cope • Ibne K. Ali

AMEBIASIS

Although there are many species of ameba that infect humans, the term "amebiasis" generally refers to human infection by the enteric protozoan *Entamoeba histolytica*. Three other *Entamoeba* species that are morphologically indistinguishable from *E. histolytica* can infect humans as well.[1] These are: *E. dispar*, *E. moshkovskii*, and *E. bangladeshi*. Among these, *E. dispar* is nonpathogenic, *E. moshkovskii* is emerging as a pathogen, and the pathogenicity of *E. bangladeshi* is yet to be investigated. Other *Entamoeba* species such *E. coli*, *E. hartmanni*, or *E. polecki* can also infect humans. However, these nonpathogenic species are distinguishable from the pathogenic *E. histolytica* by virtue of their cyst and/or trophozoite morphology and shape. Earlier studies suggest *E. histolytica* and nonpathogenic *Entamoeba dispar* infect 10% of the earth's population, with higher incidence in poor developing areas. *E. histolytica* is estimated to be the third leading parasitic cause of death worldwide.[2] Infection with *E. histolytica* or *E. dispar* readily follows ingestion of the cyst form; however, only approximately 10% of those infected with *E. histolytica* manifest the symptoms of invasive amebiasis, colitis, and liver abscess. *E. dispar* infections are generally asymptomatic. Recognition of amebic infection requires knowledge of the epidemiology of the parasite, the varied clinical presentations, and the available diagnostic methods. Therapy for amebiasis requires use of multiple antiparasitic drugs that act against amebae in the bowel lumen or invaded host tissues. Prevention of amebic infections depends on adequate sanitation and hygiene, with availability of safe water supplies and avoidance of direct fecal-oral contamination among family members or sexual partners.

LIFE CYCLE AND EPIDEMIOLOGY

Infection is contracted by ingestion of the cyst form, which by virtue of its chitinous cell wall resists desiccation in the environment and destruction by stomach acid. Cysts contain one to four nuclei; encystation occurs in the small bowel, and the trophozoite form proceeds downstream to colonize the colon. Encystment of trophozoites followed by fecal excretion of cysts completes the life cycle; trophozoites rapidly disintegrate in the environment and if immediately ingested would most likely be killed by the acid pH of the stomach. Risk factors for acquisition of *E. histolytica* infection and increased susceptibility to aggressive invasive amebiasis are summarized in Box 117-1. Infection is most prevalent in developing areas of the world including Mexico, Africa, India, Southeast Asian, and South America. In developed countries, amebic infection and disease are concentrated in high-risk groups, such as those with prior exposure to an endemic environment or those more likely to have direct fecal oral contamination because of unhygienic living conditions. People living in institutionalized settings and men who have sex with men are at risk of developing amebiasis.[3]

BOX 117-1 Epidemiologic Risk Factors that Apparently Predispose to Entamoeba Histolytica Infection and Increased Severity of Disease

Increased Prevalence

Lower socioeconomic status in endemic area, including crowding and lack of indoor plumbing
Immigrants from endemic area
People living in institutionalized settings, especially with mental disability
Communal living
Men who have sex with men (MSM)
Adult males (as opposed to females), especially for ALA

Increased Severity

Children, especially neonates
Pregnancy and postpartum states
Corticosteroid use
Malignancy
Malnutrition
Host genetics (e.g., leptin-receptor polymorphism)
Intestinal microbiome

Until recently, studies demonstrating prevalence of amebiasis have been flawed by failing to distinguish *E. histolytica* from other *Entamoeba* species. More recent studies have begun to elucidate the true prevalence of amebiasis. A past study investigating immunity to disease in Bangladesh enrolled 230 Bangladeshi children (age 2–5 years) in a 2-year observational study. Over the duration of the study, 55% of children acquired *E. histolytica* infection in this high-risk population. Of these infected children, 80% remained asymptomatic while 20% had an associated diarrhea with 4% of these meeting the definition of amebic colitis. Of interest, 17% of infected children acquired an additional *E. histolytica* infection during the 2-year study. These second infections were felt to be due to a genetically distinct strains[4]. More recently, the same research team enrolled 392 children in their first week of birth from the same underserved community to detect 32 enteropathogen gene targets by molecular assay including the *E. histolytica*.[5,6] This study detected at least one *E. histolytica* infection in approximately one in five infants $\leq$ 24 months, including 17.3% that were associated with diarrhea.

Although little has been published on distinguishing *E. histolytica* and *E. dispar* in African communities, it is clear that amebiasis is prevalent in many areas of Africa. One thorough prevalence study was conducted in school children in Cote d'lvoire where an overall prevalence of *E. histolytica* was low at 0.83%, while *E. dispar* infected 15% of the children.[7] In South Africa, an earlier study found that children living in areas with better water supply harbored both *E. dispar* and *E. histolytica* (2%), while those in the rural setting with less sanitation harbored only *E. dispar* but at a high rate (>50%).[8] A recent South African study with gastroenterology clinic patients was conducted to detect four *Entamoeba* species by PCR and sequencing.[9] Overall, *Entamoeba* species were detected in 27% of patients. *E. histolytica* was detected in 8.5% (41/484), *E. dispar* in 8% (38/484), and *E. bangladeshi* in 4.75% (23/484), but no *E. moshkovskii* was detected. This was the first study that detected *E. bangladeshi* outside of Bangladesh. Two studies in Egypt, found high rates of *E. histolytica* (20% and 57%).[10,11]

Another cross-sectional survey of children in Ecuador found asymptomatic *E. histolytica* in only 7 of 178 children. However, it was interesting to note that more than 64% of children showed high serotiters, implying current or recent infection with *E. histolytica*.[12] This high seroprevalence corresponds to another recent sero-survey conducted in Mexico.[13] The Mexico study identified some challenges in conducting prevalence studies and highlighted the question of what should be considered the true "gold standard" in investigating individuals for *E. histolytica* and *E. dispar*. Species-specific conventional PCRs and real-time PCRs are becoming method of choice for detection of *Entamoeba* species in well-resourced countries because of their increased sensitivity and specificity. However, these PCRs are not readily available in low-resourced countries because of associated costs.

A related question arises frequently in clinical practice in low prevalence areas, which receive large numbers of immigrants and refugees from high prevalence areas. Most medical screening protocols in the United States for immigrants and refugees arriving from the developing world suggest three ova and parasite examinations (O&Ps) be routinely collected.[14] This screening is conducted to enhance the individual's health, as well as to protect the public health of the community. *Entamoeba* is known to spread within families, childcare and healthcare facilities, and occasionally may cause epidemics. Stool O&Ps are relatively insensitive and they are unable to distinguish *E. histolytica* from other *Entamoeba* species. As a result, diagnostic screening of immigrants and refugees for enteric pathogens should be performed with a sensitive and specific assay such as PCR. Use of molecular assays capable of detecting multiple etiologic agents (such as bacteria, parasites, virus, fungus, etc.) in a single assay (such as multiplex real-time PCR or Luminex-based GI panel)[15] would be optimal for facilitating diagnoses.

Severe invasive amebiasis with increased mortality has been reported in the very young, during pregnancy, in association with corticosteroid administration, and in malnourished individuals. A careful epidemiological history is essential for recognition of amebic disease.

PATHOGENESIS AND HOST IMMUNE RESPONSE

The low frequency of invasive clinical disease complicating widespread *E. histolytica* infection appears to be due to the existence of distinct pathogenic and nonpathogenic species (*E. histolytica* and *E. dispar*, respectively)[16] and a complex interplay between parasite and host factors that regulate expression of invasive pathogenic activities.[17] Asymptomatic intestinal infection with *E. histolytica* does occur and is distinguished from *E. dispar* infection by the presence of serum antiamebic antibodies during pathogenic infection.[18] In addition, serum antigenemia occurs during *E. histolytica* and not *E. dispar* infection.[19,20]

Pathogenesis of invasive amebiasis requires adherence of amebae to the colonic mucus blanket by a surface lectin molecule, disruption of the colonic epithelial barrier, parasite attachment to and lysis of host epithelial and acute inflammatory cells, and resistance of trophozoites to host humoral and cell-mediated immune defense mechanisms present in tissues.[21–23] Invasive *E. histolytica* trophozoites are resistant to the lytic effects of complement, despite their activation of both alternative and classic pathways. This is apparently due to an inhibitory binding effect of the lectin molecules, preventing formation of lytic complement complexes.[24] In a nonimmune host, *E. histolytica* trophozoites are capable of killing host lymphocytes and macrophages by phagocytosis and trogocytosis.[25,26]

In humans, asymptomatic *E. histolytica* infection is generally self-limited, resolving within 8–12 months of infection; whether this results from a specific host mucosal immune response or is associated with brief immunity to subsequent intestinal infection is unknown. In contrast, cure of invasive amebiasis in humans or experimental animals is followed by resistance to recurrence. This is apparently due to development of an amebicidal cell-mediated immune response.[27]

BOX 117-2 Clinical Syndromes Associated with Entamoeba Histolytica Infection

Intestinal Disease

Asymptomatic infection
Symptomatic noinvasive infection
Acute rectocolitis (dysentery)
Fulminant colitis with perforation
Toxic megacolon
Chronic nondysenteric colitis
Ameboma
Perianal ulceration

Extraintestinal Disease

Liver abscess
Liver abscess complicated by peritonitis, empyema, and pericarditis
Brain abscess
Appendicitis
Genitourinary disease
Skin lesions

CLINICAL CHARACTERISTICS

The clinical syndromes associated with *E. histolytica* infection are listed in Box 117-2. Up to 90% of individuals infected with *E. histolytica* are asymptomatic. Many infected persons have nonspecific gastrointestinal symptoms, such as abdominal pain, bloating, or watery diarrhea, but are without evidence of invasive disease. Although the reason for their complaints may not be clear or detectable, their amebic infection should be eradicated if due to *E. histolytica*. Amebic dysentery has a subacute onset over days to weeks and is manifest as abdominal pain and bloody diarrhea; only a minority of patients are febrile. Stools almost uniformly contain occult blood; despite the inflammatory nature of the disease, fecal leukocytes may not be present. The differential diagnosis includes invasive bacterial causes of colitis such as *Campylobacter*, *Shigella*, and *Salmonella* infection, toxin-mediated *Clostridium difficile* colitis or invasive *Escherichia coli* infection (i.e., Enterohemorrhagic *E. coli*).

Amebic colitis may be fulminant, especially in the high-risk groups summarized in Box 117-1, with high fever, peritonitis, and colonic perforation resulting in high mortality. Conversion of amebic dysentery to toxic megacolon is associated with corticosteroid administration, which may result from the misdiagnosis of amebic colitis as idiopathic inflammatory bowel disease. A chronic nondysenteric syndrome is characterized by intermittent bouts of inflammatory diarrhea over a period of years. These patients have invasive amebic colitis that can be diagnosed by tissue biopsy, antigen-detection ELISA for *E. histolytica*,[28] or PCR to detect amebic DNA,[29] and the presence of serum antiamebic antibodies, yet their disease is frequently mistaken for idiopathic ulcerative colitis.[30] Ameboma is a chronic segmental lesion, usually in the cecum or ascending colon, that is characterized by abdominal pain and mass and is often confused with colonic carcinoma. Perianal ulcerative amebic lesions may develop in patients with skin maceration caused by diarrhea; squamous epithelium is usually resistant to amebic invasion.

Extraintestinal disease is overwhelmingly manifest as liver abscess and its spread to contiguous body spaces. Common symptoms of amebic liver abscess are acute right upper quadrant pain and fever, necessitating differentiation from biliary tract disease. Alternatively, liver abscess may become symptomatic over a period of weeks with pain and weight loss but without fever, a presentation more suggestive of abdominal malignancy.[31] Knowledge of epidemiological risk factors and early use of hepatic imaging are essential for diagnosis. The risk of amebic liver abscess manifesting in patients returning from an endemic area is greatest in the first 3–6 months. Occasionally an amebic liver abscess, especially in the left lobe (which may be less symptomatic), ruptures into the peritoneum. The liver abscess can also penetrate through the diaphragm into the pleural space, resulting in an empyema. Extension of a left lobe abscess into the pericardium is a rare but often fatal complication.

DIAGNOSIS

Asymptomatic amebic infection is frequently encountered when individuals receive screening for parasites by stool ova and parasite examination (stool O&P) as occurs in the United States during new refugee medical screening. Many amebic species may be encountered although most are considered non-pathogenic (i.e., *Entamoeba coli, E. hartmanni, E. polecki*) and are simply a marker of fecal-oral exposure. Quadrinucleated cysts or trophozoites are encountered in about 1–3% of newly arriving refugees, depending on the population screened. As previously mentioned, these quadrinucleated cysts cannot be morphologically distinguished from the more common *E. dispar*, or other more unusual species such as *E. moshkovski* or *E. bangladeshi*. In addition, unless the trophozoite has ingested RBCs it too is indistinguishable from the more common nonpathogenic *Entamoeba* infection. In these cases, there are currently commercially available stool antigen tests as well as species-specific PCR assays, which can distinguish the species and should be used before initiating treatment.

The occurrence of invasive colitis is indicated by the finding of trophozoites (often containing ingested erythrocytes) in stool, a positive serological test for antiamebic antibodies, and the presence of ulcerative mucosal lesions observed by lower gastrointestinal endoscopy. In this setting, amebic antigen stool testing or species-specific DNA testing by PCR should be positive for *E. histolytica*, however, when not readily available, at least three separate stool samples should be examined using permanently stained slides. Colonoscopy with biopsy is highly sensitive and definitive although caution must be used in this approach in severely ill patients as the intestinal mucosa may be fragile and perforation may result. Serological tests for *E. histolytica* become positive within 1 week of disease onset and are usually positive at the time of presentation. It should be noted that prior to the diagnosis of idiopathic inflammatory bowel disease and the corresponding commencement of corticosteroid therapy, any patient with an epidemiological risk of *E. histolytica* should have a documented negative antiamebic antibody or negative PCR result for *E. histolytica* DNA.

Patients with a clinical syndrome and epidemiological risk factors consistent with amebic liver abscess should immediately undergo ultrasonography to look for a nonhomogeneous defect in the liver

TABLE 117-1 ANTIMICROBIAL AGENTS FOR USE IN TREATING AMEBIASIS

	Drug	Adult Dosage	Pediatric Dosage
Asymptomatic			
Drug of choice:	Iodoquinol[a]	650 mg PO tid × 20 d	30–40 mg/kg/d (max 2 g) PO in 3 doses × 20 d
	OR Paromomycin[b]	25–35 mg/kg/d PO in 3 doses × 7 d	25–35 mg/kg/d PO in 3 doses × 7 d
	OR Diloxanide furoate[c,e]	500 mg PO tid × 10 d	20 mg/kg/d PO in 3 doses × 10 d
Mild to moderate intestinal disease			
Drug of choice:[d]	Metronidazole	500–750 mg PO tid × 7–10d	35–50 mg/kg/d PO in 3 doses × 7–10 d
	OR Tinidazole[e]	2 g once PO daily × 3 d	>3yrs: 50 mg/kg/d (max 2 g) PO in 1 dose × 3 d
	either followed by		
	Iodoquinol[a]	650 mg PO tid × 20 d	30–40 mg/kg/d (max 2 g) PO in 3 doses × 20 d
	OR Paromomycin[b]	25–35 mg/kg/d PO in 3 doses × 7 d	25–35 mg/kg/d PO in 3 doses × 7 d
Severe intestinal and extraintestinal disease			
Drug of choice:	Metronidazole	750 mg PO (or IV) tid × 7–10 d	35–50 mg/kg/d PO (or IV) in 3 doses × 7–10 d
	OR Tinidazole[e]	2 g once PO daily × 5 d	>3 yrs: 50 mg/kg/d (max 2 g) PO in 1 dose × 5 d
	either followed by		
	Iodoquinol[a]	650 mg PO tid × 20 d	30–40 mg/kg/d (max 2 g) PO in 3 doses × 20 d
	OR Paromomycin[b]	25–35 mg/kg/d PO in 3 doses × 7 d	25–35 mg/kg/d PO in 3 doses × 7 d

[a]Iodoquinol should be taken after meals.
[b]Paromomycin should be taken with a meal.
[c]Not available commercially. It may be obtained through compounding pharmacies. Compounding pharmacies may be found through the National Association of Compounding Pharmacies (800-687-7850) or the Professional Compounding Centers of America (800-331-2498, www.pccarx.com).
[d]Nitazoxanide may be effective against a variety of protozoan and helminth infections (DA Bobak, *Curr Infect Dis Rep.* 2006;8:91; E Diaz et al. *Am J Trop Med Hyg.* 2003;68:384). It is effective against mild to moderate amebiasis, 500 mg PO bid × 3 d (JF Rossignol et al. *Trans R Soc Trop Med Hyg.* 2007;101:1025; AE Escobedo et al. *Arch Dis Child.* 2009;94:478), but perhaps less so than metronidazole (S Becker et al. *Am J Trop Hyg.* 2011;84:581). Nitazoxanide is FDA-approved only for treatment of diarrhea caused by Giardia or Cryptosporidium (*Med Lett Drugs Ther.* 2003;45:29). It is available in 500-mg tablets and an oral suspension and should be taken with food.
[d]A nitroimidazole similar to metronidazole, tinidazole appears to be as effective as metronidazole and better tolerated (*Med Lett Drugs Ther.* 2004;46:70). It should be taken with food to minimize GI adverse effects. For children and patients unable to take tablets, a pharmacist can crush the tablets and mix them with cherry syrup (Humco and others). The syrup suspension is good for 7 days at room temperature and must be shaken before use (Fung HB, Doan TL. *Clin Ther.* 2005;27:1859). Ornidazole, a similar drug, is also used outside the United States.
[e]Not available in the US.
Source: Reproduced with permission from The Medical Letter. Drugs for parasitic infections. *Treatment Guidelines from the Medical Letter.* Vol. 11. New York: The Medical Letter; 2013.

or evidence of biliary tract disease. Ultrasonography is sensitive, noninvasive, and relatively inexpensive; computed tomography (CT) and magnetic resonance imaging are not more specific and are only slightly more sensitive. Amebic liver abscess can be difficult to distinguish from bacterial liver abscess or hepatoma by imaging. Amebic liver abscess may occur at any age in persons who do not have the risk factors commonly associated with pyogenic abscess or hepatoma; however, adult males are disproportionately affected. If antigen detection ELISA, or species-specific PCR in abscess aspirate fluid, or amebic serological testing are unavailable, ultrasonography or CT-guided fine needle aspiration can be helpful. A negative Gram's stain and culture for bacteria helps establish the diagnosis. Virtually all persons with amebic liver abscess develop serum anti-amebic antibodies but often not until a week after symptom onset.[31] Thus an initial negative serological test for *E. histolytica* can be misleading early in the course of the abscess. *E. histolytica* trophozoites or cysts can be found in the stool of only a small number of patients with amebic liver abscess.

TREATMENT

Therapy for *E. histolytica* infection is complicated by the need for different agents to treat intraluminal and tissue infestation. Table 117-1 summarizes the drugs in use, their respective sites of activity, and recommendations for drug dosage, and duration of therapy.[32] For invasive intestinal and extraintestinal disease, the preferred therapy is a nitroimidazole, usually metronidazole in the United States for 7–10 days followed by an intraluminal agent such as iodoquinol or paramomycin. Diloxanide furoate is another intraluminal agent that is highly efficacious and relatively nontoxic; however, it is not readily available in the United States. A newer broad spectrum, well-tolerated, and safe antiparasitic agent, nitazoxanide, has shown evidence of effectiveness.[33]

Resistance to metronidazole remains a concern since the trophozoites of *E. histolytica* could be adapted to grow in presence of therapeutic levels of metronidazole *in vitro*.[34] Patients with amebic liver abscess respond to metronidazole with gradual defervescence and decreased symptoms over a 3- to 5-day period. Progression of symptoms during therapy or failure of metronidazole treatment is an indication for drainage of the liver abscess by needle aspiration and continued treatment with metronidazole.[35]

PREVENTION

Prevention of *E. histolytica* infection rests on availability of safe water supplies, adequate disposal of fecal material, adequate hygiene facilities, and avoidance of practices that promote direct fecal-oral contamination. Boiling of water is a dependable means of killing *E. histolytica* cysts; use of halogen-containing tablets (e.g., chlorine, bromine, iodine) can be effective, but is dependent on provision of sufficient dose and treatment time for effective disinfection.[36] No vaccine or readily accessible chemoprophylaxis is available; however, recent research on pathogenesis and host immunity has suggested that numerous amebic proteins are viable candidates for vaccine development.

DISCLAIMER

The findings and conclusions in this report are those of the author(s) and do not necessarily represent the official position of the Centers for Disease Control and Prevention.

References

1. Ali IK. Intestinal amebae. *Clin Lab Med*. 2015;35:393–422.
2. Walsh JA. Prevalence of *Entamoeba histolytica* infections. In: Ravdin JI, ed. *Amebiasis: Human Infection by Entamoeba histolytica*. New York: Churchill Livingston; 1988:93–105.
3. Petri WA Jr. Recent advances in amebiasis. *Crit Rev Clin Lab Sci* 1996;33:1–37.
4. Haque R, Duggal P, Ali IM, et al. Innate and acquired resistance to amebiasis in Bangladeshi children. *J Infect Dis*. 2002;186(4):547–52.
5. Gilchrist CA, Petri SE, Schneider BN, et al. Role of the gut microbiota of children in diarrhea due to the protozoan parasite *Entamoeba histolytica*. *J Infect Dis*. 2016;2016:1579–85.
6. Taniuchi M, Sobuz SU, Begum S, et al. Etiology of diarrhea in Bangladeshi infants in the first year of life analyzed using molecular methods. *J Infect Dis*. 2013;208:1794–802.
7. Heckendorn F, N'Foran EK, Felger I, et al. Species-specific field testing of *Entamoeba* spp. in an area of high endemicity. *Trans R Soc Trop Med Hyg*. 2002;96:521–8.
8. Jackson TFHG, Reddy S, Fincham J, et al. A comparison of cross sectional and longitudinal seroepidemiological assessments of *Entamoeba*-infected populations in South Africa. *Arch Med Res*. 2000;31:S36–7.
9. Ngobeni R, Samie A, Moonah S, Watanabe K, Petri WAJr, Gilchrist C. *Entamoeba* species in South Africa: Correlations with the host microbiome, parasite burdens, and first description of *Entamoeba bangladeshi* outside of Asia. *J Infect Dis*. 2017;216:1592–600.
10. Abd-Alla MD, Wahib AA, Ravdin JI. Comparison of antigen-capture ELISA to stool culture methods for the detection of asymptomatic *Entamoeba* species infection in Kafer Daoud, Egypt. *Am J Trop Med Hyg*. 2000;62:579–82.
11. Abd-Alla MD, Ravdin JI. Diagnosis of amoebic colitis by antigen capture ELISA in patients presenting with acute diarrhea in Cairo, Egypt. *Trop Med Int Health*. 2002;7:365–70.
12. Gatti S, Swierczynski G, Robinson F, et al. Amebic infections due to the *Entamoeba histolytica-entamoeba dispar* complex: A study of the incidence in a remote rural area of Ecuador. *Am J Trop Med Hyg*. 2002;67:123–7.
13. Petri WA, Singh U. Diagnosis and management of amebiasis. *Clin Infect Dis*. 1999;29:1117–25.
14. Stauffer WM, Kamat D, Walker PF. Screening of international immigrants, refugees, and adoptees. *Prim Care Clin Office Pract*. 2002;29:879–905.
15. Navidad JF, Griswold DJ, Gradus MS, Bhattacharyya S. Evaluation of Luminex xTAG gastrointestinal pathogen analyte-specific reagents for high-throughput, simultaneous detection of bacteria, viruses, and parasites of clinical and public health importance. *J Clin Microbiol*. 2013;51:2018–24.
16. Diamond LS, Clark CG. A redescription of *Entamoeba histolytica* Shaudinn 1903 (amended Walker 1911) separating it from *Entamoeba dispar* (Brumpt 1925). *J Eukaryot Microbiol*. 1993;40:340.
17. Sargeaunt PG. The reliability of *Entamoeba histolytica* zymodemes in clinical diagnosis. *Parasitol Today*. 1987;3:40–3.
18. Ravdin JI, Jackson TFHG, Petri WA, et al. Association of serum antiadherence lectin antibodies with invasive amebiasis and asymptomatic pathogenic *Entamoeba histolytica* infection. *J Infect Dis*. 1990;162:768–72.
19. Abd-Alla M, Jackson TFHG, Gathirim V, et al. Differentiation of pathogenic from nonpathogenic *Entamoeba histolytica* infection by detection of galactose-inhibitable adherence protein antigen in sera and feces. *J Clin Microbiol*. 1993;31:2845–50.
20. Abou-El-Magd I, Soong CG, El-Hawey AM, et al. Humoral and mucosal IgA antibody response to a recombinant 52-kDa cysteine rich portion of the *Entamoeba histolytica* galactose-inhibitable lectin correlates with detection of native 170-kDa lectin antigen in serum of patients with amebic colitis. *J Infect Dis*. 1996;174:157–62.
21. Ravdin JI. Amebiasis, "state of the art." *Clin Infect Dis*. 1995;20:1453–66.
22. Ravdin JI. *Entamoeba histolytica*: Pathogenic mechanisms, human immune response, and vaccine development. *Clin Res*. 1990;38:215–25.
23. Leippe M, Andra J, Muller Eberhard HJ. Cytolytic and antibacterial activity of synthetic peptides derived from amoebapore, the pore-forming peptide of *Entamoeba histolytica*. *Proc Natl Acad Sci U S A*. 1994;91:2602.
24. Braga LL, Ninomiya H, McCoy JJ, et al. Inhibition of the complement membrane attack complex by the galactose-specific adhesin of *Entamoeba histolytica*. *J Clin Invest*. 1992;90:1131.
25. Ralston KS, Solga MD, Mackey-Lawrence NM, Somlata, Bhattacharya A, Petri WAJr. Trogocytosis by Entamoeba histolytica contributes to cell killing and tissue invasion. *Nature*. 2014;508:526–30.
26. Somlata, Nakada-Tsukui K, Nozaki T. AGC family kinase 1 participates in trogocytosis but not in phagocytosis in *Entamoeba histolytica*. *Nat Commun*. 2017;8:101.
27. Ravdin JI. *Entamoeba histolytica*: Pathogenic mechanisms, human immune response, and vaccine development. *Clin Res*. 1990;38:215–25.
28. Haque R, Ali IK, Akther S, Petri WA Jr. Comparison of PCR, isoenzyme analysis, and antigen detection for diagnosis of *Entamoeba histolytica* infection. *J Clin Microbiol*. 1998;36:449–52.

29. Qvarnstrom Y, James C, Xayavong M, et al. Comparison of real-time PCR protocols for differential laboratory diagnosis of amebiasis. *J Clin Microbiol.* 2005;43:5491–7.

30. Schleupner CJ, Barritt AS III. Differentiation and occurrence of amebiasis in inflammatory bowel disease. In: Ravdin JI, ed. *Amebiasis: Human Infection by Entamoeba histolytica.* New York: Churchill Livingstone; 1988:582–93.

31. Katzenstein D, Rickerson V, Braude A. New concepts of amebic liver abscess derived from hepatic imaging, serodiagnosis, and hepatic enzymes in 67 consecutive cases in San Diego. *Medicine (Baltimore).* 1982;61:237–46.

32. The Medical Letter. Drugs for parasitic infections. *Treatment Guidelines from the Medical Letter.* Vol. 11. New York: The Medical Letter; 2013.

33. Bobak DA. Use of nitazoxanide for gastrointestinal tract infections: Treatment of protozoan parasitic infection and beyond. *Curr Infect Dis Rep.* 2006;8:91–5.

34. Wassmann C, Hellberg A, Tannich E, Bruchhaus I. Metronidazole resistance in the protozoan parasite *Entamoeba histolytica* is associated with increased expression of iron-containing superoxide dismutase and peroxiredoxin and decreased expression of ferredoxin 1 and flavin reductase. *J Biol Chem.* 1999;274:26051–6.

35. Thompson JEJr, Forlenza S, Verma R. Amebic liver abscess: A therapeutic approach. *Rev Infect Dis.* 1985;7:171–9.

36. Stringer RP, Cramer WN, et al. Comparison of bromine, chlorine, and iodine as disinfectants for amoebic cysts. In: Johnson JD, ed. *Disinfection: Water and Wastewater.* Ann Arbor, MI: Ann Arbor Science Publishers, Inc.; 1975:193–209.

CHAPTER 118

Amebic Meningoencephalitis*

Jennifer R. Cope • Ibne K. Ali

AMEBIC MENINGOENCEPHALITIS

Amebic meningoencephalitis is a rare clinical syndrome caused by acquisition of free-living amebae from the environment. *Naegleria fowleri* causes primary amebic meningoencephalitis (PAM) in otherwise healthy individuals; infection with *Acanthamoeba* spp. is manifest as a subacute granulomatous amebic encephalitis (GAE) in patients with serious underlying diseases. *Balamuthia mandrillaris* can also cause GAE in both healthy and immunocompromised patients (Table 118-1). Clinicians must be familiar with the epidemiology and clinical manifestations of amebic meningoencephalitis to avoid overlooking this infection in the differential diagnosis of patients at risk, despite its low incidence. Diagnosis ultimately rests on detecting amebae in cerebrospinal fluid (CSF), brain, or other affected tissue. Frequently the diagnosis is not made until postmortem examination. Unfortunately, mortality is high for these infections, even when the diagnosis is made premortem and treatment is initiated.

LIFE CYCLE AND EPIDEMIOLOGY

N. fowleri can exist in a trophozoite or a flagellate form. The organism grows best at higher temperatures (up to 46°C) and is acquired from fresh water when water containing amebae goes up the nose and enters the brain via the olfactory nerves.[1] Encystment occurs and allows prolonged survival of the ameba at low temperatures. PAM is a rare disease despite the frequent occurrence of warm fresh water exposure during swimming, diving, or other recreational water activities in which water goes up the nose. PAM cases have also occurred in patients who used undertreated tap water for nasal rinsing, for either therapeutic or religious purposes.[2,3] The disease occurs in all areas of the world. *Acanthamoeba* spp. and *Balamuthia mandrillaris* exist in only the trophozoite and cyst forms, grow best at normal ambient temperatures (25–35°C), and may be acquired via cuts in the skin or by inhalation into the lungs.[1] While *B. mandrillaris* causes disease in both healthy and immunocompromised patients, *Acanthamoeba* spp. primarily cause disease in patients with advanced HIV infection, hematologic malignancies, and history of bone marrow or solid organ transplant.

PATHOGENESIS AND HOST IMMUNE RESPONSE

N. fowleri enters the central nervous system by penetrating the nasal mucosa and cribriform plate via the olfactory nerves. Trophozoites can be found in nerves and perivascular spaces.[1] Amebic cell lytic activity has been demonstrated in vitro. Invasion of gray matter results in purulent meningitis. Trophozoites are susceptible to complement-mediated lysis, which is potentiated by agglutinating antibody to *N. fowleri.*

In GAE, granulomatous lesions can occur throughout the central nervous system, suggesting a hematogenous route of dissemination. Further evidence for this route of spread is the occurrence of skin lesions before spread to the nervous system and other organ systems. *Acanthamoeba* spp. and *B. mandrillaris* can be differentiated from *N. fowleri* by the presence of cysts in tissue. The opportunistic nature of *Acanthamoeba* spp. infection suggests that cell-mediated mechanisms are important in resistance to disease; however, GAE in immunologically competent hosts has been reported.

CLINICAL CHARACTERISTICS

PAM presents with symptoms typical of meningitis such as headache, fever, and meningismus.[4] A fulminant illness ensues with depressed mental status, focal neurologic signs, and seizures resulting from cerebral edema that ultimately ends with brain herniation and death within 5 days of onset.

GAE is a subacute disease that manifests over a period of weeks with focal neurologic signs, mental status changes, seizures, headache, and fever.[1] The occurrence of nodular or ulcerative skin lesions containing *Acanthamoeba* spp. can be helpful in establishing the diagnosis. *Balamuthia* infection can also present with a chronic skin lesion that precedes the development of encephalitis.[5] Most patients do not have meningismus, and the disease must be differentiated from other infectious and noninfectious causes of brain lesions.

DIAGNOSIS

PAM is characterized by a neutrophilic CSF pleocytosis; elevated protein levels in the CSF, and hypoglycorrhachia are not uncommon.[4] A Gram stain of CSF negative for bacteria in a young healthy person should suggest the need to examine the CSF for motile *N. fowleri* trophozoites, which are 10–30 μm in diameter. In contrast, in GAE, amebae are generally not found in the CSF, and brain biopsy or biopsy of other affected tissue is necessary for diagnosis. CT scans of the brain reveal nonspecific findings in PAM but may show ring-enhancing lesions in GAE. In GAE, the CSF undergoes nonspecific changes such as lymphocytic pleocytosis and alterations in protein and glucose levels.[1,5] A biopsy specimen should be obtained from any suspect skin lesion and examined for *Acanthamoeba* spp.

TREATMENT

No effective treatment for amebic meningoencephalitis has been established. Treatment recommendations for PAM are based on case

*Disclaimer:** The findings and conclusions in this chapter are those of the authors and do not necessarily represent the official position of the Centers for Disease Control and Prevention.

TABLE 118-1

	Disease	Other Organ Systems Affected	Patients Affected	Incubation Period	Onset to Death[a]	CSF Profile	Diagnostic Testing	Brain Imaging	Treatment
Naegleria fowleri	Primary Amebic Meningoencephalitis (PAM)	None clinically, histopathologic evidence of amebae in other organs	Healthy children and adults with recent freshwater exposure	Median 5 days (range 1–9 days)	Median 5 days (range 1–18 days)	Neutrophilic pleocytosis, elevated protein, low glucose	Visualization of motile trophozoites in CSF, PCR on CSF	Normal early in course, cerebral edema later	Amphotericin B (intrathecal and IV), rifampin, fluconazole, azithromycin, miltefosine
Balamuthia mandrillaris	Granulomatous Amebic Encephalitis (GAE)	SkinAlso histopathologic evidence of kidneys, liver, pancreas	Immunocompetent and immunocompromised; Hispanic ethnicity	Unknown (possibly weeks or months)	Median 24 days (range 4–450 days)	Lymphocytic pleocytosis, elevated protein, low or normal glucose	Immunohistochemical testing, PCR on biopsy specimen of affected tissue (brain, skin)	Enhancing, multifocal lesions with edema, anywhere in the brain	Pentamidine, sulfadiazine, fluconazole, flucytosine, azithromycin or clarithromycin, miltefosine
Acanthamoeba spp.	Granulomatous Amebic Encephalitis (GAE)	Skin, bone, sinuses, lung, eye	Immunocompromised	Unknown (possibly weeks or months)	Median 14 days (range 2–236 days)	Lymphocytic pleocytosis, elevated protein, low or normal glucose	Immunohistochemical testing, PCR on biopsy specimen of affected tissue (brain, skin, etc.)	Enhancing, multifocal lesions with edema, anywhere in the brain	Pentamidine, sulfadiazine, fluconazole, flucytosine, miltefosine

[a]Based on cases reported to U.S. Centers for Disease Control and Prevention.

reports of the few survivors. Recent U.S. survivors received IV and intrathecal amphotericin B, rifampin, fluconazole, azithromycin, miltefosine, and dexamethasone. They were also treated aggressively for elevated intracranial pressure with CSF drainage, hyperosmolar therapy, moderate hyperventilation, and therapeutic hypothermia.[6] Successful therapy for GAE also is undetermined. Treatment recommendations for both *Acanthamoeba* spp. and *B. mandrillaris* GAE are based on *in vitro* drug testing and case reports of survivors. *Acanthamoeba* spp. infection has been successfully treated with combinations of pentamidine, sulfadiazine, flucytosine, fluconazole, and miltefosine. *B. mandrillaris* infection has been successfully treated with similar combinations with the addition of azithromycin or clarithromycin.[7,8]

PREVENTION

The only certain way to prevent PAM is to avoid getting any water up the nose that might contain *N. fowleri* (e.g., when swimming in untreated fresh water, performing nasal rinsing). Personal actions that swimmers can take to limit the amount of water going up the nose include: holding the nose shut, using nose clips, or keeping the head above water when taking part in water-related activities in bodies of warm freshwater; and not putting the head under the water in hot springs and other untreated thermal waters. When using tap water for therapeutic or ritual nasal rinsing, the water should be boiled, distilled, or filtered prior to use. *N. fowleri* and *Acanthamoeba* spp. are susceptible to chemical disinfectants such as chlorine; therefore, swimming pools, hot tubs, and drinking water systems should be maintained properly and have adequate disinfectant levels at all times. As ubiquitous environmental organisms that only rarely cause infection, there are no proven prevention measures for *B. mandrillaris* and *Acanthamoeba* spp. infections. However, immunocompromised persons should generally take precautions with regard to water use.

References

1. Visvesvara GS, Moura H, Schuster FL. Pathogenic and opportunistic free-living amoebae: *Acanthamoeba* spp., *Balamuthia mandrillaris*, *Naegleria fowleri*, and *Sappinia diploidea*. *FEMS Immunol Med Microbiol.* 2007;50:1–26.
2. Yoder JS, Straif-Bourgeois S, Roy SL, et al. Deaths from *Naegleria fowleri* associated with sinus irrigation with tap water: A review of the changing epidemiology of primary amebic meningoencephalitis. *Clin Infect Dis.* 2012;55:e79–85.
3. Centers for Disease Control and Prevention. Primary amebic meningoencephalitis associated with ritual nasal rinsing—St. Thomas, U.S. Virgin Islands, 2012. *MMWR Morb Mortal Wkly Rep.* 2013;62:903.
4. Capewell LG, Harris AM, Yoder JS, et al. Diagnosis, clinical course, and treatment of primary amoebic meningoencephalitis in the United States, 1937–2013. *J Pediatric Infect Dis Soc.* 2015;4:e68–75.
5. Bravo FG, Alvarez PJ, Gotuzzo E. *Balamuthia mandrillaris* infection of the skin and central nervous system: An emerging disease of concern to many specialties in medicine. *Curr Opin Infect Dis.* 2011;24:112–7.
6. Linam WM, Ahmed M, Cope JR, et al. Successful treatment of an adolescent with *Naegleria fowleri* primary amebic meningoencephalitis. *Pediatrics.* 2015;135:e744–8.
7. Maritschnegg P, Sovinz P, Lackner H, et al. Granulomatous amebic encephalitis in a child with acute lymphoblastic leukemia successfully treated with multimodal antimicrobial therapy and hyperbaric oxygen. *J Clin Micro.* 2011;49:446–8.
8. Deetz TR, Sawyer MH, Billman G, et al. Successful treatment of *Balamuthia* amoebic encephalitis: Presentation of 2 cases. *Clin Infect Dis.* 2003;37:1304–12.

CHAPTER

119 Yersiniosis

Louise K. Francois Watkins • Cindy R. Friedman

Over the past 30 years, *Yersinia enterocolitica, Yersinia pseudotuberculosis,* and minor *Yersinia* species have been increasingly recognized as important pathogens. *Yersinia pestis,* the agent that causes plague, is discussed in Chapter 147: Plague.

EPIDEMIOLOGY

The reported incidence of yersiniosis varies geographically; in the United States, *Y. enterocolitica* accounts for approximately 92% of speciated infections,[1] whereas in other countries, such as Japan and Russia, *Y. pseudotuberculosis* is the most commonly reported *Yersinia* species. In parts of northern Europe, Japan, and Canada, *Yersinia* have been reported as a leading cause of bacterial gastroenteritis, in contrast to other countries in Africa, Asia, and South America where *Yersinia* are less often reported. Because of the complexity in culturing the organism, the incidence of Yersinia may be an underestimate, particularly in resource-limited settings. In the United States, *Yersinia* are less commonly reported than other bacterial pathogens such as *Campylobacter, Salmonella, Shigella,* or Shiga toxin-producing *Escherichia coli*, but their incidence is rising due, in part, to increased detection as a result of culture-independent diagnostic testing (CIDT).[2] Most cases occur in the cold months, and incidence of reported infections is highest in children.[1]

A wide variety of animals, including domestic dogs, cats, sheep, cattle, and pigs, have been found to be asymptomatically infected with *Y. enterocolitica*. Although *Yersinia* has been isolated from a variety of foods, most of these isolates are nonpathogenic. In northern Europe, pathogenic strains of *Yersinia* have been frequently found in the pharynx of pigs, and in raw pork and pork products. These foods have often been implicated as a source of human disease.[3,4] The ability of *Yersinia* species to grow at 4°C may contribute to the frequency with which raw or partly cooked refrigerated meats cause sporadic cases and outbreaks.[5] In the United States, illness in black infants has been associated with pork chitterlings (intestines) being prepared in the infant's home,[3] although in recent years there has been a decline in these infections, possibly as a result of reduced contamination, educational efforts, or both.[6] Outbreaks have been associated with ingestion of milk, tofu, produce, and other foods.[7–9] Cases have also been associated with ill pets including dogs.[10] Few cases have been associated with water, even though this organism has been found in rivers, lakes, and drinking water.[7,11] Secondary cases are rare, but nosocomial and intrafamilial transmission have been reported.[7]

Y. pseudotuberculosis is widespread in the environment, and is also found in many animal species, especially rodents and other small mammals, and can cause illness in deer and other ruminants.

CLINICAL CHARACTERISTICS

Most *Yersinia enterocolitica* infections present as gastroenteritis, characterized by a febrile illness with diarrhea with abdominal pain. The diarrhea can be bloody, especially in children less than 5 years old. *Y. pseudotuberculosis* and other minor *Yersinia* species (*frederiksenii, intermedia, kristensenii, ruckeri*) also cause gastroentertitis, but affect adults more often than *Y. enterocolitica.*[12] Yersiniosis may present as acute mesenteric lymphadenitis with leukocytosis, which can be clinically indistinguishable from acute appendicitis and may result in unnecessary laparotomies[13]; this presentation is more common among older children and adults.

The incubation period of *Yersinia* infections is typically 3–7 days, and usually under 10 days. Yersiniosis sometimes has a more gradual onset than other bacterial enteric infections, and may have a longer duration of symptoms (up to several weeks). Convalescent carriage of *Yersinia* is common and can be prolonged, but secondary spread is rare.

Whereas most Yersinia infections are self-limited, some patients, particularly adults, develop postinfectious complications of reactive polyarthritis, erythema nodosum, or autoimmune diseases.[14–16] Postinfectious symptoms usually occur within 2–20 days of the onset of fever and abdominal pain and resolve within 1 month, although there have been reports of persistent gastrointestinal and joint symptoms.[14,15] Less frequently reported manifestations of *Yersinia* infections are exudative pharyngitis, septicemia, and abscesses.[8,9,17–19] *Y. pseudotuberculosis* infection has been associated with Izumi fever, Kawasaki disease, and Far East scarlet-like fever; septicemia has been reported in immunocompromised patients.[20–24] *Y. enterocolitica* sepsis has been reported after blood transfusion from asymptomatic and mildly symptomatic donors.[25]

BACTERIOLOGY

Yersinia enterocolitica can be isolated using routine stool culture techniques; however, after 24 hours of incubation, the colonies are small and can be easily overgrown by other bacteria. The use of selective media like cefsulodin irgasan novobiocin with incubation at lower than usual temperatures increases the probability of isolating of *Yersinia* species (including nonpathogenic strains) and may be of particular use in persons with low numbers of organisms in their stool, such as in patients recovering from illness. Most laboratories in the United States culture for *Y. enterocolitica* only on request because it is not cost effective to use selective media routinely for this low-prevalence organism. *Yersinia* can be isolated from blood using standard blood culture media. However, yersinosis is increasingly diagnosed by CIDTs, which have become more widely available. In 2017, more than half of all *Yersinia* cases reported by U.S. FoodNet sites were detected by CIDTs.[26] Of note, CIDT panels typically target only *Y. enterocolitica*. Prospective studies to evaluate the specificity and sensitivity of CIDT platforms have not been published and may be difficult to conduct in settings where yersiniosis is uncommon. Culture is required to determine species and antibiotic susceptibility. Serologic tests (agglutination tests or enzyme-linked immunosorbent assays) may be useful for diagnosis, particularly for culture-negative cases, and are available through some reference laboratories.

More than 50 serotypes of *Y. enterocolitica* have been described; serotypes O3, O8, and O9 are most frequently associated with human illness. Type O8 caused most U.S. outbreaks through the 1980s; O3 emerged as a major cause of *Y. enterocolitica* cases in the 1990s.[27] Isolates from ill people in Europe are usually type O3 or O9. Approximately 80% of *Y. pseudotuberculosis* infections are caused by O-group I strains.

PREVENTION

The following steps can be taken to help prevent and control *Yersinia* infections: (a) cook all meat properly before consumption; (b) use pork promptly to minimize the time kept at refrigerator temperatures; (c) wash hands well after handling raw meat/intestines; (d) prevent cross-contamination of food preparation areas; (e) take steps to prevent contamination of pork meat with bacteria in the pharynx during the butchering of pigs; (f) take steps to minimize the possibility of milk being contaminated after pasteurization; and (g) defer prospective blood donors with recent history of gastroenteritis, modify, blood handling practices, or both.[26] Guidance for the prevention of yersiniosis can be found at https://www.cdc.gov/yersinia/prevention.html.

References

1. Long C, Jones TF, Vugia DJ, et al. *Yersinia pseudotuberculosis* and *Y. enterocolitica* infections, FoodNet, 1996–2007. *Emerg Infect Dis.* 2010;16(3):566–7.
2. Marder EP, Griffin PM, Cieslak MD, et al. Preliminary incidence and trends of infections with pathogens transmitted commonly through food—Foodborne Diseases Active Surveillance Network, 10 U.S. sites, 2006–2017. *MMWR Morb Mortal Wkly Rep.* 2017;66(15):397–403.
3. Tauxe RV, Vandepitte J, Wauters G, et al. *Yersinia enterocolitica* infections and pork: The missing link. *Lancet.* 1987;1:1129–32.
4. Lee LA, Gerber AR, Lonsway DR, et al. *Yersinia enterocolitica* O:3 infections in infants and children, associated with the household preparation of chitterlings. *N Engl J Med.* 1990;322:984–7.
5. Ostroff SM, Kapperud G, Hutwagner LC, et al. Sources of sporadic *Yersinia enterocolitica* infections in Norway: A prospective case-control study. *Epidemiol Infect.* 1994;112:133–41.
6. Ong KL, Gould LH, Chen DL, et al. Changing epidemiology of *Yersinia enterocolitica* infections: Markedly decreased rates in young black children, Foodborne Diseases Active Surveillance Network (FoodNet), 1996–2009. *Clin Infect Dis.* 2012;54(Suppl 5):S385–90.
7. Rahman A, Bonny TS, Stonsaovapak S, Ananchaipattana C. *Yersinia enterocolitica*: Epidemiological studies and outbreaks. *J Pathog.* 2011;2011:239391.
8. Tacket CO, Narain JP, Sattin R, et al. A multistate outbreak of infections caused by *Yersinia enterocolitica* transmitted by pasteurized milk. *JAMA.* 1984;251(4):483–6.
9. Tacket CO, Ballard J, Harris N, et al. An outbreak of *Yersinia enterocolitica* infections caused by contaminated tofu (soybean curd). *Am J Epidemiol.* 1985;121(5):705–11.
10. Hetem DJ, Pekelharing M, Thijsen SFT. Probable transmission of *Yersinia enterocolitica* from a pet dog with diarrhea to a 1-year-old infant. *BMJ Case Rep.* 2013;2013:bcr2013200046.
11. Eden KV, Rosenberg ML, Stoopler M, et al. Waterborne gastrointestinal illness at a ski resort—Isolation of *Yersinia enterocolitica* from drinking water. *Public Health Rep.* 1977;92(3):245–250.
12. Loftus CG, Harewood GC, Cockerill FR, et al. Clinical features of patients with novel *Yersinia* species. *Dig Dis Sci.* 2002;47(12):2805–10.
13. Jones MW, Deppen JG. Pseudoappendicitis. *StatPearls [Internet].* Treasure Island, FL: StatPearls Publishing; 2018.
14. Saebo A, Lassen J. Acute and chronic gastrointestinal manifestations associated with *Yersinia* enterocolitica infection. *Ann Surg.* 1992;215:250–5.
15. Yli-Kerttula T, Tertti R, Toivanen A. Ten-year follow-up study of patients from a *Yersinia pseudotuberculosis* III outbreak. *Clin Exp Rheumatol.* 1995;13:333–7.
16. Toivanen P, Toivanen A. Does *Yersinia* induce autoimmunity? *Int Arch Allergy Immunol.* 1994;104(2):107–11.
17. Sauter M, Vavricka SR, Locher P, et al. Multilocular hepatic abscess formation and sepsis due to *Yersinia enterocolitica* in a patient with hereditary hemochromatosis and type 2 diabetes mellitus. *Case Rep Gastroenterol.* 2017;11:724–8.
18. Jensen KT, Arpi M, Frederiksen W. Contributions to microbiology and immunology: *Yersinia enterocolitica* septicemia in Denmark 1972–1991: A report of 100 cases. *Contrib Microbiol Immunol.* 1995;13:11.
19. Grigull L, Linderkamp C, Sander A, et al. Multiple spleen and liver abscesses due to *Yersinia enterocolitica* septicemia in a child with congenital sideroblastic anemia. *J Pediatr Hematol Oncol.* 2005;27(11):624–6.
20. Amphlett A. Far East scarlet-like fever: A review of the epidemiology, symptomatology, and role of superantigenic toxin: *Yersinia pseudotuberculosis*-derived mitogen A. *Open Forum Infect Dis.* 2015:3(1):ofv202.
21. Deacon AG, Hay A, Duncan J. Microbiology Laboratories and Department of General Surgery, Raigmore Hospital, Inverness, UK. Septicemia due to *Yersinia pseudotuberculosis*—A case report. *Clin Microbiol Infect.* 2003;9:1118–9.
22. Antinori A, Paglia MG, Marconi P, et al. *Yersinia pseudotuberculosis* septicemia in an HIV-infected patient failed HAART. In: *AIDS Research and Human Retroviruses.* Vol. 2, No. 7. New Rochelle, New York: Mary Ann Liebert, Inc.; 2004:709–10.
23. Roussos A, Stambori M, Aggelis P, et al. Department of Internal Medicine and Microbiology, General Hospital Sotiria Hematological Center, Areteion Hospital, Athens, Greece. Transfusion-mediated *Yersinia entercolitica* septicemia in an adult patient with betathalassemia. *Scand J Infect Dis.* 2001;33:859–60.
24. van Zonneveld M, Droogh JM, Fieren MWJA, et al. University Hospital Rotterdam, Netherlands. *Yersinia pseudotuberculosis* bacteraemia in a kidney transplant patient. *Nephrol Dial Transplant.* 2002;17:2252–4.
25. Centers for Disease Control. Update: *Yersinia enterocolitica* bacteremia and endotoxin shock associated with red blood cell transfusions—United States, 1991. *MMWR Morb Mortal Wkly Rep.* 1991;40:176–8.
26. Lee LA, Taylor J, Carter GP, et al. *Yersinia enterocolitica* O:3: An emerging cause of pediatric gastroenteritis in the United States. *J Infect Dis.* 1991;163:660–3.
27. Butler T. *Yersinia infections*: Centennial of the discovery of the plague bacillus. *Clin Infect Dis.* 1994;19:655–63.

CHAPTER 120

Syphilis*

Gail Bolan

INTRODUCTION

Syphilis is a systemic sexually transmitted infection (STI) characterized by infectious stages and periods of latency. This ancient disease, known as the Great Pox and the "great imitator," has captivated clinicians, scientists, poets, and authors for millennia.[1] Though documented by clinicians and artists for centuries, the origins of syphilis, while debated, remain a mystery. Prior to the technological advances of the late 1800s and discovery of the causative organism for gonorrhea in 1879, most doctors assumed the clinical presentations of syphilis and gonorrhea represented a single disease entity.[2] It was not until 1905 that scientists identified the causative organism for syphilis, the spirochete bacterium, *Treponema pallidum subspecies pallidum*.[3] Left untreated, syphilis infection can be lifelong. Additionally, clinical management of syphilis is complex due to the various stages and limitations of the diagnostic tests. While typically associated with disease in adults, syphilis at any stage can be vertically transmitted and is one of the oldest recognized congenital infections, first described in the fifteenth century.[4] Public health providers need to understand the pathogenesis, natural history, and clinical manifestations of syphilis in order to design effective syphilis prevention and control programs.

PATHOGENESIS AND IMMUNOLOGY

As an obligate human parasite, there are no animal or environmental reservoirs for *T. pallidum subspecies pallidum*. Therefore, humans are the only natural host for syphilis. It is believed that during sexual contact, the bacteria in infectious lesions penetrate the skin or mucosal surfaces of a sexual partner through macro- or microscopic abrasions[5,6] Of note, the other pathogenic treponemes of humans [i.e., the causative agents of yaws, endemic syphilis (bejel), and pinta] share a common mode of transmission (direct skin-to-skin contact with an infectious lesion), albeit usually during infancy or childhood and not by sexual skin to skin or mucosal contact.[7] They also share similar clinical appearances and immune responses. Within hours to days after inoculation, *T. pallidum* spreads throughout the body via the lymphatics and blood stream, involving most organ systems, including the central nervous system (CNS).[8]

It is thought that replication of this slow growing organism (generation time ~ 30–33 hours)[9] at the site of inoculation leads to the development of the lesions at the primary stage of syphilis within weeks of infection. Replication after widespread dissemination leads to the signs and symptoms of secondary syphilis within months and years later, tertiary syphilis. The most infectious syphilitic lesions are the ulcerative lesions of the primary stage and the mucous membrane lesions of the secondary stage, such as condyloma lata and mucous patches. The highest concentration of spirochetes with the characteristic morphology and motility of *T. pallidum* seen on darkfield examination[10] is from fluid obtained from condyloma lata lesions. This has led to the assumption that condyloma lata lesions are the most infectious lesions of syphilis, followed by the primary-stage chancre.

Over the course of untreated syphilis, immunity to relapses of the secondary signs and symptoms is thought to be present after 4 years. In a small study of five individuals with untreated late latent syphilis who were challenged with an infectious strain of *T. pallidum*, none developed symptomatic reinfection or an increase in nontreponemal antibody titers.[11] These data have led to the belief that untreated individuals may be resistant to reinfection. Infectious challenge studies in treated individuals, though small in number, suggest that immunity to syphilis is slow to develop, incomplete at best, and may be strain specific.[11] In addition, new cases of primary and secondary syphilis infections among men with a history of adequate syphilis treatment and ongoing risk for syphilis acquisition have been well documented.[12–14] Therefore, it is assumed that after treatment for syphilis an individual is again susceptible and can be re infected. However, it has also been postulated that the duration of infection and immunologic response before treatment may influence the clinical manifestations of a reinfection, such as if symptomatic (i.e., infectious) lesions are present in a second infection. For example, if the duration of infection prior to treatment is longer than a year, it is thought that reinfection is more likely to be an asymptomatic infection without lesions; if someone is treated for primary or secondary syphilis initially, then they would be more likely to have lesions of primary or secondary syphilis if they are reinfected. This hypothesis has led to modeling studies that have suggested the periodicity of syphilis epidemics could be dependent not only on the number of susceptible individuals in a previously uninfected population but also on the number of susceptible individuals with previously treated syphilis.[15] Although as discussed, some who were previously treated may be less likely to have symptomatic second infections as a result of a longer duration of infection before treatment, and development of some immunity. These immunologic considerations have important implications for syphilis prevention and control strategies, including mitigation of factors associated with syphilis acquisition.

T. pallidum has a mysterious ability to evade the innate host immune system and establish a chronic latent infection that can persist for years. This ability is possibly due to the relative lack of surface-exposed proteins, as the outer membrane of *T pallidum* has few membrane proteins and lacks lipopolysaccharide.[16–18] However, the

*The findings and conclusions in this chapter are those of the author and do not necessarily represent the official position of the Centers for Disease Control and Prevention.

host's immune system, especially cell-mediated immunity, still plays an important role in the pathogenesis and natural history of syphilis.[19] The immune system contributes to individual variation in the clinical features and the waxing and waning course of syphilitic infection. In animal models, T-cell infiltration occurs at the site of inoculation within 3 days, and the magnitude of infiltration correlates with the concentration of *T pallidum*.[20,21] Macrophage infiltration follows, and within days the number of treponemes at the site declines, leading to lesion resolution—presumably due to phagocytosis of the treponemes by the macrophages.[22] Selective impairment of cell-mediated immunity in these animal models can alter the clinical presentation of syphilis by shortening the incubation period, increasing the number and size of infectious lesions, and prolonging the healing time of these lesions as well as influencing other clinical manifestations.[23] As for humoral immunity, antibodies that optimize, neutralize, or immobilize *T. pallidum* have been identified, but their function in the infected host is unclear. The functional role of the antibodies detected by serologic tests for syphilis is also unknown. Although it is known that sensitized T-cells and antibodies persist years after infection and after penicillin treatment, a treated infection does not seem to produce long-lasting immunity that will prevent reinfection. Thus, the purpose of this immunologic memory response after treatment is also unknown. Evidence of macrophage-mediated bacterial clearance, the treponemicidal activity of complement-dependent antibodies, and seroreversion of nontreponemal tests to negative over time in untreated patients have led some to hypothesize that the host response can completely cure some individuals. Without better diagnostic tests to directly detect syphilitic infection during latency, however, it remains unclear whether spontaneous cures occur. Therefore, it should be assumed that all patients with untreated latent *T. pallidum* infection have chronic infection and should be treated.

Case reports of atypical clinical manifestations and of neurologic and ocular symptoms of syphilis in patients living with HIV, both suggest it is plausible that impairment of cell-mediated and humoral immunity by HIV infection could limit the host defenses against *T. pallidum*.[24–28] HIV-related meningeal inflammation may also contribute to the development of neurosyphilis by facilitating CNS invasion by *T. pallidum*. In addition, the presence of both activated T lymphocytes and macrophages at the site of primary-stage lesions may explain the role of syphilis in facilitating HIV acquisition and transmission; treponemal lipoproteins stimulate macrophages, which in turn upregulate gene expression of the HIV-1 gene and the CCR-5 co-receptor used in HIV entry of blood mononuclear cells.[29]

NATURAL HISTORY

Observations from the Oslo Study conducted from 1890 to 1910 with follow-up of over 80% of the 1978 participants from 1948 to 1951 have provided insights into the natural history of untreated syphilis.[30] The rationale for the study was to address concerns that the syphilis treatment with mercurials used at that time was more toxic than the syphilis infection itself. Patients with clinical evidence of primary or secondary syphilis were enrolled and followed, as syphilis diagnostic tests were not available. The Oslo Study quantified the clinical manifestations of syphilis over the course of untreated syphilis including the frequency of tertiary syphilis morbidity and mortality by age and gender. Gumma was identified in approximately 15% of patients mainly involving the skin and was the most frequently recognized tertiary manifestation—possibly because it is easier to diagnose than the other forms of tertiary syphilis. Both cardiovascular syphilis and neurosyphilis were more common among men than women (approximately 14% vs. 8% for cardiovascular syphilis and 9.5% vs. 5% for neurosyphilis). Although less common than gummas and cardiovascular syphilis, neurosyphilis was observed to occur at younger ages and had more significant morbidity and mortality. Overall, mortality rates from late syphilis complications were higher among men.

The Oslo Study demonstrated that most individuals with untreated syphilis lived a lifetime without any discernible adverse health outcomes of syphilis and only 28% of participants followed developed tertiary syphilis. The study also provided a better understanding of the frequency and timing of secondary syphilis relapse; approximately 25% of untreated patients had one recurrence of secondary signs or symptoms. Of those with one recurrence, approximately 25% had additional recurrences. Relapse typically occurred within the first year of infection in 90% of patients although 4% of relapses occurred one to 2 years after infection and in very rare circumstances, relapse occurred 4 years later.

In 1932, the U.S. Public Health Service conducted another syphilis natural history study in Macon County, Alabama, home of the Tuskegee Institute; originally called "the U.S Public Health Service Syphilis Study," famously known as "the Tuskegee Study" and now referred to as "the U.S. Syphilis Study." The treatment for syphilis at this time was an arsenic-based drug- arsphenamine, also known as Salvarsan or compound 606, discovered by Dr. Paul Ehrlich as the first chemotherapeutic agent ever developed which he referred to as the "magic bullet." Similar to the Oslo Study, the U.S. Syphilis Study rationale was to address concerns that this syphilis treatment was more toxic than the syphilis infection itself. There were also concerns that the Oslo study lacked a control group, underestimated the frequency of tertiary syphilis as very few autopsies were done, and that the natural history of syphilis could differ by gender and race. Enrolled in the study were 412 African American men considered noninfectious with latent syphilis as defined by a positive serologic test; some had been treated with arsphenamine for the lesions of early syphilis. Two hundred and four matched, seronegative African American men were enrolled as the control group. After an initial physical examination, lumbar puncture, and chest x-ray, all were followed from 1932 to 1972, despite the availability of effective penicillin treatment in the 1940s.[31] By the 1950s, only 10% of the enrolled men were lost to follow-up and the autopsy rate among the men who died was approximately 66%—an exceptionally high follow-up and autopsy rate by most scientific study standards.[31,32] While no final summary of the study was ever published, interim reports suggested that mortality rates were higher among individuals living with syphilis compared to controls—typically occurring in the first 20 years of follow-up—, although not all deaths could be specifically attributed to clinical manifestations of late syphilis.[31–33] By the 1960s roughly 14% of the men living with syphilis had evidence of tertiary syphilis—cardiovascular syphilis was the most common finding.[34]

These findings were published in reputable journals with the opportunity for other scientists and the public to critically review the details of the study. However, it was not until 1972 that the ethical injustices of the study were captured by the media when a public health disease investigator shared the study with an Associated Press reporter. This revelation led to a federal investigation, Senate hearings, a lawsuit, and new federal regulations about informed consent that contributed to the creation of the Belmont report and ethics training requirements for all scientists who conduct human subjects research.

The United States Public Health Service and the United States government were severely criticized on several counts for their involvement in this immoral experiment, including government malfeasance, arrogance, racism, and ethical injustices.[35–38] No informed consent was obtained, and only African American men were recruited for the study. Effective treatment with penicillin was knowingly withheld by the researchers so the study could continue to achieve the originally designed objectives. In addition, participants were led to believe they were being treated for syphilis with medications provided—in actuality, the medications given were aspirin and iron tonics. This exposure of unethical government research only perpetuated the mistrust that already existed in some racial and ethnic communities about governmental research and government run healthcare programs. In 1997, President Clinton offered an apology to the remaining survivors of the study. In addition, a National Bioethics Center at Tuskegee University was established in 1999 to teach future generations of researchers about the lessons learned from the U.S. Syphilis Study and to inform medical research going forward through an ethical lens to avoid future human subject tragedies.

A third natural history of syphilis was conducted from 1917 to 1941. Unlike the Oslo and U.S. Syphilis cohort studies, this study was a cross-sectional review of all autopsies done at Yale University School of Medicine during this period.[39] The population was 90% white and of lower socioeconomic status. Of the 4000 autopsies reviewed, 9.7% had evidence of syphilis by available clinical, lab, and postmortem data. The results were very similar to the Oslo and U.S. Syphilis Study findings despite the smaller sample size. Life expectancy was lower in those with evidence of syphilis. Sixty percent of those with syphilis had no evidence of tertiary syphilis and 80% died of causes unrelated to syphilis. Of the 40% with evidence of tertiary syphilis, 83% had evidence of cardiovascular syphilis, 8.5% had gummas and 7.6% had finding of neurosyphilis. In addition, approximately 25% of patients with evidence of tertiary syphilis on autopsy had a negative serum Venereal Disease Research Laboratory test (VDRL), confirming the decline in sensitivity of nontreponemal serologic tests in late syphilis.

CLINICAL MANAGEMENT

Syphilis in Adults

In addition to primary prevention, rapid detection (through screening programs for asymptomatic populations and correct diagnosis in patients presenting with the nonspecific signs and symptoms of primary and secondary syphilis) and timely treatment (especially of the infectious stages of syphilis) are the two other most highly effective syphilis prevention and control strategies. Thus, the healthcare system is vital to syphilis prevention and control.[40] With the decline of the public health infrastructure that includes reductions in hours or closures of STI specialty clinics since the mid-2000s[41] and the expansion of the HIV care system in the 2000s and primary healthcare system and health insurance in the late 2000s,[42,43] most individuals with syphilis are now seen in the HIV or primary healthcare system. However, because syphilis is no longer on the radar of many providers, these syphilis prevention and control strategies are currently being underutilized; patients with signs of infectious syphilis are being misdiagnosed and screening recommendations are not being followed—all contributing to further transmission in the community as patients are not receiving timely treatment. Provider knowledge of the clinical manifestations of and how to diagnose, treat, and manage patients with syphilis and their sexual partners is essential to syphilis prevention and control in the twenty-first century.[44,45]

Clinical Manifestations

Primary Syphilis

If left untreated, syphilitic infection progresses through four stages—primary syphilis, secondary syphilis, latent syphilis, and tertiary syphilis.[46–48] These stages are diagnosed based on clinical findings and used to help guide treatment and clinical and public health follow-up.[49] Although case reports have suggested that coexisting HIV infection may alter the clinical course of syphilis, large observational studies indicate that the conventional staging and treatment of syphilis does not need to be modified for those living with HIV infection.[49–51] Conventional staging of syphilis also does not need to be altered in pregnant females.

The primary stage of syphilis presents initially as one or more papules, most commonly at the site of inoculation, about 3 weeks after exposure (range of 10–90 days) depending on the inoculum size and host factors. The papule(s) quickly erode(s) into an ulcerative lesion(s). The classic primary syphilis lesion, known as a chancre, is typically a single, painless, and clean-based ulcer with a firm indurated border (Fig. 120-1A).[52] However, lesions of primary syphilis can be atypical, especially in individuals living with HIV and not virally suppressed. Chancres can be multiple and painful,[24,53] leading to incorrect diagnosis and delays in treating these highly infectious lesions and furthering the spread of syphilis in the community (Fig. 120-1B).[52] Primary lesions are not confined to the genital region and can occur at any site of sexual exposure, including the rectum and oropharyngeal cavity. Regional, nontender, shotty lymphadenopathy may also be present at the primary stage, but constitutional symptoms generally are absent. Many patients are unaware of lesions in the vagina and rectum and are not diagnosed until they progress to the secondary stage of syphilis. Primary lesions will heal within a few weeks, even without treatment, as the host response plays a very important role in the natural history of syphilis; most primary lesions resolve before the signs and symptoms of secondary syphilis develop, but in about 20% of patients, the primary and secondary stages can overlap.

The clinical characteristics of primary syphilis are rarely specific enough to lead to the correct diagnosis in a patient who presents with genital lesions, with one exception: lesions caused by herpes simplex virus start as a vesicle or vesicles and can be accompanied by constitutional symptoms. Until proven otherwise, syphilis should be in the differential diagnosis of any genital, anal, or oral lesion if there has been sexual exposure at these sites. In contrast to the early 1900s when syphilis was a common disease with an estimated prevalence in the general population of 10%, most clinicians in recent decades are no longer well trained in the clinical diagnosis of syphilis and have not had the opportunity to observe any symptomatic cases. Consequently, cases of primary syphilis have been misdiagnosed as other STIs such as herpes, scabies, chancroid, or other dermatologic conditions (i.e., fixed drug eruptions, fungal infections, trauma, psoriasis, and lichen planus). The resultant delays in diagnosis compromise timely treatment and other prevention and control efforts. Diagnosis of primary syphilis is further complicated by the fact that tests to detect *T. pallidum* directly in lesion exudates are not widely available and serologic tests are insensitive at the primary stage. For these reasons, patients from communities with a high burden of syphilis infections (e.g., gay, bisexual, and other men who have sex with men, MSM) and who present with genital lesions or lesions at other sites of sexual activity should be empirically treated for primary syphilis at the time of the clinic visit, before any test results are available.

Secondary Syphilis

The secondary stage of syphilis occurs weeks to a few months after exposure with presentation on average, approximately 6 weeks later to as long as 6 months. Secondary syphilis represents the systemic stage of the disease that results from the slow proliferation of *T. pallidum* throughout the body. This follows the hematogenous dissemination that occurs within hours of inoculation. It is believed based on animal studies and limited human data that the highest level of treponemes in the blood is identified at this secondary stage. In untreated humans, the duration of bacteremia and at what concentration and periodicity is unknown. The most common clinical manifestations of secondary syphilis involve the skin or mucous membranes—an organ system of lower temperature in which *T. pallidum* may preferentially replicate. The mucocutaneous lesions can be generalized or localized and mild or florid (Fig. 120-1C, D).[52] They can include a wide variety of rashes, typically bilaterally symmetrical and ranging from macular, papular, pustular, follicular, papulosquamous to annular, and may include the palms of the hands and soles of the feet (Fig. 120-1E, F).[52] It is believed that the initial rash is evanescent and macular and often unnoticed by a patient; it may be initially present on the palms and soles and missed by a clinician if a complete dermatologic exam is not performed. Cutaneous lesions are usually dry, rarely pruritic and not

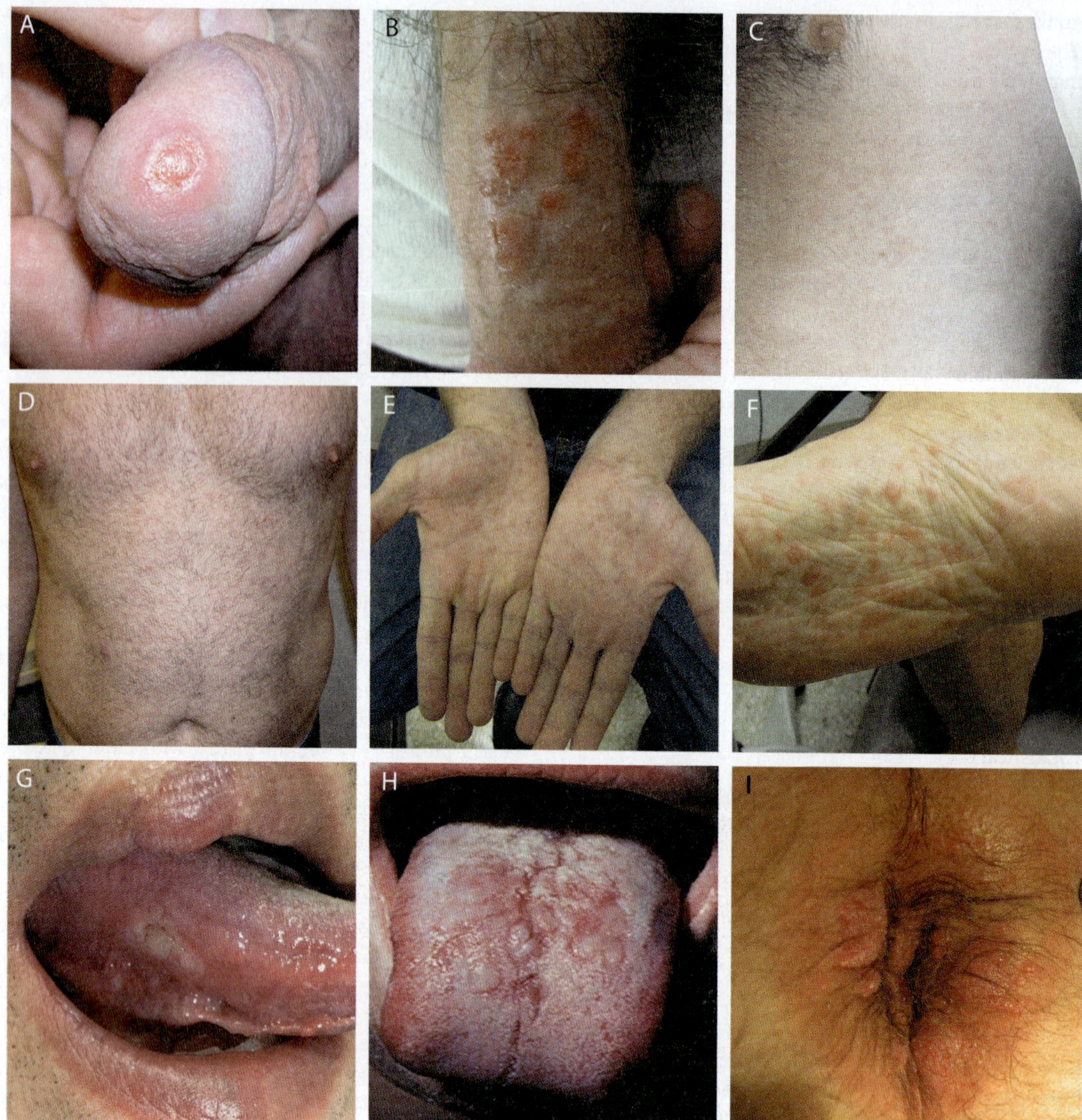

FIGURE 120-1. Primary and secondary syphilis symptoms. A: Primary syphilis, typical, indurated primary lesion. B: Primary syphilis, atypical primary lesions. C: Secondary syphilis, subtle macular torso rash. D: Secondary syphilis, macular torso rash. E: Secondary syphilis, palmar rash. F: Secondary syphilis, plantar rash. G: Secondary syphilis, mucous patch. H: Secondary syphilis, mucous patches. I: Secondary syphilis, condyloma lata. (Figure 120-01A-G and I) Source: Centers for Disease Control and Prevention. Figure 120-01H: Elsevier.

vesicular or bullous in the adult, as they can be in the neonate with congenital syphilis. The rash of secondary syphilis can mimic many dermatologic conditions and has been incorrectly managed as tinea versicolor, pityriasis rosea, scabies, fixed drug eruption, erythema multiforme, psoriasis, nummular eczema, viral exanthem, folliculitis, acute HIV infection, and mononucleosis.

Other clinical findings at this stage include constitutional symptoms such as low-grade fever, malaise, sore throat, headache, myalgias, arthralgias, and generalized lymphadenopathy. Less-common symptoms and signs that occur in approximately 25% of patients with secondary syphilis are mucosal lesions most commonly in the oropharynx (Fig. 120-1G, H),[52] known as mucous patches (small superficial ulcerated areas with grayish borders that can resemble painless aphthous ulcers or large gray plaques); condyloma lata (Fig. 120-1I),[52] (moist wart-like papules that mostly occur in the genital and perianal area but have been reported in the mouth or moist intertriginous body surfaces); and alopecia, which is typically patchy (i.e., "moth eaten") from treponemal infection of hair follicles. One to two percent of patients with secondary syphilis also present with symptomatic ocular syphilis or neurosyphilis, so careful neurologic and ocular exams are an essential part of a clinical evaluation in any suspected case of secondary syphilis. Infection of other organ systems is most often asymptomatic, but rare cases of nephrotic syndrome, hepatitis, gastritis, arthritis, and pneumonia have been reported.

Direct detection of treponemes in specimens from moist secondary lesions, such as condyloma lata, is possible, but the most sensitive diagnostic tests at the secondary stage are the serologic tests; nontreponemal and treponemal tests are positive at this stage of syphilis except in rare case reports. A resolving primary lesion at the time of development of signs and symptoms suggestive of secondary syphilis also aids in the diagnosis of the secondary stage of syphilis. To minimize misdiagnosis and treatment delays due to the nonspecific clinical presentation of secondary syphilis and for clinicians not having syphilis in their differential diagnosis, it is recommended that all sexually active adults presenting with any type of skin eruption or wart-like lesions be tested for syphilis. In adults with mononucleosis symptoms, a test for syphilis is also indicated; if these individuals are not known to be living with HIV, they should also be tested for HIV to rule out acute HIV coinfection. Like primary lesions, secondary signs and symptoms will also resolve within a few weeks to months without treatment. This resolution marks the beginning of the latent stage in most patients.

Latent Syphilis

In latent syphilis, serologic evidence of infection is found despite the absence of clinical manifestations, and infection can last a lifetime without progression to tertiary disease.[30] In the preantibiotic era, approximately one third of untreated patients developed tertiary syphilis. In the postantibiotic era, those in the latent stages rarely have further clinical problems; tertiary syphilis is rarely diagnosed and is often only an incidental finding on autopsy. It is speculated that the frequent use of antibiotics that have activity against *T. pallidum* (e.g., cephalosporins, penicillins, and macrolides) for respiratory and other infectious diseases over the lifetime is preventing tertiary disease in individuals with untreated latent infection. Sexual transmission does not occur during latency, but a pregnant woman with latent syphilis can infect her fetus, presumably due to treponemes that intermittently seed the bloodstream during the latent stage.

The latent stage of syphilis has been arbitrarily divided into early latent and late latent syphilis based on the time periods of potential infectiousness during sexual activity. In 1955, in the manual of the International Statistical Classification of Disease, Injuries and Causes of Death, the World Health Organization (WHO) conservatively defined the early latent stage as a duration of infection less than 4 years as potentially infectious syphilis, and late latent syphilis as a duration of 4 years or more as noninfectious syphilis, except in pregnant women.[54] More recently, WHO has refined the definition of the latent period of potential infectious syphilis to under 2 years for early latent and 2 years or more for late latent, noninfectious syphilis. In contrast, in the 1960s the United States Public Health Service defined potentially infectious early latent syphilis as within 1 year of infection because (1) most infectious relapse lesions occur within the first year of infection[30] and (2) epidemiologic follow-up of sexual contacts exposed beyond the first year of the infected index case identified few, if any, infectious cases, making it difficult to justify the cost of investigation of these more remote sexual contacts.

These two categories of latent syphilis have also been used to guide the duration of recommended treatment (i.e., benzathine penicillin G, 2.4 million units, IM once for syphilis of less than 1-year duration and benzathine penicillin G, 2.4 million units, IM weekly for 3 weeks for syphilis of 1-year or greater duration), despite the fact no randomized treatment trials have never been conducted to establish the duration of benzathine penicillin G treatment by stage of syphilis.

The duration of latency is also difficult to establish because current serologic tests cannot be used to measure the duration of infection; detection of IgM antibody has not been predictive of latent syphilis of less than 1-year duration. Thus, in the United States, clinical criteria are currently used by the Centers for Disease Control and Prevention (CDC) to assess evidence of infection acquired in the past 12 months and classify the stage as early latent. These clinical criteria for the diagnosis of early latent syphilis include persons who have positive syphilis nontreponemal and treponemal serologic tests; no evidence of primary or secondary syphilis after a careful physical examination, including examination of all mucocutaneous surfaces; and one of the following in the past 12 months: (1) a documented negative nontreponemal serologic test, (2) an unequivocal patient history of primary or secondary signs or symptoms, (3) a known sexual partner with early syphilis (i.e., primary, secondary, or early latent syphilis), (4) an unequivocal sexual history with the only possible sexual encounter, and (5) at least a fourfold sustained increase (greater than 2 weeks) in the nontreponemal titer in a previously treated individual.[49] However, regarding the last criterion, increasing nontreponemal titers may not unequivocally reflect a new case of early latent syphilis. Fourfold increases may be the result of fluctuation in titers due to other conditions or to a possible treatment failure. Furthermore, it is not uncommon at the time of the clinical assessment for no previous tests to have been done and for patients to be unaware of previous signs or symptoms or whether a sexual contact was diagnosed with early syphilis. In these cases, it is impossible to stage the duration of latency, especially if the risk factors were present throughout the past year; such cases should be considered latent of unknown duration. These patients should be conservatively treated for late latent infection, in case the infection was acquired more than a year previously, but could be conservatively investigated by public health as a case of early infectious syphilis with follow-up and postexposure preventive treatment of sexual partners, depending on a number of factors, such as the local syphilis epidemiology, a higher titer level (e.g., >1:8) or a Jarish-Herxheimer reaction after treatment. These public health investigation criteria should not be used for clinical staging and treatment.

It is important to note that clinical staging criteria, surveillance case definitions, and factors used to guide public health investigations do not need to be the same because each has different goals. Clinical criteria are created to ensure adequate treatment of infected patients. Surveillance case definitions are standardized with optimal sensitivity and specificity to monitor disease burden and trends in populations. Public health investigations are designed to prevent further disease transmission in a community. Surveillance case definitions are summarized in the Surveillance section, and factors guiding public health investigations are outlined in the Prevention and Control section under Partner Services.

Tertiary Syphilis

The tertiary stage of syphilis occurs decades after the primary and secondary stages, possibly due to waning host immunity and organ system damage from persisting invasive treponemes causing inflammation believed to be provoked by treponemal lipoproteins and a host delayed-hypersensitivity reaction to treponemal antigens. The late clinical manifestations of tertiary syphilis include cardiovascular features most commonly involving the walls of the aorta causing aortitis, leading to aortic aneurysms, aortic insufficiency, and/or aortic endocarditis. Cardiovascular tertiary syphilis typically occurs 30–40 years after infection and in the Oslo study, was more commonly found on autopsy than the other types of tertiary syphilis syndromes.[30] Other clinical manifestations of tertiary syphilis include late neurosyphilis, which causes general paresis with destruction of the brain parenchyma and tabes dorsalis with destruction of the dorsal roots of the spinal column. In the Oslo study, late neurosyphilis was the least common of the tertiary syphilis syndromes.[30] The time period of onset differed by type of late neurosyphilis, with general paresis occurring about 20–25 years after infection and tabes dorsalis after about 30 years. The formation of gummas, indolent but potentially destructive granulomatous lesions, can cause clinical manifestations in any organ system but most commonly involve the skin, bones, and liver. Gummas may be single or multiple lesions, ranging in size from macroscopic to large tumor-like masses, and most commonly occur in a single organ system with rare reoccurrences after resolution in the same or different organ system—like relapsing signs and symptoms of secondary syphilis in untreated patients. This type of tertiary syphilis usually occurs within the first 15 years of infection,[30] but cases have been diagnosed as early as 1 year and as late as 45 years after infection. Last, optic atrophy can also occur as a tertiary manifestation.

Neurosyphilis

Neurosyphilis, ocular syphilis, and otologic syphilis occur at sites of infection where treponemal invasion occurs early in the course of this infection, and signs and symptoms can occur at any stage of syphilis, albeit rarely at the primary stage.[55–57] Evidence for early infection of the CNS without neurologic signs or symptoms comes from clinical studies conducted in the first half of the twentieth century that examined the cerebrospinal fluid (CSF) of untreated patients with primary or secondary syphilis without neurologic symptoms. These studies identified CSF abnormalities in 13% of primary syphilis cases and 25–40% of secondary syphilis cases.[57–59] The CSF laboratory parameters examined included CSF white cell count, protein and/or glucose levels, and VDRL antibody titer. More recently, research studies with recovery of *T. pallidum* after animal inoculation with CSF or a positive experimental syphilis nucleic acid amplification test as other parameters of CNS infections, yielded similar results.[8,60,61] In these studies, approximately 15% of patients with primary syphilis and 30–40% of patients with secondary syphilis were identified with asymptomatic neurosyphilis infection; in a few of these patients, the standard CSF laboratory parameters were found to be normal. CNS invasion of *T. pallidum* was not significantly more common among those living with HIV, although the number of such study participants was small. These results document that CSF laboratory abnormalities exist early in the course of infection, are of unknown clinical significance in the absence of any neurologic clinical signs or symptoms and can resolve spontaneously or remain dormant for a lifetime depending on host factors.[62]

Like the other clinical syndromes of syphilis (e.g., primary, secondary, and tertiary syphilis), the syndromes of neurosyphilis are well described as is the timing of these neurologic syndromes.[55,57,63] Acute syphilitic meningitis and meningovascular syphilis are neurologic syndromes of early neurosyphilis, while general paresis and tabes dorsalis and are syndromes of late neurosyphilis.[63]

Acute syphilitic meningitis usually occurs within the first 2 years of infection. While approximately 10% of cases can occur at the secondary stage of syphilis, in about 25% of patients, meningitis can be the first clinical sign of syphilis. Patients present with more subacute headaches and meningeal irritation compared with other types of bacterial meningitis. A prominent finding in almost half of patients is cranial nerve abnormalities, typically involving cranial nerves at the base of the brain (especially VI, VII, and VIII).[57,63] These features of a basilar meningitis caused by inflammation of the meninges may reflect the preferential growth of *T. pallidum* at lower temperatures.

Meningovascular syphilis occurs several months to approximately 10 years after the initial infection, usually in persons less than 50 years of age. Unlike the sudden onset of thrombotic or embolic stroke syndromes, meningovascular syphilis is associated with prodromal symptoms lasting weeks to months before the more permanent focal deficits resulting from infarction from syphilitic endarteritis. Prodromal symptoms include unilateral numbness, paresthesias, extremity weakness, headache, vertigo, insomnia, and psychiatric abnormalities, such as personality changes. The symptoms present intermittently and progress slowly to more permanent stroke-like findings, including most commonly hemiparesis or hemiplegia, aphasia, and seizures.[57,63] Meningovascular syphilis of the spinal cord can occur, usually later in the course of infection (approximately a 20–25 years latent period), and presents as syphilis meningomyelitis or acute transverse myelitis.[57] Syphilis should be in the differential diagnosis of any patient, especially younger patients with symptoms of meningitis and cranial nerve palsies, stuttering stroke-like symptoms, or other symptoms suggestive of early neurosyphilis.

By contrast, late neurosyphilis is a parenchymatous form of the disease from the invasion of *T. pallidum* in the cerebrum that does not manifest until later in life. General paresis can present with symptoms like those of dementia and many psychiatric disorders such as depression, paranoia, delusions, emotional lability, and inappropriate behavior.[57] Prior to World War II, about 10% of first-time psychiatric hospital admissions were patients with general paresis, which is now rarely seen in the United States. Tabes dorsalis is associated with a triad of symptoms and signs: lightening pains, dysuria and ataxia, and the Argyll Robertson pupil (accommodation in the absence of light reaction); areflexia; and loss of proprioceptive sense, respectively.[57] Tabes dorsalis is also rarely diagnosed now in the United States.

Ocular syphilis can occur early in the course of syphilis, and the CSF evaluation can be entirely normal.[55–57] The most common presenting symptoms are changes in vision such as decreased or blurry vision and eye pain. The most common finding of ocular syphilis on ophthalmologic examination is uveitis; other findings include optic neuritis, retinitis, retinal detachment, chorioretinitis, retrobulbar neuritis, scleritis, and vitreitis. Similar to early neurosyphilis, ocular syphilis may be the initial presentation of syphilis. Otologic syphilis can also occur early in the course of the syphilis. Initial tinnitus may rapidly progress to deafness within weeks. The hearing loss generally involves higher frequencies, and vestibular abnormities are rare. Other cranial nerve abnormalities are commonly identified, but occasionally isolated cranial nerve VIII neurosensory deafness may occur. CSF evaluation in patients with otologic syphilis is usually entirely normal. Any patient presenting with inflammatory eye disease or neurosensory hearing loss should have a complete neurological and mucocutaneous examination and be tested for syphilis.

Early in the HIV epidemic, concerning case reports of early neurosyphilis and ocular and otologic syphilis led to the hypothesis that persons with untreated HIV and syphilis were more likely to develop clinically debilitating neurologic disease.[64,65] While no carefully controlled large observational studies have been done, case reports of neurosyphilis in persons living with HIV have been consistent with the clinical manifestations that have been previously described.[63] Active surveillance for neurosyphilis has not been established in the United States making it difficult to quantify the frequency and timing of neurosyphilis cases. No evidence of an increase in the rate of neurosyphilis was found in a retrospective investigation of neurosyphilis trends in San Francisco from 1985 through 1992.[66] Other limited epidemiologic data from syphilis case reporting in the United States over the past three decades suggest that neurosyphilis remains uncommon in persons living with HIV. While the magnitude of risk for neurologic complications in individuals living with HIV, especially those who have achieved viral suppression, has not been precisely determined, it is likely to be small.[27,49,62,67]

Clinical manifestations of congenital syphilis are discussed later in the chapter.

TESTING AND DETECTION METHODS

A principal challenge in diagnosing and controlling syphilis is that clinicians do not include syphilis in the differential diagnosis. Providers can be unaware of the fact that syphilis is prevalent in their communities and of its local epidemiologic features. The other challenge to the diagnosis of syphilis is that biomedical advancement in laboratory testing to detect *T. pallidum* infection has been slow for almost a century.[68–70] The nontreponemal serologic tests used today to aid in the diagnosis of syphilis were developed over 100 years ago and are only indirect antibody detection methods. The treponemal syphilis serologic test traditionally has been used to confirm a positive nontreponemal test. It is important to note that these syphilis serologic tests must be used together and can only support a presumptive laboratory diagnosis of syphilis, as clinical information is required for a more definitive syphilis diagnosis.[71]

T. pallidum cannot be easily cultured. Methods to culture it outside of animals do not yet exist, despite years of effort, although some promising *in vitro* culture systems have been recently reported.[72] Growing *T. pallidum* in rabbit testicles, while available in research laboratories, is not a feasible method for routine testing of clinical specimens. Ideally, symptomatic primary and secondary syphilis would be diagnosed by examination of lesion exudate or tissue using direct detection methods, but these methods are no longer widely available. Most infected persons identified are without symptoms or signs and are detected through screening programs in which serologic antibody tests are the only available testing option. These indirect antibody detection methods alone cannot be used to diagnose and stage syphilitic infections. Test results must be interpreted in the context of the patient's risk profile, medical history—including prior syphilis history—, and a complete physical examination.

Direct Detection Methods: Dark Field, Polymerase Chain Reaction, and Direct Fluorescent Antibody Tests

Direct detection methods include dark field microscopy, a polymerase chain reaction test (PCR), and a direct fluorescent antibody test for *T. pallidum* (DFA-TP). Direct detection methods are considered the definitive methods for diagnosing adult syphilis and congenital syphilis. Direct detection methods are particularly helpful in the evaluation of suspicious lesions of primary syphilis because serologic tests are insensitive at the primary stage.

Dark Field Testing

In a patient with a genital lesion but negative serologic results, a positive finding on a dark field or PCR test can be diagnostic for syphilis. When an experienced dark field microscopist is available and a specimen is properly collected, dark field microscopy is a sensitive and specific method.[73–75] Specimens must be examined within 15–20 minutes of collection because both morphologic and motility characteristics are needed to identify *T. pallidum*. *T. pallidum* is slender and motile with spiral-shaped coils to the end of the bacteria, characteristic bending motions, and no translational movement across the slide. Dark field testing has a sensitivity that ranges from 75% to 100%, with sensitivities > 90% if the lesion is new and the specimen is performed under optimal circumstances. Sensitivity is lower if the lesion is older (present more than 7–14 days) or if prior antimicrobial therapy or topical treatments were administered. Specificity ranges from 94% to 100%. Dark field examination of oral lesions is not recommended because saprophytic spirochetes in the mouth are difficult to distinguish from *T. pallidum*.[75] Due to the difficulties of performing this test quickly, before motility is compromised, and the lack of available dark field microscopes and adequately trained microscopists, the capacity to do dark field microscopy in the United States has become almost nonexistent.

Direct Fluorescent Antibody Test for T. pallidum

DFA-TP, a morphology-based immunofluorescent direct detection method using monoclonal or polyclonal antibodies to detect *T. pallidum* antigens, has similar performance characteristics to dark field examinations. It has the advantage of not requiring the presence of motile organisms for detecting *T. pallidum* but the disadvantage of not being a point of care test.[76] DFA-TP is no longer available in the United States because in-house or commercially available antibody reagents are not being produced.

Polymerase Chain Reaction

While there are several PCR tests for direct detection of T. *pallidum*, none is Food and Drug Administration (FDA) cleared for clinical use. Some laboratories provide locally developed and validated PCR results for the detection of *T. pallidum*. Sensitivity of these PCR tests is excellent and comparable to dark field and DFA-TP using a swab to collect material from suspicious primary syphilis lesions.[77–79] Sensitivities ranging from 72% to 95% have been reported when compared to dark field and DFA-TP methods; specificity is very high ranging from 98% to 100%. A genital ulcer disease PCR direct detection test for *T. pallidum* or a multiplex PCR test for herpes types 1 and 2 and *T. pallidum* is urgently needed because the clinician's ability to diagnose primary syphilis is hindered by the use of insensitive serologic tests.[80,81] The lack of sensitive tests to diagnose the most infectious stage of syphilis has a negative impact on public health syphilis control efforts by delaying timely diagnosis, treatment, and prevention of syphilis transmission in communities.

Serologic Tests: Nontreponemal and Treponemal Antibody Tests

Serologic tests fall into two categories: nontreponemal and treponemal antibody tests and are the cornerstone of supporting a diagnosis of syphilis because most syphilitic infections are identified at the time a person has no signs or symptoms.[70,74,75] Nontreponemal assays use cardiolipin-, lecithin-, and cholesterol-containing antigen to measure antilipoidal antibodies that develop as a result of syphilitic infections. FDA-cleared nontreponemal tests include the Rapid Plasma Reagin (RPR) and the VDRL tests. These tests are not specific to syphilis as many other infectious diseases (e.g., Lyme disease, various viral, and other bacterial infections) in addition to other conditions (e.g., injection drug use, recent immunizations, pregnancy, older age) and chronic diseases (e.g., autoimmune conditions, cancer) produce antilipoidal antibodies.[49,82,83] However, these tests have been used for decades as the initial screening test for syphilis with a reflex to a confirmatory treponemal test, if the nontreponemal test is positive.

The RPR and VDRL are equally acceptable tests, but the titers are not comparable because the testing methods used are different; RPR titers tend to be somewhat higher than VDRL titers. The VDRL test is the only nontreponemal test FDA-cleared for use on CSF specimens. The advantages of the nontreponemal tests are their low cost and quantifiable results (i.e., titers) that may correlate with disease activity.[5,74,75] Titers are used to monitor treatment success (defined by a fourfold decrease in serologic titer after treatment) and to identify reinfections or treatment failures in patients previously treated for syphilis, as evidenced by a sustained fourfold increase in titer in a serofast patient.[49,75,84,85] A serofast patient refers to someone whose nontreponemal titers do not serorevert after treatment and persist at a stable level over time. The serofast state may occur in up to one-fifth of patients after treatment for their first episode of syphilis.[85–89] The disadvantages of the nontreponemal tests are the labor and time involved in running a manual test; more subjective results due to observer differences; and false negative results from a prozone reaction. A prozone reaction refers to cases in which the specimen was not tested at enough dilution, and the undiluted nontreponemal result is falsely negative because the high concentration of antibodies inhibits the flocculation of the antigen-antibody complexes.[90] Many laboratories do not routinely perform serum dilutions on specimens submitted for nontreponemal testing unless requested by the clinician. Therefore, a specific request for dilution is needed in any suspected secondary syphilis case to avoid a possible false negative result caused by an unrecognized prozone reaction.[91]

Treponemal assays use either whole *T. pallidum*, a *T. pallidum* lysate or recombinant *T. pallidum* antigens to detect either IgM, IgG, or both antibodies.[70,74,75] The advantages of the treponemal tests are that treponemal tests are more specific than nontreponemal tests, slightly more sensitive at the primary stage of syphilis,[80,92,93] and definitively more sensitive at the tertiary stage of syphilis or latent syphilis of more than 10 years duration.[93] Two disadvantages of the treponemal tests exist.[49] The first is a lack of a quantitative result that can be used to follow treatment response. The second is the difficulty in evaluating previously treated patients for re-infection or treatment failure as treponemal antibodies generally remain positive for life in most individuals, unless the initial infection was treated very early in the course of infection. Studies have identified that approximately 15–25% of patients treated for primary syphilis will revert to a negative treponemal test result within 2–3 years after treatment; no patients treated for secondary syphilis or stages of longer duration of infection seroreverted.[85] Treponemal tests also cannot distinguish between subspecies of *T. pallidum*; positive results may reflect other endemic treponemal infections, such as yaws and pinta. In the United States, it is rare that a positive treponemal test is not from a *T. pallidum subspecies pallidum* infection. Lastly, while treponemal IgM antibody tests have been developed, ones that can specifically identify early latent syphilis do not exist as IgM antibodies can persist for longer than 1 year in adults.[94]

For years, the most common FDA-cleared treponemal tests in the United States were the manual fluorescent treponemal antibody-absorption (FTA-ABS) and the hemagglutination assays: the micro-hemagglutination assay for *T. pallidum* (MHA-TP) and the *T. pallidum* hemagglutination assay (TPHA).[70,74,75] The MHA-TP and TPHA were replaced by the *T. pallidum* particle agglutination assay (TP-PA) in the 1990s. More recently, many automated immunoassays—originally developed for blood bank screening—have been FDA-cleared with a clinical indication for syphilis screening and diagnosis.[49,68,70,93] These treponemal-based tests include various enzyme immunoassays (EIAs), chemiluminescence immunoassays (CIAs), microbead immunoassays (MBIAs) and immunoblots. Little data are available on head-to-head comparisons of these newer treponemal immunoassays by stage of syphilis.[70] The advantages of the treponemal immunoassays are their high throughput and automation resulting in lower cost, reduced labor and time, reduced occupational hazard from pipetting, more objective results, and the elimination of false negative results caused by the prozone reaction.

A head-to-head comparison of test performance of the manual and automated treponemal antibody tests was recently conducted in patients with a clinical diagnosis of syphilis and in those without evidence of syphilis infection.[93] The sensitivity and specificity of five treponemal immunoassays (ADVIA Centaur Syphilis, an automated CIA that measures IgG; Bioplex 2200 Syphilis IgG, an automated MBIA that measures IgG; INNO-LIA, a manual immunoassay that measures IgG; LIAISON Treponema Screen, an automated CIA that measures IgG and IgM; and Trep-Sure, an automated EIA that measures IgG and IgM) and the two available manual treponemal assays (FTA-ABS DS, a manual indirect fluorescence assay that measures IgG and IgM and TP-PA, a manual agglutination assay that measures IgG and IgM) were analyzed by stage of syphilis. The reference standard was a combination of clinical diagnosis [(1) current diagnosis of primary, secondary, early latent, or late latent; (2) prior treated syphilis only; and (3) no evidence of current syphilis, no prior history of syphilis, and at least four of seven treponemal tests negative] and serologic results, as no common standard for treponemal serologic test performance exists. Among the four immunoassays routinely used for screening, all performed well with high sensitivity ranging from 100% for secondary syphilis, 95.1–100% for early latent syphilis, and 94.5–96.4% for seropositive primary syphilis; these sensitivities were found to be comparable to the performance of the manual TP-PA treponemal test. Specificity was high for all treponemal tests ranging from 94.5% to 100%, except for the Trep-Sure EIA test that demonstrated specificity of 82.6%. This inferior specificity of the Trep-Sure EIA test might be explained by the signal cut off level, which optimized sensitivity but may have compromised specificity. The manual FTA-ABS test was significantly less sensitive than the other treponemal tests, especially for seropositive primary syphilis (78.2%). The TP-PA had higher overall sensitivity (95.4%) and superior overall specificity (100%) compared with the FTA-ABS (90.8% and 98%). The FTA-ABS has been considered the treponemal serologic test gold standard for decades, despite being a subjective test. Over time, quality control reagents were no longer available, and proficiency testing and quality control programs were defunded in the 1990s. Furthermore, most microbiologists with expertise in performing the subjective FTA-ABS test have retired. This study suggests the TP-PA now may be the preferred manual treponemal test and that it may be time to retire the FTS-ABS test. Overall, the data in this study were insufficient to recommend any of the immunoassays evaluated over another for use in the laboratory diagnosis of syphilis.

Laboratory considerations for treponemal test selection can include cost, labor, test volume, throughput, and turnaround time. The manual TP-PA can be used as a reflex test to confirm positive nontreponemal tests in the traditional algorithm or used to adjudicate discordant serologies (e.g., immunoassay reactive and nontreponemal test nonreactive) in the reverse sequence algorithm discussed below. The automated immunoassays also can be used as a reflex test to confirm positive nontreponemal tests in the traditional algorithm but are more commonly used as a screening test in the reverse sequence algorithm given the cost-benefit ratio.[95]

Several rapid syphilis treponemal tests including some combined with rapid HIV tests are available outside the United States and are commonly used for prenatal screening; however, they have not yet been cleared by the FDA.[96,97] As of 2019, there is only one FDA-cleared, Clinical Laboratory Improvement Amendments (CLIA) waived rapid syphilis test in the United States. A limited number of studies on this test's performance have been done in the United States.[98–101] Performance has varied by specimen type (freshly collected whole blood or frozen, archived sera), setting, and the population's prevalence of and risk factors for syphilis and healthcare seeking behaviors. The rapid syphilis treponemal tests are also limited by the same challenges of interpretation of any positive nonrapid treponemal serologic test result in a client who has a history of treated syphilis, as reinfection or treatment failure cannot be distinguished from persistent treponemal antibodies from a previously treated infection. Factors such as local rates of incident and prevalent syphilis infections and healthcare seeking behaviors of individuals to be screened should be taken into consideration when determining the net benefits and costs of a rapid syphilis test-screening program. If the currently available rapid syphilis test is used as an initial screening test in the United States, follow-up confirmation with standard nontreponemal and treponemal testing should be considered if local test performance and quality assurance data are not available.

The sensitivity of nontreponemal and treponemal tests increases with the duration of infection, ranging from about 75% in the primary stage of syphilis (with the treponemal tests having slightly higher sensitivity at this stage compared with nontreponemal tests) to essentially 100% in the secondary stage for both types of tests. In general, the treponemal tests remain positive in latent and late syphilis while the nontreponemal tests lose sensitivity over the course of infection to about 50–65% at the late latent stage or in patients with tertiary syphilis.[45,102]

Unusual serologic responses initially reported in persons living with HIV and infected with syphilis raised concerned about the accuracy of syphilis serologic tests in persons living with HIV. Since these reports appeared, it has been documented that HIV infection can cause false positive nontreponemal test results and higher than expected serofast titers after treatment in persons with syphilis and HIV infection.[83,87,89] However, false negative results and delayed seroreactivity have been found to be extremely rare.[50] Therefore, for most persons living with HIV, serologic tests for syphilis should be considered reliable and accurate for diagnosing syphilis and following their treatment response.[49] It should be noted that atypical nontreponemal test results, such as remarkably high titers or fluctuating titers, can be seen regardless of HIV status[49,50,89] and retreatment has little impact on reducing serofast titers.[103]

For decades, the traditional syphilis serologic screening algorithm started with a screening nontreponemal test (e.g., RPR or VDRL) and if positive, was reflexed to a confirmatory manual treponemal test (e.g., FTA-ABS, MHA-TP, or TP-PA). With the advent of the automated treponemal immunoassays cleared for screening and diagnosis in the mid-2000s, some laboratories began using the automated treponemal test as the screening serologic test and if positive, then reflexed to a quantitative nontreponemal test. This became known as the reverse syphilis screening algorithm.[104] This screening algorithm can identify persons with new, untreated syphilis and those with previously treated syphilis and persistent treponemal antibodies, along with biologically false positives that can occur in persons with a low likelihood of infection. Thus, the reverse sequence algorithm can present some clinical management conundrums when the initial treponemal test is discordant with the second nontreponemal test (e.g., positive treponemal immunoassay and negative RPR or VDRL) (Fig. 120-2).[105–107] If the quantitative nontreponemal test is negative after a prozone reaction has been ruled out, then a second treponemal test, preferably one with a platform using different antigens than the original treponemal test such as the TP-PA, is recommended.[49] If the second treponemal test is positive (e.g., two positive treponemal tests and a negative quantitative nontreponemal test) then the patient needs to be assessed for the possibility of a previously treated infection or if no history of syphilis treatment, then a new infection of latent syphilis is assumed. In the case of the previously treated patient, management depends on if the sexual history suggests the possibility of reinfection and the likelihood of patient follow-up. If the likelihood of reinfection is high and follow-up uncertain, treatment should be offered. If the likelihood of re-exposure is low and follow-up is certain, then education about returning immediately if any lesions or symptoms develop should be explained. Otherwise, a repeat nontreponemal test in about 3–4 weeks should identify early syphilis and treatment offered if both the nontreponemal and treponemal tests are now positive.

The reverse sequence algorithm presents even more clinical management conundrums if the second treponemal test is negative (e.g., immunoassay positive, nontreponemal test negative, and second treponemal test negative) (Fig. 120-2).[49,107,108] If the epidemiologic risk and clinical probability of syphilis are high, then the immunoassay result could be a true positive result; if low, then the result could represent a false positive. The following case reports highlight these clinical management challenges. Case reports of positive immunoassays with negative nontreponemal tests and negative second manual treponemal tests have been reported among pregnant women living in communities with low prevalence of syphilis infections who were required by law to be screened at the first prenatal visit.[109] These isolated positive immunoassays would not have been detected if the initial screening test was a nontreponemal assay. Without a gold standard to adjudicate these discordant results in pregnancy, the clinical management can be challenging, especially if the pregnant woman is allergic to penicillin. In another study, CDC analyzed syphilis screening data from five clinical laboratories that used reverse sequence screening during 2006–10.[106] The three large managed-care organization laboratories served patient populations with both high and low prevalence of syphilis, and the two public health laboratories served populations with high prevalence of syphilis, including gay, bisexual, and other MSM living with HIV. Among the 140,176 specimens screened with an EIA/CIA, 4834 (3.4%) had a reactive test result; among these reactive sera over half (56.7%) were RPR-nonreactive, of which 866 (31.6%) were also nonreactive by TP-PA or FTA-ABS testing, suggesting that the initial EIA/CIA result could be a false-positive result. The percentage with a positive EIA/CIA and nonreactive nontreponemal and TP-PA or FTA-ABS tests was 2.9 times greater in the low-prevalence population than the high-prevalence population (40.8% vs. 14.1%). Further clinical follow-up of patients with discordant results was done at one large managed-care organization.[107] Medical records of 255 patients with a reactive CIA test but a nonreactive RPR test were reviewed; clinical and demographic characteristics, prior syphilis history, CIA index values, and TP-PA status were abstracted. One hundred and eighty-four individuals had

Traditional

Quantitative RPR/VDRL

RPR/VDRL- If high vulnerability for syphilis acquisition and no signs or symptoms, repeat in 3 months

RPR/VDRL+

TP-PA or Other Treponemal Test

TP-PA- *Syphilis Unlikely* If high vulnerability for syphilis acquisition, consider repeat quantitative RPR in 3–4 weeks

TP-PA + *Syphilis (previously treated or current infection)**

Reverse Sequence

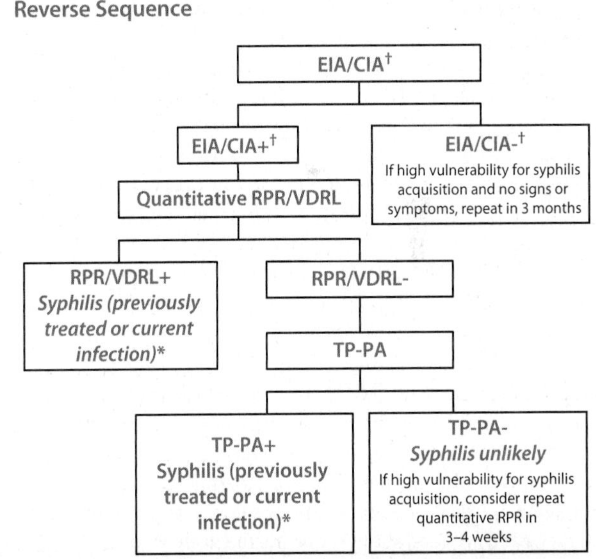

Additional Serologic Screening Considerations

* **Evaluation to determine if serologic results reflect a previous treated syphilis infection or current infection**

1. Evaluate clinically: complete medical history, including titer and treatment, full physical exam, and if they know if any of their partners were recently treated for syphilis.
2. Determine if past treatment and appropriate serological response:
   a) If there was an adequate serological response with treatment in the past and if the clinical evaluation is negative, diagnose as serofast syphilis and rescreen person per CDC screening recommendations.
   b) If inadequate or no adequate treatment documented, stage the case of syphilis and administer treatment according to CDC guidelines.

† **Or other automated treponemal tests**

FIGURE 120-2. Clinical management of syphilis serologic screening algorithms. (*Source:* Centers for Disease Control and Prevention: Syphilis testing algorithms using treponemal tests for initial screening—Four laboratories, New York City, 2005–2006. *MMWR Morb Mortal Wkly Rep*. 2008;57(32):872–5.)

a reactive TP-PA and 71 had a negative TP-PA result. After following and retesting 25 of the 71 CIA-positive, RPR-negative, TP-PA—negative patients who were not treated for the initial discordant result: 17 had no change in their test results and seven seroreverted to CIA negative, suggesting the initial CIA results were false positives. One patient seroconverted to a reactive RPR suggesting that the initial CIA result was a true positive and the patient had recently acquired syphilis. This study also found that in patients with a positive TP-PA test result, the CIA optical density index value of > 12 correlated with a positive TP-PA result.[107] In TP-PA negative patients, a CIA optical density index value of < 5 was seen in 92% of patients. Increasing signal strength values have been shown to correlate with increasing reactivity of confirmatory treponemal testing.[110–112] Thus, signal strength values could be helpful in the clinical management of discordant results in populations with low prevalence of syphilis, or some values could be used in lieu of confirmatory testing with TP-PA. These studies highlight that discordant syphilis serologic results need to be interpreted in the context of patient's medical and sexual history, physical exam, prior serologic test results, and vulnerability to syphilis acquisition. Laboratory considerations for algorithm selection can include cost, labor, test volume, throughput, turnaround time, and syphilis prevalence of populations being tested. Figure 120-2 outlines clinical management options to consider depending on the test results and which algorithm is used.[49]

CSF tests available to diagnose neurosyphilis are limited. Furthermore, no single test can be used to make the diagnosis of neurosyphilis.[55,113,114] In general, abnormal CSF laboratory results are common in early syphilis and without any neurologic signs and symptoms, are of unknown clinical significance.[49] Examination of the CSF VDRL, cell count, and protein is only recommended to help support the diagnosis of neurosyphilis in patients with reactive syphilis serologic tests and evidence of neurologic signs and symptoms on physical exam.[49,51,62] These CSF tests may also be useful in the evaluation of a possible treatment failure or tertiary syphilis, both uncommon occurrences.[49,113,114] While the FTA-ABS is not FDA-cleared for testing on CSF, some laboratories have validated the test performance characteristics of the CSF FTA-ABS; it is less specific for neurosyphilis than the CSF VDRL, but is highly sensitive. A diagnosis of neurosyphilis is highly unlikely in patients with all the following characteristics: (1) positive syphilis serologies, (2) nonspecific neurologic signs or symptoms, (3) a negative CSF VDRL, (4) mildly abnormal CSF cell count or protein, and (5) a negative CSF FTS-ABS. The role of CSF PCR to diagnosis neurosyphilis needs further study.[81]

TREATMENT

Penicillin G is the preferred drug for treating persons in all stages of syphilis and is the only drug recommended for syphilis treatment in pregnant women and for congenital, neurologic, otic, and ocular syphilis.[49] The type of Penicillin G (i.e., benzathine, procaine, or aqueous crystalline), dose, route of administration [intramuscular (IM) or intravenous (IV)], and duration of treatment depends on the stage of syphilis and sites of infection. There has never been a randomized controlled trial studying the efficacy of benzathine penicillin G dose and duration by stage of syphilis as the value of these types of clinical trials was not recognized until well after the introduction of penicillin G as a syphilis treatment. However, with decades of clinical experience since the 1940s, subsequent decreases in burden of infections, rapid resolution of clinical signs and symptoms of primary and secondary syphilis after treatment, and the return of serologic titers to negative 1–2 years after treatment in most patients with early syphilis, benzathine penicillin G is accepted worldwide as the recommended treatment for adult syphilis without neurologic, ocular or otic signs or symptoms.[115]

Benzathine penicillin G 2.4 million units IM in a single dose is the recommended treatment for primary, secondary, and early latent syphilis.[49] Longer duration of treatment is recommended for latent syphilis of greater than 1 year's duration or for tertiary syphilis. This duration is based on a theoretical concern that slower growing treponemes may survive for more than 2 weeks beyond the duration of action for one dose of benzathine penicillin G—a speculation that has not been confirmed. It is also recommended to use the longer duration of treatment if the duration of the syphilis infection is unknown to ensure adequate treatment for those who did not acquire the syphilis infection within the preceding year. Benzathine penicillin G 2.4 million units IM weekly for 3 weeks is the recommended treatment for latent syphilis of unknown duration or of greater than 1-year duration and tertiary syphilis without neurologic involvement.[49]

Preparations of penicillin G that cross the blood-brain barrier such as procaine penicillin G and aqueous crystalline penicillin G should be used for sequestered sites of infection such as the CNS and ocular aqueous humor.[49] Based on available data and published evidence-based recommendations, patients living with HIV should be treated according to the recommendations for patients without HIV.[49,51,116] Concerns about higher risk of neurologic complications in persons living with HIV were raised early in the HIV epidemic[64,65] and well before HIV treatment and viral suppression were a reality.[67] While the magnitude of this risk has not been precisely defined, it is believed to be small. In addition, no therapies other than penicillin G have proven to be more effective in preventing neurosyphilis in persons living with HIV. Accordingly, careful assessment of neurologic signs and symptoms in all patients diagnosed with syphilis; testing for syphilis in any patient who presents with symptoms or signs suggestive of neurologic, ocular, or otic syphilis; and close follow-up after treatment are probably the most important clinical strategies to identify significant neurologic complications.

Data to support alternatives to penicillin G to treat syphilis in nonpregnant, penicillin allergic patients are limited. Doxycycline has been used for many years for primary, secondary, and latent syphilis.[49,117–120] Limited studies suggest that daily ceftriaxone IM or IV for 10–14 days may effectively treat primary and secondary syphilis although the optimal dose and duration are not known.[121,122] Azithromycin in a single 2-gram dose has been studied and found to be effective for primary and secondary syphilis treatment.[123,124] However, the emergence of *T. pallidum* resistance to macrolides due to a 23S ribosomal RNA gene mutation, especially prevalent among MSM with syphilis, suggests that azithromycin is no longer a reasonable alternative.[125,126] Although limited studies of amoxicillin with probenecid has shown promise,[127,128] a double-blinded, randomized, controlled trial comparing benzathine penicillin G with and without high dose amoxicillin with probenecid in participants with early syphilis found no difference in outcomes after 12 months of follow-up.[86] If alternatives to penicillin are used, close follow-up is recommended.

Fortunately, no evidence of *T. pallidum* resistance to penicillin has been identified. Of immediate concern is the global shortages of benzathine penicillin G stocks that were first reported in 2000,[129] and in the United States in 2016.[130] As benzathine penicillin G is off patent, it sells for pennies a dose in low- and middle-income countries, but as a sterile injectable medication, it is expensive to manufacture. Several active pharmaceutical ingredient (API) manufacturers that make benzathine penicillin G's active ingredient, penicillium, and final dose formulators (FDFs) that formulate, package, and label the final product, have stopped producing benzathine penicillin G because of these economics.[129] With a highly consolidated market, alternative supplies are difficult to obtain, and risk of shortages has dramatically increased. In the United States, there is only one plant that formulates and packages the final product. Globally, the number of API manufacturers has decreased to three. This fragile benzathine penicillin G manufacturing system is threatening the global prevention and control of syphilis, including congenital syphilis and needs urgent strengthening. Furthermore, with penicillin G as the only recommended antimicrobial for syphilis treatment, more antimicrobials are urgently needed in the pipeline for syphilis treatment.

To most accurately assess treatment success as measured by a fourfold decrease in the nontreponemal test titers, titers on the day of treatment should be compared with follow-up titers obtained every 3–6 months for 1–2 years after treatment.[5,49,84,85] While a sensitive measure of neurosyphilis treatment is CSF leukocyte count,[55,61] more recent studies has demonstrated that normalization of serum RPR titers predicts the normalization of CSF parameters following neurosyphilis treatment, suggesting that follow-up lumbar punctures may be outmoded.[131] Identification of sexual contacts for evaluation including physical examination, serologic testing, and treatment, if indicated, is also an important part of the medical management for any patient with syphilis.[49] For patients with primary syphilis, all sexual contacts within 3 months before the appearance of primary lesion(s) should be evaluated. For patients with secondary syphilis, all sexual contacts within 6 months before any signs or symptoms should be evaluated. For early latent or unknown duration but a possibility of recent acquisition, all contacts within the past 12 months should be evaluated. For late latent or unknown duration but no likelihood of recent acquisition, current partners should be evaluated. All contacts whose exposure is within the past 3 months should be presumptively treated, even if serologic tests are all negative, as they may have incubating syphilis and the serologic tests are not yet are reactive.

The clinical management of adult syphilis is beyond the scope of this chapter. Evidenced-based STD Treatment Guidelines, including up-to-date syphilis management recommendations for medical providers, are published by CDC.[49] Clinical providers should use these guidelines as a reference and consult with an STI clinical specialist, if clinical questions arise, as syphilis is a complex infectious disease.

DETECTION AND TREATMENT OF SYPHILIS IN PREGNANT WOMEN

Effective prevention and detection of congenital syphilis depends on the identification of syphilis in pregnant women and, therefore, on the routine serologic screening of all pregnant women during the first prenatal visit, and at 28-week gestation and delivery for women who live in communities with high rates of syphilis or who are at increased risk of acquisition of syphilis (see Prevention and Control, Screening Programs section later in chapter). Any woman who has a fetal death after 20-week gestation should be tested for syphilis.[132] Either the traditional syphilis serologic screening algorithm (nontreponemal test followed by a treponemal test) or the reverse syphilis serologic screening algorithm (treponemal test followed by a quantitative nontreponemal test) can be used in pregnancy (see Testing and Detection Methods section). Pregnant women with both a positive treponemal and nontreponemal serologic test result should be considered infected unless an adequate treatment history is documented clearly in the medical records and sequential serologic antibody titers have declined appropriately for the stage of syphilis.[49] If the reverse sequence algorithm is used and the results for pregnant women are discrepant (positive treponemal test and a negative treponemal test), then a second treponemal test (TP-PA preferred) should be performed. If the second treponemal test is positive, untreated or previously treated syphilis needs to be confirmed. For women with a history of adequate treatment who do not have ongoing risk, no further treatment is necessary. For the other women with no evidence of syphilis treatment, they should be staged and treated accordingly. If the second treponemal test is negative, the positive treponemal test is more likely to represent a false-positive test result in a low-risk untreated woman who lacks signs or symptoms of primary syphilis and has a partner with no clinical or serologic evidence of syphilis. If follow-up is likely, repeat serologic testing within 4 weeks can be considered, in order to determine whether the treponemal test remains positive or if the nontreponemal or the TP-PA test becomes positive. If both the nontreponemal test and TP-PA remain negative, no further treatment is necessary.

Penicillin G is the only known effective treatment for treating fetal infection, and pregnant women should be treated with the penicillin regimen appropriate for their stage of infection.[49,133,134] Some evidence suggests that additional therapy is beneficial for pregnant women who have primary, secondary, or early latent syphilis, as the spirochetemia is greatest in the early stages of syphilis; a second dose of benzathine penicillin 2.4 million units IM can be administered 1 week after the initial dose.[135,136] Provider follow-up to verify treatment is crucial when prenatal care providers do not house on-site treatment and must refer patients to another healthcare facility for treatment. Pregnant women who miss any dose of therapy must repeat the full course of treatment.[49] No proven alternatives to penicillin are available for treatment of syphilis during pregnancy; erythromycin treatment failures have been reported[137] and cephalosporins and amoxicillin have not been well studied. Pregnant women who have a history of penicillin allergy should be desensitized and treated with penicillin.[49]

The clinical management of syphilis during pregnancy is beyond the scope of this chapter. Evidenced-based STD Treatment Guidelines, including up-to-date syphilis management in pregnant women, are published by CDC.[49] Prenatal care providers should use these guidelines as a reference and consult with a syphilis clinical specialist, if clinical questions arise, as syphilis is a complex infectious disease.

CONGENITAL SYPHILIS

Clinical Manifestations

Congenital syphilis is a disseminated infection. Typically, *T. pallidum* enters the bloodstream of the fetus via the placenta and can involve any fetal organ.[138–140] Less commonly, *T. pallidum* can enter the fetal circulation by infecting the fetal membranes and amniotic fluid.[141] Limited observational studies in the 1950s among pregnant women with syphilis found that congenitally acquired syphilis morbidity varied by stage of maternal syphilis during pregnancy.[142] Among women with primary or secondary syphilis, no healthy infants were identified. Approximately 50% were premature, stillborn, or died in the neonatal period; the remaining 50% developed either early or late symptomatic congenital syphilis as infants or children. For the pregnant women with early latent syphilis 20% were normal, full-term healthy infants, 40% had signs or symptoms of congenital syphilis, and 40% were premature, stillborn, or died shortly after birth. For pregnant women with late latent syphilis, 70% were normal, full-term healthy infants, 10% had congenital syphilis, and 20% were premature, stillborn, or died shortly after birth. Histopathology of fetal or congenital syphilis comprises an endarteritis with mononuclear and plasma cell infiltrates, similar to the inflammatory response seen in adult syphilis.[139,143] The histopathologic features of the placenta associated with congenital syphilis include the triad of enlarged hypercellular villi, proliferative fetal vascular changes, and acute or chronic villitis.[144,145]

Fetal syphilis is the clinical manifestations of intrauterine infection with *T. pallidum*. Fetal syphilis is not typically seen within the first 20 weeks of pregnancy, presumably because of fetal immunologic immaturity.[141,146] Appropriate maternal treatment within the first 20 weeks of pregnancy is thought to be uniformly successful in preventing fetal syphilis.[135,147] As identified by ultrasound in a retrospective study, the most common fetal abnormality is hepatomegaly (79%), followed by placentomegaly (27%), polyhydramnios (12%), and ascites (10%). Thirty three percent of cases of fetal syphilis had an abnormal middle cerebral arterial Doppler evaluation, a sign of anemia.[148] In a small prospective study of 24 pregnant women with syphilis, 17 (71%) had placentomegaly, 16 (66%) hepatomegaly, 8 (35%) thrombocytopenia, 6 (26%) anemia, and 3 (12%) ascites.[149] Ultrasound findings of fetal syphilis are associated with a higher rate of obstetric complications,[135] such as premature labor during treatment[150] and manifestations of congenital syphilis at birth, in women treated for syphilis of any stage during pregnancy.[148] In addition, a limited number of controlled studies support that intrauterine infection with *T. pallidum* identified by ultrasound is associated with prematurity, low birth weight, and small size for gestational age.[139,151,152] It is important to note that a normal ultrasound does not rule out congenital syphilis. For example, osseous lesions cannot be detected by ultrasound. In one study, 12% of neonates identified with congenital syphilis at birth occurred in mothers with a normal pretreatment ultrasound during pregnancy.[148]

Like adult syphilis, congenital syphilis is divided into stages—early and late congenital syphilis.[139] Early congenital syphilis includes clinical manifestations that present at birth, within 1 month or within the first 2 years of life. Late congenital syphilis includes signs and symptoms after 2 years, usually around puberty.[153,154] In the postantibiotic era, most cases of congenital syphilis are identified at birth, and the severe signs and symptoms seem to be less common.[155] Neonates born with symptomatic congenital syphilis have a worse prognosis, including perinatal death, than neonates born with asymptomatic congenital syphilis.[139,151]

Clinical manifestations presenting at birth[139,140,151] commonly include hepatomegaly, splenomegaly, rash (bullous lesions especially on the palms and soles, and macular, indurated plaque, desquamating, eczematoid, and impetiginous lesions), and skin petechiae. The rash of congenital syphilis is more likely to be moist and infectious compared with the dryer macular/papular rashes of adult secondary syphilis. Abnormalities of CSF cell count and protein, anemia and abnormal long bone films (osteochondritis and periostitis) may also be common. Less common manifestations include jaundice, leukocytosis, leukopenia, thrombocytopenia, pseudoparalysis, rhinitis (snuffles), laryngitis, mucous patches, and epitrochlear lymphadenopathy. Clinical meningitis may occur within a few months after birth and meningovascular syphilis toward the end of the first year of life. The longer-term sequelae of meningitis in the neonate can be obstructive hydrocephalus, seizure disorders, and impaired intellectual development. Snuffles, palmar, and plantar bullous rash, and splenomegaly have been considered by some as the "diagnostic triad" of congenital syphilis; others also include pseudoparalysis and other cutaneous manifestations (syphilids) as the "diagnostic pentad" of congenital syphilis.[2]

For infants that appear normal at birth, the diagnosis usually becomes more apparent 3–8 weeks after birth, and most cases of early congenital syphilis present within 3 months of birth.[2,48,156] For these infants with delayed signs and symptoms of early congenital syphilis, the clinical manifestations can often be very nonspecific such as failure to thrive, pneumonia (pneumonia alba), and rhinitis. Other less common delayed signs and symptoms include condyloma lata, furuncle of Barlow (violaceous nodule), nephrotic syndrome, chorioretinitis, glaucoma, and uveitis.

Late congenital syphilis is similar to tertiary syphilis in the adult and is from delayed consequences of inflammation at sites of infection early in the course of infection.[2,48,139,140,153,154] Bone, soft tissue, teeth, eyes, ears, and CNS are the most common sites of late congenital syphilis. Unlike adult tertiary syphilis, the cardiovascular system is usually spared. Stigmata include frontal bossing, saddle nose, short maxilla, high palatal arch, and rhagades—radiating furrows from scarring of mucocutaneous tissue. Sequalae of periostitis can cause saber shins. Changes in the morphologic differentiation of permanent teeth cause the Hutchison tooth—incisors widely spaced apart and shaped like a screwdriver—and the Mulberry molar—molars with tubercular projections. Interstitial keratitis is a common late congenital syphilis manifestation. The Hutchison's triad includes interstitial keratitis, neural deafness, and characteristic dental abnormalities of the incisors and molars. Clutton's joints (painless swelling of the knees), palate deformations from gummas lesions causing perforations of the soft palate and septum, and neurosyphilis manifestations similar to late neurosyphilis manifestations in adults, such as tabes dorsalis and general paresis, are also seen in late congenital syphilis. In the postantibiotic era, these complications of late congenital syphilis are rarely seen in the United States; most cases are in children born outside of the United States who recently immigrated.

Diagnosis and Treatment

Diagnosis of congenital syphilis is even more challenging than the diagnosis of syphilis in adults because of the passive transfer of maternal immunoglobulin (Ig)G antibodies across the placenta to the fetus and neonate. Maternal IgM does not cross the placenta, but no sensitive and specific IgM serologic test is currently available to diagnose active syphilitic infection in the neonate.[157,158] Nontreponemal serologic tests may detect acquired maternal antibodies up to 6 months after birth and treponemal serologic tests may remain positive from maternal antibodies for up to 15 months.[49] As a result, treponemal serologic tests are not recommended in the neonate because they cannot be titered and a 15-month follow-up period before treating an infant with possible congenital syphilis is unethical. When obtaining nontreponemal serologic tests at the time of delivery in the neonate, serum rather than cord blood is recommended because of concerns about potential maternal blood contamination causing false positive results and Wharton's jelly interfering with nontreponemal test performance in cord blood.[132] The neonate's nontreponemal antibody titer should be compared to the mother's titer at delivery.[49] A diagnosis of congenital syphilis is likely if the infant's titer is fourfold or greater than the maternal titer, even in the absence of congenital signs or symptoms. Congenital syphilis is also likely if the maternal nontreponemal and treponemal tests are reactive and the neonate has classic signs and symptoms of congenital syphilis.

Like adult syphilis, a definitive diagnosis of congenital syphilis requires direct detection of *T. pallidum*. Dark field microscopy is used to detect live treponemes in body fluids from nasal discharge, vesiculobullous skin lesions, condyloma lata, and mucous patches. Visualization of treponemes in tissue specimens such as placenta, umbilical cord, or from stillbirths by silver staining, immunofluorescence or immunocytochemistry are underutilized methods for diagnosing congenital syphilis.[159] PCR testing has proven to be useful for detection of *T. pallidum* DNA in placental tissue, skin lesions, amniotic fluid, blood, sera, and CSF in both symptomatic and asymptomatic congenital syphilis in research settings.[81,160,161] Comparable to the use of PCR tests in adults, these tests are not yet FDA-cleared for diagnosing congenital syphilis.

Given the limitations of diagnostic testing, four possible congenital syphilis diagnostic scenarios exist- proven or highly probable, possible, less likely, or unlikely to inform treatment.[49,162,163] These scenarios are dependent on the neonate's serologic titers and clinical manifestations along with the maternal serologic results and treatment status. A proven or highly probable case of congenital syphilis includes any neonate whose mother has reactive nontreponemal and treponemal test results and with either an abnormal physical examination that is consistent with congenital syphilis, a nontreponemal serologic titer that is fourfold higher than the maternal titer or a positive dark field or PCR of the placenta, lesions, or body fluids. While the signs and symptoms of congenital syphilis are diverse and can be nonspecific, many neonates with congenital syphilis have a normal physical examination and a serum quantitative nontreponemal serologic titer equal to or less than fourfold the maternal titer. Further evaluation and type of treatment recommended is complex in these infants. Additional evaluation consisting of CSF analysis, long bone radiographs, complete blood count (CBC), liver functions tests, and audiologic and ophthalmologic tests may be considered, as clinically indicated, to determine the extent of congenital syphilis or establish a possible diagnosis.

A possible case of congenital syphilis includes any neonate whose mother has reactive nontreponemal and treponemal test results and who was inadequately treated (i.e., received treatment less than 4 weeks before delivery, inadequate penicillin G treatment per national recommendations or a nonpenicillin G regimen), or has no documentation of having received treatment. Congenital syphilis is considered less likely or unlikely if the mother received adequate treatment during pregnancy greater than 4 weeks before delivery or the mother received adequate treatment before the pregnancy with a nontreponemal serologic titer that remained serofast (i.e., low and stable) before and during the pregnancy including at delivery.

Parenterally administered penicillin G is the only recommended treatment for congenital syphilis.[49] Options include aqueous crystalline penicillin G, procaine penicillin G and benzathine penicillin G depending on the likelihood of congenital syphilis. Any neonate with proven or highly probable congenital syphilis should be treated for 10 days with either aqueous crystalline penicillin G (100,000–150,000 units/kg/day, administered 50,000 units/kg/dose IV every 12 hours for 7 days and then every 8 hours thereafter for the remainder of the 10 days) or procaine penicillin G (50,000 units/kg/dose IM each day for 10 days). For a neonate with possible congenital syphilis, either of the above regimens for neonates with a high probability of congenital syphilis (i.e., aqueous crystalline penicillin G or procaine penicillin G) is an option. If a complete evaluation (i.e., CSF, long bone radiographs, and CBC) is normal and follow-up is assured, then benzathine penicillin G (50,000 units/kg/dose IM in a single dose) is another option. If congenital syphilis is less likely or unlikely, benzathine penicillin G without an evaluation is an option, especially if follow-up is uncertain. No treatment with close serologic follow-up every 2–3 months for 6 months to confirm the seroversion of a reactive nontreponemal test in the infant from maternal antibodies can be considered if the mother has an adequate fourfold serologic response after treatment but has remained serofast.

The evaluation and treatment of infants born to mothers with reactive serologic tests for syphilis is beyond the scope of this chapter. Evidence-based STD Treatment Guidelines, including up-to-date congenital syphilis management based on the most frequently encountered scenarios, are published by CDC.[49] Pediatricians should use these scenarios as reference and consult with a congenital syphilis clinical expert if questions arise as congenital syphilis diagnosis and treatment is highly individualized.

SURVEILLANCE, TRANSMISSION, AND EPIDEMIOLOGY

Surveillance

Systematic reporting of communicable diseases began in 1912 with the inception of the National Notifiable Disease Surveillance System (NNDSS) to report a few diseases of interest such as measles, poliomyelitis, influenza, tuberculosis, smallpox, and typhoid fever.[164–166] As reporting requirements evolved, additional diseases were added with syphilis case reporting beginning in 1941 in the United States (Fig. 120-3).[167]

While syphilis had been common in the United States with estimates of one in ten Americans infected in the 1930s, by 1946, reported cases of primary and secondary syphilis peaked.[167] At almost 95,000 cases, this represented the largest number of infectious cases ever reported in the United States. This peak was followed by a dramatic decline to 6392 primary and secondary cases in 1956, after penicillin treatment became widely available for syphilis in 1943.

However, in the late 1950s, the number of syphilis cases began to gradually rise. These early years of reporting did not capture the sex of recorded cases. This changed in 1963 when the sex of the reported cases was collected in the national syphilis surveillance database. From the mid-1960s to the early 1980s, the increase in syphilis cases was seen primarily among men; the number of cases remained essentially stable among women. The resultant increase in the male to female ratio of cases, which peaked at 3.5:1 in 1980,[168] suggested that the rise in male cases could be attributable to increased cases among MSM.

During this same time, from the 1950s to the 1980s, congenital syphilis in the United States declined steadily, to an all-time low of 239 cases and a rate of 6.6 per 100,000 live births reported in 1983[167]—these numbers used the less sensitive Kaufman case definition for congenital syphilis. The Kaufman criteria were based on the status of the infant and included only infants with clinical evidence of the disease or those with a persistently reactive nontreponemal serologic test 3–4 months following delivery. Stillborn infants of mothers with untreated syphilis were excluded.[169] As follow-up was needed to determine if an infant with an abnormal nontreponemal test at delivery should be counted as a case, infected infants who were lost to follow-up were also omitted. The Kaufman criteria were relatively specific but lacked sensitivity. In 1988, CDC changed the criteria used for reporting congenital syphilis, confounding the trend in congenital syphilis.[132] This change involved expanding the criteria to include maternal treatment status as a variable to consider in the case definition. Consequently, infants who had no clinical evidence or laboratory abnormalities suggestive of congenital syphilis at birth but whose mother had untreated or inadequately treated syphilis during pregnancy were now included as a possible case of congenital syphilis. As a result, the revised CDC criteria increased the sensitivity of the case definition but reduced its specificity and resulted in a spurious increase in the number of reported cases.[170,171] Congenital syphilis was not only increasing, but the downward trend in the number of syphilis cases over the previous decades had begun to stall 3 years earlier in 1986.

By 1990, primary and secondary cases of syphilis had peaked, with more than 50,000 cases reported that year.[167] This new syphilis epidemic in the United States was predominantly among heterosexuals. Cases were more common among African Americans, coinciding with the crack cocaine epidemic, and were associated with drug use and exchanging sex for drugs.[172,173] During this period, while cases of syphilis declined among MSM, possibly related to sexual behavior changes in response to the AIDS epidemic,[174] there was a striking increase in the incidence of primary and secondary syphilis in women of reproductive age—especially among females 15–29 years of age. In 1990, the highest rate of primary and secondary syphilis among women since the 1950s was reported (15 primary and secondary cases per 100,000 females and 43 primary and secondary cases per 100,000 females 15–29 years of age)—with increased cases among women of reproductive age come parallel increases in congenital syphilis. Cases of congenital syphilis surged to more than 4400 cases in 1991 (108 cases per 100,000 live births).[167]

Simultaneously as cases peaked, the CDC and the Council of State and Territorial Epidemiologists (CSTE) introduced uniform criteria for NNDSS disease reporting. In 1990, the following subtypes of syphilis cases were to be reported: primary, secondary, latent, early latent, late latent, late latent of unknown duration, neurosyphilis, syphilitic stillbirth, and congenital syphilis.[175] At that time, staging by a clinician with "expertise in syphilis" could take precedence over the standardized syphilis case definitions, possibly leading to irregularities in case reporting. In addition, for secondary syphilis, the stage of syphilis when nontreponemal tests are almost universally positive, a clinically compatible case had to have a titer of at least 1:4. Criteria for diagnosing early latent syphilis required knowledge of sexual exposure to partners with recent syphilis. The diagnosis of latent syphilis of unknown duration was based on age (13–35 years) and a nontreponemal titer (>1:16). In 1996, another subtype of syphilis was added: late with clinical manifestations other than neurosyphilis.[176]

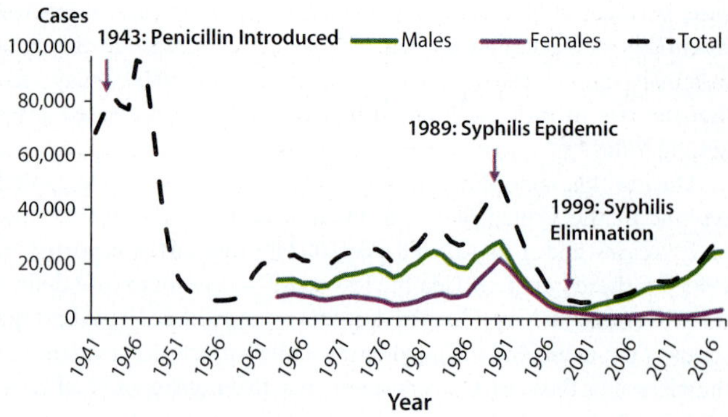

FIGURE 120-3. Primary and secondary syphilis—reported cases, United States, 1941–2017. (*Source:* Centers for Disease Control and Prevention. Sexually Transmitted Disease Surveillance 2017. Atlanta, GA: US Dept of Health and Human Services; 2018.)

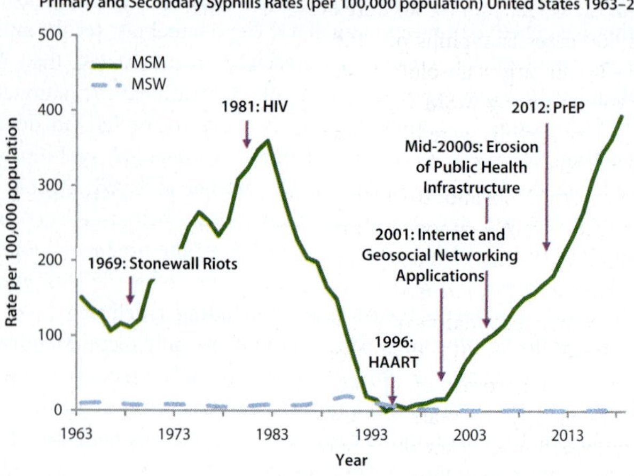

FIGURE 120-4. Drivers and determinants for the rising incidence of syphilis in men-who-have-sex-with-men. (*Sources:* Peterman TA, Su J, Bernstein KT, Weinstock H. Syphilis in the United States: on the rise? *Expert Rev Anti Infect Ther*. 2015;13(2):161–8; Heffelfinger JD, Swint EB, Berman SM, Weinstock HS. Trends in primary and secondary syphilis among men who have sex with men in the United States. *Am J Public Health*. 2007;97(6):1076–83; and Bernstein K. Drivers and determinants for the rising incidence of syphilis in men-who-have-sex-with-men. International Society for Sexually Transmitted Diseases Research; 2019; Vancouver, BC, Canada.)

Following enhanced syphilis prevention and control efforts and a simultaneous decline in crack cocaine use, reported cases of infectious syphilis declined from 43,000 cases in 1991 to 16,500 in 1995.[167] Most notably, cases of syphilis among MSM declined to the point that, in 1998, no primary or secondary cases were reported in MSM in Seattle, a previously high incidence area.[177] By 2000, primary and secondary cases reached an all-time low in the United States of 5979 cases and a national rate of 2.1 cases per 100,000 population, the lowest rate since reporting began in 1941. Over half of the cases were detected in only 28 counties, which represented less than 1% of all counties in the United States. Cases of congenitally acquired syphilis plummeted to fewer than 500 cases annually.

With almost all states reporting decreases in 2000, syphilis elimination again was envisaged, as it had once been in the 1930s[178] and the 1950s and early 1960s.[179] The argument for a syphilis elimination effort was the epidemiologic vulnerability of syphilis: (1) humans are the only reservoir; (2) the infection has a long incubation period and very limited periods of infectiousness; (3) the availability of low cost, widely available diagnostic tests and single dose, highly effective therapy; and (4) no evidence of emerging antimicrobial resistance to penicillin.[180,181]

These thoughts of elimination were short lived, as progress unraveled, and an unprecedented resurgence of syphilis cases occurred. Between 2001 and 2017, the number of primary and secondary syphilis cases in the United States increased 390%. This increase was initially seen among MSM at a time when lifesaving HIV treatments became available in the early 2000s (Fig. 120-4).[168,182–185] During 2014–15, primary and secondary syphilis cases increased in every region of the country, in every age group among those aged 15–64 years of age, in every racial/ethnic group except for American Indians and Alaska Natives, and for the first time, significantly among both men and women. By 2015, men accounted for over 90% of all cases of primary and secondary syphilis. Of those cases in men for whom the sex of the sex partner was known, 82% were MSM and approximately half of these men were living with HIV.[167]

Coinciding with the observed increases in early syphilis among MSM, case reports of ocular syphilis began to emerge in 2014[186] and the existence of a neuropathogenic strain of syphilis had been postulated. At that time, the CDC syphilis surveillance system was not well designed to capture cases of neurosyphilis or ocular syphilis in adults. A review of ocular syphilis cases reported in eight jurisdictions during 2014 and 2015, identified 388 individuals with ocular syphilis, 0.6% of total syphilis cases.[187] Molecular typing of *T. pallidum* from ocular fluid in 14 patients found no evidence that a unique strain type was responsible for these ocular syphilis cases.[188] North Carolina conducted a retrospective epidemiologic review to better understand the magnitude of and factors associated with ocular syphilis.[189] During 2014 and 2015, a total of 63 cases of ocular syphilis were identified among the total of 4234 syphilis cases reported (1.5%—well within the expected prevalence of symptomatic neurosyphilis and ocular syphilis seen in populations with early syphilis). From 2014 to 2015, ocular syphilis did increase 100%, compared with a 35% increase in syphilis cases. An ocular syphilis clinical advisory issued by CDC in April of 2015 may have contributed to increased provider recognition and, in turn, an increased number of ocular syphilis cases reported. The retrospective study found that patients with ocular syphilis were more likely to be male, white, aged 40 years or older, and living with HIV, possibly reflecting a population with ready access to care and diagnosis. Patients were identified throughout North Carolina, no patient named another ocular syphilis patient as a sexual partner, and no other epidemiologic links, such as travel, were identified. This study demonstrated that the absolute number of neurologic and ocular complications of syphilitic infections in adults will increase when syphilis increases in adults.

In 2017, there were over 30,000 reported cases of primary and secondary syphilis (rate of 9.5 per 100,000 population) in the United States[167]—a number not seen since the last syphilis epidemic in the early 1990s. Sixty-four percent of infectious syphilis cases in 2017 were among MSM only, 7% were among men who have sex with both men and women (MSMW), 17% were among men who have sex with women only (MSW), and 12% were among women. Forty-four percent of counties in the United States (1385/3142) reported at least one primary or secondary case of syphilis among MSM. These rates underscore the alarming scale of the syphilis epidemic in MSM[190] compared to the epidemic in MSW (Fig. 120-4).[168,182,183]

In 2017, one out of every 282 MSM was diagnosed with primary or secondary syphilis, and these rates in MSM were 122 times the rates in MSW. Even in the states with the most comparable rates of syphilis between MSM and MSW, there was still at least a 39-fold difference in the rate of syphilis in MSM compared to the rate in MSW, and in the state with the most disparate rate, the difference was 342-fold.[167] The state median rate ratio of MSM to MSW case rates in 2017 was 138, with rates of primary and secondary cases among MSM ranging from 56 cases per 100,000 MSM in Wyoming to 798 cases per 100,000 MSM in Nevada. Twenty-seven of 43 states with available data on the sex of the sex partner (63%) were estimated to have rates between 200 and 500 cases of syphilis per 100,000 MSM. Although white MSM make up the largest absolute number of primary and secondary cases of syphilis among MSM ($n = 7907$), in 2017 rates of primary and secondary syphilis were highest among black MSM (1054 cases per 100,000 black MSM).

Between 2000 and 2013, the number of cases of primary and secondary syphilis among women in the United States fluctuated between 1458 and 1780 cases per year, but since 2013, the numbers have substantially increased each year. From 2013 to 2017, the rate of primary and secondary syphilis among women more than doubled (Fig. 120-5).[167] In 2017, the national rate of primary and secondary syphilis among women of reproductive age was 5.1 cases per 100,000 females aged 15–44 years, representing 3750 reported cases. While 49 states reported cases of primary and secondary syphilis among females in 2017, syphilis in females is significantly more concentrated geographically than syphilis in MSM in the United States. The highest rates of primary and secondary syphilis among women are in the West and South. In 2017, 50% of all primary and secondary syphilis among women was reported from five states—Arizona, California, Florida, Louisiana, and Texas.

Similarly, the rate of congenitally acquired syphilis in 2013 marked the first increase in congenital syphilis since 2008.[167,191] The rate of 10.5 congenital syphilis cases per 100,000 live births in 2008 decreased to a rate of 8.4 in 2012. The number of congenital syphilis cases was only 334 in 2012, comparable to the 329 cases reported in 2005. The numbers of cases in 2005 and 2012 are considered the lowest level of congenitally acquired syphilis cases ever reported in the United States—the number of reported cases in the early 1980s was underestimated by approximately a factor of five with the less sensitive Kaufmann case definition.[170] Beginning in 2013, the rate of congenital syphilis has steadily increased (Fig. 120-5).[167] In 2016, among the 628 of 639 congenital syphilitic cases reported with clinical and laboratory data available, 45 (7.1%) were stillbirths or neonatal deaths, 254 (40.5%) were born alive with clinical signs and/or abnormal laboratory findings of early congenital syphilis, and 329 (52.4%) were born without any signs of congenital syphilis. In 2017, there were 918 reported cases of congenital syphilis, including 64 syphilitic stillbirths and 13 infant deaths, for a mortality rate of approximately 8.4%. The national congenital syphilis rate was 23.3 cases per 100,000 live births in 2017, representing a 44% increase relative to 2016 (16.2 cases per 100,000 live births), and a 153% increase relative to 2013 (9.2 cases per 100,000 live births); it is the highest reported rate since 1998. The geographic concentration of congenital syphilis mirrors that of primary and secondary syphilis among women. In 2017, 70% of all congenital syphilis cases was reported from the same five states that reported 50% of all primary and secondary syphilis among women. In 2017, 8.2% of counties in the United States (259/3142) reported at least one case of congenitally acquired syphilis, a 91% increase relative to 2013 when 4.3% of counties (135/3142) reported a case of congenital syphilis.

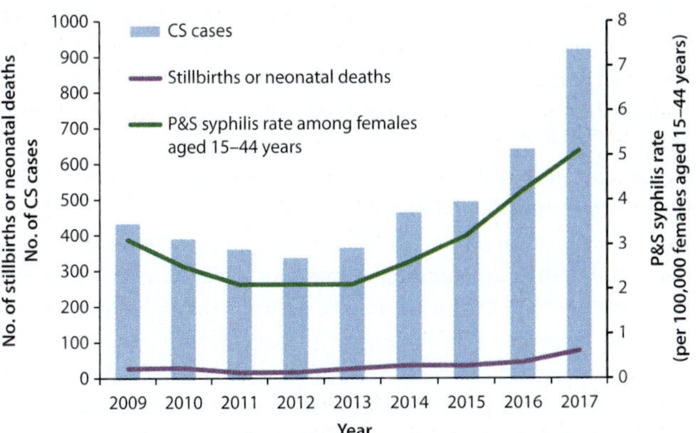

FIGURE 120-5. Congenital syphilis cases and rate of primary and secondary syphilis among females of reproductive age, U.S., 2009–17. (*Source:* Centers for Disease Control and Prevention. Sexually Transmitted Disease Surveillance 2017. Atlanta, GA: US Dept of Health and Human Services; 2018.)

Over the years, changes to syphilis case reporting have continued to occur to ensure accurate capture of cases. In the 2000s, national reporting of the sex of the partners of syphilis cases was implemented. In addition, in 2014, latent syphilis, syphilis of unknown duration, and neurosyphilis subtypes were removed.[192] Because neurosyphilis can occur at any stage of syphilis, this clinical information was to be included as part of the case report data. Also, a positive *T. pallidum* PCR test was added as a laboratory criterion for the diagnosis of primary, secondary, and congenital syphilis, and the list of treponemal tests was updated (e.g., TP-PA, EIA, CIA, and other immunoassays were added), replacing older testing methods that were no longer available (MHA-TP and microhemaglutination assay for antibody for *T. pallidum*). In 2015, CDC modified test criterion for the congenital syphilis case definition. In 2018, CDC further simplified syphilis case definitions as it is difficult to determine the duration of latent infection in a sexually active patient who has no history of serologic testing, symptoms, or epidemiologic criteria.[193] Accordingly, the early latent subtype was changed to early, nonprimary nonsecondary syphilis, and the late latent and late with clinical manifestations subtypes were changed to syphilis of unknown duration or late syphilis. All clinical manifestations of neurosyphilis, ocular and otic syphilis, and cardiovascular and gummatous syphilis were to be reported in the case report data. The specificity of the congenital syphilis case definition was also improved by adding parameters to the criteria of "elevated CSF cell count or protein (without other cause)."

Transmission

Based on one study of incubating syphilis among sexual partners of patients with primary or secondary syphilis, it has been estimated that the rate of transmission of syphilis during a single sexual contact is about 30%.[194] During the latent stage of syphilis, sexual transmission does not occur. Natural history studies from the preantibiotic era found that relapses of the secondary signs and symptoms of syphilis were seen in approximately 25% of untreated patients; 90% of relapses occurred in the first year following infection, 94% were within the first 2 years, and only rare cases occurred three to 4 years later.[30] Therefore, sexual transmission can occur during the first few years of untreated infection, providing the basis for identifying and evaluating all sexual partners within the past year of patients diagnosed with early latent syphilis, as most symptomatic relapses occur within the first year following infection.

For congenital syphilis, while a mother with an infectious genital lesion can transmit syphilis to her infant during delivery,[156,195] the most common mode of maternal transmission is by transplacental transmission of *T. pallidum* to the fetus, which can occur at any time during pregnancy.[139] The risk of fetal acquisition of syphilis is related to the stage of syphilis in the pregnant women and the level and duration of spirochetemia. Primary and secondary syphilis are the stages associated with the highest load of organisms in the bloodstream.[7,196] As a result, infants of pregnant women who acquire syphilis during pregnancy are at the highest risk for fetal and congenital syphilis. Some studies suggest this risk can be as high as 100% in pregnant women diagnosed with primary or secondary syphilis and decreases to about 40% in pregnant women with early latent syphilis.[142] After about 8 years of untreated syphilis, spirochetemia is a rare event, and the risk of congenital syphilis is small.[139,142,197] Although it was previously taught that *T. pallidum* did not cross the placenta before 18 weeks of gestation, spirochetes have been identified by histologic staining in fetal tissue at 9–10 weeks of gestation.[136,198] It is now recognized that syphilis can be a cause of first trimester spontaneous abortions, but the characteristic histopathologic response is not seen until after 18 weeks of gestation, when the fetal immune system is more mature and capable of mounting an immune response to the syphilitic infection.[146]

Epidemiology

For years, the epidemiologic risk factors for STIs, including syphilis, were seen as individual factors, such as having multiple partners, history of STIs, substance use, and transactional sex for money or drugs, along with socioeconomic factors. However, the socioepidemiologic drivers and determinants of persistent disparities in the rate of syphilis, which have existed for decades, are far more intricate. They include the intangible social determinants of health factors—cultural and political constructs of income, educational attainment, employment, accessible healthcare, insurance coverage, stigma, neighborhood/community, and social networks. Especially for racial and ethnic minorities, these are long standing factors from stubbornly entrenched systemic societal and cultural barriers to syphilis diagnosis, treatment, and prevention services.[199–203]

One hypothesis for current syphilis increases is "bridging" between MSM and heterosexual networks. Bridging refers to mixing of partnerships in different sexual networks, and recent HIV network analysis suggests that bridging between MSM and heterosexual networks may play an important role in HIV transmission.[204] HIV and syphilis are syndemics affecting similar populations. Thus, it would not be surprising that bridging between MSM and heterosexual networks could play an important role in transmission of syphilis.

Additionally, other increases in socioepidemiologic factors related to vulnerability to syphilis acquisition may best explain the epidemic among heterosexuals that began in 2013.[205] The reason why the heterosexual epidemic did not occur before 2013 could be explained by several biologic and sociobehavioral factors. One biologic difference between the transmission of syphilis and HIV in an untreated individual is that sexual transmission of syphilis requires contact with an infectious lesion. The duration of such lesions is limited, and for female partners of MSMW, exposure to an infectious rectal lesion is less likely. Thus, syphilis is more difficult to transmit than HIV and, as a result, more frequent mixing may be necessary to transmit syphilis between MSM and heterosexual networks. In addition, the prevalence of infectious syphilis in a network is likely a fundamental driver of syphilis transmission. With each sexual act, individuals in high incidence communities are more likely to encounter an infected partner than those in lower incidence communities. The number of recent sexual partners, concurrency of partnerships, rate of sex partner exchange, and condomless sex are factors that can influence an individual's chance of being exposed to infectious syphilis.[206]

Further studies of the role of networks, bridging, and other factors (e.g., sociobehavioral, biological, healthcare systems, and structural social determinants of health) influencing syphilis transmission dynamics are needed to inform network-based, cost-effective prevention approaches likely to have the highest population impact and ultimately, reduce disparities in syphilis incidence. Specific disparities leading to increased syphilis incidence for racial and ethnic minority populations, MSM, and congenital syphilis are discussed below.

Race and Ethnicity

Race and ethnicity are population characteristics that undeniably correlate with social determinants of health.[207–210] For those who are disadvantaged and cannot afford the basic necessities of life, difficulties accessing, affording and utilizing healthcare may occur.[207,211] Even when healthcare is readily available to racial and ethnic minority populations, other socioepidemiologic factors, such as fear and distrust of healthcare institutions, confidentiality concerns, embarrassment and stigma,[212,213] language barriers, differences in the quality of care provided, and the perception that provider bias and social and cultural discrimination may exist in the healthcare system can discourage individuals from seeking care.[200,214,215] All of these factors can significantly contribute to rising syphilis rates because without rapid detection and timely treatment of infectious syphilis, transmission is left unchecked in communities and sexual networks.

MSM

The drivers and determinants of the rising rates of syphilis in MSM are also complex (Fig. 120-4).[216] In the context of the AIDS epidemic, the availability since 1996 of life saving medicines has had an impact on sexual activity and sexual norms. Higher levels of condomless sex among MSM have been reported since the 2000s.[217] The more recent use of the internet[218–220] and geosocial networking apps[221,222] for meeting sexual partners may facilitate identification of partners, which in turn may support more concurrent partnerships, having an impact on the transmission of syphilis, as the likelihood of encountering a person with an infectious lesion may be greater. In 2016, almost 50% of individuals with early syphilis in San Francisco reported using a geosocial networking app to meet partners; less than 30% used the internet, less than 20% found partners at a bar/ and less than 10% at a bath house.[185] With the downturn of the economy in the late 2000s, erosion of the state and local public health infrastructure began to occur, with the closure of STI specialty clinics, settings known for serving MSM and other populations seeking confidential STI care services, and reductions in the public health staff, resulting in reduced availability of same day treatment for individuals with infectious syphilis and fewer patients and partners linked to syphilis care and treatment.[41] In addition to HIV treatment as prevention through viral suppression for those living with HIV, since 2012 pre-exposure prophylaxis (PrEP) has been available as an additional highly effective HIV biomedical prevention strategy. While some have claimed that PrEP is the reason for the rise in syphilis among MSM, the epidemic curves in Figs. 120-3 and 120-4 demonstrate that is not the case. Increases began when lifesaving antiretroviral treatment became available. HIV care settings have always presented the opportunity to detect and treat syphilis, as syphilis has been concentrated among persons living with HIV for years. PrEP now affords an additional opportunity to detect and treat more syphilis infections, as it is known that the incidence of syphilis is high among PrEP users.[223] With syphilis screening recommended as frequently as every 3 months among those most vulnerable to syphilis acquisition, the expectation is that while increases in syphilis cases may initially be seen because of increases in screening, reductions could follow.

Some of the factors associated with increasing vulnerability to acquisition of syphilis among racial and ethnic minority communities are also found in MSM communities. Behavioral health challenges, stigma, homophobia and racism, economic marginalization and discrimination in healthcare settings all make access to and utilization of prevention interventions and healthcare services more difficult.[208,215,216,224] Some MSM have more sexual partners, including concurrent partnerships, than heterosexuals, but other sociobehavioral and biobehavioral factors may potentiate vulnerability to syphilis acquisition among MSM.[217] Living in a nonaffirming society associated with stigma and discrimination creates behavioral health hardships.[216,225,226] MSM tend to have higher rates of depression, anxiety, and substance use, compared to heterosexual men.[227,228] Early childhood violence and victimization have been reported as contributing to the increased risk of acquisition of STIs among MSM.[229–231] Last, insertive and receptive anal intercourse are efficient ways to transmit syphilis, based on biologic factors.[224]

It has been well documented that black MSM have the highest rates of syphilis. The number of sexual partners and sexual practices cannot explain this disparity, as these factors do not differ among MSM by race and ethnicity.[232] In addition to the complex drivers and determinants of deep-rooted syphilis disparities in racial and ethnic minority and MSM communities, an additional factor, "assortive mixing," may further contribute to persistently higher rates of syphilis infection among black MSM.[232,233] Black MSM are more likely to be in a sexual partnership with other black MSM, all of whom live in communities with a high incidence and prevalence of syphilis, increasing the chance of infection.

Congenital Syphilis

Socioepidemiologic factors that have been associated with congenital syphilis epidemics in the past, such as poverty, unemployment, substance use, transactional sex for money or drugs, lack of prenatal care, and screening and other social disadvantages, along with fear and mistrust of government and healthcare systems,[173,234–238] may be contributing to the heterosexual and congenital syphilis epidemic that began emerging in 2013, but the drivers and determinates for these rising rates since 2013 have been less well studied.[239–242] Recent increases in syphilis infections in heterosexuals could be related to changes in social determinants of health[243] and changes in MSMW and MSW sexual networks. Based on public health case investigations of women with syphilis in the United States, risk factors for syphilis among women, especially pregnant women, in 2016 and 2017 included multiple sex partners, having a sex partner with multiple sex partners or a partner with a history of incarceration, unstable housing, substance use disorders, history of incarceration and history of exchanging sex for drugs or money.[242–244]

Substance use is an important driver of rising syphilis rates. Trends of substance use among women with syphilis, including pregnant women with syphilis, are particularly concerning. Since 2012, increases in methamphetamine, heroin, and injection drug use among women with primary or secondary syphilis have been reported. In 2017, 25% of women reported methamphetamine, heroin, and/or injection drug use and/or sex with a person who injects drugs, a 79% increase relative to 2014 (14%).[244] These increases among women were reported in every region of the country and methamphetamine was the most common drug described. Increases in drug use or sex with a partner who injects drugs have also been seen among heterosexual men with primary or secondary syphilis, although to a lesser degree (19% in 2017 and 12% in 2014). Pregnant women with substance use and syphilis may not utilize prenatal care services out of fear of drug testing and losing custody of their baby, especially if they live in states where substance use during pregnancy is legally classified as child abuse.

Congenital syphilis is entirely preventable, and every case is a sentinel event, representing a failure of the public health and/or healthcare system. Among pregnant women with syphilis, late or no prenatal care is significantly associated with delivering an infant with congenital syphilis.[245] Overall, in 2018, among mothers with a baby reported with congenital syphilis, 34% had had no prenatal care at all or prenatal care too late to screen and treat in time to prevent congenital syphilis. Eleven percent received prenatal care but were not screened; 37% were screened but not adequately treated, sometimes because benzathine penicillin G was not available at the time of the prenatal visit and they were referred for treatment but lost to follow-up; and 14% had an initial negative screening test but acquired syphilis during pregnancy and were not re-screened at 28 weeks, presumably due to a failure to identify risk.[246] The resurgence of congenital syphilis in the United States points to missed opportunities for prevention. Improvements in prenatal care utilization, screening, and treatment of pregnant women and prevention of unintended pregnancies are important to reduce congenital syphilis in the United States.[247]

PREVENTION AND CONTROL

The core strategies for a population-based STI prevention and control program were first outlined by Surgeon General Dr. Thomas Parran in "Shadow on the Land" in 1937.[248] For centuries previous approaches had focused on incarceration (isolation) for those infected and quarantine of those thought to be possibly infected (e.g., prostitutes). Tools to diagnose and treat syphilis were needed for prevention and control to become a reality, and these tools became available early in the twentieth century. At the time however, syphilis prevention, control, and public awareness were but a whisper—the subject was simply taboo in the early twentieth century. Despite this situation on the national level, California in 1912 established a law requiring physicians to report "venereal diseases" (VD), and by 1917 several other states had adopted similar measures. During World War I, venereal disease, especially syphilis, was costing the U.S. military millions in lost service days and could no longer be ignored. In 1918, the Chamberlain-Kahn Act appropriated several million dollars for the Public Health Service to assist states with venereal disease control programs.[2] However, little concerted effort was made regarding syphilis control for the 20 years prior to Dr. Parran's publication in 1937. Dr. Parran first launched a program of public education and spoke openly about syphilis to pierce the silence, despite protests. The 1938 National Venereal Disease Control Act was passed,[2] authorizing financial assistance to states for VD control, an appropriation that has continued to the present, with CDC currently distributing STD prevention and control funds to state and local health departments to, among other STD priorities, implement syphilis prevention and control strategies.

There are many themes in the Shadow on the Land that still are highly relevant to current approaches to STI prevention and control.[248] First, Dr. Parran outlined the need for a government role in the prevention and control of a private but social disease, while others argued at that time that sexual activity is a voluntary activity and that individuals should take responsibility for their actions. Global HIV prevention programs [e.g., President's Emergency Plan for AIDS Relief (PEPFAR)] are a clear example of how government support and intervention can improve the health and social wellbeing of a society. Second, Dr. Parran provided a platform for action, recognizing that while there were still many unsolved scientific questions about syphilis, diagnostic and treatment tools available at the time were good enough. He accused public health practitioners of "muddy thinking and easy talking," and for this reason, he had the Public Health Service convene a national conference of over 900 state and local health officers, VD clinic directors, syphilis specialists, medical educators, public health nurses, and social workers to draw up a plan. The plan became the platform for action and included a three-pronged approach.[248] First, every case must be located and reported, and its source ascertained, with all contacts followed-up and tested to find additional cases. Second, enough money, drugs, and doctors must be available to treat all cases, as treatment is the best control approach; treatment delays were not acceptable from a public health perspective. Efforts to raise the "index of suspicion of syphilis" among doctors were paramount. Third, public health agencies and private providers must be realigned to provide a united front, and citizens must be informed of the means to protect themselves. In addition to contact tracing programs for all reported cases, screening programs were proposed at all medical examinations and hospital admissions, as well as for employment applications, life insurance policies, and marriage licenses, to identify asymptomatic infections. VD clinics were established to treat symptomatic individuals and asymptomatic contacts.

Dr. Parran's simple formula for his platform of action was: "teamwork of government, professionals, industry and citizens + money for drugs and facilities + trained professionals for finding cases, for treating cases and for teaching the nation the importance of doing these things and doing them well = eradication of syphilis."[248] He went further, stating that "all of us, physicians, public health officials and citizens, together must learn to think of syphilis scientifically as a dangerous communicable disease rather than moralistically as a punishment for sin," which is "everybody business" in terms of "costs everyone pays for, lives that can be saved, suffering lessened and homes unbroken." In the years following the publication of the Shadow on the Land and the passage of the National Venereal Disease Control Act, the dream of syphilis eradication was thought to be a certainty. Cases declined dramatically from the 1940s to 1956, when the number of cases reported nationally increased for the first time. Many factors may have contributed to the stuttering rise in syphilis cases in the United States in the years following 1956, including public apathy related to the overoptimism generated by the availability of effective penicillin treatment; de-emphasis of syphilis control programs by both public health and medical professional organizations; and decreased appropriations in support of syphilis control. A task force report to the Surgeon General in 1962 recommended principles, methods and a feasible timeline that would lead to the eradication of syphilis by 1972, but again eradication was not achieved.[179] Following enhanced syphilis prevention efforts in heterosexual communities beginning in the 1990s and a simultaneous decline in crack cocaine use, reported cases of infectious syphilis reached an all-time low in the United States in 2000. The dream of elimination was again renewed.

In 1999, when syphilis was close to its nadir nationally, CDC launched the National Campaign to Eliminate Syphilis from the United States.[180] The rationale for elimination was that syphilis was considered epidemiologically vulnerable for reasons outlined for other infectious diseases. First, syphilis has been genetically stable, unlike gonorrhea. Second, there is no nonhuman reservoir or vector, and transmission is relatively inefficient. Last, except for pregnant women, persons with syphilis are not contagious unless they are symptomatic. There are also some important lessons learned from the smallpox eradication program. While the first smallpox strategy was mass vaccination, even in countries with high vaccine coverage (i.e., up to 95%) transmission continued. Therefore, an additional strategy was needed- a surveillance containment strategy, which included detection and isolation of active cases and intense vaccination efforts in the case household and the population surrounding the case or cases.[249] These are some commonalities with current syphilis prevention and control approaches. Rapid detection and timely treatment of infected individuals and their sexual partners has always been the main syphilis prevention and control strategy. While quarantine and isolation were used prior to the availability of syphilis treatment, it was a strategy that contributed to stigma and discrimination against vulnerable populations, such as prostitutes, in the nineteenth century.

Although no vaccine against syphilis exists, the availability of low-cost diagnostic tests, single dose therapy and the absence of antimicrobial resistance all were thought to be assets in the syphilis elimination effort.[181] The approach to syphilis elimination also supported multiple public health goals, including opportunities to improve public health infrastructure, such as infectious disease control and bioterrorism preparedness; reduce disparities; improve HIV prevention, reproductive health, and infant health; produce substantial cost savings; and address the unfinished history and broken trust resulting from the U.S. Syphilis Study in Tuskegee, Alabama. The plan was ambitious and amplified traditional approaches with community approaches to create synergies and achieve greater population-level impact. The goal was to reduce primary and secondary cases of syphilis in the United States to 1000 cases or fewer (a rate of 0.4 per 100,000 population) and increase the proportion of syphilis free counties to 90% by 2005.[180] Although the standard syphilis prevention and control strategies (enhance surveillance, expand clinical and laboratory services, enhance health promotion, strengthen community involvement and partnership, and rapid outbreak response) were intensified,[180] no new or innovative approaches were implemented.

Following implementation of the syphilis elimination effort, results were mixed, as exemplified by the "tale of two cities." In Marion County, Indiana, in 1999, the heterosexual syphilis epidemic was driven by poverty, drug use, prostitution, limited access to care, and lack of community awareness. By investing in a comprehensive health equity approach and recognizing the power of communities, appropriate media venues, the need for culturally sensitive healthcare facilities and the importance of community trust and leadership, Marion County was able to reverse its syphilis trends.[250,251] In San Francisco County, California, in 1999, on the other hand, drivers of the increase in syphilis included increasing use of the internet to identify partners and use of the private healthcare system for syphilis care rather than the STI clinic, where drop-in, confidential same day treatment and partner services were provided by syphilis clinical experts. The San Francisco approach included investments in innovations, such as offering syphilis serologic tests online, online partner services where patients could confidentially notify a partner online, and healthy penis campaigns.[252–254] Traditional contact tracing approaches seemed to have limited impact and more holistic sexual health models were emerging as possibly being more effective. Despite these investments and innovations, however, progress unraveled in San Francisco and elsewhere and an unprecedented resurgence of syphilis cases among MSM has occurred since the early 2000s. Studies suggest that the approximately 33–50% decline in syphilis cases among MSM seen in the early 1990s could be attributed to AIDS mortality.[174] By 2004, more that 60% of infectious cases of syphilis were among MSM, compared with approximately 30% of infectious cases in the early 1990s.

In 2006, CDC revised the national syphilis elimination plan.[255] New targets included an overall rate of 2.2 per 100,000 population by 2010 (4.2 per 100,000 men, and 0.38 per 100,000 women) and a rate of congenital syphilis of 3.9 per 100,000 live births. The updated plan focused on three goals: investment in and enhancement of public health services and interventions; prioritization of evidence-based, culturally competent interventions; and accountable services and interventions (Table 120-1).[255] Yet, local jurisdictions often faced differing phases of syphilis epidemics, requiring different interventions at the individual, community, and structural level, which complicated an effective national response strategy. Over time, changes in epidemiology, sexual networks, and social environments have presented challenges for any syphilis elimination efforts.[256] Syphilis is now increasingly diagnosed in the private sector, raising concerns about the impact of rapid diagnosis, timely treatment, and partner services. The STI specialty clinic infrastructure and disease investigation staff of the public sector have faced rising demands and declining resources. The social disadvantage of individuals and their communities, in addition to persistent racism, homophobia, stigma, and discrimination, continues to drive rising syphilis rates. In addition, there is a recognition that syphilis control efforts should focus more upstream in the health impact pyramid,[257] on social determinants of health,[258] on holistic sexual health approaches[224,256] and more on sexual and social networks rather than on just the infected individuals,[259–261] in order to target prevention efforts where transmission is most likely to be occurring within networks.

The goals of syphilis prevention and control have been primary prevention (i.e., preventing infection primarily through education and counseling) and secondary prevention (i.e., identifying and treating infections through screening programs, partner services and STI specialty clinic services) to prevent future infections and adverse health outcomes (i.e., disease). In 1988, the Anderson and May equation provided a framework for sexually transmitted infection prevention and control (Fig. 120-6).[262] This framework can be used to inform the selection of interventions to reduce the average number of secondary cases that arise from one primary case, known as the reproductive rate of infection or Ro. If *Ro* is >1, then the epidemic increases, if $= 1$, then the epidemic stabilizes and if < 1, an epidemic dies out. Three factors influence Ro for STI transmission in a community: transmission efficiency (beta), duration of infectiousness (*D*),

TABLE 120-1 THE 3-BY-3 APPROACH TO SYPHILIS ELIMINATION IN THE UNITED STATES

Syphilis Elimination Goal	Syphilis Elimination Strategies
Investment in, and enhancement of, public health services and interventions	1. Improve and enhance syphilis surveillance and outbreak response. 2. Improve and quality assure clinical and partner services. 3. Improve and quality assure laboratory services.
Prioritization of evidence-based, culturally competent interventions	1. Mobilization of affected communities. 2. Tailoring intervention strategies for affected populations. 3. Mobilization of, and creating alliances with health care providers.
Accountable services and interventions	1. Training and staff development. 2. Evidence-based action planning, monitoring, and evaluation. 3. Research and development.

Source: Centers for Disease Control and Prevention. Together We Can. The National Plan to Eliminate Syphilis from the United States. Atlanta, GA: US Dept of Health and Human Services; 2006.

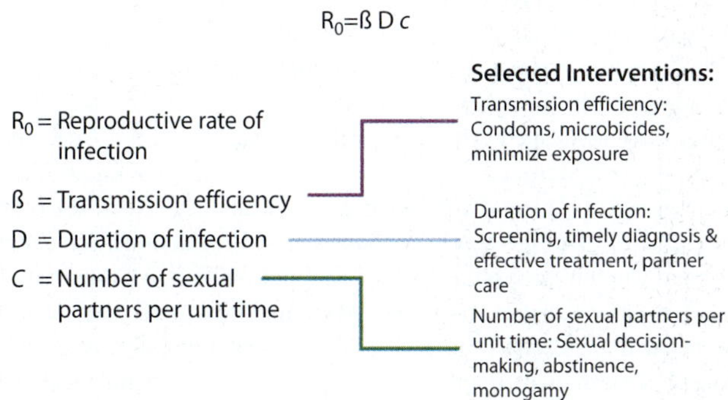

FIGURE 120-6. Selected interventions based on STI transmission dynamics at the population level. (*Source:* Anderson RM, May RM. *Infectious Diseases of Humans: Dynamics and Control*. Oxford, England: Oxford University Press; 1991.)

and the mean rate of sexual partner change per unit of time (c). Each factor gives rise to a potential intervention point; together, such interventions may have not merely an additive effect, but rather a multiplicative effect. Interventions that reduce the efficiency of transmission (beta) for each sexual partner contact, such as use of condoms or microbicides; treatment of primary or secondary syphilis lesions; or other strategies to minimize exposure to or infectiousness of lesions can impact the *Ro*. Interventions that reduce the duration of infectiousness (D), such as screening, timely diagnosis and effective treatment, as well as partner treatment, can also reduce the *Ro*. The natural history of syphilis and the host response limit the duration of infectiousness, as infectious lesions resolve even without treatment. This unique biologic characteristic of syphilis, compared to other sexually transmitted infections, renders syphilis transmission more difficult by innately reducing the duration of infectiousness. This raises the question of whether syphilis is more dependent on the number of sex partner changes per unit time (c) than chlamydia or gonorrhea infections. The mean rate of sexual partner change per unit of time (c) is influenced by the number of sexual partners per unit of time, the number of concurrent sexual partners per unit of time, and monogamy or abstinence.

Traditionally, the biomedical secondary prevention approaches of screening and partner services have been the cornerstone of syphilis prevention and control programs but have never been brought to scale. The impact of primary prevention approaches has been variable because of the influence of numerous factors, including resources at the individual, community, and societal level. The absence of a syphilis vaccine is another limitation. Until new pre- and postexposure prevention strategies, including vaccines are developed, syphilis screening and partner services will remain pivotal in identifying and treating infected individuals, because most patients infected with syphilis are unaware of their infection.

Screening Programs

Screening programs are designed to test apparently well people to find those at increased risk of a disease; earlier diagnosis improves survival or quality of life as the clinician has the time to make and manage the diagnosis before symptoms develop and the asymptomatic patient with an earlier diagnosis is willing to comply with the intervention. The effectiveness of the screening program needs to be established and the cost and accuracy of the test acceptable to the patient and society.[263,264]

As with any targeted screening program, clinician awareness of the latest surveillance and epidemiologic data for their specific patient populations and geographic area is paramount so those who can benefit from syphilis screening are tested. Community prevalence and sociodemographic factors may rapidly change over time, depending on the phase of the syphilis epidemic. Therefore, health departments must track the latest data on rates of syphilis by geographic location, subpopulations, and social factors and disseminate findings to clinicians in their jurisdictions, so that clinicians can adapt their syphilis screening criteria to match current transmission trends. Frequency of syphilis screening in those most vulnerable to syphilis acquisition must also be adapted to local syphilis rates and trends.

Nonpregnant Adult Screening

Syphilis screening, in contrast, is not as broad in population-based recommendations as chlamydia and gonorrhea screening guidelines. The USPSTF makes evidenced-based recommendations about the effectiveness of preventive clinical care services for individuals without signs or symptoms. In 2016, the USPSTF updated its 2004 recommendations on screening for syphilis in nonpregnant adults.[265,266] They found convincing evidence that syphilis screening in nonpregnant adults at increased risk of syphilis provides overall substantial health benefit. The "A" recommendation indicated that accurate screening tests were available and effective antibiotics can cure infection, prevent further transmission to others, and prevent progression to later stages of disease, with no evidence of associated harms. Screening with either nontreponemal or treponemal tests was determined to be accurate but required confirmatory testing. The evidence review identified the need for further research in three critical areas: effect of screening on clinical outcomes, effectiveness of screening strategies and harm of screening. Of note, the USPSTF does not consider cost-effectiveness in their evidence-based reviews.

The USPSTF review identified MSM, men and women living with HIV and selected racial and ethnic groups as being the groups most vulnerable to acquiring syphilis. Other risk factors identified included persons living in communities with a high prevalence of syphilis and sociodemographic risk factors, such as history of incarceration, history of commercial sex work, selected race/ethnicity, and being a male younger than 29 years of age. Furthermore, screening of those MSM most vulnerable to syphilis acquisition every 3 months enhanced detection of syphilis. The net benefit of screening persons unlikely to be at risk of syphilis was found to be low. Based on the nontreponemal and treponemal test performance characteristics in low prevalence populations, high rates of false positive test results leading to unnecessary antibiotic treatment and stigma can be harmful, so screening in low risk populations is not recommended. In general, CDC syphilis screening guidelines in nonpregnant adults mirror the USPSTF guidelines; CDC recommends at least annual syphilis screening for MSM and persons living with HIV and those who have risk factors for syphilis or live in communities with a high prevalence of infection.

MSM Screening

Despite guidelines to screen MSM annually for syphilis being in place for over 15 years, this recommended syphilis prevention strategy is still underutilized in the United States.[267] The CDC HIV Medical Monitoring Project interviews persons living with HIV to assess prevention services received and reviews their medical records to determine if STI screening is documented.[268,269] Among 2194 MSM living with HIV sampled during the 2015–16 cycle,[269] 69% had been tested for syphilis in the past 12 months. When syphilis testing rates were compared between patients receiving care at Ryan White Program (RWP)-funded facilities and those receiving care at nonfunded facilities, a significantly higher percentage of patients at RWP-funded facilities had testing in the past 12 months for syphilis (74% versus 60%, respectively). Barriers to annual syphilis screening among MSM and screening at more frequent intervals, if indicated, deserve further examination so syphilis screening rates can be optimized and brought to scale for MSM populations.

Pregnant Women Screening

Syphilis screening in pregnant women, a key component of congenital syphilis prevention strategies, has been a population-level recommendation for decades. Most states have laws requiring prenatal syphilis screening. CDC has been monitoring state statutes and regulations regarding screening for syphilis during pregnancy since 2016.[270] In 2016, only six states (12%) did not require prenatal syphilis screening. Most states ($n = 38$, 84%) with syphilis prenatal screening requirements recommended screening around the time of the first prenatal visit. An additional screening test at the beginning of the third trimester was required for all pregnant women in 12 states and was required only if the woman was at increased risk in five states. In 2016, only three states required screening for syphilis at delivery for all pregnancies, while five states required it only if the woman was at increased risk. Since then, some jurisdictions have changed prenatal syphilis regulations or laws to require screening three times in pregnancy for all pregnant women (i.e., at the first visit, at 28 weeks and at delivery) in response to the resurgence of congenital syphilis in their jurisdictions.

In 2018, the USPSTF re-reviewed the 2009 recommendation on screening for syphilis in pregnant women.[271,272] They re-affirmed the 2009 category "A" recommendation that screening for syphilis early in all pregnant women, even if a pregnant woman is at very low risk, provides substantial health benefit with small associated harms. Harms identified include false positive results in low risk pregnant women or those living in low prevalence areas, which can cause anxiety and stigma, especially for women in monogamous relationships. False positive results can also cause overtreatment, which can cause substantial harm in the penicillin-allergic pregnant women; such women need to be desensitized in an intensive-care unit to be treated.

Pregnant women should be tested for syphilis when they first present for prenatal care. CDC, the American Academy of Pediatrics (AAP) and the American College of Obstetricians and Gynecologists (ACOG) agree with this recommendation. CDC also recommends that for the women with erratic healthcare seeking behavior, the syphilis screening test should coincide with the pregnancy test, instead of waiting for the first prenatal care visit.[49] USPSTF further recommends that for pregnant women with no prenatal care, syphilis screening should occur at delivery. CDC also recommends that for pregnant women whose first healthcare encounter is when they are in labor, the woman and her infant should not be discharged from the hospital until the results of her syphilis screening tests are known.[49] The USPSTF found no studies that examined the benefits and harms of repeated testing for syphilis during pregnancy and remained silent on the frequency of screening during pregnancy after the first healthcare visit.[272] The USPSTF review also reaffirmed that the screening tests are accurate for detecting syphilis in pregnant women. Lastly, this 2018 review identified research gaps in the evidence for syphilis screening and treatment in pregnant women, including the need for evidence about the optimal use of different screening algorithms in pregnancy, rescreening intervals, the populations to rescreen, and treatment options in addition to penicillin to treat syphilis in pregnancy. Addressing these research gaps could greatly improve syphilis screening and treatment programs for pregnant women and the prevention of congenital syphilis.

Cases studies and CDC congenital syphilis surveillance data have identified pregnant women with an initial negative syphilis screening test, and who then acquired syphilis during their pregnancy, had no further screening and delivered a baby with congenital syphilis.[245,246] Given the extremely high rate of fetal infection in pregnant women with primary and secondary syphilis, these are important cases that must be identified and treated to maximize the opportunity to prevent congenital syphilis. CDC, AAP, and ACOG all recommend repeat screening for syphilis at 28 weeks of gestation and again at delivery for pregnant women who live in communities or geographic areas with a high prevalence of syphilis, those living with HIV, and those who are at increased risk of acquisition of syphilis, such as those with substance use disorders, a history of incarceration, commercial sex work or experiencing homelessness.[49] Additionally, late entry into prenatal care (first visit in the second trimester or later) or no prenatal care is significantly associated with congenital syphilis.[245] CDC, AAP, and ACOG also recommend re-testing after treatment for a known sexual exposure to a case of syphilis, if serologically negative at the time of treatment.[49] Despite guidelines, statutes and regulations, screening pregnant women for syphilis has been suboptimal in the United States and globally for decades. Improvements to maximize screening rates in these women are urgently needed.[273–276] Congenital syphilis case review boards have provided opportunities to identify gaps in syphilis prenatal screening programs and areas for program improvement.[277] Matching female syphilis and congenital syphilis surveillance data with vital statistics data along with testing all women for syphilis who deliver a stillborn baby may provide additional surveillance data on stillbirths to inform public health and healthcare prevention interventions, as syphilitic stillbirths are often undiagnosed.[278]

Partner Services

Partner services, formally referred to as contact tracing, have been the foundation of the U.S. syphilis prevention and control strategy since the 1940s.[248] Further transmission of syphilis and re-infection of patients after syphilis treatment can be reduced by timely referral of sexual partners for evaluation, testing, presumptive treatment (i.e., postexposure prophylaxis), counseling, and linkage to other care and social support services. The goal of partner services is to increase the number of infected individuals treated and to disrupt transmission networks. The essential components of partner services programs are: (1) identification of patients who may benefit from partner services; (2) identification of sexual partners who are at risk of infection or possible exposure, which is known as partner elicitation; (3) notification of partners of their possible infection; and (4) partner management.[279] The process of partner services includes efforts undertaken by the patient, medical provider, and/or the public health department. Patients may elect to notify their sexual partner(s) of the syphilis exposure, which is known as self-referral of sexual partners. Healthcare providers may elicit information about partners from their patients with syphilis and notify the partner(s), which is known as provider referral, advise patients to bring in their primary sexual partner with them when they return for treatment, or may inform their patient about health department partner services and refer them to the their local health department. For years, public health departments in most areas of the United States routinely have attempted to provide partner services for all patients reported with early syphilis (primary, secondary, and early latent syphilis) or for patients with reported laboratory results suggestive of infectious syphilis (e.g., high nontrepnomal titer > 1:16).[279,281] Health department partner services programs are voluntary and confidential. They are provided by highly trained staff, known as Disease Intervention Specialists (DIS) or Communicable Disease Investigators (CDI), with exceptional interpersonal skills in motivational interviewing, cultural humility and competency, emotional intelligence, problem solving, and active listening. These staffs understand the legal basis for partner services in the health department that has the legal authority to provide partner services, including the jurisdiction's statutory authority and case laws relevant to the protection of individual privacy and confidentiality; the duty or privilege to warn; and the protection of health department liability. Because of the health department advantage in protecting confidentiality, patients and providers may prefer to have the health department notify partners for syphilis.

Syphilis patients who warrant partner services are determined locally, depending on priorities and resources, making it necessary for healthcare providers to familiarize themselves with the partner services policies and procedures in their jurisdictions. The ultimate responsibility for ensuring the treatment of partners rests with the healthcare provider and the patient. If time is spent by providers counseling patients about the benefits of syphilis partner services, notification outcomes can be improved. Embedding syphilis DIS in clinics serving populations most vulnerable to syphilis acquisition has also improved syphilis partner elicitation and notification outcomes.[281,282] In addition, the success of partner services programs depends on effective sharing of individual-level information among health department staff to: ensure confidentiality; clear quality-assurance policies and procedures; recognize the rights of individuals with syphilis and their partners; have sensitivity to healthcare provider relationships with their patients; and engage providers and communities to increase awareness of the partner services processes.

Prioritizing syphilis patients for partner services traditionally has included consideration of clinical and socioepidemiologic factors that affect the likelihood of further transmission in a community, although pregnant women with any stage of syphilis should always be a priority. In general, the stage of syphilitic infection is used to determine the potential infectiousness of the patient and the risk of infection in their sexual partners (i.e., primary, secondary, and early latent syphilis stages). Next, the estimated duration of infectiousness is ascertained by the stage of syphilis and the duration of symptoms or signs and is used to calculate the timeframe for which contacts should be elicited, which is known as the disease interview period or contact elicitation window. For patients with primary syphilis, contacts exposed within 3 months of the patient's diagnosis plus the duration of the primary lesion(s) should be elicited; for secondary syphilis, 6 months plus the duration of secondary symptoms; and for early latent, 12 months from the first serologic evidence of syphilitic infection. Sexually active patients with insufficient information to establish the duration of infection (i.e., syphilis of unknown duration) and who are vulnerable to recent syphilis acquisition should be managed for purposes of partner services as if they have early latent syphilis. If there is evidence of syphilitic infection of greater than 1 year, then the likelihood of the patient being infectious in the past year is considered negligible and testing of their current partner is appropriate.[49] For all sexual partners who had contact with a patient with infectious syphilis within the past 90 days, CDC recommends presumptive treatment with an IM injection of Benzathine penicillin G 2.4 million units, even in the absence of clinical findings and even if serologic results are negative. If the exposure was more than 90 days in the past, which is considered the maximum incubation period for syphilis, and the serologic results are negative, then the contact is considered to be uninfected.[49] Retesting of syphilis contacts is recommended according to syphilis screening guidelines.

For populations in whom the number of anonymous sexual partners is substantial (e.g., among persons who use geosocial networking applications for identifying partners or who exchange sex for drugs, etc.), innovative screening programs,[283,284] targeted mass treatment if effective oral syphilis regimens are available,[285] or pre- or postexposure prophylaxis[286,287] may be a more effective syphilis prevention and control approach for increasing identification and treatment of infected persons and reducing community transmission rather than traditional partner notification programs.

As trends in communication and technology have advanced and more sexually active persons use technologic platforms to identify partners, health departments have begun using technology-based partner services strategies as part of the partner service program portfolio when traditional face-to-face partner services approaches are time consuming and do not elicit enough locating information to perform partner notification. Technologies such as phone calls, texting, face chat, mobile applications, and social media websites provide new, more efficient opportunities for reaching more partners at a scale not possible with face-to-face methods and existing health department staffing levels.[288,289] In some areas, patients have the option to use internet sites to send anonymous emails or text messages advising partners of their possible exposure to syphilis.[253,290–293] Whether these novel partner services methods actually result in treatment of sexual partners deserves further study, but a recent structured review shows promising results.[294] If the only alternatives are no notification versus anonymous notification, the latter could be a better option.

It should be noted that data on the cost-effectiveness of syphilis partner services to reduce the burden of infections in a community are limited and can vary by population and community sociocultural-epidemiologic factors. For MSM, the cost-effectiveness of traditional partner services at a population level remains unproven.[295] Additionally, the number of patient interviews necessary to identify an infected partner was approximately 10 in 2003,[296,297] well before the erosion of the public health infrastructure in the late 2000s. Some have suggested that partners services should be more targeted to increase efficiency[298] or focus on sexual or social network interventions rather than individual syphilis case patients' efforts.[216,260,299,300] Others have proposed that partners services for MSM with syphilis have more impact on HIV prevention outcomes than syphilis[301] and should be seen as a targeted HIV prevention strategy to identify new HIV infections and those who might benefit from PrEP because syphilis is an important biologic risk marker for HIV acquisition.[302,303] Thus, completely different syphilis prevention paradigms for MSM such as more holistic comprehensive sexual health approaches have also been recommended.[224,256,259,260,299,300] Further studies of the role of partner services approaches and more holistic comprehensive sexual health approaches influencing syphilis transmission dynamics among MSM are needed to inform cost-effective prevention strategies likely to have the highest population impact. While partner services have been widely adopted as a standard congenital syphilis prevention strategy, the utility of this approach in contributing to reduced incidence of congenital syphilis also remains unverified and deserves further study.[247,280] Partner services are not effective in reducing syphilis transmission and burden of infection in a population if the majority of partners cannot be located.

MOVING FORWARD

Despite the availability of a highly effective treatment (i.e., penicillin G), the lessons learned from the history of syphilis prevention and control efforts are that syphilis continues to thrive. Effective treatment is not enough to eliminate this infection as implementation of timely treatment is influenced by community education, awareness, and engagement; political will; access and use of clinical services; and sigma, discrimination, and social and behavioral factors. Thus, a narrowly focused biomedical testing and treatment approach has proven to have a limited and inadequate impact. An effective syphilis vaccine is critically needed to augment current screening and treatment programs to reverse current rising syphilis rates and reduce adverse health outcomes.[304–306] Other primary prevention strategies for syphilis such as individual education and counseling and social media campaigns have been under studied, under resourced, or found to only have modest, short-term benefits.[307]

In 2017, CDC releases a Call to Action, asking other federal agencies, partners, and various sectors of society to "Work Together to Stem the Tide of Rising Syphilis in the United States." The report identified specific actions that are needed for specific populations, including pregnant women; MSM; healthcare providers and healthcare systems; public health departments; biomedical scientists, universities, and industry; decision makers; and community members and leaders. The report also highlighted that new tools for syphilis prevention and control are needed to supplement those in use since the 1940s. Syphilis prevention and control efforts will require differentiating primary and secondary prevention goals for specific populations (i.e., reducing adverse health outcomes of neurosyphilis and ocular syphilis among MSM and reducing syphilis and unwanted pregnancies in women to prevent congenital syphilis). Syphilis prevention and control efforts must also address the diversity of socioepidemiologic factors and their interactions and tailor interventions accordingly. Host and biologic factors, cultural and social context, network transmission dynamics, and community burden all need to be considered in designing future syphilis prevention and control programs.

ACKNOWLEDGMENT

The author wishes to thank Amber Herald for her excellent work in helping to prepare the manuscript.

References

1. Harper KN, Zuckerman MK, Harper ML, Kingston JD, Armelagos GJ. The origin and antiquity of syphilis revisited: An appraisal of Old World pre-Columbian evidence for treponemal infection. *Am J Phys Anthropol.* 2011;146 Suppl 53:99–133.
2. US Public Health Service. *Syphilis: A Synopsis.* Vol. 1660. Atlanta, GA: Public Health Service Publication; 1968.
3. Smibert RM. Genus III. Treponema Schaudinn 1905. In: *Bergey's Manual of Systematic Bacteriology*. Vol. 1. Baltimore: Williams and Wilkins; 1984, pp. 49–57.
4. Dennie CC. *A History of Syphilis*. Springfield, Illinois: Charles C. Thomas Publishers; 1962.
5. Lafond RE, Lukehart SA. Biological basis for syphilis. *Clin Microbiol Rev.* 2006;19(1):29–49.
6. Mahoney J, Bryant K. Contact infection of rabbits in experimental syphilis. *Am J Syph.* 1933;17:188–93.
7. Radolf JD, Lukehart SA. *Pathogenic Treponema: Molecular and Cellular Biology*. Norfolk, England: Caister Academic Press; 2006.
8. Turner TB, Hardy PH, Newman B. Infectivity tests in syphilis. *Br J Vener Dis.* 1969;45(3):183–95.
9. Magnuson HJ, Eagle H, Fleischman R. The minimal infectious inoculum of Spirochaeta pallida (Nichols strain) and a consideration of its rate of multiplication in vivo. *Am J Syph Gonorrhea Vener Dis.* 1948;32(1):1–18.
10. Charon NW, Greenberg EP, Koopman MB, Limberger RJ. Spirochete chemotaxis, motility, and the structure of the spirochetal periplasmic flagella. *Res Microbiol.* 1992;143(6):597–603.
11. Magnuson HJ, Thomas EW, Olansky S, Kaplan BI, De Mello L, Cutler JC. Inoculation syphilis in human volunteers. *Medicine (Baltimore).* 1956;35(1):33–82.
12. Cohen SE, Chew Ng RA, Katz KA, et al. Repeat syphilis among men who have sex with men in California, 2002–2006: Implications for syphilis elimination efforts. *Am J Public Health.* 2012;102(1):e1–8.
13. Centers for Disease Control and Prevention. Notes from the field: Repeat syphilis infection and HIV coinfection among men who have sex with men—Baltimore, Maryland, 2010–2011. *MMWR Morb Mortal Wkly Rep.* 2013;62(32):649–50.
14. Jain J, Santos GM, Scheer S, et al. Rates and correlates of syphilis reinfection in men who have sex with men. *LGBT Health.* 2017;4(3):232–6.
15. Grassly NC, Fraser C, Garnett GP. Host immunity and synchronized epidemics of syphilis across the United States. *Nature.* 2005;433(7024):417–21.
16. Fraser CM, Norris SJ, Weinstock GM, et al. Complete genome sequence of *Treponema pallidum*, the syphilis spirochete. *Science.* 1998;281(5375):375–88.
17. Radolf JD, Norgard MV, Schulz WW. Outer membrane ultrastructure explains the limited antigenicity of virulent *Treponema pallidum*. *Proc Natl Acad Sci U S A.* 1989;86(6):2051–5.
18. Radolf JD. Role of outer membrane architecture in immune evasion by *Treponema pallidum* and *Borrelia burgdorferi*. *Trends Microbiol.* 1994;2(9):307–11.
19. Pavis CS, Folds JD, Baseman JB. Cell-mediated immunity during syphilis. *Br J Vener Dis.* 1978;54(3):144–50.
20. Lukehart S, Baker-Zander S, Lloyd R, Sell S. Immunology and pathogenesis of syphilis. In: Quinn TC, Gallin JI, Fauci AS, eds. *Sexually Transmitted Diseases*. New York: Raven Press; 1992; No. 8.
21. Lukehart SA, Baker-Zander SA, Lloyd RM, Sell S. Characterization of lymphocyte responsiveness in early experimental syphilis. II. Nature of cellular infiltration and *Treponema pallidum* distribution in testicular lesions. *J Immunol.* 1980;124(1):461–7.
22. Baker-Zander SA, Lukehart SA. Macrophage-mediated killing of opsonized *Treponema pallidum*. *J Infect Dis.* 1992;165(1):69–74.
23. Pacha J, Metzger M, Smogór W, Michalska E, Podwińska J, Ruczkowska J. Effect of immunosuppressive agents on the course of experimental syphilis in rabbits. *Arch Immunol Ther Exp (Warsz).* 1979;27(1–2):45–51.
24. Rompalo AM, Lawlor J, Seaman P, Quinn TC, Zenilman JM, Hook EW3rd. Modification of syphilitic genital ulcer manifestations by coexistent HIV infection. *Sex Transm Dis.* 2001;28(8):448–54.
25. Rompalo AM, Joesoef MR, O'Donnell JA, et al. Clinical manifestations of early syphilis by HIV status and gender: Results of the syphilis and HIV study. *Sex Transm Dis.* 2001;28(3):158–65.
26. Buchacz K, Patel P, Taylor M, et al. Syphilis increases HIV viral load and decreases CD4 cell counts in HIV-infected patients with new syphilis infections. *AIDS.* 2004;18(15):2075–9.
27. Berger JR. Neurosyphilis in human immunodeficiency virus type 1-seropositive individuals. A prospective study. *Arch Neurol.* 1991;48(7):700–2.
28. Ghanem KG, Moore RD, Rompalo AM, Erbelding EJ, Zenilman JM, Gebo KA. Neurosyphilis in a clinical cohort of HIV-1-infected patients. *AIDS.* 2008;22(10):1145–51.
29. Sellati TJ, Wilkinson DA, Sheffield JS, Koup RA, Radolf JD, Norgard MV. Virulent *Treponema pallidum*, lipoprotein, and synthetic lipopeptides induce CCR5 on human monocytes and enhance their susceptibility to infection by human immunodeficiency virus type 1. *J Infect Dis.* 2000;181(1):283–93.
30. Gjestland T. The Oslo study of untreated syphilis; an epidemiologic investigation of the natural course of the syphilitic infection based upon a re-study of the Boeck-Bruusgaard material. *Acta Derm Venereol Suppl (Stockh).* 1955;35(Suppl 34):3–368; Annex I-LVI.
31. Schuman SH, Olansky S, Rivers E, Smith CA, Rambo DS. Untreated syphilis in the male negro; background and current status of patients in the Tuskegee study. *J Chronic Dis.* 1955;2(5):543–58.
32. Olansky S, Schuman SH, Peters JJ, Smith CA, Rambo DS. Untreated syphilis in the male Negro. X. Twenty years of clinical observation of untreated syphilitic and presumably nonsyphilitic groups. *J Chronic Dis.* 1956;4(2):177–85.
33. Heller JRJr, Bruyere PT. Untreated syphilis in the male Negro; mortality during 12 years of observation. *J Vener Dis Inf.* 1946;27:34–8.
34. Rockwell DH, Yobs AR, Moore MB Jr. The Tuskegee study of untreated syphilis: The 30th year of observation. *Arch Intern Med.* 1964;114:792–8.
35. Brandt AM. Racism and research: The case of the Tuskegee syphilis study. *Hastings Cent Rep.* 1978;8(6):21–9.

36. Brandt AM. *No Magic Bullet: A Social History of Venereal Disease in the United States Since 1880*. New York: Oxford University Press; 1987.

37. Jones JH. *Bad Blood: The Tuskegee Syphilis Experiment*. New York: Free Press; 1981.

38. Reverby SM. Ethical failures and history lessons: The US Public Health Service research studies in Tuskegee and Guatemala. *Public Health Rev*. 2012;34(1):1–18.

39. Rosahn PD. Autopsy studies in syphilis *J Vener Dis Inf*. 1947:28.

40. Hsu KK. Practical considerations for health care systems involvement in a renewed syphilis initiative. *Sex Transm Dis*. 2018;45(9S Suppl 1):S93–4.

41. Leichliter JS, Heyer K, Peterman TA, et al. US public sexually transmitted disease clinical services in an era of declining public health funding: 2013–14. *Sex Transm Dis*. 2017;44(8):505–9.

42. Levi J, Segal L St Laurent R, Lang A. *Investing in America's Health: A State-by-State Look at Public Health Funding and Key Health Facts*. Washington, DC: Robert Wood Johnson Foundation; 2012.

43. Stephens SC, Cohen SE, Philip SS, Bernstein KT. Insurance among patients seeking care at a municipal sexually transmitted disease clinic: Implications for health care reform in the United States. *Sex Transm Dis*. 2014;41(4):227–32.

44. Hook EW3rd. Syphilis. *Lancet*. 2017;389(10078):1550–7.

45. Ghanem KG, Ram S, Rice PA. The modern epidemic of syphilis. *N Engl J Med*. 2020;382(9):845–54.

46. Singh AE, Romanowski B. Syphilis: Review with emphasis on clinical, epidemiologic, and some biologic features. *Clin Microbiol Rev*. 1999;12(2):187–209.

47. Sparling PF, Swartz M, Musher D, Healy B. Clinical manifestations of syphilis. In: *Sexually Transmitted Diseases*. 4th ed. New York: McGraw Hill; 2008, pp. 661–84.

48. Stokes JH. *Modern Clinical Syphilology: Diagnosis, Treatment, Case Studies*. Philadelphia and London: WB Saunders Company; 1934.

49. Workowski KA, Bolan GA. Sexually transmitted diseases treatment guidelines, 2015. *MMWR Recomm Rep*. 2015;64(Rr-03):1–137.

50. Ghanem KG, Workowski KA. Management of adult syphilis. *Clin Infect Dis*. 2011;53 Suppl 3:S110–28.

51. Ghanem KG. Management of adult syphilis: Key questions to inform the 2015 Centers for Disease Control and Prevention sexually transmitted diseases treatment guidelines. *Clin Infect Dis*. 2015;61 Suppl 8:S818–36.

52. San Francisco City Clinic. *Primary and Secondary Syphilis Symptoms*. Atlanta, GA: Centers for Disease Control and Prevention; 2020.

53. Towns JM, Leslie DE, Denham I, Azzato F, Fairley CK, Chen M. Painful and multiple anogenital lesions are common in men with *Treponema pallidum* PCR-positive primary syphilis without herpes simplex virus coinfection: A cross-sectional clinic-based study. *Sex Transm Infect*. 2016;92(2):110–5.

54. World Health Organization. Manual of the international statistical classification of diseases, injuries, and causes of death: Based on the recommendations of the seventh revision Conference, 1955, and adopted by the ninth World Health Assembly under the WHO Nomenclature Regulations. World Health Organization; 1957.

55. Ropper AH. Neurosyphilis. *N Engl J Med*. 2019;381(14):1358–63.

56. Tamesis RR, Foster CS. Ocular syphilis. *Ophthalmology*. 1990;97(10):1281–7.

57. Merritt HH, Adams RO, Solomon HC. *Neurosyphilis*. New York: Oxford University Press; 1946.

58. Mills CH. Routine examination of the cerebro-spinal fluid in syphilis: Its value in regard to more accurate knowledge, prognosis, and treatment. *Br Med J*. 1927;2(3481):527–32.

59. Moore JE, Hopkins HH. Asymptomatic neurosyphilis: VI. The prognosis of early and late asymptomatic neurosyphilis. *JAMA*. 1930;95(22):1637–41.

60. Lukehart SA, Hook EW 3rd, Baker-Zander SA, Collier AC, Critchlow CW, Handsfield HH. Invasion of the central nervous system by *Treponema pallidum*: Implications for diagnosis and treatment. *Ann Intern Med*. 1988;109(11):855–62.

61. Marra CM, Maxwell CL, Smith SL, et al. Cerebrospinal fluid abnormalities in patients with syphilis: Association with clinical and laboratory features. *J Infect Dis*. 2004;189(3):369–76.

62. Tuddenham S, Ghanem KG. Neurosyphilis: Knowledge gaps and controversies. *Sex Transm Dis*. 2018;45(3):147–51.

63. Simon RP. Neurosyphilis. *Arch Neurol*. 1985;42(6):606–13.

64. Hook EW3rd. Syphilis and HIV infection. *J Infect Dis*. 1989;160(3):530–4.

65. Marra CM, Longstreth WT Jr, Maxwell CL, Lukehart SA. Resolution of serum and cerebrospinal fluid abnormalities after treatment of neurosyphilis. Influence of concomitant human immunodeficiency virus infection. *Sex Transm Dis*. 1996;23(3):184–9.

66. Flood JM, Weinstock HS, Guroy ME, Bayne L, Simon RP, Bolan G. Neurosyphilis during the AIDS epidemic, San Francisco, 1985–1992. *J Infect Dis*. 1998;177(4):931–40.

67. Ghanem KG, Moore RD, Rompalo AM, Erbelding EJ, Zenilman JM, Gebo KA. Antiretroviral therapy is associated with reduced serologic failure rates for syphilis among HIV-infected patients. *Clin Infect Dis*. 2008;47(2):258–65.

68. Pillay A. Centers for Disease Control and Prevention Syphilis Summit—Diagnostics and laboratory issues. *Sex Transm Dis*. 2018;45(9S Suppl 1): S13–6.

69. Centers for Disease Control and Prevention. *CDC Call to Action: Let's Work Together to Stem the Tide of Rising Syphilis in the United States*. Atlanta, GA: US Dept of Health and Human Services; 2017.

70. Association of Public Health Laboratories. *Consultation on Laboratory Diagnosis of Syphilis Meeting Summary Report*. Silver Spring, MD: Association of Public Health Laboratories; 2018.

71. Hart G. Syphilis tests in diagnostic and therapeutic decision making. *Ann Intern Med*. 1986;104(3):368–76.

72. Edmondson DG, Hu B, Norris SJ. Long-term *in vitro* culture of the syphilis spirochete *Treponema pallidum* subsp. *pallidum*. *MBio*. 2018;9(3):e01153-18.

73. Kennedy EJ, Creighton ET. Darkfield microscopy for the detection and identification of *Treponema pallidum*. In: *A Manual of Tests for Syphilis*. Washington, DC: American Public Health Association; 1990.

74. Larsen SA, Pope V, Johnson RE, Kennedy EJ. *A Manual of Tests for Syphilis*. Washington, DC: American Public Health Association; 1999.

75. Larsen SA, Steiner BM, Rudolph AH. Laboratory diagnosis and interpretation of tests for syphilis. *Clin Microbiol Rev*. 1995;8(1):1–21.

76. Romanowski B, Forsey E, Prasad E, Lukehart S, Tam M, Hook EW3rd. Detection of *Treponema pallidum* by a fluorescent monoclonal antibody test. *Sex Transm Dis*. 1987;14(3):156–9.

77. Orle KA, Gates CA, Martin DH, Body BA, Weiss JB. Simultaneous PCR detection of *Haemophilus ducreyi*, *Treponema pallidum*, and herpes simplex virus types 1 and 2 from genital ulcers. *J Clin Microbiol*. 1996;34(1):49–54.

78. Heymans R, van der Helm JJ, de Vries HJ, Fennema HS, Coutinho RA, Bruisten SM. Clinical value of *Treponema pallidum* real-time PCR for diagnosis of syphilis. *J Clin Microbiol*. 2010;48(2):497–502.

79. Gayet-Ageron A, Sednaoui P, Lautenschlager S, et al. Use of *Treponema pallidum* PCR in testing of ulcers for diagnosis of primary syphilis. *Emerg Infect Dis*. 2015;21(1):127–9.

80. Creegan L, Bauer HM, Samuel MC, Klausner J, Liska S, Bolan G. An evaluation of the relative sensitivities of the venereal disease research laboratory test and the *Treponema pallidum* particle agglutination test among patients diagnosed with primary syphilis. *Sex Transm Dis*. 2007;34(12):1016–8.

81. Zhou C, Zhang X, Zhang W, Duan J, Zhao F. PCR detection for syphilis diagnosis: Status and prospects. *J Clin Lab Anal*. 2019;33(5):e22890.

82. Nandwani R, Evans DT. Are you sure it's syphilis? A review of false positive serology. *Int J STD AIDS*. 1995;6(4):241–8.

83. Rompalo AM, Cannon RO, Quinn TC, Hook EW 3rd. Association of biologic false-positive reactions for syphilis with human immunodeficiency virus infection. *J Infect Dis*. 1992;165(6):1124–6.

84. Brown ST, Zaidi A, Larsen SA, Reynolds GH. Serological response to syphilis treatment. A new analysis of old data. *JAMA*. 1985;253(9):1296–9.

85. Romanowski B, Sutherland R, Fick GH, Mooney D, Love EJ. Serologic response to treatment of infectious syphilis. *Ann Intern Med*. 1991;114(12):1005–9.

86. Rolfs RT, Joesoef MR, Hendershot EF, et al. A randomized trial of enhanced therapy for early syphilis in patients with and without human immunodeficiency virus infection. The syphilis and HIV study group. *N Engl J Med*. 1997;337(5):307–14.

87. Ghanem KG, Erbelding EJ, Wiener ZS, Rompalo AM. Serological response to syphilis treatment in HIV-positive and HIV-negative patients attending sexually transmitted diseases clinics. *Sex Transm Infect*. 2007;83(2):97–101.

88. Sena AC, Wolff M, Martin DH, et al. Predictors of serological cure and Serofast State after treatment in HIV-negative persons with early syphilis. *Clin Infect Dis*. 2011;53(11):1092–9.

89. Seña AC, Zhang XH, Li T, et al. A systematic review of syphilis serological treatment outcomes in HIV-infected and HIV-uninfected persons: Rethinking the significance of serological non-responsiveness and the serofast state after therapy. *BMC Infect Dis*. 2015;15:479.

90. Jurado RL, Campbell J, Martin PD. Prozone phenomenon in secondary syphilis. Has its time arrived? *Arch Intern Med.* 1993;153(21):2496–8.
91. Post JJ, Khor C, Furner V, Smith DE, Whybin LR, Robertson PW. Case report and evaluation of the frequency of the prozone phenomenon in syphilis serology—An infrequent but important laboratory phenomenon. *Sex Health.* 2012;9(5):488–90.
92. Huber TW, Storms S, Young P, et al. Reactivity of microhemagglutination, fluorescent treponemal antibody absorption, Venereal Disease Research Laboratory, and rapid plasma reagin tests in primary syphilis. *J Clin Microbiol.* 1983;17(3):405–9.
93. Park IU, Fakile YF, Chow JM, et al. Performance of treponemal tests for the diagnosis of syphilis. *Clin Infect Dis.* 2019;68(6):913–8.
94. Bosshard PP. Usefulness of IgM-specific enzyme immunoassays for serodiagnosis of syphilis: Comparative evaluation of three different assays. *J Infect.* 2013;67(1):35–42.
95. Owusu-Edusei K Jr, Peterman TA, Ballard RC. Serologic testing for syphilis in the United States: A cost-effectiveness analysis of two screening algorithms. *Sex Transm Dis.* 2011;38(1):1–7.
96. Kay NS, Peeling RW, Mabey DC. State of the art syphilis diagnostics: Rapid point-of-care tests. *Expert Rev Anti Infect Ther.* 2014;12(1):63–73.
97. Phang Romero Casas C, Martyn-St James M, Hamilton J, Marinho DS, Castro R, Harnan S. Rapid diagnostic test for antenatal syphilis screening in low-income and middle-income countries: A systematic review and meta-analysis. *BMJ Open.* 2018;8(2):e018132.
98. Matthias J, Dwiggins P, Totten Y, Blackmore C, Wilson C, Peterman TA. Notes from the field: Evaluation of the sensitivity and specificity of a commercially available rapid syphilis test—Escambia County, Florida, 2016. *MMWR Morb Mortal Wkly Rep.* 2016;65(42):1174–5.
99. Pereira LE, McCormick J, Dorji T, et al. Laboratory evaluation of a commercially available rapid syphilis test. *J Clin Microbiol.* 2018;56(10):e00832-18.
100. Fakile YF, Brinson M, Mobley V, Park IU, Gaynor AM. Performance of the syphilis health check in clinic and laboratory-based settings. *Sex Transm Dis.* 2019;46(4):250–3.
101. Peterman TA, Fakile YF. What is the use of rapid syphilis tests in the United States? *Sex Transm Dis.* 2016;43(3):201–3.
102. Peeling RW, Ye H. Diagnostic tools for preventing and managing maternal and congenital syphilis: An overview. *Bull World Health Organ.* 2004;82(6):439–46.
103. Sena AC, Wolff M, Behets F, et al. Response to therapy following retreatment of serofast early syphilis patients with benzathine penicillin. *Clin Infect Dis.* 2013;56(3):420–2.
104. Seña AC, White BL, Sparling PF. Novel *Treponema pallidum* serologic tests: A paradigm shift in syphilis screening for the 21st century. *Clin Infect Dis.* 2010;51(6):700–8.
105. Centers for Disease Control and Prevention. Syphilis testing algorithms using treponemal tests for initial screening—Four laboratories, New York City, 2005–2006. *MMWR Morb Mortal Wkly Rep.* 2008;57(32): 872–5.
106. Centers for Disease Control and Prevention. Discordant results from reverse sequence syphilis screening—Five laboratories, United States, 2006–2010. *MMWR Morb Mortal Wkly Rep.* 2011;60(5):133–7.
107. Park IU, Chow JM, Bolan G, Stanley M, Shieh J, Schapiro JM. Screening for syphilis with the treponemal immunoassay: Analysis of discordant serology results and implications for clinical management. *J Infect Dis.* 2011;204(9):1297–304.
108. Thorley N, Adebayo M, Smit E, Radcliffe K. The management of isolated positive syphilis enzyme immunoassay results in HIV-negative patients attending a sexual health clinic. *Int J STD AIDS.* 2016;27(9):798–800.
109. Mmeje O, Chow JM, Davidson L, Shieh J, Schapiro JM, Park IU. Discordant syphilis immunoassays in pregnancy: Perinatal outcomes and implications for clinical management. *Clin Infect Dis.* 2015;61(7):1049–53.
110. Wong EH, Klausner JD, Caguin-Grygiel G, et al. Evaluation of an IgM/IgG sensitive enzyme immunoassay and the utility of index values for the screening of syphilis infection in a high-risk population. *Sex Transm Dis.* 2011;38(6):528–32.
111. Berry GJ, Loeffelholz MJ. Use of treponemal screening assay strength of signal to avoid unnecessary confirmatory testing. *Sex Transm Dis.* 2016;43(12):737–40.
112. Fakile YF, Jost H, Hoover KW, et al. Correlation of treponemal immunoassay signal strength values with reactivity of confirmatory treponemal testing. *J Clin Microbiol.* 2018;56(1):e01165-17.
113. Jaffe HW, Larsen SA, Peters M, Jove DF, Lopez B, Schroeter AL. Tests for treponemal antibody in CSF. *Arch Intern Med.* 1978;138(2):252–5.
114. Harding AS, Ghanem KG. The performance of cerebrospinal fluid treponemal-specific antibody tests in neurosyphilis: A systematic review. *Sex Transm Dis.* 2012;39(4):291–7.
115. Nicholas L. Treatment of early infectious syphilis with benzathine penicillin G. In: *Proceedings of World Forum on Syphilis and Other Treponematoses, September 4–8, 1962, Washington, DC.* Vol Public Health Service Publication No. 997. Washington, DC: U.S. Department of Health, Education, and Welfare, Public Health Service, Communicable Disease Center, Venereal Disease Branch; 1964:296–301.
116. Yang CJ, Lee NY, Chen TC, et al. One dose versus three weekly doses of benzathine penicillin G for patients co-infected with HIV and early syphilis: A multicenter, prospective observational study. *PLoS One.* 2014;9(10):e109667.
117. Ghanem KG, Erbelding EJ, Cheng WW, Rompalo AM. Doxycycline compared with benzathine penicillin for the treatment of early syphilis. *Clin Infect Dis.* 2006;42(6):e45–9.
118. Wong T, Singh AE, De P. Primary syphilis: Serological treatment response to doxycycline/tetracycline versus benzathine penicillin. *Am J Med.* 2008;121(10):903–8.
119. Dai T, Qu R, Liu J, Zhou P, Wang Q. Efficacy of doxycycline in the treatment of syphilis. *Antimicrob Agents Chemother.* 2017;61(1):e01092-16.
120. Salado-Rasmussen K, Hoffmann S, Cowan S, et al. Serological response to treatment of syphilis with doxycycline compared with penicillin in HIV-infected individuals. *Acta Derm Venereol.* 2016;96(6):807–11.
121. Augenbraun M, Workowski K. Ceftriaxone therapy for syphilis: Report from the emerging infections network. *Clin Infect Dis.* 1999;29(5): 1337–8.
122. Hook EW 3rd, Roddy RE, Handsfield HH. Ceftriaxone therapy for incubating and early syphilis. *J Infect Dis.* 1988;158(4):881–4.
123. Hook EW 3rd, Behets F, Van Damme K, et al. A phase III equivalence trial of azithromycin versus benzathine penicillin for treatment of early syphilis. *J Infect Dis.* 2010;201(11):1729–35.
124. Riedner G, Rusizoka M, Todd J, et al. Single-dose azithromycin versus penicillin G benzathine for the treatment of early syphilis. *N Engl J Med.* 2005;353(12):1236–44.
125. A2058G Prevalence Workgroup. Prevalence of the 23S rRNA A2058G point mutation and molecular subtypes in *Treponema pallidum* in the United States, 2007 to 2009. *Sex Transm Dis.* 2012;39(10):794–8.
126. Lukehart SA, Godornes C, Molini BJ, et al. Macrolide resistance in *Treponema pallidum* in the United States and Ireland. *N Engl J Med.* 2004;351(2):154–8.
127. Faber WR, Bos JD, Rietra PJ, Fass H, Van Eijk RV. Treponemicidal levels of amoxicillin in cerebrospinal fluid after oral administration. *Sex Transm Dis.* 1983;10(3):148–50.
128. Tanizaki R, Nishijima T, Aoki T, et al. High-dose oral amoxicillin plus probenecid is highly effective for syphilis in patients with HIV infection. *Clin Infect Dis.* 2015;61(2):177–83.
129. Nurse-Findlay S, Taylor MM, Savage M, et al. Shortages of benzathine penicillin for prevention of mother-to-child transmission of syphilis: An evaluation from multi-country surveys and stakeholder interviews. *PLoS Med.* 2017;14(12):e1002473.
130. Centers for Disease Control and Prevention. *Message from CDC Regarding the Recent Shortage of Penicillin G Benzathine in the United States.* Atlanta, GA: US Dept of Health and Human Services; 2016.
131. Marra CM, Maxwell CL, Tantalo LC, Sahi SK, Lukehart SA. Normalization of serum rapid plasma reagin titer predicts normalization of cerebrospinal fluid and clinical abnormalities after treatment of neurosyphilis. *Clin Infect Dis.* 2008;47(7):893–9.
132. Centers for Disease Control and Prevention. Guidelines for the prevention and control of congenital syphilis. *MMWR Suppl.* 1988;37(1):1–13.
133. Alexander JM, Sheffield JS, Sanchez PJ, Mayfield J, Wendel GDJr. Efficacy of treatment for syphilis in pregnancy. *Obstet Gynecol.* 1999;93(1): 5–8.
134. Walker GJ. Antibiotics for syphilis diagnosed during pregnancy. *Cochrane Database Syst Rev.* 2001;(3):Cd001143.
135. Wendel GD Jr, Sheffield JS, Hollier LM, Hill JB, Ramsey PS, Sanchez PJ. Treatment of syphilis in pregnancy and prevention of congenital syphilis. *Clin Infect Dis.* 2002;35(Suppl 2):S200–9.
136. Stafford IA, Berra A, Minard CG, et al. Challenges in the contemporary management of syphilis among pregnant women in New Orleans, LA. *Infect Dis Obstet Gynecol.* 2019;2019:2613962.
137. Hashisaki P, Wertzberger GG, Conrad GL, Nichols CR. Erythromycin failure in the treatment of syphilis in a pregnant woman. *Sex Transm Dis.* 1983;10(1):36–8.

138. Benirschke K. Syphilis—The placenta and the fetus. *Am J Dis Child.* 1974;128(2):142–3.

139. Shafii T, Radolf JD, Sanchez PJ, Schulz KF, Murphy FK. Congenital syphilis. In: Holmes KK, Sparling PF, Stamm WE, Piot P, Wasserheit JN, Corey L, eds. *Sexually Transmitted Diseases*. 4th ed. New York: McGraw Hill Medical; 2008, pp. 1577–612.

140. Cooper JM, Sánchez PJ. Congenital syphilis. *Semin Perinatol.* 2018;42(3):176–84.

141. Nathan L, Bohman VR, Sanchez PJ, Leos NK, Twickler DM, Wendel GDJr. In utero infection with *Treponema pallidum* in early pregnancy. *Prenat Diagn.* 1997;17(2):119–23.

142. Fiumara NJ, Fleming WL, Downing JG, Good FL. The incidence of prenatal syphilis at the Boston City Hospital. *N Engl J Med.* 1952;247(2): 48–52.

143. Fraser JF. The pathology of congenital syphilis. *Arch Derm Syphilol.* 1920;1(5):491–514.

144. Sheffield JS, Sánchez PJ, Wendel GD Jr, et al. Placental histopathology of congenital syphilis. *Obstet Gynecol.* 2002;100(1):126–33.

145. Genest DR, Choi-Hong SR, Tate JE, Qureshi F, Jacques SM, Crum C. Diagnosis of congenital syphilis from placental examination: Comparison of histopathology, Steiner stain, and polymerase chain reaction for *Treponema pallidum* DNA. *Hum Pathol.* 1996;27(4):366–72.

146. Silverstein AM. Congenital syphilis and the timing of immunogenesis in the human foetus. *Nature.* 1962;194:196–7.

147. Rac MW, Revell PA, Eppes CS. Syphilis during pregnancy: A preventable threat to maternal-fetal health. *Am J Obstet Gynecol.* 2017;216(4): 352–63.

148. Rac MW, Bryant SN, McIntire DD, et al. Progression of ultrasound findings of fetal syphilis after maternal treatment. *Am J Obstet Gynecol.* 2014;211(4):426.e421–26.

149. Hollier LM, Harstad TW, Sanchez PJ, Twickler DM, Wendel GDJr. Fetal syphilis: Clinical and laboratory characteristics. *Obstet Gynecol.* 2001;97(6):947–53.

150. Klein VR, Cox SM, Mitchell MD, Wendel GD Jr. The Jarisch-Herxheimer reaction complicating syphilotherapy in pregnancy. *Obstet Gynecol.* 1990;75(3 Pt 1):375–80.

151. Kollmann TR, Dobson SR. Syphilis. In: Wilson CB, Nizet V, Maldonado YA, Remington JS, Klein JO, eds. *Infectious Diseases of the Fetus and Newborn Infant*. 8th ed. Philadelphia, PA: Elsevier Saunders; 2016, pp. 512–43.

152. Stoll BJ, Lee FK, Larsen S, et al. Clinical and serologic evaluation of neonates for congenital syphilis: A continuing diagnostic dilemma. *J Infect Dis.* 1993;167(5):1093–9.

153. Digre KB, White GL Jr, Cremer SA, Massanari RM. Late-onset congenital syphilis. A retrospective look at University of Iowa Hospital admissions. *J Clin Neuroophthalmol.* 1991;11(1):1–6.

154. Fiumara NJ, Lessell S. Manifestations of late congenital syphilis. An analysis of 271 patients. *Arch Dermatol.* 1970;102(1):78–83.

155. Oppenheimer EH, Hardy JB. Congenital syphilis in the newborn infant: Clinical and pathological observations in recent cases. *Johns Hopkins Med J.* 1971;129(2):63–82.

156. Dorfman DH, Glaser JH. Congenital syphilis presenting in infants after the newborn period. *N Engl J Med.* 1990;323(19):1299–302.

157. Kaufman RE, Olansky DC, Wiesner PJ. The FTA-ABS (IgM) test for neonatal congenital syphilis: A critical review. *J Am Vener Dis Assoc.* 1974;1(2):79–84.

158. Sánchez PJ, Wendel GD, Norgard MV. IgM antibody to *Treponema pallidum* in cerebrospinal fluid of infants with congenital syphilis. *Am J Dis Child.* 1992;146(10):1171–5.

159. Russell P, Altshuler G. Placental abnormalities of congenital syphilis. A neglected aid to diagnosis. *Am J Dis Child.* 1974;128(2):160–3.

160. Sánchez PJ, Wendel GD Jr, Grimprel E, et al. Evaluation of molecular methodologies and rabbit infectivity testing for the diagnosis of congenital syphilis and neonatal central nervous system invasion by *Treponema pallidum*. *J Infect Dis.* 1993;167(1):148–57.

161. Michelow IC, Wendel GD Jr, Norgard MV, et al. Central nervous system infection in congenital syphilis. *N Engl J Med.* 2002;346(23):1792–8.

162. Sheffield JS, Sánchez PJ, Morris G, et al. Congenital syphilis after maternal treatment for syphilis during pregnancy. *Am J Obstet Gynecol.* 2002;186(3):569–73.

163. Stoll BJ. Congenital syphilis: Evaluation and management of neonates born to mothers with reactive serologic tests for syphilis. *Pediatr Infect Dis J.* 1994;13(10):845–53.

164. National Office of Vital Statistics. *Reported Incidence of Selected Notifiable Disease: United States, Each Division and State, 1920–50*. Washington, DC: US Public Health Service; 1953.

165. Thacker SB, Choi K, Brachman PS. The surveillance of infectious diseases. *JAMA.* 1983;249(9):1181–5.

166. Choi BC. The past, present, and future of public health surveillance. *Scientifica (Cairo).* 2012;2012:875253.

167. Centers for Disease Control and Prevention. *Sexually Transmitted Disease Surveillance 2017*. Atlanta, GA: US Dept of Health and Human Services; 2018.

168. Peterman TA, Su J, Bernstein KT, Weinstock H. Syphilis in the United States: On the rise? *Expert Rev Anti Infect Ther.* 2015;13(2):161–8.

169. Zenker PN, Berman SM. Congenital syphilis: Trends and recommendations for evaluation and management. *Pediatr Infect Dis J.* 1991;10(7):516–22.

170. Cohen DA, Boyd D, Prabhudas I, Mascola L. The effects of case definition in maternal screening and reporting criteria on rates of congenital syphilis. *Am J Public Health.* 1990;80(3):316–7.

171. Thompson BL, Matuszak D, Dwyer DM, Nakashima A, Pearce H, Israel E. Congenital syphilis in Maryland, 1989–1991: The effect of changing the case definition and opportunities for prevention. *Sex Transm Dis.* 1995;22(6):364–9.

172. Marx R, Aral SO, Rolfs RT, Sterk CE, Kahn JG. Crack, sex, and STD. *Sex Transm Dis.* 1991;18(2):92–101.

173. Rolfs RT, Goldberg M, Sharrar RG. Risk factors for syphilis: Cocaine use and prostitution. *Am J Public Health.* 1990;80(7):853–7.

174. Chesson HW, Dee TS, Aral SO. AIDS mortality may have contributed to the decline in syphilis rates in the United States in the 1990s. *Sex Transm Dis.* 2003;30(5):419–24.

175. CDC. Syphilis (*Treponema pallidum*) 1990 Case Definition. cdc.gov. https://wwwn.cdc.gov/nndss/conditions/syphilis/case-definition/1990/. Accessed August 5, 2020.

176. CDC. Syphilis (*Treponema pallidum*) 1996 Case Definition. cdc.gov. https://wwwn.cdc.gov/nndss/conditions/syphilis/case-definition/1996/. Accessed August 5, 2020.

177. Williams LA, Klausner JD, Whittington WL, Handsfield HH, Celum C, Holmes KK. Elimination and reintroduction of primary and secondary syphilis. *Am J Public Health.* 1999;89(7):1093–7.

178. Parran T. The eradication of syphilis as a practical public health objective. *Jama.* 1931;97(2):73-77.

179. US Public Health Service. *The Eradication of Syphilis: A Task Force Report to the Surgeon General Public Health Service on Syphilis Control in the United States*. Washington, DC: U.S. Dept of Health, Education, and Welfare; 1962.

180. Centers for Disease Control and Prevention. *The National Plan to Eliminate Syphilis from the United States*. Washington, DC: US Government Printing Office; 1999.

181. Centers for Disease Control and Prevention. *Syphilis Elimination Communication Plan*. Atlanta, GA: Centers for Disease Control and Prevention; 2000.

182. Heffelfinger JD, Swint EB, Berman SM, Weinstock HS. Trends in primary and secondary syphilis among men who have sex with men in the United States. *Am J Public Health.* 2007;97(6):1076–83.

183. Bernstein K. *Drivers and Determinants for the Rising Incidence of Syphilis in Men-Who-have-Sex-with-Men*. Vancouver, BC, Canada: International Society for Sexually Transmitted Diseases Research; 2019.

184. Kahn RH, Heffelfinger JD, Berman SM. Syphilis outbreaks among men who have sex with men: A public health trend of concern. *Sex Transm Dis.* 2002;29(5):285–7.

185. Nguyen TQ, Kohn RP, Ng RC, Philip SS, Cohen SE. Historical and current trends in the epidemiology of early syphilis in San Francisco, 1955 to 2016. *Sex Transm Dis.* 2018;45(9S Suppl 1):S55–62.

186. Woolston S, Cohen SE, Fanfair RN, Lewis SC, Marra CM, Golden MR. A cluster of ocular syphilis cases—Seattle, Washington, and San Francisco, California, 2014–2015. *MMWR Morb Mortal Wkly Rep.* 2015;64(40):1150–1.

187. Oliver SE, Aubin M, Atwell L, et al. Ocular syphilis—Eight jurisdictions, United States, 2014–2015. *MMWR Morb Mortal Wkly Rep.* 2016;65(43):1185–8.

188. Oliver S, Sahi SK, Tantalo LC, et al. Molecular typing of *Treponema pallidum* in ocular syphilis. *Sex Transm Dis.* 2016;43(8):524–7.

189. Oliver SE, Cope AB, Rinsky JL, et al. Increases in ocular syphilis—North Carolina, 2014–2015. *Clin Infect Dis.* 2017;65(10):1676–82.

190. de Voux A, Kidd S, Grey JA, et al. State-specific rates of primary and secondary syphilis among men who have sex with men—United States, 2015. *MMWR Morb Mortal Wkly Rep*. 2017;66(13):349–54.

191. Su JR, Brooks LC, Davis DW, Torrone EA, Weinstock HS, Kamb ML. Congenital syphilis: Trends in mortality and morbidity in the United States, 1999 through 2013. *Am J Obstet Gynecol*. 2016;214(3):381.e381–9.

192. CDC. Syphilis (*Treponema pallidum*) 2014 Case Definition. cdc.gov. https://wwwn.cdc.gov/nndss/conditions/syphilis/case-definition/2014/. Accessed August 5, 2020.

193. CDC. Syphilis (*Treponema pallidum*) 2018 Case Definition. cdc.gov. https://wwwn.cdc.gov/nndss/conditions/syphilis/case-definition/2018/. Accessed August 5, 2020.

194. Schroeter AL, Turner RH, Lucas JB, Brown WJ. Therapy for incubating syphilis: Effectiveness of gonorrhea treatment. *JAMA*. 1971;218(5):711–3.

195. Sánchez PJ, Wendel GD, Norgard MV. Congenital syphilis associated with negative results of maternal serologic tests at delivery. *Am J Dis Child*. 1991;145(9):967–9.

196. Radolf JD, Deka RK, Anand A, Šmajs D, Norgard MV, Yang XF. *Treponema pallidum*, the syphilis spirochete: Making a living as a stealth pathogen. *Nat Rev Microbiol*. 2016;14(12):744–59.

197. Ingraham NRJr. The value of penicillin alone in the prevention and treatment of congenital syphilis. *Acta Derm Venereol Suppl (Stockh)*. 1950;31(Suppl. 24):60–87.

198. Harter C, Benirschke K. Fetal syphilis in the first trimester. *Am J Obstet Gynecol*. 1976;124(7):705–11.

199. Adimora AA, Schoenbach VJ. Contextual factors and the black-white disparity in heterosexual HIV transmission. *Epidemiology*. 2002;13(6):707–12.

200. Lichtenstein B. Stigma as a barrier to treatment of sexually transmitted infection in the American deep south: Issues of race, gender and poverty. *Soc Sci Med*. 2003;57(12):2435–45.

201. Thomas JC. From slavery to incarceration: Social forces affecting the epidemiology of sexually transmitted diseases in the rural South. *Sex Transm Dis*. 2006;33(7 Suppl):S6–10.

202. Farley TA. Sexually transmitted diseases in the Southeastern United States: Location, race, and social context. *Sex Transm Dis*. 2006;33(7 Suppl):S58–64.

203. Chesson HW, Kent CK, Owusu-Edusei K Jr, Leichliter JS, Aral SO. Disparities in sexually transmitted disease rates across the "eight Americas." *Sex Transm Dis*. 2012;39(6):458–64.

204. Oster AM, Wertheim JO, Hernandez AL, Ocfemia MC, Saduvala N, Hall HI. Using molecular HIV surveillance data to understand transmission between subpopulations in the United States. *J Acquir Immune Defic Syndr*. 2015;70(4):444–51.

205. Torrone EA, Miller WC. Congenital and heterosexual syphilis: Still part of the problem. *Sex Transm Dis*. 2018;45(9S Suppl 1):S20–2.

206. Garnett GP, Aral SO, Hoyle DV, Cates W Jr, Anderson RM. The natural history of syphilis. Implications for the transmission dynamics and control of infection. *Sex Transm Dis*. 1997;24(4):185–200.

207. Marmot M, Bell R. The socioeconomically disadvantaged. In: Levey BS, Sidel VW, eds. *Social Injustice and Public Health*. New York: Oxford University Press; 2006.

208. Millett GA, Jeffries WL, Peterson JL, et al. Common roots: A contextual review of HIV epidemics in black men who have sex with men across the African diaspora. *Lancet*. 2012;380(9839):411–23.

209. Raiford JL, Herbst JH, Carry M, Browne FA, Doherty I, Wechsberg WM. Low prospects and high risk: Structural determinants of health associated with sexual risk among young African American women residing in resource-poor communities in the south. *Am J Community Psychol*. 2014;54(3-4):243–50.

210. Boyer CB, Santiago Rivera OJ, Chiaramonte DM, Ellen JM. Examination of behavioral, social, and environmental contextual influences on sexually transmitted infections in at risk, urban, adolescents, and young adults. *Sex Transm Dis*. 2018;45(8):542–8.

211. Hardeman RR, Murphy KA, Karbeah J, Kozhimannil KB. Naming institutionalized racism in the public health literature: A systematic literature review. *Public Health Rep*. 2018;133(3):240–9.

212. Hood JE, Friedman AL. Unveiling the hidden epidemic: A review of stigma associated with sexually transmissible infections. *Sex Health*. 2011;8(2):159–70.

213. Morris JL, Lippman SA, Philip S, Bernstein K, Neilands TB, Lightfoot M. Sexually transmitted infection related stigma and shame among African American male youth: Implications for testing practices, partner notification, and treatment. *AIDS Patient Care STDS*. 2014;28(9):499–506.

214. Cooper LA, Roter DL, Carson KA, et al. The associations of clinicians' implicit attitudes about race with medical visit communication and patient ratings of interpersonal care. *Am J Public Health*. 2012;102(5):979–87.

215. Mimiaga MJ, Reisner SL, Bland S, et al. Health system and personal barriers resulting in decreased utilization of HIV and STD testing services among at-risk black men who have sex with men in Massachusetts. *AIDS Patient Care STDS*. 2009;23(10):825–35.

216. Mayer KH. Old pathogen, new challenges: A narrative review of the multilevel drivers of syphilis increasing in American men who have sex with men. *Sex Transm Dis*. 2018;45(9S Suppl 1):S38–41.

217. Paz-Bailey G, Mendoza MC, Finlayson T, et al. Trends in condom use among MSM in the United States: The role of antiretroviral therapy and seroadaptive strategies. *AIDS*. 2016;30(12):1985–90.

218. McFarlane M, Bull SS, Rietmeijer CA. The Internet as a newly emerging risk environment for sexually transmitted diseases. *JAMA*. 2000;284(4):443–6.

219. Lewnard JA, Berrang-Ford L. Internet-based partner selection and risk for unprotected anal intercourse in sexual encounters among men who have sex with men: A meta-analysis of observational studies. *Sex Transm Infect*. 2014;90(4):290–6.

220. Paz-Bailey G, Hoots BE, Xia M, Finlayson T, Prejean J, Purcell DW. Trends in Internet use among men who have sex with men in the United States. *J Acquir Immune Defic Syndr*. 2017;75(Suppl 3):S288–95.

221. Lehmiller JJ, Ioerger M. Social networking smartphone applications and sexual health outcomes among men who have sex with men. *PLoS One*. 2014;9(1):e86603.

222. Beymer MR, Weiss RE, Bolan RK, et al. Sex on demand: Geosocial networking phone apps and risk of sexually transmitted infections among a cross-sectional sample of men who have sex with men in Los Angeles County. *Sex Transm Infect*. 2014;90(7):567–72.

223. Traeger MW, Cornelisse VJ, Asselin J, et al. Association of HIV preexposure prophylaxis with incidence of sexually transmitted infections among individuals at high risk of HIV infection. *JAMA*. 2019;321(14):1380–90.

224. Wolitski RJ, Fenton KA. Sexual health, HIV, and sexually transmitted infections among gay, bisexual, and other men who have sex with men in the United States. *AIDS Behav*. 2011;15 Suppl 1:S9–17.

225. Newman BS, Muzzonigro PG. The effects of traditional family values on the coming out process of gay male adolescents. *Adolescence*. 1993;28(109):213–26.

226. Almeida J, Johnson RM, Corliss HL, Molnar BE, Azrael D. Emotional distress among LGBT youth: The influence of perceived discrimination based on sexual orientation. *J Youth Adolesc*. 2009;38(7):1001–14.

227. Stall R, Paul JP, Greenwood G., et al. Alcohol use, drug use and alcohol-related problems among men who have sex with men: The Urban Men's Health Study. *Addiction*. 2001;96(11):1589–601.

228. Mills TC, Paul J, Stall R, et al. Distress and depression in men who have sex with men: The Urban Men's Health Study. *Am J Psychiatry*. 2004;161(2):278–85.

229. Bartholow BN, Doll LS, Joy D, et al. Emotional, behavioral, and HIV risks associated with sexual abuse among adult homosexual and bisexual men. *Child Abuse Negl*. 1994;18(9):747-–61.

230. Jinich S, Paul JP, Stall R, et al. Childhood sexual abuse and HIV risk-taking behavior among gay and bisexual men. *AIDS Behav*. 1998;2:41–51.

231. Brennan DJ, Hellerstedt WL, Ross MW, Welles SL. History of childhood sexual abuse and HIV risk behaviors in homosexual and bisexual men. *Am J Public Health*. 2007;97(6):1107–12.

232. Millett GA, Peterson JL, Flores SA, et al. Comparisons of disparities and risks of HIV infection in black and other men who have sex with men in Canada, UK, and USA: A meta-analysis. *Lancet*. 2012;380(9839):341–8.

233. Mayer KH, Wang L, Koblin B, et al. Concomitant socioeconomic, behavioral, and biological factors associated with the disproportionate HIV infection burden among Black men who have sex with men in 6 U.S. cities. *PLoS One*. 2014;9(1):e87298.

234. Webber MP, Lambert G, Bateman DA, Hauser WA. Maternal risk factors for congenital syphilis: A case-control study. *Am J Epidemiol*. 1993;137(4):415–22.

235. McFarlin BL, Bottoms SF, Dock BS, Isada NB. Epidemic syphilis: Maternal factors associated with congenital infection. *Am J Obstet Gynecol*. 1994;170(2):535–40.

236. Gunn RA, Montes JM, Toomey KE, et al. Syphilis in San Diego County 1983–1992: Crack cocaine, prostitution, and the limitations of partner notification. *Sex Transm Dis*. 1995;22(1):60–6.

237. Southwick KL, Guidry HM, Weldon MM, Mert KJ, Berman SM, Levine WC. An epidemic of congenital syphilis in Jefferson County, Texas,

1994–1995: Inadequate prenatal syphilis testing after an outbreak in adults. *Am J Public Health*. 1999;89(4):557–60.

238. Warner L, Rochat RW, Fichtner RR, Stoll BJ, Nathan L, Toomey KE. Missed opportunities for congenital syphilis prevention in an urban southeastern hospital. *Sex Transm Dis*. 2001;28(2):92–8.
239. Bowen V, Su J, Torrone E, Kidd S, Weinstock H. Increase in incidence of congenital syphilis—United States, 2012–2014. *MMWR Morb Mortal Wkly Rep*. 2015;64(44):1241–5.
240. Biswas HH, Chew Ng RA, Murray EL, et al. Characteristics associated with delivery of an infant with congenital syphilis and missed opportunities for prevention—California, 2012 to 2014. *Sex Transm Dis*. 2018;45(7):435–41.
241. Slutsker JS, Hennessy RR, Schillinger JA. Factors contributing to congenital syphilis cases—New York City, 2010–2016. *MMWR Morb Mortal Wkly Rep*. 2018;67(39):1088–93.
242. DiOrio D, Kroeger K, Ross A. Social vulnerability in congenital syphilis case mothers: Qualitative assessment of cases in Indiana, 2014 to 2016. *Sex Transm Dis*. 2018;45(7):447–51.
243. Trivedi S, Williams C, Torrone E, Kidd S. National trends and reported risk factors among pregnant women with syphilis in the United States, 2012–2016. *Obstet Gynecol*. 2019;133(1):27–32.
244. Kidd SE, Grey JA, Torrone EA, Weinstock HS. Increased methamphetamine, injection drug, and heroin use among women and heterosexual men with primary and secondary syphilis—United States, 2013–2017. *MMWR Morb Mortal Wkly Rep*. 2019;68(6):144–8.
245. Kidd S, Bowen VB, Torrone EA, Bolan G. Use of national syphilis surveillance data to develop a congenital syphilis prevention cascade and estimate the number of potential congenital syphilis cases averted. *Sex Transm Dis*. 2018;45(9S Suppl 1):S23–8.
246. Kimball A, Torrone E, Miele K, et al. Missed opportunities for prevention of congenital syphilis—United States, 2018. *MMWR Morb Mortal Wkly Rep*. 2020;69(22):661–5.
247. Plotzker RE, Murphy RD, Stoltey JE. Congenital syphilis prevention: Strategies, evidence, and future directions. *Sex Transm Dis*. 2018;45 (9S Suppl 1):S29–37.
248. Parran T. *Shadow on the Land: Syphilis*. New York: Reynal and Hitchcock; 1937.
249. Foege W. Lessons and innovations from the West and Central African Smallpox Eradication Program. *Vaccine*. 2011;29 Suppl 4:D10–2.
250. Centers for Disease Control and Prevention. *Lessons Learned and Emerging Best Practices from the National Syphilis Elimination Programs Assessment*. Turlock, CA: LTG Associates, Inc.; 2004.
251. Valentine JA, DeLisle SA. Reducing disparities in sexual health: Lessons learned from the campaign to eliminate infectious syphilis from the United States. In: Aral SO, Fenton KA, Lipshutz JA, eds. *The New Public Health and STD/HIV Prevention: Personal, Public and Health Systems Approaches*. New York: Springer-Verlag; 2013.
252. Klausner JD, Kent CK, Wong W, McCright J, Katz MH. The public health response to epidemic syphilis, San Francisco, 1999–2004. *Sex Transm Dis*. 2005;32(10 Suppl):S11–8.
253. Klausner JD, Levine DK, Kent CK. Internet-based site-specific interventions for syphilis prevention among gay and bisexual men. *AIDS Care*. 2004;16(8):964–70.
254. Ahrens K, Kent CK, Montoya JA, et al. Healthy penis: San Francisco's social marketing campaign to increase syphilis testing among gay and bisexual men. *PLoS Med*. 2006;3(12):e474.
255. Centers for Disease Control and Prevention. *Together We Can. The National Plan to Eliminate Syphilis from the United States*. Atlanta, GA: US Dept of Health and Human Services; 2006.
256. Valentine JA, Bolan GA. Syphilis elimination: Lessons learned again. *Sex Transm Dis*. 2018;45(9S Suppl 1):S80–5.
257. Frieden TR. A framework for public health action: the health impact pyramid. *Am J Public Health*. 2010;100(4):590–95.
258. Williams DR, Costa MV, Odunlami AO, Mohammed SA. Moving upstream: How interventions that address the social determinants of health can improve health and reduce disparities. *J Public Health Manag Pract*. 2008;14 (6):S8–17.
259. Peterman TA, Furness BW. Public health interventions to control syphilis. *Sex Health*. 2015;12(2):126–34.
260. Golden MR, Dombrowski JC. Syphilis control in the postelimination era: Implications of a new syphilis control initiative for sexually transmitted disease/human immunodeficiency virus programs. *Sex Transm Dis*. 2018;45(9S Suppl 1):S86–92.
261. Sullivan PS. Practical considerations for implementing a new syphilis action plan. *Sex Transm Dis*. 2018;45(9S Suppl 1):S78–9.
262. Anderson RM, May RM. *Infectious Diseases of Humans: Dynamics and Control*. Oxford, England: Oxford University Press; 1991.
263. Sackett DL, Haynes RB, Guyatt GH, Tugwell P. *Clinical Epidemiology: A Basic Science for Clinical Medicine*. 2nd ed. Boston: Little Brown and Company; 1991.
264. Grimes DA, Schulz KF. Uses and abuses of screening tests. *Lancet*. 2002;359(9309):881–4.
265. Bibbins-Domingo K, Grossman DC, Curry SJ, et al. Screening for syphilis infection in nonpregnant adults and adolescents: US Preventive Services Task Force recommendation statement. *JAMA*. 2016;315(21):2321–7.
266. Cantor AG, Pappas M, Daeges M, Nelson HD. Screening for syphilis: Updated evidence report and systematic review for the US Preventive Services Task Force. *JAMA*. 2016;315(21):2328–37.
267. An Q, Wejnert C, Bernstein K, Paz-Bailey G. Syphilis screening and diagnosis among men who have sex with men, 2008–2014, 20 U.S. cities. *J Acquir Immune Defic Syndr*. 2017;75 Suppl 3:S363–9.
268. de Voux A, Bernstein KT, Bradley H, Kirkcaldy RD, Tie Y, Shouse RL. Syphilis testing among sexually active men who have sex with men and who are receiving medical care for human immunodeficiency virus in the United States: Medical monitoring project, 2013–2014. *Clin Infect Dis*. 2019;68(6):934–9.
269. Centers for Disease Control and Prevention. *Behavioral and Clinical Characteristics of Persons with Diagnosed HIV Infection—Medical Monitoring Project, United States, 2015–2016. Leveraging the HIV Prevention and Care systems to Respond to the STI Crisis*. Washington, DC: O'Neill Institute; 2019;.
270. Warren HP, Cramer R, Kidd S, Leichliter JS. State requirements for prenatal syphilis screening in the United States, 2016. *Matern Child Health J*. 2018;22(9):1227–32.
271. Curry SJ, Krist AH, Owens DK, et al. Screening for syphilis infection in pregnant women: US Preventive Services Task Force reaffirmation recommendation statement. *JAMA*. 2018;320(9):911–7.
272. Lin JS, Eder ML, Bean SI. Screening for syphilis infection in pregnant women: Updated evidence report and systematic review for the US Preventive Services Task Force. *JAMA*. 2018;320(9):918–25.
273. Neblett Fanfair R, Tao G, Owusu-Edusei K, Gift TL, Bernstein KT. Suboptimal prenatal syphilis testing among commercially insured women in the United States, 2013. *Sex Transm Dis*. 2017;44(4):219–21.
274. Matthias JM, Rahman MM, Newman DR, Peterman TA. Effectiveness of prenatal screening and treatment to prevent congenital syphilis, Louisiana and Florida, 2013–2014. *Sex Transm Dis*. 2017;44(8):498–502.
275. Hawkes S, Matin N, Broutet N, Low N. Effectiveness of interventions to improve screening for syphilis in pregnancy: A systematic review and meta-analysis. *Lancet Infect Dis*. 2011;11(9):684–91.
276. Schmid GP, Stoner BP, Hawkes S, Broutet N. The need and plan for global elimination of congenital syphilis. *Sex Transm Dis*. 2007;34(7 Suppl):S5–10.
277. Rahman MM, Hoover A, Johnson C, Peterman TA. Preventing congenital syphilis—Opportunities identified by congenital syphilis case review boards. *Sex Transm Dis*. 2019;46(2):139–42.
278. Rawstron SA, Vetrano J, Tannis G, Bromberg K. Congenital syphilis: Detection of *Treponema pallidum* in stillborns. *Clin Infect Dis*. 1997;24(1):24–7.
279. Centers for Disease Control and Prevention. Recommendations for partner services programs for HIV infection, syphilis, gonorrhea, and chlamydial infection. *MMWR Recomm Rep*. 2008;57(Rr-9):1–83; quiz CE81-84.
280. Hogben M, Collins D, Hoots B, O'Connor K. Partner services in sexually transmitted disease prevention programs: A review. *Sex Transm Dis*. 2016;43(2 Suppl 1):S53–62.
281. Taylor MM, Mickey T, Winscott M, James H, Kenney K, England B. Improving partner services by embedding disease intervention specialists in HIV-clinics. *Sex Transm Dis*. 2010;37(12):767–70.
282. Rudy ET, Aynalem G, Cross J, Ramirez F, Bolan RK, Kerndt PR. Community-embedded disease intervention specialist program for syphilis partner notification in a clinic serving men who have sex with men. *Sex Transm Dis*. 2012;39(9):701–5.
283. Blank S, McDonnell DD, Rubin SR, et al. New approaches to syphilis control. Finding opportunities for syphilis treatment and congenital syphilis prevention in a women's correctional setting. *Sex Transm Dis*. 1997;24(4):218–26.
284. Burke R, Rhodes J. Lessons learned on the implementation of jail syphilis screening in Nashville, Davidson County Jail, 1999–2005. *Sex Transm Dis*. 2009;36(2 Suppl):S14–16.
285. Rekart ML, Patrick DM, Chakraborty B, et al. Targeted mass treatment for syphilis with oral azithromycin. *Lancet*. 2003;361(9354):313–4.

286. Bolan RK, Beymer MR, Weiss RE, Flynn RP, Leibowitz AA, Klausner JD. Doxycycline prophylaxis to reduce incident syphilis among HIV-infected men who have sex with men who continue to engage in high-risk sex: A randomized, controlled pilot study. *Sex Transm Dis*. 2015;42(2):98–103.
287. Molina JM, Charreau I, Chidiac C, et al. Post-exposure prophylaxis with doxycycline to prevent sexually transmitted infections in men who have sex with men: An open-label randomised substudy of the ANRS IPERGAY trial. *Lancet Infect Dis*. 2018;18(3):308–17.
288. Heumann CL, Katz DA, Dombrowski JC, Bennett AB, Manhart LE, Golden MR. Comparison of in-person versus telephone interviews for early syphilis and human immunodeficiency virus partner services in King County, Washington (2010–2014). *Sex Transm Dis*. 2017;44(4):249–54.
289. Pennise M, Inscho R, Herpin K, et al. Using smartphone apps in STD interviews to find sexual partners. *Public Health Rep*. 2015;130(3): 245–52.
290. Centers for Disease Control and Prevention. The Toolkit for Technology-based Partner Services. cdc.gov. https://www.cdc.gov/std/program/ips/default.htm. Accessed August 8, 2020.
291. Kerani RP, Fleming M, Golden MR. Acceptability and intention to seek medical care after hypothetical receipt of patient-delivered partner therapy or electronic partner notification postcards among men who have sex with men: The partner's perspective. *Sex Transm Dis*. 2013;40(2):179–85.
292. Rietmeijer CA, Westergaard B, Mickiewicz TA, et al. Evaluation of an online partner notification program. *Sex Transm Dis*. 2011;38(5):359–64.
293. Plant A, Rotblatt H, Montoya JA, Rudy ET, Kerndt PR. Evaluation of inSPOTLA.org: An Internet partner notification service. *Sex Transm Dis*. 2012;39(5):341–5.
294. Kachur R, Hall W, Coor A, Kinsey J, Collins D, Strona FV. The use of technology for sexually transmitted disease partner services in the United States: A structured review. *Sex Transm Dis*. 2018;45(11):707–12.
295. Ferreira A, Young T, Mathews C, Zunza M, Low N. Strategies for partner notification for sexually transmitted infections, including HIV. *Cochrane Database Syst Rev*. 2013;2013(10):Cd002843.
296. Hogben M, Paffel J, Broussard D, et al. Syphilis partner notification with men who have sex with men: A review and commentary. *Sex Transm Dis*. 2005;32(10 Suppl):S43–7.
297. Brewer DD. Case-finding effectiveness of partner notification and cluster investigation for sexually transmitted diseases/HIV. *Sex Transm Dis*. 2005;32(2):78–83.
297. Hoots BE, Lewis FM, Anschuetz G, et al. Would targeting increase efficiency of syphilis partner services programs?—Data from New York City, Philadelphia, Texas, and Virginia. *Sex Transm Dis*. 2014;41(6):407–12.
299. Peterman TA, Cha S. Context-appropriate interventions to prevent syphilis: A narrative review. *Sex Transm Dis*. 2018;45(9S Suppl 1):S65–71.
300. Philip SS, Bernstein KT. Syphilis is (still) here: How must sexually transmitted disease public health programs adapt? *Sex Transm Dis*. 2018;45(9S Suppl 1):S63–64.
301. Bernstein KT, Stephens SC, Moss N, Scheer S, Parisi MK, Philip SS. Partner services as targeted HIV screening—Changing the paradigm. *Public Health Rep*. 2014;129 Suppl 1(Suppl 1):50–5.
302. Solomon MM, Mayer KH, Glidden DV, et al. Syphilis predicts HIV incidence among men and transgender women who have sex with men in a preexposure prophylaxis trial. *Clin Infect Dis*. 2014;59(7):1020–6.
303. Pathela P, Braunstein SL, Blank S, Shepard C, Schillinger JA. The high risk of an HIV diagnosis following a diagnosis of syphilis: A population-level analysis of New York City men. *Clin Infect Dis*. 2015;61(2):281–7.
304. Gottlieb SL, Deal CD, Giersing B, et al. The global roadmap for advancing development of vaccines against sexually transmitted infections: Update and next steps. *Vaccine*. 2016;34(26):2939–47.
305. Lithgow KV, Hof R, Wetherell C, Phillips D, Houston S, Cameron CE. A defined syphilis vaccine candidate inhibits dissemination of *Treponema pallidum* subspecies *pallidum*. *Nat Commun*. 2017;8:14273.
306. Cameron CE. Syphilis vaccine development: Requirements, challenges, and opportunities. *Sex Transm Dis*. 2018;45(9S Suppl 1):S17–9.
307. Darrow WW, Biersteker S. Short-term impact evaluation of a social marketing campaign to prevent syphilis among men who have sex with men. *Am J Public Health*. 2008;98(2):337–43.

CHAPTER

121 Gonorrhea

Robert D. Kirkcaldy

INTRODUCTION

Gonorrhea, caused by the bacterium *Neisseria gonorrhoeae*, is a sexually transmitted infection (STI) that occurs at the anatomic site of sexual exposure, such as the urethra, cervix, pharynx, or rectum. If untreated or inadequately treated in women, *N. gonorrhoeae* can ascend within the genital tract and cause severe reproductive health complications including pelvic inflammatory disease (PID), chronic pelvic pain, ectopic pregnancy, and tubal infertility. Infants born to mothers with untreated cervical infections are at risk of neonatal conjunctivitis and blindness.

Gonorrhea is believed to be an ancient disease: descriptions of symptoms consistent with gonorrhea such as urethral discharge have been mentioned in written texts for centuries.[1] The term *gonorrhea* is thought to have been coined by the Greek physician Galen (129 AD–c.210 AD) and derived from the erroneous belief that urethral discharge was caused by excess flow (*rrhea*) of semen (*gonos*) The causative bacterium was named in honor of Albert Neisser (1855–1916), who, as a 24-year-old German physician, identified the bacterium in 1879.[2]

MICROBIOLOGY

N. gonorrhoeae is a Gram-negative intracellular diplococcus and obligate human pathogen. Infection is facilitated by (1) adherence to host cells by pili on the surface of the bacterial cells, and (2) modulation of the host immune response by the binding of bacterial Opa proteins to receptors on host immune cells.[3–5] Pili and Opa proteins, both of which are potential targets of host immune systems, undergo frequent genetic mutation, allowing the bacteria to evade the immune system, prevent host immunological memory, and cause reinfection.[5–7] *N. gonorrhoeae* mutates rapidly and is naturally competent to acquire new DNA from other bacteria in the environment, promoting acquisition of antimicrobial resistance.[5]

EPIDEMIOLOGY AND TRENDS

Gonorrhea case reporting is mandated by legislation or regulation in all 50 U.S. states and the District of Columbia and has been a nationally notifiable disease since the 1940s. Health departments in all U.S. states and the District of Columbia voluntarily report gonorrhea cases to the Centers for Disease Control and Prevention (CDC). The demographic characteristics associated with each case that are transmitted to CDC are generally limited to the county of patient residence, age, gender, race, and ethnicity.[8] Health departments might collect additional epidemiological characteristics about each case, particularly if the health department STI program in a jurisdiction interviews gonorrhea cases for partner services or enhanced surveillance. Automatic electronic laboratory reporting (ELR) has contributed to improved completeness of case counts and timeliness of reporting, but expansions of ELR and relative infrequency of gonorrhea partner services interviews limit opportunities for jurisdictions to collect additional epidemiological data associated with cases.[9] Epidemiological data about gonorrhea cases are supplemented by CDC-supported sentinel surveillance platforms, such as the STI Surveillance Network (SSuN), described in more detail below.

In the United States, gonorrhea is the second most commonly reported notifiable disease: a total of 468,514 cases were reported in 2016.[8] Many infections, particularly asymptomatic infections, may be undetected and unreported, and CDC estimates that as many as new 820,000 gonococcal infections occur annually.[10] Reported gonorrhea case rates in the United States increased sharply during the 1960s and the early 1970s (Fig. 121-1), probably due to demographic shifts (such as greater numbers of adolescents and young adults), changes in sexual mores, and improved detection of asymptomatic infections from the introduction of modified Thayer-Martin culture media.[11,12] Implementation of a wide-scale gonorrhea screening program in the 1970s and changes in sexual behavior wrought by HIV/AIDS in the 1980s might have contributed to subsequent declines.[13] Reported gonorrhea rates remained fairly stable in the late 1990s, but reached a historic low of 98.1 per 100,000 population in 2009. Since then, rates increased to a rate of 145.8 cases per 100,000 in 2016.[8]

In 2016, the South had the highest rate of reported gonorrhea in the United States (166.8 cases per 100,000), followed by the Midwest (142.9), West (142.1), and Northeast (108.8).[8] Whereas increases were observed in all regions during 2012–16, the sharpest increase was observed in the West—the rate in the West nearly doubled from 72.1 to 142.1. The rate among women increased from 107.9 per 100,000 in 2012 to 121.0 in 2016. Steep increases in rates were observed among men—from 105.0 in 2012 to 170.7 cases in 2016—suggestive of increasing cases among gay, bisexual, and other men who have sex with men (MSM).[14] Gender of sex partner data are not routinely submitted with gonorrhea case data to CDC, so data from SSuN and the Gonococcal Isolate Surveillance Project (GISP) have proven useful for understanding gonorrhea epidemiology among MSM.

SSuN is a CDC-supported sentinel surveillance system and collaboration between CDC and selected states and independently funded cities that enhances epidemiological understanding of gonorrhea through, among other activities, health department collection of data about STI clinic attendees and interviewing of a random sample of locally reported gonorrhea cases.[8,15] Across all 10 SSuN sites that participated in 2016, 44.7% of gonorrhea cases in 2016 were estimated to be among MSM, with substantial geographic variation.[8] MSM accounted for over 81% of gonorrhea cases in San Francisco, California, but just over 16% in Baltimore, Maryland. Utilizing estimates of the size of the MSM population in the six counties that continuously participated in SSuN during 2010–15, the estimated gonorrhea incidence increased from 1368.6 cases per 100,000 MSM in

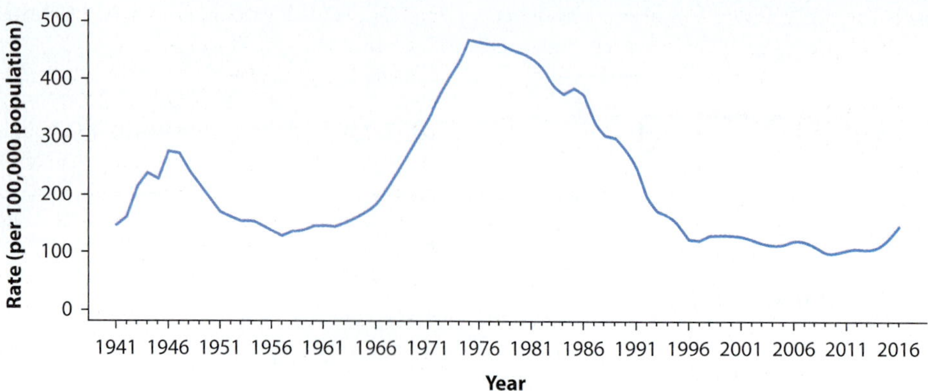

FIGURE 12-1. Rates of reported gonorrhea cases by year, United States, 1941–2016. (*Source:* Centers for Disease Control and Prevention.)

2010 to 3434.7 in 2015.[8] In addition, the percentage of urethral gonococcal infections attributable to MSM has steadily increased in GISP, a U.S.-based sentinel surveillance system that monitors gonococcal antimicrobialsusceptibility in urethral isolates.[8] Although increasing case counts among MSM might be due in part to better detection and increased case finding due to expanding gonorrhea screening at nongenital anatomic sites, the magnitude of the increases strongly suggests that gonorrhea transmission among MSM is also increasing.

Marked racial/ethnic disparities in gonorrhea cases rates are observed in the United States. The reported gonorrhea case rate among African Americans (481.2 per 100,000) was 8.6 times the rate among whites (55.7) in 2016.[8] The rates among American Indians/Alaska Natives (242.9), Native Hawaiians/Other Pacific Islanders (165.8), and Hispanics/Latinos (95.9) were substantially higher than the rate among whites. These racial and ethnic disparities are likely shaped in large part by differences in structural social determinants of health and myriad effects of institutional racism, such as differential socioeconomic status, differential access to high-quality healthcare, racial segregation, greater levels of mass incarceration within minority communities, and influences of these factors on gender dynamics, sexual network characteristics, and disease prevalence.[16]

Incarcerated men and women experience a high burden of gonorrhea, likely due to the high prevalence of individual-risk factors (such as substance abuse, commercial or transactional sex, and condomless sex) and structural-risk factors among incarcerated persons.[17–22] Among young adolescent and adult males in juvenile correctional facilities, test positivity ranged from 0.1% in 12-year-olds to 2.3% in 18-year-olds; positivity among females ranged from 2.5% in 13-year olds to 4.9% in 16-year-olds.[17] Overall positivity among adult men in corrections facilities was 1%, with the highest age-stratified positivity (1.7%) among 20-year-olds (1.7%). Overall positivity was 1.8% among adult women, with the highest positivity (4.3%) also among 20-year-olds.[17]

Worldwide, the World Health Organization (WHO) estimates a prevalence among women aged 15–49 years of 0.8% (0.6–1.0%) and among men of 0.6% (0.4–0.9%).[23] These estimates correspond to an estimated incidence of 78 million new gonococcal infections globally each year. Among women, the highest estimated incidence was in the African region (37 per 1000); among men, the highest incidence was in the Western Pacific Region (41 per 1000). The WHO bases its estimates on literature reviews of recent prevalence data among low risk or general populations.

The most proximate risk factor for infection is condomless sex with a partner infected with *N. gonorrhoeae*. Other individual-level risk factors include adolescence and young adulthood, having a new sexual partner, multiple sexual partners, or anonymous partners, substance abuse, and prior history of gonorrhea. [24–26] Residing within a geographic region with or participation in a sexual network with high prevalence of disease increases the likelihood that one's partner(s) is infected with *N. gonorrhoeae* and increases one's risk of exposure.[16] As described above, gonorrhea is associated with social determinants of health, such as low socioeconomic status and limited educational attainment.[16,27]

Few data exist on sexual transmission probabilities of *N. gonorrhoeae*. A small number of studies have estimated the probability of penile-to-vaginal transmission as approximately 50% per sex act and of vaginal-to-penile transmission as approximately 20% per act. [28–39]. These studies were limited, however, by a lack of complete enumeration of and control for the number of sexual encounters and lack of data on whether partners had been treated prior to evaluation. Very few data on oral and anal sex transmission probabilities are available; published estimates of per-act probabilities have relied on mathematical models to infer probabilities based on disease prevalence and estimates of behavior.[31] Perinatal transmission from an infected and untreated mother to her newborn is estimated to occur during 30–40% of deliveries.[32]

CLINICAL CHARACTERISTICS

Upon exposure, *N. gonorrhoeae* infects noncornified epithelium of mucosal surfaces. Infections generally remain localized to the initial anatomic sites of inoculation, such as the pharynx, urethra, cervix, and rectum. Although gonorrhea is classically associated with pain and purulent discharge, whether symptoms occur and the nature of the symptoms depend on the specific anatomic site of infection. In men, urethral infections are often symptomatic and frequently cause profuse yellow-green urethral discharge and pain with urination. Epididymitis can cause pain, tenderness, and swelling of the affected testicle. Most cervical infections in women are either asymptomatic or cause symptoms so mild as to be mistaken for urinary tract infections. When symptoms and signs of cervical infections do occur, women may experience pain with urination or sexual intercourse, intermenstrual or postcoital bleeding, and purulent or mucopurulent discharge from the cervical os. In both men and women, oropharyngeal and rectal infections are frequently asymptomatic and only detected through screening (see below). When symptoms and signs do occur, pharyngeal infections may present with throat pain, fever, and lymphadenopathy, and rectal infections may present with rectal discharge, itching, bleeding, and pain with bowel movements.

Although rare in developed countries due to maternal screening, and (in many countries) routine ophthalmic prophylaxis, maternal transmission to neonates can occur during delivery and cause ophthalmia neonatorum. Ophthalmia neonatorum causes hyperacute purulent conjunctivitis, with profuse exudate and eyelid swelling.

CONSEQUENCES OF GONORRHEA

Untreated or inadequately treated cervical infections in women can ascend to the upper genital tract, including the uterus, fallopian tubes, and ovaries, and cause serious and irreversible health sequelae, such as PID and infertility. Signs and symptoms of PID include: severe lower abdominal pain and tenderness; cervical motion, uterine, and adnexal tenderness during bimanual pelvic examination; and fever. Damage to the fallopian tubes can cause infertility and increase the risk of ectopic pregnancy. Infrequently, epididymitis can cause infertility in men.

Hematogenous spread of *N. gonorrhoeae*, or disseminated gonococcal infection (DGI), is thought to occur in 0.5–1% of patients with gonorrhea.[33,34] Patients with DGI typically present with tenosynovitis, dermatitis, polyarthalgias, or purulent septic arthritis without skin lesions.[35] Rarely, meningitis or endocarditis can occur. Apart from case reports, recent data on the epidemiology of DGI are sparse. Investigators from France found that the number of DGI cases increased from 2 in 2009 to 10 in 2011.[36] Whether this represents a true increase in DGI incidence, rather than surveillance artifact, is unclear.

If infants with ophthalmia neonatorum are not promptly treated, the infection can spread into the subconjunctival connective tissue and cornea, causing ulceration, scarring, and blindness.

Either through biological changes that result in increased HIV susceptibility or as an indicator of behavioral risk, gonorrhea is associated with heightened HIV transmission and acquisition. Among HIV-uninfected MSM in New York City, 7% of men with rectal gonorrhea at baseline acquired HIV within 12 months, compared to 2.5% among men without rectal gonorrhea.[37] Among HIV-uninfected MSM in Australia, rectal gonorrhea was associated with an HIV incidence rate of 3.4 (95% CI 2.1–5.2) per 100 person-years.[38] Investigators in San Francisco, California found that increasing numbers of rectal gonococcal or chlamydial infections in the preceding 2 years were associated with escalating risk of subsequent HIV incidence.[39]

DIAGNOSIS

Elicitation of a sexual history, with a particular focus on gender of recent sex partners, anatomic site(s) of possible exposure, recent sexual behavior (such as whether the patient was the insertive or receptive partner), and condom use, is important for appropriately evaluating a patient for gonorrhea. This information can guide both the physical examination (which should include investigation of signs of gonorrhea and other STIs) and specimen collection for laboratory-based screening from potentially exposed anatomic sites. Guidance on taking sexual histories can be found at: https://www.cdc.gov/std/treatment/sexualhistory.pdf.

Microbiological testing for *N. gonorrhoeae* is necessary to confirm a gonorrhea diagnosis. Recommended testing options include nucleic acid amplification tests (NAATs), Gram stain, and culture. NAATs amplify and detect nucleic acid sequences specific to the bacterium. Advantages of NAATs include excellent sensitivity and specificity and ease of handling (particularly as compared to culture).[40] NAAT assays have been cleared by the U.S. Food and Drug Administration (FDA) for detection of urogenital gonorrhea in men and women with and without symptoms.[40] Optimal specimen types are vaginal swabs from women and first-catch urine specimens from men, but first-catch urine in women, and endocervical, urethral, and self-collected vaginal swabs are also valid specimen types. CDC recommends NAATs for detection of oropharyngeal and rectal gonorrhea.[40] Use of pharyngeal and rectal swabs for NAATs have not been cleared by the FDA, but many laboratories have established performance specifications and met Clinical Laboratory Improvement Amendments regulatory requirements for conducting NAATS using these specimens to inform clinical management. Ease of handling of specimens collected for NAATs has facilitated expanded screening, including into nontraditional healthcare settings and mail-based testing.[41–44] A disadvantage of currently commercially available NAATs is that they do not allow reliable, well-validated, and commercially available antimicrobial susceptibility testing (AST), which at this point requires isolation of viable organisms by culture. Active research is underway to develop and operationalize reliable and well-validated molecular antimicrobial susceptibility assays that can be conducted using specimens for NAATs.[45]

Gram stain of urethral discharge collected from men is an excellent point-of-care test for gonorrhea. Demonstration of polymorphonuclear leukocytes with intracellular Gram-negative diplocci has high sensitivity and specificity and is considered diagnostic for urethral gonorrhea in symptomatic men.[40] Gram stain is not recommended for specimens collected from asymptomatic sites of infection and women. In the United States, availability of Gram stain microscopy is largely limited to specialty STI clinics.

Culture in antibiotic-containing selective media, such as modified Thayer-Martin, can be performed on specimens from all anatomic sites of infection, including blood and synovial fluid. Sensitivity varies by anatomic site of infection: sensitivities of culture of urethral specimens from men and cervical specimens from women are greater than of cultures of pharyngeal and rectal specimens (possibly due to differences by anatomic site in bacterial load).[40] As a fastidious organism, isolation of *N. gonorrhoeae* by culture requires demanding temperature and CO_2 concentration conditions. Optimal sensitivity thus relies on careful attention to specimen collection and handling. Media plates should be inoculated soon after specimen collection and placed into a temperature-controlled (35°–36.5°) and CO_2-enriched environment. Use of culture in the United States and many developed countries has declined markedly and has been largely supplanted by NAATs. The primary advantage of *N. gonorrhoeae* culture is the ability to conduct AST. In the United States, use of culture is largely limited to specialty STI clinics and used for surveillance of *N. gonorrhoeae* antimicrobial susceptibility and evaluation of patients who might have been unsuccessfully treated because of an antimicrobial-resistant infection. Because of the emerging threat of antimicrobial resistance, CDC encourages local and state public health laboratories in the United States to maintain *N. gonorrhoeae* culture and AST capabilities.[46] Clinicians and healthcare settings are encouraged to either maintain necessary supplies for collection of culture specimens or be aware of where to locally refer patients for culture and AST.[46]

Although Gram stain and culture are highly specific for *N. gonorrhoeae*, *N. meningitidis* can be indistinguishable by Gram stain and culture of urethral specimens from *N. gonorrhoeae*.[47] *N. meningitidis* has been increasingly recognized as a likely cause of urethritis.[47–49] Use of *N. gonorrhoeae* NAAT or microbiological techniques to speciation the organism (such as Analytical Profile Index Neisseria-Haemophilus strip biochemical testing [bioMérieux, Marcy l'Etoile, France] or matrix-assisted laser desorption ionization-time of flight mass spectrometry [MALDI-TOF]) can differentiate urethral *N. meningitidis* from *N. gonorrhoeae*.

SCREENING

As noted above, gonococcal infections, particularly cervical, pharyngeal, and rectal infections, may be asymptomatic and only detected through screening. Among women, the primary benefit of screening is reducing individual risk of reproductive health complications. The United States Preventive Services Task Force (USPSTF) and CDC recommend annual screening for *N. gonorrhoeae* and *C. trachomatis* in all sexually active women aged < 25 years and for older women at increased risk of infection (such as having multiple concurrent partners or an STI-infected partner).[26,50] Screening and prompt treatment of gonorrhea might also reduce the likelihood of transmission to sexual partners and continued transmission within the community.

Screening recommendations have been established for additional populations. Based on the high burden of disease among MSM and to support disease control, CDC recommends that clinicians screen sexually active MSM for gonorrhea at least annually.[50] Men who have had insertive sex in the preceding year, regardless of condom use during exposure, should be screened for urethral infections; men who have had receptive oral or anal sex, regardless of condom use, should be screened for pharyngeal or rectal infections, respectively.

CDC also recommends that all pregnant women aged < 25 years of age and older women at increased risk for gonorrhea should be screened for gonorrhea at the first prenatal visit.[50] Pregnant women who remain at high risk for gonorrhea should be retested during the third trimester to prevent postnatal complications and gonococcal infections in the newborn.[50] The Infectious Diseases Society of America (IDSA) recommends that all men and women living with HIV be screened for gonorrhea at initial presentation and then annually if at risk for infection.[51]

Screening recommendations for persons in corrections facilities have also been released. Based on high prevalence of disease in the population, CDC recommends universal chlamydia and gonorrhea screening at intake of adolescent girls in juvenile detention facilities and women ≤ 35 years of age in adult correctional facilities.[50] The National Commission on Correctional Healthcare issued a position statement in 2014 recommending that facilities offer chlamydia and gonorrhea testing to: women up to age 25, and when possible up to 35; pregnant women regardless of age; and all sexually active men up to age 25.[52]

Despite longstanding screening recommendations, widespread availability of NAATs that allow detection of both gonorrhea and chlamydia, and chlamydia screening as a Healthcare Effectiveness Data and Information Set (HEDIS) performance measure, screening rates remain suboptimal. Although not specific for gonorrhea, data from the National Survey of Family Growth (NSFG) and the National Health Interview Survey (NHIS) demonstrated that only 36.8% of 15- to 19-year-old and 54.7% of 20- to 24-year-old women who were sexually active with an opposite sex partner in the past year reported having been tested for an STI other than chlamydia.[53] Data from the Medical Monitoring Project, which samples persons in HIV care, demonstrated that only 23% of patients received a gonorrhea test in the preceding 12 months.[54] Barriers to screening may include limited physician time during clinical encounters and provider reticence to ascertain sexual histories.[55] Possible interventions to increase screening within a healthcare practice include implementation of routine patient self-collection of swabs or urine specimens and implementation of electronic medical record prompts for providers or clinical decision support tools.[56–58] Collection of NAAT specimens in settings other than traditional healthcare settings may help to reach high-risk persons who may not seek regular clinical services.[59]

TREATMENT AND RESISTANCE

Gonorrhea is treated with antimicrobial therapy, with the choice of antimicrobials based on established treatment guidelines, such as those of the CDC or WHO.[50,60] Currently, CDC recommends uncomplicated gonorrhea of the pharynx, urethra, cervix, or rectum be treated with the combination of injectable ceftriaxone 250 mg as a single intramuscular dose and oral azithromycin as a single 1 gram oral dose. The WHO, European Center for Disease Control (ECDC), and United Kingdom have released similar guidelines, though dosages of ceftriaxone or azithromycin differ from the CDC guidelines.[50–62] Per CDC guidelines, gonococcal conjunctivitis in adults should be treated with ceftriaxone 1 gram as a single intramuscular dose plus azithromycin 1 gram orally.[50] One-time lavage of the infected eye with saline solution can be considered. Treatment of DGI should include a high-dose daily parenteral cephalosporin, such as ceftriaxone 1 gram daily, plus a single dose of azithromycin; gonococcal meningitis and endocarditis should be treated with ceftriaxone 1–2 gram intravenously every 12–24 hours plus azithromycin 1 gram once orally. All *N. gonorrhoeae* isolates collected from patients with DGI should be tested for antimicrobial susceptibility. Infants with ophthalmia neonatorum should be treated with ceftriaxone 25–50 mg/kg intravenously or intramuscularly in a single dose, not to exceed 125 mg.[50]

Prior to the introduction of antimicrobial therapy in the first half of the twentieth century, gonorrhea was often treated with purgatives, diuretics and laxatives, bleeding and leeching, urethral irrigation with or topical application of mercury, and the insertion of bougies or sounds (solid rods) into the urethra to remove strictures.[1] Not only were such treatment ineffective, but it is plausible that the treatments themselves may have compounded the morbidity from the infection. The introduction of the antimicrobial sulfonamides (1936) and particularly penicillin (1943) provided safe and effective antimicrobial therapy and revolutionized gonorrhea treatment. With antimicrobial therapy, infections could be easily treated, sequelae averted, and transmission to partners prevented. Detection of infection followed by prompt and effective antimicrobial therapy has become a critical component of public health gonorrhea control efforts in the United States.

However, this component of gonorrhea control has been threatened by antimicrobial resistance. Sulfonamide resistance was identified soon after of the use of these drugs.[12] The stepwise accumulation of chromosomal mutations conferring penicillin resistance was able to be overcome with increasing dosages of penicillin and the addition of probenecid to prolong penicillin serum concentrations.[12] However, the emergence of penicillinase-producing *N. gonorrhoeae* (PPNG) in the late 1970s and the early 1980s—apparently initially in East Asia and West Africa before spreading internationally—rendered penicillin ineffective.[63] Tetracycline resistance then followed, undermining the effectiveness of minocycline and doxycycline.[64,65] Fluoroquinolone-resistant strains (QRNG) later emerged in East Asia during the 1990s.[65] As demonstrated by surveillance data from GISP, QRNG reached the United States by the 2000s, initially in Hawaii and the West Coast of the continental United States.[66] The prevalence of QRNG increased rapidly among MSM.[67] Although the prevalence of QRNG subsequently increased among men who have sex with women (MSW), the prevalence of fluoroquinolone resistance (and penicillin and tetracycline resistance) remains markedly higher among gonococcal specimens from MSM than those from MSW.[68,69] Following the emergence of QRNG and changes in CDC treatment guidelines to no longer recommend fluoroquinolones for gonorrhea treatment, third-generation or extended-spectrum cephalosporins (oral cefixime and injectable ceftriaxone) were then the only remaining antimicrobials recommended.[68]

During the past decade, the effectiveness of these drugs has been threatened by the global spread of strains with reduced cephalosporin susceptibility. Ceftriaxone-resistant infections have been identified in Japan, France, Spain, and the United Kingdom.[70–73] Data from GISP demonstrated declining cefixime and to a lesser degree, ceftriaxone susceptibility among gonococcal strains in the United States, particularly in the Western United States and among MSM.[8] Many of these isolates with reduced cephalosporin susceptibility are resistant to other previously recommended antimicrobials, such as penicillin, tetracycline, and ciprofloxacin.[8] Since 2014, susceptibility to azithromycin has declined in the United States.[8] Although the co-occurrence of reduced susceptibility to both azithromycin and cephalosporins remains rare in the United States, a small cluster of *N. gonorrhoeae* infections with high-level azithromycin resistance and decreased ceftriaxone susceptibility was identified in Hawaii in 2016.[74] In early

2018, a man in the United Kingdom who had recently returned from an Asian country was found to have a urethral and pharyngeal infection with a strain exhibiting high-level azithromycin resistance and decreased ceftriaxone susceptibility.[73] Concerningly, the pharyngeal infection was not cured despite high-dose ceftriaxone and doxycycline; three doses of intravenous ertapenem cured the infection.

Treatment guidelines are directly informed by data from clinical trials and surveillance. Traditionally, CDC has recommended antimicrobial regimens with efficacy of $\geq 95\%$ to reliably cure the infection, prevent sequelae, and prevent transmission to sex partners; treatment guidelines have been revised to no longer recommend antimicrobial agents once the prevalence of resistance exceeds 5%. Recent treatment guideline changes (such as discouraging oral cephalosporin use and adding azithromycin as dual therapy) diverged from this model because of the paucity of other treatment options and in an attempt to slow the emergence or spread of resistance to ceftriaxone.

Continuing emergence of resistance and the dwindling antibiotic pipeline have prompted experts to warn of the potential for untreatable gonorrhea.[75] Gonorrhea was designated an urgent antibiotic resistance threat by the CDC and a high priority pathogen by the WHO.[76,77] Highlighting the increasing recognition of the public health threat posed by *N. gonorrhoeae*, the U.S. White House National Strategy and National Action Plan for Combating Antibiotic-Resistant Bacteria (CARB) set a national target of maintaining the prevalence of ceftriaxone-resistance at $< 2\%$ through 2020.[7,8] Using Congressional funding allocated to support implementation of the Action Plan, CDC implemented *Strengthening U.S. Response to Resistant Bacteria* (SURRG) in 2016 in collaboration with state and local health departments. SURRG builds local capacity to rapidly detect and respond to emerging resistant gonococcal strains. Participating jurisdictions received funding to scale up collection of specimens for culture, conduct rapid AST by Etest, enhance information systems to allow rapid flow of data, build epidemiological analytic capacity, and strengthen local capacity to rapidly identify, interview, and test sexual partners to slow the spread of resistant strains. The National Institute of Allergy and Infectious Diseases (NIAID) at the National Institutes of Health (NIH) supports investigations of new antimicrobial agents and NIAID, the Biomedical Advanced Research Development Authority (BARDA), and the Wellcome Trust began a global public–private partnership called CARB-X to spur investment and research into new antimicrobials, vaccines, and diagnostics. At the time of writing, ertapenem (NCT03294395) is undergoing clinical investigation and Phase 2 studies of two new agents—gepotidicin (NCT02294682) and zoliflodacin (NCT02257918)—have been completed (www.clinicaltrials.gov).

SYNDROMIC MANAGEMENT

In low-resource countries without routine access to laboratory diagnostics, syndromic management remains the approach to individual clinical management and STI control.[79] Syndromic management involves the use of simple flowcharts for healthcare workers to choose treatment based on the most likely causes of easily identified syndromes, such as urethral discharge and genital ulcer disease. While syndromic management may assist with treatment of symptomatic men with urethral discharge, syndromic management of vaginal discharge performs poorly for correct identification and management of cervical gonococcal infections. Sensitivity suffers because of the asymptomatic nature of cervical infections and specificity suffers because syndromic evaluations cannot distinguish gonorrhea from more common infections and dysbioses, such as trichomoniasis, bacterial vaginosis, or vaginal candidiasis.[79]

FOLLOW-UP AND PARTNER MANAGEMENT

Over 10% of heterosexual men and women diagnosed with gonorrhea may become reinfected within the next several months and a substantial proportion of MSM with gonorrhea experience reinfection.[39,80] Because of the high reinfection rate, CDC recommends that persons diagnosed with and treated for gonorrhea return for retesting 3 months after treatment.[50]

An important component of preventing reinfection is ensuring that recent sex partners (from within the past 60 days) are evaluated, tested, and presumptively treated for gonorrhea. Partner notification and management has been an important aspect of United States approaches to control STIs since the 1940s.[81] Partner notification of exposure can generally be conducted in one of three ways: patient notification, in which the patient is responsible for notifying the partner; provider referral, in which a clinician or health department employee collects identifying and contact information about the partner from the patient and contacts the partner; and conditional or contract referral, in which provider referral occurs if patient notification does not occur in a defined time period. Some jurisdictions have experimented with electronic notification approaches.[82] Barriers to successful partner management include patient refusal to notify partners or provide names or locating information of partners, anonymity of partners, and challenges that partners may face accessing healthcare. An option for heterosexual partners who may be unable to unwilling to seek medical evaluation and treatment (and in geographic areas in which it is permissible) is expedited partner therapy (EPT), in which a healthcare provider offers medications or a prescription to the patient to bring to their partner(s).[50] Currently, CDC recommends the use of cefixime 400 mg and azithromycin 1 gram orally as combination therapy for EPT.[50] EPT can reduce the risk of repeated infections in the patient and might provide a marginal effect on incidence on a population level.[80,83] The continued emergence of resistance may threaten the efficacy of EPT for gonorrhea.

PREVENTION AND CONTROL

Prevention and control efforts can be considered as primary or secondary prevention. The goal of primary prevention is to prevent gonococcal infection in an individual, and the goals of secondary prevention are to avert sequelae in infected persons and prevent transmission to partners. Because of the consideration of transmission, secondary prevention in an individual to prevent transmission to others may also function as primary prevention for his or her sexual contacts.

Primary Prevention

Available approaches that reduce the likelihood of infection are abstinence or reductions in the number of sexual partners, consistent and correct use of latex condoms, and performance of nonpenetrative sex acts, such as mutual masturbation, rather than penetrative sex acts. While abstinence or mutual monogamy with an uninfected partner clearly reduce the risk of gonorrhea, these behavioral approaches may not be acceptable to all persons. Reducing the number of sexual partners and reducing concurrency of partnerships may reduce transmission risk. However, local disease prevalence can play an important role in mediating risks: persons with few partners but who are situated within a high-prevalence sexual network may experience greater risk of gonorrhea acquisition than persons with many partners but who are situated in a low-prevalence network.[15]

Correct and consistent condom use is greater than 90% effective for preventing acquisition of gonorrhea.[84,85] Inconsistent condom use with partners with whom the individual is not mutually monogamous and errors in condom use, such as late application or early removal, slippage during sex, or reuse of condoms, decrease effectiveness of condoms.[86] Although overall condom use may be increasing,[87] condom use may be declining among MSM. Reports of condomless sex at last sex increased from 34% in 2005 to 45% in 2014 among HIV-positive MSM, with increases observed in men with HIV-concordant and discordant partners.[88] The percentage of HIV-negative MSM reporting condomless sex at last anal sex increased from 29% to 41% during the same time frame.[88]

Development of a vaccine active against *N. gonorrhoeae*, even if of modest effectiveness, could play a powerful role in decreasing efficiency of transmission. The ability of the bacterium to mutate to evade the immune system, limitations of animal models, and the lack of natural host immunity have posed substantial barriers to vaccine research. Potential vaccine targets include immunogenic proteins with high degrees of antigen conservation and stable expression, such as TbpAB and the 2C7 epitope of lipooligosaccharide, and outer membrane vesicles combined with other proteins (fHBP, NHBA, and NadA) that were used in *N. meningitidis* serogroup B vaccines.[89–91] The threat of gonococcal antimicrobial resistance and recent data from New Zealand that demonstrated population-level reductions in gonorrhea following a meningococcal B vaccination campaign have reinvigorated *N. gonorrhoeae* vaccine research efforts.[92]

To prevent gonococcal ophthalmia neonatorum, pregnant women < 25 years and older women at increased risk for infection should be screened for gonorrhea at the first prenatal visit.[50] Pregnant women who remain at high risk should be retested during the third trimester to prevent maternal postnatal complications and gonococcal infection in the neonate.[50] Additionally, prophylactic erythromycin (0.5%) ophthalmic ointment should be instilled into both eyes of all newborn infants as soon as possible after delivery.[50] Ocular prophylaxis can prevent sight-threatening gonococcal ophthalmia, has an excellent safety record, and is inexpensive. If erythromycin ointment is not available, infants at risk for exposure to *N. gonorrhoeae*, such as those born to mothers at risk for gonorrhea or with no prenatal care, can receive intravenous or intramuscular ceftriaxone 25–50 mg/kg, not to exceed 125 mg in a single dose.[50] (https://www.cdc.gov/std/tg2015/references.htm#582) (https://www.cdc.gov/std/tg2015/references.htm#584) (https://www.cdc.gov/std/tg2015/references.htm#586) (https://www.cdc.gov/std/tg2015/references.htm#587) (https://www.cdc.gov/std/tg2015/references.htm#588)

Secondary Prevention

In the United States, the cornerstones of secondary prevention (often referred to as gonorrhea control) are: screening, ideally provided within the context of high-quality and culturally appropriate sexual health services provided in welcome spaces for persons of color, sexual minorities, and transgender and gender nonbinary persons; prompt and effective antimicrobial treatment of infected persons; and, given the high transmissibility of gonorrhea, treatment of the patient's recent sex partners.

As described above, gonorrhea rates have increased among men, and seemingly among MSM, and the threat of emerging resistance continues to grow. New prevention and control approaches and a more robust evidence base on effectiveness of existing approaches are needed.

CONCLUSION

Although an ancient disease, gonorrhea continues to challenge us. The specter of multidrug-resistant *N. gonorrhoeae* looms on the horizon. Advances in the understanding of epidemiology, transmission dynamics, microbiology, and mechanisms of resistance, diagnostic development, vaccine development, and development of new therapeutic candidates should provide optimism that continued efforts will allow us to stay at least a step ahead of this public health threat.

References

1. Milton JL. *On the Pathology and Treatment of Gonorrhea*. 5th ed. New York: William Wood and Company; 1884.
2. Ligon BL. Albert Ludwig Sigesmund Neisser: Discoverer of the cause of gonorrhea. *Semin Pediatr Infect Dis*. 2005;16(4):336–41.
3. Pearce WA, Buchanan TM. Attachment role of gonococcal pili: Optimum conditions and quantitation of adherence of isolated pili to human cells in vitro. *J Clin Invest*. 1978;61:931–43.
4. Sugasawara RJ, Cannon JG, Black WJ, et al. Inhibition of *Neisseria gonorrhoeae* attachment to HeLa cells with monoclonal antibody directed against a protein II. *Infect Immunol*. 1983;42:980–5.
5. Rotman E, Seifer HE. The genetics of Neisseria species. *Annu Rev Genet*. 2014;48:405–31.
6. Seifert HS, Wright CJ, Jerse AE, et al. Multiple gonococcal pilin antigenic variants are produced during experimental human infection. *J Clin Invest*. 1994;93:2744–9.
7. Black WJ, Schwalbe RS, Nachamkin I, et al. Characterization of *Neisseria gonorrhoeae* protein II phase variation by use of monoclonal antibodies. *Infect Immunol*. 1984;45:453–7.
8. Centers for Disease Control and Prevention. *Sexually Transmitted Disease Surveillance 2016*. Atlanta, Georgia: U.S. Department of Health and Human Services; 2017.
9. Overhage JM, Grannis S, McDonald CJ. A comparison of the completeness and timeliness of automated electronic laboratory reporting and spontaneous reporting of notifiable conditions. *Am J Public Health*. 2008;98(2):344–50.
10. Satterwhite CL, Torrone E, Meites E, et al. Sexually transmitted infections among US women and men: Prevalence and incidence estimates, 2008. *Sex Transm Dis*. 2013;40(3):187–93.
11. Thayer JD, Martin JE. Selective medium for the cultivation of *N. gonorrhoeae* and *N. meningitidis*. *Public Health Rep*. 1964;79:49.
12. Hook EW 3rd, Kirkcaldy RD. A brief history of evolving diagnostics and therapy in gonorrhea: Lessons learned. *Clin Infect Dis*. 2018;67(8):1294–9.
13. Peterman TA, O'Connor K, Bradley HM, Torrone EA, Bernstein KT. Gonorrhea control, United States, 1972–2015, a narrative review. *Sex Transm Dis*. 2016;43(12):725–30.
14. Weston EJ, Kirkcaldy RD, Stenger M, Llata E, Hoots B, Torrone EA. Narrative review: Assessment of *Neisseria gonorrhoeae* infections among men who have sex with men in national and sentinel surveillance systems in the United States. *Sex Transm Dis*. 2018;45(4):243–9.
15. Rietmeijer CA, Donnelly J, Bernstein KT, et al. Here comes the SSuN: Early experiences with the STD Surveillance Network. *Public Health Rep*. 2009;124 Suppl 2:72–7.
16. Hogben M, Leichliter JS. Social determinants and sexually transmitted disease disparities. *Sex Transm Dis*. 2008;35(12 Suppl):S13–18.
17. Centers for Disease Control and Prevention. *Sexually Transmitted Disease Surveillance 2011*. Atlanta, GA: U.S. Department of Health and Human Services; 2012.
18. Elkington KS, Teplin LE, Mericle AA, et al. HIV/sexually transmitted infection risk behaviors in delinquent youth with psychiatric disorders: A longitudinal study. *J Am Acad Child Adolesc Psychiatry*. 2008;47:901–11.
19. Kelly PJ, Bair RM, Baillargeon J et al. Risk behaviors and the prevalence of chlamydia in a juvenile detention facility. *Clin Pediatr*. 2000;39:521–7.
20. Teplin LA, Mericle AA, McClelland GM, et al. HIV and AIDS risk behaviors in juvenile detainees: Implications for public health policy. *Am J Public Health*. 2003;93:906Y912.
21. Mertz KJ, Schwebke JR, Gaydos CA, et al. Screening women in jails for chlamydial and gonococcal infection using urine tests: Feasibility, acceptability, prevalence, and treatment rates. *Sex Transm Dis*. 2002;29:271–6.
22. Miller JL, Samoff E, Bolan G. Implementing chlamydia screening programs in juvenile correctional settings: The California experience. *Sex Transm Dis*. 2009;36:S53–7.
23. Newman L, Rowley K, Vander Hoorn S, et al. Global estimates of the prevalence and incidence of four curable sexually transmitted infections in 2012 based on systematic review and global reporting. *PLoS One*. 2015;10(12):e0143304.
24. Hook EW3rd, Reichart CA, Upchurch DM, Ray P, Celentano D, Quinn TC. Comparative behavorial epidemiology of gonococcal and chlamydial infections among patients attending a Baltimore, Maryland, sexually transmitted disease clinic. *Am J Epidemiol*. 1992;136(6):662–72.
25. Mertz KJ, Levine WC, Mosure DJ, Berman SM, Dorian KJ, Hadgu A. Screening women for gonorrhea: Demographic screening criteria for general clinical use. *Am J Public Health*. 1997;87(9):1535–8.
26. LeFevre ML. U.S. Preventive Services Task Force. Screening for chlamydia and gonorrhea: U.S. Preventive Services Task Force recommendation statement. *Ann Intern Med*. 2014;161:902–10.
27. Klausner JD, Barrett DC, Dithmer D, Boyer CB, Brooks GF, Bolan G. Risk factors for repeated gonococcal infections: San Francisco, 1990–1992. *J Infect Dis*. 1998;177(6):1766–9.
28. Holmes KK, Johnson DW, Trostle HJ. An estimate of the risk of men acquiring gonorrhea by sexual contact with infected females. *Am J Epidemiol*. 1970;91(2):170–4.
29. Hooper RR, Reynolds GH, Jones OG, et al. Cohort study of venereal disease. I: The risk of gonorrhea transmission from infected women to men. *Am J Epidemiol*. 1978;108(2):136–44.

30. Platt R, Rice PA, McCormack WM. Risk of acquiring gonorrhea and prevalence of abnormal adnexal findings among women recently exposed to gonorrhea. *JAMA*. 1983;250(23):3205–9.
31. Hui B, Fairley CK, Chen M, et al. Oral and anal sex are key to sustaining gonorrhea at endemic levels in MSM populations: A mathematical model. *Sex Transm Infect*. 2015;91(5):365–9.
32. Alexander ER. Gonorrhea in the newborn. *Ann N Y Acad Sci*. 1988;549:180–6.
33. Noble RC, Reyes RR, Parekh MC, Haley JV. Incidence of disseminated gonococcal infection correlated with the presence of AHU auxotype in *Neisseria gonorrhoeae* in a community. *Sex Transm Dis*. 1984;11(2):68–71.
34. Tuttle CS, Van Dantzig T, Brady S, Ward J, Maguire G. The epidemiology of gonococcal arthritis in an indigenous Australian population. *Sex Transm Infect*. 2015;91(7):497–501.
35. Rice PA. Gonococcal arthritis (disseminated gonococcal infection). *Infect Dis Clin North Am*. 2005;19(4):853–61.
36. Belkacem A, Caumes E, Ouanich J, et al. Changing patterns of disseminated gonococcal infection in France: Cross-sectional data 2009–2011. *Sex Transm Infect*. 2013;89(9):613–5.
37. Pathela P, Braunstein SL, Blank S, Schillinger JA. HIV incidence among men with and those without sexually transmitted rectal infections: Estimates from matching against an HIV case registry. *Clin Infect Dis*. 2013;57(8):1203–9.
38. Cheung KT, Fairley CK, Read TR, et al. HIV incidence and predictors of HIV incidence among men who have sex with men attending a sexual health clinic in Melbourne, Australia. *PLoS One*. 2016;11(5):e0156160.
39. Bernstein KT, Marcus JL, Nieri G, Philip SS, Klausner JD. Rectal gonorrhea and chlamydia reinfection is associated with increased risk of HIV seroconversion. *J Acquir Immune Defic Syndrom*. 2010;53(4):537–43.
40. Papp JR, Schachter J, Gaydos CA, Van Der Pol B. Recommendations for the laboratory-based detection of *Chlamydia trachomatis* and *Neisseria gonorrhoeae*—2014. *MMWR Recomm Rep*. 2014;63(No. RR-2):1–19.
41. Roth AM, Goldshear JL, Martinez-Donate AP, et al. Reducing missed opportunities: Pairing sexually transmitted infection screening with syringe exchange services. *Sex Transm Dis*. 2016;43(11):706–8.
42. Donaldson AA, Burns J, Bradshaw CP, Ellen JM, Maehr J. Screening juvenile justice-involved females for sexually transmitted infection: A pilot intervention for urban females in community supervision. *J Correct Health Care*. 2013;19(4):258–68.
43. Bennett C, Knight C, Knox D, Gray J, Hartmann G, McNulty A. An alternative model of sexually transmissible infection testing in men attending a sex-on-premises venue in Sydney: A cross-sectional descriptive study. *Sex Health*. 2016 May 23 [Epub ahead of print].
44. Ladd J, Hsieh YH, Barnes M, et al. Female users of internet-based screening for rectal STIs: Descriptive statistics and correlates of positivity. *Sex Transm Infect*. 2014;90(6):485–90.
45. Allan-Blitz LT, Humphries RM, Hemarajata P, et al. Implementation of a rapid genotype assay to promote targeted ciprofloxacin therapy of *Neisseria gonorrhoeae* in a large health system. *Clin Infect Dis*. 2017;64(9):1268–70.
46. CDC. Cephalosporin-resistant *Neisseria gonorrhoeae* public health response plan. https://www.cdc.gov/std/treatment/ceph-r-responseplan-july30-2012.pdf. Accessed May 6, 2018.
47. Bazan JA, Turner AN, Kirkcaldy RD, et al. Large cluster of *Neisseria meningitidis* urethritis in Columbus, Ohio, 2015. *Clin Infect Dis*. 2017;65(1):92–9.
48. Tzeng YL, Bazan JA, Turner AN, et al. Emergence of a new *Neisseria meningitidis* clonal complex 11 lineage 11.2 clade as an effective urogenital pathogen. *Proc Natl Acad Sci U S A*. 2017;23(2):336–9.
49. Ma KC, Unemo M, Jeverica S, et al. Genomic characterization of urethritis-associated *Neisseria meningitidis* shows that a wide range of *N. meningitidis* strains can cause urethritis. *J Clin Microbiol*. 2017;55(12):3374–83.
50. Workowski KA, Bolan GA, CDC. Sexually transmitted diseases treatment guidelines, 2015. *MMWR Recomm Rep*. 2015;64(RR-03):1–137.
51. Aberg JA, Gallant JE, Ghanem KG, et al. Primary care guidelines for the management of persons infected with HIV: 2013 Update by the HIV Medicine Association of the Infectious Diseases Society of America. *Clin Infect Dis*. 2014;58(1):e1–34.
52. National Commission on Correctional Health Care. STD testing for adolescents and adults upon admission to correctional facilities. https://www.ncchc.org/std-testing-upon-admission. Accessed May 6, 2018.
53. Pazol K, Robbins CL, Black LI, et al. Receipt of selected preventive health services for women and men of reproductive age—United States, 2011–2013. *MMWR Surveill Summar*. 2017;66(No. SS-20):1–31.
54. Flagg EW, Weinstock HS, Frazier EL, et al. Bacterial sexually transmitted infections among HIV-infected patients in the United States: Estimates from the Medical Monitoring Project. *Sex Transm Dis*. 2015;42(4):171–9.
55. Carter JW, Hart-Cooper GD, Butler MO, Workowski KA, Hoover KW. Provider barriers prevent recommended sexually transmitted disease screening of HIV-infected men who have sex with men. *Sex Transm Dis*. 2014;41(2):137–42.
56. Patton ME, Kirkcaldy RD, Chang DC, et al. Increased gonorrhea screening and case finding after implementation of expanded screening criteria—Urban Indian Health Service facility in Phoenix, Arizona, 2011–2013. *Sex Transm Dis*. 2016;43(6):396–401.
57. Taylor MM, Frasure-Williams J, Burnett P, Park IU. Interventions to improve sexually transmitted disease screening in clinic-based settings. *Sex Transm Dis*. 2016;43(2Supple 1):S28–41.
58. Lutz AR. Screening for asymptomatic extragenital gonorrhea and chlamydia in men who have sex with men: Significant, recommendations, and options for overcoming barriers to testing. *LGBT Health*. 2015;2(1):27–34.
59. Bernstein KT, Chow JM, Pathela P, Gift TL. Bacterial sexually transmitted disease screening outside the clinic—Implications for the modern sexually transmitted disease program. *Sex Tranms Dis*. 2016;43(2 Suppl 1):S42–52.
60. World Health Organization. WHO guidelines for the treatment of *Neisseria gonorrhoeae*. http://apps.who.int/iris/bitstream/handle/10665/246114/9789241549691-eng.pdf;jsessionid=7A5696515FC29408DAE5408516E1FCC3?sequence=1. Accessed May 7, 2018.
61. Bignell C, Unemo M. 2012 European guideline on the diagnosis and treatment of gonorrhoea in adults. *Int J STD AIDS*. 2013;24(2):85–92.
62. Bignell C, FitzGerald M. UK national guidelines for the management of gonorrhea in adults, 2011. *Int J STD AIDS*. 2011;22:541–7.
63. Jaffe HW, Biddle JW, Johnson SR, Wiesner PJ. Infections due to penicillinase-producing *Neisseria gonorrhoeae* in the United States: 1976–1980. *J Infect Dis*. 1981;144:191–7.
64. Centers for Disease Control and Prevention. Tetracycline-resistant *Neisseria gonorrhoeae*—Georgia, Pennsylvania, New Hampshire. *MMWR Morb Mortal Wkly Rep*. 1985;34(37):563–4.
65. Unemo M, del Rio C, Shafer WM. Antimicrobial resistance expressed by *Neisseria gonorrhoeae*: A major global public health problem in the 21st century. *Microbiol Spectr*. 2016;4(3):1–18.
66. CDC. Increases in fluoroquinolone-resistant *Neisseria gonorrhoeae*—Hawaii and California, 2001. *MMWR Morb Mortal Wkly Rep*. 2002;51(46):1041–4.
67. CDC. Increases in fluoroquinolone-resistant *Neisseria gonorrhoeae* among men who have sex with men—United States, 2003, and revised recommendations for gonorrhea treatment, 2004. *MMWR Morb Mortal Wkly Rep*. 2004;53(16):335–8.
68. Kirkcaldy RD, Zaidi A, Hook EW 3rd, et al. *Neisseria gonorrhoeae* antimicrobial resistance among men who have sex with men and men who have sex exclusively with women: The Gonococcal Isolate Surveillance Project, 2005–2010. *Ann Intern Med*. 2013;158(5 Pt 1):321–8.
69. CDC. Update to CDC's sexually transmitted diseases treatment guidelines, 2006: Fluoroquinolones no longer recommended for treatment of gonococcal infections. *MMWR Morb Mortal Wkly Rep*. 2007;56(14):332–6.
70. Ohnishi M, Saika T, Hoshina S, et al. Ceftriaxone-resistant *Neisseria gonorrhoeae*, Japan. *Emerg Infect Dis*. 2011;17(1):148–9.
71. Unemo M, Golparian D, Nicholas R, Ohnishi M, Gallay A, Sednaoui P. High-level cefixime- and ceftriaxone-resistant *Neisseria gonorrhoeae* in France: Novel penA mosaic allele in a successful international clone causes treatment failure. *Antimicrob Agents Chemother*. 2012;56(3):1273–80.
72. Cámara J, Serra J, Ayats J, et al. Molecular characterization of two high-level ceftriaxone-resistant *Neisseria gonorrhoeae* isolates detected in Catalonia, Spain. *J Antimicrob Chemother*. 2012;67(8):1858–60.
73. Public Health England. Update on investigation of UK Case of *Neisseria gonorrhoeae* with high-level resistance to azithromycin and resistance to ceftriaxone acquired abroad. *Health Prot Rep*. 2018;12(14). https://assets.publishing.service.gov.uk/government/uploads/system/uploads/attachment_data/file/701185/hpr1418_MDRGC.pdf. Accessed May 7, 2018.
74. Katz AR, Komeya AY, Kirkcaldy RD, et al. Cluster of *Neisseria gonorrhoeae* isolates with high-level azithromycin resistance and decreased ceftriaxone susceptibility, Hawaii, 2016. *Clin Infect Dis*. 2017;65(6):918–23.
75. Bolan GA, Sparling PF, Wasserheit JN. The emerging threat of untreatable gonococcal infection. *N Engl J Med*. 2012;366(6):485–7.
76. CDC. Antibiotic resistance threats in the United States, 2013. https://www.cdc.gov/drugresistance/threat-report-2013/pdf/ar-threats-2013-508.pdf. Access May 7, 2018.

77. World Health Organization. Global priority list of antibiotic-resistant bacteria to guide research, discovery, and development of new antibiotics. http://www.who.int/medicines/publications/WHO-PPL-Short_Summary_25Feb-ET_NM_WHO.pdf?ua=1. Accessed May 7, 2018.

78. National Action Plan for Combating Antibiotic-Resistant Bacteria. March 2015. https://obamawhitehouse.archives.gov/sites/default/files/docs/national_action_plan_for_combating_antibotic-resistant_bacteria.pdf. Accessed May 7, 2018.

79. Low N, Broutet N, Adu-Sarkodie Y, et al. Global control of sexually transmitted infections. *Lancet.* 2006;368(9551):2001–16.

80. Golden MR, Whittington WL, Handsfield HH, et al. Effect of expedited treatment of sex partners on recurrent or persistent gonorrhea or chlamydial infection. *N Engl J Med.* 2005;352(7):676–85.

81. Parran T. *Shadow on the Land: Syphilis.* New York: Reynal & Hitchcock; 1937.

82. Kerani RP, Fleming M, Golden MR. Acceptability and intention to seek medical care after hypothetical receipt of patient-delivered partner therapy or electronic partner notification postcards among men who have sex with men: The partner's perspective. *Sex Transm Dis.* 2013;40(2):179–85.

83. Golden MR, Kerani RP, Stenger M, et al. Uptake and population-level impact of expedited partner therapy (EPT) on *Chlamydia trachomatis* and *Neisseria gonorrhoeae*: The Washington State community-level randomized trial of EPT. *PLoS Med.* 2015;12(1):e1001777.

84. Warner L, Stone KM, Macaluso H, et al. Condom use and risk of gonorrhea and chlamydia: A systematic review of design and measurement factors assessed in epidemiologic studies. *Sex Transm Dis.* 2006;33(1):36–51.

85. Mindel A, Sawleshwarkar S. Condoms for sexually transmissible infection prevention: Politics versus science. *Sex Health.* 2008;5(1):1–8.

86. Warner L, Newman DR, Kamb ML, et al. Problems with condom use among patients attending sexually transmitted disease clinics: Prevalence, predictors, and relation to incident gonorrhea and chlamydia. *Am J Epidemiol.* 2008;167(3):341–9.

87. National Survey of Family Growth. Key statistics from the National Survey of Family Growth—C. listing. http://www.cdc.gov/nchs/nsfg/key_statistics/c.htm#condomuse. Accessed May 7, 2018.

88. Paz-Bailey G, Mendoza MC, Finlayson T, et al. Trends in condom use among MSM in the United States: The role of antiretroviral therapy and seroadapative strategies. *AIDS.* 2016;30(12):1985–90.

89. Edwards JL, Jennings MP, Apicella MA, Seib KL. Is gonococcal disease preventable? The importance of understanding immunity and pathogenesis in vaccine development. *Crit Rev Microbiol.* 2016;42(6):928–41.

90. Gottlieb SL, Deal CD, Giersing B, et al. The global roadmap for advancing development of vaccines against sexually transmitted infections: update and next steps. *Vaccine.* 2016;34(26):2939–47.

91. Jerse ME, Bash MC, Russell MW. Vaccines against gonorrhea: Current status and future challenges. *Vaccine.* 2014;32(14):1579–87.

92. Petousis-Harris H, Paynter J, Morgan J, et al. Effectiveness of a group B outer membrane vesicle meningococcal vaccine against gonorrhoea in New Zealand: a retrospective case-control study. *Lancet.* 2017;390(10102):1603–10.

CHAPTER

122

Chlamydia and Other Sexually Transmitted Infections

Suzanne R. Lavoie

Three hundred and seventy-six million new cases of the four curable (chlamydia, gonorrhea, syphilis, and trichomoniasis) sexually transmitted infections (STIs) are estimated to occur each year, according to the World Health Organization (WHO).[1] This amounts to more than 1 million curable STIs occurring each day. The burden of viral STIs is similarly high, with an estimated 417 million prevalent cases of herpes simples virus infection (HSV) and approximately 291 million women infected with human papillomavirus (HPV).[1] In contrast to these infections, many countries have achieved successful control of other STIs like chancroid (etiologic agent *Haemophilus ducreyi)* and lymphogranuloma venereum or LGV (etiologic agent *Chlamydia trachomatis* serovars L1, L2, and L3).[1] In 2016, WHO released the "*Global health sector strategy on sexually transmitted infections 2016-2021,*" with a goal of ending STI epidemics as a major public health concern.[2] This strategy outlined several guiding principles including: achieving universal health coverage; use of evidence-based interventions and policies; promoting human rights, gender equality, and health equality; working through partnerships; integration across relevant sectors; and engagement and empowerment of people most affected. With this in mind, several goals to be achieved by 2030 include: $\leq$50 cases of congenital syphilis per 100,000 live births in 80% of countries; 90% reduction in *T. pallidum* incidence globally; 90% reduction in *N. gonorrhoeae* incidence globally; and 90% national vaccination coverage and at least 80% district coverage in countries with HPV vaccine in their national immunization program.[2]

Chlamydia, gonorrhea, and syphilis ranked first, second, and third among infectious diseases reportable to the U.S. National Notifiable Diseases Surveillance System in 2017, with chlamydia and gonorrhea alone accounting for 95% of these cases.[3] For nonreportable diseases such as trichomoniasis and HPV, data collection is less complete. However, estimates from alternate sources suggest that both of these diseases are even more common than chlamydia.[4] Data from 2008 estimated that 81 million Americans were living with a chronic viral STI, excluding human immunodeficiency virus (HIV).[4] Because many STIs are asymptomatic and go undiagnosed, current surveillance systems probably underestimate the actual burden of disease. In truth, the prevalence of STIs in the United States is largely unknown. However, STIs are unquestionably a substantial health and economic burden.

In 2013, the U.S. Centers for Disease Control and Prevention (CDC) estimated 20 million new STIs each year, including HIV, hepatitis B, HSV type 2, syphilis, gonorrhea, trichomoniasis, chlamydia, and HPV.[5] The economic burden of STIs is substantial, with direct medical costs estimated at 15.6 billion annually in 2008 (in year 2010 U.S. dollars).[5] These estimates do not account for indirect costs from productivity losses (lost wages) or intangible costs from pain, suffering, or diminished quality of life. Although adolescents and young adults aged 15–24 years constitute only 25% of the sexually active population, they represent over half of new STI cases, contributing disproportionately to the total economic burden of STIs. Because some STIs—especially HIV-require lifelong treatment and care, they are by far the costliest. The annual cost of curable STIs is also significant ($742 million). Among them, the most costly is chlamydia because it is the most common.[5] In this chapter, we will discuss chlamydia, LGV, chancroid, and trichomoniasis. The other major STIs including HIV/AIDS, human papilloma virus, hepatitis B, syphilis, gonorrhea, and herpes simplex virus are discussed elsewhere (chapters 87, 100, 101, 120, 121, and 123, respectively).

CHLAMYDIA

Epidemiology

Chlamydia is due to infection with *C. trachomatis* serovars B and D–K and is the most commonly reported notifiable disease in the United States. In 2017, 1,708,569 chlamydia infections were reported to CDC from 50 states and the District of Columbia, representing an incidence of 528.8 cases per 100,000 population.[3] Trends in rates of reported cases are influenced by changes in incidence of infection as well as by changes in diagnostic, screening, and reporting practices.

Since 2000, the expanded use of more sensitive diagnostic tests especially nucleic acid amplification tests (NAATs) has increased the number of infections identified. More recently, the increased use of electronic laboratory reporting has likely increased the proportion of diagnosed cases that are reported in the United States. However, infections have continued to increase yearly between 2013 and 2017 (11% increase among women and 39% increase among men). Overall, the rate of reported chlamydia in the United States increased 110% between 2000 and 2017.

In most studies, chlamydia infection is more common among females than males, although this discrepancy may simply be the result of more active surveillance (screening) of females. However, it suggests that male sex partners of women with chlamydia are not receiving a diagnosis or being reported. In 2017, women account for 66% of cases. Some of the increased rate of infection among males between 2013 and 2017 may be related to improved case identification through intensified extra-genital screening efforts among MSM.[3]

Between the years of 2013 and 2017, the rates of reported cases of chlamydia were highest among adolescents and young adults between the ages of 15 and 24 years. In 2017, the reported incidence was 2072.4/100,000 among 15–19 years olds and 2820.3/100,000 among those aged 20–24 years.[3] Among women, those aged 19–20 years had the highest incidence (5398.6–5141.4/100,000 in 2017), with over 97% of all reported cases occurring in those aged 15–44 year.

Racial and ethnic minorities are disproportionately affected, possibly reflecting a lack of access to screening and treatment programs. In 2017, reported cases of chlamydia were highest among Black, American Indian/Alaska Native (AI/AN), and Native Hawaiian/Other Pacific Islander (NHOPI) women. Overall, the reported cases of chlamydia among these race/ethnic populations was 5.6 (Black), 3.7 (AI/AN), and 3.4 (NHOPI) times that of the reported cases among Whites. The rate among Hispanics was 1.9 times that of non-Hispanic Whites. During 2013–17, rates increased among all racial and Hispanic ethnicity groups.[3]

The National Health and Nutrition Examination Survey (NHANES) is a program of studies designed to assess the health and nutritional status of adults and children in the United States. The NHANES program began in the early 1960s and has been conducted as a series of surveys focusing on different population groups or health topics. The survey examines a nationally representative sample of about 5000 persons per year. Between the years 1999 and 2016, urine samples were obtained for chlamydia testing for those 14–39 years of age. The overall prevalence of chlamydia was 1.7% during the years 2013–16. Among sexually active females aged 14–24 years, the prevalence was 4.3%.[6]

Clinical Manifestations

Chlamydial infections are frequently asymptomatic.[5,7] In a study that encompassed China, India, Peru, Russia, and Zimbabwe, the authors found a high prevalence of asymptomatic disease for chlamydia, with a range of 31–100% of both men and women reporting no symptoms. The infection can persist months to years, if untreated, and reinfections are common.

In women, infection can include urethritis, cervicitis, proctitis, and pelvic inflammatory disease (PID—which may include endometritis, salpingitis, oophoritis) and perihepatitis. Men can present with urethritis, epididymitis, and proctitis. Complications of infection are more common in women. In addition to PID, other complications include ectopic pregnancy, infertility, and chronic pelvic pain. Reactive arthritis can occur in both men and women and may be accompanied by urethritis and conjunctivitis. Infants born to untreated mothers are at risk for chlamydial conjunctivitis or pneumonia.

In a study in 2008, Geisler and associates described a prospective study of the natural history of untreated chlamydia in Jefferson County Department of Health Sexually Transmitted Diseases (STD) clinic in Birmingham, AL.[8] They identified 129 subjects who were asymptomatic and not treated empirically for chlamydia but tested positive and were asked to return for treatment. The median interval between visits was 13 days (range 4–59 days). Approximately 42% of the patients had a previous history of chlamydia. Of the 115 female patients, all but 1 had persisting infection at the time of follow up, about one quarter had newly found purulent endocervical discharge and 2 women were diagnosed with PID at the time of return. Of the 14 men who were asymptomatic but tested positive, 71% presented with new urethral discharge at the treatment visit.

In addition to frequently being asymptomatic, chlamydia infections in both men and women can clear spontaneously without treatment.[9]

Treatment

Treating chlamydia infection including asymptomatic infection prevents adverse reproductive health complications including PID, infertility, and neonatal infections. Treatment of persons infected with chlamydia and their sex partners can decrease continued sexual transmission, prevent reinfection, and infections of other partners.[10] Recommended regimens for treatment of chlamydia include the use of either azithromycin 1 gram orally or doxycycline 100 mg orally twice a day for 7 days. Alternative regimens include erythromycin, levofloxacin, or ofloxacin. To maximize adherence, onsite and directly observed single-dose therapy is preferred. Infected patients should be instructed to abstain from sexual intercourse until 7 days after an appropriate treatment course is completed and until all of their sex partners are treated. A diagnosis of chlamydia should prompt additional testing for HIV, GC, and syphilis. A test of cure is not advised for patients treated with recommended or alternative regimens unless adherence is unclear. Use of NAATs within 3 weeks of completion of therapy is not recommended because nonviable organisms' presence could lead to false-positive results.[10]

Screening

Because asymptomatic infection is common among both men and women, use of an appropriate screening program is required in order to identify infected individuals. In the United States, annual screening of all sexually active women aged < 25 years is recommended, as is screening of older women at increased risk of infection (including those with new sexual partner, more than one sex partner, a sex partner with more than one concurrent partner, or a sex partner with any STI).

While evidence for routine screening of young men is insufficient to recommend routine screening, such screening should occur in settings of high prevalence of chlamydia and in populations with high burden of infection (e.g., MSM).[10,11] Because chlamydia and gonorrhea at extragenital (rectal and pharyngeal) anatomic sites are often asymptomatic, this anatomic sites serve as a reservoir of infection. Therefore, sexually active MSM should be screened at least annually for chlamydia and gonorrhea at all exposed anatomic sites.[10,11]

LYMPHOGRANULOMA VENEREUM

Epidemiology

LGV is caused by *C. trachomatis* serovars L1, L2, and L3. LGV is traditionally most common in tropical and subtropical regions of the world, including East and West Africa, India, the Caribbean, Central America, and Southeast Asia.[12] LGV is thought to account for 2–10% of genital ulcerative disease in areas such as Southeast Asia and Africa, although these figures are based on older studies. The infection had been relatively uncommon in the United States and Europe, and sporadic cases in these geographic areas were generally considered to be imported from endemic areas.[12] From 1980 to 2003, only two clusters of LGV were described in Europe or the United States (by Scieux et al.,[13] in Paris and Bauwens et al.,[14] in Seattle). Since 2003, however, a slowly evolving epidemic of LGV anorectal infection has emerged in Western Europe and North America; LGV has become endemic among men who have sex with men (MSM), and most are coinfected with HIV.[15,16] Neither the degree of infectiousness nor the reservoir of disease has been accurately defined but transmission is attributed largely to asymptomatic carriers.

Subvariants of *C. tachomatis* serovar L2 have been described, such as L2b, which is the primary cause of infection among MSM in Europe. Heterosexual transmission of the strains found in MSM is extremely rare. While LGV, separate from *C. trachomatis*, is not nationally notifiable, it is still reportable and of local surveillance interest, especially given the disease currently found in Europe. Infections continue to occur in the United States.[16] For example, over the course of 8 months, from August 2015 through April 2016, 38 cases of LGV were reported in Michigan among MSM who were coinfected with HIV.[17,18]

Clinical Manifestations

Clinical features of LGV include asymptomatic infection, inguinal disease, proctitis, and anorectal syndrome. In MSM, about 25% of the anorectal LGV infections are asymptomatic. For those with anorectal syndrome, the usual incubation period is approximately 1–4 weeks after which three subsequent stages can follow: a primary ulcerative stage; a secondary stage with locoregional dissemination to lymph nodes and the development of buboes and fistulae; and a tertiary more complicated fibrotic stage with irreversible lymphedema.

Primary stage consists of an initial painless papule or pustule that may erode to form a small herpetiform ulcer. This ulcer often heals spontaneously and may remain unnoticed but may also present as a chancre. The location of the lesion will depend on the inoculation site but most commonly affects the rectum, and rarely the urethra or cervix. The secondary stage (or "inguinal" stage) begins several weeks after the onset of the primary lesion and causes painful inguinofemoral lymphadenopathy, which is traditionally unilateral. Along with enlargement, the lymph nodes are inflamed and ultimately may develop suppuration and abscesses that may become fluctuant and drain. This presentation (as secondary disease) is the typical one in low-income countries but is only rarely the presentation in MSM. Proctitis is the main manifestation of infection in the current LGV epidemic among MSM, and is typically associated with severe symptoms of anorectal pain, a bloody or purulent discharge, tenesmus, and constipation. The severity of symptoms varies among patients. The tertiary stage of LGV, often called the anogenitorectal syndrome, is more often present in women. Patients initially develop proctocolits followed by perirectal abscess, fistulas, strictures, and stenosis of the rectum. Without treatment, chronic progressive lymphangitis leads to edema, fibrosis, and can ultimately lead to elephantiasis. If left untreated LGV proctitis can lead to rectal strictures and other complications.

Diagnosis and Treatment

An important barrier to LGV surveillance and diagnosis includes poor laboratory capability of serotyping strains of *C. trachomatis.* Clinicians should maintain a high degree of suspicion in patients with lymphadenopathy or proctocolitis and no other etiology identified. Confirmed, probable or suspected cases should be reported to the health department. Doxycycline 100 mg twice daily for 21 days is effective treatment. Contacts should also be tested for *C. trachomatis* at the sites of exposure and, if asymptomatic, be treated presumptively with 100 mg doxycycline twice daily for 1 week.[19]

CHANCROID

Epidemiology

Chancroid, caused by *Haemophilus ducreyi,* has been a major cause of genital ulcer disease (GUD) in sub-Saharan Africa and in many parts of Southeast Asia and Latin America. The disease has always been relatively uncommon in the United States and Western Europe. In 1995, the estimated the global prevalence of chancroid was 7 million.[20] Over the last 10–20 years, there has been a substantial decline in the prevalence of chancroid in Southeast Asia and Africa; at the same time, these areas are reporting a rise in the relative prevalence of genital HSV-2 and to a lesser extent, HSV-1.[21] However, global epidemiology is poorly documented because of diagnostic challenges.

Cases of chancroid are sporadic in the United States and Western Europe. In the United States, during 2009–16, the number of reported cases ranged from 28 in 2009 to 6 in 2014. In 2017, only seven cases were reported.[3] Case reports in the United Kingdom[22] and France[23] outline recommendations for heightened awareness in cases of intractable painful genital ulcers in whom HSV has been excluded.

Clinical Manifestations

The combination of a painful genital ulcer and tender or suppurative inguinal adenopathy suggests the diagnosis of chancroid. Definitive diagnosis is difficult, but probable diagnosis can be made if the patient has a clinical presentation consistent with chancroid including typical appearance of ulcers combined with regional lymphadenopathy and the patient otherwise has no evidence of syphilis or HSV by direct examination tests [darkfield, polymerase chain reaction (PCR), culture] or serology (for syphilis).

Diagnosis and Treatment

Clinical diagnosis of chancroid is difficult and is easily confused with genital herpes. Culture of *H. ducreyi* is difficult and most labs are not equipped to do so. Finally, nucleic amplification tests such as PCR for *H. ducreyi*, are rarely available outside of national reference labs or specialized STI research setting.[22,24]

Successful treatment of chancroid can be curative and prevents transmission to others. Recommended regimens include single dose therapy with azithromycin (1 gram orally) or ceftriaxone (250 mg IM). Alternate, multiple dose regimens are effective including ciprofloxacin 500 mg twice a day for 3 days or erythromycin base 500 mg three times a day for 7 days.[10] HIV coinfected persons and uncircumcised males may not respond as well to treatment and should be followed closely for resolution of symptoms.

WHO recommendations to introduce syndromic management for treatment of GUD were fully implemented in 2000.[20,25,26] These syndromic guidelines recommend empiric treatment for syphilis with additional treatment for chancroid, granuloma inguinale, or LGV depending on local epidemiology. Use of syndromic therapy for patents presenting with GUD has led to decreases in all causes of GUD with the exception of herpes.

TRICHOMONAS

Epidemiology

Vaginal infections due to *Trichomonas vaginalis* (TV) are among the most common STIs worldwide. While the majority of TV infections are asymptomatic, TV has been associated with increased risk of HIV acquisition, preterm labor, and pelvic inflammatory disease.[27,28] The true incidence and prevalence of trichomoniasis in the United States and globally are unknown, as the infection is not reportable.[29] NHANES data from 2013 to 2014 indicated a prevalence of 0.5% among males 18–59 years and 1.8% among females,[30] with the highest prevalence observed among non-Hispanic black males (4.2%) and non-Hispanic black females (8.9%).

Clinical Manifestations

While some infected men have symptoms of urethritis, epididymitis, or prostatitis and some infected women have vaginal discharge, most infected persons have minimal or no symptoms and therefore untreated infections can last for months to years.[10]

Diagnosis

Universal, routine screening for trichomonas is not recommended. However, testing for *T. vaginalis* should be performed in women seeking care for vaginal discharge, and screening should be considered for persons receiving care in high-prevalence settings. Asymptomatic women with HIV-infection should be screened given the two- to threefold increased risk of HIV transmission.[10,31] The use of NAATs has increased the detection of up to five times more *T. vaginalis* infections than wet-mount microscopy (which has a poor sensitivity of 51–65%). In resource poor settings, the use of a testing algorithm with initial wet mount followed by NAAT if negative may improve diagnostic sensitivity.

Treatment

Treatment can reduce symptoms and signs of *T. vaginalis* infection and might reduce transmission and likelihood of adverse outcomes in women with HIV.[10] Recommended regimens include the use of one of the nitroimidazoles (metronidazole or tinidazole as a 2 gram oral single dose) Alternative regimens include the use of 500 mg of metronidazole orally twice a day for 7 days. Alcohol consumption should be avoided during treatment with these medications and for 24 hours (for metronidazole) or 72 hours (for tinidazole) after completion in order to avoid a disulfiram-like reaction. The use of metronidazole gel does not lead to therapeutic levels in the urethra or perivaginal glands and is not recommended.

CONCLUSIONS AND SUMMARY

Despite advances in knowledge related to the etiology, diagnosis, treatment, and prevention of these infections, the burden of STIs continues to be extremely high in the United States and worldwide. While decreases have occurred in some infections over the last decade, there continues to be a high number of cases for many of these infections, and in 2018, the United States experienced record numbers of STIs.[32] A comprehensive approach to achieve effective decreases in morbidity and mortality associated with them will need to include both primary and secondary prevention strategies.

Primary prevention including the regular completion by healthcare providers of an accurate risk assessment of all individuals including assessment of both behavioral and biological risks of transmission; provision of education and counseling of persons at risk on ways to avoid STDs and the use of pre-exposure vaccination of persons at risk for vaccine-preventable STDs (such as HPV). Secondary prevention includes the identification of not only symptomatically infected persons but screening for those at risk to identify those asymptomatically infected and then the provision of appropriate treatment and follow-up of those identified as infected and evaluation, treatment and counseling of their sex partners.[10] New approaches, such as expedited partner therapy, where the clinician provides prescriptions or treatment to the patient to take to their partner without having examined the partner first, are being implemented as an additional strategy for partner management, particularly for the male partners of women with chlamydia or gonorrhea infection.[33]

References

1. World Health Organization. 2018 Report on Global Sexually Transmitted Infection Surveillance. Geneva, Switzerland; 2018. https://www.who.int/reproductivehealth/publications/stis-surveillance-2018/en/.
2. World Health Organization. Global Health Sector Strategy on Sexually Transmitted Infections 2016–2021. Geneva, Switzerland; 2016. https://www.who.int/reproductivehealth/publications/rtis/ghss-stis/en/.
3. Centers for Disease Control and Prevention. Sexually Transmitted Disease Surveillance 2017. Atlanta, GA; 2018. https://www.cdc.gov/std/stats17/default.htm.
4. Satterwhite CL, Torrone E, Meites E, et al. Sexually transmitted infections among US women and men: Prevalence and incidence estimates. *Sex Transm Dis.* 2013;40(3):187–93.
5. Centers for Disease Control and Prevention. CDC Fact Sheet. Incidence, Prevalence, and Cost of Sexually Transmitted Infections in the United States. Atlanta, GA; 2013. https://www.cdc.gov/std/stats/sti-estimates-fact-sheet-feb-2013.pdf.
6. Centers for Disease Control and Prevention. NHANES—About the National Health and Nutrition Examination Survey. Atlanta, GA; 2017. http://www.cdc.gov/nchs/nhanes/about_nhanes.htm.
7. Detels R, Green AM, Klausner JD, et al. The incidence and correlates of symptomatic and asymptomatic *Chlamydia trachomatis* and *Neisseria gonorrhoeae* infections in selected populations in five countries. *Sex Transm Dis.* 2011;38(6):503–9.
8. Geisler WM, Wang C, Morrison SG, et al. The natural history of untreated *Chlamydia trachomatis* infection in the interval between screening and returning for treatment. *Sex Transm Dis.* 2008;35(2):119–23.
9. Lewis J, Price MJ, Horner PJ, White PJ. Genital *Chlamydia trachomatis* infections clear more slowly in men than women, but are less likely to become established. *J Infect Dis.* 2017;216(2):237–44.
10. Centers for Disease Control and Prevention. Sexually transmitted diseases treatment guidelines. *MMWR Morb Mortal Wkly Rep.* 2015;64 (No. RR-3):1–137.
11. Johnson Jones ML, Chapin-Bardales J, Bizune D, et al. Extragenital Chlamydia and Gonorrhea among community venue-attending men who have sex with men-five cities, United States, 2017. *MMWR Morb Mortal Wkly Rep.* 2019;68:321–5.
12. Engelkens HJ, Stolz E. Genital ulcer disease. *Int J Dermatol.* 1993;32:169–81.
13. Scieux C, Barnes R, Bianchi A, et al. Lymphogranuloma venereum: 27 Cases in Paris. *J Infect Dis.* 1989;160(4):662–8.
14. Bauwens JE, Lampe MF, Suchland RJ, et al. Infection with *Chlamydia trachomatis* lymphogranuloma venereum serovar L1 in homosexual men with proctitis: Molecular analysis of an unusual case cluster. *Clin Infect Dis.* 1995;20(3):576–81.
15. de Vries HJC, de Barbeyrac B, de Vrieze NHN, et al. 2019 European guideline on the management of lymphogranuloma venereum. *J Eur Acad Dermatol Venereol.* 2019;33(10):1821–8.
16. Pathela P, Blank S, Schillinger JA. Lymphogranuloma venereum: Old pathogen, new story. *Curr Infect Dis Rep.* 2007;9:143.
17. de Voux A, Kent JB, Macomber K, et al. Notes from the field: Cluster of lymphogranuloma venereum cases among men who have sex with men—Michigan, August 2015–April 2016. *MMWR Morb Mortal Wkly Rep.* 2016;65(34):920–1.
18. Stoner BP, Cohen SE. Lymphogranuloma venereum 2015: Clinical presentation, diagnosis, and treatment. *Clin Infect Dis.* 2015;61(S8):S865–73.
19. Workowski K, Bolan G. Sexually transmitted diseases treatment guidelines, 2015. *MMWR Morb Mortal Wkly Rep.* 2015;64(RR-03):1–37.
20. Steen R. Eradicating chancroid. *Bull World Health Organ.* 2001;79(9):818–26.
21. Lewis DA. Epidemiology, clinical features, diagnosis and treatment of *Haemophilus ducreyi*-a disappearing pathogen? *Expert Rev Anti Infect Ther.* 2014;12(6):687–96.
22. Barnes P, Chauhan M. Chancroid-desperate patient makes own diagnosis. *Intl J STD AIDS.* 2014;25(10):768–70.
23. Fouere S, Lassau F, Rousseau C, et al. First case of chancroid in 14 years at the largest STI clinic in Paris, France. *Intl J STD AIDS.* 2016;27(9):805–7.
24. González-Beiras C, Marks M, Chen CY, et al. Epidemiology of *Haemophilus ducreyi* infections. *Emerg Infect Dis.* 2016;22(1):1–8.
25. World Health Organization. Guidelines for the management of sexually transmitted infections. Geneva, Switzerland; 2004. https://www.who.int/hiv/pub/sti/pub6/en/.
26. O'Farrell N, Lazaro N. UK National guideline for the management of chancroid 2014. *Intl J STD AIDS.* 2014;25(14):975–83.
27. Laga M, Manoka A, Kivuvu M, et al. Non-ulcerative sexually transmitted diseases as risk factors for HIV-1 transmission in women: Results from a cohort study. *AIDS.* 1993;7(1):95–102.
28. McClelland RS, Sagare L, Hassan WM, et al. Infection with *Trichomonas vaginalis* increase the risk of HIV-1 acquisition. *J Infect Dis.* 2007;195:698–702.
29. Poole D, McClelland RS. Global epidemiology of *Trichomonas vaginalis*. *Sex Transm Infect.* 2013;89(6):418–22.
30. Patel EU, Gaydos CA, Packman ZR, et al. Prevalence and correlates of *Trichomonas vaginalis* infection among men and women in the United States. *Clin Infect Dis.* 2018;67(2):211–7.
31. Van Der Pol B, Kwok C, Pierre-Louis B, et al. *Trichomonas vaginalis* infection and human immunodeficiency virus acquisition in African women. *J Infect Dis.* 2008;197(4):548–54.
32. Centers for Disease Control and Prevention. CDC Fact Sheet. Reported STDs in the United States, 2018. Atlanta, GA; 2019. https://www.cdc.gov/nchhstp/newsroom/docs/factsheets/std-trends-508.pdf.
33. Centers for Disease Control and Prevention. Sexually Transmitted Diseases (STDs). Expedited Partner Therapy. Atlanta, GA; 2019. https://www.cdc.gov/std/ept/default.htm.

CHAPTER

123 Herpes Simplex Virus

Abdulsalam Alsulami • Richard J. Whitley

Herpes simplex virus (HSV) is one of the most common infections encountered by humans worldwide. As a member of the herpesvirus family *(Herpesviridae)*, it shares the unique biologic characteristic of being able to exist in a latent state and recur periodically, if not chronically, serving as a reservoir for transmission from one person to another. There are two distinct antigenic types of HSV; HSV-1 and HSV-2. HSV-1 is usually associated with infections above the belt, namely involving the oropharynx and lips; however, a large and increasing number of genital infections in the United States is attributed to HSV-1. HSV-2 routinely causes infections below the belt, involving the genitalia, buttocks, and infrequently the lower extremities. In addition, both viruses can cause infection of the newborn. The spectrum of disease caused by HSV ranges from benign and nuisance infections to those that can be life threatening.[1]

EPIDEMIOLOGY

HSV infection is transmitted by direct contact with an infected person's lesions, mucosal surfaces, or genital or oral secretions.[2] The epidemiology of infection is best defined by seroprevalence of HSV-1 and HSV-2. HSV infections remain common despite a recent steady decrease in prevalence, as shown in Fig. 123-1.[3] The seroprevalence of HSV-1 and HSV-2 increases linearly with age and is higher in females. Primary HSV-1 infections usually occur in the young child and are most often asymptomatic. During the period of 1999–2002, HSV-1 seroprevalence in U.S.-born children ages 6–13 years was 31%, progressively increasing with age.[4] In the most recent National Health and Nutrition Examination Survey (NHANES) of 2015–16, the seroprevalence in people age 14–19 years was 27%, consistent with overall trends of decreasing prevalence of HSV-1 in early childhood over the last two decades.[2] By adulthood, about half of the U.S. population (48%) has experienced HSV-1 infection.[2] HSV-1 prevalence differs by race and ethnicity, with prevalence highest in the Mexican American population and lowest in non-Hispanic whites, a finding that remains true despite a steady decline in overall prevalence in the United States. The HSV-1 contribution to genital herpetic disease has increased over the past two decades. The percentage of people who randomly tested positive for HSV-1 only and had a diagnosis of genital herpes increased to 1.8% in NHANES survey 1999–2004 when compared to 0.4% in the NHANES survey 1988–94.[5] A retrospective evaluation of college students with newly diagnosed genital infection from 1993 to 2001 showed a striking increase of HSV-1 as a cause of symptomatic genital herpes from 30.9% in 1993 to 77.6% in 2001.[6]

Geographic location, socioeconomic status, and age influence the occurrence of HSV infection, regardless of the mode of assessment. The global estimates of the incidence and prevalence of HSV-1 infections vary by region, being around 67%, and highest in African, Southeast Asian and Western Pacific countries. The prevalence of HSV-1 is higher and occurs earlier in childhood outside of Europe and the Americas, with estimates reaching 90% in Africa by 10 years of age. As noted, most of these infections are asymptomatic.

The annual global incidence of HSV-1 infections is estimated to be 2% in 2012. The contribution of HSV-1 to the incidence of genital infections is less clearly defined in the developing world since prospective studies are lacking. Estimates of HSV-1 genital infections vary by region and are also impacted by both cultural sexual practices and the prevalence of childhood HSV-1 infections. In Africa, for example, the prevalence of genital HSV-1 is estimated to be 0–0.1% (early childhood HSV-1 prevalence overall of 90%) compared to Eastern Mediterranean region with a 2–3% prevalence of genital HSV-1 (early childhood HSV-1 prevalence close to 70%).[7]

Acquisition of HSV-2 usually occurs in association with onset of sexual activity and directly correlates with the number of lifetime sexual partners. Overall, seroprevalence to HSV-2 in the United States is decreasing in recent years after a significant increase in the mid-1990s. The most recent studies showed total prevalence of 12% during 2015–16, which represent a decrease from 17% during 1999–2004. HSV-2 remains more common among women when compared to men and non-Hispanic blacks compared to other race and ethnic groups.[2,5] HSV-2 prevalence is also affected by factors such as: age (linear increase with age), poverty (higher in people below poverty line), social status (higher in those who are divorced, separated or widowed) and number of lifetime sexual partners (3.8% in people who reported one partner compared to 39.9% in people reporting ≥ 50 sexual partners lifetime).[2,5] Previous studies indicate that men who have sex with men (MSM) have an increased prevalence of HSV-2. More recently and during NHANES 2001–06, the difference in HSV-2 prevalence was not statistically different between homosexual, bisexual, and heterosexual men although the same study showed an increased prevalence in those with HIV infection and MSM compared to heterosexual men.[8] Worldwide estimates of HSV-2 infection in 2012 indicated an overall prevalence of 11.3%. Estimates vary significantly by gender and geographic area. Prevalence in females is higher, compared to males (14.8% vs. 8%), and was highest in Africa with a prevalence of 31.5%.[7] The estimated incidence of HSV-2 infections also differs by gender and geographic areas, being typically higher in the younger age groups. A decline of incidence with age was observed in areas with higher prevalence, which could be attributed to behavioral changes with age or decrease in susceptible people at older ages.[9] In general, women acquire HSV-2 infection more frequently than do men, irrespective of the number of partners.

For pregnant women, approximately 1% will excrete virus at the time of delivery. Nevertheless, the incidence of neonatal HSV infection is only approximately 1 in 1500 live born infants in the United States.[10] The incidence of neonatal HSV infection is affected by multiple factors, the most important of which is the maternal infection status. Pregnant women who contract genital HSV for the first time during the third trimester have the highest risk for transmitting infection to the fetus, as 57% of those neonates develop neonatal HSV infection. The rate of exposed neonates developing the disease

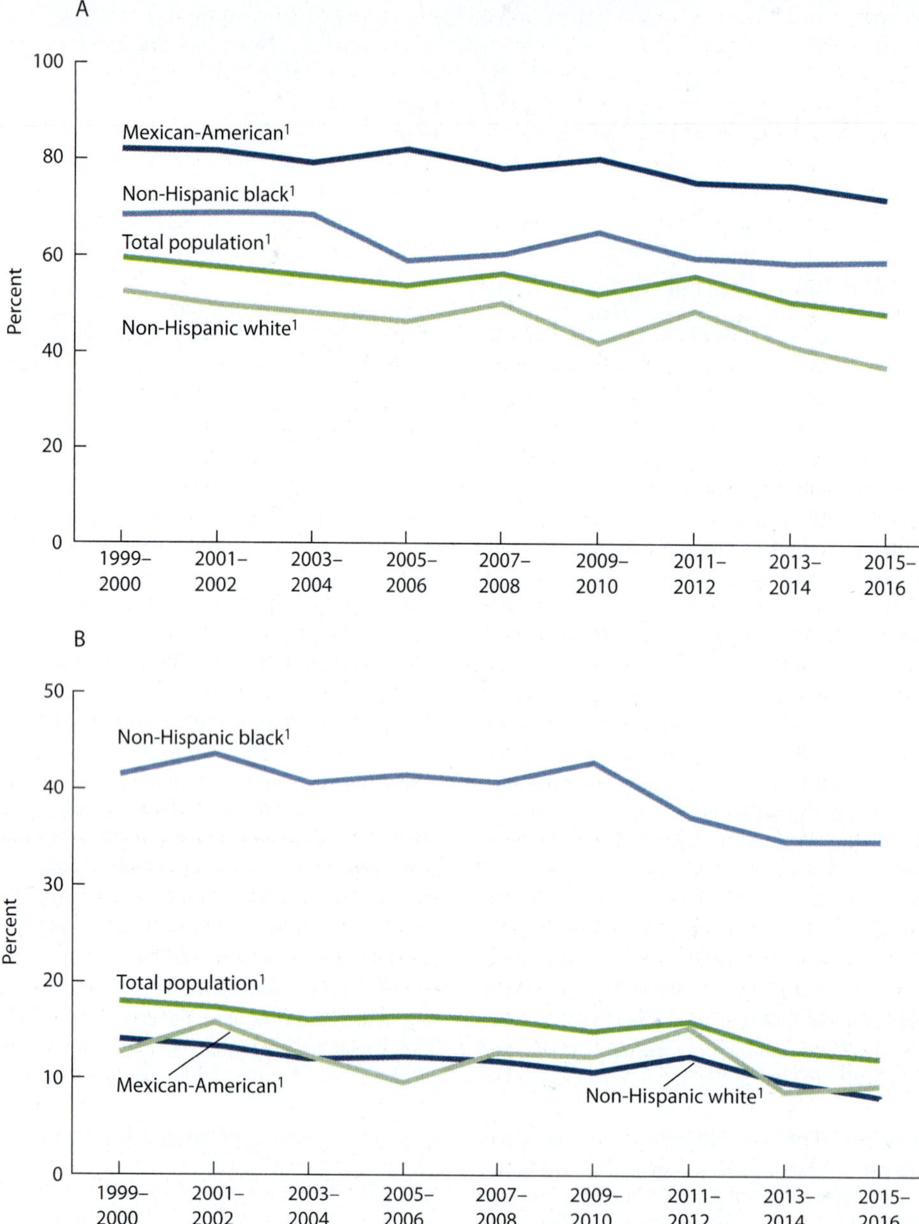

FIGURE 123-1. Downward trends of HSV-1 (A) and HSV-2 (B) age-adjusted prevalence in the U.S. population 14–49 years based on the National Health and Nutrition Examination Survey, 1999–2016. 1 significant linear trend with $p < 0.05$. (*Source:* McQuillan G, Kruszon-Moran D, Flagg EW, Paulose-Ram R. Prevalence of herpes simplex virus type 1 and type 2 in persons aged 14–49: United States, 2015–2016. *NCHS Data Brief.* 2018;(304):1–8, Figures 2 and 4.)

decreases to 25% when pregnant women contract first genital HSV but have prior history of HSV infection of the opposite type. The risk drops significantly to 2% at most, for neonates born to women with established recurrent genital HSV of either type.[11,12] The decrease in neonatal HSV infection with documented recurrent genital HSV infection is likely due to the protective transplacental antibodies. Cesarean delivery reduces the risk of neonatal HSV infection by avoiding exposure to viral shedding in maternal vaginal secretions. Other risk factors for neonatal HSV infection, particularly in women with established genital infection, include application of a fetal scalp electrode, virus type (higher risk with HSV-1 vs. HSV-2), and duration of rupture of membranes.[13,14] Global estimates of annual neonatal HSV incidence is about 14,257 neonates from 2010 to 2015 with HSV-2 being responsible for about two-thirds of the total number. The global rate of neonatal HSV is estimated to be around 10.3 per 100,000 livebirths,[9] Both HSV-1 and HSV-2 seem to contribute almost equally to neonatal HSV diseases in the United States. This is not the case in other areas of the world where childhood HSV-1 prevalence is significantly higher, as in Africa where almost all neonatal HSV cases are thought to be due to HSV-2.[7,14,15] The estimated global annual incidence of neonatal HSV disease is significantly lower than that of the United States. The reason behind this significant difference is not clear yet and further studies are needed to identify potential explanations.

Nosocomial HSV infection has been documented both in newborn nurseries as well as in intensive care units.[1] Herpetic whitlow, while decreasing in incidence, still occurs.[1]

PATHOGENESIS

Acquisition of HSV infections requires intimate contact between a person who is shedding virus and a susceptible host. After inoculation of HSV onto the skin or mucous membrane and an incubation period of 4–6 days, clinical disease may occur or, as is more common, the infection will be asymptomatic. HSV replicates in epithelial cells. As replication continues, cell lysis and local inflammation ensue, resulting in characteristic vesicles on an erythematous base.

Regional lymphatics and lymph nodes become involved; viremia and visceral dissemination may develop, depending upon the immunologic competence of the host. In all hosts, the virus generally ascends peripheral sensory nerves and reaches sensory ganglia. Replication of HSV within neural tissue is followed by retrograde axonal spread of the virus back to other mucosal and skin surfaces via the peripheral sensory nerves. Virus replicates further in the epithelial cells, reproducing the lesions of the initial infection, until infection is contained through both systemic and mucosal immune responses.

The initial host response to HSV infection is derived mainly from the innate immune system including natural killer cells (NK cells), neutrophils, B cells and T cells, as well as production of cytokines and recruitment of adaptive and humoral immune response. HSV-specific antibodies and, subsequently, CD-8 and CD-4 lymphocytes develop with time. Prevention of latent infection is not possible; thus, latency is inevitable. The production of HSV-specific neutralizing antibodies contributes to the control of infection and is also used in laboratory testing to type the viral infection.

Latency is established when HSV reaches the dorsal root ganglia after anterograde transmission via sensory nerve pathways. In its latent form, intracellular HSV DNA cannot be detected routinely unless specific molecular probes are used. The virus does not actively replicate during latency. Reactivation of latent infection result in one of two outcomes: asymptomatic viral shedding (most likely) or reactivation that results in disease with a clinical presentation similar to, but usually milder than, the original symptomatic infection. Reactivation of a latent infection may be symptomatic despite the asymptomatic nature of the original primary infection.

Rarely HSV can infect the central nervous system and cause encephalitis.[16] The focality and temporal lobe affinity suggest direct extension of virus along neural tracts. Encephalitis caused by HSV is characterized by necrosis of the inferior medial portion of the temporal lobe, initially unilaterally and then contralaterally. This necrotic process accounts for the high morbidity and mortality of infection. Specific genetic mutations in the innate immune system make affected hosts susceptible to severe or recurrent disease. For example, Toll-like receptor-3 (TLR-3) mutations have been reported to increase the risk for HSV encephalitis in pediatric and young adults.[17,18]

Infection of the neonate is usually the consequence of direct contact with infected maternal genital secretions, accounting for approximately 85% of cases of neonatal herpes. The remaining 15% are caused by in utero infection, secondary to viremia, or postnatal acquisition whereby the baby comes in contact with infectious virus in the environment.[13]

CLINICAL MANIFESTATIONS

Mucocutaneous Infections

Gingivostomatitis. Mucocutaneous infections are the most common clinical manifestations of HSV-1 and HSV-2. Gingivostomatitis is usually caused by HSV-1 and occurs most frequently in children under 5 years of age. Clinical disease is characterized by fever, sore throat, pharyngeal edema, and erythema, followed by the development of vesicular or ulcerative lesions of the oral or pharyngeal mucosa. Skin lesions are usually grouped vesicles on an erythematous base. Mucous membrane vesicles usually rupture, resulting in a painful ulcerative lesion on erythematous base, which is prone to bleeding. In children, clinical fussiness occurs and is associated with decreased oral intake that may lead to dehydration. Autoinoculation of HSV from oral lesions to fingers results in herpetic whitlow, not uncommon in the pediatric population. Another manifestation of mucocutaneous HSV is eczema herpeticum, which develops in patients with skin eczema and may not be limited to one area, but rather involves multiple patches of the skin affected by poorly controlled eczema. Mucocutaneous HSV lesions usually heal without leaving a scar at the site of infection. Recurrent HSV-1 infections of the oropharynx frequently manifest as herpes simplex labialis (cold sores) and appear on the vermilion border of the lip. Intraoral lesions, as a manifestation of recurrent disease, are uncommon in the normal host but do occur frequently in the immunocompromised host.

Genital Herpes. HSV-2 used to be the major cause of genital herpes in the past, but recent studies indicate that probably over half of new genital herpes cases are caused by HSV-1.[6,19] Primary infection in women usually involves the vulva, vagina, and cervix. In men, initial infection is most often associated with lesions on the glans penis, prepuce, or penile shaft. In individuals of either sex, primary disease is associated with fever, malaise, anorexia, and bilateral inguinal adenopathy. Women frequently have dysuria and urinary retention due to urethral involvement. As many as 10% of individuals will develop an aseptic meningitis with primary infection. Aseptic meningitis, often presenting as recurrent disease known as Mollaret's meningitis, usually presents with fever, photophobia, headache, and neck stiffness. It is more likely to happen in women with genital HSV-2 infections.[18,20] Sacral radiculomyelitis may occur in both men and women, resulting in neuralgias, urinary retention, or obstipation. The complete healing of primary infection may take several weeks. The first episode of genital infection is less severe in individuals who have had previous HSV infections at other sites, such as herpes simplex labialis. Primary genital HSV is more likely to be asymptomatic regardless of viral type. Recurrent lesions with viral shedding could also be asymptomatic, explaining the high incidence of new infections.

Recurrent genital infections in either men or women can be particularly distressing. The frequency of recurrence varies significantly from one individual to another. For those with HSV-2 infection, approximately one-third of individuals with genital herpes have virtually no recurrences, one-third have approximately three recurrences per year, and another third have more than three per year, while those individuals with HSV-1 infection are much less likely to suffer recurrences. By applying polymerase chain reaction (PCR) to genital swabs from women with a history of recurrent genital herpes, virus DNA can be detected in the absence of culture proof of infection.[21] This finding suggests the chronicity of genital herpes as opposed to a recurrent infection.

Herpetic Keratitis

HSV keratitis is usually caused by HSV-1, either primary or recurrent and is accompanied by conjunctivitis in many cases.[22] It is considered among the most common infectious causes of blindness in the United States. The characteristic lesions of herpes simplex keratoconjunctivitis are dendritic ulcers best detected by fluorescein staining. Deep stromal involvement has also been reported and may result in visual impairment. Acute necrotizing retinitis is a rare complication that leads to painless loss of vision. Chorioretinitis is another rare HSV ophthalmic complication that could develop in neonates or immunocompromised patients with HSV infections.

Other Skin Manifestations

HSV infections can manifest at any skin site. Common among healthcare workers are lesions on abraded skin of the fingers, known as herpetic whitlows. Similarly, because of physical contact, wrestlers may develop disseminated cutaneous lesions known as herpes gladiatorum. HSV infections have also been recognized as a trigger for erythema multiforme.[18]

Neonatal Herpes Simplex Virus Infection

The incidence of neonatal HSV is estimated to be 1 in 1500 live births in United States.[5,10,13] Most (85%) affected neonates acquire HSV from exposure to infected secretions during birth (intrapartum acquisition), a small number (10%) acquire the virus postnatally, and rarely (~5%) the virus will be acquired in utero, resulting in congenital HSV infection.[13,19,23] Manifestations of neonatal HSV infection can be divided into three categories: (a) skin, eye, and mouth disease (SEM) (45% of all neonatal HSV cases); (b) central nervous system (CNS) disease (30%); and (c) disseminated infection (25%). Most HSV infections during the neonatal period could present with fever, lethargy, poor feeding, skin lesions, or seizures. In SEM, as the name implies, skin, eye, and mouth disease consists of cutaneous lesions (in > 80%) and does not involve other organ systems. Involvement of the central nervous system may occur with encephalitis or disseminated infection and generally results in a diffuse encephalitis with seizures and lethargy. The cerebrospinal fluid analysis characteristically reveals an elevated protein and a mononuclear pleocytosis. Disseminated infection involves multiple organ systems and can produce disseminated intravascular coagulation, hemorrhagic pneumonitis, encephalitis, hepatitis, and cutaneous lesions. Diagnosis can be particularly difficult in the absence of skin lesions. The mortality rate for each disease classification varies from zero for skin, eye, and mouth disease to 15% for encephalitis and 60% or higher for neonates with disseminated infection in the absence of therapy. In addition to the high mortality associated with these infections, morbidity is significant in that children with encephalitis or disseminated disease develop normally in only approximately 40% of cases, even with the administration of appropriate antiviral therapy. Congenital HSV (acquired in utero, about 5% of neonatal HSV cases) manifests as a triad of skin involvement (lesions, scarring, and change of pigmentation), CNS involvement (calcifications and microcephaly), and ophthalmologic involvement (chorioretinitis and optic atrophy).[19,23] Affected neonates are usually very ill.

Herpes Simplex Encephalitis

HSV encephalitis is characterized by hemorrhagic necrosis of the inferomedial portion of the temporal lobe. Disease begins unilaterally, then spreads to the contralateral temporal lobe. It is the most common cause of focal, sporadic encephalitis in the United States today and occurs in approximately 1 in 250,000–500,000 individuals. Most cases are caused by HSV-1. The actual pathogenesis of herpes simplex encephalitis is unknown, although it has been speculated that primary or recurrent virus can reach the temporal lobe by ascending neural pathways, such as the trigeminal tracts or the olfactory nerves.

Clinical manifestations of herpes simplex encephalitis include headache, fever, altered consciousness, and abnormalities of speech and behavior. Focal seizures may also occur. The cerebrospinal fluid formulae for these patients is variable, but usually consists of a pleocytosis of monocytes. The protein concentration is characteristically elevated and glucose is usually normal. Historically, a definitive diagnosis could be achieved only by brain biopsy, since other pathogens may produce a clinically similar illness. However, the application of PCR for detection of virus DNA has replaced brain biopsy as the standard for diagnosis.[7] The mortality and morbidity are high, even when appropriate antiviral therapy is administered. At present, the mortality rate is approximately 14–19% even with appropriate intravenous (IV) acyclovir (mortality exceeds 70% without effective therapy). Approximately 50% of survivors will have significant neurologic sequelae.[24]

Herpes Simplex Virus Infections in the Immunocompromised Host

HSV infections in the immunocompromised host are clinically more severe, may be progressive, and require more time for healing. Manifestations of HSV infections in this patient population include pneumonitis, esophagitis, hepatitis, colitis, and disseminated cutaneous disease. Individuals suffering from human immunodeficiency virus infection may have extensive perineal or orofacial ulcerations. HSV infections are also noted to be of increased severity in individuals who are burned.

DIAGNOSIS

The diagnosis of HSV infections is predicated on clinical evaluation of mucocutaneous manifestations. However, confirmation of the diagnosis requires isolation of HSV in appropriate cell culture systems or the detection of viral gene products or, alternatively, the detection of viral DNA by PCR. HSV grows readily in tissue culture, producing cytopathic effects within a few days in a wide variety of mammalian cell lines. The routine typing, namely distinguishing HSV-1 from HSV-2, of the isolate is important for genital isolates as HSV-1 is much less likely to recur.

PCR is an important method for diagnosing HSV infections, particularly those involving the central nervous system. The detection of HSV DNA by PCR in the CSF has replaced brain biopsy as a method of diagnosis of central nervous system infections.

Type-specific serologic assays are commercially available. The utilization of immunoblot detection of specific glycoproteins that distinguish HSV-1 from HSV-2, namely, glycoprotein (g) G-1 and gG-2, are available for determining prior exposure to HSV-1 and HSV-2 infections.

Serologic testing is also used for population-based studies to identify the prevalence of the disease.[2,4]

Historically, Tzanck smears have been used to diagnose HSV infections. Tzanck smears are not sensitive enough for routine diagnostic purposes. However, immunofluorescent staining of cell trap preparations from lesions is both sensitive and specific for the diagnosis for HSV infections.

TREATMENT

Infections due to HSV are amenable to treatment. Acyclovir and its prodrug (valacyclovir) as well as famciclovir (prodrug of penciclovir) are the mainstays of treatment. Acyclovir works primarily by inhibiting viral DNA synthesis and acting like a substrate (after phosphorylation) for the viral DNA polymerase. Valacyclovir is a prodrug that metabolized to acyclovir and result in good serum levels, similar to levels achieved with IV acyclovir. Famciclovir undergoes metabolic conversion to penciclovir, which is active against HSV. Dose, route, and duration of therapy are very variable based on the site of infection and status of the patient. The use of high dose acyclovir and addition of suppressive therapy have improved outcomes significantly in neonatal HSV infections.

Primary mucocutaneous infections in the immunocompetent host are treated with oral acyclovir or valacyclovir for 7–10 days; famciclovir can also be used. Valacyclovir is FDA-approved in pediatric population 12 years of age or older. Recurrent orolabial HSV infection can be treated with any of these three drugs. Suppressive therapy may be considered for patients with very frequent recurrent lesions. Patients with genital HSV infection can be treated with acyclovir, valacyclovir, or famciclovir. IV acyclovir should be considered in the initial phase of treating severe orolabial disease leading to decreased oral intake in a pediatric patient or in an adult with genital herpes associated with aseptic meningitis.[18,19] Treatment of genital herpes in the HIV-infected patient may be followed by long term suppressive therapy with acyclovir, valacyclovir, or famciclovir.

Topical therapy with one of several antiviral ophthalmic preparations is appropriate for HSV keratoconjunctivitis. However, the treatment of choice is viroptic or trifluorothymidine. Secondary choices include vidarabine ophthalmic or topical idoxuridine. Consultation with an ophthalmologist for confirmation of the diagnosis and management of HSV ocular disease is indicated.

Neonatal HSV infection should always be treated with IV acyclovir. The duration of treatment varies: CNS and disseminated diseases are treated for 21 days and SEM only 14 days. All forms of neonatal HSV should be followed by minimum of 6 months of suppressive therapy with oral acyclovir. Neonatal disease involving the eyes should also be treated with topical ophthalmic drugs (trifluridine or topical ganciclovir),[19] and an ophthalmologist consulted.

IV acyclovir is the mainstay of HSV encephalitis during adulthood. Encephalitis patients require longer treatment duration for 14–21 days as compared to 7–10 days for aseptic meningitis. Acyclovir resistance can develop. Resistance is usually related to viral thymidine kinase mutations.[1,9] Treatment of choice for infections

TABLE 123-1 SUMMARY OF HSV TREATMENT

Infection	Treatment	Comments
Mucocutaneous disease		
Orolabial HSV—Primary	• Acyclovir PO 1000 mg divided three to five times per day for 7–10 days. Pediatric dose 20 mg/kg/dose (max 400 mg) four times daily • Famciclovir 500 mg bid • Valacyclovir 1000 mg bid	In the immunocompromised host, IV acyclovir may be needed in the beginning. Duration of therapy varies 7–14 days.
Orolabial HSV—Recurrent	• Acyclovir PO 400 mg five times/day for 5 days • Valacyclovir 2000 mg bid for 1 day • Famciclovir 1500 mg once	Long-term suppression is helpful in patients with prolonged immune suppression.
Genital disease		
Genital HSV—Primary	• Acyclovir 200 mg five times/day (or 400mg tid) for 7–10 days • Valacyclovir 1000 mg bid for 7–10 days • Famciclovir 250 mg tid for 7–10 days	Use of IV acyclovir may be needed for severe disease or in the immunocompromised host.
Genital HSV—Recurrent	• Acyclovir PO 200 mg five times/day (or 800 mg bid) for 5 days • Valacyclovir 500 mg bid (or 1000 mg daily) for 5 days • Famciclovir 125 mg bid for 5 days	Long-term suppression may be helpful in patients who are immunocompromised or have frequent episodes. Acyclovir PO 400 mg bid, valacyclovir 500 mg daily (or 1000 mg daily) or famciclovir 250 mg bid.
Herpetic keratitis	• Topical antiviral drugs (trifluorothymidine, vidarabine or penciclovir)	Avoid topical corticosteroids. Consult with ophthalmologist.
Herpes simplex encephalitis (HSE)	IV acyclovir 10 mg/kg/dose q8 hours	Aseptic meningitis is usually treated for 7–10 days and encephalitis for 14–21 days.
Neonatal Disease		
Central nervous system, disseminated or skin, eye and mouth disease (SEM)	• IV acyclovir 30 mg/kg/dose q 8 hours for 21 days (14 days for SEM disease)	Should be followed by oral acyclovir suppressive dose of 300 mg/m²/dose q 8 hours for 6 months after the acute treatment. Check complete blood count with differential monthly for neutropenia.

caused by acyclovir-resistant strains is foscarnet.[19] Consultation with specialists is recommended when resistance is known or suspected. See Table 123-1 for a summary of antiviral drugs recommended for treatment of various HSVs.

PREVENTION AND CONTROL

At the present, there is no licensed vaccine for the prevention for HSV infections. Consequently, prevention of HSV infections resides in the most part on knowledge of the mechanisms of transmission, including person to person as well as in the hospital environment. Individuals with known recurrent HSV infections should be counseled on the possibility of transmission of infection while lesions are present. The use of condoms for individuals with recurrent genital herpes is encouraged in that detection of HSV DNA by PCR can occur even in the absence of lesions. Similarly, for individuals who have recurrent herpes labialis, kissing should be discouraged.

There is a risk of nosocomial transmission of HSV within the hospital environment. Since many individuals excrete HSV in the absence of clinical symptoms, it is impossible to exclude all workers from the hospital environment who could transmit infection. Thus, many authorities simply recommend strict hand washing and covering of lesions, should they exist.

Finally, no data exist on the prevention of neonatal HSV infection. It has been theorized that anticipatory administration of acyclovir to babies delivered through an infected birth canal may prove of value, particularly for women who have first episode genital herpetic infection. However, no data exist to substantiate this hypothesis. Since over 1% of all women at delivery excrete HSV and the rate of neonatal HSV infection is only 1 in 1500 live born infants as noted earlier, the routine administration of acyclovir to all children born to HSV-positive women is not reasonable. Alternative approaches, namely, administration of acyclovir to known HSV-2–infected women is gaining acceptance.[9]

References

1. Roizman B, Knipe D, Whitley R. Herpes simplex viruses. In: Knipe D, Howley P, eds.Knipe D, Howley P, eds. *Fields Virology*. Vol. 2. Philadelphia: LWW; 2013, pp. 1823–97.
2. McQuillan G, Kruszon-Moran D, Flagg EW, Paulose-Ram R. Prevalence of herpes simplex virus type 1 and type 2 in persons aged 14–49: United States, 2015–2016. *NCHS Data Brief.* 2018(304):1–8.
3. NCHS. *National Health and Nutrition Examination Survey, 1999–2016.* 2017.
4. Xu F, Lee FK, Morrow RA, et al. Seroprevalence of herpes simplex virus type 1 in children in the United States. *J Pediatr*. 2007;151(4):374–7.
5. Xu F, Sternberg MR, Kottiri BJ, et al. Trends in herpes simplex virus type 1 and type 2 seroprevalence in the United States. *JAMA*. 2006;296(8): 964–73.
6. Roberts CM, Pfister JR, Spear SJ. Increasing proportion of herpes simplex virus type 1 as a cause of genital herpes infection in college students. *Sex Transm Dis*. 2003;30(10):797–800.
7. Looker KJ, Magaret AS, Turner KM, Vickerman P, Gottlieb SL, Newman LM. Global estimates of prevalent and incident herpes simplex virus type 2 infections in 2012. *PLoS One*. 2015;10(1):e114989.
8. Xu F, Sternberg MR, Markowitz LE. Men who have sex with men in the United States: Demographic and behavioral characteristics and prevalence of HIV and HSV-2 infection: Results from National Health and Nutrition Examination Survey 2001–2006. *Sex Transm Dis*. 2010;37(6): 399–405.
9. Looker KJ, Magaret AS, May MT, et al. First estimates of the global and regional incidence of neonatal herpes infection. *Lancet Glob Health*. 2017;5(3):e300–9.
10. Shah S, Hall M, Schondelmeyer A, Berry J, Kimberlin D, Mahant S. Trends in neonatal herpes simplex virus infection in the United States, 2000–2012. Paper presented at: Pediatric Hospital Medicine 2017; Nashville, TN.
11. Brown ZA, Benedetti J, Ashley R, et al. Neonatal herpes simplex virus infection in relation to asymptomatic maternal infection at the time of labor. *N Engl J Med*. 1991;324:1247–52.
12. Brown ZA, Selke S, Zeh J, et al. The acquisition of herpes simplex virus during pregnancy. *N Engl J Med*. 1997;337:509–15.
13. Kabani N, Kimberlin D. Neonatal herpes simplex virus infection. *Neoreviews*. 2018;19(2):e89–96.
14. Brown ZA, Wald A, Morrow RM, Selke S, Zeh J, Corey L. Effect of serologic status and cesarean delivery on transmission rates of herpes simplex virus from mother to infant. *JAMA*. 2003;289:203–9.
15. Handel S, Klingler EJ, Washburn K, Blank S, Schillinger JA. Population-based surveillance for neonatal herpes in New York City, April 2006–September 2010. *Sex Transm Dis*. 2011;38(8):705–11.
16. Whitley R. Herpes simplex virus. In: Scheld W, Whitley R, Marra C, eds. Scheld W, Whitley R, Marra C, eds. *Infections of the Central Nervous System*. 3rd ed. Philadelphia: LWW; 2004, pp. 123–44.

17. Lim HK, Seppanen M, Hautala T, et al. TLR3 deficiency in herpes simplex encephalitis: High allelic heterogeneity and recurrence risk. *Neurology.* 2014;83(21):1888–97.

18. Schiffer J, Corey L. Herpes simplex virus. In: Bennett J, Dolin R, Blaser M, eds. Bennett J, Dolin R, Blaser M, eds. *Mandell, Douglas and Bennett's Principles and Practice of Infectious Diseases*, 6th ed. New York: Saunders; 2015.

19. *Redbook.* 31st ed. American Academy of Pediatrics; 2018.

20. Jensenius M, Myrvang B, Storvold G, Bucher A, Hellum KB, Bruu AL. Herpes simplex virus type 2 DNA detected in cerebrospinal fluid of 9 patients with Mollaret's meningitis. *Acta Neurol Scand.* 1998;98:209–12.

21. Wald A, Zeh J, Barnum G, Davis LG, Corey L. Suppression of subclinical shedding of herpes simplex virus type 2 with acyclovir. *Ann Intern Med.* 1996;124:8–15.

22. Corey L, Spear P. Infections with herpes simplex viruses. *N Engl J Med.* 1986;314:749–57.

23. James SH, Kimberlin DW. Neonatal herpes simplex virus infection: Epidemiology and treatment. *Clin Perinatol.* 2015;42(1):47–59, viii.

24. Gnann JW Jr, Sköldenberg B, Hart J, et al. Herpsex simplex encephalitis: Lack of clinical benefit of long-term valacyclovir therapy. *Clin Infect Dis.* 2015;61(5):683–91.

CHAPTER 124

Vector-borne Filariases*

Richard S. Bradbury • Paul Cantey • Kimberly Won • Christine DuBray

The vector-borne filariases encompass a diverse range of parasitic infections, including lymphatic filariasis, onchocerciasis, mansonellosis, and loiasis. For some, such as lymphatic filariasis and onchocerciasis, large-scale World Health Organization (WHO)-supported elimination campaigns are now underway. Others, such as mansonellosis, remain neglected with limited large-scale, well-controlled clinical and epidemiologic data available. This chapter will review the common vector-borne filariases of humans. Dirofilariasis and dracunculiasis, diseases of humans also caused by filarial nematodes, are covered in Chapter 127: Tissue Nematodes chapter of this textbook.

LYMPHATIC FILARIASIS

Lymphatic filariasis is a chronic, often debilitating parasitic disease caused by infection with the filarial parasites *Wuchereria bancrofti, Brugia malayi*, and *B. timori*. It is estimated that there are currently about 68 million lymphatic filariasis cases, including 36 million people harboring active infection and 36 million living with chronic morbidity subsequent to active disease.[1,2] It is estimated that 856 million people in 72 endemic countries of the tropics and subtropics of Africa, Asia, Oceania, the Caribbean, and parts of South America are at risk for infection.[1] In 1993, the International Task Force for Disease Eradication identified lymphatic filariasis as one of six "eradicable" or "potentially eradicable" infectious diseases.[3] In 1997, the World Health Assembly (Resolution 50.29)[4] targeted lymphatic filariasis for global elimination as a public health problem by 2020. In response, in 2000, WHO launched the Global Programme to Eliminate Lymphatic Filariasis (GPELF), which aims to stop the spread of infection and alleviate suffering in affected persons.[5] Almost half of all endemic countries had initiated national control programs by the end of 2004 leading to a dramatic reduction in the prevalence of microfilaremia in the participating countries.[6]

BIOLOGY AND LIFE CYCLES

Human infection with *W. bancrofti* occurs when infective larvae penetrate the skin during the bite of a mosquito vector and migrate to the nearest lymphatic vessel. Over the course of several months, they develop into thread-like adult worms (the males are approximately 40 by 0.1 mm and the females 100 by 0.25 mm in size). The average reproductive life span of the adult worms has been estimated at 5 years.[7] Fertilized female worms produce sheathed microfilariae, which are released into the bloodstream. Circulating microfilariae are ingested by the appropriate mosquito vector intermediate host during a blood meal; they develop within the insect over the course of several weeks into infective larvae, completing the parasite life cycle.[8]

In most areas of the world, microfilariae are detectable in the peripheral blood only at night (nocturnal periodicity) based on the biting times of the *Anopheles* and *Culex* mosquito vectors. However, where *Aedes* mosquitoes are the primary vector, diurnal subperiodicity (microfilarial counts maximal during the day; parts of Polynesia) or nocturnal subperiodicity (microfilaria circulating throughout the day, with only slight increase in microfilaremia at night; some regions of South East Asia) is seen.[9]

Brugia species larvae are also introduced to human hosts via the bite of mosquito vectors. The adult worms (males 13–23 mm and females 43–55 mm) reside in the lymphatic lumen and may live for 7–10 years. Both periodic and subperiodic forms exist, with subtle morphologic, mammalian host and vector differences between the two types. The nocturnally periodic form is transmitted by *Mansonia uniformis, M. annulata,* and *M. annulifera*, as well as some other *Mansonia, Ochleratus,* and *Anopheles* species, whereas the subperiodic form is transmitted by primarily by *M. annulata, M. dives,* and *M. bonneae*, and sometimes *Coquillettidia crassipes* and *M. uniformis.*[9] The nocturnally periodic species *B. timori* has a very limited geographic range and the primary (possibly the only) vector is *Anopheles barbirostris.*[9,10]

Although experimental infection of nonhuman primates is possible, animals other than humans do not appear to be natural reservoirs of *W. bancrofti* or *B. timori*. In contrast, the subperiodic form of *B. malayi* in some parts of Malaysia is a zoonosis, where humans, leaf-eating monkeys, wild and domestic cats, civets, and pangolins may all act as zoonotic reservoirs, complicating attempts to eliminate this cause of lymphatic filariasis.[11,12,10]

Most of the filarial parasites that infect humans, including *W. bancrofti* and *Brugia spp.*, are infected with *Wolbachia*, intracellular endosymbiont bacteria that are required for filarial development, viability, and fertility.[13] These bacteria play a significant role in the pathogenesis of filarial infection and may provide targets for chemotherapy.

DISTRIBUTION

The geographic distribution of lymphatic filariasis is determined primarily by the ability of the parasite to adapt to different mosquito vectors. Consequently, *W. bancrofti*, with the widest range of potential mosquito vectors, is the most widespread of the agents of lymphatic filariasis, occurring in parts of Africa, Asia, South America, the Caribbean, and the Pacific. *B. malayi* infection is restricted

*Disclaimer: The findings and conclusions in this chapter are those of the author and do not necessarily represent the official position of the Centers for Disease Control and Prevention/the Agency for Toxic Substances and Disease Registry.

to areas of south and east Asia, including India, Sri Lanka, China, Indonesia, Malaysia, and the Philippines.[11] *B. timori* infection has been reported only from East Nusa Tengarra Province of Indonesia (West Timor, Alor, Flores, and associated smaller islands) and East Timor. Lymphatic filariasis occurs in both urban and rural settings, as mosquitoes breed in unsanitary water sources found commonly in urban environments, such as abandoned wells and septic tanks, pit latrines, and water storage tanks, as well as in rural swamps and rice paddies.

Over the past two decades, the GPELF has made great progress toward breaking transmission of lymphatic filariasis in endemic countries primarily by mass drug administration (MDA).[14,15] The program incorporates global prevalence mapping using a variety of techniques, including community surveys, global information systems, and statistical models to determine where MDAs are needed.[16] Transmission assessment surveys (TAS) are conducted to determine prevalence of antigenemia in young children. Results from these surveys are used to identify geographic areas where disease prevalence is below that at which MDAs can be stopped.[17] In 2017, 51 of the 72 countries endemic for lymphatic filariasis still required MDAs, but only five had not yet started MDA. Twenty-one countries no longer required MDA according to current GPELF criteria, including those under surveillance and those validated for meeting WHO criteria for elimination of lymphatic filariasis as a public health problem. In total, based on TAS results, an estimated 554 million persons no longer require treatment.[1]

PATHOLOGIC AND CLINICAL MANIFESTATIONS

The spectrum of clinical manifestations of lymphatic filariasis is broad and includes asymptomatic microfilaremia, acute attacks,[18] chronic lymphedema/elephantiasis, hydrocele, and tropical pulmonary eosinophilia. Whereas the host immune responses to filarial and *Wolbachia* antigens are clearly involved in determining the clinical manifestations of infection,[13,19] the determinants of these responses are complex and likely include genetic factors, as well as the timing and degree of exposure.[18,20]

Most, but not all, people living in endemic areas who acquire lymphatic filariasis are asymptomatic with circulating microfilariae detectable in the peripheral blood (microfilaremia).[21] However, despite the lack of obvious clinical signs or symptoms, pathologic changes—including alterations in lymphatic flow, as detected by lymphoscintigraphy,[22] lymphatic dilatation,[23] and renal abnormalities (hematuria and proteinuria)[24]—have been demonstrated in these individuals. In contrast to the above-described asymptomatic microfilaremic patients, the majority of visitors to endemic areas who become infected present with signs and symptoms of acute infection.[25]

Two distinct acute syndromes have been described.[18] The first, called acute filarial lymphangitis, is caused by the death of adult worm. It has a mild clinical course characterized by a circumscribed inflammatory nodule or cord in the arms, legs or the breast centered around adult worms in lymphatic vessels and rarely causes residual lymphedema. It is typically seen in patients who have been treated. Acute dermatolymphangioadenitis (ADLA), the other syndrome, is characterized by a plaque-like diffuse (sub)cutaneous inflammation. A distal skin lesion that serves as the point of entry for secondary bacterial infection can be identified in most patients. ADLA can be accompanied by systematic manifestations of bacteraemia, including, in rare cases, severe sepsis. The acute attack is often accompanied or followed by distal edema of the affected leg and recurrent ADLA is a common cause of chronic lymphedema and elephantiasis.[18,26] The lower extremities are affected more frequently than the upper extremities and breast, and in *W. bancrofti* infection, the scrotum or female external genitalia may be involved. Episodes generally last from 3 to 7 days unless they are complicated by abscess formation along the affected lymphatic, in which case healing may take several months. Additional early manifestations of *W. bancrofti* infection include orchitis and inflammation of the spermatic cord, which can lead to permanent thickening of the spermatic cord and/or hydrocele. Genital manifestations are rare in brugian filariasis.[27]

After years of infection, chronic lymphatic dysfunction caused by vessel dilatation develops in some patients. Recurrent episodes of inflammation and infection lead to irreversible enlargement of the affected area with a thickened, warty appearance of the overlying skin in advanced cases (elephantiasis, Fig. 124-1). In contrast to *W. bancrofti* infection, in which the entire limb is generally involved, the chronic lymphedema of brugian filariasis is characteristically limited to the distal portion of the involved extremity. Although elephantiasis itself is generally painless, ulceration and secondary infection are common and contribute greatly to the morbidity and mortality of lymphatic filarial infection. In the genital region, lymphatic dysfunction may lead to rupture of the dilated lymph vessels into the urinary tract and intermittent chyluria.

A minority of patients with lymphatic filariasis present with tropical pulmonary eosinophilia (TPE).[28] The clinical manifestations of TPE are predominantly pulmonary, consisting of nocturnal wheezing, cough, and dyspnea, although constitutional symptoms may be present. Laboratory studies are notable for marked eosinophilia (both in the peripheral blood and the lower respiratory tract) and elevated serum IgE and antifilarial antibody levels. Chest radiographs typically show diffuse reticulonodular infiltrates, and pulmonary function tests are consistent with a predominantly restrictive pattern. Although most patients with TPE respond rapidly to a 3-week course of diethylcarbamazine (DEC), chronic respiratory tract inflammation and mild interstitial lung disease are not uncommon. Untreated, TPE may progress to irreversible interstitial fibrosis.

As is true of helminth infections in general, filarial infection is associated with a skewing of the immune response toward a Th2 phenotype. This has led to considerable interest in the effects of chronic filarial infection on the outcome of immunizations and of concomitant infections with pathogens such as HIV and malaria, which require an effective Th1 type response. The response to tetanus vaccine does appear to be impaired in patients with lymphatic filariasis.[29] There are some data that suggest increased susceptibility of filarial-infected cells to HIV infection[30] and one prospective study in Tanzania demonstrated an increased risk of HIV acquisition among individuals with lymphatic filariasis.[31]

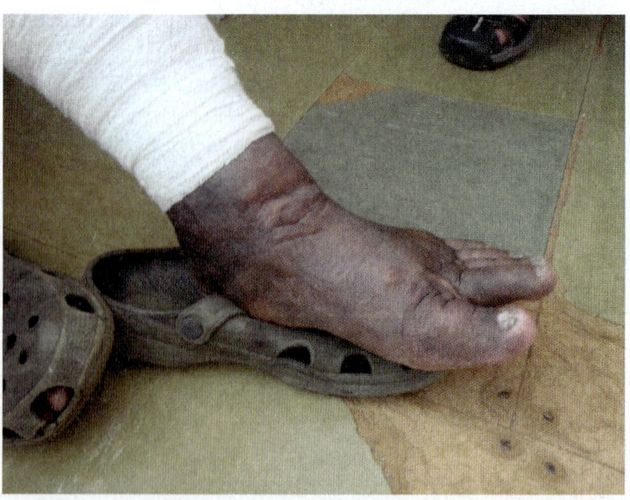

FIGURE 124-1. Elephantiasis of the foot in a case of bancroftian (*W. bancrofti*) filariasis. (Dr. Richard S. Bradbury.)

DIAGNOSIS

Until the advent of modern serologic, antigenic, and molecular tests, definitive parasitological diagnosis could only be made by demonstration of the characteristic sheathed microfilariae in a Giemsa-stained specimen of peripheral blood (Fig. 124-2), a smear made from the deposit of a Knott's microfilaria concentration blood preparation[8] or, rarely, by excision of an adult worm. More recently, polycarbonate membrane filtration filter assays for microfilaria have been used to detect circulating microfilaria.[32] Because the microfilariae exhibit periodicity in many areas of the world, the timing of blood samples for parasite detection is critical and may require collection in the middle of the night.

When definitive diagnosis of the parasite is not possible or practical, the presence of circulating filarial antigen (CFA) can serve as a proxy for *W. bancrofti* infection. CFA tests recognize parasite antigen that is highly expressed in the cuticle and reproductive organs of adult worms and is released in relatively large quantities by living worms.[33] Consequently, CFA is commonly detectable in microfilaremic individuals.[33–35] Additionally, CFA is often present in infected individuals who are amicrofilaremic and asymptomatic.[36,37] Thus, results from these tests provide a more sensitive measure of infection than tests that detect microfilariae. An additional advantage is that CFA is detectable in peripheral blood regardless of the time of day.[38]

Quantitative measures of CFA assessed by enzyme-linked immunosorbent assay (ELISA) can provide an indication of adult worm infection intensity.[33,39] Detection of CFA was simplified with the introduction of an immunochromatographic card test (ICT).[34] As with the ELISA format, the ICT was found to be sensitive and highly specific for the detection of *W. bancrofti* adult worm antigen.[40–42] However, positive ICT results have been reported among individuals infected with *Loa loa* but negative for *W. bancrofti*, thus making it difficult to discriminate between the two filarial infections.[43,44] Unlike the ELISA platform, the ICT can only provide a qualitative assessment of the presence or absence of CFA. In 2011, the ICT was reformatted, and the Filariasis Test Strip (FTS) was developed.[15] In laboratory and field evaluations, the FTS was found to be slightly more sensitive than the ICT but overall very comparable.[15,45,46] Currently, production of the ICT has been discontinued, and has been replaced solely by the FTS.[15,32,34,39,47]

Seroepidemiological surveys of children or adults, combined with molecular surveys of vectors may be used to confirm elimination of *W. bancrofti* from a given region.[48,49] The recent development of the highly sensitive and specific recombinant antigen Wb123 for the detection of antibodies to *W. bancrofti* at all stages of disease shows great promise.[50] This antigen has been adapted to both a Luciferase Immunoprecipitation System (LIPS),[50] ELISA, multiplex bead and lateral flow test strip platforms[51] and in some cases these tests have been used in the monitoring of lymphatic filariasis elimination in post-MDA areas.[51–53] Another recombinant antigen, Bm14, has been incorporated into an ELISA format that shows a high sensitivity for the detection of antibodies to both *W. bancrofti* and *Brugia* lymphatic filariasis. Cross-reaction with other filarial, but not nonfilarial parasitic, infections was noted.[54] Antifilarial antibody and antigen tests may also be used in diagnosing infection in patients with TPE and in visitors to endemic areas who have symptoms consistent with infection but no detectable microfilariae.

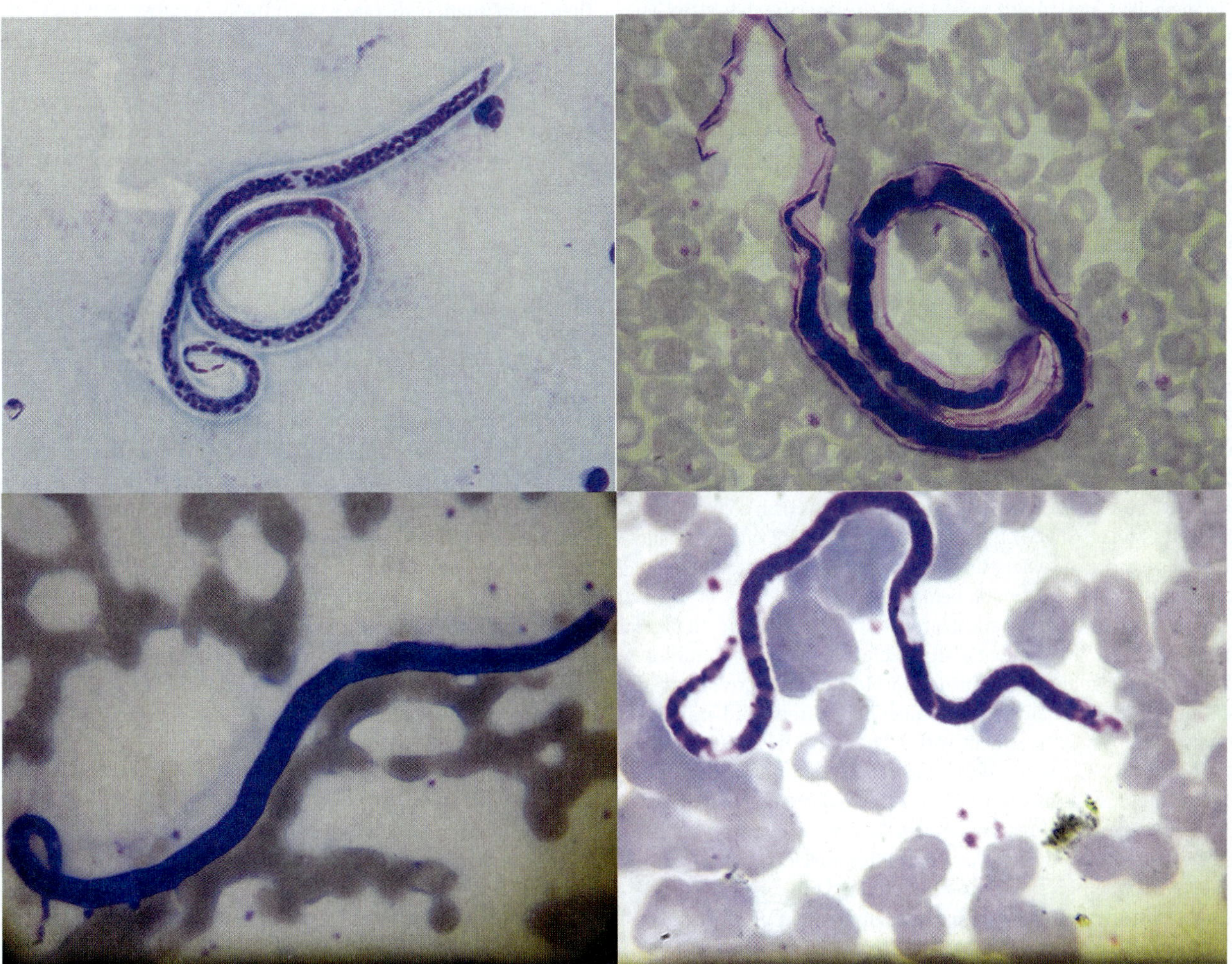

FIGURE 124-2. Common microfilaria infecting humans in Giemsa stained blood smears (clockwise from top left) *W. bancrofti*, *B. malayi*, *Loa loa*, and *M. perstans*. (Dr. Richard S. Bradbury.)

Antigen test detection assays are not available for *B. malayi* or *B. timori* infection; however, an IgG4 antibody dipstick assay based on a recombinant antigen has recently been developed and appears to be sensitive and specific for the detection of active *Brugia* infection.[55] Several DNA-based polymerase chain reaction (PCR) assays for *W. bancrofti* and *B. malayi* are comparable in sensitivity and specificity to the circulating antigen assay and antibody dipstick for detection of microfilaremia. Loop-mediated isothermal amplification (LAMP) assays for the isothermal detection of *W. bancrofti* and *B. malayi* DNA have also been recently developed.[56,57] Molecular assays such as these are more commonly applied to the xenomonitoring of infection rates in mosquitoes (see Control and Prevention) than diagnosis in humans.[48]

Ultrasonography is useful for the identification of subclinical hydrocele and can be used to make a diagnosis of lymphatic filariasis through detection of the presence of living adult worms ("filarial dance sign") in the scrotal lymphatics of male patients[58] and in the axillary, breast, uterine, femoral, and groin lymphatics of female patients.[59]

TREATMENT

The anthelminthics, DEC, ivermectin, and albendazole, have been the mainstays of treatment for lymphatic filariasis for many years. More recently, doxycycline has been shown to have antifilarial activity due to its effect on the bacterial endosymbiont, *Wolbachia*.[60,61]

DEC is a piperazine derivative with excellent microfilaricidal activity at low doses. The mechanism of action of DEC is unknown but appears to depend on the host immune response. Although adult worms are affected by DEC treatment at higher doses,[62] killing is inefficient and cure is uncommon. Ivermectin shows similar activity to DEC against microfilariae of lymphatic-dwelling filariae but has no effect on adult worms.[63] It is thought to act by blocking the neurotransmitter γ-aminobutyric acid (GABA). Albendazole is a poorly absorbed benzimidazole with activity against a wide variety of helminths, including filariae. Unlike DEC and ivermectin, albendazole has little direct activity on microfilariae, but appears to act predominantly on the adult parasite leading to decreased microfilarial production. Side effects of therapy are few when used at low doses, and because of the lack of rapid microfilaricidal activity, albendazole can be given safely to patients with *Loa loa* infection and/or onchocerciasis.

Adverse events related to DEC and ivermectin treatment, which are generally mild, include fever, headache, malaise, arthralgia, and localized swellings along the lymphatics. These are thought to be related to the release of filarial and bacterial antigens as a result of microfilarial death, and increase in severity with increasing microfilarial load.[64] Severe reactions may occur in patients with concomitant loiasis (DEC or ivermectin) or onchocerciasis (DEC only),[65–67] and individuals from areas where these infections are endemic should be screened for *Loa loa* coinfection before treatment.

In view of the recent data demonstrating pathologic changes even in asymptomatic patients, all infected individuals should be treated with the goal of preventing morbidity and decreasing disease transmission. The current recommended therapy for lymphatic filariasis is high-dose treatment with DEC. A study showed that a single dose of DEC was as effective as full 12-day course for long-term control of microfilaremia.[68] For TPE, a DEC treatment course of 21 days is generally recommended.[69] Although impractical for mass treatment, doxycycline has both microfilaricidal and adulticidal activity when given at doses of 200 mg daily for 6–8 weeks.[60] Side effects of therapy are minimal and suppression of microfilaremia is sustained for up to 14 months. Shorter course doxycycline (3 weeks) combined with single dose ivermectin/albendazole appears equally effective at reducing microfilarial loads, but has no detectable adulticidal activity.[61]

Although there is no direct evidence for the development of drug resistance in lymphatic filariasis, diminished efficacy of DEC treatment in some patients with circulating microfilariae despite adequate drug levels suggests that resistance may occur in some situations.[70] Selection for benzimidazole mutations in response to albendazole therapy has also been reported, although the clinical significance of these findings remains uncertain.[71]

For symptomatic patients with lymphedema and elephantiasis, intensive local hygiene and prompt treatment of bacterial or fungal superinfection should be instituted as this has been shown to reduce lymphedema and decrease the frequency of episodes of adenolymphangitis.[20] Hydrocelectomy should be considered for all symptomatic patients as it has been shown to improve work capacity, sexual function, and integration into community activities.[72]

CONTROL AND PREVENTION

The major goals of GPELF are infection elimination as a public health problem (control of infection) and reduction of suffering (morbidity control). Since vector control measures alone have been generally unsuccessful in decreasing the prevalence of infection, an integrated approach of (a) microfilaremia reduction through chemotherapy, (b) vector control, and (c) reduction of host–vector contact has been advocated. The optimal control strategies for a given endemic area will depend on the particular parasite and vector species involved as well as on the ecological, cultural, and political factors specific to the region.

Regimens that include combinations of single doses of albendazole (400 mg) and either DEC (6 mg/kg) or ivermectin (200 μg/kg) have all been demonstrated to have a sustained microfilaridical effect. These combination therapies are now being used in Africa (albendazole/ivermectin) and elsewhere (albendazole/DEC) for the elimination of lymphatic filariasis as a public health problem.[73] A recent clinical trial has shown that a single dose of a triple drug combination that includes ivermectin with DEC and albendazole is superior to ivermectin plus albendazole or DEC plus albendazole for clearing microfilariae from the blood.[74] In 2017, WHO recommended the use of the triple-drug therapy in selected settings where onchocerciasis is not endemic.[1,75]

Both DEC and ivermectin have been demonstrated to suppress microfilaremia (90–95% reduction) in infected patients for up to 1 year after therapy is stopped.[76] Although the addition of albendazole to ivermectin does not appear to substantially increase microfilaricidal efficacy as compared to ivermectin alone, this regimen continues to be used in areas where onchocerciasis limits the use of DEC, in part because of the broad spectrum anthelminthic benefits afforded by albendazole.[76] Options for mass treatment in areas where *Loa loa* is coendemic continue to be limited; this is an area of active research. Currently, mass administration of albendazole (400 mg every 6 months) along with provision of insecticide-treated bednets to reduce exposure to vectors of lymphatic filariasis[77,78] is recommended by WHO for interruption of transmission of lymphatic filariasis in areas where loiasis is endemic and onchocerciasis is not highly endemic.

The length of time that MDA strategies need to be implemented in endemic areas in order to achieve elimination of lymphatic filariasis as a public health problem is estimated to be 5–6 years. Additional rounds of yearly treatment may be needed in some settings, especially where baseline microfilaremia prevalence was high. In those areas, alternative strategies like triple drug therapy might reduce program duration.[79]

Vector control has played a limited role in elimination of lymphatic filariasis, primarily because of the widespread distribution of potential mosquito vectors and the ability of mosquitoes to adapt to varied ecological conditions.[80] Toxin-producing bacteria such as *Bacillus sphaericus* and *Bacillus thuringiensis*[81] and entomopathogenic fungi[82] have been used to control larvae of *Culex*, *Mansonia*, and *Anopheles* species. Breeding sites can be eliminated through the construction of improved water and sanitary facilities but is not economically feasible in many endemic regions. Reduction of host-vector contact can be achieved with the use of insect repellents and protective clothing or, in areas where vector feeding is predominantly indoors, with indoor spraying with pyrethroids and other household measures (including screens and bed nets).

Prevention of lymphatic filariasis through immunization would greatly enhance current control strategies by limiting the population at risk for infection and addressing the potential for drug resistance to develop.[83] Although evidence from both human and animal laboratory models suggests that protective immunity to filariasis may develop,[84] vaccine development has been hampered by the complexity of the human immune response to filarial infection.[83] At the time of writing, no vaccine for use in humans is yet available.

Surveillance for reintroduction or recrudescence of infection is the next challenge for countries that have been able to stop MDA. Laboratory assays that are adequately sensitive and suitable for large-scale surveillance of endemic populations and vectors are needed.[29,85,86]

Addressing lymphatic filariasis morbidity will remain a problem in the near future. Efforts to promote local hygiene and early treatment of cellulitis in symptomatic patients need to be sustained, since these have been associated with a decrease in the number of episodes of adenolymphangitis.[87] Strategies to prevent morbidity in asymptomatic infected individuals are also needed. Annual or semiannual treatment with DEC-albendazole has been shown to reverse early pathology and offers promise.[88]

Onchocerciasis

Onchocerciasis, a disease caused by the filarial worm *Onchocerca volvulus*, occurs in sub-Saharan Africa, parts of the Americas and Yemen in the Middle East. The parasite is spread by blackflies of the genus *Simulium*. It is colloquially known as "river blindness" due to its association with riverine vector breeding sites.

It is currently estimated that 205 million people live in areas where there is risk acquiring onchocerciasis.[89] Approximately 21 million people are estimated to be infected with *O. volvulus*,[90] with over 99% of these residing in 31 sub-Saharan African countries.[91] The endemic countries at the time of writing are Angola, Benin, Burkina Faso, Burundi, Cameroon, Central African Republic, Chad, Republic of Congo, Côte d'Ivoire, Democratic Republic of the Congo, Equatorial Guinea, Ethiopia, Gabon, Ghana, Guinea, Guinea-Bissau, Kenya, Liberia, Malawi, Mali, Mozambique, Niger, Nigeria, Rwanda, Senegal, Sierra Leone, South Sudan, Sudan, Togo, Uganda, and the United Republic of Tanzania.[91] In the Americas, *O. volvulus* transmission has been verified by WHO as having been eliminated in Colombia (2013), Ecuador (2014), Mexico (2015), and Guatemala (2016). The Yanomami region bordering Brazil and Venezuela is at present the last remain area in the Americas of ongoing transmission.[92,93] Transmission of disease also continues in Yemen.[94] The black fly vectors of disease are the *S. damnosum* complex[90] and *S. neavei* complex in Africa, with *S. albovirgulatum* in the central basin of the Democratic Republic of Congo,[8,95] *S. guianense* complex, *S. incrustatum*, and *S. oyapockense* complex in the remaining endemic focus of the Americas,[95,96] and *S. rasyani* in Yemen.[97]

Infective stage 3 larvae of *O. volvulus* enter the human body during a blood meal of an infective female *Simulium* black fly. Larvae molt into stage 4 larvae and then develop into adults over a 1- to 3-month period. Female adult worms grow to a length of 33–50 cm and adult males to 19–42 mm. Adults may live 15 years or more, though modelling suggests that the typical life span may be closer to 10 years. Females produce microfilariae for 9–12 years.[98] Adult worms tend to congregate in nodules. Nodules may occur anywhere in the body, but are most common over body prominences in the pelvic arch, at the junction of long bones, and in the temporal or occipital regions of the scalp. Most nodules contain multiple worms.[8] The adult worms produce 1300–1900 microfilariae per day,[99] which migrate primarily through the skin and eye. When microfilariae are ingested by the black fly, those that survive the transfer process will molt inside the fly and once they have matured to the infective stage 3 larvae, will migrate to the head of the fly and will transfer to the skin of a human during the next blood meal. Microfilariae have a life span of up to 2 years.[98] The host inflammatory response to dying microfilariae and/or the endosymbiont *Wolbachia* is thought to be the driver of most of the symptoms of onchocerciasis.[100] Manifestations may include troublesome itch, acute and chronic papular dermatitis, lichenified dermatitis (with an extreme form called Sowdah), areas of depigmentation (leopard skin), and atrophy with loss of skin elasticity (with an extreme form called hanging groin).[8,90] Invasion of the eye by microfilaria leads to ocular manifestations including punctate or sclerosing keratitis, iridocyclitis, and glaucoma, with eventual vision loss.[8] It is estimated that currently 270,000 people worldwide are blind due to the effects of *O. volvulus* infection.[90] It remains unclear if there are associations of onchocerciasis with nodding syndrome, Nakalanga syndrome, and epilepsy, which requires further investigation.[101]

Diagnosis of onchocerciasis in individuals seeking treatment outside of mass treatment programs can be complex, particularly for patients who do not live in endemic areas (e.g., expatriates and travelers). The Ov16 serologic tests may provide some assistance in diagnosis, but these were not intended to be individual diagnostic tests and there are concerns about the risk of false positive results in low-risk populations. Positive results in patients seeking treatment would be helpful in establishing a diagnosis, but negative results are probably not sufficient to exclude the diagnosis. The gold standard diagnostic test is microscopic examination of superficial skin biopsies (skin snips).

There are a variety of approaches to the diagnosis of onchocerciasis within the context of mass treatment programs. Palpation of nodules and clinical diagnosis of characteristic skin and ocular lesions are simple, if insensitive, methods of case detection often used in areas of high prevalence. Detection of microfilaria in skin snips by microscopy has good specificity, but has poor sensitivity when microfilarial density is low (Figure 124-3).[102,103] Care must be taken to differentiate microfilaria from those of *Mansonella streptocerca* in regions where the diseases overlap.[104] The use of *O. volvulus* PCR on DNA extracts from skin snips greatly improves the sensitivity of filarial detection and resolves the specificity issues associated with performing traditional microscopic methods on these specimens.[103] WHO recommends tests for use by onchocerciasis elimination programs to determine when programs may stop treatment including the anti-Ov16 recombinant antigen antibody serologic assay in humans and O-150 PCR in blackflies.[105] The serologic test comes in both ELISA and rapid test formats. Both formats typically have moderate sensitivity and high specificity,[102] but cannot distinguish between past and current infection.[102,106] Better understanding of the sensitivity and performance of the two formats in low prevalence settings is needed.[107]

Progress toward elimination of onchocerciasis has been encouraging since the first Onchocerciasis Control Program (OCP) was initiated in West Africa in 1974. The OCP is credited with preventing infection in 40 million people and preventing 600,000 cases of blindness. The economic rate of return of the program was estimated to be 20%.[108] The OCP was replaced by the African Programme for Onchocerciasis Control (APOC), which ran from 1995 to 2015. It is estimated that APOC averted 17.4 million DALYs at a cost of U.S.$27 per DALY and helped avoid U.S.$2.2 billion in productivity losses.[109] The year that the program closed more than 119 million people received ivermectin and nearly 1 million people lived in areas where it had been demonstrated that ivermectin treatment was no longer needed.[90,110] In the Americas the onchocerciasis programs have been coordinated since 1993 by the Onchocerciasis Elimination Program for the Americas (OEPA). As of 2017, transmission of onchocerciasis had been eliminated in all the foci in the region except for the Yanomami cross-border focus, shared by Venezuela and Brazil. Here, over 500,000 were no longer at risk for onchocerciasis, but approximately 30,000 people remained at risk.[111]

In 2016, the Expanded Special Project for the Elimination of neglected tropical diseases (NTDs) in Africa (ESPEN) was launched to support elimination and control of five preventive chemotherapy NTDs: onchocerciasis, lymphatic filariasis, trachoma, schistosomiasis, and soil-transmitted helminthiases. Efforts to eliminate onchocerciasis that were begun under OCP and APOC are being continued with the support of ESPEN. OEPA continues to support Brazil and Venezuela in their attempt to complete elimination and control efforts in the Americas. Yemen launched its first mass treatment campaign in 2018 and has set an elimination target. Current tools for elimination of transmission include one and twice per year mass treatment with ivermectin and limited use of vector control.

Loiasis

Loiasis, infection with the African eye worm *Loa loa*, occurs in all or parts of 11 countries in Central Africa and West Africa extending from Nigeria through to northern Angola, from South Sudan and potentially eastern Ethiopia to Chad and throughout the Democratic Republic of Congo.[112,113] The vector of loiasis is the day-biting mango fly (*Chrysops* spp.). Approximately 30 million people are at risk and 10 million people are thought to be currently infected.[114]

Patients often first become aware of infection due to the visible migration of the adult worm under the conjunctiva or on the surface of the orbit. Episodic subcutaneous nonpitting and nontender edema, called "calabar swellings" can also occur, as may urticaria, pruritis, myalgias, and arthralgias. Peripheral eosinophilia is very common in infected persons.[115,116]

Microfilaria of *L. loa* show diurnal periodicity due to the daytime biting habits of the vector fly; blood microfilaria densities are highest between 10 am and 4 pm.[114] Diagnosis has been traditionally performed via the detection of microfilaria in peripheral blood (Fig. 124-2). Methods such as Knott's concentration and polycarbonate membrane filtration may increase recovery of microfilaria in blood. More recently, molecular tests such as LAMP PCR have proved highly sensitive and specific.[114,116] Amicrofilaraemic or so-called "occult" loiasis will not be detected by these methods.[117] An *Ll*-SXP-1 antigen ELISA for the detection of antibodies to *L. loa* has been shown to be 67% sensitive and 81% specific.[116] Increased sensitivity (97–100%) and specificity (78–81%) has been demonstrated in a luciferase immunoassay (LIPS) format where only IgG4 antibodies targeting *Ll*-SXP-1 are used. The antigen has been converted to a rapid lateral flow assay with a reported sensitivity of 94% and between 82% and 87%.[116]

L. loa may be treated with DEC.[115] Severe adverse neurologic effects such as potentially fatal encephalopathy may occur in those with very high filarial counts. The possibility of severe adverse events has precluded use of DEC for lymphatic filariasis and onchocerciasis elimination in these areas.[117,118] Recently, a "LoaScope," a smart phone-based tool that detects the presence of *L. loa* microfilaria burdens of sufficiently high intensity to cause neurologic reaction to treatments was trialed in Central Africa as part of a strategy to identify and avoid treatment of individuals with high *L. loa* microfilaremia in areas where *O. volvulus* MDA is indicated.[119] Although rare, cases have occurred in travelers returning from these countries; these often receive a great deal of attention due to the psychologically disturbing nature of eyeworm disease.

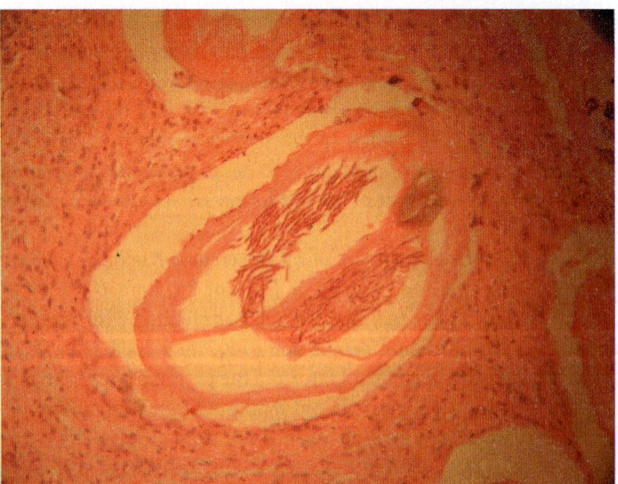

FIGURE 124-3. Histological section of a skin nodule biopsy (hematoxylin and eosin stained) from a human showing cross-section of a gravid adult female *O. volvulus*, note microfilaria within the ovary of the worm. (Dr. Richard S. Bradbury.)

Mansonellosis

Mansonellosis, human infection with one of four species of *Mansonella* genus filaria, as well as occasional zoonotic species, occurs in both Africa, the Caribbean and Latin America. Data on the prevalence and clinical presentation of human infection with *Mansonella* species are limited.[120] Vectors vary by geography and infection appears to be focal; for instance, infections with *M. ozzardi* in the Caribbean islands are restricted to a single village each on the islands of St. Vincent, St Lucia, and Nevis.[121]

M. perstans (formerly *Dipetalonema perstans*), which appears to be the most common species infecting humans, is endemic in west, central (including Uganda), and southern (to Zimbabwe) Africa, as well as the northern Amazon rainforest region of South America.[120,122] Prevalence varies widely within and between countries,[123] but average prevalence across endemic regions has been estimated at approximately 20% of the population.[124] Reports of infections from Papua New Guinea and Fiji up until the 1970s may represent spurious misidentifications of *W. bancrofti*.[120,121,123]

Based on a study in Uganda, microfilaremia was found to be somewhat subperiodic in distribution with the moderately elevated parasitemias seen in the first half of the day, peaking at around 08:00 am in the morning, but microfilaria are present in the blood at all times of the day and night.[125] Average parasitemia increases with age and is higher in males than females.[120,122] The vector insects are biting midges of the genus *Culicoides*. High parasitemia with perstans filariasis has been reported among banana plantation workers, as one vector species, *C. austeni* uses the stumps of banana trees for breeding.[120] *M. perstans* microfilaria have been recovered from gorillas, chimpanzees, and monkeys,[122,123] but humans appear to be the primary reservoirs of infection.[122] Recently a novel clade of *M. perstans*, called *Mansonella* sp. "Deux" has been described in Brazil and Gabon.[120]

Adult *M. perstans* reside in the serous body cavities, mainly the peritoneum, but also the pericardium. Clinical disease caused by *M. perstans* is not well researched or described.[120] Asymptomatic infection has been reported. Signs and symptoms that have been associated with mansonellosis perstans include eosinophilia, pruritis, joint pain, lymphadenopathy, calabar swellings, abdominal pain, headaches, and fatigue.[120,122,124] Yellowish nodules on the conjunctiva have been reported in association with *M. perstans* infection but evidence for this association was uncertain, also, rare reports of adult *M. perstans* invading the eye may represent misidentifications of other, zoonotic, and filariae.[120,122,126,127]

M. ozzardi adults reside in the mesenteries of the peritoneal cavity. Microfilaria are aperiodic and found in blood and subcutaneous tissues. The species is distributed in noncontiguous foci in Latin America and the Caribbean from southern Mexico to northwest Argentina. It has not been reported from Chile, Uruguay, or Paraguay.[120] Prevalence may reach up to 46% of people in endemic regions.[128] Humans appear to be the only reservoir host.[123] Microfilarial loads in blood are higher in adults over 30 years old.[129] *Simulium spp.* black flies and *Culicoides spp.* are vectors in Latin America. In Haiti, Trinidad, and St. Vincent, only *Culicoides* act as vectors.[120] *Leptoconops bequaerti* midges are a vector in Haiti only.[128] The vector species affects the epidemiology of infection in different geographic regions. *Mansonellosis ozzardi* is associated with rivers where *Simulium* species breed in South America, but in Trinidad, the vector *C. phlebotomus* breeds in beach sand thus infections are associated with coastal regions of the island. Infection is often asymptomatic. Signs and symptoms associated with some *M. ozzardi* infection include fatigue, headache, fever, articular pain, a feeling of coldness in the lower limbs, foot and facial edema, and skin rash.[120] Ocular lesions, including punctate keratitis, nummular keratitis, and even corneal opacity have been associated with *M. ozzardi* microfilaria invading the cornea.[120,130,131]

M. streptocerca (formerly *Dipetalonema streptocerca*) is found only in tropical rainforest areas of West and Central Africa (including western Uganda).[120] Adults reside in subcutaneous tissues of the upper trunk and shoulder girdle.[120] Humans are thought to be the main reservoir of disease,[120] though infection has also been reported in wild chimpanzees.[132] Microfilaria are found in the subdermis, not the blood. As with other *Mansonella* infections, microfilarial intensity and prevalence is highest in older adults and infection is more common in men than in women.[104,120] Very few studies of the clinical effects and prevalence of *M. streptocerca* have been performed. Hyperpigmented macules have been reported in patients in the Democratic Republic of Congo, although controlled studies have found no difference in reporting of skin ailments between infected and uninfected subjects.[120] Prevalence of infection varies greatly, with a study in western Uganda finding prevalence rates varying from 0.5% to 89%, depending on the village sampled.[123]

Traditional microscopy of blood (Fig. 124-2) or skin biopsies remain the most common tools used in the diagnosis of mansonellosis. Although microfilaria are sometimes seen on direct blood smears and thick films, the sensitivity of diagnosis of blood-borne mansonellosis may be improved by using Knott's concentration or polycarbonate membrane filtration prior to microscopy.[129] PCR techniques are increasingly used in research and epidemiologic studies, and provide improved sensitivity for detection of infections. A comparative study of diagnostic methods for the detection of *M. ozzardi* in blood using polycarbonate membrane filtration as the reference standard found that PCR had the highest sensitivity of detection (98.5%), followed by Knott concentration (83.5%).[129] PCR is useful for differentiating *M. ozzardi* and *M. streptocerca* from *O. volvulus* in epidemiological studies.

Limited data are available on the optimal treatment or control strategies for *Mansonella* species infection. Vector control specifically targeting mansonellosis has not been trialed in any region. For individual treatment, DEC in combination with mebendazole appears to be the most effective treatment for *M. perstans* infection, followed by DEC or mebendazole alone.[133] Ivermectin, albendazole, and praziquantel are not effective and provision of two doses of thiabendazole has only limited efficacy.[133] Long-term (6 weeks) doxycycline has been shown to effectively treat *M. perstans* infection, though some genotypes may not respond to this treatment, possibly due to the absence of a *Wolbachia* bacterial endosymbiont, the target of doxycycline treatment in filarial worms.[120] *M. ozzardi* may be effectively treated with ivermectin and phase III trials using ivermectin to reduce *M. ozzardi* infection at a population level are currently ongoing in the Brazilian Amazon region.[134]

Zoonotic and Otherwise Unidentified Filariases

B. pahangi,[126] a natural parasite of cats, but also dogs, wild canids, and other mammals, is closely related to *B. malayi*. *B. pahangi* has been reported infecting two humans in Kuala Lumpur, Malaysia; one patient had symptoms of descending lymphangitis of the lower limb and cellulitis while the other had foot cellulitis only.[135] Other zoonotic *Brugia* species have occasionally been reported infecting humans in both North and South America,[136] as well as other parts of the world.[126] In such cases, adult worms are recovered from the subcutaneous tissues or the conjunctiva and in most cases peripheral microfilaremia is absent. The exact agents of infection remain unknown.[126,136]

Rarely, cases of infection with zoonotic *Onchocerca* species have been reported in humans. The most common among these is *O. lupi*, a natural parasite of wolves, dogs, and cats in Europe and the United States. All cases of human disease reported from Europe have presented with ocular manifestations, with all patients having subconjunctival nodules harboring the adult worm. In the United States, cases have involved subdermal, rather than subconjunctival nodules, with half of these occurring around the cervical spine region.[137] Further occasional reports of subcutaneous nodules in humans containing zoonotic *Onchocerca* species in Japan, Europe, and Northern America have variously implicated *O. dewittei japonica* (natural reservoir wild boars), *O. gutturosa* (cattle), *O. jakutensis* (red deer), *O. cervicalis*, and *O. reticulata* (horses) and there have been several cases where the pathogen has not been identified to species level.[138] Diagnosis may be undertaken via PCR and histological examination of excised nodules.[137]

Occasional human infections with zoonotic *Mansonella* species have been reported. In a study in Gabon, 14 villagers were found to be infected with the chimpanzee parasite *M. rodhaini*. A child infected with a zoonotic filaria, most likely the squirrel parasite *M. interstitium*, has been reported from Alabama.[126] An unidentified species of microfilaria, thus far referred to as Microfilaria *bolivarensis*, has been reported infecting Amerindian villagers along the Orinoco River in Venezuela.[126] Another unidentified microfilaria recovered from the blood of villagers in Equator province, Democratic Republic of Congo is currently referred to as Microfilaria *semiclarum*.[126] Microfilariae resembling those of *M. perstans* found in the cerebrospinal fluid of a soldier in Zimbabwe during the late 1960s[127] were later identified as the zoonotic monkey parasite *Meningonema Peruzzi*.[122,126]

References

1. World Health Organisation. Global programme to eliminate lymphatic filariasis: Progress report, 2016. *Wkly Epidemiol Rec.* 2017;92:594–607.
2. Ramaiah KD, Ottesen EA. Progress and impact of 13 years of the global programme to eliminate lymphatic filariasis on reducing the burden of filarial disease. *PLoS Negl Trop Dis.* 2014;8:e3319.
3. World Health Organisation. Recommendations of the International Task Force for disease eradication. *MMWR Recomm Rep.* 1993;42:1–38.
4. World Health Organization. Elimination of lymphatic filariasis as a public health problem—Resolution of the executive board of the WHO. http://www.who.int/neglected_diseases/mediacentre/WHA_50.29_Eng.pdf. 1997.
5. World Health Organisation. Global programme to eliminate lymphatic filariasis: Progress report, 2013. *Wkly Epidemiol Rec.* 2014;89:409–18.
6. World Health Organization. Global programme to eliminate lymphatic filariasis. *Wkly Epidemiol Rec.* 2005;80:202–12.
7. Vanamail P, Ramaiah KD, Pani SP, Das PK, Grenfell BT, Bundy DA. Estimation of the fecund life span of *Wuchereria bancrofti* in an endemic area. *Trans R Soc Trop Med Hyg.* 1996;90:119–21.
8. Beaver PC, Jung RC, Cupp EW. *Clinical Parasitology*. 9th ed. Philadelphia: Lea & Febiger; 1984.
9. World Health Organization. *Lymphatic Filariasis: A Handbook of Practical Entomology for National Lymphatic Filariasis Elimination Programmes*. Geneva: World Health Organization; 2013.
10. Fischer P, Wibowo H, Pischke S, et al. PCR-based detection and identification of the filarial parasite *Brugia timori* from Alor Island, Indonesia. *Ann Trop Med Parasitol.* 2002;96:809–21.
11. Chansiri K, Brugia SA. *Molecular Detection of Human Parasitic Pathogens*. Boca Raton: CRC Press; 2013, pp. 521–8.
12. Laing AB, Edeson JF, Wharton RH. Studies on filariasis in Malaya: The vertebrate hosts of *Brugia malayi* and *B. pahangi*. *Ann Trop Med Parasitol.* 1960;54:92–9.

13. Taylor MJ, Bandi C, Hoerauf A. *Wolbachia* bacterial endosymbionts of filarial nematodes. *Adv Parasitol.* 2005;60:245–84.
14. Hooper PJ, Bradley MH, Biswas G, Ottesen EA. The global programme to eliminate lymphatic filariasis: Health impact during its first 8 years (2000–2007). *Ann Trop Med Parasitol.* 2009;103(Suppl 1):S17–21.
15. Weil GJ, Curtis KC, Fakoli L, et al. Laboratory and field evaluation of a new rapid test for detecting *Wuchereria bancrofti* antigen in human blood. *Am J Trop Med Hyg.* 2013;89:11–5.
16. Michael E, Bundy DA. Global mapping of lymphatic filariasis. *Parasitol Today.* 1997;13:472–6.
17. World Health Organisation. Transmission assessment surveys in the global programme to eliminate lymphatic filariasis: WHO position statement. *Wkly Epidemiol Rec.* 2012;87:478–82.
18. Dreyer G, Medeiros Z, Netto MJ, Leal NC, de Castro LG, Piessens WF. Acute attacks in the extremities of persons living in an area endemic for bancroftian filariasis: Differentiation of two syndromes. *Trans R Soc Trop Med Hyg.* 1999;93:413–7.
19. Hoerauf A, Satoguina J, Saeftel M, Specht S. Immunomodulation by filarial nematodes. *Parasite Immunol.* 2005;27:417–29.
20. Joseph A, Mony P, Prasad M, John S, Srikanth, Mathai D. The efficacies of affected-limb care with penicillin diethylcarbamazine, the combination of both drugs or antibiotic ointment, in the prevention of acute adenolymphangitis during bancroftian filariasis. *Ann Trop Med Parasitol.* 2004;98:685–96.
21. Weller PF, Ottesen EA, Heck L, Tere T, Neva FA. Endemic filariasis on a Pacific island. I. Clinical, epidemiologic, and parasitologic aspects. *Am J Trop Med Hyg.* 1982;31:942–52.
22. Freedman DO, de Almeido Filho PJ, Besh S, et al. Abnormal lymphatic function in presymptomatic bancroftian filariasis. *J Infect Dis.* 1995;171:997–1001.
23. Dreyer G, Addiss D, Roberts J, Noroes J. Progression of lymphatic vessel dilatation in the presence of living adult Wuchereria bancrofti. *Trans R Soc Trop Med Hyg.* 2002;96:157–61.
24. Dreyer G, Ottesen EA, Galdino E, et al. Renal abnormalities in microfilaremic patients with bancroftian filariasis. *Am J Trop Med Hyg.* 1992;46:745–51.
25. Wartman WB. Filariasis in American armed forces in World War II. *Medicine (Baltimore).* 1947;26:333–94.
26. Dreyer G, Noroes J, Figueredo-Silva J, Piessens WF. Pathogenesis of lymphatic disease in bancroftian filariasis: A clinical perspective. *Parasitol Today.* 2000;16:544–8.
27. Turner LH. Studies on filariasis in Malaya; the clinical features of filariasis due to *Wuchereria malayi. Trans R Soc Trop Med Hyg.* 1959;53:154–69.
28. Boggild AK, Keystone JS, Kain KC. Tropical pulmonary eosinophilia: A case series in a setting of nonendemicity. *Clin Infect Dis.* 2004;39:1123–8.
29. Nookala S, Srinivasan S, Kaliraj P, Narayanan RB, Nutman TB. Impairment of tetanus-specific cellular and humoral responses following tetanus vaccination in human lymphatic filariasis. *Infect Immun.* 2004;72:2598–604.
30. Gopinath R, Ostrowski M, Justement SJ, Fauci AS, Nutman TB. Filarial infections increase susceptibility to human immunodeficiency virus infection in peripheral blood mononuclear cells in vitro. *J Infect Dis.* 2000;182:1804–8.
31. Kroidl I, Saathoff E, Maganga L, et al. Effect of *Wuchereria bancrofti* infection on HIV incidence in southwest Tanzania: A prospective cohort study. *Lancet.* 2016;388:1912–20.
32. El-Moamly AA, El-Sweify MA, Hafez MA. Using the AD12-ICT rapid-format test to detect *Wuchereria bancrofti* circulating antigens in comparison to Og4C3-ELISA and nucleopore membrane filtration and microscopy techniques. *Parasitol Res.* 2012;111:1379–83.
33. Weil GJ, Liftis F. Identification and partial characterization of a parasite antigen in sera from humans infected with *Wuchereria bancrofti. J Immunol.* 1987;138:3035–41.
34. Weil GJ, Lammie PJ, Weiss N. The ICT filariasis test: A rapid-format antigen test for diagnosis of bancroftian filariasis. *Parasitol Today.* 1997;13:401–4.
35. Lammie PJ, Hightower AW, Eberhard ML. Age-specific prevalence of antigenemia in a *Wuchereria bancrofti*-exposed population. *Am J Trop Med Hyg.* 1994;51:348–55.
36. Weil GJ, Sethumadhavan KV, Santhanam S, Jain DC, Ghosh TK. Persistence of parasite antigenemia following diethylcarbamazine therapy of bancroftian filariasis. *Am J Trop Med Hyg.* 1988;38:589–95.
37. Weil GJ, Ramzy RM, Chandrashekar R, Gad AM, Lowrie RCJr, Faris R. Parasite antigenemia without microfilaremia in bancroftian filariasis. *Am J Trop Med Hyg.* 1996;55:333–7.
38. Weil GJ, Kumar H, Santhanam S, Sethumadhavan KV, Jain DC. Detection of circulating parasite antigen in bancroftian filariasis by counterimmunoelectrophoresis. *Am J Trop Med Hyg.* 1986;35:565–70.
39. More SJ, Copeman DB. A highly specific and sensitive monoclonal antibody-based ELISA for the detection of circulating antigen in bancroftian filariasis. *Trop Med Parasitol.* 1990;41:403–6.
40. Njenga SM, Wamae CN. Evaluation of ICT filariasis card test using whole capillary blood: Comparison with Knott's concentration and counting chamber methods. *J Parasitol.* 2001;87:1140–3.
41. Chandrasena TG, Premaratna R, Abeyewickrema W, de Silva NR. Evaluation of the ICT whole-blood antigen card test to detect infection due to *Wuchereria bancrofti* in Sri Lanka. *Trans R Soc Trop Med Hyg.* 2002;96:60–3.
42. Pani SP, Hoti SL, Vanamail P, Das LK. Comparison of an immunochromatographic card test with night blood smear examination for detection of *Wuchereria bancrofti* microfilaria carriers. *Natl Med J India.* 2004;17:304–6.
43. Wanji S, Amvongo-Adjia N, Koudou B, et al. Cross-reactivity of filariais ICT cards in areas of contrasting endemicity of *Loa loa* and *Mansonella perstans* in Cameroon: Implications for shrinking of the lymphatic filariasis map in the Central African region. *PLoS Negl Trop Dis.* 2015;9:e0004184.
44. Pion SD, Montavon C, Chesnais CB, et al. Positivity of antigen tests used for diagnosis of lymphatic filariasis in individuals without *Wuchereria bancrofti* infection but with high Loa loa microfilaremia. *Am J Trop Med Hyg.* 2016;95:1417–23.
45. Chesnais CB, Awaca-Uvon NP, Bolay FK, et al. A multi-center field study of two point-of-care tests for circulating *Wuchereria bancrofti* antigenemia in Africa. *PLoS Negl Trop Dis.* 2017;11:e0005703.
46. Yahathugoda TC, Supali T, Rao RU, et al. A comparison of two tests for filarial antigenemia in areas in Sri Lanka and Indonesia with low-level persistence of lymphatic filariasis following mass drug administration. *Parasit Vectors.* 2015;8:369.
47. Rocha A, Braga C, Belem M, et al. Comparison of tests for the detection of circulating filarial antigen (Og4C3-ELISA and AD12-ICT) and ultrasound in diagnosis of lymphatic filariasis in individuals with microfilariae. *Mem Inst Oswaldo Cruz.* 2009;104:621–5.
48. McCarthy JS, Lustigman S, Yang GJ, et al. A research agenda for helminth diseases of humans: Diagnostics for control and elimination programmes. *PLoS Negl Trop Dis.* 2012;6:e1601.
49. Won KY, Sambou S, Barry A, et al. Use of antibody tools to provide serologic evidence of elimination of lymphatic filariasis in the Gambia. *Am J Trop Med Hyg.* 2018;98:15–20.
50. Kubofcik J, Fink DL, Nutman TB. Identification of Wb123 as an early and specific marker of *Wuchereria bancrofti* infection. *PLoS Negl Trop Dis.* 2012;6:e1930.
51. Steel C, Golden A, Kubofcik J, et al. Rapid *Wuchereria bancrofti*-specific antigen Wb123-based IgG4 immunoassays as tools for surveillance following mass drug administration programs on lymphatic filariasis. *Clin Vaccine Immunol.* 2013;20:1155–61.
52. Arnold BF, van der Laan MJ, Hubbard AE, et al. Measuring changes in transmission of neglected tropical diseases, malaria, and enteric pathogens from quantitative antibody levels. *PLoS Negl Trop Dis.* 2017;11:e0005616.
53. de Souza DK, Owusu IO, Otchere J, et al. An evaluation of Wb123 antibody ELISA in individuals treated with ivermectin and albendazole, and implementation challenges in Africa. *Pan Afr Med J.* 2017;27:65.
54. Weil GJ, Curtis KC, Fischer PU, et al. A multicenter evaluation of a new antibody test kit for lymphatic filariasis employing recombinant Brugia malayi antigen Bm-14. *Acta Trop.* 2011;120(Suppl 1):S19–22.
55. Rahmah N, Taniawati S, Shenoy RK, et al. Specificity and sensitivity of a rapid dipstick test (Brugia Rapid) in the detection of *Brugia malayi* infection. *Trans R Soc Trop Med Hyg.* 2001;95:601–4.
56. Takagi H, Itoh M, Kasai S, Yahathugoda TC, Weerasooriya MV, Kimura E. Development of loop-mediated isothermal amplification method for detecting *Wuchereria bancrofti* DNA in human blood and vector mosquitoes. *Parasitol Int.* 2011;60:493–7.
57. Alhassan A, Li Z, Poole CB, Carlow CK. Expanding the MDx toolbox for filarial diagnosis and surveillance. *Trends Parasitol.* 2015;31:391–400.
58. Faris R, Hussain O, El Setouhy M, Ramzy RM, Weil GJ. Bancroftian filariasis in Egypt: Visualization of adult worms and subclinical lymphatic pathology by scrotal ultrasound. *Am J Trop Med Hyg.* 1998;59:864–7.
59. Mand S, Debrah A, Batsa L, Adjei O, Hoerauf A. Reliable and frequent detection of adult *Wuchereria bancrofti* in Ghanaian women by ultrasonography. *Trop Med Int Health.* 2004;9:1111–4.

60. Taylor MJ, Makunde WH, McGarry HF, Turner JD, Mand S, Hoerauf A. Macrofilaricidal activity after doxycycline treatment of *Wuchereria bancrofti*: A double-blind, randomised placebo-controlled trial. *Lancet.* 2005;365:2116–21.
61. Turner JD, Mand S, Debrah AY, et al. A randomized, double-blind clinical trial of a 3-week course of doxycycline plus albendazole and ivermectin for the treatment of *Wuchereria bancrofti* infection. *Clin Infect Dis.* 2006;42:1081–9.
62. Noroes J, Dreyer G, Santos A, Mendes VG, Medeiros Z, Addiss D. Assessment of the efficacy of diethylcarbamazine on adult *Wuchereria bancrofti* in vivo. *Trans R Soc Trop Med Hyg.* 1997;91:78–81.
63. Dreyer G, Addiss D, Noroes J, Amaral F, Rocha A, Coutinho A. Ultrasonographic assessment of the adulticidal efficacy of repeat high-dose ivermectin in bancroftian filariasis. *Trop Med Int Health.* 1996;1:427–32.
64. Budge PJ, Herbert C, Andersen B, Weil GJ. Adverse events following single dose treatment of lymphatic filariasis: Observations from a review of the literature. *PLoS Negl Trop Dis.* 2018;12:e0006454.
65. Carme B, Boulesteix J, Boutes H, Puruehnce MF. Five cases of encephalitis during treatment of loiasis with diethylcarbamazine. *Am J Trop Med Hyg.* 1991;44:684–90.
66. Bird AC, el-Sheikh H, Anderson J, Fuglsang H. Changes in visual function and in the posterior segment of the eye during treatment of onchocerciasis with diethylcarbamazine citrate. *Br J Ophthalmol.* 1980;64:191–200.
67. Gardon J, Gardon-Wendel N, Demanga N, Kamgno J, Chippaux JP, Boussinesq M. Serious reactions after mass treatment of onchocerciasis with ivermectin in an area endemic for Loa loa infection. *Lancet.* 1997;350:18–22.
68. Andrade LD, Medeiros Z, Pires ML, et al. Comparative efficacy of three different diethylcarbamazine regimens in lymphatic filariasis. *Trans R Soc Trop Med Hyg.* 1995;89:319–21.
69. Ottesen EA, Nutman TB. Tropical pulmonary eosinophilia. *Annu Rev Med.* 1992;43:417–24.
70. Eberhard ML, Lammie PJ, Dickinson CM, Roberts JM. Evidence of nonsusceptibility to diethylcarbamazine in *Wuchereria bancrofti*. *J Infect Dis.* 1991;163:1157–60.
71. Schwab AE, Boakye DA, Kyelem D, Prichard RK. Detection of benzimidazole resistance-associated mutations in the filarial nematode *Wuchereria bancrofti* and evidence for selection by albendazole and ivermectin combination treatment. *Am J Trop Med Hyg.* 2005;73:234–8.
72. Ahorlu CK, Dunyo SK, Asamoah G, Simonsen PE. Consequences of hydrocele and the benefits of hydrocelectomy: A qualitative study in lymphatic filariasis endemic communities on the coast of Ghana. *Acta tropica.* 2001;80:215–21.
73. Ichimori K, King JD, Engels D, et al. Global programme to eliminate lymphatic filariasis: The processes underlying programme success. *PLoS Negl Trop Dis.* 2014;8:e3328.
74. Thomsen EK, Sanuku N, Baea M, et al. Efficacy, safety, and pharmacokinetics of coadministered diethylcarbamazine, albendazole, and ivermectin for treatment of bancroftian filariasis. *Clin Infect Dis.* 2016;62(3):334–41.
75. WHO/Department of Control of Neglected Tropical Diseases. Global programme to eliminate lymphatic filariasis: Progress report, 2016. *Wkly Epidemiol Rec.* 2017;92(40):594–607.
76. Tisch DJ, Michael E, Kazura JW. Mass chemotherapy options to control lymphatic filariasis: A systematic review. *Lancet Infect Dis.* 2005;5:514–23.
77. Pion SDS, Chesnais CB, Weil GJ, Fischer PU, Missamou F, Boussinesq M. Effect of 3 years of biannual mass drug administration with albendazole on lymphatic filariasis and soil-transmitted helminth infections: A community-based study in Republic of the Congo. *Lancet Infect Dis.* 2017;17:763–9.
78. World Health Organizaion. Provisional strategy for interrupting lymphatic filariasis transmission in loiasis-endemic countries. In: *Report of the Meeting on Lymphatic Flariasis, Malaria and Integrated Vector Management. WHO/HTM/NTD/PCT/2012.6.* Geneva: World Health Organizaion; 2012.
79. Stolk WA, Prada JM, Smith ME, et al. Are alternative strategies required to accelerate the global elimination of lymphatic filariasis? Insights from mathematical models. *Clin Infect Dis.* 2018;66:S260–6.
80. Arata AA. Difficulties facing vector control in the 1990s. *Am J Trop Med Hyg.* 1994;50:6–10.
81. Regis L, Oliveira CM, Silva-Filha MH, Silva SB, Maciel A, Furtado AF. Efficacy of *Bacillus sphaericus* in control of the filariasis vector *Culex quinquefasciatus* in an urban area of Olinda, Brazil. *Trans R Soc Trop Med Hyg.* 2000;94:488–92.
82. Scholte EJ, Knols BG, Samson RA, Takken W. Entomopathogenic fungi for mosquito control: A review. *J Insect Sci.* 2004;4:19.
83. Babu S, Nutman TB. Immunology of lymphatic filariasis. *Parasite Immunol.* 2014;36:338–46.
84. Babayan SA, Allen JE, Taylor DW. Future prospects and challenges of vaccines against filariasis. *Parasite Immunol.* 2012;34:243–53.
85. Williams SA, Laney SJ, Bierwert LA, et al. Development and standardization of a rapid, PCR-based method for the detection of *Wuchereria bancrofti* in mosquitoes, for xenomonitoring the human prevalence of bancroftian filariasis. *Ann Trop Med Parasitol.* 2002;96 Suppl 2:S41–6.
86. Gass K, Beau de Rochars MV, Boakye D, et al. A multicenter evaluation of diagnostic tools to define endpoints for programs to eliminate bancroftian filariasis. *PLoS Negl Trop Dis.* 2012;6:e1479.
87. Stillwaggon E, Sawers L, Rout J, Addiss D, Fox L. Economic costs and benefits of a community-based lymphedema management program for lymphatic filariasis in Odisha State, India. *Am J Trop Med Hyg.* 2016;95:877–84.
88. Kar SK, Dwibedi B, Das BK, Agrawala BK, Ramachandran CP, Horton J. Lymphatic pathology in asymptomatic and symptomatic children with *Wuchereria bancrofti* infection in children from Odisha, India and its reversal with DEC and albendazole treatment. *PLoS Negl Trop Dis.* 2017;11:e0005631.
89. World Health Organization. Progress report on the elimination of human onchocerciasis, 2017–2018. *Wkly Epidem Rec.* 2018;93:633–48.
90. World Health Organization. *Onchocerciasis—Fact Sheet.* Geneva: World Health Organization; 2018.
91. World Health Organization. *Onchocerciasis Key Facts.* Geneva: World Health Organization; 2018.
92. Pan American Health Organization. *Onchcocerciasis in the Americas for Public Health Workers Fact Sheet.* Washington, DC: Pan American Health Organization; 2017.
93. World Health Organization. Progress towards eliminating onchocerciasis in the WHO region of the Americas: Advances in mapping of Yanomami focus area. *Wkly Epidemiol Rec.* 2018;93:541–4.
94. Mahdy MAK, Abdul-Ghani R, Abdulrahman TAA, et al. Onchocerca volvulus infection in Tihama region—West of Yemen: Continuing transmission in ivermectin-targeted endemic foci and unveiled endemicity in districts with previously unknown status. *PLoS Negl Trop Dis.* 2018;12:e0006329.
95. Cheke RA. Factors affecting onchocerciasis transmission: Lessons for infection control. *Expert Rev Anti Infect Ther.* 2017;15:377–86.
96. Gustavsen K, Hopkins A, Sauerbrey M. Onchocerciasis in the Americas: From arrival to (near) elimination. *Parasit Vectors.* 2011;4:205.
97. Al-Kubati AS, Mackenzie CD, Boakye D, et al. Onchocerciasis in Yemen: Moving forward towards an elimination program. *Int Health.* 2018;10:i89–96.
98. Duke BO. The effects of drugs on *Onchocerca volvulus*. 1. Methods of assessment, population dynamics of the parasite and the effects of diethylcarbamazine. *Bull World Health Organ.* 1968;39:137–46.
99. Burnham G. Onchocerciasis. *Lancet.* 1998;351:1341–6.
100. Tamarozzi F, Halliday A, Gentil K, Hoerauf A, Pearlman E, Taylor MJ. Onchocerciasis: The role of Wolbachia bacterial endosymbionts in parasite biology, disease pathogenesis, and treatment. *Clin Microbiol Rev.* 2011;24:459–68.
101. Colebunders R, Hendy A, van Oijen M. Nodding syndrome in onchocerciasis endemic areas. *Trends Parasitol.* 2016;32:581–3.
102. Vlaminck J, Fischer PU, Weil GJ. Diagnostic tools for onchocerciasis elimination programs. *Trends Parasitol.* 2015;31:571–82.
103. Thiele EA, Cama VA, Lakwo T, et al. Detection of *Onchocerca volvulus* in skin snips by microscopy and real-time polymerase chain reaction: Implications for monitoring and evaluation activities. *Am J Trop Med Hyg.* 2016;94:906–11.
104. Fischer P, Bamuhiiga J, Buttner DW. Occurrence and diagnosis of *Mansonella streptocerca* in Uganda. *Acta tropica.* 1997;63:43–55.
105. World Health Organization. Guidelines for stopping mass drug administration and verifying elimination of human onchocerciasis: Criteria and procedures. Geneva: WHO/HTM/NTD/PCT/2016.1. http://apps.who.int/iris/bitstream…; 2016.
106. Dieye Y, Storey HL, Barrett KL, et al. Feasibility of utilizing the SD BIOLINE onchocerciasis IgG4 rapid test in onchocerciasis surveillance in Senegal. *PLoS Negl Trop Dis.* 2017;11:e0005884.
107. Unnasch TR, Golden A, Cama V, Cantey PT. Diagnostics for onchocerciasis in the era of elimination. *Int Health.* 2018;10:i20–6.

108. Hodgkin C, Molyneux DH, Abiose A, et al. The future of onchocerciasis control in Africa. *PLoS Negl Trop Dis.* 2007;1:e74.
109. Coffeng LE, Stolk WA, Zoure HG, et al. African programme for onchocerciasis control 1995–2015: Model-estimated health impact and cost. *PLoS Negl Trop Dis.* 2013;7:e2032.
110. World Health Organization. Progress report on the elimination of human onchocerciasis, 2015–2016. *Wkly Epidemiol Rec.* 2016;91:505–14.
111. World Health Organization. Progress towards eliminating onchocerciasis in the WHO region of the Americas: Elimination of transmission in the north-east focus of the Bolivarian Republic of Venezuela. *Wkly Epidemiol Rec.* 2017;92:617–23.
112. World Health Organization. *Map of the Estimated Prevalence of Eye Worm History in Africa.* Geneva: World Health Organization; 2018.
113. Zoure HG, Wanji S, Noma M, et al. The geographic distribution of Loa loa in Africa: Results of large-scale implementation of the Rapid Assessment Procedure for Loiasis (RAPLOA). *PLoS Negl Trop Dis.* 2011;5:e1210.
114. Metzger WG, Mordmuller B. *Loa loa*—Does it deserve to be neglected? *Lancet Infect Dis.* 2014;14:353–7.
115. Antinori S, Schifanella L, Million M, et al. Imported *Loa loa* filariasis: Three cases and a review of cases reported in non-endemic countries in the past 25 years. *Int J Infect Dis.* 2012;16:e649–62.
116. Pedram B, Pasquetto V, Drame PM, et al. A novel rapid test for detecting antibody responses to *Loa loa* infections. *PLoS Negl Trop Dis.* 2017;11:e0005741.
117. Boussinesq M. Loiasis. *Ann Trop Med Parasitol.* 2006;100:715–31.
118. Holmes D. Loa loa: Neglected neurology and nematodes. *Lancet Neurol.* 2013;12:631–2.
119. Kamgno J, Pion SD, Chesnais CB, et al. A test-and-not-treat strategy for onchocerciasis in *Loa loa*-endemic areas. *N Engl J Med.* 2017;377:2044–52.
120. Ta-Tang TH, Crainey JL, Post RJ, Luz SL, Rubio JM. Mansonellosis: Current perspectives. *Res Rep Trop Med.* 2018;9:9–24.
121. Crainey JL, Ribeiro da Silva TR, Luz SL. Historic accounts of *Mansonella* parasitaemias in the South Pacific and their relevance to lymphatic filariasis elimination efforts today. *Asian Pac J Trop Med.* 2016;9:205–10.
122. Simonsen PE, Onapa AW, Asio SM. Mansonella perstans filariasis in Africa. *Acta Trop.* 2011;120 Suppl 1:S109–20.
123. Downes BL, Jacobsen KH. A systematic review of the epidemiology of mansonelliasis. *Afr J Infect Dis.* 2010;4:7–14.
124. Gobbi F, Beltrame A, Buonfrate D, et al. Imported Infections with *Mansonella perstans* Nematodes, Italy. *Emerg Infect Dis.* 2017;23:1539–42.
125. Asio SM, Simonsen PE, Onapa AW. Analysis of the 24-h microfilarial periodicity of *Mansonella perstans. Parsaitol Res.* 2009;104:945–8.
126. Orihel TC, Eberhard ML. Zoonotic filariasis. *Clin Microbiol Rev.* 1998;11:366–81.
127. Holmes GK, Gelfand M, Boyt W, Mackenzie P. A study to investigate the pathogenicity of a parasite resembling *Acanthocheilonema perstans. Trans R Soc Trop Med Hyg.* 1969;63:479–84.
128. Lima NF, Veggiani Aybar CA, Dantur Juri MJ, Ferreira MU. *Mansonella ozzardi*: A neglected New World filarial nematode. *Pathog Glob Health.* 2016;110:97–107.
129. Medeiros JF, Fontes G, Nascimento VLD, et al. Sensitivity of diagnostic methods for *Mansonella ozzardi* microfilariae detection in the Brazilian Amazon region. *Mem Inst Oswaldo Cruz.* 2018;113:173–7.
130. Vianna LM, Martins M, Cohen MJ, Cohen JM, Belfort RJr. *Mansonella ozzardi* corneal lesions in the Amazon: A cross-sectional study. *BMJ Open.* 2012;2(6):e001266.
131. Cohen JM, Ribeiro JA, Martins M. Ocular manifestations in mansonelliasis. *Arq Bras Oftalmol.* 2008;71:167–71.
132. Gardiner CH, Meyers WM, Lanoie LO. Recovery of intact male and female *Dipetalonema streptocerca* from man. *Am J Trop Med Hyg.* 1979;28:49–52.
133. Bregani ER, Rovellini A, Mbaidoum N, Magnini MG. Comparison of different anthelminthic drug regimens against *Mansonella perstans* filariasis. *Trans R Soc Trop Med Hyg.* 2006;100:458–63.
134. de Almeida Basano S, de Souza Almeida Aranha Camargo J, Fontes G, et al. Phase III clinical trial to evaluate Ivermectin in the reduction of *Mansonella ozzardi* infection in the Brazilian Amazon. *Am J Trop Med Hyg.* 2018;98:786–90.
135. Tan LH, Fong MY, Mahmud R, Muslim A, Lau YL, Kamarulzaman A. Zoonotic *Brugia pahangi* filariasis in a suburbia of Kuala Lumpur City, Malaysia. *Parasitol Int.* 2011;60:111–3.
136. Orihel TC, Beaver PC. Zoonotic *Brugia* infections in North and South America. *Am J Trop Med Hyg.* 1989;40:638–47.
137. Cantey PT, Weeks J, Edwards M, et al. The emergence of zoonotic *Onchocerca lupi* infection in the United States—A case-series. *Clin Infect Dis.* 2016;62:778–83.
138. Koehsler M, Soleiman A, Aspock H, Auer H, Walochnik J. *Onchocerca jakutensis* filariasis in humans. *Emerg Infect Dis.* 2007;13:1749–52.

Studies of MDA efficacy often have not considered differential efficacy of drugs used based upon the species of hookworm being treated. A review of 68 studies showed that the efficacy of albendazole for *A. duodenale* infection was far higher than for *N. americanus* (91.8% cure rate vs. 75.0% cure rate). This review also showed that while cure rates did not differ with age in *A. duodenale* infections, they were markedly lower in children (67.0%) than adults (80.9%) for *N. americanus*.[89] Single-dose mebendazole (600 mg) has shown lower efficacy than albendazole (400 mg) for *N. americanus* infection in one study, with cure rates of 11% versus 64%. In contrast, another study showed good efficacy, with cure rates of 68% for 600 mg of mebendazole.[90] Although mebendazole is ovicidal and larvicidal, albendazole kills both preintestinal and intestinal worms, but it is not known whether it affects arrested larvae of *A. duodenale*.[50] Pyrantel pamoate, oxantel pamoate, and ivermectin have also been used to treat hookworm infection.[37,91]

Concerns about the potential emergence of resistance to standard anthelmintic drugs in the hookworms are increasing, with resistance in analogous veterinary helminths having been observed for some time. This concern has been magnified by the detection of low egg reduction rates in some infections following treatment,[90] as well as diminished efficacy with repeated rounds of treatment,[92] though it is unclear if these observations reflect true drug resistance or poor drug quality. Mutant alleles in the beta-tubulin gene associated with resistance in veterinary helminths were detected in 10% of pooled adult *N. americanus* samples from Haiti and 36% of pooled samples from Pemba Island, Tanzania.[93] No further data are available on the prevalence of beta-tubulin gene mutation markers of resistance in hookworms where MDA is conducted, though some studies are underway. Some researchers have suggested that combination drug therapy may be warranted,[91] both to reduce the probability of resistance emerging and to improve cure rates.

At present no effective vaccines are available, but given the variable efficacies of anthelminthic drugs and the possibility of emerging drug resistance, a human hookworm vaccine is under development, showing cost effectiveness compared to periodic deworming.[94] A first-generation recombinant hookworm vaccine is completing phase 1 clinical trials.[95]

Hookworm infection remains a significant cause of morbidity and economic loss in many parts of the world. Recent improvements in diagnostic methodologies and greater awareness of the significance of STH disease has led to a greater interest in this problem from public health, nongovernmental, and aid agencies globally. The primary approaches taken in control efforts are education, MDA, and WASH. A vaccine is under development at the time of writing.[96] This may lead to another option for hookworm control, given current concerns about the potential for the development of anthelmintic resistance in the context of MDA, as seen in analogous veterinary helminth infections. Ultimately, the optimum pathway to the elimination of hookworm as a public health problem will be improvements in socioeconomic conditions of affected societies, leading to broadly higher levels of education, more ubiquitous use of footwear and improved sanitation and hygiene.

Disclaimer

The findings and conclusions in this book chapter are those of the author and do not necessarily represent the official position of the Centers for Disease Control and Prevention/the Agency for Toxic Substances and Disease Registry.

References

1. Bethony J, Brooker S, Albonico M, et al. Soil-transmitted helminth infections: Ascariasis, trichuriasis, and hookworm. *Lancet*. 2006;367(9521):1521–32.
2. GBD 2016 Disease and Injury Incidence and Prevalence Collaborators. Global, regional, and national incidence, prevalence, and years lived with disability for 328 diseases and injuries for 195 countries, 1990–2016: A systematic analysis for the Global Burden of Disease Study 2016. *Lancet*. 2017;390(10100):1211–59.
3. Jourdan PM, Lamberton PHL, Fenwick A, Addiss DG. Soil-transmitted helminth infections. *Lancet*. 2018;391(10117):252–65.
4. Hotez PJ, Brooker S, Bethony JM, Bottazzi ME, Loukas A, Xiao S. Hookworm infection. *N Engl J Med*. 2004;351(8):799–807.
5. Muller R. *Worms and Human Disease*. 2nd ed. Wallingford: CABI Publishing; 2002.
6. Bartsch SM, Hotez PJ, Asti L, et al. The global economic and health burden of human hookworm infection. *PLoS Negl Trop Dis*. 2016;10(9):e0004922.
7. World Health Organization. Intestinal worms—Strategy. 2018.
8. Traub RJ. *Ancylostoma ceylanicum*, a re-emerging but neglected parasitic zoonosis. *Int J Parasitol*. 2013;43(12–13):1009–15.
9. Bradbury RS, Hii SF, Harrington H, Speare R, Traub R. *Ancylostoma ceylanicum* hookworm in the Solomon Islands. *Emerg Infect Dis*. 2017;23(2):252–7.
10. Anten JF, Zuidema PJ. Hookworm infection in Dutch servicemen returning from West New Guinea. *Trop Geogr Med*. 1964;16:216–24.
11. Hoagland KE, Schad GA. *Necator americanus* and *Ancylostoma duodenale*: Life history parameters and epidemiological implications of two sympatric hookworms of humans. *Exp Parasitol*. 1978;44(1):36–49.
12. Goldsmid JM. The African hookworm problem: An overview. In: Macpherson CNL, Craig PS, eds. *Parasitic Helminths and Zoonoses in Africa*. London: Allen & Unwin; 1991:101–37.
13. Hotez P. Neglected diseases amid wealth in the United States and Europe. *Health Aff (Millwood)*. 2009;28(6):1720–5.
14. Koehler AV, Bradbury RS, Stevens MA, Haydon SR, Jex AR, Gasser RB. Genetic characterization of selected parasites from people with histories of gastrointestinal disorders using a mutation scanning-coupled approach. *Electrophoresis*. 2013;34(12):1720–8.
15. Bundy DAP, Keymer AE. The epidemiology of hookworm infection. In: Gilles HM, Ball PAJ, eds. *Hookworm Infections*. Amsterdam: Elsevier; 1991:147–78.
16. Beaver PC, Jung RC, Cupp EW. *Clinical Parasitology*. 9th ed. Philadelphia: Lea & Febiger; 1984.
17. Bradbury RS, Traub RJ. Hookworm in Oceania. In: Loukas A, ed. *Neglected Tropical Diseases—Oceania*. Cham: Springer; 2016:33–68.
18. Meurs L, Polderman AM, Vinkeles Melchers NV, et al. Diagnosing polyparasitism in a high-prevalence setting in Beira, Mozambique: Detection of intestinal parasites in fecal samples by microscopy and real-time PCR. *PLoS Negl Trop Dis*. 2017;11(1):e0005310.
19. Darling ST, Barber MA, Hacker HP. Hookworm and malaria research in Malay, Java and the Fiji islands. *Report of Uncinariasis Commission to the Orient, 1915–1917*. New York: Rockefeller Foundation; 1920:47–64.
20. Lambert SM. Medical conditions in the South Pacific. *Med J Aust*. 1928;2(12):362–78.
21. Stoll NR. *Necator americanus* and *Ancylostoma duodenale* in Guam, Leyte and Okinawa, with a note on hookworm egg sizes. *J Parasitol*. 1946;32(5):490–6.
22. Schad GA, Anderson RM. Predisposition to hookworm infection in humans. *Science*. 1985;228(4707):1537–40.
23. Gualdieri L, Rinaldi L, Petrullo L, et al. Intestinal parasites in immigrants in the city of Naples (southern Italy). *Acta Trop*. 2011;117(3):196–201.
24. Garg PK, Perry S, Dorn M, Hardcastle L, Parsonnet J. Risk of intestinal helminth and protozoan infection in a refugee population. *Am J Trop Med Hyg*. 2005;73(2):386–91.
25. Davies J, Majumdar SS, Forbes RT, Smith P, Currie BJ, Baird RW. Hookworm in the Northern Territory: Down but not out. *Med J Aust*. 2013;198(5):278–81.
26. Starr MC, Montgomery SP. Soil-transmitted Helminthiasis in the United States: A systematic review—1940–2010. *Am J Trop Med Hyg*. 2011;85(4):680–4.
27. McKenna ML, McAtee S, Bryan PE, et al. Human intestinal parasite burden and poor sanitation in rural Alabama. *Am J Trop Med Hyg*. 2017;97(5):1623–8.
28. McIntyre MG. *Notice: Environmental Study in Lowndes County, Alabama, Fails to Prove Hookworm Infection*. Montgomery, AL: Alabama Department of Public Health; 2018.
29. Bradbury RS, Arguello I, Lane M, et al. Parasitic Infection Surveillance in Mississippi Delta Children. *Am J Trop Med Hyg*. 2020;103(3):1150-3.
30. Cappello M, Clyne LP, McPhedran P, Hotez PJ. *Ancylostoma* factor Xa inhibitor: Partial purification and its identification as a major hookworm-derived anticoagulant in vitro. *J Infect Dis*. 1993;167(6):1474–7.

CHAPTER 125

31. Ranjit N, Zhan B, Hamilton B, et al. Proteolytic degradation of hemoglobin in the intestine of the human hookworm *Necator americanus*. *J Infect Dis*. 2009;199(6):904–12.
32. Schad GA. The parasite. In: Gilles HM, Ball PAJ, eds. *Hookworm Infections*. Amsterdam: Elsevier; 1991:15–49.
33. Albonico M, Stoltzfus RJ, Savioli L, et al. Epidemiological evidence for a differential effect of hookworm species, *Ancylostoma duodenale* or *Necator americanus*, on iron status of children. *Int J Epidemiol*. 1998;27(3):530–7.
34. Maguire JH. Intestinal nematodes (Roundworms). In: Mandell GL, Bennett JE, Dolin R, eds. *Mandell, Douglas and Bennett's Principles and Practice of Infectious Diseases*. 7th ed. Philadelphia: Churchill Livingstone; 2010:3577–353586.
35. Komiya Y, Yasuraoka K. The biology of hookworms. In: Morishita K, ed. *Progress of Medical Parasitology in Japan*. Tokyo: Meguro Parasitological Museum; 1966:5–114.
36. Schad GA. Hypobiosis and related phenomena in hookworm infection. In: Schad GA, Warren KS, eds. *Hookworm Disease: Current Status and New Directions*. London: Taylor & Francis; 1990:71–88.
37. Stoltzfus RJ, Dreyfuss ML, Chwaya HM, Albonico M. Hookworm control as a strategy to prevent iron deficiency. *Nutr Rev*. 1997;55(6):223-32.
38. Yu SH, Jiang ZX, Xu LQ. Infantile hookworm disease in China. A review. *Acta Trop*. 1995;59(4):265–70.
39. Stone WM, Girardeau M. Transmammary passage of *Ancylostoma caninum* larvae in dogs. *J Parasitol*. 1968;54(3):426–9.
40. Arasu P, Kwak D. Developmental arrest and pregnancy-induced transmammary transmission of *Ancylostoma caninum* larvae in the murine model. *J Parasitol*. 1999;85(5):779–84.
41. Nwosu AB. Human neonatal infections with hookworms in an endemic area of Southern Nigeria. A possible transmammary route. *Trop Geogr Med*. 1981;33(2):105–11.
42. Wang MP, Hu YF, Peng JM, Wu DL, Yao SY. Persistent migration of *Ancylostoma duodenale* larvae in human infection. *Chin Med J (Engl)*. 1984;97(2):147–9.
43. Schad GA, Chowdhury AB, Dean CG, et al. Arrested development in human hookworm infections: An adaptation to a seasonally unfavorable external environment. *Science*. 1973;180(4085):502–4.
44. Schad GA, Murrell KD, Fayer R, et al. Paratenesis in *Ancylostoma duodenale* suggests possible meat-borne human infection. *Trans R Soc Trop Med Hyg*. 1984;78(2):203–4.
45. Carroll SM, Grove DI. Experimental infection of humans with *Ancylostoma ceylanicum*: Clinical, parasitological, haematological and immunological findings. *Trop Geogr Med*. 1986;38(1):38–45.
46. Areekul S, Saenghirun C, Ukoskit K. Studies on the pathogenicity of *Ancylostoma ceylanicum*. I. Blood loss in experimental dogs. *Southeast Asian J Trop Med Public Health*. 1975;6(2):235–40.
47. Speare R, Bradbury RS, Croese J. A case of *Ancylostoma ceylanicum* infection occurring in an Australian soldier returned from Solomon Islands. *Korean J Parasitol*. 2016;54(4):533–6.
48. Kaya D, Yoshikawa M, Nakatani T, et al. *Ancylostoma ceylanicum* hookworm infection in Japanese traveler who presented chronic diarrhea after return from Lao People's Democratic Republic. *Parasitol Int*. 2016;65(6 Pt A):737–40.
49. Yoshikawa M, Ouji Y, Hirai N, et al. *Ancylostoma ceylanicum*, novel etiological agent for traveler's diarrhea-report of four Japanese patients who returned from Southeast Asia and Papua New Guinea. *Trop Med Health*. 2018;46:6.
50. Schad GA, Banwell JG.Hookworms. In: Warren KS, Mahmoud AAF, eds. *Tropical and Geographical Medicine*. New York: McGraw-Hill; 1990:379-393.
51. Koshy A, Raina V, Sharma MP, Mithal S, Tandon BN. An unusual outbreak of hookworm disease in North India. *Am J Trop Med Hyg*. 1978;27(1 Pt 1):42–5.
52. Harada Y. Wakana disease & hookworm allergy. *Yonago Acta Medica*. 1962;6(2):109–18.
53. World Health Organization. *Helminth Control in School-Aged Children: A Guide for Managers of Control Programmes*. 2nd ed. Geneva: World Health Organization; 2011.
54. Crompton DWT, McKean PG, Schad GA. Hookworm disease: Current status and new directions. *Parasitol Today*. 1989;5:1–2.
55. Lunn PG, Northrop-Clewes CA. The impact of gastrointestinal parasites on protein-energy malnutrition in man. *Proc Nutr Soc*. 1993;52(1):101–11.
56. Christian P, Khatry SK, West KP Jr. Antenatal anthelmintic treatment, birthweight, and infant survival in rural Nepal. *Lancet*. 2004;364(9438):981–3.
57. Gyorkos TW, Maheu-Giroux M, Casapia M, Joseph SA, Creed-Kanashiro H. Stunting and helminth infection in early preschool-age children in a resource-poor community in the Amazon lowlands of Peru. *Trans R Soc Trop Med Hyg*. 2011;105(4):204–8.
58. Aderoba AK, Iribhogbe OI, Olagbuji BN, Olokor OE, Ojide CK, Ande AB. Prevalence of helminth infestation during pregnancy and its association with maternal anemia and low birth weight. *Int J Gynaecol Obstet*. 2015;129(3):199–202.
59. Stoll NR. On endemic hookworm, where do we stand today? *Exp Parasitol*. 1962;12:241–52.
60. Maxwell C, Hussain R, Nutman TB, et al. The clinical and immunologic responses of normal human volunteers to low dose hookworm (*Necator americanus*) infection. *Am J Trop Med Hyg*. 1987;37(1):126–34.
61. Truant AL, Elliott SH, Kelly MT, Smith JH. Comparison of formalin-ethyl ether sedimentation, formalin-ethyl acetate sedimentation, and zinc sulfate flotation techniques for detection of intestinal parasites. *J Clin Microbiol*. 1981;13(5):882–4.
62. Inpankaew T, Schar F, Khieu V, et al. Simple fecal flotation is a superior alternative to guadruple Kato Katz smear examination for the detection of hookworm eggs in human stool. *PLoS Negl Trop Dis*. 2014;8(12):e3313.
63. Utzinger J, Rinaldi L, Lohourignon LK, et al. FLOTAC: A new sensitive technique for the diagnosis of hookworm infections in humans. *Trans R Soc Trop Med Hyg*. 2008;102(1):84–90.
64. Barda BD, Rinaldi L, Ianniello D, et al. Mini-FLOTAC, an innovative direct diagnostic technique for intestinal parasitic infections: Experience from the field. *PLoS Negl Trop Dis*. 2013;7(8):e2344.
65. Bradbury RS, Herwaldt B. Section VIII:C – Parasitic agents. In: Meecham P, Wilson D, eds. *Biosafety in Microbiological and Biomedical Laboratories*. Washington D.C.: U.S. Department of Health and Human Services; 2020:223-238.
66. Glinz D, Silue KD, Knopp S, et al. Comparing diagnostic accuracy of Kato-Katz, Koga agar plate, ether-concentration, and FLOTAC for *Schistosoma mansoni* and soil-transmitted helminths. *PLoS Negl Trop Dis*. 2010;4(7):e754.
67. Pilotte N, Papaiakovou M, Grant JR, et al. Improved PCR-based detection of soil transmitted helminth infections using a next-generation sequencing approach to assay design. *PLoS Negl Trop Dis*. 2016;10(3):e0004578.
68. Papaiakovou M, Pilotte N, Grant JR, et al. A novel, species-specific, real-time PCR assay for the detection of the emerging zoonotic parasite *Ancylostoma ceylanicum* in human stool. *PLoS Negl Trop Dis*. 2017;11(7):e0005734.
69. Wang JX, Pan CS, Cui LW. Application of a real-time PCR method for detecting and monitoring hookworm *Necator americanus* infections in Southern China. *Asian Pac J Trop Biomed*. 2012;2(12):925–9.
70. Croese J, Loukas A, Opdebeeck J, Fairley S, Prociv P. Human enteric infection with canine hookworms. *Ann Intern Med*. 1994;120(5):369–74.
71. Hotez P. Hookworm and poverty. *Ann N Y Acad Sci*. 2008;1136:38–44.
72. Miller A. Dung beetles (Coleoptera, Scarabaeidae) and other insects in relation to human feces in a hookworm area of southern Georgia. *Am J Trop Med Hyg*. 1954;3(2):372–89.
73. Sulaiman S, Sohadi AR, Yunus H, Iberahim R. The role of some cyclorrhaphan flies as carriers of human helminths in Malaysia. *Med Vet Entomol*. 1988;2(1):1–6.
74. Dipeolu OO. Laboratory investigations into the role of *Musca vicina* and *Musca domestica* in the transmission of parasitic helminth eggs and larvae. *Int J Zoonoses*. 1982;9(1):57–61.
75. Williams-Blangero S, Blangero J, Bradley M. Quantitative genetic analysis of susceptibility to hookworm infection in a population from rural Zimbabwe. *Hum Biol*. 1997;69(2):201–8.
76. Breitling LP, Wilson AJ, Raiko A, et al. Heritability of human hookworm infection in Papua New Guinea. *Parasitology*. 2008;135(12):1407–15.
77. Hominick WM, Dean CG, Schad GA. Population biology of hookworms in West Bengal: Analysis of numbers of infective larvae recovered from damp pads applied to the soil surface at defaecation sites. *Trans R Soc Trop Med Hyg*. 1987;81(6):978–86.
78. Liang S, Yang C, Zhong B, Qiu D. Re-emerging schistosomiasis in hilly and mountainous areas of Sichuan, China. *Bull World Health Organ*. 2006;84(2):139–44.
79. Hotez P. *Blue Marble Health: An Innovative Plan to Fight Diseases of the Poor Amid Wealth*. Baltimore: John Hopkins University Press; 2016.
80. Strunz EC, Addiss DG, Stocks ME, Ogden S, Utzinger J, Freeman MC. Water, sanitation, hygiene, and soil-transmitted helminth infection: A systematic review and meta-analysis. *PLoS Med*. 2014;11(3):e1001620.
81. Harrington H, Bradbury R, Taeka J, et al. Prevalence of soil-transmitted helminths in remote villages in East Kwaio, Solomon Islands. *Western Pac Surveill Response J*. 2015;6(3):51–8.

82. Clarke NE, Clements ACA, Amaral S, et al. (S)WASH-D for Worms: A pilot study investigating the differential impact of school- versus community-based integrated control programs for soil-transmitted helminths. *PLoS Negl Trop Dis*. 2018;12(5):e0006389.

83. Asaolu SO, Ofoezie IE. The role of health education and sanitation in the control of helminth infections. *Acta Trop*. 2003;86(2–3):283–94.

84. World Health Organization. *Reaching Girls and Women of Reproductive Age with Deworming. Report of the Advisory Group on Deworming in Girls and Women of Reproductive Age*. Rockefeller Foundation Bellagio Center, Bellagio, Italy 28–30 June 2017. Geneva: World Health Organization; 2018.

85. Anderson R, Truscott J, Hollingsworth TD. The coverage and frequency of mass drug administration required to eliminate persistent transmission of soil-transmitted helminths. *Philos Trans R Soc Lond B Biol Sci*. 2014;369(1645):20130435.

86. Keiser J, Utzinger J. Efficacy of current drugs against soil-transmitted helminth infections: Systematic review and meta-analysis. *JAMA*. 2008;299(16):1937–48.

87. Vaz Nery S, Qi J, Llewellyn S, et al. Use of quantitative PCR to assess the efficacy of albendazole against *Necator americanus* and *Ascaris* spp. in Manufahi District, Timor-Leste. *Parasit Vectors*. 2018;11(1):373.

88. Soukhathammavong PA, Sayasone S, Phongluxa K, et al. Low efficacy of single-dose albendazole and mebendazole against hookworm and effect on concomitant helminth infection in Lao PDR. *PLoS Negl Trop Dis*. 2012;6(1):e1417.

89. Steinmann P, Utzinger J, Du ZW, et al. Efficacy of single-dose and triple-dose albendazole and mebendazole against soil-transmitted helminths and Taenia spp.: A randomized controlled trial. *PLoS One*. 2011;6(9):e25003.

90. Horton J. Albendazole: A review of anthelmintic efficacy and safety in humans. *Parasitology*. 2000;121(Suppl):S113–32.

91. Georgiev VS. Necatoriasis: Treatment and developmental therapeutics. *Expert Opin Investig Drugs*. 2000;9(5):1065–78.

92. Clarke NE, Doi SAR, Wangdi K, Chen Y, Clements ACA, Nery SV. Efficacy of anthelminthic drugs and drug combinations against soil-transmitted helminths: A systematic review and network meta-analysis. *Clin Infect Dis*. 2018;68(1):96–105.

93. Albonico M, Bickle Q, Ramsan M, Montresor A, Savioli L, Taylor M. Efficacy of mebendazole and levamisole alone or in combination against intestinal nematode infections after repeated targeted mebendazole treatment in Zanzibar. *Bull World Health Organ*. 2003;81(5):343–52.

94. Diawara A, Schwenkenbecher JM, Kaplan RM, Prichard RK. Molecular and biological diagnostic tests for monitoring benzimidazole resistance in human soil-transmitted helminths. *Am J Trop Med Hyg*. 2013;88(6):1052–61.

95. Bartsch SM, Hotez PJ, Hertenstein DL, et al. Modeling the economic and epidemiologic impact of hookworm vaccine and mass drug administration (MDA) in Brazil, a high transmission setting. *Vaccine*. 2016;34(19):2197–206.

96. Diemert DJ, Freire J, Valente V, et al. Safety and immunogenicity of the Na-GST-1 hookworm vaccine in Brazilian and American adults. *PLoS Negl Trop Dis*. 2017;11(5):e0005574.

CHAPTER

126

Intestinal Nematode Infections*

Richard S. Bradbury • Sarah G. H. Sapp • Mary Kamb • Peter J. Hotez

Intestinal nematodes (roundworms) infect up to one-fourth of the world's population, primarily affecting people living in warm, moist climates in communities where poverty and poor sanitation favor transmission. Most helminths do not multiply in the human host (*Strongyloides stercoralis* and *Capillaria philippinensis* being notable exceptions), and thus overall worm burden reflects the extent of environmental exposure. Low-intensity infections are typically asymptomatic, while moderate or heavy intensity infections can be highly symptomatic. Heavy worm burdens may cause chronic (and sometimes severe) illness, impaired school or work performance, stunted growth in children, and a variety of unusual manifestations.[1] Through their tendency for autoinfection, *S. stercoralis* and *C. philippinensis* have the potential to cause life-threatening hyperinfections in susceptible individuals.

The intestinal nematodes vary greatly in size, life cycle, and disease manifestations. In this chapter, we review the most common intestinal nematodes, excluding the hookworms, which are discussed in the previous chapter of this textbook.

STRONGYLOIDES STERCORALIS

S. stercoralis (threadworm) occurs primarily in tropical, subtropical, and warm temperate climates where sanitation conditions are poor.[2–4] Official World Health Organization (WHO) figures estimate that between 30 and 100 million people are infected worldwide, though recognizing that prevalence data from endemic countries are sparse.[5] This estimate originally dates from 1989,[6] and since that time improvements in the sensitivity of diagnostic methods has led many experts to accept a revised prevalence figure, based on more recent and accurate studies, of approximately 370 million affected people worldwide.[2] In immunocompetent individuals, strongyloidiasis is often asymptomatic or only minimally symptomatic; however, its potential for autoinfection allows for unusually chronic infections and potential for severe hyperinfection and disseminated disease in immuncompromised hosts.[7]

The Parasite

The complex life cycle of *S. stercoralis* is distinctive amongst the intestinal nematodes (Fig. 126-1). The adult worm, a parthenogenetic female, lives within the mucosal epithelium of the human small intestine where it deposits eggs (usually fewer than 50 per day). There, the eggs hatch into noninfective rhabditiform larvae, migrate into the small intestinal lumen, and are excreted along with human feces into the soil (Fig. 126-2a). In soil the larvae develop into free-living, infective filariform larvae (direct cycle) or a free-living adult form. This single generation of free-living male and female adults reproduces sexually in the soil, amplifying the intensity of infective forms in the environment. The second generation of larvae all develops into filariform larvae and cannot differentiate further into free-living adults, ending the life cycle unless a new host is found. The larvae of this sexually reproducing stage mature into a filariform stage (indirect cycle). Human infection occurs through skin penetration or (less commonly) ingestion, and the filariform larvae then typically pass through the venous circulation to reach the lungs. Once in the lungs, the filariform larvae penetrate capillary walls, enter the alveoli, and ascend the trachea to the epiglottis where they are coughed up and swallowed. The larvae eventually burrow into the mucosa of the upper part of the small intestine where they develop into adult worms and eventually lay their eggs. Experiments in dogs have shown that some filariform larvae bypass the lungs and migrate through other host organs directly to the intestine.[7]

In the autoinfection cycle, rhabditiform larvae mature into infective filariform larvae within the human gut and then reinvade the host through the intestinal mucosa or perianal skin. This allows the infection to continue, and the parasites to multiply, without any additional exposure to soil-borne filariform larvae. Autoinfection accounts for the extremely long-lived infections that are observed in strongyloidiasis, as well as possible development of hyperinfection and disseminated strongyloidiasis in immunocompromised hosts.

Epidemiology

Strongyloidiasis is an infection of worldwide importance, particularly in settings with limited access to modern sanitation. It is endemic in almost all tropical and subtropical climates, and pockets exist in impoverished areas in some temperate climates such as Eastern and Southern Europe, Northern and Central Australia, and the Appalachian and South Eastern regions of the United States. In North America, *S. stercoralis* has been classically associated with uniformed service veterans returning from Southeast Asia or the South Pacific, but today occurs primarily in immigrants, travelers, or institutionalized populations at risk due to fecal-oral transmission or geophagia (eating dirt). Recent studies have demonstrated the existence of at least two genetic haplotypes of *S. stercoralis*, one that appears only to infect dogs and another that can infect dogs, humans and other primates.[8,9] These findings confirm strongyloidiasis as a potential canine zoonosis, which has public health implications for controlling the disease. In cats, experimental infections with *S. stercoralis* have been successful but the host competence of cats is not well understood. Natural feline infections with *Strongyloides* sp. have also occurred, but it is unknown whether these infections represent human-infecting *S. stercoralis* or a veterinary species (e.g., *S. felis*, *S. planiceps*, *S. tumefaciens*).[10]

Infection occurs through contact with soil that is contaminated with *Strongyloides* larvae, typically through walking barefoot, contact with human waste or sewage or occupational exposure (e.g., farming, coal mining). People who acquire *S. stercoralis* in endemic areas can

* The findings and conclusions in this book chapter are those of the author and do not necessarily represent the official position of the Centers for Disease Control and Prevention/the Agency for Toxic Substances and Disease Registry.

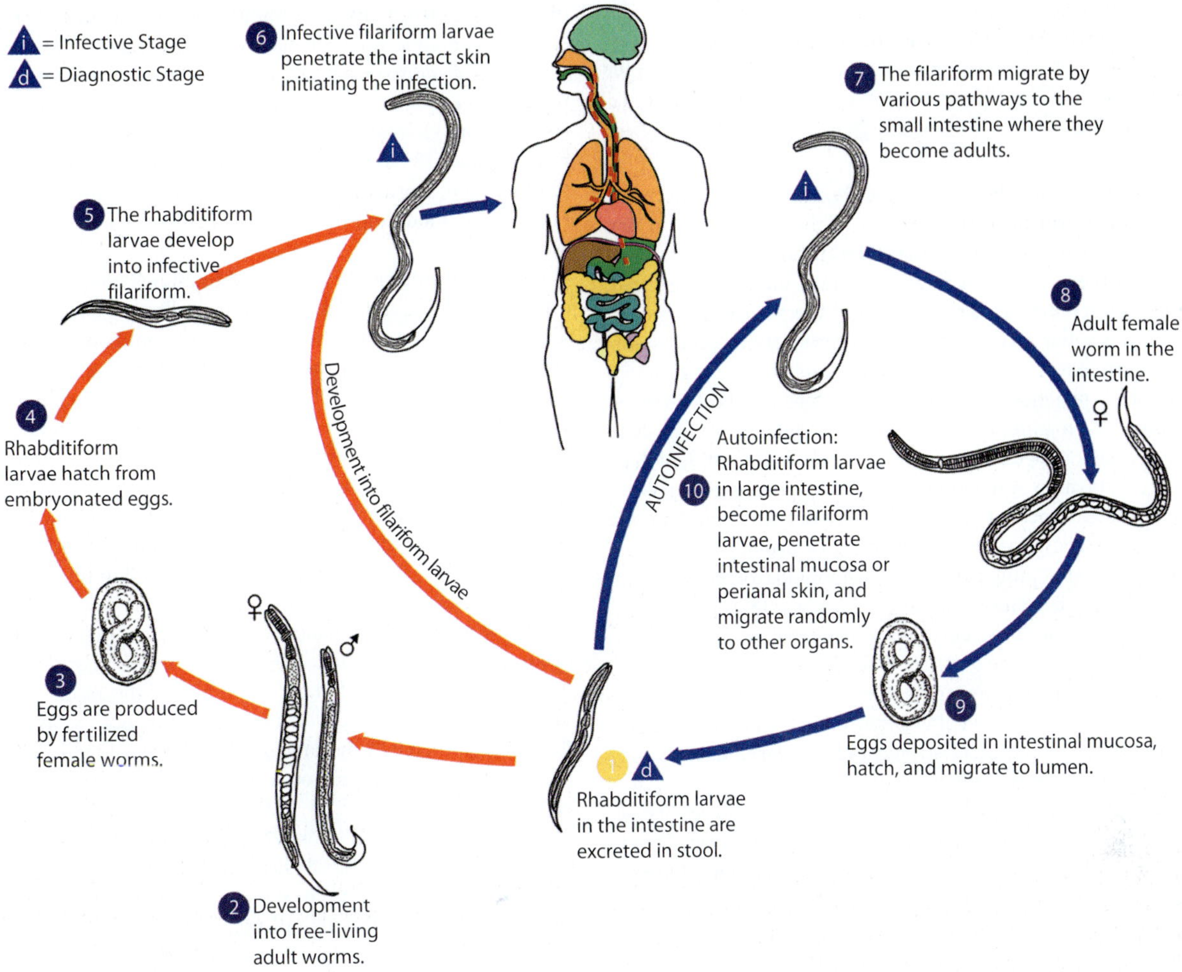

i = Infective Stage
d = Diagnostic Stage

6 Infective filariform larvae penetrate the intact skin initiating the infection.

7 The filariform migrate by various pathways to the small intestine where they become adults.

5 The rhabditiform larvae develop into infective filariform.

8 Adult female worm in the intestine.

4 Rhabditiform larvae hatch from embryonated eggs.

Development into filariform larvae

AUTOINFECTION

10 Autoinfection: Rhabditiform larvae in large intestine, become filariform larvae, penetrate intestinal mucosa or perianal skin, and migrate randomly to other organs.

3 Eggs are produced by fertilized female worms.

9 Eggs deposited in intestinal mucosa, hatch, and migrate to lumen.

1 Rhabditiform larvae in the intestine are excreted in stool.

2 Development into free-living adult worms.

FIGURE 126-1. The complex life cycle of *S. stercoralis* showing both the autoinfective (7–10), direct environmental (1 and 6), and indirect free-living environmental (1–6) pathways to infection. Note that the free-living adults (2) only exist for one generation, after which a new host must be found to continue the life cycle. (*Source:* From CDC DPDx website.)

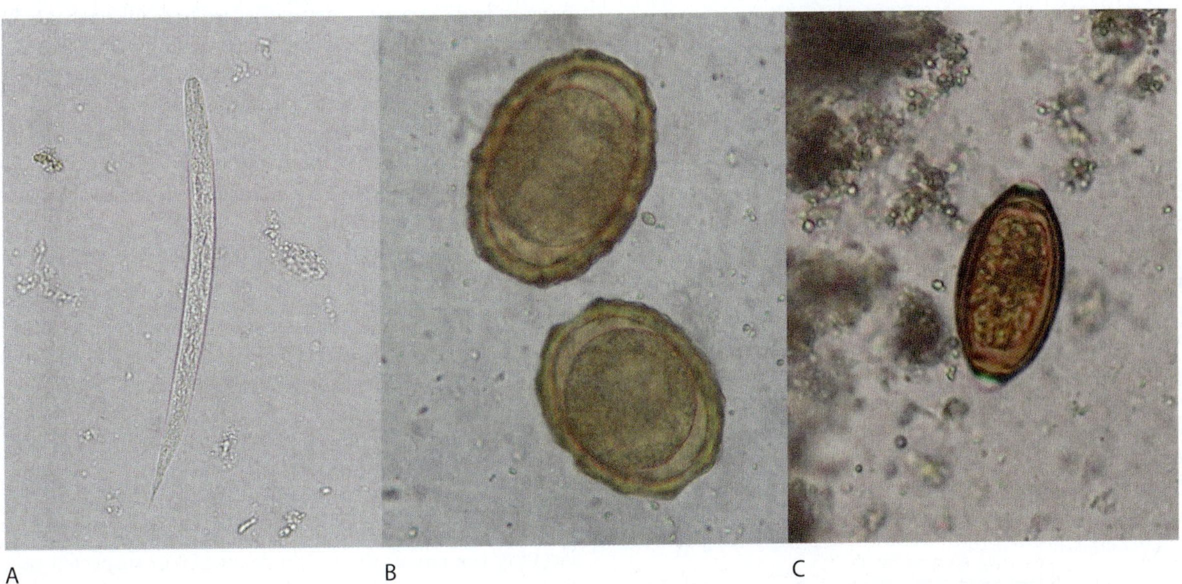

FIGURE 126-2. Stages passed in feces of some important intestinal nematodes; (left to right) L1 (rhabditiform) larva of *Strongyloide stercoralis*; corticated and fertile eggs of *Ascaris lumbricoides*; egg of *Trichuris trichiura*. (Dr. Richard S. Bradbury.)

harbor the parasite with few (if any) symptoms for decades through autoinfection. The lifelong nature of untreated disease in many patients accounts for the observation increased sdprevalence with advancing age. In settings with modern sanitation where transmission has been interrupted, older adults may still retain infection; and infections have been reported in individuals up to 60 years after their last possible exposure.[11] In addition to contact with soil or autoinfection, rare cases of person-to-person transmission of *Strongyloides* have been observed with organ transplantation or within institutions for the developmentally disabled, long-term-care facilities and day-care centers. Transmammary transmission has been observed, and *S. stercoralis* infective larvae have been recovered from breast milk of both infected humans[12] and dogs.[13]

Infection and Disease

The initial entry of the filariform larvae through the skin may produce a transient pruritus similar to that of the hookworms. A dry cough and wheezing, similar to that seen in hookworm infection, may occur as the larval forms migrate through the respiratory tree. Pulmonary symptoms are usually mild and short lived in immunocompetent hosts, but may be severe in hyperinfection and disseminated strongyloidiasis associated with immunocompromised status.

Established infection in an immunocompetent host may be asymptomatic or manifested by intermittent vague symptoms such as epigastric pain, indigestion, nausea, anorexia, or intermittent diarrhea and constipation. Uncommonly, infected people may develop more severe signs such as fecal occult blood, colonic and gastric hemorrhage, or ileus. Up to three quarters of people with chronic *Strongyloides* have a mild peripheral eosinophilia or elevated IgE levels, which may be transient findings. People with ongoing autoinfection may develop "larva currens," an urticarial, serpiginous rash that typically occurs on the buttocks or abdomen. This rapidly moving eruption (up to 5–10 cm/hr) is due to autoinfecting filariform larva migrating under the skin after penetrating the perianal surface. Considered pathognomonic of strongyloidiasis, larva currens may last days, and may resolve only to recur after months or even years. Severe strongyloidiasis may resemble inflammatory bowel disease and lead to the (disastrous) initiation of immunosuppressive therapy and subsequent hyperinfection. Children with heavy worm burdens may develop malabsorption and growth retardation.

Hyperinfection and disseminated strongyloidiasis occur when autoinfection is amplified by the presence of immunosuppressive drugs (e.g., corticosteroid therapy, chemotherapeutic agents) or chronic illnesses causing immunosuppression, such as renal failure, certain hematologic malignancies, human T-lymphocyte virus (HTLV) 1, chronic pulmonary disease or autoimmune diseases (often treated with steroids), alcoholism, tuberculosis, or malnutrition.[14] Transplant recipients are at particular risk for life-threatening infections. However, remarkably, HIV infection does not appear to confer increased risk for acquiring *Strongyloides* or having a more severe clinical course. Although cases of hyperinfection in apparently immunocompetent individuals are reported, they are rare. Hyperinfection is due to a massive parasite load as *S. stercoralis* larvae aberrantly migrate within the host. While in chronic strongyloidiasis the larvae are limited to the gastrointestinal and pulmonary systems, in disseminated disease the larvae can invade other organs including the brain and meningeal spaces, liver, heart, and other tissues. Bacteremia may occur if the larvae penetrate the gastrointestinal mucosa and carry gut flora into the bloodstream. Hyperinfection in immunosuppressed patients may manifest as an unexplained, severe gastrointestinal or pulmonary process, or a recurrent Gram-negative bacteremia or meningitis. Eosinophilia, is often absent in these seriously ill patients. Overall mortality in hyperinfection syndrome can approach 90% even with appropriate therapy.[14]

Diagnosis

There is no gold standard test for the diagnosis of *S. stercoralis* infection. Diagnosis based on direct microscopy rests on identifying the larval forms; however, eggs hatch before exiting the gut and thus are usually not found in the stool. Because of the low rate of egg production in chronic and low-grade infections, examination of a single stool specimen has low (21–56%) sensitivity.[15,16] Direct smear examination of three or more fresh stools for the presence of rhabditiform larvae greatly improves detection, although this is still a poor method for diagnosing strongyloidiasis. Specialized coprologic techniques have much higher sensitivity than traditional microscopy. The formalin-ethyl acetate concentration method removes larvae, resulting in a sensitivity of approximately 48–52% for one stool.[15,16] Baermann sedimentation has superior sensitivity (72%), Harada-Mori larval culture is slightly more sensitive (85%) while Koga agar plate culture is the most sensitive (89%) phenotypic detection method.[17] For any phenotypic method, sensitivity increases when multiple stools are analyzed. Flotation methods and Kato Katz are ineffective for the diagnosis of *Strongyloides*.

Serology using an enzyme-linked immunosorbent assay (ELISA) can be a practical initial diagnostic test, allowing diagnosis without the need to collect stool. In addition, since antibody titers decrease and may serorevert after therapy, serology can be useful in evaluating treatment efficacy. Serologic testing may also be helpful to screen patients from endemic areas prior to initiating immunosuppressive therapy or who are known to have HTLV-1 infection, certain leukemias, or lymphomas, or are being considered for organ transplantation.[18] However, in immunocompromised individuals, serology results can be falsely negative. Cross-reaction with other parasitic infections may also occur in ELISA formats and immunofluorescent antibody tests (IFATs), with a recent comprehensive study demonstrating cross reaction to another nematode or trematode infection occurring in approximately 10% of cases, on average.[19] Sensitivities of available serologic tests vary depending on the antigen employed. The comprehensive study of available serological assays included the two commercially available ELISA kits and found the In Vitro Diagnostics ELISA kit to have a sensitivity of 91.2% and specificity of 99.1%, while the Bordier ELISA had a sensitivity of 89.5% and specificity of 98.3%.[19] IFAT was found to have a sensitivity of 93.9% and specificity of 92.2%.[19] *S. stercoralis* recombinant antigens such as NIE and SSiR show promise for improved specificity of serological analyses, but at the time of this writing were not yet available in commercial test formats. The most commonly used *Strongyloides* 18s rRNA gene PCR[20] has a sensitivity ranging between 61% and 94% and a specificity between 86% and 96%, when performed on DNA extracted from feces versus agar plate culture.[21–25] The fact that PCR can be performed on appropriately preserved (e.g., ethanol, potassium dichromate, commercial fixatives for use with PCR and microscopy, but not formalin, which cross-links DNA) stool samples, whereas culture requires fresh unpreserved stool, adds to the utility of the PCR as a diagnostic test. Other tests may be helpful in the diagnosis of *Strongyloides* in specific circumstances: for example, duodenal aspirate or biopsy may reveal parasites or eosinophilic infiltration, and a wet-mount of fluid from a bronchoalveolar lavage may identify larvae in cases of hyperinfection.

Therapy

For anyone diagnosed with strongyloidiasis, even if asymptomatic, the goal of therapy is eradication of the parasite. Not treating or simply reducing worm burden is inadequate as autoinfection can allow worm burden to increase again, leaving infected individuals at risk for subsequent hyperinfection. In acute and chronic strongyloidiasis, Ivermectin (200 μg/kg orally in a single dose for 1–2 days) is the drug of first choice because it is generally well tolerated and is highly effective (>90%) even in chronic intestinal infections[18]. Ivermectin is contraindicated in children weighing less than 15 kg, pregnant or lactating women, or those with confirmed or suspected coinfection with *Loa loa*. Albendazole, 400 mg orally twice daily for 7 days is an alternative treatment that is effective and generally well tolerated except in those with hypersensitivity to benzimidazole compounds. Albendazole is recommended to be avoided in the first trimester of pregnancy.[18] In people with persistent symptoms who have a positive stool examination for *Strongyloides*, follow-up stool examinations at 2–4 weeks after treatment can confirm clearance of infection, with retreatment indicated if larvae are observed. For patients with hyperinfection syndrome (disseminated strongyloidiasis), data are limited and there is no agreed upon optimal treatment regimen. CDC guidelines recommend ivermectin, 200 mg/kg orally per day until stool or sputum exams or both are negative for two weeks (one autoinfection cycle).[18] Some patients unable to tolerate oral therapy (e.g., due to ileus, obstruction or malabsorption) have been successfully treated with rectal administration of the drug. Regardless of the anthelmintic agent used, discontinuing or reducing any immunosuppressive therapy, if possible, is an important first step.[18]

Prevention and Control

The sanitary disposal of human and dog feces is essential for the control of strongyloidiasis in endemic areas. Community control of infection in dogs is also important to prevent spread of the disease. Wearing appropriate footwear is a valuable adjunct to prevention, but may be impractical in warmer climates. Hyperinfection syndromes can be prevented by identifying and treating people with strongyloidiasis promptly. Serologic screening in patients at risk for hyperinfection (e.g., those taking or about to take steroids or other immunosuppressive therapies, patients with HTLV-1 or certain malignancies, or individuals who are going to donate or receive organ transplants) or for residents of endemic areas can identify some chronic infections and allow institution of treatment to prevent disseminated strongyloidiasis.

ASCARIS LUMBRICOIDES

Ascaris lumbricoides (intestinal roundworm) is the largest intestinal nematode infecting humans and the most common soil-transmitted helminth (STH). It is estimated to affect more than 800 million people worldwide, with most infections occurring in children under 15 years old living in sub-Saharan Africa, Southeast Asia and Latin America. The fecundity of the female ascarid and the prolonged egg survival in the soil are factors supporting *A. lumbricoides* to be among humankind's most prevalent infections. Transmission occurs primarily through ingestion of contaminated food or water. Two major haplotypes have been identified, one most commonly found in humans and one commonly found in pigs. Historically, the ascarid of pigs was referred to as *Ascaris suum*, although in recent years the status of this as a separate, valid species is questionable.[26]

The Parasite

Adult worms are 120–400 mm long and able to live within the lumen of the small intestine. Mature females produce approximately 200,000 unembryonated eggs daily (Fig. 126-2b). These eggs have a rough, mammillated coat and are discharged into the intestinal lumen and passed with the feces. Eggs of *Ascaris* are environmentally resistant and, once deposited in soil, not infectious until they embryonate, which takes 2–4 weeks. Once embryonated, *Ascaris* eggs remain viable for years despite extremes of temperature and moisture or remarkably adverse environments, including chemical methods of water purification and formalin.[27] After ingestion via contaminated soil, foods, water, or hands, the eggs hatch into larvae within the small intestine. The larvae penetrate the intestinal mucosa, invade the portal veins, and migrate through the liver and then via the bloodstream to the lungs. Once in the lung, the larvae infiltrate into the alveoli, are coughed up, swallowed, and return to the lumen of the small intestine where they develop into the adult worms (Fig. 126-3). Most worms reside in the

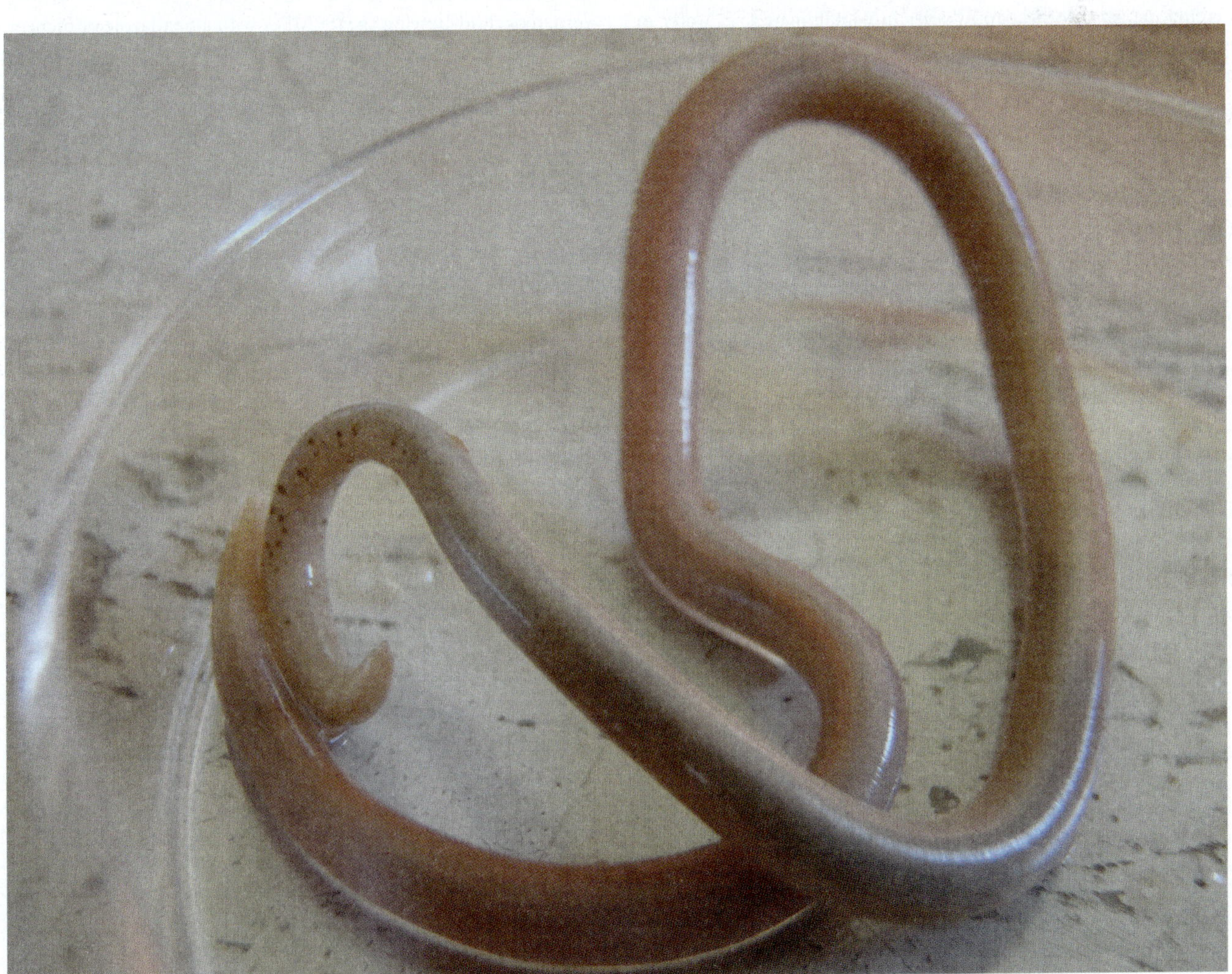

FIGURE 126-3. Adult *Ascaris lumbricoides* passed per rectum by a heavily infected patient. (Dr. Richard S. Bradbury.)

small intestine; however, they occasionally migrate to other parts of the gastrointenstinal tract or ectopic sites. Worms have a lifespan of 10 months to 2 years, after which they are defecated in the stool. As adult worms do not multiply within the human host, worm burden is dependent on intensity of an individual's exposure to infectious eggs.

Epidemiology

Ascariasis is most common in agrarian countries with inadequate human waste facilities. Infections tend to cluster in families, and are most common among young children 2–10 years old. Prevalence is particularly high in rural areas practicing subsistence agriculture, especially when human feces (night soil) is used as fertilizer. Despite association of *A. lumbricoides* infection with warmer climates, high rates of human-to-human transmission of ascariasis may occur in temperate climates where crowding, poor sanitation and inadequate waste disposal are found.[4] Rarely, individual cases and small outbreaks can occur in developed countries with good sanitation, usually associated with close contact with infected pigs.[28] Although these pig *Ascaris* were once considered to be a separate species (*Ascaris suum*), modern phylogenetic analysis has demonstrated their synonymy with *A. lumbricoides*.[26,29,30]

Although the usual mode of transmission is fecal-soil-oral via pica or contaminated hands[31], other routes including consumption of contaminated water, vegetables or fruit that have not been carefully washed (particularly those grown on fields fertilized with human waste, "night soil") and inhalation of airborne eggs in contaminated dust may also produce infection.[32] *Ascaris* eggs are covered in a sticky outer membrane[33] and some authors have suggested that infection may also be acquired from ingestion of eggs on fomites or hands after washing utensils, clothes, and bodies in contaminated sea water or using such water to season food in regions where populations use latrines that empty directly into the sea.[34,35]

Infection and Disease

Most infections with *A. lumbricoides* are asymptomatic. Clinical disease occurs mainly in heavily infected individuals, especially children. During the larval migration through the lungs in primary infection, a transient pneumonitis with eosinophilia (Loeffler's syndrome), which is more severe than the pulmonary phase of *Strongyloides* and hookworms, may be observed. Gastrointestinal symptoms of ascariasis are often mild and vague, but wandering ascarids occasionally cause severe pancreatic or hepatobiliary disease by physically blocking these organs. Peripheral eosinophilia is typically absent during asymptomatic or early symptomatic infection, but may be observed with persistent symptoms, especially pulmonary symptoms. Children with heavy infections often present with a "pot belly" and may develop bowel obstruction.[36] The role of sustained heavy *Ascaris* burdens in childhood malnutrition and developmental delays is difficult to firmly establish but probably is a contributing factor.

Diagnosis

The diagnosis of ascariasis is made by microscopy through identifying the large number of eggs in a single stool specimen. The formalin-ethyl acetate concentration technique has only a 44% sensitivity for the detection of *A. lumbricoides* eggs. Kato Katz provides a better sensitivity of 69% on a single stool test, but unfertilized eggs may dissolve if the Kato Katz preparation is not examined within an hour of preparation.[34] FLOTAC on fresh stool has a sensitivity of 72% and presents the most sensitive phenotypic method for the detection of *A. lumbricoides* infection.[37] PCR has also been applied and shows greater sensitivity than microscopy alone. Pulmonary ascariasis is occasionally diagnosed by identifying the larvae in sputum or gastric aspirates. Since pulmonary involvement and respiratory symptoms occur early, within weeks of egg ingestion, stool examination is not useful in diagnosing ascariasis at that time. However, in prolonged infections of longer than 1–2 years, adult worms may be found in the stools or emerging from the mouth or nose.

Treatment

Anthelminthic drugs can reduce the morbidity associated with intestinal ascariasis, but may not prevent reinfection. The primary drugs of choice are the benzimidazoles; mebendazole (100 mg orally twice daily for 3 days or 500 mg orally once), or albendazole (400 mg orally once on an empty stomach), which have high efficacy and relatively few side effects.[38] Although the safety of these drugs in children is not entirely described, both agents have been used in mass drug administration (MDA) campaigns in children as young as 1 or 2 years of age.[38] Limited data exist on use of either drug during pregnancy; however, WHO recommendations support the use of both drugs during the second and third trimesters of pregnancy when treatment is warranted. Other experts recommend pyrantel pamoate (11 mg/kg up to a maximum of 1 gram once) for pregnant women. Ivermectin (150–200 μg/kg once) is also an effective alternative.[38] Management of pulmonary ascariasis consists primarily of supportive care, since the efficacy of anthelminthic drugs against pulmonary larvae remains uncertain.

Prevention and Control

Proper human and pig waste disposal is essential to control ascariasis. In endemic areas, preventive strategies include avoiding exposure and ingestion of human or pig feces; washing hands with soap and water before handling food and after touching or handling pigs; washing, peeling, or cooking raw vegetables and fruits before eating; and teaching children how to wash their hands effectively.[39] *Ascaris* eggs are extremely hardy and difficult to remove from the environment.[27] The WHO has targeted STH, including ascariasis, for eradication as a public health problem by 2020. Programs designed toward reaching this goal target school aged and pre-school aged children as well as women of child-bearing age for MDA with albendazole or mebendazole, combined with community-wide education and improvements in water, sanitation and hygiene (WASH). More complete details of the WHO program for the control of STH infection are given in chapter of this textbook dealing with hookworm infections.

TRICHURIS TRICHIURA

Trichuriasis (whipworm) is an extremely common STH infection, affecting an estimated 800 million persons worldwide.[40] In endemic communities, more than 90% of residents may be infected, although most will have relatively low worm burden. Many people with trichuriasis are coinfected with other STH such as *Ascaris* or hookworm, which share a similar geographic and socioeconomic distribution. Like *Ascaris*, most infections are asymptomatic, but severe disease can occur with massive worm burdens.

The Parasite

Adult *T. trichiura* are approximately 30–50 mm long and live for years in the upper, large intestine of a human host. The posterior section of the adult worm appears thick and tapers to a long threadlike anterior structure, resembling a bull whip (hence the name whipworm). The tail of the adult male worm is coiled while the tail of the female worm is straight. Unusually among the intestinal nematodes, *T. trichiura* resides in the mucosa of the cecum or colon rather than the small intestine. The females are oviparous, producing 2000–10,000 eggs each day, which pass into the environment in feces (Fig. 126-2c). Once in the soil, the eggs mature over the next 2–4 weeks developing into infective first-stage larvae. Under conducive conditions, *Trichuris* spp. eggs may survive and remain viable in the soil for 6 years or more.[41] Once introduced into a human host through ingestion of fecally contaminated material, the first-stage larvae hatch in the small intestine and migrate to the colonic or cecal mucosa where they develop into mature worms. The life span of adult worms is 1–3 years. There is no tissue phase in the whipworm life cycle.

Epidemiology

Trichuris has a cosmopolitan geographic distribution but is more common in warm, moist regions where sanitation facilities are lacking.

Although individuals of all ages can acquire infection, children living in endemic areas are especially susceptible because behaviors that put them at risk for contact with feces. Transmission is primarily due to poor sanitation and in foci of high poverty and poor living standards where open defecation occurs.[4] The use of night soil facilitates the transmission of *T. trichiura* and the other STH. Human infections with zoonotic *Trichuris* species, such as *Trichuris vulpis* from dogs, may occasionally occur in upper-income countries with efficient sanitation.[42] Rates of *T. vulpis* infection in children of up to 11%, as determined by PCR, have been reported from some villages, suggesting that dog to human transmission may be more common than previously identified, with such infections previously identified morphologically as *T. trichiura*.[43,44]

Infection and Disease

Most *T. trichiura* infections are asymptomatic, but abdominal pain, anorexia, and diarrhea can occur. Heavy infections can produce the *Trichuris* dysentery syndrome in which whipworm infiltrates the entire lower bowel from the cecum to the rectum. The syndrome is characterized by frequent painful defecation of stools that may contain water, mucus, and blood. Symptoms may be so severe as to resemble inflammatory bowel disease and may result in anemia or rectal prolapse.[36] As with other geohelminths, younger children are most often heavily infected with *Trichuris*, and may suffer growth retardation and delayed cognitive development. *Trichuris* is usually not associated with eosinophilia.

Diagnosis

Diagnosis is made by identifying the relatively small (50–54 × 22–30 μm), but morphologically distinct, eggs in feces. The eggs have a thick, clear shell with distinctive bipolar plugs. Kato Katz (sensitivity 20%, increasing to 31% if three stools are examined) and formalin-ethyl acetate concentration (sensitivity 51%) will both improve the yield of microscopy for *T. trichiura* eggs. The most sensitive method for the detection of *T. trichiura* appears to be FLOTAC with flotation solution FS4, having a sensitivity of 78% when used on a single, fresh, stool.[37] PCR has been employed, but the eggs are difficult to break open for DNA extraction and thus special techniques involving bead beating of stool prior to DNA extraction and PCR are indicated for improving sensitivity. More than 10,000 eggs/g of stool indicate heavy infection. The diagnosis of trichuriasis is occasionally made endoscopically through direct visualization of adult worms in the colon.

Treatment

A 3-day course of mebendazole (500 mg orally once daily for 3 days, or 100 mg orally twice daily for 3 days) is the optimal therapy for treatment of trichuriasis.[45] Albendazole (400 mg orally, on an empty stomach, once daily for three days) is considered second-line treatment due to its slightly lower efficacy; however, it may be preferred in hookworm coinfections. Longer treatment regimens may be warranted for patients with heavy burden of infection (i.e., >1000 *Trichuris* eggs/g feces). Based on results of a meta-analysis of results from treatment trials, single-dose therapy had relatively low efficacy against trichuriasis, with cure rates of 42% for mebendazole and 31% for albendazole.[46] Ivermectin has some activity against *Trichuris*, but is not as effective as mebendazole or albendazole. Combining a single dose of albendazole and ivermectin was shown to be more effective than either drug alone as a single dose, making this the best choice for mass treatment campaigns.[47] Pyrantel pamoate has lower efficacy against trichuriasis than the benzimidazoles. Limited data exist on the efficacy of nitazoxanide in treating trichuriasis.

Prevention and Control

As with most STH, the primary mode of prevention is to provide the proper disposal of human feces and to avoid ingestion of soil-contaminated material through careful hand washing and food preparation (i.e., carefully washing or peeling vegetables and fruits contaminated with soil before eating). Teaching children good personal hygiene, including how to adequately wash their hands, is important in preventing infection. Reinfection following antihelminthic therapy is common in endemic areas, thus adopting these preventive behaviors is important in interrupting transmission. *T. trichiura* is targeted under the WHO goal to eliminate STH as a public health problem by 2020 through MDA, WASH, and education. Further details are available in the hookworm infection chapter of this textbook.

ENTEROBIUS VERMICULARIS

Enterobius (human pinworm) is one of the most common parasitic intestinal infections of humans, occurring in both temperate and tropical climates. The worldwide prevalence is difficult to estimate, as the infection is often asymptomatic and diagnosis is difficult. Recent prevalence studies in children from nonindustrialized or middle-income countries have found between 5% and 47% prevalence.[48–50] No recent studies of prevalence in industrialized nations have been performed; however, the Centers for Disease Control and Prevention (CDC) estimates there are 40 million infected persons in the United States alone.[51] Pinworm infection rarely results in serious illness, but frequently produces considerable morbidity and anxiety among school-age children and their parents.

The Parasite

Adult pinworms are small (females, 8–13 mm long with a long pointed tail; males, 2–3 mm in length with a blunt tail) and live in the ileum, cecum, colon, and appendix. Typical infections involve a few to several hundred adult worms. *E. vermicularis* has a relatively simple life cycle: The gravid adult female migrates out of the anus at night to lay thousands of eggs in the perianal region. The eggs are elongate, flattened on one side, with a thick clear shell. They are partially embryonated when laid and become infective within 4–6 hours at body temperature. Affected persons, typically children, scratch the area and the sticky eggs become lodged under the fingernails or on hands. Infection occurs when the eggs are ingested by eating food touched by contaminated hands, biting contaminated nails or otherwise transferring the eggs to the mouth. The eggs hatch in the small intestine to produce larvae, and pass into the colon where they molt twice as they mature into adult worms. The lifespan of the adult worm is 2–3 months.[51]

Epidemiology

Enterobiasis occurs worldwide, affecting all socioeconomic classes. It is considered to be the most common nematode infection in the United States and North Western Europe, usually involving school-aged children.[52] Amongst parents, mothers have been found to be twice as likely as fathers to be infected,[53] probably due to the traditional role as primary caregivers to children. Ingesting infective eggs via contaminated fingers, fomites (e.g., bed linens, clothes, curtains, carpets), or direct oral-anal sexual contact can lead to infection. The condition may spread rapidly within families, day-care facilities, institutions, or other crowded situations.

Infection and Disease

Most infections are asymptomatic. Pruritus or dysesthesia of the perianal and perineal areas ("pruritus ani") occurs most commonly at night, caused by an inflammatory reaction to the presence of adult worms and eggs. Severe excoriation can result in difficulty sleeping and secondary bacterial infections. Vulvovaginitis and urinary tract infection due to migration of adult worms are sometimes reported in prepubescent girls. Rarely, adult worms may traverse the fallopian tubes or move across breaks in the gut mucosa to gain access to the peritoneum and form granulomas.[52] The role of *E. vermicularis* in the etiology of appendicitis is controversial, but adult worms have been found in the appendiceal lumen in between 0.2% and 42% of cases of acute appendicitis in some pediatric populations.[54] The pinworm larval forms have been implicated in case reports as a rare cause of eosinophilic colitis resembling the trichuriasis dysentery syndrome.[55] Enterobiasis is not associated with anemia, and in most cases peripheral eosinophilia is not present.

Diagnosis

Enterobiasis diagnosis can be made by applying adhesive tape (the "cellotape test") or clear plastic paddle coated with an adhesive surface on one side (the "pinworm paddle test") to the perianal region and microscopically examining the tape or an adhesive-exposed glass slide for *E. vermicularis* eggs or adults. For the highest diagnostic sensitivity, material should be collected in the early morning prior to bathing or defecation. Examination may need to be repeated several times before infection can be conclusively excluded, but three specimens are adequate in most cases. Standard microscopic stool examination has limited sensitivity and is positive in only 5–15% of confirmed cases.[52] The highly motile adult worms are sometimes visualized as an incidental finding on colonoscopy.

Treatment

Single doses of albendazole (400 mg orally once on an empty stomach), mebendazole (100 mg orally once), or pyrantel pamoate (11 mg/kg, maximum 1 g, orally once) are all highly effective and widely used. A second dose 14 days after initial therapy is recommended because a single dose of medication does not reliably kill pinworm eggs. Reinfection, whether through self-infection or infection from close contacts, is a major problem in *E. vermicularis* therapy. In households were more than one family member is infected or where repeated infection occurs, some experts recommend that all household members be treated at the same time. When pinworm infections occur among residents in institutionalized settings, mass and simultaneous treatment may be effective. A U.S. study of infection among institutionalized children with developmental delays found mass deworming with two 100 mg doses of oral mebendazole, given 14 days apart resulted in a reduction of prevalence from 21% to 1% within 3 years.[50] A study in Korea found that mass deworming with 100 mg doses of oral albendazole, given 15 days apart reduced infection within the group to near zero at 3 and 6 months.

Prevention and Control

Enterobiasis can be prevented through proper personal hygiene practices including washing hands with soap and warm water after defecation or changing diapers and before eating or preparing foods; teaching children careful handwashing practices is also important. Other preventive measures include discouraging bare perianal scratching, changing undergarments and bedding regularly, and providing sanitary human waste disposal. Reinfection is common, and can be prevented by careful hand washing, morning showering to remove eggs (avoid cobathing with others), keeping fingernails cut short and avoiding nail biting. Washing of bed sheets, pajamas, and underwear in hot water, followed by drying in a hot tumble drier may kill any eggs remaining on these items. Treatment of cellotape positive children followed by education of parents about the epidemiology and control of enterobiasis resulted in a two-third reduction in cases after 6 months, which was less effective than blanket group treatment of children in the same school.[56]

CAPILLARIA (=PARACAPILLARIA) PHILIPPINENSIS

Intestinal capillariasis represents a severe helminthic disease acquired by the ingestion of freshwater fish containing infective larvae of *C. philippinensis*. Unlike the more common intestinal nematodes infecting humans, intestinal capillariasis almost always results in severe infection, and without treatment can lead to death. The sylvatic cycle and ecology of *C. philippinensis* is not fully understood.

The Parasites

C. philippinensis is commonly believed to exist in a fish-bird life cycle; however, it has almost never been detected in wild birds, so this assumption must be questioned.[57] Thus, the environmental reservoir host is unclear, although several species of birds, primates, and gerbils have been successfully infected in experimental trials.[58,59] Human infection occurs with ingestion of infected freshwater fish who have fed on eggs passed by the reservoir host into the environment. Larval forms of *C. philippinensis* develop within the fish, which are then consumed by a definitive host to complete the cycle. Humans become infected by ingesting raw fish or crustaceans infected with the larval forms; the eggs are not infectious to humans. Following raw fish ingestion, the adult worms develop and reside in the proximal small bowel. As with strongyloidiasis, eggs can hatch into infective larvae within the human gut and can produce autoinfection, leading to extremely high parasite burdens and severe illness.[57]

Epidemiology

C. philippinensis was originally described in 1964, and recognized as a serious pathogen following a 1967 epidemic in the northern Philippines, in which an estimated 1000 cases and 77 deaths occurred.[57] Since that time, most cases of *C. philippinensis* infections have been reported from the Philippines and Thailand. More recently, cases have been confirmed from Japan, Iran, Taiwan, Egypt, Indonesia, Korea, and India.[60–64] These importations were most likely anthropogenic and not via migration of a hypothetical avian definitive host.

Infection and Disease

Infection with *C. philippinensis* usually (if not always) leads to a severe illness characterized by abdominal pain, nausea, vomiting, borborygmi, and voluminous diarrhea. Severe chronic infection is characterized by protein-losing enteropathy leading to malabsorption, electrolyte abnormalities, wasting, cardiac disturbances, and eventual death. The mortality of untreated infection has been estimated at 10–30%. Asymptomatic infection appears uncommon.[57]

Diagnosis

The diagnosis of intestinal capillariasis in humans is usually based on the identification of thick-shelled, striated, bipolar *C. philippinensis* eggs in the feces. The eggs (35–45 μm long by 20 μm wide) somewhat resemble those of the closely related *Trichuris*. In chronic cases of *C. philippinensis*, larvae and adult worms may be seen in stool specimens. Examination of small bowel aspirates or biopsies may occasionally be helpful in making the diagnosis when stool examinations are negative. Serologic tests (indirect fluorescent antibody and ELISA) have been developed but are not widely available.

Treatment

Treatment of intestinal capillariasis includes albendazole (400 mg on an empty stomach once daily for a minimum of 10 days, often given for 30 days) or mebendazole (200 mg twice daily for 20–30 days). The previously used 30-day course of thiabendazole is too toxic for routine therapy. Shorter courses of treatment lead to an unacceptably high relapse rate and should be avoided.[65]

Prevention and Control

As with other intestinal nematodes, human capillariasis can be prevented with proper hygiene and careful disposal of contaminated fecal matter to prevent maintenance and transmission of the parasite in the environment. Latrines and water systems should be out of reach of animals. Intestinal capillariasis can be prevented by avoiding consumption of raw or undercooked fish. Fish should be cooked to an internal temperature of at least 145°F (63°C). When cases occur, prompt treatment is essential to prevent mortality and to limit possible contamination of local waters with feces, which could create local outbreaks

RARE INTESTINAL NEMATODES OF HUMANS

Strongyloides fuelleborni

Two subspecies of *S. fuelleborni* are capable of producing intestinal infections in humans. *S. fuelleborni* subsp. *fuelleborni* is widespread in wild primates in Africa and Asia. Most human cases are reported from jungle regions of central and southern Africa, with confirmed cases reported from Guinea (Conakry), Ivory Coast, Ghana, Togo, Cameroon, Gabon, Central African Republic, Republic of Congo (Brazzaville), Democratic Republic of Congo (Kinshasa),

Ethiopia, Somalia, Rwanda, Tanzania, Zambia, Malawi, Zimbabwe, and Namibia.[66–71] Recently, human infections have also been reported from Thailand.[72] In studies on *Strongyloides* spp. in Zambia, *S. f. fuelleborni* accounted for between 9.9% and 30.8% of all strongyloidiasis cases investigated.[67,73] Adults of this species are morphologically distinct from *S. stercoralis*, but disease characteristics appear to be similar. However, an important difference is that eggs containing developing larvae are commonly passed in stool, unlike *S. stercoralis* where generally only rhabditiform larvae are seen in fresh stool.[74]

S. fuelleborni subsp. *kellyi* was first identified in "*S. fuelleborni*-like" infections of infants in Papua New Guinea and presenting with acute systemic disease. This "swollen belly sickness" involved symptoms such as abdominal distention and edema, dyspnea, and gastrointestinal abnormalities, which were occasionally fatal in heavy infections.[75,76] Cases have also been reported from Papua province of Indonesia.[70] This subspecies appears to be anthroponotic in transmission, as nonhuman primates are not present on the island of Papua. The major route of infection appears to be transdermal. Transmammary infection has been postulated, although not proven. Adults appear morphologically similar to *S. f. fuelleborni*, but unlike the latter subspecies, eggs are passed trapped in clusters or strings of mucous.[70]

Trichostrongylidae

Trichostrongylids are ubiquitously distributed small, bursate nematodes of livestock and wild herbivores. Eggs are passed in the stools of infected animals, and the hatched rhabditiform larvae develop into infective filariform larvae in the environment. These sheathed larvae are rather resistant to temperature changes and desiccation, allowing them to persist on pasture for extended periods. Transmission to the definitive host occurs primarily via ingestion of filariform larvae, which mature into adults that embed headfirst in the mucosa of the jejunum and occasionally duodenum. Human infections are believed to be uncommon, but the true incidence may be underestimated given the eggs' morphologic similarity to human hookworms. Furthermore, most infections are asymptomatic, but those that are can involve diarrhea, abdominal cramping, mild anemia, occult blood in stool, and weight loss associated with inflammation of the jejunal mucosa.[77]

Most reports of human trichostrongyliasis involve species of the genus *Trichostrongylus; T. axei, T. colubriformis, T. capricola, T. orientalis,* and *T. vitrinus* are the most commonly reported. Rare human cases involving other trichostrongylids are also known, including *Haemonchus contortus, Mecistocirrus digitalis, Ostertagia* spp., and *Marshallagia marshalli.* Incidence appears highest in pastoral, livestock-rearing areas of the Middle East and Asia, although cases have been reported sporadically across the world.[77,78]

Oesophagostomum Species

Oesophagostomum spp. or "nodular worms" are strongyles of ruminants, primates, and swine. Larvae form nodules along the gastrointestinal wall, in which they develop and emerge as adults into the intestinal lumen. Like some trichostrongylids, some *Oesophagostomum* spp. (including the most commonly reported zoonotic species, *O. bifurcum*) filariform larvae show a remarkable degree of environmental resilience, capable of surviving and maintaining infectivity following periods of desiccation and freezing.[79] Transmission is via ingestion of filariform larvae, like other strongylid species. Eggs cannot be morphologically differentiated from hookworm eggs, thus larval culture is required for definitive identification.[80]

Nodules associated with *Oesophagostomum* spp. larvae are tumor-like, contain a single larva or subadult, and usually reach 1–2 cm in size; occasionally much larger sizes develop. Cases involving particularly large nodules or heavy infections with numerous nodules may present with symptomatic disease. Intense abdominal pain, intestinal blockage, and in severe cases, rupture and peritonitis can occur. Surgical intervention is required in cases where nodules occlude the small intestine or bowel.[80]

The distribution of human *Oesophagostomum* spp. infections is extremely focal. These infections are very uncommon outside of particular endemic regions of northern Ghana and Togo, where local prevalences of up to 59% have been observed. The factors driving this highly concentrated distribution are not well understood. *Oesophagostomum* spp. infections have been found to be positively correlated with hookworm infections in these endemic areas, although the two worms utilize different modes of transmission.[81]

Ternidens deminutus

Also known as the "false hookworm," *Ternidens deminutus* is a zoonotic strongylid nematode of several Old World primate species. Adult nematodes are blood feeding, and are typically found attached to the large intestinal wall (occasionally duodenal) where they create ulcerative and sometimes cystic lesions. Otherwise, the pathology, life cycle, and route of transmission are not well known; only one of many attempts to infect laboratory animals and human volunteers has been successful, via ingestion of third-stage larvae. The clinical syndrome associated with heavy *T. deminutus* infection is poorly characterized, though it seems to involve anemia and generalized weakness. Most cases are probably asymptomatic. Eggs are shed in the feces of infected hosts, and resemble human hookworm and other trichostrongylid eggs but are larger (~82 × 51 um).[82,83]

Nearly all known cases originate from eastern and southern sub-Saharan Africa. A single case report exists from south Asia[84] but this case may be a misidentification of *Oesophagostomum* spp. Whether due to a true lack of transmission or a lack of recognition, in more recent years, this species is very infrequently discussed or reported from humans. However, high (>50%) local prevalence estimates have been noted in historical reports from villages in Mozambique and Zimbabwe.[82]

References

1. World Health Organization. *Helminth Control in School-Age Children: A Guide for Managers of Control Programmes*. 2nd ed. Geneva: World Health Organization; 2011.
2. Bisoffi Z, Buonfrate D, Montresor A, et al. *Strongyloides stercoralis*: A plea for action. *PLoS Negl Trop Dis*. 2013;7:e2214.
3. Beknazarova M, Whiley H, Ross K. Strongyloidiasis: A disease of socioeconomic disadvantage. *Int J Environ Res Public Health*. 2016;13(5):517.
4. Strkolcova G, Goldova M, Bockova E, Mojzisova J. The roundworm *Strongyloides stercoralis* in children, dogs, and soil inside and outside a segregated settlement in Eastern Slovakia: Frequent but hardly detectable parasite. *Parasitol Res*. 2017;116:891–900.
5. World Health Organization. *Strongyloidiasis Fact Sheet*. Geneva: World Health Organization; 2018.
6. Genta RM. Global prevalence of strongyloidiasis: Critical review with epidemiologic insights into the prevention of disseminated disease. *Rev Infect Dis*. 1989;11:755–67.
7. Page W, Judd JA, Bradbury RS. The unique life cycle of *Strongyloides stercoralis* and implications for public health action. *Trop Med Infect Dis*. 2018;3:53.
8. Jaleta TG, Zhou S, Bemm FM, et al. Different but overlapping populations of *Strongyloides stercoralis* in dogs and humans—Dogs as a possible source for zoonotic strongyloidiasis. *PLoS Negl Trop Dis*. 2017;11:e0005752.
9. Nagayasu E, Aung M, Hortiwakul T, et al. A possible origin population of pathogenic intestinal nematodes, *Strongyloides stercoralis*, unveiled by molecular phylogeny. *Sci Rep*. 2017;7:4844.
10. Thamsborg SM, Ketzis J, Horii Y, Matthews JB. *Strongyloides* spp. infections of veterinary importance. *Parasitology*. 2017;144:274–84.
11. Robson D, Beeching NJ, Gill GV. *Strongyloides* hyperinfection syndrome in British veterans. *Ann Trop Med Parasitol*. 2009;103:145–8.
12. Brown RC, Girardeau HF. Transmammary passage of *Strongyloides* sp. larvae in the human host. *Am J Trop Med Hyg*. 1977;26:215–9.
13. Shoop WL, Michael BF, Eary CH, Haines HW. Transmammary transmission of *Strongyloides stercoralis* in dogs. *J Parasitol*. 2002;88:536–9.
14. Buonfrate D, Requena-Mendez A, Angheben A, et al. Severe strongyloidiasis: A systematic review of case reports. *BMC Infect Dis*. 2013;13:78.
15. Requena-Mendez A, Chiodini P, Bisoffi Z, Buonfrate D, Gotuzzo E, Munoz J. The laboratory diagnosis and follow up of strongyloidiasis: A systematic review. *PLoS Negl Trop Dis*. 2013;7:e2002.

16. Campo Polanco L, Gutierrez LA, Cardona Arias J. Diagnosis of *Strongyloides Stercoralis* infection: Meta-analysis on evaluation of conventional parasitological methods (1980–2013). *Rev Esp Salud Publica.* 2014;88:581–600.
17. Campo Polanco L, Gutierrez LA, Cardona Arias J. Diagnosis of *Strongyloides Stercoralis* Infection. Meta-analysis on Evaluation of Conventional Parasitological Methods (1980–2013). *Rev Esp Salud Pública.* 2014;88:581–600.
18. Centers for Disease Control and Prevention. Strongyloidiasis: Resources for Health Professionals. 2018.
19. Bisoffi Z, Buonfrate D, Sequi M, et al. Diagnostic accuracy of five serologic tests for *Strongyloides stercoralis* infection. *PLoS Negl Trop Dis.* 2014;8:e2640.
20. Verweij JJ, Canales M, Polman K, et al. Molecular diagnosis of *Strongyloides stercoralis* in faecal samples using real-time PCR. *Trans R Soc Trop Med Hyg.* 2009;103:342–6.
21. Sitta RB, Malta FM, Pinho JR, Chieffi PP, Gryschek RC, Paula FM. Conventional PCR for molecular diagnosis of human strongyloidiasis. *Parasitology.* 2014;141:716–21.
22. de Paula FM, Malta Fde M, Marques PD, et al. Molecular diagnosis of strongyloidiasis in tropical areas: A comparison of conventional and real-time polymerase chain reaction with parasitological methods. *Mem Inst Oswaldo Cruz.* 2015;110:272–4.
23. Schar F, Odermatt P, Khieu V, et al. Evaluation of real-time PCR for *Strongyloides stercoralis* and hookworm as diagnostic tool in asymptomatic schoolchildren in Cambodia. *Acta Trop.* 2013;126:89–92.
24. Saugar JM, Merino FJ, Martin-Rabadan P, et al. Application of real-time PCR for the detection of *Strongyloides* spp. in clinical samples in a reference center in Spain. *Acta Trop.* 2015;142:20–5.
25. Sharifdini M, Mirhendi H, Ashrafi K, et al. Comparison of nested polymerase chain reaction and real-time polymerase chain reaction with parasitological methods for detection of *Strongyloides stercoralis* in human fecal samples. *Am J Trop Med Hyg.* 2015;93:1285–91.
26. Leles D, Gardner SL, Reinhard K, Iniguez A, Araujo A. Are *Ascaris lumbricoides* and *Ascaris suum* a single species? *Parasit Vectors.* 2012;5:42.
27. Sandars DF. Viability of *Ascaris lumbricoides* eggs preserved in formalin. *Nature.* 1951;167:730.
28. Miller LA, Colby K, Manning SE, et al. Ascariasis in humans and pigs on small-scale farms, Maine, USA, 2010–2013. *Emerg Infect Dis.* 2015;21:332–4.
29. Shao CC, Xu MJ, Alasaad S, et al. Comparative analysis of microRNA profiles between adult *Ascaris lumbricoides* and Ascaris suum. *BMC Vet Res.* 2014;10:99.
30. Nejsum P, Hawash MB, Betson M, Stothard JR, Gasser RB, Andersen LO. Ascaris phylogeny based on multiple whole mtDNA genomes. *Infect Genet Evol.* 2017;48:4–9.
31. Jeandron A, Ensink JH, Thamsborg SM, Dalsgaard A, Sengupta ME. A quantitative assessment method for Ascaris eggs on hands. *PLoS One.* 2014;9:e96731.
32. Peng W, Zhou X, Gasser RB. *Ascaris* egg profiles in human faeces: Biological and epidemiological implications. *Parasitology.* 2003;127:283–90.
33. Nelson KL, Darby JL. Inactivation of viable *Ascaris* eggs by reagents during enumeration. *Appl Environ Microbiol.* 2001;67:5453–9.
34. Bradbury RS, Harrington H, Kekeubata E, et al. High prevalence of ascariasis on two coral atolls in the Solomon Islands. *Trans R Soc Trop Med Hyg.* 2018;112:193–9.
35 Wilson P. Maturation of *Ascaris* ova in sea water; a possible factor in dissemination of ascariasis in American Samoa. *Am J Trop Med Hyg.* 1942;1:305–7.
36. Beaver P, Jung R, Cupp E. *Clinical Parasitology.* 9th ed. Philadelphia: Lea and Febiger; 1984.
37. Glinz D, Silue KD, Knopp S, et al. Comparing diagnostic accuracy of Kato-Katz, Koga agar plate, ether-concentration, and FLOTAC for *Schistosoma mansoni* and soil-transmitted helminths. *PLoS Negl Trop Dis.* 2010;4:e754.
38. Centers for Disease Control and Prevention. Ascariasis: Resources for Health Professionals. 2018.
39. Dold C, Holland CV. Ascaris and ascariasis. *Microbes Infect.* 2011;13:632–7.
40. Vos T, Barber RM, Bell B, et al. Global, regional, and national incidence, prevalence, and years lived with disability for 301 acute and chronic diseases and injuries in 188 countries, 1990–2013: A systematic analysis for the Global Burden of Disease Study 2013. *Lancet.* 2015;386:743–800.
41. Larsen M, Roepstorff A. Seasonal variation in development and survival of *Ascaris suum* and *Trichuris suis* eggs on pastures. *Parasitology.* 1999;119:209–20.
42. Dunn JJ, Columbus ST, Aldeen WE, Davis M, Carroll KC. *Trichuris vulpis* recovered from a patient with chronic diarrhea and five dogs. *J Clin Microbiol.* 2002;40:2703–4.
43. George S, Geldhof P, Albonico M, et al. The molecular speciation of soil-transmitted helminth eggs collected from school children across six endemic countries. *Trans R Soc Trop Med Hyg.* 2016;110(11):657–63.
44. Areekul P, Putaporntip C, Pattanawong U, Sitthicharoenchai P, Jongwutiwes S. *Trichuris vulpis* and *T. trichiura* infections among schoolchildren of a rural community in northwestern Thailand: The possible role of dogs in disease transmission. *Asian Biomed.* 2010;4:49–60.
45. Centers for Disease Control and Prevention. Trichuriasis: Resources for Health Professionals. 2018.
46. Moser W, Schindler C, Keiser J. Efficacy of recommended drugs against soil transmitted helminths: Systematic review and network meta-analysis. *BMJ.* 2017;358:j4307.
47. Palmeirim MS, Hürlimann E, Knopp S, et al. Efficacy and safety of co-administered ivermectin plus albendazole for treating soil-transmitted helminths: A systematic review meta-analysis and individual patient data analysis. *PLoS Negl Trop Dis.* 2018;12:e0006458.
48. Wang S, Yao Z, Hou Y, et al. Prevalence of *Enterobius vermicularis* among preschool children in 2003 and 2013 in Xinxiang city, Henan province, Central China. *Parasite.* 2016;23:30.
49. Chai JY, Yang SK, Kim JW, et al. High prevalence of *Enterobius vermicularis* infection among schoolchildren in three townships around Yangon, Myanmar. *Korean J Parasitol.* 2015;53:771–5.
50. Lohiya GS, Tan-Figueroa L, Crinella FM, Lohiya S. Epidemiology and control of enterobiasis in a developmental center. *West J Med.* 2000; 172:305–8.
51. Centers for Disease Control and Prevention. DPDx: Enterobiasis. https://www.cdc.gov/dpdx/enterobiasis/index.html. Accessed November 30, 2018.
52. Cook GC. Enterobius vermicularis infection. *Gut.* 1994;35:1159–62.
53. Lee J, Kim K, Ryu J, Hong K, Lee H, Rim H. Pattern on *Enterobius vermicularis* in Korea. *J Agric Med Comm Health.* 1978;3:18–26.
54. Arca MJ, Gates RL, Groner JI, Hammond S, Caniano DA. Clinical manifestations of appendiceal pinworms in children: An institutional experience and a review of the literature. *Pediatr Surg Int.* 2004;20:372–5.
55. Liu LX, Chi J, Upton MP, Ash LR. Eosinophilic colitis associated with larvae of the pinworm Enterobius vermicularis. *Lancet.* 1995;346:410–2.
56. Kang IS, Kim DH, An HG, et al. Impact of health education on the prevalence of enterobiasis in Korean preschool students. *Acta Trop.* 2012;122:59–63.
57. Cross JH. Intestinal capillariasis. *Clin Microbiol Rev.* 1992;5:120–9.
58. Cross JH, Banzon T, Clarke MD, Basaca-Servilla V, Watten RH, Dizon JJ. Studies on the experimental transmission of *Capillaria philippinensis* in monkeys. *Trans R Soc Trop Med Hyg.* 1972;66:819–27.
59. Cross JH, Basaca-Sevilla V. Experimental transmission of *Capillaria philippinensis* to birds. *Trans R Soc Trop Med Hyg.* 1983;77:511–4.
60. Jung WT, Kim HJ, Min HJ, et al. An indigenous case of intestinal capillariasis with protein-losing enteropathy in Korea. *Korean J Parasitol.* 2012;50:333–7.
61. Anis MH, Shafeek H, Mansour NS, Moody A. Intestinal capillariasis as a cause of chronic diarrhoea in Egypt. *J Egypt Soc Parasitol.* 1998;28:143–7.
62. Lu LH, Lin MR, Choi WM, et al. Human intestinal capillariasis (Capillaria philippinensis) in Taiwan. *Am J Trop Med Hyg.* 2006;74:810–3.
63. Saichua P, Nithikathkul C, Kaewpitoon N. Human intestinal capillariasis in Thailand. *World J Gastroenterol.* 2008;14:506–10.
64. Wang Z, Lin X, Wang Y, Cui J. The emerging but neglected hepatic capillariasis in China. *Asian Pac J Trop Biomed.* 2013;3:146–7.
65. Cross JH, Basaca-Sevilla V. Albendazole in the treatment of intestinal capillariasis. *Southeast Asian J Trop Med Public Health.* 1987;18:507–10.
66. Pampiglione S, Ricciardi M. The presence of *Strongyloides fülleborni* von Linstow, 1905, in man in Central and East Africa. *Parassitologia.* 1971;13(1):257–269.
67. Hira P, Patel B. Human strongyloidiasis due to the primate species *Strongyloides fuelleborni. Trop Geogr Med.* 1980;32:23–9.
68. Kyrönseppä H, Goldsmid J. Studies on the intestinal parasites in African patients in Owamboland, South West Africa. *Trans R Soc Trop Med Hyg.* 1978;72:16–21.
69. Goldsmid JM. Studies on intestinal helminths in African patients at Harari Central Hospital, Rhodesia. *Trans R Soc Trop Med Hyg.* 1968;62:619–29.
70. Ashford R, Barnish G. *Strongyloides fuelleborni* and similar parasites in animals and man. In: Grove D, ed.Grove D, ed. *Strongyloidiasis: A Major Roundworm Infection of Man.* London: Taylor & Francis; 1989, pp. 271–86.

71. Hasegawa H, Sato H, Fujita S, et al. Molecular identification of the causative agent of human strongyloidiasis acquired in Tanzania: Dispersal and diversity of *Strongyloides* spp. and their hosts. *Parasitol Int.* 2010;59:407–13.
72. Thanchomnang T, Intapan PM, Sanpool O, et al. First molecular identification and genetic diversity of *Strongyloides stercoralis* and *Strongyloides fuelleborni* in human communities having contact with long-tailed macaques in Thailand. *Parasitol Res.* 2017;116:1917–23.
73. Hira P, Patel B. *Strongyloides fülleborni* infections in man in Zambia. *Am J Trop Med Hyg.* 1977;26:640–3.
74. Grove DI. Human strongyloidiasis. *Adv Parasitol.* Amsterdam, Netherlands: Elsevier; 1996, pp. 251–309.
75. Ashford R, Barnish G, Viney M. *Strongyloides fuelleborni kellyi*: Infection and disease in Papua New Guinea. *Parasitol Today.* 1992;8:314–8.
76. Ashford R, Vince J, Gratten M, Miles W. *Strongyloides* infection associated with acute infantile disease in Papua New Guinea. *Trans R Soc Trop Med Hyg.* 1978;72:554.
77. Miyazaki I. An illustrated book of helminthic zoonoses: International Medical Foundation of Japan Tokyo; 1991.
78. Bradbury R. An imported case of Trichostrongylid infection in Tasmania and a review of human Trichostrongylidiosis. *Ann ACTM.* 2006;7:25.
79. Pit DS, Blotkamp J, Polderman AM, Baeta S, Eberhard ML. The capacity of the third-stage larvae of *Oesophagostomum bifurcum* to survive adverse conditions. *Ann Trop Med Parasitol.* 2000;94:165–71.
80. Polderman A, Blotkamp J. *Oesophagostomum* infections in humans. *Parasitol Today.* 1995;11:451–6.
81. Krepel HP, Baeta S, Polderman AM. Human *Oesophagostomum* infection in northern Togo and Ghana: Epidemiological aspects. *Ann Trop Med Parasitol.* 1992;86:289–300.
82. Amberson JM, Schwarz E. *Ternidens deminutus* Railliet and Henry, a nematode parasite of man and primates. *Ann Trop Med Parasitol.* 1952;46:227–37.
83. Goldsmid JM. Studies on the life cycle and biology of *Ternidens deminutus* (Railliet & Henry, 1905) (Nematoda: Strongylidae). *J Helminthol.* 1971;45:341–52.
84. Hemsrichart V. *Ternidens deminutus* infection: First pathological report of a human case in Asia. *J Med Assoc Thai.* 2005;88:1140–3.

CHAPTER

127 Tissue Nematodes

Sarah G. H. Sapp • Richard S. Bradbury

The species discussed herein are all nematodes that invade tissues, either in their adult or larval stages. A common feature among many of these species is low host specificity, which facilitates zoonotic transmission. Associated disease varies widely by the tissue impacted, and some manifestations such as invasion of the central nervous system (CNS) may prove fatal. Diagnosis is difficult for several discussed agents due to a lack of infectious stages shed in feces or blood and relies on serology, imaging, or biopsy. Thus, the true incidence and impact of tissue nematode infections could be underestimated Table 127-1.

TOXOCARIASIS

The larvae of the common ascarid roundworms of dogs and cats, *Toxocara canis* and *Toxocara cati*, respectively, may infect humans. The adult worms live in the small intestines of their animal hosts, and eggs are shed in the feces. The eggs develop in the environment over 2–4 weeks, and both definitive and paratenic hosts (including many species of birds and mammals) may acquire infection following the ingestion of these infectious eggs. Definitive hosts may also become infected by consuming encysted larvae from tissues of an infected paratenic host. Larval migration follows a hepatotracheal route to the gastrointestinal tract in the definitive host, while somatic migration via circulation to visceral organs occurs in the paratenic host (including humans) and to some extent in the definitive host.[1] Transmission to humans primarily occurs through the fecal-oral route, from eggs in the environment or adhering to animal hair, but *Toxocara* spp. may also be a foodborne agent if undercooked meat from paratenic host tissue containing larvae is eaten. Foodborne cases have been reported after eating raw bovine and poultry livers; the liver is a common site for accumulation of larvae in paratenic hosts.[2,3] Larvae of *T. cati* in meat have been shown to be tolerant of refrigeration and short-term freezing (up to 2 weeks).[4]

The most significant clinical manifestation of human toxocariasis is visceral larva migrans (VLM) caused by mechanical damage and inflammation incurred during the migration of *Toxocara* larvae through visceral organs, particularly the liver and lungs. Migrating larvae are attacked by the host immune system and eventually become trapped in granulomas (Fig. 127-1A). Clinical symptoms and signs are fairly nonspecific. Hepatomegaly and pneumonitis may occur alone or together, and are usually accompanied by peripheral hypereosinophilia and sometimes hyperglobulinemia. Fever, malaise, and anorexia may occur. Severe cases may involve myocarditis, nephritis, and neurological manifestations if the respective organs are sufficiently impacted. Causal links between mild or subclinical cases and pulmonary insufficiency, cognitive deficits, and unexplained urticaria have been proposed.[5–7] *Toxocara* spp. larvae sometimes enter the eyes; this is referred to as ocular larva migrans (OLM). OLM is often associated with diffuse unilateral subacute neuroretinitis (DUSN), endopthalmitis, retinitis, and granuloma formation, which can result in retinal detachment and permanent vision defects.[1]

The gold standard for diagnosis of toxocariasis is the finding of larvae in biopsy sections; larvae are 15–20 μm in diameter, about 400-μm-long maximum, with single-pointed lateral alae on either side. However, the probability for larval capture in small ante-mortem biopsy specimens is quite low, and imaging techniques (e.g., CT, ultrasound) may reveal lesions that are nonspecific. Serologic diagnosis is therefore the most commonly used diagnostic tool for cases of VLM. A variety of native and recombinant *Toxocara* excretory-secretory antigens (TES) are used in ELISA and immunoblot formats for the detection of specific IgG (either total IgG or IgG_4); these are reviewed by Fillaux and Magnaval[8] and Moirera.[9] In general, sensitivity for these immunoassays is usually high (>90%) on VLM samples, but specificity varies due to cross-reactivity and can be unacceptably low in ELISA formats using native TES.[9] Therefore, patients should first be tested using ELISA and positive results should be confirmed with immunoblotting to examine specific antigen fractions.[8] A positive serologic result paired with peripheral eosinophilia in a symptomatic patient is considered sufficient for a diagnosis of active toxocariasis. In acute ocular cases, larvae are viewed using slit-lamp examination; patients are often seronegative without peripheral eosinophilia because OLM is thought to result from one or very few larvae.[8] Most cases of ocular toxocariasis are diagnosed based on presence of characteristic changes in the eye, including posterior pole granuloma or peripheral granuloma with traction bands.[10] Antibody detection in serum and/or aqueous humor may also support diagnosis.[8]

Epidemiological studies of human toxocariasis are primarily based on serologic investigation. It is believed to be prevalent infection globally; reported seroprevalence varies by geographic region and the performance characteristics of the assay used. In the United States, studies on sera banked for the National Health and Nutrition Examination Survey (NHANES) have generated prevalence estimates of 5–14% nationwide, with higher prevalence among persons in lower socioeconomic strata, males, African-American and Hispanic individuals, and pet owners.[11,12] Though most active VLM cases are diagnosed in children, the most recent survey (2011–14 NHANES) used a multiplex bead-based assay and found greater seroprevalence among adults aged 50 and up, which may reflect the longevity of the antibody response and/or repeated exposures.[12] Seroprevelance in highly developed countries is much lower (e.g., 0.7–7.5% in Australia, New Zealand, Japan, and Denmark) than in developing countries, where values of 30–81% have been noted.[13] However, despite the ubiquity of toxocariasis, its global burden and economic impacts have not been well studied.

Treatment is based on the use of anthelmintics to kill larvae or slow their migration and corticosteroids to control the host reaction. Currently, albendazole is favored, although its efficacy on tissue migratory stages remains limited with generally only half of patients in existing trials experiencing clinical improvement.[1] This phenomenon may be due to poor tissue penetrance by drugs; new formulations

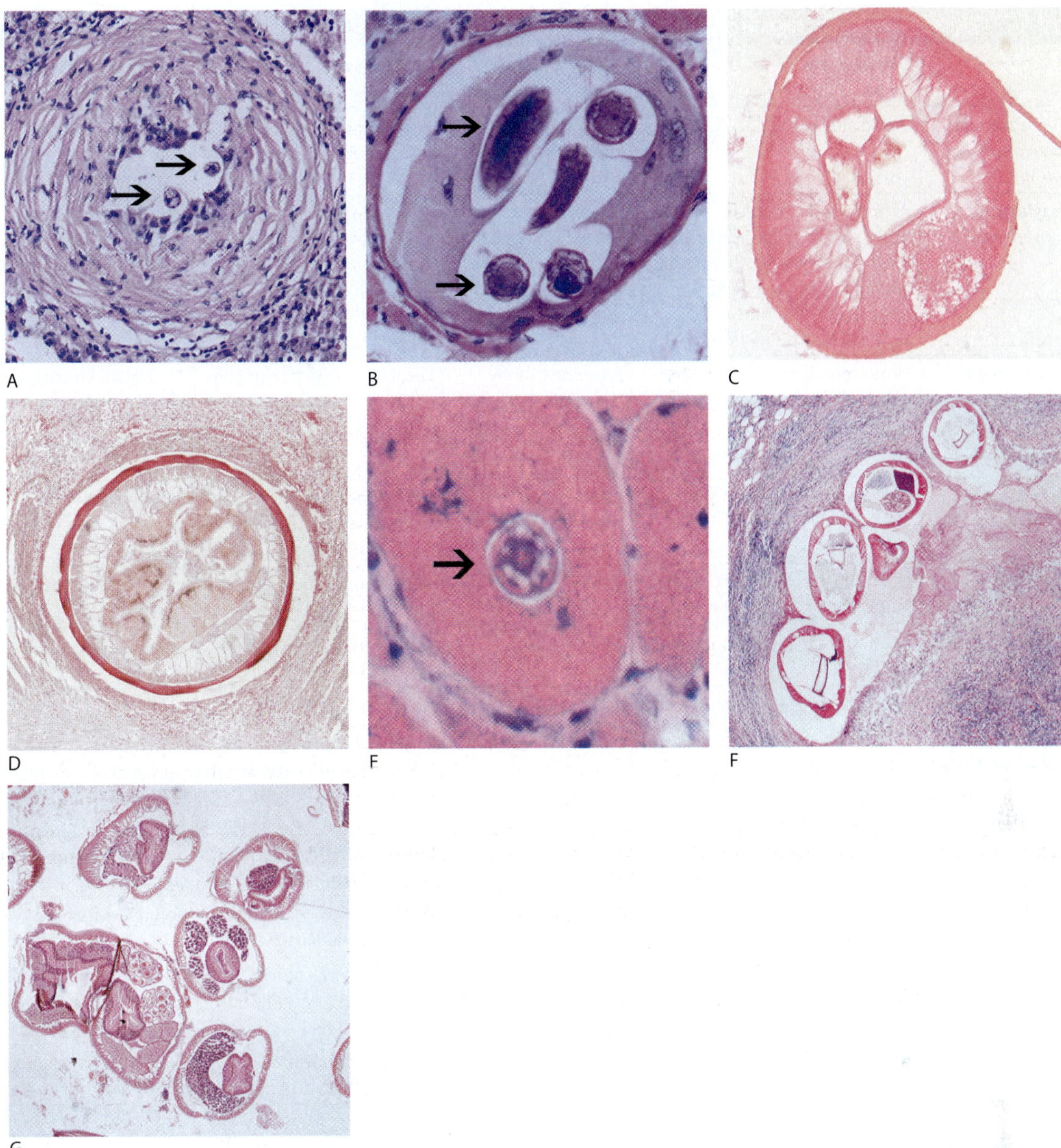

FIGURE 127-1. Appearance of some selected tissue-stage nematodes in histological sections. A. *Toxocara* sp.; B. *Trichinella spiralis*; C. *Dirofilaria tenuis*; D. *Gnathostoma spinigerum*; E. *Haycocknema perplexum*; F. *Dioctophyme renale*; and G. *Lagochilascaris* sp. (*Source:* Sarah G. H. Sapp, PhD.)

to improve drug delivery to tissues are being investigated. Novel therapeutic approaches to address immunosuppression caused by the parasite's immune evasion mechanisms are also in development.[9] For ocular cases, no standard treatment exists, but corticosteroids are generally indicated to control inflammation and help reduce the risk of permanent ocular damage.[1]

Prevention and control are of utmost importance. Treatment of pet dogs and cats with anthelmintics, of which most are effective against intestinal *Toxocara* spp., is critical in reducing environmental contamination—particularly since ascarid eggs are hardy and persistent and difficult to completely eliminate once in soil.[14] Pet feces should also be removed and disposed of promptly, particularly in public places like parks and playgrounds. Good hand hygiene should be taught to children from an early age.

TRICHINELLOSIS

Trichinellosis, also called trichinosis, is a foodborne disease caused by ingesting the larvae of the genus *Trichinella* in meat. *Trichinella* infection has been reported in almost all mammalian species as well as carnivorous marsupials, reptiles, and birds[15] (Table 127-2).

Humans are infected when they consume raw or undercooked meat of domestic and wild animals, mainly pork, but horses and wild boars are also considered important source of infection. The life cycle of *Trichinella* is unique and includes two generations in same host. The intestinal phase occurs when meat containing *Trichinella* first-stage (L1) larvae is consumed. This stage of the disease may be accompanied by abdominal pain, diarrhea, and hemorrhage.[16] The larvae molt four times to develop into adults in the duodenum, adults sexually reproduce within 7 days, and the females give birth to a new generation of larvae. At this phase, the "newborn" first-stage larvae migrate through lymphatic and blood vessels to skeletal muscle; this phase is called the "muscle phase." Typically, active muscles such as the diaphragm, biceps, gastrocnemius, and facial muscles are impacted. Larvae invade muscle cells forming structures called nurse cells, which usually become encapsulated by the host reaction, though encapsulation is not seen with *T. pseudospiralis*, *T. zimbabweensis*, and *T. papuae*. These hypobiotic muscle-stage larvae can survive for many years (up to 40 years) (Fig. 127-1B).[17]

Clinical diagnosis of disease is difficult, due to subtle clinical signs and nonspecific manifestations of disease. Typical signs of facial edema, fever, myositis, peripheral eosinophilia, and elevated muscle enzymes

TABLE 127-1 SUMMARY OF TISSUE NEMATODES DISCUSSED IN THIS CHAPTER

Agent	Distribution	Major Definitive Host	Transmission	Location in Tissue
Anisakids (*Anisakis* spp., *Pseudoterranova* spp., *Contracecum* spp.)	Worldwide	Cetaceans and pinnipeds	Foodborne: ingestion of undercooked fish	Usually gastric mucosa, sometimes other intestinal or aberrant sites
***Angiostrongylus* spp.** (=*Parastrongylus* spp.)	*A. cantonensis*: East Asia, Southeast Asia, Pacific Islands, Australia, Africa, Southeastern United States, Caribbean; *A. costaricensis:* Caribbean, Central America, South America	Rat species	Foodborne: ingestion of snail intermediate host or larvae	*A. cantonensis*: Brain, occasionally eyes; *A. costaricensis:* vessels of the intestinal wall, sometimes liver or testes
Baylisascaris procyonis	North America, Europe, Japan,	Raccoons, rarely domestic dogs	Fecal-oral: ingestion of eggs	Central nervous system, eyes, also visceral organs
Capillaria hepatica (=*Calodium hepaticum*)	Worldwide	Rodents, carnivores	Fecal-oral: ingestion of eggs	Liver parenchyma
Dioctophyme renale	Likely worldwide	Carnivores, especially mink	Likely foodborne: ingestion of larvae in undercooked fish or amphibians	Kidney, subcutaneous
***Dirofilaria* spp.**	*D. immitis*: Worldwide; *D. repens*: Europe; *D. tenuis*: North America	Canids, felids, some wild carnivores	Vector-borne: mosquitoes	Lungs, subcutaneous
Dracunculus medinensis	Isolated areas of sub-Saharan Africa	Humans, dogs	Waterborne: ingestion of copepod intermediate host	Subcutaneous
Haycocknema perplexum	Australia: Queensland and Tasmania	Unknown	Unknown	Skeletal muscle
Halicephalobus gingivalis (=*deletrix*)	Worldwide	Free-living	Unknown; organ transplant transmission has been reported	Central nervous system, heart, kidney, liver
Lagochilascaris minor	Central and South America	Wild and domestic felids	Likely foodborne: ingestion of larvae in meat	Subcutaneous in cervical and cephalic sites
***Thelazia* spp.**	Asia, Europe, parts of North America	Canids, felids, livestock species	Vector-borne: lachrymophagous flies	Conjunctiva of eye
***Toxocara* spp.**	Worldwide	Canids and felids (domestic and wild)	Fecal-oral: ingestion of eggs; foodborne: ingestion of larvae in meat	Visceral organs, eyes, sometimes central nervous system
***Trichinella* spp.**	Worldwide	Carnivores, swine	Foodborne: ingestion of larvae in meat	Skeletal muscle, rarely elsewhere

(aspartate aminotransferase and creatine kinase) are noted during the muscle phase of trichinellosis. Conjunctivitis, skin rash, and uveitis may also be seen. Infected patients may exhibit signs of larval invasion that can lead to poor muscle movement (e.g., with chewing, talking, swallowing and in some cases with breathing), cardiac or CNS disease which may occasionally lead to death.[16,18–20] The global yearly number of clinical trichinellosis has been estimated at 10,000 cases, of which an estimated 0.2% are fatal.[21] Outbreaks of multiple cases associated with a single source of contaminated meat can occur.[18,20]

The main diagnostic approaches are serological testing of potentially infected humans and animals. Various recombinant and crude antigens have been used in ELISA, EITB, or IFA formats.[22] ELISA using excretory/secretory (ES) antigens and crude antigens have equivalent sensitivity (99%), but ES antigens are more specific than crude antigens (91–96% vs. 60%, in humans) for the detection of *Trichinella* antibodies.[23] In pigs, the ES ELISA has a sensitivity of 93–99%, with a sensitivity of between 91% and 99%; the use of crude antigen tests on pig sera often results in false positives.[22] IgG antibodies are normally detectable at 3 weeks postinfection, peak around 3 months, and may remain detectable for many years afterward. Serosurveillance studies must be approached on a host-by-host basis, as antibody levels may decline more rapidly in some hosts, such as horses, and also that antibody kinetics may vary by *Trichinella* species/genotype.[22,23] The statistical positive predictive value of such testing is also influenced by the prevalence of trichinellosis in the population undergoing surveillance.[22,24] Various PCR methodologies or microscopy on digested muscle biopsies from patients or meat-associated outbreaks may also be used in diagnosis and epidemiologic investigations.[25]

Cooking meat to reach temperatures above 71°C and freezing sufficiently are considered two main mechanisms to prevent trichinellosis, with the caveat that not all species/genotypes are killed by freezing.[18] For example, while *T. spiralis* is inactivated within 12–48 hours at −10°C, the arctic species *T. nativa* may retain infectivity for up to 5 years at that temperature.[26] Pig husbandry practices impact the likelihood of *Trichinella* infection on farms, with factors such as rodent control, limitation of contact with other fauna, diet composition (i.e., inclusion of meat scraps), and free-ranging versus indoor housing all reducing the likelihood of swine becoming infected with *Trichinella*.[24] Education of hunters and others who consume game meat about risks and safety practices may also reduce the occurrence of trichinellosis.

BAYLISASCARIASIS

Baylisascaris procyonis (raccoon roundworm) is a rare but serious cause of neurological and ocular disease in humans. While several other species of *Baylisascaris* exist, it is not known if they are capable of infecting humans; cases of baylisascariasis are nearly universally assumed to be caused by *B. procyonis*.[27] The life cycle is similar to that of *Toxocara* spp. Adult *B. procyonis* are large, robust ascarid nematodes that are found in the small intestines of raccoons. Eggs are passed in the feces and require 10–14 days to embryonate and

TABLE 127-2 SUMMARY OF *TRICHINELLA* SPECIES, THEIR GEOGRAPHIC DISTRIBUTION, RESERVOIR HOSTS AND PUBLIC HEALTH IMPLICATIONS[15,17,20,24,110–112]

Species/Genotype	Estimated Percentage of Human Infections[a]	Geographic Distribution	Reservoir Hosts	Encapsulated/ Nonencapsulated	Resistance to Freezing at −18°C
***Trichinella spiralis* (T1)**	~50% of cases	Worldwide, except Australia and Antarctica	Carnivores and omnivores, especially swine	Encapsulated	Between 56 hours and 7 days, some references state up to 4 weeks
***Trichinella britovi* (T3)**	~25% of cases	Europe, North and West Africa, the Middle East and extending through the Central Asia and South Western Asia to Afghanistan	Carnivores, wild boar, horses	Encapsulated	At least 6 months
***Trichinella papuae* (T10)**	~10% of cases	South East Asia, from Thailand/ Myanmar through to Papua New Guinea, including Gabba Island in the Torres Strait (Australia)	Wild and domestic swine, salt water crocodiles, possibly turtles and lizards	Nonencapsulated	No
***Trichinella nativa* (T2)**	~5–10% of cases	Arctic and subarctic, Poland, Germany, Japan	Wild and domestic canids, raccoons, bears, and walrus	Encapsulated	At least 4 years
***Trichinella murrelli* (T5)**	~1–4% of cases	Southern Canada, the United States and possibly northern Mexico	Black bears, raccoons, wild felines, wild and domestic canids	Encapsulated	Between 56 hours and 7 days
***Trichinella pseudospiralis* (T4)**	<1% of cases	Europe (including the UK), Russia (including Siberia), the United States, Canada, and the island of Tasmania (Australia)	Carnivores, including marsupial carnivores and carnivorous birds, wild boar	Nonencapsulated	At least 4 weeks
***Trichinella* T6**	<1% of cases	Canada and the North Eastern United States, Northern California	Carnivores	Encapsulated	At least 2½ years
***Trichinella* T9**	<1% of cases	Japan	Black bears, red foxes, raccoon dogs	Encapsulated	No
***Trichinella nelsoni* (T7)**	A few unconfirmed reports of human infection	Eastern Africa from Kenya to South Africa	Lions, leopards, cheetahs, spotted hyenas, bat eared foxes, serval	Encapsulated	No
***Trichinella zimbabweensis* (T11)**	No reported cases	Ethiopia, Central and southern Africa	Nile crocodiles, monitor lizards	Nonencapsulated	No
***Trichinella patagoniensis* (T12)**	No reported cases	Argentina	Cougars	Encapsulated	No
***Trichinella* T8**	No reported cases	South Africa and Namibia	Lions, leopards, spotted hyenas	Encapsulated	No

[a]As estimated by collation of data from the International *Trichinella* Reference Center and published reports.

develop to infectivity. Infection of paratenic hosts occurs following accidental ingestion of feces containing eggs with L3 larvae.[28]

Humans are accidental paratenic hosts, and do not support the maturation of larvae to adulthood. Larvae hatch from infectious eggs in the small intestine and migrate extensively in tissues, which may cause a number of larva migrans syndromes. Neural larva migrans (NLM) occurs when larvae enter the brain or spinal cord. The primary clinical presentation is eosinophilic meningitis; onset of symptoms may be slow or follow a rapid degenerative course. Clinical disease manifestations include altered mental state, tremor, ataxia, paresis, and seizures, which may progress to coma and death. Peripheral blood and CNS eosinophilia usually occur. Neurological disease associated with *B. procyonis* is generally more severe than that associated with *Toxocara* spp. due to the more aggressive migration and the fact that *Baylisascaris* larvae grow considerably in the paratenic host (from ~200 μm in length at hatching up to 1800 μm, versus *Toxocara* spp. which generally do not exceed 300 μm), and shed antigenic material as they migrate.[28]

OLM associated with baylisascariasis, like with *Toxocara*, may result in DUSN and permanent vision defects. It can be distinguished from *Toxocara* OLM based on the much larger size of larvae.[28] A VLM syndrome may occur but has not been well described for *B. procyonis* infection in humans. Not all human infections with *Baylisascaris* become symptomatic, and infections may be subclinical as with *Toxocara* spp. This is supported by the finding of *Baylisascaris* specific antibodies in otherwise healthy individuals, and one incidental finding of a *B. procyonis* larva in the brain during autopsy of a patient who died from unrelated causes.[29,30]

As with most tissue helminths, diagnosis is difficult due to a lack of parasitic stages shed in feces or present in blood. In recent years, a Western blot based on a recombinant antigen (rBpRAG-1) has been used to detect specific *Baylisascaris* antibodies in serum and cerebrospinal fluid (CSF).[31] For confirmed diagnosis, larvae may be identified in biopsy sections, but the probability of detection is low. Known contact with raccoons or raccoon feces may suggest the possibility of *Baylisascaris* infection but its absence should not exclude consideration of baylisascariasis in areas where raccoons are known to be present.[32]

Most known cases of baylisascariasis have been in young children or developmentally disabled adults who may have intentionally ingested raccoon feces, but some more recent cases in adults are likely due to indirect routes such as contaminated soil. High doses of albendazole are preferred for baylisascariasis treatment, along with corticosteroids to control inflammation. Of the ~35 confirmed *Baylisascaris* NLM cases, about 40% were fatal. Only two full recoveries are documented[28,32]; both were likely due to the early diagnosis and initiation of aggressive treatment with albendazole. The majority of survivors are left with neurological sequelae. As awareness and diagnostic detection have improved, clinical outcomes may become more favorable.[32]

Importantly, *B. procyonis* is very common in raccoons in many parts of the United States and Canada. Prevalence may be over 80% in raccoons in areas of the upper Midwest, New England, Pacific Northwest, and on the west coast.[28] Many of the reported clinical cases occurred in these hyperendemic regions, and residence in the western region was found to be a significant risk factor for exposure (based on seropositivity) in one study on wildlife rehabilitators.[33] Due to trade of live raccoons for fur farming, hunting, or for pets, the parasite is also found throughout much of continental Europe, Japan, and China.[28] Prevention is primarily centered on good hygiene and avoiding fecal-oral transmission. Notably, inconsistent hand washing after potential contact with raccoon feces (e.g., during cage cleaning) was significantly associated with seropositivity in wildlife rehabilitators.[33] Sandboxes, outdoor fireplaces, and similar areas should be covered when not in use to prevent raccoons from defecating in them. Feeding of wild raccoons whether intentional or accidental (e.g., leaving bowls of cat food outside) should be discouraged to prevent defecation in areas with high human activity. Extreme caution should be taken when removing raccoon "latrines" (communal defecation sites) that may occur on decks, attics, logs, and crooks of trees as those often contain large numbers of infective eggs. Eggs are very hardy and are only inactivated by high heat; environmental sanitization must involve a heat source such as a propane torch or boiling water—although these approaches are not always feasible. Finally, dogs and some exotic pets (kinkajous, coatis, or other procyonids) may in rare cases act as definitive hosts for *B. procyonis* and shed eggs as do raccoons. These pets should be dewormed regularly or placed on a monthly preventive to prevent infection.[28]

NEURAL ANGIOSTRONGYLIASIS

The metastrongylid nematode *Angiostrongylus (=Parastrongylus) cantonensis* was first recognized as a human pathogen in Japan in 1944 following a case of otherwise unexplained meningitis. Initially referred to as "*Haemostrongylus ratti,*" other workers later identified it as a previously described species *Angiostrongylus cantonensis* ("rat lungworm") during investigation of an outbreak of eosinophilic meningitis in Tahiti.[34] Since the correct identification and life-cycle elucidation, *A. cantonensis* has become increasingly recognized as a frequent, if not the most common, cause of eosinophilic meningitis, particularly in its original endemic range of Southeast Asia.[35] *A. cantonensis* has dispersed far beyond Southeast Asia and is an emerging pathogen globally.[36] Autochthonous human infections have now been documented in many East Asian countries, Fiji and other Pacific Islands, India, Australia, Brazil, Egypt, Madagascar, the Caribbean, and the United States, indicating the parasite's ecological establishment.[36,37] Both the movement of "stowaway" rat definitive hosts and introduction of invasive gastropod intermediate hosts are thought to contribute to this spread.[36,38]

A. cantonensis follows a complex multihost life cycle and uses various species of rats as the normal definitive hosts, hence the common name "rat lungworm." Adult nematodes reside in the pulmonary arteries, and produce first-stage (L1) larvae, which exit the bronchioles, are swallowed, and are shed in the feces. L1 larvae are then ingested by gastropod intermediate hosts, which include a relatively wide variety of snails and slugs [e.g., giant African snail (*Lissachatina fulica*), apple snails (*Pomacea* spp.), the semislug (*Parmarion martensi*), and many more]. L1 larvae molt to reach the infective L3 stage within the gastropod tissues. Transmission to the definitive host occurs via ingestion of L3 larvae in gastropod tissue, or in the tissue of some cold-blooded paratenic or transport hosts (e.g., crabs, freshwater shrimp) that may acquire L3 larvae.[36] In the appropriate definitive host (rats and some other related rodents), L3 larvae penetrate the intestinal wall, enter circulation, and eventually arrive in the subarachnoid space of the brain. Development to L4, L5, and adult stages takes place here, and eventually the young adult worms migrate to the pulmonary artery and reproduce.[16]

Usually, human exposure follows the accidental consumption of gastropods (or tissue thereof) on unwashed produce or the intentional consumption of whole gastropods (e.g., undercooked escargot; or for perceived medicinal properties). A few cases have been linked to the consumption of paratenic hosts, including frogs, terrestrial crabs, and freshwater shrimp.[39,40] Some debate exists as to whether *A. cantonensis* L3 larvae are shed from gastropods into slime trails in sufficient enough numbers to present an infection risk. It is likely a minor to negligible route of transmission as apparently low numbers are shed from snails versus other *Angiostrongylus* species, and they survive only a few hours outside of the host.[41–43]

Neurological manifestations in humans result from the presence of larvae in the subarachnoid space. Neural angiostrongyliasis presentation nearly always (in over 90% of cases) begins with development of a headache, possibly severe, which lasts up to a week.[35] Other symptoms are typical of meningitis (e.g., neck stiffness, weakness, nausea, paresthesia, visual disturbances) and may or may not be accompanied by fever.[35] Eosinophilia of the peripheral blood and CSF are typical features. Most patients will present with substantial peripheral eosinophilia, and occasionally with substantial CSF eosinophilia.[35,37,44] *A. cantonensis* are apparently short lived in the human host, and many cases are self-limiting and resolve within a month or two.[16] However, occasionally fatal neurological sequelae may result following damage incurred by CNS inflammation.[16,36,45] While larvae may undergo a degree of maturation, even reaching the subadult stage, reproductive maturity (and shedding of L1 larvae) has never been documented in humans. In the aberrant human host, larvae/subadults may occasionally wander to the eyes and cause ocular angiostrongyliasis.[35]

Diagnosis is often based on clinical presentation and case history. Larvae and/or subadults are seldom recovered from CSF, but provide definitive confirmation of diagnosis.[36,46] PCR testing of CSF to detect *A. cantonensis* DNA has proven to be a sensitive method for confirming infection and is increasingly used in clinical diagnosis.[37,47] Serological methods are not widely available and are primarily used as adjunct tests as substantial issues with cross-reactivity exist for many antigens.[48] Treatment is typically only supportive. The use of anthelmintics in treating neural angiostrongyliasis is somewhat controversial, due to concerns about potential exacerbation of CNS symptoms following the mass killing of larvae (and release of larval antigens). Corticosteroids are usually administered to control cerebral inflammation, and removal of CSF may aid in reducing intracranial pressure.[49] Prevention is centered on safe eating habits—thorough washing of produce to remove gastropods and/or their tissues, cooking produce or pasteurization of vegetable/fruit juices that could possibly be contaminated, and avoiding the consumption of raw gastropods or paratenic hosts.[16,46]

ABDOMINAL ANGIOSTRONGYLIASIS

A second *Angiostrongylus* species, *A. costaricensis* (=*Morerastrongylus costaricensis*), was first reported as a cause of human infection in 1952 in Costa Rica and is the causative agent of abdominal angiostrongyliasis.[50] This species differs from the better-known *A. cantonensis* with respect to adult morphology, geographic distribution, migration/

localization in the host, and host specificity.[51] It is endemic throughout much of Central and South America, and has been identified in wildlife in the southern United States although there is no evidence for autochthonous zoonotic transmission in the United States.[52] Adult worms are found in the ileocecal mesenteric arteries of the definitive host. Hispid cotton rats (*Sigmodon hispidus*) are the primary host but some other rodent species including black rats (*Rattus rattus*) are capable of harboring patent infections. The intermediate hosts are slugs, most typically leatherleaf slugs (*Sarasinaula* spp.), across the primary endemic range.[51]

Transmission to humans occurs following accidental ingestion of L3 larvae or infected intermediate hosts. Larvae migrate to the ileocecal mesenteric arteries (occasionally other ectopic sites) and unlike *A. cantonensis* can achieve sexual maturity in human host.[50,53,54] The presence of parasites and eggs creates a massive inflammatory reaction in the human intestine, which can symptomatically resemble appendicitis or VLM due to *Toxocara* spp.[55] The development of an eosinophilic granuloma/pseudotumor around the parasites, which may be large enough to be palpated, is a typical outcome of this inflammatory reaction. Significant peripheral eosinophilia is nearly always present, accompanied by high fever, anorexia, and vomiting. Adult worms in the mesenteric arteries can lead to endothelial damage and associated sequelae (thrombosis, vasculitis, etc.). Note that while eggs are produced by adult worms in zoonotic infections, larval shedding in human stool has not been reported, likely because eggs and larvae are damaged extensively by the inflammatory reaction prior to exiting the host.[50,53]

Diagnosis and treatment of abdominal angiostrongyliasis are difficult. Adult worms, larvae, and/or eggs are usually detected postoperatively on biopsy specimens, and some experimental serologic tests have been used. Treatment remains symptomatic; use of anthelmintics is considered risky as it may either induce aberrant migration of worms or cause a sudden release of worm antigens, worsening the course of disease.[53] Prevention strategies are the same as for neural angiostrongyliasis (*A. cantonensis*) and involve food safety practices (e.g., washing produce, avoiding eating raw/undercooked gastropods).[16]

DIROFILARIASIS

Dirofilaria is a genus of filarial nematodes, which are typically associated with carnivorous mammal hosts and usually vectored by mosquitoes. Species of the genus *Dirofilaria* that are confirmed zoonotic agents include *D. repens, D. immitis, D. striata, D. tenuis*, and a *D. ursi/D. subdermata*-like species. Generally, humans are considered accidental hosts, but reported occurrence of microfilaraemia in some human infections could change this perception of the disease.[56–58]

Transmission of *Dirofilaria* is indirect and via an insect vector, like other filarial nematodes. Several species of mosquitoes serve as both vector and intermediate host, with the exception of *D. ursi*, which uses black flies (*Simulium* spp.). The definitive host becomes infected when vector insects feed on their blood. Third-stage larvae penetrate the skin and molt and complete their development as immature stages in subcutaneous tissues (*D. repens, D. immitis, D. ursi*); *D. immitis* further matures in the pulmonary vasculature.[59,60] In the appropriate definitive hosts, adult females produce microfilariae which are discharged into circulation.

Among *Dirofilaria* spp., only *D. immitis*, the "canine heartworm," has a nearly global distribution. In human hosts, larvae of this species create pulmonary lesions recognized in chest x-rays as a "coin lesion." The majority of these human pulmonary infections are asymptomatic, but symptoms such as cough, thoracic pain, fever, dyspnoea, hemoptysis, and bloody sputum have been reported.[16] Two cases of orbital infection of humans with *D. immitis* have been reported from Australia.[61] On very rare occasions, cardiac or pericardiac dirofilariasis have been reported, usually discovered during autopsy.[60,62]

The other five human infecting species of *Dirofilaria* belong to a different subgenus (*Nochitella*) and localize mainly in the periorbital area and subcutaneous tissues, especially in the upper half of the body in human hosts. In the Old World, subcutaneous dirofilariasis is caused by *D. repens*, and this is the most commonly diagnosed species causing human dirofilariasis globally.[63] New World species *D. tenuis, D. ursi/D. subdermata*-like species, and *D. striata* are less common causes of human subcutaneous dirofilariasis.[57] Infection is often asymptomatic or with a mild course. Subcutaneous disease usually presents with a single nodule associated with erythema or pruritus. The presence of *Dirofilaria* worms in the orbital area may be accompanied by ocular discomfort, blepharedema, and hyperemia of bulbar conjunctiva. The parasite has been known to migrate to aberrant locations, such as the peritoneal cavity or scrotum. Recently, a larva migrans syndrome caused by *D. repens* was observed in a human infection,[58,64] as were several cases of microfilaremia due to this species.[65–67] Diagnosis is typically based on recovery of the whole worm (e.g., extraction of *D. repens* from the eye) or by morphological diagnosis on lateral sections in tissue (Fig. 127-1C). Certain morphological features, such as an internal lateral ridge, characteristics of cuticular ridges, and tall muscle cells aid in generic and specific diagnosis, although parasitological expertise is required for accurate distinction of *Dirofilaria* spp. from other filarids (e.g., zoonotic *Onchocerca* or *Brugia* spp., which are covered in the vector-borne filariases chapter of this textbook).[60]

Screening, prevention, and treatment of companion animals is important in reducing the risk of zoonotic dirofilariasis. The Companion Animal Parasite Council (USA) recommends yearly screening of all dogs using antigen-based tests and microscopy to detect microfilariae in blood, and twice-yearly testing may be advised for outdoor dogs or dogs in highly endemic areas.[68] A wide variety of anthelmintic preventives have been developed for *D. immitis* prophylaxis in companion dogs and cats. Most modern chemoprophylactic agents for this purpose are macrocyclic lactones (e.g., ivermectin, moxidectin, selamectin) which are usually administered monthly in chewable or topical formulations; year-round administration is generally recommended by most veterinary professional bodies.[68,69] This is advisable not only for *D. immitis* prevention but also because many products are also labeled for the prevention of other helminth infections.[68,69] Individuals should apply insect repellant to reduce or prevent exposure through mosquito bites.[69] On a broader scale, extensive monitoring of domestic animals and wildlife along with vector control may be necessary for future public health interventions.[57]

GNATHOSTOMIASIS

Larval and sometimes subadult forms of spirurid nematodes belonging to the genus *Gnathostoma* may migrate through the subcutaneous tissues and organs of humans in a clinical condition also known as "larva migrans profundus." Adult gnathostomes are found embedded in tumor-like lesions in the gastric or esophageal wall of their normal mammalian definitive hosts (see Table 127-3), and eggs are passed through the gastrointestinal tract into the feces. Eggs entering bodies of water become embryonated and first-stage larvae hatch. The free-swimming larvae are consumed by first intermediate host *Cyclops* copepods, in which they molt to the infectious third stage. These copepods are in turn ingested by the second intermediate host (which includes a diversity of freshwater fish, eels, frogs, salamanders, snakes, some aquatic snails).[70–73] Humans are infected via the ingestion of undercooked second intermediate hosts or paratenic hosts such as rats, chickens, ducks, and piscivorous birds.[70,71,73] It may be possible for human infection to also occur via the ingestion of infected first intermediate host copepods in water, although this has not been well substantiated.

Multiple species of *Gnathostoma* may affect wildlife, but thus far only five species of *Gnathostoma* have been reported as affecting

TABLE 127-3 SUMMARY OF *GNATHOSTOMA* SPECIES REPORTED AS INFECTING HUMANS, THEIR GEOGRAPHIC DISTRIBUTION, AND DEFINITIVE HOSTS[72,113,114]

Species	Reported Geographic Distribution	Definitive Host(s)
Gnathostoma binucleatum	South and Central America, Mexico	Canids and Felids
Gnathostoma doloresi	Southeast Asia	Pigs
Gnathostoma hispidum	Southeast Asia, Australia, Europe	Pigs
Gnathostoma malaysiae[a]	Southeast Asia	Rats
Gnathostoma nipponicum	Japan	Weasels
Gnathostoma spinigerum	Asia (including India and Bangladesh), Southern Africa, Northern Australia	Canids and Felids

[a]Two possible cases of human infection with this species, acquired in Myanmar, have been reported.

humans, each with varying geographic range and definitive hosts (Table 127-3). Human disease is most prevalent in Mexico and Southeast Asia, but cases have been reported from all inhabited continents.[72] It is not clear whether or not genuine autochthonous transmission occurs in the United States. A recent case of ocular gnathostomiasis (possibly *G. binucleatum*) was diagnosed in Texas, though it is not clear whether the patient acquired the infection in the United States or during previous residence in Venezuela.[74] Early reports of *Gnathostoma spinigerum* in minks and raccoons from the United States probably represent *Gnathostoma procyonis* cases identified before description of said species; *G. procyonis* is not known to be zoonotic.[73]

Within 48 hours of ingesting an infected intermediate host, patients will often experience acute illness including vomiting, diarrhea, malaise, myalgias, fever, arthralgia, and/or epigastric pain. Later, the migration of the larva within the body most commonly presents as transient, migratory swellings and motile subcutaneous erythematous or urticarial tracks. Localizing the larva can be difficult; larvae may be able to move at approximately one cm per hour.[73] More severe symptoms occur when the larva migrate into the visceral organs; symptoms vary depending on the affected organ. *Gnathostoma* larvae are particularly known to migrate into the organs above the neck. Invasion of the eye can lead to visual impairment and orbital cellulitis, whereas neurognathostomiasis (invasion of the CNS) can lead to severe brain damage causing paralysis, seizures, and death.[72]

Peripheral eosinophilia is almost always present in cases of gnathostomiasis, and neurognathsostomiasis usually presents with eosinophilia in the CSF. Findings on magnetic resonance imaging or slit lamp examination, respectively, are particularly helpful for neurognathostomiasis and ocular gnathostomiasis. Diagnosis may be approached with a combination of clinical presentation, serologic testing, or extraction of the migrating larvae from the tissues. A crude larval 24 kDa antigen IgG4 Western blot has shown 92.9% sensitivity and 93.4% specificity for sera from *G. spinigerum* infected patients in Thailand,[75] but only 26.4% sensitivity for sera from *Gnathostoma binucleatum*-infected patients in Mexico.[76] Species may be determined by morphologic examination of extracted larvae or examination of the nuclei and structure of larval intestinal cells in histological section (Fig. 127-1D) by experienced parasitologists. PCR for eukaryotic mitochondrial genes such as ITS2 and COX1 followed by sequencing have also been used for this purpose.[72]

Gnathostomiasis has been successfully treated with albendazole, with cure rates of $> 90\%$ after 3 weeks of treatment. Albendazole treatment may cause the larvae to migrate to the skin, where spontaneous emergence or excision is possible. Ivermectin has a similar cure rate, but has been noted to cause exacerbation of cutaneous reactions during treatment. This host immunologic reaction to larval antigens presents a theoretical risk for the treatment of visceral, orbital, and neurologic disease.[71]

Adequate cooking of potential intermediate hosts is the optimal method for preventing gnathostomiasis. Experiments have shown that encysted larva in meat retain 20% infectivity rate after 48 hours at −2 to −4°C.[77] Freezing at −20°C for 3–5 days will effectively kill the larvae.[71] Marination of fish in vinegar for 6 hours or soy sauce for 12 hours will kill larvae,[73] but marination in lime juice does not kill larvae, even after 5 days.[71]

THELAZIASIS

While *Thelazia* spp. are not tissue invasive nematodes, they occupy the conjunctival sac and adjacent tissues of their definitive hosts. The larvae and adult worms of two species, *Thelazia callipaeda* and *Thelazia californiensis* are known to be causative agents of human ocular thelaziasis in Europe and Asia (*T. callipaeda*) and North America (*T. californiensis*).[16] Both species are parasites mainly of canids, but many other *Thelazia* spp. are parasites of ungulates or birds. A recent case of human infection with the cattle eyeworm, *Thelazia gulosa*, acquired in Oregon, USA has also been described.[78]

T. callipaeda has its origin in Asia, where the species is common in resource-constrained communities. However, it has recently emerged in Europe and appears to be rapidly enlarging its range on that continent.[79,80] The drosophilid flies, *Phortica variegata*, *P. okadai*, and *P. magna* serve as vectors and intermediate hosts of this worm.[81] The primary zoonotic species in the New World is *T. californiensis* ("California eyeworm") which has been reported infecting canids in the United States and Brazil. Human cases have thus far only been reported from California and Utah.[82] This species transmitted by houseflies *Fannia canicularis* and *Fannia benjamini*.[78,83] The vector of *T. gulosa* in North America is *Musca autumnalis*.[78]

Humans are infected when flies feed on lachrymal secretions from the eye. Larvae deposited into the eye develop into adults, which dwell in the conjuctival sac and tear film of definitive host. Intraocular invasion does not appear to occur. The presence of *Thelazia* adults in the conjunctiva may cause mild to severe ocular pathology, depending on the adult worm burden. In human cases, the number of worms is usually small and infection is generally noticed in the early stages of disease. Usual clinical features include hyperlacrimation, conjunctivitis, epiphora, with keratitis in prolonged cases. Prolonged, heavy, infection can also lead to blindness.[16,79,84,85]

Diagnosis requires careful ophthalmological examination following with morphological and/or molecular identification of extracted worms. Mechanical removal of the parasites is the primary treatment. The worms can be extracted with sterile tweezers or by rinsing with sterile saline solution under local anaesthesia.[79]

HEPATIC CAPILLARIASIS

Capillaria hepatica, also known as *Calodium hepaticum* in some countries, is a small nematode that infects the liver parenchyma of many animal hosts, including rodents, carnivores, swine, and primates. The adults are slender, delicate nematodes (females 50–70 mm long, 0.1–0.2 mm wide; males slightly smaller) that are buried within the liver parenchyma of the host and are very rarely seen.[16] Eggs are released into the surrounding tissue after the adult female dies and disintegrates but are not excreted—rather, the eggs are only released into the environment following either the decomposition of the first host's carcass, or predation by another suitable host and the passage of eggs through the second host's digestive tract. Transmission to a new host occurs when embryonated eggs are ingested. Larvae hatch in the small intestine and eventually migrate to the liver for maturation.[86]

In humans, hepatic capillariasis can lead to severe liver dysfunction. The inflammatory response to the eggs within the parenchyma creates extensive fibrosis and granuloma formation, with concomitant hepatomegaly and usually a persistent high fever. Cases are uncommon (72 true cases reported) and a few have proven fatal. Diagnosis can only be achieved through the visualization of eggs, or less commonly, adult worms, in a liver biopsy or autopsy specimen. Eggs superficially resemble those of *Trichuris* spp. but the double shell is distinctly pitted (has a radiating appearance when in cross section) and elliptical, and the poles do not noticeably protrude. It is important to note that occasionally *C. hepatica* eggs may be detected in human stools and that this does not indicate true infection. This is a result of spurious passage following the ingestion of infected animal liver.[86,87]

While human cases are infrequent, *C. hepatica* is common worldwide in rodents, and prevalence of close to 100% has been noted in some rodent populations.[88] Human cases are known to have occurred on all inhabited continents. There is no standard treatment protocol, but some cases have been successfully treated with benzimidazoles (thiabendazole, albendazole).[89]

ANISAKIASIS

Anisakiasis is caused by members of three species complexes: *Anisakis simplex* sensu lato, *Pseudoterranova decipiens* sensu lato, and *Contracecum osculatum* sensu lato.[90] These marine ascarids use cetaceans and pinnipeds as definitive hosts, and a variety of crustaceans and marine fishes as intermediate and paratenic hosts. Human infection is acquired by eating encysted larvae in undercooked fish. The most typical clinical presentation is the rapid onset (1–10 hours after ingestion) of nausea, vomiting, unusual throat sensations, and severe gastric pain associated with larval perforation into the gastrointestinal mucosa (usually the stomach). These symptoms may be misdiagnosed as appendicitis or peptic ulcers. Most infections spontaneously resolve (either through host immunity or if larvae are coughed up); however, infections that persist for longer than a few weeks or into deeper tissue can cause the development of eosinophilic granulomas, which can be mistaken for malignant tumors. Larvae that are embedded in mucosa can be seen by endoscopy and may also be removed in this process.[91] Identification to genus is based on features of the esophagus and intestine of larvae.[16]

Cases occur worldwide, but are particularly common in Japan and Northern Europe where dishes containing uncooked fish are popular cuisine. Infections are easily prevented by cooking fish to a temperature of 60°C throughout. Freezing to −35°C for > 15 hours or −23°C for at least 7 days renders larvae inviable; however, larval antigens that may be in the surrounding tissue are not inactivated in this process and can cause anaphylactic reactions in some individuals.[92]

DRACUNCULIASIS

The Guinea worm, *Dracunculus medinensis*, is a species of particular historical significance and has been known since antiquity. Adult female *D. medinensis* are long, slender, white worms (70–120 cm) that inhabit subcutaneous spaces of the host. Reproductively mature females eventually partially emerge from the skin, typically on the lower limbs and feet. This creates a bullous cutaneous reaction that is intensely pruritic, often compelling infected individuals to submerge affected limbs in water for relief. The gravid female extrudes her uterus into the water and releases free-swimming first-stage larvae. The larvae are infective to the copepod intermediate host (genus *Cyclops*), in which they molt to the final infective stage (third stage). Humans are infected primarily through drinking water containing infected copepods. The potential role of paratenic or transport hosts (fish, frogs) in the ecology and transmission of *D. medinensis* to humans is not well understood, though this is probably an important transmission route for other animal hosts.[93,94] The only effective means of treatment is through removal of the adult female worm, either through surgical means or through slowly winding the female around a stick as she emerges until the entire length has been extracted.[95]

Efforts to eradicate dracunculiasis/Guinea worm disease have been remarkably successful, bringing cases down from over 800,000 per year in 1989 to no more than about 30 human cases/year in recent years. The global effort was mounted in the 1980s by agencies such as the World Health Assembly and the Carter Center, and combined rigorous surveillance with strategies to break the transmission cycle of the parasite. The latter is achieved by containment of cases (occlusive bandaging, discouraging entering of water sources) and water sanitation (filtration to remove copepods). *D. medinensis* human cases now only occur in isolated pockets of the Sahel and below; since 2014 human cases have occurred in Chad, Ethiopia, Mali, and South Sudan with one case in Angola in 2018.[95] However, also in recent years, domestic and wild animals—including dogs, cats, and baboons—have been found to harbor infections with adult worms.[94,96] It is not yet clear how this challenge of an animal reservoir will impact eradication goals.

HAYCOCKNEMATOSIS

Haycocknema perplexum is a poorly understood, very rarely encountered nematode that infects and reproduces within the skeletal muscle of humans. Ten cases have been reported thus far, all from residents of either Tasmania or North Queensland (five cases each), Australia.[97] Symptom onset is insidious and occurs over 1–3 years, with patients describing increasing weight loss and decreasing muscle strength and tone. Muscle enzymes such as creatine kinase and aspartate aminotransferase are markedly elevated and all patients have peripheral eosinophilia.[97] Disease is often not diagnosed until an advanced and severe stage, when profound loss of muscle function may occur; one death has been reported.[98] Unencapsulated adult nematodes, including gravid females, migrate within and between the fibrils of the muscle, often showing serpentine appearance in both direct squash preparations and histologically stained transverse sections of muscle biopsies (Fig. 127-1E).[99] Nematodes migrate and reproduce within the muscle fibrils until they become sufficiently prevalent to be detected on muscle biopsy. One case has been diagnosed by PCR in the absence of detectable nematodes in the muscle.[97] The natural reservoir of disease and mode of transmission are unknown, though several of the cases have reported eating bush meat, hunting, or extensive interaction with Australian native animals.[99] Long-term (2–3 months) treatment with albendazole has proved effective.[98]

HALICEPHALOBIASIS

Halicephalobus gingivalis (formerly *Micronema deletrix*) is a facultative nematode pathogen that causes rapid, fatal meningoencephalitis in humans and equines.[100] Human infection is extremely rare, with only seven human cases described since the first in 1975; most cases occurred in the United States, though isolated cases have also occurred in Canada, South Australia, the United Kingdom, and Germany.[100–102] Three further cases have occurred in the United Kingdom, associated with transmission from one organ donor to two recipients, but this event was not well described in the medical literature.[102] Twenty-nine animal infections have been reported, mostly from horses, though one case each has been reported from a zebra, a donkey, and a cow.[100] Only four of these animals survived, all human cases have been fatal.[101] Treatment of one horse with both ivermectin and aggressive surgical debridement of the brain was successful.[101] Infection may be confined to the brain or may include other organs of the body (including the eyes, lungs, and kidneys). The disease is rapidly progressive and fatal in humans, with death usually occurring within 1 week of onset. On autopsy, live adult parasitic female worms, larvae, and eggs are found throughout the brain.[101]

The natural habitat and complete life cycle of the organism remains undefined, but it appears to dwell in soil or rotting vegetation and has been isolated from horse manure.[100,101] The adult parasitic female appears to reproduce parthenogenetically. Route of infection is unknown, though is it postulated to be through open wounds, or possibly invasion via the eye.[100] *H. gingivalis* have been isolated from semen and urine, and transmammary infection in a horse has been reported once. Fatal *H. gingivalis* meningoencephalitis has been reported in two organ transplant recipients, each within 2 weeks of receiving a kidney from a donor who died from undefined meningoencephalitis.[102] For cases with exposure information, infection was not associated with contact with horses.[103]

DIOCTOPHYMATOSIS

Dioctophyme (=*Dioctophyma*) *renale,* the giant kidney worm, is a remarkably large (females up to 102 cm), bright red nematode that invades the kidneys of various carnivore hosts, primarily mink and canids. The intermediate host is an aquatic oligochaete worm, and fish and amphibians are known to be paratenic hosts. Definitive hosts including humans become infected when they ingest an infected intermediate or paratenic host, the adult worm develops within the kidney. The large adult(s) eventually displace the parenchyma, which creates a hollow capsule and destroys renal function.[104] In infected dogs, hypertrophy of the unaffected kidney is often observed. Only ~15 cases have been reported in humans, usually presenting as abdominal pain and hematuria associated with passage of eggs in urine. Occasionally, larval migration to aberrant sites (e.g., subcutaneous) occurs in both the natural and aberrant definitive host.[16] The diagnosis of these such cases is usually based on examination of histological sections (Fig. 127-1F). Treatment involves nephrectomy of the affected kidney, or nephrotomy and extraction of the worm if in both kidneys although the latter situation is very rare.[105]

LAGOCHILASCARIASIS

Lagochilascaris spp. are small ascarids of wild and domestic cats in Central and South America, the best known being *L. minor*. In the natural definitive host, as well as in the known human cases, adult nematodes create nodules in subcutaneous spaces with a predilection for cervical and cephalic sites (e.g., larynx, pharynx, tongue, palate); nodules may be benign or become purulent and fistulous. Deeper migration may also occur. The approximately 60 confirmed zoonotic cases occurred in Mexico, Trinidad, Suriname, Venezuela, Colombia, Brazil, Bolivia, and Argentina, and at least one has been fatal.[106–108] Unlike other ascarids, transmission is likely solely through the consumption of undercooked paratenic host tissue (agoutis and other native rodents), as inoculation of cats with eggs in experimental trials has not resulted in infection. Autoinfection also apparently occurs, demonstrated by the finding of adult worms, larvae, and eggs in the same nodule (Fig. 127-1G).[109]

Disclaimer: The findings and conclusions in this report are those of the authors and do not necessarily represent the official position of the Centers for Disease Control and Prevention.

References

1. Magnaval J-F, Glickman LT, Dorchies P, Morassin B. Highlights of human toxocariasis. *Korean J Parasitol.* 2001;39:1–11.
2. Morimatsu Y, Akao N, Akiyoshi H, Kawazu T, Okabe Y, Aizawa H. A familial case of visceral larva migrans after ingestion of raw chicken livers: Appearance of specific antibody in bronchoalveolar lavage fluid of the patients. *Am J Trop Med Hyg.* 2006;75:303–6.
3. Yoshikawa M, Nishiofuku M, Moriya K, et al. A familial case of visceral toxocariasis due to consumption of raw bovine liver. *Parasitol Int.* 2008;57:525–9.
4. Taira K, Saitoh Y, Okada N, Sugiyama H, Kapel CMO. Tolerance to low temperatures of *Toxocara cati* larvae in chicken muscle tissue. *Vet Parasitol.* 2012;189:383–6.
5. Sharghi N, Schantz P, Hotez PJ. Toxocariasis: An occult cause of childhood neuropsychological deficits and asthma? *Seminars Pediatr Infect Dis.* 2000;4(11):257–60.
6. Sharghi N, Schantz PM, Caramico L, Ballas K, Teague BA, Hotez PJ. Environmental exposure to *Toxocara* as a possible risk factor for asthma: A clinic-based case-control study. *Clin Infect Dis.* 2001;32:e111–6.
7. Humbert P, Niezborala M, Salembier R, et al. Skin manifestations associated with toxocariasis: A case-control study. *Dermatology.* 2000;201:230–4.
8. Fillaux J, Magnaval J-F. Laboratory diagnosis of human toxocariasis. *Vet Parasitol.* 2013;193:327–36.
9. Moreira GMSG, de Lima Telmo P, Mendonça M, et al. Human toxocariasis: Current advances in diagnostics, treatment, and interventions. *Trends Parasitol.* 2014;30:456–64.
10. Woodhall D, Starr MC, Montgomery SP, et al. Ocular toxocariasis: Epidemiologic, anatomic, and therapeutic variations based on a survey of ophthalmic subspecialists. *Ophthalmology.* 2012;119:1211–7.
11. Lee RM, Moore LB, Bottazzi ME, Hotez PJ. Toxocariasis in North America: A systematic review. *PLoS Negl Trop Dis.* 2014;8:e3116.
12. Liu EW, Chastain HM, Shin SH, et al. Seroprevalence of antibodies to *Toxocara* species in the United States and associated risk factors, 2011–2014. *Clin Infect Dis.* 2017;66:206–12.
13. Macpherson CN. The epidemiology and public health importance of toxocariasis: A zoonosis of global importance. *Int J Parasitol.* 2013;43: 999–1008.
14. Lee AC, Schantz PM, Kazacos KR, Montgomery SP, Bowman DD. Epidemiologic and zoonotic aspects of ascarid infections in dogs and cats. *Trends Parasitol.* 2010;26:155–61.
15. International Commission on Trichinellosis. Species and Genotypes of *Trichinella.* 2018. http://www.trichinellosis.org/Species_and_Genotypes.html. Accessed 2019.
16. Miyazaki I. *An Illustrated Book of Helminthic Zoonoses.* Tokyo, Japan: International Medical Foundation of Japan; 1991.
17. Pozio E, Zarlenga DS. New pieces of the *Trichinella* puzzle. *Int J Parasitol.* 2013;43:983–97.
18. Gottstein B, Pozio E, Nockler K. Epidemiology, diagnosis, treatment, and control of trichinellosis. *Clin Microbiol Rev.* 2009;22:127–45, Table of Contents.
19. Hurnikova Z, Hrčková G, Ågren E, et al. First finding of *Trichinella pseudospiralis* in two Tawny Owls (Strix aluco) from Sweden. *Helminthologia.* 2014;51:190–7.
20. Tada K, Suzuki H, Sato Y, Morishima Y, Nagano I, Ishioka H, et al. Outbreak of *Trichinella* T9 infections associated with consumption of Bear Meat, Japan. *Emerg Infect Dis.* 2018;24:1532.
21. International Commission on Trichinellosis. Trichinellosis in Humans. 2018. http://www.trichinellosis.org/Trichinellosis_in_Humans.html. Accessed 2019.
22. Gamble H, Pozio E, Bruschi F, Nöckler K, Kapel C, Gajadhar A. International Commission on Trichinellosis: Recommendations on the use of serological tests for the detection of *Trichinella* infection in animals and man. *Parasite.* 2004;11:3–13.
23. Yang Y, Cai YN, Tong MW, et al. Serological tools for detection of *Trichinella* infection in animals and humans. *One Health.* 2016;2:25–30.
24. Kapel CMO. Changes in the EU legislation on *Trichinella* inspection—New challenges in the epidemiology. *Vet Parasitol.* 2005;132:189–94.
25. de Almeida M, Bishop H, Nascimento F, Mathison B, Bradbury R, da Silva A. Multiplex TaqMan qPCR assay for specific identification of encapsulated *Trichinella* species prevalent in North America. *Mem Inst Oswaldo Cruz.* 2018;113.
26. Dick TA, Pozio E. *Trichinella* spp. and trichinellosis. *Parasitic Diseases of Wild Mammals.* IA, Ames: Iowa State University Press. Vol. 2. 2001, pp. 380–96.
27. Sapp SGH, Gupta P, Martin MK, et al. Beyond the raccoon roundworm: The natural history of non-raccoon *Baylisascaris* species in the New World. Int J Parasitol Parasites Wildl. 2017;6:85–99.
28. Kazacos K. Baylisascaris Larva Migrans—Circular 1412. US Geological Survey. 2016.
29. Sapp SGH, Rascoe LN, Wilkins PP, et al. *Baylisascaris procyonis* roundworm seroprevalence among wildlife rehabilitators, United States and Canada, 2012–2015. *Emerg Infect Dis.* 2016;22:2128.
30. Hung T, Neafie RC, Mackenzie IR. *Baylisascaris procyonis* infection in elderly person, British Columbia, Canada. *Emerg Infect Dis.* 2012;18:341.
31. Rascoe LN, Santamaria C, Handali S, et al. Inter-laboratory optimization and evaluation of a serological assay for diagnosis of human baylisascariasis. *Clin Vaccine Immunol.* 2013;20:1758–63.
32. Sircar AD. Raccoon roundworm infection associated with central nervous system disease and ocular disease—Six states, 2013–2015. *MMWR Morb Mortal Wkly Rep.* 2016;65(35):930–3.

33. Sapp SGH, Murray B, Hoover ER, Green GT, Yabsley MJ. Raccoon roundworm (*Baylisascaris procyonis*) as an occupational hazard: 2. Use of personal protective equipment and infection control practices among raccoon rehabilitators. *Zoonoses Public Health*. 2018;65:490–500.

34. Alicata J. The discovery of *Angiostrongylus cantonensis* as a cause of human eosinophilic meningitis. *Parasitol Today*. 1991;7:151–3.

35. Martins YC, Tanowitz HB, Kazacos KR. Central nervous system manifestations of *Angiostrongylus cantonensis* infection. *Acta Trop*. 2015;141:46–53.

36. Barratt J, Chan D, Sandaradura I, et al. *Angiostrongylus cantonensis*: A review of its distribution, molecular biology and clinical significance as a human pathogen. *Parasitology*. 2016;143:1087–118.

37. Liu EW, Schwartz BS, Hysmith ND, et al. Rat lungworm infection associated with central nervous system disease—Eight US states, January 2011–January 2017. *Morb Mortal Wkly Rep*. 2018;67:825.

38. Kliks MM, Palumbo NE. Eosinophilic meningitis beyond the Pacific Basin: The global dispersal of a peridomestic zoonosis caused by *Angiostrongylus cantonensis*, the nematode lungworm of rats. *Soc Sci Med*. 1992;34:199–212.

39. Lai C-H, Yen C-M, Chin C, Chung H-C, Kuo H-C, Lin H-H. Eosinophilic meningitis caused by *Angiostrongylus cantonensis* after ingestion of raw frogs. *Am J Trop Med Hyg*. 2007;76:399–402.

40. Wallace GD, Rosen L. Studies on eosinophilic meningitis. 2. Experimental infection of shrimp and crabs with *Angtostrongylus cantonensis*. *Am J Epidemiol*. 1966;84:120–31.

41. Prociv P, Spratt DM, Carlisle MS. Neuro-angiostrongyliasis: Unresolved issues. *Int J Parasitol*. 2000;30:1295–303.

42. Ubelaker JE, Bullick GR, Caruso J. Emergence of third-stage larvae of *Angiostrongylus costaricensis* Morera and Cespedes 1971 from *Biomphalaria glabrata* (Say). *J Parasitol*. 1980;66:856–7.

43. Ash LR. Observations on the role of mollusks and planarians in the transmission of *Angiostrongylus cantonensis* infection to man in New Caledonia. *Rev Biol Trop*. 1976;24:163–74.

44. Tseng Y-T, Tsai H-C, Sy CL, et al. Clinical manifestations of eosinophilic meningitis caused by *Angiostrongylus cantonensis*: 18 Years' experience in a medical center in southern Taiwan. *J Microbiol Immunol Infect*. 2011;44:382–9.

45. Lindo J, Escoffery C, Reid B, Codrington G, Cunningham-Myrie C, Eberhard M. Fatal autochthonous eosinophilic meningitis in a Jamaican child caused by *Angiostrongylus cantonensis*. *Am J Trop Med Hyg*. 2004;70:425–8.

46. Cross J. Public health importance of *Angiostrongylus cantonensis* and its relatives. *Parasitol Today*. 1987;3:367–9.

47. Qvarnstrom Y, Xayavong M, da Silva ACA, et al. Real-time polymerase chain reaction detection of *Angiostrongylus cantonensis* DNA in cerebrospinal fluid from patients with eosinophilic meningitis. *Am J Trop Med Hyg*. 2016;94:176–81.

48. Wilkins PP, Qvarnstrom Y, Whelen AC, Saucier C, da Silva AJ, Eamsobhana P. The current status of laboratory diagnosis of *Angiostrongylus cantonensis* infections in humans using serologic and molecular methods. *Hawaii J Med Public Health*. 2013;72:55.

49. Centers for Disease Control and Prevention. Angiostrongyliasis: Resources for Health Professionals. 2018. https://www.cdc.gov/parasites/angiostrongylus/health_professionals/index.html#tx. Accessed January 30, 2019.

50. Morera P, Céspedes R. *Angiostrongylus costaricensis* n. sp. (Nematoda: Metastrongyloidea), a new lungworm occurring in man in Costa Rica. *Rev Biol Trop*. 1971;18:173–85.

51. Morera P. Life history and redescription of *Angiostrongylus costaricensis* Morera and Céspedes, 1971. *Am J Trop Med Hyg*. 1973;22:613–21.

52. Miller CL, Kinsella JM, Garner MM, Evans S, Gullett PA, Schmidt RE. Endemic infections of *Parastrongylus* (= *Angiostrongylus*) *costaricensis* in two species of nonhuman primates, raccoons, and an opossum from Miami, Florida. *J Parasitol*. 2006;92:406–8.

53. Rodriguez R, Dequi RM, Peruzzo L, Mesquita PM, Garcia E, Fornari F. Abdominal angiostrongyliasis: Report of two cases with different clinical presentations. *Rev Inst Med Trop Sao Paulo*. 2008;50:339–41.

54. Mota EM, Lenzi HL. *Angiostrongylus costaricensis*: Complete redescription of the migratory pathways based on experimental *Sigmodon hispidus* infection. *Mem Inst Oswaldo Cruz*. 2005;100:407–20.

55. Morera P, Perez F, Mora F, Castro L. Visceral larva migrans-like syndrome caused by *Angiostrongylus costaricensis*. *Am J Trop Med Hyg*. 1982;31:67–70.

56. Sałamatin R, Pavlikovska T, Sagach O, et al. Human dirofilariasis due to *Dirofilaria repens* in Ukraine, an emergent zoonosis: Epidemiological report of 1465 cases. *Acta Parasitol*. 2013;58:592–8.

57. Diaz JH. Increasing risks of human dirofilariasis in travelers. *J Travel Med*. 2014;22:116–23.

58. Paul M, Pielok Ł, Kłudkowska M, Frąckowiak K, Masny A, Gołąb E. An unusual clinical course of human subcutaneous dirofilariosis with intensive microfilariemia in peripheral blood. *J Trop Dis Public Health*. 2017;5:1-5.

59. Simón F, González-Miguel J, Diosdado A, Gómez PJ, Morchón R, Kartashev V. The complexity of zoonotic filariasis episystem and its consequences: A multidisciplinary view. *BioMed Res Int*. 2017;2017:6436130.

60. Orihel TC, Eberhard ML. Zoonotic filariasis. *Clin Microbiol Rev*. 1998;11:366–81.

61. Moorhouse D. *Dirofilaria immitis*: A cause of human intra-ocular infection. *Infection*. 1978;6:192–3.

62. Goldstein, JD, Smith DR. *Dirofilaria immitis* in a portacaval shunt. *Hum Pathol*. 1985;16(11),1172–3.

63. Cancrini G. Human infections due to nematode helminths nowadays: Epidemiology and diagnostic tools. *Parassitologia*. 2006;48:53–6.

64. Antolová D, Miterpáková M, Paraličová Z. Case of human *Dirofilaria repens* infection manifested by cutaneous larva migrans syndrome. *Parasitol Res*. 2015;114:2969–73.

65. Kłudkowska M, Pielok Ł, Frąckowiak K, Masny A, Gołąb E, Paul M. *Dirofilaria repens* infection as a cause of intensive peripheral microfilariemia in a Polish patient: Process description and cases review. *Acta Parasitol*. 2018;63:657–63.

66. Potters I, Vanfraechem G, Bottieau E. *Dirofilaria repens* Nematode Infection with Microfilaremia in Traveler Returning to Belgium from Senegal. *Emerg Infect Dis*. 2018;24:1761.

67. Blaizot R, Receveur M-C, Millet P, Otranto D, Malvy DJ. Systemic infection with *Dirofilaria repens* in Southwestern France. *Ann Intern Med*. 2018;168:228–9.

68. Companion Animal Parasite Council. CAPC Guidelines: Heartworm. 2016. https://capcvet.org/guidelines/heartworm/. Accessed October 7, 2019.

69. Dantas-Torres F, Otranto D. Best practices for preventing vector-borne diseases in dogs and humans. *Trends Parasitol*. 2016;32:43–55.

70. Beaver PC, Jung RC, Cupp EW, Craig CF. *Clin Parasitol*. Philadelphia: Lea & Febige; 1984.

71. Herman JS, Chiodini PL.Gnathostomiasis, another emerging imported disease. *Clin Microbiol Rev*. 2009;22:484–92.

72. Dekumyoy P, Yoonuan T, Waikagul J. Gnathostoma. *Molecular Detection of Parasitic Pathogens*. Boca Raton: CRC Press; 2013, pp. 563–70.

73. Rusnak JM, Lucey DR. Clinical gnathostomiasis: Case report and review of the English-language literature. *Clin Infect Dis*. 1993;16:33–50.

74. Benavides MA, Baldo MB, Tauber S, Figueiras SF, Incani RN, Nawa Y. Case report: Ocular gnathostomiasis in Venezuela most likely acquired in Texas. *Am J Trop Med Hyg*. 2018;99:1028–32.

75. Laummaunwai P, Sawanyawisuth K, Intapan PM, Chotmongkol V, Wongkham C, Maleewong W. Evaluation of human IgG class and subclass antibodies to a 24 kDa antigenic component of *Gnathostoma spinigerum* for the serodiagnosis of gnathostomiasis. *Parasitol Res*. 2007;101:703–8.

76. Zambrano-Zaragoza JF, de Jesús Durán-Avelar M, Messina-Robles M, Vibanco-Pérez N. Characterization of the humoral immune response against *Gnathostoma binucleatum* in patients clinically diagnosed with gnathostomiasis. *Am J Trop Med Hyg*. 2012;86:988–92.

77. Rojekittikhun W, Buchachart K. The infectivity of frozen *Gnathostoma spinigerum* encysted larvae in mice. *J Trop Med Parasitol*. 2002;25:79–82.

78. Bradbury RS, Breen KV, Bonura EM, Hoyt JW, Bishop HS. Case report: Conjunctival infestation with *Thelazia gulosa*: A novel agent of human thelaziasis in the United States. *Am J Trop Med Hyg*. 2018;98:1171–74.

79. Shen J, Gasser RB, Chu D, et al. Human thelaziosis—A neglected parasitic disease of the eye. *J Parasitol*. 2006;92:872–6.

80. Čabanová V, Miterpáková M, Oravec M, et al. Nematode *Thelazia callipaeda* is spreading across Europe. The first survey of red foxes from Slovakia. *Acta Parasitol*. 2018;63:160–6.

81. Máca J, Otranto D. Drosophilidae feeding on animals and the inherent mystery of their parasitism. *Parasites Vectors*. 2014;7:516.

82. Doezie AM, Lucius RW, Aldeen W, Hale D, Smith DR, Mamalis N. *Thelazia californiensis* conjunctival infestation. *Ophthalmic Surg Lasers Imaging Retina*. 1996;27:716–9.

83. Anderson RC. *Nematode Parasites of Vertebrates: Their Development and Transmission*. Wallingford, UK: CABI Publishing; 2000.

84. Magnis J, Naucke TJ, Mathis A, Deplazes P, Schnyder M. Local transmission of the eye worm *Thelazia callipaeda* in southern Germany. *Parasitol Res*. 2010;106:715–7.

85. Marino V, Gálvez R, Colella V, et al. Detection of *Thelazia callipaeda* in *Phortica variegata* and spread of canine thelaziosis to new areas in Spain. *Parasites Vectors.* 2018;11:195.

86. Fuehrer H-P, Igel P, Auer H. *Capillaria hepatica* in man—An overview of hepatic capillariosis and spurious infections. *Parasitol Res.* 2011;109:969–79.

87. Gonçalves AQ, Ascaso C, Santos I, Serra PT, Julião GR, Orlandi PP. *Calodium hepaticum*: Household clustering transmission and the finding of a source of human spurious infection in a community of the Amazon region. *PLoS Negl Trop Dis.* 2012;6:e1943.

88. Fuehrer H-P. An overview of the host spectrum and distribution of *Calodium hepaticum* (syn. *Capillaria hepatica*): part 1—Muroidea. *Parasitol Res.* 2014;113:619–40.

89. Pereira VG, Franca LCM. Successful treatment of *Capillaria hepatica* infection in an acutely ill adult. *Am J Trop Med Hyg.* 1983;32:1272–4.

90. Mattiucci S, Cipriani P, Webb SC, et al. Genetic and morphological approaches distinguish the three sibling species of the *Anisakis simplex* species complex, with a species designation as *Anisakis berlandi* n. sp. for *A. simplex* sp. C (Nematoda: Anisakidae). *J Parasitol.* 2014;100:199–214.

91. Sakanari J, Mckerrow JH. Anisakiasis. *Clin Microbiol Rev.* 1989;2:278–84.

92. Audicana MaT, Ansotegui IJ, de Corres LF, Kennedy MW. *Anisakis simplex*: dangerous—Dead and alive? *Trends Parasitol.* 2002;18:20–5.

93. Cleveland CA, Eberhard ML, Thompson AT, et al. Possible role of fish as transport hosts for *Dracunculus* spp. larvae. *Emerg Infect Dis.* 2017;23:1590.

94. Cleveland CA, Eberhard ML, Thompson AT, Garrett KB, Swanepoel L, Zirimwabagabo H, et al. A search for tiny dragons (*Dracunculus medinensis* third-stage larvae) in aquatic animals in Chad, Africa. *Sci Rep.* 2019;9:375.

95. Ruiz-Tiben E, Hopkins DR. Dracunculiasis (Guinea worm disease) eradication. *Adv Parasitol.* 2006;61:275–309.

96. Eberhard ML, Ruiz-Tiben E, Hopkins DR.Dogs and Guinea worm eradication. *Lancet Infect Dis.* 2016;16:1225–6.

97. Koehler A, Leung P, McEwan B, Gasser R. Using PCR-based sequencing to diagnose *Haycocknema perplexum* infection in human myositis case, Australia. *Emerg Infect Dis.* 2018;24:2368.

98. Vos LJ, Robertson T, Binotto E. *Haycocknema perplexum*: An emerging cause of parasitic myositis in Australia. *Commun Dis Intell Q Rep.* 2016;40:E496–9.

99. Koehler AV, Spratt DM, Norton R, et al. More parasitic myositis cases in humans in Australia, and the definition of genetic markers for the causative agents as a basis for molecular diagnosis. *Infect Genet Evol.* 2016;44:69–75.

100. Onyiche TE, Okute TO, Oseni OS, Okoro DO, Biu AA, Mbaya AW. Parasitic and zoonotic meningoencephalitis in humans and equids: Current knowledge and the role of *Halicephalobus gingivalis. Parasite Epidemiol Control.* 2018;3:36–42.

101. Lim CK, Crawford A, Moore CV, et al. First human case of fatal *Halicephalobus gingivalis* meningoencephalitis in Australia. *J Clin Microbiol.* 2015;53:1768–74.

102. Cooper AJ, Dholakia S, Holland CV, Friend PJ. Helminths in organ transplantation. *Lancet Infect Dis.* 2017;17:e166–76.

103. Ondrejka SL, Procop GW, Lai KK, Prayson RA. Fatal parasitic meningoencephalomyelitis caused by *Halicephalobus deletrix*: A case report and review of the literature. *Arch Pathol Lab Med.* 2010;134:625–9.

104. Mace T, Anderson R. Development of the giant kidney worm, *Dioctophyma renale* (Goeze, 1782) (Nematoda: Dioctophymatoidea). *Can J Zoo.* 1975;53:1552–68.

105. Mesquita L, Rahal SC, Faria L, et al. Pre-and post-operative evaluations of eight dogs following right nephrectomy due to *Dioctophyma renale. Vet Q.* 2014;34:167–71.

106. Botero D, Little M. Two cases of human *Lagochilascaris infection* in Colombia. *Am J Trop Med Hyg.* 1984;33:381–6.

107. Volcan GS, Ochoa FR, Medrano CE, de Valera Y. *Lagochilascaris minor* infection in Venezuela. *Am J Trop Med Hyg.* 1982;31:1111–3.

108. Rosemberg S, Lopes M, Masuda Z, Campos R, Bressan MV. Fatal encephalopathy due to *Lagochilascaris minor* infection. *Am J Trop Med Hyg.* 1986;35:575–8.

109. Paçô JM, Campos DMB, Oliveira JA. Wild rodents as experimental intermediate hosts of *Lagochilascaris minor* Leiper, 1909. *Mem Inst Oswaldo Cruz.* 1999;94:441–9.

110. Lacour SA, Heckmann A, Macé P, et al. Freeze-tolerance of *Trichinella* muscle larvae in experimentally infected wild boars. *Vet Parasitol.* 2013;194:175–8.

111. Feidas H, Kouam MK, Kantzoura V, Theodoropoulos G. Global geographic distribution of *Trichinella* species and genotypes. *Infect Genet Evol.* 2014;26:255–66.

112. Pozio E. Adaptation of *Trichinella* spp. for survival in cold climates. *Food Waterborne Parasitol.* 2016;4:4–12.

113. Nomura Y, Nagakura K, Kagei N, Tsutsumi Y, Araki K, Sugawara M. Gnathostomiasis possibly caused by *Gnathostoma malaysiae. Tokai J Exp Clin Med.* 2000;25:1–6.

114. Liu G-H, Shao R, Cai X-Q, Li W-W, Zhu X-Q. *Gnathostoma spinigerum* mitochondrial genome sequence: A novel gene arrangement and its phylogenetic position within the class Chromadorea. *Sci Rep.* 2015;5:12691.

CHAPTER

128

Schistosomiasis

Richard S. Bradbury • W. Evan Secor

Schistosomiasis, or bilharziasis, is a chronic debilitating disease associated with significant morbidity and mortality. The disease affects more than 190 million[1] people in 78 countries[2] worldwide and is second only to malaria among parasitic diseases in socioeconomic and public health importance in tropical and subtropical areas.[1] Most human disease is caused by three species of blood flukes of the genus *Schistosoma*: *S. mansoni, S. haematobium, S. japonicum. S. mekongi, S. intercalatum, S. guineensis,* and some rare zoonotic species can also infect people.

BIOLOGY AND LIFE CYCLES

The schistosome requires an intermediate and a definitive host to complete its life cycle. Asexual reproduction takes place in the molluscan intermediate host and sexual reproduction in the definitive vertebrate host. Briefly, free-swimming miracidia hatch from eggs deposited in freshwater during defecation or urination by an infected definitive host. These miracidia penetrate the snail host and develop into primary sporocysts, each of which produces multiple secondary sporocysts. Each of the secondary sporocysts produces a great number of cercariae, resulting in the production of hundreds to thousands of cercariae from an individual miracidium. The fork-tailed cercariae migrate out of the snail under appropriate environmental stimuli, usually heat and light, and move toward the surface of the water. Of note, both free living stages (miracidia and cercariae) have a limited life span in the absence of an appropriate host (6–24 hours under experimental conditions).[3] Sporocysts, on the other hand, can remain dormant in estivating snails during adverse conditions and resume cercarial production with the return of a favorable environment.

When humans contact schistosome-infested water, cercariae penetrate the skin, lose their tails, and transform into the schistosomula life stage. After several days, the schistosomula enter a venule or lymphatic vessel and migrate to the right side of the heart, then to the lungs, and finally to the liver sinusoids, where they begin to mature. On reaching maturity, adult male and female worms pair and migrate to their final destinations, which differ by schistosome species. There, eggs are released from adult females into the venules of the intestine or urinary bladder, break through the submucosa and mucosa into the lumen, and are evacuated through the feces or urine, again depending on the species, to complete the life cycle.

The size of adult schistosomes varies by species. Mature female *S. haematobium* measure up to 20 mm in length by 0.25 mm in width at the widest point, whereas the mature males measure from 10 to 15 mm in length and 0.8–1 mm in width. Adult worms of *S. mansoni* are smaller, with females measuring 7.2–17 mm long and males 6.4–12 mm in length.[4] Adult male and female schistosomes live *in copula* an average of 5–8 years but sometimes for as long as 30 years (Fig. 128-1).[5] Adult *S. japonicum* and *S. mekongi* parasites are generally found in the superior mesenteric veins and *S. mansoni* in the inferior mesenteric veins of the lower bowel. *S. haematobium* resides in the vesicular and pelvic venous plexuses around the bladder, but may ectopically migrate to the inferior venous plexus around the rectum. *S. intercalatum* and *S. guineensis* inhabit the inferior mesenteric plexus but lower in the bowel than *S. mansoni*.[6] Daily egg production also varies from approximately 1500–3000 eggs per day per worm pair in *S. japonicum* infection to approximately 250 eggs per day in *S. mansoni* infection and 50–100 eggs/day in *S. haematobium* infection. Biological differences between schistosome species impact both the clinical manifestations and infection transmission rates.

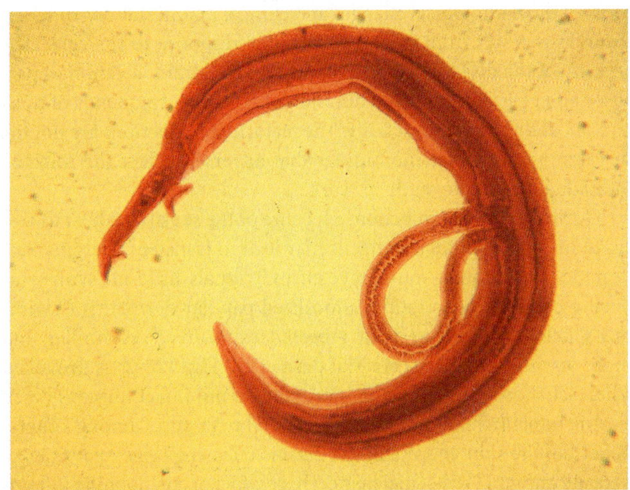

FIGURE 128-1. Adult *Schistosoma mansoni*, the smaller adult female fluke permanently resides within the gynaecophoric canal of the larger adult male fluke within the enteric venous plexus. (Dr. Richard S. Bradbury.)

DISTRIBUTION

Schistosomiasis is endemic in many tropical and subtropical countries and is a frequent reason for travel clinic visits, particularly for travelers to Africa.[7,8] The distribution of schistosomiasis is dependent on the presence of the appropriate intermediate snail host and necessary environmental conditions. *S. mansoni* (intermediate host: *Biomphalaria* spp.) has the most widespread distribution, ranging from the Arabian peninsula to South America and the Caribbean.[9] *S. japonicum* (intermediate host: *Oncomelania* spp.) is confined to the Far East, distributed in parts of China, the Indonesian island of Sulawesi (*S. japonicum*-like), and the Philippines. Japan was previously endemic for *S. japonicum* and is one of the few countries where elimination of schistosomiasis has been validated. A species related to *S. japonicum*, *S. mekongi* (intermediate host: *Neotricula* spp.), is found in Laos, Cambodia, and Thailand. *S. haematobium* (intermediate host: *Bulinus* spp.) is endemic in the Middle East and Africa.

Recently, hybrids of *S. haematobium* with *S. bovis* have been identified in infected humans in West Africa and on the French island of Corsica.[10] *S. guineensis* (intermediate host: a range of *Bulinus* spp.) occurs in São Tomé, Equatorial Guinea, Cameroon, Nigeria, and Gabon. *S. intercalatum* is found only in the Democratic Republic of Congo.[11] *Bulinus globosus* and *Bulinus wrighti* are the intermediate hosts for this species.[12]

Although natural infection of rodents and nonhuman primates with *S. mansoni* and *S. haematobium* has been described, animals other than humans do not appear to be major reservoirs of infection with these species. Important reservoir hosts for *S. japonicum* include mice, dogs, goats, rabbits, cattle, sheep, rats, pigs, horses, and buffalo.[13] Dogs and pigs may be important reservoir hosts for *S. mekongi*.

PATHOLOGICAL AND CLINICAL MANIFESTATIONS

Most of the pathological changes and clinical manifestations of schistosomiasis result from the host's immune response to the eggs. The severity of the disease depends on the species, strain, location of parasites and eggs, intensity and duration of infection, frequency of reinfection, and the host's reactivity. The majority of infections are not life threatening but cause morbidities that adversely affect the infected individual's ability to study or work.

During the initial infection, exposure of the sensitized host to cercarial or schistosomular antigens may lead to transient allergic manifestations. Although most infected individuals have no symptoms during cercarial penetration, a localized papular dermatitis ("swimmer's itch") may occur with repeated exposures.[14] A similar, but more intense, reaction (cercarial dermatitis, Fig. 128-2) is provoked when schistosome species that normally do not infect humans (such as *Australobilharzia* spp. and *Ornithobilharzia* spp., among others) penetrate the skin and die in the dermis releasing large quantities of parasite antigen.[15] Petechial hemorrhages, foci of eosinophilic inflammation, and leukocytic infiltration may be produced in the lung or in the liver when schistosomula migrate through the lungs and reach the liver. During this period, transitional symptoms of fever, malaise, cough, and a generalized allergic reaction may appear. When present, symptoms generally resolve in 5–15 days without treatment.

Acute schistosomiasis, or Katayama fever, describes an immune hypersensitivity reaction in response to migration of the schistosomula in the first weeks to months after infection. Occurring most commonly in persons with heavy *S. japonicum* or *S. mansoni* infection, the clinical manifestations are characterized by a serum sickness-like syndrome of fever, chills, cough, arthralgias and myalgias, diarrhea, eosinophilia, hepatosplenomegaly, urticaria, generalized lymphadenopathy, and patchy infiltrates that can be observed using chest radiography.[16,17] Recovery usually occurs within several weeks, but fatalities do occur. The syndrome most likely reflects the strong host immune response to egg antigens and the formation and deposition of circulating immune complexes.

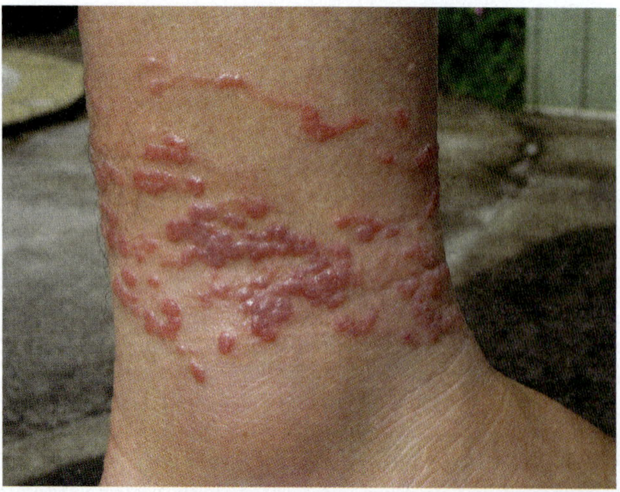

FIGURE 128-2. Cercarial dermatitis of the ankle following exposure to cercariae of bird schistosomes on the surface of a freshwater lake. (Dr. Richard S. Bradbury.)

As the infections become chronic, egg deposition and excretion increase. The intestinal schistosomes (*S. japonicum, S. mekongi, S. mansoni, S. guineensis,* and *S. intercalatum*) release eggs into the mesenteric veins. Some of these become lodged in the intestinal submucosa, where they secrete proteolytic enzymes that erode the tissue, break through the intestinal wall, enter the lumen of the gut, and pass out of the body in feces. In heavy infection, this may cause diarrhea and blood in the stool. Other eggs may be trapped at the original site or swept back into the portal blood flow and distributed to the liver, spleen, or other ectopic foci, where they provoke inflammatory tissue responses and granuloma formation. This may cause a range of symptoms including abdominal pain, fatigue, delay of physical or cognitive development, thrombosis of vessels, formation of polyps in the intestinal wall, and organomegaly. In *S. mansoni* infection, the rectum and colon are affected more frequently than other parts of the gastrointestinal tract and rectal bleeding may be observed. The severity of symptoms is correlated with the number of eggs and their anatomic location. Consequently, *S. japonicum*, which has the highest capacity for egg production and the widest egg distribution, is a more common cause of symptomatic infections than other schistosomes. Fortunately, at this stage successful treatment reverses most of the symptoms.

Although most individuals with chronic intestinal schistosomiasis have mild to moderate pathology, egg-induced granuloma formation in persons with chronic heavy infections can lead to fibrous proliferation around the portal veins and vascular occlusion. Other manifestations include inflammatory polyps, thickening of the intestinal wall and adhesions of the thickened mesentery and omentum to the intestine. Secondary intestinal obstruction and bacterial infection such as recurrent *Salmonella* bacteremia can also occur.[18] Hepatosplenomegaly may be pronounced. Over time, the liver gradually shrinks in size as a result of increasing fibrosis in a periportal distribution, a condition called Symmers' pipestem fibrosis. This may result in blockage of presinusoidal blood flow, leading to portal hypertension, ascites, collateral circulation, and esophageal varices. An association between hepatosplenic schistosomiasis and nephrotic syndrome secondary to immune complex glomerulonephritis has been well documented.[19] Once initiated, schistosome-induced fibrosis may progress despite resolution of the initial infection.[20]

Pulmonary schistosomiasis has been reported in persons infected with any of the five species that cause intestinal schistosomiasis. Eggs may be carried to the lungs by venous shunting through systemic collateral vessels formed as a result of portal hypertension or because of aberrant migration of worms into the vena caval or vertebral venous systems. The resultant granulomatous arteritis of the pulmonary capillary bed may lead to obliterative arteriolitis, dilatation of the pulmonary arteries, and pulmonary hypertension. Rarely, this leads to cor pulmonale with right-sided heart failure.

In *S. haematobium* infections, adult worms in the veins surrounding the urinary bladder deposit eggs into the vesicular plexus. These commonly cause dysuria, urinary frequency, proteinuria, and hematuria. Inflammatory polypoid masses in the bladder or ureteral walls are common early in infection and are a significant cause of obstructive uropathy. Eggs may also be carried by the venous system to the genital organs, gastrointestinal tract, lungs, and liver. As with intestinal schistosomiasis, successful treatment at this stage reverses most of the symptoms.

As urogenital schistosomiasis becomes chronic, fibrosis and calcification of the eggs in the urinary bladder may impair bladder function. Fibrosis of the neck of the bladder and of the opening of the ureter result in obstruction of urine flow and may lead to the development of hydroureter, hydronephrosis, renal stones and, rarely, renal failure. Chronic ulceration and irritation of the bladder epithelium may in time lead to malignant transformation and the development of squamous cell carcinoma of the bladder. Eggs deposited in genital tissue lead to development of female genital schistosomiasis (FGS) or male genital schistosomiasis (MGS). Development of "sandy patches" in the cervix and vaginal wall are characteristic FGS,[21] which has been associated with transmission of sexually transmitted infections, development of malignancies of the genital tract, and subfertility. Both FGS and MGS may also increase transmission of, and susceptibility to, HIV through heterosexual intercourse.

Occasionally, ectopic eggs may cause granuloma formation in the central nervous system, resulting in cerebrospinal schistosomiasis.[22] Brain involvement is most common in *S. japonicum* infection, and may present acutely as meningoencephalitis.[12,31] Seizures are the predominant manifestation. *S. mansoni* and *S. haematobium* more commonly affect the spinal cord, causing transverse myelitis.[23]

COINFECTIONS

The immune response to helminth infections, including schistosomiasis, is characterized by a Th2-type immune response with eosinophilia and elevated serum IgE levels. By contrast, viruses and protozoa generally induce Th1-type immune responses. Because of Th1/Th2 cross regulation, the immunological and clinical effects of coinfection with schistosomes and Th1-inducing pathogens reflect the balance between their opposing responses.[24–26] In some infections, such as viral hepatitis C, coinfection with schistosomes leads to more severe liver disease, with higher viral titers and increased mortality.[25] *Salmonella* species sequestered within schistosome adults may lead to prolonged shedding of typhoidal serovars of *Salmonella enterica* (S. Typhi, S. Paratyphi A, and S. Paratyphi B) as well as *S. typhimurium,* in infected hosts.[27] Urinary tract infections may also be associated with the delayed or prolonged *Salmonella* septicaemia that can occur during schistosomiasis mansoni or haematobium,[18,28,29] including protection of the bacteria within the schistosomes from some classes of antibiotics.[29] It has been suggested, though not confirmed, that the two pathogens in synergy may even augment the host immune response and resultant pathology caused by schistosomiasis. The potential immunosuppressive impact of schistosomiasis on HIV, including the reduction of CD4 cell counts, and potential decreased resistance to reinfection with schistosomes in HIV positive patients are examples of these.[30] Schistosome infections coincident with tuberculosis may cause persistent epigenetic alterations.[31]

DIAGNOSIS

Definitive diagnosis of schistosomiasis is made by identifying characteristic eggs in stool or urine samples. Eggs of *S. japonicum* are 70–100 μm long by 50–65 μm and round to suboval in shape. They possess an inconspicuous comma shaped recurved spinous process, which will only be seen when the egg is correctly oriented. *S. mekongi* have a very similar appearance but are smaller (40–45 μm in length) and possess an inconspicuous knob rather than a recurved spinous process.[4] *S. mansoni* eggs are large, 114–175 μm by 45–68 μm, with an elongate oval shape and a prominent lateral spine. *S. haematobium* eggs are 112–170 μm by 40–70 μm and have an elongate oval shape with a prominent terminal spine. *S. guineensis* and *S. intercalatum* eggs are larger than the other schistosomes that infect humans at 140–240 μm by 50–85 μm.[4] They are elongated and oval, but bilaterally taper at each end, presenting a "fluted" shape, with *S. guineensis* having slightly greater bilateral indentations than *S. intercalatum.*[12]

The quantitative Kato-Katz technique is a rapid and simple method to detect *Schistosoma* eggs in stool. This method remains widely used in surveys of prevalence. One study compared a combined reference standard of triplicate Kato Katz, single formalin-ethyl acateate concentrate and quadruplicate FLOTAC employing flotation solution 4 (FS4; sodium nitrate) and FS7 (zinc sulfate), and tested at intervals between zero and 83 days postcollection in dilute formalin or sodium acetate formalin preserved samples. This found that a single Kato-Katz slide has a sensitivity of 68% for *S. mansoni*, rising to 77% if three stools are tested whereas formalin-ethyl acateate concentration had a sensitivity of 85%. FLOTAC on fresh feces had a sensitivity of only 69%, but this rose incrementally to 75.9% if performed at 30 or 83 days post-collection on preserved samples.[32] In diagnostic settings, the formalin-ethyl acetate concentration method appears to be the most sensitive and immediate phenotypic method currently available. Multiple fecal samples should be tested in persons suspected of having infection but yielding negative results. If eggs cannot be found in someone with compatible chronic symptoms, rectal biopsy snips can be obtained, pressed between two slides and examined by light microscopy for eggs.[33] Colposcopic biopsy with histologic examination may also be useful in such instances. Although abdominal ultrasonography is sometimes helpful diagnostically, findings may be nonspecific early in infection. Consequently, it is most useful in assessing morbidity and monitoring the response to treatment in patients with chronic disease.[20]

Urine nucleopore membrane filtration followed by examination of the filter surface for trapped eggs is the optimal method for detection of *S. haematobium* eggs. Alternatively, either sedimentation or centrifugation followed by examination of the urine deposit can also be used. Because *S. haematobium* eggs are shed into the bladder following a circadian rhythm, urine samples should be obtained between 10 AM and 2 PM. Examination of large volumes (>3 liters) of urine may be needed to detect eggs in light infections. In epidemiological studies, hematuria is often used as an indirect indicator of *S. haematobium* infection; however, the diagnostic value of hematuria at the individual level is limited by large variations in the predictive value of the test between different populations.[34] Cystoscopy may reveal patches of granulomatous "sandpaper bladder" in affected patients.

Serologic testing by ELISA is highly effective for the diagnosis of schistosome infection in exposed travelers to Africa, with a reported sensitivity and specificity of 99% each.[35] Immunoblot protocols developed by the CDC in Atlanta, USA also allow differentiation of *S. haematobium* and *S. mansoni* infections.[36] Antibodies will not be detectable until 4–8 weeks after infection, when the adult schistosomes have established in the appropriate venous plexus.[17,37] The inability of these tests to distinguish between past and current infections limits their utility in endemic areas.[37,38]

More recently, schistosome antigen detection tests have been developed in which circulating cathodic antigen (CCA) or circulating anodic antigen (CAA) released from adult worms can be detected in serum and urine.[38] CCA and CAA can be detected early in infection, are correlated with the intensity of infection, and clear rapidly following successful treatment. A point-of-care (POC) CCA test is now commercially available and is very sensitive for detecting *S. mansoni* infections using a urine sample. Paradoxically, this test is less sensitive for *S. haematobium* infections because worms of this species produce less of the antigen. CAA testing of either urine or serum can be used to diagnose either *S. mansoni* or *S. haematobium* infections with high sensitivity and high specificity. However, this test includes a sample concentration step that currently limits its use in field settings.[37]

Comparison of Kato Katz microscopy and *S. mansoni* real-time polymerase chain reaction (PCR) testing for the diagnosis of schistosome infections demonstrates that PCR is more sensitive. During studies in Senegal and Kenya, PCR on a single stool sample estimated *S. mansoni* prevalence levels of 72.6% and 32.4%, respectively, compared to prevalences of 68.5% and 25.9% when microscopy on duplicate Kato Katz slides was used. However, Kato Katz microscopy detected infections that were not detected on real-time PCR, and *vice versa*, with test correlations of only 82% (Senegal) and 85% (Kenya).[39]

Similar findings were obtained when comparing real-time PCR on uncentrifuged urine to microscopy of centrifuged deposits of 10-mL urine samples.[40] More recently, a PCR method on filtered urine has shown promise for detection of either *S. mansoni* or *S. haematobium* infections.[41] *S. mansoni* loop-mediated isothermal amplification assays are available and have been shown to also have high sensitivity and specificity for the detection of schistosomiasis.[9]

TREATMENT

Praziquantel, a heterocyclic pyrazinoisoquinoline, is the drug of choice for infections with all species of schistosomes, with estimated cure rates based on egg excretion that range from 60% to 98%.[42] However, recent posttreatment studies using the more sensitive POC-CCA test suggest that praziquantel cure rates may actually be much lower.[43] The drug is well tolerated, with only mild transient side effects, including abdominal discomfort, nausea, diarrhea, headache, dizziness, drowsiness, and pruritus. Three doses of 20 mg/kg given at 4-hour intervals are recommended for treatment of *S. japonicum* and *S. mekongi* infections.[17] For most individuals, a single dose of 40 mg/kg or two doses of 20 mg/kg is sufficient for treatment of infection with other schistosome species[17,42] However, young children may require higher doses for effective treatment as drug efficacy varies with immunologic maturity.[44] Of note, HIV status does not appear to reduce the response of schistosome infections to praziquantel therapy in adults, most likely because most individuals become infected and develop an immune response to schistosome infections earlier in life relative to their exposure to HIV.[45]

Resistance to praziquantel has been induced in laboratory strains of *S. mansoni* with repeated exposure to the drug.[46,2] Praziquantel resistance has been reported in focal regions of sub-Saharan Africa, most notably in Senegal and the Nile Delta Region of Egypt.[16,47] Praziquantel resistance in *S. japonicum* has not emerged thus far in China, despite high coverage of affected populations with the drug.[16]

Concern about reliance on a single drug has led to renewed interest in alternatives to praziquantel therapy.[48] Artemisinin derivatives, including artesunate and artemether, are best known for their antimalarial properties; however, laboratory experiments and clinical trials have confirmed that these compounds also exhibit activity against all of the major schistosome species that infect humans.[49–52] Artemisinin derivatives are well tolerated and may be administered orally or by intramuscular injection. Optimal regimens for treatment of schistosomiasis with arteminsin derivatives have not yet been determined. Unlike praziquantel, which is active only against adult worms, artemisinin compounds have activity against both the immature and adult stages of the schistosome life cycle and have been proposed for chemoprophylaxis. Artemether has superior activity (85–98% adult and 70% juvenile worm burden reduction) when compared to artesunate (34–49% adult and 67–77% juvenile worm burden reduction).[48]

Oxamniquine, a tetrahydroquinoline previously used for the treatment of *S. mansoni,* has generated new interest recently with the detailed description of the basis for drug resistance.[53] This has led to studies of drug derivatives with potential for action against other schistosome species.[54]

CONTROL AND PREVENTION

Control and prevention of schistosomiasis are among the most complex problems in public health. Success in control depends on having a well-organized program based on an in depth understanding of the epidemiology of the disease, the biology, ecology, and distribution of the parasite intermediate snail host, and the geographic characteristics of the environment. Program staff also benefit from sound knowledge of local socioeconomic conditions, support from health authorities, and cooperation of the communities.

The elimination of schistosomiasis through interruption of transmission has been attempted for the last five decades. It has been successful in some countries, such as Japan and large parts of Egypt[55] and China,[56] but has proved to be beyond the resources available to many endemic areas. Furthermore, ecological changes, both natural (e.g., drought) and manmade (e.g., water resource development projects or relocation of populations for political reasons), have led to reintroduction of schistosomiasis in some regions where disease transmission was previously controlled.[57]

MASS DRUG ADMINISTRATION

The World Health Assembly (WHA) passed resolution 54.19 in 2001, calling for mass drug administration (MDA) of praziquantel to at least 75% of school-aged children at risk of morbidity.[58] While this MDA initiative will serve to reduce morbidity, MDA alone will not eliminate transmission. Countries that have successfully interrupted the transmission of schistosomiasis have done so by means of public health programs, and social as well as concurrent economic development of the population.[58] As a result, the WHA released resolution 65.21 in 2012, acknowledging that some countries had interrupted transmission and encouraging low transmission countries to attempt elimination through MDA to at risk groups or even entire communities in affected areas, combined with provision of potable water, sanitation, education, and mollusk control.[59]

SNAIL CONTROL

Molluscicides provide a rapid and effective means of reducing the snail population and decreasing disease transmission[60,61]; however, their application must take into account the focal and seasonal patterns of disease transmission. A suitable molluscicide must be safe and nontoxic to mammals and aquatic organisms, stable in storage, and simple to apply. Niclosamide, a synthetic amide that has been used since the 1960s, fulfils most of these criteria and remains the molluscicide of choice. The major limitations to its widespread use are cost and the high incidence of drug-associated fish mortality. Natural molluscicides of plant origin provide the theoretical advantage of decreased cost, local production, and low toxicity, but to date have not been as effective as niclosamide in field trials.

Long-lasting effects in the reduction of snail populations can be achieved by environmental modifications, such as the installation of overhead sprinklers and trickle-type irrigation systems, modification of canal design, alteration of water level, or lining of canals with cement. Simple methods, including weed control and drainage of unused standing water, can also reduce snail populations. Biological snail control using fish, particularly field trial of the cichlid fish *Astatoreochromis alluaudi*, have met with only limited success.[62] Field trials of biological control with competing snails of the Thiarid group appear effective, an example of which was the introduction of *Melanoides tuberculata* into Martinique, where it out-competed *Bulinus glabrata* in waterways to the point of almost total disappearance of this vector snail.[63] Biological control of *B. glabrata* and *Biomphalaria alexandrina* using the water bug insect *Shaeroderma unrinator* has shown some success in laboratory conditions,[64] as has control of *B. alexandrina* with cyanobacterium phycocyanins.[65] Release of the snail-sterilizing trematode *Ribeiroia guadeloupensis* into a pond in Guadeloupe removed *B. glabrata.*[63] However, the effects of introducing biological control agents and toxins into the wider ecosystem must be carefully and extensively assessed prior to any use or trials of such agents outside of the laboratory. For instance *R. guadeloupensis* may cause severe malformations and potentially catastrophic mortality in amphibian populations[66] where it is present and thus deleterious effect on the wider ecosystem are far more concerning than its positive capacity to control schistosome snail vectors.

EDUCATION

Health education is an integral part of any successful schistosomiasis control program and has been shown in several studies to have an effect on human behavior and ultimately on disease transmission and prevalence.[67] It is much more likely that people will minimize contact with infested water, avoid polluting water sources, and cooperate with community control programs if they understand the basic mechanism of disease transmission. Furthermore, simple and inexpensive water disinfection procedures can be instituted, such as boiling, filtering, or storing for 24 hours, after which contaminating cercariae become noninfective. Finally, people who must have contact with contaminated water can be taught personal protection measures, including the use of repellents, rubber boots, and other barrier methods (e.g., wrapping the feet with cloth or puttees smeared with powdered *Thea oleosa* fruits), which may provide partial protection against infection.

SANITATION AND WATER SUPPLY

Although expensive, the provision of safe water and adequate sanitation is crucial to the long term control of schistosomiasis. In St. Lucia, the installation of individual household water systems was associated with a 75% decrease in the incidence of new *S. mansoni* infections in children.[68] In theory, installation of latrines may protect snail-bearing waters from contamination with infectious human wastes; however, this has been less effective than provision of a safe water supply in decreasing transmission. The reason for this is likely multifactorial, and includes accessibility and social issues limiting the use of latrines in many communities. Finally, since water resource development programs may spread schistosomiasis to previously uninfected areas, an example of which is the emergence and spread of intestinal schistosomiasis and the marked increase in urinary schistosomiasis cases following construction of the Diama dam on the Senegal river basin.[69] Such programs should be planned by multidisciplinary teams, including epidemiologists, ecologists, biologists, engineers, and public health officials.

VACCINE DEVELOPMENT

The immune response to schistosome infection is extremely complex and likely depends on the intensity and timing of exposure as well as genetic factors.[70,71] Nevertheless, epidemiological studies in areas endemic for schistosomiasis suggest that acquired resistance to reinfection occurs with age. Furthermore, although vaccination of experimental animals (including nonhuman primates) with live attenuated schistosomes provides only partial immunity to reinfection (70–90% reduction in worm burden), such levels of immunity could have a significant effect on morbidity by reducing the prevalence of high intensity infections and could potentially reduce transmission.[72,73] Since the use of a live vaccine would be unethical in humans, recent attention has focused on recombinant or synthetic peptides as potential vaccine candidates and on the use of novel delivery systems (e.g., BCG) and adjuvants (e.g., IL-12) to enhance their immunogenicity.

OTHER SCHISTOSOMA SPECIES AND HYBRIDS INFECTING HUMANS

Rarely, human infections with animal schistosomes or hybrids of the *S. haematobium* complex have been recorded in Corsica[10] and Senegal.[69] Apart from presenting a diagnostic conundrum, such infections may also confuse efforts toward schistosomiasis elimination. In consideration of this, previous unconfirmed reports of *S. bovis* infecting humans in southern Africa and the Democratic Republic of Congo[4] may have some legitimacy. Natural hybridization of *S. haematobium* and *S. intercalatum* were identified in Cameroon in the 1970s.[74] Human infection with hybrids of the ruminant schistosome, *Schistosoma matheei*, and *S. haematobium* was described in the early 1930s,[75] and human passage of eggs in feces and urine of (possible hybrids) of *S. matheei* was reported in South Africa and Zimbabwe up to the 1980s.[4] Eggs of "*S. haematobium*" from human feces and urine were identified in Gimvi village, Maharashtra, and Dokur village, Andra Pradesh, India between the 1950s and 1980s.[76–80] Animal schistosomes or hybrids thereof rather than true *S. haematobium* may have caused these foci. Indeed, Chandler reported two human infections with the terminal spined dog and pig schistosome, *Schistosoma incognitum* from India in 1926.[81] Occasional reports of *S. japonicum* in Africa may be attributable to *Schistosoma margrebowei*, a parasite of antelope, horses, cattle and sheep in Central and Southern Africa with eggs almost identical to *S. japonicum*.[82] Five humans' infections with the probably synonymous *Schistosoma faradjei* were reported from the Democratic Republic of Congo.[4,82] Occasional human cases of *S. malayensis*, a rat schistosome with eggs resembling those of *S. japonicum*, occur in Peninsular Malaysia.[9]

DISCLAIMER

The findings and conclusions in this book chapter are those of the author and do not necessarily represent the official position of the Centers for Disease Control and Prevention/the Agency for Toxic Substances and Disease Registry.

References

1. Vos T, Abajobir AA, Abate KH, et al. Global, regional, and national incidence, prevalence, and years lived with disability for 328 diseases and injuries for 195 countries, 1990–2016: A systematic analysis for the Global Burden of Disease Study 2016. *Lancet*. 2017;390(10100):1211–59.
2. World Health Organization. *Schistosomiasis Fact Sheet*. Geneva: World Health Organization; 2018.
3. Arnon R. Life span of parasite in schistosomiasis patients. *Isr J Med Sci*. 1990;26(7):404–5.
4. Beaver P, Jung R, Cupp E. *Clinical Parasitology*. 9th ed. Philadelphia: Lea and Febiger; 1984.
5. Sturrock R. The intermediate hosts and host-parasite relationship. In: Jordan P, Webbe G, Sturrock R, eds.Jordan P, Webbe G, Sturrock R, eds. *Human Schistosomiasis*. Oxon: CAB International; 1993, pp. 87–158.
6. Murinello A, Germano N, Mendonça P, Campos C, Grácio A. Liver disease due to schistosoma guineensis: A review. *J Port Gastrenterol*. 2006;13(2):97–104.
7. Chitsulo L, Loverde P, Engels D. Schistosomiasis. *Nat Rev Microbiol*. 2004; 2(1):12–3.
8. Jelinek T. Imported schistosomiasis in Europe: Preliminary data for 2007 from TropNetEurop. *Euro Surveill*. 2008;13(7):8038.
9. McManus DP, Dunne DW, Sacko M, Utzinger J, Vennervald BJ, Zhou XN. Schistosomiasis. *Nat Rev Dis Primers*. 2018;4:13.
10. Mone H, Holtfreter MC, Allienne JF, et al. Introgressive hybridizations of *Schistosoma haematobium* by *Schistosoma bovis* at the origin of the first case report of schistosomiasis in Corsica (France, Europe). *Parasitol Res*. 2015;114(11):4127–33.
11. Webster BL, Southgate VR, Littlewood DT. A revision of the interrelationships of *Schistosoma* including the recently described *Schistosoma guineensis*. *Int J Parasitol*. 2006;36(8):947–55.
12. Wright CA, Southgate VR, Knowles RJ. What is *Schistosoma intercalatum* Fisher, 1934? *Trans R Soc Trop Med Hyg*. 1972;66(1):28–64.
13. Jordan P, Webbe G. Epidemiology. In: Jordan P, Webbe G, Sturrock R, eds. Jordan P, Webbe G, Sturrock R, eds. *Human Schistosomiasis*. Oxon: CAB International; 1993, pp. 87–158.
14. Hoeffler DF. Cercarial dermatitis. *Arch Environ Health*. 1974;29(4):225–9.
15. Horak P, Mikes L, Lichtenbergova L, Skala V, Soldanova M, Brant SV. Avian schistosomes and outbreaks of cercarial dermatitis. *Clin Microbiol Rev*. 2015;28(1):165–90.
16. Vale N, Gouveia MJ, Rinaldi G, Brindley PJ, Gartner F, Correia da Costa JM. Praziquantel for schistosomiasis: Single-drug metabolism revisited, mode of action, and resistance. *Antimicrob Agents Chemother*. 2017;61(5):e02582-16.
17. Sheorey H, Walker J, Biggs B. *Clinical Parasitology*. Geelong: Erudite Medical Books; 2013.
18. Rocha H, Kirk JW, Hearey CD Jr. Prolonged *Salmonella* bacteremia in patients with *Schistosoma mansoni* infection. *Arch Intern Med*. 1971;128(2):254–7.
19. Andrade ZA, Van Marck E. Schistosomal glomerular disease (a review). *Mem Inst Oswaldo Cruz*. 1984;79(4):499–506.
20 Wiest PM. The epidemiology of morbidity of schistosomiasis. *Parasitol Today*. 1996;12(6):215–20.
21. Poggensee G, Feldmeier H, Krantz I. Schistosomiasis of the female genital tract: Public health aspects. *Parasitol Today*. 1999;15(9):378–81.
22. Vale TC, de Sousa-Pereira SR, Ribas JG, Lambertucci JR. Neuroschistosomiasis mansoni: Literature review and guidelines. *Neurologist*. 2012;18(6):333–42.

23. Carod Artal FJ. Cerebral and spinal schistosomiasis. *Curr Neurol Neurosci Rep*. 2012;12(6):666–74.
24. McElroy MD, Elrefaei M, Jones N, et al. Coinfection with *Schistosoma mansoni* is associated with decreased HIV-specific cytolysis and increased IL-10 production. *J Immunol*. 2005;174(8):5119–23.
25. Kamal S, Madwar M, Bianchi L, et al. Clinical, virological and histopathological features: Long-term follow-up in patients with chronic hepatitis C co-infected with *S. mansoni*. *Liver*. 2000;20(4):281–9.
26. Rafi W, Ribeiro-Rodrigues R, Ellner JJ, Salgame P. 'Coinfection-helminthes and tuberculosis.' *Curr Opin HIV AIDS*. 2012;7(3):239–44.
27. Gendrel D. *Salmonella-Schistosoma* interactions. *Rev Prat*. 1993;43:450–2.
28. Bouree P, Botterel F, Romand S. Delayed *Salmonella* bacteriuria in a patient infected with *Schistosoma haematobium*. *J Egypt Soc Parasitol*. 2002;32(2): 355–60.
29. Barnhill AE, Novozhilova E, Day TA, Carlson SA. *Schistosoma*-associated *Salmonella* resist antibiotics via specific fimbrial attachments to the flatworm. *Parasites Vectors*. 2011;4:123.
30. Actor JK, Shirai M, Kullberg MC, Buller RM, Sher A, Berzofsky JA. Helminth infection results in decreased virus-specific CD8+ cytotoxic T-cell and Th1 cytokine responses as well as delayed virus clearance. *Proc Natl Acad Sci U S A*. 1993;90(3):948–52.
31. DiNardo AR, Nishiguchi T, Mace EM, et al. Schistosomiasis induces persistent DNA methylation and tuberculosis-specific immune changes. *J Immunol*. 2018;201(1):124–33.
32. Glinz D, Silue KD, Knopp S, et al. Comparing diagnostic accuracy of Kato-Katz, Koga agar plate, ether-concentration, and FLOTAC for *Schistosoma mansoni* and soil-transmitted helminths. *PLoS Negl Trop Dis*. 2010;4(7):e754.
33. Rabello AL, Rocha RS, de Oliveira JP, Katz N, Lambertucci JR. Stool examination and rectal biopsy in the diagnosis and evaluation of therapy of schistosomiasis mansoni. *Rev Inst Med Trop Sao Paulo*. 1992;34(6):601–8.
34. Mott KE, Dixon H, Osei-Tutu E, England EC, Ekue K, Tekle A. Evaluation of reagent strips in urine tests for detection of *Schistosoma haematobium* infection: A comparative study in Ghana and Zambia. *Bull World Health Organ*. 1985;63(1):125–33.
35. Tsang VC, Wilkins PP. Immunodiagnosis of schistosomiasis. *Immunol Invest*. 1997;26(1–2):175–88.
36. Tsang VC, Wilkins PP. Immunodiagnosis of schistosomiasis. Screen with FAST-ELISA and confirm with immunoblot. *Clin Lab Med*. 1991;11(4): 1029–39.
37. van Grootveld R, van Dam GJ, de Dood C, et al. Improved diagnosis of active Schistosoma infection in travellers and migrants using the ultra-sensitive in-house lateral flow test for detection of circulating anodic antigen (CAA) in serum. *Eur J Clin Microbiol Infect Dis*. 2018;37(9):1709–16.
38. Doenhoff MJ, Chiodini PL, Hamilton JV. Specific and sensitive diagnosis of schistosome infection: Can it be done with antibodies? *Trends Parasitol*. 2004;20(1):35–9.
39. Meurs L, Brienen E, Mbow M, et al. Is PCR the next reference standard for the diagnosis of *Schistosoma* in stool? A comparison with microscopy in Senegal and Kenya. *PLoS Negl Trop Dis*. 2015;9(7):e0003959.
40. Pillay P, Taylor M, Zulu SG, et al. Real-time polymerase chain reaction for detection of Schistosoma DNA in small-volume urine samples reflects focal distribution of urogenital Schistosomiasis in primary school girls in KwaZulu Natal, South Africa. *Am J Trop Med Hyg*. 2014;90(3):546–52.
41. Lodh N, Naples JM, Bosompem KM, Quartey J, Shiff CJ. Detection of parasite-specific DNA in urine sediment obtained by filtration differentiates between single and mixed infections of *Schistosoma mansoni* and *S. haematobium* from endemic areas in Ghana. *PLoS One*. 2014;9(3):e91144.
42. Pearson RD, Guerrant RL. Praziquantel: A major advance in anthelminthic therapy. *Ann Intern Med*. 1983;99(2):195–8.
43. Mwinzi PN, Kittur N, Ochola E, et al. Additional evaluation of the point-of-contact circulating cathodic antigen assay for *Schistosoma mansoni* infection. *Front Public Health*. 2015;3:48.
44. Bustinduy AL, Waterhouse D, de Sousa-Figueiredo JC, et al. Population pharmacokinetics and pharmacodynamics of praziquantel in Ugandan children with intestinal schistosomiasis: Higher dosages are required for maximal efficacy. *mBio*. 2016;7(4):e00227-16.
45. Karanja DM, Boyer AE, Strand M, et al. Studies on schistosomiasis in western Kenya: II. Efficacy of praziquantel for treatment of schistosomiasis in persons coinfected with human immunodeficiency virus-1. *Am J Trop Med Hyg*. 1998;59(2):307–11.
46. Fallon PG, Doenhoff MJ. Drug-resistant schistosomiasis: Resistance to praziquantel and oxamniquine induced in *Schistosoma mansoni* in mice is drug specific. *Am J Trop Med Hyg*. 1994;51(1):83–8.
47. Fallon PG. Schistosome resistance to praziquantel. *Drug Resist Updat*. 1998;1(4):236–41.
48. Bergquist R, Utzinger J, Keiser J. Controlling schistosomiasis with praziquantel: How much longer without a viable alternative? *Infect Dis Poverty*. 2017;6(1):74.
49. Inyang-Etoh PC, Ejezie GC, Useh MF, Inyang-Etoh EC. Efficacy of artesunate in the treatment of urinary schistosomiasis, in an endemic community in Nigeria. *Ann Trop Med Parasitol*. 2004;98(5):491–9.
50. Liu YX, Wu W, Liang YJ, et al. New uses for old drugs: The tale of artemisinin derivatives in the elimination of schistosomiasis japonica in China. *Molecules*. 2014;19(9):15058–74.
51. Li YS, Chen HG, He HB, Hou XY, Ellis M, McManus DP. A double-blind field trial on the effects of artemether on *Schistosoma japonicum* infection in a highly endemic focus in southern China. *Acta Tropica*. 2005;96(2–3): 184–90.
52. Utzinger J, N'Goran EK, N'Dri A, Lengeler C, Xiao S, Tanner M. Oral artemether for prevention of *Schistosoma mansoni* infection: Randomised controlled trial. *Lancet*. 2000;355(9212):1320–5.
53. Valentim CL, Cioli D, Chevalier FD, et al. Genetic and molecular basis of drug resistance and species-specific drug action in schistosome parasites. *Science*. 2013;342(6164):1385–9.
54. Taylor AB, Roberts KM, Cao X, et al. Structural and enzymatic insights into species-specific resistance to schistosome parasite drug therapy. *J Biol Chem*. 2017;292(27):11154–64.
55. Abou-El-Naga IF. Towards elimination of schistosomiasis after 5000 years of endemicity in Egypt. *Acta Trop*. 2018;181:112–21.
56. Xianyi C, Liying W, Jiming C, et al. Schistosomiasis control in China: The impact of a 10-year World Bank Loan Project (1992–2001). *Bull World Health Organ*. 2005;83(1):43–8.
57. Liang S, Yang C, Zhong B, Qiu D. Re-emerging schistosomiasis in hilly and mountainous areas of Sichuan, China. *Bull World Health Organ*. 2006;84(2):139–44.
58. Secor W, Colley DG. When should the emphasis on schistosomiasis control move to elimination? *Trop Med Infect Dis*. 2018;3(3):85.
59. World Health Organization. *Schistosomiasis—Strategy*. Geneva: World Health Organization; 2018.
60. Perrett S, Whitfield PJ. Currently available molluscicides. *Parasitol Today*. 1996;12(4):156–9.
61. King CH, Sutherland LJ, Bertsch D. Systematic review and meta-analysis of the impact of chemical-based mollusciciding for control of *Schistosoma mansoni* and *S. haematobium* transmission. *PLoS Negl Trop Dis*. 2015;9(12): e0004290.
62. Slootweg R, Malek E, McCullough F. The biological control of snail intermediate hosts of schistosomiasis by fish. *Rev Fish Biol Fish*. 1994;4:67–90.
63. Pointier JP, Jourdane J. Biological control of the snail hosts of schistosomiasis in areas of low transmission: The example of the Caribbean area. *Acta Trop*. 2000;77(1):53–60.
64. Younes A, El-Sherief H, Gawish F, Mahmoud M. Biological control of snail hosts transmitting schistosomiasis by the water bug, Sphaerodema urinator. *Parasitol Res*. 2017;116(4):1257–64.
65. Abd El-Ghany AM, Salama A, Abd El-Ghany NM, Gharieb RMA. New approach for controlling snail host *of Schistosoma mansoni*, *Biomphalaria alexandrina* with cyanobacterial strains-derived C-phycocyanin. *Vector Borne Zoonotic Dis*. 2018;18(9):464–8.
66. Johnson PT, McKenzie VJ. Effects of environmental change on helminth infections in amphibians: Exploring the emergence of *Ribeiroia* and *Echinostoma* infections in North America. *The Biology of Echinostomes: From the Molecule to the Community*. New York: Springer; 2009, pp. 249–80.
67. Hu GH, Hu J, Song KY, et al. The role of health education and health promotion in the control of schistosomiasis: Experiences from a 12-year intervention study in the Poyang Lake area. *Acta Trop*. 2005;96(2–3): 232–41.
68. Li YS, Sleigh AC, Li Y, et al. Five-year impact of repeated praziquantel treatment on subclinical morbidity due to *Schistosoma japonicum* in China. *Trans R Soc Trop Med Hyg*. 2002;96(4):438–43.
69. Sow S, de Vlas SJ, Engels D, Gryseels B. Water-related disease patterns before and after the construction of the Diama dam in northern Senegal. *Ann Trop Med Parasitol*. 2002;96(6):575–86.
70. Marquet S, Abel L, Hillaire D, et al. Genetic localization of a locus controlling the intensity of infection by *Schistosoma mansoni* on chromosome 5q31–q33. *Nat Genet*. 1996;14(2):181–4.
71. Wynn TA, Hoffmann KF. Defining a schistosomiasis vaccination strategy—Is it really Th1 versus Th2? *Parasitol Today*. 2000;16(11):497–501.

72. Eberl M, Langermans JA, Frost PA, et al. Cellular and humoral immune responses and protection against schistosomes induced by a radiation-attenuated vaccine in chimpanzees. *Infect Immun.* 2001;69(9):5352–62.
73. Bergquist NR, Leonardo LR, Mitchell GF. Vaccine-linked chemotherapy: Can schistosomiasis control benefit from an integrated approach? *Trends Parasitol.* 2005;21(3):112–7.
74. Wright CA, Southgate VR, van Wijk HB, Moore PJ. Letter: Hybrids between *Schistosoma haematobium* and *S. intercalatum* in Cameroon. *Trans R Soc Trop Med Hyg.* 1974;68(5):413–4.
75. Wright CA, Ross GC. Hybrids between *Schistosoma haematobium* and *S. mattheei* and their identification by isoelectric focusing of enzymes. *Trans R Soc Trop Med Hyg.* 1980;74(3):326–32.
76. Varma AK. Human schistosomiasis in India. *J Indian Med Assoc.* 1955; 25:173–5.
77. Southgate VR, Agrawal MC. Human schistosomiasis in India? *Parasitol Today.* 1990;6(5):166–8.
78. Sathe BD, Pandit CH, Chanderkar NG, Badade DC, Sengupta SR, Renapurkar DM. Sero-diagnosis of schistosomiasis by ELISA test in an endemic area of Gimvi village, India. *J Trop Med Hyg.* 1991;94(2):76–8.
79. Gaitonde BB, Sathe BD, Mukerji S, et al. Studies on schistosomiasis in village Gimvi of Maharashtra. *Indian J Med Res.* 1981;74:352–7.
80. Bidinger PD, Crompton DW. A possible focus of schistosomiasis in Andhra Pradesh, India. *Trans R Soc Trop Med Hyg.* 1989;83(4):526.
81. Chandler A. A new schistosome infection of man, with notes on other human fluke infections in India. *J Med Res.* 1926;14:179–83.
82. Jordan P, Webbe G. *Human Schistosomiasis.* London: Heinemann; 1969.

CHAPTER

129

Foodborne Trematode Infections*

Sarah G. H. Sapp • Sarah Anne J. Guagliardo • Richard S. Bradbury

CLONORCHIASIS AND OPISTHORCHIASIS

The trematodes *Clonorchis sinensis*, *Opisthorchis viverrini*, and *O. felineus* are members of the family Opisthorchidae and are important causes of liver disease in people within endemic areas. Notably, and somewhat uniquely among parasitic species, *C. sinensis* and *O. viverrini* are classified as group 1 carcinogens due to their association with cholangiocarcinoma and other neoplasms of the biliary system.[1] Infections with these "fishborne liver flukes" are widely distributed in countries in the Far East and Southeast Asia, and countries of the former Soviet Union. They present serious public health problems in certain localized areas of China, Korea, Thailand, Laos, Cambodia, Vietnam, and several countries of the former Soviet Union and increasingly into Europe. The most recent estimate of global burden indicates 45 million infections in the endemic Asian and European range; this includes 35 million *C. sinensis* cases, 10 million *O. viverrini* cases, and 1.2 million *O. felineus* cases.[2] Up to 680 million people may be at risk for infection.[2] Globally, clonorchiasis and opisthorciasis are associated with an estimated 522,863 and 188,346 disability-adjusted life years, which is relatively high among parasitic helminths.[3] With increased travel and migration of populations at risk and importation of indigenous uncooked foods contaminated with these parasites, infections have also occurred in nonendemic areas.

Life Cycle

The flukes *C. sinensis*, *O. viverrini*, and *O. felineus* follow a typical multi-host trematode life cycle, requiring two intermediate hosts and a definitive host to complete their life cycle. The host range for these species is summarized in Table 129-1. Infected definitive hosts pass embryonated eggs, containing miracidia, into the environment. These eggs are ingested by snails, the first intermediate hosts, and the miracidia are released. Within the snail tissues, the miracidia develop into rediae and then cercariae—long-tailed, motile forms which are infective to the second intermediate host. Cercariae emerge from the snail into water, and upon contact with a suitable intermediate host (nearly always fish of the family Cyprinidae, such as carp, true minnows, and barbs) they penetrate the skin of the fish, shed their tails, and encyst in the skeletal muscle and viscera as metacercariae. When infected raw freshwater fish containing the encysted stages of the parasite are eaten, the larvae are set free in the duodenum of the definitive host. The larvae enter the bile ducts within a few hours after being ingested.[2] In about 3–4 weeks, the hermaphroditic adult flukes (Fig. 129-1) reach maturity and begin shedding eggs into the bile ducts. The estimated daily egg output of these flukes varies substantially; the typical egg output for an individual *C. sinensis* in a human host is estimated about 4000 eggs/day, but outputs of > 400,000 eggs/day in very high burden infections have been noted.[4] Limited studies on *O. viverrini* suggest a typical egg output of anywhere between 3000 and 36,000 eggs/day.[5] The complete life cycle, from one infected person to another, requires at least 3 months. Individual *C. sinensis* flukes have can live up to 25 years in the human host, and *Opisthorchis* spp. are believed to be similarly long-lived.[6]

While these flukes follow similar life cycles, their host specificity is variable. The *Opisthorchis* species can invade only snails of the genus *Bithyna*, while *C. sinensis* has been found to infect snails across five families. The definitive host range of *C. sinensis* is broad, including humans, cats, dogs, foxes, pigs, some rodents, and possibly even

TABLE 129-1 SUMMARY OF THE PRIMARY EPIDEMIOLOGICALLY IMPORTANT HOST SPECIES OF THE FISHBORNE LIVER FLUKES DISCUSSED IN THIS CHAPTER

	First Intermediate Hosts (Snails)	Second Intermediate Hosts (Cyprinid Fishes)[a]	Definitive Hosts (Usually Carnivores)
Clonorchis sinensis	Assimineidae, Bithyniidae, Hydrobiidae, Melaniidae,Thiaridae families	Tilapia (*Oreochromis mossambicus*), grass carp (*Ctenopharyngodon idella*), stone moroko (*Pseudorasbora parva)*, Mugitsuku (*Pungtungia herzi*), *Pseudogobio esocinus*, Amur sucker (*Sarcocheilichthys sinensis*), barbel steed (*Hemibarbus labeo*), pond smelt (*Hypomesus olidus*)	Humans, domestic dogs and cats, swine, some rodents
Opisthorchis viverrini	*Bithynia* spp.	Barb (*Cyclocheilichthys* spp., *Hampala* spp.), water carp (*Puntius* spp.)	Humans, domestic cats and dogs, fishing cat (*Prionailurus viverrinus)*
Opisthorchis felineus	*Bithynia* spp.	Ide (*Leuciscus idus*), Roach (*Rutilus rutilus*), European dace (*Leuciscus leuciscus*), Tench (*Tinca tinca*), Verhovka (*Leuciscus delineatus*), Silver crucian carp (*Carassius auratus gibelio*)	Domestic dogs and cats, foxes (many species), mink, weasels, occasionally pinnipeds (sea lions, seals)

[a]Not exhaustive; only hosts of particular epidemiological importance listed.

* **Disclaimer:** The findings and conclusions in this chapter are those of the author and do not necessarily represent the official position of the Centers for Disease Control and Prevention/the Agency for Toxic Substances and Disease Registry.

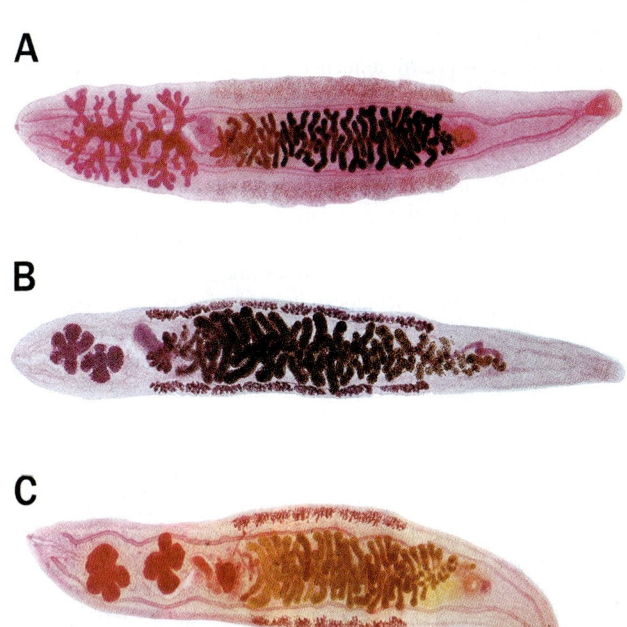

FIGURE 129-1. Adult specimens of the liver flukes (Opisthorchidae) discussed in this chapter, carmine stained. A: *Clonorchis sinensis*; B. *Opisthorchis viverrini*; C. *Opisthorchis felineus*. (Dr. Richard S. Bradbury.)

piscivorous birds. *O. viverrini* has seldom been detected in wildlife, despite its specific epithet (derived from the fishing cat, *Prionailurus viverrinus*, the host from which the original type specimen was recovered). Humans and domestic dogs and cats appear to be the major definitive hosts, maintaining a nearly completely anthropogenic cycle. Conversely, *O. felineus* is maintained in a sylvatic cycle with a variety of small wild carnivores (e.g., many fox species, weasels, mink, polecats, raccoon dogs) and occasionally rodents, and spills over into domestic dogs and cats.[6,7]

Geographic Distribution

The geographic distribution of endemic clonorchiasis or opisthorchiasis is primarily driven by three factors: (a) the presence of suitable intermediate hosts (particularly snails), (b) the preference of the people in these areas to eat raw/insufficiently cured fish, and (c) the level of contamination of aquatic environments with sewage containing parasite eggs. Therefore, while concerns over the spread of these flukes into nonendemic areas are valid, these species will not be able to become established in new environments unless suitable intermediate hosts are present (particularly for *Opisthorchis* spp., which can only use *Bithynia* snails).[8]

Clonorchis sinensis

C. sinensis infections are common in localized populations in Korea, Mainland China, Hong Kong, Taiwan, and from northern parts of Vietnam.[2,6] Reports of *C. sinensis* from Cambodia likely represent *O. viverrini*.[6] The last reported autochthonous case in Japan was in 1991.[2] Cases also occur in Eastern Russia and occasionally from India.[2]

Opisthorchis viverrini

The geographic range of *Opisthorchis* spp. is more restricted. *O. viverrini* is broadly endemic in Thailand, Laos, and parts of Cambodia, southern Vietnam, and Myanmar.[9,10] Prevalence is notably higher in northern Thailand versus southern Thailand.[11]

Opisthorchis felineus

O. felineus occupies a more northern range than *O. viverrini*, endemic across Eastern Europe through Western Siberia. Within that range, incidence in people is highest in the Volga-Kama basin, Ukraine, and Kazakhstan. *O. felineus* has been recovered from various wild hosts across a relatively broad range of Western Europe, but human cases only occasionally occur, including recent cases in Germany, Greece, and Italy.[12] A large outbreak occurred in Italy following consumption of raw tench filets.[13] Cases are also reported from travelers to these endemic areas or following consumption of imported fish.[2]

Clinical Illness

The outward signs and symptoms of clonorchiasis and opisthorchiasis are nonspecific. Most infected persons are asymptomatic and only about one-third of chronic infections are symptomatic; severity of symptoms appears directly related to fluke burden.[2,14] In patients who do have symptoms, gradual onset of discomfort in the upper abdomen, anorexia, indigestion, and abdominal pain or distention can occur. In the late stages obstructive jaundice, portal hypertension, ascites, and gastrointestinal bleeding can occur. Recurrent pyogenic cholangitis is a frequent serious acute complication of clonorchiasis and also occurs in opisthorchiasis.[2,15,16] Episodes of cholangitis can be followed by the formation of biliary stones in the gallbladder and bile ducts.[17] While the chronic course is well characterized, little is known about the presentation of acute disease. During an outbreak of *O. felineus* in Italy, acute signs and symptoms included high fever, headache, dry cough, and abdominal pain with leukocytosis, eosinophilia, and elevated liver enzymes.[13]

Pathologically, the flukes injure the bile ducts and produce chronic cholangitis characterized by marked hyperplasia of the cylindrical epithelium, frequently associated with numerous mitoses. These changes may become evident as soon as 30 days postinfection. Eventually, nonspecific changes result from chronic inflammation in response to adult flukes and eggs, and subsequent reinfections lead to a progressive fibrous thickening of the walls. This fibrosis leads to partial or complete obstruction of terminal bile ducts, pressure necrosis of the surrounding parenchyma, and in severe cases, biliary cirrhosis. In very severe, high-burden infections, the liver may reach twice the typical weight.[18] Development of cholangitic cirrhosis is enhanced by intermittent acute episodes of complicating bacterial cholangitis, especially from *Escherichia coli* and other gut flora, potentially producing abscesses that lead to chronic cholecystitis. A causal relationship between chronic clonorchiasis or opisthorchiasis and biliary tract carcinoma (cholangiocarcinoma; CCA) has been established.[2,17] The factors leading to the development of clonorchiasis/opisthorchiasis-related CCA are not completely understood, but they are believed to include a combination of parasite-specific immune responses that induce proliferative changes and host genetic background.[2] Approximately two-thirds of patients from northeastern Thailand with obstructive jaundice secondary to malignant disease have cholangiocarcinoma related to liver flukes. In contrast in persons living in Western nations, carcinoma of the head of the pancreas is by far the most frequent cause of obstructive jaundice secondary to malignant disease.[3]

Diagnosis

Diagnosis is based on recovery of typical eggs from stool specimens, although distinguishing eggs of *C. sinensis* from the *Opisthorchis* species can be difficult to impossible. Eggs of these parasites are very small, usually pale amber, and roughly sesame seed-shaped, with protruding "shoulders" flanking an operculum (cap-like structure from which the miracidum emerges) at the narrow pole. The wide pole may have a small knob or spine visible, and the shell may appear radially striated in some planes of focus. Eggs of *O. viverrini* and *O. felineus* are usually slightly smaller (19–30 × 10–12 μm) than those of *C. sinensis* (27–35 × 11–20 μm), but potential overlap makes size an unreliable diagnostic criteria. Care should be taken to distinguish eggs from those of minute intestinal flukes, such as those from the family Heterophyidae.[2] For example, many cases of *C. sinensis* in Vietnam diagnosed using egg detection may represent misidentifications of

Fascioliasis can be challenging to diagnose because the symptoms are nonspecific and some laboratory tests have limited sensitivity.[53] Diagnosis is ideally based on a combination of clinical signs and symptoms, exposure history, and laboratory tests that are specific to either the acute or chronic phase of disease.[53] Microscopy is the most commonly used laboratory method for diagnosis, and is based on the identification of eggs in the stool or in the duodenal or biliary aspirates.[54] Eggs are very large (130–150 × 60–100 μm), ellipsoid, and golden in color, with an inconspicuous operculum; they are functionally indistinguishable from those of *Fasciolopsis buski* and can be difficult to differentiate from some echinostome eggs (both discussed under "Intestinal Trematodiases").[41] Diagnosis based on microscopy is laborious, relatively insensitive, and is subject to the ability of the operator.[54] The Kato-Katz technique can be used to quantify the burden of eggs in the stool. Alternatively, more sensitive methods such as Lumbreras rapid sedimentation and Flotac, may be more appropriate for more mild infections.[55] Flotac is possibly the optimal method for *F. hepatica* egg detection in feces, with one study demonstrating a sensitivity of 92.6% on a single Flotac test, compared to 63.0–85.2% sensitivity of triplicate sedimentation for the detection of eggs in infected rat feces.[56]

Because egg production does not start until at least 3–4 months after exposure, serologic testing may be indicated during the acute phase, or during the chronic phase if egg production is low or intermittent.[53] Antibodies to *Fasciola* are detectable within 2–4 weeks following exposure, allowing serologic diagnosis during the acute phase of disease. Several immunodiagnostic tests are available, and several are highly sensitive and specific.[57–59] An IgG4 serologic assay using recombinant antigen FhSAP2 (*F. hepatica* saposin-like protein-2) in Western blot format is available at the Centers for Disease Control and Prevention (CDC) in Atlanta, Georgia, USA. This test has a demonstrated sensitivity of 94% and specificity of 98% when compared to fecal microscopy for egg production as a reference standard.[60] Serological cross-reaction in this test is relatively uncommon, with estimated occurrence of cross-reaction in approximately 11% of *Necator americanus* (hookworm) infected patient sera.[60] Nonetheless, to avoid difficulty in interpreting positive results, serologic diagnosis should only be performed in cases where travel history, potential exposures, and clinical presentation are consistent with fascioloasis. Several highly sensitive and specific PCR assays have been developed and investigated for the detection of *F. hepatica* in human feces,[61] as has a commercial coproantigen detection test[61] However, as of 2019 none of these are commercially available for human diagnosis in the United States. In addition, contrast-enhanced computed tomography (CT) may reveal hypoattenuating subcapsular tracts consistent with the diagnosis during the acute phase of disease.[62]

Triclabendazole is the drug of choice for the treatment of fascioliasis. Triclabendazole is a benzimidazole compound that is active against immature and adult *Fasciola* parasites, and therefore can be used in both the acute and chronic phases of disease. The suggested treatment regimen is one or two doses (10 mg/kg) after a meal, separated by 12–24 hours.[53] The World Health Organization currently recommends a single dose as initial treatment, and in case of a treatment failure, 20 mg/kg divided into two doses 12–24 hours apart.[63] (Treatment failure is indicated by continued presence of eggs in the stool, persistent eosinophilia, or recurrence of symptoms following treatment[64]) Some studies have indicated that two doses (10 mg/kg) of triclabendazole may be more effective as an initial treatment.[65–68] Further research is required to determine whether one or two doses is appropriate for initial treatment. Triclabendazole has not been approved by the Food and Drug Administration and currently is only available for use in the United States through the CDC's Drug Service. There are no alternative treatments that are well established in the scientific literature, however, some limited data have indicated that treatment with nitazoxanide may be effective.[69,70,71] Removal of adult flukes via endoscopic retrograde cholangiopancreatography may be indicated in some patients with biliary tract obstruction.[72]

PARAGONIMIASIS

Lung flukes of the genus *Paragonimus* may infect humans and animals in Asia, Africa, and the Americas. There are at least 50 species of *Paragonimus* worldwide,[73] including multiple species that infect humans (Table 129-2),[74] each of which present with a similar clinical picture. Approximately 293 million people are at risk[73] and an estimated 21 million people suffer from paragonimiasis worldwide.[75] Infection occurs through the ingestion of undercooked freshwater crustaceans (crabs and crayfish), though wild boar meat containing immature flukes and acting as a paratenic host[75] has also been implicated in transmission. The zoonotic reservoir of infection involves many mammals, but domestic and wild felines (including big cats) and canids are particularly implicated.[73] In some parts of Asia, pickled crab dishes such as "drunken crab" (crab in saki rice wine) are leading sources of infection.[73] In other regions, such as the United States, infection has been reported among young adult males in association with alcohol consumption at the time of ingestion of raw freshwater crayfish.[76]

Upon consumption of an infected crustacean, metacercariae within the flesh of the crustacean are released in the host duodenum and from there migrate to the lungs. The adult worms (Fig. 129-2) encyst in the lungs and mature to adulthood. Each cyst may contain one to three each of these hermaphroditic trematodes.[77,78] The worms become gravid between 9 and 13 weeks after initial infection.[73] The flukes may live for up to 20 years,[78] after which they die and calcify.[79] Eggs are coughed up in sputum, which is either spat out into the environment or swallowed, resulting in the eggs being passed in feces. Once in the environment, eggs embryonate for 2 weeks, after which the motile miracidia will hatch and infect a freshwater snail. Within the snail, the miracidia develop into sporocysts, then two rediae generations followed by maturation into ceraceriae.[73] Approximately 20 rediae are produced in every sporocyst, resulting in an amplification of parasite load in this first intermediate host.[78] *Paragonimus* spp. cercariae, unlike those of many other trematodes, are short-tailed and not effective swimmers. Thus, the second intermediate host (freshwater crustaceans) is typically infected after preying upon infected snails containing cercariae (although a small proportion of cercariae emerge from the snail and can invade the crustacean directly).[41] The cercariae then encyst as a metacercariae within the flesh of the crustacean.[73]

Clinically, pulmonary paragonimiasis is characterized by cough, with or without hemoptysis. Fever and hepatomegaly may be seen in patients with moderate to heavy pulmonary infections. Due to the similarity of symptoms, pulmonary tuberculosis should be ruled out in patients in whom paragonimiasis is being considered. Pulmonary paragonimiasis may present with cloudy infiltrates of the lungs on CT scans, with nodular shadows and calcified spots. Multiple ring-shaped opacities resembling grape clusters is a suggestive finding. Pleural effusion, thickening of the pleura and pneumothorax may be seen in some cases.[73,80] Ectopic paragonimiasis may occur at almost any anatomic site,[81] most commonly in the brain or bowel wall, but also in the subcutaneous tissues (in which lesions may be migratory)[73,80] or the urinary tract,[73] in which cases eggs may be passed in the urine.[81] The specific clinical presentation of ectopic paragonimiasis varies and is correlated to the site of infection.[73,80]

Confirmation of diagnosis may be undertaken by microscopy of sputum or feces or serology. Eggs of *Paragonimus* may be detected on standard Ziehl-Neelsen sputum smear examination.[82] Detection of the characteristic eggs on microscopy of sputum or feces is diagnostic, but not all cases of pulmonary disease produce eggs and ectopic infections do not result in release eggs into the feces or sputum.[80] Even in egg producing cases, multiple sputa may need to be examined to detect eggs, and detection may be complicated by the fact that acid-fast staining used for tuberculosis screening may destroy *Paragonimus*

TABLE 129-2 SUMMARY OF THE GEOGRAPHIC DISTRIBUTION OF *PARAGONIMUS* SPECIES LUNG FLUKES REPORTED AS INFECTING HUMANS

Species	Reported Geographic Distribution[a]	Natural Definitive Hosts[b]
Paragonimus africanus	Cameroon, Nigeria,	Cercopithecids,canids, lorids, herpestids, viverrids
Paragonimus heterotremus	China, Korea, Taiwan, Vietnam, Laos, Thailand, Myanmar, India	Cercopithecids, canids, felids, sciuruds, murids
Paragonimus kellicotti	United States of America, Canada	Didelphids, canids, felids, mustellids, tupaiids, procyonids, suids, bovids, murids
Paragonimus mexicanus[c] (Possibly including multiple species)	Latin America	Didelphids, cebids, canids, felids, mustellids, procyonids, suids
Paragonimus ohirai	China, Korea, Taiwan, Japan	Canids, felids, mustellids, suids, murids
Paragonimus pseudoheterotremus	Thailand	Felids
Paragonimus siamensis	Thailand, Sri Lanka, Papua New Guinea	
Paragonimus skrjabini subsp. *skrjabini*	China, Vietnam, India	Canids, felids, mustellids, viverrids, suids, murids
Paragonimus skrjabini subsp. *miyazakii*	Japan	Canids, felids, mustellids, suids
Paragonimus uterobilateralis	Gabon, Cameroon, Nigeria, Liberia, Ivory Coast, Equatorial Guinea, Guinea (Conakry)	Cercopithecids, canids, felids, herpestids, viverrids, mustelids, murids
Paragonimus westermani	Russia, China, Taiwan, Korea, Japan, Vietnam, Laos, India, Sri Lanka, Philippines, Malaysia	Cercopithecids, canids, felids, herpestids, viverrids, mustelids, suids, murids
Reports of undetermined *Paragonimus* species[b]	Libya, Gambia, Senegal (Casamance region), Gabon, Benin, Democratic Republic of Congo, South Africa, Nepal, Pakistan	undetermined

[a]Not exhaustive; only hosts of particular epidemiological importance listed.
[b]In many reports, the term "*P. westermani*" has been used to describe any generic *Paragonimus* infection. Therefore, many geographic reports of "*P. westermani*" most likely reflect infection with *Paragonimus* species that were not identified to species level. The geographic distributions described in this table are limited to those with molecular or morphologic confirmation of species, it is likely some species infecting humans remain undescribed and that the comprehensive geographic range of known human infecting species has not yet been fully elucidated.
[c]The taxonomy of human infecting *Paragonimus* in Latin America requires further investigation. Reports of human infections with *P. mexicanus* may include multiple species, or a species complex.

eggs. Multiple stool samples may also be required to demonstrate swallowed eggs.[75] Serology provides an excellent alternative diagnostic tool for this disease in cases where infection is suspected based on clinical presentation. Western blot serology using crude antigen derived from adult *P. westermani* is available through the U.S. CDC and has a sensitivity of 96% and specificity of 99% for *P. westermani* infections, based on sera from egg-confirmed, symptomatic cases.[83] However, the sensitivity is lower for infection with other species, including *P. kellicotti*.[76] Thus, serological results should be interpreted carefully if species other than *P. westermani* are suspected based on travel or potential exposure history. Due to the potential cross-reactivity and complications in interpretation, serological testing for paragonimiasis should only be performed when a combination of relevant travel history and clinically suggestive signs/symptoms are present.

If adult worms are recovered, species identification is possible but requires detailed examination of anatomical features by an experienced morphologist with or without molecular sequencing of mitochondrial genes. Molecular tests for the detection and identification of *Paragonimus* species, as well as species-specific recombinant antigen tests are under development, but are not available for routine clinical use at the time of writing.

Paragonimiasis may be effectively treated with oral praziquantel 25 mg/kg given three times daily for 2 consecutive days. Triclabendazole (10 mg/kg) given orally once or on 2 consecutive days has also been used.[84] Disease control involves primarily education, particularly about the need to cook foods[73] to at least 63°C[84] and avoidance of consuming raw, pickled or undercooked crustaceans or raw boar meat.[80]

INTESTINAL TREMATODIASES

The following trematodes inhabit the gastrointestinal tract of definitive hosts. Apart from heavy infections associated with some species, most cause asymptomatic infections and are thus rarely if ever screened. Therefore, the true diversity of human-infecting intestinal trematodes is likely underappreciated, particularly considering morphologic similarities among eggs across some taxa. Only selected species are discussed here.

Fasciolopsis Buski

The best studied of the human intestinal flukes, *Fasciolopsis buski* is a large fluke restricted to East and Southeast Asia. Adults are oblong, somewhat tapered on both ends, and can reach 8–10 × 1–3 cm in size (Fig. 129-2). This fluke has been detected in China, Taiwan, India, Bangladesh, Vietnam, Cambodia, Laos, Thailand, Singapore, Malaysia, and Indonesia. Within these endemic regions, the occurrence of fasciolopsiasis is often characterized by foci with very high prevalence. Infections were detected in 80% of adults and 86% of children in Chekiang Province, China, 57% of children in Tainan, China, 60% in India, and 50% in Bangladesh, and 25% in Taiwan.[41,85]

Transmission occurs in an indirect, aquatic life cycle typical of most flukes discussed in this chapter. Eggs shed in the feces of infected hosts develop in water over 2–3 weeks in typical tropical summer conditions, after which a miracidium hatches out and infects a snail intermediate host (*Gyraulus chinensis*, *Polyphylis hemisphaerula*, and *Segmentia* spp. are known competent species). Cercariae emerge from the infected snail, and encyst to infective metacercariae on the surface of aquatic plants. People and swine are infected after consuming metacercariae on plants; no other animal definitive hosts have been identified. Adult flukes develop in the small intestine, but in heavy infections can be found in the stomach and colon. Water chestnut, water caltrop, and lotus grown for consumption are often fertilized with night soil, or cultivated near where swine are kept, and are thus common vehicles for the transmission of *F. buski* to the final host.[86]

While fasciolopsiasis is rarely fatal, it is a source of considerable morbidity. Generalized symptoms such as headache, lethargy, mild anemia, peripheral eosinophilia, abdominal pain, and loose stools are usually present in light infections. With heavy infections, symptoms may be more severe and malabsorption may occur due to fluke-induced damage of the intestinal mucosa.[85] Diagnosis is based on the detection of eggs in the stool (120–130 × 70–80 μm, thin-shelled and golden in color with an inconspicuous operculum). These eggs can be difficult or impossible to distinguish from *Fasciola* spp. A single dose of praziquantel (15 mg/kg) has been shown to be an efficacious treatment amongst Thai children,[87] although infection can recur if precautions are not taken to prevent or interrupt transmission (e.g., cooking vegetables prior to eating, restricting swine from aquatic cropland, discontinuing the use of nightsoil). The CDC suggests a praziquantel dose of 75 mg/kg administered orally in three doses over a single day.[88]

Heterophyid Trematodes

Heterophyid trematodes are a diverse group. *Heterophyes heterophyes, H. nocens* (=*H. heterophyes nocens*), and *Metagonimus yokogawai* are the most medically important of these "minute intestinal flukes." These species have pear-shaped bodies covered in spines, and reach similar adult sizes of only 1–2.5 mm long to 0.3–0.75 mm in width (Fig. 129-2). Eggs are also minute, measuring 28–30 μm × 15–17 μm, and are embryonated when passed. These two species are overall quite similar in morphology, but can be distinguished based on the nature and position of the ventral sucker and genital pores.[41]

The life cycle and transmission are similar to that of the opisthorchids; metacercariae encyst in the skeletal muscle of fish and transmission to the definitive host occurs via this foodborne route. *Heterophyes* spp. occurs in brackish water environments, and the most typical fish host is a mullet (family Mugilidae). In contrast, *M. yokogawai* is a freshwater species and infects freshwater cyprinid fish; human infection is commonly linked to undercooked Ayu sweetfish (*Plecoglossus altivelis*).[41,89] Natural hosts are diverse, including cats, dogs, jackals, and fish-eating birds. The adult fluke buries deep into the small intestinal wall, which can cause significant diarrhea and colicky abdominal pain in heavy infections. Occasionally, ectopic infections can occur.[89]

The endemic range of *H. heterophyes* encompasses the Middle East and North Africa, particularly in the Nile Delta region. Once considered a subspecies of *H. heterophyes, H. nocens* is now regarded as a morphologically and geographically distinct species and is endemic to Japan and Korea.[90] One case report of a human infection with *H. dispar,* a species associated primarily with canids, exists but is of questionable validity.[91] *M. yokogawai* occurs across much of East Asia, where most human infections are reported. It is also found in its natural hosts across parts of the Middle East in some Balkan countries although human cases are less frequently reported from these locations.[41]

Echinostomid Trematodes

Flukes in the family *Echinostomatidae* are long, narrow (usually 2–10 mm long, 1–2 mm wide), and possess a characteristic spiny collar, from which the name is derived (Fig. 129-2). A large number of species across different echinostome genera have been reported from human infections, such as *Echinostoma* (*E. hortense, E. macrorchis, E. ilocanum, E. trivolis, E. caproni, E. revolutum, E. cinetorchis, etc.*), *Echinochasmus* (*E. japonicus, E. liliputianus, E. perfoliatus,* etc.), *Echinoparyphium,* and *Artyfechinostomum;* this list is not exhaustive and nomenclature is continually being revised.[41,92,93] These are normally parasites of various birds and rats, and occasionally dogs,[94] and use freshwater planorbid snails as first intermediate hosts. The typical second intermediate hosts for echinostomes are some mollusks (including other snails) and amphibians, and less commonly fish. Despite fish being a somewhat minor host, the majority of human cases have been linked to consumption of undercooked fish and not amphibians.[95] However, in some Asian countries, dishes with frog and salamander meat are popular which may present a risk of transmission. Following ingestion of undercooked meat containing metacercariae, adults mature in about 2 weeks in the small intestine and produce eggs. Eggs are rather large (96–100 × 60–71 μm; variable by species), unembryonated, golden-brown, with a shallow operculum. Large eggs outwardly resemble those of *Fasciola* spp. and *Fasciolopsis buski.*[41]

Human echinostomiasis is mostly recognized in East and Southeast Asia, and could perhaps be underrecognized in other areas given that many echinostomes (including known zoonotic agents) occur broadly across North America, South America, Europe, and Africa.[96] Clinical signs involve nonspecific gastrointestinal dysfunction, which is related to pathology associated with the fluke's attachment to the intestinal mucosa. The deep anchoring of the echinostome spiny collar is capable of creating ulcerative, inflamed lesions. Abdominal pain, cramps, anorexia, and diarrhea are usually reported.[95]

References

1. International Agency for Cancer Research. *IARC: Monograph on Biological Agents: A Review of Human Carcinogens.* Lyon, France: International Agency for Cancer Research; 2012.
2. Saijuntha W, Sithithaworn P, Kaitsopit N, Andrews RH, Petney TN. *Liver Flukes: Clonorchis and Opisthorchis. Digenetic Trematodes.* New York: Springer; 2014, pp. 153–99.
3. World Health Organization. WHO estimates of the global burden of foodborne diseases: Foodborne disease burden epidemiology reference group 2007–2015. 2015.
4. Kim J-H, Choi M-H, Bae YM, Oh J-K, Lim MK, Hong S-T. Correlation between discharged worms and fecal egg counts in human clonorchiasis. *PLoS Negl Trop Dis.* 2011;5:e1339.
5. Wykoff DE, Chittayasothorn K, Winn MM. Clinical manifestations of *Opisthorchis viverrini* infections in Thailand. *Am J Trop Med Hyg.* 1966; 15:914–8.
6. Petney TN, Andrews RH, Saijuntha W, Wenz-Mücke A, Sithithaworn P. The zoonotic, fish-borne liver flukes *Clonorchis sinensis, Opisthorchis felineus* and *Opisthorchis viverrini. Int J Parasitol.* 2013;43:1031–46.
7. Wykoff DE, Harinasuta C, Juttijudata P, Winn MM. *Opisthorchis viverrini* in Thailand: The life cycle and comparison with *O. felineus. J Parasitol.* 1965:207–14.
8. Saijuntha W, Sithithaworn P, Wongkham S, et al. Evidence of a species complex within the food-borne trematode *Opisthorchis viverrini* and possible co-evolution with their first intermediate hosts. *Int J Parasitol.* 2007;37:695–703.
9. Petney TN, Andrews RH, Saijuntha W, et al. Taxonomy, ecology and population genetics of *Opisthorchis viverrini* and its intermediate hosts. *Adv Parasitol.* 2018;101:1–39.
10. Aung WPP, Htoon TT, Tin HH, et al. First report and molecular identification of *Opisthorchis viverrini* infection in human communities from Lower Myanmar. *PLoS One.* 2017;12:e0177130.
11. Pumidonming W, Katahira H, Igarashi M, Salman D, Abdelbaset AE, Sangkaeo K. Potential risk of a liver fluke *Opisthorchis viverrini* infection brought by immigrants from prevalent areas: A case study in the lower Northern Thailand. *Acta Trop.* 2018;178:213–8.
12. Pakharukova MY, Mordvinov VA. The liver fluke *Opisthorchis felineus*: Biology, epidemiology and carcinogenic potential. *Trans R Soc Trop Med Hyg.* 2016;110:28–36.
13. Traverso A, Repetto E, Magnani S, et al. A large outbreak of *Opisthorchis felineus* in Italy suggests that opisthorchiasis develops as a febrile eosinophilic syndrome with cholestasis rather than a hepatitis-like syndrome. *Eur J Clin Microbiol Infect Dis.* 2012;31:1089–93.
14. Qian M-B, Utzinger J, Keiser J, Zhou X-N. Clonorchiasis. *Lancet.* 2016;387: 800–10.
15. Mairiang E, Mairiang P. Clinical manifestation of opisthorchiasis and treatment. *Acta Trop.* 2003;88:221–7.
16. Sun T. Pathology and immunology of *Clonorchis sinensis* infection of the liver. *Ann Clin Lab Sci.* 1984;14:208–15.
17. Sripa B, Bethony JM, Sithithaworn P, et al. Opisthorchiasis and Opisthorchis-associated cholangiocarcinoma in Thailand and Laos. *Acta Trop.* 2011; 120(Suppl 1):S158–68.
18. Sripa B. Pathobiology of opisthorchiasis: An update. *Acta Trop.* 2003; 88:209–20.
19. Doanh PN, Nawa Y. *Clonorchis sinensis* and *Opisthorchis* spp. in Vietnam: Current status and prospects. *Trans R Soc Trop Med Hyg.* 2016;110:13–20.
20. Le TH, Van De N, Blair D, Sithithaworn P, McManus DP. *Clonorchis sinensis* and *Opisthorchis viverrini*: Development of a mitochondrial-based

multiplex PCR for their identification and discrimination. *Exp Parasitol.* 2006;112:109–14.

21. Qiao T, Zheng P-M, Ma R-H, Luo X-B, Luo Z-L. Development of a real-time PCR assay for the detection of *Clonorchis sinensis* DNA in gallbladder bile and stone samples from patients with cholecystolithiasis. *Parasitol Res.* 2012;111:1497–503.
22. Lim MK, Ju Y-H, Franceschi S, et al. *Clonorchis sinensis* infection and increasing risk of cholangiocarcinoma in the Republic of Korea. *Am J Trop Med Hyg.* 2006;75:93–6.
23. Shi Y, Jiang Z, Yang Y, et al. *Clonorchis sinensis* infection and co-infection with the hepatitis B virus are important factors associated with cholangiocarcinoma and hepatocellular carcinoma. *Parasitol Res.* 2017;116:2645–9.
24. Sithithaworn P, Haswell-Elkins M. Epidemiology of *Opisthorchis viverrini. Acta Trop.* 2003;88:187–94.
25. Sripa B, Pairojkul C. Cholangiocarcinoma: Lessons from Thailand. *Curr Opin Gastroenterol.* 2008;24:349.
26. Sithithaworn P, Yongvanit P, Duenngai K, Kiatsopit N, Pairojkul C. Roles of liver fluke infection as risk factor for cholangiocarcinoma. *J Hepatobiliary Pancreat Sci.* 2014;21:301–8.
27. World Health Organization. Control of foodborne trematode infections: Report of a WHO study group. 1995.
28. Pitaksakulrat O, Kiatsopit N, Laoprom N, et al. Preliminary genetic evidence of two different populations of *Opisthorchis viverrini* in Lao PDR. *Parasitol Res.* 2017;116:1247–56.
29. Centers for Disease Control and Prevention. Opisthorchiasis: Resources for health professionals. 2018.
30. Jongsuksuntigul P, Imsomboon T. Opisthorchiasis control in Thailand. *Acta Trop.* 2003;88:229–32.
31. Kaewpitoon N, Kootanavanichpong N, Kompor P, et al. Review and current status of *Opisthorchis viverrini* infection at the community level in Thailand. *Asian Pac J Cancer Prev.* 2015;16:6825–30.
32. Grundy-Warr C, Andrews RH, Sithithaworn P, et al. Raw attitudes, wetland cultures, life-cycles: Socio-cultural dynamics relating to *Opisthorchis viverrini* in the Mekong Basin. *Parasitol Int.* 2012;61:65–70.
33. Campbell SJ, Biritwum N-K, Woods G, Velleman Y, Fleming F, Stothard JR. Tailoring water, sanitation, and hygiene (WASH) targets for soil-transmitted helminthiasis and schistosomiasis control. *Trends Parasitol.* 2018;34:53–63.
34. Aunpromma S, Tangkawattana P, Papirom P, et al. High prevalence of *Opisthorchis viverrini* infection in reservoir hosts in four districts of Khon Kaen Province, an opisthorchiasis endemic area of Thailand. *Parasitol Int.* 2012;61:60–4.
35. Enes JE, Wages AJ, Malone JB, Tesana S. Prevalence of *Opisthorchis viverrini* infection in the canine and feline hosts in three villages, Khon Kaen Province, northeastern Thailand. *Southeast Asian J Trop Med Public Health.* 2010;41:36.
36. Fürst T, Keiser J, Utzinger J. Global burden of human food-borne trematodiasis: A systematic review and meta-analysis. *Lancet Infect Dis.* 2012; 12:210–21.
37. Charlier J, Vercruysse J, Morgan E, van Dijk J, Williams DJ. Recent advances in the diagnosis, impact on production and prediction of *Fasciola hepatica* in cattle. *Parasitology.* 2014;141:326–35.
38. Mas-Coma S, Bargues MD, Valero M. Fascioliasis and other plant-borne trematode zoonoses. *Int J Parasitol.* 2005;35:1255–78.
39. Le TH, Van De N, Agatsuma T, et al. Human fascioliasis and the presence of hybrid/introgressed forms of *Fasciola hepatica* and *Fasciola gigantica* in Vietnam. *Int J Parasitol.* 2008;38:725–30.
40. Periago M, Valero M, El Sayed M, et al. First phenotypic description of *Fasciola hepatica/Fasciola gigantica* intermediate forms from the human endemic area of the Nile Delta, Egypt. *Infect Genet Evol.* 2008;8:51–8.
41. Miyazaki I. *An Illustrated Book of Helminthic Zoonoses.* Tokyo: International Medical Foundation of Japan; 1991.
42. Doy T, Hughes D. Early migration of immature *Fasciola hepatica* and associated liver pathology in cattle. *Res Vet Sci.* 1984;37:219–22.
43. Fica A, Dabanch J, Farias C, Castro M, Jercic M, Weitzel T. Acute fascioliasis—Clinical and epidemiological features of four patients in Chile. *Clin Microbiol Infect.* 2012;18:91–6.
44. Marcos LA, Tagle M, Terashima A, et al. Natural history, clinicoradiologic correlates, and response to triclabendazole in acute massive fascioliasis. *Am J Trop Med Hyg.* 2008;78:222–7.
45. Park CI, Kim H, Ro JY, Gutierrez Y. Human ectopic fascioliasis in the cecum. *Am J Surg Pathol.* 1984;8:73–7.
46. Vatsal DK, Kapoor S, Venkatesh V, Vatsal P, Husain N. Ectopic fascioliasis in the dorsal spine: Case report. *Neurosurgery.* 2006;59:E706–7; discussion E-7.
47. Mas-Coma S, Agramunt VH, Valero MA. Neurological and ocular fascioliasis in humans. *Adv Parasitol.* 2014;84:27–149.
48. Taira N, Yoshifuji H, Boray JC. Zoonotic potential of infection with *Fasciola* spp. by consumption of freshly prepared raw liver containing immature flukes. *Int J Parasitol.* 1997;27:775–9.
49. Mas-Coma S. Epidemiology of fascioliasis in human endemic areas. *J Helminthol.* 2005;79:207–16.
50. Marcos L, Maco V, Samalvides F, Terashima A, Espinoza JR, Gotuzzo E. Risk factors for *Fasciola hepatica* infection in children: A case–control study. *Trans R Soc Trop Med Hyg.* 2006;100:158–66.
51. Fentie T, Erqou S, Gedefaw M, Desta A. Epidemiology of human fascioliasis and intestinal parasitosis among schoolchildren in Lake Tana Basin, northwest Ethiopia. *Trans R Soc Trop Med Hyg.* 2013;107:480–6.
52. Curtale F, Hassanein YAW, Barduagni P, et al. Human fascioliasis infection: Gender differences within school-age children from endemic areas of the Nile Delta, Egypt. *Trans R Soc Trop Med Hyg.* 2007;101:155–60.
53. Webb CM, Cabada MM. Recent developments in the epidemiology, diagnosis, and treatment of Fasciola infection. *Curr Opin Infect Dis.* 2018; 31:409–14.
54. Mas-Coma S, Bargues MD, Valero MA. Diagnosis of human fascioliasis by stool and blood techniques: Update for the present global scenario. *Parasitology.* 2014;141:1918–46.
55. Valero MA, Perez-Crespo I, Periago MV, Khoubbane M, Mas-Coma S. Fluke egg characteristics for the diagnosis of human and animal fascioliasis by *Fasciola hepatica* and *F. gigantica. Acta Trop.* 2009;111:150–9.
56. Duthaler U, Rinaldi L, Maurelli MP, et al. *Fasciola hepatica*: Comparison of the sedimentation and FLOTAC techniques for the detection and quantification of faecal egg counts in rats. *Exp Parasitol.* 2010;126:161–6.
57. Sarkari B, Khabisi SA. Immunodiagnosis of human fascioliasis: An update of concepts and performances of the serological assays. *J Clin Diagn Res.* 2017;11:OE05–10.
58. Valero MA, Periago MV, Perez-Crespo I, et al. Assessing the validity of an ELISA test for the serological diagnosis of human fascioliasis in different epidemiological situations. *Trop Med Int Health.* 2012;17:630–6.
59. Khan MAH, Ullah R, Rehman A, Rehman L, Ahammed SPA, Abidi SMA. Immunolocalization and immunodetection of the excretory/secretory (ES) antigens of *Fasciola gigantica. PLoS One.* 2017;12:e0185870.
60. Shin SH, Hsu A, Chastain HM, et al. Development of two FhSAP2 recombinant-based assays for immunodiagnosis of human chronic fascioliasis. *Am J Trop Med Hyg.* 2016;95:852–5.
61. Keiser J, Duthaler U, Utzinger J. Update on the diagnosis and treatment of food-borne trematode infections. *Curr Opin Infect Dis.* 2010;23:513–20.
62. Patel NU, Bang TJ, Dodd 3rd GD. CT findings of human *Fasciola hepatica* infection: Case reports and review of the literature. *Clin Imaging.* 2016;40:251–5.
63. World Health Organization. *Fascioliasis Diagnosis, Treatment and Control Strategy.* Foodborne trematode infections. Geneva: World Health Organization; 2018.
64. Patrick DM, Isaac-Renton J. Praziquantel failure in the treatment of *Fasciola hepatica. Can J Infect Dis Med Microbiol.* 1992;3:33–6.
65. Keiser J, Engels D, Buscher G, Utzinger J. Triclabendazole for the treatment of fascioliasis and paragonimiasis. *Expert Opin Investig Drugs.* 2005; 14:1513–26.
66. Bosnak VK, Karaoglan I, Sahin HH, et al. Evaluation of patients diagnosed with fascioliasis: A six-year experience at a university hospital in Turkey. *J Infect Dev Ctries.* 2016;10:389–94.
67. Dauchy FA, Vincendeau P, Lifermann F. Eight cases of fascioliasis: Clinical and microbiological features. *Med Mal Infect.* 2006;36:42–6.
68. Millan JC, Mull R, Freise S, Richter J, Triclabendazole Study G. The efficacy and tolerability of triclabendazole in Cuban patients with latent and chronic *Fasciola hepatica* infection. *Am J Trop Med Hyg.* 2000;63:264–9.
69. Zumaquero-Ríos JL, Sarracent-Pérez J, Rojas-García R, et al. Fascioliasis and intestinal parasitoses affecting schoolchildren in Atlixco, Puebla State, Mexico: Epidemiology and treatment with nitazoxanide. *PLoS Negl Trop Dis.* 2013;7:e2553.
70. Favennec L, Jave Ortiz J, Gargala G, et al. Double-blind, randomized, placebo-controlled study of nitazoxanide in the treatment of fascioliasis in adults and children from northern Peru. *Aliment Pharmacol Ther.* 2003;17:265–70.
71. Rossignol JF, Abaza H, Friedman H. Successful treatment of human fascioliasis with nitazoxanide. *Trans R Soc Trop Med Hyg.* 1998;92:103–4.
72. Fox L. Infectious diseases related to travel: Fascioliasis. In: Centers for Disease Control and Prevention, ed. *CDC Yellow Book 2018: Health Information for International Travel.* New York: Oxford University Press; 2018.

73. Liu Q, Wei F, Liu W, Yang S, Zhang X. Paragonimiasis: An important food-borne zoonosis in China. *Trends Parasitol.* 2008;24:318–23.

74. Blair D, Xu Z-B, Agatsuma T. Paragonimiasis and the genus Paragonimus. *Adv Parasitol.* 1999:42;113–222.

75. Keiser J, Utzinger J. Food-borne trematodiases. *Clin Microbiol Rev.* 2009; 22:466–83.

76. Lane MA, Marcos LA, Onen NF, et al. Paragonimus kellicotti flukes in Missouri, USA. *Emerg Infect Dis.* 2012;18:1263–7.

77. Kanazawa T, Hata H, Kojima S, Yokogawa M. Paragonimus westermani: A comparative study on the migration route of the diploid and triploid types in the final hosts. *Parasitol Res.* 1987;73:140–5.

78. Beaver PC, Jung RC, Cupp EW, Craig CF. *Clinical Parasitology.* Philadelphia: Lea & Febiger; 1984.

79. Chan ED, Morales DV, Welsh CH, McDermott MT, Schwarz MI. Calcium deposition with or without bone formation in the lung. *Am J Respir Crit Care Med.* 2002;165:1654–69.

80. Blair D, Agatsuma T, Wang W. Paragonimiasis. In: Murrell KD, Fried BMurrell KD, Fried B, eds. *Food-borne Parasitic Zoonoses. World Class Parasites.* Vol. 11. Boston, MA: Springer; 2007, pp. 117–50.

81. Weinstein PP, Duman LJ, Trelawny GS, Patterson JC. Paragonimiasis: Failure of nilodin in therapy and report of one case with urinary tract involvement. *Am J Trop Med Hyg.* 1953;2:517–23.

82. Slesak G, Inthalad S, Basy P, et al. Ziehl-Neelsen staining technique can diagnose paragonimiasis. *PLoS Negl Trop Dis.* 2011;5:e1048.

83. Slemenda SB, Maddison SE, Jong EC, Moore DD. Diagnosis of paragonimiasis by immunoblot. *Am J Trop Med Hyg.* 1988;39:469–71.

84. Centers for Disease Control and Prevention. *DPDM Fact Sheet—Paragonimiasis.* Atlanta: Centers for Disease Control and Prevention; 2018.

85. Fried B, Graczyk TK, Tamang L. Food-borne intestinal trematodiases in humans. *Parasitol Res.* 2004;93:159–70.

86. Graczyk TK, Gilman RH, Fried B. Fasciolopsiasis: Is it a controllable food-borne disease? *Parasitol Res.* 2001;87:80–3.

87. Harinasuta T, Bunnag D, Radomyos P. Efficacy of praziquantel on fasciolopsiasis. *Arzneimittelforschung.* 1984;34:1214–5.

88. Centers for Disease Control and Prevention. Fasciolopsiasis: Resources for health professionals. 2018.

89. Keiser J, Utzinger J. Emerging foodborne trematodiasis. *Emerg Infect Dis.* 2005;11:1507–14.

90. Chai J-Y, Hong S-J, Shon W-M, Lee S-H, Seo B-S. Further cases of human *Heterophyes heterophyes nocens* infection in Korea. *Seoul J Med.* 1985;26(2):197–200.

91. Chai JY, Seo BS, Lee SH, Hong SJ, Sohn WM. Human infections by *Heterophyes heterophyes* and *H. dispar* imported from Saudi Arabia. *Korean J Parasitol.* 1986;24:82–6.

92. Belizario VY, Geronilla GG, Anastacio MB, et al. *Echinostoma malayanum* infection, the Philippines. *Emerg Infect Dis.* 2007;13:1130–1.

93. Chai JY, Sohn WM, Cho J, et al. *Echinostoma ilocanum* Infection in two residents of Savannakhet Province, Lao PDR. *Korean J Parasitol.* 2018;56:75–9.

94. Seo B-S, Cho S-Y, Chai J-Y. Studies on intestinal trematodes in Korea 1. A human case of *Echinostoma cinetorchis* infection with an epidemiological investigation. *Seoul J Med.* 1980;21(1):21–9.

95. Chang Y-D, Sohn W-M, Ryu J-H, Kang S-Y, Hong S-J. A human infection of *Echinostoma hortense* in duodenal bulb diagnosed by endoscopy. *Korean J Parasitol.* 2005;43:57.

96. Huffman JE, Fried B. Echinostoma and echinostomiasis. *Adv Parasitol.* 1990;29:215–69.

CHAPTER

130

Taeniasis and Cysticercosis*

Richard S. Bradbury • Sukwan Handali

Taeniasis refers to an intestinal infection with the adult stage of the beef tapeworm (*Taenia saginata*), the pork tapeworm (*T. solium*), or the Asian pork tapeworm (*T. asiatica*). Cysticercosis is the somatic infection with the larval stage of the pork tapeworm. Neurocysticercosis (NCC) is central nervous system infection with *T. solium* larvae. Both beef and pork tapeworms have been known as parasites of humans since ancient times, but infection of humans by the larval stage of the pork tapeworm was not recognized until the sixteenth century.[1]

LIFE CYCLE

Cestodes of the family Taeniidae complete their cycle in two mammalian hosts, typically a carnivore and an herbivore, between which a well-defined predator/prey relationship exists.[1,2] Humans are the definitive hosts for three species of *Taenia*: *T. saginata*, *T. solium*, and *T. asiatica*. The larval stages infect cattle (*T. saginata*) and swine (*T. solium and T. asiatica*). The larvae of *T. solium* can develop in dogs and humans.[3-5] Larval stages of *T. asiatica* are only found in pigs and it is assumed to be confined to the liver of this porcine host.[6] However, its high prevalence in some countries where raw liver is not routinely consumed suggests that *T. asiatica* may encyst in other organs.[7] The northern strain of *T. saginata*, reported only from northern Russia (Siberia), has a unique life cycle with larvae encysted in the muscles and cerebral meninges of reindeer. The transmission cycle of this strain is maintained by the local custom of eating raw reindeer brain.[8]

Humans contract taeniasis through the ingestion of infective cysticerci in raw or undercooked beef, pork, or dog meat (Fig. 130-1).[2] In the small intestine, the cysticercus inserts its scolex to attach to the mucosa and develops into the adult worm, which can survive for up to 30 years in the human intestine. Usually one tapeworm is present, but up to 25 have been reported from a single host.[9] Adult *T. saginata* usually measure 4–12 meters in length, but may reach lengths up to 25 meters, while *T. solium* grows to lengths of between 2 and 8 meters.[10] Release of segments containing eggs infective for the intermediate host begins in the human intestine after 10–12 weeks for *T. saginata*, 5–12 weeks for *T. solium, and 8–17 weeks for T. asiatica.*[6,9] A single gravid proglottid may contain between 1000 and 2000 eggs for *T. saginata*, 1000 eggs for *T. solium* and approximately 700 eggs for *T. asiatica*.[10] A tapeworm carrier releases between six and nine proglottids daily.

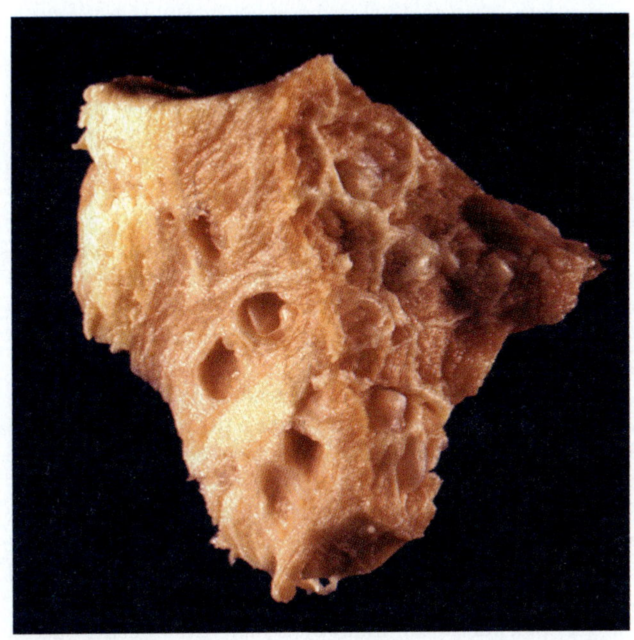

FIGURE 130-1. Cysticerci, larval forms of *T. solium*, in "measly" pork. (*Source:* Dr. Green/CDC.)

Cysticercosis is caused by infection with the larval stage of *T. solium*. Although *T. solium* taeniasis is acquired through consumption of infected pork, people who do not eat meat can acquire cysticercosis through ingestion of food or fomites contaminated with fecal matter passed by a person infected with the *T. solium* adult stage tapeworm. As an example, an outbreak of NCC was described among members of an orthodox Jewish community, likely due to transmission from a household worker with *T. solium* taeniasis.[11,12] People can also acquire cysticercosis by ingestion of *T. solium* eggs from their own stool. Internal autoinfection, in which egg containing proglottids of *T. solium* are "swept back" into the stomach by reverse peristalsis, is also possible.

DISTRIBUTION

It is estimated that 45–60 million people worldwide are infected with *T. saginata*.[13] However, many of the studies employed for this estimate did not differentiate *T. saginata* from *T. asiatica*; the latter accounting for up to 20% of taeniasis infections in some countries.[7,13] *T. solium* taeniasis is estimated to affect 2.5 million people worldwide,[14] with a population of 103 million at risk of the disease.[15] *T. saginata* is particularly common in some regions of East Africa and some Latin American countries.[10] The highest rates of human infections have been reported from Africa, among nomadic cattle herders.[1,2] *T. saginata* taeniasis is rarely reported from developed countries. However, rare

*Disclaimer:** The findings and conclusions in this book chapter are those of the author and do not necessarily represent the official position of the Centers for Disease Control and Prevention/the Agency for Toxic Substances and Disease Registry.

autochthonous transmission has occurred in Spain, Portugal, and parts of Central Europe, Eastern Europe, and Russia.[16] *T. solium* taeniasis is most prevalent in Eastern Europe, sub-Saharan Africa, India, Asia, and Latin America.[10] Immigrants from these areas who migrate to developed countries can arrive with active infections.[10] *T. asiatica* is widely distributed in East and Southeast Asia, including China, South Korea, Japan, Nepal, Thailand, the Philippines, Indonesia, and Laos.[6,7,17] *T. asiatica* is the predominant *Taenia* species infecting humans in Vietnam and northern India.[7,18] Cysticercosis is estimated to affect 2.7 million people globally.[19] It is responsible for approximately 30% of epilepsy cases in endemic areas, and an estimated -28,000 deaths annually.[14,20] Multiple genotypes of *T. solium* have been identified and it has been suggested that genetic variation may be responsible for differing prevalence of subcutaneous and muscular cysticercosis (SCC) versus NCC in different geographic regions.[21]

TABLE 130-1 CLASSIFICATION OF THE CLINICAL PRESENTATIONS OF NEUROCYSTICERCOSIS ACCORDING TO THE INFECTIOUS DISEASES SOCIETY OF AMERICA/AMERICAN SOCIETY OF TROPICAL MEDICINE AND HYGIENE GUIDELINES[29]

Parenchymal	Extraparenchymal
Nonviable calcified	Intraventricular
Single, small enhancing	Subarachnoid
Viable parenchymal	Spinal

CLINICAL PICTURE

Taeniasis in the human intestine is often asymptomatic. The symptoms, when present, are nonspecific and include abdominal pain, nausea, flatulence, diarrhea, and weight loss. Patients, especially those infected with *T. saginata*, may sense the active migration of proglottids through the anus. *T. solium* proglottids do not migrate spontaneously.

In humans, systemic infection with *T. solium* larvae causes cysticercosis. This cestode is unique in the Taeniidae family in that both stages of its life cycle can develop in a single mammalian host; the preferred sites of larvae being the central nervous system, eyes, skeletal muscle, or subcutaneous tissues.[22]

Symptoms of cysticercosis vary depending on the size, location, and number of larval cysts, as well as the host's immune response.[22] SCC is generally asymptomatic. When large numbers of cysts are present, a condition known as disseminated cysticercosis may occur. Subcutaneous cysts can be palpable and are often asymptomatic or may be painful.[23] Medical imaging may reveal large numbers of cysts in other tissues, including the muscles, brain, eye, thyroid, and pleura.[24]

Significant functional disturbances may result when cysticerci localize in tissues of the central nervous system. NCC can be associated with a variety of clinical symptoms. Seizures are the most common clinical manifestation and occur in about 80–90% of cases.[25] Intracranial hypertension, neurologic deficits, and sometimes psychiatric manifestations, including psychosis, may also occur.[22,26] Less commonly, patients will present with headache, symptoms of elevated intracranial pressure, depressed mental status (including coma), stiff neck, or focal neurologic findings. The clinical presentation depends on the location, number, and viability of the cysts as well as the host response to their presence.[25,27,28] The Infectious Diseases Society of America/American Society of Tropical Medicine and Hygiene guidelines classify NCC into three parenchymal and three extraparenchymal presentations (Table 130-1).[29] The organ tropism of cysticercosis differs geographically. In Latin America, NCC patients rarely present with evidence of SCC, whereas in Asia patients present with both forms of the disease. In Africa, SCC associated with NCC is rare in some regions, but common in others.[21] Ophthalmic cysticercosis occurs in 1–3% of patients with cysticercosis.[2]

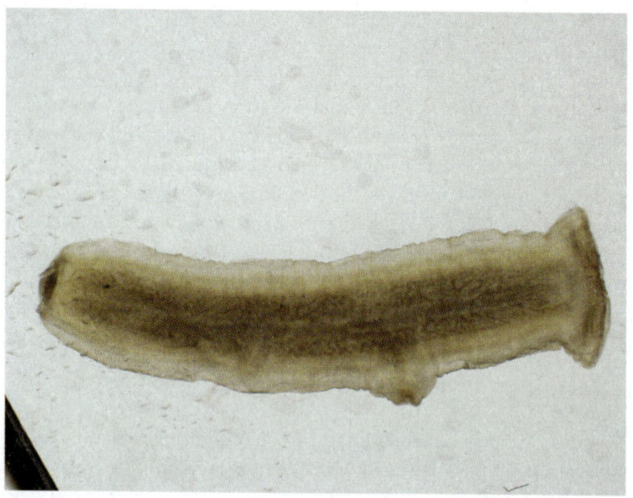

FIGURE 130-2. Gravid proglottid of *T. saginata* passed per rectum. Note the many uterine branches, which have been filled with India Ink to allow visualization. (*Source:* Sarah G. H. Sapp, PhD.)

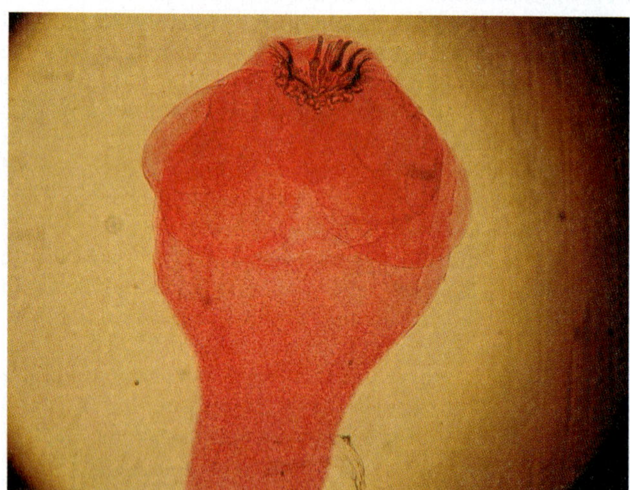

FIGURE 130-3. Scolex of *T. solium* showing for suckers and armed rostellum. (Dr. Richard S. Bradbury.)

DIAGNOSIS

The diagnosis of taeniasis is based on detection of the characteristic eggs or proglottids, or their DNA, in stool. The eggs of *T. solium* and *T. saginata* are morphologically indistinguishable, but the species can be differentiated by examination of the gravid proglottids. The number of primary uterine branches in *T. saginata* gravid proglottids is 14–32, whereas *T. solium* has 7–16 and *T. asiatica* have 11–31 branches (Fig. 130-2).[30] There are also differences in the morphology of the cirrus sac between species.[31,32] Tapeworms may be passed following treatment or detected on colonoscopy. All three species of *Taenia* may be differentiated by the distinct morphology of their scolices (Fig. 130-3), but as the scolex of an infecting worm is rarely recovered, this is often not of diagnostic utility.

Microscopy of stool has a sensitivity of 60–70% for detection of intestinal taeniasis.[33] The formalin-ethyl acetate concentration technique appears superior to Kato Katz technique for the recovery of *Taenia* eggs in stool (Fig. 130-4).[34] However, coproantigen ELISA, currently an investigative diagnostic assay for intestinal taeniasis,

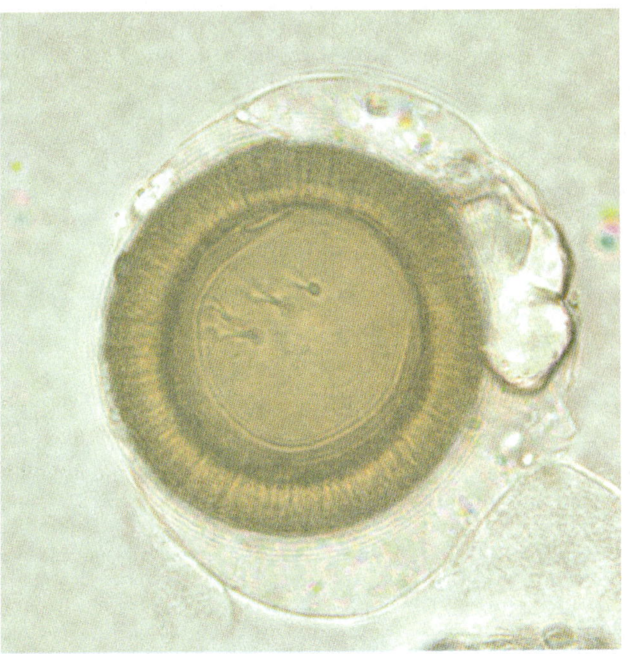

FIGURE 130-4. Egg of *Taenia* species passed in feces. (*Source:* Sarah G. H. Sapp, PhD.)

has 96% sensitivity and 100% specificity.[35] This assay was effectively used for the identification of infection clearance in patients after mass treatment during a public health program to eliminate *T. solium* from northern Peru.[36]

The use of molecular tools such as conventional, nested, and real-time polymerase chain reaction protocols has allowed highly sensitive and specific detection of *Taenia* species, as well as differentiation of species and genotypes both from eggs in infected stool and passed gravid proglottids.[37–39] In lower resourced areas, LAMP assays that will detect and differentiate *Taenia* species eggs and proglottids, have been tested and have proven effective.[40] Such tools are used in research only settings at present, but may be adopted for routine diagnostic use in the future.

The diagnosis of cysticercosis involving the central nervous system is sometimes difficult. Cysticercosis should be considered in the differential diagnosis of epilepsy, basilar meningitis, obstructive hydrocephalus, and other neurologic disorders in patients with a history of residence or travel in regions where *T. solium* is endemic.[27] A combination diagnostic algorithm incorporating a comprehensive clinical history, physical examination, and neuroradiologic techniques [such as computed tomography (CT) scanning and magnetic resonance imaging (MRI)], combined with serologic testing is recommended by the Infectious Diseases Society of America for the diagnosis of cysticercosis.[29] Cysts in the early, viable, vesicular stage will appear as circular (5–20 mm in diameter) lesions with clear margins and a thin wall (2–4 mm thick), with a density and signal intensity similar to cerebrospinal fluid (CSF) on MRI and CT.[41] Early vesicular cysts do not show contrast enhancement. A single curled, invaginated, larva (length 4–5 mm) with a discrete and eccentrically placed scolex may be identified within each cyst.[41,42] There may be a single or multiple cysts, with some cases having such intense infection that the brain has a "Swiss cheese" appearance.[41] Cysts may remain in this stage for several years.[42] As cysts degenerate and become nonviable, they tend to reduce in size and the scolex eventually disappears.[41,42] Cyst walls become thick and irregular, are enhanced by contrast and become hypodense and more hyperattenuating than CSF on CT.[42] Surrounding edema may be extensive in this stage.[41] The cyst will further degenerate into a small granulomatous lesion, which may appear nodular and have ring-like enhancement.[41] The surrounding edema will decrease, but gliosis of the surrounding parenchyma may be seen.[41,42] Finally, inactive, nonviable cysts will become calcified nodules, without surrounding edema; this stage is best detected using CT rather than MRI.[41,42] Cysticerci localized in subcutaneous tissues or skin can form palpable nodules that are readily identified by biopsy. Rarely, patients with massive deposition of cysts in their muscle will develop muscular pseudohypertrophy.

Immunodiagnostic tests for cysticercosis are available and contribute to the diagnosis of cysticercosis. The best performing assay for antibody detection currently available is the enzyme-linked immunoelectrotransfer blot method, using lentil-lectin affinity-purified glycoprotein antigens for immunodiagnosing human cysticercosis, which is 98% sensitive and 100% specific in patients with more than one viable brain cyst.[43] In patients with a single viable or degenerating cyst or only calcified cysts, the sensitivity is lower.[43,44] In general, the test is similarly sensitive for both serum and CSF samples.[43] However, detectable levels of antibody do not distinguish between active and past infection. Antigen detection has been used to determine the presence of live parasite cysts in the host, with levels of antigens dropping quickly following successful course of antiparasitic therapy.[43]

TREATMENT

Appropriately administered niclosamide (85% cure rate)[16] is effective for the treatment of intestinal taeniasis, but is often less available than praziquantel. Good results have been obtained with praziquantel (95% cure rate),[16] but due to its absorption in the gut, the use of praziquantel carries an attendant risk of inducing seizures in patients with concurrent NCC.[45] Albendazole has been used and has a 100% cure rate when correctly administered,[16] but also may induce seizures in patients with NCC.

The approach to treatment of NCC depends on the classification and staging of disease. The primary focus should be treatment to control neurologic manifestations. The use of drug therapy, either antiepileptic, anti-inflammatory, or antiparasitic, must be considered and tailored in context to the form and stage of NCC being treated. In many cases, antiparasitic treatment may not be indicated. Antiparasitic drugs are contraindicated in cases with uncontrolled increased cranial pressure and in cases where neurosurgery is indicated first. Disorders attributable to interference with the flow of cerebrospinal fluid due to extraparenchymal racemose cysticerci can sometimes be alleviated surgically by removing the cysts or by performing shunting procedures. The use of adjunct corticosteroid therapy, commonly prednisolone or dexamethasone, to reduce the immune response to the release of antigens by the dying cysticercus when antiparasitic drug therapy is used, is also suggested, and should begin 3 days prior to antiparasitic drugs first being administered.[29,46]

PREVENTION AND CONTROL

Requisite conditions for the infection of humans by *T. saginata*, *T. solium*, and *T. asiatica* are poor sanitation, access by livestock to human waste, and consumption of beef and pork insufficiently cooked to kill the cysticerci. The use of raw sewage containing infected human feces to fertilize crops can contribute to the transmission cycle of these organisms. The best preventive measures include maintaining strict personal hygiene and environmental sanitation, and protecting cattle and hogs from contact with human excretions. Individual infection is prevented by thorough cooking of beef and pork to above 60°C or freezing at −10°C for at least 10 days.[47] In endemic regions, educational programs are needed to alert the public to the risks of eating inadequately cooked beef and pork. In the United States, federal meat inspection includes direct examination for the presence of cysticerci (i.e., looking for "measly" meat).

Mass drug administration (MDA) of humans with albendazole, niclosamide, or praziquantel for the control of taeniasis and cysticercosis has been investigated in several settings with limited efficacy. Human MDA alone appears to reduce rates of taeniasis in the general population over the short term (2 years), but has little effect on rates of cysticercosis.[16] A high prevalence of taeniasis and cysticercosis remains in Latin America after widespread use of MDA during the 1980s and 1990s.[48] The use of drugs other than the relatively expensive niclosamide for MDA, carries the risk of inducing seizures in members of the community with NCC. MDA of pigs with oxfendazole effectively treats porcine cysticercosis for up to 3 months.[45] Treatment of cattle with praziquantel has been shown to also be highly effective in controlling *T. saginata* cysticerci, but no commercial bovine preparation of this drug is currently available.[16]

Recombinant antigen *T. solium* vaccines, such as TSOL 18 and SP3Vac have proved very effective in field trials for the control of cysticercosis in pigs.[16,48] Similarly, a TSA9/TSOL18 vaccine was found to be highly effective in protecting cattle from infection with larval *T. saginata*.[16] The TSOL18 vaccine has recently become commercially available and approved for use in India, while approval for use in Africa is currently pending.[16] It should be noted that vaccines will not be effective against existing cysts and the administration of oxfendazole to pigs in combination with vaccination may be advisable.[16] Combination therapy with niclosamide MDA in humans and oxfendazole MDA in pigs, followed by mass vaccination of pigs using TSOL18 eliminated *T. solium* transmission in Northern Peru.[36] This approach shows promise for the control and elimination of *T. solium* in similar highly endemic areas. Despite the efficacy of vaccination combined with MDA of pigs and humans, issues may arise in relation to cost and maintenance of the required cold chain during vaccine transport within affected developing countries.[45]

Intestinal taeniasis and cysticercosis remain significant public health problems in developing countries. While the diagnosis and treatment of intestinal taeniasis is quite straightforward, the diagnosis and treatment of cysticercosis presents a complex problem requiring input from clinical, laboratory, and medical imaging results, as well as tailoring of treatment in specific presentations. Control of these diseases with combination of strategies including MDA to human and pig populations, and pig vaccination appears to be effective.[38] Addition of education and hygiene, including avoidance of swine contact with human feces, appropriate cooking of pork and beef, good food-safety practices and hand hygiene, and inspection of carcasses for cysticerci are indicated.

ACKNOWLEDGMENTS

The authors would like to acknowledge the very helpful assistance and comments provided by Dr. Sue Montgomery of the Division of Parasitic Diseases and Malaria, Centers for Disease Control and Prevention.

References

1. Rausch RL. On the ecology and distribution of *Echinococcus* spp. (Cestoda: Taeniidae), and characteristics of their development in the intermediate host. *Ann Parasitol Hum Comp*. 1967;42:19–63.
2. Garcia HH, Gonzalez AE, Evans CA, Gilman RH. *Taenia solium* cysticercosis. *Lancet*. 2003;362:547–56.
3. Meijer WCP. Extracten unit de maand—En jaarverslagen der gouvernements en provinciale veeartsen. No. 62, I. Cysticercosis. II. Trichinosis. *Nederlandsch-Indische Bladen voor Diergeneeskunde en Dierenteelt*. 1933;14:165–75.
4. Okolo MI. Observations on Cysticercus cellulosae in the flesh of rural dogs. *Int J Zoonoses*. 1986;13:286–9.
5. Ito A, Putra MI, Subahar R, et al. Dogs as alternative intermediate hosts of *Taenia solium* in Papua (Irian Jaya), Indonesia confirmed by highly specific ELISA and immunoblot using native and recombinant antigens and mitochondrial DNA analysis. *J Helminthol*. 2002;76:311–4.
6. Ale A, Victor B, Praet N, et al. Epidemiology and genetic diversity of *Taenia asiatica*: A systematic review. *Parasit Vectors*. 2014;7:45.
7. Galan-Puchades MT, Fuentes MV. *Taenia asiatica*: The most neglected human *Taenia* and the possibility of cysticercosis. *Korean J Parasitol*. 2013;51:51–4.
8. Konyaev SV, Nakao M, Ito A, Lavikainen A. History of *Taenia saginata* tapeworms in Northern Russia. *Emerg Infect Dis*. 2018;23:2030–7.
9. Beaver PC, Jung RC, Cupp EW. *Clinical Parasitology*. 9th ed. Philadelphia: Lea & Febiger; 1984.
10. Centers for Disease Control and Prevention. Parasites—Taeniasis. Centers for Disease Control and Prevention; 2018.
11. Schantz PM, Moore AC, Munoz JL, et al. Neurocysticercosis in an Orthodox Jewish community in New York City. *N Engl J Med*. 1992;327:692–5.
12. Moore AC, Lutwick LI, Schantz PM, et al. Seroprevalence of cysticercosis in an Orthodox Jewish community. *Am J Trop Med Hyg*. 1995;53:439–42.
13. Clinton White A, Brunetti E. Cestodes. In: Godman L, Schafer A, eds. *Goldman's Cecil Medicine*. 24th ed. Philadelphia, PA: Elsevier; 2012, pp. 2052–7.
14. Aung AK, Spelman DW. *Taenia solium* taeniasis and cysticercosis in Southeast Asia. *Am J Trop Med Hyg*. 2016;94:947–54.
15. Torgerson PR, Devleesschauwer B, Praet N, et al. World Health Organization estimates of the global and regional disease burden of 11 foodborne parasitic diseases, 2010: A data synthesis. *PLoS Med*. 2015;12:e1001920.
16. Okello AL, Thomas LF. Human taeniasis: Current insights into prevention and management strategies in endemic countries. *Risk Manag Healthc Policy*. 2017;10:107–16.
17. Tsuboi M, Hayakawa K, Yamasaki H, et al. Clinical characteristics and epidemiology of intestinal tapeworm infections over the last decade in Tokyo, Japan: A retrospective review. *PLoS Negl Trop Dis*. 2018;12:e0006297.
18. Singh SK, Prasad KN, Singh AK, et al. Identification of species and genetic variation in Taenia isolates from human and swine of North India. *Parasitol Res*. 2016;115:3689–93.
19. GBD 2016 Disease and Injury Incidence and Prevalence Collaborators. Global, regional, and national incidence, prevalence, and years lived with disability for 328 diseases and injuries for 195 countries, 1990–2016: A systematic analysis for the Global Burden of Disease Study 2016. *Lancet*. 2017;390:1211–59.
20. Havelaar AH, Kirk MD, Torgerson PR, et al. World Health Organization global estimates and regional comparisons of the burden of foodborne disease in 2010. *PLoS Med*. 2015;12:e1001923.
21. Ito A, Yamasaki H, Nakao M, et al. Multiple genotypes of *Taenia solium*—Ramifications for diagnosis, treatment and control. *Acta Trop*. 2003;87:95–101.
22. Bouteille B. Epidemiology of cysticercosis and neurocysticercosis. *Med Sante Trop*. 2014;24:367–74.
23. Barro-Traore F, Ouedraogo MS, Sanou-Lamien A, et al. Disseminated subcutaneous cysticercosis: A report of six cases in Burkina Faso. *Bull Soc Pathol Exot*. 2008;101:17–9.
24. Mouhari-Toure A, N'Timon B, Kumako V, et al. Disseminated cysticercosis: Report of three cases in Togo. *Bull Soc Pathol Exot*. 2015;108:165–70.
25. White ACJr. Neurocysticercosis: A major cause of neurological disease worldwide. *Clin Infect Dis*. 1997;24:101–13; quiz 14-5.
26. Mahajan SK, Machhan PC, Sood BR, et al. Neurocysticercosis presenting with psychosis. *J Assoc Physicians India*. 2004;52:663–5.
27. Wallin MT, Kurtzke JF. Neurocysticercosis in the United States: Review of an important emerging infection. *Neurology*. 2004;63:1559–64.
28. Lotz J, Hewlett R, Alheit B, Bowen R. Neurocysticercosis: Correlative pathomorphology and MR imaging. *Neuroradiology*. 1988;30:35–41.
29. White AC, Coyle CM, Rajshekhar V, et al. Diagnosis and treatment of neurocysticercosis: 2017 Clinical practice guidelines by the Infectious Diseases Society of America (IDSA) and the American Society of Tropical Medicine and Hygiene (ASTMH). *Am J Trop Med Hyg*. 2018;98:945–66.
30. Parija SC, Ponnambath DK. Laboratory diagnosis of *Taenia asiatica* in humans and animals. *Trop Parasitol*. 2013;3:120–4.
31. Verster A. Redescription of *Taenia solium* Linnaeus, 1758 and *Taenia saginata* Goeze, 1782. *Z Parasitenkd*. 1967;29:313–28.
32. Eom KS. What is Asian *Taenia*? *Parasitol Int*. 2006;55 Suppl:S137–41.
33. McCarthy JS, Lustigman S, Yang GJ, Barakat RM, Garcia HH, Sripa B, et al. A research agenda for helminth diseases of humans: Diagnostics for control and elimination programmes. *PLoS Negl Trop Dis*. 2012;6:e1601.
34. Taye S. Comparison of Kato-Katz and Formol-Ether concentration methods for the diagnosis of intestinal helminthic infections among school children of Wonji Shoa town, Eastern Ethiopia: A school based cross-sectional study. *Am J Health Res*. 2014;2:271–4.
35. Guezala MC, Rodriguez S, Zamora H, et al. Development of a species-specific coproantigen ELISA for human *Taenia solium* taeniasis. *Am J Trop Med Hyg*. 2009;81:433–7.

36. Garcia HH, Gonzalez AE, Tsang VC, et al. Elimination of *Taenia solium* transmission in Northern Peru. *N Engl J Med.* 2016;374:2335–44.
37. Jeon HK, Chai JY, Kong Y, et al. Differential diagnosis of *Taenia asiatica* using multiplex PCR. *Exp Parasitol.* 2009;121:151–6.
38. Ng-Nguyen D, Stevenson MA, Dorny P, et al. Comparison of a new multiplex real-time PCR with the Kato Katz thick smear and copro-antigen ELISA for the detection and differentiation of *Taenia* spp. in human stools. *PLoS Negl Trop Dis.* 2017;11:e0005743.
39. Mayta H, Gilman RH, Prendergast E, et al. Nested PCR for specific diagnosis of *Taenia solium* taeniasis. *J Clin Microbiol.* 2008;46:286–9.
40. Nkouawa A, Sako Y, Okamoto M, Ito A. Simple identification of human *Taenia* species by multiplex loop-mediated isothermal amplification in combination with dot enzyme-linked immunosorbent assay. *Am J Trop Med Hyg.* 2016;94:1318–23.
41. Zhao JL, Lerner A, Shu Z, Gao XJ, Zee CS. Imaging spectrum of neurocysticercosis. *Radiol Infect Dis.* 2015;1:94–102.
42. Venkat B, Aggarwal N, Makhaik S, Sood R. A comprehensive review of imaging findings in human cysticercosis. *Jpn J Radiol.* 2016;34:241–57.
43. Garcia HH, O'Neal SE, Noh J, Handali S. Laboratory diagnosis of neurocysticercosis/*Taenia solium*. *J Clin Microbiol.* 2018;56(9):e00424-18.
44. Garcia HH, Nash TE, Del Brutto OH. Clinical symptoms, diagnosis, and treatment of neurocysticercosis. *Lancet Neurol.* 2014;13:1202–15.
45. Symeonidou I, Arsenopoulos K, Tzilves D, Soba B, Gabriel S, Papadopoulos E. Human taeniasis/cysticercosis: A potentially emerging parasitic disease in Europe. *Ann Gastroenterol.* 2018;31:406–12.
46. Gripper LB, Welburn SC. Neurocysticercosis infection and disease—A review. *Acta Trop.* 2017;166:218–24.
47. World Organization for Animal Health (OIE). Infection with *Taenia solium* (porcine cysticercosis). *Terrestrial Animal Health Code.* 27th ed. Paris: World Organisation for Animal Health; 2018, pp. 781–3.
48. Carpio A, Fleury A, Romo ML, Abraham R. Neurocysticercosis: The good, the bad, and the missing. *Expert Rev Neurother.* 2018;18:289–301.

CHAPTER

131 Zoonotic Cestodes*

Sarah G. H. Sapp • Richard S. Bradbury

HYDATID DISEASE (ECHINOCOCCOSIS)

Hydatid disease (echinococcosis) is the infection of humans by the larval stages of taeniid cestodes of the genus *Echinococcus*. Humans are incidental intermediate hosts for several *Echinococcus* species, which cause various forms of "hydatid disease," including cystic echinococcosis (CE), alveolar echinococcosis (AE), and neotropical echinococcosis [which includes polycystic (PE) and unicystic echinococcosis (UE)]. Four species/complexes of *Echinococcus* are currently recognized, of which three cause distinctive forms of human disease: *Echinococcus granulosus* sensu lato with cystic echinococcosis (CE), *Echinococcus multilocularis* with alveolar echinococcosis (AE), and *Echinococcus vogeli* with polycystic echinococcosis (PE). The fourth species, *E. oligarthrus*, has only rarely been identified in humans and is associated with unicystic echinococcosis (UE).[1] Diverse subpopulations of *E. granulosus*, distinguished by genetic, morphologic, and biologic characteristics, have long been recognized; the taxonomic significance of these differences remain unresolved and controversial.[1] However, recent demonstration of consistent genetic differences has prompted calls for splitting this species. A cause of high morbidity and with capacity for considerable pathology, *Echinococcus* spp. are collectively some of the most important zoonotic cestodes from a public health standpoint.[1,2]

Life Cycle

The life cycles of *Echinococcus* species involve carnivores as final hosts and herbivores or omnivores as intermediate hosts (Fig. 131-1). In their adult stages, *Echinococcus* species are "true tapeworms" belonging to Eucestoda (family Taeniidae) measuring 3–6 mm long (*E. granulosus* sensu lato) or 1.7–3.0 cm long (*E. multilocularis*) at maturity and possessing generally three to five proglottids with a large, oblong terminal proglottid. The scolex possesses a rostellum with two concentric rings of hooks and four suckers, and is attached to the strobila ("body") with a narrow, tapering neck.[3] All members of *Echinococcus* use carnivorous mammals as definitive hosts, where they typically localize in the lower duodenum and jejunum of the definitive host. All known human-infecting *Echinococcus* have definitive hosts that are members of the Canidae family, with the exception of the very rare *E. oligarthrus,* which uses various tropical members of Felidae. Eggs containing infective oncospheres are expelled in large numbers in feces. These eggs are immediately infectious to intermediate hosts, not requiring a period of development in the environment, and are rather hardy. Eggs have been shown to be viable for up to a year in cool, humid conditions.[3]

Following ingestion of eggs by susceptible intermediate hosts, oncospheres emerge from the egg in the small intestine and embed in the small intestinal wall where they enter host circulation. Oncospheres develop into metacestodes; the encapsulation of the metacestode by the intermediate host reaction forms a structure referred to as the hydatid cyst. Protoscolices and daughter cysts develop inside the fluid-filled cyst interior. The sites of localization and the structural characteristics of the hydatid cyst vary by parasite species; they may also be influenced by the species of the intermediate host. Generally, the liver and lungs are the most frequent sites for cyst development, with rare cerebral or other organ involvement. Intermediate hosts vary considerably depending on *Echinococcus* species, and intermediate host competence may vary across strains/genotypes of the same species. A general overview of definitive and intermediate hosts of public health-relevant *Echinococcus* species is provided in Table 131-1. Humans are an incidental intermediate host, since further development of these cestodes depends on ingestion of larval forms (hydatids) by a carnivore (definitive host).[3]

Definitive hosts consume hydatid cysts in infected intermediate host tissue. Protoscolices are liberated from the cyst during digestion, which also induces the process of evagination (release of the protoscolex, rostellum, and suckers) allowing attachment in the small intestine. Fully mature *Echinococcus* worms are found within intestinal crypts, anchored by the embedding of the rostellum in the mucosal layer and sucker adherence to the villus epithelium. This process occurs with virtually no significant pathology or inflammatory reaction; clinical signs are seldom observed in infected definitive hosts.[3]

Distribution/Epidemiology

E. Granulosus ***Sensu Lato***

E. granulosus sensu lato, causing cystic hydatid disease, has a broad global distribution and is present on all continents except for Antarctica, with highly endemic foci in Central Asia, Northern Africa, and Patagonia.[3] The movement of livestock across the globe and the low intermediate host specificity in some genotypes have allowed this parasite to become established over this large and climactically diverse range. Rare in the United States, sporadic cases may occur in the southwestern states and Alaska, although cases in the United States are primarily travel associated. Southeast Asia, New Zealand, Tasmania, Cyprus, Greenland, and Iceland are presently considered *E. granulosus*-free.[4,5] Note that distribution of specific genotypes within *E. granulosus* sensu lato is variable; see Table 131-2.

The global burden of cystic echinococcosis (CE) is estimated to be 188,000 disability-adjusted life years (DALYs) per annum, which is comparable to other parasitic neglected tropical diseases.[4,6] China and the Middle East represent the regions with the greatest socioeconomic burden as measured by DALYs. Furthermore, CE causes an estimated $2 billion loss to the livestock industry annually from

*Disclaimer: The findings and conclusions in this book chapter are those of the author and do not necessarily represent the official position of the Centers for Disease Control and Prevention/the Agency for Toxic Substances and Disease Registry.

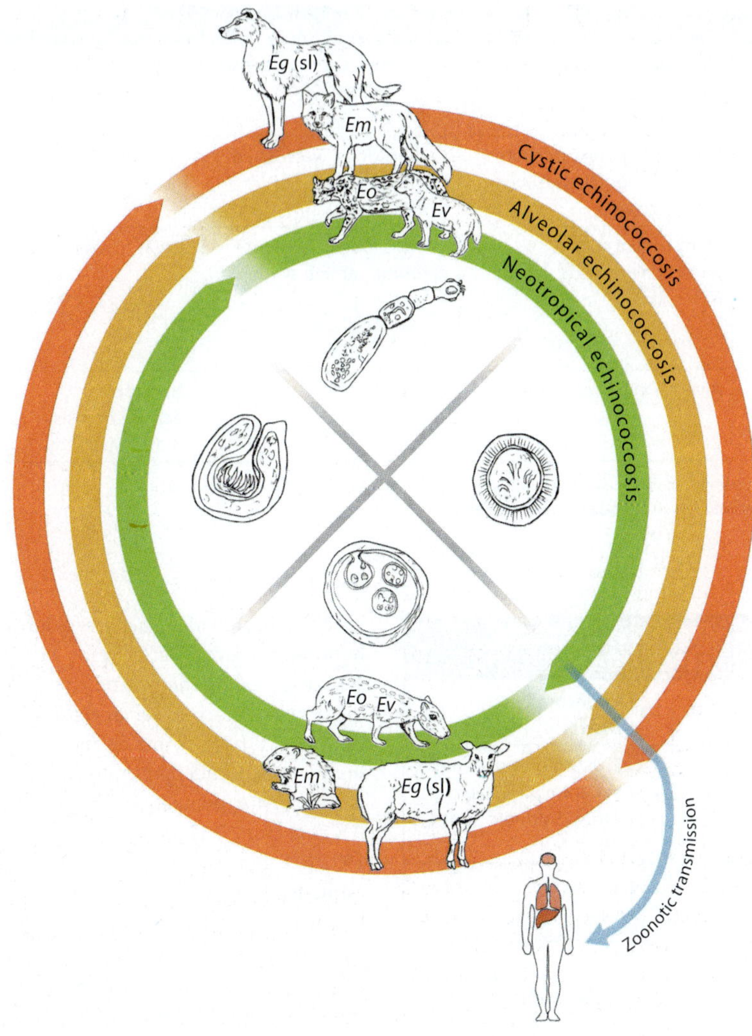

FIGURE 131-1. Generalized life cycle scheme of *Echinococcus* spp. [*Eg* (sl) = *E. granulosus* sensu lato; *Em* = *E. multilocularis*; *Eo* = *E. oligarthrus*; *Ev* = *E. vogeli*]. Clockwise from top: adult worm, egg, hydatid cyst, protoscolex.

lost wages, treatment and surveillance costs, and production impacts (liver condemnation, decreased fecundity, etc.).[7]

Characterization of *E. granulosus* genotypes based on mitochondrial markers has revealed that this grouping is a complex or assemblage of many distinct, cryptic species. Ten genotypes (G1–G10), historically referred to as "strains" prior to the advent of molecular techniques, have been identified. These include two sheep genotypes (G1, G2), two bovid genotypes (G3, G5), a horse genotype (G4), the camelid genotype (G6), two pig genotypes (G7, G9), and two cervid genotypes (G8, G10).[8] The vast majority of human CE are associated with "*E. granulosus* sensu stricto" genotypes G1, G2, and G3, with G1 "sheep strain" accounting for approximately 80% of cases globally. However, the validity of genotype G2 is now disputed, appearing to be indistinct from G3 based on the most recent phylogenetic analysis.[9] Due to the genotype-level variability in distribution, host specificity, and possibly pathogenicity, the *E. granulosus* genotypes are frequently referred to by new species names instead of genotypes, summarized in Table 131-2. Notably, genotypes G6, G7, G8, and G10 are now frequently referred to as *E. canadensis*. Based on genetic and morphologic differences, even more subdivision of *E. canadensis* has also been proposed, resurrecting the historical name *E. intermedius* for G6 and G7 and maintaining G8 and G10 as *E. canadensis*. The novel name *E. borealis* has also been proposed for G10.[10]

Zoonotic *E. granulosus* transmission is primarily associated with impoverished pastoral communities, and the presence of free-ranging dogs.[11] The common practice of feeding of infected livestock offal to farm dogs maintains domestic cycles of the parasite and patently infected dogs can lead to high levels of environmental contamination. Owners of dogs in poor rural areas may lack access to anthelmintics and commercial dog food, and also lack sufficient knowledge of the parasite, thus supporting this domestic cycle.[11,12] Northern *E. canadensis* genotypes G8 and G10 are maintained in sylvatic cycles involving wolf definitive hosts and deer, elk, and moose intermediate hosts, but feeding of this wild cervid offal to hunting and sled dogs can create a potential zoonotic risk. The domestic cycle of farmed reindeer (*Rangifer tarandus*) and herding dogs was formerly an important public health issue in relevant regions; however, the replacement of herding dogs with snowmobiles has reduced the prevalence of *E. canadensis* in domestic hosts.[13]

E. multilocularis

This parasite generally has a holarctic distribution and is most prevalent in central Asia, Russia, and eastern Europe. The global incidence is approximately 18,000 new alveolar echinococcosis (AE) cases per year with 90% of these occurring in China.[4] The severity and high mortality of AE is estimated to cause an annual loss of approximately 688,000 disability-adjusted life years; the high incidence of human cases in pastoral Tibetan communities is a major driver of this burden.[6] While rare or absent in eastern China and South Korea, *E. multilocularis* is endemic in the introduced red fox populations in northern Japan (Hokkaido).[14] *E. multilocularis* has been detected in canid hosts throughout central Asia and Siberia, although obtaining

TABLE 131-1 OVERVIEW OF MAJOR *ECHINOCOCCUS* SPECIES RELEVANT TO PUBLIC HEALTH

	Echinococcus granulosus sensu stricto	*Echinococcus multilocularis*	*Echinococcus canadensis*[a]	*Echinococcus vogeli*	*Echinococcus oligarthrus*
Primary definitive hosts	Canids (dogs, wolves)	Canids (dogs, foxes, coyotes), raccoon dogs (*Nyctereutes procyonoides*)	Canids (dogs, wolves, red fox, arctic fox)	Bush dog (*Speothos venaticus*)	Tropical felids (Ocelots, Pumas, Jaguarundis, others)
Primary intermediate hosts	Domestic ruminants (sheep, goats, camelids)	Many rodent species, particularly voles (Arvicolinae)	Cervids (deer, elk, moose, caribou), camels, swine[b]	Pacas (*Cuniculus paca*)	Pacas (*Cuniculus paca*), Agoutis (*Dasyprocta* spp.), Opossums (*Didelphis marsuipialis*), spiny rats (*Proechimys* spp.)
Associated disease	Cystic echinococcosis	Alveolar echinococcosis	Cystic echinococcosis	Neotropical echinococcosis (Polycystic)	Neotropical echinococcosis (Unicystic)

[a]"*E. canadensis*" refers to several genotypes classically included in *E. granulosus* sensu lato; see Table 131-2 for more details.
[b]Intermediate host tropism varies by genotype, see Table 131-2 for more details.

TABLE 131-2 SUMMARY OF GENOTYPES INCLUDED IN *ECHINOCOCCUS GRANULOSUS* SENSU LATO

Genotype	Name	Confirmed Distribution
G1	*Echinococcus granulosus* sensu stricto	Broad; highly endemic in Central Asia, Northern Africa, Southern South America
G2[a]	"	"
G3	"	"
G4[b]	*Echinococcus equinus* "Horse strain"	United Kingdom, Ireland, Western Europe, Northern Africa
G5	*Echinococcus ortleppi* "Cattle strain"	Argentina, Brazil, Mexico, Northern India, South Africa
G6	*Echinococcus Canadensis* "Camel strain" "*Echinococcus intermedius*"[c]	Northern and Eastern Africa, Middle East, Central Asia, South America
G7	*Echinococcus Canadensis* "Pig strain" "*Echinococcus intermedius*"[c]	Western, Central, and Eastern Europe, Russia, Brazil
G8	*Echinococcus Canadensis* "Cervid strain"	Canada, Russia, Northern United States
G9[a]	*Echinococcus Canadensis*	Poland
G10	*Echinococcus Canadensis* "*Echinococcus borealis*"[c] "Fennoscandian cervid strain"	Scandinavia, Finland, Estonia, Latvia, Western Canada, Northwestern United States

[a]Disputed validity, see reference 8 (G2) and reference 81 (G9).
[b]Not considered a zoonotic agent, although a single case in a captive primate (lemur) has been reported.[82]
[c]Proposed name as an alternative to *E. canadensis;* see reference 9.

accurate estimates of human AE cases is difficult for some of these regions. Transmission is less common in the Middle East, restricted to primarily arid, high altitude areas. This parasite is rare to absent below the Himalayas although more work is needed to define the southern border of the endemic zone.[4]

Human activities such as deforestation, agricultural activities, hunting, and even conservation may affect the balance of host species of *E. multilocularis* and the incidence of disease.[15] While the incidence is much lower in central-western Europe than in eastern Europe, AE has become an increasing public health concern, as *E. multilocularis* undergoes range expansions associated with growing urban red fox populations. In Switzerland, the annual incidence of AE rose from 0.12 to 0.15 (per 100,000) people between 1956 and 1992 to 0.26 between 2001 and 2005, with a sharp increase from the estimated 0.10 between 1993 and 2000. This increase was concomitant with a population surge of red foxes in the country during that time span; 35–65% of foxes were infected with *E. multilocularis.*[16] AE cases have been documented in Slovakia, Slovenia, Romania, Czech Republic, Hungary, the Netherlands, Belgium, Lithuania, and Poland, all of which were historically AE-free prior to 1995.[17] Additionally, incidence has increased in historically AE-endemic areas such as Austria, Switzerland, France, and Germany.[17] A dramatic rise in rates of human AE in northern Slovakia since its first detection in 1999 has been associated with a high prevalence (30.3%) of *E. multilocularis* infection in red foxes.[18] Recently, martens and raccoon dogs (*Nyctereutes procyonides*) have been identified as definitive hosts in European Russia.[19] The introduction of raccoon dogs to Eastern and Central Europe from the Far East may represent a further potential source of *E. multilocularis* infection though prevalence is still apparently low and raccoon dogs do not shed eggs to the same degree as red foxes.[20,21]

E. multilocularis is considered an emerging threat in western Canada (British Columbia, Alberta); cases were recently identified in a dog and three people in southwestern Ontario.[22] It is possible that many more autochthonous AE cases exist in Canada, particularly in northern provinces, but reporting and surveillance are limited and AE is often not differentiated from CE in hospital records.[23] The growth of urban coyote (*Canis latrans*) populations within AE endemic zones in Canada is also a cause for concern; 25% of coyotes in metropolitan Edmonton, Alberta were positive for *E. multilocularis*, mirroring the red fox situation in Europe.[24] Broadly absent from the United States, only a single autochthonous case of AE has been identified in the contiguous United States (Minnesota).[25]

Other Zoonotic *Echinococcus* spp.

E. vogeli and *E. oligarthrus* are found in Central and South America and are rare causes of human infections, causing neotropical echinococcosis [including polycystic (PE) and unicystic (UE) forms, respectively]. Their epidemiology is poorly studied and enigmatic.[12] Approximately 180 human cases of *E. vogeli* and only four cases of *E.*

oligarthrus are unequivocally species-confirmed, although these may represent emerging/underrecognized zoonoses.[26,27] The only confirmed natural definitive host for *E. vogeli* is the bush dog (*Speothos venaticus*). Experimental infection of domestic dogs with *E. vogeli* has been successful, and it is unclear if very occasional reports of human infection outside of the natural range of bush dogs and sometimes in association with domestic dogs fed pacas represent another *Echinoccocus* species or indicate a wider host range.[12] *E. oligarthrus* has been found in various wild feline definitive hosts (e.g., ocelot, puma, jaguarundi, and others).[28] Attempts to infect domestic dogs with *E. oligarthrus* have been unsuccessful and the few reported natural infections of dogs were underdeveloped; experimental infection of domestic cats has been successfully performed.[12] Both species use native rodent intermediate hosts such as pacas (*Cuniculus paca*); *E. vogeli* appears to infect pacas and agoutis exclusively[12] whereas *E. oligarthrus* has been detected in some other rodent species[26] as well as southern opossums and eastern cottontail rabbits.[12]

Clinical Features

Cystic Echinococcosis (CE)

This form of hydatid disease is characterized by large, robust, and unilocular hydatid cysts. Cysts are generally slow-growing (~1–50 mm/year), and patients may remain asymptomatic for months or years, with symptoms only arising after the cysts have grown to a sufficient size to disrupt normal organ function.[29] The liver is most commonly impacted in primary infection, followed by lungs and uncommonly other organs; in patients with multiple cysts, liver cysts typically outnumber lung cysts from 2:1 to 7:1.[30] Distribution of cysts and other clinical features are likely influenced by genotype, for example, some evidence suggests that *E. granulosus* genotype G6 has a greater affinity for the brain than G1.[31,32] Early symptoms of hepatic involvement are generally nonspecific and include abdominal pain, hepatomegaly, anorexia, and jaundice. Spontaneous rupture of cysts may release the "hydatid sand" fluid (containing protoscolices that impart a granular, sandy texture) and lead to severe anaphylaxis that is life threatening without intervention. Furthermore, rupture of cysts frequently leads to metastasis and development of additional cysts in other sites (secondary CE).[33] Potential secondary complications are numerous and include fistula formation between the cyst wall and biliary tree, bacterial superinfection, compression of visceral organs, and spontaneous fracture from the pressure exerted by cysts on or near bone.[3]

Alveolar Echinococcosis (AE)

As opposed to CE, AE involves numerous, small, and thin-walled cysts that occur in multilocular, grape-like clusters (hence the specific epithet *E. multilocularis*). These cysts grow in a proliferative, neoplastic-like manner that complicates the clinical picture and creates considerable morbidity. Patients may remain asymptomatic for 5–15 years until entering the progressive phase, which is marked by nonspecific signs and symptoms (abdominal pain, jaundice, malaise, fever) progressing to severe hepatic disease. Metastasis to other sites such as the brain, bladder, and lung occurs in some cases, although estimates of metastatic occurrence are variable across studies (ranging from ~6% to 35% of cases).[34] Without adequate treatment, mortality rates approach 90% within 10 years postdiagnosis, although spontaneous self-cure with calcification of cysts has occasionally been observed in milder/asymptomatic cases.[35]

Neotropical Echinococcosis

Infection with *E. vogeli* causes polycystic echinococcosis (PE). Cysts are most frequently in the liver and pleural cavity and are generally 4–6 cm in diameter with relatively thick walls, and may be interconnected. Like AE, aberrant sites may be involved, and many of these cases prove fatal. Infection with *E. oligarthrus* is referred to as "unicystic echinococcosis," is associated with a thinner lamina and is generally a less invasive course of disease; reports exist of cysts found in the orbit of the eye and on the heart.[1,26,36]

Diagnosis

Diagnosis of human echinococcosis is based on case history, clinical findings, imaging of cysts, and adjunct serologic or molecular testing. Known exposure to dogs or other potential definitive hosts in endemic areas is suggestive of CE. AE should be considered in patients presenting with hepatic disease in known endemic areas, but identification of potential exposures is much more difficult given the major contribution of wild hosts to its transmission.

In CE cases, both active and inactive/calcified hydatid cysts can be visualized by a variety of means, depending on the location of the cysts. Ultrasound is the mainstay for CE diagnoses in abdominal locations, including the liver, whereas CT and MRI are indicated for CE diagnoses in subdiaphragmatic, extra-abdominal, or disseminated locations, as well as in complicated cysts (e.g., cystobiliary fistulae, abscesses) and presurgical evaluations.[29] Immunodiagnostic methods can provide serologic evidence of echinococcal infection without disturbing the cyst. Serologic diagnosis of CE is primarily based on detection of IgG against antigen B (AgB), which can be either native or recombinant in origin.[1,37] The sensitivity and specificity of diagnostic platforms based on AgB is generally good, but the exact sensitivity and specificity vary with the source of AgB by intermediate host species and cyst location (maximum sensitivity of 97.8% and specificity of 97.1%, using antigen derived from human liver cysts).[38] A percentage of patients fail to seroconvert, leading to false negative serologic results; this appears to be dependent on factors such as cyst size, integrity, stage, and location.[39] Sera from polycystic echinococcosis (PE) cases will cross-react with many of the AgB subunits used in the diagnosis of CE and sensitivity is similar for both CE and PE.[40] Serology directly on hydatid cyst fluid is not recommended as specificity is low given the extensive milieu of host and parasite proteins within. Proof of the presence of protoscoleces may be obtained by microscopic examination of cyst fluid and histology, but such verification is not required for the diagnosis.[29] The invasive nature of these examinations risks cyst rupture resulting in potential hypersensitivity reaction and dissemination of the parasite. Protoscolices and free-floating hooklets (hydatid sand) can be viewed microscopically from fluid aspirated from viable cysts or withdrawn from the cyst following its surgical removal. Histologically, echinococcal cyst walls will possess a distinctive laminar membrane, allowing diagnosis even in the absence of visualized protoscolices; this laminar layer readily stains via periodic acid-Schiff.[29] PCR on hydatid cyst fluid is not typically used for diagnosis given the ease of visualizing protoscolices, but provides information on the infecting genotype and can be useful epidemiologically.[41]

In suspect cases of AE, ultrasound is often used to diagnose disease in abdominal locations. However, CT best shows the characteristic calcification pattern and MRI may show the multivesicular morphology of the AE lesions. Magnetic resonance cholangiopancreatography (MRCP) is most often used to study the biliary tree and [^{18}F] Fluoro-Deoxyflucose-Positron-Emission-Tomography (FDG-PET) scanning indirectly shows areas of parasitic activity and, therefore, may show active lesions in the absence of clinical symptoms when recurring disease is not yet detectable by other imaging techniques.[29] Imaging studies may demonstrate lesions that can be misdiagnosed, often as primary or metastatic tumors.[29,42] Diagnostic confirmation of AE can be challenging and is frequently based on histopathology and/or PCR, supported by serology.[4] AE is not reliably diagnosed using the same serologic test used to diagnose CE—the AgB immunoblot has a sensitivity of only 46% with AE cases.[40] Rather, serology for AE involves different antigen targets than those for CE (primarily Em2, Em2+, and Em18), which are generally sensitive and specific (>90%) in enzyme linked immunosorbent assay (ELISA) format.[37,43]

Currently, ELISA based on these antigens are used in clinical practice in many European countries for diagnosis and monitoring of patients; alveolar echinococcus serology is not available in the United States.[35] As with CE, false negative serologic results sometimes occur and this appears to be associated with cyst size, integrity, stage, and location.[39] Serology directly on hydatid cyst fluid is not recommended for reasons previously stated.

Treatment

Cystic Echinococcosis

The World Health Organization has developed an image-based staging system that assists in selecting among different potential case-management strategies that include observation without medical therapy, percutaneous interventions, surgical resection, benzimidazole therapy, and combinations of these strategies.[29] Surgical removal is preferred in patients with complicated cysts (e.g., ruptured cysts, infected cysts, cyst-biliary fistula, cysts compressing vital organs or vessels, hemorrhage) or cysts > 10 cm with many daughter vesicles not suitable for percutaneous treatments.[29,42] During surgical removal, it is critical to prevent the accidental release of fluid from the cyst. This is achieved through injection of a protoscolicide, such as hypertonic saline, into the cyst before surgical removal[29] as well as by perioperative benzimidazole prophylaxis beginning 1 week to 1 day before surgery and from 1 to 3 months after surgery, depending on surgical factors, such as whether the cyst was opened. If spillage has occurred or if the cyst has been incompletely resected, treatment may extend 3–6 months.[1] Adjunct praziquantel has also been given, but this needs further evaluation to assess its efficacy.[1,29] As a less invasive alternative to surgery, there are three percutaneous techniques for treating CE cysts: (1) puncture of the cyst under ultrasound guidance, aspiration of the cyst fluid, injection of a protoscolicide (either 20% saline or 95% ethanol), and reaspiration of the fluid (PAIR),[29] (2) the standard catheterization technique, and (3) the modified catheterization technique. The first two techniques chemically sterilize the cyst; these techniques are usually combined with benzimidazole treatment. The third technique also removes the parasitic membranes of the cyst in addition to chemical sterilization.[1] PAIR is used for liver and peritoneal cysts, for inoperable patients, relapses after surgery, or failure to respond to benzimidazole treatment alone. PAIR is contraindicated for lung cysts, multivesicular cysts with daughter cysts, and inactive cysts.[29] PAIR is usually combined with benzimidazole treatment, with similar timing and duration as recommended for surgery.[1] Albendazole is the first-line anthelmintic for CE. Small cysts (<5–6 cm) located in the liver and lungs may respond to treatment with albendazole, or alternatively mebendazole, alone.[1] The efficacy of combination of albendazole plus praziquantel therapy may be superior to the efficacy of albendazole alone.[3,44] However, drugs alone are not effective in treating large cysts (>10 cm) in diameter.[1,29] A "watch and wait" approach may be indicated for small, slow-growing, or apparently inactive cysts.[1]

Alveolar Echinococcosis

Treatment for AE is more complicated than for CE given the proliferative nature of cysts and the fact that symptomatic patients often have advanced disease. Aggressive and long-term anthelmintic therapy is used to limit the progression of disease; albendazole is again preferred. Radical resection is considered the most effective intervention, removing the cysts and resecting the surrounding margin of tissue and lymph nodes to reduce the risk of recrudescence.[34] With radical resection, albendazole is given for at least 2 years; in all other cases, albendazole is given for life with continual monitoring.[29] With early diagnosis, chemotherapy, and improved surgical techniques and medical treatment, the survival time for AE patients has increased and they now may experience an almost normal life expectancy.[29,42] In very advanced cases, liver transplantation may be the only option, however, data are limited on the long-term efficacy and rates of relapse.[45]

Treatment protocols and efficacy for CE, AE, and PE are reviewed extensively in references 1 and 29.

Control and Prevention

As human echinococcosis has severe clinical consequences and is potentially complicated to treat, control and prevention are of utmost importance. Control strategies for *Echinococcus* spp. involve both personal protection and interrupting transmission among wild and domestic hosts. Education and proper hand hygiene are recommended to reduce risk of exposure to infectious eggs. The transmission of livestock-associated *E. granulosus* can be limited by altering some husbandry practices, namely, avoiding the feeding of offal from slaughtered or hunted animals to dogs. These tissues should be incinerated or disposed of in a way that they are not accessible to dogs or wild definitive hosts. All dogs should be treated regularly with effective anthelmintics (e.g., praziquantel) to prevent infection and reduce environmental contamination. The Australian Pesticides and Veterinary Medicines Authority recommends treating dogs in hydatid-endemic areas every 6 weeks.[46]

Successful CE control and/or eradication campaigns have been carried out on various islands, including Iceland, Cyprus, Tasmania, the Falkland Islands, and New Zealand. Control methods typically rely on education (e.g., the distribution of informational materials in Iceland), slaughterhouse inspections, embargoed livestock imports, and treatment of dogs.[47] In Cyprus, an aggressive campaign involved tactics to control stray dog populations (sterilization and culling of stray dogs, mandated euthanasia for infected dogs) along with slaughterhouse checkpoints and public health outreach.[48] Elimination is far more complicated in nonisland nations with lower socioeconomic status where movement of domestic animals is much more difficult to track and control and resources for surveillance are limited.

An exemplar for the public health control of hydatid disease was the eradication of a highly endemic focus of disease in Tasmania, Australia in 1996. This island state, separated from mainland Australia, had reported some of the highest rates of CE disease globally 30 years prior. This remarkable feat was achieved by a combination of the examination of abattoir slaughtered sheep, fecal testing and the administration of praziquantel to rural dogs, education of farmers toward appropriate sleep slaughtering practices and toward the use of dry dog food, and legislation prohibiting the feeding of offal to dogs and requiring praziquantel administration to all dogs imported to the island.[49] Tasmanian eradication efforts were possible in part due to the almost complete absence of wild canids, a case not applicable to mainland Australia where an ongoing sylvatic cycle between macropodid marsupials (wallabies and kangaroos), wombats, feral pigs, wild dogs, foxes, and dingoes provides a significant reservoir of potential zoonotic disease.[50]

Vaccination would be another attractive option for control of CE in domestic hosts, provided the vaccine is affordable, "user friendly," and confers long-term immunity. A vaccine based on a recombinant metacestode antigen (EG95) has shown good efficacy in experimental trials in Australia, Argentina, and China, with up to 99% protection.[51,52] Two pilot studies on vaccination of dogs demonstrated varying levels of protection (70–90%), but thus far no larger trials have been conducted for assessment on a larger scale.[53,54] Despite these advancements, none of the above vaccines have been licensed and sold commercially. In addition, it is unknown if the EG95 and other vaccines are effective against other genotypes within *E. granulosus* sensu lato.

Management of wild definitive hosts is of particular importance in *E. multilocularis*, as wild canids (i.e., foxes and raccoon dogs) have a much greater host competence and contaminative potential than domestic dogs.[20] Oral praziquantel baiting campaigns in Germany,

Switzerland, France, Slovakia, and Japan have reduced local prevalence of *E. multilocularis* in some red fox populations although not all campaigns were successful. These deworming campaigns must be rigorously maintained to reduce reinfection rates in areas with extensive environmental contamination and in areas where movement of infected foxes into management areas is a possibility.[55] Other approaches to the control of wild *E. multilocularis* definitive hosts that have been proposed include reduction of populations in urban areas (either by trapping or culling) and behavioral modification (i.e., avoiding habituation of wild canids to humans).[15] Also, despite their lower contaminative potential versus wild hosts,[20] pet dogs should be treated appropriately with preventives given their close contact with domestic environments. Dogs imported from or traveling to *E. multilocularis* endemic areas should be diligently treated and monitored for shedding of eggs in feces to avoid introduction of the parasite into naïve areas.[56]

MISC. ZOONOTIC TAPEWORMS

The following cestodes are rarer causes of human infections and/or are of lesser medical importance than *Echinococcus* spp. Note that in many cases the true incidence may not be known due to the absence of formal reporting.

Hymenolepis Species

The dwarf tapeworm of humans and rodents, *Hymenolepis* (=*Rodentolepis*) *nana*, is the most common cestode infection in the United States and many other parts of the world.[57] This cyclophyllidean tapeworm is unique amongst the human-infecting cestodes in its capacity for direct fecal-oral transmission. It also employs a traditional lifecycle between a rodent (or human) definitive host and a wide range of insect intermediate hosts, including fleas and beetles.[58] The worm is 10–50 mm long, has an armed rostellum and produces distinctive eggs (30–47 μm in diameter) with a central oncosphere containing hooklets and having external bipolar filaments (Fig. 131-2A). Upon ingestion by humans, the oncosphere in the eggs will hatch into a larval cysticercoid, which develops directly within the intestinal villi and breaks open to implant as a tapeworm within 96 hours; time to patency is 3–4 weeks. Once patency is reached, many eggs implant directly into the villi during passage through the gut and this autoinfective process results in rapidly increasing parasite loads.[58]

Although globally distributed, infection is most common in tropical and subtropical regions, with children being the most commonly affected.[58] Infection in children generally self clears during adolescence so that infection in adults is rare.[57] Although very high worm burdens have been associated with abdominal cramps and diarrhea, the majority of infections are asymptomatic[57] and case-control studies have not identified any additional abdominal symptoms in infected participants.[59] Human infection with the rodent tapeworms *Hymenolepis diminuta* occasionally occurs (Fig. 131-2B)[60] and a single study in Western Australia found that four of 11 hymenolepiasis cases investigated by molecular methods were due to another rodent species, *Hymenolepis microstoma*.[61]

Diphyllobothriidae Family Tapeworms

The Diphyllobothriidae family of cyclophyllidean tapeworms includes several genera and species that have been implicated in human infection, though only some of these have been confirmed by molecular means, each having different freshwater, marine, or anadromous (fish that live in the sea, but migrate to freshwater to spawn) hosts. Recent taxonomic changes have led to the renaming of many species infecting humans (Table 131-3).[62] Many human infection reports have been spuriously attributed to *Dibothriocephalus latus* without morphologic or molecular confirmation that this species identification is correct. Infection rates have been decreasing in the United States for the past 50 years, but the recent advent of molecular identification of species has led to a greater understanding of the common infecting species.

Diphyllobothriid eggs are passed by an infected mammal (or bird in the case of *Dibothriocephalus dendriticum*) into water, releasing coracidia that are ingested by small waterborne crustaceans and therein develop to procercoid larvae. The first intermediate host crustaceans are ingested by second intermediate hosts (usually small fish), within which the larvae further develop into plerocercoid larvae; the larvae migrate to the muscles or viscera. Larger predator fish may

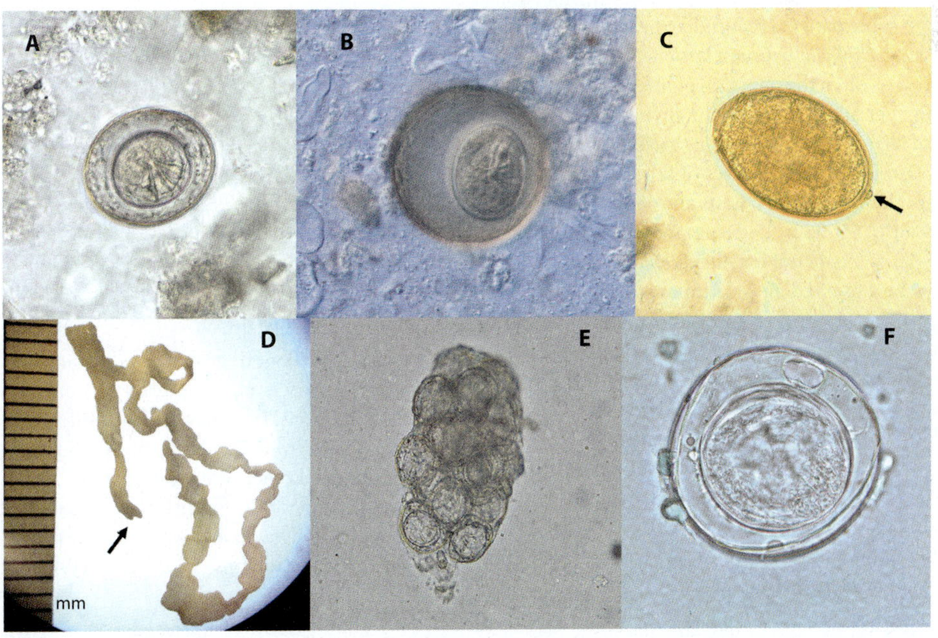

FIGURE 131-2. Selected diagnostic stages of some tapeworms discussed in this chapter, shown under light microscopy. A: *Hymenolepis nana* egg; B: *Hymenolepis diminuta* egg; C. Diphyllobothriid egg, showing abopercular knob (arrow); D: Sparganum, with developing scolex on the anterior end (arrow); E: *Dipylidium caninum* egg packet; and F: *Bertiella* sp. egg. (*Source:* Sarah G. H. Sapp, PhD.)

TABLE 131-3 TAXONOMIC CHANGES AND DISTRIBUTION OF DIPHYLLOBOTHRIID FAMILY CESTODES COMMONLY INFECTING HUMANS

Old Name(s)	Taxonomic Revision	Geographic Distribution
Diphyllobothrium latum	*Dibothriocephalus latus*	North America, Europe, eastern Russia, South America, possibly Africa
Diphyllobothrium nihonkaiense	*Dibothriocephalus nihonkaiense*	Japan, Korea, North America, eastern Russia, possibly New Zealand
Diphyllobothrium pacificum	*Adenocephalus pacificus*	Pacific coast of South America, Australia
Diphyllobothrium dendriticum	*Dibothriocephalus dendriticus*	Alaska, northern Canada, northern Russia, possibly Brazil, and central Europe
Diphyllobothrium stemmacephalum and Diphyllobothrium yonagoense	*Diphyllobothrium stemmacephalum*	Japan, Korea
Diplogonoporus grandis and Diplogonoporus balaenopterae	*Diphyllobothrium balaenopterae*	Japan, Korea

consume these smaller fish hosts and the plerocercoid larvae may remain infective in these paratenic hosts (hosts in which no critical development takes place, but which play a role in the transmission of the parasite). Consumption of second intermediate or paratenic host fish will result in intestinal infection in the definitive hosts (humans, other mammals, or birds).[63]

Diphyllobothriosis occurs commonly in cold climates of the northern hemisphere. Northern Russia, Japan, Korea, Alaska, Canada, northern states of the United States, and Scandinavian countries report the most disease.[63] Human infection has also been reported from South Australia,[64] South America, and there have been unconfirmed reports in Africa.[63] Diphyllobothriosis is clinically innocuous in 80% of cases, though some patients report diarrhea and abdominal pain. The passage of long *Diphyllobothrium* strobila, which may lead to psychological distress, is often the only sign of infection.[63,65] Egg are ovoid in shape with an operculum at the narrower end and an abopercular knob opposite of it (Fig. 131-2C). Egg size varies by species with marked crossover in size. Reported egg sizes of the three most commonly encountered species from human hosts are; 60–81 × 40–58 μm for *Dibothriocephalus latus*, 55–76 × 35–58 μm for *Dibothriocephalus nihonkaiense*, and 43–55 × 35–44 μm for *Adenocephalus pacificus*.[66,67] Eggs may not always be observed in fecal microscopy of infected patients, colonoscopy may be required to diagnose infection.[65] The reported association of *D. latum* infection with vitamin B12 deficiency appears to be overstated and only occurs in a small fraction of patients.[68] Risk factors for human infection include the consumption of raw or undercooked fish, including marinated dishes such as ceviche and carpaccio. The U.S. Food and Drug Administration recommends freezing fish at to kill plerocercoid larvae prior to consumption. Larvae may be killed by freezing at −4°F (−20°C) or below for 7 days. Cooking fish to an internal temperature of at least 145°F (63°C) will kill the infective plerocercoid larvae.[69]

Sparganum

Humans exposed to the plerocercoid larvae of Cyclophillidean cestodes of the genera *Spirometra* may develop a distinctive condition known as sparganosis whereby the tapeworm larvae migrate through the muscles and organs of the body or partially develop in a specific organ. Several species of *Spirometra* are cosmopolitan tapeworms of dogs and cats and have a life cycle broadly similar to that of the *Diphyllobothrium* tapeworms, but with a wider second intermediate host range, incorporating fish, amphibians, and reptiles. Humans may be infected by eating a paratenic host or even by transdermal migration of the plerocoercoid larvae when intermediate hosts are used as a poultice, as commonly occurs with frogs on the eye in Thailand.[70] Most human cases are reported from South East Asia,[70] though infection may occur in many parts of the world. Most commonly, sparganum larvae will migrate to cause a painful the subcutaneous nodule, but they may occur in any organ, including the eye and the brain.[63] The pathology of infection is specific to the organ affected.[63] Rarely, a proliferative form of disease (*Sparganum proliferum*) may occur, where the infecting plerocercoid larva divides and branches and buds to produce massive numbers of daughter pleroceroid larvae, with associated severe and often fatal pathology.[63] Diagnosis relies on a mix of clinical evaluation, medical imaging, and histological examination of biopsy material. Recovery of the migrating sparganum is sometimes possible, and is recognizable by a flat, ribbon-like shape, size (usually about 1–10 cm long), and the presence of a rudimentary, cleft-shaped developing scolex (Fig. 131-2D).[63]

Dipylidium Caninum

D. caninum is a ubiquitous tapeworm of domestic dogs and cats; common names include "cucumber tapeworm," "double-pored tapeworm," and "flea tapeworm." The adult tapeworm has oblong, rounded proglottids with two genital pores (versus single pores of Taeniids). Proglottids and egg packets containing multiple round eggs bound in a membrane may be passed in the stool (Fig. 131-2E). Transmission occurs in an indirect cycle involving common fleas of dogs and cats (*Ctenocephalides felis, C. canis*) and occasionally the chewing louse *Trichodectes canis*.[71] Human infections are uncommon, typically low intensity, and mostly reported in children following accidental ingestion of infected fleas; however, given the high global prevalence of this species in pet dogs and cats, zoonotic cases may be under recognized.[72,73] Monthly flea preventives to control infestations on pet cats and dogs mitigate the risk of human exposure.

Bertiella Species

Bertiella spp. are cyclophyllidean tapeworms of primates that are transmitted by ingestion of oribatid mite intermediate hosts. Two species, *B. studeri* (Old World) and *B. mucronata* (New World) are known to infect humans.[74,75] Over 80 human cases have been reported, primarily in children; infection is usually associated with contact with captive or wild primates, although a few case reports have involved possible ingestion of mites on contaminated fruit.[74,76,77] Diagnosis is typically via the visualization of eggs in stool, which are round (about 35–62 μm in diameter), containing an oncosphere with hooklets and a pyriform apparatus (Fig. 131-2E).[77]

Raillietina Species

A poorly understood group, *Raillietina* spp. are cyclophyllidean tapeworms of rodents, some primates, and fowl in warm climates. Roaches and beetles are the presumed intermediate hosts. Cases have been reported from Thailand, the Philippines, Taiwan, Indonesia, Australia, and French Polynesia, nearly always in young children. Because of taxonomic confusion and incomplete recovery of specimens, it is not always clear which species are involved; *R. sriraji, R. celebensis* (and synonyms), *R. demerariensis* have been described.[77–80]

ACKNOWLEDGMENT

The authors would like to thank Dr. Sharon Roy of the Centers for Disease Control and Prevention for providing clearance review of this manuscript.

References

1. Kern P, Menezes da Silva A, Akhan O, et al. The echinococcoses: Diagnosis, clinical management and burden of disease. *Adv Parasitol.* 2017;96:259–369.
2. Lawson JR, Gemmell MA. Hydatidosis and cysticercosis: The dynamics of transmission. *Adv Parasitol.* 1983;22:261–308.
3. Thompson RCA. Biology and systematics of *Echinococcus.* Adv Parasitol. 2017;95:65–109.
4. Deplazes P, Rinaldi L, Alvarez Rojas CA, et al. Global distribution of alveolar and cystic echinococcosis. *Adv Parasitol.* 2017;95:315–493.
5. Budke CM, Deplazes P, Torgerson PR. Global socioeconomic impact of cystic echinococcosis. *Emerg Infect Dis.* 2006;12(2):296.
6. Torgerson PR, Keller K, Magnotta M, Ragland N. The global burden of alveolar echinococcosis. *PLoS Negl Trop Dis.* 2010;4:e722.
7. Torgerson PR, Macpherson CNL. The socioeconomic burden of parasitic zoonoses: Global trends. *Vet Parasitol.* 2011;182(1):79–95.
8. Alvarez Rojas CA, Romig T, Lightowlers MW. *Echinococcus granulosus* sensu lato genotypes infecting humans—Review of current knowledge. *Int J Parasitol.* 2014;44:9–18.
9. Kinkar L, Laurimäe T, Sharbatkhori M, et al. New mitogenome and nuclear evidence on the phylogeny and taxonomy of the highly zoonotic tapeworm *Echinococcus granulosus* sensu stricto. *Infect Genet Evol.* 2017;52:52–8.
10. Lymbery AJ, Jenkins EJ, Schurer JM, Thompson RCA. *Echinococcus canadensis, E. borealis,* and *E. intermedius.* What's in a name? *Trends Parasitol.* 2015;31:23–9.
11. Otero-Abad B, Torgerson PR. A systematic review of the epidemiology of echinococcosis in domestic and wild animals. *PLoS Negl Trop Dis.* 2013;7:e2249.
12. Romig T, Deplazes P, Jenkins D, et al. Ecology and life cycle patterns of *Echinococcus* species. *Adv Parasitol.* 2017;95:213–314.
13. Oksanen A, Lavikainen A. *Echinococcus canadensis* transmission in the North. *Vet Parasitol.* 2015;213:182–6.
14. Ito A, Romig T, Takahashi K. Perspective on control options for *Echinococcus multilocularis* with particular reference to Japan. *Parasitol.* 2003;127(S1):S159–72.
15. Hegglin D, Deplazes P. Control strategy for *Echinococcus multilocularis. Emerg Infect Dis.* 2008;14(10):1626–8.
16. Schweiger A, Ammann RW, Candinas D, et al. Human alveolar echinococcosis after fox population increase, Switzerland. *Emerg Infect Dis.* 2007;13:878.
17. Vuitton DA, Demonmerot F, Knapp J, et al. Clinical epidemiology of human AE in Europe. *Vet Parasitol.* 2015;213:110–20.
18. Antolová D, Miterpáková M, Radoňak J, Hudačkova D, Szilagyiova M, Žáček M. Alveolar echinococcosis in a highly endemic area of northern Slovakia between 2000 and 2013. *Euro Surveill.* 2014;19:20882.
19. Andreyanov O. Alveolar echinococcosis at trade animals in the Ryazan region. *Russ Parasitol J.* 2011;3:7–11.
20. Kapel CMO, Torgerson PR, Thompson RCA, Deplazes P. Reproductive potential of *Echinococcus multilocularis* in experimentally infected foxes, dogs, raccoon dogs and cats. *Int J Parasitol.* 2006;36:79–86.
21. Laurimaa L, Süld K, Davison J, Moks E, Valdmann H, Saarma U. Alien species and their zoonotic parasites in native and introduced ranges: The raccoon dog example. *Vet Parasitol.* 2016;219:24–33.
22. Trotz-Williams LA, Mercer NJ, Walters JM, et al. Public health follow-up of suspected exposure to *Echinococcus multilocularis* in southwestern Ontario. *Zoonoses Public Health.* 2017;64:460–7.
23. Davidson RK, Lavikainen A, Konyaev S, et al. *Echinococcus* across the north: Current knowledge, future challenges. *Food Waterborne Parasitol.* 2016;4:39–53.
24. Catalano S, Lejeune M, Liccioli S, et al. *Echinococcus multilocularis* in urban coyotes, Alberta, Canada. *Emerg Infect Dis.* 2012;18(10):1625.
25. Gamble W, Segal M, Schantz P, Rausch R. Alveolar hydatid disease in Minnesota: First human case acquired in the contiguous United States. *JAMA.* 1979;24:904–7.
26. D'Alessandro A, Rausch RL. New aspects of neotropical polycystic (*Echinococcus vogeli*) and unicystic (*Echinococcus oligarthrus*) echinococcosis. *Clin Microbiol Rev.* 2008;21:380–401.
27. Soares M do CP, Rodrigues AL dos S, Moreira Silva CA, et al. Anatomo-clinical and molecular description of liver neotropical echinococcosis caused by *Echinococcus oligarthrus* in human host. *Acta Trop.* 2013;125:110–4.
28. Arrabal JP, Avila HG, Rivero MR, et al. *Echinococcus oligarthrus* in the subtropical region of Argentina: First integration of morphological and molecular analyses determines two distinct populations. *Vet Parasitol.* 2017;240:60–7.
29. Brunetti E, Kern P, Vuitton DA. Expert consensus for the diagnosis and treatment of cystic and alveolar echinococcosis in humans. *Acta Tropica.* 2010;114:1–16.
30. Larrieu EJ, Frider B. Human cystic echinococcosis: Contributions to the natural history of the disease. *Ann Trop Med Parasitol.* 2001;95:679–87.
31. Sadjjadi SM, Mikaeili F, Karamian M, et al. Evidence that the *Echinococcus granulosus* G6 genotype has an affinity for the brain in humans. *Int J Parasitol.* 2013;43:875–7.
32. Shirmen O, Batchuluun B, Lkhamjav A, et al. Cerebral cystic echinococcosis in Mongolian children caused by *Echinococcus canadensis. Parasitol Int.* 2018;67:584–6.
33. Eckert J, Deplazes P. Biological, epidemiological, and clinical aspects of echinococcosis, a zoonosis of increasing concern. *Clin Microbiol Rev.* 2004;17:107–35.
34. Kern P. Clinical features and treatment of alveolar echinococcosis. *Curr Opin Infect Dis.* 2010;23:505–12.
35. Kern P, Bardonnet K, Renner E, et al. European echinococcosis registry: Human alveolar echinococcosis, Europe, 1982–2000. *Emerg Infect Dis.* 2003;9:343.
36. Do Carmo Pereira Soares M, Souza de Souza AJ, Pinheiro Malheiros A, et al. Neotropical echinococcosis: Second report of *Echinococcus vogeli* natural infection in its main definitive host, the bush dog (*Speothos venaticus*). *Parasitol Int.* 2014;63:485–7.
37. Siles-Lucas M, Casulli A, Conraths FJ, Müller N. Laboratory diagnosis of *Echinococcus* spp. in human patients and infected animals. *Adv Parasitol.* 2017;96:159–257.
38. Rahimi H, Sadjjadi SM, Sarkari B. Performance of antigen B isolated from different hosts and cyst locations in diagnosis of cystic echinococcosis. *Iran J Parasitol.* 2011;6:12.
39. Lissandrin R, Tamarozzi F, Piccoli L, et al. Factors influencing the serological response in hepatic *Echinococcus granulosus* infection. *Am J Trop Med Hyg.* 2016;94:166–71.
40. De La Rue ML, Yamano K, Almeida CE, et al. Serological reactivity of patients with *Echinococcus* infections (*E. granulosus, E. vogeli,* and *E. multilocularis*) against three antigen B subunits. *Parasitol Res.* 2010;106:741–5.
41. Boubaker G, Macchiaroli N, Prada L, et al. A multiplex PCR for the simultaneous detection and genotyping of the *Echinococcus granulosus* complex. *PLoS Negl Trop Dis.* 2013;7:e2017.
42. Brunetti E, White AC. Cestode infestations: Hydatid disease and cysticercosis. *Inf Dis Clin.* 2010;26:421–35.
43. Ito A, Sako Y, Yamasaki H, et al. Development of Em18-immunoblot and Em18-ELISA for specific diagnosis of alveolar echinococcosis. *Acta Trop.* 2003;85:173–82.
44. Cobo F, Yarnoz C, Sesma B, et al. Albendazole plus praziquantel versus albendazole alone as a pre-operative treatment in intra-abdominal hydatidosis caused by *Echinococcus granulosus. Trop Med Int Heal.* 2002;3:462–6.
45. Koch S, Bresson-Hadni S, Miguet J-P, et al. Experience of liver transplantation for incurable alveolar echinococcosis: A 45-case European collaborative report. *Transplantation.* 2003;75:856–63.
46. Australian Pesticides and Veterinary Medicines Authority. Anthelmintics for dogs and cats. 2018. https://apvma.gov.au/node/917. Accessed May 30, 2018.
47. Craig PS, Larrieu E. Control of cystic echinococcosis/hydatidosis: 1863–2002. *Adv Parasitol.* 2006;61:443–508.
48. Economides P, Christofi G, Gemmell MA. Control of *Echinococcus granulosus* in Cyprus and comparison with other island models. *Vet Parasitol.* 1998;79:151–63.
49. O'Hern JA, Cooley L. A description of human hydatid disease in Tasmania in the post-eradication era. *Med J Aust.* 2013;199:117–20.
50. Jenkins DJ. *Echinococcus granulosus* in Australia, widespread and doing well. *Parasitol Int.* 2006;55:S203–6.
51. Gauci C, Heath D, Chow C, Lightowlers MW. Hydatid disease: Vaccinology and development of the EG95 recombinant vaccine. *Expert Rev Vaccines.* 2005;4:103–12.
52. Lightowlers MW, Jensen O, Fernandez E, et al. Vaccination trials in Australia and Argentina confirm the effectiveness of the EG95 hydatid vaccine in sheep. *Int J Parasitol.* 1999;29(4):531–4.

53. Zhang W, Zhang Z, Shi B, et al. Vaccination of dogs against *Echinococcus granulosus* the cause of cystic hydatid disease in humans. *J Infect Dis.* 2006;194:966–74.
54. Petavy A-F, Hormaeche C, Lahmar S, et al. An oral recombinant vaccine in dogs against *Echinococcus granulosus*, the causative agent of human hydatid disease: A pilot study. *PLoS Negl Trop Dis.* 2008;2:e125.
55. Hegglin D, Deplazes P. Control of *Echinococcus multilocularis*: Strategies, feasibility and cost-benefit analyses. *Int J Parasitol.* 2013;43:327–37.
56. European Scientific Counsel Companion Animal Parasites. ESCCAP Guideline 01: Worm Control in Dogs and Cats, 3rd ed. 2017:40.
57. Sirivichayakul C, Radomyos P, Praevanit R, Jojjaroen-Anant C, Wisetsing P. *Hymenolepis nana* infection in Thai children. *J Med Assoc Thail.* 2000;83:1035–8.
58. Craig P, Ito A. Intestinal cestodes. *Curr Opin Infect Dis.* 2007;20:524–32.
59. Chero JC, Saito M, Bustos JA, Blanco EM, Gonzalvez G, Garcia HH. *Hymenolepis nana* infection: Symptoms and response to nitazoxanide in field conditions. *Trans R Soc Trop Med Hyg.* 2007;101:203–5.
60. Bradbury RS, Barbé B, Jacobs J, et al. Enteric pathogens of food sellers in rural Gambia with incidental finding of *Myxobolus* species (Protozoa: Myxozoa). *Trans R Soc Trop Med Hyg.* 2015;109:334–9.
61. Macnish MG, Ryan UM, Behnke JM, Thompson RCA. Detection of the rodent tapeworm *Rodentolepis* (= *Hymenolepis*) *microstoma* in humans. A new zoonosis? *Int J Parasitol.* 2003;33:1079–85.
62. Waeschenbach A, Brabec J, Scholz T, Littlewood DTJ, Kuchta R. The catholic taste of broad tapeworms—Multiple routes to human infection. *Int J Parasitol.* 2017;47:831–43.
63. Kuchta R, Scholz T, Brabec J, Narduzzi-Wicht B. Chapter 17: *Diphyllobothrium, Diplogonoporus and Spirometra.* In: Xiao L, Ryan U, Feng F, eds. Biology of Foodborne Parasites. Boca Raton, FL: CRC Press; 2015:299–326.
64. Moore C V, Thompson RCA, Jabbar A, et al. Rare human infection with pacific broad tapeworm *Adenocephalus pacificus*, Australia. *Emerg Infect Dis.* 2016;22:1510.
65. Ikuno H, Akao S, Yamasaki H. Epidemiology of *Diphyllobothrium nihonkaiense* Diphyllobothriasis, Japan, 2001–2016. *Emerg Infect Dis.* 2018;24:1428–34.
66. Choi S, Cho J, Jung BK, et al. *Diphyllobothrium nihonkaiense*: Wide egg size variation in 32 molecularly confirmed adult specimens from Korea. *Parasitol Res.* 2015;114:2129–34.
67. Leštinová K, Soldánová M, Scholz T, Kuchta R. Eggs as a suitable tool for species diagnosis of causative agents of human diphyllobothriosis (Cestoda). *PLoS Negl Trop Dis.* 2016;10:e0004721.
68. Lukeš J, Kuchta R, Scholz T, Pomajbíková K. (Self-) infections with parasites: Re-interpretations for the present. *Trends Parasitol.* 2014;30:377–85.
69. Centers for Disease Control and Prevention. CDC DPDM *Diphyllobothirum* (and other species) fact sheet. 2012. https://www.cdc.gov/parasites/diphyllobothrium/faqs.html. Accessed August 28, 2018.
70. Anantaphruti MT, Nawa Y, Vanvanitchai Y. Human sparganosis in Thailand: An overview. *Acta Trop.* 2011;118:171–6.
71. Bowman DD. *Georgis' Parasitology for Veterinarians.* 10th ed. St. Louis, MI: Elsevier; 2014:496.
72. Cabello RR, Ruiz AC, Feregrino RR, Romero LC, Feregrino RR, Zavala JT. *Dipylidium caninum* infection. *BMJ Case Rep.* 2011;2011:bcr0720114510.
73. Chappell CL, Enos JP, Penn HM. *Dipylidium caninum*, an under-recognized infection in infants and children. *Pediatr Infect Dis J.* 1990;9:745–7.
74. Bhagwant S. Human *Bertiella studeri* (family Anoplocephalidae) infection of probable Southeast Asian origin in Mauritian children and an adult. *Am J Trop Med Hyg.* 2004;70:225–8.
75. Denegri G, Perez-Serrano J. Bertiellosis in man: A review of cases. *Rev Inst Med Trop São Paulo.* 1997;39:123–8.
76. Sun X, Fang Q, Chen X-Z, Hu S-F, Xia H, Wang X-M. *Bertiella studeri* infection, China. *Emerg Infect Dis.* 2006;12:176–7.
77. Sapp SGH, Bradbury RS. The forgotten exotic tapeworms: A review of uncommon zoonotic Cyclophyllidea. *Parasitology.* 2020;47:533–58.
78. Chandler AC, Pradatsundarasar A. Two cases of *Raillietina infection* in infants in Thailand, with a discussion of the taxonomy of the species of *Raillietina* (Cestoda) in man, rodents and monkeys. *J Parasitol.* 1957;43:81–8.
79. Margono SS, Handojo I, Hadidjaja P, Mahfudin H. *Raillietina* infection in children in Indonesia. *Southeast Asian J Trop Med Public Health.* 1977;8:195–9.
80. Rougier Y, Legros F, Durand JP, Cordoliani Y. Four cases of parasitic infection by *Raillietina* (*R.*) *celebensis* (Kanicki, 1902) in French Polynesia. *Trans R Soc Trop Med Hyg.* 1981;75:121.
81. Kedra AH, Swiderski Z, Tkach V V, et al. Genetic analysis of *Echinococcus granulosus* from humans and pigs in Poland, Slovakia and Ukraine. A multicenter study. *Acta Parasitol.* 1999;44:248–54.
82. Boufana B, Stidworthy MF, Bell S, et al. *Echinococcus* and *Taenia* spp. from captive mammals in the United Kingdom. *Vet Parasitol.* 2012;190:95–103.

CHAPTER

132 Chagas Disease (American Trypanosomiasis)

Italo B. Zecca • Sarah A. Hamer

CHAGAS DISEASE EPIDEMIOLOGY

The etiological agent of Chagas disease, *Trypanosoma cruzi*, is a single celled protozoal parasite primarily transmitted through the infected feces of blood feeding triatomine insects. The parasite was discovered in 1909 by a Brazilian scientist and physician named Carlos Chagas.[1] Infected humans and animals may suffer a spectrum of acute and chronic health issues including fatal cardiac disease. Domestic and wild mammals serve as reservoirs for the parasite. The triatomine insect vector, commonly known as a kissing bug, is widely dispersed throughout the Americas, including South America, Central America, Mexico, and the southern United States (U.S.). Chagas disease may be found in other areas of the world where the vector is not present due to migration or travel of infected individuals into nonendemic countries.[2]

Chagas disease is classified as a neglected tropical disease due to its distribution in tropical and subtropical climates, disproportionate impact on people living in poverty, and relative neglect from research and funding arenas.[3] Estimates by the World Health Organization suggest Chagas disease affects approximately 6–8 million individuals in Latin America,[4] and a more liberal estimate suggests 17 million people are infected and 100 million are at risk of contracting the parasite.[5] Of 21 Latin American countries, the majority of cases occur in Argentina, Brazil, and Mexico.[4,6] Active transmission of *T. cruzi* in Latin American countries places 13% of the Latin American population at risk for *T. cruzi* infection.[6] Vector transmission in the domestic environment has been interrupted or diminished in some Latin American countries through targeted vector interventions, but wildlife and sylvatic vectors in these areas maintain transmission cycles.[7] The average annual economic burden of health-care cost related to Chagas disease in Latin America is approximately U.S.$500 million.[8] In Latin America, the disease is responsible for 772,304 disability-adjusted life years (DALYs) which comprises over 95% of DALYs attributed to Chagas disease worldwide.[8]

In the United States, there is increasing recognition of Chagas disease in the human health community. The majority of human cases in the United States are identified through blood banks and occur in individuals who likely acquired the infection while living or visiting an endemic region in Latin America.[9] However, locally acquired infections in the United States are increasingly recognized.[10,11] The first documented case of locally acquired Chagas disease in the United States was in Corpus Christi, Texas in 1955.[12] The 2012 estimate of over 238,000 cases of *T. cruzi* infection in the United States may be higher when undocumented immigrant populations are considered.[13] Individuals living in impoverished and medically underserved communities along the U.S.-Mexico border may be at heightened risk for infection.[14]

VECTOR

Triatomine insects, comprised of approximately 150 species in the subfamily Triatominae, are known by many different names in Latin America and are commonly referred to as "chinche besuconas" or "vinchucas."[15] In the United States, triatomines are commonly called "kissing bugs," "cone-nosed bugs," and "reduviid bugs." Triatomine insects mainly occur in the Americas and some Caribbean islands. One species of triatomine occurs in Africa and a few occur in Australia/Indo-Pacific region.[16,17] Species of triatomines occur in parts of southeast Asia but are not known to transmit *T. cruzi*.[18] The life cycle of the usually nocturnal insect includes five flightless nymph stages that develop into adults capable of flying. All life stages are hematophagous, meaning they strictly feed on blood. Insect size and appearance is dependent on life stage and species (Fig. 132-1). Early life stages are likely to be located in nesting habitats of mammals in close proximity to blood

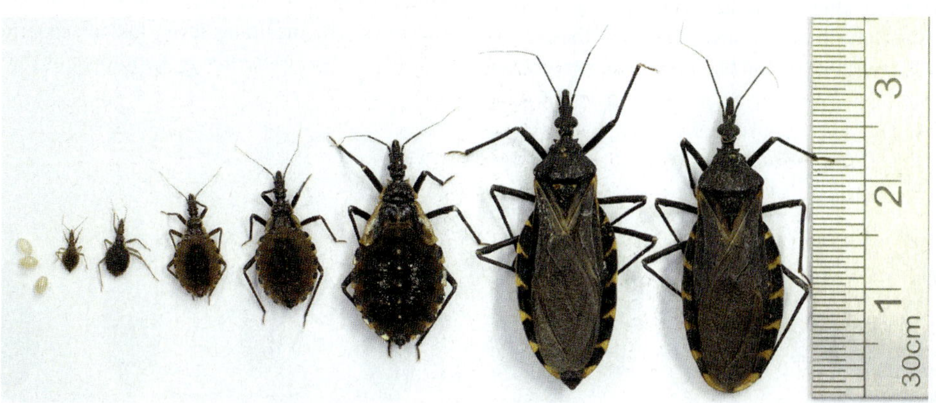

FIGURE 132-1. Triatomine life stages. From left to right, egg, nymphal instars 1–5, adult female, and adult male *Triatoma gerstaeckeri*. Photographed specimens were collected in Texas. (*Source:* Gabriel L. Hamer, PhD.)

sources. Adult triatomines may range from approximately 5–44 mm in length.[19] Triatomines in the United States range from 13 to 29 mm in length.[19] Some triatomine species favor sylvatic environments while others favor peridomiciliary structures or houses, which influence their proximity and potential infectivity to domestic animals and humans. For example, *Triatoma infestans* in South America is known to colonize and infest housing, which increases their contact with humans.[20] There are 11 species occurring in the United States (Fig. 132-2), with *Triatoma sanguisuga* the most widely distributed infective triatomine insect which often feeds on humans.[21] In a citizen science program in Texas, the majority of triatomines collected by members of the public were found in peridomestic environments including dog kennels, patios, garages, and the outside of houses.[22]

The infection prevalence of triatomine vectors in the United States varies by species and geographic area; for example, in the western United States the dominant vector *Triatoma rubida* is characterized by less than 20% infection prevalence, whereas in the south central United States over 50% of the dominant vector *Triatoma gerstaeckeri* are infected.[22–24]

ANIMAL RESERVOIRS

There is historical evidence of *T. cruzi* infection in wild and domestic animals in the southern United States.[12,14,25–27] Triatomines are often associated with the nests and burrows of wildlife hosts, including woodrats (*Neotoma* spp.). Studies conducted in domestic dog (*Canis lupus familiaris*) populations from the southern United States show exposure to *T. cruzi* (seroprevalence: 3.6–57.6%) indicating active transmission in peridomestic environments and identifying domestic dogs as key sentinel hosts. [28,29] Additionally, several species of wildlife in the United States, including raccoons (*Procyon lotor*), opossums (*Didelphis virginiana*), and coyotes (*Canis latrans*), serve as key reservoir hosts contributing to the infection cycle.[30–32] The impact this parasite has on animal populations is largely unknown, although cardiac pathology in infected wild animals and domestic dogs has been detected.[30,33,34] There is no approved treatment or vaccine for Chagas disease in animals. *Trypanosoma cruzi* is unlikely to be transmitted directly from infected animals to humans; however, infected animals signal an environment where infected triatomine insects occur and may pose risk of transmission to humans.

BIOLOGY AND TRANSMISSION

Trypanosoma cruzi undergoes various changes in stage within the vector and the host. When feeding, a triatomine insect ingests a flagellated form of the parasite (trypomastigote) from an infected mammalian host. Within the insect, the parasite then undergoes transformation to the epimastigote stage and multiplication occurs in the midgut of the insect. Transformation of the parasite occurs again in the hindgut of the insect, after which the metacyclic trypomastigote stage is passed in the feces; this is the infective stage of the parasite and is the primary source of infection to mammals. The stercorarian (vector-fecal) route of transmission occurs when the triatomine insect defecates infected feces on the host, which may self-inoculate by introducing the parasite into broken skin (bite, abrasion, cut) or mucous membranes (mouth, eyes, nose). The postfeeding defecation interval (amount of time between vector feeding and vector defecation) may be variable among vector species and is important for transmission, because a shorter interval suggests the vector is likely to still be in contact with the host when it defecates, resulting in increased risk of transmission.[35–37] Once the parasite enters the host, the trypomastigote circulates in the blood and infiltrates various tissues. Subsequent to tissue infiltration is transformation into the intracellular amastigote stage of parasite, which multiplies via binary fission. Eventually parasites burst out of the cell into the bloodstream circulation and infects other tissues.[38]

In addition to vector-fecal transmission, the parasite may be transmitted through ingestion of infected triatomine insects or foods contaminated by insects, congenitally, via infected blood transfusion or organ transplant, and through laboratory/medical accidents[39] (Fig. 132-3). There have been outbreaks of acute Chagas disease in South America associated with the consumption of food/beverages contaminated by infected triatomine insects that had been crushed in the preparation process.[40,41] Additionally, consumption of infected insects is speculated to be an important route of transmission leading to Chagas disease in domestic dogs and wildlife.[42] Additionally, there is limited evidence of parasite transmission through breastfeeding via broken skin and through sexual transmission.[43,44]

Vector-borne transmission: (1) Stercorarian (vector-fecal) transmission occurs via self-inoculation when contaminated feces enter broken skin or a mucous membrane of a host. (2) Oral transmission occurs when an infected triatomine insect contaminates a food source or when an infected insect is eaten directly by a host. Nonvector transmission: (3) Vertical transmission may occur if the mother is infected before or during pregnancy. (4) Transmission via organ transplant occurs when infected tissues are transplanted to an uninfected individual. (5) Transfusion transmission occurs when an individual receives blood from an infected donor. (6) Transmission via occupational and laboratory accidents may occur.

PATHOLOGY

Chagas disease occurs in three phases, which may be associated with inapparent or nonspecific symptoms.[38] The *acute phase* occurs when the parasite has entered the blood stream and is circulating and actively multiplying. If the host was infected via a vector, there may be swelling and inflammation at the bite site, known as a chagoma. Unilateral swelling around the eye, due to the introduction of infected triatomine feces, is the most recognizable indicator of acute Chagas disease and is commonly known as Romaña's sign.[45] Other symptoms may become present within 1–2 weeks after initial infection, including fever, loss of appetite, lethargy, malaise, and headaches. More severe symptoms of the acute phase include

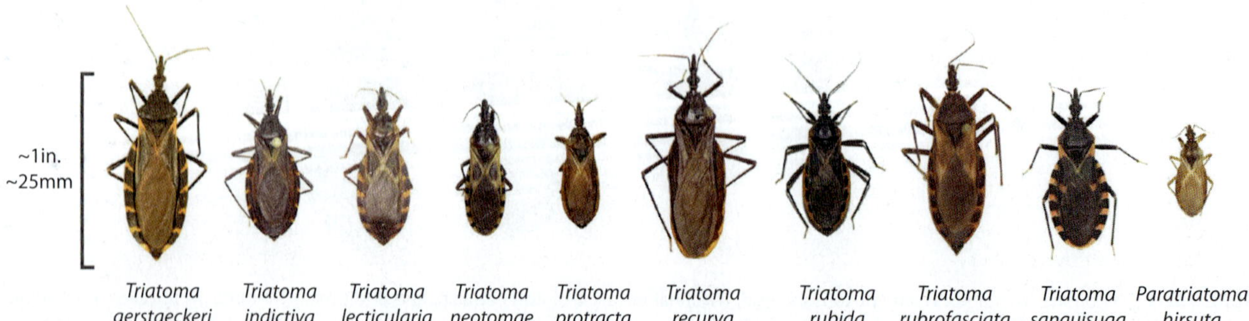

FIGURE 132-2. Adults of ten kissing bug species that occur in the United States. (*Source:* Gabriel L. Hamer, PhD.)

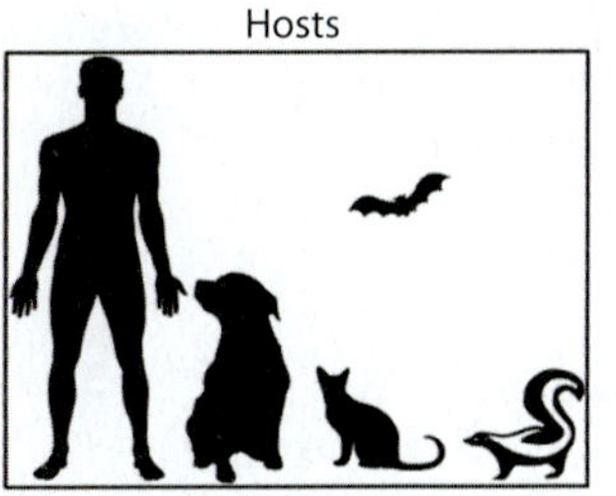

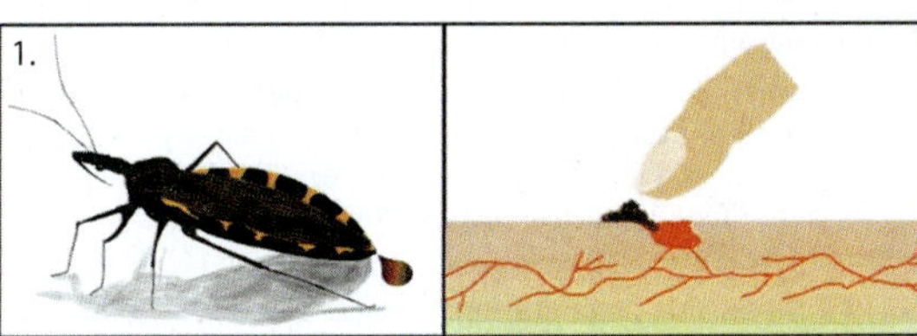

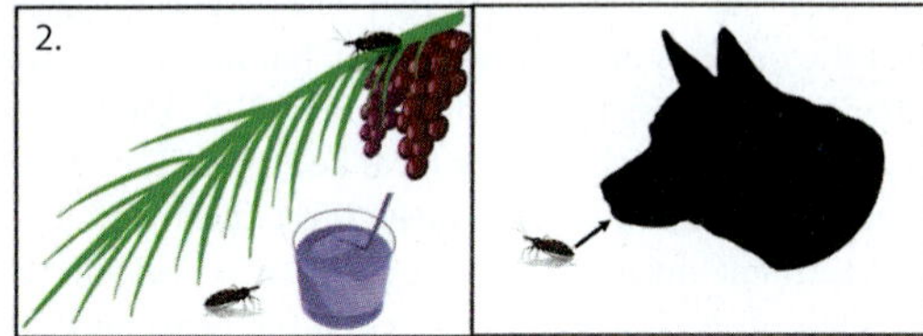

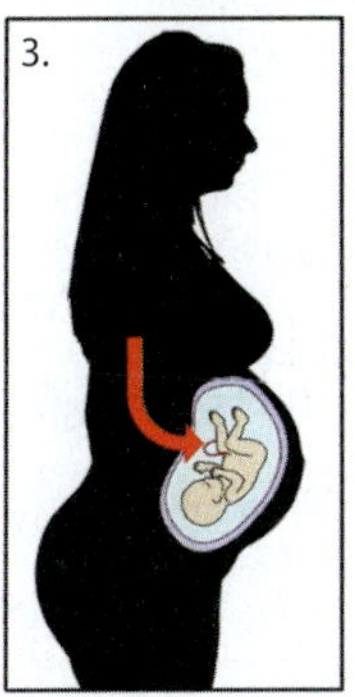

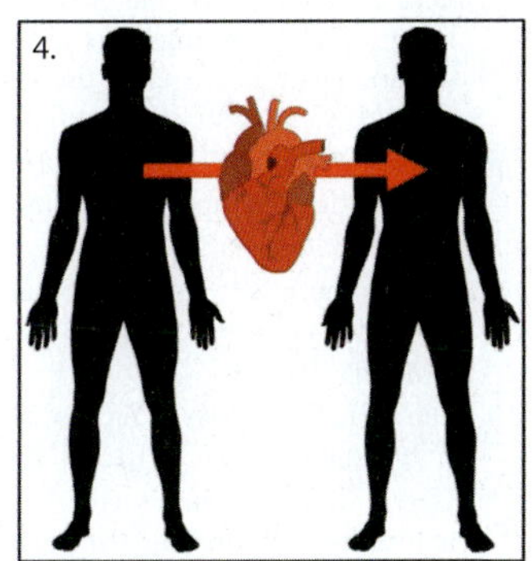

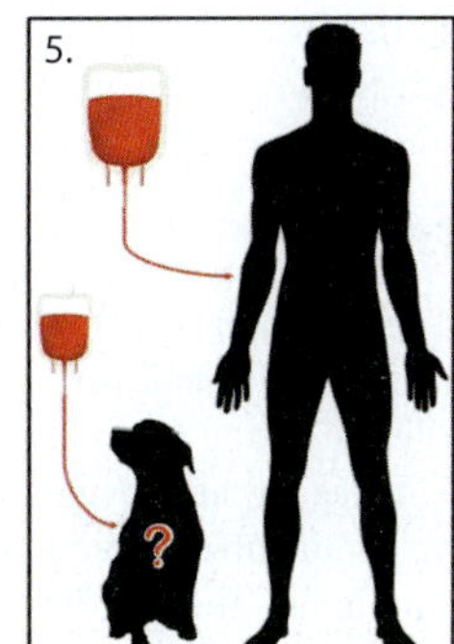

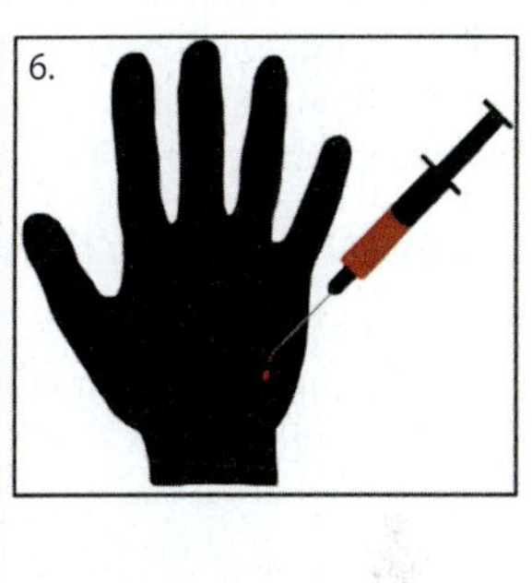

FIGURE 132-3. *Trypanosoma cruzi* transmission routes.

enlarged lymph nodes, spleen, and liver or cardiac abnormalities. Some acutely infected individuals may experience no symptoms at all. Following the acute phase, infected individuals enter the *indeterminate phase*. During this phase, which may last years to decades, the circulating parasite is diminished to low or undetectable levels, and the parasite remains in tissues with no obvious symptoms or complications. Many infected individuals may remain asymptomatic for life. Approximately 20–30% of infected individuals then enter the *chronic phase*, characterized by clinical abnormalities that may include may include severe cardiac abnormalities, such as enlargement the heart (cardiomegaly), congestive heart failure, and death.[38] Other clinical manifestations of the chronic phase include digestive complications, primarily the enlargement of the colon (megacolon) or esophagus (megaesophagus), and, less commonly, neurological complications.

The degree to which infected individuals present acute or chronic signs is likely dependent on several factors including the individual's immune system, the genetics of the infected person, and the genetics of the parasite. Coinfections, such as HIV, may increase the severity of Chagas signs and symptoms.[46] Immunocompromised individuals such as young children, the elderly, individuals taking immunosuppressants, or those with immunosuppressive diseases may experience more severe symptoms and complications.[47] There is also evidence showing that the genetics of the host is a key factor in the presentation and severity of cardiac pathology.[48] Additionally, variation in the genetic strain of the parasite (discrete typing unit) has been attributed to variation in the clinical outcome of infected persons and animals.[49] For example, in humans, the *T. cruzi* strain type TcI is more associated with cardiac pathology in comparison to TcII/V, which is associated with digestive pathology.[50] In a mouse study, cardiac pathology and survival rate was dependent *T. cruzi* strain type.[51]

DIAGNOSTICS

Diagnosis of Chagas disease is made based on the patient's clinical findings, history that suggests the patient may be at risk, and the use of multiple diagnostic tests. The approach for diagnosis of Chagas disease depends upon the phase of infection. During the acute phase when the parasite is actively circulating in the blood of the host, methods to directly detect the parasite from blood are useful. The parasite can be detected during the acute phase through microscopic assessment of blood smears. Additionally, DNA from the parasite can be amplified from the blood using polymerase chain reaction (PCR). Other diagnostic approaches that are useful during the acute phase include hemoculture (using culture media to grow parasite from a blood sample) and xenodiagnosis (in which uninfected triatomine insects feed on a host and are later assayed for infection). Unless antibody-detection assays are targeted to IgM antibodies, serological methods may be of limited utility in the acute phase, as the host may not yet have a detectable antibody response to infection.

Diagnostic tests used during the indeterminate and chronic phases are usually serological tests to detect anti-*T. cruzi* IgG antibodies, including enzyme-linked immunosorbent assays, radioimmune precipitation assay, indirect immunofluorescence assays, and more recently, lateral flow immunochromatographic assays. [52] However, each assay may be associated with cross-reaction, false positive or false negative results. For this reason, the WHO recommends confirming infection on the basis of reactivity in at least two conventional serological tests with independent antigenic principles.[53] Besides serological testing, biopsies, cardiac evaluations, and postmortem procedures may assist in diagnosis of Chagas disease in the indeterminate and chronic phases. Muscle biopsies may reveal intracellular amastigotes or inflammation when histologically observed.[54] Electrocardiograms and radiographs are often used in suspect Chagas cases to evaluate cardiac abnormalities, including arrhythmias and cardiomegaly. Postmortem gross abnormalities and histological assessments of tissues, including the heart, may confirm the presence of *T. cruzi* or associated cardiomyopathies such as lymphoplasmacytic inflammation.

TREATMENT

Two antitrypanosomal drugs, nifurtimox and benznidazole, are available for treating human Chagas disease. In 2017, the Food and Drug Administration (FDA) approved benznidazole for use in infected children (ages 2–12).[55] Nifurtimox produces more toxic side effects than benznidazole, but has shown similar effectiveness.[56] In the United States, nifurtimox is not FDA approved, but may be obtained through CDC using an investigational protocol. Both medications are used in Latin America, where they have been noted to provide significant cure rates in infants and acutely infected individuals.[57,58] Antiparasitic treatment during the chronic phase is less effective. Once the parasite causes irreparable damage to the heart and other tissues, symptomatic treatment is administered that may include pacemaker implants. The international clinical trial (BENznidazole Evaluation For Interrupting Trypanosomiasis [BENEFIT]) showed benznidazole failed to halt disease progression in patients with chronic Chagas cardiomyopathy.[59,60]

DISEASE PREVENTION AND CONTROL

There is no vaccine against Chagas disease. Vector control can reduce the risk of Chagas disease in humans and domestic animals. The Southern Cone Initiative (SCI), a coalition of South American countries (Argentina, Bolivia, Brazil, Chile, Paraguay, and Uruguay), was designed to interrupt transmission by eliminating or reducing *Triatoma infestans* vectors in at-risk communities through insecticide treatment and community engagement.[7] Residual pesticide interventions were shown to reduce or deter insects in peridomestic habitats, thus reducing the risk to domestic animals and humans.[61,62] SCI insecticide interventions were especially effective when combined with housing improvements.[61] Improvements to homes with thatched roofs and abode exteriors in endemic countries showed a reduction in triatomine infestations.[61,63] Homes with modern construction may not be as prone to triatomine infestations. However, older homes with inadequate window screening or homes with entry points due to compromised structures may allow triatomine intrusion or domiciliation.[64] Since triatomine insects are attracted to artificial light, reduction of light sources around peridomiciliary structures and homes reduce their attraction to the vectors.[65] Reduction of triatomine habitat and habitats of sylvatic hosts including wood and debris piles around homes may reduce insect numbers.[66] In addition, structural updates to compromised housing provide protection from entry by triatomines.[67]

The SCI also focused on eliminating transmission via blood product transfusions through the development of patient and product screenings. This portion of the initiative lacked compliance in some countries with high prevalence rates, such as Bolivia, where an estimated 50% of blood banks still lack serological screenings.[7] In the United States, first time blood donors are tested for anti-*T. cruzi* antibodies, but not upon subsequent donations, since the risk of local transmission is thought to be minimal. Pregnant women who were born or lived in endemic countries, as well as women who suspect having been bitten by a triatomine insect, should be screened to manage congenital transmission as early detection and treatment of congenital infections is associated with high rates of cure.[68,69]

Individuals traveling to endemic areas where triatomine insects are present should consider the use of insect repellent and mosquito nets to deter insects when sleeping in compromised housing.[70,71] A traveler should also take caution when drinking unpasteurized juices or eating uncooked foods from areas with previous food borne outbreaks of *T. cruzi*.

References

1. Chagas C. Nova tripanozomiaze humana: estudos sobre a morfolojia e o ciclo evolutivo do Schizotrypanum cruzi n. gen., n. sp., ajente etiolojico de nova entidade morbida do homem. *Mem Inst Oswaldo Cruz.* 1909;1(2):159–218.
2. Requena-Méndez A, Aldasoro E, de Lazzari E, et al. Prevalence of Chagas disease in Latin-American migrants living in Europe: A systematic review and meta-analysis. *PLoS Negl Trop Dis.* 2015;9(2):e0003540.
3. Hotez PJ, Dumonteil E, Woc-Colburn L, et al. Chagas disease: "The new HIV/AIDS of the Americas." *PLoS Negl Trop Dis.* 2012;6(5):4–7.
4. World Health Organisation. WHO Chagas disease (American trypanosomiasis) Factsheet. World Health Organisation. http://www.who.int/mediacentre/factsheets/fs340/en/. Published 2015.
5. Moncayo A, Silveira AC. Current epidemiological trends of Chagas disease in Latin America and future challenges: Epidemiology, surveillance, and health policies. In: American Trypanosomiasis Chagas Disease: One Hundred Years of Research. 2nd ed. Amsterdam: Elsevier; 2017:59–88.
6. World Health Organization. Chagas disease in Latin America: an epidemiological update based on 2010 estimates. *Wkly Epidemiol Rec.* 2015;6(90):33–44.
7. Dias JCP. Southern Cone Initiative for the elimination of domestic populations of Triatoma infestans and the interruption of transfusional Chagas disease. Historical aspects, present situation, and perspectives. *Mem Inst Oswaldo Cruz.* 2007;102(Suppl 1):11–18.
8. Lee BY, Bacon KM, Bottazzi ME, Hotez PJ. Global economic burden of Chagas disease: A computational simulation model. *Lancet Infect Dis.* 2013;13(4):342–8.
9. Montgomery SP, Starr MC, Cantey PT, Edwards MS, Meymandi SK. Neglected parasitic infections in the United States: Chagas disease. *Am J Trop Med Hyg.* 2014;90(5):814–8.
10. Dorn PL, Perniciaro L, Yabsley MJ, et al. Autochthonous transmission of *Trypanosoma cruzi*, Louisiana. *Emerg Infect Dis.* 2007;13(4):13–5.
11. Garcia MN, Aguilar D, Gorchakov R, et al. Case report: Evidence of autochthonous Chagas disease in southeastern Texas. *Am J Trop Med Hyg.* 2015;92(2):325–30.
12. Woody NC, Woody HB. American Trypanosomiasis (Chagas' disease): First indigenous case in the United States. *J Am Med Assoc.* 1955;159(7):676–7.
13. Manne-Goehler J, Umeh CA, Montgomery SP, Wirtz VJ. Estimating the burden of chagas disease in the United States. *PLoS Negl Trop Dis.* 2016;10(11):1–7.
14. Curtis-Robles R, Zecca IB, Roman-Cruz V, et al. *Trypanosoma cruzi* (agent of Chagas disease) in sympatric human and dog populations in "colonias" of the Lower Rio Grande Valley of Texas. *Am J Trop Med Hyg.* 2017;96(4):805–14.
15. Coura JR, Vĩas PA. Chagas disease: A new worldwide challenge. *Nature.* 2010;465(7301 suppl):S6–7.
16. Monteith GB. Confirmation of the presence of Triatominae (Hemiptera: Reduviidae) in Australia, with notes on indo-pacific species. *Aust J Entomol.* 1974;13(2):89–94.
17. Tartarotti E, Azeredo-Oliveira MTV, Ceron CR. Phylogenetic approach to the study of triatomines (Triatominae, Heteroptera). *Brazilian J Biol.* 2006;66(2B):703–708.
18. Patterson JS, Guhl F. Geographical distribution of Chagas disease. In: Telleria J, Tibayrenc M, eds. *American Trypanosomiasis Chagas Disease: One Hundred Years of Research.* London: Elsevier; 2010:83–114.
19. Lent H, Wygodzinsky P. Revision of the Triatominae (Hemiptera, Reduviidae), and their significance as vectors of Chagas' disease. *Bull Am Museum Nat Hist.* 1979;163(3):123–520.
20. Gürtler RE, Cecere MC, Lauricella MA, Cardinal MV, Kitron U, Cohen JE. Domestic dogs and cats as sources of *Trypanosoma cruzi* infection in rural northwestern Argentina. *Parasitology.* 2007;134(Pt 1):69–82.
21. Klotz SA, Dorn PL, Klotz JH, et al. Feeding behavior of triatomines from the southwestern United States: An update on potential risk for transmission of Chagas disease. *Acta Trop.* 2009;111(2):114–8.
22. Curtis-Robles R, Aukland LD, Snowden KF, Hamer GL, Hamer SA. Analysis of over 1500 triatomine vectors from across the US, predominantly Texas, for *Trypanosoma cruzi* infection and discrete typing units. *Infect Genet Evol.* 2018;58:171–80.
23. Kjos SA, Snowden KF, Olson JK. Biogeography and *Trypanosoma cruzi* infection prevalence of Chagas disease vectors in Texas, USA. *Vector-Borne Zoonotic Dis.* 2009;9(1):41–50.

24. Klotz SA, Dorn PL, Mosbacher M, Schmidt JO. Kissing bugs in the United States: Risk for vector-borne disease in humans. *Environ Health Insights*. 2014;8(Suppl 2):49–59.
25. Kjos SA, Marcet PL, Yabsley MJ, et al. Identification of bloodmeal sources and *Trypanosoma cruzi* infection in triatomine bugs (Hemiptera: Reduviidae) from residential settings in Texas, the United States. *J Med Entomol*. 2013;50(5):1126–39.
26. Olsen PF, Shoemaker JP, Turner HF, Hays KL. Incidence of *Trypanosoma cruzi* (Chagas) in wild vectors and reservoirs in East-Central Alabama. *J Parasitol*. 1964;50(5):599–603.
27. Garcia MN, Woc-Colburn L, Aguilar D, Hotez PJ, Murray KO. Historical perspectives on the epidemiology of human Chagas disease in Texas and recommendations for enhanced understanding of clinical Chagas disease in the Southern United States. *PLoS Negl Trop Dis*. 2015;9(11):e0003981.
28. Bradley K, Bergman D, Woods J, Crutcher J, Kirchhoff L. Prevalence of American trypanosomiasis (Chagas disease) among dogs in Oklahoma. *J Am Vet Med Assoc*. 2000;217(12):1853–7.
29. Curtis-Robles R, Snowden KF, Dominguez B, et al. Epidemiology and molecular typing of *Trypanosoma cruzi* in naturally-infected hound dogs and associated triatomine vectors in Texas, USA. *PLoS Negl Trop Dis*. 2017;11(1):e0005298.
30. Curtis-Robles R, Lewis BC, Hamer SA. High *Trypanosoma cruzi* infection prevalence associated with minimal cardiac pathology among wild carnivores in central Texas. *Int J Parasitol Parasites Wildl*. 2016;5(2):117–23.
31. Pung OJ, Banks CW, Jones DN, Krissinger MW. *Trypanosoma cruzi* in wild raccoons, opossums, and triatomine bugs in southeast Georgia, U.S.A. *J Parasitol*. 1995;81(2):324–6.
32. Hodo CL, Hamer SA. Toward an ecological framework for assessing reservoirs of vector-borne pathogens: Wildlife reservoirs of *Trypanosoma cruzi* across the southern United States. *ILAR J*. 2017;58(3):379–92.
33. Meyers AC, Meinders M, Hamer SA. Widespread *Trypanosoma cruzi* infection in government working dogs along the Texas-Mexico border: Discordant serology, parasite genotyping and associated vectors. *PLoS Negl Trop Dis*. 2017;11(8):1–19.
34. Barr S, Schmidt S, Brown C, Klei T. Pathologic features of dogs inoculated with North American *Trypanosoma cruzi* isolates. *Am J Vet Res*. 1991;52(12):2033–9.
35. Villacís AG, Arcos-Terán L, Grijalva MJ. Life cycle, feeding and defecation patterns of Rhodnius ecuadoriensis (Lent & León 1958) (Hemiptera: Reduviidae: Triatominae) under laboratory conditions. *Mem Inst Oswaldo Cruz*. 2008;103(7):690–5.
36. Zeledón R, Alvarado R, Jiron LF. Observations on the feeding and defecation patterns of three triatomine species (Hemiptera: Reduviidae). *Acta Trop*. 1977;34(1):65–77.
37. Klotz SA, Dorn PL, Klotz JH, et al. Feeding behavior of triatomines from the southwestern United States: An update on potential risk for transmission of Chagas disease. *Acta Trop*. 2009;111(2):114–8.
38. CDC. CDC—Chagas Disease. http://www.cdc.gov/parasites/chagas/health_professionals/tx.html. Published 2013.
39. Brenière SF, Waleckx E, Aznar C. Other forms of transmission: Blood transfusion, organ transplantation, laboratory accidents, oral and sexual transmission. In: *American Trypanosomiasis Chagas Disease: One Hundred Years of Research*. 2nd ed. Amsterdam: Elsevier; 2017:561–78.
40. Dias JP, Bastos C, Araújo E, et al. Acute Chagas disease outbreak associated with oral transmission Surto de doença de Chagas aguda associada à transmissão oral. *Rev Soc Bras Med Trop*. 2008;41(3):296–300.
41. Ramírez JD, Montilla M, Cucunubá ZM, Floréz AC, Zambrano P, Guhl F. Molecular epidemiology of human oral Chagas disease outbreaks in Colombia. *PLoS Negl Trop Dis*. 2013;7(2):e2041.
42. Roellig DM, Ellis AE, Yabsley MJ. Oral transmission of *Trypanosoma cruzi* with opposing evidence for the theory of carnivory. *J Parasitol*. 2009;95(2):360–4.
43. Norman FF, López-Vélez R. Chagas disease and breast-feeding. *Emerg Infect Dis*. 2013;19(10):1561–6.
44. Ribeiro M, Nitz N, Santana C, et al. Sexual transmission of *Trypanosoma cruzi* in murine model. *Exp Parasitol*. 2016;162:1–6.
45. Dias JC. Cecilio Romana, Romana's sign and Chagas' disease. *Rev Soc Bras Med Trop*. 1997;30(5):407–13.
46. Sartori AMC, Ibrahim KY, Westphalen EVN, Braz LMA, Oliveira OC, Gakiya E. Manifestations of Chagas disease (American trypanosomiasis) in patients with HIV/AIDS. *Ann Trop Med Parasitol*. 2007;101(1):31–50.
47. Simões MV, Soares FA, Marin-Neto J. Severe myocarditis and esophagitis during reversible long standing Chagas' disease recrudescence in immunocompromised host. *Int J Cardiol*. 1995;49(3):271–3.
48. Marinho CRF, Bucci DZ, Dagli MLZ, et al. Pathology affects different organs in two mouse strains chronically infected by a *Trypanosoma cruzi* clone: A model for genetic studies of Chagas' disease. *Infect Immun*. 2004;72(4):2350–7.
49. Messenger LA, Yeo M, Lewis MD, Llewellyn MS, Miles MA. Molecular genotyping of *Trypanosoma cruzi* for lineage assignment and population genetics. In: Peacock C, ed. *Parasite Genomics Protocols*. Vol. 1201. Methods in Molecular Biology. New York: Springer; 2015:297–337.
50. Miles M, Póvoa M, Prata A, Cedillos R, De Souza A, Macedo V. Do radically dissimilar *Trypanosoma cruzi* strains (zymodemes) cause Venezuelan and Brazilian forms of Chagas' disease? *Lancet*. 1981;(June 20):1338–40.
51. Bustamante JM, Rivarola HW, Fernández AR, et al. Indeterminate Chagas' disease: *Trypanosoma cruzi* strain and re-infection are factors involved in the progression of cardiopathy. *Clin Sci (Lond)*. 2003;104(4):415–20.
52. Meymandi S, Hernandez S, Park S, Sanchez DR, Forsyth C. Treatment of Chagas disease in the United States. *Neglected Trop Dis*. 2018;10(3):373–88.
53. World Health Organization. *Control of Chagas Disease: Second Report of the WHO Expert Committee World Health Organization*. Vol. 905. 2002.
54. Laguens RP, Cossio PM, Diez C, et al. Immunopathologic and morphologic studies of skeletal muscle in Chagas' disease. *Am J Pathol*. 1975;80(1):153.
55. Traynor K. Benznidazole approved for Chagas disease in children. *Am J Health Syst Pharm*. 2017;74(19):1519.
56. Urbina JA. Chemotherapy of Chagas' disease: The how and the why. *J Mol Med*. 1999;77(3):332–8.
57. Oliveira I, Torrico F, Muoz J, Gascon J. Congenital transmission of Chagas disease: A clinical approach. *Expert Rev Anti Infect Ther*. 2010;8(8):945–56.
58. Viotti R, Vigliano C, Lococo B, et al. Side effects of benznidazole as treatment in chronic Chagas disease: Fears and realities. *Expert Rev Anti Infect Ther*. 2009;7(2):157–63.
59. Marin-Neto JA, Rassi A, Morillo CA, et al. Rationale and design of a randomized placebo-controlled trial assessing the effects of etiologic treatment in Chagas' cardiomyopathy: The BENznidazole Evaluation For Interrupting Trypanosomiasis (BENEFIT). *Am Heart J*. 2008;156(1):37–43.
60. Rassi A, Marin-Neto JA, Rassi A. Chronic Chagas cardiomyopathy: A review of the main pathogenic mechanisms and the efficacy of aetiological treatment following the BENznidazole evaluation for interrupting trypanosomiasis (BENEFIT) trial. *Mem Inst Oswaldo Cruz*. 2017;112(3):224–35.
61. Gurtler R, Kitron U, Cecere M, Segura E, Cohen J. Sustainable vector control and management of Chagas disease in the Gran Chaco, Argentina. *Proc Natl Acad Sci U S A*. 2007;104(41):16194–9.
62. Lucero DE, Morrissey LA, Rizzo DM, et al. Ecohealth interventions limit triatomine reinfestation following insecticide spraying in La Brea, Guatemala. *Am J Trop Med Hyg*. 2013;88(4):630–7.
63. Rojas De Arias A, Ferro EA, Ferreira ME, Simancas LC. Chagas disease vector control through different intervention modalities in endemic localities of Paraguay. *Bull World Health Organ*. 1999;77(4):331–9.
64. Klotz SA, Shirazi FM, Boesen K, et al. Kissing bug (Triatoma spp.) intrusion into homes: Troublesome bites and domiciliation. *Environ Health Insights*. 2016;10:45–9.
65. Castro MCM, Barrett TV, Santos WS, Abad-Franch F, Rafael JA. Attraction of Chagas disease vectors (Triatominae) to artificial light sources in the canopy of primary Amazon rainforest. *Mem Inst Oswaldo Cruz*. 2010;105(8):1061–4.
66. Walter A, Lozano-Kasten F, Bosseno MF, et al. Peridomicilary habitat and risk factors for Triatoma infestation in a rural community of the Mexican occident. *Am J Trop Med Hyg*. 2007;76(3):508–5.
67. Rojas-de-Arias A. Chagas disease prevention through improved housing using an ecosystem approach to health. *Cad Saude Publica*. 2001;17:89–97.
68. Alegria I, Coll MT, Bachs MR, et al. Congenital Chagas disease: The importance of screening before the delivery. Our experience in a regional hospital in Catalonia. *Trop Med Int Health*. 2011;16:370.
69. Neto EC, Rubin R, Schulte J, Giugliani R. Newborn screening for congenital infectious diseases. *Emerg Infect Dis*. 2004;10(6):1068–73.
70. Zamora D, Klotz SA, Meister EA, Schmidt JO. Repellency of the components of the essential oil, citronella, to *Triatoma rubida*, *Triatoma protracta*, and *Triatoma recurva* (Hemiptera: Reduviidae: Triatominae). *J Med Entomol*. 2015;52(4):719–21.
71. Levy MZ, Quíspe-Machaca VR, Ylla-Velasquez JL, et al. Impregnated netting slows infestation by *Triatoma infestans*. *Am J Trop Med Hyg*. 2008;79(4):528–34.

CHAPTER

133

Human African Trypanosomiasis

Jan Van Den Abbeele

INTRODUCTION

Human African trypanosomiasis (HAT), or sleeping sickness, is a vector-borne parasitic disease that is restricted to sub-Saharan Africa. It is caused by extracellular protozoa belonging to the genus *Trypanosoma*, which are transmitted by the bite of a blood-feeding insect, the tsetse fly (Diptera; *Glossina*). Two human-pathogenic subspecies of trypanosomes, *T. brucei gambiense and T. brucei rhodesiense*, cause different forms of the disease: the slow-progressing form (gambiense-HAT) which is endemic in western and central Africa, and the faster progressing form (rhodesiense-HAT) found in eastern and southern Africa.[1] About 97% of cases of HAT are due to *T. b. gambiense*. HAT still has a severe social and economic impact in various countries in sub-Saharan Africa, with an estimated 55 million people at risk and over 10 million people living in areas where gambiense-HAT is considered a public health problem.[2] Sleeping sickness has been responsible for devastating epidemics in the twentieth century. However, due to increased disease surveillance efforts and large-scale use of control tools, major improvements have been achieved during the last two decades. Today, the number of newly reported cases is low. The World Health Organization (WHO) has targeted the elimination of HAT as a public health problem by 2020 with a target of fewer than 2000 reported cases per year.[2–5] For *T. b. rhodesiense*-HAT, sporadic cases are diagnosed outside endemic African countries, mainly among travelers from Europe and the United States returning from visits to east African game parks, as well as expatriates and migrants.[5–8]

BIOLOGY AND TRANSMISSION

T. brucei is a digenetic parasite that is transmitted between mammals by the blood feeding tsetse fly (Fig. 133-1). During its life cycle, the parasite undergoes complex developmental changes in the mammalian host and tsetse fly vector. In the mammalian bloodstream, two life cycle stages are recognized: the proliferative long slender form and the short stumpy trypanosome form. The latter is preadapted for survival in the tsetse fly midgut when ingested during the fly's blood meal. In addition to blood, *T. brucei* parasites colonize the interstitial spaces of several other tissues, including brain, adipose tissue, and skin.[9–13] When ingested by the tsetse fly through a blood meal on an infected host, the parasite must go through an obligatory and complex life cycle in the alimentary tract and salivary glands of the fly.[14] Here, the final developmental stage is the infectious metacyclic stage that is injected into the mammalian host skin through the bite of the infected fly.

Both sexes of adult tsetse feed exclusively on vertebrate blood every 2–5 days and can contribute to the transmission of the trypanosome.[15] Tsetse flies have a unique method of reproduction with the female depositing one fully developed larva every 10 days that burrows into the soil, pupates, and emerges as an adult fly a month later. The 31 species and subspecies of tsetse flies are confined to sub-Saharan Africa, and are subdivided into three groups: the fusca, palpalis, and morsitans.[16,17] The species of the palpalis group are associated with coastal habitats, degraded forests of West-Africa and riverine vegetation, as well as gallery forest. The palpalis group contains the important vectors for gambiense-HAT (*G. palpalis palpalis, G. palpalis gambiensis, G. fuscipes fuscipes*, and *G. f. quanzensis*). Tsetse species belonging the morsitans group are restricted to dryer regions such as savannah woodlands. Here, *G. morsitans* spp. and *G. pallidipes* are the most important are major vectors of rhodesiense-HAT.[18]

EPIDEMIOLOGY

The major host-to-human transmission route of the human-pathogenic trypanosomes is by bite of an infected tsetse fly. In a natural tsetse fly population, only a small proportion (less than 0.1%) are actual transmitters, carrying the final infective stage of the parasite in the salivary glands. Despite this, due to the frequent blood feeding (every 2–5 days) on multiple hosts, a single infected tsetse fly can transmit the parasite to a multitude of people during its 2- to 3-month lifespan.[19] In addition, occasional cases of congenital transmission of *T. b. gambiense* have been documented in the literature.[20–23]

Currently, gambiense-HAT is endemic in 24 countries of west and central Africa, and causes more than 97.6% of reported cases of sleeping sickness. Rhodesiense-HAT is endemic in 13 countries of eastern and southern Africa, representing about 2.4% of reported cases. Between 1999 and 2016, the reported number of new cases of gambiense-HAT fell by 92%, from 27,862 to 2131. The majority of gambiense cases continues to occur in the Democratic Republic of the Congo (83%), followed by the Central African Republic (5.8%), Guinea (5.0%), and Chad (2.5%). During the same period, the number of newly reported cases of rhodesiense-HAT fell from 619 to 53, remaining concentrated in Malawi and Uganda, which account for 69.8% and 18.9% of the WHO-reported cases, respectively.[24] Cases of HAT exported to nonendemic countries are reported from all continents. Here, most cases are due to the rhodesiense-HAT in short-term travelers who acquired the disease while visiting game-parks in eastern and southeastern Africa. Gambiense-HAT is rare among travelers but was sporadically reported in migrants and long-term expatriates living in rural settings.[7,8,25] Although epidemics have not been reported during the last decades, large outbreaks of HAT have been documented in the past.[26,27]

Gambiense-HAT is mainly considered an anthroponotic disease, with a minor role for animal reservoirs. The disease typically develops in geographically limited foci and is usually found in rural areas with suitable habitats for the tsetse fly vector and frequent human–tsetse contact. Periurban areas can also be affected, especially where riverine tsetse species have adapted to anthropic environments although its distribution has changed over time. This is likely due to the migration

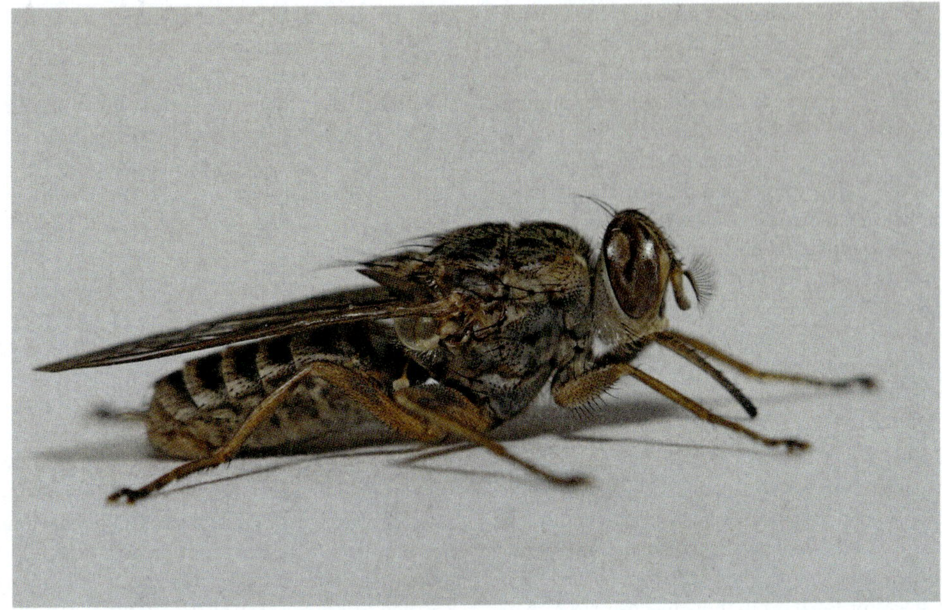

FIGURE 133-1. The tsetse fly, vector of the parasites causing human African trypanosomiasis. (*Source:* Luc Verhelst, Institute of Tropical Medicine Antwerp.)

of farmers to new areas, changing environments, population displacements, and health service disorganization resulting from conflicts, border zone proximity, and climate change. Notably, there has been a decrease in rainfall, altering the characteristics of forests and gallery-forests; the main biotope of the tsetse fly vector.[28] People can be infected while farming, fishing, hunting, collecting water or wood, or engaging in any other activity that exposes them to the bite of an infective tsetse fly. All age groups and both sexes are at risk, although prevalence is higher in adults, and sex distribution varies in relation to gender-specific at-risk activities.[5] It remains largely unknown for gambiense-HAT whether, and to what extent, the existence of latent asymptomatic human infections as well as possible animal reservoirs have an impact on its transmission and epidemiology.[29] Rhodesiense-HAT is a zoonotic disease with livestock and wildlife acting as reservoir hosts, and humans are only accidentally infected. Foci are mainly in remote areas, where a lack of diagnostic facilities and awareness of HAT are frequently reported. Many of these foci have been linked to devastating outbreaks in the past. There have been recent outbreaks, but smaller in magnitude, suggesting that the risk still exists.[30]

PATHOLOGY/CLINICAL MANIFESTATIONS

Both rhodesiense- and gambiense-HAT infections start after the injection of infective metacyclic trypanosomes with tsetse fly vector saliva into human skin. Here, they differentiate to the bloodstream stage and spread via the local draining lymph node into the vascular system. In some, but not all infections, a local skin reaction or chancre occurs at the site of inoculation approximately 1 week after the bite of an infected tsetse fly. This reaction occurs in around 20% of patients infected with *T. b. rhodesiense* but is rarely seen for gambiense-HAT. The disease further evolves in two distinct successive stages: a hemolymphatic stage followed by a meningoencephalitic stage in which trypanosomes cross the blood–brain barrier and invade the central nervous system (CNS). The major symptoms for the two disease forms are the same, but their severity and progression kinetics generally differ strongly. Rhodesiense-HAT is acute, with development of the second stage within a few weeks and death within 6 months. Gambiense-HAT follows a chronic progression for a total of nearly 3 years in the absence of treatment; although some patients survive for more than 10 years.[5] For both forms a wide spectrum of clinical symptoms, disease severity, and duration of illness has been observed with low virulence forms of *T. brucei rhodesiense* infection, as well as cases ranging from acute to asymptomatic cases for gambiense-HAT.[31,32] It is generally assumed that both forms of the disease lead to death if left untreated, although for gambiense-HAT healthy carriers and self-cure have been reported.[33]

The first stage is called the hemolymphatic or bloodstream stage. During this period, the parasites proliferate within the blood and lymphatic system. Early-stage symptoms tend to be nonspecific, with an onset 1–3 weeks after sustaining a tsetse fly bite, and include headache, malaise, arthralgia, weight loss, fatigue, intermittent fever with rigors, and generalized lymphadenopathy.[34] Immune-activation is evident from lymph node enlargement, hepatomegaly, and splenomegaly. Enlargement of the posterior cervical lymph nodes is typical of gambiense-HAT and is known as Winterbottom's sign.[35]

Once the parasites cross the blood-brain barrier, the late or meningoencephalic stage of infection coincides with a parasite invasion of the CNS. This second stage is fatal if untreated. A variety of symptoms can occur with almost all regions of the nervous system potentially involved. Mainly during this late stage, stigmatization of patients is common.[36] Major symptoms are neuropsychiatric and include sleep disturbances, abnormal movement, limb paralysis, hemiparesis, irritability, aggressive behavior, and psychotic reactions. Other common cerebral changes that are observed include emotional liability, attention deficit, indifference, apathy, stereotypic behavior, manic episodes, melancholia, and confusion.[35] Motor features may also occur in late-stage HAT. Tremors of the hands and tongue are common, choreiform movements of the head, limbs, and trunk may occur, as may pyramidal weakness of the limbs. Lower limb paralysis may occur because of spinal cord involvement (myelopathy or myelitis) or peripheral motor neuropathy.[36] The hallmark of sleeping sickness is the disruption of the sleep pattern which occur in 74% of patients according to an extensive study of 2541 patients with late-stage HAT.[37] Sleep abnormalities consist of a reversal of the normal sleep/wake cycle, with nocturnal insomnia and daytime somnolence, uncontrollable episodes of sleep, and an alteration of the structure of sleep itself, but with total time spent sleeping comparable to healthy individuals. Polysomnographic records show a disruption of the sleep–wake cycle, with frequent, short, sleep-onset rapid eye movement episodes that are equally likely to occur during day and night.[38–40] The fact that the sleep/wake cycle disruption in patients reverts to normal upon treatment, and that autopsies show that patients who die of sleeping sickness lack neurodegeneration, suggests that the presence of parasites, rather than neuronal death, is the cause of these symptoms.[41] Results of a recent experimental study in a mouse model showed that *T. brucei* infection shortens the period of the circadian activity rhythm at the organismal level, and at cellular and molecular levels. This acceleration of the host circadian clock is probably caused by the direct interaction of cells with the parasite or with a parasite molecule.[41] At the terminal phase of the disease, CNS demyelination and atrophy are accompanied by disturbances in consciousness with progressive dementia. The patient dies in a state of cachexia and afflicted with opportunistic infections.

DIAGNOSIS

Diagnosis should be made as early as possible. Presenting symptoms of HAT in the early stages are nonspecific and can easily be mistaken for those of other diseases. In rhodesiense-HAT, parasite numbers in the blood are usually high enough to allow microscopic detection in Giemsa stained thin smear or thick drop. In gambiense-HAT, parasitemia is often far below the detection limit of thin smear or thick drop preparations. Trypanosome concentration techniques such as the mini Anion Exchange Centrifugation Technique (mAECT), with a lower detection limit of < 50 parasites per mL of blood, are therefore necessary.[42–44] *T. brucei gambiense* infected persons may present with swollen cervical lymph nodes that can be punctured with a dry needle to aspirate some microliters of lymph for fresh examination under the microscope. This method is simple and cheap, and, in a considerable fraction of patients, the parasites are only detectable in the lymph and not in the blood.

Patients with strong neurological and/or serological suspicion of late-stage HAT may not have parasitological confirmation from blood or lymph. In such cases, lumbar puncture and microscopic examination of the cerebrospinal fluid may reveal the parasites that have entered the CNS.[42] Stage determination in HAT-infected persons relies on the examination of cerebrospinal fluid.[45] Patients with five or fewer white blood cells per μL and no trypanosomes in the cerebrospinal fluid are classified as first stage. Those with more than five white blood cells per μL or trypanosomes in the cerebrospinal fluid are classified as second stage.

Because of the limited sensitivity of microscopic parasite detection techniques especially for gambiense-HAT, efforts have focused on the development of indirect diagnostic tests. Reliable serodiagnostic tests exist only for *T. brucei gambiense* infection and are based on the detection of specific antibodies (Abs). No field-applicable serodiagnostic test exists for *T. brucei rhodesiense* infection. The card agglutination test for trypanosomiasis (CATT) visualizes the interaction of gambiense-specific Abs with color-dyed, freeze-dried *T. brucei gambiense* parasites.[46] CATT can be done with blood collected from a finger prick, plasma, or serum, and the agglutination reaction is scored visually after 5 min. It is particularly suited for screening of at-risk populations by mobile teams. However, with the steadily decreasing prevalence of trypanosomiasis, individual rapid diagnostic tests that can be used in primary health centers are essential. Two rapid diagnostic tests with high sensitivity and specificity were recently developed: the HAT Sero-K-SeT and the SD Bioline HAT 1.0.[47–49] Immune trypanolysis and ELISAs are applicable in laboratory conditions on serum, plasma, and dried blood spots. Their high specificity and sensitivity, their applicability to dried blood spots, and adaptability to animal specimens make them excellent tools for large-scale surveys, postelimination monitoring, and animal reservoir studies.[5]

Molecular diagnosis of HAT has been the subject of numerous investigations but should be interpreted with caution in clinical practice. Molecular diagnostics are based on detection of parasite-specific DNA or RNA in a clinical specimen from a patient, usually after enzymatic amplification of a target nucleotide sequence. So far, they have not reached the status of point-of-care test due to their cost, complexity, and requirements regarding controlled reaction temperature(s), specimen preparation, and skilled personnel.[50] Nevertheless, elimination and postelimination campaigns will need standardized high-throughput molecular test formats. In addition, monitoring infections in animals and vectors will require subspecies-specific molecular tests.[50]

TREATMENT

The earlier HAT is treated, the better the prospects of treatment tolerability and cure. The assessment of treatment outcome requires follow up of the patient for potentially 24 months, and entails laboratory exams of body fluids including cerebrospinal fluid obtained by lumbar puncture. The choice of treatment depends on the causative agent and disease stage (Table 133-1). Four drugs are registered for the treatment of HAT: pentamidine, suramin, melarsoprol, and eflornithine. A fifth drug, nifurtimox, is used in combination under special authorizations.[51] To ensure its quality and use by National Sleeping Sickness Control Programmes, drugs are provided free of charge by WHO to endemic countries with a kit containing all the material needed for its administration. Two new medications (i.e., Fexinidazole and Benzoxaborole SCYX-7158) in clinical development are administered orally and are intended for treatment of both disease stages. For both drugs, clinical trials—phase 2/3 and phase 3, respectively—are currently ongoing.[52–57]

Pentamidine (pentamidine isethionate) is the drug of choice for treatment of first-stage gambiense-HAT. The standard dosage regimen is 4 mg /kg body weight per day for 7 days. Because of the risk of hypotension after intravenous application, the drug is usually given as deep intramuscular injection. In settings where adequate nursing care and monitoring are available, an intravenous infusion in saline over 2 hours may be used as an alternative.[58] Pentamidine is well tolerated and most reactions are reversible. The intramuscular injection causes site pain and transient swelling. Abdominal pain, gastrointestinal problems, nausea, vomiting, and hypoglycemia (5–40%) are the most frequently reported adverse events.[5,58,59]

Suramin is effective in the first stage of gambiense- and rhodesiense-HAT. However, it is used only in the treatment of *T. brucei rhodesiense* infections, because of the risk of onchocerciasis co-infection in *T. brucei gambiense*-endemic areas (i.e., risk of allergic reactions arising from rapid killing of microfilaria), and because pentamidine administration is simpler. Suramin is administered as a slow intravenous infusion. The most commonly used dosage regimen consists of a test dose of 4–5 mg/kg body weight at day 1, followed by five weekly injections of 20 mg/kg body weight (e.g., days 3, 10, 17, 24, 31),

TABLE 133-1 DIFFERENT TREATMENTS AVAILABLE FOR HUMAN AFRICAN TRYPANOSOMIASIS

	Early Stage	Late Stage
First-line treatment:		
T. brucei gambiense	Pentamidine	Nifurtimox + Eflornithine (NECT)
T. brucei rhodesiense	Suramin	Melarsoprol
Second-line treatment:		
T. brucei gambiense	Suramin	Melarsoprol
T. brucei rhodesiense	Pentamidine	Not available
Clinical testing phase III:		
T. brucei gambiense	Fexinidazole	

with a maximum dose per injection of 1 gram. Some degree of kidney damage is common, but nephrotoxicity is usually mild and reversible. The first symptoms of renal impairment are albuminuria, later cylinduria and hematuria. Other adverse drug reactions reported are early hypersensitivity reactions occurring in 0.1–0.3% of cases causing nausea, circulatory collapse and urticaria, and rare late hypersensitivity reactions such as exfoliative dermatitis and hemolytic anemia, peripheral neuropathy, and bone marrow toxicity with agranulocytosis and thrombocytopenia.[58]

The treatment of second-stage HAT is more problematic than is the case for early-stage disease. Treatment success depends on drugs that cross the blood-brain barrier to reach the parasite and are more complicated to administer. The first-line treatment for second-stage *T brucei gambiense* disease is currently the *nifurtimox–eflornithine combination therapy (NECT)*. The NECT treatment consists of eflornithine 400 mg/kg per day intravenous short infusion for 7 days, plus nifurtimox 15 mg/kg orally per day (5 mg/kg every 8 hours) for 10 days. This represents a considerable simplification compared to the standard eflornithine schedule. The most common treatment-emergent adverse events are abdominal pain, vomiting, and headache. The toxicity profile replicates that of nifurtimox and eflornithine monotherapies, but with lower frequency and severity, most likely because of shorter drug exposure.[5] *Eflornithine* (α-difluoromethylornithine or DFMO) can also be used as monotherapy, but only in the second stage of *T. brucei gambiense* infection because it is not effective against disease due to *T. brucei rhodesiense*. It is a cytostatic and trypanostatic drug that requires an active immune system to achieve cure (90–95% cure rate). As monotherapy, it is given as a slow intravenous infusion for 14 days (56 infusions in total) but is cumbersome to administer and challenging in resource-poor settings. Severe catheter-related bacterial infections are an important complication risk, which can be effectively prevented by providing adequate nursing care.[60] Adverse side effects from treatment are frequent and similar to those of other cytostatics. The main adverse events are fever, pruritus, hypertension, nausea, vomiting, diarrhea, abdominal pain, headaches, and myelosuppression (i.e., anemia, leucopenia, thrombocytopenia). Another treatment option is *melarsoprol*, which is the only option in the case of *T. brucei rhodesiense*, and the second-line drug for the second stage of *T. brucei gambiense* infections. The recommended treatment schedule comprises intravenous injections of 2.2 mg/kg bodyweight per day during 10 consecutive days. The most severe and life-threatening adverse reaction is an encephalopathic syndrome (ES) which occurs in around 10% of the patients, half of whom die.[34,61] It usually occurs between 7 and 14 days after the first injection and is characterized by fever and convulsions, rapid onset of neurological disorders and progressive coma. Coadministration of prednisolone may have a protective effect against the immune reaction thought to be a component of the ES. Close monitoring of patients may allow detection of early signs, such as fever or headache, or both, leading to the cessation of melarsoprol and management with dexamethasone and diazepam. Other frequent adverse reactions include general malaise, gastrointestinal (nausea, vomiting, and diarrhea), and skin reactions (pruritus).[5] Compared with melarsoprol or eflornithine monotherapy, NECT has higher cure rates (95–98%), lower fatality rates (<1%), less severe adverse events, and simpler administration. Although it is often said that the drugs mentioned above suffer from problems of drug resistance, melarsoprol resistance is the only concrete example of clinically relevant drug-resistant parasites.[62]

PREVENTION AND CONTROL

No vaccine against HAT is available and the toxicity of existing drugs precludes the adoption of control strategies based on preventive chemotherapy. Control and surveillance of the disease includes active and passive case finding, diagnosis, treatment, follow-up, vector control, and control of the animal reservoir, if possible. These are performed at different levels and intensity, depending on the epidemiological situation, local and national capacity, and environment.[63] Although vector control is critical to achieve the elimination/eradication goals, it is very challenging to sustain control of all tsetse fly populations in all endemic countries. Therefore, gambiense-HAT control will continue to rely on surveillance, diagnosis, and treatment, both for reducing transmission and for monitoring progress toward these goals.[29] Rhodesiense-HAT represents a relatively small part of the global HAT problem. Because of its zoonotic dimension (i.e., wildlife as well as domestic animals as parasite reservoir), control of rhodesiense-HAT requires a multisectoral approach that should involve veterinary services, in addition to a strong tsetse fly control component.[30,64] Large-scale screening of populations at risk, drug donations, and efforts by national and international stakeholders have brought the epidemic under control with < 2200 cases in 2016. The WHO has set the goals of gambiense-HAT elimination as a public health problem for 2020, and of interruption of transmission to humans for 2030. In view of the global elimination of HAT, it is important to clarify the extent to which these human reservoirs contribute to the transmission of the parasite and hence to gambiense-HAT persistence and potential resurgence.[29] Long-term elimination of rhodesiense-HAT is currently not feasible due to the existence of animal reservoirs.[30]

References

1. Simarro PP, Cecchi G, Paone M, et al. The Atlas of human African trypanosomiasis: A contribution to global mapping of neglected tropical diseases. *Int J Health Geogr*. 2010;9:57.
2. Franco JR, Cecchi G, Priotto G, et al. Monitoring the elimination of human African trypanosomiasis: Update to 2014. *PLoS Negl Trop Dis*. 2017;11(5):e0005585.
3. Simarro PP, Cecchi G, Franco JR, et al. Monitoring the progress towards the elimination of gambiense human African trypanosomiasis. *PLoS Negl Trop Dis*. 2015;9(6):e0003785.
4. Franco JR, Simarro PP, Diarra A, et al. The journey towards elimination of gambiense human African trypanosomiasis: Not far, nor easy. *Parasitology*. 2014;141(6):748–60.
5. Büscher P, Cecchi G, Jamonneau V, et al. Human African trypanosomiasis. *Lancet*. 2017;390(10110):2397–409.
6. Simarro PP, Franco JR, Cecchi G, et al. Human African trypanosomiasis in non-endemic countries (2000–2010). *J Travel Med*. 2012;19(1):44–53.
7. Blum JA, Neumayr AL, Hatz CF. Human African trypanosomiasis in endemic populations and travellers. *Eur J Clin Microbiol Infect Dis*. 2012;31(6):905–13.
8. Neuberger A, Meltzer E, Leshem E, et al. The changing epidemiology of human African trypanosomiasis among patients from nonendemic countries—1902–2012. *PLoS One*. 2014;9(2):e88647.
9. Vickerman K, Tetley L, Hendry KAK, et al. Biology of African trypanosomes in the tsetse fly. *Biol Cell*. 1988;64(2):109–19.
10. Mogk S, Meiwes A, Boßelmann CM, et al. The lane to the brain: How African trypanosomes invade the CNS. *Trends Parasitol*. 2014;30(10):470–6.
11. Trindade S, Rijo-Ferreira F, Carvalho T, et al. *Trypanosoma brucei* parasites occupy and functionally adapt to the adipose tissue in mice. *Cell Host Microbe*. 2016;19(6):837–48.
12. Caljon G, Van Reet N, De Trez C, et al. The dermis as a delivery site of *Trypanosoma brucei* for tsetse flies. *PLoS Pathog*. 2016;12(7):e1005744.
13. Capewell P, Cren-Travaillé C, Marchesi F, et al. The skin is a significant but overlooked anatomical reservoir for vector-borne African trypanosomes. *eLife*. 2016;5:e17716.
14. Rotureau B, Van Den Abbeele J. Through the dark continent: African trypanosome development in the tsetse fly. *Front Cell Infect Microbiol*. 2013;3:53.
15. Leak SGA. *Tsetse Biology and Ecology: Their Role in the Epidemiology and Control of Trypanosomosis*. 1st ed. UK: CABI; 1999.
16. Gooding RH, Krafsur ES. Tsetse genetics: Contributions to biology, systematics, and control of tsetse Flies. *Annu Rev Entomol*. 2005;50:101–23.
17. Krafsur ES. Tsetse flies: Genetics, evolution, and role as vectors. *Infect Genet Evol*. 2009;9(1):124–41.
18. Van Den Abbeele J, Caljon G. Tsetse fly saliva proteins as biomarkers of vector exposure. In: Aksoy S, Wikel S, Dimopoulos G, eds. *Arthropod Vector: Controller of Disease Transmission*. Vol. 2. London: Academic Press; 2017:195.

19. Van Den Abbeele J, Caljon G, De Ridder K, et al. *Trypanosoma brucei* modifies the tsetse salivary composition, altering the fly feeding behavior that favors parasite transmission. *PLoS Pathog*. 2010;6(6):e1000926.
20. Lindner AK, Priotto G. The unknown risk of vertical transmission in sleeping sickness—A literature review. *PLoS Negl Trop Dis*. 2010;4(12):e783.
21. Gaillot K, Lauvin M-A, Cottier J-P. Vertical transmission of human African trypanosomiasis: Clinical evolution and brain MRI of a mother and her son. *PLoS Negl Trop Dis*. 2017;11(7):e0005642.
22. Lestrade-Carluer De Kyvon MA, Maakaroun-Vermesse Z, Lanotte P, et al. Congenital trypanosomiasis in child born in France to African mother. *Emerg Infect Dis*. 2016;22(5):935–7.
23. Rocha G, Martins A, Gama G, et al. Possible cases of sexual and congenital transmission of sleeping sickness. *Lancet*. 2004;363(9404):247.
24. World Health Organization: Global Health Observatory (GHO) data—Human African Trypanosomiasis. http://www.who.int/gho/neglected_diseases/human_african_trypanosomiasis/en/.
25. Sudarshi D, Brown D. Human African trypanosomiasis in non-endemic countries. *Clin Med*. 2015;15(1):70–3.
26. Franco JR, Simarro PP, Diarra A, et al. Epidemiology of human African trypanosomiasis. *Clin Epidem*. 2014;6:257–75.
27. Hide G. History of sleeping sickness in East Africa. *Clin Microbiol Rev*. 1999;12(1):112–25.
28. Courtin F, Jamonneau V, Duvallet G, et al. Sleeping sickness in West Africa (1906–2006): Changes in spatial repartition and lessons from the past. *Trop Med Int Health*. 2008;13(3):334–44.
29. Buscher P, Bart J-M, Boelaert M, et al. Do cryptic reservoirs threaten gambiense-sleeping sickness elimination? *Trends in Parasitol*. 2018;34(3):197–207.
30. Auty H, Morrison LJ, Torr SJ, Lord J. Transmission dynamics of rhodesian sleeping sickness at the interface of wildlife and livestock areas. *Trends in Parasitol*. 2016;32(8):608–21.
31. MacLean LM, Odiit M, Chisi JE, et al. Focus-specific clinical profiles in human African trypanosomiasis caused by *Trypanosoma brucei rhodesiense*. *PLoS Negl Trop Dis*. 2010;4(12):e906.
32. Sternberg JM, Maclean L. Spectrum of disease in human African trypanosomiasis: The host and parasite genetics of virulence. *Parasitology*. 2010;137(14):2007–15.
33. Jamonneau V, Ilboudo H, Kabore´ J, et al. Untreated human infections by *Trypanosoma brucei gambiense* are not 100% fatal. *PLoS Negl Trop Dis*. 2012;6(6):e1691.
34. Kennedy PGE. Clinical features, diagnosis, and treatment of human African trypanosomiasis (sleeping sickness). *Lancet Neurol*. 2013;12(2):186–94.
35. Malvy D, Chappuis F. Sleeping sickness. *Clin. Microbiol. Infect*. 2011;17(7):986–95.
36. Kennedy PGE. The continuing problem of human African trypanosomiasis (sleeping sickness). *Ann Neurol*. 2008;64:116–27.
37. Blum J, Schmid C, Burri C. Clinical aspects of 2541 patients with second stage human African trypanosomiasis. *Acta Trop*. 2006;97(1):55–64.
38. Mpandzou G, Cespuglio R, Ngampo S, et al. Polysomnography as a diagnosis and post-treatment follow-up tool in human African trypanosomiasis: A case study in an infant. *J Neurol Sci*. 2011;305(1–2):112–5.
39. Njamnshi AK, Seke Etet PF, Perrig S, et al. Actigraphy in human African trypanosomiasis as a tool for objective clinical evaluation and monitoring: A pilot study. *PLoS Negl Trop Dis*. 2012;6(2):e1525.
40. Buguet A, Bourdon L, Bouteille B, et al. The duality of sleeping sickness: Focusing on sleep. *Sleep Med Rev*. 2001;5(2):139–53.
41. Rijo-Ferreira F, Carvalho T, Afonso C, et al. Sleeping sickness is a circadian disorder. *Nat Commun*. 2018;9(1):62.
42. Buscher P. Diagnosis of African trypanosomiasis. In: Magez S, Radwanska M, eds. *Trypanosomes and Trypanosomiasis*. Wien: Springer-Verlag; 2014:189.
43. Buscher P, Mumba Ngoyi D, Kabore J, et al. Improved models of mini anion exchange centrifugation technique (mAECT) and modified single centrifugation (MSC) for sleeping sickness diagnosis and staging. *PLoS Negl Trop Dis*. 2009;3(11):e471.
44. Mumba Ngoyi D, Ali Ekangu R, Mumvemba Kodi MF, et al. Performance of parasitological and molecular techniques for the diagnosis and surveillance of gambiense sleeping sickness. *PLoS Negl Trop Dis*. 2014;8(6):e2954.
45. Mumba Ngoyi D, Menten J, Pyana PP, et al. Stage determination in sleeping sickness: Comparison of two cell counting and two parasite detection techniques. *Trop Med Int Health*. 2013;18(6):778–82.
46. Magnus E, Van Meirvenne N, Vervoort T, et al. Use of freeze-dried trypanosomes in the indirect fluorescent antibody test for the serodiagnosis of sleeping sickness. *Ann Soc Belg Méd Trop*. 1978;58(2):103–9.
47. Buscher P, Gilleman Q, Lejon V. Rapid diagnostic test for sleeping sickness. *N Engl J Med*. 2013;368(11):1069–70.
48. Bisser S, Lumbala C, Nguertoum E, et al. Sensitivity and specificity of a prototype rapid diagnostic test for the detection of *Trypanosoma brucei gambiense* infection: A multi-centric prospective study. *PLoS Negl Trop Dis*. 2016;10(4):e0004608.
49. Jamonneau V, Camara O, Ilboudo H, et al. Accuracy of individual rapid tests for serodiagnosis of gambiense sleeping sickness in West Africa. *PLoS Negl Trop Dis*. 2015;9(2):e0003480.
50. Büscher P, Deborggraeve S. How can molecular diagnostics contribute to the elimination of human African trypanosomiasis? *Expert Rev Mol Diagn*. 2015;15(5):607–15.
51. Fairlamb AH. Chemotherapy of human African trypanosomiasis: Current and future prospects. *Trends Parasitol*. 2003;19(11):488–94.
52. Tarral A, Blesson S, Mordt OV, et al. Determination of an optimal dosing regimen for fexinidazole, a novel oral drug for the treatment of human African trypanosomiasis: First-in-human studies. *Clin Pharmacokinet*. 2014;53(6):565–80.
53. Jacobs RT, Nare B, Wring SA, et al. SCYX-7158, an orally-active benzoxaborole for the treatment of stage 2 human African trypanosomiasis. *PLoS Negl Trop Dis*. 2011;5(6):e1151.
54. Drugs for Neglected Diseases Initiative. Prospective study on efficacy and safety of SCYX-7158 in patients infected by human African trypanosomiasis due to *T. b. gambiense* (OXA002). https://clinicaltrials.gov/ct2/show/NCT03087955. NLM identifier: NCT03087955.
55. Drugs for Neglected Diseases Initiative. Fexinidazole in human African trypanosomiasis due to *T. b. gambiense* at any stage. https://clinicaltrials.gov/ct2/show/NCT03025789. NLM identifier: NCT03025789.
56. Mesu VKBK, Kalonji WMK, Bardonneau C, et al. Oral fexinidazole for late-stage African *Trypanosoma brucei gambiense* trypanosomiasis: A pivotal multicentre, randomised, non-inferiority trial. *Lancet*. 2018;391(10116):144–54.
57. Chapuis F. Oral fexinidazole for human African trypanosomiasis. *Lancet*. 2018;391(10116):101–2.
58. Burri C. Chemotherapy against human African trypanosomiasis: Is there a road to success? *Parasitology*. 2010;137(14):1987–94.
59. Pohlig G, Bernhard SC, Blum J, et al. Efficacy and safety of pafuramidine versus pentamidine maleate for treatment of first stage sleeping sickness in a randomized, comparator controlled, international phase 3 clinical trial. *PLoS Negl Trop Dis*. 2016;10(2):e0004363.
60. Chappuis F, Udayraj N, Stietenroth K, et al. Eflornithine is safer than melarsoprol for the treatment of second-stage *Trypanosoma brucei gambiense* human African trypanosomiasis. *Clin Infect Dis*. 2005;41(5):748–51.
61. Schmid C, Richer M, Bilenge CM, et al. Effectiveness of a 10-day melarsoprol schedule for the treatment of late-stage human African trypanosomiasis: Confirmation from a multinational study (IMPAMEL II). *J Infect Dis*. 2005;191(11):1922–31.
62. Fairlamb AH, Horn D. Melarsoprol resistance in African trypanosomiasis. *Trends Parasitol*. 2018;34(6):481–92.
63. Simarro PP, Franco JR, Diarra A, et al. Diversity of human African trypanosomiasis epidemiological settings requires fine-tuning control strategies to facilitate disease elimination. *Res Rep Trop Med*. 2013;4:1–6.
64. Okello AL, Welburn SC. The importance of veterinary policy in preventing the emergence and reemergence of zoonotic disease: Examining the case of human African trypanosomiasis in Uganda. *Front Public Health*. 2014;2:218.

CHAPTER

134 Leishmaniasis*

Diogo G. Valadares • Godwin Kwakye-Nuako • Mary E. Wilson

INTRODUCTION

Leishmaniasis refers to a constellation of clinical syndromes caused by protozoa belonging to the genus *Leishmania*. Autocthonous acquisition of these diseases by humans occurs in more than 90 countries of the world, located in all continents except Antarctica.[1] The distribution of these diseases is determined largely by the distribution of the different species of *Leishmania*. Remarkably and despite their highly similar genomes, the different species display quite unique biological characteristics leading to differences in localization, predilection for dissemination, and pathogenicity for human and other vertebrate hosts. The incidence of cutaneous leishmaniasis (CL), the most common form of disease, ranges from 0.7 to 1.2 million new cases per year. Visceral leishmaniasis (VL), the second most common form, has been estimated up to 400,000 cases annually but recently may have dropped below 100,000 per year.[2] However, these estimates may be highly inaccurate. As an illustration, the actual incidence of VL in 14 villages in an endemic area of Bihar, India (population 26,444) according to a household survey was 8.13-fold higher than records of reporting agencies in the same 3-year period of time.[3]

Leishmaniasis has afflicted humans for centuries, documented in pre-Incan pottery from Ecuador and Peru showing cutaneous and mucosal lesions on pottery.[4] The etiologic protozoan was discovered nearly simultaneously and published in sequential months of the 1903 British Medical Journal by Sir William Boog Leishman, a British military physician, and Charles Donovan, an Irish medical officer in the Indian Medical Service, who observed the parasites microscopically in samples from fatal cases of patients with febrile illnesses, in the Indian cities of Dum Dum near Calcutta (hence the name, Dum Dum fever) and Madras, respectively.[4,5]

There are more than 20 defined species of *Leishmania* found to cause human disease, a number that expands and contracts as the taxonomic lines are redefined. Most cases of leishmaniasis are vector-borne and transmitted through the bite of a Phlebotomine sand fly, with notable exceptions now being discovered (see Transmission below). Considering the discoveries of new *Leishmania* species, new clinical forms of leishmaniasis, expanded knowledge of the spectrum of reservoirs and vectors/modes of transmission, and newly appreciated magnitude of human asymptomatic infections, the factors underlying the maintenance and expansion of leishmaniasis in human populations must be reassessed. In addition, due to imperfect diagnostic and therapeutic measures, the control of leishmaniasis at an individual and a community-wide level, remains elusive. In this chapter, we attempt to define the uncertainties and point out areas in which there are critical needs for more complete knowledge of the spectrum of leishmaniasis.[2]

LIFE CYCLE AND TAXONOMY

The different *Leishmania* species share similar life cycles and transmission characteristics (Fig. 134-1). It has been taught that most mammalian leishmaniasis, and all vector-initiated leishmaniasis is initiated by the bite of a phlebotomine sand fly vector belonging to the *Lutzomyia* spp. in the New World, or *Phlebotomus* spp. in the Old World.[6–8] The sand fly deposits the infectious promastigote form of the parasite into the skin of a susceptible mammal (Fig. 134-2). The extracellular flagellated promastigote then interacts with several cell types including epidermal keratinocytes, fibroblasts, polymorphonuclear leukocytes (neutrophils), and mononuclear phagocytes (monocytes, macrophages, dendritic cells). Parasites can be taken up after ligation of host receptors on professional phagocytic cells such as neutrophils and macrophages. They replicate in mononuclear phagocytes, so that throughout chronic infection, parasites are found primarily in tissue macrophages. There they remain quiescent, releasing cytokines and/or other factors into the host that suppress some microbicidal, yet amplify some inflammatory pathways. Once intracellular, the parasite retracts its flagellum and transforms to the obligate intracellular amastigote (Fig. 134-2). Thereafter the amastigote survives in the mammalian host as an obligate intracellular parasite primarily in macrophages.[2,9]

Human leishmaniasis is caused by protozoa belonging to three subgenera of *Leishmania: L. Leishmania* spp., *L. Viannia* spp., and the recently recognized *L. Mundinia* spp. (Table 134-1). Some parasites have been described as belonging to genetically related "complexes," a term describing categories of parasites with similar biological characteristics with respect to human disease, and (as we now realize) highly homologous genomes. Examples are the *L. (L.) donovani* complex including *L. (L.) donovani* and *L. (L.) infantum*, and the *L. (L.) mexicana* complex including *L. (L.) mexicana* complex. Members of the three subgenera differ biologically. *L. Leishmania* spp. and *L. Viannia* spp. infections are usually transmitted through the bite of a phlebotomine sand fly,[2] whereas biting midges have been implicated as vectors in the few studies of *L. Mundinia* spp. transmission.[10,11] The parasites must develop within the insect to an infectious "metacyclic" state in order to be transmitted to a mammalian host, a process that is sometimes modeled in laboratories by development from logarithmic to stationary phase in liquid medium.[12–17] Metacyclogensis must take place in a compatible insect-*Leishmania* species pair. Most often, sand fly vectors for leishmaniasis are competent to host only

*These authors made equal contributions to the work.

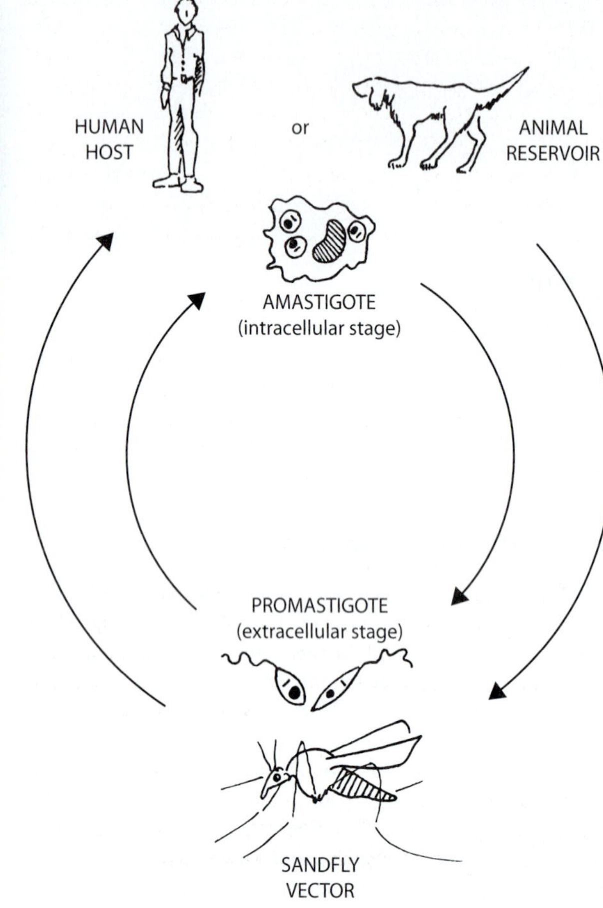

FIGURE 134-1. Leishmania life cycle.

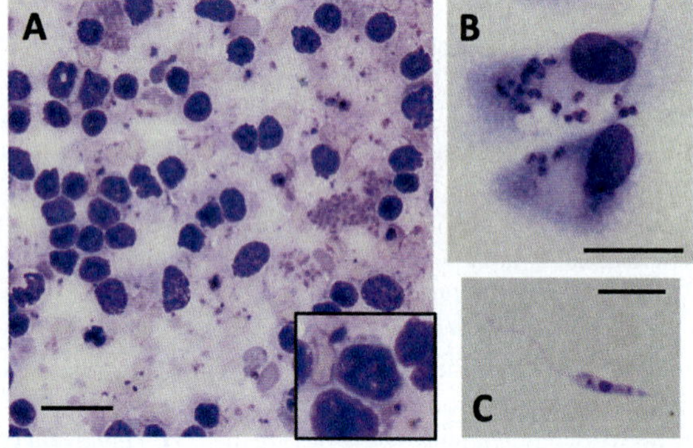

FIGURE 134-2. Intracellular amastigote and extracellular promastigote life stages of the *Leishmania spp.* protozoa. Mary E. Wilson, M.D.

TABLE 134-1 LEISHMANIA SPECIES (SUBGENUSES *L. LEISHMANIA*, *L. VIANNIA* AND *L. MUNDINIA*) COMMONLY CAUSING CLINICAL SYNDROMES IN THE NEW AND THE OLD WORLDS[a]

New World	Old World
Cutaneous leishmaniasis	
L. mexicana complex: *L. (L.) mexicana, L. (L.) venezuelensis* *L. (L.) amazonensis* ***L. Viannia subgenus:*** *L. (V.) braziliensis, L. (V.) panamensis,* *L. (V.) guyanensis, L. (V.) peruviana*	***L. Leishmania subgenus*** *L. (L.) tropica* *L. (L.) major* *L. (L.) aethiopica* ***L. Mundinia subgenus*** *L. (M.) martiniquensis* (Caribbean) *L. (M.) orientalis* (previously L. (M.) siamensis; Thailand) *L. (M.) GH* (Africa)
Disseminated leishmaniasis	
L. (V.) braziliensis	
Leishmaniasis recidivans	
	L. (L.) tropica
Diffuse cutaneous leishmaniasis	
L. (L.) mexicana, L. (V.) braziliensis	*L. (L.) aethiopica*
Mucosal leishmaniasis	
L. (V.) braziliensis, L.(V.)guyanensis	
Visceral leishmaniasis	
L. (L.) infantum,[b] rarely *L. (L.) amazonensis*	*L. (L.) donovani complex:* *L. (L.) donovani, L. (L.) infantum*[b] *L. (L.) tropica* (viscerotropic leishmaniasis)

[a]Please note that many exceptions to these generalities have been reported.
[b]The older name *L.(L.) chagasi* refers to *L. (L.) infantum* strains in the New World, found to correspond to Old World *L. (L.) infantum* MON-1. This is a strain of *L. (L.) infantum* different geographic locations, possibly imported by Europeans into South America.
Source: Mauricio et al. *Parasitol Today*. 2000;16(5):188–9.

one or a few *Leishmania* species, except *Lu. Longipalpis*, which is nearly a "universal" host for these protozoa.[18] The two well-studied *L. Mundinia* spp. will not develop to a virulent state in any sand fly species examined.[18,19]

Three to five days after being taken up by a compatible sand fly, procyclic promastigotes (low virulence, also called logarithmic phase) emerge from the blood meal and initiate a developmental process through nectomonad, leptomonad, and haptomonad and promastigote forms, culminating in the highly virulent, motile, and nonreplicative metacyclic near the insect's stomodeal valve.[20] The "plug" at the stomodeal valve includes salivary components, a tenacious parasite-derived "promastigote secretory gel," small vesicles resembling exosomes from the parasite and (presumably) fly, as well as fly gut components including local microbiota. During a blood meal the entire plug is inoculated into mammalian dermis.[21,22] Each component of the inoculated plug modifies the nature of the host immune response, and consequently the disease.[23,24]

Each of the subgenera has different biological characteristics within the vector. *L. Leishmania* spp., the longest studied of these protozoa, are taken into a blood meal and initiate development to virulence in the midgut of the sand fly vector. *L. Viannia* spp., in contrast, start developing in the hind gut of the sand fly.[25] Clinical presentations also differ. Although the vectors are not well documented in most cases, the *L. Mundinia* spp. may be the most divergent, with strong evidence that two species are transmitted by a biting midge *Culicoides sonorensis* rather than sand flies.[26,27] Whether this will hold true for all members of this subgenus, and the implications for disease spread and control, have yet to be discovered.

Because sexual replication occurs only in the insect vector, there is well-documented interspecies sexual replication in the vector, and the parasite can be maintained entirely through asexual replication, there cannot be a specific definition of species.[28] As such, the taxonomic lines have been fluctuant. For instance, *L. (L.) major* and *L. (L.) tropica* were in the past thought of as two strains of one species. More recently, genome sequencing has revealed that what had been called *L. (L.) chagasi* in South America was actually the same as one strain of *L. (L.) infantum*, MON-1, likely bequeathed to the New World by European explorers.[29]

THE SPECTRUM OF CLINICAL DISEASE

The different *Leishmania* species typically cause distinct clinical syndromes, summarized in Table 134-1. There are, however, many examples of nontraditional or unusual manifestations that have recently been reported. Examples include VL caused by *L. amazonensis*,[30] an unexpected disseminated form of leishmaniasis in military veterans termed "viscerotropic leishmaniasis," caused by *L. tropica* , after the 1990–91 Persian Gulf conflict,[31] and newly reported human infections with members of the *L. Mundinia* subgenus, which are most highly related to the parasite of lizards, *L. enriettii*.[32]

Variability in clinical presentation and disease severity is due to several factors. The most evident is the infecting species of *Leishmania*. For example, mucosal leishmaniasis (ML) occurs mostly due to *L. braziliensis*, which often causes an initial cutaneous lesion that can be accompanied by metastatic disease in mucosal tissues either simultaneously or months to years later. *L. braziliensis* is common in northeast Brazil, and countries in the Andes including Colombia, Bolivia, Ecuador, and Peru. This distribution accounts for the high incidence of ML in these areas.[33] Nonetheless host factors also contribute, favoring or disfavoring mucosal dissemination, as observed in different ethnic and racial groups.[34,35] Familial aggregation of ML is in part accounted for by genetic background and specific alleles of several loci (*TNFA, IL6*) are being reported in association with this disease.[36–38]

Cutaneous Leishmaniasis and Other Tegumentary Forms of Leishmaniasis

The classic localized ulcers of CL are often caused by *L. (L.) major*, *Leishmania (L.) tropica*, or *Leishmania (L.) aethiopica* in the Old World or by *Leishmania (L.) mexicana*, *Leishmania (V.) panamensis*, *Leishmania (L.) amazonensis*, or *Leishmania (V.) braziliensis* in the New World.[39] Newly emerging species belonging to the *L. (Mundinia)* subgenus can also cause localized ulcers, as well as other manifestations.[26,27,40–42] Different species cause disease of different severity or propensity to metastasize. The disease onset occurs between 2 weeks and several months after the sand fly bite. Cutaneous lesions often appear as chronic ulcers with raised erythematous borders and a granulomatous base. Lesions begin as papules that gradually increase in size and eventually ulcerate. Alternate forms can appear as papules, plaques, nodules, or erysipeloid lesions. Metastatic lesions in nearby skin are common, and regional adenopathy can occur particularly with disease due to *L. (V.) braziliensis*. Lesions may last for months to more than a year. Occasionally, nodules assume a sporotrichoid conformation. New World CL, particularly that caused by *L. (V.) braziliensis*, can take on more severe forms in which ulcers are deep and mutilating, and there is massive lymphadenopathy or chains of enlarged lymph nodes. Eventually most lesions heal spontaneously, leaving a flat atrophic scar. Although spontaneous healing is common, treatment can speed or ensure recovery. During disease and after recovery, patients usually exhibit strong delayed-type hypersensitivity (DTH) responses to *Leishmania* antigen, commonly called the Montenegro or leishmanin test.

Less common chronic forms of CL include diffuse cutaneous leishmaniasis (DCL) in which there are many localized papules that do not ulcerate. Satellite lesions and metastatic skin lesions arise, usually on the face and extremities. DCL is an anergic form of leishmaniasis, with a negative Montenegro response occurring primarily in South America. In contrast, leishmaniasis recidivans is a relapsing tuberculoid form of CL, usually caused by *L. tropica* in the Old World, in which lesions on the extremities or face slowly spread outward while healing in the center. This is associated with strong DTH reactivity. Each of these unusual forms of CL can lead to chronic disease lasting 20 years or more. The *L. (Viannia)* subgenus member *L. (V.) braziliensis* recently has been well documented to cause a different disseminating form of leishmaniasis called disseminated leishmaniasis, which has overtaken ML as the second most common disseminated form of *L. braziliensis* disease in regions of northeast Brazil.[39] Also new is the existence of strains of *L. (L.) infantum* leading to nonulcerating CL instead of disseminated severe VL. The fact that these parasites are found in geographically distinct regions leads scientists to hypothesis that these are strain-specific characteristics. In support of the latter hypothesis, sequence analysis of some Sri Lankan isolates revealed genomic differences including those in the A2 genes, which are thought responsible for dissemination of parasites during VL.[43]

Mucosal Leishmaniasis

Parasites belonging to the *L. Viannia* subgenus, *L. (V.) braziliensis, L. (V.) panamensis,* or *L. (V.) guyanensis,* or occasionally other *Leishmania* species are causal and 2–3% of infected individuals can develop disease at mucosal sites distant from the original cutaneous lesion. Most often, this occurs before or after healing of a cutaneous lesion, although occasionally ML is observed without a history of a CL lesion. Mucosal dissemination can occur between 1 month and more than 20 years after the original cutaneous ulcer. ML can begin with edema and erythema of mucosal sites in the nose or oropharynx. Progressive granulomatous inflammation can lead to destruction of the nose with perforation of the nasal septum, as well as to lesions involving the lips, tongue or the buccal, pharyngeal, or laryngeal mucosa. Death is rare but occurs due to involvement of the trachea or larynx and subsequent complications such as aspiration. ML is associated with strong cellular immune responses manifested as positive DTH reactivity and peripheral lymphocyte reactivity. The disease process is likely exacerbated by a hyperergic response to the parasite. Infection of *L. (V.) braziliensis* or *L. (V.) guyanensis* with RNA viruses belonging to the *Totiviridae* family, LRV1, is associated with increased severity and disseminated mucosal disease.[44]

Visceral Leishmaniasis

Visceral disease is generally caused by parasites belonging to *L. donovani* complex, including *L. (L.) donovani* and *Leishmania (L.) infantum* in the Old World and New World. New World VL [previously called *L. (L.) chagasi*] was found by sequence analysis to be identical to *L. infantum*, and specifically the MON-1 zymodeme, presumed to have been imported into South American by European explorers.[45] Classical and unusual cases of VL due to other species [*L. (L.) amazonensis, L. (L.) tropica*] have been reported.[30,46] VL is a severe form of leishmaniasis that usually begins between 3 and 8 months after the bite of an infected sand fly. Most patients develop the insidious onset of fevers, malaise, and weight loss associated with splenomegaly, hepatomegaly, anemia, leukopenia, thrombocytopenia, and hypergammaglobulinemia.[47,48] Lymphadenopathy occurs in the Sudan but is not as common in other regions.[49,50] VL can lead to progressive suppression of specific and nonspecific cell-mediated immune responses with absent Montenegro reactivity, and associated bacterial infections causing pneumonia, diarrhea, or tuberculosis are common.[51,52] These secondary infections contribute to the high mortality seen in untreated symptomatic disease. The spectrum of VL ranges from asymptomatic infection, occurring in 86–95% of infected Brazilians, to fulminant disease that may be fatal. Indeed, most fatalities due to leishmaniasis are due to the visceral form of disease.[47,53]

VL due to *L. infantum* has been reported in AIDS patients in Spain, France, and Italy as their presenting manifestation of HIV disease, often with atypical clinical presentations.[54] Additionally, visceral disease has unexpectedly been documented during infection with species that were thought to be limited to the skin, including *L. amazonensis* and *L. (L.) tropica*.[30,55] Patients with VL due to *L. amazonensis* have presented with syndromes mimicking typical VL, but *L. (L.) tropica* was found to underlie a previously unrecognized form of VL, termed "viscerotropic leishmaniasis." Viscerotropic disease was observed in U.S. troops returning from the 1990–91 Persian Gulf conflict. Although one infected soldier was asymptomatic,

symptomatic individuals had varied complaints including fever, chills, malaise, generalized lymphadenopathy, diarrhea, nausea, abdominal pain, and weight loss. Biopsy and culture of the bone marrow revealed *L. (L.) tropica*, a species previously thought only to cause cutaneous disease.[55]

Cutaneous Complications of Visceral Leishmaniasis

A proportion of patients with VL caused by *L. (L.) donovani* will develop a cutaneous syndrome termed post-kala azar dermal leishmaniasis (PKDL) after treatment. PKDL is particularly common in East Africans who do not complete a course of therapy, and on the Indian subcontinent. Since PKDL provides a source of parasites accessible in the dermis and accessible to insect vectors, it has been claimed that humans with PKDL serve as a reservoir for VL.[47] The occurrence of endemic regions for PKDL and regions of high human population density has led to the conclusion that humans are the main reservoir for *L. (L.) donovani* infection. Consequently, there are few investigations of potential alternate reservoirs that maintain the disease when incidence is at a nadir, a situation that is becoming reality now that elimination programs are underway.[56–58] Declining VL cases during the elimination program have led investigators to tackle the complex possibility of nonhuman reservoirs; results are yet to be reported.[57]

PKDL assumes two clinical forms, both disseminated through the skin. The first is a pleotropic papulonodular form called "polymorphic" or "nodular," and the second, called "macular," presents with flat, hypomelanotic macules. Lesions of polymorphic PKDL range from macules to nodules containing numerous organisms; histologic studies reveal more intense inflammatory infiltrates and higher parasite loads than macular lesions.[59] These observations led to hypotheses that polymorphic lesions may be more efficient at transmitting infection to the insect vector. Both the question of efficiency of PKDL forms in transmission to flies and whether there are nonhuman reservoirs, are best addressed with xenodiagnosis. Indeed, several ongoing xenodiagnosis studies are addressing questions related to the efficiency of parasite transmission from reservoir hosts, especially humans with or without skin lesions, to sand fly vectors. This is discussed further in "Vectors and Reservoirs" below.

Emerging Infections with *L. (Mundinia)* Subgenus Members

The newly recognized subgenus *Leishmania (Mundinia)* has led, among other things, to the recognition of additional endemic geographic regions, harboring human infections with new species of the parasite. Partly due to this, the frontiers of leishmaniasis have expanded from the previously estimated 88 to now 98 countries.[2,60] Considering both human and animal hosts, there are reports of autochthonous cases of *L. (Mundinia)* species infections across all continents except Antarctica. The emerging species, which belong to the *Leishmania* (*Mundinia*) *enriettii* complex, include *L.* (*M.*) *martiniquensis* from Martinique Island in Caribbean, *L.* (*M.*) *macropodum* from Australia, *L.* (*M.*) *orientalis* from Thailand, *L.* (*M.*) *siamensis* found in the United States, *L.* (*M.*) *enriettii* from Brazil, and the yet-to-be-named "*L.* (*M.*) GH" from Ghana.[10,26,27,40,41,61] The first of these isolates were found in nonhuman hosts. *L.* (*M.*) *enriettii* was first recognized as a pathogen affecting guinea pigs (not humans) in Brazil in 1946.[61] More recently *L.* (*M.*) *macropodum* was documented in red kangaroos in Australia, and *L.* (*M.*) *siamensis** was isolated from horses in Texas and Switzerland[32] [*L.* (*M.*) *siamensis* has now been renamed *L.* (*M.*) *orientalis*)[32]].

Most human infections due to these emerging species were recognized due to manifestations resembling typical localized CL.[26,27,63] *Leishmania* species belonging to the *L. enriettii* complex, first reported by Muniz and Medina, were not previously recognized reported to be pathogenic for humans. Based on unconvincing evidence that *Lutzomyia monticula* is its vector, the species was assigned to the *L. (Leishmania)* subgenus. More recent evidence based on sequence homology assigned the parasites to a separate subgenus, that is, the *L. (Mundinia)* spp. It is only recently that members of the *L. (Mundinia.)* species have been implicated as pathogenic for humans. Reports have attributed cases of CL and VL in Thailand, Asia, and Martinique Island in Caribbean to infection with *L. (Mundinia)* species members. The most recent isolates were derived from CL lesions in Ghana. Sequence analyses have attributed these to a newly recognized species characterized as "*L. (M.)* Ghana" or "*L. (M.)* GH." The "*L. (M.) GH*" species has yet to be taxonomically classified, hence the quotation marks. The current convincing evidence attributes CL isolates acquired in the southeastern part of Ghana to "*L. (M.) GH*."

This notwithstanding, it is not ruled out that these emerging species can disseminate into the visceral organs and to mucosal surfaces to cause lethal VL or disfiguring mucocutaneous forms. For instance, *L.* (*M.*) *martiniquensis* as well as the inadvertently named "*L.* (*M.*) *siamensis*," later corrected to *L.* (*M.*) *orientalis*, have reportedly caused disseminated manifestations in HIV patients in Martinique Island and Thailand, respectively.[26,62,63]

DIAGNOSIS

The diagnosis of either CL or VL should be considered in patients from endemic areas who present with findings suggesting these diagnoses, such as chronic painless cutaneous ulcer or fever with hepatosplenomegaly, respectively. Unfortunately, leishmaniasis is often not considered by practitioners in developed countries when considering immigrants or travelers returning from *Leishmania*-endemic countries. A diagnosis is best established by demonstration of the parasite in infected tissues (parasitological diagnosis). Cutaneous ulcers should be biopsied at lesion margins, and the parasite found either by histologic examination of sections stained with hematoxylin and eosin or with Wright-Giemsa stains, or by culture of the parasite. In the United States, the appropriate media should be obtained from the Centers for Disease Control and Prevention (CDC) prior to the biopsy procedure. Biopsy material is inoculated directly into media and sent immediately to the CDC.[64] Occasionally, parasites can be visualized in impression smears of aspirates or lesions.[65] VL is demonstrated by the finding of *Leishmania* spp. amastigotes in bone marrow biopsy or aspirate, either by histology or culture, or occasionally in the peripheral blood of patients with concurrent AIDS.[66] Practitioners in some endemic countries have diagnosed VL by microscopic examination of fine-needle aspirates from the spleen. Although this is more sensitive, the potential for hemorrhage makes this a less desirable test than a sternal marrow aspirate. Indeed, splenic aspirates are outlawed in many countries. Even when preformed for diagnostic purposes, they are discouraged in the hands of anyone other than the most highly experienced practitioner.

The less definitive constellation of positive *Leishmania* serology with compatible symptoms is accepted as adequate evidence to initiate therapy. This is most valid in individuals with VL with previously normal immune systems, although such tests are unreliable in immunocompromised states such as HIV infection. Many persons with *L. (L.) infantum* infection have underlying subtle abnormalities in cellular immunity, and the incidence of VL with HIV-1 coinfection is expanding, making serology a less reliable test than before. Serologic responses to *L. (L.) donovani* linger for years after clearance of symptomatic Indian kala-azar, diminishing the utility of elevated serology. Antibody tests include indirect fluorescent antibody (IFA) (used by CDC), enzyme-linked immunosorbent assay (ELISA), and a direct agglutination test (DAT) optimized for use in developing countries. The DAT is useful in African countries and in India due

*The species name *L.* (*M.*) *siamensis* is considered a nomen nudum for these isolates, since the name does not meet international zoologic nomenclature code.[27,32,62]

to its simplicity in field settings. However the variability and expense of antigen preparations makes this inconsistently reliable.[67] Patients with active VL usually have antibodies to the recombinant antigen K39 (rK39) and this has provided the basis for a sensitive and specific ELISA.[68,69] In South America, a rapid rK39 strip test has proven both sensitive and specific.[68,69] Unfortunately, the rK39 test remains positive for years in Indian kala-azar, meaning it is not always reflective of acute infection.[70,71]

Unfortunately, patients with CL do not reliably develop antibody responses, so serology is often not helpful in evaluating cutaneous ulcers. In addition, the few individuals documented with "viscerotropic" leishmaniasis had negative or low antibody titers, making serology an unreliable test for this form of visceral disease. Cross-reactive antibodies may occur in patients with Chagas disease or leprosy, decreasing the specificity of antibody-based testing in regions where these diseases are coendemic.

Disadvantages of all serologic tests are low responses in some individuals, persistence of serologic response after cure, and false positive reaction in some healthy individuals.[71] A number of laboratories have reported diagnosis of infection with the different *Leishmania* species using approaches based on the polymerase chain reaction (PCR). Unfortunately, PCR-based tests are not standardized and therefore not offered universally as diagnostic tests. Quantitative (q) PCR and urine antigen-based tests are being explored but are not yet standardized for clinical use. qPCR to detect parasite DNA is particularly valuable as both a diagnostic test and has been used as a test of cure in Indian subjects treated for VL, where there is a high degree of drug resistance. In addition, qPCR is used by the CDC for species identification.[72,73] Investigators are working on adapting PCR amplification methods to a low-temperature amplification system ("Loop-mediated isothermal amplification," often abbreviated as "LAMP"), which might be used in remote clinics at endemic sites without access to a reference center for diagnostics.[74,75] One caveat is that the duration of time that DNA persists in tissues after death or eradication of live organisms must be determined before PCR-based methods can be used as a test of ongoing infection.

DTH responses to intradermally administered *Leishmania* antigen (Montenegro or leishmanin test) usually develop during uncomplicated cases of CL and ML. The Montenegro test is usually positive in other forms of leishmaniasis where the immune response is exuberant, including leishmaniasis recidivans and PKDL. The Montenegro is usually negative in individuals with forms of leishmaniasis with abundant parasite growth but suppressed immune responses, including diffuse CL and acute VL. Positive reactions usually develop after cure. Thus, skin testing serves as an adjunct to clinical and parasitological diagnosis, but the test must be interpreted correctly.

Like the tuberculin skin test, results of the DTH skin test for leishmaniasis is read 48–72 hours after placement, necessitating a second and sometimes a third visit to homes in endemic regions. The test is not standardized worldwide and often not country-wide (with Brazil being a notable exception). Thus, it is difficult to generalize the implications of a positive or negative test result between distinct geographic regions, or between different species of *Leishmania* causing similar syndromes. The skin test reagent has not been approved by the U.S. Food and Drug Administration, causing it to fall out of favor with funding agencies, and consequently with investigators. It seems unlikely, therefore, that we will expand our understanding of the test and its usage in symptomatic or asymptomatic leishmaniasis. A more rapid interferon (IFN)-γ release assay (IGRA) test to detect IFN-γ producing cellular immune responses to *Leishmania* antigens, similar to the QuantiFERON-TB® test for latent tuberculosis infection (Qiagen) has been studied in endemic sites.[76–80] Although these yield positive tests in some immune subjects, there is overlap but only moderate correlation with results of the DTH.[79] The meaning of IGRA versus DTH results with regards to exposure and protective immunity, therefore, has yet to be resolved. Current efforts are aimed toward developing proteomic- or PCR-based amplification methods for circulating nucleic acids.[1]

One challenge has been the detection of asymptomatic infection, a condition that is more prevalent than symptomatic disease. Individuals with asymptomatic *L. (L.) infantum* infection present a proven risk of contaminating the blood supply, and a potential risk of serving as reservoirs transmitting *Leishmania* spp. to naïve sand flies.[53,81–83] Asymptomatic individuals who become immunocompromised are at risk for developing symptomatic disease.[54,84,85] Previously, asymptomatic infection with the VL *Leishmania* species in South America was defined as a positive DTH skin test without history or evidence of active VL. However, due to the lack of standardization, difficulty in interpretation, and unreliability in some countries such as India, replacements tests such as those named in the above paragraph are needed.[70] This is illustrated by reports that a significant proportion of healthy blood donors in a northeastern Brazilian city are asymptomatically infected with *L. (L.) infantum*.[81] Furthermore, 19.5% of U.S. troops stationed in endemic regions of Iraq were asymptomatically infected with *L. (L.) infantum*, underscoring the urgency of this need for improved diagnostics.[86]

TREATMENT

Treatment of leishmaniasis differs between the species and clinical types of leishmaniasis. A definitive summary of current recommendations of the Infectious Diseases Society of America (IDSA) and the American Society of Tropical Medicine and Hygiene (ASTMH) has been published recently, summarizing the consensus of experts in the field after an exhaustive review of literature and weighing of expert opinions.[87] The recommendations reflect the consensus of a panel of experts who spent 5 years assessing the literature and gathering opinions regarding management of the different forms of leishmaniasis.[88] The guidelines consider the contributions of *Leishmania* species, subgenus, geographic region and host health to the spectrum of leishmaniasis and implications for its diagnosis and management. Some salient points include the question of whether treatment of uncomplicated CL is necessary since most cases resolve without therapy, the need to treat disease caused by members of the *L. Viannia* subspecies since disseminated tegumentary complications are so frequent,[33] host immunity and predisposition to symptomatic disease, and the increased risk of leishmaniasis in the setting of political or social instability. Treatment is always recommended for symptomatic VL, even though asymptomatic infection with the agents of VL is more common than disease. The question of whether and how to treat asymptomatic infection is predicated on whether asymptomatic hosts pose a risk of transmission to sand flies. PKDL is thought to be a transmissible form of anthroponotic leishmaniasis that occurs during infection with *L. (L.) donovani*, particularly in the regions of northeast India and Bangladesh and sub-Saharan Africa (Sudan). Although PKDL may respond poorly to drugs, treatment is recommended.[89]

The mainstay of therapy for leishmaniasis since the 1920s has been pentavalent antimony compounds [sodium stibogluconate (SSG); Sb^V], such as sodium stibogluconate available through CDC and meglumine antimoniate available in endemic countries.[89,90] These must be administered either intravenously or intramuscularly for 10–28 days for different forms of disease. Antimonials are associated with considerable gastrointestinal, liver, pancreatic, and cardiac toxicity, which sometimes require cessation of therapy. Alternate agents for treatment of leishmaniasis include miltefosine, soluble amphotericin B deoxycholate, liposomal amphotericin B, paromomycin, pentamidine, selected imidazoles, allopurinol, topical imiquimod, and combinations of the above. Recommended regimens are highly variable depending on the disease, the causative *Leishmania* species, and local patterns of drug susceptibility, if known. Below we summarize possibilities by clinical disease type. Our summaries are not complete, and readers are advised to consult the published guidelines before making a treatment decision.[87]

Visceral Leishmaniasis

With rare exceptions, VL is caused by *L. (L.) donovani* or *L. (L.) infantum* in the Old World, and exclusively by *L. (L.) infantum* [previously called *L. (L.) chagasi*] in New World VL.[48] Pentavalent antimonials (SSGs) are still the drug of choice for treatment of symptomatic VL in most regions of the world. In recent decades, use of the SSGs for VL has been regionally limited by increasing numbers of drug-resistant *L. (L.) donovani* isolates in India, Bangladesh, and Nepal, leading in the past to treatment failures in as many as 60% of VL cases.[89] Drug-resistant *L. (L.) donovani,* defined because of lack of response to SSG, has required testing of alternate effective therapies for VL caused by *L. (L.) donovani.* Initially pentamidine was used. However, its toxicity was a deterrent, and its efficacy decreased over time such that it has been succeeded by more effective options (amphotericin B deoxycholate, liposomal amphotericin B).

Amphotericin B, used either in its soluble deoxycholate form or as liposomal amphotericin B, is highly effective for treatment of leishmaniasis.[89,91] A high frequency of renal and other toxic side effects led a group in India to a series of trials, directed by Shyam Sundar, to examine alternate treatments for resistant *L. (L.) donovani.*[89] The lipid-encapsulated formulation of amphotericin B avoids much of the renal toxicity, with the caveat that it is expensive and may be difficult to acquire in endemic regions. When available, a single dose of liposomal amphotericin B (LamB) has been highly effective in treatment of VL in endemic regions of India and Bangladesh.[92] Its efficacy is lower in East African countries, however, where the cold chain is difficult to maintain. Liposomal amphotericin B infused over days (up to 39) has been highly effective for treatment of VL in African countries, the endemic area of India, Bangladesh, and Nepal, countries surrounding the Mediterranean Sea, and nations in Central and South America. The total dose requirement for VL cure varies in different regions.[89] Coinfection with HIV and either *L. (L.) donovani* or *L. (L.) infantum* has become more common in Southern Europe, the Middle East, India, and South America, where either amphotericin B deoxycholate or LamB remain highly effective for initial treatment. Often, secondary prophylaxis with LamB every 3–4 weeks is needed to prevent relapses.[54,89,93,94]

Miltefosine is the only orally available drug for leishmaniasis. Initial trials revealed it highly effective for treatment of VL due to *L. (L.) donovani* in Bihar, India, leading to its adoption as the drug of choice in the region. However, after more than a decade of use it has become less able to prevent relapses in the region. Relapses after miltefosine have also been high in Ethiopia (~24%), and in a phase II trial in Brazil (40%). Miltefosine treatment for HIV-VL coinfected individuals has been less effective in Brazil and southern Europe, where *L. (L.) infantum* is the predominant cause of VL. Miltefosine has been effective for treating PKDL, although concerns about developing drug resistance are ongoing. Furthermore, adverse gastrointestinal side effects are frequent and it is teratogenic, limiting its utility in endemic populations.[89]

Paromomycin, an aminoglycoside, was incidentally observed to synergize with SSG for treatment of VL, in a trial of its use against diarrhea. Efficacy as a single agent against VL has shown either similar or lower efficacy than SSG alone, in Indian or East African VL. Because of the concern for breeding resistant parasites during monotherapy with an aminoglycoside, most prefer its use in combination therapy.[89]

Alternatives in the future may include paromomycin and oral sitamaquine, both of which are still under investigation.[67] Recombinant interferon gamma has been used successfully as an adjunct to antimony therapy in cases of treatment failure, but this is only available under investigation.

Cutaneous Leishmaniasis

Approaches to CL are the most highly variable of the forms of leishmaniasis. Many cases of localized CL heal spontaneously without therapy. However, appropriate therapy for localized disease is often preferred because it speeds healing. In contrast it is always recommended that complicated tegumentary leishmaniasis is treated.[87] The latter statement applies to mucosal and other localized and disseminated forms of leishmaniasis. Both systemic and local modes of treatment have been studied. In regions where *L. (V.) braziliensis* is common, which commonly causes complicated tegumentary leishmaniasis, treatment is usually recommended as an (unproven) measure to decrease the possibility of future dissemination.[95] Simple localized CL due to parasites belonging to the L. (*Leishmania*) spp. or the *L. (Viannia)* spp. subgenuses can be treated with antimony compounds, and these are recommended for *L. braziliensis* disease. Similar to VL, amphotericin B or pentamidine can be used as alternate drug choices. CL from both the Old World and the New World have responded to liposomal Amphotericin B with efficacy of more than 80%, an outcome comparable to SSG. The azoles have been tried for all forms of CL, and are attractive because of the oral route of delivery, and their extensive use for treatment of other infections.

Oral agents have been used to treat CL due to species other than *L. braziliensis.* Trials of topical paromomycin and topical imiquimod are promising. A trial of oral miltefosine for CL yielded 100% cure among *x* patients, using the highest dose. Ketoconazole may be most useful for *L. (L.) mexicana,* and oral fluconazole has been used with success against *L. major* disease.[67] Other options include local heat therapy, topical antimony, itraconazole, and allopurinol.

Miltefosine has been used with success to treat *L. (V.) braziliensis* in some settings, despite reports of some treatment failures.[87] One trial in patients with CL due to *L. (V.) braziliensis* documented a 75% response to miltefosine in contrast to a 53.3% response rate to SSG.[96] Miltefosine has also been studied for treatment of tegumentary leishmaniasis, including uncomplicated CL. There was a good response in subjects with Old World CL in 89–100% of subjects due to *L. (L.) major* and for New World CL in Colombia cause by *L. (V.) panamensis* or *L. (V.) guyanensis.*[97] In studies of subjects with New World CL in Colombia infected with *L. (V.) braziliensis, L. (V.) panamensis, or L. (V.) guyanensis,* its efficacy was acceptable.[89]

Mucosal leishmaniasis, as discussed previously, is a complication of CL. It is usually caused by infection with *L. (V.) braziliensis, L. (V.) guyanensis,* or *L. (V.) panamensis,* in which parasites disseminate to skin or mucosa distant from the original infection site. ML, diffuse CL, and leishmaniasis recidivans fall into this category. All are difficult to treat, often requiring repeated courses of the same or alternate therapies. Antimony, amphotericin B, miltefosine, and pentamidine have all been used in these situations. The combination of antimony plus either parenteral or topical granulocyte macrophage colony stimulating factor (GM-CSF) is promising for treatment of refractory CL due to *L. braziliensis.*[98] Furthermore, GM-CSF has proven useful for adjunct treatment of ML in Brazilian subjects.[98]

VECTORS AND RESERVOIRS

The most established, and probably the main route of transmission of the *Leishmania* spp. to humans or other mammals is via the bite of a phlebotomine sand fly.[99] A specific pairing of fly–parasite species is necessary for parasites to develop to a virulent state in the vector, and the developmental process (termed "metacyclogenesis") is absolutely needed for transmission to occur.[12] Biochemical lectin-like adhesion between the surface membrane of the developing parasite and the insect gut epithelium seems to be at least partially responsible for this pairing.[100,101] Recent data show that the environment within the sand fly gut, including the local microbiota content, is a requirement for parasite development to its virulent metacyclic state.[102]

The sand fly bite itself causes an inflammatory response that leads to expression of cytokines and chemokines recruiting inflammatory cells to the site.[103] Sand fly saliva contains potent molecules that inhibit hemostasis and elicit an independent immune response. The sand fly delivers not only its own salivary proteins, but also microbiota from the fly gut and released components from the parasite (exosomes, and a gelatinous "promastigote secretory gel").[104] All the above components influence the host response, and when coinoculated with *Leishmania* spp., some such as the microbiota, augment host inflammatory responses.[22,24,103,105] There is evidence that prior exposure to sand fly saliva elicits a Th1-type immune response (characterized by IFN-γ release), skewing mice to generate protection against infection via sand flies carrying live *Leishmania* spp. parasites.[103] Vaccination of Brazilian dogs with two salivary proteins followed by challenge infection with *L. (L.) infantum* introduced with *Lu. Longipalpis* salivary proteins induced a systemic immune response suggestive of a Th1-type protective immune response to parasite antigens, with elevated parasite antigen-specific IFN-γ and decreased IL-10, although no dogs became infected.[106] The possible use of combination vaccines containing sand fly salivary protein and parasite antigen(s) for prevention of VL in both dogs and humans needs further exploration.

There are recently recognized exceptions deviating from the paradigm of sand fly vector—mammalian host transmission of leishmaniasis. First, mother-to-pup transmission of *L. (L.) infantum* is a well-demonstrated means of maintaining the ongoing outbreak of visceral leishmaniosis among fox-hunting dog kennels in the United States and Canada.[107] ("Leishmaniosis" is the term used for the canine version of human VL.) Indeed, vertical transmission is likely responsible for maintenance of infection among kennels in more temperate climates.[107] The contribution of vertical transmission to disease abundance in endemic regions is difficult to quantify since vector-borne disease is so prominent. Furthermore, sexual recombination of the *Leishmania* spp. likely occurs in the insect, and the impact of bypassing the insect vector on parasite evolution is not clear. Second, transmission of *L. (M.) macropodum* among Australian kangaroos was shown to occur through the biting midge *C. sonorensis*. Parasites of the genus *Leishmania* and subgenus *Mundinia* were recently shown to cause CL in humans in Ghana; *C. sonorensis* has been implicated as the vector transmitting this species as well.[27]

Definitive proof that an animal reservoir can participate in transmission to humans, and the vectors that are competent to transmit *Leishmania* spp. requires careful study. A recent comprehensive investigation conducted in Bangladesh documented surprisingly efficient experimental transmission of *L. (L.) donovani* from patients with PKDL to sand flies.[108] Using xenodiagnosis the authors showed 27 of 47 subjects with PKDL were positive by direct xenodiagnois, and that transmission occurred more frequently from nodular than from macular PKDL lesions.[108] Similar to other infectious diseases, as the goal of elimination draws nearer, minor reservoirs become more important. Ongoing transmission of VL in India has caused groups to investigate the controversial question of occult animal reservoir hosts for *L. (L.) donovani* in the Indian subcontinent. Depending on the results, it may be necessary to adopt new approaches to elimination of VL and PKDL in the endemic region of India, Bangladesh, and Nepal.

Recent recognition that an additional *L. Mundinia* subgenus, and additional species belonging to this subgenus cause disease in humans has forced the field to divergence from the belief that phlebotomine sand flies are the only insect vectors capable of transmitting *Leishmania* spp. to humans. Although a recent study documented transmission of several *L. (Mundinia)* species from guinea pigs to *L. migonei*, findings of other investigators provide contrasting findings. Whether *L. (M.) enriettii* can be transmitted from guinea pigs to *Lutzomia* spp. in Brazil is still inconclusive.[61] In an in vitro experiment, *L. (M) enriettii* proved unable to infect *L. longipalpis*, which is the most uniformly permissive vector, whereas it was able to establish long-term infection of the *Culicoides* species biting midges.[19] Similarly, human CL isolates [termed "*L. (M) GH*"] were unable to establish infection in *Lu. longipalpis* but able to establish infection in the biting midge *Culiocoides sonorensis* [(27) and Kwakye-Nuako, Ph.D. Thesis, Lancaster University, UK, 2016]. Likewise, members of the day feeding biting midge subgenus *Culicoides Forcipoyia* spp. are implicated as the vector host for the kangaroo parasite *L. (M) macropodum* in Australia.[10] *C. sonorensis* was also implicated as the insect vector for the taxonomically related species *L. (M.) orientalis* causing human CL.[18,26] Thus, the weight of evidence implicates biting midges as vectors of this newly recognized subgenus, although the definitive proof showing maturation and transmission from *Culicoides* spp. to humans has yet to be established.

PREVENTION AND CONTROL

Control of the different forms of leishmaniasis must take into consideration whether the diseases are transmitted via anthroponotic, zoonotic, or peridomestic cycles in each endemic region. In addition, important to consider is the ease of access to local medical care. Poor access is compounded by the fact that the long-standing first-line drug regimens require lengthy parenteral administration and cause considerable toxicity, making therapy difficult to administer and monitor. In the case of anthroponotic disease such as occurs in India and possibly the Sudan, the presence of chronic cutaneous PKDL allows the disease to be maintained long-term and available for sand fly-mediated spread. Whether asymptomatic infection is a source for transmission to sand flies remains an open question, with arguments in both directions. The bulk of evidence seems to indicate that people co-infected with HIV and *L. infantum* can efficiently transmit parasites to the *Lu. longipalpis* insect vector, whereas asymptomatically infected persons infected with *L. infantum* alone only occasionally transmit parasites to the *Lu. longipalpis* vector.[109] Most certainly, improved human disease detection and treatment would help prevent new cases of disease.

Visceral Leishmaniasis

VL has long been recognized as a disease that clusters, both geographically and temporally. Within endemic regions, mini-epidemics occur in small areas such as a small village or neighborhood, with peaks and wanes in activity, and after a few years cases occur in a nearby neighborhood where disease peaks again.[110] This has made it challenging to conduct vaccine trials, as endemic regions do not present a homogeneous risk over time. Also remarkable is the temporal variation in the incidence of VL in larger regions such as states, regions, and countries. Peak incidence of symptomatic VL varies every 5–10 years in distinct endemic regions.[56] This variability has been attributed to the development of herd immunity, as well as factors related to the sand fly vector including climate change.[26] Also contributing is the improved overall health condition of the population, with improved healthcare available and adherence to routine childhood vaccines correlating with decreased symptomatic VL.[111] Asymptomatic infection seems unrelated to such regional and temporal variability, although as the disease incidence diminishes, so does the incidence of infection.[56,60]

Cutaneous Leishmaniasis

CL is more likely than VL to be transmitted through outdoor activities, elevating the importance of a wild reservoir. Wild rodent or canid reservoirs of zoonotic leishmaniasis are difficult or impossible to eradicate. Attempts to poison rodents in their burrows are impractical beyond very limited geographic regions.[112] A major reservoir of South American zoonotic VL is the domestic dog, which is available for surveillance and treatment. However, surveillance methods are far from good and even in the case of *L. infantum* the dog may not be the only disease reservoir.

Until living conditions can be improved to remove human habitat from sand fly breeding grounds and to make treatment and early disease recognition more available, the cycle is likely to be maintained.

Insect Vector

Simple barrier measures are recommended for individual travelers as a means of controlling exposure to the insect vector, and thus reducing the risk of leishmaniasis. Both effective insect repellents (DEET or permethrin) and the use of fine mesh netting at night to exclude the sand fly vector, in addition to other disease-transmitting vectors, are recommended. Although effective for individual prophylaxis, novel methods are needed for preventing leishmaniasis in a large population. The incidence of leishmaniasis decreased after spraying for mosquitoes in the "Roll Back Malaria" campaign in the 1950s, only to resurge after the discontinuation of DDT.[47] Quite effective vector control measures that decreased both malaria and VL in Brazil include active insecticide spraying of houses and the use of bed nets with or without impregnated insecticide. A greater success of these measures in controlling VL than CL stems from the fact that *L. longipalpis*, the vector transmitting VL due to *L. infantum*, has adapted to a domestic/peridomestic habitat and delivers sand fly bites most often in the home, whereas CL is often transmitted by insects feeding on wild hosts. The specific phlebotomine sand flies implicated as vectors for the different *Leishmania* species is well summarized.[113] Suffice it to say that it is advantageous to understand the habitat of the specific sand fly vector before designing an approach to interrupt vector-mediated transmission. For example, leishmaniasis is peridomestic in Nepal and the use of bed nets reduced the incidence of VL by 70%. Spraying houses with insecticide has reduced the incidence of CL in Peru and in Kabul, Afghanistan by 54% and 60%, respectively. It is not clear whether universal or targeted spraying, the latter focused in neighborhoods where disease is documented, would be more effective. Furthermore, the relative value of permethrin impregnated bed nets compared to household spraying needs to be carefully assessed.[46] The expense of insecticides, the potential transience of effect, and risk of selecting for drug-resistant insects must be weighed against the benefit to the endemic country as a long-term solution to the control of leishmaniasis.

Reservoir

Measures to control the dog reservoir for VL in South America have included the use of insecticide impregnated dog collars, treating dogs directly with insecticides, and euthanizing infected dogs. The efficacy of these measures, particularly the controversial approach taken by the government of euthanizing all infected dogs, has been debated. One thing that is evident, is that the prolonged duration of canine infection with *L. infantum*, yields a prolonged period in which dogs are infectious for sand flies. The use of geographic information systems (GIS) has documented a geographic and temporal co-occurrence of canine and human VL.[94] Due to concern about inducing drug resistance, several governments including Brazil's, prohibit the treatment of canine leishmaniosis with drugs used for humans. Compounded by a high parasite load in canine skin, proximity of humans and domestic dogs, and relative resistance to some forms of treatment, there is an urgent need for new or improved measures for prevention, early diagnosis, and treatment of canine leishmaniosis.[114]

The animal reservoir maintaining leishmaniasis varies between endemic regions, and between the different *Leishmania* species. Monitoring disease over a larger region such as a state or country shows a net peak in VL every 7–10 years. Several studies have used the combination of GIS and epidemiological data to discern the main reservoirs of infection.[111,115] These studies have shown co-occurrence of human and canine VL [usually caused by *L. infantum* (previously *L. chagasi*) in Brazil and other Central/South American countries], supporting the domestic dog as the main reservoir of human VL.[56,116] The situation differs in the Indian subcontinent and neighboring regions of Bangladesh and Nepal, where symptomatic VL due to *L. donovani* clusters with other recent cases of VL, PKDL, and asymptomatic infection, suggesting an anthroponotic cycle.[56,108] Transmission to sand flies has been shown by xenodiagnosis studies, as have several studies investigating the ability of flies to acquire infection from individuals with PKDL. Although reports are conflicting, some studies have documented low-level transmission from subjects with asymptomatic *L. donovani* infection.[108] New World VL and VL caused by *L. infantum* in Old World endemic sites have not yet been associated with anthroponotic transmission.[110]

Multipronged Approach

In 2005, the governments of India, Bangladesh, and Nepal established an agreement to eliminate VL in endemic regions, defined as less than 1 case per 10,000 population, at a subdistrict level by 2015.[92,117] Although the target date has been pushed back to 2020, elimination has remained an emphasis in all three countries. Approaches have included multiple levels of intervention. As the disease was considered exclusively anthroponotic, measures included rapid detection of human cases (VL and PKDL), as well as increased surveillance and indoor residual spraying of insecticide to decrease vector exposure in endemic regions. Near-total elimination has been reached by some, but not all areas, leading investigators to consider factors that might be responsible for ongoing transmission in the face of diminishing VL cases.[56,92,118,119] "Hotspots" of remaining disease clusters were associated with markers of poverty. As asymptomatic human infection is highly prevalent but not an indication for treatment, investigators are considering whether transmission from asymptomatically infected humans is sufficient to maintain disease in a community. Furthermore and despite long-standing beliefs to the contrary, residual disease has led some to reconsider whether there might be zoonotic transmission in endemic areas of India, which is only visible in the face of diminishing anthroponotic spread.[92,117]

Concluding Comments. Leishmaniasis refers to a set of vector-borne diseases caused by the *Leishmania* spp. protozoa in more than 90 endemic nations worldwide. Ongoing observations have revealed changing population demographics in endemic regions, newly emerging clinical presentations due to either well-recognized or novel *Leishmania* species, a new subgenus [*Leishmania (Mundinia)*_ spp.] potentially transmitted by a novel (biting midge) vector, and the clear recognition that trans-placental transmission is the main means of transmitting canine leishmaniosis in the U.S. Novel observations about disease patterns are being made due to the residual transmission of VL in the endemic region of India, Bangladesh and Nepal, where disease eradication campaigns are meeting success. These findings have required us to re-evaluate basic aspects of the disease such as the reservoir host, transmission mechanism, and pathogenesis of different forms of disease.

Lessons from the Dracunculiasis eradication and other similar program indicate that previously unrecognized minor reservoirs of infection and novel mechanisms of parasite entry into the human host emerge during eradication campaigns.[120] Similarly, surprising findings in leishmaniasis have forced scientists to adopt an open mind about the life cycle, reservoir, and mechanisms of human acquisition of leishmaniasis. The ability to discern these different patterns of disease will be essential before we can approach total eradication of leishmaniasis a goal that remains elusive despite concerted efforts in many countries.

References

1. Chappius F, Sundar S, Hailu A, et al. Visceral leishmaniasis: What are the needs for diagnosis, treatment and control? *Nat Rev Microbiol.* 2007;5:S7–16.
2. Alvar J, Velez ID, Bern C, et al. Leishmaniasis worldwide and global estimates of its incidence. *PLoS One.* 2012;7(5):e35671.
3. Singh SP, Reddy DC, Rai M, Sundar S. Serious underreporting of visceral leishmaniasis through passive case reporting in Bihar, India. *Trop Med Int Health.* 2006;11(6):899–905.

4. McCallum JE. *Military Medicine: From Ancient Times to the 21st Century.* Denver, Colorado: ABC CLIO; 2008.
5. Sir William Leishman: 1866–1926. *Lancet.* 1966;1(7432):310–1.
6. Guerin PJ, Olliaro P, Sundar S, et al. Visceral leishmaniasis: Current status of control, diagnosis, and treatment, and a proposed research and development agenda. *Lancet Infect Dis.* 2002;2:494–501.
7. Jeronimo SMB, Sousa AdQ, Pearson RD. Leishmaniasis. In: *Tropical Infectious Diseases.* 2nd ed. Philadelphia: Elsiever, Inc.; 2006.
8. Burza S, Croft SL, Boelaert M. Leishmaniasis. *Lancet.* 2018;392(10151):951–70.
9. Rittig MG, Bogdan C. *Leishmania*-host-cell interaction: Complexities and alternative views. *Parasitol Today.* 2000;16(7):292-–7.
10. Dougall AM, Alexander B, Holt DC, et al. Evidence incriminating midges (Diptera: Ceratopogonidae) as potential vectors of *Leishmania* in Australia. *Int J Parasitol.* 2011;41(5):571–9.
11. Seblova V, Sadlova J, Carpenter S, Volf P. Speculations on biting midges and other bloodsucking arthropods as alternative vectors of *Leishmania. Parasit Vectors.* 2014;7:222.
12. Sacks DL, Perkins PV. Identification of an infective stage of *Leishmania* promastigotes. *Science.* 1984;223:1417–9.
13. McKean PG, Denny PW, Knuepfer E, Keen JK, Smith DF. Phenotypic changes associated with deletion and overexpression of a stage-regulated gene family in *Leishmania. Cell Microbiol.* 2001;3(8):511–23.
14. Coulson RMR, Smith DF. Isolation of genes showing increased or unique expression in the infective promastigotes of *Leishmania major. Mol Biochem Parasitol.* 1990;40:63–76.
15. Smith DF, Gokool S, Keen JK, McKean PG, Rangarajan D. Structure and function of infective stage proteins of *Leishmania. Biochem Soc Trans.* 1994;22:286–91.
16. Flinn HM, Rangarajan D, Smith DF. Expression of a hydrophilic surface protein in infective stages of *Leishmania major. Mol Biochem Parasitol.* 1994;65:259–70.
17. Doehl JS, Sadlova J, Aslan H, et al. *Leishmania* HASP and SHERP genes are required for in vivo differentiation, parasite transmission and virulence attenuation in the host. *PLoS Pathog.* 2017;13(1):e1006130.
18. Chanmol W, Jariyapan N, Somboon P, Bates MD, Bates PA. Development of *Leishmania orientalis* in the sand fly *Lutzomyia longipalpis* (Diptera: Psychodidae) and the biting midge *Culicoides soronensis* (Diptera: Ceratopogonidae). *Acta Trop.* 2019;199:105157.
19. Seblova V, Sadlova J, Vojtkova B, et al. The miting midge *Culicoides sonorensis* (Diptera: Ceratopogonidae) is capable of developing late stage infections of *Leishmania enriettii. PLoS Negl Trop Dis.* 2015;9(9):e0004060.
20. Bates PA. Revising *Leishmania*'s life cycle. *Nat Microbiol.* 2018;3(5):529–30.
21. Rogers ME, Ilg T, Nikolaev AV, Ferguson MA, Bates PA. Transmission of cutaneous leishmaniasis by sand flies is enhanced by regurgitation of fPPG. *Nature.* 2004;430(6998):463–7.
22. Dey R, Joshi AB, Oliveira F, et al. Gut microbes egested during bites of infected sand flies augment severity of leishmaniasis via inflammasome-derived IL-1beta. *Cell Host Microbe.* 2018;23(1):134–43 e6.
23. Rogers ME, Corware K, Muller I, Bates PA. *Leishmania infantum* proteophosphoglycans regurgitated by the bite of its natural sand fly vector, *Lutzomyia longipalpis,* promote parasite establishment in mouse skin and skin-distant tissues. *Microbes Infect.* 2010;12(11):875–9.
24. Atayde VD, Aslan H, Townsend S, et al. Exosome secretion by the parasitic protozoan *Leishmania* within the sand fly midgut. *Cell Rep.* 2015;13(5):957–67.
25. Bates PA. Transmission of *Leishmania* metacyclic promastigotes by phlebotomine sand flies. *Int J Parasitol.* 2007;37(10):1097–106.
26. Jariyapan N, Daroontum T, Jaiwong K, et al. *Leishmania (Mundinia) orientalis* n. sp. (Trypanosomatidae), a parasite from Thailand responsible for localised cutaneous leishmaniasis. *Parasit Vectors.* 2018;11(1):351.
27. Kwakye-Nuako G, Mosore MT, Duplessis C, et al. First isolation of a new species of *Leishmania* responsible for human cutaneous leishmaniasis in Ghana and classification in the *Leishmania enriettii* complex. *Int J Parasitol.* 2015;45(11):679–84.
28. Akopyants NS, Kimblin N, Secundino N, et al. Demonstration of genetic exchange during cyclical development of *Leishmania* in the sand fly vector. *Science.* 2009;324(5924):265–8.
29. Kuhls K, Alam MZ, Cupolillo E, et al. Comparative microsatellite typing of new world leishmania infantum reveals low heterogeneity among populations and its recent old world origin. *PLoS Negl Trop Dis.* 2011;5(6):e1155.
30. Aleixo JA, Nascimento ET, Monteiro GR, et al. Atypical American visceral leishmaniasis causedc by disseminated *Leishmania amazonensis* infection presenting with hepatitis and adenopathy. *Trans R Soc Trop Med Hyg.* 2006;100(1):79–82.
31. Magill AJ, Gasser RA, Oster CN, Grogl M. Viscerotropic leishmaniasis in persons returning from Operation Desert Storm—1990–1991. *MMWR Morb Mortal Wkly Rep.* 1992;41:131–4.
32. Sereno D. *Leishmania (Mundinia)* spp.: From description to emergence as new human and animal *Leishmania* pathogens. *New Microbes New Infect.* 2019;30:100540.
33. Schriefer A, Wilson ME, Carvalho EM. Recent developments leading toward a paradigm switch in the diagnostic and therapeutic approach to human leishmaniasis. *Curr Opin Infect Dis.* 2008;21(5):483–8.
34. Castellucci LC, Almeida LF, Jamieson SE, et al. Host genetic factors in American cutaneous leishmaniasis: A critical appraisal of studies conducted in an endemic area of Brazil. *Mem Inst Oswaldo Cruz.* 2014;109(3):279–88.
35. Shaw MA, Davies CR, Llanos-Cuentas EA, Collins A. Human genetic susceptibility and infection with *Leishmania peruviana. Am J Hum Genet.* 1995;57:1159–68.
36. Cabrera M, Shaw MA, Sharples C, et al. Polymorphism in tumor necrosis factor genes associated with mucocutaneous leishmaniasis. *J Exp Med.* 1995;182:1259–64.
37. Castellucci L, Menezes E, Oliveira J, et al. IL6-174 G/C promoter polymorphism influences susceptibility to mucosal but not localized cutaneous leishmaniasis in Brazil. *J Infect Dis.* 2006;194(4):519–27.
38. Castellucci L, Cheng LH, Araujo C, et al. Familial aggregation of mucosal leishmaniasis in Northeast Brazil. *Am J Trop Med Hyg.* 2005;73(1):69–73.
39. Scorza BM, Carvalho EM, Wilson ME. Cutaneous manifestations of human and murine leishmaniasis. *Int J Mol Sci.* 2017;18(6):1296.
40. Dougall A, Shilton C, Low Choy J, Alexander B, Walton S. New reports of Australian cutaneous leishmaniasis in Northern Australian macropods. *Epidemiol Infect.* 2009;137(10):1516–20.
41. Desbois N, Pratlong F, Quist D, Dedet JP. *Leishmania (Leishmania) martiniquensis* n. sp. (Kinetoplastida: Trypanosomatidae), description of the parasite responsible for cutaneous leishmaniasis in Martinique Island (French West Indies). *Parasite.* 2014;21:12.
42. Paranaiba LF, Pinheiro LJ, Macedo DH, et al. An overview on *Leishmania (Mundinia) enriettii*: Biology, immunopathology, LRV and extracellular vesicles during the host-parasite interaction. *Parasitology.* 2018;145(10):1265–73.
43. Zhang WW, Mendez S, Ghosh A, et al. Comparison of the A2 gene locus in *Leishmania donovani* and *Leishmania major* and its control over cutaneous infection. *J Biol Chem.* 2003;278(37):35508–15.
44. Ives A, Ronet C, Prevel F, et al. *Leishmania* RNA virus controls the severity of mucocutaneous leishmaniasis. *Science.* 2011;331(6018):775–8.
45. Mauricio IL, Stothard JR, Miles MA. The strange case of *Leishmania chagasi. Parasitol Today.* 2000;16(5):188–9.
46. Magill AJ, Grogl M, Johnson SC, Gasser RAJr. Visceral infection due to *Leishmania tropica* in a veteran of Operation Desert Storm who presented 2 years after leaving Saudi Arabia. *Clin Infect Dis.* 1994;19:805–6.
47. Pearson RD, Sousa AdQ. Clinical spectrum of leishmaniasis. *Clin Infect Dis.* 1996;22:1–13.
48. Wilson ME, Jeronimo SMB, Pearson RD. Immunopathogenesis of infection with the visceralizing *Leishmania* species. *Microb Pathog.* 2005;38:147–60.
49. Zijlstra EE, Ali MS, El-Hassan AM, et al. Kala-azar in displaced people from Southern Sudan: Epidemiological, clinical and therapeutic findings. *Trans Roy Soc Trop Med Hyg.* 1991;85:365–9.
50. Zijlstra EE, El-Hassan AM, Ismael A, Ghalib HW. Endemic kala-azar in eastern Sudan: A longitudinal study on the incidence of clinical and subclinical infection and post-kala-azar dermal leishmaniasis. *Am J Trop Med Hyg.* 1994;51(6):826–36.
51. Barral A, Barral-Netto M, Almeida R, et al. Lymphadenopathy associated with *Leishmania braziliensis* cutaneous infection. *Am J Trop Med Hyg.* 1992;47(5):587–92.
52. Andrade TM, Carvalho EM, Rocha H. Bacterial infections in patients with visceral leishmaniasis. *J Infect Dis.* 1990;162:1354–9.
53. Lima ID, Queiroz JW, Lacerda HG, et al. *Leishmania infantum chagasi* in northeastern Brazil: Asymptomatic infection at the urban perimeter. *Am J Trop Med Hyg.* 2012;86(1):99–107.
54. Monge-Maillo B, Norman FF, Cruz I, Alvar J, Lopez-Velez R. Visceral leishmaniasis and HIV coinfection in the Mediterranean region. *PLoS Negl Trop Dis.* 2014;8(8):e3021.

55. Magill AJ, Grogl M, Gasser RA, Wellington S, Oster CN. Visceral infection caused by *Leishmania tropica* in veterans of Operation Desert Storm. *N Engl J Med.* 1993;328:1383–7.

56. Courtenay O, Peters NC, Rogers ME, Bern C. Combining epidemiology with basic biology of sand flies, parasites, and hosts to inform leishmaniasis transmission dynamics and control. *PLoS Pathog.* 2017;13(10):e1006571.

57. Bhattacharya SK, Sur D, Sinha PK, Karbwang J. Elimination of leishmaniasis (kala-azar) from the Indian subcontinent is technically feasible and operationally achievable. *Indian J Med Res.* 2006;123(3):195–6.

58. WHO/CDS. *Communicable Disease Profile in Iraq*. Geneva: World Health Organization; 2003:39–44.

59. Sengupta R, Mukherjee S, Moulik S, et al. In-situ immune profile of polymorphic vs. macular Indian post kala-azar dermal leishmaniasis. *Int J Parasitol Drugs Drug Resist.* 2019;11:166–76.

60. Roberts T, Barratt J, Sandaradura I, et al. Molecular epidemiology of imported cases of leishmaniasis in Australia from 2008 to 2014. *PLoS One.* 2015;10(3):e0119212.

61. Paranaiba LF, Pinheiro LJ, Torrecilhas AC, et al. *Leishmania enriettii* (Muniz & Medina, 1948): A highly diverse parasite is here to stay. *PLoS Pathog.* 2017;13(5):e1006303.

62. Pothirat T, Tantiworawit A, Chaiwarith R, et al. First isolation of *Leishmania* from Northern Thailand: Case report, identification as *Leishmania martiniquensis* and phylogenetic position within the *Leishmania enriettii* complex. *PLoS Negl Trop Dis.* 2014;8(12):e3339.

63. Noyes H, Pratlong F, Chance M, et al. A previously unclassified trypanosomatid responsible for human cutaneous lesions in Martinique (French West Indies) is the most divergent member of the genus *Leishmania* ss. *Parasitology.* 2002;124(Pt 1):17–24.

64. Almeida, MD. Practical guide for specimen collection and reference diagnosis of Leishmaniasis. U.S. Department of Health and Human Services, Centers for Disease Control and Prevention. https://www.cdc.gov/parasites/leishmaniasis/resources/pdf/cdc_diagnosis_guide_leishmaniasis_2016.pdf. Published 2016. Accessed.

65. Luz ZM, Silva AR, Silva Fde O, et al. Lesion aspirate culture for the diagnosis and isolation of *Leishmania* spp. from patients with cutaneous leishmaniasis. *Mem Inst Oswaldo Cruz.* 2009;104(1):62–6.

66. Alvar J. Leishmaniasis and the AIDS co-infection: The Spanish example. *Parasitol Today.* 1994;10:160–3.

67. Davies CR, Kaye PM, Croft SL, Sundar S. Leishmaniasis: New approaches to disease control. *BMJ.* 2003;326:377–82.

68. Braz RFS, Nascimento ET, Martins DRA, et al. The sensitivity and specificity of *Leishmania chagasi* recombinant K39 antigen in the diagnosis of American visceral leishmaniasis and in differentiating active from subclinical infection. *Am J Trop Med Hyg.* 2002;67:344–8.

69. Zijlstra EE, Daifalla NS, Kager PA, et al. rK39 enzyme-linked immunosorbent assay for diagnosis of *Leishmania donovani* infection. *Clin Diagn Lab Immunol.* 1998;5(5):717–20.

70. Hasker E, Malaviya P, Gidwani K, et al. Strong association between serological status and probability of progression to clinical visceral leishmaniasis in prospective cohort studies in India and Nepal. *PLoS Negl Trop Dis.* 2014;8(1):e2657.

71. Hasker E, Kansal S, Malaviya P, et al. Latent infection with *Leishmania donovani* in highly endemic villages in Bihar, India. *PLoS Negl Trop Dis.* 2013;7(2):e2053.

72. de Almeida ME, Steurer FJ, Koru O, et al. Identification of *Leishmania* spp. by molecular amplification and DNA sequencing analysis of a fragment of the rRNA Internal Transcribed Spacer 2 (ITS2). *J Clin Microbiol.* 2011;49(9):3143–9.

73. Weirather JL, Jeronimo SM, Gautam S, et al. Serial quantitative PCR assay for detection, species-discrimination and quantification of *Leishmania* spp. in human samples. *J Clin Microbiol.* 2011;49(11):3892–904.

74. Mori Y, Notomi T. Loop-mediated isothermal amplification (LAMP): A rapid, accurate, and cost-effective diagnostic method for infectious diseases. *J Infect Chemother.* 2009;15(2):62–9.

75. Tomita N, Mori Y, Kanda H, Notomi T. Loop-mediated isothermal amplification (LAMP) of gene sequences and simple visual detection of products. *Nat Protoc.* 2008;3(5):877–82.

76. Mazurek GH, Villarino ME, CDC. Guidelines for using the QuantiFERON-TB test for diagnosing latent *Mycobacterium* tuberculosis infection. Centers for Disease Control and Prevention. *MMWR Recomm Rep.* 2003;52(RR-2):15–8.

77. Chakravarty J, Hasker E, Kansal S, et al. Determinants for progression from asymptomatic infection to symptomatic visceral leishmaniasis: A cohort study. *PLoS Negl Trop Dis.* 2019;13(3):e0007216.

78. Mody RM, Lakhal-Naouar I, Sherwood JE, et al. Asymptomatic visceral *Leishmania infantum* infection in U.S. soldiers deployed to Iraq. *Clin Infect Dis.* 2019;68(12):2036–44.

79. Schnorr D, Muniz AC, Passos S, et al. IFN-gamma production to *Leishmania* antigen supplements the *Leishmania* skin test in identifying exposure to *L. braziliensis* infection. *PLoS Negl Trop Dis.* 2012; 6(12):e1947.

80. Singh OP, Sundar S. Whole blood assay and visceral leishmaniasis: Challenges and promises. *Immunobiology.* 2014;219(4):323–8.

81. Monteiro DC, Sousa AQ, Lima DM, et al. *Leishmania infantum* infection in blood donors, Northeastern Brazil. *Emerg Infect Dis.* 2016;22(4):739–40.

82. Le Fichoux Y, Quaranta J-F, Aufeuvre J-P, et al. Occurrence of *Leishmania infantum* parasitemia in asymptomatic blood donors living in an area of endemicity in Southern France. *J Clin Micro.* 1999;37(6):1953–7.

83. Costa SR, D'Oliveira AJr, Bacellar O, Carvalho EM. T cell response of asymptomatic *Leishmania chagasi* infected subjects to recombinant *Leishmania* antigens. *Mem Inst Oswaldo Cruz.* 1999;94(3):367–70.

84. Orsini M, Canela JR, Disch J, et al. High frequency of asymptomatic *Leishmania* spp. infection among HIV-infected patients living in endemic areas for visceral leishmaniasis in Brazil. *Trans R Soc Trop Med Hyg.* 2012;106(5):283–8.

85. Costa CHN, Stewart JM, Gomes RBB, et al. Asymptomatic human carriers of *Leishmania chagasi*. *Am J Trop Med Hyg.* 2002;66(4):334–7.

86. Mody RM, Lakhal-Naouar I, Sherwood JE, et al. Asymptomatic visceral *Leishmania infantum* infection in US soldiers deployed to Iraq. *Clin Infect Dis.* 2019;68(12):2036–44.

87. Aronson N, Herwaldt BL, Libman M, et al. Diagnosis and treatment of leishmaniasis: Clinical practice guidelines by the Infectious Diseases Society of America (IDSA) and the American Society of Tropical Medicine and Hygiene (ASTMH). *Clin Infect Dis.* 2016;63(12):e202–64.

88. Aronson NE. Addressing a clinical challenge: Guidelines for the diagnosis and treatment of leishmaniasis. *BMC Med.* 2017;15(1):76.

89. Chakravarty J, Sundar S. Current and emerging medications for the treatment of leishmaniasis. *Expert Opin Pharmacother.* 2019;20(10):1251–65.

90. Ponte-Sucre A, Gamarro F, Dujardin JC, et al. Drug resistance and treatment failure in leishmaniasis: A 21st century challenge. *PLoS Negl Trop Dis.* 2017;11(12):e0006052.

91. Sundar S, Singh A. Chemotherapeutics of visceral leishmaniasis: Present and future developments. *Parasitology.* 2018;145(4):481–9.

92. Bulstra CA, Le Rutte EA, Malaviya P, et al. Visceral leishmaniasis: Spatiotemporal heterogeneity and drivers underlying the hotspots in Muzaffarpur, Bihar, India. *PLoS Negl Trop Dis.* 2018;12(12):e0006888.

93. Nascimento ET, Moura ML, Queiroz JW, et al. The emergence of concurrent HIV-1/AIDS and visceral leishmaniasis in Northeast Brazil. *Trans R Soc Trop Med Hyg.* 2011;105(5):298−−300.

94. Lima ID, Lima ALM, Mendes-Aguiar CO, et al. Changing demographics of visceral leishmaniasis in northeast Brazil: Lessons for the future. *PLoS Negl Trop Dis.* 2018;12(3):e0006164.

95. Aronson NE, Joya CA. Cutaneous leishmaniasis: Updates in diagnosis and management. *Infect Dis Clin North Am.* 2019;33(1):101–17.

96. Machado PR, Ampuero J, Guimaraes LH, et al. Miltefosine in the treatment of cutaneous leishmaniasis caused by *Leishmania braziliensis* in Brazil: A randomized and controlled trial. *PLoS Negl Trop Dis.* 2010;4(12):e912.

97. Davies CR, Kaye P, Croft SL, Sundar S. Leishmaniasis: New approaches to disease control. *BMJ.* 2003;326(7385):377–82.

98. Almeida RP, Brito J, Machado PL, et al. Successful treatment of refractory cutaneous leishmaniasis with GM-CSF and antimonials. *Am J Trop Med Hyg.* 2005;73(1):79–81.

99. Abdeladhim M, Kamhawi S, Valenzuela JG. What's behind a sand fly bite? The profound effect of sand fly saliva on host hemostasis, inflammation and immunity. *Infect Genet Evol.* 2014;28:691–703.

100. Pimenta PFP, Saraiva EMB, Rowton E, et al. Evidence that the vectorial competence of phlebotomine sand flies for different species of *Leishmania* is controlled by structural polymorphisms in the surface lipophosphoglycan. *Proc Natl Acad Sci U S A.* 1994;91:9155–9.

101. Pimenta PFP, Turco SJ, McConville MJ, et al. Stage-specific adhesion of *Leishmania* promastigotes to the sandfly midgut. *Science.* 1992;256:1812–5.

102. Kelly PH, Bahr SM, Serafim TD, et al. The gut microbiome of the vector *Lutzomyia longipalpis* is essential for survival of *Leishmania infantum*. *mBio*. 2017;8(1):e01121-16.

103. Teixeira C, Gomes R, Oliveira F, et al. Characterization of the early inflammatory infiltrate at the feeding site of infected sand flies in mice protected from vector-transmitted *Leishmania major* by exposure to uninfected bites. *PLoS Negl Trop Dis*. 2014;8(4):e2781.

104. Bates PA. Transmission of *Leishmania* metacyclic promastigotes by phlebotomine sand flies. *Int J Parasitol*. 2007;37(10):1097–106.

105. Teixeira MJ, Teixeira CR, Andrade BB, Barral-Netto M, Barral A. Chemokines in host-parasite interactions in leishmaniasis. *Trends Parasitol*. 2006;22(1):32–40.

106. Abbehusen MMC, Cunha J, Suarez MS, et al. Immunization of experimental dogs with salivary proteins from *Lutzomyia longipalpis*, using DNA and recombinant Canarypox virus induces immune responses consistent with protection against *Leishmania infantum*. *Front Immunol*. 2018;9:2558.

107. Petersen CA. Leishmaniasis, an emerging disease found in companion animals in the United States. *Top Comanion Anim Med*. 2009;24(4):182–8.

108. Mondal D, Bern C, Ghosh D, et al. Quantifying the infectiousness of post-kala-azar dermal leishmaniasis toward sand flies. *Clin Infect Dis*. 2019;69(2):251–8.

109. Ferreira GR, Castelo Branco Ribeiro JC, Meneses Filho A, et al. Human competence to transmit *Leishmania infantum* to *Lutzomyia longipalpis* and the influence of human immunodeficiency virus infection. *Am J Trop Med Hyg*. 2018;98(1):126–33.

110. Jeronimo SMB, Duggal P, Braz RFS, et al. An emerging peri-urban pattern of infection with *Leishmania chagasi*, the protozoan causing visceral leishmaniasis in northeast Brazil. *Scand J Infect Dis*. 2004;36(6/7):443–9.

111. Cavalcante FRA, Cavalcante KKS, Florencio C, et al. Human visceral leishmaniasis: Epidemiological, temporal and spacial aspects in Northeast Brazil, 2003–2017. *Rev Inst Med Trop Sao Paulo*. 2020;62:e12.

112. Schonian G, Mauricio I, Gramiccia M, et al. Leishmaniases in the Mediterranean in the era of molecular epidemiology. *Trends Parasitol*. 2008;24(3):135–42.

113. Bezerra CM, Cavalcanti LP, Souza Rde C, et al. Domestic, peridomestic and wild hosts in the transmission of *Trypanosoma cruzi* in the Caatinga area colonised by *Triatoma brasiliensis*. *Mem Inst Oswaldo Cruz*. 2014;109(7):887–98.

114. Solano-Gallego L, Cardoso L, Pennisi MG, et al. Diagnostic challenges in the era of canine *Leishmania infantum* vaccines. *Trends Parasitol*. 2017;33(9):706–17.

115. do Nascimento PR, Martins DR, Monteiro GR, et al. Association of pro-inflammatory cytokines and iron regulatory protein 2 (IRP2) with *Leishmania* burden in canine visceral leishmaniasis. *PLoS One*. 2013;8(10):e73873.

116. Queiroz PV, Monteiro GR, Macedo VP, et al. Canine visceral leishmaniasis in urban and rural areas of Northeast Brazil. *Res Vet Sci*. 2009;86(2):267–73.

117. Sundar S, Singh OP, Chakravarty J. Visceral leishmaniasis elimination targets in India, strategies for preventing resurgence. *Expert Rev Anti Infect Ther*. 2018;16(11):805–12.

118. Hasker E, Malaviya P, Cloots K, et al. Visceral leishmaniasis in the Muzaffapur demographic surveillance site: A spatiotemporal analysis. *Am J Trop Med Hyg*. 2018;99(6):1555–61.

119. Olliaro PL, Shamsuzzaman TA, Marasini B, et al. Investments in research and surveillance are needed to go beyond elimination and stop transmission of *Leishmania* in the Indian subcontinent. *PLoS Negl Trop Dis*. 2017;11(1):e0005190.

120. Galan-Puchades MT. Dracunculiasis: Water-borne anthroponosis vs. food-borne zoonosis. *J Helminthol*. 2019;94:e76.

CHAPTER 135 Leprosy

Kenrad E. Nelson • David M. Scollard

Leprosy or Hansen's disease is a chronic infectious disease involving primarily the peripheral nervous system, skin, eyes, and mucous membranes. It is endemic in many countries in Asia, Africa, the Pacific Islands, Latin America, southern Europe, and the Middle East. There are endemic areas of infection in the United States as well, particularly in Gulf coast states and California. The major sequelae of leprosy are physical deformities involving the extremities, face, and eyes due primarily to damage to the sensory nerves from infection by organisms of the *Mycobacterium leprae*-complex (*M. leprae* and *M. lepromatosis*), and the immune reaction to those pathogens. The resultant deformities often lead to stigmatization that continues after the infection becomes inactive and the patient is not infectious.

Since several effective antileprosy drugs are now available, new cases of leprosy can be treated effectively and rendered noninfectious. Leprosy should not pose a significant public health problem once treatment is instituted. In fact, despite the recognized importation of 100–320 cases annually in the United States for the last few decades, the development of clinical leprosy among the contacts of these imported cases has not been documented.[1]

ETIOLOGIC AGENT

Leprosy is caused by *M. leprae and its close relative, M. lepromatosis. These are* weakly acid-fast bacteria that can be demonstrated in tissues using a modified acid-fast stain, the Fite-Faraco stain. *M. leprae* was originally identified in 1873 by Gerhard Henrik Armauer Hansen, and *M. lepromatosis* was recognized by DNA sequencing in 2008.[2] These organisms have not yet been successfully cultivated *in vitro*.

M. leprae has one of the slowest replication cycles of any known bacteria: it divides only every 10–12 days during the log phase of growth, as determined from studies in mouse footpads. The organism replicates in mouse footpads,[3] in thymectomized mice or rats, nude mice, severe combined immunodeficient mice, the nine-banded armadillo, and in several nonhuman primate species.[4] Naturally occurring leprosy infections have been documented in nine-banded armadillos (*Dasypus novemcinctus*),[5] chimpanzees, and sooty mangabeys.[6] *M. lepromatosis* has recently been found in red squirrels in the United Kingdom.[7–9] The complete genome sequences of *M. leprae* and *M. lepromatosis* have been reported, and they are very similar.[10] The *M. leprae* genome contains 3.3 million base pairs compared to 4.4 million base pairs in the *M. tuberculosis* genome. However, in contrast with the *M. tuberculosis* genome, less than half of the *M. leprae* genome encodes functional genes, but pseudogenes with intact counterparts of *M. tuberculosis* are common. Gene deletion and decay eliminated many important metabolic activities, including part of the oxidative and most of the microaerophilic and anaerobic respiratory chains and numerous catabolic systems and regulatory circuits in *M. leprae*. The reductive evolution indicated by the *M. leprae* genome's structure explains its slow growth and limited metabolic capability.[11]

Throughout the world, *M. leprae* strains are remarkably similar.[12] *M. leprae* has very little genetic diversity with single nucleotide polymorphism (SNPs) only every 28,000 base pairs; however, genetic analysis has identified four subtypes. At least 16 different genotypes have now been described using a combination of SNPs and variable number tandem repeats.[13–16] No genotypes of *M. lepromatosis* have yet been described.

CLINICAL MANIFESTATIONS

The clinical manifestations of leprosy are variable. *M. leprae* and *M. lepromatosis* present with an identical range of clinical manifestations, respond to the same treatment, and have similar risks of leprosy reactions and other complications.

The clinical presentation and course of the disease depend on the interactions between the *pathogen's* bacterial load and the host's immune system, especially the cellular immune system. The most accurate and informative system for clinical-immunologic classification of leprosy was developed by Ridley and Jopling,[17] which subdivides leprosy into five general classes: polar lepromatous leprosy (LL), borderline lepromatous (BL) leprosy, midborderline (BB) leprosy, borderline tuberculoid (BT) leprosy, and polar tuberculoid (TT) leprosy. In addition, a very early form of leprosy, not readily classified into the above groups, is called indeterminate (I) leprosy. Indeterminate leprosy is the earliest clinical evidence of infection and often resolves spontaneously without specific therapy; however, it may progress to one of the five classes. The most widely used classification system for leprosy is the one devised by the World Health Organization (WHO), which identifies only two groups: multibacillary leprosy (MB), comprising LL, BL, and BB leprosy, and paucibacillary leprosy (PB), comprising BT and TT leprosy.[18] These broader groupings are useful for therapeutic decisions, and are valuable in resource-poor settings where no doctor is available.

There is a good correlation between the clinical appearance, number of organisms and distribution and type of skin lesions, and the patient's classification according to the Ridley-Jopling criteria. Patients with TT-BT (paucibacillary) leprosy have well-defined macular skin lesions with distinct borders, which are few in number and distributed asymmetrically. Lesions increase in number and become more diffuse and smaller as the disease moves toward the lepromatous end of the spectrum. Patients with BB, BL, or LL (multibacillary) leprosy have ill-defined, sometimes nodular, skin lesions without clear borders. Conspicuous thickening of earlobes is often seen. Loss of eyebrows or hair and deformities caused by infiltration of the pinna of the ear are common in patients with lepromatous disease. Another characteristic of leprosy is hypoesthesia or anesthesia of the skin lesions. Leprosy skin lesions generally spare the body's warmer intertriginous areas. Enlargement and nodularity of the peripheral nerves, especially the ulnar, posterior tibial, and great auricular nerves, are characteristic. Patients may have corneal anesthesia and keratitis or lagophthalmos due to involvement of the facial and trigeminal nerves. Damage to the hands, feet, and eyes is characteristic of lepromatous disease. Trophic ulcers and resorption of digits may result from the sensory and motor nerve damage and the repeated trauma that these patients undergo. Early involvement of large sensory nerves is characteristic of tuberculoid leprosy.

An important clinical feature of leprosy is the occurrence of leprosy reactions, which are spontaneous episodes of enhanced immunological activity and are not drug reactions. There are two major types of leprosy reaction. Type 1 are "reversal" reactions that represent increased (or decreased in the case of downgrading reactions) cell-mediated immune responses to the organisms. Type 2 are erythema nodosum leprosum (ENL) reactions, believed to be mediated largely by humoral immune responses to *M. leprae*, leading to immune complexes. Nearly half of all leprosy patients experience a reaction during the first few years after their diagnosis.[19]

Type 1 (reversal) reactions can occur in any patient with borderline (BL, BB, or BT) leprosy; they are not seen in patients with polar lepromatous or tuberculoid leprosy. Clinically, Type 1 reactions consist of acute inflammation of pre-existing leprosy lesions, including superficial nerves, with fever and systemic symptoms that begin gradually and have a natural course of several weeks or months. Often these are very severe episodes; patients may present to the emergency room with an appearance suggestive of sepsis. Early recognition and aggressive therapy of Type 1 reactions is especially important to prevent irreversible deformity from nerve damage.

Type 2 (ENL) reactions are characteristic of and limited to patients with multibacillary leprosy. Type 2 reactions consist of the sudden appearance of crops of tender, erythematous skin nodules in sites that did not previously have leprosy lesions. These are systemic reactions, with fever, malaise, and sometimes acute neuritis, arthritis, orchitis, iritis, glomerulonephritis, myalgia, and peripheral edema. Typically, type 2 reactions have a sudden onset and may subside in several days to a few weeks, though they may cause severe nerve damage during that time. Type 2 reactions may recur over the course of a year or more, especially in patients treated with anti-inflammatory agents, after these drugs are withdrawn or tapered.

DIAGNOSIS

The diagnosis of leprosy is usually made clinically. Characteristics of leprosy are macular or nodular skin lesions that are hypoesthetic or anesthetic to light touch, enlarged nerves to palpation, lagophthalmos, and distal stocking-glove anesthesia. The diagnosis should be confirmed by skin biopsy or slit-skin smears whenever possible. When taking a punch biopsy, it is important to include specimens of the entire dermis at a lesion's active border, because the organisms are often located deep in the skin, but not found in the epidermis, and in multibacillary disease there may be a "clear zone" at the dermal-epidermal junction.

The histopathologic features of leprosy correlate well with the disease's clinical presentation. Patients with lepromatous disease have many organisms in their lesions and lack a well-developed granulomatous response due to ineffective cellular immunity to the organism. In contrast, tuberculoid patients have few (or no detectable) organisms with a well-organized granulomatous infiltrate. Lesions in the borderline types of leprosy have gradations between these two poles. In patients with tuberculoid leprosy, the leprosy granulomas are infiltrated with cells of the CD4+ T-helper memory phenotype and macrophages with a ring of CD8+ cells around the periphery. In contrast, in lepromatous lesions CD4+ T cells of the naïve phenotype and CD8+ suppressor cells are scattered randomly throughout the lesions.[20,21] Consultation for the interpretation and classification of skin biopsies or for therapeutic decisions can be obtained from the National Hansen's Disease Programs in Baton Rouge, Louisiana (https://www.hrsa.gov/hansens-disease/diagnosis/biopsy.html; Phone: 504-642-4740).

The Mitsuda lepromin skin test is not useful in making a diagnosis of *M. leprae*. The Mitsuda skin test measures the response to *M. leprae* antigens. The main use of the lepromin test in the past was to classify patients once the diagnosis had been made,[22] but this reagent is no longer available except for research purposes.

A phenolic glycolipid (PGL) that is antigenic and specific was isolated from the *M. leprae* cell wall.[23] However, serodiagnosis using PGL-1 is not sensitive enough to be a routine diagnostic adjunct, because not all untreated multibacillary patients and only 20–30% of paucibacillary patients are antibody positive. The development of a sensitive and specific serologic test remains a major goal of leprosy research, increasingly focused on the use of recombinant protein antigens.[24] Significant differences have been seen in the ratio of IP-10/IL10 in plasma[25] of leprosy patients compared to endemic controls, suggesting that cytokine-based assays may be of diagnostic value.

DISTRIBUTION

Leprosy has existed in eastern Mediterranean and Asian populations since ancient times. During the Middle Ages, leprosy became widespread in Europe. It declined in most of Europe after the sixteenth century but peaked in Norway during the nineteenth century, followed by a rapid decline during the late nineteenth and early twentieth centuries. The last known endemic case in Norway had onset about 1950.[26] The disease was introduced into the northern United States and Canada by European settlers from Norway, France, and Germany. It persisted in several clearly defined foci and within certain family groups for several decades and then disappeared.[27]

Currently leprosy is primarily epidemic in certain tropical countries in Africa, Southeast Asia, India, some Pacific Islands, and Latin America. It remains a significant endemic problem in 22 countries worldwide.[28] However, three countries—India, Brazil, and Indonesia—accounted for over 80% of the new cases registered with the WHO in 2017.[28] In seven countries (Bangladesh, Brazil, Comoros, Mozambique, Nepal, Philippines, and Sri Lanka), the annual incidence of new cases has increased between 2015 and 2016.

Over the last four decades, the estimated prevalence of leprosy has declined remarkably. In 1982, over 12 million leprosy cases were estimated to exist worldwide, and in 1992, there were an estimated 3.1 million cases.[29] By 2001, the estimate was 700,000–1,000,000 cases, and in 2017 it has dropped to 192,713 cases.[30] However, these figures are not comparable, since the earlier data included inactive cases while the data since the mid-1990s only include new active patients receiving treatment.[31] In 1981, the WHO recommended the routine treatment of all active cases with multidrug therapy (MDT) containing dapsone, rifampin, and clofazimine for a fixed time period, rather than indefinite treatment with dapsone alone, as was common practice until then. The substantial decline in the global numbers of leprosy cases is probably in part related to the widespread use of supervised MDT. MDT renders most leprosy cases noninfectious sooner after the start of therapy, in comparison to the previous monotherapy with dapsone, a bacteriostatic drug to which many *M. leprae* were resistant. Some experts believe that stricter compliance with shorter drug regimens may have decreased the rates of relapse, as well as interrupted the transmission cycle.[33] However, another factor that clearly reduced the current estimated prevalence of leprosy is the release of patients from the registry of active cases after MDT is completed and they are considered cured. Initially, dapsone monotherapy was recommended for life for multibacillary cases, and patients were never dropped from the registry even after they became inactive, or "cured." Therefore, the decreased leprosy prevalence rates are due in part to a change in the definition of what constitutes an "active case."[34]

In recent years, the WHO has shifted its emphasis to reporting the number of new cases (as a rough estimate of incidence), rather than

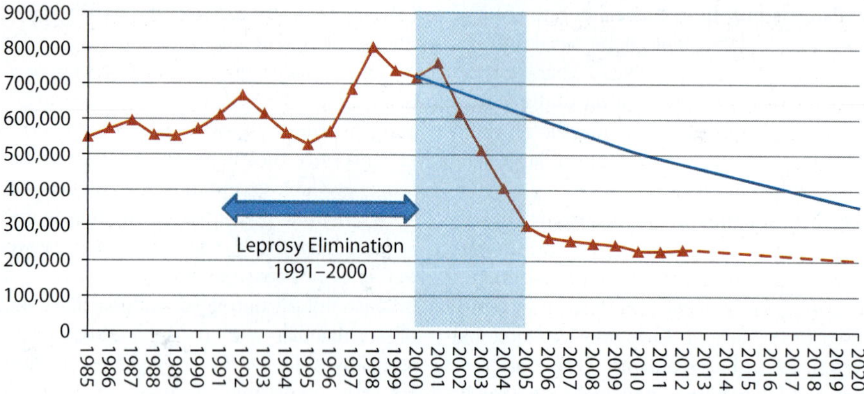

FIGURE 135-1. Number of new leprosy cases by year. The red continuous line represents the observed annual new case detection rate between 1985 and 2012, with extrapolation to 2020 based on the trend after 2005 (red dotted line). The blue continuous line is the predicted new case detection rate based on mathematical modeling, applying an intermediate scenario in the presence of an infant BCG vaccination program. (*Source:* From Smith WC, van Brakel W, Gillis T, Saunderson P, Richardus JH. The missing millions: A threat to the elimination of leprosy. *PLoS Negl Trop Dis.* 2015;9(4):e0003658.)

prevalence. In 2017, a total of 210,671 new cases[30] were reported.*[1] However, this figure for new cases is probably also a low estimate, because it is based primarily on passive case finding. Active case finding efforts in selected areas have found the number of cases to be considerably higher than expected based on WHO estimates.[35,36] Based on new-case detection data and epidemiological modelling,[37] it has been estimated that 2–4 million patients are currently undiagnosed[38] or unreported (Fig. 135-1). There is concern that this trend may continue due to the reduction or elimination of infrastructure for appropriate leprosy surveillance.

Leprosy was apparently introduced into the Americas through African and European immigration.[39] A genetic study of 175 strains of *M. leprae* found rare SNPs that allowed subclassification of the organism into four subtypes. These genetic data suggested that *M. leprae* originated as a human pathogen in East Africa or the near East.[12] Leprosy was reported in French Polynesia as the eighteenth century ended. Trade links among these islands, Easter Island, and Hawaii probably helped spread the disease.[40]

North American endemic foci are now in Gulf coast states and California. New cases in North America now occur primarily among immigrants, which occur four to five times more commonly than infections acquired among U.S. residents. Many cases in the United States come from Southeast Asia, and others from Mexico and Latin America or Africa where leprosy is endemic. Approximately 20–25% of new cases in the United States occur in native-born residents, primarily in Gulf Coast states. One of the most impressive epidemics of leprosy was reported from the island of Nauru, in the South Pacific.[41] A single case of leprosy was introduced into a population of approximately 1200 persons in 1912 and this led to an epidemic that eventually affected 30% of the population over the next 30 years. It is of interest that nearly all of the leprosy cases on Nauru were of the tuberculoid type, and only about 1% were multibacillary. The marked predominance of tuberculoid leprosy in hyperendemic populations led Newell to suggest that LL occurs only in persons with specific genetic immunological deficiencies in controlling infection with this organism, a view subsequently supported by several genetic studies.[42] It is believed that only 1–5% of the human population is susceptible to leprosy.[19]

[1] This number of new cases is greater than the point prevalence cited above, because paucibacillary patients are treated for only 6 months and many have completed treatment. They are thus "cured" and dropped from the registry by the time the number of registered cases is tabulated each year.

EPIDEMIOLOGY

Transmission. M. leprae is believed to be transmitted from person to person by close contact. However, some debate continues about the exact means of transmission. Only about 15–30% of patients with clinical leprosy who live in endemic areas have a history of close personal or household contact with a known leprosy case.[43] However, the indolent nature and the long incubation period of the disease could have led to failure to recognize or recall this exposure in many cases. Attempts to study transmission of *M. leprae* are also complicated by the inability to cultivate the organism in vitro, and by the lack of a suitable animal model in which to study transmission experimentally.

In contrast with tuberculosis, a primary site of infection in the respiratory tract has not been documented. Nevertheless, many experts believe that the infection is most often transmitted from contact with the nasal secretions of an infectious case. Studies of the nasal discharge of multibacillary cases have estimated that 10^7 bacilli per day may be contained in these secretions.[44] The polymerase chain reaction (PCR) to amplify *M. leprae* DNA, can detect the presence of the organism in the nasal secretions of leprosy cases and their household contacts.[45–47] One study of 1228 persons living in two villages in Indonesia where leprosy was endemic found 7.85% healthy persons to have nasal smears that were PCR positive.[47]

In contrast with these findings, the organism is not found in the epidermis of the intact skin, although it may be present in ulcerated lesions, usually in much lower numbers than found in nasal secretions. The organism has also been found in high concentration in the blood of lepromatous cases[48] and in the breast milk of patients with active MB disease.[49] Some investigators speculate that *M. leprae* may be infectious by direct skin contact. The more common occurrence of the initial leprosy lesions on exposed skin is sometimes cited as evidence for this site of entry of the organisms.[50] However, since the organisms are known to grow better in cooler, exposed skin, this could influence the distribution of lesions. There are reports of inoculation of *M. leprae* by tattooing or bacillus Calmette-Guérin (BCG) injection, leading to clinical leprosy at the site of inoculation, many years later.[43] Some special exposures in some populations (e.g., Micronesia) in which leprosy is epidemic, such as sharing of bamboo sleeping mats with an active case, could result in the transmission of *M. leprae* by direct inoculation of organisms from an infectious case into the skin (J. Douglas, personal communication).

Reservoir. Viable *M. leprae* have been recovered from arthropods including mosquitoes and bed bugs who have fed on lepromatous patients.[51] Cochrane noted that, even when malaria prevalence was equal in adjacent villages in India, leprosy prevalence differed significantly, suggesting that, at least anopheline transmission of *M. leprae* was not important.[52] Some investigators suggested that the original site of *M. leprae* entry could condition the host immune response to the organism; skin or upper respiratory penetration could more readily provoke a TH-1-type lymphocyte response, whereas the lower respiratory or oral route could lead to a TH-2-type lymphocyte response and progression of infection to lepromatous disease.[53]

Infectious human cases almost certainly are the most important reservoir of *M. leprae* (and *M. lepromatosis*) for human infections globally. In addition, there are reports of isolation of noncultivatable mycobacteria resembling *M. leprae* from several environmental sites, including soil, sphagnum moss, and thorns[54]; leprosy infections are also endemic in feral armadillos.[55]

Infection with *M. leprae* occurs among nine-banded armadillos (*D. novemcinctus*) in the Gulf Coast region of the United States.[14,15,56] In addition to carrying *M. leprae* genotypes seen in other parts of the world, two unique genotypes have been found in armadillos and in human patients in this region that have not been found elsewhere. Some reports indicate that the zoonosis in nine-banded armadillos also extends to Central and South America. These findings suggest that the armadillo may be an important reservoir in the western hemisphere, and that programs to control or eliminate leprosy there must consider the implications of zoonotic transmission in addition to human transmission. In addition, there is now experimental evidence that *M. leprae* can be ingested by ticks (*Amblyomma sculptum*), survive in their midgut, and infect their eggs and larvae.[57] Infected larvae were able to inoculate *M. leprae* in blood feeding on a rabbit. If confirmed, these findings indicate another potential reservoir and vector for *M. leprae* transmission, which would further complicate efforts at control and elimination of *M. leprae*.

Prevalence and Incidence. The prevalence of leprosy varies widely in different populations but generally involves 0.01–2.0% of the population in areas where the disease is endemic. Although leprosy may occur in infants and young children, it is rare in children under 7 years old; this is likely due to the long incubation period between exposure and the onset of clinical symptoms. The incubation period was estimated through military personnel and missionaries who returned to the United States or Europe from endemic areas. These data indicate that the incubation period is longer for lepromatous (median of 8–12 years) than it is for tuberculoid disease (median of 2–5 years).[58] These studies are also the basis for the estimate that only approximately 5% of the adult population may be susceptible.

The incidence of leprosy peaks between the ages of 10 years and 29 years.[43,59,60] The rates of new cases are at least 5- to 10-fold higher in persons with a close contact in the household.[43,59,60] Leprosy incidence rates rarely exceed 2 per 1000 persons per year, except in persons with a household contact with an active case. A prospective study in Malawi found the incidence to be 1.2 per 1000 persons per year and the rates were significantly higher (RR = 1.65) in persons who had not had BCG vaccination.[61] India contributes the largest number of cases annually, and a recent national survey revealed an overall new case detection rate of 27.7/100,000.[62] Notably, more than 50% of the new cases came from two provinces in North India—Uttar Pradesh and Bihar. Household crowding and a population's low socioeconomic status are important factors promoting *M. leprae* transmission and the development of clinical leprosy. A prospective study in Malawi found a lower incidence of leprosy in persons with less household crowding and higher levels of education.[63] Improving the standards of living may have been critical in the spontaneous disappearance of leprosy from several countries, such as Norway, where the disease had been endemic in the nineteenth and early twentieth centuries.[64]

It is likely that genetic susceptibility may be one of the important factors contributing to the risk of leprosy and in the type of leprosy that develops after exposure. A twin study found higher concordance rates for leprosy among 62 monozygotic twin pairs (60%) than among 40 dizygotic twin pairs (20%).[65] However, this important study may have been affected by recruitment bias, since more monozygotic than dizygotic twins were studied. Several studies of human lymphocyte antigen (HLA) distributions of leprosy patients found significant associations with certain HLA haplotypes.[66–69] A segregation analysis of leprosy in families with multiple cases suggested that the genetic susceptibility may differ between tuberculoid and lepromatous disease.[70] More recent studies linked leprosy susceptibility to the human NRAMP1 gene[71] and to the Parkinson's disease susceptibility genes PARK2 and PRCRG on chromosome 6.[72] This continues to be a very active area of investigation and has been discussed in detail by Fava and Schurr.[73] Depending on geographic location, the proportion of multibacillary and PB cases in different populations varies considerably. A much higher proportion of lepromatous cases was observed in Southeast Asia than in Africa, where most cases are tuberculoid.[74] Whether these differences are due to host differences (such as genetic or nutritional factors), epidemiological factors influencing the route or age at the time of exposure, the size of the inoculum, or to differences in the strains of *M. leprae* in different areas of the world is not known. However, as noted above, *M. leprae* strains from different areas of the world have very little genetic diversity. The inability to culture the organism and the lack of an easily manipulated animal model that develops a disease similar to that seen in humans has hindered investigations of these important scientific questions.

Interaction of HIV and Leprosy. The pandemic of human immunodeficiency virus (HIV) infection and acquired immunodeficiency syndrome (AIDS) has markedly increased the incidence of several mycobacterial infections, particularity *M. tuberculosis* and *M. avium-intracellulare*. This has led to concerns that HIV infection might also increase the rates of leprosy in areas of the world where both HIV and *M. leprae* are epidemic. Theoretically, immunosuppression from HIV could affect the transmission of *M. leprae* by increasing the prevalence of multibacillary forms of leprosy, which could be more readily transmitted. If true, the interaction between HIV infection and leprosy could produce a higher proportion of multibacillary cases, a greater incidence, and more frequent relapses after a course of therapy.[75]

Several studies of the interaction between HIV and *M. leprae* have been reported from areas of the world where both leprosy and HIV infections are common. Most of these studies have not found HIV infections to have a significant impact on the number of new leprosy cases.[76–78] Case-control studies in Malawi,[79] Uganda,[80] and Yemen[81] failed to show a significantly higher HIV antibody prevalence among leprosy patients than in control subjects. In addition, these studies did not find a higher proportion of multibacillary leprosy cases among patients infected with HIV than in those who were HIV uninfected. However, a small hospital-based study in Zambia found a higher HIV prevalence rate in leprosy patients than control subjects.[82] A larger community-based case-control study in Tanzania, in which leprosy cases and control subjects were matched by their geographic areas of residence, found an association between HIV infection and leprosy in those from rural areas and in those with multibacillary leprosy.[83]

The different findings in these studies could be explained by several factors. The rates of leprosy are higher in rural populations, whereas HIV infections often are concentrated among urban populations. Therefore, overlap between the epidemics of leprosy and HIV/AIDS may not have occurred yet in some countries where both diseases are epidemic. While the effects of HIV infection certainly are not as evident for leprosy as they have been for tuberculosis, further evaluation of this interaction is warranted before definite conclusions are drawn.

There is no evidence that active leprosy accelerates HIV progression, as has been reported in tuberculosis patients.[84] However, in coinfected individuals, antiretroviral treatment has been associated with the development of Type 1 leprosy reactions. This is considered to be an example of the immune reconstitution inflammatory syndrome in leprosy.[85,86] One intriguing study[87] in rhesus monkeys who were inoculated with *M. leprae* suggested that those monkeys who were co-infected with Simian immunodeficiency virus (SIV) were more likely to progress to LL. Nevertheless, the published studies did not report a significant interaction between HIV and *M. leprae*.

TREATMENT AND REHABILITATION

Antileprosy Drugs. At present, three drugs are commonly used for the treatment of leprosy: dapsone, rifampin, and clofazimine. The use of ethionamide-prothionamide was abandoned due to its hepatotoxicity and the availability of better alternative drugs. Dapsone and clofazimine have weak bactericidal activity against *M. leprae*, and rifampin has potent bactericidal activity against nearly all strains of the organism. However, a few strains of *M. leprae* that are resistant to rifampin have been reported.[88] Other drugs were recently shown to have good antibacterial activity against *M. leprae* including ofloxacin, moxifloxacin, minocycline, and clarithromycin. Isoniazid, an important first-line drug for treating tuberculosis, is ineffective for treating leprosy.

Dapsone. The usual dose is 100 mg daily for adults and 1.0 mg per kg per day for children. It is a safe, cheap, and effective drug for treating all types of leprosy. Strains of *M. leprae* that are fully sensitive to dapsone have a minimal inhibitory concentration (MIC) of about 0.003 mg per mL, as determined in the mouse footpad assay. Although doses of 100 mg per day of dapsone exceed the MIC by a factor of nearly 500-fold, the increasing prevalence of mild, moderate, or complete resistance to dapsone among *M. leprae* organisms, either in untreated leprosy (primary resistance) or emergence of resistance during treatment (secondary resistance), and the relatively weak bactericidal action of the drug have dictated the current recommendation for treatment at the 100-mg daily dosage. Because of the problem of dapsone resistance, the drug should always be used in combination with rifampin and/or clofazimine for treating active leprosy (Table 135-1).[32]

The most common side effect of dapsone therapy is anemia. However, this is usually very mild and well tolerated, unless the patient has a complete glucose-6-phosphate dehydrogenase (G6PD) deficiency, in which case the anemia may be more severe. Therefore, it is wise to screen patients for complete (G6PD) deficiency prior to instituting therapy with dapsone. More serious but, fortunately, very rare side effects of dapsone include agranulocytosis, exfoliative dermatitis, hepatitis, and a syndrome termed the "dapsone syndrome," which includes hepatitis and a generalized rash and can progress to exfoliation. Since these more serious toxic effects generally occur soon after initiation of therapy, patients should be seen periodically, and complete blood counts and liver enzymes should be measured after therapy has begun.

Rifampin. Because of its excellent bactericidal activity against *M. leprae*, rifampin is included in the therapy of leprosy patients. Patients with LL who are treated with a drug regimen that includes rifampin will become noncontagious after only 1 week of treatment, or less.[89] The recommended adult daily dose in the United States is 600 mg; children should be treated with 10–20 mg per kg, not to exceed 600 mg per day. In the 1980s, the cost of daily administration of rifampin was sometimes prohibitive for leprosy control programs in the developing world; however, the very slow replication of *M. leprae* permits administration of the drug once monthly. The alternative regimen recommended by WHO for leprosy control programs in developing countries includes administration of 600 mg of rifampin at monthly intervals as directly observed therapy. This regimen of monthly administration of rifampin was shown to be equivalent to daily doses. The major toxic side effect of rifampin is hepatotoxicity. Generally, rifampin should be discontinued if the alanine transaminase (ALT) (SGPT) or aspartate transaminase (AST) (SGOT) levels increase to more than 2.5–5.0 times the upper limit of normal. Rifabutin, a drug licensed for therapy of *M. avium* complex infections, also has bactericidal activity against *M. leprae*.

Clofazimine. Clofazimine is an iminophenazine dye with antimycobacterial activity roughly equivalent to that of dapsone. It is a useful drug for controlling leprosy reactions, since it also has some anti-inflammatory activity. The usual adult daily dose is 50–100 mg. Higher doses of 200–300 mg daily have more pronounced anti-inflammatory activity but are more likely to lead to gastrointestinal toxicity with long-term use. In addition, clofazimine has been used in doses of 100 mg three times weekly for the chronic treatment of leprosy. The drug is deposited in the skin and slowly released, thus providing a repository effect in chronic therapy.

The most frequent side effect of clofazimine therapy is reddish-black pigmentation of the skin. The degree of pigmentation is dose related. However, in many patients the pigmentation tends not to be uniform but is concentrated in the areas of the lesions, producing a blotchy pigmentation that many patients consider to be unsightly. Since virtually all fair-skinned patients will have some pigmentation

TABLE 135-1 MULTIDRUG REGIMENS FOR TREATMENT OF LEPROSY

Age Group	Drug	Dosage	Multibacillary Duration	Paucibacillary (PB) Duration
Adult (>15 years)	Rifampin	600 mg once a month	12 months	6 months (Clofazimine not universally used for PB patients)[a]
	Dapsone	100 mg daily		
	Clofazimine	300 mg once a month and 50 mg daily		
Children 10–14 years old	Rifampin	450 mg once a month	12 months	6 months (Clofazimine not universally used for PB patients)[a]
	Dapsone	50 mg daily		
	Clofazimine	150 mg once a month and 50 mg daily		
Children < 10 or < 40 kg	Rifampin	10 mg/kg once a month	12 months	6 months (Clofazimine not universally used for PB patients)[a]
	Dapsone	2 mg/kg daily		
	Clofazimine	6 mg/kg once a month and 1 mg/kg daily		

Source: Modified with permission from World Health Organization. Guidelines for the diagnosis, treatment and prevention of leprosy. 2018. https://zeroleprosy.org/wp-content/uploads/2018/08/WHO-Guidelines-Web-Version.pdf.

[a]Some experts are concerned about risk-benefit of clofazimine in paucibacillary patients and recommend treatment with rifampin and dapsone without clofazimine. Current U.S. guidelines are available at https://www.hrsa.gov/hansens-disease/diagnosis/recommended-treatment.html.

with clofazimine therapy, it also serves as a useful marker of drug compliance. The pigmentation is slowly cleared 6–12 months or more after therapy is discontinued.

Aside from pigmentation, the major side effects of clofazimine therapy involve the gastrointestinal tract. Patients may develop abdominal cramps, sometimes associated with nausea, vomiting, and diarrhea. On high doses of clofazimine (over 100 mg daily), these symptoms are common after more than 3–6 months of therapy. Radiographic studies of the small bowel may show a pattern compatible with malabsorption. Fortunately, these symptoms usually are reversible when the drug is discontinued.

Other side effects include anticholinergic activity, which may result in diminished sweating and tearing. Since LL can cause autonomic nerve involvement, patients commonly have ichthyosis from their decreased sweating, and this problem may be intensified by clofazimine.

Ofloxacin. A number of fluoroquinolones have been developed; many of these drugs, such as ciprofloxacin, are not active against *M. leprae*. Among those that are active against *M. leprae* are ofloxacin[90,91] and moxifloxacin. These drugs interfere with bacterial DNA replication by inhibiting the enzyme DNA gyrase. They were shown, in animal and short-term human experiments, to have good bactericidal activity against *M. leprae*. Ofloxacin is absorbed well orally and generally given in a dose of 400 mg once daily.

Minocycline. Minocycline is the only member of the tetracycline group of antibiotics that has significant bactericidal activity against *M. leprae*.[92] The standard dose is 100 mg daily, which gives a peak serum level that exceeds the MIC of minocycline against *M. leprae* by a factor of 10–20. Although the drug is tolerated relatively well, in some patients, vestibular toxicity was reported.

Clarithromycin. Among the macrolide antibiotics, clarithromycin is the only drug shown to have significant bactericidal activity against *M. leprae*. When given in a daily dose of 500 mg to patients with LL, 99% of bacilli were killed within 28 days and 99.9% were killed by 56 days.[93] The drug is relatively nontoxic; however, gastrointestinal irritation, nausea, vomiting, and diarrhea are the most common side effects.

Treatment Regimens. The standard therapy for leprosy should include MDT for all forms of the disease.[32] Prior to the early 1980s, patients were often treated with dapsone alone. This led to the emergence of dapsone resistance and rendered further dapsone therapy ineffective in many areas. In 1981, a WHO study group met to recommend new treatment regimens for leprosy control programs. The WHO study group reviewed the data on both the resistance of *M. leprae* organisms to dapsone and their sensitivity to rifampin and clofazimine and recommended that MDT be used to treat all active cases of leprosy (Table 135-1). The WHO recommended the treatment of patients with paucibacillary disease with 100 mg (1–2 mg per kg) of dapsone daily, unsupervised, and 600 mg of rifampin once a month as directly observed therapy for 6 months. Patients with multibacillary leprosy are to be treated with dapsone 100 mg daily, clofazimine 50 mg daily, both self-administered, and rifampin 600 mg once monthly and clofazimine 300 mg once monthly, both supervised for at least 2 years under the WHO protocol. Patients in whom acid-fast organisms were identified on their slit-skin smears or skin biopsies prior to treatment should be treated with the regimen for multibacillary disease. In addition, patients with currently "inactive" leprosy, who have had only monotherapy with dapsone, should be given MDT to prevent relapse.

In 2018, the WHO announced a new recommendation that all patients (PB and MB) should be treated with the three-drug combination of dapsone, clofazimine, and rifampin (U-MDT).[32,94] The recommendation is that PB patients should be treated for 6 months and MB patients treated for 12 months. The strongest evidence for the efficacy of this regimen comes from a randomized controlled trial in Brazil.[95] The three-drug, 6-month regimen is judged to be better than the two-drug, 6-month regimen, although there are concerns that the pigmentation associated with clofazimine may discourage some PB patients from taking this drug.

Trials of a single dose of a combination of rifampin, ofloxacin, and minocycline (ROM), have indicated that this regimen is not as effective as standard MDT, even in paucibacillary cases.[96,97] The possibility that multiple doses of ROM might be effective remains to be determined.

Relapse, Reaction, and Re-infection. Relapse rates have varied from 20 per 1000 person-years among patients in India with multibacillary leprosy who were treated for 2 years to 10 per 1000 person-years in persons treated until they were smear negative.[98] Higher relapse rates have been reported in patients with a high bacterial index (BI $\geq$ 4.0). In lepromatous patients with high BI, relapses have occurred in some patients as long as 15 years after completing treatment.[99] The development of new lesions after completion of treatment is much more likely to be due to reaction (~40%) than to relapse (~2–4%) or drug resistance.

Low levels of dapsone resistance are still encountered, particularly in areas where dapsone monotherapy has been used.[100] Resistance to rifampin or ofloxacin are rare, and no confirmed cases of clofazimine resistance have been observed. The WHO and the International Federation of Anti-Leprosy Organizations (ILEP) implemented a sentinel network of global surveillance for drug resistance in leprosy from 2008 to 2014.[101] This working group has now recommended testing in all countries for mutations associated with drug resistance. In the United States, all biopsies submitted to the National Hansen's Disease Programs are tested for resistance-associated mutations.

Relapses cannot be differentiated clinically from reinfection, which is problematic since patients usually continue to live in the same communities in which they were initially infected with *M. leprae*. However, recent studies using whole genome sequencing have demonstrated that reinfection with a different *M. leprae* genotype can occur and that differentiation of reinfection is technically possible in some instances.[102]

Patients should be followed at frequent intervals after treatment is started. Follow-up should include examination for new skin lesions, new areas of anesthesia, new motor deficits, enlargement or tenderness of nerves, changes in visual acuity or other ocular symptoms, and clinical evidence of reactions. In addition, annual skin biopsies are useful in documenting changes in disease status. Slit-skin smears are helpful in estimating the bacillary load of acid-fast organisms remaining in the skin. These smears are done by pinching the skin to reduce bleeding, cleaning with alcohol, and making a superficial skin slit through the epidermis with a scalpel blade and transferring the subepidermal fluid to a circular area 5–6 mm in diameter on a clean glass slide. Slit-skin smears are taken from six or more sites (e.g., earlobe, eyebrow, trunk, elbow, thigh, and knee) at 6- to 12-month intervals and stained using the Fite-Faraco acid-fast stain. The bacteriologic index (BI) is a semiquantitative logarithmic estimate of the number of organisms in the skin (Table 135-2). With effective therapy of lepromatous patients, the average BI should decrease at a rate of about 0.5–1 log each year. Failure of the BI to fall suggests poor compliance with therapy or infection with drug-resistant organisms. The National Hansen's Disease Programs in Baton Rouge, Louisiana (https://www.hrsa.gov/hansens-disease/index.html), will stain and examine slides prepared by the slit-skin smear technique. Inactive leprosy is defined as a BI of zero on slit-skin smear, no active lesions on skin biopsy, and no clinical evidence of disease activity for at least 1 year. In cases of intolerance to one of the primary drugs (i.e., dapsone, clofazimine, or rifampin) or drug-resistant organisms, one of the other antileprosy drugs can be substituted (i.e., ofloxacin, minocycline, or clarithromycin).

Treatment of Reactions. Reactions are common during leprosy treatment and complicate the outcome of therapy. Educating patients to recognize and seek prompt treatment for reactions is essential for

TABLE 135-2 THE BACTERIAL INDEX

BI	Number of Organisms
0	No bacilli in 100 OIF
1+	1–10 bacilli per 100 OIF
2+	1–10 bacilli per 10 OIF
3+	1–10 bacilli per OIF
4+	10–100 bacilli per OIF
5+	100–1000 bacilli per OIF
6+	Over 1000 bacilli per OIF

Abbreviation:OIF = oil immersion fields.

a successful therapeutic outcome. These reactions, especially those involving major nerves or the eyes, can cause permanent incapacitation if they are not promptly recognized and properly treated.

Type 1 Reactions. The most important goals in treating Type 1 reactions (reversal reactions) are to prevent nerve damage, control severe inflammation, and prevent necrosis of skin lesions.[103] Antileprosy chemotherapy should not be interrupted during the reaction. In mild reactions, especially those without neuritis or facial lesions, treatment with analgesics and anti-inflammatory agents and close observation may suffice. However, any reaction where there is evidence of acute neuritis with pain, tenderness, or loss of nerve function should be treated with corticosteroids, starting with prednisone in doses of 40–60 mg per day. It should be noted that the metabolism of prednisone is accelerated in patients who are also receiving rifampin, and it is advisable to reduce rifampin to once monthly for the duration of prednisone treatment. The patient may need hospitalization and should be closely observed with frequent voluntary muscle tests (VMTs) to evaluate nerve weakness. The dose of prednisone may be reduced by 5–10 mg every 1–2 weeks until a maintenance dose of 20–25 mg is reached. It can then be reduced slowly over the course of 6 months or more while repeating VMT and watching for the reaction to recur. In severe cases, prednisone treatment for several months may be required. Careful management of Type 1 reactions is essential to prevent long-term sequelae.

Type 2 Reactions. Although type II (ENL) reactions are important because of their frequency and potential for organ damage, mild reactions can sometimes be managed with anti-inflammatory agents, such as salicylates or nonsteroidal anti-inflammatory agents. However, severe or persistent ENL often requires therapy with corticosteroids, thalidomide, or clofazimine singly or in combination. Commonly, prednisone in doses of 40–60 mg is given, and the patient is started on 400 mg per day of thalidomide. Steroids can be reduced or withdrawn, and the ENL can be controlled in some cases with thalidomide alone. Although thalidomide is often effective in controlling ENL reactions, it cannot be given to women of childbearing age unless they are following a foolproof method of contraception, since the drug is highly teratogenic. In the United States, thalidomide is only available at selected pharmacies, through the Celgene REMS Program (http://www.thalomidrems.com/). Clofazimine in doses of 100–300 mg per day has anti-inflammatory effects, but gastrointestinal toxicity is common when the drug is continued at this dose for more than 2–3 months. Some patients will require chronic steroid therapy to suppress their ENL reaction, which can persist for several months. Alternative immunosuppressive treatment for ENL has been attempted using methotrexate, cyclosporin, and other immunosuppressive agents,[104] but none of these have been successful when used alone. However, some of these are used as steroid-sparing agents to try to reduce the dose of prednisone needed in long-term treatment of some patients.

Complications. Important complications of leprosy, such as neuritis, iridocyclitis, orchitis, and glomerulonephritis, may occur during reactions. Therefore, it is important that leprosy patients be carefully monitored at frequent intervals, especially while the disease is active. If available, baseline slit lamp examination of the eyes is recommended. Iridocyclitis commonly accompanies type II reactions and may cause blindness in leprosy. Another cause of visual damage in leprosy is keratitis secondary to lagophthalmos and corneal anesthesia arising from damage to the facial and trigeminal nerves. Acute iridocyclitis should be treated with mydriatics, such as 1% atropine or 0.25% scopolamine, and anti-inflammatory drugs, such as 1% hydrocortisone.

Patients should be trained to avoid injuries to anesthetic areas and to report injuries promptly, even in the absence of pain. Sensory loss (to the point of compromised protective sensation) is often more severe than is generally appreciated.[105] In addition to sensory loss, many leprosy patients experience neuropathic pain.[106] Frequent inspection of the feet and hands and special footwear constructed to prevent permanent damage to deformed and anesthetic feet are important aspects of the care of leprosy patients. Reconstructive surgery, such as tibialis posterior muscle transfer to correct footdrop, and temporalis muscle transplant to correct lagophthalmos, may be important in treating some patients. Patients who have ocular problems should be seen by an ophthalmologist. Patients with permanent sensory or motor loss need frequent reminders about the risk of painless injury from cuts and burns and may need special orthotics or other protective measures for life.

CONTROL AND PREVENTION

Three basic approaches have been used to control and prevent leprosy, namely:

1. Early detection and supervised chemotherapy of active cases, as described above;
2. Postexposure prophylaxis (PEP) with rifampin or dapsone; and
3. Immunization: BCG or a defined subunit vaccine (LepVax).

Active searching for cases is important for controlling leprosy where the disease is endemic. Especially important is periodic screening and follow-up of household contacts of newly diagnosed cases. In leprosy endemic areas, it is important to train healthcare professionals to recognize and treat leprosy. Healthcare facilities, such as general or skin disease clinics, can provide screening and appropriate leprosy therapy in an atmosphere that is not stigmatizing. Screening of special populations, such as school children, laborers, or military populations can be useful in detecting early leprosy in some highly endemic populations.

Children with close contact with someone with paucibacillary (tuberculoid) leprosy are also at some increased risk; however, their risk is less, so they should be examined every 6–12 months for several years after this exposure, and biopsies should be obtained of any suspicious lesions in order to detect and institute treatment soon after clinical disease appears. The rate of leprosy in household members in the 10 years after close household contacts with someone with untreated LL was reported to be about 11% after 10 years follow-up in careful studies by Worth and Hirschy in Hawaii and Hong Kong.[107,108] When the index case had tuberculoid leprosy, the incidence in household contacts was reported to be 0.5%. A study of 80,000 disease-free persons in a rural district of northern Malawi found 331 incident cases of leprosy on follow-up in the 1980s.[109] Persons having dwelling contact with a multibacillary case had an eightfold higher incidence and those whose contact was with a paucibacillary case had a twofold greater incidence than those without household contact. However, only 15% of new leprosy cases occurred in those who had household contact with leprosy.

A study of prophylaxis with dapsone, 25 mg per kg, was conducted in the Marquesas Islands in the late 1980s. Although this appeared promising at first, it was determined ultimately that this had little effect.[110] A randomized controlled study of dapsone prophylaxis, using a 50-mg daily dose for 3 years in household contacts, found a 52.5% reduction in leprosy in the 12 years after exposure in those who received dapsone.[111]

Recently, interest has grown in the use of single-dose rifampin (SDR) for PEP against leprosy.[112] A trial of SDR in contacts of new cases in Bangladesh showed a protective effect of 56% over 2 years,[113] although this benefit was not demonstrated beyond 2 years or in follow up after 6 years. Notably, as also seen in earlier dapsone prophylaxis studies, the SDR regimen had the least benefit on those most closely associated with the index case. However, several endemic countries have now implemented SDR or similar PEP regimens as research initiatives or as a national policy for leprosy prevention.[114]

Leprosy Vaccines: BCG and LepVax

The initial experimental evidence for the possible preventive efficacy of BCG was reported by Shepard in 1966.[115] He found that vaccinating mice with BCG prevented experimental infection from footpad inoculation with viable *M. leprae*. Subsequently, several randomized trials of BCG in human populations were done. A trial in Uganda, where most leprosy is tuberculoid, showed an 80% protective efficacy of BCG[116]; another trial in Karimui, New Guinea, found 48% efficacy[117]; and a third trial in Burma found an efficacy of 20% (however, the efficacy was 38% in children from 0 to 4 years of age and when a second more immunogenic lot of freeze-dried BCG was used).[118] A more recent trial of BCG in Malawi found that the incidence of leprosy was reduced by 50% after a second inoculation of BCG, but no additional efficacy was associated with inclusion of heat-killed *M. leprae* with BCG.[119] In summary, these controlled studies of BCG, together with several case-control studies,[120,121] suggest that BCG affords significant but incomplete protection against leprosy in several populations. However, vaccines prepared from heat-killed *M. leprae* were not efficacious.[20]

A new candidate leprosy vaccine, LepVax,[122] has now been developed. This is a defined subunit vaccine composed of a tetravalent fusion protein in emulsion with a Toll-like receptor (TLR-4) based adjuvant. When injected prophylactically, this vaccine reduced the *M. leprae* burden in a mouse footpad model. Immunized mice generated an interferon-γ response to crude *M. leprae* antigens. In subsequent testing in experimentally infected armadillos, this vaccine delayed conduction abnormalities in motor nerve and decreased the extent of morphological abnormalities in sensory nerves. BCG immunization of another group of armadillos did not have this beneficial effect but, instead, precipitated nerve conduction abnormalities. The new subunit vaccine is in advanced stages of Phase 1 clinical trials, and Phase 2 clinical trials are now being organized in endemic countries.

In recent years, the widespread use of effective MDT for leprosy under direct supervision, the earlier diagnosis of leprosy, the reduction of the stigma previously associated with this disease in many societies, and the routine use of BCG in many leprosy endemic countries led to a decline in new leprosy cases.[122–124] Many experts are cautiously optimistic that this trend will continue in the future and that the public health importance of leprosy will continue to decline,[124,125] as long as the effort to control this disease persists. The long-term outlook for controlling leprosy as a public health problem is good, as long as the effective prevention efforts are not abandoned prematurely. However, many experts are concerned that leprosy control efforts might be terminated too soon by assuming that a prevalence rate of under 1 per 10,000 population signifies that leprosy has been "eliminated" permanently as a public health problem.[20,32,126] A newly organized Global Partnership for Zero Leprosy (https://zeroleprosy.org/) seeks to coordinate the many antileprosy efforts that continue worldwide, aiming to standardize diagnostic techniques and treatment regimens, coordinate PEP initiatives, promote efforts at early detection and the reduction of disabilities and stigma, and encourage research on the major issues that still obstruct progress toward the control and elimination of leprosy.

References

1. Nolen L, Haberling D, Scollard D, et al. Incidence of Hansen's disease—United States, 1994–2011. *MMWR Morb Mortal Wkly Rep.* 2014;63(43):969–72.
2. Han XY, Seo YH, Sizer KC, et al. A new *Mycobacterium* species causing diffuse lepromatous leprosy. *Am J Clin Pathol.* 2008;130(6):856–64.
3. Shepard CC. The experimental disease that follows the injection of human leprosy bacilli into foot-pads of mice. *J Exp Med.* 1960;112:445–54.
4. Walsh GP, et al. Experimental leprosy, workshop 5. *Int J Lepr Other Mycobact Dis.* 1993;61(4 Suppl):733–6.
5. Kirchheimer WF, Storrs CC. Attempts to establish the armadillo (*Dasypus novemcinctus*) as a model for the study of leprosy. *Int J Lepr Other Mycobact Dis.* 1971;39:693–702.
6. Gormus BJ, Wolf RH, Baskin GB, et al. A second sooty mangabey monkey with naturally acquired leprosy. *Int J Lepr Other Mycobact Dis.* 1988;56:61–5.
7. Simpson V, Hargreaves J, Butler H, Blackett T, Stevenson K, McLuckie J. Leprosy in red squirrels on the Isle of Wight and Brownsea Island. *Vet Rec.* 2015;177(8):206–7.
8. Meredith A, Del Pozo J, Smith S, Milne E, Stevenson K, McLuckie J. Leprosy in red squirrels in Scotland. *Vet Rec.* 2014;175(11):285–6.
9. Avanzi C, Del-Pozo J, Benjak A, et al. Red squirrels in the British Isles are infected with leprosy bacilli. *Science.* 2016;354(6313):744–7.
10. Singh P, Benjak A, Schuenemann VJ, et al. Insight into the evolution and origin of leprosy bacilli from the genome sequence of *Mycobacterium lepromatosis. Proc Natl Acad Sci.* 2015;112(14):4459–64.
11. Cole ST, Eiglmeier K, Parkhill J, et al. Massive gene decay in the leprosy bacillus. *Nature.* 2001;409:107–11.
12. Monot M, Honore N, Garnier T, et al. On the origin of Leprosy. *Science.* 2005;308:1040–2.
13. Gillis T, Vissa V, Matsuoka M, et al. Characterization of short tandem repeats for genotyping *Mycobacterium leprae. Lepr Rev.* 2009;80(3):250–60.
14. Truman RW, Singh P, Sharma R, et al. Probable zoonotic leprosy in the southern United States. *N Engl J Med.* 2011;364(17):1626–33.
15. Sharma R, Singh P, Loughry WJ, et al. Zoonotic leprosy in the southeastern United States. *Emerg Infect Dis.* 2015;21(12):2127–34.
16. Kimura M, Sakamuri RM, Groathouse NA, et al. Rapid variable-number tandem-repeat genotyping for *Mycobacterium leprae* clinical specimens. *J Clin Microbiol.* 2009;47(6):1757–66.
17. Ridley DS, Jopling WH. Classification of leprosy according to immunity. A five-group system. *Int J Lepr Other Mycobact Dis.* 1966;34:255–73.
18. World Health Organization. Leprosy elimination. *Classification of Leprosy.* https://www.who.int/lep/classification/en/. 2018.
19. Scollard DM, Smith T, Bhoopat L, et al. Epidemiologic characteristics of leprosy reactions. *Int J Lepr Other Mycobact Dis.* 1994;62:559–67.
20. Scollard DM, Adams LB, Gillis TP, et al. The continuing challenge of leprosy. *Clin Micro Rev.* 2006;19:338–81.
21. Modlin RL, Melancon-Kaplan J, Young SM. Learning from lesions: Patterns of tissue inflammation in leprosy. *Proc Natl Acad Sci U S A.* 1988;85:1213–7.
22. Shepard CC, Saitz CW. Lepromin and tuberculin reactivity in adults not exposed to leprosy. *J Immunol.* 1967;99:637–42.
23. Hunter SW, Brennan PJ. A novel glycolipid from *Mycobacterium leprae* possibly involved in immunogenicity and pathogenicity. *J Bacteriol.* 1981;147:725–35.
24. Geluk A, Duthie MS, Spencer JS. Postgenomic *Mycobacterium leprae* antigens for cellular and serological diagnosis of *M. leprae* exposure, infection and leprosy disease. *Lepr Rev.* 2011;82(4):402–21.
25. Bobosha K, Tjon Kon Fat EM, van den Eeden SJ, et al. Field-evaluation of a new lateral flow assay for detection of cellular and humoral immunity against *Mycobacterium leprae. PLoS Negl Trop Dis.* 2014;8:e2845.
26. Irgens LM. Leprosy in Norway—An epidemiological study based on a national patient registry. *Lepr Rev.* 1980;51(Suppl):1–130.
27. Feldman RA, Sturdivant M. Leprosy in the United States, 1950–1969: An epidemiologic review. *South Med J.* 1976;69:920–9.
28. WHO SEARO/Department of Control of Neglected Tropical Diseases. In: Cooreman EA, ed. *Operational Manual: Global Leprosy Strategy 2016–2020; Accelerating Towards a Leprosy-free World.* WHO. 2016, Table 1, p. 2.

29. Nordeen SK. Elimination of leprosy as a public health problem. *Int J Lepr Other Mycobact Dis.* 1994;62:278–83.
30. World Health Organization. Global leprosy update, 2017: Reducing the disease burden due to leprosy. *Wkly Epidemiol Rec.* 2018;35(93):445–56.
31. Lockwood DNJ. Leprosy elimination—A virtual phenomenon or a reality. *BMJ.* 2002;324:1516–8.
32. World Health Organization. Guidelines for the diagnosis, treatment and prevention of leprosy. 2018. https://zeroleprosy.org/wp-content/uploads/2018/08/WHO-Guidelines-Web-Version.pdf.
33. Jesudasan K, Vijayakumaran P, Pannikarvk, et al. Impact of MDT on leprosy as measured by selective indicators. *Lepr Rev.* 1988;59:215–33.
34. Bechelli LM. Prospects of global elimination of leprosy as a public health problem by the year 2000. *Int J Lepr Other Mycobact Dis.* 1994;62:284–92.
35. Basel P, Pahan D, Moet FJ, Oskam L, Richardus JH. Leprosy incidence: Six years follow-up of a population cohort in Bangladesh. *Lepr Rev.* 2014;85:158–69.
36. Kumar A, Girdhar A, Chakma JK, Girdhar BK. Detection of previously undetected leprosy cases in Firozabad District (U.P.), India during 2006–2009: A short communication. *Lepr Rev.* 2013;84:124–7.
37. Meima A, Smith WC, van Oortmarssen GJ, Richardus JH, Habbema JD. The future incidence of leprosy: A scenario analysis. *Bull World Health Organ.* 2004;82:373–80.
38. Smith WC, van Brakel W, Gillis T, Saunderson P, Richardus JH. The missing millions: A threat to the elimination of leprosy. *PLoS Negl Trop Dis.* 2015;9(4):e0003658.
39 Badger LF. Leprosy in the United States. *Public Health Rep.* 1955;70(6):525–35.
40. Vigneron E. The epidemiological transition in an overseas territory: Disease mapping in French Polynesia. *Soc Sci Med.* 1989;28:913–22.
41. Wade HW, Ledowski V. The leprosy epidemic at Naura: A review with data on the status since 1937. *Int J Lepr Other Mycobact Dis.* 1952;20:1–29.
42. Newell KW. An epidemiologist's view of leprosy. *Bull World Health Organ.* 1966;34:827–57.
43. Fine PM. Leprosy: The epidemiology of a slow bacterium. *Epidemiol Rev.* 1982;4:161–88.
44. Davey TF, Rees RJW. The nasal discharge in leprosy: Clinical and bacteriological aspects. *Lepr Rev.* 1974;45:121–34.
45. Pattyn SR, Ursi D, Ieven M, et al. Detection of *Mycobacterium leprae* by the polymerase chain reaction in nasal swabs of leprosy patients and their contacts. *Int J Lepr Other Mycobact Dis.* 1993;61:389–93.
46. Gillis TT, Williams DL. Polymerase chain reaction and leprosy. *J Lepr.* 1991;59:311–6.
47. Klatser PR, van Beers S, Madjid B, et al. Detection of *Mycobacterium leprae* nasal carriers in populations for which leprosy is endemic. *J Clin Micro.* 1993;31:2947–51.
48. Drutz DJ, Chen TSN, Lu WH. The continuous bacteremia of lepromatous leprosy. *N Engl J Med.* 1972;287:159–64.
49. Pedley JC. The presence of *M. leprae* in human milk. *Lepr Rev.* 1967;38:239–4.
50. Leiker DL. On the mode of transmission of *Mycobacterium leprae. Lepr Rev.* 1977;48:9–16.
51. Kirchheimer WF. The role of arthropods in the transmission of leprosy. *Int J Lepr Other Mycobact Dis.* 1976;44:104–7.
52. Cochrane RA. Epidemiology. In: *A Practical Textbook of Leprosy*. London: Oxford University Press; 1947, pp. 10–22.
53. Challacombe SJ, Tomasi TB. Systemic tolerance and secretory immunity after oral immunization. *J Exp Med.* 1980;152:1459–72.
54. Blake LA, West BC, Cary CH, et al. Environmental non-human sources of leprosy. *Rev Infect Dis.* 1987;9:562–77.
55. Walsh GP, Storrs LE, Burchfield HP, et al. Leprosy-like disease occurring naturally in armadillos. *J Reticuloendothelial Soc.* 1975;18:347–51.
56. Domozych R, Kim E, Hart S, Greenwald J. Increasing incidence of leprosy and transmission from armadillos in Central Florida: A case series. *JAAD Case Rep.* 2016;2(3):189–92.
57. Ferreira JS, Souza DA, Santos JP, et al. Ticks as potential vectors of *Mycobacterium* 1 *leprae:* Use of their cellular machinery to culture the bacilli and generate transgenic strains. *PLoS Negl Trop Dis.* 2018;12(12):e0007001.
58. Brubaker MC, Binford CH, Trautman JR. Occurrence of leprosy in U.S. veterans after service in endemic areas aboard. *Public Health Rep.* 1969;84:1051–8.
59. Doull JA, Guinto RS, Rodriquez JN, et al. The incidence of leprosy in Cordova and Talisey, Philippines. *Int J Lepr Other Mycobact Dis.* 1942;10:107–31.
60. Doull JA, Guinto RS, Rodriquez JN, et al. Risk of attack on leprosy in relation to age at exposure. *Int J Lepr Other Mycobact Dis.* 1945;13:435–9.
61. Ponnighaus JM, Fine PEM, Sterne JAC, et al. Incidence rates of leprosy in Karonga district, Northern Malawi: Patterns by age, sex, BCG status and classification. *Int J Lepr Other Mycobact Dis.* 1994;62:10–22.
62. Katoch K, Aggarwal A, Yadav VS, Pandey A. National sample survey to assess the new case disease burden of leprosy in India. *Indian J Med Res.* 2017;146(5):585–605.
63. Ponnighaus JM, Fine PEM, Sterne JAC, et al. Extended schooling and good housing conditions are associated with reduced risk of leprosy in rural Malawi. *Int J Lepr Other Mycobact Dis.* 1994;62:345–52.
64. Irgens LM, Skjerven R. Secular trends in age at onset, sex ratio, and type of index in leprosy observed during declining incidence rates. *Am J Epidemiol.* 1985;122:695–705.
65. Chakravarti MR, Vogel F. A twin study on leprosy. *Top Hum Genet.* 1973;1:1–123.
66. DeVries RR, Fat RF, Nijenhnis LE, et al. HLA-linked genetic control of host response to *Mycobacterium leprae. Lancet.* 1976;2:1328–30.
67. Fine PEM, Wolf E, Pritchard J, et al. HLA-linked genes and leprosy: A family study in a south Indian population. *J Infect Dis.* 1979;140:152–61.
68. DeVries RR, Van Eden W, Van Rood JJ. HLA-linked control of the course of *M. leprae* infections. *Lepr Rev.* 1981;52(Suppl):109–19.
69. Schauf V, Ryan S, Scollard DM, et al. Leprosy is associated with HLA-DR2 and DQW1 in the population of northern Thailand. *Tissue Antigens.* 1985;26:243–7.
70. Wagener DK, Schauf V, Nelson KE, et al. Segregation analysis of leprosy in northern Thailand. *Genet Epidemiol.* 1988;5:95–105.
71. Abel L, Sanchez FO, Oberti J, et al. Susceptibility to leprosy is linked to the human NRAMP1 gene. *J Infect Dis.* 1998;177:133–45.
72. Mira MT, Alcais A, Van Thuc N, et al. Susceptibility to leprosy is associated with PARK2 and PACRG. *Nature.* 2004;427:636–40.
73. Fava VM, Schurr E. The complexity of the host genetic contribution to the human response to Mycobacterium leprae. In: Scollard DM, Gillis TP eds. *International Textbook of Leprosy*. Greenville, SC: American Leprosy Missions; 2016, Ch. 8.1, pp. 1–33. www.internationaltextbookofleprosy.org.
74. Noordeen SK. Epidemiology of leprosy. In: Hastings RC, ed. *Leprosy*. 2nd ed. New York: Churchill Livingston; 1985, pp. 15–30.
75. Turk JL, Rees RJW. AIDS and leprosy. *Lepr Rev.* 1988;59:193–4.
76. Ustianowski HP, Lawn SD, Lockwood DNJ. Interactions between HIV infection and leprosy: A paradox. *Lancet Infect Dis.* 2006;6:350–60.
77. Nelson KE. Leprosy and HIV infection: Rarely the twain shall meet? *Int J Lepr Other Mycobact Dis.* 2005;73:131–3.
78. Massone C, Talhari C, Ribeiro-Rodrigues R, et al. Leprosy and HIV coinfection: A critical approach. *Expert Rev Anti Infect Ther.* 2011;9(6):701–10.
79. Ponninghaus JM, Mwanjasi LJ, Fine PE, et al. Is HIV infection a risk factor for leprosy? *Int J Lepr Other Mycobact Dis.* 1991;59:221–8.
80. Kuwama HJS, Bwire R, Adatu-Engwau F. Leprosy and infection with the human immunodeficiency virus in Uganda: A case-control study. *Int J Lepr Other Mycobact Dis.* 1994;62:521–6.
81. Leonard G, Sangare A, Verdier M, et al. Prevalence of HIV infection among patients with leprosy in African countries and Yemen. *J Acquir Immune Defic Syndr.* 1990;3:1109–13.
82. Meeran K. Prevalence of HIV infection among patients with leprosy and tuberculosis in rural Zambia. *Br Med J.* 1989;298:364–5.
83. Borgdorff MW, VandenBroek J, Chum HJ, et al. HIV-1 infection as a risk factor for leprosy: A case-control study in Tanzania. *Int J Lepr Other Mycobact Dis.* 1993;61:556–62.
84. Whalen C, Horsburgh CR, Hom D, et al. Accelerated course of human immunodeficiency virus infection after tuberculosis. *Am J Respir Crit Care Med.* 1995;151:129–35.
85. Kharkar V, Bhor UH, Mahajan S, Khopkar U. Type I lepra reaction presenting as immune reconstitution inflammatory syndrome. *Indian J Dermatol Venereol Leprol.* 2007;73(4):253–6.
86. Bussone G, Charlier C, Bille E, et al. Unmasking leprosy: An unusual immune reconstitution inflammatory syndrome in a patient infected with human immunodeficiency virus. *Am J Trop Med Hyg.* 2010;83(1):13–4.
87. Gormus BJ, Murphey-Corb M, et al. Interactions between simian immunodeficiency virus and *Mycobacterium leprae* in experimentally inoculated rhesus monkeys. *J Infect Dis.* 1989;160:405–13.
88. Williams DL, Hagino T, Sharma R, Scollard D. Primary multidrug-resistant leprosy, United States. *Emerg Infect Dis.* 2013;19(1):179–81.

89. Centers for Disease Control and Prevention. Immigration requirements: Technical instructions for Hansen's disease (leprosy) for panel physicians. https://www.cdc.gov/immigrantrefugeehealth/exams/ti/panel/technical-instructions/panel-physicians/hansens-disease.html. Atlanta, GA. 2017.
90. Grosset JH, Guelpa-Laorus C, Peraai EG, et al. Clinical trials of pefloxacin and ofloxacin in the treatment of lepromatous leprosy. *Int J Lepr Other Mycobact Dis.* 1990;58:281–6.
91. Ji B, Perani EG, Petinom C, et al. Clinical trials of ofloxacin alone and in combination with dapsone plus clofazimine for treatment of lepromatous leprosy. *Antimicrob Agents Chemother.* 1994;38:662–7.
92. Gelber RH, Murray CP, Siu P, et al. Efficacy of minocycline in single dose and at 100 mg twice daily for lepromatous leprosy. *Int J Lepr Other Mycobact Dis.* 1994;64:568–73.
93. Franzblau SG, Hastings RC. In vitro and in vivo activities of macrolides against *Mycobacterium leprae. Antimicrob Agents Chemother.* 1990;34:229–31.
94. World Health Organization SEARO/Department of Control of Neglected Tropical Diseases. Guidelines for the diagnosis, treatment and prevention of leprosy. Executive summary. 2018; p. 87. http://www.searo.who.int/entity/global_leprosy_programme/approved-guidelines-leprosy-executives-summary.pdf?ua=1.
95. Penna GO, Buhrer-Sekula S, Kerr LRS, et al. Uniform multidrug therapy for leprosy patients in Brazil (U-MDT/CT-BR): Results of an open label, randomized and controlled clinical trial, among multibacillary patients. *PLoS Negl Trop Dis.* 2017;11(7):e0005725.
96. Setia MS, Shinde SS, Jerajani HR, Boivan JF. Is there a role for rifampicin, ofloxacin and minocycline (ROM) therapy in the treatment of leprosy? Systematic review and meta-analysis. *Trop Med Int Health.* 2011;16(12):1541–51.
97. Kumar A, Girdhar A, Girdhar BK. A randomized controlled trial to compare cure and relapse rate of paucibacillary multidrug therapy with monthly rifampicin, ofloxacin, and minocycline among paucibacillary leprosy patients in Agra District, India. *Indian J Dermatol Venereol Leprol.* 2015;81(4):356–62.
98. Girdhar BK, Girdhar A, Kamer A. Relapses in multibacillary leprosy patients: Effect of length of therapy. *Lepr Rev.* 2006;71:144–53.
99. Norman G, Joseph G, Richard J. Relapses in multibacillary patients treated with multidrug therapy until smear negative: Findings after twenty years. *Int J Lepr Other Mycobact Dis.* 2004;72:1–7.
100. World Health Organization. Surveillance of drug resistance in leprosy: 2010. *Wkly Epidemiol Rec.* 2011;86(23):237–40.
101. World Health Organization. Antimicrobial resistance in leprosy. Report of a global consultation. 27–28 October 2016, Kathmandu, Nepal. p. 58. http://www.searo.who.int/entity/global_leprosy_programme/documents/sea-glp-2016-5/en/.
102. Stefani MMA, Avanzi C, Bührer-Sékula S, et al. Whole genome sequencing distinguishes between relapse and reinfection in recurrent leprosy cases. *PLoS Negl Trop Dis.* 2017;11(6):e0005598.
103. Walker SL, Lockwood DN. Leprosy type 1 (reversal) reactions and their management. *Lepr Rev.* 2008;79(4):372–86.
104. Van Veen NH, Lockwood DN, van Brakel WH, Ramirez JJr, Richardus JH. Interventions for erythema nodosum leprosum. *Cochrane Database Syst Rev.* 2009;3:CD006949.
105. Bell-Krotoski J. A study of periperal nerve involvement underlying physical disability of the hand in Hansen's disease. *J Hand Ther.* 1992;5:1–10.
106. Haanpaa M, Lockwood DN, Hietaharju A. Neuropathic pain in leprosy. *Lepr Rev.* 2004;75:7–18.
107. Worth RM, Hirschy ID. A test of the infectivity of tuberculoid leprosy patients. *Hawaii Med J.* 1964;24:116–9.
108. Worth RM. Is it safe to treat the lepromatous patient at home? *Int J Lepr Other Mycobact Dis.* 1968;36:296–302.
109. Fine PEM, Sterne JAC, Ponnighaus JM, et al. Household and dwelling contact as risk factors for leprosy in northern Malawi. *Am J Epidemiol.* 1997;146:91–102.
110. Nguyen LN, Cartel JL, Grosset JH. Chemoprophylaxis of leprosy in the southern Marquesas with a single 25 mg/kg dose of rifampicin. Results after 10 years. *Lepr Rev.* 2000;71(Suppl):S33–35. discussion S35–36.
111. Nordeen SK. Chemoprophylaxis in leprosy. *Lepr India.* 1969;41:247–54.
112. Gillini L, Cooreman E, Wood T, Pemmaraju VR, Saunderson P. Global practices in regard to implementation of preventive measures for leprosy. *PLoS Negl Trop Dis.* 2017;11(5):e0005399.
113. Moet FJ, Pahan D, Oskam L, Richardus JH. Effectiveness of single dose rifampicin in preventing leprosy in close contacts of patients with newly diagnosed leprosy: Cluster randomised controlled trial. *BMJ.* 2008;336:761–4.
114. Barth-Jaeggi T, Steinmann P, Mieras L, et al. Leprosy post-exposure prophylaxis (LPEP) programme: Study protocol for evaluating the feasibility and impact on case detection rates of contact tracing and single dose rifampicin. *BMJ Open.* 2016;6(11):e013633.
115. Shepard CC. Vaccination against human leprosy bacillus infections of mice: Protection by BCG given during the incubation period. *J Immunol.* 1966;96:279–83.
116. Stanley SJ, Howland C, Stone MM, et al. BCG vaccination of children against leprosy in Uganda: Final results. *J Hyg.* 1981;87:233–48.
117. Bagshawe A, Scott GC, Russell DA, et al. BCG vaccination in leprosy: Final results of the trial in Karimui, Pagon New Guinea, 1963–1979. *Bull World Health Organ.* 1989;67:389–99.
118. Lwin K, Sundaresan T, Gyi MM, et al. BCG vaccination of children against leprosy: Fourteen-year findings of the trial in Burma. *Bull World Health Organ.* 1985;63:1069–78.
119. Karonga Prevention Trial Group. Randomized controlled trial of single BCG, repeated BCG, or combined BCG and *Mycobacterium leprae* vaccine for prevention of leprosy and tuberculosis in Malawi. *Lancet.* 1996;348:17–24.
120. Convit JC, Smith PG, Zuniga M, et al. BCG vaccination protects against leprosy in Venezuela: A case-control study. *Int J Lepr Other Mycobact Dis.* 1993;61:185–91.
121. Muliyil JP, Nelson KE, Diamond EL. Effect of BCG on the risk of leprosy in an endemic area: A case-control study. *Int J Lepr Other Mycobact Dis.* 1991;59:229–36.
122. Duthie MS, Pena MT, Ebenezer GJ, et al. LepVax, a defined subunit vaccine that provides effective pre-exposure and post-exposure prophylaxis of *M. leprae* infection. *NPJ Vaccines.* 2018;3:12. doi: 10.1038/s41541-018-0050-z,.
123. Smith TC, Richardus JH. Leprosy trends in northern Thailand: 1951–1990. *Southeast Asian J Trop Med Public Health.* 1993;24:3–10.
124. Bechelli LM. Prospects of global elimination of leprosy as a public health problem by the year 2000. *Int J Lepr Other Mycobact Dis.* 1994;62:284–92.
125. Fine PEM. Reflections on the elimination of leprosy. *Int J Lepr Other Mycobact Dis.* 1992;60:71–80.
126. Lockwood DNJ, Suneetha S. Leprosy: Too complex a disease for a simple elimination paradigm. *Bull WHO.* 2005;83:230–5.

CHAPTER

136 Buruli Ulcer

Zaal Meher-Homji • Paul D. R. Johnson

Buruli ulcer (BU) is a slowly progressive necrotizing infection of the skin and soft tissue caused by *Mycobacterium ulcerans*.[1,2] It is the third most common mycobacterial infection in otherwise healthy humans worldwide, after tuberculosis and leprosy. BU is prevalent in defined endemic regions across 33 countries, and is 1 of 19 neglected tropical diseases identified by WHO based on its morbidity and socioeconomic burden in developing countries.[3]

Sir Albert Cook, a medical missionary in Uganda, had described large ulcers with undermined edges of unknown cause on the African continent as early as 1897. The first case series of six Australian patients was published in 1948 by MacCallum et al., who identified the pathogen as a strongly acid fast mycobacterium which could only be cultured at temperatures below 37°C, and thus represented a separate entity from *Mycobacterium tuberculosis*.[4] The name BU originated from the region of Uganda where the disease was endemic in the 1960s, but is now no longer prevalent.[5] In the 1980s, the main foci of infection on the African continent shifted to Western Africa, where the majority of cases are still seen today.

From recent genetic studies, it is evident that *M. ulcerans* has evolved from a *Mycobacterium marinum* progenitor. However, the acquisition of the virulence plasmid pMUM distinguishes *M. ulcerans* from closely related *M. marinum*. pMUM encodes an enzyme which produces the toxin mycolactone, which mediates surrounding tissue necrosis and inhibits the host immune response,[6] by inhibiting molecular translocation in the host cell's endoplasmic reticulum and the subsequent the production of inflammatory cytokines including TNF, IL-6, and Cox-2.[7]

The ancestral lineage causes sporadic disease in Asia and the Americas whereas the classical lineage causes focal pockets of endemic high-burden disease in Africa and Australia. Isolates of classical lineage are closely related but can be distinguished by a small group of single nucleotide polymorphisms (SNPs). These SNPs have allowed microbial geneticists to track the historical spread of the classical lineage of *M. ulcerans*. It has been hypothesized that the *M. ulcerans* originally arrived on the Australian continent relatively recently from Papua New Guinea.[8] The genetic trail leads in a series of steps down the Australian east coast all the way to temperate Victoria, which is now experiencing major new outbreaks of human BU. The pattern or isolate relatedness now being uncovered through whole genome sequencing suggest that *M. ulcerans* appears to be introduced by some chance event and expands rapidly rather than being widely dispersed and subsequently amplified.

PATHOGENESIS

M. ulcerans is a slowly replicating mycobacterium that grows optimally at 30–32°C, which may lead it to prefer cooler parts of the body, such as the distal limbs. Alternatively, lesion distribution may reflect environmental contact; although lesions can occur anywhere on the body, they are most common on exposed skin.[9,10] The key virulence determinant, mycolactone, diffuses through tissue causing local tissue destruction and inhibition of the host immune response. Biopsies of Buruli lesions reveal large numbers of extracellular acid-fast bacilli within areas of coagulative necrosis of the dermis and septate panniculitis of the subcutaneous fat with the absence of an inflammatory response, at least in early lesions.[11] From a clinical perspective Buruli is a slowly spreading infection of subcutaneous fat leading to massive undermining and secondary destruction of the overlying skin, rather than a primary infection of the skin itself. Osteomyelitis can occur but is relatively rare, perhaps also due to the organism's preference for growth at lower temperature.

EPIDEMIOLOGY

BU has been reported in 33 countries across Africa, the Americas, Asia, and the Western Pacific.[3] The majority of cases are reported in West Africa and Australia where the disease is endemic. Outside of endemic areas sporadic cases have been documented in Japan, Southeast Asia, and South America.[12,13] Cases are often distributed in highly endemic focal areas, frequently around aquatic ecosystems such as rivers, lakes, or irrigation systems. In highly endemic regions in Ghana, the point prevalence of BU has been estimated to be as high as 150/100,000 people[14] although BU in West Africa may be beginning to abate.

In 2016, 1864 new cases of BU were reported across ten countries, with 1676 cases from eight countries in Africa.[13] The countries with the highest number of reported cases in 2016 were Côte d'Ivoire, Ghana, Benin, and Nigeria. This represents a decline in incidence by over 60% since 2009 when approximately 5000 cases were reported. The reason for the decline in African cases remains unknown; however, it may be related to increased public health awareness, effective treatment regimens, or control of the environmental reservoir.

Almost all Australian cases of BU occur currently in the temperate southeastern state of Victoria, predominantly in coastal areas near Melbourne. In contrast to global trends, the numbers of notifiable cases there have doubled between 2015 and 2017.[15] There are now two major endemic areas on the outskirts of Melbourne, the Bellarine and Mornington Peninsulas. This expansion in the number of endemic areas of BU mirrors the emergence of the disease in West Africa in the 1980s, albeit on a smaller scale.

The disease varies in the age of affected individuals based on location. In Africa, almost 50% of cases are in children under 18 years, whereas in Australia only 10% of cases affect children, with a case series describing 40% of treated patients being over the age of 65 years.[16] Another unique characteristic of Australian cases is that patients vising an endemic area for short periods of time also appear to be at risk of developing BU, while in Africa the disease only seems prevalent in long-term residents of an endemic area. The review of cases with a single visit to an endemic region in Australia has led to the estimation of an incubation period of BU of 4–5 months.[17,18]

TRANSMISSION

The exact mechanism of BU transmission remains unclear and may differ between endemic areas. The two major hypotheses include either direct inoculation of the skin from a contaminated environmental source or the indirect acquisition of the disease via an insect vector.

An outbreak of BU in Phillip Island in Victoria, Australia in the 1990s was linked to a golf course irrigation system.[19] Testing by polymerase chain reaction (PCR) of water samples from the pumping system detected the presence of *M. ulcerans*, the first time the organism had been detected in the environment.[20,21] Since then the organism has been detected by PCR in multiple animal and environmental specimens including mosquitoes,[22] soil, biofilms, and water residing biting arthropods.[23]

Risk factors for disease acquisition are mainly centered on exposure to affected water sources and biting insects. Having uncovered skin, open wounds, exposure to mosquitoes, and swimming appear to be associated with disease acquisition, whereas wearing mosquito repellent and protective clothing appears to shield against infection.[23–25] Outbreaks in the disease have been linked with environmental changes including damming, flooding, and deforestation.[23]

In Victoria, Australia, the possum (small native marsupial) population was observed to develop BU and shed high concentrations of *M. ulcerans* in feces in close proximity to human cases, suggesting the disease here may be zoonotic with humans an incidental host.[26] The finding of *M. ulcerans* in mosquitoes and a link between the proportion of captured PCR-positive mosquitoes by town and the 5-year incidence in humans living in those towns[27] has led to the development of a model linking mosquitoes, possums, and humans. A similar animal reservoir or plausible insect vector has yet to be identified in Africa.

Studies from both Cameroon and Australia have mapped the location of BU lesions on the human body and reveal similarities in ulcer location. Lesions are predominantly located on the ankles, elbows, and calves with the palms and soles rarely affected.[9,10] This finding appears to refute the direct environmental inoculation theory, and instead supports the targeted biting patterns of some insects. Males were more likely to be affected on the upper limbs compared with females, which may reflect differences in protective clothing.

CLINICAL PRESENTATION

The classical presentation is of a slowly growing ulcer with deeply undermined edges and surrounding induration (Fig. 136-1). There is usually good demarcation between the ulcer and the surrounding skin, which may be edematous. Infection typically extends beyond intact healthy skin into the subcutaneous fat, and multiple ulcers often communicate via the subcutis. The base of the ulcer may have a cotton wool like appearance secondary to tissue necrosis. The ulcer is relatively painless and odorless unless there is a bacterial coinfection. Differential diagnoses to consider include cutaneous tuberculosis, other nontuberculous mycobacteria, bacterial ulcer, leishmaniasis, yaws, malignancy, or pyoderma gangrenosum.

Importantly there are also nonulcerative cutaneous forms of BU that may confuse clinicians because of the absence, at least initially of the characteristic ulcer.

Buruli lesions are classified by WHO[3]:

- Papule: a painless raised skin lesion of less than 1 cm in diameter. Papules may be more often seen in Australia and may be mistaken initially for an insect bite.
- Nodule: a painless but often-itchy subcutaneous lesion less than 3 cm in diameter, often seen in Africa.

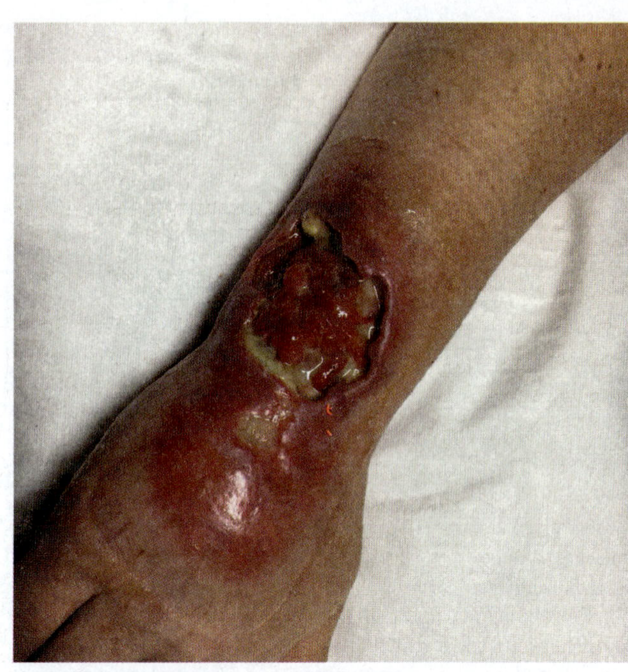

FIGURE 136-1. Buruli ulcer of the distal arm. Treatment of Mycobacterium ulcerans disease (Buruli ulcer): guidance for health workers. 2012/WHO

- Plaque: a firm painless demarcated lesion of greater than 3 cm with irregular borders, often with discolored overlying skin.
- Edema: diffuse extensive nonpitting painless edema with ill-defined margins involving part or all of a limb or body part. Ulcers that subsequently follow are often large and limb threatening.

Osteomyelitis is a complication of severe disease and is seen in up to 10% of BU cases in Benin, usually from contiguous spread of infection from an overlying subcutaneous site. However, osteomyelitis has been found to occur in distant sites via hematogenous spread, or very rarely in cases where no primary cutaneous lesion was identified.[28]

There are various ways of classifying the severity of BU; however, the most commonly used is the WHO categories I–III (Table 136-1). This classification is based on lesion size, location, and likely need for surgical management, but does not take into account the disease activity with respect to the evolution of *M. ulcerans* infection. For example, a single small nodule may fit WHO category I status but may be highly active with subsequent rapid wound breakdown and ulceration, whereas a large category III lesion may be completely inactive. Large skin defects pose the challenges of preventing secondary bacterial infection as well as primary skin closure, often achieved with skin grafting.

Long-term permanent functional morbidity is primarily seen in patients with large category III lesions, patients presenting with edema or patients with osteomyelitis.[28] This is due to eventual scarring and contracture formation leading to limb deformity. The frequency of permanent functional disability is dependent on timely access to appropriate care varies largely according to populations studied. In a large cohort in Benin, 22% of patients were deemed to have permanent functional sequelae 1-year postpresentation.[28]

DIAGNOSIS

In low resource countries, diagnosis is often made on clinical findings alone, as there is currently an absence of an accurate point of care diagnostic test that can be used in the field. Where possible, a laboratory diagnosis should be used to confirm a clinician's suspicion of BU. A sterile tissue sample either from a swab from the undermined edge of an ulcer, tissue biopsy, or fine needle aspirate is required. When sampling nonulcerative lesions, deep tissue layers must be sampled,

CHAPTER 136

TABLE 136-1 WHO CLASSIFICATION OF BU LESIONS

Category	Description
Category I	• Single small lesion < 5 cm in diameter (e.g., nodule, papule, plaque, and ulcer)
Category II	• Nonulcerative and ulcerative plaque and edematous forms • Single large ulcerative lesion 5–15 cm in diameter
Category III	• Lesions in the head and neck region • Disseminated mixed forms (including osteitis, osteomyelitis, and joint involvement) • Extensive lesions > 15 cm in diameter

Source: Used with Permission from WHO. Treatment of *Mycobacterium ulcerans* disease (Buruli ulcer): Guidance for health workers. 2012.

as most mycobacteria are located in the deeper subcutaneous layers of tissue.

M. ulcerans is distributed focally in tissue and therefore microscopic examination with Ziehl-Neelsen or auramine acid fast staining is limited by its lack of sensitivity (approximately 40–60%). Culture is very slow and insensitive compared with modern molecular methods (especially for swab and fine needle aspirate samples), and requires 6–8 weeks of incubation at 30–33°C on standard mycobacterial media. Special media such as Brown and Buckle media, which were developed especially for *M. ulcerans*, may enhance culture sensitivity.

Due to the limitations of traditional mycobacterial testing, researchers in Australia developed an *M. ulcerans*-specific PCR that targets a unique high copy-number insertion sequence IS2404.[21] The presence of this insertion sequence differentiates *M. ulcerans* from closely related *M. marinum*. The IS2404 PCR is highly sensitive and specific due to the large numbers of mycobacteria present in most lesions and the high copy number of the PCR target, making it the current gold standard for diagnosis of BU worldwide.

TREATMENT

Until 2004, the treatment of BU consisted of surgical debridement and excision although individual clinicians reported variable success with antibiotics before this.[29] Two field trials of antibiotics for BU[30,31] yielded negative or inconclusive results, one of which included rifampicin combined with dapsone. We are now aware that rifampicin is highly active against *M. ulcerans* and in hindsight a longer period of follow up may have yielded different results. Following disappointing and inconsistent results from antibiotic studies, surgical treatment with wide excision became the main treatment modality and, while effective for most patients, a significant proportion suffered relapse.[32–34] Poor availability of skilled surgery in resource limited settings, and potential disfigurement when the ulcer affected critical areas such as the face, genitals, or breast, led to a review of past anecdotal evidence of antibiotic effectiveness.[29,35,36] In addition, results of systematic animal model research using predominantly the mouse foot pad model,[37,38] and a highly influential pilot study conducted in 21 patients with BU in Ghana that demonstrated microbiological efficacy in surgically excised lesions with the combination of rifampicin plus streptomycin,[39] have strengthened an antibiotic approach.

In 2004, WHO introduced guidance recommending combination antibiotics alone (for small early lesions) or as an adjunct to surgical resection (for larger lesions).[40] Using this protocol, Chauty and colleagues reported a large case series of patients from Benin, of whom 47% were able to be cured of BU without surgery, and of those patients with ulcers less than 5 cm, 81% were cured with antibiotics alone.[41] A subsequent randomized controlled trial reported high cure rates of over 90% for patients with early (less than 6 months) and limited (less than 10 cm) lesions, treated with either rifampicin and streptomycin for 8 weeks or rifampicin and streptomycin for 4 weeks followed by rifampicin and clarithromycin for 4 weeks.[42] The WHO guidelines were updated in 2012[3] to reflect the evolving literature that supported the use of antibiotics alone for all but the most severe of BU infections.

ANTIBIOTIC REGIMENS FOR BU

All studied antibiotic regimens contain rifampicin combined with either clarithromycin, a fluoroquinolone, or streptomycin for 8 weeks. Previous WHO guidelines recommended streptomycin (an injectable agent) in combination with rifampicin as first line.[3] This combination has proven efficacy across multiple cohorts,[39,41] however the burden of daily intramuscular injections, poor availability of streptomycin and aminoglycoside toxicity are barriers to its widespread implementation. Australia's national guidelines[43] recommend oral combination antibiotics, either rifampicin and clarithromycin or rifampicin and a fluoroquinolone, based on favorable observational data[29,36,44–46] and local experience. This has the benefit of being well tolerated and more acceptable to patients. In 2017, the WHO Technical Advisory Group on BU considered clinical experience in Australia and Africa with all oral regimens, evidence of adverse effects on hearing from streptomycin even when given for only 8 weeks, and recommended rifampicin plus clarithromycin orally for 8 weeks as the primary initial regimen for BU.[47]

A 2010 randomized controlled trial comparing BU treatment regimens demonstrated equivalent clinical outcomes in patients with early and limited BU treated with 4 weeks rifampicin and streptomycin followed by 4 weeks rifampicin and clarithromycin, compared to 8 weeks of rifampicin and streptomycin.[42] In this trial, lesions from 5 of 151 patients were culture positive for *M. ulcerans* after completion of antibiotic treatment, all of whom were in the 4-week streptomycin plus 4-week clarithromycin group. This might suggest that rifampicin and streptomycin is the superior regimen for microbiological clearance, but importantly, microbiological eradication may not be necessary for clinical cure of BU, as three of these patients were fully healed at 12 months without additional treatment. An important insight from this and other studies is that healing of Buruli lesions is not complete at the end of the 2-month antibiotic therapy period. The median time to healing was 18 weeks for category I lesions to 30 weeks for larger lesions, a concept that patients and clinicians must understand in order to avoid falsely believing *M. ulcerans* infection is still active and that antibiotic therapy has failed. Despite prolonged healing time, clinical BU recurrence post 8 weeks of antibiotics is extremely rare and has not been described in trials to date.[36,42,45,46,48]

Of the oral antibiotic combinations, rifampicin and clarithromycin has been most extensively studied and was initially recommended for use in children and pregnant women, and is now the first-line recommended treatment option.[43] A cohort of 30 patients in Benin achieved 100% cure rates after 12 months of follow-up; however, 50% of patients still required some form of surgical resection.[44] Those with ulcerative WHO category I lesions were most likely to heal without surgery. The use of fluoroquinolones is based on clinical experience and efficacy in *in vitro* and mouse models[37,38,49] without clinical trial data. Moxifloxacin is currently the only fluoroquinolone recommended by WHO for BU.[3]

Premature antibiotic cessation due to intolerance or noncompliance has led to the observation that the full 8-week course of therapy may not be required to achieve clinical cure. Of 62 patients in an Australian center with predominantly WHO category I lesions, who completed less than 8 weeks of oral combination treatment, 9 of 11 patients achieved cure without surgery and 50 of 51 were cured following antibiotics and surgery.[50] No patient failed therapy when treated for 4 weeks or more, raising the question of whether WHO category I ulcerative lesions could be managed with a 4-week course of oral combination antibiotics alone.

A prolonged antibiotic course (up to 12 weeks) is recommended in patients with infection of deep structures (joint or bone) or with severe paradoxical reaction requiring prednisolone therapy.[43] However, this precautionary approach has not been studied.

Treatment failure due to antibiotic resistance has not been observed in human studies. Recent whole genome sequencing of two *M. ulcerans* strains detected only two antibiotic resistance genes (*katG* and *pncA*) out of 14 putative resistance genes.[51] Neither of these two mutations conferred resistance to the commonly used antibiotics described above. However, murine models have shown *M. ulcerans* can acquire mutations in the *rpoB* gene after monotherapy with rifampicin[52] and use of rifampicin with an active companion drug is recommended in all current guidelines.

PARADOXICAL TREATMENT REACTIONS

Similar to other mycobacterial infections, BU lesions commonly clinically worsen after initiation of appropriate antibiotic treatment, a phenomenon termed "paradoxical reaction." Such reactions include enlargement of ulcers, plaques, and edema, progression of nonulcerative to ulcerative lesions, and the emergence of new lesions. The frequency of paradoxical reactions reported varies from 21% in a retrospective Australian cohort[48] to 78% in the aforementioned randomized trial cohort in Ghana.[53] The timing of the reaction is also variable, and can occur at any time during the period of antibiotic treatment or after completion.

One proposed mechanism to explain paradoxical reactions is the progressive fall in tissue levels of mycolactone following initiation of antibiotic treatment. Dead and dying mycobacteria are intensely immunogenic[54] and falling mycolactone levels release host immune effector cells from its immunosuppressive effect.[55,56] This results in a vigorous immune response, which can be appreciated histologically. However, there is also evidence that mycolactone clears relatively slowly and is still present in lesions even after antibiotic treatment is completed.[57] It should be noted that clinically worsening lesions are not indicative of treatment failure at the microbiological level. Mycobacterial cultures are almost always negative; however, acid-fast bacilli staining and PCR will remain positive.[53,55] Management of mild reactions involves reassurance and persistence with the antibiotic regimen. Severe reactions have been successfully managed with corticosteroids (prednisolone 0.5–1 mg/kg, tapered over 4–8 weeks), and with continuation of antibiotics for up to 12 weeks.[43,58,59] Surgery may also be required in severe or destructive reactions, and for grafting to repair large defects once the Buruli infection has been controlled.

THERMOTHERAPY

M. ulcerans grows optimally at 30–33°C and not above 37°C,[1] and therefore thermotherapy has been proposed as an alternative approach to BU treatment. Recently, a single-center noncomparative clinical trial in Cameroon showed remarkable efficacy with thermotherapy alone, with a 92% primary cure rate within 6 months.[60] BU lesions were covered with sterile dressings, elastic bandage, and cotton to which the phase change material sodium acetate trihydrate in plastic bags were used to provide constant heat, with an additional foam insulation layer to reduce heat loss and stabilize the heat bags. Digital thermometers were included to monitor heat at the skin and to prevent burns with a target therapeutic range of 39–42°C. The majority of ulcers were WHO category II and the intervention was applied for a mean of 10 hours per day for 6–8 weeks. The majority of adverse effects reported were minor local blistering related to thermotherapy. Concerning however was the 26% rate of recurrence within 2 years of treatment completion, demonstrating that heat alone may not possess sufficient bactericidal properties required to eradicate *M. ulcerans* completely in at least a quarter of cases.

The role of thermotherapy in BU treatment may be best suited to instances where antibiotic therapy is poorly tolerated, incomplete, or contraindicated and where curative surgery is not available or feasible. Due to its favorable cost and safety profiles, thermotherapy in combination with regular wound care may be valuable in resource-limited settings where BU diagnostics and antibiotics are unavailable. Further research should also explore whether thermotherapy is able to reduce wound healing time when combined with standard antibiotic treatment.

ANTIBIOTIC SAFETY

The adverse effects encountered during an 8-week course of antibiotics can lead to substantial morbidity and increase risk of treatment failure. Follow up of patients treated with 4–8 weeks of streptomycin 4–6 years prior, identified significant rates of audiometric ototoxicity in both adults (29%) and children (25%).[61] This effect appears to be dose dependent in adults, with 40% of adult patients self-reporting hearing loss after treatment with an 8-week streptomycin regimen versus 25% in those treated with a 4-week regimen. Streptomycin nephrotoxicity appears to be an immediate, short-term complication, which is reversible postaminoglycoside cessation. Rifampicin can rarely cause drug-induced hepatitis, and liver function tests should be periodically monitored, with patients being informed to present immediately for testing if warning symptoms of hepatitis develop (nausea, anorexia, abdominal pain, or jaundice). There is also an uncommon fever-leukopenia reaction to rifampicin, which is reversible when the drug is withdrawn. Fluoroquinolones can cause tendinitis or spontaneous tendon rupture and an alternative agent should be prescribed if patients report symptoms on treatment.

Amongst an Australian cohort, those aged over 65 years appear to be at highest risk of antibiotic complications and treatment failure.[16] Rifampicin was associated with complications in 30% of elderly patients predominantly due to one or more of rash, gastrointestinal upset, and hepatitis. Similar rates of complications were attributed to clarithromycin and fluoroquinolones. Overall 42% of elderly patients required antibiotic cessation and 18% required hospitalization due to drug side effects. Elderly patients also appear to have more severe disease at presentation, which is likely to be due to pre-existing comorbidities including diabetes and medical immunosuppression, and increased rates of paradoxical reactions.

Drug intolerance and adverse reactions often manifest early in the treatment course. Substituting the culprit drug with an alternative agent can be considered when the offending agent is a companion drug (i.e., streptomycin, clarithromycin, or a fluoroquinolone). However, when rifampicin is the offending agent or is contraindicated there are little clinical data to guide effective alternative antibiotic combinations.[43] Mouse models suggest that a combination of clarithromycin and moxifloxacin is effective in curing BU[37]; however, the net effect on the patient's cardiac QT interval must be monitored as both of these drugs have QT prolonging properties. In patients on either clarithromycin or fluoroquinolone regimens, electrocardiograms should be obtained at baseline and 2 weeks after treatment initiation.[43]

Prior to commencing treatment, it is imperative to consider concurrent medications as there are numerous potential drug interactions due to the effects of BU antimicrobials on hepatic cytochrome p450 enzymes and the P-glycoprotein (Pgp) efflux transporter. Rifampicin is a potent inducer of several hepatic isoenzymes and Pgp, leading to a reduction in the therapeutic levels of many drugs. Clarithromycin inhibits the hepatic isoenzyme CYP3A4 and Pgp, which paradoxically increases the therapeutic levels of substrate drugs. Patients taking concomitant antiepileptic drugs, corticosteroids, anticoagulants, antiretroviral agents, or opiates should be monitored closely for signs of toxicity or withdrawal based on the expected interaction, and often pre-emptive dosing changes can be made after commencement of BU antimicrobials.

While rifampicin and clarithromycin do interact when used in combination, it has not been clinically observed to lead to excess toxicity or treatment failure. The aforementioned single randomized trial in BU antibiotic regimens[42] performed pharmacokinetic assessment of patients treated with rifampicin and clarithromycin compared to patients on rifampicin and streptomycin. Patients taking rifampicin and low-dose clarithromycin (7.5 mg/kg once daily) had 60% higher plasma rifampicin levels and a decrease in plasma clarithromycin levels.[62] No differences in the healing rates or rifampicin toxicity were seen, however these findings led to the widespread implementation of high-dose clarithromycin (7.5 mg/kg twice daily) to ensure adequate time above minimum inhibitory concentration.

SURGERY

Prior to the recent systematic use of antibiotic regimens to treat BU, surgical management was the mainstay of treatment and involved extensive debridement with wide margins, with a disappointing recurrence rate of up to 30%.[33] Risk factors for recurrence included age greater than 60 years, distal lesions, positive histological margins, immunosuppression, and duration of symptoms greater than 75 days.[33] These operations often involved need for skin grafting, with subsequent lengthy hospital stays and significant healthcare costs. In recent Australian guidelines, surgical management is limited to certain indications described below[43]:

- Small early lesions may be electively managed with curative excision and direct closure to avoid lengthy antibiotic treatment.
- In lesions with significant skin and soft tissue necrosis, conservative debridement of necrotic tissue may be performed in order to improve wound healing and prevent deformity.
- In cases where antibiotics are poorly tolerated or refused, curative surgery with wide margins should be attempted without antibiotics or with a shorter antibiotic course.
- In advanced disease where repair of large defects would aid wound closure and reduce short-term morbidity, surgery should be considered after 4–8 weeks of antibiotics have been given.

A recently published prospective randomized trial from a single center in Benin has compared delaying surgery until 14 weeks post commencement of antibiotics versus surgery at 8 weeks, where it was thought indicated by an external blinded observer.[63] In both arms rifampicin and streptomycin were used for 8 weeks. At the 12-month follow-up mark, almost all 119 enrolled patients' lesions had completely healed and those in the delayed surgical arm (33%) had a significantly lower need for surgery compared to standard care (52%). This intervention decreased hospitalization and wound dressing duration but did not alter the need for skin grafting to achieve wound closure in large lesions where active infection had resolved. The results of the study support the findings of earlier antibiotic trials and treatment cohorts that wound healing continues long after antibiotics are ceased and that patience may reduce the need for surgical intervention.

BURULI ULCER IN HIV

From a single case-control study in Benin, it appears that individuals with HIV may have a higher risk of BU acquisition, as is seen in other mycobacterial diseases. The overall HIV prevalence was 2.6% in cases with BU and 0.3% in controls, giving an odds ratio of 8.1.[64] However, other case-controlled studies have not observed this association.[65]

In a large cohort study in Benin, patients coinfected with HIV developed more severe BU lesions, with 70% of coinfected patients having category III lesions, mainly due to large and edematous lesions.[66] Coinfected patients should be offered appropriate antiretroviral therapy without delay, noting the significant interactions that exist between rifampicin and various antiretrovirals. If possible, efavirenz should be used in preference to nevirapine, and protease inhibitors should be avoided.

CONTROL AND PREVENTION

Due to the current obscurity surrounding the transmission of *M. ulcerans*, it is difficult to recommend specific strategies to reduce the environmental burden of disease or prevention among individuals in an endemic region. Case-control studies in Australia and Africa associate decreased risk of acquisition in those who report regular use of insect repellent,[25] the use protective clothing while farming, those who clean wounds thoroughly, and those who use bed nets for sleeping.[67,68]

Early Ugandan trials in the 1960s and 1970s concluded that Bacillus Calmette–Guérin (BCG) vaccination inferred partial short-term protection in preventing BU.[69,70] Follow-up times were 12–16 months, which limited the ability to assess longer-term effectiveness. More recent case-controlled studies however, have found no association,[25,65,67,68] suggesting that BCG may only possibly provide short-term prevention postvaccination. Recently, the observation that those with BCG vaccination appeared to suffer less osteomyelitis secondary to BU suggests that BCG protection may be site dependent and further work is required to confirm this finding.[71]

References

1. Farrar J, Hotez PJ, Junghanss T, Kang G, Lalloo D, White NJ. *Manson's Tropical Diseases*. Amsterdam: Elsevier Health Sciences; 2013.
2. Johnson PD, Stinear T, Pamela L, et al. Buruli ulcer (*M. ulcerans* infection): New insights, new hope for disease control. *PLoS Med*. 2005;2:e108.
3. WHO. Treatment of *Mycobacterium ulcerans* disease (Buruli ulcer): Guidance for health workers. 2012.
4. MacCallum P, Tolhurst JC, Buckle G, Sissons H. A new mycobacterial infection in man. *J Pathol*. 1948;60:93–122.
5. Clancey J, Dodge O, Lunn H, Oduori M. Mycobacterial skin ulcers in Uganda. *Lancet*. 1961;2(7209):951–4.
6. George KM, Chatterjee D, Gunawardana G, et al. Mycolactone: A polyketide toxin from *Mycobacterium ulcerans* required for virulence. *Science*. 1999;283:854–7.
7. Hall BS, Hill K, McKenna M, et al. The pathogenic mechanism of the *Mycobacterium ulcerans* virulence factor, mycolactone, depends on blockade of protein translocation into the ER. *PLoS Pathog*. 2014;10:e1004061.
8. Buultjens AH, Vandelannoote K, Meehan CJ, et al. Comparative genomics shows that *Mycobacterium ulcerans* migration and expansion preceded the rise of Buruli ulcer in southeastern Australia. *Appl Environ Microbiol*. 2018;84:e02612-17.
9. Bratschi MW, Bolz M, Minyem JC, et al. Geographic distribution, age pattern and sites of lesions in a cohort of Buruli ulcer patients from the Mapé Basin of Cameroon. *PLoS Negl Trop Dis*. 2013;7:e2252.
10. Yerramilli A, Tay EL, Stewardson AJ, et al. The location of Australian Buruli ulcer lesions—Implications for unravelling disease transmission. *PLoS Negl Trop Dis*. 2017;11:e0005800.
11. Hayman J, McQueen A. The pathology of *Mycobacterium ulcerans* infection. *Pathology*. 1985;17:594–600.
12. Nakanaga K, Hoshino Y, Yotsu RR, Makino M, Ishii N. Nineteen cases of Buruli ulcer diagnosed in Japan, 1980–2010. *J Clin Microbiol*. 2011;49(11):3829–36.
13. WHO. Number of new cases of Buruli ulcer reported: 2016. 2017.
14. Amofah G, Bonsu F, Tetteh C, et al. Buruli ulcer in Ghana: Results of a national case search. *Emerg Infect Dis*. 2002;8:167.
15. O'Brien DP, Athan E, Blasdell K, De Barro P. Tackling the worsening epidemic of Buruli ulcer in Australia in an information void: Time for an urgent scientific response. *Med J Aust*. 2018;208:287–9.
16. O'Brien DP, Friedman ND, Cowan R, et al. *Mycobacterium ulcerans* in the elderly: More severe disease and suboptimal outcomes. *PLoS Negl Trop Dis*. 2015;9:e0004253.
17. Loftus MJ, Trubiano JA, Tay EL, et al. The incubation period of Buruli ulcer (*Mycobacterium ulcerans* infection) in Victoria, Australia—Remains similar despite changing geographic distribution of disease. *PLoS Negl Trop Dis*. 2018;12:e0006323.
18. Trubiano JA, Lavender CJ, Fyfe JA, Bittmann S, Johnson PD. The incubation period of Buruli ulcer (*Mycobacterium ulcerans* infection). *PLoS Negl Trop Dis*. 2013;7:e2463.
19. Johnson P, Veitch M, Flood PE, Hayman JA. *Mycobacterium ulcerans* infection on Phillip Island, Victoria. *Med J Aust*. 1995;162:221.
20. Ross B, Johnson P, Oppedisano F, et al. Detection of *Mycobacterium ulcerans* in environmental samples during an outbreak of ulcerative disease. *Appl Environ Microbiol*. 1997;63:4135–8.

21. Ross B, Marino L, Oppedisano F, Edwards R, Robins-Browne R, Johnson P. Development of a PCR assay for rapid diagnosis of *Mycobacterium ulcerans* infection. *J Clin Microbiol.* 1997;35:1696–700.
22. Johnson PD, Azuolas J, Lavender CJ, et al. *Mycobacterium ulcerans* in mosquitoes captured during outbreak of Buruli ulcer, southeastern Australia. *Emerg Infect Dis.* 2007;13:1653.
23. Merritt RW, Walker ED, Small PL, et al. Ecology and transmission of Buruli ulcer disease: A systematic review. *PLoS Negl Trop Dis.* 2010;4:e911.
24. Debacker M, Portaels F, Aguiar J, et al. Risk factors for Buruli ulcer, Benin. *Emerg Infect Dis.* 2006;12:1325.
25. Quek TY, Athan E, Henry MJ, et al. Risk factors for *Mycobacterium ulcerans* infection, southeastern Australia. *Emerg Infect Dis.* 2007;13:1661.
26. Fyfe JA, Lavender CJ, Handasyde KA, et al. A major role for mammals in the ecology of *Mycobacterium ulcerans*. *PLoS Negl Trop Dis.* 2010;4:e791.
27. Lavender CJ, Fyfe JA, Azuolas J, et al. Risk of Buruli ulcer and detection of *Mycobacterium ulcerans* in mosquitoes in southeastern Australia. *PLoS Negl Trop Dis.* 2011;5:e1305.
28. Vincent QB, Ardant M-F, Adeye A, et al. Clinical epidemiology of laboratory-confirmed Buruli ulcer in Benin: A cohort study. *Lancet Glob Health.* 2014;2:e422–30.
29. Jenkin GA, Smith M, Fairley M, Johnson PD. Acute, oedematous *Mycobacterium ulcerans* infection in a farmer from far north Queensland. *Med J Aust.* 2002;176:180–1.
30. Espey DK, Djomand G, Diomande I, et al. Pilot study of treatment of Buruli ulcer with rifampin and dapsone. *Int J Infect Dis.* 2002;6:60–5.
31. Revill W, Morrow R, Pike M, Ateng J. A controlled trial of the treatment of *Mycobacterium ulcerans* infection with clofazimine. *Lancet.* 1973;302:873–7.
32. Amofah G, Asamoah S, Afram-Gyening C. Effectiveness of excision of pre-ulcerative Buruli lesions in field situations in a rural district in Ghana. *Trop Doct.* 1998;28:81–3.
33. O'Brien DP, Walton A, Hughes AJ, et al. Risk factors for recurrent *Mycobacterium ulcerans* disease after exclusive surgical treatment in an Australian cohort. *Med J Aust.* 2013;198:436–9.
34. Debacker M, Aguiar J, Steunou C, Zinsou C, Meyers WM, Portaels F. Buruli ulcer recurrence, Benin. *Emerg Infect Dis.* 2005;11:584.
35. Radford AJ. The surgical management of lesions of ulcerans infections due to *Mycobacterium ulcerans*, revisited. *Trans R Soc Trop Med Hyg.* 2009;103:981–4.
36. O'Brien DP, Hughes AJ, Cheng AC, et al. Outcomes for *Mycobacterium ulcerans* infection with combined surgery and antibiotic therapy: Findings from a south-eastern Australian case series. *Med J Aust.* 2007;186:58.
37. Ji B, Lefrançois S, Robert J, Chauffour A, Truffot C, Jarlier V. In vitro and in vivo activities of rifampin, streptomycin, amikacin, moxifloxacin, R207910, linezolid, and PA-824 against *Mycobacterium ulcerans*. *Antimicrob Agents Chemother.* 2006;50:1921–6.
38. Converse PJ, Xing Y, Kim KH, et al. Accelerated detection of mycolactone production and response to antibiotic treatment in a mouse model of *Mycobacterium ulcerans* disease. *PLoS Negl Trop Dis.* 2014;8:e2618.
39. Etuaful S, Carbonnelle B, Grosset J, et al. Efficacy of the combination rifampin-streptomycin in preventing growth of *Mycobacterium ulcerans* in early lesions of Buruli ulcer in humans. *Antimicrob Agents Chemother.* 2005;49:3182–6.
40. WHO. Provisional guidance on the role of specific antibiotics in the management of *Mycobacterium ulcerans* disease (Buruli ulcer). 2004.
41. Chauty A, Ardant M-F, Adeye A, et al. Promising clinical efficacy of streptomycin-rifampin combination for treatment of buruli ulcer (*Mycobacterium ulcerans* disease). *Antimicrob Agents Chemother.* 2007;51:4029–35.
42. Nienhuis WA, Stienstra Y, Thompson WA, et al. Antimicrobial treatment for early, limited *Mycobacterium ulcerans* infection: A randomised controlled trial. *Lancet.* 2010;375:664–72.
43. O'Brien DP, Jenkin G, Buntine J, et al. Treatment and prevention of *Mycobacterium ulcerans* infection (Buruli ulcer) in Australia: Guideline update. *Med J Aust.* 2014;200:267–70.
44. Chauty A, Ardant M-F, Marsollier L, et al. Oral treatment for *Mycobacterium ulcerans* infection: Results from a pilot study in Benin. *Clin Infect Dis.* 2011;52:94–6.
45. Friedman ND, Athan E, Hughes AJ, et al. *Mycobacterium ulcerans* disease: Experience with primary oral medical therapy in an Australian cohort. *PLoS Negl Trop Dis.* 2013;7:e2315.
46. Friedman ND, Athan E, Walton AL, O'Brien DP. Increasing experience with primary oral medical therapy for *Mycobacterium ulcerans* disease in an Australian cohort. *Antimicrob Agents Chemother.* 2016;60:2692–5.
47. WHO. *Report from the Meeting of the Buruli Ulcer Technical Advisory Group*. Geneva, Switzerland: World Health Organization, 2017.
48. O'Brien DP, Robson M, Friedman ND, et al. Incidence, clinical spectrum, diagnostic features, treatment and predictors of paradoxical reactions during antibiotic treatment of *Mycobacterium ulcerans* infections. *BMC Infect Dis.* 2013;13:416.
49. Thangaraj H, Adjei O, Allen B, et al. In vitro activity of ciprofloxacin, sparfloxacin, ofloxacin, amikacin and rifampicin against Ghanaian isolates of *Mycobacterium ulcerans*. *J Antimicrob Chemother.* 2000;45:231–3.
50. Cowan R, Athan E, Friedman ND, et al. *Mycobacterium ulcerans* treatment—Can antibiotic duration be reduced in selected patients? *PLoS Negl Trop Dis.* 2015;9:e0003503.
51. Gupta SK, Drancourt M, Rolain J-M. In silico prediction of antibiotic resistance in *Mycobacterium ulcerans* Agy99 through whole genome sequence analysis. *Am J Trop Med Hyg.* 2017;97:810–4.
52. Marsollier L, Honoré N, Legras P, et al. Isolation of three *Mycobacterium ulcerans* strains resistant to rifampin after experimental chemotherapy of mice. *Antimicrob Agents Chemother.* 2003;47:1228–32.
53. Nienhuis WA, Stienstra Y, Abass KM, et al. Paradoxical responses after start of antimicrobial treatment in *Mycobacterium ulcerans* infection. *Clin Infect Dis.* 2011;54:519–26.
54. Jennings VM. Review of selected adjuvants used in antibody production. *ILAR J.* 1995;37:119–25.
55. O'Brien DP, Robson ME, Callan PP, McDonald AH. "Paradoxical" immune-mediated reactions to *Mycobacterium ulcerans* during antibiotic treatment: A result of treatment success, not failure. *Med J Aust.* 2009;191(10):564–6.
56. Ruf M-T, Schütte D, Chauffour A, Jarlier V, Ji B, Pluschke G. Chemotherapy-associated changes of histopathological features of *Mycobacterium ulcerans* lesions in a Buruli ulcer mouse model. *Antimicrob Agents Chemother.* 2012;56:687–96.
57. Sarfo FS, Le Chevalier F, Phillips RO, et al. Mycolactone diffuses into the peripheral blood of Buruli ulcer patients—Implications for diagnosis and disease monitoring. *PLoS Negl Trop Dis.* 2011;5:e1237.
58. Friedman ND, McDonald AH, Robson ME, O'Brien DP. Corticosteroid use for paradoxical reactions during antibiotic treatment for *Mycobacterium ulcerans*. *PLoS Negl Trop Dis.* 2012;6:e1767.
59. Trevillyan JM, Johnson P. Steroids control paradoxical worsening of *Mycobacterium ulcerans* infection following initiation of antibiotic therapy. *Med J Aust.* 2013;198:443–4.
60. Vogel M, Bayi PF, Ruf M-T, et al. Local heat application for the treatment of Buruli ulcer: Results of a phase II open label single center non comparative clinical trial. *Clin Infect Dis.* 2015;62:342–50.
61. Klis S, Stienstra Y, Phillips RO, Abass KM, Tuah W, van der Werf TS. Long term streptomycin toxicity in the treatment of Buruli ulcer: Follow-up of participants in the BURULICO drug trial. *PLoS Negl Trop Dis.* 2014;8:e2739.
62. Alffenaar J, Nienhuis W, De Velde F, et al. Pharmacokinetics of rifampin and clarithromycin in patients treated for *Mycobacterium ulcerans* infection. *Antimicrob Agents Chemother.* 2010;54:3878–83.
63. Wadagni AC, Barogui YT, Johnson RC, et al. Delayed versus standard assessment for excision surgery in patients with Buruli ulcer in Benin: A randomised controlled trial. *Lancet Infect Dis.* 2018;18(6):650–6.
64. Johnson RC, Nackers F, Glynn JR, et al. Association of HIV infection and *Mycobacterium ulcerans* disease in Benin. *AIDS.* 2008;22:901–3.
65. Raghunathan PL, Whitney EA, Asamoa K, et al. Risk factors for Buruli ulcer disease (*Mycobacterium ulcerans* infection): Results from a case-control study in Ghana. *Clin Infect Dis.* 2005;40:1445–53.
66. Vincent QB, Ardant M-F, Marsollier L, Chauty A, Alcaïs A. HIV infection and Buruli ulcer in Africa. *Lancet Infect Dis.* 2014;14:796–7.
67. Landier J, Boisier P, Piam FF, et al. Adequate wound care and use of bed nets as protective factors against Buruli Ulcer: Results from a case control study in Cameroon. *PLoS Negl Trop Dis.* 2011;5:e1392.
68. Pouillot R, Matias G, Wondje CM, et al. Risk factors for Buruli ulcer: A case control study in Cameroon. *PLoS Negl Trop Dis.* 2007;1:e101.
69. Uganda Buruli Group. BCG vaccination against *Mycobacterium ulcerans* infection (Buruli ulcer). First results of a trial in Uganda. *Lancet.* 1969;1(7586):111–15.
70. Smith P, Revill W, Lukwago E, Rykushin Y. The protective effect of BCG against *Mycobacterium ulcerans* disease: A controlled trial in an endemic area of Uganda. *Trans R Soc Trop Med Hyg.* 1976;70:449–57.
71. Portaels F, Aguiar J, Debacker M, et al. *Mycobacterium bovis* BCG vaccination as prophylaxis against *Mycobacterium ulcerans* osteomyelitis in Buruli ulcer disease. *Infect Immun.* 2004;72:62–5.

CHAPTER

137 Trachoma

Victor H. Hu • Matthew J. Burton • Anna R. Last • David C. Mabey

INTRODUCTION

Trachoma is the leading infectious cause of blindness worldwide and is caused by recurrent episodes of infection with *Chlamydia trachomatis*. Repeat infection is characterized by inflammatory changes in the conjunctiva in children with subsequent scarring, corneal opacity, and blindness in adults. It is largely found in poor, rural areas in low-income countries. Trachoma is an ancient disease and there have been concerted efforts more recently to eliminate blindness from trachoma.

HISTORICAL PERSPECTIVE

From as early as the twenty-seventh century BC in China there have been references to trachoma.[1] The Ebers papyrus from Egypt, fifteenth-century BC, also makes reference to trachoma and epilation forceps have been discovered in tombs from the nineteenth-century BC.[2,3] At the beginning of the nineteenth-century trachoma became a major public health problem in Europe when the disease was believed to have been brought back by troops returning from the Napoleonic wars in Egypt. Many of the major ophthalmic hospitals founded in the nineteenth century were established to treat trachoma, including Moorfields Eye Hospital and Massachusetts Eye and Ear Infirmary. Immigrants to the United States were routinely screened for trachoma at the end of the nineteenth century and sent home if they had signs of the disease. Trachoma has now disappeared from developed countries (with the exception of Aboriginal communities in outback Australia), probably as a result of general improvements in living and hygiene standards.[4]

EPIDEMIOLOGY

Blinding trachoma is endemic in at least 20 countries, largely in poor and remote areas across Africa, Asia, Latin America, the Middle East, and the Pacific rim.[5,6] In 2016, there were an estimated 190 million people living in regions requiring trachoma control programs, 3.1 million who require surgery for trichiasis, and 1.9 million who are blind or have significant visual impairment from trachoma.[5–8] The vast majority of these people live in the African region.

Some caution needs to be applied when interpreting trachoma prevalence estimates as various assumptions and extrapolations are used, and there is a relative lack of data from India and China. Small changes in the prevalence of either of these countries potentially has a large effect overall. However, it is clear that the numbers estimated to be affected by trachoma have shown large reductions in recent decades and the number of countries that are thought to have eliminated trachoma (at least the active form) is increasing. This is likely a result in part of trachoma control strategies, but also general improvements in living and hygienic standards.

Loss of vision and ocular pain from trachoma leads to loss of economic productivity and quality of life, with the burden of disease estimated to be around 1.3 million disability-adjusted life years (DALY) in 2004, although this is likely to be an underestimation.[9–11] Trachoma tends to be found in remote, rural areas, is strongly associated with poverty, and perpetuates the cycle of poverty and blindness.[12,13]

CLINICAL FEATURES AND NATURAL HISTORY

Trachoma is a chronic keratoconjunctivitis caused by recurrent infection with *C. trachomatis*. Infection is most commonly found in children who manifest the "active" forms of the disease. These children are at risk of developing the scarring complications of trachoma in later life after suffering repeated episodes of reinfection. Active disease is characterized by a follicular and papillary conjunctivitis. Follicles are subepithelial collections of lymphoid cells and appear as small, yellow-white elevations on the conjunctiva of the everted upper lid (Fig. 137-1). Papillary hypertrophy (engorgement of small vessels with surrounding edema) also occurs and can obscure the deep tarsal vessels if severe enough. Pannus, a vascular infiltration of the upper cornea, may also develop in active disease, although this tends to regress. Even with marked signs of inflammation individuals are often asymptomatic. If present, symptoms are typical of those of a chronic conjunctivitis, that is, redness, discomfort, light-sensitivity and mucopurulent discharge. All children in an endemic area will be infected at some point in their life and often on multiple occasions.

The prevalence of active disease and *C. trachomatis* infection is highest in young children and declines to low levels in adulthood. Active disease can be found in up to 60% of children under the age of 5 years, and half of the community bacterial load of *C. trachomatis* has been found in children under the age of 1 year in some studies.[14–16] However, despite low levels of *C. trachomatis* infection in adults, the disease continues to progressively manifest its scarring complications. This is initially seen with conjunctival scarring in the subtarsal conjunctiva, which can range from a few linear or stellate scars to thick, distorting bands of fibrosis. Contraction of this scar tissue causes entropion (in-turning of the eyelids) and trachomatous trichiasis (eyelashes touching the eyeball). The blinding, end-stage of the disease involves corneal opacification, which is probably a result of a number of insults to the ocular surface: mechanical abrasions from in-turning lashes, secondary bacterial or fungal infection, and a dry ocular surface. In contrast to other common causes of blindness such as cataract or uncorrected refractive, blindness from trachoma can be debilitating, painful, and is essentially irreversible.

Various grading systems for trachoma have been proposed over the years.[12] The one which is currently used by trachoma control programs is the 1987 WHO simplified grading system (Table 137-1 and Fig. 137-1).[17] The five signs of the disease are independently assessed,

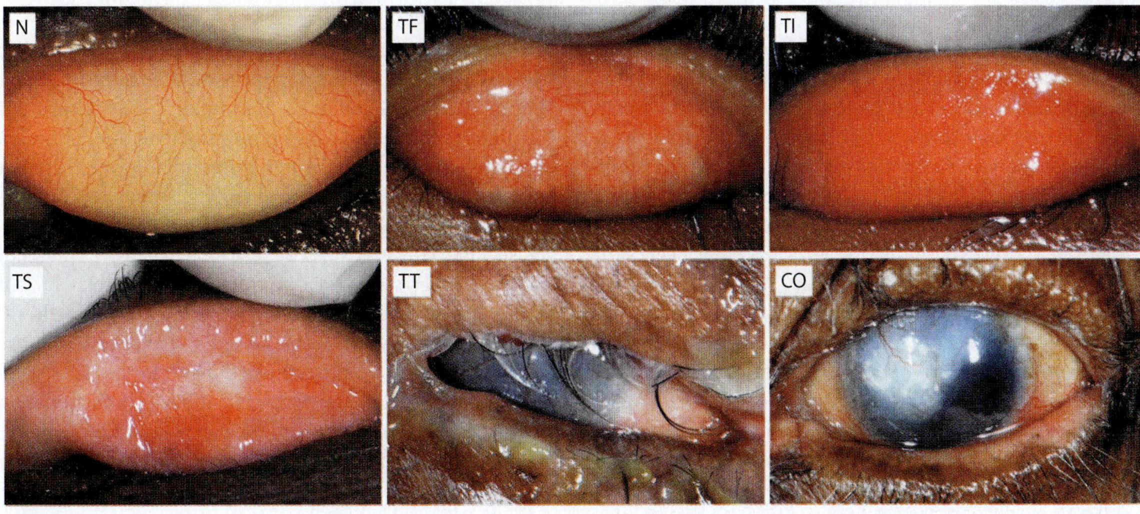

FIGURE 137-1. Clinical features and grades of trachoma. (Abbreviations: N = normal; TF = trachomatous inflammation—follicular; TI = trachomatous inflammation—intense; TS = trachomatous scarring; TT = trachomatous trichiasis; CO = corneal opacity). See also Table 137-1. McGraw Hill

TABLE 137-1 1987 WHO SIMPLIFIED TRACHOMA GRADING SYSTEM

Grade		Description
Trachomatous inflammation - Follicular	TF	The presence of 5 or more follicles (each > 0.5 mm in diameter) in the upper tarsal conjunctiva
Trachomatous inflammation - Intense	TI	Pronounced inflammatory thickening of the tarsal conjunctiva that obscures more than half of the deep normal vessels
Trachomatous scarring	TS	The presence of scarring in the tarsal conjunctiva
Trachomatous trichiasis	TT	At least one lash rubs on the eyeball
Corneal opacity	CO	Easily visible corneal opacity over the pupil

but are not mutually exclusive, and two or more features can coexist in the same eye. Examination is usually performed in the community with a 2.5 × loupe (magnifying lens) for magnification and a good light with even illumination should be used. In order to examine the tarsal conjunctiva the upper lid must be everted. The simplified system can be used by nonspecialists with some initial training and is useful for screening programs. Earlier, more detailed systems require experienced eye specialists to perform.[18]

The development of conjunctival scarring is strongly associated with previous conjunctival inflammation.[19] A subgroup of children may have persistent infection, and sustained, severe inflammation, and are at increased risk of developing scarring.[20] Estimates of the progression rate for scarring trachoma have been somewhat variable and depend on the study site, burden of disease and study methodology.[19] A strong association between progressive scarring and conjunctival inflammation is also seen, but evidence for the role of *C. trachomatis* in scarring progression is limited, with infection rarely found in adults with scarring. Part of the reason for this may be because episodes of infection in adults, with the development of some protective immunity, are shorter and more difficult to detect.[21] However, it is also thought that other factors, such as nonchlamydial bacterial infection, may be important in driving the scarring process in adults.[22]

PATHOGENESIS

Chlamydia Biology

C. trachomatis is a small, gram-negative, obligate intracellular bacterium, which only naturally infects humans. Trachoma is caused almost exclusively by the serotypes A, B, Ba, and C although the genital serotypes, D–K, can also cause a follicular "inclusion" conjunctivitis. The basis for the tissue tropism is not completely clear. Ocular serotypes have lost the ability to synthesize tryptophan, but typing of *ompA* may not be as reliable as previously thought.[20] A unique developmental life cycle involving intracellular invasion helps *C. trachomatis* to evade the host immune response. An extracellular, infectious form, the elementary body, is around 0.5 μm in diameter, is metabolically inert, and is taken up by epithelial cells into intracellular inclusion bodies. Here they transform into reticulate bodies, which are 1.5 μm in diameter, and multiply by binary fission until there are thousands of organisms in the host cell inclusion bodies. The reticulate bodies then transform back into elementary bodies and are released by lysis of the host cell. This cycle takes between 24 and 48 hours in vitro.

Histopathology

Lymphoid follicles are the clinical and pathological hallmark of trachoma. They are found in the stroma and consist largely of B cells with some macrophages and T cells with a surrounding lymphocytic mantle.[20,23] A mixed inflammatory cell infiltrate is also seen in active trachoma, with macrophages, T cells, polymorphonuclear leucocytes, dendritic cells, and plasma cells. Adults with scarring have a chronic inflammatory cell infiltrate with an abnormal or denuded epithelium. Thick, compact, and avascular scar tissue is found under the epithelium, which is firmly adherent to the tarsal plate.

Protective Immune Responses

Infection triggers an innate immune response with release of a large array of inflammatory and chemotactic cytokines, many from the conjunctival epithelium.[23] Animal models of genital tract infection suggest that clearance of infection is dependent on a Type-1 T-helper cell response mediated through IFNγ.[24,25] IFNγ has a number of antichlamydial actions including depleting the levels of the essential amino acid tryptophan and iron and upregulating inducible nitric oxide synthase. A partial, protective immune response has been found after ocular *C. trachomatis* infection, although this is only serovar specific.[23] Longitudinal studies have shown that the duration of infection and disease decrease with age, and this is probably a result of T-cell dependent immune responses. The role of humoral immunity needs to be defined.

Immunopathology

Host immune responses are central to the development of pathology in trachoma, leading to scarring complications and loss of vision. Previous lines of investigation led to the conclusion that a cell-mediated immune response to specific chlamydial antigens leads to tissue damage and fibrosis.[26,27] Animal studies suggested that chlamydial heat shock protein 60, cHsp60, may be a key antigen leading to inflammation and fibrosis, with a delayed type hypersensitivity reaction proposed.[23] However, human studies have not been supportive of the role of cHsp60 in pathogenesis. The role of infected epithelial cells driving pathogenesis through innate pathways has been supported by more recent work involving conjunctival transcriptome studies, and animal models of genital-tract infection. Epithelial cells infected with *C. trachomatis* produce a large range of proinflammatory cytokines, chemokines and growth factors. The subsequent recruitment of inflammatory immune cells, which helps to clear infection, also causes tissue damage and fibrosis.[28] Nonchlamydial bacterial pathogens have been associated with trachoma and may also stimulate innate, proinflammatory pathways leading to scarring progression.[22] Host factors are also likely to be an important, with 39% of the variability in lymphoproliferative responses to *C. trachomatis* antigens estimated to a result of host genetic factors.[29]

TRANSMISSION AND RISK FACTORS

C. trachomatis is probably transmitted between individuals by a variety of mechanisms. These include direct spread from eye to eye or indirect spread of ocular and nasal secretions on fingers, through use of contaminated fomites such as clothing and possible transmission by eye-seeking flies.[30] Trachoma is a focal disease and has been found to cluster at the level of the community, the household, and within bedrooms, reflecting the infectious nature of the disease and suggesting that prolonged contact is necessary for transmission of infection. Nonhuman reservoirs have not been found, with eye-seeking flies acting only as passive vectors.

A number of environmental, socioeconomic, and behavioral factors have been associated with trachoma, although the interpretation of studies and potential confounding factors can be complex.[12,20,23] A clean face has been strongly linked with a lower risk of trachoma whereas poor access to water increases the risk. However, how water is used and changing facial hygienic practices are complex issues with studies sometimes showing conflicting results. Overcrowding appears to be a risk factor for trachoma facilitating easier transfer of infected secretions. Women tend to have more scarring complications and this is thought to reflect increased contact with small children, the main reservoir of infection. *Musca sorbens* and other eye-seeking flies may transmit trachoma and reducing fly-eye contact through insecticide spraying or latrine provision lowers the risk, although trachoma can occur in the absence of flies.

TRACHOMA ASSESSMENT

Clinical Examination

The WHO defines trachoma as a public health problem when the prevalence of follicular trachoma, TF, is at least 10% in 1–9 years olds, or the prevalence of trachomatous trichiasis, TT, is at least 1% in over 14 years olds.[31] A population-based prevalence survey, with cluster random sampling, gives good prevalence data on active disease and trichiasis and is the gold standard for assessing where trachoma is a public health problem.[30] Clinical examination using the simplified WHO grading system is employed. The Global Trachoma Mapping Project has recently completed comprehensive global trachoma surveys to guide trachoma control programs.[32,33]

Laboratory Tests

A wide variety of approaches have been used to detect ocular *C. trachomatis* infection. These have previously included Giemsa staining and microscopy of conjunctival samples, tissue culture (highly specific but expensive and time consuming) and direct immunofluorescent cytology and enzyme immunoassay. However, these have largely been superseded by nucleic acid amplification tests. Amplification of *C. trachomatis* DNA or RNA from ocular swabs is highly sensitive and specific. However, it is also relatively expensive and requires good laboratory access. An area of concern is a mismatch, which often exists between laboratory testing and clinical examination. This mismatch is especially noticeable in low-prevalence settings and those that have received mass treatment.[22] This may be partly explained by the kinetics of the disease with a latent phase (infection before signs) and a recovery phase (infection cleared but clinical signs of active trachoma persisting for many months), and the use of simple grading systems which may miss mild disease. The much higher levels of clinically detectable active trachoma compared to actual *C. trachomatis* infection, especially after mass antibiotic treatment, has raised the question as to whether clinical examination is adequate to guide further medical management.[20,22] Hopes for an inexpensive, reliable, field-based assay have not been realized, but selective testing of representative samples and shared used of laboratory facilities with other programs may help overcome reliance on clinical grading alone.[20]

Differential Diagnosis

Conjunctival hyperemia, follicles, papillae, and scarring may have causes other than trachoma, particularly other infective agents. However, in the absence of laboratory tests, cases of follicular conjunctivitis and/or conjunctival scarring in known trachoma endemic areas, or that have risk factors for trachoma, are generally assumed to be trachoma.

TRACHOMA CONTROL: PREVENTION OF TRANSMISSION

Trachoma as a public health problem is largely addressed by preventing the transmission of *C. trachomatis* infection. The Alliance for the Global Elimination of Blinding Trachoma by the year 2020 (GET 2020) was established by the WHO in 1997 and recommends the "SAFE" strategy for trachoma control: **S**urgery, **A**ntibiotics, **F**acial Cleanliness, **E**nvironmental improvements.[34] The A, F, and E components block person-to-person transmission.

Antibiotics for *C. trachomatis* Infection

Mass antibiotic treatment of a community reduces the reservoir of *C. trachomatis* infection.[35] The WHO recommends community mass treatment of all people over 6 months of age where the prevalence of active trachoma in children aged 1–9 years is over 10% with a goal of attaining at least 80% coverage.[36] First line treatment is a single oral dose of the macrolide antibiotic azithromycin (20 mg per kg to a maximum of 1 gram), which is generally extremely safe and well tolerated. Topical tetracycline ointment is an alternative, but this requires a 6-week course and adherence to treatment is often poor. Large-scale antibiotic distribution has only been possible through a donation program from Pfizer, administered through the International Trachoma Initiative. Community mass treatment should continue until the prevalence of follicular trachoma in 1–9 years olds falls below 5%. When the starting district-level prevalence of active disease is 10–30%, mass treatment should continue for 3 years and then prevalence reassessed and with an initial prevalence above 30%, mass treatment should be continued for 5 years before reassessment. If the starting district-level prevalence is between 5% and 9%, then targeted treatment is recommended at subdistrict level. The optimal frequency and duration of treatment has generated considerable debate, prompted research studies, and the use of mathematical modelling.

In very high-prevalence communities, biannual treatment may be more effective, and in low-prevalence communities a shorter duration of treatment may be adequate. However, in the absence of widespread testing for *C. trachomatis* infection WHO guidelines remain the best guide for treatment.[20] Coverage rates in national programs may also be conspicuously lower than in research studies.

Resistance to azithromycin has not been observed in *C. trachomatis*. However, following multiple rounds of mass treatment with azithromycin, there is a shift in the prevalent *Streptococcus pneumoniae* strains carried in the nasopharynx to ones with greater macrolide resistance. This appears to be a temporary shift, with the prevalent strains tending to revert to the pattern that preceded the introduction of treatment, after the mass treatment has been discontinued.[37] Recent studies have shown that azithromycin distribution has been associated with significant reductions in diarrhea, respiratory tract infections, and a 50% reduction in childhood mortality.[22] These additional benefits need careful consideration and follow up in future studies.

Facial Cleanliness and Environmental Improvements to Interrupt *C. trachomatis* Transmission

The presence of ocular and/or nasal discharge has been consistently associated with trachoma. However, these may be a result of trachoma rather than a risk factor for transmission. While the causative relationship between dirty faces and trachoma is not completely clear, and evidence that promotion of face washing actually reduces the prevalence of active trachoma is limited, facial hygiene is generally considered an important modifiable risk factor.[38] Trachoma was once a major problem in Europe and North America and disappeared from these areas as a result of improved living conditions rather than mass antibiotic distribution. Environmental interventions involve components such as improving water and latrine access and use, reducing fly density and health education. Without addressing these underlying hygiene issues, attempts to eliminate *C. trachomatis* infection with antibiotics alone are likely to lead to recurrence once distribution ceases. However, the evidence base for environmental improvements is poor and implementation in national trachoma control programs often limited or nonexistent.[30,39] Integration with national hygiene and sanitation programs may benefit this aspect of trachoma control.[20]

TRACHOMA CONTROL: SURGERY FOR TRICHIASIS

While the prevention of infection is an integral component of trachoma control, there is also a large cohort of adults who have already had recurrent episodes of infection as children and have either developed the scarring, blinding complications, or at risk of doing so. The aim of surgery is to stop eyelashes abrading the cornea, reducing progression to corneal opacity and relieving pain. Currently the WHO recommends the use of either the bilamellar tarsal rotation or the posterior lamellar tarsal rotation procedure to correct the trichiasis, with the posterior procedure recently reported to have better outcomes.[40–42] Surgery has been shown to improve comfort, reduce ocular discharge and improve visual acuity in trichiasis cases, and is thought to reduce progression to corneal opacity. Major challenges need to be overcome for successful implementation of a trichiasis surgery program including high recurrence rates, lack of training, equipment and audit, low surgical productivity at outreach campaigns, and loss of surgeons to other jobs.[22,30] Patient barriers to surgery include fear, lack of awareness, perceived costs, transport difficulties, other responsibilities and lack of an escort. Ophthalmic nurses can be trained to deliver high-quality surgery in the community where attendance rates are greater. The use of azithromycin after surgery may help reduce recurrence. When only a few eyelashes are touching the eye then proper epilation of lashes has shown no differences compared to surgery in terms of vision or corneal opacity after 4 years, and can be considered an option where surgery is delayed, refused or not available.[43]

ELIMINATION OF TRACHOMA?

The Alliance for the Global Elimination of Blinding Trachoma by the year 2020 (GET 2020) was established by the WHO in 1997 and has helped to coordinate trachoma control efforts with some encouraging reductions in the prevalence of trachoma, particularly active disease. Ghana has recently become the first country to have eliminated trachoma as public health problem in the WHO's African Region.[45] Nepal, where trachoma was considered the second leading cause of preventable blindness in the 1980s, has similarly been validated as having eliminated trachoma.[46] These are very encouraging developments, and the recent Global Trachoma Mapping Project has established where current control efforts still need to be concentrated.[44] Concerted implementation of all components of the SAFE strategy is likely to have the most success in reducing blinding disease and integration with control strategies for other neglected tropical diseases may provide a cost-effective way forward. However, there are still major challenges facing trachoma control. Programmatic mass distribution of azithromycin in some areas may be far below the levels required, and reemergence of infection is seen in some communities. It is not clear how environmental improvements for trachoma should be implemented or what the effect of specific interventions really are. Reliance on clinical examination alone may misestimate actual levels of *C. trachomatis* infection, and a diagnostic test which can be used in the field would be tremendously helpful. There is also a very large cohort of individuals who have already been exposed to recurrent *C. trachomatis* infection and are at risk of blinding complications. Low rates of trichiasis surgery, recurrence after surgery and the difficulty of managing recurrent cases means further work needs to be done to really eliminate trachoma as a blinding problem.

References

1. al-Rifai KM. Trachoma through history. *Int Ophthalmol.* 1988;12:9–14.
2. Hirschberg J. *The History of Ophthalmology, in Eleven Volumes. 1: Antiquity*. Bonn: Wayenborg Verlag; 1982.
3. Maccallan AF. The epidemiology of trachoma. *Br J Ophthalmol.* 1931;15:369–411.
4. Cowling CS, Liu BC, Snelling TL, Ward JS, Kaldor JM, Wilson DP. Australian trachoma surveillance annual report, 2013. *Commun Dis Intell Q Rep*. 2016;40:E255–66.
5. WHO. Alliance for the Global Elimination of Trachoma by 2020. http://www.trachomacoalition.org/sites/default/files/content/resources/files/GET2020%20data%20Overview%20epidemiology%20data%20sheet_20April2017.pdf. Accessed December 21, 2017.
6. WHO. Trachoma epidemiology. http://www.who.int/trachoma/epidemiology/en/. Accessed December 21, 2017.
7. WHO. Alliance for the global elimination of trachoma by 2020: Progress report on elimination of trachoma, 2014–2016. *Wkly Epidemiol Rec.* 2017;92:359–68.
8. Flaxman SR, Bourne RRA, Resnikoff S, et al. Global causes of blindness and distance vision impairment 1990–2020: A systematic review and meta-analysis. *Lancet Glob Health.* 2017;5:e1221–34.
9. World Health Organization. *The Global Burden of Disease: 2004 Update.* Geneva: World Health Organization; 2008.
10. Frick KD, Hanson CL, Jacobson GA. Global burden of trachoma and economics of the disease. *Am J Trop Med Hyg.* 2003;69:1–10.
11. Burton MJ, Mabey DC. The global burden of trachoma: A review. *PLoS Negl Trop Dis.* 2009;3:e460.
12. Taylor HR. *Trachoma: A Blinding Scourge from the Bronze Age to the Twenty-First Century.* Melbourne: Centre for Eye Research Australia; 2008.
13. Habtamu E, Wondie T, Aweke S, et al. Trachoma and relative poverty: A case-control study. *PLoS Negl Trop Dis.* 2015;9:e0004228.
14. Solomon AW, Holland MJ, Burton MJ, et al. Strategies for control of trachoma: Observational study with quantitative PCR. *Lancet.* 2003;362:198–204.

15. West SK, Munoz B, Turner VM, Mbaga BB, Taylor HR. The epidemiology of trachoma in central Tanzania. *Int J Epidemiol.* 1991;20:1088–92.
16. Ngondi J, Onsarigo A, Adamu L, et al. The epidemiology of trachoma in Eastern Equatoria and Upper Nile States, southern Sudan. *Bull World Health Organ.* 2005;83:904–12.
17. Thylefors B, Dawson CR, Jones BR, West SK, Taylor HR. A simple system for the assessment of trachoma and its complications. *Bull World Health Organ.* 1987;65:477–83.
18. WHO. *Guide to Trachoma Control in Programs for the Prevention of Blindness.* Geneva: World Health Organization; 1981.
19. Ramadhani AM, Derrick T, Holland MJ, Burton MJ. Blinding trachoma: Systematic review of rates and risk factors for progressive disease. *PLoS Negl Trop Dis.* 2016;10:e0004859.
20. Taylor HR, Burton MJ, Haddad D, West S, Wright H. Trachoma. *Lancet.* 2014;384:2142–52.
21. Gambhir M, Basanez MG, Burton MJ, et al. The development of an age-structured model for trachoma transmission dynamics, pathogenesis and control. *PLoS Negl Trop Dis.* 2009;3:e462.
22. Bhosai SJ, Bailey RL, Gaynor BD, Lietman TM. Trachoma: An update on prevention, diagnosis, and treatment. *Curr Opin Ophthalmol.* 2012;23:288–95.
23. Hu VH, Holland MJ, Burton MJ. Trachoma: Protective and pathogenic ocular immune responses to *Chlamydia trachomatis. PLoS Negl Trop Dis.* 2013;7:e2020.
24. Rank RG, Soderberg LS, Barron AL. Chronic chlamydial genital infection in congenitally athymic nude mice. *Infect Immun.* 1985;48:847–9.
25. Ramsey KH, Rank RG. Resolution of chlamydial genital infection with antigen-specific T-lymphocyte lines. *Infect Immun.* 1991;59:925–31.
26. Darville T, Hiltke TJ. Pathogenesis of genital tract disease due to *Chlamydia trachomatis. J Infect Dis.* 2010;201(Suppl 2):S114–25.
27. Silverstein AM. The immunologic modulation of infectious disease pathogenesis. Friedenwald Lecture, 1973. *Invest Ophthalmol.* 1974;13:560–74.
28. Stephens RS. The cellular paradigm of chlamydial pathogenesis. *Trends Microbiol.* 2003;11:44–51.
29. Bailey RL, Natividad-Sancho A, Fowler A, et al. Host genetic contribution to the cellular immune response to *Chlamydia trachomatis*: Heritability estimate from a Gambian twin study. *Drugs Today (Barc).* 2009;45(Suppl B):45–50.
30. Hu VH, Harding-Esch EM, Burton MJ, Bailey RL, Kadimpeul J, Mabey DC. Epidemiology and control of trachoma: Systematic review. *Trop Med Int Health.* 2010;15:673–91.
31. WHO. *Planning for the Global Elimination of Trachoma (GET).* Geneva: World Health Organization; 1997.
32. Solomon AW, Pavluck AL, Courtright P, et al. The global trachoma mapping project: Methodology of a 34-country population-based study. *Ophthalmic Epidemiol.* 2015;22:214–25.
33. http://www.trachomaatlas.org. Accessed December 29, 2017.
34. WHO. *Global Elimination of Blinding Trachoma. World Health Assembly Resolution WHA 51.11.* Geneva: WHO; 1998. http://www.who.int/neglected_diseases/mediacentre/WHA_51.11_Eng.pdf.
35. Evans JR, Solomon AW. Antibiotics for trachoma. *Cochrane Database Syst Rev.* 2011;3:CD001860.
36. WHO. Report of the 3rd global scientific meeting on trachoma elimination, 2010. http://www.who.int/trachoma/resources/who_pbd_2.10/en/. Accessed December 31, 2017.
37. Ho DK, Sawicki C, Grassly N. Antibiotic resistance in *Streptococcus pneumoniae* after azithromycin distribution for trachoma. *J Trop Med.* 2015;2015:917370.
38. Ejere H, Alhassan MB, Rabiu M. Face washing promotion for preventing active trachoma. *Cochrane Database Syst Rev.* 2004;4:CD003659.
39. Rabiu M, Alhassan M, Ejere H. Environmental sanitary interventions for preventing active trachoma. *Cochrane Database Syst Rev.* 2007;4:CD004003.
40. Rajak SN, Collin JR, Burton MJ. Trachomatous trichiasis and its management in endemic countries. *Surv Ophthalmol.* 2012;57:105–35.
41. Burton M, Habtamu E, Ho D, Gower EW. Interventions for trachoma trichiasis. *Cochrane Database Syst Rev.* 2015;11:CD004008.
42. Habtamu E, Wondie T, Aweke S, et al. Posterior lamellar versus bilamellar tarsal rotation surgery for trachomatous trichiasis in Ethiopia: A randomised controlled trial. *Lancet Glob Health.* 2016;4:e175–84.
43. Habtamu E, Rajak SN, Tadesse Z, et al. Epilation for minor trachomatous trichiasis: Four-year results of a randomised controlled trial. *PLoS Negl Trop Dis.* 2015;9:e0003558.
44. Solomon AW, Kurylo E. The global trachoma mapping project. *Community Eye Health.* 2014;27:18.
45. http://www.who.int/neglected_diseases/news/Ghana-eliminates-trachoma-2018/en/.
46. http://www.who.int/neglected_diseases/news/Nepal-first-country-in-SEARO-validated-for-eliminating-trachoma/en/.

CHAPTER 138 Yaws

Michael Marks

INTRODUCTION

The human treponematoses remain important health problems worldwide.[1] Venereal syphilis, caused by *Treponema pallidum* subsp. *pallidum*, is a major public health challenge in both low and high-income settings whilst the three endemic (nonvenereal) endemic treponematoses remain significant problems in more focal regions of the world. Of the three endemic treponematoses (yaws, bejel, and pinta), yaws is the most prevalent globally.[2]

Yaws was previously widespread across the topics, but is now believed to be restricted to foci in West and Central Africa, South East Asia, and the Pacific). As with the other treponematoses, yaws is characterized by a multi-stage infection that predominantly affects the skin, bones, and cartilage.[3] During the twentieth-century penicillin was the mainstay of treatment,[4] but more recently azithromycin has been shown to be an effective therapy leading to renewed efforts to eradicate the disease worldwide.[5]

CAUSATIVE ORGANISM

Yaws is caused by *Treponema pallidum* subsp. *pertenue*, a gram-negative spirochete. *T. pallidum* subsp. *pertenue* is morphologically indistinguishable from *T. pallidum* subsp. *pallidum* and from the other endemic treponematoses.[6] Sequencing of a limited number of treponemal strains has shown the sequence of *T. pallidum* subsp. *pallidum* and *T. pallidum* subsp. *pertenue* are more than 99.8% identical and there is some evidence of recombination between *T. pallidum*. subsp. *pertenue* and *T. pallidum* subsp. *pallidum*.[7,8] The identified differences between the genomes are restricted to a small number of regions, which it is believed may contribute to difference in the pathogenicity between subspecies. More recently whole genome sequencing of *Treponema* directly from clinical samples has become possible[9] and it is likely that these new techniques will provide considerable new data on the relationship between Treponema subspecies.

PATHOGENESIS

Our knowledge of the pathogenesis of treponemal infections has been predominantly derived from animal models. The causative organisms are acquired by transmission through breaches in the skin or mucous membranes.[3] Soon after initial infection, the treponemes disseminate to lymph nodes where they undergo rapid multiplication. Host immune responses are responsible for most of the pathology that accompanies infection and this is mediated by both cellular and humoral immune responses. It is currently believed that there is no long-lasting acquired immunity to treponemal infections and that following successful treatment individuals are therefore at risk of reinfection.

EPIDEMIOLOGY

Yaws is restricted to warm and humid environments[4] and is the most prevalent of the three endemic treponematoses. During the twentieth century, it was believed that as many as 50 million individuals were infected by yaws. Successful control efforts in Haiti prompted the World Health Organization (WHO) to consider a global eradication effort and in 1949, the World Health Assembly passed a resolution supporting efforts for the control and elimination of the endemic treponematoses, including yaws. Between 1952 and 1964, WHO and the United Nations International Children's Emergency Fund (UNICEF) jointly led a global effort based on mass-penicillin treatment. The campaign treated approximately 300 million individuals worldwide with injectable penicillin and it is believed that this reduced the global burden of yaws by as much as 98%.[10] However, following the cessation of these control efforts the disease rebounded in a number of countries in the 1970s and a further World Health Assembly resolution for the eradication of yaws was passed in 1978. In a limited number of countries, this second resolution lead to renewed control efforts but, as with the earlier effort the disease was not eradicated. The number of reported cases globally has continued to climb in recent years, but accurate prevalence and incidence data are lacking from most countries.

Yaws is currently reported to still be endemic in at least 15 countries in the Pacific, South-East Asia, and West and Central Africa[2,11–13] (Fig. 138-1). Globally, the highest number of cases are reported from Papua New Guinea, the Solomon Islands, and Ghana. All three have reported greater than 15,000 new cases per year in recent years. Even in countries where yaws is endemic, the disease may be extremely focal in its geographic distribution. In the twentieth century, yaws was endemic in South America and the Caribbean, but it believed that the WHO/UNICEF control programs in the mid-twentieth century may have eliminated yaws from the majority of countries in the region. India interrupted transmission in 2004 and declared elimination in 2006[14] following a sustained program that began in 1996.

Transmission of yaws is via skin-to-skin contact from active infectious lesions[1] often after a cut or abrasion on a limb. The majority of active infection cases occur in children aged under 15 years. Children born to mothers with yaws are considered to be unaffected, and the majority of evidence indicates that mother-to-child transmission does not occur. In prevalence surveys it has been shown that for every clinical case of yaws there may be as many as six to ten latent cases in the community. Some studies have suggested that flies might play a role in transmission but there is no definitive proof that this occurs.[4,15,16] Closely related treponemal infections have been identified in primate populations, but zoonotic transmission to humans has not been established.[17,18]

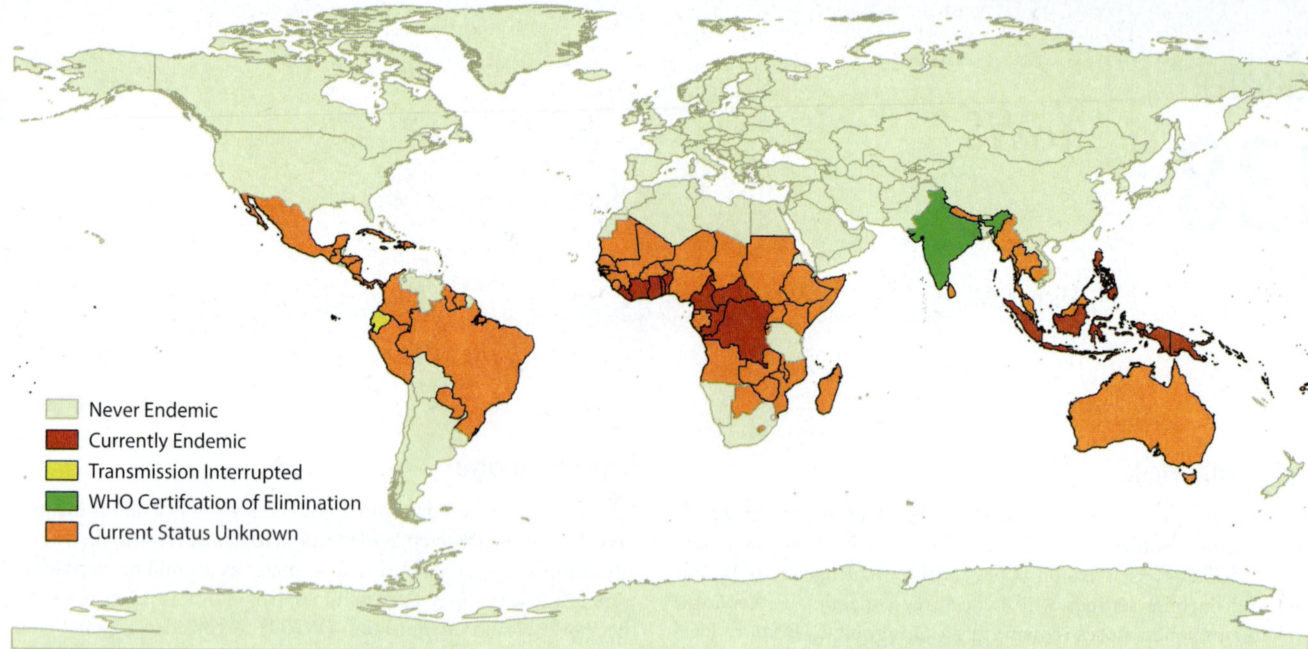

FIGURE 138-1. Worldwide distribution of yaws. (*Source:* Data taken from the World Health Organization Global Health Observatory Data Repository.)

CLINICAL FEATURES

As with the other treponematoses, yaws is characterized by a relapsing remitting multistage infection. Periods of active, infectious disease are interspersed with periods of clinical latency. If untreated the disease may progress to late-stage tertiary disease.[1,3,4]

Primary Yaws

The incubation period for primary yaws is approximately 21 days (range 9–90 days), and is characterized by a papule appearing at the site of inoculation. This initial lesion, which is often referred to as a "Mother Yaw," may evolve either into an exudative papilloma, 2–5 cm in size, or into a single, crusted, and nontender ulcer (Fig. 138-2). Primary lesions are most commonly found on the lower limbs, but all parts of the body can be affected. Unlike venereal syphilis, genital lesions are rare. If the patient is not treated then the primary lesions will heal spontaneously over a period of 3–6 months resulting in the formation of a pigmented scar. Occasionally, the primary yaws lesions may still be present at the time that secondary manifestations of yaws develop.

SECONDARY YAWS

The manifestations of secondary yaws are the result of both hematogenous and lymphatic dissemination of treponemes. Clinical features typically occur over 1–2 months, but as long as 24 months, after initial infection. The manifestations of secondary yaws predominantly involve the skin and bones, and may be accompanied by general malaise and lymphadenopathy.

As in secondary syphilis, a wide range of skin manifestations have been described in secondary yaws.[4] These range from disseminated papillomatous and ulcerative lesions, scaly macular lesions, and hyperkeratotic lesions of the palms and soles. Lesions of the soles may crack and become secondarily infected giving rise to an abnormal gait, sometimes referred to as crab yaws. Unlike venereal syphilis, mucus membrane involvement is not commonly seen in secondary yaws. Bony involvement is one of the cardinal features of secondary yaws and most commonly presents as osteoperiostitis. In the majority of individuals more than one bone is involved, most frequently the fingers (resulting in dactylitis), or the long bones (forearm, fibula, and tibia) resulting in bony swelling and pain (Fig. 138-3).

LATENT YAWS

If patients remain untreated then they develop latent infection, analogous to latent syphilis. These individuals have positive serological tests (see below) but no clinical evidence of infection. Individuals with latent yaws can relapse to active disease, usually in the first 5 years (rarely up to 10 years) after infection. These individuals therefore represent an important reservoir of disease and cause of ongoing transmission in endemic communities.[3] Relapsing lesions tend to occur around the axillae, anus, and mouth. At present, there is no test that can distinguish between latent infection and "serofast status" following successful treatment.

TERTIARY YAWS

After 5–10 years, the late-stage lesions of tertiary yaws may occur in approximately 10% of patients who remain untreated. These late-stage lesions are considered to be noninfectious. Nodular lesions may occur near joints and ulcerate, causing necrosis. Gangosa, a destructive osteitis of the palate and nasopharynx, results in mutilating facial ulceration. Goundou, which was rarely reported even when yaws was hyperendemic, is characterized by exostoses of the maxillary bones. Although some authors have suggested yaws may cause cardiovascular or neurological disease, the accepted consensus is that it does not. For reasons that are unclear, the late stage manifestations of yaws are now seen less frequently.

ATTENUATED DISEASE

In some studies, the clinical manifestations of yaws have been reported to be less florid than previously described. For example, in many Pacific countries the destructive lesions of tertiary yaws are now rare. Improving living conditions, use of antibiotics for other infections and mutations in *T. pallidum* subsp. *pertenue* have been proposed as potential explanations for why the clinical manifestations of yaws may be less severe.[19]

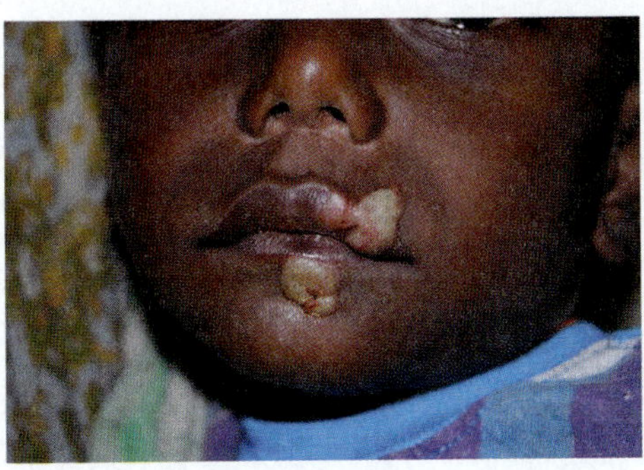
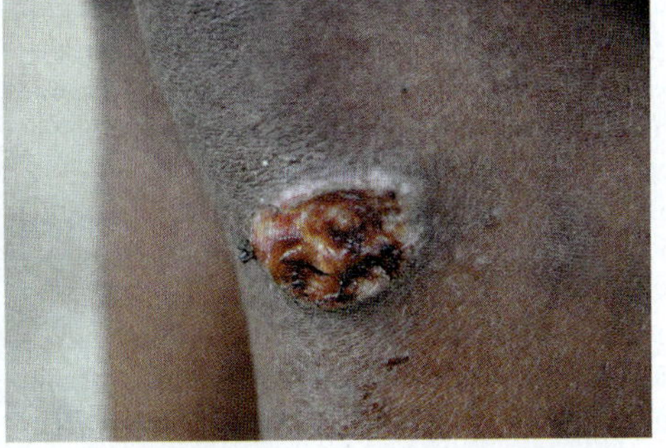

FIGURE 138-2. Lesions of primary yaws. A typical ulcer and papilloma of primary yaws. (*Source:* (a) Oriol Mitja; (b) Michael Marks.)

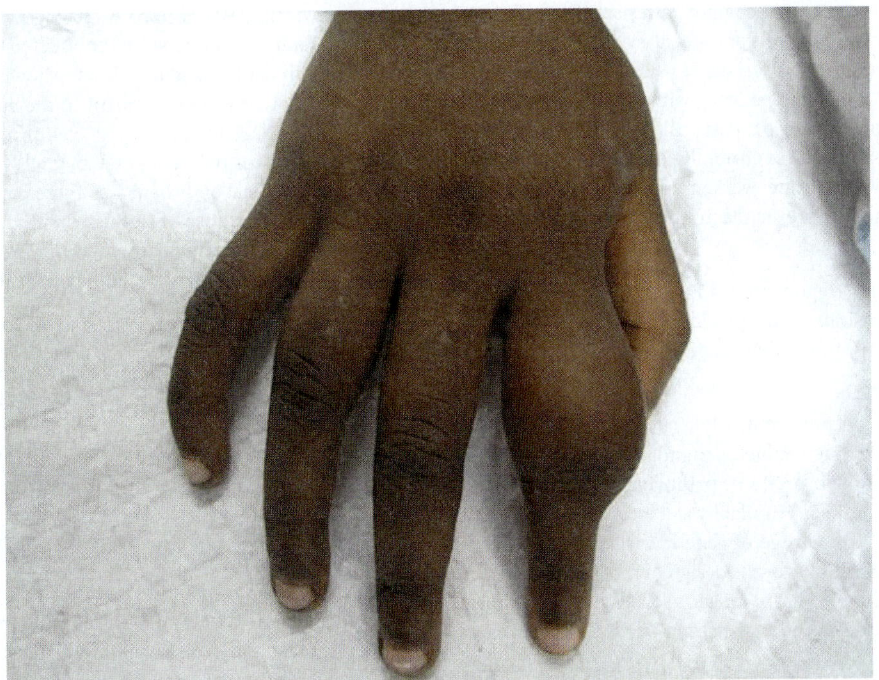

FIGURE 138-3. Bony lesions of secondary yaws. Dactylitis due to secondary yaws. (*Source:* Oriol Mitjà.)

DIFFERENTIAL DIAGNOSIS

The differential diagnosis for yaws varies with each stage of the disease. The lesions of early yaws must be distinguished from other ulcerative skin diseases including tropical ulcer, cutaneous leishmaniasis, and pyoderma. Venereal syphilis is a key differential diagnosis for secondary yaws in particular. Dactylitis due to yaws must be distinguished from that of sickle-cell disease. The late-stage manifestations of yaws diseases may be confused with those of syphilis, fungal and mycobacterial infections, psoriasis, and eczema.

Most importantly, several recent studies have demonstrated that *Haemophilus ducreyi* is an extremely common cause of nongenital skin lesions in children in yaws endemic communities.[20–22] Lesions caused by *H. ducreyi* are found in individuals who are both sero-negative and sero-positive for yaws and co-infection with *H. ducreyi* and *T. pallidum* subsp. *pertenue* is also common. Clinical features do not reliably differentiate ulcers caused by *T. pallidum.* subsp. *pertenue* and those caused by *H. ducreyi*.

DIAGNOSIS

The diagnosis of yaws is based on a combination of clinical and epidemiological features combined with microbiological evidence of infection, most frequently serology but increasingly also molecular diagnostic assays.

In highly endemic settings the diagnosis may be relatively straightforward, although the epidemiological and serological overlap with venereal syphilis remains a diagnostic challenge. Even in endemic settings clinical and serological assessment cannot reliably distinguish ulcerative lesions caused by *T. pallidum* subsp. *pertenue* from those caused by *H. ducreyi*, although both can be treated with azithromycin (see below).[23] Clinicians in nonendemic settings may encounter diagnostic difficulties when individuals who have emigrated from an endemic area are found to have reactive serology, as this may reflect either a previous infection with an endemic treponemal infection or venereal syphilis. A detailed social and medical history of the patient should be obtained and if there is clinical doubt then treatment with benzathine-penicillin should be offered.

Serology

As with venereal syphilis, serological assays remain the mainstay of diagnosis for yaws. Importantly, it should be noted that no currently available serological test can distinguish between the different human treponematoses. Standard serological testing combines a highly specific treponemal assay with a less specific nontreponemal assay. Commonly used treponemal assays include the *T. pallidum* haemagglutination (TPHA) and the *T. pallidum* particle agglutination (TPPA) assays. Both tests are specific but remain positive for life following infection. Nontreponemal tests include the venereal disease research laboratory (VDRL) and rapid plasma reagin (RPR) tests. Although nonspecific, these assays best reflect disease activity. The titer rises following infection and falls following treatment. A fourfold fall in VDRL/RPR titer (i.e., from 1:16 to 1:4) is considered serological evidence of cure. Following treatment of early diseases the VDRL/RPR titer may fall to zero but some individuals will continue to have a low-titer positive VDRL/RPR result (serofast status) which can complicate interpretation.

In most countries where yaws is endemic there is limited access to routine diagnostic testing and the majority of diagnoses are clinical. A single commercially available, rapid diagnostic test combining both a treponemal and a nontreponemal component exists. The assay was originally developed for the diagnosis of venereal syphilis and has subsequently been validated for the diagnosis of yaws. Cost-effectiveness analysis suggests that screening patients with a treponemal only rapid-syphilis test, and only testing patients positive on this initial assay with the more expensive dual test is currently the optimal strategy.[24–27] Developing appropriate healthcare worker training will be vital to ensure the benefits of these improved diagnostics are achieved.[26]

Microscopy

As with venereal syphilis, treponemes can be demonstrated in exudates from early yaws lesions by dark-field examination, but this is not routinely available in yaws-endemic countries.

Molecular Techniques

PCR-based assays have become routinely available for the diagnosis of syphilis in high-income countries. Standard commercial PCR assays cannot distinguish subspecies of pathogenic treponemes but real-time PCR assays are now available at research laboratories, which can achieve this. Knowledge of genetic variability in yaws is limited and this has implications for the design of molecular assays. A previously designed PCR assay is no longer used, as primer-binding site mutations were demonstrated in the strain of yaws circulating in parts of the Pacific.[9,28]

Antimicrobial Susceptibility

Despite use of penicillin for more than 50 years, there is no convincing evidence of resistance emerging in *T. pallidum*. However, resistance to azithromycin is well documented and now also described in yaws. Macrolide resistance is mediated by one of two mutations in the 23S rDNA. Specific molecular assays exist to detect these mutations and a scale up of laboratory capacity will be necessary to support yaws eradication efforts.[29–31]

TREATMENT

Studies conducted early in the twentieth century in Haiti demonstrated that penicillin-based therapy was highly efficacious for the treatment of yaws.[32] On the basis of this, and other data, penicillin-based treatment was subsequently adopted as the standard of care worldwide for all of the endemic treponematoses.[4] While a number of penicillin-based regimes are effective for the treatment of yaws, long acting intramuscular benzathine benzylpenicillin has been the most commonly used regime. Lower doses of benzathine benzylypenicillin than those recommended for the treatment of venereal syphilis were commonly used (1.2 million units for the treatment of adults and 0.6 million units for the treatment of children).[4] While there have been occasional rare reports of "treatment failure" with penicillin treatment, the inability to distinguish treatment failure from reinfection makes these data extremely difficult to interpret, especially in highly endemic settings.[33] While highly effective, treatment with penicillin remains challenging in many countries, especially in the context of community mass treatment. Injectable penicillin requires access to a cold chain and the availability of trained staff to administer therapy. Such issues have been compounded by challenges with the global supply chain of benzathine–benzylpenicillin in recent years.[34]

Azithromycin, an oral macrolide antibiotic, had previously been shown to be an effective treatment for venereal syphilis syphilis.[35] A landmark study was conducted in Papua New Guinea, where patients with early (primary and secondary) yaws were randomized to receive either treatment with a single dose of intramuscular benzathine benzyl–penicillin or a single, oral dose of azithromycin. The trial demonstrated clearly that azithromycin was noninferior to benzathine benzyl–penicillin with a cure rate greater than 95% in both arms.[36] A study conducted in Ghana subsequently confirmed the noninferiority of azithromycin compared to benzathine benzylpenicillin.[37]

These initial studies included patients with early (primary or secondary) yaws and used a dose of 30 mg/kg (max 2 g). In a subsequent longitudinal cohort study conducted in Papua New Guinea, treatment with azithromycin was also shown to have a cure rate for patients with latent yaws equivalent to the cure rate of patients with active yaws.[35,38,39] A lower dose of azithromycin is recommended for the treatment of trachoma (see below). In many countries, both diseases are endemic and there was therefore a need to establish the efficacy of the lower dose of azithromycin for the treatment of yaws. These doses were formally compared in a trial in patients with both early active and latent yaws, conducted in Papua New Guinea and Ghana. The clinical cure rate was equivalent in both arms. The serological cure rate in patients with active yaws was slightly lower in the low-dose arm. In patients with latent yaws, the serological cure rate was equivalent with either doses of azithromycin.[36,40] Alongside observational data (see below), this trial suggests that low-dose azithromycin is also effective in the treatment of yaws, although the 30 mg/kg dose remains the standard of care.

PREVENTION, CONTROL, AND ERADICATION

In many countries worldwide, social and economic development have contributed to a natural decline in the prevalence of yaws. Even in endemic settings the overwhelming majority of cases occur in children whilst adults appear relatively unaffected, which might suggest immunity does eventually develop. In experimental studies, there is some evidence that individuals develop some degree of protection from re-infection with homologous strains but not from infection with alternative treponemal species or subspecies.

As noted previously, yaws has been the focus of several large-scale control and eradication programs. While these programs resulted in a substantial reduction in the burden of disease worldwide, focal pockets of the disease have remained and the disease has rebounded in some settings. In recent years, both Ecuador and India have achieved local elimination of yaws, through government led mass treatment and case finding programs, demonstrating that eradication is in principle achievable.

Following the studies demonstrating the effectiveness of azithromycin in the treatment of yaws there has been renewed interest in yaws eradication. The World Health Organization launched a new strategy (the "Morges Strategy") in 2012. Several key areas will need to be addressed if the current eradication campaign is to be successful. In particular, there is a need for a significant improvement in the accuracy of information about the current epidemiology of yaws, and for studies to understand the optimal mass treatment strategy required to achieve eradication.

Community based treatment with azithromycin has been widely undertaken for the treatment of trachoma[43] and forms part of the WHO SAFE [**S**urgery for trichiasis (i.e., inturned eyelashes), **A**ntibiotics, **F**acial cleanliness, and **E**nvironmental improvement] strategy for the elimination of trachoma.[44] Mass drug administration (MDA) with azithromycin has been shown to be safe, and several other studies have suggested it may lead to significant off-target benefits, including potentially reductions in child mortality.[45]

MDA with azithromycin is central to the new WHO yaws eradication strategy. Following an initial round of MDA, it may be appropriate to conduct further rounds of MDA or depending on the diseases prevalence to switch to a strategy of treating active cases and their contacts.[46] Currently, there is no clear evidence to guide decisions about when programs should switch from MDA to a case-finding strategy but mathematical modeling studies suggest that MDA is likely to be the preferable strategy, as it is likely to achieve a higher coverage of latent yaws cases.[46,47]

Initial pilot assessment of the efficacy of azithromycin MDA has been conducted in both West Africa and the Pacific. In a study conducted in the Solomon Islands, communities received a single round of MDA of azithromycin (conducted for the elimination of trachoma as a public health problem) at a dose of 20 mg/kg and were subsequently followed up at 6 and 18 months post MDA.[41–43] Following MDA there was a significant reduction in the prevalence of both active and latent yaws. In a single district in Ghana, MDA with azithromycin (30 mg/kg max 2 g) was provided and follow-up conducted at 12 months. As in the study in the Solomon Islands, there was a significant reduction in both active and latent yaws.[12]

The largest evaluation of the WHO Morges strategy was conducted in Lihir, Papua New Guinea.[44] In this project, an initial round of MDA was undertaken followed by six-monthly rounds of surveillance. At each six-monthly survey, new cases of yaws were identified and cases and their contacts treated with azithromycin. Similar to the studies in the Solomon Islands and Ghana, there was a significant reduction in both the prevalence of active and latent yaws. However, despite this initial reduction, interruption of yaws transmission was not achieved.[45] Several factors drove ongoing transmission following the start of the control program in particular cases, arising from importation of yaws from outside the study site and from individuals who had missed the round of MDA. Three years into the program, a case of azithromycin treatment failure was detected. The patient had initially been treated at 30 months, but at the subsequent survey at month 36, had developed clinical evidence of disease progression and serological evidence of treatment failure. Molecular testing confirmed genotypic azithromycin resistance. As well as the index case, a number of cases of active yaws were detected amongst the patient's contacts at month 36 and month 42, who also had acquired azithromycin resistant yaws. Treatment with benzathine benzyl-penicillin was used to successfully ring-fence the outbreak, but the data highlight the risk of azithromycin resistance to current yaws eradication efforts.[45]

CONCLUSIONS

The last decade has seen renewed interest and considerable progress in the treatment of yaws. In particular, azithromycin has emerged as an effective oral treatment option which can be used both for the treatment of individual cases and during community MDA. The threat of azithromycin resistance highlights the need for ongoing surveillance and health systems strengthening to support yaws eradication efforts globally. Further research is needed to better inform the WHO eradication strategy, in particular defining the number of rounds and population coverage required to interrupt transmission of yaws.

References

1. Marks M, Solomon AW, Mabey DC. Endemic treponemal diseases. *Trans R Soc Trop Med Hyg*. 2014;108:601–7.
2. Mitjà O, Marks M, Konan DJP, et al. Global epidemiology of yaws: A systematic review. *Lancet Glob Health*. 2015;3:e324–31.
3. Mitjà O, Asiedu K, Mabey D. Yaws. *Lancet*. 2013;381:763–73.
4. Perine PL, Hopkins DR, Niemel PLA, St. John R, Causse G, Antal GM. *Handbook of Endemic Treponematoses : Yaws, Endemic Syphilis and Pinta*. Geneva, Switzerland: World Health Organization; 1984. http://apps.who.int/iris/handle/10665/37178?locale=en. Accessed May 2, 2013.
5. The World Health Organisation. Eradication of yaws—The Morges strategy. *Wkly Epidemiol Rec*. 2012;87:189–94.
6. Giacani L, Lukehart SA. The endemic treponematoses. *Clin Microbiol Rev*. 2014;27:89–115.
7. Cejková D, Zobaníková M, Chen L, et al. Whole genome sequences of three *Treponema pallidum* ssp. *pertenue* strains: Yaws and syphilis treponemes differ in less than 0.2% of the genome sequence. *PLoS Negl Trop Dis*. 2012;6:e1471.
8. Pětrošová H, Zobaníková M, Čejková D, et al. Whole genome sequence of *Treponema pallidum* ssp. *pallidum*, strain Mexico A, suggests recombination between yaws and syphilis strains. *PLoS Negl Trop Dis*. 2012;6:e1832.
9. Marks M, Fookes M, Wagner J, et al. Direct whole-genome sequencing of cutaneous strains of *Haemophilus ducreyi*. *Emerg Infect Dis*. 2018;24:786–9.
10. Asiedu K, Amouzou B, Dhariwal A, et al. Yaws eradication: Past efforts and future perspectives. *Bull World Health Organ*. 2008;86:499–499A.
11. Kline K, McCarthy JS, Pearson M, Loukas A, Hotez PJ. Neglected tropical diseases of Oceania: Review of their prevalence, distribution, and opportunities for control. *PLoS Negl Trop Dis*. 2013;7:e1755.
12. Abdulai AA, Agana-Nsiire P, Biney F, et al. Community-based mass treatment with azithromycin for the elimination of yaws in Ghana—Results of a pilot study. *PLoS Negl Trop Dis*. 2018;12:e0006303.
13. WHO. Yaws. http://www.who.int/mediacentre/factsheets/fs316/en/. Accessed June 10, 2013.
14. World Health Organization. Elimination of yaws in India. *Wkly Epidemiol Rec*. 2008;83:125–32.
15. Houinei W, Godornes C, Kapa A, et al. *Haemophilus ducreyi* DNA is detectable on the skin of asymptomatic children, flies and fomites in villages of Papua New Guinea. *PLoS Negl Trop Dis*. 2017;11:e0004958.
16. Knauf S, Raphael J, Mitjà O, et al. Isolation of treponema DNA from necrophagous flies in a natural ecosystem. *EBioMedicine*. 2016;11:85–90. doi:10.1016/j.ebiom.2016.07.033.
17. Knauf S, Batamuzi EK, Mlengeya T, et al. Treponema infection associated with genital ulceration in wild baboons. *Vet Pathol Online*. 2012;49:292–303.
18. Knauf S, Liu H, Harper KN. Treponemal infection in nonhuman primates as possible reservoir for human yaws. *Emerg Infect Dis*. 2013;19:2058–60.
19. Niemel PL, Brunings EA, Menke HE. Attenuated yaws in Surinam. *Br J Vener Dis*. 1979;55:99–101.
20. Marks M, Chi K-H, Vahi V, et al. *Haemophilus ducreyi* associated with skin ulcers among children, Solomon Islands. *Emerg Infect Dis*. 2014;20:1705–7.
21. Mitjà O, Lukehart SA, Pokowas G, et al. *Haemophilus ducreyi* as a cause of skin ulcers in children from a yaws-endemic area of Papua New Guinea: A prospective cohort study. *Lancet Glob Health*. 2014;2:e235–41.
22. González-Beiras C, Marks M, Chen CY, Roberts S, Mitjà O. Epidemiology of *Haemophilus ducreyi* infections. *Emerg Infect Dis*. 2016;22:1–8.
23. González-Beiras C, Kapa A, Vall-Mayans M, et al. Single-dose azithromycin for the treatment of *Haemophilus ducreyi* skin ulcers in Papua New Guinea. *Clin Infect Dis*. 2017;65:2085–90.
24. Ayove T, Houniei W, Wangnapi R, et al. Sensitivity and specificity of a rapid point-of-care test for active yaws: A comparative study. *Lancet Glob Health*. 2014;2:e415–21.
25. Fitzpatrick C, Asiedu K, Sands A, et al. The cost and cost-effectiveness of rapid testing strategies for yaws diagnosis and surveillance. *PLoS Negl Trop Dis*. 2017;11:e0005985.
26. Marks M, Goncalves A, Vahi V, et al. Evaluation of a rapid diagnostic test for yaws infection in a community surveillance setting. *PLoS Negl Trop Dis*. 2014;8:e3156.
27. Marks M, Yin Y-P, Chen X-S, et al. Metaanalysis of the performance of a combined treponemal and nontreponemal rapid diagnostic test for syphilis and yaws. *Clin Infect Dis*. 2016;63:627–33.
28. Chi K-H, Danavall D, Taleo F, et al. Molecular differentiation of *Treponema pallidum* subspecies in skin ulceration clinically suspected as yaws in Vanuatu using real-time multiplex PCR and serological methods. *Am J Trop Med Hyg*. 2015;92:134–8.
29. Grimes M, Sahi SK, Godornes BC, et al. Two mutations associated with macrolide resistance in *Treponema pallidum*: Increasing prevalence and correlation with molecular strain type in Seattle, Washington. *Sex Transm Dis*. 2012;39:954–8.
30. Lukehart SA, Godornes C, Molini BJ, et al. Macrolide resistance in *Treponema pallidum* in the United States and Ireland. *N Engl J Med*. 2004;351:154–8.

31. Chen C-Y, Chi K-H, Pillay A, Nachamkin E, Su JR, Ballard RC. Detection of the A2058G and A2059G 23S rRNA gene point mutations associated with azithromycin resistance in *Treponema pallidum* by use of a TaqMan real-time multiplex PCR assay. *J Clin Microbiol.* 2013;51:908–13.
32. Rein CR. Treatment of yaws in the Haitian peasant. *J Natl Med Assoc.* 1949;41:60–5.
33. Backhouse JL, Hudson BJ, Hamilton PA, Nesteroff SI. Failure of penicillin treatment of yaws on Karkar Island, Papua New Guinea. *Am J Trop Med Hyg.* 1998;59:388–92.
34. Nurse-Findlay S, Taylor MM, Savage M, et al. Shortages of benzathine penicillin for prevention of mother-to-child transmission of syphilis: An evaluation from multi-country surveys and stakeholder interviews. *PLoS Med.* 2017;14:e1002473.
35. Riedner G, Rusizoka M, Todd J, et al. Single-dose azithromycin versus penicillin G benzathine for the treatment of early syphilis. *N Engl J Med.* 2005;353:1236–44.
36. Mitjà O, Hays R, Ipai A, et al. Single-dose azithromycin versus benzathine benzylpenicillin for treatment of yaws in children in Papua New Guinea: An open-label, non-inferiority, randomised trial. *Lancet.* 2012;379:342–7.
37. Kwakye-Maclean C, Agana N, Gyapong J, et al. A single dose oral azithromycin versus intramuscular benzathine penicillin for the treatment of yaws—A randomized non inferiority trial in Ghana. *PLoS Negl Trop Dis.* 2017;11:e0005154.
38. Marks M, Mabey D. Single-dose azithromycin to treat latent yaws. *Lancet Glob Health.* 2017;5(12):e1172–3. doi:10.1016/S2214-109X(17)30424-2.
39. Mitjà O, González-Beiras C, Godornes C, et al. Effectiveness of single-dose azithromycin to treat latent yaws: A longitudinal comparative cohort study. *Lancet Glob Health.* 2017;5(12):e1268–74. doi:10.1016/S2214-109X(17)30388-1.
40. Marks M, Mitjà O, Bottomley C, et al. Comparative efficacy of low-dose versus standard-dose azithromycin for patients with yaws: A randomised non-inferiority trial in Ghana and Papua New Guinea. *Lancet Glob Health.* 2018;6:e401–10.
41. Marks M, Vahi V, Sokana O, et al. Mapping the epidemiology of yaws in the Solomon Islands: A cluster randomized survey. *Am J Trop Med Hyg.* 2015;92:129–33.
42. Marks M, Vahi V, Sokana O, et al. Impact of community mass treatment with azithromycin for trachoma elimination on the prevalence of yaws. *PLoS Negl Trop Dis.* 2015;9:e0003988.
43. Marks M, Sokana O, Nachamkin E, et al. Prevalence of active and latent yaws in the Solomon Islands 18 months after azithromycin mass drug administration for trachoma. *PLoS Negl Trop Dis.* 2016;10:e0004927.
44. Mitjà O, Houinei W, Moses P, et al. Mass treatment with single-dose azithromycin for yaws. *N Engl J Med.* 2015;372:703–10.
45. Mitjà O, Godornes C, Houinei W, et al. Re-emergence of yaws after single mass azithromycin treatment followed by targeted treatment: A longitudinal study. *Lancet Lond Engl.* 2018;391:1599–607.
46. Dyson L, Marks M, Crook OM, et al. Targeted Treatment of Yaws With Household Contact Tracing: How Much Do We Miss? *Am J Epidemiol* 2018; 187: 837–44.
47. Holmes A, Tildesley MJ, Solomon AW, et al. Modeling Treatment Strategies to Inform Yaws Eradication. DOI:10.3201/eid2611.191491.

CHAPTER 139

Ebola and Other Viral Hemorrhagic Fevers

Mary J. Choi • Aaron D. Kofman • James Graziano

Hemorrhagic fevers caused by viruses are generally rare diseases, but some, like Ebola, have attracted sufficient attention from the press and laypeople that they have become part of our normal vocabulary. The clinical condition known as hemorrhagic fever is quite variable and may result from infection with any one of several different viruses or bacteria. In general, they present as a febrile disease that can progress to manifest some degree of hemorrhage, often in the form of increased capillary permeability, which may lead to death in a significant proportion of those clinically ill. The number of distinct viruses able to cause hemorrhagic fevers continues to grow as we recognize new viruses, such as those associated with hantavirus pulmonary syndrome and the arenaviruses of South America (Table 139-1). All hemorrhagic fever viruses, with the possible exception of dengue viruses, are zoonotic agents that exist in nature in a silent cycle that involves nonhuman vertebrate hosts and often arthropod vectors. Transmission to humans is by the bite of an infectious vector, by small particle aerosol from infectious urine or feces of an infectious host, or through nosocomial transmission, often under conditions where routine safe hospital practices are not being followed. Hemorrhagic fever viruses do not share a common taxonomic origin; they are found among different virus families: Arenaviridae, Hantaviridae, Nairoviridae, Phenuiviridae, Filoviridae, and Flaviviridae.

ARENAVIRUSES

Until recently, only three arenaviruses were associated with hemorrhagic fever: Lassa fever caused by Lassa virus of West Africa; Argentine hemorrhagic fever (AHF) caused by Junin virus; and Bolivian hemorrhagic fever (BHF) caused by Machupo virus (MACV).[1] In the past decade, however, new pathogenic arenaviruses have been discovered, and it is likely that others will be recognized as humans continue to occupy previously sparsely populated regions of the world (Table 139-2).

Lassa Fever

First recognized in Nigeria in 1969, Lassa fever has caused nosocomial outbreaks in rural hospitals in Nigeria, Liberia, and Sierra Leone, where direct secondary transmission with high mortality occurred.[2] These outbreaks have often devastated rural hospital staff, claiming the lives of physicians and nurses as well as patients' family members, friends, and other close contacts. Additionally, Lassa fever acquired in West Africa has been detected in other countries in Europe, the Middle East, Asia, Africa, and North America. A total of 33 such cases have occurred from 1969 through 2016.[3]

Lassa fever is endemic to West Africa, occurring principally in savannah landscapes or tropical areas heavily modified by human agricultural activity.[4] The majority of cases are seen in Liberia, Sierra Leone, Guinea, and Nigeria, and account for 10% or more of admissions to some hospitals. Approximately 80% of people infected with Lassa virus have mild or no overt symptoms; in its severe form, Lassa fever is a protean febrile disease attacking many vital organs including the heart, lungs, liver, pancreas, and kidneys.[5] Jaundice is unusual but pulmonary and peritoneal effusions are common. A fulminating hemorrhagic picture with shock occurs in only about 20% of hospitalized cases. Overall, approximately 1% of all infections with Lassa virus end in death; however, approximately 15–20% of patients hospitalized with Lassa fever die from the illness. Death rates are especially high among pregnant women and their fetuses during the third trimester of pregnancy, when about 95% of fetuses of infected mothers may die. Up to 25% of maternal deaths are due to Lassa in some hospitals. Lassa virus has also been isolated from breast milk, suggesting that there is a clear risk to nursing infants. Virus is present in blood and effusions for many days and has been recovered from throat washings and urine. Deafness is a notable sequela of Lassa fever, affecting approximately one-quarter of prospectively studied cases in Sierra Leone.[6] Antibodies to Lassa virus are also more common in deaf residents of endemic areas. While no specific vaccine is available for Lassa fever, the disease has anecdotally responded well to intravenous treatment with the antiviral drug, ribavirin.[7] Unfortunately, access to this drug is significantly hampered due to lack of availability, cost, and licensure issues.

Lassa virus is maintained by peridomestic rodents of the genus *Mastomys*.[8] Original studies indicated that *M. natalensis*, also known as the multimammate rat, was the principal reservoir host, but this actually represents a complex of sibling species difficult to differentiate by physical characteristics alone. Additional species demonstrated to be reservoirs for Lassa fever include the Guinea mouse (*M. erythroleucus*) and the African wood mouse (*Hylomyscus pamfi*).[9] Indeed, many villages in eastern Sierra Leone may average one to four *Mastomys* in each house, with as many as 20% infected with Lassa virus. Mice are chronically infected and shed virus in their urine for many weeks, leading to infectious aerosol that may contaminate the environment and foodstuffs, or directly lead to infection by inhalation or contact through cuts or mucous membranes. In addition, in some areas these mice are consumed by villagers for food, leading to greater risk of Lassa infection.[10]

Prospective, laboratory-based studies of Lassa fever in eastern Sierra Leone have demonstrated that transmission is endemic, with peak activity occurring in the dry season (January–May).[5] Attack rates range up to 5 per 1000 per year, with a case-fatality rate of 18%, much lower than reported during earlier outbreaks. Epidemiological investigations conducted in villages, however, showed that up to half the population had been infected with the virus, and annual infection rates as high as 8% have been documented, giving an infection-case ratio of about 16:1.[11] Persons of all ages and both sexes are infected and may suffer severe clinical illness; why only certain individuals become very sick is still not known.

Surveillance for Lassa fever presents a difficult challenge. Because the clinical spectrum is so wide, cases are likely detected primarily when they are clinically severe, associated with clusters, or involving transmission to hospital staff. Thus, specific diagnosis is essential and best done by measurement of virus-specific IgM antibodies, which appear in patients within 7–10 days after onset of symptoms, or by direct measurement of viral antigen or nucleic acids earlier in the course of illness.[5] The potential hazards associated with laboratory work on Lassa virus and the paucity of virological laboratories in West Africa have limited the application of these technologies.

TABLE 139-1 VIRAL HEMORRHAGIC FEVERS

Family, Virus	Disease	Distribution	Means
Arenaviridae			
Lassa	Lassa fever	West Africa	Rodent
Junin	Argentine HF	Argentina	Rodent
Machupo	Bolivian HF	Bolivia	Rodent
Guanarito	Venezuelan HF	Venezuela	Rodent
Sabia	Brazilian HF	Brazil	Unknown
Filoviridae			
Marburg	Marburg HF	Sub-Saharan Africa	Bat
Ebola	Ebola HF	Sub-Saharan Africa	Bat suspected
Flaviviridae			
Dengue	Dengue fever, Dengue HF	Asia, Americas, Africa, Pacific	Mosquito
Yellow fever	Yellow fever	Tropical Americas, sub-Saharan Africa	Mosquito
Kyasanur Forest disease	Kyasanur Forest disease	India	Tick
Alkhurma	Unnamed	Saudia Arabia	Unknown
Omsk	Omsk HF	Russia	Tick, other
Bunyaviridae			
Ngari	Unnamed	Sub-Saharan Africa	Mosquito suspected
Rift Valley fever	Rift Valley fever	Sub-Saharan Africa	Mosquito
Crimean-Congo	Crimean-Congo HF	Africa, Asia, Southern Russia, NIS	Tick
Hantaan and related viruses	HF with renal syndrome, others	Asia, Balkans, Russia, Europe	Rodent

Abbreviation: NIS = newly independent states.

Persons traveling from West Africa may introduce the virus to nonendemic countries. Healthcare facilities should obtain a travel history from all patients presenting for care. In addition, contact and droplet precautions should be instituted for patients suspected of having Lassa fever, and airborne precautions should be used when performing aerosol-generating medical procedures. High-risk contacts, or those with direct, unprotected contact with patients or their body fluids, should be monitored for fever for 21 days following last direct contact with a Lassa patient. Quarantine is not indicated for contacts of Lassa patients.

Control of Lassa fever represents a major biological challenge. Vaccine development is hampered by technical problems and the absence of an economically sustainable market. Rodent control is effective in reducing virus transmission to humans, but is likewise difficult to sustain or easily applied over the broad geographical distribution of *Mastomys*.

Argentine Hemorrhagic Fever

Like Lassa fever, AHF is maintained in rodents and is transmitted to humans through direct contact with infected animals or by inhaling infectious rodent excreta or secretions. The disease is caused by Junin virus, first discovered in the 1950s in the rich agricultural pampas of Buenos Aires, Cordoba, and Santa Fe Provinces of Argentina. Outbreaks of AHF occur yearly. Historically, case counts reported during outbreaks were in excess of 1000 per year.[12] With the availability of an effective Junin virus vaccine in 2007 the number of cases has dropped to fewer than 100 cases per year.[13] There is a peak in disease incidence during the fall harvest season when agricultural workers are exposed to aerosols generated by infected mice. Adult males comprise the great majority of cases, due to their occupational exposure through farming and related agrarian activities.

The primary rodent reservoir for Junin virus is *Calomys musculinus*. However, Junin virus infections have also been reported in other rodent species including *C. laucha, Akodon azarae, Bolomys obscurus,* and *Galicitis cuja.* Infected rodents can shed the virus in their saliva, urine, and feces. Chronic viremic and viruric infection of rodents has been shown to be the principal means of virus maintenance within the reservoir host.[14] Prospective studies of *C. musculinus* suggests that most infected animals acquire the virus horizontally after weanling, although vertical transmission clearly occurs. Similar in size to house mice (*Mus musculus*), *C. musculinus* invades crops during the fall from permanent harborage along roadsides, railways, and other linear habitats. Population densities are highest in fields of maize.[15]

Onset of symptoms is usually gradual with fever and malaise progressing to myalgia, headache, and dizziness and followed by signs of central nervous system involvement such as tremor of the limbs and tongue, gastrointestinal symptoms including nausea and vomiting, and indications of vascular instability that may progress to shock. Severely ill patients may bleed from the gums, gastrointestinal tract, or mucosal surfaces, and suffer from severe neurological symptoms including coma and convulsions.[16]

Case fatality rate is from 5% to more than 15% but prompt immunotherapy may reduce the mortality rate to 1% or less. Inapparent infections rarely occur. Viremia is sporadic or of low titer and

TABLE 139-2 ARENAVIRUSES KNOWN TO CAUSE HUMAN DISEASE

Virus	Abbr.	Host	Original Isolation	Disease
Lymphocytic choriomeningitis	LCM	*Mus musculus*	USA	Lymphocytic choriomeningitis
Lassa	LAS	*Mastomys sp.*	Nigeria	Lassa Fever
Junin	JUN	*Calomys musculinus*	Argentina	Argentine hemorrhagic Fever (AHF)
Machupo	MAC	*Calomys callosus*	Bolivia	Bolivian hemorrhagic fever (BHF)
Guanarito	GUA	*Zygodontomys sp.*	Venezuela	Venezuelan hemorrhagic fever (VHF)
Sabia	SAB	Unknown	Brazil	Brazilian hemorrhagic fever

nosocomial infections, although reported, are very unusual. Attack rates may be quite high in circumscribed, small communities.

A live, attenuated vaccine, Candid 1, developed jointly by the Government of Argentina, the Pan American Health Organization, the United Nations Development Programme, and the United States Army Medical Research and Development Command, has been evaluated and found to be safe and 95% efficacious in preventing AHF. Nearly 250,000 at risk individuals in the endemic region of Argentina have now received the vaccine, leading to a dramatic drop in AHF incidence (Fig. 139-1).[13]

Bolivian Hemorrhagic Fever

BHF is caused by Machupo virus. It is similar to AHF in both the clinical manifestation and the way it is maintained in nature. The disease was first recognized in 1959, and by the early 1960s nearly 500 cases had been recorded, with a case fatality rate of approximately 30%.[17] The peak incidence is usually during the late rainy season and early dry season months of February–July. Outbreaks of BHF have been controlled and prevented by vigorous rodent control programs in affected towns and on ranches.

A pastoral rodent, *C. callosus*, is found at the edge of riverine forest-savannah formations. While *C. callosus* can be found in several South American countries (Bolivia, Brazil, Paraguay, and Argentina), MACV is only endemic to a small region of Bolivia.[18] Studies have shown that *C. callosus* rodents in this region belong to an independent monophyletic lineage, and are genetically different from other lineages in found in Bolivia and South America.[19] In 1963–64, a large outbreak occurred in Bolivia after a population explosion of the primary rodent host, *C. callosus* led to hundreds of mice invading the town, resulting in an extremely high BHF attack rate among residents.

The signs and symptoms of BHF include fever, malaise, myalgia, and headache followed by nausea, vomiting, and cutaneous hyperesthesia. Approximately a third of patients develop severe neurological or hemorrhagic symptoms, which can include intention tremors, seizures, delirium, hematemesis, melena, and coma. The convalescent phase is marked by severe fatigue, hair loss, and dizziness that can persist for several months.[18,20] The mortality rate varies between outbreaks but is estimated at 25%. Unlike AHF, nosocomial transmission has been reported.[21] The live, attenuated Junin vaccine cross protects against BHF in monkey models, and may offer an alternative to rodent control among rural populations at high risk of BHF.[22] Limited experience with the antiviral drug ribavirin in humans suggests that it may be useful in treating BHF.[23]

Venezuelan Hemorrhagic Fever

This disease was discovered when a cluster of hemorrhagic fever cases was seen in the city of Guanarito in the central Venezuelan state of Portuguesa in 1989. A total of 104 presumptive cases with 26 deaths was recorded during that outbreak.[24] Clinical disease is similar to that documented for AHF and BHF, although pharyngitis appears to be more common. Adult males comprise the great majority of cases, due to their occupational exposure through farming and related agrarian activities. Person-to-person transmission has been reported but is rare.[25] The majority of cases have occurred during the dry season from December to March and those infected are usually rural residents involved in agricultural activities. The short-tailed cane mouse, *Zygodontomys brevicauda* is the primary reservoir host, and laboratory studies have demonstrated that this rodent may sustain long-term viremia and viruria.[26]

Sabia Virus

Only four cases of Sabia virus have been recognized. Two were naturally acquired (a fatal infection of a young women hospitalized in São Paulo, Brazil in 1990,[27] another fatal infection in a coffee-grain machine operator in 1999[28]) and two laboratory-acquired infections in scientists attempting to characterize this new virus in Brazil[27] and in Connecticut.[29] Both patients with laboratory-acquired infections survived, apparently responding well to treatment with ribavirin administered soon after the diagnosis was suspected. Attempts to identify a rodent host of Sabia virus have to date been unsuccessful, and there is little known about the natural history of the virus, although it is clear from the laboratory infections that it is easily transmitted by aerosol.

Lymphocytic Choriomeningitis

Lymphocytic choriomeningitis virus (LCMV) is another member of the Arenaviridae family. It is maintained in nature through chronic infections of the peridomestic mouse, *Mus musculus*, and both the virus and vector have been recognized virtually worldwide.[30]

Unlike other arenaviruses LCMV is rarely hemorrhagic or fatal to humans.[31] Of 150 patients diagnosed with LCMV infection during hamster-associated outbreaks, about half had "flu-like" symptoms, 22% were diagnosed with aseptic meningitis, 5% with encephalitis,

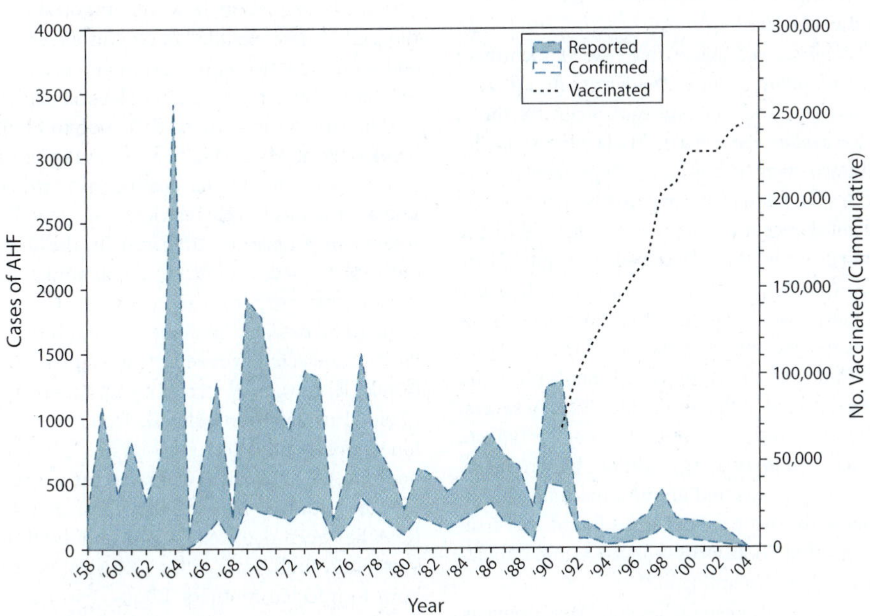

FIGURE 139-1. Reported cases of Argentine hemorrhagic fever (AHF) and number of persons vaccinated, 1958–2004.

1% with myelitis, and 23% appeared asymptomatic. Initial febrile episodes typically last from 3 to 7 days. For those who develop neurological sequelae, they typically occur during a second febrile period from 1 to 5 days after the initial febrile episode resolves. LCMV may also cause abortion in pregnant women or lead to hydrocephalus, chorioretinitis, or mental defects in the newborn child.

LCMV is maintained in nature by chronic infection of feral *Mus* mice, which can acquire it vertically from infected parent to progeny, or horizontally through contact with other infected mice.[32] Mice infected *in utero* or from maternal milk secrete significant quantities of virus in the urine from weeks to lifelong. Transmission to humans occurs upon exposure to infectious rodent urine, most commonly in the form of aerosols associated with nests. An alternate host of significance in recent years in both Europe and the United States is the Syrian hamster (*Mesocricetus auratus*).[33] Outbreaks have occurred among personnel in medical research institutions where hamsters were housed, as well as among persons keeping hamsters as pets.

Because of the variable transmission pattern of LCMV and wide range of clinical presentations, precise attack rates in human populations are difficult to determine. Infection is likely more common than is realized, since specific viral testing methods are needed to make the diagnosis. Approximately 10% of aseptic meningitis and encephalitis cases studied in one U.S. center over a period of several years were found to have been caused by LCMV.

Adults are infected more often than children, and most *Mus*-related infections occur in fall and winter. Between 1965 and 1975, hamster-related outbreaks of occurred in New York, California, and ten other states.[34] Several clusters of LCMV infection associated with solid organ transplant have occurred. In 2012, 31 employees at three commercial rodent breeding facilities tested positive for IgM and/or IgG positive for LCMV. Of the 1820 rodents that were tested at one of the facilities, 382 (21%) of mice (*Mus musculus*) had detectable IgG, and 13 (0.7%) were positive by reverse transcription PCR.[35]

There is no specific treatment and no vaccine is available for LCMV infection. Adhering to good standards of environmental sanitation and testing of hamster colonies for endemic LCMV infection represent the best currently available methods for avoiding human contact with this agent.

FILOVIRUSES

Among the most severe viral pathogens, Marburg and Ebola viruses burst on an unprepared world in 1967 and 1976, respectively. The virus family *Filoviridae* is composed of thread-like viruses from two genera, *Marburgvirus* and *Ebolavirus*.

Within the genus *Ebolavirus*, six species have been identified: *Reston ebolavirus*, *Sudan ebolavirus*, *Zaire ebolavirus*, *Bundibugyo ebolavirus*, *Tai forest ebolavirus*, and *Bombali ebolavirus*. Of these, only Sudan virus (species *Sudan ebolavirus*), Ebola virus (species *Zaire ebolavirus*), Bundibugyo virus (species *Bundibugyo ebolavirus*), and Tai Forest virus (species *Tai forest ebolavirus*) are known to cause disease in humans. The most recently recognized virus within the genus Ebolavirus is Bombali virus. First described in August 2018, the virus was detected in free-tailed bats in Sierra Leone. It is not known if Bombali virus can cause disease in either animals or people.[36] Fruit bats are the suspected reservoir host for viruses within the genus Ebolavirus. Immunoglobulin G specific for Ebola virus and Ebola virus RNA has been detected in the serum and tissue of several different bat species (*Hypsignathus monstrosus*, *Epomops franqueti*, *Eidolon helvum*, *Myonycteris torquata*).[37] In addition, experimental infections of various species of plants and animals naturally occurring in areas where Ebola outbreaks have occurred found that fruit and insectivorous bats supported Ebola virus replication and circulation of high titers of virus without becoming ill.[38]

Marburg virus (MARV) is the only virus in the genus *Marburgvirus*. Fruit bats (*Rousettus aegypticacus*) are the natural reservoirs for MARV. MARV has been isolated from the tissue of wild-caught, apparently healthy *R. aegypticacus*.[39] In addition, infected *R. aegypticacus* bats can shed the virus in their saliva, urine, and feces.

The incubation period for filovirus infection ranges from 2 to 21 days although most people develop symptoms 7–10 days after exposure to the virus. The clinical presentation of Ebola virus disease (EVD) and Marburg virus disease (MVD) can vary but in general, begins with fever, myalgia, weakness, and headache. Other reported signs and symptoms include conjunctival injection, rash, and cough. Typically, this is followed by abdominal pain, nausea, vomiting, and diarrhea. Coagulopathy usually appears late in the illness course and can include a petechial rash, ecchymosis, and sometimes overt bleeding (e.g., epistaxis, melena). Laboratory findings may include elevated liver enzymes, leukopenia, and thrombocytopenia.

During filovirus outbreaks, it is thought that there is one introduction of the virus (or spillover) from animals to humans. Any subsequent transmission events that may ensue are due to human-to-human transmission. Individuals infected with a filovirus can transmit the virus through contact, through broken skin, eyes, nose, mouth, or other mucous membranes, with a person who is ill or has died of the disease or with objects contaminated with the body fluids of a person who is ill or has died of the disease. There is no evidence that infectious aerosols play a role in human-to-human transmission of filoviruses.

Ebola Virus

An outbreak involving 318 cases and 280 deaths occurred in Yambuku, Zaire, in 1976, led to the discovery of Ebola virus. Investigations suggested that reuse of contaminated needles served to amplify the outbreak with devastating effects; all those infected by needle died.[40]

Between 1976 and July 2020, there have been 19 outbreaks due to Ebola virus (species Zaire Ebolavirus).

The major outbreaks of Ebola virus have all been associated with hospitals or clinics where nosocomial transmission was associated with reuse of needles or other unhygienic practices, from intimate contact between patients and caregivers at home, or from burial rituals that facilitated transmission. Outbreaks in Gabon and the Republic of the Congo appear to have originated following human contact with chimpanzees either killed or found dead and prepared as food.[41,42] In prior outbreaks, transmission was halted when patients were isolated, strict barrier nursing procedures implemented and safe burial practices were implemented. Isolated cases seen in modern, well-equipped medical facilities have not experienced sustained nosocomial transmission; however, importation of EVD from Liberia to the United States resulted in two instances of secondary transmission and serves as warning that given modern air travel, even an outbreak in a remote area represents a risk to all countries.[43,44]

The largest outbreak of EVD due to Ebola virus is the 2014 outbreak in West Africa (Guinea, Sierra Leone, Liberia) with 28,610 confirmed cases and 11,308 deaths. Prior this outbreak, knowledge of Ebola virus was largely restricted to a few distinct human outbreaks. Intense investigations triggered by the unprecedented 2014 Ebola outbreak has led to a great understanding of the pathogen.

After recovery from acute disease, the virus or its RNA can continue to be detected in some specific body fluids. Ebola virus RNA has been detected by reverse transcriptase polymerase chain reaction (RT-PCR) in vaginal secretions up to 33 days after onset of illness.[45] Ebola virus has been cultured from breast milk up to 15 days after illness onset and detected by RT-PCR as long as 16 months after illness onset.[46] Ebola virus can cross the placenta and pregnant women infected with the virus will likely transmit it to the fetus. Ebola virus RNA has been detected in amniotic fluid, fetal meconium, vaginal secretions, umbilical cord, and buccal swab samples from neonates born to infected mothers. Ebola virus can also persist in "immune privileged sites." Ebola virus RNA has been cultured from cerebrospinal fluid 10 months after illness onset.[47] Ebola virus has been cultured from ocular aqueous humor at 3 months after disease onset.[48] Ebola virus has been shown to persist in amniotic fluid for an unknown duration of time after negative RT-PCR tests for the virus in maternal blood.[49] Therefore proper infection control precautions should be taken when managing convalescent pregnant women. Ebola virus RNA has cultured from semen up to 82 days after illness onset[50] and detected by RT-PCR as long as 965 days after illness onset.[51]

Sexual transmission of Ebola virus has been documented following the 2014 West Africa epidemic. The first documented occurrence was reported in November of 2014 in Liberia.[52] In this instance, a male EVD survivor transmitted the virus to a female sexual partner 199 days after illness onset. Although no infectious virus was isolated from the semen, genetic analysis of the Ebola viruses recovered from the woman and from the semen of the male survivor closely matched.[53] In December 2015, a male EVD survivor in Guinea sexually transmitted Ebola virus to his female partner 470 days after onset of symptoms.[54]

In December 2019, the U.S. Federal Food and Drug Administration licensed the rVSVΔG-ZEBOV-GP Ebola vaccine (Ervebo®, Merck), a replication-competent, live, attenuated recombinant vesicular stomatitis virus-based vaccine (https://www.fda.gov/vaccines-blood-biologics/ervebo). The vaccine contains a live attenuated vesicular stomatitis virus in which the G gene of the VSV (Indiana) has been replaced with the GP gene of Ebola virus (Kikwit). Studies in nonhuman primates (NHP) have demonstrated that a single intramuscular injection of rVSV-ZEBOV elicits protective immune responses against lethal EBOV challenge when the vaccine is given at least 7 days before the challenge.[55] Complete protection has been observed when NHPs are challenged out to 42 days postvaccination but the duration of protection is unclear.[56] No serious vaccine-related adverse events were reported in published Phase 1 and Phase 2 clinical trials. However, mild to moderate transient reactogenicity was reported. The rVSV-ZEBOV vaccine was administered as part of a Phase 3 ring vaccination trial in Guinea during the 2014-16 EVD outbreak in West Africa. In this trial, all contacts and contacts to contacts of confirmed EVD patients were identified and randomly allocated to immediate or delayed vaccination. In this study zero cases of EVD occurred 10 or more days following randomization in those who were vaccinated immediately while 23 cases of EVD occurred among those randomized to delayed vaccination.[57]

There are no FDA approved treatments for EVD. However, promising results have been reported two monoclonal antibodies, REGN-EB3 and mAb114.[58,59] During the 2018 Democratic Republic of Congo EVD outbreak, a randomized clinical control trial was conducted comparing ZMapp (triple monoclonal antibody cocktail), REGN-EB3 (triple monoclonal antibody cocktail), mAb114 (single monoclonal antibody), and remdesivir (antiviral agent). REGN-EB3 and mAb114 were shown to be superior in reducing overall EVD mortality. At 28 days, the mortality rates for patients who received mAb114 was 35% and 33.5% in those who received REGN-EB3, compared to 49.7% in the ZMapp group.[101]

Reston Virus

In 1990, another Ebola virus was discovered, and like Marburg virus, it was associated with the importation of nonhuman primates for medical research. Rather than originating in Africa, these animals had been imported from the Philippines.[60] Infected monkeys suffered a severe, often fatal hemorrhagic disease, but although there is serological evidence of at least 16 human infections, none were symptomatic.[61] This strain has been named Reston virus for the northern Virginia suburb near Washington, DC where the first epizootic was discovered.

Tai Forest Virus

Tai Forest virus originated from a single human infection acquired when a primatologist studying free-living chimpanzees in the Tai Forest of western Côte d'Ivoire was infected while taking clinical specimens from a chimpanzee that had recently died of a hemorrhagic illness. This animal was one of several that had succumbed during a series of epizootics that had devastated the troop over the course of a few years. The patient suffered a febrile illness with rash, but fully recovered and it was only learned that her infection was due to a new strain of Ebola after she had been discharged from hospital. There was no indication of spread to the medical staff.[62]

Marburg Virus

Marburg virus (MARV) was first discovered following the importation of African Green Monkeys (*Cercopithecus aethiops*), into Germany and Yugoslavia from Uganda. These monkeys were used for production of kidney cells for use in preparation of poliovirus vaccine; the monkeys served as the source of MARV infection for laboratory workers initially, with secondary spread to both medical staff and family members. A total of 31 cases and 7 deaths occurred in Marburg, Germany, and another two in Belgrade, Yugoslavia, both of whom survived. Subsequent cases of Marburg infection have sporadically appeared in Zimbabwe, Democratic Republic of the Congo, Kenya, and Uganda. A large outbreak occurred in Angola in 2005, where 374 people were infected and 329 died.

BUNYAVIRUSES

The Order *Bunyavirales* is named after Bunyamwera, a town in Uganda where it was first identified.[63] Bunyaviruses include an estimated 530 viruses. Some are not associated with human disease and some cause human infection ranging from asymptomatic to fulminant hemorrhagic disease and death.[63] The rise of whole-genome sequencing has expanded the taxonomy and led to the renaming and restructuring of the Order *Bunyavirales* to 12 families and 46 genera, including the genus *Orthonairovirus*, family *Nairoviridae*, in which Crimean-Congo Hemorrhagic Fever virus is found; genus *Orthohantavirus*, family *Hantaviridae*, which contains the Hantaviruses; and the genus *Phlebovirus*, family *Phenuiviridae*, which contains Rift Valley Fever virus. The majority of the members of the Order *Bunyavirales* are arboviruses, transmitted to animals and/or humans via insect bites. The notable exception are the Hantaviruses, which are primarily found in rodents as well as shrews, moles, and bats.

Rift Valley Fever

Rift Valley fever virus, of the genus *Phlebovirus,* was discovered in 1931 during an investigation on a sheep farm in Kenya's Rift Valley, though reports of sick livestock emerged from the same area as early as 1910. Until 1977, major epizootics in eastern and southern Africa among large wild and domestic animals led to small numbers of human cases in association with outbreaks. In 1977, however, an explosive epizootic epidemic struck portions of the lower Nile River delta in Egypt with an estimated 200,000 human cases and at least 598 recorded deaths.[64] During an outbreak in Egypt in 1993, involving 6000 human cases, ocular disease was first recognized as an infrequent late manifestation of infection. Subsequent outbreaks have occurred in Kenya and Somalia, southern Saudi Arabia (884 cases, 14% mortality) and Yemen (1087 cases, 11.1% mortality).[65]

Typical RVF infection in humans presents as a self-limiting, undifferentiated acute febrile, flu-like illness marked by brief, high fever that is sometimes biphasic or cyclic every few days. Most RVF infections have no sequelae. Rare complications can include clinical ocular serous retinopathy with central scotomata in about 1% of cases, and acute fulminant, usually nonicteric hepatitis and hemorrhagic features (e.g., blood in urine, feces, and/or vomit), in approximately 1% of cases with a case-fatality of 20–50%.[66,67] Delayed neurologic symptoms including vertigo, disorientation, weakness, or partial paralysis can occur.[66]

Treatment for human disease is limited to supportive care. Antiviral drugs like ribavirin and favipiravir have shown promise for RVF as well as other viral hemorrhagic fevers.[68] Vaccines, however, remain the most promising and effective One-Health approach to prevention in both livestock and humans, and diverse attempts at vaccine development have been made.[67] They include inactivated vaccines for use in humans and livestock that generated antibody response but require multiple doses, a challenge for nomadic pastoral communities. A live attenuated vaccine (i.e., Smithburn vaccine) developed in South Africa for use in humans and animals produced immunity after a single dose but was associated with abortion in sheep, a concern with using live virus.[69] The first conditionally licensed recombinant live vaccine (MP-12) has been developed in the United States.[67] International concern over RVF is not limited to human infection. RVF can cause serious pantropic infection with significant mortality, particularly in young animals, and high rates of abortion in domestic animals such as cattle, sheep, and goats.[70] Understanding the prevalence and movement of livestock throughout and between countries is critical in preventing introduction of the disease into animal industries.

The ecology of RVF virus is relatively complex, relying on an insect reservoir (primarily *Aedes* mosquitos), with transovarial transmission facilitating viral maintenance, and amplifying hosts including wild and domestic animals. During periods of high rainfall, like those seen during an El Nino event, flooding can increase populations of *Aedes* mosquitoes, as well as other suspected vectors including *Anopheles*, *Culex*, and *Eretmapodites* mosquitoes.[71] Direct transmission to humans handling infected large animals or their carcasses via contact with infectious blood and infectious aerosols can also occur. Despite increased understanding of viral transmission and persistence, challenges remain in treatment and prevention.[67,68,70]

Due to its threat to humans and livestock, research using live virus is limited to facilities with at least a Biosafety Level 3 laboratory and is forbidden in many countries. Broad prevention efforts include mosquito abatement, syndromic surveillance in sentinel herds, and training health professionals to test and treat for Rift Valley fever virus infection.

Crimean-Congo Hemorrhagic Fever

Crimean-Congo hemorrhagic fever, CCHF, was first recognized in 1944 in Crimea during WWII and was later linked to a similar disease in 1956 in Belgian Congo [currently Democratic Republic of the Congo (DRC)], giving rise to its current name.[72] The causative agent of the disease was finally isolated in newborn mice in 1968 and found to be a member of the large Bunyaviridae family, genus *Nairovirus* (since renamed Family *Nairoviridae*, genus *Orthonairovirus*).[63] CCHF is currently regarded as the most broadly geographically distributed and genetically diverse tick-borne virus that infects humans.[73] Though ticks of the genus *Hyalomma* are the primary cause of human infections, CCHF is found in several genera of ixodid ticks (i.e., hard ticks).[73] Consequently, the possible range extends from Western China and India through the Middle East to much of Africa and Southern Europe with an expanding geographic range since first being recognized.[73–75] Emergence in previously unknown areas can be attributed to factors including tick vector expansion into suitable habitats, increased or improved surveillance, and introduction via wild animal migration expansion, including ticks transported by birds, and livestock trade practices to name a few.[76]

Presence of the tick vector alone is not indicative of the presence of CCHF. A variety of tick species has been implicated in the natural cycle and transmission to humans of CCHF virus. In Bulgaria and Russia, *Hyalomma marginatum*, is the principal vector. Immature stages parasitize small mammals and ground-feeding birds, while adults favor large domestic animals, such as cattle and sheep in addition to humans. Persons engaged in pastoral and agricultural activities are most at risk, and most cases occur during April–July, the period of peak activity of the adult ticks.[76] *H. marginatum* is also the primary tick vector in Turkey, where more than 10,000 confirmed cases (4.5% mortality) have been reported since 2002, with two-thirds of the cases occurring in rural areas, peaking in July amidst increasingly extended seasons.[77] Outbreaks in central Asia are less strongly seasonal but tend to occur most often during summer months and implicate ticks of the genera *Hyalomma, Rhipicephalus,* and *Boophilus*, which parasitize a range of hosts, most of which are large domestic animals.

CCHF is one of the most virulent viral hemorrhagic fevers and only causes clinical illness in humans despite causing viremia multiple vertebrate hosts. In addition to tick bites, contact with blood, tissue, or bodily fluids of infected animals or people is also a common source of infection. The incubation period and severity of disease can vary based on the source of exposure. Infection via tick bite has a usual incubation of 1–3 days with a maximum of 9 days and case-fatality average range of 13–25%. The incubation period associated with blood or tissue contact (often nosocomial) is usually 5–6 days up to a maximum of 13 days and nearly 40% case-fatality. Hemorrhagic manifestations, often with severe blood loss, appear after 3–7 days of illness.[78] Mild neurological manifestations can occur as well, and surviving patients occasionally suffer peripheral neuritis or emotional disturbances.[73,78]

There are no currently approved therapeutics or vaccines and supportive care is the primary treatment approach. Ribavirin may be an effective therapeutic agent, but consensus has not been reached owing to a lack of well-controlled studies.[79] Given orally, the drug may also be useful for postexposure prophylaxis of case contacts and has been used accordingly in outbreaks. Though approaches like reverse-genetics are revealing possible approaches for antivirals, the lack of an animal model of CCHF disease is an obstacle to development of a vaccine or antiviral drug. Development is slowed by the fact that work with live CCHF needs to be done in high-containment (BSL-4) laboratories. However, research using various vaccine approaches including adenovirus vectors, DNA-based vaccines as well as monoclonal antibodies used independently and in conjunction with antivirals such as favipiravir and ribavirin is ongoing.[77]

Hemorrhagic Fever with Renal Syndrome

Hemorrhagic fever with renal syndrome (HFRS) is a general term used to denote a constellation of similar clinical diseases with a range of similar symptoms caused by related viruses of the genus *Orthohantavirus*, family Hantaviridae. Many synonyms exist for these related diseases, including epidemic hemorrhagic fever, Korean hemorrhagic fever, hemorrhagic nephrosonephritis, and nephropathia epidemica.

Hantaviruses came to prominence in the 1950s during the Korean War, when United Nations soldiers were falling ill with fever, kidney failure, and shock. Approximately one-third of the over 3000 soldiers infected displayed symptoms of hemorrhagic illness and roughly 10% died.[80] It was not until 1978 that a virus was isolated in its host, *Apodemus agrarius* (striped field-mouse), and named Hantaan virus for the Hantaan River in South Korea.[80,81] Hantaviruses have since been shown to be globally distributed across all continents except Antarctica, residing in a diverse range of hosts and leading to a range of illnesses.[82,83]

The genus *Orthohantavirus* is divided into Old World and New World virus species. Old World hantaviruses are found across Asia and Europe and include Hantaan, Seoul, Dobrava, and Puumala hantaviruses among others and are associated with HFRS.[82,83] In contrast, New World hantaviruses are distributed throughout the Americas and include Sin Nombre, Black Creek Canal, and Andes hantaviruses and are associated with hantavirus pulmonary syndrome (HPS) or hantavirus cardiopulmonary syndrome (HCPS), a more severe disease with close to 40% mortality.[82]

The hantaviruses are maintained in nature by chronic infection of rodent hosts. Each hantavirus is thought to have co-evolved over a long period with a specific rodent host (e.g., Seoul orthohantavirus with *Rattus norvegicus* or Sin Nombre orthohantavirus with *Peromyscus maniculatus*) (Table 139-3).[84] Consequently, virus phylogeny mirrors rodent phylogeny consistent with the broad geographic distribution and diversity of potential rodent hosts.

Hantaan virus is the cause of HFRS, which occurs in a wide belt across Eurasia from Japan and Korea to the Ural Mountains of Russia, including much of China.[85] Humans are most frequently infected in rural areas during the harvest months of fall and early winter.[86] Other hantaviruses causing HFRS include Seoul virus,

TABLE 139-3 HANTAVIRUSES KNOWN TO CAUSE HUMAN DISEASE, THEIR PRIMARY HOSTS, AND DISTRIBUTION

Virus	Host Species[a]	Distribution of Virus	Distribution of Host Species[b]	Disease
Order: Rodentia; Family: Muridae; Subfamily: Murinae				
Hantaan[a] (HTNV)	*Apodemus agrarius*	Far Eastern Russia, Northern Asia, Balkans	Central Europe, S to Thrace, Caucasus, and Tien Mtns; Amur River through Korea, to E Xizang and E Yunnan, W Sichuan, Fujiau, Taiwan	Severe HFRS
Seoul[c] (SEOV)	*Rattus norvegicus*	Nearly worldwide	Nearly Worldwide	Mild/Moderate HFRS
Dobrava[c] (DOBV)	*Apodemus flavicollis*	Balkans	England, Wales; NW Spain, France,Denmark, S Scandinavia through European Russia, Italy, Balkans, Syria, Lebanon, Israel; Netherlands	HFRS (Severe)
Order: Rodentia; Family: Muridae; Subfamily: Arvicolinae				
Puumala[c] (PUUV)	*Clethrionomys glareolus*	Europe, Scandinavia, Russia, Balkans	France and Scandinavia to Lake Baikal, S to N Spain, N Italy, Balkans, W Turkey, N Kazakhstan; England, SW Ireland	Mild HFRS (Nephropathia epidemica)
Order: Rodentia; Family: Muridae; Subfamily: Sigmodontinae				
Sin Nombre[c] (SNV)	*Peromyscus Maniculatus;*	North America	Alaska across N Canada, S through USA to S Baja California and NC, Oaxaca, Mexico	HPS
SNV/New York[c,4] (NYV)	*Peromyscus leucopus*	East and Central USA	C and E USA into S and SE Canada, S to Yucatan Peninsula, Mexico	HPS
Black Creek Canal[c] (BCCV)	*Sigmodon hispidus (spadicipygus)*	Southern Florida	SE USA	HPS
Bayou[c] (BAYV)	*Oryzomys palustris*	Southeastern USA	SE USA	HPS
Muleshoe (MULEV)	*Sigmodon hispidus (texianus)*	Texas to Southern Nebraska	SE USA, interior Mexico to C Panama, N Columbia, and N Venezuela	HPS
Monongahela (MONV)	*Peromyscus maniculatus (nubiterrae)*	Eastern USA and Canada	Alaska across N Canada, S through USA to S Baja California and NC, Oaxaca, Mexico	HPS
Juquitiba (JUQV)	*Oligoryzomys nigripes*	Southeastern Brazil	E Brazil, E Paraguay, Uruguay, N Argentina	HPS
Araraquara (ARAV)	*Bolomys lasiurus*	Southeastern Brazil	E Bolivia, Paraguay, N Argentina, S Brazil	HPS
Castelo dos Sonhos (CASV)	*Unknown*	Central Brazil		HPS
Laguna Negra[c] (LNV)	*Calomys laucha*	Western Paraguay and Bolivia	N Argentina and Urguay, SE Boliviam W Paraguay, WC Brazil	HPS
Andes[c] (ANDV)	*Oligoryzomys longicaudatus*	Southwestern Argentina and Chile	Andes of Chile and Argentina	HPS
Order: Rodentia; Family: Muridae; Subfamily: Sigmodontinae				
Lechiguanas[c] (LECV)	*Oligoryzomys flavescens*	Central Argentina	SE Brazil, Uruguay, Argentina	HPS
Bermejo (BMJV)	*Oligoryzomys chacoensis*	Northwestern Argentina, Southern Bolivia	W Paraguay, SE Bolivia, WC Brazil, N Argentina	HPS
Oran (BMJV)	*Oligoryzomys logicaudatus*[d]	Northwestern Argentina, Southern Bolivia	Andes of Chile and Argentina	HPS
Hu39694	*Unknown*	Central Argentina		HPS
Central Plata	*Oligoryzomys flavescens*	S Uruguay	SE Brazil, Uruguay, Argentina	HPS
Choclo[c]	*Oligoryzomys fluvescens (costaricensis)*	Southwestern Panama	W and E versants of S Mexico, throughout Mesoamerica, to Ecuador, N Brazil, and Guianas in South America	HPS

[a]Subspecies are provided in parentheses for some species; distribution is for entire species.
[b]From Wilson DE and Reeder DM, eds., 1992. Mammal Species of the World: A Taxonomic and Geographic Reference 2nd ed. Smithonian Institution Press, Washington.
[c]Virus isolated in cell culture; others identified from genetic sequence.
[d]May be different species or subspecies of *Oligoryzomys longicaudatus.*
Sources: Compiled from Eisenberg JF, Redford KH. 1999. *Mammals of the Neotropics.* Vols. 1–3. Chicago: The University of Chicago Press; 1999.
Wilson DE, Ruff S. *The Smithsonian Book of North American Mammals.* Washington: Smithsonian Institution Press; 1999. Reid FA. *A Field Guide to the Mammals of Central America and Southeast Mexico.* New York: Oxford University Press; 1997.

associated with domestic rats (*Rattus rattus, R. norvegicus*) and found virtually worldwide; Puumala virus, maintained by the bank vole, *Clethrionomys glareolus*, and abundant in western Europe; and Dobrava virus, primarily in the Balkan region of Europe, and hosted by *Apodemus flavicollis*.[85,87]

Incidence rates of HFRS vary by country, the specific virus, and the abundance of their principal rodent hosts. In China, approximately 100,000 cases occur annually or about 0.1 per 1000 population. Puumala virus incidence ranges from 0.01 to greater than 0.2 per 1000, in endemic countries.[88]

Classic HFRS has a variable though potentially long incubation period of up to 4 weeks. The disease is characterized by five phases with possible overlap: (1) a *febrile phase* of 3–7 days' duration with fever, malaise, headache, abdominal pain, nausea, vomiting, facial flushing, petechiae, and conjunctival hemorrhage; (2) a *hypotensive phase* of a few hours to 3 days' duration, when hypotension, shock, visual blurring, and hemorrhagic signs occur; (3) an *oliguric phase* of 3–7 days' duration during which oliguria or anuria predominates, blood pressure returns to normal or is elevated, and hemorrhagic manifestations may worsen; (4) a *diuretic phase* of days to weeks' duration when polyuria predominates; and (5) a prolonged *convalescence phase* of weeks to months. Mortality rates for classic HFRS due to Hantaan virus range from 1% to 15%. Death typically occurs during the *hypotensive* or *oliguric* phases.[89] Seoul virus and Puumala virus cause a similar but typically milder disease with mortality rates < 1%. Seoul virus has been associated with outbreaks of HFRS traced to infected laboratory rat colonies and is also known to be abundant in urban rats in many large cities, including port cities in the United States.[88] Studies among Baltimore residents have explored the role of past infection with Seoul virus in the subsequent development of hypertensive renal disease.[90] Seoul virus has also been found in pet "fancy" rats in the United Kingdom,[91] and, more recently, Canada and in at least eleven states with 17 confirmed human infections in the United States.[92]

As with any rodent-related infectious disease, a first line of prevention relies primarily on reducing human-rodent contact through effective sanitation and waste management, and rodent exclusion from homes and buildings.

Hantavirus Pulmonary Syndrome

In 1993, an otherwise healthy Navajo couple in the Four Corners area of the United States fell ill with a severe respiratory illness of unknown etiology.[82] Not long after, researchers learned through serologic and molecular approaches that the etiologic agent was a newly identified virus in the genus *Hantavirus*, and the associated respiratory illness in humans was named HPS. The new virus species was named *Sin Nombre* and the primary host determined to be a rodent reservoir, *Peromyscus maniculatus*, or deer mouse, with a geographic range that includes most of North America,[80,93,94] HPS cases have been reported in Canada but not Mexico possibly as a result of surveillance bias.[94]

HPS surveillance began with the initial 1993 outbreak and became a nationally notifiable disease in 1995.[82] Since 1993, there have been close to 800 HPS cases reported across 39 U.S. states (31 cases were retrospectively identified through archived autopsy tissues or convalescent serum samples) with greater than 96% of the cases having occurred west of the Mississippi River. Nearly all of the HPS cases are attributed to SNV infection, however, some have been associated with other hantaviruses: Bayou (LA and TX; five cases), Black Creek Canal (FL; one case).

During the initial 1993 outbreak, HPS had a case fatality ranging from 50% to 60%, though it is currently estimated to be 35%.[80,95] The proposed mechanism of SNV infection in humans is inhalation of dried rodent excreta (e.g., urine and feces), followed by a typical incubation period of 2–3 weeks, but it can be as much as 8 weeks.[96] HPS is an aggressive clinical disease consisting of three phases: (1) prodromal, (2) cardiopulmonary, and (3) convalescent. The first phase presents with nonspecific symptoms of fever, malaise, and myalgia. The second phase, however, presents with distinctive cardiopulmonary involvement that can rapidly progress to noncardiogenic pulmonary edema and occasional renal involvement.[80,83] Asymptomatic cases are likely uncommon. For example, after a 2012 Yosemite Park outbreak where thousands of samples were tested by serology, only two cases were identified that did not report pulmonary symptoms.[97] Accordingly, the presence of cardiopulmonary symptoms is a reliably consistent and distinctive clinical feature of SNV infection.[82,96]

In HPS, histopathology displays lung inflammation and edema, but intact respiratory epithelium indicates cell-death is not the principal source of the pulmonary symptoms.[80] Treatment consists of general supportive therapy to support respiratory function, maintain fluid volume, and ensure adequate cardiac output. In the most severe HPS cases, advanced treatments such as extracorporeal membrane oxygenation (ECMO) have been used with some success.[89]

Increased risk of SNV infection is spatiotemporally related to the presence of infected rodent excrement, itself relating to high rodent density.[94] The primary route of transmission of rodents to humans is thought to be via inhalation of aerosolized rodent excrement, though risk of infection through direct inoculation from a bite or from contact of virus containing material with breaks in the skin or mucous membranes is also possible.[98,99] Consequently, behaviors and occupations such as forestry workers, construction workers, farmers, hunting/camping, and cleaning personnel are strong risk factors.[95,100] Prevention consists primarily of minimizing human exposure to rodents and their feces through sanitation and vector control.

References

1. Peters CJ. Arenaviruses. In: Belshi R, ed. *Textbook of Human Virology*. St. Louis, MO: Mosby Year Book; 1991:541–70.
2. Frame JD, Baldwin JM Jr, Gocke DJ, Troup JM. Lassa fever, a new virus disease of man from West Africa. I. Clinical description and pathological findings. *Am J Trop Med Hyg*. 1970;19(4):670–6.
3. Kofman A, Choi MJ, Rollin PE. Lassa fever in travelers from West Africa, 1969–2016. *Emerg Infect Dis*. 2019;25(2):245–8.
4. Mylne AQ, Pigott DM, Longbottom J, et al. Mapping the zoonotic niche of Lassa fever in Africa. *Trans R Soc Trop Med Hyg*. 2015;109(8):483–92.
5. Centers for Disease Control and Prevention. Lassa Fever. https://www.cdc.gov/vhf/lassa/index.html. Accessed September 10, 2019.
6. Cummins D, McCormick JB, Bennett D, et al. Acute sensorineural deafness in Lassa fever. *JAMA*. 1990;264(16):2093–6.
7. WHO. Lassa Fever. 2017. https://www.who.int/news-room/fact-sheets/detail/lassa-fever. Accessed September 10, 2019.
8. Lecompte E, Fichet-Calvet E, Daffis S, et al. Mastomys natalensis and Lassa fever, West Africa. *Emerg Infect Dis*. 2006;12(12):1971–4.
9. Mari Saez A, Cherif Haidara M, Camara A, et al. Rodent control to fight Lassa fever: Evaluation and lessons learned from a 4-year study in Upper Guinea. *PLoS Negl Trop Dis*. 2018;12(11):e0006829.
10. Ter Meulen J, Lukashevich I, Sidibe K, et al. Hunting of peridomestic rodents and consumption of their meat as possible risk factors for rodent-to-human transmission of Lassa virus in the Republic of Guinea. *Am J Trop Med Hyg*. 1996;55(6):661–6.
11. McCormick JB, King IJ, Webb PA, et al. A case-control study of the clinical diagnosis and course of Lassa fever. *J Infect Dis*. 1987;155(3):445–55.
12. Maiztegui JI. Clinical and epidemiological patterns of Argentine haemorrhagic fever. *Bull World Health Organ*. 1975;52(4-6):567–75.
13. Ambrosio A, Saavedra M, Mariani M, Gamboa G, Maiza A. Argentine hemorrhagic fever vaccines. *Hum Vaccin*. 2011;7(6):694–700.
14. Carballal G, Videla CM, Merani MS. Epidemiology of Argentine hemorrhagic fever. *Eur J Epidemiol*. 1988;4(2):259–74.
15. Mills JN, Ellis BA, Childs JE, et al. Prevalence of infection with Junin virus in rodent populations in the epidemic area of Argentine hemorrhagic fever. *Am J Trop Med Hyg*. 1994;51(5):554–62.
16. Enria DA. Arenaviral hemorrhagic fevers: Argentine hemorraghic fever and Lassa fever. In: Power C, Johnson RT, eds. *Emerging Neurological Infections (Neurological Disease and Therapy Series)*. Vol. 67. Boca Raton, FL: CRC Press; 2005, p. 505.

17. Mackenzie RB, Beye HK, Valverde L, Garron H. Epidemic hemorrhagic fever in Bolivia. I. A preliminary report of the epidemiologic and clinical findings in a new epidemic area in South America. *Am J Trop Med Hyg.* 1964;13:620–5.
18. Patterson M, Grant A, Paessler S. Epidemiology and pathogenesis of Bolivian hemorrhagic fever. *Curr Opin Virol.* 2014;5:82–90.
19. Dragoo JW, Salazar-Bravo J, Layne LJ, Yates TL. Relationships within the *Calomys callosus* species group based on amplified fragment length polymorphisms. *Biochem Syst Ecol.* 2003;31(7):703–13.
20. Stinebaugh BJ, Schloeder FX, Johnson KM, Mackenzie RB, Entwisle G, De Alba E. Bolivian hemorrhagic fever. A report of four cases. *Am J Med.* 1966;40(2):217–30.
21. Peters CJ, Kuehne RW, Mercado RR, Le Bow RH, Spertzel RO, Webb PA. Hemorrhagic fever in Cochabamba, Bolivia, 1971. *Am J Epidemiol.* 1974;99(6):425–33.
22. Jahrling PT, R Barrero O. Cross protection against Machupo virus with Candid 1 Junin virus vaccine. Paper presented at: *Proceedings of the Second International Vonference on the Impact of Viral Disease on the Development of Latin American Countries and the Caribbean Region* 1988; Mar del Plata, Argentina.
23. Kilgore PE, Ksiazek TG, Rollin PE, et al. Treatment of Bolivian hemorrhagic fever with intravenous ribavirin. *Clin Infect Dis.* 1997;24(4):718–22.
24. Salas R, de Manzione N, Tesh RB, et al. Venezuelan haemorrhagic fever. *Lancet.* 1991;338(8774):1033–6.
25. de Manzione N, Salas RA, Paredes H, et al. Venezuelan hemorrhagic fever: Clinical and epidemiological studies of 165 cases. *Clin Infect Dis.* 1998;26(2):308–13.
26. Fulhorst CF, Ksiazek TG, Peters CJ, Tesh RB. Experimental infection of the cane mouse *Zygodontomys brevicauda* (family Muridae) with guanarito virus (Arenaviridae), the etiologic agent of Venezuelan hemorrhagic fever. *J Infect Dis.* 1999;180(4):966–9.
27. Lisieux T, Coimbra M, Nassar ES, et al. New arenavirus isolated in Brazil. *Lancet.* 1994;343(8894):391–2.
28. Coimbra T. Arenavirus: A fatal outcome. *Virus Rev Res.* 2001;6(1):14.
29. Barry M, Russi M, Armstrong L, et al. Brief report: Treatment of a laboratory-acquired Sabia virus infection. *N Engl J Med.* 1995;333(5):294–6.
30. Centers for Disease Control and Prevention. Lymphocytic choriomeningitis. 2014. https://www.cdc.gov/vhf/lcm/index.html. Accessed September 10, 2019.
31. Bonthius DJ. Lymphocytic choriomeningitis virus: An underrecognized cause of neurologic disease in the fetus, child, and adult. *Semin Pediatr Neurol.* 2012;19(3):89–95.
32. Childs JE, Glass GE, Korch GW, Ksiazek TG, Leduc JW. Lymphocytic choriomeningitis virus infection and house mouse (*Mus musculus*) distribution in urban Baltimore. *Am J Trop Med Hyg.* 1992;47(1):27–34.
33. Genovesi EV, Johnson AJ, Peters CJ. Susceptibility and resistance of inbred strains of Syrian golden hamsters (*Mesocricetus auratus*) to wasting disease caused by lymphocytic choriomeningitis virus: Pathogenesis of lethal and non-lethal infections. *J Gen Virol.* 1988;69 (Pt 9):2209–20.
34. Hinman AR, Fraser DW, Douglas RG, et al. Outbreak of lymphocytic choriomeningitis virus infections in medical center personnel. *Am J Epidemiol.* 1975;101(2):103–10.
35. Knust B, Stroher U, Edison L, et al. Lymphocytic choriomeningitis virus in employees and mice at multipremises feeder-rodent operation, United States, 2012. *Emerg Infect Dis.* 2014;20(2):240–7.
36. Goldstein T, Anthony SJ, Gbakima A, et al. The discovery of Bombali virus adds further support for bats as hosts of ebolaviruses. *Nat Microbiol.* 2018;3(10):1084–9.
37. Leroy EM, Kumulungui B, Pourrut X, et al. Fruit bats as reservoirs of Ebola virus. *Nature.* 2005;438(7068):575–6.
38. Swanepoel R, Leman PA, Burt FJ, et al. Experimental inoculation of plants and animals with Ebola virus. *Emerg Infect Dis.* 1996;2(4):321–5.
39. Towner JS, Amman BR, Sealy TK, et al. Isolation of genetically diverse Marburg viruses from Egyptian fruit bats. *PLoS Pathog.* 2009;5(7):e1000536.
40. Report of an International Commission. Ebola haemorrhagic fever in Zaire, 1976. *Bull World Health Organ.* 1978;56(2):271–93.
41. Georges AJ, Leroy EM, Renaut AA, et al. Ebola hemorrhagic fever outbreaks in Gabon, 1994–1997: Epidemiologic and health control issues. *J Infect Dis.* 1999;179 Suppl 1:S65–75.
42. Maganga GD, Kapetshi J, Berthet N, et al. Ebola virus disease in the Democratic Republic of Congo. *N Engl J Med.* 2014;371(22):2083–91.
43. Liddell AM, Davey RT Jr, Mehta AK, et al. Characteristics and clinical management of a cluster of 3 patients with Ebola virus disease, including the first domestically acquired cases in the United States. *Ann Intern Med.* 2015;163(2):81–90.
44. Yacisin K, Balter S, Fine A, et al. Ebola virus disease in a humanitarian aid worker—New York City, October 2014. *MMWR Morb Mortal Wkly Rep.* 2015;64(12):321–3.
45. Rodriguez LL, De Roo A, Guimard Y, et al. Persistence and genetic stability of Ebola virus during the outbreak in Kikwit, Democratic Republic of the Congo, 1995. *J Infect Dis.* 1999;179 Suppl 1:S170–6.
46. WHO. Clinical care of survivors of Ebola virus disease interim guidance. https://www.who.int/csr/resources/publications/ebola/guidance-survivors/en/.
47. Jacobs M, Rodger A, Bell DJ, et al. Late Ebola virus relapse causing meningoencephalitis: A case report. *Lancet.* 2016;388(10043):498–503.
48. Varkey JB, Shantha JG, Crozier I, et al. Persistence of Ebola virus in ocular fluid during convalescence. *N Engl J Med.* 2015;372(25):2423–7.
49. Oduyebo T, Pineda D, Lamin M, Leung A, Corbett C, Jamieson DJ. A pregnant patient with Ebola virus disease. *Obstet Gynecol.* 2015;126(6):1273–5.
50. Uyeki TM, Erickson BR, Brown S, et al. Ebola virus persistence in semen of male survivors. *Clin Infect Dis.* 2016;62(12):1552–5.
51. Fischer WA, Brown J, Wohl DA, et al. Ebola virus ribonucleic acid detection in semen more than two years after resolution of acute Ebola virus infection. *Open Forum Infect Dis.* 2017;4(3):ofx155.
52. Christie A, Davies-Wayne GJ, Cordier-Lassalle T, et al. Possible sexual transmission of Ebola virus—Liberia, 2015. *MMWR Morb Mortal Wkly Rep.* 2015;64(17):479–81.
53. Mate SE, Kugelman JR, Nyenswah TG, et al. Molecular evidence of sexual transmission of Ebola virus. *N Engl J Med.* 2015;373(25):2448–54.
54. Diallo B, Sissoko D, Loman NJ, et al. Resurgence of Ebola virus disease in Guinea linked to a survivor with virus persistence in seminal fluid for more than 500 days. *Clin Infect Dis.* 2016;63(10):1353–6.
55. Marzi A, Robertson SJ, Haddock E, et al. EBOLA VACCINE. VSV-EBOV rapidly protects macaques against infection with the 2014/15 Ebola virus outbreak strain. *Science.* 2015;349(6249):739–42.
56. Geisbert TW, Daddario-Dicaprio KM, Lewis MG, et al. Vesicular stomatitis virus-based Ebola vaccine is well-tolerated and protects immunocompromised nonhuman primates. *PLoS Pathog.* 2008;4(11):e1000225.
57. Henao-Restrepo AM, Camacho A, Longini IM, et al. Efficacy and effectiveness of an rVSV-vectored vaccine in preventing Ebola virus disease: Final results from the Guinea ring vaccination, open-label, cluster-randomised trial (Ebola Ca Suffit!). *Lancet.* 2017;389(10068):505–18.
58. Corti D, Misasi J, Mulangu S, et al. Protective monotherapy against lethal Ebola virus infection by a potently neutralizing antibody. *Science.* 2016;351(6279):1339–42.
59. Sivapalasingam S, Kamal M, Slim R, et al. Safety, pharmacokinetics, and immunogenicity of a co-formulated cocktail of three human monoclonal antibodies targeting Ebola virus glycoprotein in healthy adults: A randomised, first-in-human phase 1 study. *Lancet Infect Dis.* 2018;18(8):884–93.
60. Jahrling PB, Geisbert TW, Dalgard DW, et al. Preliminary report: Isolation of Ebola virus from monkeys imported to USA. *Lancet.* 1990;335(8688):502–5.
61. Centers for Disease Control and Prevention. Update: Filovirus infection in animal handlers. *MMWR Morb Mortal Wkly Rep.* 1990;39(13):221.
62. Le Guenno B, Formenty P, Wyers M, Gounon P, Walker F, Boesch C. Isolation and partial characterisation of a new strain of Ebola virus. *Lancet.* 1995;345(8960):1271–4.
63. Adams MJ, Lefkowitz EJ, King AMQ, et al. Changes to taxonomy and the International Code of Virus Classification and Nomenclature ratified by the International Committee on Taxonomy of Viruses (2017). *Arch Virol.* 2017;162(8):2505–38.
64. Khan AS, Smith CV. Rift Valley fever: Still an emerging infection after 3500 years. *Lancet Glob Health.* 2016;4(11):e773–4.
65. Shoemaker T, Boulianne C, Vincent MJ, et al. Genetic analysis of viruses associated with emergence of Rift Valley fever in Saudi Arabia and Yemen, 2000–01. *Emerg Infect Dis.* 2002;8(12):1415–20.
66. Madani TA, Al-Mazrou YY, Al-Jeffri MH, et al. Rift Valley fever epidemic in Saudi Arabia: Epidemiological, clinical, and laboratory characteristics. *Clin Infect Dis.* 2003;37(8):1084–92.
67. Faburay B, LaBeaud AD, McVey DS, Wilson WC, Richt JA. Current status of Rift Valley fever vaccine development. *Vaccines (Basel).* 2017;5(3):29.
68. Atkins C, Freiberg AN. Recent advances in the development of antiviral therapeutics for Rift Valley fever virus infection. *Future Virol.* 2017;12(11):651–65.

69. Ikegami T. Rift valley fever vaccines: An overview of the safety and efficacy of the live-attenuated MP-12 vaccine candidate. *Expert Rev Vaccines.* 2017;16(6):601–11.
70. Bird BH, McElroy AK. Rift Valley fever virus: Unanswered questions. *Antiviral Res.* 2016;132:274–80. Web.
71. Bird BH, Ksiazek TG, Nichol ST, Maclachlan NJ. Rift Valley fever virus. *J Am Vet Med Assoc.* 2009;234(7):883–93.
72. Al-Abri SS, Abaidani IA, Fazlalipour M, et al. Current status of Crimean-Congo haemorrhagic fever in the World Health Organization Eastern Mediterranean region: Issues, challenges, and future directions. *Int J Infect Dis.* 2017;58:82–9.
73. Bente DA, Forrester NL, Watts DM, McAuley AJ, Whitehouse CA, Bray M. Crimean-Congo hemorrhagic fever: History, epidemiology, pathogenesis, clinical syndrome and genetic diversity. *Antiviral Res.* 2013;100(1):159–89.
74. WHO. First documented case of human Crimean-Congo Haemorrhagic Fever (CCHF) in India. 2018. http://www.searo.who.int/emerging_diseases/topics/cchf/en/. Accessed March 10, 2019.
75. Negredo, A. Brief report: Autochthonous Crimean-Congo hemorrhagic fever in Spain. *N Engl J Med.* 2017;377(2):154. *Pharma and Biotech Premium PRO.* Web.
76. Dowall SD, Carroll MW, Hewson R. Development of vaccines against Crimean-Congo haemorrhagic fever virus. *Vaccine.* 2017;35(44):6015–23.
77. Spengler JR, Bente DA, Bray M, et al. Second International Conference on Crimean-Congo hemorrhagic fever. *Antiviral Res.* 2018;150:137–47.
78. Ergönül Ö. Crimean-Congo haemorrhagic fever. *Lancet Infect Dis.* 2006;6(4):203–14.
79. Johnson S, Henschke N, Maayan N, et al. Ribavirin for treating Crimean Congo haemorrhagic fever. *Cochrane Database Syst Rev.* 2018;6:CD012713.
80. McCaughey C, Hart CA. Hantaviruses. *J Med Microbiol.* 2000;49(7):587–99.
81. Glass GE, Cheek JE, Patz JA, et al. Using remotely sensed data to identify areas at risk for hantavirus pulmonary syndrome. *Emerg Infect Dis.* 2000;6(3):238–47.
82. Knust B, Rollin PE. Twenty-year summary of surveillance for human hantavirus infections, United States. *Emerg Infect Dis.* 2013;19(12):1934–7.
83. Vaheri A, Strandin T, Hepojoki J, et al. Uncovering the mysteries of hantavirus infections. *Nat Rev Microbiol.* 2013;11(8):539–50.
84. Plyusnin A, Sironen T. Evolution of hantaviruses: Co-speciation with reservoir hosts for more than 100 MYR. *Virus Res.* 2014;187:22–6.
85. Avšič-Županc T, Saksida A, Korva M. Hantavirus infections. *Clin Microbiol Infect.* 2019;21:e6–16.
86. Zhang C, Fu X, Zhang Y, et al. Epidemiological and time series analysis of haemorrhagic fever with renal syndrome from 2004 to 2017 in Shandong Province, China. *Sci Rep.* 2019;9(1):1–9.
87. Holmes EC, Zhang YZ. The evolution and emergence of hantaviruses. *Curr Opin Virol.* 2015;10:27–33.
88. Clement J, LeDuc WJ, Lloyd G, et al. Wild rats, laboratory rats, pet rats: Global seoul hantavirus disease revisited. *Viruses.* 2019;11(7):652.
89. Rollin PE,Knust B, Nichol S. Hantaviral diseases. In: Heymann DL, ed. *Control of Communicable Diseases Manual.* 20th ed. Washington, DC: American Public Health Association; 2015.
90. Glass GE, Watson AJ, LeDuc JW, Kelen GD, Quinn TC, Childs JE. Infection with a ratborne hantavirus in US residents is consistently associated with hypertensive renal disease. *J Infect Dis.* 1993;167(3):614–20.
91. Jameson LJ, Logue CH, Atkinson B, et al. The continued emergence of hantaviruses: Isolation of a Seoul virus implicated in human disease, United Kingdom, October 2012. *Euro Surveill.* 2013;18(1):4–7.
92. Kerins JL, Koske SE, Kazmierczak J, et al. Outbreak of Seoul virus among rats and rat owners—United States and Canada, 2017. *MMWR Morb Mortal Wkly Rep.* 2018;67(4):131–4.
93. Childs JE, Ksiazek TG, Spiropoulou CF, et al. Serologic and genetic identification of *Peromyscus maniculatus* as the primary rodent reservoir for a new hantavirus in the southwestern United States. *J Infect Dis.* 1994;169(6):1271–80.
94. Mills JN, Amman BR, Glass GE. Ecology of hantaviruses and their hosts in North America. *Vector Borne Zoonotic Dis.* 2010;10(6):563–74.
95. de St Maurice A, Ervin E, Schumacher M, et al. Exposure characteristics of hantavirus pulmonary syndrome patients, United States, 1993–2015. *Emerg Infect Dis.* 2017;23(5):733–39.
96. Kitsutani PT, Denton RW, Fritz CL, et al. Acute Sin Nombre hantavirus infection without pulmonary syndrome, United States. *Emerg Infect Dis.* 1999;5(5):701–5.
97. Nunez JJ, Fritz CL, Knust B, et al. Hantavirus infections among overnight visitors to Yosemite National Park, California, USA, 2012. *Emerg Infect Dis.* 2014;20(3):386–93.
98. Carver S, Mills JN, Parmenter CA, et al. Toward a mechanistic understanding of environmentally forced zoonotic disease emergence: Sin Nombre hantavirus. *Bioscience.* 2015;65(7):651–66.
99. Mills JN, Johnson JM, Ksiazek TG, et al. A survey of hantavirus antibody in small-mammal populations in selected United States National Parks. *Am J Trop Med Hyg.* 1998;58(4):525–32.
100. Watson DC, Sargianou M, Papa A, Chra P, Starakis I, Panos G. Epidemiology of hantavirus infections in humans: A comprehensive, global overview. *Crit Rev Microbiol.* 2014;40(3):261–72.
101. Mulangu S, Dodd LE, Davey RT Jr, et al. A randomized, controlled trial of Ebola virus disease therapeutics. N Engl J Med. 2019;381(24): 2293-2303.

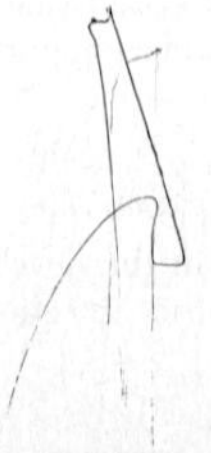

CHAPTER

140 Viral Zoonoses—Rabies

Emily G. Pieracci • Jesse D. Blanton

INTRODUCTION

Rabies is an acute progressive viral infection of the central nervous system that has affected animals and humans for millennia. The etiological agents of rabies are bullet-shaped RNA viruses in the genus *Lyssavirus*, family *Rhabdoviridae*. Currently, 16 species are recognized members of the *Lyssavirus* genus (Table 140-1).[1] Human rabies cases have been attributed to six different species, but *rabies lyssavirus* remains the leading cause of rabies globally. While most warm-blooded vertebrates have been shown to be susceptible to infection under experimental conditions,[2,3] mammals are the hosts responsible for maintaining the virus in nature. Specifically, species in the orders *Carnivora* and *Chiroptera* act as primary reservoirs.[4] Globally, the domestic dog is the primary reservoir and the species most associated with infection in humans.[5] However, multiple wildlife species have also been identified as reservoirs of specific rabies virus variants and various bat species as reservoirs of different *Lyssavirus* species. Human rabies cases are an incidental consequence of interaction with rabid animals.

DISTRIBUTION AND EPIDEMIOLOGY

Rabies is globally distributed, with the exception of Antarctica and some islands (mostly Pacific Islands).[6] Some countries such as those in Western Europe have been successful at eliminating rabies in both domestic dogs and wildlife [e.g., Arctic foxes (*Vulpes lagopus*)] populations through vaccination campaigns. While domestic dogs were targeted using historical vaccination methods (i.e., parenteral vaccines), foxes were successfully vaccinated through oral rabies vaccination campaigns.[7–9] While *Lyssaviruses* are present in European bat populations, *rabies lyssavirus* is not present in bats outside the Western hemisphere.[10]

In the United States and Canada, rabies virus was eliminated from domestic dogs through increased vaccination coverage and dog control programs that included confinement, stringent leash-laws, and destruction of stray animals.[2,11] However, both countries continue to have enzootic transmission in both bats and other wildlife species including: striped skunks (*Mephitis mephitis*), raccoons (*Procyon lotor*), Arctic foxes (*V. lagopus*), gray foxes (*Urocyon cinereoargenteus*), coati (*Nasua narica*), and mongoose (*Herpestes auropunctatus*) (Fig. 140-1).[12] Cases of human rabies associated with most of these terrestrial wildlife reservoirs are rarely reported. Bats are now the primary species associated with human rabies cases in the Western Hemisphere. However, exposure to potentially rabid animals and the need for postexposure prophylaxis (PEP) remains frequent despite the elimination of canine rabies. In the United States, the annual incidence of PEP administration is estimated to be between 8 and 11/100,000 population, but varies geographically depending on the predominant rabies reservoir present in each region.[13]

In Central and South America, wildlife as well as domestic dog rabies persists. Canine rabies vaccination programs are in place, however, achieving adequate vaccination coverage has been challenging. As a result, a small number of human deaths attributed to canine rabies occur every year in this region of the world.[4,14] Wildlife species, such as the common vampire bat (*Desmodus rotundus*), are primarily responsible for rabies transmission in livestock animals.[15]

African and Asian countries continue to have widespread rabies virus transmission, and domestic dogs are the primary contributors to the global human rabies burden.[5] Wildlife reservoirs in Africa and Asia can include: ferret badgers (*Melogale moschata*),[16] red foxes (*V. vulpes*), golden jackals (*Canis aureus*), grey wolves (*Canis lupus*),[17,18] and African jackals (*C. adustus, C. mesomelas*).[19] However, the true impact of wildlife rabies on the global rabies burden is largely uncharacterized due to limited surveillance and laboratory diagnostic capacity within many countries.[5] Approximately 96% of the estimated 59,000 global human rabies deaths annually occur in Asia and Africa specifically in countries where canine rabies remains endemic.[5,20] Another 28 million persons in this region are estimated to receive rabies PEP due to potential rabies virus exposures. However, poor surveillance for human and animal rabies makes global estimates difficult[21] resulting in broad ranges in the estimated number of cases. In comparison, developed countries in Western Europe and the Americas have largely eliminated or controlled canine rabies and consequently have observed significant decreases in the number of reported human rabies cases.[14]

TRANSMISSION

Rabies virus is transmitted most commonly through saliva from the bite or scratch of an infected animal.[22] Once introduced into the site of the wound the virus will replicate in peripheral tissues before entering the peripheral nervous system and traveling to the central nervous system, where it will begin to replicate and disseminate to the salivary glands and other organs.[14,23] Other modes of transmission may include aerosolization of virus (a potential risk in laboratory settings and possibly in caves occupied by bats), organ transplantation, and ingestion of infected meat (containing peripheral nervous tissue) and organs.[20,24–27] Infectious material from a rabid human or animal includes saliva, nervous tissue and tears; however, blood, urine, and feces are not considered infectious.[22]

DISEASE CHARACTERISTICS IN ANIMALS

Rabies virus has a variable incubation period, but clinical signs of infection are most commonly seen 1–3 months after infection.[28] The infectious period is the time period in which an infected animal is shedding virus in their saliva, and therefore capable of transmitting

TABLE 140-1 LYSSAVIRUS SPECIES

Lyssavirus Species	Distribution	Reservoirs	Comments
Rabies lyssavirus	Worldwide[a]	Chiroptera, Carnivora	Estimated > 59,000 human deaths per year
Aravan lyssavirus[b]	Eurasia	Chiroptera	No reported human cases
Australian bat lyssavirus	Australia	Chiroptera	Three reported human cases
Bokeloh bat lyssavirus	Europe	Chiroptera	No reported human cases
Duvenhage lyssavirus	Africa	Chiroptera	Three reported human cases
European bat 1 lyssavirus	Europe	Chiroptera	Two reported human cases, spillover into domestic and wild species
European bat 2 lyssavirus	Europe	Chiroptera	Two reported human cases, spillover reported in domestic and wild species
Gannoruwa bat lyssavirus	Asia	Chiroptera	No reported human cases
Ikoma lyssavirus[b]	Africa	Carnivora	No reported human cases
Khujand lyssavirus[b]	Eurasia	Chiroptera	No reported human cases
Lagos bat lyssavirus	Africa	Chiroptera	No reported human cases, spillover reported in domestic and wild species
Lleida bat lyssavirus[b]	Europe	Chiroptera	No reported human cases
Mokola lyssavirus	Africa	Shrews (*Crocidura spp.*)	Two reported human cases
Shimoni bat lyssavirus[b]	Africa	Chiroptera	No reported human cases
West Caucasian bat lyssavirus[b]	Eurasia	Chiroptera	No reported human cases

[a]Except Antarctica, Australia, and New Zealand.
[b]Only a single isolate identified.

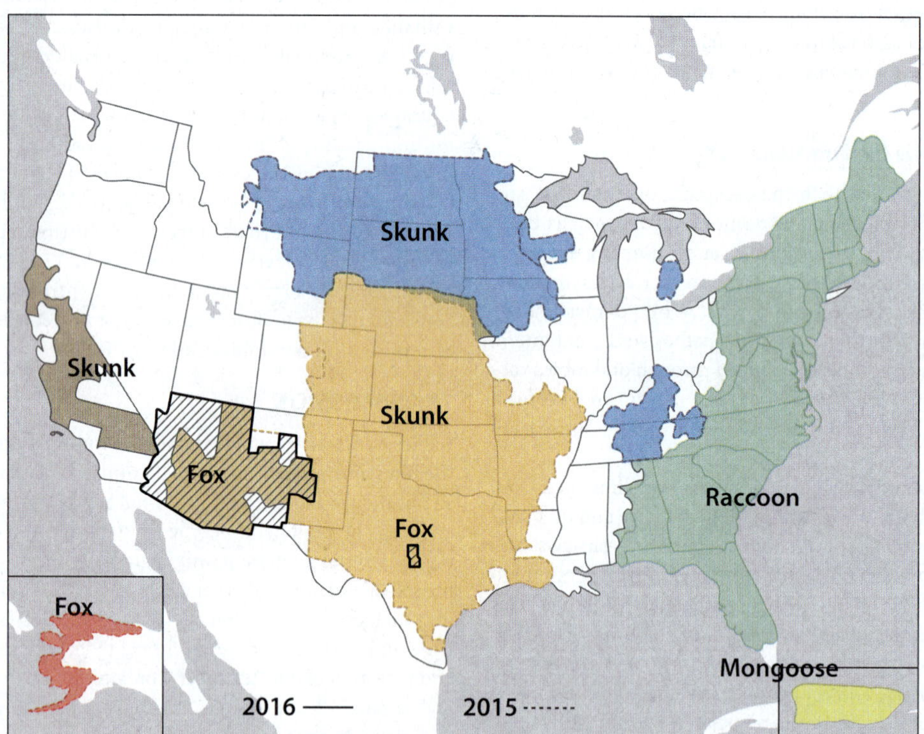

FIGURE 140-1. Distribution of major rabies virus variants (RVV) among mesocarnivores in the United States and Puerto Rico for 2011–16. Black diagonal lines represent distribution of gray fox RVV. Solid borders represent RVV distribution for 2012–16; dashed borders represent the previous 5-year distribution for 2011–15.[12] Reproduce with Permission from Ma X, Monroe BP, Cleaton JM, et al. Rabies surveillance in the United States during 2016. JAVMA 2018, 252; 8: 945–957.

the virus. Cats, dogs, and ferrets are well documented to begin shedding virus in their saliva several days before the onset of clinical signs, which is the basis for the 10-day quarantine recommendation in these species.[20] The overall infectious period extends from this presymptomatic period until the animal has died. If a person is bitten more than 10 days prior to the animal showing clinical signs of illness then PEP is not indicated or can be discontinued if already started. Some studies have shown intermittent shedding periods in rabid dogs,[29,30] but there are limited shedding studies for wildlife reservoirs and domestic livestock.[28]

Historically, rabid animals were described as having either "furious," "dumb," or "paralytic"[31] forms of the virus; however, this nomenclature does not accurately portray the varied presentations of rabies virus infections. Animals can experience a variety of clinical signs over the course of illness, such as fever, excessive salivation, hydrophobia (fear of water), aerophobia (fear of air), lethargy, change in vocalization, aggression, priapism, and sensitivities to light, movement, and sound.[28] While an animal may initially show signs of aggression, over the course of illness, the animal will become increasingly lethargic and disoriented before death occurs. The general time period from illness onset to death is 1–2 weeks.

DISEASE CHARACTERISTICS IN HUMANS

The average incubation period of rabies virus infections in humans is 1–3 months, but can range from 2 weeks to 6 years.[32] The incubation period may be dependent on several factors including, the location and severity of the wound, and the amount of virus inoculated.[20,32] Wounds to the face, head, neck, and hands can have shorter incubation periods due to decreased distance from the site of the wound to the central nervous system, as well as a greater number of neurons in those anatomical locations.[33] Illness onset has been documented in as little as 5 days in cases where severe head wounds were sustained.[20] Clinical signs of rabies virus infection in humans include: paresthesias at the site of the inoculation, fever, hydrophobia, aerophobia, excessive salivation, lethargy, painful laryngeal spasms, and eventually death.[20,34]

There is no known cure for rabies once clinical signs have begun. Palliative care can include sedation, muscle relaxants, antipyretics, respiratory support, and pain medication. Comprehensive and compassionate patient management should aim to alleviate thirst, anxiety, and epileptic fits.[35] Experimental clinical therapies have been used on an individual basis with limited success.[36,37] As of June 2017, only 14 of the 70 (20%) rabies victims that have undergone experimental treatment protocols have survived.[38,39] However, it has been suggested that the elevated survival rates are due to the intensive care provided to these patients over their months-long period of illness, and not directly correlated with the experimental clinical therapy itself.[40] This experimental treatment protocol is infrequently used in resource-limited settings. Patients that do survive rabies virus infection must overcome numerous severe, neurologic sequelae, such as involuntary movements, limb rigidity, poor swallow reflex, quadriplegia, and opisthotonoid (muscle spasm causing severe backward arching of head, neck, and spine) postures.[41,42] Very few survivors have ever completely recovered.[40,42]

DIAGNOSIS

A well-defined case definition can help identify cases of acute progressive encephalitis that are probably due to rabies. However, clinical diagnosis can be difficult and other infectious and noninfectious conditions can present with similar clinical signs to rabies.[20] Laboratory methods should be used to confirm clinically suspect or probable rabies cases whenever possible.

Laboratory diagnosis of suspect or probable cases of human or animal rabies can be performed before or after death. Ante-mortem laboratory diagnosis requires multiple diagnostic samples (i.e., CSF, saliva, serum, and a nuchal skin biopsy) to evaluate for the presence of viral antigen, viral RNA, and rabies virus-specific antibodies and is typically reserved for human rabies diagnosis. The relative sensitivity of any specific assay on a given sample depends on when samples are taken in the course of illness. For example, serological assays on serum and CSF tend to be more sensitive when performed during the later stages of illness. Postmortem detection of rabies virus in brain tissue remains the standard diagnostic assay.[20] Postmortem sampling of brain tissue remains the standard for rabies diagnosis in animals.

The direct fluorescent antibody (DFA) test is the standard assay for diagnosing rabies. The assay utilizes a rabies virus-specific antibody labeled with a fluorescent tag to detect antigen in brain tissue impressions (postmortem) or skin biopsy sections (ante mortem) under fluorescent microscopy.[20] The direct rapid immunohistochemistry test (DRIT) has the advantage of only requiring a regular light microscope and has comparable sensitivity and specificity to that of the DFA.[43] Additional characterization of positive samples is possible using specific monoclonal antibody panels using either the DFA or DRIT to identify rabies virus variants. Other assays for antigen detection (e.g., ELISA and Lateral Flow Assays) have been developed but have lower diagnostic validity compared to the DFA and DRIT and are not routinely recommended for diagnosis impacting clinical decision-making.[20,44]

Detection of viral RNA by reverse transcriptase polymerase chain reaction (RT-PCR) has been well described and—depending on the specific assay used—can be equivalent or more sensitive and specific than the DFA. RT-PCR assays have been used as primary confirmatory tests for inconclusive DFA and DRIT results. A number of recently developed real-time RT-PCR assays show promise as alternatives for primary diagnosis. Sequencing of the products from PCR amplification also allows for additional detailed analysis of viral variants and phylogenetic analysis, which can provide important information for epidemiological investigations.[20]

Serological analysis of serum and CSF can be an important tool for the detection of rabies virus infection, particularly in the later stages of illness. While detection of rabies specific antibodies in serum can be confounded by prior vaccination, detection in CSF is considered indicative of active rabies infection regardless of prior vaccination status. Virus neutralization assays (either the rapid fluorescent focus inhibition test or fluorescent antibody virus neutralization test) are preferred for diagnostic purposes or when there is a need to directly measure protective antibodies. Antibody binding assays (e.g., ELISA) are useful for more routine screening where the objective is to measure overall response to vaccination.[45]

PREVENTION

Despite the high case fatality ratio of rabies, it is essentially 100% preventable. Animal vaccination programs have been demonstrated to be the most cost-effective method for rabies prevention. The objective of these vaccination programs can be either vaccinating the target reservoir species to reduce or eliminate transmission of rabies virus or vaccinating vector species (e.g., domestic pets) to decrease the conduit of exposure from the primary reservoir species. Public awareness about behaviors that decrease the likelihood of animal bites is an important component of primary rabies prevention. Among persons with increased risk of rabies exposure, pre-exposure prophylaxis (preEP) may be considered. PEP is necessary to prevent the development of rabies in an exposed individual.

HUMAN VACCINATION

Louis Pasteur developed the first methods for PEP in the 1880s. These early vaccines utilized desiccated nerve tissue from infected rabbits, contained residual live virus, and required multiple doses because of their low potency. PEP typically required 14–21 doses administered daily using these early vaccines. Variations of this method were used widely by countries through the mid- to late 1900s and continue to be used as the primary rabies vaccine by a few countries. However, these nerve tissue vaccines were associated with severe adverse neurological reactions and the WHO has recommended discontinuation of the production of nerve tissue vaccines.[20]

The adoption of modern cell culture vaccines began in the late 1970s with the introduction of the Human Diploid Cell Vaccine. Subsequent introduction of Purified Chick Embryo Cell and Vero Cell rabies vaccines significantly increased access to high-quality cell culture vaccines. Adverse reactions to these vaccines are considerably lower and less severe than that reported for nerve tissue vaccines. Local adverse reactions (e.g., swelling and redness at injection site) were most frequently reported (30–70%) followed by systemic reactions (e.g., headache, fatigue, etc.) in 5–40%. Few cases of severe adverse reactions (e.g., Guillain-Barre syndrome) have ever been reported.[22] In addition to fewer adverse reactions, smaller doses and shorter schedules are possible using cell culture vaccines that meet WHO recommended potency levels. Global recommendations advise administration according to several acceptable schedules by either the intramuscular or intradermal route.[20]

Once a person is exposed to rabies virus and starts vaccination, a window remains in which the virus may progress toward the CNS, but before the humoral immune response begins production of neutralizing antibodies against the vaccine. Rabies immunoglobulin (RIG) is administered as part of a PEP regimen to provide immediate neutralizing antibodies, effectively closing this window. The only contraindication against RIG administration is in persons who have a prior history of rabies vaccination. It is critical to infiltrate as much of the recommended dose of RIG as possible into the bite wound or site of exposure to facilitate neutralization of the virus at the entry point. The remainder of the recommended dosage can be administered intramuscularly at a site separate from the vaccination site.[46] Human RIG is utilized in the United States and throughout most developed countries, but a heterologous Equine RIG is used as well and confers equivalent protection, albeit at a higher dosage.[20]

Wound washing alone has been determined to significantly reduce the risk of developing rabies.[20] For persons who have never been vaccinated against rabies, PEP begins with administration of RIG as described above. Vaccination is started on the same day as the RIG administration (day 0). In the United States, the Advisory Committee on Immunization Practices (ACIP) recommends four doses of rabies vaccine administered over 2 weeks (i.e., on days 0, 3, 7, and 14). A fifth dose administered on day 28 is recommended for immunocompromised persons.[22,47] Persons with a prior history of rabies vaccination (either preEV or PEP) do not receive RIG as part of subsequent PEP series. Instead, two doses of vaccine are administered on days 0 and 3.[20,22]

Rabies pre-exposure vaccination is recommended for persons with a higher risk of rabies exposure than the general population (Table 140-2). Several pre-exposure vaccination schedules have been reviewed by WHO. In the United States, the ACIP recommends three doses of rabies vaccine administered on days 0, 7, and 21 (or 28).[22] Pre-exposure vaccination simplifies PEP in the event of an exposure by reducing the total number of doses of vaccine required and eliminating the need for RIG. Periodic boosters and serological monitoring are not recommended for most persons receiving PreEV. However, certain groups with occupational exposure risks (e.g., veterinarians), may be recommended to undergo periodic serological monitoring to determine if and when booster doses may be required.

ANIMAL VACCINATION

Rabies is rare in vaccinated animals.[48,49] Parenteral vaccines are the most cost-effective vaccines available for use; however, oral rabies vaccine (ORV) baits have been successfully used in the control of wildlife rabies in some countries (e.g., foxes in Western Europe and raccoons and coyotes in the United States).[6,7] There are numerous parenteral cell culture vaccines available for use in dogs, cats, ferrets, cattle, horses, and sheep.[28] Parenteral vaccines are administered on an annual or triannual schedule depending on the species of animal and vaccine manufacturer. ORVs are available for use in the United States for several wildlife species (i.e., raccoon, fox, coyote). Currently, there are two ORV vaccines licensed for wildlife vaccination in the United States: Raboral V-RG, which is a recombinant Vaccinia vaccine, and Onrab, a recombinant human adenovirus Type 5 vaccine. Use of ORV can pose a human health risk from potential exposure. In the United States, there are estimated to be 0.07 adverse events/million ORV baits distributed. To date, there have been two adverse events linked to ORV bait distribution in the United States.[12]

SURVEILLANCE AND CONTROL

The World Health Organization, Food and Agricultural Organization, and World Organization for Animal Health have set a goal to eliminate canine-mediated human rabies deaths by 2030.[50,51] This ambitious goal will require collaboration from partners worldwide.[52] Key areas to target for success in 2030 include: surveillance, laboratory diagnostic capacity, mass canine vaccination, and community education and awareness.

Timely reporting of animal bites and suspect rabid animals to public health officials, followed by prompt investigation, quarantine, and testing of the suspect animal if indicated, and administration of PEP can reduce human rabies deaths.[53] Communication of quarantine and laboratory testing results has also been shown to increase PEP compliance in bite victims receiving rabies PEP.[54] Collaboration

TABLE 140-2 POPULATION RISK GROUPS AND PRE-EXPOSURE PROPHYLAXIS RECOMMENDATIONS*

Risk Category	Nature of Risk	Population	Pre-exposure Vaccination Recommendations
Rare	• Exposure always sporadic. • Exposure recognized. • Bite and nonbite exposure types.	• Population at large.	• Not recommended
Infrequent	• Exposure mostly sporadic. • Exposure recognized. • Bite and nonbite exposure types.	• Veterinarians and animal-care workers in low-endemic rabies areas. • Travelers visiting rabies endemic areas where access to healthcare is limited.	• Primary vaccination • No serological monitoring • No boosters
Frequent	• Exposure usually sporadic. • Exposure usually recognized • Bite, nonbite, or aerosol exposure types.	• Rabies diagnostic workers. • Veterinarians and animal-care workers in high-endemic rabies areas. • Covers. • Persons who handle bats.	• Primary vaccination • Serological monitoring every 2 years • Booster as indicated
Continuous	• Virus present continuously. • Exposures likely to go unrecognized. • Bite, nonbite, or aerosol exposure types.	• Rabies Research laboratory workers. • Rabies biologics production workers.	• Primary vaccination • Serological monitoring every 6 months • Booster as indicated

*This chart is intended as a guide, based on 2008 ACIP recommendations.[22] Centers for Disease Control and Prevention. Human rabies prevention- United States, 2008: Recommendations of the Advisory Committee on Immunization Practices. MMWR 2008; 57: (No. RR-3): [1–28]

between animal and human health has resulted in a combined One Health approach toward rabies elimination. Rabies surveillance requires information from both the human and animal health sectors to institute timely and accurate response measures.

Laboratory diagnostic capacity is a critical component of any rabies surveillance system. Without diagnostic capabilities, governments may waste millions of dollars on unnecessary PEP. Additionally, without laboratory diagnosis, people exposed to rabid animals may not be accurately informed of their risk, which could lead to thousands of unnecessary deaths from rabies. Laboratory diagnosis requires proficient staff who can process and test samples, functional laboratory equipment, an established sample transportation system, and a timely reporting system.

The World Health Organization recommends repeated vaccination campaigns reaching at least 70% of the dog population to control canine rabies.[20,55] Many countries with endemic canine rabies transmission face challenges such as low vaccination campaign turnout, poor "cold-chain" maintenance of the vaccine, and inadequate workforce capacity.[52,56] Vaccination campaigns must be tailored to a country's individual dog ecology. Ownership (i.e., sole ownership, community ownership, not owned) and confinement status (i.e., confined, semiconfined, free-roaming) of dogs impacts vaccination method success; and vaccination methods should be designed with a countries' dog ecology in mind.[57,58] Various vaccination methods (e.g., central point, door-to-door, capture-vaccinate-release) have been used to vaccinate dogs successfully.[57,58] Mixed vaccination methods that incorporate a countries' specific dog ecology may be the best way to reach consistent vaccination coverage levels of at least 70%. For example, in the United States, the majority of dogs are confined; therefore, a central point vaccination method (such as a veterinary clinic) is likely to reach the majority of dogs. However, in Africa and Asia, many dogs roam the streets making it necessary to incorporate capture-vaccinate-release in addition to central point vaccination.

Community education and awareness is improving as efforts, such as World Rabies Day (celebrated on September 28), are expanded. Global partners committed to rabies prevention continue to promote education and awareness on multiple components of rabies prevention including: responsible dog ownership, bite prevention, wound management, and novel tools for use in the rabies community. For example, mobile technology is making it easier to send and receive surveillance data, send vaccination reminders, track canine vaccination campaigns, and target vaccination campaigns in outbreak and high risk areas.[59,60] Rabies continues to be considered a global neglected disease. Increased knowledge and awareness of this devastating disease is needed in order to eliminate canine-mediated human rabies deaths by 2030.

References

1. King AMQ, Lefkowitz EJ, Mushegian AR, et al. Changes to taxonomy and the International Code of Virus Classification and Nomenclature ratified by the International Committee on Taxonomy of Viruses. *Arch Virol.* 2018;163(9):2601–31.
2. Rupprecht CE, Hanlon CA, Hemachudha T. Rabies re-examined. *Lancet Infect Dis.* 2002;2(6):327–43.
3. Baby J, Mani RS, Abraham SS, et al. Natural rabies infection in a domestic fowl (*Gallus domesticus*): A report from India. *PLoS Negl Trop Dis.* 2015;9(7):e0003942.
4. Velasco-Villa A, Escobar LE, Sanchez A, et al. Successful strategies implemented towards the elimination of canine rabies in the Western Hemisphere. *Antiviral Res.* 2017;143:1–12.
5. Hampson K, Coudeville L, Lembo T, et al. Estimating the global burden of endemic canine rabies. *PLoS Negl Trop Dis.* 2015;9(4):e0003709.
6. Freuling CM, Hampson K, Selhorst T, et al. The elimination of fox rabies from Europe: Determinants of success and lessons for the future. *Phil Trans R Soc B.* 2013;368:20120142.
7. Müller T, Demetriou P, Moynagh J, et al. Rabies elimination in Europe: A success story. In:Fooks AR, Müller T, eds. *Rabies Control: Towards Sustainable Prevention at the Source, Compendium of the OIE Global Conference on Rabies Control.* Incheon, Seoul, September 7–9, 2011, Republic of Korea Paris, France: OIE; 2012:31–44.
8. Johnson N, Un H, Fooks AR, et al. Rabies epidemiology and control in Turkey: Past and present. *Epidemiol Infect.* 2010;138:305–12.
9. Freuling CM, Hampson K, Selhorst T, et al. The elimination of fox rabies from Eureope: Determinants of success and lessons learned. *Phil Trans R Soc B.* 2013;368:20120142.
10. Kuzmin IV, Bozick B, Guagliardo SA, et al. Bats, emerging infectious diseases, and the rabies paradigm revisited, *Emerg Health Threats J.* 2011;4:7159.
11. Nicholls E, Davies J. Rabies control and management. *Can Med Assoc J.* 1982;126(11):1286.
12. Ma X, Monroe BP, Cleaton JM, et al. Rabies surveillance in the United States during 2016. *J Am Vet Med Assoc.* 2018;252(8):945–57.
13. Christian KA, Blanton JD, Auslander M, Rupprect CE. Epidemiology of rabies post-exposure prophylaxis—United States of America, 2006–2008. *Vaccine.* 2009;27(51):7156–61.
14. Vigilato MAN, Clavijo A, Knobl T, et al. Progress towards eliminating canine rabies: Policies and perspectives from Latin America and the Caribbean. *Phil Trans R Soc B.* 2013;368:20120143.
15. Johnson N, Arechiga-Ceballos N, Aguilar-Setien A. Vampire bat rabies: Ecology, epidemiology and control. *Viruses.* 2014;6:1911–28.
16. Lan Y, Wen T, Chang C, et al. Indigenous wildlife rabies in Taiwan: Ferret Badgers, a long term terrestrial reservoir. *Biomed Res Int.* 2017;2017:5491640.
17. Kuzmin IV, Botvinkin AD, McElhinney LM, et al. Molecular epidemiology of terrestrial rabies in the former Soviet Union. *J Wildl Dis.* 2004;40:617–31.
18. Aylan O, El-Sayed AF, Farahtaj F, et al. Report of the first meeting of the middle East and eastern europe rabies expert bureau, Istanbul, Turkey (June 8–9, 2010). *Adv Prev Med.* 2011;2011:812515.
19. Bingham J. Canine rabies ecology in Southern Africa. *Emerg Infect Dis.* 2005;11(9):1337–42.
20. WHO expert consultation on rabies, third report. Geneva: World Health Organization; 2018 (WHO Technical Report Series, No. 1012). License: CC BY-NC-SA 3.0 IGO.
21. Taylor LH, Knopf L, Partners for Rabies Prevention. Surveillance of human rabies by National Authorities—A global survey. *Zoonoses and Public Health.* 2015;62(7):543–52.
22. Centers for Disease Control and Prevention. Human rabies prevention—United States, 2008: Recommendations of the Advisory Committee on Immunization Practices. *MMWR.* 2008;57(RR-3):1–28.
23. Murphy FA. Rabies pathogenesis. *Arch Virol.* 1977;54:279–97.
24. Winkler WG, Fashinell TR, Leffingwell L, Howard P, Conomy JP. Airborne rabies transmission in a laboratory worker. *J Am Med Assoc.* 1973;226:1219–21.
25. Gibbons RV. Cryptogenic rabies, bats, and the question of aerosol transmission. *Ann Emerg Med.* 2002;39:528–36.
26. Javadi M, Fayaz A, Mirdehghan SA, Ainollahi B. Transmission of rabies by corneal graft. *Cornea.* 1996;15:431–3.
27. Krebs JW, Mandel EJ, Swerdlow DL, Rupprecht CE. Rabies surveillance in the United States during 2004. *J Am Vet Med Assoc.* 2005;227:1912–25.
28. National Association of State Public Health Veterinarians Committee. Compendium of animal rabies prevention and control, 2008. *J Am Vet Med Assoc.* 2008;232:1478–86.
29. Weyer J, Blumberg L. Rabies: Challenge of diagnosis in resource poor countries. *IDJP.* 2007;16(3):86–8.
30. Consales CA, Bolzan VL. Rabies review: Immunopathology, clinical aspects and treatment. *J Venom Anim Toxins Incl Trop Dis.* 2007;13(1):5–38.
31. Hemachudha T, Laothamatas J, Rupprecht CE. Human rabies: A disease of complex neuropathogenic mechanism and diagnostic challenges. *Lancet Neurol.* 2002;1:101–9.
32. Greene CE, Rupprecht CE. Rabies and other lyssavirus infections. In: Greene CE, ed. *Infectious Diseases of the Dog and Cat.* St Louis: Elsevier Saunders; 2006:167–83.
33. Singh R, Singh KP, Cherian S, et al. Rabies—Epidemiology, pathogenesis, public health concerns and advances in diagnosis and control: A comprehensive review. *Vet Q.* 2017;37(1):212–51.
34. Nigg AJ, Walker PL. Overview, prevention, and treatment of rabies. *Pharmacotherapy.* 2009;29:1182–95.

35. Tarantola A, Crabol Y, Mahendra BJ, et al. Caring for patients with rabies in developing countries-the neglected importance of palliative care. *Trop Med Int Health*. 2016;21(4):564–7.

36. Centers for Disease Control and Prevention. Recovery of a patient from clinical rabies—Wisconsin, 2004. *MMWR Morb Mortal Wkly Rep*. 2004;53(50):1171–3.

37. Willoughby REJr, Tieves KS, et al. Survival after treatment of rabies with induction of coma. *N Engl J Med*. 2005;352(24):2508–14.

38. deSouza A, Madhusudana SN. Survival from rabies encephalitis. *J Neurol Sci*. 2014;339:8–14.

39. Medical College of Wisconsin. Pediatrics: Infectious Diseases; Rabies Registry Website. https://www.mcw.edu/Pediatrics/Infectious-Diseases/Patient-Care/Rabies.htm. Accessed May 28, 2018.

40. Manesh A, Mani RS, Pichamuthu K, et al. Case report: Failure of therapeutic coma in rabies encephalitis. *Am J Trop Med Hyg*. 2018;98(1):207–10.

41. Madhusudana SN, Nagaraj D, Uday M, Ratnavalli E, Verendra Kumar M. Partial recovery from rabies in a six-year-old girl. *Int J Infect Dis*. 2002;6:85–6.

42. Weyer J, Msimang-Dermaux V, Paweska JT, et al. A case of human survival of rabies, South Africa, *S Afr J Infect Dis*. 2016;31(2):66–8.

43. Coetzer A, Sabeta CT, Markotter W, Rupprecht CE, Nel LH. Comparison of biotinylated monoclonal and polyclonal antibodies in an evaluation of a direct rapid immunohistochemical test for the routine diagnosis of rabies in Southern Africa. *PLoS Negl Trop Dis*. 2014;8(9):e3189.

44. Eggerbauer E, de Benedictis P, Hoffmann B, et al. Evaluation of six commercially available rapid immunochromatographic tests for the diagnosis of rabies in brain material. *PLoS Negl Trop Dis*. 2016;10(6):e0004776.

45. Moore SA, Gilbert A, Vos A, et al. Rabies virus antibodies from oral vaccination as a correlate of protection against lethal infection in wildlife. *Trop Med Infect Dis*. 2017;2(3):31.

46. WHO. Rabies vaccines: WHO position paper—April 2018. *Wkly Epidemiol Rec*. 2018;93:201–20.

47. Centers for Disease Control and Prevention. Use of a reduced (4-dose) vaccine schedule for postexposure prophylaxis to prevent human rabies: Recommendations of the Advisory Committee on Immunization Practices. *MMWR*. 2010;59(RR-02):1–9.

48. Murray KO, Holmes KC, Hanlon CA. Rabies in vaccinated dogs and cats in the United States, 1997–2001. *J Am Vet Med Assoc*. 2009;235:691–5.

49. Frana TS, Clough NE, Gatewood DM, et al. Postmarketing surveillance of rabies vaccines for dogs to evaluate safety and efficacy. *J Am Vet Med Assoc*. 2008;232:1000–2.

50. Scott T, Coetzer A, de Balogh K, Wright N, Nel L. The Pan-African rabies control network (PARACON): A unified approach to eliminating canine rabies in Africa. *Antiviral Res*. 2015;124:93–100.

51. Aiming for elimination of dog-mediated human rabies cases by 2030. *Vet Rec*. 2016;178(4):86–7.

52. Wallace RM, Undurraga EA, Blanton JD, Cleaton J, Franka R. Elimination of dog-mediated human rabies deaths by 2030: Needs assessment and alternatives for progress based on dog vaccination. *Front Vet Sci*. 2017;4:9.

53. Wallace RM, Reses H, Franka R, et al. Establishment of a canine rabies burden in Haiti through the implementation of a novel surveillance program. *PLoS Negl Trop Dis*. 2015;9(11):e0004245.

54. Etheart MD, Kligerman M, Augustin PD, et al. Effect of counselling on health-care-seeking behaviours and rabies vaccination adherence after dog bites in Haiti, 2014–15: A retrospective follow-up survey. *Lancet Glob Health*. 2017;5:e1017–25.

55. Coleman PG, Dye C. Immunization coverage required to prevent outbreaks of dog rabies. *Vaccine*. 1996;14(3):185–6.

56. Lankester FJ, Wouters PAWM, Czupryna A, et al. Thermotolerance of an inactivated rabies vaccine for dogs. *Vaccine*. 2016;34:5504–11.

57. Arief RA, Hampson K, Jatikusumah A, et al. Determinants of vaccination coverage and consequences for rabies control in Bali, Indonesia. *Front Vet Sci*. 2017;3:123.

58. Pimburage RMS, Harischandra PAL, Gunatilake M, Jayasinhe DN, Balasuriya A, Amunugama RMSK. A cross-sectional survey on dog ecology and dog anti-rabies vaccination coverage in selected areas in Sri Lanka. *Sri Lanka Vet J*. 2017;64(1A):1–7.

59. Cleaton JM, Wallace RM, Crowdis K, et al. Impact of community-delivered SMS alerts on dog-owner participation during a mass rabies vaccination campaign, Haiti 2017. *Vaccine*. 2018;36:2321–5.

60. Gibson AD, Ohal P, Shervell K, et al. Vaccinate-assess-move method of mass canine rabies vaccination utilising mobile technology data collection in Ranchi, India. *BMC Infect Dis*. 2015;15:589.

CHAPTER

141

Dengue, Chikungunya, and Zika Virus

Carina G. M. Blackmore

INTRODUCTION

The mosquito-borne chikungunya and Zika virus diseases have emerged from obscurity in recent years. Previously they were thought to be mild, and at most of limited geographic distribution and public health concern. Now, they are among arboviruses that are a significant public health priority worldwide. Dengue, chikungunya, and Zika viruses share the same mosquito vectors (*Aedes* subgenus stegomyia and diceromyia mosquitoes) (Fig. 141-1). The feeding and breeding behaviors of these mosquitoes greatly impact the epidemiology of the diseases they transmit. The vector mosquitoes prefer to live in subtropical and tropical regions of the world, and dengue, chikungunya, and Zika virus infections are endemic in these areas. The most important human vector for these diseases, *A. aegypti*, also called the house mosquito or yellow fever mosquito, has adapted to and lives in very close contact with humans. As a result, *A. aegypti*, together with *Anopheles gambiae and funestus*, two highly anthropomorphic malaria vector mosquito species in Africa[1] are probably the most efficient mosquito-borne disease vectors in the world. They are also among the vectors that are most difficult to control.

In areas where more than one of these diseases are endemic, they can be difficult to distinguish clinically and patients can become infected with more than one virus at the same time.[2] The public health impact of dengue, chikungunya, and Zika virus will likely increase even further as the human population in tropical and subtropical areas grows and urbanization continues. The disease incidence is predicted to increase most in areas with low or modest incomes and suboptimal housing conditions without intact walls, windows, and/or screens that can keep mosquitoes out.[3]

DENGUE VIRUS

Virus

Dengue infections are caused by dengue viruses, which are single-stranded positive-sense RNA viruses that belong to the family *Flaviviridae*, genus *Flavivirus*. They are small (50 nm in diameter), enveloped viruses with three structural proteins and seven nonstructural proteins. The *Flavivirus* genus contains more than 40 human pathogens including West Nile virus, tick-borne encephalitis virus, yellow fever virus, and Zika virus.[4] The dengue virus has four distinct but closely related dengue virus serotypes (dengue virus 1–4).[5]

Symptoms

Dengue virus infections can range from asymptomatic to a severe hemorrhagic disease with a potentially fatal outcome. After a 4- to 10-day incubation period, most persons develop a mild febrile illness or classic dengue fever (DF). Young children generally present with nonspecific fever symptoms. Older children and adults often develop classic DF, which is characterized by sudden onset of fever, severe headache, retroocular pain, and myalgias. Rash and joint pains are also common and many patients have leukopenia and thrombocytopenia. In addition, some have signs of minor hemorrhage. Symptoms generally last 3–10 days. Viremia usually lasts 5 days or less. The most severe form of dengue is called dengue hemorrhagic fever (DHF). It typically occurs in children less than 15 but can also occur in adults. It can be difficult to distinguish initially from DF. The first warning signs usually occur 3–7 days after disease onset with a decrease in temperature, and often mild petechial hemorrhage. DHF patients can develop plasma leakage and severe internal hemorrhaging (dengue shock syndrome) during this phase, which can be fatal if not identified early.[6]

While dengue viruses are primarily transmitted by mosquito bites, transmission can also occur through blood transfusion, transplantation of infected organ or tissues, and occupational exposures such as needle stick injuries. Vertical transmission during pregnancy or delivery has also been described.[7]

History

Dengue fever as a clinical syndrome has been known for several hundred years under multiple names including break bone fever and bilious remitting fever. The four virus subtypes likely evolved in Africa and Asia and circulated between *Aedes* mosquitoes and lower primates there. They spread to the Americas, along with the primary human vector *A. aegypti*, on cargo ships that transported goods and slaves.[8] The first outbreak described in the United States occurred in Philadelphia in 1780.[9] Dengue-like disease outbreaks were common in port cities of the Caribbean, North, Central, and South America during the nineteenth century. The disease also spread into the United States (Texas, Louisiana, Florida, and Georgia). The outbreaks were large, some involving several 100,000 cases. The largest disease clusters occurred in communities with mass transit hubs.[10] The last large dengue epidemics within the continental United States occurred in coastal cities of Texas in 1941 and Louisiana in 1945.

Researchers established by 1903 that dengue was mosquito-borne, and the virus was first isolated from humans in 1944 from ill soldiers in Calcutta, India, Hawaii, and New Guinea.[5] One of the strains from New Guinea (named dengue 2) was different from three other strains from India, Hawaii, and New Guinea (called dengue 1). The two additional dengue serotypes (dengue 3 and 4) were isolated during an outbreak in the Philippines in 1956.

The decline in dengue activity in the United States occurred as a result of improved housing conditions (doors, windows, screens, and air conditioning) that protect people during the peak biting times for the mosquitoes.[5] It was also impacted by *A. aegypti* control efforts in South and Central America aimed at eliminating urban yellow fever.[9] The mosquito control activities, which included fumigation and dumping standing water from containers, were initiated by William Gorgas in Havana, Cuba in 1901. His work followed in the footsteps of Walter Reed and Carlos Finlay, the researchers credited

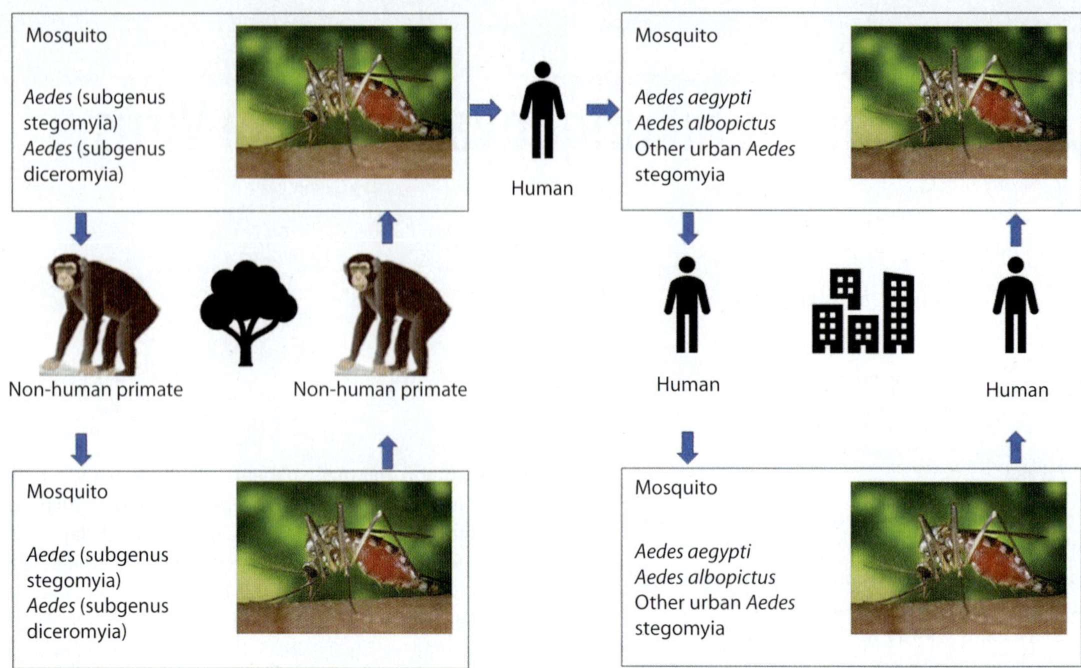

FIGURE 141-1. Sylvatic and urban dengue, chikungunya, and Zika virus transmission cycles. (*Source:* James Gathany/CDC.)

with establishing mosquitoes as disease vectors of yellow fever in 1900. The *A. aegypti* control project was later also implemented in Rio de Janeiro, Brazil. The campaign's success led to a partnership between the Rockefeller Foundation and the Brazilian government to eliminate the mosquito throughout Brazil. The control activities were adopted by neighboring countries and in 1947, the Pan American Sanitary Bureau determined that it would lead the effort to eradicate *A. aegypti* from urban areas across the South American continent. With the use of DDT, which had been discovered to be an effective insecticide during World War II, and the new 17D yellow fever vaccine,[11] the control efforts were very successful and disease rates of both yellow fever and dengue plummeted. The control efforts continued through the early 1960s after which they declined over time likely due to cost, decreased political and public support, rapidly growing urbanization, and an increase in travel and vector resistance to DDT. *A. aegypti*, which had largely remained in the Caribbean, Cuba, United States, and Venezuela slowly reestablished populations across the continent.

After more than 30 years without reported human dengue in the Americas, the disease was detected again in the late 1970s in the Caribbean and Mexico. In 1980, Texas implemented passive dengue fever surveillance and reported sporadic locally transmitted cases along the Mexico border, with cases occurring periodically ever since.[10] Autochthonous dengue transmission was also documented on three islands in Hawaii in 2001–02, with 122 confirmed cases. At the time, *A. aegypti* was not present on the islands and *A. albopictus* was implicated as the vector.[12] In 2015–16, another dengue outbreak with 264 confirmed cases occurred on the island of Hawaii. By this time *A. aegypti* mosquitoes had reinfested Hawaii and were considered the most important vector for transmission.[13] Local dengue virus outbreaks have also occurred in Florida in 2009–10 (Key West)[14] and 2013 (Martin county).[15]

The incidence of dengue worldwide has increased 30-fold over the last 50 years. Mass transit, in particular the increase in air travel since the 1960s, which moves potentially infected people quickly across the globe has contributed to the significant increase in the frequency of dengue epidemics in tropical areas.[5] Today dengue is endemic in more than 100 countries in subtropical and tropical Africa, South-East Asia, the Americas, the Caribbean, Eastern Mediterranean, and the Western Pacific. The World Health Organization (WHO)[16] estimates that about 40% (>2.5 billion) of the world population lives in geographic areas conducive to *A. aegypti* breeding year-round (Fig. 141-2). Recent estimates indicate 390 million are infected with dengue annually and 96 million (67–136 million) people become clinically ill worldwide each year.[17]

DHF, the most serious form of dengue infection, was first documented in the 1950s in Thailand and the Philippines.[18] Before the 1970's outbreaks of severe dengue were rare but the frequency and intensity has increased and WHO currently estimates that more than 500,000 people develop DHF and about 22,000 (mostly children) die from the disease annually.[19] The increase in severe dengue appears linked to the spread and cocirculation of multiple dengue serotypes in the same communities.

Clinical

Patients with immunity to one dengue serotype are at greater risk of developing DHF if they are infected by a second heterotypic serotype, especially if they are reinfected 2 or more years after the first dengue infection. Babies born with maternal antibodies to dengue virus are also at higher risk, particularly from age 6–12 months. However, only 2–4% of dengue immune patients who are exposed to a heterotypic virus will go on to develop severe dengue.[20]

The treatment for dengue is limited to supportive care. There are no approved antiviral medications for its treatment. Attempts to develop vaccine are complicated by the fact that the vaccine must protect against infections from all four virus serotypes to ensure that the vaccinated patient is less likely, not more likely, to become severely ill from a later exposure to dengue. For example, vaccination recommendations for CYD-TDC (Dengvaxia), the vaccine candidate that has come furthest to date, had to be reexamined by WHO in 2018.[21]

It is not clear how antibody cross reactivity between dengue and Zika virus will impact clinical disease among persons successively infected with both viruses. Researchers from Brazil have suggested that the large number of individuals with immunity against Zika in 2016–17 may have contributed to the smaller than expected number of dengue cases diagnosed during this time period.[22]

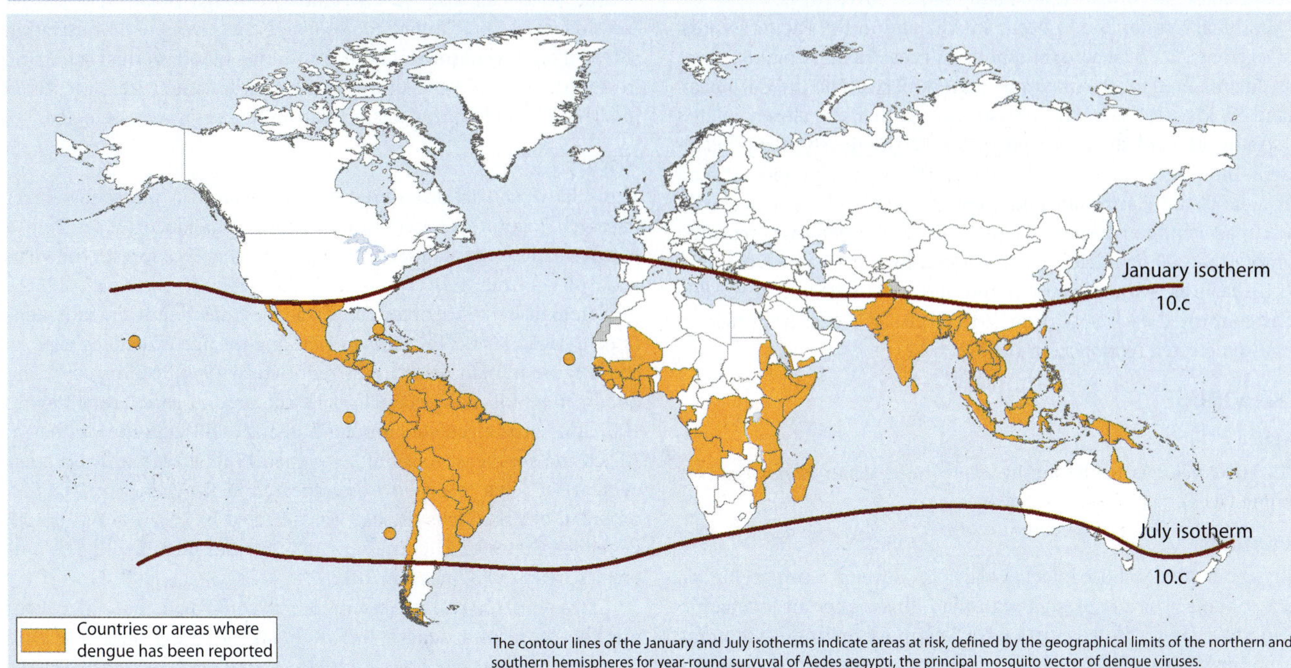

Dengue, countries or areas at risk, 2013
January isotherm
10.c
July isotherm
10.c
Countries or areas where dengue has been reported
The contour lines of the January and July isotherms indicate areas at risk, defined by the geographical limits of the northern and southern hemispheres for year-round survuval of Aedes aegypti, the principal mosquito vector of dengue viruses.
The boundaries and names shown and the designations used on this map do not imply the expression of any opinion whatsoever on the part of the World Health Organization concerning the legal status of any country, territory, city or area or of its authorities, or concerning the delimitation of its frontiers of boundaries. Dotted and dashed lines on maps represent approximate border lines for which there may not yet be full agreement.
Data Source: World Health Organization
Map Production: Health Statistics and Information Systems (HSI)
World Health Organization
World Health Organization
© WHO 2014. All rights reserved.

FIGURE 141-2. The January and July isotherms outline the subtropical and tropical parts of the world suitable for year-round breeding of *A. aegypti*, the primary human disease vector of dengue, chikungunya, and Zika viruses. (*Source:* Used with Permission from World Health Organization (WHO). Available from: http://gamapserver.who.int/mapLibrary/Files/Maps/Global_DengueTransmission_ITHRiskMap.png. July 30, 2013. Copyright © 2012.)

CHIKUNGUNYA VIRUS

Virus

Chikungunya virus is a positive-sense single-stranded RNA virus that belongs to the family *Togaviridae* and genus *Alphavirus*.[23] These are small, spherical, and enveloped viruses that are 60–70 nm in diameter.

Symptoms

Chikungunya typically presents with abrupt onset of high (>39°C, 102°F) fever and bilateral, symmetric, often severe and debilitating polyarthralgia which is often migratory and frequently involves small joints of the hands, wrists, and ankles. Large joints such as the knees or shoulders are seldom affected. Other common symptoms include headache, myalgia, maculopapular rash, conjunctivitis, and arthritis. Less common symptoms include myocarditis, hepatitis, nephritis, neurological, and ocular signs.[24] Symptoms generally resolve in 7–10 days, although some patients may have persisting rheumatologic symptoms and fatigue for months to years.[25]

The incubation period is typically 3–7 days, but can range from 1 to 12 days. The viral load is often high ($>10^9$)[26] and the majority of cases are symptomatic (>75%). The chikungunya virus can be detected during the first week of illness. The high viremia contributes to the often-explosive spread of chikungunya virus outbreaks because mosquitoes are infected more easily. Infected persons likely acquire life long immunity.

Mother to child transmission has been reported during the second trimester and half of mothers who become ill shortly before delivery may transmit the virus to their infant.[26] Disease in infants can be severe and symptoms can include encephalopathy, myocardial disease, and hemorrhage. Young children, older adults, and patients with underlying medical conditions are also at risk of severe disease. Mortality is rare but has been reported, especially among older adults.[24] Virus transmission from transfusions and transplants has not been documented.

Treatment for chikungunya is symptomatic. Nonsteroidal anti-inflammatory drugs can be used to treat the joint pain. Chikungunya and dengue are difficult to distinguish clinically, and coinfections have been reported.[27]

History

Chikungunya is a word from the Makonde language meaning "that which bends up." The term refers to the stooping posture of local chikungunya fever patients afflicted with severe, often incapacitating joint pains. The disease was named and characterized during the first documented epidemic of chikungunya in what is now Tanzania in 1952–53,[28] though clinical descriptions of nineteenth-century outbreaks suggests that the virus has long caused human disease. Outbreaks where patients developed particularly severe postillness arthralgia were likely caused by the chikungunya virus rather than dengue.[29] The 1952 outbreak in Tanzania was suspected to be mosquito-borne and an unknown virus was isolated from both humans and mosquitoes. The chikungunya virus was classified as an alphavirus a few years later. Additional studies in Africa established that the virus had a sylvatic cycle involving lower primates and aedine mosquitoes. Periodic minor outbreaks of chikungunya fever were documented throughout much of sub-Saharan Africa and Southeast Asia over the next 30 years. After a large outbreak on the Kenyan coast in 2004, the virus spread to numerous islands in the Indian Ocean, India, and in Southeast Asia between 2004 and 2008 in a series of explosive outbreaks involving millions of cases.[26]

The outbreak on La Reunion Island in 2005–06 was unique in several ways. It was the first time that neurological manifestations, fetal infections, and mortality were associated with chikungunya virus infections.[24] The outbreak-related virus strain had also undergone a mutation that resulted in higher infection rates in *A. albopictus* mosquitoes, generally considered a less effective chikungunya vector. The same virus and vector combination caused the subsequent chikungunya outbreaks in Italy (2007) and France (2010, 2014).[26]

Outbreaks continued to occur in Asia and in the Pacific Islands. In December, 2013 an autochthonous outbreak of chikungunya fever was documented for the first time in the Americas, on the Caribbean Island St. Martin.[30] Genetic analysis showed that was closely related to strains adapted to *A. aegypti* that were previously identified in China, Indonesia, and the Philippines.[31] The outbreak rapidly spread throughout the Caribbean and Central and South America with more than 1 million suspected and 25,000 confirmed cases reported in more than 40 countries between December 2013 and December 2014. The virus is now endemic in the region, with more than 100,000 cases confirmed each year from 2015 to 2017.[32] Local transmission was also detected in Florida in 2014 ($n = 12$).[33]

ZIKA VIRUS

Virus

Zika virus belongs to the family *Flaviviridae* genus *Flavivirus* (see dengue virus).

Symptoms

Only about 20% of those infected with Zika develop a clinical illness. Zika patients typically present with mild illness after an incubation period that ranges from 3 to 14 days. The most common symptoms include acute onset fever, maculopapular rash, arthralgia, or conjunctivitis.[34] The rash, which can be pruritic, is diffusely distributed and may involve the face, trunk, and extremities (including palms and soles). Arthralgia often affects the small joints in the hands and feet. Other common symptoms include myalgia and headache. Retro-orbital pain and gastrointestinal signs can also occur. Symptoms generally last for 4–7 days. Zika virus disease is self-limiting and severe symptoms requiring hospitalizations are uncommon. Fatalities are rare.[35] Guillain-Barré syndrome (GBS) has been associated with Zika infections but it is rare (0.7–1.2% of cases).[36,37]

Both asymptomatic and symptomatic Zika-infected pregnant women can transmit the virus vertically to the fetus. A series of birth defects have been described as part of the congenital Zika syndrome. The infant can have altered cranial morphology with a severe microcephaly and partially collapsed skull, a brain with thin cerebral cortices with subcortical calcification, eyes with macular scarring and focal pigmentary retinal mottling, and congenital joint contractures and marked early hypertonia with symptoms of extrapyramidal involvement.[38] Hearing loss and milder neurologic findings such as hypotonia, poor suck, or swallow have also been reported.[39]

Vertical transmission may occur throughout the pregnancy but the most severe symptoms appear to be associated with infections in the late first and early second trimester. Data from the United States indicate that 10% of pregnant women with confirmed Zika virus infection had a fetus or baby with a Zika virus-associated birth defect. The risk was 15% for women infected during the first trimester.[40] A prospective cohort study of Zika virus-infected pregnant women in the French territories showed neurologic and ocular defects in 12.7% of infants born to mothers infected in the first trimester, 3.5% in the second, and 5.3% infected in the third trimester.[41] Severe microcephaly and intracranial calcifications are often visible on ultrasound exams done mid-pregnancy.

Zika virus viremia lasts up to a week. The virus can be detected longer (8–13 weeks) in pregnant women. The reason for this is not clear but it may be related to Zika virus infections of the placenta or fetus.[42] In addition to being vertically transmitted, Zika virus can be transmitted sexually from both men and women to their partners. The virus appears to be able to persist longer in semen than in other body fluids. Viral RNA has been detected in semen 188 days after disease onset; however, studies indicate that the virus only remains infectious for a few weeks.[43]

The virus can also be transmitted through blood and platelet transfusion.[44] The United States Food and Drug Administration (FDA) issued recommendations for routine blood product screening in August 2016. Nine Zika-positive blood donations were identified in 2016–17[45] and no transfusion transmitted cases were detected.

History

The Zika virus was discovered by investigators at the Yellow Fever Research Institute[46] based near Entebbe, Uganda in 1947 from a febrile sentinel rhesus macaque placed in the Zika forest. The virus was isolated from *A. africanus* mosquitoes in the same area in 1948.[47]

Serologic evidence of human Zika virus infections were first identified in Uganda and Tanzania in 1952 and the first evidence that Zika could cause human disease was reported in 1964 by Simpson[48] who documented his own occupationally acquired disease. From 1964 to 2007, the virus circulated among humans and *Aedes* mosquitoes in Africa and southeast Asia but fewer than 15 illnesses with laboratory evidence of Zika infection were reported in the literature. The first outbreak of Zika virus disease was detected in 2007 on Yap Island, Federated States of Micronesia with 108 cases identified.[34] The outbreak spread to Polynesia in 2013–14.

In May 2015, researchers in Brazil confirmed that Zika virus was the cause of a dengue-like outbreak there that had spread to six states over the previous 3 months.[49] Phylogenetic studies of the virus strain indicated that it arrived in Brazil from French Polynesia in 2013[50] and may have been causing outbreaks in Brazil as early as in August 2014. The virus swept through Brazil during 2015–June 2016 with more than 200,000 cases of Zika virus disease, and ultimately spread throughout South America, Central America, Mexico, and the Caribbean.[51] Autochthonous transmission was also detected in Miami, Florida,[52] and in South Texas.[53] The main vector in the Americas is *A. aegypti*. However, *A. albopictus* was implicated as the primary vector in a 2007 Zika virus outbreak in Gabon.[54]

The first indication of more severe clinical sequelae from Zika was reported from French Polynesia. During a 2013–14 outbreak there which ultimately resulted in more than 41,000 reports of suspected Zika virus infections, some patients presented with neurological or autoimmune symptoms a few days after a Zika-like illness. Of these, 42 were confirmed as having GBS (five to ten times the expected baseline rate).[55] Evidence linking Zika virus with GBS and other rare neurological syndrome outcomes (myelitis, meningoencephaitis) has strengthened with the data gathered from the Zika outbreak in the Americas.[36,37,56]

Evidence establishing that Zika virus causes human birth defects emerged from Brazil in September 2015, about 6 months after the start of the outbreak. Infectious causes of birth defects are rare and flaviviruses had never been shown to cause birth defects. In addition, microcephaly can be difficult to diagnose clinically so many doubted the accuracy of the data.[57] They were concerned that the babies' head circumferences were not measured in a standardized way and that healthcare practitioners confused microcephaly with the normal compression of a baby's head circumference that occurs during the birthing process. The Brazilian Ministry of Health established a microcephaly disease registry and by mid-November 2015, they had documented that reported case numbers had doubled compared to the previous 5-year average counts. The same month Zika virus RNA was also detected in amniotic fluid samples from two pregnant women with fetuses diagnosed with microcephaly by ultrasound exams.[58] The data accumulated rapidly and by May 2016, Centers for Disease Control and Prevention (CDC) researchers concluded that the burden of proof of human teratogenicity for Zika virus had been met.[57] Retrospective studies indicate that Zika-induced microcephaly occurred during the 2013–14 outbreak in French Polynesia as well.[59]

DIFFERENTIAL DIAGNOSES

Zika, dengue, and chikungunya virus infections can be difficult to distinguish clinically.[60,61] Table 141-1 compares common clinical signs and laboratory results for the three diseases. Other differential diagnoses include yellow fever, leptospirosis, malaria, rickettsial infections, viral hepatitis, group A streptococcal disease, rubella, measles, influenza, parvovirus B19, and other enterovirus infections.

LABORATORY TESTING CONSIDERATIONS

During acute infections, dengue, Zika, and chikungunya viruses can be isolated from cell culture or detected by nucleic acid tests such as real-time polymerase chain reaction (RT-PCR) tests. Most commercially used diagnostic tests are validated for serum specimens. However, the Trioplex Real-time RT-PCR Assay developed by CDC and used by many public health laboratories in the United States can differentiate RNA from Zika, dengue, and chikungunya viruses from human sera, whole blood, and cerebrospinal fluid. This assay may also be used to detect Zika virus in urine, tissues, and amniotic fluid.[62]

Virus infections can also be diagnosed through serologic testing. Patients with acute primary infections first mount an IgM response, followed by an IgG response a few days later. Commercial laboratories perform both IgM and IgG tests. Some public health laboratories also perform the gold standard total antibody Plaque Reduction Neutralization test, which can distinguish serologic cross reactivity among the medically important flaviviruses most closely related to Zika virus.

While the sensitivity and specificity of these tests are good, both false positive and false negative results are possible. The likelihood of a true positive result (positive predictive value) and a true negative result (negative predictive value) decreases when the incidence of acute disease is low or when specimens are not collected at the optimal time frame (at the time of peak viral load). Since dengue, Zika, and chikungunya are rare diseases in temperate regions of the world, many health departments in the United States elect to have specimens that test positive in commercial laboratories forwarded to public health laboratories for additional confirmatory testing.

Serological diagnostic tests can detect chikungunya virus IgM antibodies in serum specimens from day 4 to 5 after disease onset. IgM and IgG ELISA tests are specific and cross-reactivity with other alphaviruses is limited.[24] Diagnosis can also be made by detecting a fourfold increase in specific IgG antibody in paired serum samples.

TABLE 141-1 COMPARISON OF THE CLINICAL MANIFESTATIONS AND LABORATORY TESTS FOR PERSONS INFECTED WITH DENGUE, CHIKUNGUNYA, OR ZIKA VIRUSES

Disease	Dengue	Chikungunya	Zika
Fever	+++	+++	++
Myalgia	++	+	+
Arthralgia	+	+++	++
Maculopapular rash	+	++	+++
Headache	++	++	+
Conjunctivitis	--	---	++
Hemorrhage	++	--	--
Shock	+	--	--
Leukopenia	+++	++	--
Neutropenia	+++	+	--
Lymphopenia	++	+++	--
Thrombocytopenia	+++	+	--

Source: Adapted from clinical guidance documents from CDC, WHO, and PAHO.

Studies indicate that dengue virus IgM antibodies are detectable 5–10 days postsymptom onset and persist more than 90 days after primary infections. Specific antidengue IgG antibodies are usually detectable at low levels within the first week of primary disease onset with titers rising over the following 2 weeks. The IgM response is shorter and lower, even sometimes undetectable, after a secondary dengue virus infection. Instead, these tend to induce a rapid rise of often highly cross-reactive antidengue IgG antibodies. Another test that can be used to detect acute dengue infections is the nonstructural protein 1 (NS1) ELISA test. It is commercially available and detects the presence of the NS1 protein, which is part of the dengue virus genome in the patient's blood and can be detected during approximately the same period virus is also detectable by PCR.

Zika-virus-specific IgM antibodies are typically detectable around day 4 postonset. They persist for 12 weeks or longer. A recent study from Florida concluded that more than 70% ($n = 47$) of Zika virus cases had detectable IgM antibodies 12 months or more after disease onset, including three who were still positive 18 months after having Zika disease.[63] It is therefore not possible to rely on IgM antibody test results alone to distinguish between a recent or historical Zika virus infection.

In addition to the apparent longevity of Zika virus IgM antibodies, the serologic cross reactivity between antibodies to the closely related dengue and Zika virus makes it difficult to distinguish the milder forms of disease if patients have had exposure to both.

A patient with a history of a previous dengue infection, who is subsequently infected with Zika virus may also develop higher antibody titers to dengue than Zika, a phenomenon called antigenic sin.[64] If the patient's previous history of dengue was unknown, it is likely based on the test result that the patient, who actually had Zika virus disease, would be diagnosed with acute dengue.

Since there is substantial overlap between the distribution of Zika and dengue viruses, many people have been infected with both viruses at some point. This phenomenon has significant clinical relevance, particularly for providing a reliable risk assessment for pregnant women concerned about congenital Zika syndrome.[65–67]

Prevention from Sexual Transmission of Zika

Sexual transmission of Zika virus can occur from both symptomatic and asymptomatically infected persons. To prevent infection during pregnancy, CDC recommends that men use condoms through the duration of pregnancy or for 6 months after travel or symptom onset. Condom use is also recommended for 8 weeks after travel or disease onset to prevent sexual transmission from infected women to men.

THE VECTORS

Chikungunya, dengue, and Zika viruses are transmitted by a number of aedine mosquitoes. In urban areas, *A. aegypti* (Fig. 141-3A) is the most important vector. *A. albopictus* (the Asian tiger mosquito) (Fig. 141-3B) is also a competent vector and may contribute to the propagation of outbreaks.[5,28,65] *A. hensilli* and *A. polynesiensis* were determined to be the principal vectors in the outbreaks in Yap and French Polynesia.[65]

Mosquitoes have six life stages: eggs, 1–4 instar larvae, pupae, and adults. The immature forms are aquatic. Female mosquitoes I become infected with virus when the vertebrate host they feed on is viremic. They in turn transmit the virus when they feed on another vertebrate host. Vertical transmission of the virus from the infected females to their offspring has been demonstrated for dengue, chikungunya, and Zika virus.[68,69]

Mosquitoes are not immediately infectious when they ingest an arbovirus. The virus multiplies in the tissues of the mosquito and

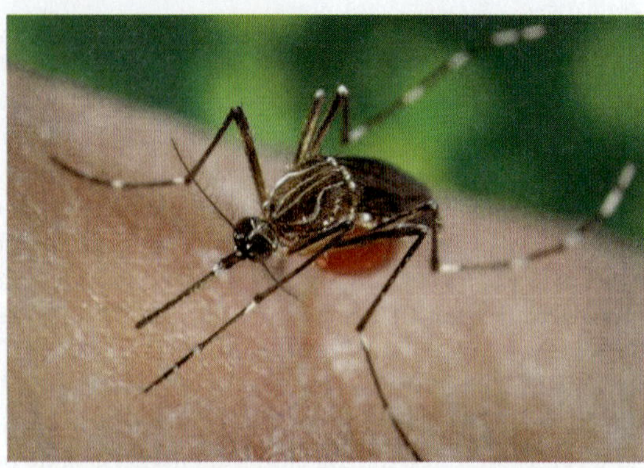

A

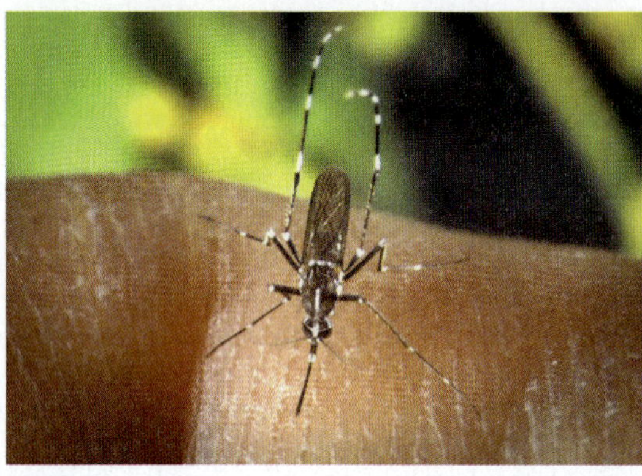

B

FIGURE 141-3A. Female *A. aegypti*. The picture highlights the characteristic lyre-shaped scutum. **B.** Female *A. albopictus*. Note the dorsal white stripe on the scutum which is used to distinguish *A. albopictus* from *A. aegypti*. (*Source:* James Gathany/CDC.)

eventually infects the insect's salivary gland. It is transmitted to the vertebrate host through the mosquito saliva, which is injected to help prevent blood coagulation when feeding. The virus developmental period in the mosquito is called the extrinsic incubation period (EIP). It is temperature (the higher temperature the shorter EIP) and vector dependent. For dengue, it appears to range from 7 to 14 days.[70]

Vector competence varies by mosquito species. There is also an infection dose threshold for competent mosquitoes. Animal populations that are more susceptible to infections and attain higher virus concentrations in their blood are therefore more effective vertebrate hosts for the particular virus. Virus transmission between vertebrates and mosquitoes is impacted by several factors including whether the vector prefers to feed on animals that are competent hosts and the herd immunity to the virus among the vertebrate host population. Species like *A. aegypti* that almost exclusively feed on people are more effective vectors of human diseases.[71] Mosquito species that are more opportunistic and willing to feed on multiple animal species, such as *A. albopictus*, are generally less effective vectors since every time the infected mosquito bites an animal that is incompatible with the virus, transmission ends.

Both *A. aegypti* and *A. albopictus* are primarily daytime biters. *A. aegypti* is found mainly in tropical and subtropical areas of the world. It prefers to breed very close to human habitations and typically flies only short distances (150 m or less) to obtain blood meals. *A. albopictus* is less dependent on humans and breeds more often in natural containers, such as tree holes. It can also survive in more temperate areas where they have acquired the ability to overwinter as eggs (diapause).[71]

HUMAN DISEASE SURVEILLANCE

Dengue, Zika, and chikungunya virus infections are nationally notifiable in a number of countries. Data come from laboratories and healthcare practitioners who report cases to public health officials. Public health authorities also receive data on positive blood product tests from blood banks, and mosquito surveillance.

PREVENTION

Mosquito-borne diseases can be prevented through personal protection, environmental modification, and mosquito control. People can avoid mosquito bites by wearing long-sleeved clothing and using a variety of effective repellents, following label instructions. In the United States, these are approved by the Environmental Protection Agency (EPA).

The effectiveness varies by concentration of the product. 10% N,N-Diethyl-3-Methylbenzamide (DEET) is generally effective for 90 minutes, a product with 30% DEET will last 5–6 hours. Products with 30% DEET or less can be used safely on children two months of age and older. (Children less than 2 months can be protected using mosquito netting.) Products with more than 50% DEET should not be applied directly to the skin.

Metofluthrin and allethrin are active ingredients found in spatial repellents available commercially. Residual pesticides applied in the home by professional pest control operators can also be effective.

Environmental control measures for individual home dwellers include eliminating mosquito breeding sites (e.g., dumping water, shredding tires, removing bromeliads), limiting dark, humid, protected resting places for mosquitoes near human dwellings (e.g., cutting vegetation, clean up trash), and ensuring intact housing with sealed or screened doors and windows. Air-conditioning use also helps limit the human risk for mosquito-borne diseases because of the low humidity that dries out the vector.

Mosquitoes are best controlled through integrated pest management performed by trained professionals. Such programs involve larval and adult mosquito surveillance activities, and based on the surveillance data, larval and adult mosquito control. Larval development can be controlled by eliminating breeding sites, as discussed above, and application of biological and chemical control agents [including *Bacillus thurigiensis* (bti)] into the water. Adult control generally requires pesticide applications. This is most effectively done through aerial application of tiny pesticide droplets that target host seeking (flying) mosquitoes. Trucks and backpack applications can also be used. Pesticides used by mosquito control must be approved. In the United States, this is handled by the EPA. Chemicals used for mosquito control generally break down very quickly in the environment and are not harmful to humans and other vertebrates.

A. aegypti and *A. albopictus* surveillance and control is challenging. The small, obscure bodies of water where these mosquitoes tend to breed are easy to miss. The adult *Aedes* can also be difficult to monitor because of their limited flight range. In addition, *A. aegypti* and *A. albopictus* are generally not attracted to traps typically used for nuisance mosquito surveillance. The limited flight range also makes it more difficult to control adult mosquitoes. Researchers have been exploring sterile insect techniques (SIT) for *A. aegypti* control since the success of the screwworm eradication in the 1960s. Historically, attempts to control mosquitoes using SIT have had limited success but the interest in these control methods have been renewed as the public health impact of diseases spread by *A. aegypti* have increased.[72]

Recent pesticide resistance testing in Florida has shown that *A. aegypti*, in particular, is increasingly resistant to pyrethroids (which are also commonly used by household pest control operators), and sometimes to organophosphate pesticide products as well. It is therefore important that the integrated pest management activities include routine pesticide resistance monitoring.[73]

References

1. Beier JC, Perkins PV, Onyango FK, et al. Characterization of malaria transmission by Anopheles (*Diptera: Culicidae*) in western Kenya in preparation for malaria vaccine trials. *J Med Entomol.* 1990;27(4):570–7.
2. Mehta R, Soares CN, Medialdea-Carrera R, et al. The spectrum of neurological disease associated with Zika and chikungunya viruses in adults in Rio de Janeiro, Brazil: A case series. *PLoS Negl Trop Dis.* 2018;12(2):e0006212.
3. Ali S, Gugliemini O, Harber S, et al. Environmental and social change drive the explosive emergence of Zika virus in the Americas. *PLoS Negl Trop Dis.* 2017;11(2):e0005135.
4. Bollati M, Alvarez K, Assenberg R, et al. Structure and functionality in flavivirus NS-proteins: Perspectives for drug design. *Antiviral Res.* 2010;87:125–48.
5. Gubler DJ. Dengue. In: Monath TP, ed. *The Arboviruses: Epidemiology and Ecology*. Vol. II. Boca Raton, FL: CRC Press; 1988:223–60.
6. World Health Organization (WHO). *Handbook for Clinical Management of Dengue*. Geneva: World Health Organization; 2012.
7. Arragain L, Dupont-Rouzeyrol M, O'Connor O, et al. Vertical transmission of dengue virus in the peripartum period and viral kinetics in newborns and breast milk: New data. *J Pediatric Infect Dis Soc.* 2017;6(4):324–31.
8. Powell JR, Tabachnick WJ. History of domestication and spread of *Aedes aegypti*—A review. *Mem Inst Oswaldo Cruz.* 2013;108(Suppl 1):11–7.
9. Brathwaite Dick O, San Martin JL, Montoya RH, et al. Review: The history of dengue outbreaks in the Americas. *Am J Trop Med Hyg.* 2012;87(4):584–93.
10. Beaumier C, Garcia MN, Murray KO. The history of dengue in the United States and its recent emergence. *Curr Trop Med Rep.* 2014;1:32–5.
11. Monath T. Yellow fever. In: Monath T, ed. *The Arboviruses, Epidemiology and Ecology*. Vol. V. Boca Raton, FL: CRC Press;1988:139–231.
12. Effler PV, Pang L, Kitsutani P, et al. Dengue fever, Hawaii, 2001–2002. *Emerg Infect Dis.* 2005;11(5):742–9.
13. Johnston D, Viray M, Ushiroda J, et al. Outbreak of locally acquired cases of dengue fever—Hawaii, 2015. *MMWR Morb Mortal Wkly Rep.* 2016;65(2):34–5.
14. Radke EG, Gregory CJ, Kintziger KW, et al. Dengue outbreak in Key West, Florida, USA, 2009. *Emerg Infect Dis.* 2012;18(1):135–7.
15. Florida Department of Health (FDOH). Dengue virus: Outbreak investigation following a cluster of three locally acquired dengue fever cases, Martin County. *Annual Morbidity Report.* 2013:105. http://www.floridahealth.gov/diseases-and-conditions/disease-reporting-and-management/disease-reporting-and-surveillance/data-and-publications/_documents/2013-section4.pdf.
16. World Health Organization (WHO). *Dengue: Guidelines for Diagnosis, Treatment Prevention and Control*. Geneva: World Health Organization; 2009.
17. Bhatt S, Gething PW, Brady OJ, et al. The global distribution and burden of dengue. *Nature.* 2013;496(7446):504–7.
18. Gyawali N, Bradbury RS, Taylor-Robinson AW. The epidemiology of dengue infection: Harnessing past experience and current knowledge to support implementation of future control strategies. *J Vector Borne Dis.* 2016;53:293–304.
19. Centers for Disease Control and Prevention (CDC). Dengue: Epidemiology. https://www.cdc.gov/dengue/epidemiology/index.html.
20. Halstead SB. Pathogenesis of dengue: Dawn of a new era. *F1000Res.* 2015;4:1353.
21. World Health Organization (WHO). Meeting of the Strategic Advisory Group of Experts on Immunization, April 2018—Conclusions and recommendations. *Wkly Epidemiol Rec.* 2018;93(23):329–44.
22. Ribeiro GS, Kikuti M, Tauro LB, et al. Does immunity after Zika virus infection cross-protect against dengue? *Lancet Glob Health.* 2018;6(2):e140–1.
23. Powers AM, Brault AC, Shirako Y, et al. Evolutionary relationships and systematics of the Alphaviruses. *J Virol.* 2001;75(21):10118–31.
24. Staples JE, Breiman RF, Powers AM. Chikungunya fever: An epidemiological review of a re-emerging infectious disease. *Clin Infect Dis.* 2009;49(6):942–8.
25. Duvignaud A, Fianu A, Bertolotti A, et al. Rheumatism and chronic fatigue, the two facets of post-chikungunya disease: The TELECHIK cohort study on Reunion Island. *Epidemiol Infect.* 2018;146(5):633–41.
26. Weaver SC, Lecuit M. Chikungunya virus and the global spread of a mosquito-borne disease. *N Engl J Med.* 2015;372:1231–9.
27. White SK, Mavian C, Elbadry MA, et al. Detection and phylogenetic characterization of arbovirus dual-infections among persons during a chikungunya fever outbreak, Haiti 2014. *PLoS Negl Trop Dis.* 2018;12(5):e0006505.
28. Jupp PG, McIntosh BM. Chikungunya virus disease. In: Monath TP, ed. *The Arboviruses: Epidemiology and Ecology*. Vol. II. Boca Raton, FL: CRC Press; 1988:137–57.
29. Halstead SB. Reappearance of chikungunya, formerly called dengue, in the Americas. *Emerg Infect Dis.* 2015;21(4):557–61.
30. Cassadou S, Boucau S, Petit-Sinturel M, Huc P, Leparc-Goffart I, Ledrans M. Emergence of chikungunya fever on the French side of Saint Martin island, October to December 2013. *Euro Surveill.* 2014;19(13):20752.
31. Leparc-Goffart I, Nougairede A, Cassadou S, Prat C, de Lamballerie X. Chikungunya in the Americas. *Lancet.* 2014;383(9916):514.
32. Pan American Health Organization (PAHO). Chikungunya: Data, maps and statistics. https://www.paho.org/hq/index.php?option=com_topics&view=readall&cid=5927&Itemid=40931&lang=en.
33. Kendrick K, Stanek D, Blackmore C. Transmission of chikungunya virus in the continental United States—Florida, 2014. *MMWR Morb Mortal Wkly Rep.* 2014;63(48):1137.
34. Duffy MR, Chen TH, Hancock WT, et al. Zika virus outbreak on Yap Island, Federated States of Micronesia. *N Engl J Med.* 2009;360(24):2536–43.
35. Mittal R, Nguyen D, Debs LH, et al. Zika virus: An emerging global health threat. *Front Cell Infect Microbiol.* 2017;7:486.
36. Barbi L, Coelho AVC, de Alencar LCA, Crovella S, et al. Prevalence of Guillain-Barré syndrome among Zika virus infected cases: A systematic review and meta-analysis. *Braz J Infect Dis.* 2018;22(2):137–41.
37. Dos Santos T, Rodriguez A, Almiron M, et al. Zika virus and the Guillain–Barré syndrome—Case series from seven countries. *N Engl J Med.* 2016;375(16):1598–601.
38. Moore CA, Staples JE, Dobyns WB, et al. Congenital Zika syndrome: Characterizing the pattern of anomalies for pediatric healthcare providers. *JAMA Pediatr.* 2017;171(3):288–95.
39. Pacheco O, Beltran M, Nelson CA, et al. Zika virus disease in Colombia—Preliminary report. *N Engl J Med.* 2020;383(6):e44.
40. Honein MA. Recognizing the global impact of Zika virus infection during pregnancy. *N Engl J Med.* 2018;378:1055–6.
41. Hoen B, Schaub B, Funk AL, et al. Pregnancy outcomes after ZIKV infection in French territories in the Americas. *N Engl J Med.* 2018;378(11):985–94.
42. Driggers RW, Ho CY, Korhonen EM, et al. Zika virus infection with prolonged maternal viremia and fetal brain abnormalities. *N Engl J Med.* 2016;374(22):2142–51.
43. Mead PS, Duggal NK, Hook SA, et al. Zika virus shedding in semen of symptomatic infected men. *N Engl J Med.* 2018;378(15):1377–85.
44. Motta IJF, Spencer BR, Cordeiro da Silva SG, et al. Evidence for transmission of Zika virus by platelet transfusion. *N Engl J Med.* 2016;375(11):1101–3.
45. Saa P, Proctor M, Foster G, et al. Investigational testing for Zika virus among U.S. blood donors. *N Engl J Med.* 2018;378(19):1778–88.
46. Uganda Virus Research Institute (UVRI). History of health research at UVRI. http://uvri.go.ug/index.php/about-uvri/history.
47. Hayes EB. Zika virus outside Africa. *Emerg Infect Dis.* 2009;15(9):1347–50.
48. Simpson DI. Zika virus infection in man. *Trans R Soc Trop Med Hyg.* 1964;58:335–8.
49. European Centre for Disease Prevention and Control (ECDC). Rapid risk assessment: Zika virus infection outbreak, Brazil and the Pacific region. Stockholm: ECDC; 25 May 2015.
50. Faria NR, Azevedo RDSDS, Kraemer MUG, et al. Zika virus in the Americas: Early epidemiological and genetic findings. *Science.* 2016;352(6283):345–9.
51. Pan American Health Organization (PAHO). Zika virus infection. https://www.paho.org/hq/index.php?option=com_content&view=article&id=11585&Itemid=41688&lang=en.
52. Likos A, Griffin I, Bingham AM, et al. Local mosquito-borne transmission of Zika virus—Miami-Dade and Broward Counties, Florida, June–August 2016. *MMWR Morb Mortal Wkly Rep.* 2016;65(38):1032–8.
53. Hall NB, Broussard K, Evert N, Canfield M. Notes from the field: Zika virus-associated neonatal birth defects surveillance—Texas, January 2016–July 2017. *MMWR Morb Mortal Wkly Rep.* 2017;66(31):835–6.
54. Grard G, Caron M, Mombo IM, et al. Zika virus in Gabon (Central Africa)—2007: A new threat from *Aedes albopictus*? *PLoS Negl Trop Dis.* 2014;8(2):e2681.

55. Mier-y-teran Romero LMT, Delorey MJ, Sejvar JJ, Johansson MA. Guillain–Barré syndrome risk among individuals infected with Zika virus: A multi-country assessment. *BMC Med.* 2018;16:67.
56. Styczynski AR, Malta JMAS, Krow-Lucal ER, et al. Increased rates of Guillain-Barré syndrome associated with Zika virus outbreak in the Salvador metropolitan area, Brazil. *PLoS Negl Trop Dis.* 2017;11(8):e0005869.
57. Rasmussen SA, Jamieson DJ, Honein MA, Petersen LR. Zika virus and birth defects—Reviewing the evidence for causality. *N Engl J Med.* 2016;374(20):1981–7.
58. Calvet G, Aguiar RS, Melo AS, et al. Detection and sequencing of Zika virus from amniotic fluid of fetuses with microcephaly in Brazil: A case study. *Lancet Infect Dis.* 2016;16(6):653–60.
59. Cauchemez S, Besnard M, Bompard P, et al. Association between Zika virus and microcephaly in French Polynesia, 2013–2015: A retrospective study. *Lancet.* 2016;387(10033):2125–32.
60. Beltrán-Silva SL, Chacón-Hernández SS, Moreno-Palacios E, et al. Clinical and differential diagnosis: Dengue, chikungunya and Zika. *Rev Med Hosp Gen Méx.* 2018;81(3):146–53.
61. Sharp TM. Differentiating chikungunya from dengue: A clinical challenge. *Medscape.* 2015. https://www.medscape.com/viewarticle/831523.
62. U.S. Food and Drug Administration (FDA). Trioplex real-time RT-PCR assay—Instructions for use—Centers for Disease Control and Prevention. https://www.fda.gov/downloads/MedicalDevices/Safety/EmergencySituations/UCM491592.pdf.
63. Griffin I, Miami-Dade County Health Department, personal comment.
64. Halstead SB, Rojanasuphot S, Sangkawibha N. Original antigenic sin in dengue. *Am J Trop Med Hyg.* 1983;32:154–6.
65. Petersen LR, Jamieson DJ, Powers AM, Honein MA. Zika virus. *N Engl J Med.* 2016;374(16):1552–63.
66. Lanciotti RS, Kosoy OL, Laven JJ, et al. Genetic and serologic properties of Zika virus associated with an epidemic, Yap State, Micronesia, 2007. *Emerg Infect Dis.* 2008;14(8):1232–9.
67. Rabe IB, Staples JE, Villanueva J, et al. Interim guidance for interpretation of Zika virus antibody test results. *MMWR Morb Mortal Wkly Rep.* 2016;65(21):543–6.
68. Ciota AT, Bialosuknia SM, Ehrbar DJ, Kramer LD. Vertical transmission of Zika virus by *Aedes aegypti* and *Ae. albopictus* mosquitoes. *Emerg Infect Dis.* 2017;23(5):880–2.
69. Ferreira-de-Lima VH, Lima-Camara TN. Natural vertical transmission of dengue virus in *Aedes aegypti* and *Aedes albopictus*: A systematic review. *Parasit Vectors.* 2018;11(1):77.
70. Tjaden NB, Thomas SM, Fischer D, Beierkuhnlein C. Extrinsic incubation period of dengue: Knowledge, backlog, and applications of temperature dependence. *PLoS Negl Trop Dis.* 2013;7(6):e2207.
71. Kauffman EB, Kramer LD. Zika virus mosquito vectors: Competence, biology, and vector control. *J Infect Dis.* 2017;216(10):S976–90.
72. Alphey L, Benedict M, Bellini R, et al. Sterile-insect methods for control of mosquito borne diseases: An analysis. *Vector-Borne Zoonotic Dis.* 2010;10(3):295–311.
73. Centers for Disease Control and Prevention (CDC). Mosquito control: Insecticide resistance. https://www.cdc.gov/zika/vector/insecticide-resistance.html.

CHAPTER 142

Diseases Transmitted Primarily by Arthropod Vectors: Viral Infections

Ingrid Rabe • Ann M. Powers • Marc Fischer

INTRODUCTION TO ARBOVIRUSES

Arthropod-borne viruses (arboviruses) are transmitted between vertebrate hosts by certain species of hematophagous insects, including mosquitoes, sand flies, midges, and ticks.[1] Although covered by the overarching term, "arbovirus," to denote the mode of transmission, these viruses belong to different taxonomic families. Transmission by arthropod vectors is biologic, rather than mechanical, in that true arboviruses replicate in arthropod tissues and salivary glands prior to transmission, rather than simply being carried by vectors.

Arbovirus infections in natural hosts typically result in development of a viremia of sufficient magnitude to infect an arthropod and propagate further vector-borne transmission. For most arboviruses, humans are not the natural host in which they ordinarily reside and propagate, and the majority of human infections do not produce clinical disease. However, in the small proportion of infected persons with clinically apparent illness, presentation typically falls into the following broad categories: generalized febrile illness, neuroinvasive disease, polyarthralgia, or hemorrhagic fever. Development of severe, possibly fatal, disease is rare and often dependent on age and underlying medical conditions. Described in separate chapters are the related diseases of dengue, Zika, chikungunya (chapter141), and arthropod-borne viral hemorrhagic fevers (Chapter 139).

CLASSIFICATION OF ARBOVIRUSES

Medically important arboviruses belong primarily to *Flaviviridae*, *Togaviridae*, *Peribunyaviridae*, *Phenuiviridae*, and *Reoviridae* families (Table 142-1). The term arbovirus covers a heterogeneous group of viruses with only broad commonalities in mode of transmission but some significant differences in viral replication strategies, ecologic dynamics, and infection outcomes. The most comprehensive list of viruses biologically transmitted by arthropods in nature and infectious for humans or domestic animals is contained in the *International Catalogue of Arboviruses*.[2] Of more than 500 viruses listed, just over 100 have been shown to cause disease in humans and only a small proportion of those are of clinical or public health importance.[3]

EPIDEMIOLOGY OF ARBOVIRUSES

The distribution and incidence of arbovirus infections are affected by epidemiological, ecological, and biological factors including geographical distribution of hosts and vectors, climate, seasonal variations, and viral survival strategies.

Geographical Distribution

Historically, geophysical barriers such as mountain ranges or bodies of water have limited vector and host distribution. These barriers may be overcome, however, by factors such as changes in modes of transportation enabling vectors and vertebrate hosts to transport viruses out of their natural habitats, and relocation of human host populations to areas in which they are exposed to unfamiliar circulating viruses. If appropriate local conditions exist, viral circulation may continue in newly introduced or inhabited areas.

Biologic barriers that may limit the geographical distribution of arbovirus infections are determined by the presence or absence of susceptible vertebrate hosts and competent arthropod vectors. Viruses that utilize avian hosts tend to be more widely distributed than those that utilize small terrestrial mammals with restricted territories and limited migration.[5] Relative nonsusceptibility of arthropod vectors or hosts to a particular virus also limits distribution. In developed countries improved sanitation, a higher standard in living conditions, and lifestyle changes have significantly decreased the prevalence of vector-borne disease.[6]

Epidemiologic evaluations also show that the distribution of a virus may be much wider than that of its recognized associated disease.[7] Explanations for these discrepancies include the following: (a) vector feeding preferences for nonhumans; (b) virus circulation in areas seldom or not frequented by human hosts; (c) existence of viral strains with reduced virulence in humans; (d) high population-level immunity; and (e) lack of recognition and reporting.

Seasonal Distribution and Chronology of Epidemics

Climate and seasonal variations play an important role in the epidemiology of arboviral infections due to the impact on vector density and activity.[3] Seasonal variations typically correspond to vector breeding cycles and periods of peak population density. In temperate zones, vector density is highest from late spring through early fall. In tropical regions, vector density is higher during the rainy seasons. Even among different arboviruses utilizing the same vector and vertebrate hosts, the seasonal distribution of human disease cases may vary due to the duration of replication, viremia, and incubation periods within the arthropod vector.

VIRUS TRANSMISSION CYCLES

Arboviral transmission cycles may be simple, involving only one host and one vector, or more complex with enzootic cycles, possibly involving multiple vector species or animal hosts.[3] Important determinants in arboviral transmission include the competence (ability to acquire, maintain, and transmit the infecting virus) and density of the arthropod vector, as well as the susceptibility, viremic potential, and abundance of the vertebrate host.

After ingestion of a blood meal from a viremic vertebrate, a competent vector develops a systemic infection that eventually leads to infection of the salivary glands.[8] This process typically lasts 1–2 weeks and is referred to as the extrinsic incubation period. Upon completion of extrinsic incubation, an arthropod is capable of transmitting the virus to a susceptible vertebrate upon taking a subsequent blood meal. Therefore, the role of the vector is biological and dynamic,

TABLE 142-1 CHARACTERISTICS OF SELECTED ARBOVIRUS BY PREDOMINANT CLINICAL SYNDROME

Virus	Vector	Viral family	Animal Hosts	Geographical Distribution	Predominant Season	Incubation
Viruses causing generalized febrile illness						
Colorado tick fever	Tick	*Reoviridae*	Small rodents	Western United States and Canada	March–November (peak May–July)	3–6 days
Oropouche fever	Midge, mosquito	*Peribunyaviridae*	Wild birds, monkeys, sloths	Amazon region of Brazil, Peru and Panama	Rainy season	4–8 days
Sandfly fever	Sandfly	*Phenuiviridae*	Unknown	Mediterranean, Middle East, Southwestern Asia	June–September (peak August)	3–8 days
Heartland	Tick	*Phenuiviridae*	Raccoons and deer?	Midwest and southern United States	Spring and summer	Unknown
Bourbon	Tick (likely)	*Orthomyxoviridae*	Unknown	Unknown; likely Midwest United States	Spring and summer	Unknown
Viruses causing acute central nervous system infections						
West Nile virus	Mosquito	*Flaviviridae*	Birds	Americas, Europe, Asia, Africa, Middle East, Australia	April–December (peak August–September) in the northern hemisphere	2–14 days
St. Louis encephalitis	Mosquito	*Flaviviridae*	Birds	Americas	June–October (peak August–September)	4–14 days
Japanese encephalitis	Mosquito	*Flaviviridae*	Pigs, birds	Asia	Temperate Zones: May–September Tropical Zones (Asia): Year-round	5–14 days
Usutu	Mosquito	*Flaviviridae*	Birds	Africa, Europe	June–October	Unknown
Powassan virus	Tick	*Flaviviridae*	Small mammals	Eastern Canada and United States	May–December	6–34 days
Tickborne encephalitis	Tick	*Flaviviridae*	Small rodents	Europe, Asia	March–November (peak June–July)	4–28 days
La Crosse	Mosquito	*Peribunyaviridae*	Small mammals	Midwest, mid-Atlantic, southern United States	July–September	5–15 days
Jamestown Canyon	Mosquito	*Peribunyaviridae*	Deer	North America	July–September	3–7 days
Cache Valley	Mosquito	*Peribunyaviridae*	Hoofed animals	North and Central America	May–October	
Toscana	Sand fly	*Phenuiviridae*	Unknown	Europe	June–October (peak August)	3–7 days
Eastern equine encephalitis	Mosquito	*Togaviridae*	Birds	Americas, Caribbean	August–September	~7 days
Venezuelan equine encephalitis	Mosquito	*Togaviridae*	Birds, rodents	Americas	Rainy season	1–6 days
Western equine encephalitis	Mosquito	*Togaviridae*	Birds	Americas	April–September (peak July–August)	~7 days
Viruses causing polyarthralgia						
Ross River	Mosquito	Togaviridae	Marsupials	Australia, South Pacific	March–May	7–11 days
Sindbis	Mosquito	Togaviridae	Birds	Europe, Asia, Africa, Oceania	Summer-Fall	~7 days
Mayaro	Mosquito	Togaviridae	Nonhuman primates	South America, Caribbean?	Rainy season	3–11 days

because active viral replication occurs within the vector providing a secondary reservoir for amplification. The viral biology creates a highly efficient means for transmission: a small inoculum of virus into an arthropod vector can be greatly amplified.

Several factors related specifically to the vector, such as abundance, longevity, and host preference, determine the rate of viral transmission and the risk of epidemics. Vector abundance depends on factors that affect breeding and survival. For example, variations in weather and environmental conditions dramatically impact vector abundance accounting for many of the seasonal variations in arboviral infections.[9] Longevity is critical, since even a brief prolongation in vector lifespan may increase the proportion of the vector population capable of transmitting virus. The host preference of a vector species also is epidemiologically important, since vectors that are strongly attracted to reservoir hosts and are highly anthropophilic are ideal vectors for transmission of a zoonotic virus to humans. Host preferences may change during a season: the vectors of western equine encephalitis and St. Louis encephalitis viruses shift from predominant feeding on avian amplifying hosts in early summer to mammals, including humans, in late summer.[10]

Important Vectors: Mosquitoes and Ticks

Mosquitoes transmit arboviruses from different families. Viruses that utilize mosquito vectors adapted to habitats that are in close proximity to human populations tend to be responsible for the major epidemic diseases. Mosquitoes require aquatic habitats for oviposition (laying of eggs) and larval development.[11] Suitable habitats that promote breeding vary by species, but are typically characterized by the presence of standing water. Natural habitats include salt- and freshwater marshes, mangroves, swamps, lakes, ponds, streams, rain pools, and tree holes. Manmade mosquito habitats include storm water control ditches, floodwaters, irrigation system runoff, and receptacles, such as discarded tires and other refuse.

Ticks transmit the widest variety of pathogens of any blood-feeding arthropod.[12] They have complicated life cycles that optimize contact with susceptible hosts at various stages. During the larval, nymph, and adult stages, the tick may seek a different host, which adds to the complexity of the transmission cycle. In addition, some infected ticks may transfer certain viruses directly to co-feeding uninfected ticks via the host's tissue lymphatics and macrophages without the need for vertebrate host viremia or viral replication.

Important Hosts: Wild Birds, Rodents, and Domesticated Animals

Various vertebrate hosts play a role in arbovirus ecology.[13,14] Wild birds are important vertebrate hosts in the transmission cycles of many mosquito-borne arboviruses, and some ground-dwelling birds may also play a role in tick-borne infections. This is particularly relevant to human infections because of the proximity to large bird populations in residential and agricultural settings. Due to migration patterns, avian hosts also affect the transportation, dissemination, and reintroduction of viruses over large geographical areas. During the spring and summer, nestling birds that are relatively defenseless against mosquito bites often support higher levels of viremia than adults and are considered important hosts for some viruses.

Birds generally develop viremia within the first 2 days after inoculation by an infected arthropod. The viremia may last only a few days or be prolonged depending on the specific viral species. For most arboviruses, infected birds remain asymptomatic and viremia is followed by the appearance of specific antibodies.[15] However, outbreaks of symptomatic avian arboviral disease have occurred and significant avian mortality has been noted in susceptible species, exemplified by the dramatic occurrence of corvid deaths following West Nile virus introduction to the United States in 1999.[16]

Rodents are the principal hosts for nearly a dozen mosquito- and tick-borne arboviruses.[17] General characteristics of rodent hosts that affect viral transmission rates include high reproductive capacity and population turnover, limited movement and dispersal, and specific habitat requirements. These factors favor restricted viral transmission and enzootic maintenance of the virus, although focal epidemics can occur. Rodents tend to be hosts for the larval and nymph stages of tick vectors, whereas the tick adult stage generally feed on large animals, including humans.

Domestic animals are effective viremic hosts for a limited number of arboviruses, serving not only as a source for viral amplification and vector feeding, but in some cases showing overt clinical manifestations of disease. Since viral amplification in livestock precedes spillover to the human population, epizootic infections can portend an impending epidemic. Japanese encephalitis virus is a notable example, in which swine are efficient amplifying hosts that develop a spectrum of clinical manifestations dependent on the age of the infected animal, with important public health and agricultural economic ramifications.[18] Although not discussed in this chapter, nonhuman primates also have a notable role in maintenance of sylvatic cycles of arbovirus transmission, such as yellow fever virus.

Viral Survival Strategies

Virus survival is threatened during the winter and dry months when arthropod vector densities decrease and viral transmission and amplification is slowed or interrupted.[4] Overwintering is an important concept in the epidemiology of vector-borne disease and includes known and speculative strategies for local survival or reintroduction. Overwintering may depend on the level of viral activity during the preceding summer and fall, accounting for arboviral outbreaks that commonly occur in two or more successive years. Strategies include hibernation, chronically infected reservoirs, transovarial infection, and reintroduction.[19]

Hibernation of arboviruses in the primary arthropod vector through adverse survival periods has been well documented in nymph and adult ticks. Hibernation as a survival strategy in mosquito vectors is less clear. Survival through chronically infected vertebrate reservoirs to span periods of vector hibernation or quiescence has been speculated as a possible recrudescence strategy for arboviruses but clear evidence of chronically infected animals that maintain arbovirus viremia in nature is lacking.[20] Transovarial transmission is a common and efficient method for transmission of some arboviruses from adult mosquito or tick vectors to their progeny.[21] Viruses also can be reintroduced to a habitat by migratory vertebrates. Transport of viruses over long distances by migratory birds occasionally has been documented, but is generally not considered to be an important mechanism for the annual recrudescence of viral activity.[22]

SURVEILLANCE

The purpose of arboviral disease surveillance is to (1) quantify disease burden and identify seasonal, geographic, and demographic patterns in human morbidity and mortality, and (2) detect increases in virus transmission activity and respond with effective, disease-reducing interventions.[11] Successful implementation requires coordinated efforts of health agencies at the local, regional, and national levels, and support from the communities they serve. While specific surveillance activities vary based on local resources and population needs, most programs include monitoring of human disease cases, vector population density, and vector infection rates. Data on nonhuman vertebrate hosts, landscape ecology, season, climate, and weather also may be evaluated.

Human Surveillance

Human disease surveillance typically entails reporting of cases to regional health authorities as mandated by notifiable disease reporting policies and legislation. In general, healthcare providers or testing laboratories are responsible for reporting, and accurate quantification of disease burden is dependent upon clinician recognition of disease, appropriate diagnostic confirmation, and compliance with notification procedures. In the United States, under the National Notifiable Diseases Surveillance System, arboviral disease case definitions are developed and published by the Council for State and Territorial Epidemiologists.[23] These definitions include specific clinical and laboratory criteria for reporting of cases to the Centers for Disease Control and Prevention (CDC) through ArboNET, a comprehensive surveillance data capture platform that can receive human and nonhuman surveillance data.[24] Human surveillance activities also may be intensified when an outbreak is suspected or anticipated. Possible strategies include active hospital and clinic surveillance of specific syndromes, as well as alerting and educating local healthcare providers of testing and reporting procedures.

Environmental Surveillance

Environmental surveillance of nonhuman arbovirus activity may enable earlier detection of impending human epidemics, since transmission cycles of arboviruses require cumulative infection of vectors and amplifying vertebrate hosts before the virus can spill over into human populations.[3] Mosquito surveillance involves identifying and mapping larval habitats and monitoring adult mosquito activity. Specific indices based on data from mosquito pool testing are useful for determining trends in viral activity, provided surveillance efforts have remained consistent over time. Monitoring infection rates in sentinel host species (e.g., birds, horses) can be a useful adjunct to vector data in certain circumstances.

DIAGNOSIS OF ARBOVIRAL DISEASES

Arboviral infections are typically confirmed by detection of virus-specific antibody in serum or cerebrospinal fluid (CSF), usually using an enzyme immunoassay.[25,26] Acute-phase serum specimens should be tested for virus-specific immunoglobulin (Ig) M antibody. If correlated with clinical findings and exposure history, a positive IgM test result has good diagnostic predictive value, but cross-reaction with related arboviruses from the same viral family can occur.[4] For most arboviral infections, IgM is detectable within the first week after onset of illness and remain detectable for 30–90 days, but longer persistence has been documented.[27] Therefore, a positive IgM test result on serum occasionally may reflect a prior infection. IgM may be detected in CSF within a week of illness onset and may persist for several weeks to months, or even years.[28] Serum collected within 7 days of illness onset may not have detectable IgM, and the test should be repeated on a convalescent sample. IgG antibody generally is detectable in serum shortly after IgM and persists for years. A plaque-reduction neutralization test can be performed to measure virus-specific neutralizing antibodies and to discriminate between cross-reacting antibodies, particularly in primary arboviral infections.[29] Either seroconversion or a fourfold or greater increase in virus-specific neutralizing antibodies between acute- and convalescent-phase serum specimens can be used to confirm recent infection.

In patients who have been immunized against or infected with another arbovirus from the same virus family in the past, cross-reactive antibodies in both the IgM and neutralizing antibody assays may complicate identification of the specific arbovirus causing the patient's illness; this is noted most commonly among flaviviruses but occurs in other viral families also. For some tick-borne infections (e.g., Colorado tick fever), the immune response may be delayed, with prolonged viremia, absence of detectable IgM antibodies until 2–3 weeks after onset of illness, and neutralizing antibodies taking up to a month to develop.[30] Patients with significant immunosuppression may have a delayed or blunted serologic response. Immunization history, date of symptom onset, immune competence, and information regarding other arboviruses known to circulate in the geographic area that may cross-react in serologic assays should be considered when interpreting results.

Viral culture and nucleic acid amplification tests (NAATs) for viral RNA can be performed on acute-phase serum, CSF, or tissue specimens.[31] Arboviruses that are more likely to be detected using culture or NAATs early in the illness include Colorado tick fever, chikungunya, dengue, yellow fever, and Zika viruses. For other arboviruses, results of these tests often are negative even early in the clinical course because of the relatively short duration of viremia. Immunohistochemical staining can detect specific viral antigen in fixed tissue.

Antibody testing for common domestic arboviral diseases is performed in most state public health laboratories and many commercial laboratories. Confirmatory plaque-reduction neutralization tests, viral culture, NAATs, immunohistochemical staining, and testing for less common domestic and international arboviruses are performed at the CDC in Fort Collins, Colorado, and selected other reference laboratories.

CLASSIFICATION OF ARBOVIRUSES BY PREDOMINANT DISEASE PATTERN

Although most infections are subclinical, symptomatic illness usually manifests as one of three primary clinical syndromes: generalized febrile illness, acute central nervous system infections, or polyarthralgia. Dengue and yellow fever viruses can cause hemorrhage or shock, and are covered in other chapters.

Most medically important arboviruses are capable of causing generalized febrile illness that often includes headache, arthralgia, myalgia, and rash. Symptoms generally last for a few days to a week. Most patients recover completely, but fatigue, malaise, arthralgia, and weakness can linger for weeks or months.

For arboviruses causing neuroinvasive disease, most infections are asymptomatic or limited to the aforementioned febrile illness; however, some patients will develop aseptic meningitis, encephalitis, or acute flaccid paralysis.[32] Illness usually presents with a prodrome similar to the systemic febrile illness, followed by neurologic symptoms. The specific symptoms vary by virus but can include vomiting, stiff neck, mental status changes, seizures, or focal neurologic deficits. The severity and long-term outcome of arboviral neuroinvasive disease varies by etiologic agent and the underlying characteristics of the host, such as age, immune status, and preexisting medical condition.

Several arboviral infections, particularly the alphaviruses, manifest with acute febrile illness and polyarthralgia or arthritis.[33] Clinical features include joint pain, periarticular swelling, and less commonly, joint effusions. The differential diagnosis for arboviral disease is broad and includes other viral, bacterial, and parasitic infections, depending on the geographic locations of exposure. Chikungunya virus is discussed in a separate chapter together with other *Aedes* species mosquito-borne arboviral infections.

Viruses Causing Generalized Febrile Illness

Colorado Tick Fever Virus

Colorado tick fever virus is a double-stranded RNA virus in the genus *Coltivirus*, family *Reoviridae*. The geographic distribution of the virus corresponds to that of the primary tick vector, *Dermacentor andersoni* (Rocky Mountain wood tick) in the western United States and Canada at 4000- to 10,000-foot elevations.[34,35] Small mammals, such as chipmunks and ground squirrels, serve as the amplifying host for the immature forms of the tick; adult ticks feed on larger mammals. Infections are acquired through recreational and occupational pursuits in tick habitats. Person-to-person transmission through blood transfusion has also been described.[36] In a review of human cases diagnosed at the CDC from 2002 through 2012, 75 Colorado tick fever cases were identified with a median of five cases per year; 80% of cases occurred from May through July. Up to 90% of patients report a tick bite or tick exposure.

The incubation period following a tick bite is usually 3–6 days, followed by fever, headache, myalgia, and fatigue that can persist for several weeks.[34] Leukopenia and thrombocytopenia also may develop. Less common clinical manifestations include meningitis, encephalitis, and bleeding disorders; the latter being the main presentation in three reported pediatric deaths. Diagnostic considerations unique to Colorado tick fever virus are that serologic tests are often not positive for up to 2 weeks after symptom onset, and due to viral infection of marrow erythrocytic precursors, PCR can detect viral RNA for a prolonged period following infection.[30]

Oropouche Virus

Oropouche virus is a single-stranded RNA virus in the genus *Orthobunyavirus*, family *Peribunyaviridae*. The virus was initially identified in a patient in Trinidad; however, the impact of its epidemic potential is most notable in the Amazon region of Brazil and Peru, as well as Panama, where it has caused $>$ 30 recognized outbreaks of febrile illness during the rainy season.[37] It is suspected that viral circulation includes both epidemic and sylvatic cycles.[38] In the epidemic cycle, humans are the amplifying vertebrate host and the biting midge (*Culicoides paraensis*) is the principal arthropod vector. In the sylvatic cycle, primates, sloths, and perhaps birds are the vertebrate hosts, although a definitive arthropod vector has not been identified.[39] Disease outbreaks are often characterized by high attack rates in affected localities. Infections through percutaneous and inhalational laboratory exposure have been described.[40]

Approximately two-thirds of infections are symptomatic.[39] Following an incubation period of 4–8 days, symptoms include abrupt onset of fever, severe headache, myalgia, arthralgia, chills, dizziness, photophobia, nausea, and vomiting; rash is infrequently reported. Illness typically lasts 3–6 days.[38] A brief recurrence of symptoms may occur in up to 60% of cases. Aseptic meningitis is an uncommon complication.

Sandfly Fever Viruses

Sandfly fever is caused by a group of serologically distinct, single-stranded RNA viruses belonging to the genus *Phlebovirus*, family *Phenuiviridae*. Viruses include the sandfly fever Naples serocomplex, Salehabad serocomplex, and Sicilian serocomplex.[41] They are distributed through the Mediterranean area extending from the Balkans into China, as well as into the Middle East and southwestern Asia. Human disease cases in endemic areas typically occur from May to October, with peak incidence in August.[42] The vectors, *Phlebotomus* species sandflies, are nocturnal with limited flight range and small size enabling them to penetrate screens and mosquito nets.[43] The most common vector, *P. papatasi*, breeds in both rural and urban habitats. Sandfly fever viruses are transmitted transovarially by female sandflies to their progeny, and transstadially between life stages. No vertebrate reservoir has been definitively demonstrated. Humans are a dead-end host.

In endemic regions, seroprevalence rates are high and infection is usually acquired in childhood when disease is mild or inapparent. High attack rates may occur among immunologically naïve tourists and visiting military personnel. Previously termed a "3-day fever," "papataci fever," or "phlebotomus fever," clinical disease consists of a brief, debilitating febrile illness without rash. Complete recovery is typical.

Heartland Virus

Heartland virus is a single-stranded RNA virus in the genus *Phlebovirus*, family *Phenuiviridae*. Heartland virus disease was first identified in two patients with febrile illness in Missouri in 2009, and subsequent cases have been diagnosed in several Midwestern and Southern states.[44,45] Recent studies have shown that *Amblyomma americanum* (Lone Star tick) is the likely vector.[46] Raccoons and deer have antibodies against the virus and are possible vertebrate hosts.[47]

Patients typically present with fever, fatigue, anorexia, headache, nausea, and myalgia or arthralgia.[45] Additional laboratory findings have included leukopenia, thrombocytopenia, and mild to moderate elevation of liver transaminases. Because of the similarity of these findings to other bacterial and parasitic tick-borne diseases, Heartland virus disease should be considered in patients being treated for ehrlichiosis who do not respond to treatment with doxycycline. Although most patients recover, fatalities have been reported, typically in older patients with underlying medical conditions.

Bourbon Virus

Bourbon virus is a novel single-stranded RNA virus in the genus *Thogotovirus*, family *Orthomyxoviridae*, that was first identified in Bourbon County, Kansas in 2014.[48] Transmission is assumed to be through the bite of an infected tick, and the virus has been isolated from ticks collected in Missouri.[49] Limited numbers of cases and entomologic data thus far preclude any certainty about the distribution of the virus. As of mid-2017, a limited number of Bourbon virus disease cases had been identified in the Midwest and southern United States. Most patients reported exposure to ticks prior to becoming ill. Patients typically presented with fever, fatigue, anorexia, nausea, vomiting, and maculopapular rash. Additional laboratory findings include thrombocytopenia and leukopenia. Some people who were infected later died.

Viruses Causing Acute Central Nervous System Infections

West Nile Virus

West Nile virus is a single-stranded, enveloped virus in the Japanese encephalitis serogroup of the genus *Flavirus*, family *Flaviviridae*. Transmission has been documented on every continent except Antarctica. Since the 1990s, the largest outbreaks of West Nile virus neuroinvasive disease have occurred in the Middle East, Europe, and North America. The first reported case in the United States was in New York in 1999, and the virus subsequently spread across the continental United States and Canada. Reported numbers of West Nile virus neuroinvasive disease cases fluctuate annually, and peak incidence rates occurred in 2002 (1.0 per 100,000 population), 2003 (1.0 per 100,000 population), and 2012 (0.9 per 100,000 population). It remains the leading cause of neuroinvasive arboviral disease in the United States.[50,51]

West Nile virus is transmitted primarily by *Culex* species mosquitoes and is maintained in nature in a cycle with wild birds as amplifying hosts. Humans do not develop sufficient viremia to serve as a source of infection for subsequently feeding mosquitoes, and are considered "dead-end hosts." In temperate and subtropical regions, most human West Nile virus infections occur in summer or early autumn. Nearly all human infections are acquired through mosquito bites, but transmission has also been documented through blood transfusion, organ transplantation, transplacental transmission, breastfeeding, and percutaneous exposure.[52] The incubation period following mosquito bites usually is 2–6 days but ranges from 2 to 14 days and can be prolonged in immunocompromised people.

West Nile virus causes both sporadic cases as well as epidemics. Serologic surveys suggest that 70–80% of infections are asymptomatic, 20–30% present with undifferentiated febrile illness, and less than 1% present with neuroinvasive disease.[53,54] In addition to elevated body temperature, West Nile fever is characterized by headache, myalgia, arthralgia, vomiting, diarrhea, or a transient maculopapular rash. West Nile virus meningitis may occur in younger age groups and is indistinguishable clinically from aseptic meningitis caused by other viruses. Patients with West Nile virus encephalitis, which is more common in the elderly, usually present with high fever, headache, seizures, mental status changes, focal neurologic deficits including paralysis, or movement disorders such as tremor. Patients with West Nile virus acute flaccid paralysis due to anterior horn cell damage present with the same neurological features as poliovirus-associated myelitis, with risk of respiratory paralysis requiring mechanical ventilation. West Nile virus-associated Guillain-Barré syndrome also has been reported and can be distinguished from West Nile virus acute flaccid paralysis by clinical manifestations and electrophysiologic testing. Rare clinical manifestations include cardiac dysrhythmias, myocarditis, rhabdomyolysis, optic neuritis, uveitis, chorioretinitis, orchitis, pancreatitis, and hepatitis. Risk factors for development of severe disease include chronic renal failure, history of cancer, history of alcohol abuse, diabetes, and hypertension.[55]

Patients with West Nile fever generally have a full recovery. However, for patients with neuroinvasive disease, neurological and psychiatric sequelae have been reported and the case-fatality rate is approximately 10%. Mortality is significantly higher in West Nile virus encephalitis and myelitis than in West Nile virus meningitis.

St. Louis Encephalitis Virus

St. Louis encephalitis virus is a single-stranded, enveloped virus in the Japanese encephalitis serogroup of the genus *Flavirus*, family *Flaviviridae*. Virus distribution is limited to the Americas, where activity has been reported from Southern Canada to Argentina.[56] A closely related virus, Rocio virus, was first isolated from a fatal case of encephalitis in the Rocio district in São Paulo, Brazil but has rarely been reported since then, and not from any other country.[57] The life cycle of St. Louis encephalitis virus includes wild birds and several species of *Culex* mosquitoes. St. Louis encephalitis virus previously was the leading cause of arboviral encephalitis in the United States, causing periodic large urban outbreaks occurring in 10- to 20-year cycles. However, since the introduction and spread of West Nile virus, St. Louis encephalitis virus disease incidence has decreased and few outbreaks have been reported. The largest outbreak of St. Louis encephalitis virus disease was in the central United States in 1975 and resulted in about 2000 reported neuroinvasive disease cases. Subsequent focal outbreaks of St. Louis encephalitis virus disease occurred in Florida in 1977 and 1990, Louisiana in 2001, and Argentina in 2005. The most recent identified outbreak in the United States occurred in Arizona in 2015, included 23 confirmed St. Louis encephalitis virus cases, and was notable for its occurrence with a concurrent West Nile virus outbreak.[58] St. Louis encephalitis virus infections occur in the summer months and early autumn, with peak incidence in August and September. Possible transmission of infection through blood transfusion has been described.[59]

Overt clinical manifestations of disease are rare with older age being an important risk factor. Disease severity also increases with age.[60] The spectrum of clinical illness includes mild febrile disease, aseptic meningitis, and meningoencephalitis. The incubation period for St. Louis encephalitis virus is estimated to be 4–14 days. Meningitis is clinically similar to other viral meningitides, with clinical features including fever, headache, neck stiffness, and other meningeal signs. Analysis of CSF shows a moderately elevated white blood cell count and protein. Clinical outcome is generally favorable. Encephalitis caused by St. Louis encephalitis virus infection may result in altered mental status, ataxia, tremors, seizures, or other neurologic signs. Hyponatremia due to a syndrome of inappropriate secretion of antidiuretic hormone (SIADH) has been documented in up to 30% of patients. The case-fatality rate in patients with St. Louis encephalitis virus encephalitis ranges from 5% to 20%; it is higher in older age groups and in patients with underlying hypertension.

Japanese Encephalitis Virus

Japanese encephalitis virus is a single-stranded, enveloped virus in the Japanese encephalitis serogroup of the genus *Flavirus*, family *Flaviviridae*. It is endemic throughout most of Asia and parts of the western Pacific.[61] In temperate areas of Asia, transmission is seasonal, and human disease usually peaks in summer and fall. In the subtropics and tropics, transmission may occur year-round, with peaks during monsoon rains. The virus is maintained in an enzootic cycle between mosquitoes and amplifying vertebrate hosts, primarily pigs and wading birds. The principal vectors are *Culex* species mosquitoes, particularly *C. tritaeniorhynchus*, although other mosquito species may be of importance in certain regions. *C. tritaeniorhynchus* breeds in rice paddy habitats and in areas with standing water (as may be present in flood irrigation systems), and is a night-time outdoor feeder. Pigs are an important amplifying host because they develop high viremic titers, are bred in proximity to human populations, and have a high population turnover with frequent production of large numbers of susceptible offspring.[62] Intrauterine infection of swine with Japanese encephalitis virus can result in abortion or stillbirth. Rare instances of other modes of transmission (i.e., intrauterine or blood product transfusion) have been documented in humans. Humans are incidental or dead-end hosts, because they usually do not develop a level or duration of viremia sufficient to infect mosquitoes.

In endemic areas where adults have been previously exposed and immunity is high, the disease primarily affects young children. The overall incidence of Japanese encephalitis among people from non-endemic countries traveling to Asia is estimated to be < 1 case per 1 million travelers.[63] However, expatriates and travelers who stay for prolonged periods in rural areas with active Japanese encephalitis virus transmission might be at similar risk as the susceptible pediatric resident population (5–10 cases per 100,000 children per year).

The majority of Japanese encephalitis viral infections are asymptomatic.[64] Mild disease is typically undetected and includes aseptic meningitis and febrile illness with headache after an incubation period of 5–15 days, and symptoms resolve within 5–7 days. Encephalitis tends to be more severe with seizures occurring in up to 85% of children and 10% of adults. Other typical neurological features include motor disturbances, Parkinsonism, and psychiatric abnormalities. Common laboratory findings include moderate leukocytosis, mild anemia, and hyponatremia. CSF typically has a mild to moderate pleocytosis with a lymphocytic predominance, slightly elevated protein, and normal glucose. The case-fatality ratio is approximately 20–30%. Among survivors, 30–50% have serious neurologic, cognitive, or psychiatric sequelae.

Usutu Virus

Usutu virus is a single-stranded, enveloped virus in the genus *Flavivirus*, family *Flaviviridae*. It was first identified in Africa in patients with febrile rash illness.[65] More recently, Usutu virus epizootics have been reported among birds in Europe.[66] Human cases of Usutu virus neurologic disease have been diagnosed, often during surveillance for West Nile virus infections, and through routine diagnostic testing because of increasing clinician awareness of Usutu virus epidemiology. The virus is maintained in nature in a cycle between *Culex* species mosquitoes and amplifying avian hosts. Humans are incidental dead-end hosts.

Infected persons may be asymptomatic or have mild to moderate symptoms including fever, rash, and headache. For those who progress to neurologic involvement, clinical manifestations typically include aseptic meningitis and meningoencephalitis; one case of facial paralysis has been described.[67–69] Most descriptions of severe disease have been in immunosuppressed patients. No fatalities have been reported.

Powassan Virus

Powassan virus is a single-stranded, enveloped virus in the tick-borne encephalitis serogroup of the genus *Flavirus*, family *Flaviviridae*. It is an uncommon but increasingly recognized cause of encephalitis in eastern Canada and the United States.[70] Increased awareness has facilitated more requests for Powassan diagnostic testing. The virus is primarily transmitted by *Ixodes* species ticks, including *I. cookei*, *I. marxi*, and *I. scapularis*. Hosts include small to medium sized mammals such as squirrels, groundhogs, and mice. Two distinct viral lineages are recognized, namely lineage I (Powassan virus) and lineage II (deer tick virus).[71] The incubation period can range from 1 to 5 weeks. Human infections occur from May through December after outdoor exposure to ticks. There were 99 cases of Powassan virus disease reported in the United States from 2006 to 2016.[72] Asymptomatic infection has been documented. In patients with neuroinvasive disease, encephalitis is the typical manifestation although aseptic meningitis has been described. Encephalitis, which typically begins with a febrile prodrome, is severe and case fatality rate is 10%; neurologic sequelae are noted in over half of survivors.

Tick-borne Encephalitis Viruses

Tick-borne encephalitis viruses are single-stranded, enveloped viruses in the genus *Flavirus*, family *Flaviviridae*. Infections are caused by three viral subtypes namely, Far Eastern, Siberian, and European.[73] The disease is endemic in focal areas of Europe and Asia, from eastern France to northern Japan and from northern Russia to Albania. Approximately 5000–13,000 tick-borne encephalitis cases are reported each year, with large annual fluctuations. The risk of infection for most travelers to endemic areas is low, particularly if their itineraries do not involve extensive activities with potential for tick bites.[74] The principal vectors are *Ixodes* ticks, which act as both vector and virus reservoir. *I. ricinis* is the primary vector for the European subtype, and *I. persulcatus* for the Far Eastern and Siberian subtypes. Small rodents are the primary amplifying host. Ticks can acquire infection through feeding on amplifying vertebrate hosts, vertical transmission, or cofeeding with infected ticks.[75] Tick-borne encephalitis virus also can be transmitted through ingestion of unpasteurized dairy products (such as milk and cheese) from infected goats, sheep, or cows. Additional, though infrequent, routes of transmission include laboratory exposure and slaughtering of viremic animals. Direct person-to-person spread of tick-borne encephalitis virus occurs only rarely, through blood transfusion, solid organ transplantation, or breastfeeding.

Approximately one third of infections are symptomatic and the most common clinical presentation is with acute neuroinvasive disease.[73] The median incubation period for tick-transmitted tick-borne encephalitis virus infection is 8 days (range, 4 days–4 weeks), and for milk-borne exposure it is 3–4 days. Although the most common clinical presentation is acute encephalitis, tick-borne encephalitis virus disease may be milder or demonstrate a biphasic course. The first phase is characterized by nonspecific febrile illness with headache, myalgia, and fatigue lasting several days; this may be followed by an afebrile and relatively asymptomatic period. Up to two-thirds of patients recover without any further illness. For those with disease progression, the second phase consists of central nervous system involvement resulting in aseptic meningitis, encephalitis, or myelitis. Findings include meningeal signs, altered mental status, cognitive dysfunction, ataxia, rigidity, seizures, tremors, cranial nerve palsies, and limb paresis. The European subtype causes milder disease, with a case-fatality ratio of < 2%, and neurologic sequelae in up to 30% of patients. The Far Eastern subtype is often associated with greater severity and a case-fatality ratio of 20–40% and higher rates of severe neurologic sequelae. The Siberian subtype has a reported case-fatality ratio of 2–3%.

La Crosse Virus

La Crosse virus is a single-stranded, enveloped virus in the California encephalitis serogroup of the genus *Orthobunyavirus*, family *Peribunyaviridae*. It has only been identified in North America and is the leading cause of pediatric arboviral neuroinvasive disease in the United States.[76] From 2007 to 2016, a median of 59 cases of La Crosse virus disease were reported annually and cases were most frequently reported from high-incidence areas in upper Midwestern, mid-Atlantic, and southeastern states.[77] In recent years, the main burden of infections has shifted from the upper Midwest to the Appalachian region, including West Virginia, Tennessee, North Carolina, and Ohio. In these endemic areas, the virus circulates in deciduous forests, where the primary vector is the daytime biting *A. triseriatus* (the eastern treehole mosquito) and the main amplifying hosts are small mammals (e.g., squirrels and chipmunks). La Crosse virus is transmitted transovarially from a female mosquito to her progeny, and can survive the winter in the mosquito eggs that will hatch into infected mosquitoes in the spring. Most cases occur from late spring through early autumn.

The majority of infections are subclinical. Disease manifestations include aseptic meningitis to severe and occasionally fatal encephalitis.[78] The incubation period is 5–15 days. Onset of neurologic disease is typically sudden, but may be preceded by a prodrome. Significant neurological dysfunction is common with up to 6–15% having residual neurologic sequelae, including seizures. The overall reported case-fatality was < 1% in cases notified to CDC.

Jamestown Canyon Virus

Jamestown Canyon virus is a single-stranded, enveloped virus in the California encephalitis serogroup of the genus *Orthobunyavirus*, family *Peribunyaviridae*. It is distributed throughout much of the United States and Canada.[79,80] The virus was first recovered from a *Culiseta* species mosquito pool in the state of Colorado in 1961, and was subsequently isolated from various mosquito species across temperate areas of North America. Seropositivity has been documented in several vertebrate species across a broad geographic distribution, although deer likely are the primary vertebrate hosts.[81] Human disease cases increasingly have been identified as a result of expanded testing for Jamestown Canyon virus.[82] The seasonal distribution of cases commences in May–June, a few months earlier than many other arboviruses, reflecting earlier mosquito vector activity in association with snowmelt breeding sites. A review of laboratory-confirmed cases of Jamestown Canyon virus disease reported in the United States during 2000–13 described 31 human disease cases across 13 states.[80] Symptomatic patients typically present with an acute febrile illness, meningitis, or meningoencephalitis. Headache is notable and several case reports have described initial attribution of symptoms to complex migraine. Most reported cases in the United States have occurred in adults (median age 48 years), with only half requiring hospital admission, and rare fatalities.

Cache Valley Virus

Cache valley virus is a single-stranded, enveloped virus in the genus *Orthobunyavirus*, family *Peribunyaviridae*. Although the virus has been recovered from several mosquito species (including *Anopheles*, *Culiseta*, *Coquillettidia*, and *Aedes* spp.), the primary vector is not known.[83] The main vertebrate hosts likely include larger hoofed animals such as deer, cattle, horses, and sheep. The virus is widely distributed in mosquito populations in North America and in parts of Central America.[84] Human Cache Valley virus disease cases have only rarely been reported (<10 cases) and have occurred from late spring through early fall. However, the disease is likely under-recognized. Initial symptoms of Cache Valley virus disease include fever, headache, nausea, vomiting, fatigue, and sometimes rash. In cases with progression to neurologic disease, clinical presentation has ranged from aseptic meningitis to fatal encephalitis.[85,86] One case report described protracted, progressive course of illness in an adult with X-linked agammaglobulinemia.[87]

Toscana Virus

Toscana virus is a single-stranded, enveloped virus in the *Phlebotomus* fever serogroup of the genus *Phlebovirus*, family *Phenuiviridae*. The virus is an important cause of summertime meningitis and, to a lesser extent, encephalitis in southern Europe from Spain to Turkey.[43] Italy has had several outbreaks in recent years.[88] *Phlebotomus* species sandflies are the primary vector for Toscana virus; no natural vertebrate host has been identified. Young adults are predominately affected and typically present with an initial mild febrile illness after an incubation period of 3–7 days. Most do not progress to nervous system involvement, however, in those that do complaints include headache, fever, nausea, vomiting, and myalgia.[89] Physical examination may reveal signs of meningismus and in some cases unconsciousness, tremors, paresis, and nystagmus. CSF analysis in patients with meningitis usually shows > 5 white cells/mL with normal levels of glucose and proteins. Leukopenia or leukocytosis has been reported. More severe encephalitis and encephalomyelitis, as well as atypical neurological presentations have been reported. Patients generally recover without sequelae and fatalities are rare.

Eastern Equine Encephalitis Virus

Eastern equine encephalitis virus is a single-stranded, enveloped virus, among the New World viruses in the genus *Alphavirus*, family *Togaviridae*.[90] It is distributed throughout the Atlantic and Gulf states of North America. Madariaga virus, a closely related virus, circulates in South America and causes milder disease.[91,92] Eastern equine encephalitis virus is maintained in nature in a cycle between *C. melanura* mosquitoes and birds residing in freshwater hardwood swamps. Transmission to other vertebrate species may occur through bridging vectors such as *Coquillettidia* and *Aedes* species mosquitoes; however, these vertebrates do not develop sufficient viremia to sustain further transmission. In the southern United States, cycles involving mosquitoes and wading birds, as well as reptiles, have been postulated as means of virus overwintering.[93] Person-to-person transmission through solid organ transplantation was described recently.[94] In a report summarizing eastern equine encephalitis virus surveillance data in the United States from 2003 to 2016, 121 cases were identified, with a median of eight cases reported annually.[7] Human disease cases were reported from 20 states and occurred predominantly along the Atlantic and Gulf coasts. Cases typically occur in July–September.

Asymptomatic infection is common.[90] Neuroinvasive disease occurs in $< 5\%$ of eastern equine encephalitis virus infections, with the youngest and oldest age groups at highest risk for severe clinical course. After a 1-week incubation period, the initial clinical manifestations consist of a prodrome with fever, headache, nausea, and vomiting. Neurological disease is severe and typically includes development of headache, confusion, focal neurologic deficits, meningismus, seizures, or coma. While infection is rare, eastern equine encephalitis virus is one of the most severe arboviral diseases in North America, with approximately 30% fatality among reported neurological disease cases. Even in survivors, complete recovery is uncommon. Sequelae include seizure disorders, hemiplegia, and cognitive dysfunction.

Venezuelan Equine Encephalitis Virus

Venezuelan equine encephalitis virus is a single-stranded, enveloped virus in the genus *Alphavirus*, family *Togaviridae*. It has only been identified in the Americas. After initial descriptions of human disease in Venezuala, large epidemics were reported several countries in South and Central America, with cases reported as far north as Texas and Florida.[3,95] Respective viral variants are associated with either enzootic or epizootic foci, with differences in mosquito vectors and primary amplifying vertebrate hosts (equines in epizootic, and rodents and birds in enzootic foci). In areas of enzootic transmission, human cases occur only sporadically, or in small localized clusters and this is attributed to accidental intrusion into an area of sylvatic transmission. Disease is usually limited to mild febrile illness and neurologic involvement is rare. Epizootics, by contrast, move across larger geographic areas with high attack rates in equines, followed by human infections around 2 weeks later. This tends to occur during the rainy season in tropical and subtropical America. Symptomatic persons typically have a self-limited flu like illness, although 4–14% may develop neuroinvasive disease and the case fatality rate is $< 1\%$. Young children are at higher risk for severe, and possibly fatal, encephalitis. Neuropsychiatric sequelae have been reported.[96]

Western Equine Encephalitis Virus

Western equine encephalitis virus is a single-stranded, enveloped virus, among the New World viruses in the genus *Alphavirus*, family *Togaviridae*. It is found in North America, west of the Mississippi River, and in South America.[97] In the United States, the virus is maintained in a cycle between *C. tarsalis* mosquitoes and wild birds, especially house finches and house sparrows. In midsummer, *Cx. tarsalis* feeding shifts to mammals, which coincides with peak timing for equine and human infections.[10]

Horses and humans are dead-end hosts that do not develop sufficient viremias to infect mosquito vectors. Flooding due to irrigation or heavy snowmelt promotes higher vector density and may precipitate summer outbreaks. Reported numbers of western equine encephalitis virus disease cases have waned in recent decades, with the last human case in the United States reported in the 1990s. The reasons for this decline in incidence are unclear; animal studies comparing strains isolated across several decades suggest this is not related to a decrease in the pathogen's virulence.[98] Genetic sequencing analyses suggest reduction in the number of lineages in circulation.[99] Mutagenesis studies suggest the presence of a particular glycoprotein mutation that is necessary for mosquito infectivity is also associated with decreased virulence in vertebrates.[100]

Most cases of human infection are asymptomatic or very mild. For symptomatic cases, after an incubation period of about 1 week, initial symptoms include a prodrome of stiff neck, headache, backache, and vomiting. Restlessness, irritability, and neurologic sequelae such as seizures are more common in children. The development of neurologic symptoms and severity of disease is increased in children, as is the frequency of neurologic and psychiatric sequelae.[78]

Viruses Causing Polyarthralgia

Ross River Virus Infection

Ross River virus is a single-stranded, enveloped virus, among the Old World viruses in the genus *Alphavirus*, family *Togaviridae*. Ross River virus causes epidemic polyarthritis and is distributed across Australia and the western South Pacific.[101] Infection is most common in spring and summer, and outbreaks have occurred in diverse ecological settings from tropical to arid environments. Principal rural vectors include *Ochlerotatus camptorhynchus* and *O. vigilax* in coastal regions, *C. annulirostris* in inland and coastal areas, and *A. notoscriptus*, a container-inhabiting species, in urban areas.[102] The main amplifying vertebrate hosts appear to be marsupials, notably kangaroos and wallabies, and perhaps possums and horses. Humans may play a minor role in low-level viral amplification and introduction into new geographic areas. In Australia over the past decade, an average of 5400 cases were reported annually.[101]

The predominant clinical manifestation of severe joint pain occurs after a 7- to 11-day incubation period. A sparse maculopapular rash may occur in 50% of patients. Constitutional symptoms, including fever, are not prominent and only reported in half of cases. Rheumatologic symptoms involve the wrist, ankle, metacarpalphalangeal, interphalangeal, and knee joints.[33] Joint involvement is symmetric although severity of inflammation may be asymmetric. Periarticular swelling and tenosynovitis are common; a third of patients will have true arthritis. Joint symptoms often persist for months.[103]

Sindbis Virus

Sindbis virus is a single-stranded, enveloped virus, among the Old World viruses in the genus *Alphavirus*, family *Togaviridae*. It was initially identified in mosquitoes in Egypt, and diagnosed as the cause of human febrile illness in Uganda.[104] Sindbis outbreaks involving hundreds of cases have subsequently been reported in Europe, Africa, Asia, and Oceania. The terminology for the clinical disease produced differs depending on the region of occurrence, referred to in Sweden as Ockelbo disease, in Finland as Pogosta disease, and in Russia as Karelian fever. The virus is maintained through an avian-*Culex* mosquito transmission cycle. Humans are dead-end hosts.

Symptomatic patients present with sudden onset of fever and maculopapular rash, which is often pruritic.[105] Papules, which sometimes vesiculate over pressure points, have also been described. Patients complain of pain in the small joints of hands and feet, as well as frequent involvement of the larger joints of arms and legs. Joint pain may persist for months, and possibly years in some patients.

Mayaro Virus

Mayaro virus is a single-stranded, enveloped virus in the genus *Alphavirus*, family *Togaviridae*. Since its discovery in Trinidad, cases have been reported in several South American countries.[106,107] More recently, the report of a case of laboratory-confirmed acute Mayaro virus infection in a child in Haiti suggests that distribution may extend into the Caribbean.[108] The virus is maintained in a cycle between *Haemagogus* species mosquitoes and nonhuman primates.

Clinical manifestations are typically of a nonfatal, dengue-like illness with fever, chills, headache, eye pain, generalized myalgia, arthralgia, diarrhea, vomiting, and rash lasting several days to a week. Most patients recover from their acute illness but a substantial proportion may have prolonged arthralgia.[107]

TREATMENT, PREVENTION, AND CONTROL

Treatment

There is no specific treatment for infection with any of the arboviruses mentioned. Management is supportive and directed at the predominant clinical features. In the acute phase, fever and pain can be managed with analgesics and nonsteroidal anti-inflammatory medications; however, if the patient may have dengue, nonsteroidal drugs should be avoided until dengue virus infection is ruled out. For patients with arboviral encephalitis, attention should be given to possible complications of recurrent seizures, cerebral edema, and SIADH. Long-term neurologic and psychiatric sequelae may occur and require continued monitoring and supportive care. Patients with prolonged joint pains following infection with arthritogenic alphaviruses may need continued rheumatological care.

Prevention and Control

Personal Protective Methods

Personal protective measures include various strategies for arthropod vector avoidance and bite prevention.[109] Interventions include use of Environmental Protection Agency-approved insecticides and repellents, avoidance of exposure to arthropods at peak times of vector feeding, wearing appropriate clothing to cover exposed skin, performing checks for tick attachment, and use of bednets. In addition, persons at risk for infection should be educated to recognize signs and symptoms of arboviral diseases.

Effective human vaccines have been developed for a limited number of arbovirus infections and several are undergoing preliminary trials. One Japanese encephalitis vaccine, an inactivated Vero cell culture-derived vaccine (Ixiaro), is licensed and available in the United States for use in travelers aged $\geq$2 months.[110] The CDC Advisory Committee on Immunization Practices recommends use of this vaccine for some travelers to Asia depending on their planned itinerary, including travel location, duration, activities, and seasonal patterns of disease in the areas to be visited.[64] Other inactivated and live attenuated Japanese encephalitis vaccines are manufactured and used in other countries but are not licensed for use in the United States. Inactivated tick-borne encephalitis vaccines are available in Europe and Russia. In some endemic regions, routine population based vaccination is employed. Tick-borne encephalitis virus vaccines are not available in the United States. Travelers anticipating high-risk exposures in tick-borne virus-endemic areas (e.g., living, working, or recreating in forested areas) for an extended period of time, may wish to be vaccinated in Europe.[111] Candidate West Nile virus vaccines are being evaluated, but none are licensed for use in humans.

Several veterinary arboviral vaccines are available, particularly for arboviruses causing neuroinvasive disease in horses (i.e., West Nile and equine encephalitis viruses). These vaccines have been used successfully in equines in areas at high risk for infection.

Community Based Control Interventions

Surveillance for human disease cases and nonhuman arboviral activity should guide public health efforts to prevent or mitigate outbreaks.[11] This is best achieved through integrated vector management programs in conjunction with education of healthcare providers and the public about personal protective measures and disease recognition.[112]

Mosquitoes are generally more amenable to vector control interventions than other arthropod vectors. Comprehensive programs include source reduction, control of mosquito larvae, control of adult mosquitoes, and community education. Source reduction involves the elimination or reduction of mosquito larval breeding habitats. Methods of source reduction include education of property owners on how to identify and eliminate reservoirs of standing water, regional water management programs, and sanitation projects. Effective elimination or reduction in breeding habitats can substantially reduce mosquito population densities and help to reduce the need for insecticides.

While source reduction is the least invasive method to reduce mosquito breeding sites and larval development, this is not always feasible or successful and it may be necessary to employ larval control methods, including application of chemical pesticides or use of biological controls (e.g., *Bacillus thuringiensis* or lavivorous fish).[113] Applications can be limited to known mosquito breeding habitats or vector species, and are therefore more target-specific. Larval mosquito control is used to manage mosquito populations before they emerge as adults and can be effective when larval habitats are readily accessible. However, larval control alone is not able to stop outbreaks once virus amplification has reached levels causing human infections.

Adult mosquito control is needed to the reduce numbers of mosquitoes laying eggs, and the presence of infected adults that may bite humans. It should be added to larval control when surveillance indicates adult mosquito population pose a health risk to communities. Pesticide selection and timing of application are based on the specific distribution and behaviors of the target mosquito species. These can be applied from hand-held application devices, or from trucks or aircraft. Hand-held or truck-based applications are useful to manage relatively small areas, but are limited in their capacity to treat large areas quickly during an outbreak. In addition, gaps in coverage may occur during truck-based applications due to limitations of the road infrastructure. Aerial application of mosquito control adulticides is required when large areas must be treated quickly.

Chemical control methods should be integrated with a resistance management program to prevent or delay the development of insecticide resistance in vector populations.[114] Resistance management requires annual monitoring of target populations to track resistance patterns. These data facilitate the use of appropriate insecticides at the lowest effective concentrations.

For arboviruses implicated in transfusion or transplant transmission of infection, interventions depend on disease prevalence and utility of screening procedures. Blood donations in several West Nile virus endemic countries are routinely screened for West Nile virus RNA. Transmission of Colorado tick fever, Ross River, and Japanese encephalitis virus through blood transfusion has been documented but there is no donor screening for these infections; persons who have been infected should be deferred from blood donation for the maximum estimated period of transmissibility (usually 4–6 months, depending on the virus). Similarly, there is no routine laboratory screening for West Nile virus and eastern equine encephalitis in organ donors, although clinicians are advised to consider the presence of neuroinvasive pathogens when there is a history of neurologic illness at the time of death.

SUMMARY

More than 100 arboviruses are known to cause human disease. These viruses are primarily transmitted by mosquitoes and ticks, and a small subset of them are significant causes of morbidity and mortality in pathogen-specific geographic distributions across the globe. The epidemiology and clinical manifestations of arboviruses depend on complex interactions between the virus, vectors, animal hosts, and ecologic conditions. Several of these viruses have been recently identified or are increasing in incidence or geographic distribution. There is no specific treatment for any arboviral infection and vaccines are available for only a few; the mainstay of disease prevention remains reduction of infective vector bites through adherence to personal protective measures and vector control.

References

1. Brés P. Impact of arboviruses on human and animal health. In: Monath TP, ed. *The Arboviruses: Epidemiology and Ecology*. Vol. 1. Boca Raton, FL: CRC Press; 1988:1–18.
2. Center for Diseases Control and Prevention. Arbovirus Catalogue. https://wwwn.cdc.gov/arbocat/. Accessed May 15, 2018.
3. Weaver SC, Reisen WK. Present and future arboviral threats. *Antiviral Res*. 2010;85(2):328–45.
4. Calisher CH. Medically important arboviruses of the United States and Canada. *Clin Microbiol Rev*. 1994;7:89–116.

5. Weaver SC. Host range, amplification and arboviral disease emergence. *Arch Virol Suppl.* 2005;19:33–44.
6. Vitek CJ, Gutierrez JA, Dirrigl FJ Jr. Dengue vectors, human activity, and dengue virus transmission potential in the lower Rio Grande Valley, Texas, United States. *J Med Entomol.* 2014;51(5):1019–28.
7. Lindsey NP, Staples JE, Fischer M. Eastern equine encephalitis virus in the United States, 2003–2016. *Am J Trop Med Hyg.* 2018;98(5):1472–7.
8. Hardy, JL, Houk FJ, Kramer LD, et al. Intrinsic factors affecting vector competence of mosquitoes for arboviruses. *Annu Rev Entomol.* 1983;28:229–62.
9. Reisen WK, Fang Y, Martinez VM. Effects of temperature on the transmission of West Nile virus by *Culex tarsalis* (Diptera: Culicidae). *J Med Entomol.* 2006;43(2):309–17.
10. Reisen WK, Hardy JL, Presser SB, et al. Seasonal variation in the vector competence of *Culex tarsalis* (Diptera: Culicidae) from the Coachella Valley of California for western equine encephalomyelitis and St. Louis encephalitis viruses. *J Med Entomol.* 1996;33(3):433–7.
11. Centers for Disease Control and Prevention. West Nile virus in the United States: Guidelines for surveillance, prevention, and control. Revised 2013. https://www.cdc.gov/westnile/resources/pdfs/wnvGuidelines.pdf. Accessed May 15, 2018.
12. Kazimírová M, Thangamani S, Bartíková P, et al. Tick-borne viruses and biological processes at the tick-host-virus interface. *Front Cell Infect Microbiol.* 2017;7:339.
13. Kuno G, Chang GJ. Biological transmission of arboviruses: Reexamination of and new insights into components, mechanisms, and unique traits as well as their evolutionary trends. *Clin Microbiol Rev.* 2005;18(4):608–37.
14. van der Meulen KM, Pensaert MB, Nauwynck HJ. West Nile virus in the vertebrate world: Brief review. *Arch Virol.* 2005;150:637–57.
15. Ahlers LRH, Goodman AG. The immune responses of the animal hosts of West Nile virus: A comparison of insects, birds, and mammals. *Front Cell Infect Microbiol.* 2018;8:96.
16. Eidson M, Komar N, Sorhage F, et al. Crow deaths as a sentinel surveillance system for West Nile virus in the northeastern United States, 1999. *Emerg Infect Dis.* 2001;7(4):615–20.
17. Gubler DJ, Reiter P, Ebi KL, et al. Climate variability and change in the United States: Potential impacts on vector- and rodent-borne diseases. *Environ Health Perspect.* 2001;109(Suppl 2):223–33.
18. Yamada M, Nakamura K, Yoshi M, Kaku Y. Nonsuppurative encephalitis in piglets after experimental inoculation of Japanese encephalitis flavivirus isolated from pigs. *Vet Pathol.* 2004;41:62–7.
19. Rosen L. Overwintering mechanisms of mosquito-borne arboviruses in temperate climates. *Am J Trop Med Hyg.* 1987;37:69S–76S.
20. Kuno G, Mackenzie JS, Junglen S, et al. Vertebrate reservoirs of arboviruses: Myth, synonym of amplifier, or reality? *Viruses.* 2017;9(7):185.
21. Miller BR, DeFoliart GR, Yuill TM. Vertical transmission of La Crosse virus (California encephalitis group): Transovarial and filial infection rates in *Aedes triseriatus* (Diptera: Culicidae). *J Med Entomol.* 1977;14(4):437–40.
22. Sellers RF, Maarouf AR. Weather factors in the prediction of western equine encephalitis epidemics in Manitoba. *Epidemiol Infect.* 1993;111(2):373–90.
23. Council of State and Territorial Epidemiologists. Arboviral diseases, neuroinvasive and non-neuroinvasive. 2015 case definition. https://wwwn.cdc.gov/nndss/conditions/arboviral-diseases-neuroinvasive-and-non-neuroinvasive/case-definition/2015/. Accessed May 15, 2018.
24. Lindsey NP, Brown JA, Kightlinger L, et al. State health department perceived utility of and satisfaction with ArboNET, the U.S. national arboviral surveillance system. *Public Health Rep.* 2012;127(4):383–90.
25. Calisher CH, Pretzman CI, Muth DJ, et al. Serodiagnosis of La Crosse virus infections in humans by detection of immunoglobulin M class antibodies. *J Clin Microbiol.* 1986;23(4):667–71.
26. Martin DA, Biggerstaff BJ, Allen B, et al. Use of immunoglobulin m cross-reactions in differential diagnosis of human flaviviral encephalitis infections in the United States. *Clin Diagn Lab Immunol.* 2002;9(3):544–9.
27. Roehrig JT, Nash D, Maldin B, et al. Persistence of virus-reactive serum immunoglobulin m antibody in confirmed West Nile virus encephalitis cases. *Emerg Infect Dis.* 2003;9(3):376–9.
28. Kapoor H, Signs K, Somsel P, et al. Persistence of West Nile Virus (WNV) IgM antibodies in cerebrospinal fluid from patients with CNS disease. *J Clin Virol.* 2004;31(4):289–91.
29. Calisher CH, Karabatsos N, Dalrymple JM, et al. Antigenic relationships between flaviviruses as determined by cross-neutralization tests with polyclonal antisera. *J Gen Virol.* 1989;70:37–43.
30. Lambert AJ, Kosoy O, Velez JO, et al. Detection of Colorado tick fever viral RNA in acute human serum samples by a quantitative real-time RT-PCR assay. *J Virol Methods.* 2007;140(1-2):140–8.
31. Lanciotti RS. Molecular amplification assays for the detection of flaviviruses. *Adv Virus Res.* 2003;61:67–99.
32. Beckham JD, Tyler KL. Arbovirus infections. *Continuum (Minneap Minn).* 2015;21(6 Neuroinfectious Disease):1599–611.
33. Suhrbier A, Jaffar-Bandjee MC, Gasque P. Arthritogenic alphaviruses—An overview. *Nat Rev Rheumatol.* 2012;8(7):420–9.
34. Brackney MM, Marfin AA, Staples JE, et al. Epidemiology of Colorado tick fever in Montana, Utah, and Wyoming, 1995–2003. *Vector Borne Zoonotic Dis.* 2010;10:381–5.
35. Yendell SJ, Fischer M, Staples JE. Colorado tick fever in the United States, 2002–2012. *Vector Borne Zoonotic Dis.* 2015;15(5):311–6.
36. Centers for Disease Control and Prevention. Transmission of Colorado tick fever virus by blood transfusion—Montana. *MMWR Morb Mortal Wkly Rep.* 1975;24:422–7.
37. LeDuc JW, Hoch AL, Pinheiro FP, Travassos da Rosa APA. Epidemic Oropouche virus disease in northern Brazil. *Bull Pan Am Health Organ.* 1981;15(2):97–103.
38. Travassos da Rosa JF, de Souza WM, Pinheiro FP, et al. Oropouche virus: Clinical, epidemiological, and molecular aspects of a neglected orthobunyavirus. *Am J Trop Med Hyg.* 2017;96(5):1019–30.
39. Romero-Alvarez D, Escobar LE. Oropouche fever, an emergent disease from the Americas. *Microbes Infect.* 2018;20(3):135–46.
40. Pinheiro FP, Travassos da Rosa APA, Travassos da Rosa JFS, et al. Oropouche virus. I. A review of clinical, epidemiological, and ecological findings. *Am J Trop Med Hyg.* 1981;30:149–60.
41. Moriconi M, Rugna G, Calzolari M, et al. Phlebotomine sand fly-borne pathogens in the Mediterranean Basin: Human leishmaniasis and phlebovirus infections. *PLoS Negl Trop Dis.* 2017;11(8):e0005660.
42. Guler S, Guler E, Caglayik DY, et al. A sandfly fever virus outbreak in the East Mediterranean region of Turkey. *Int J Infect Dis.* 2012;16(4):e244–6.
43. Alkan C, Bichaud L, de Lamballerie X, et al. Sandfly-borne phleboviruses of Eurasia and Africa: Epidemiology, genetic diversity, geographic range, control measures. *Antiviral Res.* 2013;100(1):54–74.
44. McMullan LK, Folk SM, Kelly AJ, et al. A new phlebovirus associated with severe febrile illness in Missouri. *N Engl J Med.* 2012;367:834–41.
45. Pastula DM, Turabelidze G, Yates KF, et al. Heartland virus disease—United States, 2012–2013. *MMWR Morb Mortal Wkly Rep.* 2014;63:270–1.
46. Savage HM, Godsey MS Jr, Panella NA, et al. Surveillance for heartland virus (Bunyaviridae: Phlebovirus) in Missouri during 2013: First detection of virus in adults of *Amblyomma americanum* (Acari: Ixodidae). *J Med Entomol.* 2016;53(3):607–12.
47. Bosco-Lauth AM, Panella NA, Root JJ, et al. Serological investigation of heartland virus (Bunyaviridae: Phlebovirus) exposure in wild and domestic animals adjacent to human case sites in Missouri 2012–2013. *Am J Trop Med Hyg.* 2015;92:1163–7.
48. Lambert AJ, Velez JO, Brault AC, et al. Molecular, serological and *in vitro* culture-based characterization of Bourbon virus, a newly described human pathogen of the genus *Thogotovirus*. *J Clin Virol.* 2015;73:127–32.
49. Savage HM, Burkhalter KL, Godsey MS, et al. Bourbon virus in field-collected ticks, Missouri, USA. *Emerg Infect Dis.* 2017;23(12):2017–22.
50. Burakoff A, Lehman J, Fischer M, Staples JE, Lindsey NP. West Nile virus and other nationally notifiable arboviral diseases—United States, 2016. *MMWR Morb Mortal Wkly Rep.* 2018;67:13–7.
51. Reimann CA, Hayes EB, DiGuiseppi C, et al. Epidemiology of neuroinvasive arboviral disease in the United States, 1999–2007. *Am J Trop Med Hyg.* 2008;79:974–9.
52. Petersen LR, Brault AC, Nasci RS. West Nile virus: Review of the literature. *JAMA.* 2013;310(3):308–15.
53. Petersen LR, Carson PJ, Biggerstaff BJ, et al. Estimated cumulative incidence of West Nile virus infection in US adults, 1999–2010. *Epidemiol Infect.* 2013;141(3):591–5.
54. Zou S, Foster GA, Dodd RY, Petersen LR, Stramer SL. West Nile fever characteristics among viremic persons identified through blood donor screening. *J Infect Dis.* 2010;202(9):1354–61.
55. Lindsey NP, Staples JE, Lehman JA, Fischer M. Medical risk factors for severe West Nile Virus disease, United States, 2008–2010. *Am J Trop Med Hyg.* 2012;87(1):179–84.
56. Reisen WK. Epidemiology of St. Louis encephalitis virus. *Adv Virus Res.* 2003;61:139–83.

57. de Souza Lopes O, de Abreu Sacchetta L, Coimbra TL, Pinto GH, Glasser CM. Emergence of a new arbovirus disease in Brazil. II. Epidemiological studies on 1975 epidemic. *Am J Epidemiol.* 1978;108:394–401.
58. Venkat H, Krow-Lucal E, Hennessey M, et al. Concurrent outbreaks of St. Louis encephalitis virus and West Nile virus disease — Arizona, 2015. *MMWR Morb Mortal Wkly Rep.* 2015;64(48):1349–50.
59. Venkat H, Adams L, Sunenshine R, et al. St. Louis encephalitis virus possibly transmitted through blood transfusion — Arizona, 2015. *Transfusion.* 2017;57(12):2987–94.
60. Tsai TF, Mitchell CJ. St Louis encephalitis. In: Monath TP, ed. *The Arboviruses: Epidemiology and Ecology.* Vol. 4. Boca Raton, FL: CRC Press; 1988:113–44.
61. Endy TP, Nisalak A. Japanese encephalitis virus: Ecology and epidemiology. *Curr Top Microbiol Immunol.* 2002;267:11–48.
62. Ricklin ME, Garcìa-Nicolàs O, Brechbühl D, et al. Japanese encephalitis virus tropism in experimentally infected pigs. *Vet Res.* 2016;47:34.
63. Hills SL, Griggs AC, Fischer M. Japanese encephalitis in travelers from non-endemic countries, 1973–2008. *Am J Trop Med Hyg.* 2010;82:930–6.
64. Fischer M, Lindsey N, Staples JE, Hills S. Japanese encephalitis vaccines: Recommendations of the Advisory Committee on Immunization Practices (ACIP). *MMWR Recomm Rep.* 2010;59(RR-1):1–27.
65. Giabani P, Rossini G. An overview of Usutu virus. *Microbes Infect.* 2017;19:382–7.
66. Cadar D, Lühken R, van der Jeugd H, et al. Widespread activity of multiple lineages of Usutu virus, western Europe, 2016. *Euro Surveill.* 2017;22(4):30452.
67. Pecorari M, Longo G, Gennari W, et al. First human case of Usutu virus neuroinvasive infection, Italy, August–September 2009. *Euro Surveill.* 2009;14(50):19446.
68. Santini M, Vilibic-Cavlek T, Barsic B, et al. First cases of human Usutu virus neuroinvasive infection in Croatia, August–September 2013: Clinical and laboratory features. *J Neurovirol.* 2015;21(1):92–7.
69. Simonin Y, Sillam O, Carles MJ, et al. Human Usutu virus infection with atypical neurologic presentation, Montpellier, France, 2016. *Emerg Infect Dis.* 2018;24(5):875–8.
70. Hermance ME, Thangamani S. Powassan virus: An emerging arbovirus of public health concern in North America. *Vector Borne Zoonotic Dis.* 2017;17(7):453–62.
71. Dupuis AP, Peters RJ, Prusinski MA, et al. Isolation of deer tick virus (Powassan virus, lineage II) from *Ixodes scapularis* and detection of antibody in vertebrate hosts sampled in the Hudson Valley, New York State. *Parasit Vectors.* 2013;6:185.
72. Krow-Lucal ER, Lindsey NP, Fischer M, Hills SL. Powassan virus disease in the United States, 2006–2016. *Vector Borne Zoonotic Dis.* 2018;18(6):286–90.
73. Suss J. Tick-borne encephalitis 2010: Epidemiology, risk areas, and virus strains in Europe and Asia—An overview. *Ticks Tick Borne Dis.* 2011;2(1):2–15.
74. Centers for Disease Control and Prevention. Tick-borne encephalitis among US travelers to Europe and Asia—2000–2009. *MMWR Morb Mortal Wkly Rep.* 2010;59(11):335–8.
75. Labuda M, Danielova V, Jones LD, et al. Amplification of tick-borne encephalitis virus infection during co-feeding of ticks. *Med Vet Entomol.* 1993;7(4):339–42.
76. Gaensbauer JT, Lindsey NP, Messacar K, Staples JE, Fischer M. Neuroinvasive arboviral disease in the United States: 2003 to 2012. *Pediatrics.* 2014;134(3):e642–50.
77. Centers for Disease Control and Prevention. La Crosse encephalitis: Epidemiology & geographic distribution. https://www.cdc.gov/lac/tech/epi.html. Accessed January 30, 2018.
78. McJunkin JE, Khan RR, Tsai TF. California-La Crosse encephalitis. *Infect Dis Clin North Am.* 1998;12(1):83–93.
79. Centers for Disease Control and Prevention. Human Jamestown Canyon virus infection—Montana, 2009. *MMWR Morb Mortal Wkly Rep.* 2011;60:652–5.
80. Pastula DM, Hoang Johnson DK, White JL, et al. Jamestown Canyon virus disease in the United States—2000–2013. *Am J Trop Med Hyg.* 2015;93(2):384–9.
81. Patriquin G, Drebot M, Cole T, et al. High seroprevalence of Jamestown Canyon virus among deer and humans, Nova Scotia, Canada. *Emerg Infect Dis.* 2018;24(1):118–21.
82. Kulkarni MA, Berrang-Ford L, Buck PA, et al. Major emerging vector-borne zoonotic diseases of public health importance in Canada. *Emerg Microbes Infect.* 2015;4:e33.
83. Calisher CH, Francy DB, Smith GC, et al. Distribution of Bunyamwera serogroup viruses in North America, 1956–1984. *Am J Trop Med Hyg.* 1986;35:429–43.
84. Mangiafico JA, Sanchez JL, Figueiredo LT, et al. Isolation of a newly recognized Bunyamwera serogroup virus from a febrile human in Panama. *Am J Trop Med Hyg.* 1988;39(6):593–6.
85. Sexton DJ, Rollin PE, Breitschwerdt EB, et al. Life-threatening Cache Valley virus infection. *N Engl J Med.* 1997;336:547–9.
86. Campbell GL, Mataczynski JD, Reisdorf ES, et al. Second human case of Cache Valley virus disease. *Emerg Infect Dis.* 2006;12(5):854–6.
87. Wilson MR, Suan D, Duggins A, et al. A novel cause of chronic viral meningoencephalitis: Cache Valley virus. *Ann Neurol.* 2017;82(1):105–14.
88. Dupouey J, Bichaud L, Ninove L, et al. Toscana virus infections: A case series from France. *J Infect.* 2014;68(3):290–5.
89. Powers AM, Brault AC, Shirako Y, et al. Evolutionary relationships and systematics of the alphaviruses. *J Virol.* 2001;75(21):10118–31.
90. Morris CD. Eastern equine encephalitis. In: Monath TP, ed. *The Arboviruses: Epidemiology and Ecology.* Vol. 3. Boca Raton, FL: CRC Press; 1988:1–20.
91. Molaei G, Armstrong PM, Abadam CF, Akaratovic KI, Kiser JP, Andreadis TG. Vector-host interactions of *Culiseta melanura* in a focus of eastern equine encephalitis virus activity in southeastern Virginia. *PLoS One.* 2015;10(9):e0136743.
92. Arrigo NC, Adams AP, Weaver SC. Evolutionary patterns of eastern equine encephalitis virus in North versus South America suggest ecological differences and taxonomic revision. *J Virol.* 2010;84(2):1014–25.
93. Bingham AM, Burkett-Cadena ND, Hassan HK, et al. Field investigations of winter transmission of eastern equine encephalitis virus in Florida. *Am J Trop Med Hyg.* 2014;91(4):685–93.
94. Pouch SM, Katugaha SB, Shieh W, et al. Transmission of eastern equine encephalitis virus from an organ donor to three transplant recipients. *Clin Infect Dis.* 2019;69(3):450–8.
95. Kubes V, Ríos FA. The causative agent of infectious equine encephalomyelitis in Venezuela. *Science.* 1939;90(2323):20–1.
96. Ronca SE, Dineley KT, Paessler S. Neurological sequelae resulting from encephalitic alphavirus infection. *Front Microbiol.* 2016;7:959.
97. Weaver SC, Kang W, Shirako Y, et al. Recombinational history and molecular evolution of western equine encephalomyelitis complex alphaviruses. *J Virol.* 1997;71(1):613–23.
98. Forrester NL, Kenney JL, Deardorff E, Wang E, Weaver SC. Western equine encephalitis submergence: Lack of evidence for a decline in virus virulence. *Virology.* 2008;380(2):170–2.
99. Bergren NA, Auguste AJ, Forrester NL, Negi SS, Braun WA, Weaver SC. Western equine encephalitis virus: Evolutionary analysis of a declining alphavirus based on complete genome sequences. *J Virol.* 2014;88(16):9260–7.
100. Mossel EC, Ledermann JP, Phillips AT, et al. Molecular determinants of mouse neurovirulence and mosquito infection for Western equine encephalitis virus. *PLoS One.* 2013;8(3):e60427.
101. Mackenzie JS, Lindsay MDA, Smith DW, Imrie A. The ecology and epidemiology of Ross River and Murray Valley encephalitis viruses in Western Australia: Examples of one health in action. *Trans R Soc Trop Med Hyg.* 2017;111(6):248–54.
102. Claflin SB, Webb CE. Ross River virus: Many vectors and unusual hosts make for an unpredictable pathogen. *PLoS Pathog.* 2015;11(9):e1005070.
103. Condon RJ, Rouse IL, et al. Acute symptoms and sequelae of Ross River virus infection in South-Western Australia: A follow-up study. *Clin Diagn Virol.* 1995;3(3):273–84.
104. Niklasson B. Sindbis and Sindbis-like viruses. In: Monath TP, ed. *The Arboviruses: Epidemiology and Ecology.* Vol. 4. Boca Raton, FL: CRC Press; 1988:1–20.
105. Laine M, Luukkainen R, Toivanen A. Sindbis viruses and other alphaviruses as cause of human arthritic disease. *J Intern Med.* 2004;256(6):457–71.
106. Tesh RB, Watts DM, Russell KL, et al. Mayaro virus disease: An emerging mosquito-borne zoonosis in tropical South America. *Clin Infect Dis.* 1999;28:67–73.
107. Halsey ES, Siles C, Guevara C, et al. Mayaro virus infection, Amazon Basin region, Peru, 2010–2013. *Emerg Infect Dis.* 2013;19(11):1839–42.
108. Lednicky J, De Rochars V, Elbadry M, et al. Mayaro virus in child with acute febrile illness, Haiti, 2015. *Emerg Infect Dis.* 2016;22(11):2000–2.
109. Mutebi JP, Hawley WA, Brogdon WG. Protection against mosquitoes, ticks, and other arthropods. In: *Health Information for International*

Travel. CDC. 2018. https://wwwnc.cdc.gov/travel/yellowbook/2018/the-pre-travel-consultation/protection-against-mosquitoes-ticks-other-arthropods.

110. Centers for Disease Control and Prevention. Use of Japanese encephalitis vaccine in children: Recommendations of the advisory committee on immunization practices, 2013. *MMWR Morb Mortal Wkly Rep.* 2013;62(45):898–900.
111. Fischer M, Rabe I, Rollin P. Tickborne encephalitis. In: *Health Information for International Travel.* CDC. 2018. https://wwwnc.cdc.gov/travel/yellowbook/2018/infectious-diseases-related-to-travel/tickborne-encephalitis. Accessed May 15, 2018.
112. World Health Organization. *Handbook for Integrated Vector Management.* Geneva: World Health Organization; 2012. http://apps.who.int/iris/bitstream/handle/10665/44768/9789241502801_eng.pdf;sequence=1.
113. Rose RI. Pesticides and public health: Integrated methods of mosquito management. *Emerg Infect Dis.* 2001;7(1):17–23.
114. Liu N.Insecticide resistance in mosquitoes: Impact, mechanisms, and research directions. *Annu Rev Entomol.* 2015;60:537–59.

CHAPTER

143

Lyme Disease and Other Borrelia Infections

Stefanie Campbell • Alison Hinckley

INTRODUCTION

Lyme disease (also called Lyme borreliosis) is the most common illness resulting from infection with spirochetes of the *Borrelia* genus.[1,2] Lyme disease predominantly occurs in North America and Europe following the bite of infected *Ixodes* spp. (hard-bodied) ticks. *B. miyamotoi* is a recently recognized pathogen that causes a relapsing fever illness and is also transmitted by *Ixodes* ticks.[3] Given the common vector, disease resulting from this infection likely occurs in the same geographic regions as Lyme disease.[4] Tick-borne relapsing fever (TBRF) and louse-borne relapsing fever (LBRF) are caused by infection with several species from the relapsing fever group of *Borrelia*. Whereas TBRF is endemic on most continents and most often follows the bite of infected *Ornithodoros spp.* (soft-bodied) ticks, LBRF occurs only in the Horn of Africa and is transmitted by lice (*Pediculus humanus*).[5] Patients who are ill due to these *Borrelia* infections most often present with acute fever (without typical symptoms of viral respiratory infection or gastroenteritis), and possibly skin rash. Southern Tick-Associated Rash Illness (STARI) is clinically similar to early Lyme disease, but occurs after the bite of a lone star tick.[6] Knowledge regarding geographic location and possibility of exposure to potential vectors, as well as certain risk factors, can inform the differential diagnosis. Methods for prevention of these diseases vary according to the vector of transmission.

LYME DISEASE

Lyme disease is the most commonly reported vector-borne disease in the United States and Europe and is caused by specific genospecies in the *B. burgdorferi* sensu lato complex.[1,2,7] In the United States, it is a considerable public health problem in the upper Midwest, northeast, and mid-Atlantic regions. The distribution of reported cases has expanded significantly in these geographic regions and the incidence of human cases continues to rise in both new and established foci of infection.[8,9] It is transmitted throughout the northern hemisphere by *Ixodes spp.* ticks. The ecology and epidemiology of Lyme disease are complex, and practical methods for prevention and control on a large scale are currently lacking.

AGENT

Borreliae are flexible helical cells comprised of a protoplasmic cylinder surrounded by a cell membrane, periplasmic flagella, and an outer membrane that is loosely associated with the underlying structures.[10] A number of genospecies have been described among the *B. burgdorferi* sensu lato complex. The primary genospecies infecting humans and causing Lyme disease in the United States is *B. burgdorferi* sensu stricto (hereafter referred to as *B. burgdorferi*). Recently, the genetically distinct *B. mayonii* has also been found to cause Lyme disease, with a small number of people affected in the upper Midwestern United States.[11] The dominant genospecies in Europe and Asia are *B. garinii* and *B. afzelii*; although, *B. burgdorferi* also contributes to the overall incidence of Lyme borreliosis.[11,12] While all four species typically cause the same initial disease expression, manifesting with fever and skin lesion or erythema migrans (EM) at the location of the tick bite, they appear to have somewhat different disease courses. Arthritis occurs more frequently following infection with *B. burgdorferi*; neurologic manifestations are more common with *B. garinii* infection; and cutaneous manifestations occur more frequently with *B. afzelii* infection.[13] Very little is known about any unique clinical manifestations associated with *B. mayonii* infections.[11]

TRANSMISSION

Lyme disease is transmitted to humans through the saliva of an attached feeding tick. *I. scapularis* (also known as the black-legged tick) is the principal vector of *B. burgdorferi* in the northeast, mid-Atlantic, and upper Midwest United States. It is also known to transmit *B. mayonii* in the upper Midwest.[11] *I. scapularis* ticks also transmit other tick-borne pathogens including *Babesia microti*, the causative agent of babesiosis, *Anaplasma phagocytophilum*, the causative agent of anaplasmosis, *Ehrlichia muris* eauclairensis, one of the causes of ehrlichiosis, and Powassan virus.[14] The geographic range of *I. scapularis* extends into some southern states, where Lyme disease is uncommon. In these areas, however, the risk to humans is low because *I. scapularis* has a low *B. burgdorferi* infection rate and rarely feeds on humans.[15,16] *I. pacificus* is the principal vector of *B. burgdorferi* in the western United States and British Columbia, Canada.[17] *I. ricinus* is the primary vector in western and central Europe extending into parts of Asia and, *I. persulcatus* is the main vector in central and eastern Russia, China, and Japan.[15,18]

Transmission of *B. burgdorferi* occurs most commonly through the bite of juvenile (nymphal) ticks. Due to their smaller size, nymphs more often escape detection, which may allow for the extended feeding time (36–48 hours) necessary for transmission to occur.[19] Infection rates in nymphal ticks vary by region. Nymphal infection rates with *B. burgdorferi* have been found to be $> 23\%$ in New York and $> 13\%$ in northern California.[20,21]

In humans, transplacental transmission of *B. burgdorferi* has been reported, although this has not been demonstrated as a definitive cause of adverse outcomes (including intrauterine death or congenital malformation).[22–24] In addition, no serious effects on the fetus have been found in cases where the mother receives appropriate antibiotic treatment for Lyme disease. In general, treatment for pregnant women with Lyme disease is similar to that of nonpregnant adults. Certain antibiotics, such as doxycycline, are not recommended because they can affect fetal development. [25] Laboratory-adapted strains of *B. burgdorferi* have been shown to survive in blood that is stored for donation, however, no human infections with naturally occurring strains have been documented as being acquired through transfusions.[26] Similarly, there is no evidence that *B. burgdorferi* can be transmitted through sexual contact or breast milk.[27]

LIFE CYCLE AND VERTEBRATE HOSTS

The life cycle of the *Ixodes* tick spans a 2- or 3-year period (Fig. 143-1). The basic elements involved in this cycle in North America include three stages of the tick (larva, nymph, adult), each of which typically takes one blood meal, and several reservoir hosts. Larvae and nymphal ticks have a wide host range including rodents, insectivores, birds, lagomorphs, and ungulates. In the endemic northeastern United States, the white-footed mouse (*Peromyscus leucopus*), serves as the preferred vertebrate host for the immature stages of the tick vector, and is the most competent vertebrate reservoir of *B. burgdorferi*, typically with infection rates of up to 75%.[28] The chipmunk is also a competent reservoir host in the eastern United States and may be more important than the white-footed mouse in maintaining cycles of infection in the upper Midwest region.[29] In addition, several bird species serve as maintenance hosts for vector ticks, and some, such as robins, may serve as lesser reservoir hosts of *B. burgdorferi*.[30] Lizards are not competent reservoirs for *B. burgdorferi*, and thus act as zooprophylactic hosts.[31] This may explain low infection rates of *Ixodes* vectors in the southern and western regions of the United States where ticks preferentially feed on lizards.

Adult ticks prefer medium to large size mammals, particularly white-tailed deer. Deer have an essential role in the enzootic cycle of Lyme disease in North America, acting as the principal host for adult *Ixodes spp.* ticks.[14,32] However, deer do not appear to be an important reservoir for *B. burgdorferi* as cervid serum has borreliacidal properties.[33]

Larvae most frequently feed in the summer from July through September, and nymphs typically feed from May to July. This reversed feeding pattern aids in the transmission of pathogens, such as *B. burgdorferi*, since nymphs feeding in the spring may infect rodents that later in the year will serve as a source of infection for the larvae. Adult females feed mainly during the fall, but can also feed throughout winter and early spring. Transstadial transmission of *B. burgdorferi* from larva to nymph to adult helps maintain the infective cycle. Transovarial transmission of *B. burgdorferi* from an infected female adult tick to her eggs, while previously reported in the literature, likely does not occur.[34,35]

In Eurasia, the cycle is similar, although the bank vole (*Clethrionomys glareolus*) and wood mouse (*Apodemus sp.*) serve as principal rodent reservoirs of infection, and the roe deer and other cervids typically serve as maintenance hosts for vector ticks.[36]

GEOGRAPHIC DISTRIBUTION

In the United States, the highest incidence of Lyme disease is in the upper Midwest, northeast, and mid-Atlantic states. When cases occur outside of these states, there is often a travel history to a high incidence area. Outside of the United States, Lyme disease occurs in Southern Canada, the British Isles, Scandinavia, other parts of Europe, and Asia. The incidence of the disease in Europe is greatest in the central and northeast regions.[15] It has also been reported from northeast China and eastern regions of Japan.[37]

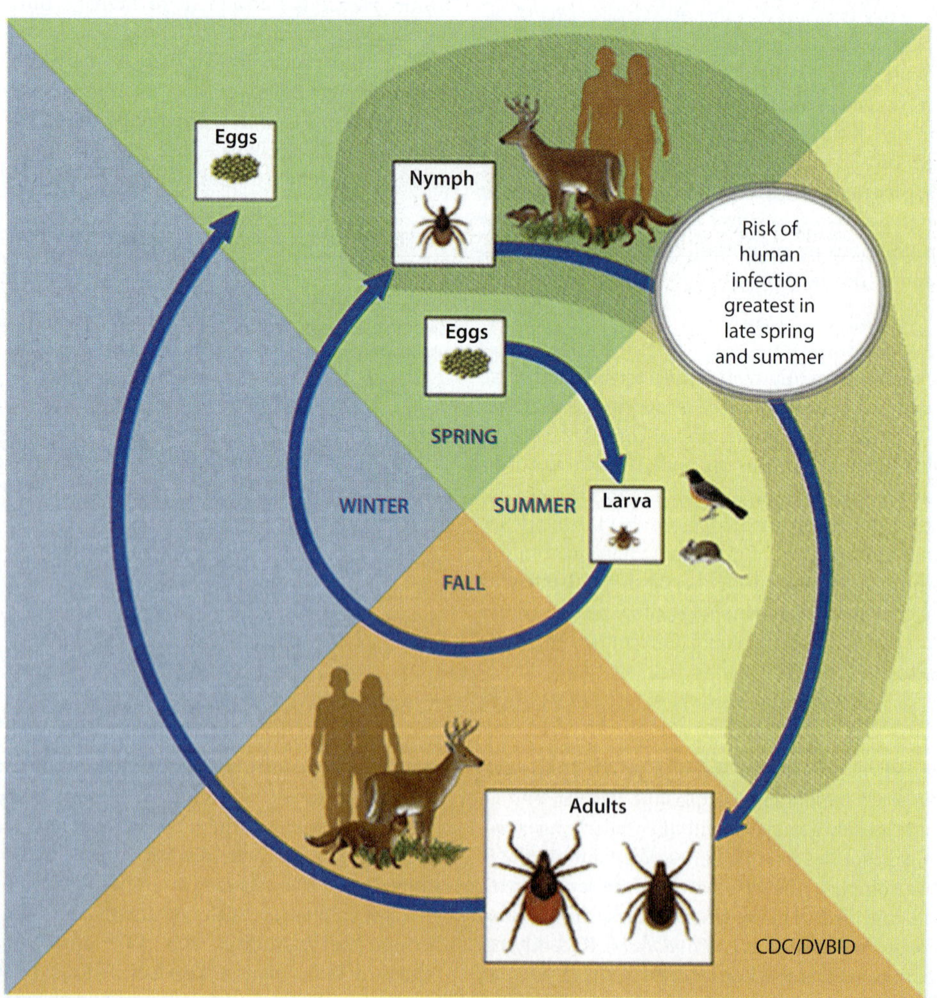

FIGURE 143-1. This diagram shows the life cycle of black-legged ticks that can transmit anaplasmosis, babesiosis, and Lyme disease.

CLINICAL MANIFESTATIONS

Lyme disease morbidity is variable, ranging from inapparent or mild illness to severe, chronic, and disabling, especially if the disease is not treated in its early stages. Lyme disease is rarely a cause of death.[38] In general, signs and symptoms of Lyme disease can be classified as early (3–30 days after tick bite) or late (days to months after tick bite) and localized or disseminated.[39]

Early localized: EM rash occurs early and begins at the site of the tick bite in approximately 80% of cases in the United States.[40,41] The rash expands gradually over a period of days, is annular, and may feel warm to the touch. In many cases, the rash is accompanied by constitutional symptoms including fever, headache, myalgia, arthralgia, and occasionally by regional lymphadenopathy. The portal of entry for *B. burgdorferi* is the dermis and the spirochete will live primarily as an extracellular pathogen.[42] Following inoculation, infection spreads by cutaneous, lymphatic, and hematogenous routes.

Early disseminated: Early disseminated infection usually occurs within days to weeks after the onset of localized infection. The skin, nervous system, musculoskeletal system, and heart may be affected. Lyme neuroborreliosis patients manifest with neurologic signs and symptoms, most commonly aseptic (lymphocytic) meningitis, cranial neuropathy, or radiculoneuritis. Many patients also describe migratory musculoskeletal pains in joints, bursae, tendon, muscle, or bone. Persons with early disseminated Lyme disease may also develop cardiac conduction abnormalities. Although typically mild, Lyme carditis has been associated with sudden cardiac death following third-degree atrioventricular conduction block.[39,43]

Late disseminated: Manifestations of late disseminated disease occur weeks to months after infection in some untreated patients. The most common late-stage manifestation in the United States is arthritis in one or a few joints; usually large, weight-bearing joints, such as the knee. Lyme arthritis usually resolves following appropriate antimicrobial therapy.[44] In Europe, arthritis can occur in some cases but a skin lesion, acrodermatitis chronica atrophicans, is a more common sequelae associated with *B. afzelii*. The lesion is described as slow and progressive affecting the extensor surfaces of extremities.[39]

Following antibiotic therapy, some patients may experience postinfectious signs or symptoms including fatigue, pain, joint, and muscle aches. Antibiotic-refractory Lyme arthritis is the only well-characterized postinfectious manifestation that can persist, despite apparent spirochetal killing following antimicrobials.[45] Chronic Lyme disease is a term that has been used to describe patients with unexplained symptoms or patients without objective evidence of current or past *Borrelia* infection.[46,47]

The rate of asymptomatic seroconversion, indicating exposure to *B. burgdorferi* without illness, has been reported as 11%.[48] Infection does not confer lasting protective immunity, and more than one occurrence of Lyme disease is possible, particularly among persons at high environmental risk.[49] Given the potential for *Ixodes* ticks to harbor multiple pathogens, concurrent infections are also possible. Coinfection with *B. burgdorferi* and *B. microti* (the agent of babesiosis) has been associated with a severity and duration of illness greater than expected for either infection alone.[50]

DIAGNOSIS

A diagnosis of Lyme disease can be made based on clinical signs (EM rash) and exposure history to potential tick habitats in high-incidence areas.[51] As mentioned previously, the STARI rash can be indistinguishable from the EM rash of Lyme disease. In southern and southeast areas of the United States where Lyme disease is rare, patients who present with a bull's-eye rash and no travel history would be more likely to have STARI.[6]

Serodiagnostic testing may be indicated for patients with clinical signs typical of Lyme disease and a likely exposure history. The recommended test protocol utilizes a two-tier testing approach with a sensitive first test, either enzyme-linked immunosorbent assay or indirect fluorescent antibody testing, followed by Western immunoblotting (WB) of serum specimens found to be equivocal or positive in the first test. Negative specimens do not require further testing. Specific WB banding criteria have been recommended for detection of IgM and IgG antibodies.[52] IgM antibodies typically appear within the first several weeks after exposure, and this response may persist for months or years. IgG antibodies can be detected in most patients within 1 month of active infection, and likewise may persist for years after treatment and after symptoms have resolved.[15,53] In patients with illness that has lasted longer than 1 month, a positive IgM and negative IgG is suggestive of a false positive IgM result.[54] There is currently no test to indicate a resolution of disease or cure.[55,56]

An important consideration in Lyme disease diagnostics is the predictive value of both clinical signs and laboratory testing. The likelihood of Lyme disease will be associated with regional disease prevalence (high or low incidence). In a high-incidence setting, the predictive value of clinical signs, including skin rash, or positive serology is good. In a low-incidence setting, the negative predictive value of testing is high: if a patient's test is negative then it strongly indicates that the patient does not have Lyme disease. In this same low-incidence setting, the predictive value of a positive test is low and even patients with a skin lesion or positive serology may be misdiagnosed as having Lyme disease.[57,58] Although not generally recommended or cleared by the US Food and Drug Administration (FDA), alternative tests [e.g., polymerase chain reaction (PCR), urine antigen test] are used by some providers.[59]

CLINICAL MANAGEMENT

Proven antibiotic treatment modalities should be administered to Lyme disease patients according to clinical signs and duration of illness.[60] Untreated and inadequately treated infection may result in microbial persistence with subsequent cardiac, dermatologic, neurologic, or musculoskeletal sequelae. Several antibiotics including doxycycline, cefuroxime axetil, and amoxicillin, are recommended for the treatment of adult patients with early localized or early disseminated Lyme disease (<21-day duration) without complicated neurologic or severe cardiac manifestations.[61] In children, doxycycline or amoxicillin are recommended for the treatment of early localized disease.[62] Doxycycline is contraindicated during pregnancy and lactation, and other antimicrobials are preferred for these patients. Oral therapy is recommended for most manifestations including EM, cranial nerve palsy, mild cardiac disease, and arthritis. Intravenous therapy is sometimes recommended for meningitis, radiculopathy, more severe cardiac disease, and arthritis refractory to the first course of antibiotics.[61]

Antibiotic prophylaxis for tick bites is generally not recommended. In areas of high risk for Lyme disease, chemoprophylaxis with a single dose of doxycycline may be beneficial when: (1) the tick can be identified as *Ixodes scapularis*, (2) the tick is engorged or has been attached for ≥ 36 hours, and (3) prophylaxis can be started within 72 hours of the tick being removed.[63,64] In a national survey of healthcare providers, over 50% reported prescribing tick bite prophylaxis sometime during the previous year, even in areas where Lyme disease is rare.[65]

SURVEILLANCE STATISTICS FOR THE UNITED STATES

Lyme disease was made a nationally notifiable disease in 1991 and a uniform national case definition was adopted for surveillance purposes at that time.[66] The case definition was updated in 2008 and most recently in 2017.[67] During 2008–15, a total of 275,589 cases of Lyme disease were reported to CDC. Lyme disease affects persons in all age groups, but the highest rates are found in children aged 5–9 years and adults aged 50–55 years. The majority of cases are male (56.7%) and white (89.7%).[1]

Surveillance data provides valuable information on demographics, geographic distribution, and seasonality of Lyme disease trends over time. Differences in reporting practices between states and characteristics of the surveillance case definition result in a smaller number of cases reported through surveillance than truly exist. In 2010, 22,561 cases of Lyme disease were reported, compared to an analysis of health insurance claim data from 2005 to 2010 showing an estimated 329,000 clinician-diagnosed cases per year in the United States.[68,69] In addition, an assessment of large commercial laboratory data from four states in 2008 provided an estimate of 288,000 U.S. patients in that year.[59]

LYME DISEASE EMERGENCE AND RISK FACTORS FOR INFECTION

Environmental change influences the distribution of *I. scapularis* ticks. In recent times, agricultural land in the Northeast and upper Midwest was converted to suburban land that is becoming re-forested.[14] This habitat is ideal as *I. scapularis* ticks require shade and a high humidity in their microenvironment to prevent dessication.[70]

The possibility of Lyme disease emergence continues to exist outside of known high-incidence areas due primarily to growing deer populations that support the *Ixodes* tick vector, increased residential development of wooded areas, and tick dispersal to new areas.[9,14] Contiguous spread arising from movement of deer and increased reforestation are the principal factors in geographic spread of Lyme disease.[14,71] Studies mapping the distribution of ticks, seropositivity of animals, and the incidence of human cases over time provide information on the spread of Lyme disease in the United States. Seropositivity of dogs has been used as an epidemiologic marker of the geographic distribution of *B. burgdorferi*.[72] Considerations for using these data include small sample sizes, travel-related exposures, and testing of dogs with potential for previous exposure that may not be representative of true local risk.[73,74]

The introduction and geographic expansion of Lyme disease within some states and regions is a considerable problem. This occurrence has been most pronounced in northeast states where counties identified as having high incidence of Lyme disease increased > 320% from[43] (1993–97) to 183 (2008–12).[75] Similar trends have been identified in the North Central states where counties with high incidence of Lyme disease increased > 250% from[22] (1993–97) to 182 (2008–12).[75]

The principal risk factor for Lyme disease in the United States is living in or visiting an area with an abundance of infected *Ixodes* ticks. The greatest risk occurs in the peridomestic environment, principally in or near the woods that may surround human homes. Current understanding of risk for tick exposure is based primarily on ecologic and entomologic studies. *Ixodes* ticks were observed in 10 of 11 yards of patients with Lyme disease in New York.[76,77] The ecotone area of a yard is where the lawn and woods converge. This area has been identified as a high tick area in the peridomestic setting. [78] Pet ownership may increase the risk for tick encounters and tick-borne disease. In one study, owners of dogs or cats had 1.8 times the risk of finding ticks crawling and 1.5 times the risk of finding ticks attached to household members compared to households without pets.[79] While the mechanism for this increased risk remains unclear, it is possible that pets may bring ticks on the property and into the home. It is also possible that pet owners spend more time outdoors and in tick habitats compared to nonpet owners. Pet owners should perform daily tick checks of pets and household members and consult their veterinarian regarding appropriate tick prevention products.[79]

Recreational activities, such as hiking, camping, fishing, and hunting potentially expose persons to tick bites, especially during the late spring and summer months. In addition, outdoor occupations, such as landscaping, brush clearing, forestry, and wildlife and parks management, may place persons at higher risk. Outdoor use of maintained trails for more than 5 hours per week and gardening for more than 4 hours per week have been shown to be risk factors for infection with Lyme disease.[80]

PREVENTION

There is currently no Lyme disease vaccine available for humans. Therefore, in areas endemic for Lyme disease, reducing exposure to the tick vector is an important means of prevention, which requires a multipronged approach. This can include personal protection measures, residential modification, and community efforts.[78]

Personal protective measures: The public should be informed about tick-infested areas in endemic regions and should be encouraged to avoid risky exposures (grassy, brushy, wooded areas), especially in spring and summer.[81] Using Environmental Protection Agency (EPA)-registered repellents (https://www.epa.gov/insect-repellents) and treating clothing and gear with permethrin are strategies for tick-bite prevention.

Early detection and proper removal of attached ticks is one of the most important Lyme disease prevention strategies. When in high-risk areas, a daily check for ticks and their proper removal is an important measure to prevent infection as studies have shown that transmission of *B. burgdorferi* from an infected tick is unlikely to occur before at least 24 hours of attachment.[82,83] Fine-tipped tweezers should be used to grasp the tick mouthparts, removing the tick by steady, gentle traction. In addition, placing clothing in a dryer on high heat after spending time outdoors is an effective strategy to kill *I. scapularis* ticks.[84,85]

Residential modifications: In the residential environment, landscape management is the practice of making the environment less suitable for tick survival and tick hosts. This can include, removing leaf litter and woodpiles, and clearing trees and brush around houses and yard edges. In addition, consistent mowing can limit habitat suitable for deer, ticks, and rodent reservoirs. Deer management can include fencing, repellents, and deer resistant plants.[86]

Other strategies to combat the *Ixodes* tick directly or indirectly have been evaluated with mixed results. The application of synthetic chemical acaricides (tick-specific pesticides) to residential areas, while effective at reducing tick populations, may not prevent human disease.[87] Acaricides will not completely eliminate a tick population, so human exposure to infected nymphs will still occur if this is the sole reduction measure.[88] In addition, application of many of these products is not always practical (e.g., they cannot be applied near bodies of water).[87,89]

Several approaches have been designed to interrupt the transmission cycle at the level of the rodent reservoir. The distribution in yards of acaricide impregnated cotton balls, which mice then use for nest building, has not been shown to reduce the number of infected, host-seeking *I. scapularis* nymphs.[90] A product in which mice are treated with an acaricide, upon entering a bait box initially demonstrated a reduction in tick infestations on white-footed mice, but more recent studies have shown a questionable effect.[91,92] Treated bait products for oral ingestion by rodents require additional evaluation.[89,93,94]

Community interventions: Community control measures are similar to residential ones, including deer control and wide scale pesticide applications. Deer reduction and deer exclusion via fencing have shown to be effective in reducing tick populations in certain situations. On islands or in isolated settings, removing deer can significantly reduce host seeking nymphal ticks.[95] The density to which deer need to be reduced to have this effect is not known. [89,95] In addition, this strategy is controversial and often not feasible for communities.[95] Community-wide education has been evaluated with some success. For example, after an intensive educational intervention in Connecticut, recommendations were made to focus on promotion of measures likely to be accepted and incorporated into routine behaviors (e.g., showering).[96]

Borrelia miyamotoi

The recently discovered *B. miyamotoi* is one cause of a relapsing fever-like illness. It has been detected in all tick species that are vectors of Lyme disease. The prevalence of *B. miyamotoi* in *Ixodes spp*. ticks has been reported as less than 1% and up to 10.5%, in certain geographic areas.[3,4,97] The seroprevalence of *B. miyamotoi* in one study among people living in the northeast United States has been reported as 10%, suggesting that it may have been present in the environment for years before detection.[4]

There is limited information available regarding the clinical spectrum of infection with *B. miyamotoi*. Patients may present with acute headache, fever, and chills and have evidence of leukopenia, thrombocytopenia, and elevated aminotransferase levels.[98] The few *B. miyamotoi* cases described in the literature have been older and had severe CSF disease among those with immunocompromising conditions.[99]

Serology with antibody-based tests, including enzyme-linked immunoassay and separate IgG and IgM Western blots as well as PCR testing are currently available through a limited number of laboratories.[4,100,101] Treatment regimens for *B. miyamotoi* are the same as for other tick-borne disease and typically include doxycycline (2–4 weeks), or amoxicillin.[98]

It is likely that risk factors described for Lyme disease are similar for *B. miyamotoi*. *B. miyamotoi* can be transmitted within the first 24 hours of tick attachment (vs. 36–48 hours for *B. burgdorferi*).[100,102] The probability of transmission increases with every day an infected tick remains attached. In addition, most known cases of *B. miyamotoi* have occurred in July and August, later than the onset of most Lyme disease cases, and suggestive of *B. miyamotoi* transmission through larval, rather than nymphal, ticks.[100] Unlike *B. burgdorferi*, *B. miyamotoi* can be transmitted transovarially from female tick to larvae.[3,34,35]

People living in areas where black-legged ticks are common should take appropriate precautions against tick bites and seek medical care if they experience illness after a tick bite or after spending time in tick habitat.

TICK-BORNE AND LOUSE-BORNE RELAPSING FEVER BORRELIA

TBRF and LBRF are caused by several species of spirochetes in the genus *Borrelia*.[103] TBRF is endemic on most continents and follows the bite of infected soft-bodied ticks (*Ornithodoros spp.*). There are several species of *Borrelia* that cause TBRF, each transmitted by a different *Ornithodoros spp.* tick. In contrast, LBRF is geographically limited to the Horn of Africa and is caused by a single species, *B. recurrentis*, which is transmitted by lice (*P. humanus*).[5] Disease caused by relapsing fever *Borrelia* is likely under recognized and underreported due to its rare occurrence and nonspecific symptoms.

The relapsing fever *Borrelia* spp. are helical spirochete agents, similar to *B. burgdorferi* (Fig. 143-2). They range from 3 to 25 μm long and 0.2 to 0.5 μm wide with a loose coil appearance. The bacteria have the ability to undergo antigenic variation with the appearance of new outer surface proteins. This alteration in proteins causes repeated stimulation of the host immune system, causing the characteristic symptoms of relapsing fever.[104] In addition, the bacteria simultaneously replicates in the blood, sometimes causing high burdens of spirochetemia.[105]

Infection with TBRF or LBRF *Borrelia* may result in a wide range of nonspecific symptoms. The most commonly reported symptoms of TBRF include high fever, headache, chills, muscle, and joint aches. In addition, nausea, arthralgia, vomiting, or abdominal pain can occur.[104] Severity of illness can be variable and some patients may have jaundice, hepatosplenomegaly, meningismus, and photophobia.[104] Also notable, there is evidence that infection with *B. turicatae* more often results in neurologic involvement.[106] Symptoms usually occur 1 week following a tick bite. A symptomatic period will occur

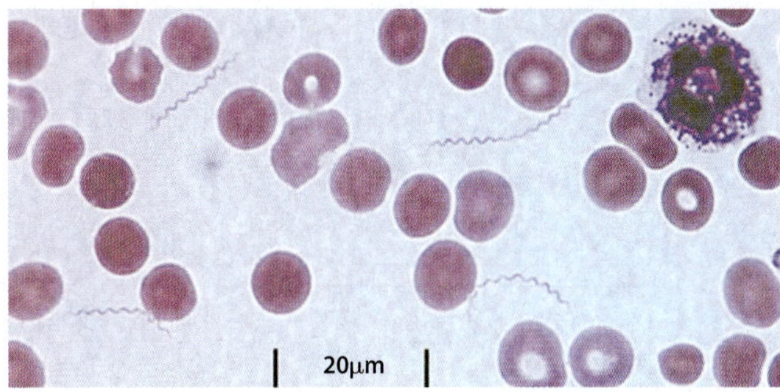

FIGURE 143-2. Peripheral blood smear. The TBRF bacteria are long and spiral-shaped. The circular objects are red blood cells. The irregular purple object in the top right corner is a white blood cell. *Source*: Centers for Disease Control and Prevention.

followed by a few days of recovery. This cycle of symptoms and relief can reoccur up to a dozen times, although 1–3 relapses is more typical. The clinical manifestations of LBRF and TBRF are similar, although LBRF is usually associated with a single relapse, whereas multiple relapses are more common with TBRF.[107]

There are several laboratory tests that can be used to diagnose TBRF and LBRF. During a febrile period, when there are high concentrations of spirochetes in the blood, microscopy can be used for diagnosis by visually observing the spirochetes. Blood samples obtained prior to antibiotic treatment can be cultured.[104] Serologic testing is the most common diagnostic tool used. Acute and convalescent samples should be taken within 1 week and at least 3 weeks following symptom onset to assess seroconversion.[108] Serology cannot differentiate between species of relapsing fever *Borrelia*; therefore, it is important to consider the likely geographic location of exposure. Patients with TBRF may have false-positive tests for Lyme disease because of the similarity of proteins between the two organisms.[109]

Relapsing fever *Borrelia* are susceptible to several classes of antibiotics. The preferred treatment for adults is: tetracycline 500 mg every 6 hours for 10 days. The occurrence of a Jarish-Herxheimer reaction has been documented in up to 50% of people with TBRF.[104] This reaction is described as an initial worsening of symptoms or development of new symptoms including rigors, hypotension, and high fever following treatment. The reaction is reportedly more severe during treatment of LBRF as compared to TBRF, with death occurring in some cases.[104] Given appropriate supportive care, most patients recover within a week.

TBRF VECTOR, ECOLOGY, AND PREVENTION

TBRF was first described in 1905 in the United States, more than half a century before Lyme disease.[110] The major *Borrelia* species that cause TBRF in North America are: *B. hermsii* and *B. turicatae*. *B. parkeri* is considered a possible cause of TBRF but no human isolate has been documented. The TBRF causing *Borrelia* are transmitted by soft ticks of the genus *Ornithodoros*. Each different species of *Ornithodoros* tick can carry a strain of *Borrelia* that is specific to that tick.[105]

The vector of TBRF, the *Ornithodoros* soft tick, belongs to the family Argasidae. There are several notable differences between soft ticks and the more familiar hard ticks. Unlike the *Ixodes* tick, *Ornithodoros* ticks have two or more nymphal stages (Fig. 143-3), each of which requires a blood meal. Soft ticks are faster feeders and the bite is brief, usually less than half an hour and as fast as 30 seconds.[105] The *Borrelia* bacteria colonize the salivary glands of the *Ornithodoros* tick, which enables quick transmission of the pathogen from vector to host.[105] Soft ticks can live up to 10 years and will survive without a blood meal for several years. It is common for *Ornithodoros* ticks to pass the *Borrelia* bacteria through their eggs via transovarial transmission. These factors maintain spirochete presence in an environment for

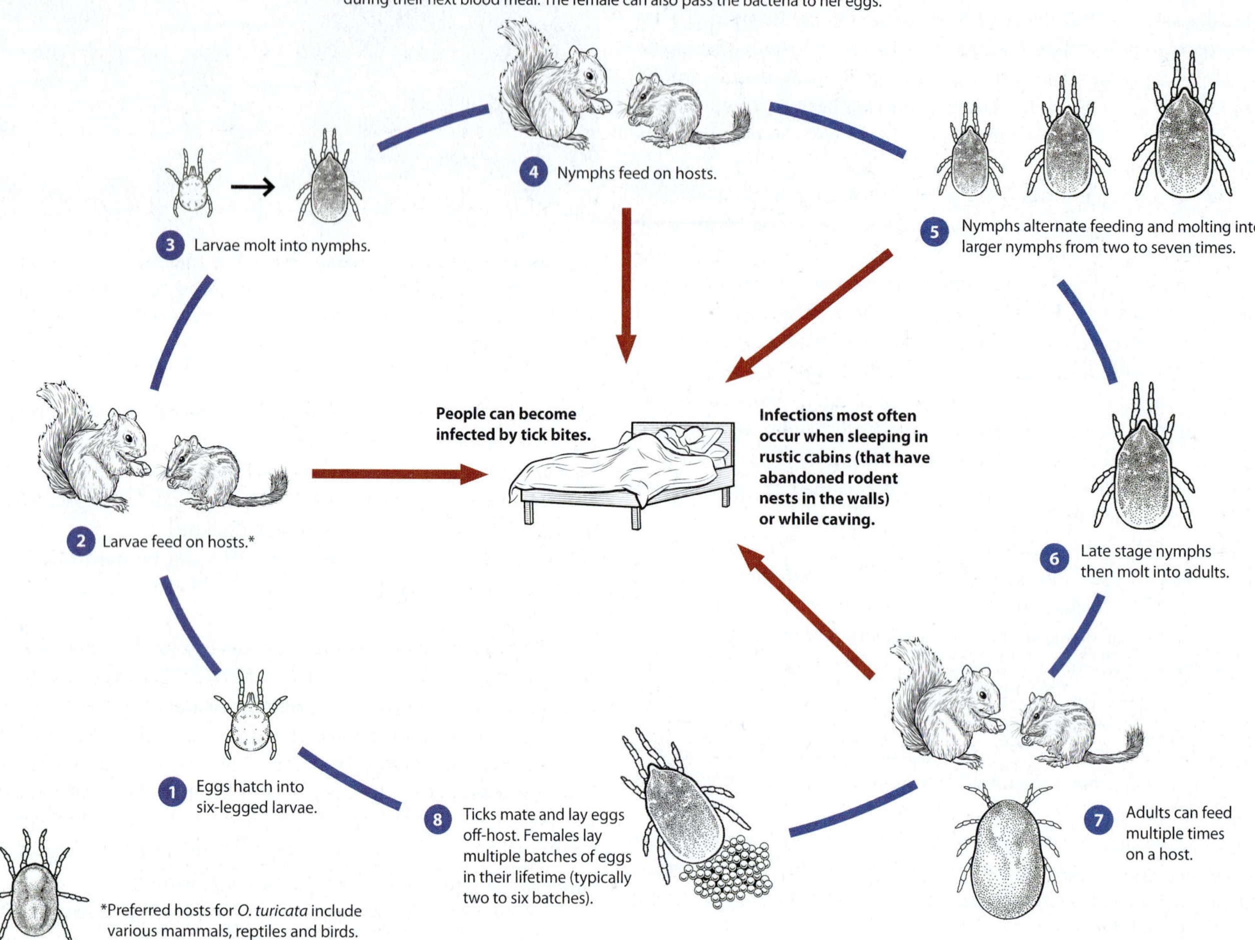
Life cycle of Ornithodoros hermsi and O. turicata ticks
Ticks can acquire the bacteria that cause tick-borne relapsing fever while feeding on infected rodents. They maintain the bacteria during the molt and can transmit infection to rodents (or people) during their next blood meal. The female can also pass the bacteria to her eggs.
4 Nymphs feed on hosts.
3 Larvae molt into nymphs.
5 Nymphs alternate feeding and molting into larger nymphs from two to seven times.
People can become infected by tick bites.
Infections most often occur when sleeping in rustic cabins (that have abandoned rodent nests in the walls) or while caving.
2 Larvae feed on hosts.*
6 Late stage nymphs then molt into adults.
1 Eggs hatch into six-legged larvae.
8 Ticks mate and lay eggs off-host. Females lay multiple batches of eggs in their lifetime (typically two to six batches).
7 Adults can feed multiple times on a host.
*Preferred hosts for O. turicata include various mammals, reptiles and birds.

FIGURE 143-3. This diagram shows the life cycle of *Ornithodoros hermsi* and *O. turicata* ticks.

long periods of time.[103] Soft ticks do not search for prey in tall grass or brush, like hard ticks. They are opportunistic and have been shown to feed off of many animal species.

The *Ornithodoros* ticks are distributed in endemic foci of the United States and western Canada as well as in other parts of the world, particularly Africa.[105,111] *O. hermsii* tends to be found in western states and at higher altitudes (1500–8000 feet). The ticks feed on ground or tree squirrels, chipmunks, and other small mammals. *O. parkeri* are also found in western states but live in grassland, sagebrush, and burrows and are associated with lagomorphs and rodents.[112] *O. turicata* are found at lower altitudes and inhabit caves and burrows in Texas and gopher tortoise dens in Florida. *O. turicata* are particularly nonselective and promiscuous feeders. These ticks can go 5 years or more without feeding and remain infectious upon the next feeding. They also maintain the *Borrelia* bacteria transovarially.[105] The species of *Ornithodoros* ticks in Africa differ from those in the United States and these ticks transmit different species of relapsing fever causing *Borrelia* bacteria. In Africa, the ticks also live in rodent burrows, which can be found inside or near households.[111]

TBRF spirochetes circulate in enzootic cycles between ticks and animals. *Ornithodoros* ticks obtain blood meals from squirrels, chipmunks, lagomorphs, rodents, opossums, wild canids, and likely many others.[112] Humans come into contact with these ticks when they sleep in rodent infested cabins, enter caves or come in contact with animal burrows. In Texas, vertebrate species that live in or near caves make for ideal blood sources for the ticks.[105,113] There is limited information regarding vertebrate hosts of the above mentioned *Ornithodoros* ticks in Africa. Rodents, chickens, and swine living in close proximity to humans may be competent hosts.[111]

Known risk factors for TBRF include spending time in wilderness areas in western states, especially cabins with rodent infestations.[114–118] In addition, caves have been identified as a risk factor for *B. turicatae* in Texas.[104,119–121] Outbreaks of TBRF often follow recent exposure to cabins. In this setting, ticks inhabit the nests of rodents in cabins and can bite humans sleeping in the cabin at night. Groups of people can become infected and multiple cases of TBRF can occur from the same exposure setting. LBRF outbreaks in contrast, most often occur in overcrowded, impoverished areas.[111]

Congenital transmission of relapsing fever spirochetes has been reported infrequently.[122] Infection with a relapsing fever bacteria during pregnancy can lead to poor outcomes for the mother and fetus, including: respiratory distress syndrome, Jarish-Herxheimer reaction, premature delivery, or death.[123–125]

Efficacy of tick prevention products, including permethrin and repellents, against *Ornithodoros* ticks is unknown. To treat structures, such as cabins, an appropriate pesticide should be applied, and rodent exclusion should take place. Sleeping areas in cabins should be inspected for any cracks or gaps in the walls or ceilings and baseboards where ticks could gain entry. If found, they should be filled in. In order to limit soft tick access to bedding, move beds away from walls and do not to allow bed sheets to touch the ground.[126] If entering caves or areas with rodent burrows, long clothing should be worn and contact with the cave floor or burrow should be minimized.

LBRF VECTOR AND ECOLOGY

LBRF is caused by the bacteria *B. recurrentis* and is similar to the TBRF causing *Borrelia spp*.

The vector of LBRF is *P. humanus humanus*, the body louse, and infrequently *P. humanus capitis*, the head louse. When feeding on an infected human, the body louse will ingest *B. recurrentis*. Transmission occurs when the louse is crushed and the bacteria are released onto the human skin. *B. recurrentis* can penetrate intact mucosa and skin.[127] The only known host of *P. humanus* is humans.[127] LBRF occurs in the highlands of Ethiopia during the rainy season when the cold and wet climate causes overcrowding and lice infestation.[128] In addition, LBRF outbreaks occur in other congested, high louse density areas.[111]

The life cycle of the body louse has three stages: egg, nymph, and adult. The adult louse is about the size of a sesame seed, has six legs (each with claws), and is tan to grayish-white.[129] Females are usually larger than males and can lay up to eight nits per day.[130] Adult lice can live up to 30 days on a person's body and adult lice need to feed on blood several times daily or they will die within 1–2 days off the host.[130]

LBRF prevention should focus on avoidance of the louse vector. This can be done by minimizing overcrowded situations, improving hygiene and access to washing facilities.[103] Shaving and the application of topical medications (permethrin, pyrethrins, benzyl alcohol, ivermectin, malathion, spinosad) can be used to treat existing infestations.[130]

References

1. Schwartz AM, Hinckley AF, Mead PS, Hook SA, Kugeler KJ. Surveillance for Lyme disease—United States, 2008–2015. *MMWR Surveill Summ.* 2017;66(22):1–12.
2. CDC. Data and Statistics. 2015. http://www.cdc.gov/lyme/stats/index.html. Accessed July 31, 2018.
3. Scoles GA, Papero M, Beati L, Fish D. A relapsing fever group spirochete transmitted by Ixodes scapularis ticks. *Vector Borne Zoonotic Dis.* 2001;1(1):21–34.
4. Krause PJ, Narasimhan S, Wormser GP, et al. *Borrelia miyamotoi* sensu lato seroreactivity and seroprevalence in the northeastern United States. *Emerg Infect Dis.* 2014;20(7):1183–90.
5. Cutler SJ, Moss J, Fukunaga M, et al. *Borrelia recurrentis* characterization and comparison with relapsing-fever, Lyme-associated, and other Borrelia spp. *Int J Syst Bacteriol.* 1997;47(4):958–68.
6. Blanton L, Keith B, Brzezinski W. Southern tick-associated rash illness: Erythema migrans is not always Lyme disease. *South Med J.* 2008;101(7):759–60.
7. Prevention CfDCa. Data and Statistics. 2015. http://www.cdc.gov/lyme/stats/index.html.
8. Rosenberg R, Lindsey NP, Fischer M, et al. Vital signs: Trends in reported vectorborne disease cases—United States and territories, 2004–2016. *MMWR Morb Mortal Wkly Rep.* 2018;67(17):496–501.
9. Ogden NH, Feil EJ, Leighton PA, et al. Evolutionary aspects of emerging Lyme disease in Canada. *Appl Environ Microbiol.* 2015;81(21):7350–9.
10. Johnson RCHF, Rumpel CM. Taxonomy of the Lyme disease spirochetes. *Yale J Biol Med.* 1984;57:529–37.
11. Pritt BS, Mead PS, Johnson DKH, et al. Identification of a novel pathogenic Borrelia species causing Lyme borreliosis with unusually high spirochaetaemia: A descriptive study. *Lancet Infect Dis.* 2016;16(5):556–64.
12. Baranton G, Postic D, Girons I, et al. Delineation of *Borrelia burgdorferi sensu stricto, Borrelia garinii* sp. nov., and group VS461 associated with Lyme borreliosis. *Int J Syst Bacteriol.* 1992;42(3):378–83.
13. Brouqui P, Bacellar F, Baranton G, et al. Guidelines for the diagnosis of tick-borne bacterial diseases in Europe. *Clin Microbiol Infect Dis.* 2004;10(12):1108–32.
14. Eisen RJ, Eisen L. The blacklegged tick, *Ixodes scapularis*: An increasing public health concern. *Trends Parasitol.* 2018;34(4):295–309.
15. Mead PS. Epidemiology of Lyme disease. *Infect Dis Clin North Am.* 2015;29(2):187–210.
16. Eisen RJ, Eisen L. Spatial modeling of human risk of exposure to vector-borne pathogens based on epidemiological versus arthropod vector data. *J Med Entomol.* 2008;45(2):181–92.
17. Mak S, Morshed M, Henry B. Ecological niche modeling of Lyme disease in British Columbia, Canada. *J Med Entomol.* 2010;47(1):99–105.
18. Lane RSPJ, Burgdorfer W. Lyme borreliosis: Relation of its causative agent to its vectors and hosts in North America and Europe. *Annu Rev Entomol.* 1991;36:587–609.
19. Piesman J, Mather TN, Sinsky RJ, Spielman A. Duration of tick attachment and *Borrelia burgdorferi* transmission. *J Clin Microbiol.* 1987;25(3):557–8.
20. Feldman KA, Connally NP, Hojgaard A, et al. Abundance and infection rates of *Ixodes scapularis* nymphs collected from residential properties in Lyme disease-endemic areas of Connecticut, Maryland, and New York. *J Vector Ecol.* 2015;40(1):198–201.
21. Clover J, Lane R. Evidence implicating nymphal *Ixodes pacificus* (Acari: Ixodidae) in the epidemiology of Lyme disease in California. *Am J Trop Med Hyg.* 1995;53(3):237–40.
22. Elliott D, Eppes S, Klein J. Teratogen update: Lyme disease. *Teratology.* 2001;64:276–81.
23. Weber K, Bratzke HJ, Neubert U, Wilske B, Duray PH. *Borrelia burgdorferi* in a newborn despite oral penicillin for Lyme borreliosis during pregnancy. *Pediatr Infect Dis J.* 1988;7(4):286–9.
24. Waddell LA, Greig J, Lindsay LR, Hinckley AF, Ogden NH. A systematic review on the impact of gestational Lyme disease in humans on the fetus and newborn. *PLoS One.* 2018;13(11):e0207067.
25. Walsh CA, Mayer EW, Baxi LV. Lyme disease in pregnancy: Case report and review of the literature. *Obstet Gynecol Surv.* 2007;62(1):41–50.
26. Cable R, Leiby D. Risk and prevention of transfusion-transmitted babesiosis and other tick-borne diseases. *Curr Opin Hematol.* 2003;10(6):405–11.
27. Shapiro ED. Lyme disease in children. *Am J Med.* 1995;98(4A):69S–73S.
28. Bunikis J, Tsao J, Luke C, et al. *Borrelia burgdorferi* infection in a natural population of *Peromyscus leucopus* mice: A longitudinal study in an area where Lyme borreliosis is highly endemic. *J Infect Dis.* 2004;189:1515–23.
29. Slajchert T, Kittron U, Jones C, Mannelli A. Role of the eastern chipmunk (*Tamias striatus*) in the epizootiology of Lyme borreliosis in northwestern Illinois, USA. *J Wildl Dis.* 1997;33(1):40–6.
30. Richter D, Spielman A, Komar N, Matuschka F. Competence of American robins as reservoir hosts for Lyme disease spirochetes. *Emerg Infect Dis.* 2000;6(2):133–8.
31. Piesman J. Lyme borreliosis: Biology, epidemiology, and control. In: Gray J, Kahl O, Lane R, Stanek G, eds. *Ecology of Borrelia burgdorferi* sensu lato *in North America.* Wallingford, England: CABI Publishing; 2002:223–49.
32. Piesman J, Spielman A, Etkind P, Ruebush TK 2nd, Juranek DD. Role of deer in the epizootiology of *Babesia microti* in Massachusetts, USA. *J Med Entomol.* 1979;15(5–6):537–40.
33. Nelson D, Rooney S, Miller N, Mather T. Complement-mediated killing of *Borrelia burgdorferi* by nonimmune sera from sika deer. *J Parasitol.* 2000;86(6):1232–8.
34. Rollend L, Fish D, Childs JE. Transovarial transmission of *Borrelia* spirochetes by *Ixodes scapularis*: A summary of the literature and recent observations. *Ticks Tick Borne Dis.* 2013;4(1–2):46–51.
35. Breuner NE, Hojgaard A, Replogle AJ, Boegler KA, Eisen L. Transmission of the relapsing fever spirochete, *Borrelia miyamotoi*, by single transovarially-infected larval *Ixodes scapularis* ticks. *Ticks Tick Borne Dis.* 2018;9(6):1464–7.
36. Piesman J, Gern L. Lyme borreliosis in Europe and North America. *Parasitology.* 2004;129:S191–220.
37. Dennis DT. *Epidemiology*. St. Louis, MO: Mosby Year Book; 1993.
38. Kugeler KJ, Griffith KS, Gould LH, et al. A review of death certificates listing Lyme disease as a cause of death in the United States. *Clin Infect Dis.* 2011;52(3):364–7.
39. Steere AC, Strle F, Wormser GP, et al. Lyme borreliosis. *Nat Rev Dis Primers.* 2016;2:16090.
40. Steere ACBT, Malawista SE. Erythema chronicum migrans and Lyme arthritis: Epidemiologic evidence for a tick vector. *Am J Epidemiol.* 1978;108(4):312–21.
41. Steere AC. Lyme disease. *N Engl J Med.* 1989;321(9):586–96.
42. Fraser CM, Casjens S, Huang WM, et al. Genomic sequence of a Lyme disease spirochete, *Borrelia burgdorferi. Nature.* 1997;390:580–91.
43. Forrester JD, Mead P. Third-degree heart block associated with Lyme carditis: Review of published cases. *Clin Infect Dis.* 2014;59(7):996–1000.

44. Hu L. Lyme arthritis. *Infect Dis Clin North Am.* 2005;19(4):947–61.
45. Steere AC, Arvikar SL. Editorial commentary: What constitutes appropriate treatment of post-Lyme disease symptoms and other pain and fatigue syndromes? *Clin Infect Dis.* 2015;60(12):1783–5.
46. Marques A. Chronic Lyme disease: A review. *Infect Dis Clin North Am.* 2008;22(2):341–60, vii-viii.
47. Lantos PM. Chronic Lyme disease: The controversies and the science. *Expert Rev Anti Infect Ther.* 2011;9(7):787–97.
48. Steere AC, Sikand VK, Schoen RT, Nowakowski J. Asymptomatic infection with *Borrelia burgdorferi. Clin Infect Dis.* 2003;37(4):528–32.
49. Nowakowski J, Nadelman R, Sell R, et al. Long-term follow-up of patients with culture-confirmed Lyme disease. *Am J Med.* 2003;115:91–6.
50. Krause P, Telford S, Spielman A, et al. Concurrent Lyme disease and babesiosis. *J Am Med Assoc.* 1996;275(21):1657–60.
51. Blackmore C, Hinckley A, Moncayo A, Brown J. A modification of the exposure criteria used as part of the case definition to help classify cases of Lyme disease. In. *CSTE.org.* 2016:1–9.
52. CDC. Notice to readers recommendations for test performance and interpretation from the Second National Conference on Serologic Diagnosis of Lyme Disease. *MMWR Morb Mortal Wkly Rep.* 1995;44(31):590–1.
53. Reed KD. Laboratory testing for Lyme disease: Possibilities and practicalities. *J Clin Microbiol.* 2002;40(2):319–24.
54. Dressler F, Whalen JA, Reinhardt BN, Steere AC. Western blotting in the serodiagnosis of Lyme disease. *J Infect Dis.* 1993;167(2):392–400.
55. Ramsey AH, Belongia EA, Chyou PH, Davis JP. Appropriateness of Lyme disease serologic testing. *Ann Fam Med.* 2004;2(4):341–4.
56. Littman MP, Goldstein RE, Labato MA, Lappin MR, Moore GE. ACVIM small animal consensus statement on Lyme disease in dogs: Diagnosis, treatment, and prevention. *J Vet Intern Med.* 2006;20(2):422–34.
57. Tugwell P, Dennis DT, Weinstein A, et al. Laboratory evaluation in the diagnosis of Lyme disease. *Ann Intern Med.* 1997;127(12):1109–23.
58. Forrester JD, Brett M, Matthias J, et al. Epidemiology of Lyme disease in low-incidence states. *Ticks Tick Borne Dis.* 2015;6(6):721–3.
59. Hinckley AF, Connally NP, Meek JI, et al. Lyme disease testing by large commercial laboratories in the United States. *Clin Infect Dis.* 2014;59(5):676–81.
60. Wormser G, Nadelman R, Dattwyler R, et al. Practice guidelines for the treatment of Lyme disease. *Clin Infect Dis.* 2000;31:S1–14.
61. Wormser GP, Dattwyler RJ, Shapiro ED, et al. The clinical assessment, treatment, and prevention of Lyme disease, human granulocytic anaplasmosis, and babesiosis: Clinical practice guidelines by the Infectious Diseases Society of America. *Clin Infect Dis.* 2006;43(9):1089–134.
62. Kimberlin D, Brady M, Jackson M, Long S, eds. *Red Book: 2018–2021 Report of the Committee on Infectious Diseases.* 31st ed. Itasca, IL: American Academy of Pediatrics; 2018.
63. American Academy of Pediatrics. Lyme disease. In: Kimberlin D, Brady M, Jackson M, Long S, eds. *Red Book: 2018 Report of the Committee on Infectious Diseases.* Vol. 200. 31st ed. Itasca, IL: American Academy of Pediatrics; 2018:515–23.
64. Nadelman R, Nowakowski J, Fish D, et al. Prophylaxis with single-dose doxycycline for the prevention of Lyme disease after an *Ixodes scapularis* tick bite. *N Engl J Med.* 2001;345:79–84.
65. Perea AE, Hinckley AF, Mead PS. Tick bite prophylaxis: Results from a 2012 survey of healthcare providers. *Zoonoses Public Health.* 2015;62(5):388–92.
66. CDC. Lyme disease—United States, 2001–2002. *MMWR Morb Mortal Wkly Rep.* 2004;53(17):365–9.
67. CDC. Lyme Disease (*Borrelia burgdorferi*) 2017 Case Definition 2017; National Notifiable Diseases Surveillance System (NNDSS). https://wwwn.cdc.gov/nndss/conditions/lyme-disease/case-definition/2017/. Accessed October 1, 2018.
68. CDC. Lyme disease data tables. 2017; Reported cases of Lyme disease by state or locality, 2006–2016. https://www.cdc.gov/lyme/stats/tables.html#modalIdString_CDCTable_0. Accessed September 5, 2018.
69. Nelson CA, Saha S, Kugeler KJ, et al. Incidence of clinician-diagnosed Lyme disease, United States, 2005–2010. *Emerg Infect Dis.* 2015;21(9):1625–31.
70. Stafford K. Survival of immature *Ixodes scapularis* (Acari: Ixodidae) at different relative humidities. *J Med Entomol.* 1994;31(2):310–4.
71. Spielman A. The emergence of Lyme disease and human babesiosis in a changing environment. *Ann N Y Acad Sci.* 1994;740:146–56.
72. Duncan A, Correa M, Levine J, Breitschwerdt E. The dog as a sentinel for human infection: Prevalence of *Borrelia burgdorferi* C6 antibodies in dogs from southeastern and mid-Atlantic states. *Vector Borne Zoonotic Dis.* 2005;5(2):101–9.
73. Mead P, Goel R, Kugeler K. Canine serology as adjunct to human Lyme disease surveillance. *Emerg Infect Dis.* 2011;17(9):1710–2.
74. Millen K, Kugeler KJ, Hinckley AF, Lawaczeck EW, Mead PS. Elevated Lyme disease seroprevalence among dogs in a nonendemic county: Harbinger or artifact? *Vector Borne Zoonotic Dis.* 2013;13(5):340–41.
75. Kugeler KJ, Farley GM, Forrester JD, Mead PS. Geographic distribution and expansion of human Lyme disease, United States. *Emerg Infect Dis.* 2015;21(8):1455–7.
76. Falco RC, Fish D. Prevalence of *Ixodes dammini* near the homes of Lyme disease patients in Westchester County, New York. *Am J Epidemiol.* 1988;127(4):826–30.
77. Mead P, Hook S, Niesobecki S, et al. Risk factors for tick exposure in suburban settings in the Northeastern United States. *Ticks Tick Borne Dis.* 2018;9(2):319–24.
78. Connally NP, Durante AJ, Yousey-Hindes KM, et al. Peridomestic Lyme disease prevention: Results of a population-based case-control study. *Am J Prev Med.* 2009;37(3):201–6.
79. Jones EH, Hinckley AF, Hook SA, et al. Pet ownership increases human risk of encountering ticks. *Zoonoses Public Health.* 2018;65(1):74–9.
80. Ley COE, Reingold AL. Case-control study of risk factors for incident Lyme disease in California. *Am J Epidemiol.* 1995;142(9):S39–47.
81. Hayes E, Piesman J. How can we prevent Lyme disease? *N Engl J Med.* 2003;348(24):2424–30.
82. des Vignes F, Piesman J, Heffernan R, et al. Effect of tick removal on transmission of *Borrelia burgdorferi* and *Ehrlichia phagocytophila* by *Ixodes scapularis* nymphs. *J Infect Dis.* 2001;183:773–8.
83. Piesman J, Dolan M. Protection against Lyme disease spirochete transmission provided by prompt removal of nymphal *Ixodes scapularis* (Acari: Ixodidae). *J Med Entomol.* 2002;39(3):509–12.
84. Carroll JF. A cautionary note: Survival of nymphs of two species of ticks (Acari: Ixodidae) among clothes laundered in an automatic washer. *J Med Entomol.* 2003;40(5):732–6.
85. Nelson CA, Hayes CM, Markowitz MA, et al. The heat is on: Killing blacklegged ticks in residential washers and dryers to prevent tickborne diseases. *Ticks Tick Borne Dis.* 2016;7(5):958–63.
86. Stafford K. *Tick Management Handbook.* New Haven, Connecticut: Connecticut Agricultural Experiment Station; 2007.
87. Hinckley AF, Meek JI, Ray JA, et al. Effectiveness of residential acaricides to prevent Lyme and other tick-borne diseases in humans. *J Infect Dis.* 2016;214(2):182–8.
88. Eisen RJ, Piesman J, Zielinski-Gutierrez E, Eisen L. What do we need to know about disease ecology to prevent Lyme disease in the northeastern United States? *J Med Entomol.* 2012;49(1):11–22.
89. Eisen L, Dolan MC. Evidence for personal protective measures to reduce human contact with blacklegged ticks and for environmentally based control methods to suppress host-seeking blacklegged ticks and reduce infection with Lyme disease spirochetes in tick vectors and rodent reservoirs. *J Med Entomol.* 2016;53(5):1063–92.
90. Hornbostel VL, Ostfeld RS, Benjamin MA. Effectiveness of *Metarhizium anisopliae* (Deuteromycetes) against *Ixodes scapularis* (Acari: Ixodidae) engorging on *Peromnyscus leucopus. J Vector Ecol.* 2005;30(1):91–101.
91. Dolan MC, Maupin GO, Schneider BS, et al. Control of immature *Ixodes scapularis* (Acari: Ixodidae) on rodent reservoirs of *Borrelia burgdorferi* in a residential community of southeastern Connecticut. *J Med Entomol.* 2004;41(6):1043–54.
92. Williams SC, Little EAH, Stafford KC 3rd, Molaei G, Linske MA. Integrated control of juvenile *Ixodes scapularis* parasitizing *Peromyscus leucopus* in residential settings in Connecticut, United States. *Ticks Tick Borne Dis.* 2018;9(5):1310–6.
93. Meirelles R, Aroso M, Contente-Cuomo T, Ivanova L, Gomes-Solecki M. Reservoir targeted vaccine for Lyme borreliosis induces a yearlong, neutralizing antibody response to OspA in white-footed mice. *Clin Vaccine Immunol.* 2011;18(11):1809–16.
94. Gomes-Solecki M. Blocking pathogen transmission at the source: Reservoir targeted OspA-based vaccines against *Borrelia burgdorferi. Front Cell Infect Microbiol.* 2014;4:136.
95. Kugeler KJ, Jordan RA, Schulze TL, Griffith KS, Mead PS. Will culling white-tailed deer prevent Lyme disease? *Zoonoses Public Health.* 2016;63(5):337–45.
96. Gould LH, Nelson RS, Griffith KS, et al. Knowledge, attitudes, and behaviors regarding Lyme disease prevention among Connecticut residents, 1999–2004. *Vector Borne Zoonotic Dis.* 2008;8(6):769–76.

97. Barbour AG, Bunikis J, Travinsky B, et al. Niche partitioning of *Borrelia burgdorferi* and *Borrelia miyamotoi* in the same tick vector and mammalian reservoir species. *Am J Trop Med Hyg.* 2009;81(6):1120–31.
98. Molloy PJ, Telford SR 3rd, Chowdri HR, et al. *Borrelia miyamotoi* disease in the northeastern United States: A case series. *Ann Intern Med.* 2015;163(2):91–8.
99. Wormser GP, Pritt B. Update and commentary on four emerging tick-borne infections: *Ehrlichia muris*-like agent, *Borrelia miyamotoi*, deer tick virus, heartland virus, and whether ticks play a role in transmission of *Bartonella henselae*. *Infect Dis Clin North Am.* 2015;29(2):371–81.
100. Krause PJ, Narasimhan S, Wormser GP, et al. Human *Borrelia miyamotoi* infection in the United States. *N Engl J Med.* 2013;368(3):291–3.
101. Molloy PJ, Weeks KE, Todd B, Wormser GP. Seroreactivity to the C6 peptide in *Borrelia miyamotoi* infections occurring in the northeastern United States. *Clin Infect Dis.* 2018;66(9):1407–10.
102. Breuner NE, Dolan MC, Replogle AJ, et al. Transmission of *Borrelia miyamotoi* sensu lato relapsing fever group spirochetes in relation to duration of attachment by *Ixodes scapularis* nymphs. *Ticks Tick Borne Dis.* 2017;8(5):677–81.
103. Barbour A. Relapsing fever In: Goodman J, Dennis D, Sonenshine D, eds. *Tick-Borne Diseases of Humans.* Washington, DC: ASM Press; 2005:268--84.
104. Dworkin MS, Schwan TG, Anderson DE Jr, Borchardt SM. Tick-borne relapsing fever. *Infect Dis Clin North Am.* 2008;22(3):449–68.
105. Boyle WK, Wilder HK, Lawrence AM, Lopez JE. Transmission dynamics of *Borrelia turicatae* from the arthropod vector. *PLoS Negl Trop Dis.* 2014;8(4):e2767.
106. Sethi N, Sondey M, Bai Y, Kim KS, Cadavid D. Interaction of a neurotropic strain of *Borrelia turicatae* with the cerebral microcirculation system. *Infect Immun.* 2006;74(11):6408–18.
107. Remington J, Klein J, Wilson C, Nizet V, Maldonado Y, eds. *Infectious Diseases of the Fetus and Newborn: Borrelia Infections.* Amsterdam: Elsevier Inc.; 2011.
108. Roscoe C, Epperly T. Tick-borne relapsing fever. *Am Fam Physician.* 2005;72(10):2039–44.
109. Rath PM, Rogler G, Schonberg A, Pohle HD, Fehrenbach FJ. Relapsing fever and its serological discrimination from Lyme borreliosis. *Infection.* 1992;20(5):283–6.
110. Weller B, Graham GM. Relapsing fever in central Texas. *J Am Med Assoc.* 1930;95:1834–5.
111. Cutler SJ, Abdissa A, Trape JF. New concepts for the old challenge of African relapsing fever borreliosis. *Clin Microbiol Infect.* 2009;15(5):400–6.
112. Dworkin MS, Schwan TG, Anderson DE Jr. Tick-borne relapsing fever in North America. *Med Clin North Am.* 2002;86(2):417–33.
113. Lopez JE, Krishnavahjala A, Garcia MN, Bermudez S. Tick-borne relapsing fever spirochetes in the Americas. *Vet Sci.* 2016;3(3):16.
114. Paul WS, Maupin G, Scott-Wright AO, Craven RB, Dennis DT. Outbreak of tick-borne relapsing fever at the north rim of the Grand Canyon: Evidence for effectiveness of preventive measures. *Am J Trop Med Hyg.* 2002;66(1):71–5.
115. Jones JM, Hranac CR, Schumacher M, et al. Tick-borne relapsing fever outbreak among a high school football team at an outdoor education camping trip, Arizona, 2014. *Am J Trop Med Hyg.* 2016;95(3):546–50.
116. CDC. Tickborne relapsing fever outbreak after a family gathering—New Mexico, August 2002. *MMWR Morb Mortal Wkly Rep.* 2003;52(34):809–12.
117. Schwan TG, Policastro PF, Miller Z, et al. Tick-borne relapsing fever caused by *Borrelia hermsii*, Montana. *Emerg Infect Dis.* 2003;9(9):1151–4.
118. Trevejo RT, Schriefer ME, Gage KL, et al. An interstate outbreak of tick-borne relapsing fever among vacationers at a Rocky Mountain cabin. *Am J Trop Med Hyg.* 1998;58(6):743–7.
119. Rawlings JA. An overview of tick-borne relapsing fever with emphasis on outbreaks in Texas. *Tex Med.* 1995;91(5):56--9.
120. Wilder HK, Wozniak E, Huddleston E, et al. Case report: A retrospective serological analysis indicating human exposure to tick-borne relapsing fever spirochetes in Texas. *PLoS Negl Trop Dis.* 2015;9(4):e0003617.
121. Forrester JD, Kjemtrup AM, Fritz CL, et al. Tickborne relapsing fever—United States, 1990–2011. *MMWR Morb Mortal Wkly Rep.* 2015;64(3):58–60.
122. Jongen VH, van Roosmalen J, Tiems J, Van Holten J, Wetsteyn JC. Tick-borne relapsing fever and pregnancy outcome in rural Tanzania. *Acta Obstet Gynecol Scand.* 1997;76(9):834–8.
123. Davis RD, Burke JP, Wright LJ. Relapsing fever associated with ARDS in a parturient woman. A case report and review of the literature. *Chest.* 1992;102(2):630–2.
124. Guggenheim JN, Haverkamp AD. Tick-borne relapsing fever during pregnancy: A case report. *J Reprod Med.* 2005;50(9):727–9.
125. Fuchs PC, Oyama AA. Neonatal relapsing fever due to transplacental transmission of Borrelia. *JAMA.* 1969;208(4):690–2.
126. CDC. Recommendations for Reducing Risk of Tick-Borne Relapsing Fever. 2017. https://www.cdc.gov/relapsing-fever/prevention/index.html. Accessed October 1, 2018.
127. Cutler SJ. Relapsing fever borreliae: A global review. *Clin Lab Med.* 2015;35(4):847–65.
128. Warrell DA. Relapsing fevers. In: Cohen J, Powderly WG, Opal SM, eds. *Infectious Diseases.* 4th ed. London, UK: Elsevier; 2017:1105–9.
129. Bonilla DL, Durden LA, Eremeeva ME, Dasch GA. The biology and taxonomy of head and body lice—Implications for louse-borne disease prevention. *PLoS Pathog.* 2013;9(11):e1003724.
130. CDC. Pediculosis. 2009. http://zcs.k12.in.us/sites/default/files/Documents/Health/CDClice.pdf. Accessed October 1, 2018.

CHAPTER 144 Rickettsial Infections

Amy Peterson • Caitlin Cotter • Gilbert J. Kersh

OVERVIEW

Introduction

Rickettsial diseases include a wide range of infections caused by alphaproteobacteria in the Order Rickettsiales. The Order Rickettsiales consists of two families, with the family *Rickettsiaceae* containing the genera *Rickettsia* and *Orientia*. The other family, *Anaplasmataceae,* contains the genera *Ehrlichia*, *Anaplasma*, *Neorickettsia*, and *Wolbachia*. All of these organisms are obligate intracellular bacteria, with the *Rickettsiaceae* growing in host cell cytoplasm, and *Anaplasmataceae* growing within host cell vacuolar structures.

There are at least 27 agents within the Order Rickettsiales that can infect humans (Table 144-1). Within the *Rickettsiaceae*, the typhus group (TG) rickettsia include *R. typhi* (endemic typhus), *R. prowazekii* (epidemic typhus), and *O. tsutsugamushi* (scrub typhus). The spotted fever group (SFG) includes a variety of rickettsia species including *R. rickettsii* (Rocky Mountain spotted fever, RMSF), *R. conorii* (Mediterranean spotted fever, MSF), and *R. africae*.[1] In the family *Anaplasmataceae*, the *Wolbachia* are not known to infect humans and will not be discussed here. Multiple species within the *Ehrlichia* genus can cause human ehrlichiosis, with *E. chaffeensis* being the most prominent. The genus *Anaplasma* contains pathogens of veterinary importance, but *A. phagocytophilum* is the most common etiologic agent of human anaplasmosis. *Neorickettsia* includes the pathogenic species *N. sennetsu* that causes sennetsu fever.

These diseases are widely distributed throughout the world and are a significant cause of illness and death within the human population. Most are zoonotic diseases maintained in the environment through complex cycles involving mammalian reservoirs and invertebrate vectors that can also serve as reservoirs. These pathogens are transmitted to humans by vectors that include ticks, lice, fleas, and mites. Spotted fever rickettsioses, anaplasmosis, and ehrlichiosis are notifiable conditions in the United States, but passive surveillance likely underestimates the true incidence and prevalence of these diseases due to their nonspecific clinical presentations and difficulties in laboratory diagnosis and interpretation of results.

HISTORY

Rickettsial diseases are of great historical significance. Epidemic typhus, caused by *R. prowazekii* and transmitted by body lice, has been a major factor in human conflicts over the last 500 years. The first written description of the disease appears to be in an account of the 1489 siege of Granada by the Spanish army.[2] Notably, epidemic typhus killed large numbers of soldiers in World Wars I and II, and in various other conflicts.[2] Crowded environments where good hygiene practices are not possible are likely to have led to its notable impacts during wartime. Delousing and the widespread use of DDT led to great reductions in the incidence of epidemic typhus.[2]

Scrub typhus, caused by *O. tsutsugamushi* and transmitted by mites, was originally described in the 1930s. This disease had significant impacts during World War II.[3] Scrub typhus is primarily found in southern Asia, and military operations in the region led to outbreaks among soldiers. Scrub typhus continues to be a public health threat in southern Asia.[4]

RMSF, caused by infection with *R. rickettsii*, was first identified in the western United States early in the twentieth century. The etiology of the disease, and its transmission by ticks slowly unfolded over the first half of the twentieth century as a result of investigations at the Rocky Mountain Laboratories in Hamilton, Montana, a research station set up by the U.S. Public Health Service with the primary goal of understanding and preventing RMSF.[5] The disease had a high case fatality rate (CFR) in the early part of the twentieth century and was most common in the western states of Idaho, Montana, Wyoming, and Nevada. Today, RMSF is more commonly found in the southeastern United States, with cases also appearing in Arizona and Northern Mexico.[6,7]

Human pathogens among the *Anaplasmataceae* have been more recently discovered. Human ehrlichiosis was first described in the United States in the 1980s.[8] Infection of animals with *Anaplasma* spp. was described more than 100 years ago, but infection of humans with *A. phagocytophilum* was first described in the 1990s as human granulocytic ehrlichiosis, but is now called anaplasmosis.[9]

EPIDEMIOLOGY

Overview

Rickettsial diseases are transmitted to humans by multiple vectors. Rickettsial pathogens discussed here are classified into the SFG rickettsiae, mainly transmitted by ticks; the TG rickettsiae, transmitted infected fleas, lice, and mites; and the transitional group (TRG) containing rickettsialpox, which is transmitted by infected mites.[10] Within the *Anaplasmataceae* family, human infections are caused by species within the genus *Ehrlichia* and the genus *Anaplasma*.

Tick-borne rickettsial pathogens are maintained in natural cycles involving domestic or wild vertebrates and primarily hard-bodied ticks. The epidemiology of each tick-borne rickettsial disease reflects the geographic distribution and seasonal activities of the tick vectors and vertebrate hosts involved in their transmission, as well as the human behaviors that place persons at risk for exposure to ticks and infection. The distribution of tick-borne rickettsial diseases varies geographically both globally and in the United States and approximates the primary tick vector distributions, making it important for healthcare providers to be familiar with the regions where tick-borne rickettsial diseases are common.

Tick-borne rickettsial diseases in humans often share similar clinical features yet are epidemiologically and etiologically distinct. In the United States, these diseases include RMSF, caused by *R. rickettsii*,

TABLE 144-1 RICKETTSIALES CAUSING INFECTION IN HUMANS

Disease	Etiologic Agent	Principal Vector(s)	Natural Hosts of Vector(s)	Geographic Distribution
Rocky Mountain spotted fever	*Rickettsia rickettsii*	*Dermacentor* and *Rhipicephalus* tick species	Various small mammals including rodents, lagomorphs, dogs	North and South America
Rickettsialpox	*Rickettsia akari*	*Mouse mite (Allodermanyssus sanguineus)*	House mouse (*Mus musculus*); other rodents	Worldwide
Rickettsia parkeri rickettsiosis	*Rickettsia parkeri*	Gulf Coast tick (*Amblyomma maculatum*)	Rodents, birds, large mammals	Western hemisphere
Mediterranean spotted fever/ boutonneuse fever/Israeli spotted fever /Astrakahn spotted fever/ Indian tick typhus/Kenyan tick typhus	*Rickettsia conorii*	*Rhipicephalus* tick species	Dogs, small mammals	Mediterranean region, Africa, Black Sea region, Israel, India
African tick bite fever	*Rickettsia africae*	*Amblyomma* tick species	Cattle and wild ungulates	Sub-Saharan Africa, Caribbean
Pacific Coast tick fever	*Rickettsia species 364D*	Pacific Coast tick (*Dermacentor occidentalis*)	Mammals	California
North Asian tick typhus	*Rickettsia sibirica*	*Dermacentor, Haemaphysalis, Rhipicephalus* tick species	Livestock, small mammals (rodents)	Northern Asia, China, Pakistan
Lymphangitis-associated rickettsiosis	*Rickettsia sibirica mongolitimonae*	*Hyalomma* tick species	Cattle, migratory birds	Sub-Saharan Africa, France, Spain, China
Queensland tick typhus	*Rickettsia australis*	*Ixodes* tick species, especially *I. holocyclus*	Small marsupials, rodents	Eastern Australia
Flinders Island spotted fever	*Rickettsia honei*	*Aponomma hydrosauri; Ixodes, Rhipacephalus,* and *Amblyomma* tick species	Reptiles, rodents, cattle, small mammals	Australia, southeast Asia, North America
Japanese spotted fever	*Rickettsia japonica*	Ticks—multiple species	rodents	Japan
Rickettsia heilongjangensis infection	*Rickettsia heilongjangensis*	*Dermacentor* tick species	Mammals	Eastern Asia
Flea-borne spotted fever	*Rickettsia felis*	Cat flea (*Ctenocephalides felis*)	Opossums, cats, rodents	North and South America, Europe, Africa, Asia
DEBONEL/TIBOLA	*Rickettsia slovaca/ Rickettsia raoultii*	*Dermacentor* tick species	Mammals	Europe
Rickettsia helvetica infection	*Rickettsia helvetica*	*Ixodes* tick species	Rodents	Europe, Asia
Rickettsia massiliae infection	*Rickettsia massiliae*	*Rhipicephalus* tick species	Dogs, small mammals	Europe, Africa
Rickettsia monacensis infection	*Rickettsia monacensis*	*Ixodes* tick species		Europe
Rickettsia aeschlimannii infection	*Rickettsia aeschlimannii*	*Hyalomma, Rhipicephalus* tick species	Cattle, sheep, boars, migratory birds (?)	Mediterranean region, eastern Europe, Africa
Rickettsia tamurae infection	*Rickettsia tamurae*	*Amblyomma testudinarium*		Japan
Epidemic typhus/louse-borne typhus	*Rickettsia prowazekii*	Human body louse (*Pediculus humanis corporis*)	Humans, flying squirrels	Africa, Central and South America, Asia
Murine typhus/endemic typhus	*Rickettsia typhi*	Oriental rat flea (*Xenopsylla cheopis*)	*Rattus* species, cats, opossums	Worldwide
Scrub typhus	*Orientia tsutsugamushi*	Larval trombiculid mites (*Leptotrombidium* species)	Small wild rodents, birds	Southeast Asia, Australia, Pacific islands
Ehrlichiosis (*Ehrlichia chaffeensis* infection)	*Ehrlichia chaffeensis*	Lone star ticks (*Amblyomma americanum*)	White-tailed deer	United States, Korea
Ehrlichiosis (*Ehrlichia ewingii* infection)	*Ehrlichia ewingii*	Lone star ticks (*Amblyomma americanum*)	Dogs, white-tailed deer	United States
Ehrlichiosis (*Ehrlichia muris eauclairensis* infection)	*Ehrlichia muris eauclairensis*	*Ixodes scapularis* ticks	Rodents, white-tailed deer	Wisconsin and Minnesota
Anaplasmosis	*Anaplasma phagocytophilum*	*Ixodes scapularis, I. pacificus, I. ricinus*	Rodents, white-tailed deer	United States, Europe
Sennetsu fever	*Neorickettsia sennetsu*	Trematodes	Fish	Japan

and other SFG rickettsioses, caused by *R. parkeri* and *Rickettsia* species 364D. Globally, tick-borne rickettsial infections include African tick bite fever (ATBF); MSF, also known as Boutonneuse fever; and other diseases such as Japanese spotted fever (JSF).[11]

Spotted Fever Group Rickettsiae

Rocky Mountain Spotted Fever

RMSF, caused by *R. rickettsii*, is the best known and most severe of the tick-borne rickettsioses. RMSF has been recognized as a distinct entity in the United States since the late 1800s; various researchers, including Ricketts in Montana (1906), defined the disease and described the natural cycle of the agent. RMSF is the rickettsiosis in the United States that is associated with the highest rates of severe and fatal outcomes. It is also the etiologic agent of spotted fevers in Central and South America.

The vectors of *R. rickettsii* organisms are various ixodid ticks, which also serve as a reservoir for *R. rickettsii* because of the passage of the RMSF agent by transovarial transmission. Ticks may also become infected by feeding on rickettsemic vertebrate hosts such as rodents, small- and medium-sized mammals, and dogs.

In the United States, the tick species that is most frequently associated with transmission of *R. rickettsii* is the American dog tick, *Dermacentor variabilis*. This tick is found primarily in the eastern, central, and Pacific coastal United States. The Rocky Mountain wood tick, *Dermacentor andersoni*, is associated with transmission in the western United States. *D. variabilis* ticks often are encountered in wooded, shrubby, and grassy areas and tend to congregate along walkways and trails. These ticks also can be found in residential areas and city parks. Larval and nymphal stages of most *Dermacentor* spp. ticks in the United States usually do not bite humans. Although adult *D. variabilis* and *D. andersoni* ticks bite humans, the principal hosts tend to be deer, dogs, and livestock. Adult *Dermacentor* ticks are active from spring through autumn, with maximum activity during late spring through early summer.

The brown dog tick, *Rhipicephalus sanguineus*, was recognized as a vector of *R. rickettsii* in Mexico as early as the 1940s.[12] It is located throughout the United States, and is recognized as an important vector in parts of Arizona and along the U.S.-Mexico border.[6,7] In the United States, *Rhipicephalus*-transmitted *R. rickettsii* was not identified until 2003, when it was confirmed in a child on tribal lands in Arizona.[7] Commonly, domestic dogs are the preferred hosts for the brown dog tick in all of its life stages. Humans are often bitten incidentally from coming into contact with tick-infested dogs or environments such as yards or houses. Heavily parasitized dogs, as well as sizable infestations of brown dog ticks in and around homes, have been found in affected communities with *Rhipicephalus*-transmitted *R. rickettsii*.[7,13,14] Infection can be clustered in affected communities as a result of free-roaming dogs spreading infected ticks within their range. Children aged < 10 years represent more than half of reported cases in Arizona.[7,15] The majority of human cases of RMSF occur during July–October after seasonal monsoon rains; however, cases have been reported every month of the year.[15].[16,17] *Rh. sanguineus* is found worldwide and it could also play a role in transmission of RMSF in regions of South America.[18,19]

Other Spotted Fever Rickettsioses

A recently recognized spotted fever rickettsiosis in North America is caused by *Rickettia parkeri*. *R. parkeri* rickettsiosis has similar signs and symptoms to RMSF, including fever, rash, and headache, as well as an eschar typically at the site of the tick bite.[20] It was originally isolated from *Amblyomma maculatum*, the Gulf Coast tick, in Texas in 1939.[21] In 2002, *R. parkeri* was cultured and identified from patient specimens.[20] *R. parkeri* has also been detected in Uruguay in *A. triste*, a tick species that feeds on humans, and may be responsible for cases in South America.[22] In the United States, *A. maculatum* is distributed throughout all the states bordering the Gulf of Mexico, and extends into southern, mid-Atlantic, and central states. *R. parkeri* has been detected in ticks from many of these states. *R. parkeri* rickettsiosis can resemble other SFG rickettsioses such as RMSF, and can also resemble rickettsialpox.[23]

During the early part of this century, ATBF was recognized as a rural tick-borne disease of the African continent, and at the time was considered synonymous with MSF. However, two distinct clinical presentations of rash-like illness occurring after tick bites were noted during the 1930s in southern Africa.[24] One was consistent with MSF, which was usually associated with urban environments, but the other was found in patients with a history of travel into the bush and contact with game, cattle, and ticks. In 1992, after a human case of ATBF was diagnosed in Zimbabwe, the strain was characterized as *R. africae*.[25] The most important vectors and reservoirs of ATBF are *Amblyomma* ticks, principally *A. hebraeum* in southern Africa, and *A. variegatum* in central, west, and east Africa. The major hosts of *Amblyomma* ticks are cattle and wild ungulates, but these ticks will feed on any available host. Most reported cases of ATBF have been diagnosed in travelers returning from trips to Africa, although less than 50% reported tick bites.[26] *R. africae* has also been detected in *A. variegatum* in several islands of the West Indies.

In the United States, the number of travelers to Africa have been increasing over the last decade, and in 2015 almost 1 million persons from the United States traveled to Africa.[27] Globally, ATBF is the second most commonly reported cause of febrile illness in travelers returning from sub-Saharan Africa after malaria.[28] ATBF can present with multiple eschars, and cases can occur in clusters.[28] Activities such as working on a farm or walking in a game park have been linked to clusters of infected persons.[29]

MSF, also known as Boutonneuse fever, is caused by *R. conorii* and has been reported from southern Europe, Asia, the Middle East, India, and Africa.[26,30] Strains closely related to MSF include Kenya tick typhus, Astrakhan fever, Israeli tick typhus, and Indian tick typhus. The brown dog tick, *R. sanguineus*, is the principal vector and reservoir of MSF.[31] Adult *R. sanguineus* ticks preferentially feed on dogs, and are found in the peridomestic environment, including houses and kennels. The immature stages may be more likely to feed on other hosts in addition to dogs, and human cases usually occur during late spring, summer, and early fall when all stages of *R. sanguineus* are abundant. Patients with MSF usually give a history of exposure to high grass or bushes and contact with dogs, although a history of tick bite is often not reported.

Another rickettsiosis of the SFG caused by *R. japonica*, has been described in Japan.[32] JSF can cause fever, headache, and a characteristic rash with 90% of cases reporting an eschar.[33] The most probable vectors of *R. japonica* are *Haemaphysalis flava* and *longicornis*, and *Ixodes ovatus*. In Australia, *R. australis* has been identified as the etiologic agent of North Queensland tick typhus which has been found to occur along the eastern coast. The only two tick vectors currently identified are *I. holocyclus* and *I. tasmani*.[34]

Pacific Coast tick fever is a SFG rickettsiosis found in California and caused by infection with *Rickettsia* species 364D.[35] The Pacific Coast tick (*Dermacentor occidentalis*), one of the most widely distributed and frequently encountered tick species in California, is its primary vector.[36] Important questions still remain regarding its classification and taxonomic status. Potential genotypic variations among different strains of this species may influence its pathogenicity.

Typhus Group

Scrub Typhus

Scrub typhus (also known as tsutsugamushi disease, mite-borne typhus, Japanese-river fever, tropical typhus, and rural typhus) is caused by *O. tsutsugamushi* (formerly *R. tsutsugamushi*), which exhibits genetic, antigenic, and pathogenic diversity with numerous serotypes recognized.[37] *O. tsutsugamushi* strains are distributed widely throughout southeastern Asia, the islands of the western Pacific, and northern Australia. Scrub typhus was a frequent source of illness in U.S. troops during World War II in the South Pacific and during the Vietnam conflict. It is transmitted to humans by larval mites, also referred to as chiggers.[38]

Globally, scrub typhus remains a leading cause of illness in indigenous populations throughout endemic areas, especially in rural areas of Southeast Asia, Indonesia, China, Japan, India, and northern Australia. Cases of scrub typhus most frequently occur among farmers, forestry workers, and others involved in outdoor occupations or recreational activities.[38] In North America, scrub typhus is primarily diagnosed among returning travelers.[39] There has been a reemergence of scrub typhus in recent years. Recent outbreaks have occurred in Nepal, Bhutan, India, China, Australia, Thailand, and the Solomon Islands.[38]

Scrub typhus is transmitted to humans following the bite of trombiculid mites, also known as chiggers. The agent is found in the feces and saliva of the larval mites and enters the body through abraded skin after the mites feed. Trombiculid mites of the subgenus *Leptotrombidium* serve as both vectors and reservoirs due to transovarial transmission of *O. tsutsugamushi*. Their normal hosts are wild rodent species that have also been found to be reservoirs for the agent. Transmission may be affected by seasonal exposure of humans, or by chigger activity that is dependent on temperature, humidity, and availability of rodent hosts. No person-to-person transmission has been documented.[38]

Endemic Typhus

Murine typhus (also known as endemic or flea-borne typhus) is caused by the agent *R. typhi*, which is transmitted by the Oriental rat flea *Xenopsylla cheopis*. The reservoir of *R. typhi* is *Rattus rattus* and other rodent species. Murine typhus occurs in tropical, subtropical, and temperate zones throughout the world, principally in Southeast Asia, Africa, Central America, and the Mediterranean region.[40] In the United States, it is most prevalent in Texas, southern California, and Hawaii.[41] While rates of murine typhus declined in the United States after efforts to control rat fleas were introduced in the 1940s, it now appears to be increasing, especially from southern Texas and California.[42] In these cases, the agent appears to be transmitted by the cat flea, *Ctenocephalides felis*. Murine typhus occurs primarily in seaports, urban areas, and certain rural settings infested by wild rats (e.g., grain-storage facilities). A seasonal incidence peak occurs in late summer and fall, although the disease peaks in late spring and early summer along the Gulf Coast. The main life cycle involves a reservoir of rodents (principally *R. rattus* and *R. norvegicus*) and the vector, *X. cheopis*. The rat flea acquires *R. typhi* by feeding on an infected host, remains infected for life, and is capable of transmitting the rickettsiae to its offspring. *R. typhi* multiplies in the flea and is excreted in the feces, which can contaminate skin breaks or mucous membranes. Direct flea bites or inhalation of aerosolized feces may also cause infection. The human flea, *Pulex irritans*, and the human body louse may also play a role in transmission. Numerous wild vertebrates are natural hosts and may bring infected fleas into close proximity to humans. Dog and cat fleas have been suspected as occasional vectors for humans. There is no documented person-to-person transmission. In the United States, transmission of *R. typhi* involving the cat flea as the principal vector and the opossum (*Didelphis virginiana*) as well as *Rattus* spp. as the reservoirs has been demonstrated in suburban areas.[42]

Epidemic Typhus

Epidemic typhus, also called louse-borne typhus, is an uncommon disease caused by infection with *R. prowazekii*. Epidemic typhus is spread to people through contact with infected body lice. It is the only rickettsial disease that has been associated with explosive outbreaks in the past.[43] Though epidemic typhus was responsible for millions of deaths in previous centuries, it is now rare. Occasionally, cases occur in areas with extreme overcrowding. This disease has disappeared from much of the world except in remote areas of Africa, Asia, and Central and South America. It may, however, reappear under conditions of war or natural disasters where crowding and unsanitary conditions may prevail.

In the United States, rare cases of epidemic typhus, called sylvatic typhus, can occur.[44] These cases of epidemic typhus have been associated with exposure to flying squirrels or their nests. Fleas and lice carried by the squirrels become naturally infected with *R. prowazekii*; however, the exact mechanism of transmission remains unknown.

R. prowazekii is transmitted by the human body louse, *Pediculus humanus corporis*. Lice become infected when feeding on actively infected humans. The rickettsiae multiply within the louse and are excreted in the feces. There is no transovarial or transtadial transmission. Humans become infected when the organisms enter the body through the bite lesion or through skin abraded from scratching. Other potential mechanisms of infection include mucosal contact or inhalation of dried louse feces. The lice die within 10–12 days of infection; however, *R. prowazekii* may remain viable for up to 100 days in the dried state. Transmission between humans usually requires close personal contact or exposure to contaminated clothing or bedding. The agent is not shed in human secretions, so there is no direct person-to-person transmission.

Humans are the main reservoir of epidemic *R. prowazekii*.[45] The southern flying squirrel, *Glaucomys volans*, found in the eastern United States, has also been implicated as an animal reservoir.[44] Flea species that parasitize rodents have been found to be infected with *R. prowazekii*; however, no specific arthropod vectors have been identified. This flying squirrel-associated typhus agent may have a lower virulence than the louse-borne variant, and better health, hygiene and living conditions, and appropriate antimicrobial treatment might also explain the decreased (<1%) CFR.[45]

Transitional Group

Rickettsialpox

R. akari, the causative agent of rickettsialpox, is transmitted by house-mouse mites, and is known to circulate in mainly urban centers in Ukraine, South Africa, Korea, the Balkan states, and the United States. Outbreaks of rickettsialpox most often occur after contact with infected rodents and their mites, especially during natural die-offs or exterminations of infected rodents that cause the mites to seek out new hosts, including humans.[46] The agent may spill over and occasionally be found in other wild rodent populations. Rickettsialpox or vesicular rickettsiosis was first recognized as a distinct clinical entity in apartment dwellers in New York City in 1946. Cases were subsequently detected in several other cities in the northeastern United States, with an annual incidence of nearly 200 cases.[47] In the last few decades, only a few cases per year have been confirmed in the United States. The mite also serves as a reservoir since transstadial and transovarial transmission of the agent has been documented. Rickettsialpox is a relatively mild disease.

Anaplasmatacea

Overview Human ehrlichiosis cases are primarily caused by *E. chaffeensis*, *E. ewingii*, **or** *E. muris eauclairensis* in the United States. These bacteria are primarily spread to people by the bite of an infected tick. Anaplasmosis, also known as human granulocytic anaplasmosis, is also tick-borne, and is caused by the bacterium *A. phagocytophilum*. There are reports of other primarily animal *Ehrlichia* species that may cause disease in humans including *E. canis*, the agent of canine monocytic ehrlichiosis, among others.[10] Each ehrlichial species targets different cells, such as neutrophils, monocytes, erythrocytes, platelets, and endothelial cells. They cause mild to severe febrile illness with occasional rash; however, in elderly or immunocompromised persons, the illness may be severe and result in multiorgan failure.

The geographic range of ehrlichiosis cases depends highly on the species of *Ehrlichia* causing illness. *E. chaffeensis* and *E. ewingii* infections occur primarily in south-central, southeastern, and mid-Atlantic States. *E. muris eauclairensis* infections have been reported from Wisconsin and Minnesota. The majority of cases reported to CDC have an illness onset during the summer months with a peak in cases typically occurring in June and July.[48–50]

Ehrlichiosis, previously referred to as human monocytic ehrlichiosis (HME), was first recognized as a human disease in the United States in the late 1980s but did not become a reportable disease until 1999. In the United States, the majority of reported cases are due to infection by *E. chaffeensis*.

Ehrlichia Chafeensis

In 1987, an acute, febrile syndrome similar to RMSF was first reported in humans. The etiologic agent of HME was identified as *E. chaffeensis*[51] and found to be transmitted by the vector, *A. americanum*, the lone star tick.[52] The definitive host of *A. americanum* is the white-tailed deer, *Odocoileus virginianus*, which has also been found to be the principal wildlife reservoir for *E. chaffeensis*. There is transstadial transmission of *E. chaffeensis* in *A. americanum*, but transovarial transmission has not been proven. Numerous wild and domestic mammals serve as hosts for the immature stages of the vector tick; however, their roles as reservoirs have not been well studied.

The number of ehrlichiosis cases due to *E. chaffeensis* reported in the United States has increased steadily since the disease reporting began. In 2000, only 200 cases of ehrlichiosis were reported, while in 2016 more than 1377 cases were reported.[53] The number of cases and disease incidence has risen since 2000; however, the CFR has declined since then. The published CFR of ehrlichiosis remains at roughly 1%.[54]

Cases of ehrlichiosis can occur during any month of the year; however, the majority of cases reported in the United States occur during the summer months with a peak in cases typically occurring in June and July. This coincides with the season for increased numbers of adult and nymphal lone star ticks. All stages of this tick feed on humans; however, only adult and nymphal ticks spread *E. chaffeensis* to humans.[54]

Ehrlichiosis is most frequently reported from the southeastern and south-central United States, from the Eastern Coast extending westward to Texas. These areas align with the geographic distribution of the lone star tick. In 2016, four states (Missouri, Arkansas, New York, and Virginia) accounted for 50% of all reported cases of ehrlichiosis in the United States.

Ehrlichia Muris Eauclairensis

An *E. muris*-like agent (EMLA), now called *E. muris eauclairensis*, causes a novel form of human ehrlichiosis in the upper Midwestern United States.[50,55] To date, all infected tick and vertebrate hosts of this pathogen have originated from Minnesota and Wisconsin, and it is transmitted by *I. scapularis* ticks.[49]

Anaplasmosis

A. phagocytophilum causes human anaplasmosis, which was previously known as both human granulocytic anaplasmosis and human granulocytic ehrlichiosis. Anaplasmosis was first characterized in the United States in 1992 when an agent resembling *E. equi* and *E. phagocytophila* was found to cause disease in humans.[9] These were subsequently reclassified into a single species, *A. phagocytophilum*.[56] It did not become a reportable disease in the United States until 1999.

The number of anaplasmosis cases reported in the United States has increased steadily from 348 cases in 2000, to 4151 cases in 2016. The incidence of anaplasmosis has also increased, from 1.4 cases per million persons in 2000 to 6.1 cases per million persons in 2010.[57] Reported cases are highest in the northeastern and upper Midwestern states, and the geographic range of anaplasmosis appears to be expanding.[57,58] The reported case-fatality rate during 2008–12 was 0.3% and was higher among persons aged $\geq$ 70 years and those with immunosuppression.[57]

A. phagocytophilum is transmitted by *I. scapularis*, the deer or black-legged tick. The tick vector in California is *I. pacificus*. The white-footed mouse, *Peromyscus leucopus*, is believed to be the principal reservoir, in addition to other mammals such as gray squirrels, raccoons, striped skunks, and opossums. Cases of anaplasmosis have also been diagnosed in Europe, where the principal tick vector is *I. ricinus*.[59]

Although cases of anaplasmosis can occur during any month, the majority occur during the summer months, typically with a peak in June and July. This corresponds to the period of increased numbers of nymphal black-legged ticks, which is the primary life stage of this tick that bites humans and can transmit the pathogen, are also found. A second, smaller peak occurs in October and November and matches the period of increased adult blacklegged tick activity.[57,60]

CLINICAL MANIFESTATIONS

SFG Rickettsiae

General symptoms shared amongst the Spotted Fever Group Rickettsioses (SFGR) include fever, rash, and nausea. The rash is variable but can sometimes help to differentiate the SFGR diseases from one another. Ocular manifestations of SFGRs (including conjunctivitis, anterior uveitis, and retinitis) are common, but they are frequently asymptomatic or self-limited, and so they may be overlooked.[61]

Rocky Mountain Spotted Fever

Symptoms of RMSF typically appear 3–12 days after the bite of an infected tick.[62] The incubation period is generally shorter (5 days or less) in patients who develop severe disease.[63] Initial symptoms include sudden onset of fever, severe headache, chills, malaise, and myalgia. Other early symptoms can include nausea or vomiting, abdominal pain, anorexia, and photophobia. A rash typically appears 2–4 days after the onset of fever; however, most patients initially seek healthcare before appearance of a rash.[64–66] The classic triad of fever, rash, and reported tick bite is present in only a minority of patients during initial presentation[64,67]; therefore, healthcare providers should not wait for development of this triad before considering a diagnosis of RMSF.

The RMSF rash typically begins as small (1–5 mm in diameter), blanching, pink macules on the ankles, wrists, or forearms that subsequently spread to the palms, soles, arms, legs, and trunk, usually sparing the face. The classic spotted or generalized petechial rash, including involvement of the palms and soles and sometimes associated with edema,[68] can appear by day 5 or 6 and is indicative of advanced disease. Absence of rash should not preclude consideration of RMSF; $<$ 50% of patients have a rash in the first 3 days of illness, and a smaller percentage of patients never develop a rash.[64,67] The rash might be atypical, localized, faint, or evanescent,[69] and skin pigmentation might make a rash difficult to recognize. The rash may be easily confused with those of other infectious or noninfectious etiologies. Children aged $<$ 15 years more frequently have a rash than older patients and develop the rash earlier in the course of illness.[67,70,71] Lack of rash or late-onset rash in RMSF has been associated with delays in diagnosis and increased mortality.[65,67,72] Unlike some SFG rickettsioses, an inoculation eschar is rarely present with RMSF.[73,74] Thrombocytopenia, anemia, elevated liver function tests, coagulopathy, renal failure, pulmonary edema, and involvement of all organ systems may be seen. Other clinical features that have been observed in association with RMSF include abdominal pain that mimics acute appendicitis,[75] cholecystitis,[76] or gastroenteritis; diarrhea; conjunctival suffusion; periorbital and peripheral edema (more common in children); calf pain; acute transient hearing loss; hepatomegaly; and splenomegaly.[67,77]

Severe, late-stage manifestations of RMSF can include meningoencephalitis, acute renal failure, acute respiratory distress syndrome

(ARDS), cutaneous necrosis, shock, arrhythmia, and seizures. Focal neurologic deficits can occur, including cranial or peripheral motor nerve paralysis, or sudden transient hearing loss;[78–80] long-term neurological sequelae can also be observed.[81]

Clinical suspicion for RMSF should be maintained in cases of nonspecific febrile illness and sepsis of unclear etiology, particularly during spring and summer months. Delay in diagnosis and treatment is the most important factor associated with increased likelihood of death, and early empiric therapy is the best way to prevent RMSF progression. Without treatment, RMSF progresses rapidly. Patients treated after the fifth day of illness are more likely to die than those treated earlier in the course of illness.[65,82–84] The frequency of hospital admission, intensive-care unit admission, and death increases with time from symptom onset to initiation of appropriate antibacterial treatment.[83] Delays in diagnosis and initiation of antirickettsial therapy have been associated with seeking healthcare early in the course of the illness due to the nonspecific nature of early symptoms.[65,70] Other factors associated with delayed diagnosis and therapy include late-onset or absence of rash,[67,83] and nonspecific or atypical early manifestations, such as gastrointestinal symptoms[66,83] or absence of headache.[84] Epidemiologic factors associated with increased risk for death include disease that occurs early or late in the typical tick season[65] and the lack of a report of a tick bite.[66,82,84]

RMSF is the most frequently fatal rickettsial illness in the United States; the case-fatality rate in the preantibiotic era was approximately 25%.[85–87] Present-day case-fatality rates, estimated at 5–10% overall, depend in part on the timing of initiation of appropriate treatment; case-fatality rates of 40–50% among patients treated on day 8 or 9 of illness have been described.[18] Additional risk factors for fatal RMSF include age $\geq$40 years, age $<$10 years, and alcohol abuse.[83,84,88,89] Glucose-6-phosphate dehydrogenase deficiency is a risk factor for fulminant RMSF, and death can occur in $\leq$5 days.[90] Experimental and accumulated anecdotal clinical data suggest that treatment of patients with RMSF using a sulfonamide antimicrobial can result in increased disease severity and death.[91,92]

Long-term neurologic sequelae of RMSF include cognitive impairment; paraparesis; hearing loss; blindness; peripheral neuropathy; bowel and bladder incontinence; cerebellar, vestibular, and motor dysfunction; and speech disorders.[78,93,94] These complications are observed most frequently in persons recovering from severe, life-threatening disease, often after lengthy hospitalizations, and are most likely the result of *R. rickettsii*-induced vasculopathy. Cutaneous necrosis and gangrene might result in amputation of digits or limbs.[77] Long-term or persistent infection by *R. rickettsii* has not been observed.

Mediterranean Spotted Fever R. Conorii

MSF is a mild to moderately severe illness with an incubation period ranging from 6 to 10 days. It is less frequently associated with the progressive, hemorrhagic tendency of RMSF. An abrupt onset of high fever may be accompanied by headache, arthralgia, and myalgia lasting a few days to 2 weeks.[95,96] A maculopapular rash appears by approximately the third day in 96% of cases. It can persist for 6–7 days and is usually generalized. A single eschar (tache noir) is present at the site of tick attachment in 30–90% of cases. Antibiotic therapy shortens the course and severity of the illness. The disease is usually self-limited, but 10% of cases may have severe complications such as neurological involvement or multiorgan failure, with an overall CFR of 2.5%.

African Tick Bite Fever

Patients with ATBF typically have fever, headache, myalgia, one or more inoculation eschars, regional lymphadenopathy, and sometimes maculopapular or vesicular rash.[97,98] The incubation period is typically 5–7 days but can be up to 10 days after the bite of an infected *A. hebraeum* or *A. variegatum* tick.[97,98] The course of illness is usually mild. Complications are rare and no fatal cases have been reported.

Rickettsia Parkeri

A newly recognized spotted fever rickettsiosis in North and South America is caused by *R. parkeri*, which has been associated with fever, headache, myalgia, fatigue, an eschar, regional lymphadenopathy, and a generalized rash appearing 6–10 days after tick attachment.[99] The rash is normally present on the trunk, extremities, palms, and soles. Symptoms of *R. parkeri* are similar to RMSF, but *R. parkeri* patients often present with an eschar at the site of tick attachment. A mild fever can be seen with this disease, a low hospitalization rate has been seen, and no case fatalities have been reported.[23]

Rickettsia Japonica and Others

JSF was described in 1984 as an emerging SFG rickettsiosis from Japan and South Korea. It has been found to cause fever, headache, and the characteristic rash, with 90% of cases reporting an eschar.[32,33] The incubation period is 2–8 days, with rash first on extremities and then spreading to the trunk. Patients can develop acute infectious purpura fulminans,[100] and disease can be severe or fatal. *R. slovaca* infection has been described in Spain as "Dermacentor-borne necrosis erythema lymphadenopathy" (DEBONEL). After a median incubation period of 4–5 days, disease presents with a necrotic eschar at the site of a *Dermacentor marginatus* tick bite, surrounding erythema, and painful regional lymphadenopathy.[101–103] *R. sibirica mongolotimonae* has been found in *Hyalomma* species ticks and humans in China, Niger, France, and South Africa. Symptoms include one or two inoculation eschars, fever, maculopapular rash, and lymphangitis.[104] Infection with *R. helvetica* in Europe and Asia has presented clinically as a mild febrile illness with no cutaneous rash.[105,106] *R. heilongjiangensis* has been isolated in China in *D. sylvarum* ticks and has been found to cause rickettsial-like disease in humans in eastern Russia.[107] *Rickettsia* species 364D, initially identified in California ticks, displays generally mild clinical features characterized by eschar, fever, headache, malaise, and lymphadenopathy.[108]

Typhus Group

Scrub Typhus

The clinical spectrum of scrub typhus is broad, with most infections of mild to moderate severity. After an incubation period of 7–21 days, the first sign of disease in 85–90% of patients is a vesicular lesion at the site of mite feeding, which later becomes an eschar or ulcer, with regional lymphadenopathy. Fever commences a few days later, generally accompanied by headache, myalgia, and occasionally conjunctivitis or cough. A maculopapular rash may appear at the end of the first week, starting on the chest, abdomen, and trunk, and spreading to involve the proximal arms and legs. Rarely, the rash may spread to the face, palms, and soles. In severe cases, pneumonitis, encephalitis, cardiomyopathy, and septic shock may occur,[109] with mortality ranging from 5% to 40% if no antibiotic therapy is given. The course of the disease and prognosis may vary depending on the strain. Infection with one strain provides only short-term immunity against subsequent infection by others, and immunity even to homologous strains lasts for only 1–3 years. Nevertheless, second and even third attacks may be milder or atypical.

Murine Typhus (Rickettsia Typhi)

The incubation period for *R. typhi* is 1–2 weeks. Disease is characterized by an abrupt onset of symptoms, usually fever and severe headache. Fever lasts 1–2 weeks, often accompanied by persistent headache, myalgia, vomiting, abdominal pains, conjunctivitis, splenomegaly, and pneumonitis; delirium, stupor, or coma occurs rarely. Between the fifth and seventh day a macular rash usually appears in 50–80% of the patients, starting on the chest and abdomen, and spreading to the back and proximal limbs over 2–3 days. Fever subsides within 2–3 days after initiation of treatment. Without treatment, symptoms may resolve within 2 weeks. Death occurs in approximately 1% of cases, and a single attack confers immunity. Delayed neurologic sequelae can occasionally occur and may resolve over time.

Epidemic Typhus (Rickettsia Prowazekii)

After an incubation period of 1–2 weeks, clinical symptoms of epidemic typhus usually appear abruptly with the onset of fever, chills, headache, muscle aches, and generalized weakness. Approximately 5 days later, a maculopapular rash can develop, beginning on the trunk and spreading to the limbs. The rash may become darker and confluent, covering the entire body, but usually sparing the face, palms, and soles. During the second week, neurological symptoms may develop resulting in delirium or coma. The CFR in untreated cases can exceed 10–15%.[110] Chronic infection or late relapse and long-term persistence in lymph nodes or other tissues have been documented.[111] Epidemic typhus may recur decades later in recovered patients—as an illness known as Brill-Zinsser disease, which usually has a milder presentation with little or no rash.

Transitional Group

Rickettsialpox

After an incubation period of 9–14 days, a papular lesion with surrounding erythema develops at the site of mite feeding, accompanied by regional lymphadenopathy. The papule ulcerates centrally, forming an eschar. Systemic symptoms, including fever, headache, backache, myalgias, and occasionally photophobia, develop approximately 1 week after the initial lesion. Within a few days of the onset of symptoms, a generalized maculopapular rash develops on the face, trunk, and extremities, but not on the palms and soles. The rash, which can resemble chickenpox, becomes vesicular, and eventually heals without scarring. Rickettsialpox is a relatively mild disease. Symptoms resolve within 6–10 days and recovery can occur without treatment.

Anaplasmataceae

Symptoms of infections with agents of the Anaplasmataceae family generally include nonspecific signs such as headache, myalgia, malaise, and fever. Other symptoms can include arthralgia, nausea, and cough. Rash only occurs in about 10% of patients.[112,113] The severity of ehrlichiosis could be related, in part, to host factors such as age and the immune status of the patient. Ehrlichial species cause mild to severe febrile illness with occasional rash; however, in elderly or immunocompromised persons, the illness may be severe and result in multiorgan failure. Between 2008 and 2012, the hospitalization rate for ehrlichiosis was 57% and the CFR was 1%. Children aged < 5 years had the highest CFR, at 4%.[114]

Signs and symptoms commonly seen with ehrlichiosis include fever, chills, headache, malaise, muscle pain, gastrointestinal symptoms (nausea, vomiting, diarrhea, anorexia), altered mental status, and rash (more commonly reported among children). It is important to note that few people will exhibit all symptoms, and the number and combination of symptoms varies greatly from person to person.

Ehrlichia Chaffeensis Erlichiosis

Symptoms of *E. chaffeensis* ehrlichiosis typically appear after a mean incubation period of 7–9 days (range: 5–14 days) following the bite of an infected tick.[115] Fever (96%), headache (72%), malaise (77%), and myalgia (68%) are common signs and symptoms. Gastrointestinal signs such as nausea (57%), vomiting (47%), and diarrhea (25%) can be prominent.[112] Gastrointestinal manifestations may be more common among children,[116] although ehrlichiosis has been mistaken for acute appendicitis during pregnancy.[117] Approximately one-third of patients develop a skin rash during the course of illness; rash occurs more frequently in children than in adults. Rash patterns vary in character from petechial or maculopapular to diffuse erythema[115,118] and typically occur a median of 5 days after illness onset.[8] The rash typically involves the extremities and trunk but can affect the palms, soles, or face.[119] Cough or respiratory symptoms are reported in approximately 28% of patients and are more common among adults.[8,112,120] Central nervous system involvement, such as meningitis or meningoencephalitis, is present in approximately 20% of patients.[121]

Other severe manifestations include ARDS, toxic shock-like or septic shock-like syndromes, renal failure, hepatic failure, coagulopathies, and occasionally, hemorrhagic manifestations.[118] *E. chaffeensis* infection can rarely trigger hemophagocytic lymphohistiocytosis.[122–125] Severe cases have been mistaken for thrombotic thrombocytopenic purpura[126] and fulminant hepatitis.[127]

E. chaffeensis ehrlichiosis can cause severe disease or death, although at lower rates than have been observed for RMSF. Approximately 3% of patients with symptoms severe enough to seek medical attention die from the infection.[115,120] More than 40% of *E. chaffeensis* cases require hospitalization. On the basis of U.S. passive surveillance and some case series reports, case-fatality rates among persons who are immunosuppressed may be higher than those among the general population[54,128,129]; delays in recognition and initiation of appropriate antibacterial treatment in this population can contribute to increased mortality.[130] Although older age (≥60 years) and immunosuppression are risk factors for severe ehrlichiosis,[8,54,128] many cases of severe or fatal ehrlichiosis have been described in previously healthy children and young adults.[115] Pediatric patients frequently have an asymptomatic or a mild infection[115,120]; however, children aged <10 years have the highest case-fatality rate among passively reported cases.[54,128] Severe ehrlichial illness may occur after treatment of the infection with a sulfonamide antimicrobial agent.[131–133] Confirmed reinfection with *E. chaffeensis* has been described in an immunosuppressed patient[134]; but, the frequency of reinfection in immunocompetent persons is unknown.

Erlichia Ewingii

E. ewingii has been recognized as a cause of ehrlichiosis in humans, especially among those that are immunosuppressed. Symptoms generally begin 7–14 days after exposure to an infected tick.[114] Rash is rare.[71] Leukopenia, thrombocytopenia, and elevations in serum hepatic aminotransferase levels are frequent laboratory findings.[112] Severe illness may include cough, diarrhea, confusion, and lymphadenopathy in adults, and edema of the hands or feet in children.[112] When left untreated or when treatment is delayed, severe complications such as ARDS, a disseminated intravascular coagulation-like syndrome (DIC), central nervous system involvement, and renal failure[112,128] may occur. Infection by *E. ewingii* usually results in milder illness than *E. chaffeensis*, and no *E. ewingii* deaths have been reported.[71,115]

Ehrlichia Muris Subsp. Eauclairensis

Human infection with *E. muris* subsp. *eauclairensis* causes an illness characterized by fever, headache, myalgias, lymphopenia, and thrombocytopenia.[50] Although fatal cases of disease caused by *E. chaffeensis* have been reported, no deaths have been reported due to *E. ewingii* or *E. muris* subsp. *eauclairensis*.

Anaplasma Phagocytophilum

Symptoms of anaplasmosis typically appear 5–14 days after the bite of an infected tick and usually include fever (92–100%), headache (82%), malaise (97%), myalgia (77%), and shaking chills.[112] Other symptoms include arthralgia, nausea, and cough. Rash is rare (<10% of patients), and compared with *E. chaffeensis* ehrlichiosis and RMSF, gastrointestinal symptoms are less frequent and central nervous system involvement is rare.[112,113] Patients with anaplasmosis typically seek medical care 4–8 days after onset, which is later in the course of illness than patients with other tick-borne rickettsial diseases (2–4 days after onset).[135] Once hospitalized, approximately 7% of patients will require admission to an intensive care unit.[60,128]

In most cases, anaplasmosis is a self-limiting illness. In healthy adults, the disease is usually mild and may be asymptomatic. However, in the elderly or immunocompromised, anaplasmosis may be severe with multiorgan failure. Severe or life-threatening manifestations are less frequent with anaplasmosis than with RMSF or *E. chaffeensis* ehrlichiosis; however, ARDS, peripheral neuropathies,

DIC-like coagulopathies, hemorrhagic manifestations, rhabdomyolysis, pancreatitis, and acute renal failure have been reported. Severe anaplasmosis can also resemble toxic shock syndrome, thrombotic thrombocytopenic purpura,[136] or hemophagocytic syndromes.[137] Serious and fatal opportunistic viral and fungal infections during the course of anaplasmosis infection have been described. The case-fatality rate among patients who seek healthcare for anaplasmosis is < 1%. Predictors of severe anaplasmosis include advanced patient age, immunosuppression, comorbid medical conditions such as diabetes, and delay in diagnosis and treatment.[60]

DIAGNOSIS

SFG Rickettsiae

Indirect immunofluorescence antibody (IFA) assays using paired acute and convalescent sera are the reference standard for serologic confirmation of rickettsial infection.[138] The IFA assay consists of rickettsial antigens fixed on a slide and then detected by specific antibodies in patient serum, which can then be identified by a fluorescein-labeled conjugate. IFA assays for immunoglobulin G (IgG) antibodies, the recommended serologic method for confirming tick-borne rickettsial disease in the United States,[139,140] are insensitive during the first week of rickettsial infection, when most patients seek medical attention and have specimens collected for evaluation.[141] As the illness progresses past 7 days, pathogen-specific antibody production increases, and the sensitivity of IFA assays generally improves.[141] Since IFA assays are most sensitive 2–3 weeks after illness onset, results of assays on serum samples collected in the acute and convalescent (2–4 weeks later) phases of illness are best interpreted in tandem.[142,143] IgG IFA testing of at least two serum samples collected, ideally, 2–4 weeks apart, during acute and convalescent phases of illness, is recommended serologic confirmation of SFG rickettsioses, ehrlichioses, or anaplasmosis.[139,140,144] The diagnosis is confirmed if a fourfold or greater increase in antibody titer between these two samples is seen.[139,140] The diagnosis can be supported by one or more samples with an IgG antibody reciprocal titer $\geq$ 64 in patients with a clinically compatible acute illness.[139,140] A single elevated antibody titer is never sufficient to confirm acute infection with a rickettsial pathogen.

Culture generally represents the reference standard for microbiological diagnosis[145]; however, rickettsial agents are obligate intracellular pathogens and must be isolated from patient samples using cell culture techniques that are not widely available. Theoretically, any laboratory capable of performing routine viral isolations has the expertise to isolate these pathogens; however, *R. rickettsii* is classified as a biosafety level 3 (BSL-3) agent, and attempts to isolate this agent should be made only in laboratories equipped for and with laboratorians trained to work with BSL-3 pathogens.[146] Clinical specimens used to inoculate cell cultures should be collected before the start of appropriate antibacterial therapy and preferably not frozen.

Diagnostic assays should always be ordered and interpreted in the context of a compatible illness and appropriate epidemiologic setting to obtain optimal positive and negative predictive values.[144] Misuse of specialized assays for patients with a low pretest probability of a rickettsial disease can result in confusion. For example, antirickettsial antibodies can remain detectable for months to years after infection,[142,147] and in the absence of a clinically compatible acute illness, detectable antibodies are not an indication for treatment for tick-borne rickettsial disease.

Some commercial laboratories offer serologic testing in the easier, higher-throughput, enzyme-linked immunosorbent assay (ELISA) format. These ELISA tests offer only qualitative results (i.e., antibody presence or absence relative to a threshold value) and do not provide a quantitative method of demonstrating increases or decreases in antibody levels. Confirmation of an acute infection by documenting the rise in antibody titer between the acute and convalescent serum samples is therefore impossible, and this is the most useful serologic strategy for evaluating etiology of potential rickettsial disease.

The majority of commercial reference laboratories test for IgG antibodies to rickettsial pathogens. Some commercial laboratories also perform IFA assays and other serologic testing for IgM antibodies. However, IgM antibodies against RMSF have been detected in patients for whom no evidence for rickettsial disease can be detected by properly timed acute and convalescent IgG titers or PCR, and they can persist in serum for at least 1 year.[148] IgM antibodies against ehrlichiae and *A. phagocytophilum* are likely less specific than IgG antibodies.[149] In this context, IgM antibody titers should be interpreted carefully and should not be used as a stand-alone method for diagnosis or public health reporting of tick-borne rickettsial diseases.

Cross-reactive immune responses to rickettsial antigens are typically group-specific for tick-borne rickettsial pathogens.[138] Antibodies reactive with *R. rickettsii* often cross-react with other SFG rickettsiae. Similarly, antibodies can be cross-reactive between *E. chaffeensis* and *A. phagocytophilum*, which can impede epidemiologic distinction between these infections.[149,150]

The Weil-Felix reaction is a nonspecific agglutination test for rickettsial antibodies. Although it lacks sensitivity, it is used extensively in some countries. Due to its low specificity, a fourfold rise in titer detected by this technique is not considered diagnostic.

Immunohistochemistry (IHC), where available, may demonstrate organisms in skin lesions such as a rash or eschar. It can rapidly confirm a suspected diagnosis, may provide immediate confirmation, and is 100% specific and 70% sensitive in diagnosing RMSF.[151] Due to increased concentration of organisms in eschar tissues, sensitivities might be higher for tests using eschars than for those using rash lesions.[138] Bone marrow biopsies often are performed to investigate cytopenias, and IHC of these specimens can be diagnostic for ehrlichiosis or anaplasmosis.[152] IHC can be particularly useful for diagnosing fatal tick-borne rickettsial diseases in tissue specimens after death from patients whose serological results had not been conclusive.[7,126,153] IHC for SFG rickettsiae, *E. chaffeensis*, and *A. phagocytophilum* is offered by CDC and some academic hospitals. This method is most likely to reveal organisms in patients before or within the first 48 hours after initiating appropriate antibacterial therapy.

Polymerase chain reaction (PCR) can be used for amplification of DNA extracted from rickettsioses in tissue or whole blood, and can confirm diagnosis if samples were obtained before treatment was initiated. PCR assays may yield a rapid diagnosis during severe infection, and it is available through reference laboratories or at the CDC. Although PCR can be timely in severe acute infection, most laboratory diagnoses of rickettsial diseases are made retrospectively by documenting a fourfold or equivalent rise in titer between acute and convalescent serum samples. A fourfold rise in titer by IFA serology in acute and convalescent samples and PCR performed on blood or tissue are both confirmatory. PCR on whole blood is effective for ehrlichiosis and anaplasmosis diagnosis.

Rocky Mountain Spotted Fever

Since the majority of patients are seronegative during the acute phase of illness, early diagnosis must be based on clinical and epidemiological risk factors. Clinical observations suggest that very early therapy with a tetracycline-class drug could potentially diminish or delay the development of antibodies in RMSF[154]; however, this should not dissuade appropriate serologic testing.

Detectable IgG titers for *R. rickettsii* have been seen to persist for >1 year after primary infection in some patients.[142] In the United States, IgG antibodies reactive with antigens of *R. rickettsii* at reciprocal titers $\geq$ 64 can be found in 5–10% of the population,[147,155,156] and this prevalence may be higher in certain regions.

African Tick Bite Fever

Although the majority of patients have increased IgG titers by the second week of the illness, persons infected with certain *Rickettsia* species might have delayed development of significant antibody titers. For example, patients infected with *R. africae* might not show seroconversion until 4 weeks after illness onset.[157] Antigen-specific assays are not available commercially in the United States for *R. africae*. However, commercially available tests using *R. conorii* or *R. rickettsii* antigens frequently cross-react with *R. africae* and can therefore provide utility as screening tests.[144] Alternatively, pathogen-specific testing may be submitted to CDC through the state public health laboratories.

Typhus Group

Murine Typhus

Serological diagnosis can be difficult due to cross-reactivity between *R. typhi* and *R. prowazekii*. Western blot may be more sensitive in distinguishing murine typhus from epidemic typhus, but this can be resource-intensive. PCR assays performed on whole blood or skin biopsies may also yield a confirmatory diagnosis.[158]

Anaplasmataceae

Diagnosis can be made through serology (IFA), culture, microscopic detection of morulae within granulocytes, or PCR. As with other rickettsioses, serologic diagnosis of anaplasmataceae is often confounded by the occurrence of pre-existing cross-reactive antibodies.[159] PCR on whole blood is commonly used to confirm anaplasmosis and ehrlichiosis.[160]

Ehrlichiosis

PCR on whole blood can be used to diagnose ehrlichiosis during the first week of illness. Sensitivity is decreased by delayed blood draws and initiation of doxycycline treatment. Patients with *E. ewingii* infections can develop antibodies that react with *E. chaffeensis* and, less commonly, *A. phagocytophilum* antigens.[129] Careful microscopic examination of blood smears or buffy-coat preparations stained with eosin-azure–type dyes (e.g., Wright-Giemsa stains) during the first week of illness might reveal morulae in the cytoplasm of infected circulating leukocytes of patients with *E. chaffeensis* ehrlichiosis[161] or anaplasmosis.[60] Observation of morulae is highly suggestive of infection by ehrlichiae or anaplasmae. However, blood-smear examination is a relatively insensitive and inconsistent technique and should be performed by experienced microscopists, who must distinguish morulae from other intraleukocytic structures. Blood-smear examination is not useful for diagnosis of RMSF or other SFG rickettsioses. PCR can distinguish *E. ewingii*, *E. chaffeensis*, and *E. muris euclairensis* infections.[162]

Anaplasmosis

PCR is very effective for anaplasmosis diagnosis during the first week of illness. The duration that antibodies persist after recovery from rickettsial infections varies, and depends on the pathogen and host factors. In certain persons, high titers of antibodies against *A. phagocytophilum* have been observed for over 4 years after the acute illness.[163]

TREATMENT

Antibiotic treatment with tetracyclines, especially doxycycline, is usually effective if started early in the course of rickettsial disease. Antibacterial treatment should never be delayed while awaiting laboratory confirmation of rickettsial illness, nor should treatment be discontinued solely on the basis of a negative test result with an acute phase specimen. Delay in the initiation of proper antibiotic therapy may lead to complications, such as neurologic manifestations, pneumonitis, myocarditis, and renal failure, long-term sequelae, or death.[65,88,164] The recommended dose of doxycycline for the treatment of tick-borne rickettsial diseases is 100 mg twice daily (orally or intravenously) for adults and 2.2 mg/kg body weight twice daily (orally or intravenously) for children weighing $<$ 100 lbs (45 kg).[71] Oral therapy is appropriate for patients with early-stage disease who can be treated as outpatients. Intravenous therapy might be indicated for more severely ill patients who require hospitalization, particularly in patients who are vomiting or obtunded. Patients should be monitored closely, since poorly treated patients, especially those with RMSF, have the potential to undergo rapid decline.

Doxycycline is the drug of choice for treatment of all tick-borne rickettsial diseases in patients of all ages, including children aged $<$ 8 years, and treatment should be initiated immediately in persons with signs and symptoms of rickettsial disease.[71,165] The American Academy of Pediatrics and CDC recommend doxycycline as the treatment of choice for all children with suspected tick-borne rickettsial disease.[165,166] Previous concerns about tooth staining in children aged $<$ 8 years stem from experience with older tetracycline-class drugs that bind more readily to calcium than do newer members of the drug class, such as doxycycline.[167] More recent studies found no evidence of dental staining in children treated with doxycycline for rickettsial infection.[168,169]

Controlled studies to assess the safety of doxycycline use in pregnant women have not been conducted, and available data are primarily observational. An expert review on doxycycline use during pregnancy concluded that therapeutic doses were unlikely to pose a substantial teratogenic risk; however, the data were insufficient to conclude that no risk exists.[170,171] Recent reviews reported no evidence of teratogenicity associated with doxycycline use during pregnancy; however, limited data and a lack of controlled studies were limitations.[170–172]

Tetracyclines, including doxycycline, are the only antibacterial agents recommended for treatment of all tick-borne rickettsial diseases. Many classes of broad-spectrum antibacterial agents that are used empirically to treat febrile patients, such as beta-lactams, macrolides, aminoglycosides, and sulfonamides, are not effective against tick-borne rickettsial diseases.[83,173] Although some fluoroquinolones have *in vitro* activity against rickettsiae,[174] their use for treatment of certain rickettsial infections has been associated with delayed subsidence of fever, increased disease severity, and longer hospital stay.[175,176] Sulfonamide antimicrobials are associated with increased severity of tick-borne rickettsial diseases, including RMSF and ehrlichiosis.[91]

Severe doxycycline or tetracycline allergy in a patient with a suspected rickettsial disease poses a challenge because of the lack of equally effective alternative antimicrobial agents. In a patient reporting an allergy to a tetracycline-class drug, determining the type of adverse drug reaction and whether it is potentially life threatening (e.g., anaphylaxis or Stevens-Johnson syndrome) by history or medical documentation is important. In patients with nonlife-threatening tetracycline-class drug reactions, administering doxycycline in an observed setting is an option; however, the risks and benefits should be evaluated on a case-by-case basis. In patients with a life-threatening tetracycline allergy, options include use of alternative antibacterial agents discussed in the preceding section or, possibly for immediate hypersensitivity reactions, rapid doxycycline desensitization in consultation with an allergy and immunology specialist.

Studies of preventive antibacterial therapy for rickettsial infection in humans are limited. Available data[177] do not support prophylactic treatment for rickettsial diseases in persons who have had recent tick bites and are not ill.

SFG Rickettsiae

The recommended duration of therapy for RMSF is at least 3 days after subsidence of fever and until evidence of clinical improvement is noted.[165,166] The minimum total course of treatment is typically 5–7 days, but severe or complicated disease could require longer treatment courses.

Fever typically subsides within 24–48 hours of treatment with doxycycline, if it was initiated within 4–5 days of illness onset. Lack of a clinical response within 48 hours of early treatment with doxycycline could be an indication that the condition is not a tick-borne rickettsial disease, and alternative diagnoses or coinfection should be considered. Severely ill patients might require > 48 hours of treatment before clinical improvement is noted, especially if multiple organ dysfunction is present. Signs and symptoms of tick-borne rickettsial diseases are generally nonspecific, and early empiric treatment often needs to be combined with treatment for the other possible etiologic differentials.

Rocky Mountain Spotted Fever

Treatment of RMSF should be initiated promptly on the basis of epidemiological setting and clinical suspicion without waiting for laboratory confirmation. Supportive care is important in the management of the complications of RMSF. Patients with evidence of organ dysfunction, severe thrombocytopenia, mental status changes, or the need for supportive therapy should be hospitalized. Other important considerations for hospitalization include social factors, the likelihood that the patient can and will take oral medications, and existing comorbid conditions, including the patient's immune status.

Chloramphenicol is the only alternative drug that has been used to treat RMSF; however, epidemiologic studies using CDC case report data suggest that patients with RMSF treated with chloramphenicol are at higher risk for death than persons who received a tetracycline.[82,84] Chloramphenicol is a potential alternative treatment for RMSF during pregnancy; however, care must be used when administering the drug late during the third trimester of pregnancy because of the theoretical risk for gray baby syndrome.[178] Chloramphenicol is no longer available in the oral form in the United States, and the intravenous form is not readily available at all institutions. Chloramphenicol is associated with adverse hematologic effects (i.e., aplastic anemia), which have resulted in its limited use in the United States.

Typhus Group

Doxycycline for 1 week is the recommended treatment for uncomplicated cases of scrub typhus. If treatment is not initiated, the fever and symptoms may persist for more than 3 weeks. Because of possible antibiotic resistance to doxycycline, the use of macrolide antibiotics can be considered.[179] A single dose of 500 mg azithromycin has been found to be effective in the treatment of mild scrub typhus.[180] For murine typhus, the antibiotic of choice is doxycycline. Ciprofloxacin has also been found to be effective.[181] For epidemic typhus doxycycline is the antibiotic of choice for treatment and is usually curative if given early in the course of the disease. A single dose of doxycycline (100 mg) has been found to be effective for treating symptomatic cases and this may be the most practical approach when dealing with large epidemics.

Anaplasmataceae

While the recommended treatment for Anaplasmataceae is doxycycline, Rifamycins demonstrate *in vitro* activity against *E. chaffeensis* and *A. phagocytophilum*.[182] Small numbers of children also have been treated successfully for anaplasmosis using rifampin[183]; however, no clinical trials demonstrating *in vivo* efficacy of rifampin in the treatment of anaplasmosis or ehrlichiosis have been conducted. Rifampin can be an alternative for the treatment of mild illness due to anaplasmosis in the case of pregnancy or documented allergy to tetracycline-class drugs.[184] The dose of rifampin is 300 mg orally twice daily for adults or 10 mg/kg of body weight for children (not to exceed 300 mg/dose).[113]

Although *A. phagocytophilum* is susceptible to levofloxacin *in vitro*,[185] relapse of infection after treatment with levofloxacin has been reported,[186] and, as with the other tick-borne rickettsial diseases, fluoroquinolones are not recommended for treatment of anaplasmosis.[184] Chloramphenicol is not an alternative for the treatment of ehrlichiosis or anaplasmosis.[182]

Ehrlichiosis

The recommended duration of doxycycline therapy for ehrlichiosis is also at least 3 days after subsidence of fever and until evidence of clinical improvement is noted.[165] Cases of severe or fatal ehrlichiosis have been associated with the use of trimethoprim-sulfamethoxazole.[131–133]

Anaplasmosis

Doxycycline is the recommended treatment for anaplsmosis for a duration of 7–10 days, or until 3–5 days after fever has subsided. To provide appropriate length of therapy for possible coinfection with *B. burgdorferi*, patients with anaplasmosis may be treated with doxycycline for 10 days.[184] Children aged < 8 years with anaplasmosis in whom concurrent Lyme disease is not suspected can be treated for a duration similar to that for other tick-borne rickettsial diseases.[165] Limited case report data document favorable maternal and pregnancy outcomes in small numbers of pregnant women treated with rifampin for anaplasmosis.[187,188]

PREVENTION AND CONTROL

Prevention and control of rickettsial and ehrlichial diseases rely on avoidance of vector-infested sites, and vector and reservoir host control by habitat modification or use of appropriate pesticides. If exposure is unavoidable, appropriate clothing should be worn, such as long-sleeved shirts and long pants, which may be pretreated with permethrin products. N,N-diethyl-meta-toluamide (DEET)-containing repellants should be applied to exposed skin following directions on the label. In tick-infested areas, persons should check themselves frequently for the presence of ticks. Attached ticks should be removed carefully with tweezers and exposure to fluids of the ticks should be minimized with the use of gloves. In the United States, most cases of rickettsial diseases are associated with occupational or recreational exposures to the vectors. These diseases are also being increasingly recognized in international travelers visiting remote areas of endemicity. Travelers should be aware of the diseases to which they may be exposed and the appropriate methods for decreasing exposures. No vaccines are currently available for prevention of these diseases.

Rickettsialpox is recognized as an urban disease occurring in large cities with crowded areas infested with rodents. Residual insecticides and rodent-control measures may limit or eliminate the vector and reservoir, and thus rickettsial transmission to humans.

Prevention of epidemic typhus is accomplished primarily by elimination of the louse vector through application of insecticides to individuals and their clothing, and to the bedding on which the eggs are laid and lice reside. Several applications may be required periodically, since the eggs are resistant to most insecticides and continue to hatch. Clothes and bedding can also be washed in hot water (≥130°F) to kill lice and eggs. Head lice and pubic lice should also be treated if present. Similar treatment of family or other close contacts is advisable. Once deloused, the patient need not be quarantined, but others who have been exposed should remain under surveillance for the disease for 2 weeks. In epidemic settings, treatment of the entire community with insecticide is often the most practical and effective approach to eliminate the louse vector.

To prevent infection by *O. tsutsugamushi* in local populations, focal areas known to be endemic should be avoided. In addition, vertebrate hosts and protective vegetation can be eliminated and the area can be treated with pesticides. For travelers, personal prophylaxis with protective clothing, treatment of clothing with insecticides and application of mite repellants such as DEET to the skin is useful.[189] Prophylactic use of doxycycline at a weekly dose of 200 mg for short-term exposures has been shown to be effective.[190] There is no commercial vaccine for scrub typhus.

Prevention of murine typhus requires ongoing control of the natural host and vector, rodent-control measures, and use of appropriate insecticides. Local public health authorities should be consulted for advice on approved residual-action insecticides to apply to rat habitats. Flea control should be achieved initially, followed by rat trapping and poisoning, rodent-proofing of buildings, and elimination of rodent shelter and food attractants. Failure to control the flea population initially may lead to human outbreaks as the infected fleas move from dying rats to humans.

References

1. Jensenius M, Fournier PE, Vene S, et al. African tick bite fever in travelers to rural sub-Equatorial Africa. *Clin Infect Dis*. 2003;36(11):1411–7.
2. Snyder JC. Typhus fever in the Second World War. *Calif Med*. 1947;66(1):3–10.
3. Megaw JW. Scrub typhus as a war disease. *Br Med J*. 1945;2(4412):109–12.
4. Shrestha P, Roberts T, Homsana A, et al. Febrile illness in Asia: Gaps in epidemiology, diagnosis and management for informing health policy. *Clin Microbiol Infect*. 2018;24(8):815–26.
5. Harden VA. *Rocky Mountain Spotted Fever. History of a Twentieth-Century Disease*. Baltimore, MD: The Johns Hopkins University Press; 1990.
6. Álvarez-Hernández G, Roldán JFG, Milan NSH, Lash RR, Behravesh CB, Paddock CD. Rocky Mountain spotted fever in Mexico: Past, present, and future. *Lancet Infect Dis*. 2017;17(6):e189–96.
7. Demma LJ, Traeger MS, Nicholson WL, et al. Rocky Mountain spotted fever from an unexpected tick vector in Arizona. *N Engl J Med*. 2005;353(6):587–94.
8. Fishbein DB, Dawson JE, Robinson LE. Human ehrlichiosis in the United States, 1985 to 1990. *Ann Intern Med*. 1994;120(9):736–43.
9. Chen SM, Dumler JS, Bakken JS, Walker DH. Identification of a granulocytotropic *Ehrlichia* species as the etiologic agent of human disease. *J Clin Microbiol*. 1994;32(3):589–95.
10. Guillemi EC, Tomassone L, Farber MD. Tick-borne Rickettsiales: Molecular tools for the study of an emergent group of pathogens. *J Microbiol Methods*. 2015;119:87–97.
11. Parola P, Paddock CD, Socolovschi C, et al. Update on tick-borne rickettsioses around the world: A geographic approach. *Clin Microbiol Rev*. 2013;26(4):657–702.
12. Delgado-De la Mora L-E, Leyva-Gastelum M, Licona-Enríquez JD, Delgado-De la Mora D, Rascón-Alcantar A, Álvarez-Hernández G. Una serie de casos fatales de fiebre manchada de las Montanas Rocosas en Sonora, Mexico. *Biomedica*. 2018;38(1).
13. Drexler NA, Miller M, Gerding J, et al. Community-based control of the brown dog tick in a region with high rates of Rocky Mountain spotted fever, 2012–2013. *PLoS One*. 2014;9(12):e112368.
14. Nicholson WL, Paddock CD, Demma L, et al. Rocky Mountain spotted fever in Arizona: Documentation of heavy environmental infestations of *Rhipicephalus sanguineus* at an endemic site. *Ann N Y Acad Sci*. 2006;1078(1):338–41.
15. Traeger MS, Regan JJ, Humpherys D, et al. Rocky Mountain spotted fever characterization and comparison to similar illnesses in a highly endemic area—Arizona, 2002–2011. *Clin Infect Dis*. 2015;60(11):1650–8.
16. Alvarez-Hernandez G, Murillo-Benitez C, Candia-Plata Mdel C, Moro M. Clinical profile and predictors of fatal Rocky Mountain spotted fever in children from Sonora, Mexico. *Pediatr Infect Dis J*. 2015;34(2):125–30.
17. Eremeeva ME, Zambrano ML, Anaya L, et al. *Rickettsia rickettsii* in Rhipicephalus ticks, Mexicali, Mexico. *J Med Entomol*. 2011;48(2):418–21.
18. Moraes-Filho J, Pinter A, Pacheco RC, et al. New epidemiological data on Brazilian spotted fever in an endemic area of the state of Sao Paulo, Brazil. *Vector Borne Zoonotic Dis*. 2009;9(1):73–8.
19. Pacheco RC, Moraes-Filho J, Guedes E, et al. Rickettsial infections of dogs, horses and ticks in Juiz de Fora, southeastern Brazil, and isolation of *Rickettsia rickettsii* from Rhipicephalus sanguineus ticks. *Med Vet Entomol*. 2011;25(2):148–55.
20. Paddock CD, Sumner JW, Comer JA, et al. *Rickettsia parkeri*: A newly recognized cause of spotted fever rickettsiosis in the United States. *Clin Infect Dis*. 2004;38(6):805–11.
21. Parker RR. A pathogenic rickettsia from the Gulf Coast tick, Amblyomma maculatum. *Report of the Proceedings of the Third International Congress for Microbiology*. New York: International Association of Microbiologists; 1940:390–1.
22. Venzal JM, Portillo A, Estrada-Pena A, et al. *Rickettsia parkeri* in Amblyomma triste from Uruguay. *Emerg Infect Dis*. 2004;10(8):1493–5.
23. Paddock C, Finley R, Wright C, et al. *Rickettsia parkeri* rickettsiosis and its clinical distinction from Rocky Mountain spotted fever. *Clin Infect Dis*. 2008;47(9):1188–96.
24. Pjiper A, Crocker GC. Rickettsioses of South Africa. *S Afr Med J*. 1938;12:613–30.
25. Kelly PJ, Beati L, Matthewman LA, et al. A new pathogenic spotted fever group rickettsia from Africa. *J Trop Med Hyg*. 1994;97(3):129–37.
26. McQuiston J, Paddock C, Singleton J, et al. Imported spotted fever rickettsioses in United States travelers returning from Africa: A summary of cases confirmed by laboratory testing at the Centers for Disease Control and Prevention, 1999–2002. *Am J Trop Med Hyg*. 2004;70(1):98–101.
27. Cherry CC, Denison AM, Kato CY, Thornton K, Paddock CD. Diagnosis of spotted fever froup rickettsioses in U.S. travelers returning from Africa, 2007–2016. *Am J Trop Med Hyg*. 2018;99(1):136–42.
28. Albizuri Prado F, Sanchez A, Feito M, et al. Fever and multiple eschars after an African safari: Report of three cases. *Pediatr Dermatol*. 2017;34(4):e179–81.
29. Althaus F, Greub G, Raoult D, Genton B. African tick-bite fever: A new entity in the differential diagnosis of multiple eschars in travelers. Description of five cases imported from South Africa to Switzerland. *Int J Infect Dis*. 2010;14(Suppl 3):e274–6.
30. Jensenius M, Fournier PE, Raoult D. Tick-borne rickettsioses in international travellers. *Int J Infect Dis*. 2004;8(3):139–46.
31. Parola P. Tick-borne rickettsial diseases: Emerging risks in Europe. *Comp Immunol Microbiol Infect Dis*. 2004;27(5):297–304.
32. Uchida T, Uchiyama T, Kumano K, Walker DH. *Rickettsia japonica* sp. nov., the etiological agent of spotted fever group rickettsiosis in Japan. *Int J Syst Bacteriol*. 1992;42(2):303–5.
33. Mahara F. Japanese spotted fever: Report of 31 cases and review of the literature. *Emerg Infect Dis*. 1997;3(2):105–11.
34. Sexton DJ, Dwyer B, Kemp R, Graves S. Spotted fever group rickettsial infections in Australia. *Rev Infect Dis*. 1991;13(5):876–86.
35. Shapiro MR, Fritz CL, Tait K, et al. Rickettsia 364D: A newly recognized cause of eschar-associated illness in California. *Clin Infect Dis*. 2010;50(4):541–8.
36. Padgett KA, Bonilla D, Eremeeva ME, et al. The eco-epidemiology of Pacific Coast tick fever in California. *PLoS Negl Trop Dis*. 2016;10(10):e0005020.
37. Tamura A, Ohashi N, Urakami H, Miyamura S. Classification of *Rickettsia tsutsugamushi* in a new genus, Orientia gen. nov., as *Orientia tsutsugamushi* comb. nov. *Int J Syst Bacteriol*. 1995;45(3):589–91.
38. Xu G, Walker DH, Jupiter D, Melby PC, Arcari CM. A review of the global epidemiology of scrub typhus. *PLoS Negl Trop Dis*. 2017;11(11):e0006062.
39. McDonald JC, MacLean JD, McDade JE. Imported rickettsial disease: Clinical and epidemiologic features. *Am J Med*. 1988;85(6):799–805.
40. Civen R, Ngo V. Murine typhus: An unrecognized suburban vectorborne disease. *Clin Infect Dis*. 2008;46(6):913–8.
41. Adjemian J, Parks S, McElroy K, et al. Murine typhus in Austin, Texas, USA, 2008. *Emerg Infect Dis*. 2010;16(3):412–7.
42. Afzal Z, Kallumadanda S, Wang F, Hemmige V, Musher D. Acute febrile illness and complications due to murine typhus, Texas, USA. *Emerg Infect Dis*. 2017;23(8):1268–73.
43. Angelakis E, Bechah Y, Raoult D. The history of epidemic typhus. *Microbiol Spectr*. 2016;4(4).
44. Prusinski MA, White JL, Wong SJ, et al. Sylvatic typhus associated with flying squirrels (*Glaucomys volans*) in New York State, United States. *Vector Borne Zoonotic Dis*. 2014;14(4):240–4.
45. Bechah Y, Capo C, Mege JL, Raoult D. Epidemic typhus. *Lancet Infect Dis*. 2008;8(7):417–26.
46. Comer JA, Paddock CD, Childs JE. Urban zoonoses caused by *Bartonella*, *Coxiella*, *Ehrlichia*, and *Rickettsia* species. *Vector Borne Zoonotic Dis*. 2001;1(2):91–118.
47. Lackman DB. A review of information on ricketsialpox in the United States. *Clin Pediatr (Phila)*. 1963;2:296–301.
48. Dahlgren FS, Mandel EJ, Krebs JW, Massung RF, McQuiston JH. Increasing incidence of *Ehrlichia chaffeensis* and *Anaplasma phagocytophilum* in the United States, 2000–2007. *Am J Trop Med Hyg*. 2011;85(1):124–31.
49. Johnson DK, Schiffman EK, Davis JP, et al. Human infection with *Ehrlichia muris*-like pathogen, United States, 2007–2013. *Emerg Infect Dis*. 2015;21(10):1794–9.
50. Pritt BS, Sloan LM, Johnson DK, et al. Emergence of a new pathogenic *Ehrlichia* species, Wisconsin and Minnesota, 2009. *N Engl J Med*. 2011;365(5):422–9.
51. Dawson JE, Anderson BE, Fishbein DB, et al. Isolation and characterization of an *Ehrlichia* sp. from a patient diagnosed with human ehrlichiosis. *J Clin Microbiol*. 1991;29(12):2741–5.

52. Anderson BE, Sims KG, Olson JG, et al. *Amblyomma americanum*: A potential vector of human ehrlichiosis. *Am J Trop Med Hyg.* 1993;49(2):239–44.
53. Rosenberg R, Lindsey NP, Fischer M, et al. Vital signs: Trends in reported vectorborne disease cases—United States and territories, 2004–2016. *MMWR Morb Mortal Wkly Rep.* 2018;67(17):496–501.
54. Nichols Heitman K, Dahlgren FS, Drexler NA, Massung RF, Behravesh CB. Increasing incidence of ehrlichiosis in the United States: A summary of national surveillance of *Ehrlichia chaffeensis* and *Ehrlichia ewingii* infections in the United States, 2008–2012. *Am J Trop Med Hyg.* 2016;94(1):52–60.
55. Pritt B, Allerdice MEJ, Sloan LM, et al. Proposal to reclassify *Ehrlichia muris* as *Ehrlichia muris* subsp. *muris* subsp. nov. and description of *Ehrlichia muris* subsp. *eauclairensis* subsp. nov., a newly recognized tick-borne pathogen of humans. *Int J Syst Evol Microbiol.* 2017;67(7):2121–6.
56. Dumler JS, Barbet AF, Bekker CP, et al. Reorganization of genera in the families Rickettsiaceae and Anaplasmataceae in the order Rickettsiales: Unification of some species of *Ehrlichia* with *Anaplasma*, *Cowdria* with *Ehrlichia* and *Ehrlichia* with *Neorickettsia*, descriptions of six new species combinations and designation of *Ehrlichia* equi and 'HGE agent' as subjective synonyms of *Ehrlichia phagocytophila*. *Int J Syst Evol Microbiol.* 2001;51(Pt 6):2145–65.
57. Dahlgren FS, Heitman KN, Drexler NA, Massung RF, Behravesh CB. Human granulocytic anaplasmosis in the United States from 2008 to 2012: A summary of national surveillance data. *Am J Trop Med Hyg.* 2015;93(1):66–72.
58. Robinson SJ, Neitzel DF, Moen RA, et al. Disease risk in a dynamic environment: The spread of tick-borne pathogens in Minnesota, USA. *Ecohealth.* 2015;12(1):152–63.
59. Lillini E, Macri G, Proietti G, Scarpulla M. New findings on anaplasmosis caused by infection with *Anaplasma phagocytophilum*. *Ann N Y Acad Sci.* 2006;1081:360–70.
60. Bakken JS, Dumler S. Human granulocytic anaplasmosis. *Infect Dis Clin North Am.* 2008;22(3):433–48.
61. Abroug N, Khochtali S, Kahloun R, Mahmoud A, Attia S, Khairallah M. Ocular manifestations of rickettsial disease. *J Infect Dis Ther.* 2014;2:3.
62. Wolbach SB. Studies on Rocky Mountain spotted fever. *J Med Res.* 1919;41(1):1–198.141.
63. Harrell GT. George T. Harrell (1908-). Rocky Mountain spotted fever. 1949. *Medicine.* 1992;71(4):333–70.
64. Traeger MS, Regan J, Humpherys D, et al. Rocky Mountain spotted fever characterization and comparison to similar illnesses in a highly endemic area: Arizona, 2002–2011. *Clin Infect Dis.* 2015;60(11):1650–8.
65. Kirkland KB, Wilkinson WE, Sexton DJ. Therapeutic delay and mortality in cases of Rocky Mountain spotted fever. *Clin Infect Dis.* 1995;20(5):1118–21.
66. Hattwick MA, Retailliau H, O'Brien RJ, et al. Fatal rocky mountain spotted fever. *JAMA.* 1978;240(14):1499–503.
67. Helmick CG, Bernard KW, D'Angelo LJ. Rocky Mountain spotted fever: Clinical, laboratory, and epidemiological features of 262 cases. *J Infect Dis.* 1984;150(4):480–88.
68. Thorner A, Walker D, Petri W Jr. Rocky Mountain spotted fever. *Clin Infect Dis.* 1998;27(6):1353–9.
69. Sexton DJ, Corey GR. Rocky Mountain "spotless" and "almost spotless" fever: A wolf in sheep's clothing. *Clin Infect Dis.* 1992;15(3):439–48.
70. Buckingham SC, Marshall GS, Schutze GE, et al. Clinical and laboratory features, hospital course, and outcome of Rocky Mountain spotted fever in children. *J Pediatr.* 2007;150(2):180–4.e181.
71. Centers for Disease Control and Prevention Tickborne Rickettsial Diseases Working Group. Diagnosis and management of tickborne rickettsial diseases: Rocky Mountain spotted fever, ehrlichioses, and anaplasmosis—United States: A practical guide for physicians and other health-care and public health professionals. *MMWR Recomm Rep.* 2006;55(RR-4):1–27.
72. Regan JJ, Traeger MS, Humpherys D, et al. Risk factors for fatal outcome from Rocky Mountain spotted fever in a highly endemic area: Arizona, 2002–2011. *Clin Infect Dis.* 2015;60(11):1659–66.
73. Walker DH, Gay RM, Valdes-Dapena M. The occurrence of eschars in Rocky Mountain spotted fever. *J Am Acad Dermatol.* 1981;4(5):571–6.
74. Arguello AP, Hun L, Rivera P, Taylor L. A fatal urban case of Rocky Mountain spotted fever presenting an eschar in San Jose, Costa Rica. *Am J Trop Med Hyg.* 2012;87(2):345–8.
75. Walker DH, Henderson FW, Hutchins GM. Rocky Mountain spotted fever: Mimicry of appendicitis or acute surgical abdomen? *Am J Dis Child.* 1986;140(8):742–4.
76. Walker DH, Lesesne HR, Varma VA, Thacker WC. Rocky Mountain spotted fever mimicking acute cholecystitis. *Arch Intern Med.* 1985;145(12):2194–6.
77. Walker DH, Blanton LS. *Rickettsia rickettsii* and other spotted fever group rickettsiae (Rocky Mountain spotted fever and other spotted fevers). In: Bennett JE, Dolin R, Blaser MJ, eds. *Mandell, Douglas, and Bennett's Principles and Practice of Infectious Diseases.* Philadelphia, PA: Elsevier Saunders; 2015:2198–205.
78. Archibald LK, Sexton DJ. Long-term sequelae of Rocky Mountain spotted fever. *Clin Infect Dis.* 1995;20(5):1122–5.
79. Massey EW, Thames T, Coffey CE, Gallis HA. Neurologic complications of Rocky Mountain spotted fever. *South Med J.* 1985;78(11):1288–90, 1303.
80. Bleck TP. Central nervous system involvement in rickettsial diseases. *Neurol Clin.* 1999;17(4):801–12.
81. Archibald LK, Sexton DJ. Long-term sequelae of Rocky Mountain spotted fever. *Clin Infect Dis.* 1995;20(5):1122–5.
82. Dalton M, Clarke M, Holman R, et al. National surveillance for Rocky Mountain spotted fever, 1981–1992: Epidemiologic summary and evaluation of risk factors for fatal outcome. *Am J Trop Med Hyg.* 1995;52(5):405–13.
83. Regan J, Traeger M, Humpherys D, et al. Risk factors for fatal outcome from Rocky Mountain spotted fever in a highly endemic area: Arizona, 2002–2011. *Clin Infect Dis.* 2015;60(11):1659–66.
84. Holman RC, Paddock CD, Curns AT, et al. Analysis of risk factors for fatal Rocky Mountain Spotted fever: Evidence for superiority of tetracyclines for therapy. *J Infect Dis.* 2001;184(11):1437–44.
85. Childs JE, Paddock CD. Passive surveillance as an instrument to identify risk factors for fatal Rocky Mountain spotted fever: Is there more to learn? *Am J Trop Med Hyg.* 2002;66(5):450–7.
86. Smadel JE. Status of the rickettsioses in the United States. *Ann Intern Med.* 1959;51(3):421–35.
87. Topping NH. Rocky Mountain spotted fever: A note on some aspects of its epidemiology. *Public Health Rep.* 1941;56(34):1699–703.
88. Dahlgren FS, Holman RC, Paddock CD, Callinan LS, McQuiston JH. Fatal Rocky Mountain spotted fever in the United States, 1999–2007. *Am J Trop Med Hyg.* 2012;86(4):713–9.
89. Walker DH. The role of host factors in the severity of spotted fever and typhus rickettsioses. *Ann N Y Acad Sci.* 1990;590(1):10–9.
90. Walker DH, Hawkins HK, Hudson P. Fulminant Rocky Mountain spotted fever. Its pathologic characteristics associated with glucose-6-phosphate dehydrogenase deficiency. *Arch Pathol Lab Med.* 1983;107(3):121–5.
91. Topping NH. Experimental Rocky Mountain spotted fever and endemic typhus treated with prontosil or sulfapyridine. *Public Health Rep.* 1939;54(26):1143–7.
92. Harrell GT. Rocky Mountain spotted fever. 1949;*Medicine.* 28(4):333–70.
93. Bergeron JW, Braddom RL, Kaelin DL. Persisting impairment following Rocky Mountain spotted fever: A case report. *Arch Phys Med Rehabil.* 1997;78(11):1277–80.
94. Wright L. Intellectual sequelae of Rocky Mountain spotted fever. *J Abnorm Psychol.* 1972;80(3):315–6.
95. Raoult D, Weiller PJ, Chagnon A, et al. Mediterranean spotted fever: Clinical, laboratory and epidemiological features of 199 cases. *Am J Trop Med Hyg.* 1986;35(4):845–50.
96. Anton E, Font B, Munoz T, Sanfeliu I, Segura F. Clinical and laboratory characteristics of 144 patients with Mediterranean spotted fever. *Eur J Clin Microbiol Infect Dis.* 2003;22(2):126–8.
97. Raoult D, Fournier PE, Fenollar F, et al. *Rickettsia africae*, a tick-borne pathogen in travelers to sub-Saharan Africa. *N Engl J Med.* 2001;344(20):1504–10.
98. Jensenius M, Fournier PE, Kelly P, Myrvang B, Raoult D. African tick bite fever. *Lancet Infect Dis.* 2003;3(9):557–64.
99. Kelman P, Thompson CW, Hynes W, et al. *Rickettsia parkeri* infections diagnosed by eschar biopsy, Virginia, USA. *Infection.* 2018;46(4):559–63.
100. National Institute of Infectious Diseases. Scrub typhus and Japanese spotted fever in Japan 2007–2016. *Infect Agents Surveill Rep.* 2017;38:(448).
101. Raoult D, Lakos A, Fenollar F, et al. Spotless rickettsiosis caused by *Rickettsia slovaca* and associated with Dermacentor ticks. *Clin Infect Dis.* 2002;34(10):1331–6.
102. Oteo JA, Ibarra V, Blanco JR, et al. Dermacentor-borne necrosis erythema and lymphadenopathy: Clinical and epidemiological features of a new tick-borne disease. *Clin Microbiol Infect.* 2004;10(4):327–31.

103. Ibarra V, Oteo JA, Portillo A, et al. *Rickettsia slovaca* infection: DEBONEL/TIBOLA. *Ann N Y Acad Sci*. 2006;1078:206–14.

104. Fournier PE, Gouriet F, Brouqui P, Lucht F, Raoult D. Lymphangitis-associated rickettsiosis, a new rickettsiosis caused by *Rickettsia sibirica* mongolotimonae: Seven new cases and review of the literature. *Clin Infect Dis*. 2005;40(10):1435–44.

105. Parola P, Davoust B, Raoult D. Tick- and flea-borne rickettsial emerging zoonoses. *Vet Res*. 2005;36(3):469–92.

106. Fournier PE, Allombert C, Supputamongkol Y, et al. Aneruptive fever associated with antibodies to *Rickettsia helvetica* in Europe and Thailand. *J Clin Microbiol*. 2004;42(2):816–8.

107. Mediannikov OY, Sidelnikov Y, Ivanov L, et al. Acute tick-borne rickettsiosis caused by *Rickettsia heilongjiangensis* in Russian Far East. *Emerg Infect Dis*. 2004;10(5):810–7.

108. Johnston SH, Glaser CA, Padgett K, et al. *Rickettsia* spp. 364D causing a cluster of eschar-associated illness, California. *Pediatr Infect Dis J*. 2013;32(9):1036–9.

109. Tsay RW, Chang FY. Serious complications in scrub typhus. *J Microbiol Immunol Infect*. 1998;31(4):240–4.

110. Raoult D, Woodward T, Dumler JS. The history of epidemic typhus. *Infect Dis Clin North Am*. 2004;18(1):127–40.

111. Walker DH, Fishbein DB. Epidemiology of rickettsial diseases. *Eur J Epidemiol*. 1991;7(3):237–45.

112. Dumler JS, Walker DH. *Ehrlichia chaffeensis* (human monocytotropic ehrlichiosis), *Anaplasma phagocytophilum* (human granulocytic anaplasmosis), and other Anaplasmataceae. In: Dumler J, Walker D, eds. *Mandell, Douglas, and Bennett's Principles and Practice of Diseases*. Vol. 2. Philadelphia, PA: Elsevier; 2014:2227–33.

113. Dumler JS, Madigan JE, Pusterla N, Bakken JS. Ehrlichioses in humans: Epidemiology, clinical presentation, diagnosis, and treatment. *Clin Infect Dis*. 2007;45(Suppl 1):S45–51.

114. Heitman KN, Dahlgren FS, Drexler NA, Massung RF, Behravesh CB. Increasing incidence of ehrlichiosis in the United States: A summary of national surveillance of *Ehrlichia chaffeensis* and *Ehrlichia ewingii* infections in the United States, 2008–2012. *Am J Trop Med Hyg*. 2016;94(1):52–60.

115. Paddock CD, Childs JE. *Ehrlichia chaffeensis*: A prototypical emerging pathogen. *Clin Microbiol Rev*. 2003;16(1):37–64.

116. Schutze GE, Jacobs RF. Human monocytic ehrlichiosis in children. *Pediatrics*. 1997;100(1):art. no.-e10.

117. Smith Sehdev AE, Sehdev PS, Jacobs R, Dumler JS. Human monocytic ehrlichiosis presenting as acute appendicitis during pregnancy. *Clin Infect Dis*. 2002;35(9):e99–102.

118. Fichtenbaum CJ, Peterson LR, Weil GJ. Ehrlichiosis presenting as a life-threatening illness with features of the toxic shock syndrome. *Am J Med*. 1993;95(4):351–7.

119. Harkess JR, Ewing SA, Brumit T, Mettry CR. Ehrlichiosis in children. *Pediatrics*. 1991;87(2):199–203.

120. Olano JP, Masters E, Hogrefe W, Walker DH. Human monocytotropic ehrlichiosis, Missouri. *Emerg Infect Dis*. 2003;9(12):1579–86.

121. Ratnasamy N, Everett ED, Roland WE, McDonald G, Caldwell CW. Central nervous system manifestations of human ehrlichiosis. *Clin Infect Dis*. 1996;23(2):314–9.

122. Abbott KC, Vukelja SJ, Smith CE, et al. Hemophagocytic syndrome: A cause of pancytopenia in human ehrlichiosis. *Am J Hematol*. 1991;38(3):230–4.

123. Burns S, Saylors R, Mian A. Hemophagocytic lymphohistiocytosis secondary to *Ehrlichia chaffeensis* infection: A case report. *J Pediatr Hematol Oncol*. 2010;32(4):e142–3.

124. Vijayan V, Thambundit A, Sukumaran S. Hemophagocytic lymphohistiocytosis secondary to ehrlichiosis in a child. *Clin Pediatr*. 2015;54(1):84–6.

125. Pandey R, Kochar R, Kemp S, Rotaru D, Shah SV. Ehrlichiosis presenting with toxic shock-like syndrome and secondary hemophagocytic lymphohistiocytosis. *J Ark Med Soc*. 2013;109(13):280–2.

126. Marty AM, Dumler JS, Imes G, et al. Ehrlichiosis mimicking thrombotic thrombocytopenic purpura. Case report and pathological correlation. *Hum Pathol*. 26(8):920–5, 1995.

127. Smith Sehdev AE, Dumler JS. Hepatic pathology in human monocytic ehrlichiosis. *Ehrlichia chaffeensis* infection. *Am J Clin Pathol*. 2003;119(6):859–65.

128. Dahlgren FS, Mandel EJ, Krebs JW, Massung RF, McQuiston JH. Increasing incidence of *Ehrlichia chaffeensis* and *Anaplasma phagocytophilum* in the United States, 2000–2007. *Am J Trop Med Hyg*. 2011;85(1):124–31.

129. Paddock CD, Folk SM, Shore GM, et al. Infections with *Ehrlichia chaffeensis* and *Ehrlichia ewingii* in persons coinfected with human immunodeficiency virus. *Clin Infect Dis*. 2001;33(9):1586–94.

130. Thomas LD, Hongo I, Bloch KC, Tang YW, Dummer S. Human ehrlichiosis in transplant recipients. *Am J Transplant*. 2007;7(6):1641–7.

131. Peters TR, Edwards KM, Standaert SM. Severe ehrlichiosis in an adolescent taking trimethoprim-sulfamethoxazole. *Pediatr Infect Dis J*. 2000;19(2):170–2.

132. Brantley RK. Trimethoprim-sulfamethoxazole and fulminant ehrlichiosis. *Pediatr Infect Dis J*. 2001;20(2):231.

133. Seema UN, Gary LS. Myocarditis after trimethoprim/sulfamethoxazole treatment for ehrlichiosis. *Emerg Infect Dis J*. 2013;19(12):1975.

134. Liddell AM, Sumner JW, Paddock CD, et al. Reinfection with *Ehrlichia chaffeensis* in a liver transplant recipient. *Clin Infect Dis*. 2002;34(12):1644–7.

135. Bakken JS, Krueth J, Wilson-Nordskog C, et al. Clinical and laboratory characteristics of human granulocytic ehrlichiosis. *JAMA*. 1996;275(3):199–205.

136. Bellone M, Chiang J, Ahmed T, Galanakis D, Senzel L. Thrombotic thrombocytopenic purpura and its look-alikes: A single institution experience. *Transfus Apher Sci*. 2012;46(1):59–64.

137. Dumler JS. The biological basis of severe outcomes in *Anaplasma phagocytophilum* infection. *FEMS Immunol Med Microbiol*. 2012;64(1):13–20.

138. Walker D, DH B. Rickettsia and *Orientsia*. In: Jorgensen JH, Pfaller MA, Carroll KC, eds. *Manual of Clinical Microbiology*, 11th ed. Washington, DC: American Society of Microbiology Press; 2015:1122–34.

139. Council of State and Territorial Epidemiologists. Public health reporting and national notification for spotted fever rickettsioses (including Rocky Mountain spotted fever) position statement. Paper presented at: *Council of State and Territorial Epidemiologists Annual Conference 2009*; Buffalo, NY.

140. Engel J BK, Swerdlow D, et al. Position statement 07-ID-03, Revision of the national surveillance case definition for ehrlichiosis (ehrlichiosis/anaplasmosis). http://c.ymcdn.com/sites/www.cste.org/resource/resmgr/PS/07-ID-03.pdf. Atlanta, GA. 2007.

141. Walker D, Dumler J. Rickettsiae: Spotted fever and typhus group. In: Lennette EH, Lennette DA, Lennette ET, eds. *Diagnostic Procedures for Viral, Rickettsial, and Chlamydial Infections*. 7th ed. Washington, DC: American Public Health Association; 1995:575–81.

142. Clements ML, Dumler JS, Fiset P, et al. Serodiagnosis of Rocky Mountain spotted fever: Comparison of IgM and IgG enzyme-linked immunosorbent assays and indirect fluorescent antibody test. *J Infect Dis*. 1983;148(5):876–80.

143. Newhouse VF, Shepard CC, Redus MD, Tzianabos T, McDade JE. A comparison of the complement fixation, indirect fluorescent antibody, and microagglutination tests for the serological diagnosis of rickettsial diseases. *Am J Trop Med Hyg*. 1979;28:387–95.

144. Dumler J. Indirect fluorescent-antibody test. In: Isenberg H, ed. *Clinical Microbiology Procedures Handbook*. 2nd ed. Washington, DC: American Society for Microbiology Press; 2004.

145. Lagier JC, Edouard S, Pagnier I, et al. Current and past strategies for bacterial culture in clinical microbiology. *Clin Microbiol Rev*. 2015;28(1):208–36.

146. CDC. *Biosafety in Microbiological and Biomedical Laboratories (BMBL)*. 5th ed. Washington, DC: US Department of Health and Human Services, CDC; National Institutes of Health; 2009.

147. Wilfert CM, MacCormack JN, Kleeman K, et al. The prevalence of antibodies to *Rickettsia rickettsii* in an area endemic for Rocky Mountain spotted fever. *J Infect Dis*. 1985;151(5):823–31.

148. McQuiston JH, Wiedeman C, Singleton J, et al. Inadequacy of IgM antibody tests for diagnosis of Rocky Mountain spotted fever. *Am J Trop Med Hyg*. 2014;91(4):767–70.

149. Walls JJ, Aguero-Rosenfeld M, Bakken JS, et al. Inter- and intralaboratory comparison of *Ehrlichia equi* and human granulocytic ehrlichiosis (HGE) agent strains for serodiagnosis of HGE by the immunofluorescent-antibody test. *J Clin Microbiol*. 1999;37(9):2968–73.

150. Comer JA, Nicholson WL, Olson JG, Childs JE. Serologic testing for human granulocytic ehrlichiosis at a national referral center. *J Clin Microbiol*. 1999;37(3):558–64.

151. Walker DH, Burday MS, Folds JD. Laboratory diagnosis of Rocky Mountain spotted fever. *South Med J*. 1980;73(11):1443–6, 1449.

152. Allen MB, Pritt BS, Sloan LM, et al. First reported case of *Ehrlichia ewingii* involving human bone marrow. *J Clin Microbiol*. 2014;58(11): 4102–4.

153. Dawson JE, Paddock CD, Warner CK, et al. Tissue diagnosis of *Ehrlichia chaffeensis* in patients with fatal ehrlichiosis by use of immunohistochemistry, in situ hybridization, and polymerase chain reaction. *Am J Trop Med Hyg*. 2001;65(5):603–9.
154. Philip RN, Casper EA, MacCormack JN, et al. A comparison of serologic methods for diagnosis of Rocky Mountain spotted fever. *Am J Epidemiol*. 1977;105(1):56–67.
155. Hilton E, DeVoti J, Benach J, et al. Seroprevalence and seroconversion for tick-borne diseases in a high-risk population in the northeast United States. *Am J Med*. 1999;106(4):404–9.
156. Marshall GS, Stout GG, Jacobs RF, et al. Antibodies reactive to *Rickettsia rickettsii* among children living in the southeast and south central regions of the United States. *Arch Pediat Adol Med*. 2003;157(5):443–8.
157. Fournier PE, Jensenius M, Laferl H, Vene S, Raoult D. Kinetics of antibody responses in *Rickettsia africae* and *Rickettsia conorii* infections. *Clin Diagn Lab Immunol*. 2002;9(2):324–8.
158. La Scola B, Rydkina L, Ndihokubwayo JB, Vene S, Raoult D. Serological differentiation of murine typhus and epidemic typhus using cross-adsorption and Western blotting. *Clin Diagn Lab Immunol*. 2000;7(4):612–6.
159. Bakken JS, Goellner P, Van Etten M, et al. Seroprevalence of human granulocytic ehrlichiosis among permanent residents of Northwestern Wisconsin. *Clin Infect Dis*. 1998;27(6):1491–6.
160. Centers for Disease Control and Prevention. Anaplasmosis and ehrlichiosis—Maine, 2008. *MMWR Morb Mortal Wkly Rep*. 2009;58(37):1033–6.
161. Hamilton KS, Standaert SM, Kinney MC. Characteristic peripheral blood findings in human ehrlichiosis. *Mod Pathol*. 2004;17:512.
162. Allerdice MEJ, Pritt BS, Sloan LM, Paddock CD, Karpathy SE. A real-time PCR assay for detection of the *Ehrlichia muris*-like agent, a newly recognized pathogen of humans in the upper Midwestern United States. *Ticks Tick Borne Dis*. 2016;7(1):146–9.
163. Bakken JS, Haller I, Riddell D, Walls JJ, Dumler JS. The serological response of patients infected with the agent of human granulocytic ehrlichiosis. *Clin Infect Dis*. 2002;34(1):22–7.
164. Centers for Disease Control and Prevention. Consequences of delayed diagnosis of Rocky Mountain spotted fever in children—West Virginia, Michigan, Tennessee, and Oklahoma, May–July 2000. *MMWR Morb Mortal Wkly Rep*. 2000;49(39):885–8.
165. American Academy of Pediatrics. *Ehrlichia, Anaplasma*, and related infections (human ehrlichiosis, anaplasmosis, and related infections). In: Kimberlin DW, Brady MT, Jackson MA, Long SS, eds. *Red Book: 2015 Report of the Committee on Infectious Diseases*. 30th ed. Elk Grove Village, IL: American Academy of Pediatrics; 2015:329–33.
166. Chapman AS, Bakken JS, Folk SM, et al. Diagnosis and management of tickborne rickettsial diseases: Rocky Mountain spotted fever, ehrlichioses, and anaplasmosis—United States: A practical guide for physicians and other health-care and public health professionals. *MMWR Recomm Rep*. 2006;55(Rr-4):1–27.
167. Von Wittenau MS. Some pharmacokinetic aspects of doxycycline metabolism in man. *Chemotherapy*. 1968;13(suppl 1)(Suppl. 1):41–50.
168. Todd SR, Dahlgren FS, Traeger MS, et al. No visible dental staining in children treated with doxycycline for suspected Rocky Mountain spotted Fever. *J Pediatr*. 2015;166(5):1246–51.
169. Volovitz B, Shkap R, Amir J, et al. Absence of tooth staining with doxycycline treatment in young children. *Clin Pediatr*. 2007;46(2):121–6.
170. Friedman JM, Polifka JE. *Teratogenic Effects of Drugs: A Resource for Clinicians (TERIS)*. 2nd ed. Baltimore, MD: The Johns Hopkins University Press; 2000.
171. FDA.gov. Doxycycline (vibramycin, monodox, doryx, doxy, atridox, periodox, vibra-tabs) use by pregnant and lactating women. http://www.fda.gov/Drugs/EmergencyPreparedness/BioterrorismandDrugPreparedness/ucm131011.htm. Silver Spring, MD. 2015.
172. Cross R, Ling C, Day NP, McGready R, Paris DH. Revisiting doxycycline in pregnancy and early childhood—Time to rebuild its reputation? *Expert Opin Drug Saf*. 2016;15(3):367–82.
173. Walker DH. Rocky Mountain spotted fever: A seasonal alert. *Clin Infect Dis*. 1995;20(5):1111–7.
174. Rolain JM, Maurin M, Vestris G, Raoult D. In vitro susceptibilities of 27 rickettsiae to 13 antimicrobials. *Antimicrob Agents Chemother*. 1998;42(7):1537–41.
175. Botelho-Nevers E, Rovery C, Richet H, Raoult D. Analysis of risk factors for malignant Mediterranean spotted fever indicates that fluoroquinolone treatment has a deleterious effect. *J Antimicrob Chemother*. 2011;66(8):1821–30.
176. Gudiol F, Pallares R, Carratala J, et al. Randomized double-blind evaluation of ciprofloxacin and doxycycline for Mediterranean spotted fever. *Antimicrob Agents Chemother*. 1989;33(6):987–8.
177. Kenyon RH, Williams RG, Oster CN, Pedersen CEJr. Prophylactic treatment of Rocky Mountain spotted fever. *J Clin Microbiol*. 1978;8(1):102–4.
178. Meaney-Delman D, Rasmussen SA, Beigi RH, et al. Prophylaxis and treatment of anthrax in pregnant women. *Obstet Gynecol*. 2013;122(4):885–900.
179. Tanskul P, Linthicum KJ, Watcharapichat P, et al. A new ecology for scrub typhus associated with a focus of antibiotic resistance in rice farmers in Thailand. *J Med Entomol*. 1998;35(4):551–5.
180. Kim YS, Yun HJ, Shim SK, et al. A comparative trial of a single dose of azithromycin versus doxycycline for the treatment of mild scrub typhus. *Clin Infect Dis*. 2004;39(9):1329–35.
181. Strand O, Stromberg A. Ciprofloxacin treatment of murine typhus. *Scand J Infect Dis*. 1990;22(4):503–4.
182. Brouqui P, Raoult D. In vitro antibiotic susceptibility of the newly recognized agent of ehrlichiosis in humans, *Ehrlichia chaffeensis*. *Antimicrob Agents Chemother*. 1992;36(12):2799–803.
183. Krause PJ, Corrow CL, Bakken JS. Successful treatment of human granulocytic ehrlichiosis in children using rifampin. *Pediatrics*. 2003;112 (3 Pt 1):e252–3.
184. Wormser GP, Dattwyler RJ, Shapiro ED, et al. The clinical assessment, treatment, and prevention of Lyme disease, human granulocytic anaplasmosis, and babesiosis: Clinical practice guidelines by the Infectious Diseases Society of America. *Clin Infect Dis*. 2006;43(9):1089–134.
185. Maurin M, Bakken JS, Dumler JS. Antibiotic susceptibilities of *Anaplasma (Ehrlichia)* phagocytophilum strains from various geographic areas in the United States. *Antimicrob Agents Chemother*. 2003;47(1):413–5.
186. Wormser GP, Filozov A, Telford SR3rd, et al. Dissociation between inhibition and killing by levofloxacin in human granulocytic anaplasmosis. *Vector Borne Zoonotic Dis*. 2006;6(4):388–94.
187. Buitrago MI, Ijdo JW, Rinaudo P, et al. Human granulocytic ehrlichiosis during pregnancy treated successfully with rifampin. *Clin Infect Dis*. 1998;27(1):213–5.
188. Dhand A, Nadelman RB, Aguero-Rosenfeld M, et al. Human granulocytic anaplasmosis during pregnancy: Case series and literature review. *Clin Infect Dis*. 2007;45(5):589–93.
189. Tilak R, Tilak VW, Yadav JD. Laboratory evaluation of repellents against *Leptotrombidium deliense*, vector of scrub typhus. *Indian J Med Res*. 2001;113:98–102.
190. Olson JG, Bourgeois AL, Fang RC, Coolbaugh JC, Dennis DT. Prevention of scrub typhus. Prophylactic administration of doxycycline in a randomized double blind trial. *Am J Trop Med Hyg*. 1980;29(5):989–97.

CHAPTER

145 Q Fever

Cara Cherry • Gilbert J. Kersh

INTRODUCTION

Q fever in humans is caused by infection with the gram-negative bacterium *Coxiella burnetii*. The organism grows intracellularly in a parasitophorous vacuole at acidic pH (4.75).[1] *C. burnetii* is a member of the gammaproteobacteria and is classified in the order *Legionellales*, family *Coxiellaceae*. This bacterium infects a broad range of animal species, and is thought to be transmitted primarily by inhalation, but tick transmission could play a role in maintaining the bacteria in wildlife. Q fever is a zoonosis, and humans usually acquire the disease via inhalation of contaminated dust or dried material from animal waste, with a small number of organisms (<10) thought to be able to initiate an infection.[2] Infected livestock, such as cattle, sheep, and goats are the primary reservoirs for human exposure. The organism can grow to very high densities in the placenta of infected livestock. Therefore, these animals shed the largest amounts of *C. burnetii* during parturition. The replicative form of *C. burnetii* has been described as the "large cell variant" (LCV), whereas nonreplicating *C. burnetii* will form a spore-like "small cell variant" (SCV).[3] The SCV is resistant to heat and desiccation resulting in impressive stability in the environment.[4] The environmental stability, transmission by inhalation, and low infectious dose have led to classification of *C. burnetii* as a potential bioweapon and inclusion on the list of select agents maintained by the U.S. Department of Health and Human Services.

HISTORY

Q fever was first described in Australian abattoir workers in the 1930s by Derrick, with characterization of the causative agent by Burnet and Freeman. Between 1936 and 1938, Davis and Cox discovered the Nine Mile agent in a pool of ticks while studying the ecology of Rocky Mountain spotted fever at the Rocky Mountain laboratories in Hamilton, MT.[5,6] The agent was first described as a Rickettsia, and later determined to be the same agent that was causing Q fever in Australia. The designation as *C. burnetii* to honor the contributions of Cox and Burnet gained widespread use in the 1960s. More recent genomic analysis indicates that *C. burnetii* is not closely related to the Rickettsiales, but is a close relative of *Legionella* species.[7] Q fever has primarily been considered an occupational disease, with outbreaks occurring among people that work with animals, and in research institutions that work with livestock.[8] A series of large outbreaks occurred in the Netherlands between 2007 and 2010.[9] These outbreaks were linked to infected goats. *C. burnetii* spread from these goats through the air to the surrounding population resulting in over 4000 symptomatic infections. The outbreaks were halted by culling of infected goats and vaccination of other goats in the affected areas.[10]

EPIDEMIOLOGY

C. burnetii is endemic in the United States, though outbreaks of coxiellosis in livestock species are sporadic. While *C. burnetii* has been detected in many mammalian species, U.S. outbreaks are typically associated with livestock. Nationally representative prevalence studies estimate that *C. burnetii* seroprevalence for sheep was 2.7% in 2011[11] and that 76.9% of dairy bulk milk tanks were positive for *C. burnetii* in 2007.[12] Various smaller scale studies have found seroprevalence in goats ranging from 1.2% to 24%.[13,14] Though the most common mode of transmission to humans is from inhalation of infectious aerosol of infected birth fluids, less frequent routes of transmission include consumption of unpasteurized milk and dairy products as well fomite transmission from contaminated clothing.[15,16] Lack of direct contact with animals should not preclude healthcare providers from considering a diagnosis of Q fever, as airborne transmission of *C. burnetii* is possible.[17]

Q fever became a nationally notifiable disease in the United States in 1999.[18] From 2000 to 2016, 2139 cases of Q fever were reported to the Centers for Disease Control and Prevention.[19,20] An average of 126 cases were reported each year (range: 21–192). Cases were reported from all 50 states with the highest case count in California and Texas. Persons with reported Q fever were predominately male (73.5%) and the mean age was 51.2 years (range: 0–95).[19,20] Thirty-nine percent of cases occurred in April, May, or June. For more than half of the reported cases, there was no noted exposure to animals.[21] In 2008, the case definition for reporting Q fever was updated to divide reporting categories into acute Q fever and chronic Q fever.[22] From 2008 to 2016, there were 1133 reported cases of acute Q fever and 226 reported cases of chronic Q fever.

Q fever is a rare disease in the United States. The 2016 annual incidence rate was 0.05 cases/100,000 persons.[20] However, passive national surveillance underestimates the true burden of disease and there are likely additional cases missed because of underreporting and underdiagnosis.[23] A national seroprevalence study estimated the overall seroprevalence of Q fever in the United States was 3.1%, which is larger than expected based on national surveillance data.[24] Seroprevalence is higher in certain at-risk occupations; 22.2% of veterinarians, 10% of military personnel deployed to Iraq, and 6% of laboratory animal technicians were seropositive for *C. burnetii* antibodies.[25–27]

CLINICAL MANIFESTATIONS

Acute Q fever

The incubation period is typically 2–3 weeks, but varies depending on the inoculum dose.[15,16] The primary infection may be asymptomatic or mild in up to 60% of patients with evidence of seroconversion. Acute Q fever symptoms vary widely, but common presentations are influenza-like febrile illness, hepatitis, or pneumonia. Other symptoms include rigors, myalgia, malaise, severe retrobulbar headache, fatigue, night-sweats, dyspnea, confusion, nausea, diarrhea, abdominal pain, vomiting, nonproductive cough, and chest pain. Women who develop Q fever infections in pregnancy or shortly before conception are at risk for fetal death and abortion.[15]

Chronic Q fever

Chronic Q fever is a rare disease affecting <5% of patients with acute infections.[15] Chronic Q fever occurs months to years after primary infection. Chronic Q fever patients have a persistent, focalized infection with *C. burnetii*.[16] Risk factors associated with progression to chronic Q fever include: valvular heart disease, vascular defects, immunosuppression, and pregnancy during acute infection. Though culture-negative endocarditis is the most common clinical presentation for chronic Q, other manifestations include: infections of aneurysms and vascular prostheses, chronic hepatitis, osteomyelitis, osteoarthritis, and pneumonitis. Q fever endocarditis usually is fatal without proper treatment.[15]

Q Fever Fatigue Syndrome

Q fever fatigue syndrome (QFS) is characterized as persistent fatigue following acute Q fever and is the most common chronic outcome after acute infection.[15,28] QFS has been reported in up to 20–30% of acute Q fever patients.[29] In some patients, fatigue may last for several years to life.[15,29] However, QFS lacks an international uniform definition and differentiating fatigue caused by *C. burnetii* from other postinfective fatigue syndromes and chronic fatigue syndrome might be difficult.[29] There is no consensus on the pathogenesis of QFS.[15,28]

DIAGNOSIS

Acute Q Fever

Diagnosis of acute Q fever is achieved with a combination of PCR and serology. PCR is effective during the first week after symptom onset, either before or within 24–48 hours of antibiotic administration.[30] Serology testing, using the immunofluorescence assay, is the most common laboratory diagnostic technique used for Q fever. Serology requires analysis of acute and convalescent serum samples for confirmation. Antigens used for Q fever serology are derived from two antigenic phases of the Nine Mile strain of *C. burnetii*. Phase 1 has complex LPS side chains and is virulent in animal infections, whereas Phase 2 has a truncated LPS and low virulence in animal infections.[31] In acute infection, the initial antibody reactivity detected by IFA is primarily directed against Phase 2 antigen, though Phase 1 titers may be elevated as well. To confirm diagnosis of acute Q fever by serology, a fourfold rise in Phase 2 IgG between acute and convalescent serology is needed.[15] Phase 2 reactivity in a single serum sample is not sufficient to confirm diagnosis and could represent previous infection. Ideally, the acute specimen is collected in the first week of illness, followed by a convalescent specimen 3–6 weeks later.[15] Phase 2 antibodies are usually not detectable until 1–2 weeks after onset of clinical symptoms, and diagnosis in the first week of illness requires PCR.[30]

Chronic Q Fever

The large number of chronic Q fever cases in the Netherlands that have been analyzed since 2007 have resulted in the Dutch consensus guidelines for chronic Q fever diagnosis.[32] These guidelines require the identification of a nidus of infection by either (1) meeting the modified Duke criteria for endocarditis, or (2) positive PCR on blood or tissue (in absence of acute infection), or (3) demonstration of a vascular or other infection by imaging. In addition to the focus of infection, an IgG serum antibody titer against Phase 1 *C. burnetii* ≥ 1:1024 should be present. For vascular infections, ^{18}F-FDG-PET/CT imaging has proven to be particularly valuable in identifying infectious foci.[33] Direct detection by methods other than PCR can also be used. Immunohistochemistry can be performed on formalin-fixed, paraffin-embedded tissues, such as excised heart valve tissue, to detect the presence of *C. burnetii* antigen. Isolation of *C. burnetii* can be confirmatory for chronic infection, but is not recommended for routine diagnosis. Culture is difficult and requires a biosafety level 3 laboratory. A negative culture does not rule out *C. burnetii* infection.[15]

TREATMENT

The recommended treatment for acute Q fever in adults is doxycycline for 14 days at a dose of 100 mg twice daily. Alternatives when doxycycline is contraindicated include cotrimoxazole, rifampin, and some quinolones.[15] For children, there could be some risk of dental staining with a 2-week course of doxycycline. Short courses (5 days) of doxycycline are not associated with dental staining in children but longer courses are less well studied.[34] For cases with severe disease, effective treatment with doxycycline may outweigh the risk of dental staining. Children should receive a doxycycline dose of 2.2 mg/kg twice per day with a maximum of 100 mg per dose. For mild illness, cotrimoxazole is a good alternative. For adults with chronic Q fever the most effective treatment is doxycycline at 100 mg twice per day in combination with hydroxychloroquine at 200 mg three times per day.[15] Hydroxychloroquine raises the pH of the parasitophorous vacuole where *C. burnetii* replicates. Because *C. burnetii* requires an environment with low pH to replicate, raising the pH of the vacuoles is bacteriostatic for *C. burnetii*.[35] Because doxycycline is also bacteriostatic, and *C. burnetii* can persist for long periods without replication, treatment for chronic Q fever should continue for at least 18 months. Some cases require even longer treatment such as infected prosthetic heart valves. Recovery from chronic Q fever infections is typically aided by surgical removal of the infected tissue.[36] Phase 1 IgG titers should be monitored monthly during chronic infection and should decrease at least fourfold in response to treatment.[15] Resistance to doxycycline is rare in *C. burnetii* infections, but it has been shown that serum levels of doxycycline should be maintained at ≥ 5 μg/mL for effective treatment.[37]

PREVENTION

There are no human or animal vaccines to prevent Q fever available in the United States. A Phase 1 *C. burnetii* vaccine for humans (Q-Vax, CSL Limited) is available in Australia for those at occupational risk for Q fever.[16] A Phase 1 *C. burnetii* vaccine for goats and cattle (Coxevac®, CEVA Sante Animale) is available in Europe. The animal vaccine has been used as an element of outbreak control strategies and to prevent economic losses from abortion.[38]

Certain occupations are at increased risk of exposure to *C. burnetii*, including veterinarians, dairy workers, meat processing plant workers, livestock farmers, and researchers at facilities housing sheep and goats. Q fever education should be provided to employees in high-risk occupations, describing transmission and clinical features of Q fever. Gloves, N95 respirator, protective clothing (e.g., washable or disposable coveralls), and eye protection should be used when assisting with delivery of animals and cleaning up birthing products or in other scenarios where exposure to *C. burnetti* is of concern.[15] *C. burnetii* has been noted to have resistance to some disinfectants.[39] An effective disinfectant for *C. burnetii* is 5% Microchem Plus.[39] The organisms are also susceptible to 70% ethanol, but rapid evaporation makes this a suboptimal choice for surface disinfection.[39]

SPECIAL CONSIDERATIONS

C. burnetii is recognized as a potential biological warfare weapon.[40] The characteristics of low infectious dose, transmission by inhalation of aerosols, and stability in the environment made it a candidate for biological weapon research in the 1950s and 1960s.[41] It was studied by both the U.S. and Soviet biological weapons programs. As part of these studies, use of human volunteers established the very low infective dose of one to ten organisms.[2] These programs were dismantled in the early 1970s and offensive bioweapon research was officially terminated with the passage of the Biological Weapons Convention in 1972. Currently, *C. burnetii* is considered a Category B agent of bioterrorism, and is on the Health and Human Services list of select agents. As a select agent, there are strict rules that govern possession and transport of the agent, and strict reporting requirements if the agent is identified in clinical, animal, or environmental samples.

CONCLUSIONS

C. burnetii, a zoonosis found throughout the world, causes Q fever in humans. Transmission is by inhalation, and human infections usually follow contact with domestic livestock and are more common in rural endemic areas. The illness is usually mild but can become chronic and severe. Endocarditis occurs among patients with underlying heart disease, in particular valvular disease, and cure requires long-term multidrug therapy often accompanied by surgical intervention. Laboratory confirmation of acute Q fever can be achieved by PCR detection in serum or blood, or by titer changes between acute and convalescent serology. Chronic infection is diagnosed by a combination of clinical signs and high titers against Phase 1 *C. burnetii*. Because of the aerosol transmission and impressive durability of the nonreplicating small cell variant form, *C. burnetii* is a potential agent of bioterrorism which has been weaponized in the past. Because the disease is often not suspected, diagnosed, or reported, educational efforts to increase awareness of the disease and improvements in diagnostic capabilities and surveillance are needed to increase the ability to identify and respond to natural and manmade outbreaks in the future.

References

1. Voth DE, Heinzen RA. Lounging in a lysosome: The intracellular lifestyle of *Coxiella burnetii*. *Cell Microbiol*. 2007;9(4):829–40.
2. Tigertt WD, Benenson AS, Gochenour WS. Airborne Q fever. *Bacteriol Rev*. 1961;25:285–93.
3. Coleman SA, Fischer ER, Howe D, Mead DJ, Heinzen RA. Temporal analysis of *Coxiella burnetii* morphological differentiation. *J Bacteriol*. 2004;186(21):7344–52.
4. Kersh GJ, Fitzpatrick KA, Self JS, et al. Presence and persistence of *Coxiella burnetii* in the environments of goat farms associated with a Q fever outbreak. *Appl Environ Microbiol*. 2013;79(5):1697–703.
5. Cox HR. A filter-passing infectious agent isolated from ticks III. Description of organism and cultivation experiments. *Public Health Rep*. 1938;53(52):2270–6.
6. Davis GE, Cox HR, Parker RR, Dyer RE. A filter-passing infectious agent isolated from ticks I. Isolation from *Dermacentor andersoni*, reactions in animals, and filtration experiments. *Public Health Rep*. 1938;53(52):2259–67.
7. Seshadri R, Paulsen IT, Eisen JA, et al. Complete genome sequence of the Q-fever pathogen *Coxiella burnetii*. *Proc Natl Acad Sci U S A*. 2003;100(9):5455–60.
8. McQuiston JH, Childs JE. Q fever in humans and animals in the United States. *Vector Borne Zoonotic Dis*. 2002;2(3):179–91.
9. Delsing CE, Kullberg BJ, Bleeker-Rovers CP. Q fever in the Netherlands from 2007 to 2010. *Neth J Med*. 2010;68(12):382–7.
10. van der Hoek W, Morroy G, Renders NH, et al. Epidemic Q fever in humans in the Netherlands. *Adv Exp Med Biol*. 2012;984:329–64.
11. Oliveira RD, Mousel MR, Pabilonia KL, et al. Domestic sheep show average *Coxiella burnetii* seropositivity generations after a sheep-associated human Q fever outbreak and lack detectable shedding by placental, vaginal, and fecal routes. *PLoS One*. 2017;12(11):e0188054.
12. USDA. Prevalence of Coxiella burnetii in Bulk-tank Milk on U.S. Dairy Operations, 2007. 2011. https://www.aphis.usda.gov/animal_health/nahms/dairy/downloads/dairy07/Dairy07_is_Coxiella.pdf. Accessed June 11, 2018.
13. Baker MD, Pithua PO. Low seroprevalence of *Coxiella burnetii* in Boer goats in Missouri. *BMC Res Notes*. 2014;7:421.
14. Ruppanner R, Riemann HP, Farver TB, West G, Behymer DE, Wijayasinghe C. Prevalence of *Coxiella burnetii* (Q fever) and *Toxoplasma gondii* among dairy goats in California. *Am J Vet Res*. 1978;39(5):867–70.
15. Anderson A, Bijlmer H, Fournier PE, et al. Diagnosis and management of Q fever—United States, 2013: Recommendations from CDC and the Q Fever Working Group. *MMWR Recomm Rep*. 2013;62(RR-03):1–30.
16. Eldin C, Melenotte C, Mediannikov O, et al. From Q fever to *Coxiella burnetii* infection: A paradigm change. *Clin Microbiol Rev*. 2017;30(1):115–90.
17. Tissot-Dupont H, Amadei MA, Nezri M, Raoult D. Wind in November, Q fever in December. *Emerg Infect Dis*. 2004;10(7):1264–9.
18. CSTE. Placing Q Fever (Coxiella burnetii) Under National Surveillance in the United States under the National Public Health Surveillance System (NPHSS). 1999. https://c.ymcdn.com/sites/www.cste.org/resource/resmgr/PS/1999-ID-1.pdf. Accessed June 1, 2018.
19. CDC. MMWR: Summary of Notifiable Infectious Diseases. 2017. https://www.cdc.gov/mmwr/mmwr_nd/index.html. Accessed May 31, 2018.
20. CDC. Notifiable Infectious Diseases and Conditions Data Tables. 2018. https://wwwn.cdc.gov/nndss/infectious-tables.html. Accessed May 31, 2018.
21. Dahlgren FS, McQuiston JH, Massung RF, Anderson AD. Q fever in the United States: Summary of case reports from two national surveillance systems, 2000–2012. *Am J Trop Med Hyg*. 2015;92(2):247–55.
22. CSTE. 08-ID-06 Revision of the Surveillance Case Definition for Q fever. 2008. https://c.ymcdn.com/sites/www.cste.org/resource/resmgr/PS/08-ID-06.pdf. Accessed June 1, 2018.
23. Dahlgren FS, Haberling DL, McQuiston JH. Q fever is underestimated in the United States: A comparison of fatal Q fever cases from two national reporting systems. *Am J Trop Med Hyg*. 2015;92(2):244–6.
24. Anderson AD, Kruszon-Moran D, Loftis AD, et al. Seroprevalence of Q fever in the United States, 2003–2004. *Am J Trop Med Hyg*. 2009;81(4):691–4.
25. Whitney EA, Massung RF, Kersh GJ, et al. Survey of laboratory animal technicians in the United States for *Coxiella burnetii* antibodies and exploration of risk factors for exposure. *J Am Assoc Lab Anim Sci*. 2013;52(6):725–31.
26. Anderson AD, Baker TR, Littrell AC, Mott RL, Niebuhr DW, Smoak BL. Seroepidemiologic survey for *Coxiella burnetii* among hospitalized US troops deployed to Iraq. *Zoonoses Public Health*. 2011;58(4):276–83.
27. Whitney EA, Massung RF, Candee AJ, et al. Seroepidemiologic and occupational risk survey for *Coxiella burnetii* antibodies among US veterinarians. *Clin Infect Dis*. 2009;48(5):550–7.
28. Keijmel SP, Delsing CE, Sprong T, et al. The Qure study: Q fever fatigue syndrome—Response to treatment; a randomized placebo-controlled trial. *BMC Infect Dis*. 2013;13:157.
29. Morroy G, Keijmel SP, Delsing CE, et al. Fatigue following acute Q-fever: A systematic literature review. *PLoS One*. 2016;11(5):e0155884.
30. Schneeberger PM, Hermans MH, van Hannen EJ, Schellekens JJ, Leenders AC, Wever PC. Real-time PCR with serum samples is indispensable for early diagnosis of acute Q fever. *Clin Vaccine Immunol*. 2010;17(2):286–90.
31. Stoker MG, Fiset P. Phase variation of the Nine Mile and other strains of *Rickettsia burneti*. *Can J Microbiol*. 1956;2(3):310–21.
32. Kampschreur LM, Wegdam-Blans MC, Wever PC, et al. Chronic Q fever diagnosis—Consensus guideline versus expert opinion. *Emerg Infect Dis*. 2015;21(7):1183–8.
33. Kouijzer I, Kampschreur L, Wever P, et al. The value of 18F-FDG-PET/CT in diagnosis and during follow-up in 273 patients with chronic Q fever. *J Nucl Med*. 2018;59(1):127–33.
34. Todd SR, Dahlgren FS, Traeger MS, et al. No visible dental staining in children treated with doxycycline for suspected Rocky Mountain spotted fever. *J Pediatr*. 2015;166(5):1246–51.
35. Raoult D, Drancourt M, Vestris G. Bactericidal effect of doxycycline associated with lysosomotropic agents on *Coxiella burnetii* in P388D1 cells. *Antimicrob Agents Chemother*. 1990;34(8):1512–4.
36. Million M, Thuny F, Richet H, Raoult D. Long-term outcome of Q fever endocarditis: A 26-year personal survey. *Lancet Infect Dis*. 2010;10(8):527–35.
37. Rolain JM, Mallet MN, Raoult D. Correlation between serum doxycycline concentrations and serologic evolution in patients with *Coxiella burnetii* endocarditis. *J Infect Dis*. 2003;188(9):1322–5.
38. Hogerwerf L, van den Brom R, Roest HI, et al. Reduction of *Coxiella burnetii* prevalence by vaccination of goats and sheep, The Netherlands. *Emerg Infect Dis*. 2011;17(3):379–86.
39. Scott GH, Williams JC. Susceptibility of *Coxiella burnetii* to chemical disinfectants. *Ann N Y Acad Sci*. 1990;590:291–6.
40. Madariaga MG, Rezai K, Trenholme GM, Weinstein RA. Q fever: A biological weapon in your backyard. *Lancet Infect Dis*. 2003;3(11):709–21.
41. Riedel S. Biological warfare and bioterrorism: A historical review. *Proceedings*. 2004;17(4):400–6.

CHAPTER

146 Tularemia*

Diseases Transmitted Primarily from Animals to Humans (Zoonoses)

Paul S. Mead

Tularemia is an uncommon but potentially serious bacterial zoonosis caused by *Francisella tularensis*. Transmission to humans occurs through arthropod bites, ingestion of contaminated food or water, inhalation of contaminated aerosols, or handling of infected animal tissues. Clinical manifestations are variable and depend on the route of inoculation, the dose, and the virulence of the organism. Most commonly, the disease presents in humans as an indolent ulcer at the site of cutaneous inoculation accompanied by regional lymphadenitis (ulceroglandular form). Other forms include glandular, oculoglandular, oropharyngeal, gastrointestinal, septic, and pneumonic tularemia. Although uncommon, tularemia occurs widely in temperate and subarctic regions of North America and Eurasia. Currently in the United States, fewer than 200 cases are reported annually.[1] *F. tularensis* is classified as a Tier 1 Select Agent and has been evaluated as a potential weapon by several countries.

AGENT

F. tularensis is a small (0.2 by 0.2–0.7 μm), nonmotile, pleomorphic, gram-negative coccobacillus. Although nonsporulating and strictly aerobic, the bacterium is a hardy saprophyte that can survive in water, moist soil, and in decaying animal carcasses. In the laboratory, *F. tularensis* is fastidious, slow growing, and requires cysteine, cystine, or other sulfhydryl containing media.

Isolates of *F. tularensis* can be divided into several subspecies based on virulence testing, biochemical reactions, PCR, and epidemiologic features. Two subspecies account for most human illness: *F. tularensis* subspecies *tularensis* (Jellison Type A) and *F. tularensis* subspecies *holarctica* (formerly *paleartica*, Jellison Type B). Type A strains have an LD_{50} in rabbits of fewer than ten organisms and are generally considered more virulent. They are found almost exclusively in North America. Type B strains have an LD_{50} of more than 10^7 organisms in rabbits and are found in both North America and Eurasia. Further discrimination of isolates can be achieved using a variety of molecular assays, including pulsed-field gel electrophoresis, multiple-locus variable-number tandem repeat analysis, single-nucleotide polymorphisms, and whole-genome microarray.[2,3]

LIFE CYCLE OF *F. TULARENSIS*

F. tularensis has been isolated from more than 100 species of wild mammals, at least 9 species of domestic animals (including cattle, dogs, cats), 25 species of birds, amphibians, fish, and more than 50 species of arthropods. However, many of these animals may be colonized or infected only incidentally. Actual maintenance cycles, although incompletely defined, appear to differ among *F. tularensis* subspecies. Type A *F. tularensis* is believed to occur primarily in rabbits with transmission by ticks (*Demacentor* spp, *Amblyomma* spp, *Ixodes* spp) and tabanid or deer flies (*Cysops discalis*). Type B infections are often associated with aquatic environments and rodents such as beaver, muskrats, and voles. Transmission among these animals may occur through ingestion of contaminated water, soil, or food. Epidemiological studies have also implicated mosquitoes as a potential mode of Type B transmission to humans in Europe.[4] *F. tularensis* has been shown to survive within free living amoeba, suggesting that protozoa might also play a role in the life cycle of this organism.[5]

EPIDEMIOLOGY

Geographic Distribution

Tularemia is endemic throughout much of the northern hemisphere including North America from the Arctic Circle to Mexico, continental Europe, states of the Russian Federation, China, and Japan.[6] In the United States, incidence is generally highest in the South-central and Great Plains regions, and on the island of Martha's Vineyard, Massachusetts (Fig. 146-1).[1] In Eurasia, reported incidence is highest in Sweden, Finland, and Russia. Although the southern hemisphere has long been considered free of tularemia, recent reports have documented rare cases in Tasmainia associated with exposure to ringtail possums (*Pseudocheirus peregrinus*), from which *F. tularensis* subspecies *holarctica* has been isolated.[7]

Populations Affected

Tularemia is a primarily a disease of rural areas. Persons at increased risk of infection include hunters, trappers, and wildlife specialists who handle potentially infected animals, persons in contact with water and soils contaminated by wild animals, persons exposed to bites of certain hard ticks and biting flies, and landscapers who mow or cut brush.[8] Over time, these associations have generated various descriptive terms, including "wild hare disease," "rabbit fever," "deerfly fever," and "lawnmower tularemia." In addition, laboratory workers who work with cultures of *F. tularensis* can be at high risk of infection if proper laboratory precautions are not observed.

In the United States, 1208 tularemia cases were reported during 2001–10, with a median of 126 cases per year.[1] This compares with a high of 2291 reported cases in 1939.[1] Incidence is highest among children 5–9 years old and adult men aged 65–69 years. A significant majority of cases occur among whites; however, incidence is highest among American Indians/Alaskan Natives at 0.3 per 100,000, as compared with 0.04 per 100,000 among the overall population. Recent case counts by state are available at https://www.cdc.gov/Tularemia. Although cases have been reported from all states other than Hawaii,

*Note: The findings and conclusions in this chapter are those of the author and do not necessarily represent the views of the Centers for Disease Control and Prevention.

the states of Arkansas, Missouri, and Oklahoma regularly account for more than half of reported cases in the United States (Fig. 146-1).

Sources of Infection

Tularemia is notable for having an especially wide array of potential sources and modes of transmission; the risk posed by any particular source often varies by season and location. In general, arthropod bites and animal contact are believed to be the most common sources of infection. In North American, vector tick species include the American dog tick (*Dermacentor variabilis*), the lone star tick (*A. americanum*), and the Rocky Mountain wood tick (*D. andersoni*).[6,8] Outbreaks due to bites by American dog ticks have occurred repeatedly in spring and early summer among native Americans in Great Plains states of the United States.[9] Lone star ticks are thought to account for most cases in south-central states, and the wood tick accounts for scattered human cases across the western United States.[8] Biting flies have been identified as the source of both outbreaks and sporadic cases in western states, especially semiarid areas of Utah, Nevada, California, and Wyoming.[10,11] Mosquitoes, although not established as a vector in North America, are believed to be important in transmitting the disease to humans in forested Scandinavian and Baltic regions, and mosquito-borne outbreaks have been reported from Sweden and Finland.[12]

Direct contact with animals, especially wild rabbits, hares, and rodents, is also an important source of human infection. In Japan, tularemia has long been associated with the hunting and eating of rabbits,[13] and direct contact with rabbits still accounts for many cases in the southeastern United States. Water-loving rodents such as muskrats and beaver are commonly infected, and contact with these animals has been associated with large outbreaks among trappers.[14] At least one sporadic case has been linked to a fishhook injury.[15] Contact with domesticated cats[16] and dogs, as well as commercially distributed pets such as prairie dogs[17,18] and hamsters[19] have been identified as sources of outbreaks and sporadic cases of human infection.

Although uncommon, ingestion of contaminated food or water has occasionally lead to substantial outbreaks, especially in Europe.[20] Following a decade long conflict in the 1990s, a large outbreak in Kosovo was attributed to contaminated food and water supplies.[21] More recently an outbreak in Germany was linked to drinking freshly pressed must (juice) made from mechanically harvested wine grapes; in addition to *F. tularensis*, molecular analysis of the must detected evidence of wood mouse DNA, suggesting a likely reason for the contmination.[22]

Aerosolization of *F. tularensis* can occur in certain settings and may result in primary pneumonic tularemia. This has been a particular problem for laboratorians working with live cultures, leading to the requirement that *F. tularensis* be handled with BSL-3 level precautions. It has also been described following exposures to contaminated stored and fresh mown hay, and among workers in factories exposed to contaminated water sprays. In Sweden, a large outbreak of pneumonic tularemia occurred among farm workers exposed to hay contaminated by field voles.[23] Cases of pneumonic tularemia on Martha's Vineyard, Massachusetts, have been linked to landscaping practices, especially mowing, cutting brush, and using power blowers.[24,25]

THE DISEASE

Clinical Manifestations

The signs and symptoms of tularemia vary depending on route of exposure. The major clinical forms are: ulceroglandular (45–85% of cases); glandular (10–25%); oculoglandular (<5%); septic (<5%); oropharyngeal (<5%); and pneumonic (<5%). The usual incubation period is 3–5 days after exposure, with a range of 1–21 days. All forms are accompanied by similar nonspecific symptoms of fever (38–40°C), chills, headache, cough, and generalized body aches.[26,27] Without treatment, nonspecific symptoms may persist for several weeks and result in weight loss. Any of the principal forms of tularemia may be complicated by bacteremic spread, leading variously to sepsis, tularemic pneumonia, and meningitis.

Ulceroglandular disease is characterized by a local papule that appears at the site of inoculation within a few days of the onset of generalized symptoms. This papule usually becomes pustular, and then ulcerates about 4 days after it first appears. The ulcer may take the appearance of an eschar but usually has an indolent character. Lymphadenitis with pain, tenderness, and swelling of one or more regional nodes is usually apparent by the time of ulceration. Epitrochlear and axillary nodes are most commonly affected in persons infected through handling of contaminated materials. Children infected through arthropod bites often have cervical lymphadenopathy, while adults usually have femoral/inguinal adenopathy; these distributions reflect differences in the most common sites of arthropod bites.[27] In rare cases, abscessed nodes may suppurate and discharge purulent material.

Glandular tularemia is very similar to the ulceroglandular form except that there is no cutaneous ulceration. In oculoglandular disease, which follows contamination of the eye by infectious fluids, ulceration is localized to the conjunctiva, and the cervical and preauricular nodes become enlarged.

Tularemia sepsis, or so-called "typhoidal" tularemia, presents as an acute, sometimes fulminant illness without localizing signs; the diagnosis is most often made by identifying *F. tularensis* in cultures of the blood. The systemic inflammatory response syndrome may ensue accompanied by any of its usual complications. Hematogenous spread to other organ systems may lead to pneumonia, involvement of the kidneys, and to meningitis.

Oropharyngeal tularemia is acquired by ingesting contaminated food (almost always inadequately cooked meat) or water. Typically, the patient develops exudative pharyngitis or tonsillitis, sometimes with ulceration, and cervical lymphadenopathy. Stomatitis occasionally occurs. Infrequently, the upper gastrointestinal tract may become involved, leading to persistent diarrhea.

Pneumonic tularemia can arise as a secondary complication of other forms of tularemia or, less frequently, as a primary pneumonia from exposure to an infective aerosol. Pneumonic infiltrates of varying character may be seen in one or more lobes, and are often accompanied by pleural effusion, and by hilar lymphadenopathy.[28] Lung abscesses are sometimes seen. Pulmonic manifestations include cough (usually with minimal sputum production), sometimes pleuritic pain, and rarely, dyspnea.

Prior to the use of antibiotics, overall mortality from infections with Type A *F. tularensis* was in the range of 5–10%, but with fatality rates of 40–60% for septicemic and pneumonic forms of disease. Infection with Type B strains was associated with a fatality rate of only 1–3%. However, recent studies indicate that some Type A strains are associated with lower mortality in humans than Type B strains.[29] In 2000–01, there were 3 fatalities reported among 271 case reported in the United States, for an overall fatality rate of 1.1%.[30]

Diagnosis

The diagnosis of tularemia is made by clinical findings combined with information on potentially infective exposures. Differential diagnostic possibilities are many: in persons with glandular disease they include plague, sporotrichosis, lymphogranuloma venereum, chancre, and chancroid; in persons with oropharyngeal tularemia, other bacterial and viral causes of stomatitis, pharyngitis and cervical adenitis must be considered; in persons with pneumonia, they include legionnaires disease, histoplasmosis, and tuberculosis; and, in persons with tularemia sepsis, typhoid fever, and other causes of systemic inflammatory response syndrome.

The diagnosis of tularemia is confirmed by isolation of *F. tularensis*. Suspicion of tularemia should be conveyed to the microbiology laboratory to guide selection of appropriate media and to protect the

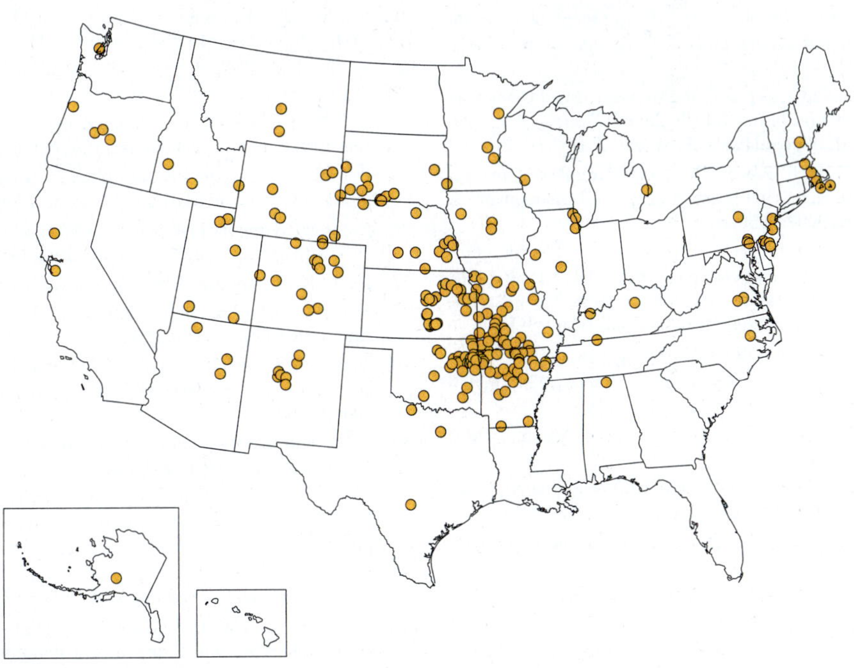

FIGURE 146-1. Reported cases of tularemia, by State, United States, 2016.

safety of laboratory workers. Appropriate media for isolation from clinical specimens include Thayer-Martin agar, chocolate agar, cysteine heart agar with 9% chocolatized blood (CHAB), buffered charcoal-yeast extract agar, and thyoglycollate broth.[31] Inoculated plates should be incubated at 37°C and held for up to 14 days. Colonies are pinpoint after 24 hours of incubation, and may be only 3 mm in diameter at 96 hours. Because of its slow growth, *F. tularensis* may be obscured in culture by more rapidly growing organisms. Isolation from contaminated materials can be achieved by passage through laboratory mice in specialized laboratories or by growth on enriched cysteine heart agar blood culture medium supplemented with antibiotics (CHAB-A).[32]

In addition to culture, materials other than blood should be streaked on glass slides for examination by fluorescent antibody testing. Other potentially useful rapid diagnostic procedures include enzyme-linked immunoassay and immunoblotting for IgM antibodies, polymerase chain reaction assays, and DNA probes; however, these are not routine. The agglutination reaction for combined IgM and IgG immunoglobulins is the routine immunodiagnostic procedure in use in most laboratories. Reference laboratories use microagglutination methods that are more sensitive than tube agglutination procedures.

Many routine diagnostic laboratories have policies that exclude work on *F. tularensis*, since it readily aerosolizes and is a notorious cause of laboratory-acquired infections. Biosafety level 2 precautions are essential for routine diagnostic procedures, and biosafety level 3 precautions are needed for culture or animal studies.[33] In the United States, the national diagnostic and reference laboratory for tularemia is located at the Centers for Disease Control and Prevention, Division of Vector-Borne Infectious Diseases, Fort Collins, Colorado. Identification by automated systems can be unreliable and is potentially dangerous.

Treatment

Streptomycin is the drug of choice based on experience, efficacy, and FDA approval. Gentamicin is considered an acceptable alternative, but some series have reported a lower primary success rate and some relapses.[34] Treatment with aminoglycosides should be continued for 10 days.[35] Tetracycline may be a suitable alternative to aminoglycosides for less severely ill patients, but must be given for at least 14 days as relapses can occur. Ciprofloxacin is not FDA approved for treatment of tularemia but has shown good efficacy in vitro, in animals, and in humans.[34,36–39]

Although *F. tularensis* Type B strains from Eastern Europe are commonly resistant to macrolides, azithromycin has activity *in vitro* against other strains, and may be useful for treatment in patients for whom other treatments are contraindicated.[40,41] Despite some supporting in vitro suceptablility data, use of cephalosporins has been associated with frequent treatment failures.[34]

Prevention and Control

Prevention of tularemia is best achieved by avoiding exposure to bites of ticks and blood-feeding flies, and by avoiding direct contact with wild animal tissues. Persons exposed to biting fly- and tick-infested areas should when feasible wear protective clothing, tuck pants legs into socks, and apply repellents containing DEET to skin and clothing as directed by the manufacturer. Permethrin-based acaricides can be applied to clothing to kill ticks on contact. Frequent examinations should be made for ticks on clothing and skin, and attached ticks should be promptly removed. Persons should avoid contact with sick or dead animals, and hunters and trappers should always handle animal carcasses with impervious gloves. In order to reduce tick infestations in residential areas, pet dogs and cats should be restrained and kept tick-free using appropriate acaricides. A live attenuated vaccine has been used previously to protect laboratory personnel who routinely work with *F. tularensis*, however, is not widely available. Antibiotic prophylaxis is not recommended for persons having exposure to patients with pneumonic tularemia, since person-to-person respiratory spread has not been documented. Recommendations for management of exposed laboratory personnel are available at: https://www.cdc.gov/tularemia/laboratoryexposure/index.html.

References

1. CDC. Tularemia—United States, 2001-2010. *MMWR Morb Mortal Wkly Rep.* 2013;62:963–6.
2. Johansson A, Forsman M, Sjostedt A. The development of tools for diagnosis of tularemia and typing of *Francisella tularensis. APMIS.* 2004;112:898–907.
3. Birdsell DN, Vogler AJ, Buchhagen J, et al. TaqMan real-rime PCR assasys for single-nucleotide polymorhpisms withich identify *Francisella tularensis* and its subspecies and subpopulations. *PLoS One.* 2014;9:e107964.
4. Eliasson H, Lindback J, Nuorti JP, et al. The 2000 tularemia outbreak: A case-control study of risk factors in disease-endemic and emergent areas, Sweden. *Emerg Infect Dis.* 2002;8:956–60.
5. Beier CL, Horn M, Michel R, et al. The genus *Caedibacter* comprises endosymbionts of *Paramecium* spp. related to the Rickettsiales (Alphaproteobacteria) and to *Francisella tularensis* (Gammaproteobacteria). *Appl Environ Microbiol.* 2002;68:6043–50.
6. Hopla CE. The ecology of tularemia. *Adv Vet Sci Comp Med.* 1974;18:25–53.
7. Eden J, Rose K, Ng J, et al. *Francisella tularensis* ssp. *holarctica* in Ringtail Possums, Australia. *Emerg Infect Dis.* 2017;23:1198–201.
8. Jellison WL. *Tularemia in North America, 1930–1974.* Missoula, MT: University of Montana; 1974.
9. Markowitz LE, Hynes NA, de la Cruz P, et al. Tick-borne tularemia. An outbreak of lymphadenopathy in children. *JAMA.* 1985;254:2922–5.
10. Klock LE, Olsen PF, Fukushima T. Tularemia epidemic associated with the deerfly. *JAMA.* 1973;226:149–52.
11. CDC. Tularemia transmitted by insect bites—Wyoming, 2001–2003. *MMWR Morb Mortal Wkly Rep.* 2005;54:170–3.
12. Tarnvik A, Priebe HS, Grunow R. Tularaemia in Europe: An epidemiological overview. *Scand J Infect Dis.* 2004;36:350–5.
13. Ohara Y, Sato T, Homma M. Epidemiological analysis of tularemia in Japan (yato-byo). *FEMS Immunol Med Microbiol.* 1996;13:185–9.
14. Young LS, Bickness DS, Archer BG, et al. Tularemia epidemia: Vermont, 1968. Forty-seven cases linked to contact with muskrats. *N Engl J Med.* 1969;280:1253–60.
15. Whitten T, Bjork J, Neitzel D, Smith K, Sullivan M, Scheftel J. Notes from the field: *Francisella tularensis* type B infection from a fish hook injury—Minnesota, 2016. *MMWR Morb Mortal Wkly Rep.* 2017;66:194.
16. Capellan J, Fong IW. Tularemia from a cat bite: Case report and review of feline-associated tularemia. *Clin Infect Dis.* 1993;16:472–5.
17. Avashia SB, Petersen JM, Lindley CM, et al. First reported prairie dog-to-human tularemia transmission, Texas, 2002. *Emerg Infect Dis.* 2004;10:483–6.
18. Petersen JM, Schriefer ME, Carter LG, et al. Laboratory analysis of tularemia in wild-trapped, commercially traded prairie dogs, Texas, 2002. *Emerg Infect Dis.* 2004;10:419–25.
19. CDC. Tularemia associated with a hamster bite—Colorado, 2004. *MMWR Morb Mortal Wkly Rep.* 2005;53:1202–3.
20. Aktas D, Celebi B, Isik ME, et al. Oropharyngeal tularemia outbreak associated with drinking contaminated tap water, Turkey, July–September 2013. *Emerg Infect Dis.* 2015;21:2194–6.
21. Reintjes R, Dedushaj I, Gjini A, et al. Tularemia outbreak investigation in Kosovo: Case control and environmental studies. *Emerg Infect Dis.* 2002;8:69–73.
22. Bruckhardt F, Hoffmann D, Jahn K, et al. Oropharyngeal tularemia from freshly pressed grape must. *New Engl J Med.* 2018;379:197–9.
23. Syrjala H, Kujala P, Myllyla V, et al. Airborne transmission of tularemia in farmers. *Scand J Infect Dis.* 1985;17:371–5.
24. Feldman KA, Stiles-Enos D, Julian K, et al. Tularemia on Martha's Vineyard: Seroprevalence and occupational risk. *Emerg Infect Dis.* 2003;9:350–4.
25. Feldman KA, Enscore RE, Lathrop SL, et al. An outbreak of primary pneumonic tularemia on Martha's Vineyard. *N Engl J Med.* 2001;345:1601–6.
26. Evans ME, Gregory DW, Schaffner W, et al. Tularemia: A 30-year experience with 88 cases. *Medicine (Baltimore).* 1985;64:251–69.
27. Jacobs RF. Tularemia. *Adv Pediatr Infect Dis.* 1996;12:55–69.
28. Miller RP, Bates JH. Pleuropulmonary tularemia. A review of 29 patients. *Am Rev Respir Dis.* 1969;99:31–41.
29. Staples JE, Kubota KA, Chalcraft LG, et al. Epidemiologic and molecular analysis of human tularemia, United States, 1964–2004. *Emerg Infect Dis.* 2006;12:1113–8.
30. CDC. Summary of notifiable diseases—United States, 2003. *MMWR Morb Mortal Wkly Rep.* 2005;52:78.
31. Chu M, Weyant R. *Franscisella* and *Brucella*. In: Murray PR, ed. *Manual of Clinical Microbiology*, 8th ed. Washington, DC: ASM Press; 2003, pp. 789–808.
32. Petersen JM, Schriefer ME, Gage KL, et al. Methods for enhanced culture recovery of *Francisella tularensis. Appl Environ Microbiol.* 2004;70:3733–5.
33. U.S. Department of Health and Human Services. Biosafety in Microbiological and Biomedical Laboratories. 5th Edition. Revised December 2009. https://www.cdc.gov/biosafety/publications/bmbl5/.
34. Enderlin G, Morales L, Jacobs RF, et al. Streptomycin and alternative agents for the treatment of tularemia: Review of the literature. *Clin Infect Dis.* 1994;19:42–7.
35 Dennis DT, Inglesby TV, Henderson DA, et al. Tularemia as a biological weapon: Medical and public health management. *JAMA.* 2001;285:2763–73.
36. Syrjala H, Schildt R, Raisainen S. In vitro susceptibility of *Francisella tularensis* to fluoroquinolones and treatment of tularemia with norfloxacin and ciprofloxacin. *Eur J Clin Microbiol Infect Dis.* 1991;10:68–70.
37. Russell P, Eley SM, Fulop MJ, et al. The efficacy of ciprofloxacin and doxycycline against experimental tularaemia. *J Antimicrob Chemother.* 1998;41:461–5.
38. Limaye AP, Hooper CJ. Treatment of tularemia with fluoroquinolones: Two cases and review. *Clin Infect Dis.* 1999;29:922–4.
39. Johansson A, Berglund L, Gothefors L, et al. Ciprofloxacin for treatment of tularemia in children. *Pediatr Infect Dis J.* 2000;19:449–53.
40. Ahmad S, Hunter L, Qin A, Mann BJ, van Hoek ML. Azithromycin effectiveness against intracellular infections of *Francisella. BMC Microbiol.* 2010;10:123.
41. Dentan C, Pavese P, Pelloux I, Boisset S, Brion JP, Stahl JP, Maurin M. Treatment of tularemia in pregnant woman, France. *Emerg Infect Dis.* 2013;19:996–8.

CHAPTER

147 Plague

Kiersten J. Kugeler

INTRODUCTION

Plague is a highly virulent zoonosis that has claimed hundreds of millions of lives over recorded history.[1-3] The etiologic agent, *Yersinia pestis*, persists in complex enzootic cycles of rodents and fleas in discrete geographic foci in Asia, Africa, and the Americas. Humans are incidental hosts, most often infected by flea bites, but also by direct contact with infected animal tissues or inhalation of infectious respiratory droplets. The clinical syndrome varies with route of inoculation of the bacterium, resulting in three primary clinical forms, bubonic, septicemic, and pneumonic plague. Although most cases of plague are sporadic and effective therapy exists, periodic outbreaks can generate fear among the public, driven by misinformation. Plague remains a persistent public health concern due to its rapid clinical course, high mortality, and potential for epidemic spread. *Y. pestis* is currently classified as a Tier 1 select agent, subject to high-level regulation and oversight, due to both its past and potential use as a bioweapon.[4]

HISTORY

During the course of recorded history, plague caused three deadly pandemics, collectively giving rise to a notorious reputation in modern society.[1-3] Although possible epidemics occurring before 1000 BC have been described, the first well-recorded plague pandemic began in AD 542. The associated cumulative death toll is highly debatable, but most historians agree that roughly half of the population was lost during the series of epidemics that occurred over the ensuing 150 years.[1] This event is often referred to as the Justinian Plague, named after the Byzantine emperor under whose rule the most consequential effects of the pandemic were felt. The pandemic affected the entire "known" world at the time—primarily the Mediterranean basin, but also central and southern Asia.

Plague retreated at the close of the first pandemic only to emerge several centuries later, spreading along trade routes from central Asia.[1] After reaching Europe in AD 1347, plague decimated one-third to one-half of Europe's population in a few short years in what is now referred to as the "Black Death."[2,5] Ongoing epidemics continued for the next three centuries, not only in Europe but also in the Mediterranean basin and central Asia. The second pandemic has earned an important place in human history due to its consequential effect on the economics, labor markets, culture, art, religion, and politics in medieval Europe.[1,5] The origin of public health practice dates from this time, when administrative functions of governments expanded to institute quarantines and barriers to trade to limit the spread of disease.[5]

The third pandemic began in China during the mid-to-late 1800s, and spread to the port of Hong Kong in 1894, presumably accelerated by troop movement. Soon thereafter, plague rapidly spread worldwide by way of new steamships, and was introduced into 77 different port cities on five continents, ultimately becoming entrenched on all continents except Australia.[1-3] Shipborne spread of plague ceased after a few decades following intense rat-proofing and rat control efforts in ports throughout the world.[6]

Plague entered the United States via the port of San Francisco, with the first autochthonous cases occurring in the Chinatown district in March of 1900.[2,3] In the following two decades, cases occurred in multiple port cities along the Pacific and Gulf Coasts, including Seattle, Los Angeles, and New Orleans.[3] During this time, plague became entrenched in discrete foci worldwide, but also became manageable with environmental controls and effective antimicrobial treatment.[1,2]

Discovery and early research into the plague bacterium and its association with rats and fleas occurred at the outset of the third pandemic.[1] Observations during extensive pneumonic plague outbreaks in Manchuria in the early 1900s generated much of the modern knowledge on primary pneumonic plague, including its incubation period, duration and distance of infectivity, and the effectiveness of gauze and cotton masks for preventing infection.[7-9] The cumulative death toll during the third pandemic is estimated at ~12 million.[1]

Modern plague is marked by sporadic cases and small outbreaks in discrete foci in Africa, Asia, and the Americas. Lengthy quiescent periods between epizootics can lull governments and public health authorities into complacency and result in loss of institutional knowledge regarding how to detect, treat, and prevent plague. Epidemics can generate an inappropriate level of panic, fueled by fear and misinformation, such as in India in 1994 and Madagascar in 2017.[10,11] Poor diagnostics and nonspecific case definitions challenge interpretation regarding scope and extent of actual plague infection in these settings. For example, in 1994 in Surat, India, roughly 500,000 people fled the city, products and travelers were quarantined, and tourism to India diminished, all resulting in billions of dollars in economic loss. After the dust settled, there was minimal evidence that the outbreak was due to *Y. pestis*.[8,11,12] The modern experience of plague is tinged with concern over its potential use as a bioweapon.[13] This concern is not only due to its infectivity and high mortality, but its historical use as a weapon in diverse circumstances, from the catapulting of corpses of plague victims over city walls during the siege on Kaffa in central Asia (in modern day Ukraine) in the 1300s, to the dropping of infected fleas from airplanes during World War II.[4,14] After World War II, bioweapons programs in both the United States and the Soviet Union developed methods to aerosolize *Y. pestis*.[4]

AGENT

Yersinia pestis is an aerobic, gram-negative, nonmotile, nonsporulating coccobacillus in the family *Enterobacteriaceae*.[1,15] *Y. pestis* is among the most invasive bacteria known. Molecular evolutionary research has suggested *Y. pestis* diverged from its close relative, the enteric bacterium *Y. pseudotuberculosis,* as recently as 1500–20,000 years ago.[16] *Y. pestis* isolates are divided into three main biovars based on biochemical reactivity, *Antiqua, Medievalis,* and *Orientalis.* Although it has been suggested that these three biovars were clones that resulted in the three pandemics, respectively, and *Orientalis* strains appear to have emerged and spread from China in the late 1800s, there is no clear evidence that Antiqua and *Medievalis biovars* caused the first and second pandemics.[16]

Yersinia pestis is nonfastidious and characteristic growth occurs slowly, with pinpoint colonies visible after 24–48 hours on many types of culture media, including blood and MacConkey agar. Colonies grown on blood agar display a "hammered copper" appearance, and after 72 hours, "fried egg" morphology.[15] A highly immunogenic and specific envelope glycoprotein (fraction 1 or F1) is expressed at high levels when the organism is grown at greater than 30°C. Staining rarely occurs in modern practice, but under polychromatic stains such as Wayson or Giemsa, cells exhibit bipolar staining that resembles a closed safety pin.[1,15] Highly virulent strains have three plasmids that encode a variety of virulence factors responsible for flea-borne transmission, utilization of host nutrients, evasion of phagocytosis, and initiation of cellular damage, among other processes.[1,15] All biovars appear to be equally virulent for mammalian hosts.

Investigators have used many different subtyping methods to differentiate *Y. pestis* strains for varied purposes, ranging from species identification to individual strain differentiation.[17] Overall, *Y. pestis* strains are less genetically diverse than other bacteria. Recent work has demonstrated single nucleotide polymorphisms, variable number tandem repeat analysis, and multilocus sequence typing (MLST) to be useful subtyping approaches, depending on the scientific question.[17] Whole genome MLST (wgMLST) is a single platform approach used to simultaneously capture multiple sequence features and holds promise as the tool of choice for most applied public health questions.[18]

ECOLOGY

Y. pestis is maintained in nature in complex and incompletely understood cycles of rodents and their fleas.[19] Enzootic (maintenance) cycles necessarily involve heterogeneously susceptible populations of wild rodent hosts and varied flea species. Although the dynamics of long-term plague foci are poorly defined, their distribution appears linked to climate and presence of distinct vector species rather than of rodent species.[20,21] Most foci are found in semiarid areas with low annual precipitation but not extreme desert-like conditions.[22]

Fleas acquire *Y. pestis* from feeding on an infected rodent host; transovarial transmission in the flea does not occur. Although over 80 flea species have been found infected with *Y. pestis,* the potential for various species to serve as important enzootic or bridging vectors depends on several factors including temperature, their feeding style and frequency, and host preferences.[20,23] Although rodent infection may occasionally occur by direct contact or ingestion, flea-borne transmission between rodents is critical to maintenance in nature.[19,20] Spillover into more universally susceptible species results in geographically localized amplification of the cycle characterized by high mortality, termed an epizootic. Almost all mammals can become infected,[19] including canids, lagomorphs, and humans; most are incidental hosts and do not contribute to ongoing maintenance. Although possible for incidental hosts to become infected by contact with enzootic plague cycles, contact seems to occur most often in concert with rapid spread indicative of epizootic activity, as large numbers of infected fleas search for alternative blood meal hosts due to the substantial mortality of their preferred hosts.

Rodent and flea species involved in plague cycles vary across different parts of the world.[23] The species culpable for human infection in many parts of the world are the mainly peridomestic black rat (*Rattus rattus*) and the rat fleas *Xenopsylla cheopis* and *X. brasiliensis.* In the western United States, plague is maintained in small rodents with spillover into prairie dogs, wood rats, and ground squirrels. In this setting, diverse flea species have been linked to human infection given the variability of involved rodent species in any given epizootic.[23] Human ectoparasites, primarily the flea *Pulex irritans* and the body louse, *Pediculus humanus,* have been subject to speculation and study regarding their potential role in fostering rapid transmission during the Black Death.[24–26] However, their potential to serve as efficient vectors is not well documented and their possible role in modern plague epidemics appears to be minor.[25]

Since first described in 1914, the mechanism by which *Y. pestis* amplified in nature was explained solely by a "blocked" flea paradigm.[23,27] In this scenario, *Y. pestis* multiplies extensively in the proventriculus (or "fore gut") of the flea, ultimately creating a biofilm that functionally prevents blood meals from digesting within the flea. Absent digestible nutrients, the flea then begins to starve and repeatedly seeks additional blood meals, regurgitating *Y. pestis* into each attempted blood meal source. Although well demonstrated, this system seemed discordant with rapidly spreading epizootics because of the time required for biofilm formation to occur, 5 days to 3 weeks postflea infection. Recent research has yielded an alternate paradigm, termed early-phase transmission, in which fleas are able to successfully transmit *Y. pestis* infection as early as 3 hours postinfection and in the absence of any blockage. Although demonstrated for a handful of North American flea species to date, the biologic mechanism for early-phase transmission has not been fully described. Nevertheless, it seems possible that the blocked flea paradigm supports enzootic transmission, whereas early-phase transmission may better explain epizootic transmission.[20,28] As a nonspore forming organism, *Y. pestis* does not survive well outside hosts. However, sporadic reports have found evidence of survival in amebae and soil, which could also contribute to long-term maintenance.[19,20,29]

The factors that contribute to distribution of enzootic and epizootic plague are poorly defined but likely include an abundance of highly susceptible hosts and climatic factors such as temperature and precipitation that may contribute to rodent abundance and flea survival.[19,30] Recent studies have defined landscape, elevation, and climatic conditions associated with plague occurrence, mainly in North America and sub-Saharan Africa.[31–33] In the United States, human cases in semienzootic foci appear to be linked to moderate temperatures and follow wetter periods, supporting a trophic cascade hypothesis in which increased precipitation in turn leads to more vegetation that then supports increased rodent populations.[30] In northwestern Uganda, localized plague risk is associated with elevation above 1300 m, increased rainfall, and patterns associated with planting of agricultural crops that may foster increased rodent populations at certain times of year.[33]

EPIDEMIOLOGY

Although a major cause of worldwide morbidity and mortality for millennia, the advent of antibiotics and improvements in sanitation and living conditions in many parts of the world have resulted in a decline in human plague over recent decades.[34] Plague was one of three diseases subject to international quarantine under the International Health Regulations (IHR) adopted in 1969; reporting to the World Health Organization (WHO) was mandatory.[35] The 2005 revision of the IHR shifted focus away from specific pathogens or diseases toward a more holistic and flexible approach to protecting public health worldwide by encouraging development of rapid detection and response capacity for both recognized and emerging public health issues among all WHO member states.[36] From 1954 to 1997, an average of 1800 cases occurred worldwide each year, with some years substantially higher—the highest number (6004) was reported in 1967.[34] During 2004–09, an average of ~ 2000 cases were reported each year worldwide, and during 2010–15, an average of 541 cases were reported to WHO per year (Fig. 147-1). However, given the lack of mandatory reporting under the revised IHR, it is unclear if the most recent decline in cases is real or due to reporting bias.[37] Outbreaks of plague in North Africa after decades of quiescence demonstrate the cyclical and unpredictable nature of plague foci.[38,39]

In the United States, during the early part of the twentieth century when plague was repeatedly imported into Pacific and Gulf Coast port cities, a median of 3.5 cases occurred each year, with a wide range from 0 to 191 per year. Plague began circulating in native wild rodents outside the urban setting on the Pacific Coast within a few years, and then rapidly spread to its natural boundary at approximately the 100th meridian, east of which plague appears unable to survive in enzootic cycles.[6,40] Plague became a constant but rare occurrence throughout western states.[40] The last year without at least one case of human plague in the United States was 1964. During 1970–2016, a median of nine human cases were reported each year (range: 1–17 cases) (Fig. 147-2).

African countries account for > 95% of all human plague reported in recent decades, with Madagascar and the Democratic Republic of Congo (DRC) particularly affected.[37,41] Underreporting and over-reporting both likely occur, adding complexity to interpretation of worldwide trends. In the absence of adequate laboratory capacity and reporting infrastructures in many countries, clinically suspect cases likely undergo no diagnostic testing and their occurrence may not be transmitted into national systems and represented accordingly.[34] In contrast, of 255 suspect cases in an endemic area of Uganda, approximately 45% had confirmed or presumptive laboratory evidence of *Y. pestis* infection, despite specimens from nearly all patients being subjected to diagnostic tests. In the same case series, the case-fatality proportion was 26% among those with laboratory confirmed plague, but 7% among suspect cases lacking any positive laboratory evidence of *Y. pestis* infection.[42] Following a pneumonic plague outbreak in DRC in 2004, retrospective analysis demonstrated leptospirosis as a likely cause of illness among a substantial portion of the 130 suspect plague cases.[43,44]

All persons, regardless of age or sex are susceptible to *Y. pestis* infections.[2] Differences in age, sex, or racial or ethnic distribution are seemingly a product of differential exposure to the bacterium. For example, in the United States, male patients have predominated among reported cases, whereas in some countries in Uganda and Tanzania, adult females and children of both sexes are most common among reported cases.[40,42,45]

In endemic foci, regardless of whether temperate or tropical in climate, there is clear seasonality associated with plague, likely tied to rainfall and temperature, and corresponding changes in rodent and flea abundance. Risk of infection is tied not only to these factors that contribute to epizootics, but to human behavioral practices that foster close contact with epizootic activity. This could include practices related to agricultural harvest, food storage, refuse disposal, sleeping arrangements in underresourced settings, and hunting, skinning, and consumption of infected animals.[40,46,47] In the United States, although human cases have occurred year round, most cases occur in the warmer spring and summer months.[40] Although traditionally considered a disease of poverty, as human suburban and exurban development encroaches on enzootic cycles in the United States, areas with human plague in New Mexico are becoming increasingly affluent.[48]

HUMAN ILLNESS

Humans can become infected with the plague bacterium through various modes of transmission. Human plague is characterized by the rapid onset of high fever and a variety of other potential clinical signs and symptoms depending on the route by which *Y. pestis* enters the body.[2,34] Untreated, the infection can disseminate broadly causing septicemia, pneumonia, and more rarely meningitis.[49] Plague is a severe infection that can be rapidly fatal if effective antimicrobial therapy is not initiated in the first few days of illness. With the advent of antibiotics, overall mortality due to plague in the United States fell from 66% to 16%.[40] Among records from the United States that contained treatment and illness outcome information, mortality was 9% among those that received at least one dose of an antibiotic, whereas was 52% for those that received either no treatment or ineffective treatment. In recent years, several notable fatal plague cases have occurred in the United States, all characterized by lack of early and appropriate therapy, including a wildlife biologist in Grand Canyon National Park[50] and a teenager in Colorado (CDC, unpublished data).

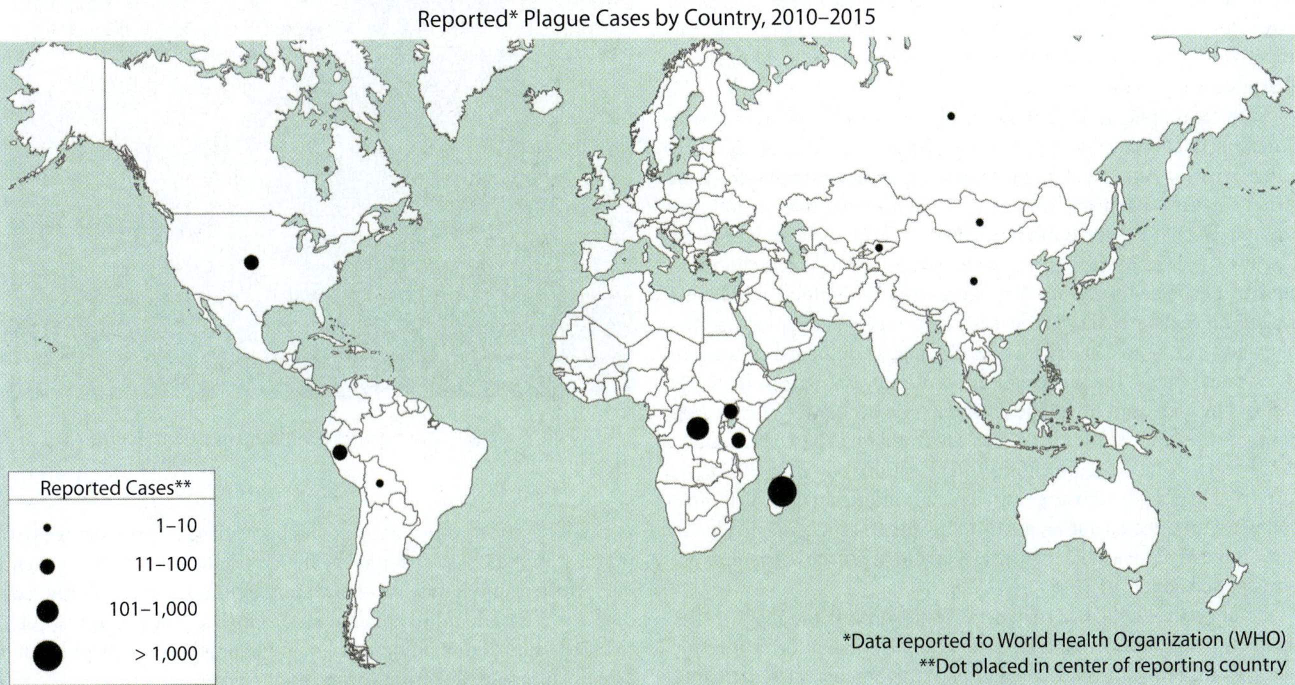

FIGURE 147-1. Suspect, probable, and confirmed plague cases reported the World Health Organization by country during 2010–15. Plague in the United States, Centers for Disease Control and Prevention. https://www.cdc.gov/plague/maps/index.html. Published November 25, 2019. Accessed December 24, 2020.

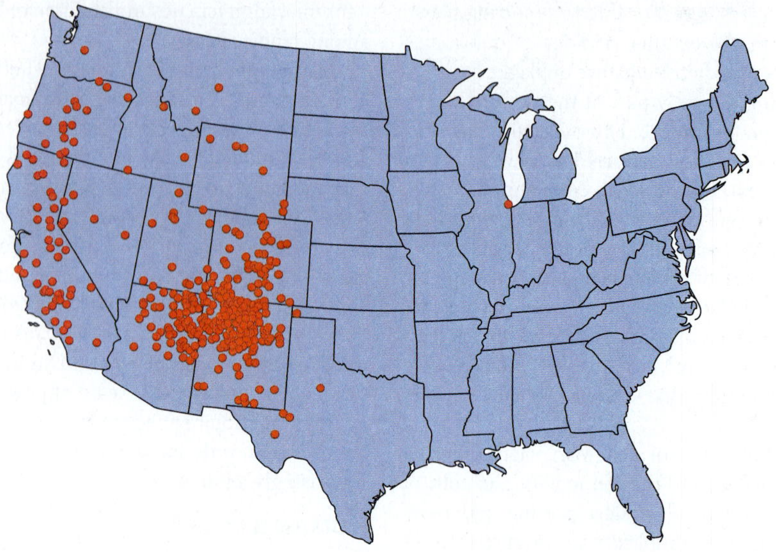

Reported cases of human plague—United States, 1970–2016
1 dot placed randomly in most likely county of exposure for each confirmed Plague case

FIGURE 147-2. Human plague in the United States, 1970–2016. The case in Louisiana was laboratory acquired.[68] Plague in the United States, Centers for Disease Control and Prevention. https://www.cdc.gov/plague/maps/index.html. Published November 25, 2019. Accessed December 24, 2020.

The most common and classic clinical manifestation is bubonic plague, in which the sudden onset of high fever is accompanied, sometimes at a delay, by a swollen and very painful lymph node (bubo)[22,49] (Fig. 147-3). This manifestation occurs following cutaneous inoculation, usually a flea bite.[2] The incubation period is generally 2–6 days, with a range up to 2 weeks. Lymphadenopathy occurs in the lymph nodes nearest the site of dermal exposure, typically inguinal or femoral nodes for bites on legs, but axillary and cervical lymphadenopathy are also common. Occasionally a vesicle or papule can form at the site of the flea bite, and more rarely ulcerate. In a review of all human plague cases in the United States from the first case in 1900–2012, 82% of 913 cases were bubonic.[40] Mortality among U.S. bubonic cases was 66% before the advent of effective antibiotics, and fell to 13% with availability of effective therapy.

Septicemic plague is characterized by a severe systemic febrile illness in the absence of apparent lymphadenopathy or other localizing signs.[49,51] Patients often present with gastrointestinal symptoms such as nausea, vomiting, diarrhea, and abdominal pain in addition to high fever. As with bubonic plague, lack of early and effective therapy can lead to dissemination as well as septic shock and rapid clinical decline. Absent any hallmark clinical findings, septicemic plague presents a challenge for early and accurate diagnosis and is often not considered until *Y. pestis* is isolated on blood culture. In the United States, primary septicemic plague was rare in the early 1900s, but increased in frequency over time accounting for $> 15\%$ of cases in recent decades. This increase could be due to better detection of such a nonspecific clinical presentation, but also potentially due to changes in exposures fostered by different types of human contact with infected animals. Mortality due to septicemic plague in the United States was 89% before availability of effective therapy, but remains substantial at 27%.

Pneumonic plague occurs when *Y. pestis* infects the lungs, either through hematogenous spread of untreated bubonic or septicemic plague, or directly through inhalation of the organism from another pneumonic plague patient or other infected animal. Secondary pneumonic plague, which occurs following untreated infection and spread to the lungs from other parts of the body, is often the beginning of plague outbreaks accompanied by high mortality among many members of the same family or community before the cause of the epidemic is realized and treatment and prophylaxis measures instituted to halt its spread. Pneumonic plague is the only form of plague that is directly transmissible from person to person.[8]

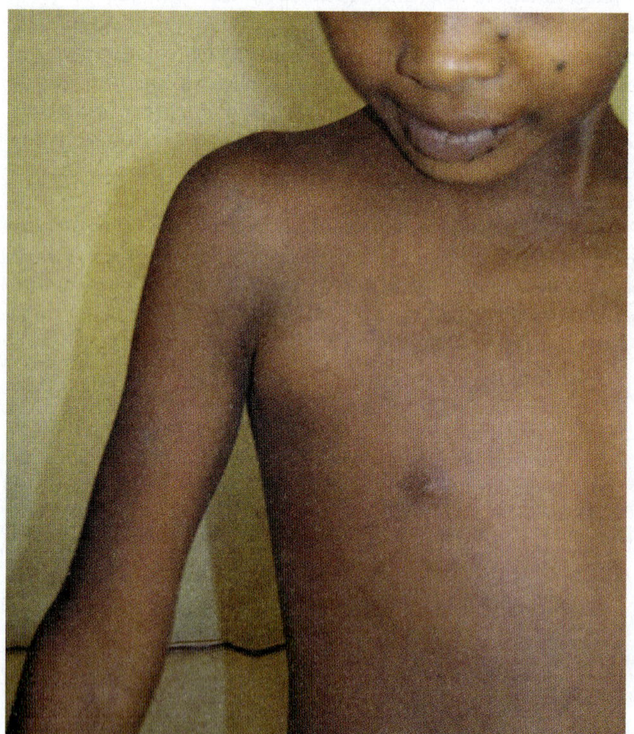

FIGURE 147-3. Axillary bubo in a young plague patient. *Source*: CDC.

Primary pneumonic plague usually occurs 1–4 days after inhalation of infectious droplets, is the most fulminant form of plague, and can be rapidly fatal if treatment is not initiated in the first ~ 24 hours of illness.[49] Primary pneumonic plague often begins with headache, malaise, and elevated heart and respiratory rates coincident with unilobar involvement. A dry cough and high fever typically follow these initial symptoms. The cough becomes increasingly productive, and initially contains no blood, but progressively becomes blood-tinged. A few hours prior to death, the terminal patient coughs copious amounts of bloody sputum containing numerous *Y. pestis* bacteria.[8,9] Untreated, pneumonic plague is nearly always fatal within 1–3 days of symptom onset. The rapid onset and progression, in addition to presence of bloody sputum in the hours near death, should collectively raise clinical suspicion of pneumonic plague vs. other respiratory conditions.[8] Primary pneumonic plague has accounted for ~ 10% of all human plague cases that have occurred in the United States.[40] The vast majority of these occurred in the first two decades of the twentieth century in urban port cities. Mortality due to primary pneumonic plague in the United States was 93% in the era before effective antibiotics, and approximately one-third of all primary pneumonic cases since that time have died.

DIAGNOSIS AND TREATMENT

Plague is a fulminant, invasive illness that can be rapidly fatal if not treated early and appropriately.[49] When plague is suspected based on the clinical picture and careful assessment of potential exposures, clinical specimens should be collected as soon as possible, but preferably prior to prompt administration of empiric therapy. Public health laboratories in each U.S. state have capacity to perform *Y. pestis* diagnostics through the Laboratory Response Network (LRN) and forward specimens to CDC for advanced analyses.[52]

Blood is a highly sensitive diagnostic specimen, as symptomatic human plague infections of all clinical forms are associated with bacteremia.[15] Other appropriate diagnostic specimen types depend upon the clinical manifestation. In areas where blood culture may not be routine, aspiration of a bubo with ~ 1 mL of saline appears quite sensitive for specimen type for bubonic plague. In circumstances of fulminant pneumonia, sputum can also be used to support diagnosis.

Y. pestis can be cultured from these varied specimen types, and isolation of the organism and subsequent lysis by specific bacteriophage is considered confirmatory. Bacterial growth is usually evident after 24–48 hours of incubation at 37°C.[15] Clinical specimens from patients with suspect plague should be handled under routine biosafety precautions. Processing of specimens should occur in a Biosafety Level 2 environment, although culture manipulation is best performed under Biosafety Level 3 precautions. Automated systems can complicate the laboratory recognition of rare bacteria including *Y. pestis*, resulting in delay of effective antimicrobial therapy and unintended potential laboratory and healthcare exposures.[53,54] Fourfold change in specific antibody titer between acute and convalescent sera collected at least 2 weeks apart is also confirmatory evidence of recent *Y. pestis* infection. Most patients seroconvert within 1–2 weeks postillness onset.[15]

Presumptive tests that can provide earlier results include fluorescent antibody assays directed at F1 antigen, molecular assays, and rapid lateral flow or "dipstick" tests. Molecular assays are in use in the United States through the LRN, and some assays are now commercially available. Rapid tests developed and produced by the Institut Pasteur Madagascar have been in use in that country for several years, and have been utilized in plague outbreak responses in other countries as well.[38,44,55] Other rapid tests have been developed and manufactured and are under evaluation. Their utility is most helpful in guiding clinical care in settings with possible plague that lack laboratory capacity for other recommended tests. However, results should be verified with reference laboratories, as rapid tests can be prone to overreading and generation of false-positive results, which in turn create unnecessary fear and panic among healthcare providers.[10]

Treatment

Historically, streptomycin has been the drug of choice for treatment of plague, but due to its substantial toxicity profile and limited availability, other options have been explored and appear equally as effective. Gentamicin is an acceptable alternative aminoglycoside although is not approved for plague treatment by the U.S. Food and Drug Administration (FDA).[4] Clinical experience with gentamicin and tetracyclines is positive.[56,57] Doxycycline is the preferred tetracycline for plague due to its absorption, high peak serum concentration, and convenient dosing.[49] Doxycycline or tetracycline can also be used to complete a treatment course initiated with an aminoglycoside. Chloramphenicol has been the antibiotic agent of choice for plague meningitis and other rare complications due to its high tissue penetration. In more recent years, fluoroquinolones have been explored and levofloxacin, ciprofloxacin, and moxifloxacin have been approved by the FDA for treatment of plague based on animal studies.[58–60] Clinical experience is more limited, but appears positive, including for pneumonic illness.[61,62] As bactericidal agents, the fluoroquinolones have the potential to provide improved outcomes compared even to tetracyclines, which are bacteriostatic in nature. Trimethoprim-sulfamethoxozole has been used to successfully treat bubonic plague but is not considered first-line therapy. In general, regardless of choice, antibiotics are usually given for a minimum of 10 days, or until 3 days postdefervescence.[4] Patients initially given intravenous therapy may be switched to oral therapy after clinical improvement. Although isolated reports of in vitro multidrug resistant isolates from Madagascar have been published, clinical failures with first line agents have not been documented.[63–65] Buboes have the potential to persist for days or even weeks after defervesence and can ultimately require surgical drainage.[49]

TRANSMISSION TO HUMANS

Most human infections worldwide are due to flea-borne transmission. Flea bites occur during close physical contact with enzootic or epizootic activity, such that humans become incidental blood meal hosts for infected fleas whose primary rodent hosts have succumbed to plague. In the United States, this occurs in rural and semirural settings through routine outdoor activities such as hiking, camping, or even chopping wood on one's own property. Additionally, persons can be exposed to infected fleas on animal carcasses if handling carcasses without sufficient protective clothing and gloves. In other parts of the world, exposure typically occurs in settings where humans live in close contact with rodents and their fleas. When flea bites are the route of plague transmission, bubonic plague is typically the resulting clinical form, but in a comprehensive review of human plague cases in the United States, 10% of all plague patients that had a known flea bite presented with primary septicemic plague.[40]

Direct contact with infected animal tissues or fluids can lead to direct inoculation of the bacterium without flea-borne transmission. Notably, the mortality rate among U.S. patients with a history of direct animal contact is significantly higher than among persons with a recognized flea bite, even after controlling for receipt of effective antibiotics, a finding that supports hypotheses regarding differential pathogenesis between infections with and without mediating vectors.[40] Consumption of infected animal meat is also a documented route of human infection.[46]

Pneumonic plague transmission occurs following inhalation of infectious droplets from a human or animal gravely ill with plague pneumonia. This typically requires close, often prolonged, contact (< 2 m) with droplets coughed by the sick rather than smaller particles that remain airborne (droplet nuclei). Person-to-person transmission of pneumonic plague is the source of rapidly spreading outbreaks with extremely high mortality prior to detection. Yet, due to the requirement for close contact, pneumonic plague transmission chains are easy to break. Transmissibility of pneumonic plague has been the subject of study, as it pertains to not only naturally occurring outbreaks but also to potential use of plague as a bioweapon.[8,66,67] Persons with close contact with a pneumonic plague patient when that patient is coughing sputum are often the victims of transmission. Conversely, persons residing in the same home, even the same room, but who lacked that close caregiver contact have escaped infection.[8,9] Simple respiratory barrier ("droplet") precautions greatly reduce the likelihood of transmission. Even in the absence of surgical masks, healthcare workers have protected themselves sufficiently simply by avoiding direct face-to-face contact and instead examining patients from behind.[8] Patients in the early stages of pneumonic plague are coughing negligible *Y. pestis*, and thus present a minimal risk of transmission.[2,8] Modeling studies have documented the reproductive number (R_0) from pneumonic plague epidemics, including pneumonic cases absent secondary transmission, to be near 1.[66,67] Infections among laboratorians are now exceedingly rare, but a fatal infection occurred in 2009 in a researcher with undiagnosed hereditary hemochromatosis using an otherwise attenuated strain.[68]

The first ~ 25 years of the plague experience in the United States was characterized by multiple pneumonic plague outbreaks in the urban settings of port cities on the Pacific and Gulf Coasts. The last documented case of person-to-person transmission of plague in the United States occurred in 1924.[40] Primary pneumonic plague cases since that time have been predominantly associated with cat-to-human but also dog-to-human droplet transmission to owners and veterinary personnel.[40,69] Although cats are highly susceptible to plague, dogs can also become ill, although often not as severely.[70] A potential pneumonic transmission event occurred in 2014 in Colorado, in the circumstances of an outbreak linked to a domestic dog. The dog died of plague; the owners, a husband and wife, as well as two veterinary personnel were infected. The wife had some contact with the ill dog, but it is quite possible that her infection could have occurred during close contact with her ill husband.[53]

Domestic animals can also indirectly facilitate human exposure to the bacterium.[69,71–74] This can include bringing infected fleas into the home and bringing infected animal carcasses into the home environment that in turn necessitate human intervention for proper disposal. In one matched case-control study in New Mexico and Colorado, allowing a dog to sleep in the owner's bed was a risk factor for human plague after controlling for other possible modes of dog-mediated infection.[74]

RESPONSE, PREVENTION, AND CONTROL

In endemic areas, risk of plague is low, but ever-present. Surveillance, education, and environmental control remain the primary components of effective plague prevention and response.[34] In the scenario of a single case or cluster of suspect plague, the immediate goals are to: ensure prompt and effective therapy to those with suggestive clinical illness; provide prophylaxis to persons after thorough evaluation of potential high-risk exposures to pneumonic patients; ensure appropriate collection and testing of clinical specimens to confirm the diagnosis; mitigate environmental risk to prevent further bubonic cases from occurring; and disseminate appropriate clinical and public education to ensure at-risk communities can recognize the signs of plague and promptly seek and receive appropriate therapy.

All suspect cases should be reported immediately to local health authorities, who can in turn assist with laboratory and epidemiologic investigations, and ensure adequate public health follow-up. Travel-associated plague can arise in persons exposed in endemic areas, but who fall ill after returning to places in which plague is not typically considered in ill persons. Thus, travel history anywhere in the western U.S. should raise suspicion of plague in a patient with clinically compatible illness. Patients with suspected plague of any clinical form should be placed into respiratory isolation to prevent droplet transmission until pneumonic involvement has been ruled out or the patient has been on effective therapy for at least 48 hours. In the absence of pneumonic involvement, standard precautions are sufficient.

In some circumstances oral postexposure prophylaxis with doxycycline or ciprofloxacin could be indicated, such as in laboratory, veterinary, or clinical settings when events likely to produce droplets or aerosols occurred absent glove, surgical mask, or eye protection.[4,75] In adults, prophylaxis options include doxycycline 100 mg twice daily, or ciprofloxacin 500 mg twice daily, both for 7 days. In children, ciprofloxacin and doxycycline are also viable prophylactic options, with dosing according to weight.[4] Given the effectiveness of therapy, fever watch for 14 days is often a reasonable choice following exposures of seemingly moderate to low risk. Pre-exposure prophylaxis is unwarranted except in the rarest of circumstances, such as for someone providing direct clinical care in an outbreak setting in an underresourced area lacking sufficient gloves or masks.

As domestic pets can not only serve as sentinels for plague activity in an area but can also facilitate human illness, suspected plague in a dog or cat should also be reported immediately to local health authorities so follow-up investigation and risk mitigation activities can ensue. Owners of plague-infected animals should be advised that their risks of contracting plague depend on the type of interaction they had with the ill animal, and public health officials should assess the risk and provide guidance accordingly. Consistent flea prevention on indoor/outdoor domestic animals can reduce the likelihood of those pets bringing infected fleas into the home. Occupational exposures have been well documented and consequently persons with exposure to wild or domestic animals should take precaution, including use of gloves, masks, and eye protection, depending on the nature of the interaction.

Elimination of rodent habitat in the peridomestic environment reduces the risk that humans will come into contact with enzootic or epizootic plague activity. Physical rodent removal via trapping or poisoning is extremely labor intensive and difficult to fully achieve, and thus is an ineffective means of environmental plague risk reduction. Additionally, removal of living rodents, some of which may be newly immune to infection in an ongoing epizootic, could exacerbate an existing problem by in turn promoting immigration of fully susceptible rodent hosts. Use of insecticides to control on-host and off-host fleas in epizootic situations appears to the most effective means to prevent human infection. This can include dusting of rodent burrows or indoor residual spraying in situations where the rodents and fleas are in the home, such as in plague foci in sub-Saharan Africa and Madagascar (Fig. 147-4). An "early-warning" surveillance system, such as watching for rodent die-off to initiate insecticide measures can be used even in underresourced settings, to mitigate morbidity and mortality due to plague.[76]

Additional prevention activities include rodent proofing of housing and out-buildings, avoidance of areas with evidence of a recent animal die-off such as quiet prairie dog towns, routine use of insect repellent when engaging in outdoor activity, and use of gloves and long sleeves when handling animal carcasses. Vaccines effective against bubonic but not pneumonic plague were previously in use by the U.S. military and laboratory researchers, but are no longer available.[4] Interest in next-generation vaccines is ongoing, but given the rare and sporadic nature of plague in the world, it is difficult to conceive of plague vaccine as an important component of plague prevention from a public health perspective.

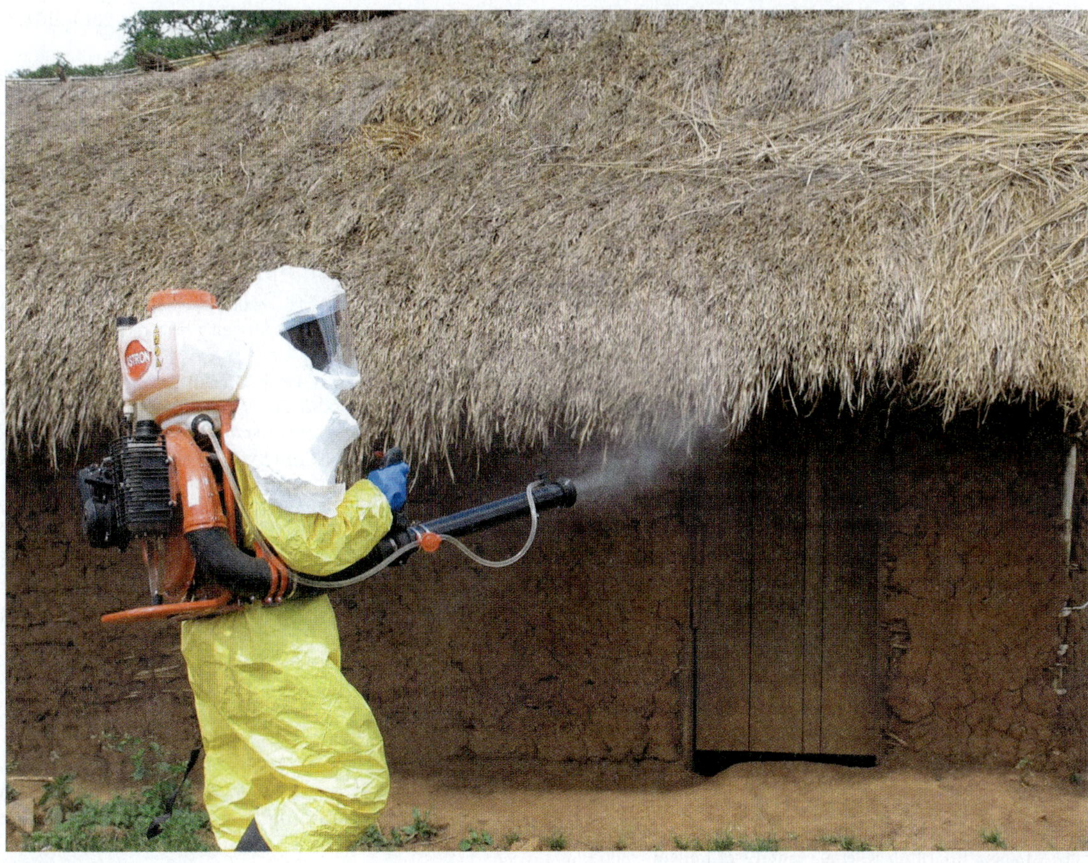

FIGURE 147-4. Insecticide spraying by trained applicators to mitigate human plague risk during an epizootic in the West Nile region of Uganda. *Source*: CDC.

References

1. Perry RD, Fetherston JD. *Yersinia pestis*—Etiologic agent of plague. *Clin Microbiol Rev*. 1997;10(1):35–66.
2. Pollitzer R. *Plague*. Geneva, Switzerland: World Health Organization; 1954.
3. Link VB. A history of plague in United States of America. *Public Health Monogr*. 1955;26:1–120.
4. Inglesby TV, Dennis DT, Henderson DA, et al. Plague as a biological weapon: Medical and public health management. Working Group on Civilian Biodefense. *JAMA*. 2000;283(17):2281–90.
5. Slack P. The Black Death past and present 2, some historical problems. *Trans R Soc Trop Med Hyg*. 1989;83:461–3.
6. Caten JL, Kartman L. Human Plague in the United States: 1900–1966. *JAMA*. 1968;205(6):81–4.
7. Lien Teh W, Litt D. Plague in the orient with special reference to the Manchurian outbreaks. *J Hyg (Lond)*. 1922;21(1):62–76.
8. Kool JL. Risk of person-to-person transmission of pneumonic plague. *Clin Infect Dis*. 2005;40(8):1166–72.
9. Lien-Teh W, Chun JWH, Pollitzer R, Wu CY. *A Treatise on Pneumonic Plague*. Geneva: League of Nations; 1926.
10. Mead PS. Plague in Madagascar—A tragic opportunity for improving public health. *N Engl J Med*. 2018;378(2):106–8.
11. Campbell GL, Hughes JM. Plague in India: A new warning from an old nemesis. *Ann Intern Med*. 1995;122(2):151–3.
12. Mavalankar DV. Indian 'plague' epidemic: Unanswered questions and key lessons. *J R Soc Med*. 1995;88(10):547–51.
13. Centers for Disease Control and Prevention and United States Department of Agriculture. Federal Select Agent Program 2018. https://www.selectagents.gov/index.html.
14. Koirala J. Plague: Disease, management, and recognition of act of terrorism. *Infect Dis Clin North Am*. 2006;20(2):273–87, viii.
15. Centers for Disease Control and Prevention. Laboratory Manual of Plague Diagnostic Tests. Geneva, Switzerland: U.S. Dept. Health Human Services and World Health Organization; 2000, pp. 1–129.
16. Achtman M, Morelli G, Zhu P, et al. Microevolution and history of the plague bacillus, Yersinia pestis. *Proc Natl Acad Sci U S A*. 2004;101(51):17837–42.
17. Vogler AJ, Keim P, Wagner DM. A review of methods for subtyping *Yersinia pestis*: From phenotypes to whole genome sequencing. *Infect Genet Evol*. 2016;37:21–36.
18. Kingry LC, Rowe LA, Respicio-Kingry LB, Beard CB, Schriefer ME, Petersen JM. Whole genome multilocus sequence typing as an epidemiologic tool for *Yersinia pestis*. *Diagn Microbiol Infect Dis*. 2016;84(4):275–80.
19. Gage KL, Kosoy MY. Natural history of plague: Perspectives from more than a century of research. *Annu Rev Entomol*. 2005;50:505–28.
20. Eisen RJ, Gage KL. Adaptive strategies of *Yersinia pestis* to persist during inter-epizootic and epizootic periods. *Vet Res*. 2009;40(2):1.
21. Ben Ari T, Gershunov A, Gage KL, et al. Human plague in the USA: The importance of regional and local climate. *Biol Lett*. 2008;4(6):737–40.
22. Dennis DT, Gage KL, Gratz ND, Poland JD, Tikhomirov E. *Plague Manual: Epidemiology, Distribution, Surveillance and Control*. Geneva, Switzerland: World Health Organization; 1999.
23. Eisen RJ, Gage K. Transmission of flea-borne zoonotic agents. *Annu Rev Entomol*. 2012;57:61–82.
24. Ayyadurai S, Sebbane F, Raoult D, Drancourt M. Body lice, *Yersinia pestis* orientalis, and Black Death. *Emerg Infect Dis*. 2010;16(5):892–3.
25. Dean KR, Krauer F, Walloe L, et al. Human ectoparasites and the spread of plague in Europe during the Second Pandemic. *Proc Natl Acad Sci U S A*. 2018;115(6):1304–9.
26. Drancourt M, Houhamdi L, Raoult D. *Yersinia pestis* as a telluric, human ectoparasite-borne organism. *Lancet Infect Dis*. 2006;6(4):234–41.
27. Bacot AW, Martin CJ. Observations on the mechanism of transmission of plague by fleas. *J Hyg*. 1914;13 (Plague Suppl. III):423–39.
28. Eisen RJ, Bearden SW, Wilder AP, Montenieri JA, Antolin MF, Gage KL. Early-phase transmission of *Yersinia pestis* by unblocked fleas as a mechanism explaining rapidly spreading plague epizootics. *Proc Natl Acad Sci U S A*. 2006;103(42):15380–5.

29. Eisen RJ, Petersen JM, Higgins CL, et al. Persistence of *Yersinia pestis* in soil under natural conditions. *Emerg Infect Dis.* 2008;14(6):941–3.
30. Parmenter RR, Yadav EP, Parmenter CA, Ettestad P, Gage KL. Incidence of plague associated with increased winter-spring precipitation in New Mexico. *Am J Trop Med Hyg.* 1999;61(5):814–21.
31. Neerinckx SB, Peterson AT, Gulinck H, Deckers J, Leirs H. Geographic distribution and ecological niche of plague in sub-Saharan Africa. *Int J Health Geogr.* 2008;7:54.
32. Eisen RJ, Enscore RE, Biggerstaff BJ, et al. Human plague in the southwestern United States, 1957–2004: Spatial models of elevated risk of human exposure to Yersinia pestis. *J Med Entomol.* 2007;44(3):530–7.
33. Eisen RJ, Griffith KS, Borchert JN, et al. Assessing human risk of exposure to plague bacteria in northwestern Uganda based on remotely sensed predictors. *Am J Trop Med Hyg.* 2010;82(5):904–11.
34. Plague manual—Epidemiology, distribution, surveillance and control. *Wkly Epidemiol Rec.* 1999;74(51–52):447.
35. World Health Organization. International Health Regulations, 1969 Geneva. http://www.who.int/ihr/current/en/.
36. World Health Organization. International Health Regulations, 2005 Geneva. http://www.who.int/ihr/publications/9789241580496/en/.
37. World Health Organization. Human plague: Review of regional morbidity and mortality, 2004–2009. *Wkly Epidemiol Rec.* 2009;85(6):40–5.
38. Bertherat E, Bekhoucha S, Chougrani S, et al. Plague reappearance in Algeria after 50 years, 2003. *Emerg Infect Dis.* 2007;13(10):1459–62.
39. Cabanel N, Leclercq A, Chenal-Francisque V, et al. Plague outbreak in Libya, 2009, unrelated to plague in Algeria. *Emerg Infect Dis.* 2013;19:230–6.
40. Kugeler KJ, Staples JE, Hinckley AF, Gage KL, Mead PS. Epidemiology of human plague in the United States, 1900–2012. *Emerg Infect Dis.* 2015;21(1):16–22.
41. World Health Organization. Plague around the world, 2010–2015. *Wkly Epidemiol Rec.* 2016;91:89–104.
42. Forrester JD, Apangu T, Griffith K, et al. Patterns of human plague in Uganda, 2008–2016. *Emerg Infect Dis.* 2017;23(9):1517–21.
43. Bertherat E, Mueller MJ, Shako JC, Picardeau M. Discovery of a leptospirosis cluster amidst a pneumonic plague outbreak in a miners' camp in the Democratic Republic of the Congo. *Int J Environ Res Public Health.* 2014;11:1824–33.
44. Bertherat E, Thullier P, Shako JC, et al. Lessons learned about pneumonic plague diagnosis from 2 outbreaks, Democratic Republic of the Congo. *Emerg Infect Dis.* 2011;17(5):778–84.
45. Davis S, Makundi RH, Machang'u RS, Leirs H. Demographic and spatio-temporal variation in human plague at a persistent focus in Tanzania. *Acta Trop.* 2006;100(1–2):133–41.
46. Bin Saeed AA, Al-Hamdan NA, Fontaine RE. Plague from eating raw camel liver. *Emerg Infect Dis.* 2005;11(9):1456–7.
47. Eisen RJ, MacMillan K, Atiku LA, et al. Identification of risk factors for plague in the West Nile region of Uganda. *Am J Trop Med Hyg.* 2014;90(6):1047–58.
48. Schotthoefer AM, Eisen RJ, Kugeler KJ, et al. Changing socioeconomic indicators of human plague, New Mexico, USA. *Emerg Infect Dis.* 2012;18(7):1151–4.
49. Mead PS. *Yersinia* species (including plague). In: Bennett JE, Dolin R, Blaser MJ, eds. *Principles and Practice of Infectious Diseases. 2.* 8th ed. Philadelphia: Elsevier; 2015, pp. 2607–18.
50. Wong D, Wild MA, Walburger MA, et al. Primary pneumonic plague contracted from a mountain lion carcass. *Clin Infect Dis.* 2009;49(3):e33–8.
51. Hull HF, Montes JM, Mann JM. Septicemic plague in New Mexico. *J Infect Dis.* 1987;155(1):113–8.
52. Centers for Disease Control and Prevention. Emergency Preparedness and Response, the Laboratory Response Network 2018. https://emergency.cdc.gov/lrn/index.asp.
53. Runfola JK, House J, Miller L, et al. Outbreak of human pneumonic plague with dog-to-human and possible human-to-human transmission—Colorado, June–July 2014. *MMWR Morb Mortal Wkly Rep.* 2015;64(16):429–34.
54. Tourdjman M, Ibraheem M, Brett M, et al. Misidentification of *Yersinia pestis* by automated systems, resulting in delayed diagnoses of human plague infections—Oregon and New Mexico, 2010–2011. *Clin Infect Dis.* 2012;55(7):e58–60.
55. Chanteau S, Rahalison L, Ralafiarisoa L, et al. Development and testing of a rapid diagnostic test for bubonic and pneumonic plague. *Lancet.* 2003;361(9353):211–6.
56. Boulanger LL, Ettestad P, Fogarty JD, Dennis DT, Romig D, Mertz G. Gentamicin and tetracyclines for the treatment of human plague: Review of 75 cases in new Mexico, 1985–1999. *Clin Infect Dis.* 2004;38(5):663–9.
57. Mwengee W, Butler T, Mgema S, et al. Treatment of plague with gentamicin or doxycycline in a randomized clinical trial in Tanzania. *Clin Infect Dis.* 2006;42(5):614–21.
58. Layton RC, Mega W, McDonald JD, et al. Levofloxacin cures experimental pneumonic plague in African green monkeys. *PLoS Negl Trop Dis.* 2011;5(2):e959.
59. Peterson JW, Moen ST, Healy D, et al. Protection afforded by fluoroquinolones in animal models of respiratory infections with *Bacillus anthracis, Yersinia pestis,* and *Francisella tularensis. Open Microbiol J.* 2010;4:34–46.
60. Rosenzweig JA, Brackman SM, Kirtley ML, et al. Cethromycin-mediated protection against the plague pathogen *Yersinia pestis* in a rat model of infection and comparison with levofloxacin. *Antimicrob Agents Chemother.* 2011;55(11):5034–42.
61. Apangu T, Griffith K, Abaru J, et al. Successful treatment of human plague with oral ciprofloxacin. *Emerg Infect Dis.* 2017;23(3).
62. Kuberski T, Robinson L, Schurgin A. A case of plague successfully treated with ciprofloxacin and sympathetic blockade for treatment of gangrene. *Clin Infect Dis.* 2003;36(4):521–3.
63. Guiyoule A, Gerbaud G, Buchrieser C, et al. Transferable plasmid-mediated resistance to streptomycin in a clinical isolate of *Yersinia pestis. Emerg Infect Dis.* 2001;7(1):43–8.
64. Urich SK, Chalcraft L, Schriefer ME, Yockey BM, Petersen JM. Lack of antimicrobial resistance in *Yersinia pestis* isolates from 17 countries in the Americas, Africa, and Asia. *Antimicrob Agents Chemother.* 2012;56(1):555–8.
65. Galimand M, Guiyoule A, Gerbaud G, et al. Multidrug resistance in *Yersinia pestis* mediated by a transferable plasmid. *N Engl J Med.* 1997;337(10):677–80.
66. Hinckley AF, Biggerstaff BJ, Griffith KS, Mead PS. Transmission dynamics of primary pneumonic plague in the USA. *Epidemiol Infect.* 2012;140(3):554–60.
67. Gani R, Leach S. Epidemiologic determinants for modeling pneumonic plague outbreaks. *Emerg Infect Dis.* 2004;10(4):608–14.
68. Centers for Disease Control and Prevention. Fatal laboratory-acquired infection with an attenuated *Yersinia pestis* strain—Chicago, Illinois, 2009. *MMWR Morb Mortal Wkly Rep.* 2011;60(7):201–5.
69. Gage KL, Dennis DT, Orloski KA, et al. Cases of cat-associated human plague in the western US, 1977–1998. *Clin Infect Dis.* 2000;30(6):893–900.
70. Nichols MC, Ettestad PJ, Vinhatton ES, et al. Yersinia pestis infection in dogs: 62 Cases (2003–2011). *J Am Vet Med Assoc.* 2014;244(10):1176–80.
71. Rust JH Jr, Miller BE, Bahmanyar M, et al. The role of domestic animals in the epidemiology of plague. II. Antibody to *Yersinia pestis* in sera of dogs and cats. *J Infect Dis.* 1971;124(5):527–31.
72. Eidson M, Tierney LA, Rollag OJ, Becker T, Brown T, Hull HF. Feline plague in New Mexico: Risk factors and transmission to humans. *Am J Public Health.* 1988;78(10):1333–5.
73. von Reyn CF, Weber NS, Tempest B, et al. Epidemiologic and clinical features of an outbreak of bubonic plague in New Mexico. *J Infect Dis.* 1977;136(4):489–94.
74. Gould LH, Pape J, Ettestad P, Griffith KS, Mead PS. Dog-associated risk factors for human plague. *Zoonoses Public Health.* 2008;55(8–10):448–54.
75. Centers for Disease Control and Prevention. Plague: Information for healthcare professionals 2018. https://www.cdc.gov/plague/healthcare/index.html.
76. Boegler KA, Atiku LA, Enscore RE, et al. Rat fall surveillance coupled with vector control and community education as a plague prevention strategy in the West Nile Region, Uganda. *Am J Trop Med Hyg.* 2018;98(1):238–47.

CHAPTER 148 Anthrax*

Katherine A. Hendricks • Antonio Vieira

Background. Anthrax, caused by the bacterium *Bacillus anthracis*, has been recognized as an infectious disease of both humans and animals for many centuries. While no longer causing substantial disease in the United States, it occurs in multiple countries worldwide and is a major bioterrorist threat. The name of the disease, "anthrax," is derived from the Greek word *anthrakos*, meaning charcoal or carbuncle, and refers to the black skin lesions commonly seen with cutaneous anthrax infection.[1] Anthrax is likely to have originated over 6000 years ago in ancient Mesopotamia and Egypt, where it may have caused the fifth plague of Egypt in which the "horses, donkeys, and camels and cattle, sheep, and goats" of the Egyptians died the same day.[2] However it may have existed as long as 12,000 years ago, when livestock were first domesticated.[1,3] The Roman poet Virgil described an anthrax epizootic, observing that eating meat or wearing clothes made from the wool or hides of infected animals resulted in human anthrax.[4] Devastating epizootics of anthrax were described in the middle ages, and an outbreak of anthrax referred to as the "black bain" is reported to have killed 60,000 people in Europe in 1613.[5] A number of notable historical[6–8] as well as recent[9,10] outbreaks have occurred in the wake of famines or food shortages.

In nineteenth century Europe, anthrax outbreaks resulted in significant loss of livestock. In France, at least 20–30% of the sheep and cattle died of anthrax each year.[3] This devastating effect of anthrax stimulated microbiological studies of the disease in the mid-1800s. Delafond, Rayer, Daviane, and others described "bodies" or "little rods" in the blood of animals, which died of the disease, and in the 1860s Davaine demonstrated that anthrax could be transmitted to healthy animals through the inoculation of blood from anthrax-affected sick or dead animals.[3,11] Robert Koch was able to grow the anthrax bacillus in a sterile medium outside of an animal host and then infect mice with the resulting spores—thus first demonstrating in 1877 what have become known as Koch's postulates, and making anthrax the first disease for which a single microorganism was proven to be the etiological agent. Louis Pasteur was the first to develop an effective vaccine for a bacterial disease, demonstrating his anthrax vaccine in 1881.[3]

In the middle of the nineteenth century, inhalation anthrax, or "woolsorter's disease," was recognized as an occupationally acquired disease of textile workers in England who sorted imported mohair and alpaca hair. It was not until 1879, over 30 years after the disease was first recognized, that John Bell determined that woolsorter's disease was what we now refer to as inhalation anthrax. Recommendations were made the following year for the cleaning of imported mohair, and later these "Bradford Rules," named for the English city, which was the center of the mohair wool industry, were improved by calling for ventilation to protect workers from contaminated dust. The Bradford Rules were codified in 1897, followed by the Anthrax Prevention Act in 1919, which called for formaldehyde disinfection of potentially infected imported mohair and wool.[11] These rules and laws dramatically decreased the incidence of disease. In the United States, improvements in industrial hygiene; a decrease in the use of imported, contaminated, raw animal materials; and immunization of at-risk workers helped to limit industrial inhalation anthrax,[12] and during the twentieth century there were only 18 reported inhalation anthrax cases in the United States.[13]

Historically, cutaneous anthrax is the most common type of endemic and epidemic anthrax in humans. An outbreak of cutaneous anthrax from *B. anthracis*-contaminated shaving brushes occurred in American servicemen and civilians during World War I following disruption of the supply chain of Russian badger hair normally used in brushes; concurrent cases were also reported from England and Canada. This outbreak abated following 1918 and 1920 edicts from the Surgeon General and New York City Board of Health that mandated ways to disinfect brushes and that only ["sterilized"] brushes be sold.[14]

Since the late nineteenth century, livestock vaccination has helped to reduce the impact of the disease on livestock, thereby diminishing its spread to humans. However, epizootics of anthrax still occur worldwide, especially in areas where vaccine use is not comprehensive, and these are frequently associated with cases of anthrax among persons exposed to infected animals.

Anthrax is one of the most serious of biowarfare or bioterrorism agents. It was used by Germany during World War I against livestock and draft animals, and Japan conducted field trials with anthrax in Manchuria during World War II.[15] The United States and Britain conducted anthrax weapon research during World War II, and the Soviet Union, Iraq, and others nations did so afterward.[15,16] In 1979, at least 75 cases of inhalation anthrax occurred in the Soviet city of Sverdlovsk, following an accidental release from a military microbiologic facility.[17] In 2001, 22 confirmed or suspected cases of anthrax occurred in the United States after bioterrorists sent *B. anthracis* through the mail in powder-containing envelopes; half were inhalation anthrax and half were cutaneous anthrax.[18] Twenty of the cases occurred in mail handlers or persons exposed to buildings where contaminated mail was processed or received. The source of exposure was unknown in two of the fatal inhalation anthrax cases; however, it is suspected that the cases were exposed through cross-contaminated mail.[18]

Injection anthrax was first described by Ringertz in 2000 in a 49-year-old Norwegian described as a "heroin skin popper." The patient presented with a 4-day history of infection in one buttock but was not admitted. When brought to the hospital a few days later, he was hypothermic, comatose, and in shock. A Gram stain of his CSF revealed Gram positive rods with spores, and within days he

*The findings and conclusions in this chapter are those of the authors and do not necessarily represent the official position of the Centers for Disease Control and Prevention.

succumbed to his illness.[19] It was almost a decade before more cases were found, this time in Scotland. From December 2009 to July 2010, 119 cases of injection anthrax were identified in Scotland; 47 were categorized as confirmed; 35 as probable; and 37 as possible.[20] A total of 14 of 119 (11.8%) died. During the same timeframe, at least five cases were identified in England and two in Germany. Cases were twice as likely to occur in males as females, and had an average age in the mid-30s. Although all were heroin users, and a majority injected it, at least two confirmed and three probable cases occurred in patients who stated that they only smoked or snorted heroin.[20] Duration of opioid use and alcohol consumption appeared to be risk factors for illness[21] and alcohol use was a risk factor for fatal illness.[22]

Underdiagnosis and underreporting of animal and human cases, especially in developing countries, limit knowledge of the true burden of the disease. In Zimbabwe, a reanalysis of data from 1978 through 1984 suggests that there were more than 17,000 human cases with 200 deaths.[23] The same authors hypothesize that the number of cattle deaths could have been ten times that number. During this period, prolonged political instability and armed conflict disrupted animal anthrax control activities. In some countries with significant epizootic anthrax such as exists in sub-Saharan Africa and Asia, several hundred cases occur each year. In the United States, anthrax infection in humans is rare. From 1992 through 2000, only one case of cutaneous anthrax was reported in the United States, in association with an epizootic in cattle,[24] and the last fatal case of anthrax prior to the bioterrorist attacks of 2001 occurred in 1976, in a home craftsman who died of inhalation anthrax after working with yarn imported from Pakistan.[13]

The Agent. *B. anthracis*, the etiologic agent of anthrax, is a large, Gram-positive, nonmotile, spore-forming bacterial rod. The bacillus grows well on a variety of bacterial culture media, with optimal growth at 37°C. On blood agar plates, it forms large, nonhemolytic, grey or white-colored colonies. The tenacious character of these colonies can be demonstrated when lifted by an inoculating loop and has been described as standing up like "beaten egg whites."[12] The virulence of *B. anthracis* is dependent on three plasmid-mediated virulence factors: edema toxin, lethal toxin, and a poly-D-glutamic acid capsule.[25] The antiphagocytic poly-D-glutamic acid capsule is encoded for by the pXO2 plasmid.[26] The pXO1 plasmid encodes for three exotoxin components—edema factor, lethal factor, and protective antigen (PA). Edema factor combines with PA to form edema toxin, which causes edema and inhibits neutrophil function, which may contribute to host-susceptibility to infection with *B. anthracis*.[27,28] Lethal factor combines with PA to form lethal toxin, which causes shock and death. Injection of lethal factor in the mouse model has been shown to result in hypoxic tissue injury and liver failure, and death with shock-like manifestations.[29]

Human Anthrax. There are four main types of anthrax that correspond to the routes of transmission: cutaneous, inhalation, ingestion, and injection. Spores introduced through the skin cause cutaneous anthrax; spores that are respired generally cause inhalation anthrax; spores that are swallowed cause ingestion anthrax; and those that are introduced percutaneously into deeper soft tissue cause injection anthrax. Cutaneous anthrax is by far the most common manifestation of infection with *B. anthracis*.

CUTANEOUS ANTHRAX

Cutaneous anthrax is associated with a characteristic skin lesion that usually develops 5–7 days after subcutaneous introduction of *B. anthracis* spores (range 1–17 days),[30–32] frequently from contact with infected animals or their by-products. Cuts or abrasions increase susceptibility to cutaneous infection. Close to 90% of the cutaneous anthrax lesions occur on exposed areas such as the face, neck, arms, and hands.[33,34] The lesion begins as a small, painless, but often pruritic papule, which quickly enlarges and develops a central vesicle or bulla. The vesicle ruptures or erodes, leaving an underlying necrotic ulcer. A characteristic black eschar develops over the surface of the ulcer. Satellite vesicles and ulcers may also form.[35–37] Edematous swelling of the surrounding tissues is present, often with regional lymphadenopathy and lymphangitis.[38,39] Historically, almost a quarter of patients died without appropriate treatment[40]; however, the case fatality rate is less than 2% with antimicrobial therapy.[34]

INHALATION ANTHRAX

Naturally occurring inhalation anthrax results from the inhalation of *B. anthracis* spores aerosolized through industrial processing of animal hair, fleeces, or hides. Inhalation disease can also result from the inhalation of intentionally aerosolized spores. Whether natural or intentional, spore-containing particles that escape via mechanisms such as coughing, sneezing, and ciliary action, are inhaled and deposited in the alveoli. Although larger particles can reach the alveoli, particles 5 μm in size or less are most easily deposited in the alveolar ducts or alveoli and have the lowest lethal dose.[41] The spores are phagocytosed by alveolar macrophages and dendritic cells.[42] Those that escape macrophage defense mechanisms are transported to mediastinal lymph nodes where they germinate, multiply, and release toxins, resulting in hemorrhagic necrosis of the thoracic lymph nodes and a hemorrhagic mediastinitis. Necrotizing pneumonia may also develop at the portal of entry in the lungs.[43] The incubation period for inhalation anthrax is typically 1–7 days; however, incubation periods as long as 42 days were reported in the 1979 outbreak in Sverdlosk.[17] During the 2001 bioterrorism event in the United States, the time between exposure and symptom onset ranged from 4 to 6 days.[18] Inhalation anthrax has developed in experimentally infected primates up to 58 days after aerosol exposure despite receipt of 5 days of postexposure antimicrobials.[44]

Inhalation anthrax, which is primarily a mediastinitis, is often described as biphasic. Early prodromal symptoms are nonspecific and include fatigue and fever with or without chills. Pulmonary symptoms such as cough, chest pain, and dyspnea follow in a day or two, as may nausea and abdominal pain. Diaphoresis is not uncommon. Pulmonary auscultation and mental status are often abnormal when patients present for care. In the absence of diagnostic testing or epi-linkage to other cases, inhalation anthrax is easily confused with respiratory illnesses such as influenza and pneumonia. Some extrathoracic presentations (i.e., primary meningitis,[45] nasopharyngeal anthrax,[45] and occasional gastrointestinal cases[41,46]) may also be caused by the inhalation of spores. Bacteremia may result in lesions in other organ systems, including hemorrhagic meningitis and submucosal gastrointestinal lesions.[43]

Untreated inhalation anthrax is almost always fatal. In the twentieth-century treatment did little to improve survival. The case fatality rate for the 18 twentieth-century cases from the United States was 89%.[47,48] Similarly, the case fatality rate for the 75 cases of inhalation anthrax reported in the 1979 Sverdlosk outbreak was 88%.[17] However, therapy can be successful, especially if combination antimicrobials and drainage of pleural fluid are initiated early in the course of disease.[49] With early initiation of treatment, 6 of the 11 (55%) inhalation anthrax cases associated with the 2001 bioterrorism event in the United States survived.[47,48]

Inhalation anthrax causes a hemorrhagic mediastinitis, and mediastinal widening on chest radiographs is considered pathognomonic. However only half of the 26 patients with inhalation anthrax described in the English literature from 1880 through 2013 had mediastinal widening at presentation; a larger proportion—two-thirds—had pleural effusion, and one-third had consolidation.

Several studies have attempted to identify signs and symptoms that could distinguish inhalation anthrax from cases of influenza-like illness or pneumonia during a bioterrorist event.[50–54] Most schema included complaints of dyspnea, chest pain, nausea/vomiting, and diaphoresis accompanied by abnormal radiographs or white counts. The Centers for Disease Control and Prevention (CDC) recently developed triage recommendations for use following a *B. anthracis* wide area aerosol release: anthrax cases in need of hospitalization (i.e., cases of systemic anthrax) could be identified by (1) tachycardia (>110 beats/min), tachypnea, or altered mental status; (2) tachycardia (>100 beats/min), diaphoresis, dyspnea, abdominal pain, or severe headache accompanied by abnormal lung or heart sounds or increasing girth; or (3) skin lesions with characteristic features. In 2014, the CDC published recommendations for antimicrobial post-exposure prophylaxis (PEP) and antimicrobial and antitoxin treatment options for persons with anthrax[40]: https://wwwnc.cdc.gov/eid/article/20/2/13-0687_article.

INGESTION ANTHRAX

Ingestion anthrax develops following the consumption of undercooked meat from animals sick or dead as a result of anthrax, and tends to occur in family clusters or point source outbreaks, often accompanied by cutaneous anthrax cases acquired through the butchering and handling of infected meat. The median incubation period for ingestion anthrax is 3.5 days with a range of 1–16 days.[55,56] Mortality is estimated to range from 25% to 60%.[12] There are two clinical forms of ingestion anthrax–oropharyngeal and gastrointestinal; both may be present in the same individual. The oropharyngeal form develops following infection of the oropharyngeal epithelium. Edematous lesions develop on the epithelium and progress to necrotic ulcers with a pseudomembrane. Profound edema develops in the oropharynx and neck, and cervical lymphadenopathy, pharyngitis, and fever develop.[57–59] Patients complain of sore throat and difficulty swallowing and may develop respiratory distress. The gastrointestinal form develops following infection of the gastric or intestinal mucosa. The infected intestinal segments become edematous, lesions may become necrotic and ulcerated, and draining mesenteric lymph nodes become infected and enlarged.[25,56] Abdominal pain with ascites is the norm and diarrhea is present about half the time.

INJECTION ANTHRAX

The incubation period for injection anthrax ranges from a day or less to more than 10 days,[20,60] with most cases occurring 3–4 days after exposure. Patients often are afebrile, and have far less pain than the degree of swelling would suggest.[61] An eschar is generally not present.[20]

Diagnosis. Preliminary diagnostic testing such as blood cultures or cultures and Gram stains of cerebrospinal fluid, pleural fluid, ascites, or swabs from under the eschar can be performed in hospital laboratories. However, confirmatory tests should be performed by Laboratory Response Network (LRN) laboratories. The LRN has been established by the Association of Public Health Laboratories and the CDC to provide the appropriate laboratory response for acts of bioterrorism, and includes the state public health laboratories. Guidelines for the collection of specimens and testing procedures for each type of anthrax can be found at https://www.cdc.gov/anthrax/specificgroups/lab-professionals/recommended-specimen.html/.

Reporting. Immediate notification should be made to the local or state health department and public health laboratory. Diagnostic laboratories receiving specimens associated with potential bioterrorist events should contact an LRN laboratory for instructions on testing and handling the specimen.

Treatment. Successful treatment of anthrax with the use of antiserum was demonstrated in 1903, neoarsphenamine was added in 1926, and penicillin treatment was first reported in 1944.[3,62,63] *B. anthracis* is usually susceptible to a variety of antimicrobials including penicillin, chloramphenicol, tetracycline, erythromycin, streptomycin, and the fluoroquinolones.[64,65] Testing of the isolates from the bioterrorism-related cases in the United States in 2001 showed susceptibility in vitro to rifampin, vancomycin, chloramphenicol, imipenem, clindamycin, and clarithromycin. Although the isolates were sensitive to penicillin and ampicillin, the presence of inducible beta-lactamases led the CDC to advise against the use of either of these drugs alone for therapy of anthrax cases associated with the 2001 bioterrorism event.

All patients with anthrax should be assessed for evidence of meningitis, as it may complicate any type of anthrax, including cutaneous anthrax—and its presence changes the number and duration of antimicrobials that are advised. Both animal and human data suggest that therapy with combination antimicrobials confers a survival advantage for systemic disease.[66,67] Treatment may need to commence prior to confirmation if there is a high clinical suspicion for systemic anthrax regardless of the mode of transmission, as a delay in treatment may prove fatal.

Three articles summarize guidelines for anthrax PEP and antimicrobial treatment options for adults (Tables 148-1 and 148-2),[40] pregnant women,[68] and children.[69] Antitoxin use is also addressed in each of the three articles.

Uncomplicated cutaneous anthrax (single < 4 cm lesion not on the head or neck and lacking evidence of edema, bullae, and lymphadenopathy) in an afebrile person unlikely to have been exposed to aerosolized *B. anthracis* may be treated with a 7- to 10-day course of oral monotherapy with ciprofloxacin or doxycycline; amoxicillin or penicillin may be used if the organism is susceptible. Antimicrobial treatment does not prevent progression to the eschar phase. Surgical excision of the cutaneous lesions is not recommended. Follow up PEP to finish out a 60-day course of antimicrobials is only indicated if concurrent aerosol exposure is thought to have occurred.[40]

More complicated (i.e., systemic) cutaneous cases, and cases of ingestion and inhalation anthrax should be treated with three or more antimicrobials—two bactericidal agents including both a fluoroquinolone and a beta-lactam and also a protein-synthesis inhibitor—if meningitis is present or suspected.[67,70] Two or more antimicrobials should be given—a bactericidal agent and a protein synthesis inhibitor—if there are no signs of meningitis.[40] Suggested bactericidal agents include the fluoroquinolones ciprofloxacin, levofloxacin, and moxifloxacin and the beta-lactams meropenem, imipenem, doripenem, penicillin, and ampicillin. Suggested protein synthesis inhibitors include linezolid, clindamycin, rifampin, and chloramphenicol. Because of the seriousness of the disease and exposure, treatment with ciprofloxacin or doxycycline is also recommended for children and pregnant women, despite usual contraindications against their use.

Injection anthrax is treated with broad spectrum antimicrobials that include a combination of ciprofloxacin, clindamycin, an additional agent to provide coverage for potential central nervous system infection with *B. anthracis*, and flucloxacillin and metronidazole for necrotizing fasciitis.[61,71] Animal origin antiserum was previously used successfully in the treatment of anthrax.[63,72] In animal models, passive immunization with immune serum containing antibodies against PA administered up to 24 hours after exposure proved effective in preventing infection,[73] and high-affinity antibodies from persons immunized against anthrax protected rats from injection of anthrax toxin.[74] Two antitoxins that were approved by the Food and Drug Administration (FDA) under the animal rule[75] are available through the Strategic National Stockpile (SNS) for the treatment of inhalation anthrax in adult and pediatric patients: Anthrasil™ (anthrax immune globulin, human)[76] and raxibacumab[77]; both can also be given under an investigational new drug application for noninhalation systemic anthrax. Antitoxins should be given in combination with appropriate antimicrobials. Both of the antitoxins have been shown to be superior to placebo when administered postexposure as monotherapy to toxemic monkeys. Marginal efficacy was shown postexposure in toxemic rabbits for both antitoxins when coadministered with levofloxacin compared to levofloxacin alone [82% vs. 65% ($p = 0.09$) survival for raxibacumab and 58% vs. 39% ($p = 0.14$, Z-test) for Anthrasil].[76,77]

TABLE 148-1 INTRAVENOUS ANTIMICROBIALS FOR SEVERE ANTHRAX* IN ADULTS WITH/WITHOUT POSSIBLE MENINGITIS

Triple Therapy for Cases with Possible or Confirmed Meningitis	Dual Therapy for Cases in Which Meningitis Has Been Excluded
1. Bactericidal Agent (Fluoroquinolone)	**1. Bactericidal Agent**
ciprofloxacin 400 mg Q8H **OR** levofloxacin 750 mg Q24H **OR** moxifloxacin 400 mg Q24H	a. For all strains, regardless of penicillin susceptibility or if susceptibility is unknown
PLUS	**ciprofloxacin 400 mg Q8H** **OR** levofloxacin 750 mg Q24H **OR** moxifloxacin 400 mg Q24H **OR** meropenem 2 g Q8H **OR** imipenem[a] 1 g Q6H **OR** doripenem 500 mg Q8H **OR** vancomycin 60 mg/kg/day divided Q8H (maintain serum trough concentrations of 15–20 µg/mL)
2. Bactericidal Agent (Beta-Lactam)	
a. For all strains, regardless of penicillin susceptibility or if susceptibility is unknown **meropenem 2 g Q8H** **OR** imipenem[a] 1 g Q6H **OR** doripenem 500 mg Q8H	
OR	**OR**
b. Alternatives for penicillin-susceptible strainspenicillin G 4 million units Q4H **OR** ampicillin 3 g Q6H	c. Alternatives for penicillin-susceptible strainspenicillin G 4 million units Q4H **OR** ampicillin 3 g Q6H
PLUS	**PLUS**
3. Protein Synthesis Inhibitor	**2. Protein Synthesis Inhibitor**
Linezolid[b] 600 mg Q12H **OR** clindamycin 900 mg Q8H **OR** rifampin[c] 600 mg Q12H **OR** Chloramphenicol[d] 1 g Q6-8H	**clindamycin 900 mg Q8H** **OR** **Linezolid[b] 600 mg Q12H** **OR** Doxycycline[c] 200 mg initially, then 100 mg Q12H **OR** Rifampin[d] 600 mg Q12H
Duration of Therapy: for 2–3 weeks or greater, until clinical criteria for stability are met. Patients exposed to aerosolized spores will require prophylaxis to complete an antimicrobial course of up to 60 days from onset of illness (see Table 148-2. Postexposure Prophylaxis)	**Duration of Therapy:** for 10–14 days or until clinical criteria for stability are met. Patient exposed to aerosolized spores will require prophylaxis to complete an antimicrobial course of up to 60 days from onset of illness (see Table 148-2. Postexposure Prophylaxis)
*Severe anthrax includes anthrax meningitis, inhalation, injection, and gastrointestinal anthrax; and cutaneous anthrax with systemic involvement, extensive edema, or lesions of the head or neck.	*Severe anthrax includes anthrax meningitis, inhalation, injection, and gastrointestinal anthrax; and cutaneous anthrax with systemic involvement, extensive edema, or lesions of the head or neck.
Bold Font: Preferred agent.	**Bold Font:** Preferred agent.
Normal Font: Alternative selections are listed in order of preference for therapy for patients who cannot tolerate first-line therapy, or if first-line therapy is unavailable.	Normal Font: Alternative selections are listed in order of preference for therapy for patients who cannot tolerate first-line therapy, or if first-line therapy is unavailable.
[a]Increased risk of seizures associated with imipenem/cilastatin therapy.	[a]Increased risk of seizures associated with imipenem/cilastatin therapy.
[b]Linezolid should be used with caution in patients with thrombocytopenia, as it may exacerbate it. Linezolid use for >14 days carries additional hematopoietic toxicity.	[b]Linezolid should be used with caution in patients with thrombocytopenia, as it may exacerbate it. Linezolid use for >14 days carries additional hematopoietic toxicity.
[c]Rifampin is not a protein synthesis inhibitor, it may also be used in combination therapy based on *in vitro* synergy.	[c]A single 10–14 day course of doxycycline is not routinely associated with tooth-staining.
[d]Should only be used if other options are not available, due to toxicity concerns.	[d]Rifampin is not a protein synthesis inhibitor, but it may also be used in combination therapy based on *in vitro* synergy.

TABLE 148-2 ORAL ANTIMICROBIALS FOR SEVERE ANTHRAX FOLLOWING INTRAVENOUS THERAPY, CUTANEOUS ANTHRAX LACKING SYSTEMIC INVOLVEMENT, AND FOR POSTEXPOSURE PROPHYLAXIS

Oral Therapy for Severe Anthrax[a] Following Intravenous Therapy	Oral Therapy for Cutaneous Anthrax Lacking Systemic Involvement	Oral Postexposure Prophylaxis for *Bacillus anthracis*
a. For all strains, regardless of penicillin susceptibility or if susceptibility is unknown	a. For all strains, regardless of penicillin susceptibility or if susceptibility is unknown	a. For all strains, regardless of penicillin susceptibility or if susceptibility is unknown
ciprofloxacin 500 mg Q12H **OR** **doxycycline 100 mg Q12H** **OR** levofloxacin 750 mg Q24H **OR** moxifloxacin 400 mg Q24H **OR** clindamycin[b] 600 mg Q8H **OR**	**ciprofloxacin 500 mg Q12H** **OR** **doxycycline 100 mg Q12H** **OR** **levofloxacin 750 mg Q24H** **OR** **moxifloxacin 400 mg Q24H** **OR** clindamycinb 600 mg Q8H **OR**	**ciprofloxacin 500 mg Q12H** **OR** **doxycycline 100 mg Q12H** **OR** levofloxacin 750 mg Q24H **OR** moxifloxacin 400 mg Q24H **OR** clindamycinb 600 mg Q8H **OR**
b. Alternatives for penicillin-susceptible strains	b. Alternatives for penicillin-susceptible strains	b. Alternatives for penicillin-susceptible strains
amoxicillin 1 g Q8H **OR** penicillin VK 500 mg Q6H	amoxicillin 1 g Q8H **OR** penicillin VK 500 mg Q6H	amoxicillin 1 g Q8H **OR** penicillin VK 500 mg Q6H
Duration of Therapy: After finishing treatment, patients who were exposed to aerosolized spores should finish out a 60-day course of oral antimicrobials (i.e., 60 days minus the duration of treatment)	**Duration of Therapy:** For bioterrorism-related cases: 60 days For naturally acquired cases: 7–10 days	**Duration of Therapy:** With or without AVA: 60 days

[a]Severe anthrax includes anthrax meningitis, inhalation, injection, and gastrointestinal anthrax; and cutaneous anthrax with systemic involvement, extensive edema, or lesions of the head or neck.
[b]Based on in vitro susceptibility data, rather than studies of clinical efficacy.
Bold Font: Preferred agent.
Normal Font: Alternative selections are listed in order of preference for therapy for patients who cannot tolerate first-line therapy, or if first-line therapy is unavailable.

Drainage of pleural fluid and ascites is believed to reduce the toxin level and was positively associated with survival in a systematic review of inhalation anthrax cases from 1900 to 2005.[49] In contrast to cutaneous anthrax in which the lesion should generally be left alone, for injection anthrax, debridement of affected tissue is advised—as it may serve as a nidus for release of toxin. Compartment syndrome is not uncommon with injection anthrax.

PREVENTION AND CONTROL

Postexposure Prophylaxis. In a study setting, attempts to successfully prophylax animals that had been exposed to aerosolized *B. anthracis* spores in high doses proved futile when monotherapy was used; success was only achieved when vaccine and antimicrobials were combined (Figs. 148-1).[44,78] Once begun, the antimicrobials provide protection until vaccine-induced immunity can develop. Long-term immunity is needed because spores can be retained in the lungs for months or more,[44] and human cases of inhalation anthrax have occurred up to 42 days after exposure.[17] If there were to be a purposeful mass exposure, spores that settled to the ground could potentially be re-aerosolized from the environment.

Three oral antimicrobials have been approved by the Food and Drug Administration (FDA) for postexposure prophylaxis (AbxPEP) in persons with suspected or confirmed exposure to aerosolized *B. anthracis* (Table 148-2). Ciprofloxacin[79] and doxycycline[80] are approved for use in adults and children, and levofloxacin[81] is approved for use in adults 18 and older. Alternative antimicrobials that may be used for AbxPEP include levofloxacin; moxifloxacin; amoxicillin and penicillin VK, if the isolate is susceptible; and clindamycin. Currently, the recommended duration of AbxPEP for aerosol exposures is 60 days. The antitoxin raxibacumab is also FDA approved for the prophylaxis of inhalation anthrax when alternative therapies are not available or are not appropriate.

Anthrax vaccine adsorbed (BioThrax, BioPort, Lansing, MI) is the only licensed human anthrax vaccine in the United States.[82] Anthrax vaccine is indicated for the active immunization for the prevention of disease caused by *B. anthracis* in persons 18–65 years of age. It can be used for both postexposure prophylaxis (VxPEP) and pre-exposure prophylaxis (PrEP). It is available for VxPEP through an investigational new drug application for children and persons over 65 years of age. When used as a component of PEP, it must be given in conjunction with an appropriate antimicrobial (Table 148-2), as immunity takes a few weeks to develop and most cases occur during the first few weeks after exposure. Vaccine given for VxPEP should be administered subcutaneously at 0, 2, and 4 weeks in conjunction with an antimicrobial that continues for at least 7–14 days following the last vaccine dose.[82] Vaccine and antimicrobials for PEP are available to local public health entities through the SNS. Pre-exposure vaccination is recommended for "laboratorians at risk for repeated exposure to fully virulent *B. anthracis* spores, such as those who (1) work with high concentrations of spores with potential for aerosol production; (2) handle environmental samples that might contain powders and are associated with anthrax investigations; (3) routinely work with pure cultures of *B. anthracis*; (4) frequently work in spore-contaminated areas after a bioterrorism attack; or (5) work in other settings where repeated exposures to *B. anthracis* aerosols may occur," as well as for military "personnel determined by DoD to have a calculable risk for exposure to aerosolized *B. anthracis* spores…."[82]

The dosing for PrEP of at-risk workers is 1/2 mL intramuscularly at 0, 1, and 6 months to complete the initial series, then 6 and 12 months after the completion of the primary series, and at 12-month intervals thereafter.[83]

In endemic areas, prevention of human anthrax infection is primarily dependent on the control of the disease in animals, especially livestock. Annual immunization of livestock in areas of endemic anthrax is recommended. The animal anthrax vaccine that is most commonly used is the avirulent Sterne strain live spore vaccine.[84] Livestock should be vaccinated 2–4 weeks before the start of the season when outbreaks may be expected.

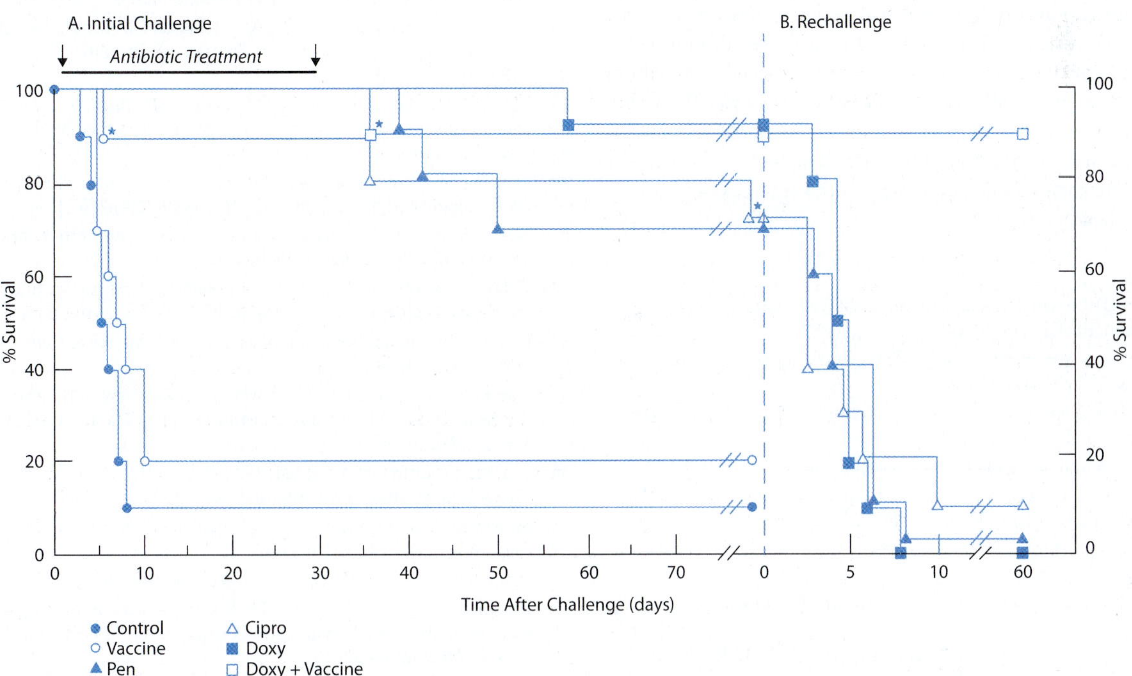

FIGURE 148-1. Postexposure prophylaxis of nonhuman primates with antibiotics and vaccine for inhalation anthrax. (A) Groups of ten nonhuman primates were exposed to aerosolized anthrax spores on day 0 and were left untreated (controls); given vaccine only on days 1 and 15; treated with penicillin (pen), ciprofloxacin (cipro), or doxycycline (doxy); or treated with doxy plus vaccine. Antibiotics were given from days 1 through 30. (B) Survivors were rechallenged by aerosol on days 13–142 (day 0, B). Percentage survival is plotted by day after initial challenge (A) or rechallenge (B). *The three animals that died of causes other than anthrax. (*Source:* Reproduced with Permission from Friedlander AM, Welkos SL, Pitt ML, et al. Postexposure prophylaxis against experimental inhalation anthrax. *J Infect Dis.* 1993;167(5):1239-1243.)

Animal anthrax cases and outbreaks should be reported to agriculture and public health officials. Affected premises or areas should be quarantined and any slaughter, butchering, and marketing of infected animals or their parts prevented. Antibiotic treatment of affected animals and immunization of all susceptible livestock on affected and surrounding premises is recommended. Investigation for sources of infection other than contaminated pastures may identify other sources, such as contaminated bone meal or feed, which should be eliminated to prevent further infection. Carcasses of animals that die of anthrax, bedding, and other contaminated material should be either buried deeply or burned completely. Regulation of the processing, importation, and use of bones or bone meal for use in animal feeds or fertilizer requires heating at sufficiently high temperatures to ensure destruction of anthrax spores. Herds in an outbreak area should be placed under surveillance and vaccination of healthy animals should be initiated if the herd has not been immunized before.

Disinfection of materials and surfaces contaminated with *B. anthracis* is complicated by the resistance of the spore. Surface decontamination of the soil requires significant resources and effort,[8] and the decontamination of buildings or facilities that have been contaminated with *B. anthracis* spores is a substantial and costly effort. A variety of procedures are effective for the decontamination of small items or equipment. These include dry heat, steam under pressure, formaldehyde soaking or vapor exposure, ethylene oxide gas exposure, hypochlorite solution soaking, and gamma-irradiation, and some of these measures have been applied to the decontamination of contaminated buildings or areas. The potential risks associated with disinfection methods, such as the use of formaldehyde or ethylene oxide, need to be weighed against the potential risk for anthrax infection when considering the decontamination method of choice. The effectiveness of disinfection should be verified by appropriate cultures and quality-control procedures.

Outbreaks of naturally occurring anthrax continue to occur worldwide, although they are relatively infrequent in developed countries, and parts of the world have been declared to be free of the disease. Intentional anthrax infection resulting from bioterrorist activities has occurred and continues to be a threat. Prompt identification and treatment of anthrax infection, especially inhalation anthrax infection, is essential to improve patient survival. The ability to recognize anthrax infection and an understanding of the epidemiology of the disease is necessary for timely diagnosis and treatment of cases, and for early identification of potential outbreaks and appropriate public health response.

References

1. Whitford HW, Hugh-Jones ME. In: Beran GW, ed. *Handbook of Zoonoses*. Boca Raton, FL: CRC Press; 1994.
2. Bible. *Exodus. New International Version*. Grand Rapids, MI: Zondervan Academic; 1978:3–6, Chapter 9.
3. Klemm DM, Klemm WR. A history of anthrax. *J Am Vet Med Assoc*. 1959;135:458–62.
4. Dirckx JH. Virgil on anthrax. *Am J Dermatopathol*. 1981;3(2):191–5.
5. Stein CD. In: Hull TG, ed. *Diseases Transmitted from Animals to Man*. Springfield, IL: Charles C Thomas; 1963:82–125.
6. Eusebius. *The Church History*. In. Maier PL, trans. Grand Rapids, MI: Kregel, Inc.; 1999:292.
7. Ziegler M. Famine and epidemic anthrax, Saint-Domingue (Haiti), 1770. *Contagions*. Vol. 2018.
8. Guillemin J. *Anthrax: The Investigation of a Deadly Outbreak*. Berkley, CA: University of California Press; 1999.
9. Lehman MW, Craig AS, Malama C, et al. Role of food insecurity in outbreak of anthrax infections among humans and hippopotamuses living in a game reserve area, rural Zambia. *Emerg Infect Dis*. 2017;23(9):1471–7.
10. Kohout E, Sehat A, Ashraf M. Anthrax: A continous problem in southwest Iran. *Am J Med Sci*. 1964;247:565–75.
11. Laforce FM. Woolsorters' disease in England. *Bull N Y Acad Med*. 1978;54(10):956–63.
12. Brachman PS, Kaufmann AF. In: Evans AS, Brachman PS, eds. *Bacterial Infections of Humans: Epidemiology and Control*. 3rd ed. New York: Plenum Publishing; 1998:95–107.
13. Brachman PS. Inhalation anthrax. *Ann N Y Acad Sci*. 1980;353:83–93.
14. Szablewski CM, Hendricks K, Bower WA, Shadomy SV, Hupert N. Anthrax cases associated with animal-hair shaving brushes. *Emerg Infect Dis*. 2017;23(5):806–8.
15. Cohen WS. In: Lederburg, ed. *Biological Weapons: Limiting the Threat*. Cambridge, Massachusetts: MIT Press; 1999:XI-XVI.
16. Manchee RJ, Broster MG, Melling J, Henstridge RM, Stagg AJ. *Bacillus anthracis* on Gruinard Island. *Nature*. 1981;294(5838):254–5.
17. Meselson M, Guillemin J, Hugh-Jones M, et al. The Sverdlovsk anthrax outbreak of 1979. *Science*. 1994;266(5188):1202–8.
18. Jernigan DB, Raghunathan PL, Bell BP, et al. Investigation of bioterrorism-related anthrax, United States, 2001: Epidemiologic findings. *Emerg Infect Dis*. 2002;8(10):1019–28.
19. Ringertz SH, Hoiby EA, Jensenius M, et al. Injectional anthrax in a heroin skin-popper. *Lancet*. 2000;356(9241):1574–5.
20. Health Protection Scotland. *National Anthrax Outbreak Control Team. An Outbreak of Anthrax Among Drug Users in Scotland, December 2009 to December 2010*. Glasgow, Scotland: Health Protection Scotland; December 2011.
21. Palmateer NE, Ramsay CN, Browning L, Goldberg DJ, Hutchinson SJ. Anthrax infection among heroin users in Scotland during 2009–2010: A case-control study by linkage to a national drug treatment database. *Clin Infect Dis*. 2012;55(5):706–10.
22. Booth M, Donaldson L, Cui X, et al. Confirmed *Bacillus anthracis* infection among persons who inject drugs, Scotland, 2009–2010. *Emerg Infect Dis*. 2014;20(9):1452–63.
23. Wilson JM, Brediger W, Albright TP, Smith-Gagen J. Reanalysis of the anthrax epidemic in Rhodesia, 1978–1984. *PeerJ*. 2016;4:e2686.
24. CDC. Human anthrax associated with an epizootic among livestock—North Dakota, 2000. *MMWR Morb Mortal Wkly Rep*. 2001;50(32):677–80.
25. Hausler WJ, Collier L, Balows A, Sussman M, eds. *Topley and Wilson's Microbiology and Microbial Infection*. Vol. III. Bacterial Infections. 9th ed. London: Edward Arnold; 1998:799–818.
26. Green BD, Battisti L, Koehler TM, Thorne CB, Ivins BE. Demonstration of a capsule plasmid in *Bacillus anthracis*. *Infect Immun*. 1985;49(2):291–7.
27. Leppla SH. *Bacillus anthracis* calmodulin-dependent adenylate cyclase: Chemical and enzymatic properties and interactions with eucaryotic cells. *Adv Cyclic Nucleotide Protein Phosphorylation Res*. 1984;17:189–98.
28. O'Brien J, Friedlander A, Dreier T, Ezzell J, Leppla S. Effects of anthrax toxin components on human neutrophils. *Infect Immun*. 1985;47(1):306–10.
29. Moayeri M, Haines D, Young HA, Leppla SH. *Bacillus anthracis* lethal toxin induces TNF-alpha-independent hypoxia-mediated toxicity in mice. *J Clin Invest*. 2003;112(5):670–82.
30. Dennett CG. Anthrax at Camp Dodge, Iowa: Report of three cases, with bacteriologic and blood studies. *JAMA*. 1919;72(4):270–2.
31. Doganay M, Metan G, Alp E. A review of cutaneous anthrax and its outcome. *J Infect Public Health*. 2010;3(3):98–105.
32. Gelaw Y, Asaminew T. Periocular cutaneous anthrax in Jimma Zone, Southwest Ethiopia: A case series. *BMC Res Notes*. 2013;6:313.
33. Davies JC. A major epidemic of anthrax in Zimbabwe. *Cent Afr J Med*. 1982;28(12):291–8.
34. Davies JC. A major epidemic of anthrax in Zimbabwe. The experience at the Beatrice Road Infectious Diseases Hospital, Harare. *Cent Afr J Med*. 1985;31(9):176–80.
35. Fox MD, Kaufmann AF, Zendel SA, et al. Anthrax in Louisiana, 1971: Epizootiologic study. *J Am Vet Med Assoc*. 1973;163(5):446–51.
36. Swartz MN. Recognition and management of anthrax—An update. *N Engl J Med*. 2001;345(22):1621–6.
37. Wenner KA, Kenner JR. Anthrax. *Dermatol Clin*. 2004;22(3):247–56, v.
38. Brachman PS, Gold H, Plotkin SA, Fekety FR, Werrin M, Ingraham NR. Field evaluation of a human anthrax vaccine. *Am J Public Health Nations Health*. 1962;52(4):632–45.
39. Carucci JA, McGovern TW, Norton SA, et al. Cutaneous anthrax management algorithm. *J Am Acad Dermatol*. 2002;47(5):766–9.
40. Hendricks KA, Wright ME, Shadomy SV, et al. Centers for disease control and prevention expert panel meetings on prevention and treatment of anthrax in adults. *Emerg Infect Dis*. 2014;20(2):e130687.
41. Thomas R, Davies C, Nunez A, et al. Influence of particle size on the pathology and efficacy of vaccination in a murine model of inhalational anthrax. *J Med Microbiol*. 2010;59(Pt 12):1415–27.

42. Weiner ZP, Glomski IJ. Updating perspectives on the initiation of *Bacillus anthracis* growth and dissemination through its host. *Infect Immun.* 2012;80(5):1626–33.
43. Abramova FA, Grinberg LM, Yampolskaya OV, Walker DH. Pathology of inhalational anthrax in 42 cases from the Sverdlovsk outbreak of 1979. *Proc Natl Acad Sci U S A.* 1993;90(6):2291–4.
44. Henderson DW, Peacock S, Belton FC. Observations on the prophylaxis of experimental pulmonary anthrax in the monkey. *J Hyg (Lond).* 1956;54(1):28–36.
45. Holty JE, Kim RY, Bravata DM. Anthrax: A systematic review of atypical presentations. *Ann Emerg Med.* 2006;48(2):200–11.
46. Klempner MS, Talbot EA, Lee SI, Zaki S, Ferraro MJ. Case records of the Massachusetts General Hospital. Case 25-2010. A 24-year-old woman with abdominal pain and shock. *N Engl J Med.* 2010;363(8):766–77.
47. Barakat LA, Quentzel HL, Jernigan JA, et al. Fatal inhalational anthrax in a 94-year-old Connecticut woman. *JAMA.* 2002;287(7):863–8.
48. Jernigan JA, Stephens DS, Ashford DA, et al. Bioterrorism-related inhalational anthrax: The first 10 cases reported in the United States. *Emerg Infect Dis.* 2001;7(6):933–44.
49. Holty JE, Bravata DM, Liu H, Olshen RA, McDonald KM, Owens DK. Systematic review: A century of inhalational anthrax cases from 1900 to 2005. *Ann Intern Med.* 2006;144(4):270–80.
50. Cinti SK, Saravolatz L, Nafziger D, Sunstrum J, Blackburn G. Differentiating inhalational anthrax from other influenza-like illnesses in the setting of a national or regional anthrax outbreak. *Arch Intern Med.* 2004;164(6):674–6.
51. Hupert N, Bearman GM, Mushlin AI, Callahan MA. Accuracy of screening for inhalational anthrax after a bioterrorist attack. *Ann Intern Med.* 2003;139(5 Pt 1):337–45.
52. Kuehnert MJ, Doyle TJ, Hill HA, et al. Clinical features that discriminate inhalational anthrax from other acute respiratory illnesses. *Clin Infect Dis.* 2003;36(3):328–36.
53. Kyriacou DN, Stein AC, Yarnold PR, et al. Clinical predictors of bioterrorism-related inhalational anthrax. *Lance.* 2004;364(9432):449–52.
54. Mayer TA, Morrison A, Bersoff-Matcha S, et al. Inhalational anthrax due to bioterrorism: Would current Centers for Disease Control and Prevention guidelines have identified the 11 patients with inhalational anthrax from October through November 2001? *Clin Infect Dis.* 2003;36(10):1275–83.
55. Navacharoen N, Sirisanthana T, Navacharoen W, Ruckphaopunt K. Oropharyngeal anthrax. *J Laryngol Otol.* 1985;99(12):1293–5.
56. Kanafani ZA, Ghossain A, Sharara AI, Hatem JM, Kanj SS. Endemic gastrointestinal anthrax in 1960s Lebanon: Clinical manifestations and surgical findings. *Emerg Infect Dis.* 2003;9(5):520–5.
57. Beatty ME, Ashford DA, Griffin PM, Tauxe RV, Sobel J. Gastrointestinal anthrax: Review of the literature. *Arch Intern Med.* 2003;163(20):2527–31.
58. Sirisanthana T, Brown AE. Anthrax of the gastrointestinal tract. *Emerg Infect Dis.* 2002;8(7):649–51.
59. Sirisanthana T, Navachareon N, Tharavichitkul P, Sirisanthana V, Brown AE. Outbreak of oral-oropharyngeal anthrax: An unusual manifestation of human infection with *Bacillus anthracis. Am J Trop Med Hyg.* 1984;33(1):144–50.
60. Cui X, Nolen LD, Sun J, et al. Analysis of anthrax immune globulin intravenous with antimicrobial treatment in injection drug users, Scotland, 2009–2010. *Emerg Infect Dis.* 2017;23(1):56–65.
61. Abbara A, Brooks T, Taylor GP, et al. Lessons for control of heroin-associated anthrax in Europe from 2009–2010 outbreak case studies, London, UK. *Emerg Infect Dis.* 2014;20(7):1115–22.
62. Murphy C, LaBocetta AC, Lockwood JA. Treatment of human anthrax with penicillin: Report of three cases. *J Amer Vet Med Assoc.* 1944;126(15):948–50.
63. Lucchessi PF, Gildersleeve N. The treatment of anthrax. *JAMA.* 1941;116(14):1506–8.
64. Lightfoot NF, Scott RJD, Turnbull PCB. Antimicrobial susceptibility of *Bacillus anthracis. Salisbury Med Suppl.* 1990;68:95–8.
65. Doganay M, Aydin N. Antimicrobial susceptibility of *Bacillus anthracis. Scand J Infect Dis.* 1991;23(3):333–5.
66. Lincoln RE, Klein F, Walker JS, et al. Successful treatment of rhesus monkeys for septicemia anthrax. *Antimicrob Agents Chemother (Bethesda).* 1964;10:759–63.
67. Katharios-Lanwermeyer S, Holty JE, Person M, et al. Identifying meningitis during an anthrax mass casualty incident: Systematic review of systemic anthrax since 1880. *Clin Infect Dis.* 2016;62(12):1537–45.
68. Meaney-Delman D, Rasmussen SA, Beigi RH, et al. Prophylaxis and treatment of anthrax in pregnant women. *Obstet Gynecol.* 2013;122(4):885–900.
69. Bradley JS, Peacock G, Krug SE, et al. Pediatric anthrax clinical management. *Pediatrics.* 2014;133(5):e1411–36.
70. Pillai SK, Huang E, Guarnizo JT, et al. Antimicrobial treatment for systemic anthrax: Analysis of cases from 1945 to 2014 identified through a systematic literature review. *Health Secur.* 2015;13(6):355–64.
71. Veitch J, Kansara A, Bailey D, Kustos I. Severe systemic *Bacillus anthracis* infection in an intravenous drug user. *BMJ Case Rep.* 2014;2014:bcr2013201921.
72. Knudson GB. Treatment of anthrax in man: History and current concepts. *Mil Med.* 1986;151(2):71–7.
73. Kobiler D, Gozes Y, Rosenberg H, Marcus D, Reuveny S, Altboum Z. Efficiency of protection of guinea pigs against infection with *Bacillus anthracis* spores by passive immunization. *Infect Immun.* 2002;70(2):544–60.
74. Wild MA, Xin H, Maruyama T, et al. Human antibodies from immunized donors are protective against anthrax toxin in vivo. *Nat Biotechnol.* 2003;21(11):1305–6.
75. Langford MJ, Myers RC. Difficulties associated with the development and licensing of vaccines for protection against bio-warfare and bio-terrorism. *Dev Biol (Basel).* 2002;110:107–12.
76. Emergent Biosolutions. Highlights of prescribing information: Anthrasil [Anthrax Immune Globulin (Human)], sterile solution for infusion [Package Insert]. March 2015, pp. 1–25. https://www.fda.gov/downloads/BiologicsBloodVaccines/Vaccines/ApprovedProducts/UCM439812.pdf.
77. GlaxoSmithKline. Highlights of prescribing information: Raxibacumab injection. December 2012, pp. 1–14. https://www.accessdata.fda.gov/drugsatfda_docs/label/2012/125349s000lbl.pdf.
78. Friedlander AM, Welkos SL, Pitt ML, et al. Postexposure prophylaxis against experimental inhalation anthrax. *J Infect Dis.* 1993;167(5):1239–43.
79. Bayer Healthcare Pharmaceuticals I. Highlights of prescribing information: Cipro. 2016. https://www.accessdata.fda.gov/drugsatfda_docs/label/2016/019537s086lbl.pdf.
80. Warner Chilcott. Highlights of prescribing information: Doxycycline hyclate. 2008, pp. 1–18. https://www.accessdata.fda.gov/drugsatfda_docs/label/2008/050795s005lbl.pdf. Accessed May 23, 2018.
81. Janssen Pharmaceuticals I. Highlights of prescribing information: Levaquin. 2017. https://www.janssenmd.com/pdf/levaquin/levaquin_pi.pdf.
82. Wright JG, Quinn CP, Shadomy S, Messonnier N. Use of anthrax vaccine in the United States: Recommendations of the Advisory Committee on Immunization Practices (ACIP), 2009. *MMWR Recomm Rep.* 2010;59(Rr-6):1–30.
83. Emergent Biosolutions. Highlights of prescribing information: BiothraxR (Anthrax Vaccine Adsorbed). 2015. https://www.fda.gov/downloads/BiologicsBloodVaccines/BloodBloodProducts/ApprovedProducts/LicensedProductsBLAs/UCM074923.pdf. Accessed May 23, 2018.
84. Kaufmann AF, Fox MD, Kolb RC. Anthrax in Louisiana, 1971: An evaluation of the Sterne strain anthrax vaccine. *J Am Vet Med Assoc.* 1973;163(5):442–5.

CHAPTER

149 Brucellosis

María E. Negrón Sureda

BACKGROUND

Brucellosis, a bacterial zoonotic disease that affects humans, domesticated livestock and wildlife, is considered one of the most common and economically important zoonoses globally. Brucellosis infection in humans, also known as undulant fever, Mediterranean fever or Malta fever, is a debilitating disease that occurs from exposure to infected animals or contaminated animal products such as unpasteurized milk or dairy products. The disease is misdiagnosed often due to the resemblance with other acute febrile illnesses.

Analysis of cheese and skeletal remains from the town of Herculaneum during the Roman Empire suggest this bacterium has been affecting humans for millennia.[1] However, it was not until the nineteenth century during the British occupation of the island of Malta that Sir Arthur Bruce first identified what is now known as *Brucella melitensis.* There were many theories as to how the disease caused by *Micrococcus melitensis*, the name given to the bacteria by Sir Arthur Bruce, was acquired by humans. It was not until the early 1900s that by serendipity the organism was discovered in Maltese goats' blood and milk with contaminated milk identified as the source of human infection.[2] These findings led to public health campaigns banning goat milk consumption by military authorities thereby eradicating the disease from the military base. During the same period, Bernhard Bang isolated what he referred to as *Bacillus abortus*, from the uterus of an infected cow and was able to reproduce the disease by experimentally inoculating naïve animals. However, it was not until 1918 that Alice Evans determined that *Micococcus melitensis* and *B. abortus* were closely related.[3] Since then, a number of *Brucella* spp. have been identified from a wide variety of animals.

AGENT

Brucella spp. are classified as α-Proteobacteria, and their closest relatives are the *Ochrobactrum* spp. that are known to cause opportunistic infections in humans. *Brucella* sp. are characterized as small, facultative, nonmotile, nonspore forming Gram-negative intracellular coccobacilli. The original classification of the genus *Brucella* was based on phenotypic characteristics and species were named according to the animal they were first isolated from. Based on genomic analyses, the genus *Brucella* is considered a single population that evolved in different hosts with distinct phenotypic characteristics. Currently, there are 12 recognized *Brucella* spp. with a primary animal host preference and secondary hosts having a lesser role in maintenance and or transmission (Table 149-1). The most commonly known *Brucella* species to cause infections in humans are *B. melitensis*, *B. abortus*, *B. suis*, and *B. canis*; but human infections caused by other *Brucella* spp. have been identified (Table 149-1).

The cell wall lipopolysaccharide (LPS) in *Brucella sp* is classified as smooth or rough based on the presence or absence of the O-polysaccharide. *B. melitensis*, *abortus*, *suis*, *ceti*, and *pinnipedialis* are classified as smooth *Brucella* species, because they contain the O-polysaccharide. *B. canis* and *ovis*, and *B. abortus* strain RB51 are classified as rough *Brucella* species. The classification of smooth versus rough LPS correlates with disease severity in humans. Infections in humans caused by rough species are less severe when compared to infections caused by smooth *Brucella* spp. This is in part because, despite the absence of the O-polysacchardide influencing the uptake of the bacteria by cells, rough LPS *Brucellae* are less successful in surviving inside cells.

Survival of the bacteria outside the body has been documented to be as little as 4 hours to as long as 8 months or more.[4] This extensive range is due to survival in different substrates (i.e., dust, fecal material, water slurry, aborted fetuses, soil, meat, and dairy products) and other variables such as number of organisms, temperature, pH, and sunlight.[4]

Disease in Humans

Brucellosis in humans is characterized by nonspecific symptoms, typically presenting as an acute febrile illness. The incubation period is typically 2–4 weeks with a range of 5 to as long as 6 months. Fever is the most common clinical manifestation reported by over 75% of patients.[5] Thus, in brucellosis endemic countries, the disease should be included as part of the differential diagnosis for fevers of unknown origin. Other common, but nonspecific brucellosis symptoms include night sweats, malaise, arthralgia, myalgia, chills, fatigue headache, and back pain. Osteoarticular complications (i.e., arthritis, sacroiliitis, and spondylitis) are the most common in humans. Epididymo-orchitis is the most common genitourinary complication, experienced by approximately one in ten males.[5,6] Abortion, mainly during the first and second trimester is the most commonly reported adverse pregnancy outcome, followed by preterm delivery.[6]

Transmission to Humans

Humans are incidental hosts for *Brucella* sp. and the vast majority of human cases are caused by consumption of unpasteurized dairy products. The organism is present in the genital tract, reproductive tissues, and birth products of infected animals at very high concentrations. The tissues and fluids associated with birth can contain up to 10^{10} organisms per mL. In addition, the organism remains viable in desiccated placental remains for up to 20 weeks. Between 12% and 44% of infected cattle and up to 66% of infected goats will shed the bacteria in milk. Survival of the bacteria in dairy products is quite variable. Survival has been reported to be as short as minutes and up to months, depending on type of dairy product and temperature.[7] Muscle tissue does not present as high of a risk as milk as long as the meat is properly cooked and stored. *Brucella* spp. can survive drying, salting, smoking, refrigeration, and freezing.

Brucellosis is a significant occupational hazard for persons working closely with live animals or carcasses as direct or indirect

TABLE 149-1 HOST PREFERENCE AND ZOONOTIC POTENTIAL FOR EACH OF THE *BRUCELLA* SPECIES RECOGNIZED

Species	Main Host	Human infections diagnosed
B. melitensis	Sheep, goats	Yes
B. abortus	Cattle	Yes
B. suis	Swine (biovars 1–3), reindeer/caribou (biovar 4), rodent (biovar 5)	Yes
B. canis	Dog	Yes
B. ceti	Cetaceans (i.e., dolphins, porpoises, whales)	Yes
B. pinnipedialis	Pinnipeds (i.e., seal)	Yes
B. innopinata	Unknown	Yes
B. neotomae	Desert wood rat	Yes
B. microti	Common vole	No
B. ovis	Sheep	No
B. papionis	Baboons	No
B. vulpis	Foxes	No

exposure via broken skin, mucous membranes, inhalation, or contact with infected placenta, aborted fetuses, and contaminated fomites. Contamination of skin wounds or accidental ingestion of bacteria may be a problem for persons working in slaughterhouses or meat packing plants, veterinarians and hunters. The average infectious aerosol dose in humans is relatively small, only 100–1000 organisms, thus 1 mL of such fluid may contain many logs above an infectious dose. Therefore, inhalation of *Brucella* organisms can be a significant hazard for people in certain occupations, such as those working in laboratories, or those performing aerosol-generating tasks such as carcass dressing by slaughterhouse workers or hunters. Brucellosis is the most common laboratory acquired infection because clinical specimens were not handled under appropriate biosafety practices.[8]

Person-to-person transmission is extremely rare; mechanisms can include vertical transmission, blood transfusion, bone marrow transplant, and rarely sexual or close household contact.[9] Mother-to-child transmission is possible by transplacental transmission or by breast milk. Although rare, physicians assisting infected women during parturition are at risk of developing brucellosis.[10]

Diagnosis

Diagnosis of brucellosis cannot be accomplished based on symptoms alone as the disease can affect any body organ or system and patients can present with a wide spectrum of nonspecific symptoms. As there are no pathognomonic symptoms, diagnosis is often delayed or missed.

Infections can be diagnosed by direct detection of the bacteria or by the detection of immune response against the pathogen. Bacterial culture is the "gold standard" for diagnosing human brucellosis. Appropriate specimens for culture include bone marrow, blood, abscess material, and tissue samples. Direct microscopic examination of samples with Gram stain is not feasible given the small number of bacteria present in human clinical specimens. Samples grow best at 35–37°C at a neutral pH and CO_2 enrichment between 5% and 10%. The average time to detection of *Brucella* spp. growth in culture is 7 days (range of 5–12 days).[11] Cultures from suspect brucellosis patients should be incubated for 2–4 weeks before discarding as negative.[11] Isolation rates can vary between 25% and 80% depending on the stage of disease (blood samples collected during the febrile phase are most likely to yield positive results), previous use of antibiotics, type and volume of clinical specimen, and culture methods used. If a focal infection is suspected, it is recommended to collect samples from the affected area (e.g., CSF, joint aspirate, urine, to increase the likelihood of positive culture). Presumptive identification of the bacteria includes the observation of small, circular, smooth, nonhemolitic, and translucent to white-cream colored colonies which are oxidase and catalase positive, nitrate reduction, and urease positive within 2 hours; H_2S production is variable. In the United States, a presumptive or confirmatory *Brucella* spp. by culture requires notification to the Laboratory Response Network (LRN) within 2 hours (Tables 149-2 and 149-3).[12,13] The LRN is a national network of federal, state, and local public health, military, food testing, environmental, veterinary, and international laboratories whose mission is to respond quickly to biological and chemical public health emergencies.[13]

Serological tests are commonly used for diagnosis of human brucellosis to circumvent some of the difficulties around culture pf the organism like low sensitivity, delayed diagnosis, and the need to grow the organism under biosafety level 3 laboratory conditions. The majority of serological tests use a whole cell antigen preparation from a *B. abortus* strain, which cross-reacts with other smooth *Brucella* spp. (*B. abortus*, *B. melitesnis*, and *B. suis*). Furthermore, the antigen used shows variable levels of cross-reactivity with other Gram-negative bacteria such as *Yersinia enterocolitica*, *E coli O:157*, *Franciscella tularensis*, *Salmonella*, and *Vibrio cholera*. Agglutination tests, such as Serum Agglutination Test (SAT), Rose Bengal Test (RBT), and Coombs Test, are the most commonly used and detect the presence of IgM, IgG, or IgA *Brucella* antibodies. The SAT is considered the reference serological test and the *Brucella* microagglutination test (BMAT) is a modified version of SAT used at the CDC. This test identifies both IgM and IgG antibodies to smooth-*Brucella* sp. The addition of 2-mercaptoetanol as a second step increases the specificity of the test by breaking disulfide bonds and depolymerizing IgM antibodies without affecting IgG, allowing the comparison of total antibody level versus IgG levels.[14] The Rose Bengal Test is used as a screening test in endemic countries as it is quick and relatively inexpensive to perform. However, antigen quality can vary depending on where it was produced and the test has poor specificity as, like the SAT, it cross-reacts with other Gram-Negative bacteria. False-negative results can occur due to the prozone effect, which happens when an excess of antibodies inhibits agglutination in low dilutions.[15] The Coombs test or BrucellaCapt detect nonagglutinating antibodies, which are the predominating antibody type 6–12 months after infection. The use of ELISAs have increased in popularity given their quick turnaround time, less training needed compared to agglutinations tests, and ability to differentiate between antibody classes. ELISA tests have high sensitivity and specificity and depending on the test, ELISAs may detect total and specific immunoglobulins (e.g., IgM, IgG, and IgA). A positive IgM ELISA test result on its own is not sufficient to diagnose brucellosis and it should be supplemented with other tests such as IgG ELISA.[16]

Several factors must be taken into consideration when interpreting serological test results. Exposure history can narrow down the most likely infecting *Brucellae*, as commercially available antibody tests do not identify detect rough *Brucella* like *B. canis* or *B. abortus* RB51. In these situations, culture should be performed in order to properly diagnose an infection. Timing of exposure and development of symptoms will assist in determining the classes of antibodies expected as well as the presence of agglutinating or nonagglutinating antibodies. IgM antibodies appear the first weeks after infection and IgG antibodies begin to appear after the second week and both IgM and IgG peak 1 month after infection.[14] The presence of antibodies itself is not enough to warrant antimicrobial treatment as *Brucella* antibodies can persist for over a year postinfection despite successful antibiotic treatment. Thus, the decision to start a patient on treatment should take into consideration clinical presentation, symptom onset, and exposure history. It is not uncommon to find background levels

TABLE 149-2 COUNCIL OF STATE AND TERRITORIAL EPIDEMIOLOGISTS (CSTE) 2010 BRUCELLOSIS CASE DEFINITION*,[28]

Laboratory Criteria for Diagnosis		Case Classification	
Definitive	• Culture and identification of *Brucella* spp. from clinical specimens • Evidence of a fourfold or greater rise in *Brucella* antibody titer between acute- and convalescent-phase serum specimens obtained greater than or equal to 2 weeks apart	**Confirmed**	• A clinically compatible illness with definitive laboratory evidence of *Brucella* infection
Presumptive	• *Brucella* total antibody titer of greater than or equal to 160 by standard tube agglutination test (SAT) or *Brucella* microagglutination test (BMAT) in one or more serum specimens obtained after onset of symptoms • Detection of *Brucella* DNA in a clinical specimen by PCR assay	**Probable**	• A clinically compatible illness with at least one of the following: • Epidemiologically linked to a confirmed human or animal brucellosis case • Presumptive laboratory evidence, but without definitive laboratory evidence, of *Brucella* infection

*This is the official case definition used in the United States by States and Federal government.
Note: Clinical description: An illness characterized by acute or insidious onset of fever and one or more of the following: night sweats, arthralgia, headache, fatigue, anorexia, myalgia, weight loss, arthritis/spondylitis, meningitis, or focal organ involvement (endocarditis, orchitis/epididymitis, hepatomegaly, splenomegaly).
Statement. CP. Brucellosis (Brucella sp) 2010 Case definition. Surveillance Case Definition 2010. Cited May 2018. Available from: https://wwwn.cdc.gov/nndss/conditions/brucellosis/case-definition/2010/.

TABLE 149-3 WHO BRUCELLOSIS CASE DEFINITION[29]

Laboratory Criteria for Diagnosis		Case Classification	
Confirmatory	• Culture and identification of *Brucella* spp. from clinical specimens • A presumptive laboratory diagnosis based on detection of agglutinating antibodies (i.e. rose Bengal test, serum agglutination test) combined with detection of non-agglutinating antibodies through ELISA IgG test or Coombs IgG.	**Suspected**	• A case that is compatible with the clinical description and is epidemiologically linked to suspected/confirmed animal cases or contaminated animal products.
Presumptive	• Positive Rose Bengal Test • Positive Standard Agglutination Test	**Probable**	• A suspected case with presumptive laboratory diagnosis
		Confirmed	• A suspected or probable case with confirmatory laboratory diagnosis

Note: Clinical Description: Acute or insidious onset, with continued, intermitted, or irregular fever of variable duration, profuse sweating, fatigue, anorexia, weight loss, headache, arthralgia, and generalized aching. Abscess formation is a rare complication.

of reactive antibodies in continuously exposed populations in brucellosis endemic countries.

Detection of *Brucella* spp. DNA in clinical specimens is frequently used in combination with other diagnostic tests and can add valuable information to patient diagnosis, animals disease status and laboratory surveillance.[10–12] PCR is simple, fast, more sensitive, and safer than culture. However, patients who have been successfully treated can remain PCR positive for over 2 years.[17] Similarly, a negative result on PCR does not indicate absence of infection by *Brucella* spp.

Treatment

Brucellosis treatment depends on the presence of complications, patient allergies, or existing conditions that could make some treatment choices contraindicated, or whether the disease is caused by *B. abortus* RB51. The treatment of choice is doxycycline (2–4 mg/kg/day, twice a day) and rifampin (15–20 mg/kg/day, once a day) for at least 6 weeks. Another treatment option is to replace rifampin with streptomycin (15 mg/kg/day, intramuscularly once a day) or gentamycin (3–5 mg/kg, intravenous or intramuscularly) for 2–3 weeks. A doxycycline/streptomycin regimen is considered superior to doxycycline/rifampin as the latter is associated with higher risk of treatment failure, and minor adverse reactions.[18–20] However, access to care and cost are important factors amongst clinicians when deciding between the two treatments regimens. Because of this, the doxycycline/rifampin combination is the most common choice administered for uncomplicated brucellosis as doxycycline and rifampin can be taken orally, while streptomycin s administered intramuscularly. Streptomycin (or gentamicin) along with doxycycline for 4–6 months is recommended for complicated brucellosis, defined as the presence of endocarditis, meningitis osteomyelitis, or other invasive disease. In children < 8 years of age, trimethoprim-sulfamethoxazole (TMP-SMZ) is recommended instead of doxycycline in dual drug regimens. In situations where *B. abortus* RB51 is the infecting bacterial strain, the treatment of choice is TMP-SMZ in combination with doxycycline for 6 weeks. The RB51 strain is resistant to rifampin, tetracycline, thus these two antibiotics should be avoided. Trimethoprim-sulfamethoxazole (TMP-SMZ) or quinolones like ciprofloxacin and ofloxacin can be used if there is a contraindication for any of the previously mentioned drugs.

There are two key factors associated with relapse: inadequate duration of treatment, due to lack of adherence or inadequate prescription, and the use monotherapy. Lack of adherence is particularly a problem as duration of treatment brucellosis treatment is particularly long. This will result in the need to change the antibiotic regime, to most likely a less effective combination, or early termination of therapy, increasing the probability of a relapse. Current recommendations include the use of two or more antibiotics in order to decrease the probability of relapse as studies demonstrate that between 2% and 39% of patients treated with monotherapy relapse. Approximately 80% of relapses occur within the first 3 months and almost all occur within the first 6 months after discontinuation of therapy.[20]

Prevention

Brucellosis is the classical bacterial zoonosis where controlling or eliminating the disease in animals is the most effective way of decreasing human disease burden via vaccination of animals (there is no human vaccine available) and pasteurization of dairy products. To ensure safety, all milk should be processed by heating to a temperature of 80–85°C and holding for several minutes.

Vaccines commercially available exist for only two *Brucella* spp.: *B. melitensis* and *B. abortus*. Rev-1 was developed in the mid-1950s and is the only commercially available vaccine for *B. melitensis* in small ruminants. There are two widely used *B. abortus* vaccines, S19 and RB51. S19 was developed in 1930s and is currently used in many parts of the world for the control of bovine brucellosis. The RB51 vaccine is the only available vaccine in the United States to vaccinate cattle against *B. abortus*. All three vaccines are considered abortigenic (RB51 to a lesser degree) and can be shed in milk. Human illness due to vaccine strains occurs most commonly in veterinarians and veterinary technicians when accidentally exposed.

Infection cause by the RB51 vaccine strain can only be diagnosed by culturing the organism.[21] The RB51 strain is rifampin resistant, and, physicians should consider combination regimen with doxycycline and trimethoprim/sulfamethoxazole for postexposure prophylaxis (PEP) and treatment.

Brucellosis is one of the top diseases acquired in the laboratory. Birth products suspected to contain pathogenic *Brucella* and all manipulations of culture of *Brucella* spp. should be handled under BSL-3 conditions.[22] In situations where a potential exposure has been identified, the first step is to determine what activities may have led to the exposure, identify who was at the laboratory while those activities were performed and their distance from the exposure.[23] Postexposure recommendations vary depending on the risk level [i.e., minimal (but not zero), low, and high risk] ranging from possible symptom watch to symptom watch, serological monitoring, and PEP.[23]

Bioterrorism Potential

B. suis was the first biological agent weaponized in 1952. Several biological and pathological properties makes these three *Brucella* species good biological weapon candidates. They can be easily obtained from areas where the disease is endemic, bulk-produced, and aerosolized. Humans are susceptible to most routes of infection and may become infected with as little as 10–100 microorganisms. Although the disease has a long incubation period, which could be a drawback, once established in the body, *Brucella* successfully evades the immune system and it is very difficult to diagnose because it presents as a flu-like illness. Finally, there are no human vaccines available or adequate medical countermeasures.[24]

In the United States, the Department of Health and Human Services (HHS) and the United States Department of Agriculture (USDA) are required by law to create and regulate a list of biological agents and toxins with the potential to pose a severe threat of public health and animal, plant, and animal or plant product safety. *B. abortus*, *B. melitensis*, and *B. suis* are categorized as a Category B Pathogen ("moderately easy to disseminate, causes moderate morbidity and low mortality and specific enhancements are needed for diagnostic capacity and surveillance").[25] As a select agent, anyone who identifies any of these three *Brucella* sp. is required to notify the Division of Select Agents and Toxins (DSAT) at CDC.

Brucellosis in the United States

Brucellosis has a worldwide distribution. There are over 500,000 new human cases annually worldwide[26]; however, this number is likely an underestimation as brucellosis is easily misdiagnosed.

Brucellosis is reportable disease in all U.S. states and territories, with voluntary reporting to CDC. In the United States, the cattle brucellosis control and eradication program began in 1930s and human brucellosis became a nationally notifiable disease in 1944. A sharp decline has since been observed in both cattle and humans. Human cases dropped from over 3000 cases per year in early 1950s to approximately 100–120 cases per year now.[27] As a result of the near elimination of bovine brucellosis in the United States, pasteurization, and increase in international travel, the epidemiology of brucellosis in the United States has changed dramatically. Approximately 70–75% of the brucellosis cases reported annually in the United States are now people who visited or brought back unpasteurized dairy products from locations where the disease is highly endemic in animals. Hunting is the second most commonly reported exposures, primarily through dressing feral swine or caribou. Physicians should also be aware of the possibility of *B. suis* or *B. canis* infection as these two *Brucella* species are present in swine (*B. suis*) and canine (*B. canis*) populations worldwide.

References

1. Capasso L. Bacteria in two-millennia-old cheese, and related epizoonoses in roman populations. *J Infect*. 2002;45(2):122–7.
2. Vassallo DJ. The saga of brucellosis: Controversy over credit for linking Malta fever with goats' milk. *Lancet*. 1996;348(9030):804–8.
3. Evans AC. Further studies on bacterium abortus and related bacteria: III Bacterium abortus and related bacteria in cow's milk. *J Infect Dis*. 1918;23(4):354–72.
4. Corbel MJ. *Brucellosis in Humans and Animals*. Geneva: World Health Organization; 2006.
5. Dean AS, Crump L, Greter H, Hattendorf J, Schelling E, Zinsstag J. Clinical manisfestations of human brucellosis: A systematic review and meta-analysis. *PLoS Negl Trop Dis*. 2012;6(12):e1929.
6. Arenas-Gamboa AM, Rossetti CA, Chaki SP, Garcia-Gonzalez DG, Adams LG, Ficht TA. Human brucellosis and adverse pregnancy outcomes. *Curr Trop Med Rep*. 2016 Dec;3(4):164–72.
7. Rowe MT. Brucella—Problems with dairy products. In: *Encyclopedia of Food Microbiology*. 2nd ed. London: Academic Press; 2014:340–3.
8. Traxler RM, Lehman MW, Bosserman EA, Guerra MA, Smith TL. A literature review of laboratory-acquired brucellosis. *J Clin Microbiol*. 2013 Sep;51(9):3055–62.
9. Tuon FF, Gondolfo RB, Cerchiari N. Human-to-human transmission of Brucella—A systematic review. *Trop Med Int Health*. 2017 May;22(5):539–46.
10. Mesner O, Riesenberg K, Biliar N, et al. The many faces of human-to-human transmission of brucellosis: Congenital infection and outbreak of nosocomial disease related to an unrecognized clinical case. *Clin Infect Dis*. 2007 Dec 15;45(12):e135–40.
11. Al Dahouk S, Tomaso H, Nockler K, Neubauer H, Frangoulidis D. Laboratory-based diagnosis of brucellosis—A review of the literature. Part I: Techiniques for direct detection and identification of *Brucella* spp. *Clin Lab*. 2003;49:487–505.
12. Centers for Disease Control and Prevention. National Center for Emerging and Zoonotic Infectious Diseases. Brucellosis Reference Guide: Exposures, Testing, and Prevention. 2017.
13. Centers for Disease Control and Prevention. Laboratory Response Network. https://emergency.cdc.gov/lrn/index.asp.
14. Al Dahouk S, Tomaso H, Nockler K, Neubauer H, Frangoulidis D. Laboratory-based diagnosis of brucellosis—A review of the literature. Part II: Serological tests for brucellosis. *Clin Lab*. 2003;49:577–89.
15. Mahon CR, Lehman DC, Manuselis G. *Textbook of Diagnostic Microbiology*. 4th ed. Maryland Heights, MO: Elsevier Saunders; 2011.
16. Solis Garcia Del Pozo J, Lorente Ortuno S, Navarro E, Solera J. Detection of IgM antibrucella antibody in the absence of IgGs: A challenge for the clinical interpretation of *Brucella* serology. *PLoS Negl Trop Dis*. 2014;8(12):e3390.
17. Vrioni G, Pappas G, Priavali E, Gartzonika C, Levidiotou S. An eternal microbe: *Brucella* DNA load persists for years after clinical cure. *Clin Infect Dis*. 2008;46(12):e131–6.
18. Skalsky K, Yahav D, Bishara J, Pitlik S, Leibovici L, Paul M. Treatment of human brucellosis: Systematic review and meta-analysis of randomised controlled trials. *BMJ*. 2008;336(7646):701–4.
19. Meng F, Pan X, Tong W. Rifampicin versus streptomycin for brucellosis treatment in humans: A meta-analysis of randomized controlled trials. *PLoS One*. 2018;13(2):e0191993.
20. Yousefi-Nooraie R, Mortaz-Hejri S, Mehrani M, Sadeghipour P. Antibiotics for treating human brucellosis. *Cochrane Database Syst Rev*. 2012;10:CD007179.

21. Olsen SC, Stoffregen WS. Essential roles of vaccines in brucellosis control and eradication programs for livestock. *Expert Rev Vaccines.* 2005;4(6):915–28.
22. US Department of Health and Human Services. *Biosafety in Microbiological and Biomedical Laboratories (BMBL).* 5th ed. Washington, DC: US Government Printing Office; 2009.
23. Bacterial Special Pathogens Branch. *Brucellosis Reference Guide: Exposures, Testing and Prevention.* Atlanta, GA: Centers for Disease Control and Prevention; 2017.
24. Pappas G, Panagopoulou P, Christou L, Akritidis N. Brucella as a biological weapon. *Cell Mol Life Sci.* 2006 Oct;63(19–20):2229–36.
25. Animal and Plant Health Inspection Service Centers for Disease Control and Prevention. National Select Agent Registry. https://www.selectagents.gov/.
26. Pappas G, Papadimitriou P, Akritidis N, Christou L, Tsianos EV. The new global map of human brucellosis. *Lancet Infect Dis.* 2006;6(2):91–9.
27. Glynn MK, Lynn TV. Brucellosis. *J Am Vet Med Assoc.* 2008;233(6):900–7.
28. Statement. CP. Brucellosis (*Brucella* sp) 2010 Case definition. Surveillance Case Definition 2010. Cited May 2018. https://wwwn.cdc.gov/nndss/conditions/brucellosis/case-definition/2010/.
29. WHO. *Brucellosis in Humans and Animals.* Washington, DC: World Health Organization/American Public Health Association; 2005.

CHAPTER

150 Leptospirosis

John R. Dunn • Mary-Margaret Fill

Leptospirosis is a zoonotic bacterial infection with a ubiquitous worldwide distribution. Weil's disease, or severe icteric leptospirosis associated with renal failure, was first described in 1886. However, reports of illnesses that most likely representing leptospiral jaundice date back to the early 1800s. The causative organism of leptospirosis, *Leptospira* species, was recognized independently in Japan and Germany in 1915 through the investigation of illnesses related to occupational and environmental exposures.[1] Leptospirosis is the likely etiology for other long recognized occupational hazards among rice field workers in China and Japan, and was referred to as "Autumn Fever."[1] Now considered an emerging neglected infectious disease, it is estimated to cause 1 million severe cases and 60,000 deaths annually.[2] Prompt recognition and treatment of leptospirosis continue to be problematic due to the wide spectrum of clinical manifestations and imperfect diagnostic tests. Due to the complexity of the organism, global distribution, and the lack of robust surveillance data, the reported burden of leptospirosis worldwide is underestimated and the epidemiology poorly described.

THE AGENT

Leptospires are slow growing, obligate aerobe, flagellated, and highly motile spirochetes.[1] They have a distinct morphologic appearance, which resulted in the species nomenclature of "*interrogans*," due to their question mark-like microscopic appearance (Fig. 150-1). Surface lipopolysaccharides (LPS) contribute to host immune response, facilitate characterization of antigenically related serovars of *Leptospira* into serogroups, and have a role in virulence.[1,3,4] Virulence traits of Lepotspires are not well described but include LPS and hemolysins, among others. Based on phenotypic LPS characterization, the genus *Leptospira* has historically been divided into two species: *Leptospira biflexa*, containing the nonpathogenic serovars, and *Leptospira interrogans*, containing more than 200 known pathogenic serovars comprising 24 serogroups.[5,6]

More recently, *Leptospira* have been classified into 22 distinct genomospecies based on DNA relatedness, 10 of which are pathogenic.[6,7] Genomospecies do not equate with traditional serovar and serogroup classifications, or with the traditional species divisions. Genomospecies may contain both pathogenic and nonpathogenic serovars of *Leptospira*, as well as serovars from more than one serogroup. Serovar and serogroup designations will likely remain in use, therefore, as they are valuable in both the serologic diagnosis and epidemiologic characterization of leptospirosis. The complexity of phenotypic characterization and lack of a standardized molecular subtyping method limit public health investigation and response. Traditional temporal, spatial, and epidemiological determinants most often identify outbreaks rather than use of molecular subtyping.

Molecular typing methods have been applied to leptospires. Pulsed-field gel electrophoresis and other genetic subtyping methods, including whole genome sequencing, hold promise as clinically and epidemiologically relevant techniques for identification and subtyping of leptospiral strains in the future.[6]

Historical discovery and diagnosis of Leptospirosis was via microscopy. Identification of Leptospires by darkfield microscopy remains a component of common testing practice and is included in the U.S. Centers for Disease Control and Prevention (CDC) case definition.[7] Leptospirosis is definitively diagnosed by isolation of the organism in culture from clinical or autopsy specimens; however, the sensitivity of culture is only 5–50%.[8] Leptospiremia precedes symptom onset and generally lasts through the first week of illness. Leptospires survive in blood culture media for several days, though blood should be inoculated into semisolid media as soon as possible to increase the likelihood of isolating the bacteria.[9–11] Culture of cerebrospinal fluid during the first week of illness may also yield leptospires. Leptospiruria generally begins during the second week of illness and may be prolonged (≤30 days).[11] Survival of leptospires in voided urine is limited, and urine should be processed and inoculated into semisolid media as quickly as possible. Leptospires grow slowly, so cultures should be incubated and examined weekly for up to 13 weeks before discarding.[9–11] Environmental isolation to support epidemiological investigations is challenging due to the ubiquity and diversity of environmental leptospires.

In clinical practice, routine diagnosis continues to rely on serology. Microscopic agglutination testing (MAT) is the reference serologic method, in which sera from patients are reacted with a panel of live antigen suspensions using a variety of leptospiral serovars.[1,9,12] Serial dilution of sera is performed, and the serum-antigen mixtures incubated and examined by dark-field microscopy for agglutination. The highest titer at which 50% agglutination occurs is the end-point. Agglutinating antibodies consist of IgM, IgG, and IgA, and become detectable approximately 5–7 days after symptom onset, though the sensitivity is highest after 10–14 days. Due to cross-reactivity of antibodies among antigenically related serovars, MAT is considered a serogroup-specific test. In general, at least one serovar from a wide range of serogroups is included on an MAT panel, as are all locally important serovars. A large and diverse antigen panel increases the likelihood of detecting infections with rare or new serovars, but adds to the complexity of interpreting the assay as it increases the likelihood of detecting cross-reacting antibodies. MAT requires technical expertise, maintenance and weekly subculturing of live antigen stocks, and considerable effort to minimize inter- and intraobserver variation in interpretation of results. Reference laboratory services, including MAT, are available at several World Health Organization (WHO) Collaborating Centers for Leptospirosis around the world, including CDC.[13,14] CDC recommends collection of acute and convalescent serum samples 7–14 days apart or if a single sample is collected that it ideally be collected 7–10 days after illness onset.[13]

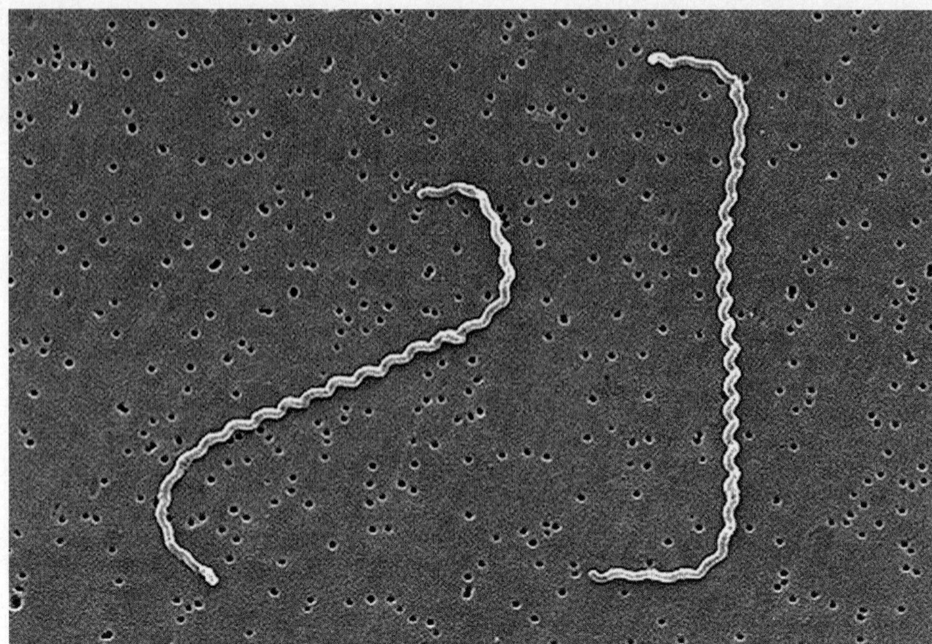

FIGURE 150-1. Scanning electron microscopic (SEM) image of *Leptospira interrogans*. (*Source:* Janice Haney Carr/NCID/HIP/CDC.)

In the context of a compatible febrile illness, a single high titer by MAT (≥800) or demonstration of a fourfold or greater rise in titer between acute and convalescent sera confirm the diagnosis serologically.[7] Patient sera may demonstrate elevated titers to more than one serovar, resulting from cross reactivity. The serovar to which the highest antibody titer is detected is generally considered the infecting serogroup. Patients who have past infection with a different leptospiral serovar may demonstrate an anamnestic response, in which the initial rising antibody titer resulting from the current infection is directed toward the previous serovar.[6,9,15] Antibody titers specific to the current infecting serovar subsequently develop. Interpretation of MAT is complicated and even in the absence of antibody cross reactions and paradoxical responses, results correlate only moderately with definitive isolation of serovars by culture and identification by cross-agglutinin absorption.[9,16] Consequently, definitive serogroup and serovar determination requires isolation of leptospires in culture. MAT results can provide epidemiological insights by identifying likely serogroups, and therefore animal reservoirs and potential sources of infection, in populations. Notably, MAT titers may be very high and take months or years to fall following infection, making it a useful tool for epidemiologic serosurveys.[6,9]

Rapid screening serologic tests are important for clinical management due to the complexity of MAT and molecular testing methods.[9,17,18] Most rapid test formats use enzyme-linked immunosorbent assay (ELISA) methods to detect IgM. IgM antibodies are produced and become detectable early during illness (around day 3). IgM detection is more sensitive than MAT when employed on specimens obtained in the acute phase of illness, making these tests useful for diagnosing leptospirosis and initiating early and effective treatment.[9] However, IgM antibodies may persist for many months following onset of illness, making interpretation of positive IgM assay results problematic in endemic areas, especially when only a single specimen is available to be tested.[19] IgM assays have many forms, including a dot-ELISA dipstick test, and are broadly reactive and genus specific, in contrast to MAT. Development of rapid tests and evaluation is needed, particular in endemic areas.[18] Polymerase chain reaction (PCR) techniques have been applied to detection of leptospires, using a variety of primers and clinical specimen sources.[6,9] PCR availability has increased and can provide a sensitive, specific, and rapid means of detecting leptospires in clinical specimens, before the development of antileptospiral antibodies. PCR, however, is not currently capable of identifying the infecting serovar. For PCR testing, CDC recommends collection of whole blood (within the first week but ideally within 4 days of illness onset), urine (collected within 1 week of illness onset), cerebrospinal fluid, or fresh frozen kidney (preferred) or liver from deceased patients. Other detection methods include pathology using immunohistochemical staining of tissue, and visualization by direct microscopy, though the latter is difficult and prone to both false positive and false negative readings. Postmortem tissues for immunohistochemistry at CDC include kidney (preferred), liver, lung, heart, or spleen.[13]

THE DISEASE

Recent studies have estimated the tremendous yet underappreciated burden and impact of leptospirosis on populations globally.[2,20] For the infected individual, the spectrum of symptoms and clinical presentations in leptospirosis is broad and nonspecific, resembling many other "influenza-like illnesses." While most cases have generalized "influenza-like illness" with fever, chills, muscle aches, and headaches, others have more specific symptoms including conjunctivitis, vomiting, diarrhea, stomach pain, jaundice, cough, and rarely a skin rash. Severe disease occurs in an estimated 10% of cases with progression to kidney or liver failure, meningitis, difficulty breathing, bleeding, and meningitis. A total of 5–15% of cases with the classic Weil disease, consisting of renal and liver failure, die.[21] The clinical course is biphasic and follows a 2- to 20-day incubation period. The acute, leptospiremic phase lasts about 1 week, followed by an immune phase of up to 30 days or more that coincides with localization of leptospires in the kidneys and development of leptospiruria. Fortunately, most cases have increased antibody production and resolution of symptoms during the immune phase rather than progression to severe disease. Localization of leptospires in various tissues results in specific organ manifestations or severe multiorgan failure and death.

Leptospirosis is categorized into anicteric and icteric forms. The majority of infections with leptospires are anicteric, and most are subclinical or mildly symptomatic and self-limited.[1,9] Symptomatic infections classically present with an acute febrile illness of sudden onset. Headache, myalgias, and conjunctival suffusion are reported in the majority of cases. Myalgias are often prominent and frequently affect the lower back, thighs, and calves. Headache is reported to be severe and often includes retro-orbital pain and photophobia. Nausea, abdominal pain, diarrhea, and arthralgias occur less frequently, reported in less than 50% of cases. Mortality is very low with an anicteric clinical course.

In contrast to the anicteric form, 5–10% of cases develop severe and sometimes rapidly fatal icteric leptospirosis, as mentioned.[1] Acute renal failure and subsequent oliguria are associated with increased case fatality.[1,22] A pulmonary syndrome consisting of cough, dyspnea, and hemoptysis associated with intra-alveolar hemorrhage has been increasingly recognized in both outbreaks and sporadic cases.[1,23] It occurs in up to two-thirds of severe cases, and may progress to acute respiratory distress syndrome. Cardiac involvement is probably more common than has been traditionally described. EKG abnormalities are present in almost half of patients when cardiac monitoring is performed.[1,24] Myocarditis, arrhythmias, and repolarization abnormalities are associated with increased mortality.[22,25] Leptospirosis during pregnancy can lead to abortion or fetal death. Aseptic meningitis, cerebrovascular accident, cranial nerve palsies, and reactive arthritis are also reported leptospirosis manifestations. Notably, ocular manifestations are present in the majority of cases of icteric leptospirosis and may include conjunctival suffusion with scleral icterus.[1] Recurrent anterior uveitis may occur during recovery in rare cases.[1,26]

The differential diagnosis of leptospirosis includes numerous other viral, bacterial, mycotic, rickettsial, and parasitic infections of the tropics.[27] Febrile diseases that mimic leptospirosis include brucellosis, dengue fever, yellow fever, viral hemorrhagic fevers, typhoid fever, disseminated histoplasmosis, louse- or tick-borne relapsing fever, malaria, and other vector-borne disease. Because of the nonspecific signs and symptoms of leptospirosis, misdiagnosis is common. In developing countries, limited diagnostic testing options contribute to misdiagnosis while in temperate climates and developed countries, a lack of clinical suspicion contributes. In either scenario, misdiagnosis results in delayed treatment with appropriate antibiotics and worse outcomes. Misdiagnosis, as well as poor public health surveillance infrastructure, lead to delayed recognition of and response to outbreaks.[23,27]

Treatment of leptospirosis differs based on clinical presentation. Many patients with mild anicteric leptospirosis recover with symptomatic treatment and no antibiotic treatment. Worsening symptoms or the development of jaundice indicates more severe manifestations and potentially multisystem involvement. Doxycycline is the drug of choice (100 mg orally, twice daily for 7 days) but is not recommended for pregnant women or children aged < 8 years. Alternative options include ampicillin and amoxicillin. Intravenous penicillin (1.5 MU every 6 hours) is a drug of choice for patients with severe leptospirosis, and ceftriaxone has been shown to be equally effective.[1,9,21,28] Specific antibiotic treatment should be initiated as soon as possible for optimal treatment efficacy. Empirical treatment should be initiated based on clinical suspicion if timely diagnostic testing is unavailable or inconclusive. Severe icteric leptospirosis often requires intensive care and dialysis for renal failure. Intensive care and dialysis can require several weeks. Cardiac monitoring is also encouraged initially in severe icteric cases.

MODE OF TRANSMISSION

Pathogenic leptospires have zoonotic reservoirs in wild, domestic, and peridomestic mammals.[5,29,30], These zoonotic reservoir species are referred to as maintenance hosts in contrast to accidental hosts, such as humans. Many leptospires are highly adapted to their maintenance hosts, such as icterohaemorrhagiae with rats and mice. Historically, the rat (*Rattus norvegicus*) has played a prominent role in leptospirosis transmission.[1,30] Serovar Pomona is strongly associated with cattle and swine.[5,31] Infection in these animals by host-adapted serovars is usually enzootic and asymptomatic. Maintenance hosts typically acquire leptospirosis early in life through animal-to-animal contact, and develop chronic infection of the renal tubules with shedding of leptospires into the environment. This is a classic One Health example of the interrelationship of animal health, human health, and environmental health.[2,29] The impact of multiple factors such as climate, population density, interaction of various animal maintenance hosts influence leptospirosis risk. For example, recent expansion of feral swine in the United States show how an introduced maintenance host can have environmental impacts leading to introduction of pathogenic leptospires into areas populated by humans.[32] As mentioned, humans are nonadapted accidental hosts and develop symptomatic and sometimes severe leptospirosis without persistent renal infection and shedding. Humans do not contribute significantly to transmission as accidental hosts but can impact habitat and zoonotic reservoir maintenance hosts affecting the risk of leptospirosis.[29,30,32] Animals may be maintenance hosts for some serovars and accidental hosts for others, and geographic variations in maintenance hosts and their associated serovars are observed throughout the world. Understanding the prevalent serovars and their maintenance hosts is essential in understanding the local epidemiology of leptospirosis and its prevention.

Humans most commonly acquire infection with leptospires through contact with the urine of leptospiruric animals. Infection may be acquired through direct contact with infected animal tissues or body fluids. Infections may be sporadic or outbreak-associated, and can result from occupational, recreational, or avocational exposures.[1,9] Occupational exposure has been recognized for centuries as a risk factor among groups who work with animals. Increased risk of leptospirosis from direct exposure to animals or animal urine is well described. Additionally, infection can also occur indirectly, through exposure to leptospires in urine-contaminated soil and surface water. As mentioned, sewer workers and rice-field workers were some of the earliest occupational risks described for leptospirosis.[1] Gardeners or those who swim or raft in contaminated rivers are at increased risk of infection through indirect exposure. The route of entry is usually through breaks in the skin, though mucous membrane contact, inhalation, and prolonged immersion or ingestion of contaminated water. Interestingly, numerous adventure races have resulted in sporadic cases and outbreaks of leptospirosis due the prolonged contact with soil and water throughout the race course.[33,34] Infection has also been described following contact with animal bites, and consumption of contaminated food and water.[35–37] Human-to-human and sexual transmission of leptospires has been documented, though the risk is considered to be very low.

OCCURRENCE

Leptospirosis is a global health problem reported most commonly in tropical regions. Surveillance data on leptospirosis is limited, leading to reduced ability to ascertain the true incidence and burden. Leptospirosis is considered a neglected and underreported infection.[2,14,27] In tropical, warm climates there are increased numbers of maintenance hosts and leptospiral serovars and increased survival of leptospires in the environment. These factors increase the frequency of exposure to environmental leptospires during activities of daily living resulting in increased incidence of human infection. In temperate climates, disease is more common during late summer and early fall, while infections in tropical areas tend to increase in number during rainy seasons. Urban, primarily rat-associated leptospirosis, has also been described.[31,40,41] This is a growing concern in many parts of the world where large urban slums are expanding.[38–41] Leptospirosis is an important risk to consider following large or localized flooding events.[32,42–44] A recent meta-analysis of risk factors post-flood identified positive associations of male sex, livestock exposure, and having a lacerated wound with leptospirosis.[42] As mentioned, recent outbreaks related to recreational water and soil exposures, such as occur during adventure travel or races, have been reported with increasing frequency.[33,34,45,46] Historically, a male predominance has been noted, though this is likely to be a result of the association of leptospirosis with many traditionally male occupations, such as farming, mining, and emergency response, rather than differential risks based on gender alone. More recently, cases associated with recreational exposures and among females and younger age groups have been described.[47–49]

PREVENTION AND CONTROL

Leptospirosis risks are reduced by avoiding water potentially contaminated with animal urine, or by limiting contact with potentially infected animals. Known occupational risks can be reduced by wearing protective clothing and footwear to reduce exposure to contaminated water or soil. Efforts to control and prevent leptospirosis can be thought of in three interventional categories: the source or reservoir of infection, the route of transmission, or the human host.

Because humans acquire infection primarily from animals shedding leptospires in their urine, it is critical to understand local or regional reservoirs and serovars. Domestic, agricultural, feral, or nuisance animals all serve as reservoirs for leptospires. In small or well-defined animal populations such as dogs or farm herds, infected animals may be treated with antibiotics to control leptospiral shedding. Animal vaccines are available and may be useful, but vaccine-induced immunity is serovar specific, requires frequent revaccination, and protects against symptomatic disease but not necessarily against infection or urinary shedding.[1] When rodents, feral swine, or other feral or invasive animals are known or suspected to be reservoirs affecting humans, they should be reduced or eliminated through integrated wildlife management approaches.[29,30,32] Access of maintenance reservoir animals to food and water sources should be considered and limited, and strict environmental hygiene employed.

Interrupting transmission routes is another approach to prevention and control. Exposures to infected animals, tissues, or body fluids should be minimized or personal protective equipment worn when exposures are unavoidable such as in occupational settings. Contact with water sources known or suspected to be contaminated with leptospires should be avoided, but if contact is unavoidable, any open wounds present on the skin should be covered with occlusive dressings. Care should be taken to prevent submersion of the face, and washing or showering is recommended following exposure. CDC has provided specific recommendations to minimize risks for adventure travelers and racers including avoiding environments potentially contaminated with animal urine, avoiding swallowing water from lakes, rivers, or swamps while swimming, avoiding adventure racing if you have any cuts or abrasion of the skin, and wearing protective clothing and shoes.[50]

Finally, and perhaps most challenging, interventions may be aimed at human populations. In endemic areas, educational campaigns should be conducted to promote awareness of the clinical manifestations, healthcare seeking behaviors, and prevention of leptospirosis among at-risk groups. The general public should be made aware of risk avoidance measures, especially when specific risks are known. Healthcare professionals should consider leptospirosis, and should inquire into occupational, avocational, and recreational exposures, animal contacts, and travel histories. Antibiotic prophylaxis for travelers to endemic areas for whom exposure to infected animals or contaminated environments is unavoidable can be considered but must be balanced with antibiotic stewardship concerns.[9,51] Doxycycline 200 mg in one dose or once weekly may prevent symptomatic infection and reduce mortality when used during brief, high-risk exposures in endemic areas, wet environments, or following floods.[9,51]

Prompt reporting of leptospirosis cases to public health officials can initiate investigation facilitating identification of the source of infection and implementation of prevention efforts aimed at reducing ongoing risk to populations. Enhanced surveillance efforts and thorough investigation of outbreaks will improve understanding of the epidemiology and control of endemic leptospirosis. Continued efforts are needed to develop simple, rapid, and clinically useful diagnostic tests and improve molecular strain typing methods to assist in describing transmission risks for leptospirosis and help target prevention strategies.

References

1. Levett PN. Leptospirosis. *Clin Microbio Rev.* 2001;14:296–326.
2. Costa F, Hagan JE, Calcagno J, et al. Global morbidity and mortality of leptospirosis, a systematic review. *PLoS Negl Trop Dis.* 2015;9(9):e0003898.
3. Dikken H, Kmety E. Serological typing methods of leptospires. In: Bergan T, Norris JR, eds. *Methods in Microbiology*. Vol. 11. London: Academic Press; 1978, pp. 259–307.
4. Kmety E, Dikken H. *Classification of the Species Leptospira Interrogans and History of its Serovars*. Groningen: University Press Groningen; 1993.
5. Bharti AR, Nally JE, Ricaldi JN, et al. Leptospirosis: A zoonotic disease of global importance. [see comment]. *Lancet Infect Dis.* 2003;3(12):757–71.
6. Marquez A, Djelouadji Z, Lattard V, Kodjo A. Overview of laboratory methods to diagnose leptospirosis and to identify and to type leptospires. *Int Microbiol.* 2017;20:184–93.
7. Centers for Disease Control and Prevention. Leptospirosis 2013 case definition. https://wwwn.cdc.gov/nndss/conditions/leptospirosis/case-definition/2013/. Atlanta, GA. 2019.
8. Katz AR, Ansdell VE, Effler PV, et al. Assessment of the clinical presentation and treatment of 353 cases of laboratory-confirmed leptospirosis in Hawaii, 1974–1998. *Clin Infect Dis.* 2001;33:1834–41.
9. Haake DA, Levett PN. Leptospirosis in humans. *Curr Top Microbiol Immunol.* 2015;387:65–97.
10. Palmer M, Waitkins SA, Zochowski W. Survival of leptospires in commercial blood culture systems. *Zentralblatt Bakteriol, Mikrobiol Hyg [A].* 1984;257:480–7.
11. Sulzer CR, Jones WL. *Leptospirosis: Methods in Laboratory Diagnosis.* Atlanta, GA: U.S. Department of Health, Education and Welfare; 1978.
12. Turner LH. Leptospirosis II. Serology. *Trans R Soc Trop Med Hyg.* 1968;62:880–9.
13. Centers for Disease Control and Prevention. Leptospirosis. https://www.cdc.gov/leptospirosis/index.html. Atlanta, GA. 2019.
14. World Health Organization. Leptospirosis. https://www.who.int/topics/leptospirosis/en/. Geneva. 2019.
15. Lupidi R, Cinco M, Balanzin D, et al. Serological follow-up of patients in a localized outbreak of leptospirosis. *J Clin Microbiol.* 1991;29:805–9.
16. Katz AR, Effler PV, Ansdell VE. Comparison of serology and isolates for the identification of infecting leptospiral serogroups in Hawaii, 1979–1998. *Trop Med Int Health.* 2003;8:639–42.
17. Picardeau M, Bertherat E, Jancloes M, et al. Rapid tests for diagnosis of leptospirosis: Current tools and emerging technologies. *Diagn Microbiol Infect Dis.* 2014;78(1):1–8.
18. Alia SN, Joseph N, Philip N, et al. Diagnostic accuracy of rapid diagnostic tests for the early detection of leptospirosis. *J Infect Public Health.* 2019;12(2):263–9.
19. Bajani MD, Ashford DA, Bragg SL, et al. Evaluation of four commercially available rapid serologic tests for diagnosis of leptospirosis. *J Clin Microbiol.* 2003;41:803–9.
20. Torgerson PR, Hagan JE, Costa F, et al. Global burden of leptospirosis: Estimated in terms of disability adjusted life years. *PLoS Negl Trop Dis.* 2015;9(10):e0004122.
21. Centers for Disease Control and Prevention. Chapter 3 Infectious Diseases Related to Travel Leptospirosis. https://wwwnc.cdc.gov/travel/yellowbook/2018/infectious-diseases-related-to-travel/leptospirosis. Atlanta, GA. 2019.
22. Daher E, Zanetta DM, Cavalcante MB, et al. Risk factors for death and changing patterns in leptospirosis acute renal failure. *Am J Trop Med Hyg.* 1999;61:630–4.
23. Trevejo RT, Rigau-Perez JG, Ashford DA, et al. Epidemic leptospirosis associated with pulmonary hemorrhage-Nicaragua, 1995. *J Infect Dis.* 1998;178:1457–63.
24. Rajiv C, Manjuran RJ, Sudhayakumar N, et al. Cardiovascular involvement in leptospirosis. *Indian Heart J.* 1996;48:691–4.
25. Watt G, Padre LP, Tuazon M, Caluaquib C. Skeletal and cardiac muscle involvement in severe, late leptospirosis. *J Infect Dis.* 1990;162:266–9.

26. Watt G. Leptospirosis as a cause of uveitis. *Arch Intern Med.* 1990; 150:1130–2.
27. Crump JA, Morrissey AB, Nicholson WL, et al. Etiology of severe non-malaria febrile illness in Northern Tanzania: A prospective cohort study. *PLoS Negl Trop Dis.* 2013;7(7):e2324.
28. McClain JBL, Ballou WR, Harrison SM, et al. Doxycycline therapy for leptospirosis. *Ann Intern Med.* 1984;100:696–8.
29. Goarant C. Leptospirosis: Risk factors and management challenges in developing countries. *Res Rep Trop Med.* 2016;7:49–62.
30. Costa F, Ribeiro GS, Felzemburgh RDM, et al. Influence of household rat infestation on *Leptospira* transmission in the urban slum environment. *PLoS Negl Trop Dis.* 2014;8(12):e3338.
31. Bolin C. Leptospirosis. In: Brown C, Bolin C, eds. *Emerging Diseases of Animals*. Washington, DC: ASM Press; 2000, pp. 185–200.
32. Frawley AA, Schafer IJ, Galloway R, et al. Notes from the field: Postflooding leptospirosis—Louisiana, 2016. *MMWR Morb Mortal Wkly Rep.* 2017;66:1158–9.
33. Schmalzle SA, Tabatabai A, Mazzeffi M, et al. Recreational 'mud fever': *Leptospira interrogans* induced diffuse alveolar hemorrhage and severe acute respiratory distress syndrome in a U.S. Navy seaman following 'mud-run' in Hawaii. *IDCases.* 2019;15:e00529.
34. Sejvar J, Bancroft E, Winthrop K, et al. Leptospirosis in "Eco-Challenge" athletes, Malaysian Borneo, 2000. *Emerg Infect Dis.* 2003;9(6):702–7.
35. Luzzi GA, Milne LM, Waitkins SA. Rat-bite acquired leptospirosis. *J Infect.* 1987;15:57–60.
36. Wynwood SJ, Graham GC, Weier SL, Collet TA, McKay DB, Craig SB. Leptospirosis from water sources. *Pathog Glob Health.* 2014;108(7):334–8.
37. Cacciapuoti B, Ciceroni L, Maffei C, et al. A waterborne outbreak of leptospirosis. *Am J Epidemiol.* 1987;126:535–45.
38. Felzemburgh RD, Ribeiro GS, Costa F, et al. Prospective study of leptospirosis transmission in an urban slum community: Role of poor environment in repeated exposures to the *Leptospira* agent. *PLoS Negl Trop Dis.* 2014;8(5):e2927.
39. Hagan JE, Moraga P, Costa F, et al. Spatiotemporal determinants of urban leptospirosis yransmission: Four-year prospective cohort study of slum residents in Brazil. *PLoS Negl Trop Dis.* 2016;10(1):e0004275.
40. Vinetz JM, Glass GE, Flexner CE, et al. Sporadic urban leptospirosis. *Ann Intern Med.* 1996;125:794–8.
41. Ko AI, Galvao Reis M, et al. Urban epidemic of severe leptospirosis in Brazil. *Lancet.* 1999;354:820–5.
42. Naing C, Reid SA, Aye SN, et al. Risk factors for human leptospirosis following flooding: A meta-analysis of observational studies. *PLoS One.* 2019 May 29;14(5):e0217643. doi: 10.1371/journal.pone.0217643. eCollection 2019.
43. Togami E, Kama M, Goarant C, et al. A large leptospirosis outbreak following successive severe floods in Fiji, 2012. *Am J Trop Med Hyg.* 2018 Oct;99(4):849–51. doi: 10.4269/ajtmh.18-0335.
44. Fuortes L, Nettleman M. Leptospirosis: A consequence of the Iowa flood. *Iowa Med.* 1994;84:449–50.
45. Morgan J, Bornstein SL, Karpati AM, et al. Outbreak of leptospirosis among triathlon participants and community residents in Springfield, Illinois, 1998. *Clin Infect Dis.* 2002;34:1593–9.
46. Centers for Disease Control and Prevention. Outbreak of leptospirosis among white-water rafters—Costa Rica, 1996. *MMWR Morb Mortal Wkly Rep.* 1997;46:577–9.
47. Johnson MA, Smith H, Joeph P, et al. Environmental exposure and leptospirosis, Peru. *Emerg Infect Dis.* 2004;10(6):1016–22.
48. Meites E, Jay MT, Deresinski S, et al. Reemerging leptospirosis, California. *Emerg Infect Dis.* 2004;10(3):406–12.
49. Katz AR, Ansdell VE, Effler PV, et al. Leptospirosis in Hawaii, 1974–1998: Epidemiologic analysis of 353 laboratory-confirmed cases. *Am J Trop Med Hyg.* 2002;66:61–70.
50. Centers for Disease Control and Prevention. Adventure Racing and Leptospirosis. https://www.cdc.gov/leptospirosis/features/adventure-racing.html. Atlanta, GA. 2019.
51. Sehgal SC, Sugunan AP, Murhekar MV, et al. Randomized controlled trial of doxycycline prophylaxis against leptospirosis in an endemic area. *Int J Antimicrob Agents.* 2000;13:249–55.

CHAPTER

151 Toxoplasmosis

Anne Straily

Toxoplasma gondii, the etiologic agent of toxoplasmosis, is one of the most common protozoan parasites of humans. *T. gondii* was described in 1908, both by Nicolle and Manceaux at the Pasteur Institute in Tunis from gondis (a type of small rodent) used as laboratory animals in typhus research, and by Splendore at the Hygiene Institute in Sao Paulo, Brazil, from a laboratory rabbit. Human infection was first discovered in 1924 in the eye of an infant by Janku in Czechoslovakia. This was followed, starting in 1937, by several diagnoses in infants by Wolf, Cowan, and Paige at Colombia University in New York City. After the development of a serologic test, the dye test by Sabin and Feldman in 1948, it became clear that infections in humans and animals were found worldwide and were highly prevalent in many areas. The identification of the sexual cycle of *Toxoplasma* in cats led to its classification as a coccidian.[32] It became clear then that the infections of gondis and rabbits were linked to cats, which at the time were kept in laboratories to catch wild rodents and laboratory animals that had escaped.

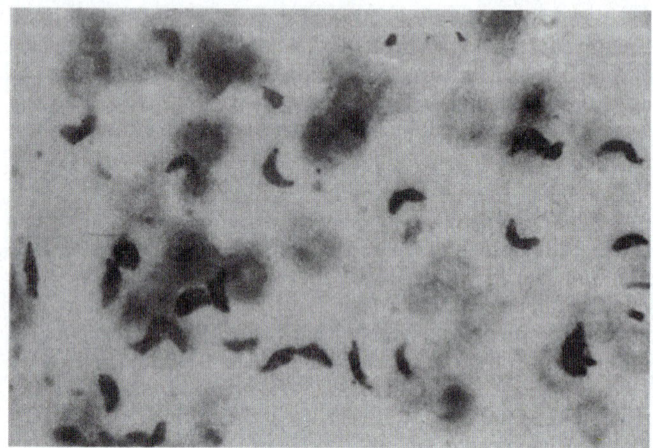

FIGURE 151-1. Tachyzoites of *Toxoplasma gondii* in smear of mouse peritoneal fluid. (Giemsa stain, × 1200.)

LIFE CYCLE AND MODES OF TRANSMISSION

Felines, including domestic cats and wild felids, are the definitive host for *T. gondii*; sexual reproduction of the parasite occurs only in the feline small intestine, producing oocysts that are shed in the feces. These oocysts are unsporulated when passed and are not immediately infective, requiring between 1 and 5 days in the environment to sporulate and become infective. An intermediate host, which can be any warm-blooded animal, can ingest soil, water, or plant material contaminated with these sporulated oocysts. Shortly after ingestion, the sporozoites in the oocyst are released and transform into tachyzoites (Fig. 151-1), the rapidly proliferating intracellular form. Tachyzoites localize primarily in brain, eye, heart muscle, and skeletal muscle or other low mitotic tissues where they transform into bradyzoites. Bradyzoites multiply slowly and form cysts (Fig. 151-2) in the tissues where they may persist for years, possibly for the life of the host.[32]

T. gondii is adapted to spread naturally among felids by predation. Cats acquire infection by ingesting bradyzoites in fresh tissues from infected prey animals and rarely from tachyzoites or sporulated oocysts. *Toxoplasma* damages the brain of infected rodents, making them less neophobic and less fearful of cat odors, enhancing their chances of becoming prey to a cat and ensuring that the parasite completes its life cycle.[1] Cats infected by ingesting tissue cysts are much more likely to develop a patent infection (and subsequently shed oocysts) than cats infected through ingestion of tachyzoites or sporulated oocysts. The prepatent period of infection (the time between ingestion of infective stages and the passage of oocysts in the feces) may be as short as 3–10 days when bradyzoites are ingested, or 21–40 days after either tachyzoites or mature oocysts are ingested. Cats shed oocysts in their feces for 1–3 weeks following the initial infection but may shed millions of oocysts during that time. Cats that have recovered from toxoplasmosis may become reinfected if exposed, but their immunity either arrests the infection before oocyst formation or greatly reduces oocyst shedding.

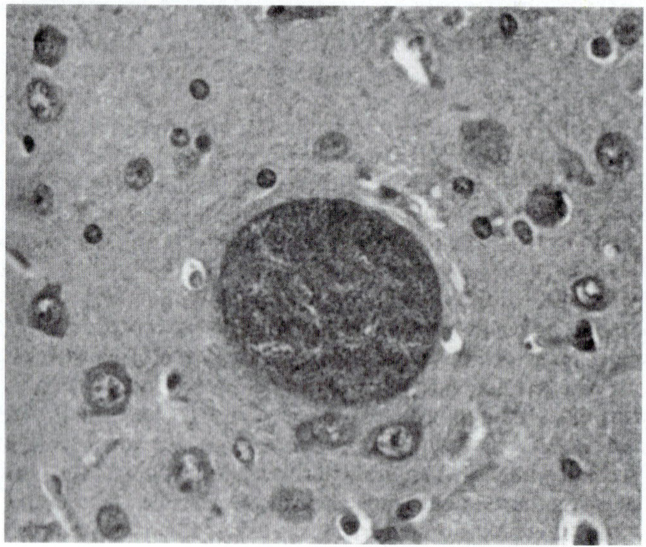

FIGURE 151-2. Section of mouse brain showing a cyst of *Toxoplasma gondii* containing hundreds of bradyzoites. (Hematoxylin and Eeosin stain, × 480.)

All warm-blooded animals are susceptible to infection by *T. gondii*. Intermediate hosts acquire infection by ingesting soil, plant matter, or

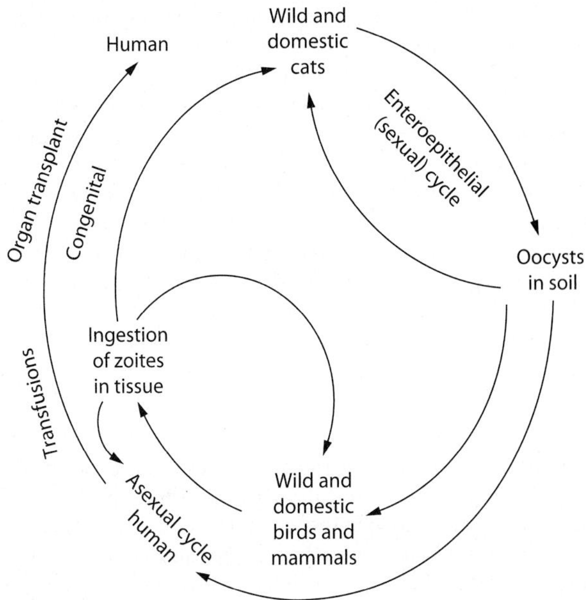

FIGURE 151-3. Transmission of *Toxoplasma gondii* in nature involves two main cycles: (a) from cats to intermediate hosts and back to cats and to humans through fecal contamination of the environment with oocysts that are generated during the enteroepithelial cycle in the cat, mature in the outside environment, and are taken up in contaminated foods or water, and (b) from intermediate hosts to cats and to intermediate hosts (and humans) when zoites (tachyzoites and bradyzoites, generally the latter) that are generated in extraintestinal tissues by asexual reproduction (endodyogeny) are ingested. Except for congenital transmission, blood or cell transfusion, or organ transplant, the place of humans in either of these two cycles is that of a dead-end intermediate host. Predation and cannibalism among intermediate hosts, though not essential to enzooticity, are factors of great significance.

water contaminated with oocysts or through consumption of other animals infected with tissue cysts. Human infection can result from ingestion of the tissue cysts from undercooked or raw meat and shellfish, from ingestion of the sporulated oocysts in contaminated food or water, or indirectly from the soil. Transplacental infection (from mother to fetus) is also possible in humans, as is transmission by organ transplantation or blood transfusion.

T. gondii is one of the most common protozoan parasites of animals and humans. Survival of the species is assured because: (a) it infects a wide range of hosts; (b) many hosts survive infection; (c) it can persist in its host for many years so that predators can acquire infection; (d) infected felids produce millions of oocysts which are hardy and can remain infective in the environment for long periods, and although of lesser epidemiological importance; and (e) it can be transmitted transplacentally in certain hosts (see lifecycle, Fig. 151-3).

CLINICAL CHARACTERISTICS

In humans, clinical manifestation of toxoplasmosis is dependent upon whether the infection was acquired congenitally or postnatally and the person's immune status. Illness in immunocompetent persons with postnatally acquired infection is usually asymptomatic or has such mild transient manifestations that it goes unrecognized. It is estimated that clinical illness develops in only 10–20% of acutely infected immunocompetent individuals. Symptoms can include generalized or local lymphadenopathy (most commonly the cervical nodes), fever, sore throat, myalgia, a maculopapular rash sparing the palms and soles, abdominal pain, hepatosplenomegaly, and atypical lymphocytosis suggestive of infectious mononucleosis. In rare acute cases, more severe manifestations such as pneumonitis, myocarditis, pericarditis, hepatitis, polymyositis, encephalitis, and meningoencephalitis have been reported. In uncomplicated acute infections, symptoms are generally self-limited and resolve without treatment, although lymphadenopathy may persist for many months. Studies in laboratory animals have demonstrated the persistence of cysts in brain and skeletal muscle for long periods after the initial acute infection, but data on the proportion of recovered human cases with persistent cysts are not available. In immunocompetent individuals, a chronic retinochoroiditis may be the only manifestation of toxoplasmosis.[2] Lesions may be unilateral or bilateral, may be recurrent, and may consist of active lesions without a scar, old scars with active satellite lesions, or inactive scars.

Congenital toxoplasmosis can only occur when a woman acquires her initial infection during pregnancy. Although the infection is usually unapparent in the woman, the lesions in the fetus show a wide degree of severity, depending on the gestational age at which transplacental transmission occurred. The risk of congenital transmission is decreased if maternal infection is acquired earlier in gestation, but fetal damage is usually more severe the earlier during gestation transmission occurs.[3] Outcomes of congenital transmission can include (a) spontaneous abortion of a severely damaged fetus, (b) a fully developed stillborn infant with evidence of severe lesions, (c) a live infant with classic signs, such as hydrocephalus or microcephalus, cerebral calcifications, and retinochoroiditis, (d) a premature infant who fails to thrive or in whom retinochoroiditis or other symptoms of central nervous system involvement may be found, or (e) a seemingly normal infant in whom retinochoroiditis or symptoms of central nervous system involvement develop later.[4] Evidence suggests that if a woman becomes infected a few weeks before conception, it is unlikely that the infant will be born infected. Women infected at least 3 months before conception will develop antibodies that subsequently protect the fetus from infection.[5] Since physical examinations and antibody titers of infants born to women who acquired *Toxoplasma* infection during pregnancy may be inconclusive, these infants should be observed over a period of one year for the development of antibodies, or the development of lesions such as retinochoroiditis or cerebral calcifications. If found, or suspected to be, infected, prompt therapy should be given in an attempt to prevent more serious injury to the brain and retina.[6]

Toxoplasmosis is considerably more severe in the immunodeficient patient and can develop from either newly acquired infection or recrudescence of a latent infection. Individuals with HIV infection and who have not previously been infected with *Toxoplasma* are more likely to develop a severe primary infection with this organism. The most common clinical manifestation is a life-threatening toxoplasmic encephalitis.[7] However, with the advent of prophylactic medication and highly effective antiretroviral therapy in the mid-1990s, the frequency of toxoplasmic encephalitis among persons with AIDS has been reduced.[7,8] Ocular lesions are less common than encephalitis in HIV-infected persons, but can lead to blindness. Involvement of other organs has occasionally also been described. Patients who receive organ transplants, particularly heart transplants, may acquire *T. gondii* infection from the donor organ or through recrudescence of latent infection as a result of antirejection immunosuppressive therapy.[9]

EPIDEMIOLOGY

T. gondii is found everywhere that cats are found, and human infection has been documented in nearly every country.[10,11] Prevalence of infection is highest in hot, humid climates, which favor oocyst survival, and lowest in dry or cold climates and at high altitudes. Cats usually cover their feces with sand or soil, thus protecting the oocysts, which measure 10 μm by 13 μm and may remain viable for up to a year or more in moist soil. An area where cats abound may be contaminated continually with infective oocysts as generations of cats inhabit the area. In spite of the fact that felids are the definitive hosts for this parasite, cat ownership alone has not been shown to be correlated with the prevalence of human infection in most studies.[6,12] Exposure to three or more kittens was determined to be a significant risk factor for toxoplasmosis in one study, but not exposure to adult cats or cat feces.[13] Cats often become infected with toxoplasmosis as kittens when they are weaned and develop hunting skills; because cats only shed oocysts during their initial infection, it is plausible that kittens pose a greater risk of transmission than adult cats.

In the United States, foodborne toxoplasmosis is estimated to result in over 86,000 infections annually, making it the most common parasitic cause of foodborne illness.[14] A recent national survey of pregnant women indicated that although they were well informed about the risk directly from cats, they were relatively unaware of the risk of toxoplasmosis from undercooked meat and other food-related risk factors.[15] Food-related risk factors for toxoplasmosis include consumption of undercooked or raw meat, consumption of raw shellfish, working with raw meat, eating locally produced, cured, dried, or smoked meats; and drinking unpasteurized goat's milk.[13] Different food animals have different risks for and prevalence of toxoplasmosis. Prevalence of *T. gondii* is greater in pigs, sheep, and poultry than in cattle.[16] Risk factors for exposure in livestock include farm type, feed source, presence of cats, methods of rodent and bird control, carcass handling, and water quality.[17,18] Prevalence of *T. gondii* is also higher in meat products from animals raised under organic farming conditions than conventional systems; this is attributable to outdoor access, which allows for exposure to infected rodents and wildlife, and feed, water, or environments contaminated with oocysts.[17,18] Where domestic water supplies are not filtered, *Toxoplasma* oocysts may contaminate drinking water for humans.[19]

A population-based study conducted in the United States from 2011 to 2014 showed that 10.4% of the population $\geq$ 6 years of age, and 7.5% of women 15–44 years old, were infected with *T. gondii* as determined by the presence of IgG antibodies.[20] This study and others have demonstrated that the percentage of seropositive persons increases with age, indicating continued exposure throughout life.[20–22] Nevertheless, seroprevalence rates in the United States have steadily declined over the years and this decrease is thought to be attributable to reduction of *T. gondii* in meats such as pork, due to changes in animal husbandry,[16] or less exposure from meat due to changes in preparation or freezing practices.[21] Although data regarding the incidence of congenital transmission in the United States are limited because prenatal screening of pregnant women is not routinely performed, incidence rates of congenital transmission appear to be decreasing, in line with the decrease in the percentage of seropositive adults.[6] Serologic surveys from other countries have shown that up to 90% of some populations worldwide have been infected with *Toxoplasma*.[11]

DIAGNOSIS

Toxoplasmosis can be diagnosed by serology; histopathology of bone marrow, lymph nodes, brain, placenta, or other tissues; examination of CSF; isolation of the organism via inoculation of cell cultures or weanling mice; or identification of parasite DNA through polymerase chain reaction (PCR) testing. Serology is by far the most common diagnostic method used and several tests are available: the dye test, indirect fluorescent antibody test (IFA), and enzyme immunoassays (ELISA, immunoblots) can all detect specific IgG, IgM, or IgA titers within several weeks of infection. IgM and IgA levels rise first and will decline to below the level of detection within 1–2 years. IgG titers rise later and decline significantly more slowly and may remain detectable at low levels for the patient's lifetime. Determination of an acute infection cannot be made on the basis of IgM or IgA levels alone because of the ability for these antibodies to persist for 12–18 months or more.[5,23] Additional testing, including IgG avidity testing and differential agglutination tests are often required to determine acute versus chronic infection, especially in the pregnant patient, when the risk of adverse outcomes is high. Such tests are available at reference laboratories.

Serologic tests are sometimes unreliable in immunosuppressed patients; tests for *Toxoplasma* DNA are available at some laboratories and may be useful in some patients. However, in immunosuppressed patients both positive PCR and serologic results must be interpreted in relation to the patient's clinical presentation because of the persistence of *Toxoplasma* cysts and antibody in asymptomatic chronic latent infections. Histologic examination of a tissue biopsy can often help to distinguish active from latent toxoplasmosis. *Toxoplasma* PCR performed on amnioitic fluid has been shown to be helpful in determining fetal infection following acute acquired infection in the mother.

TREATMENT

Most immunocompetent individuals recover from the acute phase of toxoplasmosis without treatment. The combination of pyrimethamine, sulfadiazine, and folinic acid is a standard component of therapy. Where sulfadiazine is unavailable or the patient cannot tolerate it, clindamycin or the fixed combination of trimethoprim with sulfamethoxazole can be substituted.[24] Pyrimethamine works by inhibiting the parasite's folate-metabolizing enzymes and can cause dose-related suppression of the bone marrow in persons receiving this treatment. Folinic acid (not folic acid), administered in combination with pyrimethamine protects the bone marrow from these toxic effects, but frequent differential blood and platelet counts are still recommended to monitor for bone marrow toxicity. Ocular toxoplasmosis is treated with the same combination therapy, sometimes with the addition of corticosteroids to combat inflammation.[25]

Treatment during pregnancy, and of the newborn and infant, has been successfully carried out in immunocompetent individuals, although this treatment does not eliminate the parasite completely.[4,6,26,27] Women who are suspected to be acutely infected with *T. gondii* during pregnancy would ideally receive an amniocentesis and PCR test of amniotic fluid at $\geq$ 18 weeks gestation to determine if the infant is infected with *T. gondii*.[28] When a pregnant woman is found to be acutely infected with toxoplasmosis, spiramycin is given prior to amniocentesis in an effort to prevent infection of the fetus, and if the fetus is not found to be infected at the time of amniocentesis, throughout the pregnancy.[6,28] If the pregnant woman acquires her infection after 18 weeks gestation or amniocentesis or fetal ultrasound indicates the fetus is likely infected, combination therapy with pyrimethamine, sulfadiazine, and folinic acid is recommended until delivery.[6] Congenitally infected newborns are treated with this same combination for the first 12 months of life.[6]

Toxoplasmosis in immunodeficient patients is often fatal if not treated. Severely immunosuppressed HIV-infected adults and adolescents who have never had an active *T. gondii* infection, but are *T. gondii* antibody seropositive, should receive primary preventive therapy with trimethoprim-sulfamethoxazole or alternative medications.[33] Treatment of clinical toxoplasmosis in the immunodeficient patient is done using the same combination therapy as for the immunocompetent patient. Continuation of therapy is recommended for at least 4–6 weeks beyond the point where significant clinical improvement has been achieved and may be required for 6 months or more as relapses are known to occur.[33] Reactivation and progression of ocular or cerebral toxoplasmic lesions in AIDS patients after therapy is discontinued has been reported.[29]

PREVENTIVE MEASURES

Preventive measures are identical for both immunosuppressed and immunocompetent individuals, including pregnant women. Although hard freezing of meat kills most *Toxoplasma* stages, occasionally organisms can survive. Meat should always be thoroughly cooked to recommended temperatures, as measured using a food thermometer placed in the thickest part of the meat. Consumption of raw or undercooked shellfish has also been shown to be a risk factor for toxoplasmosis and should be avoided. Pregnant women in particular should not eat raw or undercooked meat or shellfish. Pregnant women should also be advised to wash their hands after contact with meat, soil, kittens and outdoor cats, litter boxes, and before eating. Because some dogs have the habit of eating or rolling in cat feces, hand washing after contact with dogs is also recommended.[30] Contact with soil should be avoided by wearing gloves when working in the garden, and then thoroughly scrubbing one's hands afterward, including under the nails. Cats do not recognize property lines and a neighbor's cats may use the yard of another, especially if the soil is well cultivated for flowers or vegetables. Children's sandboxes should be covered when not in use. Cat litter boxes should be cleaned daily because *T. gondii* oocysts take more than 1 day to sporulate and become infectious. Feed cats only cooked meat or commercially prepared dried or canned food. Stray cats should be controlled. If possible, pet cats should be kept indoors to prevent them from hunting. To prevent transmission through blood transfusion or organ transplantation, the donor's and recipient's blood should be serologically tested prior to transfusion or transplantation and appropriate prophylactic medications given to the recipient if applicable.[31]

There is currently no vaccine available to prevent infection in humans. A vaccine for sheep has been licensed to reduce abortions due to *Toxoplasma*; it contains a live, incomplete strain of *Toxoplasma* that has lost its ability to develop tissue cysts. An oral live vaccine consisting of a mutant strain of *Toxoplasma* was previously developed for use in cats to prevent oocyst shedding; however, its production was discontinued because it had a short shelf life and needed to be kept frozen until just before use, it was expensive, and there was poor acceptance by cat owners.[34]

References

1. Vyas A, Kim S-K, Giacomini N, Boothroyd JC, Sapolsky RM. Behavioral changes induced by Toxoplasma infection of rodents are highly specific to aversion of cat odors. *Proc Natl Acad Sci U S A.* 2007;104(15):6442–7.
2. Holland GN. Ocular toxoplasmosis: A global reassessment. Part I: Epidemiology and course of disease. *Am J Ophthalmol.* 2003;136(6):973–88.
3. Dunn D, Wallon M, Peyron F, Petersen E, Peckham C, Gilbert R. Mother-to-child transmission of toxoplasmosis: Risk estimates for clinical counselling. *Lancet.* 1999;353(9167):1829–33.
4. Desmonts G, Couvreur J. Congenital toxoplasmosis. A prospective study of 378 pregnancies. *N Engl J Med.* 1974;290(20):1110–6.
5. Montoya JG, Liesenfeld O. Toxoplasmosis. *Lancet.* 2004;363(9425):1965–76.
6. Maldonado YA, Read JS. Diagnosis, treatment, and prevention of congenital toxoplasmosis in the United States. *Pediatrics.* 2017;139(2):e20163860.
7. Jones JL, Hanson DL, Dworkin MS, et al. Surveillance for AIDS-defining opportunistic illnesses, 1992–1997. *MMWR CDC Surveill Summ.* 1999;48(2):1–22.
8. Jones JL, Roberts JM. Toxoplasmosis hospitalizations in the United States, 2008, and trends, 1993–2008. *Clin Infect Dis.* 2012;54(7):e58–61.
9. Fernandez-Sabe N, Cervera C, Fariñas MC, et al. Risk factors, clinical features, and outcomes of toxoplasmosis in solid-organ transplant recipients: A matched case-control study. *Clin Infect Dis.* 2012;54(3):355–61.
10. Torgerson PR, Mastroiacovo P. The global burden of congenital toxoplasmosis: A systematic review. *Bull World Health Organ.* 2013;91(7):501–8.
11. Pappas G, Roussos N, Falagas ME. Toxoplasmosis snapshots: Global status of *Toxoplasma gondii* seroprevalence and implications for pregnancy and congenital toxoplasmosis. *Int J Parasitol.* 2009;39(12):1385–94.
12. Boyer K, Hill D, Mui E, et al. Unrecognized ingestion of *Toxoplasma gondii* oocysts leads to congenital toxoplasmosis and causes epidemics in North America. *Clin Infect Dis.* 2011;53(11):1081–9.
13. Jones JL, Dargelas V, Roberts J, Press C, Remington JS, Montoya JG. Risk factors for *Toxoplasma gondii* infection in the United States. *Clin Infect Dis.* 2009;49(6):878–84.
14. Scallan E, Hoekstra RM, Angulo FJ, et al. Foodborne illness acquired in the United States—Major pathogens. *Emerg Infect Dis.* 2011;17(1):7–15.
15. Jones JL, Ogunmodede F, Scheftel J, et al. Toxoplasmosis-related knowledge and practices among pregnant women in the United States. *Infect Dis Obstet Gynecol.* 2003;11(3):139–45.
16. Hill DE, Dubey JP. *Toxoplasma gondii* prevalence in farm animals in the United States. *Int J Parasitol.* 2013;43(2):107–13.
17. Belluco S, Mancin M, Conficoni D, et al. Investigating the determinants of *Toxoplasma gondii* Prevalence in meat: A systematic review and meta-regression. *PLoS One.* 2016;11(4):e0153856.
18. Guo M, Dubey JP, Hill D, et al. Prevalence and risk factors for *Toxoplasma gondii* infection in meat animals and meat products destined for human consumption. *J Food Prot.* 2015;78(2):457–76.
19. Bowie WR, King AS, Werker DH, et al. Outbreak of toxoplasmosis associated with municipal drinking water. The BC Toxoplasma Investigation Team. *Lancet.* 1997;350(9072):173–7.
20. Jones JL, Kruszon-Moran D, Elder S, et al. *Toxoplasma gondii* infection in the United States, 2011–2014. *Am J Trop Med Hyg.* 2018;98(2):551–7.
21. Jones JL, Kruszon-Moran D, Rivera HN, Price C, Wilkins PP. *Toxoplasma gondii* seroprevalence in the United States 2009–2010 and comparison with the past two decades. *Am J Trop Med Hyg.* 2014;90(6):1135–9.
22. Sousa OE, Saenz RE, Frenkel JK. Toxoplasmosis in Panama: A 10-year study. *Am J Trop Med Hyg.* 1988;38(2):315–22.
23. Dhakal R, Gajurel K, Pomares C, Talucod J, Press CJ, Montoya JG. Significance of a positive Toxoplasma immunoglobulin M test result in the United States. *J Clin Microbiol.* 2015;53(11):3601–5.
24. Cohn JA, McMeeking A, Cohen W, Jacobs J, Holzman RS. Evaluation of the policy of empiric treatment of suspected Toxoplasma encephalitis in patients with the acquired immunodeficiency syndrome. *Am J Med.* 1989;86(5):521–7.
25. de-la-Torre A, Stanford M, Curi A, Jaffe GJ, Gomez-Marin JE. Therapy for ocular toxoplasmosis. *Ocul Immunol Inflamm.* 2011;19(5):314–20.
26. Guerina NG, Hsu HW, Meissner HC, et al. Neonatal serologic screening and early treatment for congenital *Toxoplasma gondii* infection. The New England Regional Toxoplasma Working Group. *N Engl J Med.* 1994;330(26):1858–63.
27. Roizen N, Swisher CN, Stein MA, et al. Neurologic and developmental outcome in treated congenital toxoplasmosis. *Pediatrics.* 1995;95(1):11–20.
28. Montoya JG, Remington JS. Management of *Toxoplasma gondii* infection during pregnancy. *Clin Infect Dis.* 2008;47(4):554–66.
29. Holland GN, Engstrom RE Jr, Glasgow BJ, et al. Ocular toxoplasmosis in patients with the acquired immunodeficiency syndrome. *Am J Ophthalmol.* 1988;106(6):653–67.
30. Frenkel JK, Hassanein KM, Hassanein RS, Brown E, Thulliez P, Quintero-Nunez R. Transmission of *Toxoplasma gondii* in Panama City, Panama: A five-year prospective cohort study of children, cats, rodents, birds, and soil. *Am J Trop Med Hyg.* 1995;53(5):458–68.

31 Schaffner A. Pretransplant evaluation for infections in donors and recipients of solid organs. *Clin Infect Dis.* 2001;33 Suppl 1:S9–14.

32 Toxoplasmosis Frenkel JK. Parasite life cycle, pathology, and immunology. In: Hammond DM, Long PL, eds. *The Coccidia.* Baltimore: University Park Press; 1973, pp. 343–410.

33 Guidelines for Prevention and Treatment of Opportunistic Infections in HIV-infected Adults and Adolescents. 2015. https://aidsinfo.nih.gov/guidelines/html/5/pediatric-opportunistic-infection/418/toxoplasmosis. Accessed May 23, 2018.

34 Dubey JP. *Toxoplasmosis of Animals and Humans.* 2nd ed. Boca Raton, FL: CRC Press; 2010.

CHAPTER 152

Control of Infections in Institutions: Healthcare-Associated Infections*

Belinda Ostrowsky • Joseph F. Perz

INTRODUCTION

Healthcare-Associated Infections (HAIs) are a major but preventable patient safety threat. Based on 2002 data, HAIs were estimated to affect approximately 1.7 million persons and contribute to approximately 99,000 deaths annually in the United States.[1–3] The annual economic burden of these infections in the United States was estimated at $6.7 billion per year, in 2002 dollars.[2]

Since no single U.S. surveillance system could provide more refined and updated estimates, a prevalence survey of 10 geographically diverse states that were a part of the Emerging Infections Program, was conducted from 2009 to 2011 in 183 hospitals.[4] From this survey, it was projected that 648,000 patients with 721,000 infections were seen among inpatients in 2011. Approximately 4% of the patients had one or more HAIs. The most common types were pneumonia (21.8%), surgical site infections (SSI; 21.8%), and gastrointestinal infections (17.1%). The most common pathogen reported was *Clostridioides difficile (C. difficile)*.[4]

A repeat survey to assess changes in the prevalence of HAIs showed fewer patients had HAIs in 2015 [394 patients (3.2%; 95% confidence interval {CI}, 2.9–3.5)] than in 2011 [452 (4.0%; 95% CI, 3.7–4.4)] ($p < 0.001$), largely owing to reductions in the prevalence of surgical-site and urinary tract infections (UTIs). Pneumonia, gastrointestinal infections, most of which were due to *C. difficile,* and surgical-site infections were the most common HAIs. Patients' risk of having a HAI was 16% lower in 2015 than in 2011 (risk ratio, 0.84; 95% CI, 0.74–0.95; $p = 0.005$), after adjustment for age, presence of devices, days from admission to survey, and status of being in a large hospital.[4,5]

Healthcare in the United States has been increasingly delivered in outpatient, long-term care, and home health settings. Invasive procedures are now frequently performed on an outpatient basis. Although the U.S. population has grown about 38% since the 1970s, the number of hospital admissions remains at 1975 levels (36.3 million in 2002 compared to 36.2 million in 1975); in contrast, the number of outpatient visits has increased 2.5 times (to 640.5 million from 254.8 million).[6] Further, the number of certified ambulatory surgical centers increased more than tenfold, from 336 in 1985 to over 5300 in 2013.[7] These changes result in an inpatient population that is more likely to have severe illnesses[8] and be older.[6] Because of this evolution in healthcare, the term "healthcare-associated infection" has become more appropriate and is preferred over "nosocomial infection" or "hospital-acquired infection," since these latter terms are restricted to the hospital setting.

The epidemiology of HAI in the past was best described in hospital intensive-care units (ICUs); within hospitals, for many years, the highest rates of infections were observed in ICUs.[9–11] However, there has been increasing recognition that procedures and exposures, which pose risks of infection, such as the use of central venous catheters (CVC), are also frequent outside ICUs. One study involving six medical centers revealed that 29% of 2459 patients had CVCs including 7–39% (mean 24%) of non-ICU patients.[12] Given the recognition that there are significant risks beyond the ICU and the extension of surveillance and prevention activities to more patient-care locations, this chapter will address this larger landscape for HAIs.[13]

In general, HAIs are infections that are not present or incubating at the time of admission to the hospital or entry to a healthcare facility.[13,14] Infections are the most frequent adverse event in healthcare.[1,15,16] Development of an HAI is often associated with an increased length of hospital stay, prolonged therapy,[17,18] and increased costs.[19] Mortality is high: 26.6% of all deaths in a multihospital study were associated with an HAI.[20] Among persons with a healthcare-associated bloodstream infection (BSI), the attributable mortality can be even higher (35%).[21–23]

In the mid-1970s, data from the Study on the Efficacy of Nosocomial Infection Control (SENIC) suggested that about a third of hospital-associated infections could have been prevented if effective infection control programs were in place.[24] While many gains have been made, recent studies suggest that a sizeable fraction of preventable infections remains.[25–29] In fact, for some types of HAI such as blood-borne pathogen infections (e.g., hepatitis stemming from mishandling of injection supplies or blood glucose monitoring equipment), the expectation is 100% preventability and zero infections.[30]

Given the high cost of HAIs and increases in overall healthcare expenditures in the United States, there are strong financial incentives and benefits for hospitals to implement and maintain an effective infection control program.[28] In addition, the healthcare and quality landscapes have changed in that HAI measures have become part of public reporting.[13,26] Likewise, HAI measures have been tied to reimbursement, affecting healthcare system access to crucial federal funds. Most of the newer reporting requirements use standard definitions and collection methods based on the Centers for Disease Control and Prevention (CDC) National Healthcare Safety Network (NHSN), the nation's most widely used HAI surveillance system.[13] The Hospital Acquired Conditions (HAC) Reduction Program administered by Centers for Medicare and Medicaid Services (CMS) allows for 1% reductions in payment to hospitals in the worst performing quartiles for specific safety and HAI measures.[31] These types of programs have raised awareness among hospital leaders and administrators. This has helped to shift the dynamics beyond counting HAIs to focusing on ways to prevent these infections.[31]

*The findings and conclusions in this chapter are those of the authors and do not necessarily represent the official position of the Centers for Disease Control and Prevention (CDC).

It is important to place the scope of HAIs in additional context since response activities provide one indication of the volume of public health activity in this area. Recently, HAI programs, based within state health departments and several large cities, were asked to assess the burden of HAI outbreaks and resources needed to support their investigation and control. For the calendar year 2015, there were more than 6000 HAI-related outbreaks or clusters investigated by 55 HAI programs (median 58, mean 123 per program). These investigations included some combination of technical support for healthcare facilities, onsite and laboratory support, and/or surveillance activities.[32]

This chapter will review recent trends in HAI, general principles in HAI transmission, surveillance and prevention, common HAIs by type of infection, and describe the components of HAI programs and their interaction with the public health system.

GENERAL PRINCIPLES

General risk factors for HAIs include issues related to the patient, the disease or condition that the patient is presenting with, and the practices and procedures used for their management and treatment.[33] As in other settings, three elements are needed for transmission of infection in healthcare: a source of the pathogen, a susceptible host, and a mode of transmission.[34] In healthcare, the source is frequently a human (e.g., flora from the patient, another patient, or possibly a healthcare provider) and, less frequently, originates in the environment.[35] Pathogens that are associated with water, such as *Legionella* spp. and nontuberculous mycobacteria, are examples of the latter. Infections such as *C. difficile* and *Candida auris* highlight the role of the environment and inanimate surfaces as an intermediary in potential HAI transmission and illustrate the need for adequate cleaning of environmental services and equipment as part of successful infection prevention.[36,37] Host susceptibility varies, and may be influenced by characteristics such as age, nutritional status, comorbidities, and severity of underlying disease. Diagnostic procedures, various medical devices, and medical or surgical therapy may breach the normal host defenses, presenting unique opportunities for patients' exposure to pathogens that result in infections. Potent immunosuppressives, chemotherapy, and antibiotics may affect the host's normal colonizing flora, cause skin and mucosal membrane breakdown, and impair immune system function.[38]

Substantial attention has been focused in recent years on improving infection prevention practices within acute-care hospitals to optimize patient safety; many of these practices also need to be applied across multiple aspects of patient care.[39] Adherence to infection prevention and control practices is essential to providing safe and high-quality patient care across all settings where healthcare is delivered.

A number of core practices are recommended by CDC and considered standards of care and/or accepted practices (e.g., aseptic technique, hand hygiene before patient contact) to prevent infection in healthcare settings.[39] These widely agreed upon practices are elements of care that are not expected to change based on additional research, either because of an overwhelming preponderance of evidence (e.g., hand-hygiene requirements), or in some cases due to ethical concerns (e.g., randomizing patients to procedures performed by trained versus untrained personnel). Therefore, these accepted practices are categorized as strong recommendations, even when high-quality randomized controlled trials are not available to support them. In an effort to streamline and systematize the process for updating existing guidelines without recreating the analytic process for each of these accepted/core practices, CDC charged Healthcare Infection Control Practices Advisory Committee (HICPAC) to review existing CDC guidelines and identify all recommendations that warrant inclusion as core practices.[39] The resulting compilation of core practices included: (1) leadership support, (2) education and training of healthcare personnel on infection prevention, (3) patient, family and caregiver education, (4) performance monitoring and feedback, (5) Standard Precautions, including hand hygiene, environmental cleaning and disinfection, and injection and medication safety, risk assessment with appropriate use of personal protective equipment (PPE), minimizing potential exposures, reprocessing of reusable medical equipment, (6) transmission-based precautions, (7) temporary invasive medical devices for clinical management, and (8) occupational health.[39]

Standard Precautions help ensure proper selection and use of PPE based on the nature of the patient interaction and potential for exposure to blood, body fluids and/or infectious material. Transmission-Based Precautions (i.e., Contact, Droplet, and/or Airborne Precautions) are implemented for patients with a documented or suspected diagnose where contact with the patient, their body fluids, or their environment presents substantial additional transmission risk. In other words, Transmission-Based Precautions are used to supplement Standard Precautions when the route(s) of transmission for a particular pathogen is (are) not completely interrupted using Standard Precautions alone.[34,39] One example is the use of Contact Precautions, which triggers the use of gowns and gloves by healthcare workers, when caring for patients with *C. difficile*, norovirus and other intestinal tract pathogens, where there is potential for extensive environmental contamination. Detailed guidance on the application of Transmission-Based Precautions, including a list of pathogens and recommended precautions, is available from CDC and HICPAC.[34]

REVIEW OF COMMON HAI TYPES

In the following sections common HAI are reviewed, including a summary of risk factors, trends in data over time, and successful strategies for prevention.

Urinary Tract Infections

UTI is one of the most common HAIs. The greatest risk factor for UTIs is the use of urinary catheters with 70–80% of these infections attributable to an indwelling urethral catheter. Older estimates were that 12–16% of adult hospital inpatients would have a urinary catheter at some time during their admission.[36,40–44] With more recent focus on requiring valid justification for urinary catheters insertion and continuation, the use of urinary catheters appears to be decreasing.[45]

CDC's National Healthcare Safety Network (NHSN) has been trending data for catheter-associated UTI (CAUTI) for the last several years. A definitional change removed those cultures growing a yeast in 2016. In tracking CAUTIs from 2009 to 2016 (regardless of this change in definition), there has been consistent year-to-year decline in CAUTI incidence. This was evident in both ICU and non-ICU wards for 2012–16 as measured by the standardized infection ratio, or SIR, which decreased from 0.97 in 2012 to 0.66 (HAI story success CDC web/2015 report).[46]

Prevention of UTI starts with limiting the use of urinary catheters to necessary clinical indications and not for convenience of care.[41] Consideration of the risks and benefits of catheterization has led to development of more limited indications for its use. Alternative approaches to catheterization have included patient training and biofeedback, medications, surgery, and use of special clothes and pads. If a urinary catheter must be used, minimizing the duration of catheterization and maintaining a closed drainage system are recommended measures to prevent bacteriuria. Aseptic technique is recommended during insertion, as is securing the catheter after insertion to prevent movement and urethral traction.[41] Several studies have demonstrated effectiveness of using urinary catheters impregnated with silver, in order to prevent UTI; this may be a supplemental strategy in select patient populations.[47,48] However, good hand hygiene after caring for each patient remains the single measure most likely to prevent cross transmission of urinary pathogens.[49,50].

A summary of practical recommendations for UTI prevention in acute-care hospitals was published in 2014 by the Society for

Healthcare Epidemiologists of America and Infectious Diseases Society of America (SHEA/IDSA) as part of a larger compendium of HAI prevention strategies.[41] The document reviews literature, including recommendations from a series of prior guidelines. Recommendations are categorized as basic practices that should be adopted by all acute-care hospitals or special approaches for use in particular locations or populations within hospitals when HAIs are not controlled by basic practices. The basic practices for prevention included infrastructure for preventing CAUTI such as: written guidelines for catheter use; insertion and maintenance; ensuring skill of those who insert catheters; supply availability for aseptic insertion; systems to document insertion and tracking of catheter use; performing surveillance for CAUTI; providing healthcare worker education; and ensuring appropriate technique for insertion and management of indwelling catheters. Restricting collection of urine cultures to those patients with appropriate symptoms or indications may also play a role. Special approaches for CAUTI prevention include: risk assessments in facility areas or populations with high SIRs despite basic prevention strategies; development of protocols for management of postoperative urinary retention; including nurse-directed use of intermittent catheterization and use of bladder scanners; and establishing a system for analyzing and reporting data on catheter use and adverse events from catheter use.[41]

Surgical-Site Infections

SSIs constitute a common category of adverse events, occurring historically in 2–5% of patients undergoing inpatient surgery.[3,51–53] SSIs result in increased morbidity, prolonged hospital stays, and increased direct costs.[52,53] Rates of infection after surgery vary widely by surgical procedure[26,27,51]; feedback on infection rates is helpful in preventing infections.[24] Patient factors and surgical wound characteristics affect the risk of infection. Adjustment of SSI rates to account for underlying risk is both necessary and challenging; this requires the collection of additional information, such as wound classification (clean, clean-contaminated, contaminated, or dirty-infected), the physical status of the patient (using the American Society of Anesthesiology score ranging from one or healthy to five or moribund), and duration of the operative procedure.[13] Most SSIs become evident after discharge,[54,55] therefore postdischarge surveillance is essential.

As the number of surgical procedures performed in the United States continues to rise, attention to SSI prevention is increasingly important. Requirements for public reporting include process measures, and have been expanded to encompass outcome measures (e.g., rates of SSI and comparative SIR for such procedures as colon resections and cardiac bypass surgeries), and other quality improvement metrics. Reimbursements for treating SSIs are being reduced or denied. It has been estimated that approximately half of SSIs are preventable by application of currently recommended evidence-based strategies.[51]

Guidelines for preventing SSIs were updated in 2017 by CDC with its HICPAC Group[56,57]; general recommendations based on the strongest scientific evidence include: postponing surgery until any remote site infections are resolved; not removing hair preoperatively; administration of the appropriate prophylactic antimicrobials only if necessary; and administration of intravenous antimicrobials timed to ensure bactericidal levels from the time the incision is made to hours after the incision is closed (and not much beyond). Other factors that have warranted attention include perioperative glycemic and normothermic control.[56,57]

The SHEA/IDSA Compendium Strategies for Prevention of SSIs distinguishes basic approaches from special approaches for use in situations when the basic approaches have not reduced SSI rates.[51] Basic practices from the Compendium, beyond the guidance and strategies summarized above, include: antimicrobial prophylaxis dosing for obesity; redosing for long procedures or those with excessive blood loss; use of alcohol-containing preoperative skin preparatory agents if no contraindication; use of impervious plastic wound protectors for gastrointestinal and biliary tract surgery; use of World Health Organization (WHO)-based checklist lists to improve surgical patient safety; performing SSI surveillance and providing feedback to surgeons and perioperative personnel on this surveillance (with their rates compared to that of other facilities and their peers within their facility), and educating providers, patients, and families on SSI prevention measures. Some of the special or supplemental approaches outlined in the Compendium include: screening for *S. aureus* and decolonization; antiseptic wound lavage; performing SSI risk assessments; observing operating room personnel and environment of care of the operating rooms. Approaches that were not supported for SSI prevention were routine use of vancomycin for antimicrobial prophylaxis, or antiseptic-impregnated sutures and drapes. Some areas that are presently unresolved include preoperative bathing, intranasal and pharyngeal treatment with chlorhexidine-containing products, gentamicin-collagen sponges, and "bundles" to ensure best practices. Although the latter (use of bundled approaches) is in common practice, there is no consensus on bundle components or the attributable contribution from any single intervention. Of note, a useful feature in the Compendium is a section on implementation of the strategies in real-world facility settings.[51]

Bloodstream Infections

An estimated one-half of all BSIs are healthcare-associated and are often CVC associated.[58] As described in a CDC Vital Signs report, this translates into estimates of approximately 23,000 central line-associated bloodstream infections (CLABSIs) in inpatients and 37,000 CLABSIs among patients receiving hemodialysis. The mean cost of a BSI is about $35,000.[59] Mortality is high: an estimated 14% of hospital deaths may be associated with BSIs,[60] and the attributable mortality is about 23%.[22]

BSIs can be primary, when the isolation of a bacterial bloodstream pathogen occurs in the absence of an infection at another site, or secondary, when bacteria are isolated from the blood subsequent to another site of infection such as a UTI. Most primary BSIs are associated with the use of CVCs. Thus, prevention has focused efforts to restrict use of catheters and remove catheters that are no longer necessary. For example, in dialysis patients, rates of BSI are lower among patients with fistula and graft vascular access compared to those with catheters.[61–64] Other important prevention recommendations are described in guidelines developed by HICPAC and others.[62] These include: training of healthcare workers; improving hand hygiene; implementing aseptic catheter insertion techniques including the use of maximal barrier precautions; optimizing selection of the catheter insertion site and site-care practices; and the use of check lists to standardize and track line insertion and maintenance practices. Traditionally, most BSI surveillance was conducted in ICUs, but recent expansion to non-ICU locations has generated data highlighting the need for prevention efforts to address a much larger area of the hospital environment.[65] The SHEA/IDSA Compendium for CLABSI prevention also includes special approaches to consider when the basic approaches are unable to reduce CLABSI rates. These include: antiseptic- or antimicrobial-impregnated CVCs in adults; antiseptic-containing hub/connector cap/port protector to cover connectors; silver-zeolite-impregnated umbilical catheters in preterm infants (in countries where it is approved for use in children); and use of antibiotics locks for CVCs.[66]

CDC's Annual *National and State Healthcare-Associated Infections Progress Report*[67] describes national and state progress in preventing HAIs. Among national acute-care hospitals, this report showed that hospitals have made significant progress in preventing CLABSIs nationally, with a roughly 50% drop in CLABSIs between 2008 and 2016. The data are combined with declining SIRs and change in relation to the number of CLABSIs per central line days. These data show declines in the device (i.e., central line) use ratio on wards, and especially neonatal intensive-care units (NICUs), highlighting the net benefit to patients afforded by both safer and reduced central-line use.[67]

The pathogens associated with CLABSI have changed over time.[62–64] For example, among adult ICU patients, declines in CLABSIs caused by *Staphylococcus* and *Enterococcus* spp. have outpaced declines in infections caused by gram negative and fungal pathogens. The frequency of CLABSI associated with antimicrobial-resistant organisms is increasing.[62–64,67]

Pneumonia (Emphasis on Ventilator-associated Pneumonia and Ventilator-associated Events)

Pneumonia and lower respiratory infections are associated with significant morbidity, mortality, and costs.[68,69] The greatest risk factor for healthcare-associated pneumonia is the use of mechanical ventilation.[70,71] The true incidence of ventilator-associated pneumonia (VAP) is difficult to determine since surveillance definitions are nonspecific. Historically, 10–20% of ventilated patients have developed VAP. More recent reports suggest much lower rates, but it is unclear to what extent these lower rates reflect better care versus stricter application of subjective surveillance criteria.[69,72]

Patients on mechanical ventilation are at risk for a variety of serious complications in addition to pneumonia. These include acute respiratory distress syndrome, pneumothorax, pulmonary embolism, lobar atelectasis, and pulmonary edema.[68,69] CDC released new surveillance definitions for ventilator-associated event (VAE) designed to make surveillance more objective and to expand surveillance from VAP alone to include other complications of mechanical ventilation. VAE definitions include criteria for ventilator-associated conditions (VACs), infection-related ventilator-associated complications (IVACs), possible pneumonia, and probable pneumonia.[13,69,72]

Multiple factors are associated with development of VAP. Risk factors for VAP include comorbid conditions such as burn, trauma, central nervous system disease, and cardiac and respiratory disease.[71] Strategies to prevent VAP and other acute respiratory infections were identified by HICPAC.[68,69] These include appropriate use and reprocessing of equipment and devices, hand hygiene, and other aspects of Standard Precautions. The guidelines also address prevention of VAP and other infections outside of acute-care hospitals; notably, vaccination for primary prevention of influenza and pneumococcus.

The SHEA/APIC Compendium for VAP[72] discusses basic strategies such as: avoidance of mechanical ventilation, using noninvasive positive pressure ventilation when feasible; minimizing sedation; regularly assessing readiness for extubation; maintaining physical conditioning; minimizing pooling of secretions above the endotracheal tube cuff; and elevating the head of the bed. Additional special measures include: oral chlorhexidine washes; prophylactic probiotics; ultrathin polyurethane endotracheal tube cuffs; and automated control of endotracheal tube cuff pressure.

THE SHIFTING LANDSCAPE IN HEALTHCARE

With the delivery of healthcare expanding to a variety of settings outside of short stay acute-care hospitals as noted earlier, there has been increased recognition of the need for infection control programs and activities beyond acute-care settings. The National Action Plan to Prevent Health Care-Associated Infections: Road Map to Elimination, first published in 2009 with a focus on acute-care hospitals, was subsequently expanded to address HAI prevention across a larger span of the healthcare continuum.[73] The various components of the National HAI Action Plan provide useful summaries of policy directions, quality improvement guidelines, prevention initiatives, and research needs. In the following sections, we will provide a brief overview of some of the HAI challenges and promising developments in long-term care, dialysis centers, ambulatory care, and home health.

Long-term-care Facilities

In the United States approximately 4 million persons annually are admitted to or reside in nursing homes and skilled nursing facilities, and nearly 1 million persons reside in assisted living facilities.[74] Data about infections in long-term care facilities (LTCFs) are limited, but it has been estimated that 1–3 million infections occur each year in these facilities.[74] Common HAIs in LTCFs are UTIs, lower respiratory tract infections, skin and soft tissue infections, and diarrheal diseases; antibiotic-resistant pathogens are commonly encountered including methicillin-resistant *Staphylococcus aureus* (MRSA), *C. difficile*, and resistant gram-negative pathogens. Infections are a major cause of hospitalization and death for LTCF residents and upward of 380,000 people die from infections in LTCFs every year.[74,75]

Care for elderly patients is complicated; susceptibility to HAIs is facilitated by the interaction of multiple factors, including age and its associated decrease in immunity[76]; multiple comorbidities, including cognitive impairment[77]; decreased functional status (e.g., urinary and fecal incontinence, immobility)[78]; and long-term exposure to medical devices (e.g., urinary catheters). LTCFs are congregational environments that support routine group activities such as dining, recreation, and physical therapy. These characteristics, along with shared healthcare staff and limited resources for infection prevention and control, can facilitate exposure to and spread of infectious agents.

1. The National HAI Prevention Action Plan chapter on LTCFs focused on nursing homes and skilled nursing facilities and reviewed the epidemiology of infection risks in these environments, emphasizing antibiotic use and resistance.[73] Antimicrobials account for approximately 40% of all systemic drugs prescribed in LTCFs with over half of residents receiving at least one course of a systemic antimicrobial agent each year. Associated risks include complications such as *C. difficile* infection (CDI) and the emergence of multidrug-resistant organisms. The Action Plan highlighted priorities that include: improving surveillance for HAIs (e.g., participation in NHSN); efforts for *C. difficile* prevention; improvements in rates of resident and healthcare worker influenza vaccination, addressing UTIs, CAUTI prevention and processes for catheter care.[73] CDC and other partners have responded by developing and expanding resource offerings, which include CDI prevention materials, Core Elements of Antibiotic Stewardship for Nursing Homes, a large quality-care collaborative, and support for LTCF enrolment in NHSN.[79,80]

Outpatient Dialysis Centers

Over 425,000 patients rely on chronic hemodialysis patients in the United States.[81,82] In 2008, an estimated 37,000 BSIs occurred among kidney dialysis patients with central lines.[82] Dialysis patients are at high risk for HAI for several reasons[83]: they require vascular access for prolonged periods during hemodialysis; they are immunosuppressed and more susceptible to infection; they require frequent hospitalizations and surgery; and often have comorbidities.[81] Antimicrobial resistance (AR) is an important issue for dialysis patients because they commonly receive antimicrobials including vancomycin; five of the first six patients with vancomycin intermediate or fully resistant *S. aureus* were dialysis patients.[84] Vascular access is the strongest risk factor for infection; grafts and fistulas should be preferred over temporary and permanent catheters[62]; other recommendations to prevent infections have been developed for peritoneal and hemodialysis patients.[61,62,83–85]

CDC has organized a comprehensive approach to hemodialysis infection prevention, with a strong focus on BSI prevention. This includes core activities such as surveillance and feedback using the NHSN, hand hygiene observations, catheter and vascular access care observations, staff education and competency, patient education and engagement, catheter reduction, chlorhexidine skin antisepsis, catheter hub disinfection, and antimicrobial ointments each with tools and audit systems. Collaborative partnerships have shown sustained reductions in CLABSIs in this vulnerable dialysis population,[86–88] and these successes are driving a National Coalition that was formed in 2016.

Outpatient Settings and Home Care

Outpatient care is delivered in a wide range of settings. These include primary-care physician office practices, dental clinics and offices, public health clinics, and urgent-care clinics. Outpatient care also extends to various medical specialty clinics, and office-based surgery, and ambulatory surgical centers. In 2002, about half of the U.S. population made at least one visit to a doctor's office or emergency room or had a home healthcare visit.[6] Of all surgical procedures in community hospitals in 2002, 63% were on outpatients compared with 16% on outpatients in 1980.[6] In addition, home health and hospice services represent another area of continued growth. For example, 1.3 million patients were enrolled in home care in 2000, with even larger estimates by more recent CDC statistics.[6,89] According to a national study of long-term-care providers, in 2014 there were nearly 14,000 home health agencies in the United States.[74,75]

Although patients receiving care in outpatient settings might not experience the same level of exposure to HAIs as inpatient or long-term-care populations, invasive procedures (including injections) are common and carry risks of infection. There is little in the way of routine surveillance for HAI in outpatient settings beyond dialysis clinics (as described above). However, numerous outbreaks are reported each year. These are usually related to gaps in basic infection control. Unsafe injection practices, including reuse of syringes, and contamination of medication vials, have been associated with large outbreaks of viral hepatitis (e.g., hepatitis C virus following alternative medicine infusion therapies), bacterial infections (e.g., septic arthritis following joint injections), and even fungal infections (e.g., BSIs among cancer clinic patients).[90–92] The *One & Only Campaign* is a public health campaign, led by the CDC and the Safe Injection Practices Coalition (SIPC), to raise awareness among patients and healthcare providers about safe injection practices. The Campaign aims to eliminate infections resulting from unsafe injection practices.[92] Of note, intravenous infusion therapy also has been identified as an important risk for infections in home-care patients.[93]

Compared to inpatient acute-care settings, ambulatory-care settings have traditionally lacked infrastructure and resources to support infection control and surveillance activities. Many outpatient facilities continue to operate independently of hospital-based systems and relatively few are Medicare-certified, accredited, or state-licensed. As a result, active oversight of these facilities in the form of periodic on-site inspections or surveys is very limited. Similarly, detailed infection prevention and safety standards, such as those that apply to Medicare-certified hospitals, nursing homes, dialysis clinics, and ambulatory surgery centers, are lacking for many providers on the outpatient continuum. These issues are addressed as part of the Outpatient Policy Options resource on CDC's Outpatient Settings website. This site also houses the Guide to Infection Prevention in Outpatient Settings: Minimum Expectations for Safe Care, which includes a checklist that can be used to assess infection prevention practices and policies. This guide is based heavily on Standard Precautions and the HICPAC Core Measures, which are applicable to a wide range of outpatient care encounters. In addition, guides are now available specifically for oncology, podiatry, dental, pain, and orthopedic clinics.[39,94]

While efforts to achieve the goal of reducing CLABSIs have been focused primarily on the acute-care and dialysis settings, the substantial number of patients discharged from hospital to their home or an LTCF with central lines in place represents an area of concern. A limited body of studies has defined the number of peripherally inserted central catheter (PICC) lines and evaluated the extent of CLABSIs outside the acute-care hospital setting.[95–97] Among the research conducted in this area are two studies that focused on patients given home parenteral nutrition (HPN) delivered through PICC lines. The first compared the PICC line group to those receiving HPN through other central venous access devices; those in the PICC line group had a significantly higher CLABSI rate.[95] The second study used a retrospective chart review to quantify complications related to HPN, and found that patients who experienced catheter complications (including CLABSIs) had more PICC line days and more hospital admissions than those without complications.[96] One of the challenges facing healthcare providers is that home-care staff, partnering with patients and/or family caregivers, become responsible for safely maintaining central lines inserted in the acute-care setting, without having a clear standard for that maintenance. A toolkit from the United Hospital Fund and two healthcare systems in New York offers some practical tools for prevention of central-line-associated infections[95–97]:

ANTIMICROBIAL RESISTANCE AND EMERGING INFECTIONS

HAIs associated with resistant pathogens have increased substantially; these infections are frequently associated with increased mortality, morbidity, and costs.[98] The factors contributing to increasing resistance are complex.[98] To control resistance, it is necessary to employ a strategy that includes a monitoring system for antimicrobial use and associated outcomes, development of guidelines for control of antimicrobial use, and appropriate implementation of infection control measures.[99] During the last several decades, the prevalence of multidrug-resistant organisms in U.S. hospitals and medical centers has increased steadily. Methicillin-resistant *S. aureus* (MRSA), first recognized in the 1960s, became endemic in many hospitals during the 1990s.

In recent years, other emerging AR threats have taken center stage, such as multidrug-resistant gram-negative and fungal pathogens. In 2013, CDC published a comprehensive analysis ranking the top 18 antibiotic-resistant threats in the United States titled, *Antibiotic Resistance Threats in the United States, 2013.*[100] The report categorized these AR threats, based on level of concern to human health, as urgent, serious, or concerning. The AR Threat Report also established estimates for morbidity and mortality, identified patients at risk, and gaps in knowledge for these pathogens. The report outlined the core actions needed at the local, regional, and national levels, to prevent infections caused by AR bacteria and slow spread of resistance.[100]

CDC and other public health partners are supporting AR threat "containment" activities, as part of a more active and coordinated strategy to address AR.[101] Containment complements foundational public health strategies, including improving antibiotic use and preventing infections, and builds on existing HAI/AR detection and response structures. The goal is to limit the impact and spread of urgent threats such as carbapenem-resistant Enterobacteriaceae (CRE) and *Candida auris*, acting aggressively while their presence remains localized. Typically, containment relies on: rapid identification; targeted infection control assessments; colonization screenings; coordinated response between facilities; and continued assessments and screenings until spread is controlled. Three response tiers help health departments tailor and organize containment activities once a threat is confirmed by laboratory partners, as follows[100,101]:

- Tier 1 Containment Response: Genes and organisms never seen in the United States and/or pan-resistant organisms.
- Tier 2 Containment Response: Genes and organisms never or rarely seen in a geographic area.
- Tier 3 Containment Response: Genes and organisms that are known threats in a geographic area, but are not endemic.

CDC's April 2018 *Vital Signs* and the Interim Guidance for a Health Response to Contain Novel or Targeted Multidrug-resistant Organisms (MDROs) illustrated the rationale for and details of the containment strategy including utilizing regional approaches.[101,102] This included roles for CDC/federal partners, state and local health departments and healthcare facility partners. Federal partners are tasked with monitoring resistance, sharing information on new pathogens and expanding access to testing (e.g., for a wider array of pathogens and resistance mechanisms), and supporting infection control and prevention efforts. State and local health departments can inform healthcare facility partners regarding public health laboratory support that has been made available through the Antimicrobial Resistance Laboratory Network Laboratory (ARLN). Likewise, health departments have increased capacities to: provide advice on which types of isolates to send for testing; assess the quality and consistency of infection control in healthcare facilities; coordinate information and activities across facilities; and provide timely lab results and recommendations. Healthcare facilities can plan for and help address resistance. For example, acute-care facilities are called upon to identify a multidisciplinary team, with engagement of facility, leadership, laboratories, and infection control experts. Antibiotic resistance threats vary by state, thus the details of the response may vary and be scaled within this framework.[101,102]

PROGRAMMATIC ACTVITIES

Components of Effective Infection Control Programs

Infection control programs have long been required in acute-care facilities; these programs, or their components, are increasingly being specified as part of regulatory requirements, for example, as part of Medicare-certification. A model infection control program, recommended by CDC, the American Hospital Association, and The Joint Commission, was adopted in principle by many U.S. hospitals by the mid-1970s.[103–105] CDC conducted the SENIC study in the late 1970s to evaluate the effectiveness of hospital infection control programs.[103] This study demonstrated that hospitals with active surveillance and control programs had significantly fewer infections than did hospitals without such programs. The SENIC study also found that four elements were associated with effective programs: an active infection surveillance system with reporting of results to staff members; presence of vigorous control measures designed to eliminate recognized hazards; at least one full-time infection control practitioner for every 250 beds; and a physician on the staff knowledgeable about hospital-associated infections who took an active part in the infection control program.

Most infection control teams in U.S. hospitals now consist of a hospital epidemiologist and one or more infection control preventionists.[106] The traditional duties of the infection control team include the collection and analysis of surveillance data, assisting in the development of infection control policies and procedures, and providing education and consultation to other hospital personnel. The team also plays a critical role in advising the hospital's medical staff and administration about the clinical implications of patient-care practices, occupational infections, and quality improvement. Changes in the healthcare delivery system, the emergence of new infections, the emphasis on antimicrobial stewardship and bioterrorism have added even more activities and responsibilities to the infection control team. Reporting and accrediting mandates, as well as increased expectations to conduct compliance audits and lead performance improvement initiatives, have placed additional strain on hospital infection prevention teams.[106]

Surveillance

Surveillance is a first step in describing any public health event, and, in the area of HAI, its implementation has been associated with declines in infection rates.[105] Healthcare system surveillance has expanded to capture events associated not only with infections but also with medical errors and a wide array of quality measures.

The National Nosocomial Infection Surveillance System (NNIS), a hospital-based, systematic, voluntary, and confidential reporting system,[15,107–109] was started in 1970 as a partnership between CDC and volunteer hospitals in the United States.[107] Protocols and definitions were developed, and prospective, hospital-wide surveillance for HAIs was initiated. In the 1980s, focus shifted to patient-care areas with the highest infection rates, including risk adjustment to facilitate comparison of rates across hospitals.[108–112]

In 2005, NNIS was revamped and integrated with two other small voluntary systems for dialysis and healthcare worker surveillance to form the National Healthcare Safety Network (NHSN).[112,13,113] Beginning with only 300 participating hospitals and several dozen dialysis clinics, NHSN participation grew quickly to include over 17,000 medical facilities by the mid-2010s. Much of this growth was driven by state public reporting mandates and CMS incentives. Current participants include acute-care hospitals, long-term acute-care hospitals, psychiatric hospitals, rehabilitation hospitals, outpatient dialysis centers, ambulatory surgery centers, and nursing homes. Hospitals and dialysis facilities represent the majority of participating facilities.

NHSN provides standard national measures for HAIs as well as analytic tools that enable each facility to assess its progress and identify where additional efforts are needed. One widely used tool is the SIR,[114] which is a summary measure used to track different HAIs at a national, state, local or facility level. The SIR adjusts for various facility and/or patient-level factors that contribute to facility HAI risks. It was modeled loosely on the Standardized Mortality Ratio (SMR), a summary statistic widely used in public health to analyze mortality data. In HAI data analysis, the SIR compares the actual number of HAIs reported in NHSN to the number predicted for that facility/location and infection type using prior experience from a baseline calendar year (akin to the SMR's use of a standard population), adjusting for selected factors that have been found to affect infection incidence. Interpretation of SIRs is straightforward; an SIR greater than 1.0 indicates that more HAIs were observed than predicted; conversely, an SIR less than 1.0 indicates that fewer HAIs were observed than predicted. SIRs are currently calculated in NHSN for the following HAI types: CLABSI, mucosal barrier injury laboratory-confirmed BSIs (MBI-LCBI), CAUTI, SSI, CDI, MRSA, and VAE.

In the past few years, efforts to improve the efficiency of surveillance have included increasing use of computer algorithms and electronic medical and laboratory data systems to identify patients likely to have acquired an HAI.[115,116] As an example, the sensitivity of surveillance for SSIs has improved by using electronic data.[117] These practices help to further standardize case finding and the application of surveillance definitions. In addition, the effort required to review medical records by surveillance personnel is lessened, making the process more efficient.[118] Of note, a comprehensive review by Woeltje et al., summarizes electronic surveillance methods, advanced informatics, and their applicability to HAI surveillance and ICP programs.[119]

Infection Control and Prevention—Emphasis on "Prevention"

Preventing HAIs is an integral part of the national safety agenda.[120,121] Data from NNIS showed that during 1990–99, risk-adjusted infection rates in ICUs decreased for respiratory tract, urinary tract, and BSIs; BSI rates decreased substantially in medical ICUs (44%), coronary ICUs (43%), pediatric ICUs (32%), and surgical ICUs (31%).[9] In the era of NHSN, we have had even greater improvements and new, increasingly ambitious, goals as described in the HHS HAI Action Plans that was highlighted earlier.[26,29]

There has been movement toward adoption of HAI elimination and "zero" preventable infections as a goal.[120] Most HAIs are related to specific patient-care practices, and should be preventable with increased adherence to available guidelines.[39,54,57,62] Continuous quality improvement efforts, which focus on a continuous cycle of event tracking and process improvement, have been shown to reduce serious medication errors.[15] A similar approach to HAI prevention, with attention to individual infections, analyzing for opportunities that could have led to transmission events as safety signals, could yield positive results.[121] A recent systematic review and meta-analysis examined studies published between 2005 and 2016 assessing multifaceted interventions aimed at reducing CAUTI, CLABSI, SSI, or VAP. Each of these outcomes was associated with a mean pooled decrease in incidence ranging from approximately 30–50%. Even in high-income countries such as the United States, there remain many untapped opportunities to further reduce HAIs; with an ever-increasing population of vulnerable patients and care volumes, our work is far from done.[29]

The Targeted Assessment for Prevention (TAP) Tools in NHSN were designed to identify and prioritize healthcare facilities and/or locations where prevention efforts can yield the largest impact. The Cumulative Attributable Difference (CAD) is the metric used to rank facilities or facility locations within the TAP Report to help guide interventions and deployments of prevention resources.[122]

Public Health Investments in HAI Programs and Prevention

There has been growing recognition that Public Health and Healthcare must work together in an active and collaborative manner if we are to succeed in meeting the challenges posed by HAI risk and AR threats. Since 2009, health departments have received funding and other support from CDC's Division of Healthcare Quality Promotion (DHQP) as part of the Epidemiology and Laboratory Capacity Cooperative Agreement (ELC). The original stated objective of this support was "Building and Sustaining State Programs to Prevent Healthcare-associated Infections," in line with overall ELC goals.[123] In 2009, 51 programs (49 states plus DC and Puerto Rico) were funded using a $40 million allocation from the American Recovery and Reinvestment Act. This initial funding provided support for an HAI Coordinator staff position and required the formation of a multidisciplinary advisory groups, which typically included state hospital associations and healthcare delivery partners, CMS-funded quality improvement organizations, and other stakeholders. These efforts were enhanced by a separate requirement for each state to develop its own HAI Plan to maintain eligibility for Preventive Health and Health Services Block Grant funds. Through the Affordable Care Act of 2010, funding was maintained at roughly baseline levels, with expansion of program goals related to address HAI prevention needs across the healthcare continuum, moving beyond the initial focus on hospital settings. During the 5-year ELC cycle, which began in 2014, the goals and scope of the HAI/AR Programs grew to include antibiotic stewardship as well as prevention and containment of novel pathogens and emerging AR threats.[123]

The 2015 ELC Ebola Supplement ($85 million) included Ebola and other preparedness elements, HAI Plan revisions, outbreak reporting and response capacity assessments, and on-site infection control assessments in >3000 healthcare facilities. Regular ELC HAI/AR Program funding reached new levels beginning in 2016 with funds appropriated to CDC as part of the National Action Plan for Combating Antibiotic-Resistant Bacteria; over $110 million was disbursed over project years 3 and 4.

As of 2018, there were 57 HAI/AR programs with over 500 staff positions that are at least partially funded through the ELC mechanism. Funding now offers support for the HAI Coordinator as well as AR Expert and AR Laboratory Expert positions.[32] As a testament to this investment in infrastructure at state and local health departments for HAI prevention, all 50 states have meaningful activities in infection prevention (such as implementation of the TAP strategy) and control, with a growing collection of success stories.[26]

HAI Outbreak Response Activities

Despite significant progress, patients still experience preventable harms in the form of outbreaks and adverse events due to delayed recognition of emerging infectious diseases, unsafe healthcare practices, and contaminated drugs, and medical device risks. The volume of joint health department and healthcare investigation activity is very high. In 2015, 55 ELC-funded HAI/AR Programs reported more than 6000 investigations, many of which involved on-site technical and/or laboratory assistance. For these reasons, healthcare outbreak response activities are being elevated and recognized as a core component of HAI/AR prevention and containment strategies. The Council for Outbreak Response: Healthcare-Associated Infections & Antibiotic-Resistant Pathogens (CORHA)[124] provides a forum for public health and healthcare partners to collaborate to improve practices and policies for detection, investigation, and control of HAI/AR outbreaks. Response refers to efforts to assist with assessment and investigation of specific, acute HAI/AR risks which can present as clusters of infections, sentinel cases (e.g., HAI or emerging AR threat), or even simply as a serious breach in infection control practice (e.g., syringe reuse). Healthcare response activities include assessing for and controlling deficient or risky practices and ruling out a larger problem (e.g., via case finding activities). CORHA has highlighted the fact that the types of events that might signal potential outbreaks, are neither limited to HAIs for which there is routine surveillance, nor to infections/conditions that are routinely reportable to public health authorities. More systematic and consistent approaches to healthcare outbreak response are needed, from signal detection to investigation and control.

Response to Challenges Enriches Healthcare and Public Health Partnerships

Infection prevention and control programs—at both the healthcare facility and public health levels—have been important in the control of emerging threats. Following the terrorist attacks on September 11, 2001, and the subsequent outbreak of anthrax, healthcare facilities developed plans to enhance bioterrorism preparedness. In 2003, healthcare facilities were at the center of the severe acute respiratory syndrome (SARS) outbreak—a newly discovered respiratory disease caused by SARS-coronavirus that emerged in China and spread globally.[125] The healthcare infection prevention and control community proved to be a pivotal partner to public health in 2009–10 during the H1N1 influenza pandemic, and in 2013–16 during the domestic Ebola response.[125] The infection control issues to be addressed in response to natural epidemic or intentional infectious threats include identifying persons who may be infected or exposed; preventing transmission among patients, healthcare personnel, and visitors; providing treatment and prophylaxis; protecting the environment; and providing appropriate staffing. The public health-healthcare interface comes into prominence during such events, given the need for close collaboration and coordination.

CONCLUSION

This chapter has reviewed high-level trends and developments in HAI surveillance, prevention, and control. This included general concepts in pathogen transmission and HAI epidemiology, common types of HAIs by body site along with associated targeted prevention efforts, complex populations, and issues in HAI prevention and control such as AR, the infrastructure and key functions of HAI programs and their interactions with the public health system. The section below summarizes additional resources organized by key stakeholders in the public health system and professional organizations with expertise in these topics.

RESOURCES FOR SURVEILLANCE, PREVENTION, AND CONTROL OF HAI

- Centers for Disease Control and Prevention:
  - Rates of HAI, device utilization, resistant pathogens, and use of antimicrobials are published intermittently in journals such

as the American Journal of Infection Control and are available from the CDC HAI Data Portal website: www.cdc.gov/hai/data/portal/index.html.

- Other resources on the CDC website include:
- Guidelines for prevention and control of HAI are developed in partnership with HICPAC (https://www.cdc.gov/hicpac/index.html).
- Core Infection Prevention and Control Practices for Safe Healthcare Delivery in All Settings—Recommendations of the Healthcare Infection Control Practices Advisory Committee (HICPAC) (https://www.cdc.gov/hicpac/recommendations/core-practices.html).
- Guidance and educational materials for improving hand hygiene are also available: www.cdc.gov/handwashing.
- Outpatient Resources—The Guide to Infection Prevention for Outpatient Settings, its companion Checklist (appendix A) (https://www.cdc.gov/hai/settings/outpatient/outpatient-care-guidelines.html) and the Outpatient Settings Infection Control Assessment Tool (available at: https://www.cdc.gov/hai/prevent/infection-control-assessment-tools.html), were developed and standardized to assist health departments in evaluating practices in outpatient settings.
- In addition, CDC provides technical assistance with outbreaks of HAI and protocols for monitoring and reporting novel multidrug-resistant organisms. The CDC AR Threats Report available at: https://www.cdc.gov/drugresistance/threat-report-2013/pdf/ar-threats-2013-508.pdf.

Tools for assisting in the response to resistant pathogens https://www.cdc.gov/hai/containment/what-can-be-done.html.

- The Association for Professionals in Infection Control and Epidemiology (APIC; https://apic.org/) and the Society for Healthcare Epidemiology in America (SHEA; http://www.shea-online.org) are professional organizations of persons working in healthcare epidemiology and infection control. Both conduct training activities in infection control and surveillance for HAI.
  - The SHEA/ IDSA Compendium resources are available at: https://www.shea-online.org/index.php/practice-resources/priority-topics/compendium-of-strategies-to-prevent-hais.
  - The SHEA White Paper for IPC Infrastructure available at: https://www.cambridge.org/core/journals/infection-control-and-hospital-epidemiology/article/requirements-for-infrastructure-and-essential-activities-of-infection-control-and-epidemiology-in-hospitals-a-consensus-panel-report/4124C97AE2017326759E3D126B916FB2.
- The Joint Commission on Accreditation of Healthcare Organizations (JCAHO) requires that accredited hospitals have an active infection control program, an infection control committee, and specific written infection control policies and procedures for each of the hospital's departments. The JCAHO also requires written definitions of nosocomial infections, a system for reporting of infections, laboratory support for infection control, an active employee health program, and review of antibiotic use.
- The American Hospital Association's Committee on Infections within Hospitals has published guidelines for establishing infection control programs.
- State health departments and universities provide training courses and advice or assistance in conducting epidemiological investigations. A state-by-state compendium of HAI Activities at: www.cdc.gov/hai/state-based/index.html.
  - A wide variety of HAI/AR related trainings are available on the TRAIN Learning Network site: www.train.org.

References

1. Klevens RM, Edwards JR, Richards CL, et al. Estimating healthcare-associated infections and deaths in U.S. hospitals, 2002. *Public Health Rep.* 2007;122:160–66.
2. Graves N. Economics and preventing hospital-acquired infections. *Emerg Infect Dis.* 2004;10:561–66.
3. Leape LL, Brennan TA, Laird N, et al. The nature of adverse events in hospitalized patients: Results of the Harvard Medical Practice Study II. *N Engl J Med.* 1991;324:377–84.
4. Magill SS, Edwards JR, Bamberg W, et al. Multistate point prevalence survey of healthcare associated infections. *N Engl J Med.* 2014;370:1198–208. https://www.nejm.org/doi/full/10.1056/NEJMoa1306801.
5. Magill SS, O'Leary E, Janelle SJ, et al. Changes in prevalence of health care-associated infections in U.S. hospitals. *N Engl J Med.* 2018;379:1732–44.
6. National Center for Health Statistics. *Health, United States, 2004 with Chartbook on Trends in the Health of Americans.* Hyattsville, MD: NCHS; 2004.
7. U.S. Department of Health and Human Services. National Action Plan to Prevent Health Care-Associated Infections: Road Map to Elimination. 2013. Part 4. Phase two—Outpatient Settings and Influenza Vaccination of Healthcare Personnel. Chapter 5: Ambulatory Surgical Centers. https://health.gov/hcq/pdfs/hai-action-plan-asc.pdf.
8. Jarvis WR. Infection control and changing health-care delivery systems. *Emerg Infect Dis.* 2001;7:170–73.
9. Centers for Disease Control and Prevention. Monitoring hospital-acquired infections to promote patient safety—United States, 1990–1999. *MMWR Morb Mortal Wkly Rep.* 2000;49:149–53.
10. Vincent JL, Bihari DJ, Suter PM, et al. The prevalence of nosocomial infection in intensive care units in Europe. Results of the European Prevalence of Infection in Intensive Care (EPIC) Study. EPIC International Advisory Committee. *JAMA.* 1995;274:639–44.
11. Morris JG, Shay DK, Hebden JN, et al. Enterococci resistant to multiple antimicrobial agents, including vancomycin. Establishment of endemicity in a university medical center. *Ann Intern Med.* 1995;123:250–59.
12. Climo M, Dickema D, Warren DK, et al. Prevalence of the use of central venous access devices within and outside of the intensive care unit: Results of a survey among hospitals in the prevention epicenter program of the Centers for Disease Control and Prevention. *Infect Control Hosp Epidemiol.* 2003;24:942–45.
13. National Healthcare Safety Network (NHSN) Home page, CDC. https://www.cdc.gov/nhsn/index.html.
14. Horan TC, Emori TG. Definitions of key terms used in the NNIS system. *Am J Infect Control.* 1997;25:112–16.
15. Burke JP. Infection control—A problem for patient safety. *N Engl J Med.* 2003;348:651–56.
16. Sohn AH, Garrett DO, Sinkowitz-Cochran RL, et al. Prevalence of nosocomial infections in neonatal intensive care unit patients: Results from the first national point-prevalence survey. *J Pediatr.* 2001;139:821–27.
17. Wenzel RP. The mortality of hospital-acquired bloodstream infections: Need for a new vital statistic? *Int J Epidemiol.* 1988;17:225–27.
18. Townsend TR, Wenzel RP. Nosocomial bloodstream infections in a newborn intensive care unit: A case-controlled matched study of morbidity, mortality, and risk. *Am J Epidemiol.* 1981;14:73–80.
19. Digiovine B, Chenoweth C, Watts C, et al. The attributable mortality and costs of primary nosocomial bloodstream infections in the intensive care unit. *Am J Respir Crit Care Med.* 1999;160:976–81.
20. Kaoutar B, Joly C, Heriteau FL, et al. Nosocomial infections and hospital mortality: A multicenter epidemiological study. *J Hosp Infect.* 2004;58:268–75.
21. Laupland KB, Zygun DA, Davies HD, et al. Population-based assessment of intensive care unit-acquired bloodstream infections in adults: Incidence, risk factors, and associated mortality rate. *Crit Care Med.* 2002;30:2462–67.
22. Diekema DJ, Beekmann SE, Chapin KC, et al. Epidemiology and outcome of nosocomial and community-onset bloodstream infection. *J Clin Microbiol.* 2003;41:3655–60.
23. Pittet D, Tarara D, Wenzel RP. Nosocomial bloodstream infection in critically ill patients. Excess length of stay, extra costs, and attributable mortality. *JAMA.* 1994;271:1598–601.
24. Haley RW, Culver DH, White J, et al. The efficacy of infection surveillance and control programs in preventing nosocomial infections in U.S. hospitals. *Am J Epidemiol.* 1985;121:182–205.

25. Harbarth S, Sax H, Gastmeier P. The preventable proportion of nosocomial infections: An overview of published reports. *J Hosp Infect.* 2003;54:258–66.
26. National and State Healthcare Associated Infections 2016 Progress Report. https://www.cdc.gov/HAI/pdfs/progress-report/hai-progress-report.pdf.
27. National Healthcare Safety Network (NHSN) 2017 Reports. On CDC webpages. https://www.cdc.gov/nhsn/datastat/index.html.
28. Centers for Disease Control and Prevention. Public health focus: Surveillance, prevention, and control of nosocomial infections. *MMWR Morb Mortal Wkly Rep.* 1992;41:783–7.
29. Schreiber PW, Sax H, Wolfensberger A, Clack L, Kuster SP, Swissnoso. The preventable proportion of healthcare-associated infections 2005–2016: Systematic review and meta-analysis. *Infect Control Hosp Epidemiol.* 2018;39(11):1277–95.
30. Perz JF, Thompson ND, Schaefer MK, Patel PR. US outbreak investigations highlight the need for safe injection practices and basic infection control. *Clin Liver Dis.* 2010;14(1):137–51.
31. Centers for Medicare and Medicaid Services. Hospital-Acquired Condition Reduction Program (HACRP). https://www.cms.gov/Medicare/Medicare-Fee-for-Service-Payment/AcuteInpatientPPS/HAC-Reduction-Program.html.
32. Taylor D, Rebmann C, Ashley M, et al. Evolution of ELC Healthcare-Associated Infections/Antimicrobial Resistance (HAI/AR) Programs, 2009–2018. Paper presented at the *Council of State and Territorial Epidemiologists Annual Conference.* June 11, 2018. https://cste.confex.com/cste/2018/meetingapp.cgi/Paper/9828. Accessed May 27, 2020.
33. Vincent JL. Infection control in the intensive-care unit. *Expert Rev Anti Infect Ther.* 2004;2:795–805.
34. Siegel JD, Rhinehart E, Jackson M, Chiarello L, The Healthcare Infection Control Practices Advisory Committee. Guideline for Isolation Precautions: Preventing Transmission of Infectious Agents in Healthcare Settings. 2007. https://www.cdc.gov/infectioncontrol/guidelines/isolation/executive-summary.html.
35. Hota B. Contamination, disinfection, and cross-colonization: Are hospital surfaces reservoirs for nosocomial infection? *Clin Infect Dis.* 2004;39:1182–9.
36. McDonald LC, Gerding DN, Johnson S, et al. Clinical practice guidelines for *Clostridium difficile* infection in adults and children: 2017 Update by the Infectious Diseases Society of America (IDSA) and Society for Healthcare Epidemiology of America (SHEA). *Clin Infect Dis.* 2018;66(7):e1–48.
37. Welsh RM, Bentz ML, Shams A, et al. Survival, persistence, and isolation of the emerging multidrug-resistant pathogenic yeast *Candida auris* on a plastic healthcare surface. *J Clin Microbiol.* 2017;55(10):2996–3005.
38. Centers for Disease Control. Nosocomial infection rates for interhospital comparison: Limitations and possible solutions. *Infect Control Hosp Epidemiol.* 1991;12:609–21.
39. CDC. Core Infection Prevention and Control Practices for Safe Healthcare Delivery in All Settings—Recommendations of the Healthcare Infection Control Practices Advisory Committee (HICPAC). https://www.cdc.gov/hicpac/pdf/core-practices.pdf.
40. Wong ES, Hooton TM. *Guideline for Prevention of Catheter-Associated Urinary Tract Infections.*, Atlanta, GA: Centers for Disease Control, U.S. Department of Health and Human Services, Public Health Service; 1981 (Replacing with new guideline).
41. Lo E, Nicolle LE, Coffin SE, et al. Strategies to prevent catheter-associated urinary tract infections in acute care hospitals: 2014 Update. *Infect Control Hosp Epidemiol.* 2014;35(5):464–79.
42. Saint S, Chenoweth CE. Biofilms and catheter-associated urinary tract infections. *Infect Dis Clin North Am.* 2003;17:411–32.
43. Weber DJ, Sickbert-Bennett EE, Gould CV, Brown VM, Huslage K, Rutala WA. Incidence of catheter-associated and non-cath-eter-associated urinary tract infections in a healthcare system. *Infect Control Hosp Epidemiol.* 2011;32:822–3.
44. Weinstein JW, Mazon D, Pantelick E, Reagan-Cirincione P, Dembry LM, Hierholzer WJ. A decade of prevalence surveys in a tertiary-care center: Trends in nosocomial infection rates, device utilization, and patient acuity. *Infect Control Hosp Epidemiol.* 1999;20:543–8.
45. CDC. Data Summary of HAIs in the US: Assessing Progress 2006–2016. https://www.cdc.gov/hai/data/archive/data-summary-assessing-progress.html.
46. CDC. SIR Reference—SIR. https://www.cdc.gov/nhsn/pdfs/ps-analysis-resources/nhsn-sir-guide.pdf.
47. Rupp ME, Fitzgerald T, Marion N, et al. Effect of silver-coated urinary catheters: Efficacy, cost-effectiveness, and antimicrobial resistance. *Am J Infect Control.* 2004;32:445–50.
48. Brosnahan J, Jull A, Tracy C. Types of urethral catheters for management of short-term voiding problems in hospitalised adults. *Cochrane Database Syst Rev.* 2004;(1):CD004013.
49. Doebbeling BN, Stanley GL, Sheetz CT, et al. Comparative efficacy of alternative hand-washing agents in reducing nosocomial infections in intensive care units. *N Engl J Med.* 1992;327:88–93.
50. Casewell M, Phillips I. Hands as route of transmission for *Klebsiella* species. *Br Med J.* 1977;2:1315–7.
51. Anderson D, Kaye KS, Classen D, et al. Strategies to prevent surgical site infections in acute care hospitals. *Infect Control Hosp Epidemiol.* 2008;29(suppl 1):S51–61. https://www.cambridge.org/core/journals/infection-control-and-hospital-epidemiology/article/strategies-to-prevent-surgical-site-infections-in-acute-care-hospitals-2014-update/EE4D1EC09206F231C69CB0E1A3F4EAC9.
52. Green JW, Wenzel RP. Postoperative wound infection: A controlled study of the increased duration of hospital stay and direct cost of hospitalization. *Ann Surg.* 1977;185:264–8.
53. Gaynes RP, Culver DH, Horan TC, et al. Surgical site infection rates in the United States, 1992–1998: The National Nosocomial Infections Surveillance System basic SSI risk index. *Clin Infect Dis.* 2001;33:S69–77.
54. Manian F, Meyer L. Adjunctive use of monthly physician questionnaires for surveillance of surgical site infections after hospital discharge and in ambulatory surgical patients: Report of a seven year experience. *Am J Infect Control.* 1997;25:390–4.
55. Sands K, Vineyard G, Platt R. Surgical site infections occurring after hospital discharge. *J Infect Dis.* 1996;173:963–70.
56. Mangram AJ, Horan TC, Pearson ML, et al. The Hospital Infection Control Practices Advisory Committee. Guideline for prevention of surgical site infection, 1999. *Infect Control Hosp Epidemiol.* 1999;20:248–80.
57. Barrios-Torres SI, Umscheid CA, Bratzler DW, et al. Centers for Disease Control and Prevention Guideline for the Prevention of surgical site infection, 2017. *JAMA Surg.* 2017;152(8):784–91.
58. Weinstein MP, Towns ML, Quartey SM, et al. The clinical significance of positive blood cultures in the 1990s: A prospective comprehensive evaluation of the microbiology, epidemiology, and outcome of bacteremia and fungemia in adults. *Clin Infect Dis.* 1997;24:584–602.
59. Stone PW, Larson E, Najib Kawar L. A systematic audit of economic evidence linking nosocomial infections and infection control interventions: 1990–2000. *Am J Infect Control.* 2002;30:145–52.
60. Pittet D, Wenzel RP. Nosocomial bloodstream infections. Secular trends in rates, mortality, and contribution to total hospital deaths. *Arch Intern Med.* 1995;155:1177–84.
61. Alter MJ, Tokars JI, Arduino MJ, et al. Nosocomial infections associated with hemodialysis. In: Mayhall CG, ed. *Hospital Epidemiology and Infection Control,* 3rd ed. Philadelphia: Lippincott Williams & Wilkins; 2004, pp. 1139–60.
62. Centers for Disease Control and Prevention. Guidelines for the prevention of intravascular catheter-related infections. *MMWR Morb Mortal Wkly Rep.* 2002;51(RR-10):1–28.
63. Wisplinghoff H, Bischoff T, Tallent SM, et al. Nosocomial bloodstream infections in U.S. hospitals: Analysis of 24,179 cases from a prospective nationwide surveillance study. *Clin Infect Dis.* 2004;39:309–17.
64. Fagan RP, Edwards JR, Park BJ, Fridkin SK, Magill SS. Incidence trends in pathogen-specific central line-associated bloodstream infections in US intensive care units, 1990–2010. *Infect Control Hosp Epidemiol.* 2013;34(9):893–9.
65. Climo M, Diekema D, Warren DK, et al. Prevalence of the use of central venous access devices within and outside of the intensive care unit: Results of a survey among hospitals in the prevention epicenter program of the Centers for Disease Control and Prevention. *Infect Control Hosp Epidemiol.* 2003;24:942–5.
66. Marschall J, Mermel LA, Fakih M, et al. Strategies to prevent central line-associated bloodstream infections in acute care hospitals: 2014 Update. *Infect Control Hosp Epidemiol.* 2007;28:905–9.
67. CDC Vital Signs. Making healthcare saget: Reducing bloodstream infections. March 2011. https://www.cdc.gov/vitalsigns/pdf/2011-03-vitalsigns.pdf.
68. Centers for Disease Control and Prevention. Guidelines for preventing health care-associated pneumonia, 2003: Recommendations of CDC and the Healthcare Infection Control Practices Advisory Committee. *MMWR Morb Mortal Wkly Rep.* 2004;53(RR-3):1–36.

69. Kalil AC, Metersky ML, Klompas M, et al. Management of adults with hospital-acquired and ventilator-associated pneumonia: 2016 Clinical practice guidelines by the Infectious Diseases Society of America and the American Thoracic Society. *Clin Infect Dis.* 2016;63(5):e61–111.
70. Bergmans DCJ, Bonten MJM. Nosocomial pneumonia. In: Mayhall CG, ed. *Hospital Epidemiology and Infection Control*, 3rd ed. Philadelphia: Lippincott Williams & Wilkins; 2004, pp. 311–40.
71. Cook DJ, Walter SD, Cook RJ, et al. Incidence of and risk factors for ventilator-associated pneumonia in critically ill patients. *Ann Intern Med.* 1998;129:433–40.
72. Klompas M, Branson R, Eichenwald EC, et al. Strategies to prevent ventilator-associated pneumonia in acute care hospitals: 2014 Update. *Infect Control Hosp Epidemiol.* 2014;35(8):915–36.
73. U.S. Department of Health and Human Services. National action plan to prevent health care-associated infections: Road map to elimination. 2013. https://health.gov/hcq/pdfs/hai-action-plan-cover-toc.pdf.
74. CDC. Nursing home and assisted living facilities (LTCF) Page. https://www.cdc.gov/longtermcare/index.html.
75. Harris-Kojetin L, Sengupta M, Park-Lee E, et al. Long-term care providers and services users in the United States: Data from the National Study of Long-Term Care Providers, 2013–2014. National Center for Health Statistics. *Vital Health Stat 3.* 2016;(38):1–105. https://www.cdc.gov/nchs/data/series/sr_03/sr03_038.pdf.
76. Khanna KV, Markham RB. A perspective on cellular immunity in the elderly. *Clin Infect Dis.* 1999;28(4):710–3.
77. Richards C. Infections in residents of long-term care facilities: An agenda for research. *J Am Geriatr Soc.* 2002;50:570–6.
78. High KP, Bradley S, Loeb M, et al. A new paradigm for clinical investigation of infectious syndromes in older adults: Assessment of functional status as a risk factor and outcome measure. *Clin Infect Dis.* 2005;40:114–22.
79. CDC. Nursing homes and assisted living (Long term care facilities [LTCF]). Prevention tools. https://www.cdc.gov/longtermcare/prevention/index.html.
80. Quality Improvement Organizations. QIO New. National nursing home quality care collaborative aims to create lasting improvements. May 2015. https://qioprogram.org/qionews/articles/national-nursing-home-quality-care-collaborative-aims-create-lasting-improvements.
81. U.S. Renal Data System, USRDS 2003. *Annual Data Report: Atlas of End-Stage Renal Disease in the United States.* Bethesda, MD: National Institutes of Health, National Institute of Diabetes and Digestive and Kidney Diseases; 2003.
82. CDC. Vital signs. Making healthcare safer. Reducing bloodstream infections. https://www.cdc.gov/vitalsigns/pdf/2011-03-vitalsigns.pdf.
83. Centers for Disease Control and Prevention. Recommendations for preventing transmission of infections among chronic hemodialysis patients. *MMWR Morb Mortal Wkly Report.* 2001;50(RR-5):1–43.
84. Fridkin SK. Vancomycin-intermediate and resistant *Staphylococcus aureus*: What the infectious disease specialist needs to know. *Clin Infect Dis.* 2001;32:108–15.
85. Berns JS, Tokars JI. Preventing bacterial infections and antimicrobial resistance in dialysis patients. *Am J Kidney Dis.* 2002;40(5):886–98.
86. CDC. CDC Approach to BSI prevention in dialysis facilities. Reviewed June 15, 2016. https://www.cdc.gov/dialysis/prevention-tools/core-interventions.html.
87 Yi SH, Kallen AJ, Hess S, et al. Sustained infection reduction in outpatient hemodialysis centers participating in a collaborative bloodstream infection prevention effort. *Infect Control Hosp Epidemiol.* 2016;37(7):863–6.
88. Patel PR, Yi SH, Booth S, et.al. Bloodstream infection rates in outpatient hemodialysis facilities participating in a collaborative prevention effort: A quality improvement report. *Am J Kidney Dis.* 2013;62(2):322–30.
89. Kossover RA, Chi CJ, Wise ME, et al. Infection prevention and control standards in assisted living facilities: Are residents' needs being met? *J Am Med Dir Assoc.* 2014;15:47–53.
90. Centers for Disease Control and Prevention. Transmission of hepatitis B and C viruses in outpatient settings—New York, Oklahoma, and Nebraska, 2000–2002. *MMWR Morb Mortal Wkly Rep.* 2003;52:901–4.
91. Wade BH. Outpatient/out of hospital care issues. In: Wenzel RP, ed. *Prevention and Control of Nosocomial Infections*, 3rd ed. Baltimore: Williams & Wilkins; 1997, pp. 243–60.
92. CDC. One & Only Campaign. 2009. http://www.oneandonlycampaign.org/about/the-campaign.
93. Danzig LE, Short LJ, Collins K, et al. Bloodstream infections associated with a needleless intravenous infusion system in patients receiving home infusion therapy. *JAMA.* 1995;273:1862–4.
94. CDC. Healthcare associated infections in outpatient settings. https://www.cdc.gov/hai/settings/outpatient/outpatient-settings.html and dental outpatient resources: https://www.cdc.gov/oralhealth/infectioncontrol/index.html.
95. Szeinbach SL, Pauline J, Villa KF, Commerford SR, Collins A, Seoane-Vazquez E. Evaluating catheter complications and outcomes in patients receiving home parenteral nutrition. *J Eval Clin Pract.* 2015;21(1):153–9.
96. Van Winkle P, Whiffen T, Liu IL. Experience using peripherally inserted central venous catheters for outpatient parenteral antibiotic therapy in children at a community hospital. *Pediatr Infect Dis J.* 2008;27(12):1069–72.
97. UHF. Toolkit. Preventing Central Line-Associated Bloodstream Infection (CLABSI) in the Home Care Setting. 2016. file:///Users/belindaostrowsky/Downloads/PICC-LineToolkit_FINAL_(004)%20(1).pdf (fixing link).
98. Smolinski MS, Hamburg MA, Lederberg J, eds. *Microbial Threats to Health: Emergence, Detection, and Response.* Washington, DC: Institute of Medicine, National Academy of Sciences; 2003, pp. 32–41.
99. Shlaes DM, Gerding DN, John JF, et al. Society for Healthcare Epidemiology of America and Infectious Diseases Society of America Joint Committee on the Prevention of Antimicrobial Resistance: Guidelines for the prevention of antimicrobial resistance in hospitals. *Infect Control Hosp Epidemiol.* 1997;18:275–91.
100. CDC. Antibiotic resistance threats in the United States 2013. https://www.cdc.gov/drugresistance/threat-report-2013/pdf/ar-threats-2013-508.pdf.
101. Woodworth KR, Walters MS, Weiner LM. Vital signs issue details: Containment of novel multidrug-resistant organisms and resistance mechanisms—United States, 2006–2017. *MMWR Morb Mortal Wkly Rep.* 2018:67(13);396–401. https://www.cdc.gov/mmwr/volumes/67/wr/mm6713e1.htm?s_cid=mm6713e1_w.
102. CDC. Interim guidance for a public health response to contain novel or targeted MDROs. https://www.cdc.gov/hai/outbreaks/docs/Health-Response-Contain-MDRO.pdf.
103. Haley RW, Schachtman RH. The emergence of infection surveillance and control programs in U.S. hospitals: An assessment, 1976. *Am J Epidemiol.* 1980;11:574–91.
104. O'Boyle C, Jackson M, Henly SJ. Staffing requirements for infection control programs in U.S. health care facilities: Delphi project. *Am J Infect Control.* 2002;30:321–33.
105. Gaynes RP, Solomon S. Improving hospital-acquired infection rates: The CDC experience. *Jt Comm J Qual Improv.* 1996;22:457–67.
106. Bryant KA, Harris AD, Gould CV, et al. Necessary infrastructure of infection prevention and healthcare epidemiology programs: A review. *Infect Control Hosp Epidemiol.* 2016;37:371–80.
107. Sartor C, Edwards JR, Gaynes RP, Culver DH. Evolution of hospital participation in the National Nosocomial Infections Surveillance System, 1986–1993. *Am J Infect Control.* 1995;23:364–8.
108. Gaynes R, Richards C, Edwards J, et al. Feeding back surveillance data to prevent hospital-acquired infections. *Emerg Infect Dis.* 2001;7:295–8.
109. Leape LL. Reporting of adverse events. *N Engl J Med.* 2002;347:1633–8.
110. Healthcare Infection Control Practices Advisory Committee (HICPAC). Guidance on public reporting of healthcare-associated infections. https://www.cdc.gov/hicpac/recommendations/index.html#PubReportingHAI.
111. Horan TC, Gaynes RP. Surveillance of nosocomial infections. In: Mayhall CG, ed. *Hospital Epidemiology and Infection Control*, 3rd ed. Philadelphia: Lippincott Williams & Wilkins; 2004, pp. 1659–702.
112. Tokars JI, Richards C, Andrus M, et al. The changing face of surveillance for health care-associated infections. *Clin Infect Dis.* 2004;39:1347–52.
113. CDC. About NHSN. https://www.cdc.gov/nhsn/about-nhsn/index.html.
114. CDC. The NSHN standardized infection ratio (SIR)—A guide to SIR. March 2018. https://www.cdc.gov/nhsn/pdfs/ps-analysis-resources/nhsn-sir-guide.pdf.
115. Broderick A, Mori M, Nettleman MD, et al. Nosocomial infections: Validation of surveillance and computer modeling to identify patients at risk. *Am J Epidemiol.* 1990;131:734–42.
116. Trick WE, Zagorski BM, Tokars JI, et al. Computer algorithms to detect bloodstream infections. *Emerg Infect Dis.* 2004;10:1612–20.
117. Yokoe DS, Noskin GA, Cunningham SM, et al. Enhanced identification of postoperative infections among inpatients. *Emerg Infect Dis.* 2004;10:1924–30.

118. Shepard J, Hadhazy E, Frederick J, et al. Using electronic medical records to increase the efficiency of catheter-associated urinary tract infection surveillance for National Health and Safety Network reporting. *Am J Infect Control.* 2014;42:e33–6.

119. Woeltje KF, Lautenbach E. Informatics and epidemiology in infection control. *Infect Dis Clin North Am.* 2011;25:261–70.

120. Cardo D, Dennehy PH, Halverson P, et al. Moving toward elimination of healthcare-associated infections: A call to action. *Am J Infect Control.* 2010;38:671–5. http://www.apic.org/Resource_/TinyMceFileManager/Advocacy-PDFs/AJIC_Elimin.pdf.

121. CDC. Safe healthcare blog. https://blogs.cdc.gov/safehealthcare/341-days-without-a-c-difficile-infection-how-mercy-health-st-anne-hospital-reduced-c-difficile-infection-rates-to-zero/.

122. Soe M, Gould CV, Pollock D, Edwards J. Targeted assessment for prevention of healthcare-associated infections: A new prioritization metric. *Infect Control Hosp Epidemiol.* 2015;36(12):1379–84.

123. Taylor D, Rebmann C, Ashley M, et al. Evolution of ELC healthcare-associated infections/antimicrobial resistance (HAI/AR) programs, 2009–2018. Paper presented at the *Council of State and Territorial Epidemiologists Annual Conference.* June 11. 2018. https://cste.confex.com/cste/2018/meetingapp.cgi/Paper/9828. Accessed May 27, 2020.

124. Council for Outbreak Response. Healthcare-Associated Infections (HAIs) and Antimicrobial-Resistant Pathogens (AR). http://corha.org/.

125. Ksiazek TG, Erdman D, Goldsmith CS, et al. A novel coronovirus associated with severe acute respiratory syndrome. *N Engl J Med.* 2003;348:1953–66.

CHAPTER 153

Antibiotic Resistance and Stewardship

Amanda Beaudoin • Laura E. Norton

ANTIBIOTIC RESISTANCE (AR)

Overview of the Problem

History of Antibiotics and AR

Antibiotics are chemical substances, usually produced by living microorganisms, which kill or inhibit the growth of other microorganisms.[1] Many antibiotics are naturally produced by bacteria or fungi. In natural environments, these compounds are produced at subinhibitory concentrations to facilitate interaction and communication with, and protection against, other microbes. Antibiotic resistance (AR), the ability of microorganisms to remain viable and multiply in the presence of antibiotics, is a natural phenomenon, driven by the ability of microorganisms to adapt to environmental pressures through genetic mutations and sharing of genetic material.[2] Adaptation to the selective pressure of antibiotics can occur *in vivo* as well as in built and natural environments.[2] Bacteria have developed AR characteristics throughout history, and genes conferring resistance to antibiotics that are used clinically today have been identified in DNA obtained from 30,000-year-old Beringian permafrost sediments and cave environments.[3,4] Antibiotics are a type of antimicrobial, which is a broader group of agents used to treat infections caused by microorganisms (e.g., bacteria, viruses, fungi). Although antimicrobial resistance of other types can present clinical and public health challenges, this chapter will focus on antibiotics.

Human discovery of antibiotics revolutionized medicine, providing a cure for many previously fatal and debilitating infectious diseases. It was not long after the discovery of antibiotics that the medical community became aware that the use of antibiotics was associated with consequences. Sir Alexander Fleming received the Nobel Prize in 1945 for his discovery of penicillin. That same year, Fleming warned of the risk of bacteria becoming resistant to penicillin and cautioned the medical community to be thoughtful in its use.[5,6] In modern times, a widespread AR crisis that significantly impacts our ability to treat infections is driven by the massive and at times inappropriate use of antibiotics. Because AR can be directly and indirectly influenced by antibiotic exposure, the problem of AR parallels the use patterns of clinically important drugs. Clinical resistance can appear within a few years of a drug's introduction.[7,8] The nature of this adaptation means that we need to continuously develop new antibiotics. At the current pace of spread, the global problem of AR is estimated to result in millions of deaths and US$100 trillion of expense by 2050.[9] This crisis highlights the need for judicious use of antibiotics, development of new antibiotics, and alternative approaches to killing or slowing the growth of bacteria.

Genetics of AR

Acquired Resistance

Bacteria acquire resistance through two mechanisms: point mutation and horizontal gene transfer (HGT) as described below.

Spontaneous Mutation Point mutation, or changes to individual DNA base pairs, contributes to bacterial genetic variability and drives bacterial adaptation to external stressors like antibiotics. Clonal replication of organisms with advantageous mutations allows persistence and spread of resistant phenotypes. Given the rapidity with which bacteria replicate (e.g., *Staphylococcus aureus* divides approximately every 30 minutes, yielding over one million replicates in <12 hours), the chance of beneficial mutations emerging is apparent.[10]

Resistance of *Mycobacterium tuberculosis* (causative agent of TB) develops exclusively by spontaneous mutation in response to antibiotic exposure.[11] A disease for which elimination optimism was high, tuberculosis now impacts 25% of the world's population.[12] MDR *M. tuberculosis* is resistance to first-line drugs isoniazid and rifampin, and extremely drug-resistant (XDR) *M. tuberculosis* is defined as MDR-TB plus resistance to at least one drug in both the fluoroquinolone class and the group of second-line injectable agents (amikacin, capreomycin, kanamycin).[13] Although *M. tuberculosis* acquires resistance by spontaneous mutation in an individual patient, once MDR or XDR organisms develop, they can be transmitted among people by using the same transmission routes as non-MDR *M. tuberculosis*. Of an estimated 558,000 new tuberculosis cases globally in 2017 that were resistant to rifampin, the most effective first-line drug, 82% were MDR.[13] Almost half (47%) of those cases were in India, China, and the Russian Federation.

Horizontal Gene Transfer In addition to accumulation of point mutations in response to antibiotic exposure, AR traits can be acquired through HGT, the transfer of genetic material among bacteria. Acquired genes that provide a selective advantage or have a neutral effect on the recipient organism can remain for prolonged periods within the clonal lineage.[14,15] Bacterial HGT occurs by three main processes: conjugation (direct cell-to-cell transfer of genetic material), transduction (bacteriophage-mediated gene transfer), and transformation (uptake of extracellular genetic material). The genetic tools required for completion of HGT include plasmids, transposons, insertion sequences, and integrons. Some bacteria are more able to acquire genetic elements than others, likely because of the differences in cell structure (e.g., cell wall) and variability of HGT genetic functions.[16] HGT can occur between bacteria of differing species and genera.[17,18]

Plasmids are autonomously replicating, circular pieces of DNA in which antibiotic resistance genes (ARG) can be embedded. They play an important role in HGT. Plasmids store additional, nonchromosomal, genetic information and are transmissible from one bacterium to another by the processes of conjugation and transformation. Plasmids are either conjugative, mobilizable, or nonmobilizable.[19] Conjugative plasmids possess genes that facilitate development of a direct connection between two bacterial cell membranes, allowing transfer of single-stranded plasmid DNA from one cytoplasm to the other. Mobilizable and nonmobilizable plasmids are capable of moving from one bacterium to another in the presence of or assisted by a conjugative plasmid.[20]

An important characteristic of plasmids is their ability to serve as a framework on which genes can assemble and spread. Since the start of the antibiotic drug era, the frequency of bacterial plasmid carriage has increased.[21,22] Increased plasmid availability might influence the frequency with which chromosomal resistance genes mobilize to plasmids. In turn, antibiotic exposures provide selective pressures needed to maintain these mobile resistance determinants. Chromosomal bla_{CTX-M} (beta-lactamase) gene mobilizations might exemplify this theory, as they have become increasingly plasmid-associated and have transitioned from incidental organisms associated with humans to common human and animal pathogens, like *E. coli*.[21]

Transposable genetic elements (transposons and insertion sequences) are DNA segments capable of insertion into chromosome or plasmid DNA, independent of homologous recombination processes.[16] Transposons that carry ARG are flanked by insertion sequences, which facilitate the insertion and excision processes. Some transposable genetic elements are conjugative and capable of facilitating their own movement from one bacterial cell to another. Unlike plasmids, transposons and insertion sequences cannot replicate on their own and rely on chromosome or plasmid replication.[20] Recombination events can involve large DNA sequences and lead to rapid emergence of multidrug resistance in clinically important bacteria, and Gram-negative bacteria, in particular.[16] Beyond conferring AR, transposable genetic elements can have other impacts on the bacterial genome. In some cases, recombination events lead to loss of gene function and loss of overall fitness.[23,24]

Also contributing to the transfer and spread of ARG are integrons, which provide targets for insertion of ARG. These genetic elements are characterized by the inclusion of insertion and integrase genes and the ability to acquire and transcribe ARG in expression cassettes.[25,26] Integrons are not independently mobile but can contribute to the spread of AR by linkages to transposons, insertion sequences, and plasmids.[27] Of the five classes of integrons that can be mobilized, class 1 integrons are the most important to the clinical issue of AR and have been found to carry many different ARG cassettes, including those granting resistance to β-lactams, aminoglycosides, chloramphenicol, trimethoprim, rifampin, erythromycin, fosfomycin, lincomycin, and quaternary-ammonium-compound antiseptics.[27]

Bacteria can take up DNA directly from the external environment (transformation) and from bacteriophages (transduction).[28] Recent study of these mechanisms has focused on the role of the natural and built environments in the spread of resistance and the development of novel methods of treatment for resistant infections.[29–31]

These HGT mechanisms heavily influence the AR patterns encountered in clinical medicine. One example of considerable clinical significance now is β-lactam resistance in the Enterobacteriaceae family.[11] Plasmid-associated extended-spectrum β-lactamase (ESBL) and carbapenemase genes have been implicated in conferring resistance to critical antibiotic classes, such as cephalosporins and carbapenems.

Intrinsic Resistance

In addition to acquiring resistance by genetic mutation or HGT, members of a given bacterial species can have universal genome-based resistance (e.g., lack the target for an antibiotic's mechanism of action), which is termed "intrinsic resistance." The presence of intrinsic resistance guides some of the general principles of antibacterial therapy. For example, Gram-negative bacteria possess an outer membrane and express efflux pumps, providing reduced permeability and preventing the accumulation of sufficient intracellular drug concentrations, respectively.[32]

The widespread emergence of MDR Gram-negative bacteria has led to the increasing consideration of colistin as last-line treatment for Gram-negative infections.[33] After falling out of use because of toxicity, the polymixin antibiotics colistin and polymixin B are again in the spotlight because of their ability to disrupt key intrinsic resistance mechanisms of Gram-negative bacteria.[34] With emerging resistance to polymixins, including transmissible plasmid-conferred *mcr* resistance, treatment of MDR Gram-negative infections will continue to be a challenge.[35]

Mechanisms of AR

"Mechanisms" of resistance are cellular functions that enable bacteria to resist the effects of an antibiotic. These mechanisms can be grouped broadly as: (1) restriction of antibiotic access to its target; (2) inactivation of the antibiotic compound; and (3) alteration of the antibiotic target. A single bacterial cell might employ multiple resistance mechanisms, and drug classes are often thwarted with more than one approach.[36] Resistance mechanisms for important AR threats will be highlighted in the following sections.

Important AR Threats

AR is a serious threat to the health of people in the United States and around the world. In recent years, many pathogens have become increasingly difficult to treat. The most concerning of these are identified in the 2013 Centers for Disease Control and Prevention (CDC) report, *Antibiotic Resistance Threats in the United States, 2013* and in the *World Health Organization Global Priority List of AR Bacteria to Guide Research, Discovery, and Development of New Antibiotics* (Table 153-1).[7,37] The epidemiology of AR is not homogenous and, at national and global levels, reports such as these are essential to increase awareness and prioritize action.

In this section we will provide examples of AR in a few organisms. Please see organism-specific chapters for more detailed discussion.

Gram-Positive Threats

Staphylococcus Aureus *S. aureus* is common skin flora, frequently associated with asymptomatic nasal carriage and superficial skin infections, such as impetigo. *S. aureus* is also among the most common causes of more severe and invasive infections, such as skin and soft tissue infection, sepsis, pneumonia, and endocarditis.[38,39] Methicillin-resistant *S. aureus* (MRSA) has been recognized as a concern in healthcare facilities in Europe and the United States since the 1960s, causing serious disease and presenting therapeutic challenges,[40] and infections in community settings since the late 1990s. Methicillin resistance results from expression of the *mecA* gene, which is carried on a larger chromosomal genetic element (SCCmec) and encodes penicillin binding protein (PBP) 2a (PBP2a). In susceptible *S. aureus*, cellular PBP binds to beta-lactam antibiotics, which are then incorporated as a substrate of cell wall biosynthesis, leading to defective cell wall structure and subsequent death during replication. PBP2a of MRSA binds to beta-lactam antibiotics with less affinity, precluding the inclusion of the antibiotic in cell wall development.[41] With *mecA* and PBP2a, *S. aureus* is capable of avoiding the impact of beta-lactam antibiotics, including methicillin, nafcillin, oxacillin, and almost all cephalosporins.[20]

MRSA infections are characterized as healthcare-associated (HA) and community-associated (CA). These categories are distinguished by epidemiologic and microbiologic characteristics, including exposure history and clonal type and toxin profile of the isolate.[38,42–44] CA-MRSA is a frequent cause of *S. aureus* skin and soft tissue infections, and is typically identified as USA300 strain.[45,46] In the United States, CDC tracks invasive MRSA infection (MRSA cultured from normally sterile body sites such as blood or pleural fluid).[47] In 2014, an estimated 72,444 invasive MRSA cases occurred, resulting in an incidence rate of 22.7 cases/100,000 population (95% CI 19.56–26.61).[48] The contributions of CA and HA-MRSA to the estimated 2014 MRSA burden were approximately 24% and 76%, respectively, with most infections being healthcare-associated with onset in the community (rather than hospital onset).

TABLE 153-1 AR PRIORITIES IDENTIFIED BY U.S. CENTERS FOR DISEASE CONTROL AND PREVENTION (CDC) AND WORLD HEALTH ORGANIZATION (WHO)

CDC: Antibiotic Resistance Threats in the United States, 2013		WHO: Global Priority List of AR Bacteria to Guide Research, Discovery, and Development of New Antibiotics, 2017
Urgent Threat Level	**Estimated No. Cases (Deaths) per Year**	**Priority 1: Critical**
Clostridium difficile	500,000 (29,000)(267)	Carbapenem-resistant *Acinetobacter baumannii*
Carbapenem-resistant Enterobacteriaceae	9,300 (610)	Carbapenem-resistant *Pseudomonas aeruginosa*
Drug-resistant *Neisseria gonorrhoeae*	246,000 (<5)	Carbapenem-resistant, 3rd-generation cephalosporin-resistant Enterobacteriaceae
Serious Threat Level		**Priority 2: High**
Multidrug-resistant *Acinetobacter*	7,300 (500)	Vancomycin-resistant *Enterococcus faecium*
Drug-resistant *Campylobacter*	310,000 (28)	Methicillin-resistant, vancomycin-intermediate and vancomycin-resistant *Staphylococcus aureus*
Fluconazole-resistant *Candida*	3,400 (220)	Clarithromycin-resistant *Helicobacter pylori*
Extended spectrum β-lactamase producing Enterobacteriaceae	26,000 (1,700)	Fluoroquinolone-resistant *Campylobacter*
Vancomycin-resistant *Enterococcus*	20,000 (1,300)	Fluoroquinolone-resistant *Salmonella*
Multidrug-resistant *Pseudomonas aeruginosa*	6,700 (440)	3rd-generation cephalosporin-resistant and fluoroquinolone-resistant *Neisseria gonorrhoeae*
Drug-resistant nontyphoidal *Salmonella*	100,000 (40)	**Priority 3: Medium**
Drug-resistant *Salmonella* Typhi	3,800 (<5)	Penicillin nonsusceptible *Streptococcus pneumoniae*
Drug-resistant *Shigella*	27,000 (<5)	Ampicillin-resistant *Haemophilus influenzae*
Methicillin-resistant *Staphylococcus aureus*	80,000 (11,000)	Fluoroquinolone-resistant *Shigella spp.*
Drug-resistant *Streptococcus pneumoniae*	1,200,000 (7,000)	
Drug-resistant tuberculosis	1,042 (50)	
Concerning Threat Level		
Vancomycin-resistant *Staphylococcus aureus*	<5 (<5)	
Erythromycin-resistant Group A *Streptococcus*	1,300 (160)	
Clindamycin-resistant Group B *Streptococcus*	7,600 (440)	

Note: Except where otherwise referenced, CDC estimates of cases and deaths are taken from the report Antibiotic Resistance Threats in the United States, 2013.[7] Surveillance data used for CDC estimates differ for each organism. Full estimation methodology can be found in the report index.

Vancomycin is a first-line treatment for MRSA infections. However, several cases of vancomycin-resistant *S. aureus* (VRSA) have been detected in the United States and elsewhere.[7] Genomic studies show that VRSA isolates have independently acquired the vancomycin-resistant transposon (and VanA phenotype) from enterococcal benefactors.[49,50] When MRSA is also resistant to vancomycin, there can be limited treatment options. Fortunately, all VRSA isolates detected in the United States to date have been susceptible to other FDA-approved drugs.[51]

Enterococcus *Enterococcus* spp. are commensal organisms of human and animal gastrointestinal tracts, plants, and the natural environment.[52] Enterococcal diversity is considerable in natural settings, and the organisms play an important role in the microflora of people and animals. Clinical infection is most often caused by *Enterococcus faecalis* and *Enterococcus faecium* and occurs primarily among patients with weakened immune systems, medical devices, or healthcare exposure. Enterococci demonstrate intrinsic resistance to beta-lactam antibiotics (by low-affinity PBP), aminoglycosides (prevention of drug entry into the cell), and trimethoprim-sulfamethoxazole (bypassing drug's effect by another cellular pathway). Beta-lactam-aminoglycoside combination therapy facilitates higher intracellular levels of the aminoglycoside and has been a standard treatment for enterococcal infections.[53] Enterococci are also intrinsically resistant to lincosamides and streptogramins, perhaps by a drug efflux mechanism.[54] Intrinsic resistance is supplemented by acquired resistance to beta-lactams (e.g., beta-lactamase production, PBP mutations), high-level acquired resistance to aminoglycosides (e.g., genes encoding phosphorylases), and glycopeptides, such as vancomycin (e.g., altered affinity of antibiotic target associated with the enzymatic actions conferred by the VanA or VanB operon).[54]

First noted in 1988, vancomycin resistance is not uncommon in *E. faecalis* (3.5–9.8%) and *E. faecium* (58–85%) organisms causing healthcare-associated infections in the United States, with the likelihood of resistance varying by infection type (i.e., central-line-associated bloodstream infection, catheter-associated urinary tract infection, skin and soft tissue infection).[55] Enterococci have been noted to rapidly develop resistance to new antimicrobial drugs intended to treat Gram-positive infections.[56]

Group A Streptococcus Group A Streptococcus (GAS, *Streptococcus pyogenes*) is a common cause of upper respiratory tract infection, including pharyngitis, and can cause a range of skin and soft tissue infections, varying in severity from impetigo to cellulitis and necrotizing fasciitis. GAS is also a cause of streptococcal toxic shock syndrome (STSS). GAS isolates currently do not demonstrate resistance to penicillin, the recommended first-line treatment for GAS infections. However, through the national Active Bacterial Core Surveillance (ABCs) program, CDC has found that 10% of invasive GAS isolates in the United States are resistant to erythromycin.[7] Resistance to erythromycin also confers resistance to azithromycin, a common antibiotic alternative for patients with penicillin allergy. CDC also reports 3.4% of invasive GAS isolates are resistant to clindamycin, an antibiotic commonly used in cases of STSS and necrotizing fasciitis to supplement treatment with penicillin, because of its antitoxin properties.[7,57] These emerging resistance profiles make it more difficult to treat GAS infections.

The major mechanisms of GAS macrolide resistance are target site modification by ribosomal methylation (conferred by chromosomal *ermB* and *ermTR* genes) and active drug efflux by transmembrane pump (conferred by *mefA*).[58,59] Because the drugs demonstrate functional overlap, *ermB* and *ermTR* genes can confer resistance to macrolide, lincosamide, and streptogramin B antibiotics, in what are referred to as MLS_B phenotypes.[60–63] In the constitutive MLS ($cMLS_B$) phenotype, which is associated with *ermB*, resistance to both erythromycin and clindamycin is present. The inducible MLS ($iMLS_B$) phenotype, associated with *ermTR*, is defined by erythromycin resistance with inducible clindamycin resistance. However, inducible resistance might mutate to constitutive expression. Resistance to some macrolides and not clindamycin is conferred by *mefA* a membrane protein gene and referred to as the M phenotype.[64,65]

Group B Streptococcus In the United States, Group B Streptococcus (GBS, *Streptococcus agalactiae*) is perhaps best known for its ability to cause sepsis in newborns but can also be a cause of invasive disease in adults, especially those with comorbidities, pregnant women, and the elderly, and GBS infection disproportionally affects African Americans.[66,67] In 2016, estimated rates of invasive GBS infection in neonates <7 days old were 0.24/1000 live births over all U.S. births and 0.51/1000 for African American births.[68] There is a growing concern about GBS resistance to clindamycin and vancomycin.[7] In 2015, 42% of isolates tested in ABCs were resistant to clindamycin. Mechanisms of GBS resistance to erythromycin and clindamycin are similar to those for GAS and are generally mediated by *erm* and *mef* genes, although it is thought that the cMLS phenotype is not limited to isolates expressing *ermB*, and the M phenotype can be encoded by *mefA* and *mefE*.[69,70]

In 2014, two nonepidemiologically linked cases of vancomycin-resistant GBS were detected in New York and New Mexico.[71] Sufficient divergence in the gene sequences of the two isolates indicates that each acquired vancomycin resistance independently and perhaps by horizontal gene transfer from *Enterococcus faecalis*. Rare isolates with decreased susceptibility to penicillin, associated with mutations in PBPs have been detected.[72] The rates of AR in GBS have increased, and continued surveillance is essential.[73]

Streptococcus Pneumoniae *Streptococcus pneumoniae*, or pneumococcus, is the leading cause of bacterial pneumonia and meningitis in the United States and is an important cause of bloodstream, ear, and sinus infections.[7] Resistance has been seen in particular to penicillin and macrolide antibiotics. Penicillin resistance is driven by decreased PBP affinity for penicillin and, depending on which of the six *S. pneumoniae* PBP is altered, can be low-level or high-level resistance.[74,75] Resistance determinants, including those from nonpathogenic pneumococci and other *Streptococcus* species (e.g., *Streptococcus mitis*), can be obtained by clinically relevant pneumococcal serotypes through transformation. These gene transfers can facilitate incremental transition of a clone from low- to high-level resistance.[76–78] As a result of horizontal *pbp* gene spread and accumulation of additional point mutations, a diversity of resistance profiles can be observed within pneumococcal serotypes, including resistance to other beta-lactams, like cephalosporins.[79]

Macrolide antibiotics block pneumococcal protein assembly by binding to 23S ribosomal RNA in the 50S-ribosome subunit.[80,81] *ErmB*, *mefA/E*, and *mel* genes confer resistance primarily by facilitating drug target site alteration (*ermB*) and efflux from the bacterial cell (*mefA/E*, *mel*).[81–83]

Because of growing resistance of *S. pneumoniae* to beta-lactam and macrolide antibiotics, respiratory fluoroquinolones have been recommended for treatment of community-acquired pneumonia. As overall use of fluoroquinolones has increased, pneumococcal fluoroquinolone resistance has emerged and threatens to impact utility of this drug class for this pathogen. In North America, *S. pneumoniae* resistance is <1% for the respiratory fluoroquinolones (levofloxacin, moxifloxacin, gemifloxacin), and ciprofloxacin resistance is <2%.[84,85] Rates of resistance in other parts of the world are higher.[86] Given the problem of beta-lactam and macrolide resistance, surveillance to identify changes in fluoroquinolone resistance is essential.

In 2016, there were estimated to be about 30,000 cases of invasive pneumococcal disease in the United States with > 3500 deaths.[87] Pneumococcal bacteria are resistant at least one antibiotic in 30% of cases.[7,88] Prior to the year 2000, pneumococcus caused 60,000 cases of invasive disease each year, and up to 40% were infections resistant to one or more antibiotic.[89] The decline in the number of pneumococcal disease cases, and proportion of resistant infections, is primarily a result of the 7-valent pneumococcal conjugate vaccine (PCV7, Prevnar®), which was introduced for use in the United States in 2000. PCV7 incorporates the serotypes that most commonly cause drug-resistant *S. pneumoniae* (6A, 6B, 9V, 14, 19A, 19F, 23F). A newer 13-valent pneumococcal conjugate vaccine (PCV13, Prevnar 13®) has been used since 2010. In countries where pneumococcal conjugate vaccines have been used, many drug-resistant pneumococcal infections have been prevented, and it is estimated that with universal PCV vaccination globally, 11.4 million antibiotic days could be avoided each year.[90]

Gram-Negative Threats

Extended-Spectrum Beta-lactamases and Carbapenemases The movement of resistance genes, accumulation of genes conferring cross-drug class resistance on single genetic elements, and intrinsic resistance characteristics have led to a dire situation for treatment of Gram-negative infections.[16,91]

Beta-lactamase genes, encoding enzymes that inactivate beta-lactam antibiotics, are a critical concern, especially regarding AR of Gram-negative organisms. Beta-lactamase production can lead to bacterial resistance to beta-lactam-class antibiotics, including penicillin, cephalosporins, monobactams, and carbapenems. The complexities of beta-lactamase classification and their history have been recently summarized.[92,93] Within two broad beta-lactamase classes (metallo-beta-lactamases and serine-beta-lactamases) are functional groups that demonstrate differing spectrums of beta-lactam inactivation. These groups are also variably impacted by beta-lactamase inhibitors, which are often used in clinical treatment to augment the activity of beta-lactam antibiotics. AmpC cephalosporinases inactivate penicillins as well as first- and second-generation cephalosporins and beta-lactam inhibitor combinations.[94] Genes encoding AmpC beta-lactamases are primarily chromosomally encoded but have also been identified on transmissible plasmids.[94] Extended-spectrum beta-lactamases (ESBL) are able to inactivate a wide range of beta-lactam class antibiotics, including penicillins, early and later-generation cephalosporins, and aztreonam.[95] Examples of clinically important, plasmid-mediated ESBL are TEM, SHV, and CTX-M.[96] Carbapenemases are beta-lactamases capable of inactivating carbapenem antibiotics (as well as penicillins, cephalosporins, and, variably, aztreonam). Because carbapenems are often last-line antibiotics for resistant Gram-negative infections, carbapenemases are a current, critical concern in healthcare. Clinically important carbapenemases, including KPC, NDM, IMP, VIM, and OXA, are discussed further below.[97] Beta-lactamases are also present in Gram-positive bacteria, including penicillinases, which were responsible for early penicillin resistance in *S. aureus* and are found in environmental bacilli.[92]

While many beta-lactamase genes are chromosomally encoded, ESBL and carbapenemase genes are often associated with plasmids, which facilitate transmission of these resistance genes among bacteria, including among different bacterial species. This has led to widespread emergence of beta-lactam resistance among Gram-negative bacteria.[92] Although emergence began within hospital settings, the epidemiology of ESBL and carbapenemases has expanded to include both healthcare and community settings.[97–99]

Enterobacteriaceae Enterobacteriaceae are a family of Gram-negative bacteria that includes *Escherichia coli*, *Klebsiella*, *Salmonella*, *Shigella*, *Enterobacter*, *Proteus*, *Serratia*, and others. Carbapenem-resistant Enterobacteriaceae (CRE) have been of mounting global concern over recent decades.[100] Carbapenem resistance can be mediated by decreased antibiotic penetrability of bacteria, coupled with beta-lactamase production, or by production of carbapenemases, which directly hydrolyze drugs like imipenem, meropenem, and ertapenem.[100,101] Enterobacteriaceae are also frequently resistant to multiple classes of beta-lactam antibiotics, including third-generation cephalosporins and aztreonam, and, as a result of gene colocation, aminoglycosides and quinolones.[100,102–104] Emerging carbapenem resistance is, thus, accompanied by the threat of extreme or pan-resistant Gram-negative bacteria. CRE infections are associated with mortality as high as 40–50%.[105,106]

Carbapenemase genes are often encoded within plasmids (primarily) and other transmissible genetic elements. The most commonly identified carbapenemases include those in beta-lactamase Ambler Class A (*Klebsiella pneumoniae* carbapenemase, KPC), Class B (New Delhi metallo-beta-lactamase, NDM; Verona integron-encoded, VIM; and metallo-beta-lactamase IMP), and Class D (oxacillinase, OXA), each of which has individual biochemical intricacies that influence treatment options as well as a characteristic global distribution.[93,107,108] KPC carbapenemase genes are endemic in the United States, several South American countries, Greece, Italy, Israel, and China.[109] NDM has become established primarily in China and in India and its surrounding countries. In the U.S. patients with non-KPC, carbapenemase-producing CRE often have received healthcare services abroad, but this epidemiology, including that of NDM, is changing as carbapenemases become more widespread. Globally, the most common Enterobacteriaceae species containing plasmid-associated carbapenemase genes is *Klebsiella pneumoniae*.

Active surveillance of CRE conducted by CDC during 2012–2013 in seven U.S. states (defined as carbapenem-nonsusceptible and extended-cephalosporin-resistant *Escherichia coli*, *Enterobacter aerogenes*, *Enterobacter cloacae* complex, *Klebsiella pneumoniae*, or *Klebsiella oxytoca* recovered from sterile-site or urine cultures) identified a rate of 2.93 cases/100,000 population and major risk factors of frequent prior hospitalization or indwelling medical devices, and discharge to long-term care facilities.[110] Among 188 isolates submitted to CDC for characterization, KPC was the only carbapenemase detected. As of December 2017, KPC carbapenemases have been identified in all 50 states, NDM in 33 states, OXA-48 in 27 states, VIM in 11 states, and IMP in 13 states.[111] Exposure to antibiotics, including but not limited to carbapenems, has also been identified as a risk factor for CRE colonization and infection.[100]

Pseudomonas Aeruginosa *Pseudomonas aeruginosa*, an opportunistic environmental pathogen, is one of the most common causes of HAI, causing >50,000 HAI, including pneumonia and surgical site, urinary tract, and bloodstream infections, each year in the United States.[7] Approximately 6000 (13%) of these HAI are MDR, causing over 400 deaths per year. *P. aeruginosa* is the second most common pathogen associated with ventilator-associated pneumonia (VAP) across all measured healthcare types and is the most common cause of VAP and catheter-associated urinary tract infections in long-term acute care hospitals.[55,112] Patients with cystic fibrosis are at particularly high risk of infection, including infection with MDR organisms.[113] *P. aeruginosa* is a common cause of infections in immune-compromised hosts and, less frequently, of infections in healthy persons, such as folliculitis after exposure to inadequately maintained chlorinated water.

P. aeruginosa demonstrates acquired resistance (e.g., ESBL and carbapenemases), as well as considerable intrinsic resistance, with a remarkably impermeable outer membrane, production of a chromosomally encoded AmpC cephalosporinase, and drug efflux pumps.[32,114] The organism has shown resistance to beta-lactams, including carbapenems, tetracyclines, chloramphenicol, and fluoroquinolones. During 2017, 107 patients with carbapenemase-producing *P. aeruginosa* were reported in states across the United States through CDC surveillance.[115] VIM ($n = 86$) was the most commonly identified carbapenemase, followed by IMP ($n = 8$), NDM ($n = 7$), and KPC ($n = 6$). Because the array of intrinsic and acquired resistance mechanisms in *P. aeruginosa* is so broad, selection of MDR organisms in the presence of antibiotic use is of great concern.[116]

Acinetobacter Baumannii Bacteria in the *Acinetobacter* genus are ubiquitous in the environment. MDR *Acinetobacter baumannii* does not typically cause infections in the immunocompetent host but is a considerable AMR threat in healthcare facilities globally, with intensive care units (ICU) at particular risk.[37,117] In the United States, VAP-associated *Acinetobacter* spp. are frequently MDR (63%) and carbapenem-resistant (63%), as are *Acinetobacter* organisms isolated from catheter-associated urinary tract infections (69% and 76%, respectively).[55] Widespread resistance in *A. baumannii* developed rapidly, with a change from widespread susceptibility in the 1970s to the considerable resistance seen today.[16] One reported resistance island, located on the *A. baumannii* chromosome, is composed of transposons, insertion sequences, and 46 antibiotic and antimicrobial resistance genes conferring resistance to early disinfectants, some sulfonamides, penicillins, extended-spectrum beta-lactams, cephalosporins, aminoglycosides, tetracyclines, chloramphenicol, and trimethoprim.[16]

A. baumannii presents challenges for control, with a reputation for tenacity in the healthcare environment.[118–120] Persistence is at least in part driven by biofilm formation, which facilitates longer colonization of the respiratory tract, medical devices, and the healthcare environment.[121,122] Caring for patients with MDR infection, contact with patient bed rails, and care of wounds and endotracheal tubes have been associated with *A. baumannii* contamination of healthcare worker hands in ICU and intermediate care unit settings.[123] There is evidence that concerted infection prevention practices and reductions in medical device use can influence *Acinetobacter* control.[124]

AR Ecology

Because of its complexity, exploring dynamics of AR from the viewpoint of ecology (the science concerned with the interrelationship of organisms and their environments) is essential.[125] Among the nuances that must be elucidated are: natural and anthropogenic elements that contribute to antibiotic use, resistance, and HGT; confounding factors that influence the evolution of AR and our ability to measure the emergence of resistance; environmental niches that sustain AR; and the relationship between exposure and infection.

Direct and Indirect Effects of Antibiotic Use on Resistance

At the population level, the problem of AR is directly and indirectly influenced by antibiotic use. Lipsitch and Samore present four key ways that antibiotic use leads to resistance: emergence of resistance by point mutation in a patient receiving insufficient antibiotic treatment, with subsequent transmission of the resistant pathogen to others (e.g., MDR tuberculosis); reduction in the proportion of susceptible bacteria in a treated patient, which increases the probability that other individuals will be exposed to (and infected by) resistant bacteria (e.g., MRSA, *S. pneumoniae*); reduction of susceptible bacteria in a treated patient, making that patient more susceptible to infection with a new pathogen, which might be resistant (e.g., *C. difficile*); and development of resistant infection in an individual harboring (colonized with) a resistant strain prior to antibiotic treatment [e.g., vancomycin-resistant Enterococcus (VRE), *C. difficile*].[126]

Once acquired by mutation or HGT, resistance elements are maintained and spread by the direct and indirect selective pressures of clinical antibiotic use. This is especially relevant for nonobligate organisms, such as MRSA and *S. pneumoniae*. Because the influence of an antibiotic is not limited to just one bacterial species in one body site, many nontarget bacteria, including those in our normal gut and skin microbiome, are impacted by antibiotic selective pressures. This occurrence has been termed "bystander selection."[127] As a result, across a patient's exposed bacterial population, susceptible bacteria are eliminated and resistant bacteria (both target and nontarget species) can proliferate. Thus, the problem of resistance is not just defined by presence or absence of a resistant organism, but also proportions of susceptible and resistant organisms and microbial balance. When resistant bacteria proliferate in the presence of a declining susceptible population, the proportion of resistant bacteria exceeds that of susceptible bacteria. This proportional advantage becomes important when considering the risk of resistant pathogen transmission. Under the selective power of antibiotics, there is a higher likelihood that a resistant organism (as compared to a susceptible organism) will be passed from the patient to another individual, from the patient to a healthcare facility surface, or from the patient into the natural environment in fecal or medical waste.

The Environment as a Reservoir of Resistance

Our built and natural environments are reservoirs of resistant bacteria and resistance genes, which can be acquired by people, animals, or fomites (e.g., healthcare surfaces and equipment), through direct contact. Many environments can act as resistance "pawn shops," facilitating the exchange of resistance genes among bacteria. The term "antibiotic resistome" has been used to describe the "...collection of all the genetic elements that contribute to blocking the action of molecules toxic to bacteria."[128] The resistome within a healthcare setting is supported by the continual presence of antibiotic selective pressure among clinical patients. In the natural environment, the resistome is supported by antibiotics and antibiotic metabolites present in urban and rural waterways and soils.

Illustrative of the fact that our built-environments have their own AR ecology is the finding that within healthcare facilities, the risk of resistant infection (and asymptomatic colonization with resistant organisms) is influenced by overall antibiotic use patterns.[129,130] As compared to nursing homes using few antibiotics, nursing homes with high antibiotic use rates have more frequent antibiotic-related adverse outcomes for both treated and untreated residents.[130] Because of their selective pressure and influence on the proportion of resistant bacteria in a healthcare setting, high antibiotic use leads to increased risk for antibiotic-resistant infections and *C. difficile* infections for all individuals, regardless of direct antibiotic exposure. Preventive measures can also benefit from the complex and interconnected nature of AR. Improvement in unnecessary or inappropriate antibiotic use will not only reduce resistance in target organisms, but will also minimize impacts on bystander organisms, reducing the reservoir of resistant gene donors, and will reduce susceptibility to opportunistic infections by preservation of healthy gut flora.[127]

The role of the natural environment in the maintenance and spread of ARG and bacteria has yet to be adequately elucidated. Of late, this area of study has received increased attention.[131–134] Numerous anthropogenic factors contribute to the presence of antibiotics, antibiotic metabolites, resistance genes, and antibiotic-resistant bacteria in the natural environment. These factors include everyday life, inpatient and outpatient healthcare, agriculture (animal, crop, and aquatic), and industrial processes. Antibiotics and other pharmaceuticals have been found in U.S. surface and ground waters.[135–137] Waste from municipal treatment processes, landfills, agricultural runoff, and industrial facilities end up on land and in waterways, which has the potential to harm humans, domestic animals, and wildlife.[138,139] Assuming they are not otherwise at a survival disadvantage, once in the environment, antibiotic-resistant bacteria can expand clonally and share ARG by HGT. Systematic reviews have identified an unquestionable need for additional research to quantify the role of the environment, and environmental antibiotic contamination, in the overall problem of AR and the risk to individual and public health.[139,140]

Detection of AR

Standardized antimicrobial susceptibility testing (AST) methodologies are critical to the clinical treatment of infections as well as to AR surveillance. Phenotypic AST methods quantify a cultured organism's *in vitro* response to antibiotic exposure. The most commonly used phenotypic AST methods are broth microdilution, disk diffusion, and gradient diffusion and include both manual and automated approaches. The principles of these methods have been reviewed.[141] The minimum inhibitory concentration (MIC) is central to AST, as it defines the minimum antibiotic concentration at which the replication of an organism is inhibited. Two major organizations, the Clinical and Laboratory Standards Institute (CLSI) and the European Committee on Antimicrobial Susceptibility Testing (EUCAST), provide standardized guidance for conducting AST and for interpretation of results.[142,143] Standardized breakpoints from CLSI and EUCAST are used to relate quantitative MIC results to "susceptible," "intermediate," or "resistant" interpretation. These breakpoints differ for each organism-antibiotic combination.

Genotyping methods are frequently used in tandem with phenotypic AST. One example is detection of carbapenemase genes within an organism that has shown resistance to carbapenem antibiotics on AST. Polymerase chain reaction (PCR)–based detection of carbapenemases is important to guide treatment, as effective antibiotic therapy can vary by carbapenemase type. Whole genome sequencing is increasingly used to identify related infections and to track resistant organisms within healthcare facilities, across geographic areas, and over time.

AR Surveillance

United States

In the United States, healthcare and community-associated AR is tracked within several active, population-based surveillance programs. The Emerging Infections Program (EIP), which includes the Active Bacterial Core Surveillance (ABCs) and Healthcare-Associated Infections-Community Interface (HAIC) projects, uses national laboratory-based surveillance to collect and track pathogen and clinical information.[144] EIP surveillance is conducted within a network of 10 state health departments in collaboration with academic partners, with catchment areas that are representative of the wider U.S. population. The ABCs program collects data on GAS, GBS, *Haemophilus influenzae*, *Legionella* spp., MRSA, *Neisseria meningiditis*, and *S. pneumoniae*.[145] HAIC collects data on infections caused by *C. difficile*, MRSA, *Candida* bloodstream infections, and MDR Gram-negative bacteria, including CRE, carbapenem-resistant *Acinetobacter*, and carbapenem-resistant *P. aeruginosa*.[146] The National AR Laboratory Network (ARLN) supports laboratory capacity through seven regional laboratories that coordinate and complement activities conducted in all states.[147] These regional laboratories have training and equipment to ensure that cutting edge laboratory capacity is available beyond CDC. They also contribute to the ability to react rapidly to novel MDR organisms and assist healthcare facilities and health departments to proactively respond to even single isolates of concern through enhanced detection by screening of patients at risk of transmission.[148]

AR is closely associated with healthcare settings, and patients admitted to inpatient facilities are at increased risk of contracting a resistant infection. The National Healthcare Safety Network (NHSN) is a CDC-driven system to track healthcare-associated infections (HAI), including those caused by MDR organisms and *C. difficile*.[149] During 2009–2010, the overall percent (20%) of resistance among HAI was similar to the 2 years prior, but the organism distribution changed. MRSA infection rates declined, while MDR Gram-negative bacteria were shown to be of growing concern and not limited to a small number of hospitals.[150] NHSN data can be informative to understand the impact of AR interventions. A 2018 report described a marked decline in the proportion of *E. coli* or *K. pneumoniae* having a CRE phenotype (8.8% in 2006 to 3.1% in 2015), while the proportion with ESBL phenotype remained fairly stable (17.6% in 2006 to 16.5% in 2015).[148] Epidemiologists at CDC attribute this difference, at least in part, to targeted efforts (including support from ARLN regional laboratories) to slow the spread of CRE once identified in a healthcare facility.

The National Antimicrobial Resistance Monitoring System (NARMS) is an integrated system that tracks phenotypic and genotypic AR characteristics of nontyphoidal *Salmonella* and *Campylobacter,* two food-borne pathogens, and two indicator organisms (*Enterococcus* and *E. coli*) in human, animal, and retail meat specimens.[151] Representative isolates from food-borne and zoonotic disease outbreaks are also tested in the NARMS system.

Global AR Surveillance

The World Health Organization (WHO) has established the Global Antimicrobial Resistance Surveillance System (GLASS), which provides a standardized platform for compiling AR data. As of December 2017, 50 countries, which represent more than 25% of WHO member states were enrolled in GLASS.[152,153] During the GLASS early implementation stage (2015–2019), priority pathogens are *Acinetobacter* spp., *E. coli, K. pneumoniae, N. gonorrhea, Salmonella* spp., *Shigella* spp., *S. aureus*, and *S. pneumoniae*. Priority specimens include blood, urine, stool, and cervical and urethral samples. Not all enrolled countries submit data on all specimens, nor on all priority organisms or antibiotics, but as AR laboratory and clinical capacity and urgency grow around the world, so too will the quantity and quality of data.

Approaches to AR Prevention

The four core actions identified by CDC to fight AR[7] including, infection prevention, surveillance, improved prescribing, and development of new treatments and diagnostics, are described briefly here.

Prevention of Infection Infection prevention is an essential component of the approach to AR. For any infection that is prevented, antibiotic use is avoided. In addition, the prevention of resistant infections eliminates an opportunity for an additional host to enable the replication and shedding of the resistant organism. Hand hygiene, vaccination, staying home when ill, and safe food handling are important in the community setting. MDR organisms (MDRO), including CRE, can be difficult to control in healthcare settings. For CRE, the overall goals are to prevent direct (patient-to-patient) and indirect (via healthcare workers or environment) transmission of CRE from an infected patient to others, and to detect MDRO infection and colonization among patients within a healthcare facility. Measures are focused on surveillance (which might include diagnostic testing for patients in contact with CRE-infected patients and admission screening), infection prevention and control practices (including hand hygiene, use of gown and gloves when in contact with a CRE patient and patient environment, patient isolation or cohorting, and staff cohorting), environmental cleaning, chlorhexidine bathing of patients, antibiotic stewardship, and strong clinical-laboratory relationships.[154] Regional control methods can also play a role in prevention of transmission of CRE among individual healthcare facilities, including hospitals and long-term care facilities.[155]

Surveillance Surveillance within healthcare facilities and across health systems, as well as at the state, national, and global levels, is essential to combatting AR. Tracking AR facilitates the recognition of current threats and provides opportunities to target preventive measures and assess the impact of interventions.

Improved Prescribing The development of AR is complex and, to a great extent, the exact combination of pathways that lead to the current state of clinical resistance is unknown. As could be expected, the pathway to elimination of current resistant phenotypes and resolution of the larger AR problem is complex and incredibly challenging to predict. If resistant bacteria do not possess any survival advantage over susceptible bacteria, as antibiotic use and pressure decreases, it could be expected that susceptible bacteria would potentially outcompete resistant strains. Although there are examples of the impact of large-scale changes in antibiotic use on AR (e.g., removal of avoparcin from animal agriculture in the EU led to a decrease in VRE from animal sources; removal of fluoroquinolones from use in U.S. poultry led to a decrease in ciprofloxacin and nalidixic acid resistance in poultry *Salmonella* organisms), return to susceptible phenotypes is not always as easy as simply removing an antibiotic from use.[151] After an over 97% reduction in sulfonamide use in the United Kingdom during the 1990s, sulfonamide resistance in *E. coli* remained prevalent, likely because of coselection for sulfonamide resistance by other antibiotics still widely used, the location of *sul2*, an important sulfonamide resistance gene, on transmissible plasmids, and a lack of selective disadvantage (fitness cost) for carriage of *sul2*.[156–158] Despite these complexities, antibiotic prescribing is a factor that is modifiable, and antibiotic stewardship is recognized as the most important action needed to slow the spread of AR. This topic is covered extensively below.

Development of New Treatments and Diagnostics The development of AR is a natural selective process that humans cannot prevent completely. Accordingly, there is an immediate need for new antibiotics to address our current AR threats. Although the pace of antibiotic production has slowed in recent decades, the clinical AR crisis has led to renewed emphasis on antibiotic production for critical infections. Over the last 5 years, several new antibiotics with resistant Gram-negative coverage have been approved.[159] Although the individual coverage of each of these antibiotics differs, as a group they have provided new treatment options for ESBL, KPC, OXA, and NDM-producing bacteria, as well as for MDR *Acinetobacter* and *Pseudomonas aeruginosa*.

Antibiotic alternatives are an important area of research today, and novel approaches are becoming more numerous, including those that influence the immune system and host microbial communities.[160] One such approach, phage therapy, which uses targeted bacteriophages to treat bacterial infections, has received considerable research attention and is garnering excitement in clinical and public health sectors.[161]

Development of rapid diagnostics are also an essential aspect of AR prevention. Earlier identification of an infection's etiology and susceptibility profile facilitates the earlier selection of appropriate, targeted treatment. Rapid tests are often antigen-based or molecular (e.g., PCR) tests that are conducted independently of bacterial culture.[162] These tests can be conducted quickly and with high sensitivity, even for multiple pathogens, and they are an important option to identify infection with organisms for which there are no existing culture-based tests available. Although rapid diagnostic tests are positively transforming the approach to treatment at the bedside, culture-independent testing has presented new challenges for the existing public health surveillance paradigm. Surveillance programs such as EIP, NARMS, and PulseNet are dependent upon the availability of bacterial isolates to distinguish strains and subtypes and to conduct whole genome sequencing. Attention has been focused on how to ensure that clinical diagnostics and public health surveillance continue to move forward in tandem.[162–164]

ANTIBIOTIC STEWARDSHIP

Definition

Antibiotic stewardship (AS) is defined as "coordinated interventions designed to improve and measure the appropriate use of antimicrobial agents by promoting the selection of the optimal antimicrobial drug regimen including dosing, duration of therapy, and route of administration."[165]

History of AS

The concept of AS evolved to address and limit the consequences of antibiotic use. The term antimicrobial stewardship began to appear in publications in the late 1990s, although the concept of using an interdisciplinary approach to streamline antibiotic therapy was published earlier.[166,167] In 1997, the Society for Healthcare Epidemiology of America (SHEA) and the Infectious Diseases Society of America (IDSA) published guidelines for the prevention and reduction of AR in hospitals, which stated appropriate AS would slow the emergence of resistant microorganisms.[168] Following the position paper, studies were published demonstrating a variety of effective strategies to reduce antibiotic use, slow development of resistance, and save on antibiotic costs.[169–172] Available evidence and expert opinion were used by SHEA and IDSA to create guidelines for developing an institutional AS program (ASP), which were published in 2007.[173]

Studies suggest that 20–50% of antibiotic use for hospitalized patients is unnecessary or inappropriate.[174–177] The need for programs to address this inappropriate use was increasingly recognized prompting SHEA, IDSA, and the Pediatric Infectious Diseases Society (PIDS) to publish a policy statement in 2012, which recommended mandating the implementation of AS throughout healthcare and pushed for public policy on the issue.[165] CDC supported the recommendation that all hospitals implement an ASP and published the Core Elements of Hospital Antibiotic Stewardship Programs in 2014.[174,178] In 2015, the White House issued the National Action Plan for Combating Antibiotic-Resistant Bacteria, which set a goal to establish ASP in all acute care hospitals by 2020.[179]

The body of evidence demonstrating the impact of hospital-based ASP continues to grow. In June 2016, Centers for Medicare and Medicaid Services (CMS) proposed a rule that requires hospitals to establish an ASP as a condition of participation.[180] Effective January 1, 2017 the Joint Commission requires all hospitals, critical access hospitals, and nursing care centers to have an AS program.[181] Antibiotic use is common in nursing homes and an estimated 45–70% of antibiotic prescriptions are inappropriate in these facilities.[182,183] CDC published the Core Elements of Antibiotic Stewardship for Nursing Homes in 2015 to guide expansion of stewardship beyond hospitals to long-term care facilities and nursing homes.[184] In 2016, CMS finalized a new rule that requires long-term care facilities implement an antibiotic stewardship program (ASP) that includes antibiotic use protocols and a system to monitor use as a requirement for participation.[185]

Ambulatory healthcare represents another opportunity for antibiotic stewardship efforts. The majority of healthcare-related antibiotic expenditures in the United States occur in the outpatient setting with $33.2 billion spent on antibiotics in the outpatient setting between 2010 and 2015.[186] It is estimated that more than 25% of ambulatory antibiotic prescriptions are unnecessary or inappropriate.[187,188] The White House National Action Plan established a goal of 50% reduction in inappropriate antibiotic use in outpatient settings by 2020.[179] CDC released a report of the core elements of outpatient antibiotic stewardship in 2016.[189]

General Principles of Appropriate Antibiotic Use in Humans

Antibiotics should only be prescribed for the treatment of suspected or confirmed bacterial infections and for the prevention of bacterial infections in certain high-risk patients. The identification of the causative pathogen of a suspected bacterial infection and the pathogen's susceptibility to antibiotics are frequently unknown to the prescriber at the time of antibiotic initiation and in some cases are never definitively identified. Therefore, decisions regarding antibiotic selection are often made empirically using available evidence and experience. There are a number of patient-related and pathogen-related factors to consider when prescribing antibiotics (Box 153-1).[190]

BOX 153-1 Considerations When Selecting Antibiotic Therapy[190]

1. Define the disease process
   - Site(s) of infection
   - Likely pathogen(s)
   - Severity of illness
2. Assess host factors
   - Age
   - Immune status
   - Comorbid conditions (underlying diseases, implantable devices)
   - Exposure history (healthcare and antibiotic exposure, communicable disease exposure, travel history)
   - Drug allergies
3. Perform diagnostic testing when indicated
4. Consider pathogen factors
   - Antibiotic resistance patterns
5. Understand antibiotic properties
   - Spectrum of activity
   - Pharmacokinetics/pharmacodynamics
   - Routes of administration
   - Adverse effect profile
6. Adjust empiric therapy to appropriate definitive therapy
7. Define duration

The first step in determining optimal antibiotic therapy for an infection is defining the disease process, including the site of infection. Knowledge of the common pathogens causing infection in an affected anatomic site allows the prescriber to predict likely pathogen(s). Understanding pharmacokinetic and pharmacodynamic properties of antibiotics allows the prescriber to select and dose an antibiotic to ensure expected activity at the infection site. Host-related factors that affect an individual's susceptibility to infection include alterations in the development and function of the immune system (e.g., age/maturity, congenital or acquired disorders, immunocompromising conditions and therapies). Defects in specific functions of innate immunity, adaptive immunity, or physical barriers to infection (e.g., skin) lead to increased susceptibility to infection with specific pathogens.[191]

Medication interactions and drug allergies must also be considered. Antibiotic allergies are commonly reported, but many of these do not represent true drug hypersensitivity.[192,193] Some patients with IgE-mediated hypersensitivity lose sensitivity over time and many patients with a "penicillin allergy" can safely tolerate beta-lactam antibiotics.[194,195] Accurate classification of antibiotic allergies has important implications for healthcare resource utilization and outcomes. Patients with beta-lactam allergy labels have increased prevalence of *C. difficile* infections, MRSA, and VRE.[196] Avoidance of beta-lactam therapy in patients with reported beta-lactam allergies is associated with prolonged time to first dose of antibiotic therapy, prolonged hospitalization, increased risk for adverse events, and higher healthcare costs.[196–200]

Knowledge of the local antibiotic susceptibility profile of common pathogens should also guide empiric antibiotic selection. An antibiogram is a profile of cumulative antibiotic susceptibility reports generated by compiling aggregate data of isolates cultured from a group of patients.[201] Healthcare institution-specific antibiograms, created using guidelines from CLSI, monitor trends in AR and guide prescribers when selecting empiric antibiotic treatment. CLSI advises that institutional antibiogram data are analyzed and presented at least annually because MDRO prevalence varies across geographic regions and healthcare settings and has risen over the past few decades.[202–208]

Accurate infection diagnosis facilitates optimized care, including avoidance of wasteful and potentially harmful treatment and testing.

Laboratory evaluation and radiological studies aid in the diagnosis of bacterial infections. Recovery of the causative pathogen by culture in the microbiology laboratory allows antibiotic susceptibility testing to optimize antibiotic selection. Lack of growth of bacteria from sampled body fluids rules out bacterial infection in some patients and avoids unnecessary antibiotic therapy. Decisions regarding the use of diagnostic testing to confirm or exclude the presence of a bacterial infection should factor in the sensitivity, specificity, predictive value, turn-around time, and cost of this testing. Laboratories specializing in microbiology and infectious diseases diagnostics assist medical providers in patient evaluation for infections. Clinical interpretation of test results in the context of a patient's history and findings is needed to avoid misdiagnosis and nonindicated therapies. Identification of contaminating or colonizing bacteria, for example, identification of bacteria in urine of asymptomatic patients, can lead to unnecessary antibiotic exposure. Use of diagnostic testing for infection should be judicious to reduce healthcare waste and avoid confusion in interpretation of test results.

When empiric antibiotic therapy is initiated, the need for this therapy should be reassessed throughout the treatment course, taking into account the patient's clinical response and results of diagnostic evaluation. Empiric antibiotic therapy can be safely discontinued for some patients while in some patients, the antibiotic selected for empiric therapy is continued for the duration of treatment. In other patients, empiric therapy is adjusted to definitive therapy once the causative bacteria is identified. When selecting definitive antibiotic therapy, consideration should be given to selecting the narrowest efficacious option available to minimize impact on the microbiome and development of AR. The shortest effective duration of antibiotic therapy should be chosen to limit consequences of antibiotic exposure.[209] Evidence-based treatment guidelines with recommendations for duration of antibiotic therapy are available for many common infections to guide prescribers.

Components of Hospital Antibiotic Stewardship Programs

The structure of an ASP depends on facility size, patient characteristics, laboratory services, personnel, and information technology services. The guidelines from IDSA and SHEA for developing an institutional ASP and CDC's report of the seven core AS elements (Box 153-2)[178] are helpful resources for facilities during implementation and maintenance of an institutional ASP.[173,178]

BOX 153-2 Summary of CDC's Core Elements of Hospital Antibiotic Stewardship Programs[178]

1. Leadership Commitment: Support of program and dedication of necessary resources
2. Accountability: Appointment of single leader responsible for program outcomes
3. Drug Expertise: Appointment of pharmacy leader
4. Action: Implementation of policies or interventions
5. Tracking: Measuring antibiotic use and defined outcomes
6. Reporting: Sharing antibiotic use outcome metrics data with prescribers regularly
7. Education: Teaching clinicians about optimal antibiotic use

Leadership Commitment

Support of hospital/institutional leaders is essential to ensure an ASP has sufficient staffing, training, technology, and financing to operate successfully. Substantial anti-infective cost savings, more than US$1million, have been reported following implementation of institutional ASPs.[210–212] Anti-infective cost savings provided by ASP activities can be used to justify salary support for the ASP to institutional leaders. Leadership support of an ASP encourages clinician buy-in for the program. An element of performance for the Joint Commission's Antimicrobial Stewardship Standard is prioritization of AS by hospital leaders.[181]

Key Collaborators

Infection control programs share many similarities with stewardship programs including a common goal to reduce the incidence and spread of antibiotic resistant infections. Collaboration between the ASP team and the institution's infection control team enhances stewardship programs. Infection preventionists and hospital epidemiologists assist with surveillance of AR and *C. difficile* infection (CDI) incidence, outcomes which can be used to measure the impact of targeted stewardship interventions. Hospital epidemiologists also support ASPs by sharing resources and collaborating on educational programs.[213]

Partnership with clinical laboratory staff, including a clinical microbiologist, advances AS efforts. Laboratory staff employ policies for appropriate specimen management to ensure accurate diagnostic results. Presentation of laboratory data in a manner that encourages optimal antibiotic use also supports the work of the ASP. Examples of such presentation include cascade reporting of susceptibility test results, suppression of antibiotic results based on intrinsic resistance, and reporting commensal flora without identification and susceptibility information. Laboratory support is imperative in the creation of an institution-specific antibiogram to guide prescribers in antibiotic selection.

Information technology (IT) support assists stewardship programs with collection of antibiotic use data. IT staff are also needed to incorporate stewardship tools into the institution's existing workflow, for example, incorporating clinical decision support into the computerized order entry process or making clinical practice guidelines readily available in the electronic health record.

Front-line healthcare providers, including nursing staff, are integral to effective AS. The American Nurses Association and CDC endorse engagement of registered nurses in AS practices.[214] Since bedside nurses are primarily responsible for administering inpatient medications, including antibiotics, they play an important role in monitoring antibiotic administration practices. Nurses inform antibiotic prescribing by recognizing early signs of infection and inform decisions about de-escalating therapy or changing route of administration by updating prescribers about changes in patients' clinical status. Nurses are often responsible for obtaining specimens (e.g., blood, urine) for culture and can ensure appropriate cultures are obtained before antibiotic therapy is initiated. Nursing communication with patients and families also provides an opportunity for community education about appropriate antibiotic use.

Accountability and Drug Expertise

A program leader, responsible for ASP outcomes, should be identified. Physicians frequently fill this leadership role. Identification of a pharmacist to colead the ASP is also recommended. Pharmacists contribute knowledge of pharmacokinetic and pharmacodynamic properties of antibiotics to optimize dosing. Pharmacists also provide direct knowledge of the function of the institution's pharmacy and information on current antibiotic supplies that might affect antibiotic prescribing decisions. At many institutions, ASP leadership includes an infectious diseases physician and a clinical pharmacist. Hospitalists lead stewardship programs at some institutions.[215] The exact composition of an ASP team is based on available staff support at each institution, but formal infectious diseases training or AS training for ASP leaders is beneficial. AS courses and certificate programs are available through professional organizations.

Action

ASPs should implement at least one action to improve antibiotic use. These actions might include policies that support optimal antibiotic use or specific interventions based on institutional needs and availability of resources. Required documentation of dose, duration, and indication for all prescribed antibiotics is an example of a policy supporting optimal antibiotic use. CDC recommends against implementation of too many policies and specific interventions simultaneously.

Institutions select interventions based on available expertise and resources with a goal to target identified opportunities. CDC categorizes ASP interventions into three categories: broad, pharmacy-driven, or infection/syndrome specific.

Broad Interventions The term "antibiotic time-out" is used to describe reassessment of antibiotic appropriateness after an initial period of administration. During the initial window of empiric antibiotic administration, collection of clinical and laboratory data, including microbiological data, allows clinicians to make an informed decision about antibiotic needs for each patient. CDC recommends that all clinicians perform a reassessment of antibiotics 48 hours after initiation for hospitalized patients. The use of a 48 hour window is supported by evidence that few true blood stream infections are detected after more than 48 hours of blood culture incubation.[216]

During the antibiotic time-out, clinicians should address whether or not the patient has an infection that will respond to antibiotics. If the patient does not have an infection that will respond to antibiotics, antibiotics should be discontinued. If the patient has an infection that will respond to antibiotics, the antibiotic selection should be reviewed to determine whether a more targeted antibiotic would be appropriate. The dose and route of administration should also be reviewed during the time-out to determine whether these are optimal for the defined infection. Finally, the antibiotic time-out provides an opportunity to define for what duration the patient should receive the antibiotic. Implementation of antibiotic time-outs might lead to improved antibiotic use and antibiotic cost savings.[217] Use of clinical informatics support might increase provider confidence in antibiotic de-escalation decisions during these time-outs.[218]

Guidelines from IDSA and SHEA also recommend that hospitals implement preauthorization or prospective audit with feedback protocols. Preauthorization refers to restriction on prescribing certain antibiotics until approval is given by the institution's AS team. This type of intervention is associated with decreased antibiotic use and decreased AR without adverse patient outcomes.[219-221] Factors to consider when developing a preauthorization intervention include availability and skills of the person(s) providing approval, method and accuracy of communication of the clinical information from the prescriber to the stewardship team, and impact restriction of certain antibiotics has on use of nonrestricted agents.

Prospective audit with feedback refers to the process of external review of antibiotic therapy by staff, generally an expert in antibiotic therapy, with feedback provided to clinicians after antibiotics are prescribed. Prospective audit with feedback is an effective strategy to improve antibiotic use and decrease consequences of antibiotic use including AR and CDI.[169,222,223] Prospective audit with feedback requires availability of experts in antibiotic use to perform reviews and give feedback. This process can be time and labor intensive. Limited studies have compared outcomes between preauthorization interventions and prospective audit with feedback interventions. CDC and IDSA do not recommend one of these strategies over the other. Some institutions implement a combination of preauthorization and prospective audit with feedback.

Pharmacy-driven Interventions Many stewardship strategies are delivered by pharmacy programs and staff. Therapeutic drug monitoring with dose optimization, directed by pharmacists, can reduce risk for antibiotic-associated nephrotoxicity.[224-226] Pharmacists at some institutions direct conversion from intravenous to oral antibiotic therapy when appropriate. Increased use of oral antibiotic therapy can be associated with decreased costs, reduced length of hospitalization, and lower incidence of intravenous line complications.[227,228] Allergy assessments and penicillin skin testing, when appropriate, should be promoted by ASPs to facilitate use of first-line antibiotics.[209] Pharmacists effectively manage allergy assessment and skin testing at some institutions.[229,230] Health information technology resources can be leveraged to assist pharmacy-driven interventions such as automated, time-sensitive antibiotic stop orders, detection and notification of antibiotic-related drug-drug interactions, and alerts when antibiotic therapy is duplicative or mismatched with the organism detected from microbiological testing ("bug-drug mismatch").

Syndrome-specific Interventions In addition to the broad interventions described above, ASPs should implement interventions to target improvement in prescribing for commonly encountered infectious disease syndromes such as pneumonia, bacteremia, urinary tract infection, skin and soft tissue infections. These interventions might focus on improving diagnostic accuracy, optimizing antibiotic selection based on local antibiotic susceptibilities, and providing correct treatment duration. Implementation of facility-specific clinical pathways or practice guidelines has been associated with reductions in mortality, adverse events, and treatment costs.[231-233] Additional syndrome-specific interventions with evidence support include electronic order sets, care bundles, and use of best practice alerts and clinical decision support.[234,235] ASPs should design and adapt targeted interventions based on assessment of local needs and available resources.

Additional Stewardship Strategies Optimal antibiotic use begins with accurate diagnosis of infections. Diagnostic stewardship refers to the judicious use of diagnostic testing to guide patient management and is an important component of AS efforts.[236] Testing should be appropriate for the clinical scenario with timely results. Modifications to processes for ordering and performing diagnostic tests facilitate optimal use of diagnostic tests. The electronic health record can be used to create clinical decision support tools and to implement minimum requirements for testing, such as presence of pyuria prior to urine culture.[237] Microbiology laboratories can implement practices to reject specimens that are inappropriately collected or do not meet established criteria, such as rejecting specimens for *C. difficile* testing that do not conform to the shape of the container. Development of new infectious diseases diagnostics, including rapid and molecular techniques, provides future opportunities for ASPs to design strategies that improve antibiotic use.

Optimal antibiotic use includes appropriate storage and disposal of antibiotic waste. Healthcare facilities are responsible for disposing of pharmaceutical waste according to federal and state regulations. Antibiotic residues from healthcare facilities enter municipal sewage and are present in hospital solid wastes.[238] ARG are also detectable in municipal, hospital, and industrial wastewater.[239] Wastewater treatment plants might provide an environment for transfer of resistance genes between bacteria contributing to the AR profile, or resistome, in the environment.[239] Antibiotics, including synthetic, human-use antibiotics, are also present in lake sediment supplied by wastewater effluents and agricultural activities.[240] Although, antibiotics are classified as nonhazardous pharmaceutical waste by the Environmental Protection Agency, proper disposal limits environmental impact. Patients can also contribute to AS efforts by disposing of unused antibiotics through collection boxes and take-back programs instead of flushing unused antibiotics or disposing of them in the household trash. Patients should also be discouraged from keeping unused antibiotics for use by themselves or others during future illnesses.

Tracking and Reporting

Measurement is an important aspect of antibiotic stewardship work. Process and outcome measures, followed over time, assess the impact of ASP efforts. Measurement is also used to identify targets for future efforts, and to provide feedback to prescribers. Measurement of compliance with hospital policies, for example, documentation of antibiotic indication and duration, provide evaluation of processes.

Periodic audits of the quality of antibiotic use are also recommended. Evaluation of diagnostic criteria prior to antibiotic prescribing and compliance with clinical guidelines measure impact of targeted interventions. Tracking antibiotic expenditures also reflect impact of ASP interventions.

Measurement of Antibiotic Use Antibiotic use can be measured using a variety of methods depending on an institution's resources. Drug utilization evaluations of specific antibiotics can identify high use units or clinical services. Length of therapy analyses can be used to assess interventions that target optimal antibiotic duration. Point prevalence surveys can be used to provide a cross-sectional evaluation of antibiotic consumption in an institution at a single point in time. These surveys provide assessment of multiple antibiotic classes and frequently include the indication for antibiotic use. Large point prevalence surveys can be used to assess and compare antibiotic use in multiple facilities.[9,241]

Measurement of aggregate antibiotic use can be tracked over time and used to compare antibiotic use between institutions. The standardized units most commonly used to measure aggregate antibiotic use are defined daily dose (DDD) and days of therapy (DOT). DDD is calculated by aggregating total grams of each antibiotic purchased, dispensed, or administered during a defined period of time, divided by the World Health Organization-assigned DDD.[178] DDD is often calculated using readily available purchasing data. DOT is calculated by summing the days any amount of a specific antibiotic is administered or dispensed to a patient (e.g., if a patient receives two different antibiotics for 4 days this equals eight DOT). DOT can be measured from billing data, dispensing data, and bar code administration data.[242] Unlike DDD, DOT is not affected by dose adjustment and is applicable in pediatrics where weight-based dosing is used.[209] DOT calculations require patient-level data, which might not be available at some facilities. Both DDD and DOT allow tracking of antibiotic use over time within a facility, unit, or for individual prescribers.

For comparison between facilities, DDD and DOT can be expressed as a proportion using a standardized denominator. Patient days normalized to 1000 patients (1000 patient days) is a commonly used denominator. CDC's NHSN created the Antimicrobial Use and Resistance (AUR) module to facilitate benchmarking of antibiotic use and AR.[243] Participation in the Antimicrobial Use (AU) Option facilitates inter- and intrafacility comparison and tracking of antibiotic use over time. DOT per 1000 days present is the primary metric reported to the AU Option.

Accurate comparison of antibiotic use between facilities requires adjustment for differences in patient mix. CDC developed the Standardized Antimicrobial Administration Ratio (SAAR) to analyze risk-adjusted antibiotic use.[244] The SAAR is calculated by dividing observed antibiotic use by predicted antibiotic use. Predicted use is calculated by CDC using predictive models based on nationally aggregated AU data. A high SAAR might indicate excessive antibiotic use and a low SAAR might indicate underutilization of antibiotics. SAARs are generated for specific antibiotic groupings and specific patient care locations.

Other Measures of Antibiotic Stewardship Achievement Patient-centered outcomes such as adverse drug events, days of hospitalization avoided, CDI rates, and drug-bug mismatches can be measured to assess impact of targeted ASP interventions. Tracking AR patterns over time also reflects impact of ASP efforts. ASP impact on AR patterns is not predictable, but reduction in resistance of Gram-positive and Gram-negative organisms has been observed following implementation of ASPs.[209]

Education

ASPs must provide regular education to prescribers on antibiotic-related topics such as AR, infection management, and antibiotic use. The Joint Commission's Antimicrobial Stewardship Standard includes education of staff and practitioners who order, dispense, administer, and monitor antibiotics as an element of performance.[181] Education alone does not result in as much sustained improvement in prescribing as education paired with other interventions. Didactic presentations, academic detailing, and electronic communications have been used for prescriber education. Online educational resources are available to assist with content development for prescriber education.

Patient and community education about appropriate antibiotic use is another important aspect of AS. CDC offers print materials and references for clinicians to use in education of patients about antibiotics and AR. CDC created a national educational campaign called "Be Antibiotics Aware" to raise awareness about the importance of appropriate antibiotic use.[245] CDC also partners with organizations in the annual observance of U.S. Antibiotic Awareness Week.

Antibiotic Stewardship in Other Healthcare Settings

AS strategies should extend outside the hospital to nursing homes, skilled nursing facilities, and outpatient healthcare. The CDC's report on core elements of antibiotic stewardship for nursing homes provides practical stewardship guidance for nursing homes. The structure of nursing homes care creates opportunity to develop unique stewardship models that differ from hospital stewardship programs. Nursing home medical directors and nursing directors should set standards for providers to ensure assessment and antibiotic prescribing are appropriate. Partnership with health departments and consultants (pharmacists and infectious diseases physicians) on stewardship activities is encouraged. Residents and their families should be educated about antibiotic use.

CDC's Core Elements of Outpatient Antibiotic Stewardship (Box 153-3)[189] are intended for use by healthcare providers in a variety of ambulatory care settings including emergency departments, primary care and specialty medical clinics, retail and urgent care clinics, and dental clinics. CDC also provides a checklist for clinicians and facilities to use in assessment of their outpatient antibiotic stewardship activities. ASPs in outpatient settings have been shown to improve prescribing without adverse effects on patient outcomes, but most studied programs target prescribing for respiratory tract infections.[246] Future research is needed to assess effective outpatient stewardship interventions in nonrespiratory infections and long-term sustainability of outpatient stewardship interventions.

Transitions of care (e.g., discharge from inpatient admission to outpatient or long-term care) provide another opportunity for stewardship efforts. In a study from one large institution, despite presence of a robust hospital ASP the majority of antibiotic prescriptions at discharge were inappropriate in dose, selection, or duration.[247] Additional study is needed to determine effective stewardship strategies at care transitions.

Public Health Role in Antibiotic Stewardship

Antibiotic misuse affects population health by driving the spread of antibiotic resistant organisms. The promotion of AS aligns with the essential services of public health organizations.[248] Engagement of state health departments in stewardship activities is recommended by the Council of State and Territorial Epidemiologists (CSTE) and

BOX 153-3 Summary of CDC's Core Elements of Outpatient Antibiotic Stewardship[189]

1. Commitment: Demonstrate dedication and accountability
2. Action for policy and practice: Implement, assess, and modify as needed
3. Tracking and reporting: Monitor prescribing practices with feedback or self-assessment
4. Education and expertise: Provide resources to prescribers and patients, and access to expertise

the Association of State and Territorial Health Officials (ASTHO).[249] Public health organizations are in a position to emphasize AS across care transitions, and to coordinate approaches to stewardship within and across states. Partnership between healthcare institutions and public health organizations allows sharing of assessment tools and resources. Collection of antibiotic use and susceptibility data by public health organizations allows for creation of region-specific reports to guide local practice. Many state health departments collaborate with healthcare institutions on AS activities, such as trainings, surveys, site visits, and collaboratives.[248]

Public health organizations are also positioned to increase public awareness of the importance of appropriate antibiotic use. Many state health departments, in partnership with community organizations, participate in consumer-based educational campaigns.[248–250] Public health organizations also inform the legislative process by educating policymakers about judicious antibiotic use.

Antibiotic Stewardship as a One Health Issue

Because of its complexity, the actions directed at detection, prevention, and control of AR must incorporate an ecological view of the problem and incorporate human, animal, and environmental components. The understanding that human, animal, and environmental health are connected is referred to as "One Health." In practice, CDC identifies One Health as a "collaborative, multisectoral, and trans-disciplinary approach…with the goal of achieving optimal health outcomes recognizing the interconnection between people, animals, plants, and their shared environment."[251] AR is a One Health issue and a collaborative, One Health approach to AS efforts is ideal. The Netherlands observed success using One Health interventions to combat AR.[252,253] All the countries in the European Union have committed to a One Health approach to AR and support for this approach is increasing in the United States.[252–254]

Antibiotics are used in more sectors than just healthcare, including small animal and large animal veterinary medicine, aquaculture, bee production, crop-based agriculture (particularly in apple and pear production), and industries such as ethanol and pharmaceutical production. Medically important antibiotics (MIA), from the human health perspective, are used in animal agriculture systems and in clinic-based veterinary medicine.[255–258] In animal agriculture settings, antibiotic stewardship occurs at two levels: clinical decision making and regulation. As in other areas of veterinary medicine, clinical decision-making is based on clinical signs of animal illness, herd/flock history, and laboratory diagnostic data. Food animal producers should work closely with veterinarians to ensure that antibiotics are used only when needed, and are selected and used appropriately. Use of antibiotics in animal agriculture is also largely influenced by state- and federal-level regulations and inspection processes. FDA has outlined specifics for how MIA can be used in U.S. animal agriculture by the oral (feed and water) routes.[259] Three areas receiving considerable attention in regard to agricultural antibiotic use are definition of use duration for some older antibiotics where no duration is labeled by FDA, refinement of preventive antibiotic uses in herd/flock settings, and identification of antibiotic alternatives.[260,261] Because food animals are raised in groups and are often exposed to production-related stressors (e.g., weaning, transport, insect vectors), antibiotics can be important to prevent predictable morbidity related to opportunistic pathogens.[262] Continued improvement of overall animal health, identification of other preventive measures (e.g., management changes) that lessen the need for preventive antibiotic use, and refinement of preventive antibiotic use guidelines are essential parts of stewardship in food animal veterinary medicine.

MIA are also used in clinic-based veterinary medicine (e.g., canine, feline, equine). Because humans experience close direct contact with these species and have been shown to share microbiota, it is essential to conduct surveillance for AR and ARG in these species and to integrate antibiotic stewardship into daily practices.[263,264] Companion animal antibiotic stewardship is a growing focus for the American Veterinary Medical Association and FDA, and evidence-based approaches from healthcare are increasingly explored in this field.[265,266, 267]

Because all antibiotic use has the potential to contribute to AR, critical assessment and judicious use must occur in all sectors. A multidisciplinary approach is important because exposure to resistant bacteria or ARG is not limited only to the sector from which they emerge. AR threats that began in the hospital now pose a risk in community settings, and AR that emerges on farms or in veterinary clinics can lead to exposure in homes. Resistant bacteria can persist in varied settings. Key methods of AR prevention (infection prevention, surveillance, improved prescribing, development of new drugs and diagnostics) are similar across health disciplines and effective tools and approaches developed in one setting can be modified and shared with others.[7]

References

1. The Editors of Encyclopaedia Britannica. Antibiotic. *Encyclopaedia Britannica* 2018. Available at https://www.britannica.com/science/antibiotic. Accessed November 19, 2018.
2. Gabani P, Prakash D, Singh OV. Emergence of antibiotic-resistant extremophiles (AREs). *Extremophiles.* 2012;16(5):697–713.
3. D'Costa VM, King CE, Kalan L, et al. Antibiotic resistance is ancient. *Nature.* 2011;477(7365):457–61.
4. Pawlowski AC, Wang W, Koteva K, et al. A diverse intrinsic antibiotic resistome from a cave bacterium. *Nat Commun.* 2016;7:13803.
5. Centers for Disease Control and Prevention. Antibiotic/antimicrobial resistance. Available at https://www.cdc.gov/drugresistance/about.html. Accessed June 18, 2018.
6. Penicillin's Finder Assays Its Future. *New York Times.* June 26, 1945.
7. Centers for Disease Control and Prevention (CDC). *Antibiotic resistance threats in the United States, 2013.* Atlanta, GA: CDC; 2013.
8. Clatworthy AE, Pierson E, Hung DT. Targeting virulence: A new paradigm for antimicrobial therapy. *Nat Chem Biol.* 2007;3(9):541–8.
9. Singh N, Muller A, Levy Hara G, Luis Castro J, Ramon-Pardo P. Antibiotic awareness week and hospital antimicrobial use point prevalence study. *Infect Control Hosp Epidemiol.* 2017;38(12):149–500.
10. Pray L. Antibiotic resistance, mutation rates and MRSA. *Nature Education.* 2008;1(1):30.
11. Davies J, Davies D. Origins and evolution of antibiotic resistance. *Microbiol Mol Biol Rev.* 2010;74(3):417–33.
12. Centers for Disease Control and Prevention (CDC). Tuberculosis data and statistics. 2018. Available at https://www.cdc.gov/tb/statistics/default.htm. Accessed November 10, 2018.
13. World Health Organization (WHO). *Global Tuberculosis Report, 2018.* Geneva; 2018.
14. Gogarten JP, Townsend JP. Horizontal gene transfer, genome innovation and evolution. *Nat Rev Microbiol.* 2005;3(9):679–87.
15. Soucy SM, Huang J, Gogarten JP. Horizontal gene transfer: Building the web of life. *Nat Rev Genet.* 2015;16(8):472–82.
16. Toleman MA, Walsh TR. Combinatorial events of insertion sequences and ICE in Gram-negative bacteria. *FEMS Microbiol Rev.* 2011;35(5):912–35.
17. Brisson-Noel A, Arthur M, Courvalin P. Evidence for natural gene transfer from gram-positive cocci to Escherichia coli. *J Bacteriol.* 1988;170(4):1739–45.
18. Tompkins LS, Plorde JJ, Falkow S. Molecular analysis of R-factors from multiresistant nosocomial isolates. *J Infect Dis.* 1980;141(5):625–36.
19. Smillie C, Garcillan-Barcia MP, Francia MV, Rocha EP, de la Cruz F. Mobility of plasmids. *Microbiol Mol Biol Rev.* 2010;74(3):434–52.
20. Opal SM, Pop-Vicas A. Molecular mechanisms of antibiotic resistance in bacteria. In: Bennett JE, Dolin R, Blaser MJ, Mandell GL, Douglas RG, eds. *Mandell, Douglas, and Bennett's Principles and Practice of Infectious Diseases.* Vol 1. 8th ed.; 2015, pp. 235–51.
21. Barlow M, Reik RA, Jacobs SD, et al. High rate of mobilization for blaCTX-Ms. *Emerg Infect Dis.* 2008;14(3):423–8.
22. Souza V, Rocha M, Valera A, Eguiarte LE. Genetic structure of natural populations of Escherichia coli in wild hosts on different continents. *Appl Environ Microbiol.* 1999;65(8):3373–85.
23. Cole ST, Eiglmeier K, Parkhill J, et al. Massive gene decay in the leprosy bacillus. *Nature.* 2001;409(6823):1007–11.

24. Shapiro JA. Mutations caused by the insertion of genetic material into the galactose operon of Escherichia coli. *J Mol Biol*. 1969;40(1):93–105.
25. Recchia GD, Hall RM. Gene cassettes: A new class of mobile element. *Microbiology*. 1995;141(Pt 12):3015–27.
26. Stokes HW, Hall RM. A novel family of potentially mobile DNA elements encoding site-specific gene-integration functions: Integrons. *Mol Microbiol*. 1989;3(12):1669–83.
27. Mazel D. Integrons: Agents of bacterial evolution. *Nat Rev Microbiol*. 2006;4(8):608–20.
28. Johnston C, Martin B, Fichant G, Polard P, Claverys JP. Bacterial transformation: Distribution, shared mechanisms and divergent control. *Nat Rev Microbiol*. 2014;12(3):181–96.
29. Anand T, Bera BC, Vaid RK, et al. Abundance of antibiotic resistance genes in environmental bacteriophages. *J Gen Virol*. 2016;97(12):3458–66.
30. Shao S, Hu Y, Cheng J, Chen Y. Research progress on distribution, migration, transformation of antibiotics and antibiotic resistance genes (ARGs) in aquatic environment. *Crit Rev Biotechnol*. 2018;38(8):1195–208.
31. Wilharm G, Piesker J, Laue M, Skiebe E. DNA uptake by the nosocomial pathogen Acinetobacter baumannii occurs during movement along wet surfaces. *J Bacteriol*. 2013;195(18):4146–53.
32. Cox G, Wright GD. Intrinsic antibiotic resistance: Mechanisms, origins, challenges and solutions. *Int J Med Microbiol*. 2013;303(6-7):287–92.
33. Gregoire N, Aranzana-Climent V, Magreault S, Marchand S, Couet W. Clinical pharmacokinetics and pharmacodynamics of colistin. *Clin Pharmacokinet*. 2017;56(12):1441–60.
34. Vaara M. Agents that increase the permeability of the outer membrane. *Microbiol Rev*. 1992;56(3):395–411.
35. Liu YY, Wang Y, Walsh TR, et al. Emergence of plasmid-mediated colistin resistance mechanism MCR-1 in animals and human beings in China: A microbiological and molecular biological study. *Lancet Infect Dis*. 2016;16(2):161–8.
36. Munita JM, Arias CA. Mechanisms of antibiotic resistance. *Microbiol Spectr*. 2016;4(2).
37. World Health Organization (WHO). *Global priority list of antibiotic-resistant bacteria to guide research, discovery, and development of new antibiotics*. February 27, 2017.
38. Klevens RM, Morrison MA, Nadle J, et al. Invasive methicillin-resistant Staphylococcus aureus infections in the United States. *JAMA*. 2007;298(15):1763–71.
39. Tong SY, Davis JS, Eichenberger E, Holland TL, Fowler VGJr. Staphylococcus aureus infections: Epidemiology, pathophysiology, clinical manifestations, and management. *Clin Microbiol Rev*. 2015;28(3):603–61.
40. Barrett FF, McGehee RFJr, Finland M. Methicillin-resistant Staphylococcus aureus at Boston City Hospital. Bacteriologic and epidemiologic observations. *N Engl J Med*. 1968;279(9):441–8.
41. Peacock SJ, Paterson GK. Mechanisms of methicillin resistance in Staphylococcus aureus. *Annu Rev Biochem*. 2015;84:577–601.
42. David MZ, Daum RS. Community-associated methicillin-resistant Staphylococcus aureus: Epidemiology and clinical consequences of an emerging epidemic. *Clin Microbiol Rev*. 2010;23(3):616–87.
43. Fridkin SK, Hageman JC, Morrison M, et al. Methicillin-resistant Staphylococcus aureus disease in three communities. *N Engl J Med*. 2005;352(14):1436–44.
44. Naimi TS, LeDell KH, Como-Sabetti K, et al. Comparison of community- and health care-associated methicillin-resistant Staphylococcus aureus infection. *JAMA*. 2003;290(22):2976–84.
45. King MD, Humphrey BJ, Wang YF, et al. Emergence of community-acquired methicillin-resistant Staphylococcus aureus USA 300 clone as the predominant cause of skin and soft-tissue infections. *Ann Intern Med*. 2006;144(5):309–17.
46. McDougal LK, Steward CD, Killgore GE, et al. Pulsed-field gel electrophoresis typing of oxacillin-resistant Staphylococcus aureus isolates from the United States: Establishing a national database. *J Clin Microbiol*. 2003;41(11):5113–20.
47. Centers for Disease Control and Prevention (CDC). Active Bacterial Core surveillance (ABCs) surveillance reports. 2018. Available at http://www.cdc.gov/abcs/reports-findings/surv-reports.html. Accessed November 19, 2018.
48. Centers for Disease Control and Prevention (CDC). *Active bacterial core surveillance report, Emerging Infections program network, methicillin-resistant Staphylococcus aureus, 2014*. Atlanta, GA: CDC; 2014.
49. Kos VN, Desjardins CA, Griggs A, et al. Comparative genomics of vancomycin-resistant Staphylococcus aureus strains and their positions within the clade most commonly associated with Methicillin-resistant S. aureus hospital-acquired infection in the United States. *MBio*. 2012;3(3).
50. Sievert DM, Rudrik JT, Patel JB, et al. Vancomycin-resistant Staphylococcus aureus in the United States, 2002–2006. *Clin Infect Dis*. 2008;46(5):668–74.
51. Centers for Disease Control and Prevention (CDC). VISA/VRSA in healthcare settings. 2015. Available at https://www.cdc.gov/hai/organisms/visa_vrsa/visa_vrsa.html. Accessed November 26, 2018.
52. Fisher K, Phillips C. The ecology, epidemiology and virulence of Enterococcus. *Microbiology*. 2009;155(Pt 6):1749–57.
53. Leone S, Noviello S, Esposito S. Combination antibiotic therapy for the treatment of infective endocarditis due to enterococci. *Infection*. 2016;44(3):273–81.
54. Hollenbeck BL, Rice LB. Intrinsic and acquired resistance mechanisms in enterococcus. *Virulence*. 2012;3(5):421–33.
55. Weiner LM, Webb AK, Limbago B, et al. Antimicrobial-resistant pathogens associated with healthcare-associated infections: Summary of data reported to the National Healthcare Safety Network at the Centers for Disease Control and Prevention, 2011–2014. *Infect Control Hosp Epidemiol*. 2016;37(11):1288–301.
56. Miller WR, Munita JM, Arias CA. Mechanisms of antibiotic resistance in enterococci. *Expert Rev Anti Infect Ther*. 2014;12(10):1221–36.
57. Stevens DL, Gibbons AE, Bergstrom R, Winn V. The Eagle effect revisited: Efficacy of clindamycin, erythromycin, and penicillin in the treatment of streptococcal myositis. *J Infect Dis*. 1988;158(1):23–28.
58. Bemer-Melchior P, Juvin ME, Tassin S, et al. In vitro activity of the new ketolide telithromycin compared with those of macrolides against Streptococcus pyogenes: Influences of resistance mechanisms and methodological factors. *Antimicrob Agents Chemother*. 2000;44(11):2999–3002.
59. Michos AG, Bakoula CG, Braoudaki M, et al. Macrolide resistance in Streptococcus pyogenes: Prevalence, resistance determinants, and emm types. *Diagn Microbiol Infect Dis*. 2009;64(3):295–9.
60. Hyder SL, Streitfeld MM. Inducible and constitutive resistance to macrolide antibiotics and lincomycin in clinically isolated strains of Streptococcus pyogenes. *Antimicrob Agents Chemother*. 1973;4(3):327–31.
61. Leclercq R, Courvalin P. Bacterial resistance to macrolide, lincosamide, and streptogramin antibiotics by target modification. *Antimicrob Agents Chemother*. 1991;35(7):1267–72.
62. Seppala H, Skurnik M, Soini H, Roberts MC, Huovinen P. A novel erythromycin resistance methylase gene (ermTR) in Streptococcus pyogenes. *Antimicrob Agents Chemother*. 1998;42(2):257–62.
63. Weisblum B. Erythromycin resistance by ribosome modification. *Antimicrob Agents Chemother*. 1995;39(3):577–85.
64. Clancy J, Petitpas J, Dib-Hajj F, et al. Molecular cloning and functional analysis of a novel macrolide-resistance determinant, mefA, from Streptococcus pyogenes. *Mol Microbiol*. 1996;22(5):867–79.
65. Sutcliffe J, Tait-Kamradt A, Wondrack L. Streptococcus pneumoniae and Streptococcus pyogenes resistant to macrolides but sensitive to clindamycin: A common resistance pattern mediated by an efflux system. *Antimicrob Agents Chemother*. 1996;40(8):1817–24.
66. Centers for Disease Control and Prevention (CDC). Group B Strep (GBS): Clinical overview. 2018. Available at https://www.cdc.gov/groupbstrep/clinicians/clinical-overview.html. Accessed November 20, 2018.
67. Le Doare K, Heath PT. An overview of global GBS epidemiology. *Vaccine*. 2013;31(Suppl 4):D7–12.
68. Centers for Disease Control and Prevention (CDC). *Active Bacterial Core Surveillance Report, Emerging Infections Program Network, Group B Streptococcus, 2016*. 2016.
69. Arpin C, Daube H, Tessier F, Quentin C. Presence of mefA and mefE genes in Streptococcus agalactiae. *Antimicrob Agents Chemother*. 1999;43(4):944–6.
70. Heelan JS, Hasenbein ME, McAdam AJ. Resistance of group B Streptococcus to selected antibiotics, including erythromycin and clindamycin. *J Clin Microbiol*. 2004;42(3):1263–4.
71. Park C, Nichols M, Schrag SJ. Two cases of invasive vancomycin-resistant group B streptococcus infection. *N Engl J Med*. 2014;370(9):885–6.
72. Metcalf BJ, Chochua S, Gertz REJr, et al. Short-read whole genome sequencing for determination of antimicrobial resistance mechanisms and capsular serotypes of current invasive Streptococcus agalactiae recovered in the USA. *Clinical Microbiology and Infection: The Official Publication of the European Society of Clinical Microbiology and Infectious Diseases*. 2017;23(8):574 e577–574 e514.
73. Centers for Disease Control and Prevention (CDC). Active Bacterial Core surveillance (ABCs): Bact facts interactive. 2018. Available at https://www.cdc.gov/abcs/bact-facts-interactive.html. Accessed November 20, 2018.

74. Cherazard R, Epstein M, Doan TL, et al. Antimicrobial resistant Streptococcus pneumoniae: Prevalence, mechanisms, and clinical implications. *Am J Ther*. 2017;24(3):e361–9.
75. Nichol KA, Zhanel GG, Hoban DJ. Penicillin-binding protein 1A, 2B, and 2X alterations in Canadian isolates of penicillin-resistant Streptococcus pneumoniae. *Antimicrob Agents Chemother*. 2002;46(10):3261–4.
76. Dowson CG, Coffey TJ, Kell C, Whiley RA. Evolution of penicillin resistance in Streptococcus pneumoniae; the role of Streptococcus mitis in the formation of a low affinity PBP2B in S. pneumoniae. *Mol Microbiol*. 1993;9(3):635–43.
77. Hauser C, Aebi S, Muhlemann K. An internationally spread clone of Streptococcus pneumoniae evolves from low-level to higher-level penicillin resistance by uptake of penicillin-binding protein gene fragments from nonencapsulated pneumococci. *Antimicrob Agents Chemother*. 2004;48(9):3563–6.
78. Whatmore AM, Efstratiou A, Pickerill AP, et al. Genetic relationships between clinical isolates of Streptococcus pneumoniae, Streptococcus oralis, and Streptococcus mitis: Characterization of "Atypical" pneumococci and organisms allied to S. mitis harboring S. pneumoniae virulence factor-encoding genes. *Infect Immun*. 2000;68(3):1374–82.
79. McDougal LK, Rasheed JK, Biddle JW, Tenover FC. Identification of multiple clones of extended-spectrum cephalosporin-resistant Streptococcus pneumoniae isolates in the United States. *Antimicrob Agents Chemother*. 1995;39(10):2282–8.
80. Brisson-Noel A, Trieu-Cuot P, Courvalin P. Mechanism of action of spiramycin and other macrolides. *J Antimicrob Chemother*. 1988;22(Suppl B):13–23.
81. Zhanel GG, Dueck M, Hoban DJ, et al. Review of macrolides and ketolides: Focus on respiratory tract infections. *Drugs*. 2001;61(4):443–98.
82. Janoff EN, Musher DM. Streptococcus pneumoniae. In: Bennett JE, Dolin R, Blaser MJ, Mandell GL, Douglas RG, eds. *Mandell, Douglas, and Bennett's Principles and Practice of Infectious Diseases*. Vol 2. 8th ed.; 2015, 2310–27.
83. Schroeder MR, Stephens DS. Macrolide resistance in Streptococcus pneumoniae. *Front Cell Infect Microbiol*. 2016;6:98.
84. Jenkins SG, Brown SD, Farrell DJ. Trends in antibacterial resistance among Streptococcus pneumoniae isolated in the USA: Update from PROTEKT US Years 1-4. *Ann Clin Microbiol Antimicrob*. 2008;7:1.
85. Patel SN, McGeer A, Melano R, et al. Susceptibility of Streptococcus pneumoniae to fluoroquinolones in Canada. *Antimicrob Agents Chemother*. 2011;55(8):3703–8.
86. Kim ES, Hooper DC. Clinical importance and epidemiology of quinolone resistance. *Infect Chemother*. 2014;46(4):226–38.
87. Centers for Disease Control and Prevention (CDC). *Active Bacterial Core Surveillance Report, Emerging Infections Program Network, Streptococcus pneumoniae, 2016*. 2016.
88. Kim L, McGee L, Tomczyk S, Beall B. Biological and epidemiological features of antibiotic-resistant Streptococcus pneumoniae in pre- and post-conjugate vaccine eras: A United States perspective. *Clin Microbiol Rev*. 2016;29(3):525–52.
89. Centers for Disease Control and Prevention (CDC). Pneumococcal disease: Drug resistance. 2018. Available at https://www.cdc.gov/pneumococcal/drug-resistance.html. Accessed November 20, 2018.
90. Laxminarayan R, Matsoso P, Pant S, et al. Access to effective antimicrobials: A worldwide challenge. *Lancet*. 2016;387(10014):168–75.
91. Exner M, Bhattacharya S, Christiansen B, et al. Antibiotic resistance: What is so special about multidrug-resistant Gram-negative bacteria? *GMS Hyg Infect Control*. 2017;12:Doc05.
92. Bueno I, Williams-Nguyen J, Hwang H, et al. Systematic review: Impact of point sources on antibiotic-resistant bacteria in the natural environment. *Zoonoses Public Health*. 2018;65(1):e162–84.
93. Bush K. Proliferation and significance of clinically relevant beta-lactamases. *Ann N Y Acad Sci*. 2013;1277:84–90.
94. Jacoby GA. AmpC beta-lactamases. *Clin Microbiol Rev*. 2009;22(1):161–82, Table of Contents.
95. Akinci E, Vahaboglu H. Minor extended-spectrum beta-lactamases. *Expert Rev Anti Infect Ther*. 2010;8(11):1251–8.
96. Bonnet R. Growing group of extended-spectrum beta-lactamases: The CTX-M enzymes. *Antimicrob Agents Chemother*. 2004;48(1):1–14.
97. Doi Y, Paterson DL. Carbapenemase-producing Enterobacteriaceae. *Semin Respir Crit Care Med*. 2015;36(1):74–84.
98. Kelly AM, Mathema B, Larson EL. Carbapenem-resistant Enterobacteriaceae in the community: A scoping review. *Int J Antimicrob Agents*. 2017;50(2):127–34.
99. Pitout JD, Nordmann P, Laupland KB, Poirel L. Emergence of Enterobacteriaceae producing extended-spectrum beta-lactamases (ESBLs) in the community. *J Antimicrob Chemother*. 2005;56(1):52–9.
100. Guh AY, Limbago BM, Kallen AJ. Epidemiology and prevention of carbapenem-resistant Enterobacteriaceae in the United States. *Expert Rev Anti Infect Ther*. 2014;12(5):565–80.
101. MacKenzie FM, Forbes KJ, Dorai-John T, Amyes SG, Gould IM. Emergence of a carbapenem-resistant Klebsiella pneumoniae. *Lancet*. 1997;350(9080):783.
102. Elemam A, Rahimian J, Mandell W. Infection with panresistant Klebsiella pneumoniae: A report of 2 cases and a brief review of the literature. *Clin Infect Dis*. 2009;49(2):271–4.
103. Jacoby GA, Munoz-Price LS. The new beta-lactamases. *N Engl J Med*. 2005;352(4):380–91.
104. Rice LB, Carias LL, Hutton RA, et al. The KQ element, a complex genetic region conferring transferable resistance to carbapenems, aminoglycosides, and fluoroquinolones in Klebsiella pneumoniae. *Antimicrob Agents Chemother*. 2008;52(9):3427–9.
105. Patel G, Huprikar S, Factor SH, Jenkins SG, Calfee DP. Outcomes of carbapenem-resistant Klebsiella pneumoniae infection and the impact of antimicrobial and adjunctive therapies. *Infect Control Hosp Epidemiol*. 2008;29(12):1099–106.
106. Schwaber MJ, Klarfeld-Lidji S, Navon-Venezia S, et al. Predictors of carbapenem-resistant Klebsiella pneumoniae acquisition among hospitalized adults and effect of acquisition on mortality. *Antimicrob Agents Chemother*. 2008;52(3):1028–33.
107. Mathers A. Mobilization of carbapenemase-mediated resistance in Enterobacteriaceae. *Microbiol Spectr*. 2016;4(3).
108. van Duin D, Bonomo RA. Ceftazidime/avibactam and ceftolozane/tazobactam: Second-generation beta-lactam/beta-lactamase inhibitor combinations. *Clin Infect Dis*. 2016;63(2):234–41.
109. Logan LK, Weinstein RA. The epidemiology of carbapenem-resistant Enterobacteriaceae: The impact and evolution of a global menace. *J Infect Dis*. 2017;215(suppl_1):S28–36.
110. Guh AY, Bulens SN, Mu Y, et al. Epidemiology of carbapenem-resistant Enterobacteriaceae in 7 US communities, 2012–2013. *JAMA*. 2015;314(14):1479–87.
111. Centers for Disease Control and Prevention (CDC). Healthcare-associated infections: tracking CRE. 2018. Available at https://www.cdc.gov/hai/organisms/cre/TrackingCRE.html. Accessed November 20, 2018.
112. Chitnis AS, Edwards JR, Ricks PM, et al. Device-associated infection rates, device utilization, and antimicrobial resistance in long-term acute care hospitals reporting to the National Healthcare Safety Network, 2010. *Infect Control Hosp Epidemiol*. 2012;33(10):993–1000.
113. Parkins MD, Somayaji R, Waters VJ. Epidemiology, biology, and impact of clonal Pseudomonas aeruginosa infections in cystic fibrosis. *Clin Microbiol Rev*. 2018;31(4):e00019-18.
114. Potron A, Poirel L, Nordmann P. Emerging broad-spectrum resistance in Pseudomonas aeruginosa and Acinetobacter baumannii: Mechanisms and epidemiology. *Int J Antimicrob Agents*. 2015;45(6):568–85.
115. Centers for Disease Control and Prevention (CDC). Healthcare-associated infections: Tracking carbapenem-resistant Pseudomonas aeruginosa. 2018. Available at https://www.cdc.gov/hai/organisms/pseudomonas/tracking.html. Accessed November 20, 2018.
116. Nguyen L, Garcia J, Gruenberg K, MacDougall C. Multidrug-resistant Pseudomonas infections: Hard to treat, but hope on the horizon? *Curr Infect Dis Rep*. 2018;20(8):23.
117. Centers for Disease Control and Prevention (CDC). Healthcare-associated infections: Acinetobacter in healthcare settings. 2018. Available at https://www.cdc.gov/HAI/organisms/acinetobacter.html. Accessed November 20, 2018.
118. Lambiase A, Piazza O, Rossano F, et al. Persistence of carbapenem-resistant Acinetobacter baumannii strains in an Italian intensive care unit during a forty-six month study period. *New Microbiol*. 2012;35(2):199–206.
119. Landman D, Quale JM, Mayorga D, et al. Citywide clonal outbreak of multiresistant Acinetobacter baumannii and Pseudomonas aeruginosa in Brooklyn, NY: The preantibiotic era has returned. *Arch Intern Med*. 2002;162(13):1515–20.
120. Sung JY, Koo SH, Kim S, Kwon GC. Persistence of multidrug-resistant Acinetobacter baumannii isolates harboring blaOXA-23 and bap for 5 years. *J Microbiol Biotechnol*. 2016;26(8):1481–9.
121. Greene C, Vadlamudi G, Newton D, Foxman B, Xi C. The influence of biofilm formation and multidrug resistance on environmental survival

of clinical and environmental isolates of Acinetobacter baumannii. *Am J Infect Control*. 2016;44(5):e65–71.

122. Ryu SY, Baek WK, Kim HA. Association of biofilm production with colonization among clinical isolates of Acinetobacter baumannii. *Korean J Intern Med*. 2017;32(2):345–51.
123. Thom KA, Rock C, Jackson SS, et al. Factors leading to transmission risk of Acinetobacter baumannii. *Crit Care Med*. 2017;45(7):e633–9.
124. Abdallah M, Olafisoye O, Cortes C, et al. Reduction in the prevalence of carbapenem-resistant Acinetobacter baumannii and Pseudomonas aeruginosa in New York City. *Am J Infect Control*. 2015;43(6):650–2.
125. Merriam-Webster.com. Ecology. In: Merriam-Webster; 2018.
126. Lipsitch M, Samore MH. Antimicrobial use and antimicrobial resistance: A population perspective. *Emerg Infect Dis*. 2002;8(4):347–54.
127. Tedijanto C, Olesen S, Grad Y, Lipsitch M. Estimating the proportion of bystander selection for antibiotic resistance among potentially pathogenic bacterial flora. *bioRxiv 288704*. 2018.
128. Gaze WH, Krone SM, Larsson DG, et al. Influence of humans on evolution and mobilization of environmental antibiotic resistome. *Emerg Infect Dis*. 2013;19(7).
129. Almagor J, Temkin E, Benenson I, et al. The impact of antibiotic use on transmission of resistant bacteria in hospitals: Insights from an agent-based model. *PLoS One*. 2018;13(5):e0197111.
130. Daneman N, Bronskill SE, Gruneir A, et al. Variability in antibiotic use across nursing homes and the risk of antibiotic-related adverse outcomes for individual residents. *JAMA Intern Med*. 2015;175(8):1331–39.
131. Berendonk TU, Manaia CM, Merlin C, et al. Tackling antibiotic resistance: The environmental framework. *Nat Rev Microbiol*. 2015;13(5):310–17.
132. Singer RS, Ward MP, Maldonado G. Can landscape ecology untangle the complexity of antibiotic resistance? *Nat Rev Microbiol*. 2006;4(12):943–52.
133. Wooldridge M. Evidence for the circulation of antimicrobial-resistant strains and genes in nature and especially between humans and animals. *Rev Sci Tech*. 2012;31(1):231–47.
134. Woolhouse M, Ward M, van Bunnik B, Farrar J. Antimicrobial resistance in humans, livestock and the wider environment. *Philos Trans R Soc Lond B Biol Sci*. 2015;370(1670):20140083.
135. Barber LB, Murphy SF, Verplanck PL, et al. Chemical loading into surface water along a hydrological, biogeochemical, and land use gradient: A holistic watershed approach. *Environ Sci Technol*. 2006;40(2):475–86.
136. Barnes KK, Kolpin DW, Furlong ET, et al. A national reconnaissance of pharmaceuticals and other organic wastewater contaminants in the United States—I) groundwater. *Sci Total Environ*. 2008;402(2-3):192–200.
137. Kolpin DW, Furlong ET, Meyer MT, et al. Pharmaceuticals, hormones, and other organic wastewater contaminants in U.S. streams, 1999–2000: A national reconnaissance. *Environ Sci Technol*. 2002;36(6):1202–11.
138. Ashbolt NJ, Amezquita A, Backhaus T, et al. Human Health Risk Assessment (HHRA) for environmental development and transfer of antibiotic resistance. *Environ Health Perspect*. 2013;121(9):993–1001.
139. Huijbers PM, Blaak H, de Jong MC, et al. Role of the environment in the transmission of antimicrobial resistance to humans: A review. *Environ Sci Technol*. 2015;49(20):11993–2004.
140. Bueno I, Williams-Nguyen J, Hwang H, et al. Impact of point sources on antibiotic resistance genes in the natural environment: A systematic review of the evidence. *Anim Health Res Rev*. 2017;18(2):112–27.
141. Jorgensen JH, Ferraro MJ. Antimicrobial susceptibility testing: A review of general principles and contemporary practices. *Clin Infect Dis*. 2009;49(11):1749–55.
142. Clinical and Laboratory Standards Institute (CLSI). 2018. Available at https://clsi.org/. Accessed November 20, 2018.
143. European Committee on Antimicrobial Susceptibility Testing (EUCAST). 2018. Available at http://www.eucast.org/. Accessed November 20, 2018.
144. Centers for Disease Control and Prevention (CDC). Division of Preparedness and Emerging Infections (DPEI): Emerging Infections program. 2018. Available at https://www.cdc.gov/ncezid/dpei/eip/index.html. Accessed November 20, 2018.
145. Centers for Disease Control and Prevention (CDC). Active Bacterial Core surveillance (ABCs). 2018. Available at https://www.cdc.gov/abcs/index.html. Accessed November 20, 2018.
146. Centers for Disease Control and Prevention (CDC). Healthcare-Associated Infections-Community Interface (HAIC). 2018. Available at https://www.cdc.gov/hai/eip/index.html. Accessed November 20, 2018.
147. Centers for Disease Control and Prevention (CDC). Antibiotic/Antimicrobial Resistance (AR/AMR): Lab Capacity: Antibiotic Resistance Laboratory Network (AR Lab Network). 2018. Available at https://www.cdc.gov/drugresistance/solutions-initiative/ar-lab-network.html. Accessed November 20, 2018.
148. Woodworth KR, Walters MS, Weiner LM, et al. Vital signs: Containment of novel multidrug-resistant organisms and resistance mechanisms—United States, 2006–2017. *MMWR Morb Mortal Wkly Rep*. 2018;67(13):396–401.
149. Centers for Disease Control and Prevention (CDC). National Healthcare Safety Network (NHSN). 2018. Available at https://www.cdc.gov/nhsn/index.html. Accessed November 20, 2018.
150. Sievert DM, Ricks P, Edwards JR, et al. Antimicrobial-resistant pathogens associated with healthcare-associated infections: Summary of data reported to the National Healthcare Safety Network at the Centers for Disease Control and Prevention, 2009–2010. *Infect Control Hosp Epidemiol*. 2013;34(1):1–14.
151. Food and Drug Administration. *NARMS Integrated Report: 2014*. 2014.
152. Tornimbene B, Eremin S, Escher M, et al. WHO Global Antimicrobial Resistance Surveillance System early implementation 2016–17. *Lancet Infect Dis*. 2018;18(3):241–2.
153. World Health Organization. *Global antimicrobial resistance surveillance system (GLASS) report: Early implementation 2016–2017*. Geneva; 2017.
154. Centers for Disease Control and Prevention (CDC). *Facility Guidance for Control of Carbapenem-resistant Enterobacteriaceae (CRE)*. 2015.
155. Slayton RB, Toth D, Lee BY, et al. Vital signs: Estimated effects of a coordinated approach for action to reduce antibiotic-resistant infections in health care facilities—United States. *MMWR Morb Mortal Wkly Rep*. 2015;64(30):826–31.
156. Allen RC, Engelstadter J, Bonhoeffer S, McDonald BA, Hall AR. Reversing resistance: Different routes and common themes across pathogens. *Proc Biol Sci*. 2017;284(1863).
157. Bean DC, Livermore DM, Hall LM. Plasmids imparting sulfonamide resistance in Escherichia coli: Implications for persistence. *Antimicrob Agents Chemother*. 2009;53(3):1088–93.
158. Enne VI, Livermore DM, Stephens P, Hall LM. Persistence of sulphonamide resistance in Escherichia coli in the UK despite national prescribing restriction. *Lancet*. 2001;357(9265):1325–8.
159. Food and Drug Administration. New drugs at FDA: CDER's new molecular entities and new therapeutic biological products. 2018. Available at https://www.fda.gov/Drugs/DevelopmentApprovalProcess/DrugInnovation/default.htm. Accessed November 20, 2018.
160. Marston HD, Dixon DM, Knisely JM, Palmore TN, Fauci AS. Antimicrobial resistance. *JAMA*. 2016;316(11):1193–204.
161. Lin DM, Koskella B, Lin HC. Phage therapy: An alternative to antibiotics in the age of multi-drug resistance. *World J Gastrointest Pharmacol Ther*. 2017;8(3):162–73.
162. Langley G, Besser J, Iwamoto M, et al. Effect of culture-independent diagnostic tests on future emerging infections program surveillance. *Emerg Infect Dis*. 2015;21(9):1582–8.
163. Iwamoto M, Huang JY, Cronquist AB, et al. Bacterial enteric infections detected by culture-independent diagnostic tests—FoodNet, United States, 2012–2014. *MMWR Morb Mortal Wkly Rep*. 2015;64(9):252–7.
164. Shea S, Kubota KA, Maguire H, et al. Clinical microbiology laboratories' adoption of culture-independent diagnostic tests is a threat to foodborne-disease surveillance in the United States. *J Clin Microbiol*. 2017;55(1):10–19.
165. Fishman N, Patterson J, Saiman L, et al. Policy statement on antimicrobial stewardship by the Society for Healthcare Epidemiology of America (SHEA), the Infectious Diseases Society of America (IDSA), and the Pediatric Infectious Diseases Society (PIDS). *Infect Control Hosp Epidemiol*. 2012;33(4):322–7.
166. Briceland LL, Nightingale CH, Quintiliani R, Cooper BW, Smith KS. Antibiotic streamlining from combination therapy to monotherapy utilizing an interdisciplinary approach. *Arch Intern Med*. 1988;148(9):2019–22.
167. McGowan JEJr, Gerding DN. Does antibiotic restriction prevent resistance? *New Horiz*. 1996;4(3):370–6.
168. Shlaes DM, Gerding DN, John JFJr, et al. Society for Healthcare Epidemiology of America and Infectious Diseases Society of America Joint Committee on the Prevention of Antimicrobial Resistance: Guidelines for the prevention of antimicrobial resistance in hospitals. *Infect Control Hosp Epidemiol*. 1997;18(4):275–91.
169. Carling P, Fung T, Killion A, Terrin N, Barza M. Favorable impact of a multidisciplinary antibiotic management program conducted during 7 years. *Infect Control Hosp Epidemiol*. 2003;24(9):699–706.
170. Ansari F, Gray K, Nathwani D, et al. Outcomes of an intervention to improve hospital antibiotic prescribing: Interrupted time series with segmented regression analysis. *J Antimicrob Chemother*. 2003;52(5):842–8.
171. Ruttimann S, Keck B, Hartmeier C, Maetzel A, Bucher HC. Long-term antibiotic cost savings from a comprehensive intervention program in a medical department of a university-affiliated teaching hospital. *Clin Infect Dis*. 2004;38(3):348–56.

172. MacDougall C, Polk RE. Antimicrobial stewardship programs in health care systems. *Clin Microbiol Rev*. 2005;18(4):638–56.
173. Dellit TH, Owens RC, McGowan JEJr, et al. Infectious Diseases Society of America and the Society for Healthcare Epidemiology of America guidelines for developing an institutional program to enhance antimicrobial stewardship. *Clin Infect Dis*. 2007;44(2):159–77.
174. Fridkin S, Baggs J, Fagan R, et al. Vital signs: Improving antibiotic use among hospitalized patients. *MMWR Morb Mortal Wkly Rep*. 2014;63(9):194–200.
175. Levin PD, Idrees S, Sprung CL, et al. Antimicrobial use in the ICU: Indications and accuracy—an observational trial. *J Hosp Med*. 2012;7(9):672–8.
176. Patel SJ, Oshodi A, Prasad P, et al. Antibiotic use in neonatal intensive care units and adherence with Centers for Disease Control and Prevention 12 Step Campaign to Prevent Antimicrobial Resistance. *Pediatr Infect Dis J*. 2009;28(12):1047–51.
177. Walsh TL, Chan L, Konopka CI, et al. Appropriateness of antibiotic management of uncomplicated skin and soft tissue infections in hospitalized adult patients. *BMC Infect Dis*. 2016;16(1):721.
178. Pollack LA, Srinivasan A. Core elements of hospital antibiotic stewardship programs from the Centers for Disease Control and Prevention. *Clin Infect Dis*. 2014;59(Suppl 3):S97–100.
179. The White House. National action plan for combating antibiotic-resistant bacteria. 2015. Available at https://www.whitehouse.gov/sites/default/files/docs/national_action_plan_for_combating_antibotic-resistant_bacteria.pdf. Accessed July 24, 2018.
180. Centers for Medicare & Medicaid Services (CMS). Medicare and Medicaid Programs; Hospital and Critical Access Hospital (CAH) Changes to Promote Innovation, Flexibility, and Improvement in Patient Care In: U.S. Federal Register, ed. Vol 42 CFR 482, 42 CFR 485.
181. Joint Commission on Hospital A. APPROVED: New Antimicrobial Stewardship Standard. *Jt Comm Perspect*. 2016;36(7):1, 3, 4, 8.
182. Lim CJ, Kong DC, Stuart RL. Reducing inappropriate antibiotic prescribing in the residential care setting: Current perspectives. *Clin Interv Aging*. 2014;9:165–77.
183. Nicolle LE, Bentley DW, Garibaldi R, Neuhaus EG, Smith PW. Antimicrobial use in long-term-care facilities. SHEA Long-Term-Care Committee. *Infect Control Hosp Epidemiol*. 2000;21(8):537–45.
184. Centers for Disease Control and Prevention (CDC). The core elements of antibiotic stewardship for nursing homes. 2015. Available at http://www.cdc.gov/longtermcare/prevention/antibiotic-stewardship.html. Accessed November 29, 2018.
185. U.S. Federal Register. Medicare and Medicaid Programs; Reform of Requirements for LongTerm Care Facilities In: (CMS). CfMMS, HHS, eds. Vol 42 CFR 405, 42 CFR 431, 42 CFR 447, 42 CFR 482, 42 CFR 483, 42 CFR 485, 42 CFR 488, 42 CFR 489.2016:68688-68872.
186. Suda KJ, Hicks LA, Roberts RM, et al. Antibiotic expenditures by medication, class, and healthcare setting in the United States, 2010–2015. *Clin Infect Dis*. 2018;66(2):185–90.
187. Shapiro DJ, Hicks LA, Pavia AT, Hersh AL. Antibiotic prescribing for adults in ambulatory care in the USA, 2007–09. *J Antimicrob Chemother*. 2014;69(1):234–40.
188. Fleming-Dutra KE, Hersh AL, Shapiro DJ, et al. Prevalence of inappropriate antibiotic prescriptions among US ambulatory care visits, 2010–2011. *JAMA*. 2016;315(17):1864–73.
189. Sanchez GV, Fleming-Dutra KE, Roberts RM, Hicks LA. Core elements of outpatient antibiotic stewardship. *MMWR Recomm Rep*. 2016;65(6):1–12.
190. Bradley J, Long S. Principles of anti-infective therapy. In: *Principles and Practice of Pediatric Infectious Diseases*. 5th ed. Elsevier, Inc.; 2018.
191. Dropulic LK, Lederman HM. Overview of infections in the immunocompromised host. *Microbiol Spectr*. 2016;4(4).
192. Joint Task Force on Practice Parameters. Drug allergy: An updated practice parameter. *Ann Allergy Asthma Immunol*. 2010;105(4):259–73.
193. Rubio M, Bousquet PJ, Gomes E, Romano A, Demoly P. Results of drug hypersensitivity evaluations in a large group of children and adults. *Clin Exp Allergy*. 2012;42(1):123–30.
194. Gadde J, Spence M, Wheeler B, Adkinson NFJr. Clinical experience with penicillin skin testing in a large inner-city STD clinic. *JAMA*. 1993;270(20):2456–63.
195. Blanca M, Torres MJ, Garcia JJ, et al. Natural evolution of skin test sensitivity in patients allergic to beta-lactam antibiotics. *J Allergy Clin Immunol*. 1999;103(5 Pt 1):918–24.
196. Macy E, Contreras R. Health care use and serious infection prevalence associated with penicillin "allergy" in hospitalized patients: A cohort study. *J Allergy Clin Immunol*. 2014;133(3):790–6.
197. MacFadden DR, LaDelfa A, Leen J, et al. Impact of reported beta-lactam allergy on inpatient outcomes: A multicenter prospective cohort study. *Clin Infect Dis*. 2016;63(7):904–10.
198. Conway EL, Lin K, Sellick JA, et al. Impact of penicillin allergy on time to first dose of antimicrobial therapy and clinical outcomes. *Clin Ther*. 2017;39(11):2276–83.
199. Huang KG, Cluzet V, Hamilton K, Fadugba O. The impact of reported beta-lactam allergy in hospitalized patients with hematologic malignancies requiring antibiotics. *Clin Infect Dis*. 2018;67(1):27–33.
200. Mattingly TJ 2nd, Fulton A, Lumish RA, et al. The cost of self-reported penicillin allergy: A systematic review. *J Allergy Clin Immunol Pract*. 2018;6(5):1649–54.
201. Minnesota Department of Health. About antibiograms fact sheet. 2014. Available at http://www.health.state.mn.us/divs/idepc/dtopics/antibioticresistance/abx/antibiograms.pdf. Accessed June 18, 2018.
202. NCCLS. Analysis and Presentation of Cumulative Antimicrobial Susceptibility Test Data; Approved Guideline—Fourth Edition. CLSI document M39-A4. In. Wayne, PA: Clinical and Laboratory Standards Institute; 2014.
203. Harbarth S, Albrich W, Goldmann DA, Huebner J. Control of multiply resistant cocci: Do international comparisons help? *Lancet Infect Dis*. 2001;1(4):251–61.
204. Zinn CS, Westh H, Rosdahl VT, Sarisa Study G. An international multicenter study of antimicrobial resistance and typing of hospital Staphylococcus aureus isolates from 21 laboratories in 19 countries or states. *Microb Drug Resist*. 2004;10(2):160–8.
205. McKinnell JA, Miller LG, Singh R, et al. Prevalence of and factors associated with Multidrug Resistant Organism (MDRO) colonization in 3 nursing homes. *Infect Control Hosp Epidemiol*. 2016;37(12):1485–8.
206. Nellums LB, Thompson H, Holmes A, et al. Antimicrobial resistance among migrants in Europe: A systematic review and meta-analysis. *Lancet Infect Dis*. 2018;18(7):796–811.
207. Gaynes R, Edwards JR, National Nosocomial Infections Surveillance S. Overview of nosocomial infections caused by Gram-negative bacilli. *Clin Infect Dis*. 2005;41(6):848–54.
208. Klevens RM, Edwards JR, Tenover FC, et al. Changes in the epidemiology of methicillin-resistant Staphylococcus aureus in intensive care units in US hospitals, 1992–2003. *Clin Infect Dis*. 2006;42(3):389–91.
209. Barlam TF, Cosgrove SE, Abbo LM, et al. Implementing an antibiotic stewardship program: Guidelines by the Infectious Diseases Society of America and the Society for Healthcare Epidemiology of America. *Clin Infect Dis*. 2016;62(10):e51–77.
210. Nowak MA, Nelson RE, Breidenbach JL, Thompson PA, Carson PJ. Clinical and economic outcomes of a prospective antimicrobial stewardship program. *Am J Health Syst Pharm*. 2012;69(17):1500–8.
211. Parker SK, Hurst AL, Thurm C, et al. Anti-infective acquisition costs for a stewardship program: Getting to the bottom line. *Clin Infect Dis*. 2017;65(10):1632–7.
212. Beardsley JR, Williamson JC, Johnson JW, et al. Show me the money: Long-term financial impact of an antimicrobial stewardship program. *Infect Control Hosp Epidemiol*. 2012;33(4):398–400.
213. Abbas S, Stevens MP. The role of the hospital epidemiologist in antibiotic stewardship. *Med Clin North Am*. 2018;102(5):873–82.
214. American Nurses Association; Centers for Disease Control and Prevention. Redefining the antibiotic stewardship team: Recommendations from the American Nurses Association/Centers for Disease Control and Prevention workgroup on the role of registered nurses in hospital antibiotic stewardship practices. Available at https://www.cdc.gov/getsmart/healthcare/pdfs/ANA-CDC-whitepaper.pdf. Accessed September 28, 2018.
215. Rohde JM, Jacobsen D, Rosenberg DJ. Role of the hospitalist in antimicrobial stewardship: A review of work completed and description of a multisite collaborative. *Clin Ther*. 2013;35(6):751–7.
216. Pardo J, Klinker KP, Borgert SJ, et al. Time to positivity of blood cultures supports antibiotic de-escalation at 48 hours. *Ann Pharmacother*. 2014;48(1):33–40.
217. Lee TC, Frenette C, Jayaraman D, Green L, Pilote L. Antibiotic self-stewardship: Trainee-led structured antibiotic time-outs to improve antimicrobial use. *Ann Intern Med*. 2014;161(10 Suppl):S53–8.
218. Graber CJ, Jones MM, Glassman PA, et al. Taking an antibiotic time-out: Utilization and usability of a self-stewardship time-out program for renewal of vancomycin and piperacillin-tazobactam. *Hosp Pharm*. 2015;50(11):1011–24.
219. White ACJr, Atmar RL, Wilson J, et al. Effects of requiring prior authorization for selected antimicrobials: Expenditures, susceptibilities, and clinical outcomes. *Clin Infect Dis*. 1997;25(2):230–9.

220. Pakyz AL, Oinonen M, Polk RE. Relationship of carbapenem restriction in 22 university teaching hospitals to carbapenem use and carbapenem-resistant Pseudomonas aeruginosa. *Antimicrob Agents Chemother.* 2009;53(5):1983–6.

221. Buising KL, Thursky KA, Robertson MB, et al. Electronic antibiotic stewardship—Reduced consumption of broad-spectrum antibiotics using a computerized antimicrobial approval system in a hospital setting. *J Antimicrob Chemother.* 2008;62(3):608–16.

222. DiazGranados CA. Prospective audit for antimicrobial stewardship in intensive care: Impact on resistance and clinical outcomes. *Am J Infect Control.* 2012;40(6):526–9.

223. Elligsen M, Walker SA, Pinto R, et al. Audit and feedback to reduce broad-spectrum antibiotic use among intensive care unit patients: A controlled interrupted time series analysis. *Infect Control Hosp Epidemiol.* 2012;33(4):354–61.

224. Schuts EC, Hulscher M, Mouton JW, et al. Current evidence on hospital antimicrobial stewardship objectives: A systematic review and meta-analysis. *Lancet Infect Dis.* 2016;16(7):847–56.

225. Streetman DS, Nafziger AN, Destache CJ, Bertino ASJr. Individualized pharmacokinetic monitoring results in less aminoglycoside-associated nephrotoxicity and fewer associated costs. *Pharmacotherapy.* 2001;21(4):443–51.

226. Bond CA, Raehl CL. Clinical and economic outcomes of pharmacist-managed aminoglycoside or vancomycin therapy. *Am J Health Syst Pharm.* 2005;62(15):1596–605.

227. Sevinc F, Prins JM, Koopmans RP, et al. Early switch from intravenous to oral antibiotics: Guidelines and implementation in a large teaching hospital. *J Antimicrob Chemother.* 1999;43(4):601–6.

228. Laing RB, Mackenzie AR, Shaw H, Gould IM, Douglas JG. The effect of intravenous-to-oral switch guidelines on the use of parenteral antimicrobials in medical wards. *J Antimicrob Chemother.* 1998;42(1):107–11.

229. Wall GC, Peters L, Leaders CB, Wille JA. Pharmacist-managed service providing penicillin allergy skin tests. *Am J Health Syst Pharm.* 2004;61(12):1271–5.

230. Gugkaeva Z, Crago JS, Yasnogorodsky M. Next step in antibiotic stewardship: Pharmacist-provided penicillin allergy testing. *J Clin Pharm Ther.* 2017;42(4):509–12.

231. Hauck LD, Adler LM, Mulla ZD. Clinical pathway care improves outcomes among patients hospitalized for community-acquired pneumonia. *Ann Epidemiol.* 2004;14(9):669–75.

232. Carratala J, Garcia-Vidal C, Ortega L, et al. Effect of a 3-step critical pathway to reduce duration of intravenous antibiotic therapy and length of stay in community-acquired pneumonia: A randomized controlled trial. *Arch Intern Med.* 2012;172(12):922–8.

233. Worrall CL, Anger BP, Simpson KN, Leon SM. Impact of a hospital-acquired/ventilator-associated/healthcare-associated pneumonia practice guideline on outcomes in surgical trauma patients. *J Trauma.* 2010;68(2):382–6.

234. Schulz L, Osterby K, Fox B. The use of best practice alerts with the development of an antimicrobial stewardship navigator to promote antibiotic de-escalation in the electronic medical record. *Infect Control Hosp Epidemiol.* 2013;34(12):1259–65.

235. Jenkins TC, Knepper BC, Sabel AL, et al. Decreased antibiotic utilization after implementation of a guideline for inpatient cellulitis and cutaneous abscess. *Arch Intern Med.* 2011;171(12):1072–9.

236. Patel R, Fang FC. Diagnostic stewardship: Opportunity for a laboratory-infectious diseases partnership. *Clin Infect Dis.* 2018;67(5):799–801.

237. Morgan DJ, Malani P, Diekema DJ. Diagnostic stewardship-leveraging the laboratory to improve antimicrobial use. *JAMA.* 2017;318(7):607–8.

238. Pruden A, Larsson DG, Amezquita A, et al. Management options for reducing the release of antibiotics and antibiotic resistance genes to the environment. *Environ Health Perspect.* 2013;121(8):878–85.

239. Karkman A, Do TT, Walsh F, Virta MPJ. Antibiotic-resistance genes in waste water. *Trends Microbiol.* 2018;26(3):220–8.

240. Kerrigan JF, Sandberg KD, Engstrom DR, LaPara TM, Arnold WA. Sedimentary record of antibiotic accumulation in Minnesota lakes. *Sci Total Environ.* 2018;621:970–9.

241. Magill SS, Edwards JR, Beldavs ZG, et al. Prevalence of antimicrobial use in US acute care hospitals, May–September 2011. *JAMA.* 2014;312(14):1438–46.

242. Ibrahim OM, Polk RE. Antimicrobial use metrics and benchmarking to improve stewardship outcomes: Methodology, opportunities, and challenges. *Infect Dis Clin North Am.* 2014;28(2):195–214.

243. Centers for Disease Control and Prevention (CDC). National Healthcare Safety Network. Surveillance for antimicrobial use and antimicrobial resistance options. January 2019. Accessed December 17, 2018.

244. van Santen KL, Edwards JR, Webb AK, et al. The Standardized Antimicrobial Administration Ratio: A new metric for measuring and comparing antibiotic use. *Clin Infect Dis.* 2018;67(2):179–85.

245. Centers for Disease Control and Prevention (CDC). Be antibiotics aware: Smart use, best care. Available at https://www.cdc.gov/features/antibioticuse/index.html. Accessed November 23, 2018.

246. Drekonja DM, Filice GA, Greer N, et al. Antimicrobial stewardship in outpatient settings: A systematic review. *Infect Control Hosp Epidemiol.* 2015;36(2):142–52.

247. Scarpato SJ, Timko DR, Cluzet VC, et al. An evaluation of antibiotic prescribing practices upon hospital discharge. *Infect Control Hosp Epidemiol.* 2017;38(3):353–5.

248. Trivedi KK, Pollack LA. The role of public health in antimicrobial stewardship in healthcare. *Clin Infect Dis.* 2014;59(Suppl 3):S101–3.

249. Centers for Disease Control and Prevention (CDC). Antibiotic prescribing and use in doctor's offices: Antibiotic stewardship implementation framework for health departments. Available at https://www.cdc.gov/antibiotic-use/community/programs-measurement/state-local-activities/framework.html. Accessed November 23, 2018.

250. Centers for Disease Control and Prevention (CDC). Antibiotic prescribing and use in doctor's offices: State efforts. Available at https://www.cdc.gov/antibiotic-use/community/programs-measurement/state-local-activities/state-activities.html. Accessed November 23, 2018.

251. Centers for Disease Control and Prevention (CDC). One Health. 2018. Available at https://www.cdc.gov/onehealth/index.html. Accessed November 20, 2018.

252. Sheldon T. Saving antibiotics for when they are really needed: The Dutch example. *BMJ.* 2016;354:i4192.

253. Lammie SL, Hughes JM. Antimicrobial resistance, food safety, and One Health: The need for convergence. *Annu Rev Food Sci Technol.* 2016;7:287–312.

254. Ogawa VA, Shah CM, Hughes JM, King LJ. Prioritizing a One Health approach in the immediate fight against antimicrobial resistance. *Ecohealth.* 2018;16(3):410–3.

255. Food and Drug Administration. *Guidance for Industry #152: Evaluating the Safety of Antimicrobial New Animal Drugs with Regard to Their Microbiological Effects on Bacteria of Human Health Concern.* 2003.

256. Food and Drug Administration. *Guidance for Industry #209: The Judicious Use of Medically Important Antimicrobial Drugs in Food-Producing Animals.* 2012.

257. Food and Drug Administration. *Guidance for Industry #213: New Animal Drugs and New Animal Drug Combination Products Administered in or on Medicated Feed or Drinking Water of Food-Producing Animals: Recommendations for Drug Sponsors for Voluntarily Aligning Product Use Conditions with GFI #209* 2013.

258. World Health Organization. *Critically important antimicrobials for human medicine—5th rev.* Geneva, 2017.

259. U.S. Federal Register. Veterinary Feed Directive. In: Food and Drug Administration, ed. Vol 21 CFR 514, 21 CFR 5582015.

260. Pew Charitable Trusts. *Alternatives to Antibiotics in Animal Agriculture.* 2017.

261. U.S. Federal Register. The Judicious Use of Medically Important Antimicrobial Drugs in Food-Producing Animals; Establishing Appropriate Durations of Therapeutic Administration; Request for Comments. In: Food and Drug Administration, ed. *81 FR 631872*016:63187-63191.

262. Abell KM, Theurer ME, Larson RL, White BJ, Apley M. A mixed treatment comparison meta-analysis of metaphylaxis treatments for bovine respiratory disease in beef cattle. *J Anim Sci.* 2017;95(2):626–35.

263. Song SJ, Lauber C, Costello EK, et al. Cohabiting family members share microbiota with one another and with their dogs. *Elife.* 2013;2:e00458.

264. Tun HM, Konya T, Takaro TK, et al. Exposure to household furry pets influences the gut microbiota of infant at 3-4 months following various birth scenarios. *Microbiome.* 2017;5(1):40.

265. American Veterinary Medical Association. *Antimicrobial Stewardship in Companion Animal Practice (2016).* 2016.

266. Food and Drug Administration. *Supporting Antimicrobial Stewardship in Veterinary Settings Goals For Fiscal Years 2019–2023.* 2018.

267. Lessa FC, Mu Y, Bamberg WM, et al. Burden of Clostridium difficile infection in the United States. *N Engl J Med.* 2015;372(9):825–34.

CHAPTER

154 *Staphylococcus aureus*

Michael Z. David

BACKGROUND

The bacterium *Staphylococcus aureus* is among the most common causes of human infection requiring medical care across the lifespan, and among the most common causes of skin, bone, and bloodstream infections globally.[1] It is also a pathogen of agricultural importance, particularly in dairy cows and poultry.[2] *S. aureus* is generally a commensal organism, and it has been recovered in tests of asymptomatic nasal colonization from 23% to 41% of human populations in studies throughout the world.[3–10] *S. aureus* is often part of the human skin and gut microbiome, and it is transmitted from person to person by direct contact. *S. aureus* can also spread between animals and humans.

S. aureus has been the target of antibiotic development since the 1930s, when sulfonamides were first introduced.[11] However, well-documented resistance emerged to each new class of antibiotics that has been developed to combat this pathogen. Most notably, methicillin-resistant *S. aureus* (MRSA) strains are resistant to nearly all antibiotics related to penicillins, a large group of drugs that are known as ß-lactam antibiotics.[1,12]

S. aureus is a public health threat because it is spread from person to person inside and outside of the healthcare arena, causes thousands of fatal infections each year in the United States alone, and is an increasingly important cause of antimicrobial-resistant infections. However, the most important public health challenge of *S. aureus* lies in the fact that we have yet to develop adequate interventions to recognize and control the spread of virulent strains among humans and animals in order to prevent infections and to protect vulnerable populations. No vaccine exists to prevent *S. aureus* infections, and therefore approaches to infection prevention have focused on the interruption of transmission in healthcare facilities and less commonly in households and other community settings, decolonization of chronic carriers, and suppression of colonization prior to high-risk surgical procedures.

Although the vast majority of human infections caused by *S. aureus* are skin and soft tissue infections (SSTIs), the bacterium also causes invasive disease, particularly among individuals with certain risk factors. People at high risk of invasive infection include those with an intravenous catheter, chronic skin disease, recent surgery, hemodialysis, recent hospitalization, endotracheal intubation, or an immunocompromised state due to human immunodeficiency virus infection, immunosuppressive medications, or cancer. Patients with diabetes mellitus are also at elevated risk of *S. aureus* infection. *S. aureus* is a common cause of human surgical-site infections, bacteremia, osteomyelitis, joint infections, pneumonia, infective endocarditis, and abscesses in internal organs after dissemination in blood. It is a rare cause of urinary tract and central nervous system infections except those that occur after surgical procedures (Table 154-1).[1] Infection is almost always preceded by asymptomatic colonization which is a risk factor for infection.[15,16]

S. aureus is a Gram-positive, nonmotile, coagulase- and catalase-positive bacterium that usually reduces nitrate and is a facultative anaerobe. Under microscopy, the bacterium typically appears as a cluster of round-shaped bacteria, and when grown on solid agar the colonies have a golden yellow color. It was named because of these two attributes: *Staphylococcus*, from the Greek σταφυλόκοκκος (*stafilokokkos*), meaning a *grape-cluster ball* or *berry*; and *aureus*, from the Latin word *aurum*, meaning *gold*. It is readily cultured from sources of infection or asymptomatic colonization in people or animals, and from surfaces in the environment of a colonized human or animal host.

Because of the long evolutionary history of *S. aureus* as a human commensal organism, it has acquired numerous virulence factors and mechanisms of immune evasion in people. This results in sometimes prolonged, and even indefinite, asymptomatic carriage of the bacterium on the skin or mucous membranes and the possibility of recurrent infections caused by a single clonal strain.[17] Genetic variation in the species has been studied extensively, and many strain types have been identified with defined phylogenetic lineages. While nearly every strain type of *S. aureus* may cause infection, there is wide variation among strains in their carriage of virulence factors.

Since the discovery of *S. aureus* in 1881, more than 80 species or subspecies of *Staphylococcus* have been identified.[18] The coagulase-positive species *S. aureus* is importantly distinguished from many coagulase-negative staphylococcal species (CONS), such as *S. epidermidis* and *S. hominis*, which are likely carried by all people. The CONS species are far less pathogenic, rarely infecting people without the presence of a foreign body, such as a vascular catheter, a pacemaker, or a prosthetic joint.

In livestock, *S. aureus* is an important cause of economically important infections such as mastitis in cows, exudative dermatitis in pigs, and bumblefoot (chondronecrosis with osteomyelitis) in turkeys. It can spread rapidly in livestock herds, and livestock may serve as a large reservoir for pathogenic *S. aureus* strains or for genes coding for resistance to antimicrobials that may impact human health.[2,19,20]

HISTORY AND EPIDEMIOLOGY

S. aureus was discovered by Alexander Ogston, a Scottish surgeon who identified the bacterium in pus from a septic knee in 1880 and in a series of 65 acute skin abscesses in 1881,[21] relatively early in the era of bacterial discovery that marked the Bacteriological Revolution. Friedrich Julius Rosenbach in 1884 distinguished *S. aureus* from "*S. albus*," likely a CONS species.[22] After these pioneering discoveries, it quickly became clear that *S. aureus* causes a variety of infections ranging from minor infections of the skin, such as folliculitis or impetigo, to bloodstream infections, which were nearly uniformly fatal before antibiotics were introduced.

TABLE 154-1 COMMON *S. AUREUS* CLINICAL SYNDROMES

Syndrome	Notes
Skin and soft tissue infections (SSTIs)	Most common type of *S. aureus* infection. Wide range of severity. Includes folliculitis, impetigo, abscess, cellulitis, surgical-site infections, and necrotizing fasciitis. Skin abscesses often require incision and drainage. Folliculitis and impetigo are usually treated topically or only symptomatically.
Bacteremia	Risk factors include invasive medical procedures, injection drug use, hemodialysis, chronic indwelling intravascular catheters, and immunocompromised conditions. Mortality remains high even with optimal medical care.
Endocarditis	Infection of a heart valve and/or the cardiac muscle. Risk factors include injection drug use and bacteremia from any cause. Often requires valve replacement. May lead to cardiac conduction abnormalities, metastatic infection of internal organs, stroke, septic emboli of lungs, vertebral osteomyelitis and discitis, or epidural abscess.
Pneumonia	Risk factors include prior viral upper respiratory infection, especially influenza, endotracheal intubation, and chronic lung disease.
Osteomyelitis	Risk factors include prior surgery, endocarditis, or deep soft tissue infections. Often treated with prolonged antibiotic therapy alone.
Septic arthritis	Occurs by hematogenous spread or by direct extension from another site of infection. Often requires surgical drainage and antimicrobial therapy. Complications include severe damage to the infected joint, including frozen joints.
Gastroenteritis	Caused by ingestion of preformed *S. aureus* toxin with food; common cause of foodborne outbreaks worldwide.
Pyomyositis	Infection of skeletal muscle, often with abscess formation. Most common site is the pelvic muscles. Risk factor is prior bacteremia.
Toxic shock syndrome	Life-threatening systemic syndrome caused by toxic shock syndrome toxin production by *S. aureus* causing an infection or with a focus of colonization associated with the mucous membranes or a wound. The case definition[13] is as follows:
	A. Clinical Criteria: An illness with the following manifestations:
	Fever: temperature >= 102.0°F (>= 38.9°C)
	Rash: diffuse macular erythroderma
	Desquamation: 1–2 weeks after onset of rash
	Hypotension: systolic blood pressure <= 90 mm Hg for adults or < 5th percentile by age for children < 16 years
	Multisystem involvement (>=3 of the following organ systems):
	Gastrointestinal: vomiting or diarrhea at onset of illness
	Muscular: severe myalgia or CPK at least twice ULN
	Mucous membrane: vaginal, oropharyngeal, or conjunctival hyperemia
	Renal: BUN or creatinine at least twice the ULN or urinary sediment with pyuria (>= 5 leukocytes per high-power field) in the absence of urinary tract infection
	Hepatic: total bilirubin, ALT, or AST at least twice the ULN
	Hematologic: platelets < 100,000/mm^3
	Central nervous system: disorientation or alterations in consciousness without focal neurologic signs when fever and
	hypotension are absent
	B. Laboratory Criteria: If obtained, negative results on:
	Blood or cerebrospinal fluid cultures (blood may be positive for *S. aureus*)
	Negative serologies for Rocky Mountain spotted fever, leptospirosis, or measles
	Case Classification
	Probable
	A case which meets the laboratory criteria and in which four of the five clinical criteria above are present
	Confirmed
	A case which meets the laboratory criteria and in which all five of the clinical criteria above are present, including desquamation, unless the patient dies before desquamation occurs
Scalded skin syndrome	A syndrome caused by exfoliative toxin A or B. Associated with sloughing of skin, positive Nikolsky's sign, tender erythema, and absence of mucosal involvement. Case fatality rate is 10% in children and 40–63% in adults.[14]
Parotitis	Infection of the parotid gland. Often cured by antimicrobial therapy alone.
Ocular infections	Includes orbital cellulitis, endophthalmitis, and panophthalmitis. Can be caused by hematogenous seeding or by direct spread from a soft tissue or sinus infection.
Lung abscess	Complication of pneumonia or of bacteremia.
Organ abscess	Most often a complication of bacteremia or surgery.
Central nervous system infection	Rare without presence of a foreign body or after a surgical procedure
Urinary tract infection	Unusual site for *S. aureus* infection

Abbreviations: ALT = alanine aminotransferase; AST = aspartate aminotransferase; BUN = Blood urea nitrogen; CPK = creatinine phosphokinase; ULN = upper limit of normal.

S. aureus is a leading cause of human bacterial infections for which people seek medical care. In 2001–11 in New Zealand, a single-center study estimated an annual incidence for all *S. aureus* infections of 360–412 per 100,000 population.[23] Among U.S. veterans in Maryland during 1999–2008, the mean annual incidence of all *S. aureus* infections was 749 per 100,000.[24] Although there are no large-scale surveillance programs to estimate the incidence of SSTIs definitively in human populations, in a health system in California, an SSTI was diagnosed in 496 per 100,000 person-years, and *S. aureus* was isolated in 81% of pathogen-positive SSTI cultures.[25] In a population of retired and active U.S. military personnel and their dependents, the incidence of *S. aureus* SSTIs was estimated to be 122.7–168.9 per 100,000 person-years.[26]

S. aureus is also a common cause of invasive bacterial infectious syndromes. The estimated incidence of *S. aureus* bacteremia is 10–30 per 100,000, with variation by country.[1] In 2017, about 117,247

S. aureus bloodstream infections were treated in the United States.[27] *S. aureus* is the second most common cause of bacteremia and the cause of 25–30% of infective endocarditis.[28] Mortality from *S. aureus* bacteremia varies in recent studies from 15% to 50%.[1] The rate of invasive *S. aureus* infections is higher among black than white populations in the United States.[29] Invasive MRSA infections (i.e., those occurring in normally sterile sites) in the United States in 2005 had an estimated incidence of 31.8 per 100,000,[30] but the incidence then decreased by 31% between 2005 and 2011,[31] a change largely due to a decrease in healthcare-associated infections. For example, hospital-onset invasive MRSA infections decreased 28% between 2005 and 2008.[32] In 2014–15 in two counties in Minnesota, consistent with this trend, the incidence of invasive MRSA infections was 13.1 per 100,000; invasive methicillin-susceptible *S. aureus* (MSSA) infections during the same period had an incidence of 27.1 per 100,000.[33]

S. aureus is a leading cause of hospital-onset pneumonia.[34] In the United States, data from the National Inpatient Sample (NIS) showed that the incidence of MRSA pneumonia among hospitalized patients between 2009 and 2012 decreased from 75.6 to 56.6 per 100,000 hospital discharges. Case fatality rates for MRSA pneumonia decreased in this period from 7.9% to 6.4%, while for MSSA pneumonia, they decreased from 6.9% to 4.7%.[35] Outside of hospitals, *S. aureus* was estimated to account for 12.6–30.8% of community-acquired pneumonia, with great variation by continent.[36] *S. aureus* is especially common as a cause of bacterial superinfection of influenza and other upper respiratory virus infections. A meta-analysis showed that *S. aureus* caused about 28% of bacterial superinfections complicating influenza,[37] while in a U.S. multicenter study of influenza among intensive care unit (ICU) patients, 9.3% had a *S. aureus* pneumonia or bacteremia.[38]

While the nares are the most common site of asymptomatic *S. aureus* carriage, screening of the nares likely misses about one-third of S. *aureus* carriers. Other common sites of colonization are the throat, the gut, and the perineal skin.[39,40] Colonization of the throat may be a risk factor for prolonged MRSA carriage.[41,42]

S. aureus infections appear to be seasonal in incidence, with an increased rate of infection in the warmer months. As noted, SSTIs are frequently caused by *S. aureus*. Among children with Medicaid insurance in a county in Arizona in 2005–08, the annual peak total SSTI incidence was in early September.[43] Similar seasonal variation was identified in the epidemiology of SSTIs in both adults and children at an academic medical center in Chicago in 2006–14.[44] In a separate study, all MRSA infections occurring in the community in people without healthcare risk factors (community-associated), regardless of anatomic site, were more common in the third and fourth quarters of the year in adults and children at a U.S. medical center in 2001–10.[45] In a study of administrative data for the United States in 1998–2011, surgical-site infections were found to vary by month of the year, perhaps also due to seasonal variation in *S. aureus* infection incidence, peaking in August.[46] The seasonal variability may be due increased *S. aureus* skin colonization in the warmer months, but the underlying reason for this consistent pattern in the literature has not been determined.

Antimicrobial Resistance in *S. aureus*

The history of *S. aureus* epidemiology since the 1940s has been marked by an increasing trend toward antimicrobial resistance. There are myriad mechanisms of resistance to antibiotics in *S. aureus*, dictated by the mechanism of action of each antibiotic class (see Table 154-2).[47] A series of epidemic waves of discrete strain types with distinct antimicrobial susceptibility profiles have been posited to underlie epidemiologic change during the twentieth and early twenty-first centuries.[48] Although very rarely is a single strain resistant to all available classes of antistaphylococcal antimicrobials, *S. aureus* has acquired clinically significant resistance to every newly introduced class of antibiotics, including penicillin, semisynthetic "antistaphylococcal" penicillins, cephalosporins, sulfa drugs, glycopeptides, tetracyclines, dihydrofolate reductase inhibitors, aminoglycosides, rifamycins, fluoroquinolones, oxazolidinones, and lipoglycopeptides.[47]

TABLE 154-2 SELECTED MECHANISMS OF RESISTANCE TO CLASSES OF ANTIMICROBIALS USED IN THE TREATMENT OF *S. AUREUS* INFECTIONS

Drug Class	Common Genes Associated with Resistance	Common Mechanism of Resistance	Site/Mechanism of Drug Action
Penicillins	ß-lactamases	Drug inactivation	Cell membrane; peptidoglycan synthesis
Methicillin (MRSA)	*mecA*	Low-affinity binding	Cell membrane; peptidoglycan synthesis
Fluoroquinolones	*gyrA, gyrB,* parC, pare, *NorA*	Mutations in DNA topoisomerase-IV or gyrase genes; efflux pumps	DNA replication
Clindamycin/Lincosamides	*erm*, MLS_B	Ribosomal methylase; target modification	Protein synthesis
Tetracyclines	tet(A), tet(B)	Drug efflux pumps	Protein synthesis
Sulfonamides	Dihydropteroate synthetase	Mutations of target	Folate synthesis
Rifampin		Mutations of target, efflux	Transcription
Trimethoprim	Dihydrofolate reductase	Mutations of target	Folate synthesis
Aminoglycosides	*aacA-aphD*	Drug modification	Protein synthesis
Oxazolidinones	*cfr*	Mutations of target ribosomal proteins; 23S rRNA methyl transferase (*cfr*)	Protein synthesis
Vancomycin	*vanA*	Peptidoglycan biosynthesis	Cell wall; blocks PBP2 and PBP2a
Daptomycin	*mprF*	Change in cell membrane charge	Cell wall damage
Ceftaroline	Altered PBP2a	Mutations of target	Cell membrane
Mupirocin	*mupA, ileRS*	Mutations in target; Enzyme replacement	Protein synthesis
Pleuromutilins/Retapamulin	*cfr*	23S rRNA methyl transferase	Protein synthesis

A particular phenotype of *S. aureus* that demonstrates resistance to nearly all ß-lactam antimicrobial drugs (i.e., penicillins, cephalosporins, and carbapenems) was first recognized in 1960.[49] This phenotype was termed MRSA after methicillin, the first semisynthetic penicillinase-resistant ß-lactam drug, which is no longer in clinical use. MRSA strains carry a mobile genetic element known as the staphylococcal chromosome cassette *mec* (SCC*mec*), which is uniformly inserted in a specific chromosomal site, orfX. SCC*mec* elements have been incorporated into many previously MSSA strains, and therefore there is wide genetic variation in circulating MRSA strains around the world. SCC*mec* carries a ccR gene complex, which codes for the excision of SCC*mec* from and insertion of SCC*mec* into the chromosome, as well as the *mecA* gene, which codes for a protein known as penicillin binding protein 2a (PBP2a).[12] PBP2a, like other penicillin binding proteins, is inserted into the staphylococcal cell wall; PBPs are usually the targets of ß-lactam antibiotics, but in the presence of PBP2a, *S. aureus* strains are resistant to almost all ß-lactams.[47] The hundreds of genetically distinct MRSA strains identified worldwide since 1961 have variable antimicrobial-resistance patterns and geographic variability in their global distribution (see Table 154-3).

In the 1960s, MRSA strains of *S. aureus* became increasingly common in the United Kingdom in large hospitals and then later in smaller hospitals. These strains caused infections in patients with impaired immunity or breaches in skin or impairment of other barriers to infection. In 1968, the first outbreak of MRSA infections was reported in the United States in at the Boston Children's Hospital.[51] In the course of the 1970s and more rapidly in the 1980s and 1990s, MRSA began to replace MSSA strains, initially in ICUs and later in other wards.[12] In the United States, the proportion of MRSA among *S. aureus* infections with onset in the healthcare setting increased from 2% in 1975 to 29% in 1991[52] and then to 42% in non-ICU hospital units in 2003.[53] Between 1993 and 2005, according to data from the NIS, the absolute number of MRSA infections increased nearly 10 times in U.S. hospitals, from approximately 38,100 to 368,600, with males comprising a significantly higher percentage of the total than females.[54] In Canada, the pattern of emergence of MRSA was similar.[55] In continental Europe, MRSA gradually became common in hospitals during the 1980s; hospital incidence has long been higher in southern than in northern European countries.[56–58] In Australia, a distinctive pattern of emergence was documented. First in eastern Australia in the 1980s, there were hospital MRSA outbreaks, and eventually multidrug-resistant MRSA strains became established as endemic hospital pathogens across much of Australia. However, in Western Australia (WA) the incidence of MRSA infections was very low until 1995 when there was a rapid increase in gentamicin-susceptible "WA-MRSA" infections.[59,60] In several countries of northern Europe, "Search and Destroy" public health programs, which included patient and household member decolonization, were instituted to prevent the spread of MRSA, and the incidence of MRSA infection has remained very low there.[61,62] In China, Japan, Taiwan, and Korea by the 2010s, the incidence of healthcare associated (HA)-MRSA infections was high.[63]

Starting in the 1980s, a novel public health problem emerged when, for the first time, scattered reports of MRSA infections diagnosed in patients with no known healthcare exposures were published in the United States,[64] Canada,[65] and especially in Australia.[59,66,67] In the late 1990s, additional reports appeared among indigenous populations.[68] By 2005, so-called "community-associated" (CA)—MRSA infections were a common occurrence in the United States, Australia, and Canada. Although not as common as in North America, in the early 2000s they were increasingly recognized in nearly every region of the world.[69]

In the United States, the incidence of MRSA increased substantially between 1998 and 2006, as evidenced by reports of increasing numbers of patients with SSTIs cared for in emergency departments,[70] ambulatory care,[71,72] and hospitals.[73,74] The change was rapid,[75] and a similar rise occurred in Canada.[55] In California among children, the incidence of hospitalization for a *S. aureus* infection increased from 49 per 100,000 in 1985 to 83 per 100,000 in 2006.[76] The incidence of MRSA infections among children admitted to U.S. hospitals increased from 6.7 to 21.1 cases per 1000 admissions between 2002 and 2007.[77] At Kaiser Permanente of Northern California, a large, integrated health plan, the percentage of *S. aureus* isolates that were MRSA increased from 9% in 1998 to 20% in 2001, and further to 49% in 2005. The change was driven by increasing numbers of community-onset MRSA infections.[24,78,79] Many studies from North America provide evidence that the increased incidence of MRSA infections in 1998–2010 was due to the emergence of novel MRSA strains, particularly USA300, defined by pulsed field gel electrotropheresis (PFGE, see below) typing, that initially caused a great number of MRSA infections in the community (CA-MRSA strains).[55,80–84] By 2011, USA300 was the predominant type among all MRSA isolates causing infections at 43 U.S. medical centers.[85] In San Francisco, a study of 549 USA300 MRSA bacteremia cases suggested that frequently the source of bacteremia was an SSTI, raising concern that the frequent USA300 MRSA SSTIs were a harbinger of more invasive infections.[86]

Since 2010 in many countries, and earlier in Australia[87] and Taiwan,[88] studies have suggested the incidence of MRSA SSTIs and invasive infections, including both CA-MRSA and HA-MRSA infections, have decreased.[26,78,89–93] The reasons for the decrease in MRSA infection incidence are not precisely known, but improved infection control protocols in acute healthcare facilities likely contributed in some countries.[89] A change in the molecular epidemiology of *S. aureus* or in host herd immunity may also have played a role although neither of these hypotheses is yet supported by studies. The number of MRSA-related hospitalizations in the United States decreased by about 15.8% between 2010 and 2014.[93] Among veterans in Atlanta, the incidence of community-onset MRSA infections decreased between 2007 and 2011 from 5.45 to 3.14 per 1000 veterans per year.[94] This nationwide trend has likely resulted in the observed decreased incidence of medically attended SSTIs from all causes in the United States. This is supported by a study of visits to emergency departments at academic medical centers in the United States, where the proportion of visits for an SSTI decreased by 16% between 2006 and 2014.[44] USA100 is the predominant HA-MRSA strain type in the United States. The Centers for Disease Control and Prevention (CDC) Emerging Infections Program (EIP) surveillance data found an overall 60% decrease in USA100 MRSA bacteremia between 2005 and 2013, and the decrease occurred particularly with hospital-onset MRSA bacteremia (a 21% modeled annual decrease of 6.1–0.9 per 100,000 population). During the same period, there was a 13% modeled annual decrease in hospital-onset USA300 MRSA bacteremic infections (1.5–0.6 per 100,000 population), but no statistically significant decrease in USA300 MRSA bacteremia occurring in patients with healthcare risk factors but with onset of infection in the community nor in USA300 CA-MRSA bacteremia.[92] Continued surveillance of MRSA strain types causing invasive infections may provide essential data for the control of emerging or especially virulent strain types of *S. aureus* in the future, as we do not understand the reasons for the rapid emergence or decline of various *S. aureus* strains.

Taxonomy and Molecular Epidemiology

Since the 1930s, it has been known that there is variation in toxin production and virulence in different *S. aureus* strains, but such distinctions were not very useful in developing taxonomic schemes to classify strain types. Beginning in the 1940s and then more systematically in the 1950s, *S. aureus* strains were distinguished with a classification system based on lysis of the bacteria using a series of specific viruses that infect bacteria, called bacteriophages.[95] This phage typing system was used to identify a specific emergent strain known as the 80/81 phage type that caused hospital outbreaks in the

TABLE 154-3 MAJOR MRSA STRAIN TYPES WORLDWIDE, INDICATING TYPICAL SCC*MEC* TYPES, AND GEOGRAPHIC DISTRIBUTION

Strain MLST [Clonal Cluster (CC)]; Related Clone Names[a]	Usual SCC*mec* Type	Typical *spa* Types	Countries or Continents Where Most Prevalent; Animal Species Listed for LA-MRSA
Community-associated MRSA (typically carry Panton Valentine leukocidin genes unless otherwise noted)			
ST1 (CC1), USA400, CMRSA7, WAMRSA1	IV	t127	Worldwide
ST8 (CC8), USA300, CMRSA10, WAMRSA12	IVa	t008, t064, t121, t723	United States, Canada, Europe, Japan
ST8 (CC8), USA500, CMRSA5 (PVL-)	IV	t008, t064	
ST8 (CC8), USA300-Latin American variant		t008	South America
ST30 (CC30), USA1100, SWP clone, WSPP clone	IV/IVa	t012, t018, t019, t021, t755	Worldwide except Africa
ST59 (CC59), USA1000	IV	t216, t316, t437, t441, t3485	Asia, Australia, United States
ST59 (CC59), WAMRSA9 (PVL-)	V	t437	Asia, Australia
ST59 (CC59)	V_T	t437, t441, t1950, t2365	Taiwan, Australia
ST72 (CC72), USA700 (PVL-)	IVa/IVc	t126, t148, t324, t664, t791, t2431, t2461	Europe, South Korea
ST72 (CC72), WAMRSA91	V/V(5C)	t3092	Africa, Cuba, Europe
ST75 (CC75),[b] WAMRSA79, WAMRSA8 (PVL-)	IV		Australia
ST78 (CC88), WAMRSA2 (PVL-)	IVa	t3205	Australia
ST80 (CC80), European CA-MRSA clone, FIN-11	IV	t044, t131, t376, t455	Europe, Africa, Middle East
ST88 (CC88)	IV/V	t186, t325, t690, t786, t1764, t1814, t1951, t2592, t2649, t5348	Africa, Asia, Europe
ST88 (CC88)	III/IIIA	t1376	China
ST93 (CC93); Queensland clone	IVa	t202, t4178	Australia, New Zealand China, France
ST97 (CC97), WAMRSA54	IV/V	t267, t359, t521	Worldwide
ST152 (CC152), WAMRSA89	V	t355	Europe, Australia
ST188 (CC1), WAMRSA38, WAMRSA78 (usually PVL-)	IV/V	t189	Asia, South America
ST772 (CC1, but have agr group II); Bengal Bay clone, WAMRSA-60	V	t345, t657, t1387, t3387	India, Pakistan, Malaysia, Australia
Healthcare-associated MRSA (typically lack the PVL genes)			
ST5 (CC5), USA100, CMRSA2, EMRSA-3, Rhine-Hesse Epidemic Strain	II	t002, t003, t105	Worldwide
ST5 (CC5), USA800, Pediatric clone, WAMRSA3	IV	t002, t105, t688	United States, Europe, South America, Angola
ST22 (CC22), EMRSA-15, CMRSA8, Barnim Epidemic Strain	IVh	t022, t032, t379, t515, t747, t1214, t2357	Europe
ST22 (CC22)	IVa	t223, t474	Europe, Middle East
ST30 (CC30)	IVc	t012, t018, t019, t021	Europe, South America, China. Australia
ST36 (CC30), EMRSA-16, USA200, FIN-6, CMRSA4	II	t018, t021	Europe, South Africa, United States
ST45 (CC45), Berlin clone, USA600, FIN-10, WAMRSA23, WAMRSA75	IV	t004, t015, t026, t038, t740, t1081	Europe, Asia, Australia
ST89 (CC89)	I/II/IIb	t375, t8841	Japan, South Korea, Taiwan
ST121 (CC121)	IV	t159, t645	Asia, Middle East, Europe, South America, United States
ST121 (CC121)	V	t5110, t10641	Japan
ST125 (CC5)	IVa/IVc	t002, t067, t010, t2220	Europe
ST146 (CC5)	IV	t002, t010, t067	Portugal, Spain
ST225 (CC5)	II	t003, t014, t045	Europe, United States
ST228 (CC5), southern German clone	I	t001, t041, t109, t744	Europe
ST239 (CC239; related to CC8, but 20% of genome derived from a CC30 precursor), Brazilian/Portuguese clone, Hungarian clone, Vienna clone, EMRSA-1, -4, -7, -9, or -11	III/IIIA	t030, t037, t138, t388, t421, t459, t461, t632, t1152, t2270, t2760, t4150, t4410	Asia, Europe, Middle East, South America, Australia, Africa
ST247 (CC8), EMRSA-5, -7, Iberian clone, North German Epidemic Strain, Rome clone	I	t051, t052, t303	Europe, Africa (common in the 1960s–1990s)

TABLE 154-3 MAJOR MRSA STRAIN TYPES WORLDWIDE, INDICATING TYPICAL SCC*MEC* TYPES, AND GEOGRAPHIC DISTRIBUTION

Strain MLST [Clonal Cluster (CC)]; Related Clone Names[a]	Usual SCC*mec* Type	Typical *spa* Types	Countries or Continents Where Most Prevalent; Animal Species Listed for LA-MRSA
ST250 (CC8), First MRSA; also called Archaic, Early or Ancestral MRSA	I	t008, t051, t211	Europe, Africa, Australia (more common in 1960s)
ST254 (CC8), EMRSA10, Hannover Epidemic strain	I/IV	t009, t036, t139	Europe, Korea, Taiwan (more common before 2000)
Livestock-associated MRSA (typically lack the PVL genes)			
ST9 (CC9)	IVb/V	t899, t1430	Pigs, turkeys, chickens
ST130 (CC130)	XI (*mecC*)	t843, t1736, t1773, t3256	Cows, cats, horses, hares, humans
ST133 (CC133)	IV		Sheep, goats, cows
ST398 (CC398)	V	t011, t034, t571	Pigs, horses, cattle, poultry
ST425 (CC425)	XI (*mecC*)	t742, t6292, t6300, t11212	Rabbits, cows, boars, deer
ST612 (CC8), WAMRSA20	IV/IVa	t064, t1257, t1443	Horses, humans

[a]Strain names here reflect national or regional nomenclature for strains; "USA-" designations were developed by the U.S. Centers for Disease Control and Prevention (CDC) are determined by PFGE type; "EMRSA-" designations are from the United Kingdom; "FIN-" designations used in Finland; "CMRSA-" designations are used in Canada; and "WAMRSA-" designations are used in Western Australia.
[b]Now designated as a separate species, *S. argenteus*.[50]
Abbreviations: MLST = multilocus sequence type; MRSA = methicillin-resistant *S. aureus*; PVL = Panton-Valentine leukocidin; SCC*mec* = staphylococcal cassette chromosome *mec*.

1950s, especially in newborn hospital units in the United Kingdom, Australia, the United States, and France. The 80/81 epidemic suddenly subsided in the early 1960s for unknown reasons.[96,97] Phage typing studies, performed well into the 1980s, were hampered by the fact that a substantial proportion of isolates were untypeable using the technique.[98]

In the 1990s, PFGE was developed using restriction endonucleases isolated from other species of bacteria. These endonucleases cut genomic DNA into segments at specific DNA sequences, resulting in a reproducible series of DNA fragments. The DNA is run on a gel with an electric current to separate fragments into a reproducible pattern that enables comparison of strains to assess their relatedness.[99] PFGE was applied to many bacterial species and used in *S. aureus* hospital outbreak investigations as well as public health studies. Separate standardized PFGE nomenclature systems were developed for MRSA strains circulating in the United States,[100] Canada,[101] and Europe,[102] among other countries and regions.

It quickly became clear that the CA-MRSA infections outside of the healthcare setting in the late 1990s and early 2000s were usually caused by strain types of MRSA, defined by PFGE, that were distinct from the HA-MRSA strain types typically circulating in medical institutions.[103,104] The new CA-MRSA strains were also distinguished by almost always carrying the Panton Valentine leukocidin (PVL) toxin genes (Table 154-4) and the SCC*mec* type IV or V elements, being susceptible to most non-ß-lactam drugs, and causing predominantly SSTIs, usually in children and young adults. In contrast, the HA-MRSA strains tended to cause invasive, healthcare-associated infections (HAIs), were more likely to be multidrug resistant, lacked carriage of the PVL genes, differed in SCC*mec* type, and infected older people.[69] The CDC created narrowly defined epidemiological criteria for CA-MRSA infections, which identified a group of infections that almost certainly had onset in the community. Non-CA-MRSA infections were further stratified into two categories, hospital-onset-MRSA and healthcare-associated, community-onset (HACO-) MRSA (i.e., infections with onset in the community in people with certain prior healthcare exposures).[30,32] However, a number of studies in the United States and Europe soon demonstrated that the application of the epidemiological criteria for CA-MRSA infections did not accurately identify all patients who were infected with the novel CA-MRSA strains. This is because these CA-MRSA strains after their appearance in the community quickly began to cause infections in hospitalized patients as well.[112–114]

TABLE 154-4 SELECTED *S. AUREUS* TOXINS IMPORTANT IN HUMAN INFECTIONS

Toxin	Toxicity	Reference
Toxic shock toxin-1	Superantigen that nonspecifically actives T cells	105
SEA, SEB, SEC, SED, SEE, SEF, SEG, SHE, SEI, SEJ, SEK, SEL, SEM, SEN, SEO, SEP, SEQ, SER, SET	Staphylococcal enterotoxins that cause gastroenteritis or emesis (SEG, SEH, SEI, SER, SES, and SET). The enterotoxins are resistant to heat and to low pH. SEA and SEB are superantigens that can cause shock.	106,107
Exfoliative toxin A, B, and D	Causes staphylococcal scalded skin syndrome (SSSS)	14,105
Panton Valentine leukocidin (PVL)	Pore-forming toxin that kills human white blood cells	108
Alpha toxin	Lyses red blood cells and neutrophils; disrupts epithelial barriers by binding ADAM-10	109
Leukocidin AB (LukAB), leukocidin ED (LukED), gamma-hemolysin AB (HlgAB), and gamma-hemolysin CB (HlgCB)	ß-barrel, 2-component, pore-forming leukocidins	110
hemolysin-ß	Lyses cell membranes, kills neutrophils, monocytes, and T cells	105
Phenol-soluble modulins (psms)	Disrupt cell membranes in a receptor-independent manner	111

PFGE has been used for decades. However, because the technique is labor intensive and complex to analyze, after 2003, DNA sequence-based typing schemes gradually replaced PFGE for most epidemiologic studies. The two most common sequence-based techniques used to genotype *S. aureus* are multilocus sequence typing (MLST),[115] and *spa* typing.[116] MLST has been applied to many bacterial species while *spa* typing is unique to *S. aureus*. MLST for *S. aureus* is defined by a combination of allelic variants of portions of seven housekeeping genes, each of which is sequenced, and each variant sequence is designated by a unique number. The combination of the seven numbers, one for each of the seven housekeeping gene variants, determines the ST. For example, the set of allelic variants 1-1-1-1-1-1-1 is designated as "ST1." Because of the number of allelic variants in each of the seven genes is great, there have been > 5200 MLSTs defined (https://pubmlst.org/saureus/). These sequence types are arbitrarily designated by a serial number, starting with ST1, then ST2, etc. In contrast, *spa* typing is determined by the identity and order of repeat sequences in a part of a single gene, called *spa*, which codes for staphylococcal Protein A (see Table 154-5).[117,118] The number and order of the repeat sequences varies, and so > 18,600 *spa* types have been defined (https://www.spaserver.ridom.de/). As new types are identified, they are arbitrarily given a serial number designation following the letter "t" in the following format: t001, t002, t003, etc. In both *spa* typing and MLST, individual types can be combined into related groups by similarities and shared sequences presumed to be evolutionarily related. These are called clonal complexes (CCs). The older PFGE-based strain nomenclatures often, but not always, correlate with specific MLST and *spa* designations. For example, the USA300 strain type defined by PFGE is usually found to be ST8 by MLST and t008 by *spa* typing.

The molecular epidemiology of MRSA has been studied much more carefully than that of MSSA. The major strain types of MRSA worldwide, designated by older PFGE as well as MLST and *spa* type designations, are summarized in Table 154-3, indicating CA-MRSA isolates, HA-MRSA isolates, and livestock-associated (LA-) MRSA isolates. Among CA-MRSA isolates, as noted above, the virulent ST8 USA300 strain type predominates in North America, ST80 in Europe, the Middle East and North Africa, ST59 in China and Taiwan, PVL-negative ST72 in South Korea, ST772 in India, and ST93 in Australia.[69,119,120] Interestingly, USA300 MRSA has been reported in countries worldwide,[121] but outside of North America, its introduction typically results in limited local spread.[122–124] Among HA-MRSA isolates, ST5- (SCC*mec* type) II (USA100 by PFGE) predominates in North America, and ST22-IV is frequently isolated in the United Kingdom and Ireland, while ST239-III is common in much of the rest of the world (Table 154-3). There have been many recorded instances of strain replacement at individual medical centers, in regions, and in entire countries[125–131] in the span of several years to a decade. There is evidence from some studies that ST239-III may be waning in prevalence in many parts of the world.

LA-MRSA strains, described later in the chapter, have been shown in several cases to have developed specific genetic adaptations after a host jump from humans to an animal species or vice versa.[18,19,132] *mecC*, a *mecA* homologue that also confers methicillin resistance, first described in 2011,[133] has been identified almost exclusively in Europe. It is most often found in isolates obtained from livestock and wild animals in LA-MRSA genetic backgrounds (especially in clonal clusters CC130, CC425, and CC599).[134–150] *mecC*-positive MRSA was also isolated from a domestic cat in Melbourne, Australia.[151] There is a risk that *mec*-containing MRSA strains may sometimes be misclassified, using standard methods in human clinical microbiology practice, as MSSA.[152]

MSSA strain genotypes have greater variability compared with MRSA strain genotypes in any given setting. CC30 and CC45 tend to be common clonal complexes among MSSA worldwide although the molecular epidemiology of MSSA is less well described than that of MRSA. Several large studies of human colonization and infection

TABLE 154-5 SELECTED IMMUNE EVASION MECHANISMS OF *S. AUREUS*

Protein	Gene Name	Mechanism
Collagen-binding protein	*cna*	Collagen-binding surface protein
Staphylokinase (protease III)	*sak*	Plasminogen activator, which cleaves fibrin and extracellular matrix proteins
Staphylocoagulase	*coa*	With prothrombin, makes an enzyme complex that cleaves fibrinogen to produce a fibrin coat that blocks phagocytosis
Staphylococcal Protein A	*spa*	Binds antibodies; binds B lymphocytes to cause proliferation and class switching as well as secretion of nonspecific antibodies; B-cell apoptosis
Staphylococcal complement inhibitor family	SCIN, SCIN-B, SCIN-C	Inhibit complement by binding C3 convertase and C3b; induce convertase dimerization to prevent phagocytosis
Chemotaxis inhibitory protein of *S. aureus*	CHIPS	Impairs chemoattraction of neutrophils and monocytes by binding C5aR1 and the formyl peptide receptor 1
Extracellular adherence proteins	Eap, EapH1, and EapH2	Cause bacterial agglutination and binding to host tissues; inhibit neutrophil serine proteases
Staphyococcal superantigens	SAgs	Bind T lymphocyte receptors and antigen-presenting cells, cause shock
Staphylococcal superantigen-like proteins	SSLs[1–14]	Multiple functions; SSL2 and SSL3 inhibit TLR2
Extracellular fibrinogen-binding protein	*Efb, Ecb*	Efb binds fibrinogen to form a shield over complement bound to bacterial cell surface; Efb and Ecb inhibit complement by binding C3d
Staphylococcal nuclease	SNase	Breaks down neutrophil extracellular traps (NETs); induces macrophage apoptosis
Phenol soluble modulins	PSMs	Small peptide molecules that disrupt cell membranes in a receptor-independent, detergent-like fashion; upregulated by agr system
Second immunoglobulin-binding protein	*sbi*	Binds to IgG Fc domain; inhibits complement activation by binding to C3 and factor H
FPR2 inhibitory protein	FLIPr	Impairs chemoattraction of neutrophils and monocytes by blocking formyl peptide receptors; similar in structure to CHIPS
Von Willebrand factor-binding protein	vWbp	With prothrombin, makes an enzyme complex that cleaves fibrinogen to produce a fibrin coat that blocks phagocytosis
Staphyloxanthin		Antioxidant; protects against neutrophil respiratory burst
Staphylococcal proteases, including aureolysin	several	Inhibit complement and break down other host proteins, including antimicrobial peptides

by MSSA strain genotypes have been published, demonstrating that no single ST accounts for >20% of a local circulating population. The MSSA population is often dominated by STs included in the CC1, CC5, CC8, CC30, CC45, CC15, CC121, CC22, CC7, CC398, CC25, and CC12 clonal complexes.[3,4,6,8,153,154] Livestock-associated MSSA strain types described commonly include CC1, CC5, CC121, CC130, CC133, CC398, and CC425.[19]

ST398 MSSA strains are common causes of human colonization and infection in many regions of the world, reported in China,[155–157] the Caribbean,[158,159] among the Dominican population of New York City,[160] and in inmates at the Dallas County Jail.[161] Unlike ST398 MRSA, these MSSA strains may not be associated with livestock. A phylogenetic study of local ST398 MSSA isolates from New York City, for example, suggested that this lineage and LA-MRSA ST398 diverged in the mid-1970s.[159]

In 2001, the first two whole genome sequences (WGS) were completed for *S. aureus*.[162] With a rapid decrease in the cost of genome sequencing and analysis in the era of next-generation sequencing technologies, >43,000 *S. aureus* isolates were sequenced by 2018.[163] Because the MLST and *spa* type of a *S. aureus* isolate can be determined reliably from the WGS, this technique is likely to replace other genotyping methods. The core genome of the single bacterial chromosome of *S. aureus* includes approximately 2.6 million base pairs of DNA; these code for about 2500 open reading frames (i.e., genes). In the *S. aureus* genome, lateral gene transfer plays a critical role in shaping the diversity of strain types. The "core variable genome" includes genes that are frequently carried by most strain types. The "accessory genome," which is made up of mobile genetic elements (MGEs) and can comprise 20% of the *S. aureus* genome, varies widely from strain to strain. These MGEs include transposons, pathogenicity islands, plasmids, bacteriophages (called prophages when embedded in the chromosome), and staphylococcal cassette chromosomes,[18] all of which may be transmitted from one strain of *S. aureus* to another, resulting in evolutionary adaptation, including acquisition of antimicrobial resistance.[164] Plasmids are MGEs that are small, circular extrachromosomal DNA structures that may carry genes for virulence factors or for proteins responsible for antimicrobial resistance. Bacteriophages and pathogenicity islands may carry toxins, such as the genes for PVL, or other virulence factors. Recombination in the *S. aureus* genome occurs, but relatively rarely; however, it can sometimes be a critical factor in driving evolution in the accessory genome.[18]

Next-generation genome sequencing platforms have decreased the cost of WGS to the point where it can be used as a public health tool. By approximately 2012, genomics had revolutionized the ability of public health institutions to track the large- and small-scale epidemiology of pathogens. Recent studies demonstrated the value of routine WGS of MRSA from cities[165] or larger regions.[166–168] Such studies have provided insights into the evolution of pathogens over the timescale of years, decades, and even centuries. WGS has also revealed the importance of MGEs; the distribution of strains across reservoirs and the size of these reservoirs; the geographic spread of a clone in outbreaks; the intrahost evolution of pathogens during colonization and infection;[17,169,170] and the source of outbreaks in healthcare settings and the community.[171] Further insights include host adaptation to different animal species,[18] novel mechanisms of virulence, and determination of antimicrobial resistance.[172,173] WGS is likely to transform the practice of outbreak investigation and the tracking of emerging strains.[174] Remarkably, WGS has demonstrated that MRSA strains first emerged in the mid-1940s,[175] two decades prior to their detection in clinical practice.

USA300 MRSA has been examined extensively by WGS. In a study of 224 ST8 genomes, the evolutionary history of the USA300 MRSA was reconstructed. The authors concluded, based on these genomes that a likely ancestor of USA300 emerged from Central Europe in the mid-nineteenth century. The strain was transmitted to the Americas in the early 1900s and there, successively acquired the PVL genes, SCC*mec*, the arginine catabolic mobile element (ACME), and a distinctive *cap5E* mutation. USA300 was then exported worldwide out of North America.[176] Analysis of genetic variation among 357 USA300 MRSA isolates assessed the range expansion of the strain within the United States, with an origin in Pennsylvania.[177] Shifting to focus on individuals, intrahost evolution of USA300 MRSA during recurrent SSTIs over several years was demonstrated, with changing susceptibility patterns and acquisition and loss of MGEs.[17] In another study, USA300 MRSA from infections and colonization clustered within households, showing person-to-person transmission and prolonged persistence of clones.[178] USA300 isolates collected in 2009–13 from two hospitals in Chicago, Illinois, showed that USA300 MRSA strains from nosocomial and community infections arose from a single reservoir of MRSA, suggesting importation of community clones into the healthcare setting.[179] Recent studies from Europe, where USA300 is relatively rare, demonstrated that the USA300 strain was introduced repeatedly followed by limited clonal spread in Switzerland,[124] East England,[123] and France.[122]

MRSA has been studied with WGS to assess suspected hospital and community outbreaks. For example, an outbreak in a neonatal unit in Cambridge, England in 2011 was determined to be caused by an ST2371 strain involving community transmission, mothers, infants, and a healthcare worker.[180] An outbreak in a neonatal unit involving 12 patients in 2009 was proven to be caused by an ST22 strain.[173] In the United States, spread of both ST225/t045 and ST8/t008 MRSA clones was documented in a Florida neonatal unit in 2008–10.[181] A foodborne outbreak of CC75 MRSA (*S. argenteus*) in Japan was documented by WGS of two strains, which carried an SEB-like enterotoxin gene in a *S. aureus* pathogenicity island.[182] In Copenhagen, Denmark, routine surveillance with characterization by WGS of MRSA strains cultured in 2011–12 from clinical samples was performed. This surveillance revealed a neonatal hospital outbreak caused by 34 isolates of a ST6/t304 strain, which were genetically distinct from 21 other ST6/t304 isolates from the city.[165]

The use of WGS for routine clinical and epidemiologic studies is limited by the cost of sequencing, although this has rapidly decreased. A more important limitation is that interpretation of WGS data requires expertise in bioinformatics as there are few available software pipelines that can be used with no prior training. In addition, there are not yet standards that define clonality of strains that would uniformly rule in or rule out a local outbreak. It is likely that each of these limitations will be overcome within several years.[174]

PATHOGENESIS AND IMMUNE EVASION

It is believed that a clinically apparent *S. aureus* infection usually occurs only after prior colonization of a person's body.[7,183] Colonization is dependent upon attachment of the bacterium to the mucous membranes or skin of the patient. This is accomplished by the binding of one or more of at least nine cell-surface proteins known as microbial surface components recognizing adhesive matrix molecules (MSCRAMMs) to specific host epithelial cell surface receptors. Prominent MSCRAMMs include clumping factor A (ClfA) and clumping factor B (ClfB). These bacterial proteins are not merely the means of attachment of *S. aureus* to host cells; they serve other functions as well in the pathogenesis of *S. aureus* infection. There are a great number of additional *S. aureus* proteins that interact with human cells to attach and invade.[184] An injury to a colonized person's skin or mucous membranes after attachment may afford the opportunity for *S. aureus* to invade, which is made easier by certain bacterial virulence factors.

Survival on the skin and within human tissues requires a complex interplay between *S. aureus* and host proteins. On the skin, the USA300 MRSA strain's survival, for example, is enhanced by carriage of ACME.[185] ACME codes for a number of proteins including *speG*, which enables *S. aureus* to survive in the presence of usually toxic amines produced by human cells,[186] and *arcA*, which improves the ability of *S. aureus* to live in acidic environments.[185] USA300 MRSA may have differing colonization dynamics and a lower within-host single nucleotide variability compared with MSSA strains, although the mechanisms underlying these differences are not yet fully defined.[159] Interestingly, ST398 MSSA isolates have been found to have an enhanced ability to adhere to human skin keratinocytes and keratin compared with ST398 LA-MRSA isolates[158]; this may put ST398 MSSA at an advantage in spreading among humans.

Once an infection has been initiated, *S. aureus* relies upon a number of virulence strategies to maintain the infection, some of which result in damage to host tissues. For example, PVL has been associated with necrotic skin lesions as well as destructive necrotizing pneumonia.[187] While a complete discussion of these virulence mechanisms is beyond the scope of the present chapter, among the most important mechanisms are the production of biofilms in the presence of foreign bodies,[188,189] the use of toxins to breach barriers and combat immune effector cells (see below), survival against neutrophil killing,[118] and intracellular survival (Table 154-4).

S. aureus has evolved mechanisms to sense and respond to stimuli in its environment, including quorum-sensing systems to assess the local population size of *S. aureus*.[190] Similar to many other Gram-positive bacteria, among the most important mechanisms that *S. aureus* has for responding to environmental changes or specific stimuli at the cell surface are the two-component signal transduction systems (TCSTSs), such as VraRS, WalKR, and GraRS. These TCSTSs sense a stimulus with one component (e.g., VraS, for "sensor kinase") and then increase or decrease gene expression, often of many genes, via binding of the effector component (e.g., VraR, for "regulator") to specific sites on chromosomal DNA. *S. aureus* also has so-called "master switch" or transcriptional regulatory operons, for example, agr (accessory gene regulator) and *Sae* (*S. aureus* exoprotein expression). These gene systems turn on and off large numbers of virulence genes, enabling the bacterium in the course of an infection to enhance survival, persist, or penetrate barriers as needed in different conditions.[191]

Among its armamentarium of toxins, *S. aureus* may elaborate proteins known as superantigens that nonspecifically stimulate T cells and lead to a cascade of T-cell activation, resulting in shock. These superantigens include certain staphylococcal enterotoxins (e.g., SEA, SEB) and the toxic shock syndrome toxin (*tst-1*).[105] In the late 1970s, there was a sharp increase in the incidence of a potentially fatal disease caused by *S. aureus*, called toxic shock syndrome (TSS) (see Table 154-1). TSS is caused by strains of *S. aureus* carrying *tst-1*, which is encoded in a chromosomal pathogenicity island. TSS may occur in the absence of infection when toxin-bearing strains grow in large quantities in direct contact with host mucous membranes. For example, the outbreak of TSS in the 1970s was associated with the use of newly introduced superabsorbent tampons.[192,193] The incidence of TSS quickly decreased when certain brands of tampons were removed from the market.[194]

Evasion of the human innate and adaptive immune response is critical to the ability of *S. aureus* to infect a person or animal and impair the development of immune memory responses, enabling *S. aureus* to cause recurrent infections (Table 154-5). Under certain conditions, *S. aureus* induces inflammation during an infection, but it also acts against many activities of the immune system. *S. aureus* impairs immune function by producing virulence factors that block host receptors; binding host antibodies (Protein A and sbi); shielding itself from host proteins; preventing opsonization (e.g., SSL7); and inhibiting complement activation (e.g., *sbi*, *Efb*, and SCIN); inhibiting antimicrobial peptides (e.g., aureolysin, a protease); inhibiting neutrophil recruitment (e.g., SEIX and the protease Staphopain A), activation (e.g., CHIPs), and extravasation (SSL5). *S. aureus* also inhibits monocyte responses (e.g., CHIPs); degrades host proteins with proteases, including complement components and antibodies; binds neutrophils to prevent interaction with P-selectin (e.g., SSL11); binds and inhibits Toll-like receptors, including TLR2 (SSL4); and directly kills neutrophils (with toxins including PVL). *S. aureus* produces factors that can activate B cells and T cells; that interfere with coagulation by enhancing or inhibiting platelets (e.g., SSL5) or clotting factors (e.g., SSL10), and by breaking down fibrin (e.g., staphylokinase); that inhibit antibodies such as IgG1 (e.g., SSL10); and that affect the normal response of epithelial cells. It also can cause potentially fatal shock by activating T cells indiscriminately thereby preventing a usual immune response to infection.[117]

In addition, *S. aureus* can develop small colony variants, which are very slow-growing, usually nutritionally variant mutants that may enable it to persist in host tissues for prolonged periods.[188]

TREATMENT

The treatment of *S. aureus* infections is based on principles of source control and antimicrobial therapy.[195–198] *S. aureus* is notorious for causing purulence at sites of infection, and usually to cure an infection, this pus must be drained. In the case of an infection involving a foreign body, removal of the foreign body is often required to achieve a cure. *S. aureus* can infect any organ in the human body, and it is likely the most common cause of cultured human SSTIs.[25] Common sites of infection by *S. aureus* are shown in Table 154-1. The choice of an antimicrobial drug is based on the anatomic site of infection, local *S. aureus* antibiotic-resistance patterns, patient allergies, adverse drug effects, and the results of antimicrobial susceptibility testing of an isolate cultured from the site of infection.

SSTIs are the most common type of *S. aureus* infection, and they range from impetigo, which is a very superficial infection of the skin treated by topical agents[199] to deep-seated infections of the muscle that require surgical drainage and intravenous antibiotics. In SSTIs, a drainage procedure is generally necessary in purulent lesions > 5 cm in diameter, and studies have shown that antibiotics after drainage of even small abscesses increase the likelihood of cure.[200] Many define an uncomplicated SSTI as one without systemic signs of infection, such as rapid heart rate, rapid respiratory rate, low blood pressure, or fever.[195] If an SSTI occurs on the genitals or on the face, or if there are any of the listed systemic signs, then it is often considered complicated, and treatment may require a surgical procedure. Oral antibiotics are generally adequate to cure uncomplicated SSTIs after drainage. Antistaphylococcal penicillins (such as cloxacillin or dicloxacillin) or oral cephalosporins, such as cephalexin, are used for MSSA SSTIs. For uncomplicated MRSA SSTIs, common antibiotic choices are oral trimethoprim-sulfamethoxazole, clindamycin, or doxycycline (Table 154-6).[195,196,201] For complicated MSSA infections, intravenous cephalosporins, such as cefazolin, or intravenous antistaphylococcal penicillins, such as oxacillin or nafcillin, are often used. In cases of allergy or an adverse reaction to ß-lactam drugs and for complicated MRSA SSTIs (defined as causing vital sign abnormalities, infection in an immunocompromised host, infection spreading rapidly, or suspected bacteremia), intravenous vancomycin is the first-line therapy. Length of therapy, treatment of special populations, such as the immunocompromised, and switch from intravenous to oral agents is discussed in the relevant guidelines.[195,196] When vancomycin cannot be tolerated, alternatives include daptomycin, linezolid, or tedizolid (Table 154-1). In the case of a vancomycin-intermediate *S. aureus* (VISA) or if the minimum inhibitory concentration of vancomycin is rising on therapy, daptomycin is not an appropriate alternative as there is cross-resistance between vancomycin and daptomycin. In these cases, therefore, linezolid or tedizolid may be optimal, and some have used daptomycin in addition to ceftaroline with success.[202] The long-acting lipoglycopeptide drugs, oritavancin and dalbovancin (Table 154-6), have been approved by the U.S. Food and Drug Administration (FDA) to treat SSTIs, but they are not used frequently for this indication due to availability of alternative agents.

TABLE 154-6 ANTIBIOTIC CLASSES USED IN THE THERAPY OF *S. AUREUS* INFECTIONS INDICATING ADVANTAGES AND ADVERSE EFFECTS

Drug/Drug Class	Route of Administration	Advantages	Common Adverse Effects, Disadvantages
Antistaphylococcal penicillins	IV or oral	Safe	Seizures at very high doses; GI
Cephalosporins, first, second and third generation	IV or oral	Safe	Seizures at very high doses; GI
Trimethoprim-sulfamethoxazole	IV or oral	Effective for SSTIs; resistance is rare	Renal, bone marrow toxicity
Doxycycline	IV or oral	Effective for SSTIs	Rash with sun exposure; cannot be used by young children or pregnant women
Minocycline	Oral	Effective for SSTIs	Rash with sun exposure; nail discoloration; cannot be used by young children or pregnant women
Clindamycin	IV or oral	Effective for SSTIs; antiribosomal so decreases toxin production; active against anaerobes	GI toxicity; risk of *Clostridioides difficile*-associated diarrhea
Gentamicin	IV only	Resistance is rare	Renal and ototoxicity; not used alone
Rifampin	IV or oral	Effective at penetration of biofilms in foreign body infections; resistance is rare	Liver toxicity; not used alone as there is a low barrier to resistance
Vancomycin	IV only for treatment of *S. aureus*	First-line therapy for invasive MRSA infections	Renal and ototoxicty; rare bone marrow toxicity
Daptomycin	IV only	Safe and noninferior to vancomycin for bacteremia and right-sided endocarditis; unlike vancomycin, dosing is typically daily and does not require monitoring of serum concentration	Rhabdomyolysis; inactivated by pulmonary surfactant, so it cannot be used to treat pneumonia; rare eosinophilic pneumonitis
Linezolid	IV or oral	Resistance rare; antiribosomal so decreases toxin production; active against anaerobes; twice daily doing	Bone marrow toxicity; interacts with SSRIs and other medication, may lead to serotonin syndrome
Tedizolid	IV or oral	Resistance rare; antiribosomal so decreases toxin production; daily dosing; fewer toxicities than linezolid	Bone marrow toxicity; interacts with SSRIs and other medication, may lead to serotonin syndrome; toxicities less common than linezolid; FDA approved only for skin and soft tissue infections
Tigecycline	IV only	Active against MRSA; approved for complicated skin infections and intra-abdominal infections	Increased risk of death in studies; used only when few other choices available; derivative of minocycline
Ceftaroline/Ceftobiprole	IV only	Safe; active against MRSA	Few studies in invasive MRSA infections; FDA approved only for skin and soft tissue infections
Telavancin	IV only	Effective against MRSA; approved for skin infections and hospital-acquired pneumonia	Must avoid in patients with renal dysfunction
Oritavancin	IV only	Single dose for SSTIs; effective against MRSA	Cannot remove by dialysis if an adverse effect occurs; FDA approved only for skin and soft tissue infections
Dalbavancin	IV only	Single dose for SSTIs; effective against MRSA	Cannot remove by dialysis if an adverse effect occurs; FDA approved only for skin and soft tissue infections

Abbreviations: FDA = Food and Drug Administration; GI = gastrointestinal; IV = intravenous; MRSA = methicillin-resistant *S. aureus*; SSTIs = skin and soft tissue infections.

While they may be convenient to dose, there are few data available on the efficacy of dalbavancin and oritavancin in the treatment of invasive infections, such as osteomyelitis and endocarditis.[203]

When *S. aureus* causes invasive infections, it is important that the source of the infection be identified and addressed appropriately to optimize the chance of cure and to prevent recurrence. Infections of the blood, a bone or joint, or an internal organ are not infrequent, and these are often treated with intravenous medications for the entirety or part of the course of therapy. In general, for invasive MSSA infections, intravenous cephalosporins, such as cefazolin, or intravenous antistaphylococcal penicillins are often used. A study of MSSA bacteremia showed that cefazolin is superior to oxacillin and nafcillin, and thus should be the preferred agent.[204] In cases of allergy to ß-lactam drugs and for invasive MRSA infections, intravenous vancomycin is the first-line therapy. Specific recommendations for the treatment of each type of invasive syndrome is derived from extensive literature although randomized trials are lacking for the treatment of many specific sites of *S. aureus* infection.[195,201]

S. aureus infections in certain conditions are particularly difficult to treat, such as infective endocarditis in the injection drug user[205]; pneumonia in patients with cystic fibrosis[206] or bronchiectasis; and skin infections in patients with hidradenitis suppurativa, hyper-IgE syndrome, or eczema. Patients with frequent recurrences of *S. aureus* skin abscesses (furunculosis) are challenging.[207] Such patients are often treated by an interdisciplinary team, which includes a specialist in infectious diseases.

ENVIRONMENTAL RESERVOIRS OF *S. AUREUS*

There is limited conclusive evidence that *S. aureus* is spread by fomites from one host to another, but there are several lines of circumstantial evidence to support this intuitively likely mode of transmission of *S. aureus* and other pathogenic bacteria.[208] *S. aureus* can contaminate a variety of surfaces and inanimate objects,[209–216] including pagers,[217] computer keyboards,[218] faucet handles,[219] and many other fomites[220] in hospitals. Dry mops contaminated with MRSA continued to have MRSA cultured from them for 4–8 weeks.[214] *S. aureus* can survive desiccation for up to 6 months, and there may be strain-related differences in survival on fomites.[221,222] MRSA could be transferred easily from a variety of fomites to pigskin in an experimental model,[223] suggesting that fomite-to-skin transmission is possible. People shed their commensal *S. aureus* into the environment.[224,225] A study found that environmental contamination was more frequent when patients in a hospital room had a MRSA wound or urine infection (36% of tested surfaces) than if they had other sites of infection (6%),[226] demonstrating that fomite contamination directly from free body fluids is common. A study of a MRSA outbreak on a U.S. professional football team by the CDC showed that sharing of fomites having common skin contact, such as towels, was associated with risk of developing a MRSA infection.[227] Therefore, fomites can act as a reservoir and as a vector for transmission of MRSA in healthcare and community settings.

Environmental cleaning in hospitals is often emphasized as an important element of infection control programs to prevent spread of MRSA and other nosocomial pathogens,[228] and studies suggest that it may reduce MRSA transmission from person to person.[212,224,229–232] Resistance to some biocides used in hospital cleaning has been reported among MRSA isolates, and resistant mutants could be generated in laboratory experiments.[233] Methods used to clean the environment in hospitals vary, and studies have shown a wide variety of outcomes in the efficacy of decontamination protocols.[234] In addition to traditional manual cleaning methods, therefore, a variety of newer cleaning methods have been used during the past decade in an attempt to enhance decontamination of fomites, including ultraviolet light,[235] ozone, steam cleaning,[229] and airborne hydrogen peroxide.[235,236] Limited evidence supports the efficacy of each of these novel approaches to eliminate MRSA from hospital rooms.

In some cases, spread of MRSA from a person occurs by the airborne route,[237] and may be enhanced during bedmaking in a hospital.[238] Airborne MRSA transmission was demonstrated both from pig-to-pig in a model system[239] and from pig-to-human in a study of volunteers visiting a pig farm who had no direct contact with pigs.[240] Airborne transmission may be enhanced by contaminated dust.[241–244]

The importance of fomites in MRSA transmission has also been suggested by studies in households.[245–247] For example, in each of 350 households in a study, one individual had been treated for an SSTI caused by a genotyped *S. aureus* index infection isolate a mean of 18 days prior to enrollment. These index patients and all household contacts (HCs) were tested for *S. aureus* colonization in the nares, throat, and perirectal region at baseline, 3 months later, and 6 months later. Environmental contamination with the *S. aureus* strain type of the index infection isolate was associated with risk of later SSTIs among household members. However, colonization of a person's body with the same strain type in that household was not associated with risk of infection in the subsequent 6 months.[245]

EPIDEMIOLOGY AND APPROACHES TO PREVENTION OF MRSA INFECTION IN SPECIFIC SETTINGS

High-risk groups for any *S. aureus* infection include patients with diabetes mellitus, a break in the skin or mucous membranes, certain chronic skin diseases, cystic fibrosis, and a weakened immune system. High-risk groups for MRSA colonization and infections are shown in Table 154-7. Since the 1970s in many countries of the world, patients exposed to healthcare settings have been at risk for MRSA infection. After the emergence of CA-MRSA strains, the groups at risk expanded to include those exposed to certain institutions or environments in the community and those with specific habits or behaviors, such as injection drug use or frequent use of gyms or health clubs.[69] Below, the epidemiology of MRSA and approaches to prevention of MRSA infections are described in a number of high-risk settings.

CA-MRSA strains outside of healthcare facilities tend to spread and cause infections most commonly among people living in poverty and crowded conditions, persons experiencing homelessness, athletes, military recruits, persons who inject drugs, and HIV-infected people. Soon after their appearance in the community, CA-MRSA strains also began to cause nosocomial infections.[92,298] LA-MRSA strains are most often spread among those with livestock exposure (Table 154-7), and are discussed later.

Much less attention in the literature has been paid to MSSA transmission from person to person. MRSA has been regarded as a greater risk to human health than MSSA in part because invasive MRSA infections may be more difficult to treat and may have worse

TABLE 154-7 HIGH-RISK GROUPS OR SITES FOR MRSA INFECTION OR COLONIZATION IN THE UNITED STATES

Group at High Risk	Example References	Typical MRSA Strain Type(s) (CA, HA, or LA)
Hospitalized patients	30,32,92	HA
Stay in a hospital room previously occupied by a MRSA carrier	248	HA or CA
Recent surgery	249	HA
Hemodialysis	250	HA
Indwelling vascular catheters	251	HA or CA
Nursing home residents	252	HA
HIV-infected patients	253–255	HA or CA
Cystic fibrosis patients	206,256	HA or CA
Soldiers in a military training facility	257–260	CA
Gym/health club/locker room users	227,261	CA
Athletes	227,262,263	CA
Household contact of a MRSA carrier	264–266	
Homeless shelter resident	267–269	CA
Exposure to a farm with large animal livestock	20,270	LA
Slaughterhouse workers	270–275	LA
Veterinarians and veterinary clinic or hospital workers	276–280	LA
Jail or prison detainee	259,281–287	CA
History of MRSA infection	288	CA or HA
Immunocompromised host	251	CA or HA
Atopic dermatitis or eczema patient	289,290	CA or HA
Aboriginal/Native peoples (American Indian, Pacific Islander, First Nations people, Native Alaskans, Maori, and others)	68,291–293	CA
People who inject drugs	205,294–297	CA

Abbreviations: CA = community-associated; HA = healthcare-associated; LA = livestock-associated; MRSA = methicillin-resistant *S. aureus*; US = United States of America.

outcomes.[299–304] Further research is necessary to better define risk factors for transmission of and infection by virulent MSSA strains.[305]

Hospitals

S. aureus infections in hospitals have been occurring in surgical and other vulnerable patients for centuries. It has been estimated that there were about 171,000 nosocomial MRSA infections in the European Union, Iceland, and Norway in 2008, resulting in a cost of 380 million Euros.[306] In the United States in 2010, it was estimated that about 4% of hospitalized patients had a HAI, and *S. aureus* was the second most common pathogen reported.[307] Control of HAIs is discussed in detail in Chapter Healthcare Associated Infections. During the second half of the twentieth century, infection control programs developed around the world to decrease the risk of pathogen transmission and infections occurring in healthcare facilities. Infection control is a multidisciplinary field carried out in large hospitals by a team of infection control practitioners, microbiologists, and infectious disease specialists. These teams work not only to reduce infection risk, but also to monitor their medical facility for patterns of infection to detect clusters, perform outbreak investigations within the medical centers, and, when required, report infections and trends to state regulatory authorities. The most common interventions to prevent the transmission of MRSA in hospitals are shown in Table 154-8.

Traditionally, there has been a distinction between "vertical" and "horizontal" infection control interventions. Vertical interventions (e.g., nares MRSA screening) target a single organism. Horizontal interventions (e.g., hand hygiene) target multiple pathogens at once. This distinction is artificial because many interventions aimed a single organism will affect the epidemiology of other organisms as well (e.g., disposable gowns and gloves for the prevention of MRSA transmission).

A fundamental conundrum in the prevention of *S. aureus* infections in the healthcare setting is that the origin of the bacterium may be most commonly from a patient's endogenous flora or it may be introduced to the patient's body after admission to a medical facility. It has been shown that patients shed and contaminate their hospital environment with *S. aureus*, as noted above,[226,323] which may begin a direct or an indirect pathway for transmission to others. The primary intervention utilized to combat *S. aureus* infections for the first case (endogenous) is suppression of endogenous colonization in patients prior to a procedure or on admission to a facility. Disagreement remains as to whether such suppressive regimens are indicated for all patients admitted to a facility (universal) or if they should be limited to only high-risk patients or proven carriers identified through either targeted or universal screening. For the second case (spread from others), in order to prevent new transmission, healthcare facilities frequently use improved hygiene, especially thorough washing of the hands among healthcare workers, sometimes combined with recommendations related to choice of clothing. Other interventions include contact precautions with removable gowns and gloves at every patient contact, use of prophylactic antibiotics before invasive procedures, and improved environmental and equipment cleaning. The approaches to addressing the risk of *S. aureus* and especially MRSA infections in hospitals differ markedly by country.[312,324–326] Hand hygiene is likely the most important single intervention to prevent the spread of MRSA from one patient to another.[308,309]

While healthcare infection control engages with the work of public health in the larger sphere, the specific programs and controversies in healthcare epidemiology related to *S. aureus* control are beyond the scope of this chapter. However, some recent findings in the literature will be discussed, and recent reviews and guidelines provide more detailed summaries of the literature.[306] There are controversies about who should be screened for MRSA carriage, how they should be screened, and what to do when a patient is identified as a MRSA carrier or as having a MRSA infection. The risk factors for colonization with MRSA at hospital admission are recent prior hospitalization, nursing home (NH) exposure, and history of exposure to MRSA, *Clostridioides difficile*, or vancomycin-resistant *Enterococcus* (VRE). MRSA colonization in hospitalized patients has also been associated with having congestive heart failure, lung disease, an immunocompromised state, diabetes mellitus, or renal failure.[327]

TABLE 154-8 MAJOR INTERVENTIONS USED TO CONTROL MRSA TRANSMISSION AND INFECTION IN HOSPITALS

Intervention	Primary Target/Agent of Intervention	Example References
Hand hygiene	Healthcare workers	308,309
Contact precautions	Healthcare workers	310
Cohorting/Isolation	Administration/Patient	311
Recording prior MRSA colonization or infection	Infection control staff/ Electronic medical record	
Screening for colonization		
Targeted	Patient	312
Universal	Patient	313
Decolonization		
Targeted	Patient	313
Universal	Patient	313,314
Equipment cleaning	Environmental services/ Healthcare workers	
Environmental cleaning		
Daily	Environmental services	232,315,316
Terminal	Environmental services	224
Ultraviolet (UV) room disinfection	Environmental services	235
Hydrogen peroxide cleaning	Environmental services	236
Bare below the elbows policy	Healthcare workers	317,318
Screening of healthcare workers for colonization	Healthcare workers	319,320
Outbreak investigations	Infection control staff	173,180
Antimicrobial stewardship	Stewardship staff	321,322

Abbreviation: MRSA = methicillin-resistant *S. aureus*.

Experts in many countries have published guidelines for the control of MRSA in the healthcare setting,[306,328–333] and they differ in their approaches to control. These differences are related to the local epidemiology of MRSA, historical approaches to MRSA control, the structure and legal authority of national health authorities to regulate hospital practices, and changing evidence for various approaches to infection control. In the United States, for example, where the incidence of MRSA infection is high, guidelines of two national professional organizations, the Society for Healthcare Epidemiology of America (SHEA) and the Association of Professionals in Infection Control (APIC), as well as guidance from the U.S. CDC, are generally followed. However, practices even among U.S. hospitals vary greatly as these guidelines do not have the force of law. Some states, however, have passed legislation requiring testing for MRSA in high-risk inpatients.[334] In contrast, in northern European countries, as noted above, public health workers have long practiced a "Search and Destroy" policy for MRSA. This means that when a patient is found to have a MRSA infection or colonization, he or she and their household members undergo decolonization (if colonized), in an effort to eliminate

MRSA from the household. With this program, in the Netherlands, 86% of MRSA carriers were decolonized successfully.[335] This program has resulted in a very low prevalence (0.13%) of MRSA colonization among Dutch patients admitted to the hospital.[336] In low burden countries such as Denmark and the Netherlands, the emergence of CA-MRSA and LA-MRSA, with origin outside of hospitals, has led to an increase in MRSA infection incidence and colonization as their major control efforts are based on MRSA detection among hospitalized patients.[165,337]

Healthcare workers often suspect that they are at very high risk of MRSA carriage, but in surveys in nonoutbreak settings, typically only $< 7\%$ are found to be colonized with MRSA.[320,338,339] For example, in Germany, only 1 of 149 HCWs with direct patient exposure was found to carry MRSA in the nares.[340] Occasionally studies have shown a higher prevalence, but these seem exceptional.

Antimicrobial stewardship programs in the acute-care hospital setting, encouraging avoidance of unnecessary antibiotic use, may limit the dissemination of MRSA and other multidrug-resistant pathogens in the healthcare setting through decreasing selective pressure.[321,322]

While there is concern about person-to-person transmission of *S. aureus* in hospitals, one study from the United Kingdom suggested that this is infrequent in an ICU setting. WGS was performed on isolates obtained from regular colonization cultures from 1181 ICU patients during 13 months; 680 patients had repeat sampling. The authors found 44 acquisitions of *S. aureus* in 41 patients, and only 7 (2 MSSA and 5 MRSA isolates) were closely related to a *S. aureus* isolate carried by another patient in the ICU.[341] This study had limitations in that it was only performed at a single site and only the nares were sampled. However, the findings did suggest that *S. aureus* transmission in an ICU may not be common. If this is true, infection prevention activities perhaps need to focus on decolonization of carriers rather than exclusively on prevention of transmission.

Below are a number of topics addressed by infection control practitioners related to *S. aureus* infection prevention and recent studies to support them.

Bundled Intervention in Acute-care Hospitals

A prominent intervention to limit the incidence of MRSA infections in acute-care hospitals was introduced as a bundle in the U.S. Veterans Affairs medical system in 2007. The initiative required screening of patients upon admission, unit-to-unit transfer, and discharge to any acute-care hospital; use of contact precautions for any patients with MRSA colonization or infection; a campaign to improve hand hygiene; and an institutional culture change to improve MRSA prevention efforts.[342] With this approach, theoretically every hospitalized person colonized with MRSA in the nares would be identified and placed in contact precautions at the time of admission, breaking the chain of transmission. With the introduction of this bundle, eventually resulting in 92% adherence with the admission nasal screen, by September 2015 the incidence of HAIs decreased by 87% in ICUs, and 80.1% in non-ICU units.[343] These impressive results may reflect the efficacy of any or all of the elements in the "MRSA bundle." As there were no simultaneous controls in this study, it may also be that the decrease in incidence of HAIs was related to a secular trend resulting in a decreased incidence of MRSA infections in the United States overall during the study period. Notably, one statistical modeling study of the VA bundle's screening and contact precaution intervention found that this intervention was unlikely to have been responsible for the observed decrease in MRSA infections.[344]

Universal Decolonization of Intensive Care Unit Patients

Chlorhexidine gluconate bathing (washing of the skin) in ICU patients was found in a meta-analysis of the literature to be effective at reducing the risk of catheter-related bloodstream infections, MRSA colonization, and MRSA bacteremia in these patients.[345] In another meta-analysis of seven trials, acquisition of MRSA colonization in ICUs was reduced by daily chlorhexidine bathing (RR 0.67, 95% CI 0.59–0.77, $p < 0.001$).[346] In the REDUCE MRSA study, Huang et al. randomized 74 ICUs in 43 U.S. hospitals for an 18-month trial to one of the three arms: (1) MRSA nares screening and contact precautions if MRSA-positive, (2) MRSA nares screening with contact precautions and chlorhexidine gluconate decolonization if the screening test was positive for MRSA, and (3) universal chlorhexidine decolonization on admission. Compared with baseline incidence (i.e., 12 months prior to the initiation of the interventions), the universal decolonization arm showed a significant and more substantial decrease in rate of culturing of MRSA clinical isolates than did the targeted decolonization arm, although there was also significant reduction from baseline in the targeted arm. The screening and contact precautions arm showed no significant change from baseline practice in the rate of MRSA clinical isolate cultures. The study thus supported the practice of universal chlorhexidine gluconate decolonization, suggesting it was superior to MRSA screening plus directed decolonization in U.S. ICUs.[313] One weakness of the study was that only the nares were screened, and thus some MRSA carriers were likely missed. Concerns also remain that universal decolonization may lead to elevated risk of chlorhexidine resistance in *S. aureus*; currently, the prevalence of chlorhexidine resistance is fairly low.[347]

Decolonization of Proven MRSA-colonized Patients after Hospital Discharge

A randomized, controlled trial (Project CLEAR) of 2121 U.S. patients colonized with MRSA during admission to a hospital or NH demonstrated that decolonization was effective in reducing the incidence of MRSA infections after discharge. A postdischarge intervention of education plus a decolonization regimen, compared with the educational intervention alone, resulted in a 30% reduction in risk of postdischarge MRSA infection. The decolonization regimen consisted of chlorhexidine mouthwash and baths for 5 days each month for 6 months after discharge.[348]

Use of Contact Precautions

It seems intuitive that wearing clean or disposable gowns and gloves by healthcare workers entering rooms occupied by a MRSA-colonized patient would reduce the likelihood of transmission from patient to patient in a hospital. However, there are few data to support this practice, which is commonly used in many countries, including the United States. Some have argued that without active surveillance, contact precautions will not be effective because lacking a screening program would result in the precautions not being applied to many colonized patients.[349] In a case-control study of universal contact precautions carried out in 20 medical and surgical ICUs in 2012, each ICU was randomized to universal gown and glove use or usual care, which involved placement of patients on contact precautions only when they were identified as a carrier of MRSA, VRE, or another antibiotic-resistant organism. The primary endpoint was a decrease in MRSA and VRE colonization; these were tested for at admission and discharge. There was no difference in combined MRSA or VRE transmission risk in the two groups.[310] A Cochrane review of the literature in 2015 found no studies to support the use of gowns and gloves to reduce MRSA transmission in hospitals.[350] A separate, thorough literature review published in 2016 similarly found no evidence that contact precautions reduced the incidence of MRSA infections in hospitals.[351]

In another study, contact precautions were discontinued in a single hospital. The authors found that the mean positive clinical culture rates for MRSA before and after discontinuing contact precautions were 0.40 and 0.32 cultures per 100 admissions ($p = 0.09$), respectively, showing no statistically significant difference. With the end of contact precautions, the health system saved $643,776 in one year. This total did not count the estimated nursing time spent donning and doffing personal protective equipment for MRSA or VRE before the change, which would have occupied nurses for approximately 45,277 hours per year and incurred an estimated cost of $4.6 million.[352]

Surveillance Screening and Subsequent Isolation of Colonized Intensive Care Unit Patients

In the STAR-ICU trial in 10 intervention ICUs in the United States, universal surveillance for nasal MRSA and rectal VRE screening and initial universal gloving (i.e., until a negative test result was returned) was compared with eight control ICUs, where the same screening cultures were obtained but the results were not reported to the ICU staff. In the control ICUs, patients were placed on contact precautions only if they had a history of VRE or MRSA colonization or infection, as per usual hospital protocols. There was no significant difference in the two groups in MRSA or VRE colonization or infection. However, the staff did not adhere strictly to the contact precautions protocols in either the intervention or control ICUs, complicating the interpretation of the study.[353]

Screening for MRSA Carriage with Decolonization Prior to Surgical Procedures

Decolonization of *S. aureus* carriers prior to surgery is an effective method of reducing the risk of postoperative infection. Nasal *S. aureus* colonization prior to surgery is a risk factor for postoperative surgical-site infection.[354–356] Decolonization is supported by a number of studies, especially prior to orthopedic[357–363] and cardiac[361,362,364,365] surgical procedures. Some experts recommend a bundle of interventions, including the use of intranasal mupirocin along with chlorhexidine body washes prior to surgery.[366] A systematic literature review found that in 10 of 19 studies, preoperative decolonization regimens consisting of chlorhexidine baths and mupirocin applied to the nares were associated with a decreased incidence of *S. aureus* surgical-site infections and a decrease in nosocomial MRSA infections.[367] There is controversy about the need to test patients prior to preoperative decolonization rather than using a universal decolonization approach, which some argue is superior.[314] If mupirocin is used too widely for this indication, there is a risk that more frequent *S. aureus* mupirocin resistance may emerge as a limitation to its use.[368]

Households

Although with the emergence of CA-MRSA strains in the late 1990s, most attention was paid to jails, athletic facilities, military training facilities, and farms to study the dynamics of transmission and to introduce preventive measures,[69] the household is likely to be the most common site of CA-MRSA transmission in the United States. An agent-based model of the city of Chicago suggested that the majority of CA-MRSA transmission occurred in the household, where high-touch items are frequently shared and person-to-person contact is common. Furthermore, the model showed that the majority of transmission occurred from colonized people to others, and did not originate from people with an active infection.[369]

North America: CA-MRSA in Household Transmission

MRSA asymptomatic colonization of HCs of patients with a recent MRSA SSTI is common, suggesting that MRSA can spread readily in households from person to person.[264,265,370–372] One study in Missouri in 2008–9 found that 58% of such households had one or more members who were colonized in the nares with MRSA. In contrast, in control households with no known CA-MRSA infections, only 6.9% were colonized with MRSA.[372] Risk factors for MRSA colonization among HCs of children with a CA-*S. aureus* SSTI (70% of which were MRSA), included having had an SSTI in the past year, being a parent of the index patient, and being $<$ 5 years or $>$ 10 years of age different from the index patient. Other risk factors included the index patient being colonized at two or three body sites (when three body sites were tested), and a higher household colonization pressure.[370]

A study was conducted in Los Angeles and Chicago in 2008–10 of 350 patients who had an index *S. aureus* infection and their 803 HCs. Index patients and HCs were cultured in the nares, perirectal region, and throat at enrollment (a mean of 18 days after the index infection) and then at 3 months and 6 months after enrollment. At enrollment, 40% of index patients and 50% of HCs had *S. aureus* colonization. In addition, 17 fomites were tested at baseline and again 3 months later. Risk factors for colonization of HCs with the same strain type that caused the index infection included the HC having had an SSTI in the prior 3 months, a USA300 index infection strain, or cephalexin use in past year.[264] Among index patients, 51% had a recurrent SSTI within 6 months after the index infection, and among HCs, 13% had infection. Risk of recurrent SSTIs in an index patient included a recent hospitalization and household fomite MRSA contamination. During the 6-month follow-up period, risk of an SSTI in a HC of a patient with an index SSTI included Chicago site (vs. LA), antibiotic use in past year, and skin infection in the prior 3 months. Interestingly, risk of SSTI during the 6-month study was not associated with colonization of an individual at enrollment.[373] In a sample of 29 households having a USA300 MRSA index infection strain and USA300 MRSA colonizing at least one person during the 6-month study, a monophyletic group of USA300 was identified in 23 of the households using WGS. This suggested that USA300 MRSA colonization in U.S. households is clonal and shared among household residents. Phylogenetic data suggested that a single USA300 MRSA clone could persist in a household for up to 8 years or longer.[178]

At enrollment in the Los Angeles/Chicago study, risk factors for contamination of a household fomite with the index infection strain type included body colonization by someone in household with the index infection strain type, higher housing density, and, counterintuitively, more frequent reported household cleaning. Three months after the enrollment visit contamination of a household fomite with the index infection strain type was more common if the index infection strain was USA300 MRSA.[245]

A WGS study of ST398 MSSA from human colonization and environmental surfaces in households in New York City in 2010–13 demonstrated clear clustering of clonally related strains by household. This reflected local person-to-person MSSA spread and suggested the involvement of fomites as a possible reservoir. Related MSSA clusters were identified within social networks in the community across households,[159] demonstrating the risk of social networks in the transmission of MSSA beyond households.

In summary, households are likely the primary place for USA300 MRSA transmission in North America, and fomites may play an important role in household transmission. USA300 MRSA, compared with other index infection strain types, likely persists on fomites longer and causes more frequent HC colonization after causing an index infection in a household member. USA300 MRSA may remain in a household for many years. The presence of young children, household crowding, previous use of cephalexin, and previous skin infections are risk factors for persistence of a virulent MRSA in a household.[264,265,370] Fomite contamination with MRSA is likely a risk factor for persistence of MRSA as well, suggesting that cleaning of fomites is an important element in a household decolonization protocol (see later discussion) although self-reported increased cleaning was not effective at reducing fomite *S. aureus* contamination in one study.[245] Few genotyping studies of MSSA strains colonizing people in households have been performed, but evidence suggests that MSSA is spread from person to person within households as well.[159]

Risk of MRSA Acquisition from HCs with Livestock Contact

As ST398 MRSA and other CC398 strain types became more common causes of infection in Europe, studies have demonstrated that they were likely transmitted from veterinarians to their HCs in both Germany[374] and the Netherlands.[375,376] HCs of farmers in the Netherlands were found to be at risk of colonization with CC398 MRSA or MRSA more generally.[377,378]

Risk of Acquisition from HCs Who Are Healthcare Workers

There has been household transmission of USA300[123] and ST22 MRSA[379] documented in England by WGS, and in other countries where CA-MRSA is less common than in North America. There is concern that one source of MRSA introduction to households could be healthcare workers who acquire MRSA colonization in their workplace.[380,381] There are few studies of healthcare worker colonization in high incidence countries such as Taiwan, the United States, or Canada. However, in the available studies, the prevalence of nasal MRSA colonization in this population, while usually 0–7%, has occasionally been as high as 15%.[320,338–340,382–388] More study is required to assess the importance of and to prevent this possible route of MRSA spread.

Strategies to Prevent Household Transmission for Patients with MRSA Infections

Prevention strategies for recurrent MRSA infections in the household have been developed in several European countries with a low prevalence of MRSA and have shown great efficacy in limiting the spread of MRSA. In the Netherlands, an iterative household-based outpatient decolonization program, with up to three repeated decolonization regimens, was reported to eliminate colonization in 86% of people.[335] In Denmark and the Netherlands, these "Search and Destroy" public health programs have prevented widespread dissemination of MRSA.[61,62] In North America, the circulating strain types differ from European countries that have low prevalence of MRSA infection (Table 154-3), raising the possibility that the same regimens may not be effective in both continents.

Guidelines in the United States suggest MRSA decolonization be considered in the case of recurrent MRSA SSTIs.[195] Two randomized, controlled trials in the United States in the USA300 MRSA era have shown some promise for decolonization regimens for *S. aureus* SSTI patients. The first study showed that a 5-day regimen of dilute bleach baths was superior to topical chlorhexidine body washes in decolonizing subjects when either was combined with intranasal mupirocin.[389] The second U.S. study found that decolonization of all members of the household was superior in preventing recurrent SSTIs in a household during the subsequent 12 months in comparison with decolonizing only an index patient who had a *S. aureus* SSTI, using the same 5-day duration.[390] In the United States, such regimens are generally selectively used for patients with recurrent infections, unlike the "Search and Destroy" policies in use in northern European countries.[207] A study in Pennsylvania showed, in a secondary outcome, that successful decolonization (using intranasal mupirocin and chlorhexidine baths) of HCs of 243 index subjects with MRSA SSTIs in 2010–12 was more likely when people were strictly compliant with the decolonization regimen, suggesting that it was effective.[391]

Recurrent infections likely increase the likelihood of household transmission. Although many *S. aureus* SSTIs resolve with drainage alone, there is evidence that therapy with an antibiotic in addition to an incision and drainage procedure reduces the likelihood of a recurrent infection.[200,207,392] Also, clindamycin therapy may be more likely to prevent a recurrent SSTI than treatment with trimethoprim-sulfamethoxazole.[200,393]

Often daily cleaning of high-touch environmental household surfaces with bleach and frequent washing of underclothes, towels, and bedclothes in hot water during the decolonization regimen is recommended,[389,390] in addition to decolonization of people in a household, although evidence is scarce to support the independent value of environmental interventions.[207] Other topical medications, such as intranasal retapamulin, alcohol, and povidone-iodine may be useful for decolonization in place of mupirocin, but there are limited data available to support their use. Few adverse effects have been reported with topical chlorhexidine, mupirocin, iodine products, or retapamulin.[207]

Ideally, any underlying high-risk behavior or modifiable condition should be addressed before attempting decolonization. Decolonization will likely have a greater chance of success if it is performed in the absence of any active purulent skin lesion. For complex cases of recurrent MRSA skin infections, consultation with an infectious disease expert is recommended.

Public Institutions

Jails and Prisons

Infection control in jails and prisons is complex due to the physical layout of the facilities, security concerns, the need to move detainees from place to place unexpectedly, barriers to accessing medical care, and the high prevalence of mental illness among detainees.[394] At the end of 2016, 1.5 million people were held in state and federal prisons in the United States, with 450 per 100,000 population sentenced,[395] in addition to 740,700 more in local jails.[396] Outbreaks of MRSA SSTIs in prisons were among the first reports of MRSA infections in the United States outside of healthcare institutions.[284,285] Few studies reporting MRSA infection in places of incarceration outside of the United States have been published,[397] and thus it is not known if imprisonment is associated with MRSA risk in many countries. There were 10,942 cases of MRSA infection recorded in Texas state prisons between 1996 and mid-2002, and 94.6% were confirmed to be SSTIs.[285] It is likely that frequent homelessness among admitted detainees[398] and high rates of prior drug use[399] and HIV infection place new detainees in U.S. jails at high risk of MRSA colonization prior to imprisonment.[400] High rates of incarceration may accelerate MRSA transmission in a city or region outside of jails and prisons.[401,402] While there is certainly some transmission of MRSA in places of incarceration,[161] limited evidence suggests that *S. aureus* may not be frequently transmitted among detainees in prisons[403] or jails.[404]

Reported MRSA colonization prevalence in prisons has varied, is more common in women, and increased during the first decade of the twenty-first century. In 2000, after a Mississippi prison MRSA outbreak was detected, 5.9% of women and 2.5% of men had MRSA nares colonization.[284] In two New York maximum-security state prisons, a study in 2005–6 showed that 20.0% of women and 2.9% of men had nasal MRSA colonization.[405] A second study, among 830 inmates in 2009–11 tested in the nares and oropharynx as they entered the same prisons, the prevalence was 10.6% in women and 5.9% in men.[286] In female prisoners, obesity was independently associated with *S. aureus* colonization.[406]

Incidence and risk factors have been studied for MRSA infections in prisons, where unlike jails, detainees are held only after sentencing. USA300 typically predominates among infecting MRSA isolates in U.S. prisons.[405] In Texas prisons, it was estimated that there were 12 MRSA infections per 1000 prisoner person-years in 1999–2001,[287] and the incidence of MRSA infection was 327.9 per 100,000 inmates.[407] HIV infection, diabetes mellitus, and skin, cardiovascular, liver, and end-stage renal disease were risk factors for MRSA infections,[287] likely reflecting a risk of healthcare exposure. In a Texas prison in 2000, MRSA SSTI risk was associated with previous SSTI and contact with a person who had a MRSA infection. In a Georgia prison in 2002, risk factors for a MRSA SSTI were prior recent antibiotics, intravenous drug use, lacerations of the skin, washing of clothes by hand, self-draining of boils, sharing soap, and recent arrival to prison.[285]

Detainees in local U.S. jails, who are typically being held prior to and during trials, have been found to have frequent MRSA colonization. In 2009 in the Dallas County Jail, the prevalence of nasal MRSA colonization was 6.3% and prevalence of MRSA hand colonization, 4.1%.[404] In the Los Angeles County Jail in 2006–7, 25% of 60 patients who had a MRSA SSTI in the jail and 11% of 102 control subjects who did not have an SSTI were colonized by MRSA. Nasal colonization was associated with current skin infection, not having showered daily in the prior week, and receiving antimicrobials during the prior 12 months.[408]

There has been a high and increasing incidence of MRSA SSTIs, usually caused by USA300 MRSA, among jail detainees during the CA-MRSA era.[409,410] For example, the percent of *S. aureus* SSTIs that were MRSA in the San Francisco County Jail increased from 29% in 1997 to 74% in 2002.[282] Among 502 MRSA isolates obtained in the Jail between 2000 and 2007, 82.1% had the USA300 MRSA strain type.[411] In a study of an 18-month period during 2004–05 in the Cook County Jail in Chicago, 378 cultured SSTIs from different detainees were studied, and MRSA grew from 63.5% of infections. MSSA grew from only 11.4%, demonstrating that MRSA had come to dominate as a cause of SSTIs in detainees by 2005.[283] Risk factors for MRSA SSTIs in the Los Angeles County Jail in 2006–07 included MRSA nares colonization, lower level of educational attainment, SSTI in the previous 3 months, less frequent showering in jail, sharing soap with other detainees, a lower level of knowledge about MRSA infections, and no contact with the healthcare system in the 3 months prior to incarceration.[408] In a 2012 study in Omaha, Nebraska in a county jail, 132 detainees likely had an SSTI. This cohort had a high prevalence of many of the risk factors identified in other studies. They had a median length of stay of 86 days, 8.6% were homeless prior to incarceration, 12.9% had been hospitalized in the previous 12 months, 39.4% had a psychiatric illness, and 25.6% presented to jail with a skin lesion. Interestingly, only 2.3% had diabetes mellitus.[412]

The importance in places of incarceration of the environment as a reservoir for MRSA has not been adequately studied. It is possible that improved environmental cleaning could decrease MRSA transmission among detainees, but data are scant. A 2009 study in a Texas jail with no known MRSA outbreak at the time revealed MRSA contamination of 6.1% of 132 surface cultures.[413] In contrast, only 1 of 283 cultured surfaces were contaminated with MRSA in a study comparing environments of detainees with and without culture-proven *S. aureus* SSTIs in two New York state prisons with a high prevalence of prisoner MRSA body colonization (higher contamination with MSSA was found).[414] The authors did not specifically evaluate environmental cleaning but wondered whether there may have been differential cleaning for those with known SSTIs.

Optimal protocols for prevention of the spread of MRSA and the development of MRSA SSTIs in places of incarceration require additional study. Guidelines in the United States, based largely on expert opinion, have been prepared by the Federal Bureau of Prisons,[415] states, and local governmental bodies that run city or county jails. Studies of various interventions or bundles aimed at decreasing the incidence of MRSA SSTIs or decreasing colonization in jails since 2002 have had varying levels of success.[410,412,416–418] Successful infection control programs in jails and prisons will likely require tailoring of guidelines to local conditions, especially to specific security protocols. The Federal[415] and several state guidelines provide excellent outlines for the development of local jail protocols. Preventive programs may include employee and detainee education; improved access to clean clothes washed by machine, soap, showers, and urgent medical care for immediate diagnosis and treatment of SSTIs; improved hand hygiene; discouraging sharing of personal items and self-treatment of SSTIs; and improved wound care programs.[281,394]

Homeless Shelters

Persons experiencing homelessness have been found to have an elevated risk of colonization with MRSA. For example, in a study of 194 homeless persons in 2015 in Boston, Massachusetts, 8.3% were colonized with MRSA in the nares. Colonization was associated with poor hygiene, recent hospitalization, and heavy alcohol use.[267] In another study from the Midwestern United States in 2012–14, a homeless cohort of 285 people had a 9.8% prevalence of MRSA nares colonization.[268] Among 215 homeless individuals in Ohio, the prevalence of nares MRSA colonization was 25.6%. Colonization was associated in a multivariable analysis with recent antibiotic use, a history of alcoholism, and decreased frequency of having stayed with a friend in the previous 30 days.[269] Because of the high prevalence of MRSA colonization in this disadvantaged group, educational interventions at shelters and clinics serving homeless populations may lead to prevention of and earlier care for suspected MRSA infections.

Athletics and Athletic Facilities

Spread of pathogens causing SSTIs among athletes has long been a concern in children[419] and adults.[263,420] After the emergence of CA-MRSA strains in the 1990s, MRSA infections among high school[421–429]; college and university[262,425,426,430–434]; club[435]; and professional[227,436,437] athletes were reported.[69,438] A French rugby team reported an outbreak of PVL-containing MSSA SSTIs in 2010–11,[439] as did a U.S. college football team in 2007,[440] suggesting that the PVL toxin may play a role in the spread of CA-MRSA and MSSA among athletes.

Student athletes in the United States, especially wrestlers and football players, are at risk for *S. aureus* SSTIs, although that risk has likely decreased since 2015. In U.S. high schools and universities in 2015–16, the incidence of CA-MRSA infections was estimated at 26.8 per 10,000 athletes, decreasing in 2016–17 to 20.3 per 10,000. Among wrestlers, the incidence was higher in both 2015–16 and 2016–17 (248.3 and 100.0 per 10,000, respectively) than among football players (71.0 and 81.8 per 10,000, respectively).[425] Among college wrestlers in the United States in 2009–14 monitored by the National Collegiate Athletic Association (NCAA) Injury Surveillance Program during 35 team-seasons, overall there were 14.23 SSTIs per 10,000 athlete exposures [95% confidence intervals (CI), 11.59, 16.86], and viral SSTIs (44.6%, $n = 50$) were more common than bacterial SSTIs (25.9%, $n = 29$).[431]

MRSA colonization of athletes in the United States, especially in contact sports,[441,442] while not detected in all studies,[443] is more common than in other countries that have available data. For example, in a longitudinal study of 186 U.S. varsity athletes in college in 2008–10 initially not colonized with *S. aureus*, 40 (22%) became colonized with MRSA, and new colonization with *S. aureus* was more common among athletes in contact sports (odds ratio, 2.36; 95% CI, 1.13–4.93).[444] Among 223 student athletes and support staff at a single U.S. university in 2007–08 who were tested for nasal, axillary, and inguinal colonization each week for 12 weeks, 35% were colonized with MRSA at least once. Wrestlers and baseball players were most likely to be colonized, and 47% of carriers had exclusively extranasal colonization.[445] In contrast to these U.S. studies, in Taiwan among 259 college students in 2013, only 1.5% carried MRSA in the nares, and there was no significant difference in carriage prevalence between athletes and nonathletes.[446] In a survey of nasal colonization in France of 300 athletes in 2011, although 61% were *S. aureus*-colonized, only one carried MRSA.[447]

Fomites in athletic areas have been contaminated with MRSA, including whirlpools and other surfaces in athletic training rooms,[448,449] locker room surfaces,[227,450] and fomites in wrestling facilities.[450,451] Cleaning of high-touch fomites and surfaces is likely an important means of reducing person-to-person spread of *S. aureus*. It is recommended that disinfectant cleaning products be used according to their label directions. More research is needed to determine the optimal means of decolonizing fomites in gyms, health clubs, locker rooms, and other athletic facilities.

Preventive measures are recommended for *S. aureus* SSTIs in guidelines prepared by the NCAA,[452] the National Federation of State High School Associations,[453] and the National Athletic Trainers' Association (NATA).[454] These guidelines recommend return to play for MRSA SSTI patients only when skin lesions are no longer actively draining, and only > 72 hours after an incision and drainage procedure[453] or after > 72 hours of therapy with antibiotics.[452,454] Return to play guidelines after an SSTI are critically important in reducing the risk of *S. aureus* spread, and upon return, an occlusive dressing is recommended over skin lesions.[455] The NCAA and NATA guidelines provide guidance for cleaning of athletic equipment.[452,454] The NATA guideline recommends attention to handwashing, personal attention to hygiene by the athletes, institutional attention to infection control, and prompt reporting of skin lesions to healthcare professionals, among other interventions.[454] The U.S. CDC on its website also offers guidance to athletes and athletics programs related to *S. aureus* skin infections.[456]

In a trial carried out among 474 high school wrestlers, use of either soap and water wipes or 70% isopropyl alcohol wipes after competition were associated with a lower risk of developing any SSTI than among controls with no intervention.[457] While such interventions are not recommended in the listed guidelines, use of similar wipes may decrease the risk of MRSA transmission. In a meta-analysis of the literature, decolonization of athletes who were colonized with MRSA was found to be effective at reducing the risk of SSTIs.[261] Further research is needed to determine which athletes benefit from decolonization and which decolonization regimen is optimal in the setting of a team or school outbreak of MRSA infections.

Nursing Homes

NHs are reservoirs of MRSA within the healthcare system. More study is needed to understand the risk factors for transmission within NHs and to identify effective interventions that reduce transmission and prevent infections among residents. It is clear that typical infection control interventions used in acute-care hospitals to prevent MRSA spread are not appropriate for NHs, where residents live for prolonged periods of time. All MRSA infections in NH patients are considered to be healthcare-associated infections by U.S. CDC criteria.

During 2009–13, the U.S. CDC conducted a study of NHs in 33 counties in 9 states, as part of the EIP surveillance on invasive MRSA infections. They identified 4607 residents with invasive MRSA infection with onset in the NH (or within 3 days of hospitalization, termed "NH onset") and another 4344 NH patients who had an invasive MRSA infection that had onset after 3 days of hospitalization (considered "NH hospital onset," or NH-HO); approximately 20% of each group died. It was very common for the NH residents to have devices in place (24% of the NH onset and 35% of the NH-HO had a central venous catheter, and 24% of NH onset and 12% of NH-HO were on hemodialysis); also 50% of NH onset and 40% of NH-HO had chronic medical conditions. Additionally, 32% of the NH onset and 27% of the NH-HO MRSA patients had a known history of MRSA colonization or infection, and 22% of the NH onset and 11% of NH-HO cases had decubitus ulcers.[458]

In studies to date, the prevalence of MRSA colonization in U.S. NHs is high compared with other U.S. populations, usually ranging from 22% to 30%. USA300 has been identified as a common strain type in NHs, although few NHs studies include genotyping data. An early study was from Michigan in 1990, when 341 NH residents were tested for MRSA colonization monthly for a year; the mean monthly colonization prevalence was 23% $\pm$ 1.0%.[459] Fourteen years later, in 2003–04 in Michigan MRSA was more prevalent; 52% of NH residents with an invasive device and 29% of those without an invasive device were colonized by MRSA.[460] In California in 2008–11, the mean MRSA prevalence was 22% in 26 NHs, and risk factors for colonization included, consistent with the findings in Michigan, the presence of an indwelling device. There was a higher transmission risk if there was a higher proportion of diabetics or lower level of social engagement in a NH.[461] In Orange County, California in 26 NHs in 2009–11, the admission prevalence of MRSA colonization was 16% and the point prevalence was 26%, suggesting relatively common transmission in the NH or longer stays for colonized residents.[462] Among NH residents in Baltimore, Maryland, the MRSA prevalence was 18% in 2003–07,[463] and a study of 129 of the residents identified no significant difference in duration of colonization with USA300 MRSA or other strain types.[464] The MRSA prevalence was 27.5% in NH residents in Queens County, New York, and carriage prevalence was higher among those hospitalized in the previous 3 years, those with renal insufficiency, Asian residents, and those who had received a greater number of antibiotic courses in the previous year.[465] In a national study of U.S. Veterans Affairs NHs, admitted residents from 2009 to 2012 were tested for MRSA nasal carriage. The admission prevalence ranged from 23.2% to 28.7% by year. The prevalence decreased over time by 36%, likely reflecting the introduction of the Veterans Affairs MRSA prevention bundle into both the acute-care and long-term-care settings.[466]

In Europe, the prevalence of MRSA in NHs tends to be somewhat lower in than in the United States, and CA-MRSA strain types are rarely identified. For example, among 2908 residents of 24 NHs in Belgium in 2000, the MRSA carriage prevalence was 7.1%,[467] and a later study in Belgium from 2015 showed a prevalence of 9.0%.[468] In Saarland, Germany in 2013–14, only 4.8% of 2858 NH residents were MRSA colonized. Risk factors for colonization included the presence of a urinary catheter, an ulcer or deep SSTI, or prior MRSA decolonization.[469] In the United Kingdom 22% of older residents (median age 85 years, range 61–103 years) of NHs were colonized. Risk factors for colonization included a low ratio of nurses to patients in the home, male sex, location of the NH in a deprived area, presence of an invasive device, and hospitalization for $>$ 10 days in prior 2 years.[470] Similarly, in 2006–09, the prevalence of MRSA in Leeds, U.K. NHs was 19–22% with no PVL-containing MRSA identified.[471] Remarkably, and consistent with the very low prevalence of MRSA in the country, a study in the central Netherlands showed that 0% of 125 tested residents in 5 NHs and 2 rehabilitation wards had MRSA colonization.[472] However, there was a reported outbreak of ST398 MRSA in a NH in 2010–11 in the southeastern region of the country where there is a concentration of pig farms. The outbreak affected seven NH residents and four healthcare workers. Twelve of 16 isolates were closely related by PFGE. Hand hygiene was improved, and the outbreak ended. Interestingly, the outbreak strain was not directly linked to pig contact.[473]

There are few studies of MRSA in NHs in Asia. In Shanghai, China in 2014, the MRSA prevalence was 10.6% in seven NHs.[474] Risk factors for colonization included previous hospitalization, an invasive device, chloramphenicol or macrolide therapy, and poor sanitary conditions in the home.[475]

To summarize, risk factors for MRSA colonization in NHs around the world in available data seem consistent. Studies suggest that MRSA colonization is common in most of the world in NH residents. Recent hospitalization, the presence of an indwelling device, a low staff-to-patient ratio, previous antibiotic use, and a skin ulcer are strong predictors of risk. Modifiable predictors include the devices, which can perhaps be removed, the staffing, which can be improved, and better care can be provided for decubitus ulcers.

Control measures for MRSA in NHs have been introduced as part of research studies. Most, but not all of these studies have shown that the tested interventions have failed to decrease the prevalence of MRSA colonization. In one randomized control trial of 36 elderly care homes in Hong Kong, a hygiene bundle was tested, including improved hand hygiene and environmental hygiene, as well as modified contact precautions. The study failed to show a significant difference in MRSA prevalence in the two arms.[476] Another unsuccessful intervention was attempted in Switzerland in a randomized controlled trial in 104 NHs. Universal screening and decolonization for MRSA was instituted compared with usual care. The prevalence of MRSA was not significantly different in the intervention arm.[477] A study testing an educational initiative for infection control among staff had no impact on MRSA prevalence in 16 randomized NHs in the United Kingdom.[478] In contrast, in Michigan in 2010–13 an infection control bundle including pre-emptive barrier precautions, enhanced staff education, and active surveillance for MDROs was tested. It did decrease new MRSA acquisitions and MDRO prevalence among residents with indwelling devices.[479] Another successful bundle intervention was tested in three NHs in Illinois beginning in 2011. The intervention involved routine nasal surveillance for MRSA detection, decolonization, education of staff, and enhanced environmental cleaning. This bundle led to a decrease in MRSA transmission over 2 years; MRSA colonization prevalence decreased from 16.64% to 10.55%.[480]

MRSA in Animals and Human Exposure to Animal Reservoirs

Livestock Animals

S. aureus infections in cattle and poultry have long been recognized as an economically important problem. Therefore, *S. aureus* represents a critical intersection in animal and human health and is a target of One Health programs.[19,481,482] *S. aureus* causes mastitis in dairy cows, among other milk-producing animals, leading to the contamination of milk and other dairy products.[483,484] The bacterium can cause SSTIs in a wide variety of livestock animals including sheep (impetigo, scalded skin syndrome), goats (often complicating prior fungal or viral skin infections), pigs (exudative epidermitis or greasy pig disease), and cattle (udder impetigo).[485] The emergence and persistence of MRSA strains in livestock animals may be driven by overuse of antibiotics.[486] The use of zinc additives in animal feed for growth enhancement likely co-selects for zinc- and antibiotic-resistant strains of bacteria.[487,488]

MRSA strains in the food chain may place the human population at risk in two ways. First, MRSA may be transmitted directly via livestock animals to farm workers and from meat to food handlers. Second, a large reservoir of MRSA on farms in the setting of frequent antibiotic use may breed novel reservoirs of antimicrobial resistance genes that can spread to human host-adapted *S. aureus* strains types.[489] Overuse worldwide has led the World Health Organization to recognize agricultural antibiotics as a major threat to human health, and it has also led to increasing governmental regulation of antibiotic use for farming in many countries, including Denmark, the European Union, the United States, and China.[490] The use of antibiotics as growth stimulators has been phased out in some countries, including the United States.

MRSA was first detected in a livestock animal in cattle in the early 1970s,[491] and then rarely identified for three decades. In 2004, MRSA ST398 was found to be a common colonizer of pigs in the Netherlands,[492,493] and soon thereafter in the United States[494] and other countries, including 17 of 24 European Union countries by 2008.[20,495–498] ST398 was identified as a common pig-adapted MRSA strain type, which can spread quickly among pigs in a herd, causing 4–100% colonization prevalence.[499,500] Notably, in Norway[501] and Sweden,[502] which have very low incidence of human MRSA infection, MRSA in pigs has been rarely identified.

In Europe, livestock other than pigs have frequent asymptomatic MRSA colonization, including dairy cows,[135,141,150,503–507] chickens and turkeys,[508–513] goats,[514] rabbits,[144,515] sheep,[141] and horses.[503,516–518] There are distinct genomic and phenotypic characteristics that can distinguish strains adapted to a particular hosts species, including level of adhesion to host cells.[519] In addition to ST398, other likely host-adapted MRSA strain types, including ST1, CC5, CC97, ST121, CC126, CC130, CC133, ST425, ST1464, and ST612 have been identified in various livestock species globally.[2,19,132]

It is believed that ST398 originated in humans and spread to livestock as an MSSA precursor, adapting to live on animals in part by losing the human "immune evasion cluster" of genes [usually defined as the following three genes: *scn* (staphylococcal complement inhibitor), *chp* (chemotaxis inhibitory protein precursor), and *sak* (see Table 154-5)] and eventually developing additional antimicrobial resistance with the acquisition of SCC*mec* and tetracycline-resistance genes.[20,520,521] CC398 strain types rarely carry the PVL genes and are a rare cause of infections among livestock workers despite their frequent carriage of the strains.[270,492]

ST398 MRSA has spread to populations having no known direct contact with livestock, and increasingly colonizing[522] and infecting isolates among people in Europe[473,523–529] especially in Germany,[530] and also in Australia.[531] Remarkably, ST398 was the most common MRSA strain type isolated from people in 2017 in Denmark,[532] a country with a low prevalence of MRSA. A study of genomes of 12 CC398 isolates in the United Kingdom in 2013–15 showed that there were multiple introductions of CC398 MRSA to the United Kingdom. Therefore, effective interventions to prevent future spread of these strains to the United Kingdom may optimally focus upon routes of international importation.[533] Although widespread in pig farming, human ST398 MRSA infections have only rarely been reported in North America.[534] Surgical-site infections were occasionally caused by ST398 MRSA in China in 2013–14[535]; it is not known whether these infections were related to livestock contact.

Workers on pig farms have frequent nasal colonization with ST398 MRSA, sometimes with a prevalence $> 50\%$, in continental Europe and North America[497,536–544] and with ST9 in China, Korea, and Taiwan.[496,535,545–548] Strong evidence of direct transmission of MRSA from a farm animal to a human[514,549] supports the idea that MRSA transmission may be common with routine exposure to colonized livestock. Increased duration of exposure to livestock among farm workers is associated with the risk of long-term LA-MRSA colonization.[241,377,550] Dust from pig farms can harbor MRSA for a half-life of 5 days,[242] and may transmit MRSA to workers indirectly.[241] Although there is some evidence that LA-MRSA colonization is more likely to be transient than with human-adapted MRSA strains, LA-MRSA colonization in industrial hog operation workers may persist for 14 days even after a 96-hour absence from work.[551] LA-MRSA carriage may be more common among workers at industrial hog operations than among antibiotic-free livestock operation workers in the United States[552] and workers on "organic farms" in Korea.[496] As regulations change on the use of preventive antibiotics in agriculture, however, new studies will be needed to reassess these differences.[553] Interestingly, in Australia, farm workers having direct exposure to pigs were more likely than other farm workers to carry ST93 MRSA, the most common Australian CA-MRSA strain type.[542] In addition to animal to human transmission of MRSA, there are reports of animals thought to have been colonized with MRSA originating from a human,[554,555] an example of a "humanosis."[556] It is possible that farm workers could acquire MRSA colonization by human-adapted strains from livestock after the animals acquire it from other people.

MRSA can be spread by means of pigs transferred from one farm to another,[557,558] but this is likely not the only driver for rapid spread of MRSA among pig farms.[559] Another contributing factor may be transmission among pigs on different farms by large-animal veterinarians, who are at high risk of LA-MRSA colonization,[20,276–280,560,561] and even by rats living on farms, which have tested positive for MRSA colonization.[562–565]

MRSA has been isolated from 0.9% to 85% of pigs handled at slaughterhouses worldwide,[500] including in the Netherlands,[566] Italy,[497] Germany,[567] Korea,[272] China,[568,569] Canada,[570] and the United States.[571] Slaughterhouses may be a site of transmission of *S. aureus* among animals or from workers to animals or to meat products.[572] Slaughterhouse workers, particularly those in contact with pigs, have been found frequently to be colonized with LA-MRSA stra ins.[271–275,497,573] A study in the United States showed no such colonization in 137 tested beefpacking workers,[574] suggesting that, at least in the United States, cattle may be less likely than pigs to carry and transmit MRSA to slaughterhouse workers. Routine use of plastic gloves by slaughterhouse workers may protect them from MRSA colonization,[274] but few studies address prevention of MRSA transmission to these workers.

Through environmental contamination and perhaps the local spread of CC398 MRSA via dust, populations living near large pig farming facilities may face an elevated risk of MRSA infections. In a Dutch high-density pig-farm area, a study identified patients with ST398 MRSA colonization and a wide range of infectious syndromes caused by ST398 MRSA.[575] Among veterans in Iowa, living within one mile of a large pig farm increased the risk of colonization by MRSA by nearly two times.[576] In a large cohort of patients from Pennsylvania in 2005–10, proximity of a person's domicile to a field with swine manure used as fertilizer was associated with an increased risk of a MRSA infection.[577] In contrast, a nationwide study in Denmark of people living in three regions with a high concentration of pig farms did not identify an association between proximity of a person's domicile to a pig farm and risk of a CC398 infection. The authors found, however, that living in rural areas more generally did increase the risk of infection with CC398 MRSA.[578] In China in 2015, backyard pig farming was associated with high risk of the spread of pig-adapted MRSA strains to humans and transmission of typical human-adapted CA-MRSA strains to pigs.[579]

The prevention of the spread of *S. aureus* to people in livestock agriculture is difficult. Hand hygiene is the most important intervention recommended.[270] Use of a face mask while working on pig farms may decrease the likelihood of persistent MRSA colonization and spread to HCs,[580,581] especially if there is frequent pig contact. However, there have not been adequate studies to support the universal use of masks in pig farming.[582] Because it is recognized that livestock workers are at high risk of colonization, some experts in Europe have suggested that they be screened prior to elective surgical procedures and undergo decolonization, if necessary.[270] A simulation study applied to Danish pig farms demonstrated that a combination of two or more of the following interventions may substantially decrease the prevalence of MRSA colonization on farms: (1) reduction in antimicrobial use in animals, (2) eradication of MRSA among 5–7.5% of pig herds, (3) restriction of movement of pigs from farm to farm, and (4) introduction of effective interventions to decrease the risk of MRSA transmission between farms by people.[583] In slaughterhouses, techniques such as singeing and scalding are used to decontaminate meat.[500]

There are few examples of successful eradication of MRSA from a pig farm; one instance in Norway required extensive and interdisciplinary outbreak investigation,[501] reflecting the national "One Health" approach to MRSA.[481] In Sweden, all nucleus and breeding pig herds were tested and found to have no MRSA colonization in both 2011 and 2014. Swedish pigs have been almost entirely free of MRSA. Such surveillance at the top of the breeding pyramid may be useful in very low-incidence countries to monitor risk of MRSA spread among pigs.[502]

Prevention of MRSA among animals in any country or region will ultimately likely require a One Health approach to infection prevention, with coordination between animal and human medical infrastructures. This would include improved surveillance for resistant organisms, improved infection control in the veterinary and human healthcare settings, more judicious use of antimicrobial drugs and inclusion of rapid diagnostic tests, new approaches to infection prevention and control in farming, surveillance in wild animal populations (see below), development of novel antimicrobials, and widespread implementation of educational programs for professionals and the public.[482,584]

Wild Animals

Wild animals have been studied for MRSA colonization almost exclusively in Europe, and they tend to carry strain types not often identified in humans. MRSA carriage has been found in the Iberian ibex,[585] otter,[140] hedgehog,[140,143,148,586] birds,[138,149,585,587–589] red fox,[589] European brown hare,[140,589] European rabbit,[148] red deer,[137] fallow deer,[147,589] wild boars,[147,585] Alpine chamois,[590] yellow-necked mouse,[145] a harbor seal,[591] and rats.[563,592–594] These animals may serve as a reservoir of antibiotic-resistant strains of *S. aureus*, and they may serve as a reservoir of staphylococcal-resistance genes. Animals in European and North American zoos have also been found to carry MRSA strains.[595–597]

Wild animals exposed to human populations and their waste may be colonized by human-adapted MRSA strains. For example, urban rats were colonized with USA300 MRSA in a study in Vancouver, Canada in 2011–12, with an increased prevalence associated with higher body weight, and with the winter and spring seasons. WGS revealed that USA300 MRSA in rats was clustered by neighborhood, and in one city neighborhood closely resembled MRSA carried by people in the area.[592] Colonization with MRSA in urban Norway rats in the study was associated with a low level of precipitation in the previous 15 days, and living on a block with food gardens and institutions.[565] MRSA colonization prevalence in urban rats in Vancouver in 2016–17 was not impacted by a kill-trapping program,[594] suggesting that alternative means may be required to control the potential reservoir of MRSA strains carried by urban rats.

More study is necessary to understand the role of wild animals in general and among urban and farm rats specifically in the maintenance and transmission of MRSA among humans, free-living wild animals, and livestock animals.

Companion Animals and Horses

U.S. households in 2012 owned more than 69 million dogs and 74 million cats.[598] These and other companion animals are capable of carrying and being infected by *S. aureus*, including MRSA strains. Domestic pets may serve as a reservoir for *S. aureus* in homes, independent of human carriage. However, there is only limited direct evidence to support this contention.[584,599,600] When dogs and cats develop SSTIs, including surgical-site infections, *S. aureus* is an unusual cause. More often other *Staphylococcus* species are cultured from infection and colonization cultures from dogs and cats. For example, in a study of methicillin-resistant staphylococci causing nares colonization of 131 rabbits, dogs, and cats in Austria, no MRSA was isolated. Instead, *S. epidermidis*, *S. pseudintermedius*, *S. warneri*, *S. hominis*, and four other species were cultured.[601] *S. pseudintermedius*, a rare human pathogen, is a particularly common cause of methicillin-resistant staphylococcal infection in dogs.[602] It was the most common cause of respiratory infection in dogs in a recent European survey.[603]

However, there have been MRSA infections and outbreaks among cats[604–608] and dogs.[605,607–617] *S. aureus* was identified in wounds of cats (12.2%), dogs (5.8%), and horses (22.8%) in 5229 cultures from animal wounds in German veterinary practices in 2010–12. In cats, 46.4% of *S. aureus* were MRSA; in dogs, 62.7% were MRSA; and in horses, 41.3% were MRSA.[618] Risk factors for MRSA (as compared with MSSA) infection in companion animals in Germany included the following: a greater number of workers in a veterinary facility, recent antibiotic therapy in the animal, and presence of a surgical-site infection.[619] In most studies in veterinary practice, MRSA carriage in dogs and cats usually ranges from approximately 0.5% to 10%.[611,612,620–623] In a prospective study of colonization in 506 dogs admitted to a veterinary hospital, 1.4% acquired MRSA colonization.[624] One longitudinal study of surfaces and fomites in a U.S. university small animal veterinary hospital found that a single PFGE type of MRSA, USA100 (see Table 154-3), was present for 5 months on a variety of fomites and was recovered from dogs that were patients there.[615] This suggests that the environment may serve as a reservoir for MRSA in veterinary hospitals. Cleaning of fomites, as in human hospitals, therefore, may reduce the risk of nosocomial transmission.

Transmission of MRSA between animal patients and veterinary hospital staff has been reported.[604,614,625] For example, MRSA transmission from dogs with surgical-site infections to a veterinary surgeon was reported in Ireland.[626] A study in Germany found the same strain type of MRSA (ST22-IV) commonly colonizing veterinary personnel and infecting dogs in a veterinary hospital in 2003–04.[627] More research is necessary to determine how frequently MRSA is transmitted from animals to people and vice versa in veterinary clinical settings and the optimal methods to prevent this.

The MRSA isolated from cats and dogs worldwide in households and in veterinary practice is usually related to common local human strain types,[614,615,620,621,623,627–635] and only rarely is it CC398,[610,636–639] which has been found in these animals especially on farms.[504,562] Pets and their human companions can transmit MRSA to one another, as shown in numerous small studies.[640–647] Transmission from a human to companion animals may be more common when a human in a household has a MRSA SSTI.[642] Cats living in a U.S. NH were found to carry the USA100 strain (see Table 154-3),[648] raising concern that cats could spread MRSA among residents. Companion animals have also been found in rare cases to carry *mecC*-positive MRSA in Europe,[142,649,650] perhaps due to exposure to a wildlife reservoir. In Japan, one study found that, among a great variety of *S. aureus* strain types, cats commonly carried ST133 *S. aureus*, and the authors suggested that it may be a species-adapted strain.[651]

Horses in veterinary and nonveterinary settings have been infected and asymptomatically colonized with MRSA in many countries.[519,609,631,652–662] In contrast to other companion animals, horses predominantly carry ST398 MRSA strains,[618,660,663] and a specific sublineage may be common among horse-associated ST398 MRSA.[503,516–518] Horses colonized with MRSA carrying *mecC* were reported in France.[139] Outbreaks of MRSA infections and spread of colonization have occurred among thoroughbreds, including racehorses,[658,664,665] demonstrating the great potential financial implications of MRSA infections. Furthermore, horses colonized with MRSA may pose an important risk of transmission to people in close contact with them. Further study is needed to reduce this risk.

Interventions for the prevention of transmission from companion animals to humans first should rely on trying to prevent colonization of the companion animals. This requires avoidance of pets contacting open wounds, bandages, and pus when a human has an SSTI. Routine decolonization of pets is generally not recommended if MRSA is found, as there are few tested protocols available. In the event that a companion animal has a bacterial SSTI, it is recommended that antimicrobials be used to treat the infection. Additional recommendations for prevention have been discussed in a position paper.[584]

Food and Foodborne Outbreaks of *S. aureus* Infection

S. aureus is an important cause of food poisoning and is a common etiology identified in public health investigations of foodborne outbreaks around the world. Given the problem of MRSA in livestock discussed above, in the animal-based food chain around the world, concern about *S. aureus* contamination has led to numerous studies to assess for contamination of retail foodstuffs derived from the cattle, pork, poultry, fish, and dairy industries. In the United States, approximately 241,000 cases of foodborne disease caused by *S. aureus* occur each year.[666] It has been estimated that foodborne staphylococcal infections cost more than $167 million per year in the United States.[667] *S. aureus* was the third most common etiology of bacterial gastroenteritis in a study in China.[668] *S. aureus* gastrointestinal disease is usually mediated by a preformed bacterial enterotoxin (often SEA or SEB, see Table 154-4) in food prior to consumption, and only a very small inoculum of toxin is likely required to cause disease.[669] Genes for enterotoxins are often carried by MGEs, including plasmids, *S. aureus* pathogenicity islands, or prophages in *S. aureus*, and therefore these genes can be exchanged and carried by many different genetic lineages.[107]

Contamination of food prepared in advance of a meal by a communal kitchen, food service, caterer, or retail food establishment or served at communal gatherings, such as parties, weddings, and picnics, is the typical scenario of an outbreak of *S. aureus*-associated gastroenteritis. A wide variety of foods may be associated with outbreaks, including meats, salads, sandwich fillings, and pastries filled with cream. The risk of *S. aureus* disease is commonly associated with improper refrigeration of food prior to consumption.[670,671] Fermented foods may rarely be responsible for *S. aureus* outbreaks.[672] Food produced from raw milk from goats, sheep, or cows also pose a risk of *S. aureus* infections.[673–676] Typical symptoms of staphylococcal food poisoning include abrupt onset of severe nausea, abdominal cramping, vomiting, malaise, and often diarrhea, starting approximately 3–5 hours after ingestion of the contaminated food and usually resolving after 24–48 hours.[107] Fever is typically absent or low-grade. The disease is usually self-limited and is not treated with antibiotics.

Investigations of *S. aureus* food poisoning outbreaks by public health authorities can involve isolation of enterotoxin-producing *S. aureus* from feces or vomitus of patients. Food can be tested for preformed staphylococcal enterotoxins and cultured for *S. aureus*. *S. aureus* can also be isolated from kitchen surfaces or fomites, or the bodies of food preparers or handlers, who are often identified as the source of food contamination.[107] The first community MRSA foodborne outbreak in the United States, for example, was caused by shredded pork barbeque, contaminated by MRSA from the hands of a food preparer at a convenience store.[677] Increasingly, genotyping can be used to determine relatedness of isolates to document a source and define the specific enterotoxin-causing disease, which can be essential to implementing control measures. In China, ST6 strains have often been identified as the causative strain.[678,679] In Korea,[680] Japan,[681–683] and Europe[675,684–686] *S. aureus* isolates from outbreaks have varied widely in their genetic backgrounds. Interventions to prevent outbreaks include improved refrigeration policies, improved personal and food hygiene practices by food preparers and handlers, and use of gloves by food handlers. Decolonization of food service workers may have a role in the prevention of outbreaks, but this has not been clearly shown.

Retail meats have been contaminated with MRSA even prior to reaching a kitchen, and it is possible that this may result in the risk of transmission to food workers, people cooking at home, and consumers, potentially resulting in foodborne outbreaks and/or spread of human colonization. For example, MRSA has been isolated from beef in North America,[687–689] Europe,[690–692] Korea,[693,694] and China[695]; veal in Europe[690,692,696]; pork and pork products in Europe,[567,690,697–703] North America,[688,704–708] Korea,[693,694] and China[569,695,709]; and poultry in Europe,[690,691,699,710–713] Korea,[613,693] Japan,[714] China,[695,709,715] North America,[687,688,716] and North Africa.[717] The prevalence of MRSA isolation from retail pork has ranged from 1.8% to 21.5% in various studies.[500] MRSA has been isolated from lamb or mutton[690] and fish.[718–720] The contaminating MRSA isolates tend to be related to CC398 in North America and Europe while in China either CC398 or CC9,[721] which are typical LA-MRSA clonal clusters, have been isolated. CC398 MRSA have been identified that carry enterotoxin genes. Contamination of retail meat and meat products may result from asymptomatic colonization of livestock, cross contamination of meat in a slaughterhouse, or contamination by food workers in the retail meat industry.

Dairy products have been contaminated with MRSA, especially cheeses[702,722,723] and cow milk worldwide.[133,504,507,692,709,724–735] Contaminated milk samples have been isolated both from cows with known clinical mastitis and from bulk tank cow milk; the prevalence of MRSA has varied widely in these studies. MRSA, including one *mecA*- and one *mecC*-positive isolate was isolated from 2 (0.7%) of 286 tested bulk tank milk samples from dairy sheep farms in central Italy in 2012.[136] A study of retail raw milk products in England were found to have contamination by coagulase-positive staphylococci in 15.4% (139/902) of tested samples.[736] A study by the U.S. Department of Agriculture in 2007 in 17 dairy states from 542 operations demonstrated no MRSA in bulk tank milk samples from 542 operations.[737] *S. aureus* is killed by pasteurization, and this is the major intervention to prevent its transmission through milk and dairy products to consumers.

There have not been many cross-sectional studies of *S. aureus* colonization in food handlers. In Germany, however, 286 butchers and meat retail salespeople as well as 319 cooks underwent nasal culture, with 26.2% and 16.6% carrying MSSA, respectively. Only one of the butchers and one of the retail meat salespeople, both of whom were female and neither of whom had recent healthcare exposure, carried MRSA. Both MRSA isolates were *spa* type t032/CC22 (see Table 154-3), which is not a typical LA-MRSA strain type.[738]

Prevention of contamination of meat and milk requires a comprehensive approach to hygiene along the food chain with surveillance and, if indicated, outbreak investigations. Treatment of bovine mastitis and other livestock infections now relies largely on antimicrobial therapy.[739] Recommendations for the diagnosis and treatment of infectious diarrhea is provided in a 2017 IDSA guideline.[740] Control of MRSA transmission among livestock is a challenge as addressed above. Careful hygiene in meat and milk processing and packaging plants, at dairies, and at butchers is essential to prevent additional spread among food products prior to retail sale.[741] Raw milk and dairy products pose a particular challenge, as they may contain *S. aureus* and other human pathogens, and unpasteurized foods should be avoided. Appropriate refrigeration of meat and dairy products along the food chain from slaughterhouse or dairy farm to consumer, pasteurization of milk and its products, and thorough cooking of meat prior to consumption are critically important in the prevention of *S. aureus* gastroenteritis related to these products.

National, state, and local regulations and public health surveillance of food retailers and restaurants are essential for the prevention of *S. aureus* foodborne infections. Surveillance and investigation by national public health authorities are sometimes necessary to rapidly identify and stop large foodborne *S. aureus* outbreaks. In the United States, the CDC tracks foodborne illnesses through the Foodborne Disease Outbreak Surveillance System, part of the National Outbreak Reporting System (NORS), and has published an annual report since 2011.[742] Starting in 2014, the CDC added a new reporting system for outbreaks involving retail food establishments.[743] A global laboratory-based network for foodborne disease surveillance, called PulseNet International, has been initiated using WGS to detect outbreaks due to *Salmonella enterica*, *Shigella*, *E. coli*, *Campylobacter*, *Listeria*, and *Vibrio*.[744] Additional information on foodborne outbreaks can be found in Chapter 110: Diseases Spread by Food and Water.

SURVEILLANCE PROGRAMS FOR *S. AUREUS* INFECTIONS

Many countries have instituted some form of surveillance to document trends in incidence of antimicrobial resistance in bacterial or other pathogens, and these often include *S. aureus* infections. Most *S. aureus* surveillance programs focus on MRSA. One exception is in Denmark, where since 1957 all *S. aureus* bacteremia cases have been reported.[745] A surveillance program called the Danish Integrated Antimicrobial Resistance Monitoring and Research Program (DANMAP) now tracks antimicrobial use as well as the incidence of human and animal infections with MRSA.[746] In the United Kingdom, mandatory surveillance for MRSA bacteremia was instituted in 2003, and collection began of associated demographic and clinical information in 2005.[747] Mandatory reporting for invasive MRSA infections began in Germany in 2009 and 27,706 cases were reported in 2009–16.[748] Many other individual European countries have an independent surveillance system for human infectious diseases,[326] as does the European Centre for Diseases Prevention and Control through the European Antimicrobial Resistance Surveillance Network (EARS-Net).[749] There are also a variety of surveillance programs for antimicrobial resistance in livestock animals and meat in Europe.[750]

In the United States, CDC initiated laboratory and population-based surveillance for invasive MRSA infections in 2005 as part of the Emerging Infections Program (EIP).[30–32,92] HAIs, including nosocomial MRSA bacteremia, pneumonia, and UTIs are tracked by the U.S. CDC through the National Healthcare Safety Network.[751] In Canada, the CANWARD study assesses antimicrobial resistance in human pathogens in both inpatient and outpatient settings,[752] and the Canadian Nosocomial Infection Surveillance Program directed by the Public Health Agency of Canada estimates MRSA colonization and infection rates.[55,101]

Most surveillance systems focus on invasive rather than noninvasive *S. aureus* infections, such as SSTIs. One exception is the SENTRY antimicrobial surveillance program run by JMI Laboratories in the United States. This program has tracked the susceptibilities of many pathogens, including sequential isolates of *S. aureus*, since 1997 from 427 centers in 45 countries and published results on 191,460 isolates collected between 1997 and 2016.[753]

PROMISE OF A *S. AUREUS* VACCINE

There is no licensed vaccine against *S. aureus*. A vaccine that would prevent infections, or perhaps even better, one that would also prevent colonization, could revolutionize the approach to *S. aureus* control. It could potentially save tens of thousands of lives worldwide and prevent hundreds of thousands of costly and debilitating invasive infections each year, particularly in immunocompromised hosts and elderly people.

The approach taken to vaccinate against many pathogens has involved preparation of one or more antigenic proteins or other molecules to produce protective antibodies against the organism (e.g., influenza, rabies, measles, polio, hepatitis A, or hepatitis B), or against a toxin produced by the organism (e.g., diphtheria and tetanus). For some vaccines, antigens are conjugated to an immunogenic molecule (*Haemophilus influenzae* and *Streptococcus pneumoniae* conjugate vaccines). Increasing evidence suggests that this model of producing protective antibodies alone may not be adequate for the prevention of *S. aureus* infections. Instead, eliciting an appropriate T-cell response may be necessary.[754] A recent study demonstrated that most people likely carry measurable antibodies to surface and secreted *S. aureus* antigens,[755] and for this reason, it may be difficult to detect easily a correlate of immunity. As noted above, in contrast to many pathogens, even a natural infection does not result in immunity to a specific strain of *S. aureus*.[17] The broad array of immune evasion mechanisms possessed by *S. aureus* (see Table 154-5) probably interferes with the establishment of durable immunity to vaccines tested to date.

Before the 1970s, many whole-cell killed *S. aureus* vaccines were used, some of them derived from the patient's own infecting strain, but large, controlled studies were never conducted using these preparations.[756–758] Passive vaccination with antistaphylococcal antibodies has been considered, but this approach has not reached advanced clinical trials.[759] Among the most promising antigens tested in candidate vaccines have included the iron-scavenging protein IsdB and the capsular polysaccharides CP5 and CP8, which prevent phagocytosis.[760,761] Interestingly, most *S. aureus* strain types make a capsule of either type CP5 or type CP8, but the USA300 MRSA strain does not produce capsule,[762] and therefore it is not clear that a capsular polysaccharide vaccine would be effective against USA300.

Three vaccines have been tested since 2000 in clinical trials in different human populations, but as of 2019, no vaccine has demonstrated efficacy and safety.[754,763,764] IsdB and CP5 with CP8 were tested in animal models and then used in the development of human vaccines named V710 (IsdB) and Staphvax (CP5/CP8). Both produced vigorous antibody responses in early-phase human trials. The V710 vaccine phase III trial was conducted in approximately 8000 cardiothoracic surgery patients. The study was stopped prematurely due to an interim safety analysis that demonstrated increased mortality in subjects receiving the vaccine who developed a *S. aureus* infection.[765]

The StaphVax vaccine was evaluated in two phase III trials. In the second phase III trial, carried out in 3600 end-stage renal disease patients on hemodialysis, there was no significant difference in bacteremia incidence among vaccinated subjects and controls.[766] A third vaccine, produced by Pfizer, consisted of four antigens (Clfa, MntC, CP5, and CP8). It was tested in the phase 2B STRIVE trial in patients undergoing spinal fusion surgery.[759] The trial was discontinued early due to futility.[763]

There are now a number of novel multiantigen vaccines in development. These include one with four antigens (FhuD2, CSA1A, and a fused chimeric protein combining EsxA and EsxB) owned by Glaxo-Smith-Kline (GSK), a second vaccine developed by GSK (CP5, CP8, ClfA, and detoxified alpha-toxin), and another candidate single-antigen vaccine developed by NovaDigm Therapeutics called NDV3 consisting of a surface protein derived from *Candida albicans*.[759,767] Other *S. aureus* antigens, including MntC, manganese transport protein C[768]; Luk-S-PV, a component of PVL; and a mutant version of Protein A (Table 154-4) have been proposed as candidate vaccine antigens.[764] Many of the *S. aureus* antigens proposed for use in vaccine development have been studied in detail. For example, clumping factor A, ClfA, binds fibrin and fibrinogen, among other human ligands, and aids the bacterium in attachment to human epithelial cells.[184] Detoxified alpha toxin is a mutant version of a toxin that hemolyzes red blood cells, among other functions (Table 154-4), and is carried by most *S. aureus* strains.[109] EsxA and EsxB influence the regulation of dendritic cell cytokine responses and apoptosis.[769]

Strategies to develop an effective vaccine will require the choice of an appropriate target subject group for a clinical trial. For new vaccine trials, one or more of the high-risk populations listed in Table 154-7 may be chosen, and a relatively healthy population may be optimal.[757,764] The target group should be at high risk for *S. aureus* infections, be likely to be evaluable in follow-up, and have strong immunologic responses to vaccines. Important to recognize, immune responses to a vaccine may protect against infection at some anatomic sites and not others. For example, a vaccine may protect against bacteremia but not pneumonia, osteomyelitis, or an SSTI, because the immune response differs in infections of various human tissues. Therefore, the choice of outcome (especially the anatomic site of infection) in a vaccine trial is critically important and may be challenging. A new vaccine many differ in its efficacy for different strain types of *S. aureus*, and so it may be important to know which strain types circulate in regions where a vaccine trial is performed. Evaluation of *S. aureus* isolated from cases of vaccine failure (i.e., *S. aureus* infections) may point to strain types that are not well covered by a vaccine. Of course, the choice of vaccine antigens and the choice of adjuvant that is bound to these antigens will play a critical role in the success or failure of a vaccine.

In summary, the development of a *S. aureus* vaccine may provide the best means of preventing the spread of *S. aureus*, the worsening of antimicrobial resistance in this species, and morbidity and mortality due to noninvasive and invasive *S. aureus* infections. The development of an effective vaccine will require large and expensive trials and an improved understanding of the immunology and molecular epidemiology of *S. aureus* colonization and infection.

References

1. Tong SY, Davis JS, Eichenberger E, Holland TL, Fowler VG Jr. *Staphylococcus aureus* infections: Epidemiology, pathophysiology, clinical manifestations, and management. *Clin Microbiol Rev*. 2015;28(3):603–61.
2. Aires-de-Sousa M. Methicillin-resistant *Staphylococcus aureus* among animals: Current overview. *Clin Microbiol Infect*. 2017;23(6):373–80.
3. Becker K, Schaumburg F, Fegeler C, Friedrich AW, Köck R; Prevalence of Multiresistant Microorganisms PMM Study. *Staphylococcus aureus* from the German general population is highly diverse. *Int J Med Microbiol*. 2017;307(1):21–7.
4. Donker GA, Deurenberg RH, Driessen C, Sebastian S, Nys S, Stobberingh EE. The population structure of *Staphylococcus aureus* among general practice patients from The Netherlands. *Clin Microbiol Infect*. 2009;15(2):137–43.
5. Gorwitz RJ, Kruszon-Moran D, McAllister SK, et al. Changes in the prevalence of nasal colonization with *Staphylococcus aureus* in the United States, 2001–2004. *J Infect Dis*. 2008;197(9):1226–34.
6. Holtfreter S, Grumann D, Balau V, et al. Molecular epidemiology of *Staphylococcus aureus* in the general population in northeast Germany: Results of the study of health in Pomerania (SHIP-TREND-0). *J Clin Microbiol*. 2016;54(11):2774–85.
7. Kluytmans J, van Belkum A, Verbrugh H: Nasal carriage of *Staphylococcus aureus*: Epidemiology, underlying mechanisms, and associated risks. *Clin Microbiol Rev*. 1997;10(3):505–20.
8. Miller RR, Walker AS, Godwin H, et al. Dynamics of acquisition and loss of carriage of *Staphylococcus aureus* strains in the community: The effect of clonal complex. *J Infect*. 2014;68(5):426–39.
9. Munckhof WJ, Nimmo GR, Schooneveldt JM, et al. Nasal carriage of *Staphylococcus aureus*, including community-associated methicillin-resistant strains, in Queensland adults. *Clin Microbiol Infect*. 2009;15(2):149–55.
10. Noble WC, Valkenburg HA, Wolters CH. Carriage of *Staphylococcus aureus* in random samples of a normal population. *J Hyg (Lond)*. 1967;65(4):567–73.
11. Feldman HA. The beginning of antimicrobial therapy: Introduction of the sulfonamides and penicillins. *J Infect Dis*. 1972;125:Suppl:22–46.
12. Lakhundi S, Zhang K. Methicillin-resistant *Staphylococcus aureus*: Molecular characterization, evolution, and epidemiology. *Clin Microbiol Rev*. 2018;31(4):e00020-18.
13. Centers for Disease Control and Prevention (CDC). Toxic shock syndrome (other than streptococcal) (TSS) 2011 case definition. https://wwwn.cdc.gov/nndss/conditions/toxic-shock-syndrome-other-than-streptococcal/case-definition/2011/. Accessed May 2, 2019.
14. Handler MZ, Schwartz RA. Staphylococcal scalded skin syndrome: Diagnosis and management in children and adults. *J Eur Acad Dermatol Venereol*. 2014;28(11):1418–23.
15. Paling FP, Olsen K, Ohneberg K, et al. Risk prediction for *Staphylococcus aureus* surgical site infection following cardiothoracic surgery: A secondary analysis of the V710-P003 trial. *PLoS One*. 2018;13(3):e0193445.
16. Ridgway JP, Peterson LR, Brown EC, et al. Clinical significance of methicillin-resistant *Staphylococcus aureus* colonization on hospital admission: One-year infection risk. *PLoS One*. 2013;8(11):e79716.
17. Azarian T, Daum RS, Petty LA, et al. Intrahost evolution of methicillin-resistant *Staphylococcus aureus* USA300 among individuals with reoccurring skin and soft-tissue infections. *J Infect Dis*. 2016;214(6):895–905.
18. Fitzgerald JR, Holden MT. Genomics of natural populations of *Staphylococcus aureus*. *Annu Rev Microbiol*. 2016;70:459–78.
19. Fitzgerald JR. Livestock-associated *Staphylococcus aureus*: Origin, evolution and public health threat. *Trends Microbiol*. 2012;20(4):192–8.
20. Smith TC, Pearson N. The emergence of *Staphylococcus aureus* ST398. *Vector Borne Zoonotic Dis*. 2011;11(4):327–39.
21. Ogston A. Report upon micro-organisms in surgical diseases. *Br Med J*. 1881;1(1054):369.b2–375.
22. Rosenbach, AJ. *Mikro-Organismen bei den Wund-Infections-Krankheiten des Menschen*. Wiesbaden: J.F. Bergmann; 1884.
23. Williamson DA, Lim A, Thomas MG, et al. Incidence, trends and demographics of *Staphylococcus aureus* infections in Auckland, New Zealand, 2001–2011. *BMC Infect Dis*. 2013;13:569.
24. Tracy LA, Furuno JP, Harris AD, Singer M, Langenberg P, Roghmann MC. *Staphylococcus aureus* infections in US veterans, Maryland, USA, 1999–2008. *Emerg Infect Dis*. 2011;17(3):441–8.
25. Ray GT, Suaya JA, Baxter R. Incidence, microbiology, and patient characteristics of skin and soft-tissue infections in a U.S. population: A retrospective population-based study. *BMC Infect Dis*. 2013;13:252.
26. Landrum ML, Neumann C, Cook C, et al. Epidemiology of *Staphylococcus aureus* blood and skin and soft tissue infections in the US military health system, 2005–2010. *JAMA*. 2012;308(1):50–9.
27. Kourtis AP, Hatfield K, Baggs J, et al. Vital signs: Epidemiology and recent trends in methicillin-resistant and in methicillin-susceptible *Staphylococcus aureus* bloodstream infections—United States. *MMWR Morb Mortal Wkly Rep*. 2019;68(9):214–9.
28. Saeed K, Bal AM, Gould IM, et al. An update on *Staphylococcus aureus* infective endocarditis from the International Society of Antimicrobial Chemotherapy (ISAC). *Int J Antimicrob Agents*. 2019;53(1):9–15.
29. Gualandi N, Mu Y, Bamberg WM, et al. Racial disparities in invasive methicillin-resistant *Staphylococcus aureus* infections, 2005–2014. *Clin Infect Dis*. 2018;67(8):1175–81.

30. Klevens RM, Morrison MA, Nadle J, et al. Invasive methicillin-resistant *Staphylococcus aureus* infections in the United States. *JAMA.* 2007;298(15):1763–71.
31. Dantes R, Mu Y, Belflower R, et al. National burden of invasive methicillin-resistant *Staphylococcus aureus* infections, United States, 2011. *JAMA Intern Med.* 2013;173(21):1970–8.
32. Kallen AJ, Mu Y, Bulens S, et al. Health care-associated invasive MRSA infections, 2005–2008. *JAMA.* 2010;304(6):641–8.
33. Koeck M, Como-Sabetti K, Boxrud D, et al. Burdens of invasive methicillin-susceptible and methicillin-resistant *Staphylococcus aureus* disease, Minnesota, USA. *Emerg Infect Dis.* 2019;25(1):171–4.
34. Woods C, Colice G. Methicillin-resistant *Staphylococcus aureus* pneumonia in adults. Expert Rev *Respir Med.* 2014;8(5):641–51.
35. Jacobs DM, Shaver A. Prevalence of and outcomes from *Staphylococcus aureus* pneumonia among hospitalized patients in the United States, 2009–2012. *Am J Infect Control.* 2017;45(4):404–9.
36. Aliberti S, Reyes LF, Faverio P, et al. Global initiative for meticillin-resistant *Staphylococcus aureus* pneumonia (GLIMP): An international, observational cohort study. *Lancet Infect Dis.* 2016;16(12):1364–76.
37. Klein EY, Monteforte B, Gupta A, et al. The frequency of influenza and bacterial coinfection: A systematic review and meta-analysis. *Influenza Other Respir Viruses.* 2016;10(5):394–403.
38. Shah NS, Greenberg JA, McNulty MC, et al. Bacterial and viral co-infections complicating severe influenza: Incidence and impact among 507 U.S. patients, 2013–14. *J Clin Virol.* 2016;80:12–9.
39. Ahmad A, Teoh KH, Lau L, Cheng N, Evans AR. Can we reduce the number of MRSA screening site swabs in elective orthopedic patients? *J Orthop Surg (Hong Kong).* 2019;27(2):2309499019847068.
40. McKinnell JA, Huang SS, Eells SJ, Cui E, Miller LG. Quantifying the impact of extranasal testing of body sites for methicillin-resistant *Staphylococcus aureus* colonization at the time of hospital or intensive care unit admission. *Infect Control Hosp Epidemiol.* 2013;34(2):161–70.
41. Ammerlaan HS, Kluytmans JA, Berkhout H, et al. Eradication of carriage with methicillin-resistant *Staphylococcus aureus*: Determinants of treatment failure. *J Antimicrob Chemother.* 2011;66(10):2418–24.
42. Jörgensen J, Månsson F, Janson H, Petersson AC, Nilsson AC. The majority of MRSA colonized children not given eradication treatment are still colonized one year later. Systemic antibiotics improve the eradication rate. *Infect Dis (Lond).* 2018;50(9):687–96.
43. Wang X, Towers S, Panchanathan S, Chowell G. A population based study of seasonality of skin and soft tissue infections: Implications for the spread of CA-MRSA. *PLoS One.* 2013;8(4):e60872.
44. Morgan E, Daum RS, David MZ. Decreasing incidence of skin and soft tissue infections with a seasonal pattern at an academic medical center, 2006–2014. *Open Forum Infect Dis.* 2016;3(4):ofw179.
45. Mermel LA, Machan JT, Parenteau S. Seasonality of MRSA infections. *PLoS One.* 2011;6(3):e17925.
46. Anthony CA, Peterson RA, Polgreen LA, Sewell DK, Polgreen PM. The seasonal variability in surgical site infections and the association with warmer weather: A population-based investigation. *Infect Control Hosp Epidemiol.* 2017;38(7):809–16.
47. Foster TJ. Antibiotic resistance in *Staphylococcus aureus.* Current status and future prospects. *FEMS Microbiol Rev.* 2017;41(3):430–49.
48. Chambers HF, Deleo FR. Waves of resistance: *Staphylococcus aureus* in the antibiotic era. *Nat Rev Microbiol.* 2009;7(9):629–41.
49. Jevons MP. Celbenin-resistant Staphylococci. *Br Med J.* 1961;1(5912): 124–5.
50. Tong SY, Sharma-Kuinkel BK, Thaden JT, et al. Virulence of endemic nonpigmented northern Australian *Staphylococcus aureus* clone (clonal complex 75, *S. argenteus*) is not augmented by staphyloxanthin. *J Infect Dis.* 2013;208(3):520–7.
51. Barrett FF, McGehee RFJr, Finland M. Methicillin-resistant *Staphylococcus aureus* at Boston City Hospital. Bacteriologic and epidemiologic observations. *N Engl J Med.* 1968;279(9):441–8.
52. Panlilio AL, Culver DH, Gaynes RP, et al. Methicillin-resistant *Staphylococcus aureus* in U.S. hospitals, 1975–1991. *Infect Control Hosp Epidemiol.* 1992;13(10):582–6.
53. NNIS System. National Nosocomial Infections Surveillance (NNIS) System Report, data summary from January 1992 through June 2003, issued August 2003. *Am J Infect Control.* 2003;31(8):481–98.
54. Elixhauser A. Infections with methicillin-resistant *Staphylococcus aureus* (MRSA) in U.S. hospitals, 1993–2005. HCUP Statistical Brief #35. July 2007. Agency for Healthcare Research and Quality, Rockville, MD. http://www.hcup-us.ahrq.gov/reports/statbrief/sb35.pdf.
55. Simor AE, Gilbert NL, Gravel D, et al. Methicillin-resistant *Staphylococcus aureus* colonization or infection in Canada: National surveillance and changing epidemiology, 1995–2007. *Infect Control Hosp Epidemiol.* 2010;31(4):348–56.
56. Bouchiat C, Curtis S, Spiliopoulou I, et al. MRSA infections among patients in the emergency department: A European multicentre study. *J Antimicrob Chemother.* 2017;72(2):372–5.
57. Köck R, Becker K, Cookson B, et al. Methicillin-resistant *Staphylococcus aureus* (MRSA): Burden of disease and control challenges in Europe. *Euro Surveill.* 2010;15(41):19688. Erratum in: *Euro Surveill.* 2010; 15(42).
58. Stefani S, Varaldo PE. Epidemiology of methicillin-resistant staphylococci in Europe. *Clin Microbiol Infect.* 2003;9(12):1179–86.
59. Dailey L, Coombs GW, O'Brien FG, et al. Methicillin-resistant *Staphylococcus aureus*, Western Australia. *Emerg Infect Dis.* 2005;11(10):1584–90.
60. Williamson DA, Coombs GW, Nimmo GR. *Staphylococcus aureus* 'Down Under': Contemporary epidemiology of *S. aureus* in Australia, New Zealand, and the South West Pacific. *Clin Microbiol Infect.* 2014;20(7):597–604.
61. Bartels MD, Kristoffersen K, Boye K, Westh H. Rise and subsequent decline of community-associated methicillin resistant *Staphylococcus aureus* ST30-IVc in Copenhagen, Denmark through an effective search and destroy policy. *Clin Microbiol Infect.* 2010;16(1):78–83.
62. Wertheim HF, Vos MC, Boelens HA, et al. Low prevalence of methicillin-resistant *Staphylococcus aureus* (MRSA) at hospital admission in the Netherlands: The value of search and destroy and restrictive antibiotic use. *J Hosp Infect.* 2004;56(4):321–5.
63. Chen CJ, Huang YC. New epidemiology of *Staphylococcus aureus* infection in Asia. *Clin Microbiol Infect.* 2014;20(7):605–23.
64. Saravolatz LD, Pohlod DJ, Arking LM. Community-acquired methicillin-resistant *Staphylococcus aureus* infections: A new source for nosocomial outbreaks. *Ann Intern Med.* 1982;97(3):325–9.
65. Embil J, Ramotar K, Romance L, et al. Methicillin-resistant *Staphylococcus aureus* in tertiary care institutions on the Canadian prairies 1990–1992. *Infect Control Hosp Epidemiol.* 1994;15(10):646–51.
66. Nimmo GR, Schooneveldt J, O'Kane G, McCall B, Vickery A. Community acquisition of gentamicin-sensitive methicillin-resistant *Staphylococcus aureus* in southeast Queensland, Australia. *J Clin Microbiol.* 2000;38(11):3926–31.
67. Nimmo GR, Coombs GW. Community-associated methicillin-resistant *Staphylococcus aureus* (MRSA) in Australia. *Int J Antimicrob Agents.* 2008;31(5):401–10.
68. Groom AV, Wolsey DH, Naimi TS, et al. Community-acquired methicillin-resistant *Staphylococcus aureus* in a rural American Indian community. 2001;*JAMA.* 286(10):1201–5.
69. David MZ, Daum RS. Community-associated methicillin-resistant *Staphylococcus aureus*: Epidemiology and clinical consequences of an emerging epidemic. *Clin Microbiol Rev.* 2010;23(3):616–87.
70. Pallin DJ, Egan DJ, Pelletier AJ, Espinola JA, Hooper DC, Camargo CAJr. Increased US emergency department visits for skin and soft tissue infections, and changes in antibiotic choices, during the emergence of community-associated methicillin-resistant *Staphylococcus aureus. Ann Emerg Med.* 2008;51(3):291–8.
71. Hersh AL, Chambers HF, Maselli JH, Gonzales R. National trends in ambulatory visits and antibiotic prescribing for skin and soft-tissue infections. *Arch Intern Med.* 2008;168(14):1585–91.
72. Klein E, Smith DL, Laxminarayan R. Community-associated methicillin-resistant *Staphylococcus aureus* in outpatients, United States, 1999–2006. *Emerg Infect Dis.* 2009;15(12):1925–30.
73. Lautz TB, Raval MV, Barsness KA. Increasing national burden of hospitalizations for skin and soft tissue infections in children. *J Pediatr Surg.* 2011;46(10):1935–41.
74. Suaya JA, Mera RM, Cassidy A, et al Incidence and cost of hospitalizations associated with *Staphylococcus aureus* skin and soft tissue infections in the United States from 2001 through 2009. *BMC Infect Dis.* 2014; 14:296.
75. Chambers HF. The changing epidemiology of *Staphylococcus aureus*? *Emerg Infect Dis.* 2001;7(2):178–82.
76. Gutierrez K, Halpern MS, Sarnquist C, Soni S, Arroyo AC, Maldonado Y. Staphylococcal infections in children, California, USA, 1985–2009. *Emerg Infect Dis.* 2013;19(1):10–20.
77. Gerber JS, Coffin SE, Smathers SA, Zaoutis TE. Trends in the incidence of methicillin-resistant *Staphylococcus aureus* infection in children's hospitals in the United States. *Clin Infect Dis.* 2009;49(1):65–71.

78. Ray GT, Suaya JA, Baxter R. Trends and characteristics of culture-confirmed *Staphylococcus aureus* infections in a large U.S. integrated health care organization. *J Clin Microbiol.* 2012;50(6):1950–7.

79. Johnson JK, Khoie T, Shurland S, Kreisel K, Stine OC, Roghmann MC. Skin and soft tissue infections caused by methicillin-resistant *Staphylococcus aureus* USA300 clone. *Emerg Infect Dis.* 2007;13(8):1195–200.

80. Casey JA, Cosgrove SE, Stewart WF, Pollak J, Schwartz BS. A population-based study of the epidemiology and clinical features of methicillin-resistant *Staphylococcus aureus* infection in Pennsylvania, 2001–2010. *Epidemiol Infect.* 2013;141 (6):1166–79.

81. Van De Griend P, Herwaldt LA, Alvis B, et al. Community-associated methicillin-resistant *Staphylococcus aureus*, Iowa, USA. *Emerg Infect Dis.* 2009;15(10):1582–9.

82. Kim J, Ferrato C, Golding GR, et al. Changing epidemiology of methicillin-resistant *Staphylococcus aureus* in Alberta, Canada: Population-based surveillance, 2005–2008. *Epidemiol Infect.* 2011;139(7):1009–18.

83. Tenover FC, McAllister S, Fosheim G, et al. Characterization of *Staphylococcus aureus* isolates from nasal cultures collected from individuals in the United States in 2001 to 2004. *J Clin Microbiol.* 2008;46(9):2837–41.

84. Como-Sabetti K, Harriman KH, Buck JM, Glennen A, Boxrud DJ, Lynfield R. Community-associated methicillin-resistant *Staphylococcus aureus*: Trends in case and isolate characteristics from six years of prospective surveillance. *Public Health Rep.* 2009;124(3):427–35.

85. Diekema DJ, Richter SS, Heilmann KP, et al. Continued emergence of USA300 methicillin-resistant *Staphylococcus aureus* in the United States: Results from a nationwide surveillance study. *Infect Control Hosp Epidemiol.* 2014;35(3):285–92.

86. Tattevin P, Schwartz BS, Graber CJ, et al. Concurrent epidemics of skin and soft tissue infection and bloodstream infection due to community-associated methicillin-resistant *Staphylococcus aureus*. *Clin Infect Dis.* 2012;55(6):781–8.

87. Mitchell BG, Collignon PJ, McCann R, Wilkinson IJ, Wells A. A major reduction in hospital-onset *Staphylococcus aureus* bacteremia in Australia-12 years of progress: An observational study. *Clin Infect Dis.* 2014;59(7):969–75.

88. Lai CC, Chen YH, Lin SH, at al. Changing aetiology of healthcare-associated bloodstream infections at three medical centres in Taiwan, 2000–2011. *Epidemiol Infect.* 2014;142(10):2180–5.

89. Duerden B, Fry C, Johnson AP, Wilcox MH. The control of methicillin-resistant *Staphylococcus aureus* blood stream infections in England. *Open Forum Infect Dis.* 2015;2(2):ofv035.

90. Meyer E, Schröder C, Gastmeier P, Geffers C. The reduction of nosocomial MRSA infection in Germany: An analysis of data from the Hospital Infection Surveillance System (KISS) between 2007 and 2012. *Dtsch Arztebl Int.* 2014;111(19):331–6.

91. Nichol KA, Adam HJ, Roscoe DL, et al. Changing epidemiology of methicillin-resistant *Staphylococcus aureus* in Canada. *J Antimicrob Chemother.* 2013;68 Suppl 1:i47–55.

92. See I, Mu Y, Albrecht V, et al. Trends in incidence of methicillin-resistant *Staphylococcus aureus* bloodstream infections differ by strain type and healthcare exposure, United States, 2005–2013. *Clin Infect Dis.* 2020;70(1):19–25.

93. Klein EY, Mojica N, Jiang W, et al. Trends in methicillin-resistant *Staphylococcus aureus* hospitalizations in the United States, 2010–2014. *Clin Infect Dis.* 2017;65(11):1921–3.

94. Stenehjem E, Stafford C, Rimland D. Reduction of methicillin-resistant *Staphylococcus aureus* infection among veterans in Atlanta. *Infect Control Hosp Epidemiol.* 2013;34(1):62–8.

95. Williams RE, Rippon JE. Bacteriophage typing of *Staphylococcus aureus*. *J Hyg (Lond).* 1952;50(3):320–53.

96. DeLeo FR, Kennedy AD, Chen L, et al. Molecular differentiation of historic phage-type 80/81 and contemporary epidemic *Staphylococcus aureus*. *Proc Natl Acad Sci U S A.* 2011;108(44):18091–6.

97. Rountree PM, Asheshov EH. Further observations on changes in the phage-typing pattern of phage type 80/81 staphylococci. *J Gen Microbiol.* 1961;26:111–22.

98. Anderson ES, Williams RE. Bacteriophage typing of enteric pathogens and staphylococci and its use in epidemiology. *J Clin Pathol.* 1956;9(2):94–127.

99. Tenover FC, Arbeit R, Archer G, et al. Comparison of traditional and molecular methods of typing isolates of *Staphylococcus aureus*. *J Clin Microbiol.* 1994;32(2):407–15.

100. McDougal LK, Steward CD, Killgore GE, Chaitram JM, McAllister SK, Tenover FC. Pulsed-field gel electrophoresis typing of oxacillin-resistant *Staphylococcus aureus* isolates from the United States: Establishing a national database. *J Clin Microbiol.* 2003;41(11):5113–20.

101. Simor AE, Ofner-Agostini M, Bryce E, McGeer A, Paton S, Mulvey MR. Laboratory characterization of methicillin-resistant *Staphylococcus aureus* in Canadian hospitals: Results of 5 years of National Surveillance, 1995–1999. *J Infect Dis.* 2002;186(5):652–60.

102. Murchan S, Kaufmann ME, Deplano A, et al. Harmonization of pulsed-field gel electrophoresis protocols for epidemiological typing of strains of methicillin-resistant *Staphylococcus aureus*: A single approach developed by consensus in 10 European laboratories and its application for tracing the spread of related strains. *J Clin Microbiol.* 2003;41(4):1574–85.

103. Naimi TS, LeDell KH, Como-Sabetti K, et al. Comparison of community- and health care-associated methicillin-resistant *Staphylococcus aureus* infection. *JAMA.* 2003;290(22):2976–84.

104. Herold BC, Immergluck LC, Maranan MC, et al. Community-acquired methicillin-resistant *Staphylococcus aureus* in children with no identified predisposing risk. *JAMA.* 1998;279(8):593–8.

105. Oliveira D, Borges A, Simões M. *Staphylococcus aureus* toxins and their molecular activity in infectious diseases. *Toxins (Basel).* 2018;10(6):252.

106. Pinchuk IV, Beswick EJ, Reyes VE. Staphylococcal enterotoxins. *Toxins (Basel).* 2010;2(8):2177–97.

107. Argudín MÁ, Mendoza MC, Rodicio MR. Food poisoning and *Staphylococcus aureus* enterotoxins. *Toxins (Basel).* 2010;2(7):1751–73.

108. Boyle-Vavra S, Daum RS. Community-acquired methicillin-resistant *Staphylococcus aureus*: The role of Panton-Valentine leukocidin. *Lab Invest.* 2007;87(1):3–9.

109. Bubeck Wardenburg J, Bae T, Otto M, Deleo FR, Schneewind O. Poring over pores: Alpha-hemolysin and Panton-Valentine leukocidin in *Staphylococcus aureus* pneumonia. *Nat Med.* 2007;13(12):1405-6.

110. Spaan AN, van Strijp JAG, Torres VJ. Leukocidins: Staphylococcal bi-component pore-forming toxins find their receptors. *Nat Rev Microbiol.* 2017;15(7):435–47.

111. Otto M. *Staphylococcus aureus* toxins. *Curr Opin Microbiol.* 2014;17:32–7.

112. David MZ, Glikman D, Crawford SE, et al. What is community-associated methicillin-resistant *Staphylococcus aureus*? *J Infect Dis.* 2008;197(9):1235–43.

113. Otter JA, French GL. The emergence of community-associated methicillin-resistant *Staphylococcus aureus* at a London teaching hospital, 2000–2006. *Clin Microbiol Infect.* 2008;14(7):670–6.

114. Seybold U, Kourbatova EV, Johnson JG, et al. Emergence of community-associated methicillin-resistant *Staphylococcus aureus* USA300 genotype as a major cause of health care-associated blood stream infections. *Clin Infect Dis.* 2006;42(5):647–56.

115. Enright MC, Day NP, Davies CE, Peacock SJ, Spratt BG. Multilocus sequence typing for characterization of methicillin-resistant and methicillin-susceptible clones of *Staphylococcus aureus*. *J Clin Microbiol.* 2000;38(3):1008–15.

116. Harmsen D, Claus H, Witte W, et al. Typing of methicillin-resistant *Staphylococcus aureus* in a university hospital setting by using novel software for *spa* repeat determination and database management. *J Clin Microbiol.* 2003;41(12):5442–8.

117. Koymans KJ, Vrieling M, Gorham RD Jr, van Strijp JAG. Staphylococcal immune evasion proteins: Structure, function, and host adaptation. *Curr Top Microbiol Immunol.* 2017;409:441–89.

118. Spaan AN, Surewaard BG, Nijland R, van Strijp JA. Neutrophils versus *Staphylococcus aureus*: A biological tug of war. *Annu Rev Microbiol.* 2013;67:629–50.

119. Otter JA, French GL. Molecular epidemiology of community-associated meticillin-resistant *Staphylococcus aureus* in Europe. *Lancet Infect Dis.* 2010;10(4):227–39.

120. Tristan A, Bes M, Meugnier H, et al. Global distribution of Panton-Valentine leukocidin—Positive methicillin-resistant *Staphylococcus aureus*, 2006. *Emerg Infect Dis.* 2007;13(4):594–600.

121. Nimmo GR. USA300 abroad: Global spread of a virulent strain of community-associated methicillin-resistant *Staphylococcus aureus*. *Clin Microbiol Infect.* 2012;18(8):725–34.

122. Glaser P, Martins-Simões P, Villain A, et al. Demography and intercontinental spread of the USA300 community-acquired methicillin-resistant *Staphylococcus aureus* lineage. *MBio.* 2016;7(1):e02183-15.

123. Toleman MS, Reuter S, Coll F, et al. Systematic surveillance detects multiple silent introductions and household transmission of methicillin-resistant *Staphylococcus aureus* USA300 in the East of England. *J Infect Dis.* 2016;214(3):447–53.

124. Von Dach E, Diene SM, Fankhauser C, Schrenzel J, Harbarth S, François P. Comparative genomics of community-associated methicillin-resistant *Staphylococcus aureus* shows the emergence of clone ST8-USA300 in Geneva, Switzerland. *J Infect Dis.* 2016;213(9):1370–9.

125. Aires-de-Sousa M, Correia B, de Lencastre H; Multilaboratory Project Collaborators. Changing patterns in frequency of recovery of five methicillin-resistant *Staphylococcus aureus* clones in Portuguese hospitals: Surveillance over a 16-year period. *J Clin Microbiol.* 2008;46(9):2912–7.

126. Brauner J, Hallin M, Deplano A, et al. Community-acquired methicillin-resistant *Staphylococcus aureus* clones circulating in Belgium from 2005 to 2009: Changing epidemiology. *Eur J Clin Microbiol Infect Dis.* 2013;32(5):613–20.

127. Ellington MJ, Hope R, Livermore DM, et al. Decline of EMRSA-16 amongst methicillin-resistant *Staphylococcus aureus* causing bacteraemias in the UK between 2001 and 2007. *J Antimicrob Chemother.* 2010;65(3):446–8.

128. Laine J, Huttunen R, Vuento R, et al. Methicillin-resistant *Staphylococcus aureus* epidemic restricted to one health district in Finland: A population-based descriptive study in Pirkanmaa, Finland, years 2001–2011. *Scand J Infect Dis.* 2013;45(1):45–53.

129. Li S, Sun S, Yang C, et al. The changing pattern of population structure of *Staphylococcus aureus* from bacteremia in China from 2013 to 2016: ST239-030-MRSA replaced by ST59-t437. *Front Microbiol.* 2018;9:332.

130. Schaumburg F, Köck R, Mellmann A, et al. Population dynamics among methicillin-resistant *Staphylococcus aureus* isolates in Germany during a 6-year period. *J Clin Microbiol.* 2012;50(10):3186–92.

131. Williamson DA, Roberts SA, Ritchie SR, Coombs GW, Fraser JD, Heffernan H. Clinical and molecular epidemiology of methicillin-resistant *Staphylococcus aureus* in New Zealand: Rapid emergence of sequence type 5 (ST5)-SCC*mec*-IV as the dominant community-associated MRSA clone. *PLoS One.* 2013;8(4):e62020.

132. Guinane CM, Ben Zakour NL, Tormo-Mas MA, et al. Evolutionary genomics of *Staphylococcus aureus* reveals insights into the origin and molecular basis of ruminant host adaptation. *Genome Biol Evol.* 2010;2:454–66.

133. García-Álvarez L, Holden MT, Lindsay H, et al. Meticillin-resistant *Staphylococcus aureus* with a novel *mecA* homologue in human and bovine populations in the UK and Denmark: A descriptive study. *Lancet Infect Dis.* 2011;11(8):595–603.

134. Angen Ø, Stegger M, Larsen J, et al. Report of *mecC*-carrying MRSA in domestic swine. *J Antimicrob Chemother.* 2017;72(1):60–3.

135. Bietrix J, Kolenda C, Sapin A, et al. Persistence and diffusion of *mecC*-positive CC130 MRSA isolates in dairy farms in Meurthe-et-Moselle County (France). *Front Microbiol.* 2019;10:47.

136. Giacinti G, Carfora V, Caprioli A, et al. Prevalence and characterization of methicillin-resistant *Staphylococcus aureus* carrying *mecA* or *mecC* and methicillin-susceptible *Staphylococcus aureus* in dairy sheep farms in central Italy. *J Dairy Sci.* 2017;100(10):7857–63.

137. Gómez P, Lozano C, González-Barrio D, Zarazaga M, Ruiz-Fons F, Torres C. High prevalence of methicillin-resistant *Staphylococcus aureus* (MRSA) carrying the *mecC* gene in a semi-extensive red deer (*Cervus elaphus hispanicus*) farm in Southern Spain. *Vet Microbiol.* 2015;177(3–4):326–31.

138. Gómez P, Lozano C, Camacho MC, et al. Detection of MRSA ST3061-t843-*mecC* and ST398-t011-*mecA* in white stork nestlings exposed to human residues. *J Antimicrob Chemother.* 2016;71(1):53–7.

139. Haenni M, Châtre P, Dupieux C, et al. *mecC*-positive MRSA in horses. *J Antimicrob Chemother.* 2015;70(12):3401–2.

140. Loncaric I, Kübber-Heiss A, Posautz A, et al. Characterization of methicillin-resistant *Staphylococcus spp.* carrying the *mecC* gene, isolated from wildlife. *J Antimicrob Chemother.* 2013;68(10):2222–5.

141. Loncaric I, Kübber-Heiss A, Posautz A, et al. *mecC*- and *mecA*-positive meticillin-resistant *Staphylococcus aureus* (MRSA) isolated from livestock sharing habitat with wildlife previously tested positive for *mecC*-positive MRSA. *Vet Dermatol.* 2014;25(2):147–8.

142. Medhus A, Slettemeås JS, Marstein L, Larssen KW, Sunde M. Methicillin-resistant *Staphylococcus aureus* with the novel *mecC* gene variant isolated from a cat suffering from chronic conjunctivitis. *J Antimicrob Chemother.* 2013;68(4):968–9.

143. Monecke S, Gavier-Widen D, Mattsson R, et al. Detection of *mecC*-positive *Staphylococcus aureus* (CC130-MRSA-XI) in diseased European hedgehogs (*Erinaceus europaeus*) in Sweden. *PLoS One.* 2013;8(6):e66166.

144. Moreno-Grúa E, Pérez-Fuentes S, Muñoz-Silvestre A, et al. Characterization of livestock-associated methicillin-resistant *Staphylococcus aureus* isolates obtained from commercial rabbitries located in the Iberian Peninsula. *Front Microbiol.* 2018;9:1812.

145. Mrochen DM, Schulz D, Fischer S, et al. Wild rodents and shrews are natural hosts of *Staphylococcus aureus. Int J Med Microbiol.* 2018;308(6):590–7.

146. Lindgren AK, Gustafsson E, Petersson AC, Melander E. Methicillin-resistant *Staphylococcus aureus* with *mecC*: A description of 45 human cases in southern Sweden. *Eur J Clin Microbiol Infect Dis.* 2016;35(6):971–5.

147. Porrero MC, Valverde A, Fernández-Llario P, et al. *Staphylococcus aureus* carrying *mecC* gene in animals and urban wastewater, Spain. *Emerg Infect Dis.* 2014;20(5):899–901.

148. Ruiz-Ripa L, Alcalá L, Simón C, et al. Diversity of Staphylococcus aureus clones in wild mammals in Aragon, Spain, with detection of MRSA ST130-*mecC* in wild rabbits. *J Appl Microbiol.* 2019;127(1):284–91.

149. Ruiz-Ripa L, Gómez P, Alonso CA, et al. Detection of MRSA of lineages CC130-*mecC* and CC398-*mecA* and *Staphylococcus delphini-lnu(A)* in magpies and cinereous vultures in Spain. *Microb Ecol.* 2019;78(2):409–15.

150. van Duijkeren E, Hengeveld PD, Albers M, et al. Prevalence of methicillin-resistant *Staphylococcus aureus* carrying *mecA* or *mecC* in dairy cattle. *Vet Microbiol.* 2014;171(3–4):364–7.

151. Worthing KA, Coombs GW, Pang S, et al. Isolation of *mecC* MRSA in Australia. *J Antimicrob Chemother.* 2016;71(8):2348–9.

152. Paterson GK, Harrison EM, Holmes MA. The emergence of *mecC* methicillin-resistant *Staphylococcus aureus. Trends Microbiol.* 2014;22(1):42–7.

153. Grundmann H, Aanensen DM, van den Wijngaard CC, Spratt BG, Harmsen D, Friedrich AW. Geographic distribution of *Staphylococcus aureus* causing invasive infections in Europe: A molecular-epidemiological analysis. *PLoS Med.* 2010;7(1):e1000215.

154. Olsen K, Sangvik M, Simonsen GS, et al. Prevalence and population structure of *Staphylococcus aureus* nasal carriage in healthcare workers in a general population. The Tromsø Staph and Skin Study. *Epidemiol Infect.* 2013;141(1):143–52.

155. Chen H, Liu Y, Jiang X, Chen M, Wang H. Rapid change of methicillin-resistant *Staphylococcus aureus* clones in a Chinese tertiary care hospital over a 15-year period. *Antimicrob Agents Chemother.* 2010;54(5):1842–7.

156. Li X, Zhou Y, Zhan X, Huang W, Wang X. Breast milk is a potential reservoir for livestock-associated *Staphylococcus aureus* and community-associated *Staphylococcus aureus* in Shanghai, China. *Front Microbiol.* 2018;8:2639.

157. Zhao C, Liu Y, Zhao M, et al. Characterization of community acquired *Staphylococcus aureus* associated with skin and soft tissue infection in Beijing: High prevalence of PVL+ ST398. *PLoS One.* 2012;7(6):e38577.

158. Uhlemann AC, Porcella SF, Trivedi S, et al. Identification of a highly transmissible animal-independent *Staphylococcus aureus* ST398 clone with distinct genomic and cell adhesion properties. *MBio.* 2012;3(2):e00027-12.

159. Uhlemann AC, McAdam PR, Sullivan SB, et al. Evolutionary dynamics of pandemic methicillin-sensitive *Staphylococcus aureus* ST398 and its international spread via routes of human migration. *MBio.* 2017;8(1):e01375-16.

160. Mediavilla JR, Chen L, Uhlemann AC, et al. Methicillin-susceptible *Staphylococcus aureus* ST398, New York and New Jersey, USA. *Emerg Infect Dis.* 2012;18(4):700–2.

161. David MZ, Siegel J, Lowy FD, et al. Asymptomatic carriage of sequence type 398, *spa* type t571 methicillin-susceptible *Staphylococcus aureus* in an urban jail: A newly emerging, transmissible pathogenic strain. *J Clin Microbiol.* 2013;51(7):2443–7.

162. Kuroda M, Ohta T, Uchiyama I, et al. Whole genome sequencing of meticillin-resistant *Staphylococcus aureus. Lancet.* 2001;357(9264):1225–40.

163. Petit RA 3rd, Read TD. *Staphylococcus aureus* viewed from the perspective of 40,000+ genomes. *PeerJ.* 2018;6:e5261.

164. Lindsay JA. *Staphylococcus aureus* genomics and the impact of horizontal gene transfer. *Int J Med Microbiol.* 2014;304(2):103–9.

165. Bartels MD, Larner-Svensson H, Meiniche H, et al. Monitoring meticillin resistant *Staphylococcus aureus* and its spread in Copenhagen, Denmark, 2013, through routine whole genome sequencing. *Euro Surveill.* 2015;20(17):21112.

166. Aanensen DM, Feil EJ, Holden MT, et al. Whole-genome sequencing for routine pathogen surveillance in public health: A population snapshot of invasive *Staphylococcus aureus* in Europe. *MBio.* 2016;7(3):e00444-16.

167. Reuter S, Török ME, Holden MT, et al. Building a genomic framework for prospective MRSA surveillance in the United Kingdom and the Republic of Ireland. *Genome Res.* 2016;26(2):263–70.

168. Toleman MS, Reuter S, Jamrozy D, et al. Prospective genomic surveillance of methicillin-resistant *Staphylococcus aureus* (MRSA) associated with bloodstream infection, England, 1 October 2012 to 30 September 2013. *Euro Surveill.* 2019;24(4):1800215.

169. Mwangi MM, Wu SW, Zhou Y, et al. Tracking the in vivo evolution of multidrug resistance in *Staphylococcus aureus* by whole-genome sequencing. *Proc Natl Acad Sci U S A.* 2007;104(22):9451–6.

170. Read TD, Petit RA 3rd, Yin Z, Montgomery T, McNulty MC, David MZ. USA300 *Staphylococcus aureus* persists on multiple body sites following an infection. *BMC Microbiol.* 2018;18(1):206.

171. Durand G, Javerliat F, Bes M, et al. Routine whole-genome sequencing for outbreak investigations of *Staphylococcus aureus* in a National Reference Center. *Front Microbiol.* 2018;9:511.

172. Holden MT, Hsu LY, Kurt K, et al. A genomic portrait of the emergence, evolution, and global spread of a methicillin-resistant *Staphylococcus aureus* pandemic. *Genome Res.* 2013;23(4):653–64.

173. Köser CU, Holden MT, Ellington MJ, et al. Rapid whole-genome sequencing for investigation of a neonatal MRSA outbreak. *N Engl J Med.* 2012;366(24):2267–75.

174. Humphreys H, Coleman DC. Contribution of whole-genome sequencing to understanding of the epidemiology and control of meticillin-resistant *Staphylococcus aureus. J Hosp Infect.* 2019;102(2):189–99.

175. Harkins CP, Pichon B, Doumith M, et al. Methicillin-resistant *Staphylococcus aureus* emerged long before the introduction of methicillin into clinical practice. *Genome Biol.* 2017;18(1):130.

176. Strauß L, Stegger M, Akpaka PE, et al. Origin, evolution, and global transmission of community-acquired *Staphylococcus aureus* ST8. *Proc Natl Acad Sci U S A.* 2017;114(49):E10596–604.

177. Challagundla L, Luo X, Tickler IA, et al. Range expansion and the origin of USA300 North American epidemic methicillin-resistant *Staphylococcus aureus. MBio.* 2018;9(1):e02016-17.

178. Alam MT, Read TD, Petit RA 3rd, et al. Transmission and microevolution of USA300 MRSA in U.S. households: Evidence from whole-genome sequencing. *MBio.* 2015;6(2):e00054.

179. Popovich KJ, Snitkin ES, Hota B, et al. Genomic and epidemiological evidence for community origins of hospital onset methicillin-resistant *Staphylococcus aureus* bloodstream infections. *J Infect Dis.* 2017;215(11):1640–7.

180. Harris SR, Cartwright EJ, Török ME, et al. Whole-genome sequencing for analysis of an outbreak of meticillin-resistant *Staphylococcus aureus*: A descriptive study. *Lancet Infect Dis.* 2013;13(2):130–6.

181. Azarian T, Maraqa NF, Cook RL, et al. Genomic epidemiology of methicillin-resistant *Staphylococcus aureus* in a neonatal intensive care unit. *PLoS One.* 2016;11(10):e0164397.

182. Suzuki Y, Kubota H, Ono HK, et al. Food poisoning outbreak in Tokyo, Japan caused by *Staphylococcus argenteus. Int J Food Microbiol.* 2017;262:31–7.

183. Thomsen IP, Kadari P, Soper NR, et al. Molecular epidemiology of invasive *Staphylococcus aureus* infections and concordance with colonization isolates. *J Pediatr.* 2019;210:173–7.

184. Geoghegan JA, Foster TJ. Cell wall-anchored surface proteins of *Staphylococcus aureus*: Many proteins, multiple functions. *Curr Top Microbiol Immunol.* 2017;409:95–120.

185. Diep BA, Gill SR, Chang RF, et al. Complete genome sequence of USA300, an epidemic clone of community-acquired meticillin-resistant *Staphylococcus aureus. Lancet.* 2006;367(9512):731–9.

186. Joshi GS, Spontak JS, Klapper DG, Richardson AR. Arginine catabolic mobile element encoded *speG* abrogates the unique hypersensitivity of *Staphylococcus aureus* to exogenous polyamines. *Mol Microbiol.* 2011;82(1):9–20.

187. Lina G, Piémont Y, Godail-Gamot F, et al. Involvement of Panton-Valentine leukocidin-producing *Staphylococcus aureus* in primary skin infections and pneumonia. *Clin Infect Dis.* 1999;29(5):1128–32.

188. Bui LM, Conlon BP, Kidd SP. Antibiotic tolerance and the alternative lifestyles of *Staphylococcus aureus. Essays Biochem.* 2017;61(1):71–9.

189. Otto M. Staphylococcal biofilms. *Microbiol Spectr.* 2018;6(4).

190. Balasubramanian D, Harper L, Shopsin B, Torres VJ. *Staphylococcus aureus* pathogenesis in diverse host environments. *Pathog Dis.* 2017;75(1):ftx005.

191. Hao H, Dai M, Wang Y, Huang L, Yuan Z. Key genetic elements and regulation systems in methicillin-resistant *Staphylococcus aureus. Future Microbiol.* 2012;7(11):1315–29.

192. Centers for Disease Control (CDC). Toxic-shock syndrome, United States, 1970–1982. *MMWR Morb Mortal Wkly Rep.* 1982;31(16):201–4.

193. Schlech WF 3rd, Shands KN, Reingold AL, et al. Risk factors for development of toxic shock syndrome. Association with a tampon brand. *JAMA.* 1982;248(7):835–9.

194. Berkley SF, Hightower AW, Broome CV, Reingold AL. The relationship of tampon characteristics to menstrual toxic shock syndrome. *JAMA.* 1987;258(7):917–20.

195. Liu C, Bayer A, Cosgrove SE, Daum RS, et al. Clinical practice guidelines by the Infectious Diseases Society of America for the treatment of methicillin-resistant *Staphylococcus aureus* infections in adults and children. *Clin Infect Dis.* 2011;52(3):e18–55.

196. Stevens DL, Bisno AL, Chambers HF, et al. Practice guidelines for the diagnosis and management of skin and soft tissue infections: 2014 update by the Infectious Diseases Society of America. *Clin Infect Dis.* 2014;59(2):e10–52.

197. Galli L, Venturini E, Bassi A, et al. Common community-acquired bacterial skin and soft-tissue infections in children: An intersociety consensus on impetigo, abscess, and cellulitis treatment. *Clin Ther.* 2019;41(3):532–51.e17.

198. Gould FK, Brindle R, Chadwick PR, et al. Guidelines (2008) for the prophylaxis and treatment of methicillin-resistant *Staphylococcus aureus* (MRSA) infections in the United Kingdom. *J Antimicrob Chemother.* 2009;63(5):849–61.

199. Bowen AC, Mahé A, Hay RJ, et al. The global epidemiology of impetigo: A systematic review of the population prevalence of impetigo and pyoderma. *PLoS One.* 2015;10(8):e0136789.

200. Daum RS, Miller LG, Immergluck L, et al. A placebo-controlled trial of antibiotics for smaller skin abscesses. *N Engl J Med.* 2017;376(26):2545–55.

201. David MZ, Daum RS. Treatment of *Staphylococcus aureus* infections. *Curr Top Microbiol Immunol.* 2017;409:325–83.

202. Cunha BA, Gran A. Successful treatment of meticillin-resistant *Staphylococcus aureus* (MRSA) aortic prosthetic valve endocarditis with prolonged high-dose daptomycin plus ceftaroline therapy. *Int J Antimicrob Agents.* 2015;46(2):225–6.

203. Bal AM, David MZ, Garau J, et al. Future trends in the treatment of methicillin-resistant *Staphylococcus aureus* (MRSA) infection: An in-depth review of newer antibiotics active against an enduring pathogen. *J Glob Antimicrob Resist.* 2017;10:295–303.

204. McDanel JS, Roghmann MC, Perencevich EN, et al. Comparative effectiveness of cefazolin versus nafcillin or oxacillin for treatment of methicillin-susceptible *Staphylococcus aureus* infections complicated by bacteremia: A nationwide cohort study. *Clin Infect Dis.* 2017; 65(1):100–6.

205. Sousa C, Botelho C, Rodrigues D, Azeredo J, Oliveira R. Infective endocarditis in intravenous drug abusers: An update. *Eur J Clin Microbiol Infect Dis.* 2012;31(11):2905–10.

206. Muhlebach MS. Methicillin-resistant *Staphylococcus aureus* in cystic fibrosis: How should it be managed? *Curr Opin Pulm Med.* 2017;23(6):544–50.

207. McNeil JC, Fritz SA. Prevention strategies for recurrent community-associated *Staphylococcus aureus* skin and soft tissue infections. *Curr Infect Dis Rep.* 2019;21(4):12.

208. Huijbers PM, Blaak H, de Jong MC, Graat EA, Vandenbroucke-Grauls CM, de Roda Husman AM. Role of the environment in the transmission of antimicrobial resistance to humans: A review. *Environ Sci Technol.* 2015;49(20):11993–2004.

209. Blythe D, Keenlyside D, Dawson SJ, Galloway A. Environmental contamination due to methicillin-resistant *Staphylococcus aureus* (MRSA). *J Hosp Infect.* 1998;38(1):67–9.

210. Colbeck JC. Environmental aspects of staphylococcal infections acquired in hospitals. I. The hospital environment—Its place in the hospital *Staphylococcus* infections problem. *Am J Public Health Nations Health.* 1960;50:468–73.

211. Dietze B, Rath A, Wendt C, Martiny H. Survival of MRSA on sterile goods packaging. *J Hosp Infect.* 2001;49(4):255–61.

212. Ndawula EM, Brown L. Mattresses as reservoirs of epidemic methicillin-resistant *Staphylococcus aureus. Lancet.* 1991;337(8739):488.

213. Neely AN, Maley MP. Survival of enterococci and staphylococci on hospital fabrics and plastic. *J Clin Microbiol.* 2000;38(2):724–6.

214. Oie S, Kamiya A. Survival of methicillin-resistant *Staphylococcus aureus* (MRSA) on naturally contaminated dry mops. *J Hosp Infect.* 1996;34(2):145–9.

215. Oie S, Hosokawa I, Kamiya A. Contamination of room door handles by methicillin-sensitive/methicillin-resistant *Staphylococcus aureus. J Hosp Infect.* 2002;51(2):140–3.

216. Stacey A, Burden P, Croton C, Jones E. Contamination of television sets by methicillin-resistant *Staphylococcus aureus* (MRSA). *J Hosp Infect.* 1998;39(3):243–4.

217. Beer D, Vandermeer B, Brosnikoff C, Shokoples S, Rennie R, Forgie S. Bacterial contamination of health care workers' pagers and the efficacy of various disinfecting agents. *Pediatr Infect Dis J.* 2006;25(11):1074–5.

218. Wilson AP, Hayman S, Folan P, et al. Computer keyboards and the spread of MRSA. *J Hosp Infect.* 2006;62(3):390–2.

219. Bures S, Fishbain JT, Uyehara CF, Parker JM, Berg BW. Computer keyboards and faucet handles as reservoirs of nosocomial pathogens in the intensive care unit. *Am J Infect Control.* 2000;28(6):465–71.

220. Cimolai N. MRSA and the environment: Implications for comprehensive control measures. *Eur J Clin Microbiol Infect Dis.* 2008;27(7):481–93.

221. Rountree PM. The effect of dessication on the viability of *Staphylococcus aureus*. *J Hyg (Lond).* 1963;61:265–72.

222. Wagenvoort JH, Sluijsmans W, Penders RJ. Better environmental survival of outbreak vs. sporadic MRSA isolates. *J Hosp Infect.* 2000;45(3):231–4.

223. Desai R, Pannaraj PS, Agopian J, Sugar CA, Liu GY, Miller LG. Survival and transmission of community-associated methicillin-resistant *Staphylococcus aureus* from fomites. *Am J Infect Control.* 2011;39(3):219–25.

224. Hardy KJ, Oppenheim BA, Gossain S, Gao F, Hawkey PM. A study of the relationship between environmental contamination with methicillin-resistant *Staphylococcus aureus* (MRSA) and patients' acquisition of MRSA. *Infect Control Hosp Epidemiol.* 2006;27(2):127–32.

225. Rutala WA, Katz EB, Sherertz RJ, Sarubbi FA Jr. Environmental study of a methicillin-resistant *Staphylococcus aureus* epidemic in a burn unit. *J Clin Microbiol.* 1983;18(3):683–8.

226. Boyce JM, Potter-Bynoe G, Chenevert C, King T. Environmental contamination due to methicillin-resistant *Staphylococcus aureus*: Possible infection control implications. *Infect Control Hosp Epidemiol.* 1997;18(9):622–7.

227. Kazakova SV, Hageman JC, Matava M, et al. A clone of methicillin-resistant *Staphylococcus aureus* among professional football players. *N Engl J Med.* 2005;352(5):468–75.

228. Weber DJ, Anderson D, Rutala WA. The role of the surface environment in healthcare-associated infections. *Curr Opin Infect Dis.* 2013;26(4):338–44.

229. Dancer SJ. Controlling hospital-acquired infection: Focus on the role of the environment and new technologies for decontamination. *Clin Microbiol Rev.* 2014;27(4):665–90.

230. Kumari DN, Haji TC, Keer V, Hawkey PM, Duncanson V, Flower E. Ventilation grilles as a potential source of methicillin-resistant *Staphylococcus aureus* causing an outbreak in an orthopaedic ward at a district general hospital. *J Hosp Infect.* 1998;39(2):127–33.

231. Layton MC, Perez M, Heald P, Patterson JE. An outbreak of mupirocin-resistant *Staphylococcus aureus* on a dermatology ward associated with an environmental reservoir. *Infect Control Hosp Epidemiol.* 1993;14(7):369–75.

232. Rampling A, Wiseman S, Davis L, et al. Evidence that hospital hygiene is important in the control of methicillin-resistant *Staphylococcus aureus*. *J Hosp Infect.* 2001;49(2):109–16.

233. Fraise AP. Susceptibility of antibiotic-resistant cocci to biocides. *J Appl Microbiol.* 2002;92 Suppl:158S–62S.

234. Han JH, Sullivan N, Leas BF, Pegues DA, Kaczmarek JL, Umscheid CA. Cleaning hospital room surfaces to prevent health care-associated infections: A technical brief. *Ann Intern Med.* 2015;163(8):598–607.

235. Weber DJ, Rutala WA, Anderson DJ, Chen LF, Sickbert-Bennett EE, Boyce JM. Effectiveness of ultraviolet devices and hydrogen peroxide systems for terminal room decontamination: Focus on clinical trials. *Am J Infect Control.* 2016;44(5 Suppl):e77–84.

236. Falagas ME, Thomaidis PC, Kotsantis IK, Sgouros K, Samonis G, Karageorgopoulos DE. Airborne hydrogen peroxide for disinfection of the hospital environment and infection control: A systematic review. *J Hosp Infect.* 2011;78(3):171–7.

237. Shiomori T, Miyamoto H, Makishima K. Significance of airborne transmission of methicillin-resistant *Staphylococcus aureus* in an otolaryngology-head and neck surgery unit. *Arch Otolaryngol Head Neck Surg.* 2001;127(6):644–8.

238. Shiomori T, Miyamoto H, Makishima K, et al. Evaluation of bedmaking-related airborne and surface methicillin-resistant *Staphylococcus aureus* contamination. *J Hosp Infect.* 2002;50(1):30–5.

239. Rosen K, Roesler U, Merle R, Friese A. Persistent and transient airborne MRSA colonization of piglets in a newly established animal model. *Front Microbiol.* 2018;9:1542.

240. Angen Ø, Feld L, Larsen J, Rostgaard K, Skov R, Madsen AM, Larsen AR. Transmission of methicillin-resistant *Staphylococcus aureus* to human volunteers visiting a swine farm. *Appl Environ Microbiol.* 2017;83(23):e01489-17.

241. Bos ME, Verstappen KM, van Cleef BA, et al. Transmission through air as a possible route of exposure for MRSA. *J Expo Sci Environ Epidemiol.* 2016;26(3):263–9.

242. Feld L, Bay H, Angen Ø, Larsen AR, Madsen AM. Survival of LA-MRSA in dust from swine farms. *Ann Work Expo Health.* 2018;62(2):147–56.

243. Ferguson DD, Smith TC, Hanson BM, Wardyn SE, Donham KJ. Detection of airborne methicillin-resistant *Staphylococcus aureus* inside and downwind of a swine building, and in animal feed: Potential occupational, animal health, and environmental implications. *J Agromedicine.* 2016;21(2):149–53.

244. Madsen AM, Kurdi I, Feld L, Tendal K. Airborne MRSA and total *Staphylococcus aureus* as associated with particles of different sizes on pig farms. *Ann Work Expo Health.* 2018;62(8):966–77.

245. Eells SJ, David MZ, Taylor A, et al. Persistent environmental contamination with USA300 methicillin-resistant *Staphylococcus aureus* and other pathogenic strain types in households with *S. aureus* skin infections. *Infect Control Hosp Epidemiol.* 2014;35(11):1373–82.

246. Knox J, Uhlemann AC, Miller M, et al. Environmental contamination as a risk factor for intra-household *Staphylococcus aureus* transmission. *PLoS One.* 2012;7(11):e49900.

247. Knox J, Sullivan SB, Urena J, et al. Association of environmental contamination in the home with the risk for recurrent community-associated, methicillin-resistant *Staphylococcus aureus* infection. *JAMA Intern Med.* 2016;176(6):807–15.

248. Huang SS, Datta R, Platt R. Risk of acquiring antibiotic-resistant bacteria from prior room occupants. *Arch Intern Med.* 2006;166(18):1945–51.

249. Humphreys H, Becker K, Dohmen PM, et al. *Staphylococcus aureus* and surgical site infections: Benefits of screening and decolonization before surgery. *J Hosp Infect.* 2016;94(3):295–304.

250. Suzuki M, Satoh N, Nakamura M, Horita S, Seki G, Moriya K. Bacteremia in hemodialysis patients. *World J Nephrol.* 2016;5(6):489–96.

251. Turner NA, Sharma-Kuinkel BK, Maskarinec SA, et al. Methicillin-resistant *Staphylococcus aureus*: An overview of basic and clinical research. *Nat Rev Microbiol.* 2019;17(4):203–18.

252. McKinnell JA, Singh RD, Miller LG, et al. The SHIELD Orange County Project-multi drug-resistant organism (MDRO) prevalence in 21 nursing homes and long term acute care facilities in southern California. *Clin Infect Dis.* 2019;69(9):1566–73.

253. Popovich KJ, Hota B, Aroutcheva A, et al. Community-associated methicillin-resistant *Staphylococcus aureus* colonization burden in HIV-infected patients. *Clin Infect Dis.* 2013;56(8):1067–74.

254. Sabbagh P, Riahi SM, Gamble HR, Rostami A. The global and regional prevalence, burden, and risk factors for methicillin-resistant *Staphylococcus aureus* colonization in HIV-infected people: A systematic review and meta-analysis. *Am J Infect Control.* 2019;47(3):323–33.

255. Shadyab AH, Crum-Cianflone NF. Methicillin-resistant *Staphylococcus aureus* (MRSA) infections among HIV-infected persons in the era of highly active antiretroviral therapy: A review of the literature. *HIV Med.* 2012;13(6):319–32.

256. Dasenbrook EC. Update on methicillin-resistant *Staphylococcus aureus* in cystic fibrosis. *Curr Opin Pulm Med.* 2011;17(6):437–41.

257. Ellis MW, Hospenthal DR, Dooley DP, Gray PJ, Murray CK. Natural history of community-acquired methicillin-resistant *Staphylococcus aureus* colonization and infection in soldiers. *Clin Infect Dis.* 2004;39(7):971–9.

258. Millar EV, Rice GK, Elassal EM, et al. Genomic characterization of USA300 methicillin-resistant *Staphylococcus aureus* (MRSA) to evaluate intraclass transmission and recurrence of skin and soft tissue infection (SSTI) among high-risk military trainees. *Clin Infect Dis.* 2017;65(3):461–8.

259. Aiello AE, Lowy FD, Wright LN, Larson EL. Meticillin-resistant *Staphylococcus aureus* among US prisoners and military personnel: Review and recommendations for future studies. *Lancet Infect Dis.* 2006; 6(6):335–41.

260. Morrison-Rodriguez SM, Pacha LA, Patrick JE, Jordan NN. Community-associated methicillin-resistant *Staphylococcus aureus* infections at an Army training installation. *Epidemiol Infect.* 2010;138(5):721–9.

261. Karanika S, Kinamon T, Grigoras C, Mylonakis E. Colonization with methicillin-resistant *Staphylococcus aureus* and risk for infection among asymptomatic athletes: A systematic review and metaanalysis. *Clin Infect Dis.* 2016;63(2):195–204.

262. Begier EM, Frenette K, Barrett NL, et al. A high-morbidity outbreak of methicillin-resistant *Staphylococcus aureus* among players on a college football team, facilitated by cosmetic body shaving and turf burns. *Clin Infect Dis*. 2004;39(10):1446–53.

263. Grosset-Janin A, Nicolas X, Saraux A. Sport and infectious risk: A systematic review of the literature over 20 years. *Med Mal Infect*. 2012;42(11):533–44.

264. Miller LG, Eells SJ, Taylor AR, et al. *Staphylococcus aureus* colonization among household contacts of patients with skin infections: Risk factors, strain discordance, and complex ecology. *Clin Infect Dis*. 2012;54(11):1523–35.

265. Knox J, Van Rijen M, Uhlemann AC, et al. Community-associated methicillin-resistant *Staphylococcus aureus* transmission in households of infected cases: A pooled analysis of primary data from three studies across international settings. *Epidemiol Infect*. 2015;143(2):354–65.

266. Davis MF, Iverson SA, Baron P, et al. Household transmission of meticillin-resistant *Staphylococcus aureus* and other staphylococci. *Lancet Infect Dis*. 2012;12(9):703–16.

267. Leibler JH, León C, Cardoso LJP, et al. Prevalence and risk factors for MRSA nasal colonization among persons experiencing homelessness in Boston, MA. *J Med Microbiol*. 2017;66(8):1183–8.

268. Ottomeyer M, Graham CD, Legg AD, et al. Prevalence of nasal colonization by methicillin-resistant *Staphylococcus aureus* in persons using a homeless shelter in Kansas City. *Front Public Health*. 2016;4:234.

269. Landers TF, Harris RE, Wittum TE, Stevenson KB. Colonization with *Staphylococcus aureus* and methicillin-resistant *S. aureus* among a sample of homeless individuals, Ohio. *Infect Control Hosp Epidemiol*. 2009;30(8):801–3.

270. Goerge T, Lorenz MB, van Alen S, Hübner NO, Becker K, Köck R. MRSA colonization and infection among persons with occupational livestock exposure in Europe: Prevalence, preventive options and evidence. *Vet Microbiol*. 2017;200:6–12.

271. Normanno G, Dambrosio A, Lorusso V, Samoilis G, Di Taranto P, Parisi A. Methicillin-resistant *Staphylococcus aureus* (MRSA) in slaughtered pigs and abattoir workers in Italy. *Food Microbiol*. 2015;51:51–6.

272. Moon DC, Tamang MD, Nam HM, et al. Identification of livestock-associated methicillin-resistant *Staphylococcus aureus* isolates in Korea and molecular comparison between isolates from animal carcasses and slaughterhouse workers. *Foodborne Pathog Dis*. 2015;12(4):327–34.

273. Gilbert MJ, Bos ME, Duim B, et al. Livestock-associated MRSA ST398 carriage in pig slaughterhouse workers related to quantitative environmental exposure. *Occup Environ Med*. 2012;69(7):472–8.

274. Van Cleef BA, Broens EM, Voss A, et al. High prevalence of nasal MRSA carriage in slaughterhouse workers in contact with live pigs in The Netherlands. *Epidemiol Infect*. 2010;138(5):756–63.

275. Wang XL, Li L, Li SM, et al. Phenotypic and molecular characteristics of *Staphylococcus aureus* and methicillin-resistant *Staphylococcus aureus* in slaughterhouse pig-related workers and control workers in Guangdong Province, China. *Epidemiol Infect*. 2017;145(9):1843–51.

276. Wulf M, van Nes A, Eikelenboom-Boskamp A, et al. Methicillin-resistant *Staphylococcus aureus* in veterinary doctors and students, the Netherlands. *Emerg Infect Dis*. 2006;12(12):1939–41.

277. Anderson ME, Lefebvre SL, Weese JS. Evaluation of prevalence and risk factors for methicillin-resistant *Staphylococcus aureus* colonization in veterinary personnel attending an international equine veterinary conference. *Vet Microbiol*. 2008;129(3–4):410–7.

278. Huber H, Giezendanner N, Stephan R, Zweifel C. Genotypes, antibiotic resistance profiles and microarray-based characterization of methicillin-resistant *Staphylococcus aureus* strains isolated from livestock and veterinarians in Switzerland. *Zoonoses Public Health*. 2011;58(5):343–9.

279. Garcia-Graells C, Antoine J, Larsen J, Catry B, Skov R, Denis O. Livestock veterinarians at high risk of acquiring methicillin-resistant *Staphylococcus aureus* ST398. *Epidemiol Infect*. 2012;140(3):383–9.

280. Cuny C, Nathaus R, Layer F, Strommenger B, Altmann D, Witte W. Nasal colonization of humans with methicillin-resistant *Staphylococcus aureus* (MRSA) CC398 with and without exposure to pigs. *PLoS One*. 2009;4(8):e6800.

281. Haysom L, Cross M, Anastasas R, Moore E, Hampton S. Prevalence and risk factors for methicillin-resistant *Staphylococcus aureus* (MRSA) infections in custodial populations: A systematic review. *J Correct Health Care*. 2018;24(2):197–213.

282. Pan ES, Diep BA, Carleton HA, et al. Increasing prevalence of methicillin-resistant *Staphylococcus aureus* infection in California jails. *Clin Infect Dis*. 2003;37(10):1384–8.

283. David MZ, Mennella C, Mansour M, Boyle-Vavra S, Daum RS. Predominance of methicillin-resistant *Staphylococcus aureus* among pathogens causing skin and soft tissue infections in a large urban jail: Risk factors and recurrence rates. *J Clin Microbiol*. 2008;46(10):3222–7.

284. Centers for Disease Control and Prevention (CDC). Methicillin-resistant *Staphylococcus aureus* skin or soft tissue infections in a state prison—Mississippi, 2000. *MMWR Morb Mortal Wkly Rep*. 2001;50(42):919–22.

285. Centers for Disease Control and Prevention (CDC). Methicillin-resistant *Staphylococcus aureus* infections in correctional facilities—Georgia, California, and Texas, 2001–2003. *MMWR Morb Mortal Wkly Rep*. 2003;52(41):992–6.

286. Mukherjee DV, Herzig CT, Jeon CY, et al. Prevalence and risk factors for *Staphylococcus aureus* colonization in individuals entering maximum-security prisons. *Epidemiol Infect*. 2014;142(3):484–93.

287. Baillargeon J, Kelley MF, Leach CT, Baillargeon G, Pollock BH. Methicillin-resistant *Staphylococcus aureus* infection in the Texas prison system. *Clin Infect Dis*. 2004;38(9):e92–5.

288. Montgomery CP, David MZ, Daum RS. Host factors that contribute to recurrent staphylococcal skin infection. *Curr Opin Infect Dis*. 2015;28(3):253–8.

289. Narla S, Silverberg JI. Association between atopic dermatitis and serious cutaneous, multiorgan and systemic infections in US adults. *Ann Allergy Asthma Immunol*. 2018;120(1):66–72.e11.

290. Geoghegan JA, Irvine AD, Foster TJ. *Staphylococcus aureus* and atopic dermatitis: A complex and evolving relationship. *Trends Microbiol*. 2018;26(6):484–97.

291. Tong SY, Varrone L, Chatfield MD, Beaman M, Giffard PM. Progressive increase in community-associated methicillin-resistant *Staphylococcus aureus* in Indigenous populations in northern Australia from 1993 to 2012. *Epidemiol Infect*. 2015;143(7):1519–23.

292. Tong SY, Bishop EJ, Lilliebridge RA, et al. Community-associated strains of methicillin-resistant *Staphylococcus aureus* and methicillin-susceptible *S. aureus* in indigenous Northern Australia: Epidemiology and outcomes. *J Infect Dis*. 2009;199(10):1461–70.

293. Stevens AM, Hennessy T, Baggett HC, Bruden D, Parks D, Klejka J. Methicillin-resistant *Staphylococcus aureus* carriage and risk factors for skin infections, Southwestern Alaska, USA. *Emerg Infect Dis*. 2010;16(5):797–803.

294. Leung NS, Padgett P, Robinson DA, Brown EL. Prevalence and behavioural risk factors of *Staphylococcus aureus* nasal colonization in community-based injection drug users. *Epidemiol Infect*. 2015;143(11):2430–9.

295. Packer S, Pichon B, Thompson S, et al. Clonal expansion of community-associated meticillin-resistant *Staphylococcus aureus* (MRSA) in people who inject drugs (PWID): Prevalence, risk factors and molecular epidemiology, Bristol, United Kingdom, 2012 to 2017. *Euro Surveill*. 2019;24(13):1800124.

296. Colombo C, Senn G, Bürgel A, Ruef C. Clearance of an epidemic clone of methicillin-resistant *Staphylococcus aureus* in a drug-use network: A follow-up study in Switzerland. *Scand J Infect Dis*. 2012;44(9):650–5.

297. Kreisel KM, Johnson JK, Stine OC, et al. Illicit drug use and risk for USA300 methicillin-resistant *Staphylococcus aureus* infections with bacteremia. *Emerg Infect Dis*. 2010;16(9):1419–27.

298. Bruzzese S, Bush K, Leal J, et al. Comparing the epidemiology of hospital-acquired methicillin-resistant *Staphylococcus aureus* clone groups in Alberta, Canada. *Epidemiol Infect*. 2016;144(10):2184–90.

299. Cosgrove SE, Sakoulas G, Perencevich EN, Schwaber MJ, Karchmer AW, Carmeli Y. Comparison of mortality associated with methicillin-resistant and methicillin-susceptible *Staphylococcus aureus* bacteremia: A meta-analysis. *Clin Infect Dis*. 2003;36(1):53–9.

300. Davis WT, Gilbert SR. Comparison of methicillin-resistant versus susceptible *Staphylococcus aureus* pediatric osteomyelitis. *J Pediatr Orthop*. 2018;38(5):e285–91.

301. Inagaki K, Lucar J, Blackshear C, Hobbs CV. Methicillin-susceptible and methicillin-resistant *Staphylococcus aureus* bacteremia—Nationwide estimates of 30-day readmission, in-hospital mortality, length of stay, and cost in the US. *Clin Infect Dis*. 2019;69(12):2112–8.

302. Jokinen E, Laine J, Huttunen R, et al. Comparison of outcome and clinical characteristics of bacteremia caused by methicillin-resistant, penicillin-resistant and penicillin-susceptible *Staphylococcus aureus* strains. *Infect Dis (Lond)*. 2017;49(7):493–500.

303. Joo EJ, Park DA, Kang CI, et al. Reevaluation of the impact of methicillin-resistance on outcomes in patients with *Staphylococcus aureus* bacteremia and endocarditis. *Korean J Intern Med*. 2019;34(6):1347–62.

304. Wang JT, Hsu LY, Lauderdale TL, Fan WC, Wang FD. Comparison of outcomes among adult patients with nosocomial bacteremia caused by methicillin-susceptible and methicillin-resistant *Staphylococcus aureus*: A retrospective cohort study. *PLoS One*. 2015;10(12):e0144710.

305. Lepelletier D, Lucet JC. Controlling meticillin-susceptible *Staphylococcus aureus*: Not simply meticillin-resistant *S. aureus* revisited. *J Hosp Infect*. 2013;84(1):13–21.

306. Kock R, Friedrich A, On Behalf of The Original Author Group C. Systematic literature analysis and review of targeted preventive measures to limit healthcare-associated infections by meticillin-resistant *Staphylococcus aureus*. *Euro Surveill*. 2014;19(37):20902.

307. Magill SS, Edwards JR, Bamberg W, et al. Multistate point-prevalence survey of health care-associated infections. *N Engl J Med*. 2014;370(13):1198–208.

308. World Health Organization. *WHO Guidelines on Hand Hygiene in Health Care: First Global Patient Safety Challenge Clean Care is Safer Care*. Geneva: World Health Organization; 2009.

309. Marimuthu K, Pittet D, Harbarth S. The effect of improved hand hygiene on nosocomial MRSA control. *Antimicrob Resist Infect Control*. 2014;3:34.

310. Harris AD, Pineles L, Belton B, et al. Universal glove and gown use and acquisition of antibiotic-resistant bacteria in the ICU: A randomized trial. *JAMA*. 2013;310(15):1571–80.

311. Kabbani D, Weir SK, Berg G, Chien GC, Strymish J, Gupta K. Cohorting based on nasal methicillin-resistant *Staphylococcus aureus* status: An opportunity to share more than a room. *Am J Infect Control*. 2013;41(5):401–4.

312. Lee AS, Huttner B, Harbarth S. Prevention and control of methicillin-resistant *Staphylococcus aureus* in acute care settings. *Infect Dis Clin North Am*. 2016;30(4):931–52.

313. Huang SS, Septimus E, Kleinman K, et al. Targeted versus universal decolonization to prevent ICU infection. *N Engl J Med*. 2013;368(24):2255–65. Erratum in: *N Engl J Med*. 2013;369(6):587. *N Engl J Med*. 2014;370(9):886.

314. Hetem DJ, Bootsma MC, Bonten MJ. Prevention of surgical site infections: Decontamination with mupirocin based on preoperative screening for *Staphylococcus aureus* carriers or universal decontamination? *Clin Infect Dis*. 2016;62(5):631–6.

315. Noone P, Shafi MS. Controlling infection in a district general hospital. *J Clin Pathol*. 1973;26(2):140–5.

316. Dancer SJ. Importance of the environment in meticillin-resistant *Staphylococcus aureus* acquisition: The case for hospital cleaning. *Lancet Infect Dis*. 2008;8(2):101–13.

317. Godbout EJ, Masroor N, Doll M, Edmond MB, Bearman G, Stevens MP. Bare below the elbows in an academic medical center. *Am J Infect Control*. 2019;47(8):1030–1.

318. Collins AM, Connaughton J, Ridgway PF. Bare below the elbows: A comparative study of a tertiary and district general hospital. *Ir Med J*. 2013;106(9):272–5.

319. Papastergiou P, Tsiouli E. Healthcare-associated transmission of Panton-Valentine leucocidin positive methicillin resistant *Staphylococcus aureus*: The value of screening asymptomatic healthcare workers. *BMC Infect Dis*. 2018;18(1):484.

320. Dulon M, Peters C, Schablon A, Nienhaus A. MRSA carriage among healthcare workers in non-outbreak settings in Europe and the United States: A systematic review. *BMC Infect Dis*. 2014;14:363.

321. Nathwani D, Varghese D, Stephens J, Ansari W, Martin S, Charbonneau C. Value of hospital antimicrobial stewardship programs [ASPs]: A systematic review. *Antimicrob Resist Infect Control*. 2019;8:35.

322. Cunha CB, Opal SM. Antibiotic stewardship: Strategies to minimize antibiotic resistance while maximizing antibiotic effectiveness. *Med Clin North Am*. 2018;102(5):831–43.

323. Sexton T, Clarke P, O'Neill E, Dillane T, Humphreys H. Environmental reservoirs of methicillin-resistant *Staphylococcus aureus* in isolation rooms: Correlation with patient isolates and implications for hospital hygiene. *J Hosp Infect*. 2006;62(2):187–94.

324. Fernando SA, Gray TJ, Gottlieb T. Healthcare-acquired infections: Prevention strategies. *Intern Med J*. 2017;47(12):1341–51.

325. Larsen J, David MZ, Vos MC, et al. Preventing the introduction of meticillin-resistant *Staphylococcus aureus* into hospitals. *J Glob Antimicrob Resist*. 2014;2(4):260–8.

326. Kinoshita T, Tokumasu H, Tanaka S, Kramer A, Kawakami K. Policy implementation for methicillin-resistant *Staphylococcus aureus* in seven European countries: A comparative analysis from 1999 to 2015. *J Mark Access Health Policy*. 2017;5(1):1351293.

327. McKinnell JA, Miller LG, Eells SJ, Cui E, Huang SS. A systematic literature review and meta-analysis of factors associated with methicillin-resistant *Staphylococcus aureus* colonization at time of hospital or intensive care unit admission. *Infect Control Hosp Epidemiol*. 2013;34(10):1077–86.

328. APIC. *Guide to the Elimination of Methicillin-resistant Staphylococcus aureus (MRSA) Transmission in Hospital Settings*. 2nd ed. Washington, DC: APIC; 2010.

329. Calfee DP, Salgado CD, Classen D, et al. Strategies to prevent transmission of methicillin-resistant *Staphylococcus aureus* in acute care hospitals. *Infect Control Hosp Epidemiol*. 2008;29 Suppl 1:S62–80.

330. Calfee DP, Salgado CD, Milstone AM, et al. Strategies to prevent methicillin-resistant *Staphylococcus aureus* transmission and infection in acute care hospitals: 2014 update. *Infect Control Hosp Epidemiol*. 2014;35 Suppl 2:S108–32.

331. Coia JE, Duckworth GJ, Edwards DI, et al. Guidelines for the control and prevention of meticillin-resistant *Staphylococcus aureus* (MRSA) in healthcare facilities. *J Hosp Infect*. 2006;63 Suppl 1:S1–44. Erratum in: *J Hosp Infect*. 2006;64(1):97–8.

332. Department of Health expert advisory committee on Antimicrobial Resistance and Healthcare Associated Infection (ARHAI): Implementation of modified admission MRSA screening guidance for NHS, 2014. https://assets.publishing.service.gov.uk/government/uploads/system/uploads/attachment_data/file/345144/Implementation_of_modified_admission_MRSA_screening_guidance_for_NHS.pdf. Accessed April 8, 2019.

333. Humphreys H, Grundmann H, Skov R, Lucet JC, Cauda R. Prevention and control of methicillin-resistant *Staphylococcus aureus*. *Clin Microbiol Infect*. 2009;15(2):120–4.

334. Weber SG, Huang SS, Oriola S, et al. Legislative mandates for use of active surveillance cultures to screen formethicillin-resistant *Staphylococcus aureus* and vancomycin-resistant enterococci: Position statement from the Joint SHEA and APIC Task Force. *Am J Infect Control*. 2007;35(2):73–85.

335. Ammerlaan HS, Kluytmans JA, Berkhout H, et al. Eradication of carriage with methicillin-resistant *Staphylococcus aureus*: Effectiveness of a national guideline. *J Antimicrob Chemother*. 2011;66(10):2409–17.

336. Weterings V, Veenemans J, van Rijen M, Kluytmans J. Prevalence of nasal carriage of methicillin-resistant *Staphylococcus aureus* in patients at hospital admission in the Netherlands, 2010–2017: An observational study. *Clin Microbiol Infect*. 2019;25(11):1428.e1–e5.

337. Lekkerkerk WSN, Haenen A, van der Sande MAB, et al. Newly identified risk factors for MRSA carriage in The Netherlands. *PLoS One*. 2017;12(11):e0188502.

338. Albrich WC, Harbarth S. Health-care workers: Source, vector, or victim of MRSA? *Lancet Infect Dis*. 2008;8(5):289–301.

339. Montoya A, Schildhouse R, Goyal A, et al. How often are health care personnel hands colonized with multidrug-resistant organisms? A systematic review and meta-analysis. *Am J Infect Control*. 2019;47(6):693–703.

340. Schubert M, Kämpf D, Jatzwauk L, et al. Prevalence and predictors of MRSA carriage among employees in a non-outbreak setting: A cross-sectional study in an acute care hospital. *J Occup Med Toxicol*. 2019;14:7.

341. Price JR, Golubchik T, Cole K, et al. Whole-genome sequencing shows that patient-to-patient transmission rarely accounts for acquisition of *Staphylococcus aureus* in an intensive care unit. *Clin Infect Dis*. 2014;58(5):609–18.

342. Jain R, Kralovic SM, Evans ME, et al. Veterans Affairs initiative to prevent methicillin-resistant *Staphylococcus aureus* infections. *N Engl J Med*. 2011;364(15):1419–30.

343. Evans ME, Kralovic SM, Simbartl LA, Jain R, Roselle GA. Eight years of decreased methicillin-resistant *Staphylococcus aureus* health care-associated infections associated with a Veterans Affairs prevention initiative. *Am J Infect Control*. 2017;45(1):13–16.

344. Gurieva T, Bootsma MC, Bonten MJ. Successful Veterans Affairs initiative to prevent methicillin-resistant *Staphylococcus aureus* infections revisited. *Clin Infect Dis*. 2012;54(11):1618–20.

345. Frost SA, Alogso MC, Metcalfe L, et al. Chlorhexidine bathing and health care-associated infections among adult intensive care patients: A systematic review and meta-analysis. *Crit Care*. 2016;20(1):379.

346. Kim HY, Lee WK, Na S, Roh YH, Shin CS, Kim J. The effects of chlorhexidine gluconate bathing on health care-associated infection in intensive care units: A meta-analysis. *J Crit Care*. 2016;32:126–37.

347. Milstone AM, Passaretti CL, Perl TM. Chlorhexidine: Expanding the armamentarium for infection control and prevention. *Clin Infect Dis*. 2008;46(2):274–81.

348. Huang SS, Singh R, McKinnell JA, et al. Decolonization to reduce postdischarge infection risk among MRSA carriers. *N Engl J Med.* 2019;380(7):638–50.

349. Muto CA, Jernigan JA, Ostrowsky BE, et al. SHEA guideline for preventing nosocomial transmission of multidrug-resistant strains of *Staphylococcus aureus* and *Enterococcus*. *Infect Control Hosp Epidemiol.* 2003;24(5):362–86.

350. López-Alcalde J, Mateos-Mazón M, Guevara M, et al. Gloves, gowns and masks for reducing the transmission of meticillin-resistant *Staphylococcus aureus* (MRSA) in the hospital setting. *Cochrane Database Syst Rev.* 2015;(7):CD007087.

351. Kullar R, Vassallo A, Turkel S, Chopra T, Kaye KS, Dhar S. Degowning the controversies of contact precautions for methicillin-resistant *Staphylococcus aureus*: A review. *Am J Infect Control.* 2016;44(1):97–103.

352. Martin EM, Russell D, Rubin Z, et al. Elimination of routine contact precautions for endemic methicillin-resistant *Staphylococcus aureus* and vancomycin-resistant *Enterococcus*: A retrospective quasi-experimental study. *Infect Control Hosp Epidemiol.* 2016;37(11):1323–30.

353. Huskins WC, Huckabee CM, O'Grady NP, et al. Intervention to reduce transmission of resistant bacteria in intensive care. *N Engl J Med.* 2011;364(15):1407–18.

354. Kalra L, Camacho F, Whitener CJ, et al. Risk of methicillin-resistant *Staphylococcus aureus* surgical site infection in patients with nasal MRSA colonization. *Am J Infect Control.* 2013;41(12):1253–7.

355. Rennert-May E, Bush K, Vickers D, Smith S. Use of a provincial surveillance system to characterize postoperative surgical site infections after primary hip and knee arthroplasty in Alberta, Canada. *Am J Infect Control.* 2016;44(11):1310–4.

356. Thakkar V, Ghobrial GM, Maulucci CM, et al. Nasal MRSA colonization: Impact on surgical site infection following spine surgery. *Clin Neurol Neurosurg.* 2014;125:94–7.

357. Mehta S, Hadley S, Hutzler L, Slover J, Phillips M, Bosco JA3rd. Impact of preoperative MRSA screening and decolonization on hospital-acquired MRSA burden. *Clin Orthop Relat Res.* 2013;471(7):2367–71. Erratum in: *Clin Orthop Relat Res.* 2013;471(6):2044.

358. Peng HM, Wang LC, Zhai JL, Weng XS, Feng B, Wang W. Effectiveness of preoperative decolonization with nasal povidone iodine in Chinese patients undergoing elective orthopedic surgery: A prospective cross-sectional study. *Braz J Med Biol Res.* 2017;51(2):e6736.

359. Rezapoor M, Nicholson T, Tabatabaee RM, Chen AF, Maltenfort MG, Parvizi J. Povidone-iodine-based solutions for decolonization of nasal *Staphylococcus aureus*: A randomized, prospective, placebo-controlled study. *J Arthroplasty.* 2017;32(9):2815–9.

360. Sadigursky D, Pires HS, Rios SAC, Rodrigues Filho FLB, Queiroz GC, Azi ML. Prophylaxis with nasal decolonization in patients submitted to total knee and hip arthroplasty: Systematic review and meta-analysis. *Rev Bras Ortop.* 2017;52(6):631–7.

361. Schweizer M, Perencevich E, McDanel J, et al. Effectiveness of a bundled intervention of decolonization and prophylaxis to decrease Gram positive surgical site infections after cardiac or orthopedic surgery: Systematic review and meta-analysis. *BMJ.* 2013;346:f2743.

362. Schweizer ML, Chiang HY, Septimus E, et al. Association of a bundled intervention with surgical site infections among patients undergoing cardiac, hip, or knee surgery. *JAMA.* 2015;313(21):2162–71.

363. Tsang STJ, McHugh MP, Guerendiain D, et al. Evaluation of *Staphylococcus aureus* eradication therapy in orthopaedic surgery. *J Med Microbiol.* 2018;67(6):893–901.

364. Saraswat MK, Magruder JT, Crawford TC, et al. Preoperative *Staphylococcus aureus* screening and targeted decolonization in cardiac surgery. *Ann Thorac Surg.* 2017;104(4):1349–56.

365. Tom TS, Kruse MW, Reichman RT. Update: Methicillin-resistant *Staphylococcus aureus* screening and decolonization in cardiac surgery. *Ann Thorac Surg.* 2009;88(2):695–702.

366. Schweizer ML, Herwaldt LA. Surgical site infections and their prevention. *Curr Opin Infect Dis.* 2012;25(4):378–84.

367. George S, Leasure AR, Horstmanshof D. Effectiveness of decolonization with chlorhexidine and mupirocin in reducing surgical site infections: A systematic review. *Dimens Crit Care Nurs.* 2016;35(4):204–22.

368. Poovelikunnel T, Gethin G, Humphreys H. Mupirocin resistance: Clinical implications and potential alternatives for the eradication of MRSA. *J Antimicrob Chemother.* 2015;70(10):2681–92.

369. Macal CM, North MJ, Collier N, et al. Modeling the transmission of community-associated methicillin-resistant *Staphylococcus aureus*: A dynamic agent-based simulation. *J Transl Med.* 2014;12:124.

370. Fritz SA, Hogan PG, Hayek G, et al. *Staphylococcus aureus* colonization in children with community-associated *Staphylococcus aureus* skin infections and their household contacts. *Arch Pediatr Adolesc Med.* 2012;166(6):551–7.

371. Cluzet VC, Gerber JS, Nachamkin I, et al. Duration of colonization and determinants of earlier clearance of colonization with methicillin-resistant *Staphylococcus aureus*. *Clin Infect Dis.* 2015;60(10):1489–96.

372. Rafee Y, Abdel-Haq N, Asmar B, et al. Increased prevalence of methicillin-resistant *Staphylococcus aureus* nasal colonization in household contacts of children with community acquired disease. *BMC Infect Dis.* 2012;12:45.

373. Miller LG, Eells SJ, David MZ, et al. *Staphylococcus aureus* skin infection recurrences among household members: An examination of host, behavioral, and pathogen-level predictors. *Clin Infect Dis.* 2015;60(5):753–63.

374. Walter J, Espelage W, Adlhoch C, et al. Persistence of nasal colonisation with methicillin resistant *Staphylococcus aureus* CC398 among participants of veterinary conferences and occurrence among their household members: A prospective cohort study, Germany 2008–2014. *Vet Microbiol.* 2017;200:13–18.

375. Bosch T, Verkade E, van Luit M, Landman F, Kluytmans J, Schouls LM. Transmission and persistence of livestock-associated methicillin-resistant *Staphylococcus aureus* among veterinarians and their household members. *Appl Environ Microbiol.* 2015;81(1):124–9.

376. Verkade E, Kluytmans-van den Bergh M, van Benthem B, et al. Transmission of methicillin-resistant *Staphylococcus aureus* CC398 from livestock veterinarians to their household members. *PLoS One.* 2014;9(7):e100823.

377. Dorado-García A, Bos ME, Graveland H, et al. Risk factors for persistence of livestock-associated MRSA and environmental exposure in veal calf farmers and their family members: An observational longitudinal study. *BMJ Open.* 2013;3(9):e003272.

378. van Cleef BA, van Benthem BH, Verkade EJ, et al. Livestock-associated MRSA in household members of pig farmers: Transmission and dynamics of carriage, a prospective cohort study. *PLoS One.* 2015;10(5):e0127190.

379. Toleman MS, Watkins ER, Williams T, et al. Investigation of a cluster of sequence type 22 methicillin-resistant *Staphylococcus aureus* transmission in a community setting. *Clin Infect Dis.* 2017;65(12):2069–77.

380. Eveillard M, Martin Y, Hidri N, Boussougant Y, Joly-Guillou ML. Carriage of methicillin-resistant *Staphylococcus aureus* among hospital employees: Prevalence, duration, and transmission to households. *Infect Control Hosp Epidemiol.* 2004;25(2):114–20.

381. Sassmannshausen R, Deurenberg RH, Köck R, et al. MRSA prevalence and associated risk factors among health-care workers in non-outbreak situations in the Dutch-German EUREGIO. *Front Microbiol.* 2016;7:1273.

382. Suffoletto BP, Cannon EH, Ilkhanipour K, Yealy DM. Prevalence of *Staphylococcus aureus* nasal colonization in emergency department personnel. *Ann Emerg Med.* 2008;52(5):529–33.

383. Bisaga A, Paquette K, Sabatini L, Lovell EO. A prevalence study of methicillin-resistant *Staphylococcus aureus* colonization in emergency department health care workers. *Ann Emerg Med.* 2008;52(5):525–8.

384. Ibarra M, Flatt T, Van Maele D, Ahmed A, Fergie J, Purcell K. Prevalence of methicillin-resistant *Staphylococcus aureus* nasal carriage in healthcare workers. *Pediatr Infect Dis J.* 2008;27(12):1109–11.

385. Elie-Turenne MC, Fernandes H, Mediavilla JR, et al. Prevalence and characteristics of *Staphylococcus aureus* colonization among healthcare professionals in an urban teaching hospital. *Infect Control Hosp Epidemiol.* 2010;31(6):574–80.

386. Schwarzkopf R, Takemoto RC, Immerman I, Slover JD, Bosco JA. Prevalence of *Staphylococcus aureus* colonization in orthopaedic surgeons and their patients: A prospective cohort controlled study. *J Bone Joint Surg Am.* 2010;92(9):1815–9.

387. Saito G, Thom J, Wei Y, et al. Methicillin-resistant *Staphylococcus aureus* colonization among health care workers in a downtown emergency department in Toronto, Ontario. *Can J Infect Dis Med Microbiol.* 2013;24(3):e57––60.

388. Huang YC, Su LH, Lin TY. Nasal carriage of methicillin-resistant *Staphylococcus aureus* among pediatricians in Taiwan. *PLoS One.* 2013;8(11):e82472.

389. Fritz SA, Camins BC, Eisenstein KA, et al. Effectiveness of measures to eradicate *Staphylococcus aureus* carriage in patients with community-associated skin and soft-tissue infections: A randomized trial. *Infect Control Hosp Epidemiol.* 2011;32(9):872–80.

390. Fritz SA, Hogan PG, Hayek G, et al. Household versus individual approaches to eradication of community-associated *Staphylococcus aureus* in children: A randomized trial. *Clin Infect Dis*. 2012;54(6):743–51.

391. Cluzet VC, Gerber JS, Metlay JP, et al. The effect of total household decolonization on clearance of colonization with methicillin-resistant *Staphylococcus aureus*. *Infect Control Hosp Epidemiol*. 2016;37(10):1226–33.

392. Talan DA, Mower WR, Krishnadasan A, et al. Trimethoprim-sulfamethoxazole versus placebo for uncomplicated skin abscess. *N Engl J Med*. 2016;374(9):823–32.

393. Williams DJ, Cooper WO, Kaltenbach LA, et al. Comparative effectiveness of antibiotic treatment strategies for pediatric skin and soft-tissue infections. *Pediatrics*. 2011;128(3):e479–87.

394. Bick JA. Infection control in jails and prisons. *Clin Infect Dis*. 2007;45(8):1047–55.

395. Carson EA. Prisoners in 2016. U.S. Department of Justice. Office of Justice Programs. Bureau of Justice Statistics. January 2018, NCJ 251149 (updated August 7, 2018). https://www.bjs.gov/content/pub/pdf/p16.pdf. Accessed April 12, 2019.

396. Zeng Z. Jail inmates in 2016. U.S. Department of Justice. Office of Justice Programs. Bureau of Justice Statistics. February 22, 2018, NCJ 251210. https://www.bjs.gov/index.cfm?ty=pbdetail&iid=6186. Accessed April 12, 2019.

397. Ma XX, Galiana A, Pedreira W, et al. Community-acquired methicillin-resistant *Staphylococcus aureus*, Uruguay. *Emerg Infect Dis*. 2005;11(6):973–6. Erratum in: *Emerg Infect Dis*. 2005;11(8):1329.

398. Greenberg G, Rosenheck R. Jail incarceration, homelessness, and mental health: A national study. *Psychiatr Serv*. 2008;59(2):170–7.

399. Binswanger IA, Stern MF, Yamashita TE, Mueller SR, Baggett TP, Blatchford PJ. Clinical risk factors for death after release from prison in Washington State: A nested case-control study. *Addiction*. 2016;111(3):499–510.

400. Farley JE, Ross T, Stamper P, Baucom S, Larson E, Carroll KC. Prevalence, risk factors, and molecular epidemiology of methicillin-resistant *Staphylococcus aureus* among newly arrested men in Baltimore, Maryland. *Am J Infect Control*. 2008;36(9):644–50.

401. Hota B, Ellenbogen C, Hayden MK, Aroutcheva A, Rice TW, Weinstein RA. Community-associated methicillin-resistant *Staphylococcus aureus* skin and soft tissue infections at a public hospital: Do public housing and incarceration amplify transmission? *Arch Intern Med*. 2007;167(10):1026–33.

402. Okano JT, Blower S. Are correctional facilities amplifying the epidemic of community-acquired methicillin-resistant *Staphylococcus aureus*? *Nat Rev Microbiol*. 2010;8(1):83.

403. Befus M, Mukherjee DV, Herzig CTA, Lowy FD, Larson E. Correspondence analysis to evaluate the transmission of *Staphylococcus aureus* strains in two New York State maximum-security prisons. *Epidemiol Infect*. 2017;145(10):2161–5.

404. David MZ, Siegel JD, Henderson J, et al. Hand and nasal carriage of discordant *Staphylococcus aureus* isolates among urban jail detainees. *J Clin Microbiol*. 2014;52(9):3422–5.

405. Lowy FD, Aiello AE, Bhat M, et al. *Staphylococcus aureus* colonization and infection in New York State prisons. *J Infect Dis*. 2007;196(6):911–8.

406. Befus M, Lowy FD, Miko BA, Mukherjee DV, Herzig CT, Larson EL. Obesity as a determinant of *Staphylococcus aureus* colonization among inmates in maximum-security prisons in New York state. *Am J Epidemiol*. 2015;182(6):494–502.

407. Baillargeon J, Black SA, Leach CT, et al. The infectious disease profile of Texas prison inmates. *Prev Med*. 2004;38(5):607–12.

408. Maree CL, Eells SJ, Tan J, et al. Risk factors for infection and colonization with community-associated methicillin-resistant *Staphylococcus aureus* in the Los Angeles County jail: A case-control study. *Clin Infect Dis*. 2010;51(11):1248–57.

409. Tanner J, Lin Y, Kornblum J, et al. Molecular characterization of methicillin-resistant *Staphylococcus aureus* clinical isolates obtained from the Rikers Island Jail System from 2009 to 2013. *J Clin Microbiol*. 2014;52(8):3091–4.

410. Elias AF, Chaussee MS, McDowell EJ, Huntington MK. Community-based intervention to manage an outbreak of MRSA skin infections in a county jail. *J Correct Health Care*. 2010;16(3):205–15.

411. Tattevin P, Diep BA, Jula M, Perdreau-Remington F. Long-term follow-up of methicillin-resistant *Staphylococcus aureus* molecular epidemiology after emergence of clone USA300 in San Francisco jail populations. *J Clin Microbiol*. 2008;46(12):4056–7.

412. Deger GE, Quick DW. The enduring menace of MRSA: Incidence, treatment, and prevention in a county jail. *J Correct Health Care*. 2009;15(3):174–8.

413. Felkner M, Andrews K, Field LH, et al. Detection of *Staphylococcus aureus* including MRSA on environmental surfaces in a jail setting. *J Correct Health Care*. 2009;15(4):310–7.

414. Miko BA, Herzig CT, Mukherjee DV, et al. Is environmental contamination associated with *Staphylococcus aureus* clinical infection in maximum security prisons? *Infect Control Hosp Epidemiol*. 2013;34(5):540–2.

415. Federal Bureau of Prisons. Management of methicillin-resistant *Staphylococcus aureus* (MRSA) infections, April 2012. Clinical Practice Guidelines, 2012. https://www.bop.gov/resources/pdfs/mrsa.pdf. Accessed April 12, 2019.

416. David MZ, Siegel JD, Henderson J, et al. A randomized, controlled trial of chlorhexidine-soaked cloths to reduce methicillin-resistant and methicillin-susceptible *Staphylococcus aureus* carriage prevalence in an urban jail. *Infect Control Hosp Epidemiol*. 2014;35(12):1466–73.

417. Mullen LA, O'Keefe C. Management of skin and soft tissue infections in a county correctional center: A quality improvement project. *J Correct Health Care*. 2015;21(4):355–64.

418. Wootton SH, Arnold K, Hill HA, et al. Intervention to reduce the incidence of methicillin-resistant *Staphylococcus aureus* skin infections in a correctional facility in Georgia. *Infect Control Hosp Epidemiol*. 2004;25(5):402–7.

419. Davies HD, Jackson MA, Rice SG; Committee on Infectious Diseases; Council on sports medicine and fitness. Infectious diseases associated with organized sports and outbreak control. *Pediatrics*. 2017;140(4):e20172477.

420. Harris MD. Infectious disease in athletes. *Curr Sports Med Rep*. 2011;10(2):84–9.

421. Ashack KA, Burton KA, Johnson TR, Currie DW, Comstock RD, Dellavalle RP. Skin infections among US high school athletes: A national survey. *J Am Acad Dermatol*. 2016;74(4):679–84.e1.

422. Barr B, Felkner M, Diamond PM. High school athletic departments as sentinel surveillance sites for community-associated methicillin-resistant staphylococcal infections. *Tex Med*. 2006;102(4):56–61.

423. Buss BF, Mueller SW, Theis M, Keyser A, Safranek TJ. Population-based estimates of methicillin-resistant *Staphylococcus areus* [sic] (MRSA) infections among high school athletes—Nebraska, 2006–2008. *J Sch Nurs*. 2009;25(4):282–91.

424. Buss BF, Connolly S. Surveillance of physician-diagnosed skin and soft tissue infections consistent with methicillin-resistant *Staphylococcus aureus* (MRSA) among Nebraska high school athletes, 2008–2012. *J Sch Nurs*. 2014;30(1):42–8.

425. Braun T, Kahanov L. Community-associated methicillin-resistant *Staphylococcus aureus* infection rates and management among student-athletes. *Med Sci Sports Exerc*. 2018;50(9):1802–9.

426. Centers for Disease Control and Prevention (CDC). Methicillin-resistant *Staphylococcus aureus* infections among competitive sports participants—Colorado, Indiana, Pennsylvania, and Los Angeles County, 2000–2003. *MMWR Morb Mortal Wkly Rep*. 2003;52(33):793–5.

427. Pedersen M, Doyle MR, Beste A, Diekema DJ, Zimmerman MB, Herwaldt LA. Survey of high school athletic programs in Iowa regarding infections and infection prevention policies and practices. *Iowa Orthop J*. 2013;33:107–13.

428. Rihn JA, Posfay-Barbe K, Harner CD, et al. Community-acquired methicillin-resistant *Staphylococcus aureus* outbreak in a local high school football team unsuccessful interventions. *Pediatr Infect Dis J*. 2005;24(9):841–3.

429. Williams C, Wells J, Klein R, Sylvester T, Sunenshine R; Centers for Disease Control and Prevention (CDC). Notes from the field: Outbreak of skin lesions among high school wrestlers—Arizona, 2014. *MMWR Morb Mortal Wkly Rep*. 2015;64(20):559–60.

430. Archibald LK, Shapiro J, Pass A, Rand K, Southwick F. Methicillin-resistant *Staphylococcus aureus* infection in a college football team: Risk factors outside the locker room and playing field. *Infect Control Hosp Epidemiol*. 2008;29(5):450–3.

431. Herzog MM, Fraser MA, Register-Mihalik JK, Kerr ZY. Epidemiology of skin infections in men's wrestling: Analysis of 2009–2010 through 2013–2014 National Collegiate Athletic Association surveillance data. *J Athl Train*. 2017;52(5):457–63.

432. Romano R, Lu D, Holtom P. Outbreak of community-acquired methicillin-resistant *Staphylococcus aureus* skin infections among a collegiate football team. *J Athl Train*. 2006;41(2):141–5.

433. Sanders JC. Reducing MRSA infections in college student athletes: Implementation of a prevention program. *J Community Health Nurs*. 2009;26(4):161–72.

434. Sutton SS, Stacy JJ, Mensch J, Torres-McGehee T, Bennett CL. Tackling community-acquired methicillin-resistant *Staphylococcus aureus* in collegiate football players following implementation of an anti-MRSA programme. *Br J Sports Med.* 2014;48(4):284–5.

435. Huijsdens XW, van Lier AM, van Kregten E, et al. Methicillin-resistant *Staphylococcus aureus* in Dutch soccer team. *Emerg Infect Dis.* 2006;12(10):1584–6.

436. Garza D, Sungar G, Johnston T, Rolston B, Ferguson JD, Matheson GO. Ineffectiveness of surveillance to control community-acquired methicillin-resistant *Staphylococcus aureus* in a professional football team. *Clin J Sport Med.* 2009;19(6):498–501.

437. Stacey AR, Endersby KE, Chan PC, Marples RR. An outbreak of methicillin resistant *Staphylococcus aureus* infection in a rugby football team. *Br J Sports Med.* 1998;32(2):153–4.

438. Pulido Pérez A, Baniandrés Rodríguez O, Ceballos Rodríguez MC, Mendoza Cembranos MD, Campos Domínguez M, Suárez Fernández R. Skin infections caused by community-acquired methicillin-resistant *Staphylococcus aureus*: Clinical and microbiological characteristics of 11 cases. *Actas Dermosifiliogr.* 2014;105(2):150–8.

439. Couvé-Deacon E, Tristan A, Pestourie N, et al. Outbreak of Panton-Valentine leukocidin associated methicillin-susceptible *Staphylococcus aureus* infection in a rugby team, France, 2010–2011. *Emerg Infect Dis.* 2016;22(1):96–9.

440. Fontanilla JM, Kirkland KB, Talbot EA, et al. Outbreak of skin infections in college football team members due to an unusual strain of community-acquired methicillin-susceptible *Staphylococcus aureus. J Clin Microbiol.* 2010;48(2):609–11.

441. Creech CB, Saye E, McKenna BD, et al. One-year surveillance of methicillin-resistant *Staphylococcus aureus* nasal colonization and skin and soft tissue infections in collegiate athletes. *Arch Pediatr Adolesc Med.* 2010;164(7):615–20.

442. Rackham DM, Ray SM, Franks AS, Bielak KM, Pinn TM. Community-associated methicillin-resistant *Staphylococcus aureus* nasal carriage in a college student athlete population. *Clin J Sport Med.* 2010;20(3):185–8.

443. Lear A, McCord G, Peiffer J, Watkins RR, Parikh A, Warrington S. Incidence of *Staphylococcus aureus* nasal colonization and soft tissue infection among high school football players. *J Am Board Fam Med.* 2011;24(4):429–35.

444. Jiménez-Truque N, Saye EJ, Soper N, et al. Association between contact sports and colonization with *Staphylococcus aureus* in a prospective cohort of collegiate athletes. *Sports Med.* 2017;47(5):1011–9.

445. Champion AE, Goodwin TA, Brolinson PG, Werre SR, Prater MR, Inzana TJ. Prevalence and characterization of methicillin-resistant *Staphylococcus aureus* isolates from healthy university student athletes. *Ann Clin Microbiol Antimicrob.* 2014;13:33.

446. Wang HK, Huang CY, Chen CJ, Huang YC. Nasal *Staphylococcus aureus* and methicillin-resistant *Staphylococcus aureus* carriage among college student athletes in northern Taiwan. *J Microbiol Immunol Infect.* 2017;50(4):537–40.

447. Couvé-Deacon E, Postil D, Barraud O, et al. *Staphylococcus aureus* carriage in French athletes at risk of CA-MRSA infection: A prospective, cross-sectional study. *Sports Med Open.* 2017;3(1):28.

448. Kahanov L, Kim YK, Eberman L, Dannelly K, Kaur H, Ramalinga A. *Staphylococcus aureus* and community-associated methicillin-resistant *Staphylococcus aureus* (CA-MRSA) in and around therapeutic whirlpools in college athletic training rooms. *J Athl Train.* 2015;50(4):432–7.

449. Montgomery K, Ryan TJ, Krause A, Starkey C. Assessment of athletic health care facility surfaces for MRSA in the secondary school setting. *J Environ Health.* 2010;72(6):8--11.

450. Oller AR, Province L, Curless B. *Staphylococcus aureus* recovery from environmental and human locations in 2 collegiate athletic teams. *J Athl Train.* 2010;45(3):222–9.

451. Stanforth B, Krause A, Starkey C, Ryan TJ. Prevalence of community-associated methicillin-resistant *Staphylococcus aureus* in high school wrestling environments. *J Environ Health.* 2010;72(6):12–6.

452. The National Collegiate Athletic Association. *2014–15 NCAA Sport Medicine Handbook.* 25th ed. Indianapolis, IN: The National Collegiate Athletic Association; 2014, pp. 65–71. http://www.ncaa.org/sport-science-institute/2014-15-ncaa-sports-medicine-handbook. Accessed April 16, 2019.

453. National Federation of State High School Associations (NFHS), Sports Medicine Advisory Committee (SMAC). Sports-Related Skin Infections, revised April 2018. https://www.nfhs.org/media/1014740/sports_related_skin_infections_position_statement_and_guidelines_-final-april-2018.pdf. Accessed April 16, 2019.

454. Zinder SM, Basler RS, Foley J, Scarlata C, Vasily DB. National Athletic Trainers' Association position statement: Skin diseases. *J Athl Train.* 2010;45(4):411–28.

455. Likness LP. Common dermatologic infections in athletes and return-to-play guidelines. *J Am Osteopath Assoc.* 2011;111(6):373–9.

456. Centers for Disease Control and Prevention (CDC). MRSA, For Coaches and Athletic Directors, page last reviewed January 25, 2019. https://www.cdc.gov/mrsa/community/team-hc-providers/index.html. Accessed April 16, 2019.

457. Anderson BJ. Effectiveness of body wipes as an adjunct to reducing skin infections in high school wrestlers. *Clin J Sport Med.* 2012;22(5):424–9.

458. Grigg C, Palms D, Stone ND, et al. Burden of invasive methicillin-resistant *Staphylococcus aureus* infections in nursing home residents. *J Am Geriatr Soc.* 2018;66(8):1581–6.

459. Bradley SF, Terpenning MS, Ramsey MA, et al. Methicillin-resistant *Staphylococcus aureus*: Colonization and infection in a long-term care facility. *Ann Intern Med.* 1991;115(6):417–22.

460. Mody L, Kauffman CA, Donabedian S, Zervos M, Bradley SF. Epidemiology of *Staphylococcus aureus* colonization in nursing home residents. *Clin Infect Dis.* 2008;46(9):1368–73.

461. Murphy CR, Quan V, Kim D, et al. Nursing home characteristics associated with methicillin-resistant *Staphylococcus aureus* (MRSA) burden and transmission. *BMC Infect Dis.* 2012;12:269.

462. Hudson LO, Reynolds C, Spratt BG, et al. Diversity of methicillin-resistant *Staphylococcus aureus* strains isolated from residents of 26 nursing homes in Orange County, California. *J Clin Microbiol.* 2013; 51(11):3788–95.

463. Shurland SM, Stine OC, Venezia RA, et al. USA300 methicillin-resistant *S. aureus* (USA300 MRSA) colonization and the risk of MRSA infection in residents of extended-care facilities. *Epidemiol Infect.* 2012;140(3):390–9.

464. Shurland SM, Stine OC, Venezia RA, et al. Prolonged colonization with the methicillin-resistant *Staphylococcus aureus* strain USA300 among residents of extended care facilities. *Infect Control Hosp Epidemiol.* 2010;31(8):838–41.

465. Garazi M, Edwards B, Caccavale D, Auerbach C, Wolf-Klein G. Nursing homes as reservoirs of MRSA: Myth or reality? *J Am Med Dir Assoc.* 2009;10(6):414–8.

466. Evans ME, Kralovic SM, Simbartl LA, et al. Nationwide reduction of health care-associated methicillin-resistant *Staphylococcus aureus* infections in Veterans Affairs long-term care facilities. *Am J Infect Control.* 2014;42(1):60–2.

467. Suetens C, Niclaes L, Jans B, et al. Determinants of methicillin-resistant *Staphylococcus aureus* carriage in nursing homes. *Age Ageing.* 2007;36(3):327–30.

468. Latour K, Huang TD, Jans B, et al. Prevalence of multidrug-resistant organisms in nursing homes in Belgium in 2015. *PLoS One.* 2019;14(3):e0214327.

469. Nillius D, von Müller L, Wagenpfeil S, Klein R, Herrmann M. Methicillin-resistant *Staphylococcus aureus* in Saarland, Germany: The Long-Term Care Facility Study. *PLoS One.* 2016;11(4):e0153030.

470. Barr B, Wilcox MH, Brady A, Parnell P, Darby B, Tompkins D. Prevalence of methicillin-resistant *Staphylococcus aureus* colonization among older residents of care homes in the United Kingdom. *Infect Control Hosp Epidemiol.* 2007;28(7):853–9.

471. Horner C, Parnell P, Hall D, Kearns A, Heritage J, Wilcox M. Meticillin-resistant *Staphylococcus aureus* in elderly residents of care homes: Colonization rates and molecular epidemiology. *J Hosp Infect.* 2013;83(3):212–8.

472. Hoogendoorn M, Smalbrugge M, Stobberingh EE, van Rossum SV, Vlaminckx BJ, Thijsen SF. Prevalence of antibiotic resistance of the commensal flora in Dutch nursing homes. *J Am Med Dir Assoc.* 2013;14(5):336–9.

473. Verkade E, Bosch T, Hendriks Y, Kluytmans J. Outbreak of methicillin-resistant *Staphylococcus aureus* ST398 in a Dutch nursing home. *Infect Control Hosp Epidemiol.* 2012;33(6):624–6.

474. Zhang J, Gu FF, Zhao SY, et al. Prevalence and molecular epidemiology of *Staphylococcus aureus* among residents of seven nursing homes in Shanghai. *PLoS One.* 2015;10(9):e0137593.

475. Gu FF, Zhang J, Zhao SY, et al. Risk factors for methicillin-resistant *Staphylococcus aureus* carriage among residents in 7 nursing homes in Shanghai, China. *Am J Infect Control.* 2016;44(7):805–8.

476. Chuang VW, Tsang IH, Keung JP, et al. Infection control intervention on meticillin resistant *Staphylococcus aureus* transmission in residential care homes for the elderly. *J Infect Prev.* 2015;16(2):58–66.

477. Bellini C, Petignat C, Masserey E, et al. Universal screening and decolonization for control of MRSA in nursing homes: A cluster randomized controlled study. *Infect Control Hosp Epidemiol.* 2015;36(4):401–8.

478. Baldwin NS, Gilpin DF, Tunney MM, et al. Cluster randomised controlled trial of an infection control education and training intervention programme focusing on meticillin-resistant *Staphylococcus aureus* in nursing homes for older people. *J Hosp Infect.* 2010;76(1):36–41.

479. Mody L, Krein SL, Saint S, et al. A targeted infection prevention intervention in nursing home residents with indwelling devices: A randomized clinical trial. JAMA Intern Med. 2015;175(5):714–23. Erratum in: *JAMA Intern Med.* 2015;175(7):1247.

480. Schora DM, Boehm S, Das S, et al. Impact of Detection, Education, Research and Decolonization without Isolation in Long-term care (DERAIL) on methicillin-resistant *Staphylococcus aureus* colonization and transmission at 3 long-term care facilities. *Am J Infect Control.* 2014;42(10 Suppl):S269–73.

481. Grøntvedt CA, Elstrøm P, Stegger M, et al. Methicillin-resistant *Staphylococcus aureus* CC398 in humans and pigs in Norway: A "One Health" perspective on introduction and transmission. *Clin Infect Dis.* 2016;63(11):1431–8.

482. Lammie SL, Hughes JM. Antimicrobial resistance, food safety, and One Health: The need for convergence. *Annu Rev Food Sci Technol.* 2016;7:287–312.

483. Petersson-Wolfe CS, Leslie KE, Swartz TH. An update on the effect of clinical mastitis on the welfare of dairy cows and potential therapies. *Vet Clin North Am Food Anim Pract.* 2018;34(3):525–35.

484. Ruegg PL. A 100-year review: Mastitis detection, management, and prevention. *J Dairy Sci.* 2017;100(12):10381–97.

485. Foster AP. Staphylococcal skin disease in livestock. *Vet Dermatol.* 2012;23(4):342–51, e63.

486. Woolhouse M, Ward M, van Bunnik B, Farrar J. Antimicrobial resistance in humans, livestock and the wider environment. *Philos Trans R Soc Lond B Biol Sci.* 2015;370(1670):20140083.

487. Dweba CC, Zishiri OT, El Zowalaty ME. Methicillin-resistant *Staphylococcus aureus*: Livestock-associated, antimicrobial, and heavy metal resistance. *Infect Drug Resist.* 2018;11:2497–509.

488. van Alen S, Kaspar U, Idelevich EA, Köck R, Becker K. Increase of zinc resistance in German human derived livestock-associated MRSA between 2000 and 2014. *Vet Microbiol.* 2018;214:7–12.

489. Alban L, Ellis-Iversen J, Andreasen M, Dahl J, Sönksen UW. Assessment of the risk to public health due to use of antimicrobials in pigs—An example of pleuromutilins in Denmark. *Front Vet Sci.* 2017;4:74.

490. Martin MJ, Thottathil SE, Newman TB. Antibiotics overuse in animal agriculture: A call to action for health care providers. *Am J Public Health.* 2015;105(12):2409–10.

491. Devriese LA, Hommez J. Epidemiology of methicillin-resistant *Staphylococcus aureus* in dairy herds. *Res Vet Sci.* 1975;19(1):23–7.

492. Cuny C, Wieler LH, Witte W. Livestock-associated MRSA: The impact on humans. *Antibiotics (Basel).* 2015;4(4):521–43.

493. Huijsdens XW, van Dijke BJ, Spalburg E, et al. Community-acquired MRSA and pig-farming. *Ann Clin Microbiol Antimicrob.* 2006;5:26.

494. Smith TC, Male MJ, Harper AL, et al. Methicillin-resistant *Staphylococcus aureus* (MRSA) strain ST398 is present in midwestern U.S. swine and swine workers. *PLoS One.* 2009;4(1):e4258.

495. Dressler AE, Scheibel RP, Wardyn S, et al. Prevalence, antibiotic resistance and molecular characterisation of *Staphylococcus aureus* in pigs at agricultural fairs in the USA. *Vet Rec.* 2012;170(19):495.

496. Moon DC, Jeong SK, Hyun BH, Lim SK. Prevalence and characteristics of methicillin-resistant *Staphylococcus aureus* isolates in pigs and pig farmers in Korea. *Foodborne Pathog Dis.* 2019;16(4):256–61.

497. Parisi A, Caruso M, Normanno G, et al. MRSA in swine, farmers and abattoir workers in Southern Italy. *Food Microbiol.* 2019;82:287–93.

498. European Food Safety Authority. Analysis of the baseline survey on the prevalence of methicillin-resistant *Staphylococcus aureus* (MRSA) in holdings with breeding pigs, in the EU, 2008, Part A: MRSA prevalence estimates; on request from the European Commission. *EFSA J.* 2009;7(11):1376.

499. Conceição T, de Lencastre H, Aires-de-Sousa M. Frequent isolation of methicillin resistant *Staphylococcus aureus* (MRSA) ST398 among healthy pigs in Portugal. *PLoS One.* 2017;12(4):e0175340.

500. Lassok B, Tenhagen BA. From pig to pork: Methicillin-resistant *Staphylococcus aureus* in the pork production chain. *J Food Prot.* 2013;76(6):1095–108.

501. Elstrøm P, Grøntvedt CA, Gabrielsen C, et al. Livestock-associated MRSA CC1 in Norway; introduction to pig farms, zoonotic transmission, and eradication. *Front Microbiol.* 2019;10:139.

502. Unnerstad HE, Wahlström H, Molander B, Bengtsson B. Methicillin-resistant *Staphylococcus aureus* not detected in Swedish nucleus and multiplying pig herds. *Infect Ecol Epidemiol.* 2017;7(1):1313068.

503. Abdelbary MM, Wittenberg A, Cuny C, et al. Phylogenetic analysis of *Staphylococcus aureus* CC398 reveals a sub-lineage epidemiologically associated with infections in horses. *PLoS One.* 2014;9(2):e88083.

504. Fessler AT, Olde Riekerink RG, Rothkamp A, et al. Characterization of methicillin-resistant *Staphylococcus aureus* CC398 obtained from humans and animals on dairy farms. *Vet Microbiol.* 2012;160(1–2):77–84.

505. Nemeghaire S, Argudín MA, Haesebrouck F, Butaye P. Epidemiology and molecular characterization of methicillin-resistant *Staphylococcus aureus* nasal carriage isolates from bovines. *BMC Vet Res.* 2014;10:153.

506. Spohr M, Rau J, Friedrich A, et al. Methicillin-resistant *Staphylococcus aureus* (MRSA) in three dairy herds in southwest Germany. *Zoonoses Public Health.* 2011;58(4):252–61.

507. Tavakol M, Riekerink RG, Sampimon OC, van Wamel WJ, van Belkum A, Lam TJ. Bovine-associated MRSA ST398 in the Netherlands. *Acta Vet Scand.* 2012;54:28.

508. Mulders MN, Haenen AP, Geenen PL, et al. Prevalence of livestock-associated MRSA in broiler flocks and riskfactors for slaughterhouse personnel in The Netherlands. *Epidemiol Infect.* 2010;138(5):743–55.

509. Nemati M, Hermans K, Lipinska U, et al. Antimicrobial resistance of old and recent *Staphylococcus aureus* isolates from poultry: First detection of livestock-associated methicillin-resistant strain ST398. *Antimicrob Agents Chemother.* 2008;52(10):3817–9.

510. Nemeghaire S, Roelandt S, Argudín MA, Haesebrouck F, Butaye P. Characterization of methicillin-resistant *Staphylococcus aureus* from healthy carrier chickens. *Avian Pathol.* 2013;42(4):342–6.

511. Persoons D, Van Hoorebeke S, Hermans K, et al. Methicillin-resistant *Staphylococcus aureus* in poultry. *Emerg Infect Dis.* 2009;15(3):452–3.

512. Richter A, Sting R, Popp C, et al. Prevalence of types of methicillin-resistant *Staphylococcus aureus* in turkey flocks and personnel attending the animals. *Epidemiol Infect.* 2012;140(12):2223–32.

513. Wendlandt S, Kadlec K, Feßler AT, et al. Resistance phenotypes and genotypes of methicillin-resistant *Staphylococcus aureus* isolates from broiler chickens at slaughter and abattoir workers. *J Antimicrob Chemother.* 2013;68(11):2458–63.

514. Loncaric I, Brunthaler R, Spergser J. Suspected goat-to-human transmission of methicillin-resistant *Staphylococcus aureus* sequence type 398. *J Clin Microbiol.* 2013;51(5):1625–6.

515. Agnoletti F, Mazzolini E, Bacchin C, et al. First reporting of methicillin-resistant *Staphylococcus aureus* (MRSA) ST398 in an industrial rabbit holding and in farm-related people. *Vet Microbiol.* 2014;170(1–2):172–7.

516. Parisi A, Caruso M, Normanno G, et al. High occcurrence of methicillin-resistant *Staphylococcus aureus* in horses at slaughterhouses compared with those for recreational activities: A professional and food safety concern? *Foodborne Pathog Dis.* 2017;14(12):735–41.

517. Walther B, Klein KS, Barton AK, et al. Equine methicillin-resistant sequence type 398 *Staphylococcus aureus* (MRSA) harbor mobile genetic elements promoting host adaptation. *Front Microbiol.* 2018;9:2516.

518. van Duijkeren E, Moleman M, Sloet van Oldruitenborgh-Oosterbaan MM, et al. Methicillin-resistant *Staphylococcus aureus* in horses and horse personnel: An investigation of several outbreaks. *Vet Microbiol.* 2010;141(1–2):96–102.

519. Moodley A, Espinosa-Gongora C, Nielsen SS, McCarthy AJ, Lindsay JA, Guardabassi L. Comparative host specificity of human- and pig-associated *Staphylococcus aureus* clonal lineages. *PLoS One.* 2012;7(11):e49344.

520. Price LB, Stegger M, Hasman H, et al. *Staphylococcus aureus* CC398: Host adaptation and emergence of methicillin resistance in livestock. *MBio.* 2012;3(1):e00305-11.

521. Ward MJ, Gibbons CL, McAdam PR, et al. Time-scaled evolutionary analysis of the transmission and antibiotic resistance dynamics of *Staphylococcus aureus* clonal complex 398. *Appl Environ Microbiol.* 2014;80(23):7275–82.

522. van Rijen MM, Bosch T, Verkade EJ, Schouls L, Kluytmans JA; CAM Study Group. Livestock-associated MRSA carriage in patients without direct contact with livestock. *PLoS One.* 2014;9(6):e100294.

523. Bosch T, van Luit M, Pluister GN, et al. Changing characteristics of livestock-associated meticillin-resistant *Staphylococcus aureus* isolated from humans—Emergence of a subclade transmitted without livestock exposure, the Netherlands, 2003 to 2014. *Euro Surveill.* 2016;21(21).

524. Kinross P, Petersen A, Skov R, et al. Livestock-associated meticillin-resistant *Staphylococcus aureus* (MRSA) among human MRSA isolates, European Union/European Economic Area countries, 2013. *Euro Surveill.* 2017;22(44):16-00696.

525. Larsen J, Petersen A, Larsen AR, et al. Emergence of livestock-associated methicillin-resistant *Staphylococcus aureus* bloodstream infections in Denmark. *Clin Infect Dis.* 2017;65(7):1072–6.

526. Nielsen RT, Kemp M, Holm A, et al. Fatal septicemia linked to transmission of MRSA clonal complex 398 in hospital and nursing home, Denmark. *Emerg Infect Dis.* 2016;22(5):900–2.

527. Valentin-Domelier AS, Girard M, Bertrand X, et al. Methicillin-susceptible ST398 *Staphylococcus aureus* responsible for bloodstream infections: An emerging human-adapted subclone? *PLoS One.* 2011;6(12):e28369.

528. van Cleef BA, Monnet DL, Voss A, et al. Livestock-associated methicillin-resistant *Staphylococcus aureus* in humans, Europe. *Emerg Infect Dis.* 2011;17(3):502–5.

529. Wulf MW, Markestein A, van der Linden FT, Voss A, Klaassen C, Verduin CM. First outbreak of methicillin-resistant *Staphylococcus aureus* ST398 in a Dutch hospital, June 2007. *Euro Surveill.* 2008;13(9).

530. van Alen S, Ballhausen B, Peters G, et al. In the centre of an epidemic: Fifteen years of LA-MRSA CC398 at the University Hospital Münster. *Vet Microbiol.* 2017;200:19–24.

531. Coombs GW, Pang S, Daley DA, Lee YT, Abraham S, Leroi M. Severe disease caused by community-associated MRSA ST398 type V, Australia, 2017. *Emerg Infect Dis.* 2019;25(1):190–2.

532. DANMAP. DANMAP 2017—Use of antimicrobial agents and occurrence of antimicrobial resistance in bacteria from food animals, food and humans in Denmark. https://www.danmap.org/-/media/arkiv/projekt-sites/danmap/danmap-reports/danmap-2017/danmap2017.pdf?la=en. Accessed April 7, 2019.

533. Sharma M, Nunez-Garcia J, Kearns AM, et al. Livestock-associated methicillin resistant *Staphylococcus aureus* (LA-MRSA) clonal complex (CC) 398 isolated from UK animals belong to European lineages. *Front Microbiol.* 2016;7:1741.

534. Golding GR, Bryden L, Levett PN, et al. Whole-genome sequence of livestock-associated ST398 methicillin-resistant *Staphylococcus aureus* isolated from humans in Canada. *J Bacteriol.* 2012;194(23):6627–8.

535. Sun L, Chen Y, Wang D, et al. Surgical site infections caused by highly virulent methicillin-resistant *Staphylococcus aureus* sequence type 398, China. *Emerg Infect Dis.* 2019;25(1):157–60.

536. Dahms C, Hübner NO, Cuny C, Kramer A. Occurrence of methicillin-resistant *Staphylococcus aureus* in farm workers and the livestock environment in Mecklenburg-Western Pomerania, Germany. *Acta Vet Scand.* 2014;56:53.

537. Hatcher SM, Rhodes SM, Stewart JR, et al. The prevalence of antibiotic-resistant *Staphylococcus aureus* nasal carriage among industrial hog operation workers, community residents, and children living in their households: North Carolina, USA. *Environ Health Perspect.* 2017;125(4):560–9.

538. Khanna T, Friendship R, Dewey C, Weese JS. Methicillin resistant *Staphylococcus aureus* colonization in pigs and pig farmers. *Vet Microbiol.* 2008;128(3–4):298–303.

539. Locatelli C, Cremonesi P, Caprioli A, et al. Occurrence of methicillin-resistant *Staphylococcus aureus* in dairy cattle herds, related swine farms, and humans in contact with herds. *J Dairy Sci.* 2017;100(1):608–19.

540. Mascaro V, Leonetti M, Nobile CGA, et al. Prevalence of livestock-associated methicillin-resistant *Staphylococcus aureus* (LA-MRSA) among farm and slaughterhouse workers in Italy. *J Occup Environ Med.* 2018;60(8):e416–25.

541. Reynaga E, Navarro M, Vilamala A, et al. Prevalence of colonization by methicillin-resistant *Staphylococcus aureus* ST398 in pigs and pig farm workers in an area of Catalonia, Spain. *BMC Infect Dis.* 2016; 16(1):716.

542. Sahibzada S, Abraham S, Coombs GW, et al. Transmission of highly virulent community-associated MRSA ST93 and livestock-associated MRSA ST398 between humans and pigs in Australia. *Sci Rep.* 2017;7(1):5273.

543. Smith TC, Gebreyes WA, Abley MJ, et al. Methicillin-resistant *Staphylococcus aureus* in pigs and farm workers on conventional and antibiotic-free swine farms in the USA. *PLoS One.* 2013;8(5):e63704.

544. You Y, Song L, Nonyane BAS, Price LB, Silbergeld EK. Genomic differences between nasal *Staphylococcus aureus* from hog slaughterhouse workers and their communities. *PLoS One.* 2018;13(3):e0193820.

545. Cui S, Li J, Hu C, et al. Isolation and characterization of methicillin-resistant *Staphylococcus aureus* from swine and workers in China. *J Antimicrob Chemother.* 2009;64(4):680–3.

546. Fang HW, Chiang PH, Huang YC. Livestock-associated methicillin-resistant *Staphylococcus aureus* ST9 in pigs and related personnel in Taiwan. *PLoS One.* 2014;9(2):e88826.

547. Ye X, Liu W, Fan Y, et al. Frequency-risk and duration-risk relations between occupational livestock contact and methicillin-resistant *Staphylococcus aureus* carriage among workers in Guangdong, China. *Am J Infect Control.* 2015;43(7):676–81.

548. Zhou W, Li X, Osmundson T, Shi L, Ren J, Yan H. WGS analysis of ST9-MRSA-XII isolates from live pigs in China provides insights into transmission among porcine, human and bovine hosts. *J Antimicrob Chemother.* 2018;73(10):2652–61.

549. van Duijkeren E, Ten Horn L, Wagenaar JA, et al. Suspected horse-to-human transmission of MRSA ST398. *Emerg Infect Dis.* 2011;17(6):1137–9.

550. Graveland H, Wagenaar JA, Heesterbeek H, Mevius D, van Duijkeren E, Heederik D. Methicillin resistant *Staphylococcus aureus* ST398 in veal calf farming: Human MRSA carriage related with animal antimicrobial usage and farm hygiene. *PLoS One.* 2010;5(6):e10990.

551. Nadimpalli M, Rinsky JL, Wing S, et al. Persistence of livestock-associated antibiotic-resistant *Staphylococcus aureus* among industrial hog operation workers in North Carolina over 14 days. *Occup Environ Med.* 2015;72(2):90–9.

552. Rinsky JL, Nadimpalli M, Wing S, et al. Livestock-associated methicillin and multidrug resistant *Staphylococcus aureus* is present among industrial, not antibiotic-free livestock operation workers in North Carolina. *PLoS One.* 2013;8(7):e67641.

553. Food and Drug Administration. Center for Veterinary Medicine. New Animal Drugs and New Animal Drug Combination Products Administered in or on Medicated Feed or Drinking Water of FoodProducing Animals: Recommendations for Drug Sponsors for Voluntarily Aligning Product Use Conditions with GFI #209. FDA, Rockville, MD, December 2013. https://www.fda.gov/media/83488/download. Accessed May 7, 2019.

554. Messenger AM, Barnes AN, Gray GC. Reverse zoonotic disease transmission (zooanthroponosis): A systematic review of seldom-documented human biological threats to animals. *PLoS One.* 2014;9(2):e89055.

555. Unnerstad HE, Mieziewska K, Börjesson S, et al. Suspected transmission and subsequent spread of MRSA from farmer to dairy cows. *Vet Microbiol.* 2018;225:114–9.

556. Morgan M. Methicillin-resistant *Staphylococcus aureus* and animals: Zoonosis or humanosis? *J Antimicrob Chemother.* 2008;62(6):1181–7.

557. Sieber RN, Skov RL, Nielsen J, et al. Drivers and dynamics of methicillin-resistant livestock-associated *Staphylococcus aureus* CC398 in pigs and humans in Denmark. *MBio.* 2018;9(6):e02142-18.

558. van Duijkeren E, Ikawaty R, Broekhuizen-Stins MJ, et al. Transmission of methicillin-resistant *Staphylococcus aureus* strains between different kinds of pig farms. *Vet Microbiol.* 2008;126(4):383–9.

559. Schulz J, Boklund A, Toft N, Halasa T. Drivers for livestock-associated methicillin-resistant *Staphylococcus aureus* spread among Danish pig herds—A simulation study. *Sci Rep.* 2018;8(1):16962.

560. Hanselman BA, Kruth SA, Rousseau J, et al. Methicillin-resistant *Staphylococcus aureus* colonization in veterinary personnel. *Emerg Infect Dis.* 2006;12(12):1933–8.

561. Wulf MW, Sørum M, van Nes A, et al. Prevalence of methicillin-resistant *Staphylococcus aureus* among veterinarians: An international study. *Clin Microbiol Infect.* 2008;14(1):29–34.

562. Pletinckx LJ, Verhegghe M, Crombé F, et al. Evidence of possible methicillin-resistant *Staphylococcus aureus* ST398 spread between pigs and other animals and people residing on the same farm. *Prev Vet Med.* 2013;109(3–4):293–303.

563. Rothenburger JL, Rousseau JD, Weese JS, Jardine CM. Livestock-associated methicillin-resistant *Staphylococcus aureus* and *Clostridium difficile* in wild Norway rats (*Rattus norvegicus*) from Ontario swine farms. *Can J Vet Res.* 2018;82(1):66–9.

564. van de Giessen AW, van Santen-Verheuvel MG, Hengeveld PD, Bosch T, Broens EM, Reusken CB. Occurrence of methicillin-resistant *Staphylococcus aureus* in rats living on pig farms. *Prev Vet Med.* 2009;91 (2–4):270–3.

565. Rothenburger JL, Himsworth CG, Nemeth NM, Pearl DL, Jardine CM. Environmental factors associated with the carriage of bacterial pathogens in Norway rats. *Ecohealth.* 2018;15(1):82–95.

566. de Neeling AJ, van den Broek MJ, Spalburg EC, et al. High prevalence of methicillin resistant *Staphylococcus aureus* in pigs. *Vet Microbiol.* 2007;122(3–4):366–72.

567. Beneke B, Klees S, Stührenberg B, Fetsch A, Kraushaar B, Tenhagen BA. Prevalence of methicillin-resistant *Staphylococcus aureus* in a fresh meat pork production chain. *J Food Prot.* 2011;74(1):126–9.

568. Li J, Jiang N, Ke Y, et al. Characterization of pig-associated methicillin-resistant *Staphylococcus aureus*. *Vet Microbiol*. 2017;201:183–7.
569. Sun C, Chen B, Hulth A, et al. Genomic analysis of *Staphylococcus aureus* along a pork production chain and in the community, Shandong Province, China. *Int J Antimicrob Agents*. 2019;54(1):8–15.
570. Narvaez-Bravo C, Toufeer M, Weese SJ, et al. Prevalence of methicillin-resistant *Staphylococcus aureus* in Canadian commercial pork processing plants. *J Appl Microbiol*. 2016;120(3):770–80.
571. Molla B, Byrne M, Abley M, et al. Epidemiology and genotypic characteristics of methicillin-resistant *Staphylococcus aureus* strains of porcine origin. *J Clin Microbiol*. 2012;50(11):3687–93.
572. Yan X, Yu X, Tao X, et al. *Staphylococcus aureus* ST398 from slaughter pigs in northeast China. *Int J Med Microbiol*. 2014;304(3–4):379–83.
573. Ivbule M, Miklaševičs E, Čupāne L, Bērziņa L, Bālinš A, Valdovska A. Presence of methicillin-resistant *Staphylococcus aureus* in slaughterhouse environment, pigs, carcasses, and workers. *J Vet Res*. 2017;61(3):267–77.
574. Leibler JH, Jordan JA, Brownstein K, Lander L, Price LB, Perry MJ. *Staphylococcus aureus* nasal carriage among beefpacking workers in a Midwestern United States slaughterhouse. *PLoS One*. 2016;11(2):e0148789.
575. Wulf MW, Verduin CM, van Nes A, Huijsdens X, Voss A. Infection and colonization with methicillin resistant *Staphylococcus aureus* ST398 versus other MRSA in an area with a high density of pig farms. *Eur J Clin Microbiol Infect Dis*. 2012;31(1):61–5.
576. Carrel M, Schweizer ML, Sarrazin MV, Smith TC, Perencevich EN. Residential proximity to large numbers of swine in feeding operations is associated with increased risk of methicillin-resistant *Staphylococcus aureus* colonization at time of hospital admission in rural Iowa veterans. *Infect Control Hosp Epidemiol*. 2014;35(2):190–3.
577. Casey JA, Curriero FC, Cosgrove SE, Nachman KE, Schwartz BS. High-density livestock operations, crop field application of manure, and risk of community-associated methicillin-resistant *Staphylococcus aureus* infection in Pennsylvania. *JAMA Intern Med*. 2013;173(21):1980–90.
578. Anker JCH, Koch A, Ethelberg S, Mølbak K, Larsen J, Jepsen MR. Distance to pig farms as risk factor for community-onset livestock-associated MRSA CC398 infection in persons without known contact to pig farms-A nationwide study. *Zoonoses Public Health*. 2018;65(3):352–60.
579. Bi Z, Sun C, Börjesson S, et al. Identical genotypes of community-associated MRSA (ST59) and livestock-associated MRSA (ST9) in humans and pigs in rural China. *Zoonoses Public Health*. 2018;65(3):367–71.
580. Angen Ø, Skade L, Urth TR, Andersson M, Bækbo P, Larsen AR. Controlling transmission of MRSA to humans during short-term visits to swine farms using dust masks. *Front Microbiol*. 2019;9:3361.
581. Nadimpalli ML, Stewart JR, Pierce E, et al. Face mask use and persistence of livestock-associated *Staphylococcus aureus* nasal carriage among industrial hog operation workers and household contacts, USA. *Environ Health Perspect*. 2018;126(12):127005.
582. van Cleef BA, van Benthem BH, Verkade EJ, et al. Dynamics of methicillin-resistant *Staphylococcus aureus* and methicillin-susceptible *Staphylococcus aureus* carriage in pig farmers: A prospective cohort study. *Clin Microbiol Infect*. 2014;20(10):O764–71.
583. Schulz J, Boklund A, Toft N, Halasa T. Effects of control measures on the spread of LA-MRSA among Danish pig herds between 2006 and 2015—A simulation study. *Sci Rep*. 2019;9(1):691.
584. Catry B, Van Duijkeren E, Pomba MC, et al. Reflection paper on MRSA in food-producing and companion animals: Epidemiology and control options for human and animal health. *Epidemiol Infect*. 2010;138(5):626–44.
585. Porrero MC, Mentaberre G, Sánchez S, et al. Methicillin resistant *Staphylococcus aureus* (MRSA) carriage in different free-living wild animal species in Spain. *Vet J*. 2013;198(1):127–30.
586. Bengtsson B, Persson L, Ekström K, Unnerstad HE, Uhlhorn H, Börjesson S. High occurrence of *mecC*-MRSA in wild hedgehogs (*Erinaceus europaeus*) in Sweden. *Vet Microbiol*. 2017;207:103–7.
587. Loncaric I, Stalder GL, Mehinagic K, et al. Comparison of ESBL—And AmpC producing Enterobacteriaceae and methicillin-resistant *Staphylococcus aureus* (MRSA) isolated from migratory and resident population of rooks (*Corvus frugilegus*) in Austria. *PLoS One*. 2013;8(12):e84048.
588. Robb A, Pennycott T, Duncan G, Foster G. *Staphylococcus aureus* carrying divergent *mecA* homologue (*mecA* LGA251) isolated from a free-ranging wild bird. *Vet Microbiol*. 2013;162(1):300–1.
589. Monecke S, Gavier-Widén D, Hotzel H, et al. Diversity of *Staphylococcus aureus* isolates in European wildlife. *PLoS One*. 2016;11(12):e0168433.
590. Luzzago C, Locatelli C, Franco A, et al. Clonal diversity, virulence-associated genes and antimicrobial resistance profile of *Staphylococcus aureus* isolates from nasal cavities and soft tissue infections in wild ruminants in Italian Alps. *Vet Microbiol*. 2014;170(1–2):157–61.
591. Fravel V, Van Bonn W, Rios C, Gulland F. Meticillin-resistant *Staphylococcus aureus* in a arbor seal (*Phoca vitulina*). *Vet Rec*. 2011;169(6):155.
592. Himsworth CG, Miller RR, Montoya V, et al. Carriage of methicillin-resistant *Staphylococcus aureus* by wild urban Norway rats (*Rattus norvegicus*). *PLoS One*. 2014;9(2):e87983.
593. Jamrozy DM, Fielder MD, Butaye P, Coldham NG. Comparative genotypic and phenotypic haracterization of methicillin-resistant *Staphylococcus aureus* ST398 isolated from animals and humans. *PloS One*. 2012;7(7):e40458.
594. Lee MJ, Byers KA, Donovan CM, et al. Methicillin-resistant *Staphylococcus aureus* in urban Norway rat (*Rattus norvegicus*) populations: Epidemiology and the impacts of kill-trapping. *Zoonoses Public Health*. 2019;66(3):343–8.
595. Bortolami A, Verin R, Chantrey J, et al. Characterization of livestock-associated methicillin-resistant *Staphylococcus aureus* CC398 and *mecC*-positive CC130 from zoo animals in the United Kingdom. *Microb Drug Resist*. 2017;23(7):908–14.
596. Centers for Disease Control and Prevention (CDC). Methicillin-resistant *Staphylococcus aureus* skin infections from an elephant calf—San Diego, California, 2008. *MMWR Morb Mortal Wkly Rep*. 2009;58(8):194–8.
597. Espinosa-Gongora C, Harrison EM, Moodley A, Guardabassi L, Holmes MA. MRSA carrying *mecC* in captive mara. *J Antimicrob Chemother*. 2015;70(6):1622–4.
598. American Veterinary Medical Association. U.S. Pet Ownership & Demographics Sourcebook. Schaumburg, Illinois, AVMA, 2012.
599. Leonard FC, Markey BK. Meticillin-resistant *Staphylococcus aureus* in animals: A review. *Vet J*. 2008;175(1):27–36.
600. Petinaki E, Spiliopoulou I. Methicillin-resistant *Staphylococcus aureus* colonization and infection risks from companion animals: Current perspectives. *Vet Med (Auckl)*. 2015;6:373–82.
601. Loncaric I, Tichy A, Handler S, et al. Prevalence of methicillin-resistant *Staphylococcus sp*. (MRS) in different companion animals and determination of risk factors for colonization with MRS. *Antibiotics (Basel)*. 2019;8(2):36.
602. Pires Dos Santos T, Damborg P, Moodley A, Guardabassi L. Systematic review on global epidemiology of methicillin-resistant *Staphylococcus pseudintermedius*: Inference of population structure from multilocus sequence typing data. *Front Microbiol*. 2016;7:1599.
603. Moyaert H, de Jong A, Simjee S, et al. Survey of antimicrobial susceptibility of bacterial pathogens isolated from dogs and cats with respiratory tract infections in Europe: ComPath results. *J Appl Microbiol*. 2019;127(1):29–46.
604. Allen JL, Abraham LA, Thompson K, Browning GF. Methicillin-resistant *Staphylococcus aureus*: An issue for veterinary hospitals. *Aust Vet J*. 2013;91(6):215–9.
605. Faires MC, Gard S, Aucoin D, Weese JS. Inducible clindamycin-resistance in methicillin-resistant *Staphylococcus aureus* and methicillin-resistant *Staphylococcus pseudintermedius* isolates from dogs and cats. *Vet Microbiol*. 2009;139(3–4):419–20.
606. Grinberg A, Kingsbury DD, Gibson IR, Kirby BM, Mack HJ, Morrison D. Clinically overt infections with methicillin-resistant *Staphylococcus aureus* in animals in New Zealand: A pilot study. *N Z Vet J*. 2008;56(5):237–42.
607. Haenni M, Saras E, Châtre P, et al. A USA300 variant and other human-related methicillin-resistant *Staphylococcus aureus* strains infecting cats and dogs in France. *J Antimicrob Chemother*. 2012;67(2):326–9.
608. Moodley A, Stegger M, Bagcigil AF, et al. *spa* typing of methicillin-resistant *Staphylococcus aureus* isolated from domestic animals and veterinary staff in the UK and Ireland. *J Antimicrob Chemother*. 2006;58(6):1118–23.
609. Abbott Y, Leonard FC, Markey BK. Detection of three distinct genetic lineages in methicillin-resistant *Staphylococcus aureus* (MRSA) isolates from animals and veterinary personnel. *Epidemiol Infect*. 2010;138(5):764–71.
610. Floras A, Lawn K, Slavic D, Golding GR, Mulvey MR, Weese JS. Sequence type 398 meticillin-resistant *Staphylococcus aureus* infection and colonisation in dogs. *Vet Rec*. 2010;166(26):826–7.
611. Ishihara K, Saito M, Shimokubo N, Muramatsu Y, Maetani S, Tamura Y. Methicillin-resistant *Staphylococcus aureus* carriage among veterinary staff and dogs in private veterinary clinics in Hokkaido, Japan. *Microbiol Immunol*. 2014;58(3):149–54.
612. Hoet AE, van Balen J, Nava-Hoet RC, et al. Epidemiological profiling of methicillin-resistant *Staphylococcus aureus*-positive dogs arriving at a veterinary teaching hospital. *Vector Borne Zoonotic Dis*. 2013;13(6):385–93.

613. Kwon NH, Park KT, Jung WK, et al. Characteristics of methicillin resistant *Staphylococcus aureus* isolated from chicken meat and hospitalized dogs in Korea and their epidemiological relatedness. *Vet Microbiol.* 2006;117(2–4):304–12.

614. Paterson GK, Harrison EM, Murray GG, et al. Capturing the cloud of diversity reveals complexity and heterogeneity of MRSA carriage, infection and transmission. *Nat Commun.* 2015;6:6560.

615. van Balen J, Kelley C, Nava-Hoet RC, et al. Presence, distribution, and molecular epidemiology of methicillin-resistant *Staphylococcus aureus* in a small animal teaching hospital: A year-long active surveillance targeting dogs and their environment. *Vector Borne Zoonotic Dis.* 2013;13(5):299–311.

616. Vanderhaeghen W, Van de Velde E, Crombé F, et al. Screening for methicillin-resistant staphylococci in dogs admitted to a veterinary teaching hospital. *Res Vet Sci.* 2012;93(1):133–6.

617. Weese JS, Faires M, Rousseau J, Bersenas AM, Mathews KA. Cluster of methicillin-resistant *Staphylococcus aureus* colonization in a small animal intensive care unit. *J Am Vet Med Assoc.* 2007;231(9):1361–4.

618. Vincze S, Stamm I, Kopp PA, et al. Alarming proportions of methicillin-resistant *Staphylococcus aureus* (MRSA) in wound samples from companion animals, Germany 2010–2012. *PLoS One.* 2014;9(1):e85656.

619. Vincze S, Brandenburg AG, Espelage W, et al. Risk factors for MRSA infection in companion animals: Results from a case-control study within Germany. *Int J Med Microbiol.* 2014;304(7):787–93.

620. Coelho C, Torres C, Radhouani H, et al. Molecular detection and characterization of methicillin-resistant *Staphylococcus aureus* (MRSA) isolates from dogs in Portugal. *Microb Drug Resist.* 2011;17(2):333–7.

621. Davis JA, Jackson CR, Fedorka-Cray PJ, et al. Carriage of methicillin-resistant staphylococci by healthy companion animals in the US. *Lett Appl Microbiol.* 2014;59(1):1–8.

622. Hanselman BA, Kruth S, Weese JS. Methicillin-resistant staphylococcal colonization in dogs entering a veterinary teaching hospital. *Vet Microbiol.* 2008;126(1–3):277–81.

623. Wedley AL, Dawson S, Maddox TW, et al. Carriage of *Staphylococcus* species in the veterinary visiting dog population in mainland UK: Molecular characterisation of resistance and virulence. *Vet Microbiol.* 2014;170(1–2):81–8.

624. Hamilton E, Kruger JM, Schall W, Beal M, Manning SD, Kaneene JB. Acquisition and persistence of antimicrobial-resistant bacteria isolated from dogs and cats admitted to a veterinary teaching hospital. *J Am Vet Med Assoc.* 2013;243(7):990–1000.

625. Grönlund Andersson U, Wallensten A, Hæggman S, et al. Outbreaks of methicillin-resistant *Staphylococcus aureus* among staff and dogs in Swedish small animal hospitals. *Scand J Infect Dis.* 2014;46(4):310–4.

626. Leonard FC, Abbott Y, Rossney A, Quinn PJ, O'Mahony R, Markey BK. Methicillin-resistant *Staphylococcus aureus* isolated from a veterinary surgeon and five dogs in one practice. *Vet Rec.* 2006;158(5):155–9.

627. Walther B, Wieler LH, Friedrich AW, Kohn B, Brunnberg L, Lübke-Becker A. *Staphylococcus aureus* and MRSA colonization rates among personnel and dogs in a small animal hospital: Association with nosocomial infections. *Berl Munch Tierarztl Wochenschr.* 2009;122(5–6):178–85.

628. Baptiste KE, Williams K, Willams NJ, et al. Methicillin-resistant staphylococci in companion animals. *Emerg Infect Dis.* 2005;11(12):1942–4.

629. Enoch DA, Karas JA, Slater JD, Emery MM, Kearns AM, Farrington M. MRSA carriage in a pet therapy dog. *J Hosp Infect.* 2005;60(2):186–8.

630. Harrison EM, Weinert LA, Holden MT, et al. A shared population of epidemic methicillin-resistant *Staphylococcus aureus* 15 circulates in humans and companion animals. *MBio.* 2014;5(3):e00985-13.

631. Lin Y, Barker E, Kislow J, et al. Evidence of multiple virulence subtypes in nosocomial and community-associated MRSA genotypes in companion animals from the upper midwestern and northeastern United States. *Clin Med Res.* 2011;9(1):7–16.

632. Malik S, Coombs GW, O'Brien FG, Peng H, Barton MD. Molecular typing of methicillin-resistant staphylococci isolated from cats and dogs. *J Antimicrob Chemother.* 2006;58(2):428–31.

633. Strommenger B, Kehrenberg C, Kettlitz C, et al. Molecular characterization of methicillin-resistant *Staphylococcus aureus* strains from pet animals and their relationship to human isolates. *J Antimicrob Chemother.* 2006;57(3):461–5.

634. Walther B, Wieler LH, Friedrich AW, et al. Methicillin-resistant *Staphylococcus aureus* (MRSA) isolated from small and exotic animals at a university hospital during routine microbiological examinations. *Vet Microbiol.* 2008;127(1–2):171–8.

635. Wan MT, Fu SY, Lo YP, Huang TM, Cheng MM, Chou CC. Heterogeneity and phylogenetic relationships of community-associated methicillin-sensitive/resistant *Staphylococcus aureus* isolates in healthy dogs, cats and their owners. *J Appl Microbiol.* 2012;112(1):205–13.

636. Quitoco IM, Ramundo MS, Silva-Carvalho MC, et al. First report in South America of companion animal colonization by the USA1100 clone of community-acquired ethicillin-resistant *Staphylococcus aureus* (ST30) and by the European clone of methicillin-resistant *Staphylococcus pseudintermedius* (ST71). *BMC Res Notes.* 2013;6:336.

637. Zhang W, Hao Z, Wang Y, et al. Molecular characterization of methicillin-resistant *Staphylococcus aureus* strains from pet animals and veterinary staff in China. *Vet J.* 2011;190(2):e125-9.

638. Weiss S, Kadlec K, Fessler AT, Schwarz S. Identification and characterization of methicillin-resistant *Staphylococcus aureus, Staphylococcus epidermidis, Staphylococcus haemolyticus* and *Staphylococcus pettenkoferi* from a small animal clinic. *Vet Microbiol.* 2013;167 (3–4):680–5.

639. Witte W, Strommenger B, Stanek C, Cuny C. Methicillin-resistant *Staphylococcus aureus* ST398 in humans and animals, Central Europe. *Emerg Infect Dis.* 2007;13(2):255–8.

640. Bender JB, Waters KC, Nerby J, Olsen KE, Jawahir S. Methicillin-resistant *Staphylococcus aureus* (MRSA) isolated from pets living in households with MRSA-infected children. *Clin Infect Dis.* 2012;54(3):449–50.

641. Faires MC, Tater KC, Weese JS. An investigation of methicillin-resistant *Staphylococcus aureus* colonization in people and pets in the same household with an infected person or infected pet. *J Am Vet Med Assoc.* 2009;235(5):540–3.

642. Ferreira JP, Anderson KL, Correa MT, et al. Transmission of MRSA between companion animals and infected human patients presenting to outpatient medical care facilities. *PLoS One.* 2011;6(11):e26978.

643. Nienhoff U, Kadlec K, Chaberny IF, et al. Transmission of methicillin-resistant *Staphylococcus aureus* strains between humans and dogs: Two case reports. *J Antimicrob Chemother.* 2009;64(3):660–2.

644. Rutland BE, Weese JS, Bolin C, Au J, Malani AN. Human-to-dog transmission of methicillin-resistant *Staphylococcus aureus. Emerg Infect Dis.* 2009;15(8):1328–30.

645. Sing A, Tuschak C, Hörmansdorfer S. Methicillin-resistant *Staphylococcus aureus* in a family and its pet cat. *N Engl J Med.* 2008;358(11):1200–1.

646. Vitale CB, Gross TL, Weese JS. Methicillin-resistant *Staphylococcus aureus* in cat and owner. *Emerg Infect Dis.* 2006;12(12):1998–2000.

647. Weese JS, Dick H, Willey BM, et al. Suspected transmission of methicillin-resistant *Staphylococcus aureus* between domestic pets and humans in veterinary clinics and in the household. *Vet Microbiol.* 2006;115(1–3): 148–55.

648. Coughlan K, Olsen KE, Boxrud D, Bender JB. Methicillin-resistant *Staphylococcus aureus* in resident animals of a long-term care facility. *Zoonoses Public Health.* 2010;57(3):220–6.

649. Paterson GK, Larsen AR, Robb A, et al. The newly described *mecA* homologue, mecALGA251, is present in methicillin-resistant *Staphylococcus aureus* isolates from a diverse range of host species. *J Antimicrob Chemother.* 2012;67(12):2809–13.

650. Walther B, Wieler LH, Vincze S, et al. MRSA variant in companion animals. *Emerg Infect Dis.* 2012;18(12):2017–20.

651. Sasaki T, Tsubakishita S, Tanaka Y, et al. Population genetic structures of *Staphylococcus aureus* isolates from cats and dogs in Japan. *J Clin Microbiol.* 2012;50(6):2152–5.

652. Axon JE, Carrick JB, Barton MD, et al. Methicillin-resistant *Staphylococcus aureus* in a population of horses in Australia. *Aust Vet J.* 2011;89(6):221–5.

653. Bergström K, Aspan A, Landén A, Johnston C, Grönlund-Andersson U. The first nosocomial outbreak of methicillin-resistant *Staphylococcus aureus* in horses in Sweden. *Acta Vet Scand.* 2012;54:11.

654. Cuny C, Strommenger B, Witte W, Stanek C. Clusters of infections in horses with MRSA ST1, ST254, and ST398 in a veterinary hospital. *Microb Drug Resist.* 2008;14(4):307–10.

655. Gómez-Sanz E, Simón C, Ortega C, et al. First detection of methicillin-resistant *Staphylococcus aureus* ST398 and *Staphylococcus pseudintermedius* ST68 from hospitalized equines in Spain. *Zoonoses Public Health.* 2014;61(3):192–201.

656. Haenni M, Targant H, Forest K, et al. Retrospective study of necropsy-associated coagulase-positive staphylococci in horses. *J Vet Diagn Invest.* 2010;22(6):953–6.

657. Karkaba A, Benschop J, Hill KE, Grinberg A. Characterisation of methicillin-resistant *Staphylococcus aureus* clinical isolates from animals in New Zealand, 2012–2013, and subclinical colonisation in dogs and cats in Auckland. *N Z Vet J.* 2017;65(2):78–83.

658. Kuroda T, Kinoshita Y, Niwa H, et al. Meticillin-resistant *Staphylococcus aureus* colonisation and infection in thoroughbred racehorses and veterinarians in Japan. *Vet Rec.* 2016;178(19):473.

659. Panchaud Y, Gerber V, Rossano A, Perreten V. Bacterial infections in horses: A retrospective study at the University Equine Clinic of Bern. *Schweiz Arch Tierheilkd.* 2010;152(4):176–82.

660. Van den Eede A, Martens A, Lipinska U, et al. High occurrence of methicillin-resistant *Staphylococcus aureus* ST398 in equine nasal samples. *Vet Microbiol.* 2009;133(1–2):138–44.

661. Van den Eede A, Martens A, Feryn I, et al. Low MRSA prevalence in horses at farm level. *BMC Vet Res.* 2012;8:213.

662. Weese JS, Archambault M, Willey BM, et al. Methicillin-resistant *Staphylococcus aureus* in horses and horse personnel, 2000–2002. *Emerg Infect Dis.* 2005;11(3):430–5.

663. Loncaric I, Künzel F, Licka T, Simhofer H, Spergser J, Rosengarten R. Identification and characterization of methicillin-resistant *Staphylococcus aureus* (MRSA) from Austrian companion animals and horses. *Vet Microbiol.* 2014;168(2–4):381–7.

664. Kuroda T, Kinoshita Y, Niwa H, et al. Methicillin-resistant *Staphylococcus aureus* ulcerative keratitis in a thoroughbred racehorse. *J Equine Sci.* 2015;26(3):95–8.

665. Peterson AE, Davis MF, Awantang G, Limbago B, Fosheim GE, Silbergeld EK. Correlation between animal nasal carriage and environmental methicillin-resistant *Staphylococcus aureus* isolates at U.S. horse and cattle farms. *Vet Microbiol.* 2012;160(3–4):539–43.

666. Scallan E, Hoekstra RM, Angulo FJ, et al. Foodborne illness acquired in the United States—Major pathogens. *Emerg Infect Dis.* 2011;17(1):7–15.

667. Kadariya J, Smith TC, Thapaliya D. *Staphylococcus aureus* and staphylococcal food-borne disease: An ongoing challenge in public health. *Biomed Res Int.* 2014;2014:827965.

668. Liu J, Bai L, Li W, et al. Trends of foodborne diseases in China: Lessons from laboratory-based surveillance since 2011. *Front Med.* 2018;12(1):48–57.

669. Evenson ML, Hinds MW, Bernstein RS, Bergdoll MS. Estimation of human dose of staphylococcal enterotoxin A from a large outbreak of staphylococcal food poisoning involving chocolate milk. *Int J Food Microbiol.* 1988;7(4):311–6.

670. Guidi F, Duranti A, Gallina S, et al. Characterization of a staphylococcal food poisoning outbreak in a workplace canteen during the post-earthquake reconstruction of central Italy. *Toxins (Basel).* 2018;10(12):523.

671. Le Loir Y, Baron F, Gautier M. *Staphylococcus aureus* and food poisoning. *Genet Mol Res.* 2003;2(1):63–76.

672. Sivamaruthi BS, Kesika P, Chaiyasut C. Toxins in fermented foods: Prevalence and preventions-a mini review. *Toxins (Basel).* 2018;11(1):4.

673. De Buyser ML, Dufour B, Maire M, Lafarge V. Implication of milk and milk products in food-borne diseases in France and in different industrialised countries. *Int J Food Microbiol.* 2001;67(1–2):1–17.

674. Giezendanner N, Meyer B, Gort M, Müller P, Zweifel C. [Raw milk-associated *Staphylococcus aureus* intoxication in children]. *Schweiz Arch Tierheilkd.* 2009;151(7):329–31.

675. Johler S, Weder D, Bridy C, et al. Outbreak of staphylococcal food poisoning among children and staff at a Swiss boarding school due to soft cheese made from raw milk. *J Dairy Sci.* 2015;98(5):2944–8.

676. Ostyn A, De Buyser ML, Guillier F, et al. First evidence of a food poisoning outbreak due to staphylococcal enterotoxin type E, France, 2009. *Euro Surveill.* 2010;15(13):19528.

677. Jones TF, Kellum ME, Porter SS, Bell M, Schaffner W. An outbreak of community-acquired foodborne illness caused by methicillin-resistant *Staphylococcus aureus*. *Emerg Infect Dis.* 2002;8(1):82–4.

678. Li G, Wu S, Luo W, Su Y, Luan Y, Wang X. *Staphylococcus aureus* ST6-t701 isolates from food-poisoning outbreaks (2006–2013) in Xi'an, China. *Foodborne Pathog Dis.* 2015;12(3):203–6.

679. Yan X, Wang B, Tao X, et al. Characterization of *Staphylococcus aureus* strains associated with food poisoning in Shenzhen, China. *Appl Environ Microbiol.* 2012;78(18):6637–42.

680. Cha JO, Lee JK, Jung YH, et al. Molecular analysis of *Staphylococcus aureus* isolates associated with staphylococcal food poisoning in South Korea. *J Appl Microbiol.* 2006;101(4):864–71.

681. Sato'o Y, Omoe K, Naito I, et al. Molecular epidemiology and identification of a *Staphylococcus aureus* clone causing food poisoning outbreaks in Japan. *J Clin Microbiol.* 2014;52(7):2637–40.

682. Suzuki Y, Omoe K, Hu DL, et al. Molecular epidemiological characterization of *Staphylococcus aureus* isolates originating from food poisoning outbreaks that occurred in Tokyo, Japan. *Microbiol Immunol.* 2014;58(10):570–80.

683. Umeda K, Nakamura H, Yamamoto K, et al. Molecular and epidemiological characterization of staphylococcal foodborne outbreak of *Staphylococcus aureus* harboring *seg, sei, sem, sen, seo,* and *selu* genes without production of classical enterotoxins. *Int J Food Microbiol.* 2017;256:30–5.

684. Kérouanton A, Hennekinne JA, Letertre C, et al. Characterization of *Staphylococcus aureus* strains associated with food poisoning outbreaks in France. *Int J Food Microbiol.* 2007;115(3):369–75.

685. Mossong J, Decruyenaere F, Moris G, et al. Investigation of a staphylococcal food poisoning outbreak combining case-control, traditional typing and whole genome sequencing methods, Luxembourg, June 2014. *Euro Surveill.* 2015;20(45).

686. Wattinger L, Stephan R, Layer F, Johler S. Comparison of *Staphylococcus aureus* isolates associated with food intoxication with isolates from human nasal carriers and human infections. *Eur J Clin Microbiol Infect Dis.* 2012;31(4):455–64.

687. Bhargava K, Wang X, Donabedian S, Zervos M, de Rocha L, Zhang Y. Methicillin-resistant *Staphylococcus aureus* in retail meat, Detroit, Michigan, USA. *Emerg Infect Dis.* 2011;17(6):1135–7.

688. Ge B, Mukherjee S, Hsu CH, et al. MRSA and multidrug-resistant *Staphylococcus aureus* in U.S. retail meats, 2010–2011. *Food Microbiol.* 2017;62:289–97.

689. Weese JS, Avery BP, Reid-Smith RJ. Detection and quantification of methicillin-resistant *Staphylococcus aureus* (MRSA) clones in retail meat products. *Lett Appl Microbiol.* 2010;51(3):338–42.

690. de Boer E, Zwartkruis-Nahuis JT, Wit B, et al. Prevalence of methicillin-resistant *Staphylococcus aureus* in meat. *Int J Food Microbiol.* 2009;134(1–2):52–6.

691. Dhup V, Kearns AM, Pichon B, Foster HA. First report of identification of livestock-associated MRSA ST9 in retail meat in England. *Epidemiol Infect.* 2015;143(14):2989–92.

692. Tenhagen BA, Vossenkuhl B, Käsbohrer A, et al. Methicillin-resistant *Staphylococcus aureus* in cattle food chains—Prevalence, diversity, and antimicrobial resistance in Germany. *J Anim Sci.* 2014;92(6):2741–51.

693. Kim YJ, Oh DH, Song BR, et al. Molecular characterization, antibiotic resistance, and virulence factors of methicillin-resistant *Staphylococcus aureus* strains isolated from imported and domestic meat in Korea. *Foodborne Pathog Dis.* 2015;12(5):390–8.

694. Lim SK, Nam HM, Park HJ, et al. Prevalence and characterization of methicillin-resistant *Staphylococcus aureus* in raw meat in Korea. *J Microbiol Biotechnol.* 2010;20(4):775–8.

695. Boost MV, Wong A, Ho J, O'Donoghue M. Isolation of methicillin-resistant *Staphylococcus aureus* (MRSA) from retail meats in Hong Kong. *Foodborne Pathog Dis.* 2013;10(8):705–10.

696. Vandendriessche S, Vanderhaeghen W, Soares FV, et al. Prevalence, risk factors and genetic diversity of methicillin-resistant *Staphylococcus aureus* carried by humans and animals across livestock production sectors. *J Antimicrob Chemother.* 2013;68(7):1510–6.

697. Benito D, Gómez P, Lozano C, et al. Genetic lineages, antimicrobial resistance, and virulence in *Staphylococcus aureus* of meat samples in Spain: Analysis of immune evasion cluster (IEC) genes. *Foodborne Pathog Dis.* 2014;11(5):354–6.

698. Bystroń J, Podkowik M, Korzekwa K, Lis E, Molenda J, Bania J. Characterization of borderline oxacillin-resistant *Staphylococcus aureus* isolated from food of animal origin. *J Food Prot.* 2010;73(7):1325–7.

699. Fox A, Pichon B, Wilkinson H, et al. Detection and molecular characterization of livestock-associated MRSA in raw meat on retail sale in North West England. *Lett Appl Microbiol.* 2017;64(3):239–45.

700. Hadjirin NF, Lay EM, Paterson GK, et al. Detection of livestock-associated meticillin-resistant *Staphylococcus aureus* CC398 in retail pork, United Kingdom, February 2015. *Euro Surveill.* 2015;20(24):21156.

701. Oniciuc EA, Ariza-Miguel J, Bolocan AS, et al. Foods from black market at EU border as a neglected route of potential methicillin-resistant *Staphylococcus aureus* transmission. *Int J Food Microbiol.* 2015;209:34–8.

702. Rodríguez-Lázaro D, Ariza-Miguel J, Diez-Valcarce M, Fernández-Natal I, Hernández M, Rovira J. Foods confiscated from non-EU flights as a neglected route of potential methicillin-resistant *Staphylococcus aureus* transmission. *Int J Food Microbiol.* 2015;209:29–33.

703. Vestergaard M, Cavaco LM, Sirichote P, et al. SCC*mec* type IX element in methicillin resistant *Staphylococcus aureus spa* type t337 (CC9) isolated from pigs and pork in Thailand. *Front Microbiol.* 2012;3:103.

704. Buyukcangaz E, Velasco V, Sherwood JS, Stepan RM, Koslofsky RJ, Logue CM. Molecular typing of *Staphylococcus aureus* and methicillin-resistant

S. aureus (MRSA) isolated from animals and retail meat in North Dakota, United States. *Foodborne Pathog Dis.* 2013;10(7):608–17.

705. Hanson BM, Dressler AE, Harper AL, et al. Prevalence of *Staphylococcus aureus* and methicillin-resistant *Staphylococcus aureus* (MRSA) on retail meat in Iowa. *J Infect Public Health.* 2011;4(4):169–74.
706. Jackson CR, Davis JA, Barrett JB. Prevalence and characterization of methicillin-resistant *Staphylococcus aureus* isolates from retail meat and humans in Georgia. *J Clin Microbiol.* 2013;51(4):1199–207.
707. O'Brien AM, Hanson BM, Farina SA, et al. MRSA in conventional and alternative retail pork products. *PLoS One.* 2012;7(1):e30092.
708. Weese JS, Reid-Smith R, Rousseau J, Avery B. Methicillin-resistant *Staphylococcus aureus* (MRSA) contamination of retail pork. *Can Vet J.* 2010;51(7):749–52.
709. Wang X, Li G, Xia X, Yang B, Xi M, Meng J. Antimicrobial susceptibility and molecular typing of methicillin-resistant *Staphylococcus aureus* in retail foods in Shaanxi, China. *Foodborne Pathog Dis.* 2014;11(4):281–6.
710. Agersø Y, Hasman H, Cavaco LM, Pedersen K, Aarestrup FM. Study of methicillin resistant *Staphylococcus aureus* (MRSA) in Danish pigs at slaughter and in imported retail meat reveals a novel MRSA type in slaughter pigs. *Vet Microbiol.* 2012;157(1–2):246–50.
711. Fessler AT, Kadlec K, Hassel M, et al. Characterization of methicillin-resistant *Staphylococcus aureus* isolates from food and food products of poultry origin in Germany. *Appl Environ Microbiol.* 2011;77(20):7151–7.
712. Lozano C, López M, Gómez-Sanz E, Ruiz-Larrea F, Torres C, Zarazaga M. Detection of methicillin-resistant *Staphylococcus aureus* ST398 in food samples of animal origin in Spain. *J Antimicrob Chemother.* 2009;64(6):1325–6.
713. Vossenkuhl B, Brandt J, Fetsch A, et al. Comparison of *spa* types, SCC*mec* types and antimicrobial resistance profiles of MRSA isolated from turkeys at farm, slaughter and from retail meat indicates transmission along the production chain. *PLoS One.* 2014;9(5):e96308.
714. Ogata K, Narimatsu H, Suzuki M, Higuchi W, Yamamoto T, Taniguchi H. [Molecular epidemiological study of community-acquired methicillin-resistant *Staphylococcus aureus* (CA-MRSA)—An examination of commercially distributed meat as a possible vehicle for CA-MRSA]. *J UOEH.* 2014;36(3):179–90.
715. Li Q, Li Y, Tang Y, Meng C, Ingmer H, Jiao X. Prevalence and characterization of *Staphylococcus aureus* and *Staphylococcus argenteus* in chicken from retail markets in China. *Food Control.* 2019;96:158–64.
716. Abdalrahman LS, Stanley A, Wells H, Fakhr MK. Isolation, virulence, and antimicrobial resistance of methicillin-resistant *Staphylococcus aureus* (MRSA) and methicillin sensitive *Staphylococcus aureus* (MSSA) strains from Oklahoma retail poultry meats. *Int J Environ Res Public Health.* 2015;12(6):6148–61.
717. Chairat S, Gharsa H, Lozano C, et al. Characterization of *Staphylococcus aureus* from raw meat samples in Tunisia: Detection of clonal lineage ST398 from the African continent. *Foodborne Pathog Dis.* 2015;12(8):686–92.
718. Hammad AM, Watanabe W, Fujii T, Shimamoto T. Occurrence and characteristics of methicillin-resistant and -susceptible *Staphylococcus aureus* and methicillin-resistant coagulase-negative staphylococci from Japanese retail ready-to-eat raw fish. *Int J Food Microbiol.* 2012;156(3):286–9.
719. Rhee CH, Woo GJ. Emergence and characterization of foodborne methicillin-resistant *Staphylococcus aureus* in Korea. *J Food Prot.* 2010;73(12):2285–90.
720. Sergelidis D, Abrahim A, Papadopoulos T, et al. Isolation of methicillin-resistant *Staphylococcus spp.* From ready-to-eat fish products. *Lett Appl Microbiol.* 2014;59(5):500–6.
721. Wu S, Huang J, Zhang F, et al. Prevalence and characterization of food-related methicillin-resistant *Staphylococcus aureus* (MRSA) in China. *Front Microbiol.* 2019;10:304.
722. Adame-Gómez R, Toribio-Jimenez J, Vences-Velazquez A, Rodríguez-Bataz E, Santiago Dionisio MC, Ramirez-Peralta A. Methicillin-resistant *Staphylococcus aureus* (MRSA) in artisanal cheeses in México. *Int J Microbiol.* 2018;2018:8760357.
723. Hummerjohann J, Naskova J, Baumgartner A, Graber HU. Enterotoxin-producing *Staphylococcus aureus* genotype B as a major contaminant in Swiss raw milk cheese. *J Dairy Sci.* 2014;97(3):1305–12.
724. Chao G, Bao G, Jiao X. Molecular epidemiological characteristics and clonal genetic diversity of *Staphylococcus aureus* with different origins in China. *Foodborne Pathog Dis.* 2014;11(7):503–10.
725. Cortimiglia C, Bianchini V, Franco A, et al. Short communication: Prevalence of *Staphylococcus aureus* and methicillin-resistant *S. aureus* in bulk tank milk from dairy goat farms in Northern Italy. *J Dairy Sci.* 2015;98(4):2307–11.
726. Haran KP, Godden SM, Boxrud D, Jawahir S, Bender JB, Sreevatsan S. Prevalence and characterization of *Staphylococcus aureus*, including methicillin-resistant *Staphylococcus aureus*, isolated from bulk tank milk from Minnesota dairy farms. *J Clin Microbiol.* 2012;50(3):688–95.
727. Juhász-Kaszanyitzky E, Jánosi S, Somogyi P, et al. MRSA transmission between cows and humans. *Emerg Infect Dis.* 2007;13(4):630–2.
728. Kreausukon K, Fetsch A, Kraushaar B, et al. Prevalence, antimicrobial resistance, and molecular characterization of methicillin-resistant *Staphylococcus aureus* from bulk tank milk of dairy herds. *J Dairy Sci.* 2012;95(8):4382–8.
729. Li T, Lu H, Wang X, et al. Molecular characteristics of *Staphylococcus aureus* causing bovine mastitis between 2014 and 2015. *Front Cell Infect Microbiol.* 2017;7:127.
730. Luini M, Cremonesi P, Magro G, et al. Methicillin-resistant *Staphylococcus aureus* (MRSA) is associated with low within-herd prevalence of intra-mammary infections in dairy cows: Genotyping of isolates. *Vet Microbiol.* 2015;178(3–4):270–4.
731. Nam HM, Lee AL, Jung SC, et al. Antimicrobial susceptibility of *Staphylococcus aureus* and characterization of methicillin-resistant *Staphylococcus aureus* isolated from bovine mastitis in Korea. *Foodborne Pathog Dis.* 2011;8(2):231–8.
732. Oliveira CJ, Tiao N, de Sousa FG, et al. Methicillin-resistant *Staphylococcus aureus* from Brazilian dairy farms and identification of novel sequence types. *Zoonoses Public Health.* 2016;63(2):97–105.
733. Paterson GK, Larsen J, Harrison EM, et al. First detection of livestock-associated meticillin-resistant *Staphylococcus aureus* CC398 in bulk tank milk in the United Kingdom, January to July 2012. *Euro Surveill.* 2012;17(50):pii: 20337.
734. Traversa A, Gariano GR, Gallina S, et al. Methicillin resistance in *Staphylococcus aureus* strains isolated from food and wild animal carcasses in Italy. *Food Microbiol.* 2015;52:154–8.
735. Wang D, Wang Z, Yan Z, et al. Bovine mastitis *Staphylococcus aureus*: Antibiotic susceptibility profile, resistance genes and molecular typing of methicillin-resistant and methicillin-sensitive strains in China. *Infect Genet Evol.* 2015;31:9–16.
736. Willis C, Jørgensen F, Aird H, et al. An assessment of the microbiological quality and safety of raw drinking milk on retail sale in England. *J Appl Microbiol.* 2018;124(2):535–46.
737. Veterinary Services, Centers for Epidemiology and Animal Health, APHIS, US Department of Agriculture. Methicillin resistant Staphylococcus aureus in bulk-tank milk on U.S. dairy operations, 2007. Technical Brief, March 2011.
738. Cuny C, Layer F, Hansen S, Werner G, Witte W. Nasal colonization of humans with occupational exposure to raw meat and to raw meat products with methicillin-susceptible and methicillin-resistant *Staphylococcus aureus*. *Toxins (Basel).* 2019;11(4):190.
739. Gomes F, Henriques M. Control of bovine mastitis: Old and recent therapeutic approaches. *Curr Microbiol.* 2016;72(4):377–82.
740. Shane AL, Mody RK, Crump JA, et al. 2017 Infectious Diseases Society of America clinical practice guidelines for the diagnosis and management of infectious diarrhea. *Clin Infect Dis.* 2017;65(12):1963–73.
741. Doyle ME, Hartmann FA, Lee Wong AC. Methicillin-resistant staphylococci: Implications for our food supply? *Anim Health Res Rev.* 2012;13(2):157–80.
742. Centers for Disease Control and Prevention (CDC). Surveillance for Foodborne Disease Outbreaks, United States, 2016, Annual Report. Atlanta, Georgia: U.S. Department of Health and Human Services, CDC, 2018.
743. Lipcsei LE, Brown LG, Coleman EW, et al. Foodborne illness outbreaks at retail establishments—National Environmental Assessment Reporting System, 16 state and local health departments, 2014–2016. *MMWR Surveill Summ.* 2019;68(1):1–20.
744. Nadon C, Van Walle I, Gerner-Smidt P, et al. PulseNet International: Vision for the implementation of whole genome sequencing (WGS) for global food-borne disease surveillance. *Euro Surveill.* 2017;22(23):30544.
745. Oestergaard LB, Schmiegelow MD, Bruun NE, et al. The associations between socioeconomic status and risk of *Staphylococcus aureus* bacteremia and subsequent endocarditis—A Danish nationwide cohort study. *BMC Infect Dis.* 2017;17(1):589.
746. Hammerum AM, Heuer OE, Emborg HD, et al. Danish integrated antimicrobial resistance monitoring and research program. *Emerg Infect Dis.* 2007;13(11):1632–9.

747. Johnson AP, Davies J, Guy R, et al. Mandatory surveillance of methicillin-resistant *Staphylococcus aureus* (MRSA) bacteraemia in England: The first 10 years. *J Antimicrob Chemother.* 2012;67(4):802–9.

748. Schönfeld V, Diercke M, Gilsdorf A, Eckmanns T, Walter J. Evaluation of the statutory surveillance system for invasive MRSA infections in Germany, 2016–2017. *BMC Public Health.* 2018;18(1):1063.

749. European Centre for Disease Prevention and Control. European Antimicrobial Resistance Surveillance Network (EARS-Net), accessed on May 7, 2019. https://ecdc.europa.eu/en/about-us/partnerships-and-networks/disease-and-laboratory-networks/ears-net.

750. Schrijver R, Stijntjes M, Rodríguez-Baño J, Tacconelli E, Babu Rajendran N, Voss A. Review of antimicrobial resistance surveillance programmes in livestock and meat in EU with focus on humans. *Clin Microbiol Infect.* 2018;24(6):577–90.

751. Centers for Disease Control and Prevention (CDC). 2017 National and State Healthcare-Associated Infections Progress Report. Last updated March 19, 2019. https://www.cdc.gov/hai/data/portal/progress-report.html. Accessed April 8, 2019.

752. Hoban DJ, Zhanel GG. Introduction to the CANWARD study (2007–11). *J Antimicrob Chemother.* 2013;68 Suppl 1:i3–5.

753. Diekema DJ, Pfaller MA, Shortridge D, Zervos M, Jones RN. Twenty-year trends in antimicrobial susceptibilities among Staphylococcus aureus from the SENTRY Antimicrobial Surveillance Program. *Open Forum Infect Dis.* 2019;6(Suppl 1):S47–53.

754. Daum RS, Spellberg B. Progress toward a *Staphylococcus aureus* vaccine. *Clin Infect Dis.* 2012;54(4):560–7.

755. Rigat F, Bartolini E, Dalsass M, et al. Retrospective identification of a broad IgG repertoire differentiating patients with *S. aureus* skin and soft tissue infections from controls. *Front Immunol.* 2019;10:114.

756. Kelly BC. On the administration and dose of *Staphylococcus* vaccine. *Br Med J.* 1908;2(2494):1150.

757. Missiakas D, Schneewind O. *Staphylococcus aureus* vaccines: Deviating from the carol. *J Exp Med.* 2016;213(9):1645–53.

758. Wright AE. On the treatment of acne, furunculosis, and sycosis by therapeutic inoculations of *Staphylococcus* vaccine. *Br Med J.* 1904;1(2262):1075–7.

759. Giersing BK, Dastgheyb SS, Modjarrad K, Moorthy V. Status of vaccine research and development of vaccines for *Staphylococcus aureus. Vaccine.* 2016;34(26):2962–6.

760. Thakker M, Park JS, Carey V, Lee JC. *Staphylococcus aureus* serotype 5 capsular polysaccharide is antiphagocytic and enhances bacterial virulence in a murine bacteremia model. *Infect Immun.* 1998;66(11):5183–9.

761. Xu S, Arbeit RD, Lee JC. Phagocytic killing of encapsulated and microencapsulated *Staphylococcus aureus* by human polymorphonuclear leukocytes. *Infect Immun.* 1992;60(4):1358–62.

762. Boyle-Vavra S, Li X, Alam MT, et al. USA300 and USA500 clonal lineages of *Staphylococcus aureus* do not produce a capsular polysaccharide due to conserved mutations in the cap5 locus. *MBio.* 2015;6(2):e02585-14.

763. Pfizer. Independent data monitoring committee recommends discontinuation of the phase 2B STRIVE clinical trial of *Staphylococcus aureus* vaccine following planned interim analysis, December 20, 2018. https://investors.pfizer.com/investor-news/press-release-details/2018/Independent-Data-Monitoring-Committee-Recommends-Discontinuation-of-the-Phase-2b-STRIVE-Clinical-Trial-of-Staphylococcus-aureus-Vaccine-Following-Planned-Interim-Analysis/default.aspx. Accessed May 7, 2019.

764. Pozzi C, Olaniyi R, Liljeroos L, Galgani I, Rappuoli R, Bagnoli F. Vaccines for *Staphylococcus aureus* and target populations. *Curr Top Microbiol Immunol.* 2017;409:491–528.

765. Fowler VG, Allen KB, Moreira ED, et al. Effect of an investigational vaccine for preventing *Staphylococcus aureus* infections after cardiothoracic surgery: A randomized trial. *JAMA.* 2013;309(13):1368–78.

766. Fattom A, Matalon A, Buerkert J, Taylor K, Damaso S, Boutriau D. Efficacy profile of a bivalent *Staphylococcus aureus* glycoconjugated vaccine in adults on hemodialysis: Phase III randomized study. *Hum Vaccin Immunother.* 2015;11(3):632–41.

767. Yeaman MR, Filler SG, Chaili S, et al. Mechanisms of NDV-3 vaccine efficacy in MRSA skin versus invasive infection. *Proc Natl Acad Sci U S A.* 2014;111(51):E5555–63.

768. Handke LD, Gribenko AV, Timofeyeva Y, Scully IL, Anderson AS. MntC-dependent manganese transport is essential for *Staphylococcus aureus* oxidative stress resistance and virulence. *mSphere.* 2018;3(4):e00336-18.

769. Cruciani M, Etna MP, Camilli R, et al. *Staphylococcus aureus* Esx factors control human dendritic cell functions conditioning Th1/Th17 response. *Front Cell Infect Microbiol.* 2017;7:330.

CHAPTER 155

The Group A *Streptococcus**

Emily Mosites • Edward L. Kaplan • Yuan L. Li • Chris A. Van Beneden

INTRODUCTION

The group A *Streptococcus* (GAS), a β-hemolytic *Streptococcus*, presents significant clinical and public health challenges throughout the world. The magnitude of disease burden varies not only by geographic region and within countries, but also between distinct populations within regional or national borders. Currently, more than 600 million cases of GAS pharyngitis and 162 million cases of impetigo—a common presentation of GAS infection—are estimated to occur worldwide each year.[1,2] Although less common, invasive GAS infections, such as necrotizing fasciitis and streptococcal toxic shock syndrome (STSS), can result in death in 20–25% of cases.[3] Nonsuppurative sequelae of GAS infection, such as acute rheumatic fever (ARF) and poststreptococcal glomerulonephritis (PSGN), are also major contributors to disease burden. A systematic review published in 2005 estimated that approximately 470,000 cases each of PSGN and ARF occur globally every year and between 15.6 and 19.6 million people were estimated to have rheumatic heart disease (RHD), a severe and chronic complication of ARF.[1] RHD is the leading cause of death from acquired heart disease among persons under 50 years of age, and from all cardiovascular disease among children in low income countries.[4–6] Because of the immense burden of disease, GAS continues to be an important target for prevention and public health control [7].

Following a brief discussion of other groups of β-hemolytic streptococci, this chapter addresses the relevant basic biology, epidemiology, clinical manifestations, immune responses, treatment, and public health approaches to prevention and control of GAS infection in humans.

GROUPS OF B-HEMOLYTIC STREPTOCOCCI IN HUMANS AND ANIMALS

GAS is one of approximately 20 serogroups of β-hemolytic streptococci. Group classifications were developed by Rebecca Lancefield in the 1920s based on cell wall carbohydrate antigens.[8,9] The groups of public health importance are summarized in Table 155-1. Some species of streptococci express more than one group-specific antigen and are therefore included in more than one group category. For example, *S. dysgalactiae* subspecies *equisimilis* can express group A, C, G, and L antigens.[10] While GAS colonizes or infects humans (although it has been reported to cause "big foot disease" in field voles and has very rarely been isolated from the throats of dogs[11,12]), the other serogroups exhibit variable pathogenicity to humans and animals. Understanding the potential for zoonotic transmission of some β-hemolytic streptococcal serogroups is important for accurate diagnosis and appropriate clinical and public health management of streptococcal disease.

TABLE 155-1 GROUPS OF BETA HEMOLYTIC STREPTOCOCCI OF PUBLIC HEALTH IMPORTANCE

Serogroup (Species)	Human Diseases	Animal Diseases
Group A (primarily *Streptococcus pyogenes*; also, *S. dysgalactiae* subspecies *equisimilis*, *S. anginosus*)	Pharyngitis/tonsillitis, skin infection, invasive disease, immune-mediated sequelae	None/rare
Group B (*Streptococcus agalactiae*)	Neonatal sepsis, adult sepsis, urinary tract infections	Mastitis (cattle)
Group C (*S. dysgalactiae*, *S. dysgalactiae* subsp. dysgalactiae, *S. dysgalactiae* subsp. equisimilis, *S. equi*, *S. equisimilis*, *S. zooepidemicus*, *S. phocae*)	Pharyngitis, sepsis, endocarditis, immune-mediated sequelae	Strangles (horses)
Group G (*S. canis*, *S. dysgalactiae* subsp. equisimilis)	Pharyngitis, sepsis	Pharyngitis (dogs)
Group F (*S. phocae*, *S. anginosus*)	Abscesses, bacteremia	Pneumonia, bacteremia (marine mammals)

Group B streptococci (GBS) can colonize the human genital and gastrointestinal tracts.[13,14] Infection with GBS often manifests as meningitis, pneumonia, or sepsis in humans. It is a leading cause of neonatal morbidity and mortality globally but can also cause disease in adults with comorbid conditions, particularly diabetes.[15–17] Please see Chapter 156 for further discussion of GBS disease in humans. GBS is also a pathogen of cattle (causing mastitis) and infections have been reported in pets.[18,19] However, the risk of zoonotic transmission has been largely eliminated by the pasteurization process for milk.

Group C streptococci include species that can colonize and infect humans and other mammals. In humans, group C streptococci can colonize the human pharynx, similar to GAS.[20] Group C streptococci also cause pharyngitis and invasive disease.[21] Group C streptococci have been identified in the throat of approximately 6% of patients with pharyngitis in some outpatient settings and a small percentage of blood cultures in patients with bacteremia.[22] Rare cases of RHD and PSGN have been associated with group C streptococcal infection although further study is needed to confirm group C streptococci

*Disclaimer: The findings and conclusions in this chapter are those of the authors and do not necessarily represent the official position of the Centers for Disease Control and Prevention/the Agency for Toxic Substances and Disease Registry. Use of trade names is for identification only and does not imply endorsement by the Public Health Service or by the U.S. Department of Health and Human Services.

as the actual cause of these sequelae.[23,24] Some group C streptococci cause morbidity in dogs, cats, horses, bats and other animals; zoonotic transmission does occur.[25–27]

Group F streptococci are considered a commensal organism of the human upper respiratory and gastrointestinal tract and are a potential cause of abscesses and bacteremia.[28] Up to 2% of streptococcal bacteremia isolates in humans may be group F streptococci.[29] Infections caused by group F strains have also been identified in other mammals.[30,31]

Group G streptococci are commensal organisms of the human upper respiratory tract, skin, gastrointestinal tract, and genital tract. However, like group A and group C streptococci, these strains can also cause pharyngitis and invasive disease in humans.[32] Foodborne outbreaks due to group G streptococci are rare but have been reported.[33] Group G streptococci can also be part of the normal skin and mucosal flora of dogs and cats but can also cause opportunistic infections in these animals.[34,35]

GROUP A STREPTOCOCCI: THE ORGANISM

GAS are structurally and functionally complex microorganisms. Although the group A antigen has been found in *S. anginosus* and in rare isolates of *S. dysgalactiae* subsp. *equisimilis*, the majority of bacteria with group A antigens are *S. pyogenes* (for the remainder of this chapter, GAS refers to *S. pyogenes*). *S. pyogenes* is a facultative, gram-positive coccus. GAS grows optimally in an environment of 10% carbon dioxide, and typically appears as whitish colonies surrounded by a zone of complete (beta) hemolysis on blood agar culture plates containing 5% sheep blood. Thick hyaluronic capsules in some colonies can cause them to appear mucoid. Human blood agar plates are not recommended for culturing GAS; they can inhibit growth due to the presence of antibiotics and change the typical colony and pericolonial appearance because beta hemolysis is not present.

CHARACTERIZATION OF SUBTYPES WITHIN GAS

The *S. pyogenes* genome exhibits very high sequence diversity and harbors a wide variety of virulence factors. Molecular typing (or subtyping) of GAS isolates combined with epidemiological data can help confirm whether a strain could be the cause of a suspected disease cluster, trace the origin and evolution of a disease cluster, monitor the dynamics of strain distribution, and identify lineages associated with increased virulence.

Serotyping

Historically, *S. pyogenes* strains were subtyped using serological phenotypes of cell surface proteins. The target cell surface proteins in serotyping methods include the M protein, the T-antigen, and the serum opacity factor (SOF). M-typing is based on antibodies directed against the variable M proteins of different isolates and was first developed during the 1920s by Lancefield.[9] M types are of public health importance because protective immunity to *S. pyogenes* infection is generally M-type-specific. SOF-typing is based on a serum opacity reaction induced by the *S. pyogenes* SOF protein; the reaction can be neutralized by antiserum produced in animals.[36] T-typing is based on binding of the T-antigen on trypsin-treated *S. pyogenes* cells by hyper immune rabbit serum, as originally described by Griffin in England.[37]

Molecular Typing

Molecular methods have generally replaced serologic methods for subtyping. The most common molecular subtyping methods are *emm* typing, multilocus sequence typing, and whole genome sequence typing (described in detail below). Molecular characterization by SOF and T-antigen are less common. Not all *S. pyogenes* strains produce SOF, and *sof* genotyping is less developed than *emm* typing. The T-Antigen is encoded by a genomic region commonly described as FCT (fibronectin-binding, collagen-binding, T-antigen). A consensus on the genotyping scheme for the FCT region is in development.

Emm Typing

The nucleotide sequence-based *emm* typing, which generates results accurately indicating the M serotypes,[38] has now largely replaced the use of antibodies for M-typing in laboratories. In addition, multiple *emm* types have now been recognized for which an M type has not been assigned because type-specific antibodies have not been identified. The *emm* typing scheme is based on nucleotide sequence of the 5' variable region of the M protein gene.[39] The sequence is obtained through specific amplification of the target in a polymerase chain reaction (PCR) followed by sequencing of the PCR product. Each unique sequence is then assigned an *emm* type. *Emm* typing currently is the most widely used method to define *S. pyogenes* strains, with more than 250 different *emm*-types reported worldwide. Isolates of the same *emm* type tend to share similar virulence factors and antibiotic resistance genes. A cumulated database of all *emm*-types is hosted by the U.S. Centers for Disease Control and Prevention (https://www2a.cdc.gov/ncidod/biotech/strepblast.asp). This source provides strain information of previously identified *emm*-types for comparison. The resolution of *emm* typing is limited because it uses a single target. As a result, if an *emm* type becomes endemic within a geographic area, as has been noted by invasive GAS disease surveillance in the United States (https://www.cdc.gov/abcs/reports-findings/surv-reports.htm), it can be difficult to determine epidemiologic relatedness of isolates based on *emm* type alone.

Multilocus Sequence Typing (MLST)

The MLST scheme is based on nucleotide sequences of conserved regions in seven core metabolic "housekeeping" genes.[40,41] These sequences are determined by target-specific PCR and sequencing. The sequence at each of the seven loci is assigned an allele number and the combined seven allele numbers define an MLST number. Stable associations between *emm* type and MLST have been documented, yet MLST provides higher resolution in differentiating isolates within *emm* type.[40,42] As of early 2019, the *S. pyogenes* MLST database (https://pubmlst.org/spyogenes/) contained 976 unique MLST values from 3888 isolates, representing a worldwide diversity of the organism.

Whole Genome Sequencing (WGS)

WGS has emerged as a powerful, all-inclusive tool for characterizing *S. pyogenes* isolates.[42] Developments in the next-generation sequencing technology have substantially reduced sequencing cost; near-complete bacterial genome sequences can now be routinely obtained through WGS (https://doi.org/10.1016/j.clinmicnews.2016.10.001). Genome sequences unambiguously define the genetic relatedness between strains. Therefore, WGS is increasingly used to assist investigations of invasive GAS disease outbreaks.[43–45] In addition, WGS allows sequence-based prediction of almost all important strain features, including *emm* type, MLST, antimicrobial resistance, important surface proteins, secreted virulence proteins, and other virulence-related characteristics.[42] Longitudinal analyses of GAS WGS results have identified molecular evolutionary events that were associated with emergence of new strains found to have enhanced strain transmission and virulence in animal models.[46–48] WGS "typing" is generally only available in reference laboratories.[49]

SPECTRUM OF DISEASE

Interactions between GAS and the human host may lead to multiple outcomes, including asymptomatic carriage, infection (which can result in mild to invasive disease), and postinfection suppurative and nonsuppurative sequelae. The spectrum of GAS interactions with humans is shown in Fig. 155-1 (modified from ref. 54).

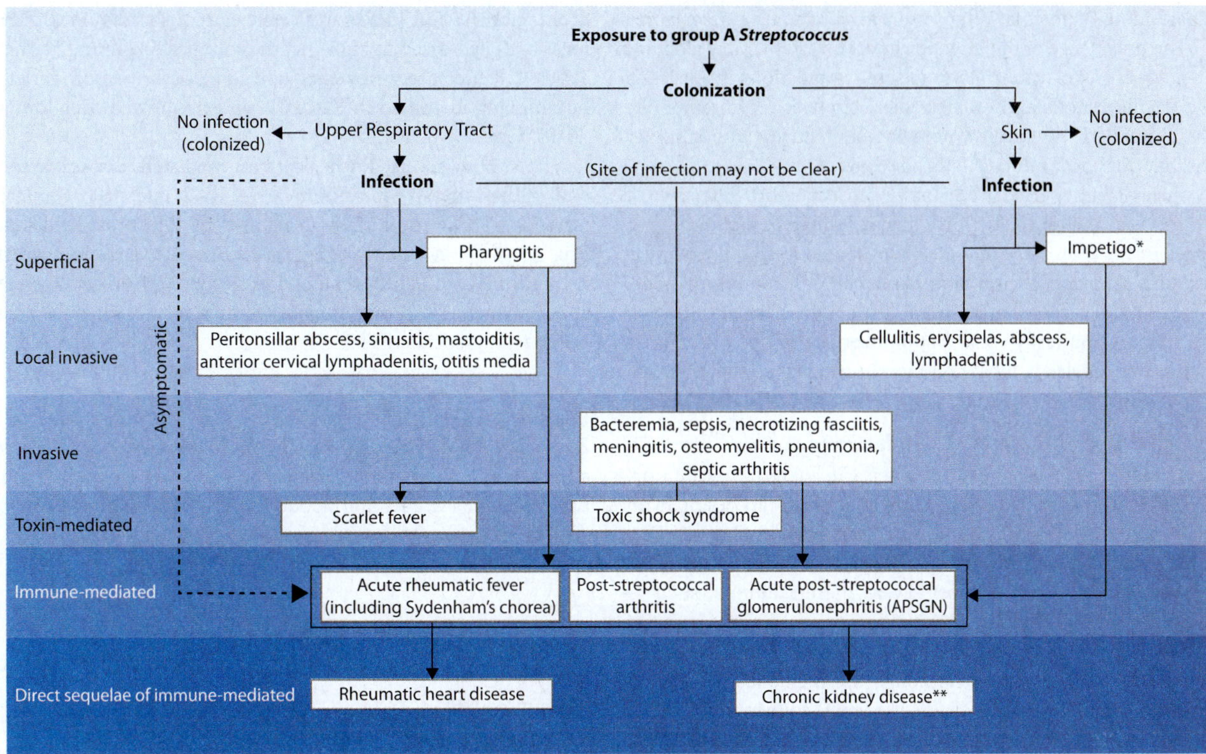

FIGURE 155-1. Spectrum of group A streptococcal disease. *Some have suggested that impetigo may lead to acute rheumatic fever.[50] **Chronic kidney disease following APSGN has been reported in adults but less often in children.[51–53] (*Source:* Adapted from Cannon JW et al. An economic case for a vaccine to prevent group A *Streptococcus* skin infections. Vaccine. 2018;36(46):6968–78.)

Carriage

Defining carriage of GAS and differentiating people who are upper respiratory tract GAS carriers from those who are infected is challenging. A frequently used but incomplete definition of a human upper respiratory tract GAS carrier is an individual in whom this bacterium is detected in the pharynx but who does not have clinical symptoms of disease, such as fever, sore throat, or inflammation and therefore is not considered infected.[55–57] However, determining carrier status solely based on clinical presentation may lead to inaccurate categorization. For example, it has been demonstrated that approximately one-third of people with ARF did not have preceding clinical symptoms of pharyngitis, suggesting that they were "infected" with GAS while asymptomatic.[58] Therefore, a subgroup of asymptomatically "infected" individuals exists.

A more accurate definition of a GAS upper respiratory tract carrier is a person from whom GAS is detected in the upper respiratory tract, but who does not demonstrate laboratory evidence of a host immune response to either somatic or extracellular GAS antigens. However, laboratory evidence of immune response is not commonly available. Additionally, newly recognized GAS antigens and associated immune responses have been documented,[59] but their pathogenic significance is unclear and the majority can currently only be detected in research laboratories.

Carriers are considerably less likely than persons who have symptomatic infection to spread GAS to contacts or to develop nonsuppurative sequelae such as ARF. However, when developing disease control measures during GAS infection outbreaks, it is important to remember that carriers can still transmit streptococci to others.

GAS carriage can be transient or can persist for more than 6 months.[60,65] Certain groups are more likely to harbor GAS than others. A meta-analysis of 18 prevalence studies showed that up to 12% of children harbored GAS asymptomatically, but the asymptomatic presence of GAS in the throats of adults is generally much less common.[61–64] Additionally, children who have a sibling who is a GAS carrier are more likely to be carriers themselves.[65] Carriage also appears to be more prevalent among people in close contact with other persons who are also carriers, particularly in crowded conditions such as military barracks.[66]

Superficial and Locally Invasive GAS Infections

The most common manifestations of acute GAS infection are noninvasive or superficial diseases, such as such as pharyngitis and impetigo. These usually mild GAS infections are easily transmitted.

GAS is estimated to be responsible for 15–30% of pharyngitis cases in children and 5–20% of cases among adults.[67] GAS pharyngitis is most prevalent among school age children (5–15 years) and, in temperate climates, most commonly occurs during the winter and early spring.[68] The incubation period is usually 2–5 days. Typical clinical presentation includes the sudden onset of a very sore throat, odynophagia, and fever. Other symptoms may include headache, abdominal pain, nausea, and vomiting. Patients with GAS pharyngitis typically do *not* have cough, rhinorrhea, hoarseness, oral ulcers, or conjunctivitis—symptoms more suggestive of viral pharyngitis. On clinical exam, persons with GAS pharyngitis usually have pharyngeal and tonsillar erythema, tonsillar hypertrophy with or without exudates, palatal petechiae and anterior cervical lymphadenitis.[69] Potential suppurative sequelae of pharyngitis include peritonsillar abscesses.

Impetigo (also called pyoderma or *impetigo contagiosa*) involves discrete purulent lesions of the keratin layer of the skin. Nonbullous impetigo is caused by GAS, *Staphylococcus aureus*, or both.[70] Streptococcal impetigo typically begins as papules that evolve into vesicles, surrounded by an area of erythema. The vesicles give rise to pustules that gradually enlarge then break down to form characteristic thick crusts. GAS impetigo appears most frequently on the lower extremities or face. Impetigo is most common in children aged 2–5 years, but also occurs among older children and adults who participate in activities that often result in cutaneous cuts or abrasions.[70] The prevalence of impetigo in children varies widely globally, with the highest reported estimates in some populations in Australia and the Pacific Islands and other tropical climates.[2,71] In temperate climates, impetigo is typically more frequent during the summer months, but does occur during fall and winter.[72]

Erysipelas is a superficial but locally invasive GAS infection of the dermis accompanied by prominent lymphatic involvement. The edges of these lesions are typically raised above the level of the surrounding skin and a clear line demarcates the infected tissue. The affected skin is a brilliant salmon-red color. Erysipelas is often noted as having "butterfly" distribution over the bridge of the nose and cheeks. Erysipelas is most common in infants, young children, and older adults.[70]

Invasive and Toxin-Mediated GAS Infections

GAS may result in invasive disease when the bacteria invade normally sterile body sites. Invasive GAS infections can result from infection or colonization of skin (e.g., wounds) or the pharynx. The resulting clinical manifestations include cellulitis, septic arthritis, pneumonia, sepsis, and the most severe manifestations, such as necrotizing fasciitis.[3] In high income countries, the incidence of invasive GAS infection usually ranges from two to four cases per 100,000 population per year,[3,73] although the incidence has gradually increased over the past few years in several countries.[74,75] In the United States, incidence has steadily increased since 2014, reaching 7.26 cases per 100,000 population in 2017.[75] The precise burden of GAS invasive disease in low- and middle-income countries is unclear but has been estimated to be two to three times that in high-income countries.[1,76]

In the United States, the most common manifestations of invasive GAS disease include cellulitis or other skin and soft tissue infections with bacteremia (~40% of reported invasive infections), bacteremia without focus (~20%), and pneumonia (14–16%). Less frequent are septic arthritis (~10%) and necrotizing fasciitis (5–8%).[3,77–79] Risk factors for invasive disease include skin breakdown, older age, immunocompromising conditions, diabetes, alcohol-use disorder, and influenza infection.[80–83]

GAS necrotizing fasciitis is an infection that involves the deeper, subcutaneous tissue and superficial or deep fascia. It is characterized by rapid progression and extensive destruction of muscle fascia and overlying subcutaneous fat. In its later stages, necrotizing fasciitis involves all layers of the skin and muscle.[70] Necrotizing fasciitis often presents as a soft tissue infection (erythema, edema, warmth) with extreme pain. Flu-like symptoms are commonly present early in the course of disease and include fever, malaise, myalgias, and anorexia. Illness progresses rapidly over several days. Skin over the affected area changes from red-purple to blue-gray; skin breakdown with bullae often occurs. Hemodynamic instability often results. Early recognition of necrotizing infection is essential to effective treatment; limb amputation may be required, and case-fatality is substantial (20–29% in the United States).[3] In several descriptive studies of invasive infections in North America and Europe, approximately 50% of patients with GAS necrotizing fasciitis infections also developed STSS, a severe toxin-mediated disease (described below). M protein or *emm* types 1 and 3 have often been reported to be the most common types among GAS causing necrotizing fasciitis.[84–86]

Toxin-mediated scarlet fever occurs when GAS releases pyrogenic exotoxins in the course of an infection. Scarlet fever is usually associated with pharyngeal infections but may also follow wound infections or puerperal sepsis.[70] The scarlatina rash typically appears on the second day of illness and is a diffuse red rash, with areas of deeper red that blanch on pressure. It often begins on the upper chest, and then spreads over the trunk and to the neck and extremities. The palms, soles, and usually the face are spared. Skin folds in the neck, axillae, groin, elbows, and knees are a deeper red (Pastia's lines).[70] Scarlet fever rates decreased in high-income countries beginning in the mid-1900s, but increased incidence and large outbreaks of scarlet fever began being identified in East Asia and the United Kingdom in the 2010s.[73,87–89]

STSS is a severe form of toxin-mediated disease associated with either invasive or noninvasive GAS infection. Clinical criteria for STSS were initially developed in 1993 and are detailed in Box 155-1.[90,91] A rapidly progressive clinical course is characteristic, and the case fatality rate can exceed 50%. In the United States, approximately 3–5% of patients with invasive GAS disease are diagnosed with associated STSS.[3]

Immune-Mediated Disease and Sequelae

Immune-mediated sequelae of acute GAS infections include ARF, RHD, and PSGN (Fig. 155-1). These sequelae follow a latent period after acute GAS infection. For example, PSGN onset occurs 10–14 days after pharyngitis and about 3 weeks after impetigo onset, and ARF onset occurs 1–5 weeks after GAS pharyngitis.[92]

BOX 155-1 Working Group Definition for Streptococcal Toxic Shock Syndrome[90,91]

Clinical Criteria

An illness with the following clinical manifestations:

- Hypotension defined by a systolic blood pressure ≤ 90 mm Hg for adults or ≤ fifth percentile by age for children aged ≤16 years.
- Multiorgan involvement characterized by ≥ 2 of the following:
  - *Renal impairment*: creatinine ≥ 2 mg/dL (≥177 μmol/L) for adults or ≥ twice the upper limit of normal for age. In patients with pre-existing renal disease, a twofold or more elevation over the baseline level.
  - *Coagulopathy*: Platelets ≤100,000/mm^3 (≤100 × 106/L) or disseminated intravascular coagulation, defined by prolonged clotting times, low fibrinogen level, and the presence of fibrin degradation products.
  - *Liver involvement*: Alanine aminotransferase, aspartate aminotransferase, or total bilirubin levels twofold or more the upper limit of normal for the patient's age. In patients with pre-existing liver disease, a more than twofold increase over the baseline level.
  - *Acute respiratory distress syndrome*: defined by
  - Acute onset of diffuse pulmonary infiltrates and hypoxemia in the absence of cardiac failure,
  - *Or* by evidence of diffuse capillary leak manifested by acute onset of generalized edema,
  - *Or* pleural or peritoneal effusions with hypoalbuminemia.
  - A generalized erythematous macular rash that may desquamate.
  - Soft-tissue necrosis, including necrotizing fasciitis or myositis, or gangrene.

Case Classification

Probable

A case that meets the clinical case definition in the absence of another identified etiology for the illness and with isolation of group A *Streptococcus* from a nonsterile site (e.g., throat, sputum, vagina, superficial skin lesion).

Confirmed

A case that meets the clinical case definition and with isolation of group A *Streptococcus* from a normally sterile site (e.g., blood or cerebrospinal fluid or, less commonly, joint, pleural, pericardial fluid, surgical wound).

ARF is a multisystemic, nonsuppurative delayed response to GAS infection that can involve the heart, joints, skin, and central nervous system.[93] The attack rate of ARF among people with untreated GAS pharyngitis has been estimated to range from 0.3% to 3%.[94,95] In the United States, the incidence of ARF markedly decreased by the early 1960s, from 20 cases to less than 1 case per 100,000 people per year.[96] Hypotheses for this observation is overall improvements in access to healthcare and use of antibiotics, in addition to reduced prevalence of some specific M types of GAS, suggesting that some strains (referred to as "rheumatogenic" strains) are more likely than others to lead to development of ARF.[97,98] However, specific rheumatogenic properties associated with these strains have not been identified. It is generally believed that ARF follows only GAS pharyngitis; whether it can follow GAS skin infection remains controversial.[50]

The most important complication of ARF is RHD, in which heart valves are damaged. While the exact pathogenic mechanisms leading to RHD have not been fully defined, it is universally agreed that the pathology is not related to direct infection of the heart by the GAS, but rather is the result of an immunologic response that takes place following untreated or inadequately treated pharyngitis in approximately 3% of patients with true GAS infection. The most frequent damage is to the mitral valve. Aortic valve involvement, when it occurs, is usually associated with concomitant mitral valve disease; isolated aortic valve disease rarely occurs with RHD. In some cases of longstanding RHD, the tricuspid or the pulmonary valve may be involved. Whether the myocardium itself is involved in the pathogenetic process remains controversial. It is clear, however, that any decrease in myocardial function that occurs in those with advanced valvular heart disease is largely the result of hemodynamic abnormalities with subsequent stress on the myocardium and not directly caused by recurrent GAS infection.

In the 2010s, advances in the use of 2D, continuous-wave and color-Doppler echocardiography to screen for RHD have augmented diagnostic capacity for identifying cardiac complications of ARF, including valvular and myocardial abnormalities. In 2012, the World Heart Federation published standardized echocardiographic criteria for RHD diagnosis.[99] In 2015, the criteria for diagnosis of ARF were revised to support the use of Doppler echocardiography in the diagnosis of ARF carditis[93] (Table 155-2).

PSGN is another nonsuppurative sequelae to GAS infection. This complication differs from ARF in several ways. First, epidemiologic data support that only certain ("nephritogenic") strains of GAS (e.g., M type 49) appear capable of initiating this immunologic process. In addition, PSGN can follow GAS infection of either the skin (e.g., impetigo) or the throat (e.g., pharyngitis). While there is clear evidence that treatment of the preceding GAS infection can prevent development of rheumatic fever, there is not sufficient evidence that antibiotic therapy of streptococcal impetigo can prevent the development of PSGN.

Relationships between GAS infections and other nonsuppurative conditions have been proposed but have not been adequately established; in some cases, available data conflict. These conditions include Jaccoud's arthritis, hemolytic uremic syndrome, and pediatric acute-onset neuropsychiatric syndrome (PANS).[100,101]

TABLE 155-2 REVISED JONES CRITERIA FOR DIAGNOSING ACUTE RHEUMATIC FEVER[93]

Part A. For all patient populations with evidence of preceding group A streptococcal infection		
Diagnosis: Initial ARF	2 major manifestations *or* 1 major plus 2 minor manifestations	
Diagnosis: Recurrent ARF	2 major manifestations *or* 1 major plus 2 minor manifestations *or* 3 minor manifestations	
	Low-risk populations[a]	**Moderate- and high-risk populations[a]**
Part B. Major manifestations	Carditis[b] • Clinical and/or subclinical Arthritis • Polyarthritis only Chorea Erythema marginatum Subcutaneous nodules	Carditis[b] • Clinical and/or subclinical Arthritis • Monoarthritis or polyarthritis • Polyarthralgia (if other causes have been excluded) Chorea Erythema marginatum Subcutaneous nodules
Part C. Minor manifestations	Polyarthralgia Fever (≥38.5°C) ESR ≥ 60 mm in the first hour and/or CRP ≥ 3.0 mg/dL Prolonged PR interval on electrocardiography, after accounting for age variability (unless carditis is a major criterion)	Monoarthralgia Fever (≥38°C) ESR ≥ 30 mm/hr and/or CRP ≥ 3.0 mg/dL Prolonged PR interval on electrocardiography, after accounting for age variability (unless carditis is a major criterion)

Abbreviations: ARF = acute rheumatic fever; CRP = C-reactive protein; mm = millimeters; mg/dL = milligrams per deciliter; ESR = erythrocyte sedimentation rate.

[a]Low-risk population is defined as an acute rheumatic fever incidence of < 2 per 100,000 school-aged children or all-age rheumatic heart disease prevalence of ≤ 1 per 1000 population per year. Those not included in the low-risk population are defined as moderate or high risk depending upon their reference population.

[b]Subclinical carditis indicates echocardiographic valvulitis.

HOST IMMUNE RESPONSES TO GAS INFECTION

Measurement of immune responses to GAS can be used to reveal evidence of streptococcal exposure, making it an essential tool for understanding GAS infections in the population. Documentation of an immune response to one or more of the somatic or extracellular streptococcal antigens, in addition to isolation of the organism, has been thought to be necessary to confirm true infection. Absence of an immune response in someone from whom GAS has been isolated has been postulated to reflect the GAS "carrier state" (see above). Differentiation between true infection and carriage is important for understanding the epidemiology of GAS infections and their sequelae and to inform public health prevention efforts.

Numerous variables influence human immune responses to GAS extracellular antigens. Examples of variables include the site of infection (e.g., skin versus upper respiratory tract), season of the year (because of differences in peak seasonal periods of GAS infections, especially in temperate climates), the age distribution of the population or cohort being observed, and the specific antigens or antibodies being examined (because of the unique immunokinetics of the host response to each antigen).

Commonly Studied Group A Streptococcal Antigens

The somatic and extracellular GAS antigens which have been most frequently examined in clinical and epidemiologic studies include streptolysin O, streptococcal deoxyribonuclease B, streptococcal hyaluronidase, and streptococcal group A carbohydrate (from the streptococcal cell wall). Antibodies to streptolysin O and streptococcal deoxyribonuclease B can be identified through commercially available test kits. A test for multiple unspecified GAS antibodies is the commercially available Streptozyme® test; however, published data suggest that the reagents are difficult to standardize which compromises the reliability of the test.[55] Of the antibodies listed in Table 155-3, streptolysin O is most commonly measured and utilized clinically. However, serogroups A, C, and G beta hemolytic streptococci produce

TABLE 155-3 MOST FREQUENTLY ASSESSED GROUP A STREPTOCOCCAL ANTIGENS AND ANTIBODIES

Antigen	Somatic or Extracellular	Time to Reach Peak Titer[a]	Commercial Test Kit Availability	Availability of Population or Age-based Distributions
Streptolysin O	Extracellular (ASO or ASLO)	3–6 weeks	Multiple kits available	Probably the most complete available data for any of the streptococcal antibodies
Deoxyribonuclease B	Extracellular (anti-DNase B or ADB)	6–8 weeks	Varies by country	Multiple reference population values available
Streptokinase	Extracellular (ASK)	3–4 weeks	Varies by country	Limited data available
Streptococcal hyaluronidase	Somatic (AH)	2–4 weeks	No longer commercially available	Limited data available
Nicotinamide adenine di-nucleosidase	Extracellular (anti-NADase)	3–6 weeks	Available in specific research laboratories	Limited data available
Group A carbohydrate	Somatic (ACHO)	4–6 weeks	Available in specific research laboratories	Limited data available
Group A streptococcal M-protein	Somatic anti-M antibody or type specific antibody.)	Approximately 6–8 weeks	Available only in research laboratories	Limited data available
C5A peptidase	Extracellular (anti-SCPA)	4–8 weeks	Available only in specific research laboratories	Limited data available

[a]Does not include anamnestic responses; may be affected if patient is treated with antibiotics.

identical streptolysin O, therefore the presence of an elevated or a rising anti-streptolysin O titer is not specific for GAS infection.

Immune Responses as Evidence of Infection

A greater number of different GAS antibodies detected in the serum of a given patient increases the likelihood that the person is experiencing a *bona fide* GAS infection.[102,103] However, it is difficult to identify which specific GAS antigens (other than M protein, as discussed below) are responsible for conferring host protection and which simply stimulate a nonprotective immune response. Recent studies have confirmed that numerous GAS antigens evoke antibody responses, but the full significance of these antibodies is incompletely understood.[59] The most commonly studied immune responses to GAS antigens are outlined in Table 155-3.

Measurement of antibody to GAS M protein has been very useful in epidemiologic studies. These type-specific anti-M protein antibodies are considered protective against reinfection with GAS of the homologous M type. Antibodies to GAS M proteins have been demonstrated to persist in the serum of previously infected individuals for 30 or more years.[104,105] Measurement of M protein antibodies is primarily limited to research laboratories.

When studying the immune responses of individuals within a defined study population, serial collection of blood specimens is necessary. Understanding the immunokinetics of each specific antibody response is essential for accurate data interpretation. Examples of prospectively obtained serial antibody responses to streptolysin O and to streptococcal deoxyribonuclease B, along with the respective interpretations, are shown in Fig. 155-2 (A and B).[60] The results from throat cultures collected monthly from individual pediatric study participants followed during a 2-year prospective study are temporally coordinated with antibody determinations from serial collections of serum from these participants. If a participating child developed symptoms of GAS infection between scheduled visits, additional throat cultures and serum samples were collected. Figure 155-3 illustrates another important consideration in interpreting antibody data obtained from prospective GAS studies. The figure presents an example of the variation in mean streptococcal antibody titers in a defined North American cohort over the course of 2 years, demonstrating that, even within the same population, mean streptococcal antibody titers may vary significantly by season of the year. These significant differences in mean titers reflect the differences in seasonality of pediatric GAS infections within this population.[106]

EPIDEMIOLOGY OF GROUP A *STREPTOCOCCUS*

Transmission of GAS

GAS can be transmitted through respiratory droplets or direct skin contact. Foodborne transmission from infected food handlers has also been implicated in outbreaks of streptococcal pharyngitis.[107–111] Although carriers are less likely than persons with symptomatic infection to transmit GAS, carriers can serve as a reservoir for transmission during outbreaks.[112–115]

Population Dynamics of Transmission

Incidence rates of acute GAS infection vary by demographics as well as by molecular differences in the bacteria across geographic areas and time. Although incidence rates of invasive GAS disease have decreased since the mid-1900s in high-income countries (as a result of improved hygiene and less crowding), periodic waves of increased incidence continue to be documented.[73] These waves are thought to be the result of the introduction of newly introduced strains against which limited immunity is present in the affected population (i.e., a lack of "herd immunity"). Alternatively, these could be the result of changes in the prevalence of risk factors for GAS infection, which facilitate spread, such as increased drug use or homelessness in the population.[46,116] As an example of the former, over 100 cases of ARF occurred among middle class families in the Salt Lake City, Utah area in each 1985–86 and 1997–98. The increased incidence was noted to be temporally associated with the introduction of mucoid strains, primarily M type 18 streptococci, into the population.[117]

Smaller scale outbreaks also continue to occur in a wide variety of settings. Settings for invasive GAS outbreak investigations occurring during 2013–18 and described in the published scientific literature include long-term care facilities (LTCF); a telephone factory; tertiary-care hospitals; a podiatry clinic; an ear, nose, and throat ward; an outpatient liposuction facility; and a trauma center; community-based outbreaks were also described among persons who inject drug and persons who are experiencing homelessness.[43,118–125] During the same period, large pharyngitis outbreaks (~30–300 cases) have been described in Peru, Japan, China, the United States, and Spain.[108,110,126–129] Surges in scarlet fever infections have been reported in east Asia (e.g., China, Hong Kong, South Korea) and England.[130–132] Outbreaks of ARF have been reported in northeast Italy.[133] A poststreptococcal glomerulonephritis outbreak was reported from Western Australia.[134] These

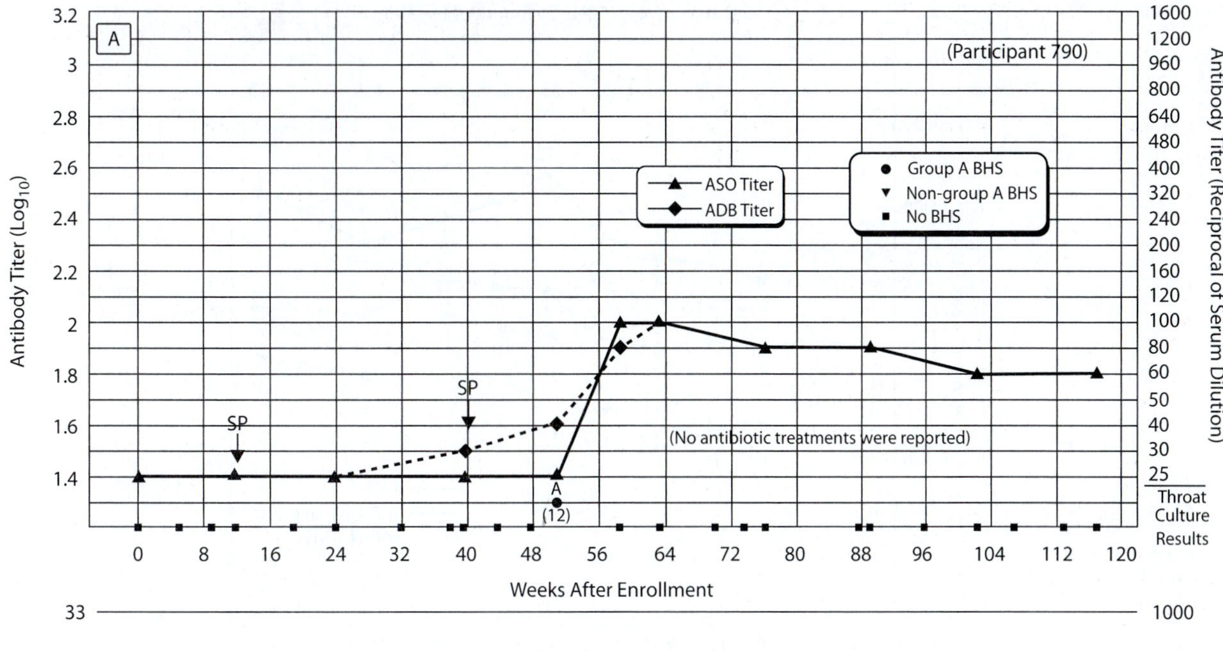

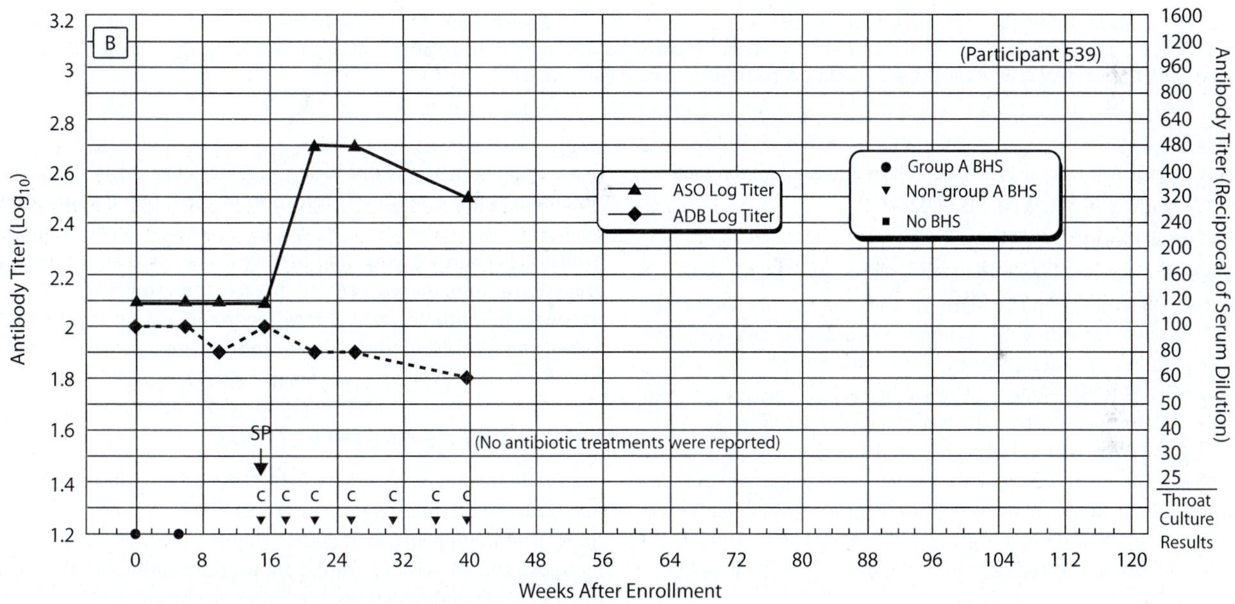

FIGURE 155-2. Serial antibody responses to streptolysin O and to streptococcal deoxyribonuclease B among children followed during a 2-year study with monthly throat cultures and blood samples obtained every 13 weeks. Panel A: The solid lines represent the antistreptolysin O (ASO) titer ($\log_{10}$) changes, and the dashed lines represents the anti-DNase B-titers ($\log_{10}$) changes. The letter "A" indicates the beta hemolytic serogroup; SP = symptomatic pharyngitis. Both the ASO and the anti-DNase B titers rise concomitant with an initial isolation of GAS from the subject's pharynx. The slope of the ASO titer rise is steeper than the slope of the rise for anti-DNase B titer compatible with an earlier rise in ASO than in anti-DNase B. The titer values remain elevated for both the ASO and the anti-DNase B despite the fact that there are no subsequent GAS isolations from the pharynx. These data emphasize that it is the *change* in serial antibody titers that is more important than the specific individual titer value itself to indicate infection. Panel B: The solid lines represent the antistreptolysin O (ASO) titer ($\log_{10}$) changes, and the dashed lines represents the anti-DNase B-titers ($\log_{10}$) changes. The letter "C" indicates the beta hemolytic serogroup; SP = symptomatic pharyngitis. There is a prompt immune response in antistreptolysin O titer but no demonstrated immunologic response to streptococcal DNase B when group C streptococci were initially isolated from the subject's throat. Group C streptococci do *not* produce streptococcal nuclease B. (Panels A and B reproduced with permission from Johnson DR, Kurlan R, Leckman J, Kaplan EL. The human immune response to streptococcal extracellular antigens: Clinical, diagnostic and potential pathogenetic implications. *Clin Infect Dis.* 2010;50:481–90.)

outbreaks likely represent only a small proportion of the true number of outbreaks, given that many outbreaks are not reported nor investigated.

At-Risk Populations

Several specific population groups are at increased risk of GAS infections compared to the general population as a result of crowded living conditions or other underlying risk factors for streptococcal infection. Some of these groups at high risk are described below.

School Children

School-aged children between 5 and 15 years of age often carry GAS in their upper respiratory tracts and are at risk for GAS infections and suppurative, nonsuppurative, and immune-mediated sequelae.[65,135] Incidence of pharyngitis and ARF are higher in this age group than other age groups. Studies have shown that the presence of school-aged children is also a risk factor for household spread of GAS,[136,137]

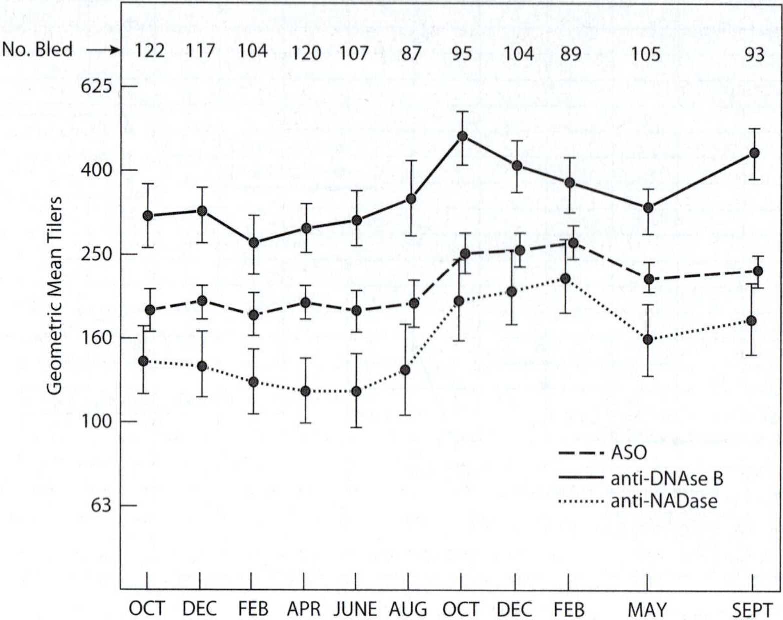

FIGURE 155-3. Mean streptococcal antibody titers in a defined cohort over 2 years. (*Source:* Reproduced with permission from From Kaplan EL, Anthony BF, Ayoub EM, Wannamaker LW: A two-year longitudinal study of streptococcal infections in an isolated community: Antibody dynamics. In: *Streptococcal Disease and the Community*. Haverkorn MJ, ed. Excerpta Medica Press, Amsterdam, 1974.)

with the risk of invasive disease in children and adults increased by the presence of children in the household.[80,138]

Military Personnel

Historically, military personnel have experienced a high burden of respiratory infections,[139] particularly among new recruits. Outbreaks of GAS disease, including pharyngitis, pneumonia, and cellulitis, have frequently been identified. Increased risk for infection among military recruits is likely due to crowded barracks living quarters and a rapid influx of persons from diverse geographic locations with low immunity to newly acquired M types.[140,141] Parenthetically, because of the high burden of disease and the contained populations, military personnel have also served as an opportune group for epidemiologic and outbreak prevention investigations. Much has been learned from classic epidemiological studies of GAS in military populations.[141–146]

Residents of Long-term Care Facilities

Residents of LTCF are also at an increased risk of invasive GAS infections. The incidence of invasive GAS disease among LTCF residents has been estimated to be six times that of elderly people of the same age living in the community.[147] Advanced age, communal living setting, exposure to ill or colonized healthcare workers, exposure to ill visitors, frequent presence of wounds, and chronic medical conditions contribute to this risk.[121,123,148,149]

Indigenous Communities

High rates of invasive GAS infection have been reported among indigenous communities in the United States (Native Americans and Alaska Native people), Australia (Indigenous Australians), New Zealand (Māori), and Canada (Native Canadians).[150–154] The introduction of previously absent GAS types into such communities has been associated with spread of GAS disease.[155] These high rates have been considered by some as a marker of social disadvantage[152] and may also be associated with high prevalence of underlying risk factors for disease.[150]

Persons experiencing homelessness and persons who inject drugs

Persons experiencing homelessness and persons who inject drugs are at an increased risk of invasive GAS disease.[74,156–160] Persons who inject drugs may have reduced access to hygiene resources and spend time in crowded conditions. Infection in these populations is facilitated by the injection of drugs, which creates a portal of entry for the bacteria. Persons experiencing homelessness often suffer from skin breakdown, unmanaged chronic disease, undernutrition, substance use, mental health disorders, crowding in shelters, and limited access to hygiene resources, all of which can increase their risk of invasive GAS.[161,162]

TREATMENT OF GAS INFECTIONS

Successful treatment of acute GAS infections, from the usually milder manifestations of pharyngitis and impetigo to very severe manifestations including pneumonia, necrotizing fasciitis and STSS, relies on the rapid and effective use of the appropriate antibiotics.[69,163] Formal treatment recommendations for primary clinical syndromes often differ between various professional societies and organizations in multiple countries.[164] We describe some general treatment principles for important GAS clinical syndromes below.

Pharyngitis and Impetigo

Prompt administration of appropriate antibiotics for GAS pharyngitis shortens the clinical course, especially in children, decreases disease transmission, decreases risk of suppurative sequelae, and, if administered up to 9 days after illness onset, prevents ARF.[163,165] The drug of choice for pharyngitis is typically a penicillin or amoxicillin to promote bacterial eradication.[164,166] Narrow-spectrum first-generation cephalosporins are indicated for patients with a history of non-anaphylactic allergy to penicillin. Patients with anaphylactic or type 1 hypersensitivity to penicillin can be treated with clindamycin, macrolides (erythromycin), or azalides (azithromycin and clarithromycin), if the isolate is sensitive to these antibiotics.[101,163,166,167] Recommended first line treatment of limited non-bullous impetigo includes topical mupirocin or retapamulin ointment.[69] Oral antimicrobial agents active against both GAS and *S. aureus* should be used to treat impetigo in persons with multiple lesions and in outbreaks (e.g., within households, child-care centers, athletic teams).[101] If GAS is confirmed, oral penicillin is preferred.[69]

Invasive Infections

Management of severe systemic infection and associated toxin-mediated disease—including sepsis, STSS, and necrotizing fasciitis—requires rapid evaluation, hemodynamic support, initial broad-spectrum empiric treatment, and prompt surgical debridement of deep-seated infection.

For necrotizing fasciitis, radiologic assessment (e.g., computer tomography or magnetic resonance imaging) may not always be definitive to diagnosis this infection. Emergent surgical exploration is imperative and is used to confirm the diagnosis, to perform aggressive debridement of all necrotic or devitalized tissue, and to obtain tissue for microbiologic testing.[69] Repeat debridement is frequently necessary.

Once GAS is identified as the etiology in cases of septic shock, STSS or necrotizing fasciitis, penicillin and clindamycin are the recommended antibiotics. Penicillin, which inhibits bacterial cell wall synthesis is most effective against rapidly growing bacteria. Clindamycin, a protein synthesis-inhibitor, suppresses the synthesis of some streptococcal toxins and cytokines and is not affected by the inoculum size or the stage of bacterial growth.[168] Penicillin should be used in conjunction with clindamycin because of potential GAS resistance to clindamycin.[69]

Various studies have been undertaken to assess the potential benefit of intravenous immunoglobulin (IVIG) in the treatment of STSS.[169–172] However, the definitive answer remains elusive. An observational study which demonstrated better outcomes in patients who received IVIG was subject to confounding, because patients receiving IVIG were more likely to have had surgery and to have received clindamycin than historical controls.[84] A randomized, double-blind, placebo-controlled trial performed by a multi-country research group in Northern Europe did not show a statistically significant improvement in survival with IVIG but may have been limited by small sample sizes.[69,171,172] Recently, however, support for the use of IVIG in STSS has increased following publication of a systematic review and meta-analysis that studied the effect of IVIG on mortality in clindamycin-treated STSS and concluded that use of IVIG was associated with a reduction in mortality from 33.7% to 15.7%.[173]

Management of Group A Streptococcal Carriers

Eradication of GAS colonization in GAS carriers is not usually attempted in normal circumstances. However, eradication of colonization may be considered in several specific settings, including: localized outbreaks of GAS sequelae, such as ARF and AGN; outbreaks of pharyngitis in closed or semi-closed communities; households in which a family member has had rheumatic fever or has evidence of RHD; or, households in which multiple episodes of symptomatic GAS pharyngitis continue to occur despite administration of appropriate antibiotics.[174] Public health officials may also recommend eradication of GAS colonization during outbreaks of severe GAS infections among residents of LTCFs and in other scenarios (see below).

No randomized, controlled studies measuring the effectiveness of chemoprophylaxis in preventing secondary (or "subsequent") cases of invasive GAS disease have been completed to date, although prophylaxis has been used to successfully control GAS outbreaks in LTCFs.[13,175–177] Recommended regimens to prevent colonized or recently exposed individuals from contracting GAS infection in higher risk populations have been extrapolated from studies of eradication of colonization.[178]

A regimen of benzathine penicillin G (BPG) and oral rifampin has been shown to be effective in eradication of GAS colonization and was reported to be significantly more effective than BPG alone.[179] First-generation cephalosporins have also been shown to be effective in eradicating GAS colonization.[178,180,181] First-generation cephalosporins can be considered for patients allergic to penicillin whose allergic reactions are not anaphylactic.[182] Depending on resistance profiles, macrolides and azalides are acceptable alternatives. The list of recommended antibiotics may change as additional studies on effectiveness of various regimens are completed. See Table 155-4 for several regimens currently recommended in the United States and Canada[182,183] as of 2019.

Antimicrobial Resistance

Fortunately, no clinical GAS isolate demonstrating resistance to penicillin or other beta-lactams has been identified to date. However, a rare pbp2x missense mutation which led to elevated β-lactam minimum inhibitory concentrations among two U.S. patients has recently been identified.[184] Levels of macrolide and clindamycin resistance vary by geographic area and time; resistance to these agents can be > 10% in a community[178,182] and inducible clindamycin resistance may be a concern. Therefore, local antibiotic resistance profiles should always be considered when prescribing macrolides or azalides. Testing GAS isolates for clindamycin susceptibility, including both constitutive and inducible resistance,[185] should be considered in areas of high clindamycin resistance when treating invasive infections.

PREVENTION AND CONTROL OF GAS

In the absence of an effective GAS vaccine, opportunities for disease prevention and control are limited. Given that humans are the only natural reservoir for GAS, prevention can be achieved only by interrupting transmission of the bacteria from an infected or colonized person to another susceptible person.

General approaches to disease prevention and control therefore include implementation of appropriate hand hygiene, environmental cleaning, and other general infection control practices such as transmission-based precautions (droplet precautions) and cohorting of ill persons in facilities (e.g., hospitals, nursing homes). In many settings, educating vulnerable persons and hospital or residence facility staff about the early signs and symptoms of GAS infection (e.g., fever, sore throat, early evidence of skin infection) can increase the speed of recognition of an infection, leading to timely evaluation and management by healthcare providers. Other important tenets of general GAS control include: reducing crowding when possible (e.g., among military recruits); controlling skin lesions through wound management (particularly in nursing homes),[149] varicella vaccination, and scabies control[186]; and preventing other respiratory infections (e.g., influenza) that increase the risk of GAS infections through influenza vaccination and cough etiquette.

Targeted approaches to prevention of new GAS infections in the setting of an outbreak include eradication of GAS colonization and rapid identification and treatment of those with GAS infections to reduce the risk of additional GAS infections among close contacts, including residents and staff.

Public health authorities and professional societies from multiple countries have developed guidance for public health responses to GAS infections.[178,182,187] Specific steps differ by country and by public health organization. However, development of effective public health guidance typically takes into consideration the following factors: burden and severity of the disease, including the urgency of disease control; evidence supporting effectiveness of any proposed intervention; cost effectiveness (e.g., direct costs, human resources); potential adverse effects; and feasibility of implementing a proposed intervention. Several settings, typically those that are closed or semi-closed, offer an opportunity for efficient control—particularly once an infection cluster is identified. These settings include households, hospitals and other acute care facilities, LTCFs, schools, and military recruit bases or ships at sea.

Examples of current public health guidance for select settings are described below.

Healthcare-associated Infections

GAS infections are typically defined as healthcare-associated if they are associated with admission to a healthcare facility (e.g., hospitals,

TABLE 155-4 NORTH AMERICAN REGIMENS FOR CHEMOPROPHYLAXIS TO PREVENT INVASIVE GROUP A STREPTOCOCCAL INFECTIONS AMONG CLOSE CONTACTS**

Antibiotic	Dosage(s)	Duration	Reference
BPG plus rifampin[a]	BPG: 600,000 U IM in 1 dose for patients weighing < 27 kg or 1,200,000 U IM in 1 dose for patients weighing ≥ 27 kg; rifampin: 20 mg/kg/day po (max. daily dose, 600 mg) in 2 divided doses per day	4 days (rifampin)	(182)
Clindamycin[b]	U.S.: 20 mg/kg/day po (max. daily dose, 900 mg) in 3 divided doses per day; Canada: (CCDR: Children: 8 to 16 mg/kg daily divided into 3 or 4 equal doses (max: 150 mg every 6 hours). Adults: 150 mg every 6 hours	10 days	(182,183)
Azithromycin[b]	12 mg/kg/day po (max. daily dose, 500 mg/day) in a single dose per day	5 days	(182)
First-generation cephalosporins: cephalexin, cephadroxil, cephradine	Children and adults: 25–50 mg/kg daily (max. 1 g/day in 2–4 divided doses)	10 days	(183)
Erythromycin[b]	Children: 5–7.5 mg/kg every 6 hours or 10–15 mg/kg every 12 hours (base) (not to exceed maximum of adult dose) Adults: 500 mg every 12 hours (base)	10 days	(183)
Clarithromycin[a]	Children: 15 mg/kg daily in divided doses every 12 hours (max: 250 mg po bid); Adults: 250 mg po bid	10 days	(183)

Abbreviations: BPG = benzathine penicillin G; max. = maximum; IM = intramuscular; po = orally/by mouth; bid = twice a day; CDC = U.S. Centers for Disease Control and Prevention; PHAC = Public Health Agency of Canada.
**This list of recommended regimens is not exhaustive; it reflects public health recommendations in Canada and the United States.
[a]Rifampin and clarithromycin are not recommended for pregnant women.
[b]Sensitivity testing is necessary in areas where high macrolide or clindamycin resistance is documented.

nursing homes) or with an intervention performed in a healthcare facility. Healthcare-associated infections found in nursing homes are discussed in more depth below. To distinguish from community-acquired infections, GAS infections have been considered healthcare-associated if illness onset occurs >48 hours after admission and up to 7 days after discharge from a healthcare facility.[73] GAS infections are typically defined as postpartum infections when they occur in a new mother up to 7 days following delivery or hospital discharge.[73,182] Both postsurgical and postpartum patients are likely at increased risk for GAS infection in healthcare settings because of the presence of surgical wounds and exposure to multiple medical personnel who may unknowingly harbor GAS. GAS healthcare-associated infections occur at a low frequency in acute care facilities, likely due to existing standards of infection control and short duration of hospitalization.[188] However, clusters still occur. Investigations of healthcare-associate GAS clusters have identified both healthcare personnel (HCP)-to-patient and patient-to-patient transmission.[73,189]

Asymptomatic HCPs have been documented to be colonized with outbreak strains of GAS in body sites including the oropharynx (most common), nonintact skin, the rectum, and the vagina.[73,182] Colonized HCPs who are epidemiologically linked to confirmed healthcare-associated cases provide a potential means for targeted intervention. Some recommendations in the United States promote enhanced surveillance for GAS infections in a healthcare facility after a single postpartum or postsurgical case is identified, and screening for GAS colonization among all epidemiologically linked HCP after a potential cluster (two or more cases of the same GAS strain) is identified.[182] In such circumstances, existing recommendations indicate that HCPs found to harbor the organism should be treated with antibiotics and suspended from direct patient care for at least the first 24 hours of administration of an appropriate antibiotic and while symptomatic[190]; some experts suggest that personnel with direct patient contact in high-risk settings such as operating rooms be suspended from patient care responsibilities for at least 24 hours, but longer if the HCP remains ill or febrile. Some guidelines suggest that the duration of exclusion from work should be decided on a case-by-case basis if HCP carriage is confirmed to be linked to an outbreak—depending on the clinical situation, the likelihood of further transmission, colonization site, and evidence of previous transmission.[191] If epidemiologically linked cases continue to occur, it has been recommended that household members of colonized or ill HCPs should be screened for GAS[182]; for example, specimens collected from the throat and skin lesions should be cultured for GAS to detect potential colonization.

Food service workers can also be a source of GAS transmission in healthcare settings and other facilities such as schools. Recommendations from the U.S. Food and Drug Administration indicate that those with positive GAS cultures should be treated and restricted from food service or food preparation until they have been on appropriate antibiotics for more than 24 hours, have at least one negative GAS throat culture, or are determined by a provider to be free of GAS infection (https://www.fda.gov/food/fda-food-code/food-code-2017).

Long-term Care Facilities

People residing in assisted living facilities or nursing homes are at increased risk for both acquiring and dying from GAS infections as a result of multiple risk factors: advanced age, crowding, presence of nonintact skin, increased frequency of influenza infection, and other underlying chronic medical conditions.[147,149] In such facilities, GAS may be introduced through new residents, staff, and visitors who are either colonized or infected.[121,149] In some instances, staff work while ill with pharyngitis, often because of inadequate sick leave policies.[192] This increases risk of transmission. Once introduced, disease transmission among this vulnerable population is often aided by substandard infection control practices.[44,149,193] Transmission is typically person-to-person. Multiple outbreaks in the United States have occurred among nursing home residents with wounds; in these settings, additional transmission is thought to have occurred as a result of inadequate infection control.[43,194]

In general, recommendations indicate that active surveillance for GAS infections should be initiated among both residents and facility staff and infection control practices should be critically assessed and lapses corrected as soon as a potential GAS outbreak is identified. Focus for active case finding and for investigation of appropriate infection control practices should be placed on residents with wounds, especially open wounds. Screening for colonization among staff or residents should start with focused, limited screening for colonization among residents and staff with epidemiologic links to infected residents (e.g., residents on the same ward or floor, and staff working directly with GAS-infected residents) and subsequent use of antibiotic prophylaxis among those found to be GAS-colonized. In some residential settings, more extensive screening and prophylaxis of both residents and staff may be necessary, depending on evidence for ongoing transmission, effectiveness of initial efforts at disease control, and local resource capacity.[178,183] In-service education sessions for care providers, staff and food service workers are an important component of prevention and response activities.

Household Settings

Studies conducted in multiple countries have attempted to quantify the risk of secondary severe (invasive) infections among household contacts. Household contacts were typically defined as those who spent > 24 hours in the same house as an index case during the 7 days prior to symptom onset. In the United States, Canada, the United Kingdom, and Australia the background incidence of sporadic invasive GAS infections when these studies were conducted ranged from 2.4 to 3.5 per 100,000 population per year. The attack rate of invasive disease among household contacts in the 30 days following exposure to the index case ranged from 804 to 5468 cases per 100,000 person-years (pooled attack rate: 2681 per 100,000 person-years). However, it must be noted that these numbers are based on a total of only 13 secondary GAS infections among household contacts in four countries.[170,193,195–197]

Published recommendations for managing household contacts of patients with invasive GAS disease vary by country. Recommendations from the U.S. Centers for Disease Control and Prevention published in 2002 do not advocate for routine use of antibiotics among all household contacts; however, they state that healthcare providers may consider offering prophylaxis to contacts who are at increased risk for severe disease (e.g., elderly, persons with chronic underlying conditions such as diabetes). Guidance from the United Kingdom's Health Protection Agency published in 2004 recommends that routine antibiotic prophylaxis be given to mothers and their infants if either develops GAS infection during the neonatal period.[187] In Canada, the Ontario Group A Streptococcal Study Group Recommendations published in 2006 state that antibiotics should be offered to household contacts who were in close contact with any index patient with confirmed severe disease (e.g., STSS, necrotizing fasciitis, or meningitis) during the week before onset of illness in the index patient.[183] As additional evidence becomes available to quantify the risk of disease in household contacts and the benefits of prophylaxis, or to identify subgroups of household contacts at particularly increased risk for secondary infection, it may be possible to refine these recommendations.

Although recommendations vary across countries, all endorse educating exposed household contacts about the early signs and symptoms of infection and the need to rapidly seek appropriate medical care. Heightened suspicion for disease should be maintained for at least 30 days after contact with the index case while the index case is ill with GAS infection.[182] Some experts recommend that all household contacts of invasive cases receive prophylaxis and that special attention should be paid to school-aged children who are household contacts, as they often harbor the organism and may serve as a source of GAS disease spread.

Other Congregate Settings: Schools, Daycare, and Military

Outbreaks of pharyngitis, scarlet fever, and impetigo are common and occur mostly among school and preschool populations.[67,196,198] Disease control efforts focus on improved hand-hygiene and exclusion from school until effective antibiotics have been administered for ≥ 12 hours and the child is afebrile and otherwise well-appearing.[101,199] In some populations, scabies treatment also may improve control of impetigo.[200]

Outbreaks of invasive GAS disease in daycare or other childcare centers are rare but are documented. Because varicella infection (chicken pox) significantly increases the risk of invasive GAS disease, routine varicella vaccination protocols are recommended where available. In two Canadian studies conducted before nationwide use of varicella vaccine, 15–25% of invasive GAS infections among children were associated with antecedent varicella infection.[201,202] The risk is significantly increased in the 2 weeks immediately following onset of varicella infection.[202] In all outbreaks, schools should inform parents and guardians about the signs and symptoms of GAS infection. Canadian recommendations published in 2006 suggest chemoprophylaxis be administered to all children and staff among family or home day care centers if one severe infection (defined as meningitis, STSS, and/or soft tissue necrosis) in a child attending this type of childcare setting is identified.[183] In group or institutional childcare centers and preschools, chemoprophylaxis is not generally recommended following an invasive infection unless more than one case is identified within 1 month, or a concurrent outbreak of varicella is identified.[183]

Outbreaks of GAS infections, including scarlet fever, cellulitis, GAS pneumonia, and ARF, have impacted the military population for decades in many countries. A significant burden of GAS infections has occurred among military recruit training bases during the first month of training.[203] Due to the frequency and severity of GAS outbreaks in training centers, preventive measures have been employed, including engineering controls such as enhanced air ventilation, head-to-foot bed orientation in the barracks, and increasing space per occupant.[204] Intramuscular BPG has been used extensively by the U.S. military since the mid-1950s to prevent and to control GAS outbreaks.[205,206] Extensive studies of military recruits occurred during the late 1940s and early 1950s at the U.S. Francis E. Warren Air Force Base, where the efficacy of penicillin in preventing rheumatic fever was established.[207] The most commonly employed strategy among military populations is to provide chemoprophylaxis (e.g., BPG, azithromycin [where resistance not found]) to incoming recruits.[205] Beginning in the early 1980s, both the U.S. Navy Training Center in San Diego and all U.S. Army basic training centers stopped prophylaxis, based on a perception of low GAS disease risk. However, in 1986, ten recruits at the San Diego facility developed ARF and six developed GAS pneumonia.[208] In addition, between 1988 and 1991, five outbreaks of GAS infection occurred among recruits in Army training centers.[205] As a result, prophylaxis was reinitiated in many training centers. During 2005–06, several outbreaks occurred during periods of BPG shortages.[209]

In response to global BPG shortages in 2016 and 2017, military preventive medicine and infectious disease authorities in San Antonio and San Diego reviewed the use of routine prophylaxis in the U.S. military. In 2017, the U.S. military deferred routine GAS chemoprophylaxis decisions to individual training centers to be based on local GAS epidemiology and directed by the military preventive medicine authority.[205,210] In recruiting centers using intramuscular BPG, recruits with a penicillin allergy were prescribed weekly oral azithromycin or erythromycin.[205] Use of the two latter alternative antibiotics is dependent on the local antibiotic susceptibility patterns.

Periodic shortages of BPG[211] such as these have led to interest in the use of other antibiotics for chemoprophylaxis in the military. However, several historic studies have documented the advantage of long acting BPG over oral penicillin at a dose of 1.2 million units intramuscularly for adults.[206,212] Macrolide antibiotics, the preferred alternative to BPG, have three important disadvantages: potential decreased efficacy due to antibiotic resistance; potential for overuse and antimicrobial resistance in other pathogens such as *S. pneumoniae*[213]; and rare occurrence of prolongation of the QT interval on the electrocardiogram with associated fatal arrhythmias.[205] Effective GAS vaccines could provide the most effective preventive tool for military training centers, but such vaccines are not yet available.

Secondary Prevention of RHD

Since the etiologic role of GAS in the pathogenesis of rheumatic fever (and subsequent rheumatic valvular heart disease) is accepted, continuous use of an antibiotic by individuals who have had an initial attack of ARF ("secondary prophylaxis") to prevent recurrent streptococcal infections has been the worldwide standard for more than half a century. Numerous comparative studies have confirmed that secondary antibiotic prophylaxis is very effective. Comparative studies in several locales have demonstrated that repository BPG is more effective than oral penicillin preparations and more effective than sulfadiazine for the prevention of recurrent infection.[214,215]

Use of Targeted Measures and Mass Antibiotic Prophylaxis for Outbreak Control

Targeted measures often used to successfully control GAS outbreaks include rapid identification and treatment of new infections, screening and antibiotic treatment of asymptomatic GAS colonization, and identification and remediation of lapses in infection control in closed or semi-closed facilities (e.g., hospital ward, nursing homes). In some situations, an outbreak continues despite these measures. Reasons for failure of targeted antibiotics include: failure to identify (false negative test results or incomplete screening) and treat all GAS-colonized persons; failure of the antibiotic regimen to eradicate colonization; failures of infection control; and ping-pong transmission of GAS from a person who is colonized to a previously noncolonized person prior to antibiotic treatment.

Mass prophylaxis—administering prophylactic antibiotics to an entire cohort of persons at increased risk for infection—is typically undertaken to stop persistent, ongoing disease transmission or sequelae when more targeted methods (e.g., providing antibiotics only to persons who are found to be ill with or colonized with GAS upon screening) to control disease have failed. Factors that would justify the use of mass prophylaxis include a failure of targeted antibiotic treatment to stop an outbreak in a semiclosed facility (e.g., LTCFs, schools, or military recruits) or a rapidly progressing outbreak. Mass prophylaxis has been shown to successfully control prolonged or recurrent GAS outbreaks among residents of LTCFs.[175,216]

GAS VACCINES: POSSIBILITIES FOR THE FUTURE

Research on the development of GAS vaccine candidates has intensified following the revocation in 2006 of a 1979 U.S. FDA resolution that prohibited the use of GAS organisms or their derivatives in any bacterial vaccine.[217,218] This resolution was based on concerns about the theoretical risk of autoimmunity that were raised by a single study in 1969 using a relatively impure type 3 M protein vaccine. In that study, ARF occurred in three vaccinated children who already had documented GAS infection one to 5 months prior to receiving the vaccine and were siblings of ARF patients.[217,219] No similar adverse events have been identified in the limited number of studies completed since vaccine development research resumed[217]; recent studies have reported use of more purified antigens than were used in the 1969 study.

Two candidate vaccines were under evaluation in human trials as of early 2021: MJ8VAX, a 29-amino acid long peptide (J8) from the conserved carboxyl terminus of the M protein,[220] and 30-valent StreptAnova®, an M protein-based vaccine with 4 recombinant subunits of N-terminal fragments of 30 diverse *emm* types linked in tandem.[221] The 30-valent vaccine is an advanced formulation of a 26-valent M protein that was reported to be safe and immunogenic in healthy adults.[222] Based on growing knowledge of *emm* diversity globally, the vaccine was expanded to include 30 *emm* types.[223] The coverage of the 30-valent vaccine may be even greater than 30 *emm* types; evidence for cross-opsonic antibodies against nonvaccine serotypes has been demonstrated *in vitro* following vaccination with the 30-valent vaccine, although the clinical significance of this remains to be determined.[221] Other antigen discovery efforts are also underway.[220]

Recently, development of GAS vaccines has received coordinated, global support. In 2014, the World Health Organization (WHO) product development for vaccines advisory committee (PD-VAC) prioritized the development of GAS vaccines.[224] The governments of Australia and New Zealand also jointly funded the formation of the Coalition to Advance New Vaccines for Group A Streptococcus (CANVAS), which proposes to accelerate the development of GAS vaccines for these two countries with high rates of ARF among their indigenous populations and other high-risk settings.[217] In a 2018 resolution on RHD, the World Health Assembly highlighted the interest in GAS vaccines to complement available control strategies (71st WHA).[225] In 2019 a Strep A Vaccine Consortium (named SAVAC) was formed with support by the Wellcome Trust. SAVAC is working with the WHO to outline the global health investment benefits and the industry business case for a GAS vaccine through development of a Public Health Value Proposition.[226]

The WHO recently published preferred product characteristics for GAS vaccines and a research and development technology roadmap. These two documents provide regulatory and policy decision-makers with an actionable framework for vaccine development. WHO proposes that key near-term strategic goals include early demonstration of vaccine efficacy against pharyngitis and skin infections.[220] Surveillance using *emm* typing will be important to help estimate the efficacy of experimental multivalent M protein-based vaccines.[38]

References

1. Carapetis JR, Steer AC, Mulholland EK, Weber M. The global burden of group A streptococcal diseases. *Lancet Infect Dis.* 2005;5(11):685–94.
2. Bowen AC, Mahe A, Hay RJ, et al. The global epidemiology of impetigo: A systematic review of the population prevalence of impetigo and pyoderma. *PLoS One.* 2015;10(8):e0136789.
3. Nelson GE, Pondo T, Toews KA, et al. Epidemiology of invasive group A streptococcal infections in the United States, 2005–2012. *Clin Infect Dis.* 2016;63(4):478–86.
4. Martins TB, Veasy LG, Hill HR. Antibody responses to group A streptococcal infections in acute rheumatic fever. *Pediatr Infect Dis J.* 2006;25(9):832–7.
5. Soler-Soler J, Galve E. Worldwide perspective of valve disease. *Heart.* 2000;83(6):721–5.
6. Bessen DE, Smeesters PR, Beall BW. Molecular epidemiology, ecology, and evolution of group A streptococci. *Microbiol Spectr.* 2018;6(5).
7. Kaplan E. Global assessment of rheumatic fever and rheumatic heart disease at the close of the century. Influences and dynamics of populations and pathogens: A failure to realize prevention? *Circulation.* 1993;88:1964–72.
8. Lancefield RC. The immunological relationships of *Streptococcus viridans* and certain of its chemical fractions: I. Serological reactions obtained with antibacterial sera. *J Exp Med.* 1925;42(3):377–95.
9. Lancefield RC. Current knowledge of type-specific M antigens of group A streptococci. *J Immunol.* 1962;89:307–13.
10. Facklam R. What happened to the streptococci: Overview of taxonomic and nomenclature changes. *Clin Microbiol Rev.* 2002;15(4):613–30.
11. Hook EW, Wagner RR, Lancefield RC. An epizootic in swiss mice caused by a group A *Streptococcus*, newly designated type 501. *Am J Epid.* 1960;72(1):111–9.
12. Wilson KS, Maroney SA, Gander RM. The family pet as an unlikely source of group A beta-hemolytic streptococcal infection in humans. *Pediatr Infect Dis J.* 1995;14(5):372–5.
13. Hansen SM, Uldbjerg N, Kilian M, Sorensen UB.: Dynamics of *Streptococcus agalactiae* colonization in women during and after pregnancy and in their infants. *J Clin Microbiol.* 2004;42(1):83–9.
14. Hickman ME, Rench MA, Ferrieri P, Baker CJ. Changing epidemiology of group B streptococcal colonization. *Pediatrics.* 1999;104(2 Pt 1):203–9.
15. Centers for Disease Control and Prevention (CDC). Trends in perinatal group B streptococcal disease—United States, 2000–2006. *MMWR Morb Mortal Wkly Rep.* 2009;58(5):109–12.
16. Johri AK, Lata H, Yadav P, et al. Epidemiology of group B *Streptococcus* in developing countries. *Vaccine.* 2013;31(Suppl 4):D43–5.
17. Pitts SI, Maruthur NM, Langley GE, et al. Obesity, diabetes, and the risk of invasive group B streptococcal disease in nonpregnant adults in the United States. *Open Forum Infect Dis.* 2018;5(6):ofy030.
18. Fortin M, Higgins R. Mixed infection associated with a group B *Streptococcus* in a dog. *Can Vet J.* 2001;42(9):730.

19. Lyhs U, Kulkas L, Katholm J, et al. *Streptococcus agalactiae* serotype IV in humans and cattle, Northern Europe. *Emerg Infect Dis.* 2016;22(12):2097–103.
20. Belard S, Toepfner N, Arnold B, Alabi AS, Berner R. Beta-hemolytic streptococcal throat carriage and tonsillopharyngitis: A cross-sectional prevalence study in Gabon, Central Africa. *Infection.* 2015;43(2):177–83.
21. Rantala S. *Streptococcus dysgalactiae* subsp. equisimilis bacteremia: An emerging infection. *Eur J Clin Microbiol Infect Dis.* 2014;33(8):1303–10.
22. Rossler S, Berner R, Jacobs E, Toepfner N. Prevalence and molecular diversity of invasive *Streptococcus dysgalactiae* and *Streptococcus pyogenes* in a German tertiary care medical centre. *Eur J Clin Microbiol Infect Dis.* 2018;37(7):1325–32.
23. Chandnani HK, Jain R, Patamasucon P. Group C *Streptococcus* causing rheumatic heart disease in a child. *J Emerg Med.* 2015;49(1):12–4.
24. Pinto SW, Mastroianni-Kirsztajn G, Sesso R. Ten-year follow-up of patients with epidemic post infectious glomerulonephritis. *PLoS One.* 2015;10(5):e0125313.
25. Mioni MSR, Castro FFC, Moreno LZ, et al. Septicemia due to *Streptococcus dysgalactiae* subspecies *dysgalactiae* in vampire bats (*Desmodus rotundus*). *Sci Rep.* 2018;8(1):9772.
26. Pesavento PA, Hurley KF, Bannasch MJ, Artiushin S, Timoney JF. A clonal outbreak of acute fatal hemorrhagic pneumonia in intensively housed (shelter) dogs caused by *Streptococcus equi* subsp. *zooepidemicus*. *Vet Pathol.* 2008;45(1):51–3.
27. Schrieber L, Towers R, Muscatellö G, Speare R. Transmission of *Streptococcus dysgalactiae* subsp. *equisimilis* between child and dog in an aboriginal Australian community. *Zoonosis Public Health.* 2014;61(2):145–8.
28. DeAngelo AJ, Dooley DP, Skidmore PJ, Kopecky CT. Group F streptococcal bacteremia complicating a Bartholin's abscess. *Infect Dis Obstet Gynecol.* 2001;9(1):55–7.
29. Libertin CR, Hermans PE, Washington JA 2nd. Beta-hemolytic group f streptococcal bacteremia: A study and review of the literature. *Rev Infect Dis.* 1985;7(4):498–503.
30. Taurisano ND, Butler BP, Stone D, et al. *Streptococcus phocae* in marine mammals of Northeastern Pacific and Arctic Canada: A retrospective analysis of 85 postmortem investigations. *J Wildl Dis.* 2018;54(1):101–11.
31. Ihms EA, Daniels JB, Koivisto CS, Barrie MT, Russell DS. Fatal *Streptococcus anginosus*-associated pneumonia in a captive sumatran orangutan (*Pongo abelii*). *J Med Primatol.* 2014;43(1):48–51.
32. Broyles LN, Van Beneden C, Beall B, et al. Population-based study of invasive disease due to beta-hemolytic streptococci of groups other than A and B. *Clin Infect Dis.* 2009;48(6):706–12.
33. Yamaguchi T, Kawahara R, Katsukawa C, et al. Foodborne outbreak of group G streptococcal pharyngitis in a school dormitory in Osaka, Japan. *J Clin Microbiol.* 2018;56(5):e01884-17.
34. Miller CW, Prescott JF, Mathews KA, et al. Streptococcal toxic shock syndrome in dogs. *J Am Vet Med Assoc.* 1996;209(8):1421–6.
35. Tsuyuki Y, Kurita G, Murata Y, Goto M, Takahashi T. Identification of group G streptococcal isolates from companion animals in Japan and their antimicrobial resistance patterns. *Jpn J Infect Dis.* 2017;70(4):394–8.
36. Maxted WR, Widdowson JP, Fraser CAM, Ball LC, Bassett DCJ. The use of the serum opacity reaction in the typing of group A streptococci. *J Med Microbiol.* 1973;6(1):83–90.
37. Griffith F. The serological classification of *Streptococcus pyogenes*. *J Hyg.* 1934;34(04):542–84.
38. Sanderson-Smith M, De Oliveira DMP, Guglielmini J, et al. A systematic and functional classification of *Streptococcus pyogenes* that serves as a new tool for molecular typing and vaccine development. *J Infect Dis.* 2014;210(8):1325–38.
39. Beall B, Facklam R, Thompson T. Sequencing *emm*-specific pcr products for routine and accurate typing of group A streptococci. *J Clin Microbiol.* 1996;34(4):953–8.
40. Enright MC, Spratt BG, Kalia A, Cross JH, Bessen DE. Multilocus sequence typing of *Streptococcus pyogenes* and the relationships between *emm* type and clone. *Infect Immun.* 2001;69(4):2416–27.
41. Maiden MCJ, Bygraves JA, Feil E, et al. Multilocus sequence typing: A portable approach to the identification of clones within populations of pathogenic microorganisms. *Proc Natl Acad Sci U S A.* 1998;95(6):3140–5.
42. Chochua S, Metcalf BJ, Li Z, et al. Population and whole genome sequence based characterization of invasive group A streptococci recovered in the United States during 2015. *mBio.* 2017;8(5):e01422-17.
43. Nanduri SA, Metcalf BJ, Arwady MA, et al. Prolonged and large outbreak of invasive group A *Streptococcus* disease within a nursing home: Repeated intrafacility transmission of a single strain. *Clin Microbiol Infect.* 2019;25(2):248.e1–7.
44. Mosites E, Frick A, Gounder P, et al. Outbreak of invasive infections from subtype *emm* 26.3 group A *Streptococcus* among homeless adults—Anchorage, Alaska, 2016–2017. *Clin Infect Dis.* 2017;66(7):1068–74.
45. Turner CE, Bedford L, Brown NM, et al. Community outbreaks of group A *Streptococcus* revealed by genome sequencing. *Sci Rep.* 2017;7(1):8554.
46. Zhu L, Olsen RJ, Nasser W, et al. A molecular trigger for intercontinental epidemics of group A *Streptococcus*. *J Clin Invest.* 2015;125(9):3545–59.
47. Zhu L, Olsen RJ, Nasser W, de la Riva Morales I, Musser JM. Trading capsule for increased cytotoxin production: Contribution to virulence of a newly emerged clade of *emm* 89 *Streptococcus pyogenes*. *mBio.* 2015;6(5):e01378-15.
48. Nasser W, Beres SB, Olsen RJ, et al. Evolutionary pathway to increased virulence and epidemic group A *Streptococcus* disease derived from 3,615 genome sequences. *Proc Natl Acad Sci U S A.* 2014;111:E1768–76.
49. Gargis AS, Kalman L, Lubin IM. Assuring the quality of next-generation sequencing in clinical microbiology and public health laboratories. *J Clin Microbiol.* 2016;54(12):2857–65.
50. Parks T, Smeesters PR, Steer AC. Streptococcal skin infection and rheumatic heart disease. *Curr Opin Infect Dis.* 2012;25(2):145–53.
51. Baldwin DS. Chronic glomerulonephritis: Nonimmunologic mechanisms of progressive glomerular damage. *Kidney Int.* 1982;21(1):109–20.
52. Lien JW, Mathew TH, Meadows R. Acute post-streptococcal glomerulonephritis in adults: A long-term study. *Q J Med.* 1979;48(189):99–111.
53. Hoy WE, White AV, Dowling A, et al. Post-streptococcal glomerulonephritis is a strong risk factor for chronic kidney disease in later life. *Kidney Int.* 2012;81(10):1026–32.
54. Cannon JW, Jack S, Wu Y, et al. An economic case for a vaccine to prevent group A *Streptococcus* skin infections. *Vaccine.* 2018;36(46):6968–78.
55. Kaplan E, Kunde C. A quantitative evaluation of variation in composition of the streptozyme agglutination reagent for detection of antibodies to group A streptococcal extracellular antigens. *J Clin Microbiol.* 1981;14(6):678–80.
56. Martin JM. The *Streptococcus pyogenes* carrier state. In: Ferretti J, Stevens D, Fischetti V, eds. *Streptococcus Pyogenes: Basic Biology to Clinical Manifestations*. Oklahoma City: University of Oklahoma Health Sciences Center; 2016.
57. Kaplan E. The group A streptococcal upper respiratory tract carrier state: An enigma. *J Ped.* 1980;97(3):337–45.
58. Gordis L, Lilienfeld A, Rodriguez R. Studies in the epidemiology and preventability of rheumatic fever. I. Demographic factors and the incidence of acute attacks. *J Chronic Dis.* 1969;21(9):645–54.
59. Hysmith ND, Kaplan EL, Cleary PP, Johnson DR, Penfound TA, Dale JB. Prospective longitudinal analysis of immune responses in pediatric subjects after pharyngeal acquisition of group A streptococci. *J Ped Infect Dis.* 2017;6(2):187–96.
60. Johnson DR, Kurlan R, Leckman J, Kaplan EL. The human immune response to streptococcal extracellular antigens: Clinical, diagnostic, and potential pathogenetic implications. *Clin Infect Dis.* 2010;50(4):481–90.
61. Shaikh N, Leonard E, Martin JM. Prevalence of streptococcal pharyngitis and streptococcal carriage in children: A meta-analysis. *Pediatrics.* 2010;126(3):e557–64.
62. Ditchburn R, Ditchburn J. Rate of carriage of group A beta haemolytic streptococci. *BMJ.* 1995;311(6998):193.
63. Jounio U, Juvonen R, Bloigu A, et al. Pneumococcal carriage is more common in asthmatic than in non-asthmatic young men. *Clin Respir J.* 2010;4(4):222–9.
64. Spitzer J, Hennessy E, Neville L. High group A streptococcal carriage in the orthodox Jewish community of North Hackney. *Br J Gen Pract.* 2001;51(463):101–5.
65. Martin JM, Green M, Barbadora KA, Wald ER. Group A streptococci among school-aged children: Clinical characteristics and the carrier state. *Pediatrics.* 2004;114(5):1212–9.
66. Wannamaker LW. The epidemiology of streptococcal infections. In: *Streptococcal Infections*. New York: Columbia University Press; 1954.
67. Efstratiou A, Lamagni T. Epidemiology of *Streptococcus pyogenes*. In: Ferretti JJ, Stevens DL, Fischetti VA, eds. *Streptococcus Pyogenes: Basic Biology to Clinical Manifestations*. Oklahoma City, OK: University of Oklahoma Health Sciences Center; 2016.
68. Wannamaker LW. Perplexity and precision in the diagnosis of streptococcal pharyngitis. *Am J Dis Child.* 1972;124(3):352–8.
69. Stevens DL, Bisno AL, Chambers HF, et al. Executive summary: Practice guidelines for the diagnosis and management of skin and soft tissue

infections: 2014 Update by the Infectious Diseases Society of America. *Clin Infect Dis*. 2014;59(2):147–59.

70. Stevens D, Bryant A. Impetigo, erysipelas and cellulitis. In: Ferretti JJ, Stevens DL, Fischetti VA, eds. *Streptococcus Pyogenes: Basic Biology to Clinical Manifestations*. Oklahoma City, OK: University of Oklahoma Health Sciences Center; 2016.
71. Romani L, Steer AC, Whitfeld MJ, Kaldor JM. Prevalence of scabies and impetigo worldwide: A systematic review. *Lancet Infect Dis*. 2015;15(8):960–7.
72. Loffeld A, Davies P, Lewis A, Moss C. Seasonal occurrence of impetigo: a retrospective 8-year review (1996-2003). *Clin Exp Dermatol*. 2005;30(5):512–4. doi:10.1111/j.1365-2230.2005.01847.x. PMID: 16045681.
73. Steer AC, Lamagni T, Curtis N, Carapetis JR. Invasive group A streptococcal disease: Epidemiology, pathogenesis and management. *Drugs*. 2012;72(9):1213–27.
74. Teatero S, McGeer A, Tyrrell GJ, et al. Canada-wide epidemic of *emm*74 group A *Streptococcus* invasive disease. *Open Forum Infect Dis*. 2018;5(5):ofy085.
75. Centers for Disease Control and Prevention. Active Bacterial Core surveillance report, Emerging Infections Program network, group A Streptococcus, 2017. 2016.
76. Seale AC, Davies MR, Anampiu K, et al. Invasive group A *Streptococcus* infection among children, rural Kenya. *Emerg Infect Dis*. 2016;22(2):224–32.
77. Centers for Disease Control and Prevention. Active Bacterial Core surveillance report, Emerging Infections Program network, group A Streptococcus, 2014. 2014.
78. Centers for Disease Control and Prevention. Active Bacterial Core surveillance report, Emerging Infections Program network, group A Streptococcus, 2015. 2015.
79. Centers for Disease Control and Prevention. Active Bacterial Core surveillance report, Emerging Infections Program network, group A Streptococcus, 2016. 2016.
80. Factor SH, Levine OS, Schwartz B, et al. Invasive group A streptococcal disease: Risk factors for adults. *Emerg Infect Dis*. 2003;9(8):970–7.
81. Langley G, Hao Y, Pondo T, et al. The impact of obesity and diabetes on the risk of disease and death due to invasive group A *Streptococcus* infections in adults. *Clin Infect Dis*. 2016;62(7):845–52.
82. Linder KA, Alkhouli L, Ramesh M, Alangaden GA, Kauffman CA, Miceli MH. Effect of underlying immune compromise on the manifestations and outcomes of group A streptococcal bacteremia. *J Infect*. 2017;74(5):450–5.
83. Saavedra-Campos M, Simone B, Balasegaram S, Wright A, Usdin M, Lamagni T. Estimating the risk of invasive group A *Streptococcus* infection in care home residents in England, 2009–2010. *Epidemiol Infect*. 2017;145(13):2759–65.
84. Kaul R, McGeer A, Low DE, Green K, Schwartz B. Population-based surveillance for group A streptococcal necrotizing fasciitis: Clinical features, prognostic indicators, and microbiologic analysis of seventy-seven cases. Ontario Group A Streptococcal Study. *Am J Med*. 1997;103(1):18–24.
85. Darenberg J, Luca-Harari B, Jasir A, et al. Molecular and clinical characteristics of invasive group A streptococcal infection in Sweden. *Clin Infect Dis*. 2007;45(4):450–8.
86. Chelsom J, Halstensen A, Haga T, Hoiby EA. Necrotising fasciitis due to group A streptococci in western Norway: Incidence and clinical features. *Lancet*. 1994;344(8930):1111–5.
87. Lamagni T, Guy R, Chand M, et al. Resurgence of scarlet fever in England, 2014–16: A population-based surveillance study. *Lancet Infect Dis*. 2018;18(2):180–7.
88. You Y, Davies MR, Protani M, McIntyre L, Walker MJ, Zhang J. Scarlet fever epidemic in China caused by *Streptococcus pyogenes* serotype m12: Epidemiologic and molecular analysis. *EBioMedicine*. 2018;28:128–35.
89. Yung CF, Thoon KC. A 12 year outbreak of scarlet fever in Singapore. *Lancet Infect Dis*. 2018;18(9):942.
90. Working Group on Severe Streptococcal Infections. Defining the group A streptococcal toxic shock syndrome. Rationale and consensus definition. The working group on severe streptococcal infections. *JAMA*. 1993;269(3):390–1.
91. Centers for Disease Control and Prevention. Streptococcal toxic shock syndrome (STSS) (Streptococcus pyogenes) 2010 case definition. 2010. https://wwwn.cdc.gov/nndss/conditions/streptococcal-toxic-shock-syndrome/case-definition/2010/.
92. Schulman S, Bisno A. Nonsuppurative poststreptococcal sequelae: Rheumatic fever and glomerulonephritis. In: Bennett J, Dolin R, Blaser M, eds. *Bennett's Principles and Practice of Infectious Diseases*. Vol. 2. Philadelphia, PA: Elsevier; 2015:2300–9.
93. Gewitz MH, Baltimore RS, Tani LY, et al. Revision of the Jones criteria for the diagnosis of acute rheumatic fever in the era of Doppler echocardiography: A scientific statement from the American Heart Association. *Circulation*. 2015;131(20):1806–18.
94. Siegel A, Johnson E, Stollerman G. Controlled studies of streptococcal pharyngitis in a pediatric population. *N Engl J Med*. 1961;265:559–66.
95. Rammelkamp C, Denny F, Wannamaker L. Studies on the epidemiology of rheumatic fever in the armed services. In: *Rheumatic Fever*. Minneapolis, MN: University of Minnesota Press; 1952.
96. Land MA, Bisno AL. Acute rheumatic fever. A vanishing disease in suburbia. *JAMA*. 1983;249(7):895–8.
97. Shulman ST, Stollerman G, Beall B, Dale JB, Tanz RR. Temporal changes in streptococcal M protein types and the near-disappearance of a cute rheumatic fever in the United States. *Clin Infect Dis*. 2006;42(4): 441–7.
98. Gray BM, Stevens DL. Streptococcal infections. In: Brachman PS, Abrutyn E, eds. *Bacterial Infections of Humans: Epidemiology and Control*. 4th ed. New York: Springer; 2009.
99. Remenyi B, Wilson N, Steer A, et al. World heart federation criteria for echocardiographic diagnosis of rheumatic heart disease—An evidence-based guideline. *Nat Rev Cardiol*. 2012;9(5):297–309.
100. Nielsen MO, Kohler-Forsberg O, Hjorthoj C, Benros ME, Nordentoft M, Orlovska-Waast S. Streptococcal infections and exacerbations in pandas: A systematic review and meta-analysis. *Pediatr Infect Dis J*. 2019;38(2):189–94.
101. American Academy of Pediatrics. *Red Book: 2018 Report of the Committee on Infectious Diseases*. Elk Grove Village, IL: American Academy of Pediatrics; 2018.
102. Stollerman GH, Lewis AJ, Schultz I, Taranta A. Relationship of immune response to group A streptococci to the course of acute, chronic and recurrent rheumatic fever. *Am J Med*. 1956;20(2):163–9.
103. Wannamaker LW, Ayoub EM. Antibody titers in acute rheumatic fever. *Circulation*. 1960;21(4):598–614.
104. Bencivenga JF, Johnson DR, Kaplan E. Determination of group A streptococcal anti-M type-specific antibody in sera of rheumatic fever patients after 45 years. *Clin Infect Dis*. 2009;49:1237–9.
105. Lancefield RC. Persistence of type-specific antibodies in man following infection with group A streptococci. *J Exp Med*. 1959;110(2):271–92.
106. Kaplan E, Anthony B, Ayoub E, Wannamaker L. A two year longitudinal study of streptococcal infections in an isolated community: Antibody dynamics. In: Haverkorn M, ed. *Streptococcal Disease and the Community*. Amsterdam: Exerpta Medica Press; 1974.
107. Asteberg I, Andersson Y, Dotevall L, et al. A food-borne streptococcal sore throat outbreak in a small community. *Scand J Infect Dis*. 2006;38(11–12):988–94.
108. Culqui DR, Manzanares-Laya S, Van Der Sluis SL, et al. Group A beta-hemolytic streptococcal pharyngotonsillitis outbreak. *Rev Saude Publica*. 2014;48(2):322–5.
109. Decker MD, Lavely GB, Hutcheson RH Jr, Schaffner W. Food-borne streptococcal pharyngitis in a hospital pediatrics clinic. *JAMA*. 1985;253(5):679–81.
110. Kemble SK, Westbrook A, Lynfield R, et al. Foodborne outbreak of group A *Streptococcus* pharyngitis associated with a high school dance team banquet—Minnesota, 2012. *Clin Infect Dis*. 2013;57(5):648–54.
111. Linhart Y, Amitai Z, Lewis M, Katser S, Sheffer A, Shohat T. A food-borne outbreak of streptococcal pharyngitis. *Isr Med Assoc J*. 2008;10(8–9):617–20.
112. Arnold KE, Schweitzer JL, Wallace B, et al. Tightly clustered outbreak of group A streptococcal disease at a long-term care facility. *Infect Control Hosp Epidemiol*. 2006;27(12):1377–84.
113. Cockerill FR 3rd, MacDonald KL, Thompson RL, et al. An outbreak of invasive group A streptococcal disease associated with high carriage rates of the invasive clone among school-aged children. *JAMA*. 1997;277(1):38–43.
114. Feeney KT, Dowse GK, Keil AD, Mackaay C, McLellan D. Epidemiological features and control of an outbreak of scarlet fever in a perth primary school. *Commun Dis Intell Q Rep*. 2005;29(4):386–90.
115. Weiss K, Laverdiere M, Lovgren M, Delorme J, Poirier L, Beliveau C. Group A *Streptococcus* carriage among close contacts of patients with invasive infections. *Am J Epidemiol*. 1999;149(9):863–8.

116. Engelthaler DM, Valentine M, Bowers J, et al. Hypervirulent *emm* 59 clone in invasive group A *Streptococcus* outbreak, Southwestern United States. *Emerg Infect Dis.* 2016;22(4):734–8.
117. Veasy LG, Tani LY, Daly JA, et al. Temporal association of the appearance of mucoid strains of *Streptococcus pyogenes* with a continuing high incidence of rheumatic fever in Utah. *Pediatrics.* 2004;113(3 Pt 1):e168–72.
118. Beaudoin AL, Torso L, Richards K, et al. Invasive group A *Streptococcus* infections associated with liposuction surgery at outpatient facilities not subject to state or federal regulation. *JAMA Intern Med.* 2014;174(7):1136–42.
119. Cornick JE, Kiran AM, Vivancos R, et al. Epidemiological and molecular characterization of an invasive group A *Streptococcus emm* 32.2 outbreak. *J Clin Microbiol.* 2017;55(6):1837–46.
120. Ibrahim LA, Sellick JA, Watson EL, et al. An outbreak of severe group A *Streptococcus* infections associated with podiatric application of a biologic dermal substitute. *Infect Control Hosp Epidemiol.* 2016;37(3):306–12.
121. Kobayashi M, Lyman MM, Francois Watkins LK, et al. A cluster of group A streptococcal infections in a skilled nursing facility—The potential role of healthcare worker presenteeism. *J Am Geriatr Soc.* 2016;64(12):e279–84.
122. Mahida N, Beal A, Trigg D, Vaughan N, Boswell T. Outbreak of invasive group A *Streptococcus* infection: Contaminated patient curtains and cross-infection on an ear, nose and throat ward. *J Hosp Infect.* 2014;87(3):141–4.
123. Olufon O, Iyanger N, Cleary V, Lamagni T. An outbreak of invasive group A streptococcal infection among elderly patients receiving care from a district nursing team, October 2013—May 2014. *J Infect Prev.* 2015;16(4):174–7.
124. Qing-Zeng C, Yun-Bo S, Shi-Hai L, et al. Outbreak of infections caused by group A *Streptococcus* after modified radical mastectomy. *Surg Infect (Larchmt).* 2013;14(4):385–8.
125. Chen M, Wang W, Tu L, et al. An *emm* 5 group A streptococcal outbreak among workers in a factory manufacturing telephone accessories. *Front Microbiol.* 2017;8:1156.
126. Aoki A, Ashizawa T, Ebata A, Nasu Y, Fujii T. Group A *Streptococcus* pharyngitis outbreak among university students in a Judo club. *J Infect Chemother.* 2014;20(3):190–3.
127. Liu YM, Zhao JZ, Li BB, et al. A report on the first outbreak of a single clone group A *Streptococcus* (*emm*-type 89) tonsillopharyngitis in China. *J Microbiol Immunol Infect.* 2014;47(6):542–5.
128. Okamoto F, Murakami K, Maeda E, et al. A foodborne outbreak of group A streptococcal infection in Fukuoka Prefecture, Japan. *Jpn J Infect Dis.* 2014;67(4):321–2.
129. Ramos M, Valle R, Reaves EJ, et al. Outbreak of group A beta hemolytic *Streptococcus* pharyngitis in a Peruvian military facility, April 2012. *MSMR.* 2013;20(6):14–7.
130. Guy R, Williams C, Irvine N, et al. Increase in scarlet fever notifications in the United Kingdom, 2013/2014. *Euro Surveill.* 2014;19(12):20749.
131. Lee CF, Cowling BJ, Lau EHY. Epidemiology of reemerging scarlet fever, Hong Kong, 2005–2015. *Emerg Infect Dis.* 2017;23(10):1707–10.
132. Yang P, Peng X, Zhang D, et al. Characteristics of group A *Streptococcus* strains circulating during scarlet fever epidemic, Beijing, China, 2011. *Emerg Infect Dis.* 2013;19(6):909–15.
133. Gaibani P, Scaltriti E, Foschi C, et al. Matrix-assisted laser desorption ionization-time of flight and comparative genomic analysis of m-18 group A *Streptococcus* strains associated with an acute rheumatic fever outbreak in Northeast Italy in 2012 and 2013. *J Clin Microbiol.* 2015;53(5):1562–72.
134. Speers DJ, Levy A, Gichamo A, Eastwood A, Leung MJ. M protein gene (*emm* type) analysis of group A *Streptococcus* isolates recovered during an acute glomerulonephritis outbreak in northern Western Australia. *Pathology.* 2017;49(7):765–9.
135. Schroeder BM. Diagnosis and management of group A streptococcal pharyngitis. *Am Fam Physician.* 2003;67(4):880, 883–4.
136. Badger GF, Dingle JH, Feller AE, Hodges RG, Jordan WS Jr, Rammelkamp CH Jr. A study of illness in a group of Cleveland families: IV. The spread of respiratory infections within the home. *Am J Hyg.* 1953;58(2):174–8.
137. Woods WA, Carter CT, Stack M, Connors AF Jr, Schlager TA. Group A streptococcal pharyngitis in adults 30 to 65 years of age. *South Med J.* 1999;92(5):491–2.
138. Factor SH, Levine OS, Harrison LH, et al. Risk factors for pediatric invasive group A streptococcal disease. *Emerg Infect Dis.* 2005;11(7):1062–6.
139. Ottolini MG, Burnett MW. History of U.S. Military contributions to the study of respiratory infections. *Mil Med.* 2005;170(4 Suppl):66–70.
140. Centers for Disease Control and Prevention. Outbreak of group A streptococcal pneumonia among marine corps recruits—California, November 1–December 20, 2002. *JAMA.* 2003;289(11):1373–5.
141. Crum NF, Russell KL, Kaplan EL, et al. Pneumonia outbreak associated with group A *Streptococcus* species at a military training facility. *Clin Infect Dis.* 2005;40(4):511–8.
142. Brundage JF, Gunzenhauser JD, Longfield JN, et al. Epidemiology and control of acute respiratory diseases with emphasis on group A betahemolytic *Streptococcus*: A decade of U.S. Army experience. *Pediatrics.* 1996;97(6 Pt 2):964–70.
143. Hoe NP, Fullerton KE, Liu M, et al. Molecular genetic analysis of 675 group A *Streptococcus* isolates collected in a carrier study at Lackland Air Force Base, San Antonio, Texas. *J Infect Dis.* 2003;188(6):818–27.
144. Lee SE, Eick A, Bloom MS, Brundage JF. Influenza immunization and subsequent diagnoses of group A *Streptococcus*-illnesses among U.S. Army trainees, 2002–2006. *Vaccine.* 2008;26(27–28):3383–6.
145. Lee SE, Eick A, Ciminera P. Respiratory disease in army recruits: Surveillance program overview, 1995–2006. *Am J Prev Med.* 2008;34(5):389–95.
146. Pearson M, Fallowfield JL, Davey T, et al. Asymptomatic group A streptococcal throat carriage in royal marines recruits and young officers. *J Infect.* 2017;74(6):585–9.
147. Thigpen MC, Richards CL Jr, Lynfield R, et al. Invasive group A streptococcal infection in older adults in long-term care facilities and the community, United States, 1998–2003. *Emerg Infect Dis.* 2007;13(12):1852–9.
148. Rainbow J, Jewell B, Danila RN, et al. Invasive group A streptococcal disease in nursing homes, Minnesota, 1995–2006. *Emerg Infect Dis.* 2008;14(5):772–7.
149. Jordan HT, Richards CL Jr, Burton DC, Thigpen MC, Van Beneden CA. Group A streptococcal disease in long-term care facilities: Descriptive epidemiology and potential control measures. *Clin Infect Dis.* 2007;45(6):742–52.
150. Bocking N, Matsumoto CL, Loewen K, et al. High incidence of invasive group A streptococcal infections in remote indigenous communities in Northwestern Ontario, Canada. *Open Forum Infect Dis.* 2017;4(1):ofw243.
151. Boyd R, Patel M, Currie BJ, Holt DC, Harris T, Krause V. High burden of invasive group A streptococcal disease in the Northern Territory of Australia. *Epidemiol Infect.* 2016;144(5):1018–27.
152. May PJ, Bowen AC, Carapetis JR. The inequitable burden of group A streptococcal diseases in indigenous Australians. *Med J Aust.* 2016;205(5):201–3.
153. Rudolph K, Bruce MG, Bruden D, et al. Epidemiology of invasive group A streptococcal disease in Alaska, 2001 to 2013. *J Clin Microbiol.* 2016;54(1):134–41.
154. Williamson DA, Morgan J, Hope V, et al. Increasing incidence of invasive group A *Streptococcus* disease in New Zealand, 2002–2012: A national population-based study. *J Infect.* 2015;70(2):127–34.
155. Anthony BF, Kaplan EL, Wannamaker LW, Chapman SS. The dynamics of streptococcal infections in a defined population of children: Serotypes associated with skin and respiratory infections. *Am J Epidemiol.* 1976;104(6):652–66.
156. Bundle N, Bubba L, Coelho J, et al. Ongoing outbreak of invasive and non-invasive disease due to group A *Streptococcus* (GAS) type *emm* 66 among homeless and people who inject drugs in England and Wales, January to December 2016. *Euro Surveill.* 2017;22(3):30446.
157. Mosites E, Frick A, Gounder P, et al. Outbreak of invasive infections from subtype *emm*26.3 group A *Streptococcus* among homeless adults—Anchorage, Alaska, 2016–2017. *Clin Infect Dis.* 2018;66(7):1068–74.
158. Sierra JM, Sanchez F, Castro P, et al. Group A streptococcal infections in injection drug users in Barcelona, Spain: Epidemiologic, clinical, and microbiologic analysis of 3 clusters of cases from 2000 to 2003. *Medicine (Baltimore).* 2006;85(3):139–46.
159. Valenciano SJ, McMullen C, Torres S, Smelser C, Matanock A, Van Beneden C. Notes from the field: Identifying risk behaviors for invasive group A *Streptococcus* infections among persons who inject drugs and persons experiencing homelessness—New Mexico, May 2018. *MMWR Morb Mortal Wkly Rep.* 2019;68(8):205–6.
160. Valenciano SJ, Onukwube J, Spiller MW, et al. Invasive group A streptococcal infections among people who inject drugs and people experiencing homelessness in the United States, 2010–2017. *Clin Infect Dis.* 2020;ciaa787, https://doi.org/10.1093/cid/ciaa787.
161. Aldridge RW, Story A, Hwang SW, et al. Morbidity and mortality in homeless individuals, prisoners, sex workers, and individuals with substance use disorders in high-income countries: A systematic review and meta-analysis. *Lancet.* 2018;391(10117):241–50.

162. Fazel S, Geddes JR, Kushel M. The health of homeless people in high-income countries: Descriptive epidemiology, health consequences, and clinical and policy recommendations. *Lancet*. 2014;384(9953):1529–40.
163. Shulman ST, Bisno AL, Clegg HW, et al. Executive summary: Clinical practice guideline for the diagnosis and management of group A streptococcal pharyngitis: 2012 Update by the Infectious Diseases Society of America. *Clin Infect Dis*. 2012;55(10):1279–82.
164. Matthys J, De Meyere M, van Driel ML, De Sutter A. Differences among international pharyngitis guidelines: Not just academic. *Ann Fam Med*. 2007;5(5):436–43.
165. Tanz RR, Gewitz M, Kaplan E, Shulman ST. Stay the course: Targeted evaluation, accurate diagnosis, and treatment of streptococcal pharyngitis prevent acute rheumatic fever. *J Pediatr*. 2020;216:208–12.
166. Gerber MA. Five vs ten days of penicillin v therapy for streptococcal pharyngitis. *Arch Pediatr Adolesc Med*. 1987;141(2):224.
167. Harris AM, Hicks LA, Qaseem A. Appropriate antibiotic use for acute respiratory tract infection in adults: Advice for high-value care from the American College of Physicians and the Centers for Disease Control and Prevention. *Ann Intern Med*. 2016;164(6):425–34.
168. Stevens DL. Group A beta-hemolytic streptococci: Virulence factors, pathogenesis, and spectrum of clinical infections. In: Stevens D, Kaplan E, eds. *Streptococcal Infections. Clinical Aspects, Microbiology' and Molecular Pathogenesis*. New York: Oxford University Press; 2000.
169. Linner A, Darenberg J, Sjolin J, Henriques-Normark B, Norrby-Teglund A. Clinical efficacy of polyspecific intravenous immunoglobulin therapy in patients with streptococcal toxic shock syndrome: A comparative observational study. *Clin Infect Dis*. 2014;59(6):851–7.
170. Carapetis JR, Jacoby P, Carville K, Ang SJJ, Curtis N, Andrews R. Effectiveness of clindamycin and intravenous immunoglobulin, and risk of disease in contacts, in invasive group A streptococcal infections. *Clin Infect Dis*. 2014;59(3):358–65.
171. Darenberg J, Ihendyane N, Sjolin J, et al. Intravenous immunoglobulin g therapy in streptococcal toxic shock syndrome: A European randomized, double-blind, placebo-controlled trial. *Clin Infect Dis*. 2003;37(3):333–40.
172. Kaul R, McGeer A, Norrby-Teglund A, et al. Intravenous immunoglobulin therapy for streptococcal toxic shock syndrome—A comparative observational study. *Clin Infect Dis*. 1999;28(4):800–7.
173. Parks T, Wilson C, Curtis N, Norrby-Teglund A, Sriskandan S. Polyspecific intravenous immunoglobulin in clindamycin-treated patients with streptococcal toxic shock syndrome: A systematic review and meta-analysis. *Clin Infect Dis*. 2018;67(9):1434–6.
174. American Academy of Pediatrics. Group A streptococcal infections. In: Kimberlin D, Brady M, Jackson M, Long S, eds. *Red Book: 2018 Report of the Committee on Infectious Diseases*. Itasca, IL: American Academy of Pediatrics; 2018:748.
175. Smith A, Li A, Tolomeo O, Tyrrell GJ, Jamieson F, Fisman D. Mass antibiotic treatment for group A *Streptococcus* outbreaks in two long-term care facilities. *Emerg Infect Dis*. 2003;9(10):1260–5.
176. Greene C, Vanbeneden C, Javadi M, et al. Cluster of deaths from group A *Streptococcus* in a long-term care facility, Georgia, 2001. *Am J Infect Control*. 2005;33(2):108–13.
177. Auerbach SB, Schwartz B, Williams D, et al. Outbreak of invasive group A streptococcal infections in a nursing home: Lessons on prevention and control. *Arch Intern Med*. 1992;152(5):1017–22.
178. Li YA, Martin I, Tsang R, Squires SG, Demczuk W, Desai S. Invasive bacterial diseases in Northern Canada, 2006-2013. *Can Commun Dis Rep*. 2016;42(4):74–80.
179. Tanz RR, Shulman ST, Barthel MJ, Willert C, Yogev R. Penicillin plus rifampin eradicates pharyngeal carriage of group A streptococci. *J Pediatr*. 1985;106(6):876–80.
180. Casey JR, Pichichero ME. Meta-analysis of cephalosporins versus penicillin for treatment of group A streptococcal tonsillopharyngitis in adults. *Clin Infect Dis*. 2004;38(11):1526–34.
181. Casey JR, Pichichero ME. Meta-analysis of cephalosporin versus penicillin treatment of group A streptococcal tonsillopharyngitis in children. *Pediatrics*. 2004;113(4):866–82.
182. Prevention of invasive group A streptococcal disease among household contacts of case patients and among postpartum and postsurgical patients: Recommendations from the Centers for Disease Control and Prevention. *Clin Infect Dis*. 2002;35(8):950–9.
183. Public Health Agency of Canada. Guidelines for the prevention and control of invasive group A streptococcal disease. CCDR. 2006.
184. Vannice KS, Ricaldi J, Nanduri S, et al. Streptococcus pyogenes pbp2x mutation confers reduced susceptibility to β-lactam antibiotics. *Clin Infect Dis*. 2020;71(1):201–4. doi:10.1093/cid/ciz1000. Erratum in: *Clin Infect Dis*. 2020;70(6):1265. PMID: 31630171; PMCID: PMC7167332.
185. Leclercq R. Mechanisms of resistance to macrolides and lincosamides: Nature of the resistance elements and their clinical implications. *Clin Infect Dis*. 2002;34(4):482–92.
186. Heukelbach J, Mazigo HD, Ugbomoiko US. Impact of scabies in resource-poor communities. *Curr Opin Infect Dis*. 2013;26(2):127–32.
187. Health Protection Agency, Group A Streptococcus Working Group. Interim UK guidelines for management of close community contacts of invasive group A streptococcal disease. 2004.
188. de Almeida Torres RS, dos Santos TZ, Torres RA, et al. Management of contacts of patients with severe invasive group A streptococcal infection. *J Pediatric Infect Dis Soc*. 2016;5(1):47–52.
189. Daneman N, Green KA, Low DE, et al. Surveillance for hospital outbreaks of invasive group A streptococcal infections in Ontario, Canada, 1992 to 2000. *Ann Intern Med*. 2007;147(4):234.
190. US Public Health Service and Food and Drug Administration. Food code. Recommendations of the US Public Health Service and Food and Drug Administration. 2017. https://www.fda.gov/media/110822/download. 5/10/19.
191. Steer JA, Lamagni T, Healy B, et al. Guidelines for prevention and control of group A streptococcal infection in acute healthcare and maternity settings in the UK. *J Infect*. 2012;64(1):1–18.
192. Kobayashi M, Lyman MM, Francois Watkins LK, et al. A cluster of group A streptococcal infections in a skilled nursing facility—The potential role of healthcare worker presenteeism. *J Am Geriatr Soc*. 2016;64(12):e279–84.
193. Robinson KA, Rothrock G, Phan Q, et al. Risk for severe group A streptococcal disease among patients' household contacts. *Emerg Infect Dis*. 2003;9(4):443–7.
194. Ahmed S, Diebold K, Brandvold JM, et al. The role of wound care in two group A streptococcal outbreaks in a Chicago skilled nursing facility, 2015-2016. *Open Forum Infect Dis*. 2018;5(7):ofy145.
195. Mearkle R, Saavedra-Campos M, Lamagni T, et al. Household transmission of invasive group A *Streptococcus* infections in England: A population-based study, 2009, 2011 to 2013. *Euro Surveil*. 2017;22(19):30532.
196. Lamagni TL, Oliver I, Stuart JM. Global assessment of invasive group A *Streptococcus* infection risk in household contacts. *Clin Infect Dis*. 2014;60(1):166–7.
197. Davies HD, McGeer A, Schwartz B, et al. Invasive group A streptococcal infections in Ontario, Canada. Ontario group A streptococcal study group. *N Engl J Med*. 1996;335(8):547–54.
198. Smith T, WIlkinson V, Kaplan E. Group A. *Streptococcus*-associated upper respiratory tract infections in a day care center. *Pediatrics*. 1989;83:380–4.
199. Snellman L, Stang H, Johnson D, Kaplan E. Duration of positive throat cultures for group A streptococci after initiation of antibiotic therapy. *Pediatrics*. 1993;91:1166–70.
200. Andrews RM, McCarthy J, Carapetis JR, Currie BJ. Skin disorders, including pyoderma, scabies, and tinea infections. *Pediatr Clin North Am*. 2009;56(6):1421–40.
201. Tyrrell GJ, Lovgren M, Kress B, Grimsrud K. Invasive group A streptococcal disease in Alberta, Canada (2000 to 2002). *J Clin Microbiol*. 2005;43(4):1678–83.
202. Laupland KB, Davies HD, Low DE, Schwartz B, Green K, McGeer A. Invasive group A streptococcal disease in children and association with varicella-zoster virus infection. *Pediatrics*. 2000;105(5):e60.
203. Sanchez JL, Cooper MJ, Myers CA, et al. Respiratory infections in the U.S. Military: Recent experience and control. *Clin Microbiol Rev*. 2015;28(3):743–800.
204. Lee T, Jordan NN, Sanchez JL, Gaydos JC. Selected nonvaccine interventions to prevent infectious acute respiratory disease. *Am J Prev Med*. 2005;28(3):305–16.
205. Webber BJ, Kieffer JW, White BK, Hawksworth AW, Graf PCF, Yun HC. Chemoprophylaxis against group A *Streptococcus* during military training. *Prev Med*. 2019;118:142–9.
206. MacFarland RB, Colvin VG, Seal JR. Mass prophylaxis of epidemic streptococcal infections with benzathine penicillin G. II. Experience at a naval training center during the winter of 1956–57. *N Engl J Med*. 1958;258(26):1277–84.
207. Wannamaker LW, Rammelkamp CH, Denny FW, et al. Prophylaxis of acute rheumatic fever. *Am J Med*. 1951;10(6):673–95.
208. Leads from the MMWR. Acute rheumatic fever at a navy training center—San Diego, California. *JAMA*. 1988;259(12):1782, 1787.

209. S-E Lee, Eick A, Ciminera P. Respiratory disease in army recruits. *Am J Prev Med*. 2008;34(5):389–95.
210. Headquarters, Department of the Army, the Navy, the Air Force, and the Coast Guard. Immunization and chemoprophylaxis for the prevention of infectious diseases. 2013.
211. Nurse-Findlay S, Taylor MM, Savage M, et al. Shortages of benzathine penicillin for prevention of mother-to-child transmission of syphilis: An evaluation from multi-country surveys and stakeholder interviews. *PLoS Med*. 2017;14(12):e1002473.
212. Schreier AJ, Hockett VE, Seal JR. Mass prophylaxis of epidemic streptococcal infections with benzathine penicillin G. *N Engl J Med*. 1958;258(25):1231–8.
213. Guchev Igor A, Gray Gregory C, Klochkov Oleg I. Two regimens of azithromycin prophylaxis against community-acquired respiratory and skin/soft-tissue infections among military trainees. *Clin Infect Dis*. 2004;38(8):1095–101.
214. Gerber MA, Baltimore RS, Eaton CB, et al. Prevention of rheumatic fever and diagnosis and treatment of acute streptococcal pharyngitis: A scientific statement from the American Heart Association Rheumatic Fever, Endocarditis, and Kawasaki Disease Committee of the Council on Cardiovascular Disease in the Young, The Interdisciplinary Council on Functional Genomics and Translational Biology, and The Interdisciplinary Council on Quality of Care and Outcomes Research: Endorsed by the American Academy of Pediatrics. *Circulation*. 2009;119(11):1541–51.
215. Carapetis JR, Beaton A, Cunningham MW, et al. Acute rheumatic fever and rheumatic heart disease. *Nat Rev Dis Primers*. 2016;2:15084.
216. Dooling KL, Crist MB, Nguyen DB, et al. Investigation of a prolonged group A streptococcal outbreak among residents of a skilled nursing facility, Georgia, 2009–2012. *Clin Infect Dis*. 2013;57(11):1562–7.
217. Sheel M, Moreland NJ, Fraser JD, Carapetis J. Development of group A streptococcal vaccines: An unmet global health need. *Expert Rev Vaccines*. 2015;15(2):227–38.
218. Dale JB, Batzloff MR, Cleary PP, et al. Current approaches to group A streptococcal vaccine development. In: Ferretti JJ, Stevens DL, Fischetti VA, eds. *Streptococcus Pyogenes: Basic Biology to Clinical Manifestations*. Oklahoma City, OK: University of Oklahoma Health Sciences Center; 2016.
219. Massell BF. Rheumatic fever following streptococcal vaccination. *JAMA*. 1969;207(6):1115.
220. Vekemans J, Gouvea-Reis F, Kim JH, et al. The path to group A *Streptococcus* vaccines: WHO research and development technology roadmap and preferred product characteristics. *Clin Infect Dis*. 2019;69(5):877–83.
221. Dale JB, Penfound TA, Chiang EY, Walton WJ. New 30-valent m protein-based vaccine evokes cross-opsonic antibodies against non-vaccine serotypes of group A streptococci. *Vaccine*. 2011;29(46):8175–8.
222. McNeil SA, Halperin SA, Langley JM, et al. Safety immunogenicity of 26-valent group A *Streptococcus* vaccine in healthy adult volunteers. *Clin Infect Dis*. 2005;41(8):1114–22.
223. Steer AC, Law I, Matatolu L, Beall BW, Carapetis JR. Global *emm* type distribution of group A streptococci: Systematic review and implications for vaccine development. *Lancet Infect Dis*. 2009;9(10):611–6.
224. World Health Organization. WHO product development for vaccines advisory committee meeting—2014. 2014. https://www.who.int/immunization/research/meetings_workshops/pdvac_2014/en/.
225. Beaton A, Kamalembo FB, Dale J, et al. The American Heart Association's Call to Action for Reducing the Global Burden of Rheumatic Heart Disease: A policy statement from the American Heart Association. *Circulation*. 2020;142(20):e358–68. doi:10.1161/CIR.0000000000000922. Epub 2020 Oct 19. PMID: 33070654.
226. Dale JB, Walker MJ. Update on group A streptococcal vaccine development. *Curr Opin Infect Dis*. 2020;33(3):244–50. doi:10.1097/QCO.0000000000000644. PMID: 32304470; PMCID: PMC7326309.

CHAPTER

156 *Streptococcus agalactiae* (Group B Streptococcal) Disease

Monica M. Farley

BACKGROUND

Streptococcus agalactiae, or Group B *Streptococcus* (GBS), was first identified as a pathogen in cattle, associated with bovine mastitis.[1,2] Widespread recognition of GBS as a significant human pathogen occurred in the 1960s–1970s, when it emerged as the most common cause of neonatal sepsis and an important cause of bacterial meningitis in infants less than 3 months of age in the United States.[3–5] It was later shown that maternal colonization with GBS in the genital or gastrointestinal track represented the most important risk factor for early-onset (between 0 and 6 days of life) GBS disease in the newborn[6,7] and that administration of intrapartum antibiotics to colonized women could prevent most cases of early-onset neonatal GBS infections.[8,9] Consensus guidelines for the prevention of neonatal GBS disease, developed through collaboration between public health, academic investigators, and professional organizations including obstetricians and pediatricians, with the strong support of parent advocacy groups, were first published in 1996.[10–12] These guidelines, revised in 2002 to include universal screening of pregnant women for GBS colonization, resulted in dramatic declines in early-onset GBS disease in the United States.[13] However, early-onset cases still occur and rates of late-onset GBS disease (between 7 and 89 days of life) have not declined despite relatively high uptake and implementation of the guidelines.[14] At least ten capsular serotypes have been described; serotypes Ia, Ib, II, III, IV, and V are the most common in the United States.

EPIDEMIOLOGY AND CLINICAL MANIFESTATIONS

GBS infections remain a leading cause of morbidity and mortality in infants in the United States and worldwide.[14,16] Early-onset disease occurs in the first week of life (most in the first 48 hours of life) and often manifests as sepsis, pneumonia, and less frequently as meningitis.[14,15,17] More than a quarter of cases are in preterm infants.[15] Late-onset disease occurs between 7 and 89 days of life and almost a third will present with meningitis. Other presentations include bacteremia without focus (61–65%), and rarely cellulitis and pneumonia.[15,17] In the era since introduction of intrapartum antibiotic prophylaxis (IAP) in the United States, the rate of early-onset GBS infection in newborns declined to 0.23/1000 live births and late-onset disease remained stable at 0.31/1000 live births in 2015.[15] More than 99% of the isolates from neonatal disease fell into six common serotypes (Ia, Ib, II, III, IV, and V). Serotype III accounted for more than half (56.2%) of late-onset neonatal infections in the United States.[15] In a worldwide, systematic review and meta-analysis performed by an international Infant GBS Investigator Group, the pooled incidence of invasive GBS disease in neonates was 0.41/1000 live births for early-onset disease and 0.26/1000 live births for late-onset disease. Rates were highest in Africa (1.12) and lowest in Asia (0.30). These pooled rates were considered to be underestimated given significant constraints in case identification and availability of optimal diagnostic capacity in low- and middle-income settings.[16] Serotype III was the most prevalent neonatal serotype worldwide and five serotypes (Ia, Ib, II, III, and V) accounted for 97% of the isolates in this global analysis.[16]

The primary risk factor for early-onset GBS infection is maternal intrapartum vaginal/rectal colonization, resulting in a > 25-fold increased risk of delivering an infant with early-onset disease compared to pregnant women with negative prenatal cultures.[14] Heavy GBS colonization and GBS from a urine culture during pregnancy further increases the risk of early-onset neonatal disease.[18,19] Other risk factors include previous delivery of an infant with invasive GBS disease, prolonged rupture of membranes, premature delivery, intrapartum fever, young maternal age, black race, and low levels of maternal antibodies to GBS capsule.[20,21]

Pregnancy-related maternal infections represent less than 5% of all invasive GBS disease in adults (>15 years of age) in the era of IAP in the United States.[22] The most common maternal invasive GBS manifestations include chorioamnionitis, postpartum endometritis, and bacteremia. Serious complications including endocarditis and meningitis occur rarely in pregnancy-associated GBS disease. Invasive infection involving the upper genital tract, placenta, or amniotic sac has been associated with spontaneous abortion or a stillborn infant in more than half the cases.[17] Postpartum endometritis may follow caesarean delivery. GBS endocarditis, meningitis, and septic arthritis have all been reported following elective abortions.[23–25] Wound infections, cellulitis, fasciitis, pneumonia, infections of ventriculoperitoneal shunts, bone and joint infections, and deep abscess formation (including epidural abscess) may occur. Urinary tract infections are the most common manifestation of noninvasive, pregnancy-associated disease and GBS bacteriuria has been shown to be a marker for heavy GBS genital and/or gastrointestinal colonization in a pregnant woman.[14,19]

With the decline in early-onset neonatal disease due to the effectiveness of IAP, now more than 80% of invasive GBS disease occurs in nonpregnant adolescents and adults[17] and adult disease rates are increasing.[26,27] Disease may occur in adults of all ages, but rates are highest in older adults with a median age of 64 years and nearly half of all disease occurs in those aged 65 years and older.[27] Invasive GBS infection rates remain significantly higher in blacks than in whites in the United States.[26] The most common clinical manifestations of invasive GBS infections in nonpregnant adults include skin and soft tissue infections, bacteremia without an obvious focus, osteomyelitis, pneumonia, and septic arthritis. Endocarditis and meningitis are less common but severe clinical syndromes and can result in higher morbidity and mortality.[26–28] Toxic shock and necrotizing fasciitis have also been reported.[26,29] Urinary tract infections are the most common form of noninvasive disease in nonpregnant adults.[28,30,31]

Most nonpregnant adults with invasive GBS disease have significant underlying diseases including the presence of diabetes mellitus and/or obesity in over half the cases.[27] In a multivariable analysis of population-based GBS surveillance, the adjusted relative risk of invasive GBS infection in adults with diabetes and morbid obesity was 6.04 and 8.97, respectively.[32] Among diabetic patients with invasive GBS disease, skin, soft tissue, and bone infections are more common compared with those without diabetes.[26] Obesity has also been associated with GBS colonization in pregnancy. A retrospective analysis of pregnant women determined that those who were obese had a higher incidence of either vaginal or rectal GBS colonization when compared to those who were not.[33] Additional pre-existing conditions that have been associated with increased risk of serious GBS disease include: cirrhosis, history of stroke, breast cancer, decubitus ulcer, and neurogenic bladder.[28,34] Nursing home residents are at significantly greater risk of invasive GBS infection than community-dwelling individuals of similar age.[26]

The case fatality rate in nonpregnant adults has improved from a rate of almost 24% in 1990 to 6% in recent years in the United States.[27] GBS bacteremia may be polymicrobial in a subset of patients, most often in association with Staphylococcal species.[28] Approximately 7% of invasive GBS infections in adults represent a recurrent episode of disease, most often associated with skin and soft tissue disease in patients with diabetes, obesity, kidney disease, and chronic skin conditions.[27,35] Blood cultures are the most common site of isolation of GBS in invasive disease (>80%), followed by bone and joint fluid cultures. Urine cultures are the most common site of isolation of GBS from noninvasive adult disease. Capsule serotype distribution among invasive GBS infections in nonpregnant adults has been changing in the United States. Although serotypes Ia and V remain the predominant serotypes associated with nonpregnant adult GBS disease in the United States, the rates of these serotypes are decreasing while rates of serotypes Ib, II, and IV increased substantially between 2008 and 2106.[27] Serotypes III, II, and Ib are also common globally in various orders of frequency depending on the geographic location. A small but growing proportion of nonpregnant adult disease in North America is attributable to serotype IV[27]; serotype IV represented approximately 4.6% of isolates from nonpregnant adults in United States in 2008 surveillance compared with 11.3% in 2016.[27] In surveillance conducted in two Canadian provinces from 2010 to 2014, ~17% of adult invasive disease was due to serotype IV.[36]

A large foodborne outbreak of severe GBS infections in nonpregnant adults due to a zoonotic GBS serotype III Sequence Type 283 (ST283) clone was investigated in Singapore and traced to consumption of raw farmed freshwater fish that were colonized or infected with the ST283 GBS clone.[37] Patients with disease due to ST283 were more likely to be younger adults, be of Chinese ethnicity, and have meningoencephalitis or septic arthritis. GBS serotype III ST283 associated with severe disease in nonpregnant adults has also been reported from Hong Kong.[38]

PATHOGENESIS

Asymptomatic colonization with GBS may occur in the gastrointestinal tract, the perineal area, vagina, cervix, or urethra, and occasionally the skin and throat. Co-colonization with identical GBS isolates may occur in sexual partners.[39] Male and female college students living in dormitories were frequently colonized (20–34%) with GBS; the anal orifice was the most common site followed by the vagina, urine, and throat.[40] The gastrointestinal track is likely the main reservoir for GBS and the source for vaginal colonization. It has been estimated that an average of 18% of all pregnant women worldwide have vaginal and/or rectal colonization with GBS,[41] with estimates near 25% in the United States.[14] Colonization late in pregnancy represents the most important risk factor for early-onset GBS disease in the newborn.[14,18] Vaginal colonization near the time of delivery, particularly heavy colonization, is also a risk factor for intra-amniotic infection and postpartum endometritis in pregnant women. GBS bacteriuria, present in 2–10% of pregnant women, is a marker for heavy vaginal colonization, and has been identified as a risk factor for both early- and late-onset disease in infants.[19]

For early-onset disease, transmission of GBS from mother to infant is thought to occur by inhalation of GBS-contaminated amniotic or vaginal fluid during delivery and subsequent translocation across the respiratory mucosa leading to systemic disease.[42] The route of transmission for late-onset disease is less clear but may involve persistence of asymptomatic gastrointestinal colonization acquired at the time of birth, which may result in translocation across the intestinal mucosa to the bloodstream.[43] Once in the bloodstream, the GBS sialic acid/polysaccharide capsule and other complement-inhibitory factors are antiphagocytic and allow for survival in the bloodstream.[44] The presence of high GBS capsule serotype-specific maternal antibodies correlate with protection against early-onset infection in the infant.[45] A GBS surface glycoprotein, call Srr-1, facilitates crossing of the blood brain barrier in mice and promotes adhesion to and invasion of human brain microvascular endothelial cells.[46] An additional virulence factor, called hypervirulent GBS adhesion (HvgA), has been linked to the GBS clone ST-17 that is strongly associated with late-onset neonatal meningitis. This surface-anchored HvgA protein promotes neonatal intestinal colonization and translocation of both the intestinal epithelium and the blood brain barrier.[47]

A study of healthy adults $\geq$ 65 years of age noted that almost a quarter had GBS colonization in the rectum, vagina, or urine and nearly half of the isolates were serotype V, an important cause of invasive disease in the elderly.[48] Skin and/or mucous membrane disruption, compromised blood flow or lymphatic drainage, and peripheral neuropathy may predispose to GBS infection, particularly skin and soft tissue infections, in nonpregnant adults. Specific examples include chronic foot ulcers and neuropathy associated with diabetes, pressure-related skin breakdown, postsurgical lymphatic disruption, radiation damage, and peripheral vascular disease. Unrecognized deep-seated infections (e.g., osteomyelitis, endocarditis) may result in recurrent episodes of invasive GBS disease.[35]

DIAGNOSIS

GBS are encapsulated gram-positive cocci that form pairs or short chains in culture media. They form gray-white colonies on sheep's blood agar plates and demonstrate narrow zones of β-hemolysis and are rarely nonhemolytic. Serologic determination of the presence of the Lancefield group B antigen on the surface of the bacteria can provide definitive diagnosis. Latex slide agglutination using group B specific antisera is a commonly used technique. Hydrolysis of hippurate and a positive CAMP test are additional characteristics that can be used to distinguish GBS from other *Streptococci*. GBS can be identified using nucleic acid amplification testing (NAAT), such as commercially available PCR assays, in laboratories that have performed appropriate validation measures and quality controls.[14]

Screening for GBS colonization in pregnant women should be performed on vaginal and rectal swabs (or a single combined swab) collected at 35- to 37-week gestation. Specimens should be incubated for 18–24 hours at 35–37°C in either nonpigmented selective enrichment broth or enrichment broth incorporating GBS indicator pigments. Nonpigmented broth and pigmented broths with no color detection should be further evaluated with agar subculture or NAAT after the initial incubation period is complete. In penicillin-allergic women at high risk for anaphylaxis, antimicrobial susceptibility testing should be performed, including testing for inducible clindamycin resistance on GBS isolates that are susceptible to clindamycin but resistant to erythromycin.[14]

TREATMENT AND ANTIBIOTIC RESISTANCE

GBS isolates are generally susceptible to penicillin, ampicillin, and other beta-lactam antibiotics. Penicillin or ampicillin remains the drugs of choice in nonallergic patients. Gentamicin may be added in serious neonatal infections such as meningitis, endocarditis, and sepsis, although discontinuation is recommended once the infection is under control. Cefazolin and ceftriaxone are also effective against GBS. For patients with significant penicillin allergies, clindamycin can be considered only if susceptibility is documented. Vancomycin is another alternative for those with penicillin allergies. IAP recommendations are discussed below (GBS Prevention Strategies).

A small number of GBS isolates with reduced susceptibility to one or more beta-lactam antibiotics associated with changes within the transpeptidase domain of the penicillin binding protein 2x (PBP2x) have been identified in the United States, Japan, and elsewhere.[49–52] The prevalence remains < 1% in the United States but has been increasing in Japan (from 4.5% in 2007 to 6.6% in 2013). Prevalence of clindamycin and erythromycin resistance is high in the United States, noted to be 21% and 45%, respectively, in Active Bacterial Core surveillance (ABCs) in 2015.[15] Fluoroquinolone resistance remains low in the United States (1.2%) but a highly clonal fluoroquinolone resistant serotype Ib GBS strain is responsible for up to a third of invasive GBS cases in Japan and South Korea.[53,54] Vancomycin resistance has been reported rarely.[55]

GBS PREVENTION STRATEGIES

IAP is indicated for any pregnant woman with a positive GBS vaginal-rectal screening culture optimally obtained at 35- to 37-week gestation. It is also routinely recommended for any pregnant woman with a prior history of giving birth to an infant with invasive GBS disease or with GBS bacteriuria during any trimester of the current pregnancy. For women presenting in labor with an unknown GBS colonization status, IAP should be given in the presence of any of the following GBS risk factors including delivery at <37-week gestation, prolonged rupture of membranes (≥18 hours), intrapartum fever, or a positive intrapartum NAAT for GBS if such testing is available.[14] The recommended regimen for IAP is penicillin or ampicillin given intravenously on presentation in labor and repeated every 4 hours until delivery. Penicillin-allergic individuals who are considered at high risk for anaphylaxis (i.e., prior anaphylaxis, angioedema, respiratory distress, or urticaria following penicillin or a cephalosporin) should receive clindamycin every 8 hours until delivery if clindamycin susceptibility of the GBS isolate has been documented or vancomycin every 12 hours if susceptibility results are not available. For those with a history of a less-severe penicillin reaction, cefazolin given every 8 hours until delivery is recommended.[14] The approach to perinatal GBS disease prevention is currently being reviewed by the American College of Obstetricians and Gynecologists, the American Academy of Pediatrics and the American Society of Microbiology, with refinements expected to be released in 2019.

Despite the success of IAP in the United States, early-onset cases still occur and there has been no impact on late-onset GBS disease. In low- and middle-income countries, limitations in access to prenatal care and laboratory facilities for GBS screening, and the increased frequency of home deliveries make IAP more difficult to implement. In addition, in all settings, relatively broad antibiotic exposure with resulting impact on the microbiome and the potential for emerging antibiotic resistance remain a concern. GBS prevention through maternal immunization is an active area of research but no vaccine is currently available. Capsular polysaccharide (CPS)-protein conjugate vaccines using tetanus toxoid or CRM_{197}, a genetically detoxified form of diphtheria toxin, as carrier proteins to enhance immunogenicity are in various stages of development. Preclinical and Phase 1 and 2 human trials of prototypic monovalent and bivalent CPS conjugate vaccines have been conducted in adults and found to be well tolerated and immunogenic.[56,57]

More recently, trivalent conjugate vaccines designed to protect against serotypes Ia, Ib, and III have been developed and tested in Phase 1/Phase 2 clinical trials in pregnant women and women of child-bearing age. Trivalent CPS-conjugate vaccines produced significant antibody responses to the vaccine serotypes, antibodies were transferred to the infants of pregnant women, and there were no safety concerns.[58,59] In a trivalent CPS-CRM_{197} (Ia, Ib, and III) vaccine trial in healthy pregnant women, vaccine-specific anti-CPS antibodies persisted in the infant until 90 days of life and did not affect immune responses to infant diphtheria toxoid and the pneumococcal vaccine.[60] Higher baseline GBS antibodies resulted in a better response to the vaccine. In a vaccine trial in HIV-infected and HIV-uninfected pregnant women in Malawi and South Africa, antibody responses in HIV-positive women were found to be lower than in HIV-negative women.[61] Despite general concerns about immunizing pregnant women, none of these trials identified significant safety signals. A Phase 1/2 clinical trial of a six-valent polysaccharide-protein conjugate vaccine in healthy adults 18–49 years of age is underway (ClinicalTrials.gov). In an effort to develop a protein-based vaccine, a recombinant fusion protein antigen (GBS-NN) composed of N-terminal regions of two highly conserved surface proteins, Rib and alpha C protein, has been designed and found to be immunogenic and cross-protective in preclinical and a Phase 1 human trial in healthy adult women.[62,63] Vaccines under development for the prevention of neonatal GBS may have application in adult populations, particularly those at high risk for GBS disease such as adults with diabetes or morbid obesity.

References

1. Ayers HS, Mudge CS. The *Streptococci* of the bovine udder: IV. Studies of the *Streptococci*. *J Infect Dis*. 1922;31(1):40–50.
2. El Ghoroury AA. Comparative studies of group "B" *Streptococci* of human and bovine origin: I. Cultural and biochemical characters. *Am J Public Health Nations Health*. 1950;40(10):1273–7.
3. Eickhoff TC, Klein JO, Daly KA, Ingall D, Findland M. Neonatal sepsis and other infections due to group B beta-hemolytic *Streptococci*. *N Engl J Med*. 1964;271:1221–8.
4. Baker CJ, Barrett FF. Group B streptococcal infections in infants. The importance of the various serotypes. *JAMA*. 1974;230(8):1158–60.
5. McCracken GH Jr. Group B *Streptococci*: The new challenge in neonatal infections. *J Pediatr*. 1973;82:703–6.
6. Allardice JG, Baskett TF, Seshia MM, Bowman N, Malazdrewicz R. Perinatal group B streptococcal colonization and infection. *Am J Obstet Gynecol*. 1982;142:617–20.
7. Schuchat A, Wenger JD. Epidemiology of group B streptococcal disease. Risk factors, prevention strategies, and vaccine development. *Epidemiol Rev*. 1994;16(2):374–402.
8. Boyer KM, Gotoff SP. Prevention of early-onset neonatal group B streptococcal diseases with selective intrapartum chemoprophylaxis. *N Engl J Med*. 1986;314(26):1665–9.
9. Tuppurainen N, Hallman M. Prevention of neonatal group B streptococcal disease: Intrapartum detection and chemoprophylaxis of heavily colonized parturients. *Obstet Gynecol*. 1989;73(4):583–7.
10. American College of Obstetricians and Gynecologists. ACOG committee opinion. Prevention of early-onset group B streptococcal disease in newborns. Committee on Obstetric Practice. American College of Obstetrics and Gynecologists. *Int J Gynaecol Obstet*. 1996;54(173):197–205.
11. CDC. Prevention of perinatal group B streptococcal disease: A public health perspective. *MMWR Recomm Rep*. 1996;45(RR-7):1–24.
12. American Academy of Pediatrics. Revised guidelines for prevention of early-onset group B streptococcal (GBS) infection. American Academy of Pediatrics Committee on Infectious Diseases and Committee on Fetus and Newborn. *Pediatrics*. 1997;99:489–96.
13. Jordan HT, Farley MM, Craig A, et al. Revisiting the need for vaccine prevention of late-onset neonatal group B streptococcal disease: A multistate, population-based analysis. *Pediatr Infect Dis J*. 2008;27(12):1057–64.
14. CDC. Prevention of perinatal group B streptococcal disease. Revised Guidelines from CDC, 2010. *MMWR Recomm Rep*. 2010;59(RR-10):1–32.
15. Nanduri SA, Petit S, Smelser C, et al. Epidemiology of invasive early-and late-onset group B streptococcal diseases in the United States: Multistate laboratory- and population-based surveillance report, 2006–2015. *JAMA Pediatr*. 2019;173(3):224–33.

16. Madrid L, Seale AC, Kohli-Lynch M, et al. Infant group B streptococcal diseases incidence and serotypes worldwide: Systematic review and meta-analyses. *Clin Infect Dis.* 2017;65(Suppl 2):S160–72.
17. Phares CR, Lunfield R, Farley MM, et al. Epidemiology of invasive group B streptococcal disease in the United States, 1999–2005. *JAMA.* 2008;299:2056–65.
18. Regan JA, Klebanoff MA, Nugent RP, et al. Colonization with group B *Streptococci* in pregnancy and adverse outcome. VIP Study Group. *Am J Obstet Gynecol.* 1996;174(4):1354–60.
19. Wood EG, Dillon HC Jr. A prospective study of group B streptococcal bacteriuria in pregnancy. *Am J Obstet Gynecol.* 1981;140:515–20.
20. Schuchat A, Deaver-Robinson K, Plikaytis BD, Zangwill KM, Mohle-Boetani J, Wenger JD. Multistate case-control study of maternal risk factors for neonatal group B streptococcal disease. The Active Surveillance Study Group. *Pediatr Infect Dis J.* 1994;13:623–9.
21. Baker CJ, Edwards MS, Kasper DL. Role of antibody to native type III polysaccharide of group B *Streptococcus* in infant infection. *Pediatrics.* 1981;68:544–9.
22. Schrag SJ, Zywicki S, Farley MM, et al. Group B streptococcal disease in the era of intrapartum antibiotic prophylaxis. *N Engl J Med.* 2000;342:15–20.
23. Camarillo D, Banerjee R, Greenhow TL, Tureen JH. Group B streptococcal endocarditis after elective abortion in an adolescent. *Pediatr Infect Dis J.* 2009;28(1):67–9.
24. Dezial PJ, McGuire N, Brown PD. Group B streptococcal meningitis complicating elective abortion: Report of 2 cases. *Clin Infect Dis.* 2000;31(5):E23–5.
25. DeNoble PH, Gonzalez D. Septic arthritis of the shoulder following elective termination of pregnancy. *J Shoulder Elbow Surg.* 2009;18:e5–6.
26. Skoff TH, Farley MM, Petit S, et al. Increasing burden of invasive group B streptococcal disease in nonpregnant adults, 1990–2007. *Clin Infect Dis.* 2009;49:85–92.
27. Watkins LKF, McGee L, Schrag SJ. Epidemiology of invasive group B streptococcal infections among nonpregnant adults—United States, 2008–2016. *JAMA Intern Med.* 2019;179(4):479–88.
28. Farley MM, Harvey CR, Stull T, et al. A population-based assessment of invasive disease due to group B *Streptococcus* in nonpregnant adults. *N Engl J Med.* 1993;328(25):1807–11.
29. Ikebe T, Chiba K, Shima T, et al. Evaluation of streptococcal toxic shock-like syndrome caused by group B *Streptococcus* in adults in Japan between 2009 and 2013. *J Infect Chemother.* 2015;21(3):207–11.
30. Ulett KB, Benjamin WH Jr, Xiao M, et al. Diversity of group B *Streptococcus* serotypes causing urinary tract infection in adults. *J Clin Microbiol.* 2009;47(7):2055–60.
31. Edwards MS, Baker CJ. Group B streptococcal infections in elderly adults. *Clin Infect Dis.* 2005;41:839–47.
32. Pitts SL, Maruthur NM, Langley GE, et al. Obesity, diabetes, and the risk of invasive group B streptococcal diseases in nonpregnant adults in the United States. *Open Forum Infect Dis.* 2018;5(6):1–7.
33. Kleweis SM, Cahill AG, Odibo AO, Tuuli MG. Maternal obesity and rectovaginal group B *Streptococcus* colonization at term. *Infect Dis Obstet Gynecol.* 2015;2015:586767.
34. Jackson LA, Hilsdon R, Farley MM. Risk factors for the group B streptococcal diseases in adults. *Ann Intern Med.* 1995;123(6):415–20.
35. Harrison LH, Ali A, Dwyer DM, et al. Relapsing invasive group B streptococcal infection in adults. *Ann Intern Med.* 1995;123(6):421–7.
36. Teatero S, Athey TBT, Caseseele PV, et al. Emergence of serotype IV group B *Streptococcus* adult invasive disease in Manitoba and Saskatchewan, Canada, is driven by clonal sequence type 459 strains. *J Clin Microbiol.* 2015;53(9):2919–26.
37. Kalimuddin S, Chen SL, Lim CTK, et al. 2015 Epidemic of severe *Streptococcal agalactiae* sequence type 283 infections in Singapore associated with the consumption of raw freshwater fish: A detailed analysis of clinical, epidemiological, and bacterial sequencing data. *Clin Infect Dis.* 2017;64(Suppl-2):S145–52.
38. Ip M, Cheuk ESC, Tsui MHY, Kong F, Leung TN, Gilbert GL. Identification of a *Streptococcus agalactiae* serotype III subtype 4 clone in association with adult invasive disease in Hong Kong. *J Clin Microbiol.* 2006;44:4252–4.
39. Manning SD, Tallman P, Baker CJ, Gillespie B, Marrs CF, Foxman B. Determinants of co-colonization with group B *Streptococcus* among heterosexual college couples. *Epidemiology.* 2002;13:533–9.
40. Manning SD, Neighbors K, Tallman PA, et al. Prevalence of group B *Streptococcus* colonization and potential for transmission by casual contact in healthy young men and women. *Clin Infect Dis.* 2004;39:380–8.
41. Russell NJ, Seale AC, O'Driscoll M, et al. Maternal colonization with group B *Streptococcus* and serotype distribution worldwide: Systematic review and meta-analysis. *Clin Infect Dis.* 2017;65(Suppl 2):S100–11.
42. Edwards MS, Nizet V, Baker CJ. Group B streptococcal infections. In: Remington JS, Wilson CB, Klein JO, Baker CJ, eds. *Infectious Diseases of the Fetus and Newborn Infant.* Philadelphia: Elsevier; 2006, pp. 403–64.
43. Hansen SM, Uldbjerg N, Kilian M, Sorensen UB. Dynamics of *Streptococcus agalactiae* colonization in women during and after pregnancy and in their infants. *J Clin Microbiol.* 2004;42:83–9.
44. Maisey HC, Doran KS, Nizel V. Recent advances in understanding the molecular basis of group B *Streptococcus* virulence. *Exp Rev Mol Med.* 2008;10:1–16.
45. Baker CJ, Carey VJ, Rench MA, et al. Maternal antibody at delivery protects neonates from early onset group B streptococcal disease. *J Infect Dis.* 2014;209:781–8.
46. van Sorge NM, Quach D, Gurney MA, Sullam PM, Nizet V, Doran KS. The group B streptococcal serine-rich repeat 1 glycoprotein mediates penetration of the blood-brain barrier. *J Infect Dis.* 2009;199:1479–87.
47. Tazi A, Disson O, Bellais S, et al. The surface protein HvgA mediates group B *Streptococcus* hypervirulence and meningeal tropism in neonates. *J Exp Med.* 2010;207:2313–22.
48. Edwards MS, Rench MA, Palazzi DL, Baker CJ. Group B streptococcal colonization and serotype-specific immunity in healthy elderly persons. *Clin Infect Dis.* 2005;40:352–7.
49. Kimura K, Suzuki S, Wachino J, et al. First molecular characterization of group B *Streptococci* with reduced penicillin susceptibility. *Antimicrob Agents Chemother.* 2008;52(8):2890–27.
50. Longtin J, Vermeiren C, Shahinas D, et al. Novel mutations in a patient isolate of *Streptococcus agalactiae* with reduced penicillin susceptibility emerging after long-term oral suppressive therapy. *Antimicrob Agents Chemother.* 2011;55(6):2983–5.
51. Dahesh S, Hensler ME, Van Sorge NM, et al. Point mutation in the group B streptococcal pbp2x gene conferring decreased susceptibility to beta-lactam antibiotics. *Antimicrob Agents Chemother.* 2008;52(8):2915–8.
52. Metcalf BJ, Chochua S, Gertz RE Jr, et al. Short-read whole genome sequencing for determination of antimicrobial resistance mechanisms and capsular serotypes of current invasive *Streptococcus agalactiae* recovered in the USA. *Clin Microbiol Infect.* 2017;23(8):547.e7–14.
53. Ryu H, Park YJ, Kim YK, et al. Dominance of clonal complex 10 among the levofloxacin-resistant *Streptococcus agalactiae* isolated from bacteremic patients in a Korean hospital. *J Infect Chemother.* 2014;20:509–11.
54. Murayama SY, Seki C, Sakata H, et al. Capsular type and antibiotic resistance in *Streptococcus agalactiae* isolates from patients, ranging from newborns to the elderly, with invasive infections. *Antimicrob Agents Chemother.* 2009;53:2650–3.
55. Park C, Nichols M, Schrag SJ. Two cases of invasive vancomycin-resistant group B *Streptococcus* infection. *N Engl J Med.* 2014;370(9):885–6.
56. Baker CJ, Paoletti LC, Wessels MR, et al. Safety and immunogenicity of capsular polysaccharide-tetanus toxoid conjugate vaccines for group B streptococcal types Ia and Ib. *J Infect Dis.* 1999;179:142–50.
57. Baker CJ, Rench MA, Fernandez M, et al. Safety and immunogenicity of a bivalent group B streptococcal conjugate vaccine for serotypes II and III. *J Infect Dis.* 2003;188(1):66–73.
58. Donders GG, Halperin SA, Devlieger R, et al. Maternal immunization with an investigational trivalent group B streptococcal vaccine: A randomized controlled trial. *Obstet Gynecol.* 2016;127:213–21.
59. Madhi SA, Cutland CL, Jose L, et al. Safety and immunogenicity of an investigational maternal trivalent group B *Streptococcus* vaccine in healthy women and their infants: A randomised phase 1b/2 trial. *Lancet Infect Dis.* 2016;16:923–34.
60. Madhi SA, Koen A, Cutland CL. Antibody kinetics and response to routine vaccinations in infants born to women who received an investigational trivalent group B *Streptococcus* polysaccharide CRM197-conjugate vaccine during pregnancy. *Clin Infect Dis.* 2017;65:1897–904.
61. Heyderman RS, Madhi SA, French N, et al. Group B *Streptococcus* vaccination in pregnant women with or without HIV in Africa: A non-randomised phase 2, open-label, multicentre trial. *Lancet Infect Dis.* 2016;16:546–55.
62. Stalhammar-Carlemalm M, Waldemarsson J, Johnsson E, Areschoug T, Lindahl G. Nonimmunodominant regions are effective as building blocks in a streptococcal fusion protein vaccine. *Cell Host Microbe.* 2007;2:427–34.
63. Rose F, Roovers S, Fano M, et al. Temperature-induced self-assembly of the group B *Streptococcus* (GBS) fusion antigen GBS-NN. *Mol Pharm.* 2018;15:2584–93.

CHAPTER 157

Clostridioides difficile Infection

Dimitri Drekonja • Stacy Holzbauer

INTRODUCTION

Clostridioides difficile (formerly known as *Clostridium difficile*) infection (CDI) has emerged as a pathogen of major importance among hospitalized and ambulatory patients. It now rivals methicillin-resistant *Staphylococcus aureus* (MRSA) as the leading cause of nosocomial infections,[1] and is increasingly encountered among ambulatory patients,[2] often with little to no prior contact with the healthcare system. Because of increased incidence and severity, and the high likelihood of recurrent disease after initial successful treatment, CDI has imposed a large burden on healthcare systems across the world. This burden is manifested by a high rate of morbidity and mortality, financial costs, and a high consumption of healthcare time and effort devoted to testing, infection control, cleaning, and reporting.[3] Because of this substantial impact on the healthcare system, the United States Centers for Diseases Control and Prevention (CDC) designated *C. difficile* as one of five "urgent" threats in its 2019 Antimicrobial Resistance Threat Report,[4] joining drug-resistant *Neisseria gonorrhoeae*, carbapenem-resistant Enterobacteriaceae, carbapenem-resistant *Acinetobacter*, and *Candida auris* in this top tier. Challenges and controversies regarding epidemiology, testing, treatment, prevention, and transmission of *C. difficile* have emerged (and sometimes re-emerged) over the past two decades, creating difficulties for clinicians and persisting questions for researchers studying CDI.

HISTORY OF CDI

Originally deemed a harmless colonizer of human neonatal intestinal flora when first isolated by Hall and O'Toole in 1934,[5] there was a hint of the potential virulence of *C. difficile* when they described themselves as "surprised to find the new bacillus highly pathogenic for guinea-pigs and rabbits." However, the change in perspective about *C. difficile* as a neonatal colonizer to one of the most important causes of healthcare-associated gastrointestinal infection took several decades. With the advent of antimicrobial therapy, there was an increase in pseudomembranous colitis, a severe gastrointestinal condition that had no clear etiology. The introduction of clindamycin and lincomycin was noted to be associated with pseudomembranous colitis, and several groups worked to determine a specific microbial cause. Several lines of research eventually led to the discovery of *C. difficile* as the offending agent. One group described a cytopathic effect of stool from patients with pseudomembranous colitis in tissue culture, and postulated the presence of an unidentified toxin.[6] Another line of investigation demonstrated that clindamycin-induced overgrowth of *Clostridium* species in hamster colonic flora, and that enterocolitis could be induced by intracecal injection of a cell-free filtrate of this clostridial strain.[7] Subsequently, stool from patients with pseudomembranous colitis or antibiotic-associated diarrhea was investigated, and *C. difficile* was isolated from the pseudomembranous colitis patients (and from one of the antibiotic-associated diarrhea patients) that produced cytotoxic changes on tissue culture and induced enterocolitis in a hamster model. Finally, both the cytotoxicity and enterocolitis were neutralized by gas-gangrene antitoxin, implicating toxin-producing *C. difficile* as the cause of illness.[8]

In the early 2000s, clinicians reported an increase in the incidence of fulminant CDI, with patients needing emergent colectomy despite initiation of appropriate antibiotic therapy.[9] Concomitantly, the overall incidence of CDI began to rise.[9] This combination of increased incidence and severity of CDI was attributed to the emergence of a specific *C. difficile* clone, variously designated as the North American pulsed-field type 1 (NAP1), BI, and 027 by pulsed-field gel electrophoresis, restriction endonuclease analysis, and polymerase chain reaction (PCR)-ribotyping, respectively.[10–12] Characteristics of this strain, which is still in circulation, include increased toxin production, fluoroquinolone resistance, and increased sporulation. Spread of the NAP1 clone was well documented, with investigators reporting emergence of the strain across all continents, including both high- and low-resource settings.[13–17] The exact cause (or combination of causes) responsible for this rapid worldwide spread is unknown. Various hypotheses for the detected increase include widespread fluoroquinolone use,[18,19] increased antibiotic use in general,[20] introduction of more sensitive testing methods, and increased CDI surveillance.[21] CDI prevalence has increased worldwide, including occurring in populations without extensive healthcare exposure.

Identifying the casual organism allowed for targeted antimicrobial therapy. Less than a year after identification of *C. difficile* as the cause of pseudomembranous colitis, a small trial of vancomycin versus placebo was published, demonstrating that antimicrobial therapy led to restoration of normal bowel function, eliminated *C. difficile*, and cleared fecal toxins.[22] Other trials established several additional antibiotics as effective therapy for CDI, including metronidazole, bacitracin, teicoplanin, fusidic acid, fidaxomicin, and others.[23–30] All agents seemed to achieve clinical cure in most patients. A variety of treatment recommendations have been released; the most recent in 2018 by the Infectious Disease Society of America (IDSA), which recommended oral vancomycin or fidaxomicin as first-line therapy for an initial episode (see later discussion on treatment).[31]

As of 2018, CDI is the most common identified cause of infectious diarrhea among hospitalized patients,[32] and an increasing cause of diarrhea in ambulatory patients.[2] In both groups of patients, the major clinical challenge is recurrent infection, which occurs in 20–35% of those with an initial episode of CDI,[33,34] and increases with each subsequent episode.[35] This has spurred interest in new treatment modalities, including new antimicrobials, immune therapy, fecal microbiota transplantation (FMT), and stool-derived products. Research to prevent CDI through improved infection control methods, environmental cleaning, source identification, and vaccination has also seen substantial advances, offering some hope that CDI may step down from its ranking as the most common cause of nosocomial infection.[36]

VIRULENCE FACTORS AND TOXINS

C. difficile is a gram-positive, spore-forming anaerobe with several virulence factors and toxins that are important for infectivity and pathogenesis. Among the virulence factors described, potentially the most important in terms of enabling spread of *C. difficile* is the ability to form a protective spore, which can survive for months under a variety of conditions, including desiccation, heat, radiation, and exposure to many cleaning agents.[37] Various lines of evidence point to the importance of spores in the transmission of CDI, including infection prevention studies documenting high rates of spore contamination in rooms of patients with CDI,[38] increased risk of CDI for the next patients occupying a room previously occupied by a CDI patient,[39,40] and animal data demonstrating that *C. difficile* strains deficient in a spore-regulation gene (Spo0A) were poorly transmitted and failed to cause relapse in an animal transmission model.[41] The ability to shed large numbers of spores into an environment where they persist until they come into contact with a susceptible host is key to CDI transmission, and provides significant challenges for healthcare infection prevention and environmental cleaning personnel.

Other virulence properties include mechanisms that lead to enhanced bacterial adhesion to the gut epithelium. These mechanisms include cell surface layers which appear to enhance adhesion and possibly modulate the immune response of the host, fimbriae which may play a role in adhesion, flagella which provide motility and may aid in pathogenesis, and other similar proteins and polysaccharides whose exact role in pathogenesis is unknown.[37]

Toxins are the major factors influencing the pathogenesis and severity of CDI.[42,43] In contrast to spore formation, which precedes a time of dormancy and exposure to a nonhospitable environment, toxin production is characteristic of vegetative growth and a metabolically active state, such as when *C. difficile* is ingested by a patient with altered gastrointestinal flora, usually due to recent antimicrobial use or some other perturbation of the intestinal flora. The necessity of toxin production for the development of CDI has been demonstrated by a variety of study designs, ranging from *in vitro* studies of toxin effects in cell cultures,[44] administration of toxin-producing strains of *C. difficile* in animal models,[45,46] and finally demonstration that *C. difficile* strains producing toxin induced manifestations of CDI in humans, whereas nontoxin-producing strains induced no signs of illness, and indeed later showed some evidence of protection.[47]

The primary toxins of *C. difficile* are two large molecular weight toxins, TcdA and TcdB, designated enterotoxin (or toxin A) and cytotoxin (or toxin B), respectively. There is considerable homology, with approximately 65% amino acid similarity.[48] Genes encoding these toxins, in addition to three other genes encoding regulatory proteins TcdR (transcription regulator), TcdC (membrane protein), and TcdE (toxin-secretion regulator) are located within a pathogenicity locus on the bacterial chromosome. This gene-clustering arrangement has led to investigation regarding the ability of horizontal gene transfer to enable nontoxigenic strains of *C. difficile* to acquire the ability to produce toxins and cause clinical illness.[49] Both the enterotoxin and the cytotoxin are produced by the bacterium and released into intestinal lumen, where they undergo endocytosis into intestinal epithelial cells.[50] Intracellularly, changes in pH facilitate protein conformational changes and autocatalytic cleavage, resulting in release of a protein fragment capable of inactivating members of the Rho family of small guanosine triphosphate-binding proteins and leading to alterations in the epithelial cell cytoskeleton.[51] These changes interfere with the cell's ability to maintain both internal structure and structural integrity of intestinal tight junctions with neighboring cells, causing increases in intestinal permeability and fluid accumulation, which manifest clinically as diarrhea. In addition to these direct toxic effects, both toxin A and B can activate cytokine production and immune cell recruitment via multiple pathways, leading to a profound proinflammatory state.[52] The degree of inflammation may be an important variable affecting clinical severity and outcomes.

The relative importance ascribed to toxins A and B in the pathogenesis of CDI has shifted over time. Initially, toxin A was believed to be more important than toxin B, based on oral administration of the toxin in hamsters leading to diarrhea, intestinal inflammation, and death.[45] In contrast, toxin B administration appeared benign, unless there was coadministration of toxin A or prior intestinal damage.[46] Support for this view was provided by studies demonstrating that treatment with antibodies against toxin A provided passive protection to animals.[53] The relative importance of toxin A was challenged by the identification of *C. difficile* strains that produced toxin B, but not A, and yet caused severe CDI.[54] This was followed by experiments using isogenic toxin gene mutants, in which strains that were designed to express exclusively toxin A or B were tested in animal models. Strains expressing toxin A led to approximately 20% mortality, whereas those expressing toxin B caused > 90% mortality.[55] In contrast, animals challenged by a strain with a double toxin knockout (producing neither toxin A or B) all survived.[56] As further clinical isolates producing only toxin B were reported, the consensus regarding the relative importance of toxins A and B coalesced around toxin B as the most significant and universal of the *C. difficile* toxin-based virulence factors.

In addition to the large molecular weight toxins A and B, *C. difficile* transferase, also known as binary toxin, has been identified as a potentially important virulence factor, especially among NAP1 strains.[57,58] First characterized in 1988, binary toxin comprises an enzymatic and a binding component, and appears to act by ribosylating intracellular actin, thus interfering with the cell's cytoskeleton, signaling, and other metabolic and functional processes.[59] The clinical significance of binary toxin is not clear. Early reports suggested that it was associated with strains causing more severe and fulminant disease, including the epidemic NAP1 and ribotype 078 strains. However, no reliable diagnostic test for binary toxin is available for clinical use, leading to speculation that the prevalence of strains expressing binary toxin is underestimated.

EPIDEMIOLOGY

The burden and scope of CDI in the United States and worldwide increased in the early 2000s, first heralded by reports from Quebec, Canada.[9] This increase led to a retrospective analysis of cases in that region over the preceding decade and demonstrated a fourfold increased incidence in that time.[60] Data from the United States affixed startlingly high numbers to CDI in 2011. Epidemiologists used data from the Emerging Infections Program, an active surveillance system in ten states, and applied regression modeling to develop estimates for incident CDI, recurrence, and mortality.[32] The number of incident cases in the United States was estimated at 453,000 [95% confidence intervals (CIs) 397,100, 508,500], with 83,000 first recurrence episodes (95% CI 57,000, 108,900) and an estimated 29,300 deaths (95% CI 16,500, 42,100). The epidemic NAP1 strain implicated in the emergence of epidemic CDI in the early 2000s was common, although not responsible for most of the cases where strain data were available (30.7% in hospitalized patients, and 18.8% in community-associated cases).[32] Similar percentages for the NAP1 strain were reported in other studies, including just under 30% in Canada in 2015,[61] and 22% in the United States Veterans Affairs system from 2012 through 2016.[62]

Historically, most CDI cases occurred in hospital settings, where broad-spectrum antimicrobial use is common and patients with risk factors for CDI are plentiful. Known risks for CDI include antimicrobial use,[63,64] older age,[63,65] proton-pump inhibitor use,[63,66] previous or prolonged hospitalization,[67] and medical comorbidities.[63] Other conditions with an association with CDI include inflammatory bowel disease[68,69] and severe liver disease,[70] although in these patients with diarrhea as a feature of their underlying illness (inflammatory bowel disease) or as a common side effect of promotility agents given to avoid hepatic encephalopathy (cirrhosis), it can be difficult to differentiate diarrhea from these causes if these patients become colonized with *C. difficile* versus true CDI.

Community-associated infection, generally defined as CDI in patients not hospitalized in the preceding 12 weeks as per current IDSA guidelines,[31] has changed from a rare occurrence to comprising one-third to one-half of CDI cases.[2,71] In an analysis of community-associated cases of CDI, 36% of cases received no antimicrobials, and 58% had no or low-level outpatient exposure to the healthcare system (with low-level defined as an outpatient visit with a physician or dentist).[2] The lack of antimicrobial exposure in such a sizable portion of cases questioned the ability to limit CDI cases with improved antimicrobial prescribing alone and suggested that ineffective infection control practices in outpatient settings might be leading to exposure to *C. difficile*. Risk factor studies in adult community-associated cases of CDI found prior antibiotic use was a common risk factor associated with infection along with emergency department visits and underlying conditions such as cardiac disease, chronic kidney disease, and inflammatory bowel disease when compared to healthy adults.[72] The increase in CDI among outpatients triggered a search for other reservoirs of *C. difficile*, including input from food sources, the environment, and transmission from index CDI patients to household contacts, including pets. Food products were hypothesized as a possible source of *C. difficile*.[73] However, studies have generally found only a small percentage of samples to be harboring *C. difficile*,[74–77] suggesting that food is at most a low-level source of exposure. Household transmission of *C. difficile* from recently treated patients to other household members has been documented (13%), with the same households demonstrating evidence of colonization in household pets (27%).[78] The advent of whole genome sequencing (WGS) has highlighted the diversity of *C. difficile* and has further complicated the understanding of *C. difficile* acquisition. In the United Kingdom, a population-based study of 1250 CDI healthcare and community-associated cases found that 45% were genetically distinct from all previous cases.[79] A point prevalence study and subsequent WGS analysis of *C. difficile* isolates across 482 European hospitals observed two distinct patterns of spread, a predominate clustering with healthcare facilities (i.e., a dominant healthcare clone) or a Europe-wide dissemination via other routes or sources.[80] Ultimately, the endemicity of these two patterns can make the distinction of healthcare and community-associated CDI less useful and emphasizes the importance of meticulous infection prevention and antimicrobial stewardship in a variety of settings.

DIAGNOSIS

Diagnostic testing for *C. difficile* has shifted from an initial culture-based technique with subsequent testing for the presence of toxin production, to enzyme immunoassays (EIAs) for the presence of specific toxins, to PCR tests (also known as nucleic acid amplification tests, or NAAT) for the presence of the genetic material encoding the toxin. Both the immunoassays and PCR-based tests provide considerably faster results than do culture-based techniques, making the latter of little clinical relevance. The institution of PCR/NAAT diagnostics has resulted in a significant increase in the number of positive tests[81] leading to considerable debate regarding the issue of overdiagnosis. This led to updated guidelines from IDSA[31] and the European Society of Clinical Microbiology and Infectious Diseases (ESCMID)[82]; each offering two different testing strategies, both including PCR and immunoassay-based testing, but with differing recommendations for the sequence in which they should be performed, and whether these tests are necessary.

Traditional culture methods typically use selective media such as cycloserine-cefoxitin-frutose agar followed by anaerobic incubation. Once growth appears, biochemical testing or newer methods such as matrix-assisted laser desorption ionization time of flight (MALDI-TOF) are used to identify the organism. After identification, further testing is needed to confirm the presence of toxin; historically, this was done by exposing a cell-line monolayer to a filtrate from the culture and looking for characteristic cytopathic effects, but now more direct immunoassays for the presence of toxin are used. Because of the requirement to prepare and maintain specialized media, the time needed for bacterial growth, the need for anaerobic culture facilities, and the labor-intensive toxin testing, culture-based testing became too costly and cumbersome to be of clinical utility. By the time results are reported, generally several days after a stool sample has been submitted, the decision to administer treatment has already been made. However, culture enables growth of an isolate, which is used for genetic characterization in research studies, public health surveillance, and outbreak investigations.

Direct detection of toxin A initially, and later of toxins A and B, became available in the late 1980s. Their ease of use and rapid turnaround time led to widespread use in most facilities. Direct toxin tests used EIAs to detect preformed toxin in stool, using labeled antibodies directed at toxins A and B that could subsequently be detected by immunofluorescence or colorimetry, depending on the specific test. Numerous commercial assays became available, all with similar sensitivity and specificity. Later versions, including those available currently, are generally more sensitive than earlier versions. Several systematic reviews and meta-analyses reported sensitivity of approximately 75–80%, with specificity in the mid-to-high 90% range.[83] Clinically, this lack of sensitivity led to concern of false negative testing, especially in the early 2000s when CDI was occurring with increased frequency and severity. With cases of fulminant CDI increasing, clinicians were understandably reluctant to rely on a test that had a false negative rate of 25%. One strategy that was adopted was the use of serial stool testing, with the rationale that repeated testing would decrease the number of missed CDI cases. One group reported a 12% increase in sensitivity by adopting repeat testing, and the practice became widespread.[84] However, this strategy fails to consider the decreasing probability of true CDI with each negative test, or the possibility of some substance in the stool possibly interfering with the test. Utilizing typical sensitivity and specificity values for EIA tests, along with a standard estimate of the proportion of tested patients with true CDI, Peterson et al. demonstrated that by the second round of testing, any positive result was more likely to be a false positive than a true positive and concluded that this strategy could not be recommended.[85]

With increasing recognition that EIA testing was too insensitive for use in the era of increasing CDI, PCR-based tests for CDI seemed to be the solution.[86] Available clinically in the early 2000s, PCR testing was reported to be highly sensitive and specific, with estimates for both in the high 90% range. In addition to superior performance characteristics, PCR testing was rapidly automated into user-friendly systems that required minimal laboratory technician time and provided rapid turn-around time. More recently, the same PCR-based technique for identifying the presence of the gene encoding *C. difficile* toxin B has been incorporated into a multiple-pathogen panel that tests for *C. difficile* as well as more than 20 other causes of infectious diarrhea. Based on these characteristics, PCR-based testing was widely adopted, and the *C. difficile* testing landscape went from most facilities in the United States using an EIA method in 2008, to most using PCR now. A consistent finding of moving from EIA to PCR-based testing was an approximately 25% increase in the incidence of CDI.[87–89] This could be interpreted in several ways, the more optimistic of which was to label the 25% increase in cases as CDI cases that were previously missed by EIA testing. An alternative explanation, however, was that some of the increase was due to identifying carriers of *C. difficile* and subsequently labeling them as having CDI. Because PCR testing identifies the presence of genetic material that encodes a toxin, and not the toxin itself, a positive result could not differentiate between carriage of *C. difficile* with the capability to produce toxin, residual genetic material from nonviable organisms, and active CDI with a toxin-producing strain.

Investigators explored the possibility of some PCR positive patients having no toxin present by evaluating patients with both EIA and PCR tests and evaluating the outcomes among those: positive by both methods, with discordant results (all PCR positive but EIA negative), and negative by both methods. Those with discordant results (genetic material encoding the toxin present, but no evidence of toxin itself present) appeared similar to those who were negative by both tests and had similar outcomes. In contrast, the subjects with detectable toxin by EIA and a positive PCR both appeared more ill and had worse outcomes.[90] These results suggested that detection of the genetic material encoding toxin B (i.e., a positive PCR test) might be overly sensitive for diagnosing CDI.

Recent IDSA and ESCMID guidelines have taken two approaches to the diagnosis of CDI. The ESCMID guidelines propose two algorithms (Fig. 157-1), one starting with a highly sensitive test such as PCR/NAAT or glutamate dehydrogenase (GDH), an enzyme expressed by both toxigenic and nontoxigenic strains of *C. difficile*.[82] A positive result from a highly sensitive test is then followed by testing with a more specific test for the presence of the actual toxin, such as an EIA. A positive result from the EIA is interpreted as CDI likely to be present, whereas a negative EIA combined with a positive PCR or GDH requires clinical evaluation for CDI or carriage of *C. difficile*, with optional use of a third test to aid in this evaluation. A negative PCR or GDH test at the outset requires no further testing, and implies CDI is unlikely to be present. The second proposed algorithm starts with two tests, a GDH and an EIA. If both are positive, CDI is likely, and no further testing is recommended. Similarly, if both are negative, CDI is unlikely, and again no further testing is recommended. In the case of discordant results, PCR or toxigenic culture can be used, with a negative test suggesting CDI is unlikely and a positive test requiring clinical evaluation for CDI versus carriage of a toxigenic strain.

In contrast, IDSA guidelines for CDI testing propose a different strategy.[31] Their proposed algorithm starts with an institutional commitment to not submit stool specimens for *C. difficile* testing from patients receiving laxatives, and to only submit specimens from patients with unexplained new onset of at least three unformed stools in a 24-hour period (Fig. 157-2). If such a commitment is in place, PCR/NAAT testing alone or a stool toxin test (EIA) as part of a multiple step algorithm including a GDH or PCR is suggested. If no such institutional commitment is in place, a stool toxin test (EIA) as part of a multiple-step algorithm including a GDH or PCR is suggested, rather than PCR testing alone.

The choice between using a single highly sensitive test (PCR) versus a two-step process combining a sensitive and more specific test has been the subject of debate.[91] In addition to the concerns most often cited, which include overtreatment of patients who are just carriers of *C. difficile* if using an overly sensitive test and missing a true case of CDI using a combined approach, practical considerations also come into consideration. Using two tests adds work for laboratory staff, both for running additional tests and for maintaining quality controls and competency in an additional test. Similarly, utilizing an institutional commitment to ensure appropriate ordering of stool tests requires ongoing monitoring and education, which can be particularly challenging at teaching institutions with multiple trainees rotating in and out of the facility. Ultimately, clinicians need to be aware that whichever test is utilized, making the diagnosis of CDI starts with an assessment of the patient's risk for CDI and their clinical manifestations. A patient with recent use of clindamycin or another high-risk antimicrobial with severe manifestations of CDI and no alternative explanation should be treated for CDI regardless of any test result, as the pre- and posttest probability of disease is high, and the clinical outcomes of severe CDI are serious. Alternatively, a patient with minimal symptoms and no clear risk factor for CDI should probably not be tested, but instead be evaluated for other causes of mild gastrointestinal symptoms.

ESCMID and IDSA guidelines also differ on who should be tested. The ESCMID guidelines suggest testing of "all submitted unformed stool samples from patients 3 years or older," whereas the IDSA guidelines state that "patients with unexplained and new-onset of three or more unformed stools in 24 hours are the preferred target population for testing for CDI." Both qualify their recommendations as weak, based on low or very low quality of evidence. Most institutions in the United States use similar criteria to those recommended by the IDSA—encouraging CDI testing in patients with three or more stools daily, without a clear alternative explanation, and assessing their pretest probability by inquiring about prior CDI episodes, antimicrobial exposure, and other risk factors. Testing of patients receiving laxatives and enteral feedings should be discouraged in most circumstances.

CLINICAL MANIFESTATIONS

The classic symptoms and signs of CDI include watery diarrhea, abdominal pain and cramping, and occasionally fever (typically low-grade).[92] However, the range of clinical manifestations is broad, ranging from asymptomatic carriage that is detected only by screening studies or inappropriate clinical testing, to fulminant CDI that typically consists of ileus, toxic megacolon, and sepsis physiology, and carries a high mortality rate.[93] Why some patients are colonized asymptomatically, whereas others have diarrhea, and a small minority experience fulminant CDI is not known. Host and pathogen factors may be involved, including the effects of the colonic microbiome and any perturbations to the microbiome composition from medications, diet, and other influences. Because outcomes differ based on disease severity, an attempt at disease classification should be part of the evaluation of any patient with CDI. However, this is currently limited by the lack of a prospectively validated scoring system that reliably identifies severe disease. The clinical manifestations of CDI of varying severity will be discussed here, but it is important to note that the differentiation between mild, moderate, and severe disease is not precise, and can vary between clinicians.

Asymptomatic Carriage

Among hospitalized patients, rectal swab cultures demonstrate up to 20% of patients harbor *C. difficile* but do not have clinical manifestations of CDI.[47,94,95] On testing, more than half of the colonizing strains are capable of producing the toxins associated with clinical illness.[47] Treating such asymptomatic carriers does not prevent subsequent illness, but paradoxically increases the percentage of patients with persistent carriage.[96] Among nonhospitalized individuals, colonization rates are considerably lower (1–6%)[97,98] likely reflecting the decreased intensity of antimicrobial use in this population, relative to hospitalized patients.

There is no protective effect of *C. difficile* carriage from the occasional episode of diarrhea from other causes, whether it is infectious, induced by diet or medications, or idiopathic. Testing of such individuals for CDI can be limited by policies restricting testing to those with three or more unformed stools and without other more likely causes of diarrhea. However, even with such restrictions some patients with asymptomatic carriage and an unrelated bout of diarrhea will be identified as having CDI. Unfortunately, there is no reliable method of differentiating a patient with CDI from one with asymptomatic

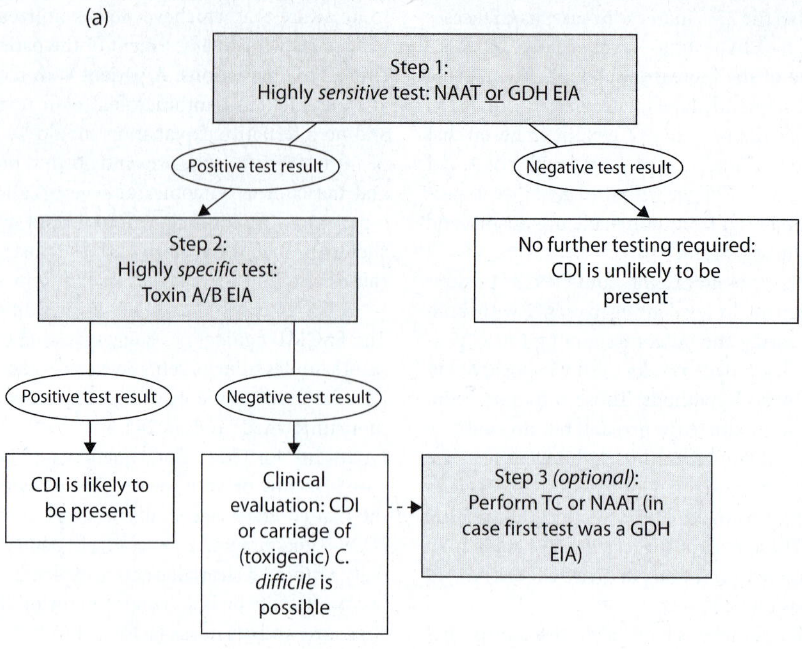

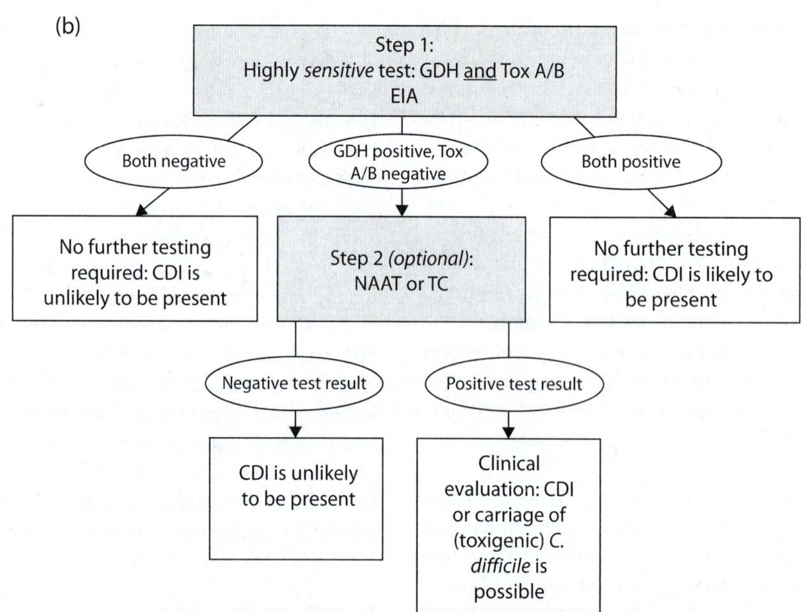

FIGURE 157-1. Diagnosis schematic adapted from the European Society of Clinical Microbiology and Infectious Diseases guidelines. Recommended algorithms for CDI testing. (a) GDH or NAAT Tox A/B algorithm. (b) GDH and Tox A/B NAAT/TC algorithm. (Abbreviations: CDI = *Clostridium difficile* infection; GDH = glutamate dehydrogenase; NAAT = nucleic acid amplification test; TC = toxigenic culture; Tox A/B = toxin A/B; EIA = enzyme immunoassay.) (*Source:* Reproduced with Permission from Crobach MJT, Planche T, Eckert C, et al. European Society of Clinical Microbiology and Infectious Diseases: Update of the diagnostic guidance document for *Clostridium difficile* infection. *Clin Microbiol Infect.* 2016;22(S4):S63–81, Fig. 3.)

carriage plus unrelated diarrhea, whether by symptoms, exam findings, laboratory investigation, or a combination thereof. As the prevalence of CDI has increased and testing has become more sensitive, this has been an increasingly common problem facing clinicians.

Mild and Moderate Disease

Mild and moderate CDI are discussed together because there is no consensus or commonly used criteria to differentiate between the two. Symptoms of mild or moderate (alternatively, nonsevere) CDI include watery diarrhea, cramping abdominal pain, low-grade fever, anorexia, and nausea. Less common manifestations are vomiting and bloody stools. Physical exam may demonstrate abdominal tenderness, usually in the lower quadrants. Expected lab findings include a leukocytosis with neutrophil predominance, mild creatinine elevation, and a positive stool test for *C. difficile*. Commonly used definitions of severe CDI include a white blood cell count greater than 15,000 cells/mL and a creatinine over 1.5 mg/dL,[99,100] but these definitions are not prospectively validated, and most clinicians will encounter patients with values above those cutoffs who otherwise appear to have mild to moderate disease. Imaging, if obtained, may show colonic thickening with a nonspecific bowel gas pattern, but no evidence of large bowel dilatation. Endoscopy is rarely performed in the setting of CDI, since

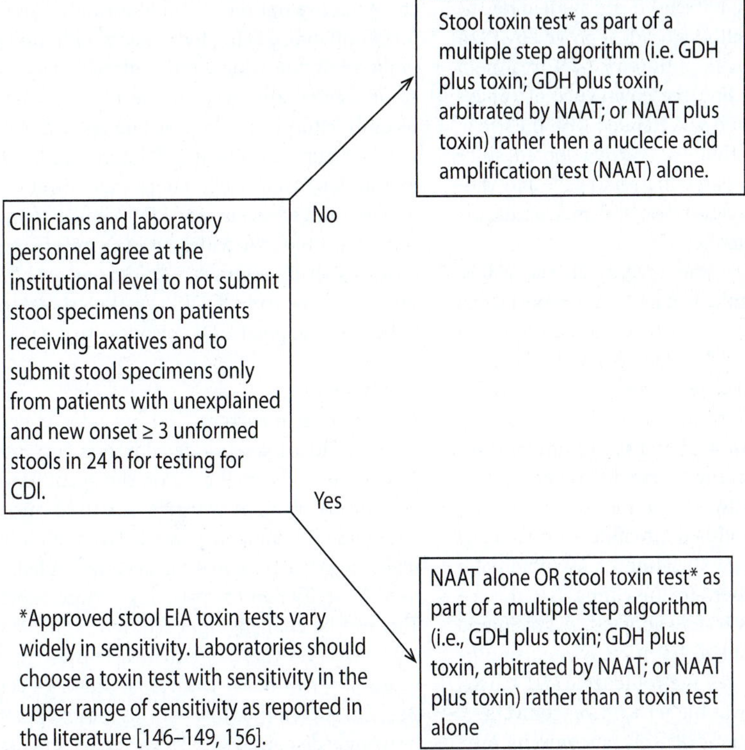

Stool toxin test* as part of a multiple step algorithm (i.e. GDH plus toxin; GDH plus toxin, arbitrated by NAAT; or NAAT plus toxin) rather then a nuclecie acid amplification test (NAAT) alone.
No
Clinicians and laboratory personnel agree at the institutional level to not submit stool specimens on patients receiving laxatives and to submit stool specimens only from patients with unexplained and new onset ≥ 3 unformed stools in 24 h for testing for CDI.
Yes
NAAT alone OR stool toxin test* as part of a multiple step algorithm (i.e., GDH plus toxin; GDH plus toxin, arbitrated by NAAT; or NAAT plus toxin) rather than a toxin test alone
*Approved stool EIA toxin tests vary widely in sensitivity. Laboratories should choose a toxin test with sensitivity in the upper range of sensitivity as reported in the literature [146–149, 156].

FIGURE 157-2. Diagnosis schematic adapted from the Infectious Disease Society of America guidelines. *C. difficile* infection laboratory test recommendations based on preagreed institutional criteria for patient stool submission. (Abbreviations: CDI = *Clostridium difficile* infection; EIA = enzyme immunoassay; GDH = glutamate dehydrogenase; NAAT = nucleic acid amplification test.) (*Source:* Reproduced with Permission from McDonald LC, Gerding DN, Johnson S, et al. Clinical Practice Guidelines for *Clostridium difficile* infection in adults and children: 2017 Update by the Infectious Diseases Society of America (IDSA) and Society for Healthcare Epidemiology of America (SHEA). *Clin Infect Dis.* 2018;66(7):987–94, Fig. 2.)

rapid and sensitive testing combined with an increasing awareness of CDI as a common cause of diarrhea usually leads to a prompt diagnosis. If performed, findings include edematous mucosa, erythema, and pseudomembrane formation.

Severe Disease

Severe CDI is a medical emergency, with mortality rates of 30–50%.[101,102] Presenting symptoms and exam findings include the diarrhea and abdominal pain expected in nonsevere disease, but also include more worrisome findings such as hypotension, abdominal distention, decreased or absent bowel sounds, and altered mental status. Additionally, worsening disease can lead to colonic dysfunction and dilatation, which can initially present as a decrease in the amount and frequency of diarrhea and give false reassurance that the patient is clinically improving. Laboratory findings include leukocytosis of greater than 15,000 cells/mL, but often a marked leukocytosis of 25,000 cells/mL or higher, and a positive stool test for *C. difficile.* Other common findings include an increase in serum creatinine and a decrease in albumin. Imaging findings suggesting severe disease include diffuse colonic thickening, colonic dilatation, and occasionally the presence of free intra-abdominal air due to colonic perforation. Any of these findings should prompt clinicians to consider the diagnosis of severe CDI, with prompt initiation of antimicrobial therapy, aggressive supportive cares, and infectious disease and surgical consultation.

TREATMENT

Several therapies have activity against *C. difficile* and have been tested in clinical trials. However, some are not available in the United States, and others are rarely used due to a combination of limited availability, cost, minimal evidence for efficacy, and the widespread availability of effective and well-tolerated first-line options. With the increase in CDI incidence and severity in the 2000s, new therapies have received approval from the U.S. Food and Drug administration (FDA), while others are still in development or awaiting regulatory clarification. Because patients with CDI are so prone to recurrence, CDI treatment is now often viewed as a two-step process: initial cure of the acute episode, and prevention of subsequent recurrence. All new CDI treatments are evaluated on both their ability to achieve initial clinical cure, and how frequently recurrence occurs. Interestingly, some therapy is now given exclusively to prevent recurrence, and can be thought of as adjunctive therapy to the primary treatment for the acute CDI episode. Therapies in this category include monoclonal antibodies against toxin B and FMT—although this has also been administered for the treatment of acute CDI, including severe disease. In addition to FMT performed via the administration of donor stool that is minimally processed, pharmaceutical companies are developing stool-derived therapies, wherein specific organisms present in the donor stool are selectively cultivated, processed, and administered.

Antimicrobial Therapy

Traditional antimicrobials that have evidence from clinical trials supporting their efficacy against acute CDI include metronidazole, vancomycin, fidaxomicin, nitazoxanide, bacitracin, fusidic acid, teicoplanin, and the combination of metronidazole and rifampin. Oral vancomycin is the only antimicrobial to be compared to placebo in a clinical trial,[22] and has since been evaluated in comparison to most of the other agents. It was initially used to treat pseudomembranous colitis prior to the discovery of *C. difficile* as the etiology of the disease and had favorable pharmacokinetics in that it had little to no systemic absorption, and thus was ideal for treating a disease of the intestinal lumen. With the discovery of an anaerobic organism as the cause of CDI, metronidazole began to be used and studied for the treatment of CDI.[23,25] Metronidazole, although not approved by FDA for this indication, became the preferred option for CDI treatment after the CDC raised concerns regarding the emergence of vancomycin-resistant enterococci that might be accelerated with the use of oral vancomycin.[103] This recommendation was widely adopted, since the few small studies that directly compared metronidazole and vancomycin showed nearly identical success rates, and metronidazole was inexpensive and relatively well tolerated.

When CDI increased in incidence and severity in the 2000s, decreasing success with metronidazole began to be reported in observational studies. The first trial evidence of metronidazole as less effective than vancomycin emerged in 2005, when Zar and colleagues reported the results of their trial stratified by disease severity—mild or moderate versus severe.[100] Their initial results showed no significant difference between treatment arms overall, but a significant increase in clinical success with vancomycin in the severe disease group was observed. Although the difference between the metronidazole and vancomycin groups shrank when a modified intention-to-treat analysis was conducted and outcome reclassification of asymptomatic carriers was changed in response to letters-to-the-editor,[104–106] the use of vancomycin for severe disease was widely adopted. A systematic review of CDI therapy in 2011 concluded that there was no significant difference in clinical success between metronidazole and vancomycin, although numerically success was higher with vancomycin.[107] Ultimately, the evidence for the superiority of vancomycin over metronidazole that is reflected in the most recent IDSA treatment guidelines came from an unlikely source—an industry-funded trial of tolevamer versus metronidazole versus vancomycin.[108] Although a negative trial from the standpoint of tolevamer, a toxin-binding resin designed to clear toxin from the intestinal lumen, the metronidazole versus vancomycin comparison was the largest single trial comparing the two drugs, and when pooled with the prior three trials comparing the same drugs demonstrated a significant improvement in initial cure with the use of vancomycin. Although the difference in efficacy between metronidazole and vancomycin is small, current IDSA guidelines suggest metronidazole only be used when recommended agents (currently vancomycin and fidaxomicin) are not available or not tolerated, although it likely is still adequate therapy for mild disease.[31]

Vancomycin is the preferred agent for fulminant CDI—generally defined as CDI with ileus, colonic dilatation, and severe sepsis physiology. Given the extremely high morbidity of this condition, vancomycin at a higher dose than that conventionally used (500 mg versus 125 mg, both four times daily) is suggested, although when compared directly in nonfulminant CDI there was no observable benefit to the higher dose.[109] Other methods to try to deliver therapy to an inflamed colon in the setting of decreased motility include delivery of vancomycin by enema, and the coadministration of intravenous metronidazole.[31,101] Other critical adjuncts include fluid resuscitation and surgical evaluation for possible colectomy or colonic decompression.

Fidaxomicin was specifically developed for the treatment of CDI after the increase in incidence and severity in the 2000s. It is a macrocyclic antibiotic with minimal absorption, potent activity against *C. difficile*, and minimal activity against typical colonic flora. Studied in two large multicenter trials with vancomycin as the comparator, initial cure rates were similar between treatment groups.[33,99] However, recurrence was significantly less frequent with fidaxomicin than with vancomycin—15% versus 25%. This absolute difference of 10% translates to a number-needed-to-treat of ten; which although lower than many commonly accepted practices, still means that nine of ten recipients receive no benefit from its use compared to use of vancomycin. Price concerns led to slow uptake of fidaxomicin, with multiple publications analyzing the cost-effectiveness of the drug, and most concluding that substantial reductions were needed before it became a cost-effective option.[110,111] Interestingly, this situation has led to most fidaxomicin use being for patients with multiple CDI recurrences—a population for which little efficacy data exists. Fidaxomicin, the second agent approved by the FDA for the treatment of CDI, was recently endorsed as a first-line agent for CDI by the most recent IDSA treatment guidelines.[31] Future studies are needed to determine its role for severe CDI, where vancomycin remains the mainstay of therapy, and for recurrent CDI. Similar to tapering regimens of vancomycin, which are widely used despite being only supported by case series, tapering regimens of fidaxomicin have been used with some success for recurrent CDI.[112] Antimicrobial treatment options for initial and subsequent CDI episodes are detailed in Table 157-1.

Recurrence

Treatment of recurrent CDI episodes is generally similar to treatment of the initial episode, although current recommendations suggest some variation, based on the agent used for the initial episode. Specifically, if metronidazole was used initially, vancomycin is recommended. If vancomycin was used initially, a tapered vancomycin regimen or fidaxomicin is recommended. Importantly, clinicians need to verify that the patient is indeed experiencing recurrent CDI. This can be challenging, because *C. difficile* can persist posttherapy, and even if no viable organisms are present, the genetic material that is tested for in many clinical laboratories can remain detectable for weeks and even months. For this reason, posttreatment "test-of-cure" is strongly discouraged.[31] However, patients are often counseled about the high risk of recurrence, and frequently present for care reporting new onset of diarrhea with the passage of a single unformed stool. In the absence of other signs of CDI (multiple diarrheal stools, abdominal pain, leukocytosis, fever), this is unlikely to represent recurrent CDI—but stool testing is often performed, and a positive result is common (regardless of whether the test is a stool toxin EIA or a PCR). Further complicating matters, postinfectious motility disorders are common, such that clinicians are often faced with the dilemma of a patient presenting with multiple unformed stools, minimal or no abdominal pain, without a leukocytosis or fever—but with a positive test for CDI. There is currently no reliable method for differentiating recurrent CDI from colonization combined with postinfectious motility issues. Stool testing for markers of inflammation may offer some help, but robust evidence supporting their use is lacking.

Because of the high rate of recurrent CDI, and the difficulty differentiating it from colonization, considerable effort has been invested into methods for preventing recurrence. In addition to the options discussed above using different antimicrobials and dosing regiments, several more novel options are available. These include inexpensive and widely available interventions such as the administration of probiotic formulations, use of combination or sequential antimicrobial therapy, FDA-approved therapy such as infusion of monoclonal antibodies targeting toxin B, and FMT and various stool-derived products, which are in different stages of development and regulatory oversight.

Probiotics are widely used by patients and recommended by practicing physicians, both for primary prevention of CDI (discussed later), and for the prevention of subsequent recurrence. Current guidelines do not support probiotic use for CDI prevention, for a variety of reasons.[31] The evidence supporting them is largely from small industry-sponsored trials, some with extremely high rates of CDI in the control groups.[113,114] Additional issues include the lack of any regulatory oversight guaranteeing the contents of a specific product, the multiple strains included in different formulations, and the uncertainty as to the required dose. The evidence for probiotics for preventing subsequent episodes of CDI is mixed. *Saccharomyces boulardii* is the organism with the most rigorous data supporting its use,[115] whereas other preparations (including probiotic containing foods such as kefir) have weaker supporting evidence.[116] In the nonimmune compromised host, the harms of probiotics are likely

TABLE 157-1 TREATMENT OPTIONS FOR INITIAL AND RECURRENT CASES OF *CLOSTRIDIODES DIFFICILE* INFECTION

Agent	Adult Dose and Route[a]	Comments
Treatment Options for Initial Cases of *C. difficile* Infection		
Agent	**Adult Dose and Route[a]**	**Comments**
Vancomycin	125 mg orally 4× daily (500 mg used for fulminant disease)	Available in capsules but also can be compounded from intravenous vancomycin. FDA approved for *C. difficile* infection.
Fidaxomicin	200 mg orally 2× daily	Reduction in recurrence versus vancomycin must be weighed against high cost. FDA approved for *C. difficile* infection.
Metronidazole	500 mg orally or intravenously 3× daily	Slightly less effective than vancomycin. Intravenous administration with oral vancomycin may have role in fulminant disease.
Nitazoxanide	500 mg orally 2× daily	Studied in two small trials with similar effectiveness to vancomycin and metronidazole.
Bacitracin	20,000–25,000 units orally 4× daily	Rarely used and not generally available in this formulation.
Teicoplanin	400 mg orally 2× daily	Not available in the United States; glycopeptide antimicrobial.
Fusidic acid	500 mg orally 3× daily	Not available in the United States.
Treatment Options for Recurrent Cases of *C. difficile* Infection		
Agent	Dose and Route	Comments
Vancomycin	125 mg orally 4× daily; may be given for a prolonged course with a tapering regimen	If vancomycin was used for the initial episode, most clinicians would opt for a longer course with a taper (i.e., moving to 3× daily, then 2× daily, then daily). If another agent was used, a nontapering course is usually tried.
Fidaxomicin	200 mg orally 2× daily	Some case reports of using a longer duration with a taper.
Rifaximin	200–400 mg orally 2× daily	Given after a course of vancomycin.
Fecal microbiota transplantation (FMT)	Varied doses, routes of administration, and frequency	When FMT should be tried is not settled. Has been used as early as the initial episode of CDI. Availability variable, regulatory status uncertain.

[a]Please see Table 2 in the Infectious Disease Society of America Guidelines [McDonald LC, Gerding DN, Johnson S, et al. Clinical Practice Guidelines for *Clostridium difficile* infection in adults and children: 2017 Update by the Infectious Diseases Society of America (IDSA) and Society for Healthcare Epidemiology of America (SHEA). *Clin Infect Dis*. 2018;66(7):987–94] for recommendations and dosing in children, or the most recent edition of the American Academy of Pediatrics, Report of the Committee of Infectious Diseases (Red Book).

minimal, and their potential use can be discussed with patients as a possible adjunct for prevention of recurrence.

Sequential combination therapy has been studied for the prevention of subsequent recurrence, albeit in nonrandomized, noncontrolled studies. The drugs most commonly used are an initial treatment course of vancomycin, followed afterward by a course of rifaximin, a minimally absorbed rifamycin derivative that is active against *C. difficile*. Most patients in these small series remained free of recurrent disease; however, high-level rifaximin resistance was observed, despite the relatively small sample size.[117,118] This raises concern that widespread adoption of this strategy might lead to similarly widespread rates of rifaximin resistance, and the loss of this as a viable option. Accordingly, this remains a relatively uncommon method of prevention but one that might be useful in the setting of multiple recurrences.

Another option for prevention of recurrent CDI is the infusion of monoclonal antibodies against toxin B. Observations that patients with lower levels of naturally occurring antibodies against CDI had higher rates of recurrence than those with higher levels led to the development of this product, currently FDA approved as bezlotoxumab. Initial studies included antibodies to both toxins A and B, but efficacy was limited to infusions containing antibodies to toxin B, so the toxin A antibody (actoxumab) was subsequently dropped from further development. Phase 3 trials showed that infusion of bezlotoxumab during their standard-of-care antimicrobial therapy for CDI led to a reduction in subsequent recurrence.[119] The reduction in recurrence was 10%, similar in magnitude to the reduction seen with the use of fidaxomicin when compared to vancomycin. It is unknown whether the combination of fidaxomicin plus bezlotoxumab would have an additional benefit to that seen with either drug alone. Since this is an agent administered via intravenous infusion during the treatment of CDI, it is likely to be used primarily in the inpatient setting, or at stand-alone infusion centers. Currently, there is insufficient experience with bezlotoxumab outside of clinical trials to comment further on the role that it may have for prevention of recurrence.

A last approach to prevention of recurrent CDI is the administration of fecal material from a healthy donor, to repopulate the microbiome of a patient with recurrent CDI. In theory, the administration of the fecal material (also known as fecal microbiota transplantation) should reconstitute the diverse normal microbiome of a healthy colon, which is believed to confer some degree of protection from CDI (and possibly other intestinal infections) by occupying the ecologic niche of the environment. Reference to administration of fecal material to ill patients is found in Chinese medical writings from the fourth century,[120] albeit with some dispute as to what ailment it was purported to cure,[121] and in the modern medical literature dating to the 1950s.[122] The literature supporting FMT as a treatment for prevention of recurrent CDI (and at times, for the treatment of the acute CDI) consisted of case reports and small case series until the epidemic of CDI that occurred in the early 2000s. With the increase in CDI incidence and severity, interest in alternative treatments grew, and there was a flurry of studies reporting on the use of FMT for prevention of recurrent CDI—including several randomized controlled trials. In addition to trials administering minimally processed donor stool to patients, there have also been studies using stool-derived products, which may eliminate the variability and the lack of standardization between different donors.

Initial case reports and case series of FMT were largely favorable, reporting high rates of success and minimal complications.[123–125] However, it was difficult to interpret this literature, since there was little standardization regarding route of administration, optimal FMT dose, donor source, definition of recurrence, follow-up time, and other variables. Route of FMT administration was of particular interest since some routes (via colonoscopy and nasogastric tube) required an endoscopist or trained personnel and imaging services, whereas others (enema or oral ingestion of encapsulated material) were able to be used without such expertise. Although the literature on FMT seemed promising, with efficacy of preventing recurrent CDI after a single administration of FMT of 85%,[126] few studies included a concurrent control group, and even fewer were able to blind participants to the treatment received. Since the primary manifestation of recurrent CDI is abnormal stool frequency and consistency (something that can be influenced by a wide variety of factors), combined with a positive laboratory test indicating the presence of *C. difficile* (knowing that many tests for *C. difficile* can remain positive for a prolonged period), this lack of a blinded control group is concerning. More robust data regarding FMT has begun to emerge, including several randomized control trials (RCTs). Some of the RCTs compared different routes of FMT administration,[127] or the difference between fresh and frozen material,[128,129] and thus provide little information regarding the benefits of FMT relative to non-FMT therapy. However, others have included non-FMT control arms, including one where the participants were blinded by administration of either donor feces or their own recently passed feces,[130] both administered via colonoscopy. The data regarding FMT efficacy from these trials has been largely favorable, but there have been some findings that merit consideration.

The first reported trial of FMT compared to two vancomycin-based control arms showed a high success rate in the FMT arm, whereas both control groups had strikingly high rates of recurrence, leading to early termination of the trial.[131] A second RCT comparing FMT to vancomycin had similar high success rates in the FMT group (90%) relative to the vancomycin group (26%), with the trial also stopped prematurely.[132] The aforementioned trial of FMT versus autologous feces administration via colonoscopy similarly had an overall positive result, with 91% of FMT recipients being free of recurrent CDI, compared to 63% among those receiving their own feces. However, there was an interesting site effect, with one of the two sites having nearly identical success rates (92% vs. 90%), whereas the other had markedly differing success rates (90% vs. 43%).[130] In contrast to these studies, a recent trial of FMT versus a tapered vancomycin regimen was also stopped prematurely, but not because of efficacy, but rather futility. In this study, the subjects receiving tapered vancomycin had higher rates of success (defined as remaining recurrence free), with 58% success in the vancomycin group compared to 44% in the FMT group.[133] Combined, these trials suggest that FMT may have a sizable effect on reducing recurrence of CDI, but with the relatively small sample sizes and some negative results, there is still uncertainty as to whether FMT is effective at preventing recurrent CDI compared to medical therapy alone. Indeed, it is difficult to determine what medical therapy should be compared to FMT. Ideally, a trial comparing FMT versus placebo, both administered after optimal medical therapy for the acute CDI episode, would be performed. Whether optimal medical therapy should be mandated to include fidaxomicin or bezlotoxumab is uncertain—trial data would support this, but real-world usage suggests that this would not reflect current clinical reality. In the interim, FMT can be administered to patients for the prevention of recurrent CDI under an enforcement discretion policy by the FDA, provided that written informed consent is obtained and the patient is aware that FMT is considered experimental and not FDA approved. In 2019, the FDA issued a safety alert regarding two patients who developed infections caused by multidrug-resistant organisms that were transmitted via FMT from a donor colonized with the identical strain.[134] There are several commercial entities studying products initially derived from human fecal material, but subsequently processed to enrich the composition of certain bacterial species and to standardize the administered product. Such a product would have the advantage of eliminating the variability between individual donors, and indeed the variability between the same donor at different time points. It may also lead to some regulatory clarity, since the difficulty in characterizing FMT and the variability between donors has been a barrier to consistent regulatory oversight. Preliminary studies of such products have been mixed, with some showing favorable results from phase II trials,[135,136] but confirmatory phase III trials are lacking.

Other agents for CDI are in various stages of development and may emerge as viable alternatives in the future. Surotomycin is an analog of daptomycin, orally administered and minimally absorbed. It appears highly active against *C. difficile*, yet minimally active against other components of the fecal flora. However, only one of two preliminary studies against vancomycin met noninferiority criteria.[137,138] Ridinilazole is another novel nonabsorbable antimicrobial with a low minimum inhibitory concentration for *C. difficile*[139] and purportedly less activity against other fecal bacteria. A favorable phase II study versus vancomycin has been reported,[140] and phase III studies are underway.

INFECTION CONTROL

Given the challenges of treating CDI, the ability of the bacterium to persist in the environment, and the high use of antimicrobial use in healthcare facilities (thus leading to a high rate of intestinal disruption and opportunity for *C. difficile* to establish a foothold), CDI is a major focus of healthcare facility infection prevention and control departments. Data regarding the optimal infection control practices to prevent acquisition and spread of CDI are largely from non-RCT studies, including observational studies utilizing pre-post design, and more robust analysis methods such as interrupted times series to assess for the effect of temporal trends that might affect the results. Broadly speaking, infection control objectives regarding *C. difficile* include preventing patients from newly acquiring the bacterium (whether from the healthcare environment, another patient, or a hospital employee), limiting the reservoir of *C. difficile* in the hospital environment, and identifying and limiting sources of *C. difficile*.

The tools available for addressing these challenges vary from the most basic tenants of infection control, including scrupulous hand hygiene and the use of gloves when contact with fecal material is possible, to high-tech methods such as robotic cleaning systems and whole-genome sequencing to clearly elucidate chains of transmission within the facility. In many cases, there is not strong comparative evidence supporting which methods should be widely adopted, and when there is evidence it is often supporting a "bundled" intervention which may lack evidence for the individual components.[141] Core recommendations that are central to infection control involving all infectious agents include universal adherence to hand hygiene and use of gloves when potentially encountering fecal material.[142] Unfortunately, alcohol hand sanitizers, which offer convenience and are typically associated with higher rates of hand hygiene compliance, do not reliably kill *C. difficile*—in particular, the spore form. Because of this, hand washing with soap and water is the recommended method of hand hygiene after contact with a patient with CDI.[143] However, if this recommendation results in a decrease in the overall rate of hand hygiene compliance, the benefit of hand washing may be overwhelmed by the higher rate of hand-hygiene noncompliance.

Other widely accepted practices include eliminating the use of reusable rectal thermometers,[144] use of private rooms for patients with CDI, and using a terminal room cleaning method that is effective at killing *C. difficile* spores. The most widely used method of terminal cleaning (the deep clean performed after a patient vacates the room) is bleach-based cleaning, typically a 10% hypochlorite solution.[145] Other methods that have data supporting their use include the use of automated systems such as ultraviolet light devices[146] and utilizing aerosolized hydrogen peroxide.[147] The importance of terminal room cleaning is highlighted by studies that showed higher rates of CDI in subsequent room occupants when the prior occupant had CDI, presumably due to residual viable *C. difficile* in the room.[39,40]

Some infection control interventions (hand hygiene, room cleaning) are achievable in all settings, including long-term-care facilities and clinics. More resource intensive efforts such as automated systems for room disinfection and WGS to elucidate transmission chains are likely only available in hospitals. With patients often transitioning from ambulatory, hospital, and long-term-care settings, attention to limiting the spread of *C. difficile* in each setting is needed. Unfortunately, effective infection control requires significant resources, which may not be readily available in clinics and long-term-care facilities.

A topic of recent interest has been the role of patients colonized with *C. difficile*, but without symptoms of infection. Prior studies had suggested that these patients are at heightened risk of developing CDI themselves, but more recently there has been concern that these patients may serve as a reservoir for the spread of *C. difficile*, since they are typically not on contact precautions or identified as patients where hand washing is preferred over alcohol hand sanitizer use.[148] Testing patients for the presence of *C. difficile* in the absence of symptoms raises several issues. Even if it was certain that isolation of colonized patients conferred clinical benefit in terms of reduced transmission, other potential harms should be considered. One such potential harm is that patients with a positive CDI test will likely have a high probability of receiving therapy, whether simply because the positive test is noted by a clinician or because a nonspecific or transitory change in bowel habits is classified as diarrhea. Another concern is that if special precautions are needed to prevent the spread of *C. difficile* from asymptomatic carriers to other patients, then potentially the performance of standard infection control measures, such as hand hygiene and use of gloves when handling body fluids, is suboptimal and needs improvement. Until there are data, which support identification and isolation of patients with asymptomatic colonization, there is no recommendation for this practice.[31]

PREVENTION

Prevention of CDI can be achieved through a multipronged approach. Some have already been discussed but will be reemphasized here to highlight the preventive aspects of each approach. Already discussed options include selection of antimicrobials to treat CDI that result in fewer episodes of recurrence, using adjunctive therapy such as FMT or bezlotoxumab during or shortly after CDI treatment, appropriately testing only symptomatic patients for CDI, and limiting in-hospital transmission and reservoirs via effective infection control practices. All play some role in limiting CDI episodes, although most are focused on secondary, not primary prevention. The most notable exception is infection control, which can limit new-onset CDI in patients,[40] and presumably also limit new episodes of colonization among healthcare personnel which theoretically will lead to new episodes of primary CDI, although direct evidence for this is lacking. Methods for primary prevention for CDI not addressed thus far include improved antimicrobial stewardship, better understanding of which antimicrobials are higher risk for triggering CDI, probiotic administration with antimicrobials, identifying and minimizing environmental sources of *C. difficile* organisms, vaccine development, and other potential methods to protect the microbiome from the perturbations that increase risk for CDI.

Improved antimicrobial stewardship has great potential for prevention of CDI. Various estimates of the percentage of antimicrobial use that is unnecessary range from 30% to over 50%.[149,150] Although some of this unnecessary use represents excessive treatment duration, which may not confer as much CDI risk as a treatment course that is completely unnecessary, driving down unnecessary antimicrobial use of any type should theoretically decrease the disruption of the microbiome and lead to fewer episodes of CDI. One study modeling community-associated CDI demonstrated that a 10% decrease in antibiotic prescribing could lead to a 17% decrease in CDI.[151] Ideally, stewardship should be targeting all types of antimicrobial prescribing, but with finite time and resources targeting high-yield areas is recommended. These include areas with high rates of antimicrobial prescribing—particularly if the agents are high risk for triggering CDI—and areas where a sizeable proportion of the use is inappropriate. This is discussed in detail in the chapter on Antibiotic Resistance and Stewardship (Chapter 153: Antibiotic Resistance and Stewardship). Respiratory infections and urinary tract infections are leading causes of antimicrobial use, but often are over- and misdiagnosed and therefore leading drivers of inappropriate use.[152] Working to reduce misdiagnoses would eliminate a considerable amount of microbiome disruption and CDI episodes, especially since agents commonly used to treat pneumonia and urinary tract infection include broad spectrum agents that are at high risk for triggering CDI, including fluoroquinolones and cephalosporins. Another high-yield area for stewardship to reduce unnecessary antimicrobial use is the use of antimicrobials prescribed before or after dental procedures, with growing evidence that much of that use is inappropriate.[153,154]

The use of probiotics for the primary prevention of CDI has gained considerable interest in the past few years. Several systematic reviews suggested that the administration of probiotics with antimicrobial therapy had a sizable and significant decrease in the rate of subsequent CDI.[113,114] Unfortunately, while there is a substantial number of trials comparing probiotic versus placebo administration during antimicrobial therapy for the prevention of CDI, there are multiple reasons to be cautious of the findings when they are combined. Many of the studies are small and funded by the probiotic manufacturer, and the interventions are a heterogeneous mixture of organisms at varying doses. Most concerning is the fact that in several of the trials reporting a benefit, the rate of CDI in the control group was much higher than that seen in typical practice. Whereas most U.S. hospitals see 1–3% of patients receiving antimicrobials subsequently develop CDI, in these trials rates were in the 15–25% range.[155,156] When limiting the analysis to just hospitals having CDI rates in the placebo groups that are in line with those seen in most facilities, any benefit of probiotics lost statistical significance.[113] Finally, the single largest trial of probiotics versus placebo for the prevention of CDI, which was independently funded, showed no benefit to probiotic administration.[157] Because of the weak evidence for benefit, and the variability and unregulated nature of probiotics in the United States, it is difficult to recommend their use for the prevention of CDI. Ingestion of probiotics via dietary sources such as yogurt, kefir, and other fermented foods has some support from observational data,[116] so if they happen to fall within the dietary preferences of the patient, encouraging their intake may be helpful, and avoids the additional pill-burden of probiotics administered via capsules or tablets.

Identifying environmental sources of *C. difficile* is an ongoing effort of many researchers. Dietary intake has been postulated, but sampling of various animal sources has thus far not identified a specific food of animal origin consistently contaminated with *C. difficile*.[74–77] One identifiable source of *C. difficile* is in the homes of patients recently treated for CDI,[78] in particular those with multiple recurrences.[158] Whether being able to detect organisms in the home leads to increased rates of reinfection, transmission, or other clinical outcomes needs further study, as does the question of which interventions might lead to reductions in these outcomes. Although strong data are lacking, advising patients to clean their homes (especially high-touch areas) may provide benefit, with little chance of harm.

The most efficient method of prevention for CDI, as for many infectious diseases, may ultimately lie with the development of a safe and effective active vaccination strategy. Although no vaccine is currently available, numerous candidate vaccines are underdevelopment.[159] The types of vaccine currently being studied include toxoid preparations, whereby purified toxins A and B are inactivated and then administered via injection,[160] and more novel preparations such as administration of nontoxigenic strains of *C. difficile* and the development of recombinant toxin-based peptides. Other strategies being studied include vaccines utilizing surface proteins to generate an immune response, although these are still in the preliminary phases of animal studies. In contrast, there is some preliminary human experience with toxoid-based vaccines, which have been studied in phase I trials for dose finding and safety assessments, and demonstrated ability to induce high titers against toxins A and B.[161,162] A final method of prevention, which could be classified as an oral vaccine or as a stool-derived product, is the administration of spores of a nontoxigenic strain of *C. difficile*. This has been the topic of investigation for several decades,[163] and culminated with a clinical trial that demonstrated safety, ability for the spores to colonize the digestive tract, and decreased recurrence relative to placebo when administered to patients recently treated for CDI.[164] Despite this, at the current time products based on nontoxigenic strains are not licensed or available for clinical use.

CONCLUSIONS

The last two decades have seen dramatic increases in the incidence and severity of CDI, such that it has become one of the most important infectious diseases of hospitalized and ambulatory patients. The high rate of recurrence, the ability of the organism to survive for extended periods of time in the environment, and the potential for catastrophic illness has forced nearly all clinicians and healthcare systems to confront this organism. Promising developments include the approval of several new agents, the emerging science of microbiome-based interventions, and the availability of rapid, sensitive, and specific tests. Furthermore, better understanding of effective infection control interventions and increased attention to antimicrobial stewardship are also helping to stem the tide on an epidemic that seemed to be exploding in the early 2000s but has since stabilized. Current challenges that need to be addressed include further understanding of the acquisition of CDI, the optimal laboratory approach to diagnosing CDI, how to differentiate chronic colonization from recurrent infection, effective and sustainable infection prevention practices outside of acute-care settings, and the development of a safe and effective vaccine that could be administered to at-risk patients to prevent the cycle of infection and recurrence.

References

1. Miller BA, Chen LF, Sexton DJ, Anderson DJ. Comparison of the burdens of hospital-onset, healthcare facility-associated *Clostridium difficile* infection and of healthcare-associated infection due to methicillin-resistant *Staphylococcus aureus* in community hospitals. *Infect Control Hosp Epidemiol.* 2011;32(4):387–90.
2. Chitnis AS, Holzbauer SM, Belflower RM, et al. Epidemiology of community-associated *Clostridium difficile* infection, 2009 through 2011. *JAMA Intern Med.* 2013;173(14):1359–67.
3. Dubberke ER, Olsen MA. Burden of *Clostridium difficile* on the healthcare system. *Clin Infect Dis.* 2012;55(Suppl 2):S88–92.
4. CDC. *Antibiotic Resistance Threats in the United States, 2019.* Atlanta, GA: U.S. Department of Health and Human Services, CDC; 2019.
5. Hall IC, O'Toole E. Intestinal flora in newborn infants with a description of a new pathogenic anaerobe, *Bacillus difficilis. Am J Dis Child.* 1935;49(49):390–402.
6. Larson HE, Price AB, Honour P, Borriello SP. *Clostridium difficile* and the aetiology of pseudomembranous colitis. *Lancet.* 1978;1(8073):1063–6.
7. Bartlett JG, Chang TW, Gurwith M, Gorbach SL, Onderdonk AB. Antibiotic-associated pseudomembranous colitis due to toxin-producing clostridia. *N Engl J Med.* 1978;298(10):531–4.
8. Bartlett JG, Moon N, Chang TW, Taylor N, Onderdonk AB. Role of *Clostridium difficile* in antibiotic-associated pseudomembranous colitis. *Gastroenterology.* 1978;75(5):778–82.
9. Loo VG, Poirier L, Miller MA, et al. A predominantly clonal multi-institutional outbreak of *Clostridium difficile*-associated diarrhea with high morbidity and mortality. *N Engl J Med.* 2005;353(23):2442–9.
10. McDonald LC, Killgore GE, Thompson A, et al. An epidemic, toxin gene-variant strain of *Clostridium difficile. N Engl J Med.* 2005;353(23):2433–41.
11. Pepin J, Valiquette L, Cossette B. Mortality attributable to nosocomial *Clostridium difficile*-associated disease during an epidemic caused by a hypervirulent strain in Quebec. *CMAJ.* 2005;173(9):1037–42.
12. Goorhuis A, Van der Kooi T, Vaessen N, et al. Spread and epidemiology of *Clostridium difficile* polymerase chain reaction ribotype 027/toxinotype III in the Netherlands. *Clin Infect Dis.* 2007;45(6):695–703.
13. Joseph R, Demeyer D, Vanrenterghem D, van den Berg R, Kuijper E, Delmee M. First isolation of *Clostridium difficile* PCR ribotype 027, toxinotype III in Belgium. *Euro Surveill.* 2005;10(10):E051020.4.
14. Riley TV, Thean S, Hool G, Golledge CL. First Australian isolation of epidemic *Clostridium difficile* PCR ribotype 027. *Med J Aust.* 2009;190(12):706–8.
15. Coignard B, Barbut F, Blanckaert K, et al. Emergence of *Clostridium difficile* toxinotype III, PCR-ribotype 027-associated disease, France, 2006. *Euro Surveill.* 2006;11(9):E060914.1.
16. Rupnik M, Tambic Andrasevic A, Trajkovska Dokic E, et al. Distribution of *Clostridium difficile* PCR ribotypes and high proportion of 027 and 176 in some hospitals in four South Eastern European countries. *Anaerobe.* 2016;42:142–4.
17. Tae CH, Jung SA, Song HJ, et al. The first case of antibiotic-associated colitis by *Clostridium difficile* PCR ribotype 027 in Korea. *J Korean Med Sci.* 2009;24(3):520–4.
18. Muto CA, Pokrywka M, Shutt K, et al. A large outbreak of *Clostridium difficile*-associated disease with an unexpected proportion of deaths and colectomies at a teaching hospital following increased fluoroquinolone use. *Infect Control Hosp Epidemiol.* 2005;26(3):273–80.
19. McFarland LV. Update on the changing epidemiology of *Clostridium difficile*-associated disease. *Nat Clin Pract Gastroenterol Hepatol.* 2008;5(1):40–8.
20. Fowler S, Webber A, Cooper BS, et al. Successful use of feedback to improve antibiotic prescribing and reduce *Clostridium difficile* infection: A controlled interrupted time series. *J Antimicrob Chemother.* 2007;59(5):990–5.
21. McDonald LC, Coignard B, Dubberke E, Song X, Horan T, Kutty PK. Recommendations for surveillance of *Clostridium difficile*-associated disease. *Infect Control Hosp Epidemiol.* 2007;28(2):140–5.
22. Keighley MR, Burdon DW, Arabi Y, et al. Randomised controlled trial of vancomycin for pseudomembranous colitis and postoperative diarrhoea. *Br Med J.* 1978;2(6153):1667–9.
23. Wenisch C, Parschalk B, Hasenhundl M, Hirschl AM, Graninger W. Comparison of vancomycin, teicoplanin, metronidazole, and fusidic acid for the treatment of *Clostridium difficile*-associated diarrhea. *Clin Infect Dis.* 1996;22(5):813–8.
24. Young GP, Ward PB, Bayley N, et al. Antibiotic-associated colitis due to *Clostridium difficile*: Double-blind comparison of vancomycin with bacitracin. *Gastroenterology.* 1985;89(5):1038–45.
25. Teasley DG, Gerding DN, Olson MM, et al. Prospective randomised trial of metronidazole versus vancomycin for *Clostridium-difficile*-associated diarrhoea and colitis. *Lancet.* 1983;2(8358):1043–6.
26. Wullt M, Odenholt I. A double-blind randomized controlled trial of fusidic acid and metronidazole for treatment of an initial episode of *Clostridium difficile*-associated diarrhoea. *J Antimicrob Chemother.* 2004;54(1):211–6.
27. Dudley MN, McLaughlin JC, Carrington G, Frick J, Nightingale CH, Quintiliani R. Oral bacitracin vs vancomycin therapy for *Clostridium difficile*-induced diarrhea. A randomized double-blind trial. *Arch Intern Med.* 1986;146(6):1101–4.
28. de Lalla F, Nicolin R, Rinaldi E, et al. Prospective study of oral teicoplanin versus oral vancomycin for therapy of pseudomembranous colitis and *Clostridium difficile*-associated diarrhea. *Antimicrob Agents Chemother.* 1992;36(10):2192–6.
29. Musher DM, Logan N, Bressler AM, Johnson DP, Rossignol JF. Nitazoxanide versus vancomycin in *Clostridium difficile* infection: A randomized, double-blind study. *Clin Infect Dis.* 2009;48(4):e41–6.
30. Musher DM, Logan N, Hamill RJ, et al. Nitazoxanide for the treatment of *Clostridium difficile* colitis. *Clin Infect Dis.* 2006;43(4):421–7.
31. McDonald LC, Gerding DN, Johnson S, et al. Clinical practice guidelines for *Clostridium difficile* infection in adults and children: 2017 Update by the Infectious Diseases Society of America (IDSA) and Society for Healthcare Epidemiology of America (SHEA). *Clin Infect Dis.* 2018;66(7):987–94.
32. Lessa FC, Mu Y, Bamberg WM, et al. Burden of *Clostridium difficile* infection in the United States. *N Engl J Med.* 2015;372(9):825–34.
33. Cornely OA, Crook DW, Esposito R, et al. Fidaxomicin versus vancomycin for infection with *Clostridium difficile* in Europe, Canada, and the USA: A double-blind, non-inferiority, randomised controlled trial. *Lancet Infect Dis.* 2012;12(4):281–9.

34. Louie TJ, Miller MA, Mullane KM, et al. Fidaxomicin versus vancomycin for *Clostridium difficile* infection. *N Engl J Med.* 2011;364(5):422–31.
35. Johnson S. Recurrent *Clostridium difficile* infection: A review of risk factors, treatments, and outcomes. *J Infect.* 2009;58(6):403–10.
36. Leffler DA, Lamont JT. *Clostridium difficile* infection. *N Engl J Med.* 2015;372(16):1539–48.
37. Awad MM, Johanesen PA, Carter GP, Rose E, Lyras D. *Clostridium difficile* virulence factors: Insights into an anaerobic spore-forming pathogen. *Gut Microbes.* 2014;5(5):579–93.
38. Verity P, Wilcox MH, Fawley W, Parnell P. Prospective evaluation of environmental contamination by *Clostridium difficile* in isolation side rooms. *J Hosp Infect.* 2001;49(3):204–9.
39. Freedberg DE, Salmasian H, Cohen B, Abrams JA, Larson EL. Receipt of antibiotics in hospitalized patients and risk for *Clostridium difficile* infection in subsequent patients who occupy the same bed. *JAMA Intern Med.* 2016;176(12):1801–8.
40. Shaughnessy MK, Micielli RL, DePestel DD, et al. Evaluation of hospital room assignment and acquisition of *Clostridium difficile* infection. *Infect Control Hosp Epidemiol.* 2011;32(3):201–6.
41. Deakin LJ, Clare S, Fagan RP, et al. The *Clostridium difficile* spo0A gene is a persistence and transmission factor. *Infect Immun.* 2012;80(8):2704–11.
42. Kyne L, Warny M, Qamar A, Kelly CP. Association between antibody response to toxin A and protection against recurrent *Clostridium difficile* diarrhoea. *Lancet.* 2001;357(9251):189–93.
43. Lanis JM, Heinlen LD, James JA, Ballard JD. *Clostridium difficile* 027/BI/NAP1 encodes a hypertoxic and antigenically variable form of TcdB. *PLoS Pathog.* 2013;9(8):e1003523.
44. Gerhard R, Nottrott S, Schoentaube J, Tatge H, Olling A, Just I. Glucosylation of Rho GTPases by *Clostridium difficile* toxin A triggers apoptosis in intestinal epithelial cells. *J Med Microbiol.* 2008;57(Pt 6):765–70.
45. Lyerly DM, Saum KE, MacDonald DK, Wilkins TD. Effects of *Clostridium difficile* toxins given intragastrically to animals. *Infect Immun.* 1985;47(2):349–52.
46. Mitchell TJ, Ketley JM, Haslam SC, et al. Effect of toxin A and B of *Clostridium difficile* on rabbit ileum and colon. *Gut.* 1986;27(1):78–85.
47. Shim JK, Johnson S, Samore MH, Bliss DZ, Gerding DN. Primary symptomless colonisation by *Clostridium difficile* and decreased risk of subsequent diarrhoea. *Lancet.* 1998;351(9103):633–6.
48. von Eichel-Streiber C, Laufenberg-Feldmann R, Sartingen S, Schulze J, Sauerborn M. Comparative sequence analysis of the *Clostridium difficile* toxins A and B. *Mol Gen Genet.* 1992;233(1–2):260–8.
49. Brouwer MS, Roberts AP, Hussain H, Williams RJ, Allan E, Mullany P. Horizontal gene transfer converts non-toxigenic *Clostridium difficile* strains into toxin producers. *Nat Commun.* 2013;4:2601.
50. Papatheodorou P, Zamboglou C, Genisyuerek S, Guttenberg G, Aktories K. Clostridial glucosylating toxins enter cells via clathrin-mediated endocytosis. *PLoS One.* 2010;5(5):e10673.
51. Carter GP, Rood JI, Lyras D. The role of toxin A and toxin B in the virulence of *Clostridium difficile*. *Trends Microbiol.* 2012;20(1):21–9.
52. Ng J, Hirota SA, Gross O, et al. *Clostridium difficile* toxin-induced inflammation and intestinal injury are mediated by the inflammasome. *Gastroenterology.* 2010;139(2):542–52, 552.e1–3.
53. Kim PH, Iaconis JP, Rolfe RD. Immunization of adult hamsters against *Clostridium difficile*-associated ileocecitis and transfer of protection to infant hamsters. *Infect Immun.* 1987;55(12):2984–92.
54. Drudy D, Fanning S, Kyne L. Toxin A-negative, toxin B-positive *Clostridium difficile*. *Int J Infect Dis.* 2007;11(1):5–10.
55. Lyras D, O'Connor JR, Howarth PM, et al. Toxin B is essential for virulence of *Clostridium difficile*. *Nature.* 2009;458(7242):1176–9.
56. Kuehne SA, Cartman ST, Heap JT, Kelly ML, Cockayne A, Minton NP. The role of toxin A and toxin B in *Clostridium difficile* infection. *Nature.* 2010;467(7316):711–3.
57. Stubbs S, Rupnik M, Gibert M, Brazier J, Duerden B, Popoff M. Production of actin-specific ADP-ribosyltransferase (binary toxin) by strains of *Clostridium difficile*. *FEMS Microbiol Lett.* 2000;186(2):307–12.
58. Bacci S, Molbak K, Kjeldsen MK, Olsen KE. Binary toxin and death after *Clostridium difficile* infection. *Emerg Infect Dis.* 2011;17(6):976–82.
59. Popoff MR, Rubin EJ, Gill DM, Boquet P. Actin-specific ADP-ribosyltransferase produced by a *Clostridium difficile* strain. *Infect Immun.* 1988;56(9):2299–306.
60. Pepin J, Valiquette L, Alary ME, et al. *Clostridium difficile*-associated diarrhea in a region of Quebec from 1991 to 2003: A changing pattern of disease severity. *CMAJ.* 2004;171(5):466–72.
61. Katz KC, Golding GR, Choi KB, et al. The evolving epidemiology of *Clostridium difficile* infection in Canadian hospitals during a postepidemic period (2009–2015). *CMAJ.* 2018;190(25):E758–65.
62. Giancola SE, Williams RJ2nd, Gentry CA. Prevalence of the *Clostridium difficile* BI/NAP1/027 strain across the United States Veterans Health Administration. *Clin Microbiol Infect.* 2018;24(8):877–81.
63. Loo VG, Bourgault AM, Poirier L, et al. Host and pathogen factors for *Clostridium difficile* infection and colonization. *N Engl J Med.* 2011;365(18):1693–703.
64. Thomas C, Stevenson M, Riley TV. Antibiotics and hospital-acquired *Clostridium difficile*-associated diarrhoea: A systematic review. *J Antimicrob Chemother.* 2003;51(6):1339–50.
65. Hu MY, Katchar K, Kyne L, et al. Prospective derivation and validation of a clinical prediction rule for recurrent *Clostridium difficile* infection. *Gastroenterology.* 2009;136(4):1206–14.
66. Linsky A, Gupta K, Lawler EV, Fonda JR, Hermos JA. Proton pump inhibitors and risk for recurrent *Clostridium difficile* infection. *Arch Intern Med.* 2010;170(9):772–8.
67. Huang H, Wu S, Chen R, et al. Risk factors of *Clostridium difficile* infections among patients in a university hospital in Shanghai, China. *Anaerobe.* 2014;30:65–9.
68. Rodemann JF, Dubberke ER, Reske KA, Seo DH, Stone CD. Incidence of *Clostridium difficile* infection in inflammatory bowel disease. *Clin Gastroenterol Hepatol.* 2007;5(3):339–44.
69. Singh H, Nugent Z, Yu BN, Lix LM, Targownik LE, Bernstein CN. Higher incidence of *Clostridium difficile* infection among individuals with inflammatory bowel disease. *Gastroenterology.* 2017;153(2):430–8.e2.
70. Yan D, Chen Y, Lv T, et al. *Clostridium difficile* colonization and infection in patients with hepatic cirrhosis. *J Med Microbiol.* 2017;66(10):1483–8.
71. Khanna S, Pardi DS, Aronson SL, et al. The epidemiology of community-acquired *Clostridium difficile* infection: A population-based study. *Am J Gastroenterol.* 2012;107(1):89–95.
72. Guh AY, Adkins SH, Li Q, et al. Risk factors for community-associated *Clostridium difficile* infection in adults: A case-control study. *Open Forum Infect Dis.* 2017;4(4):ofx171.
73. Gould LH, Limbago B. *Clostridium difficile* in food and domestic animals: A new foodborne pathogen? *Clin Infect Dis.* 2010;51(5):577–82.
74. Shaughnessy MK, Snider T, Sepulveda R, et al. Prevalence and molecular characteristics of *Clostridium difficile* in retail meats, food-producing and companion animals, and humans in Minnesota. *J Food Prot.* 2018;81(10):1635–42.
75. de Boer E, Zwartkruis-Nahuis A, Heuvelink AE, Harmanus C, Kuijper EJ. Prevalence of *Clostridium difficile* in retailed meat in the Netherlands. *Int J Food Microbiol.* 2011;144(3):561–4.
76. Hoffer E, Haechler H, Frei R, Stephan R. Low occurrence of *Clostridium difficile* in fecal samples of healthy calves and pigs at slaughter and in minced meat in Switzerland. *J Food Prot.* 2010;73(5):973–5.
77. Hensgens MP, Keessen EC, Squire MM, et al. *Clostridium difficile* infection in the community: A zoonotic disease? *Clin Microbiol Infect.* 2012;18(7):635–45.
78. Loo VG, Brassard P, Miller MA. Household transmission of *Clostridium difficile* to family members and domestic pets. *Infect Control Hosp Epidemiol.* 2016;37(11):1342–8.
79. Eyre DW, Cule ML, Wilson DJ, et al. Diverse sources of *C. difficile* infection identified on whole-genome sequencing. *N Engl J Med.* 2013;369(13):1195–205.
80. Eyre DW, Davies KA, Davis G, et al. Two distinct patterns of *Clostridium difficile* diversity across Europe indicating contrasting routes of spread. *Clin Infect Dis.* 2018;67(7):1035–44.
81. Cohen J, Limbago B, Dumyati G, et al. Impact of changes in *Clostridium difficile* testing practices on stool rejection policies and *C. difficile* positivity rates across multiple laboratories in the United States. *J Clin Microbiol.* 2014;52(2):632–4.
82. Crobach MJ, Planche T, Eckert C, et al. European Society of Clinical Microbiology and Infectious Diseases: Update of the diagnostic guidance document for *Clostridium difficile* infection. *Clin Microbiol Infect.* 2016;22(Suppl 4):S63–81.
83. Planche T, Aghaizu A, Holliman R, et al. Diagnosis of *Clostridium difficile* infection by toxin detection kits: A systematic review. *Lancet Infect Dis.* 2008;8(12):777–84.
84. Manabe YC, Vinetz JM, Moore RD, Merz C, Charache P, Bartlett JG. *Clostridium difficile* colitis: An efficient clinical approach to diagnosis. *Ann Intern Med.* 1995;123(11):835–40.
85. Peterson LR, Robicsek A. Does my patient have *Clostridium difficile* infection? *Ann Intern Med.* 2009;151(3):176–9.

86. Tenover FC, Baron EJ, Peterson LR, Persing DH. Laboratory diagnosis of *Clostridium difficile* infection can molecular amplification methods move us out of uncertainty? *J Mol Diagn*. 2011;13(6):573–82.

87. Longtin Y, Trottier S, Brochu G, et al. Impact of the type of diagnostic assay on *Clostridium difficile* infection and complication rates in a mandatory reporting program. *Clin Infect Dis*. 2013;56(1):67–73.

88. Moehring RW, Lofgren ET, Anderson DJ. Impact of change to molecular testing for *Clostridium difficile* infection on healthcare facility-associated incidence rates. *Infect Control Hosp Epidemiol*. 2013;34(10):1055–61.

89. Koo HL, Van JN, Zhao M, et al. Real-time polymerase chain reaction detection of asymptomatic *Clostridium difficile* colonization and rising *C. difficile*-associated disease rates. *Infect Control Hosp Epidemiol*. 2014;35(6):667–73.

90. Polage CR, Gyorke CE, Kennedy MA, et al. Overdiagnosis of *Clostridium difficile* infection in the molecular test era. *JAMA Intern Med*. 2015;175(11):1792–801.

91. Fang FC, Polage CR, Wilcox MH. Point-counterpoint: What is the optimal approach for detection of *Clostridium difficile* infection? *J Clin Microbiol*. 2017;55(3):670–80.

92. Bagdasarian N, Rao K, Malani PN. Diagnosis and treatment of *Clostridium difficile* in adults: A systematic review. *JAMA*. 2015;313(4):398–408.

93. Rubin MS, Bodenstein LE, Kent KC. Severe *Clostridium difficile* colitis. *Dis Colon Rectum*. 1995;38(4):350–4.

94. Leekha S, Aronhalt KC, Sloan LM, Patel R, Orenstein R. Asymptomatic *Clostridium difficile* colonization in a tertiary care hospital: Admission prevalence and risk factors. *Am J Infect Control*. 2013;41(5):390–3.

95. Johnson S, Clabots CR, Linn FV, Olson MM, Peterson LR, Gerding DN. Nosocomial *Clostridium difficile* colonisation and disease. *Lancet*. 1990;336(8707):97–100.

96. Johnson S, Homann SR, Bettin KM, et al. Treatment of asymptomatic *Clostridium difficile* carriers (fecal excretors) with vancomycin or metronidazole. A randomized, placebo-controlled trial. *Ann Intern Med*. 1992;117(4):297–302.

97. Galdys AL, Nelson JS, Shutt KA, et al. Prevalence and duration of asymptomatic *Clostridium difficile* carriage among healthy subjects in Pittsburgh, Pennsylvania. *J Clin Microbiol*. 2014;52(7):2406–9.

98. Zomer TP, Duijkeren E VAN, Wielders CCH, et al. Prevalence and risk factors for colonization of *Clostridium difficile* among adults living near livestock farms in the Netherlands. *Epidemiol Infect*. 2017;145(13):2745–9.

99. Louie TJ, Miller MA, Mullane KM, et al. Fidaxomicin versus vancomycin for *Clostridium difficile* infection. *N Engl J Med*. 2011;364:422–31.

100. Zar FA, Bakkanagari SR, Moorthi KM, Davis MB. A comparison of vancomycin and metronidazole for the treatment of *Clostridium difficile*-associated diarrhea, stratified by disease severity. *Clin Infect Dis*. 2007;45(3):302–7.

101. Rokas KE, Johnson JW, Beardsley JR, Ohl CA, Luther VP, Williamson JC. The addition of intravenous metronidazole to oral vancomycin is associated with improved mortality in critically ill patients with *Clostridium difficile* infection. *Clin Infect Dis*. 2015;61(6):934–41.

102. Longo WE, Mazuski JE, Virgo KS, Lee P, Bahadursingh AN, Johnson FE. Outcome after colectomy for *Clostridium difficile* colitis. *Dis Colon Rectum*. 2004;47(10):1620–6.

103. CDC issues recommendations for preventing spread of vancomycin resistance. *Am J Health Syst Pharm*. 1995;52(12):1272–4.

104. Zar FA, Davis MB. Reply to Bishara et al., Huggan et al., and Lawrence et al. *Clin Infect Dis*. 2007;45(12):1649–51.

105. Bishara J, Wattad M, Paul M. Vancomycin and metronidazole for the treatment of *Clostridium difficile*-associated diarrhea. *Clin Infect Dis*. 2007;45(12):1646–7; author reply 1649–51.

106. Huggan PJ, Murdoch DR. Vancomycin therapy for severe *Clostridium difficile*-associated diarrhea. *Clin Infect Dis*. 2007;45(12):1647–8; author reply 1649–51.

107. Drekonja DM, Butler M, MacDonald R, et al. Comparative effectiveness of *Clostridium difficile* treatments: A systematic review. *Ann Intern Med*. 2011;155(12):839–47.

108. Johnson S, Louie TJ, Gerding DN, et al. Vancomycin, metronidazole, or tolevamer for *Clostridium difficile* infection: Results from two multinational, randomized, controlled trials. *Clin Infect Dis*. 2014;59(3):345–54.

109. Fekety R, Silva J, Kauffman C, Buggy B, Deery HG. Treatment of antibiotic-associated *Clostridium difficile* colitis with oral vancomycin: Comparison of two dosage regimens. *Am J Med*. 1989;86(1):15–9.

110. Lam SW, Neuner EA, Fraser TG, Delgado D, Chalfin DB. Cost-effectiveness of three different strategies for the treatment of first recurrent *Clostridium difficile* infection diagnosed in a community setting. *Infect Control Hosp Epidemiol*. 2018;39(8):924–30.

111. Bartsch SM, Umscheid CA, Fishman N, Lee BY. Is fidaxomicin worth the cost? An economic analysis. *Clin Infect Dis*. 2013;57(4):555–61.

112. Soriano MM, Danziger LH, Gerding DN, Johnson S. Novel fidaxomicin treatment regimens for patients with multiple *Clostridium difficile* infection recurrences that are refractory to standard therapies. *Open Forum Infect Dis*. 2014;1(2):ofu069.

113. Goldenberg JZ, Mertz D, Johnston BC. Probiotics to prevent *Clostridium difficile* infection in patients receiving antibiotics. *JAMA*. 2018;320(5):499–500.

114. Johnston BC, Ma SS, Goldenberg JZ, et al. Probiotics for the prevention of *Clostridium difficile*-associated diarrhea: A systematic review and meta-analysis. *Ann Intern Med*. 2012;157(12):878–88.

115. Surawicz CM, McFarland LV, Greenberg RN, et al. The search for a better treatment for recurrent *Clostridium difficile* disease: Use of high-dose vancomycin combined with *Saccharomyces boulardii*. *Clin Infect Dis*. 2000;31(4):1012–7.

116. Bakken JS. Staggered and tapered antibiotic withdrawal with administration of kefir for recurrent *Clostridium difficile* infection. *Clin Infect Dis*. 2014;59(6):858–61.

117. Johnson S, Schriever C, Galang M, Kelly CP, Gerding DN. Interruption of recurrent *Clostridium difficile*-associated diarrhea episodes by serial therapy with vancomycin and rifaximin. *Clin Infect Dis*. 2007;44(6):846–8.

118. Johnson S, Schriever C, Patel U, Patel T, Hecht DW, Gerding DN. Rifaximin redux: Treatment of recurrent *Clostridium difficile* infections with rifaximin immediately post-vancomycin treatment. *Anaerobe*. 2009;15(6):290–1.

119. Wilcox MH, Gerding DN, Poxton IR, et al. Bezlotoxumab for prevention of recurrent *Clostridium difficile* infection. *N Engl J Med*. 2017;376(4):305–17.

120. Zhang F, Luo W, Shi Y, Fan Z, Ji G. Should we standardize the 1,700-year-old fecal microbiota transplantation? *Am J Gastroenterol*. 2012;107(11):1755; author reply 1755–6.

121. Jia N. A misleading reference for fecal microbiota transplant. *Am J Gastroenterol*. 2015;110(12):1731.

122. Eiseman B, Silen W, Bascom GS, Kauvar AJ. Fecal enema as an adjunct in the treatment of pseudomembranous enterocolitis. *Surgery*. 1958;44(5):854–9.

123. Aas J, Gessert CE, Bakken JS. Recurrent *Clostridium difficile* colitis: Case series involving 18 patients treated with donor stool administered via a nasogastric tube. *Clin Infect Dis*. 2003;36(5):580–5.

124. Bakken JS. Fecal bacteriotherapy for recurrent *Clostridium difficile* infection. *Anaerobe*. 2009;15(6):285–9.

125. Borody TJ, Warren EF, Leis SM, Surace R, Ashman O, Siarakas S. Bacteriotherapy using fecal flora: Toying with human motions. *J Clin Gastroenterol*. 2004;38(6):475–83.

126. Drekonja DM, Reich J, Gezahegn S, et al. Fecal microbiota transplantation for *Clostridium difficile* infection—A systematic review. *Ann Intern Med*. 2015;162(9):630–8.

127. Kao D, Roach B, Silva M, et al. Effect of oral capsule- vs colonoscopy-delivered fecal microbiota transplantation on recurrent *Clostridium difficile* infection: A randomized clinical trial. *JAMA*. 2017;318(20):1985–93.

128. Jiang ZD, Ajami NJ, Petrosino JF, et al. Randomised clinical trial: Faecal microbiota transplantation for recurrent *Clostridium difficile* infection—Fresh, or frozen, or lyophilised microbiota from a small pool of healthy donors delivered by colonoscopy. *Aliment Pharmacol Ther*. 2017;45(7):899–908.

129. Lee CH, Steiner T, Petrof EO, et al. Frozen vs fresh fecal microbiota transplantation and clinical resolution of diarrhea in patients with recurrent *Clostridium difficile* infection: A randomized clinical trial. *JAMA*. 2016;315(2):142–9.

130. Kelly CR, Khoruts A, Staley C, et al. Effect of fecal microbiota transplantation on recurrence in multiply recurrent *Clostridium difficile* infection: A randomized trial. *Ann Intern Med*. 2016;165(9):609–16.

131. van Nood E, Vrieze A, Nieuwdorp M, et al. Duodenal infusion of donor feces for recurrent *Clostridium difficile*. *N Engl J Med*. 2013;368(5):407–15.

132. Cammarota G, Masucci L, Ianiro G, et al. Randomised clinical trial: Faecal microbiota transplantation by colonoscopy vs. vancomycin for the treatment of recurrent *Clostridium difficile* infection. *Aliment Pharmacol Ther*. 2015;41(9):835–43.

133. Hota SS, Sales V, Tomlinson G, et al. Oral vancomycin followed by fecal transplantation versus tapering oral vancomycin treatment for recurrent *Clostridium difficile* infection: An open-label, randomized controlled trial. *Clin Infect Dis*. 2017;64(3):265–71.

134. DeFilipp Z, Bloom PP, Torres Soto M, et al. Drug-resistant *E. coli* bacteremia transmitted by fecal microbiota transplant. *N Engl J Med.* 2019;381(21):2043–50.

135. Orenstein R, Dubberke E, Hardi R, et al. Safety and durability of RBX2660 (microbiota suspension) for recurrent *Clostridium difficile* infection: Results of the PUNCH CD study. *Clin Infect Dis.* 2016;62(5):596–602.

136. Khanna S, Pardi DS, Kelly CR, et al. A novel microbiome therapeutic increases gut microbial diversity and prevents recurrent *Clostridium difficile* infection. *J Infect Dis.* 2016;214(2):173–81.

137. Daley P, Louie T, Lutz JE, et al. Surotomycin versus vancomycin in adults with *Clostridium difficile* infection: Primary clinical outcomes from the second pivotal, randomized, double-blind, Phase 3 trial. *J Antimicrob Chemother.* 2017;72(12):3462–70.

138. Boix V, Fedorak RN, Mullane KM, et al. Primary outcomes from a phase 3, randomized, double-blind, active-controlled trial of surotomycin in subjects with *Clostridium difficile* infection. *Open Forum Infect Dis.* 2017;4(1):ofw275.

139. Vickers RJ, Tillotson G, Goldstein EJ, Citron DM, Garey KW, Wilcox MH. Ridinilazole: A novel therapy for *Clostridium difficile* infection. *Int J Antimicrob Agents.* 2016;48(2):137–43.

140. Vickers RJ, Tillotson GS, Nathan R, et al. Efficacy and safety of ridinilazole compared with vancomycin for the treatment of *Clostridium difficile* infection: A phase 2, randomised, double-blind, active-controlled, non-inferiority study. *Lancet Infect Dis.* 2017;17(7):735–44.

141. Barker AK, Ngam C, Musuuza JS, Vaughn VM, Safdar N. Reducing *Clostridium difficile* in the inpatient setting: A systematic review of the adherence to and effectiveness of *C. difficile* prevention bundles. *Infect Control Hosp Epidemiol.* 2017;38(6):639–50.

142. Johnson S, Gerding DN, Olson MM, et al. Prospective, controlled study of vinyl glove use to interrupt *Clostridium difficile* nosocomial transmission. *Am J Med.* 1990;88(2):137–40.

143. Pittet D, Allegranzi B, Boyce J, World Health Organization World Alliance for Patient Safety First Global Patient Safety Challenge Core Group of Experts. The World Health Organization guidelines on hand hygiene in health care and their consensus recommendations. *Infect Control Hosp Epidemiol.* 2009;30(7):611–22.

144. Brooks SE, Veal RO, Kramer M, Dore L, Schupf N, Adachi M. Reduction in the incidence of *Clostridium difficile*-associated diarrhea in an acute care hospital and a skilled nursing facility following replacement of electronic thermometers with single-use disposables. *Infect Control Hosp Epidemiol.* 1992;13(2):98–103.

145. Anderson DJ, Chen LF, Weber DJ, et al. Enhanced terminal room disinfection and acquisition and infection caused by multidrug-resistant organisms and *Clostridium difficile* (the benefits of enhanced terminal room disinfection study): A cluster-randomised, multicentre, crossover study. *Lancet.* 2017;389(10071):805–14.

146. Ali S, Yui S, Muzslay M, Wilson APR. Comparison of two whole-room ultraviolet irradiation systems for enhanced disinfection of contaminated hospital patient rooms. *J Hosp Infect.* 2017;97(2):180–4.

147. Boyce JM, Guercia KA, Sullivan L, et al. Prospective cluster controlled crossover trial to compare the impact of an improved hydrogen peroxide disinfectant and a quaternary ammonium-based disinfectant on surface contamination and health care outcomes. *Am J Infect Control.* 2017;45(9):1006–10.

148. Donskey CJ, Sunkesula VCK, Stone ND, et al. Transmission of *Clostridium difficile* from asymptomatically colonized or infected long-term care facility residents. *Infect Control Hosp Epidemiol.* 2018;39(8):909–16.

149. Fleming-Dutra KE, Hersh AL, Shapiro DJ, et al. Prevalence of inappropriate antibiotic prescriptions among US ambulatory care visits, 2010–2011. *JAMA.* 2016;315(17):1864–73.

150. Gonzales R, Steiner JF, Sande MA. Antibiotic prescribing for adults with colds, upper respiratory tract infections, and bronchitis by ambulatory care physicians. *JAMA.* 1997;278(11):901–4.

151. Dantes R, Mu Y, Hicks LA, et al. Association between outpatient antibiotic prescribing practices and community-associated *Clostridium difficile* infection. *Open Forum Infect Dis.* 2015;2(3):ofv113.

152. Filice GA, Drekonja DM, Thurn JR, Hamann GM, Masoud BT, Johnson JR. Diagnostic errors that lead to inappropriate antimicrobial use. *Infect Control Hosp Epidemiol.* 2015;36(8):949–56.

153. Koyuncuoglu CZ, Aydin M, Kirmizi NI, et al. Rational use of medicine in dentistry: Do dentists prescribe antibiotics in appropriate indications? *Eur J Clin Pharmacol.* 2017;73(8):1027–32.

154. Durkin MJ, Hsueh K, Sallah YH, et al. An evaluation of dental antibiotic prescribing practices in the United States. *J Am Dent Assoc.* 2017;148(12):878–86.e1.

155. Gao XW, Mubasher M, Fang CY, Reifer C, Miller LE. Dose-response efficacy of a proprietary probiotic formula of *Lactobacillus acidophilus* CL1285 and *Lactobacillus casei* LBC80R for antibiotic-associated diarrhea and *Clostridium difficile*-associated diarrhea prophylaxis in adult patients. *Am J Gastroenterol.* 2010;105(7):1636–41.

156. Beausoleil M, Fortier N, Guenette S, et al. Effect of a fermented milk combining *Lactobacillus acidophilus* Cl1285 and *Lactobacillus casei* in the prevention of antibiotic-associated diarrhea: A randomized, double-blind, placebo-controlled trial. *Can J Gastroenterol.* 2007;21(11):732–6.

157. Allen SJ, Wareham K, Wang D, et al. *Lactobacilli* and bifidobacteria in the prevention of antibiotic-associated diarrhoea and *Clostridium difficile* diarrhoea in older inpatients (PLACIDE): A randomised, double-blind, placebo-controlled, multicentre trial. *Lancet.* 2013;382(9900):1249–57.

158. Shaughnessy MK, Bobr A, Kuskowski MA, et al. Environmental contamination in households of patients with recurrent *Clostridium difficile* infection. *Appl Environ Microbiol.* 2016;82(9):2686–92.

159. Ghose C, Kelly CP. The prospect for vaccines to prevent *Clostridium difficile* infection. *Infect Dis Clin North Am.* 2015;29(1):145–62.

160. Quemeneur L, Petiot N, Arnaud-Barbe N, Hessler C, Pietrobon PJ, Londono-Hayes P. *Clostridium difficile* toxoid vaccine candidate confers broad protection against a range of prevalent circulating strains in a nonclinical setting. *Infect Immun.* 2018;86(6):e00742-17.

161. Bezay N, Ayad A, Dubischar K, et al. Safety, immunogenicity and dose response of VLA84, a new vaccine candidate against *Clostridium difficile*, in healthy volunteers. *Vaccine.* 2016;34(23):2585–92.

162. Sheldon E, Kitchin N, Peng Y, et al. A phase 1, placebo-controlled, randomized study of the safety, tolerability, and immunogenicity of a *Clostridium difficile* vaccine administered with or without aluminum hydroxide in healthy adults. *Vaccine.* 2016;34(18):2082–91.

163. Gerding DN, Sambol SP, Johnson S. Non-toxigenic *Clostridioides* (formerly *Clostridium*) *difficile* for prevention of *C. difficile* infection: From bench to bedside back to bench and back to bedside. *Front Microbiol.* 2018;9:1700.

164. Gerding DN, Meyer T, Lee C, et al. Administration of spores of nontoxigenic *Clostridium difficile* strain M3 for prevention of recurrent *C. difficile* infection: A randomized clinical trial. *JAMA.* 2015;313(17):1719–27.

CHAPTER

158 Hepatitis C

Alfred DeMaria, Jr.

Hepatitis C is a major public health challenge worldwide. It has evolved from a diagnosis of exclusion designated as "non-A, non-B hepatitis,"[1] and principally associated with posttransfusion hepatitis, to an etiologically distinct disease; a major cause of cirrhosis, liver failure and hepatocellular carcinoma. The World Health Organization (WHO) estimates there are 71 million people infected with hepatitis C virus (HCV) worldwide, with 1,750,000 new infections in 2015 and about 400,000 deaths from the complications of infection.[2] Others have estimated a much higher and increasing global prevalence, with 2.8% of the world's population infected, translating to 185,000,000 infections, and substantially more disability and mortality than earlier estimates.[3] The U.S. Centers for Disease Control and Prevention (CDC) notes that hepatitis C is now the leading cause of liver cancer and liver transplant in the United States, and that by 2013 the number of deaths associated with hepatitis C was greater than the mortality associated with 60 other nationally notifiable conditions combined.[4]

ETIOLOGIC AGENT

The identification of the hepatitis B virus led to the availability of serologic markers for hepatitis B, so that hepatitis C could be recognized as a form of "serum hepatitis" distinct from hepatitis B.[5] The etiologic agent of hepatitis C was characterized only so far as it could be demonstrated to be transmissible and associated with chronic infection, particularly in posttransfusion hepatitis. It was differentiated from hepatitis A on the basis of epidemiological evidence and incubation period, as well as lack of serologic evidence of hepatitis A among cases.[1]

A putative antigen marker associated with non-A, non-B hepatitis was identified in 1979 using antibody in serum obtained from people who were convalescing from acute hepatitis. In 1989, Choo et al.,[6] using blind recombinant immunoscreening, identified single-stranded RNA coding for an antigen in a patient with non-A, non-B hepatitis. The genetic sequences identified suggested that the virus was of the family Togoviridae or Flaviviridae. The genome was further characterized and was recognized to be a flavivirus (Flaviviridae) and was given the name HCV, eventually assigned to a new genus, Hepacivirus.[7] HCV was once the only species in this genus, but closely related hepaciviruses have been identified in other primates, dogs, rodents, cows, bats, and even sharks, with the virus most closely related to human HCV being the equine hepacivirus.[8]

The HCV genome consists of single-stranded, positive-sense RNA of approximately 9.6 kilobases (kb). The genome is an open reading frame that codes a single polyprotein of approximately 3,000 amino acids that is cleaved into 10 protein products by cellular and viral proteases. The products include a core protein, two envelope surface glycopeptides (E1, E2), and nonstructural proteins designated p7, NS2, NS3, NS4A, NS4B, NS5A, and NS5B. The nonstructural proteins have a variety of enzymatic and replication functions; and have been the targets for therapeutic agents (see Table 158-1). The virus replicates in the hepatocyte, but may also replicate in other cells, possibly circulating mononuclear cells.

The identification of hepatitis C specific antibody using an HCV recombinant polypeptide target provided a diagnostic test reagent to identify anti-HCV specific antibody in a majority of patients with posttransfusion hepatitis and non-A, non-B hepatitis of unidentified exposure.[9] Subsequently, growth of the virus in cell culture allowed for the elucidation of the mechanisms of action of the viral proteins and refinement of test reagents for diagnostic tests.[10] This also allowed investigation of inhibitors of the mechanisms of action of the nonstructural protein enzymes.

There are 7 (6 major) genotypes of HCV numbered 1–7, with 67 or more subtypes indicated with a, b, c, etc.[11,12] Genotypes differ at the nucleotide level by 30% or more, while subtypes vary by 15–25%. Genome sequencing results differ depending on what portion of the genome is sequenced, but it appears that the major genotypes evolved from a common genotype 1b ancestor virus within the past 200–400 years.[13] Infections due to various HCV genotypes vary in prognosis and response to therapy. Simultaneous infection with more than one genotype is possible, but such coinfection may result in the ultimate, competitive exclusion of one of the infecting strains.[14] Genotype 1 accounts for approximately half of infections worldwide, but distribution of genotypes varies around the world (Fig. 158-1). Genotypes 1a and 1b predominate in North America (75%), followed by genotypes 3 and 2 (10% each). In Europe, genotypes 1 (64%) and 3 (25%) predominate. In Asia, genotype 1 is most frequent (47%), with genotype 3 (22%) and genotype 2 (19%) accounting for most of the rest of infections. Genotype 6 has its highest prevalence in Asia (7%). Genotype 4 accounts for most of the infections in Africa, in large part due to high prevalence in Egypt and other countries in which contaminated medical injection equipment led to widespread, unrecognized transmission. Genotype 7 was recently identified in Central Africa.[15]

As with other RNA viruses, poor RNA-dependent RNA-polymerase (NS5B) proofreading results in high mutation rates. Over the course of HCV infection, this results in a cloud of "quasispecies" viruses representing those viruses with mutations that still permit replication. The quasispecies evolve under the selective pressure of the host's immune system. Limited degree of divergence (smaller size of the quasispecies cloud) in acute infection is associated with successful clearance of virus. If the infecting virus cannot escape selective pressure of the host immune response by variation in its surface envelope proteins, especially E2, then resolution of infection is more likely; more diversity in quasispecies is associated with more likely chronic infection.[16] Higher quasispecies diversity has also been associated with more severe liver damage.[17]

TABLE 158-1 GENE PRODUCTS OF THE HEPATITIS C VIRUS AND THEIR FUNCTION

Designation	Other Designation[a]	Function	Comment
Structural proteins			
Core (C)	p22	Nucleocapsid	Epitopes added to NS3-4 peptides in second-generation EIA test for anti-HCV antibody
Envelope 1 (E1)	gp35	Envelope fusion	
Envelope 2 (E2)	gp70	Receptor binding	
Nonstructural proteins			
NS1	p7	Important in formation of the complete virus, calcium ion channel	
NS2	p23	Protease	
NS3	p70	Serine proteinase, helicase	Epitopes from NS3 and NS4 used in second-generation EIA test for anti-HCV antibody.Target of some DAAs
NS4A	p8	Co-factor for NS3 proteinase	Recombinant C100-3 peptide of first-generation EIA test for anti-HCV antibody generated from NS-3/4 sequence,Target of some DAAs
NS4B	p27	Recruitment of viral proteins	
NS5A	p56/58	Viral replication	Important in interferon response Epitope included with second-generation antigens for third-generation EIA test for anti-HCV antibody.Target of some DAAs
NS5B	p68	RNA-dependent RNA polymerase	Target of some DAAs

[a]Protein/glycoprotein—approximate molecular weight (kDa)
Abbreviation: NS = nonstructural.

HCV is an enveloped virus, and therefore is generally susceptible to almost all common disinfectant agents. However, studies have demonstrated that HCV can remain infectious at room temperature in dried blood plasma and can persist in dried blood serum on inanimate surfaces for hours to days.[18,19] Such demonstrations have been made with many viruses, without correlation with risk for transmission. However, in the case of HCV, these observations and observations of viral stability in drug use paraphernalia, rapidity with which infection occurs after initiation of injection drug use and environmental contamination contribution to transmission and outbreaks, suggest that stability in the environment may be important in the epidemiology of HCV infection.[20,21]

EPIDEMIOLOGY

HCV is a bloodborne virus, transmitted primarily when infected blood comes in contact with a susceptible individual in a way that allows the virus access to the circulation. Once the etiologic agent of hepatitis C was identified and characterized with a serologic assay, a number of studies demonstrated hepatitis C specific antibodies in various cohorts of non-A, non-B hepatitis patients and individuals with underlying conditions and exposures that had been recognized to put them at risk for non-A, non-B hepatitis, such as injection drug use, hemophilia and dialysis. In the past, transfusion was a major source of HCV infection. The serologic assay permitted the screening of blood donors for hepatitis C.[9] Blood donors in the United States are currently screened for both anti-HCV antibody and HCV RNA, and posttransfusion hepatitis C is very rare. Diagnosis of HCV infection also allowed for its distinction from enterically transmitted non-A, non-B hepatitis, designated hepatitis E.

Currently, most infections arise from injection drug use or use of contaminated injection equipment in the course of formal or informal medical care. While sexual transmission of hepatitis C occurs, and HCV RNA has been detected in semen, vaginal fluid, and other body fluids, sexual transmission seems to be inefficient and associated primarily with certain high-risk behaviors.[22,23] Hepatitis C is also transmitted perinatally from mother to infant, with an estimated rate of 5.8% in the case of HCV-infected women without HIV infection, and 10.8% in women who are coinfected.[24]

The earliest identified exposure risk for hepatitis C (then known as non-A, non-B hepatitis) was in recipients of blood products.[25] Posttransfusion hepatitis was very common before the identification and detection of hepatitis B and C viruses. In the 1980s, prior to the identification of HCV and availability of a screening test for evidence of infection, blood donors were screened for evidence of liver disease with testing for evidence of elevated levels of alanine aminotransferase (ALT) and for prior hepatitis B with tests for hepatitis B surface antigen (HBsAg) and antibody to the hepatitis B core antigen (anti-HBc) as surrogates of risk for any cause of hepatitis, with resulting reduction in posttransfusion hepatitis.[26] Cohorts of patient who received blood products contaminated with a hepatitis-causing agent were followed for clinical outcome, and subsequent testing for specific infectious agents.[27] One group that was at particular high risk for HCV infection from exposure to blood products were people with hemophilia and other hereditary bleeding disorders who received clotting factors prepared from pooled donor plasma before effective screening and pasteurization of clotting factor products essentially eliminated the risk.[28,29]

Contaminated medical equipment, particularly injection equipment used for necessary or unnecessary treatment, has been implicated in transmission of HCV.[30] In the developing world, limited resources led to the reuse of needles and syringes in many circumstances, while effective screening of blood donors was also a challenge. Egypt has the highest HCV population prevalence in the world at 14.7%, with over 90% of the infections due to genotype 4.[31] Cross-contamination of injection equipment used for the parenteral therapy of schistosomiasis during the 1960s–1980s has been implicated as the cause of many of these infections.[32] Molecular clock investigations of viruses infecting older people in Africa have demonstrated evidence of broad diversification and exponential growth of the infected population originating in the colonial period of the 1920s–1960s.[33] The high population prevalence of infection fuels ongoing transmission,

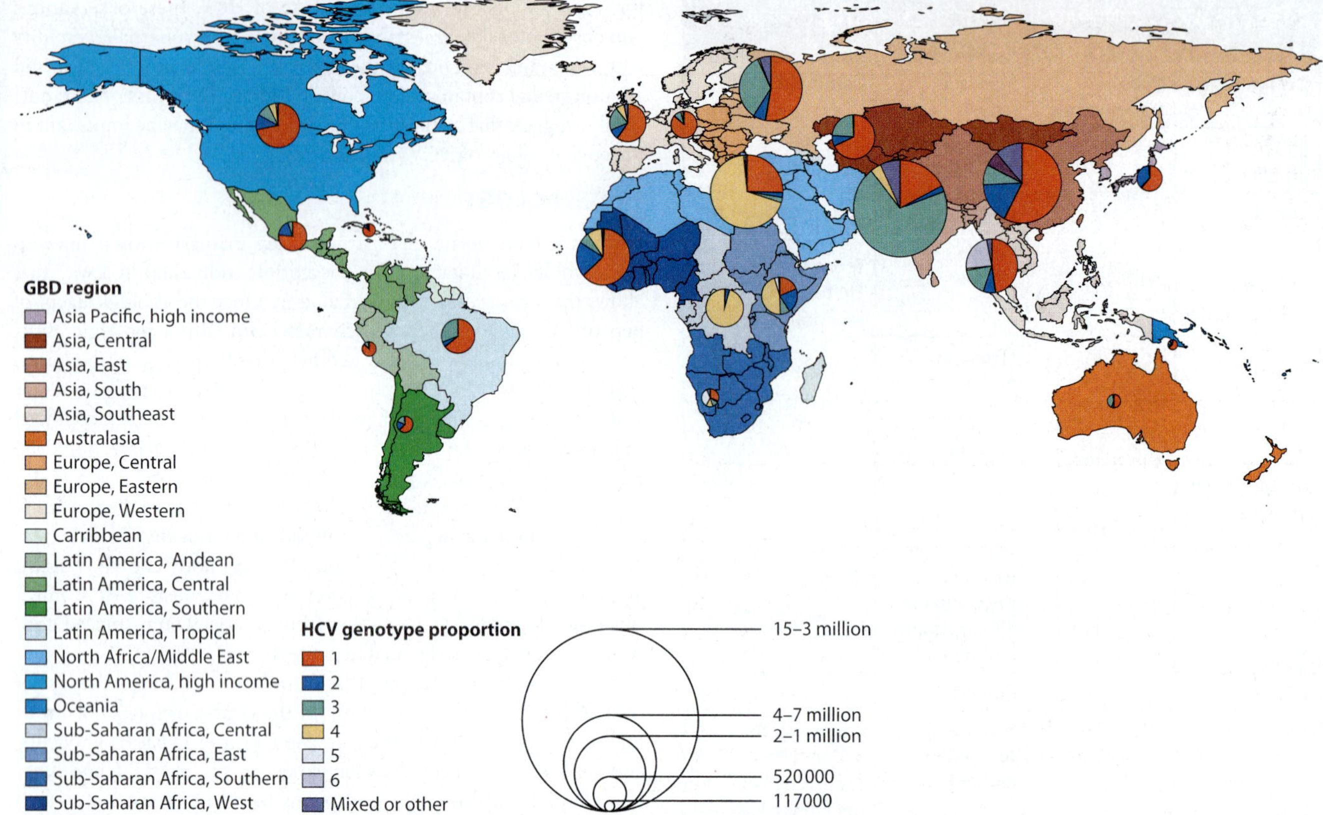

FIGURE 158-1. Global distribution of population with hepatitis C and distribution of genotypes of hepatitis C virus. (*Source:* Reprinted from Polaris Observatory HCV Collaborators. Global prevalence and genotype distribution of hepatitis C virus infection in 2015: A modelling study. *Lancet Gastroenterol Hepatol*. 2017;2(3):161–76, with permission from Elsevier.)

with healthcare-associated transmission still an important factor.[34] Similar iatrogenic epidemics of hepatitis C have occurred in many other parts of the world and in earlier times, accounting for a proportion of the global burden of infection.[34–37] Healthcare-associated transmission of hepatitis C also occurs in the developed world. A number of recognized outbreaks in clinical settings have been associated with poor infection control practices and drug diversion resulting in contaminated drugs, devices, and equipment.[38–41]

While the healthcare-associated outbreaks are often dramatic, sporadic cases of transmission occur, but these are much harder to document. Hemodialysis requires frequent bloodstream access, with potential for exposure to blood and body fluids, and contamination of equipment and the environment. Hemodialysis patients are a population in which risk for sporadic HCV transmission is high. Patients undergoing hemodialysis have a higher prevalence of HCV infection associated with location (including specific dialysis unit), prevalence of hepatitis C in the dialyzed population, understaffing, and certain practices, such as preparation of medications adjacent to the hemodialysis machine, multidose medication vials and using nondisposable container for priming the dialyzer.[42–44] In response to the potential for HCV transmission in the course of hemodialysis, infection control recommendations now include exclusive employment of single-dose medication vials, retesting HCV negative hemodialysis patients every 6–12 months, and treatment of hepatitis C in dialysis patients.[45,46] Treatment of HCV infection in hemodialysis patients lowers prevalence of infection among the population, and therefore, lowers the risk for transmission.[47] There has been increasing evidence of the effectiveness and safety of newer directly acting anti-HCV medications in renal transplant patients.

Occupational exposure has been associated with transmission of HCV to healthcare workers as a result of percutaneous injury involving infected blood. The risk for HCV infection associated with such exposure is generally in the range of 0–2%, but studies have varied in risk estimation. The type of exposure is probably the most important factor, with greater depth of injury and higher amounts of blood contamination conveying more risk.[48] A recent review of over 1300 exposures at one medical center suggested a rate closer to 0.1%.[49] Early studies of postexposure prophylaxis with interferon, with or without ribavirin, were inconclusive. Interferon-based therapy is not effective until infection is established, and with a low rate of infection, most exposed will not develop infection, and a proportion of those who do become infected spontaneously clear infection. Infection that does result from exposure can be identified by monitoring and is responsive to therapy in the acute phase. These considerations led to a lack of enthusiasm for interferon-based prophylaxis.[50,51] DAAs may offer more effective postexposure prophylaxis for occupational and other exposures to infection, but data relating to benefit will take substantial time to accrue. Transmission of HCV infection from healthcare worker to patient has been rarely described. The typical circumstance is transmission in the course of surgical procedures with patient exposure to an infected surgeon, anesthesiologist, or surgical technician.[52]

Early studies after anti-HCV antibody testing became available documented seropositivity in up to 85% of intravenous drug users.[53] In a retrospective study done on serum samples collected from 2523 patients seen in a Baltimore, Maryland emergency department over a 6-week period in 1988, 16% of all patients and 83% of injection drug users were positive for anti-HCV antibody.[54] Studies of time to HCV seroconversion among injection drug users have suggested that seroconversion occurs early after initiation of injection drug use and transmission results from the "works" used to prepare drugs for injection, such as "cookers" and cotton, as well as contaminated needles and syringes. Among a cohort of young injection drug users in Baltimore enrolled for longitudinal follow-up from 1994 to 1996, 49% of those who injected for $\geq$ 2 years were HCV-seropositive, compared to 21% of those injecting for $<$ 2 years; the incidence rate for those who entered the study HCV-seronegative was 16.0 per 100 person-years.[55] These investigators were able to associate infection with reuse of syringes, injecting with someone older by 5 years or more, and injecting cocaine and speedball. A meta-regression study using data from 72 published hepatitis C prevalence studies in injection drug users found higher prevalence of infection in injection drug users in earlier studies and in developing and transitional countries, with a median prevalence of infection across all studies of 66%.[56] In developed countries, post-1995, the model produced a mean prevalence of infection at 1 year of 32% and 53% at 5 years; in developing/transitional countries, it was 59% at 1 year. Cumulative incidence was 27.6% at 1 year. The authors concluded that transmission was slowing down in developed countries and transmission in less developed countries was at a level that was experienced earlier in the developed world. In regard to prevalence of infection, it has been estimated that there are approximately 10 million injection drug users positive for anti-HCV antibody in the world, with a 60% to more than 80% mid-point prevalence of evidence of infection (HCV RNA present) depending on the country.[57]

There have been numerous studies of risk factors for acquisition of hepatitis C in the course of injection drug use. Shared needles and syringes can become contaminated with virus and transmit infection. The preparation of drugs for injection and "works" that injection drug users employ to prepare their drugs for injection, such as "backloading" of the syringe, cotton filters, cookers, and rinse water can result in virus transmission.[58,59] HCV is more efficiently transmitted than other bloodborne viruses and smaller networks of injectors can sustain transmission.[60] Despite the ease of transmission of HCV, new infections in the United States were probably decreasing beginning in the 1980s with prevention efforts directed to HIV infection. In the United States, hepatitis C was primarily diagnosed in "baby boomers," people born roughly between 1945 and 1965, with this aging cohort of infected individuals apparent in population-based serosurveys,[61–63] while incidence of infection among recent injection drug users was apparently going down.[64] The picture began to change in the beginning of the twenty-first century, with an increasing number of infections identified in young injection drug users driven by increasing use of prescription opioids, often by injection, and injection of heroin and fentanyl.[65,66] The large increase in use of opiates and opioids, especially prescription opioids, in a population new to injection drug use, has been associated with increased incidence of hepatitis C and HIV infection.[67,68]

In addition to injection drug use, nasal inhalation of drugs has been associated with risk for hepatitis C.[69] In a study of blood donors early in the course of donor screening, intranasal cocaine use was independently associated with an eightfold increase risk for having a confirmed positive anti-HCV antibody.[70] Higher risk for hepatitis C in noninjection drug users has also been associated with sharing crack cocaine inhalation equipment.[71] However, results from other studies have been mixed. While almost all studies identify an association of HCV infection with noninjection drug use, some have demonstrated an association with inhalational use of cocaine and or smoking of crack cocaine,[72,73] while others have not.[74,75]

HCV RNA has been identified in a variety of body fluids, including semen and vaginal fluid, but the role of sexual transmission of hepatitis C is still unclear. Studies of cohorts of sexually transmitted infection clinic patients suggested a risk associated with sexual contact in noninjections drug users, although other factors may have played a role.[76,77] In addition, population-based studies in the United States have suggested that individuals with multiple sexual partners are at increased risk for hepatitis C.[61,62] However, the body of evidence suggests that heterosexual sex per se does not involve a higher risk for transmission within stable sexual partnerships.[78] Large studies among infection-discordant, long-term heterosexual couples, have found that estimated risk for transmission of HCV was very low, ranging from 0.37 to 1.07 per 1000 person-years of exposure.[79,80] It is likely that transmission in individuals with multiple sex partners and patients seeking services for sexually transmitted infections is related to the nature of the sexual contact or other factors affecting the sexual partners.

While there is low risk for sexual transmission of HCV during most heterosexual sex, men who have sex with men may experience higher risk for infection with higher risk sexual behavior,[81–83] but risk for sexual transmission is much higher in men who have sex with men who are concomitantly infected with HIV.[84,85] Unsafe sexual practices, sexually transmitted infections and substance use, injecting and non-injecting, contribute to increased risk.[86] Concomitant HIV infection can be associated with high HCV viral load, enhanced infectiousness, and more rapid hepatitis C disease progression making transmission more likely. Reinfection after treatment or after spontaneous clearing of infection is a concern with higher risk individuals living with HIV infection requiring more intensive preventive intervention work and scale up of treatment to reduce the pool of infected individuals.[87] In some European countries, there have been dramatic and persistent increases in hepatitis C among men who have sex with men.[88,89] Testing for HCV infection, at least on an annual basis is recommended for sexually active MSM with HIV infection, and more frequent testing in those who also use drugs, and periodic testing should be considered in at-risk MSM without HIV infection.

Perinatal HCV transmission occurs with virus transmitted from infected mothers to newborns, but with less efficiency than in the case of vertical transmission of HIV infection. The rate of transmission is estimated to be 5–6%, but is higher with higher viral load and HIV coinfection (11%).[24] With the increase in injection drug use in younger individuals in the United States in the past 15–20 years, there has been an increase in the numbers of reproductive-aged women with HCV infection, and therefore, an increase in the numbers of exposed infants.[90] Many of these infections are not diagnosed prenatally in the mothers and the exposure in the infant is often not recognized nor is the exposed infant tested.[91,92] This has raised the question of the utility and cost-effectiveness of prenatal screening for HCV infection. The increase in HCV-exposed infants has also revealed a lack of evidence-based testing algorithms for infants.[93]

Skin tattooing and body piercing involve breaks in the integrity of the skin with potential for contamination with bloodborne pathogens, such as HCV. The risk is minimal in controlled circumstances with standard precautions and sterile equipment, but tattooing outside of such controlled circumstances has been associated with HCV transmission.[94–96] However, the contribution of tattooing and body piercing to transmission of hepatitis C is not clearly defined, and this is partially due to the difficulties studying the contribution in populations who may have other risks for infection receiving tattoos in nonprofessional environments. Much of the data relating tattooing and body piercing to risk for infection has been generated from incarcerated populations, among whom other risks for infection are common. The high rate of HCV infection in prison populations (15–30%) is primarily a result of the high incarceration rate of those with substance use disorders, particularly people who inject drugs. Nonetheless, any break in the integrity of the skin or mucous membranes could be a route for infection if nonsterile equipment is used or appropriate precautions are not in place, and this can also include transmission from shared razors, nail clippers, or other sharp objects. This is also an issue in a variety of noncorrectional congregate living settings, such as group homes and assisted living facilities, as well as in poorly regulated personal service establishments providing hair cutting, manicure, pedicure, and other comparable services.

The estimation of population prevalence of hepatitis C suffers from the historical lack of widespread screening in the developed world, the even greater lack of data in the developing world, and the fact that hepatitis C is an infection that does not typically draw attention by manifesting clinical signs or symptoms. The National Health and Nutrition Examination Survey (NHANES) has been interviewing a representative sample of Americans in the United States since the 1960s. With the availability of a PCR test for hepatitis C RNA, banked serum specimens on NHANES participants could be tested for infection. This resulted in an estimate of 2.7 million people in the United States chronically infected with HCV based on a seroprevalence of 1.8% in samples collected in 1988–94.[61] Serosurvey of the NHANES cohort of 1999–2002 suggested an infected population of 3.2 million, and another study covering the years 2003–10 estimated 2.7 million infections, 500,000 less than the previous estimate.[62,63] These serial population-based studies found that HCV infection was most associated with substance use and injecting drugs and was more likely in males, persons 40 years of age and older, non-Hispanic blacks, people who were U.S. born, and those in lower socioeconomic and education attainment groups. However, the NHANES excludes the homeless, incarcerated and otherwise institutionalized, including many at high risk for HCV infection. Taking that into consideration, a better (but still conservative) estimate for infection prevalence in 2003–10 in the United States may be 3.5 million (2.5–4.7 million).[97] While estimation of the prevalence of infection is difficult, determination of incidence of acute hepatitis C through public health surveillance, even based on clinical recognition of symptomatic disease, is even more challenging due to difficulties collecting the information needed for classification of cases.[98]

Widespread transmission of HCV by the routes described above occurred for many years before the identification of HCV. This has resulted in the highest prevalence of infection in many developed countries to be in the "baby boomers" born between 1945 and 1965, and in developing world populations those exposed by iatrogenic means and otherwise before and after the Second World War. The incidence of acute hepatitis C in the United States went down between 1982 and 2006.[99] The opiate/opioid use epidemic that has been occurring in widespread parts of the United States and in other countries has changed the trajectory and has resulted in a concomitant epidemic of hepatitis C in young injecting drug users[66,100] recently exacerbated by the increased frequency of injection, particularly related to fentanyl and prescription opioid use,[101] and wide sharing of injection equipment.[67] On a global basis, more widespread injection drug use is resulting in increased risk for new HCV infections.[102] The increases in hepatitis C in younger individuals amounts to a second wave of prevalent infection following the post-WWII baby boomer wave.

CLINICAL ILLNESS, IMMUNE RESPONSE, PATHOGENESIS, NATURAL HISTORY

Acute hepatitis C occurs when HCV gains access to the circulation, and successfully infects liver cells either directly or possibly carried by infected mononuclear cells. The acute infection evolves over 6 months, with most infected individuals being asymptomatic; symptoms occur in only 15–30% of acute infections. The symptoms can span the entire spectrum for acute hepatitis of any cause, from malaise and fatigue, to nausea, vomiting, abdominal pain; to overt jaundice; and rarely, fulminant hepatitis, but symptoms are usually mild when they do occur. Liver function test results also span a spectrum of abnormalities, beginning 4–12 weeks after infection, with elevated aminotransferases of varying degree in all cases, and less commonly, hyperbilirubinemia of significant level. HCV RNA appears first before evidence of liver damage, followed by anti-HCV antibody. Unless HCV RNA can be detected in the absence of anti-HCV antibody, or seroconversion of anti-HCV antibody from undetectable to detectable can be demonstrated, differentiation of acute hepatitis C from chronic infection, with or without superimposed liver damage from other causes, is difficult. Clues to acute HCV infection include fluctuating ALT levels, and low and varying HCV viral loads,[103] with viral load settling down to a relatively stable level with the development of chronic infection. In other viral infections, early appearance and decline of IgM antibodies are indicators of acute viral infection. IgM antibody tests indicating acute infection are not available for hepatitis C, as they are for hepatitis A and B. Antibody avidity, the strength with which antibody binds to target antigen sites, can be used to assess recency of infection. Early responses to infection produce low avidity antibody and antibody avidity increases as infection persists; assay of avidity can provide an indication of how recent infection occurred. Both IgM antibody and antibody avidity tests are being investigated for use in diagnosing acute hepatitis C.[104]

Most acute HCV infections result in chronic infection, but roughly 15–30% of people with acute hepatitis C clear their infection, with one systematic study calculating a weighted rate of 26% clearance.[105] Symptomatic acute hepatitis C is associated with a higher rate of clearance.[106–108] Younger age and female gender are also associated with higher rates of spontaneous viral clearance,[105,108–110] as is non-black race.[111] Immune status is a critical element in clearance of infection. Lower likelihood of clearance of infection is associated with concurrent HIV infection and lack of an effective helper T-cell response to the nonstructural protein 3.[111,112] A single nucleotide polymorphism in the IFNL4 (formerly IL28B) gene that codes interferon lambda designated the CC allele has been associated with an enhanced response to interferon-based therapy of hepatitis C. The CC allele is also associated with increased likelihood of spontaneous viral clearance.[113] Reinfection with HCV, after clearance of infection, is associated with a higher rate of reclearance than in primary infection, consistent with an enhanced immune response that was correlated with female gender and IFNL4 CC genotype.[114] Clearance of infection may result in loss of anti-HCV antibody over time, with past infection only evident on laboratory testing by assays of HCV-specific T-lymphocytes.[115]

The majority of acute infections with HCV result in chronic infection, and if clearance of infection does not occur within the first 6 months of infection, chronic infection appears to be lifelong in the absence of curative treatment. The course of infection is highly variable and difficult to predict in the individual patient. Many of those infected will not have clinical consequences in their lifetime, but population studies among exposed (as opposed to those presenting with clinical signs and symptoms) are limited.[116,117] There are hepatic and nonhepatic manifestations of infection. Infection-induced damage to hepatocytes stimulates fibrosis, and progression of fibrosis results in most of the hepatic manifestations of cirrhosis, hepatic failure, and portal hypertension. Progression of fibrosis continues, usually silently, over the course of infection, with evidence of cirrhosis in 15–20% at an estimated 20-year duration of infection.[118] Symptoms in chronic infection, when they are recognized, are usually related to the degree of fibrosis and the effect on hepatic function. These symptoms may be very nonspecific, such as fatigue and depression. Factors that are associated with more rapid progression of fibrosis are older age at infection, male gender, concomitant hepatic damage due to alcohol or drugs, fatty liver related to obesity and diabetes, HIV infection and immunosuppression.[119,120] Hepatitis B coinfection also can also accelerate progression of liver damage and worsen outcome of hepatitis C.[121] Marijuana use has been associated with fibrosis progression, while coffee intake appeared to be protective.[122,123] Infection with HCV genotype 3 is also associated with more rapid progression of fibrosis.[124]

Many individuals at risk for HCV infection, particularly people who inject drugs (PWID) and MSM, are also at risk for HIV infection, so coinfection is common. HIV-infected individuals are less likely to clear HCV infection and more likely (in a small number of cases) to have active HCV infection without detectable anti-HCV antibody.[125,126] The impact of HCV infection on HIV infection and progression of HIV disease is unclear.[127] There is more evidence that HIV coinfection increases the risk for progression to cirrhosis and decompensated liver disease despite successful treatment with highly active antiretroviral therapy, which made treatment of HCV infection in those with HIV infection a priority even in the era of interferon-based therapy.[128,129] Pre-existing HIV infection has also been identified as a factor in rapid progression of fibrosis after acute HCV infection.[130] In developed world populations, a trend toward liver disease becoming the leading cause of death among people living with HIV infection has been observed, and increased all-cause mortality is associated with HCV infection even in the era of highly active antiretroviral therapy for HIV infection.[131,132]

Hepatic fibrosis is assessed and monitored through direct and indirect measures. Liver function tests may be abnormal at any stage of infection or fibrosis, and ALT has not proven useful to stage disease,[133] although elevated ALT may be the first indication that infection exists and testing should be done. Other liver function tests are generally normal until hepatic dysfunction sets in. Traditionally, the most definitive way to stage fibrosis was the liver biopsy, with histology graded as to degree of fibrosis and inflammation. A variety of scoring systems based on histology of the liver have been used, including the METAVIR, Knodell, Batts-Ludwig, and others, that categorize various levels of severity. The METAVIR scoring system assigns grades for degree of inflammation (grades A0–A3, none to severe) and assigns stages of fibrosis (F0–F4, none to cirrhosis). In the era of long-course, interferon-based therapy, liver biopsy was used to stage liver disease to allow for delay in treatment of those with earlier stages of fibrosis, exclusion of patients with fully developed cirrhosis from treatment because of poor response, and prioritization for treatment of later stages at more risk for decompensation. However, liver biopsy is invasive and a sample of tissue representative of the entire organ is not always achieved leading to misclassification. The availability of direct acting antiviral agents, with limited toxicity and adverse events, and the capacity to cure infection with a relatively short course of therapy has favored noninvasive measures of fibrosis.

The available noninvasive fibrosis staging methods include those based on laboratory tests and those based on imaging and physical properties of the fibrotic liver.[134] The simplest measure, using readily available routine blood test results, is the aspartate aminotransferase-to-platelet ratio index. Other tests, using a variety of laboratory and anthropometric data to calculate scores, include the FIB-4, HepaScore, Forns Index, and FibroIndex. These tests have relatively low sensitivity and specificity. They can serve to differentiate mild from severe fibrosis, but are not as good at discriminating levels of fibrosis between extremes.[135] The FibroSure test, or FibroTest/ActiTest, depending on where marketed, uses a more sophisticated combination of laboratory and anthropometric data applied to a proprietary algorithm. It is mainly helpful to ruling cirrhosis in or out. There are also tests that detect substances in the blood that are directly related to fibrosis, such as tissue inhibitors of metalloproteinase and hyaluronic acid. The FIBROSpect II is such a test, but like the indirect methods is not very discriminating along the spectrum of severity of fibrosis.[136] The Child-Pugh score, based on laboratory tests and the presence of ascites and encephalopathy, is used primarily to predict prognosis in advanced chronic liver disease.

Hepatic ultrasound can reveal considerable information about the state of the liver, the presence of cirrhosis, nodularity, and hepatocellular cancer. Transient elastography and shear wave elastography using ultrasound (FibroScan and ShearWave) measure the stiffness of the liver by measuring the velocity and character of the return of sound pulses generated by the device used.[137] Transient elastography has been shown to predict fibrosis similar to examination of biopsy specimens.[138] Magnetic resonance elastography is a similar ultrasound-based method, but uses MRI to measure echo sequences. Most evaluation of liver fibrosis and inflammation involves more than one method to try to best determine the extent of liver disease.

In most people with hepatitis C, progression of fibrosis is slow enough that they will go through their life without clinical disease becoming evident, but others will progress to cirrhosis and end stage liver disease. While there are some factors that correlate with progression of disease, noted above, outcome for the individual patient cannot be accurately predicted. End stage liver disease is complicated by metabolic consequences for multiple organ systems, and fibrotic impingement on blood vessels results in portal hypertension leading to the potential for gastrointestinal variceal hemorrhage. The tendency to bleeding is made worse by liver decompensation and failure of coagulation factor synthesis. The ascites arising from portal hypertension puts patients at risk for hepatorenal syndrome and hyponatremia. Failure of the normal mechanisms of clearing microorganisms from the blood stream puts patients at risk for spontaneous bacterial peritonitis. The metabolic effects of liver failure can lead to hepatic encephalopathy. End stage liver disease caused by hepatitis C has become the most frequent indication for liver transplant in the United States. Infected patients who receive transplants almost always develop infection of the new organ and more rapid progression of disease. Currently, much research is being directed toward cure of infection in the transplant recipient using directly active agents.

Chronic hepatitis C can lead to hepatocellular cancer (HCC). HCC arises as a complication of chronic liver disease, fibrosis, and cirrhosis due to hepatitis C, as well as a variety of other infections (particularly hepatitis B) and noninfectious agents (alcohol, aflatoxins, porphyria, hemochromatosis, etc.). The inflammation of the liver resulting from HCV infection, the effect of HCV replication in the liver cells, the effect of infection on immune response, and the enhanced proliferation of hepatic cells in response to damage provide a stimulus to, and favorable conditions for, the development of HCC.[139] The risk for HCC increases with increasing degrees of fibrosis, as well as with the presence of cofactors, such as alcohol consumption, diabetes, obesity (hepatic steatosis), and HIV infection. The high prevalence of hepatitis C in the baby boomer generation in the United States has contributed to an average increase of about 2% per year in mortality related to HCC from 1992 through 2015,[140] despite success in vaccinating against hepatitis B (a major risk factor for HCC), which is just starting to reduce its contribution to HCC incidence. Worldwide, liver cancer is the second most common cause of cancer death (9.1%), although causes other than hepatitis C play a larger role in incidence and prognosis in much of the world.[141] Treatment of HCC usually involves a combination of resection or ablation, with chemotherapy, or liver transplantation. Successful treatment of hepatitis C, with resulting sustained virologic response (SVR, undetectable HCV RNA for at least 6 months after treatment), can significantly reduce increased risk for HCC when treatment is administered prior to later stages of fibrosis, but in patients with established cirrhosis and advanced fibrosis a higher risk remains, requiring monitoring for potential cancerous lesions with liver ultrasonography.[142]

Hepatitis C has also been associated with an increased risk for lymphoproliferative disorders and B-cell non-Hodgkin's lymphoma[143] and other extra-hepatic manifestations.[144] HCV infection may result in autoimmune syndromes (vasculitis, polyarteritis nodosa, sicca syndrome, immune thrombocytopenia) and the production of autoantibodies, including mixed cryoglobulins, rheumatoid factor, antinuclear antibodies, and others. Most of the autoantibodies produced are not associated with characteristic clinical syndromes, except for cryoglobulins. HCV infection is the major cause of cryoglobulin-associated vasculitis that can affect skin, kidneys, and other organs. Cryoglobulinemia can precipitate glomerulonephritis (most often membranoproliferative) resulting in proteinuria, hematuria, and renal insufficiency. On occasion, the severity can be such as to lead to overt nephritis or nephrotic syndrome associated with degrees of chronic renal insufficiency and hypertension. Persistent inflammation in chronic hepatitis C appears to exacerbate atherosclerotic cardiovascular disease, with resultant increased risk for coronary artery disease and stroke.[145,146] Chronic hepatitis C is associated with insulin resistance, with an increased risk for type-2 diabetes mellitus related to liver dysfunction and a direct effect of infection.[147]

The impact of hepatitis C on premature mortality had not been fully appreciated until recently. The mortality associated with HCV infection documented on death certificates increased by 6.2% per year in the United States between 2003 and 2013, notwithstanding hepatitis C being underdocumented on death certificates.[4,148] All-cause mortality in people with HCV infection in a U.S. survey cohort was twice that than in those who did not have HCV infection, with approximately 58% attributable to HCV infection.[149] In a Taiwan population-based study, mortality due to hepatic and extrahepatic disease was almost two times higher in those with a positive anti-HCV antibody versus a negative anti-HCV antibody, and over two times higher in those with a positive anti-HCV antibody and a positive HCV RNA (active infection) than in those with a positive anti-HCV antibody and nondetectable RNA (cleared infection); the latter having a hazard of mortality similar to those with a negative anti-HCV antibody.[150]

TREATMENT

Exogenous interferon was first suggested for the treatment of chronic hepatitis B based on experiments in chimpanzees.[151] Initial clinical trials of treatment of chronic hepatitis B and non-A, non-B hepatitis were done with alpha-interferon derived from human fibroblasts and leucocytes. Lymphoblastoid and recombinant interferon (which became available in the 1980s) and was used to treat chronic non-A, non-B hepatitis, with control of disease activity evident in reduced levels of aminotransferases and improvement on biopsy.[152,153] Treatment of individuals with posttransfusion hepatitis, with and without evidence of hepatitis C as determined by presence of anti-HCV antibody, resulted in sustained response (which was defined as normalization of serum ALT levels) among approximately one-third of patients who responded.[154] By 1990, recombinant alpha-interferon monotherapy for 6–18 months was becoming the treatment of choice for chronic hepatitis C, with success measured by ALT response and changes in histology on biopsy, but with sustained response only in about 15% of those treated.[155] Response to alpha-interferon therapy was subsequently associated with disappearance of HCV RNA (SVR) in a small proportion of responders on long-term follow-up.[156]

Ribavirin was considered as a therapeutic agent for hepatitis C in the early 1990s, with some effect on disease activity of limited duration when used as a sole agent.[157,158] Combining alpha-interferon and ribavirin was then demonstrated to have a synergistic effect, with sustained biochemical and virologic response in some patients who did not respond to alpha-interferon alone,[159,160] and comparative trials demonstrated superiority of the combination over alpha-interferon alone.[161,162] A number of studies were done in treatment naïve patients, responders to interferon monotherapy who relapsed, nonresponders to interferon monotherapy, as well as various populations at risk for hepatitis C (hemophilia, injecting drug use, blood product recipients, etc.), all demonstrating the superiority of combined interferon and ribavirin. Rates of sustained virologic response went from 15–20% to 30–40%. However, the 24–48 weeks of therapy required (and for patients with the most prevalent genotype 1 infection it was 48 weeks) was associated with adverse events related to thrice weekly injection of interferon (primarily systemic symptoms of myalgia, fever, etc., and neuropsychiatric effects, such as depression and psychosis) and daily oral ribavirin (hemolytic anemia). Patients with acute hepatitis C responded to interferon therapy, with or without ribavirin, at a higher rate of SVR than observed in patients with chronic HCV infection.[51] However, the difficulty of identifying acute infection limited application.

The introduction of polyethylene glycol formulated alpha-interferon, pegylated interferon alfa-2b (PEG-IFN-α2b) in 2001 and pegylated interferon alfa-2a (PEG-IFN-α2a) in 2002, allowed for once weekly dosing of parenteral interferon combined with ribavirin as the treatment of choice. The interferon still caused systemic symptoms over a 24- to 48-week course, but the convenience of dosing and the improved pharmacokinetics leading to increased efficacy over nonpegylated interferons were a definite advance. Ever increasing numbers of patients with sustained absence of viral RNA in their blood led to a consensus that SVR, originally defined as absence of viral RNA for at least 6 months, actually amounted to cure of HCV infection.

The ability to propagate HCV in cell culture allowed for the expression of the viral genome and the study of the activities of the viral nonstructural proteins. One such protein, the HCV NS3/4A serine protease, cleaves the large polyprotein precursor molecule of the replicating virus into its component parts. Research directed at the development of small molecule inhibitors of this protease resulted in the first oral, direct acting antiviral agents for hepatitis C treatment. The serine protease inhibitors, telaprevir and boceprevir, were approved for use in combination with pegylated interferon and ribavirin in the treatment of HCV genotype 1 infection in 2011. These combinations raised the SVR rate to the range of 65–75%, but were associated with adverse events, particularly anemia and rash. Other NS3/4A protease inhibitors have been licensed (simeprevir, grazoprevir, paritaprevir) since the first two, and still others are in development. These drugs all enhanced activity against HCV genotype 1 infection when combined with pegylated interferon and ribavirin. They are now used in combination with other directly acting agents for genotypes 1 and 4 infections.

A nucleotide analog inhibitor of the HCV polymerase (nonstructural protein 5b, or NS5B), sofosbuvir, was licensed in the United States in 2013 for use in combination with ribavirin alone or pegylated interferon and ribavirin for HCV infection caused by genotypes 1, 2, 3, and 4. Treatment duration could be reduced to 12–24 weeks with sofosbuvir combined with PEG-IFN plus RBV, and response rates in the range of 70% to >95% were observed depending on the genotype being treated. A nonnucleoside NS5B inhibitor, dasabuvir, was also introduced. NS5B inhibitors are no longer used with PEG-IFN plus RBV, but in combination with other oral agents depending on the genotype being treated.

Another protease of HCV, the NS5A protease, plays a role in replication and was identified as an excellent target for inhibition. The NS5A inhibitors, daclatasvir, edipasvir, elbasvir, ombitasvir, velpatasvir, and odalasvir, have varying patterns of activity by genotype. Their development ushered in the first two all oral combinations of agents active in genotype 1 infection, ledipasvir/sofosbuvir (Harvoni™) and ombitasvir/paritaprevir/ritonavir and dasabuvir (Viekira Pak™). These combinations were better tolerated and resulted in SVR rates reliably greater than 90%. Since these directly acting agent (DAA) combinations were introduced, six other highly effective combinations of NS3A, NS5B, and NS5A inhibitors, sometimes combined with ribavirin, have been introduced with variable coverage of HCV genotypes 1–6 and entail 12 weeks of treatment, although shorter courses under various circumstances appear to be equally effective (see Table 158-2). The DAAs have revolutionized the treatment of hepatitis C.

Achieving SVR with antiviral therapy (interferon-based treatment or DAAs) results in cure of infection, arrested progression of liver disease and other consequences of infection, improved health-related quality of life and survival, and economic benefit.[163] Even in the treatment of patients with little or no hepatic fibrosis, SVR results in

TABLE 158-2 FDA (U.S.) APPROVED DIRECT-ACTING AGENTS FOR THE TREATMENT OF HEPATITIS C (AS OF 2018)

Drug(s)	Brand Name	Activity	Genotypes	Manufacturer	Indications/Comment
Simeprevir	Olysio	NS3/4A protease inhibitor	1	Janssen	Used as a component of combination therapy.
Sofosbuvir	Sovaldi	NS5B polymerase inhibitor		Gilead	Used as a component of combination therapy.
Ledipasvir, sofosbuvir	Harvoni	NS5A inhibitor, NS5B polymerase inhibitor	1, 4, 5, 6	Gilead	Fixed-dose combination.
Ombitasvir, paritaprevir, ritonavir, copackaged with dasabuvir	Viekira PakViekira XR	NS5A inhibitor, NS3/4A protease inhibitor, CYP3A inhibitor,[a] NS5B polymerase inhibitor	1	AbbVie	May be used with or without ribavirin.Viekira Pak is being replaced by Viekira XR, a coformulated combination of the same drugs as extended-release tablets.12-week course for 1a without cirrhosis and 1b; 24-week course for 1a with cirrhosis.
Ombitasvir, paritaprevir, ritonavir	Technivie	NS5A inhibitor, NS3/4A protease inhibitor, CYP3A inhibitor[a]	4	AbbVie	Fixed-dose combination.Indicated combined with ribavirin, 12-week course.
Daclatasvir	Daklinza	NS5A inhibitor	1, 3	Bristol-Myers Squibb	Used with sofosbuvir, with or without ribavirin.
Elbasvir, grazoprevir	Zepatier	NS5A inhibitor, NS3/4A protease inhibitor	1, 4	Merck Sharp Dohme	Fixed-dose combination.12- to 16-week course of treatment depending on past treatment and polymorphisms in NS5A.
Sofosbuvir, velpatasvir	Epclusa	NS5B polymerase inhibitor, NS5A inhibitor	1, 2, 3, 4, 5, 6	Gilead	Fixed-dose combinationMay be used with ribavirin in patients with advanced liver disease.12-week course of treatment.
Sofosbuvir, velpatasvir, voxilaprevir	Vosevi	NS5B polymerase inhibitor, NS5A inhibitor, NS3/4A protease inhibitor	1, 2, 3, 4, 5, 6	Gilead	Fixed-dose combination.12-week course of treatment.
Glecaprevir, pibrentasvir	Mavyret	NS3/4A protease inhibitor, NS5A inhibitor	1, 2, 3, 4, 5, 6	AbbVie	Fixed-dose combinationTreatment naïve without cirrhosis 8-week course of treatment, with cirrhosis 12-week.Previously treated 8–16 weeks depending on previous therapy.

[a]Used to potentiate levels of drugs active against HCV.

significant improvements in patient reported outcomes.[164] The initial high cost of the DAAs challenged access to widespread treatment, but as new regimens have come to market, prices have begun to come down, and volume purchase has offered further reduction of cost for large insurers or healthcare providers. Because of the current unpredictable nature of cost-of-treatment trends, cost-effectiveness studies depend on assumptions about price. Cost-effectiveness studies of DAAs in treatment of PWID have indicated that treating all stages of liver damage is cost effective compared to waiting to treat until more advanced liver disease occurs.[165] Other studies, considering a broader population of those with HCV infection, have demonstrated cost-effectiveness depending on genotype (treatment of genotypes 1 and 3 versus genotype 2).[166] Treatment can result in improved health outcomes and be cost effective, but yet be costly, especially at treatment program start-up.[167,168] Considering the most frequent genotype in the United States, genotype 1, alone, treating only more advanced disease was found to be cost ineffective compared with treating all patients.[169] However, as multiple regimens with pan-genotype effectiveness have been introduced, differences in incremental cost-effectiveness would be expected to decrease across the spectrum of genotypes.

PWID are at the highest risk of having and transmitting HCV infection, and acquiring primary infection, superinfection or reinfection. Treatment of PWID who were actively using drugs with interferon-based regimens was not routinely initiated. Healthcare providers and insurers were wary of initiating treatment in those actively using drugs and covering the cost of such treatment because of the extended treatment period, the commitment required and the consequences of loss of treatment continuity. Therapy was typically withheld until active drug use stopped. There were often restrictions based on fibrosis score. This denial of treatment was brought into question on moral grounds early on in the history of treatment of HCV infection.[170] With the DAA's ease of administration, lower incidence of adverse events and shorter courses of therapy, treatment of active drug users has been re-evaluated. Restrictions on covering the cost of treatment based on use of drugs and progression of liver disease have generally been lifted in many parts of the world. However, barriers to treatment remain, including access to screening and care, as well as misperceptions related to treatment, insurance coverage, and eligibility.[171,172] Studies of treatment in patients with recent or concurrent drug use on opioid substitution therapy suggest satisfactory levels of SVR can be achieved in those with or without HIV coinfection.[173,174] The goal of hepatitis C elimination would be best met by reducing transmission among PWID, the population with the highest risk for transmission (see Prevention and control, below).

Treatment with DAAs is highly effective in achieving SVR in well over 90% of patients treated, with definite survival benefit in patients with advanced liver disease who achieve SVR.[175] There is mounting evidence that treatment with DAAs resulting in SVR is associated with benefit in terms of survival even in patients who have early, nonadvanced liver disease with limited fibrosis. A large U.S. Veterans Affairs study demonstrated a 56% reduction in mortality in patients achieving SVR compared to those who did not achieve SVR, and a

68% reduction compared to untreated patients.[176] Past infection and coinfection with hepatitis B virus is common with HCV infection, and reactivation of hepatitis B in patients treated with DAAs has been observed in about a quarter of patients who are hepatitis B surface antigen (HBsAg) positive, but less often (1–2%) among those who are HBsAg negative (with serologic evidence of past hepatitis B infection).[177,178] This led the U.S. Food and Drug Administration to require a "black box" warning on the package inserts for DAAs. As noted above, successful treatment of HCV infection reduces the risk for HCC, but does not eliminate the risk, requiring monitoring for early detection in treated patients who had advanced liver disease at the time of treatment.

The clinical management of hepatitis C involves more than the treatment of the infection. Pending treatment and with residual damage after treatment patients with hepatitis C are at higher risk for consequences from other sources of damage. Patients with hepatitis C should be counseled about exposure to hepatotoxins, especially alcohol, as these can exacerbate the damage to the liver induced by HCV. There are drugs and popular food supplements that need to be avoided or taken with precautions because they may have a deleterious effect on the liver (acetaminophen and acetaminophen-containing products, iron and iron-containing multivitamins), may cause adverse reactions without established benefit (licorice root, colloidal silver) and may precipitate drug interactions (St. John's wort, red yeast rice extract). All drugs, vitamins, and supplements taken by the patient should be reviewed for possible adverse effects or drug interactions. If the patient is obese, counseling and interventions for weight reduction should be initiated to reduce the risk for steatohepatitis and additional liver damage. Patients should be vaccinated against hepatitis A and B, if they did not have previous infection or have not been vaccinated previously. Hepatitis A or B superimposed on hepatitis C can be more severe and even life threatening. There is evidence that epidemics of hepatitis E in low and middle-income countries can cause severe hepatic deterioration and disease when superimposed on chronic hepatitis, but a vaccine for hepatitis E is not yet available.[179] Patients at risk for reinfection, particularly those with substance use disorders and MSM, need ongoing risk-reduction education and support to reduce the risk for reinfection. Individualized risk-reduction plans are generally more effective than general counseling.

In the era of liver biopsy to stage liver disease interferon-based and year-long treatment, care for people living with HCV infection was primarily the responsibility of specialists. Project ECHO (Extension for Community Healthcare Outcomes) demonstrated that primary-care providers could provide HCV care with specialist back-up.[180] The availability and high effectiveness of DAAs in achieving cure has increased the desirability of treating as many infected individuals as possible, at all stages of disease, as quickly as possible. This has resulted in increased interest in primary-care-based management of hepatitis C.[181] There are now easily accessible and frequently updated, online resources for both primary- and specialty-care providers. The CDC-funded Hepatitis C Online produced by the University of Washington and the University of Alabama provides educational modules and guidelines for the management of hepatitis C. The American Society for the Study of Liver Disease and the Infectious Diseases Society of America provide online guidelines: *HCV Guidance: Recommendations for Testing, Managing, and Treating Hepatitis C.*

DIAGNOSIS

Most individuals with hepatitis C are asymptomatic and disease is inapparent. Clinical disease characteristic of hepatitis C when it occurs is nonspecific and consistent with acute and chronic hepatitis of almost any cause. Hepatitis C is therefore diagnosed in the laboratory, primarily by serologic and nucleic acid testing (NAT). The NAT test usually involves polymerase chain reaction (PCR) and other methods to detect HCV RNA. The initial first-generation enzyme-linked immunoassay (EIA) for anti-HCV antibodies, which used a recombinant HCV C100-3 peptide[9] from nonstructural regions NS4A to detect antibody, was supplanted by a second-generation test in 1992 that was more sensitive and specific which used the recombinant antigen from NS3/4 combined with antigen from the core region.[182,183] It became clear that there were still false positive and false negative EIA results and a supplementary test, the recombinant immunoblot assay (RIBA), was used to determine if a positive result represented a true positive antibody test or a cross-reacting antibody to a non-HCV antigen. A third-generation EIA, with an epitope from the NS5 protein represented in addition to the epitopes that had been in the second-generation test, had higher sensitivity (98%) and specificity (99%) and is now used routinely in the United States. Chemiluminescent immunoassay (CMIA) and rapid point-of-care serologic tests provide alternatives to the EIA.

Interpretation of an EIA test is dependent on the ratio between the optical density of the signal in the reaction with the patient's serum compared to the negative control; the cutoff ratio. Experience with the EIA led to the use of the quantitative value of the "signal-to-cutoff ratio" to classify a more robust positive result as more likely to be true positive. A ratio significantly higher than that required for a positive result suggests higher titers of specific antibody. That signal-to-cutoff ratio varied with the specific test platform being used and was not standardized. The signal-to-cutoff ratio is no longer recommended as an indicator of specificity of antibody and the RIBA is no longer available, both supplanted by NAT tests for HCV RNA. NAT testing for HCV RNA is a test specific for active HCV infection, and can be done using a qualitative test (detecting the presence of specific HCV RNA) or a quantitative test (real-time PCR providing a viral load determination).

Rapid result, point-of-care tests for both anti-HCV antibody and HCV RNA have been developed. These tests offer a result while the subject of the test is still present, with immediate engagement in care or referral possible. Studies suggest that rapid point-of-care testing is acceptable, and perhaps preferable, to PWID utilizing needle and syringe exchange programs.[184] Point-of-care tests for HCV RNA are becoming available and offer the advantage of immediate confirmation of active infection.[185]

Hepatitis C core antigen is a nucleocapsid peptide that is present in the serum before detectable anti-HCV antibodies appear and throughout active infection. A variety of tests to detect core antigen have been in use outside the United States. While NAT tests for HCV RNA are more sensitive, studies have indicated that an easier to perform HCV core antigen test might be more economical and, in high prevalence populations, could replace the NAT for some purposes.[186] These tests may also be used in the future for quantitative HCV viral load determination to follow response to treatment.

The CDC published updated recommendations for testing for HCV infection in 2013.[187] These guidelines took into consideration changes in the utilization and availability of tests, eliminating recommendations for using the signal-to-cutoff ratio and RIBA. The guidelines recommend NAT testing for HCV RNA for confirmation of active infection following a positive screening test for anti-HCV antibody. The current recommended algorithm for screening and diagnostic testing is presented in Fig. 158-2.

WHOM TO TEST

Screening for HCV infection is recommended in the United States specifically for those identified to be at risk of exposure to the virus and generally for the population born from 1945 through 1965 (the "baby boomers") regardless of screening for risk history (see Table 158-3). Those considered at risk for exposure to HCV include anyone currently injecting drugs or who has ever injected drugs, even once; anyone with a persistently abnormal ALT; anyone

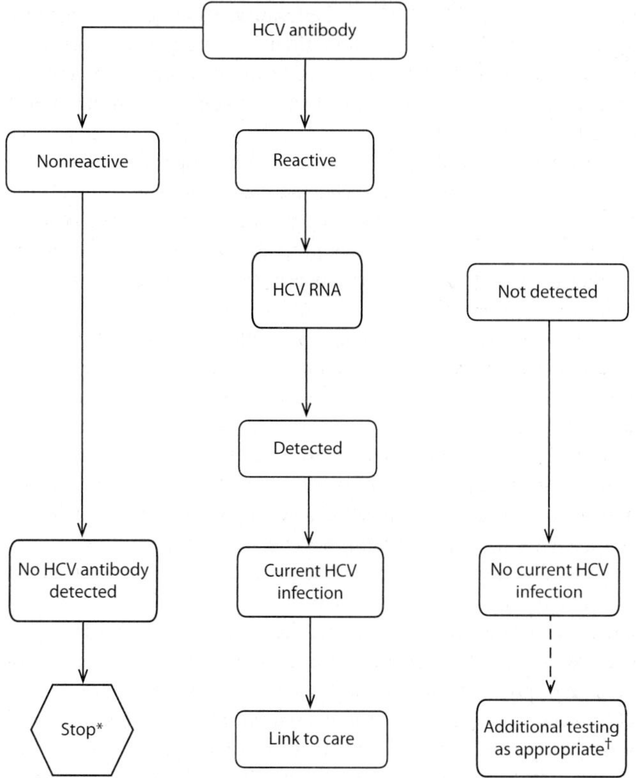

FIGURE 158-2. Recommended algorithm for screening and diagnosis of HCV infection. (*Source:* Centers for Disease Control and Prevention. Testing for HCV infection: An update of guidance for clinicians and laboratorians. *MMWR Morb Mortal Wkly Rep.* 2013;62(18):362–5.) *Testing for HCV RNA or follow-up testing for HCV antibody for persons who might have been exposed to HCV within the past 6 months is recommended. Consider testing for HCV RNA for persons who are immunocompromised. †Testing with another HCV antibody assay can be considered to differentiate past infection from a false positive and repeat HCV RNA testing if the person tested is suspected to have had HCV exposure within the past 6 months or has clinical evidence of HCV disease, or if there is concern regarding the handling or storage of the test specimen.

who has received long-term hemodialysis; anyone who has received clotting factors prior to 1987 (when heat processing was introduced), or transfusion or organ transplant prior to 1992 (when third-generation anti-HCV antibody testing was introduced); anyone with HIV infection; children born to HCV-infected mothers; and anyone with a recognized exposure to infected or potentially infected blood (sharps injury, needlestick, mucosal splash). Although data are limited and sometimes inconsistent, many consider intranasal cocaine use, tattoos, multiple sex partners, and a known HCV-infected sex partner to be associated with risk for infection (see Epidemiology). Re-evaluation of those with defined risk for infection, with retesting for continued or recurrent risk, is recommended. Since sufficient antibody production to result in a positive anti-HCV antibody test may take up to 6 months, if suspected exposure is within 6 months NAT testing may be done.

The recommendation for routine, one-time testing of everyone born during or between 1945 and 1965, has been made by the CDC[188] and the U.S. Preventive Services Task Force in 2012.[189] These recommendations were grounded on evidence that risk assessment and testing based on the elicitation of risk for HCV infection was not successful in identifying those with infection acquired in the past. Since, at the time of analysis, the baby boomers made up the majority of those living with HCV infection without knowledge of their infection, and interventions and effective treatment to reduce morbidity and mortality were becoming increasingly available, routine screening was more effective than risk assessment in identifying those with infection. Evidence suggests that these recommendations were followed by an increase in testing of the target population.[190] Evaluation of the full benefit of routine age-cohort screening remains to be completed.

The opiate/opioid use epidemic, occurring in widespread parts of the United States, has resulted in a concomitant epidemic of hepatitis C in young injecting drug users that is exacerbated by the increased frequency of injection, particularly related to fentanyl and prescription opioid use, and expansive sharing of injection equipment.[65–67] The increasing numbers of HCV infections in younger individuals has raised the question of broader routine screening recommendations beyond the baby boomer cohort. Testing in the younger age group based on ability to ascertain risk is not very effective. The cost-effectiveness of universal routine screening, similar to the one-time universal screening of all adolescents and adults in the United States for HIV infection, is an area of active discussion. It has been suggested that universal screening in the setting of access to treatment with DAAs would be more cost effective than birth cohort or risk-based screening and that one-time universal screening would be within accepted bounds of cost-effectiveness.[191,192]

Incarcerated populations have a higher prevalence of hepatitis C primarily related to a history of injection drug use. The prevalence of hepatitis C in U.S. prison inmates has been estimated to be over 17%, and approximately 30% of people with HCV infection spend some time incarcerated.[193] Risk activity that often precipitates incarceration puts newly admitted inmates at a higher risk for having acute HCV infection, especially with recent increases in the prevalence and frequency of injection drug use.[194] Screening of inmates, with education, risk-reduction interventions, and curative treatment would reach a very high-risk population in a custodial setting. Universal HCV screening (and treatment) in prisons has been proposed as cost-effective with consideration of the societal benefit of reduced transmission.[195] The implementation costs of such screening and treatment programs, even more than the ongoing costs, are a significant challenge for the introduction of such programs despite ample demonstration of benefit to individuals and society.

Current recommendations for whom to screen for hepatitis C are summarized in Table 158-3.

PREVENTION AND CONTROL

In the absence of an effective vaccine, prevention of hepatitis C is dependent on personal and institutional measures to reduce risk, and application of effective infection control practices. What to do to have the greatest impact on risk for HCV transmission is straightforward; eliminate blood-to-blood transmission among injection drug users and others with substance use and eliminate opportunities for contamination in the course of medical care, dental care, or cosmetic procedures.

In the case of HCV exposure in the course of medical or cosmetic procedures, assurance that only sterile equipment and only sterile injectable drugs are used and maintaining appropriate infection control to prevent cross-contamination are effective in preventing infection in patients and healthcare workers. Guidelines produced by professional societies, standard-setting organizations, patient safety groups, and government agencies for policies and procedures to address prevention of transmission of bloodborne pathogens are available for a variety of settings. The Safe Injection Global Network (SIGN) was established in 1999 as a multinational collaboration under the leadership of the WHO to improve the quality and safety of injection devices. In the United States, the CDC launched the "One & One Only" campaign to eliminate unsafe injections.

Accomplishing elimination of HCV transmission among people who inject drugs is more difficult and requires harm-reduction strategies, especially when opioid substitution therapy or other ways of discontinuing injection drug use are not possible or successful.

TABLE 158-3	INDIVIDUALS AND POPULATIONS WHO SHOULD BE SCREENED AND CONSIDERED FOR SCREENING FOR HCV INFECTION
By risk for exposure	Ever injected illegal drugs or other substances. Received a transfusion of blood or blood components before July 1992. Received an organ transplant before July 1992. Received clotting factors produced before 1987. Needlestick, sharps, or mucosal exposures to HCV-positive/potentially positive blood. Tattoos, piercing, and other body art received in a nonprofessional or unsafe setting. Born to an HCV-positive woman Medical care, with injections, under potentially unsafe conditions.
As a member of a population group that may have a higher prevalence of infection in all or some situations	Born during 1945–65 (one-time testing). Ever on chronic (long-term) hemodialysis. Living with HIV infection. Men who have sex with men. Ever incarcerated. Noninjection drug use. Having multiple sexual partners.
On clinical grounds	Persistently abnormal alanine aminotransferase level.Evidence of liver disease, otherwise unexplained.

Harm-reduction interventions are designed to reduce negative consequences of drug use, including infection, and have been effective in reducing transmission of HIV among injection drug users. Psychosocial interventions are basic, mainly involving educating people who inject drugs about ways to prevent transmission and acquisition of bloodborne viruses, and can be effective in reducing risk.[196] The rapid acquisition of HCV infection after initiation of injection presents a challenge in providing educational interventions early enough. Syringe and needle exchange programs have been used for decades to reduce HIV transmission and as a way of reaching people who inject drugs with harm-reduction education and information on treatment options. Evidence is increasing that provision of support for safe injection, especially combined with availability of treatment for substance use disorder, particularly opioid substitution therapy, can reduce HCV transmission.[197,198]

The effectiveness of directly acting anti-HCV agents presents the possibility of treatment as prevention. Early identification of infection and treatment is the mainstay of control of sexually transmitted infections and "treatment as prevention" is a now a phrase commonly associated with efforts to eliminate HIV transmission. The effectiveness of the DAAs in curing HCV infection in approximately 95% of those treated, regardless of genotype, means that individuals who were capable of transmitting the virus can be rendered noninfectious. The WHO published a plan in 2016, endorsed by the World Health Assembly, to eliminate hepatitis C (and hepatitis B) as a public health threat by 2030 through enhanced prevention, harm reduction, diagnosis, and treatment, with a reduction goal of 90% for incidence and 65% for mortality.[199] Mathematical models of HCV transmission have suggested that even modest levels of treatment and treatment scale-up, combined with prevention and harm reduction can have significant effects on transmission of virus among those at high risk for infection (PWID) and be cost effective, with reduction in incidence and prevalence.[200–202] Unrestricted access to DAAs in the Netherlands, and high uptake of treatment with high cure rates among HIV/HCV coinfected MSM, resulted in a 51% decrease in acute infections despite ongoing risk behavior indicated by increased rates of syphilis and gonorrhea.[203,204] "Test and treat" strategies, combining scale-up of screening with universal treatment of infected PWID, can improve patient outcomes and reduce transmission, and have been proposed for national programs.[205–209] Such scale-up of prevention interventions, including harm reduction and treatment of HCV infection, has been proposed in response to the epidemic of hepatitis C associated with the epidemic of opioid use in the United States.[210]

Treatment as prevention strategies must include recognition of the risk for reinfection, since risk behaviors may continue or restart, and HCV infection does not induce sterilizing immunity. Reinfection rates among men who have sex with men and PWID in the DAA era are in the range of two to five reinfections per 100 person-years and can be higher in relapsing PWID.[211] Reinfection has been associated with HIV coinfection and spontaneous clearance of HCV infection (vs. SVR due to treatment), but continued opioid substitution treatment and mental health services were associated with lower risk of reinfection.[212] One study of HIV-infected MSM in Europe reported a reinfection rate of 7.3 per 100 person-years after treatment or spontaneous clearance.[213] In any strategy of treatment as prevention, those treated must be recognized to be at risk for reinfection and supportive services, including substance use and mental health treatment, must continue.

The most effective preventive intervention for an infectious disease is a protective vaccine. Early in the characterization of HCV, it was recognized that its genetic diversity and the variation of the nucleocapsid proteins among and within genotypes would make vaccine development challenging.[214] This has been borne out over the decades since. HCV is highly effective in evading the immune response and reinfection may occur even after spontaneous clearance of virus (i.e., a successful immune response to an initial infection). However, there is also evidence that clearance of reinfection may be more likely than clearance of primary infection.[114,215] This appears to be due to a broad T-cell response to the primary infection.[216] A vaccine that induces a good cellular immune T-cell response may provide some protection. A number of vaccine candidates targeting the viral envelope E1 and E2 proteins essential for cell entry, as well as the core protein, have been studied in animals and in early human trials.[217] Other investigational approaches have utilized DNA vaccines (DNA coding viral antigens that cause cells to express the antigens and stimulate an immune response), viral vectors (such as adenovirus and vaccinia virus) expressing HCV antigens, and virus-like particles similar to those used for human papillomavirus vaccine. These are all in early stage of development with both positive and mixed results. A successful vaccine may be available someday, but it would have to induce a broad cellular and humoral immune response, as well as being safe.

Monoclonal antibodies against conserved regions of HCV envelope proteins have been developed primarily to prevent reinfection of transplanted livers. One monoclonal antibody specific for a region of the E2 protein has been studied in liver transplant patients. While it delayed the viral rebound seen in infected patients after transplant, virus variants with mutations allowing escape from antibody neutralization were selected and emerged.[218] Further research on monoclonal antibodies capable of neutralizing virus may be useful for identifying vaccine targets. Research on targeting host cell receptors used by HCV has resulted in promising results with a potential for a role in the immunotherapy of infection.[219]

Hepatitis C presents a major global challenge. Much has been learned about pathogenesis, natural history, and prevention since the first recognition of non-A, non-B hepatitis and the identification of HCV as the cause, but there are still aspects of the virus and the diseases it causes that are not fully understood. Now, with effective therapy for cure with directly acting agents, the long-term complications of hepatitis C are preventable. The effectiveness of therapy also provides the promise of treatment as prevention and elimination of HCV transmission. The success of the global initiative for elimination will depend on continued progress in research, effective screening strategies for those at risk, assuring access to curative therapy, and applying the political will to get the work done.

References

1. Alter HJ, Holland PV, Morrow AG, et al. Clinical and serological analysis of transfusion-associated hepatitis. *Lancet*. 1975;2(7940):838–41.
2. World Health Organization. *Global Hepatitis Report 2017*. Geneva: World Health Organization; 2017.
3. Mohd Hanafiah K, Groeger J, Flaxman AD, Wiersma ST. Global epidemiology of hepatitis C virus infection: New estimates of age-specific antibody to HCV seroprevalence. *Hepatology*. 2013;57:1333–42.
4. Ly KN, Hughes EM, Jiles RB, Holmberg SD. Rising mortality associated with hepatitis C virus in the United States, 2003–2013. *Clin Infect Dis*. 2016;62(10):1287–8.
5. Prince AM, Brotman B, Grady GF, et al. Long-incubation post-transfusion hepatitis without serological evidence of exposure to hepatitis-B virus. *Lancet*. 1974;2(7875):241–6.
6. Choo QL, Kuo G, Weiner AJ, Overby LR, Bradley DW, Houghton M. Isolation of a cDNA clone derived from a blood-borne non-A, non-B viral hepatitis genome. *Science*. 1989;244(4902):359–62.
7. Choo QL, Weiner AJ, Overby LR, Kuo G, Houghton M, Bradley DW. Hepatitis C virus: The major causative agent of viral non-A, non-B hepatitis. *Br Med Bull*. 1990;46(2):423–41.
8. Hartlage AS, Cullen JM, Kapoor A. The strange, expanding world of animal hepaciviruses. *Annu Rev Virol*. 2016;3(1):53–75.
9. Kuo G, Choo QL, Alter HJ, et al. An assay for circulating antibodies to a major etiologic virus of human non-A, non-B hepatitis. *Science*. 1989;244(4902):362–4.
10. Shimizu YK, Iwamoto A, Hijikata M, Purcell RH, Yoshikura H. Evidence for in vitro replication of hepatitis C virus genome in a human T-cell line. *Proc Natl Acad Sci U S A*. 1992;89(12):5477–81.
11. Simmonds P, Bukh J, Combet C, et al. Consensus proposals for a unified system of nomenclature of hepatitis C virus genotypes. *Hepatology*. 2005;42(4):962–73.
12. Smith DB, Bukh J, Kuiken C, et al. Expanded classification of hepatitis C virus into 7 genotypes and 67 subtypes: Updated criteria and genotype assignment web resource. *Hepatology*. 2014;59:318–27.
13. Sarwar MT, Kausar H, Ijaz B, et al. NS4A protein as a marker of HCV history suggests that different HCV genotypes originally evolved from genotype 1b. *Virol J*. 2011;8:317.
14. Laskus T, Wang LF, Radkowski M, et al. Exposure of hepatitis C virus (HCV) RNA-positive recipients to HCV RNA-positive blood donors results in rapid predominance of a single donor strain and exclusion and/or suppression of the recipient strain. *J Virol*. 2001;75(5):2059–66.
15. Murphy DG, Sablon E, Chamberland J, Fournier E, Dandavino R, Tremblay CL. Hepatitis C virus genotype 7, a new genotype originating from central Africa. *J Clin Microbiol*. 2015;53(3):967–72.
16. Farci P, Shimoda A, Coiana A, et al. The outcome of acute hepatitis C predicted by the evolution of the viral quasispecies. *Science*. 2000;288(5464):339–44.
17. Hayashi J, Kishihara Y, Yamaji K, et al. Hepatitis C viral quasispecies and liver damage in patients with chronic hepatitis C virus infection. *Hepatology*. 1997;25(3):697–701.
18. Kamili S, Krawczynski K, McCaustland K, Li X, Alter MJ. Infectivity of hepatitis C virus in plasma after drying and storing at room temperature. *Infect Control Hosp Epidemiol*. 2007;28(5):519–24.
19. Doerrbecker J, Friesland M, Ciesek S, et al. Inactivation and survival of hepatitis C virus on inanimate surfaces. *J Infect Dis*. 2011;204(12):1830–8.
20. Paintsil E, He H, Peters C, Lindenbach BD, Heimer R. Survival of hepatitis C virus in syringes: Implication for transmission among injection drug users. *J Infect Dis*. 2010;202(7):984–90.
21. Doerrbecker J, Behrendt P, Mateu-Gelabert P, et al. Transmission of hepatitis C virus among people who inject drugs: Viral stability and association with drug preparation equipment. *J Infect Dis*. 2013;207(2):281–7.
22. Bradshaw D, Lamoury F, Catlett B, et al. A comparison of seminal hepatitis C virus (HCV) RNA levels during recent and chronic HCV infection in HIV-infected and HIV-uninfected individuals. *J Infect Dis*. 2015;211(5):736–43.
23. Nowicki MJ, Laskus T, Nikolopoulou G, et al. Presence of hepatitis C virus (HCV) RNA in the genital tracts of HCV/HIV-1-coinfected women. *J Infect Dis*. 2005;192(9):1557––65.
24. Benova L, Mohamoud YA, Calvert C, Abu-Raddad LJ. Vertical transmission of hepatitis C virus: Systematic review and meta-analysis. *Clin Infect Dis*. 2014;59(6):765–73.
25. Alter HJ. The dominant role of non-A, non-B in the pathogenesis of post-transfusion hepatitis: A clinical assessment. *Clin Gastroenterol*. 1980;9(1):155–70.
26. Donahue JG, Muñoz A, Ness PM, et al. The declining risk of post-transfusion hepatitis C virus infection. *N Engl J Med*. 1992;327(6):369–73.
27. Seeff LB, Hollinger FB, Alter HJ, et al. Long-term mortality and morbidity of transfusion-associated non-A, non-B, and type C hepatitis: A National Heart, Lung, and Blood Institute collaborative study. *Hepatology*. 2001;33(2):455–63.
28. Fransen van de Putte DE, Makris M, Fischer K, et al. Long-term follow-up of hepatitis C infection in a large cohort of patients with inherited bleeding disorders. *J Hepatol*. 2014;60(1):39–45.
29. Papadopoulos N, Argiana V, Deutsch M. Hepatitis C infection in patients with hereditary bleeding disorders: Epidemiology, natural history, and management. *Ann Gastroenterol*. 2018;31(1):35–41.
30. Simonsen L, Kane A, Lloyd J, Zaffran M, Kane M. Unsafe injections in the developing world and transmission of bloodborne pathogens: A review. *Bull World Health Organ*. 1999;77(10):789–800.
31. Kouyoumjian SP, Chemaitelly H, Abu-Raddad LJ. Characterizing hepatitis C virus epidemiology in Egypt: Systematic reviews, meta-analyses, and meta-regressions. *Sci Rep*. 2018;8(1):1661.
32. Frank C, Mohamed MK, Strickland GT, et al. The role of parenteral antischistosomal therapy in the spread of hepatitis C virus in Egypt. *Lancet*. 2000;355(9207):887–91.
33. Pépin J, Lavoie M, Pybus OG, et al. Risk factors for hepatitis C virus transmission in colonial Cameroon. *Clin Infect Dis*. 2010;51(7):768–76.
34. Singh S, Dwivedi SN, Sood R, Wali JP. Hepatitis B, C and human immunodeficiency virus infections in multiply-injected kala-azar patients in Delhi. *Scand J Infect Dis*. 2000;32:3–6.
35. Di Stefano R, Stroffolini T, Ferraro D, et al. Endemic hepatitis C virus infection in a Sicilian town: Further evidence for iatrogenic transmission. *J Med Virol*. 2002;67:339–44.
36. Sun CA, Chen HC, Lu CF, et al. Transmission of hepatitis C virus in Taiwan: Prevalence and risk factors based on a nationwide survey. *J Med Virol*. 1999;59:290–6.
37. Abergel A, Ughetto S, Dubost S, et al. The epidemiology and virology of hepatitis C virus genotype 5 in central France. *Aliment Pharmacol Ther*. 2007;26:1437–46.
38. Germain JM, Carbonne A, Thiers V, et al. Patient-to-patient transmission of hepatitis C virus through the use of multidose vials during general anesthesia. *Infect Control Hosp Epidemiol*. 2005;26:789–92.
39. Perz JF, Thompson ND, Schaefer MK, Patel PR. US outbreak investigations highlight the need for safe injection practices and basic infection control. *Clin Liver Dis*. 2010;14:137–51.
40. Moore ZS, Schaefer MK, Hoffmann KK, et al. Transmission of hepatitis C virus during myocardial perfusion imaging in an outpatient clinic. *Am J Cardiol*. 2011;108:126–32.
41. Fischer GE, Schaefer MK, Labus BJ, et al. Hepatitis C virus infections from unsafe injection practices at an endoscopy clinic in Las Vegas, Nevada, 2007–2008. *Clin Infect Dis*. 2010;51:267–73.
42. Finelli L, Miller JT, Tokars JI, Alter MJ, Arduino MJ. National surveillance of dialysis-associated diseases in the United States, 2002. *Semin Dial*. 2005;18(1):52–61.
43. Petrosillo N, Gilli P, Serraino D, et al. Prevalence of infected patients and understaffing have a role in hepatitis C virus transmission in dialysis. *Am J Kidney Dis*. 2001;37(5):1004–10.
44. Fissell RB, Bragg-Gresham JL, Woods JD, et al. Patterns of hepatitis C prevalence and seroconversion in hemodialysis units from three continents: The DOPPS. *Kidney Int*. 2004;65(6):2335–42.
45. Gordon CE, Balk EM, Becker BN, et al. KDOQI US commentary on the KDIGO clinical practice guideline for the prevention, diagnosis, evaluation, and treatment of hepatitis C in CKD. *Am J Kidney Dis*. 2008;52(5):811–25.
46. Mbaeyi C, Thompson ND. Hepatitis C virus screening and management of seroconversions in hemodialysis facilities. *Semin Dial*. 2013;26(4):439–46.
47. Al-Rabadi L, Box T, Singhania G, et al. Rationale for treatment of hepatitis C virus infection in end-stage renal disease patients who are not kidney transplant candidates. *Hemodial Int*. 2018;22 Suppl 1:S45–52.
48. Yazdanpanah Y, De Carli G, Migueres B, et al. Risk factors for hepatitis C virus transmission to health care workers after occupational exposure: A European case-control study. *Clin Infect Dis*. 2005;41(10):1423–30.
49. Egro FM, Nwaiwu CA, Smith S, Harper JD, Spiess AM. Seroconversion rates among health care workers exposed to hepatitis C virus-contaminated body fluids: The University of Pittsburgh 13-year experience. *Am J Infect Control*. 2017;45(9):1001–5.

50. Corey KE, Servoss JC, Casson DR, et al. Pilot study of postexposure prophylaxis for hepatitis C virus in healthcare workers. *Infect Control Hosp Epidemiol.* 2009;30(10):1000–5.
51. Gerlach JT, Diepolder HM, Zachoval R, et al. Acute hepatitis C: High rate of both spontaneous and treatment-induced viral clearance. *Gastroenterology.* 2003;125(1):80–8.
52. Pozzetto B, Memmi M, Garraud O, Roblin X, Berthelot P. Health care-associated hepatitis C virus infection. *World J Gastroenterol.* 2014;20(46):17265–78.
53. Donahue JG, Nelson KE, Muñoz A, et al. Antibody to hepatitis C virus among cardiac surgery patients, homosexual men, and intravenous drug users in Baltimore, Maryland. *Am J Epidemiol.* 1991;134(10):1206–11.
54. Kelen GD, Green GB, Purcell RH, et al. Hepatitis B and hepatitis C in emergency department patients. *N Engl J Med.* 1992;326(21):1399–404.
55. Garfein RS, Doherty MC, Monterroso ER, Thomas DL, Nelson KE, Vlahov D. Prevalence and incidence of hepatitis C virus infection among young adult injection drug users. *J Acquir Immune Defic Syndr Hum Retrovirol.* 1998;18 Suppl 1:S11–9.
56. Hagan H, Pouget ER, Des Jarlais DC, Lelutiu-Weinberger C. Meta-regression of hepatitis C virus infection in relation to time since onset of illicit drug injection: The influence of time and place. *Am J Epidemiol.* 2008;168(10):1099–109.
57. Nelson PK, Mathers BM, Cowie B, et al. Global epidemiology of hepatitis B and hepatitis C in people who inject drugs: Results of systematic reviews. *Lancet.* 2011;378(9791):571–83.
58. Thorpe LE, Ouellet LJ, Hershow R, et al. Risk of hepatitis C virus infection among young adult injection drug users who share injection equipment. *Am J Epidemiol.* 2002;155(7):645–53.
59. Hahn JA, Page-Shafer K, Lum PJ, et al. Hepatitis C virus seroconversion among young injection drug users: Relationships and risks. *J Infect Dis.* 2002;186(11):1558–64.
60. Murray JM, Law MG, Gao Z, Kaldor JM. The impact of behavioural changes on the prevalence of human immunodeficiency virus and hepatitis C among injecting drug users. *Int J Epidemiol.* 2003;32(5):708–14.
61. Alter MJ, Kruszon-Moran D, Nainan OV, et al. The prevalence of hepatitis C virus infection in the United States, 1988 through 1994. *N Engl J Med.* 1999;341(8):556–62.
62. Armstrong GL, Wasley A, Simard EP, McQuillan GM, Kuhnert WL, Alter MJ. The prevalence of hepatitis C virus infection in the United States, 1999 through 2002. *Ann Intern Med.* 2006;144(10):705–14.
63. Denniston MM, Jiles RB, Drobeniuc J, et al. Chronic hepatitis C virus infection in the United States, National Health and Nutrition Examination Survey 2003 to 2010. *Ann Intern Med.* 2014;160(5):293–300.
64. Amon JJ, Garfein RS, Ahdieh-Grant L, et al. Prevalence of hepatitis C virus infection among injection drug users in the United States, 1994–2004. *Clin Infect Dis.* 2008;46(12):1852–8.
65. Centers for Disease Control and Prevention (CDC). Notes from the field: Risk factors for hepatitis C virus infections among young adults—Massachusetts, 2010. *MMWR Morb Mortal Wkly Rep.* 2011;60(42):1457–8.
66. Suryaprasad AG, White JZ, Xu F, et al. Emerging epidemic of hepatitis C virus infections among young nonurban persons who inject drugs in the United States, 2006–2012. *Clin Infect Dis.* 2014;59(10):1411–9.
67. Zibbell JE, Asher AK, Patel RC, et al. Increases in acute hepatitis C virus infection related to a growing opioid epidemic and associated injection drug use, United States, 2004 to 2014. *Am J Public Health.* 2018;108(2):175–81.
68. Peters PJ, Pontones P, Hoover KW, et al. HIV infection linked to injection use of oxymorphone in Indiana, 2014–2015. *N Engl J Med.* 2016;375(3):229–39.
69. Koblin BA, Factor SH, Wu Y, Vlahov D. Hepatitis C virus infection among noninjecting drug users in New York City. *J Med Virol.* 2003;70(3):387–90.
70. Conry-Cantilena C, VanRaden M, Gibble J, et al. Routes of infection, viremia, and liver disease in blood donors found to have hepatitis C virus infection. *N Engl J Med.* 1996;334(26):1691–6.
71. Macías J, Palacios RB, Claro E, et al. High prevalence of hepatitis C virus infection among noninjecting drug users: Association with sharing the inhalation implements of crack. *Liver Int.* 2008;28(6):781–6.
72. Karmochkine M, Carrat F, Dos Santos O, Cacoub P, Raguin G. A case-control study of risk factors for hepatitis C infection in patients with unexplained routes of infection. *J Viral Hepat.* 2006;13(11):775–82.
73. Allison RD, Conry-Cantilena C, Koziol D, et al. A 25-year study of the clinical and histologic outcomes of hepatitis C virus infection and its modes of transmission in a cohort of initially asymptomatic blood donors. *J Infect Dis.* 2012;206(5):654–61.
74. Novais AC, Lopes CL, Reis NR, Silva AM, Martins RM, Souto FJ. Prevalence of hepatitis C virus infection and associated factors among male illicit drug users in Cuiabá, Mato Grosso, Brazil. *Mem Inst Oswaldo Cruz.* 2009;104(6):892–6.
75. Gelberg L, Robertson MJ, Arangua L, et al. Prevalence, distribution, and correlates of hepatitis C virus infection among homeless adults in Los Angeles. *Public Health Rep.* 2012;127(4):407–21.
76. Giuliani M, Caprilli F, Gentili G, et al. Incidence and determinants of hepatitis C virus infection among individuals at risk of sexually transmitted diseases attending a human immunodeficiency virus type 1 testing program. *Sex Transm Dis.* 1997;24(9):533–7.
77. Thomas DL, Zenilman JM, Alter HJ, et al. Sexual transmission of hepatitis C virus among patients attending sexually transmitted diseases clinics in Baltimore—An analysis of 309 sex partnerships. *J Infect Dis.* 1995;171(4):768–75.
78. Tohme RA, Holmberg SD. Is sexual contact a major mode of hepatitis C virus transmission? *Hepatology.* 2010;52(4):1497–505.
79. Vandelli C, Renzo F, Romanò L, et al. Lack of evidence of sexual transmission of hepatitis C among monogamous couples: Results of a 10-year prospective follow-up study. *Am J Gastroenterol.* 2004;99(5):855–9.
80. Terrault NA, Dodge JL, Murphy EL, et al. Sexual transmission of hepatitis C virus among monogamous heterosexual couples: The HCV partners study. *Hepatology.* 2013;57(3):881–9.
81. Cohen DE, Russell CJ, Golub SA, Mayer KH. Prevalence of hepatitis C virus infection among men who have sex with men at a Boston community health center and its association with markers of high-risk behavior. *AIDS Patient Care STDS.* 2006;20(8):557–64.
82. Richardson D, Fisher M, Sabin CA. Sexual transmission of hepatitis C in MSM may not be confined to those with HIV infection. *J Infect Dis.* 2008;197(8):1213–4.
83. McFaul K, Maghlaoui A, Nzuruba M, et al. Acute hepatitis C infection in HIV-negative men who have sex with men. *J Viral Hepat.* 2015;22(6):535–8.
84. Yaphe S, Bozinoff N, Kyle R, Shivkumar S, Pai NP, Klein, M. Incidence of acute hepatitis C virus infection among men who have sex with men with and without HIV infection: A systematic review. *Sex Transm Infect.* 2012;88:558–64.
85. Chan DP, Sun HY, Wong HT, Lee SS, Hung CC. Sexually acquired hepatitis C virus infection: A review. *Int J Infect Dis.* 2016;49:47–58.
86. Garg S, Taylor LE, Grasso C, Mayer KH. Prevalent and incident hepatitis C virus infection among HIV-infected men who have sex with men engaged in primary care in a Boston community health center. *Clin Infect Dis.* 2013;56(10):1480–7.
87. Martin NK, Thornton A, Hickman M, et al. Can hepatitis C Virus (HCV) direct-acting antiviral treatment as prevention reverse the HCV epidemic among men who have sex with men in the United Kingdom? Epidemiological and modeling insights. *Clin Infect Dis.* 2016;62(9):1072–80.
88. European Centre for Disease Prevention and Control. Hepatitis C. In: *ECDC. Annual Epidemiological Report for 2015.* Stockholm: ECDC; 2017.
89. Pradat P, Huleux T, Raffi F, et al. Incidence of new hepatitis C virus infection is still increasing in French MSM living with HIV. *AIDS.* 2018;32(8):1077–82.
90. Ly KN, Jiles RB, Teshale EH, Foster MA, Pesano RL, Holmberg SD. Hepatitis C virus infection among reproductive-aged women and children in the United States, 2006 to 2014. *Ann Intern Med.* 2017;166(11):775–82.
91. Kuncio DE, Newbern EC, Johnson CC, Viner KM. Failure to test and identify perinatally infected children born to hepatitis C virus-infected women. *Clin Infect Dis.* 2016;62(8):980–5.
92. Watts T, Stockman L, Martin J, Guilfoyle S, Vergeront JM. Increased risk for mother-to-infant transmission of hepatitis C virus among medicaid recipients—Wisconsin, 2011–2015. *MMWR Morb Mortal Wkly Rep.* 2017;66(42):1136–9.
93. Bal A, Petrova A. Single clinical practice's report of testing initiation, antibody clearance, and transmission of hepatitis C virus (HCV) in infants of chronically HCV-infected mothers. *Open Forum Infect Dis.* 2016 Feb 8;3(1):ofw021.
94. Howe CJ, Fuller CM, Ompad DC, et al. Association of sex, hygiene and drug equipment sharing with hepatitis C virus infection among non-injecting drug users in New York City. *Drug Alcohol Depend.* 2005;79(3):389–95.
95. Samuel MC, Doherty PM, Bulterys M, Jenison SA. Association between heroin use, needle sharing and tattoos received in prison with hepatitis

B and C positivity among street-recruited injecting drug users in New Mexico, USA. *Epidemiol Infect*. 2001;127:475–84.

96. Tohme RA, Holmberg SD. Transmission of hepatitis C virus infection through tattooing and piercing: A critical review. *Clin Infect Dis*. 2012;54(8):1167–78.
97. Edlin BR, Eckhardt BJ, Shu MA, Holmberg SD, Swan T. Toward a more accurate estimate of the prevalence of hepatitis C in the United States. *Hepatology*. 2015;62(5):1353–63.
98. Onofrey S, Aneja J, Haney GA, et al. Underascertainment of acute hepatitis C virus infections in the U.S. surveillance system: A case series and chart review. *Ann Intern Med*. 2015;163(4):254–61.
99. Williams IT, Bell BP, Kuhnert W, Alter MJ. Incidence and transmission patterns of acute hepatitis C in the United States, 1982–2006. *Arch Intern Med*. 2011;171(3):242–8.
100. Centers for Disease Control and Prevention. Hepatitis C virus infection among adolescents and young adults: Massachusetts, 2002–2009. *MMWR Morb Mortal Wkly Rep*. 2011;60:537–41.
101. Zibbell JE, Hart-Malloy R, Barry J, Fan L, Flanigan C. Risk factors for HCV infection among young adults in rural New York who inject prescription opioid analgesics. *Am J Public Health*. 2014;104(11):2226–32.
102. Degenhardt L, Peacock A, Colledge S, et al. Global prevalence of injecting drug use and sociodemographic characteristics and prevalence of HIV, HBV, and HCV in people who inject drugs: A multistage systematic review. *Lancet Glob Health*. 2017 Dec;5(12):e1192–207.
103. McGovern BH, Birch CE, Bowen MJ, et al. Improving the diagnosis of acute hepatitis C virus infection with expanded viral load criteria. *Clin Infect Dis*. 2009;49(7):1051–60.
104. Sagnelli E, Tonziello G, Pisaturo M, Sagnelli C, Coppola N. Clinical applications of antibody avidity and immunoglobulin M testing in acute HCV infection. *Antivir Ther*. 2012;17(7 Pt B):453–8.
105. Micallef JM, Kaldor JM, Dore GJ. Spontaneous viral clearance following acute hepatitis C infection: A systematic review of longitudinal studies. *J Viral Hepat*. 2006;13(1):34–41.
106. Gerlach JT, Diepolder HM, Zachoval R, et al. Acute hepatitis C: High rate of both spontaneous and treatment-induced viral clearance. *Gastroenterology*. 2003;125(1):80–8.
107. Sharaf Eldin N, Ismail S, Mansour H, et al. Symptomatic acute hepatitis C in Egypt: Diagnosis, spontaneous viral clearance, and delayed treatment with 12 weeks of pegylated interferon alfa-2a. *PLoS One*. 2008;3(12):e4085.
108. Wang CC, Krantz E, Klarquist J, et al. Acute hepatitis C in a contemporary US cohort: Modes of acquisition and factors influencing viral clearance. *J Infect Dis*. 2007;196(10):1474–82.
109. Grebely J, Page K, Sacks-Davis R, et al. The effects of female sex, viral genotype, and IL28B genotype on spontaneous clearance of acute hepatitis C virus infection. *Hepatology*. 2014;59(1):109–20.
110. Vogt M, Lang T, Frösner G, et al. Prevalence and clinical outcome of hepatitis C infection in children who underwent cardiac surgery before the implementation of blood-donor screening. *N Engl J Med*. 1999;341(12):866–70.
111. Thomas DL, Astemborski J, Rai RM, et al. The natural history of hepatitis C virus infection: Host, viral, and environmental factors. *JAMA*. 2000;284(4):450–6.
112. Diepolder HM, Zachoval R, Hoffmann RM, et al. Possible mechanism involving T-lymphocyte response to non-structural protein 3 in viral clearance in acute hepatitis C virus infection. *Lancet*. 1995;346(8981):1006–7.
113. Thomas DL, Thio CL, Martin MP, et al. Genetic variation in IL28B and spontaneous clearance of hepatitis C virus. *Nature*. 2009;461(7265):798–801.
114. Sacks-Davis R, Grebely J, Dore GJ, et al. Hepatitis C virus reinfection and spontaneous clearance of reinfection—The InC3 Study. *J Infect Dis*. 2015;212(9):1407–19.
115. Takaki A, Wiese M, Maertens G, et al. Cellular immune responses persist and humoral responses decrease two decades after recovery from a single-source outbreak of hepatitis C. *Nat Med*. 2000;6(5):578–82.
116. Seeff LB, Miller RN, Rabkin CS, et al. 45-Year follow-up of hepatitis C virus infection in healthy young adults. *Ann Intern Med*. 2000;132(2):105–11.
117. Allison RD, Conry-Cantilena C, Koziol D, et al. A 25-year study of the clinical and histologic outcomes of hepatitis C virus infection and its modes of transmission in a cohort of initially asymptomatic blood donors. *J Infect Dis*. 2012;206(5):654–61.
118. Thein HH, Yi Q, Dore GJ, Krahn MD. Estimation of stage-specific fibrosis progression rates in chronic hepatitis C virus infection: a meta-analysis and meta-regression. *Hepatology*. 2008;48(2):418–31.
119. Poynard T, Ratziu V, Benmanov Y, Di Martino V, Bedossa P, Opolon P. Fibrosis in patients with chronic hepatitis C: Detection and significance. *Semin Liver Dis*. 2000;20(1):47–55.
120. Massard J, Ratziu V, Thabut D, et al. Natural history and predictors of disease severity in chronic hepatitis C. *J Hepatol*. 2006;44(1 Suppl):S19–24.
121. Wang H, Swann R, Thomas E, et al. Impact of previous hepatitis B infection on the clinical outcomes from chronic hepatitis C? A population-level analysis. *J Viral Hepat*. Mar 25 2018;25(8):930–8. doi: 10.1111/jvh.12897.
122. Hézode C, Roudot-Thoraval F, Nguyen S, et al. Daily cannabis smoking as a risk factor for progression of fibrosis in chronic hepatitis C. *Hepatology*. 2005;42:63–71.
123. Freedman ND, Everhart JE, Lindsay KL, et al. Coffee intake is associated with lower rates of liver disease progression in chronic hepatitis C. *Hepatology*. 2009;50:1360–9.
124. Bochud PY, Cai T, Overbeck K, et al. Genotype 3 is associated with accelerated fibrosis progression in chronic hepatitis C. *J Hepatol*. 2009;51(4):655–66.
125. Chamie G, Bonacini M, Bangsberg DR, et al. Factors associated with seronegative chronic hepatitis C virus infection in HIV infection. *Clin Infect Dis*. 2007;44(4):577–83.
126. Danta M, Semmo N, Fabris P, et al. Impact of HIV on host-virus interactions during early hepatitis C virus infection. *J Infect Dis*. 2008;197(11):1558–66.
127. Sulkowski MS, Thomas DL. Hepatitis C in the HIV-infected person. *Ann Intern Med*. 2003;138(3):197–207.
128. Graham CS, Baden LR, Yu E, et al. Influence of human immunodeficiency virus infection on the course of hepatitis C virus infection: a meta-analysis. *Clin Infect Dis*. 2001;33(4):562–9.
129. Lo Re V 3rd, Kallan MJ, Tate JP, et al. Hepatic decompensation in antiretroviral-treated patients co-infected with HIV and hepatitis C virus compared with hepatitis C virus-monoinfected patients: A cohort study. *Ann Intern Med*. 2014;160(6):369–79.
130. Fierer DS, Dieterich DT, Fiel MI, et al. Rapid progression to decompensated cirrhosis, liver transplant, and death in HIV-infected men after primary hepatitis C virus infection. *Clin Infect Dis*. 2013;56(7):1038–43.
131. Bica I, McGovern B, Dhar R, et al. Increasing mortality due to end-stage liver disease in patients with human immunodeficiency virus infection. *Clin Infect Dis*. 2001;32(3):492–7.
132. Chen TY, Ding EL, Seage III GR, Kim AY. Meta-analysis: Increased mortality associated with hepatitis C in HIV-infected persons is unrelated to HIV disease progression. *Clin Infect Dis*. 2009;49(10):1605–15.
133. Shakil AO, Conry-Cantilena C, Alter HJ, et al. Volunteer blood donors with antibody to hepatitis C virus: Clinical, biochemical, virologic, and histologic features. The Hepatitis C Study Group. *Ann Intern Med*. 1995;123(5):330–7.
134. Castera L. Noninvasive methods to assess liver disease in patients with hepatitis B or C. *Gastroenterology*. 2012;142(6):1293–302.
135. Holmberg SD, Lu M, Rupp LB, et al. Noninvasive serum fibrosis markers for screening and staging chronic hepatitis C virus patients in a large US cohort. *Clin Infect Dis*. 2013;57:240–6.
136. Patel K, Benhamou Y, Yoshida EM, et al. An independent and prospective comparison of two commercial fibrosis marker panels (HCV FibroSURE and FIBROSpect II) during albinterferon alfa-2b combination therapy for chronic hepatitis C. *J Viral Hepat*. 2009;16:178–86.
137. Steadman R, Myers RP, Leggett L, et al. A health technology assessment of transient elastography in adult liver disease. *Can J Gastroenterol*. 2013;27:149–58.
138. Kirk GD, Astemborski J, Mehta SH, et al. Assessment of liver fibrosis by transient elastography in persons with hepatitis C virus infection or HIV-hepatitis C virus coinfection. *Clin Infect Dis*. 2009;48(7):963–72.
139. Vescovo T, Refolo G, Vitagliano G, Fimia GM, Piacentini M. Molecular mechanisms of hepatitis C virus-induced hepatocellular carcinoma. *Clin Microbiol Infect*. 2016 Oct;22(10):853–61.
140. Noone AM, Howlader N, Krapcho M, et al., eds. *SEER Cancer Statistics Review, 1975–2015*. Bethesda, MD: National Cancer Institute. https://seer.cancer.gov/csr/1975_2015. Accessed May 12, 2018.
141. Ferlay J, Soerjomataram I, Ervik M, et al. *GLOBOCAN 2012 v1.0, Cancer Incidence and Mortality Worldwide: IARC Cancer Base No. 11*. Lyon, France: International Agency for Research on Cancer; 2013. http://globocan.iarc.fr. Accessed May 12, 2018.

142. Kanwal F, Kramer J, Asch SM, Chayanupatkul M, Cao Y, El-Serag HB. Risk of hepatocellular cancer in HCV patients treated with direct-acting antiviral agents. *Gastroenterology*. 2017;153(4):996–1005.
143. Dal Maso L, Franceschi S. Hepatitis C virus and risk of lymphoma and other lymphoid neoplasms: A meta-analysis of epidemiologic studies. *Cancer Epidemiol Biomarkers Prev*. 2006;15(11):2078–85.
144. Cacoub P, Gragnani L, Comarmond C, Zignego AL. Extrahepatic manifestations of chronic hepatitis C virus infection. *Dig Liver Dis*. 2014;46 Suppl 5:S165–7.
145. Butt AA, Xiaoqiang W, Budoff M, Leaf D, Kuller LH, Justice AC. Hepatitis C virus infection and the risk of coronary disease. *Clin Infect Dis*. 2009;49(2):225–32.
146. Hsu YC, Lin JT, Ho HJ, et al. Antiviral treatment for hepatitis C virus infection is associated with improved renal and cardiovascular outcomes in diabetic patients. *Hepatology*. 2014;59(4):1293–302.
147. Mason AL, Lau JY, Hoang N, et al. Association of diabetes mellitus and chronic hepatitis C virus infection. *Hepatology*. 1999;29(2):328–33.
148. Mahajan R, Xing J, Liu SJ, et al. Mortality among persons in care with hepatitis C virus infection: The Chronic Hepatitis Cohort Study (CHeCS), 2006–2010. *Clin Infect Dis*. 2014;58(8):1055–61.
149. El-Kamary SS, Jhaveri R, Shardell MD. All-cause, liver-related, and non-liver-related mortality among HCV-infected individuals in the general US population. *Clin Infect Dis*. 2011;53(2):150–7.
150. Lee MH, Yang HI, Lu SN, et al. Chronic hepatitis C virus infection increases mortality from hepatic and extrahepatic diseases: A community-based long-term prospective study. *J Infect Dis*. 2012;206(4):469–77.
151. Purcell RH, London WT, McAuliffe VJ, et al. Modification of chronic hepatitis-B virus infection in chimpanzees by administration of an interferon inducer. *Lancet*. 1976;2(7989):757–61.
152. Hoofnagle JH, Mullen KD, Jones DB, et al. Treatment of chronic non-A, non-B hepatitis with recombinant human alpha interferon. A preliminary report. *N Engl J Med*. 1986;315(25):1575–8.
153. Thomson BJ, Doran M, Lever AM, Webster AD. Alpha-interferon therapy for non-A, non-B hepatitis transmitted by gammaglobulin replacement therapy. *Lancet*. 1987;1(8532):539–41.
154. Schvarcz R, Weiland O, Wejstål R, Norkrans G, Frydén A, Foberg U. A randomized controlled open study of interferon alpha-2b treatment of chronic non-A, non-B posttransfusion hepatitis: No correlation of outcome to presence of hepatitis C virus antibodies. *Scand J Infect Dis*. 1989;21(6):617–25.
155. Davis G. Recombinant alpha-interferon treatment of non-A, and non-B (type C) hepatitis: Review of studies and recommendations for treatment. *J Hepatol*. 1990;11 Suppl 1:S72–7.
156. Shindo M, Di Bisceglie AM, Hoofnagle JH. Long-term follow-up of patients with chronic hepatitis C treated with alpha-interferon. *Hepatology*. 1992;15(6):1013–6.
157. Reichard O, Andersson J, Schvarcz R, Weiland O. Ribavirin treatment for chronic hepatitis C. *Lancet*. 1991;337(8749):1058–61.
158. Di Bisceglie AM, Shindo M, Fong TL, et al. A pilot study of ribavirin therapy for chronic hepatitis C. *Hepatology*. 1992;16(3):649–54.
159. Brillanti S, Garson J, Foli M, et al. A pilot study of combination therapy with ribavirin plus interferon alfa for interferon alfa-resistant chronic hepatitis C. *Gastroenterology*. 1994;107(3):812–7.
160. Braconier JH, Paulsen O, Engman K, Widell A. Combined alpha-interferon and ribavirin treatment in chronic hepatitis C: A pilot study. *Scand J Infect Dis*. 1995;27(4):325–9.
161. Reichard O, Norkrans G, Frydén A, Braconier JH, Sönnerborg A, Weiland O. Randomised, double-blind, placebo-controlled trial of interferon alpha-2b with and without ribavirin for chronic hepatitis C. The Swedish Study Group. *Lancet*. 1998;351(9096):83–7.
162. Davis GL, Esteban-Mur R, Rustgi V, et al. Interferon alfa-2b alone or in combination with ribavirin for the treatment of relapse of chronic hepatitis C. International Hepatitis Interventional Therapy Group. *N Engl J Med*. 1998;339(21):1493–9.
163. Smith-Palmer J, Cerri K, Valentine W. Achieving sustained virologic response in hepatitis C: A systematic review of the clinical, economic and quality of life benefits. *BMC Infect Dis*. 2015;15:19.
164. Younossi ZM, Stepanova M, Asselah T, et al. Hepatitis C in patients with minimal or no hepatic fibrosis: The impact of treatment and sustained virologic response on patient-reported outcomes. *Clin Infect Dis*. 2018;66(11):1742–50.
165. Martin NK, Vickerman P, Dore GJ, et al. Prioritization of HCV treatment in the direct-acting antiviral era: An economic evaluation. *J Hepatol*. 2016;65:17–25.
166. Najafzadeh M, Andersson K, Shrank WH, et al. Cost-effectiveness of novel regimens for the treatment of hepatitis C virus. *Ann Intern Med*. 2015;162(6):407–19.
167. Rein DB, Wittenborn JS, Smith BD, Liffmann DK, Ward JW. The cost-effectiveness, health benefits, and financial costs of new antiviral treatments for hepatitis C virus. *Clin Infect Dis*. 2015;61(2):157–68.
168. Chahal HS, Marseille EA, Tice JA, et al. Cost-effectiveness of early treatment of hepatitis C virus genotype 1 by stage of liver fibrosis in a US treatment-naive population. *JAMA Intern Med*. 2016;176(1):65–73.
169. Linas BP, Morgan JR, Pho MT, et al. cost effectiveness and cost containment in the era of interferon-free therapies to treat hepatitis C virus genotype 1. *Open Forum Infect Dis*. 2016 Dec 27;4(1):ofw266. doi: 10.1093/ofid/ofw266.
170. Edlin BR, Seal KH, Lorvick J, et al. Is it justifiable to withhold treatment for hepatitis C from illicit-drug users? *N Engl J Med*. 2001;345(3):211–5.
171. Clements KM, Clark RE, Lavitas P, et al. Access to new medications for hepatitis C for Medicaid members: A retrospective cohort study. *J Manag Care Spec Pharm*. 2016;22(6):714–22b.
172. Gowda C, Lott S, Grigorian M, et al. Absolute insurer denial of direct-acting antiviral therapy for hepatitis C: A national specialty pharmacy cohort study. *Open Forum Infect Dis*. 2018 June 1;5(6):ofy076.
173. Martinello M, Dore GJ, Matthews GV, Grebely J. Strategies to reduce hepatitis C virus reinfection in people who inject drugs. *Infect Dis Clin North Am*. 2018;32(2):371–93.
174. Martinello M, Hajarizadeh B, Grebely J, Dore GJ, Matthews GV. HCV cure and reinfection among people with HIV/HCV coinfection and people who inject drugs. *Curr HIV/AIDS Rep*. 2017;14(3):110–21.
175. Backus LI, Belperio PS, Shahoumian TA, Mole LA. Impact of sustained virologic response with direct-acting antiviral treatment on mortality in patients with advanced liver disease. *Hepatology*. 2019;69(2):487–97. doi: 10.1002/hep.29408.
176. Backus LI, Belperio PS, Shahoumian TA, Mole LA. Direct-acting antiviral sustained virologic response: Impact on mortality in patients without advanced liver disease. *Hepatology*. 2018;68(3):827–38. doi: 10.1002/hep.29811.
177. Bersoff-Matcha SJ, Cao K, Jason M, et al. Hepatitis B virus reactivation associated with direct-acting antiviral therapy for chronic hepatitis C virus: A review of cases reported to the U.S. Food and Drug Administration Adverse Event Reporting System. *Ann Intern Med*. 2017;166(11):792–8.
178. Mücke MM, Backus LI, Mücke VT, et al. Hepatitis B virus reactivation during direct-acting antiviral therapy for hepatitis C: A systematic review and meta-analysis. *Lancet Gastroenterol Hepatol*. 2018;3(3):172–80.
179. Kumar A, Saraswat VA. Hepatitis E and acute-on-chronic liver failure. *J Clin Exp Hepatol*. 2013;3(3):225–30.
180. Arora S, Thornton K, Murata G, et al. Outcomes of treatment for hepatitis C virus infection by primary care providers. *N Engl J Med*. 2011;364(23):2199–207.
181. Kattakuzhy S, Gross C, Emmanuel B, et al. Expansion of treatment for hepatitis C Virus infection by task shifting to community-based non-specialist providers: A nonrandomized clinical trial. *Ann Intern Med*. 2017;167(5):311–8.
182. Aach RD, Stevens CE, Hollinger FB, et al. Hepatitis C virus infection in post-transfusion hepatitis. An analysis with first- and second-generation assays. *N Engl J Med*. 1991;325(19):1325–9.
183. Alter HJ. New kit on the block: Evaluation of second-generation assays for detection of antibody to the hepatitis C virus. *Hepatology*. 1992;15(2):350–3.
184. Barocas JA, Linas BP, Kim AY, Fangman J, Westergaard RP. Acceptability of rapid point-of-care hepatitis C tests among people who inject drugs and utilize syringe-exchange programs. *Open Forum Infect Dis*. 2016 Apr 6;3(2):ofw075.
185. Lamoury FMJ, Bajis S, Hajarizadeh B, et al. Evaluation of the Xpert HCV viral load finger-stick point-of-care assay. *J Infect Dis*. 2018;217(12):1889–96.
186. Freiman JM, Tran TM, Schumacher SG, et al. Hepatitis C core antigen testing for diagnosis of hepatitis C virus infection: A systematic review and meta-analysis. *Ann Intern Med*. 2016;165(5):345–55.
187. Centers for Disease Control and Prevention (CDC). Testing for HCV infection: An update of guidance for clinicians and laboratorians. *MMWR Morb Mortal Wkly Rep*. 2013;62(18):362–5.
188. Smith BD, Morgan RL, Beckett GA, et al. Recommendations for the identification of chronic hepatitis C virus infection among persons born during 1945–1965. *MMWR Recomm Rep*. 2012;61(RR-4):1–32.

189. Moyer VA. U.S. Preventive Services Task Force: Screening for hepatitis C virus infection in adults: U.S. Preventive Services Task Force recommendation statement. *Ann Intern Med*. 2013;159(5):349–57.

190. Barocas JA, Wang J, White LF, et al. Hepatitis C testing increased among baby boomers following the 2012 change to CDC testing recommendations. *Health Aff (Millwood)*. 2017;36(12):2142–50.

191. Younossi Z, Blissett D, Blissett R, et al. In an era of highly effective treatment, hepatitis C screening of the United States general population should be considered. *Liver Int*. 2018 Feb;38(2):258–65.

192. Barocas JA, Tasillo A, Eftekhari Yazdi G, et al. Population level outcomes and cost-effectiveness of expanding the recommendation for age-based hepatitis C testing in the United States. *Clin Infect Dis*. 2018 Feb 6;67(4):549–56. doi: 10.1093/cid/ciy098.

193. Varan AK, Mercer DW, Stein MS, Spaulding AC. Hepatitis C seroprevalence among prison inmates since 2001: Still high but declining. *Public Health Rep*. 2014;129(2):187–95.

194. Kim AY, Nagami EH, Birch CE, Bowen MJ, Lauer GM, McGovern BH. A simple strategy to identify acute hepatitis C virus infection among newly incarcerated injection drug users. *Hepatology*. 2013;57(3):944–52.

195. He T, Li K, Roberts MS, et al. Prevention of hepatitis C by screening and treatment in U.S. prisons. *Ann Intern Med*. 2016;164(2):84–92.

196. Gilchrist G, Swan D, Widyaratna K, et al. A systematic review and meta-analysis of psychosocial interventions to reduce drug and sexual blood borne virus risk behaviours among people who inject drugs. *AIDS Behav*. 2017;21(7):1791–811.

197. Hagan H, Pouget ER, Des Jarlais DC. A systematic review and meta-analysis of interventions to prevent hepatitis C virus infection in people who inject drugs. *J Infect Dis*. 2011;204(1):74–83.

198. Platt L, Minozzi S, Reed J, et al. Needle and syringe programmes and opioid substitution therapy for preventing HCV transmission among people who inject drugs: Findings from a Cochrane Review and meta-analysis. *Addiction*. 2018;113(3):545–63.

199. World Health Organization. Draft global health sector strategy on viral hepatitis, 2016–2021—The first of it's kind. 2015.

200. Martin NK, Vickerman P, Foster GR, Hutchinson SJ, Goldberg DJ, Hickman M. Can antiviral therapy for hepatitis C reduce the prevalence of HCV among injecting drug user populations? A modeling analysis of its prevention utility. *J Hepatol*. 2011;54(6):1137–44.

201. Martin NK, Hickman M, Hutchinson SJ, Goldberg DJ, Vickerman P. Combination interventions to prevent HCV transmission among people who inject drugs: modeling the impact of antiviral treatment, needle and syringe programs, and opiate substitution therapy. *Clin Infect Dis*. 2013;57 Suppl 2:S39–45.

202. Echevarria D, Gutfraind A, Boodram B, et al. Mathematical modeling of hepatitis C prevalence reduction with antiviral treatment scale-up in persons who inject drugs in metropolitan Chicago. *PLoS One*. 2015 Aug 21;10(8):e0135901.

203. Boerekamps A, Newsum AM, Smit C, et al. High treatment uptake in human immunodeficiency virus/hepatitis C virus-coinfected patients after unrestricted access to direct-acting antivirals in the Netherlands. *Clin Infect Dis*. 2018;66(9):1352–9.

204. Boerekamps A, van den Berk GE, Lauw FN, et al. Declining hepatitis C virus (HCV) incidence in Dutch human immunodeficiency virus-positive men who have sex with men after unrestricted access to HCV therapy. *Clin Infect Dis*. 2018 Apr 17;66(9):1360–5.

205. Durham DP, Skrip LA, Bruce RD, et al. The impact of enhanced screening and treatment on hepatitis C in the United States. *Clin Infect Dis*. 2016;62(3):298–304.

206. Scott N, Iser DM, Thompson AJ, Doyle JS, Hellard ME. Cost-effectiveness of treating chronic hepatitis C virus with direct-acting antivirals in people who inject drugs in Australia. *J Gastroenterol Hepatol*. 2016;31(4):872–82.

207. Cousien A, Tran VC, Deuffic-Burban S, et al. Effectiveness and cost-effectiveness of interventions targeting harm reduction and chronic hepatitis C cascade of care in people who inject drugs: The case of France. *J Viral Hepat*. 2018 Apr 16;25(10):1197–207. doi: 10.1111/jvh.12919.

208. Mabileau G, Scutelniciuc O, Tsereteli M, et al. Intervention packages to reduce the impact of HIV and HCV infections among people who inject drugs in Eastern Europe and Central Asia: A modeling and cost-effectiveness study. *Open Forum Infect Dis*. 2018 Feb 17;5(3):ofy040.

209. Scott N, Ólafsson S, Gottfreðsson M, et al. Modelling the elimination of hepatitis C as a public health threat in Iceland: A goal attainable by 2020. *J Hepatol*. 2018;68(5):932–9.

210. Fraser H, Zibbell J, Hoerger T, et al. Scaling-up HCV prevention and treatment interventions in rural United States—Model projections for tackling an increasing epidemic. *Addiction*. 2018;113(1):173–82.

211. Falade-Nwulia O, Sulkowski MS, Merkow A, Latkin C, Mehta SH. Understanding and addressing hepatitis C reinfection in the oral direct-acting antiviral era. *J Viral Hepat*. 2018;25(3):220–7.

212. Islam N, Krajden M, Shoveller J, et al. Incidence, risk factors, and prevention of hepatitis C reinfection: A population-based cohort study. *Lancet Gastroenterol Hepatol*. 2017;2(3):200–10.

213. Ingiliz P, Martin TC, Rodger A, et al. HCV reinfection incidence and spontaneous clearance rates in HIV-positive men who have sex with men in Western Europe. *J Hepatol*. 2017;66(2):282–7.

214. Choo QL, Richman KH, Han JH, et al. Genetic organization and diversity of the hepatitis C virus. *Proc Natl Acad Sci U S A*. 1991;88:2451–5.

215. Page K, Hahn JA, Evans J, et al. Acute hepatitis C virus infection in young adult injection drug users: A prospective study of incident infection, resolution, and reinfection. *J Infect Dis*. 2009;200(8):1216–26.

216. Osburn WO, Fisher BE, Dowd KA, et al. Spontaneous control of primary hepatitis C virus infection and immunity against persistent reinfection. *Gastroenterology*. 2010;138:315–24.

217. Ghasemi F, Rostami S, Meshkat Z. Progress in the development of vaccines for hepatitis C virus infection. *World J Gastroenterol*. 2015;21(42):11984–2002.

218. Chung RT, Gordon FD, Curry MP, et al. Human monoclonal antibody MBL-HCV1 delays HCV viral rebound following liver transplantation: A randomized controlled study. *Am J Transplant*. 2013;13(4):1047–54.

219. Tabll A, Abbas AT, El-Kafrawy S, Wahid A. Monoclonal antibodies: Principles and applications of immmunodiagnosis and immunotherapy for hepatitis C virus. *World J Hepatol*. 2015;7(22):2369–83.

CHAPTER

159

Introduction to Infectious Disease Modeling

Andrew F. Brouwer • Rafael Meza • Jon Zelner • Marisa C. Eisenberg

OVERVIEW

Infectious disease models are tools that are increasingly used to inform public health and preventive medicine research, policy, and practice. Although implementing infectious disease models requires a certain level of theoretical background and computational experience, the basic principles are easy to grasp. This chapter is a first introduction to infectious disease models and is intended to demystify models and the modeling process. In this chapter, we first highlight some uses and limitations of infectious disease models. Next, we discuss some of the main concepts underlying infectious disease modeling. Then, we introduce the foundational infectious disease model, the SIR model (or susceptible, infectious, recovered model) and its compartmental model extensions. We next discuss network and agent-based models, which are used to explore the importance of individual-level characteristics (such as superspreading). Finally, we briefly discuss the connection between data and models. After reading this chapter, you will understand the basics of infectious disease modeling, allowing you to engage with and interrogate the assumptions and conclusions of infectious disease modeling research.

INTRODUCTION

Why Use Mathematical Models?

Patterns of health and disease arise from complex interactions of biological, social, and environmental factors. Disentangling these factors to understand the underlying causal processes is difficult, particularly as these factors often involve feedback loops playing out over time (and space). For instance, when a new respiratory pathogen is introduced in a population, it will first propagate freely without interference, but once discovered, interventions, such as social distancing and decontamination of surfaces, and changes in human behavior will affect how the pathogen continues to propagate, perhaps slowing transmission. This in turn might affect how the risk of infection is perceived, eventually leading to a return to *business as usual*, which might again facilitate the propagation of the pathogen. To make sense of these complex systems, we use models—simplifications of the real world that help us make sense of what we see. Models take many forms, from cartoon diagrams and verbal descriptions of a process ("if this, then that..."), to complex simulation models. We reason about the rules and processes that underlie health all the time—whether it's reasoning about a possible diagnosis or the likely transmission modes in an outbreak, we rely on mental models of the system in question. Mathematics and statistics provide a way to formalize this kind of reasoning and to interrogate the processes and mechanisms that drive disease spread, thereby helping to improve public health responses. For instance, models were used to help quantify the potential impact of social distancing measures in slowing the rate of transmission of pH1N1 during the 2009 pandemic (see shaded box in section "The Basic Reproduction Number").

BOX159-1 Mathematical Modeling of the 2013–2016 Ebola Epidemic in West Africa

The 2013–2016 West African outbreak was the largest Ebola virus disease (EVD) epidemic to date, resulting in over 28,000 cases and 11,000 deaths. Mathematical modeling was used to assist in predicting the course of the epidemic and determining which interventions would be most effective,[2] and "helped to inspire and inform" the strong international response to the epidemic.[7] However, different models generated widely varying predictions for incidence and mortality, particularly early in the epidemic,[2,7,8] with several prominent models seeming to overpredict the number of cases and deaths, drawing criticism.[9] This underscores the importance of understanding the uncertainty and limitations involved in mathematical models, particularly when the data are limited. This epidemic also highlights the importance of model comparison efforts—in spite of the range of predictions of numbers of cases and deaths, most models agreed on which intervention approaches would be effective in reducing the spread of disease,[8] illustrating how, even in the presence of uncertainty, models can (when carefully deployed) be used to help inform response efforts.

Mathematical models and statistical models are not truly distinct classes (as many models are both mathematical and statistical), but there are some broad general distinctions between the two. Statistical models are typically used to examine associations and account for observed variation—and when possible, to infer causality. However, most statistical models don't account for the underlying mechanisms at work—they might describe an association or even a causal relationship between two variables but typically not the process underlying that association. Mathematical modeling, on the other hand, typically focuses more on mechanisms, dynamics, and understanding the "how" as well as the "what." Because of their mechanistic focus, mathematical models are particularly useful for:

- **Understanding how the system works.** We often want to use models to infer or understand mechanistic processes underlying transmission and how they might affect health outcomes. For example, we might use associational studies to show that a vaccine is protective, but if we want to understand the relative contributions of direct protection and herd protection, we might instead use a mathematical model that accounts for the transmission process and models transmission from one person to the next.
- **Examining counterfactuals, making predictions, and selecting interventions.** Because mathematical models include mechanisms, we can alter or adjust those mechanistic processes and see how things play out. This allows us to test out alternative intervention

strategies and make predictions under new conditions, examining questions such as, "What would have happened if we had not intervened?," "What might happen if we change our intervention strategy?," or (e.g.) "What might happen to patterns of malaria incidence if climate change affects mosquito populations?."

- **Exploring the unexpected.** Mathematical models can also be used to examine how the complex interactions between different factors can lead to the emergence of unexpected patterns and behaviors. Because the processes underlying health and public health are so complex, it is difficult to know what might happen when a given change or intervention takes place. For example, ecological interventions (such as gene editing of mosquitoes) can have far reaching consequences on the ecological networks that include both human and animal hosts,[1] leading to many efforts to understand the joint "one health" of human and animal populations (see Chapter 84, One Health: A New Paradigm for Disease Prevention and Control). Similarly, even fairly standard interventions can interact with human behavior and culture in unexpected ways, sometimes leading to unintended (and potentially serious) consequences (e.g., vaccine hesitancy or noncompliance with interventions).[2–6] Unexpected patterns can emerge from these complex systems, and models can be used to help explore the range of behaviors one might expect to see.

As computational power and data collection have increased, models have become increasingly useful, and are now part of the suite of tools used by the Centers for Disease Control and Prevention (CDC), the World Health Organizations (WHO), and other major public health agencies for planning in response to infectious diseases.[10–14] They are used in practice at levels ranging from local or state health departments, to international outbreak response.[14–17]

In the subsequent sections, we will discuss the basic concepts, methods, and approaches for mathematical models. Keep an eye out for the shaded boxes—these will include specific examples of models being used in practice, as well as key ideas and questions to help the reader think through the modeling process.

Limitations of Mathematical Models

Mathematical models are highly useful, but they come with perils and potential pitfalls too. It is often easy to "bake in" particular answers to a question—and, more dangerously, not always easy to see when this is the case. Mathematical models can be adapted in nearly limitless ways, which makes it all the more critical to be careful to balance mechanistic detail with enough simplicity that we can still understand what is going on. Mathematical models are often highly uncertain, in their parameters, predictions, and even their structure, and understanding and quantifying these uncertainties is critical to using them responsibly.

As an example to illustrate these issues, let us consider modeling a new outbreak of disease, using the data shown in Fig. 159-1. Many outbreaks follow a predictable pattern: initial fluctuations when the disease is first introduced, followed by an exponential growth phase, and then a peak and a downturn. We often want to predict the eventual size and timing of an outbreak (e.g., timing of the peak) when it is still in the growth phase, but even seemingly minor differences in model assumptions can result in different predictions for the peak and downturn. For example, a model might predict that nearly the entire susceptible population must be infected before the epidemic will extinguish, while other models might hypothesize that the epidemic will lose steam without infecting all susceptible individuals, petering out with only a fraction of the total population infected. These different models can give very different predictions of the epidemic turnover, that will nonetheless both match equally well to the initial epidemic growth. Without collecting more data (e.g., data on contact networks, the response to interventions, or continued tracking of the incidence) and without knowledge of critical aspects such

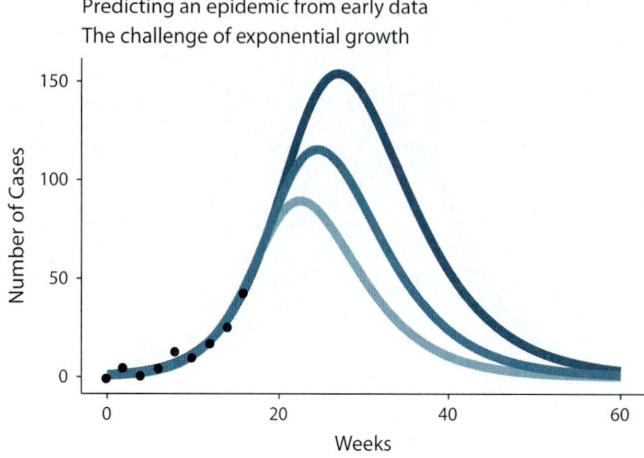

FIGURE 159-1. Example of incidence data (black circles) fit with three different models (lines). The three models agree during the initial exponential growth portion (black line), but then diverge to generate different predictions. Because all three fit the initial data equally well, we cannot know which model is making the correct prediction without additional data (either on the epidemic time course or on the different mechanisms and parameters underlying the models).

as the rate of asymptomatic transmission, the mutation rate of the pathogen, or the level of individual immunity post infection, as is usual the case during an emergent disease epidemic, we can't know which model (if any) is the best match.

OVERARCHING CONCEPTS IN MATHEMATICAL MODELING

Getting Started: Identifying Processes and Assumptions

Mathematical modeling is the process—part algorithm, part art—of abstracting and translating our assumptions about the underlying mechanisms of real-world process into mathematical language. For infectious disease modeling, the two fundamental processes are transmission and recovery. Transmission is the process of a susceptible person contracting a disease from an infectious person. Although this process seems simple, a great deal of complexity can arise from the fact that two people need to come into contact (directly or indirectly) for transmission to occur. In models of infectious disease transmission dynamics, we need to specify how fast and how effective the transmission process is, which is usually done through a transmission parameter, denoted β. Recovery, where an individual stops being infectious, is a comparatively simpler process because it involves only a single individual. The recovery rate is usually written γ. Much of infectious disease modeling involves deciding what additional processes and assumptions should be considered in order to describe a given disease and population with reasonable accuracy. In the following sections, we describe some common assumptions that are made, additional process that might be considered, and how they translate into mathematical models.

Mathematical Models Describe Dynamical Systems

In infectious disease models, we are usually interested in how the number of people infected changes over time. We develop models to describe the longitudinal dynamics of the disease as it spreads through a population. The mathematical study of how quantities change over time is called dynamical systems.

When modeling dynamical systems, there are several different choices that may need to be made about how we implement our models. A key choice is whether to use a *stochastic* or *deterministic* implementation of the model. Stochastic processes are used when we want to highlight the importance of randomness in the system, such as when the at-risk population is small or when some processes are rare. In *deterministic* models, the simulation outputs are completely

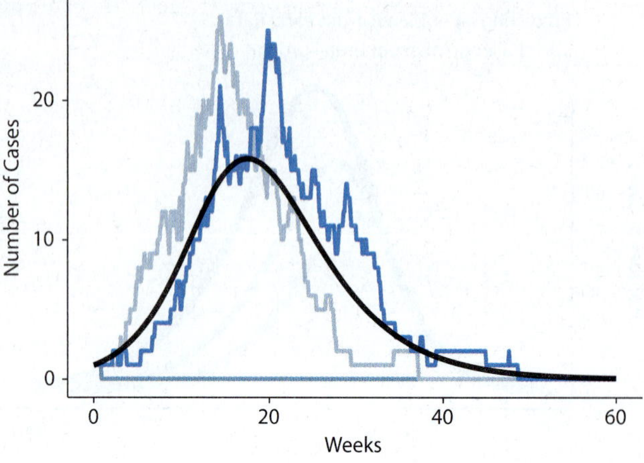

FIGURE 159-2. Two ways to simulate an epidemic using an infectious disease model: the thick black line shows a deterministic (nonrandom) simulation of total current cases using an infectious disease model, while the three blue lines show different stochastic (random) simulations of the same model. The stochastic simulations vary randomly from one simulation to the next, showing fluctuations and also the potential for the epidemic to randomly extinguish early on (note the blue-gray line at the bottom of the graph).

determined by the model configuration and parameters, whereas *stochastic* models give different answers every time that you run a new simulation (even if the parameters are the same). These stochastic differences occur because the modeled randomness of the constituent processes (transmission, recovery, etc.) causes events to occur in different orders. But, stochastic does not mean arbitrary—stochastic processes still have to have the same average behavior, for example. The difference between a stochastic and deterministic implementation of the same model is illustrated in Fig. 159-2.

Deterministic and stochastic implementations have their own strengths and weaknesses and should be chosen based on the situation. Models of larger populations where we care about average behavior are suited to deterministic implementations (which are often simpler to code and more efficient to run), whereas smaller populations with rare events are better suited to stochastic implementations.

One popular deterministic implementation of dynamical systems models is with ordinary differential equations (ODEs), which depend on the concept of the derivative from calculus. In brief, a derivative describes how fast a quantity is changing at a certain point in time. By writing mathematical equations for these derivatives, we can describe how a number of different quantities that all depend on one another change over time. In the next sections, we'll explore several different ODE models of infectious disease dynamics.

Many models (whether deterministic or stochastic) must also choose a time scale for which they'll update the variables in their model—do you want to update the number of disease cases in your model hourly, daily, or weekly? The choice will depend on the situation and type of disease that you are modeling (e.g., respiratory vs. sexually transmitted versus vectorborne) and perhaps on the type of data available. This time scale determines what we call the model time-step Δt. Choosing a model time-step means that the model is *discrete* in time—we only see the output on the time steps and never in between. By contrast, *continuous* time models allow events to occur at any point in time rather than on specified time steps. Similarly, many modeling frameworks require a choice of either discrete or continuous values for the modeled quantities we're examining (each of which may make more sense for different variables, for example, numbers of infectious individuals vs. fraction of the population that is infectious).

It can sometimes be useful to convert between deterministic and stochastic implementations of a model. ODE models usually work with constant event rates, such as the recovery rate γ, introduced above. An important property of models using constant event rates is that the average time between events that happen at rate α is exactly $1/\alpha$—in other words, if the average duration of infectiousness (time to recovery) is 5 days, then the rate for recovery is $\alpha = 1/(5 \text{ days}) = 0.2/\text{day}$. This is helpful as it is usually relatively easy to obtain data on the duration of symptoms or infection of patients, which can then be analyzed to estimate average duration times and thus recovery rates, which can then in turn be incorporated into transmission models.

BOX 159-2. A Brief History of Mathematical Models of Infectious Disease

The first infectious disease model dates back to the 1760s! At the time, smallpox (Variola) was a devastating disease. The act of variolation—inoculation with material taken from a sick person in the hope that a mild, protective form of the disease would result, a kind of precursor to vaccination—was highly controversial. Bernoulli developed a mathematical model in support of the practice,[18] which is widely credited as the first epidemiological model of infectious disease.[19,20] Epidemic models as we know them today were introduced in the 1920s by Kermack and McKendrick (deterministic)[21] and Reed and Frost (stochastic).[22] The use of mathematical models in epidemiology was popularized in the 1980s by Anderson and May.[23] Advances in theory and computation continue to increase the usefulness and applicability of models today.

Discrete time stochastic models need to convert these rates into probabilities based on the time step chosen for the model. There is a convenient formula to convert a constant rate α of an event into a probability (p_α) that that event takes place over the time step:

$$p_\alpha(\Delta t) = 1 - \exp(-\alpha \Delta t). \tag{1}$$

To put this all together, let's look at an example. Suppose that for a particular disease, individuals recover after 10 days of being infectious. Then in an ODE model we could set the exponential rate for recovery to be $\gamma = 1/(10 \text{ days}) = 0.1/\text{day}$. In a discrete time stochastic model, plugging this in to Eq. (1) would mean that the probability of an individual recovering in the next day ($\Delta t = 1$) is about 10%, while the probability of recovering in the next week ($\Delta t = 7$) is 50%. For other processes such as transmission, the rate that people move from susceptible to infectious may not be a constant (like the γ we used for recovery above), but instead will change over time as the number of infectious individuals in the population changes.

In the next sections, we describe three distinct kinds of models that are most commonly used in infectious disease modeling: compartmental models, network models, and individual/agent-based models. Any of these model types can be built using either deterministic or stochastic frameworks, although individual and agent-based models are almost always stochastic.

COMPARTMENTAL MODELS

Introduction to the Susceptible-Infectious-Recovered (SIR) Model

Fundamentally, compartmental models describe partitions of populations into distinct groups based on their disease status (and possibly other characteristics). Because disease status can change, our goal as modelers is to track how people move between these groups of people over time and the resulting changing total numbers of people in each group. The seminal compartmental infectious disease model, from which most other compartmental disease models are derived, is the SIR model, named for its partition of the population into three groups: individuals who are susceptible to infection (S), infectious individuals (I), and recovered individuals (R).[21] In the SIR model, susceptible people can become infectious when a currently infectious person transmits the disease to them, and an infectious person will recover after a period of time. Then, the basic accounting of the infectious disease model is the following:

$$\begin{aligned}
\text{Change in number of susceptibles} &= -\,\text{number of new infections},\\
\text{Change in number of infectious} &= +\,\text{number of new infections}\\
&\quad -\,\text{number of recoveries},\\
\text{Change in number of recovered} &= +\,\text{number of recoveries}. \qquad (2)
\end{aligned}$$

To turn this into a model, we need to figure out how to represent the number of new infections and the number of recoveries. The canonical form of the SIR model turns the equations above into rates of change per unit time like this:

$$\begin{aligned}
\frac{dS}{dt} &= \underbrace{-\beta\cdot\frac{1}{N}\cdot S}_{\text{new infections}},\\
\frac{dI}{dt} &= \underbrace{-\beta\cdot\frac{1}{N}\cdot S}_{\text{new infections}} - \underbrace{\gamma\cdot I}_{\text{recoveries}}\\
\frac{dR}{dt} &= \underbrace{\gamma\cdot I}_{\text{recoveries}}. \qquad (3)
\end{aligned}$$

These equations capture the same flows that we outlined above—the $\beta\frac{1}{N}S$ term represents the movement of susceptible individuals becoming infectious (people/time moving from S to I) and the γI term represents the recovery of infectious individuals (people/per time moving from I to R). Also note that we've written the variables simply as S, I, and R here for simplicity, but each of these does change with time—sometimes we will write the variables as $S(t)$, $I(t)$, and $R(t)$ to more explicitly indicate this. In the next section, we'll explore why we choose these specific terms to represent each process—in brief, the transmission term for new infections depends on both S and I because we need susceptible and infectious individuals to interact for this process to occur, while the term for recovery depends only on I because each infectious individual recovers independently of the number of people in the other compartments.

In general, when designing an infectious disease model, one of the first steps is to illustrate the movement between compartments with a model diagram. The black arrows in Fig. 159-3a represent this movement of people between compartments, with the labels indicating the rates at which individuals move from one compartment to another. For example, the label $\beta\frac{1}{N}$ indicates the rate that susceptible individuals become infected—in other words, the total people per unit time moving from S to I is given by $\left(\beta\frac{1}{N}\right)\cdot S$ By assigning values to the parameters for movement between the compartments, we can simulate the model and observe in Fig. 159-3b how the number of people in each compartment change over time.

The epidemic curves generated by the SIR model have a canonical shape: although the specific numbers change depending on context (e.g., recovery rates vary by disease, population sizes differ, etc.), the qualitative shapes generated by this model stay the same. Notice that the dynamic pattern of infectious individuals in Fig. 159-3b captures the classic shape of an epidemic—early exponential growth followed by a peak and then decline. We'll explore how variations of the basic SIR model can capture other common disease dynamics in section "Extending the SIR Model: Relaxing Assumptions and Modeling Other Processes" below.

Digging into the Details

Compartmental models explain how the numbers of individuals in each of the compartments change over time. Let's see what that looks like for the SIR model—in this section, we'll dig into the details on how to move from the idea behind the SIR model expressed in Eq. (2) to the ordinary differential equation model given in Eq. (3).

First, two important assumptions of compartmental models in general are that everyone in a compartment is essentially identical and that they interact with others entirely at random. These assumptions are sometimes called the homogeneity and well-mixedness assumptions, in a nod to earlier models of chemical reactions, where all molecules in a compartment are thought of as identical and completely well mixed (i.e., evenly and randomly distributed such that we can assume the bump into one another at random). The homogeneity and well-mixedness assumptions can be easily violated by real populations for many diseases, so further partitioning of the population may be needed to more accurately explain the disease processes, as we'll discuss in more detail in a later section (section "Extending the SIR Model: Relaxing Assumptions and Modeling Other Processes").

With those assumptions out of the way, let's examine the SIR model in more detail. First, let us consider the transmission process and count the number of people who become infected in some time interval Δt. Think of a single susceptible person contacting other people at rate κ. Their probability of contacting another person (infectious or not) in time Δt is $p_{\kappa}(\Delta t)$ [see Eq. (1)]. Assuming that everyone is contacting everyone else at the same rate, the probability that each of this person's contact is infectious (as opposed to susceptible or recovered) is exactly the fraction of the population that is infectious at time t, or $I(t)/N$, where N is the total size of the initially at-risk population. But, not every contact with an infectious person results

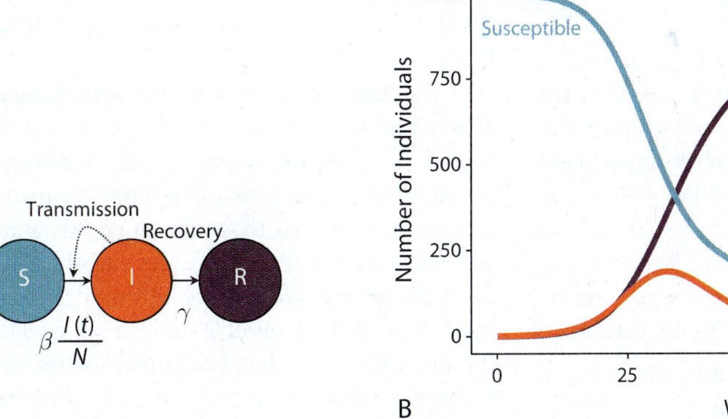

FIGURE 159-3. (A) Compartmental model diagram for the SIR (susceptible, infectious, recovered) model, with transmission rate $\beta I(t)/N$ and recovery rate γ. (B) The epidemic curves trace out the number of people in each of the S, I, and R compartments over time.

in disease transmission; we'll say that transmission occurs with probability π. Thus, the probability that out susceptible person becomes infected in time Δt is $\pi \cdot p_k(\Delta t) \cdot \frac{I(t)}{N(t)}$. Because of the homogeneity assumption, this individual is representative of every susceptible person. So, we can get the expected number of people that become infected in this time interval by multiplying the probability of contacting someone, the probability that that contact is infectious, the probability that the infectious contact results in transmission, and the number of susceptible people, $\pi \cdot p_k(\Delta t) \cdot \frac{I(t)}{N} \cdot S(t)$.

Next, let's think about how many people recover over the Δt time interval. If an individual recovers at a constant rate γ, then the probability that any given infectious person recovers is $p_\gamma(\Delta t)$. So, the expected number of people who recover will be the probability of recovering times that number of people who could recover, $p_\gamma(\Delta t)\ldots I(t)$.

Putting this all together, we can track the changes in the number of people in each of the susceptible, infectious, and recovered compartments at time t over the next Δt time:

Change in number of susceptibles

$$\text{Change in number of susceptibles} = -\pi \cdot p_k(\Delta t) \cdot \frac{I(t)}{N} \cdot S(t)$$
$$= \pi \cdot p_k(\Delta t) \cdot \frac{I(t)}{N} \cdot S(t) - p_\gamma(\Delta t) \cdot I(t), \quad (4)$$

Change in number of infectious,

Change in number of recovered $= p_\gamma(\Delta t)\ldots I(t)$.

##We have to be careful though! If the numbers of people in these compartments change drastically over the Δt time interval, you'll introduce error into your predictions. Thus, it is very important to pick the right step size if you're using a discrete-time model. One way to avoid this error is to convert these heuristic equations into the ordinary differential equations that we discussed above. To do this, we take the limit as the time interval Δt gets smaller and smaller. We won't do those calculations here, but they are straightforward if you'd like to refresh your calculus concepts of limits and derivatives.[24]

The corresponding system of ordinary differential equation for the SIR model [the same as those in Eq. (3)] tell us how the derivatives of the numbers of people in each compartment (i.e., dS/dt, dI/dt, and dR/dt) change as a function of the number of people in each of the compartments. Here, we typically combine the contact rate κ and infection probability π into a single transmission rate $\beta = \pi\ldots\kappa$.

$$\frac{dS}{dt} = -\beta \cdot \frac{1}{N} \cdot S,$$
$$\frac{dI}{dt} = \beta \cdot \frac{1}{N} \cdot S - \gamma \cdot I,$$
$$\frac{dR}{dt} = \gamma \cdot I. \quad (5)$$

Notice that the right side of these equations are very similar to the discrete time equations above, but the $p{\cdot}\Delta t$ terms are replaced by the corresponding rates. When simulating these differential equations, we also have to specify how many people are in each compartment at the start of the simulation, called the initial conditions $S(0)$, $I(0)$, and $R(0)$.

The solutions to these equations tell us how S, I, and R change over time. These longitudinal trajectories have well-known shapes, and are often referred to as called *epidemic curves* (Fig. 159-3b). Because S is initially large typically, the rate of people being infected $\beta \frac{1}{N} S$ is higher than the rate of people recovering γI. Thus, we see positive, exponential growth in number of infectious people the early phase of the epidemic. Eventually, though, so many people have been infected that infectious people are contacting infectious or recovered people more and susceptible people less. At this time, the epidemic stops growing and the recovery term begins to take over. This phenomenon is called epidemic turnover, and we refer to the decreasing number of susceptible people leading up to epidemic turnover as susceptible burnout. Note that not every susceptible necessarily becomes infected, just enough that the group of infectious people are no longer replenishing themselves by transmitting new infections. Indeed, notice that the number or fraction of recovered people at the end of the epidemic—sometimes called the cumulative incidence $Z = R(\infty)$ or the attack ratio—is actually less than the total population (Fig. 159-3b), meaning that not everyone was eventually infected before the epidemic died out.

BOX 159-3. When Do Outbreaks Spontaneously Die Out?

Sometimes, outbreaks die out even when we expect them to spread. If there are only a small number of infected people at the start of an outbreak, there is a chance that each of them could recover before infecting anyone else. If we want to account for this possibility, which we usually need to do for small population sizes, we have to use a stochastic model. This phenomenon is a function of random chance and cannot occur in a deterministic model. Once an epidemic ensues, or if there is certainty that an epidemic will occur, deterministic models are a reasonable option to model the dynamics of disease transmission.

Compartmental Model Diagrams

One way that modelers quickly convey information about the assumptions and implications of compartmental models is with a model diagram like the one in Fig. 159-3a. It is important to be able to glean important aspects of a model from its diagram, and to know how to create a diagram that clearly communicates the essential aspects of your own model. An effective diagram succinctly summarizes all model processes through interconnected circles and arrows. Every circle represents a single compartment. In the SIR model (Fig. 159-3a), we have three circles for the S, I, and R compartments. A model diagram also has arrows that represent the flow of individuals between compartments. In the SIR model, we have two processes: transmission, which moves people from the susceptible to the infectious compartments, and recovery, which moves people from the infectious to the recovered compartment.

It is also important to indicate nonlinearities in the model, that is, when the flow from a given compartment also depends on another compartment. In the SIR model, the flow out of the susceptible compartment S is affected by the infectious compartment I [since we have an I in the $\beta(I/N)S$ term]. We might visualize this with an arrow from the I compartment to the flow that it affects. It is a good idea to visually differentiate these kinds of arrows, such as with solid and dotted lines.

These kinds of arrows are not always used, though, as they can clutter the diagram (as we will see in section "Extending the SIR Model: Relaxing Assumptions and Modeling Other Processes"), so it's important to also look at a model's equations. In particular, you don't need to include these lines if you are annotating your flow lines with their rates. For example, the rate of leaving the susceptible class for the infectious class in the SIR model is $\beta I(t)/N$ because it is the coefficient on the S variable in the dS/dt equation [Eq. (3)]. Similarly, the rate of leaving the infectious class for the recovered class is γ because γ is the coefficient on I in the dI/dt equation.

Ideally, the model diagram should contain all of the information you would need to write down the model equations. This is not always possible in practice, particularly for complex models. In these cases, the model diagram can be thought of as an illustrative accompaniment to both text description of the model and the model equations. We will see more examples of model diagrams later in the compartmental model section when we discuss expanding beyond the SIR model and modifying the basic assumptions (section "Extending the SIR Model: Relaxing Assumptions and Modeling Other Processes").

The Basic Reproduction Number

The basic reproduction number, or R_0, is a fundamental concept in mathematical infectious disease epidemiology.[25,26] It is defined as the expected number of people a single infectious person in an otherwise susceptible population is expected to infect over their infectious lifetime.

Let's break this definition down a bit. First, note that the definition describes what happens to a single infectious person in an otherwise susceptible population. Hence, the basic reproduction number describes what happens at the very beginning of an outbreak (although we shall see that it affects all aspects of the outbreak). Second, it describes the expected number of new infectious people. That means that it describes what happens in an average scenario; of course, any given person may infect more or fewer people. Third, R_0 describes what happens over a person's infectious lifetime. Because people's infectious lifetimes may differ, the concept of average is important again here.

R_0 is particularly important to understanding the early dynamics of an outbreak. We can see why as follows: if on average, an individual generates more than 1 new case over their lifetime, this means that they are making enough new cases to more than replace themselves after their infectious period is complete—in other words, this means the outbreak will tend to grow into a larger epidemic. By contrast if, on average, each person generates less than one case over their infectious lifetime, this means that most people who are infected are unlikely to generate a new case, and so the outbreak will tend to die out. Thus, the threshold of $R_0 = 1$ is an important one—if $R_0 > 1$ the outbreak will tend to grow in the early phase, while if $R_0 < 1$ the outbreak will tend to die out before really taking off.

It is relatively straightforward to determine the value of R_0 for a given model from the model's parameters. We refer the reader to references on the Next Generation Method[27,28] if the need to calculate an R_0 arises. But as an example, let's examine the basic reproduction number of the classic SIR model [Eq. (3)], given by β/γ. Let's see why this makes sense. Near the beginning of an outbreak, $I \approx 1$ and $S \approx N$, so the rate that patient zero is infecting people is $\beta \frac{}{N} I S \approx \beta$, and the rate of people recovering is $\gamma I \approx \gamma$. Because γ is a constant rate, as we said above, the average duration of being infectious is $1/\gamma$. If patient zero is infecting an average of β people per day for $1/\gamma$ days, then they'd expect to infect β/γ people over their infectious lifetime. It's important to note that the basic reproduction number will depend on both the disease and the population involved. R_0 can range from as little to just above 1 (for some respiratory viruses) to up to 20 (for measles).[29]

While the basic reproduction number is defined around the early outbreak phase, it can be used to determine a lot of the dynamics of outbreaks, such as whether the outbreak is long and slow (small R_0) or short and fast (large R_0). The growth in the number of infected person during the exponential phase of an outbreak is given by $\exp(\gamma(R_0 - 1))$. R_0 often can also tell us about the total percentage of individuals who will be infected over the course of the outbreak (in the absence of interventions), also called the attack rate. For the SIR model, there is a formula for the attack rate Z in terms of the basic reproduction number[30,31]:

$$Z = 1 - \exp(R_0 Z) \tag{6}$$

There is also an analogous concept, called the effective reproduction number R_{eff}, that describes what the current expected number of infections generated by a single person over their infectious period; this number changes over the course of the outbreak and takes into account the relative number of susceptible and infectious people. In discussions of outbreak control, we often discuss trying to get the effective reproduction number below 1, so that the outbreak will die out.

BOX 159-4. Curbing Fear in the 2009 Influenza Pandemic

Mathematical models played an important role during the response to the 2009 influenza pandemic. At the beginning of the outbreak, when it was discovered that a new strain of influenza A was circulating, mathematical models and data on the number of cases per week were used to estimate the basic reproductive number (R_0) and other disease characteristics such as the rate of recovery, γ. This was important since there were a lot of concerns with this virus given that it was a recombination of avian, swine, and human influenza and initially it was reported to be of high virulence with a considerable number of cases developing complications and dying from the disease. Using data initially from Mexico and then from other countries, the analyses showed that the R_0 of the pandemic 2009 virus was similar to that of seasonal flu, alleviating some of the earlier concerns of a fast, highly transmissible disease[17] of a fast, highly transmissible disease.[17]

One possible control strategy is vaccination, that is, turning susceptible people into recovered/immune people before they can become infected (we discuss other control strategies in section "Modeling Interventions and Other Control Strategies"). This is where the concept of *herd immunity* comes from.[29] Not everyone in a population has to be immune to interrupt infection—only enough people that the effective reproduction number goes below 1, so infectious people tend to recover before they contact a susceptible person at random. If enough individuals are vaccinated, an infectious person becomes more likely to contact vaccinated individuals (who are protected from the disease), and less likely to contact susceptible individuals—thereby preventing the disease from spreading further and potentially protecting susceptible individuals from becoming infected. Herd immunity is a very important epidemiological phenomenon as not everyone can be immunized, either for medical or logistical reasons. The level of vaccination needed to engage herd immunity to eliminate a disease, known as the critical vaccination theshold H, differs from disease to disease based on the basic reproduction number:

$$H = 1 - \frac{1}{R_0}. \tag{7}$$

So, some strains of the flu need little more than 50% of people to be vaccinated, while more infectious disease need upward of 95%. Keep in mind that these compartmental models are assuming homogeneity and well-mixedness, however. If populations are clustered or assortative (i.e., if people tend to contact mostly people like them), or if there is significant variation in susceptibility and infectiousness, then herd immunity becomes more complicated.[35] Nonetheless, this formula is a good reference point to give a rough sense of the vaccination targets for diseases for which the R_0 is known.

Extending the SIR Model: Relaxing Assumptions and Modeling Other Processes

Although the classical SIR model has been hugely important for understanding the dynamics of and the mechanistic processes underlying infectious disease outbreaks, particularly for single outbreaks of a directly transmitted (i.e., person-to-person) disease, its simplistic assumptions are soon violated once we start trying to understand specific diseases and specific contexts. In this section, we outline some of the most common adjustments that modelers make to the SIR model to better capture the intricacies of specific diseases.

We illustrate these extensions in the model diagrams in Fig. 159-5. Although we present these changes in the context of deterministic compartmental models, analogous changes can be made to SIR network and agentbased models as well (introduced in section "Network and Agent-based Models").

Determining the relevant mechanistic process to include in a model is always an important preliminary step in model, one which may require interdisciplinary collaboration between modelers, biologists, and medical professionals. Ultimately, every modeler is responsible for both understanding the assumptions of their model and for ensuring that they are appropriate to the context.

Immunity

The strength of the immune response generated by a disease can vary greatly and impact the populationlevel dynamics of its spread. In some cases, we assume that a disease does not induce any natural immunity (often assumed for some sexually transmitted infections like chlamydia and gonorrhea). In other cases, we might assume lifelong immunity (e.g., measles). For many diseases, immunity, whether natural or vaccineinduced, wanes over time (e.g., influenza).[36]

To capture waning immunity, we can extend the SIR model to an SIRS model by including a term representing the movement of recovered individuals back into the susceptible class (at rate ω) Models with waning immunity can produce a range of commonly observed infectious disease patterns, as we show in Fig. 159-4, including:

- Epidemics that start with exponential growth, then peak, then turn over;
- Regular or semiregular periodic epidemics (e.g., annual epidemics); and
- Endemic disease, where the disease remains in the population and never dies out completely.

The basic SIRS model equations are given below—note that the model is the same as the original SIR model [Eq. (3)], with an additional term to account for waning immunity, that is, a return from recovered (immune) to susceptible:

$$\frac{dS}{dt} = -\beta\left(\frac{1}{N}\right)S \underbrace{+\omega R,}_{\text{waning immunity}}$$
$$\frac{dI}{dt} = \beta\left(\frac{1}{N}\right)S - \gamma I,$$
$$\frac{dR}{dt} = \gamma I \underbrace{-\omega R,}_{\text{waning immunity}} \tag{8}$$

Latent Period

One of the first assumptions in the SIR model that is violated when we want to capture the dynamics of a specific disease is the assumption that an infected person is immediately infectious. Instead, most diseases have a latent period, during which individuals are infected but not yet infectious.[37] It turns out that including a latent period in an infectious disease model can change the dynamics in important ways, allowing us to fit outbreak shapes that cannot be explained well by the classic SIR model.[38]

The SIR model with an additional latent compartment is shown in Fig. 159-5a, and sometimes termed the SLIR model. The latent compartment is denoted L for latent, with $1/\sigma$ giving the average length of the latency period. However, often this compartment is instead denoted E for "exposed" and the entire model called an SEIR model

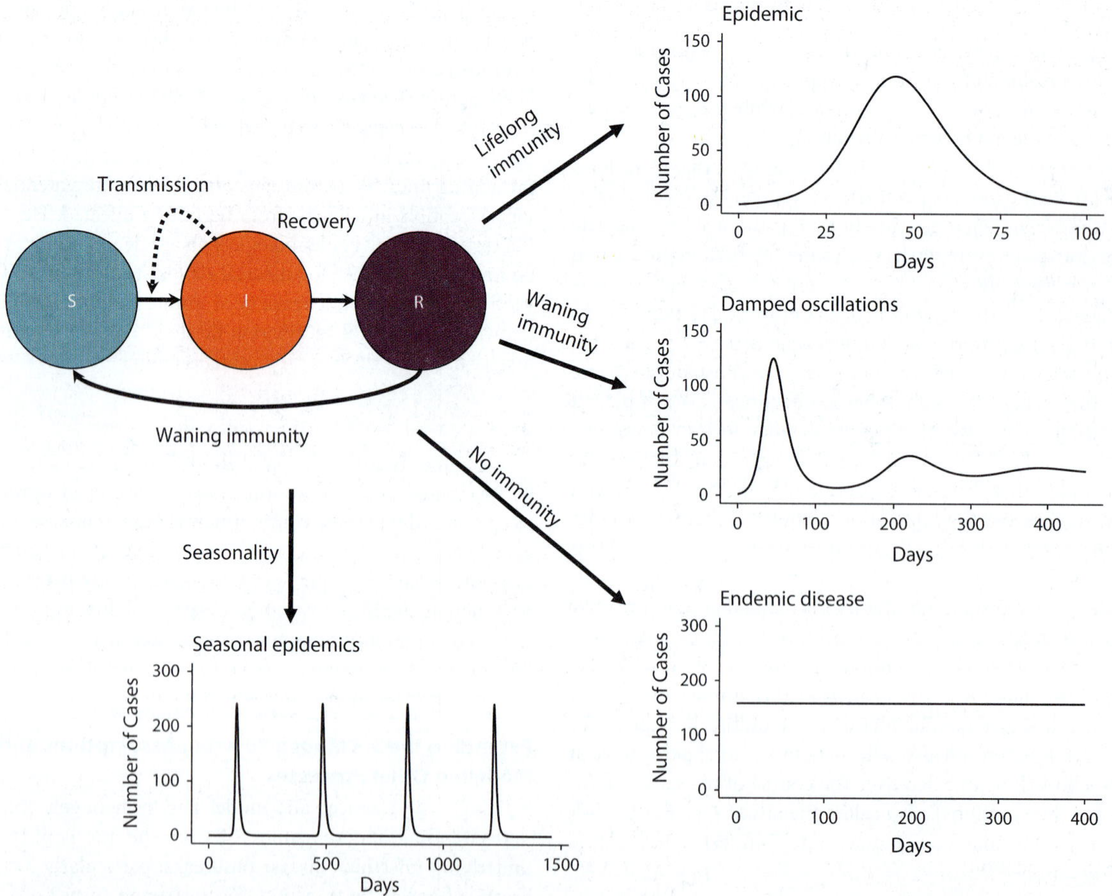

FIGURE 159-4. The SIRS model extends the SIR model by including waning immunity. Although this extension seems relatively simple, depending on the parameters, this model can produce a variety of dynamics observed in the real world, including single epidemics (e.g., if there is no loss of immunity, i.e., the classic SIR model), periodic declining epidemics (e.g., if immunity wanes over time), endemic disease (e.g., if there is rapid loss of immunity or no immunity), and regular seasonal epidemics (e.g., if there are seasonal changes in contact such as school-year increases in interaction).

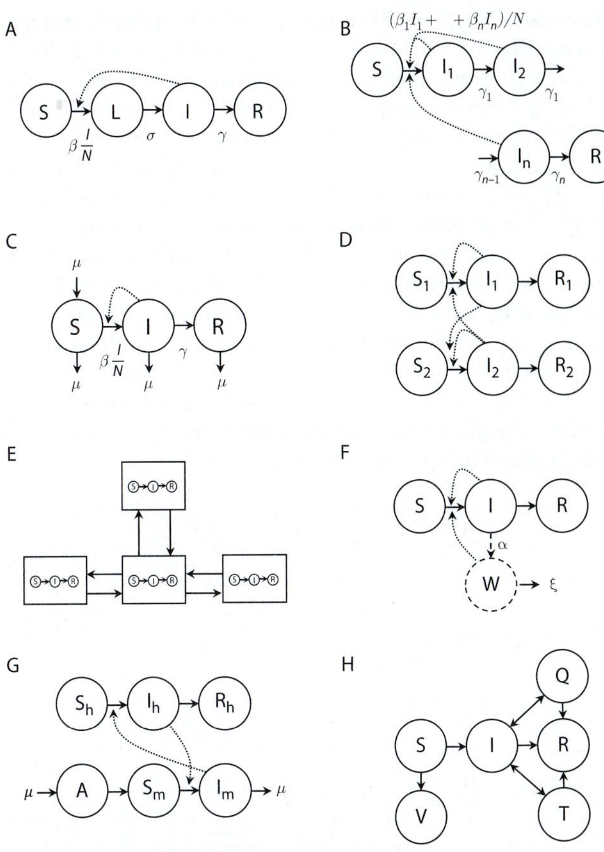

FIGURE 159-5. Extended compartmental model diagrams illustrating (A) a latent compartment, (B) stage progression, (C) birth and death, (D) subpopulation interactions, (E) metapopulation interactions, (F) environmentally mediated transmission, (G) vector mediated transmission, and (H) assorted control strategies including vaccination, quarantine, and treatment.

BOX 159-5.	Measles, Herd Immunity, and Vaccine Hesitancy

Measles is a highly contagious respiratory disease. Once considered eliminated in the United States, it has been making a comeback in recent years. Why? Measles is controlled by vaccination, but it is so infectious that at least 95% of people in an area need to be vaccinated before herd immunity can be achieved. Rising rates of vaccine hesistancy have caused vaccination coverage to drop in some regions and for some subgroups, allowing measles to spread explosively once introduced.[32–34]

instead of an SLIR model. Although the community is slowly moving to adopt the L notation (because latent is a more accurate description, medically speaking), it's useful to be aware of both notations. The model equations are given by:

$$\begin{aligned}
\frac{dS}{dt} &= -\beta\left(\frac{1}{N}\right)S, \\
\frac{dL}{dt} &= \beta\left(\frac{1}{N}\right)S \underbrace{-\sigma L,}_{\text{latent to infectious}} \\
\frac{dI}{dt} &= \underbrace{+\sigma L,}_{\text{latent to infectious}} - \gamma I, \\
\frac{dR}{dt} &= \gamma I.
\end{aligned} \tag{9}$$

Stage Progression

A natural extension or generalization of the SLIR model is the stage progression model, shown in Fig. 159-5b. We use a stage progression model when the well-mixedness assumption of the infectious compartment I breaks down because of differences in symptoms or behavior over the disease progression. Stage progression models may be used, for example, for Ebola, which has distinct clinical stages with different degrees of infectiousness.[39] HIV infection also has a pronounced stage progression from acute to asymptomatic to AIDS.[40] Infected people are more infectious in the acute phase shortly after infection, when viral titers are high, than the later, longer asymptomatic chronic phase.[41]

The model equations are given by:

$$\begin{aligned}
\frac{dS}{dt} &= \underbrace{-\left(\beta_1\frac{I_1}{N} + \cdots + \beta_n\frac{I_n}{N}\right)S,}_{\text{transmission from each infection stage}} \\
\frac{dI_1}{dt} &= \left(\beta_1\frac{I_1}{N} + \cdots \beta_n\frac{I_n}{N}\right)S \quad \underbrace{-\gamma_1 I,}_{\text{progression to stage 2}} \\
\frac{dI_2}{dt} &= +\gamma_1 I \quad \underbrace{-\gamma_2 I_2,}_{\text{progression to stage 3}} \\
&\vdots \\
\frac{dI_n}{dt} &= \gamma_{n-1} I_{n-1} \quad \underbrace{-\gamma_n I_n,}_{\text{progression to } R} \\
\frac{dR}{dt} &= \gamma I_n,
\end{aligned} \tag{10}$$

where each stage of infection is modeled as a separate compartment $I_1, I_2, \ldots, I_n$, and has its own transmission parameter (the β_i terms in the S equation, and stage progression rate (the γ_i terms in each stage of infection).

Birth, Death, and Demographic Considerations

Classic SIR dynamics may work well for certain epidemics considered in isolation, but basic models cannot capture repeated epidemics or long-term endemic behavior without a mechanism to replenish the number of susceptible people in the population.[42] On longer time scales, we must consider birth and death processes. In models, we include a flow μN into the susceptible compartment,[38] where N is the total population in the model (potentially changing over time). For convenience of keeping the total population size fixed, we will often set the death rate to μ as well, although it can also be modeled as a different rate. In this case, we note that the total death rate across all three equations is $\mu S + \mu I + \mu R = \mu N$, so that the births and deaths precisely cancel out, leaving us with a constant total population. One could also imagine that people who are infected or have recovered from a disease (or some subset of recovered people) might have a different background death rate due to disease-induced morbidities (e.g., polio-induced paralysis), which can be accounted for as well (making the population nonconstant). The basic, constant population form of the model is shown in Fig. 159-5c and the equations are given by:

$$\begin{aligned}
\frac{dS}{dt} &= \underbrace{\mu N}_{\text{births}} - \beta\left(\frac{1}{N}\right)S - \underbrace{\mu S,}_{\text{deaths}} \\
\frac{dI}{dt} &= \beta\left(\frac{I}{N}\right)S - \gamma I - \underbrace{\mu I,}_{\text{deaths}} \\
\frac{dR}{dt} &= \gamma I - \underbrace{\mu R.}_{\text{deaths}}
\end{aligned} \tag{11}$$

Density- vs. Frequency-dependent Transmission

In the previous section on demographic considerations, we introduced the idea that the total population size N could change over

BOX 159-6 Accounting for Environmental Transmission: Cholera Epidemics and Interventions

Environmental transmission pathways are increasingly being recognized as important targets for intervention, and thus important components to include in mathematical models. Since the 2010 cholera epidemic in Haiti,[58,59] environmental pathways have been broadly used to model cholera epidemics in a range of settings.[14,60–63] One example comes from a recent cholera vaccination campaign in Maela refugee camp.[64,65] Maela refugee camp is located in northwest Thailand, along the Burma (Myanmar) border, and had previously experienced semiregular cholera epidemics. In 2013, a cholera vaccination campaign was implemented as a critical addition to existing water, sanitation, and hygiene efforts to reduce cholera transmission in Maela. Mathematical models were used to assist in evaluating the campaign and testing whether a booster campaign was needed in the following year.[60] These models accounted for both person-to-person and environmentally mediated transmission, which was particularly important given Models were used to assess alternative dosing strategies and to evaluate the minimum doses needed to ensure effective cholera prevention, and were used in the subsequent year to evaluate whether a booster campaign was needed (based on potential loss of immunity and population turnover/migration/births/deaths).

time. Does the rate of contacting other people change as the population size changes? It may or may not, depending on the scenario.

If the contact rate does not depend on the population size (i.e., if each person contacts the same number of individuals regardless of the total number of people in the population), we say transmission is *frequency dependent*. In this situation, we can imagine a population that takes up as much space as it needs to keep the population density and contact rate constant. Or, consider a scenario in which the number of people we contact doesn't change with the number of people in the population, as could be the case for sexually transmitted infections. In either of these cases, we would expect the probability of becoming infected should depend on the fraction of the population that is infected (I/N) rather than the number of individuals who are infected (I), as is the case in Eq. (3).

If the contact rate is proportional to the population size $\kappa = \kappa_0 N(t)$, we say that transmission is *density dependent*. Think about a population of people who live in a fixed area; when there are more people living in the area, the population is denser, and contacts happen more frequently. In this case, the transmission rate simplifies: $\pi \kappa_0 \cdot N(t) \cdot (I(t)/N(t)) = \pi \kappa_0 \cdot I(t) = \beta I(t)$. Here, transmission depends on the actual *number* of infectious people, not just the *fraction* of people infected. Of course, the contact rate could depend on the population size in a nonlinear way; in these cases, one would just adjust the equations accordingly. The density-dependent version of the SIR model in Eq. (3) is given by:

$$\frac{dS}{dt} = -\beta IS, \quad \frac{dI}{dt} = \beta IS - \gamma I, \quad \frac{dR}{dt} = \gamma I. \tag{12}$$

Subpopulation Models

As we discussed above, the well-mixed assumption of compartmental models is usually too strong. Well-mixedness, for example, is often insufficient to describe sexually transmitted infections (in which some individuals may have much higher numbers of partners than average)[43] and may be better treated with network or agent-based models (e.g., ref. 44). In many cases, however, it is sufficient to account for different subgroups of a population by including multiple kinds of S, I, and R compartments. By splitting along demographic (e.g., age, race) or behavioral lines, we can account for more complex contact patterns such as assortativity (i.e., people most often associate with people similar to them) and analyze how disease spreads through subpopulations. When we subdivide the population, we have to include not only the process of transmission within these subpopulations, but also transmission across subpopulations.[45] For example, models of respiratory viruses (influenza, respiratory syncytial virus, etc.) may need to be age-structured to account for transmission among infants and school-aged children[46]; this younger age group can drive infection in adults and in elderly people who are more at risk for complications. A simple subpopulation model with two groups is shown in Fig. 159-5d, with equations:

$$\begin{aligned}
\frac{dS_1}{dt} &= -\left(\underbrace{\beta_{11}\frac{I_1}{N}}_{I_1 \text{ tranmits to } S_1} + \underbrace{\beta_{21}\frac{I_2}{N}}_{I_2 \text{ tranmits to } S_1}\right) S_1, \\
\frac{dI_1}{dt} &= \left(\beta_{11}\frac{I_1}{N} + \beta_{21}\frac{I_2}{N}\right) S_1 - \gamma I_1, \\
\frac{dR_1}{dt} &= \gamma I_1, \\
\frac{dS_2}{dt} &= -\left(\underbrace{\beta_{11}\frac{I_1}{N}}_{I_1 \text{ tranmits to } S_2} + \underbrace{\beta_{21}\frac{I_2}{N}}_{I_2 \text{ tranmits to } S_2}\right) S_2, \\
\frac{dI_2}{dt} &= \left(\beta_{22}\frac{I_2}{N} + \beta_{12}\frac{I_1}{N}\right) S_2 - \gamma I_2, \\
\frac{dR_2}{dt} &= \gamma I_2.
\end{aligned} \tag{13}$$

Metapopulation and Multiple Population Models

If subpopulation models represent a finer population scale, metapopulation models and other multiple community models represent a coarser scale, zoomed out to view multiple populations simultaneously. At this scale, we are often interested in how diseases move between population hubs, across countries, or even internationally. We may be interested in commuting/traveling[47,48] (i.e., accounting for people who go back and forth between populations) or migration[49] (i.e., accounting for people moving permanently) depending on the time scales and the disease scenario. Operationally, we need to decide how populations are connected (e.g., can anyone go anywhere, or just to the neighboring population centers) and how we want to model the movement. Popular ways of parameterizing movement include gravity models[50] (where the probability of movement or transmission between two cities is proportional to their sizes but inversely proportional to their distance from one another), flight patterns,[51,52] and cell phone records,[53,54] among others. Metapopulation models have been used to investigate the impact of human mobility for a variety of diseases and scenarios (e.g., refs. 39 and 55–58). Because there is not a standard way to model multiple populations, we omit equations here, however a model diagram for a simple multiple population model is shown in Fig. 159-5e.

Environmentally Mediated Transmission

Some pathogens are spread through the environment (such as through contaminated water) in addition to or instead of directly person-to-person.[66–68] Models for environmental disease transmission such as the SIWR model in Fig. 159-5f are often used for gastrointestinal disease in low income countries with unimproved water and sanitation infrastructure. Indeed, SIWR-style models (W for water or, more broadly, an environmental compartment) were used effectively

BOX 159-7 How will Climate Change Affect Infectious Diseases?

Climate change is expected to make some areas warmer, some cooler, some wetter,and some drier. How will these changes affect the global burden of infectious disease? Vectorborne diseases are likely to be appear in new regions, for example, as climate change opens up new areas to mosquitoes, ticks, and other vectors. But there are many interrelated factors at work.[75,76] Approaching this complicated question requires a systems perspective and the answers may not always be intuitive. For example, climate change may increase the burden of bacterial gastroinestinal disease but reduce the burden of viral gastroinestinal disease.[77]

in the analysis of the 2010 cholera outbreak in Haiti, highlighting their strengths and popularizing their use (e.g., refs. 58 and 59).

Several new processes need to be incorporated in models of environmental transmission that were not part of the SIR model. First, we need to account for contact with the environment (typically thought of as ingestion) and the probability that the contact successfully causes infection. In order to do this, we need to be aware of the connection between the amount of pathogen ingested (dose) and the probability of infection (response). Although in most cases doses can be considered low enough that the response is linear, we have to be cognizant of both the likely doses people in the model are encountering and the dynamic consequences of our choices of model.[69]

A second process we have to consider is the death of pathogens in the environment (with constant rate ξ). Many pathogens require a host to replicate in and can survive in the environment for only a finite amount of time. It has been shown that diseases with environmental transmission of pathogens that can only live in the environment for a short amount of time have dynamics that look very similar those of diseases with person-to-person transmission.[67,68,70] Pathogens that can last a long time in the environment have dynamics that cannot be replicated by models without an environmental compartment. It is also important to remember that for our compartmental models that in general all flows are assumed to be based on a constant transition rate, which results in exponential decay in the number of individuals in a compartment; while many pathogens do appear to decay exponentially in the environment, not all do (*Escherichia coli* is one example).[71,72] Some pathogens, such as *Vibrio cholerae* can even grow in the environment.[73]

A third process we must consider is shedding of pathogens into the environment (represented by a linear rate α in Fig. 159-5f). The shedding rate is often very difficult to parameterize with data, particularly if we want to model concentration instead number of pathogens (accounting for the size of the environment). Fortunately, there are ways to scale the environment in ways that we can wrap up the shedding rate with other parameters.[74] The model equations for the SIWR model shown in Fig. 159-5f are:

$$
\begin{aligned}
\frac{dS}{dt} &= \underbrace{-\beta_W W_S}_{\text{environmental transmission}} \quad \underbrace{-\beta_I \frac{1}{N} S,}_{\text{human transmission}} \\
\frac{dI}{dt} &= \beta_W WS - \beta_I \frac{1}{N} S - \gamma I, \\
\frac{dR}{dt} &= \gamma I, \\
\frac{dW}{dt} &= \underbrace{\alpha I}_{\text{shedding}} \; - \underbrace{\xi W.}_{\text{decay}}
\end{aligned}
\tag{14}
$$

Vector Mediated Transmission

There are entire classes of pathogens, such as arboviruses, that cannot be transmitted directly between two human hosts but instead rely on an intermediate, or vector, for transmission. Globally, the most important class of vectorborne diseases are carried by mosquitoes, mostly the *Anopheles* and *Aedes* genuses. Mosquitoes carry the pathogens responsible for malaria (*Plasmodium* spp.), dengue, chikungunya, Zika, and others.[78] Other vectors carry Chagas disease, leishmaniasis, and schistosomiasis.[78] Ticks are vectors for Lyme disease and many emerging diseases, particularly in the United States.[79]

Many processes of the vectors themselves—their births and maturation, their contact with humans, their own disease progression, and their deaths (usually fast enough that we don't consider recovered classes of vectors)—need to be considered when modeling vectorborne disease dynamics. Consequently, even relatively simple vector models can add significant complexity to your model. Depending on the level of specificity and realism desired, one can include additional processes in the model, such as seasonal cycles in vector population, gonotrophic cycles or other breeding dynamics of mosquitoes, or the presence of other hosts. Some vectorborne model extensions may be better suited to an agent-based model than a compartmental model, particularly once one is modeling detailed spatial processes with high heterogeneity between individuals (e.g., distinct contact or travel patterns, etc.). Nonetheless, a simple vectorborne disease model that forms the basis of many models used in practice[80–83] is:

$$
\begin{aligned}
\frac{dS_h}{dt} &= \underbrace{-\beta_{vh} \frac{I_v S_h}{N_h}}_{\text{vector infects humans}} \qquad \frac{dS_v}{dt} = \mu N_v \; \underbrace{-\beta_{hv} \frac{I_h S_v,}{N_h}}_{\text{vector infected by human}} \; - \mu S_v \\
\frac{dI_h}{dt} &= \beta_{vh} \frac{I_v S_h}{N_h} - \gamma_h I_h, \quad \frac{dI_v}{dt} = \beta_{hv} \frac{I_h S_v}{N_h} - \mu I_m, \\
\frac{dR_h}{dt} &= \gamma I_h,
\end{aligned}
\tag{15}
$$

where the subscript h denotes humans and the subscript v denotes vectors. This model can be extended to include an aquatic, immature phase of the mosquito (A), as shown in Fig. 159-5g. While highly simplified, these models and others like them have been used to examine the dynamics and evaluate interventions for a range of mosquito-borne diseases, such as dengue, chikungunya, and Zika.[82–88]

Other Disease Dynamics

Many other processes can be represented in compartmental models. One might be interested in modeling infection-related death (could be of interest for modeling Ebola, influenza, diarrheal disease, tuberculosis, and more, depending on the scenario and time scales of interest). Multiple circulating strains may need to be considered simultaneously, particularly in the case of dengue, where infections by a second strain can have more severe symptoms.[89] Seasonally varying parameters are also often of interest, both as temperature and humidity change (particularly for vectorborne diseases) and also when considering differences in transmission due to school calendars.[90] Although seasonality is often modeled with sinusoidal functions, approximate step-functions may be more appropriate for modeling more abrupt transitions (such as school closures).

Behavior

Critically intertwined with infectious disease processes are behavioral processes—from social distancing, to vaccine hesitancy, to disease-related stigma—social and behavioral processes can have an enormous impact on transmission patterns and intervention success. While many social behavioral processes are often modeled implicitly (e.g., as part of the parameter values for the model), there has been increasing recognition of the importance of modeling behavior patterns and behavior change explicitly as well.[6,91–93] Behavioral models may use tools from economics, game theory, and decision theory, or may build more heuristically based on studies of human behavior in response to disease processes.[6,91,94,95] Often, these models include feedback processes between the dynamics of the disease and those of behavior—disease risk affects behavior (e.g., condom-use might increase across when STI risk is perceived to be high, as has been observed for HIV risk[96,97]), but behavior also affects disease (as increased condom use will reduce transmission).[98] This feedback loop can affect prediction and intervention efforts and is an active area of development in mathematical modeling.

Modeling Interventions and Other Control Strategies

The models above can also be adapted to examine intervention and control strategies, as illustrated in Fig. 159-5h. Modeling can be used to estimate the effectiveness of interventions before allocating resources, potentially avoiding costly but ineffective efforts,[99] to try out alternative intervention strategies, or to compare intervention simulations with counterfactuals that may not be testable in the real world, such as not intervening. From the public health perspective, interventions are usually categorized by scale—from the individual to the community level. For mathematical models, it is equally critical to understand how the intervention works mechanistically in the model:

- **Interventions can add new processes to the system.** Vaccination is one of the most frequently modeled interventions. It is typically modeled as a flow from the susceptible compartment to an immune compartment (either the existing recovered compartment or a new vaccinated compartment, depending on the disease specifics). The constant rate assumption can be easily violated for vaccination, as in the case of pulsed vaccination,[100] but alternative vaccination schedules can usually be modeled as specific simulations. Other interventions that sometimes warrant the introduction of a new process include quarantine[101] and treatment (such as antiretroviral therapy for people with HIV[102]). Some environmental interventions, such as surface decontamination, could also be considered a new process that kills some percentage of pathogens at certain times.[103]
- **Interventions can modify existing processes.** Many interventions can be considered to modify processes that are already being modeled. For example, your intervention may reduce the transmission rate, acting either on the contact rate (e.g., mosquito bed nets, encouraging sick people to stay home) or by reducing the probability of transmission when contact occurs (e.g., condoms, prophylaxis, water treatment devices).

In either case, we have to be sure whether the way that we implement the intervention in the model, given the model assumptions (e.g., well-mixed compartments and exponential rates), is a reasonably accurate abstraction of reality. Because the exact effects of an intervention are usually not known precisely (e.g., will the intervention reduce transmission by 25% or 50%?), model studies aimed at assessing interventions usually focus on quantifying the uncertainty on outcomes of interest (often number of cases averted) given a reasonable range of intervention effectiveness.

NETWORK AND AGENT-BASED MODELS

Introduction to Network and Agent-based Models

While flexible in many ways, compartmental models assume that any individual in a given class or compartment can interact with all individuals in a connected compartment (well-mixedness/homogeneous mixing). In addition, compartmental models are limited in their ability to simultaneously incorporate multiple characteristics (covariates) or other sources of heterogeneity into the analysis. While theoretically plausible, in practice this usually requires increasing the number of compartments in the model beyond what is feasible, for example, if breaking the population into multiple subgroups (e.g, by age, sex, race, level of connectivity, etc.).[104]

As an alternative, network or agent-based models can be used to explicitly track the contacts and disease states of discrete *individuals* (as illustrated in Fig. 159-6). This opens the door to models that can account for *heterogeneity* that may have important implications for both individual and population-level risk. Because they allow for the representation of individuals rather than subpopulations (unlike compartmental models), network and agent-based models can easily incorporate additional characteristics that may impact risks of infection without dramatically increasing the complexity of the model. Additionally, as mentioned above, most network or agent-based models are stochastic in nature, meaning that the process of disease transmission from one individual to another in the model involves randomness.

When Should Models Account for Heterogeneity?

As we've seen from the discussion of compartmental modeling in section "Extending the SIR Model: Relaxing Assumptions and Modeling

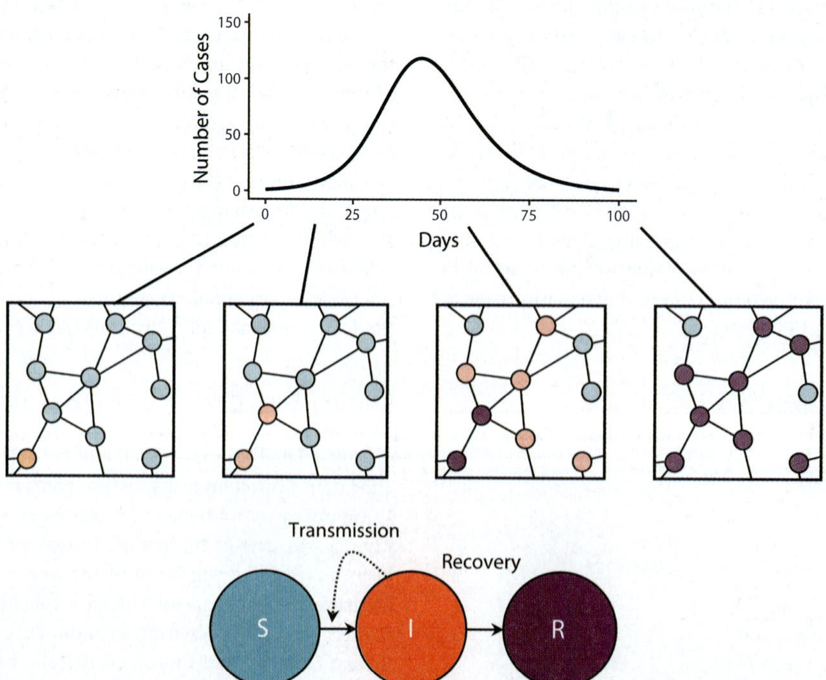

FIGURE 159-6. Visualization of infectious disease spread on a network. As the epidemic progresses, susceptible individuals (blue) within the network become infectious (red) after transmission from an infectious contact, and eventually recover from the disease (dark purple).

Other Processes" above, simplifying assumptions about individual behavior and contact are often adequate to address population-level questions. However, if we are interested in understanding how heterogeneous traits and behaviors of individuals impact those around them and the disease system as a whole, we might then approach the problem with a network or agent-based model that will let us more explicitly represent these mechanisms. For example, it has been shown that as individual heterogeneity in transmission probability increases, outbreaks become less likely. However, when outbreak do stochastically arise, they tend to be more explosive.[107] Without models that can account for this random variation, it is difficult to make important decisions during critical public health emergencies. For example, this randomness has been shown to make it difficult to evaluate the risk of large-scale outbreaks of emerging infectious diseases such as Ebola,[108] monkeypox, and pandemic influenza. Similarly, such models have also been used to address the impact of heterogeneity on preventing the resurgence of infectious diseases such as measles[109] in settings where they are presently well-controlled.

Models that explicitly represent this kind of variation are also necessary to identify and target so-called *superspreaders* who are much more infectious or have many more contacts than the average person. Such individuals have been identified as key to understanding and effectively intervening on the transmission dynamics of a wide range of pathogens from noroviruses,[110] which can cause epidemic gastroenteritis, to tuberculosis,[111] HIV, and pandemic influenza. Recent advances in both mathematical modeling as well as the use of whole-genome sequencing and other methods of pathogen genotyping are now making it possible to identify and incorporate key sources of individual-level variability into models, with greater accuracy than had previously been possible.[112–115]

In short, heterogeneity should be accounted for when we can characterize it and know that it is relevant to one or more disease processes. In general, this kind of modeling is more useful for exploring the effects of different assumptions rather than when trying to explain a specific data set, as it can be difficult to make inferences about heterogeneity from longitudinal case data alone.

BOX 159-8 The Outbreak Ended, So the Intervention Worked—or Did It?

We often attribute the end of an outbreak to interventions, when in fact the outbreak may have naturally ended due to, for example, the exhaustion of susceptible individuals or simply random chance. This overestimation is a problem because resources may be spent on strategies that we mistakenly think will control later outbreaks. Mathematical models have been used to show that this problem can arise in part from selection bias. Pathogens like norovirus or MRSA, for example, are relatively commonplace, usually causing sporadic cases and sometimes triggering larger (but likely short-lived) outbreaks. However, interventions are typically only triggered when outbreaks reach a critical threshold. Mathematical models have been used to demonstrate that this selection bias alone can lead to overly confident estimates of intervention effectiveness.[105,106]

Contact Network Models

Contact network models represent a population as a collection of nodes (corresponding to individuals) and edges or links (corresponding to connections between individuals).[116] In infectious disease epidemiology, such contact networks are used as the basis for modeling disease transmission. These models assume that infectious individuals can transmit the disease directly only to their contacts. Depending on the specific disease being modeled, we might treat these connections as static (staying the same over time, e.g., for home and work contacts) or dynamic (changing over time, e.g., for short-term sexual partners). Network models of transmission have increased in popularity in recent years, driven in part by the development of network theory in mathematics, statistics, physics, and computing science[117,118] and also by the improvements in computational power, which have made it feasible to simulate networks with millions of individuals and connections.[119–121]

To develop a network model of disease transmission, the first task is to select a network (i.e., a set of nodes and edges). Researchers use either stylized networks (networks defined by the distribution of the number of contacts in the population) or empirical networks (networks inferred from an observed sample of individuals, or empirical simulations of a community, city or even a country). Depending on the infectious disease in question, different types of networks might be more appropriate to model the transmission process, for example, a network of contacts relevant to the transmission of a sexually transmitted infection will be likely very different from a contact network for transmission of a respiratory disease. In a broader setting, networks can also be used to capture larger scale interactions such as movement patterns between cities and communities (such as with the compartmental models described above). Two such networks are illustrated in Fig. 159-7.

Agent-based Models

Like network models, agent-based models (ABMs)[122–124] have the ability to represent discrete individuals, but they do not require a contact network. Indeed, they are very flexible models that are often well suited to capture complex dynamics and emergent behaviors, although this flexibility comes at the cost of additional model complexity and, consequently, often a lack tractability. For the purpose of this discussion, we will make a distinction between *individual-based* models, which includes many network models as well as other types of transmission models where we are concerned with the *state* of individuals but less

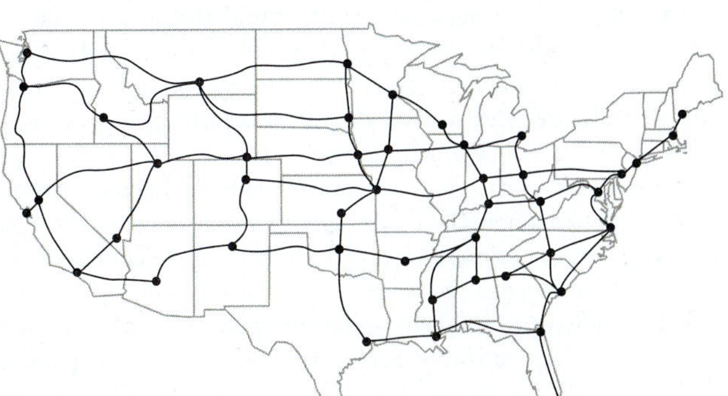

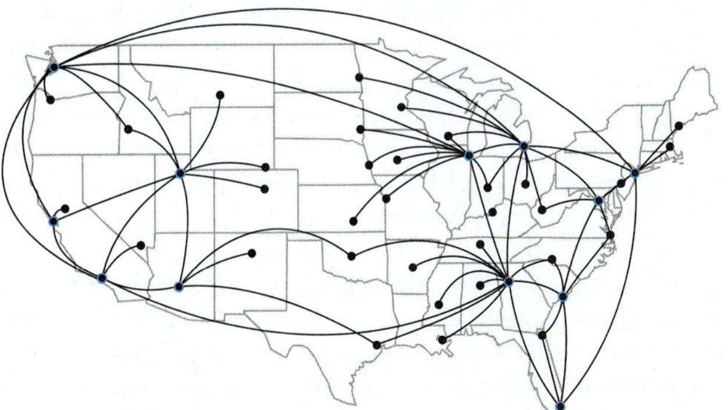

FIGURE 159-7. Different kinds of networks have different patterns of connectedness. In road networks (left), most nodes (cities) have similar degrees (i.e., the number of other cities they are connected to). By contrast, in air travel networks (right), most nodes have very low degree, but a few cities act as hubs and have high degree.

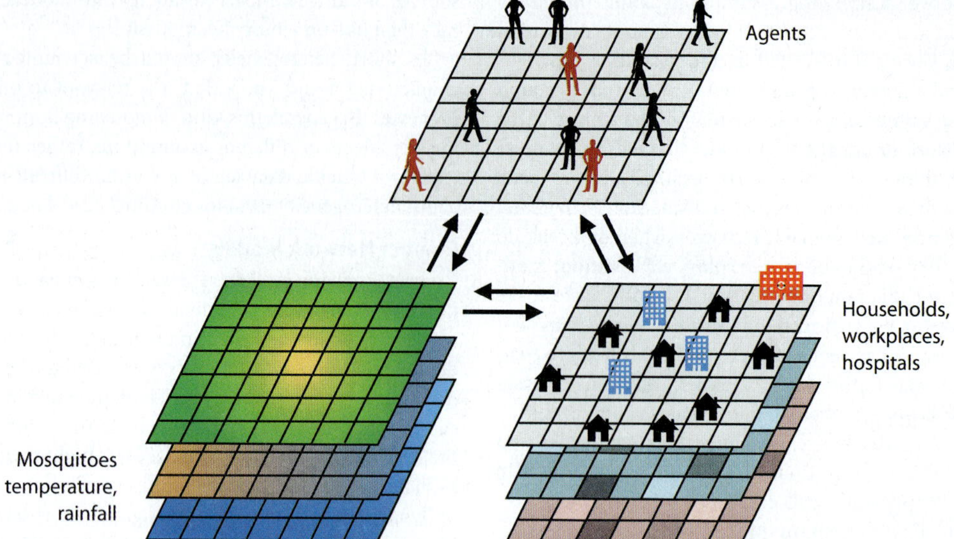

FIGURE 159-8. Example of an agent-based model of vectorborne disease transmission. The model is built on a spatial grid with layers for different model features. Top: human agents in the model (with disease status indicated by agent colors). Left: mosquito-related variables such as mosquito density and weather drivers (temperature and rainfall). Right: behavior and built environment variables such as workplaces (blue buildings), homes (black buildings), and hospitals (red building), as well as other spatial variables (indicated by the cyan and pink layers underneath). All of these different variables interact to generate the overall disease dynamics in the model.

BOX 159-9 Like Attracts Like: Assortativity in Sexual Networks

Racial disparities in sexually transmitted infections have persisted, and traditional risk factors—such as a large number of sexual partners and lack of condom use—do not explain these disparities. One alternate explanation suggests that sexual assortativity, that is, the preference to have sex with people of the same group, coupled with higher rates of concurrent partnerships could be responsible. It is hard to imagine the epidemiological study that could easily test this hypothesis, but network-based mathematical models have shown that these mechanisms are a potential explanation for this type of persistent disparity.[44]

concerned with their individual behavior, and *agent-based* models, in which individuals act depending on their environment, internal state, or interactions with other agents (as illustrated in Fig. 159-8). Some of the earliest examples of agent-based models were focused on understanding how collective dynamics may emerge from individual behavior. For example, the synchronized flight of a flock of birds or school of fish may be explained by a set of simple rules regarding the way individual agents modify their movement based on the movement of their nearest neighbors. In the context of infectious disease transmission, ABMs may allow us to understand how individual behaviors collectively result in population-level dynamics. For example, individuals with an influenza infection are likely reduce their rate of contact with people in the community when they perceive an increased risk of disease, that is, by seeing people in their contact network becoming ill, and they may stay home to reduce risk of transmitting to others when they are symptomatic.[125–128]

Incorporating these mechanisms has been shown to be important for understanding how seemingly irrational, suboptimal behaviors may emerge. For example, in one study, individuals in a simulated community used information on illness among their contacts in the previous influenza season to decide whether to get a flu shot in the current season. This resulted in the most-connected individuals being more likely to choose to vaccinate than less-connected individuals, resulting in vaccination coverage insufficient to have a significant impact on transmission.[132] A key use of ABMs is understanding the potential implications individual behavior for the efficacy of policies or interventions. For example, one study explored the implications of pediatricians dismissing vaccine-refusing families from their practice on overall measles vaccination coverage and outbreak risk.[133] They found that such policies were unlikely to change behavior and were in fact likely to concentrate susceptible, unvaccinated children in a small set of tolerant practices, potentially increasing the contact rate between them and the likelihood of outbreaks among these children if one of them was exposed to a measles case.

CONNECTING MATHEMATICAL MODELS WITH DATA

A key step of the modeling process (whether for statistical or mathematical models) is connecting the model with data. Parameter estimation for mathematical models can take many forms, from direct measurement of the parameters from experiments or field studies, to indirect estimation of the parameters from surveillance and other disease data (e.g., incidence curves). Connecting models with data allows us to establish values or distributions for epidemiologically important parameters (such as R_0) and make realistic predictions or forecasts of the system's behavior.

In many cases, some model parameters can be estimated from data from previous experiments or observations. For example, the length of the latent and infectious periods of a disease are usually known. However, we must always be careful that a new outbreak is not substantially different in some way, for example, if it is being transmitted in a vulnerable population that may have longer infectious periods. In general, data can often directly give us starting points for our model parameters.

In other cases, we want to estimate the model parameters given a set of data, often longitudinal case data. Here, we may not know the parameters ahead of time, but we can use statistical techniques to say what values of the parameters are most consistent with the observed data. This indirect use of data can be very powerful. There are three important concepts involved here: identifiability ("can the parameters be uniquely determined"), parameter estimation ("what are the most likely values of the parameters"), and uncertainty quantification ("what range of parameter values are consistent with the data").[136] By doing this kind of indirect estimation, we can gain insight into the mechanisms of the disease process.

BOX 159-10 Combating Healthcare Acquired Infections (HCAIs)

Nosocomial infections—those acquired in a hospital or other healthcare setting—remain a serious concern in both developing and developed countries. Pathogens like MRSA and *C. difficile* have been difficult to combat because of the rise of antibiotic resistance, asymptomatic carriers, and environmental persistence.[129] Agent-based models are well suited to studying HCAIs because transmission can depend on the actions and movement of individual healthcare providers and patients, as well as the specific rooms in which they work and stay.[130,131]

BOX 159-11 Environmental Surveillance: A New Tool

Many pathogens (other than sexually transmitted infections) have an environmental component to their transmission, even when we think of them as transmitted person-to-person. Technological advances are making it easier to detect and even quantify pathogen levels in environments such as drinking or wastewater, air, and household objects. This kind of surveillance is especially helpful when detecting asymptomatic infections. For example, the 2013 polio outbreak in Israel was detected early in wastewater, allowing vaccines to be distributed before there were any cases of paralysis.[134,135]

CONCLUSION

Infectious disease modeling is a tool used to systematically explore the larger public health implications of what we know about a disease and how it is spread. Modeling is an essentially *integrative* activity: By bringing together what we know about the pathophysiology of infection, with processes of contact, and other environmental and social dynamics, we can understand the implications of the interactions between all of these moving parts. This is especially useful for understanding the potential impact of changes in policy or practice. However, the quality of conclusions of modeling studies depends entirely on the quality of its inputs and the thoughtfulness with the model is constructed. So, it is imperative to critically assess a model's underlying assumptions and that data it is built upon when using infectious disease modeling research to guide clinical practice and policymaking.

References

1. Webber BL, Raghu S, Edwards OR. Opinion: Is CRISPR-based gene drive a biocontrol silver bullet or global conservation threat? *Proc Natl Acad Sci U S A*. 2015;112(34):10565–7.
2. Chretien JP, Riley S, George DB. Mathematical modeling of the West Africa Ebola epidemic. *Elife*. 2015;4:e09186.
3. May RM. Uses and abuses of mathematics in biology. *Science*. 2004;303(5659):790–3.
4. Dub´e E, Laberge C, Guay M, Bramadat P, Roy R, Bettinger JA. Vaccine hesitancy: An overview. *Hum Vaccin Immunother*. 2013;9(8):1763–73.
5. Sharareh N, Sabounchi NS, Sayama H, MacDonald R. The ebola crisis and the corresponding public behavior: A system dynamics approach. *PLoS Curr*. 2016;8.
6. Funk S, Salathé M, Jansen VA. Modelling the influence of human behaviour on the spread of infectious diseases: A review. *J R Soc Interface*. 2010;7(50):1247–56.
7. Rivers CM. Ebola: Models do more than forecast. *Nature*. 2014; 515(7528):492.
8. Li SL, Bjørnstad ON, Ferrari MJ, et al. Essential information: Uncertainty and optimal control of Ebola outbreaks. *Proc Natl Acad Sci U S A*. 2017;114(22):5659–64.
9. Butler D. Models overestimate Ebola cases. *Nat News*. 2014;515(7525):18.
10. CDC Division of Preparedness and Emerging Infections. Published Models and Tools; 2018. https://www.cdc.gov/ncezid/dpei/hemu/published-models-tools.html. Accessed Feb. 14, 2020.
11. Fischer LS, Santibanez S, Hatchett RJ, et al. CDC grand rounds: Modeling and public health decision-making. *MMWR Morb Mort Wkly Rep*. 2016;65(48):1374–7.
12. Reich NG, Brooks LC, Fox SJ, et al. A collaborative multiyear, multimodel assessment of seasonal influenza forecasting in the United States. *Proc Natl Acad Sci U S A*. 2019;116(8):3146–54.
13. Lutz CS, Huynh MP, Schroeder M, et al. Applying infectious disease forecasting to public health: A path forward using influenza forecasting examples. *BMC Public Health*. 2019;19(1):1659.
14. Date KA, Vicari A, Hyde TB, et al. Considerations for oral cholera vaccine use during outbreak after earthquake in Haiti, 2010–2011. *Emerg Infect Dis*. 2011;17(11):2105.
15. Castro LA, Fox SJ, Chen X, et al. Assessing real-time Zika risk in the United States. *BMC Infect Dis*. 2017;17(1):284.
16. Gicquelais RE, Foxman B, Coyle J, Eisenberg MC. Hepatitis C transmission in young people who inject drugs: Insights using a dynamic model informed by state public health surveillance. *Epidemics*. 2019;27:86–95.
17. Fraser C, Donnelly CA, Cauchemez S, et al. Pandemic potential of a strain of influenza A (H1N1): Early findings. *Science*. 2009;324(5934):1557–61.
18. Bernoulli D. Essai D'une nouvelle analyse de la mortalite cause par la petite verole et des a vantages de Finoculation pour la prevenir. *Mem Math Phys Acad Roy Sci*. 1766;1.
19. Dietz K, Heesterbeek J. Daniel Bernoulli's epidemiological model revisited. *Math Biosci*. 2002;180(1–2):1–21.
20. Colombo C, Diamanti M. The smallpox vaccine: The dispute between Bernoulli and d'Alembert and the calculus of probabilities. *Lett Mate*. 2015;2(4):185–92.
21. Kermack WO, McKendrick AG. A contribution to the mathematical theory of epidemics. *Proc R Soc Lond A*. 1927;115(772):700–21.
22. Abbey H. An examination of the Reed-Frost theory of epidemics. *Hum Biol*. 1952;24(3):201. Last updated—Feb. 24, 2013.
23. Anderson RM, May RM. *Infectious Diseases of Humans: Dynamics and Control*. Oxford: Oxford University Press; 1992.
24. Stewart J. *Single Variable Calculus: Early Transcendentals*. Boston, MA: Cengage Learning; 2015.
25. Diekmann O, Heesterbeek JA, Metz JA. On the definition and the computation of the basic reproduction ratio R_0 in models for infectious diseases in heterogeneous populations. *J Math Biol*. 1990;28(4):365–82.
26. Heesterbeek J, Dietz K. The concept of R_0 in epidemic theory. *Stat Neerl*. 1996;50(1):89–110.
27. Van Den Driessche P, Watmough J. Reproduction numbers and sub-threshold endemic equilibria for compartmental models of disease transmission. *Math Biosci*. 2002;180:29–48.
28. Diekmann O, Heesterbeek JAP, Roberts MG. The construction of next-generation matrices for compartmental epidemic models. *J R Soc Interface*. 2010;7(47):873–85.
29. Fine PE. Herd immunity: History, theory, practice. *Epidemiol Rev*. 1993;15(2):265–302.
30. Ma J, Earn DJD. Generality of the final size formula for an epidemic of a newly invading infectious disease. *Bull Math Biol*. 2006;68(3):679–702.
31. Miller JC. A note on the derivation of epidemic final sizes. *Bull Math Biol*. 2012;74(9):2125–41.
32. Dub´e E, Gagnon D, Nickels E, Jeram S, Schuster M. Mapping vaccine hesitancy—Country-specific characteristics of a global phenomenon. *Vaccine*. 2014;32(49):6649–54.
33. Lo NC, Hotez PJ. Public health and economic consequences of vaccine hesitancy for measles in the United States. *JAMA Pediatr*. 2017;171(9): 887–92.
34. Mellerson JL, Maxwell CB, Knighton CL, Kriss JL, Seither R, Black CL. Vaccination coverage for selected vaccines and exemption rates among children in kindergarten—United States, 2017–18 School Year. *MMWR Morb Mortal Wkly Rep*. 2018;67(40):1115.
35. Peeples L. Rethinking herd immunity. *Nat Med*. 2019;25(8):1178.
36. Heffernan J, Keeling M. Implications of vaccination and waning immunity. *Proc Biol Sci*. 2009;276(1664):2071–80.
37. Sartwell PE. The distribution of incubation periods of infectious diseases. *Am J Hyg*. 1950;51(3):310–8.
38. Brauer F, van den Driessche P, Wu J, eds. Mathematical epidemiology. *Lecture Notes in Mathematics*. Vol. 1945. Berlin, Heidelberg: Springer; 2008.
39. D'Silva JP, Eisenberg MC. Modeling spatial invasion of Ebola in West Africa. *J Theor Biol*. 2017;428(7):65–75.
40. Hyman JM, Li J, Stanley EA. The differential infectivity and staged progression models for the transmission of HIV. *Math Biosci*. 1999;155(2):77–109.

41. Fauci AS, Pantaleo G, Stanley S, Weissman D. Immunopathogenic mechanisms of HIV infection. *Ann Intern Med.* 1996;124(7):654–63.
42. Scott S, Duncan CJ. *Human Demography and Disease.* Cambridge: Cambridge University Press; 2005.
43. Dietz K, Hadeler KP. Epidemiological models for sexually transmitted diseases. *J Math Biol.* 1988;26(1):1–25.
44. Morris M, Kurth AE, Hamilton DT, Moody J, Wakefield S. Concurrent partnerships and HIV prevalence disparities by race: Linking science and public health practice. *Am J Public Health.* 2009;99(6):1023–31.
45. Mossong J, Hens N, Jit M, et al. Social contacts and mixing patterns relevant to the spread of infectious diseases. *PLoS Med.* 2008;5(3):0381–91.
46. Yamin D, Jones FK, DeVincenzo JP, et al. Vaccination strategies against respiratory syncytial virus. *Proc Natl Acad Sci U S A.* 2016;113(46):13239–44.
47. Keeling MJ, Rohani P. Estimating spatial coupling in epidemiological systems: A mechanistic approach. *Ecol Lett.* 2002;5(1):20–9.
48. Arino J, Van den Driessche P. A multi-city epidemic model. *Math Popul Stud.* 2003;10(3):175–93.
49. Arino J. Diseases in metapopulations. *Modeling and Dynamics of Infectious Diseases.* Beijing: World Scientific Publisher, Higher Ed. Press; 2009:64–122.
50. Truscott J, Ferguson NM. Evaluating the adequacy of gravity models as a description of human mobility for epidemic modelling. *PLoS Comput Biol.* 2012;8(10):e1002699.
51. Balcan D, Gonçalves B, Hu H, Ramasco JJ, Colizza V, Vespignani A. Modeling the spatial spread of infectious diseases: The GLobal Epidemic and Mobility computational model. *J Comput Sci.* 2010;1(3):132–45.
52. Lawyer G. Measuring the potential of individual airports for pandemic spread over the world airline network. *BMC Infect Dis.* 2015;16(1):70.
53. Tizzoni M, Bajardi P, Decuyper A, et al. On the use of human mobility proxies for modeling epidemics. *PLoS Comput Biol.* 2014;10(7):e1003716.
54. Wesolowski A, Stresman G, Eagle N, et al. Quantifying travel behavior for infectious disease research: A comparison of data from surveys and mobile phones. *Sci Rep.* 2014;4:5678.
55. Wesolowski A, Eagle N, Tatem AJ, et al. Quantifying the impact of human mobility on malaria. *Science.* 2012;338(6104):267–70.
56. Dalziel BD, Pourbohloul B, Ellner SP. Human mobility patterns predict divergent epidemic dynamics among cities. *Proc Biol Sci.* 2013;280(1766):20130763.
57. Kraay ANMM, Trostle J, Brouwer AF, Cevallos W, Eisenberg JNSS. Determinants of short-term movement in a developing region and implications for disease transmission. *Epidemiology.* 2018;29(1):117–25.
58. Tuite AR, Tien J, Eisenberg M, Earn DJDD, Ma J, Fisman DN. Cholera epidemic in Haiti, 2010: Using a transmission model to explain spatial spread of disease and identify optimal control interventions. *Ann Intern Med.* 2011;154(9):593–601.
59. Rinaldo A, Bertuzzo E, Mari L, et al. Reassessment of the 2010–2011 Haiti cholera outbreak and rainfall-driven multiseason projections. *Proc Natl Acad Sci U S A.* 2012;109(17):6602–7.
60. Havumaki J, Meza R, Phares CR, Date K, Eisenberg MC. Comparing alternative cholera vaccination strategies in Maela refugee camp: Using a transmission model in public health practice. *BMC Infect Dis.* 2019;19(1):1–17.
61. Capasso V, Paveri-Fontana S. A mathematical model for the 1973 cholera epidemic in the European Mediterranean region. *Rev Epidemiol Sante Publique.* 1979;27(2):121–32.
62. Mukandavire Z, Liao S, Wang J, Gaff H, Smith DL, Morris JG. Estimating the reproductive numbers for the 2008–2009 cholera outbreaks in Zimbabwe. *Proc Natl Acad Sci U S A.* 2011;108(21):8767–72.
63. Reiner RC, King AA, Emch M, Yunus M, Faruque A, Pascual M. Highly localized sensitivity to climate forcing drives endemic cholera in a megacity. *Proc Natl Acad Sci.* 2012;109(6):2033–6.
64. Phares CR, Date K, Travers P, et al. Mass vaccination with a two-dose oral cholera vaccine in a long-standing refugee camp, Thailand. *Vaccine.* 2016;34(1):128–33.
65. Scobie HM, Phares CR, Wannemuehler KA, et al. Use of oral cholera vaccine and knowledge, attitudes, and practices regarding safe water, sanitation and hygiene in a long-standing refugee camp, Thailand, 2012–2014. *PLoS Negl Trop Dis.* 2016;10(12):e0005210.
66. Chick SE, Koopman JS, Soorapanth S, Brown ME. Infection transmission system models for microbial risk assessment. *Sci Total Environ.* 2001;274(1–3):197–207.
67. Li S, Spicknall IH, Koopman JS, Eisenberg JNS. Dynamics and control of infections transmitted from person to person through the environment. *Am J Epidemiol.* 2009;170(2):257–65.
68. Tien JH, Earn DJD. Multiple transmission pathways and disease dynamics in a waterborne pathogen model. *Bull Math Biol.* 2010;72(6):1506–33.
69. Brouwer AF, Weir MH, Eisenberg MC, et al. 2017 B. Dose-response relationships for environmentally mediated infectious disease transmission models. *PLoS Comput Biol.* 2017;13(4):e1005481.
70. Cortez MH, Weitz JS. Distinguishing between indirect and direct modes of transmission using epidemiological time series. *Am Nat.* 2013;181(2):E43–54.
71. Brouwer AF, Eisenberg MC, Remais JV, Collender PA, Meza R, Eisenberg JNS. Modeling biphasic environmental decay of pathogens and implications for risk analysis. *Environ Sci Technol.* 2017;51(4):2186–96.
72. Brouwer AF, Eisenberg MC, Love NG, Eisenberg JNS. Phenotypic variations in persistence and infectivity between and within environmentally transmitted pathogen populations impact population-level epidemic dynamics. *BMC Infect Dis.* 2019;19(1):449.
73. Codeço CT. Endemic and epidemic dynamics of cholera: The role of the aquatic reservoir. *BMC Infect Dis.* 2001;1(1):1.
74. Eisenberg MC, Robertson SL, Tien JH. Identifiability and estimation of multiple transmission pathways in cholera and waterborne disease. *J Theor Biol.* 2013;324:84–102.
75. Campbell-Lendrum D, Manga L, Bagayoko M, Sommerfeld J. Climate change and vector-borne diseases: What are the implications for public health research and policy? *Philos Trans R Soc Lond B Biol Sci.* 2015;370(1665):20130552.
76. Parham PE, Waldock J, Christophides GK, et al. Climate, environmental and socio-economic change: Weighing up the balance in vector-borne disease transmission. *Philos Trans R Soc Lond B Biol Sci.* 2015;370(1665):20130551.
77. Levy K, Woster AP, Goldstein RS, Carlton EJ. Untangling the impacts of climate change on waterborne diseases: A systematic review of relationships between diarrheal diseases and temperature, rainfall, flooding, and drought. *Environ Sci Technol.* 2016;50(10):4905–22.
78. World Health Organization. Vector-borne diseases; 2017.
79. Beard CB, Eisen R, Barker C, et al. Ch. 5: Vectorborne diseases. US Global Change Research Program, Washington, DC; 2016.
80. Brauer F, van den Driessche P, Wu J. *Lecture Notes in Mathematical Epidemiology.* Berlin, Germany: Springer; 2008.
81. Nishiura H, et al. Mathematical and statistical analyses of the spread of Dengue. WHO Regional Office for South-East Asia. 2006. https://apps.who.int/iris/handle/10665/170261.
82. Gao D, Lou Y, He D, et al. Prevention and control of Zika as a mosquito-borne and sexually transmitted disease: A mathematical modeling analysis. *Sci Rep.* 2016;6:28070.
83. Kao YH, Eisenberg MC. Practical unidentifiability of a simple vector-borne disease model: Implications for parameter estimation and intervention assessment. *Epidemics.* 2018;25:89–100.
84. Caminade C, Turner J, Metelmann S, et al. Global risk model for vector-borne transmission of Zika virus reveals the role of El Nino 2015. *Proc Natl Acad Sci.* 2017;114(1):119–24.
85. Cauchemez S, Besnard M, Bompard P, et al. Association between Zika virus and microcephaly in French Polynesia, 2013–15: A retrospective study. *Lancet.* 2016;387(10033):2125–32.
86. Christofferson RC, Mores CN, Wearing HJ. Bridging the gap between experimental data and model parameterization for chikungunya virus transmission predictions. *J Infect Dis.* 2016;214(suppl 5):S466–70.
87. Manore CA, Hickmann KS, Xu S, Wearing HJ, Hyman JM. Comparing dengue and chikungunya emergence and endemic transmission in *A. aegypti* and *A. albopictus. J Theor Biol.* 2014;356:174–91.
88. Wearing HJ, Rohani P. Ecological and immunological determinants of dengue epidemics. *Proc Natl Acad Sci U S A.* 2006;103(31):11802–7.
89. Tsang TK, Ghebremariam SL, Gresh L, et al. Effects of infection history on dengue virus infection and pathogenicity. *Nat Commun.* 2019;10(1):1–9.
90. Altizer S, Dobson A, Hosseini P, Hudson P, Pascual M, Rohani P. Seasonality and the dynamics of infectious diseases. *Ecol Lett.* 2006;9(4):467–84.
91. Bauch CT, Earn DJ. Vaccination and the theory of games. *Proc Natl Acad Sci.* 2004;101(36):13391–94.
92. Reluga TC. Game theory of social distancing in response to an epidemic. *PLoS Comput Biol.* 2010;6(5):e1000793.
93. Conrad JR, Xue L, Dewar J, Hyman JM. Modeling the impact of behavior change on the spread of Ebola. *Mathematical and Statistical Modeling for Emerging and Re-emerging Infectious Diseases.* New York: Springer; 2016:5–23.
94. Hayashi MA, Eisenberg MC, Eisenberg JN. Linking decision theory and quantitative microbial risk assessment: Tradeoffs between compliance and efficacy for waterborne disease interventions. *Risk Anal.* 2019;39(10):2214–26.

95. Ross EL, Cinti SK, Hutton DW. Implementation and operational research: A cost-effective, clinically actionable strategy for targeting HIV preexposure prophylaxis to high-risk men who have sex with men. *J Acquir Immune Defic Syndr*. 2016;72(3):e61–7.
96. Ahituv A, Hotz VJ, Philipson T. The responsiveness of the demand for condoms to the local prevalence of AIDS. *J Hum Resour*. 1996:869–97.
97. Bankole A, Darroch JE, Singh S. Determinants of trends in condom use in the United States, 1988–1995. *Fam Plann Perspect*. 1999:264–71.
98. Hayashi MA, Eisenberg MC. Effects of adaptive protective behavior on the dynamics of sexually transmitted infections. *J Theor Biol*. 2016;388:119–30.
99. Halloran ME, Longini IM. Emerging, evolving, and established infectious diseases and interventions. *Science*. 2014;345(6202):1292–4.
100. d'Onofrio A. Stability properties of pulse vaccination strategy in SEIR epidemic model. *Math Biosci*. 2002;179(1):57–72.
101. Yan X, Zou Y. Optimal and sub-optimal quarantine and isolation control in SARS epidemics. *Math Comput Model*. 2008;47(1-2):235–45.
102. Huo HF, Chen R, Wang XY. Modelling and stability of HIV/AIDS epidemic model with treatment. *Appl Math Model*. 2016;40(13-14):6550–9.
103. Kraay AN, Hayashi MA, Hernandez-Ceron N, et al. Fomitemediated transmission as a sufficient pathway: A comparative analysis across three viral pathogens. *BMC Infect Dis*. 2018;18(1):540.
104. Siebert U, Alagoz O, Bayoumi AM, et al. State-transition modeling: A report of the ISPOR-SMDM modeling good research practices task force–3. *Med Decis Making*. 2012;32(5):690–700.
105. Zelner J, Adams C, Havumaki J, Lopman B. Understanding the importance of contact heterogeneity and variable infectiousness in the dynamics of a large Norovirus outbreak. *Clin Infect Dis*. 2020;70(3):493–500.
106. Cooper BS, Stone S, Kibbler C, et al. Systematic review of isolation policies in the hospital management of methicillin-resistant Staphylococcus aureus: A review of the literature with epidemiological and economic modelling. *Health Technol Assess*. 2003;7(39):1–194.
107. Lloyd-Smith JO, Schreiber SJ, Kopp PE, Getz WM. Superspreading and the effect of individual variation on disease emergence. *Nature*. 2005;438(7066):355–9.
108. Lau MS, Dalziel BD, Funk S, et al. Spatial and temporal dynamics of superspreading events in the 2014–2015 West Africa Ebola epidemic. *Proc Natl Acad Sci*. 2017;114(9):2337–42.
109. Blumberg S, Enanoria WT, Lloyd-Smith JO, Lietman TM, Porco TC. Identifying postelimination trends for the introduction and transmissibility of measles in the United States. *Am J Epidemiol*. 2014;179(11):1375–82.
110. Zelner J, Adams C, Havumaki J, Lopman B. Understanding the importance of contact heterogeneity and variable infectiousness in the dynamics of a large norovirus outbreak. *Clin Infect Dis*. 2020;70(3):493–500.
111. Ypma RJF, Korthals Altes H, van Soolingen D, Wallinga J, van Ballegooijen WM. A sign of suprespreading in tuberculosis: Highly skewed distribution of genotypic cluster sizes. *Epidemiology*. 2013;24(3):395–400.
112. Stimson J, Gardy J, Mathema B, Crudu V, Cohen T, Colijn C. Beyond the SNP threshold: Identifying outbreak clusters using inferred transmissions. *Mol Biol Evol*. 2019;36(3):587–603.
113. Volz EM, Pond SLK, Ward MJ, Brown AJL, Frost SD. Phylodynamics of infectious disease epidemics. *Genetics*. 2009;183(4):1421–30.
114. Kretzschmar M, Gomes MGM, Coutinho RA, Koopman JS. Unlocking pathogen genotyping information for public health by mathematical modeling. *Trends Microbiol*. 2010;18(9):406–12.
115. Volz EM, Ionides E, Romero-Severson EO, Brandt MG, Mokotoff E, Koopman JS. HIV-1 transmission during early infection in men who have sex with men: A phylodynamic analysis. *PLoS Med*. 2013;10(12):e1001568.
116. Newman ME. Spread of epidemic disease on networks. *Phys Rev E*. 2002;66(1):016128.
117. Newman M. *Networks*. Oxford: Oxford University Press; 2018.
118. Vespignani A. Twenty years of network science. *Nature*. 2018;558(7711):528–9.
119. Meyers LA, Pourbohloul B, Newman ME, Skowronski DM, Brunham RC. Network theory and SARS: Predicting outbreak diversity. *J Theor Biol*. 2005;232(1):71–81.
120. Liu QH, Ajelli M, Aleta A, Merler S, Moreno Y, Vespignani A. Measurability of the epidemic reproduction number in data-driven contact networks. *Proc Natl Acad Sci*. 2018;115(50):12680–5.
121. Colizza V, Barrat A, Barthelemy M, Valleron AJ, Vespignani A. Modeling the worldwide spread of pandemic influenza: Baseline case and containment interventions. *PLoS Med*. 2007;4(1):e13.
122. Tracy M, Cerda M, Keyes KM. Agent-based modeling in public health: Current applications and future directions. *Annu Rev Public Health*. 2018;39:77–94.
123. Hammond RA. Considerations and best practices in agent-based modeling to inform policy. *Assessing the Use of Agent-Based Models for Tobacco Regulation*. Washington, DC: National Academies Press (US); 2015.
124. Merler S, Ajelli M, Fumanelli L, et al. Spatiotemporal spread of the 2014 outbreak of Ebola virus disease in Liberia and the effectiveness of non-pharmaceutical interventions: A computational modelling analysis. *Lancet Infect Dis*. 2015;15(2):204–11.
125. Sadique MZ, Edmunds WJ, Smith RD, et al. Precautionary behavior in response to perceived threat of pandemic influenza. *Emerg Infect Dis*. 2007;13(9):1307–13.
126. Halloran ME, Ferguson NM, Eubank S, et al. Modeling targeted layered containment of an influenza pandemic in the United States. *Proc Natl Acad Sci*. 2008;105(12):4639–44.
127. Eubank S, Guclu H, Kumar VA, et al. Modelling disease outbreaks in realistic urban social networks. *Nature*. 2004;429(6988):180–4.
128. Epstein JM. Modelling to contain pandemics. *Nature*. 2009;460(7256):687.
129. van Kleef E, Robotham JV, Jit M, Deeny SR, Edmunds WJ. Modelling the transmission of healthcare associated infections: A systematic review. *BMC Infect Dis*. 2013;13(1):294.
130. Lee BY, McGlone SM, Wong KF, et al. Modeling the spread of methicillinresistant Staphylococcus aureus (MRSA) outbreaks throughout the hospitals in Orange County, California. *Infect Control Hosp Epidemiol*. 2011;32(6):562–72.
131. Lee BY, Yilmaz SL, Wong KF, et al. Modeling the regional spread and control of vancomycin-resistant enterococci. *Am J Infect Control*. 2013;41(8):668–73.
132. Cornforth DM, Reluga TC, Shim E, Bauch CT, Galvani AP, Meyers LA. Erratic flu vaccination emerges from short-sighted behavior in contact networks. *PLoS Comput Biol*. 2011;7(1):e1001062.
133. Buttenheim AM, Asch DA. Making vaccine refusal less of a free ride. *Hum Vaccin Immunother*. 2013;9(12):2674–5.
134. Manor Y, Shulman LM, Kaliner E, et al. Intensified environmental surveillance supporting the response to wild poliovirus type 1 silent circulation in Israel, 2013. *Euro Surveill*. 2014;19(7):20708.
135. Brouwer AF, Eisenberg JNS, Pomeroy CD, et al. Epidemiology of the silent polio outbreak in Rahat, Israel, based on modeling of environmental surveillance data. *Proc Natl Acad Sci*. 2018;115(45):E10625–33.
136. Smith RC. *Uncertainty Quantification: Theory, Implementation, and Applications*. Vol. 12. Philadelphia, PA: SIAM; 2013.

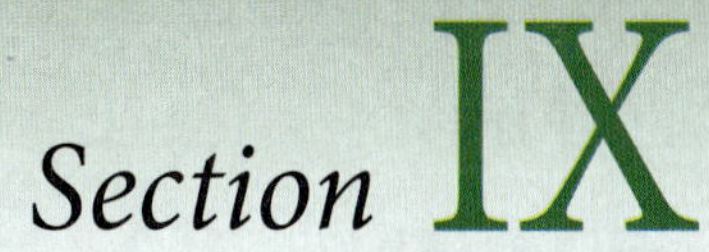

Section Editor
Sandro Galea

Mental Health and Substance Use

CHAPTER

160 Developmental Disabilities

Nigel Paneth

INTRODUCTION

The human species is altricial in comparison to other large mammals, including large primates, and has only a modest supply of motor and cognitive skills at birth. The anatomic substrates of cognition, behavior, and movement are largely set down in utero, but their full functional expression takes many years. Alterations in patterns of in-utero brain development, whether fashioned by genetic abnormalities, by damage from environmental exposures, or by the interaction of these two forces, can damage this anatomic substrate without altering early developmental trajectories in any substantial way. Children born lacking major cortical structures, as in hydranencephaly, are often incapable of expressing the full repertoire of typical human newborn behavior.[1]

Disorders of development, which by convention refer nearly exclusively to development of the nervous system, are thus almost never diagnosed at birth, but are recognized when milestones expected of typical human behavior are not met. Unlike diagnostic categories in adults, or those involving organ systems in children that do not have as prolonged a postnatal developmental trajectory as the brain, recognition of developmental disorders, and assessment of their impact on the child, is entirely age dependent. Widely used measures such as IQ have no real meaning until at least early childhood, and the firm diagnosis of cerebral palsy (CP) requires a child to be at least 18–24 months old. Learning disabilities, by definition, cannot be diagnosed until school age.

The topic of this chapter is developmental *disabilities*. As is appropriate for a text-book of public health, the focus of this chapter is on those developmental disorders that are not just present, but that are disabling, meaning that they exact a price in terms of human functionality, that represent a personal, familial, and societal burden, and that require a substantial investment of familial and societal resources for their amelioration and prevention. Thus, I exclude from consideration in this chapter a number of disorders of development that do not reach the threshold of having public health implications, either because of their rarity or because they do not convey major disability to affected individuals. I focus on six disorders, three of which (severe intellectual disability [ID], autism spectrum disorder [ASD], and CP) are clearly disabling, while the other three (mild ID, learning disability [LD], and attention deficit/hyperactivity disorder [ADHD]) occur with relatively high frequency in the population, and interfere in a measurable way with quality of life.[2,3]

One way of looking at developmental disabilities is to distinguish the conditions that are rare and severe, and those that are fairly common and present somewhat fewer difficulties to affected individuals and their families. CP and severe ID together rarely exceed a prevalence of 5–6/1000 live births, but, as will be detailed below, they entail heavy burdens in terms of medical expenditure, family caregiving needs, and foregone earnings. ASD is more common, perhaps affecting as many as 1–1.5% of the population, and also carries a substantial burden at the severe end of the spectrum where it is often comorbid with ID. The three less severe disabilities, mild ID, ADHD, and LD are not at all rare. As many as 10–15% of U.S. children have one or more of these disabilities.

If all developmental disabilities are added together, the size of the public health burden becomes evident. In the United States, at least one in six children, and perhaps as many as one in five, has a diagnosed or diagnosable developmental disability. And many of these children grow up to be adults with disabilities. Estimates of the current U.S. prevalence rates in childhood of each of the conditions under consideration are provided in Table 160-1.

A socioeconomic gradient in the three severe conditions exists, but it is not very marked. CP has been found to be somewhat more common in low-income settings,[4,5] while ASD, if anything, may be diagnosed more frequently in affluent families, as shown, for example, by the higher prevalence in U.S. non-Hispanic White children than in non-Hispanic Black and Hispanic children.[6] But all three of the milder conditions have pronounced social class gradients, as will be detailed below, with poverty and resource lack prominent as risk factors, most notably for mild ID. To illustrate this epidemiologic distinction between the two sets of disabilities, in a study of more than a third of a million linked birth-education records in Florida, low SES was associated with a 1.8 relative risk of profound ID, a 2.5 relative risk of moderate to severe ID, but an 8.9 relative risk of mild ID.[7]

This chapter focuses largely on the situation in higher income countries with the resources to offer prenatal and neonatal screening programs, perinatal medical care, early educational interventions, appropriate immunizations, effective diets, and other benefits that can reduce the overall burden of developmental disabilities. Needless to say, such programs are lacking in many parts of the globe.

TABLE 160-1 ESTIMATES OF THE PREVALENCE OF DEVELOPMENTAL DISABILITIES IN THE UNITED STATES

Disability	Prevalence
Severe intellectual disability	3–5 per 1000 live births
Mild intellectual disability	1–1.7% of the child population
Autism spectrum disorder	Between 1% and 1.5% of U.S. children now carry the diagnostic label of ASD
Cerebral palsy	1.5–4 per 1000 live births
Attention deficit/hyperactivity disorder	5–7%
Learning disabilities	9–10%
Total (allowing for overlap among disabilities)	15–20%

In addition, a range of insults infrequently encountered in high-income countries can lead to impairments of cognitive and behavioral function in resource-poor locations. The overall situation for developmental disabilities in lower income countries is not fully understood. On the one hand, a range of exposures that can damage the prenatal and infant brain (such as cerebral malaria) are more common in low-income countries, but on the other hand, early mortality is high. The consensus, however, is that several of the disorders reviewed in this chapter are considerably commoner in low-income countries.[8,9]

OVERVIEW OF THE DEVELOPMENTAL DISABILITIES

Terminology

The language used to describe the developmental disabilities is complex and changing. In part this is due to the evolving sensibilities of our culture. The term "*mental retardation*" was introduced in the early twentieth century to humanely replace categorizations of cognitive dysfunction used by professionals such as "*imbecile*" and "*idiot*," as recently as the 1960s.[10] But the term mental retardation has in turn been replaced. The most prominent U.S. advocacy organization for people with developmental disorders of intellectual function was named, in 1953, *The National Association for Retarded Children (NARC)*. In 1973 the C in the acronym came to stand for *Citizens*, and in 1992, the organization become known as *The ARC for People with Intellectual and Developmental Disabilities*.[11] In 2010, federal legislation required removal of the term "*mental retardation*" from federal records, replacing it with "*intellectual disability*,"[12] a usage adopted in 2013 in the fifth edition of *The Diagnostic and Statistical Manual of Mental Disorders*.[13] The term "*cognitive impairment*" has also been applied to developmental disorders, but since this term is widely used to describe a common disorder of elderly adults, and because impairment, unlike disability, does not imply problems in functioning, the term *intellectual disability* (ID) is the one I will use in this chapter.

The term autism has also undergone considerable mutation, but for other reasons. Originally viewed as describing a rare and distinct disorder of communication and interpersonal interaction, with variable levels of associated ID,[14] the term has been expanded to include groups of people with behavioral disorders of lesser severity, and also to include other individuals formerly classified by their cognitive, rather than their behavioral disability. A milder form of behavioral difficulty, described at about the same time as autism,[15] came to be called "*Asperger's syndrome*" and was incorporated into the fourth edition of the DSM in 1994,[16] only to be removed from the fifth edition in 2013,[13] which incorporated all forms of autism and autism-like conditions into the broad term "*autism spectrum disorders (ASD)*."

CP, the major neurodevelopmental disorder, is for the most part excluded from consideration by the several editions of DSM, and perhaps therefore has retained more stability in nomenclature and usage. CP, however, at times presents difficulties in diagnosis, largely at the milder end, and with younger children, where atypical motor signs and reflexes can suggest CP, but subsequent development shows otherwise. Moreover, the term CP is an inaccurate descriptor of the condition, since palsy means paralysis, or inability to move, a finding rarely present in this disorder. That this term, which dates back to the nineteenth century, has survived to the present day, no doubt reflects widespread public recognition of the term CP.

Considerable effort was put into a 2005[17] (updated in 2007[18]) re-definition and re-classification of CP by an international committee which resolved a number of difficulties, including providing a clearer separation of progressive genetic disorders with motor dysfunction from CP; a requirement for evidence of disability for the diagnosis to be made; and recognition that since brain imaging studies have shown that CP can be due to cerebral anomalies, especially migration disorders, that exclusion of malformations from the rubric is no longer justified.

Recognition that some children did poorly in school in spite of apparently typical cognitive and behavioral skills was late in coming; only a handful of references to "learning disability" can be found in PUBMED prior to 1970. Social and cultural forces were influential, particularly their influence on legislation affecting schools. The first guarantee of public education to children with disabilities of any kind in the United States was the 1975 *Education of All Handicapped Children Act (Public Law 94-142)*, which focused largely on children who had been segregated from mainstream public education, largely those with severe CP and/or ID. The 1994 reworking of that act, renamed the *Individuals with Disabilities Education Act (IDEA)*, and especially the 2004 update, expanded the scope of the guarantee of appropriate and targeted public education to children who were not doing well in school, even if they did not have a diagnosis of a developmental disability.

In parallel, educators and healthcare providers came to recognize that an entity existed that caused difficulties in learning in children with apparently normal cognitive function. The term *learning disability* was coined to describe this entity, originally as a single diagnosis, but later formulated as a family of *specific learning disabilities* (e.g., *dyscalculia and dyslexia*) whose names indicate the specific deficit that impairs learning.

Attention deficit/hyperactivity disorder evolved from another cause of school difficulties, initially referred to as *hyperactivity*, which only came to be viewed as a disorder in the 1960s. The availability of effective treatment, in the form of methylphenidate, increased the extent of diagnosis, but with enormous variability in practice. DSM II (1968)[19] refers briefly to *hyperkinetic reaction of childhood*, which is described as "*characterized by overactivity, restlessness, distractibility, and short attention span*." Recognition that failure of focused attention was the central feature of this condition led the authors of DSM—III (1980) to move away from the centrality of hyperactivity by naming the entity *attention deficit disorder (ADD) (with or without hyperactivity)*. A compromise between the two features was reached in DSM-IV (1994), which coined the term in current use *attention deficit/hyperactivity disorder*.

Epidemiologic Considerations

For two related reasons, epidemiologists who study the developmental disorders generally use the term prevalence rate and not incidence rate to describe the frequency of these conditions. The first reason is that these disabilities are generally once-only disorders whose origins are prenatal or in early childhood. The severe disabilities are generally lifelong. The less severe disabilities—ADHD and learning disorders—may in some sense be viewed as curable, but not as recurrent. Thus, there is only one period of risk—early development—and by the time the disorder is diagnosed, that period is over.

When the frequency of a developmental disability is denominatored to children of the same age in the same population, it is evident that one is describing a prevalence figure obtained from cross-sectional data. Somewhat subtler is the use of prevalence when live births are the denominator, the latter a common practice. But since the number of births does not give a formal indication of time, that denominator cannot be viewed as a form of person-years at risk, as in incidence. The risk of CP, say, is no different if expressed per thousand births that took place over 1 year or over 5 years.

The social nexus in many which developmental disabilities are found makes uncovering environmental influences difficult, because confounding is hard to exclude. Both lead ingestion and IQ are strongly linked to socioeconomic status, and thus separating the effects of lead from the effects of social context in which lead exposure occurs is challenging.

Cause and effect can be difficult to separate in a situation where both the disorder and the risk factor are in dynamic competition. Thus, lead exposure may lead to intellectual impairment, but children with ID are more likely to ingest lead. Similarly, a concussion history was found more commonly in adolescents with learning disabilities and/or attention deficit/hyperactivity disorder, suggesting a causal role for head injury in these disabilities. But the time order suggested that in some cases the disabilities preceded the concussions and may indeed have predisposed to them.[20]

Impact on Society

An important feature of the developmental disabilities is their disproportionate impact on families, and thus on society, as compared to their frequency. In developed countries, the formerly high mortality rate in infancy and childhood of the severely disabled has largely been eliminated, and developmental disorders have become lifelong conditions in the past half-century. Most affected individuals will have a normal or close to normal life span.[21,22]

Nearly all of the premature loss of life in children with severe CP and/or ID occurs in the first year or so of life, before the age at which these diagnoses are usually made. Thus, these deaths are to children thought probably to have these disorders, either because of their evident severity or their association with conditions, such as some chromosomal disorders, where the prevalence of developmental disability is nearly universal. But because their deaths occur before the condition can be formally diagnosed, they are rarely included in prevalence figures.

Severe ID in a child creates care burdens similar to those of Alzheimer's disease (AD) in the elderly, but the mean time between AD diagnosis and death is 3–5 years,[23] whereas survival is now very much longer among people with severe ID. Estimates of the lifelong costs—both direct medical and educational costs, and indirect costs from loss of productivity to the affected individual and to his or her parents—were estimated in the first decade of the twenty-first century in the United States to be just under $1 million[24] for each case of CP, and above $1M for each case of ID.[25] A U.S. estimate from 2014 puts the lifetime cost of autism at between $1.2 and $2.4 million, depending on the absence or presence of associated ID.[26]

In addition, the burden on families is very substantial, frequently causing sleep disruption and depression in mothers,[27] and often altering life trajectories for family members, by reducing maternal employment and family income.[28] Thus, the developmental disabilities are an important public health priority, especially since several prevention modalities are available, as outlined below.

The commoner disabilities also carry burdens, and these are often felt by the broader society. Of particular concern to young adults with any of the three conditions are the reduction in educational opportunities; the burden of unemployment; and the increased risk of incarceration and involvement with the criminal justice system.

Individuals with DD, both as children and adults, face substantial barriers in obtaining healthcare,[29] including mental healthcare.[30] Fragmentation of care is the rule rather than the exception. Developmental disabilities can present obstacles to the communication of symptoms to health providers, and to the assessment and recognition of signs of illness. A recent issue of the journal Psychiatric Quarterly was devoted to mental health problems in DD.[31] Aggressive behaviors are often the first behavioral issue to be noted in people with DD, both self-injury and mutilation (as in the Lesch-Nyhan syndrome[32]) and aggression toward others. The latter can exert a major toll in terms of social isolation, need for psychotropic medication, or even physical constraint.[33] However, mood disorders have been identified as the commonest problem affecting people with DD.[34] Anxiety is also commonly found in people with DD,[35] but frank psychosis is unusual.

A common dual diagnosis, of public health importance because of its frequency, is the combination of ADHD and substance abuse disorder, with some 20–30% of people with opiate dependency having ADHD.[36–38] Concern has been expressed that use of stimulant medication in ADHD may be abused, and may even predispose to substance abuse. In Norway, stimulant medication is proscribed in individuals with both opiate dependence and ADHD.[39]

THE MAJOR DISABILITIES OF COGNITION AND BEHAVIOR

Intellectual Disability

Definition

ID is defined first, by results of IQ tests, and second, by evidence that the tested child indeed has difficulties in adapting to societal expectations, especially in relation to school. Individuals with IQs more than 2 standard deviations below the mean, or below 70 for tests with a mean of 100 and a standard deviation of 15, are considered to have ID. The International Classification of Disease, Ninth Edition, Clinical Modification (ICD-9-CM) categorizes ID as mild (IQ of 50–70), moderate (IQ of 35–49), severe (an IQ of 20–34), or profound (IQ of < 20). It is also common to see ID more simply categorized as severe when IQ is below 50. It must also be shown that the affected individual has difficulties with age-appropriate tasks that require cognitive input. Individuals with IQs between one and two standard deviations below the population mean (70–85) have sometimes been labeled as having "*borderline intellectual dysfunction*"[40] but there is not yet strong evidence that this entity is a stable enough or severe enough to be considered a developmental disability.

Prevalence and Time Trends

The epidemiology of severe ID (IQ scores below 50) and mild ID (scores between 50 and 69) are quite distinct, as shown by the pioneering work of Susser and Stein, summarized in a previous edition of this text,[41] and more recently by Drews et al.[42] Briefly, people with IQs below 50 often have recognizable inherited conditions, chromosomal defects, neuromotor disabilities, and/or brain malformations. Advanced maternal age is commonly a risk factor. Severe ID is relatively rare, with a prevalence amounting to about 3–4/1000 live births, but population prevalences as high as 5.1/1000 have been recorded.[43] The prevalence of severe ID, however, is dependent on the extent of antepartum screening and therapeutic abortion in the population.[44]

By contrast, people with IQs between 50 and 70 seem to emerge largely from adverse socioeconomic circumstances. Low maternal education is a particular risk factor.[42] Where fertility is high, the later-born children in large poor families are especially susceptible.[45]

The frequency of mild ID in any society is thus very dependent on the social circumstances of that society. It has been widely assumed that people scoring low on IQ tests, who tend also to do more poorly in school, have been deprived of some of the cognitive stimulation that most children receive, especially in early childhood. When IQ tests were first developed, they were standardized so that about 2.5% of the population (two SDs below the mean) had IQ scores below 70, the vast majority between 50 and 70.

When socioeconomic circumstances improve, the prevalence of mild ID drops considerably. In the most recent data from the Developmental Disabilities Surveillance Program in Metropolitan Atlanta, the prevalence of ID, during the last decade of the twentieth century and the first decade of the twenty-first century, ranged from about 1.0% to 1.5%, with no clear time trend.[46] In Scandinavian countries with comprehensive social services and educational opportunities, the condition has become rare.[47]

Risk Factors and Preventability

Severe ID is composed of a variety of conditions, many of genetic origin. Many phenotypically identifiable congenital syndromes have been recognized in which ID is a prominent feature including eponymic syndromes (e.g., Prader-Willi, Cornelia de Lange, Williams); syndromes whose names represent clinical features (e.g., Cri-du-chat; Cretinism); or syndromes defined by the metabolic defect responsible for the disability (e.g., Phenylketonuria). Chromosomal abnormalities are major contributors, especially Down's syndrome and the Fragile X syndrome, but many individually rare chromosomal rearrangements and deletions are found among people with severe ID.

Prenatal screening for Down's syndrome is now widely accepted in most parts of the developed world, and is often followed by therapeutic abortion, although therapeutic abortion for a fetus with Down's syndrome was made illegal in the state of Ohio in 2017,[48] following similar legislation in North Dakota and Indiana. The other major prenatal screening target is neural tube defects. It has been shown that programs to detect these syndromes leading to ID, followed by therapeutic abortion, have reduced the birth prevalence of both conditions.[49,50]

However, not all severe ID is of genetic origin. Congenital viral infections, most notably cytomegalovirus[51] and rubella,[52] can cause brain damage in utero sufficiently severe to manifest as ID. Severe deficiency of iodine in pregnancy causes the syndrome known as endemic cretinism, which manifests as ID with sensorineural hearing loss, at times accompanied by a motor disorder very much like CP (endemic neurological cretinism). Iodine deficiency remains the major remediable contributor to ID in the world.[53] Although once though conquered in high-income countries, a steady decline in iodine sufficiency in women of child-bearing ages has been noted in several developed nations.[54] It is likely that this disorder results from iodine deficiency in pregnancy leading to maternal hypothyroidism. The fetus produces little thyroid hormone and is largely dependent on maternal supplies of thyroxine, perhaps the single most important hormone in brain development.[55] Thus in-utero iodine deficiency, with consequent maternal hypothyroidism, is an underlying cause of prenatal brain damage. Postnatal supplementation with iodine or thyroid hormone is not effective.

Phenylketonuria (PKU) was the first metabolic disorder to be firmly linked to ID, by Folling in Norway in 1934,[56] and screening for PKU at birth initiated the era of newborn genetic screening. Not all the disorders screened for lead to ID; much screening is to detect metabolic disorders that threaten the life of the infant. After PKU, the most prominent agent of ID screened for in the newborn is either thyroxine or thyroid-stimulating hormone,[57] each used an indicator of a nonfunctional thyroid gland. Failure to supplement the hypothyroxinemic infant with thyroid hormone as soon as possible after birth places the affected infant at high risk of ID. Congenital hypothyroidism occurs as a defect in babies, and is not a result of maternal deficiency, and is therefore remediable with postnatal treatment.

Folic acid deficiency in the diet, easily treatable by provision of preconceptional supplementation,[58] is a major cause of neural tube defects, which are often accompanied by developmental disorders. Mandatory supplementation of flour with folate in the United States, but unfortunately not yet in most of Europe, has been effective in reducing the birth prevalence of this group of defects.[59]

Whether environmental chemicals are implicated in ID is an unresolved question, for three reasons. First, nearly all of the epidemiologic work on such agents as lead, mercury, PCBs, and similar toxic exposures has focused on deviations of IQ within the normal range. However, in one of the few studies of this topic, a record linkage study of more than 80,000 children with both blood lead levels and diagnoses of ID, found a relative risk of 1.5 for ID when blood lead levels were over 5 μg/L.[60]

Second, one cannot fully exclude the possibility that children with ID may be more likely to ingest or otherwise acquire exposures to environmental agents. This issue is particularly a concern with lead exposure inasmuch as the behavioral trait referred to as "pica," the tendency to ingest non-nutrient items such as paint chips, is often strongly manifest in children with ID.[61]

Third, while the development of cognitive capacities can be affected by environmental chemicals such as lead or by nutritional deficiencies such as iodine, cognitive development is entirely dependent on the child having a social, psychological, and emotional environment that promotes cognitive development. The very strong association of mild ID with low socioeconomic status has led to the entity being described as "the cultural-familial syndrome."[62] Where there is poverty and resource lack, the child must struggle harder to obtain the optimum environment for cognition to fully develop, and this is reflected in the sharp social gradient in IQ in the United States.

A substantial body of knowledge indicates that societies can choose to allocate resources to programs—in the form of structured nursery and preschool experiences for children from poor families,[63] or parental support programs[64]—that can do much to prevent the common developmental disorders, especially mild ID. The prevalence of mild ID, for example, was reduced in Sweden to as low as 0.4 per 1000 school-age children by the 1960s.[47] This prevalence is less than 20% of that expected from the normal IQ distribution, and about a third of the most recent estimate in the United States. Even in rural Sweden, mild ID is as rare as severe ID.[65]

Autism Spectrum Disorder

Definition

ASD is fundamentally a disorder of behavior, characterized especially by difficulties in communication and social interactions. Obsessive features, such as persistent repeating of words or behaviors, intense focusing on inanimate objects, and difficulty adapting to a nonstereotyped environment are common. Cognitive and learning difficulties are frequently, but not universally, associated with ASD. ASD is diagnosed most securely using one of two instruments, the Autism Diagnostic Observation Schedule (ADOS)[66] or the Autism Diagnostic Interview-Revised (ADIR).[67] Both instruments require qualified individuals and are time-consuming. Screening tools have been proposed, but cannot substitute for a firm diagnosis made by professionals.[68] It is likely that diagnoses used in the epidemiologic literature, which is often based on medical records, contain many children in whom the diagnosis is recorded who have not been fully evaluated, but nevertheless, in at least some record systems, the administrative diagnosis has considerable validity.

Prevalence and Time Trends

The recorded prevalence of ASD has been rising steadily in recent decades in all high-income countries, and a major controversy is whether this increase is real, or reflects improvements in diagnostic sensitivity or shifting diagnostic categories. Two concerns have arisen. The first is that children who have both cognitive and behavioral disorders in the past were more likely to be classified by the cognitive disorder. Shattuck[69] and Shattuck and Durkin[70] have shown that from 1994 to 2003, in 44 of 50 states, the increase in autism was completely offset by a decrease in the prevalence of children considered "cognitively disabled" or "learning disabled." The second concern is that children with mild ASD symptomatology, who previously were not considered to qualify for the diagnostic label of autism, are now being included under that label, especially with the expansion of the rubric into the broader category of ASD. An answer might be provided to this dilemma if successive population-representative cohorts of children could be assessed using the same criteria, but that exercise has not yet been undertaken. In the meantime, time-trends in autism prevalence should be treated with caution, since the limitations of extant data prevent firm conclusions. As the eminent autism epidemiologist Craig Newschaffer argued in 2006, "*we are not likely to develop a conclusive body of evidence to either fully support or fully refute the notion that there has been some real increase in autism risk over the past 2 decades.*"[71] The situation is no clearer now.

Risk Factors and Preventability

A genetic component to ASD has been suggested by the increased risk in siblings. Relative risks as high as 15 have been found for children with an elder sibling with autism,[72] although the largest study ever done, in the population of Denmark, found a relative risk of about 7.[73] Ascertainment bias in assessing younger siblings cannot fully be ruled out. Attempts to identify specific genetic loci linked to ASD, however, have been only moderately successful, with about 11%

of cases having a suspected molecular genetic basis, based on whole genome sequencing.[74] Many ASD-associated genetic loci appear to be associated with other developmental and psychiatric disorders as well.[75] A striking male excess in risk has been found nearly universally, with the relative risk in males some three to four times that in females.[76]

An extraordinary number of prenatal and perinatal environmental risk factors have been linked to ASD, usually with modest effect sizes (odds ratios 0.7–1.5).[77] Sociodemographic risk factors such as advanced parental age and education, likely reflect in part access to diagnostic services. Several maternal life-style and dietary factors (pregnancy smoking and alcohol use and fish consumption) have largely been exonerated,[78] but associations with maternal obesity[79] and low intake of omega-3 fatty acids are more suggestive.[80]

The intersection of epidemiologic interest in the effect of environmental chemicals on health and concerns about a possible rise in ASD prevalence has stimulated much research into the potential relationships of ASD to early-life exposures to heavy metals, air pollution, polychlorinated biphenyls, endocrine-disrupting chemicals, and other environmental agents.[78] Studies have frequently lacked formal ASD diagnoses and findings have generally been inconsistent, although the link with exposure to organophosphate insecticides may be more persuasive.[81]

Some potentially modifiable risk factors stand out, however, either because of their consistency and strong effects or their modifiability. Among these are periconceptional folate and vitamin intake, preterm birth and low birthweight, and disorders of thyroid hormone/iodine intake.

In several studies, mothers who took periconceptional folic acid and/or vitamins had offspring with lower risks of ASD,[82–84] with the caution that one study found hints of an increased risk with higher doses of multivitamins.[85] Preterm birth has repeatedly been found to be associated with ASD,[86–88] and risk increases steadily with decreasing gestational age at birth. In a study where the ASD diagnosis was based on a full ADOS assessment, infants born before 28 weeks of gestation had an ASD prevalence of 7%, increasing to 15% for infants 25–26 weeks.[89] Low birthweight (<2500 g) is also consistently linked to ASD, as it is to most neurodevelopmental disorders, and the claim has been made that poor fetal growth, per se, is a risk factor for ASD.[90]

Hypothyroxinemia in pregnancy, whether assessed by measurement of TSH,[91] or by formal medical diagnosis,[92] has been associated with ASD in two large European studies. Earlier in this chapter, the role of iodine deficiency in many parts of the world as an important cause of ID was noted. A strong link of iodine deficiency to ASD has been found in Egypt, a country in which iodine deficiency is highly prevalent,[93] and in Poland, where iodine deficiency disorders are rarer.[94]

Cerebral Palsy

Definition

In 2007, the Executive Committee on the Definition and Classification of Cerebral Palsy issued its final report[18] providing the following definition of the disorder:

> *"Cerebral Palsy (CP) describes group of permanent disorders of the development of movement and posture, causing activity limitation, that are attributed to nonprogressive disturbances that occurred in the developing fetal or infant brain. The motor disorders of cerebral palsy are often accompanied by disturbances of sensation, perception, cognition, communication, and behaviour, by epilepsy, and by secondary musculoskeletal problems."*

The definition was accompanied by the detailed annotation and explanation of no less than 21 of the 58 words in the definition, giving a sense of how difficult it is to capture in words the precise demarcation of a complex syndrome, particularly a syndrome such as CP which is often accompanied by other neurodevelopmental disorders, but can also be a solitary motor disability. About 40% of affected children cannot walk independently,[95,96] a third have epilepsy,[97] up to a third may be nonverbal,[98,99] and about half have some degree of cognitive impairment.[100,101] The inclusion of a requirement for activity limitation, the term now preferred by the WHO to disability, indicates that to assign a CP diagnosis, more is required than just the presence of neurological findings. The affected individual must also have some demonstrable interference with usually expected daily tasks such as walking, stair-climbing, or writing. This definition thus excludes the several minor motor abnormalities, often self-correcting, found during development, particularly in infants at risk, such as survivors of premature birth. CP is generally classified by the type of motor disorder—spastic, choreoathetotic, and ataxic. Most children with choreoathetosis (writhing movements) has spasticity, while ataxic CP is very rare. Thus 80–90% of CP children have spasticity, which is conventionally categorized as either diplegic (predominantly involving the legs), quadriplegic (all four limbs), or hemiplegic (one side).

Most clinicians with experience working with CP avoid making a firm diagnosis until the age of 18–24 months. Recent literature has suggested, however, that the absence of fidgety movements in infants younger than 6 months is an accurate predictor of CP. This promising approach, however, has so far only been examined in infants at high risk for CP.[102,103]

Evidence for the effectiveness of early intervention in CP is lacking,[104] but recent developments in neuroimaging and early identification of children at high risk of CP may permit better selection of candidates for early intervention in future trials.[105] Constraint of the unaffected arm or increased active movement of the affected arm in hemiplegic CP can substantially improve motor function and control in the affected arm and hand,[106] suggesting that motor regions affected by CP are susceptible to improved function if activity can be increased.

Prevalence and Time Trends

CP is the commonest permanent motor disorder of childhood, occurring in at least 2/1000 live births in most populations, but prevalences as high as 4/1000 have occasionally been recorded. Most CP prevalence studies, many of which are based on national registries, denominator CP to live births, but some studies describe a prevalence per school-age children. This difference matters only if infant mortality is high. Thus, the two numbers differ substantially for extremely low birthweight infants, but not for the general population in high-income countries.

The usually cited prevalence rate for CP is between 2 and 3/1000 live births, as has been reported recently from South Korea[107] and Japan.[108] But considerable variability is found in cross-national comparisons, some of which may be due to reporting practices. Prevalence rates below 2/1000 have been reported recently from Europe,[109] while prevalences above 3/1000 have been reported from Taiwan,[110] Egypt,[111] Uganda,[112] and the United States.[95,113] In the latter studies, prevalence in African American children was found to be 20% higher than in White children, and the prevalence of severe CP, 70% higher.[114] Prevalence rates in parts of rural Africa might be considerably higher.[115]

CP prevalence was clearly increasing in high-income countries in the final third of the 20th century, as newborn intensive care permitted the survival of severely premature babies at high risk of CP. There is now evidence, principally from Europe, than this trend has leveled off and may be dropping.

Because CP is the developmental disability most closely linked to birth events and to perinatal management, interest in assessing its prevalence and time trends has always been high. Several European countries (e.g., Denmark, Norway, and Ireland) have national CP registries, and regional registries exist in many other parts of Europe and Asia.

Risk Factors and Preventability

Familial clustering of CP has been described, with relative risks for CP of between 4 and 9.[116–118] However, even these relative risks translate to an absolute risk of CP for case siblings of about 1–2%. Apolipoprotein E is a lipid transport protein abundant in the brain, and the e4 allele coding for this protein has been associated with several neurological conditions, most notably Alzheimer's disease. An elevated relative risk for CP has been found with the e4 allele in three studies[119–121] but these findings were not replicated in three other studies.[122–124] Males are at slightly higher risk of CP than females, but the excess risk is modest.

The known etiologic factors in CP fall into two broad categories, those affecting premature infants and those affecting infants born at term. Preterm birth is the major single risk factor for CP in all countries where there is appreciable survival of premature infants. Tellingly, in a recent survey in rural Uganda, just 2% of all cases of CP had been born prematurely, while in high-income countries, the proportion is often nearer 50%. The risk of CP increases linearly as a function of number of weeks born prematurely, from a risk near 1/1000 at term, to as much as 10% in births prior to 28 weeks. Among preterm infants, cranial ultrasound patterns indicative of white matter injury in the first days or weeks of life are powerful predictors of risk of CP.[125] Other risk factors include duration and pattern of mechanical ventilation, especially if accompanied by prolonged hypocapnea;[126] evidence of infection or inflammation;[127] and lung or gut complications.[128,129] Fetal growth retardation also contributes to risk of CP in both preterm and term-born infants.[130]

If preterm birth could be prevented, much CP would disappear in parallel. But as yet, there is no well-established way to prevent preterm birth and the prevalence of prematurity has not changed substantially in high-income countries over the past half-century.

Among term births, the presence of neonatal encephalopathy as indicated by lack of responsiveness, need for mechanical ventilation, or seizures is the single most powerful predictor of CP. At times, this clinical picture follows a difficult labor with evidence of prolonged birth asphyxia, but it is likely neonatal encephalopathy can have other causes.[131] Asphyxiated babies who do not manifest any signs of neonatal encephalopathy are at very low risk of CP.[132]

After accounting for preterm birth and neonatal encephalopathy, much of CP remains unexplained. Intrauterine or perinatal strokes can occur, and, as in adults, a hemiplegic pattern is commonly seen.[133] Unconjugated bilirubin is a potent neurotoxin in the newborn period, and the control of severe neonatal jaundice through exchange transfusion and phototherapy has led to a gratifying decline in the choreoathetotic form of CP most closely linked to brain damage causes by bilirubin.[134] Occasional cases of CP can be linked to congenital infection with rubella or cytomegalovirus.

Two effective approaches to the prevention of CP have been established in recent decades, one for preterm and one for term-born infants. Several trials have documented that provision of magnesium sulfate in labor occurring at 32 weeks of gestation or earlier reduces the risk of CP in surviving infants by nearly a third.[135] Another set of very consistent trials have shown that head or body cooling (by 2°C for 72 h) can reduce the risk of CP in term-born asphyxiated infants with severe neonatal encephalopathy by 25%.[136]

There have been suggestions that two other interventions, both in premature infants, might also be effective in reducing the burden of CP in this vulnerable population. Corticosteroids are given in labor when premature birth is imminent to mature the lungs and to reduce neonatal mortality. This effective intervention has been shown to reduce the risk of brain lesions that are precursors to CP, but the evidence that they reduce the risk of CP is less clear.[137] Caffeine treatment is given to prematures postnatally to reduce the number of apneic episodes. In one large, but as yet unreplicated, randomized trial, the risk of CP was nearly halved in treated infants.[138]

LESS SEVERE DEVELOPMENTAL DISABILITIES

Attention Deficit/Hyperactivity Disorder

Definition

ADHD, the most common neurobehavioral disorder in childhood, is characterized by inattention, hyperactivity, impulsivity, low frustration tolerance, and a lack of organizational behavior disproportionate to age.[139] The formal diagnosis requires the presence of five to six (depending on age) or more symptoms in each of the categories of inattention and hyperactivity/impulsivity. If the threshold is reached in both categories, the individual is recognized as having a combined presentation; if only in one of the two domains as "predominantly inattentive" or "predominantly hyperactive/impulsive." Several of the symptoms must have been present before the age of 12 years, and symptoms must be noted in more than one setting, e.g., both in school and at home. In addition, there must be evidence of interference with functioning in school or home or other setting.

ADHD is conventionally recognized as a disorder of childhood, and ADHD prevalence tends to diminish with age. However, it has become increasingly recognized that in many individuals the disorder persists into adult life, and interferes with work. ADHD is an important risk factor for a number of adverse outcomes, including failure to complete high school, having other mental health or substance use disorders, entry into the criminal justice system and unemployment.[140]

A considerable number of children continue to exhibit symptoms of ADHD into adulthood. While only 15% of children will continue to have the full-fledged ADHD picture as adults, 65% will continue to show some symptomatology.[141] The risk of ADHD continuing into adult life increases with increasing severity of symptoms, history of treatment with medication, and co-occurring psychiatric disorders.[142]

Prevalence and Time Trends

Most reviews of the prevalence of ADHD have been performed in school-age children. Thomas et al. have performed the most detailed recent meta-analysis of studies from all over the world, finding a pooled prevalence of 7.1%.[143] However, even in studies judged relatively free of bias, prevalence estimates ranged from 1% to 20%. Their data suggest an increasing prevalence between 1975 and 2013, with some impact, not statistically significant, of changes in DSM criteria from the third to the fourth edition. This prevalence estimate was slightly higher than the 5.3% prevalence found by Polancyk et al., who found, in contrast, that ADHD prevalence had been stable over the previous three decades, at least in studies that used standardized diagnostic criteria.[144] A meta-analysis of 67 studies in China found a pooled prevalence between these two estimates of 6.2%[145]

A feature of ADHD that distinguishes it from the other disabilities described in this chapter is that its symptoms are controllable via medication. Stimulant medications, especially Ritalin, have been found to substantially reduce the burden of symptoms.[146] It is not possible to fully ignore the effect of the availability of stimulant medication on the diagnosis of ADHD. Effective treatment must inevitably raise the profile of a condition, and ADHD is no exception. In a Michigan study, the diagnosis was found to vary tenfold in adjacent, socioeconomically similar counties, but with different physician prescribing patterns for Ritalin.[147]

Risk Factors and Preventability

Familial occurrence of ADHD has been noted, with relative risks in affected siblings and parents estimated at two to eight times the prevalence in children without affected family members.[148]

But familial occurrence can reflect the social and economic environment and these in turn are reflected in prevalence rates of ADHD. In a large national U.S. sample, lower family income increased the risk of ADHD by 33%, while living in a two-parent home and with parents having a college education each reduced the risk by about 30%.[149] These social factors, which must include both parental recognition and concern about symptoms and access to diagnostic services, make assessment of racial differences in risk difficult. It appears that in the United States, Black children have more ADHD symptoms, but are diagnosed with ADHD less frequently.[150,151] Boys are more frequently affected by ADHD than girls, with a relative risk of 2–3.[152,153]

A large number of environmental variables have been suggested to influence the risk of ADHD. Prematurely born and low birth weight children have about a threefold excess risk of ADHD.[154] Maternal smoking in utero is more strongly supported as a risk factor for ADHD than is maternal alcohol ingestion during pregnancy.[155] Much popular attention has focused on the possibility that food additives or other dietary factors might be involved in ADHD. One factor promoting this hypothesis is perhaps the often-noted association of ADHD with obesity,[156] although whether ADHD causes obesity or the reverse, or whether they have a third common cause, has yet to be sorted out.

Trials of dietary interventions show mixed results for eliminating food additives or adding polyunsaturated fats to the diet.[157] A trial of reducing the range of foods (oligoantigenic diet) provided to affected young children showed some promising results, but evaluators were not blinded to treatment, the sample was not very representative of the general population, and a large number of children did not complete the protocol.[158]

Environmental chemicals have also been a source of concern. Lead exposure has consistently been associated with ADHD,[159] with relative risks ranging from 1.8 to 6.0 in several studies with different designs.[160] Most impressive is the finding of a fourfold range, from the highest to lowest blood lead quintile, in parentally reported ADHD in the nationally representative National Health and Nutrition Examination Survey (NHANES) database.[161] A weaker link was found in this same database for the effect of urinary markers of PCB exposure, where a tenfold range of urinary values was linked to a risk increase of 1.5.[162]

The NHANES data have also been used to examine whether persistent organic pollutants (POPS) measured in serum, and phthalates measured in urine are associated with ADHD. Children aged 12–15 with any measurable level of POPS had a RR for ADHD ranging from 2.3 to 3.4, depending on the specific chemical assayed, compared to children without any measurable POPS in their serum.[163] The authors controlled for sex, race/ethnicity, age, poverty, birth weight, maternal age, cigarette smoking during pregnancy, body mass, and saturated fat intake. Urinary phthalates were likewise associated with ADHD, with ORs of between 2.1 and 2.7 depending on the compound, in children ages 6–15, controlling for sex, age, race, household income, blood lead, and maternal smoking during pregnancy.[164] Neither exposure to fluorine compounds or to fluoride were found to be associated with ADHD.[165,166]

Learning Disability

Definition

DSM-V describes learning disabilities as conditions that impede the ability to learn or to use specific basic academic skills, such as reading, writing, or arithmetic, which are needed for future success in school. It is assumed that these disabilities occur in children with essentially normal IQ, although the diagnosis is now made without formal reference to an IQ score. The clinical DSM diagnosis may not precisely parallel the educational diagnosis, and varying prevalences have been found from school district to school district.[167] In general, the DSM diagnosis is more restrictive, and virtually all children fitting the DSM-V diagnostic criteria will be so diagnosed in the school system.

DSM-V recognizes that learning disabilities are specific. *Dyslexia* refers to learning difficulties related to word recognition, decoding and spelling. *Dyscalculia* is a term used to describe difficulties performing mathematical calculations, memorizing mathematical facts, or using mathematical reasoning for problem solving. At least one difficulty in any of the following six areas must have been present for at least six months—reading, understanding what is read, spelling, written expression, mathematical concepts, or mathematical reasoning.

Prevalence and Time Trends

Assessments of the population prevalence of specific learning disabilities based on diagnostic criteria and formal assessments are not available. In the National Health Interview Survey, some 9% of children were reported by their parents to have a learning disability, which was associated with ADHD nearly half the time.[168] A similar estimate of 9.7% was found in an analysis based on the 2003 National Survey of Children's Health, another nationally representative sample, also based on parental report.[169] There seems to be no suggestion of any major secular trends in the United States.

Risk Factors and Preventability

Because ADHD and LD overlap considerably, we here review environmental factors found in children with LD, but not ADHD. Boys are at excess risk of LD, but the excess is not as large as in ASD or ADHD, ranging between 1.3[153] and 1.8[152] in two large nationally representative studies.

In the National Health Interview Survey, having Medicaid insurance, an indicator of lower socioeconomic status, approximately doubled the risk of parental report of LD, while a mother with a bachelor's degree lowered the risk by some 40% compared to have a less educated mother. Interestingly, race and ethnicity had virtually no effect on the risk of ADHD. The study based on the National Survey of Child Health assessed a different set of socioeconomic indicators. Children from single parent families had relative risks of LD from 60% to 90% higher than children from two-parent families. The multivariate relative risk of having a smoker in the house or having a mother who did not finish high school was both about 1.6. Adopted children had a nearly 2.5 relative risk of having LD.

The NHANES data cited above to examine environmental pollutants and ADHD also examined LD in the same population, but did not find any significant association with POPS or phthalates (Table 160-2).[163]

MANAGEMENT OF DEVELOPMENTAL DISABILITIES IN THE COMMUNITY

To effectively manage the health and developmental problems of children with developmental disabilities, a wide range of medical, educational, and social services must be available. Many such services are provided in higher income countries to help children with developmental disabilities grow to their fullest potential. Medical interventions include surgery, largely for CP management, and medication use, especially methylphenidate and allied stimulant medications, in ADHD. Physical therapy is used frequently in CP. Nutritional plans are developed for children with phenylketonuria who must adhere to a phenylalanine free diet. Speech and language therapies are often used by children with specific learning disabilities and/or ID. Applied behavioral therapy has become the most widely used intervention to improve function in children with ASD. Preschool-enhanced education programs appear to reduce the frequency of mild ID.

But it should not be surprising to learn that the complexity of services for the developmentally disabled, their expense, the frequent lack of coordination among disciplines, and the at-times heroic efforts needed by parents to access them indicate that services for the developmentally disabled are often seen by families as inadequate. In many jurisdictions, services are under at least partial control or funding by public health authorities, so that improvement of service provision for the developmentally disabled must, along with prevention, be seen as a public health priority.

As children with developmental disabilities age and begin the transition from school to the workplace, occupational therapy and job counseling become paramount. This transition is often difficult,

TABLE 160-2 INTERVENTIONS TO PREVENT DEVELOPMENTAL DISABILITIES

Approach	Target Conditions	Pathway to Prevention
Rubella immunization	ID	Brain damage in congenital rubella syndrome can manifest as ID and CP.[177]
Folic acid supplementation	ID, CP, ASD	Periconceptional intake of folic acid can reduce the risk of neural tube defects by 60–70%. Some 15–20% of affected children have ID[178] and close to 10% have CP.[179] Folic acid may also prevent ASD.[82]
Iodine supplementation	ID, CP	Endemic cretinism leading to severe ID, and sometimes to CP, remains a public health issue in several regions of the world.[180]
Newborn genetic screening	ID	Screening for phenylketonuria[181] and for congenital hypothyroidism[182] reduces the prevalence of ID.
Prenatal screening	ID	Prenatal diagnosis can reduce the contribution of chromosomal and other conditions to ID.[44]
Magnesium sulfate in labor	CP	Several trials confirm 30–35% reduction in CP in infants <32 weeks gestation.[135]
Head or body cooling	CP	Several trials confirm 25% reduction in CP in infants with neonatal encephalopathy and birth asphyxia.[136]
Early education	Mild ID	Randomized trials of enhanced early education have shown improved school and cognitive performance in children.[63]

but there has been a welcome increase in resources spent on transition programs in communities, and in research into the most cost-effective ways to manage such programs.[170]

FUTURE PUBLIC HEALTH DIRECTIONS

Both the prevention and the management of developmental disorders often fall under the aegis of public health agencies. Every state in the United States maintains public health laboratories for testing newborn blood collected on filter papers to detect phenylketonuria, congenital hypothyroidism, and other disorders that lead to premature death or brain damage. Many states also take responsibility for laboratory testing of antenatal specimens assessed for chromosomal disorders or alpha-fetoprotein, an indicator of the presence of a neural tube defect. State and local public health programs that support vaccination efforts and nutritional support likewise contribute to DD prevention.

Historically, public health and allied mental health agencies were often heavily engaged in providing services to children with the severer forms of DD, often under the aegis of "*Crippled Children's Programs*" or by supporting state institutions that housed severely developmentally delayed children. In more recent times in the United States, such activities have been moving steadily into the private sector, but with considerable public funding. As responsibilities for the care and management of children with DD become more of a private responsibility, with perhaps less public health oversight than in the past, it will be important for the public, especially the families of children with DD, to be vigilant and outspoken when needed.

Prevention of DD is, or should be, a widespread public responsibility. The role of public health agencies has been highlighted above, and another critically important sector in this task is education. Wider adoption of preschool and very early educational programs, with outreach to resource-poor communities is likely to substantially reduce the frequency of mild ID, and perhaps may also play a role in the prevention of ADHD and learning disabilities. The sustained effort of the March of Dimes Foundation to publicize the importance, to women of child-bearing age, of taking folate supplements is an illustration of what the nonprofit sector can contribute.

The obstetric community must be alert to opportunities for prevention such as providing preconceptional rubella immunization where needed, encouraging folate use, providing access to antenatal screening services where possible, and administering magnesium sulfate to laboring mothers at less than 32 complete weeks of gestation. The neonatal community should emphasize the importance of treating infants with neonatal encephalopathy of presumed asphyxial origin with head and body cooling, and continue its ongoing research into broader application of this effective and generalizable low-technology intervention.[171]

Scientific research continues into the origins of all forms of disability and their most effective remediation. Technical advances in gene therapy, molecular imaging, and stem cell research hold considerable promise, but it would be unwise to neglect research into the mechanisms behind the profound social gradient in many developmental disabilities, and the best ways to address it. As reviewed above, environmental pollutants may injure the developing nervous system and be implicated in DD, especially ADHD.

Very large pregnancy cohort studies, designed and powered to examine the antenatal antecedents of severe developmental disabilities, have been mounted in Norway,[172] Denmark,[173] Japan,[174] and the United States[175] in recent decades. Some promising findings have been noted earlier in this chapter, but the greatest promise lies ahead, when the full value of these cohorts, with their archived specimens and interviews, can be fully exploited.

A pressing need remains to better understand the situation for DD in lower income countries. Pioneering research has been done using simple measures to assess development in less developed countries,[176] and sophisticated surveys have been performed in sub-Saharan Africa.[112] Yet there is room for additional careful assessment of the frequency of DDs and their preventability around the globe. It is likely that much can be done, using simple interventions that address specific infections and nutritional agents, to substantially improve the development and life prospects of children and their families.

References

1. Andre M, Plenat F, Floquet J, et al. Hydranencephaly. Major cerebral lesions with normal neonatal neurologic behavior. *Arch Fr Pediatr*. 1975;32(10):915–24.
2. Pinho TD, Manz PH, DuPaul GJ, et al. Predictors and moderators of quality of life among college students with ADHD. *J Atten Disord*. 2019;23(14):1736–45.
3. Hubert-Dibon G, Bru M, Gras Le Guen C, et al. Health-related quality of life for children and adolescents with specific language impairment. *PLoS One*. 2016;11(11):e0166541.
4. Dowding VM, Barry C. Cerebral palsy: Social class differences in prevalence in relation to birthweight and severity of disability. *J Epidemiol Community Health*. 1990;44:191–5.
5. Spencer NJ, Blackburn CM, Read JM. Disabling chronic conditions in childhood and socioeconomic disadvantage: A systematic review and meta-analyses of observational studies. *BMJ Open*. 2015;5(9):e007062.

6. Christensen DL, Baio J, Van Naarden Braun K. Prevalence and Characteristics of Autism Spectrum Disorder Among Children Aged 8 Years—Autism and Developmental Disabilities Monitoring Network, 11 Sites, United States, 2012. *MMWR Surveill Summ*. 2018;65(13):1–23.
7. Chapman DA, Scott KG, Stanton-Chapman TL. Public health approach to the study of mental retardation. *Am J Ment Retard*. 2008;113(2):102–16.
8. Durkin M. The epidemiology of developmental disabilities in low-income countries. *Ment Retard Dev Disabil Res Rev*. 2002;8(3):206–11.
9. Bergen DC. Effects of poverty on cognitive function—A hidden neurologic epidemic. *Clinical Neurology*. 2008; 71:447–51.
10. Goodman N, Tizard J. Prevalence of imbecility and idiocy among children. *Br Med J*. 1962;1(5273):216–9.
11. Available at http://www.thearc.org/who-we-are/history/name-change.
12. Available at https://www.federalregister.gov/documents/2013/08/01/2013-18552/change-in-terminology-mental-retardation-to-intellectual-disability.
13. American Psychiatric Association. *Diagnostic and Statistical Manual of Mental Disorders*. 5th ed. Arlington, VA: American Psychiatric Association; 2013.
14. Kanner L. Autistic disturbances of affective contact. *Nervous Child*. 1943;2:217–50.
15. Asperger H. Die "Autistischen Psychopathen" im Kindesalter. *Archiv für Psychiatrie und Nervenkrankheiten*. 1944;117:76–136.
16. American Psychiatric Association Committee on Nomenclature and Statistics. *Diagnostic and Statistical Manual of Mental Disorders (DSM-III)*. Washington, DC: American Psychiatric Association; 1994.
17. Bax M, Goldstein M, Rosenbaum P, et al. Proposed definition and classification of cerebral palsy, April 2005. *Dev Med Child Neurol*. 2005;47(8):571–6.
18. Rosenbaum P, Paneth N, Leviton A, et al. A report: The definition and classification of cerebral palsy April 2006. *Dev Med Child Neurol Suppl*. 2007;109:8–14.
19. American Psychiatric Association. *Diagnostic and Statistical Manual of Mental Disorders*. 2nd ed. Arlington, VA: American Psychiatric Association; 1968.
20. Nelson LD, Guskiewicz KM, Marshall SW. Multiple self-reported concussions are more prevalent in athletes with ADHD and learning disability. *Clin J Sport Med*. 2016;26(2):120–7.
21. Dieckmann F, Giovis C, Offergeld J. The life expectancy of people with intellectual disabilities in Germany. *J Appl Res Intellect Disabil*. 2015;28(5):373–82.
22. Coppus AM. People with intellectual disability: What do we know about adulthood and life expectancy? *Dev Disabil Res Rev*. 2013;18(1):6–16.
23. Larson EB, Shadlen MF, Wang L, et al. Survival after initial diagnosis of Alzheimer disease. *Ann Intern Med*. 2004;140(7):501–9.
24. Kruse M, Michelsen SI, Flachs EM, et al. Lifetime costs of cerebral palsy. *Dev Med Child Neurol*. 2009;51(8):622–8.
25. Centers for Disease Control and Prevention (CDC). Economic costs associated with mental retardation, cerebral palsy, hearing loss, and vision impairment—United States, 2003. *MMWR Morb Mortal Wkly Rep*. 2004;53:57–9.
26. Buescher AV, Cidav Z, Knapp M, et al. Costs of autism spectrum disorders in the United Kingdom and the United States. *JAMA Pediatr*. 2014;168(8):721–8.
27. Lee J. Maternal stress, well-being, and impaired sleep in mothers of children with developmental disabilities: A literature review. *Res Dev Disabil*. 2013;34(11):4255–73.
28. Heller T, Caldwell J, Factor A. Aging family caregivers: Policies and practices. *Ment Retard Dev Disabil Res Rev*. 2007;13(2):136–42.
29. Ervin DA, Hennen B, Merrick J, et al. Healthcare for persons with intellectual and developmental disability in the community. *Front Public Health*. 2014;2(83):1–8.
30. Ervin DA, Hennen B, Merrick J, et al. Primary care: Mental and behavioral health and persons with intellectual and developmental disabilities. *Front Public Health*. 2014;2(76):1–5.
31. Saeed SA. Working with individuals with mental illness and developmental disabilities: Synthesizing the best information for the practicing clinician. *Psychiatr Q*. 2008;79:153–5.
32. Harris JC. Lesch-Nyhan syndrome and its variants: Examining the behavioral and neurocognitive phenotype. *Curr Opin Psychiatry*. 2018;31(2):96–102.
33. Antonacci DJ, Manuel C, Davis E. Diagnosis and treatment of aggression in individuals with developmental disabilities. *Psychiatr Q*. 2008;79(3):225–47.
34. Antonacci DJ, Attiah N. Diagnosis and treatment of mood disorders in adults with developmental disabilities. *Psychiatr Q*. 2008; 79(3):171–92.
35. Davis E, Saeed SA, Antonacci DJ. Anxiety disorders in persons with developmental disabilities: Empirically informed diagnosis and treatment. Reviews literature on anxiety disorders in DD population with practical take-home messages for the clinician. *Psychiatr Q*. 2008;79(3):249–63.
36. Zulauf CA, Sprich SE, Safren SA, et al. The complicated relationship between attention deficit/hyperactivity disorder and substance use disorders. *Curr Psychiatry Rep*. 2014 Mar;16(3):436.
37. Carpentier PJ, van Gogh MT, Knapen LJ. Influence of attention deficit hyperactivity disorder and conduct disorder on opioid dependence severity and psychiatric comorbidity in chronic methadone-maintained patients. *Eur Addict Res*. 2011;17(1):10–20.
38. Lugoboni F, Levin FR, Pieri MC. Co-occurring attention deficit hyperactivity disorder symptoms in adults affected by heroin dependence: Patients characteristics and treatment needs. *Psychiatry Res*. 2017;250:210–6.
39. Abel KF, Bramness JG, Martinsen EW. Stimulant medication for ADHD in opioid maintenance treatment. *J Dual Diagn*. 2014;10(1):32–8.
40. Peltopuro M, Ahonen T, Kaartinen J, et al. Borderline intellectual functioning: A systematic literature review. *Intellect Dev Disabil*. 2014;52(6):419–43.
41. Stein and Susser in Last 13th edition, 1980.
42. Drews CD, Yeargin-Allsopp M, Decouflé P, et al. Variation in the influence of selected sociodemographic risk factors for mental retardation. *Am J Public Health*. 1995 Mar;85(3):329–34.
43. van Bakel M, Einarsson I, Arnaud C, et al. Monitoring the prevalence of severe intellectual disability in children across Europe: Feasibility of a common database. *Dev Med Child Neurol*. 2014;56(4):361–9.
44. Soler-Casas A, Sánchez-Díaz A, Morales-Peydró C. The impact of prenatal diagnosis on the prevention of chromosomal mental retardation. Chromosomal alterations that can be detected by prenatal diagnosis. *Rev Neurol*. 2006;42(Suppl 1):S27–32.
45. Belmont L, Stein ZA, Wittes JT. Birth order, family size and school failure. *Dev Med Child Neurol*. 1976;18(4):421–30.
46. Van Naarden Braun K, Christensen D, Doernberg N, et al. Trends in the prevalence of autism spectrum disorder, cerebral palsy, hearing loss, intellectual disability, and vision impairment, Metropolitan Atlanta, 1991–2010. *PLoS One*. 2015;10(4):e0124120.
47. Hagberg B, Hagberg G, Lewerth A. Mild mental retardation in Swedish school children. I. Prevalence. *Acta Paediatr Scand*. 1981;70(4): 441–4.
48. Available at https://www.legislature.ohio.gov/legislation/legislation-summary?id=GA131-HB-135.
49. de Graaf G, Buckley F, Skotko BG. Estimates of the live births, natural losses, and elective terminations with Down syndrome in the United States. *Am J Med Genet A*. 2015;167A(4):756–67.
50. Cragan JD, Roberts HE, Edmonds LD. Surveillance for anencephaly and spina bifida and the impact of prenatal diagnosis—United States, 1985–1994. *MMWR CDC Surveill Summ*. 1995;44(4):1–13.
51. Swanson EC, Schleiss MR. Congenital cytomegalovirus infection: New prospects for prevention and therapy. *Pediatr Clin North Am*. 2013;60(2):335–49.
52. Thompson KM, Simons EA, Badizadegan K. Characterization of the risks of adverse outcomes following Rubella infection in pregnancy. *Risk Anal*. 2016;36(7):1315–31.
53. Delange F, de Benoist B, Pretell E. Iodine deficiency in the world: Where do we stand at the turn of the century? *Thyroid*. 2001;11(5):437–47.
54. Pearce EN, Andersson M, Zimmermann MB. Global iodine nutrition: Where do we stand in 2013? *Thyroid*. 2013;23(5):523–8.
55. de Escobar GM, Obregón MJ, del Rey FE. Maternal thyroid hormones early in pregnancy and fetal brain development. *Best Pract Res Clin Endocrinol Metab*. 2004;18(2):225–48.
56. Følling A. Über Ausscheidung von Phenylbrenztraubensäure in den Harn als Stoffwechselanomalie in Verbindung mit Imbezillität. *Zeitschrift für physiologische Chemie*. 1934:227(1–4):169––81.
57. Grosse SD, Van Vliet G. Prevention of intellectual disability through screening for congenital hypothyroidism: How much and at what level? *Arch Dis Child*. 2011;96(4):374–9.
58. Prevention of neural tube defects: Results of the Medical Research Council vitamin study. MRC Vitamin Study Research Group. *Lancet*. 1991;338(8760):131–7.

59. Atta CA, Fiest KM, Frolkis AD. Global birth prevalence of spina bifida by folic acid fortification status: A systematic review and meta-analysis. *Am J Public Health*. 2016;106(1):e24–34.
60. Delgado CF, Ullery MA, Jordan M. Lead exposure and developmental disabilities in preschool-aged children. *J Public Health Manag Pract*. 2018;24(2):e10–17.
61. Matson JL, Hattier MA, Belva B. Pica in persons with developmental disabilities: Approaches to treatment. *Res Dev Disabil*. 2013;34(9):2564–71.
62. Stein Z. Strategies for the prevention of mental retardation. *Bull N Y Acad Med*. 1975;51(1):130–42.
63. Ramey CT, Ramey SL. Prevention of intellectual disabilities: Early interventions to improve cognitive development. *Prev Med*. 1998;27(2):224–32.
64. Olds DL, Kitzman H, Cole R. Effects of nurse home-visiting on maternal life course and child development: Age 6 follow-up results of a randomized trial. *Pediatrics*. 2004;114(6):1550–9.
65. Blomquist HK, Gustavson KH, Holmgren G. Mild mental retardation in children in a northern Swedish county. *J Ment Defic Res*. 1981;25(Pt 3):169–86.
66. Lord C, Rutter M, Goode S, et al. Autism diagnostic observation schedule: A standardized observation of communicative and social behavior. *J Autism Dev Disord*. 1989:19 (2):185–212.
67. Lord C, Rutter M, Le Couteur A. Autism diagnostic interview-revised: A revised version of a diagnostic interview for caregivers of individuals with possible pervasive developmental disorders. *J Autism Dev Disord*. 1994;24(5):659–85.
68. García-Primo P, Hellendoorn A, Charman T. Screening for autism spectrum disorders: State of the art in Europe. *Eur Child Adolesc Psychiatry*. 2014;23(11):1005–21.
69. Shattuck PT. The contribution of diagnostic substitution to the growing administrative prevalence of autism in US special education. *Pediatrics*. 2006;117(4):1028–37.
70. Shattuck PT, Durkin M. A Spectrum of Disputes, Op-ed, New York Times, June 11, 2007. Available at http://www.nytimes.com/2007/06/11/opinion/11shattuck.html. Accessed Jan 28, 2018.
71. Newschaffer CJ. Investigating diagnostic substitution and autism prevalence trends. *Pediatrics*. 2006;117(4):1436–7.
72. Xie F, Peltier M, Getahun D. Is the risk of autism in younger siblings of affected children moderated by sex, race/ethnicity, or gestational age? *J Dev Behav Pediatr*. 2016;37(8):603–9.
73. Grønborg TK, Schendel DE, Parner ET. Recurrence of autism spectrum disorders in full- and half-siblings and trends over time: A population-based cohort study. *JAMA Pediatr*. 2013;167(10):947–53.
74. Yuen RKC, Merico D, Bookman M, et al. Whole genome sequencing resource identifies 18 new candidate genes for autism spectrum disorder. *Nat Neurosci*. 2017;20(4):602–11.
75. De Rubeis S, Buxbaum JD. Genetics and genomics of autism spectrum disorder: Embracing complexity. *Hum Mol Genet*. 2015;24(R1):R24–31.
76. Loomes R, Hull L, Mandy WPL, et al. What is the male-to-female ratio in autism spectrum disorder? A systematic review and meta-analysis. *J Am Acad Child Adolesc Psychiatry*. 2017;56(6):466–74.
77. Wang C, Geng H, Liu W, et al. Prenatal, perinatal, and postnatal factors associated with autism: A meta-analysis. *Medicine (Baltimore)*. 2017;96(18):e6696.
78. Schmidt RJ, Lyall K, Hertz-Picciotto I. Environment and autism: Current state of the science. *Cut Edge Psychiatry Pract*. 2014;1(4):21–38.
79. Mehta SH, Kerver JM, Sokol RJ, et al. The association between maternal obesity and neurodevelopmental outcomes of offspring. *J Pediatr*. 2014;165(5):891–6.
80. Lyall K, Munger KL, O'Reilly EJ, et al. Maternal dietary fat intake in association with autism spectrum disorders. *Am J Epidemiol*. 2013;178(2):209–20.
81. Shelton JF, Hertz-Picciotto I, Pessah IN. Tipping the balance of autism risk: Potential mechanisms linking pesticides and autism. *Environ Health Perspect*. 2012;120(7):944–51.
82. Surén P, Roth C, Bresnahan M. Association between maternal use of folic acid supplements and risk of autism spectrum disorders in children. *JAMA*. 2013;309(6):570–7.
83. Schmidt RJ, Tancredi DJ, Ozonoff S. Maternal periconceptional folic acid intake and risk of autism spectrum disorders and developmental delay in the CHARGE (CHildhood Autism Risks from Genetics and Environment) case-control study. *Am J Clin Nutr*. 2012;96(1):80–9.
84. Levine SZ, Kodesh A, Viktorin A. Association of maternal use of folic acid and multivitamin supplements in the periods before and during pregnancy with the risk of autism spectrum disorder in offspring. *JAMA Psychiatry*. 2018;75(2):176–84.
85. Raghavan R, Riley AW, Volk H. Maternal multivitamin intake, plasma folate and vitamin B12 levels and autism spectrum disorder risk in offspring. *Paediatr Perinat Epidemiol*. 2018;32(1):100–11.
86. Pinto-Martin JA, Levy SE, Feldman JF, et al. Prevalence of autism spectrum disorder in adolescents born weighing <2000 grams. *Pediatrics*. 2011;128(5):883–91.
87. Kuzniewicz MW, Wi S, Qian Y. Prevalence and neonatal factors associated with autism spectrum disorders in preterm infants. *J Pediatr*. 2014;164(1):20–5.
88. Hwang YS, Weng SF, Cho CY. Higher prevalence of autism in Taiwanese children born prematurely: A nationwide population-based study. *Res Dev Disabil*. 2013;34(9):2462–8.
89. Joseph RM, O'Shea TM, Allred EN. Prevalence and associated features of autism spectrum disorder in extremely low gestational age newborns at age 10 years. *Autism Res*. 2017;10(2):224–32.
90. Class QA, Rickert ME, Larsson H, et al. Fetal growth and psychiatric and socioeconomic problems: Population-based sibling comparison. *Br J Psychiatry*. 2014;205(5):355–61.
91. Román GC, Ghassabian A, Bongers-Schokking JJ, et al. Association of gestational maternal hypothyroxinemia and increased autism risk. *Ann Neurol*. 2013;74(5):733–42.
92. Andersen SL, Laurberg P, Wu CS, et al. Attention deficit hyperactivity disorder and autism spectrum disorder in children born to mothers with thyroid dysfunction: A Danish nationwide cohort study. *BJOG*. 2014;121(11):1365–74.
93. Hamza RT, Hewedi DH, Sallam MT. Iodine deficiency in Egyptian autistic children and their mothers: Relation to disease severity. *Arch Med Res*. 2013;44(7):555–61.
94. Błażewicz A, Makarewicz A, Korona-Glowniak I, et al. Iodine in autism spectrum disorders. *J Trace Elem Med Biol*. 2016;34:32–7.
95. Kirby RS, Wingate MS, Van Naarden Braun K, et al. Prevalence and functioning of children with cerebral palsy in four areas of the United States in 2006: A report from the Autism and Developmental Disabilities Monitoring Network. *Res Dev Disabil*. 2011;32:462–9.
96. Christensen, D, Van Naarden Braun K, Doernberg NS, et al. Prevalence of cerebral palsy, co-occurring autism spectrum disorders, and motor functioning—Autism and Developmental Disabilities Monitoring Network, USA, 2008. *Dev Med Child Neurol*. 2014;56:59–65.
97. Reid SM, Meehan E, McIntyre S, et al. Temporal trends in cerebral palsy by impairment severity and birth gestation. *Dev Med Child Neurol*. 2016;58(Suppl 2):25–35.
98. Zhang JY, Oskoui M, Shevell, M. A population-based study of communication impairment in cerebral palsy. *J Child Neurol*. 2015;30:277–84.
99. Mei C, Reilly S, Reddihough D, et al. Language outcomes of children with cerebral palsy aged 5 years and 6 years: A population-based study. *Dev Med Child Neurol*. 2016;58:605–11.
100. Levy SE, Giarelli E, Lee LC, et al. Autism spectrum disorder and co-occurring developmental, psychiatric, and medical conditions among children in multiple populations of the United States. *J Dev Behav Pediatr*. 2010;31:267–75.
101. Pakula AT, Van Naarden Braun K, Yeargin-Allsopp M, et al. Cerebral palsy: Classification and epidemiology. *Phys Med Rehabil Clin N Am*. 2010;20:425–52.
102. Morgan C, Crowle C, Goyen TA, et al. Sensitivity and specificity of General Movements Assessment for diagnostic accuracy of detecting cerebral palsy early in an Australian context. *J Paediatr Child Health*. 2016;52(1):54–9.
103. Bosanquet M, Copeland L, Ware R, et al. A systematic review of tests to predict cerebral palsy in young children. *Dev Med Child Neurol*. 2013;55(5):418–26.
104. Blauw-Hospers CH, Hadders-Algra M. A systematic review of the effects of early intervention on motor development. *Dev Med Child Neurol*. 2005;47:421–32.
105. Herskind A, Greisen G, Nielsen JB. Early identification and intervention in cerebral palsy. *Dev Med Child Neurol*. 2015;57:29–36.
106. Chiu HC, Ada L. Constraint-induced movement therapy improves upper limb activity and participation in hemiplegic cerebral palsy: A systematic review. *J Physiother*. 2016;62(3):130–7.
107. Park MS, Kim SJ, Chung CY, et al. Prevalence and lifetime healthcare cost of cerebral palsy in South Korea. *Health Policy*. 2011;100:234–8.
108. Toyokawa S, Maeda E, Kobayashi Y. Estimation of the number of children with cerebral palsy using nationwide health insurance claims data in Japan. *Dev Med Child Neurol*. 2017;59:317–21.

109. Sellier E, Platt MJ, Andersen GL, et al. Decreasing prevalence in cerebral palsy: A multi-site European population-based study, 1980 to 2003. *Dev Med Child Neurol.* 2016;58(1):85–92.
110. Chang MJ, Ma HI, Lu TH. Estimating the prevalence of cerebral palsy in Taiwan: A comparison of different case definitions. *Res Dev Disabil.* 2014;36C:207–12.
111. El-Tallawy HN, Farghaly WM, Shehata GA, et al. Cerebral palsy in Al-Quseir City, Egypt: Prevalence, subtypes, and risk factors. *Neuropsychiatr Dis Treat.* 2014;10:1267–72.
112. Kakooza-Mwesige A, Andrews C, Peterson S, et al. Prevalence of cerebral palsy in Uganda: A population-based study. *Lancet Global health.* 2017;5:e1275–82.
113. Maenner MJ, Blumberg SJ, Kogan MD, et al. Prevalence of cerebral palsy and intellectual disability among children identified in two U.S. National Surveys, 2011–2013. *Ann Epidemiol.* 2016;26:222–6.
114. Maenner MJ, Benedict RE, Arneson CL, et al. Children with cerebral palsy: Racial disparities in functional limitations. *Epidemiology.* 2012;23(1):35–43.
115. Couper J. Prevalence of childhood disability in rural KwaZulu-Natal. *S Afr Med J.* 2002;92:549–52.
116. O'Callaghan ME, MacLennan AH, Gibson CS, et al. Epidemiologic associations with cerebral palsy. *Obstet Gynecol.* 2011;118:576–82.
117. Hemminki K, Li X, Sundquist K, et al. High familial risks for cerebral palsy implicate partial heritable aetiology. *Paediatr Perinat Epidemiol.* 2007;21:235–41.
118. Tollanes, MC, Wilcox A J, Lie RT, et al. Familial risk of cerebral palsy: Population based cohort study. *BMJ.* 2014;349:g4294.
119. Meirelles Kalil Pessoa de B, Rodrigues, CJ, de Barros TE, et al. Presence of apolipoprotein E epsilon4 allele in cerebral palsy. *J Pediatr Orthop.* 2000;20:786–9.
120. Kuroda MM, Weck ME, Sarwark JF, et al. Association of apolipoprotein E genotype and cerebral palsy in children. *Pediatrics.* 2007;119:306–13.
121. Wu YW, Croen LA, Vanderwerf A, et al. Candidate genes and risk for CP: A population-based study. *Pediatr Res.* 2011;70:642–6.
122. McMichael GL, Gibson CS, Goldwater PN, et al. Association between Apolipoprotein E genotype and cerebral palsy is not confirmed in a Caucasian population. *Human Genetics.* 2008;124:411–16.
123. O'Callaghan ME, Maclennan AH, Gibson CS, et al. Fetal and maternal candidate single nucleotide polymorphism associations with cerebral palsy: A case-control study. *Pediatrics.* 2012;129:e414–23.
124. Xu Y, Wang H, Sun Y, et al. The association of apolipoprotein E gene polymorphisms with cerebral palsy in Chinese infants. *Molecular Genetics and Genomics.* 2014;289:411–16.
125. Pinto-Martin Pediatrics Pinto-Martin J, Riolo S, Cnaan A, Holzman C, Susser MW, Paneth N. Cranial ultrasound prediction of disabling and non-disabling cerebral palsy in a low birthweight population. *Pediatrics.* 1995;95:249–54.
126. Collins M Pediatric Research Collins M, Paneth N, Lorenz J. Hypocapnia and other ventilation-related risk factors for disabling cerebral palsy in low birth weight infants. *Pediatric Research.* 2001;50:712–9.
127. Kuban KC, O'Shea TM, Allred EN, et al. Systemic inflammation and cerebral palsy risk in extremely preterm infants. *J Child Neurol.* 2014;29(12):1692–8.
128. Skidmore MD, Rivers A, Hack M. Increased risk of cerebral palsy among very low-birthweight infants with chronic lung disease. *Dev Med Child Neurol.* 1990;32(4):325–32.
129. Fullerton BS, Hong CR, Velazco CS, et al. Severe neurodevelopmental disability and healthcare needs among survivors of medical and surgical necrotizing enterocolitis: A prospective cohort study. *J Pediatr Surg.* 2017;S0022-3468(17):30651–6.
130. Jarvis S, Glinianaia SV, Torrioli MG, et al. Cerebral palsy and intrauterine growth in single births: European collaborative study. *Lancet.* 2003;362(9390):1106–11.
131. Adamson SJ, Alessandri LM, Badawi N, et al. Predictors of neonatal encephalopathy in full-term infants. *BMJ.* 1995;311(7005):598–602.
132. Freeman JM, Nelson KB. Intrapartum asphyxia and cerebral palsy. *Pediatrics.* 1988;82(2):240–9.
133. Raju TN, Nelson KB, Ferriero D, et al. Ischemic perinatal stroke: Summary of a workshop sponsored by the National Institute of Child Health and Human Development and the National Institute of Neurological Disorders and Stroke. *Pediatrics.* 2007;120(3):609–16.
134. Rose J, Vassar R. Movement disorders due to bilirubin toxicity. *Semin Fetal Neonatal Med.* 2015;20(1):20–25.
135. Doyle LW, Crowther CA, Middleton P. Antenatal magnesium sulfate and neurologic outcome in preterm infants: A systematic review. *Obstet Gynecol.* 2009;113(6):1327–33.
136. Jacobs SE, Berg M, Hunt R. Cooling for newborns with hypoxic ischaemic encephalopathy. *Cochrane Database Syst Rev.* 2013;(1):CD003311.
137. Roberts D, Dalziel S. Antenatal corticosteroids for accelerating fetal lung maturation for women at risk of preterm birth. *Cochrane Database Syst Rev.* 2006;(3):CD004454.
138. Schmidt B, Roberts RS, Davis P, et al. Long-term effects of caffeine therapy for apnea of prematurity. *N Engl J Med.* 2007;357(19):1893–902.
139. American Psychiatric Association. *Diagnostic and Statistical Manual of Mental Disorders.* 5th ed. Arlington, VA: American Psychiatric Association; 2013.
140. Erskine HE, Norman RE, Ferrari AJ, et al. Long-term outcomes of attention-deficit/hyperactivity disorder and conduct disorder: A systematic review and meta-analysis. *J Am Acad Child Adolesc Psychiatry.* 2016;55(10):841–50.
141. Faraone SV, Biederman J, Mick E. The age-dependent decline of attention deficit hyperactivity disorder: A meta-analysis of follow-up studies. *Psychol Med.* 2006;36(2):159–65.
142. Caye A, Spadini AV, Karam RG, et al. Predictors of persistence of ADHD into adulthood: A systematic review of the literature and meta-analysis. *Eur Child Adolesc Psychiatry.* 2016;25(11):1151–9.
143. Thomas R, Sanders S, Doust J, et al. Prevalence of attention-deficit/hyperactivity disorder: A systematic review and meta-analysis. *Pediatrics.* 2015;135(4):e994–1001.
144. Polanczyk G, de Lima MS, Horta BL, et al. The worldwide prevalence of ADHD: A systematic review and metaregression analysis. *Am J Psychiatry.* 2007;164(6):942–8.
145. Wang T, Liu K, Li Z, et al. Prevalence of attention deficit/hyperactivity disorder among children and adolescents in China: A systematic review and meta-analysis. *BMC Psychiatry.* 2017;17(1):32.
146. Chan E, Fogler JM, Hammerness PG. Treatment of attention-deficit/hyperactivity disorder in adolescents: A systematic review. *JAMA.* 2016;315(18):1997–2008.
147. Rappley MD, Gardiner JC, Jetton JR. The use of methylphenidate in Michigan. *Arch Pediatr Adolesc Med.* 1995;149(6):675–9.
148. Banerjee TD, Middleton F, Faraone SV. Environmental risk factors for attention-deficit hyperactivity disorder. *Acta Paediatr.* 2007;96(9):1269–74.
149. Lingineni RK, Biswas S, Ahmad N. Factors associated with attention deficit/hyperactivity disorder among US children: Results from a national survey. *BMC Pediatr.* 2012;12:50.
150. Miller TW, Nigg JT, Miller RL. Attention deficit hyperactivity disorder in African American children: What can be concluded from the past ten years? *Clin Psychol Rev.* 2009;29(1):77–86.
151. Morgan PL, Staff J, Hillemeier MM. Racial and ethnic disparities in ADHD diagnosis from kindergarten to eighth grade. *Pediatrics.* 2013;132(1):85–93.
152. Altarac M, Saroha E. Lifetime prevalence of learning disability among US children pediatrics. 2007;119(Supplement 1):S77–8.
153. Pastor PN, Reuben CA. Diagnosed attention deficit hyperactivity disorder and learning disability: United States, 2004–2006. National Center for Health Statistics. *Vital Health Stat.* 2008;10(237).
154. Franz AP, Bolat GU, Bolat H, et al. Attention-deficit/hyperactivity disorder and very preterm/very low birth weight: A meta-analysis. *Pediatrics.* 2018;141(1). pii: e20171645.
155. Linnet KM, Dalsgaard S, Obel C, et al. Maternal lifestyle factors in pregnancy risk of attention deficit hyperactivity disorder and associated behaviors: Review of the current evidence. *Am J Psychiatry.* 2003;160(6):1028–40.
156. Cortese S, Moreira-Maia CR, St Fleur D. Association between ADHD and obesity: A systematic review and meta-analysis. *Am J Psychiatry.* 2016;173(1):34–43.
157. Pelsser LM, Frankena K, Toorman J, et al. Diet and ADHD, reviewing the evidence: A systematic review of meta-analyses of double-blind placebo-controlled trials evaluating the efficacy of diet interventions on the behavior of children with ADHD. *PLoS One.* 2017;12(1):e0169277.
158. Pelsser LM, Frankena K, Toorman J, et al. Effects of a restricted elimination diet on the behaviour of children with attention-deficit hyperactivity disorder (INCA study): A randomised controlled trial. *Lancet.* 2011;377(9764):494–503.

159. Goodlad JK, Marcus DK, Fulton JJ. Lead and attention-deficit/hyperactivity disorder (ADHD) symptoms: A meta-analysis. *Clin Psychol Rev.* 2013;33(3):417–25.
160. Eubig PA, Aguiar A, Schantz SL. Lead and PCBs as risk factors for attention deficit/hyperactivity disorder. *Environ Health Perspect.* 2010;118(12):1654–67.
161. Braun JM, Kahn RS, Froehlich T. Exposures to environmental toxicants and attention deficit hyperactivity disorder in U.S. children. *Environ Health Perspect.* 2006;114(12):1904–9.
162. Bouchard MF, Bellinger DC, Wright RO, et al. Attention-deficit/hyperactivity disorder and urinary metabolites of organophosphate pesticides. *Pediatrics.* 2010;125(6):e1270–7.
163. Lee DH, Jacobs DR, Porta M. Association of serum concentrations of persistent organic pollutants with the prevalence of learning disability and attention deficit disorder. *J Epidemiol Community Health.* 2007;61(7):591–6.
164. Chopra V, Harley K, Lahiff M. Association between phthalates and attention deficit disorder and learning disability in U.S. children, 6–15 years. *Environ Res.* 2014;128:64–9.
165. Abid Z, Roy A, Herbstman JB, et al. Urinary polycyclic aromatic hydrocarbon metabolites and attention/deficit hyperactivity disorder, learning disability, and special education in U.S. children aged 6 to 15. *J Environ Public Health.* 2014;2014:628508.
166. Barberio AM, Quiñonez C, Hosein FS, et al. Fluoride exposure and reported learning disability diagnosis among Canadian children: Implications for community water fluoridation. *Can J Public Health.* 2017;108(3):e229–39.
167. MacMillan DL, Gresham FM, Bocian KM. Discrepancy between definitions of learning disabilities and school practices: An empirical investigation. *J Learn Disabil.* 1998;31(4):314–26.
168. Pastor PN, Reuben CA. Diagnosed attention deficit hyperactivity disorder and learning disability: United States, 2004–2006. *Vital Health Stat 10.* 2008;(237):1–14.
169. Altarac M, Saroha E. Lifetime prevalence of learning disability among US children. *Pediatrics.* 2007;119(Suppl 1):S77–83.
170. Nord D, Luecking R, Mank D. The state of the science of employment and economic self-sufficiency for people with intellectual and developmental disabilities. *Intellect Dev Disabil.* 2013;51(5):376–84.
171. Shabeer MP, Abiramalatha T, Smith A. Comparison of two low-cost methods of cooling neonates with hypoxic ischemic encephalopathy. *J Trop Pediatr.* 2017;63(3):174–81.
172. Magnus P, Birke C, Vejrup K, et al. Cohort profile update: The Norwegian mother and child cohort study (MoBa). *Int J Epidemiol.* 2016;45(2):382–8.
173. Tollånes MC, Strandberg-Larsen K, Forthun I, et al. Cohort profile: Cerebral palsy in the Norwegian and Danish birth cohorts (MOBAND-CP). *BMJ Open.* 2016;6(9):e012777.
174. Ishitsuka K, Nakayama SF, Kishi R, et al. Japan Environment and Children's Study: Backgrounds, activities, and future directions in global perspectives. *Environ Health Prev Med.* 2017;22(1):61.
175. Gillman MW, Blaisdell CJ. Environmental influences on Child Health Outcomes, a Research Program of the National Institutes of Health. *Curr Opin Pediatr.* 2018;30(2):260–2.
176. Stein Z, Belmont L, Durkin M. Mild mental retardation and severe mental retardation compared: Experiences in eight less developed countries. *Ups J Med Sci Suppl.* 1987;44:89–96.
177. Yoshimura M, Tohyama J, Maegaki Y. Computed tomography and magnetic resonance imaging of the brain in congenital rubella syndrome. *No To Hattatsu.* 1996;28(5):385–90.
178. Sutton M, Daly LE, Kirke PN. Survival and disability in a cohort of neural tube defect births in Dublin, Ireland. *Birth Defects Res A Clin Mol Teratol.* 2008;82(10):701–9.
179. Ozaras N, Yalcin S, Ofluoglu D. Are some cases of spina bifida combined with cerebral palsy? A study of 28 cases. *Eura Medicophys.* 2005;41(3):239–42.
180. Glinoer D. Feto-maternal repercussions of iodine deficiency during pregnancy. An update. *Ann Endocrinol (Paris).* 2003;64(1):37–44.
181. van Wegberg AMJ, MacDonald A, Ahring K. The complete European guidelines on phenylketonuria: Diagnosis and treatment. *Orphanet J Rare Dis.* 2017;12(1):162.
182. Grosse SD, Van Vliet G. Prevention of intellectual disability through screening for congenital hypothyroidism: How much and at what level? *Arch Dis Child.* 2011;96(4):374–9.

CHAPTER

161 Neurocognitive Disorder and Cognitive Decline

Rhoda Au • Ryan J. Piers • Ting Fang Ang

INTRODUCTION

The global prevalence of dementia is over 24 million.[1] This number is expected to reach over 81 million by the year 2040.[1] The most common type of dementia is Alzheimer's disease (AD) In the United States, it is estimated that more than 5.4 million people are living with AD, with approximately 5.2 million over the age of 65.[2,3] Approximately 10.5% of 65-year-olds will develop AD dementia at some point in their life.[4] There is evidence that after reaching the age of 65, the incidence of AD doubles every 5 years.[5] The prevalence of AD is expected to increase rapidly as the "baby boomer generation" enters old age.[2] The financial burden of caring for 5.2 million people with AD is $214 billion.[6] This number will rise to $1.2 trillion by 2050 if the projected tripling to 16 million cases occurs.[7] Importantly, these estimates are likely conservative, given the numerous causes of dementia. All of these factors underscore the critical importance of developing effective treatments.

Dementia is relentless and devastating. A host of cognitive capacities, as well as the ability to perform activities of daily living (e.g., washing, eating, dressing), are affected. Watching a loved one struggle with dementia can take an incredible emotional toll on family members and caretakers.[8] According to the Alzheimer's Association, in the United States alone 14.9 million family members and caretakers put forth approximately 17 billion hours of unpaid care every year.[9] Due to the physically demanding and time-consuming nature of providing care, it is not uncommon for family members to experience depression and loneliness.[10,11]

The purpose of this chapter is to provide a brief overview of age-related neurocognitive disorders with a particular focus on AD. We also forecast how future advances in technology may enable earlier detection for potentially more effective intervention strategies, as well as promote disease prevention and preservation of brain health.

DEMENTIA

Introduction

Dementia is a broad diagnostic category characterized by a change in cognitive and behavioral functioning. The presentation of dementia is heterogeneous, and involves impairment in multiple domains of functioning, including memory, executive function, attention, visuospatial ability, and language.[12] Dementia is typically associated with a change in personality (e.g., difficulty controlling emotions, loss of interest in hobbies), impairment or an inability to perform activities of daily living (e.g., cooking, paying bills), and difficulty in social situations (e.g., maintaining or following conversation, social inappropriateness). Dementia diagnosis is made when the cognitive and behavioral symptoms cause significant interference with activities of daily living or occupation.[12] Diagnosis is dependent on self-report accuracy by the patient and/or informant (e.g., family member), the availability of medical or personal records documenting the symptoms over time, the correct administration and interpretation of neurocognitive tests, and the judgment of the clinician.[12] In making the diagnosis, it is important to conclude that the symptoms of dementia are not better explained by other neurological (e.g., traumatic brain injury, TBI) or psychiatric conditions (e.g., depression, other mental health disorders), the side effects of medications, or exposure to toxins.

Within the broad diagnosis of dementia, there are varying degrees of impairment: mild, moderate, or severe. Determination of severity depends on a number of factors, including the level of interference with occupation or activities of daily living and the degree to which cognition has deteriorated from their normal baseline.[12] McKhann et al. (2011)[12] provides an in-depth description of the current Alzheimer's Association's diagnostic criteria for dementia.

Despite the serious economic and healthcare-associated impact posed by the aging "baby boomer" generation, there is some evidence that the incidence of dementia has declined over the past 30 years.[13] Interestingly, the observed decline in prevalence of vascular risk factors (systolic blood pressure, use of antihypertensive medications, smoking, atrial fibrillation, and heart disease) did not explain the decline in the incidence of dementia. This suggests that other lifestyle and genetic factors may be playing a role.

Detection and Diagnosis

Cognitive Screening Tools

In the primary-care setting, it is common for brief neurocognitive tools to be administered to assess cognitive impairment.[14,15] The Mini Mental State Examination (MMSE) is a commonly used evaluation of global cognitive ability. The MMSE is inexpensive, brief, and easy to administer. There is evidence of excellent test–retest and interrater reliability, as well as good concurrent validity when compared to the Verbal and Performance Intellectual Quotient (WAIS).[16] However, research indicates that the MMSE is insensitive in measuring cognitive impairment, especially in the earliest stages of the disease,[17] particularly among those with higher levels of education. A study by Nasreddine et al. (2005) found that the Montreal Cognitive Assessment (MoCA), a separate brief global cognitive assessment, was superior in detecting more subtle cognitive impairment as compared to the MMSE (90% and 18%, respectively).[18] The MoCA may be more sensitive in detecting cognitive impairment because of the inclusion of several executive function tasks that are not included in the MMSE.[19] Both of these cognitive screening tests have been criticized for having ceiling effects, although the MoCA is less prone to them.[18,19]

Medical History

Medical history and family interview data often provide important historical context to the cognitive symptoms. For example, psychiatric conditions such as depression[20] or environmental exposures to toxins, such as lead[21,22] can have a detriment effect on performance on cognitive tasks unrelated to a neurodegenerative disease process. Family members may notice subtle changes in behavior that formal assessments may not be sufficiently sensitive to detect.

Neurological Examination

The neurological examination entails a comprehensive review of sensory and motor functions, which is intended to rule out other neurologic disorders that could account for cognitive dysfunction (e.g., stroke, Parkinson's disease). From the information gathered during the interview and mental status examination, physicians score the patients' level of functioning in domains of memory, orientation, judgment and problem solving, community affairs, home of hobbies, and personal care. Each domain is scored based on the physician's clinical judgment of the level of impairment: 0 (none), 0.5 (questionable), 1 (mild), 2 (moderate), and 3 (severe). Lastly, a clinical dementia rating (CDR) is often reported as a single score to summarize overall impairment.[23] Although there is evidence that the CDR has high reliability and validity in detecting cognitive impairment and dementia, it has been criticized for its reliance on the subjective assessment by clinicians.[24] McCarten (2013)[25] provides a description of the prototypical neurologic exam. Resources are also available on the American Academy for Neurology website (see Chapter 1: The Neurologic Examination).

Neuropsychological Examination

A neuropsychological examination is a series of tests designed to assess an individual's level of functioning in a specific cognitive domain (e.g., memory, attention, executive functioning, abstract reasoning, language, processing speed, visuospatial, visuoperceptual, and visuoconstruction ability). These tests have been used to diagnose brain injury[26,27] and developmental disorders,[28] but they are most commonly used for the diagnosis of neurodegenerative disorders such as AD.[29,30] For a review of the clinical applications of neuropsychological assessment, see Harvey (2012).[31]

There is evidence that the Boston Process Approach (BPA) to neuropsychological assessment enhances the detection and evaluation of cognitive impairment and dementia.[32] Those who practice the BPA contend that cognition cannot captured by a single score on a test. Although quantitative scores can be informative, it is the careful observation and documentation of an individual during the entire problem-solving activity, which provides the best evaluation of the domain in question. Furthermore, two people could earn the same score on a test, but the nature of their errors could reveal that they used very different strategies. As the famed neuropsychologist, Edith Kaplan, Ph.D. observed, "the patient who misplaces one of nine blocks on a difficult Block Design item receives the same 'zero' score as the patient who throws or eats the blocks."[33]

ALZHEIMER'S DISEASE

Introduction

Dementia from Alzheimer's disease is the most common type of progressive dementia, accounting for approximately 60–80% of cases.[2] AD typically has an insidious onset and is characterized by slow, progressive cognitive, and behavioral decline.[12] Unlike TBI or stroke, there are no fixed experiences or exposures that catalyze symptoms and associated brain pathology.[34] However, cognitive decline is often apparent to family members, and to the individuals themselves.[12]

Diagnosis

To meet the diagnostic criteria for AD dementia, patients must first meet criteria for dementia. The cognitive impairment can either have an amnestic presentation or a nonamnestic presentation. The amnestic presentation of AD dementia is more common and includes memory dysfunction (i.e., difficulty remembering new information), as well as cognitive decline in at least one other domain, such as executive function, attention, visuospatial function, or language.[12] The nonamnestic presentation of AD dementia does not include memory dysfunction, but does include dysfunction in at least one other domain.[12]

The diagnosis of "definite AD dementia" requires autopsy data revealing widespread distribution of amyloid plaques and neurofibrillary tangles for diagnosis. Prior to death, patients are diagnosed as "probable or possible AD dementia."[12,35] Individuals are diagnosed with "possible AD dementia" if: (a) cognitive impairment has a sudden onset, (b) there is insufficient documentation of a progressive course and/or history of cognitive impairment, or (c) the disorder has an etiologically mixed presentation (e.g., there is evidence other factors or conditions contributing to cognitive decline).[12] "Probable AD dementia" requires evidence of insidious onset and slow, progressive cognitive and behavioral decline[12] in the absence of any other factors that can account for these changes. For diagnostic purposes, it should be noted that repeated neurocognitive testing that documents decline over the course of several years is preferable to comparing an individual's performance at a single time point to normative data. For a discussion of the limitations of normative comparison and unfairness in testing, see Berry, Clark, and McClure (2011)[36] and Helms (2006).[37] Atrophy documented via brain MRI scans are commonly used in tandem with other clinical data (e.g., neuropsychological test performance) to inform diagnosis and monitoring disease progression.[38]

It has been well documented that sporadic AD is a heterogeneous disease,[39] characterized by a variable profile in which indices of the neurodegenerative processes (as indicated by changes in cognitive and brain structure) may precede the advent of amyloid-beta plaques.[40] Au, Piers, and Lancashire (2015) contend that AD clinical trial studies have largely failed because AD has been conceptualized as a single disease[41] when in fact the heterogeneity suggests it may be multiple diseases. The path to effective treatment of AD may lie in the identification of Alzheimer's "diseases," potentially resulting in multiple drug targets as opposed to one.

Biomarkers

Positron Emission Tomography and Cerebral Spinal Fluid

The pathological hallmarks for AD are the accumulation of amyloid-beta plaques and neurofibrillary tau tangles in the brain.[12,42–44] These pathologies can be observed via positron emission tomography (PET).[45] Early in the disease process, pathology is seen in areas of the brain associated with memory function, such as the hippocampus and entorhinal cortex.[42,43,46,47] As the disease progresses, pathology is seen increasingly in the cerebral cortex.[42,43] At this time, other major domains of cognitive functioning become impaired including abstract reasoning, language ability, attention, and executive functioning.[43,48]

While there is evidence of an association between increased amyloid deposition and cognitive decline,[49–54] there is still much debate about whether the amyloid deposition is causing the cognitive decline or a byproduct of a still unknown mechanism. More consistent has been the relationship between neurofibrillary tau tangles and cognition.[55,56] One AD autopsy study found that the density of neurofibrillary tangles mediated the association between amyloid-beta deposition and level of cognitive function.[56]

AD biomarkers are also measured in cerebral spinal fluid (CSF),[57] represented by levels of amyloid ($A\beta_{1\text{-}42}$) and tau (Total tau, phosphorated tau 181).[58] In order to obtain CSF, a lumbar puncture must be performed, a procedure that is invasive and not well tolerated by the general population.[59] A recent meta-analysis found that CSF $A\beta_{1\text{-}42}$ levels demonstrated high accuracy in the differential diagnosis of AD patients compared to normal controls.[60] However, CSF biomarkers have been criticized for their lack of specificity in differentiating AD from non-AD dementias overall.[58]

There is evidence that AD biomarkers (as measured by CSF and PET imaging) can be found in both cognitively intact and demented individuals.[61–65] It is estimated that between 20% and 40%

of cognitively intact elderly have significant amyloid deposition.[63-65] While it is acknowledged that in vivo AD biomarkers may aid in the valid identification of an AD pathophysiological process, because of inconsistent findings the Alzheimer's Association recommends that biomarker evidence be used in conjunction with neuropsychological testing in the diagnosis of AD, and not as a stand-alone solution.[12]

Inflammation and Other Biomarkers

Biomarkers related to AD include lipid profile,[66] blood glucose,[67] C-reactive protein,[68] Interleukin 6,[69,70] isoprostanes,[71] and insulin.[72,73] Neurotrophic factors have been associated with preclinical dementia,[74-79] brain morphology,[80,81] and cognitive function.[82-90]

Risk Factors

Vascular

There are many risk factors that have been associated with AD. Most commonly studied are vascular risk factors, which have been shown to increase risk.[91,92] There is evidence demonstrating an association between vascular risk factors and cognitive decline, as well as differences in brain volume. The Framingham Stroke Risk Profile (which factors age, systolic blood pressure, antihypertensive medication, diabetes, cigarette smoking, cardiovascular disease, atrial fibrillation) has been associated with cognitive decline[93,94] and differences in brain volume.[95] Individual vascular risk factors, such as atrial fibrillation, diabetes, hypertension, obesity, cardiovascular disease, and cigarette smoking have been associated with cognitive decline[96-103] and differences in brain volume.[97,104,105] There is evidence that the impact of vascular risk increases risk for AD earlier in adult life[106] and that it is progressive.[98]

APOE4 (Genetic, Nonfamilial)

Apolipoprotein E4 (APOE4) is the most well-documented genetic risk factor for AD.[107] An individual can be a carrier of one or two APOE4 alleles, and the risk of development of AD is higher among those who are homogygotes. APOE2 and APOE3 alleles also exist. One study reported that the lifetime risk of AD is between 51% and 60% for men and women who are carriers of two APOE4 alleles and between 23% and 30% for men and women who are carriers of one APOE4 allele and one APOE3 allele.[108] APOE2 has been reported to have a neuroprotective effect.[109]

APP, PSEN1, PSEN2 (Genetic, Familial)

It is estimated that 85–90% of AD cases are sporadic.[110] That is, for the vast majority of cases of AD, there is no single cause. For sporadic AD, cognitive symptoms related to the disease typically begin after the age of 65 and are characterized by a slow, progressive decline.[12,110] Alternatively, familial AD (also known as autosomal dominant AD), is associated with early onset of cognitive symptoms and a more rapid decline.[110,111] Mutations in three genes are now widely recognized as the cause of autosomal dominant AD: presenilin1 (PSEN1), presenilin2 (PSEN2), and the amyloid precursor protein (APP).[111] These mutations are passed down from generation to generation.[111-113] If one parent has the PSEN1, PSEN2, or APP mutation, his/her child will inherit it and with certainty develop familial AD.

Protective Factors

Environment

Numerous studies have found that environmental factors play a large role in brain health and development.[114-116] Researchers have observed neurogenesis in mice exposed to enriched environments and physical activity, particularly in the hippocampus[117] and dentate gyrus.[118] In humans, there is evidence that a high level of complex mental activity is protective against hippocampal atrophy over time.[119] Furthermore, a cross-sectional PET study found that higher involvement in cognitively stimulating activities throughout life (e.g., reading books, writing emails or letters, playing games), was associated with lower amyloid-beta deposition in cognitively intact elderly (average age = 76.1).[120] Interestingly, intact elderly who scored in the highest cognitive activity tertile had amyloid-beta deposition similar to young controls (average age = 24.5), while intact elderly who scored in the lowest cognitive activity tertile had amyloid-beta deposition similar to AD patients.[120] These results suggest that lifetime cognitive engagement is neuroprotective against AD pathology.

There is evidence that the number of leisure activities that one engages in during old age reduces dementia risk.[121] In one longitudinal study, a "high" number of leisure activities was classified as seven or more activities in the preceding month.[121] Activities included "knitting or music or other hobby, walking for pleasure or excursion, visiting friends or relatives, being visited by relatives or friends, physical conditioning, going to movies or restaurants or sporting events, reading magazines or newspapers or books, watching television or listening to the radio, doing unpaid community volunteer work, playing cards or games or bingo, going to a club or center, going to classes, and going to church or synagogue or temple (p. 2238)."[121] In this nondemented sample of individuals 65 years of age and older, those who reported "high" number of leisure activities had a 38% lower risk of developing dementia as compared to those who reported a "low" (or less than seven) number of leisure activities.[121]

APOE2

Apolipoprotein E2 (APOE2) is potentially neuroprotective.[109] Relative to APOE3 (78.6%) and APOE4 (13.5%), APOE2 occurs with the lowest frequency (7.5%).[122] One longitudinal study investigated the effect of APOE status on cognitive function in nondemented adults 65 years of age or older.[123] APOE2 (2/2, 2/3) was associated with a net annual increase in memory scores over an 8-year period. APOE3 (3/3) and APOE4 (3/4, 4/4) carriers, on the other hand, experienced an annual decrease in memory scores (APOE4 worse than APOE3).

Chiang et al. (2010) found that, over a 2-year period, cognitively intact elderly APOE2 carriers (2/2 or 2/3) displayed slower rates of hippocampal atrophy than cognitively intact elderly APOE3 homozygotes (3/3).[124] While the literature does not link APOE3 homozygotes to an increased risk for AD, the study suggests one potential mechanism for how APOE2 guards against the cognitive effects of AD.

Shaw et al. (2007) investigated the impact of APOE status on cortical morphology in children and adolescents.[125] In the left entorhinal cortex, medial temporal cortex, and orbitofrontal cortex, the researchers observed that APOE2 (2/3) carriers had the greatest cortical thickness, followed by APOE3 homozygotes, and APOE4 carriers had the thinnest cortical volume. The increased cortical thickness observed in APOE2 carriers could serve as another possible explanation for the neuroprotective features of APOE2.

Finally, APOE2 also appears to guard against the accumulation of both amyloid plaques and neurofibrillary tau tangles.[126]

Education

Recent evidence suggests that high educational attainment may delay cognitive decline in individuals with AD by up to 7 years.[127] Unlike lower education groups who experience cognitive symptoms at the onset of AD pathology (amyloid-beta plaques and neurofibrillary tau tangles), higher education groups have cognitive reserve, which allows them to maintain their functioning for a longer period of time.

In familial AD (Colombian Kindred cohort, PSEN1 E280A mutation), higher educational attainment was seen to be protective and associated with a delay in cognitive decline by 3 years.[128] However, participants with higher education level experienced steeper cognitive decline after symptom onset than those with lower education level.

Cognitive Reserve

The concept of cognitive reserve stems from the observation that some individuals with high levels of brain pathology (i.e., amyloid-beta plaques and neurofibrillary tau tangles) do not experience cognitive consequences.[129] It is not uncommon for individuals with no lifetime history of significant cognitive impairment to be diagnosed with AD at autopsy.[130] Factors that have been associated with increased cognitive reserve include high educational attainment, occupational success, and participation in leisure activities in old age.[121,129,131] One study found that the risk of developing dementia was 2.2 times higher in individuals with less than 8 years of education.[131] This same study found that the risk of developing dementia was 2.25 times higher in individuals with low lifetime occupational attainment, defined as "unskilled/semiskilled, skilled trade or craft, and clerical/office worker (p. 1006)."[131] Individuals who met criteria for both "low education" and "low occupation" had the highest risk of developing dementia.[131] Interestingly, a separate study found that the association between low occupation-based SES and increased risk of dementia became insignificant after educational attainment was entered into the model.[132] This finding lends further support on the relationship between education and the cognitive reserve hypothesis.

Treatment

To date there are no disease-modifying medications. The presumption is that the vast number of failed clinical trial studies are the result of interventions coming too late in the course of the disease.[133] As a result, current AD research includes significant effort to identify biomarkers decades before the threshold for a clinical diagnosis of dementia is crossed.[4,41,61,64,134] This "preclinical AD" phase is being targeted as a promising path for effective treatments that can either attenuate or disrupt disease progression.[41]

VASCULAR DEMENTIA

Vascular dementia (VaD) is the second most common cause of dementia after Alzheimer's disease (AD), affecting about 15% of the dementia cases, with its risk doubling every 5 years of age.[135,136] Its prevalence reaches 30% among 3-month poststroke individuals.[137] Unlike AD, the diagnosis of VaD is less defined. Even the word "dementia" is a point of controversy as experts argue that the cognitive dysfunction of VaD lies on a spectrum rather than discrete cut-offs. Due to the lack of a common consensus regarding the diagnosis of VaD, researchers have been using different diagnostic criteria.[138–142] The National Institute of Neurological Disorders and Stroke and the Association Internationale pour la Recherche et l'Enseignement en Neurosciences (NINDS-AIREN) criteria is widely accepted as the benchmark due to its high specificity, although some studies employed the Diagnostic and Statistical Manual of Mental Disorders (DSM) or Alzheimer's Disease Diagnostic and Treatment Centers (ADDTC) criteria as they are more sensitive.[143,144]

As the name implies, VaD is due to brain vascular pathology, which presents as hemorrhages, ischemia, or the combination of both.[145] In the case of ischemia, it can be broadly subdivided into large vessel and small vessel diseases, with age-related, hypertension-related, and cerebral amyloid angiopathy making up the majority for the latter.[146] Given its pronounced association with the circulatory system, the onset of VaD can be sudden or gradual, a stark difference from AD, where the onset is never sudden. Poststroke dementia is the classic example an acute onset dementia subtype. Likewise, the risk factors for VaD closely resemble those for cardiovascular disease and stroke. Besides the common atherosclerotic risk factors,[147] namely, advanced age, male gender, cigarette smoking, hypertension, hyperlipidemias and diabetes mellitus, autoimmune, and infective vasculitides, such as lupus erythematosus and Lyme disease, respectively, result in vasculopathy that leads to VaD.[148]

The diverse clinical presentation of VaD is a major contributing factor to the ongoing debate, regarding the most ideal classification, among the research community. Although the cognitive impairment of VaD subjects is wide-ranging, most typically present with attention and executive function deficits initially,[149,150] as opposed to memory dysfunction, which is often associated with early AD.[151] Hence, standardized tests, like the MMSE,[16] which focus much on short-term memory, have been shown to be insensitive to detecting cognitive abnormalities in early stages of VaD.[152] On the contrary, neuropsychological tests that assess the executive function—Trail-Making Test and the Clock Drawing Test, for example—are especially important in the diagnosis for VaD.[150]

More important than neuropsychological assessment is the presence of cerebrovascular disease on neuroimaging—a hallmark feature of VaD.[139] Generally, this will show up as strategic lacunar strokes, multiple cortical or subcortical strokes, and extensive white matter lesions on the scans.[153] Another pertinent radiological feature is hippocampal atrophy, which is suggestive of underlying cognitive impairment, this however is more frequently observed in AD.[154] Under the NINDS-AIREN criteria,[139] evidence from neuroimaging is a sine qua nonelement; evaluation would be impossible without it.

Similar to AD, the clinical intervention for VaD requires early and accurate diagnosis, treating underlying comorbidities and managing patients' and caregivers' expectations. The current standard pharmacotherapy for VaD is cholinesterase inhibitors[155] and memantine,[156,157] medications that were initially studied and used in AD. The efficacy of these modalities had been lackluster, showing minimal to no benefits to global function.[158] In fact, instead of tackling the cognitive impairment aspect, clinicians have shifted their treatment focus to manage the underlying comorbidities (such as hypertension, hyperlipidemia, and diabetes mellitus) for individuals with VaD. The survival from dementia onset to death for subjects with VaD was 3.9 years, as compared to 7.1 years for those with AD; the former usually died from cerebrovascular disease while the latter died from dementia or failure to thrive.[159]

Prevention is the key to counter the increasing global burden of VaD. A person at risk of cardiovascular disease and/or stroke is a person at risk for VaD. Many modifiable risk factors, including hypertension, cigarette smoking, hyperlipidemias, and diabetes mellitus, have been thoroughly studied and there is a repertoire of preventive measures that could be implemented at population level, to reduce the incidence of VaD. Of note, hypertension is arguably the most important risk factor to control, as it elevates stroke risk significantly throughout life,[160] which may give rise to poststroke VaD. Several studies have demonstrated that with appropriate antihypertensive interventions, the risk of dementia would drastically reduced.[161–163] Even among individuals who previous strokes, secondary prevention using antiplatelet medications is beneficial in minimizing stroke recurrence.[164]

Likewise, the main rationale for prevention or treatment of hyperlipidemias and diabetes mellitus is to reduce the risk of cardiovascular disease and/or stroke. Large-scale studies reported that optimal control of hyperlipidemias markedly lowers stroke risk.[165,166] In addition to stroke prevention, statins exhibited neuroprotective effects of endothelial nitric oxide synthase enhancement and down regulation of proinflammatory cytokines.[167] Besides the use of statins, lifestyle modifications such as dietary fat restriction and increase consumption of food that is rich in omega fatty acids (i.e., fish and olive oil) should be part of ongoing public health campaigns, in an effort to educate the masses. Diabetes affects both the large and small vessels,[168] both of which constitute the bulk of the brain vascular pathologies for VaD. The long-term goal for diabetic subjects is to maintain good glycemic control. This can be achieved not just by medications, but the combination of diet modifications, maintaining normal body mass index and adequate exercise. Hence, organized efforts to heighten the awareness of healthy lifestyle among the public is quintessential.

More research efforts need to be put in for VaD, especially to better define the diagnostic criteria and develop new treatment options. Researchers should appreciate the differences between VaD and AD and design their studies accordingly, to accurately assess the cognitive status of affected individuals and provide fair measurements for clinical trials.

PARKINSON'S DISEASE DEMENTIA

Motor-related neurodegenerative symptoms, such as tremors, bradykinesia, rigidity, and postural instability, are well-established characteristics of Parkinson's disease (PD). In the face of the dementia epidemic, the less-discussed cognitive impairment due to PD—Parkinson's disease dementia (PD-D)—has since gained more attention. It is estimated that prevalence of dementia among subject with PD is about 30% and this escalates to nearly 75% in 10-years-or-more survivors.[169] The mean duration from onset of PD to dementia occurrence is about 10 years,[170,171] although this fluctuates widely.[172] Movement Disorder Society (MDS)-proposed clinical diagnostic criteria[173] is now the widely accepted standard for PD-D diagnosis, replacing the generic DSM-IV criteria[141] (currently known as DSM-V). A condition tantamount to PD-D is Lewy Body Dementia (LBD). The distinguishing feature between these two conditions is the temporal relationship of dementia to Parkinsonism. In LBD, the symptoms of dementia and Parkinsonism emerge within 1 year of each other, while PD-D patients exhibit more than 1 year of levodopa-responsive symptoms before developing dementia.

In Aarsland et al. study,[169,172] they showed that individual chronological age, rather than the age of onset of PD, significantly affects the development of dementia; hence not all PD subjects end up with dementia—about 25% remain nondemented after more than 10 years with the disease. Risk factors for PD-D includes advanced age, severe Parkinsonism and mild cognitive impairment (MCI) at onset of PD. Firstly, similar to other types of dementia, advanced age is an important factor to consider in the dementia risk assessment of PD subjects.[172] Secondly, individuals with severe motor dysfunction, postural instability, and gait disorder in particular, were found to have increased risk for dementia.[174,175] Lastly, it is not uncommon for individuals to exhibit MCI right from the onset of PD.[176] Studies have demonstrated that subjects with Parkinson's disease MCI (PD-MCI) were at higher risk of developing dementia over time.[177] Apart from the above-mentioned risk factors, PD subjects with visual hallucinations were also found to have higher incidence of dementia.[170]

The onset of PD-D is always insidious and generally it affects the executive, visuospatial, and memory functions. Akin to VaD, PD-D predominately affects individuals' executive function.[178,179] Common neuropsychological tests that can be used to elicit these impaired responses include verbal fluency, digit span backward, Wisconsin Card Sorting Test, Stroop Test, and Trail Making Test.[180] Visuospatial function is also much more affected in PD-D subjects, as compared to AD subjects,[181,182] with the former performing much worse in visual discrimination, object-form, and space-motion perception. PD-D subjects typically also present with memory impairment—isolated short-term memory; it is however not as severe as that of AD.[182,183] In addition, unlike AD, the amnesic component of PD was thought to be more of a retrieval problem, rather than encoding and storage.[184] When PD subjects convert to PD-D, this distinction becomes blurred, as they too are unable to recall with cues.[185]

Besides the motor-related and impaired cognitive symptoms, individuals with PD-D also commonly present with neuropsychiatric and sleep symptoms. Hallucinations are frequently reported psychotic symptoms, affecting as many as 65% of the PD-D cases.[186] As mentioned earlier, the presence of hallucinations in PD nondemented subjects increases their dementia risk.[170] These hallucinations are often described as colorful and involving well-formed people and animals.[187] In addition, mood symptoms such as depression[186] and anxiety[188] affect as many as 50% of the PD-D subjects. It is also widely accepted that REM sleep behavior disorder (RBD) is associated with PD-D.[189]

Given the myriad of symptoms a PD-D patient can present with, a holistic clinical approach is imperative. Levodopa remains the mainstay of the therapy cocktail for individuals with PD-D. Although it has minimal effect on cognitive impairment, much of the decline in quality of life (QOL) in PD-D subjects arise from the worsening of motor-related symptoms, caused by the progressive neurodegeneration process of PD. Nonetheless, the cognitive impairment component of PD-D is equally debilitating, but there is currently no treatment modality that can retard its progress. Like VaD, clinicians resort to use medications like cholinesterase inhibitors[190] and memantine[191] to alleviate the cognitive symptoms. Even though the cholinesterase inhibitors manage to improve the symptoms in nonsevere PD-D, the efficacy of memantine remains questionable. Apart from the motor and cognitive symptoms, intervention is also required for the neuropsychiatric symptoms—a rather unique set of problems for the both the patient and caregivers. A thorough clinic interview of both parties is paramount in this regard, as the patient cannot provide the full history, especially when it comes to hallucination and RBD.

Unfortunately, as the exact pathogenesis of Parkinson's is still a mystery, there are no evidence-based preventive measures available.

CHRONIC TRAUMATIC ENCEPHALOPATHY

Chronic traumatic encephalopathy (CTE) has created quite a buzz not just within the research community but also among the general public in the past few years. This condition, previously known as *dementia pugilistica*, that was first noted in professional boxers and described by Harrison S. Martland in his JAMA article—titled "Punch Drunk"—in 1928.[192] Recently, growing number of studies revealed that CTE is not unique to the boxing profession, as it also affects several other contact sports such as football, soccer, and ice hockey.[193,194] It is hence clear to the experts that CTE is a sequela to multiple TBIs.

TBI is a major public health issue. An estimated 1.7 million people sustain a TBI annually in the United States, among which 52,000 are fatal,[195] and the prevalence is even higher in the developing countries.[196] These numbers are certainly underestimates as a large portion of mild TBI goes unreported since the acute symptoms are generally self-limiting and affected individuals tend to self-aid. Despite the staggering statistics, the societal and economic burden of TBI is underappreciated. TBI remains the leading cause of death and disability for persons aged 1–44 years, and an estimate of 5.3 million Americans live with long-term disabilities due to a prior TBI.[197] Several studies revealed that TBI itself is a risk factor for incident non-CTE dementia.[198]

Currently, the diagnosis of CTE is consider a diagnosis of exclusion, where it is predominately made in young patients, who presents with progressive neurocognitive decline and prior TBI exposure, with all other etiologies ruled out. Even then, like AD, the CTE diagnosis can only be confirmed after death, during autopsy. Although signs and symptoms of early CTE has yet to be defined since the clinical research is still in the infancy, many researchers hypothesize that they would be very similar to those observed in combat veterans with posttraumatic stress disorder (PTSD), as they drew parallel with the condition *Shell shock*, a term coined after World War I.[199] In addition, the accounts from combatants, who suffered from PTSD, seem to overlap with those of professional athletes with CTE diagnosed at autopsy. The common physical symptoms include difficulty in concentrating, persistent headaches, and sleep disturbances, while the cognitive and behavioral symptoms are impaired memory, attention deficits, depression, and abrupt mood swings.

Besides symptomatic relief, there is currently no treatment for CTE. However, unlike all the other dementia types, CTE is a class of its own, as TBI—the necessary cause in its causal pathway—is purely an environmental-based risk factor. Therefore, theoretically speaking, CTE is highly preventable. Given the high interest about the general public, public health officials should make sure of this opportunity to reach out to the masses, to raise awareness regarding CTE and advocate safety measures in sports. The rule of thumb is to prevent, if not reduce, additional TBI after a concussion. If an individual is suspect to suffer from concussion, remove him/her from the stimulus and seek early medical attention. The use of sport-specific helmets may reduce the impact of the concussion; however, it is still unknown if it can prevent CTE in the long term.

MILD COGNITIVE IMPAIRMENT

MCI is part of the progression of symptoms in neurodegenerative disease and is most consistently linked to AD. It is also a diagnosis given for nondemented individuals with nonprogressive cognitive impairment, such as resulting from a head injury.[200,201] When originally conceived, MCI was seen as a distinct clinical state on the continuum of cognitive dysfunction, as opposed to a separate disorder.[202] For example, because AD typically has an insidious onset and is characterized by slow, progressive cognitive and behavioral decline, there is a distinct period of time when milder cognitive dysfunction is observed before the individual reaches the threshold of clinical dementia.[12,34] Those individuals with amnestic MCI, characterized by a difficulty with new learning and poor recall of learned information, are thought to be at increased risk of developing AD dementia.[203]

According to the NIA and Alzheimer's Association's (NIA-AA) guidelines for MCI due to Alzheimer's disease[12] require (1) concern expressed by the patient, family member, or informant; (2) cognitive impairment evident in one or more domains of functioning (e.g., memory, attention, executive functioning, language, visuospatial skills); and (3) the individual still able to perform their activities of daily living (e.g., cooking, cleaning, paying bills) independently.

In the United States, it is estimated that approximately 22.2% of individuals aged 71 years or older have MCI, and the prevalence increases with age.[204] There are currently no effective drug treatments for MCI.[205] One recent public health concern that has been raised surrounding MCI is impairment in ability to drive an automotive vehicle.[206] It is recommended that visuospatial and executive function tests be administered to individuals to determine if they are cognitively competent to drive.[207]

NEUROCOGNITIVE DISEASE VERSUS BRAIN HEALTH: FUTURE CONSIDERATIONS AND PUBLIC HEALTH IMPLICATIONS

The current public health approach to preventing neurocognitive disorders relies on the preventive medicine model.[208] As briefly reviewed above, numerous research studies seek to identify risk factors for dementia, including those that are and are not modifiable,[49–56,91–108,110,111,147,160,172,174,175,198,203] The compendium of dementia-related cohort studies relies on standard bear epidemiologic methods that were long ago defined by seminal studies such as the Framingham Heart Study (FHS), which not only coined the original term and concept of risk factors, but also essentially laid the foundation for the field of preventive medicine.[209] Even nearly 70 years later, researchers of all types of chronic diseases worldwide seek to establish their own "Framingham-like" study and continue to hold these well-defined public health methods as the gold standard for studying disease prevention. The most important takeaway to consider is the persistent emphasis on disease, which in turn translates into a drive to find effective treatments. Case in point is that despite numerous failed clinical trial studies,[210–213] finding a cure for AD garners far greater research support than finding a way to prevent it. As noted earlier, the current and projected costs of AD are staggering and without any solutions, going to become an increasingly significant economic drag on many countries worldwide.[1–7] In his 2015 State of the Union Address, President Obama announced the need to accelerate the progress of precision medicine. National Institute of Health Director Francis Collins translated this vision into the Precision Medicine Initiative (PMI) research strategy.[214] In tandem, the National Institute on Aging NIA established an ambitious plan for finding effective interventions for AD by 2025. Precision medicine is emerging as the path of healthcare's future, further highlighting the bias toward thinking of populations as patients rather than as people.

As discussed earlier, all progressive neurocognitive disorders including the major ones highlighted above are insidious in onset.[12,34] Current practice is for prospective surveillance for the emergence of symptoms such as change in cognitive status. FHS like many other epidemiologic studies use cognitive screening tools such as the MMSE to monitor for threshold levels of decline in performance.[14–16] Application of diagnostic criteria are applied to identify cases that meet definition for disease and risk prediction models are built to determine factors that differentiate between those at higher and lower risk for the disease.[61,62] The public health challenge for the future is to shift away from the medically driven presumption of precision medicine and bring forward what is potentially a much more transformative focus on precision health.

The distinction between precision medicine and precision health is not clearly made and is even used interchangeably. This lack of clarity impedes the critical role that public health needs to play in leading a major paradigm shift that can solve the persistent U.S. problem of high healthcare costs and low health quality.[215] Core assumptions to precision medicine are that there are clinical symptoms, followed by diagnostic testing to determine if disease criteria are met and if so, a treatment protocol is established and followed. Since 86% of diseases in the United States are chronic,[216] the high-cost/low-quality conundrum endures because the practice is to wait till disease is evident and then treat it, often for the remainder of a patient's lifespan. Precision medicine seeks to find customized treatments that will be more responsive at the individual level, but does not challenge the presupposition of symptoms, diagnosis, and treatment.

In fact, the health continuum begins at conception and continues until death. Since most diseases are chronic and insidious in their onset and progression, significant symptom severity for diagnosis appears further downstream along the continuous health spectrum. Given that most people are free of disease in the earliest years of life, the concept of precision health is that it precedes the need for precision medicine, and seeks to find personalized methods for optimizing a person's health across the entire lifespan. Precision health also offers the opportunity to move from a physician-centric model for disease prevention to a person-centered one.

To make the case for the promise of precision health, we apply it to neurocognitive disorders and offer a futuristic vision that could dramatically alter customary practice. Current methods for testing cognitive capabilities as described earlier rely on administration of a range of neuropsychological tests that together test skills in different domains (e.g., memory, attention, executive function, visuospatial, etc.). For many years, measuring cognitive function has used paper-pencil tests. Computerization of these tests is the modernized version of this long-standing system, and still requires a health professional to be involved in administration and/or interpretation of findings. The majority of neurocognitive disorders are tied to older age, but attention deficit disorders or learning disabilities are developmental conditions in which cognitive testing is frequently done with children.[217–220] Regardless of the age, the relevant point is that neuropsychologist testing is done to identify impairments. Further, these assessments are conducted at one or more sporadic points in time and much is interpreted from it. Yet, it is well recognized that cognitive capabilities fluctuate and a myriad of internal and external factors can influence performance. In reality, neuropsychological test scores are relatively crude measures of cognition, and to account for natural variability in performance, it is common practice to administer multiple tests that often can take up to hours to administer.

Technological advances provide the means to revolutionize how cognition is monitored. Consider first that everything a person does involves the brain. Every movement, from physical gestures to spoken responses, reflect an individual's cognitive capabilities.[221,222] Imagine being able to track continuous measures of behavior, behaviors that are all mediated through the brain. The internet of things has opened up a world of possibilities for tracking cognition in a person's natural environment through wearables, smartphone applications, and smart home devices. Using algorithms derived from advanced machine learning techniques that can automatically and simultaneously account for factors of variability, accurate cognitive profiles can be generated through the integration of multisensor signals across smart monitoring devices.

Continuous monitoring of behaviors that reflect cognitive capabilities enable the ability to detect a negative trajectory of change well within the realm of normal. Research has shown that delaying onset of symptoms by 5 years can reduce the risk of AD by 50%.[223] Given the numerous studies that also indicate modifiable risk factors for AD, intervention at the preclinical state is currently the best hope for changing the trajectory of this disease. In principle, the need for traditional neuropsychological tests could be replaced by a smart brain health monitoring system. As subtle changes in cognition are detected, automated feedback mechanisms could be instituted that help a person manage causal indices such as cardiovascular risk factors. The impact of intervention early enough may result in not simply attenuating progressive decline, but eliminating it altogether.

What does all this mean for public health? Catalyzing groundbreaking discoveries for cognitive impairment prevention by identifying determinants of progressive dementing disorders, such as AD, will inform new strategies for sustained lifelong cognitive health. The opportunity for public health is to play a pivotal role in driving forward precision health as the key solution that is more than complementary to the goals of precision medicine. Along the lifespan continuum of brain health, public health should be embracing the new technological advances and considering how it should alter its own methods in order to go well beyond monitoring for prevalence and incidence of disease. Further, long-standing traditional statistical approaches for identifying specific risk factors to cognitive-related disorders as has been typically used in many epidemiologic studies needs to make way for the analytic capabilities of data science and the results derived from them. It is also the case that driving forward precision health related to cognitive-related outcomes can serve as a model that can apply across all chronic diseases. Thus, most importantly, public health needs to lead the charge of sustaining brain health as the primary objective in place of tracking and treating neurocognitive disorders such as AD. Only in this way can precision health bring a seismic shift from an emphasis on disease to prevention. In tandem, public health will also be providing key solutions to fixing the U.S. healthcare system and the economic consequences tied to it.

References

1. Ferri CP, Prince M, Brayne C, et al. Global prevalence of dementia: A Delphi consensus study. *Lancet.* 2005;366:2112–7.
2. Alzheimer's Association. 2016. Alzheimer's disease facts and figures. https://www.alz.org/documents_custom/2016-facts-and-figures.pdf. Accessed November 6, 2017.
3. Hebert LE, Bienias JL, Aggarwal NT, et al. Change in risk of Alzheimer disease over time. *Neurology.* 2010;75:786–91.
4. Sperling RA, Aisen PS, Beckett LA, et al. Toward defining the preclinical stages of Alzheimer's disease: Recommendations from the National Institute on Aging-Alzheimer's Association workgroups on diagnostic guidelines for Alzheimer's disease. *Alzheimers Dement.* 2011;7:280–92.
5. Kukull WA, Ganguli M. Epidemiology of dementia: Concepts and overview. *Neurol Clin.* 2000;18:923–50.
6. Hurd MD, Martorell P, Delavande A, et al. Monetary costs of dementia in the United States. *N Engl J Med.* 2013;368:1326–34.
7. Hebert LE, Weuve J, Scherr PA, et al. Alzheimer disease in the United States (2010–2050) estimated using the 2010 Census. *Neurology.* 2013;80:1778–83.
8. Beinart N, Weinman J, Wade D, et al. Caregiver burden and psychoeducational interventions in Alzheimer's disease: A review. *Dement Geriatr Cogn Dis Extra.* 2012;2:638–48.
9. Alzheimer's Association; Thies W, Bleiler L. Alzheimer's disease facts and figures. *Alzheimers Dement.* 2011;7:208–44.
10. Schulz R, McGinnis KA, Zhang S, et al. Dementia patient suffering and caregiver depression. *Alzheimer Dis Assoc Disord.* 2008;22:170–6.
11. Beeson R, Horton-Deutsch S, Farran C, et al. Loneliness and depression in caregivers of persons with Alzheimer's disease or related disorders. *Issues Ment Health Nurs.* 2000;21:779–806.
12. McKhann GM, Knopman DS, Chertkow H, et al. The diagnosis of dementia due to Alzheimer's disease: Recommendations from the National Institute on Aging-Alzheimer's association workgroups on diagnostic guidelines for Alzheimer's disease. *Alzheimers Dement.* 2011;7:263–9.
13. Satizabal CL, Beiser AS, Chouraki V, et al. Incidence of dementia over three decades in the Framingham heart study. *N Engl J Med.* 2016;374:523–32.
14. Sheehan B. Assessment scales in dementia. *Ther Adv Neurol Disord.* 2012;5:349–58.
15. Cullen B, O'Neill B, Evans JJ, et al. A review of screening tests for cognitive impairment. *J Neurol Neurosurg Psychiatry.* 2007;78:790–9.
16. Folstein MF, Folstein SE, McHugh PR. "Mini-mental state." A practical method for grading the cognitive state of patients for the clinician. *J Psychiatr Res.* 1975;12:189–98.
17. Naugle RI, Kawczak K. Limitations of the mini-mental state examination. *Cleve Clin J Med.* 1989;56:277–81.
18. Nasreddine ZS, Phillips NA, Bedirian V, et al. The Montreal cognitive assessment, MoCA: A brief screening tool for mild cognitive impairment. *J Am Geriatr Soc.* 2005;53:695–9.
19. Trzepacz PT, Hochstetler H, Wang S, et al. Relationship between the Montreal cognitive assessment and mini-mental state examination for assessment of mild cognitive impairment in older adults. *BMC Geriatr.* 2015;15:107.
20. Gonda X, Pompili M, Serafini G, et al. The role of cognitive dysfunction in the symptoms and remission from depression. *Ann Gen Psychiatry.* 2015;14:27.
21. Fiedler N, Weisel C, Lynch R, et al. Cognitive effects of chronic exposure to lead and solvents. *Am J Ind Med.* 2003;44:413–23.
22. Weisskopf MG, Wright RO, Schwartz J, et al. Cumulative lead exposure and prospective change in cognition among elderly men: The VA Normative aging study. *Am J Epidemiol.* 2004;160:1184–93.
23. Hughes CP, Berg L, Danziger WL, et al. A new clinical scale for the staging of dementia. *Br J Psychiatry.* 1982;140:566–72.
24. Rikkert MG, Tona KD, Janssen L, et al. Validity, reliability, and feasibility of clinical staging scales in dementia: A systematic review. *Am J Alzheimers Dis Other Demen.* 2011;26:357–65.
25. McCarten JR. Clinical evaluation of early cognitive symptoms. *Clin Geriatr Med.* 2013;29:791–807.
26. Podell K, Gifford K, Bougakov D, et al. Neuropsychological assessment in traumatic brain injury. *Psychiatr Clin North Am.* 2010;33:855–76.
27. Brenner LA. Neuropsychological and neuroimaging findings in traumatic brain injury and post-traumatic stress disorder. *Dialogues Clin Neurosci.* 2011;13:311–23.
28. Castles A, Kohnen S, Nickels L, et al. Developmental disorders: What can be learned from cognitive neuropsychology? *Philos Trans R Soc Lond B Biol Sci.* 2014;369:20130407.
29. Salmon DP, Bondi MW. Neuropsychological assessment of dementia. *Annu Rev Psychol.* 2009;60:257–82.
30. Weintraub S, Wicklund AH, Salmon DP. The neuropsychological profile of Alzheimer disease. *Cold Spring Harb Perspect Med.* 2012;2:a006171.
31. Harvey PD. Clinical applications of neuropsychological assessment. *Dialogues Clin Neurosci.* 2012;14:91–9.
32. Au R, Piers RJ, Devine S. How technology is reshaping cognitive assessment: Lessons from the Framingham heart study. *Neuropsychology.* 2017 Nov;31(8):846–61.
33. Bauer RM, Bowers D. Intellectual antecedents to the Boston process approach to neuropsychological assessment. In: Ashendorf L, Swenson R, Libon D, eds. *The Boston Process Approach to Neuropsychological Assessment: A Practitioner's Guide.* New York: Oxford University Press; 2013.
34. Albert MS, DeKosky ST, Dickson D, et al. The diagnosis of mild cognitive impairment due to Alzheimer's disease: Recommendations from the National Institute on Aging-Alzheimer's Association workgroups on diagnostic guidelines for Alzheimer's disease. *Alzheimers Dement.* 2011;7:270–9.
35. Hyman BT, Trojanowski JQ. Consensus recommendations for the postmortem diagnosis of Alzheimer disease from the National Institute on Aging and the Reagan Institute Working Group on diagnostic criteria

for the neuropathological assessment of Alzheimer disease. *J Neuropathol Exp Neurol*. 1997;56:1095–7.

36. Berry CM, Clark MA, McClure TK. Racial/ethnic differences in the criterion-related validity of cognitive ability tests: A qualitative and quantitative review. *J Appl Psychol*. 2011;96:881–906.
37. Helms JE. *Fairness* is not validity or cultural bias in racial-group assessment: A quantitative perspective. *Am Psychol*. 2006;61:845–59.
38. Walhovd KB, Fjell AM, Brewer J, et al. Combining MR imaging, positron-emission tomography, and CSF biomarkers in the diagnosis and prognosis of Alzheimer disease. *Am J Neuroradiol*. 2010;31:347–54.
39. Lam B, Masellis M, Freedman M, et al. Clinical, imaging, and pathological heterogeneity of the Alzheimer's disease syndrome. *Alzheimers Res Ther*. 2013;5:1.
40. McEvoy LK, Brewer JB. Biomarkers for the clinical evaluation of the cognitively impaired elderly: Amyloid is not enough. *Imaging Med*. 2012;4:343–57.
41. Au R, Piers RJ, Lancashire L. Back to the future: Alzheimer's disease heterogeneity revisited. *Alzheimers Dement (Amst)*. 2015;1:368–70.
42. Serrano-Pozo A, Frosch MP, Masliah E, et al. Neuropathological alterations in Alzheimer disease. *Cold Spring Harb Perspect Med*. 2011;1:a006189.
43. Nelson PT, Braak H, Markesbery WR. Neuropathology and cognitive impairment in Alzheimer disease: A complex but coherent relationship. *J Neuropathol Exp Neurol*. 2009;68:1–14.
44. Braak H, Braak E. Staging of Alzheimer's disease-related neurofibrillary changes. *Neurobiol Aging*. 1995;16:271–8.
45. Chetelat G, Villemagne VL, Bourgeat P, et al. Relationship between atrophy and beta-amyloid deposition in Alzheimer disease. *Ann Neurol*. 2010;67:317–24.
46. Van Hoesen GW, Hyman BT, Damasio AR. Entorhinal cortex pathology in Alzheimer's disease. *Hippocampus*. 1991;1:1–8.
47. Frisoni GB, Laakso MP, Beltramello A, et al. Hippocampal and entorhinal cortex atrophy in frontotemporal dementia and Alzheimer's disease. *Neurology*. 1999;52:91–100.
48. Van Der Flier WM, Van Den Heuvel DM, Weverling-Rijnsburger AW, et al. Cognitive decline in AD and mild cognitive impairment is associated with global brain damage. *Neurology*. 2002;59:874–9.
49. Lim YY, Maruff P, Pietrzak RH, et al. Effect of amyloid on memory and non-memory decline from preclinical to clinical Alzheimer's disease. *Brain*. 2014;137:221–31.
50. Lim YY, Ellis KA, Harrington K, et al. Cognitive decline in adults with mild cognitive impairment and high Ab amyloid: Prodromal Alzheimer's disease? *J Alzheimers Dis*. 2013;33:1167–76.
51. Lim YY, Pietrzak RH, Ellis KA, et al. Rapid decline in episodic memory in healthy older adults with high amyloid-b. *J Alzheimers Dis*. 2013;33:675–9.
52. Ellis KA, Lim YY, Harrington K, et al. Decline in cognitive function over 18 months in healthy older adults with high amyloid-b. *J Alzheimers Dis*. 2013;34:861–71.
53. Lim YY, Ellis KA, Pietrzak RH, et al. Stronger effect of amyloid load than APOE genotype on cognitive decline in healthy older adults. *Neurology*. 2012;79:1645–52.
54. Villemagne VL, Pike KE, Chetelat G, et al. Longitudinal assessment of Aβ and cognition in aging and Alzheimer disease. *Ann Neurol*. 2011;69:181–92.
55. Nelson PT, Alafuzoff I, Bigio EH, et al. Correlation of Alzheimer disease neuropathologic changes with cognitive status: A review of the literature. *J Neuropathol Exp Neurol*. 2012;71:362–81.
56. Bennett DA, Schneider JA, Wilson RS, et al. Neurofibrillary tangles mediate the association of amyloid load with clinical Alzheimer disease and level of cognitive function. *Arch Neurol*. 2004;61:378–84.
57. Hampel H, Burger K, Teipel SJ, et al. Core candidate neurochemical and imaging biomarkers of Alzheimer's disease. *Alzheimers Dement*. 2008;4:38–48.
58. Khan TK, Alkon DL. Peripheral biomarkers of Alzheimer's disease. *J Alzheimers Dis*. 2015;44:729–44.
59. Menendez-Gonzalez M. Routine lumbar puncture for the early diagnosis of Alzheimer's disease. Is it safe? *Front Aging Neurosci*. 2014;6:65.
60. Mo JA, Lim JH, Sul AR, et al. Cerebrospinal fluid β-amyloid1-42 levels in the differential diagnosis of Alzheimer's disease—Systematic review and meta-analysis. *PLoS One*. 2015;10:e0116802.
61. Jack CR Jr, Knopman DS, Jagust WJ, et al. Hypothetical model of dynamic biomarkers of the Alzheimer's pathological cascade. *Lancet Neurol*. 2010;9:119–28.
62. Jack CR Jr, Knopman DS, Jagust WJ, et al. Tracking pathophysiological processes in Alzheimer's disease: An updated hypothetical model of dynamic biomarkers. *Lancet Neurol*. 2013;12:207–16.
63. Rowe CC, Ellis KA, Rimajova M, et al. Amyloid imaging results from the Australian Imaging, Biomarkers and Lifestyle (AIBL) study of aging. *Neurobiol Aging*. 2010;31:1275–83.
64. Mintun MA, Larossa GN, Sheline YI, et al. [11C]PIB in a nondemented population: Potential antecedent marker of Alzheimer disease. *Neurology*. 2006;67:446–52.
65. Mielke MM, Wiste HJ, Weigand SD, et al. Indicators of amyloid burden in a population-based study of cognitively normal elderly. *Neurology*. 2012;79:1570–7.
66. Presecki P, Muck-Seler D, Mimica N, et al. Serum lipid levels in patients with Alzheimer's disease. *Coll Antropol*. 2011;35:115–20.
67. Crane PK, Walker R, Hubbard RA, et al. Glucose levels and risk of dementia. *N Engl J Med*. 2013;369:540–8.
68. O'Bryant SE, Waring SC, Hobson V, et al. Decreased C-reactive protein levels in Alzheimer disease. *J Geriatr Psychiatry Neurol*. 2010;23:49–53.
69. Cojocaru IM, Cojocaru M, Miu G, et al. Study of interleukin-6 production in Alzheimer's disease. *Rom J Intern Med*. 2011;49:55–8.
70. Licastro F, Grimaldi LM, Bonafe M, et al. Interleukin-6 gene alleles affect the risk of Alzheimer's disease and levels of the cytokine in blood and brain. *Neurobiol Aging*. 2003;24:921–6.
71. Pratico D. The neurobiology of isoprostanes and Alzheimer's disease. *Biochim Biophys Acta*. 2010;1801:930–3.
72. Morris JK, Burns JM. Insulin: An emerging treatment for Alzheimer's disease dementia? *Curr Neurol Neurosci Rep*. 2012;12:520–7.
73. Watson GS, Craft S. The role of insulin resistance in the pathogenesis of Alzheimer's disease: Implications for treatment. *CNS Drugs*. 2003;17:27–45.
74. Qin XY, Cao C, Cawley NX, et al. Decreased peripheral brain-derived neurotrophic factor levels in Alzheimer's disease: A meta-analysis study ($N = 7277$). *Mol Psychiatry*. 2017;22:312–20.
75. Michalski B, Corrada M, Kawas CH, et al. Brain-derived neurotrophic factor and TrkB expression in the "oldest-old," the 90+ Study: Correlation with cognitive status and levels of soluble amyloid-beta. *Neurobiol Aging*. 2015;36:3130–9.
76. Forlenza OV, Diniz BS, Teixeira AL, et al. Lower cerebrospinal fluid concentration of brain-derived neurotrophic factor predicts progression from mild cognitive impairment to Alzheimer's disease. *Neuromolecular Med*. 2015;17:326–32.
77. Faria MC, Goncalves GS, Rocha NP, et al. Increased plasma levels of BDNF and inflammatory markers in Alzheimer's disease. *J Pyschiatr Res*. 2014;53:166–72.
78. Weinstein G, Beiser AS, Choi SH, et al. Serum brain-derived neurotrophic factor and the risk for dementia: The Framingham heart study. *JAMA Neurol*. 2014;71:55–61.
79. Adamczuk K, De Weer AS, Nelissen N, et al. Polymorphism of brain derived neurotrophic factor influences β amyloid load in cognitively intact apolipoprotein E ε4 carriers. *Neuroimage Clin*. 2013;2:512–20.
80. Wang C, Zhang Y, Liu B, et al. Dosage effects of BDNF Val66Met polymorphism on cortical surface area and functional connectivity. *J Neurosci*. 2014;34:2645–51.
81. Borroni B, Bianchi M, Premi E, et al. The brain-derived neurotrophic factor Val66Met polymorphism is associated with reduced hippocampus perfusion in frontotemporal lobar degeneration. *J Alzheimers Dis*. 2012;31:243–51.
82. Azeredo LA, De Nardi T, Levandowski ML, et al. The brain-derived neurotrophic factor (BDNF) gene Val66Met polymorphism affects memory performance in older adults. *Rev Bras Psiquiatr*. 2017;39:90–4.
83. Sapkota S, Backman L, Dixon RA. Executive function performance and change in aging is predicted by apolipoprotein E, intensified by catechol-O-methyltransferase and brain-derived neurotrophic factor, and moderated by age and lifestyle. *Neurobiol Aging*. 2017;52:81–9.
84. Forlenza OV, Teixeira AL, Miranda AS, et al. Decreased neurotrophic support is associated with cognitive decline in non-demented subjects. *J Alzheimers Dis*. 2015;46:423–9.
85. Lim YY, Villemagne VL, Laws SM, et al. APOE and BDNF polymorphisms moderate amyloid β-related cognitive decline in preclinical Alzheimer's disease. *Mol Psychiatry*. 2015;20:1322–8.
86. Shimada H, Makizako H, Doi T, et al. A large, cross-sectional observational study of serum BDNF, cognitive function, and mild cognitive impairment in the elderly. *Front Aging Neurosci*. 2014;6:69.

87. Whiteman AS, Young DE, He X, et al. Interaction between serum BDNF and aerobic fitness predicts recognition memory in healthy young adults. *Behav Brain Res.* 2014;259:302–12.
88. Estrada JA, Contreras I, Pliego-Rivero FB, et al. Molecular mechanisms of cognitive impairment in iron deficiency: Alterations in brain-derived neurotrophic factor and Insulin-like growth factor expression and function in the central nervous system. *Nutr Neurosci.* 2014;17:193–206.
89. Rendeiro C, Vauzour D, Rattray M, et al. Dietary levels of pure flavonoids improve spatial memory performance and increase hippocampal brain-derived neurotrophic factor. *PLoS One.* 2013;8:e63535.
90. Gajewski PD, Hengstler JG, Golka K, et al. The Met-genotype of the BDNF Val66Met polymorphism is associated with reduced Stroop interference in elderly. *Neuropsychologia.* 2012;50:3554–63.
91. O'Brien JT, Markus HS. Vascular risk factors and Alzheimer's disease. *BMC Med.* 2014;12:218.
92. de Bruijn RF, Ikram MA. Cardiovascular risk factors and future Alzheimer's disease risk. *BMC Med.* 2014;12:130.
93. Jefferson AL, Hohman TJ, Liu D, et al. Adverse vascular risk is related to cognitive decline in older adults. *J Alzheimers Dis.* 2015;44:1361–73.
94. Elias MF, Sullivan LM, D'Agostino RB, et al. Framingham stroke risk profile and lowered cognitive performance. *Stroke.* 2004;35:404–9.
95. Seshadri S, Wolf PA, Beiser A, et al. Stroke risk profile, brain volume, and cognitive function: The Framingham offspring study. *Neurology.* 2004;63:1591–9.
96. Nishtala A, Piers RJ, Himali JJ, et al. Atrial fibrillation and cognitive decline in the Framingham heart study. *Heart Rhythm.* 2018 Feb;15(2):166–72.
97. Nation DA, Preis SR, Beiser A, et al. Pulse pressure is associated with early brain atrophy and cognitive decline: Modifying effects of APOE4. *Alzheimer Dis Assoc Disord.* 2016;30:210–5.
98. Bangen KJ, Beiser A, Delano-Wood L, et al. APOE genotype modifies the relationship between midlife vascular risk factors and later cognitive decline. *J Stroke Cerebrovasc Dis.* 2013;22:1361–9.
99. Wolf PA, Beiser A, Elias MF, et al. Relation of obesity to cognitive function: Importance of central obesity and synergistic influence of concomitant hypertension. The Framingham heart study. *Curr Alzheimer Res.* 2007;4:111–6.
100. Elias MF, Sullivan LM, Elias PK, et al. Left ventricular mass, blood pressure, and lowered cognitive performance in the Framingham offspring. *Hypertension.* 2007;49:439–45.
101. Elias MF, Elias PK, Sullivan LM, et al. Obesity, diabetes and cognitive deficit: The Framingham heart study. *Neurobiol Aging.* 2005;26:11–6.
102. Arvanitakis Z, Wilson RS, Bienias JL, et al. Diabetes mellitus and risk of Alzheimer disease and decline in cognitive function. *Arch Neurol.* 2004;61:661–6.
103. Elias MF, Elias PK, Sullivan LM, et al. Lower cognitive function in the presence of obesity and hypertension: The Framingham heart study. *Int J Obes Relat Metab Disord.* 2003;27:260–8.
104. Piers RJ, Nishtala A, Preis SR, et al. Association between atrial fibrillation and volumetric magnetic resonance imaging brain measures: Framingham offspring study. *Heart Rhythm.* 2016;13:2020–4.
105. Zade D, Beiser A, McGlinchey R, et al. Interactive effects of apolipoprotein E type 4 genotype and cerebrovascular risk on neuropsychological performance and structural brain changes. *J Stroke Cerebrovasc Dis.* 2010;19:261–8.
106. Maillard P, Seshadri S, Beiser A, et al. Effects of systolic blood pressure on white-matter integrity in young adults in the Framingham Heart Study: A cross-sectional study. *Lancet Neurol* 2012;11:1039–47.
107. Saunders AM, Strittmatter WJ, Schmechel D, et al. Association of apolipoprotein E allele epsilon 4 with late-onset familial and sporadic Alzheimer's disease. *Neurology.* 1993;43:1467–72.
108. Genin E, Hannequin D, Wallon D, et al. APOE and Alzheimer disease: A major gene with semi-dominant inheritance. *Mol Psychiatry.* 2011;16:903–7.
109. Wu L, Zhao L. ApoE2 and Alzheimer's disease: Time to take a closer look. *Neural Regen Res.* 2016;11:412–3.
110. Awada AA. Early and late-onset Alzheimer's disease: What are the differences? *J Neurosci Rural Pract.* 2015;6:455–6.
111. Bertram L, Tanzi RE. Thirty years of Alzheimer's disease genetics: The implications of systematic meta-analyses. *Nat Rev Neurosci.* 2008;9: 768–78.
112. Bertram L, Tanzi RE. The genetic epidemiology of neurodegenerative disease. *J Clin Invest.* 2005;115:1449–57.
113. Tanzi RE, Bertram L. Twenty years of the Alzheimer's disease amyloid hypothesis: A genetic perspective. *Cell.* 2005;120:545–55.
114. Rutter M, O'Connor TG; English and Romanian Adoptees (ERA) Study Team. Are there biological programming effects for psychological development? Findings from a study of Romanian adoptees. *Dev Psychol.* 2004;40:81–94.
115. Lebel C, Mattson SN, Riley EP, et al. A longitudinal study of the long-term consequences of drinking during pregnancy: Heavy in utero alcohol exposure disrupts the normal processes of brain development. *J Neurosci.* 2012;32:15243–51.
116. Sameroff A. A unified theory of development: A dialectic integration of nature and nurture. *Child Dev.* 2010;81:6–22.
117. Brown J, Cooper-Kuhn CM, Kemperman G, et al. Enriched environment and physical activity stimulate hippocampal but not olfactory bulb neurogenesis. *Eur J Neurosci.* 2003;17:2042–6.
118. van Praag H, Kemperman G, Gage FH. Running increases cell proliferation and neurogenesis in the adult mouse dentate gyrus. *Nat Neurosci.* 1999;2:266–70.
119. Valenzuela MJ, Sachdev P, Wen W, et al. Lifespan mental activity predicts diminished rate of hippocampal atrophy. *PLoS One.* 2008;3:e2598.
120. Landau SM, Marks SM, Mormino EC, et al. Association of lifetime cognitive engagement and low β-amyloid deposition. *Arch Neurol.* 2012;69:623–9.
121. Scarmeas N, Levy G, Tang MX, et al. Influence of leisure activity on the incidence of Alzheimer's disease. *Neurology.* 2001;57:2236–42.
122. Ordovas JM, Litwack-Klein L, Wilson PW, et al. Apolipoprotein E isoform phenotyping methodology and population frequency with identification of apoE1 and apoE5 isoforms. *J Lipid Res.* 1987;28:371–80.
123. Wilson RS, Bienias JL, Berry-Kravis E, et al. The apolipoprotein E epsilon 2 allele and decline in episodic memory. *J Neurol Neurosurg Psychiatry.* 2002;73:672–7.
124. Chiang GC, Insel PS, Tosun D, et al. Hippocampal atrophy rates and CSF biomarkers in elderly APOE2 normal subjects. *Neurology.* 2010;75: 1976–81.
125. Shaw P, Lerch JP, Pruessner JC, et al. Cortical morphology in children and adolescents with different apolipoprotein E gene polymorphisms: An observational study. *Lancet Neurol.* 2007;6:494–500.
126. Nagy Z, Esiri MM, Jobst KA, et al. Influence of the apolipoprotein E genotype on amyloid deposition and neurofibrillary tangle formation in Alzheimer's disease. *Neuroscience.* 1995;69:757–61.
127. Amieva H, Mokri H, LeGoff M, et al. Compensatory mechanisms in higher-educated subjects with Alzheimer's disease: A study of 20 years of cognitive decline. *Brain.* 2014;137:1167–75.
128. Aguirre-Acevedo DC, Lopera F, Henao E, et al. Cognitive decline in a Colombian kindred with autosomal dominant Alzheimer disease: A retrospective cohort study. *JAMA Neurol.* 2016;73:431–8.
129. Stern Y. Cognitive reserve in ageing and Alzheimer's disease. *Lancet Neurol.* 2012;11:1006–12.
130. SantaCruz KS, Sonnen JA, Pezhouh MK, et al. Alzheimer disease pathology in subjects without dementia in 2 studies of aging: The Nun Study and the Adult Changes in Thought Study. *J Neuropathol Exp Neurol.* 2011;70:832–40.
131. Stern Y, Gurland B, Tatemichi TK, et al. Influence of education and occupation on the incidence of Alzheimer's disease. *JAMA.* 1994;271: 1004–10.
132. Karp A, Kareholt I, Qiu C, et al. Relation of education and occupation-based socioeconomic status to incident Alzheimer's disease. *Am J Epidemiol.* 2004;159:175–83.
133. Sperling RA, Karlawish J, Johnson KA. Preclinical Alzheimer disease—The challenges ahead. *Nat Rev Neurol.* 2013;9:54–8.
134. Aisen PS. Alzheimer's disease therapeutic research: The path forward. *Alzheimers Res Ther.* 2009;1:2.
135. Jorm AF, Jolley D. The incidence of dementia A meta-analysis. *Neurology.* 1998;51:728–33.
136. Plassman BL, Langa KM, Fisher GG, et al. Prevalence of dementia in the United States: The aging, demographics, and memory study. *Neuroepidemiology.* 2007;29:125–32.
137. Pendlebury ST, Rothwell PM. Prevalence, incidence, and factors associated with pre-stroke and post-stroke dementia: A systematic review and meta-analysis. *Lancet Neurol.* 2009;8:1006–18.
138. World Health Organization. *The ICD-10 Classification of Mental and Behavioural Disorders: Clinical Descriptions and Diagnostic Guidelines.* Geneva: WHO; 1992.

139. Román GC, Tatemichi TK, Erkinjuntti T, et al. Vascular dementia diagnostic criteria for research studies: Report of the NINDS-AIREN International Workshop. *Neurology.* 1993;43:250–60.

140. Chui HC, Victoroff JI, Margolin D, et al. Criteria for the diagnosis of ischemic vascular dementia proposed by the State of California Alzheimer's Disease Diagnostic and Treatment Centers. *Neurology.* 1992;42:473–80.

141. American Psychiatric Association. *Diagnostic and Statistical Manual of Mental Disorders (DSM-5®).* Washington, DC: American Psychiatric Association; 2013.

142. Pantoni L, Inzitari D. Hachinski's ischemic score and the diagnosis of vascular dementia: A review. *Italian J Neurol Sci.* 1993;14:539–46.

143. Wetterling T, Kanitz RD, Borgis KJ. Comparison of different diagnostic criteria for vascular dementia (ADDTC, DSM-IV, ICD-10, NINDS-AIREN). *Stroke.* 1996;27:30–6.

144. Gold G, Bouras C, Canuto A, et al. Clinicopathological validation study of four sets of clinical criteria for vascular dementia. *Am J Psychiatry.* 2002;159:82–7.

145. Román GC. Vascular dementia revisited: Diagnosis, pathogenesis, treatment, and prevention. *Med Clin North Am.* 2002;86:477–99.

146. Pantoni L. Cerebral small vessel disease: From pathogenesis and clinical characteristics to therapeutic challenges. *Lancet Neurol.* 2010;9:689–701.

147. Gorelick PB. Risk factors for vascular dementia and Alzheimer disease. *Stroke.* 2004;35:2620–2.

148. Geldmacher DS, Whitehouse PJ. Evaluation of dementia. *N Engl J Med.* 1996;335:330–6.

149. T O'Brien J, Erkinjuntti T, Reisberg B, et al. Vascular cognitive impairment. *Lancet Neurol.* 2003;2:89–98.

150. Román GC, Royall DR. Executive control function: A rational basis for the diagnosis of vascular dementia. *Alzheimer Dis Assoc Disord.* 1998;13:S69–80.

151. Looi JCL, Sachdev PS. Differentiation of vascular dementia from AD on neuropsychological tests. *Neurology.* 1999;53:670–8.

152. Royall DR, Lauterbach EC, Cummings JL, et al. Executive control function: A review of its promise and challenges for clinical research. A report from the Committee on Research of the American Neuropsychiatric Association. *J Neuropsychiatry Clin Neurosci.* 2002;14:377–405.

153. Price CC, Jefferson AL, Merino JG, et al. Subcortical vascular dementia integrating neuropsychological and neuroradiologic data. *Neurology.* 2005;65:376–82.

154. Mungas D, Jagust WJ, Reed BR, et al. MRI predictors of cognition in subcortical ischemic vascular disease and Alzheimer's disease. *Neurology.* 2001;57:2229–35.

155. Amenta F, Di Tullio MA, Tomassoni D. The cholinergic approach for the treatment of vascular dementia: Evidence from pre-clinical and clinical studies. *Clin Exp Hypertens.* 2002;24:697–713.

156. Wilcock G, Möbius HJ, Stöffler A. A double-blind, placebo-controlled multicentre study of memantine in mild to moderate vascular dementia (MMM500). *Int Clin Psychopharmacol.* 2002;17:297–305.

157. Orgogozo JM, Rigaud AS, Stöffler A, et al. Efficacy and safety of memantine in patients with mild to moderate vascular dementia. *Stroke.* 2002;33:1834–9.

158. Kavirajan H, Schneider LS. Efficacy and adverse effects of cholinesterase inhibitors and memantine in vascular dementia: A meta-analysis of randomised controlled trials. *Lancet Neurol.* 2007;6:782–92.

159. Fitzpatrick AL, Kuller LH, Lopez OL, et al. Survival following dementia onset: Alzheimer's disease and vascular dementia. *J Neurol Sci.* 2005;229:43–9.

160. Harmsen P, Lappas G, Rosengren A, et al. Long-term risk factors for stroke. *Stroke.* 2006;37:1663–7.

161. Forette F, Seux ML, Staessen JA, et al. The prevention of dementia with antihypertensive treatment: New evidence from the systolic hypertension in Europe (Syst-Eur) study. *Arch Intern Med.* 2002;162:2046–52.

162. Murray MD, Lane KA, Gao S, et al. Preservation of cognitive function with antihypertensive medications: A longitudinal analysis of a community-based sample of African Americans. *Arch Intern Med.* 2002;162:2090–6.

163. Collaborative PR, Neal B, MacMahon S. Effects of blood pressure lowering with perindopril and indapamide therapy on dementia and cognitive decline in patients with cerebrovascular disease. *Arch Intern Med.* 2003;163:1069–75.

164. Baigent C, Blackwell L, Collins R, et al. Aspirin in the primary and secondary prevention of vascular disease: Collaborative meta-analysis of individual participant data from randomised trials. *Lancet.* 2009:373:1849–60.

165. Scandinavian Simvastatin Survival Study Group. Randomised trial of cholesterol lowering in 4444 patients with coronary heart disease: The Scandinavian Simvastatin Survival Study (4S). *Lancet.* 1994;344:1383–9.

166. Amarenco P, Labreuche J. Lipid management in the prevention of stroke: Review and updated meta-analysis of statins for stroke prevention. *Lancet Neurol.* 2009;8:453–63.

167. Hess DC, Demchuk AM, Brass LM, et al. HMG-CoA reductase inhibitors (statins) A promising approach to stroke prevention. *Neurology.* 2000;54:790–6.

168. Emerging Risk Factors Collaboration. Diabetes mellitus, fasting blood glucose concentration, and risk of vascular disease: A collaborative meta-analysis of 102 prospective studies. *Lancet.* 2010;375:2215–22.

169. Aarsland D, Kurz MW. The epidemiology of dementia associated with Parkinson disease. *J Neurol Sci.* 2010;289:18–22.

170. Aarsland D, Andersen K, Larsen JP, et al. Prevalence and characteristics of dementia in Parkinson disease: An 8-year prospective study. *Arch Neurol.* 2003;60:387–92.

171. Hughes TA, Ross HF, Musa S, et al. A 10-year study of the incidence of and factors predicting dementia in Parkinson's disease. *Neurology.* 2000;54:1596–603.

172. Aarsland D, Kvaløy JT, Andersen K, et al. The effect of age of onset of PD on risk of dementia. *J Neurol.* 2007;254:38–45.

173. Emre M, Aarsland D, Brown R, et al. Clinical diagnostic criteria for dementia associated with Parkinson's disease. *Mov Disord.* 2007;22:1689–707.

174. Alves G, Larsen JP, Emre M, et al. Changes in motor subtype and risk for incident dementia in Parkinson's disease. *Mov Disord.* 2006;21:1123–30.

175. Burn DJ, Rowan EN, Allan LM, et al. Motor subtype and cognitive decline in Parkinson's disease, Parkinson's disease with dementia, and dementia with Lewy bodies. *J Neurol Neurosurg Psychiatry.* 2006; 77:585–9.

176. Foltynie T, Brayne CE, Robbins TW, et al. The cognitive ability of an incident cohort of Parkinson's patients in the UK. The CamPaIGN study. *Brain.* 2004;127:550–60.

177. Litvan I, Aarsland D, Adler CH, et al. MDS task force on mild cognitive impairment in Parkinson's disease: Critical review of PD-MCI. *Mov Disord.* 2011;26:1814–24.

178. Pillon B, Dubois B, Ploska A, et al. Severity and specificity of cognitive impairment in Alzheimer's, Huntington's, and Parkinson's diseases and progressive supranuclear palsy. *Neurology.* 1991;41:634–43.

179. Litvan I, Mohr E, Williams J, et al. Differential memory and executive functions in demented patients with Parkinson's and Alzheimer's disease. J Neurol *Neurosurg Psychiatry.* 1991;54:25–9.

180. Kudlicka A, Clare L, Hindle JV. Executive functions in Parkinson's disease: Systematic review and meta-analysis. *Mov Disord.* 2011;26:2305–15.

181. Starkstein SE, Sabe L, Petracca G, et al. Neuropsychological and psychiatric differences between Alzheimer's disease and Parkinson's disease with dementia. *J Neurol Neurosurg Psychiatry.* 1996;61:381–7.

182. Mosimann UP, Mather G, Wesnes KA, et al. Visual perception in Parkinson disease dementia and dementia with Lewy bodies. *Neurology.* 2004;63:2091–6.

183. Helkala EL, Laulumaa V, Soininen H, et al. Different error pattern of episodic and semantic memory in Alzheimer's disease and Parkinson's disease with dementia. *Neuropsychologia.* 1989;27:1241–8.

184. Pillon B, Deweer B, Agid Y, et al. Explicit memory in Alzheimer's, Huntington's, and Parkinson's diseases. *Arch Neurol.* 1993;50:374–9.

185. Higginson CI, Wheelock VL, Carroll KE, et al. Recognition memory in Parkinson's disease with and without dementia: Evidence inconsistent with the retrieval deficit hypothesis. *J Clin Exp Neuropsychol.* 2005;27:516–28.

186. Aarsland D, Ballard C, Larsen JP, et al. A comparative study of psychiatric symptoms in dementia with Lewy bodies and Parkinson's disease with and without dementia. *Int J Geriatr Psychiatry.* 2001;16:528–36.

187. Janvin CC, Larsen JP, Salmon DP, et al. Cognitive profiles of individual patients with Parkinson's disease and dementia: Comparison with dementia with Lewy bodies and Alzheimer's disease. *Mov Disord.* 2006;21:337–42.

188. Bronnick K, Aarsland D, Larsen JP. Neuropsychiatric disturbances in Parkinson's disease clusters in five groups with different prevalence of dementia. *Acta Psychiatr Scand.* 2005;112:201–7.

189. Gagnon JF, Vendette M, Postuma RB, et al. Mild cognitive impairment in rapid eye movement sleep behavior disorder and Parkinson's disease. *Ann Neurol.* 2009;66:39–47.

190. Emre M, Aarsland D, Albanese A, et al. Rivastigmine for dementia associated with Parkinson's disease. *N Engl J Med.* 2004;351:2509–18.

191. Aarsland D, Ballard C, Walker Z, et al. Memantine in patients with Parkinson's disease dementia or dementia with Lewy bodies: A double-blind, placebo-controlled, multicentre trial. *Lancet Neurol.* 2009;8:613–8.
192. Martland HS. Punch drunk. *J Am Med Assoc.* 1928;91:1103–7.
193. McKee AC, Cantu RC, Nowinski CJ, et al. Chronic traumatic encephalopathy in athletes: Progressive tauopathy after repetitive head injury. *J Neuropathol Exp Neurol.* 2009;68:709–35.
194. Mez J, Daneshvar DH, Kiernan PT, et al. Clinicopathological evaluation of chronic traumatic encephalopathy in players of American football. *JAMA.* 2017;318:360–70.
195. Faul M, Xu L, Wald MM, et al. *Traumatic Brain Injury in the United States.* Atlanta, GA: Centers for Disease Control and Prevention, National Center for Injury Prevention and Control. 2010.
196. Thurman DJ, Coronado V, Selassie A. The epidemiology of TBI: Implications for public health. In: Zasler ND, Katz DI, Zafonte RD, eds. *Brain Injury Medicine: Principles and Practice.* New York: Demos; 2007, pp. 45–55.
197. Thurman DJ, Alverson C, Dunn KA, et al. Traumatic brain injury in the United States: A public health perspective. *J Head Trauma Rehab.* 1999;14:602–15.
198. Plassman BL, Havlik RJ, Steffens DC, et al. Documented head injury in early adulthood and risk of Alzheimer's disease and other dementias. *Neurology.* 2000;55:1158–66.
199. Mott FW. The effects of high explosives upon the central nervous system. *Lancet.* 1916;1:331–8.
200. Kelley BJ, Petersen RC. Alzheimer's disease and mild cognitive impairment. *Neurol Clin.* 2007;25:577–609.
201. Lyketsos C, Colenda C, Beck C, et al. Position statement of the American Association for Geriatric Psychiatry regarding principles of care for patients with dementia resulting from Alzheimer's disease. *Am J Geriatr Psychiatry.* 2006;14:561–72.
202. Langa KM, Levine DA. The diagnosis and management of mild cognitive impairment: A clinical review. *JAMA.* 2014;312:2551–61.
203. Petersen RC, Doody R, Kurz A, et al. Current concepts in mild cognitive impairment. *Arch Neurol.* 2001;58:1985–92.
204. Plassman BL, Langa KM, Fisher GG, et al. Prevalence of cognitive impairment without dementia in the United States. *Ann Intern Med.* 2008;148:427–34.
205. Karakaya T, Fuber F, Schroder J, et al. Pharmacological treatment of mild cognitive impairment as a prodromal syndrome of Alzheimer's disease. *Curr Neuropharmacol.* 2013;11:102–8.
206. Carr DB, Ott BR. The older adult driver with cognitive impairment: "It's a very frustrating life." *JAMA.* 2010;303:1632–41.
207. Rapoport MJ, Naglie G, Herrmann N, et al. Developing physician consensus on the reporting of patients with mild cognitive impairment and mild dementia to transportation authorities in a region with mandatory reporting legislation. *Am J Geriatr Psychiatry.* 2014;22:1530–43.
208. Solomon A, Mangialasche F, Richard E, et al. Advances in the prevention of Alzheimer's disease and dementia. *J Intern Med.* 2014;275:229–50.
209. Wolf PA. Contributions of the Framingham heart study to stroke and dementia epidemiologic research at 60 years. *Arch Neurol.* 2012;69:567–71.
210. Salloway S, Sperling R, Fox NC, et al. Two phase 3 trials of bapineuzumab in mild-to-moderate Alzheimer's disease. *N Engl J Med.* 2014;370:322–33.
211. Doody RS, Thomas RG, Farlow M, et al. Phase 3 trials of solanezumab for mild-to-moderate Alzheimer's disease. *N Engl J Med.* 2014;370:311–21.
212. Carroll J. 2017, February 15. Another Alzheimer's drug flops in pivotal clinical trial. http://www.sciencemag.org/news/2017/02/another-alzheimers-drug-flops-pivotal-clinical-trial.
213. Abbott A, Dolgin E. 2016, November 23. Failed Alzheimer's trial does not kill leading theory of disease. https://www.nature.com/news/failed-alzheimer-s-trial-does-not-kill-leading-theory-of-disease-1.21045.
214. Collins FS, Varmus H. A new initiative on precision medicine. *N Engl J Med.* 2015;372:793–5.
215. Squires D, Anderson C. U.S. health care from a global perspective: Spending, use of services, prices, and health in 13 countries. *Issue Brief (Commonw Fund).* 2015;15:1–15.
216. National Center for Chronic Disease Prevention and Health Promotion. At A Glance 2015. 2015. https://www.cdc.gov/chronicdisease/resources/publications/aag/pdf/2015/nccdphp-aag.pdf.
217. Colvin MK, Stern TA. Diagnosis, evaluation, and treatment of attention-deficit/hyperactivity disorder. *J Clin Psychiatry.* 2015;76:e1148.
218. Ahmadi N, Mohammadi MR, Araghi SM, et al. Neurocognitive profile of children with attention deficit hyperactivity disorders (ADHD): A comparison between subtypes. *Iran J Psychiatry.* 2014;9:197–202.
219. Silver CH, Ruff RM, Iverson GL, et al. Learning disabilities: The need for neuropsychological evaluation. *Arch Clin Neuropsychol.* 2008;23:217–9.
220. Silver CH, Blackburn LB, Arffa S, et al. The importance of neuropsychological assessment for the evaluation of childhood learning disorders NAN Policy and Planning Committee. *Arch Clin Neuropsychol.* 2006;21:741–4.
221. Alhanai T, Au R, Glass J. "Spoken Language Biomarkers for Detecting Cognitive Impairment." *IEEE Workshop on Speech Recognition and Understanding, 2017.* https://arxiv.org/abs/1710.07551.
222. Souillard-Mandar W, Davis R, Rudin C, et al. Learning classification models of cognitive conditions from subtle behaviors in the digital clock drawing test. *Mach Learn.* 2016;102:393–441.
223. Seshadri S, Beiser A, Kelly-Hayes M, et al. The lifetime risk of stroke: Estimates from the Framingham study. *Stroke.* 2006;37:345–50.

CHAPTER

162

A Public Health Approach to Severe Mental Illness

Lawrence Yang • Drew Blasco • Lily Kamalyan • Saige Stortz

INTRODUCTION

Severe mental illness (SMI) is defined as "a mental, behavior, or emotional disorder" diagnosable according to the Diagnostic and Statistical Manual (DSM) that results in significant functional impairment.[2,3] A traditional focus for public mental health systems has been to treat SMI, which account for a disproportionate amount of disability among all mental disorders.[1] However, public health approaches to treat mental illness have gradually shifted toward progressively earlier identification and treatment strategies, including preventive strategies. Most of these efforts have been on SMIs such as bipolar disorder and psychotic disorders (including schizophrenia); accordingly, this review focuses on these disorders.

GLOBAL BURDEN OF SERIOUS MENTAL ILLNESS

Because many SMI are chronic in nature, these disorders constitute some of the most debilitating illnesses globally.[1] Mental illness and substance use disorders accounted for 7.4% of worldwide Disability Adjusted Life Years (DALYs) in 2010, a measure of disease burden.[1] Of the proportion of DALY's accounted for by mental and substance use disorders globally, schizophrenia accounted for 7.4% and bipolar disorder accounted for 7.0%.[1] SMI thus severely and adversely impacts an individual's functioning and life chances.[2]

Bipolar disorder and schizophrenia are considered major types of SMI due to their resulting impairment.[3] In addition to other criteria, those diagnosed with bipolar disorder experience the occurrence of a manic episode in which a person experiences elevated mood and energy levels lasting most of the day for most days out of at least 1 week.[5] Worldwide, lifetime prevalence of bipolar I disorder was found to be approximately 0.6%.[6] In the United States, data from the National Comorbidity Survey Replication estimated lifetime prevalence of bipolar I to be 1%.[7]

A diagnosis of schizophrenia is characterized by the occurrence of two or more of the following symptoms occurring during a time period of 1 month and for a significant amount of time: delusions, hallucinations, disorganized speech, disorganized or catatonic behavior, or negative symptoms.[5]Additionally, one or more of the symptoms experienced must include delusions, hallucinations, or disorganized speech.[5] These symptoms must persist over a 6-month period, although only 1 month of active symptoms is required, and are not explainable by other factors (e.g., organic cause or substance abuse).[5] To be diagnosed, significant disturbances in functioning (i.e., at work, relationships, etc.) must be present.[5] While variation in prevalence exists, the average point prevalence for schizophrenia is estimated to be 4.6 per 1000 people.[8] Several large-scale studies have found 12-month prevalence estimates to range from 0.5% to 1.1% in the United States.[9–11] Key to early intervention strategies, onset of schizophrenia and bipolar disorders is typically in late adolescence and early adulthood with the greatest burden occurring during ages 25–50,[1] when work and marriage typically occur. Finally, the financial burden associated with schizophrenia is severe, with global economic costs ranging from $94 million to $102 billion per country, accounting for 0.02–5.46% of the Gross Domestic Product (GDP) of countries surveyed.[12]

HISTORICAL PERSPECTIVE ON TREATMENT

While schizophrenia and bipolar disorder are considered distinct diagnoses, they often share symptomatic experiences, including psychosis. Psychosis refers to experiences of hallucinations, delusional beliefs, disorganized thoughts, and/or disorganized behavior, which cause significant loss of functioning. Psychosis is recognized as cutting across these disorders,[13] and has emerged as a common target to intervene with these conditions. Psychosis symptoms are typically accompanied with little or no insight,[14] which has historically led to an undervaluing of the sick individual's participation in treatment. For much of the nineteenth and twentieth centuries, care for individuals with psychosis focused on tertiary intervention, consisting of long-term management of chronic illness.[15] Treatment frequently occurred in inpatient settings (e.g., asylums), which were known for being underfunded, understaffed, and providing harsh treatment.[16,17] Yet at this time, the inpatient-care model was considered the most effective way to care for those with SMI.

CHANGING CARE MODELS: INPATIENT CARE TO DEINSTITUTIONALIZATION

In the 1950s, the number of psychiatric beds in the United States totaled close to 560,000, with similar figures in other countries (Fig. 162-1).[18–20] In the United States, there were a limited number of mental health professionals available, with estimates of approximately 7000 psychiatrists, 13,500 psychologists, and 20,000 social workers (Fig. 162-1).[18,19] With the groundbreaking advancement of pharmacological treatments such as chlorpromazine in 1954 and the political, social, economic, and moral arguments made against asylum-based care, a shift toward community-based care began.

Community-based care refers to when an individual's residential community provides the source of support and treatment for an individual with mental illness. Care includes not only outpatient mental health treatment, but also other necessary resources including housing, employment, and recreation.[21] Mental health services may be provided by government-funded agencies that would provide services for individuals within a designated region or catchment area. For example, "Assertive Community Treatment" involves collaborative care from a multidisciplinary team, including a psychiatrist, case managers or service coordinators, social workers, nurses, substance use specialists, vocational rehabilitation specialists, and peer supporters.[22] This shift to community-based care was legislated with the Community Mental Health Care Construction Act in 1954,

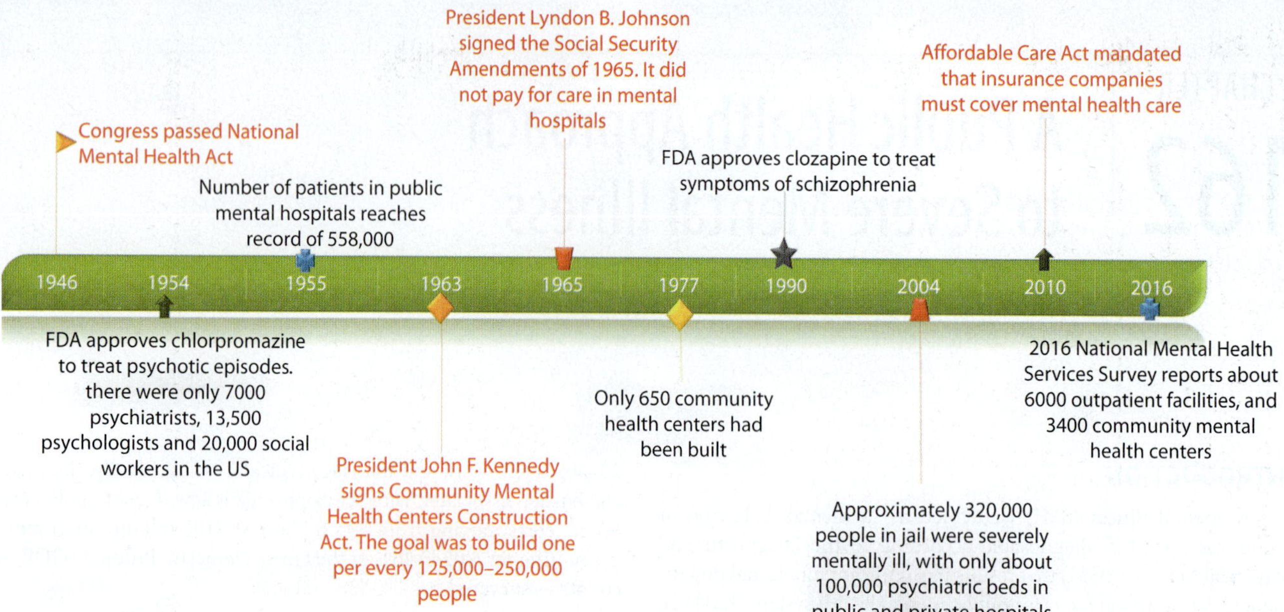

FIGURE 162-1. Timeline of deinstitutionalization and mental healthcare in the United States.

which aimed to build one center for every 125,000–250,000 people (Fig. 162-1),[18,19] thus marking the beginning of deinstitutionalization.

Although deinstitutionalization focused care in the community, in some cases it left patients without access to coordinated care. By 1977, only about 650 community mental health centers had been built in the United States (Fig. 162-1).[18,19] While serving to reintegrate people with SMI into their communities, critics of deinstitutionalization noted a failure to detect individuals who had newly developed SMI as well as those who showed comorbid substance abuse or other debilitating health concerns. These critics argued that these individuals may have been disproportionately sent to prison, become homeless, or were cared for by the forensic psychiatry system which did not service all of their needs.[23]

LIMITATIONS OF STANDARD CARE SERVICES FOR SERIOUS MENTAL ILLNESS

Even with access to community mental health services, more than 70% of first-episode patients (FEP), or patients with a psychotic episode who are receiving their first treatment, are still admitted to psychiatric hospital, either as an inpatient or an outpatient. Worldwide, multiple studies have observed an average delay of 2 years between the appearance of psychotic symptoms and initiation of appropriate treatment.[24] An outpatient psychiatrist will typically initiate antipsychotic medications and when available, psychological interventions (e.g., behavioral psychoeducation or cognitive behavioral therapy). Two classes of antipsychotic drugs exist: (1) "typical" or first-generation antipsychotics that were created in the 1950s; and (2) "atypical" or second-generation antipsychotics that were developed in the 1990s due to the side effects linked with typical antipsychotics (e.g., extrapyramidal symptoms, or motor side effects).[25] Both types of antipsychotics are effective in reducing the positive symptoms of psychosis (e.g., hallucinations, delusions) in a short time span.[26] Yet antipsychotics are only partially or minimally effective in approximately 40% of cases and result in side effects such as abnormal motor symptoms and weight gain.[27]

One major critique is that care for psychosis primarily consisted of tertiary care that focused on managing chronic illness rather than seeking to ameliorate illness chronicity or being preventative in nature.[28] Further, this care showed only modest efficacy; up to 70% of individuals with schizophrenia fail to stick to treatment plans,[29] and approximately 20% will relapse in 1 year.[30] The substantial heterogeneity shown in treatment adherence and outcomes for standard care indicated a great need to develop empirically based treatments for psychosis.

DEVELOPMENT OF EVIDENCE-BASED PRACTICES TO TREAT SCHIZOPHRENIA

The Schizophrenia Patient Outcomes Research Team (PORT) was created in 1992 by a consortium of U.S. researchers to improve common psychiatric practices and evidence-based psychosocial interventions.[4] Via intensive literature review up through 2009, the team has reported treatment recommendations for: case management, psychotherapy, family support/education, education and employment support, and pharmacotherapy, among others. In 2003, PORT published the second edition of recommendations on the traditional course of treating positive symptoms of schizophrenia with psychopharmacology, resulting in guidelines for treatment of acute positive symptoms in treatment-responsive patients, daily dosages, maintenance pharmacotherapy, treating intermittent symptoms, treating treatment-resistant patients, and many other circumstances.[31] However, psychopharmacology mostly focused on symptom reduction and relapse prevention, and did not include possible beneficial effects of psychosocial interventions.

In their most updated report in 2009, the third revision of PORT sought to update recommendations to integrate psychosocial interventions into treatment plans. This update offers recommendations for those who are at risk for repeated hospitalization or have been recently homeless to receive Assertive Community Treatment (ACT). ACT has been found to significantly improve these outcomes. ACT programs emphasize clients' strengths to better adapt to community life by providing support with their families, employers, friends and peers, and community agencies. Medication adherence is also emphasized by the multidisciplinary team, which includes a psychiatrist, strives for high frequency of client contact via active outreach, and has low client-to-staff ratios. ACT has shown effectiveness when expanded to other outcomes, including employment. Recommended practices for supported employment for persons with SMI include individually tailored job development, rapid job search, and providing job support. Crucially, integration of these supported employment programs with other interventions may improve long-term job retention and economic self-sufficiency.[4]

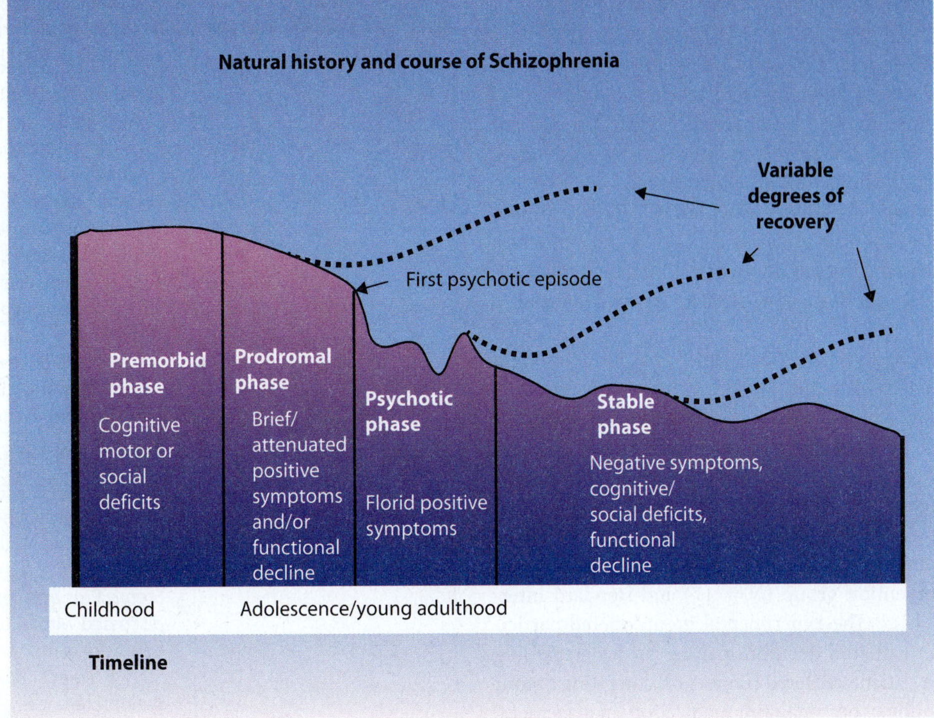

FIGURE 162-2. Natural history and course of schizophrenia. Reproduced with Permission from Tandon R, Nasrallah HA, Keshavan MS. Schizophrenia," just the facts" 4. Clinical features and conceptualization. *Schizophr Res*. 2009;110(1):1–23.

The third revision of PORT also recommends cognitive behavior therapy to reduce the severity of symptoms for persons with SMI. This therapy allows clients to identify target problems and develop specific coping strategies, and has been shown to improve delusions, hallucinations, negative and overall symptoms, and social functioning.[4] Effective family interventions include psychoeducation, crisis intervention, emotional support, and training in coping with symptoms.[31] Integration of family interventions can improve relationships with family and decrease illness burden, while also improving treatment adherence, functional and vocational status, and treatment satisfaction.[4] While further outcomes remain to be evaluated (e.g., relapse), these recommendations constitute a foundation of evidence-based practices for psychosis.

EVOLVING CONCEPTUALIZATIONS OF PSYCHOSIS AND ITS IMPACTS ON TREATMENT APPROACHES

As evidence-based treatments have evolved, concurrent recognition that psychosis progresses in stages has played a substantial role in shaping treatment for psychotic conditions. The term "first-episode psychosis" (FEP) appeared around the late 1980s as a way to classify the first episode of a psychotic disorder. This contemporary understanding of psychosis now reflects a "lifetime illness trajectory" (Fig. 162-2).[32]

This model proposes that psychosis exhibits signs as early as childhood during the "premorbid" phase, with clients presenting with symptoms of subtle thought, motor, and/or social dysfunction.[32,33] This is followed by a "prodromal" phase typically seen in adolescence, characterized by attenuated positive symptoms (delusions or hallucinations) and declining cognition and social functioning.[34,35] This "prodromal" phase serves as the target for preventative intervention for the "clinical high-risk state for psychosis" (CHR; described later). FEP occurs when criteria for a full psychotic disorder (e.g., bipolar disorder with psychotic features, schizophrenia) is met. Recognition of FEP typically occurs via first contact with a medical professional or psychiatric hospitalization.[36]

ADOPTING EVIDENCE-BASED PRACTICES FOR FIRST-EPISODE PSYCHOSIS TREATMENT

PORT not only established evidence-based practices for the treatment of chronic schizophrenia[4]; researchers then built upon these well-established evidence-based practices to treat FEP individuals. The novelty of these FEP programs was to apply these practices to an earlier stage of psychosis to reduce illness chronicity and morbidity. A "common-elements approach" has been taken to the designation of evidence-based practices for FEP.[37] This approach indicates that a multicomponent, team-based approach is needed, with some flexibility in adapting components to the specific situation. "Core" components are considered case management, psychotherapy, family support and/or education, education and employment support, and pharmacotherapy. In the United States, these multimethod components have shown evidence-based support for early psychosis intervention and are now referred to as "coordinated specialty care." A recent review indicates that "coordinated specialty care" holds substantial benefits for symptoms, functioning, and quality of life for individuals with FEP.[38]

International Examples of FEP Programs

Specialized treatment programs for FEP have developed throughout the 1990s and early 2000s[39] and include programs in Australia, Canada, Europe (e.g., Sweden, Norway, and Amsterdam), and Asia (e.g., Hong Kong).[40–43] While programs differ in duration and staff composition, many of these programs bundle and deliver several of the "core" components of coordinated specialty care identified above. One main predictor of recovery from FEP is the time from which psychotic symptoms start to when appropriate treatment is accessed (i.e., typically ranging from 1 to 2 years). Given that a longer duration of untreated psychosis is associated with more impaired function overall and a longer length in stabilizing psychotic symptoms,[44] these programs prioritize provision of rapid identification and treatment.

Development and Implementation of FEP Services in the United States

To illuminate the development of early-intervention services, we illustrate how FEP treatment programs were developed in the United States. The National Institute of Mental Health (NIMH) sponsored the *Recovery After an Initial Schizophrenia Episode* (RAISE) project[39] to in support of research about FEP programs in the United States. The RAISE project sought to answer whether: (1) FEP treatment worked better than treatment as usual, and (2) to identify the best way for community-based clinics to implement FEP treatment.[45]

To assess the first question, the RAISE study evaluated a four-component intervention, called NAVIGATE, which provided participants at minimum 2 years of treatment.[45] NAVIGATE sought to help consumers cope with the initial confusion that typically accompanies psychotic symptoms via collaboration with a specialized treatment team to help negotiate the mental healthcare system.[39] The RAISE study was conducted in 34 community mental health centers (CMHCs) throughout 21 states that were intended to represent "real-world" CMHCs in the United States (i.e., were not specialized academic research centers). These CMHCs were randomized into an experimental intervention group ($N = 17$) and standard intervention group ($N = 17$).[45] The experimental group offered participants participation in a shared decision-making process regarding their treatment, and a patient-centered framework consisting of four NAVIGATE interventions: personalized medication management, family psychoeducation, resilience-focused individual therapy, and supported employment and education.[45] Participants in the control group received treatment as usual. Participants were tracked monthly in their use of the four NAVIGATE interventions.[45]

RAISE aimed to decrease likelihood of future episodes of psychosis and long-term disability by helping people to achieve crucial developmental goals during recovery.[4] Experimental group participants showed improvement in sense of purpose, motivation, curiosity, and emotional engagement.[45] They also showed an increase in engagement of "common activities," such as a higher proportion of participants working or going to school.[45] Further, there was improvement in overall positive and negative symptoms and depression.[45] These encouraging results led to the New York State Office of Mental Health (OMH) to provide funds to develop a FEP program, named OnTrackNY that would use and refine these identified best practices in treating FEP.[47] We highlight the OnTrackNY program as an example of a community-based FEP program as a case study for other FEP programs worldwide.[47]

Development of OnTrackNY

OnTrackNY was implemented throughout New York,[46] with 13 OnTrackNY programs in place in September 2016 and 21 programs expected to be fully operational by the end of 2016.[47] As of 2016, these programs serviced a total of 376 clients. While these programs sought to ascertain consumers from outside the mental healthcare system, the majority still came from mental health treatment centers; 40% were referred from inpatient psychiatric units, 20% from outpatient mental health settings or self- and family-referred, while the rest were from school systems, community organizations, and emergency departments.[47] An emphasis was to decrease duration of untreated psychosis; in OnTrackNY, this figure ranges from 4.3 to 15.6 months, averaging 7.2 months. Once treatment is initiated, continued enrollment remains high, averaging 99% at 3 months and 82% at 12-month follow-up.[47]

OnTrackNY utilizes components derived from NAVIGATE including standards of shared decision making, active and focused treatment, flexible and consistent treatment, and fostering autonomy to maximize recovery[48] (see Table 162-1 for definitions). Recovery focuses on restoring capacities in four life domains: health, home, purpose, and community.[48] Because of OnTrackNY's multicomponent nature—consisting of evidence-based psychopharmacology, an emphasis on primary-care coordination, case management, two cognitive behavioral therapy components, individualized psychotherapy, and family support and education—this program requires a collaborative team.[47] This team consists of two licensed clinicians who fill three roles (i.e., primary clinician, outreach and recruitment coordinator, and team leader) an education and employment specialist, a peer specialist, a prescriber, and a nurse.[47] Lastly, OnTrackNY integrates another evidence-based practice, that of Critical Time

TABLE 162-1 COMPONENTS IN ONTRACKNY

Recovery Orientation	Four Dimensions for Recovery: 1. Health: help client and family make informed decisions in managing symptoms and support physical and mental health 2. Home: help client with management services like insurance, entitlements, and a stable and safe place to live 3. Purpose: help client to clarify and meet personal work and school goals 4. Community: responsiveness to client's desired level of interaction with family and friends and develop involvement in community groups
Shared Decision-Making	Client and Clinician "Disagreement" to "Compromise" in 5 Steps: • Step 1: Client defines the problem or decision to be made • Step 2: Options are outlined • Step 3: Pros and cons for options discussed with information and educational materials • Step 4: Client and clinician express their preferences • Step 5: Negotiation of disagreements until compromise is reached
Active and Focused Treatment	Active Treatment: • Providing all relevant treatment information for client to consider • Proactive in connecting with client and their family members Focused Treatment: • Team addresses intervention areas while helping client partner with community partners
Flexible and Consistent Treatment	Flexible Treatment: • Flexibility allows team to adjust plan accordingly, respond to clients on as-needed basis, and treat clients differently based on client's strengths and difficulties Consistent Treatment: • Team members are consistent as people and professionals
Fostering Autonomy and Remaining Available	Responsiveness and Independence: • Early treatment involves meeting frequently and high involvement in facilitating care. Over time, client and family take increasing responsibility for care and finding responsibilities • Throughout treatment, team members balance between giving clients more autonomy and providing greater support when needed

Intervention, or CTI, which enhances continuity of support for people during critical periods of time.[48,49] CTI is crucial to OnTrackNY because it adds three key components: (1) ongoing assessment and treatment planning; (2) incorporation of family involvement; and (3) recognition of client diversity[48] that are delivered during distinct phases of "initial engagement" (months 1–3), "ongoing intervention" (months 4–18), and finally, "service transition" (months 19 and on).

Evaluation and Implementation of OnTrackNY

While the RAISE study, upon which OnTrackNY is based, systematically evaluated outcomes, a randomized controlled trial of OnTrackNY has not been conducted. Nonetheless, evaluation of this early intervention program has been promising. Initial evaluation based on follow-up data on nearly 2/3 of OnTrackNY clients showed decreasing use of hospitalization; participants who reported one hospitalization decreased from 73% at baseline to 11% in the most recent 3-month follow-up.[47] A similar improvement manifested in enrollment in school or employment over time, with 45% of clients at baseline being in school or employed increasing to 74% in the most recent 3-month follow-up.[47] This focus on vocational participation might help to prevent disability, as rates of enrollment in disability programs (i.e., Supplemental Security Income/Social Security Disability Insurance) remained relatively low for participants over the 2-year program (2.5% at baseline to 18.3% at 2 years).[50] This relatively low rate of disability evidenced in OnTrackNY appears even more beneficial than the rates of disability shown in the RAISE study (where up to 34.1% of all study participants received benefits during the 2-year study period),[51] although sample differences between studies limit direct comparisons. Because OnTrackNY collects outcome and care process data from all sites, more studies evaluating outcomes are expected shortly, which will be of great value to policy makers.

Barriers to implementation of OnTrackNY exist, reflecting challenges to a public health approach. The ability to effectively implement OnTrackNY in a particular CMHC depends on the recovery orientation skills of the individual clinicians, clients, and organization as a whole, as well as staff turnover. Additional barriers include limitations in available transportation, availability of host agency resources to provide a flexible intervention (e.g., ability to provide 24/7 coverage), availability of first-line antipsychotic medications, use of technology (e.g., telemedicine), and ensuring community buy-in of mental health services. These issues are particularly salient in rural areas, which grapple with stigma and limits to confidentiality that are endemic to small communities where young adults with FEP are trying to secure employment. Regardless, OnTrackNY offers these advantages: (1) an evidence-based program which has reported high rates of engagement among clients and improvements in symptoms and functional outcomes[52]; (2) serves regions of New York State by collaborating with government mental health authorities[53]; (3) is practical and scalable with good fidelity.

CONCEPTUALIZATION OF CHR AND FOCUS ON PREVENTION

Concurrent with efforts to treat psychosis in its earlier stages, there has been a landmark shift to identify and treat youth who show subthreshold psychotic symptoms, who *show early symptoms that may occur before full development of psychosis*. To reduce the burden associated with development of schizophrenia or other psychotic disorders, early intervention during what is considered the prodromal phase is imperative.[54] The CHR was developed from evidence that 80–90% of individuals with schizophrenia reported prodromal, or subacute symptoms including changes in thinking, perception, and behavior before experiencing full psychosis. The CHR is a systematic attempt to operationalize these prodromal symptoms to identify those at high risk of developing psychosis.[55] This approach holds great promise in initiating treatment at the earliest signs of psychosis and possibly preventing the advent of a psychotic disorder in some cases. Accordingly, CHR services are distinct in that they target the identification of those who are at *high risk* for developing psychosis, in contrast to FEP services described above which seek to reduce the burden of symptoms for those who had already developed a first episode of psychosis.[56–58]

A main advance of the CHR approach is its focus on preventing the development of more serious mental illness symptoms. Specialized CHR clinics focus on *secondary prevention*, which is characterized by CHR interventions aiming to limit the progression of psychotic-like symptoms to full psychotic symptoms.[58] CHR clinics engage in secondary prevention by carefully monitoring and treating individuals with the aim to reduce overall incidence of psychosis, and improving overall symptoms and functioning.[58] Reducing symptoms and preventing conversion to psychosis is crucial considering the significant financial, social, and life costs associated with developing a full psychotic disorder.[58] CHR is thus one of the few approaches to secondary prevention in mental health that has received empirical evaluation.

The CHR approach originated in Melbourne, Australia, where the Personal Assessment and Crisis Evaluation (PACE) clinic was created to treat those presenting with potential subthreshold psychotic symptoms.[59–61] Like many subsequent CHR services, the PACE clinic broadened the comprehensive care provided by an affiliated FEP treatment program by targeting those at high risk to develop psychosis.[62,63] CHR programs have since proliferated worldwide.[64,65] In the United States, CHR clinics often partner with academic institutions or hospitals[65]; often, treatment is provided for free with individuals being compensated for their participation in research.[66] Two examples of major CHR consortia include the eight-site North American Prodrome Longitudinal Study (NAPLS) and the six-site Early Detection and Intervention for the Prevention of Psychosis (EDIPPP).[67–69] The National Institute of Mental Health has also proposed the creation of a worldwide consortium of CHR sites.

CHR IDENTIFICATION STATE

One major contribution of the CHR identification was to operationalize a "high-risk" state for psychosis.[60,70] The CHR in North America and Europe is primarily assessed using the Structured Interview for Prodromal Symptoms (SIPS) criteria, a structured interview used to identify prodromal criteria.[60,70] Crucially, the originators of the CHR identification established that approximately 35% of individuals identified as CHR will convert to psychosis within 12 months of diagnosis.[72] Other meta-analyses have confirmed similar rates of psychosis conversion within 2 years of identification, including the North American Prodrome Longitudinal Study.[64]

CHR criteria can be met by recent development of positive symptoms at a full psychotic level for very brief durations (i.e., several minutes a day; termed "Brief Intermittent Psychosis Syndrome"), or by having a first degree relative with a diagnosed psychotic disorder in conjunction with a significant decrease in functioning over the past year (i.e., termed "Genetic Risk and Deterioration").[71] Yet most individuals meet criteria for CHR by showing the presence of one or more positive symptoms (e.g., "unusual thought content" or "perceptual abnormalities") at a prodromal rating which in the past year developed or began to worsen (termed "attenuated psychotic symptom syndrome").[71] While requiring specialized training, the SIPS has shown good interrater reliability as well as predictive validity for future conversion to psychosis.[71]

These CHR criteria enable identification of "high-risk" psychosis symptoms (which consist of positive, negative, disorganized, and general symptoms) from those that meet a fully psychotic level.[71] An example of a mild or attenuated psychosis symptom includes an individual experiencing perceptual abnormalities who might hear someone calling their name when in fact no one said their name.[71] CHR symptoms also differ from full psychotic symptoms in that the individual still has insight into the possibility that their experiences may not be real.[71] In contrast, an individual meets diagnostic criteria for a psychotic disorder when they have conviction that their symptoms are real.[71] CHR is thus a "high-risk" identification that emphasizes secondary prevention to reduce development of full psychosis symptoms.[58,71]

CHR PROGRAMS AND COMMUNITY ASCERTAINMENT

CHR clinics typically target identification among adolescents and young adults with existing mental health difficulties, who are at highest risk of conversion to psychosis.[60] While CHR clinics typically consist of a multidisciplinary team including psychiatrists, psychologists, therapists, and researchers who provide comprehensive evaluation, monitoring, and treatment, team members also perform active community outreach.[66] CHR clinics ascertain heavily from the community for referrals.[64,73] Typically, individuals are enrolled from a number of sources including schools and other mental health agencies,[64] bolstered by outreach and community education to identify individuals who may meet CHR criteria in the community.[73,74] The primary aim is to ascertain individuals currently outside of the traditional, tertiary mental healthcare system, to prevent worsening symptoms and illness course.[75] Because the underlying risk factors associated with psychosis development is still unknown, primary prevention is unachievable; therefore, secondary prevention remains the most effective way to reduce incidence and burden of psychotic disorders.[75]

Example of Community Referral for CHR

We highlight the Portland Identification and Early Referral program (PIER) as an example of a community-based CHR program.[73] Prior to recruitment, PIER undertook a large-scale effort to educate the community both within and outside mental health services to increase CHR identification.[73] The goal was to identify and treat all consenting individuals identified as at-risk for psychosis (ages 12–35) in the Portland area.[73] PIER targeted a wide variety of community professionals—including school and college counselors, other health professionals, primary-care and mental health clinicians, and others working with young people (see Fig. 162-3)—to increase the referral network.[73] PIER staff completed outreach using standardized material via on-site visits, presentations, and education.[73] In conjunction, PIER conducted a public education campaign targeting friends and family of young adults to improve recognition of early signs of psychosis to increase referrals.[73] Multiple outreach methods were used, including TV and radio advertisements, customized websites, and brochures.[73] About 74% of the professionals PIER educated about CHR symptoms were from outside the mental healthcare system, resulting in > 50% of referrals originating from outside traditional mental healthcare agencies.[73] Overall, 37% of referrals formally screened were determined to meet CHR criteria,[73] similar to the rate reported by NAPLS.[64] Final analyses indicated a positive effect of the education and outreach intervention on clinic referrals, although there was about a 6-month lag between outreach and impact on referrals.[73]

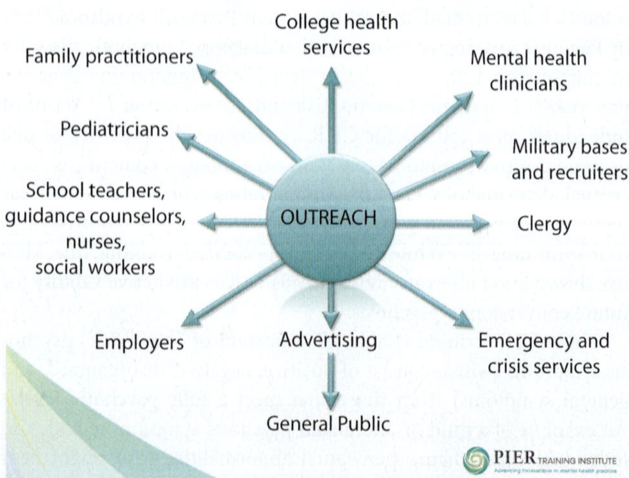

FIGURE 162-3. Example of community ascertainment from PIER. Used with Permission from PIER Training Institute.

A study by PIER also indicated that implementation of CHR services acts to reduce incidence of psychosis in that catchment area. McFarlane et al. compared rates of psychosis-related hospitalizations for the PIER catchment area (experimental group) and comparable regions of Maine without CHR programs (control group), before and after PIER was implemented.[76] Results indicated a 26% decrease in psychosis-related hospitalization rates for the experimental area and an 8% increase in the control area.[76] This suggests the effectiveness of the PIER program in decreasing hospitalization rates through effective monitoring and treatment of high-risk individuals.[76] This is a crucial development for public mental health in the United States, as this shows that implementation of a CHR program can have significant community-level impacts on reducing transition to psychosis.[76]

EVIDENCE-BASED TREATMENTS FOR CHR

While programs focus primarily on treating CHR symptoms, individuals with CHR also commonly experience mental illness comorbidities such as depression, anxiety, and substance use.[60] Additionally, patients often exhibit functional impairments in academic and/or work performance, interpersonal relationships, and psychosocial functioning.[60] Depending on the clinic, psychotherapy may include: cognitive therapy, family psychoeducation, or other psychosocial interventions. Only in the most advanced cases where development of a full psychotic disorder is imminent (or has already developed) is the use of antipsychotic drug treatment advocated; otherwise, adjunctive nonpsychotic medication treatment is used when warranted.[64,73]

Although research is ongoing, studies have indicated that specialized CHR treatment is associated with a reduced risk of full development of psychosis when compared with treatment as usual or no treatment.[60,64,77] Further, a systematic review of 11 intervention trials suggests that prevention of psychosis may be possible; however, more evidence is needed to determine what interventions are best for those at high risk.[78] As per above, in CHR clinics, antipsychotics are generally not the first line of treatment,[64] and the available literature has not shown effectiveness of antipsychotics in preventing psychosis.[78] A randomized control trial has shown efficacy of cognitive therapy in decreasing conversion to psychosis among CHR individuals.[79] Additionally, Stafford et al. (2013) determined that a number of CBT trials had a moderate effect on preventing development of psychosis, while further research is needed to ascertain the benefits of family-based interventions. Finally, one study has revealed the possibility of nutritional supplements such as omega-3 acids in reducing the risk of conversion, although more robust research is needed due to the small number of participants included.[78,80] As evidence-based treatments for CHR advance, the possibility of further decreasing incidence and burden of psychosis on a population-level increases.[81]

STIGMA AS A BARRIER TO THE PUBLIC HEALTH BENEFIT OF CHR

Despite the beneficial effects of early intervention with CHR, being identified as at high psychosis risk may elicit stigma by conveying an added psychiatric "label"[82] by initiating pejorative stereotypes associated with psychosis (e.g., "dangerous").[83] Since only about 35% of youth identified as CHR may develop psychosis within 2 years, a majority could be subject to risk for stigma for a condition that never develops.[84] This is of particular importance because stigma in CHR youth has been linked with worse psychosocial well-being both cross-sectionally and longitudinally.[85–87] More recently, efforts have been made to parse out the effects of stigma that are associated with the CHR identification itself (i.e., the CHR "label") versus the symptoms that CHR individuals experience,[82] as the latter is expected to be minimized as CHR symptoms themselves are reduced via early intervention. Future investigations regarding the impact of the CHR "label" itself will then shed insight regarding to what extent stigma might impede the public health benefit for the CHR identification, and what strategies might be taken to mitigate any such "labeling-related" stigma if it indeed exists.

CONCLUSION

This chapter has traced the development of public health approaches to SMI, which have evolved from tertiary treatment provided in psychiatric hospitals and asylums to approaches including FEP treatment to reduce illness chronicity and CHR treatment focusing on secondary prevention to limit the progression of subthreshold psychosis symptoms. In conjunction with the movement toward earlier treatment, the continuing shift toward identification, treatment, and rehabilitation of SMI in the community promises to enhance recovery, thereby reducing morbidity and societal burden of these disorders. Future public health effects may be enhanced by expanding the current emphasis on psychosis and schizophrenia to including other common mental disorders such as depressive and anxiety disorders, which also cause substantial functional impairment. While early intervention approaches are primarily located within specialty treatment centers, as evidence for their efficacy increases, it is hoped that these interventions will be adopted into mainstream mental healthcare systems worldwide to maximize their public health impact.

References

1. Whiteford HA, Degenhardt L, Rehm J, et al. Global burden of disease attributable to mental and substance use disorders: Findings from the Global Burden of Disease Study 2010. *Lancet.* 2013;382(9904):1575–86.
2. Center for Behavioral Health Statistics and Quality. Key substance use and mental health indicators in the United States: Results from the 2015 National Survey on Drug Use and Health. http://www.samhsa.gov/data/.
3. Kessler RC, Berglund PA, Bruce ML, et al. The prevalence and correlates of untreated serious mental illness. *Health Serv Res.* 2001;36(6 Pt 1):987–1007.
4. Dixon LB, Dickerson F, Bellack AS, et al. The 2009 schizophrenia PORT psychosocial treatment recommendations and summary statements. *Schizophr Bull.* 2009;36(1):48–70.
5. American Psychiatric Association. *Diagnostic and Statistical Manual of Mental Disorders: DSM-5*, 5th ed. Arlington, VA: American Psychiatric Association; 2013.
6. Merikangas KR, Jin R, He JP, et al. Prevalence and correlates of bipolar spectrum disorder in the world mental health survey initiative. *Arch Gen Psychiatry.* 2011;68(3):241–51.
7. Merikangas KR, Akiskal HS, Angst J, et al. Lifetime and 12-month prevalence of bipolar spectrum disorder in the National Comorbidity Survey replication. *Arch Gen Psychiatry.* 2007;64(5):543–52.
8. Saha S, Chant D, Welham J, McGrath J. A systematic review of the prevalence of schizophrenia. *PLoS Med.* 2005;2(5):e141.
9. Kessler RC, McGonagle KA, Zhao S, et al. Lifetime and 12-month prevalence of DSM-III-R psychiatric disorders in the United States: Results from the National Comorbidity Survey. *Arch Gen Psychiatry.* 1994;51(1):8–19.
10. Narrow WE, Rae DS, Robins LN, Regier DA. Revised prevalence estimates of mental disorders in the United States: Using a clinical significance criterion to reconcile 2 surveys' estimates. *Arch Gen Psychiatry.* 2002;59(2):115–23.
11. Regier DA, Narrow WE, Rae DS, Manderscheid RW, Locke BZ, Goodwin FK. The de facto US mental and addictive disorders service system: Epidemiologic Catchment Area prospective 1-year prevalence rates of disorders and services. *Arch Gen Psychiatry.* 1993;50(2):85–94.
12. Chong HY, Teoh SL, Wu DB, Kotirum S, Chiou CF, Chaiyakunapruk N.. Global economic burden of schizophrenia: A systematic review. *Neuropsychiatr Dis Treat.* 2016;12:357.
13. Tamminga CA, Pearlson G, Keshavan M, Sweeney J, Clementz B, Thaker G. Bipolar and schizophrenia network for intermediate phenotypes: Outcomes across the psychosis continuum. *Schizophr Bull.* 2014;40(Suppl_2):S131–7.
14. Del-Ben CM, Rufino AC, Azevedo-Marques JM, Menezes PR. Differential diagnosis of first episode psychosis: Importance of optimal approach in psychiatric emergencies. *Braz J Psychiatry.* 2010;32:78–86.
15. Goldston SE. *Concepts of Primary Prevention: A Framework for Program Development.* Sacramento: California Department of Mental Health; 1987.
16. Novella EJ. Mental health care and the politics of inclusion: A social systems account of psychiatric deinstitutionalization. *Theor Med Bioeth.* 2010;31(6):411–27.
17. Knapp M, Beecham J, McDaid D, Matosevic T, Smith M. The economic consequences of deinstitutionalisation of mental health services: Lessons from a systematic review of European experience. *Health Soc Care Community.* 2011;19(2):113–25.
18. Pan D. TIMELINE: Deinstitutionalization and Its Consequences. Mother Jones, Mother Jones and the Foundation for National Progress, 2017. www.motherjones.com/politics/2013/04/timeline-mental-health-america/.
19. Department of Health and Human Services. 2016 National Mental Health Services Survey (N-MHSS): 2016 Data on Mental Health Treatment Facilities. https://www.samhsa.gov/data/sites/default/files/2016_National_Mental_Health_Services_Survey.pdf.
20. Eisenberg L, Guttmacher LB. Were we all asleep at the switch? A personal reminiscence of psychiatry from 1940 to 2010. *Acta Psychiatr Scand.* 2010;122(2):89–102.
21. Bentley KJ. Supports for community-based mental health care: An optimistic review of federal legislation. *Health Soc Work.* 1994;19(4):288–94.
22. Kent A, Burns T. Setting up an assertive community treatment service. *Adv Psychiatr Treat.* 1996;2:143–50.
23. Fakhoury W, Priebe S. Deinstitutionalization and reinstitutionalization: Major changes in the provision of mental healthcare. *Psychiatry.* 2007;6(8):313–6.
24. Marshall M, Lewis S, Lockwood A, Drake R, Jones P, Croudace T. Association between duration of untreated psychosis and outcome in cohorts of first-episode patients: A systematic review. *Arch Gen Psychiatry.* 2005;62(9):975–83.
25. Schennach R, Riedel M, Musil R, Möller HJ. Treatment response in first-episode schizophrenia. *Clin Psychopharmacol Neurosci.* 2012;10(2):78–87.
26. Adams CE. Schizophrenia. Full National Clinical Guideline on Core Interventions in Primary and Secondary Care National Collaborating Centre for Mental Health. *Psychiatr Bull.* 2004;28(9):351.
27. Crossley NA, Constante M, McGuire P, Power P. Efficacy of atypical v. typical antipsychotics in the treatment of early psychosis: Meta-analysis. *Br J Psychiatry.* 2010;196(6):434–9.
28 Clark DW. Preventive medicine for the doctor in his community. An epidemiologic approach. *Am J Public Health Nations Health.* 1958;48(7):947.
29. Leucht C, Heres S, Kane JM, Kissling W, Davis JM, Leucht S. Oral versus depot antipsychotic drugs for schizophrenia—A critical systematic review and meta-analysis of randomised long-term trials. *Schizophr Res.* 2011;127(1):83–92.
30. Kishimoto T, Agarwal V, Kishi T, Leucht S, Kane JM, Correll CU. Relapse prevention in schizophrenia: A systematic review and meta-analysis of second-generation antipsychotics versus first-generation antipsychotics. *Mol Psychiatry.* 2013;18(1):53–66.
31. Lehman AF, Kreyenbuhl J, Buchanan RW, et al. The schizophrenia patient outcomes research team (PORT): Updated treatment recommendations 2003. *Schizophr Bull.* 2003;30(2):193–217.
32. Tandon R, Nasrallah HA, Keshavan MS. Schizophrenia, "just the facts" 4. Clinical features and conceptualization. *Schizophr Res.* 2009;110(1):1–23.
33. Schenkel LS, Silverstein SM. Dimensions of premorbid functioning in schizophrenia: A review of neuromotor, cognitive, social, and behavioral domains. *Genet Soc Gen Psychol Monogr.* 2004;130(3):241–72.
34. Riecher-Rössler A, Rössler W. The course of schizophrenic psychoses: What do we really know? A selective review from an epidemiological perspective. *Eur Arch Psychiatry Clin Neurosci.* 1998;248(4):189–202.
35. Schultze-Lutter F. Subjective symptoms of schizophrenia in research and the clinic: The basic symptom concept. *Schizophr Bull.* 2009;35(1):5–8.
36. Beiser M, Erickson D, Fleming JA, Iacono WG. Establishing the onset of psychotic illness. *Am J Psychiatry.* 1993;150:9.
37. Dixon LB, Goldman HH, Srihari VH, Kane JM. Transforming the treatment of schizophrenia in the US: The RAISE initiative. *Annu Rev Clin Psychol.* 2018;14:237–58.
38. Heinssen RK, Goldstein AB, Azrin ST. Evidence-based treatments for first episode psychosis: Components of coordinated specialty care. NIMH White Pap. 2014.

39. Mueser KT, Penn DL, Addington J, et al. The NAVIGATE program for first-episode psychosis: Rationale, overview, and description of psychosocial components. *Psychiatr Serv*. 2015;66(7):680–90.
40. Cullberg J, Levander S, Holmqvist R, Mattsson M, Wieselgren IM. One-year outcome in first episode psychosis patients in the Swedish Parachute project. *Acta Psychiatr Scand*. 2002;106(4):276–85.
41. Grawe RW, Falloon IR, Widen JH, Skogvoll E. Two years of continued early treatment for recent-onset schizophrenia: A randomised controlled study. *Acta Psychiatr Scand*. 2006;114(5):328–36.
42. Tang JY, Wong GH, Hui CL, et al. Early intervention for psychosis in Hong Kong—The EASY programme. *Early Interv Psychiatry*. 2010;4(3):214–9.
43. Linszen D, Dingemans P, Lenior M. Early intervention and a five year follow up in young adults with a short duration of untreated psychosis: Ethical implications. *Schizophr Res*. 2001;51(1):55–61.
44. Mueser KT, Gringerich S, Addington J, et al. *The NAVIGATE Team Members' Guide*. Concord, NH: Dartmouth Psychiatric Research Center; 2014, pp. 1–63.
45. Kane JM, Robinson DG, Schooler NR, et al. Comprehensive versus usual community care for first-episode psychosis: 2-Year outcomes from the NIMH RAISE early treatment program. *Am J Psychiatry*. 2015;173(4):362–72.
46. "RAISE Questions and Answers." National Institute of Mental Health, U.S. Department of Health and Human Services. www.nimh.nih.gov/health/topics/schizophrenia/raise/raise-questions-and-answers.shtml.
47. Bello I, Lee R, Malinovsky I, et al. OnTrackNY: The development of a coordinated specialty care program for individuals experiencing early psychosis. *Psychiatr Serv*. 2017;68(4):318–20.
48. Goldberg R, Bennett M, Sikich L. *OnTrackNY: My health. My choices. My future. Team Manual*. New York: Center for Practice Innovations; 2017, pp. 1–97.
49. Susser E, Valencia E, Conover S, Felix A, Tsai WY, Wyatt RJ. Preventing recurrent homelessness among mentally ill men: A "critical time" intervention after discharge from a shelter. *Am J Public Health*. 1997;(2):256–62.
50. Humensky J, Scodes J, Wall M, et al. Disability enrollment in a community-based coordinated specialty care program. *Am J Psychiatry*. 2017;174(12):1224.
51. Rosenheck RA, Estroff SE, Sint K, et al. Incomes and outcomes: Social security disability benefits in first-episode psychosis. *Am J Psychiatry*. 2017;174(9):886–94.
52. Dixon LB, Goldman HH, Bennett ME, et al. Implementing coordinated specialty care for early psychosis: The RAISE Connection Program. *Psychiatr Serv*. 2015;66(7):691–8.
53. Essock SM, Goldman HH, Hogan MF, Hepburn BM, Sederer LI, Dixon LB. State partnerships for first-episode psychosis services. *Psychiatr Serv*. 2015;66(7):671–3.
54. Addington J, Heinssen R. Prediction and prevention of psychosis in youth at clinical high risk. *Annu Rev Clin Psychol*. 2012;8:269–89.
55. McGorry P. Early psychosis prevention and intervention centre. *Australas Psychiatry*. 1993;1(1):32–4.
56. McGorry PD, Edwards J, Mihalopoulos C, Harrigan SM, Jackson HJ. EPPIC: An evolving system of early detection and optimal management. *Schizophr Bull*. 1996;22(2):305.
57. Yung AR, McGorry PD, McFarlane CA, Jackson HJ, Patton GC, Rakkar A. Monitoring and care of young people at incipient risk of psychosis. *Focus (Am Psychiatr Publ)*. 2004;2(1):158–74.
58. McGlashan TH, Walsh BC, Woods SW. *The Psychosis-Risk Syndrome: Handbook for Diagnosis and Follow-Up*. Oxford, MS: Oxford University Press; 2010, p. 256.
59. Addington J. The prodromal stage of psychotic illness: Observation, detection or intervention? *J Psychiatry Neurosci*. 2003;28(2):93–7.
60. Fusar-Poli P, Borgwardt S, Bechdolf A, et al. The psychosis high-risk state: A comprehensive state-of-the-art review. *JAMA Psychiatry*. 2013;70(1):107–20.
61. Yung AR, Yuen HP, Mcgorry PD, et al. Mapping the onset of psychosis: The comprehensive assessment of at-risk mental states. *Aust N Z J Psychiatry*. 2005;39(11–12):964–71.
62. Orygen Youth Health: Our Story. http://oyh.org.au/about-us/our-story.
63. Yung AR, McGorry PD, McFarlane CA, Jackson HJ, Patton GC, Rakkar A. Monitoring and care of young people at incipient risk of psychosis. *Focus (Am Psychiatr Publ)*. 2004;2(1):158–74.
64. Cannon TD, Cadenhead K, Cornblatt B, et al. Prediction of psychosis in youth at high clinical risk: A multisite longitudinal study in North America. *Arch Gen Psychiatry*. 2008;65(1):28–37.
65. McGorry PD, Killackey E, Yung A. Early intervention in psychosis: Concepts, evidence and future directions. *World Psychiatry*. 2008;7(3):148–56.
66. Compton MT, Goulding SM, Ramsay CE, Addington J, Corcoran C, Walker EF. Early detection and intervention for psychosis: Perspectives from North America. *Clin Neuropsychiatry*. 2008;5(6):263.
67. Addington J, Cadenhead KS, Cannon TD, et al. North American Prodrome Longitudinal Study: A collaborative multisite approach to prodromal schizophrenia research. *Schizophr Bull*. 2007;33(3):665–72.
68. McFarlane WR. Prevention of the first episode of psychosis. *Psychiatr Clin North Am*. 2011;34(1):95–107.
69. McFarlane WR, Levin B, Travis L, et al. Clinical and functional outcomes after 2 years in the early detection and intervention for the prevention of psychosis multisite effectiveness trial. *Schizophr Bull*. 2014;41(1):30–43.
70. Yung AR, McGorry PD. The prodromal phase of first-episode psychosis: Past and current conceptualizations. *Schizophr Bull*. 1996;22(2):353–70.
71. Miller TJ, McGlashan TH, Rosen JL, et al. Prodromal assessment with the structured interview for prodromal syndromes and the scale of prodromal symptoms: Predictive validity, interrater reliability, and training to reliability. *Schizophr Bull*. 2003;29(4):703.
72. Yung AR, McGorry PD, Francey SM, et al. PACE: A specialised service for young people at risk of psychotic disorders. *Med J Aust*. 2007;187 (7 Suppl):S43–6.
73. McFarlane WR, Cook WL, Downing D, Verdi MB, Woodberry KA, Ruff A. Portland identification and early referral: A community-based system for identifying and treating youths at high risk of psychosis. *Psychiatr Serv*. 2010;61(5):512–5.
74. McGlashan TH, Addington J, Cannon T, et al. Recruitment and treatment practices for help-seeking "prodromal" patients. *Schizophr Bull*. 2007;33(3):715–26.
75. McGorry PD, Killackey E, Yung A. Early intervention in psychosis: Concepts, evidence and future directions. *World Psychiatry*. 2008;7(3):148–56.
76. McFarlane WR, Susser E, McCleary R, et al. Reduction in incidence of hospitalizations for psychotic episodes through early identification and intervention. *Psychiatr Serv*. 2014;65(10):1194–200.
77. Preti A, Cella M. Randomized-controlled trials in people at ultra high risk of psychosis: A review of treatment effectiveness. *Schizophr Res*. 2010;123(1):30–6.
78. Stafford MR, Jackson H, Mayo-Wilson E, Morrison AP, Kendall T. Early interventions to prevent psychosis: Systematic review and meta-analysis. *BMJ*. 2013;346:f185.
79. Morrison AP, French P, Walford L, et al Cognitive therapy for the prevention of psychosis in people at ultra-high risk. *Br J Psychiatry*. 2004;185(4):291–7.
80. Amminger GP, Schäfer MR, Papageorgiou K, et al. Long-chain ω-3 fatty acids for indicated prevention of psychotic disorders: A randomized, placebo-controlled trial. *Arch Gen Psychiatry*. 2010;67(2):146–54.
81. Testimony before the Committee on Health, Education, Labor, and Pensions United States Senate. https://www.nih.gov/sites/default/files/institutes/olpa/20151029-senate-testimony-insel.pdf.
82. Yang LH, Link BG, Ben-David S, et al. Stigma related to labels and symptoms in individuals at clinical high-risk for psychosis. *Schizophr Res*. 2015;168(1):9–15.
83. Yang LH, Wonpat-Borja AJ, Opler MG, Corcoran CM. Potential stigma associated with inclusion of the psychosis risk syndrome in the DSM-V: An empirical question. *Schizophr Res*. 2010;120(1):42–8.
84. Fusar-Poli P, Bonoldi I, Yung AR, et al. Predicting psychosis: Meta-analysis of transition outcomes in individuals at high clinical risk. *Arch Gen Psychiatry*. 2012;69(3):220–9.
85. Rüsch N, Corrigan PW, Heekeren K, et al. Well-being among persons at risk of psychosis: The role of self-labeling, shame, and stigma stress. *Psychiatr Serv*. 2014;65(4):483–9.
86. Rüsch N, Müller M, Heekeren K, et al. Longitudinal course of self-labeling, stigma stress and well-being among young people at risk of psychosis. *Schizophr Res*. 2014;158(1):82–4.
87. Rüsch N, Heekeren K, Theodoridou A, et al. Stigma as a stressor and transition to schizophrenia after one year among young people at risk of psychosis. *Schizophr Res*. 2015;166(1):43–8.

CHAPTER

163 Mood Disorders

Rachel S. Bergmans • Liming Dong • Natalie Bareis • Kara Zivin • Briana Mezuk

DESCRIPTIVE EPIDEMIOLOGY OF MOOD DISORDERS

Mood disorders (e.g., depressive disorders, bipolar spectrum disorders) are leading causes of morbidity and mortality worldwide.[1] The primary symptom feature of these group of psychiatric disorders are a disturbance in affect.[2] Symptoms often first manifest in adolescence, but onset can occur throughout lifespan into later adulthood; appropriate diagnosis, particularly for bipolar spectrum disorders, may not occur until early adulthood. Mood disturbance can range from mild to severe, on a spectrum of depression to mania, and may be accompanied by psychosis.

This chapter takes a public health approach to mood disorders. This approach is one that emphasizes the role that "upstream" factors play in increasing (and decreasing) risk of mood disorders in the population. This includes the need for strategies to target the underlying causes of mental disorders from a systems perspective, one that recognizes how relatively weak but common risk (and protective) factors work together to shift population health outcomes.[3] It is now appreciated that mood disorders, like most complex diseases, emerge from a pluripotent set of predictors; none of these factors, in and of themselves, is either necessary or sufficient to cause psychopathology. Recent decades have emphasized the population burden of mood disorders and the need to identify modifiable determinants of these conditions to and develop effective interventions.[4]

Depressive Disorders

Major Depressive Disorder. Major depressive disorder (MDD) is the most prevalent mood disorder globally, affecting approximately 4.7% of the world's population at any given time.[1] MDD is a syndrome characterized by core feelings of sadness or low mood, and disinterest or anhedonia, accompanied by sleep disturbances (either sleeping too much or too little); changes in appetite or weight (either increases or decreases); fatigue or low energy; problems concentrating; psychomotor agitation or retardation; feelings of worthlessness, hopelessness or guilt; and preoccupation with death or suicidal thoughts.[5,6] To have a MDD diagnosis, an individual must experience symptoms nearly every day for at least 2 weeks, and these symptoms must be associated with functional impairment. The 2012 revision of the Diagnostic and Statistical Manual of Mental Disorders (DSM-5), removed the so-called "bereavement exclusion" (i.e., a criterion stating if this syndrome developed immediately after death of a loved one, it would not qualify as MDD, but would instead be understood as a "normative" grief reaction); this change was the subject of intense scientific and philosophical debate.[7]

The projected lifetime risk MDD is 23.2%, with median age of onset at 32 years.[8] However, many cases develop earlier in the life course. During childhood, the point prevalence of depressive episode is only 1–3%; however, this increases to 5–7% by adolescence and remains about this level throughout adulthood.[9] There are significant sex differences in risk of MDD; women have significantly higher risk than men starting in adolescence. In a national survey, the cumulative incidence of MDD among females was 5.2% as compared to 2.0% in males at age 12; between the ages of 12 and 17, females had a cumulative incidence of 36.1% compared to 13.6% among males.[10] Even among adults, the risk of depression is twice as high for females than males.[11] Inflammatory processes,[12] gonadal steroids,[13] personality, and social roles[14] are among the biological and psychosocial factors suspected to play a role in sex differences of depression prevalence.

MDD can have an episodic or chronic course, although approximately 50% of cases appear to be a single episode.[15] Following an initial episode of MDD, rate of recurrence is 50% and likely to take place within 5 years. After a second episode, recurrence rate increases to 80%. Those with a history of MDD have, on average, between five and nine major depressive episodes in their lifetime, and recovery from a single episode can continue past 10 years.[16] Those with recurring depression tend to experience more severe symptoms and have a higher rate of comorbidity with other psychiatric disorders.[17] Recurrent MDD is strongly associated with familial and genetic influences.[18]

For some, an initial episode of MDD may not occur until later in life, known as late-onset depression.[19] These individuals are less likely to have a family history of depression or comorbid psychiatric conditions, and are more likely to have physical comorbidities.[20] Lifetime prevalence of MDD declines with age, and it is uncertain how much of this decline reflects cohort effects, measurement issues, or survival bias.[21,22] For example, a community sample of Dutch adults over 55 years old, only 2.0–3.5% of women and 0.5–1.2% of men had MDD.[23] However, late-life MDD is common among medical inpatients (10–12%), and those living in long-term care facilities (14–42%).[24]

Dysthymia. As with MDD, the cardinal symptom of dysthymia is sadness or low mood; what distinguishes dysthymia from MDD is severity and chronicity.[6] Whereas MDD requires at least five (out of nine) symptom groups to be endorsed, dysthymia requires only three. Additionally, dysthymia must be present for at least 2 years in adults (or 1 year in children), compared to 2 weeks for MDD. Although dysthymia may be considered a milder form of depression, the course of this illness can include periods of MDD and high healthcare utilization.[25] Lifetime risk for dysthymia is much lower than MDD, at only 3.4%, with a similar median age of onset at 31 years.[8] Dysthymia is often comorbid with MDD (called "double depression"), anxiety disorders, and substance abuse syndromes.[26] Similar to MDD, dysthymia is more common among women and those under 65 years of age.[25]

Subthreshold Depression. There is increasing attention among researchers and clinicians to the impact of subsyndromal/subthreshold depression.[27] Subthreshold depression is a syndrome that is either shorter duration, fewer symptoms, or less impairing then MDD, but is far more common.[28] Indeed, approximately 50% of adolescents and 20% of adults endorse depressive symptoms when assessed in epidemiological community surveys.[29] As with MDD and dysthymia, subthreshold MDD is more common among women relative to men.

Although subthreshold depression is less impairing than MDD, it is associated with risk of developing more severe forms of psychopathology. In a study of adolescents across 11 countries, 29.2% experienced subthreshold depression and had elevated risk of suicidality, despite not meeting criteria for MDD.[30] In a New Zealand birth cohort, subthreshold depression at 17–18 years was associated with great risk of MDD by age 25 as well as risk of suicidal behaviors.[31] In a review of studies within older adults,[32] subthreshold depression was two to three times more common than MDD, 8–10% went on to have a major depressive episode, and only 27% experienced remission of symptoms after 1 year. Older adults who experience subthreshold depression are at a heightened risk of suicidality[33] and face a greater risk of disability.[34]

Pre- and Postpartum Depression. Pre- (e.g., perinatal) and postpartum depression refers to depressive episodes that occur during pregnancy through the 12-month period following childbirth. Postpartum depression affects 9–21% of women in the general population.[35,36] Although it is not included as a separate category in the DSM, "postpartum onset" of depressive disorders refers to onset within 4 weeks of childbirth.[5] In addition, up to 50% of women experience postpartum dysphoric syndrome,[37] colloquially known as the "baby blues." However, these milder postpartum blues usually resolve without requiring intervention.[38] Postpartum depression is more common among mothers who experience stressful life events during pregnancy or shortly after birth, have low levels of social support, have a history of depression, or who experience anxiety or depression during pregnancy.[39] It is estimated that 10–12% of those with postpartum depression have prepartum onset.[40,41]

Research on prepartum depression is more limited than that on the postpartum period, but it is estimated to affect approximately 9–11% of women, and can have detrimental consequences for both the mother and her child. Prepartum depression is associated with an increased risk of spontaneous preterm birth,[42] and infant low birthweight[43] and behavioral problems in the child.[44] Prepartum depression can be masked by other symptoms of pregnancy, including loss of energy, weight gain, and trouble sleeping.[45] Prepartum depression is most common among mothers with low socioeconomic status, who have a lack of social support, and who experience domestic violence.[46]

Bipolar Disorders

Bipolar Disorder I and II. The hallmark of bipolar disorder is oscillation in mood, energy, and functional capacity. There are two primary classifications of bipolar disorder: bipolar I and bipolar II. To be diagnosed with bipolar I, patients must have experienced at least one manic episode.[6] Mania is characterized by elevated, expansive, or irritable mood, and increased energy. In addition, at least three of the following symptoms must co-occur: impulsivity, decreased need for sleep, racing thoughts or speech, inflated self-esteem, increased motivation, and distractibility. Manic episodes last at least 7 days and result in severe cognitive or functional impairment, often including psychosis (e.g., delusions or hallucinations) or hospitalization. Although individuals with bipolar I may also experience episodes of major depression, this is not a diagnostic criterion. In contrast, a bipolar II diagnosis requires periods of depression which cycle with periods of hypomania (e.g., milder, shorter periods of elevated mood that does not involve psychosis, severe functional impairment, or require hospitalization) rather than episodes of mania.[6] Finally, so-called "mixed states" (e.g., episodes that involve manic-like symptoms of hyperactivity and speech that occur in the context of low or depressive mood) occur in both bipolar I and II.

The prevalence of bipolar I is relatively consistent worldwide, ranging from 0.1% in Japan to 1.5% in Hungary.[47,48] Bipolar I is equally common in men and women, however, there are sex differences in clinical features. Women are more likely than men to experience rapid cycling (78% vs. 28%),[49] defined as at least four major affective episodes within a year. Women also tend to have greater depressive symptoms and mixed episodes.[50] Men have an earlier onset of mania and bipolar disorder than women.[51] Although some studies report that bipolar II is more common in women versus men, this finding is not consistent, and may be due to sex differences regarding who seeks clinical care.[52] Previous findings also suggest that psychiatric comorbidities are more common among women with bipolar II,[53] whereas substance abuse is more common among men with this condition.[54] There is some evidence to indicate that a substantial portion of individuals diagnosed with MDD may instead have unrecognized bipolar II disorder.[55]

Collectively, the lifetime risk for bipolar I or II is approximately 5.1%, with a median age of onset of 25 years.[8] Those diagnosed before 18 years of age tend to have higher psychiatric morbidity including more rapid cycling, suicidal ideation, and substance abuse disorders.[56] Unlike MDD, which tends to be more prevalent among those of lower socioeconomic status, bipolar disorder appears to be more common among those with greater educational attainment and higher social status.[57]

Other Bipolar Disorders. Cyclothymic disorder is also considered a bipolar disorder.[6] This is a chronic condition lasting at least 2 years in adults and 1 year in children. Cyclothymic disorder entails cycling between periods of subclinical depressive symptoms and mood elevation, and euthymic periods lasting no longer than 2 months. The DSM 5 also recognizes other specified bipolar and related disorder and unspecified bipolar and related disorder,[5] which apply to those with manic or hypomanic and depressive symptoms that do not meet the diagnostic criteria for any other depressive or bipolar disorder.[6]

Relationship between Mood and Anxiety Disorders

Anxiety disorders are a broad class of conditions characterized primarily by feelings of fear, worry, anxiety, panic attacks, as well as coping behaviors intended to help individuals manage or avoid these feelings.[6] Anxiety tends to have an earlier age of onset relative to mood disorders, with some symptoms occurring in childhood and some disorders (e.g., separation anxiety disorder) defined by early onset.[58] Both MDD and bipolar disorders have high comorbidity with anxiety. Among adolescents with depressive disorders, anxiety is considered the most prevalent comorbid psychiatric condition with estimates ranging widely from 15% to 75%.[59] In a study of 87 adult patients,[60] comorbid anxiety was present within 92% of MDD cases, 79% of bipolar patients, and 88% of those with dysthymia. Those with comorbid anxiety and depressive disorder are more likely to have an earlier age of onset than those with depressive disorder alone, as well as greater dysfunction and suicidality.[61]

Suicide

Suicide is currently the tenth leading cause of death in the United States.[62] In 2015, the World Health Organization estimated that there were 788,000 suicide deaths worldwide.[63] An additional 10–20 times more people attempt suicide each year and survive than those who die by suicide.[64] Suicidal behavior is strongly associated with history of psychiatric and substance use disorders—including MDD and bipolar disorders; physical health problems; social isolation; major life disruptions; and functional impairment and decline.[65] Previously attempting suicide is among the strongest predictor of committing suicide, especially within the following year.[66] Although suicidal behavior is heightened by ongoing health and social problems, it is estimated that 20–30% of suicide attempts are impulsive acts; in a sample of 153 persons aged 13–35 years that had attempted suicide and survived,[67] 24% reported attempting suicide within 5 minutes of their decision to do so; and 70% attempted suicide within an hour of their decision.

Paralleling gender differences in MDD, women are more likely to report suicidal ideation and to attempt suicide. However, men are substantially more likely to complete suicide; rates of suicide in males exceeds that of females everywhere in the world except China and Bangladesh.[63] Gender differences in suicide completion are attributable, in part, to differential use of lethal means of self-harm.[68] In Western countries, men are far more likely to die by suicide using firearms or suffocation (mostly hanging), whereas women are more likely to attempt by poisoning (e.g., intentional medication overdose), which has a greater chance of rescue or resuscitation. In contrast, in many Asian countries, women use more lethal methods of suicide, including jumping, drowning, hanging, and self-immolation[69]; in these countries, suicide rates among women are higher and closer to that of men. Other factors, such as cultural norms and religious preferences, also contribute to geographic differences in the rate of suicide (both within countries and across nations).[64]

CONCEPTUAL FRAMEWORKS FOR UNDERSTANDING THE CAUSES OF MOOD DISORDERS OVER THE LIFESPAN

The Stress-Diathesis Model

Stressors, defined generally as any threat to homeostasis (whether biological or psychological), play an essential role in the development of all forms of psychopathology, but particularly MDD.[70] Twin studies and natural experiments have shown both that negative life events (e.g., getting divorced, losing a job) are causally associated with risk of developing MDD in the following year among adults,[71] and that alleviating chronic stressors (e.g., moving out of poverty) are causally associated with lower risk of behavioral problems in children.[72] However, there are several elements that complicate the stress-psychopathology relationship: (1) stressors may be qualitatively different (e.g., some stressors are "positive" events such as getting married, birth of a child, getting a promotion, whereas others negative, such as experiencing death of a loved one); (2) that the timing of events may influence their impact on mental health (e.g., unexpected pregnancy in adolescence versus a planned pregnancy in a stable relationship); (3) stressful events may foster effective coping strategies that protect against developing psychopathology later (e.g., resilience)[73]; and (4) even when exposed to the same extreme stressor (e.g., physical and emotional neglect in childhood; being in a natural disaster), not all individuals develop MDD. To explain this individual variability in the relationship between stress and psychopathology, psychologists have developed the *Stress-Diathesis Model*. This model incorporates individual variability in diathesis (e.g., genetic liability, personality traits) to explain why individuals exposed to the same stressor differ in their probability of developing psychopathology. Although there are several variations on this conceptual model, and emerging research on the ways stressors influence epigenetic changes (both within a single lifetime and across generations) calls into question the degree to which "stress" and "diathesis" are distinct constructs, the essential concept is that individuals vary in the threshold above which stressors cause psychopathology.

For example, Caspi et al. (2003) showed that the relationship between stressful life events and MDD was moderated by a functional polymorphism in the promoter region of the serotonin transporter gene (5-HTTLPR).[74] There are two common polymorphisms of 5-HTTLPR: long and short, having 16- and 14-repeat units, respectively.[75] Compared to the long allele, the short allele is associated with lower 5-HTT protein levels, less serotonin re-uptake, and diminished 5-HTT transcription.[76] Individuals with more short alleles of the 5-HTTLPR genotype were more likely to MDD at the same level of stressors as those with the long allele. However, in the absence of stress, 5-HTTLPR was not associated with risk of MDD. More recent evidence from brain imaging studies show that compared to long-allele carriers of the 5-HTTLPR genotype, individuals with short alleles have less gray matter, which is critical for negative emotion regulation.[77] Thus, the diathesis may be expressed as changed in brain anatomy that influences cognitive processing, and imparts higher risk for MDD in the face of stressful events.

Expanding on the Stress-diathesis Model: Differential Sensitivity Hypothesis

Mitchell et al. (2013) theorize that genetic factors moderate the influence of environmental stressors on brain development and the onset of mood disorders through differential sensitivity to social environments. Specifically, genetic traits can make individuals more sensitive to *both* unfavorable and favorable environmental influences.[78,79] This implies that some individuals have more flexibility to adapt to their environments, and that through these environments genetic traits translate into advantages or disadvantages. This differs from the Stress-Diathesis Model, where individuals with "risky" genotypes are more susceptible to poor psychiatric outcomes subsequent to negative exposures, but respond similarly to those with "protective" genotypes to protective or positive exposures.[78] For example, the short allele of the 5-HTTLPR has been associated with hyperreactivity of the hypothalamus-pituitary-adrenal axis in response to environmental stressors.[80] In a cohort of Taiwanese older adults, those with at least one short allele were more likely to experience depressive symptoms following a traumatic event compared to those homozygous for the long allele.[75] However, according to the differential sensitivity hypothesis, a "risky" allele may also enhance the protective influences provided by positive environments and exposures; for example, one study showed that among adults exposed to a supportive environment early in life, those homozygous for short 5-HTTLPR alleles had less depressive symptomatology compared to those with at least one long allele.[81] That is, harmful exposures (e.g., negative life events) had a more detrimental effect, but protective exposures (e.g., parental support) had a more positive effect, on later development of MDD as a function of genotype.

The Developmental Framework

As illustrated by the Stress-Diathesis Model, a developmental framework is a useful lens for understanding the etiology of mood disorders. That is, that the risk of MDD or bipolar disorders is not simply an additive relationship of risk factors minus protective ones; instead, these risk and protective factors should be understood as proxy indicators of underlying processes that locate individuals on trajectories of higher or lower risk of developing of mood disorders that manifest over time. By emphasizing risk (and protective) trajectories, rather than discrete factors, the developmental framework highlights the interconnectedness of predictors not as a statistical nuisance (i.e., multicollinearity) but as theoretically relevant indicators of underlying etiologic processes. Moreover, the developmental framework demands explicit consideration of three elements that are often de-emphasized in traditional risk factor epidemiology: (1) the timing of events, including "sensitive" periods during which events have more potent influence on developmental trajectories; (2) the accumulation of risk (or resilience) over time; (3) consideration of multiple pathways to the same outcome as a function of contextual factors (i.e., multifinality); and (4) that the relationship between stress and diathesis can change over the development. For example, the kindling hypothesis of MDD posits that individuals become sensitized to depression after the first onset, and subsequently become more prone to depression with lower level of stress.[82]

Sensitive Periods and Cumulative Exposure

Although incidence of mood disorders peaks in early adulthood, the trajectories that place individuals at higher risk of these disorders have their origins much earlier in the life course. Infancy through childhood represents a significant period in brain development when exposure to stressors can have lifelong consequences for mental health. During the first 3 years of life, the brain reaches 80% of its adult weight through the production of neurons, synaptogenesis, synaptic pruning, and axonal and dendritic growth.[83] Exposure to stressors during windows of activity in brain development can induce neurobiological changes and increase the risk of mood disorders that begin to emerge during adolescence.[84] For example, child sexual abuse is one of the strongest predictors of adult MDD,[85] however studies in young adults and animal models demonstrate its influence on brain morphology varies by age of abuse.[86–89] Psychiatric symptoms can also vary due to timing of abuse. Those exposed at ages 3–6 were more likely to experience depressive symptoms, whereas those exposed at ages 9–10 were more likely to experience symptoms of posttraumatic stress disorder.[89] Moreover, studies of identical twins discordant for history of abuse show persistent epigenetic changes that have implications for health in general, not just risk of mood disorders.[90]

Beyond sensitive periods of development, exposure to multiple stressors or traumatic life experiences, regardless of age group, heightens risk of developing mood disorders in a dose-response manner.[91–94] This relationship may reflect the intersection of biological, psychological, and social factors. Negative experiences illicit a stress-response in the body which may have lasting effects on neurobiology. These processes may be mediated by neuroendocrine systems including the hypothalamic-pituitary-adrenal (HPA)-axis, the immune system, and related physiologic systems.[95] Stressors also tax psychological coping resources (e.g., self-efficacy) and influence health behaviors (e.g., sleep, tobacco and alcohol use) that in turn influence risk of mood disorders.[96] Finally, there are qualitative differences in the types of stressors that more strongly predict mood disorders; stressors that involve entrapment (e.g., domestic violence, poverty) or feelings of shame, guilt, or rejection (e.g., romantic breakup, being fired from a job) are more likely to predict MDD than stressors that involve danger (e.g., being in a natural disaster).[97] These former stressors are also intrinsically social experiences—that is, they involve interacting with other people. In this way, MDD can be conceptualized as the biological expression of a social disruption.

RISK FACTORS

Consequentialist epidemiology[98] calls for a renewed focus on the responsibility of epidemiological researchers to go beyond identifying risk factors or describing population distributions to propose specific interventions to prevent and/or control disease. Identifying novel prevention and intervention strategies is of particular importance for mood disorders since MDD is projected to be the leading cause of morbidity and mortality worldwide by 2030 (it is already among the top 15 causes).[99] In the spirit of consequentialist epidemiology, this section discusses three broad classes of risk factors for mood disorders—nutrition, neighborhood context, and occupational strain—that are both clinically significant and are potentially modifiable by programs, policies, and interventions at the individual, community, and/or population level.

Nutrition and Dietary Behaviors

Diet and nutrition have a significant influence on development and management of chronic diseases such as cardiovascular disease,[100] type 2 diabetes,[101] and certain types of cancer.[102] In response, nutritional protocols and dietary recommendations are implicit within preventative strategies and treatment protocols for these illnesses.[103] However, dietary and nutritional interventions are not included in standard care guidelines for mood disorders,[104] and are instead categorized as complementary or alternative medicine.[105] Indeed, nutrition and diet have a complex but important relationship with mood disorders. However, to date, research and clinical care has focused on the high comorbidity between mood disorders and eating disorders, including anorexia nervosa,[106,107] bulimia nervosa,[108] and binge eating disorder.[109] Only relatively recently has there been concerted effort by public health researchers to examine the biological mechanisms linking nutrition and mental health more broadly.[110] With a shift toward understanding the underlying neurobiology of mood disorders,[111] an emerging body of literature has drawn attention to the pathogenic role of nutrition and dietary behaviors.

Specific Nutrient Deficiencies

Evidence that nutrient deficiencies may be associated with mood disorders goes back as far as 1905, when a physician at a psychiatric-care facility observed that anemia (i.e., iron deficiency) was often proceeded by symptoms of mood disorders, possibly indicating a common cause.[112] Over 100 years later, contemporary research has identified specific micronutrients that may be of critical importance to mood, including folate, vitamin B12, and polyunsaturated fatty acids.

Folate (i.e., vitamin B9) is water-soluble with high concentrations found in beets, avocado, and legumes like pinto beans.[113] In the late 1960s, researchers observed that those with psychiatric disorders may be more likely to have low levels of serum folate concentrations.[114] Whether folate deficiency simply reflects poor diet among individuals with mood disorders, or represents an etiologic mechanism linking nutrition and mood disorders, is not yet established. In the body, folate is metabolized to S-adenosylmethionine, which may be important for the synthesis of neurotransmitters including dopamine, norepinephrine, and serotonin.[115] Folate is important for metabolizing homocysteine, high concentrations of which can lead to neuronal injury and cell death.[116] Hyperhomocysteinemia has been associated with symptom severity among those with MDD[117] and bipolar disorder.[118,119] In response, researchers have tested whether increased consumption of folate may benefit those suffering from mood disorders via dietary changes or consumption of supplements and fortified foods containing folic acid, folinic acid, and 5-methyltetrahydrofolate , which are commercially available forms of folate.[120] In a 10-week randomized and placebo-controlled trial, folic acid supplementation enhanced the antidepressant effects of fluoxetine, a selective serotonin reuptake inhibitor commonly used to treat MDD, supporting the hypothesized role of folate metabolism in treating depressed mood.[121] However, the efficacy may vary by the type of folate supplementation used and whether a patient carries the C677T polymorphism, which influences metabolism of this nutrient. In addition, excessive intake of folic acid has been associated with health risks including increasing the incidence of certain types of cancer, masking B12 deficiency and possibly increasing depressive symptoms. These limitations emphasize the need for further evidence regarding who folate supplementation is suitable for among patients with mood disorders as well as appropriate dosage.[120]

Similar to folate, B12 is an essential vitamin that is also critical for preventing homocysteine toxicity.[122] Likewise, lower levels of B12 are associated with depression.[123] Almeida et al. conducted a systematic review and meta-analysis of randomized placebo-controlled trials of folate and vitamin B12 for MDD[124]; they concluded evidence does not support use of folate or B12 supplementation to decrease depression severity in the short term. However, folate and B12 may be effective for managing depressive symptoms and preventing relapse over longer periods of time.

An emerging area of research in nutrition and mood disorders revolves around polyunsaturated acids (PUFAs), including n-3 and n-6. Evidence suggests that PUFAs, especially n-3 PUFA, play a key role in mood and depressive symptoms.[125–127] While the mechanisms are not clear, PUFA have an established influence on gut microbiota composition and systemic inflammation.[128,129] Gut dysbiosis, the underrepresentation of microbial species typically dominant in the gastrointestinal tract of healthy adults, is one of the modifiable factors that likely contributes to systemic inflammation in those with mood disorders,[130] and it is hypothesized to offer an opportunity for intervention.[131] In vitro studies demonstrate the ability of PUFAs to modulate bacterial species adherence to a mucosal surface[132] and alter the expression of proteins involved in maintaining tight junctions and intestinal integrity[129]—two mechanisms linked to inflammatory pathways.[133] Scientific evidence supporting the use of essential fatty acids as a treatment for mood disorders is inconclusive; however, this has largely focused on supplementation of n-3 PUFA, primarily eicosapentaenoic and docosahexaenoic enriched in fish oils.[125,126] Further evidence suggests that the balance of n-6 to n-3 may influence the pathogenesis of mood disorders, independent of total PUFA intake. Berger et al.[134] conducted a longitudinal study to determine whether the ratio of n-6 to n-3 may influence the onset of mood disorders. Those with a higher n-6/3 PUFA ratio at baseline had a higher incidence of any mood disorder diagnosis at follow-up (median of 7 years). It is hypothesized that a lower n-6/3 PUFA ratio maintains ideal physiological membrane properties important for serotonin neurotransmission and decreased neurogenesis.

Unhealthy Dietary Patterns

A limitation of examining the effect of specific nutrients on health outcomes, including mood disorders, is that this approach does not account for the fact that foods have properties beyond specific nutritional content.[135] As an alternative, researchers have investigated the role of dietary patterns, which refers to the aggregate composition of foods and nutrients. Common dietary patterns are defined by geographic regions and include the Western diet (often characterized as high in saturated fat, red meat, and refined grains), and the Mediterranean diet (often characterized as high in olive oil, whole grains, vegetables, and fish). A number of studies have demonstrated a link between dietary patterns and the prevalence of mood disorders.[136,137] For example, a longitudinal cohort of Spanish university students showed that greater adherence to a Mediterranean diet was associated with lower incidence of MDD (median follow-up: 4.4 years).[138]

Although studies that assess the relationship between geographically defined dietary patterns and mood disorders are informative in terms of eating behaviors that may be beneficial, insight into underlying mechanisms is lacking. One hypothesis is that dietary consumption can stimulate inflammatory pathways associated with the neurobiology of mood disorders.[139] Shivappa et al. developed a novel strategy to quantify the total inflammatory potential of diet via the Dietary Inflammatory Index (DII).[140,141] Based on a literature review that assessed the overall influence of individual food parameters on circulating levels of proinflammatory cytokines [i.e., C-reactive protein, interleukin (IL) 1β, IL-4, IL-6, IL-10, and tumor necrosis factor α], the DII estimates the degree to which an individual's diet induces or suppresses proinflammatory pathways from dietary intake data (e.g., food frequency questionnaires). The DII has been validated in a multiple study populations using circulating levels of C-reactive protein and IL-6,[142–145] and is associated with a number of chronic conditions where systemic inflammation may play an etiologic role, including MDD.[146–148] The relationship between dietary inflammatory potential and MDD has also been demonstrated using reduced-rank regression to identify a dietary pattern associated with inflammatory markers within a longitudinal cohort of female nurses.[149] However, most of this information stems from observational studies; large, randomized clinical trials of dietary change and prevention or management of mood disorders have not yet been conducted.

Neighborhood Environment

Researchers have studied the association between the contextual ("neighborhood") environment and mental health for decades. As early as 1939, Farris and Dunham investigated the relationship between urbanicity and bipolar disorder.[150] More recently there has been an interest in the potential of neighborhood characteristics to serve as an important source of social and physical resources that influence mental health.[151] Physical neighborhood features include quality of the built environment, such as broken windows or trash; access to resources like public transportation or green space; and other characteristics, including housing vacancy, traffic, noise, and walkability. Social neighborhood features include crime, violence, collective efficacy, social capital, population density, ethnic and racial diversity, and family structure.

Most research on neighborhood environments and mood disorders focuses on depression and depressive symptoms.[152–154] For example, Ross (2000) assessed the influence of census-tract poverty and family structure on depressive symptoms among Chicago adults; even after accounting for individual-level socioeconomic status (i.e., education level, household income, and employment), those living in census tracts with a higher proportion of poverty and single female-headed households had more depressive symptomology. Within a longitudinal sample of primarily current or former drug users, Latkin and Curry (2003) found that perceived neighborhood features were predictive of depressive symptoms prospectively, even after account for individual-level risk factors. Galea et al. (2005) investigation of the relationship between objective measures of neighborhood characteristics and MDD within 59 community districts of New York City. Those living in community districts with poorer built environment features were more likely to have MDD in the previous 6 months and to report ever having MDD in their lifetime. Although it has been the subject of far fewer investigations, there is little evidence that neighborhood features are related to mania or bipolar disorders,[150,155–157] consistent with Faris and Dunham's 1939 observation.

To date, a small number of neighborhood-level interventions to improve mental health have been tested. The Moving to Opportunity (MTO) study[158] was the first to provide experimental evidence that neighborhood residence may have a causal impact on mental health. MTO was a randomized controlled trial where 550 urban families were randomized to either remained in their current residence, receive a Section 8 housing voucher, or receive a voucher to move to a low-poverty neighborhood. Adults that moved to low-poverty neighborhoods reported fewer depressive symptoms than those that remained in place; adults that moved into Section 8 housing did not experience any mental health benefit. Another study[159] evaluated postrelocation depressive symptomology among a sample of primarily African American female-headed households ($n = 127$). Following relocation from socioeconomically disadvantaged areas and poorly maintained public housing to less distressed areas, 60% of respondents reported fewer depressive symptoms.

There are several explanatory models of the apparent relationship linking the neighborhood environment with mood disorders. Stressors, particularly those related to social features of neighborhoods, are hypothesized to be a key mediator.[160–162] For example, using longitudinal panel data, Dustmann and Fasani showed that exposure to violent crime is associated with greater levels of depressive symptomology, especially when individuals are exposed frequently (e.g., during daily routines such as traveling to work).[163] Other explanatory models emphasize neighborhoods not as sources of stress, but as sources of positive resources to cope with stress.[164] For example, there is some evidence that living in an ethnic enclave (e.g., a neighborhood with a high density of people of one's same background) is associated with lower risk of MDD among immigrants; perhaps reflecting social cohesion and capital.[165,166] Most recently, Erdem et al. suggest that ethnic-diversity may have ethnic-specific effects, beneficial for some groups and not others.[167] Finally, other environmental exposures that tend to cluster with lower socioeconomic areas, known as concentrated disadvantage,[154] may contribute to the relationship between neighborhoods and mood disorders, such as air pollution and ambient noise.[168,169]

When reviewing existing evidence regarding the relationship between neighborhood environments and mood disorders, Diez et al. (2010) report that perceptions of neighborhood disorganization, quality of neighborhood built environment, walkability, exposure to violence, and social capital tend to be associated with depression and depressive symptoms. In contrast, studies evaluating the effect of residential instability and racial/ethnic composition are less conclusive. Overall there appears to be a modest relationship between neighborhood effects and MDD when accounting for individual- and household-level factors.[151,170–173] This literature is limited in several ways: (1) variation in the measurement of neighborhood features limits comparisons across studies; (2) self-selection (e.g., downward drift of individuals predisposed to mood disorders into disadvantaged neighborhoods) is a major concern, particularly of cross-sectional studies; and (3) certain studies define neighborhood characteristics, such as socioeconomic status, using aggregate data from residents, which must also be accounted for at the individual level within statistical models. This raises methodological concerns since it is not well established whether these effects can be empirically separated in a meaningful way.[174] Despite these limitations, policies and programs that influence neighborhood factors associated with poor mental health provide a unique opportunity to test hypothesized interventions of how contextual factors influence mood disorders, and health more generally.

Occupational Characteristics and Job Strain

The work environment is where most people spend a significant amount of their waking time during the adulthood. As a result, occupational characteristics can have a profound influence on trajectories of risk of mood disorders. The relationship between work and psychiatric disorders is multifactorial: although unemployed adults have higher prevalence of mood disorders relative to their employed counterparts,[175] among workers the prevalence of mood disorders varies as a function of occupation,[176] and mood disorders are among the leading cause of lost productivity and disability leave across occupations.[177] On the other hand, work is an effective means to promote mental health (e.g., job training programs are effective and reducing psychiatric hospitalizations for persons with serious mental illness)[178] and workplaces increasingly offer programs to promote mental health or facilitate access to psychiatric care among workers (e.g., Employee Assistance Programs). Finally, one of the most well-studied risk factors for risk of mood disorders is job strain.[179]

Conceptual Frameworks for How Work Influences Mental Health

Job strain is a construct that embodies the discrepancy between job demands and a worker's capacity to meet those demands. Factors contributing to job strain include, but not limited to, excessive workload, low levels of autonomy, and lack of workplace support. In the late 1970s, Karasek (1979) proposed the *Demand-Control Model*, which focused on the intersection of job demands (e.g., workload and pace of work) and job control (e.g., decision authority and skill discretion) as two essential elements in the work environment that increase risk of psychopathology.[180] Jobs with high demands and low control (e.g., waitresses, telephone operators) are classified as high strain jobs, and associated with higher risk of MDD.[181] Elaborations to the *Demand-Control Model* have incorporated elements of workplace social support,[182] which extends the concept of job strain to incorporate the effect of isolated versus collective work environment. Another influential job stress model is *Effort-Reward Imbalance*,[183] which centers on whether psychological needs are supported (or impaired) by work, such as a sense of security, self-esteem, and social belonging, though the balance of workers' efforts spent to meet the job demands and received rewards (e.g., financial gains, appreciation, and career opportunities). Finally, the *Demand-Resource Model* incorporates a broader range of working conditions and classifies workplace factors into two general categories: job demands and job resources.[184] Job demands refer to any job characteristics associated with physiological and psychological costs, and job resources refer to any factors that help with achieving work goals, reducing the physiological and psychological costs and stimulating personal development, including autonomy, social support, and rewards.[184] It proposes dual psychological processes, the health impairment process which leads to exhaustion and illness through high job demands, and the motivation process which leads to disengagement through low job resources.[185] The interaction between job demands and resources determines the occurrence of job strain as well as burnout, a state characterized by exhaustion, cynicism, and inefficacy in work.[186]

Occupational Exposures and Mood Disorders

For decades, these conceptual models have been used to study the impacts of job characteristics on mental health, particularly risk of MDD. Numerous population-based studies show that high job strain (in the demand-control formulation) is associated with MDD, and have shown that specific occupational features including skill discretion, decision authority, psychological demand, job insecurity, physical exertion, and social support[181] are independent risk factor for onset of MDD.[187–190] Adverse impacts of job stressors may persist postretirement[191]; however, on average, depression risk is lower during retirement transition.[192]

The underlying mechanisms linking job strain and MDD remain unclear.[190] Burnout, a process that begins with exhaustion due to excessive demands and mental strain associated it, then withdrawal behaviors when resources available to meet the demands are insufficient, and finally disengagement from work, has been identified as a mediator the relationship between occupational stress and MDD.[185,193–197] Linking to the Stress-Diathesis Model described above, there is suggestive evidence that individuals with more susceptibility (e.g., neurotic or Type A personality characteristics) to workplace adversity are more like to develop burnout and experience MDD.[198]

Managing job stress in the workplace is of significance for promoting public mental health, given its chronic and substantial adverse effects. Providing workplace support in terms of positive psychological feedback, collaboration and resources may buffer the perceived job stress,[199] improve engagement in work activities, reduce job-related burnout and therefore prevent onset of MDD for working-age individuals. Beyond job stress, other occupational characteristics such as physical environment and chemical exposures also contribute to the development of mood disorders.[200] For instance, occupational lead exposure has been shown to overstimulate protein kinase C activity in the prefrontal cortex, impair behavior regulations, and may increase risk of bipolar disorders for individuals with genetic vulnerability.[201]

TREATMENT FOR MOOD DISORDERS

History

Although there are numerous effective nonpharmacological treatments for mood disorders (e.g., various forms of psychotherapy, exercise), by far the most common treatment of mood disorders in the United States involves psychotropic medications.[202,203] However, until the early twentieth century, treatment for mood disorders did not involve medications. Many individuals were institutionalized in state psychiatric hospitals that often did little to promote their health and well-being. For example, hydrotherapy (i.e., immersion in warm or cool baths for extended periods of time) was used to calm psychiatric patients.[204] Electroconvulsive Therapy (ECT)—a procedure that is still used today particularly for cases of mood disorders that do not respond to pharmacotherapy—was one of the first effective treatments used for many forms of psychiatric disorders that allowed individuals to be discharged from hospital and live in the general community.[205,206] Memory loss is a side effect of ECT, particularly for repeated treatments.[206,207]

Lithium, a naturally occurring salt, was the first medication identified to help individuals with psychiatric illness, and then specifically mood disorders. As early as 1847, a hint of the psychotherapeutic properties of lithium were identified by Alfred Baring Garrod. An internist in London, Garrod identified the healing properties of lithium for gout, including "brain gout."[208] It was then characterized as having anticonvulsant and hypnotic properties, and was used to treat general "nervousness." In 1871 William Hammond became the first physician to recommend lithium specifically for mania.[209] Today, lithium is still the most effective mood stabilizer for bipolar disorder. However, the narrow therapeutic index between clinically effective levels and overdose necessitates careful monitoring by psychiatrists and their patients.[210,211] In addition, lithium can lead to kidney damage and cannot be taken by individuals with decreased kidney function.[212]

Moving from Crisis-Management to a Chronic-care Model

Effective medications and psychotherapy have transformed management of mood disorders from one of crisis-management (e.g., emergency treatment or hospitalization after a suicide attempt) to a chronic disease model. For example, in the U.S. primary-care providers, not mental health specialists, prescribe over 60% of antidepressants.[213] However, this shift requires new models of person-centered care. For example, long-term use of atypical antipsychotic medications, which is common among individuals with bipolar disorder[214] and treatment-resistant MDD,[215] is associated with metabolic syndrome and development of type 2 diabetes.[216,217] Similarly, long-term use of mood stabilizers is associated with risk of cardiovascular and cerebrovascular disease.[218] These risks require continual dialogue between patients and providers as to how best reduce psychiatric symptoms while managing adverse effects of medications, which together support the common goal of promoting overall functioning. This requires novel conceptualizations of person-centered care to individualize treatment plans. Kraemer et al., 2011, indicates specific strategies to evaluate patients' responses to different choices of treatments based on their clinical significance rather than on objective measures alone. Integrating not only the clinicians' perspectives of their patients' response to treatment but the net benefit identified by the patients themselves is a way to bridge this gap toward effective person-centered care.[219] Morselli et al. (2003) identified that individuals' perspective of their treatment of depression, improved functioning and management of adverse events were most important to their perceived benefit from treatment.[220]

Pharmacologic Treatments for MDD

The earliest medications effective at treating MDD target three neurotransmitters (called amines): serotonin, dopamine, and norepinephrine. The first medication marketed as an antidepressant in the United States was the monoamine oxidase inhibitor (MAOI) iproniazid in the 1950s.[18] MAOIs targeted all three neurotransmitters simultaneously, as well as many other systems[221] by inhibiting MAO, which led to severe side with core physiologic functions.[222] To avoid the side-effects of MAOIs, later antidepressants became more targeted to specific neurotransmitters. First, the tricyclic and tetracyclic antidepressants targeted only norepinephrine and/or serotonin; later, selective serotonin reuptake inhibitors (SSRIs) targeted serotonin only. These have become the first-line treatment for individuals with MDD.[221] STAR*D was a large clinical trial conducted to establish treatment guidelines for MDD; it found that approximately 37% of individuals respond to first-line medication treatment, but that the likelihood of responding after a second trial is substantially lower, and that there is little benefit to switching medications within a class (e.g., to another SSRI) versus across classes (e.g., from a SSRI to a TCA).[223,224] Finally, as discussed above, anxiety disorders commonly co-occur with mood disorders. If antidepressants are not fully effective in treating anxiety, anxiolytics are often added as an adjuvant treatment to manage these symptoms.[225]

Pharmacologic Treatments for Bipolar Disorder

Although lithium remains a standard treatment for bipolar disorders, newer classes of mood stabilizers, including antiepileptic mediations, are effective at managing manic symptoms in individuals with bipolar disorder.[226,227] These mood stabilizers, particularly antiepileptics, are often effective in decreasing the severity of depressive episodes as well.[228] Atypical antipsychotic medications are often added to treatment regimens for bipolar disorder to manage treatment resistant depression and acute mania.[227,229] Psychiatric polypharmacy (e.g., taking four or more psychotropic mediations) is common among persons with bipolar disorder (i.e., on average, three different psychiatric medications in their daily regimens),[230] and it is not uncommon for individuals with bipolar disorder to take five or more psychiatric medications concurrently.[231]

Antidepressants and Suicidality

In 2004, based on reports from 24 clinical trials of antidepressants in children and adolescents that showed a greater prevalence of suicidal ideation among those receiving SSRIs in the active treatment arm relative to the placebo,[232] the U.S. Food and Drug Administration (FDA) mandated a "black box" warning indicating this effect for children; this was updated in 2007 to include young adults aged 18–24 years. There were no completed suicides in any of these medication trials; however, because suicide is a rare event, the proxy indicator of suicidal ideation was used as justification for the warning. At the time, providers expressed concerns that the warning would have an unintended deleterious effect, where young individuals who needed treatment with antidepressants were less likely receive a prescription. Although psychotherapy is an effective alternative treatment, access to psychotherapy is far more limited than pharmacotherapy[233,234] and is less well-covered by insurance plans, and thus there was concern that the net result of the warning would be to reduce access to effective psychiatric treatment. Indeed, a Swedish study showed that in the 5 years following the black box warning, completed suicides increased by 60% among children, adolescents, and young adults who were not prescribed antidepressants.[235] Debate is ongoing regarding the utility of this black box warning.[236]

CONCLUSION

The goal of this chapter was to address the question: What is the role of public health in mood disorders? This question was answered by highlighting major conceptual models of the etiology of mood disorders (i.e., stress-diathesis) and the importance of a life course framework for understanding the development of these conditions. The chapter also discussed three emerging—and modifiable—risk factors for mood disorders: diet, neighborhood context, and occupational characteristics. Finally, the most common therapies for mood disorders were discussed, including the ongoing controversy surrounding the safety of antidepressants for adolescents. This chapter is not exhaustive in its discussion of any of these components. For example, several forms of psychotherapy have been shown to be effective at treating mood disorders[237,238]; however, these treatments are less available, and less affordable, than pharmacologic ones in the United States[239] and thus were not discussed at length.

This chapter highlights the potential for a public health approach to address the burden of mood disorders. This does not preclude, nor should it de-emphasize, the need to develop more effective clinical treatments for mood disorders. Similarly, while not a focus of this discussion, government stakeholders and advocates should consider how the concepts discussed here intersect with mental health policy recommendations. Finally, beyond understanding etiology and developing effective treatments, fully reducing the public health burden of mood disorders will require tackling issues of social stigma and treatment accessibility.

References

1. Whiteford HA, Degenhardt L, Rehm J, et al. Global burden of disease attributable to mental and substance use disorders: Findings from the Global Burden of Disease Study 2010. *Lancet*. 2013;382(9904):1575–86.
2. World Health Organization. *The ICD-10 Classification of Mental and Behavioural Disorders: Clinical Descriptions and Diagnostic Guidelines*. Geneva: World Health Organization; 2017.
3. Rose G. Sick individuals and sick populations. *Int J Epidemiol*. 2001;30(3):427–32; discussion 433–4.
4. Lindert J, Bilsen J, Jakubauskiene M. Public mental health. *Eur J Public Health*. 2017;27(suppl_4):32–5.
5. American Psychiatric Association. *Diagnostic and Statistical Manual of Mental Disorders DSM-5*. 5th ed. Washington, DC: American Psychiatric Publishing; 2013.
6. Roberts LW, Louie AK. *Study Guide to DSM-5®*. Arlington, VA: American Psychiatric Pub; 2014.
7. Zachar P, First MB, Kendler KS. The bereavement exclusion debate in the DSM-5: A history. *Clin Psychol Sci*. 2017;5(5):890–906.
8. Kessler RC, Berglund P, Demler O, Jin R, Merikangas KR, Walters EE. Lifetime prevalence and age-of-onset distributions of DSM-IV disorders in the National Comorbidity Survey replication. *Arch Gen Psychiatry*. 2005;62(6):593–602.
9. Wilson S, Hicks BM, Foster KT, McGue M, Iacono WG. Age of onset and course of major depressive disorder: Associations with psychosocial functioning outcomes in adulthood. *Psychol Med*. 2015;45(3):505–14.
10. Breslau J, Gilman SE, Stein BD, Ruder T, Gmelin T, Miller E. Sex differences in recent first-onset depression in an epidemiological sample of adolescents. *Transl Psychiatry*. 2017;7(5):e1139.
11. Kessler RC, McGonagle KA, Swartz M, Blazer DG, Nelson CB. Sex and depression in the National Comorbidity Survey. I: Lifetime prevalence, chronicity and recurrence. *J Affect Disord*. 1993;29(2–3):85–96.
12. Moieni M, Irwin MR, Jevtic I, Olmstead R, Breen EC, Eisenberger NI. Sex differences in depressive and socioemotional responses to an inflammatory challenge: Implications for sex differences in depression. *Neuropsychopharmacology*. 2015;40(7):1709–16.
13. Young E, Korszun A. Sex, trauma, stress hormones and depression. *Mol Psychiatry*. 2010;15(1):23.
14. Kendler KS, Gardner CO. Sex differences in the pathways to major depression: A study of opposite-sex twin pairs. *Am J Psychiatry*. 2014; 171(4):426–35.
15. Burcusa SL, Iacono WG. Risk for recurrence in depression. *Clin Psychol Rev*. 2007;27(8):959–85.
16. Mueller TI, Keller MB, Leon AC, et al. Recovery after 5 years of unremitting major depressive disorder. *Arch Gen Psychiatry*. 1996;53(9):794–9.
17. Melartin TK, Rytsälä HJ, Leskelä US, Lestelä-Mielonen PS, Sokero TP, Isometsä ET. Severity and comorbidity predict episode duration and recurrence of DSM-IV major depressive disorder. *J Clin Psychiatry*. 2004;65(6):810–9.
18. Sullivan PF, Neale MC, Kendler KS. Genetic epidemiology of major depression: Review and meta-analysis. *Am J Psychiatry*. 2000;157(10):1552–62.
19. Korten NC, Comijs HC, Lamers F, Penninx BW. Early and late onset depression in young and middle aged adults: Differential symptomatology, characteristics and risk factors? *J Affect Disord*. 2012;138(3):259–67.
20. Ballmaier M, Narr KL, Toga AW, et al. Hippocampal morphology and distinguishing late-onset from early-onset elderly depression. *Am J Psychiatry*. 2008;165(2):229–37.
21. Jorm AF. Does old age reduce the risk of anxiety and depression? A review of epidemiological studies across the adult life span. *Psychol Med*. 2000;30(1):11–22.
22. Jokela M, Batty GD, Kivimäki M. Ageing and the prevalence and treatment of mental health problems. *Psychol Med*. 2013;43(10):2037–45.
23. Penninx BWJH, Comijs HC. Depression and other common mental health disorders in old age. In: Newman A, Cauley JA, eds. *The Epidemiology of Aging*. Amsterdam, The Netherlands: Springer Science & Business Media; 2012.
24. Fiske A, Wetherell JL, Gatz M. Depression in older adults. *Annu Rev Clin Psychol*. 2009;5:363–89.
25. Weissman MM, Leaf PJ, Bruce ML, Florio L. The epidemiology of dysthymia in five communities: Rates, risks, comorbidity, and treatment. *Am J Psychiatry Wash*. 1988;145(7):815–9.
26. Blanco C, Okuda M, Markowitz JC, Liu S-M, Grant BF, Hasin DS. The epidemiology of chronic major depressive disorder and dysthymic disorder: Results from the National Epidemiologic Survey on Alcohol and Related Conditions. *J Clin Psychiatry*. 2010;71(12):1645–56.
27. Pietrzak RH, Kinley J, Afifi TO, Enns MW, Fawcett J, Sareen J. Subsyndromal depression in the United States: Prevalence, course, and risk for incident psychiatric outcomes. *Psychol Med*. 2013;43(7):1401–14.
28. Cohen NL. *Public Health Perspectives on Depressive Disorders*. Baltimore, MD: JHU Press; 2017.
29. Kessler RC, Bromet EJ. The epidemiology of depression across cultures. *Annu Rev Public Health*. 2013;34(1):119–38.
30. Balázs J, Miklósi M, Keresztény Á, et al. Adolescent subthreshold-depression and anxiety: Psychopathology, functional impairment and increased suicide risk. *J Child Psychol Psychiatry*. 2013;54(6):670–7.
31. Fergusson DM, Horwood LJ, Ridder EM, Beautrais AL. Subthreshold depression in adolescence and mental health outcomes in adulthood. *Arch Gen Psychiatry*. 2005;62(1):66–72.
32. Meeks T, Vahia I, Lavretsky H, Kulkarni G, Jeste D. A tune in "a minor" can "B major": A review of epidemiology, illness course, and public health implications of subthreshold depression in older adults. *J Affect Disord*. 2011;129(1–3):126–42.
33. Montross LP, Kasckow J, Golshan S, Solorzano E, Lehman D, Zisook S. Suicidal ideation and suicide attempts among middle-aged and older patients with schizophrenia spectrum disorders and concurrent subsyndromal depression. *J Nerv Ment Dis*. 2008;196(12):884–90.
34. Li LW, Conwell Y. Effects of changes in depressive symptoms and cognitive functioning on physical disability in home care elders. *J Gerontol A Biol Sci Med Sci*. 2009;64A(2):230–6.
35. Angst J, Gamma A, Gastpar M, et al. Gender differences in depression. Epidemiological findings from the European DEPRES I and II studies. *Eur Arch Psychiatry Clin Neurosci*. 2002;252(5):201–9.
36. Ryba MM, Hopko DR. Gender differences in depression: Assessing mediational effects of overt behaviors and environmental reward through daily diary monitoring. *Depress Res Treat*. 2012;2012:865679.
37. Rauh C, Beetz A, Burger P, et al. Delivery mode and the course of pre- and postpartum depression. *Arch Gynecol Obstet*. 2012;286(6):1407–12.
38. O'Hara MW. Postpartum depression: What we know. *J Clin Psychol*. 2009;65(12):1258–69.
39. Robertson E, Celasun N, Stewart D. Risk factors for postpartum depression. In: Stewart D, Robertson E, Dennis C-L, Grace S, Wallington T, eds. *Postpartum Depression: Literature Review of Risk Factors and Interventions*; 2003.
40. Gotlib IH, Whiffen VE, Mount JH, Milne K, Cordy NI. Prevalence rates and demographic characteristics associated with depression in pregnancy and the postpartum. *J Consult Clin Psychol*. 1989;57(2):269–74.
41. Stowe ZN, Hostetter AL, Newport DJ. The onset of postpartum depression: Implications for clinical screening in obstetrical and primary care. *Am J Obstet Gynecol*. 2005;192(2):522–6.
42. Davalos DB, Yadon CA, Tregellas HC. Untreated prenatal maternal depression and the potential risks to offspring: a review. *Arch Womens Ment Health*. 2012;15(1):1–14.
43. Grote NK, Bridge JA, Gavin AR, Melville JL, Iyengar S, Katon WJ. A meta-analysis of depression during pregnancy and the risk of preterm birth, low birth weight, and intrauterine growth restriction. *Arch Gen Psychiatry*. 2010;67(10):1012–24.
44. Field T. Prenatal depression effects on early development: A review. *Infant Behav Dev*. 2011;34(1):1–14.
45. Scrandis DA, Langenberg P, Tonelli LH, et al. Prepartum depressive symptoms correlate positively with C-reactive protein levels and negatively with tryptophan levels: A preliminary report. *Int J Child Health Hum Dev IJCHD*. 2008;1(2):167–74.
46. Lancaster CA, Gold KJ, Flynn HA, Yoo H, Marcus SM, Davis MM. Risk factors for depressive symptoms during pregnancy: A systematic review. *Am J Obstet Gynecol*. 2010;202(1):5–14.
47. Weissman MM, Bland RC, Canino GJ, et al. Cross-national epidemiology of major depression and bipolar disorder. *JAMA*. 1996;276(4):293–9.
48. Johnson KR, Johnson SL. Cross-national prevalence and cultural correlates of bipolar I disorder. *Soc Psychiatry Psychiatr Epidemiol*. 2014;49(7):1111–7.
49. Tondo L, Baldessarini RJ. Rapid cycling in women and men with bipolar manic-depressive disorders. *Am J Psychiatry*. 1998;155(10):1434–6.
50. Goodwin FK, Jamison KR. *Manic-Depressive Illness: Bipolar Disorders and Recurrent Depression*. Oxford, MS: Oxford University Press; 2007.
51. Kennedy N, Boydell J, Kalidindi S, et al. Gender differences in incidence and age at onset of mania and bipolar disorder over a 35-year period in Camberwell, England. *Am J Psychiatry*. 2005;162(2):257–62.
52. Kawa I, Carter JD, Joyce PR, et al. Gender differences in bipolar disorder: Age of onset, course, comorbidity, and symptom presentation. *Bipolar Disord*. 2005;7(2):119–25.

53. Benazzi F. Gender differences in bipolar II and unipolar depressed outpatients: A 557-case study. *Ann Clin Psychiatry*. 1999;11(2):55–9.
54. Robb JC, Young LT, Cooke RG, Joffe RT. Gender differences in patients with bipolar disorder influence outcome in the medical outcomes survey (SF-20) subscale scores. *J Affect Disord*. 1998;49(3):189–93.
55. Bauer M, Pfennig A. Epidemiology of bipolar disorders. *Epilepsia*. 2005;46:8–13.
56. Cate Carter TD, Mundo E, Parikh SV, Kennedy JL. Early age at onset as a risk factor for poor outcome of bipolar disorder. *J Psychiatr Res*. 2003;37(4):297–303.
57. Bebbington P, Ramana R. The epidemiology of bipolar affective disorder. *Soc Psychiatry Psychiatr Epidemiol*. 1995;30(6):279–92.
58. Merikangas KR, He J, Burstein M, et al. Lifetime prevalence of mental disorders in US adolescents: Results from the National Comorbidity Study-Adolescent Supplement (NCS-A). *J Am Acad Child Adolesc Psychiatry*. 2010;49(10):980–9.
59. Cummings CM, Caporino NE, Kendall PC. Comorbidity of anxiety and depression in children and adolescents: 20 Years after. *Psychol Bull*. 2014;140(3):816–45.
60. Pini S, Cassano BG, Simonini E, Savino M, Russo A, A Montgomery S. Prevalence of anxiety disorders comorbidity in bipolar depression, unipolar depression and dysthymia. *J Affect Disord*. 1997;42:145–53.
61. Adams GC, Balbuena L, Meng X, Asmundson GJG. When social anxiety and depression go together: A population study of comorbidity and associated consequences. *J Affect Disord*. 2016;206(Supplement C):48–54.
62. Kochanek KD, Murphy SL, Xu J, Arias E. Mortality in the United States, 2013. *NCHS Data Brief*. 2014;(178):1–8.
63. World Health Organization. *The 2016 Update, Global Health Workforce Statistics*. Geneva: World Health Organization; 2016.
64. Bertolote JM, Fleischmann A. A global perspective in the epidemiology of suicide. *Suicidologi*. 2002;7(2):628.
65. Goldman-Mellor SJ, Caspi A, Harrington H, et al. Suicide attempt in young people: A signal for long-term health care and social needs. *JAMA Psychiatry*. 2014;71(2):119–27.
66. Brown GK, Beck AT, Steer RA, Grisham JR. Risk factors for suicide in psychiatric outpatients: A 20-year prospective study. *J Consult Clin Psychol*. 2000;68(3):371.
67. Simon OR, Swann AC, Powell KE, Potter LB, Kresnow MJ, O'Carroll PW. Characteristics of impulsive suicide attempts and attempters. *Suicide Life Threat Behav*. 2001;32(1 Suppl):49–59.
68. J Callanan V, Davis M. Gender differences in suicide methods. *Soc Psychiatry Psychiatr Epidemiol*. 2011;47:857–69.
69. Wu KC-C, Chen Y-Y, Yip PSF. Suicide methods in Asia: Implications in suicide prevention. *Int J Environ Res Public Health*. 2012;9(4):1135–58.
70. Belmaker RH, Agam G. Major depressive disorder. *N Engl J Med*. 2008;358(1):55–68.
71. Kendler KS, Karkowski LM, Prescott CA. Causal relationship between stressful life events and the onset of major depression. *Am J Psychiatry*. 1999;156(6):837–41.
72. Costello EJ, Compton SN, Keeler G, Angold A. Relationships between poverty and psychopathology: A natural experiment. *JAMA*. 2003;290(15):2023–9.
73. Southwick SM, Vythilingam M, Charney DS. The psychobiology of depression and resilience to stress: Implications for prevention and treatment. *Annu Rev Clin Psychol*. 2005;1:255–91.
74. Caspi A, Sugden K, Moffitt TE, et al. Influence of life stress on depression: Moderation by a polymorphism in the 5-HTT gene. *Science*. 2003;301(5631):386–9.
75. Goldman N, Glei DA, Lin Y-H, Weinstein M. The serotonin transporter polymorphism (5-HTTLPR): Allelic variation and links with depressive symptoms. *Depress Anxiety*. 2010;27(3):260–9.
76. Kochanska G, Philibert RA, Barry RA. Interplay of genes and early mother-child relationship in the development of self-regulation from toddler to preschool age. *J Child Psychol Psychiatry*. 2009;50(11):1331–8.
77. Pezawas L, Meyer-Lindenberg A, Drabant EM, et al. 5-HTTLPR polymorphism impacts human cingulate-amygdala interactions: A genetic susceptibility mechanism for depression. *Nat Neurosci*. 2005;8(6):828–34.
78. Belsky J, Pluess M. Beyond diathesis stress: Differential susceptibility to environmental influences. *Psychol Bull*. 2009;135(6):885–908.
79. Mitchell C, McLanahan S, Brooks-Gunn J, Garfinkel I, Hobcraft J, Notterman D. Genetic differential sensitivity to social environments: Implications for research. *Am J Public Health*. 2013;103 Suppl 1:S102–10.
80. Caspi A, Hariri AR, Holmes A, Uher R, Moffitt TE. Genetic sensitivity to the environment: The case of the serotonin transporter gene and its implications for studying complex diseases and traits. *Am J Psychiatry*. 2010;167(5):509–27.
81. Taylor SE, Way BM, Welch WT, Hilmert CJ, Lehman BJ, Eisenberger NI. Early family environment, current adversity, the serotonin transporter promoter polymorphism, and depressive symptomatology. *Biol Psychiatry*. 2006;60(7):671–6.
82. Segal ZV, Williams J, Teasdale J, Gemar M. A cognitive science perspective on kindling and episode sensitization in recurrent affective disorder. *Psychol Med*. 1996;26(2):371–80.
83. Shonkoff JP, Boyce W, McEwen BS. Neuroscience, molecular biology, and the childhood roots of health disparities: Building a new framework for health promotion and disease prevention. *JAMA*. 2009;301(21):2252–9.
84. Andersen SL, Teicher MH. Stress, sensitive periods and maturational events in adolescent depression. *Trends Neurosci*. 2008;31(4):183–91.
85. Putnam FW. Ten-year research update review: Child sexual abuse. *J Am Acad Child Adolesc Psychiatry*. 2003;42(3):269–78.
86. Andersen SL, Teicher MH. Delayed effects of early stress on hippocampal development. *Neuropsychopharmacol Off Publ Am Coll Neuropsychopharmacol*. 2004;29(11):1988–93.
87. Teicher MH, Tomoda A, Andersen SL. Neurobiological consequences of early stress and childhood maltreatment: Are results from human and animal studies comparable? *Ann N Y Acad Sci*. 2006;1071:313–23.
88. Leussis MP, Lawson K, Stone K, Andersen SL. The enduring effects of an adolescent social stressor on synaptic density, part II: Poststress reversal of synaptic loss in the cortex by adinazolam and MK-801. *Synap N Y N*. 2008;62(3):185–92.
89. Andersen SL, Tomada A, Vincow ES, Valente E, Polcari A, Teicher MH. Preliminary evidence for sensitive periods in the effect of childhood sexual abuse on regional brain development. *J Neuropsychiatry Clin Neurosci*. 2008;20(3):292–301.
90. Ouellet-Morin I, Wong CCY, Danese A, et al. Increased serotonin transporter gene (SERT) DNA methylation is associated with bullying victimization and blunted cortisol response to stress in childhood: A longitudinal study of discordant monozygotic twins. *Psychol Med*. 2013;43(9):1813–23.
91. Hammen C. Stress and depression. *Annu Rev Clin Psychol*. 2005; 1(1):293–319.
92. Lu W, Mueser KT, Rosenberg SD, Jankowski MK. Correlates of adverse childhood experiences among adults with severe mood disorders. *Psychiatr Serv Wash DC*. 2008;59(9):1018–26.
93. Suliman S, Mkabile SG, Fincham DS, Ahmed R, Stein DJ, Seedat S. Cumulative effect of multiple trauma on symptoms of posttraumatic stress disorder, anxiety, and depression in adolescents. *Compr Psychiatry*. 2009;50(2):121–7.
94. Estrada-Martínez LM, Caldwell CH, Bauermeister JA, Zimmerman MA. Stressors in multiple life-domains and the risk for externalizing and internalizing behaviors among African Americans during emerging adulthood. *J Youth Adolesc*. 2012;41(12):1600–12.
95. Frodl T, O'Keane V. How does the brain deal with cumulative stress? A review with focus on developmental stress, HPA axis function and hippocampal structure in humans. *Neurobiol Dis*. 2013;52(Supplement C):24–37.
96. Bandura A. Self-efficacy: Toward a unifying theory of behavioral change. *Psychol Rev*. 1977;84(2):191–215.
97. Kendler KS, Hettema JM, Butera F, Gardner CO, Prescott CA. Life event dimensions of loss, humiliation, entrapment, and danger in the prediction of onsets of major depression and generalized anxiety. *Arch Gen Psychiatry*. 2003;60(8):789–96.
98. Galea S. An argument for a consequentialist epidemiology. *Am J Epidemiol*. 2013;178(8):1185–91.
99. Mathers CD, Loncar D. Projections of global mortality and burden of disease from 2002 to 2030. *PLoS Med*. 2006;3(11):e442.
100. Castelli WP. Epidemiology of coronary heart disease: The Framingham study. *Am J Med*. 1984;76(2, Part A):4–12.
101. Mann JI. Diet and diabetes. *Diabetologia*. 1980;18(2):89–95.
102. Hirayama T. Diet and cancer. *Nutr Cancer*. 1979;1(3):67–81.
103. Eyre H, Kahn R, Robertson RM, et al. Preventing cancer, cardiovascular disease, and diabetes: A common agenda for the American Cancer Society, the American Diabetes Association, and the American Heart Association. *Circulation*. 2004;109(25):3244–55.
104. American Psychiatric Association. *American Psychiatric Association Practice Guidelines for the Treatment of Psychiatric Disorders: Compendium 2006*. Arlington, VA: American Psychiatric Pub; 2006.
105. Freeman MP, Fava M, Lake J, Trivedi MH, Wisner KL, Mischoulon D. Complementary and alternative medicine in major depressive disorder:

The American Psychiatric Association Task Force report. *J Clin Psychiatry*. 2010;71(6):669–81.

106. García-Alba C. Anorexia and depression: Depressive comorbidity in anorexic adolescents. *Span J Psychol*. 2004;7(1):40–52.
107. Tetsuka S, Otsuka M, Hashimoto R, Kato H. Anorexia due to depression in the elderly from the viewpoint of primary care. *J Med Cases*. 2017;8(4):119–23.
108. Lunde AV, Fasmer OB, Akiskal KK, Akiskal HS, Oedegaard KJ. The relationship of bulimia and anorexia nervosa with bipolar disorder and its temperamental foundations. *J Affect Disord*. 2009;115(3):309–14.
109. Yanovski SZ, Nelson JE, Dubbert BK, Spitzer RL. Association of binge eating disorder and psychiatric comorbidity in obese subjects. *Am J Psychiatry Wash*. 1993;150(10):1472–9.
110. Cuthbert BN, Kozak MJ. Constructing constructs for psychopathology: The NIMH research domain criteria. *J Abnorm Psychol*. 2013;122(3):928–37.
111. Marchand WR, Dilda V, Jensen CR, Wahlen GE. Neurobiology of mood disorders. *Hosp Physician*. 2005;41(9):17.
112. Langdon FW. Nervous and mental manifestations of pre-pernicious anemia. *J Am Med Assoc*. 1905;XLV(22):1635–8.
113. Lucock M. Folic acid: Nutritional biochemistry, molecular biology, and role in disease processes. *Mol Genet Metab*. 2000;71(1–2):121–38.
114. Reynolds EH, Preece JM, Bailey J, Coppen A. Folate deficiency in depressive illness. *Br J Psychiatry*. 1970;117(538):287–92.
115. Bender A, Hagan KE, Kingston N. The association of folate and depression: A meta-analysis. *J Psychiatr Res*. 2017;95(Supplement C):9–18.
116. Bottiglieri T. Homocysteine and folate metabolism in depression. *Prog Neuropsychopharmacol Biol Psychiatry*. 2005;29(7):1103–12.
117. Nabi H, Bochud M, Glaus J, et al. Association of serum homocysteine with major depressive disorder: Results from a large population-based study. *Psychoneuroendocrinology*. 2013;38(10):2309–18.
118. Osher Y, Sela B-A, Levine J, Belmaker RH. Elevated homocysteine levels in euthymic bipolar disorder patients showing functional deterioration. *Bipolar Disord*. 2004;6(1):82–6.
119. Salagre E, Fernanda Vizuete A, Leite M, et al. Homocysteine as a peripheral biomarker in bipolar disorder: A meta-analysis. *Eur Psychiatry*. 2017;43:81–91.
120. Fava M, Mischoulon D. Folate in depression: Efficacy, safety, differences in formulations, and clinical issues. *J Clin Psychiatry*. 2009;70 Suppl 5:12–7.
121. Coppen A, Bailey J. Enhancement of the antidepressant action of fluoxetine by folic acid: A randomised, placebo controlled trial. *J Affect Disord*. 2000;60(2):121–30.
122. Bhatia P, Singh N. Homocysteine excess: Delineating the possible mechanism of neurotoxicity and depression. *Fundam Clin Pharmacol*. 2015;29(6):522–8.
123. Petridou ET, Kousoulis AA, Michelakos T, et al. Folate and B12 serum levels in association with depression in the aged: A systematic review and meta-analysis. *Aging Ment Health*. 2016;20(9):965–73.
124. Almeida OP, Ford AH, Flicker L. Systematic review and meta-analysis of randomized placebo-controlled trials of folate and vitamin B12 for depression. *Int Psychogeriatr*. 2015;27(5):727–37.
125. Lopez-Huertas E. The effect of EPA and DHA on metabolic syndrome patients: A systematic review of randomised controlled trials. *Br J Nutr*. 2012;107 Suppl 2:S185–94.
126. Bloch MH, Hannestad J. Omega-3 fatty acids for the treatment of depression: Systematic review and meta-analysis. *Mol Psychiatry*. 2012;17(12):1272–82.
127. Mickelson MJ, Klipstein FA. Enterotoxigenic intestinal bacteria in tropical sprue. IV. Effect of linoleic acid on growth interrelationships of Lactobacillus acidophilus and Klebsiella pneumoniae. *Infect Immun*. 1975;12(5):1121–6.
128. Ghosh S, Molcan E, DeCoffe D, Dai C, Gibson DL. Diets rich in n-6 PUFA induce intestinal microbial dysbiosis in aged mice. *Br J Nutr*. 2013;110(3):515–23.
129. Miyamoto J, Mizukure T, Park S-B, et al. A gut microbial metabolite of linoleic acid, 10-hydroxy-cis-12-octadecenoic acid, ameliorates intestinal epithelial barrier impairment partially via GPR40-MEK-ERK pathway. *J Biol Chem*. 2015;290(5):2902–18.
130. Kaplan BJ, Rucklidge JJ, Romijn A, McLeod K. The emerging field of nutritional mental health inflammation, the microbiome, oxidative stress, and mitochondrial function. *Clin Psychol Sci*. 2015;3(6):964–80.
131. Rogers GB, Keating DJ, Young RL, Wong M-L, Licinio J, Wesselingh S. From gut dysbiosis to altered brain function and mental illness: Mechanisms and pathways. *Mol Psychiatry*. 2016;21(6):738–48.
132. Kankaanpää PE, Salminen SJ, Isolauri E, Lee YK. The influence of polyunsaturated fatty acids on probiotic growth and adhesion. *FEMS Microbiol Lett*. 2001;194(2):149–53.
133. Bischoff SC, Barbara G, Buurman W, et al. Intestinal permeability—A new target for disease prevention and therapy. *BMC Gastroenterol*. 2014;14:189.
134. Berger ME, Smesny S, Kim S-W, et al. Omega-6 to omega-3 polyunsaturated fatty acid ratio and subsequent mood disorders in young people with at-risk mental states: A 7-year longitudinal study. *Transl Psychiatry*. 2017;7(8):e1220.
135. Jacobs DR, Steffen LM. Nutrients, foods, and dietary patterns as exposures in research: A framework for food synergy. *Am J Clin Nutr*. 2003;78(3):508S–13S.
136. Jacka FN, Pasco JA, Mykletun A, et al. Association of western and traditional diets with depression and anxiety in women. *Am J Psychiatry*. 2010;167(3):305–11.
137. Jacka FN, Pasco JA, Mykletun A, et al. Diet quality in bipolar disorder in a population-based sample of women. *J Affect Disord*. 2011;129(1):332–7.
138. Sánchez-Villegas A, Henríquez-Sánchez P, Ruiz-Canela M, et al. A longitudinal analysis of diet quality scores and the risk of incident depression in the SUN Project. *BMC Med*. 2015;13:197.
139. Miller AH, Maletic V, Raison CL. Inflammation and its discontents: The role of cytokines in the pathophysiology of major depression. *Biol Psychiatry*. 2009;65(9):732–41.
140. Cavicchia PP, Steck SE, Hurley TG, et al. A new dietary inflammatory index predicts interval changes in serum high-sensitivity C-reactive protein. *J Nutr*. 2009;139(12):2365–72.
141. Shivappa N, Steck SE, Hurley TG, Hussey JR, Hébert JR. Designing and developing a literature-derived, population-based dietary inflammatory index. *Public Health Nutr*. 2014;17(8):1689–96.
142. Shivappa N, Steck SE, Hurley TG, et al. A population-based dietary inflammatory index predicts levels of C-reactive protein in the Seasonal Variation of Blood Cholesterol Study (SEASONS). *Public Health Nutr*. 2014;17(8):1825–33.
143. Tabung FK, Steck SE, Zhang J, et al. Construct validation of the dietary inflammatory index among postmenopausal women. *Ann Epidemiol*. 2015;25(6):398–405.
144. Wirth MD, Shivappa N, Davis L, et al. Construct validation of the dietary inflammatory index among African Americans. *J Nutr Health Aging*. 2017;21(5):487–91.
145. Shivappa N, Wirth MD, Hurley TG, Hébert JR. Association between the dietary inflammatory index (DII) and telomere length and C-reactive protein from the National Health and Nutrition Examination Survey-1999–2002. *Mol Nutr Food Res*. 2017;61(4).
146. Sánchez-Villegas A, Ruíz-Canela M, de la Fuente-Arrillaga C, et al. Dietary inflammatory index, cardiometabolic conditions and depression in the Seguimiento Universidad de Navarra cohort study. *Br J Nutr*. 2015;114(09):1471–9.
147. Akbaraly TN, Kerlau C, Wyart M, et al. Dietary inflammatory index and recurrence of depressive symptoms results from the Whitehall II study. *Clin Psychol Sci*. 2016;4(6):1125–34.
148. Bergmans RS, Malecki KM. The association of dietary inflammatory potential with depression and mental well-being among US adults. *Prev Med*. 2017;99:313–9.
149. Lucas M, Chocano-Bedoya P, Schulze MB, et al. Inflammatory dietary pattern and risk of depression among women. *Brain Behav Immun*. 2014;36:46–53.
150. Faris ELR, Warren Dunham H. Mental disorders in urban areas: An ecological study of schizophrenia and other psychoses. *JAMA*. 1939;112(4):331–2.
151. Diez Roux AV, Mair C. Neighborhoods and health. *Ann N Y Acad Sci*. 2010;1186(1):125–45.
152. Ross CE. Neighborhood disadvantage and adult depression. *J Health Soc Behav*. 2000;41(2):177–87.
153. Latkin CA, Curry AD. Stressful neighborhoods and depression: A prospective study of the impact of neighborhood disorder. *J Health Soc Behav*. 2003;44(1):34–44.
154. Galea S, Ahern J, Rudenstine S, Wallace Z, Vlahov D. Urban built environment and depression: A multilevel analysis. *J Epidemiol Community Health*. 2005;59(10):822–7.

155. Pedersen CB, Mortensen PB. Urbanicity during upbringing and bipolar affective disorders in Denmark. *Bipolar Disord.* 2006;8(3):242–7.

156. Kirkbride JB, Fearon P, Morgan C, et al. Neighbourhood variation in the incidence of psychotic disorders in Southeast London. *Soc Psychiatry Psychiatr Epidemiol.* 2007;42(6):438–45.

157. Kirkbride JB, Jones PB, Ullrich S, Coid JW. Social deprivation, inequality, and the neighborhood-level incidence of psychotic syndromes in East London. *Schizophr Bull.* 2014;40(1):169–80.

158. Leventhal T, Brooks-Gunn J. Moving to opportunity: An experimental study of neighborhood effects on mental health. *Am J Public Health.* 2003;93(9):1576–82.

159. Webb MD, Rohe WM, Nguyen MT, Frescoln K, Donegan M, Han H-S. Finding HOPE: Changes in depressive symptomology following relocation from distressed public housing. *Soc Sci Med.* 2017;190(Supplement C): 165–73.

160. Ellicott A, Harnincn C, Gitlin M, Brown G, Jamison K. Life events and the course of bipolar disorder. *Am J Psychiatry.* 1990;147(9):1194–8.

161. Kessler RC. The effects of stressful life events on depression. *Annu Rev Psychol.* 1997;48:191–214.

162. Mitchell PB, Parker GB, Gladstone GL, Wilhelm K, Austin MPV. Severity of stressful life events in first and subsequent episodes of depression: The relevance of depressive subtype. *J Affect Disord.* 2003;73(3):245–52.

163. Dustmann C, Fasani F. The effect of local area crime on mental health. *Econ J.* 2016;126(593):978–1017.

164. Kawachi I, Berkman LF. Social ties and mental health. *J Urban Health Bull N Y Acad Med.* 2001;78(3):458–67.

165. Putnam RD. E Pluribus Unum: Diversity and community in the twenty-first century. The 2006 Johan Skytte Prize Lecture. *Scand Polit Stud.* 2007;30(2):137–74.

166. Bécares L, Stafford M, Laurence J, Nazroo J. Composition, concentration and deprivation: Exploring their association with social cohesion among different ethnic groups in the UK. *Urban Stud Edinb Scotl.* 2011;48(13):2771–87.

167. Erdem Ö, Burdorf A, Van Lenthe FJ. Ethnic inequalities in psychological distress among urban residents in the Netherlands: A moderating role of neighborhood ethnic diversity? *Health Place.* 2017;46(Supplement C):175–82.

168. Tzivian L, Winkler A, Dlugaj M, et al. Effect of long-term outdoor air pollution and noise on cognitive and psychological functions in adults. *Int J Hyg Environ Health.* 2015;218(1):1–11.

169. Ragguett R-M, Cha DS, Subramaniapillai M, et al. Air pollution, aeroallergens and suicidality: A review of the effects of air pollution and aeroallergens on suicidal behavior and an exploration of possible mechanisms. *Rev Environ Health.* 2017;32(4):343–59.

170. Truong K, Ma S. A systematic review of relations between neighborhoods and mental health. *J Ment Health Policy Econ.* 2006;9(3):137–54.

171. Mair C, Diez Roux AV, Galea S. Are neighbourhood characteristics associated with depressive symptoms? A review of evidence. *J Epidemiol Community Health.* 2008;62(11):940–6, 8 p following 946.

172. Kim D. Blues from the neighborhood? Neighborhood characteristics and depression. *Epidemiol Rev.* 2008;30(1):101–17.

173. Gruebner O, A. Rapp M, Adli M, Kluge U, Galea S, Heinz A. Cities and mental health. *Dtsch Ärztebl Int.* 2017;114(8):121–7.

174. Oakes JM. The (mis)estimation of neighborhood effects: Causal inference for a practicable social epidemiology. *Soc Sci Med 1982.* 2004;58(10):1929–52.

175. Artazcoz L, Benach J, Borrell C, Cortès I. Unemployment and mental health: Understanding the interactions among gender, family roles, and social class. *Am J Public Health.* 2004;94(1):82–8.

176. Eaton WW, Anthony JC, Mandel W, Garrison R. Occupations and the prevalence of major depressive disorder. *J Occup Environ Med.* 1990;32(11):1079.

177. Henderson M, Harvey SB, Overland S, Mykletun A, Hotopf M. Work and common psychiatric disorders. *J R Soc Med.* 2011;104(5):198–207.

178. Bond GR. Supported employment: Evidence for an evidence-based practice. *Psychiatr Rehabil J.* 2004;27(4):345–59.

179. Bonde JPE. Psychosocial factors at work and risk of depression: A systematic review of the epidemiological evidence. *Occup Environ Med.* 2008;65(7):438–45.

180. Karasek R. Job demands, job decision latitude, and mental strain: Implications for job redesign. *Adm Sci Q.* 1979;24:285–308.

181. Karasek R, Brisson C, Kawakami N, Houtman I, Bongers P, Amick B. The job content questionnaire (JCQ): An instrument for internationally comparative assessments of psychosocial job characteristics. *J Occup Health Psychol.* 1998;3(4):322.

182. Johnson JV, Hall EM. Job strain, work place social support, and cardiovascular disease: A cross-sectional study of a random sample of the Swedish working population. *Am J Public Health.* 1988;78(10):1336–42.

183. Siegrist J, Siegrist K, Weber I. Sociological concepts in the etiology of chronic disease: The case of ischemic heart disease. *Soc Sci Med.* 1986;22(2):247–53.

184. Bakker AB, Demerouti E. The job demands-resources model: State of the art. *J Manag Psychol.* 2007;22(3):309–28.

185. Demerouti E, Bakker AB, Nachreiner F, Schaufeli WB. The job demands-resources model of burnout. *J Appl Psychol.* 2001;86(3):499.

186. Maslach C, Schaufeli WB, Leiter MP. Job burnout. *Annu Rev Psychol.* 2001;52(1):397–422.

187. Wang J. Work stress as a risk factor for major depressive episode (s). *Psychol Med.* 2005;35(6):865–71.

188. Wang J, Lesage A, Schmitz N, Drapeau A. The relationship between work stress and mental disorders in men and women: Findings from a population-based study. *J Epidemiol Community Health.* 2008;62(1):42–7.

189. Smith PM, Bielecky A. The impact of changes in job strain and its components on the risk of depression. *Am J Public Health.* 2012;102(2):352–8.

190. Madsen IE, Nyberg ST, Hanson LM, et al. Job strain as a risk factor for clinical depression: Systematic review and meta-analysis with additional individual participant data. *Psychol Med.* 2017;47(8):1342–56.

191. Virtanen M, Ferrie JE, Batty GD, et al. Socioeconomic and psychosocial adversity in midlife and depressive symptoms post retirement: A 21-year follow-up of the Whitehall II Study. *Am J Geriatr Psychiatry.* 2015;23(1):99–109.e1.

192. Kim JE, Moen P. Retirement transitions, gender, and psychological well-being: A life-course, ecological model. *J Gerontol B Psychol Sci Soc Sci.* 2002;57(3):P212–22.

193. Ahola K, Honkonen T, Isometsä E, et al. The relationship between job-related burnout and depressive disorders—Results from the Finnish Health 2000 Study. *J Affect Disord.* 2005;88(1):55–62.

194. Ahola K, Honkonen T, Kivimäki M, et al. Contribution of burnout to the association between job strain and depression: The health 2000 study. *J Occup Environ Med.* 2006;48(10):1023–30.

195. Ahola K, Hakanen J. Job strain, burnout, and depressive symptoms: A prospective study among dentists. *J Affect Disord.* 2007;104(1):103–10.

196. Hakanen JJ, Schaufeli WB, Ahola K. The job demands-resources model: A three-year cross-lagged study of burnout, depression, commitment, and work engagement. *Work Stress.* 2008;22(3):224–41.

197. Schonfeld IS, Bianchi R. Burnout and depression: Two entities or one? *J Clin Psychol.* 2016;72(1):22–37.

198. Iacovides A, Fountoulakis K, Kaprinis S, Kaprinis G. The relationship between job stress, burnout and clinical depression. *J Affect Disord.* 2003;75(3):209–21.

199. Cohen S, Wills TA. Stress, social support, and the buffering hypothesis. *Psychol Bull.* 1985;98(2):310.

200. Woo J-M, Postolache TT. The impact of work environment on mood disorders and suicide: Evidence and implications. *Int J Disabil Hum Dev IJDHD.* 2008;7(2):185–200.

201. Birnbaum SG, Yuan PX, Wang M, et al. Protein kinase C overactivity impairs prefrontal cortical regulation of working memory. *Science.* 2004;306(5697):882–4.

202. Olfson M, Marcus SC, Druss B, Elinson L, Tanielian T, Pincus HA. National trends in the outpatient treatment of depression. *JAMA.* 2002;287(2):203–9.

203. Fountoulakis KN, Vieta E, Sanchez-Moreno J, Kaprinis SG, Goikolea JM, Kaprinis GS. Treatment guidelines for bipolar disorder: A critical review. *J Affect Disord.* 2005;86(1):1–10.

204. Cawte J. Mania pre-lithium. *Aust N Z J Psychiatry.* 1999;33(1_suppl): S7–23.

205. Adams J. British nurses' attitudes to electroconvulsive therapy, 1945–2000. *J Adv Nurs.* 2015;71(10):2393–401.

206. Hirshbein L. Historical essay: Electroconvulsive therapy, memory, and self in America. *J Hist Neurosci.* 2012;21(2):147–69.

207. Semkovska M, McLoughlin DM. Measuring retrograde autobiographical amnesia following electroconvulsive therapy: Historical perspective and current issues. *J ECT.* 2013;29(2):127–33.

208. Shorter E. The history of lithium therapy. *Bipolar Disord.* 2009;11:4–9.

209. Ruffalo ML. A brief history of lithium treatment in psychiatry: (Brief report). *Prim Care Companion CNS Disord.* 2017;19(05):17br02140.

210. Kansagra AJ, Yang E, Nambiar S, Patel PS, Karetzky MS. A rare case of acute respiratory distress syndrome secondary to acute lithium intoxication. *Am J Ther.* 2014;21(2):e31–4.

211. Gitlin M. Lithium side effects and toxicity: Prevalence and management strategies. *Int J Bipolar Disord.* 2016;4(1):27.

212. Bradberry S. Lithium. *Medicine (Baltimore).* 2016;44(3):180–1.

213. Alson AR, Robinson DM, Ivanova D, et al. Depression in primary care: Strategies for a psychiatry-scarce environment. *Int J Psychiatry Med.* 2016;51(2):182–200.

214. Gao K, Gajwani P, Elhaj O, Calabrese JR. Typical and atypical antipsychotics in bipolar depression. *J Clin Psychiatry.* 2005;66(11):1376–85.

215. Zhou X, Keitner GI, Qin B, et al. Atypical antipsychotic augmentation for treatment-resistant depression: A systematic review and network meta-analysis. *Int J Neuropsychopharmacol.* 2015;18(11):pyv060.

216. Perez Rodriguez A, Tajima-Pozo K, Lewczuk A, Montañes-Rada F. Atypical antipsychotics and metabolic syndrome. *Cardiovasc Endocrinol.* 2015;4(4):132–7.

217. Correll CU, Ng-Mak DS, Stafkey-Mailey D, Farrelly E, Rajagopalan K, Loebel A. Cardiometabolic comorbidities, readmission, and costs in schizophrenia and bipolar disorder: A real-world analysis. *Ann Gen Psychiatry Lond.* 2017;16:9.

218. Correll CU, Detraux J, De Lepeleire J, De Hert M. Effects of antipsychotics, antidepressants and mood stabilizers on risk for physical diseases in people with schizophrenia, depression and bipolar disorder. *World Psychiatry.* 2015;14(2):119–36.

219. Kraemer HC, Frank E, Kupfer DJ. How to assess the clinical impact of treatments on patients, rather than the statistical impact of treatments on measures. *Int J Methods Psychiatr Res.* 2011;20(2):63–72.

220. Morselli PL, Elgie R. GAMIAN-Europe*/BEAM survey I—Global analysis of a patient questionnaire circulated to 3450 members of 12 European advocacy groups operating in the field of mood disorders. *Bipolar Disord.* 2003;5(4):265–78.

221. Liebelt EL. An update on antidepressant toxicity: An evolution of unique toxicities to master. *Clin Pediatr Emerg Med.* 2008;9(1):24–34.

222. Youdim MBH, Finberg JPM, Tipton KF. Monoamine oxidase. In: Trendelenburg U, Weiner U, eds. *Advances in Experimental Pharmacology. Catecholamine. II.* Berlin: Springer-Verlag; 1988, pp. 119–92.

223. Rush AJ, Trivedi MH, Wisniewski SR, et al. Acute and longer-term outcomes in depressed outpatients requiring one or several treatment steps: A STAR*D Report. *Am J Psychiatry.* 2006;163(11):1905–17.

224. Feinstein R, Connelly J, Feinstein M. *Integrating Behavioral Health and Primary Care.* Oxford, MS: Oxford University Press; 2017.

225. Dunlop BW, Davis PG. Combination treatment with benzodiazepines and SSRIs for comorbid anxiety and depression: A review. *Prim Care Companion J Clin Psychiatry.* 2008;10(3):222–8.

226. Geddes JR, Burgess S, Hawton K, Jamison K, Goodwin GM. Long-term lithium therapy for bipolar disorder: Systematic review and meta-analysis of randomized controlled trials. *Am J Psychiatry.* 2004;161(2):217–22.

227. Lindström L, Lindström E, Nilsson M, Höistad M. Maintenance therapy with second generation antipsychotics for bipolar disorder—A systematic review and meta-analysis. *J Affect Disord.* 2017;213(Supplement C):138–50.

228. Bowden CL, Calabrese JR, Sachs G, et al. A placebo-controlled 18-month trial of lamotrigine and lithium maintenance treatment in recently manic or hypomanic patients with bipolar I disorder. *Arch Gen Psychiatry.* 2003;60(4):392–400.

229. Hochman E, Krivoy A, Schaffer A, Weizman A, Valevski A. Antipsychotic adjunctive therapy to mood stabilizers and 1-year rehospitalization rates in bipolar disorder: A cohort study. *Bipolar Disord.* 2016;18(8):684–91.

230. Peselow ED, Naghdechi L, Pizano D, IsHak WW. Polypharmacy in maintenance of bipolar disorder. *Clin Neuropharmacol.* 2016;39(3):132–4.

231. Weinstock LM, Gaudiano BA, Epstein-Lubow G, Tezanos K, Celis-de-Hoyos CE, Miller IW. Medication burden in bipolar disorder: A chart review of patients at psychiatric hospital admission. *Psychiatry Res.* 2014;216(1):24–30.

232. Hammad TA, Laughren T, Racoosin J. Suicidality in pediatric patients treated with antidepressant drugs. *Arch Gen Psychiatry.* 2006;63(3):332–9.

233. Olfson M, Marcus SC, Druss B, Elinson L, Tanielian T, Pincus HA. National trends in the outpatient treatment of depression. *JAMA.* 2002;287(2):203–9.

234. Olfson M, Blanco C, Marcus SC. Treatment of adult depression in the United States. *JAMA Intern Med.* 2016;176(10):1482–91.

235. Isacsson G, Ahlner J. Antidepressants and the risk of suicide in young persons—Prescription trends and toxicological analyses. *Acta Psychiatr Scand.* 2014;129(4):296–302.

236. Licinio J, Wong M-L. Depression, antidepressants and suicidality: A critical appraisal. *Nat Rev Drug Discov.* 2005;4(2):nrd1634.

237. Hollon SD, Ponniah K. A review of empirically supported psychological therapies for mood disorders in adults. *Depress Anxiety.* 2010;27(10):891–932.

238. Picardi A, Gaetano P. Psychotherapy of mood disorders. *Clin Pract Epidemiol Ment Health CP EMH.* 2014;10:140–58.

239. Mojtabai R, Olfson M. National trends in psychotherapy by office-based psychiatrists. *Arch Gen Psychiatry.* 2008;65(8):962–70.

CHAPTER

164 Anxiety Disorders

Beyon Miloyan • William W. Eaton

INTRODUCTION

A case description of anxiety disorder can first be found in the Ancient Greek physician Hippocrates' eponymous medical corpus.[1] Ancient perspectives on the trait anxiety—as expressed, for instance, by the Ancient Roman Stoic philosopher Seneca the Younger—are also compatible with modern views. In the nineteenth century, Charles Darwin observed similarities in the physical expression of fear and anxiety among mammalian species, and suggested that these constitute phylogenetically ancient and adaptively significant traits.[2] From this perspective, anxiety is viewed as a survival behavior that facilitates the detection and management of anticipated hazards.[3–5] Today, anxiety is defined as constituting a disorder inasmuch as it is regarded by the individual as excessive, and a cause for distress or impairment.[6,7] This chapter addresses the neuroanatomy, classification, assessment, and epidemiology, and treatment of anxiety disorders.

NEUROANATOMY

In 1949, António Egas Moniz was awarded the Nobel Prize in Medicine for his discovery of the prefrontal leucotomy as a simple, safe, and effective treatment for mental disorders,[8] and this procedure was used to treat anxiety disorders.[9] More recent studies of combat veterans have reported that those with damage to the ventromedial prefrontal cortex are resistant to developing posttraumatic stress disorder and major depression,[10,11] and a case study of a patient with focal bilateral lesions to the amygdalae reveal an absence of fear and anxiety.[12] These findings suggest that the ventromedial prefrontal cortex and amygdala are critically involved in the expression of anxiety and its disorders.[13] Recent studies have revealed, however, that despite reducing distress, damage to these brain regions can have important adverse consequences.[14] The ventromedial prefrontal cortex, for example, is involved in a number of adaptive goal-oriented and social behaviors,[15] and damage to the amygdala is associated with a lack of appropriate caution that is necessary for the effective regulation of behavior.[12] In treating anxiety disorders, it is equally important not to abolish otherwise useful and adaptive traits.

CLASSIFICATION

The Diagnostic and Statistical Manual of Mental Disorders (DSM) classifies anxiety disorders into the following five subtypes: panic disorder, agoraphobia, specific phobia, social anxiety disorder, and generalized anxiety disorder.[6] We review these in turn, first describing the core symptoms that characterize each subtype, then describing the criteria for diagnosis, and finally describing symptom patterns.

Panic Disorder

The core feature of panic disorder is the occurrence of panic attacks, defined as the sudden, unexpected, and brief onset of terror. The panic attack is defined by the occurrence of at least four physical or mental symptoms that include heart palpitations, sweating, trembling, chest pain, dizziness, nausea, chills or hot flashes, numbness or tingling, shortness of breath or choking, and a feeling of loss of control, desensitization, or a fear of death. The recurrence of panic attacks, combined with persistent concerns about the possibility of additional panic attacks, occurring for a period of at least 1 month are integral to a diagnosis of panic disorder. In the context of panic disorder, there is evidence that panic symptoms cluster to form at least two distinguishable subtypes, characterized by predominantly respiratory and nonrespiratory (somatic) symptom presentations.[16–18] Older age is associated with fewer and less severe panic symptoms, and less frequent panic disorder.[19–21]

Agoraphobia

The core feature of agoraphobia is the fear or avoidance of situations from which escape is difficult. The diagnosis requires a fear or avoidance of at least two of the following specific situations: public transportation, open spaces, closed spaces, crowds, or being alone in public. The presence of these fears is also associated with panic disorder and specific phobia. A distinguishing factor between agoraphobia and panic disorder or specific phobia pertains to the frequency of the aforementioned fears; individuals with more of these fears tend to be classified as having agoraphobia.[22]

Specific Phobia

The core feature of specific phobia is the fear or avoidance of specific objects or situations. These fears or situations usually include, but are not limited to, the following categories: animals, typically snakes or insects; the natural environment, typically storms, water, or heights; situations, typically closed or open spaces; and, importantly, blood, injections, or injury. In order to constitute a diagnosis of specific phobia, the individual must recognize that the fear or avoidance is unreasonable, and regard it as distressing or interfering with everyday life. The most common fears reported by adults involve animals, heights, and flying,[23–25] although older adults frequently report situational fears.[26] An individual who meets the criterion for having a specific fear is also likely to report having other specific fears.[24,27]

Social Anxiety Disorder

The core feature of social anxiety disorder is the fear or avoidance of social situations. The fear or avoidance concerns the possibility of negative evaluation, for example, resulting in embarrassment or humiliation. The subject of the social anxiety may be limited to particular social settings or situations, such as small or large group settings, at work or with strangers, or the anxiety may generalize to a variety of social situations. Common social fears include public speaking, or being confronted or criticized by other people.[28] There may be age invariant distinguishing features of social anxiety disorder, including, in addition to discomfort and avoidance of social situations, and experiencing anxiety when thinking about social situations.[29]

Generalized Anxiety Disorder

Worry, defined as repetitive thinking about potentially harmful future events, is the core feature of generalized anxiety disorder. Worries tend revolve around everyday concerns, and involve attempts to minimize the likelihood or consequences of disadvantageous outcomes. Although some degree of worry is recognized as helpful,[30] when the individual reports experiencing excessive and uncontrollable worry for a period of 6 months or more, this may constitute a diagnosis of generalized anxiety disorder if it is also regarded by the individual as causing distress or impairment. Common worries concern work, finances, and personal relationships, although there are age-related changes in the phenomenology of worries depending on the life circumstances of the individual.[31–33]

ASSESSMENT

Structured Interviews

The standard for anxiety disorder assessment is the structured diagnostic interview administered by a trained professional. The structured interview consists of a set of predetermined questions that assess for the presence of the required symptoms for the relevant diagnostic criteria. For example, an interview for panic disorder would start by querying the individual about the presence of a panic attack within a specified period of time. If this is answered affirmatively, the assessor would then query the individual about the presence of the various panic symptoms. If the individual responds affirmatively to the minimum number of panic symptoms required for a diagnosis of panic disorder, the individual is then queried about the presence of distress or impairment due to the panic attacks. The advantage of the structured interview is that the standardized administration, procedure, and scoring minimize the role of bias and error in the assessment. Two commonly used structured interviews for the assessment of mental disorders in general are the *Diagnostic Interview Schedule (DIS)*,[34] and the *Composite International Diagnostic Interview (CIDI)*,[35] and a structured interview developed specifically for the anxiety disorders is the *Anxiety Disorders Interview Schedule (ADIS)*.[36] These instruments rely on the report of the individual and can be administered using computers and/or by trained lay persons. They are routinely revised based on updates to diagnostic criteria, and can vary based on the amount of structure that they provide. Due to the time-consuming nature of the structured interview, short versions such as the *Mini-International Neuropsychiatric Interview (MINI)*[37] have been developed. The examination modality of assessment contrasts with the interview technique in that the person conducting the assessment, typically a trained clinician, decides about the presence or absence of a symptom, instead of relying on the report of the individual. For example, the *Structured Clinical Interview for the DSM (SCID)*[38] and the *Schedules for Clinical Assessment in Neuropsychiatry (SCAN)*[39] are examples of semistructured interview/examinations that allow the clinician to take a more flexible approach to the interview while retaining some degree of structure. Although structured interviews and semistructured examinations are generally time consuming and not always practical to use, they play an essential role in validating briefer, easier to administer, and more widely used questionnaires and screening tools for use in particular contexts.

Rating Scales

The Generalized Anxiety Disorder 7-item (GAD-7) scale is a brief, self-administered questionnaire designed for use in general medical settings, to assess for generalized anxiety disorder based on the assessment of symptoms occurring in the preceding 2 weeks of the respondent's life.[40,41] Items are rated on a four-point scale (0–3) yielding a total score of 21. A raw score of ten or greater indicates a probable diagnosis of generalized anxiety disorder based on validation against the psychiatrist-administered SCID.[41]

The Panic Disorder Severity Scale (PDSS) is a brief, self-administered screening instrument for panic disorder.[42] There are seven items, each rated on a 5-point scale (0–4) yielding a total score of 28. A raw score of eight or greater indicates a probable diagnosis of panic disorder based on validation against the ADIS or the psychiatrist-administered SCID.[43]

The Social Phobia Inventory (SPIN) is a self-administered screening instrument for social anxiety disorder.[44] There are 17 items, each rated on a 5-point scale (0–4), yielding a total score of 68. A raw score of 19 or above indicates a probable diagnosis of social anxiety disorder based on validation against a psychiatric interview. The Mini-SPIN is a three-item version of the original questionnaire, on which a score of six or above indicates a probable diagnosis of social anxiety disorder based on validation against the ADIS or the psychiatrist-administered SCID.[45,46]

There are currently no validated rating scales for the assessment of specific phobia or agoraphobia. However, the assessment of specific phobia is more straightforward than the assessment of the other anxiety subtypes. Screening involves establishing whether the individual currently fears or avoids any specific stimulus or situation, whether the individual recognizes that the fear or avoidance is unreasonable, and regards it as distressing or as interfering with life.

The Overall Anxiety Severity and Impairment Scale (OASIS) is a brief, transdiagnostic screening tool designed to assess for the severity of anxiety in the past week of the individual's life.[47] There are five items, each rated on a 5-point scale (0–4), yielding a total score of 20. A raw score of eight or above indicates the presence of anxiety disorder based on validation against anxiety disorder diagnosis using the psychiatrist-administered SCID.[48] Raw scores of 10 and 12 indicate the presence of marked and severe anxiety, respectively, based on validation against the clinician-rated Clinical Global Impression-Severity (CGI-S) scale in a sample of individuals with any anxiety disorder ascertained using the MINI.[49]

EPIDEMIOLOGY

There has been decades of research on the epidemiology and natural history of the anxiety disorders. We describe the population prevalence and incidence of the anxiety disorders, and review the results of population-based studies on course and consequence, comorbidity, and risk factors.

Prevalence

The population prevalence of anxiety disorder is an estimate of the proportion of people in the population who meet diagnostic criteria for anxiety disorders, overall or by subtype, in a given period. The present analysis focuses on estimates of the prevalence of anxiety disorders within the past year of the life of respondents of surveys of nationally representative samples of the USA population.

Anxiety disorders have a higher overall prevalence than all other psychiatric disorders in adults.[50,51] The most prevalent subtypes are, in descending order, the specific phobias, social anxiety disorder, generalized anxiety disorder, panic disorder, and agoraphobia. Table 164-1 displays the 1-year prevalence of anxiety disorders, both overall and by subtype, in the National Epidemiologic Survey on Alcohol and Related Conditions (NESARC) and the Collaborative Psychiatric Epidemiology Surveys (CPES) of the United States. The prevalence of anxiety disorders is higher among females relative to males, and the prevalence of all anxiety subtypes is lower among persons aged 65 years or older. Previous studies report that there are also ethnic differences in anxiety disorder prevalence, such that Native and White Americans have the highest overall prevalence, and Hispanic and Asian Americans have the lowest overall prevalence.[52] The prevalence of anxiety disorders among Black Americans depends on the subtype:

estimates of specific phobias and generalized anxiety disorder prevalence are comparable to those of Native and White Americans, whereas estimates of panic disorder, agoraphobia, and social anxiety disorder are closer to those observed in Hispanic and Asian Americans (not shown). The prevalence of anxiety disorders does not vary substantially by educational attainment or marital status, although being widowed, divorced, or separated may be associated with slightly higher prevalence and higher educational attainment may be associated with slightly lower prevalence.

Incidence

The incidence of anxiety disorder is defined as the rate at which new cases occur in a given period, overall or by subtype. In contrast to prevalence estimates that are often based on measurements at a single time point, the incidence estimates require measurement at more than one time-point. The individuals at time one who do not meet criteria for an anxiety disorder are the "risk set" and form the denominator of the incidence ratio, and the individuals at time two or later who meet criteria for an anxiety disorder form the numerator. Therefore, the first lifetime incidence of anxiety disorder captures the force of morbidity in the population.

Similar to the prevalence estimates, the overall incidence of anxiety disorders is higher than other psychiatric disorders,[53] and the subtypes, in descending order of incidence, are specific phobia, social anxiety disorder, panic disorder, agoraphobia, and generalized anxiety disorder.[54,55] Data from the Epidemiologic Catchment Area (ECA) study and National Comorbidity Survey (NCS) samples of the USA indicate that there is a higher incidence in females relative to males.[56] Similar trends are observed in The Netherlands Mental Health Survey and Incidence Study (NEMESIS), in which sex differences for the specific subtypes range from 1.5 times higher for females for social anxiety disorder to four times higher for panic disorder.[57]

Data from the Early Developmental Stages of Psychopathology (EDSP) study, based on a sample of adolescents and young adults in Germany, are useful for assessing the incidence of anxiety disorders in early life. These data indicate that the age-of-onset of specific phobias peaks in early childhood, before all of the other subtypes, followed by social phobia in early adolescence, and panic disorder, agoraphobia, and generalized anxiety disorder, which begin to peak in late adolescence and early adulthood.[54] In the ECA, NCS, and NEMESIS samples, the highest overall incidence rates are observed in young adulthood (18–24 years), with a second peak in middle-age[45–64] that occurs earlier among males[45–54] than females.[55–64] [55,56]

Course

The chronicity of anxiety disorders is the persistence of the disorder over a given period. It is defined here as the percentage of respondents meeting diagnostic criteria for an anxiety disorder at baseline who meet criteria again at a follow-up interview. Data from the NESARC and NCS indicate that approximately 25% of people who

TABLE 164-1 TWELVE-MONTH PREVALENCE (%) OF ANXIETY DISORDER, OVERALL AND BY SUBTYPE, IN TWO NATIONAL SAMPLES OF THE USA

	Specific Phobia		Social Anxiety Disorder		Generalized Anxiety Disorder		Panic Disorder		Any anxiety disorder	
	NESARC	CPES[a]	NESARC	CPES	NESARC	CPES	NESARC	CPES	NESARC	CPES[b]
Total	7	9	3	6	2	4	2	3	11	10
Age 18–29 30–44 45–64 ≥65	8885	101094	3332	8862	2321	3551	2231	2431	1212127	1113114
Sex Male Female	510	512	23	67	13	35	13	24	815	812
Education Less than high school Completed high school Some college Bachelor's degree	7786	12987	3332	7676	2222	4444	3232	3232	12121310	11101110
Marital status Married or cohabiting Widowed, divorced, or separated Never married	787	8109	333	588	242	364	232	243	111311	91412

[a]Specific phobia was assessed in a subsample of 9282 respondents from the NCS-R.
[b]Specific phobia was not included in the overall anxiety disorder estimate for the CPES.

TABLE 164-2 TWELVE-MONTH PREVALENCE AND PERSISTENCE OF ANXIETY DISORDERS OVER 3-YEAR (NESARC) AND 10-YEAR (NCS) FOLLOW-UP PERIODS PERCENT

	NESARC		NCS	
	Baseline Prevalence	3-Year Persistence	Baseline Prevalence	10-Year Persistence
Specific phobia	7	28	8	37
Social anxiety disorder	3	24	8	30
Panic disorder	2	15	3	13
Generalized anxiety disorder	2	28	2	15
Any anxiety disorder	11	23	15	28

meet diagnostic criteria for any anxiety disorder at baseline experience chronicity (see Table 164-2). The overall chronicity of anxiety disorders and for individual subtypes is quite similar over the different periods of follow-up that were assessed (3 years for the NESARC and 10 years for the NCS). Specific phobia and social anxiety disorder are the most persistent subtypes, followed by generalized anxiety disorder and panic disorder. Similar estimates are observed in the Baltimore ECA sample that was assessed over 24 years of follow-up.[56]

Data from the NESARC indicate that there is high co-occurrence between anxiety and other mental disorders, and among the anxiety subtypes.[57] Data from the National Comorbidity Survey Replication (NCS-R) indicate that panic disorder, with or without agoraphobia, is most strongly associated with other anxiety disorders, especially generalized anxiety disorder, posttraumatic stress disorder, and mood disorders, especially bipolar disorder, as well as substance disorders, such as alcohol and illicit drug use disorders.[58] In adolescence, when the peak incidence of social anxiety disorder occurs, there are strong associations with other anxiety subtypes, especially phobias; mood disorders, especially persistent depressive disorder (dysthymia); and substance disorders, mainly for alcohol and nicotine.[59–61] In adults, there are relatively stronger associations between social anxiety disorder, generalized anxiety disorder, and bipolar disorder.[62] Generalized anxiety disorder has strong associations with mood disorders, especially major depressive disorder; substance disorders, especially nicotine; and other anxiety disorders, especially panic.[63,64] Finally, specific phobias have strong associations with other anxiety subtypes, especially social anxiety disorder; and mood disorders, especially major depressive disorder.[65] Overall, anxiety disorders frequently precede, co-occur, and follow other mental disorders. These patterns generally persist with the advancing age of study samples, and particularly in older adults.[66]

Data from the National Comorbidity Survey (NCS) of the United States suggest that anxiety disorders are associated with various physical conditions.[67] Panic attacks with or without agoraphobia are associated with vascular conditions, specific phobias with respiratory conditions, and social anxiety disorder with metabolic conditions. Blood-injection phobia is an important subtype of specific phobia that can interfere with medical care. The Baltimore ECA study reports an association between blood-injection phobia and vascular complications among individuals with diabetes.[68] In a German sample, blood-injection phobia is associated with respiratory conditions,[69] similar to the data on overall phobias in the NCS sample. Older adults with blood-injection phobia, with prevalence estimates ranging from 4% to 8%, also have an increased risk of hypertension relative to older adults without blood-injection phobia.[27,70] This increased risk might be related to the physiological aspects of anxiety, or possibly to avoidance of medical care and associated medications for lowering blood pressure.

Consequences

Anxiety disorders are, by definition, deemed by the individual to be distressing and/or to interfere with daily life. In the NEMESIS study, a diagnosis of anxiety disorder at baseline was associated with more suicidal ideation and a higher number of suicide attempts at 3 year follow-up, after adjustment for demographic characteristics and a history of mental disorders.[71] Similar findings were observed in the Christchurch Health and Development Study (CHDS) of New Zealander adolescents and young adults over 25 years of follow-up assessment,[72] and in cross-sectional studies of the NESARC and NCS-R samples of U.S. residing adults.[73]

Importantly, the findings of a recent systematic review and meta-analysis of prospective, longitudinal studies suggest that a diagnosis of any anxiety disorder at baseline is not associated with increased risk of all-cause mortality at follow-up.[74] In a population-based study of a 1946 U.K. birth cohort, lower levels of trait anxiety in adolescence were associated with higher risk of accident mortality at follow-up,[75] and in a population-based Norwegian

TABLE 164-3 ADVERSE LIFE EVENTS AT BASELINE AS PREDICTORS OF ANXIETY DISORDERS OVER 3 YEARS OF FOLLOW-UP IN THE NATIONAL EPIDEMIOLOGICAL SURVEY ON ALCOHOL AND RELATED CONDITIONS (NESARC), ADJUSTING FOR BASELINE SOCIODEMOGRAPHIC AND PSYCHIATRIC CHARACTERISTICS (*n* = 34,653)

	Odds Ratio (and 95% confidence interval)				
	Specific Phobia	Social Anxiety Disorder	Panic Disorder	Generalized anxiety Disorder	Any anxiety disorder
Age	0.99 (0.98–0.99)	0.98 (0.98–0.99)	0.98 (0.98–0.99)	0.99 (0.98–0.99)	0.99 (0.98–0.99)
Sex Male Female	Reference 2.00 (1.82–2.21)	Reference 1.18 (1.01–1.37)	Reference 1.79 (1.46–2.20)	Reference 1.96 (1.66–2.31)	Reference 1.87 (1.73–2.03)
Education Bachelor's degree or higher Some college Completed high school Did not complete high school	Reference 1.20 (1.06–1.37)1.22 (1.05–1.41)1.45 (1.21–1.72)	Reference 1.46 (1.18–1.80)1.65 (1.33–2.04)1.42 (1.07–1.88)	Reference 1.52 (1.20–1.93)1.30 (1.00–1.67)1.75 (1.31–2.34)	Reference 1.26 (1.04–1.54)1.10 (0.92–1.32)1.40 (1.11–1.77)	Reference 1.27 (1.15–1.39)1.22 (1.09–1.37)1.40 (1.22–1.61)
Relationship status Married or cohabiting Widowed Divorced or separated Never married	Reference 0.95 (0.77–1.19)1.13 (0.99–1.30)1.03 (0.90–1.18)	Reference 1.18 (0.80–1.77)1.48 (1.19–1.85)1.25 (1.03–1.52)	Reference 0.93 (0.57–1.53)1.00 (0.77–1.28)0.78 (0.60–1.01)	Reference 0.75 (0.55–1.04)1.09 (0.92–1.29)0.82 (0.67–0.99)	Reference 0.93 (0.77–1.12)1.11 (0.99–1.25)0.97 (0.87–1.07)
Any mood disorder Absent Present	Reference 2.24 (2.00–2.50)	Reference 3.87 (3.21–4.67)	Reference 2.52 (2.09–3.04)	Reference 3.70 (3.18–4.32)	Reference 2.77 (2.51–3.06)
Alcohol use disorder Absent Present	Reference 0.95 (0.80–1.13)	Reference 0.96 (0.73–1.28)	Reference 1.44 (1.07–1.93)	Reference 1.14 (0.90–1.43)	Reference 1.10 (0.96–1.26)
Any adverse event[a] Absent Present	Reference 1.26 (1.14–1.40)	Reference 1.04 (0.87–1.25)	Reference 1.55 (1.27–1.90)	Reference 1.29 (1.11–s1.50)	Reference 1.30 (1.20–1.42)

[a]Adverse events include the illness, injury, or death of a loved one, being fired or laid off, experiencing a financial crisis, being a victim of crime, or experiencing the dissolution of a relationship.

sample higher anxiety symptoms were associated with lower mortality among depressed individuals,[76] suggesting that some degree of anxiety is beneficial. A possible explanation for the apparent advantages of having some degree of anxiety may be that it plays a role in encouraging the individual to engage in preventive health behaviors: for example, women who worry about the possibility of breast cancer are more likely to seek routine screening,[77] people who are more worry-prone are likelier to vaccinate than those who worry less,[78] and smokers with higher worries about their health have been found to be likelier to quit.[79] In sum, excessive and insufficient levels of anxiety are both consequential, and should be assessed.

Risk Factors, Risk Assessment, and Prevention

The two strongest and most consistently observed risk factors for anxiety disorders in adulthood are female sex and younger age.[53,80] Retrospective reporting of childhood adversity has also been found to constitute a risk factor for anxiety disorder in cross-sectional studies.[81] A major modifiable risk factor that is associated with anxiety disorder onset is cigarette smoking,[82] and smoking cessation is associated with reduced anxiety[83] suggesting that smoking interventions would have a nontrivial effect on anxiety disorder onset. An important risk factor, as identified by longitudinal studies that assess anxiety disorder incidence as the outcome variable, is the occurrence of adverse life events, such as the dissolution of a relationship, or the injury, illness, or death of a loved one.[84-86] Table 164-3 displays odds ratios obtained from a set of five binary logistic regression analyses assessing the association of past-year adverse events at baseline as a predictor of anxiety disorders occurring within a 3-year follow-up period. The odds ratio relates the presence of any adverse event at baseline to the presence of any anxiety disorder at follow-up. The numerator of the odds ratio is the ratio of those who experienced an adverse event and developed an anxiety disorder to those who experienced an adverse event and did not develop an anxiety disorder. The denominator of the odds ratio is the ratio of those who did not experience an adverse event but developed an anxiety disorder to those who did not experience an adverse event and did not develop an anxiety disorder. Odds ratios greater than one indicate a higher risk of anxiety disorder and odds ratios below one indicate a lower risk of anxiety disorder.

The presence of adverse events at baseline is associated with an increased risk of overall anxiety disorder onset and for all subtypes with the exception of social anxiety disorder. As above, female sex and a history of any mood disorder at baseline are also associated with higher risk of anxiety disorder onset at follow-up. Although levels of educational attainment did not explain differences in the prevalence of anxiety disorders in Table 164-1, these results indicate that relatively lower educational attainment is associated with higher risk of anxiety disorder onset at follow-up. The combination of these results for prevalence and incidence suggests that the situation of less control of the individual's environment, experienced by those in lower levels of socioeconomic status, is a causal factor for anxiety disorder; but that the anxiety disorders among this group are more transient or more likely to remit. Excessive anxiety may be a result of licit or illicit substance use or abuse.[87-89] Anxiety disorders are also associated with increased substance use,[90] commonly interpreted as a form of self-medication for emotional distress.[91] Prescription medications may also include side effects that cause anxiety and should be carefully assessed, and recent withdrawal from the aforementioned substances can also be a cause of short-term anxiety.

TREATMENT

We now review the available evidence base for the treatment of anxiety disorders. We give first preference to recent studies that address the comparative effectiveness of different treatments by using the appropriate techniques of evidence synthesis (i.e., systematic reviews and network meta-analyses). If this information is unavailable, we rely on studies that address the effectiveness of treatments relative to nontreatment control groups by using techniques of evidence synthesis (i.e., systematic reviews and fixed or random-effects meta-analyses). In the case of specific phobia, for which there is a paucity of recent evidence, we also rely on some individual studies.

Panic Disorder with or without Agoraphobia

A recent Cochrane systematic review compared the comparative effectiveness of eight different psychological therapies and three different control conditions based on a network meta-analysis of 54 intervention studies.[92] Psychological therapy was found to be generally more effective than nontreatment for treatment response and remission. Although Cognitive Behavioral Therapy (CBT) was found to be mildly more effective than other forms of therapy, the strength of this evidence was considered weak due to various biases associated with the available studies. The investigators subsequently compared the association of CBT components with treatment response in these studies. They found that face-to-face administration of therapy (as compared to self-help modalities) and graded interoceptive exposure to the bodily sensations that accompany panic responses constitute relatively effective features of CBT treatments for panic disorder.[93] Virtual-reality exposure to scenarios that simulate real-life threats and progressive or applied muscle relaxation were found to reduce the probability of treatment response. There are ongoing efforts aimed at identifying the relative effectiveness of pharmacological interventions for panic disorder.[94]

Social Anxiety Disorder

A systematic review and network-meta analysis compared the effectiveness of 41 interventions and 17 control conditions. Individual CBT was strongly found to be the superior intervention for acute treatment of social anxiety disorder.[95] Selective Serotonin Reuptake Inhibitors (SSRIs) and Selective Norepinephrine Reuptake Inhibitors (SNRIs) are the most effective forms of pharmacotherapy. The National Institute of Health and Care Excellence (NICE) of the United Kingdom provides guidelines and recommendations for identifying, managing, and treating social anxiety disorder in children and adults.[96]

Generalized Anxiety Disorder

Two systematic reviews and meta-analyses reported that psychological therapy for generalized anxiety disorder has great short-term efficacy than nontreatment in younger and older adults.[97,98] A recent systematic review and network meta-analysis of 27 randomized, double blind, placebo-controlled studies compared the relative effectiveness of nine pharmacological treatments of generalized anxiety disorder.[99] Fluoxetine was found to be the superior choice for treatment response and remission, although sertraline was found to be the most tolerable medication. Sertraline has also been found to be the most cost-effective pharmacological treatment of generalized anxiety disorder, due in part to its tolerability.[100]

Specific Phobias

Exposure therapy is the treatment of choice for specific phobias.[101,102] The standard form of exposure therapy is the *in vivo* approach, which involves real-life exposure to phobic stimuli or situations. *Virtual reality* exposure therapy was first introduced over two decades ago as a treatment option for the fear of heights[103] and has since been found to show promise.[104] A one-session exposure therapy treatment for specific phobias was pioneered almost three decades ago,[105] although consideration is needed in choosing the appropriate number of sessions for particular patients.[106]

Pharmacotherapy is an uncommon treatment option for specific phobias. However, recent studies have investigated pharmacological augmentation of exposure therapy based on the administration of cortisol (thought to interfere with fear memories),[107,108] or D-cycloserine [thought to facilitate fear extinction due to its role as an *N*-methyl D-aspartate (NMDA) receptor agonist].[109,110] We focus here on the particular case of D-cylcoserine, because it is important to trade off any marginal benefit[111] against the risk of accelerating antibiotic resistance posed by the increasing administration of low doses of antibiotics in the population.[112,113]

CONCLUSION

Anxiety disorders have the highest prevalence of all mental disorders. The anxiety disorders are all associated with a higher engagement of threat detection or response mechanisms. The threats in question can be specific or diffuse, for example, in the cases of specific phobia and generalized anxiety disorder, respectively. Female sex is the most consistent and pronounced risk factor for anxiety disorders, and older adulthood may be a consistent protective factor against emotional distress. Adverse life events are also an important risk factor, and cigarette smoking is a key modifiable risk factor. The anxiety disorders have considerable chronicity and are associated with suicidal thoughts and behaviors, and should therefore be carefully assessed with the best available instruments. However, the absence of anxiety has also been observed to have adverse consequences, suggesting that a challenge of interventions is to reduce the anxiety to a sufficient but not excessive degree. The high prevalence of anxiety disorders, combined with their strong association with emotional distress, suggests the importance of efforts aimed at preventing new onsets in the population. There is mounting evidence for the effectiveness of short-term treatment options of anxiety disorder subtypes; however, little is currently known about the long-term efficacy of interventions.

References

1. Crocq M-A. A history of anxiety: From Hippocrates to DSM. *Dialogues Clin Neurosci.* 2015;17(3):319–25.
2. Darwin C. *The Expression of Emotion in Man and Animals.* United Kingdom: John Murray; 1872.
3. Bateson M, Brilot B, Nettle D. Anxiety: An evolutionary approach. *Can J Psychiatry.* 2011;56:707–15.
4. Marks IFM, Nesse RM. Fear and fitness: An evolutionary analysis of anxiety disorders. *Ethol Sociobiol.* 1994;15(5):247–61.
5. Miloyan B, Bulley A, Suddendorf T. Episodic foresight and anxiety: Proximate and ultimate perspectives. *Br J Clin Psychol.* 2016;55(1):4–22.
6. American Psychiatric Association. *Diagnostic and Statistical Manual of Mental Disorders.* 5th ed. Arlington, VA: American Psychiatric Association; 2013.
7. World Health Organization. *ICD-10 Classification of Mental and Behavioral Disorders—Diagnostic Criteria for Research.* 10th ed. Geneva: World Health Organization; 1993.
8. Moniz E. Prefrontal leucotomy in the treatment of mental disorders. *Am J Psychiatry.* 1937;93(6):1379–85.
9. Steele GDF. Persistent anxiety and tachycardia successfully treated by prefrontal leucotomy. *Br Med J.* 1951;2(4723):84–6.
10. Koenigs M, Huey ED, Calamia M, Raymont V, Tranel D, Grafman J. Distinct regions of prefrontal cortex mediate resistance and vulnerability to depression. *J Neurosci.* 2008;28(47):12341–8.
11. Koenigs M, Huey ED, Raymont V, et al. Focal brain damage protects against post-traumatic stress disorder in combat veterans. *Nat Neurosci.* 2008;11(2):232–7.
12. Feinstein JS, Adolphs R, Damasio A, Tranel D. The human amygdala and the induction and experience of fear. *Curr Biol.* 2011;21(1):34–8.
13. Myers-Schulz B, Koenigs M. Functional anatomy of ventromedial prefrontal cortex: Implications for mood and anxiety disorders. *Mol Psychiatry.* 2012;17(2):132–41.
14. Damasio A. *Descartes' Error.* New York: Putnam; 1994, p. 312.
15. Schneider B, Koenigs M. Human lesion studies of ventromedial prefrontal cortex. *Neuropsychologia.* 2017;107:84–93.
16. Bovasso G, Eaton W. Types of panic attacks and their association with psychiatric disorder and physical illness. *Compr Psychiatry.* 1999;40(6):469–77.
17. Briggs AC, Stretch DD, Brandon S. Subtyping of panic disorder by symptom profile. *Br J Psychiatry.* 1993;163(2):201–9.
18. Roberson-Nay R, Kendler KS. Panic disorder and its subtypes: A comprehensive analysis of panic symptom heterogeneity using epidemiological and treatment seeking samples. *Psychol Med.* 2011;41(11):2411–21.
19. Keyl PM, Eaton WW. Risk factors for the onset of panic disorder and other panic attacks in a prospective, population-based study. *Am J Epidemiol.* 1990;131(2):301–11.
20. McCabe L, Cairney J, Veldhuizen S, Herrmann N, Streiner DL. Prevalence and correlates of agoraphobia in older adults. *Am J Geriatr Psychiatry.* 2006;14(6):515–22.
21. Sheikh JI, Swales PJ, Carlson EB, Lindley SE. Aging and panic disorder: Phenomenology, comorbidity, and risk factors. *Am Geriatr Psychiatry.* 2004;12(1):102–9.
22. Wittchen HU, Reed V, Kessler RC. The relationship of agoraphobia and panic in a community sample of adolescents and young adults. *Arch Gen Psychiatry.* 1998;55(11):1017–24.
23. Depla MFIA, ten Have ML, van Balkom AJLM, de Graaf R. Specific fears and phobias in the general population: Results from the Netherlands Mental Health Survey and Incidence Study (NEMESIS). *Soc Psychiatry Psychiatr Epidemiol.* 2008;43(3):200–8.
24. Magee WJ, Eaton WW, Wittchen HU, McGonagle KA, Kessler RC. Agoraphobia, simple phobia, and social phobia in the National Comorbidity Survey. *Arch Gen Psychiatry.* 1996;53(2):159–68.
25. Stinson FS, Dawson DA, Patricia Chou S, et al. The epidemiology of DSM-IV specific phobia in the USA: Results from the National Epidemiologic Survey on Alcohol and Related Conditions. *Psychol Med.* 2007;37(7):1047–59.
26. Grenier S, Schuurmans J, Goldfarb M, et al. The epidemiology of specific phobia and subthreshold fear subtypes in a community-based sample of older adults. *Depress Anxiety.* 2011;28(6):456–63.
27. Miloyan B, Eaton WW. Blood-injection-injury phobia in older adults. *Int Psychogeriatr.* 2016;28(6):897–902.
28. Gretarsdottir E, Woodruff-Borden J, Meeks S, Depp CA. Social anxiety in older adults: Phenomenology, prevalence, and measurement. *Behav Res Ther.* 2004;42(4):459–75.
29. Miloyan B, Bulley A, Pachana NA, Byrne GJ. Social phobia symptoms across the adult lifespan. *J Affect Disord.* 2014;168:86–90.
30. Watkins ER. Constructive and unconstructive repetitive thought. *Psycholog Bull.* 2008;134(2):163–206.
31. Gonçalves DC, Byrne GJ. Who worries most? Worry prevalence and patterns across the lifespan. *Int J Geriatr Psychiatry.* 2013;28(1):41–9.
32. Lindesay J, Baillon S, Brugha T, et al. Worry content across the lifespan: An analysis of 16- to 74-year-old participants in the British National Survey of Psychiatric Morbidity 2000. *Psycholog Med.* 2006;36(11):1625–33.
33. Miloyan B, Bulley A. Worry in later life. In: Pachana NA, ed. *Encyclopedia of Geropsychology.* Singapore: Springer; 2017.
34. Robins LN, Helzer JE, Croughan J, Ratcliff KS. National Institute of Mental Health Diagnostic interview schedule. Its history, characteristics, and validity. *Arch Gen Psychiatry.* 1981;38(4):381–9.
35. Kessler RC, Ustün TB. The World Mental Health (WMH) Survey Initiative Version of the World Health Organization (WHO) Composite International Diagnostic Interview (CIDI). *Int J Methods Psychiatr Res.* 2004;13(2):93–121.
36. Di Nardo PA, O'Brien GT, Barlow DH, Waddell MT, Blanchard EB. Reliability of DSM-III anxiety disorder categories using a new structured interview. *Arch Gen Psychiatry.* 1983;40(10):1070–4.
37. Sheehan DV, Lecrubier Y, Sheehan KH, et al. The Mini-International Neuropsychiatric Interview (M.I.N.I.): The development and validation of a structured diagnostic psychiatric interview for DSM-IV and ICD-10. *J Clin Psychiatry.* 1998;59(Suppl 20):22–33, quiz 34–57.
38. Williams JB, Gibbon M, First MB, et al. The Structured Clinical Interview for DSM-III-R (SCID). II. Multisite test-retest reliability. *Arch Gen Psychiatry.* 1992;49(8):630–6.
39. Wing JK, Babor T, Brugha T, et al. SCAN. Schedules for clinical assessment in neuropsychiatry. *Arch Gen Psychiatry.* 1990;47(6):589–93.
40. Kroenke K, Spitzer RL, Williams JBW, Monahan PO, Löwe B. Anxiety disorders in primary care: Prevalence, impairment, comorbidity, and detection. *Ann Intern Med.* 2007;146(5):317–25.
41. Spitzer RL, Kroenke K, Williams JBW, Löwe B. A brief measure for assessing generalized anxiety disorder: The GAD-7. *Arch Intern Med.* 2006;166(10):1092–7.
42. Shear MK, Brown TA, Barlow DH, et al. Multicenter collaborative Panic Disorder Severity Scale. *Am J Psychiatry.* 1997;154(11):1571–5.

43. Shear MK, Rucci P, Williams J, et al. Reliability and validity of the Panic Disorder Severity Scale: Replication and extension. *J Psychiatr Res.* 2001;35(5):293–6.
44. Connor KM, Davidson JRT, Churchill LE, Sherwood A, Weisler RH, Foa E. Psychometric properties of the Social Phobia Inventory (SPIN): New self-rating scale. *Br J Psychiatry.* 2000;176(4):379–86.
45. Connor KM, Kobak KA, Churchill LE, Katzelnick D, Davidson JRT. Mini-SPIN: A brief screening assessment for generalized social anxiety disorder. *Depress Anxiety.* 2001;14(2):137–40.
46. Seeley-Wait E, Abbott MJ, Rapee RM. Psychometric properties of the Mini-Social Phobia Inventory. *Prim Care Companion J Clin Psychiatry.* 2009;11(5):231–6.
47. Norman SB, Cissell SH, Means-Christensen AJ, Stein MB. Development and validation of an Overall Anxiety Severity and Impairment Scale (OASIS). *Depress Anxiety.* 2006;23(4):245–9.
48. Norman SB, Campbell-Sills L, Hitchcock CA, et al. Psychometrics of a brief measure of anxiety to detect severity and impairment: The Overall Anxiety Severity and Impairment Scale (OASIS). *J Psychiatr Res.* 2011;45(2):262–8.
49. Bragdon LB, Diefenbach GJ, Hannan S, Tolin DF. Psychometric properties of the Overall Anxiety Severity and Impairment Scale (OASIS) among psychiatric outpatients. *J Affect Disord.* 2016;201(Suppl C): 112–5.
50. Eaton WW, Martins SS, Nestadt G, Bienvenu OJ, Clarke D, Alexandre P. The burden of mental disorders. *Epidemiol Rev.* 2008;30(1):1–14.
51. Kessler RC, Aguilar-Gaxiola S, Alonso J, et al. The global burden of mental disorders: An update from the WHO World Mental Health (WMH) Surveys. *Epidemiol Psichiatr Soc.* 2009;18(1):23–33.
52. Asnaani A, Richey JA, Dimaite R, Hinton DE, Hofmann SG. A cross-ethnic comparison of lifetime prevalence rates of anxiety disorders. *J Nerv Ment Dis.* 2010;198(8):551–5.
53. Grant B, Goldstein RB, Chou SP, et al. Sociodemographic and psychopathologic predictors of first incidence of DSM-IV substance use, mood and anxiety disorders: Results from the Wave 2 National Epidemiologic Survey on Alcohol and Related Conditions. *Mol Psychiatry.* 2009; 14(11):1051–66.
54. Beesdo K, Pine DS, Lieb R, Wittchen H-U. Incidence and risk patterns of anxiety and depressive disorders and categorization of generalized anxiety disorder. *Arch Gen Psychiatry.* 2010;67(1):47–57.
55. Bijl RV, De Graaf R, Ravelli A, Smit F, Vollebergh WAM, Netherlands Mental Health Survey and Incidence Study. Gender and age-specific first incidence of DSM-III-R psychiatric disorders in the general population. Results from the Netherlands Mental Health Survey and Incidence Study (NEMESIS). *Soc Psychiatry Psychiatr Epidemiol.* 2002;37(8):372–9.
56. Eaton WW, Alexandre P, Kessler RC, et al. The population dynamics of mental disorders. In: Eaton WW, ed. *Public Mental Health.* New York: Oxford University Press; 2012.
57. Grant B, Stinson FS, Dawson DA, et al. Prevalence and co-occurrence of substance use disorders and independent mood and anxiety disorders: Results from the National Epidemiologic Survey on Alcohol and Related Conditions. *Arch Gen Psychiatry.* 2004;61(8):807–16.
58. Kessler RC, Chiu WT, Jin R, Ruscio AM, Shear K, Walters EE. The epidemiology of panic attacks, panic disorder, and agoraphobia in the National Comorbidity Survey Replication. *Arch Gen Psychiatry.* 2006;63(4):415–24.
59. Schry AR, White SW. Understanding the relationship between social anxiety and alcohol use in college students: A meta-analysis. *Addict Behav.* 2013;38(11):2690–706.
60. Wittchen HU, Stein MB, Kessler RC. Social fears and social phobia in a community sample of adolescents and young adults: Prevalence, risk factors and co-morbidity. *Psychol Med.* 1999;29(2):309–23.
61. Wittchen HU, Fehm L. Epidemiology and natural course of social fears and social phobia. *Acta Psychiatr Scand Suppl.* 2003;(417):4–18.
62. Grant B, Hasin DS, Blanco C, et al. The epidemiology of social anxiety disorder in the United States: Results from the National Epidemiologic Survey on Alcohol and Related Conditions. *J Clin Psychiatry.* 2005;66(11):1351–61.
63. Grant B, Hasin DS, Stinson FS, et al. Prevalence, correlates, co-morbidity, and comparative disability of DSM-IV generalized anxiety disorder in the USA: Results from the National Epidemiologic Survey on Alcohol and Related Conditions. *Psychol Med.* 2005;35(12):1747–59.
64. Miloyan B, Byrne GJ, Pachana NA. Threshold and subthreshold generalized anxiety disorder in later life. *Am J Geriatr Psychiatry.* 2015;23(6):633–41.
65. Wardenaar KJ, Lim CCW, Al-Hamzawi AO, et al. The cross-national epidemiology of specific phobia in the World Mental Health Surveys. *Psychol Med.* 2017;47(10):1744–60.
66. Miloyan B, Byrne GJ, Pachana NA. Late-life anxiety. In: Pachana NA, Laidlaw K, eds. *The Oxford Handbook of Clinical Geropsychology.* United Kingdom: Oxford University Press; 2015, pp. 470–89.
67. Sareen J, Cox BJ, Clara I, Asmundson GJG. The relationship between anxiety disorders and physical disorders in the U.S. National Comorbidity Survey. *Depress Anxiety.* 2005;21(4):193–202.
68. Bienvenu OJ, Eaton WW. The epidemiology of blood-injection-injury phobia. *Psychol Med.* 1998;28(5):1129–36.
69. Witthauer C, Ajdacic-Gross V, Meyer AH, et al. Associations of specific phobia and its subtypes with physical diseases: An adult community study. *BMC Psychiatry.* 2016;16:155.
70. Sigström R, Östling S, Karlsson B, Waern M, Gustafson D, Skoog I. A population-based study on phobic fears and DSM-IV specific phobia in 70-year olds. *J Anxiety Disord.* 2011;25(1):148–53.
71. Sareen J, Cox BJ, Afifi TO, et al. Anxiety disorders and risk for suicidal ideation and suicide attempts: A population-based longitudinal study of adults. *Arch Gen Psychiatry.* 2005;62(11):1249–57.
72. Boden JM, Fergusson DM, Horwood LJ. Associations between exposure to stressful life events and alcohol use disorder in a longitudinal birth cohort studied to age 30. *Drug Alcohol Depend.* 2014;142:154–60.
73. Thibodeau MA, Welch PG, Sareen J, Asmundson GJG. Anxiety disorders are independently associated with suicide ideation and attempts: Propensity score matching in two epidemiological samples. *Depress Anxiety.* 2013;30(10):947–54.
74. Miloyan B, Bulley A, Bandeen-Roche K, Eaton WW, Gonçalves-Bradley DC. Anxiety disorders and all-cause mortality: Systematic review and meta-analysis. *Soc Psychiatry Psychiatr Epidemiol.* 2016;51(11):1467–75.
75. Lee WE, Wadsworth MEJ, Hotopf M. The protective role of trait anxiety: A longitudinal cohort study. *Psychol Med.* 2006;36(3):345–51.
76. Mykletun A, Bjerkeset O, Overland S, Prince M, Dewey M, Stewart R. Levels of anxiety and depression as predictors of mortality: The HUNT study. *Br J Psychiatry.* 2009;195(2):118–25.
77. Hay JL, McCaul KD, Magnan RE. Does worry about breast cancer predict screening behaviors? A meta-analysis of the prospective evidence. *Prev Med.* 2006;42(6):401–8.
78. Chapman GB, Coups EJ. Emotions and preventive health behavior: Worry, regret, and influenza vaccination. *Health Psychol.* 2006;25(1):82–90.
79. Dijkstra A, Brosschot J. Worry about health in smoking behaviour change. *Behav Res Ther.* 2003;41(9):1081–92.
80. Hasin DS, Grant B. The National Epidemiologic Survey on Alcohol and Related Conditions (NESARC) Waves 1 and 2: Review and summary of findings. *Soc Psychiatry Psychiatr Epidemiol.* 2015;50(11):1609–40.
81. McLaughlin KA, Conron KJ, Koenen KC, Gilman SE. Childhood adversity, adult stressful life events, and risk of past-year psychiatric disorder: A test of the stress sensitization hypothesis in a population-based sample of adults. *Psychol Med.* 2010;40(10):1647–58.
82. Mojtabai R, Crum RM. Cigarette smoking and onset of mood and anxiety disorders. *Am J Public Health.* 2013;103(9):1656–65.
83. Taylor G, McNeill A, Girling A, Farley A, Lindson-Hawley N, Aveyard P. Change in mental health after smoking cessation: Systematic review and meta-analysis. *BMJ.* 2014;348:g1151.
84. Francis JL, Moitra E, Dyck I, Keller MB. The impact of stressful life events on relapse of generalized anxiety disorder. *Depress Anxiety.* 2012;29(5):386–91.
85. Keyes KM, Pratt C, Galea S, McLaughlin KA, Koenen KC, Shear MK. The burden of loss: Unexpected death of a loved one and psychiatric disorders across the life course in a national study. *Am J Psychiatry.* 2014;171(8):864–71.
86. Taher D, Mahmud N, Amin R. The effect of stressful life events on generalized anxiety disorder. *Eur Psychiatry.* 2015;30:543.
87. Fenton MC, Keyes KM, Martins SS, Hasin DS. The role of a prescription in anxiety medication use, abuse, and dependence. *Am J Psychiatry.* 2010;167(10):1247–53.
88. Martins SS, Fenton MC, Keyes KM, Blanco C, Zhu H, Storr CL. Mood and anxiety disorders and their association with non-medical prescription opioid use and prescription opioid-use disorder: Longitudinal evidence from the National Epidemiologic Study on Alcohol and Related Conditions. *Psychol Med.* 2012;42(6):1261–72.
89. Melchior M, Prokofyeva E, Younès N, Surkan PJ, Martins SS. Treatment for illegal drug use disorders: The role of comorbid mood and anxiety disorders. *BMC Psychiatry.* 2014;14:89.

90. Martins SS, Gorelick DA. Conditional substance abuse and dependence by diagnosis of mood or anxiety disorder or schizophrenia in the U.S. population. *Drug Alcohol Depend.* 2011;119(1–2):28–36.
91. Khantzian EJ. The self-medication hypothesis of addictive disorders: Focus on heroin and cocaine dependence. *Am J Psychiatry.* 1985;142(11):1259–64.
92. Pompoli A, Furukawa TA, Imai H, Tajika A, Efthimiou O, Salanti G. Psychological therapies for panic disorder with or without agoraphobia in adults: A network meta-analysis. *Cochrane Database Syst Rev.* 2016;4:CD011004.
93. Pompoli A, Furukawa TA, Efthimiou O, Imai H, Tajika A, Salanti G. Dismantling cognitive-behaviour therapy for panic disorder: A systematic review and component network meta-analysis. *Psychol Med.* 2018;48(12):1945–53.
94. Guaiana G, Barbui C, Caldwell DM, et al. Antidepressants, benzodiazepines and azapirones for panic disorder in adults: A network meta-analysis. *Cochrane Database Syst Rev.* 2017;(7):CD012729.
95. Mayo-Wilson E, Dias S, Mavranezouli I, et al. Psychological and pharmacological interventions for social anxiety disorder in adults: A systematic review and network meta-analysis. *Lancet Psychiatry.* 2014;1(5):368–76.
96. Pilling S, Mayo-Wilson E, Mavranezouli I, Kew K, Taylor C, Clark DM. Recognition, assessment and treatment of social anxiety disorder: Summary of NICE guidance. *BMJ.* 2013;346:f2541.
97. Cuijpers P, Sijbrandij M, Koole S, Huibers M, Berking M, Andersson G. Psychological treatment of generalized anxiety disorder: A meta-analysis. *Clin Psychol Rev.* 2014;34(2):130–40.
98. Hall J, Kellett S, Berrios R, Bains MK, Scott S. Efficacy of cognitive behavioral therapy for generalized anxiety disorder in older adults: Systematic review, meta-analysis, and meta-regression. *Am J Geriatr Psychiatry.* 2016;24(11):1063–73.
99. Baldwin D, Woods R, Lawson R, Taylor D. Efficacy of drug treatments for generalised anxiety disorder: Systematic review and meta-analysis. *BMJ.* 2011;342:d1199.
100. Mavranezouli I, Meader N, Cape J, Kendall T. The cost effectiveness of pharmacological treatments for generalized anxiety disorder. *Pharmacoeconomics.* 2013;31(4):317–33.
101. Choy Y, Fyer AJ, Lipsitz JD. Treatment of specific phobia in adults. *Clin Psychol Rev.* 2007;27(3):266–86.
102. Wolitzky-Taylor KB, Horowitz JD, Powers MB, Telch MJ. Psychological approaches in the treatment of specific phobias: A meta-analysis. *Clin Psychol Rev.* 2008;28(6):1021–37.
103. Rothbaum BO, Hodges LF, Kooper R, Opdyke D, Williford JS, North M. Effectiveness of computer-generated (virtual reality) graded exposure in the treatment of acrophobia. *Am J Psychiatry.* 1995;152(4):626–8.
104. Arroll B, Wallace HB, Mount V, Humm SP, Kingsford DW. A systematic review and meta-analysis of treatments for acrophobia. *Med J Aust.* 2017;206(6):263–7.
105. Ost LG. One-session treatment for specific phobias. *Behav Res Ther.* 1989;27(1):1–7.
106. Abramowitz JS. The practice of exposure therapy: Relevance of cognitive-behavioral theory and extinction theory. *Behav Ther.* 2013; 44(4):548–58.
107. de Quervain DJ-F, Bentz D, Michael T, et al. Glucocorticoids enhance extinction-based psychotherapy. *Proc Natl Acad Sci U S A.* 2011;108(16):6621–5.
108. Soravia LM, Heinrichs M, Winzeler L, et al. Glucocorticoids enhance in vivo exposure-based therapy of spider phobia. *Depress Anxiety.* 2014;31(5):429–35.
109. Davis M. Role of NMDA receptors and MAP kinase in the amygdala in extinction of fear: Clinical implications for exposure therapy. *Eur J Neurosci.* 2002;16(3):395–8.
110. Ressler KJ, Rothbaum BO, Tannenbaum L, et al. Cognitive enhancers as adjuncts to psychotherapy: Use of D-cycloserine in phobic individuals to facilitate extinction of fear. *Arch Gen Psychiatry.* 2004;61(11):1136–44.
111. Mataix-Cols D, Fernández de la Cruz L, Monzani B, et al. D-cycloserine augmentation of exposure-based cognitive behavior therapy for anxiety, obsessive-compulsive, and posttraumatic stress disorders: A systematic review and meta-analysis of individual participant data. *JAMA Psychiatry.* 2017;74(5):501–10.
112. Opatowski L, Mandel J, Varon E, Boëlle P-Y, Temime L, Guillemot D. Antibiotic dose impact on resistance selection in the community: A mathematical model of beta-lactams and *Streptococcus pneumoniae* dynamics. *Antimicrob Agents Chemother.* 2010;54(6):2330–7.
113. Roberts JA, Kruger P, Paterson DL, Lipman J. Antibiotic resistance—What's dosing got to do with it? *Crit Care Med.* 2008;36(8):2433–40.

CHAPTER 165

Trauma- and Stressor-Related Disorders

Sarah R. Lowe • Jessica L. Bonumwezi • Veronica A. Pear • Magdalena Cerdá

INTRODUCTION

Trauma- and stressor-related disorders (TSRDs) are mental health conditions in which exposure to a triggering event is explicitly part of the diagnostic criteria. The most recent edition of the *Diagnostic and Statistical Manual of Mental Disorders*, the DSM-5,[1] contains five specific disorders in this category: posttraumatic stress disorder (PTSD), acute stress disorder (ASD), reactive attachment disorder (RAD), disinhibited social engagement disorder (DSED), and adjustment disorder (AD). Additionally, persistent complex bereavement disorder (PCBD) was added to the *DSM-5* as a condition for further study and is conceptualized as a TSRD, given that it would be diagnosed after a triggering event, the death of someone with whom the individual had a close relationship.

The purpose of this chapter is to review the public health literature on TSRDs. We begin by summarizing the empirical research on the prevalence and predictors of TSRDs. The vast majority of this literature has focused on the epidemiology of potentially traumatic events (PTEs) and PTSD and, as such comprise the bulk of our review. Subsequently, we review the literature on public health practices to decrease exposure to traumatic events and stressors, as well as to prevent and mitigate TSRDs. We conclude by making suggestions for future research and practice based on our review.

PTE EXPOSURE AND PTSD

PTEs are defined in the DSM-5 as experiences involving actual or threatened death, serious injury, or sexual violence.[1] PTEs can involve direct experiences of the event, witnessing the event occurring to someone else, learning that a relative or close friend was exposed to the event, or being exposed to aversive details of the event, typically through duties.[1] Along with PTE exposure, the diagnosis of PTSD requires at least one intrusion symptom (e.g., distressing dreams, dissociative reactions), one avoidance symptom (e.g., avoidance of trauma-related memories or situations), two symptoms indicating negative alterations of cognition and mood (e.g., inability to remember important parts of the event, feelings of detachment from others), and two arousal symptoms (e.g., hypervigilance, sleep disturbances). These symptoms must be present for at least 1 month and be associated with significant distress or impairment, and cannot be due to the effects of a substance or other medical condition. Slightly different criteria are applied for children age 6 and younger.[1]

Several changes were made to the DSM-5 diagnostic criteria for PTSD from prior versions of the DSM. Many of these changes center on how PTEs are defined. Whereas in the DSM-III and DSM-III-R, PTEs were defined as events occurring "outside the range of human experience," in the DSM-IV and DSM-IV-R they were described as involving "actual or threatened death or serious injury, or threat to the physical integrity of self or others" (criterion A1), as well as an emotional response of "fear, helplessness, or horror" (criterion A2). DSM-5 retained criterion A1, but dropped criterion A2. Further changes included the addition of the negative alterations and cognition and mood symptom cluster, and several minor revisions to the wording of symptoms in concordance with their typical expression.[2] These alterations are important to keep in mind insofar as they could affect prevalence estimates and patterns of predictors documented by studies using older versions of the DSM.

The epidemiologic literature on PTE exposure and PTSD using nationally representative samples is summarized in Table 165-1. In our review, we identified 38 studies from 27 countries. The majority of these studies ($n = 30$) included predominantly adult samples, for example, including participants over the age of 18 or within an age range covering early, middle, and older adulthood (e.g., refs. 3 and 34). The remainder ($n = 8$) focused on PTE exposure in PTSD among nationally representative samples of adolescents (e.g., refs. 11 and 39). The countries included cover low ($n = 1$), middle ($n = 6$), and high ($n = 19$) income countries, as classified by the World Bank. We draw on these studies when summarizing the prevalence of PTE exposure and PTSD. In examining the epidemiologic literature on predictors of PTEs and PTSD, we widened the scope of our review to include the more extensive body of literature using regionally representative samples in order to better document the breadth of factors that have been associated with each outcome.

PTE Prevalence

The prevalence of PTE exposure was documented in 25 of the 38 studies in Table 165-1. Lifetime exposure to PTEs among full samples (i.e., not broken down by gender or type of PTE exposure) ranged from 23.8% among Germans ages 14–93[13] to 86.9% among United States Americans ages 18–99.[35] Despite this variability, in most cases, the majority of study participants reported exposure to at least one traumatic event, and this was consistent across high-income countries, such as Australia,[4] Canada,[9] and the Netherlands,[20] and middle-income countries, such as Lebanon[8] and South Africa.[24] In addition to the aforementioned study in Germany,[13] only three investigations documented PTE prevalence estimates less than 50%, with 39.7% of persons ages 15–64 or older in Chile, 33.3% of adults ages 18–64 in South Korea,[25] 35.1% of 10- to 16-year-olds in the United States reporting at least one PTE. Notably, PTE prevalence estimates were not reported in the one country in our review classified as low income.

Several factors could account for the variability in PTE prevalence across studies. First, the variability could represent real cross-national differences in PTE exposure. Second, cross-national differences could reflect the extent to which different life experiences are perceived as traumatic in different contexts, or variation in participants' comfort with reporting PTEs. Third, the age range of participants included is likely to influence prevalences, such that older samples have had more time to experience a PTE. Notably, however, prevalence estimates above 50% have been documented among nationally representative adolescent samples, for example, in Denmark[11] and the United States.[39] Finally, a major consideration is variability in the number of events included across investigations. A trend across the studies was that those assessing fewer events tended to report lower prevalence estimates. For example, the four studies reporting prevalence estimates less than 50% each included fewer than 15 PTEs. It is worth noting, however, the large variation in prevalence estimates even across studies with a narrower range of PTEs assessed: for example, among those including 25 or more events, PTE prevalence ranged from 54% in Spain[26] to 86.9% in the United States.[35]

Predictors of PTE Exposure

Extant research has identified several factors that influence an individual's likelihood of being exposed to PTEs. These include demographic characteristics, social contextual factors, previous PTE exposure, and pre-existing mental health conditions.

Demographic characteristics. Some PTEs, such as childhood physical and sexual abuse, are inherently linked to age. However, the likelihood of exposure to other PTEs has been found to vary by age. In general, research suggests that PTE exposure decreases with age, with the exception of some types of traumatic events.[41] For example, a survey of Detroit residents found that risk of exposure to assaultive violence, injuries, and trauma to a close friend or family member was at its highest between the ages of 16 and 20, whereas the risk of exposure to the unexpected death of a loved one peaked between the ages of 40 and 45.[42]

The risk of exposure to different PTEs also varies by gender. Several studies have examined these gender differences in children and adolescents. For instance, girls have been found to be at an increased risk for interpersonal PTEs, such as sexual abuse and assault, physical assault by an intimate partner, stalking, and bereavement.[19,39] In contrast, boys have been shown to be at increased risk for exposure to nonsexual physical violence,[19,28] witnessing violence,[11,28] and serious accidents,[39] as well as a greater overall number of PTEs (e.g., refs. 43 and 44).

Epidemiologic studies have also found that race or ethnicity shape the risk of exposure, depending on the type of PTE. For instance, studies of adolescents showed that African American youth were more likely to be exposed to physical assault, unexpected death of a friend or family member, stalking, accidents, and witnessing violence, and that Hispanic children were more likely to experience intimate partner violence, stalking, accidents, and witnessing violence, compared to non-Hispanic White children.[32,39] Similar variation has been documented in adult samples. In a nationally representative sample of United States American adults, for example, non-Hispanic Whites were at increased risk of any direct or indirect PTE exposures, as well as exposure to bereavement, whereas non-Hispanic Blacks and Hispanics were at increased risk of childhood maltreatment and witnessing domestic violence, compared to their counterparts.[45]

Social contextual factors. Adolescents' risk of PTE exposure has been shown to be influenced by several social contextual factors. Three factors that have been consistently supported by the literature are lower household income (e.g., ref. 32), lower parental education (e.g., ref. 28), and parental unemployment (e.g., refs. 11 and 28). Moreover, some studies have found that children who do not live with both biological parents[28,39] are exposed to more traumatic events compared to other children.

In adults, income and education have also been found to be related to risk of PTEs. For example, one epidemiological study of adults living in urban areas of Mexico found that lower income and education were linked to higher risk of sexual assault, physical assault, and combat exposure, but lower risk of exposure to accidents, and threats with weapons.[44] Findings in the United States similarly suggest that urban adults of low socioeconomic status are at particularly high risk of assaultive violence.[42]

Other social contextual factors, such as community characteristics, have also been found to influence risk of exposure to traumatic events.[30,44] For instance, individuals living in urban areas show greater exposure to assaultive violence than those living in suburban areas.[42] Adolescents living in an urban environment have been shown to be at greater risk for physical abuse by a caregiver and for reporting that a loved one had experienced a PTE, but lower risk for car accidents.[39] Living in an area of higher socioeconomic status has also been found to decrease risk for any PTE exposure, and in particular assaultive PTE exposure.[6]

Prior PTE exposure and pre-existing mental health conditions. Epidemiologic studies have consistently found that prior PTE exposure is predictive of subsequent exposure, using both retrospective and prospective designs (e.g., refs. 30 and 46). Other research has linked different types of pre-existing mental health conditions to PTE exposure. For instance, PTSD symptoms have been linked to rape, and depression and drug use to physical assault.[47,48] Other studies have found anxiety disorders and drug use to predict exposure to both assaultive and sexual trauma trauma.[49] Additionally, more general classes of symptoms have been found to predict trauma exposure. For example, Breslau et al.[50] found that externalizing behaviors at age 6 predicted later exposure to assaultive violence. Similarly, Koenen et al.[51] found that difficult temperament, hyperactivity, antisocial behavior, and misconduct in childhood increased risk for PTE later in life.

PTSD Prevalence

PTSD prevalence was reported in all but 2 of the 38 nationally representative studies summarized in Table 165-1. As shown, there was substantial variability across the studies reviewed in the timeframe in which PTSD symptoms were assessed, ranging from current to lifetime. Among those assessing lifetime PTSD ($n = 19$), the prevalence ranged from 1.7% among adults ages 18–64 in South Korean[25] to 9.2% among adults ages 18 and older in Canada.[9] The prevalence in studies using a timeframe ranging from the past 6 months to the past year ($n = 21$) ranged from 0.4% past-year reported among adults in Israel, Italy, and Romania[8] to 4.7% past-year among adults in the United States.[40] Lastly, in studies that assessed PTSD up to the prior month ($n = 9$), prevalence estimates ranged from 1.3% past-month among adults in the Netherlands[21] to 44% past-month among adults ages 18 and older in Liberia.[18]

The latter findings are unexpected in that one would expect smallest estimates under the shortest timeframe. This pattern is likely in large part due to the differences in where past-year versus past-month PTSD was assessed (e.g., one would expect a higher maximum past-year and lifetime PTSD prevalence estimates had these timeframes been assessed in Liberia), but could also be due to other sources of variation across the studies, four of which were noted in our review. First, a variety of measures were used to assess PTSD across studies, including the World Mental Health Organization Composite International Diagnostic Interview (CIDI), PTSD Symptom Scale (PSS), and Harvard Trauma Questionnaire (HTQ). Subtle differences in the phrasing of items and response options could potentially affect prevalence estimates. Second, although all studies used the DSM classification system, there was variability in which version of the DSM was used, ranging from the DSM-III to DSM-5. This is significant given the aforementioned changes in the diagnostic criteria for PTSD, which have been shown to affect prevalence estimates of both PTE exposure and PTSD (e.g., refs. 52 and 53). Third, studies varied in their "reference event," that is, the PTE in which participants are to connect, or "anchor," any PTSD symptoms. Whereas some studies asked participants to report on PTSD symptoms in reference to the PTE identified as the "worst," that is, the most distressing or upsetting, others asked participants to report on symptoms in reference to all PTEs endured simultaneously. Investigators have noted that the former approach could lead to biased estimates of PTSD,[16,42] and therefore other studies, including those under the World Mental

TABLE 165-1 SUMMARY OF NATIONALLY REPRESENTATIVE STUDIES OF POTENTIALLY TRAUMATIC EVENT EXPOSURE AND POSTTRAUMATIC STRESS DISORDER

Author, Year	*Country*	*Study Name; N; Age Range*	*PTE Prevalence (# of PTEs Assessed)*	*PTSD Assessment (Instrument; Criteria; Index Event)*	*PTSD Prevalence (Timeframe)*
Chapman et al., 2013[3]; Mills et al., 2011[4]	Australia	2007 National Survey of Mental Health and Wellbeing; 8841; 18–65	74.9% (29)	CIDI, modified; DSM-IV; worst	7.2% (Lifetime); 4.4% (Past-year)
Creamer et al., 2001[5]; Rosenman, 2002[6]	Australia	1997 National Survey of Mental Health and Wellbeing; 10,641; 18+	57.4% (10)	CIDI, modified; DSM-IV, ICD-10; worst	1.3–1.5% (Past-year, DSM-IV); 3.6% (Past-year, ICD-10)
Darves-Bornoz et al., 2008[7]	Belgium	European Study of the Epidemiology of Mental Disorders; 1043; 18+	--	CIDI; DSM-IV; worst	0.8% (Past-year)
Karam et al., 2014[8]	Bulgaria	Bulgaria National Survey of Health and Stress; 2233; 18–98	--	CIDI; DSM-IV; worst and random	0.9% (Past-year)
Van Ameringen et al., 2008[9]	Canada	-- ; 2991; 18+	75.9% (18)	Canadian Community Health Survey (based on CIDI); DSM-IV; worst	9.2% (Lifetime); 2.4% (Current)
Benitez et al., 2009[10]	Chile	-- ; 2,978; 15–64+	39.7% (11)	CIDI; DSM-III-R; unspecified	4.4% (Lifetime)
Elklit, 2002[11]	Denmark	-- ; 390; 13–15	87% [girls], 78% [boys] (20)	HTQ; DSM-III-R; worst	9.0% (Lifetime)
Darves-Bornoz et al., 2008[7]; Husky et al., 2015[12]	France	European Study of the Epidemiology of Mental Disorders; 1436; 18+	72.7% (28)	CIDI; DSM-IV; worst and random	3.9% (Lifetime); 2.3% (Past-year)
Hauffa et al., 2011[13]	Germany	-- ; 2510; 14–93	23.8% (11)	PSS; DSM-IV; worst	2.9% (Current)
Darves-Bornoz et al., 2008[7]	Germany	European Study of the Epidemiology of Mental Disorders; 1323; 18+	--	CIDI; DSM-IV; worst and random	0.7% (Past-year)
Bödvarsdóttir and Elklit, 2007[14]	Iceland	-- ; 206; 13–15	77% [direct events], 79% [indirect events] (20)	HTQ; DSM-IV; worst	--
Alhasnawi et al., 2009[15]	Iraq	Iraq Mental Health Survey; 4332; 18+	--	CIDI; DSM-IV; unspecified	2.5% (Lifetime); 1.1% (Past-year)
Karam et al., 2014[8]	Israel	Israel National Health Survey; 4849; 21–98	--	CIDI; DSM-IV; worst and random	0.4% (Past-year)
Carmassi et al., 2014[16]; Darves-Bornoz et al., 2008[7]; Karam et al., 2014[8]	Italy	European Study of the Epidemiology of Mental Disorders; 1779, 18–100	56.1% (28)	CIDI; DSM-IV; worst and random	2.4% (Lifetime); 0.4–0.7% (Past-year)
Karam et al., 2014[8]; Karam et al., 2008[17]	Lebanon	Lebanese Evaluation of the Burden of Ailments and Needs of the Nation; 2857; 18–94	68.8% (10)	CIDI; DSM-IV; worst and random	3.4% (Lifetime); 1.6% (Past-year)
Johnson et al., 2008[18]	Liberia	-- ; 1666; 18+	--	PSS, modified; DSM-IV; unspecified	44% (Past-month)
Domanskaité-Gota et al., 2009[19]	Lithuania	-- ; 183; 13–17	80.2% (20)	HTQ; DSM-IV; worst	6.1% (Lifetime)
Bronner et al., 2009[20]	Netherlands	-- ; 2238; 18+	52.2% (12)	SRS-PTSD; DSM-IV; worst	3.8% (Current)
de Vries and Olff, 2009[21]	Netherlands	-- ; 1087; 18–80	80.7% (36)	CIDI; DSM-IV; worst	7.4% (Lifetime); 3.3% (Past-year); 1.3% (Past-month)
Darves-Bornoz et al., 2008[7]	Netherlands	European Study of the Epidemiology of Mental Disorders; 1094; 18+	--	CIDI; DSM-IV; worst	2.6% (Past-year)
Karam et al., 2014[8]	New Zealand	New Zealand Mental Health Survey; 7312; 18–98	--	CIDI; DSM-IV; worst and random	2.1% (Past-year)
de Albuquerque et al., 2003[22]	Portugal	-- ; 2606; 18–99	75.7% (10)	Short Screening Scale; DSM-IV; worst	7.9% (Lifetime); 5.3% (Current)
Florescu et al., 2009[23]; Karam et al., 2014[8]	Romania	Mental Health Study in Romania; 2357; 18–96	--	CIDI; DSM-IV; worst and random	0.4-0.7% (Past-year)

(*Continued*)

TABLE 165-1 SUMMARY OF NATIONALLY REPRESENTATIVE STUDIES OF POTENTIALLY TRAUMATIC EVENT EXPOSURE AND POSTTRAUMATIC STRESS DISORDER (*Continued*)

Author, Year	*Country*	*Study Name; N; Age Range*	*PTE Prevalence (# of PTEs Assessed)*	*PTSD Assessment (Instrument; Criteria; Index Event)*	*PTSD Prevalence (Timeframe)*
Atwoli et al., 2013[24]; Karam et al., 2014[8]	South Africa	South African Stress and Health Study; 4315; 18–92	73.8% (28)	CIDI; DSM-IV; worst and random	2.3% (Lifetime); 0.4–0.7% (Past-year)
Jeon et al., 2007[25]	South Korea	Korean Epidemiologic Catchment Area; 6258; 18–64	33.3% (11)	CIDI, Korean version; DSM-IV; worst	1.7% (Lifetime)
Karam et al., 2014[8]; Olaya et al., 2015[26]	Spain	European Study of the Epidemiology of Mental Disorders; 2121; 18–98	54% (28)	CIDI; DSM-IV; worst and random	2.2% (Lifetime); 0.6% (Past-year)
Frans et al., 2005[27]	Sweden	-- ; 1824; 18–70	80.8% (7)	PCL; DSM-IV; worst	5.6% (Current)
Landolt et al., 2013[28]	Switzerland	-- ; 6787; 9th graders (97% ages 14–17)	56.1% (13)	UCLA-RI, adolescent version; DSM-IV-TR; unspecified	4.2% (Current)
Karam et al., 2014[8]	Ukraine	Comorbid Mental Disorders during Periods of Social Disruption; 1719; 18–91	--	CIDI; DSM-IV; worst and random	2.0% (Past-year)
Weich et al., 2011[29]	United Kingdom	Adult Psychiatric Morbidity Survey 2007; 7325; 16+	--	Trauma Screening Questionnaire; DSM-IV; unspecified	2.9% (Past-week)
Finkelhor and Dziuba-Leatherman, 1994[30]	United States	National Youth Victimization Prevention Study; 2000; 10–16	35.1% (6)	--	--
Kessler et al., 1995[31]	United States	National Comorbidity Survey; 5877; 15–54	51.2% [women], 60.7% [men] (12)	Revised DIS, CIDI; DSM-III-R; worst	7.8% (Lifetime)
Rheingold et al., 2004[32]; Ford et al., 2010[33]	United States	National Survey of Adolescents; 4023; 12–17	83.3% (24)	Modified PTSD module from the National Women's Study; DSM-IV; unspecified	5.0% (Past-6-month)
Kessler et al., 2005[34]; Nickerson et al., 2012[35]; Karam et al., 2014[8]	United States	National Comorbidity Survey Replication; 5692; 18–99	86.9% (26)	CIDI; DSM-IV; worst and random	2.5–3.5% (Past-year)
McCauley et al., 2010[36]; Cisler et al., 2011[37]	United States	National Survey of Adolescents-Replication; 3614; 12–17	--	PTSD module of the National Survey of Adolescents and National Women's Study; DSM-IV; unspecified	7.0% (Lifetime); 3.9% (Past-6-months)
Pietrzak et al., 2011[38]	United States	National Epidemiological Survey on Alcohol and Related Conditions—Wave 2; 34,653; 18+	--	Module from the Alcohol Use Disorders and Associated Disabilities Interview Schedule; DSM-IV; worst	6.4% (Lifetime)
McLaughlin et al., 2013[39]	United States	National Comorbidity Survey Replication Adolescent Supplement; 10,123; 13–17	61.8% (19)	CIDI; DSM-IV; worst	4.7% (Lifetime)
Goldstein et al., 2016[40]	United States	National Epidemiologic Survey on Alcohol and Related Conditions-III; 36,309; 18+	68.6% (32)	AUDADIS-5; DSM-5; worst	6.1% (Lifetime); 4.7% (Past-year)

Note. When multiple studies were available for a given country, these are arranged sequentially. Abbreviations: AUDADIS = Alcohol Use Disorder and Associated Disabilities Interview Schedule; CIDI = World Health Organization Composite International Diagnostic Interview; DIS = Diagnostic Interview Schedule; DSM = *Diagnostic and Statistical Manual of Mental Disorders*; HTQ = Harvard Trauma Questionnaire; ICD = International Statistical Classification of Diseases and Related Health Problems; MINI = Mini International Neuropsychiatric Interview; PSS = PTSD Symptom Scale; PTE = potentially traumatic event; PTSD = posttraumatic stress disorder; SRS = Self-Rating Scale.

Health Survey Initiative (e.g., ref. 8) have used an approach to estimating PTSD for participants who have experienced multiple PTEs that combines self-reported symptoms in reference to the worst PTE as well as another randomly selected PTE, and weights estimates by the total number of PTEs endured. Lastly, the variability in the number of PTEs assessed could influence the prevalence of PTSD insofar as that participants typically only report on PTSD symptoms if they endorsed one or more PTE; studies using shorter PTE inventories could inadvertently exclude participants suffering from PTSD in reference to an excluded PTE.

Predictors of PTSD

Several of the demographic, social contextual, and mental health-related factors that are risk factors for exposure to PTEs are also risk factors for PTSD. Characteristics of PTE exposure have been linked to PTSD risk.

Demographic characteristics and social contextual factors. Findings regarding variation by age in risk for PTSD have been mixed. Among studies of children and adolescents, for example, some have found that older children and children who experience traumatic events later in childhood have an increased risk for PTSD,[54,55] whereas other have found that younger children have a higher risk for hyperarousal symptoms specifically.[11,19] Similar variability in risk for PTSD by age is found among adult samples.[6,13] In contrast, the literature has consistently identified female gender as a risk factor for PTSD across the lifespan (e.g., refs. 9, 25, 28, 31, 38, and 39). Additional demographic characteristic that have been linked to PTSD risk are first-generation immigration status,[39] and being previously married (i.e., divorced, separated, or widowed; e.g., refs. 9 and 38).

Factors indicative of low socioeconomic status at the individual level, including low parental education, living in a single parent household, low income and receipt of government assistance, increase the risk of both PTSD onset and chronicity.[19,38,39,55,56] Elevated rates of PTSD have also been documented among persons living in communities with low socioeconomic status.[6]

Pre-existing mental health conditions. Pre-existing trauma- and stress-related disorders, mood disorders, anxiety disorders, and substance use disorders have been found to increase the risk of developing PTSD after PTE exposure.[8,39,58] Additionally, mental health conditions in family members have been shown to be linked to increased PTSD risk in children.[55,57,59]

PTE characteristics and stressors. Characteristics of the traumatic events also shape PTSD risk. For example, different types of traumatic events differentially predict PTSD. Traumatic events that involve interpersonal violence, such as sexual assault, rape, physical assault, and child physical abuse, tend to confer the greatest risk for PTSD.[8,11,19,31,42,60] Among those experiencing the same PTE, more severe exposure to the event and greater postevent life disruption both increase PTSD risk.[61–63] For sexual assault specifically, survivors are most likely to develop PTSD when they were injured during the assault and when the perpetrator was someone they know.[64,65] Additional trauma exposure, both prior to and after the reference event, increases risk for PTSD onset and persistence (e.g., refs. 19, 39, and 66). Similarly, numerous studies have documented that experiencing a higher number of traumatic events in general increases PTSD risk (e.g., refs. 6, 9, 19, and 28). Experiencing a greater number of stressful life events (e.g., financial strain, relationship problems) following trauma exposure is associated with more severe PTSD symptomatology (e.g., refs. 67 and 68).

OTHER TSRDs

The epidemiologic literature on the prevalence and predictors of other TSRDs is scant compared to that on PTSD. Indeed, we know of no study investigating the prevalence and predictors of other TSRDs using nationally representative samples. In the following sections, we summarize the literature on other TSRDs using other epidemiologic methodologies and attend to factors that could perhaps account for why the research on these disorders is more limited.

Acute Stress Disorder

The DSM-5 diagnosis of ASD requires exposure to a PTE, and the presence of nine or more symptoms across five clusters (intrusion, negative mood, dissociation, avoidance, and arousal). The key differentiating factors between ASD and PTSD is symptom duration: for ASD, symptoms must be present for at least 3 days for up to 1 month after exposure to a PTE.[1] As with PTSD, the requirement of feelings of fear, helplessness or horror during PTE exposure (i.e., criterion A2) was dropped from the diagnostic criteria for ASD in DSM-5. Additionally, whereas DSM-IV required symptoms across four clusters (at least three dissociative, one intrusion, one avoidance, and one arousal symptom), DSM-5 allows for the nine required symptoms to be from any of the clusters. These changes are noteworthy given that only one epidemiologic study to our knowledge has assessed ASD using DSM-5 criteria.[69]

The short-term nature of ASD poses challenges to researchers seeking to document its prevalence and predictors. As discussed elsewhere,[70] such challenges include: the likelihood that only a few participants would have experienced a traumatic event during the prior month in general population samples; potential retrospective bias in having trauma-exposed participants report on their initial post-trauma symptoms; and difficulty securing funding and resources to assess a representative sample of survivors of the same mass traumatic event (i.e., an event that affects members of an entire community).

Despite these challenges, two studies to our knowledge have conducted studies of ASD using representative samples. First, Cohen and Yahav[71] conducted a population-based survey in northern and central Israel during the second Lebanon war in 2006, and found that 6.8% of the northern sample and 3.9% of the central sample met DSM-IV criteria for ASD. A further analysis of data from the study found that, among the northern sample, 20.3% of Arab participants met criteria for ASD, compared to 5.5% of Jewish participants.[72] Second, DSM-5 ASD was assessed in a representative sample of residents in the Philippines surveyed 3 weeks after a category 5 typhoon that struck the island in 2013.[69] The prevalence of ASD in this study was not reported, but participants meeting full criteria for the disorder had significantly higher psychological distress than those who did not.

An alternative approach to examining ASD is to assess consecutively admitted patients in the aftermath of a mass traumatic event. Notably, this approach does not capture representative samples, as survivors who present to the hospital are likely to have faced higher levels of exposure than those who do not, but does allow for explorations of the prevalence and predictors of ASD symptoms in the population of hospital admits. Liu and colleagues[73] conducted a study using this approach in the aftermath of the Wenchuan earthquake. Participants ($N = 118$) were consecutive admissions ages 5–18 at a local pediatric surgery department and, among them, 54.3% screened positive for DSM-IV ASD. Prevalence estimates were significantly higher among girls versus boys. In a multivariable model, indicators of more severe exposure and injuries (whether the participant was buried in the earthquake; whether the participant had a parent or relatives who was injured or killed during the earthquake; and whether the participants' injuries necessitated amputation or operation) were associated with more severe ASD symptoms.

A larger body of research has drawn on consecutive hospital admissions in a normative context—that is, not in the aftermath of a mass traumatic event—to estimate the prevalence and predictors of ASD.[74–85] Again, such studies are not representative of all trauma survivors, including survivors of trauma-related injuries that do not require immediate medical care and survivors of PTEs that generally do not result in injuries (e.g., bereavement, witnessing violence), but nonetheless provide insight into this topic. The prevalence of DSM-IV ASD across these studies ranged from 1.0% among admissions to a Level 1 trauma center in Australia[83] to 24% among victims of violence presenting at one of two emergency wards at a hospital in Denmark.[75] Significant predictors of ASD across these studies include a history of prior trauma exposure, pretrauma mental health problems, peritraumatic emotional responses (e.g., feelings of shock or hopelessness), more severe injuries, and lack of social support.[75,76,79,80,84]

Reactive Attachment Disorder and Disinhibited Social Engagement Disorder

RAD and DSED are conditions following extremes of insufficient care in childhood, including severe neglect and institutionalization.[1] RAD is an enduring pattern of social, emotional, and behavioral disturbance characterized by inhibition, emotional withdrawal, low positive affect, reduced responsiveness to others, and periods of irritability, sadness, or fearfulness. DSED, in contrast, is described as a behavioral pattern in which a child indiscriminately approaches and interacts with unfamiliar adults, with little or no reticence and with excessive familiarity. Both RAD and DSED require that the child be at least 9 months of age for diagnosis, and symptoms must be present by age 5 for RAD. In the DSM-5, RAD and DSED are listed as separate disorders with identical criteria for insufficient care, whereas the DSM-IV had inhibited and uninhibited subtypes under a single RAD diagnosis. For this reason, we have paired these two disorders in our review.

Two epidemiologic studies to our knowledge have shed light on the prevalence of RAD and DSED. First, using data from the Copenhagen County Child Cohort study, Skovgaard[86] found the prevalence of RAD to be 0.9% among 18-month-old infants. RAD in this study was diagnosed using criteria from the tenth edition of the International Statistical Classification of Diseases and Related Health Problems (ICD-10),[87] which, like the DSM-5, distinguishes between RAD and DSED. Second, in a study of all schoolchildren ages 6–8 in a deprived sector of a city in the United Kingdom, wherein it was assumed that child maltreatment would be higher than in the city as a whole, Minnis et al.[88] found the prevalence of DSM-IV RAD to be 1.4%; prevalence estimates for inhibited and disinhibited subtypes were not reported.

Additional epidemiologic studies of at-risk populations have used factor analytic methods to demonstrate the distinctiveness of RAD and DSED symptoms, suggesting that the prevalence of each DSM-5 disorder would be lower than the prevalence of DSM-IV RAD.[89–91] For example, a study of all Norwegian children ages 6–10 in long-term foster care provided support for a two-factor model with RAD symptom loading on one factor and DSED symptoms loading on the other.[91] Descriptively, the sample reported higher DSED symptoms than RAD symptoms, indicating that the latter are less common in this population. RAD and DSED factors were significantly and positively correlated, and both were associated with functional impairment and help-seeking behaviors.

Adjustment Disorder

DSM-5 AD is defined by emotional and behavioral symptoms associated with significant distress or impairment, occurring within 3 months of an identifiable stressor and not persisting for more than 6 months after the stressor has terminated.[1] Notably, the DSM-IV did not require a stressor for an AD diagnosis, such that AD could be given in cases of clinically significant distress that did not meet criteria for another diagnosis. Stressors specified in the DSM-5 include single events (e.g., divorce), multiple events (e.g., divorce and unemployment experienced simultaneously), recurrent problems (e.g., seasonal employment-related difficulties), continuous issues (e.g., living in neighborhood with high levels of crime), community-level events (e.g., natural disasters), developmental transitions (e.g., parenthood), and bereavement.[1] For a diagnosis of AD, stress-related symptoms must not meet criteria for another psychiatric disorder, cannot be an exacerbation of a pre-existing disorder, and are not indicative of socially normative bereavement. The DSM-5 further includes specifiers to delineate the nature of stress-related symptoms, for example, whether depressed mood, anxiety, or conduct problems are predominant, but no specific symptoms are required for an AD diagnosis. This lack of specificity is thought to have clinical utility in that the AD diagnosis can be given to a range of presentations that do not meet criteria for other disorders, but that nonetheless warrant clinical attention, yet has precluded systematic research on its prevalence and predictors.[92]

It is therefore not surprising that few studies have investigated AD in the general population. One study randomly sampled patients from primary-care centers in Catalonia, Spain, and found the prevalence of AD as defined in the DSM-IV to be 2.9%, with the majority of AD cases having either depressed mood or anxiety.[93] The results, of course, do not generalize to Catalonia residents who do not seek primary care. A study by Casey et al.[94] did not suffer from the same limitation, using data from a representative sample of urban and rural sites within Ireland, Britain, Norway, and Finland, and an urban site within Spain. The prevalence of AD in this study was only 0.3%. This study used ICD-10 criteria, which has considerable overlap with DSM-IV criteria.

In contrast, other researchers have explored the prevalence of AD using a markedly different conceptualization than in the DSM-5. More specifically, Maercker et al.[95] have proposed a *stress response model* wherein AD is defined by the presence of three clusters of symptoms (intrusion, avoidance, and failure to adapt) in the aftermath of a nonlife-threatening psychosocial stressor, and can be comorbid with other mental health conditions. The prevalence of AD under this model has been found to be 2.3% among a representative sample of Zurich, Switzerland residents aged 65–96,[96] and 0.9% among a representative sample of Germans aged 18–64.[97] Using data from the latter study, Glaesmer et al.[98] assessed AD using similar criteria—the proposed criteria for ICD-11, which consists of preoccupation with the stressor, failure to adapt, and symptoms of avoidance, depression, anxiety, and impulsivity. Under this definition, the prevalence was 2.0%.

Other epidemiologic research has focused on the prevalence of AD in at-risk populations. For example, a multisite study in Germany of consecutively enrolled patients with cancer found the DSM-IV prevalence of AD to be 12.4%, with increased risk among women, patients with higher education, and patients whose tumors had metastasized.[99] A further multisite study in Australia of consecutively enrolled injury patients found the prevalence of AD as defined in the DSM-5 to be 19% at 3 months postinjury and 16% at 12 months postinjury. AD at 3 months was predictive of AD as well as any non-AD psychiatric disorder at 12 months. A latent class analysis did not support the specifiers listed in DSM-5, but rather suggested that groups of participants were differentiated by symptom severity. Lastly, Dobricki, Komproe, de Jong, and Maercker[100] explored AD using the stress response model in four postconflict settings, and found that its prevalence ranged from 6% in Ethiopia to 40% in Algeria.

Persistent Complex Bereavement Disorder

PCBD was introduced to the DSM-5 as a condition for further study, informed by literature on how normal grief after the death of a loved one becomes pathological, including research on complicated grief (CG). PCBD is defined by clinically significant preoccupation, distress, and social or identity disruption following the death of a loved one that is out of proportion to cultural, religious, or age-appropriate norms, persisting for at least 12 months for bereaved adults and 6 months for bereaved children.[1]

Although no published epidemiological studies have explored the prevalence of PCBD as proposed in the DSM-5, at least five studies have investigated CG in general population samples and shed some light onto this issue. First, a study of the general German population reported a 3.7% prevalence of CG, assessed via the Inventory of Complicated Grief-Revised (ICG-R),[101] with significant predictors of CG risk being older age, female gender, lower income, having lost a child or spouse, and having experienced a death due to cancer.[102] Second, a 4.8% prevalence of CG was found among Dutch older adults using the ICG-R.[103] Significant predictors of CG in this study were older age, the death of a spouse or child, residence in a nursing home, lower education, and cognitive impairment. Third, a study of Swiss older adults found the prevalence of CG to be 4.2% using the Complicated Grief Module,[104] and 0.9% using the Inventory of Traumatic Grief-Revised.[105] Fourth, using the Brief Grief Questionnaire (BGQ),[106] a study of bereaved Japanese adults ages 40–79 found 2.4% to have CG,[107] with significant predictors being the relationship with the deceased, type of illness, time spent with the deceased, and unexpectedness of the death. Lastly, in a nationally representative study of Japanese adults ages 18 and older, Mizuno et al.[108] found the prevalence of CG, assessed with the BGQ to be 2.5%

among those who had experienced a significant loss. Female gender and less time since the death were associated with increased risk for CG. Taken together, the findings suggest that PCBD may be quite common and, like PTSD, related to demographic, trauma-related, and psychological characteristics. The studies also underscore that variability in prevalence estimates depend on the measure employed.

Other epidemiologic research has explored CG specifically in the aftermath of natural disasters. One study of first-degree relatives of the 84 Norwegians who lost their lives during the 2004 Southeast Asian tsunami found the prevalence of CG, assessed with the ICG, to be 47.4%, with significant predictors being female gender, predisaster unemployment, previous losses, disaster exposure, loss of a child, more time until the death was confirmed, and low social support.[109] Another study explored CG in a representative sample of Hurricane Katrina survivors—notably in relation to any significant loss, not exclusively bereavement.[110] The prevalence of CG in this study was 15.3% in the full sample, and 26.1% among participants who reported a significant loss. Bereavement had the highest conditional probability of CG relative to other losses (e.g., tangible losses, work/financial losses), and other significant predictors of CG included a greater number of hurricane-related stressors and predisaster psychopathology.

PREVENTION AND TREATMENT APPROACHES FOR TSRDS

Three general approaches are used to address PTEs, stressors, and TSRDs from a public health perspective. These include primary, secondary, and tertiary prevention.

Primary Prevention

Primary prevention strategies aim to either prevent PTEs from occurring or TSRDs from developing. General strategies include education, environmental change, and legislation and public policies. Education approaches aim to change social mores and norms through raising awareness. The evidence is limited about the effectiveness of this type of approach to reduce the occurrence of PTEs. For example, for the prevention of sexual violence, most psychoeducational interventions focused on increasing awareness or changing attitudes have not been effective.[111] However, school-based interventions that focus not only on changing norms, but also building skills have shown promising effects on violence.[112,113] For example, Safe Dates, a program that targeted eighth graders through theater and 45-minute classes with health and physical education teachers, and taught adolescents ways to communicate with their partners, verbal and nonverbal cues that their partner was not ready for sex, and dating tips to protect themselves from sexual dating violence, was associated with reduced risk of dating violence victimization and perpetration.[114]

In contrast, environmental change approaches, such as crime prevention through environmental design, treat PTEs as public health issues that can be prevented through investments in physical infrastructure and improvements to the physical environment.[115–117] Central principles[115,117,118] include that neighborhood designs should increase visibility through better lighting, more windows overlooking sidewalks, more pedestrian walkways, and fewer fences, and that physical deterioration of public spaces should be kept to a minimum. Findings on these types of approaches are promising: street lighting interventions,[119] remediation of blighted lots and buildings,[120] and other types of neighborhood infrastructure changes[118,121,122] have been associated with reduced crime and violence—PTEs associated with particularly high rates of TSRDs (e.g., refs. 8 and 31). Under similar principles, design of housing, neighborhoods, and cities to protect residents from infrastructure damage associated with major natural disasters, such as hurricanes and earthquakes, should prevent exposure to PTEs and stressors, such as bereavement, physical injury, and property loss.

Legislation and public policies also have the potential to reduce the incidence of PTEs, by banning or restricting risky behavior that is deemed to be unacceptable or to have an outsized cost, and by protecting local populations from the potential impact of PTEs. One of the leading types of legislative approaches to reduce exposure to violence, for example, has been legislation on the manufacture of, sales of, and access to firearms. The simultaneous implementation of laws targeting multiple elements of firearms regulations, including the ban of certain types of firearms, requirement of additional licenses per each firearm owned, mandated background checks, minimum age requirements for purchases, safer firearm storage regulations, and waiting periods, have been associated with reduced rates of firearm violence.[123] Legislation that assigns responsibility to perpetrators and other entities that have caused harm could also influence the likelihood that such events reoccur.[124] For example, the Violence Against Women Act (VAWA) criminalized acts of violence against women (e.g., stalking, intimate partner violence, acquaintance rape) and increased prosecution and penalties for these crimes. It also increased the amount of research on the causes and consequences of violence against women. VAWA grants to local governments have been associated with reductions in rape and assault.[125] In the case of natural disasters, sound plans for evacuation of residents in high-risk areas and transfer of medical care can prevent exposure to disaster-related PTEs and stressors.

Of course, trauma exposure cannot be eliminated completely and, as such, other primary prevention strategies focus on preventing trauma-related disorders after an event has occurred through early intervention. Early pharmacologic interventions have been used to prevent PTSD and ASD in individuals after PTE exposure. These include the administration of hydrocortisone, beta blockers, escitalopram, and temazepam, among others. Systematic reviews and meta-analyses of intervention evaluations suggest moderate support for the efficacy of hydrocortisone in preventing PTSD.[126,127] Recent studies of trauma-exposed emergency room patients have also provided evidence for the promise of early cognitive behavioral interventions and similar approaches such as "prolonged exposure" to prevent symptom development.[128,129]

Secondary Prevention

Unlike primary prevention efforts to prevent trauma and the development of TSRDs, secondary prevention aims to reduce TSRD symptoms in individuals with early signs of these disorders. A major aspect of secondary prevention consists of accurate identification of cases, which can be challenging in the early stages of TSRDs. Clinicians' assessment of patients' history of exposure to PTEs and stressors in initial evaluations to determine whether presenting problems are indicative of a TSRD are essential to case identification. Since many people suffering from TSRDs will not seek mental health treatment, other practitioners such as primary care and specialty physicians and personnel at social service agencies, should be educated about the psychological effects of PTEs and stressors and how to screen for TSRDs. Collaborative medical teams including physicians, social workers, and psychologists would also facilitate referrals for identified cases.

Once cases are identified, empirically supported treatments could be employed to reduce trauma-related psychopathology. To date, several treatments have received limited empirical support for reducing TSRD symptoms.[130,131] These include educational interventions, stepped collaborative care, psychotherapeutic interventions, and psychopharmacological therapies. Educational interventions attempt to normalize responses to PTEs and stressors. For example, clinic-based interventions aimed at parents and children after the child experienced traumatic injury, usually using educational booklets for parents and websites for children, have been associated with reduced anxiety symptoms in children, although evidence is inconsistent.[132,133] Stepped collaborative care interventions for acutely injured trauma survivors involve multicomponent interventions, including combined case management, pharmacotherapy, and psychotherapy, in trauma-care systems, and aim to integrate mental health interventions with acute injury care. Whereas collaborative-care interventions have evidence of effectiveness at improving depression, anxiety, and alcohol disorders,[134–136] little information is available on their effectiveness in reducing symptoms of TSRDs. One trial conducted among adults admitted to a level 1 trauma center found that, compared with usual care, patients randomized to collaborative care had a lower prevalence of PTSD.[137]

Early psychotherapeutic interventions aim to treat acute trauma- and stressor-related symptoms. While various psychotherapeutic interventions have been implemented within 3 months of a PTE to treat acute traumatic stress reactions, only trauma-focused cognitive behavioral interventions were found effective at reducing the likelihood of subsequent PTSD in this type of population.[138] Finally, early and brief administration of selective serotonin reuptake inhibitors (SSRIs) in the first month before the diagnosis and for 2–4 months following diagnosis of PTSD has been proposed as a way to alter the trajectory of the disorder. Although evidence is quite limited, one randomized controlled trial found that early administration of escitalopram, an SSRI, in the first month following a PTE did not prevent PTSD, but slightly decreased its severity, was associated with better quality of sleep, and was potentially beneficial for individuals exposed to intentional trauma.[139]

Tertiary Prevention

Finally, tertiary prevention involves methods to reduce the negative impact of existent disease by restoring functioning and reducing disease-related complications. As with secondary prevention, a major facet of tertiary prevention is the identification of PTSD and other TSRDs. Once cases are identified, tertiary prevention strategies include empirically supported treatments to decrease trauma-related symptom severity. Existing approaches include trauma-focused cognitive behavioral therapy (CBT), methylenedioxymethamphetamine (MDMA)-assisted psychotherapy for PTSD, psychotherapeutic approaches to complicated grief, and SSRIs to treat comorbid depression in cases of complicated grief. CBT approaches typically involve confrontation of memories or triggers related to the traumatic event (i.e., exposure therapy), and developing skills to manage anxiety and challenge distorted cognitions (i.e., cognitive restructuring).[130,131] Meta-analyses of randomized trials have found an improvement of PTSD treatment among those exposed to CBT.[140,141] Administration of MDMA along with psychotherapy has recently emerged as a novel treatment option, although the evidence is preliminary. A meta-analysis comparing MDMA-assisted psychotherapy with prolonged exposure therapy found that MDMA-assisted psychotherapy had a larger effect in clinician observed and self-reported outcomes, and lower dropout rates.[142] Promising psychotherapeutic approaches to treat PCBD specifically include CBT, supportive counseling interventions, or short-term group therapy. A meta-analysis suggested that such treatment interventions were efficacious in the alleviation of CG symptoms.[143] Finally, use of SSRIs in conjunction with psychotherapy for PCBD treatment may be effective in relieving comorbid depressive symptoms.[144]

An important consideration in the treatment of TSRDs is the occurrence of comorbid conditions. Whereas integrated treatments, in which the provider targets and attends to links between PTSD and any comorbid conditions, are generally recommended, in some cases, treatment of comorbid conditions should be prioritized to restore a level of functioning necessary to support the efficacy of trauma-focused therapies.[145,146] Similarly, interventions to address safety issues, barriers to mental health service utilization, and functional impairments could address pressing concerns that prevent patients from facing their traumatic experiences.[147,148] Collaboration between mental health practitioners and other professionals, including social workers and physicians, as well as engagement of loved ones in treatment, are essential to tertiary prevention.

CONCLUSION

This chapter reviewed the prevalence and risk factors for TSRDs, as well as approaches to prevent PTEs from occurring and TSRDs from developing, interventions to reduce TSRD symptoms in individuals with early signs of these disorders, and treatments to reduce the severity of symptoms among those with existing disorders. Our review highlights several key priorities for future research. First, while our review covered the range of TSRDs, the bulk of our understanding of these types of disorders is focused on PTSD. Hence, more research is needed to understand the magnitude of other TSRDs, including ASD, RAD, DSED, AD, and PCBD in the general population, how they develop over the lifecourse, who they affect, and what types of individual- and community-level features increase the risk of onset and persistence of these disorders. Second, differences in measurement of PTEs and instruments used to identify individuals meeting criteria for TSRDs likely lead to the marked variation found in the prevalence of TSRDs across different contexts. Multisite research consortia that use common instruments to measure the onset and prevalence of these disorders could improve our understanding of the public health burden posed by TSRDs. Third, limited evidence suggests that primary prevention approaches including skills-building educational interventions, environmental change approaches, and legislation have the potential to reduce the incidence of PTEs, while trauma-focused cognitive behavioral interventions have been found to be effective in reducing the likelihood and severity of PTSD. However, given the low to moderate quality of the evidence, investment is needed in quasiexperimental designs and randomized controlled trials to identify the types of prevention and treatment approaches that are most effective at reducing the onset and severity of the full range of TSRDs.

References

1. American Psychiatric Association. *Diagnostic and Statistical Manual of Mental Disorders*. 5th ed. Washington, DC: American Psychiatric Association; 2013.
2. Weathers FW, Marx BP, Friedman MJ, Schnurr PP. Posttraumatic stress disorder in DSM-5: New criteria, new measures, and implications for assessment. *Psychol Inj Law* 2014;7:93–107.
3. Chapman C, Mills K, Slade T, et al. Remission from post-traumatic stress disorder in the general population. *Psychol Med.* 2012;42(8):1695–703.
4. Mills KL, McFarlane AC, Slade T, et al. Assessing the prevalence of trauma exposure in epidemiological surveys. *Aust N Z J Psychiatry.* 2011;45:407–15.
5. Creamer M, Burgess P, McFarlane AC. Post-traumatic stress disorder: Findings from the Australian National Survey of Mental Health and Well-being. *Psychol Med.* 2001;31(7):1237–47.
6. Rosenman S. Trauma and posttraumatic stress disorder in Australia: Findings in the population sample of the Australian National Survey on Health and Wellbeing. *Aust N Z J Psychiatry.* 2002;36:515–20.
7. Darves-Bornoz JM, Alonso J, de Girolamo G, et al. Main traumatic events in Europe: PTSD in the European study of the epidemiology of mental disorders survey. *J Trauma Stress.* 2008;21:455–62.
8. Karam EG, Friedman MJ, Hill ED, et al. Cumulative traumas and risk thresholds: 12-Month PTSD in the World Mental Health (WMH) surveys. *Depress Anxiety.* 2014;00:1–13.
9. Van Ameringen M, Mancini C, Patterson B, Boyle MH. Post-traumatic stress disorder in Canada. *CNS Neurosci Ther.* 2008;14:171–81.
10. Benitez CP, Vicente B, Zlotnick C, et al. Estudio epidemiológico de sucesos traumáticos, trastorno de estrés post-traumático y otros trastornos psiquiátricos en una muestra representativa de Chile. *Salud Ment.* 2009;31:145–53.
11. Elklit A. Victimization and PTSD in a Danish national youth probability sample. *J Am Acad Child Adolesc Psychiatry.* 2002;41:174–81.
12. Husky MM, Lépine JP, Gasquet I, Kovess-Masfety V. Exposure to traumatic events and posttraumatic stress disorder in France: Results from the WMH survey. *J Trauma Stress.* 2015;28:275–82.
13. Hauffa R, Rief W, Brähler E, Martin A, Mewes R, Glaesmer H. Lifetime traumatic experiences and posttraumatic disorder in the German population. *J Nerv Ment Dis.* 2011;199(12):934–9.
14. Bödvarsdóttir Í, Elklit A. Victimization and PTSD-like states in an Icelandic youth probability sample. *BMC Psychiatry.* 2007;7:51.

15. Alhasnawi S, Sadik S, Rasheed M, Baban A, Al-Alak MM, Othman AY; the Iraq Mental Health Survey Study Group. The prevalence and correlates of DSM-IV in the Iraq Mental Health Survey (IMHS). *World Psychiatry.* 2009;8:97–109.
16. Carmassi C, Dell'Osso L, Manni C, et al. Frequency of trauma exposure and post-traumatic stress disorder in Italy: Analysis from the World Mental Health Survey Initiative. *J Psychiatr Res.* 2014;59:77–84.
17. Karam EG, Mneimneh ZN, Dimassi H, et al. Lifetime prevalence of mental disorders in Lebanon: First onset, treatment, and exposure to war. *PLoS Med.* 2008;5(4):0579–86.
18. Johnson K, Asher J, Rosborough S, et al. Association of combatant status and sexual violence with health and mental health outcomes in postconflict Liberia. *J Am Med Assoc.* 2008;300:676–90.
19. Domanskaité-Gota V, Elklit A, Christiansen DM. Victimization and PTSD in a Lithuanian national youth probability sample. *Nord Psychol.* 2009;61:66–81.
20. Bronner MB, Peek N, de Vries M, Bronner AE, Last BF, Grootenhuis MA. A community-based survey of posttraumatic stress disorder in the community. *J Trauma Stress.* 2009;22:74–8.
21. de Vries G, Olff M. The prevalence of traumatic events and posttraumatic stress disorder in the Netherlands. *J Trauma Stress.* 2009;22:259–67.
22. de Albuquerque A, Soares C, de Jesus PM, Alves C. Perturbação póstraumática do stress (PTSD): Avaliação da taxa de ocorrência na população adulta portuguesa. *Acta Méd Port.* 2003;16:309–20.
23. Florescu S, Moldovan M, Mihaescu-Pintia C, Ciutan M, Sorel GE. The Mental Health Study Romania 2007: Prevalence, severity, and treatment of 12-month DSM-IV disorders. *Manag Health.* 2009;4:23–31.
24. Atwoli L, Stein DJ, Williams DR, et al. Trauma and posttraumatic stress disorder in South Africa: Analysis from the South African stress and health study. *BMC Psychiatry.* 2013;13:182.
25. Jeon HJ, Suh T, Lee HJ, et al. Partial versus full PTSD in the Korean community: Prevalence, duration, correlates, comorbidity, and dysfunctions. *Depress Anxiety.* 2007;24:577–85.
26. Olaya B, Alonso J, Atwoli L, Kessler RC, Vilagut G, Haro JM. Association between traumatic events and post-traumatic stress disorder: Results from the ESEMeD-Spain study. *Epidemiol Psychiatr Sci.* 2015;24(2):172–83.
27. Frans O, Rimmo PA, Aberg L, Frederickson M. Trauma exposure and post-traumatic stress disorder in the general population. *Acta Psychiatr Scand.* 2005;111:29–299.
28. Landolt MA, Schnyder U, Maier T, Schoenbucher V, Mohler-Kuo M. Traumatic exposure and posttraumatic stress disorder in adolescents: A national study in Switzerland. *J Trauma Stress.* 2013;26:209–16.
29. Weich S, McBride O, Hussey D, Exeter D, Brugha T, McManus S. Latent class analysis of co-morbidity in the Adult Psychiatric Morbidity Survey in England 2007: Implications for DSM-V and ICD-11. *Psychol Med.* 2011;41:2201–12.
30. Finkelhor D, Dziuba-Leatherman J. Children as victims of violence: A national survey. *Pediatrics.* 1994;94:413–20.
31. Kessler RC, Sonnega A, Bromet E, Hughes M, Nelson CB. Posttraumatic stress disorder in the National Comorbidity Survey. *Arch Gen Psychiatry.* 1995;52:1048–60.
32. Rheingold AA, Smith DW, Ruggiero KJ, Saunders BE, Kilpatrick DG, Resnick HS. Loss, trauma exposure, and mental health in a representative sample of 12-17-year-old youth: Data from the national survey of adolescents. *J Loss Trauma.* 2004;9:1–19.
33. Ford JD, Elhai JD, Connor DF, Frueh BC. Poly-victimization and risk of posttraumatic, depressive, and substance use disorders and involvement in delinquency in a national sample of adolescents. *J Adolesc Health.* 2010;46:545–52.
34. Kessler RC, Chiu WT, Demler O, Walters EE. Prevalence, severity, and comorbidity of 12-month DSM-IV disorders in the National Comorbidity Survey Replication. *Arch Gen Psychiatry.* 2005;62:617–27.
35. Nickerson A, Aderka IM, Bryant RA, Hoffman, SG. The relationship between childhood exposure to trauma and intermittent explosive disorder. *Psychiatry Res.* 2012;197:128–34.
36. McCauley JL, Danielson CK, Amstadter AB, et al. The role of traumatic event history in non-medical use of prescription drugs among a nationally representative sample of US adolescents. *J Child Psychol Psychiatry.* 2010;51:84–93.
37. Cisler JM, Amstadter AB, Begle AM, et al. A prospective examination of the relationship between PTSD, exposure to assaultive violence, and cigarette smoking among a national sample of adolescents. *Addict Behav.* 2011;36:994–1000.
38. Pietrzak RH, Goldstein RB, Southwick SM, Grant BF. Prevalence and Axis I comorbidity of full and partial posttraumatic stress disorder in the United States: Results from Wave 2 of the National Epidemiological Survey on Alcohol and Related Conditions. *J Anxiety Disord.* 2011;25:456–65.
39. McLaughlin KA, Koenen KC, Hill ED, et al. Trauma exposure and posttraumatic stress disorder in a nationally representative sample of adolescents. *J Am Acad Child Adolesc Psychiatry.* 2013;52:815–30.
40. Goldstein RB, Smith SM, Chou SP, et al. The epidemiology of DSM-5 posttraumatic stress disorder in the United States: Results from the National Epidemiologic Survey on Alcohol and Related Conditions-III. *Soc Psychiatry Psychiatr Epidemiol.* 2016;51:1137–48.
41. Norris FH. Epidemiology of trauma: Frequency and impact of different potentially traumatic events on different demographic groups. *J Consult Clin Psychol.* 1992;60:409–18.
42. Breslau N, Kessler RC, Chilcoat HD, Schultz LR, Davis GC, Andreski P. Trauma and posttraumatic stress disorder in the community. *Arch Gen Psychiatry.* 1998;55:626–32.
43. Bunting BP, Ferry FR, Murphy SD, O'Neill SM, Bolton D. Trauma associated with civil conflict and posttraumatic stress disorder: Evidence from the Northern Ireland Study of Health and Stress. *J Trauma Stress.* 2013;26:134–41.
44. Norris FH, Murphy AD, Baker CK, Perilla JL, Rodriguez FG, Rodriguez JJG. Epidemiology of trauma and posttraumatic stress disorder in Mexico. *J Abnorm Psychol.* 2003;112:646–56.
45. Roberts AL, Gilman SE, Breslau J, Breslau N, Koenen KC. Race/ethnic differences in exposure to traumatic events, development of post-traumatic stress disorder, and treatment seeking for post-traumatic stress disorder in the United States. *Psychol Med.* 2011;41:71–83.
46. Finkelhor D, Ormrod RK, Turner HA. Re-victimization patterns in a national longitudinal sample of children and youth. *Child Abuse Negl.* 2007b;31:479–502.
47. Acierno R, Kilpatrick DG, Resnick H, Saunders B, de Arellano M, Best C. Assault, PTSD, family substance use, and depression as risk factors for cigarette use in youth: Findings from the National Survey of Adolescents. *J Trauma Stress.* 2000;13:381–96.
48. Acierno R, Resnick H, Kilpatrick DG, Saunder B, Best CL. Risk factors for rape, physical assault, and posttraumatic stress disorder in women: Examination of differential multivariate relationships. *J Anxiety Disord.* 1999;13:541–63.
49. Stein MB, Höfler M, Perkonigg A, et al. Patterns of incidence and psychiatric risk factors for traumatic events. *Int J Methods Psychiatr Res.* 2002;11:143–53.
50. Breslau N, Luca VC, Alvarado GF. Intelligence and other predisposing factors in exposure to trauma and posttraumatic stress disorder: A follow-up study at age 17 years. *Arch Gen Psychiatry.* 2006;63:1238–45.
51. Koenen KC, Moffitt TE, Poulton R, Martin J, Caspi A. Early childhood factors associated with the development of post-traumatic stress disorder: Results from a longitudinal birth cohort. *Psychol Med.* 2007;37:181–92.
52. Breslau N, Kessler RC. The stressor criterion in DSM-IV posttraumatic stress disorder: An empirical investigation. *Biol Psychiatry.* 2001;50:699–704.
53. Miller MW, Wolf EJ, Kilpatrick D, et al. The prevalence and latent structure of proposed DSM-5 posttraumatic stress disorder symptoms in U.S. national and veteran sample. *Psychol Trauma.* 2013;5:501–12.
54. Copeland WE, Keeler G, Angold A, Costello EJ. Traumatic events and posttraumatic stress in childhood. *Arch Gen Psychiatry.* 2007;64:577–84.
55. Hanson RF, Self-Brown S, Fricker-Elhai A, Kilpatrick DG, Saunders BE, Resnick H. Relations among parental substance use, violence exposure and mental health: The national survey of adolescents. *Addict Behav.* 2006;31:1988–2001.
56. Ahmad A, von Knorring A, Sundelin-Wahlsten V. Traumatic experiences and post-traumatic stress disorder in Kurdistanian children and their parents in homeland and exile: An epidemiological approach. *Nord J Psychiatry.* 2008;62:457–63.
57. Khamis V. Post-traumatic stress disorder among school age Palestinian children. *Child Abuse Negl.* 2005;29:81–95.
58. Thabet AA, Ibraheem AN, Shivram R, Winter EA, Vostanis P. Parenting support and PTSD in children of a war zone. *Int J Soc Psychiatry.* 2009;55:226–37.
59. Sack WH, Clarke GN, Seeley J. Posttraumatic stress disorder across two generations of Cambodian refugees. *J Am Acad Child Adolesc Psychiatry.* 1995;34:1160–6.
60. Resnick HS, Kilpatrick DG, Dansky BS, Saunders BE, Best CL. Prevalence of civilian trauma and posttraumatic stress disorder in a representative sample of women. *J Consult Clin Psychol.* 1993;61:984–91.
61. Ying L, Wu X, Lin C, Chen C. Prevalence and predictors of posttraumatic stress disorder and depressive symptoms among child survivors

1 year following the Wenchuan earthquake in China. *Eur Child Adolesc Psychiatry.* 2013;22:567–75.

62. Rosen CS, Cohen M. Subgroups of New York City children at high risk of PTSD after the September 11 attacks: A signal detection analysis. *Psychiatr Serv.* 2010;61:64–9.
63. Comer JS, Fan B, Duarte CS, et al. Attack-related life disruption and child psychopathology in New York City public schoolchildren 6-months post-9/11. *J Clin Child Adolesc Psychol.* 2010;39:460–9.
64. Broman-Fulks JJ, Ruggiero KJ, Hanson RF, et al. Sexual assault disclosure in relation to adolescent mental health: Results from the national survey of adolescents. *J Clin Child Adolesc Psychol.* 2007;36:260–6.
65. Lawyer SR, Ruggiero KJ, Resnick HS, Kilpatrick DG, Saunders BE. Mental health correlates of the victim-perpetrator relationship among interpersonally victimized adolescents. *J Interpers Violence.* 2006;21:1333–53.
66. Copeland WE, Keeler G, Angold A, Costello EJ. Traumatic events and posttraumatic stress in childhood. *Arch Gen Psychiatry.* 2007;64:577–84.
67. Lowe SR, Joshi S, Galea S, et al. Pathways from assaultive violence to post-traumatic stress, depression, and generalized anxiety symptoms through stressful life events: Longitudinal mediation models. *Psychol Med.* 2017;47(14):2556–66.
68. Tracy M, Norris FH, Galea S. Differences in the determinants of posttraumatic stress disorder and depression after a mass traumatic event. *Depress Anxiety.* 2011;28:666–7.
69. Lavenda O, Grossman ES, Ben-Ezra M, Hoffman Y. Exploring DSM-5 criterion A in acute stress disorder symptoms following natural disaster. *Psychiatry Res.* 2017;256:458–60.
70. Lowe SR, Blachman-Forshay J, Koenen KC. Epidemiology of trauma and trauma-related disorders: Trauma as a public health issue. In: Schnyder U, Cloitre M, eds. *Evidence-based Treatments for Trauma-related Psychological Disorders: A Practical Guide for Clinicians.* New York: Springer; 2015, p. 11.
71. Cohen M, Yahav R. Acute stress symptoms during the Second Lebanon War in a random sample of Israeli citizens. *J Trauma Stress.* 2008;21:118–21.
72. Yahav R, Cohen M. Symptoms of acute stress in Jewish and Arab Israeli citizens during the Second Lebanon War. *Soc Psychiatry Psychiatr Epidemiol.* 2007;42:830–6.
73. Liu K, Liang X, Guo L, et al. Acute stress disorder in the pediatric surgical children and adolescents injured during the Wenchuan earthquake in China. *Stress Health.* 2009;26:262–9.
74. Bryant RA, Creamer M, O'Donnell ML, Silove D, McFarlane AC. A multisite study of the capacity of acute stress disorder diagnosis to predict posttraumatic stress disorder. *J Clin Psychiatry.* 2008;69(6):923–9.
75. Elklit A, Brink O. Acute stress disorder in physical assault victims visiting a Danish emergency ward. *Violence Vict.* 2003;18:461–72.
76. Fugslang AK, Moergeli H, Hepp-Beg S, Schnyder U. Who develops acute stress disorder after accidental injuries. *Psychother Psychosom.* 2002;71:214–22.
77. Hamanaka S, Asukai N, Kamijo Y, Hatta K, Kishimoto J, Miyaoka H. Acute stress disorder and posttraumatic stress disorder symptoms among patients severely injured in motor vehicle accidents in Japan. *Gen Hosp Psychiatry.* 2006;28:234–41.
78. Harvey AG, Bryant RA. The relationship between acute stress disorder and posttraumatic stress disorder: A prospective evaluation of motor vehicle accident survivors. *J Consult Clin Psychol.* 1998;66:507–12.
79. Harvey AG, Bryant RA. Acute stress disorder across trauma populations. *J Nerv Ment Dis.* 1999;187:443–6.
80. Harvey AG, Bryant RA. Dissociative symptoms in acute stress disorder. *J Trauma Stress.* 1999;12:673–80.
81. Harvey AG, Bryant RA. Predictors of acute stress following motor vehicle accidents. *J Trauma Stress.* 1999;12:519–25.
82. Harvey AG, Bryant RA. The relationship between acute stress disorder and posttraumatic stress disorder: A 2-year prospective evaluation. *J Consult Clin Psychol.* 1999;67:985–8.
83. Creamer M, O'Donnell ML, Pattison P. The relationship between acute stress disorder and posttraumatic stress disorder in severely injured trauma survivors. *Behav Res Ther.* 2004;42:315–28.
84. Holeva V, Tarrier N, Wells A. Prevalence and predictors of acute stress disorder and PTSD following road traffic accidents: Thought control strategies and social support. *Behav Ther.* 2001;32:65–83.
85. Kassam-Adams N, Winston FK. Predicting child PTSD: The relationship between acute stress disorder and PTSD in injured children. *J Am Acad Child Adolesc Psychiatry.* 2004;43:403–11.
86. Skovgaard AM. Mental health problems and psychopathology in infancy and early childhood. *Dan Med Bul.* 2010;57:1–30.
87. World Health Organization: *The ICD-10 Classification of Mental and Behavioural Disorders: Clinical Descriptions and Diagnostic Guidelines.* Geneva: World Health Organization; 1992.
88. Minnis H, Macmillan S, Pritchett R, et al. Prevalence of reactive attachment disorder in a deprived population. *Br J Psychiatry.* 2013;202: 342–6.
89. Elovainio M, Raaska H, Sinkkonen J, Mäkipää S, Lapinleimu H. Associations between attachment-related symptoms and later psychological problems among international adoptees: Results from the FinAdo study. *Scand J Psychol.* 2015;56:53–61.
90. Kay C, Green J. Reactive attachment disorder following early maltreatment: Systematic evidence beyond the institution. *J Abnorm Child Psychol.* 2013;41:571–81.
91. Lehmann S, Breivik K, Heiervang ER, Havik T, Havik OE. Reactive attachment disorder and disinhibited social engagement disorder in school-aged foster children—A confirmatory approach to dimensional measures. *J Abnorm Child Psychol.* 2016;44:445–57.
92. Strain JJ, Friedman MJ. Considering adjustment disorders as stress response syndromes for DSM-5. *Depress Anxiety.* 2011;28(9):818–23.
93. Fernández A, Mendive JM, Salvador-Carulla L, et al. Adjustment disorders in primary care: Prevalence, recognition and use of services. *Br J Psychiatry.* 2012;201:137–42.
94. Casey P, Maracy M, Kelly BD, et al. Can adjustment disorder and depressive episode be distinguished? Results from ODIN. *J Affect Disord.* 2006;92:291–7.
95. Maercker A, Einsle F, Köllner V. Adjustment disorders as stress response syndromes: A new diagnostic concept and its exploration in a medical sample. *Psychopathology.* 2007;40:135–46.
96. Maercker A, Forstmeier S, Wagner B, Glaesmer H, Brähler E. Adjustment disorders, posttraumatic stress disorder, and depressive disorders in old age: Findings from a community survey. *Comp Psychiatry.* 2008;49:113–20.
97. Maercker A, Forstmeier S, Pielmaier L, Spangenberg L, Brähler E, Glaesmer H. Adjustment disorders: Prevalence in a representative nationwide survey in Germany. *Soc Psychiatry Psychiatr Epidemiol.* 2012;47: 1745–52.
98. Glaesmer H, Romppel M, Brähler E, Hinz A, Maercker A. Adjustment disorder as proposed for ICD-11: Dimensionality and symptom differentiation. *Psychiatry Res.* 2015;229:940–8.
99. Hund B, Reuter K, Härter M, et al. Stressors, symptom profile, and predictors of adjustment disorder in cancer patients. Results from an epidemiological study with the composite international diagnostic interview, adaptation for oncology (CIDI-O). *Depress Anxiety.* 2016;33:153–61.
100. Dobricki M, Komproe IH, de Jong JTVM, Maercker A. Adjustment disorders after severe life-events in four postconflict settings. *Soc Psychiat Epidemiol.* 2010;45:39–46.
101. Prigerson HG, Maciejewski PK, Reynolds CF, et al. Inventory of complicated grief: A scale to measure maladaptive symptoms of loss. *Psychiatry Res.* 1995;59:65–79.
102. Kersting A, Brähler E, Glaesmer H, Wagner B. Prevalence of complicated grief in a representative population-based sample. *J Affect Disord.* 2011;131:339–43.
103. Newson RS, Boelen PA, Hek K, Hofman A, Tiemeier H. The prevalence and characteristics of complicated grief in older adults. *J Affect Disord.* 2011;132:231–8.
104. Horowitz MJ, Siegel B, Holen A, Bonanno GA, Milbrath C, Stinson CH. Diagnostic criteria for complicated grief disorder. *Am J Psychiatry.* 1997;154(7):904–10.
105. Forstmeier S, Maercker A. Comparison of two diagnostic systems for complicated grief. *J Affect Disord.* 2006;99:203–11.
106. Shear KM, Jackson CT, Essock SM, Donahue SA, Felton CJ. Screening for complicated grief among Project Liberty service recipients 18 months after September 11, 2001. *Psychiatr Serv.* 2006;57:1291–7.
107. Fujisawa D, Miyashita M, Nakajima S, Ito M, Kato M, Kim Y. Prevalence and determinants of complicated grief in a general population. *J Affect Disord.* 2010;127:352–8.
108. Mizuno Y, Kishimoto J, Asukai N. A nationwide random sampling survey of potential complicated grief in Japan. *Death Stud.* 2012;36: 447–61.
109. Kristensen P, Weisæth L, Heir T. Predictors of complicated grief after a natural disaster: A population study two years after the 2004 South-East Asian tsunami. *Death Stud.* 2010;34:137–50.
110. Shear MK, Mclaughlin KA, Ghesquiere A, Gruber MJ, Sampson NA, Kessler RC. Complicated grief associated with hurricane Katrina. *Depress Anxiety.* 2011;28:648–57.

111. DeGue S, Valle LA, Holt MK, Massetti GM, Matjasko JL, Tharp AT. A systematic review of primary prevention strategies for sexual violence perpetration. *Aggress Violent Behav.* 2014;19(4):346–62.
112. Wolfe DA, Crooks C, Jaffe P, et al. A school-based program to prevent adolescent dating violence: A cluster randomized trial. *Arch Pediatr Adolesc Med.* 2009;163(8):692–9.
113. Rue LDL, Polanin JR, Espelage DL, Pigott TD. A meta-analysis of school-based interventions aimed to prevent or reduce violence in teen dating relationships. *Rev Educ Res.* 2017;87(1):7–34.
114. Foshee VA, Bauman KE, Ennett ST, Linder GF, Benefield T, Suchindran C. Assessing the long-term effects of the safe dates program and a booster in preventing and reducing adolescent dating violence victimization and perpetration. *Amer J Public Health.* 2004;94(4):619–24.
115. Jeffrey CR. *Crime Prevention through Environmental Design.* Beverly Hills, CA: Sage Publications; 1977.
116. Jeffrey CR. *Crime Prevention through Environmental Design.* Beverly Hills, CA: Sage Publications; 1971.
117. National Crime Prevention Council. *Best Practices for Using Crime Prevention through Environmental Design in Weed and Seed Sites.* Arlington, VA: National Crime Prevention Council; 2009.
118. Carter SP, Carter SL, Dannenberg AL. Zoning out crime and improving community health in Sarasota, Florida: "Crime prevention through environmental design." *Amer J Public Health* 2003;93(9):1442–5.
119. Welsh BC, Farrington DP. Effects of improved street lighting on crime. *Campbell Syst Rev.* 2008;13:1–51.
120. Painter K, Farrington DP. Street lighting and crime: Diffusion of benefits in the Stoke-on-Trent project. *Surveillance of Public Space: CCTV, Street Lighting and Crime Prevention.* Monsey, NY: Criminal Justice Press; 1999, pp. 77–122.
121. Foster S, Knuiman M, Villanueva K, Wood L, Christian H, Giles-Corti B. Does walkable neighbourhood design influence the association between objective crime and walking? *Int J Behav Nutr Phys Act.* 2014;11(1):100.
122. Painter K. The influence of street lighting improvements on crime, fear and pedestrian street use, after dark. *Landsc Urban Plan.* 1996;35(2):193–201.
123. Santaella-Tenorio J, Cerda M, Villaveces A, Galea S. What do we know about the association between firearm legislation and firearm-related injuries? *Epidemiol Rev.* 2016;38(1):140–57.
124. Sorenson S. Preventing traumatic stress: Public health approaches. *J Trauma Stress.* 2002;15(1):3–7.
125. Boba R, Lilley D. Violence Against Women Act (VAWA) funding: A nationwide assessment of effects on rape and assault. *Violence Against Women.* 2009;15(2):168–85.
126. Amos T, Stein DJ, Ipser JC. Pharmacological interventions for preventing post-traumatic stress disorder (PTSD). *Cochrane Database Syst Rev.* 2014;(7):CD006239.
127. Sijbrandij M, Kleiboer A, Bisson JI, Barbui C, Cuijpers P. Pharmacological prevention of post-traumatic stress disorder and acute stress disorder: A systematic review and meta-analysis. *Lancet Psychiatry.* 2015;2(5):413–21.
128. Bryant RA, Mastrodomenico J, Felmingham KL, et al. Treatment of acute stress disorder: A randomized controlled trial. *Arch Gen Psychiatry.* 2008;65(6):659–67.
129. Rothbaum BO, Kearns MC, Price M, et al. Early intervention may prevent the development of PTSD: A randomized pilot civilian study with modified prolonged exposure. *Biol Psychiatry.* 2012;72(11):957–63.
130. Schnyer U, Cloire M, eds. *Evidence Based Treatment for Trauma-related Psychological Disorders.* New York: Springer; 2015.
131. Foa E, Keane T, eds. *Effective Treatments for PTSD.* 2nd ed. New York: Guilford; 2008.
132. Cox CM, Kenardy JA, Hendrikz JK. A randomized controlled trial of a web-based early intervention for children and their parents following unintentional injury. *J Pediatr Psychol.* 2010;35(6):581–92.
133. Kenardy J, Thompson K, Le Brocque R, Olsson K. Information-provision intervention for children and their parents following pediatric accidental injury. *Eur Child Adolesc Psychiatry.* 2008;17(5):316–25.
134. Badamgarav E, Weingarten SR, Henning JM, et al. Effectiveness of disease management programs in depression: A systematic review. *Am J Psychiatry.* 2003;160(12):2080–90.
135. Williams JW Jr, Gerrity M, Holsinger T, Dobscha S, Gaynes B, Dietrich A. Systematic review of multifaceted interventions to improve depression care. *Gen Hosp Psychiatry.* 2007;29(2):91–116.
136. Oslin DW, Lynch KG, Maisto SA, et al. A randomized clinical trial of alcohol care management delivered in Department of Veterans Affairs primary care clinics versus specialty addiction treatment. *J Gen Intern Med.* 2014;29(1):162–8.
137. Zatzick D, Roy-Byrne P, Russo J, et al. A randomized effectiveness trial of stepped collaborative care for acutely injured trauma survivors. *Arch Gen Psychiatry.* 2004;61(5):498–506.
138. Roberts NP, Kitchiner NJ, Kenardy J, Bisson JI. Early psychological interventions to treat acute traumatic stress symptoms. *Cochrane Database Syst Rev.* 2010;(3):CD007944.
139. Zohar J, Fostick L, Juven-Wetzler A, et al. Secondary prevention of chronic PTSD by early and short-term administration of escitalopram: A prospective randomized, placebo-controlled, double-blind trial. *J Clin Psychiatry.* 2017;79(2):16m10730.
140. Bradley R, Greene J, Russ E, Dutra L, Westen D. A multidimensional meta-analysis of psychotherapy for PTSD. *Am J Psychiatry.* 2005;162(2):214–27.
141. Barrera TL, Mott JM, Hofstein RF, Teng EJ. A meta-analytic review of exposure in group cognitive behavioral therapy for posttraumatic stress disorder. *Clin Psychol Rev.* 2013;33(1):24–32.
142. Amoroso T, Workman M. Treating posttraumatic stress disorder with MDMA-assisted psychotherapy: A preliminary meta-analysis and comparison to prolonged exposure therapy. *J Psychopharmacol.* 2016;30(7):595–600.
143. Wittouck C, Van Autreve S, De Jaegere E, Portzky G, van Heeringen K. The prevention and treatment of complicated grief: A meta-analysis. *Clin Psychol Rev.* 2011;31(1):69–78.
144. Shear M, Reynolds CF3rd, Simon NM, et al. Optimizing treatment of complicated grief: A randomized clinical trial. *JAMA Psychiatry.* 2016;73(7):685–94.
145. Najavits L, Ryngala D, Back S, Bolton E, Mueser K, Brady K. Treatment of PTSD and comorbid disorders. In: Foa E, Keane T, Friedman M, Cohen J, eds. *Effective Treatments for PTSD.* 2nd ed. New York: Guilford; 2009.
146. Foa E, Chrestman K, Gilboa-Schechtman E. *Prolonged Exposure Therapy for Adolescents with PTSD.* New York: Oxford University Press; 2009.
147. Riggs D, Monson CM, Glynn S, Canterino J. In: Foa E, Keane T, eds. *Couple and Family Therapy for Adults, in Effective treatments for PTSD.* 2nd ed. New York: Guilford; 2008.
148. Lanktree C, Briere J. *Treating Complex Trauma in Children and Their Families: An Integrative Approach.* Los Angeles, CA: Sage; 2017.

CHAPTER

166 Tobacco Use and Tobacco Use Disorder

Renee D. Goodwin • Daniel Giovenco • Joanna M. Streck • Christine E. Sheffer • Jonathan M. Platt • Cristine D. Delnevo

Tobacco use remains a persistent human-made epidemic.[1,2] While a remarkable diversity of tobacco products is emerging, combustible tobacco products, cigarettes in particular, are responsible for the vast majority of tobacco-related disease and death. Indeed, cigarette smoking remains the leading preventable cause of disease and premature mortality[1,3] and the mortality risk from smoking has increased over time.[1,4] At current consumption rates, about 400 million adults worldwide will be killed by smoking between 2010 and 2050. Half a million adults die from smoking-related causes every year in the United States alone.[1,5,6] Smoking affects nearly every organ of the body and causes wide range of diseases and other adverse health effects. Smoking causes or contributes to nearly all the major causes of death in the U.S. including 16 different cancers, heart disease, chronic respiratory disease, cerebrovascular disease, diabetes, chronic liver disease, and kidney disease.[1]

Tobacco control efforts have dramatically decreased the prevalence of cigarette smoking in the United States, but the benefits of tobacco control efforts are not equitably distributed and remarkable tobacco-related cancer health disparities have emerged.[1,7] Tobacco-related disparities include a higher prevalence of daily smoking, lower rates of quitting, poorer responses to standard evidence-based treatments, less access to treatment, variation in healthcare providers' delivery of evidence-based tobacco use treatment, and an increased burden of tobacco-related cancers and other tobacco-related diseases.[1,8–11] For instance, individuals of lower socioeconomic status (SES) smoke at nearly three times the prevalence rate of higher SES individuals.[12] Cigarette-smoking rates for adults who are uninsured or on Medicaid are more than twice those for adults with private health insurance.[13] In 2015, 16.7% of non-Hispanic Black adults in the United States smoked cigarettes, compared with 15.1% of U.S. adults overall.[14] Higher tobacco use prevalence rates exist among sexual minorities,[15,16] persons with physical and intellectual disabilities,[17] serious mental illnesses,[1] and active military and veteran groups.[18] The prevalence of cigarette smoking among individuals in recovery from substance use disorders (SUDs) is two to four times greater than the prevalence of smoking in the general population.[19–21] All of these groups suffer disproportionately from tobacco-related disease. For instance, even after controlling for exposure levels, women are more likely to suffer from tobacco-related disease including lung cancer[22] and chronic obstructive pulmonary disease.[23] More than half of individuals who attain sustained remission from SUDs will die of tobacco-related diseases.[24,25] These tobacco-related disparities have a significant, and preventable, impact on the health and well-being of these vulnerable groups.

EPIDEMIOLOGY OF TOBACCO USE

First cultivated in the pre-Columbian Americas, tobacco was used for centuries by Native Americans in ceremonial and social gatherings. After the arrival of Europeans in the New World, the crop became a major global industry. In the United States, a wide variety of tobacco products were consumed, with chewing tobacco, pipes, and cigars becoming common products. Prior to the industrialization of cigarette rolling machines, other forms of tobacco use were prevalent. It was not until the early twentieth century that the popularity of cigarettes began to rise. The invention of the cigarette-rolling machine enabled the mass-production of cigarettes and revolutionized the commercialization and accessibility of tobacco products. From the 1940s onward, cigarettes were the dominant form of tobacco consumption. This has been shifting in recent years with increases in cigars as well as moist snuff. While e-cigarette consumption data are not available for comparison, the increase in electronic nicotine delivery systems (ENDS) has resulted in a highly diverse and complex tobacco marketplace.

Through widespread, targeted, and often deceptive marketing strategies, tobacco companies rapidly ascended to become a wealthy and powerful industry that addicted millions of users to its products.[26] By the 1960s, cigarette smoking was widespread across the U.S. and Europe. Indeed, nearly half of adults in the United States and the United Kingdom (U.K.) smoked cigarettes at that time.[27,28]

The epidemiological studies of Sir Richard Doll in the 1950s[29] and the 1964 U.S. Surgeon General's Report on Smoking and Health[30] are often credited with first publicizing the health risks of cigarettes and serving as catalysts for the subsequent decline in smoking prevalence. Indeed, as shown in Fig. 166-1, a number of major events are associated with decreases in per capita cigarette consumption—including more recently the 1998 Master Settlement Agreement and in 2009 the signing of the Family Smoking Prevention and Tobacco Control Act, which gave the FDA authority over cigarettes.

Despite notable decreases in rates of smoking over the past few decades,[31] tobacco remains a leading cause of death and disease worldwide. Moreover, significant disparities exist in tobacco use behaviors and tobacco-related health outcomes, with poorer individuals, those with mental health problems, and members of certain ethnic groups being disproportionately affected.[12,32] A growing concern is the shifting tobacco retail landscape and the recent popularity of noncigarette tobacco products,[33] which threaten the progress made by public health initiatives to combat smoking. This chapter provides an overview of common types of tobacco products, the epidemiology of tobacco use, effective tobacco control policies, and treatment of tobacco use disorders (TUDs).

TOBACCO PRODUCT CATEGORIES

Tobacco products exist on a risk continuum. The tobacco marketplace is more diverse than ever, but nearly all of today's tobacco products share an important unifying characteristic: nicotine. Moreover, important differences between tobacco product classes lie in the mechanisms and modes by which nicotine is delivered to the user.

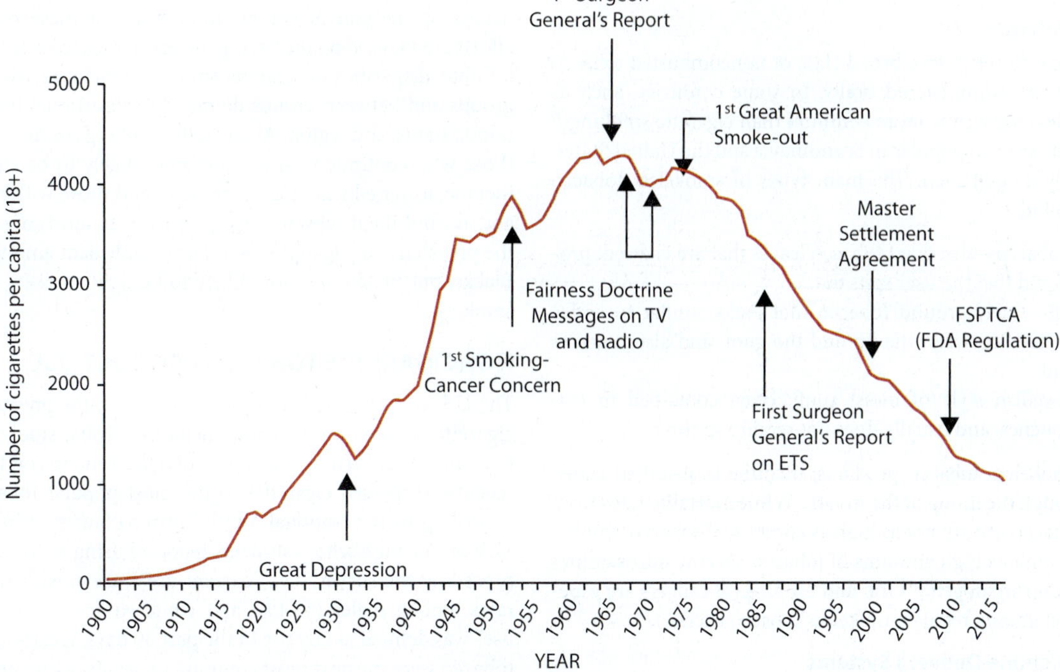

FIGURE 166-1. Adult per capita cigarette consumption and major smoking and health events—United States, 1900–2016. (*Source:* Adapted by C. Delnevo from Warner KE. *N Engl J Med.* 1985;312(6):384–8. Data prior to 2007 are abstracted from USDA Tobacco Outlook report, data from 2007 to date are abstracted from the Tobacco Tax Bureau (TTB).)

Though an extremely addictive chemical, nicotine itself is not particularly dangerous. Rather, exposure to other tobacco byproducts (e.g., tar, carbon monoxide, tobacco-specific nitrosamines, heavy metals) is primarily responsible for tobacco-related disease.[34] Indeed, the premise of medically approved nicotine replacement therapies is to satisfy the user's nicotine addiction while eliminating harmful tobacco constituents during a quit attempt. While no tobacco product is safe, it is generally accepted by medical and scientific communities that combustible products (i.e., those that are burned and inhaled) pose greater health risks to the user compared to noncombustible products, a result of the hundreds of toxins and carcinogens released during the combustion process.[1] Below are descriptions of the most popular combustible and noncombustible tobacco products in today's marketplace and population patterns in their use.

COMBUSTIBLE TOBACCO PRODUCTS

Cigarettes

Cigarettes, finely cut tobacco rolled in paper, are the most popular form of tobacco consumption and the primary contributors to the global disease burden of tobacco use.[1,35,36] Both cigarette smoking and exposure to second-hand smoke are causally linked to heart disease, lung disease, and several types of cancer.[37] Although the global prevalence of cigarette smoking has decreased in recent years to about 31% of men and 6% of women,[31] smoking rates remain much higher in certain parts of the world, including Russia, China, and many countries in Eastern Europe and Southeast Asia. For example, in 2015, over 65% of Indonesian males reported smoking.[38] Socioeconomic disparities exist in rates of cigarette smoking in the United States, as well as within low- and middle-income countries. That is, poorer individuals are more likely to smoke compared to those with greater wealth.[39] As a result of strict tobacco control regulations, such as smoke-free air policies and high taxation, the smoking prevalence has fallen to less than 20% in the United States, Canada, countries in Western Europe, and other high-income countries, but the tobacco industry is increasingly marketing its products in the developing world to maintain its consumer base.[35]

Cigars

Cigars are rolls of tobacco tightly wrapped in a tobacco leaf or in "reconstituted" paper that contains tobacco. The products vary widely in size and include large, traditional cigars, mid-sized "cigarillos," and filtered cigars that closely resemble cigarettes. Cigars have been used for centuries in Europe and the Americas, but experienced a resurgence in consumption beginning in the 1990s.[40] In the United States, for example, cigar sales have steadily risen over the last three decades, largely attributed to inexpensive, mass-produced cigars with filters that face weaker regulations compared to cigarettes.[41] In some Western countries, adolescents and young adults are known to use cigars and their wrappers as "blunts" to administer marijuana.[42,43] Despite some users' beliefs that cigar smoking is less risky than cigarette smoking, cigars contain the same cancer-causing toxins as cigarettes (often in higher volumes) and expose the user to carbon monoxide, tar, and carcinogenic nitrosamines. Although the two products are equally as hazardous from a chemical perspective, cigar smokers typically do not inhale and tend to use cigars less frequently, which may partially explain cigar users' lower rates of heart and lung disease compared to cigarette smokers.[44,45]

Hookah/Waterpipes

Originating in the Middle East, hookah use involves inhaling the smoke from a type of tobacco called "shisha" through a large waterpipe. Because the smoke passes through a water-filled chamber before it is inhaled, some users falsely believe that the smoke is "filtered" and therefore less risky.[46] In fact, it is well documented that hookah carries health risks that are similar to (and potentially worse than) other forms of combusted tobacco.[47] Hookah has become a global phenomenon, particularly among youth and young adults, and poses a serious public health concern. Contributing factors to the rise in hookah use include the widespread availability and popularity of flavored shisha, a thriving hookah bar/café culture, and weak tobacco control regulations.[48] Like cigar smoking, daily hookah use is uncommon and more typically occurs intermittently and in social settings.[48]

NONCOMBUSTIBLE TOBACCO PRODUCTS

Smokeless Tobacco

Smokeless tobacco refers to a broad class of noncombusted tobacco products that are administered orally. In some countries, such as India, smokeless tobacco is more common than cigarette smoking.[49] These products are also popular in Scandinavia and the United States, predominantly among men. The main types of smokeless tobacco worldwide include:

- Chewing tobacco—shredded tobacco leaves that are chewed, producing a liquid that the user spits out;
- Moist snuff—finely ground tobacco that looks similar to coffee grounds, placed between the lip and the gum, and also requires spitting; and
- Snus—a Swedish style of moist snuff, often contained in teabag-like pouches, and usually does not require spitting.

For all smokeless tobacco products, nicotine is absorbed transdermally through the lining of the mouth. While mortality rates from smokeless tobacco use are not as high as combusted tobacco, smokeless tobacco contains high amounts of tobacco-specific nitrosamines and is a known carcinogen.[50] Oral and esophageal cancers are especially common among regular smokeless tobacco users.[51]

Electronic Nicotine Delivery Systems

The newest class of tobacco products, and perhaps the category that has evolved most rapidly, are electronic nicotine delivery systems (ENDS). Known by a variety of terms including electronic cigarettes, e-cigarettes, vape pens, and vaporizers, ENDS entered mainstream retail markets in the late 2000s and quickly became a multibillion-dollar industry.[52] ENDS vary widely, ranging from small, cylindrical sticks that resemble cigarettes (often called "cigalikes") to complex devices that enable users to alter the battery power and add their own "e-liquid" with customized nicotine doses. Medical and scientific experts are beginning to reach consensus that ENDS are generally less risky than combusted cigarettes,[53,54] but the heterogeneity in device types, content of "e-liquids" and flavorings, as well as the relative novelty of ENDS, make it difficult to state their health risks with any precision. Studies on the efficacy of ENDS for smoking cessation have been mixed,[54] but emerging evidence suggests that frequent ENDS use is associated with higher odds of quitting cigarettes.[55,56] Some countries, such as England, have already begun recommending the devices to smokers who cannot quit using traditional methods.[57] ENDS use is most prevalent among current smokers and smokers who have recently quit, and is uncommon among individuals who have never used other types of tobacco.[54]

EPIDEMIOLOGY OF TOBACCO USE

Cigarette Smoking

In the United States, the prevalence of current cigarette smoking has declined considerably in the last half century.[14] Estimates indicate that overall approximately 20.9% of the U.S. population identified as smokers in 2005 dropping to an overall 15.1% self-identifying as smokers in 2015. It should be noted that a variety of tobacco surveillance systems monitor patterns in cigarette smoking, yielding varying estimates of behavior, we focus here on overall patterns of use. For example, consistent with patterns in developed nations, the prevalence of current cigarette smoking in the United States declined first among men and then later among women. Moreover, for much of the twentieth century, cigarette smoking was primarily defined as a daily pattern of use. However, in the early 1990s, nondaily cigarette smoking emerged as a stable pattern of use, and the proportion of nondaily cigarette smokers increased. Additionally, the proportion of daily smokers who report that they are light smokers (defined as smoking fewer than five to ten cigarettes per day) has also increased markedly over the last few decades. Historically, cigarette-smoking initiation occurs during adolescence and progression to regular smoking occurs by the end of young adulthood. For these reasons, recent efforts are focused on increasing the age of tobacco sale from 18 to 21. Of note, disparities in cigarette smoking remain across racial/ethnic groups and between groups defined by educational level, socioeconomic status, and region. As cigarette smoking continues to decrease, those who continue to smoke are more likely to be adults of lower income, lower educational attainment, and those with mental health and alcohol/illicit substance use problems. In terms of race/ethnicity, the prevalence of cigarette use is fairly equivalent among Whites and Blacks, but Blacks are more likely to be light smokers and menthol smokers.

NONCIGARETTE TOBACCO PRODUCT USE

The U.S. collects detailed population data on the prevalence of noncigarette tobacco product use, including cigars, smokeless tobacco, hookah, and electronic-cigarettes (ENDS). Among youth, ENDS have recently surpassed cigarettes as the most popular tobacco product, according to the National Youth Tobacco Survey.[58] In 2016, nearly 12% of U.S. high school students reported using ENDS in the 30 days preceding the survey (i.e., "current use") users, with slightly higher rates among males (13.1%) and white students (13.7%). "Current use" was defined as any use in the past 30 days. Cigars and smokeless tobacco were the next most common products, with current use rates of 7.7% and 5.8%, respectively. One exception to these patterns was seen among African American youth. Among these students, cigars and cigarillos were the most popular products (9.5%). Overall, youth frequently reported use of more than one tobacco product. The prevalence of polytobacco use among U.S. high school students in 2016 was approximately 8%. Noncigarette tobacco product use among youth in the United States appears to be higher compared to other high-income countries. For example, only 2% of youth in the United Kingdom and 5.7% of youth in Canada were current ENDS users in 2016.[59,60]

Among adults in the United States, cigarettes remain the most popular tobacco product, but rates of ENDS use have increased in recent years. The National Health Interview Survey revealed that in 2014, 3.5% of U.S. adults were current ENDS users.[61] "Current use" was defined as using the products every day or some days. ENDS use was significantly more common, however, among adults with a history of tobacco use. For example, 15% of current smokers were also current ENDS users in 2014.[62] Among former smokers who quit in the past year, the prevalence of current ENDS use was 18%.[62] Current use of other tobacco products, including smokeless tobacco (2.3%), cigars (3.4%), and hookah (1.2%) is more uncommon, but is considerably higher among young adults compared to the overall population.[61] As an example, 3.4% of 18- to 24-year olds in the United States are current hookah users, compared to an overall prevalence of 1.2%. For most tobacco products, patterns of use follow a socioeconomic gradient, with the highest rates of use reported among those at the lowest income level. Current use is rare among those at the highest income level.[61] Table 166-1 presents prevalence estimates of tobacco product use among adults in the United States. In the United Kingdom, use of ENDS is slightly higher than in the United States (5.7% among adults in 2016),[60] perhaps a result of Public Health England's endorsement of ENDS as a smoking cessation tool[63] (Table 166-2).

TRENDS IN TOBACCO USE

In recent years, there are increasing data to suggest that not only has the prevalence of cigarette use declined overall, but the amount/frequency of cigarette use (number of cigarettes per day (CPD) has also declined.[64] This is encouraging in that reducing the number of cigarettes consumed can lower risk of tobacco-related disease to some degree, although maximal benefits are only obtained when

TABLE 166-1 PREVALENCE OF CURRENT CIGARETTE USE (PAST 30 DAYS) AMONG U.S. PERSONS AGES 12 AND OLDER, 2015 NATIONAL SURVEY ON DRUG USE AND HEALTH

Characteristics	Overall (*N* = 57,146)	Current Smoker (*N* = 9826)	Former Smoker (*N* = 5705)	Never Smoker (*N* = 38,875)
	%	%	%	%
Age				
12–17	9.3	1.08	0.07	14.51
18–25	13.04	15.14	2.02	14.57
26–34	14.32	21.69	8.23	13.34
35–49	22.58	27.9	19.95	21.91
50–64	23.31	26.5	33.07	20.14
65 and older	17.45	7.69	36.66	15.54
Gender				
Male	48.46	55.11	55.79	44.16
Female	51.54	44.89	44.21	55.84
Total annual family income (USD)				
<$20,000	17.75	26.63	11.43	16.66
$20,000–$49,999	29.86	33.15	30.9	28.54
$50,000–$74,999	16.46	15.56	19.55	15.92
>=$75,000	35.93	24.67	38.12	38.87
Education				
Less than high school	12.82	18.44	12.11	11.36
High school graduate	23.03	33.1	25.55	19.23
Some college	27.69	34.01	30.51	24.66
College graduate	27.16	13.37	31.76	30.24
12–17 years old*	9.3	1.08	0.07	14.51
Race				
Non-Hispanic white	63.71	70.52	79.39	57.62
Non-Hispanic black	11.98	12.14	5.88	13.54
Non-Hispanic Native American/Alaskan Native	0.53	0.79	0.48	0.44
Non-Hispanic Native Hawaiian/Other Pacific Islander	0.28	0.22	0.13	0.34
Non-Hispanic Asian	5.45	2.8	2.1	7.29
Non-Hispanic more than one race	1.78	2.43	1.64	1.6
Hispanic	16.27	11.11	10.38	19.18
Marital status				
Married	47.81	37.48	65.62	46.54
Widowed, separated, or divorced	18.3	26.74	23.91	14.48
Never been married	24.59	34.7	10.4	24.47
12–17 years old	9.3	1.08	0.07	14.51

an individual quits entirely. While CPD has declined, possibly due to the increases in cost, recent data suggest that the prevalence of dependence on nicotine, or nicotine addiction (at least as measured by time to first cigarette in the morning on awakening), has increased over time among remaining smokers especially among those who are smoking fewer cigarettes,[64] suggesting that while persons have cut down increasingly on the number, they remain addicted to nicotine. Heavy or daily smoking have been a primary target of tobacco control for many years—and justifiably so—though increasingly evidence suggests that those who smoke fewer cigarettes or less frequently may emerge as an important target group for bringing the prevalence lower.

TOBACCO USE DISORDER

TUD is considered a mental disorder according to the American Psychiatric Association and the DSM-5.[65] TUD is characterized by a problematic pattern of tobacco use leading to clinically significant impairment or distress, as manifested by at least two of the following

TABLE 166-2 PREVALENCE OF CURRENT TOBACCO PRODUCT USE ("EVERY DAY" OR "SOME DAYS") AMONG U.S. ADULTS, 2015 NATIONAL HEALTH INTERVIEW SURVEY

	Cigarettes	Cigars/Cigarillos	Hookah/Waterpipe	Smokeless Tobacco[a]	ENDS[b]
Overall	15.1	3.4	1.2	2.3	3.5
Sex					
Male	16.7	6.0	1.8	4.4	4.3
Female	13.6	1.1	0.6	0.2	2.6
Age group					
18–24	13.0	4.2	3.4	3.2	5.2
25–44	17.7	3.9	1.3	2.7	4.3
45–64	17.0	3.7	0.5	2.1	3.3
≥65	8.4	1.7	0.6	1.2	1.1
Race/ethnicity					
White, non-Hispanic	16.6	3.7	1.2	3.2	4.1
Black, non-Hispanic	16.7	4.8	1.4	0.7	1.9
Hispanic	10.1	1.9	0.8	0.4	2.0
Asian, non-Hispanic	7.0	0.9	--	--	2.3
Other, non-Hispanic	20.8	6.8	--	--	7.1
Annual household income[d]					
<35,000	23.3	3.8	1.6	2.1	4.6
35,000–74,999	16.6	2.9	1.2	2.3	3.5
75,000–99,999	11.9	3.7	--	2.7	4.2
≥100,000	7.1	3.8	1.2	2.3	2.3

[a]Includes snus, snuff, chewing tobacco, or dip.
[b]ENDS: Electronic nicotine delivery systems.
[c]Estimate not presented due to small sample size.
[d]Income in U.S. dollars.

symptoms occurring within the past year: Tobacco is taken in larger amounts or over a longer period of time than intended, persistent desire or unsuccessful efforts to cut down/control use, large portion of time spent in activities to obtain or use tobacco, craving/desire to smoke, failure to fulfill major role obligations (i.e., clinical interference), important social, occupational or recreational activities are given up or reduced because of tobacco use, use of tobacco in situations when it is physically hazardous, continued use despite knowledge of physical or psychological problem that is likely to have been cause or made worse by tobacco use, tolerance, and tobacco withdrawal.[65] The diagnostic criteria for TUD are nearly identical to those for alcohol and illicit drug use disorders with key criteria including repeated use, unsuccessful attempts to quit, using more than intended, craving, tolerance, and withdrawal symptoms, though not all need to be present for a diagnosis. Historically, it has been thought that that TUD, formerly called "nicotine dependence" in DSM-IV[66] occurred either exclusively or primarily among heavy or daily smokers. Yet, recent data suggest that it is increasingly common among those smoking few cigarettes per day (e.g., 1–5) and among those who do not smoke daily.[64] This is positive news from a harm reduction perspective, as fewer cigarettes are being consumed. This change may be attributable to increased taxation, conscious attempts to reduce and/or smoke-free laws, but that there is an increasing proportion of the population who may meet criteria for TUD, though they may be neither daily smokers nor "heavy smokers."

EPIDEMIOLOGY OF TOBACCO USE DISORDER

Approximately 20% of persons ages 18 and older in the United States meet criteria for TUD, as of national U.S. data from the National Epidemiologic Survey on Alcohol and Related Conditions (NESARC-III). Relative to those without TUD, those with TUD are more likely to be male, younger, NH White and NH Native American and less likely to be Hispanic. Those with TUD are less likely to be married, tend to have incomes in the lowest group, and are less likely to have incomes in the highest group. Lower levels of educational attainment, and less likely to live in urban settings. Prevalence of any mental disorder, any mood disorder, and any anxiety disorder are substantially higher in TUD. Alcohol and illicit drug use disorder is almost twice as high among those with TUD; over half of those with TUD had lifetime alcohol use disorders and over 40% lifetime illicit drug use disorders (see Table 166-3). Persons with TUD are a vulnerable group—this is relevant because TUD is increasing even among lighter smokers[61] and traditional tobacco control efforts have not reached these groups. Therefore, to bring the overall prevalence lower, efforts that address these specific groups in novel ways may be needed.

ETIOLOGY OF TOBACCO USE DISORDER

Primary and established exposures associated with increased risk for tobacco use disorder include genetics,[67–73] parental smoking,[74–79] and prenatal exposure to tobacco,[80–82] psychiatric disorders (e.g., depression, anxiety),[76,83–89] age of onset of tobacco use,[68,90–96] other substance use including alcohol use,[31,97–106] and finally, peer smoking and social influence.[76,107–110]

GENETIC RISK

Twin studies have demonstrated a substantial amount of heritability of cigarette smoking including level of nicotine dependence and number of cigarettes smoked per day.[70] Nicotine withdrawal and associated symptoms following cessation have also been shown to be heritable with 31% and 51% of the variance in risk for withdrawal and failed cessation accounted for by genetics.[73] Genome-wide association

TABLE 166-3 TOBACCO USE DISORDER AMONG ADULTS 18 AND OLDER, BY DEMOGRAPHIC CATEGORIES, FROM THE NESARC III

	With TUD		Without TUD		
	n	%	*n*	%	chi-sq *p* value
Total	7,303	20.0	29,006	80.0	<.0001
Gender					
Men	3,804	55.9	12,058	46.1	<.0001
Women	3,499	44.1	16,948	53.9	
Age					
18–29	1,799	25.7	6,327	20.7	<.0001
30–44	2,257	30.1	7,878	24.6	
45–64	2,714	36.8	9,528	34.6	
65+	533	7.4	5,273	20.1	
Race/Ethnicity					
NH White	4,480	73.7	14,714	64.3	<.0001
NH Black	1,596	11.8	6,170	11.8	
NH Native American/AK Native	150	2.3	361	1.4	
NH Asian/Pacific Islander	198	3.2	1,603	6.4	
Hispanic	879	8.9	6,158	16.2	
Marital status					
Current	2,773	48.3	14,021	60.2	<.0001
Widowed, separated, divorced	2,205	24.7	7,218	18.4	
Never	2,325	27.0	7,767	21.4	
Personal income					
$0–19,999	3,978	53.0	12,950	42.2	<.0001
$20–34,999	1,646	21.3	6,440	20.5	
$35–69,999	1,303	19.1	6,465	23.3	
$70,000+	376	6.6	3,151	14.0	
Education					
Less than HS degree	1,416	18.2	4,074	11.7	<.0001
High school degree	4,226	57.9	13,555	44.8	
More than HS	1,661	24.0	11,377	43.5	
Urbanicity					
Urban	5,750	73.3	24,443	80.1	<.0001
Rural	1,553	26.7	4,563	19.9	
Psychiatric and substance use disorders					
Any lifetime mood disorder	2,356	32.3	5,697	19.8	<.0001
Any lifetime anxiety disorder	866	11.9	1,842	6.6	<.0001
Any lifetime mental disorder	627	8.4	1,965	6.8	<.0001
Any lifetime alcohol abuse/dependence	3,769	53.2	6,232	23.0	<.0001
Any lifetime drug use disorder	3,127	41.3	5,632	20.7	<.0001

studies have pointed to genes within the $\alpha_5/\alpha_3/\beta_4$ nicotinic cholinergic receptor gene complex on chromosome 15.[67,69,71,72]

ENVIRONMENTAL RISK

Risk of regular smoking and onset of a TUD in adolescence and adulthood is increased by maternal smoking during pregnancy, with a dose response relationship between the amount of prenatal nicotine exposure and subsequent risk of smoking among offspring.[80–82] Parental smoking has also been associated with future smoking and early onset of TUD in offspring.[74–79] Age of reaching specific smoking milestones such as age at first use of cigarettes is a risk factor for subsequent TUD.[90–96] Peer and/or social influence has been consistently identified as a predictor of development of a TUD in adolescence.[76,107–110] Finally, lower levels of educational attainment have also been associated with persistent smoking and onset of TUD.[76,100,111] Taken together, there are several prominent environmental risk factors for TUD, which are often targets of preventive interventions.

MENTAL DISORDERS AND SUBSTANCE USE

There is a strong association between mental disorders and SUDs and TUD. As can be seen in Table 166-3, mental disorders and SUDs are substantially more common among those with TUD, compared with those without, and recent evidence suggests that the prevalence of common mental disorders (e.g., depression) and substance use (e.g., cannabis use) is increasingly common among cigarette smokers. Mental disorders have been shown to both predict persistent smoking and are associated with increased risk for onset of TUD.[76,83–89] In terms of SUDs, including alcohol use disorders, both cross-sectional and longitudinal studies have demonstrated that SUDS are associated with increased likelihood of the onset of TUD and overall smoking initiation.[31,97–106] In sum, it would appear that a complex bidirectional relationship exists between TUD and mental health/SUDs. Ongoing research to understand how to best approach the integration of treatment for tobacco use and mental health/substance use is an active area of investigation.

TREATMENT FOR TOBACCO USE DISORDER

TUD occurs when individuals become dependent on tobacco products. In the DSM-5, TUD (305.1) is characterized with 3 criteria and 15 subfeatures. Specifiers include mild (ICD Z72.0: 2–3 symptoms), moderate (ICD F17.200: 4–5 symptoms), or severe (ICD F17.200: ≥ 6 symptoms). Determining the severity of TUD has implications for how it is treated. More severe presentations generally require more intensive, chronic treatment. Established standards for the evidence-based treatment of TUD are found in national clinical practice guidelines,[112–115] but are often supplemented by guidelines developed for specific populations, such as cancer patients[116] and pregnant women.[117]

ASSESSMENT

Treatment for TUD is ideally preceded by a thorough assessment of the physiological, psychological, social, and environmental factors associated with the maintenance of TUD. The results of the assessment help to tailor treatment of TUD to individuals' presentation. Assessment batteries are often tailored to setting, but often include the assessment of nicotine dependence and stress levels, motivation or readiness to quit, self-efficacy for achieving long-term abstinence, and history of psychiatric disorders. Recent research has highlighted the role of delay discounting[118] and impulsiveness,[119] but these elements are yet to be routinely incorporated into the clinical assessment of TUD. Because the occurrence of major depressive disorder and other SUDs are significantly associated with poor TUD outcomes, depression, and substance use screening measures are often used to determine potential past or current depressive diagnoses. Alcohol and other drug use is often assessed because even at low levels, substance use can affect individuals' success achieving long-term cessation.[120] Environmental factors often include partner or spouse smoking status, perceived social support for quitting, and tobacco use policies in the home.[121,122] Integrating the information from a multicomponent assessment ideally guides the development of a multicomponent evidence-based treatment plan for individuals with TUD.

The evidence-based treatment of tobacco dependence includes two basic components. cognitive-behavioral treatment (CBT) primarily addresses the psychological, social, behavioral, and environmental characteristics of the disorder. Pharmacotherapy addresses the physiological experience of withdrawal and/or blocks the pleasurable effects of tobacco use both of which function to reduce the negative and positive reinforcement of tobacco use. Optimally, treatment includes both CBT and pharmacotherapy because together they are much more effective than either one alone.[112]

CBT can be delivered in varying intensities, but all evidence-based "counseling" interventions for TUD are based on cognitive-behavioral principles.[123,124] CBT promotes understanding of the cue-urge-response cycle, awareness of conditioned internal and external cues encountered in daily life, and the development of strategies to manage urges to use tobacco.[123,124] As part of this process, CBT incorporates learning self-control over one's thoughts, behaviors, and feelings as reactions and emotions are monitored and thoughts and reactions are restructured (cognitive restructuring) as well as learning to activate specific behaviors in a range of contexts through anticipation of high-risk situations and planning (behavioral activation).[123,125] The acquired skills are often singularly described as self-monitoring, impulse control, stimulus control, stress management, problem solving, etc.

As evidenced by the high proportion of those who attempt to quit every year (>50%) compared with those who achieve abstinence (<10%) and the mean number of mean attempts (>20 per individual), the extended process of achieving long-term abstinence is fraught with relapse and motivational ambivalence.[126] Although not effective as a treatment in and of itself specifically for TUD, motivational interviewing is an evidence-based intervention for enhancing motivation for and readiness to quit, a necessary element for individuals to initiate and persevere throughout the process of achieving long-term abstinence.[127,128]

Cognitive-behavioral treatment manuals are often used to ensure patients are exposed to multiple components of treatment in a logical, programmatic manner, and to standardize treatment delivery. Many treatment manuals have been refined through decades of research, but essentially treatment sessions are offered weekly over 6–8 weeks as individuals are exposed to content and treatment-related activities in a step-by-step manner.[129,130]

CBT can be delivered efficaciously to individuals with TUD in groups, individually, and over the telephone. CBT is efficacious for the cessation of cigarettes as well as smokeless tobacco products.[131–133] Each treatment modality has unique strengths and weaknesses. When the same treatment content is delivered in different modalities no differences in long-term treatment outcomes are observed.[129,134] At present, free treatment for tobacco dependence is available by telephone in every state in the United States through state-funded *Quitlines*.[135,136] Treatment delivered by Quitlines has demonstrated scalability, reaching an unprecedented 1% of all U.S. smokers each year.[135,137,138] Detailed reports of Quitline services are published by the North American Quitline Association and are easily accessible (NAQC: http://www.naquitline.org/).

Pharmacotherapy options currently approved by the Federal Drug Administration (FDA) for smoking cessation include nicotine replacement therapy (NRT), bupropion Hcl, and varenicline.[112] These medications are deemed safe and effective for the treatment of TUD, except in the presence of contraindications or with specific population for which there is insufficient evidence for effectiveness (e.g., pregnant women, smokeless tobacco users, adolescents). [112] NRT is available in a transdermal patch, polacrilex gum, inhaler, lozenge, and nasal spray. The patch, gum, and lozenge are available over-the-counter. Similar to nicotine from tobacco, NRT appears to stimulate nicotinic receptors in the brain's ventral tegmental area (VTA), resulting in a release of dopamine in the nucleus accumbens (NA). NRT delivers nicotine more slowly than tobacco and thus does not completely replicate the pleasurable feelings associated with tobacco use and/or completely eliminate withdrawal.[139] The primary purpose of NRT is to maintain a constant level of nicotine in the body to alleviate withdrawal symptoms, but NRT can also be used as in combination with the other medications to effectively manage "breakthrough" urges and cravings. [140] Initiation of NRT before the quit date and among smokers who are not ready to quit has been shown to improve long-term treatment outcomes. Nonnicotine medications for smoking cessation include bupropion Hcl and varenicline tartrate. Bupropion, approved by the FDA for the treatment of depression in 1989, appears to be a weak dopamine re-uptake inhibitor in the NA, increasing levels of dopamine and norepinephrine in the brain. In addition, a metabolite of bupropion, hydroxybupropion, appears to act as a nicotinic receptor antagonist, blocking the pleasurable effects of nicotine. Varenicline tartrate is nicotinic receptor partial agonist-antagonist, weakly stimulating nicotinic receptors in the VTA while at the same time blocking the pleasurable effects of nicotine. Bupropion and varenicline should both be initiated at least 2 weeks before the quit date. Extended use of nicotine patch, bupropion, and varenicline has shown improved efficacy. Improved efficacy has also been observed for multiple combinations of these medications, including NRT+NRT, varenicline + bupropion, bupropion + NRT, and varenicline + NRT.[141–144] Long-term efficacy of pharmacotherapy for the cessation of tobacco products other than cigarettes has not been observed.

Traditionally, the treatment of TUD has been classified by level of intensity ranging from self-help to highly individualized, long-term treatment provided by certified Tobacco Treatment Specialists. Level of intensity is positively associated with effect size.[112] Clinically, the results of an initial assessment combined with patient preference should dictate the level and course of treatment with less complex TUD presentations candidates for less intensive approaches. In a population approach, however, lower intensity approaches often have a greater reach and potential overall impact, but are unlikely to be effective for more complex TUD presentations. Ideally, more intensive clinical approaches and less-intensive population approaches work together within a comprehensive tobacco control program.

Self-help interventions are the lowest intensity treatments but have, of course, the lowest effect size. The Forever Free booklets, specific print-based self-help materials for relapse prevention provided to newly quit smokers, have a modest long-term effect size. [107,145] Brief interventions are often provided in primary care or other healthcare settings focused on the treatment of other disorders and include systematically identifying tobacco users, providing brief advice, and referring and/or providing medication assistance and brief counseling and follow-up.[112] Brief interventions systematically provided in healthcare settings often have a strong reach into the tobacco using population with modest effect sizes. Combining brief interventions with automatic referral to the state Quitline facilitated with the electronic medical record can significantly increase the reach and impact of services.[146,147] Treatment provided over the telephone, in-person, or in groups can range from brief to intensive treatment depending on the content provided.

Innovative research is currently underway in development new methods to deliver CBT for TUD and in the examination of pharmaceutical preparations of cytisine, a naturally occurring partial agonist found in several plants species.[148] Novel methods to reach, motivate, and support tobacco users' efforts to quit tobacco include texting, online programs, and smart phone applications. Although many of these efforts are promising, conclusions about efficacy are forthcoming. In addition, while evidence-based treatment for TUD appears to be efficacious for all populations, some populations, including a wide variety of groups of lower socioeconomic status, do not benefit equally from these treatments. Innovative treatment adaptions intended to better meet the needs of tobacco users from disparate groups are also under development.

SUMMARY

Despite declines in cigarette use, it remains the leading preventable cause of death and disease in this country. There are a number of future directions that are promising in moving the prevalence even lower. First, an increasing number of efficacious treatments for tobacco are available. Yet, implementation has lagged far behind. Efforts to develop innovative strategies to improve accessibility and availability to these treatments, especially for those who need it most, are needed. Second, emerging areas in tobacco control include the rapid increase in the use of alternative tobacco products, such as ENDS, especially in young people, with very little accompanying data on either potential harm of these products themselves as well as their potential risk in the development of other forms of tobacco use, including cigarettes. Alternatively, these products may effect harm reduction though there is no conclusive evidence yet on this question. Finally, increased attention to reducing the increasing socioeconomic and mental health/substance use disparities in cigarette and other tobacco use is urgently needed.

References

1. USDHHS. *The Health Consequences of Smoking—50 Years of Progress: A Report of the Surgeon General, 2014*. Atlanta, GA: Centers for Disease Control and Prevention (US); 2014.
2. Centers for Disease Control and Prevention. Smoking & Tobacco Use. 2017. www.cdc.gov/tobacco/data_statistics/fact_sheets/fast_facts/index.htm.
3. WHO. *WHO Global Report: Mortality Attributable to Tobacco*. Geneva, Switzerland: WHO Press; 2012.
4. Mehta N, Preston, S. Continued increases in the relative risk of death from smoking. *Am J Public Health*. 2012;102:2181–6.
5. Carter BD, Abnet CC, Feskanich D, et al. Smoking and mortality—Beyond established causes. *N Engl J Med*. 2015;372(7):631–40.
6. Jha P. Avoidable deaths from smoking: A global perspective. *Public Health Rev*. 2011;33(2):569–600.
7. Legacy. *Tobacco Control in Low SES Populations*. Washington, DC. 2013.
8. ACS. *Cancer Facts and Figures 2016*. Atlanta, GA: American Cancer Society; 2016.
9. Park ER, Japuntich SJ, Traeger L, Cannon S, Pajolek H. Disparities between blacks and whites in tobacco and lung cancer treatment. *Oncologist*. 2011;16(10):1428–34.
10. Fagan. Eliminating tobacco-related health disparities: Directions for future research. *Am J Public Health*. 2004;94(2):211–7.
11. Fagan. Identifying health disparities across the tobacco continuum. *Addiction*. 2007;102(Suppl 2):5–29.
12. Centers for Disease Control and Prevention. Tobacco-Related Disparities. 2016. https://www.cdc.gov/tobacco/disparities/index.htm.
13. CDC. Current cigarette smoking among adults—United States, 2005–2014. *MMWR Morb Mortal Wkly Rep*. 2015;64(44):1233–40.
14. Jamal A. Current cigarette smoking among adults—United States, 2005–2015. *MMWR Morb Mortal Wkly Rep*. 2016;65(44):1205–11.
15. Ryan H, Wortley PM, Easton A, Pederson L, Greenwood G. Smoking among lesbians, gays, and bisexuals: A review of the literature. *Am J Prev Med*. 2001;21(2):142–9.
16. Tang H, Greenwood GL, Cowling DW, Lloyd JC, Roeseler AG, Bal DG. Cigarette smoking among lesbians, gays, and bisexuals: How serious a problem? (United States). *Cancer Causes Control*. 2004;15(8):797–803.
17. Steinberg ML, Heimlich L, Williams JM. Tobacco use among individuals with intellectual or developmental disabilities: A brief review. *Intellect Dev Disabil*. 2009;47(3):197–207.
18. Odani S, Agaku IT, Graffunder CM, Tynan MA, Armour BS. Tobacco product use among military veterans—United States, 2010–2015. *MMWR Morb Mortal Wkly Rep*. 2018;67(1):7–12.
19. Guydish J, Passalacqua E, Tajima B, Chan M, Chun J, Bostrom A. Smoking prevalence in addiction treatment: A review. *Nicotine Tob Res*. 2011;13(6):401–11.
20. Guydish J, Passalacqua E, Pagano A, et al. An international systematic review of smoking prevalence in addiction treatment. *Addiction*. 2016;111(2):220–30.
21. Kalman D, Morissette SB, George TP. Co-morbidity of smoking in patients with psychiatric and substance use disorders. *Am J Addict*. 2005;14(2):106–23.
22. Gasperino J, Rom WN. Gender and lung cancer. *Clin Lung Cancer*. 2004;5(6):353–9.
23. Han MK, Postma D, Mannino DM, et al. Gender and chronic obstructive pulmonary disease: Why it matters. *Am J Respir Crit Care Med*. 2007;176(12):1179–84.
24. Hurt RD, Offord KP, Croghan IT, et al. Mortality following inpatient addictions treatment. Role of tobacco use in a community-based cohort. *JAMA*. 1996;275(14):1097–103.
25. Hser YI, McCarthy WJ, Anglin MD. Tobacco use as a distal predictor of mortality among long-term narcotics addicts. *Prev Med*. 1994;23(1):61–9.
26. Bates C, Rowell A. Tobacco explained: The truth about the tobacco industry… in its own words. 1998. http://www.who.int/tobacco/media/en/TobaccoExplained.pdf.
27. UK Office for National Statistics. Adult smoking habits in the UK: 2016. 2017. https://www.ons.gov.uk/peoplepopulationandcommunity/healthandsocialcare/healthandlifeexpectancies/bulletins/adultsmokinghabitsingreatbritain/2016#smoking-habits-in-great-britain-using-data-

from-the-opinions-and-lifestyle-survey-1974-to-2016-adults-aged-16-and-over.

28. US Centers for Disease Control and Prevention. Trends in Current Cigarette Smoking Among High School Students and Adults, United States, 1965–2014. 2016.
29. Doll R, Hill AB. The mortality of doctors in relation to their smoking habits: A preliminary report. 1954. *BMJ*. 2004;328(7455):1529–33; discussion 1533.
30. Office of the Surgeon General. *Smoking and Health: Report of the Advisory Committee to the Surgeon General of the Public Health Service*. 1964.
31. Peters EN, Schwartz RP, Wang S, O'Grady KE, Blanco C. Psychiatric, psychosocial, and physical health correlates of co-occurring cannabis use disorders and nicotine dependence. *Drug Alcohol Depend*. 2014;134:228–34.
32. World Health Organization. *WHO Report on the Global Tobacco Epidemic*. Geneva: World Health Organization; 2008.
33. O'Connor RJ. Non-cigarette tobacco products: What have we learnt and where are we headed? *Tob Control*. 2012;21(2):181–90.
34. Fagerstrom KO, Bridgman K. Tobacco harm reduction: The need for new products that can compete with cigarettes. *Addict Behav*. 2014;39(3):507–11.
35. Reitsma MBFN, Ng M, Salama JS, Abajobir A, Abate KH. Smoking prevalence and attributable disease burden in 195 countries and territories, 1990–2015: A systematic analysis from the Global Burden of Disease Study 2015. *Lancet*. 2017;389(10082):1885–906.
36. World Health Organization. *Tobacco: Deadly in Any Form or Disguise*. Geneva: World Health Organization; 2008.
37. Centers for Disease Control and Prevention. Health Effects of Cigarette Smoking. 2017. https://www.cdc.gov/tobacco/data_statistics/fact_sheets/health_effects/effects_cig_smoking/index.htm.
38. World Health Organization. Prevalence of tobacco smoking. 2016. http://gamapserver.who.int/gho/interactive_charts/tobacco/use/atlas.html.
39. World Lung Foundation. The Tobacco Atlas: Cigarette Use Globally. 2016. http://www.tobaccoatlas.org/topic/cigarette-use-globally/.
40. Delnevo CD. Smokers' choice: What explains the steady growth of cigar use in the U.S.? *Public Health Rep*. 2006;121(2):116–9.
41. Delnevo CD, Giovenco DP, Miller Lo EJ. Changes in the mass-merchandise cigar market since the Tobacco Control Act. *Tob Regul Sci*. 2017;3(2):8–16.
42. Schauer GL, Rosenberry ZR, Peters EN. Marijuana and tobacco co-administration in blunts, spliffs, and mulled cigarettes: A systematic literature review. *Addict Behav*. 2017;64:200–11.
43. Giovenco DP, Casseus M, Duncan DT, Coups EJ, Lewis MJ, Delnevo CD. Association between electronic cigarette marketing near schools and e-cigarette use among youth. *J Adolesc Health*. 2016;59(6):627–34.
44. National Cancer Institute. U.S. National Institutes of Health. Cigar smoking and cancer. 2016. https://www.cancer.gov/about-cancer/causes-prevention/risk/tobacco/cigars-fact-sheet.
45. Chang CM, Corey CG, Rostron BL, Apelberg BJ. Systematic review of cigar smoking and all cause and smoking related mortality. *BMC Public Health*. 2015;15(1):390.
46. Kadhum M, Sweidan A, Jaffery AE, Al-Saadi A, Madden B. A review of the health effects of smoking shisha. *Clin Med (Lond)*. 2015;15(3):263–6.
47. Akl EA, Gaddam S, Gunukula SK, Honeine R, Jaoude PA, Irani J. The effects of waterpipe tobacco smoking on health outcomes: A systematic review. *Int J Epidemiol*. 2010;39(3):834–57.
48. Maziak W, Taleb ZB, Bahelah R, et al. The global epidemiology of waterpipe smoking. *Tob Control*. 2015;24(Suppl 1):i3–12.
49. Ministry of Health and Family Welfare. Government of India. *Smokeless Tobacco and Public Health in India*. 2012.
50. World Health Organization. International Agency for Research on Cancer. *Smokeless Tobacco and Some Tobacco-Specific N-Nitrosamines*. 2007.
51. National Cancer Institute. U.S. National Institutes of Health. Smokeless Tobacco and Cancer. 2010. https://www.cancer.gov/about-cancer/causes-prevention/risk/tobacco/smokeless-fact-sheet.
52. Giovenco DP, Hammond D, Corey CG, Ambrose BK, Delnevo CD. E-cigarette market trends in traditional U.S. retail channels, 2012–2013. *Nicotine Tob Res*. 2015;17(10):1279–83.
53. Dinakar C, O'Connor GT. The health effects of electronic cigarettes. *N Engl J Med*. 2016;375(14):1372–81.
54. Glasser AM, Collins L, Pearson JL, et al. Overview of electronic nicotine delivery systems: A systematic review. *Am J Prev Med*. 2017;52(2):e33–66.
55. Schoenborn CA, Gindi RM. Electronic cigarette use among adults: United States, 2014. *NCHS Data Brief*. 2015;(217):1–8.
56. Giovenco DP, Delnevo CD. Prevalence of population smoking cessation by electronic cigarette use status in a national sample of recent smokers. *Addict Behav*. 2018;76:129–34.
57. McNeill A, Brose L, Calder R, Hitchman S, Hajek P, McRobbie H. E-cigarettes: An evidence update. *Public Health Engl*. 2015;386(1000).
58. Jamal A. Tobacco use among middle and high school students—United States, 2011–2016. *MMWR Morb Mortal Wkly Rep*. 2017;66(23):597–603.
59. Montreuil A, MacDonald M, Asbridge M, et al. Prevalence and correlates of electronic cigarette use among Canadian students: Cross-sectional findings from the 2014/15 Canadian Student Tobacco, Alcohol and Drugs Survey. *CMAJ Open*. 2017;5(2):E460–7.
60. Action on Smoking and Health. Use of e-cigarettes among adults in Great Britain 2017. 2017.
61. Phillips EWT, Husten CG, et al. Tobacco product use among adults—United States, 2015. *MMWR Morb Mortal Wkly Rep*. 2017;66:1209–15.
62. Delnevo CD, Giovenco DP, Steinberg MB, et al. Patterns of electronic cigarette use among adults in the United States. *Nicotine Tob Res*. 2016;18(5):715–9.
63. Public Health England. E-cigarettes: An evidence update. 2015.
64. Goodwin RD, Wall MM, Gbedemah M, et al. Trends in cigarette consumption and time to first cigarette on awakening from 2002 to 2015 in the USA: New insights into the ongoing tobacco epidemic. *Tob Control*. 2018;27(4):379–84.
65. APA. *Diagnostic and Statistical Manual of Mental Disorders: DSM-5*. 5th ed. Arlington, VA: American Psychiatric Association; 2013.
66. APA. *Diagnostic and Statistical Manual of Mental Disorders: DSM-IV-TR*. 4th, Text Revision ed. Washington, DC: American Psychiatric Association; 2000.
67. Benowitz NL. Nicotine Addiction. *N Engl J Med*. 2010;362(24):2295–303.
68. Lynch BBR. *Growing Up Tobacco Free—Preventing Nicotine Addiction in Children and Youths*. Washington, DC: National Academy Press; 1994.
69. Bierut LJ, Madden PAF, Breslau N, et al. Novel genes identified in a high density genome wide association study for nicotine dependence. *Hum Mol Genet*. 2007;16(1):24–35.
70. Lessov-Schlaggar CN, Pergadia ML, Khroyan TV, Swan GE. Genetics of nicotine dependence and pharmacotherapy. *Biochem Pharmacol*. 2008;75(1):178–95.
71. Saccone SF, Hinrichs AL, Saccone NL, et al. Cholinergic nicotinic receptor genes implicated in a nicotine dependence association study targeting 348 candidate genes with 3713 SNPs. *Hum Mol Genet*. 2007;16(1):36–49.
72. Uhl GR, Liu Q-R, Drgon T, Johnson C, Walther D, Rose JE. Molecular genetics of nicotine dependence and abstinence: Whole genome association using 520,000 SNPs. *BMC Genet*. 2007;8(1):10.
73. Xian H, Scherrer JF, Madden PAF, et al. Latent class typology of nicotine withdrawal: Genetic contributions and association with failed smoking cessation and psychiatric disorders. *Psychol Med*. 2005;35(3):409–19.
74. Avenevoli S, Merikangas KR. Familial influences on adolescent smoking. *Addiction*. 2003;98(Suppl 1):1–20.
75. Fergusson DM, Horwood LJ, Boden JM, Jenkin G. Childhood social disadvantage and smoking in adulthood: Results of a 25-year longitudinal study. *Addiction*. 2007;102(3):475–82.
76. Hu M-C, Davies M, Kandel DB. Epidemiology and correlates of daily smoking and nicotine dependence among young adults in the United States. *Am J Public Health*. 2006;96(2):299–308.
77. Kardia SLR, Pomerleau CS, Rozek LS, Marks JL. Association of parental smoking history with nicotine dependence, smoking rate, and psychological cofactors in adult smokers. *Addict Behav*. 2003;28(8):1447–52.
78. Levin ED, Lawrence S, Petro A, Horton K, Seidler FJ, Slotkin TA. Increased nicotine self-administration following prenatal exposure in female rats. *Pharmacol Biochem Behav*. 2006;85(3):669–74.
79. Selya AS, Dierker LC, Rose JS, Hedeker D, Mermelstein RJ. Risk factors for adolescent smoking: Parental smoking and the mediating role of nicotine dependence. *Drug Alcohol Depend*. 2012;124(3):311–8.
80. Kandel DB, Wu P, Davies M. Maternal smoking during pregnancy and smoking by adolescent daughters. *Am J Public Health*. 1994;84(9):1407–13.
81. Niaura R, Bock B, Lloyd EE, Brown R, Lipsitt LP, Buka S. Maternal transmission of nicotine dependence: Psychiatric, neurocognitive and prenatal factors. *Am J Addict*. 2001;10(1):16–29.
82. Shenassa ED, Papandonatos GD, Rogers ML, Buka SL. Elevated risk of nicotine dependence among sib-pairs discordant for maternal smoking during pregnancy: Evidence from a 40-year longitudinal study. *Epidemiology*. 2015;26(3):441–7.
83. Dierker L, Rose J, Selya A, Piasecki TM, Hedeker D, Mermelstein R. Depression and nicotine dependence from adolescence to young adulthood. *Addict Behav*. 2015;41:124–8.
84. Alvarado GF, Breslau N. Smoking and young people's mental health. *Curr Opin Psychiatry*. 2005;18(4):397–400.

85. Griesler PC, Hu M-C, Schaffran C, Kandel DB. Comorbidity of psychiatric disorders and nicotine dependence among adolescents: Findings from a prospective, longitudinal study. *J Am Acad Child Adolesc Psychiatry*. 2008;47(11):1340–50.

86. Isensee B, Wittchen H-U, Stein MB, Höfler M, Lieb R. Smoking increases the risk of panic: Findings from a prospective community study. *Arch Gen Psychiatry*. 2003;60(7):692–700.

87. Kollins SH, McClernon FJ, Fuemmeler BF. Association between smoking and attention-deficit/hyperactivity disorder symptoms in a population-based sample of young adults. *Arch Gen Psychiatry*. 2005;62(10):1142–7.

88. Kushner MG, Menary KR, Maurer EW, Thuras P. Greater elevation in risk for nicotine dependence per pack of cigarettes smoked among those with an anxiety disorder. *J Stud Alcohol Drugs*. 2012;73(6):920–4.

89. Matthies S, Holzner S, Feige B, et al. ADHD as a serious risk factor for early smoking and nicotine dependence in adulthood. *J Atten Disord*. 2013;17(3):176–86.

90. Behrendt S, Wittchen HU, Höfler M, Lieb R, Beesdo K. Transitions from first substance use to substance use disorders in adolescence: Is early onset associated with a rapid escalation? *Drug Alcohol Depend*. 2009;99(1-3):68–78.

91. Breslau N, Fenn N, Peterson EL. Early smoking initiation and nicotine dependence in a cohort of young adults. *Drug Alcohol Depend*. 1993;33(2):129–37.

92. Dierker L, He J, Kalaydjian A, et al. The importance of timing of transitions for risk of regular smoking and nicotine dependence. *Ann Behav Med*. 2008;36(1):87–92.

93. Kendler KS, Myers J, Damaj MI, Chen X. Early smoking onset and risk for subsequent nicotine dependence: A monozygotic co-twin control study. *Am J Psychiatry*. 2013;170(4):408–13.

94. Lanza ST, Vasilenko SA. New methods shed light on age of onset as a risk factor for nicotine dependence. *Addict Behav*. 2015;50:161–4.

95. Pierce JP, Choi WS, Gilpin EA, Farkas AJ, Merritt RK. Validation of susceptibility as a predictor of which adolescents take up smoking in the United States. *Health Psychol*. 1996;15(5):355–61.

96. Storr CL, Zhou H, Liang K-Y, Anthony JC. Empirically derived latent classes of tobacco dependence syndromes observed in recent-onset tobacco smokers: Epidemiological evidence from a national probability sample survey. *Nicotine Tob Res*. 2004;6(3):533–45.

97. Dierker L, Selya A, Rose J, Hedeker D, Mermelstein R. Nicotine dependence and alcohol problems from adolescence to young adulthood. *Dual Diagn (Foster City)*. 2016;1(2):9.

98. García-Rodríguez O, Blanco C, Wall MM, Wang S, Jin CJ, Kendler KS. Toward a comprehensive developmental model of smoking initiation and nicotine dependence. *Drug Alcohol Depend*. 2014;144:160–9.

99. Goodwin RD, Kim JH, Weinberger AH, Taha F, Galea S, Martins SS. Symptoms of alcohol dependence and smoking initiation and persistence: A longitudinal study among US adults. *Drug Alcohol Depend*. 2013;133(2):718–23.

100. Goodwin RD, Pagura J, Spiwak R, Lemeshow A, Sareen J. Predictors of persistent nicotine dependence among adults in the United States. *Drug Alcohol Depend*. 2011;118(2–3):127–33.

101. Hasin D, Fenton MC, Skodol A, et al. Personality disorders and the 3-year course of alcohol, drug, and nicotine use disorders. *Arch Gen Psychiatry*. 2011;68(11):1158–67.

102. Ulrich J, Meyer C, Rumpf H-J, Hapke U. Probabilities of alcohol high-risk drinking, abuse or dependence estimated on grounds of tobacco smoking and nicotine dependence. *Addiction*. 2003;98(6):805–14.

103. Lopez-Quintero C, Hasin DS, de Los Cobos JP, et al. Probability and predictors of remission from life-time nicotine, alcohol, cannabis or cocaine dependence: Results from the National Epidemiologic Survey on Alcohol and Related Conditions. *Addiction*. 2011;106(3):657–69.

104. Lopez-Quintero C, Pérez de los Cobos J, Hasin DS, et al. Probability and predictors of transition from first use to dependence on nicotine, alcohol, cannabis, and cocaine: Results of the National Epidemiologic Survey on Alcohol and Related Conditions (NESARC). *Drug Alcohol Depend*. 2011;115(1–2):120–30.

105. Patton GC, Coffey C, Carlin JB, Sawyer SM, Lynskey M. Reverse gateways? Frequent cannabis use as a predictor of tobacco initiation and nicotine dependence. *Addiction*. 2005;100(10):1518–25.

106. Swendsen J, Conway KP, Degenhardt L, et al. Mental disorders as risk factors for substance use, abuse and dependence: Results from the 10-year follow-up of the National Comorbidity Survey. *Addiction*. 2010;105(6):1117–28.

107. Baker TB, Brandon TH, Chassin L. Motivational influences on cigarette smoking. *Annu Rev Psychol*. 2004;55:463–91.

108. Conrad KM, Flay BR, Hill D. Why children start smoking cigarettes: Predictors of onset. *Br J Addict*. 1992;87(12):1711–24.

109. Derzon JH, Lipsey MW. Predicting tobacco use to age 18: A synthesis of longitudinal research. *Addiction*. 1999;94(7):995–1006.

110. Engels RC, Knibbe RA, Drop MJ, de Haan YT. Homogeneity of cigarette smoking within peer groups: Influence or selection? *Health Educ Behav*. 1997;24(6):801–11.

111. Kurti AN, Klemperer EM, Zvorsky I, Redner R, Priest JS, Higgins ST. Some context for understanding the place of the general educational development degree in the relationship between educational attainment and smoking prevalence. *Prev Med*. 2016;92:141–7.

112. Fiore MC, Jaén CR, Baker TB, et al. *Treating Tobacco Use and Dependence: 2008 Update. Clinical Practice Guideline*. Rockville, MD: US Department of Public Health Service; 2008.

113. CAN-ADAPTT. *Canadian Smoking Cessation Clinical Practice Guideline*. Toronto, Canada: Action Network for the Advancement, Dissemination and Adoption of Practice-informed Tobacco Treatment, Centre for Addiction and Mental Health; 2011.

114. National Institute for Health and Clinical Excellence (NICE). *Smoking Cessation: Supporting People to Stop Smoking*. Manchester, UK: National Institute for Health and Clinical Excellence; 2013.

115. Ministry of Health Mo. *New Zealand Smoking Cessation Guidelines*. Wellington: Ministry of Health; 2007.

116. National Comprehensive Cancer Network. *National Comprehensive Cancer Network Clinical Practice Guidelines in Oncology for Smoking Cessation*. 2016.

117. Committee on Obstetric Practice. Smoking cessation during pregnacy. *ACOG Committee Opinion*. 2017:e200–4. https://www.acog.org/Resources-And-Publications/Committee-Opinions/Committee-on-Obstetric-Practice/Smoking-Cessation-During-Pregnancy.

118. Sheffer CE, Christensen DR, Landes R, Carter LP, Jackson L, Bickel WK. Delay discounting rates: A strong prognostic indicator of smoking relapse. *Addict Behav*. 2014;39(11):1682–9.

119. Flory JD, Manuck SB. Impulsiveness and cigarette smoking. *Psychosom Med*. 2009;71(4):431–7.

120. Cook JW, Fucito LM, Piasecki TM, et al. Relations of alcohol consumption with smoking cessation milestones and tobacco dependence. *J Consult Clin Psychol*. 2012;80(6):1075–85.

121. Homish GG, Leonard KE. Spousal influence on smoking behaviors in a US community sample of newly married couples. *Soc Sci Med*. 2005;61(12):2557–67.

122. Shopland DR, Anderson CM, Burns DM. Association between home smoking restrictions and changes in smoking behaviour among employed women. *J Epidemiol Community Health*. 2006;60 Suppl 2:44–50.

123. Perkins KA, Conklin CA, Levine MD. *Cognitive-Behavioral Therapy for Smoking Cessation: A Practical Guidebook to the Most Effective Treatments*. New York: Routledge; 2008.

124. Abrams DB, Niaura R, Brown RA, Emmons KM, Goldstein MG, Monti PM. *The Tobacco Dependence Treatment Handbook: A Guide to Best Practices*. New York: Guilford Press; 2003.

125. Beck AT, Rush AJ, Shaw BF, Emery G. *Cognitive Therapy for Depression*. New York: Guilford; 1979.

126. Babb S, Malarcher A, Schauer G, Asman K, Jamal A. Quitting smoking among adults—United States, 2000–2015. *MMWR Morb Mortal Wkly Rep*. 2017;65(52):1457–64.

127. Miller WR, Rollnick S. *Motivational Interviewing: Helping People Change*. 3rd ed. New York: Guilford Press; 2012.

128. Hettema J, Steele J, Miller WR. Motivational interviewing. *Ann Rev Clin Psychol*. 2005;1:91–111.

129. Sheffer C, Stitzer M, Landes R, Brackman SL, Munn T. In-person and telephone treatment of tobacco dependence: A comparison of treatment outcomes and participant characteristics. *Am J Public Health*. 2013;103(8):e74–82.

130. RA B. Intensive behavioral treatment. In: Abrams DNR, Brown RA, Emmons KM, Goldstein MG, Monti PM, eds. *The Tobacco Dependence Treatment Handbook*. New York: The Guilford Press; 2003:118–77.

131. Danaher BG, Severson HH, Zhu SH, et al. Randomized controlled tof the combined effects of web and Quitline interventions for smokeless tobacco cessation. *Internet Interv*. 2015;2(2):143–51.

132. Danaher BG, Severson HH, Andrews JA, et al. Randomized controlled trial of MyLastDip: A web-based smokeless tobacco cessation program for chewers ages 14–25. *Nicotine Tob Res*. 2013;15(9):1502–10.

133. Severson HH, Danaher BG, Ebbert JO, et al. Randomized trial of nicotine lozenges and phone counseling for smokeless tobacco cessation. *Nicotine Tob Res.* 2015;17(3):309–15.

134. Ramos M, Ripoll J, Estrades T, et al. Effectiveness of intensive group and individual interventions for smoking cessation in primary health care settings: A randomized trial. *BMC Public Health.* 2010;10:89.

135. Cummins SE, Bailey L, Campbell S, Koon-Kirby C, Zhu SH. Tobacco cessation Quitlines in North America: A descriptive study. *Tob Control.* 2007;16(Suppl 1):i9–15.

136. Bernstein SL, Rosner JM, Toll B. Cell phone ownership and service plans Among low-income smokers: The hidden cost of Quitlines. *Nicotine Tob Res.* 2016;18(8):1791–3.

137. Lichtenstein E, Zhu SH, Tedeschi GJ. Smoking cessation Quitlines: An underrecognized intervention success story. *Am Psychol.* 2010;65(4):252–61.

138. Rudie M. Results from the FY2015 NAQC Annual Survey of Quitlines. Moving Quitlines Forward: North American Quitline Consortium; 2016.

139. Balfour DJ, Fagerstrom KO. Pharmacology of nicotine and its therapeutic use in smoking cessation and neurodegenerative disorders. *Pharmacol Ther.* 1996;72(1):51–81.

140. Ebbert JO, Burke MV, Hays JT, Hurt RD. Combination treatment with varenicline and nicotine replacement therapy. *Nicotine Tob Res.* 2009;11(5):572–6.

141. Ebbert JO, Hays JT, Hurt RD. Combination pharmacotherapy for stopping smoking: What advantages does it offer? *Drugs.* 2010;70(6):643–50.

142. Ebbert JO, Hatsukami DK, Croghan IT, et al. Combination varenicline and bupropion SR for tobacco-dependence treatment in cigarette smokers: A randomized trial. *JAMA.* 2014;311(2):155–63.

143. Ebbert JO, Croghan IT, Sood A, Schroeder DR, Hays JT, Hurt RD. Varenicline and bupropion sustained-release combination therapy for smoking cessation. *Nicotine Tob Res.* 2009;11(3):234–9.

144. Koegelenberg CF, Noor F, Bateman ED, et al. Efficacy of varenicline combined with nicotine replacement therapy vs varenicline alone for smoking cessation: A randomized clinical trial. *JAMA.* 2014;312(2):155–61.

145. Brandon TH, Collins BN, Juliano LM, Lazev AB. Preventing relapse among former smokers: A comparison of minimal interventions through telephone and mail. *J Consult Clin Psychol.* 2000;68(1):103–13.

146. Vidrine JI, Shete S, Li Y, et al. The Ask-Advise-Connect approach for smokers in a safety net healthcare system: A group-randomized trial. *Am J Prev Med.* 2013;45(6):737–41.

147. Vidrine JI, Shete S, Cao Y, et al. Ask-Advise-Connect: A new approach to smoking treatment delivery in health care settings. *JAMA Intern Med.* 2013;173(6):458–64.

148. Walker N, Howe C, Glover M, et al. Cytisine versus nicotine for smoking cessation. *N Engl J Med.* 2014;371(25):2353–62.

CHAPTER

167 Alcohol and Health

Emily Oot • Richard Saitz

INTRODUCTION

Sixty-nine percent of adult Americans—some 169 million people—report past-year alcohol use, dwarfing national rates of other substance use.[1] While this high prevalence of drinking amplifies alcohol's public health impact, it also helps normalize a range of drinking patterns. Drinking alcohol as normative behavior may explain, at least in part, the public's lower perceived risk of harm from heavy alcohol use relative to even infrequent use of other drugs, some of which have fewer health consequences.[1] Regardless, alcohol contributes to an estimated 88,000 deaths each year in the United States, making it the third leading cause of preventable death.[2] Its impact also creates a significant drain on the economy, costing the U.S.$249 billion in 2010 (about U.S.$2 per drink).[3] While it is possible to drink at a low-risk level, many Americans drink amounts that expose them to risk for a variety of negative health consequences, even if they do not meet criteria for an alcohol use disorder or have not yet experienced any negative consequences. It is therefore important to begin by defining different levels of consumption and their associations with health consequences.

DEFINITIONS

Some alcohol use beyond abstinence may be considered low-risk use, although certain risks (such as cancers) may occur even with lower consumption. The National Institute on Alcohol Abuse and Alcoholism (NIAAA) defines low-risk consumption as no more than 4 drinks in a day and no more than 14 drinks per week on average for men, and no more than 3 drinks in a day, and no more than 7 drinks per week on average for women. These guidelines provide a useful framework, but drinking can be risky even within these limits under certain conditions (e.g., before driving or while taking a medication that may interact with alcohol) or for certain groups (e.g., children and adolescents, pregnant women, people with a family history of an alcohol use disorder, or people with medical conditions caused or affected by alcohol).[4]

Higher levels of alcohol consumption with or without consequences constitute unhealthy alcohol use, which is defined as any use that risks (or is accompanied by) a health consequence. Unhealthy use can be further stratified into risky use and alcohol use disorder (see Fig. 167-1).

Risky use is defined as use that increases the probability or risk of a negative consequence but has not necessarily yet resulted in one. Risky use is determined by either consumption levels (above the risk thresholds described above) or by any use by those at particular risk (e.g., family history of a disorder, as above). Alcohol use disorder, on the other hand, is determined by the recurrent consequences or symptoms experienced.

A diagnosis of alcohol use disorder (AUD) based on the *Diagnostic and Statistical Manual of Mental Disorders, fifth edition* (DSM-5) requires two or more symptoms be experienced (such as craving, withdrawal, or drinking despite alcohol causing social or interpersonal problems), along with some level of functional impairment. In the previous version of the manual, DSM-IV, alcohol use disorder was divided into alcohol abuse and alcohol dependence, with the latter diagnosis reserved as indicative of compulsive use and/or physiological dependence symptoms, such as withdrawal and tolerance. However, research does not support the idea that these are two separate diagnoses. The DSM-5, published in 2013, has combined the two terms into a spectrum of alcohol use disorder, with severity ranging from mild to moderate to severe depending on the number of symptom criteria met. Alcohol use disorder can also be diagnosed with the World Health Organization's International Classification of Diseases 10 (ICD-10) criteria, which, similar to the DSM-IV, has two diagnoses: "Harmful use of alcohol" and "Alcohol dependence syndrome." Additionally, "hazardous use," while not a diagnosis in any currently accepted classification system (it is being considered for ICD-11), has been described and refers to use with increased risk of consequences or with consequences that do not meet criteria for a disorder.

From a public health or population perspective, we are interested in the full spectrum of *unhealthy alcohol use*, from at-risk to disorder. Some interventions and approaches will affect the full spectrum, while others are targeted to and affect one end of the spectrum or the other.

EPIDEMIOLOGY

Epidemiology of Alcohol Use

According to the 2016 National Survey on Drug Use and Health (NSDUH), 169 million Americans, 69% of those 18 and older, reported consuming alcohol in the past year. The same year, 26% of adults also reported at least one episode of heavy (also more colloquially and in Centers for Disease Control literature called "binge") drinking in the past month.[1] While acceptable, the term "binge" drinking is sometimes avoided because its meaning is unclear. Some interpret it to mean drinking heavily and continuously for several days, while others use it to describe a single heavy-drinking episode.

Heavy episodic drinking is more common among men than among women, more common among people 18–34 years old than any other age group, more common among whites, and among those with $75,000 or more annual income. Ninety percent of alcohol consumed by youth is consumed during heavy-drinking episodes. Among adults, the majority of those who report heavy-drinking episodes are do not meet criteria for alcohol dependence (DSM-IV).

Past year prevalence of use among adults was higher for men (73%) than women (66%), a pattern that has been consistent over time. Past-year use data by race for those 18 and older indicated the greatest prevalence of use among whites (74%). Asians reported the lowest prevalence (51%), with Native Hawaiians or other Pacific

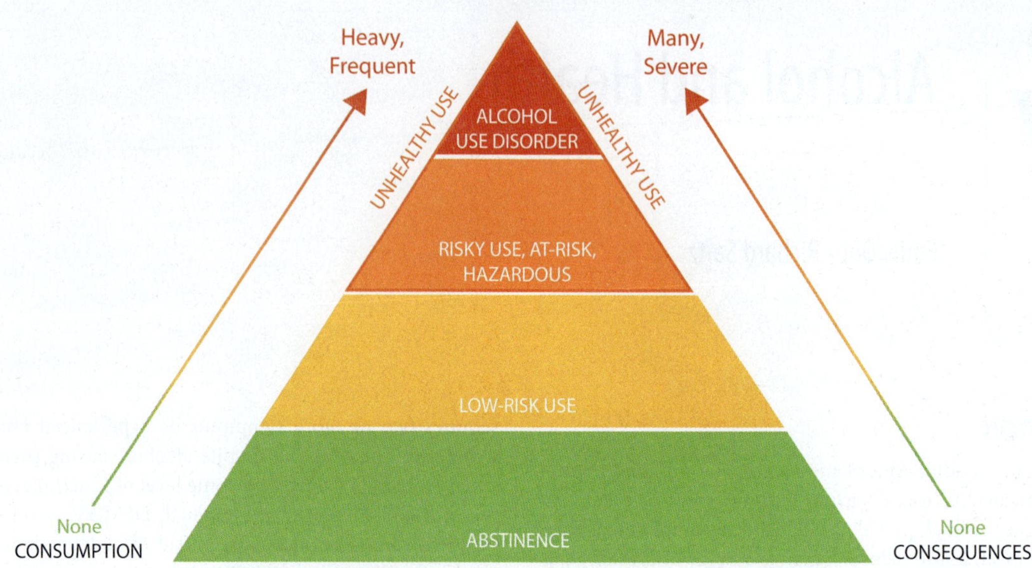

FIGURE 167-1. Unhealthy alcohol use. (*Source:* Modified from Saitz R. *New Engl J Med.* 2005;352:598.)

Islanders (56%), blacks or African Americans (60%), and "American Indians" or Alaska Natives (61%) in between. Adults of Hispanic or Latino ethnicity reported lower past-year use (64%) than did those without Hispanic or Latino ethnicity (70%).[1]

With respect to socioeconomic status, rates of use increase as the percentage of the poverty level exceeded increases. Fifty-five percent of adults at less than 100% of the poverty level reported past-year use, compared to 59% at 100–199% of the poverty level, and 75% at 200% or more of the poverty level.[1]

Epidemiology of AUD

The same 2016 survey reported diagnoses of alcohol use disorder (defined as meeting criteria for DSM-IV abuse or dependence) in 6% of people age 18 and older, or 15 million people.[1] Data from another population-based survey, the National Epidemiologic Survey on Alcohol and Related Conditions (NESARC) III, using DSM-5 criteria, reported an AUD prevalence of 13.9% among adults in 2013.[5] NESARC also reported a substantial increase in DSM-IV alcohol use disorder from 8.5% to 12.7% over the decade ending 2013.[6]

In the NSDUH, the prevalence of AUD is higher in emerging adulthood, ages 18–25, at 11% than in those 26 and older (5.2%). Among adults, prevalence is higher in men (8%) than women (4%). Racial breakdowns for AUD roughly parallel prevalence of use statistics, with the exception of American Indians and Alaska Natives, whose rates of AUD at 10% are higher than those for whites (6%) and Blacks (6%). Asians (3%) and Native Hawaiians or other Pacific Islanders (4%) again had the lowest prevalence.[1]

AUD prevalence by socioeconomic status also diverges from use statistics. The highest prevalence of AUD (7%) was among adults at less than 100% of the poverty level (prevalence at 100–199% is 5.4%, and at 200% or more, 5.8%). This discrepancy highlights an increased vulnerability to developing the disorder among those with the lowest income.[1]

ETIOLOGY OF AUD

There is no single factor that determines risk for AUD. Etiology for the disorder is complex and multifactorial. Risk factors include genetics, environment, as well as demographic characteristics.

Genetics

Most of what we know about the genetics of alcohol use disorder revolves around the central role of the enzymes alcohol dehydrogenase (ADH) and aldehyde dehydrogenase (ALDH) in metabolizing alcohol in the liver (and, to a lesser extent, in the stomach and intestines). Activity of these enzymes is associated with adverse reactions to alcohol (e.g., facial flushing, nausea) and can also impede the development of tolerance, thereby diminishing the risk that a person would increase alcohol consumption to the levels associated with higher risk of consequences. Unsurprisingly then, the genetic variants most clearly linked to alcohol use disorder are found in and around the *ADH* and *ALDH* genes (specifically alleles of *ADH1A*, *ADH1B*, *ADH1C*, *ADH2*, and *ADH4* encoding ADH and the alleles of *ALDH2* encoding ALDH). Protective *ADH* and *ALDH* alleles occurring primarily in Asian and Polynesian populations help explain the lower prevalence of alcohol use disorders in these populations relative to other racial groups.[7]

More recently, Genome Wide Association Studies (GWASs) using large databases have attempted to identify novel genetic markers of AUD susceptibility. However, there has been little overlap across studies, making results difficult to interpret, and beyond *ADH* and *ALDH*, only a handful were replicated in independent studies. Positive findings for *CDH13*, the gene responsible for encoding the protein cadherin 13, were replicated across four studies (more than any other gene). Findings for eight other genes were replicated in independent studies up to three times.[8]

While replication of GWAS findings has been limited, these studies nevertheless indicate a role for genetics in influencing alcohol-related behaviors. Taken together with other genetic approaches they demonstrate that more complex relationships exist between AUD and a host of other genes beyond *ADH* and *ALDH*. It is estimated based on twin and other epidemiological studies that genetics account for approximately 50–60% of the variance in risk for AUD.[9] Although it is difficult to generalize risk-ratio findings across studies (due in part to differences in the estimated AUD prevalence statistics used in these calculations), twin studies consistently show an increased relative risk of AUD for the twins of those with the disorder, and this relative risk is consistently higher for monozygotic twins than it is for dizygotic twins, reinforcing the clear evidence for the role of genetics in AUD etiology.[10]

Environment

Environmental factors are also implicated in the etiology of alcohol use disorder. Exposure to alcohol itself is, of course, necessary but not sufficient for manifesting the disorder. More specifically, timing of first exposure has been shown to be a significant factor, as has exposure to early childhood stress.

Data from the National Epidemiologic Survey on Alcohol and Related Conditions (NESARC, 2001–02) and from its predecessor, the National Longitudinal Alcohol Epidemiologic Survey (NLAES, 1991–92), consistently indicate that the prevalence of lifetime alcohol dependence (DSM-IV) decreases with later age of first drink.[11,12] A study analyzing the NESARC data found that 47% of respondents who began drinking before age 14 experienced lifetime dependence, compared with just 9% of those who did not begin drinking until age 21 or older. Earlier age of first drink increased the odds of experiencing longer dependence episodes, and of experiencing higher numbers of dependence symptoms.[11]

The mechanism for the increased risk associated with early-onset drinking remains poorly understood, however. There is evidence to support the hypothesis that early drinking precipitates neurobiological changes, which increases risk for the development of alcohol use disorder.[13] It is also possible, however, that common genetic factors and environmental exposures can explain risk for both early onset and for later AUD, and that the relationship between the two is therefore not causal.[14]

In addition to age of first drink, stress represents another important environmental risk factor for alcohol use and for the development of AUD. Childhood maltreatment and other adverse childhood experiences have been shown to be significantly associated with drinking outcomes later in life, including earlier age of drinking onset and greater severity of alcohol dependence.[15–17]

Demographic Risk Factors

Additional risk factors for AUD beyond genetics and environmental exposures include demographic and family history characteristics. Increased risk from a family history of AUD has been well established across various types of studies. Even more compelling, magnitude of this risk has been shown to increase as a function of family history density. A study analyzing data from the National Health Interview Survey found that having a positive family history only in second- or third-degree relatives increased odds of alcohol dependence by 45%, relative to those with a negative family history. Odds increased by 86% among those with a positive family history in only first-degree relatives, and by 167% among those with a positive family history in both first- and second- or third-degree relatives.[18] As is the case for age of first drink, the exact mechanism for the risk associated with a positive family history of AUD is unclear, since both genetics and environment are implicated in familial associations. However, studies comparing the adopted children of biological parent(s) with AUD to their nonadopted siblings found elevated but similar proportions of AUD within both the adopted and nonadopted groups, supporting genetic heritability as the primary mechanism at play in family history risk.[19,20]

Mental health comorbidities, primarily diagnoses of depression and anxiety, also appear to be contributing factors in the development of many cases of AUD. One study examining survey data on 12-month-olds of DSM-IV alcohol use disorders and independent mood and anxiety disorders found any alcohol use disorder (abuse or dependence) was significantly associated with any mood disorder (ORs 2.3–2.9) and with any anxiety disorder (ORs 1.5–2.0).[21] Longitudinal studies suggest these relationships are reciprocal, with mental health diagnoses increasing risk for alcohol use disorders and vice versa.[22]

Other risk factors include demographic variables, many of which were highlighted in the epidemiology section earlier in this chapter. The "gender gap" refers to the notable disparity in alcohol use and AUD between men and women. While trend data suggest this gap has narrowed over time, men remain significantly more at risk for the development of AUD than women.[23] Past-year prevalence of AUD among men in 2016 was twice as high as prevalence among women (at 7.8% and 4.2%, respectively).[1] Race also plays a role. As reviewed in this chapter's discussion of genetics, having Asian or Polynesian heritage decreases risk for AUD, likely due to the higher prevalence of protective *ADH* and *ALDH* alleles in these groups.[7] Past year AUD among adults in these populations (at 3.2 and 3.8%, respectively) is about half as common as it is among their European- or African-descendant counterparts. Conversely, American Indians are at increased risk for developing AUD with a prevalence of 9.8%, which is more than 50% higher than European- (6.2%) and African-descendant (6.1%) groups.[1] Lastly, socioeconomic status (SES) contributes to the likelihood of AUD diagnosis, with individuals below the poverty level most afflicted despite lower prevalence of use.[1]

Theories

A variety of theories have been proposed in an attempt to explain the complex basis of alcohol use disorder. Once stigmatized as a character flaw or moral failing, AUD is now recognized as a medical condition by scientists, clinicians, and, increasingly, the general public. However, theories aimed at elucidating its origins and mechanisms remain less established. While there is no one unifying theory, several have merit and contribute to our overall understanding.

The self-medication hypothesis, championed by psychiatrist Edward Khantzian, proposes that individuals with AUD rely on alcohol to help alleviate chronic mood or other psychiatric symptoms.[24] This theory draws support from the overwhelming comorbidities between AUD and other mental health conditions, but critics counter that evidence of a causal relationship between negative affect and drinking behaviors remains limited.

More recently, several neurobiological theories have emerged and gained traction, proposing that addiction of all types is a brain disease characterized by dysfunction of the reward system. Alcohol, like many other drugs favored for recreational use, triggers the release of dopamine in the brain, resulting in subjective feelings of pleasure or reward. Prominent neurobiological theories therefore posit that, combined with certain neurobiological characteristics (namely, hypoactive dopamine neurotransmission), alcohol can "hijack" the brain's reward system and override normal impulse inhibition responses, resulting in compulsive use.[25,26]

A separate but related neurobiological theory proposes other, more negative forces at play beyond the rewarding effects of dopamine release. This view supports the hypothesis that compulsive drinking has its basis not only in reward-seeking, but also in stress avoidance. Progressive increases in alcohol consumption lead to tolerance and, when these increases cannot be maintained, to withdrawal symptoms. This view suggests that individuals with AUD are motivated to continue drinking because stopping precipitates extreme physical discomfort as well as mood dysregulation.[27] Beyond the experience of pain and discomfort, alcohol withdrawal can also cause severe health consequences, including delirium tremens, seizures, and even death.

Other theories prioritize the central role that choice or rational agency play in addiction. Some schools of the choice model run parallel to the brain disease model however, supporting the central role of brain health, but adding that dysfunction may lie primarily in impaired valuation of reward. Addicted individuals may thereby make a "rational" choice to use substances because they have discounted other less-immediate rewards and consequences.[28]

Lastly, the socioecological model offers insight into understanding alcohol use and alcohol use disorder. The model posits that alcohol and other drug use is related to societal, community, relationship, and individual contexts.[29] For example, the social environment can be stressful or devoid of its own natural rewards, making intoxication a particularly compelling alternative. Such context can help explain the increased prevalence of AUD among those with lower socioeconomic status.

It is most likely the case, however, that all of these theories can help to partially explain addiction, and may apply more or less to specific individuals. As such they are best viewed as complementary parts to a whole picture.

PUBLIC HEALTH IMPACT

Alcohol's substantial public health impact can be traced to its role in a myriad of health consequences across nearly every system of the human body. Although the public health focus tends to be on alcohol's negative effects, some research also points to a range of possible benefits associated with particular levels of intake. Here we review these possible health benefits of alcohol use as well as established harms.

Possible Benefits

Acute effects of alcohol intake may include stimulation as well as alleviation of tension and negative mood. Possibly related to these positive feelings, some studies have linked moderate consumption to higher self-reported quality of life and physical health.[30,31] We note, however, that the word "moderate" implies an amount that is healthy, and that may not be the case, as we shall discuss shortly.

Perhaps most the most reported and widely accepted of alcohol's possible benefits are the effects of lower-risk drinking amounts on cardiovascular health. Several studies indicate that light to moderate alcohol intake (i.e., below risky drinking thresholds set by public health agencies) is inversely associated with risk of cardiovascular mortality.[32,33] The proposed mechanism for this effect is alcohol's positive impact on lipoprotein profiles (most notably on elevating levels of high-density lipoprotein), which in turn reduce risk for atherosclerosis and then myocardial infarction. There are effects on inflammatory markers as well, though these are inconsistent, and all of the effects on biomarkers combined appear to be insufficient to explain the magnitude of reductions in risk seen in observational studies.[34] Researchers are careful to point out, however, that this inverse relationship between alcohol intake and cardiovascular mortality is dose dependent and not linear, and that higher levels of alcohol consumption actually increase risk for cardiovascular disease and mortality, resulting in a U- or J-shaped curve. Individuals with the lowest risk may be those consuming < 1 drink per day,[35] calling into question whether the effect is biologically plausible and whether there exists any public health benefit of promoting "moderate" use for cardiovascular protection (particularly since even low amounts are carcinogenic, see below). Even viewed within this limited context, the results of these studies should be interpreted with caution, given the presence of systematic methodological errors in many observational studies,[36] most notably a disregard or inability to adjust for the confounding effects of risk factors unrelated to alcohol use that tend to be far more prevalent in people who do not drink than in those who report drinking "moderate" amounts.[37] A genetic randomization study has failed to support any cardiovascular benefit.[38]

A similar U- or J-shaped curve may exist for the relationship between alcohol intake and the cognitive impairment associated with dementia,[39] whereby low to "moderate" levels of drinking reduce risk, while higher levels increase risk.[40] Other possible neurological benefits have been reported as well, including reduced risk of total stroke, ischemic stroke, and stroke mortality at low levels ($<$15 g/d) of drinking relative to nondrinking.[41] High intake of $>$ 30 g/d, however, has been associated with increased risk for total stroke, and even "moderate" use may have negative neurological consequences (discussed in the *Harms* section). Moreover, further research may be needed on findings of neurological benefits to rule out the same methodological concerns observed in those studies reporting cardiovascular benefits.

Beneficial associations have also been reported across several other health outcomes with low to "moderate" alcohol consumption. Intake at the rate of ~1–3 drinks per day may lower risk of diabetes,[42] but again the curve for this relationship is U-shaped, with use above ~ 3 drinks/day conferring no benefit.[43] There is also an inverse relationship between alcohol consumption and risk of gallstone disease and cholecystectomy.[44–46] Unlike most other benefits reported, this association appears close to linear, rather than U-shaped, and prevented cholelithiasis is the only category of health effects that subtracts from the CDC's estimation of alcohol-attributable deaths across the United States.[2] However, the fact that "moderate" drinking appears to be associated with unrelated conditions via disparate purported mechanisms and differently shaped dose-response curves lends further credence to the idea that observed associations are not causal.

Lastly and perhaps most importantly, low-risk intake has been associated with reduced total mortality.[47–51] However, a recent review and meta-analysis identified common methodological errors and confounding factors in studies of alcohol and mortality risk, including misclassifying former and occasional drinkers as abstainers. After adjusting for these biases, the meta-analysis showed no reduction in mortality risk for low-volume drinkers.[52] Additionally, much of the purported reduced total mortality is attributed to reduced risk of myocardial infarction and, as mentioned above, a Mendelian randomization analysis failed to support this cardiovascular benefit.[38] Mendelian randomization studies have also called into question the causality of the association between HDL cholesterol and myocardial infarction, the purported mechanism for alcohol's beneficial cardiovascular effects.[53] Together these studies strongly suggest that the decreased total mortality that has been associated with "moderate" alcohol consumption is due to confounding and other biases, and that "moderate" alcohol use does not in fact confer any total mortality benefit.

Harms

Death

Alcohol is responsible for an estimated 88,129 deaths annually, nearly three times as many deaths as are due to opioid overdose during the current epidemic. The most significant chronic causes contributing to this statistic include alcoholic liver disease (14,695) and liver cirrhosis (7847), followed by alcohol use disorder (5750), hemorrhagic stroke (1643), and hypertension (1603). Acute causes of death are dominated by motor vehicle traffic crashes (12,460), followed by non-alcohol poisoning (8404), suicide (8179), homicide (7756), and fall injuries (7541). Alcohol poisoning accounts for 1647 deaths annually.[2] Excessive drinking is responsible for one in ten deaths among working adults.

In addition to the number of deaths, it is worth noting that alcohol is also responsible for an average of 2.5 million years of potential life lost annually between 2006 and 2010 (about 30 years per life lost).[54] This speaks to alcohol's role in an overwhelming number of premature deaths in young people.

Injury and Violence

As common sense might suggest, alcohol intoxication increases risk of accidental injury. Globally, anywhere between 6% and 45% of injury cases involve alcohol.[55] Nine percent of all MVA injuries are from alcohol-related crashes, as are 41% of all fatal MVA injuries.[56] Results of a meta-analysis showed a strong dose-response curve between alcohol consumption and both fall injuries and motor vehicle accident (MVA) injuries.[57] The odds ratio for non-MVA injury reached 24.2 at the maximum dose examined (140 g alcohol), and even higher, 52, for MVA injury at its maximum dose (120 g alcohol). Notably, even "moderate" doses of 24 g/day produced ORs of 1.79 for non-MVA and 2.20 for MVA injury.

It is also well established that alcohol has aggressogenic effects, and that alcohol use increases perpetration of violence such as child abuse, domestic abuse, and homicide.[58,59] Epidemiological statistics are striking, with perpetrators in up to 86% of homicides, 37% of assaults, 60% of sexual assaults, and 13% of child abuse cases having been drinking at the time of the offense.[60]

Interestingly, alcohol use in the victims of violence, not just the perpetrators, is also prevalent. Studies of blood alcohol concentrations (BACs) in assault victim emergency department visits report estimated positive BACs in the range of 43–51% of these cases.[61] Those reporting to the emergency department for violence-related injuries are also more likely than those with other injuries to report frequent heavy drinking, consequences of drinking, and prior AUD symptoms or treatment.[62] Animal models help explain this phenomenon in both acute and chronic drinking contexts, demonstrating that intoxicated individuals are more likely to produce social signals that provoke attacks,[63–65] and also that victims of chronic environmental stressors, such as aggression, consume more alcohol.[66] It is therefore unsurprising that patients presenting to the emergency department for violence-related injuries are more likely to have alcohol detected in blood or breath than emergency department patients with other injuries.[61] Additionally, women who have recently experienced domestic violence are more likely to have an alcohol use disorder, and are also more likely to have a partner with an alcohol or other drug use disorder.[67]

Alcohol consumption (both acute intoxication and chronic heavy drinking) has also been linked to suicide.[68–70] Possible mechanisms for the influence of acute intoxication on suicidal behaviors include alcohol-induced dysphoria, disinhibition, impulsivity, and suicidal ideation. Regular, long-term drinking, on the other hand, may exert its influence on suicide via the reciprocal relationship between alcohol use disorders and other mental health conditions like depression, or via disruption of interpersonal connections which may increase social stress and, in turn, suicide risk. Alcohol policies have been shown to influence societal drinking levels and associated behaviors, and literature suggests such policies could be employed to influence alcohol-related suicide rates.[70]

Cardiovascular

Deleterious effects of alcohol on the cardiovascular system are well established, but also highly dose-dependent. Heavy drinking is clearly linked to cardiomyopathy and atrial fibrillation, as well as to coronary artery disease, stroke, and heart failure.

One-third to one-half of dilated cardiomyopathies worldwide are attributable to alcohol, making alcohol the leading secondary cause.[71,72] Alcohol negatively impacts left ventricular (LV) ejection, the hallmark of cardiomyopathy, and as many as one third of people with AUD present with asymptomatic LV dysfunction. Chronic heavy drinking ultimately leads to four-chamber cardiac enlargement and loss of LV systolic function. Drinking > 90 g/d for > 5 years is associated with asymptomatic cardiomyopathy, and with increasing duration is associated with the development of symptomatic cardiomyopathy.[72] Prognosis for alcoholic cardiomyopathy can be dramatically improved by abstinence. Continued use, on the other hand, has been shown to predict worse outcome.

Another well-recognized cardiovascular health consequence of alcohol is atrial fibrillation, or irregular heartbeat. As with cardiomyopathy, the relationship between atrial fibrillation and heavy alcohol use is well established, but its relationship with lower consumption is less clear-cut. It is possible that low-risk alcohol use does not contribute to risk for atrial fibrillation, but some research suggests the relationship is linear, with any use incurring risk and with that risk increasing with the amount used.[73]

Alcohol use is also linked to coronary artery disease and its consequences: myocardial infarction and cardiac mortality. It is likely that the mechanism that increases this risk relates to the coronary artery calcification associated with heavy drinking. Cardiovascular mortality in people who drink surpasses that in those who abstain at approximately 25 g/d, with the heaviest drinking associated with the greatest risk.[74]

Hepatic

Liver disease represents another high impact and high prevalence health consequence of alcohol use. Toxic effects of alcohol on the liver are well established, and several epidemiologic studies demonstrate that the prevalence of liver disease and related mortality are closely related to population levels of alcohol consumption.[75–77]

Alcoholic liver disease comprises a spectrum of pathologies, most notably hepatitis and cirrhosis. Alcoholic hepatitis, inflammation of the liver, develops in approximately one-third of people who drink heavily and regularly for years.[78] Cirrhosis—a less common, but more severe manifestation of alcoholic liver disease marked by scarring of liver tissue and liver dysfunction—is observed in approximately 10% of heavy drinkers.[79] Cirrhosis may be a consequence of recurrent alcoholic hepatitis or of hepatitis C (for which individuals with AUD are at increased risk), or simply a consequence of consumption itself.

As with other health effects of alcohol, risk for alcoholic liver disease is observed above a particular threshold of consumption. Amounts as low as two to three drinks per day have been associated with an increase in incidence of cirrhosis.[80,81] More commonly, however, cirrhosis is associated with consumption above ~ 40 g/d for men or ~ 20 g/d for women over an extended period (10 years or more), and both the amount and duration of drinking appear to influence risk.[82–84] Most cases of cirrhosis occur at even higher levels of consumption, ~ 100 g/d, where risk rises to ~ 50%.[82,85]

Neurologic

An abundance of evidence has linked heavy alcohol use to brain damage, giving rise to the term "alcohol-related dementia" or ARD (sometimes also referred to as "alcohol-related brain damage"). Structural brain scans show reduced gray matter volumes with heavy drinking, indicative of brain atrophy.[86,87] People with AUD also have impaired neuropsychological profiles even when dementia per se is not present.[88]

Severe cases of AUD are also responsible for the vast majority of a particular subset of dementias: Wernicke encephalopathy, and the related Korsakoff syndrome (together referred to as Wernicke-Korsakoff syndrome, or WKS). Wernicke encephalopathy (WE) is caused by thiamine deficiency, which, in developed countries, is almost always linked to alcohol use disorder. Classic signs of WE include confusion, lack of voluntary coordination of muscle movements, and paralysis or weakness of eye muscles. Diagnosis is often missed during life, but postmortem studies that can rely on biomarkers of the disease (most notably atrophied mammillary bodies) indicate a prevalence of 1–2% in the general population, but 12–14% in people with AUD.[89] Eighty percent of people with AUD and WE progress to Korsakoff syndrome, a debilitating and largely irreversible condition characterized by significant anterograde and retrograde amnesia.[90]

A separate condition even more common among individuals with AUD, also thought to be caused by the thiamine deficiency associated with heavy alcohol use, is cerebellar degeneration.[90] As the name implies, the condition is characterized by atrophy of the cerebellum, a brain structure responsible for coordination of movement. Accordingly, symptoms include impaired motor coordination, loss of balance, and involuntary eye movements. Although cerebellar degeneration typically only develops after long-term heavy drinking (10+ years), postmortem indications of the disease are observed in up to 42% of individuals with AUD.[91]

While heavy drinking has long been known to have negative neurologic consequences, "moderate" levels of alcohol consumption were considered harmless to brain function until very recently, when evidence emerged linking lower rates of use to specific structural and functional brain damage. Most notably, atrophy of the hippocampus (the brain region responsible for consolidation of memory) has been reported even in people who drink lower amounts (112 to < 168 g/week, i.e., just over one drink a day), with damage increasing linearly with consumption.[92] The same study also found a linear relationship between consumption and both white matter integrity and lexical fluency. Both of these negative associations were also detected even at moderate consumption levels.

Alcohol's neurologic consequences extend to the peripheral nervous system as well, where damage to peripheral nerve tissue can result in alcoholic neuropathy. Neuropathy is present in 25–66% of individuals with long-term AUD (and is more prevalent in long-term, regular heavy drinkers than in more episodic drinkers). Alcoholic neuropathy is characterized by pain and strange sensations in the extremities, and can be incapacitating. Unfortunately, the primary risk factors and the etiology for the condition are not well understood, and there are no reliable treatments.[93]

Gastrointestinal

The link between alcohol intake and gastrointestinal (GI) dysfunction and bleeding was reported for the first time nearly two centuries ago. Alcohol is directly toxic to the gastric mucosa, and consumption increases risk for gastritis.[94] Gastritis symptoms may include vomiting, which in turn can lead to acute problems such as Mallory-Weiss tears, upper GI hemorrhage, and hematemesis. Acute and chronic alcohol consumption also impairs motility of the esophagus and stomach through both direct and systemic effects.[95,96]

Respiratory

Alcohol use depresses respiratory function, which can impair airway clearance and increase risk of aspiration of microbes. Together these effects help explain why AUD is a significant risk factor for the development of pneumonia,[97] and in very large doses (poisoning, overdose), respiratory failure.

Renal/Metabolic

Kidney function is compromised secondarily by alcohol's effects on muscle (see below) and volume status (prerenal azotemia from vomiting and diarrhea). Heavy consumption is associated with acid-base disturbances, both alkalemia and acidemia (lactic and keto-acidosis), and electrolyte abnormalities such as hypokalemia, hypomagnesemia, hypocalcemia, and hypophosphatemia.[98]

Hematological

Alcohol also negatively impacts blood cell production (hematopoiesis), such that frequent long-term heavy use can cause pancytopenia or isolated anemia, leukopenia, or thrombocytopenia. Impaired hematopoiesis can be due to alcohol's direct toxic effects on the bone marrow reducing counts of blood cell precursors and otherwise impeding maturation of these cells into functional mature blood cells. However, folic acid and B12 deficiencies can play a role as well.[99]

Musculoskeletal

The prevalence of myopathy, both acute and chronic, is significantly increased in individuals with AUD relative to the general population. There is also evidence that nearly half of individuals with AUD who do not have a myopathy diagnosis still present with subclinical myopathic symptoms and muscle changes. Chronic cases are associated with heavy lifetime use, while acute cases are associated with a recent heavy-drinking episode (e.g., four to five drinks). Acute cases may also be accompanied by rhabdomyolysis, muscle breakdown that can cause kidney failure.[100]

Sleep

Alcohol consumption before bed may initially facilitate sleep, but at higher doses it disrupts the second half of nocturnal sleep. Thus, many individuals with AUD who use alcohol for help with trouble falling asleep actually decrease the quality of their rest. Alcohol use also interacts with other determinants of sleepiness (e.g., sleep deprivation) to exacerbate their effect, further impairing alertness and attention.[101] This compounding effect on drowsiness has important implications for determining low-risk consumption levels when sleep deprivation is at play, especially for activities like driving.[102]

Cancer

The link between alcohol and cancer is strong—4% of all cancers are attributable to alcohol. Separate reports from the World Cancer Research Fund/the American Institute for Cancer Research and from the International Agency for Research on Cancer came to virtually identical conclusions: that the evidence supports a causal role for alcohol in cancer of the oral cavity, pharynx, larynx, esophagus, breast, colorectum, and liver (i.e., hepatocellular carcinoma).[103] Another meta-analysis suggests alcohol also increases risk of cancers of the stomach, lung, ovary, and prostate.[104] Risk for all cancers from alcohol is dose-dependent, with increasing amounts and durations of drinking associated with increasing risk. While clear associations exist between heavy use and risk for all cancers identified, risks for some cancers are apparent even at lower levels (e.g., less than one to two standard drinks per day, on average, in the case of breast cancer).[105] It remains unclear whether there is any threshold of alcohol consumption below which no increased risk of cancer is evident.

Infectious Disease

Heavy drinking puts people at increased risk for infectious diseases. Direct biological effects of alcohol exposure on the immune system reduce both the frequency and the functional effectiveness of the body's immune cells (e.g., neutrophils, monocytes, and macrophages), thereby weakening immune responses.[106] They can also impair specific defenses such as the gag reflex and respiratory clearance. Alcohol may also increase risk for infectious disease through behavioral effects, such as by interfering with motivation to seek medical care or by compromising treatment adherence.[107] Likely due to the combined effects of these diverse mechanisms, alcohol consumption has been shown to significantly increase risk and severity of infections from HIV, HCV, and *Mycobacterium tuberculosis* [the bacterium that causes tuberculosis (TB)], among others. For example, a meta-analysis found a threefold increase in active TB for individuals who drink more than 40 g/day or have AUD.[108]

Fetal Consequences

Alcohol is teratogenic, and heavy prenatal alcohol exposure has been associated with a fourfold increase in birth defects.[109] While chronic heavy episodic drinking is associated with the greatest risk and most severe consequences of birth defects, risk is present even with less use, and there is no clear consumption threshold below which risk for birth defects are not elevated,[110,111] though some studies of low consumption have failed to show associations with adverse birth outcomes. Birth defects from prenatal alcohol exposure (collectively termed Fetal Alcohol Spectrum Disorders) include brain damage with related behavioral and cognitive impairments, as well as the more severe Fetal Alcohol Syndrome (FAS), characterized by CNS abnormalities, a specific pattern of facial abnormalities, and growth deficits. Alcohol is the leading cause of "birth defects" (physical disability, deformity, and intellectual disability) in the United States.

PREVENTION

Concepts

Public health organizations and medical treatment settings have developed programs and guidelines aimed at curbing the incidence of alcohol use disorder and preventing the harms associated with risky use in the general population. These efforts can be categorized into three types based on their target audience: *universal* (i.e., applying to everyone), *selective* (i.e., applying only to those identified as being at greater risk), and *indicated* (i.e., treatment targeted at preventing progression of the disorder for those already demonstrating symptoms).

Youth Alcohol Use

Universal prevention of alcohol use disorders is generally implemented with youth under the legal drinking age of 21, given that early initiation of drinking is associated with heightened risk of developing AUD later in life, as well as with heightened risk of acute harms. Prevention of underage drinking has, however, proven to be a difficult public health goal to address systematically. Different approaches include school-based, family-based, and community-based programs.

School Based

There are varieties of different methods used in school-based prevention programs. Models relying purely on education about alcohol use harms have proven ineffective and have largely been (or should be) abandoned. A prominent example is Drug Abuse Resistance Education (DARE), a school-based program launched in 1983 whose original approach centered on uniformed police officers visiting schools to raise awareness about the dangers of drugs and alcohol. After multiple trials and meta-analyses found there was no evidence to suggest DARE. was effective, DARE abandoned its original curriculum in 2009.[112,113]

Newer efficacious approaches to school-based prevention programs include social resistance skills training, normative education, and competence enhancement. Social resistance skills training strive to improve students' awareness of influences from peers and the media, and to increase their specific skill set in responding to and resisting those influences. Normative education focuses on survey statistics to help re-establish social norms (i.e., to remind students that not all of their peers are drinking and/or using drugs, and that in many cases only a small minority are). Competence enhancement teaches general life skills in problem solving and decision-making and is meant to enhance characteristics considered to be protective against early substance use or mental health conditions, such as self-confidence and self-esteem. The key observation is that risk and resilience factors related to drinking alcohol are also related to many other health risks and related behaviors beyond alcohol use.

There is a dearth of systematic research on the effectiveness of these programs, but a Cochrane Review of school-based programs in the United Kingdom found positive effects on some drinking outcomes (namely drunkenness and binge drinking) in 6 out of 11 alcohol-specific prevention programs reviewed, and in 15 out of 39 generic alcohol and drug prevention programs.[114] The review suggests that generic programs based in psychosocial or developmental approaches (e.g., life skills) showed more significant effects over time than usual education or other interventions. Botvin's life skills training program is such an example.[115] However, there are no clear defining characteristics for optimizing success of interventions. More research is needed to establish clear guidelines for effective school-based prevention programs.

Family Based

Family-based prevention programs may include classes and workshops for parents without their child present, or may incorporate curriculum that involves the child's participation as well. These programs generally aim to educate parents about how to communicate with their child around alcohol use and how to help their child develop social resistance skills. Family-based programs may also encourage parental monitoring and supervision, and provide guidelines for rule-setting, positive reinforcement, and discipline.[116]

Community Based

Community-based programs are often a collaborative effort driven by community leaders, parents, teachers, administrators, and policy makers. These programs may involve a combination of school-based and family-based approaches, and may also incorporate other approaches, such as media campaigns (e.g., public service announcements) or policy changes (e.g., measures designed to restrict youth access to alcohol). A successful example is "Communities that Care," an intervention that organized and trained a coalition of community members to first identify risk factors for multiple behavior problems among youth in the community, and then implement a selection of relevant evidence-based interventions. Students who participated in Communities that Care were significantly more likely than controls to have abstained from alcohol, cigarette, and other drug use at follow-up 8 years after the intervention began.[117]

Fetal Alcohol Exposure

Efforts to prevent fetal alcohol exposure represent a selective approach, where pregnant women are targeted due to the increased risk associated with alcohol use during pregnancy. Given that drinking during pregnancy causes birth defects and there is no known threshold under which consumption is safe, guidelines for prevention of Fetal Alcohol Spectrum Disorders (FASD) recommend abstinence for the duration of the pregnancy. The American College of Obstetricians and Gynecologists outlines three steps for prevention of FASD: 91) use of effective birth control if you drink, are having sexual intercourse, and do not wish to become pregnant; (2) not drinking if you are trying to become pregnant; and (3) stopping drinking immediately if you have been drinking and discover you are pregnant.[118] Physicians are directed to screen pregnant women for alcohol use, to counsel them not to drink, and to refer them to treatment as indicated. Other public health efforts focus on promoting awareness of risks among the general public via, for example, media campaigns and labeling alcohol containers with warnings for pregnant women. Unfortunately, there has been limited systematic research or evaluation regarding the effectiveness of these campaigns,[119] and fetal alcohol exposure remains the leading cause of preventable birth defects. One challenge is that much exposure to alcohol occurs before women are aware of a pregnancy.

Individual Prevention

Prevention at the individual level means identifying and intervening with those who are at heightened risk for unhealthy alcohol use or who have already had consequences of hazardous use or symptoms of alcohol use disorder (i.e., indicated cases). This process relies heavily on screening and brief intervention (which may, in some cases, be augmented with a referral to other services). The U.S. Substance Abuse and Mental Health Services Administration has disseminated its version of screening and brief intervention known as Screening, Brief Intervention, and Referral to Treatment, or SBIRT, which can be incorporated into primary-care visits or done in other general health settings. SBIRT begins with screening patients by asking them about their alcohol use using a validated screening tool such as the AUDIT-C or a single-item screening question [e.g., "How many times in the past year have you had five or more drinks in a day?" (four for women)]. In cases where patients report unhealthy use, a brief intervention is conducted in which the patient is counseled in a nonjudgmental fashion (often based on the principles of motivational interviewing), offered education about the risks associated with use, and given recommendations for changing their consumption patterns. If the patient is identified as having a disorder, treatment or referral for it is the next step.

Evidence supports the utility of SBIRT for reducing self-reported consumption in less severe cases where patients are engaging in risky drinking or have experienced limited harms from their alcohol use. Brief education on the risks associated with their drinking as well as encouragement and guidelines for cutting down may be sufficient to change behavior in such cases.[120,121] However, systematic reviews have not found consistent effects on any biological, behavioral, or health-care utilization outcomes. Specifically, screening and brief intervention has been shown to be of limited, if any, effectiveness for either linking people to further care or changing use and consequences when the target of the intervention is diagnosed AUD,[122] or when there are other drug use or psychiatric comorbidities. In these cases, more intensive treatment is generally indicated.

Preventive Policies

Policy-level prevention strategies are discussed at the end of the chapter, in the *Prevention* section.

TREATMENT

Treatment for alcohol use disorder can be broadly divided into two categories: counseling/behavioral therapy, and medications. [Note: medication treatment or medication for alcohol use disorder treatment is sometimes referred to as medication-*assisted* treatment (MAT), though this term is not preferred.] These therapeutic approaches can be used independently or in combination with one another.

Counseling/Behavioral Therapy

The following approaches to counseling/behavioral therapy are evidence-based strategies that have demonstrated their effectiveness in treating AUD.[123]

12-step Facilitation

By far the most common and widely available model for behavioral treatment of AUD in the United States is psychoeducation delivered by counselors, who are deemed qualified both by their training and certification largely in the 12-step approach to AUD, as well as by their personal experience with AUD; efficacy has not been established and often the approach has been the "usual care" control group in treatment trials. However, 12-step facilitation, or TSF, which likewise has its basis in the principles of Alcoholics Anonymous (AA), was codified (manualized) into a formal treatment approach in 1999 to be included in Project MATCH (a major multisite trial of behavioral treatments for AUD led by the National Institute on Alcohol Abuse and Alcoholism). Unlike other treatments studied in project MATCH, TSF was included not because it was developed based on scientific evidence or because it had proven its effectiveness in clinical trials, but because its principles were already widely in use via Alcoholics Anonymous. Since its formal codification, however, it has been studied alongside other evidence-based approaches, and has demonstrated similar (and, for some outcomes, better) results in treating AUD.[124]

As the name would suggest, TSF is based on the 12 steps originally established by the Alcoholics Anonymous founders. The key tenets of these steps involve assessment and overview (inventory), acceptance, surrender, and getting active. The treatment approach relies on a highly structured manual used by a trained counselor to link the patient to AA meetings and to guide the patient through these steps over a 12- to 24-week period. Unlike AA, TSF is administered by a therapist (rather than peer-led mutual-help), but engagement in self/mutual-help groups like AA is a central component.

Motivational Interviewing

Motivational Interviewing (MI) is designed to help patients to resolve ambivalence they may have about change and to engage in realizing personal goals. MI can be used as counseling for various types of behavior change, but it was originally developed to help patients with alcohol and substance use disorders, and has demonstrated its effectiveness in this context. MI was standardized into a manual-based approach as motivational enhancement therapy (MET) in project MATCH, and was briefer but just as effective as the other behavioral treatments. While MI is generally used in conjunction with other behavioral therapies, it is often a useful first step for engaging people in treatment and helping define treatment goals early on. MI can be used throughout the course of treatment to help improve treatment adherence, reduce drug and alcohol use, and maintain patient investment in making health behavior changes.

Cognitive Behavioral Therapy (CBT)

Cognitive Behavioral Therapy is a broad term encompassing a range of goal-directed approaches to cognitive and behavioral change. Collectively, these approaches are designed to help identify circumstances, thoughts, and interpersonal situations that may trigger unwanted behavioral responses (in this case, alcohol use) and to practice changing unhealthy thought and behavior patterns. Patients are coached on not only identifying and anticipating the triggers, but also on developing specific coping skills to respond more adaptively. Multiple meta-analyses provide strong evidence for the efficacy of CBT in treating alcohol and other addictive disorders.[125,126] The following nine behavioral therapies are specific strategies that fall under the umbrella of CBTs.

Community Reinforcement Approach

The underlying principle of the Community Reinforcement Approach (CRA) is to eliminate positive reinforcement for drinking and enhance positive reinforcement for sobriety. Strategies utilized by CRA therapists include "increasing the client's motivation to stop drinking, initiating a trial period of sobriety, performing a functional analysis of the client's drinking behavior, increasing positive reinforcement through various measures, rehearsing new coping behaviors, and involving the client's significant others."[127]

Contingency Management

Contingency management involves monitoring the patient closely to test for alcohol use (e.g., using breath or blood tests, or urinalysis), and then using reward and punishment to encourage or maintain positive outcomes (i.e., testing negative for alcohol use). Rewards often include cash or vouchers, and punishment may be the simple withholding of the reward, or could include negative reports distributed to interested parties such as family members or parole officers.[128] The approach has not been as well studied or implemented for alcohol as it has for other drugs because of limitations in testing.

Systematic Desensitization

Systematic desensitization, a technique originally developed for use with posttraumatic stress disorder, allows patients to mentally prepare for real-world situations likely to be stressful or intolerable, while still in the safe and supportive environment of treatment. Patients are asked to rank potential environments or experiences that they would consider overwhelming to face while sober (e.g., a work holiday party, or a first date). Starting with the easiest and working toward the most difficult, they are coached through imagined exposures to help think through and practice how to approach these situations. Training in relaxation skills, techniques for managing craving states, and drink refusal skills are built into this process.

Cue Exposure Therapy

Cue exposure therapy is premised on the idea that cues historically associated with alcohol use can induce conditioned responses, triggering craving and relapse.[129] Cue exposure therapy, by extension, exposes individuals with AUD to their favorite alcoholic drink or other related triggers, again in a safe and controlled environment. This approach brings the patient into direct contact with craving states and teaches them skills to manage these states.

Interpersonal Skills Training

Many people with AUD have difficulty in interpersonal relationships. Key family and peer relationships may be impoverished or full of conflict, or patients may have trauma histories impairing their interpersonal behaviors. Helping patients improve their relationships with other human beings can increase support and reduce stress, and can help them to devalue the role of alcohol in their life.

Relapse Prevention

Relapse prevention is a treatment model that is often incorporated into the other approaches discussed here. The goal of this approach is to help the individual identify both immediate determinants (such as high-risk situations) and covert antecedents (such as lifestyle factors) that may precipitate relapse. Together the therapist and patient address each step of the relapse process and enhance the patient's skills for coping with these situations, and also managing lapses should they occur.[130]

Dialectical Behavioral Therapy

Dialectical behavioral therapy (DBT) was originally designed for people with mood disorders or borderline personality disorder. Over the last decade, a DBT specifically for alcohol/substance use disorders has been developed and tested, demonstrating its efficacy in this application. DBT for AUD tackles three domains: interpersonal effectiveness, distress tolerance, and affect management. As a whole, it is designed to help patients manage the mood states that may underlie alcohol/substance use conditions.

Acceptance and Commitment Therapy

Acceptance and commitment therapy coaches individuals with AUD to not feel compelled to avoid the feelings that make them want to drink. Instead, the treatment approach helps them accept and tolerate these feelings, and focuses on helping them act in accordance with their values.

Behavioral Marital Therapy and Family Behavioral Therapy

Much like interpersonal skills training, behavioral marital therapy and family behavioral therapy are premised on the idea that relationships can be a trigger or a resource. These approaches help significant others to become engaged in new and more productive ways, and help the patient practice skills and improve his/her relationship(s).

Combining Behavioral Therapies

Although many of these techniques have efficacy on their own, they are often used together to try to achieve greater effect (e.g., MI and CBT in a combined behavioral approach, along with elements of TSF). Combinations have not been studied widely, but some evidence exists for an addiction-specific combined MI and CBT therapy, and effects of these behavioral therapy combinations are likely also enhanced by medications.[131]

Medications

There are currently three FDA-approved pharmacotherapies for the treatment of alcohol use disorder: acamprosate, naltrexone (two medication preparations), and disulfiram. Topiramate, a medication approved for the treatment of epilepsy, also has proven efficacy for treating AUD, though it is not currently FDA-approved for this indication. All four are available in daily oral form, though one challenge to this form is adherence to medication. Naltrexone is also available as an extended-release monthly injection, which may help with adherence (at least initially), since its effects last almost 1 month.

All four have been shown in some clinical trials to modestly increase rates of abstinence and decrease incidence or frequency of heavy drinking. One potential challenge for prescribers and patients, however, is that in some cases it is required or recommended that patients be abstinent before beginning these pharmacotherapies. Acamprosate, for example, is only approved for patients who are abstinent at the time they begin the medication. Likewise, naltrexone has been shown to be more effective in study subjects who abstained from alcohol use for 4–7 days before treatment. Topiramate, the epilepsy medication, is an exception: it has been shown effective in study volunteers who were still drinking.[132]

Acamprosate

Acamprosate appears to act on the GABA and glutamate neurotransmitter systems; however, its exact mechanism of action is unclear.[133] It is believed to decrease relapse by mitigating the symptoms of the protracted abstinence syndrome, including insomnia, anxiety, and dysphoria. Its main side effect is diarrhea, which resolves with continued use of the medication.

Naltrexone

Naltrexone blocks opioid receptors, tamping down cravings for alcohol and the euphoric sensations (reward) associated with drinking. Two reviews of more than 50 randomized trials found that oral naltrexone decreased heavy drinking.[134,135] One of these reviews found that oral naltrexone also increased rates of abstinence.[134] Both reviews found injectable naltrexone ineffective; the FDA approved it based on a pivotal randomized placebo-controlled trial.[136] Naltrexone's main side effects are nausea, dizziness, and dysphoria, and it cannot be used in people who are taking opioids.

Disulfiram

Taking disulfiram makes drinking alcohol very unpleasant. The medication interferes with the metabolism of alcohol, allowing acetaldehyde to accumulate which produces severe reactions that include nausea, flushing, and palpitations.[132] A notable drawback of disulfiram is that adherence is generally poor, except in controlled environments.[137] Supervised administration (directly observed by a clinician or significant other) has greatest efficacy. A main side effect is idiosyncratic liver damage.

Topiramate

Topiramate, an anticonvulsant, has been shown in some trials to decrease heavy-drinking days and to increase rates of abstinence.[138] However, results are mixed, and a randomized trial showed no difference in alcohol consumption for topiramate relative to placebo.[139] Topiramate's mechanism of action in treatment of AUD is not well understood, and symptomatic side effects are substantial (e.g., anorexia).

SELF- AND MUTUAL-HELP

In addition to professional treatment, many individuals with alcohol use disorder may choose to attend self- or mutual-help groups. The most well known and popular of these is Alcoholics Anonymous, or AA. The group, which identifies as a fellowship, was established in 1939 on the simple premise that people in recovery could benefit from a network of social support for one another. Participation in AA involves attending meetings, which are held regularly in practically every corner of the country. There is no central governing body of the organization, and meetings are peer-led by members in recovery rather than by therapists or professionals. Meetings are meant to provide a sober environment for members to feel safe, as well as a forum for sharing stories and experiences without judgment. The founders (known as Bill W. and Dr. Bob) also established 12 steps and 12 traditions, two of the more structured elements of the program. The traditions represent guidelines for meetings, while the steps are the necessary actions for members to take to participate in the program. The process of "working the steps" involves admitting lack of control over addiction, recognizing that a higher power can give you strength to achieve sobriety, examining past mistakes, making amends, learning to live life with a new code and helping others (among other steps).

Although the design of AA at its inception was not based on any empiric evidence, several components of the program have therapeutic value. New members are encouraged to get a sponsor who will help coach them through challenges of early recovery and also provide a sense of accountability. Members are also recognized for sobriety anniversaries and given chips to reward their progress. But while many individuals with AUD find AA to be a helpful and encouraging environment, others may find certain aspects of the program to be alienating, such as the emphasis on religion and spirituality, the heavy focus on abstinence only (which sometimes extends to a culture of general disapproval toward medications for addictive disorders), or the need to acknowledge your own powerlessness and relinquish a sense of agency over your life in order to work the steps as they are written.

Although AA is not for everyone, it is a helpful resource when used voluntarily for those who find it beneficial, given that it is free, accessible, and very widespread. What began as a modest initiative is now a massive network that has maintained its popularity for decades. In the United States alone, there are over 61,000 groups, with a total of nearly 1.3 million members (worldwide these numbers climb to ~118,000 and 2.1 million, respectively).[140]

While Alcoholics Anonymous is by far the most popular and widespread of the self- and mutual-help groups, other groups with their own particular goals and nuances have emerged over time. There are additional 12-step self-help groups in the mold of AA for practically every class of substance use disorder (e.g., narcotics anonymous, cocaine anonymous, marijuana anonymous, and nicotine anonymous). There are also groups that intentionally diverge from the 12-step model such as Secular Organizations for Sobriety (SOS) and Self-Management and Recovery Training (SMART), both of which do not have a religious focus (and the latter of which attempts instead to focus meetings on skills training from the latest evidence-based research in addiction recovery). Another alternative is Moderation Management (MM), which, unlike AA, does not view abstinence as a necessary goal. All other self- and mutual-help groups are much smaller than AA (and therefore offer many fewer meetings relative to AA) and none have been empirically studied.

Although AA is difficult to study, some research on its utility has been conducted. Multiple studies indicate a relationship between self-selected participation in 12-step mutual support groups and increased likelihood of sobriety at follow-up, relative to those who did not (and chose not to) participate in groups.[140,141] Additional research conducted on TSF through the MATCH study supports a beneficial role for 12-step participation in recovery, even over evidence-based therapy like CBT for selected outcomes and participants.[124]

It is worth noting that other self-help alternatives beyond mutual support groups like AA are available and relatively accessible as well. These may take the form of books or Internet-screening tools, both of which can help an individual identify if he or she is drinking at unhealthy levels, and can offer resources, support, and sometimes even a brief intervention and linkage to in-person care.

TREATMENT SYSTEM

Alcohol use disorder is associated with devastating consequences to the individual (e.g., job loss, health harms, legal problems, and homelessness), and to society (e.g., motor vehicle accidents, violence, economic costs). It is therefore unsurprising, though unfortunate, that much of the general public has long-held negative biases toward individuals with alcohol and other substance use disorders (SUDs). Historically, individuals with AUD and SUD have been stereotyped as deceitful, prone to theft, violent, and generally immoral and, as a result of this stigma, have been ostracized from traditional medical treatment settings. Instead, a separate treatment system for use disorders developed in parallel.

At its inception, this parallel "treatment" system addressed individuals with AUD or SUD primarily via the justice system, social sanctions, or moral instruction, and offerings for therapeutic care were virtually nonexistent. Although the founders of the social network Alcoholics Anonymous and the American Medical Association (as of 1956), among others, recognized AUD and SUDs as medical conditions, society at large did not. This public view and the related approach to "treatment" proved unsustainable, however, when overwhelming numbers of veterans returned from the Vietnam War over the course of the 1960s and 1970s addicted to alcohol or other drugs. A new precedent was set in this climate for therapeutic rehabilitation to be made available to those with alcohol and other substance use disorders. However stigma persisted, and the separation of addiction treatment from general medical care had already been established and engrained. Rather than integrate with mainstream medical care or draw down its resources, addiction treatment was administered by individuals who had use disorders themselves but were no longer using substances. Therapy offerings consisted of a prescribed milieu, groups with other people seeking treatment for use disorders, and educational lectures, all led by staff in recovery and often offered at remote residential facilities culturally and physically separated from the rest of the patient's life. This model gave rise to addiction "rehab," and is still a predominant addiction treatment model offered today.

Also unique to the addiction treatment system in place today is its financing. Addiction treatment in the United States is mostly publicly funded, paid for by block federal grants to the state, which are then distributed to treatment facilities. Private programs often do not accept or are not covered by health insurance. Public funding currently supports over 14,000 treatment programs, which may take the form of inpatient (residential) treatment, or outpatient treatment (where the patient can live at home but attends treatment for most of the day). Unfortunately, today's addiction treatment system is rife with dropout and relapse, and remains in place largely because of inertia rather than any evidence that the system is optimal for either patients or society.

Fortunately, however, the last decade has seen a slow but meaningful shift in attitudes and practices surrounding the management of addiction treatment. There is a current trend toward integrating addiction care into general health settings, as well as toward coverage of addiction as a medical condition (and, increasingly, as a chronic illness). Accountable Care Organizations (ACOs) are likewise focusing more on coordinating care for people rather than just acute medical treatment episodes. They are recognizing that to better manage care in terms of cost and quality, services need to be accessible and integrated, including care for alcohol and other drug use disorders. The myth that stand-alone rehabilitation programs are the superior (or only) recourse for individuals with severe use disorders has been debunked (see the book Inside Rehab[142]), and instead there has been an increase in outpatient medical treatment offerings using evidence-based practices and treatments. Resources for navigating the changing system are becoming more available, too: just in 2017, the NIAAA launched its Treatment Navigator tool on its website (https://alcoholtreatment.niaaa.nih.gov/) to help patients and families sift through treatment options and connect with quality care.

POLICY

Alcohol-related public policy has the potential to affect large-scale change in patterns of alcohol consumption and unhealthy use. While the widespread and normative use of alcohol in the United States makes eliminating alcohol-related risk from society virtually impossible, several policies have demonstrated their efficacy in reducing certain harms.

Taxes

Research clearly indicates that rates of alcohol consumption are sensitive to alcohol price, allowing tax policy to help limit sales and thereby curb consumption.[143] Indeed, a review found that alcohol prices and taxes were inversely related to indices of sales or consumption.[144] A separate meta-analysis also concluded that policies affecting alcohol price have significant effects on rates of alcohol-related disease and injury, and that doubling the tax would reduce alcohol-related mortality by an average of 35%, making a clear case for the practical public health utility of such a policy.[145]

Driving Laws

Policies enforcing impaired driving laws have likewise proven effective. A study evaluating three laws targeting driving while intoxicated [administrative license revocation laws, 1.0 illegal per se laws, and 0.08 illegal per se laws (meaning that impaired driving need not be proven; the level is sufficient evidence)] found that each of the three had a significant relationship to the downward trend in fatal alcohol-related motor vehicle crashes.[146] Additionally, while not specifically alcohol-related policy, graduated driver licensing (GDL) laws that incrementally increase driving privileges of new, young drivers have been shown to be impactful in youth alcohol-related risky behavior. A regression model combining statistics on state GDL laws and youth behaviors found that restrictive GDL laws were related to reduced alcohol use behaviors and reduced risky driving behaviors among youth.[147] This study provides encouraging evidence that alcohol-related harms may be reduced through a variety of policy approaches that may not necessarily be alcohol-specific.

Drinking Age

The minimum legal drinking age (MLDA) has been studied extensively for its role in influencing youth alcohol consumption and alcohol-related harms.[148] A series of studies by Waagenar and colleagues thoroughly demonstrated that changes in state MLDAs (which were ongoing up until 1984, when 21 became the uniform standard) were significantly temporally related to alcohol use and consequences, such that when a state raised its MLDA, use and problems decreased, and vice versa.[149,150] Another study also found that the risks associated with a lower MLDA had long-term implications, such that adults who had been legally allowed to purchase alcohol before age 21 in the 70s and 80s were more likely to meet criteria for past-year alcohol use disorder when assessed between 1991 and 2001.[151] This finding helps highlight the impactful role that policy can have on long-term culture and behavior patterns.

Restricting Access/Sales

As common sense might suggest, limiting access to alcohol is another effective way to limit sales and consumption. This can be achieved through state policies, which may regulate the type, number, and locations of alcohol outlets.[152] The potential impact of these restrictions is supported by findings that per capita numbers of outlets are correlated with both prevalence of alcohol use disorder and acute alcohol-related harms[153,154]; however it is difficult to test whether this relationship is causal. In addition to locations, states can also legally restrict the hours and days that alcohol may be sold. These restrictions are less likely to have a large-scale impact on consumption, however, since individuals may simply buy alcohol in advance of when they consume it, or displace their drinking to other days/times of the week. Studies on the overall impact of these regulations on drinking behavior are difficult to conduct, and therefore limited, and results have been mixed.[152]

Community Interventions

It is worth mentioning that in addition to changes in state policies, community interventions can be effective. In one such example, a community undertook a campaign to mobilize its members around policies affecting risky drinking behaviors. Specifically, their goals included promoting responsible beverage service, restricting underage access to alcohol, increasing law enforcement of drinking and driving laws, and using zoning to limit overall community access to alcohol. Results of a longitudinal study indicated that, after the intervention, self-reported occasions of excessive alcohol use, as well as amount of use per occasion declined significantly (by 49% and 6%, respectively). Additionally, both self-report and traffic data indicated a decrease in drinking and driving in the wake of the intervention.[155] A separate but similar intervention targeted increasing substance use disorder treatment and reducing alcohol availability in the community. This intervention also proved successful in decreasing alcohol-related harm outcomes: the study reported significant decreases in alcohol-related motor vehicle fatalities.[156] These studies suggest community interventions may be an effective alternative to formal policy changes in influencing public health.

SUMMARY

Alcohol's public health impact is significant. While chronic heavy use is associated with the most severe negative health consequences, widespread normative consumption also contributes to these consequences, and on a much larger scale. A successful public health strategy mitigating alcohol's negative impact must therefore incorporate both universal and selective prevention efforts, as well as initiatives to improve the quality and availability of treatment for indicated cases. While more research is needed to determine best practices for integrating various public health approaches, encouraging data exist suggesting a role for alcohol-related public policy; school-, community-, and family-based prevention initiatives; as well as large-scale changes to the alcohol use disorder treatment system.

References

1. Center for Behavioral Health Statistics and Quality. *2016 National Survey on Drug Use and Health: Detailed Tables*. Rockville, MD: Substance Abuse and Mental Health Services Administration; 2017.
2. Centers for Disease Control and Prevention. Alcohol Related Disease Impact (ARDI) application. 2013.
3. Sacks JJ, Gonzales KR, Bouchery EE, Tomedi LE, Brewer RD. 2010 National and State Costs of Excessive Alcohol Consumption. *Am J Prev Med*. 2015;49(5):e73–9.
4. National Institute on Alcohol Abuse and Alcoholism. *Rethinking Drinking: Alcohol and Your Health*. Bethesda, MD: Department of Health and Human Services, NIH, National Institute on Alcohol Abuse and Alcoholism; 2016.
5. Grant BF, Goldstein RB, Saha TD, et al. Epidemiology of DSM-5 alcohol use disorder: Results from the National Epidemiologic Survey on Alcohol and Related Conditions III. *JAMA Psychiatry*. 2015;72(8):757–66.
6. Grant BF, Chou SP, Saha TD, et al. Prevalence of 12-month alcohol use, high-risk drinking, and DSM-IV alcohol use disorder in the United States, 2001–2002 to 2012–2013: Results from the National Epidemiologic Survey on Alcohol and Related Conditions. *JAMA Psychiatry*. 2017;74(9):911–23.
7. Morozova TV, Mackay TF, Anholt RR. Genetics and genomics of alcohol sensitivity. *Mol Genet Genomics*. 2014;289(3):253–69.
8. Morozova TV, Goldman D, Mackay TF, Anholt RR. The genetic basis of alcoholism: Multiple phenotypes, many genes, complex networks. *Genome Biol*. 2012;13(2):239.
9. Enoch MA, Goldman D. The genetics of alcoholism and alcohol abuse. *Curr Psychiatry Rep*. 2001;3(2):144–51.
10. Heath AC. Genetic influences on alcoholism risk: a review of adoption and twin studies. *Alcohol Health Res World*. 1995;19:166–71.
11. Hingson RW, Heeren T, Winter MR. Age at drinking onset and alcohol dependence: Age at onset, duration, and severity. *Arch Pediatr Adolesc Med*. 2006;160(7):739–46.
12. Grant BF, Dawson DA. Age at onset of alcohol use and its association with DSM-IV alcohol abuse and dependence: Results from the National Longitudinal Alcohol Epidemiologic Survey. *J Subst Abuse*. 1997;9:103–10.
13. Zeigler DW, Wang CC, Yoast RA, et al. The neurocognitive effects of alcohol on adolescents and college students. *Prev Med*. 2005;40(1):23–32.
14. Ystrom E, Kendler KS, Reichborn-Kjennerud T. Early age of alcohol initiation is not the cause of alcohol use disorders in adulthood, but is a major indicator of genetic risk. A population-based twin study. *Addiction*. 2014;109(11):1824–32.
15. Enoch MA. The role of early life stress as a predictor for alcohol and drug dependence. *Psychopharmacology (Berl)*. 2011;214(1):17–31.
16. Rothman EF, Edwards EM, Heeren T, Hingson RW. Adverse childhood experiences predict earlier age of drinking onset: Results from a representative US sample of current or former drinkers. *Pediatrics*. 2008;122(2):e298–304.
17. Schwandt ML, Heilig M, Hommer DW, George DT, Ramchandani VA. Childhood trauma exposure and alcohol dependence severity in adulthood: Mediation by emotional abuse severity and neuroticism. *Alcohol Clin Exp Res*. 2013;37(6):984–92.
18. Dawson DA, Harford TC, Grant BF. Family history as a predictor of alcohol dependence. *Alcohol Clin Exp Res*. 1992;16(3):572–5.
19. Goodwin DW, Schulsinger F, Hermansen L, Guze SB, Winokur G. Alcohol problems in adoptees raised apart from alcoholic biological parents. *Arch Gen Psychiatry*. 1973;28(2):238–43.
20. Goodwin DW, Schulsinger F, Moller N, Hermansen L, Winokur G, Guze SB. Drinking problems in adopted and nonadopted sons of alcoholics. *Arch Gen Psychiatry*. 1974;31(2):164–9.
21. Grant BF, Stinson FS, Dawson DA, et al. Prevalence and co-occurrence of substance use disorders and independent mood and anxiety disorders:

Results from the National Epidemiologic Survey on Alcohol and Related Conditions. *Arch Gen Psychiatry.* 2004;61(8):807–16.

22. Marmorstein NR. Longitudinal associations between alcohol problems and depressive symptoms: Early adolescence through early adulthood. *Alcohol Clin Exp Res.* 2009;33(1):49–59.
23. White A, Castle IJ, Chen CM, Shirley M, Roach D, Hingson R. Converging patterns of alcohol use and related outcomes among females and males in the United States, 2002 to 2012. *Alcohol Clin Exp Res.* 2015;39(9):1712–26.
24. Khantzian EJ. Self-regulation and self-medication factors in alcoholism and the addictions. Similarities and differences. *Recent Dev Alcohol.* 1990;8:255–71.
25. Koob GF. Theoretical frameworks and mechanistic aspects of alcohol addiction: Alcohol addiction as a reward deficit disorder. *Curr Top Behav Neurosci.* 2013;13:3–30.
26. Volkow ND, Fowler JS, Wang GJ, Swanson JM. Dopamine in drug abuse and addiction: Results from imaging studies and treatment implications. *Mol Psychiatry.* 2004;9(6):557–69.
27. Koob GF, Buck CL, Cohen A, et al. Addiction as a stress surfeit disorder. *Neuropharmacology.* 2014;76 Pt B:370–82.
28. Bickel WK, Koffarnus MN, Moody L, Wilson AG. The behavioral- and neuro-economic process of temporal discounting: A candidate behavioral marker of addiction. *Neuropharmacology.* 2014;76 Pt B:518–27.
29. Centers for Disease Control and Prevention. The Social-Ecological Model: A Framework for Prevention. 2015. https://www.cdc.gov/violenceprevention/overview/social-ecologicalmodel.html.
30. Gonzalez-Rubio E, San Mauro I, Lopez-Ruiz C, Diaz-Prieto LE, Marcos A, Nova E. Relationship of moderate alcohol intake and type of beverage with health behaviors and quality of life in elderly subjects. *Qual Life Res.* 2016;25(8):1931–42.
31. Schrieks IC, Wei MY, Rimm EB, et al. Bidirectional associations between alcohol consumption and health-related quality of life amongst young and middle-aged women. *J Intern Med.* 2016;279(4):376–87.
32. Jackson R, Scragg R, Beaglehole R. Alcohol consumption and risk of coronary heart disease. *BMJ.* 1991;303(6796):211–6.
33. Malinski MK, Sesso HD, Lopez-Jimenez F, Buring JE, Gaziano JM. Alcohol consumption and cardiovascular disease mortality in hypertensive men. *Arch Intern Med.* 2004;164(6):623–8.
34. Brien SE, Ronksley PE, Turner BJ, Mukamal KJ, Ghali WA. Effect of alcohol consumption on biological markers associated with risk of coronary heart disease: Systematic review and meta-analysis of interventional studies. *BMJ.* 2011;342:d636.
35. Di Castelnuovo A, Costanzo S, di Giuseppe R, de Gaetano G, Iacoviello L. Alcohol consumption and cardiovascular risk: Mechanisms of action and epidemiologic perspectives. *Future Cardiol.* 2009;5(5):467–77.
36. Fillmore KM, Stockwell T, Chikritzhs T, Bostrom A, Kerr W. Moderate alcohol use and reduced mortality risk: Systematic error in prospective studies and new hypotheses. *Ann Epidemiol.* 2007;17(5 Suppl):S16–23.
37. Naimi TS, Brown DW, Brewer RD, et al. Cardiovascular risk factors and confounders among nondrinking and moderate-drinking U.S. adults. *Am J Prev Med.* 2005;28(4):369–73.
38. Holmes MV, Dale CE, Zuccolo L, et al. Association between alcohol and cardiovascular disease: Mendelian randomisation analysis based on individual participant data. *BMJ.* 2014;349:g4164.
39. Solfrizzi V, D'Introno A, Colacicco AM, et al. Alcohol consumption, mild cognitive impairment, and progression to dementia. *Neurology.* 2007;68(21):1790–9.
40. Woods AJ, Porges EC, Bryant VE, et al. Current heavy alcohol consumption is associated with greater cognitive impairment in older adults. *Alcohol Clin Exp Res.* 2016;40(11):2435–44.
41. Zhang C, Qin YY, Chen Q, et al. Alcohol intake and risk of stroke: A dose-response meta-analysis of prospective studies. *Int J Cardiol.* 2014;174(3):669–77.
42. Howard AA, Arnsten JH, Gourevitch MN. Effect of alcohol consumption on diabetes mellitus: A systematic review. *Ann Intern Med.* 2004;140(3):211–9.
43. Koppes LL, Dekker JM, Hendriks HF, Bouter LM, Heine RJ. Moderate alcohol consumption lowers the risk of type 2 diabetes: A meta-analysis of prospective observational studies. *Diabetes Care.* 2005;28(3):719–25.
44. Leitzmann MF, Giovannucci EL, Stampfer MJ, et al. Prospective study of alcohol consumption patterns in relation to symptomatic gallstone disease in men. *Alcohol Clin Exp Res.* 1999;23(5):835–41.
45. Leitzmann MF, Tsai CJ, Stampfer MJ, et al. Alcohol consumption in relation to risk of cholecystectomy in women. *Am J Clin Nutr.* 2003;78(2):339–47.
46. Wang J, Duan X, Li B, Jiang X. Alcohol consumption and risk of gallstone disease: A meta-analysis. *Eur J Gastroenterol Hepatol.* 2017;29(4):e19–28.
47. de Groot LC, Zock PL. Moderate alcohol intake and mortality. *Nutr Rev.* 1998;56(1 Pt 1):25–6.
48. Di Castelnuovo A, Costanzo S, Bagnardi V, Donati MB, Iacoviello L, de Gaetano G. Alcohol dosing and total mortality in men and women: An updated meta-analysis of 34 prospective studies. *Arch Intern Med.* 2006;166(22):2437–45.
49. Doll R. The benefit of alcohol in moderation. *Drug Alcohol Rev.* 1998;17(4):353–63.
50. Ford ES, Zhao G, Tsai J, Li C. Low-risk lifestyle behaviors and all-cause mortality: Findings from the National Health and Nutrition Examination Survey III Mortality Study. *Am J Public Health.* 2011;101(10):1922–9.
51. Lee SJ, Sudore RL, Williams BA, Lindquist K, Chen HL, Covinsky KE. Functional limitations, socioeconomic status, and all-cause mortality in moderate alcohol drinkers. *J Am Geriatr Soc.* 2009;57(6):955–62.
52. Stockwell T, Zhao J, Panwar S, Roemer A, Naimi T, Chikritzhs T. Do "moderate" drinkers have reduced mortality risk? A systematic review and meta-analysis of alcohol consumption and all-cause mortality. *J Stud Alcohol Drugs.* 2016;77(2):185–98.
53. Voight BF, Peloso GM, Orho-Melander M, et al. Plasma HDL cholesterol and risk of myocardial infarction: A Mendelian randomisation study. *Lancet.* 2012;380(9841):572–80.
54. Centers for Disease Control and Prevention. Alcohol-attributable deaths and years of potential life lost—11 States, 2006–2010. *MMWR Morb Mortal Wkly Rep.* 2014;63(10):213–6.
55. World Health Organization. *Alcohol and Injury in Emergency Departments: Summary of the Report from the WHO Collaborative Study on Alcohol and Injuries.* Geneva, Switzerland: World Health Organization; 2007.
56. Hingson R, Winter M. Epidemiology and consequences of drinking and driving. *Alcohol Res Health.* 2003;27(1):63–78.
57. Taylor B, Irving HM, Kanteres F, et al. The more you drink, the harder you fall: A systematic review and meta-analysis of how acute alcohol consumption and injury or collision risk increase together. *Drug Alcohol Depend.* 2010;110(1–2):108–16.
58. Heinz AJ, Beck A, Meyer-Lindenberg A, Sterzer P, Heinz A. Cognitive and neurobiological mechanisms of alcohol-related aggression. *Nat Rev Neurosci.* 2011;12(7):400–13.
59. Miczek KA, DeBold JF, Hwa LS, Newman EL, de Almeida RM. Alcohol and violence: Neuropeptidergic modulation of monoamine systems. *Ann N Y Acad Sci.* 2015;1349:96–118.
60. National Institute on Alcohol Abuse and Alcoholism. National Institute on Alcohol Abuse and Alcoholism No. 38. Alcohol, Violence, and Aggression. *Alcohol Alert.* 1997.
61. Cherpitel CJ. Alcohol and injuries resulting from violence: A review of emergency room studies. *Addiction.* 1994;89(2):157–65.
62. Cherpitel CJ. Alcohol and violence-related injuries: An emergency room study. *Addiction.* 1993;88(1):79–88.
63. Yoshimura H, Ogawa N. [Pharmaco-ethological analysis of agonistic behavior between resident and intruder mice: Effects of ethylalcohol]. *Nihon Yakurigaku Zasshi.* 1983;81(2):135–41.
64. Miczek KA, Winslow JT, DeBold JF. Heightened aggressive behavior by animals interacting with alcohol-treated conspecifics: Studies with mice, rats and squirrel monkeys. *Pharmacol Biochem Behav.* 1984;20(3):349–53.
65. Miczek KA, Barry H3rd. Effects of alcohol on attack and defensive-submissive reactions in rats. *Psychopharmacology (Berl).* 1977;52(3):231–7.
66. Sinha R. How does stress increase risk of drug abuse and relapse? *Psychopharmacology (Berl).* 2001;158(4):343–59.
67. McCauley J, Kern DE, Kolodner K, et al. The "battering syndrome": Prevalence and clinical characteristics of domestic violence in primary care internal medicine practices. *Ann Intern Med.* 1995;123(10):737–46.
68. Bagge CL, Lee HJ, Schumacher JA, Gratz KL, Krull JL, Holloman G Jr. Alcohol as an acute risk factor for recent suicide attempts: A case-crossover analysis. *J Stud Alcohol Drugs.* 2013;74(4):552–8.
69. Berglund M, Ojehagen A. The influence of alcohol drinking and alcohol use disorders on psychiatric disorders and suicidal behavior. *Alcohol Clin Exp Res.* 1998;22(7 Suppl):333S–45S.
70. Xuan Z, Naimi TS, Kaplan MS, et al. Alcohol policies and suicide: A review of the literature. *Alcohol Clin Exp Res.* 2016;40(10):2043–55.
71. Regan TJ. Alcoholic cardiomyopathy. *Prog Cardiovasc Dis.* 1984;27(3):141–52.
72. Piano MR. Alcoholic cardiomyopathy: Incidence, clinical characteristics, and pathophysiology. *Chest.* 2002;121(5):1638–50.

73. Kodama S, Saito K, Tanaka S, et al. Alcohol consumption and risk of atrial fibrillation: A meta-analysis. *J Am Coll Cardiol.* 2011;57(4):427–36.

74. Costanzo S, Di Castelnuovo A, Donati MB, Iacoviello L, de Gaetano G. Alcohol consumption and mortality in patients with cardiovascular disease: A meta-analysis. *J Am Coll Cardiol.* 2010;55(13):1339–47.

75. Ramstedt M. Per capita alcohol consumption and liver cirrhosis mortality in 14 European countries. *Addiction.* 2001;96 Suppl 1:S19–33.

76. John U, Hanke M. Liver cirrhosis mortality, alcohol consumption and tobacco consumption over a 62 year period in a high alcohol consumption country: A trend analysis. *BMC Res Notes.* 2015;8:822.

77. Deleuran T, Vilstrup H, Becker U, Jepsen P. Epidemiology of alcoholic liver disease in Denmark 2006–2011: A population-based study. *Alcohol Alcohol.* 2015;50(3):352–7.

78. Singal AK, Kodali S, Vucovich LA, Darley-Usmar V, Schiano TD. Diagnosis and treatment of alcoholic hepatitis: A systematic review. *Alcohol Clin Exp Res.* 2016;40(7):1390–402.

79. Grant BF, Dufour MC, Harford TC. Epidemiology of alcoholic liver disease. *Semin Liver Dis.* 1988;8(1):12–25.

80. Thun MJ, Peto R, Lopez AD, et al. Alcohol consumption and mortality among middle-aged and elderly U.S. adults. *N Engl J Med.* 1997;337(24):1705–14.

81. Holman CD, English DR, Milne E, Winter MG. Meta-analysis of alcohol and all-cause mortality: A validation of NHMRC recommendations. *Med J Aust.* 1996;164(3):141–5.

82. Pequignot G, Tuyns AJ, Berta JL. Ascitic cirrhosis in relation to alcohol consumption. *Int J Epidemiol.* 1978;7(2):113–20.

83. Parrish KM, Dufour MC, Stinson FS, Harford TC. Average daily alcohol consumption during adult life among decedents with and without cirrhosis: The 1986 National Mortality Followback Survey. *J Stud Alcohol.* 1993;54(4):450–6.

84. Norton R, Batey R, Dwyer T, MacMahon S. Alcohol consumption and the risk of alcohol related cirrhosis in women. *Br Med J (Clin Res Ed).* 1987;295 (6590):80–2.

85. Batey RG, Burns T, Benson RJ, Byth K. Alcohol consumption and the risk of cirrhosis. *Med J Aust.* 1992;156(6):413–6.

86. Carlen PL, Wortzman G, Holgate RC, Wilkinson DA, Rankin JC. Reversible cerebral atrophy in recently abstinent chronic alcoholics measured by computed tomography scans. *Science.* 1978;200(4345):1076–8.

87. Fein G, Di Sclafani V, Cardenas VA, Goldmann H, Tolou-Shams M, Meyerhoff DJ. Cortical gray matter loss in treatment-naive alcohol dependent individuals. *Alcohol Clin Exp Res.* 2002;26(4):558–64.

88. Oscar-Berman M, Valmas MM, Sawyer KS, Ruiz SM, Luhar RB, Gravitz ZR. Profiles of impaired, spared, and recovered neuropsychologic processes in alcoholism. *Handb Clin Neurol.* 2014;125:183–210.

89. Kopelman MD, Thomson AD, Guerrini I, Marshall EJ. The Korsakoff syndrome: Clinical aspects, psychology and treatment. *Alcohol Alcohol.* 2009;44(2):148–54.

90. Martin PR, Singleton CK, Hiller-Sturmhofel S. The role of thiamine deficiency in alcoholic brain disease. *Alcohol Res Health.* 2003;27(2):134–42.

91. Torvik A. Brain lesions in alcoholics: Neuropathological observations. *Acta Med Scand Suppl.* 1987;717:47–54.

92. Topiwala A, Allan CL, Valkanova V, et al. Moderate alcohol consumption as risk factor for adverse brain outcomes and cognitive decline: Longitudinal cohort study. *BMJ.* 2017;357:j2353.

93. Chopra K, Tiwari V. Alcoholic neuropathy: Possible mechanisms and future treatment possibilities. *Br J Clin Pharmacol.* 2012;73(3):348–62.

94. Knoll MR, Kolbel CB, Teyssen S, Singer MV. Action of pure ethanol and some alcoholic beverages on the gastric mucosa in healthy humans: A descriptive endoscopic study. *Endoscopy.* 1998;30(3):293–301.

95. Teyssen S, Singer MV. Alcohol-related diseases of the oesophagus and stomach. *Best Pract Res Clin Gastroenterol.* 2003;17(4):557–73.

96. Rocco A, Compare D, Angrisani D, Sanduzzi Zamparelli M, Nardone G. Alcoholic disease: Liver and beyond. *World J Gastroenterol.* 2014;20(40):14652–9.

97. Kershaw CD, Guidot DM. Alcoholic lung disease. *Alcohol Res Health.* 2008;31(1):66–75.

98. Epstein M. Alcohol's impact on kidney function. *Alcohol Health Res World.* 1997;21(1):84–92.

99. Ballard HS. The hematological complications of alcoholism. *Alcohol Health Res World.* 1997;21(1):42–52.

100. Simon L, Jolley SE, Molina PE. Alcoholic myopathy: Pathophysiologic mechanisms and clinical implications. *Alcohol Res.* 2017;38(2):207–17.

101. Roehrs T, Roth T. Sleep, sleepiness, and alcohol use. *Alcohol Res Health.* 2001;25(2):101–9.

102. Banks S, Catcheside P, Lack L, Grunstein RR, McEvoy RD. Low levels of alcohol impair driving simulator performance and reduce perception of crash risk in partially sleep deprived subjects. *Sleep.* 2004;27(6):1063–7.

103. LoConte NK, Brewster AM, Kaur JS, Merrill JK, Alberg AJ. Alcohol and cancer: A statement of the American Society of Clinical Oncology. *J Clin Oncol.* 2017;36(1):83–93.

104. Bagnardi V, Blangiardo M, La Vecchia C, Corrao G. Alcohol consumption and the risk of cancer: A meta-analysis. *Alcohol Res Health.* 2001;25(4):263–70.

105. Chen WY, Rosner B, Hankinson SE, Colditz GA, Willett WC. Moderate alcohol consumption during adult life, drinking patterns, and breast cancer risk. *JAMA.* 2011;306(17):1884–90.

106. Szabo G, Saha B. Alcohol's effect on host defense. *Alcohol Res.* 2015;37(2):159–70.

107. Parry C, Rehm J, Poznyak V, Room R. Alcohol and infectious diseases: An overlooked causal linkage? *Addiction.* 2009;104(3):331–2.

108. Lonnroth K, Williams BG, Stadlin S, Jaramillo E, Dye C. Alcohol use as a risk factor for tuberculosis—A systematic review. *BMC Public Health.* 2008;8:289.

109. O'Leary CM, Nassar N, Kurinczuk JJ, et al. Prenatal alcohol exposure and risk of birth defects. *Pediatrics.* 2010;126(4):e843–50.

110. Maier SE, West JR. Drinking patterns and alcohol-related birth defects. *Alcohol Res Health.* 2001;25(3):168–74.

111. Day NL, Helsel A, Sonon K, Goldschmidt L. The association between prenatal alcohol exposure and behavior at 22 years of age. *Alcohol Clin Exp Res.* 2013;37(7):1171–8.

112. Pan W, Bai H. A multivariate approach to a meta-analytic review of the effectiveness of the D.A.R.E. program. *Int J Environ Res Public Health.* 2009;6(1):267–77.

113. Nordum A. The New D.A.R.E. Program—This One Works. *Scientific American.* 2014.

114. Foxcroft DR, Tsertsvadze A. Universal school-based prevention programs for alcohol misuse in young people. *Cochrane Database Syst Rev.* 2011;(5):CD009113.

115. Kreutter KJ, Gewirtz H, Davenny JE, Love C. Drug and alcohol prevention project for sixth graders: First-year findings. *Adolescence.* 1991;26(102):287–93.

116. National Institute on Drug Abuse. Lessons from Prevention Research. *DrugFacts.* 2014. https://www.drugabuse.gov/publications/drugfacts/lessons-prevention-research.

117. Hawkins JD, Oesterle S, Brown EC, Abbott RD, Catalano RF. Youth problem behaviors 8 years after implementing the communities that care prevention system: A community-randomized trial. *JAMA Pediatr.* 2014;168(2):122–9.

118. The American College of Obstetricians and Gynecologists. Alcohol and Women. *Frequently Asked Questions Women's Health.* Vol. 68. 2015.

119. Roozen S, Black D, Peters GY, et al. Fetal alcohol spectrum disorders (FASD): An Approach to effective Prevention. *Curr Dev Disord Rep.* 2016;3(4):229–34.

120. Kaner EF, Dickinson HO, Beyer F, et al. The effectiveness of brief alcohol interventions in primary care settings: A systematic review. *Drug Alcohol Rev.* 2009;28(3):301–23.

121. Jonas DE, Garbutt JC, Amick HR, et al. Behavioral counseling after screening for alcohol misuse in primary care: A systematic review and meta-analysis for the U.S. Preventive Services Task Force. *Ann Intern Med.* 2012;157(9):645–54.

122. Saitz R. Alcohol screening and brief intervention in primary care: Absence of evidence for efficacy in people with dependence or very heavy drinking. *Drug Alcohol Rev.* 2010;29(6):631–40.

123. Wilkens C. What kind of behavioral treatments are delivered in treatment programs? Paper presented at: *40th Annual Research Society on Alcoholism Scientific Meeting*; June 27, 2017, Denver, CO.

124. Project MATCH Research Group. Matching alcoholism treatments to client heterogeneity: Project MATCH three-year drinking outcomes. *Alcohol Clin Exp Res.* 1998;22(6):1300–11.

125. Magill M, Ray LA. Cognitive-behavioral treatment with adult alcohol and illicit drug users: A meta-analysis of randomized controlled trials. *J Stud Alcohol Drugs.* 2009;70(4):516–27.

126. Dutra L, Stathopoulou G, Basden SL, Leyro TM, Powers MB, Otto MW. A meta-analytic review of psychosocial interventions for substance use disorders. *Am J Psychiatry.* 2008;165(2):179–87.

127. Miller WR, Meyers RJ, Hiller-Sturmhofel S. The community-reinforcement approach. *Alcohol Res Health.* 1999;23(2):116–21.

128. Witkiewitz K, Marlatt A. Behavioral therapy across the spectrum. *Alcohol Res Health.* 2011;33(4):313–9.

129. Monti PM, Rohsenow DJ. Coping-skills training and cue-exposure therapy in the treatment of alcoholism. *Alcohol Res Health.* 1999;23(2):107–15.
130. Larimer ME, Palmer RS, Marlatt GA. Relapse prevention. An overview of Marlatt's cognitive-behavioral model. *Alcohol Res Health.* 1999;23(2):151–60.
131. Anton RF, O'Malley SS, Ciraulo DA, et al. Combined pharmacotherapies and behavioral interventions for alcohol dependence: The COMBINE study: A randomized controlled trial. *JAMA.* 2006;295(17):2003–17.
132. National Institute on Alcohol Abuse and Alcoholism. Helping Patients Who Drink Too Much: A Clinician's Guide. Rockville, MD: U.S. Dept. of Health and Human Services, National Institutes of Health, National Institute on Alcohol Abuse and Alcoholism; 2007. https://pubs.niaaa.nih.gov/publications/Practitioner/CliniciansGuide2005/PrescribingMeds.pdf.
133. Yahn SL, Watterson LR, Olive MF. Safety and efficacy of acamprosate for the treatment of alcohol dependence. *Subst Abuse.* 2013;6:1–12.
134. Jonas DE, Amick HR, Feltner C, et al. Pharmacotherapy for adults with alcohol use disorders in outpatient settings: A systematic review and meta-analysis. *JAMA.* 2014;311(18):1889–900.
135. Rosner S, Hackl-Herrwerth A, Leucht S, Vecchi S, Srisurapanont M, Soyka M. Opioid antagonists for alcohol dependence. *Cochrane Database Syst Rev.* 2010;(12):CD001867.
136. Garbutt JC, Kranzler HR, O'Malley SS, et al. Efficacy and tolerability of long-acting injectable naltrexone for alcohol dependence: A randomized controlled trial. *JAMA.* 2005;293(13):1617–25.
137. Fuller RK, Gordis E. Does disulfiram have a role in alcoholism treatment today? *Addiction.* 2004;99(1):21–4.
138. Winslow BT, Onysko M, Hebert M. Medications for alcohol use disorder. *Am Fam Physician.* 2016;93(6):457–65.
139. Likhitsathian S, Uttawichai K, Booncharoen H, Wittayanookulluk A, Angkurawaranon C, Srisurapanont M. Topiramate treatment for alcoholic outpatients recently receiving residential treatment programs: A 12-week, randomized, placebo-controlled trial. *Drug Alcohol Depend.* 2013;133(2):440–6.
140. Ouimette PC, Moos RH, Finney JW. Influence of outpatient treatment and 12-step group involvement on one-year substance abuse treatment outcomes. *J Stud Alcohol.* 1998;59(5):513–22.
141. Moos RH, Moos BS. Rates and predictors of relapse after natural and treated remission from alcohol use disorders. *Addiction.* 2006;101(2):212–22.
142. Fletcher AM. *Inside Rehab: The Surprising Truth about Addiction Treatment: And How to Get Help That Works.* New York: Penguin Books; 2013.
143. Voas RB, Fell JC. Preventing alcohol-related problems through health policy research. *Alcohol Res Health.* 2010;33(1–2):18–28.
144. Elder RW, Lawrence B, Ferguson A, et al. The effectiveness of tax policy interventions for reducing excessive alcohol consumption and related harms. *Am J Prev Med.* 2010;38(2):217–29.
145. Wagenaar AC, Tobler AL, Komro KA. Effects of alcohol tax and price policies on morbidity and mortality: A systematic review. *Am J Public Health.* 2010;100(11):2270–8.
146. Voas RB, Tippetts AS, Fell J. The relationship of alcohol safety laws to drinking drivers in fatal crashes. *Accid Anal Prev.* 2000;32(4):483–92.
147. Cavazos-Rehg PA, Housten AJ, Krauss MJ, et al. Selected state policies and associations with alcohol use behaviors and risky driving behaviors among youth: Findings from monitoring the future study. *Alcohol Clin Exp Res.* 2016;40(5):1030–6.
148. DeJong W, Blanchette J. Case closed: Research evidence on the positive public health impact of the age 21 minimum legal drinking age in the United States. *J Stud Alcohol Drugs Suppl.* 2014;75 Suppl 17:108–15.
149. O'Malley PM, Wagenaar AC. Effects of minimum drinking age laws on alcohol use, related behaviors and traffic crash involvement among American youth: 1976–1987. *J Stud Alcohol.* 1991;52(5):478–91.
150. Wagenaar AC, Toomey TL. Effects of minimum drinking age laws: Review and analyses of the literature from 1960 to 2000. *J Stud Alcohol Suppl.* 2002;(14):206–25.
151. Norberg KE, Bierut LJ, Grucza RA. Long-term effects of minimum drinking age laws on past-year alcohol and drug use disorders. *Alcohol Clin Exp Res.* 2009;33(12):2180–90.
152. Gruenewald PJ. Regulating availability: How access to alcohol affects drinking and problems in youth and adults. *Alcohol Res Health.* 2011;34(2):248–56.
153. Colon I, Cutter HS, Jones WC. Prediction of alcoholism from alcohol availability, alcohol consumption and demographic data. *J Stud Alcohol.* 1982;43(11):1199–213.
154. Watts RK, Rabow J. Alcohol availability and alcohol-related problems in 213 California cities. *Alcohol Clin Exp Res.* 1983;7(1):47–58.
155. Holder HD, Gruenewald PJ, Ponicki WR, et al. Effect of community-based interventions on high-risk drinking and alcohol-related injuries. *JAMA.* 2000;284(18):2341–7.
156. Hingson RW, Zakocs RC, Heeren T, Winter MR, Rosenbloom D, DeJong W. Effects on alcohol related fatal crashes of a community based initiative to increase substance abuse treatment and reduce alcohol availability. *Inj Prev.* 2005;11(2):84–90.

CHAPTER 168

Marijuana Use in the U.S.: Trends, Consequences, Changing Laws

Deborah S. Hasin • Hillary Samples

INTRODUCTION

This chapter aims to provide a broad overview of marijuana use and related disorders. The chapter begins with two sections, one providing historical background information and the other, current context in terms of public attitudes and laws. The next section reviews evidence for additional adverse health effects associated with marijuana use, including physical, mental, and psychosocial outcomes,[1] while considering the strength of research findings to date. The following section provides information on recent trends in perceptions of harmfulness, cannabis potency, trends in adolescent use and the relationship of this to changing marijuana laws, and corresponding information about adult use and specific subgroups. Finally, clinical implications are presented in the context of current epidemiologic evidence and trends over time in an evolving legal and social landscape.

The chapter focuses primarily on information about marijuana use in the United States. Clearly, marijuana is widely used around the world,[2,3] and is associated with risk for many adverse health and social consequences.[3] However, cross-national prevalence comparisons, policy analyses and other projects such as estimating the global burden of disease due to cannabis are considerably hampered by cross-national differences in many factors,[4] including methodological differences in survey methods that can have a substantial impact on prevalence estimates, different meaning of chronological age in terms of life course (e.g., adolescence),[5] and many other cultural differences. Further, the preponderance of high-quality evidence about cannabis and its consequences comes from a limited number of high-income countries,[5] particularly the United States. Therefore, this chapter focuses primarily on information about marijuana use and its consequences in the United States. The research studies reviewed here can be taken as examples that would be very useful to replicate or expand in other countries.

HISTORICAL PERSPECTIVE

Marijuana has had a long and controversial history in the United States, with marked fluctuations in public attitudes toward the acceptability and potential harms associated with its use.[6] The hemp plant, from which cannabis is produced, was brought to North America as a fiber crop (e.g., for rope) by Jamestown settlers in the early 1600s, and hemp products were part of the colonial economy. An early notation of medical use appeared in 1850, when Extractum Cannabis (extract of hemp) was listed in the United States Pharmacopoeia as a treatment for numerous disorders, including neuralgia, tetanus, typhus, cholera, rabies, dysentery, alcoholism, opiate addiction, anthrax, leprosy, incontinence, gout, convulsive disorders, tonsillitis, insanity, excessive menstrual bleeding, and uterine bleeding.[7] A subsequent record of marijuana as a treatment is found in the Pure Food and Drug Act of 1906, which required that any product containing "cannabis indica" be labeled as such.[8] While marijuana had largely been imported to the United States from India prior to the 1900s, the U.S. Department of Agriculture Bureau of Plant Industry announced it had succeeded in growing domestic cannabis of equal quality in 1913.

Recreational marijuana use was mentioned in only a few anecdotal reports in the late 1800s and early 1900s.[9] During that time, antidrug and alcohol sentiments were growing in the United States, and several states passed laws banning marijuana amid the many state-level bans on alcohol sales that ultimately led to national alcohol Prohibition (January 1919–33).[9] Little evidence is available on recreational use of marijuana until the end of alcohol Prohibition, when marijuana use was brought to public attention through sensationalized newspaper reports (supported by the Federal Bureau of Narcotics) connecting marijuana use to violence, insanity, and Mexican immigrants. The influence of the concept of "Reefer Madness" is seen in a 1936 article in the *American Journal of Nursing*, which states that a marijuana user "...will suddenly turn with murderous violence upon whomever is nearest to him. He will run amuck with knife, ax, gun, or anything else that is close at hand, and will kill or maim without any reason."[10] This media campaign contributed to the passage of the 1937 Marijuana Tax Act,[11] which criminalized possession and sale of marijuana. Despite opposition from the American Medical Association (AMA),[12] the law also imposed such strict requirements on physicians recommending marijuana for medical purposes that such recommendations became too burdensome for busy professionals, in effect suppressing its medical use altogether.

During the 1950s, laws were passed and then increased in severity regarding mandatory minimum sentences for marijuana and other drug violations.[13,14] However, condemnation of marijuana peaked during the Nixon administration's War on Drugs. The Comprehensive Drug Abuse Prevention and Control Act became law in 1970, creating five schedules, or classes, of substances.[15] Marijuana was classified under Schedule I (the same category that was used for heroin), meaning no accepted medical use and a high potential for abuse.[16] This definition restricted access to marijuana not only for private individuals, but also for public health and medical scientists as well as pharmaceutical developers. These restrictions were and remain an impediment to research. The 1970 law also created a National Commission on Marijuana and Drug Abuse, which was tasked with reporting to the government and the public on marijuana use, outcomes, and the effectiveness of marijuana laws at the time. The 1972 report on marijuana included recommendations to redefine marijuana in order to distinguish it from narcotics, to expand support for research on potential medicinal applications, and to decriminalize personal use and possession.[17] Although the Federal administration rejected many of the recommendations made in the report, state-level changes began to arise as a result of support by citizens and advocacy groups.

Throughout the 1970s, states began passing decriminalization laws. These laws did not make marijuana legal, but reduced legal penalties, for example, from prison terms to fines. In addition, during this time, a recognition of potential medicinal uses of marijuana use reemerged. In the months before Nixon resigned as president in 1974, Congress amended the Drug Abuse Prevention and Control Act to establish the National Institute on Drug Abuse (NIDA) as one of the research institutes of the National Institutes of Health (NIH).[18] NIDA became the single overseer of marijuana research, including legal growth for research purposes in the United States. By the end of the 1970s, NIDA was also distributing marijuana for medicinal purposes to a very small number of Americans who qualified for special access to drugs not approved by the Food and Drug Administration (FDA) under a program that was later discontinued for marijuana.

During the decade of the 1980s, antidrug sentiment once again surged. Although marijuana use was a relatively minor concern compared to cocaine and its variant, crack, the Reagan administration intensified mandatory minimums for marijuana along with sentences for other drugs.[19] Yet, a legal pathway for medicinal marijuana use also became available in the mid-1980s, when the FDA approved a synthetic form, Marinol®, of the primary psychoactive component of cannabis (delta-9-tetrahydrocannabinol, THC) to combat nausea from chemotherapy and appetite suppression from AIDS that leads to weight loss.[20] While the development of Marinol® was groundbreaking in a sense, the capsule formulation approved for use had a long delay between administration and onset of the THC effects, during which time much of the drug was metabolized or failed to be absorbed into the blood,[21] in effect reducing the dose. This delay and relative ineffectiveness compared with inhaled marijuana, and the persistent complexity of the legal and regulatory environment, is one explanation for the sustained push to legalize marijuana for medical use.

CURRENT CONTEXT

Since the 1990s, state laws about the legal use of marijuana both for medical and recreational purposes have evolved, as have public attitudes about the safety and acceptability of such use. In 1996, California passed the first state medical marijuana law (MML). Since then, 28 additional states and the District of Columbia have passed MMLs. State MMLs share a common feature in that they permit legal marijuana use to treat medical conditions if the user has obtained medical authorization; however, the specific provisions of MMLs vary considerably.[22] For example, the range and specificity of the medical conditions permitted for use, the provisions for distribution through dispensaries, allowable amounts per patient, and the degree of restrictiveness or "medicalization" of these laws varies.[23,24] Figure 168-1 shows aspects of MMLs that vary from state to state. Each of these aspects has the potential to modify the effects of MMLs, although between-state variability in the quality and quantity of available data presents challenges to research on the differential effects of these variations (Table 168-1). Additionally, because early and later MMLs were passed in differing national normative contexts (i.e., different proportions of states that already had MML; nationally decreased perceptions of harm associated with marijuana use), the effects of MMLs may vary over time, particularly among the states that passed MMLs relatively early.[25]

The primary concerns about MMLs include their potential to increase problematic marijuana use in the general population; this could occur through several mechanisms, including greater access to marijuana through dispensaries or home cultivation, reductions in perceived harmfulness, and normalization of use.[22,26] In states with less restrictive MMLs (generally the states that passed earlier laws), the possibility that medical marijuana was obtained for recreational use is supported by research showing greater similarities between medical users and recreational users than between medical users and individuals with medical illness.[27–30] Alternatively, nationally representative findings indicate that while medical and recreational marijuana users may be similar in terms of some demographic and clinical characteristics, medical marijuana users are more likely to be older and to have initiated marijuana use later in life, more likely to report poor health or disability, and less likely to have a substance use disorder,[31,32] suggesting a greater likelihood of medical rather than recreational motives for obtaining medical marijuana. Nonetheless, the percentage of marijuana users who report using for medical purposes is almost twice as high in states with MMLs (17%)[31] than in the general population (9.8%).[32]

By 2012, states with MMLs began passing laws to allow marijuana use for recreational purposes. Recreational marijuana laws (RMLs) permit legal sale and use of marijuana without the need for medical justification or authorization. In total, eight states have now passed RMLs: Colorado and Washington in 2012, Alaska and Oregon in 2014, and California, Nevada, Massachusetts, and Maine in 2016. Consequently, at the time of this writing (December 2017), 21% of the U.S. population is living in states where recreational use is legal.

Arguments in favor of RMLs center on their potential to create business opportunities and jobs while generating tax revenues,[33–35] as exemplified by Colorado[36] and Washington,[37] where cannabis is now

TABLE 168-1 FEATURES OF MML THAT MAY INFLUENCE THEIR EFFECTS
Features Pertaining to Patients
Permitted medical conditions and/or symptoms
Qualifications (e.g., age limits, residency)
Registration and ID card requirements
Payment provisions (e.g., insurance coverage, subsidized payments)
Permitted activities (e.g., cultivation, possession)
Health Professionals Providing Authorization
Qualifications
Practice requirements (e.g., established patient, medical history review, screening/diagnostic tests)
Documentation requirements
Caregivers
Qualifications
Registration requirements
Number of patients permitted
Permitted activities (e.g., cultivation, possession, payment)
Products
Cultivation (e.g., restrictions on commercial/private entities, quantity, potency, location)
Form (e.g., smoked, edibles)
Properties (e.g., formulations, purity, lab testing requirements)
Advertising regulations (e.g., content, placement, displays)
Production (e.g., taxes, packaging/labeling)
Distribution methods (e.g., government/private, identification and tracking rules)
Dispensaries, If Permitted
Settings (e.g., limits on location and/or density)
Operations (e.g., functional status, permitted activities such as on- and off-premises cultivation and consumption)
Fees and pricing (e.g., taxes, price controls, for-profit status restrictions)
Personnel (e.g., in-house physician or medical professional requirements)

a billion-dollar-a-year business.[38] They may also reduce discriminatory arrests of minorities due to biased enforcement of criminal marijuana statutes.[39,40] However, RMLs are considered likely to reduce the price of marijuana and increase availability, advertising, and accepting attitudes toward marijuana use, all of which may enlarge the population of marijuana users, raise rates of adverse health and psychosocial consequences, and produce unintended effects related to use of other substances.[40,41] Because RMLs have been passed relatively recently, little is known about their impact on public health, and aside from Colorado and Washington, laws have not yet been enacted in the states that passed them. Recognizing this, NIDA has made studies of state marijuana laws a priority as data accumulates.[42]

One issue to take into account in considering potential influences of MMLs is shifts in Federal policy short of re-scheduling marijuana or legalizing use at a national level. Before 2009, the discrepancy between Federal and state positions meant that individuals using marijuana as specified by a state MML remained vulnerable to federal prosecution. However, in 2009, the U.S. Attorney General issued a memorandum instructing federal prosecutors not to prioritize prosecution of individuals who were compliant with state MMLs.[43] This gave more flexibility to states with MMLs,[44] with particularly high impact in Colorado[25,45–47] and California,[25] where dispensaries proliferated. Furthermore, the memo may have eased concerns in states without MMLs, as the percentage of Americans living in states with MMLs has increased from 19% in 2001 to 34% in 2012 and 63% in 2016.

HEALTH RISKS ASSOCIATED WITH MARIJUANA USE

Cannabis Use Disorders

The *Diagnostic and Statistical Manual of Mental Disorders* (DSM) of the American Psychiatric Association provides specific diagnostic criteria to use in diagnosing substance use and mental disorders with periodic updates to reflect new knowledge. The fourth edition of the DSM, DSM-IV,[48] was published in 1994 and provided definitions of cannabis use disorder (CUD), including categories for abuse and dependence, that were in use until 2013. These formed the basis of a large body of research. In 2013, DSM-5 was published, which defines the current diagnostic criteria.[49] The substance use disorder category underwent considerable revision between DSM-IV and DSM-5. Abuse and dependence criteria were combined into a single disorder in DSM-5; the DSM-IV legal-problems criterion for abuse was dropped, while a criterion for craving was added across all substances; and cannabis withdrawal was newly added in DSM-5 (for a comparison of DSM-IV and DSM-5 diagnostic criteria, see Fig. 168-2). Thus, the total number of criteria available to make a CUD diagnosis is now 11, with a threshold of 2 or more required for the diagnosis (Table 168-2).

The psychiatric and substance use disorder categories in the *International Classification of Diseases* (ICD), published by the World Health Organization, are the international counterpart to the American DSM. The research version of the tenth revision of ICD (ICD-10)[50] includes diagnostic criteria for substance dependence and for a category called harmful use.[51] Diagnostic criteria in DSM-IV and DSM-5 have some overlap with ICD criteria for substance use disorders, including cannabis use disorders, but differences have emerged as each system has developed. Dependence criteria in DSM-IV and ICD-10 showed high empirical agreement,[52–57] while the DSM-IV abuse category and the parallel ICD-10 category, harmful use, agreed poorly. A new version of ICD, ICD-11 is anticipated in the next few years. In contrast to DSM-5, ICD-11 will retain dependence as the "master" substance use disorder diagnosis, likely to generate debate and further research.[58]

An important new feature of the DSM-5 substance use disorder category is the severity specifier (Fig. 168-2). According to this specifier, individuals with two to three CUD criteria have a "mild" disorder, those with four to five criteria have a disorder of "moderate" severity, and those with six or more have a "severe" disorder. The "severe" level has been noted as the equivalent of addiction,[59] although those with chronic CUD at the moderate level of severity may also be considered to have a marijuana addiction (as indicated by substantial loss of self-control and compulsive drug-taking despite the desire to quit).[59]

Another important addition to DSM-5 diagnostic criteria is withdrawal. While withdrawal from other substances (e.g., alcohol, opioids) is widely recognized,[60] little was known about cannabis withdrawal when DSM-IV was published. Since then, preclinical,[61–64] clinical,[61–63,65–69] and epidemiologic[67,69] studies have identified a cannabis

TABLE 168-2 COMPARISON OF CURRENT AND FORMER CRITERIA FOR CANNABIS USE DISORDER

DSM-5 Cannabis Use Disorder	Criteria	DSM-IV Cannabis Abuse
X	Failure to fulfill role obligations	X
X	Recurrent use in hazardous situations (e.g. driving)	X
X	Continued use despite social/interpersonal problems	X
–	Marijuana-related legal problems	X
		DSM-IV Cannabis Dependence
X	Tolerance	X
X	Used more/longer than intended	X
X	Prolonged desire to quit/repeated unsuccessful attempts to reduce use	X
X	Significant time spent on marijuana-related activities	X
X	Physical/psychological problems do not deter use	X
X	Activities given up due to marijuana use	X
X	Withdrawal	–
X	Craving	–

DSM-5 Cannabis Use Disorder (all 11 criteria): ≥2 criteria required

DSM-IV Cannabis Abuse: ≥1 criteria required + no dependence

DSM-IV Cannabis Dependence: ≥3 criteria required

Notes: Dashes indicate that criteria were not included in the definition of a Cannabis Use Disorder for the specified edition of DSM. Each relevant criterion must be met within a 12-month period.

withdrawal syndrome following cessation. In addition, statistical modeling suggests withdrawal is an important component of analyses that incorporate other CUD criteria.[70]

Withdrawal is defined as three or more of the following symptoms after cessation of prolonged marijuana use: (1) anxiety, restlessness; (2) depression, irritability; (3) insomnia, odd dreams; (4) physical symptoms (e.g., tremors); and (5) decreased appetite.[49] This syndrome is most intense during the first week of abstinence, but can persist as long as a month after use[1,61,71–74] and has pharmacological specificity.[64,75,76] Since many withdrawal symptoms overlap with symptoms of depressive or anxiety disorders and many professionals and members of the general public may still be unaware of cannabis withdrawal,[77] potential confusion could arise about marijuana use as treatment or self-medication for symptoms of anxiety or depressive disorders.

Withdrawal is reported by up to one-third of regular marijuana users in the general population[66,67,69] and by 50–95% among heavy users in treatment or research studies.[61,68,78,79] The clinical significance of withdrawal is demonstrated by its association with difficulty quitting,[61,78,80] with use of marijuana or other substances for relief, with impairment,[81] and with worse treatment outcomes.[68,79,81,82] In terms of etiology, marijuana withdrawal is moderately heritable,[83] implicating both genetic and environmental factors.

A common assumption about the risk for CUDs among marijuana users is that such risk is rare, based on findings from 25 years ago that few users developed CUD.[21,84] However, in more recent U.S. national data, three out of ten users developed DSM-IV CUD.[85] Moreover, 19.5% of lifetime users met criteria for DSM-5 CUD, of whom 23% were symptomatically severe ($\geq$6 criteria).[86] Of these, 48% were not functioning in *any* major role (e.g., work). Thus, CUD in users is not rare and can be serious.

In terms of causality, marijuana use is clearly a necessary condition for CUD, but since not all users develop CUD, use alone is not sufficient. The etiology of CUD is complex,[87–90] involving both genetic[91] and environmental factors. Social-ecological models of substance use assume that increased use is related to increased availability and desirability, which normalizes use and reduces perception of harm.[92–96] If these environmental factors also increase the prevalence of heavy or frequent marijuana users, then they are likely to increase risk for CUD.

Addiction to Marijuana and Comorbid Substance Use Disorders

Addiction is one of the primary concerns of marijuana use, and research has revealed strong associations between marijuana use and addiction or cannabis use disorders (for definitions of cannabis use disorders, see Fig. 168-2). Evidence suggests regular or heavy users as well as those who begin using marijuana in adolescence or young adulthood may be particularly likely to develop dependence on marijuana or other drugs.[41,97,98] Furthermore, studies examining co-occurring behavioral health conditions have shown a relationship between CUDs and alcohol, tobacco, and drug use disorders.[86,99–101]

The association between marijuana and tobacco use disorders merits attention due to their shared common route of administration (smoking) and the potential for combined use to intensify the effects of marijuana.[102–104] Individuals who use both marijuana and tobacco also have elevated risk of respiratory distress compared to marijuana or tobacco users alone.[105] The co-occurrence of marijuana and tobacco use could be explained by predisposing biological factors or by social and environmental factors.[105]

The link between marijuana and alcohol use is less clear. Some studies show that medical marijuana clients use marijuana in place of alcohol.[28,106–109] In analyses of data from 1990 to 2010, passage of MML was followed by decreases in alcohol-related traffic fatalities[110] and binge drinking,[110] suggesting that marijuana was substituted for alcohol in these states. A state-level study using data from 1985 to 2014 also showed that passage of MML was followed by decreases in overall traffic fatalities, but the effects were heterogeneous since they were limited to seven states and adults 25–44 years old.[111] In contrast, other research has shown that passage of MML was followed by increases in alcohol use and adverse alcohol-related outcomes, including any drinking,[112] binge drinking[26,110,113]; and alcohol-related treatment admissions among states in which dispensaries are permitted.[112] Inconsistent findings might be explained by differences in the outcomes studied (e.g., light use vs. use with the intent of intoxication, as in binge drinking) and state-level control variables used across studies.[113] Cumulatively, these studies indicate the need for further exploration using research designs that could clarify the conflicting results.

Speculation about RML effects largely assume that substituting marijuana for alcohol will be better for public health.[114,115] While some experts assume RML will lead to substitution of marijuana for alcohol,[114,116] others are less certain.[40,117–119] Whether marijuana will actually be substituted for alcohol after passage of RML, and whether the effects of any such substitution on public health will be positive, negative or neutral is currently unknown.

Mental Health

Substance use research, including studies specifically addressing marijuana use, often incorporate measures of mental health to understand comorbid conditions. Research has shown that marijuana use among adolescents and young adults is associated with lower life satisfaction,[120] but evidence for strong associations between CUDs and other mental health problems extends beyond life satisfaction.

Using diagnoses based on diagnostic criteria from the DSM-IV and DSM-5, studies have detected relationships between CUDs and mood, anxiety, and personality disorders.[86,99,100] Applying DSM-5 definitions of mild, moderate, and severe disorders, associations with psychiatric disorders were stronger at more severe CUD levels.[86] Using diagnostic criteria from the ICD, 9th Revision, Clinical Modification (ICD-9-CM), CUDs were associated with schizoaffective and mood disorders in a national database of hospitalized patients.[101] In military veterans with ICD-9-CM CUDs who were treated in the Veterans Health Administration, PTSD was the most common psychiatric comorbidity.[121]

Whether the relationships between marijuana use or disorders and comorbid mental illnesses are causal is not clear.[122] Marijuana use or disorders could lead to mental illness, but the reverse may also be true. Furthermore, significant associations between CUDs and mental disorders could arise from common causes. A prospective study controlling for many potential cofounders suggested that marijuana use predicted incidence of other substance use disorders but not mood or anxiety disorders.[123] Genetic research findings indicate that marijuana use or disorders share genetic risk with major depression.[91,124,125] Alternatively, other genetic studies indicate a possible causal effect of CUD on major depression,[126] including a study of identical twins discordant for marijuana use, which is a strong design for sorting out causal and noncausal relationships.[127] Thus, the nature of the relationship between marijuana use or disorders and psychiatric comorbidity remains a topic of debate.

Marijuana use or disorders have also been associated with psychosis.[101] For example, higher rates of marijuana use or disorders among individuals with ultra-high-risk (UHR) for psychosis (i.e., subclinical psychotic symptoms and/or genetic risk and impaired functioning) and a reciprocal relationship of higher rates of psychotic symptoms among UHR individuals who used marijuana compared to those who did not use marijuana.[128] Epidemiologic efforts to determine causation have focused on long-term prospective studies in which the chronological order of marijuana use and onset of psychosis can be determined. Some research supports a causal relationship between marijuana use and development of psychotic symptoms.[129–131] Other research challenges a causal interpretation of the relationship between marijuana use and psychosis, although largely shows that CUD is a predictor of subsequent psychosis.[132] Although some debate remains about the link between marijuana and psychosis,[133] marijuana use, and particularly heavy use, is not only likely to increase risk for psychosis[134] but also has been characterized as one of the strongest modifiable risk factors for developing a psychotic disorder.[135] Both bodies of evidence have raised concerns about elevated risk in relation to increasing marijuana potency in a changing legal environment.[131,132,136]

Effects on Development

Studies of the association between marijuana use and developmental outcomes often focus on early exposures. Prospective research has shown associations between prenatal marijuana exposure and restricted fetal growth,[137] which is consistent with a recent meta-analysis indicating that infants born to prenatal marijuana users were more likely than others to be anemic, have low birth weight, and require neonatal intensive care.[138]

This body of research also emphasizes the potential impact of marijuana use on brain development, examining brain structure and functional outcomes such as intelligence and cognition. Among children, those with prenatal exposures to marijuana have greater frontal cortical thickness than those without prenatal exposures.[137] Among adults, marijuana use has been associated with reduced brain connectivity and cognitive impairment, particularly among those with heavy or long-term use and those who began using marijuana at younger ages.[41,139–141]

Evidence of the relationship between marijuana use and development is concerning, but also inconclusive.[134] Research on prenatal exposures is complicated by the fact that most pregnant marijuana users in existing studies also used other substances, limiting knowledge about effects that are specific to marijuana.[134,142] Research on adolescent and adult exposures could indicate that marijuana use leads to cognitive impairments, but other plausible relationships can explain the findings to date. For example, shared risk factors could be responsible both for early marijuana use and impairments shown later.[41] Further, impairment could predate initial marijuana use.

Effects on Educational and Professional Achievement

Structural and functional outcomes may be related to impairments in memory and attention, which could in turn impact achievement. Prenatal marijuana exposure is linked not only to altered brain development, but also to subsequent impaired executive functioning in school.[143] Marijuana use by adolescents and young adults has also been associated with lower educational and professional achievement[130,144] and school drop-out,[145] especially with regular or heavy use.

Mortality

There are no known cases of fatal overdose from marijuana use in the epidemiologic literature.[1,146] Some research has shown an association between past marijuana use and overall mortality years later, but these data and study designs are problematic and make determination of a causal relationship difficult.[134]

Although death may not result directly from marijuana use, research has shown that marijuana has a causal link with increased risk for fatality or injury resulting from intoxication while driving.[1] The primary psychoactive component of marijuana, delta-9-THC, impairs the motor and cognitive functions needed for safe driving.[147,148] Marijuana use while driving has been shown to substantially increase the risk for motor vehicle crashes[134,148–151] and has been implicated in fatal and nonfatal crashes.[147,149–153] Injury and fatality risk for crashes may be further increased by the connection between marijuana use and failure to use seatbelts.[154] In addition to motor vehicle crashes, marijuana has been implicated in fatal injuries among U.S. pilots.[155]

RECENT TRENDS

Perceptions

Perceived harmfulness has long been considered an important factor in preventing marijuana use, particularly among adolescents.[156–159] Early evidence of an inverse relationship between perceived harmfulness and marijuana use[160–162] has now been shown repeatedly in studies of adolescents,[163,164] adults,[165] and international samples.[159] Among U.S. adolescents, the perception that regular marijuana use is risky has declined substantially since 2004–05, with reductions ranging from 50% to 80%.[166] In 2016, only about 30% of 12th graders perceived such risk. The perception that marijuana use is risky also declined among adults, from 50% in 2002 to 33% in 2014, while the perception that use involves no risk increased from about 6% to 15%.[165]

Potency of Illicit Marijuana and Retail Products

Over the past four decades, marijuana potency (measured by THC content in seized samples) has approximately doubled worldwide,[167] including in the United States.[168] In the early 1990s, the average THC content in confiscated U.S. marijuana samples was about 3.7%, while in 2014, it was about 6.1%.[169] This increase is relevant to research on trends in problems associated with marijuana use because higher THC concentrations are more likely to increase the risks associated with use.[170] However, in states that legalize marijuana use, the potency of legally purchased marijuana may be more relevant to public health than the potency of illegal samples.

Among samples of illegal marijuana seized by law enforcement between 1990 and 2010, the average THC potency was 9.1% in states that eventually passed MMLs and 5.6% in other states.[171] Findings showed that the association between MMLs and increased potency was no longer significant after controlling for potential confounders, but the association remained significant in states with legally operating dispensaries, in which THC potency increased by about 1%. As more states pass recreational marijuana laws, the THC potency of illicit marijuana in MML states may no longer be such a salient issue.

In Washington (where recreational marijuana use was legalized in 2012), the average potency of marijuana in one Seattle-based retailer was 21.2% in 2015.[172] In Colorado, where the potency of legal marijuana can range considerably, some strains have THC potencies of 28–32%.[173] In 2016, Colorado legislators attempted to limit THC content of marketed cannabis to 16%, but this attempt failed, indicating local support for continued availability of stronger marijuana products. While smoking remains the most common route of administration,[1] newly popular routes of administration offer even higher THC doses.[1] These include edibles, vaping (inhaled vapor of heated e-liquids analogous to e-cigarettes), and dabbing (inhaled vapor from heating highly concentrated forms of marijuana or hashish). The health effects of these methods are not yet known, but warrant monitoring.[169]

Marijuana Use and Related Outcomes: Trends in Adolescents

Recreational marijuana use almost always begins in adolescence, with "early-onset" generally referring to early adolescence. Data from the national Monitoring The Future study (MTF; Table 168-3) show that the rate of past-month marijuana use among eighth graders (who are generally ages 13–14 years) was 5.4% in 2016.[166] When older adolescents are included in representative samples, estimated rates of marijuana use are somewhat higher. Among National Survey on Drug Use and Health (NSDUH; Table 168-3) participants ages 12–17 years, the prevalence of past-month marijuana use was 7.4% in 2014.[174,175]

Notably, neither the MTF nor the NSDUH show increasing national trends in adolescent marijuana use over time. Findings from the NSDUH indicate stable rates between 2002 and 2014.[174,175] Findings from the MTF when all teens are aggregated together show fluctuating rates, with some increases until around 2010, and either stabilization (12th graders) or decreases (eighth and tenth graders) between 2010 and 2016.[166] A recent report that examined 2005–16 MTF data on teens who were cigarette smokers versus nonsmokers indicated that rates of marijuana use actually increased somewhat in both groups.[176] However, because adolescent cigarette smokers make a disproportionately large contribution to overall adolescent rates of marijuana use, and because teen rates of cigarette smoking declined

TABLE 168-3 NATIONALLY REPRESENTATIVE SURVEY SOURCES OF TIME TREND DATA ON MARIJUANA USE AND DISORDERS

	Survey				
	Monitoring the Future (MTF)	**National Survey on Drug Use and Health (NSDUH)**	**National Longitudinal Alcohol Epidemiologic Survey (NLAES)**	**National Epidemiologic Survey on Alcohol and Related Conditions (NESARC)**	**National Epidemiologic Survey on Alcohol and Related Conditions-III (NESARC-III)**
Study period	1991–present, repeated yearly	2002–present, repeated yearly	1991–92	2001–02	2012–13
N	~50,000/year	~70,000/year	42,862	43,093	36,309
Sample	Adolescents (8th, 10th, and 12th grade)	Adolescents and adults (≥12 years)	Adults (≥18 years)	Adults (≥18 years)	Adults (≥18 years)
Setting	School[a]	Home	Home	Home	Home
Format	Questionnaire	Interview	Interview	Interview	Interview
Administration mode	Self	Interviewer + self	Interviewer	Interviewer	Interviewer
Marijuana measures	Current and past use, current perceived risk, disapproval, availability	Current use, perceived risk, availability; current DSM-IV abuse, dependence, CUD	Current, past, and lifetime use; DSM-IV[b] abuse, dependence, CUD	Current, past, and lifetime use; DSM-IV[b] abuse, dependence, CUD	Current, past, and lifetime use; DSM-IV abuse, dependence, CUD; DSM-5[c] CUD
Sponsor	NIDA[d]	SAMHSA[e]	Co-sponsored by NIAAA[f] and NIDA[d]	Co-sponsored by NIAAA[f] and NIDA[d]	Co-sponsored by NIAAA[f] and NIDA[d]

[a]Data not available to teachers.
[b]*Diagnostic and Statistical Manual of Mental Disorders*, 4th edition.
[c]*Diagnostic and Statistical Manual of Mental Disorders*, 5th edition.
[d]National Institute on Drug Abuse, National Institutes of Health.
[e]Substance Abuse and Mental Health Services Administration.
[f]National Institute on Alcohol Abuse and Alcoholism, National Institutes of Health.

so sharply over this period, rates of marijuana use overall did not increase. Whether the stabilization/decrease in rates of marijuana use was actually due to changes in smoking cigarettes or was due to other factors (e.g., decreasing time spent face-to-face with friends, more time on the internet or social media) is currently an issue of debate.

Between 2002 and 2013, research shows that the prevalence of CUD decreased among adolescents, indicating that marijuana use disorders also have not risen among young people in recent years.[177]

Influence of Changing Marijuana Laws on Adolescent Marijuana Use and Related Outcomes

A large number of studies have been conducted on the relationship between MMLs and adolescent marijuana use. One cross-sectional study found higher rates of adolescent marijuana use in states with MMLs.[178] However, cross-sectional associations do not necessarily indicate a causal relationship between MMLs and increases in adolescent marijuana use because states with MMLs could have had higher rates of use prior to MML passage (i.e., reverse causation). Simply studying pre-post MML differences in states that passed such laws might be misleading because any increases found might reflect overall national trends rather than state-specific effects.

Experiments that randomly assign MML status to states would provide greater clarity about whether MMLs cause changes in rates of adolescent marijuana use, but such assignment is clearly impossible. Therefore, studies have examined differences in rates of adolescent marijuana use before and after MML passage, comparing pre-post MML changes in states that passed MMLs to contemporaneous change in states without MMLs using multilevel modeling and what is called difference-in-differences statistical methodology.[179–182] Using data across multiple time periods and controlling for many state- and individual-level confounders, an overwhelming majority of these studies indicated that MMLs did not lead to increases in adolescent marijuana use,[22,26,158,183–188] as confirmed by meta-analysis of 11 of these studies.[188] Therefore, MMLs have not led to increases in adolescent marijuana use, at least up to now.

Laws permitting marijuana use for recreational purposes may have different effects on adolescent use because commercialization efforts will be directed to increasing desirability and general availability, even if sales to minors remain prohibited. Extrapolating from results on adults, one study speculated that RMLs may have further effects on adolescent use in states that already have MML.[25] Analyses of MTF data show that perceived harmfulness of marijuana use decreased while marijuana use itself increased following RML passage in Washington.[189] However, perceived harmfulness of marijuana and rates of use did not change among adolescents in Colorado[189]; clearly more research is needed as data accumulate in these and the other states that have legalized recreational marijuana use.

Marijuana Use and Related Outcomes: Trends in Adults

In contrast to adolescents, rates of marijuana use have increased among adults. One main source of information on this is the set of NSDUH surveys (Table 168-3). Between 2002 and 2014, past-month marijuana use in NSDUH participants ages 18–25 years old increased significantly, from 17.3% in 2002 to 19.6% in 2014, with most of the increase occurring since 2007.[174] Among NSDUH participants 26 years and older, past-month use also increased significantly between 2002 and 2014, from 4.0% to 6.6%.[174] In this age group, the increase started in 2008.[165] Increases occurred across gender, region, educational level, and employment status, with higher rates in males and unemployed participants.[174] Other indicators of adult marijuana use also showed significant increases among NSDUH participants during this period, including first-time use and daily/near-daily use.[165] Additional studies of NSDUH data showed greater increases in marijuana use among males, especially those with lower incomes.[190]

Another source of data on trends in adult marijuana use showed increases in marijuana use consistent with NSDUH findings. The

National Institute on Alcohol Abuse and Alcoholism (NIAAA) conducted the National Epidemiologic Survey on Alcohol and Related Conditions (NESARC) in 2001–02 and the NESARC-III in 2012–13 (see Table 168-3 for more information about the NIAAA surveys). The past-year prevalence of marijuana use more than doubled, from 4.1% in NESARC to 9.5% NESARC-III.[25,85] Significant increases in marijuana use were also found across demographic subgroups, including sex, age, race/ethnicity, education, marital status, income, urban/rural, and region.

Table 168-4 shows national trends over this general time period in several additional marijuana-related outcomes, including substantial increases in the rates of marijuana detected in roadside surveys of weekend night-time drivers[191] and among decedents of fatal motor vehicle[149] and airplane crashes.[155] National roadside surveys conducted by the U.S. National Highway Traffic Safety Administration indicate that the prevalence of THC detected in saliva or blood of night-time drivers increased by approximately 50% (from 8.6% to 12.6%) between 2007 and 2013–14.[192]

Higher population prevalence of substance use is generally associated with increased population rates of substance use disorders. Indeed, several studies have shown significant increases in adult CUD, including in the U.S. adult general population[25,85] and in several national studies of patient populations, including those seen in emergency rooms,[153] hospital inpatients,[101,193] and veterans treated in the Veterans Health Administration.[194] Large local studies of adult patient samples have also shown increasing rates of CUD over time, including among patients in treatment for gastroenterological problems[195] and for burns.[196] Curiously, one large national survey shows no increases over time in the prevalence of adult CUD.[165] Methodological differences may explain the discrepancy between this survey and the other studies.[165,197,198] However, the consistency of findings on the increased prevalence of CUDs in adults are consistent with other national trends in marijuana-related problems over the same period (Table 168-4), suggesting that increased rates of CUD are valid.[199]

Influence of Changing Marijuana Laws on Adult Marijuana Use and Related Outcomes

Compared to the large number of studies on MML and adolescents, fewer studies are available on the relationship of MMLs to marijuana outcomes in adults (see Table 168-3 for information on the large-scale national surveys that have contributed the existing information on this point). As is the case with adolescent data, cross-sectional survey data on adults show that living in a state with a MML is associated with the risk for adult marijuana use and for DSM-IV CUD.[200] Studies of national data using multilevel modeling and difference-in-differences statistical tests show that in contrast to the lack of MML effects in adolescents, post-MML increases were seen in adult marijuana use, daily or near-daily use, and marijuana use disorders, compared to contemporaneous changes in states that did not pass MMLs.[25,26,185] Further, increases in adult marijuana use and disorders were greater in states that passed MMLs later (e.g., after 2001) compared to states passing MMLs earlier.[25] In addition, studies have found post-MML increases in marijuana possession arrests in major cities[201] and first-time hospital admissions for marijuana, and attributed these changesto MML passage.[201] While the literature on the relationship of MMLs to adult cannabis outcomes is not extensive, the studies that have been conducted to date are consistent in showing post-MML increases in marijuana-related outcomes among adults. Additional studies are clearly needed to determine the robustness of this relationship, including whether it extends to other marijuana outcomes (e.g., driving under the influence) and whether specific population subgroups are especially vulnerable to these influences. Further, research to date has not yet examined the relationship of RMLs to adult outcomes, an area that is clearly in need of studies as data become available.

Marijuana Use and Related Outcomes: Trends in Vulnerable Groups

Children: Among children, the main type of cannabis exposure is unintentional, often resulting from ingestion of marijuana or an edible marijuana product. Accidental exposures among children have

TABLE 168-4 ADDITIONAL SOURCES OF INFORMATION ON TIME TRENDS IN MARIJUANA-RELATED OUTCOMES

Data Source	Format	Study Period	*N*	Sample	Marijuana Measures
California Roadside Surveys[191]	Interview, survey, drug screening	2010	1,707	Adolescent and adult drivers (≥16 years)	Marijuana use, measured by saliva tests
Civil Aerospace toxicology database; National Transportation Safety Board aviation accidents[155]	Pilot characteristics, drug screening	1990–2012	6,677	Pilot decedents (average age = 50 years)	Marijuana use, measured by blood and tissue tests for cannabinol
Drug Abuse Warning Network[153]	Patient characteristics, clinical data	2004–11	2,823,321	Adolescent and adult emergency department patients (≥12 years)	Marijuana use, measured by urine tests for cannabis
Fatality Analysis Reporting System[149]	Driver characteristics, drug screening	1999–2010	23,591	Adolescent and adult driver decedents (≥15 years)	Marijuana use, measured by blood tests for cannabinol
Massachusetts General Hospital gastroenterology clinic patients[195]	Patient characteristics, clinical data	1986–2013	190,303	Gastroenterology patients (average age = 47 years)	ICD-9-CM cannabis use disorders
National Burn Repository[196]	Patient characteristics, clinical data	2002–11	73,725	Adolescent and adult burn patients (≥12 years)	Marijuana use, measured by urine tests for marijuana, cannabinoids, or THC
Nationwide Hospital Inpatient Sample[101]	Patient characteristics, clinical data	2002–11	2,833,567	Adults (≥18 years)	ICD-9-CM Cannabis Use Disorders
State Inpatient Databases[193]	State characteristics, clinical data	1997–2014	382 state-years	States (9 of 27 with medical marijuana laws)	ICD-9-CM Cannabis Use Disorders
Veterans Administration, National Patient Care Databases[194]	Patient characteristics, clinical data	2002, 2008, 2009	1,141,690	Adult veterans (average age = 53 years)	ICD-9-CM Cannabis Use Disorders

increased in recent years.[202] The literature does not show evidence of fatal exposures at any age, but acute symptoms in children can include lethargy, ataxia, dizziness, and respiratory depression[134] and can require emergency treatment.

Pregnant women: According to NSDUH data from 2007 to 2012, 3.9% of pregnant women reported past-month marijuana use, 7.0% reported past-year use, and among past-year users, 16.2% used near-daily.[203] Further, the estimated prevalence of past-month marijuana use among pregnant women 18–44 years old increased 62% between 2002 and 2014, from 2.4% to 3.9%.[204] In 2014, the rate of past-month marijuana use was highest among young pregnant women ages 18–25 years, at 7.5%.[204]

Influence of Changing Marijuana Laws on Marijuana Use and Related Outcomes in Vulnerable Groups

Children: The increase in childhood marijuana exposures is especially pronounced in states with legalized use.[134] A study of calls to poison centers for unintentional pediatric exposures from 2005 to 2011 showed little increase in states without MMLs, an increase of 11.5% in states passing MMLs during the study period, and an increase of 30.3% in states that passed MMLs before 2005.[205] Among unintentional pediatric exposures, children in states with pre-2005 MML passage had more negative outcomes, as they were more likely to be evaluated in a healthcare facility, to experience moderate or serious effects, and to be admitted to critical-care units.[205]

During a period marked by proliferation of medical dispensaries and legalization of recreational marijuana use, another study found that 2009–15 calls to Colorado poison control centers for unintentional pediatric exposures to marijuana increased by a significantly greater annual percentage than calls to poison control centers in other states.[206] A further breakdown of Colorado poison control center calls showed greater increases among children under 18 after recreational use was legalized in 2014 compared to the significant increases observed after liberalization of MMLs in 2010.[38]

Pregnant women: While studies examining the impact of MMLs and RMLs on marijuana outcomes among pregnant women have yet to emerge, unpublished results from one study suggest that rates of marijuana use among pregnant women were similar in MML and non-MML states.[204]

IMPLICATIONS FOR CLINICAL PRACTICE

Substance Use Treatment

Treatment for substance use disorders in general, and for marijuana use disorders specifically, is rare. Data from 2001 to 2002 show that only 6.4% of those with current DSM-IV cannabis abuse and 18.1% of those with current DSM-IV cannabis dependence received any kind of intervention for drug use problems.[99] Lifetime rates are only slightly higher, with 9.8% of those with cannabis abuse and 34.7% of those with cannabis dependence ever receiving any type of drug-related intervention. Furthermore, those with drug treatment may not have received services focused on CUDs. More recent data from 2012 to 2013 are similarly discouraging, showing that among those with DSM-5 current and lifetime CUDs, 7.2% and 13.7% received any type of intervention specifically for marijuana problems.[86] Further, despite the clear increases in adult marijuana use and related problems in the general population, the proportion of patients in substance use treatment whose primary substance was marijuana did not increase between 2003 (16%) and 2013 (17%).[207] Thus, CUDs remain seriously under-treated in the U.S. general population.

Use of Marijuana for Pain

Chronic pain is common in U.S. adults.[208–211] While opioids are an important treatment for acute pain, they are also widely prescribed for chronic pain[212,213] despite inconsistent evidence for clinical benefits[214] and established evidence for serious risks,[213–215] such as physical dependence, addiction, transition to heroin, and overdose.[216–218] Medical marijuana is associated with numerous problems (cognitive/motor impairments,[219] side effects,[220] no standard product formulations[221]). However, importantly, its advantages (analgesia,[220] lack of fatal overdose,[222] lack of transition to heroin) have led to professional calls to substitute medical marijuana for opioids.[223] This debate is ongoing.[224]

Meanwhile, studies at the individual level have shown that many of the patients who obtain marijuana for medical purposes use it for pain relief. Some use marijuana as a partial or complete substitute for opioids[28,106–108,225–227] and others use it simultaneously with opioids. This occurs not only in states with MMLs, but in other states as well.[228] More research on substitution/complementarity of marijuana and opioids is needed, including the relationship with marijuana laws. At the ecological level (i.e., comparing state rates of various opioid-related outcomes between states with and without MMLs), several studies have been conducted on the premise that access to marijuana will reduce opioid use and misuse. Some studies showed that MMLs led to lower rates of opioid prescriptions in Medicaid[229] and Medicare,[230] hospitalization for opioid use disorders,[193,231] and overdose.[232] Other studies demonstrate more limited support for the relationship between MMLs and overdoses[233] and for detection of opioids in some fatally injured drivers (e.g., testing the relationship in multiple age groups but finding a relationship only in adults ages 21–40 years old).[234]

Psychiatric Conditions

Depression and anxiety disorders: Personal and anecdotal testimonies suggest that marijuana use is effective for treating symptoms of depression and anxiety,[235,236] and surveys of medical marijuana patients confirm that many use marijuana to treat these symptoms.[28,29,108,225,237–239] Yet, when medical marijuana patients are asked about actual symptom relief, less than half report such relief.[237] Other medical marijuana users report return of anxiety symptoms on cessation of use,[240] suggesting the symptoms might be due to withdrawal.[238] Because many withdrawal criteria consist of depression/anxiety symptoms,[49] regular users may seek marijuana for short-term symptom relief, unaware that their use could perpetuate a longer-term withdrawal problem.

While theoretical models suggest that synthetic oral cannabinoids may be helpful for treating some aspects of Posttraumatic Stress Disorder (PTSD),[133] scientific reviews of studies to date find no evidence for the efficacy of cannabinoids in the treatment of depression or anxiety disorders.[134,220,238] In contrast, prospective studies show adverse effects of marijuana on the course of depression[241] and PTSD.[242] Nevertheless, medical marijuana is authorized as a treatment for PTSD in 21 states, and in many other states, permitted conditions are vague enough that use for depression or anxiety may also be authorized.

Although marijuana users clearly self-medicate for depression and anxiety symptoms, survey data are mixed on the relationship between MMLs and rates of self-medication.[228,243] However, administrative data demonstrate a relationship between MMLs and lower rates of antidepressant and antianxiety prescriptions.[229,230] Substituting marijuana for FDA-approved medication would be a positive public health development if marijuana products were effective treatments for depression or anxiety disorders (e.g., by reducing medical costs).[244] Since evidence on efficacy suggests otherwise,[134,220,238] and since marijuana use may result from confusion between withdrawal and depressive/anxiety disorders,[240] such shifts in clinical care are a cause for concern.

Psychosis: Marijuana use has been characterized as one of the strongest modifiable risk factors for developing a psychotic disorder. Therefore, researchers have recommended that children and adolescents with a family history of psychosis or prodromal symptoms should be informed of the risks and counseled strongly not to use marijuana.[135]

Pregnancy

Consistent with concerns about marijuana use during pregnancy and possible harm to the fetus,[142] the American College of Obstetricians and Gynecologists recommends advising women who are pregnant or contemplating pregnancy about the potential risks of prenatal marijuana use in order to discourage use.[245]

SUMMARY

Changing laws, attitudes, and prevalence of marijuana use have implications for clinicians in addition to policy makers and the public. Despite a low risk for fatal overdose or transition to heroin from marijuana use, conveying information that marijuana is not harmless and can lead to adverse health outcomes becomes more important as the public and many professionals see marijuana as a natural, harmless substance that can be used for multiple purposes. Clinicians, especially those treating younger patients or patients with symptoms of mental illness, should consider screening their patients for marijuana use and criteria for CUDs to determine if a disorder is present and explore with patients whether a marijuana use/withdrawal cycle may be perpetuating depressive or anxiety symptoms. Some patients may not be receptive to the idea that marijuana is causing or contributing to their symptoms or problems rather than alleviating them. However, continued respectful and empathic discussion and perhaps some self-monitoring may be helpful in this regard.

Finally, the strengths and limitations in the evidence base need to be understood. Further research is needed to identify risk factors for adverse marijuana-related outcomes and changes in such risk factors amid a changing legal and social landscape. Studies are also needed to provide information on the effectiveness of interventions aimed at increasing awareness of marijuana risks and reducing use, particularly among those with higher likelihood of adverse consequences. Studies are also needed to understand the relationships between marijuana use and:

1. Changes in cognitive functioning resulting from both short- and long-term use, including longitudinal studies beginning prior to marijuana exposure.
2. Marijuana withdrawal, including diagnoses of depressive and anxiety disorders, self-medication with marijuana, and utilization of psychiatric medication.
3. Opioid use, particularly individual-level studies that can control for both individual characteristics (i.e., demographic and clinical variables) and state-level covariates, such as marijuana laws, in addition to differentiating between medical and nonmedical substance use.[40,229,244,246,247]
4. Mental health treatment, particularly individual-level studies that can control for both individual variables and relevant state factors.[229]
5. Postnatal outcomes related to use during pregnancy, accounting for the high prevalence of polysubstance use by studying marijuana use in the absence of other substance use. For better or worse, such studies may be easier now than they were in previous years if more women who would not consider drinking alcohol or smoking cigarettes during pregnancy see marijuana as a harmless way to treat pregnancy-related symptoms.[248]

Although much has been learned about marijuana, its use and its consequences in recent years, much remains to be learned in order to advance the evidence base for clinical care aimed at preventing negative outcomes alongside rapidly evolving social norms and laws.

References

1. World Health Organization. *The Health and Social Effects of Nonmedical Cannabis Use*. Geneva, Switzerland: WHO Document Production Services; 2016. http://www.who.int/substance_abuse/publications/msbcannabis.pdf.
2. Imtiaz S, Shield KD, Roerecke M, et al. The burden of disease attributable to cannabis use in Canada in 2012. *Addiction*. 2016;111(4):653–62.
3. Degenhardt L, Whiteford HA, Ferrari AJ, et al. Global burden of disease attributable to illicit drug use and dependence: Findings from the Global Burden of Disease Study 2010. *Lancet*. 2013;382(9904):1564–74.
4. Giommoni L, Reuter P, Kilmer B. Exploring the perils of cross-national comparisons of drug prevalence: The effect of survey modality. *Drug Alcohol Depend*. 2017;181:194–9.
5. Hall WD, Patton G, Stockings E, et al. Why young people's substance use matters for global health. *Lancet Psychiatry*. 2016;3(3):265–79.
6. Musto DF. Opium, cocaine and marijuana in American history. *Sci Am*. 1991;265(1):40–7.
7. United States Pharmacopoeial Convention. *Pharmacopoeia of the United States of America (The United States pharmacopeia)*. Easton, PA: United States Pharmacopoeial Convention; 1820.
8. Pure Food and Drug Act, Pub. L. 59-384, 34 Stat. 768, 1906.
9. Gieringer DH. The forgotten origins of cannabis prohibition in California. *Contemp Drug Probl*. 1999;26(2):237–88.
10. Lewitus V. Marihuana. *Am J Nursing*. 1936;36(7):677–8.
11. Marihuana Tax Act of 1937, Pub. L. 75-238, 50 Stat. 551, 1937.
12. Taxation of Marihuana: Hearing before a Subcommittee of the Committee on Finance. U.S. Senate; 75th Cong., 1st session; July 12, 1937.
13. Narcotic Law Violation Penalties, Pub. L. 82-255, 65 Stat. 767, 1951.
14. Narcotic Control Act of 1956, Pub. L. 84-728, 70 Stat. 567, 1956.
15. Comprehensive Drug Abuse Prevention and Control Act of 1970, Pub. L. 91-513, 84 Stat. 1236, 1970.
16. U.S. Department of Justice, Drug Enforcement Administration. Controlled substance schedules. 2017. https://www.deadiversion.usdoj.gov/schedules/. Accessed March 15, 2017.
17. United States Commission on Marihuana and Drug Abuse. *Marihuana: A Signal of Misunderstanding*. New York: The New American Library, Inc.; 1972.
18. Comprehensive Alcohol Abuse and Alcoholism Prevention, Treatment, and Rehabilitation Act Amendments of 1974, Pub. L. 93-282, 88 Stat. 125, 1974.
19. Anti-Drug Abuse Act of 1986, Pub. L. 99-570, 100 Stat. 3207, 1986.
20. U.S. Food and Drug Administration. New drug approvals. *FDA Consum*. 1985;19:35.
21. Institute of Medicine. *Marijuana and Medicine: Assessing the Science Base*. Washington, DC: The National Academies Press; 1999.
22. Pacula RL, Powell D, Heaton P, Sevigny EL. Assessing the effects of medical marijuana laws on marijuana use: The devil is in the details. *J Policy Anal Manage*. 2015;34(1):7–31.
23. Williams AR, Santaella-Tenorio J, Mauro CM, Levin FR, Martins SS. Loose regulation of medical marijuana programs associated with higher rates of adult marijuana use but not cannabis use disorder. *Addiction*. 2017;112(11):1985–91.
24. Williams AR, Olfson M, Kim JH, Martins SS, Kleber HD. Older, less regulated medical marijuana programs have much greater enrollment rates than newer 'medicalized' programs. *Health Aff (Millwood)*. 2016;35(3):480–8.
25. Hasin DS, Sarvet AL, Cerda M, et al. US adult illicit cannabis use, cannabis use disorder, and medical marijuana laws: 1991–1992 to 2012–2013. *JAMA Psychiatry*. 2017;74(6):579–88.
26. Wen H, Hockenberry JM, Cummings JR. The effect of medical marijuana laws on adolescent and adult use of marijuana, alcohol, and other substances. *J Health Econ*. 2015;42:64–80.
27. Haug NA, Padula CB, Sottile JE, Vandrey R, Heinz AJ, Bonn-Miller MO. Cannabis use patterns and motives: A comparison of younger, middle-aged, and older medical cannabis dispensary patients. *Addict Behav*. 2017;72:14–20.
28. Reinarman C, Nunberg H, Lanthier F, Heddleston T. Who are medical marijuana patients? Population characteristics from nine California assessment clinics. *J Psychoactive Drugs*. 2011;43(2):128–35.
29. Harris D, Jones RT, Shank R, et al. Self-reported marijuana effects and characteristics of 100 San Francisco medical marijuana club members. *J Addict Dis*. 2000;19(3):89–103.
30. Walsh Z, Callaway R, Belle-Isle L, et al. Cannabis for therapeutic purposes: Patient characteristics, access, and reasons for use. *Int J Drug Policy*. 2013;24(6):511–6.
31. Lin LA, Ilgen MA, Jannausch M, Bohnert KM. Comparing adults who use cannabis medically with those who use recreationally: Results from a national sample. *Addict Behav*. 2016;61:99–103.
32. Compton WM, Han B, Hughes A, Jones CM, Blanco C. Use of marijuana for medical purposes among adults in the United States. *JAMA*. 2017;317(2):209–11.

33. McGinty EE, Samples H, Bandara SN, Saloner B, Bachhuber MA, Barry CL. The emerging public discourse on state legalization of marijuana for recreational use in the US: Analysis of news media coverage, 2010–2014. *Prev Med.* 2016;90:114–20.
34. McGinty EE, Niederdeppe J, Heley K, Barry CL. Public perceptions of arguments supporting and opposing recreational marijuana legalization. *Prev Med.* 2017;99:80–6.
35. Borchardt D. $1 Billion in marijuana taxes is addictive to state governors. Forbes. 2017. https://www.forbes.com/sites/debraborchardt/2017/04/11/1-billion-in-marijuana-taxes-is-addicting-to-state-governors/#5b-20042d2c3b. Accessed June 30, 2017.
36. Huddleston T. Colorado topped $1 billion in legal marijuana sales in 2016. Fortune. 2016. http://www.fortune.com/2016/12/13/colorado-billion-legal-marijuana-sales/?_sm_au_=iVVwFVZDW6Q7kD46. Accessed June 30, 2017.
37. Blake A. Marijuana sales in Washington state top $1 billion: Report. The Washington Times. 2016. http://www.washingtontimes.com/news/2016/jul/8/marijuana-sales-washington-top-1-billion-report/?_sm_au_=iVVwFVZDW6Q7kD46.
38. Wang GS, Hall K, Vigil D, Banerji S, Monte A, VanDyke M. Marijuana and acute health care contacts in Colorado. *Prev Med.* 2017;104:24–30.
39. Palamar JJ, Ompad DC, Petkova E. Correlates of intentions to use cannabis among US high school seniors in the case of cannabis legalization. *Int J Drug Policy.* 2014;25(3):424–35.
40. Hall W, Lynskey M. Evaluating the public health impacts of legalizing recreational cannabis use in the United States. *Addiction.* 2016;111(10):1764–73.
41. Volkow ND, Baler RD, Compton WM, Weiss SR. Adverse health effects of marijuana use. *N Engl J Med.* 2014;370(23):2219–27.
42. National Institute on Drug Abuse, National Institutes of Health, U.S. Department of Health and Human Services. *2016-2020 NIDA Strategic Plan: Advancing Addiction Science.* National Institute on Drug Abuse; 2015. https://www.drugabuse.gov/sites/default/files/nida_2016strategicplan_032316.pdf.
43. Ogden D. *Memorandum for Selected United States Attorneys: Investigations and Prosecutions in States Authorizing the Medical Use of Marijuana.* Washington, DC: The United States Department of Justice Archives; 2009. https://www.justice.gov/archives/opa/blog/memorandum-selected-united-state-attorneys-investigations-and-prosecutions-states.
44. Cambron C, Guttmannova K, Fleming CB. State and national contexts in evaluating cannabis laws: A case study of Washington state. *J Drug Issues.* 2017;47(1):74–90.
45. Davis JM, Mendelson B, Berkes JJ, Suleta K, Corsi KF, Booth RE. Public health effects of medical marijuana legalization in Colorado. *Am J Prev Med.* 2016;50(3):373–9.
46. Schuermeyer J, Salomonsen-Sautel S, Price RK, et al. Temporal trends in marijuana attitudes, availability and use in Colorado compared to non-medical marijuana states: 2003–11. *Drug Alcohol Depend.* 2014;140:145–55.
47. Salomonsen-Sautel S, Min SJ, Sakai JT, Thurstone C, Hopfer C. Trends in fatal motor vehicle crashes before and after marijuana commercialization in Colorado. *Drug Alcohol Depend.* 2014;140:137–44.
48. American Psychiatric Association. *Diagnostic and Statistical Manual of Mental Disorders*, 4th ed. Washington, DC: American Psychiatric Association; 1994.
49. American Psychiatric Association. *Diagnostic and Statistical Manual of Mental Disorders*, 5th ed. Washington, DC: American Psychiatric Association; 2013.
50. World Health Organization. *International Statistical Classification of Diseases and Related Health Problems.* 10th ed. Geneva, Switzerland: World Health Organization; 1992.
51. World Health Organization. *The ICD-10 Classification of Mental and Behavioural Disorders: Diagnostic Criteria for Research.* Geneva, Switzerland: World Health Organization; 1993.
52. Grant BF. DSM-IV, DSM-III-R, and ICD-10 alcohol and drug abuse/harmful use and dependence, United States, 1992: A nosological comparison. *Alcohol Clin Exp Res.* 1996;20(8):1481–8.
53. Hasin D, Grant BF, Cottler L, et al. Nosological comparisons of alcohol and drug diagnoses: A multisite, multi-instrument international study. *Drug Alcohol Depend.* 1997;47(3):217–26.
54. Pull CB, Saunders JB, Mavreas V, et al. Concordance between ICD-10 alcohol and drug use disorder criteria and diagnoses as measured by the AUDADIS-ADR, CIDI and SCAN: Results of a cross-national study. *Drug Alcohol Depend.* 1997;47(3):207–16.
55. Rounsaville BJ, Bryant K, Babor T, Kranzler H, Kadden R. Cross system agreement for substance use disorders: DSM-III-R, DSM-IV and ICD-10. *Addiction.* 1993;88(3):337–48.
56. Ustun B, Compton W, Mager D, et al. WHO study on the reliability and validity of the alcohol and drug use disorder instruments: Overview of methods and results. *Drug Alcohol Depend.* 1997;47(3):161–9.
57. Hasin D, Hatzenbuehler ML, Keyes K, Ogburn E. Substance use disorders: Diagnostic and Statistical Manual of Mental Disorders, fourth edition (DSM-IV) and International Classification of Diseases, tenth edition (ICD-10). *Addiction.* 2006;101(Suppl 1):59–75.
58. Saunders JB. Substance use and addictive disorders in DSM-5 and ICD 10 and the draft ICD 11. *Curr Opin Psychiatry.* 2017;30(4):227–37.
59. Volkow ND, Koob GF, McLellan AT. Neurobiologic advances from the brain disease model of addiction. *N Engl J Med.* 2016;374(4):363–71.
60. Stern TA, Gross AF, Stern TW, Nejad SH, Maldonado JR. Current approaches to the recognition and treatment of alcohol withdrawal and delirium tremens: "Old wine in new bottles" or "new wine in old bottles." *Prim Care Companion J Clin Psychiatry.* 2010;12(3):PCC.10r00991.
61. Copersino ML, Boyd SJ, Tashkin DP, et al. Cannabis withdrawal among non-treatment-seeking adult cannabis users. *Am J Addict.* 2006;15(1):8–14.
62. Martinez D, Kim JH, Krystal J, Abi-Dargham A. Imaging the neurochemistry of alcohol and substance abuse. *Neuroimaging Clin N Am.* 2007;17(4):539–55, x.
63. Goldstein RZ, Volkow ND. Dysfunction of the prefrontal cortex in addiction: Neuroimaging findings and clinical implications. *Nat Rev Neurosci.* 2011;12(11):652–69.
64. Haney M, Hart CL, Vosburg SK, et al. Marijuana withdrawal in humans: Effects of oral THC or divalproex. *Neuropsychopharmacology.* 2004;29(1):158–70.
65. Budney AJ, Hughes JR, Moore BA, Vandrey R. Review of the validity and significance of cannabis withdrawal syndrome. *Am J Psychiatry.* 2004;161(11):1967–77.
66. Budney AJ, Hughes JR. The cannabis withdrawal syndrome. *Curr Opin Psychiatry.* 2006;19(3):233–8.
67. Agrawal A, Pergadia ML, Lynskey MT. Is there evidence for symptoms of cannabis withdrawal in the national epidemiologic survey of alcohol and related conditions? *Am J Addict.* 2008;17(3):199–208.
68. Chung T, Martin CS, Cornelius JR, Clark DB. Cannabis withdrawal predicts severity of cannabis involvement at 1-year follow-up among treated adolescents. *Addiction.* 2008;103(5):787–99.
69. Hasin DS, Keyes KM, Alderson D, Wang S, Aharonovich E, Grant BF. Cannabis withdrawal in the United States: Results from NESARC. *J Clin Psychiatry.* 2008;69(9):1354–63.
70. Agrawal A, Lynskey MT. Does gender contribute to heterogeneity in criteria for cannabis abuse and dependence? Results from the national epidemiological survey on alcohol and related conditions. *Drug Alcohol Depend.* 2007;88(2–3):300–7.
71. Budney AJ, Moore BA, Vandrey RG, Hughes JR. The time course and significance of cannabis withdrawal. *J Abnorm Psychol.* 2003;112(3):393–402.
72. Milin R, Manion I, Dare G, Walker S. Prospective assessment of cannabis withdrawal in adolescents with cannabis dependence: A pilot study. *J Am Acad Child Adolesc Psychiatry.* 2008;47(2):174–8.
73. Kouri EM, Pope HG. Abstinence symptoms during withdrawal from chronic marijuana use. *Exp Clin Psychopharmacol.* 2000;8(4):483–92.
74. Elkashef A, Vocci F, Huestis M, et al. Marijuana neurobiology and treatment. *Subst Abus.* 2008;29(3):17–29.
75. Budney AJ, Vandrey RG, Hughes JR, Moore BA, Bahrenburg B. Oral delta-9-tetrahydrocannabinol suppresses cannabis withdrawal symptoms. *Drug Alcohol Depend.* 2007;86(1):22–9.
76. Lichtman AH, Martin BR. Marijuana withdrawal syndrome in the animal model. *J Clin Pharmacol.* 2002;42(11 Suppl):20S–7S.
77. Katz G, Lobel T, Tetelbaum A, Raskin S. Cannabis withdrawal: A new diagnostic category in DSM-5. *Isr J Psychiatry Relat Sci.* 2014;51(4):270–5.
78. Levin KH, Copersino ML, Heishman SJ, et al. Cannabis withdrawal symptoms in non-treatment-seeking adult cannabis smokers. *Drug Alcohol Depend.* 2010;111(1-2):120–7.
79. Cornelius JR, Chung T, Martin C, Wood DS, Clark DB. Cannabis withdrawal is common among treatment-seeking adolescents with cannabis dependence and major depression, and is associated with rapid relapse to dependence. *Addict Behav.* 2008;33(11):1500–5.
80. Budney AJ, Vandrey RG, Hughes JR, Thostenson JD, Bursac Z. Comparison of cannabis and tobacco withdrawal: Severity and contribution to relapse. *J Subst Abuse Treat.* 2008;35(4):362–8.
81. Allsop DJ, Copeland J, Norberg MM, et al. Quantifying the clinical significance of cannabis withdrawal. *PLoS One.* 2012;7(9):e44864.
82. Greene MC, Kelly JF. The prevalence of cannabis withdrawal and its influence on adolescents' treatment response and outcomes: A 12-month prospective investigation. *J Addict Med.* 2014;8(5):359–67.

83. Verweij KJ, Agrawal A, Nat NO, et al. A genetic perspective on the proposed inclusion of cannabis withdrawal in DSM-5. *Psychol Med.* 2013;43(8):1713–22.
84. Anthony JC, Warner LA, Kessler RC. Comparative epidemiology of dependence on tobacco, alcohol, controlled substances, and inhalants: Basic findings from the National Comorbidity Survey. *Exp Clin Psychopharmacol.* 1994;2(3):244–68.
85. Hasin DS, Saha TD, Kerridge BT, et al. Prevalence of marijuana use disorders in the United States between 2001–2002 and 2012–2013. *JAMA Psychiatry.* 2015;72(12):1235–42.
86. Hasin DS, Kerridge BT, Saha TD, et al. Prevalence and correlates of DSM-5 cannabis use disorder, 2012–2013: Findings from the National Epidemiologic Survey on Alcohol and Related Conditions-III. *Am J Psychiatry.* 2016;173(6):588–99.
87. Bogdan R, Winstone JM, Agrawal A. Genetic and environmental factors associated with cannabis involvement. *Curr Addict Rep.* 2016;3(2): 199–213.
88. Verweij KJ, Vinkhuyzen AA, Benyamin B, et al. The genetic aetiology of cannabis use initiation: A meta-analysis of genome-wide association studies and a SNP-based heritability estimation. *Addict Biol.* 2013;18(5):846–50.
89. Agrawal A, Lynskey MT. The genetic epidemiology of cannabis use, abuse and dependence. *Addiction.* 2006;101(6):801–12.
90. Haberstick BC, Zeiger JS, Corley RP, et al. Common and drug-specific genetic influences on subjective effects to alcohol, tobacco and marijuana use. *Addiction.* 2011;106(1):215–24.
91. Sherva R, Wang Q, Kranzler H, et al. Genome-wide association study of cannabis dependence severity, novel risk variants, and shared genetic risks. *JAMA Psychiatry.* 2016;73(5):472–80.
92. Babor T. *Alcohol: No Ordinary Commodity: Research and Public Policy.* 2nd ed. New York: Oxford University Press; 2010.
93. Gruenewald PJ. Regulating availability: How access to alcohol affects drinking and problems in youth and adults. *Alcohol Res Health.* 2011;34(2): 248–56.
94. Gruenewald PJ, Remer LG, LaScala EA. Testing a social ecological model of alcohol use: The California 50-city study. *Addiction.* 2014;109(5):736–45.
95. Connell CM, Gilreath TD, Aklin WM, Brex RA. Social-ecological influences on patterns of substance use among non-metropolitan high school students. *Am J Community Psychol.* 2010;45(1-2):36–48.
96. Corbett KK. Susceptibility of youth to tobacco: A social ecological framework for prevention. *Respir Physiol.* 2001;128(1):103–18.
97. Chen CY, Storr CL, Anthony JC. Early-onset drug use and risk for drug dependence problems. *Addict Behav.* 2009;34(3):319–22.
98. Agrawal A, Neale MC, Prescott CA, Kendler KS. A twin study of early cannabis use and subsequent use and abuse/dependence of other illicit drugs. *Psychol Med.* 2004;34(7):1227–37.
99. Stinson FS, Ruan WJ, Pickering R, Grant BF. Cannabis use disorders in the USA: Prevalence, correlates and co-morbidity. *Psychol Med.* 2006;36(10):1447–60.
100. Wu LT, Zhu H, Mannelli P, Swartz MS. Prevalence and correlates of treatment utilization among adults with cannabis use disorder in the United States. *Drug Alcohol Depend.* 2017;177:153–62.
101. Charilaou P, Agnihotri K, Garcia P, Badheka A, Frenia D, Yegneswaran B. Trends of cannabis use disorder in the inpatient: 2002 to 2011. *Am J Med.* 2017;130(6):678–87.
102. Penetar DM, Kouri EM, Gross MM, et al. Transdermal nicotine alters some of marihuana's effects in male and female volunteers. *Drug Alcohol Depend.* 2005;79(2):211–23.
103. Rabin RA, George TP. A review of co-morbid tobacco and cannabis use disorders: Possible mechanisms to explain high rates of co-use. *Am J Addict.* 2015;24(2):105–16.
104. Wang JB, Ramo DE, Lisha NE, Cataldo JK. Medical marijuana legalization and cigarette and marijuana co-use in adolescents and adults. *Drug Alcohol Depend.* 2016;166:32–8.
105. Agrawal A, Budney AJ, Lynskey MT. The co-occurring use and misuse of cannabis and tobacco: A review. *Addiction.* 2012;107(7):1221–33.
106. Lucas P, Walsh Z. Medical cannabis access, use, and substitution for prescription opioids and other substances: A survey of authorized medical cannabis patients. *Int J Drug Policy.* 2017;42:30–5.
107. Lucas P, Walsh Z, Crosby K, et al. Substituting cannabis for prescription drugs, alcohol and other substances among medical cannabis patients: The impact of contextual factors. *Drug Alcohol Rev.* 2016;35(3):326–33.
108. Nunberg H, Kilmer B, Pacula RL, Burgdorf J. An analysis of applicants presenting to a medical marijuana specialty practice in California. *J Drug Policy Anal.* 2011;4(1):1.
109. Reiman A. Cannabis as a substitute for alcohol and other drugs. *Harm Reduct J.* 2009;6:35.
110. Anderson DM, Hansen B, Rees DI. Medical marijuana laws, traffic fatalities, and alcohol consumption. *J Law Econ.* 2013;56(2):333–69.
111. Santaella-Tenorio J, Mauro CM, Wall MM, et al. US traffic fatalities, 1985–2014, and their relationship to medical marijuana laws. *Am J Public Health.* 2017;107(2):336–42.
112. Pacula RL, Powell D, Heaton P, Sevigny EL. *Assessing the Effects of Marijuana on Marijuana and Alcohol Use: The Devil is in the Details.* Cambridge, MA: National Bureau of Economic Research; 2013. http://www.nber.org/papers/w19302.pdf.
113. Guttmannova K, Lee CM, Kilmer JR, et al. Impacts of changing marijuana policies on alcohol use in the United States. *Alcohol Clin Exp Res.* 2016;40(1):33–46.
114. Anderson DM, Rees DI. The legalization of recreational marijuana: How likely is the worst-case scenario? *J Policy Anal Manage.* 2014;33(1):221–32.
115. Carnevale JT, Kagan R, Murphy PJ, Esrick J. A practical framework for regulating for-profit recreational marijuana in US States: Lessons from Colorado and Washington. *Int J Drug Policy.* 2017;42:71–85.
116. Kilmer B. Recreational cannabis: Minimizing the health risks from legalization. *N Engl J Med.* 2017;376(8):705–7.
117. Edwards G. Cannabis and the criteria for legalisation of a currently prohibited recreational drug: Groundwork for a debate. *Acta Psychiatr Scand Suppl.* 1974;251:1–62.
118. Hawken A, Caulkins J, Kilmer B, Kleiman M. Quasi-legal cannabis in Colorado and Washington: Local and national implications. *Addiction.* 2013;108(5):837–8.
119. Pacula RL, Sevigny EL. Natural experiments in a complex and dynamic environment: The need for a measured assessment of the evidence. *J Policy Anal Manage.* 2014;33(1):232–5.
120. Fergusson DM, Boden JM. Cannabis use and later life outcomes. *Addiction.* 2008;103(6):969–76; discussion 977–8.
121. Bujarski SJ, Galang JN, Short NA, et al. Cannabis use disorder treatment barriers and facilitators among veterans with PTSD. *Psychol Addict Behav.* 2016;30(1):73–81.
122. Agrawal A, Lynskey MT. Cannabis controversies: How genetics can inform the study of comorbidity. *Addiction.* 2014;109(3):360–70.
123. Blanco C, Hasin DS, Wall MM, et al. Cannabis use and risk of psychiatric disorders: Prospective evidence from a US national longitudinal study. *JAMA Psychiatry.* 2016;73(4):388–95.
124. Carey CE, Agrawal A, Bucholz KK, et al. Associations between polygenic risk for psychiatric disorders and substance involvement. *Front Genet.* 2016;7:149.
125. Hodgson K, Almasy L, Knowles EE, et al. The genetic basis of the comorbidity between cannabis use and major depression. *Addiction.* 2017;112(1): 113–23.
126. Smolkina M, Morley KI, Rijsdijk F, et al. Cannabis and depression: A twin model approach to co-morbidity. *Behav Genet.* 2017;47(4):394–404.
127. Agrawal A, Nelson EC, Bucholz KK, et al. Major depressive disorder, suicidal thoughts and behaviours, and cannabis involvement in discordant twins: A retrospective cohort study. *Lancet Psychiatry.* 2017;4(9):706–14.
128. Carney R, Cotter J, Firth J, Bradshaw T, Yung AR. Cannabis use and symptom severity in individuals at ultra high risk for psychosis: A meta-analysis. *Acta Psychiatr Scand.* 2017;136(1):5–15.
129. Boden JM, Fergusson DM, Horwood LJ. Anxiety disorders and suicidal behaviours in adolescence and young adulthood: Findings from a longitudinal study. *Psychol Med.* 2007;37(3):431–40.
130. Fergusson DM, Boden JM, Horwood LJ. Psychosocial sequelae of cannabis use and implications for policy: Findings from the Christchurch Health and Development Study. *Soc Psychiatry Psychiatr Epidemiol.* 2015;50(9):1317–26.
131. Gage SH, Hickman M, Zammit S. Association between cannabis and psychosis: Epidemiologic evidence. *Biol Psychiatry.* 2016;79(7):549–56.
132. Kraan T, Velthorst E, Koenders L, et al. Cannabis use and transition to psychosis in individuals at ultra-high risk: Review and meta-analysis. *Psychol Med.* 2016;46(4):673–81.
133. Haney M, Evins AE. Does cannabis cause, exacerbate or ameliorate psychiatric disorders? An oversimplified debate discussed. *Neuropsychopharmacology.* 2016;41(2):393–401.
134. National Academies of Sciences, Engineering, and Medicine. *The Health Effects of Cannabis and Cannabinoids: The Current State of Evidence and Recommendations for Research.* Washington, DC: The National Academies Press; 2017.
135. Weiss SRB, Blanco C, Wargo EM. Clarifying the link between cannabis use and risk for psychosis. *Acta Psychiatr Scand.* 2017;136(1):3–4.

136. Baumann A, Scheinbaum C. Weed rosin is changing the way we get high. Bloomberg Businessweek. 2016. https://www.bloomberg.com/news/articles/2016-03-23/weed-rosin-is-changing-the-way-we-get-high. Accessed July 3, 2017.
137. El Marroun H, Tiemeier H, Franken IH, et al. Prenatal cannabis and tobacco exposure in relation to brain morphology: A prospective neuroimaging study in young children. *Biol Psychiatry*. 2016;79(12):971–9.
138. Gunn JK, Rosales CB, Center KE, et al. Prenatal exposure to cannabis and maternal and child health outcomes: A systematic review and meta-analysis. *BMJ Open*. 2016;6(4):e009986.
139. Zalesky A, Solowij N, Yucel M, et al. Effect of long-term cannabis use on axonal fibre connectivity. *Brain*. 2012;135(Pt 7):2245–55.
140. Meier MH, Caspi A, Ambler A, et al. Persistent cannabis users show neuropsychological decline from childhood to midlife. *Proc Natl Acad Sci U S A*. 2012;109(40):E2657–64.
141. Batalla A, Bhattacharyya S, Yucel M, et al. Structural and functional imaging studies in chronic cannabis users: A systematic review of adolescent and adult findings. *PLoS One*. 2013;8(2):e55821.
142. Volkow ND, Compton WM, Wargo EM. The risks of marijuana use during pregnancy. *JAMA*. 2017;317(2):129–30.
143. Wu CS, Jew CP, Lu HC. Lasting impacts of prenatal cannabis exposure and the role of endogenous cannabinoids in the developing brain. *Future Neurol*. 2011;6(4):459–80.
144. Cerda M, Moffitt TE, Meier MH, et al. Persistent cannabis dependence and alcohol dependence represent risks for midlife economic and social problems. *Clin Psychol Sci*. 2016;4(6):1028–46.
145. Townsend L, Flisher AJ, King G. A systematic review of the relationship between high school dropout and substance use. *Clin Child Fam Psychol Rev*. 2007;10(4):295–317.
146. Calabria B, Degenhardt L, Hall W, Lynskey M. Does cannabis use increase the risk of death? Systematic review of epidemiological evidence on adverse effects of cannabis use. *Drug Alcohol Rev*. 2010;29(3):318–30.
147. Ramaekers JG, Berghaus G, van Laar M, Drummer OH. Dose related risk of motor vehicle crashes after cannabis use. *Drug Alcohol Depend*. 2004;73(2):109–19.
148. Rogeberg O, Elvik R. The effects of cannabis intoxication on motor vehicle collision revisited and revised. *Addiction*. 2016;111(8):1348–59.
149. Brady JE, Li G. Trends in alcohol and other drugs detected in fatally injured drivers in the United States, 1999–2010. *Am J Epidemiol*. 2014;179(6):692–9.
150. Asbridge M, Hayden JA, Cartwright JL. Acute cannabis consumption and motor vehicle collision risk: Systematic review of observational studies and meta-analysis. *BMJ*. 2012;344:e536.
151. Li MC, Brady JE, DiMaggio CJ, Lusardi AR, Tzong KY, Li G. Marijuana use and motor vehicle crashes. *Epidemiol Rev*. 2012;34:65–72.
152. Hartman RL, Huestis MA. Cannabis effects on driving skills. *Clin Chem*. 2013;59(3):478–92.
153. Zhu H, Wu LT. Trends and correlates of cannabis-involved emergency department visits: 2004 to 2011. *J Addict Med*. 2016;10(6):429–36.
154. Liu C, Huang Y, Pressley JC. Restraint use and risky driving behaviors across drug types and drug and alcohol combinations for drivers involved in a fatal motor vehicle collision on U.S. roadways. *Inj Epidemiol*. 2016;3:9.
155. McKay MP, Groff L. 23 years of toxicology testing fatally injured pilots: Implications for aviation and other modes of transportation. *Accid Anal Prev*. 2016;90:108–17.
156. Janz NK, Becker MH. The health belief model: A decade later. *Health Educ Q*. 1984;11(1):1–47.
157. Schmidt LA, Jacobs LM, Spetz J. Young people's more permissive views about marijuana: Local impact of state laws or national trend? *Am J Public Health*. 2016;106(8):1498–503.
158. Keyes KM, Wall M, Cerda M, et al. How does state marijuana policy affect US youth? Medical marijuana laws, marijuana use and perceived harmfulness: 1991–2014. *Addiction*. 2016;111(12):2187–95.
159. Piontek D, Kraus L, Bjarnason T, Demetrovics Z, Ramstedt M. Individual and country-level effects of cannabis-related perceptions on cannabis use. A multilevel study among adolescents in 32 European countries. *J Adolesc Health*. 2013;52(4):473–9.
160. Johnston LD, Bachman JG, O'Malley PM. *Highlights from Student Drug Use in America, 1975–1980*. Rockville, MD: National Institute on Drug Abuse; 1981.
161. Bachman JG, Johnston LD, O'Malley PM, Humphrey RH. Explaining the recent decline in marijuana use: Differentiating the effects of perceived risks, disapproval, and general lifestyle factors. *J Health Soc Behav*. 1988;29:92–112.
162. Bachman JG, Johnson LD, O'Malley PM. Explaining recent increases in students' marijuana use: Impacts of perceived risks and disapproval, 1976 through 1996. *Am J Public Health*. 1998;88(6):887–92.
163. Swaim RC. Individual and school level effects of perceived harm, perceived availability, and community size on marijuana use among 12th-grade students: A random effects model. *Prev Sci*. 2003;4(2):89–98.
164. Pacek LR, Mauro PM, Martins SS. Perceived risk of regular cannabis use in the United States from 2002 to 2012: Differences by sex, age, and race/ethnicity. *Drug Alcohol Depend*. 2015;149:232–44.
165. Compton WM, Han B, Jones CM, Blanco C, Hughes A. Marijuana use and use disorders in adults in the USA, 2002–14: Analysis of annual cross-sectional surveys. *Lancet Psychiatry*. 2016;3(10):954–64.
166. Monitoring the Future Study, University of Michigan. Figures 3 and 4. Marijuana: Trends in annual/daily use in grades 8, 10 and 12. 2016. http://www.monitoringthefuture.org/data/16data.html. Accessed March 22, 2017.
167. Cascini F, Aiello C, Di Tanna G. Increasing delta-9-tetrahydrocannabinol (Delta-9-THC) content in herbal cannabis over time: Systematic review and meta-analysis. *Curr Drug Abuse Rev*. 2012;5(1):32–40.
168. ElSohly MA, Mehmedic Z, Foster S, Gon C, Chandra S, Church JC. Changes in cannabis potency over the last 2 decades (1995–2014): Analysis of current data in the United States. *Biol Psychiatry*. 2016;79(7):613–9.
169. National Institute on Drug Abuse. *Is Marijuana Addictive*. National Institute on Drug Abuse; 2017. https://www.drugabuse.gov/publications/research-reports/marijuana/marijuana-addictive.
170. Englund A, Freeman TP, Murray RM, McGuire P. Can we make cannabis safer? *Lancet Psychiatry*. 2017;4(8):643–8.
171. Sevigny EL, Pacula RL, Heaton P. The effects of medical marijuana laws on potency. *Int J Drug Policy*. 2014;25(2):308–19.
172. Northwest High Intensity Drug Trafficking Area. *Washington State Marijuana Impact Report*. Seattle, WA: Northwest HIDTA; 2016. http://www.riag.ri.gov/documents/NWHIDTAMarijuanaImpactReportVolume1.pdf.
173. Cabrera A. Colorado marijuana's potency getting 'higher'. CNN. 2016. http://www.cnn.com/2016/10/21/health/colorado-marijuana-potency-above-national-average/index.html?_sm_au_=iVVwFVZDW6Q7kD46. Accessed July 2, 2017.
174. Azofeifa A, Mattson ME, Schauer G, McAfee T, Grant A, Lyerla R. National estimates of marijuana use and related indicators: National Survey on Drug Use and Health, United States, 2002–2014. *MMWR Surveill Summ*. 2016;65(11):1–28.
175. Azofeifa A, Mattson ME, Grant A. Monitoring marijuana use in the United States: Challenges in an evolving environment. *JAMA*. 2016;316(17):1765–6.
176. Miech R, Johnston L, O'Malley PM. Prevalence and attitudes regarding marijuana use among adolescents over the past decade. *Pediatrics*. 2017;140(6):e20170982.
177. Grucza RA, Agrawal A, Krauss MJ, et al. Declining prevalence of marijuana use disorders among adolescents in the United States, 2002 to 2013. *J Am Acad Child Adolesc Psychiatry*. 2016;55(6):487–94.
178. Wall MM, Poh E, Cerda M, Keyes KM, Galea S, Hasin DS. Adolescent marijuana use from 2002 to 2008: Higher in states with medical marijuana laws, cause still unclear. *Ann Epidemiol*. 2011;21(9):714–6.
179. Imbens GW, Wooldridge JM. Recent developments in the econometrics of program evaluation. *J Econ Lit*. 2009;47(1):5–86.
180. Angrist JD, Pischke JS. *Mostly Harmless Econometrics: An Empiricist's Companion*. Princeton, NJ: Princeton University Press; 2009.
181. Hunt PE, Miles J. The impact of legalizing and regulating weed: Issues with study design and emerging findings in the USA. *Curr Top Behav Neurosci*. 2017;34:173–98.
182. Angrist J, Krueger AB. Empirical strategies in labor economics. In: Ashenfelter O, Card D, eds. *Handbook of Labor Economics*. Vol. 3. Amsterdam, The Netherlands: Elsevier Science; 1999:1277–366.
183. Hasin DS, Wall M, Keyes KM, et al. Medical marijuana laws and adolescent marijuana use in the USA from 1991 to 2014: Results from annual, repeated cross-sectional surveys. *Lancet Psychiatry*. 2015;2(7):601–8.
184. Choi A. The impact of medical marijuana laws on marijuana use and other risky health behaviors. Paper presented at Health & Healthcare in America: From Economics to Policy; June 23, 2014; Los Angeles, CA.
185. Martins SS, Mauro CM, Santaella-Tenorio J, et al. State-level medical marijuana laws, marijuana use and perceived availability of marijuana among the general U.S. population. *Drug Alcohol Depend*. 2016;169:26–32.
186. Anderson DM, Hansen B, Rees DI. Medical marijuana laws and teen marijuana use. *Am Law Econ Rev*. 2015;17(2):495–528.

187. Smart R. The kids aren't alright but older adults are just fine: Effects of medical marijuana market growth on substance use and abuse. Social Science Research Network. 2015. https://papers.ssrn.com/sol3/papers.cfm?abstract_id=2574915.

188. Sarvet AL, Wall MM, Fink DS, et al. Medical marijuana laws and adolescent marijuana use in the United States: A systematic review and meta-analysis. *Addiction*. 2018;113(6):1003–16.

189. Cerda M, Wall M, Feng T, et al. Association of state recreational marijuana laws with adolescent marijuana use. *JAMA Pediatr*. 2017;171(2):142–9.

190. Carliner H, Mauro PM, Brown QL, et al. The widening gender gap in marijuana use prevalence in the U.S. during a period of economic change, 2002–2014. *Drug Alcohol Depend*. 2017;170:51–8.

191. Johnson MB, Kelley-Baker T, Voas RB, Lacey JH. The prevalence of cannabis-involved driving in California. *Drug Alcohol Depend*. 2012;123(1–3):105–9.

192. Berning A, Compton R, Wochinger K. *Results of the 2013–2014 National Roadside Survey of Alcohol and Drug Use by Drivers*. Washington, DC: Administration NHTS; 2015. DOT HS 812 118. https://www.nhtsa.gov/sites/nhtsa.dot.gov/files/812118-roadside_survey_2014.pdf.

193. Shi Y. Medical marijuana policies and hospitalizations related to marijuana and opioid pain reliever. *Drug Alcohol Depend*. 2017;173:144–50.

194. Bonn-Miller MO, Harris AH, Trafton JA. Prevalence of cannabis use disorder diagnoses among veterans in 2002, 2008, and 2009. *Psychol Serv*. 2012;9(4):404–16.

195. Gubatan J, Staller K, Barshop K, Kuo B. Cannabis abuse is increasing and associated with increased emergency department utilization in gastroenterology patients. *Dig Dis Sci*. 2016;61(7):1844–52.

196. Jehle CCJr, Nazir N, Bhavsar D. The rapidly increasing trend of cannabis use in burn injury. *J Burn Care Res*. 2015;36(1):e12–7.

197. Grucza RA, Agrawal A, Krauss MJ, Cavazos-Rehg PA, Bierut LJ. Recent trends in the prevalence of marijuana use and associated disorders in the United States. *JAMA Psychiatry*. 2016;73(3):300–1.

198. Grucza RA, Agrawal A, Bierut LJ. NESARC findings on increased prevalence of marijuana use disorders: Reply: Consistent with other sources of information. *JAMA Psychiatry*. 2016;73(5):532–3.

199. Hasin DS, Grant B. NESARC findings on increased prevalence of marijuana use disorders: Consistent with other sources of information. *JAMA Psychiatry*. 2016;73(5):532.

200. Cerda M, Wall M, Keyes KM, Galea S, Hasin D. Medical marijuana laws in 50 states: Investigating the relationship between state legalization of medical marijuana and marijuana use, abuse and dependence. *Drug Alcohol Depend*. 2012;120(1–3):22–7.

201. Chu YW. The effects of medical marijuana laws on illegal marijuana use. *J Health Econ*. 2014;38:43–61.

202. Onders B, Casavant MJ, Spiller HA, Chounthirath T, Smith GA. Marijuana exposure among children younger than six years in the United States. *Clin Pediatr (Phila)*. 2016;55(5):428–36.

203. Ko JY, Farr SL, Tong VT, Creanga AA, Callaghan WM. Prevalence and patterns of marijuana use among pregnant and nonpregnant women of reproductive age. *Am J Obstet Gynecol*. 2015;213(2):201 e201–10.

204. Brown QL, Sarvet AL, Shmulewitz D, Martins SS, Wall MM, Hasin DS. Trends in marijuana use among pregnant and nonpregnant reproductive-aged women, 2002–2014. *JAMA*. 2017;317(2):207–9.

205. Wang GS, Roosevelt G, Le Lait MC, et al. Association of unintentional pediatric exposures with decriminalization of marijuana in the United States. *Ann Emerg Med*. 2014;63(6):684–9.

206. Wang GS, Le Lait MC, Deakyne SJ, Bronstein AC, Bajaj L, Roosevelt G. Unintentional pediatric exposures to marijuana in Colorado, 2009–2015. *JAMA Pediatr*. 2016;170(9):e160971.

207. Substance Abuse and Mental Health Services Administration, Center for Behavioral Health Statistics and Quality. *Treatment Episode Data Set (TEDS) 2003–2013: National Admissions to Substance Abuse Treatment Services*. Rockville, MD: Substance Abuse and Mental Health Services Administration; 2015. https://www.samhsa.gov/data/sites/default/files/2013_Treatment_Episode_Data_Set_National/2013_Treatment_Episode_Data_Set_National.pdf.

208. Hardt J, Jacobsen C, Goldberg J, Nickel R, Buchwald D. Prevalence of chronic pain in a representative sample in the United States. *Pain Med*. 2008;9(7):803–12.

209. Tsang A, Von Korff M, Lee S, et al. Common chronic pain conditions in developed and developing countries: Gender and age differences and comorbidity with depression-anxiety disorders. *J Pain*. 2008;9(10):883–91.

210. Nahin RL. Estimates of pain prevalence and severity in adults: United States, 2012. *J Pain*. 2015;16(8):769–80.

211. Institute of Medicine. *Relieving Pain in America: A Blueprint for Transforming Prevention, Care, Education, and Research*. Washington, DC: National Academies Press (US); 2011.

212. Levy B, Paulozzi L, Mack KA, Jones CM. Trends in opioid analgesic-prescribing rates by specialty, U.S., 2007–2012. *Am J Prev Med*. 2015;49(3):409–13.

213. Volkow ND, McLellan AT. Opioid abuse in chronic pain: Misconceptions and mitigation strategies. *N Engl J Med*. 2016;374(13):1253–63.

214. Chou R, Deyo R, Devine B, et al. *The Effectiveness and Risks of Long-term Opioid Treatment of Chronic Pain*. Rockville, MD: Agency for Healthcare Research and Quality; 2014. AHRQ Publication No. 14-E005-EF. www.effectivehealthcare.ahrq.gov/reports/final.cfm.

215. Volkow N, Benveniste H, McLellan AT. Use and misuse of opioids in chronic pain. *Annu Rev Med*. 2017;69(1):451–65.

216. Paulozzi LJ, Kilbourne EM, Shah NG, et al. A history of being prescribed controlled substances and risk of drug overdose death. *Pain Med*. 2012;13(1):87–95.

217. Okie S. A flood of opioids, a rising tide of deaths. *N Engl J Med*. 2010;363(21):1981–5.

218. Rudd RA, Aleshire N, Zibbell JE, Gladden RM. Increases in drug and opioid overdose deaths: United States, 2000–2014. *MMWR Morb Mortal Wkly Rep*. 2016;64(50–51):1378–82.

219. Volkow ND, Swanson JM, Evins AE, et al. Effects of cannabis use on human behavior, including cognition, motivation, and psychosis: A review. *JAMA Psychiatry*. 2016;73(3):292–7.

220. Whiting PF, Wolff RF, Deshpande S, et al. Cannabinoids for medical use: A systematic review and meta-analysis. *JAMA*. 2015;313(24):2456–73.

221. Thomas BF, Pollard GT. Preparation and distribution of cannabis and cannabis-derived dosage formulations for investigational and therapeutic use in the United States. *Front Pharmacol*. 2016;7:285.

222. Hall W. Alcohol and cannabis: Comparing their adverse health effects and regulatory regimes. *Int J Drug Policy*. 2017;42:57–62.

223. Choo EK, Feldstein Ewing SW, Lovejoy TI. Opioids out, cannabis in: Negotiating the unknowns in patient care for chronic pain. *JAMA*. 2016;316(17):1763–4.

224. Saxon AJ, Browne KW. Marijuana not ready for prime time as an analgesic. *Gen Hosp Psychiatry*. 2014;36(1):4–6.

225. Piper BJ, DeKeuster RM, Beals ML, et al. Substitution of medical cannabis for pharmaceutical agents for pain, anxiety, and sleep. *J Psychopharmacol*. 2017;31(5):569–75.

226. Boehnke KF, Litinas E, Clauw DJ. Medical cannabis use is associated with decreased opiate medication use in a retrospective cross-sectional survey of patients with chronic pain. *J Pain*. 2016;17(6):739–44.

227. Davis AK, Bonar EE, Ilgen MA, Walton MA, Perron BE, Chermack ST. Factors associated with having a medical marijuana card among Veterans with recent substance use in VA outpatient treatment. *Addict Behav*. 2016;63:132–6.

228. Corroon JMJr, Mischley LK, Sexton M. Cannabis as a substitute for prescription drugs: A cross-sectional study. *J Pain Res*. 2017;10:989–98.

229. Bradford AC, Bradford WD. Medical marijuana laws may be associated with a decline in the number of prescriptions for Medicaid enrollees. *Health Aff (Millwood)*. 2017;36(5):945–51.

230. Bradford AC, Bradford WD. Medical marijuana laws reduce prescription medication use in Medicare Part D. *Health Aff (Millwood)*. 2016;35(7):1230–6.

231. Powell D, Pacula R, Jacobson M. Do medical marijuana laws reduce addictions and deaths related to pain killers. *J Health Econ*. 2018;58:29–42.

232. Pardo B. Do more robust prescription drug monitoring programs reduce prescription opioid overdose? *Addiction*. 2017;112(10):1773–83.

233. Bachhuber MA, Saloner B, Cunningham CO, Barry CL. Medical cannabis laws and opioid analgesic overdose mortality in the United States, 1999–2010. *JAMA Intern Med*. 2014;174(10):1668–73.

234. Kim JH, Santaella-Tenorio J, Mauro C, et al. State medical marijuana laws and the prevalence of opioids detected among fatally injured drivers. *Am J Public Health*. 2016;106(11):2032–7.

235. Squires B. Why people smoke weed to treat depression. Broadly; Vice Magazine. 2016. https://broadly.vice.com/en_us/article/bmwwmz/why-people-smoke-weed-to-treat-depression.

236. Marijuana cured my depression. Grasscity Forums. 2010. https://forum.grasscity.com/threads/marijuana-cured-my-depression.683017/?_sm_au_=iVVN7Zq5H3sKjdZq. Accessed June 29, 2017.

237. Bonn-Miller MO, Boden MT, Bucossi MM, Babson KA. Self-reported cannabis use characteristics, patterns and helpfulness among medical cannabis users. *Am J Drug Alcohol Abuse*. 2014;40(1):23–30.

238. Walsh Z, Gonzalez R, Crosby K, M ST, Carroll C, Bonn-Miller MO. Medical cannabis and mental health: A guided systematic review. *Clin Psychol Rev*. 2017;51:15–29.

239. Bohnert KM, Perron BE, Ashrafioun L, Kleinberg F, Jannausch M, Ilgen MA. Positive posttraumatic stress disorder screens among first-time medical cannabis patients: Prevalence and association with other substance use. *Addict Behav*. 2014;39(10):1414–7.

240. Swift W, Gates P, Dillon P. Survey of Australians using cannabis for medical purposes. *Harm Reduct J*. 2005;2:18.

241. Bahorik AL, Leibowitz A, Sterling SA, Travis A, Weisner C, Satre DD. Patterns of marijuana use among psychiatry patients with depression and its impact on recovery. *J Affect Disord*. 2017;213:168–71.

242. Wilkinson ST, Stefanovics E, Rosenheck RA. Marijuana use is associated with worse outcomes in symptom severity and violent behavior in patients with posttraumatic stress disorder. *J Clin Psychiatry*. 2015;76(9):1174–80.

243. Sarvet A, Wall M, Keyes KM, Olfson M, Cerdá M, Hasin DS. Self-medication of mood and anxiety disorders with marijuana: Higher in states with medical marijuana laws. *Drug Alcohol Depend*. 2018;186:10–15.

244. Bradford AC, Bradford WD. Medical marijuana laws: The authors reply. *Health Aff (Millwood)*. 2016;35(10):1937.

245. American College of Obstetricians, Gynecologists Committee on Obstetric Practice. Committee Opinion No. 637: Marijuana use during pregnancy and lactation. *Obstet Gynecol*. 2015;126(1):234–8.

246. Hayes MJ, Brown MS. Legalization of medical marijuana and incidence of opioid mortality. *JAMA Intern Med*. 2014;174(10):1673–4.

247. Finney JW, Humphreys K, Harris AH. What ecologic analyses cannot tell us about medical marijuana legalization and opioid pain medication mortality. *JAMA Intern Med*. 2015;175(4):655–6.

248. Saint Louis C. A balm when you're expecting: Sometimes pot does the trick. New York Times. 2017. https://www.nytimes.com/2017/02/20/health/marijuana-pregnancy-mothers.html.

CHAPTER

169

Prescription Drug Use and Misuse

Danielle C. Ompad • Simon Sandh

INTRODUCTION

In 2015, prescription psychotherapeutic drugs such as pain relievers, tranquilizers, stimulants, and sedatives were used by 119 million Americans aged 12 and older—representing 44.5% of the population.[1] In the same year, approximately 18.9 million Americans (or 7.1% of the population) *misused* psychotherapeutic drugs; thus, a majority of people who used prescriptions drugs did not misuse them. Prescription pain relievers are the mostly commonly misused prescription drug (4.7%), followed by tranquilizers (2.3%), stimulants (2.0%), and sedatives (0.6%). For those who misuse prescription drugs, this misuse may result in substantial morbidity and mortality. In addition, prescription drug use and misuse may result in the disruption of social ties and engagement with the criminal justice system. Here we briefly review the pharmacology of different prescription drug classes, the epidemiology of prescription drug misuse as well as the medical consequences of misuse and evidence-based interventions for harm reduction and treatment.

PHARMACOLOGY OF PRESCRIPTION DRUGS USED FOR NONMEDICAL PURPOSES

A wide variety of prescription psychotherapeutic drugs are used for nonmedical purposes and several drug classes are represented. Pain relievers, tranquilizers, stimulants, and sedatives are the most commonly misused drugs.

Pain Relievers

Pain relievers include both opioid and nonopioid medications, but the focus of most surveillance systems are the opioid analgesic pain relievers including hydrocodone, oxycodone, tramadol, codeine, morphine, fentanyl, buprenorphine, oxymorphone, Demerol, hydromorpone, and methadone.[2] The opioid analgesics bind to the delta, kappa, and/or mu opioid receptors as agonists, partial agonists, and antagonists.[3]

Tranquilizers

Tranquilizers include benzodiazepines and muscle relaxants. Tranquilizers are distinguished from sedatives because they are typically prescribed as an anxiolytic or to relieve muscle spasms.[2] Benzodiazepines are sedative-hypnotics that modulate gamma-aminobutyric acid (GABA) receptors.[4] Common benzodiazepines include chlordiazepoxide, diazepam, lorazepam, oxezepam, and clonazempa.[2,5] Some benzodiazepines function as muscle relaxants.[5] Many of the other muscle relaxants, such as carisoprodol, are central nervous system (CNS) depressants.[4] Carisoprodol also affects GABA receptors.[4]

Stimulants

Stimulants include amphetamine, methamphetamine, methylphenidate, anorectic stimulants (e.g., benzphetamine, diethylpropion, phendimetrazine, phentermine), and modafinil.[2] Amphetamine, methamphetamine, and methylphenidate are CNS stimulants that modulate catecholamine (i.e., noradrenaline and dopamine) reuptake and release.[5]

Sedatives

Sedatives include zolpidem, eszopiclone, zaleplon, benzodiazepine sedatives (e.g., flurazepam, temazepam, and triazolam), and barbiturates (e.g., phenobarbital, secobarbital).[2] Sedatives are distinguished from tranquilizers because they are typically prescribed for insomnia.[2] Zolpidem, eszopiclone, zaleplon, and barbiturates are nonbenzodiazepine sedative-hypnotics. Like benzodiazepines, these sedatives modulate GABA receptors.

EPIDEMIOLOGY OF NONMEDICAL PRESCRIPTION DRUG USE

Prevalence and Incidence

In 2015, prescription psychotherapeutic drugs were misused by 18.9 million Americans (or 7.1% of the population).[1] Globally, estimates are more difficult to summarize, due to different reporting conventions across countries. According to the United Nations Office on Drugs and Crime, there were 35 million past-year opioid users (including heroin) and 37 million amphetamine and prescription stimulant users globally in 2015; sedative and tranquilizer prevalence was not estimated.[6]

With respect to past-year initiation of nonmedical use of psychotherapeutics in the United States, there were 2.13 million past-year initiates of pain reliever misuse (0.8% of the total U.S. population), 1.44 million initiates of tranquillizer misuse (0.5%), 1.23 million initiates of stimulant misuse (0.5%), and 425,000 initiates of sedative misuse (0.2%) in 2015.[7] The mean age at first misuse of psychotherapeutics was 25.8 years for pain relievers, 25.9 for tranquilizers, 22.3 for stimulants, and 28.3 for sedatives.[7] Like prevalence estimates, global estimates of incidence are elusive.

There have been reports of misuse of other prescription drugs, although many of these drugs are not tracked via surveillance systems. For example, misuse of the anticonvulsants pregabalin and gabapentin has recently been reported,[8] with one study estimating 1% general population prevalence of gabapentin misuse.[9]

Global Burden of Disease (DALYs)

Globally, illicit drug use accounts from 20 million disability-adjusted life years (DALYs), which is equivalent to 0.8% of the global all-cause DALYs.[10] The 2010 Global Burden of Disease Study is unable to disaggregate nonmedical use of psychotherapeutics from DALY estimates for opioids, amphetamines, and other drug use disorders. Thus, the global burden of disease attributable to nonmedical use of psychotherapeutics cannot be estimated. Using the available broad categories of drugs, opioids account for 9.2 million DALYs, amphetamines for 2.62 million DALYs, and other drug use disorders for 5.06 million DALYs.[10]

Key Risk Factors for Nonmedical Prescription Drug Use

Prescription drugs can be misused to get high or enhance social interactions, but are also used to self-medicate physical and psychological symptoms (e.g., pain, insomnia, anxiety, inattention, etc.).[11] Among youth, prescription stimulant misuse is sometimes motivated by a desire to improve academic performance.[12] Sociodemographic risk factors for nonmedical prescription drug use vary by specific drugs, but in the United States, Asians and Blacks generally have the lowest prevalence of nonmedical prescription drug use overall and by specific drugs[7] and gender differences tend to be small.[11] Cross-cutting risk factors include polysubstance use and comorbid mental health conditions.[12–15] Upstream determinants of nonmedical prescription drug use should not be overlooked, particularly an increase in the prescribing of opioids, benzodiazepines, and stimulants.[12,16,17]

MEDICAL CONSEQUENCES OF NONMEDICAL PRESCRIPTION DRUG USE

While prescriptions drugs are intended to treat ailments, the misuse of prescription drugs can have opposite effects. The misuse of prescription drugs can lead to a variety of negative outcomes including sexual risk behavior, substance dependence, overdose, and increased risk for HIV, other sexually transmitted infections (STIs), and hepatitis C.

Sexual Risk Behavior and Infectious Diseases

Nonmedical prescription drug use is associated with sexual risk behaviors including sex under the influence of drugs, condomless sex, and multiple sex partners, which are in turn associated with risk for HIV and other STIs.[18–20] There is increased risk for HIV as well as hepatitis C among individuals who inject prescription opioids, as highlighted by the 2015 Scott County, Indiana HIV outbreak.[21]

Opioid Dependence and the Transition to Heroin

The misuse of prescription opioids is linked to the development of opioid dependence, which may lead to heroin use.[22] Among recent heroin users, 79.5% initiated the use of heroin after nonmedical use of prescription opioids.[23]

Overdose

Nonmedical prescription drug use may result in overdose, alone or in combination with other substances. The USA is experiencing an opioid crisis, with a 2.6-fold increase in prescription opioid overdose deaths between 2002–2003 and 2014–2015[24] and a 4.3-fold increase in the rate of deaths involving benzodiazepines between 1996 and 2012.[17] Among the top drugs involved in overdoses deaths in the United States for 2014, seven of the top ten were prescription drugs (#3 oxycodone, #4 alprazolam, #5 fentanyl, #6 morphine, #8 methadone, #9 hydrocodone, and #10 diazepam).[25] Other countries have also seen increases in prescription drug-related mortality including Australia,[26] Canada,[27] and England and Wales.[28] In Croatia, Denmark, France, and Ireland methadone-related deaths exceeded the number of heroin deaths.[29]

EVIDENCE-BASED INTERVENTIONS

Screening

The first step in providing treatment to those who misuse prescription drugs is identification of misuse. In primary-care settings, medical-care providers can identify misuse through a variety of validated screening tools such as the Drug Abuse Screening Test (DAST-10)[30] or Alcohol, Smoking, and Substance Involvement Screening Test (ASSIST).[31] These screenings may be paired with clinical observations of symptoms and urine drug testing.[32,33]

Harm Reduction

Harm reduction includes policies and interventions aimed at reducing the harms (i.e., morbidity and mortality as well as social and criminal consequences) related to substance use.[34] Harm-reduction strategies may include syringe exchange and condom provision, screening and prevention for infectious diseases, and overdose prevention. An important feature of harm reduction is that abstinence is not the only goal of interest.

Syringe exchange programs (SEPs) typically provide sterile syringes and condoms to people who inject drugs, which minimize the transmission of HIV and other blood-borne pathogens. It is noteworthy to mention that access to sterile syringes does not increase injection drug use, it simply provides an opportunity for safer administration of the drugs.[32] SEPs often provide HIV, HCV, and STI testing along with referrals for medical and drug treatment.

Naloxone, an opioid antagonist, is used to treat opioid overdoses and is available in an injectable pen or as a nasal spray. Introduction of overdose education and naloxone distribution programs in various cities have been shown to decrease opioid overdose mortality rates.[35] Naloxone is available in healthcare settings but is also distributed to first responders as well as people who use drugs and their friends and families.

Treatment

Drug treatment is a multistep process that may include one or more of the following components: detoxification, behavioral counseling, medication, assessment and treatment of comorbid mental health conditions, and relapse prevention.[36] Comprehensive drug treatment should include access to other health and social services such as educational, family, financial, legal, and vocational services; child care; housing and transportation; and medical and psychiatric care, including HIV/AIDS treatment.[36]

Mediation-assisted treatment (MAT) opioid dependence includes counseling or behavioral therapy combined with the prescription of an opioid agonist or antagonist such buprenorphine, diacetylmorphine (i.e., prescription heroin), methadone, and naltrexone.[37] MAT aims to eliminate opioid cravings. MAT is effective and suitable for long-term treatment; however, individuals may opt to taper off the opioid substitution and replace it with naltrexone. Maintenance programs may be coupled with psychosocial interventions such as counseling. Counseling or behavioral therapy seems to provide added benefits only to those with severe opioid use including the use of heroin.[16] MAT is not available in all countries (e.g., the Russian Federation does not have MAT) and specific treatment availability also varies by country. Specific FDA-approved pharmacotherapies are not available for tranquilizers, stimulants, and sedatives.

Most trials of behavioral therapies for drug use have been conducted among people who use illicit substances such as cocaine, heroin, methamphetamine, or unspecified opioid or stimulants rather than prescription drugs specifically. With respect to behavioral therapy, several modalities have demonstrated efficacy such as cognitive behavioral therapy (CBT), contingency management, and the Matrix Model.[36] CBT aids individuals in identifying and correcting problem behaviors. In contingency management, tangible incentives are provided to reinforce abstinence. The Matrix Model was specifically developed for stimulant use disorders. A therapist provides education on addiction and relapse issues, as well as coaching and support for behavior change.

SUMMARY

As with many medications, the goal is to maximize the benefits and minimize the harms. Prescription pain relievers, tranquilizers, stimulants, and sedatives are important medications in the modern pharmacopeia and are key to the treatment of a variety of physical and mental health conditions. These medications are also misused, and this misuse contributes to substantial morbidity and mortality globally. Trends in North America and Europe point to an increasing burden of nonmedical prescription drug use and concomitant harms. Implementation of prevention and treatment programming can disruption these concerning trends.

References

1. Hughes A, Williams MR, Lipari RN, Bose J, Copello EAP, Kroutil LA. *Prescription drug use and misuse in the United States: Results from the 2015 National Survey on Drug Use and Health.* NSDUH Data Review. 2016. https://www.samhsa.gov/data/.
2. Center for Behavioral Health Statistics and Quality. *2016 National Survey on Drug Use and Health: Methodological summary and definitions.* Rockville, MD: Substance Abuse and Mental Health Services Administration; 2017.
3. Pathan H, Williams J. Basic opioid pharmacology: An update. *Br J Pain.* 2012;6(1):11–16.
4. Horsfall JT, Sprague JE. The pharmacology and toxicology of the 'holy trinity'. *Basic Clin Pharmacol Toxicol.* 2017;120(2):115–9.
5. Meyer JS, Quenzer LF. *Psychopharmacology: Drugs, the Brain, and Behavior.* 2nd ed. Sunderland, MA: Sinauer Associates; 2013.
6. United Nations Office on Drugs and Crime. *World Drug Report 2017.* Vienna, Austria: United Nations; 2017.
7. Center for Behavioral Health Statistics and Quality. *2016 National Survey on Drug Use and Health: Detailed Tables.* Rockville, MD: Substance Abuse and Mental Health Services Administration; 2017.
8. Evoy KE, Morrison MD, Saklad SR. Abuse and misuse of pregabalin and gabapentin. *Drugs.* 2017;77(4):403–26.
9. Kapil V, Green JL, Le Lait MC, Wood DM, Dargan PI. Misuse of the gamma-aminobutyric acid analogues baclofen, gabapentin and pregabalin in the UK. *Br J Clin Pharmacol.* 2014;78(1):190–1.
10. Degenhardt L, Whiteford HA, Ferrari AJ, et al. Global burden of disease attributable to illicit drug use and dependence: Findings from the Global Burden of Disease Study 2010. *Lancet.* 2013;382(9904):1564–74.
11. McHugh RK, Nielsen S, Weiss RD. Prescription drug abuse: From epidemiology to public policy. *J Subst Abuse Treat.* 2015;48(1):1–7.
12. Benson K, Flory K, Humphreys KL, Lee SS. Misuse of stimulant medication among college students: A comprehensive review and meta-analysis. *Clin Child Fam Psychol Rev.* 2015;18(1):50–76.
13. Murphy Y, Wilson E, Goldner EM, Fischer B. Benzodiazepine use, misuse, and harm at the population level in Canada: A comprehensive narrative review of data and developments since 1995. *Clin Drug Investig.* 2016;36(7):519–30.
14. Tetrault JM, Butner JL. Non-medical prescription opioid use and prescription opioid use disorder: A review. *Yale J Biol Med.* 2015;88(3):227–33.
15. Nargiso JE, Ballard EL, Skeer MR. A systematic review of risk and protective factors associated with nonmedical use of prescription drugs among youth in the United States: A social ecological perspective. *J Stud Alcohol Drugs.* 2015;76(1):5–20.
16. Brady KT, McCauley JL, Back SE. Prescription opioid misuse, abuse, and treatment in the United States: An update. *Am J Psychiatry.* 2016;173(1):18–26.
17. Bachhuber MA, Hennessy S, Cunningham CO, Starrels JL. Increasing benzodiazepine prescriptions and overdose mortality in the United States, 1996–2013. *Am J Public Health.* 2016;106(4):686–8.
18. Clayton HB, Lowry R, August E, Jones SE. Nonmedical use of prescription drugs and sexual risk behaviors. *Pediatrics.* 2016;137(1).
19. Kecojevic A, Silva K, Sell RL, Lankenau SE. Prescription drug misuse and sexual risk behaviors among young men who have sex with men (YMSM) in Philadelphia. *AIDS Behav.* 2015;19(5):847–56.
20. Wells BE, Kelly BC, Rendina HJ, Parsons JT. Prescription drug misuse and sexual behavior among young adults. *J Sex Res.* 2015;52(6):659–68.
21. Peters PJ, Pontones P, Hoover KW, et al. HIV infection linked to injection use of oxymorphone in Indiana, 2014–2015. *N Engl J Med.* 2016;375(3):229–39.
22. Harocopos A, Allen B, Paone D. Circumstances and contexts of heroin initiation following non-medical opioid analgesic use in New York City. *Int J Drug Policy.* 2016;28:106–12.
23. Compton WM, Jones CM, Baldwin GT. Relationship between nonmedical prescription-opioid use and heroin use. *N Engl J Med.* 2016;374(2):154–63.
24. Kandel DB, Hu MC, Griesler P, Wall M. Increases from 2002 to 2015 in prescription opioid overdose deaths in combination with other substances. *Drug Alcohol Depend.* 2017;178:501–11.
25. Warner M, Trinidad JP, Bastian BA, Minino AM, Hedegaard H. Drugs most frequently involved in drug overdose deaths: United States, 2010–2014. *Natl Vital Stat Rep.* 2016;65(10):1–15.
26. Roxburgh A, Hall WD, Dobbins T, et al. Trends in heroin and pharmaceutical opioid overdose deaths in Australia. *Drug Alcohol Depend.* 2017;179:291–8.
27. Imtiaz S, Rehm J. The impact of prescription opioids on all-cause mortality in Canada. *Subst Abuse Treat Prev Policy.* 2016;11(1):27.
28. UK Office for National Statistics. *Deaths related to drug poisoning in England and Wales: 2016 registrations.* London. 2017.
29. European Monitoring Centre for Drugs and Drug Addiction. *European Drug Report 2017: Trends and Developments.* Luxembourg: Publications Office of the European Union; 2017.
30. Skinner HA. The drug abuse screening test. *Addict Behav.* 1982; 7(4):363–71.
31. Ali R, Awwad E, Babor T, et al. The Alcohol, Smoking and Substance Involvement Screening Test (ASSIST): Development, reliability and feasibility. *Addiction (Abingdon, England).* 2002;97(9):1183–94.
32. Bowman S, Eiserman J, Beletsky L, Stancliff S, Bruce RD. Reducing the health consequences of opioid addiction in primary care. *Am J Med.* 2013;126(7):565–71.
33. Rastegar DA, Kunins HV, Tetrault JM, Walley AY, Gordon AJ. 2012 Update in addiction medicine for the generalist. *Addict Sci Clin Pract.* 2013;8(1):6.
34. Ritter A, Cameron J. A review of the efficacy and effectiveness of harm reduction strategies for alcohol, tobacco and illicit drugs. *Drug Alcohol Rev.* 2006;25(6):611–24.
35. Mueller SR, Walley AY, Calcaterra SL, Glanz JM, Binswanger IA. A review of opioid overdose prevention and naloxone prescribing: Implications for translating community programming into clinical practice. *Subst Abus.* 2015;36(2):240–53.
36. National Institute on Drug Abuse. *Principles of Drug Addiction Treatment: A Research-based Guide.* 3rd ed. Rockville, MD: National Institute on Drug Abuse, National Institutes of Health, U.S. Department of Health and Human Services; 2012.
37. Connery HS. Medication-assisted treatment of opioid use disorder: Review of the evidence and future directions. *Harv Rev Psychiatry.* 2015;23(2):63–75.

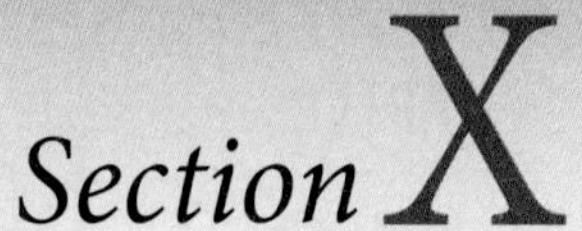

Section Editors
Grant Baldwin and James Mercy

Injury and Violence

CHAPTER 170

Road Safety and Injury Prevention*

Ann M. Dellinger • Merissa A. Yellman

INTRODUCTION

General Orientation to the Problem

Roadway use and health are closely linked. Road traffic injuries are a leading cause of death worldwide and the number one cause of death among people 5–29 years of age.[1] Approximately 1.35 million people die each year on the world's roads, and 20–50 million sustain nonfatal injuries.[1,2] Risk of death and injury show large disparities across the globe; low- and middle-income countries (LMICs) contain 60% of the world's vehicles but account for 93% of road traffic deaths. Low-income countries alone contain only 1% of the world's vehicles but account for 13% of road traffic deaths.[1] In addition to the public health burden of lives lost, LMICs lose approximately 3–5% of GDP to the consequences of these crashes.[2]

High-income countries have death rates that are about half those seen in LMICs, but within this group there are also important differences.[1,2] For example, a 2016 CDC report compared the United States with 19 other high-income countries and determined that the United States had the highest number of motor vehicle crash deaths per 100,000 population (a typical public health measure), and per 10,000 registered vehicles (a typical traffic safety measure).[3] Moreover, recent trends do not show evidence of significant improvements. In 2018, a total of 36,560 people were killed in car crashes in the United States; a 2.4% decrease from the 37,473 people killed in 2018.[4]

Approximately 100 people die and thousands more are injured in motor vehicle crashes every day in the United States.[4,5] As a leading cause of death, road traffic injuries represent a critical public health problem (Table 170-1), but what makes this issue even more compelling is the variety of highly effective strategies to reduce this burden.

Focus of the Chapter

In this chapter we focus on the road safety situation in the United States, but also provide information at the global level to provide context and examine similarities and differences across different parts of the world. Particular attention is paid to solutions to the road safety problem that have behavioral components; these behavioral components can then be addressed in a health framework. For instance, there are behavioral components to crash risk such as alcohol-impaired driving and driving too fast for conditions, and to injury risk factors such as child safety seat (CSS) or bicycle helmet use. Factors related to vehicle safety (e.g., electronic stability control and automatic braking), and road engineering (e.g., roundabouts, speed bumps) will not be addressed.

Americans value independence and self-sufficiency,[6] and for many Americans, the ability to drive is an important component of these values. The motor vehicle dominates all other modes of travel in the United States. In the span of 100+ years, the number of registered automobiles has grown from 1.3 million in 1913 to 273 million in 2017.[7] In 2017, 21% of households had at least three vehicles available, and less than 9% had zero vehicles.[8] A high degree of mobility is integral to the American lifestyle. There are more than 221 million licensed drivers in the United States, and they drive an average of 14,000 miles per year on over 4 million miles of roads.[9] Accordingly, over two thirds of traffic crash victims in the United States are drivers or passengers of motor vehicles.[4,5]

In contrast, different road use patterns tend to dominate in other parts of the world. For example, walking and cycling are a dominant form of mobility in Africa. In Southeast Asia and the Western Pacific region, motorcycles are often the predominant form of motorized transportation.[1,2] Road traffic deaths mirror these road use patterns, with over half of deaths on the world's roads occurring among pedestrians, cyclists, and motorcyclists.[1,2]

NATURE AND BURDEN OF THE PROBLEM

One of the challenges in public health is to have as great an impact as possible on the populations we serve. For road safety this means preventing as many deaths as possible, preventing as many nonfatal injuries as possible, and saving dollars spent on medical care. Prevention in road safety is generally focused at two levels: primary prevention that will prevent crashes and secondary prevention that will prevent deaths and injuries when crashes occur. For instance, reducing speed and reducing alcohol-impaired driving will reduce the occurrence of crashes, as will graduated driver's licensing systems for new teen drivers; increasing seat belt, CSS, and helmet use will reduce the likelihood of injury once a crash has occurred. Consequently, there are several ways to reduce the burden of road traffic injury: reduce risk factors (e.g., speeding), increase protective factors (e.g., use of CSSs), or reduce exposure (e.g., time on the road). A third level, tertiary prevention, is concerned with reducing the negative consequences of road traffic injury, for example, rehabilitation services to prevent or minimize disability.

In the United States, exposure has increased over time. In 1995 there were 4 trillion person-miles of travel, and in 2016 this had risen to 4.6 trillion, a 14% increase; each *vehicle* on the road travels an average of 12,000 miles a year.[9] While exposure to the road environment has increased, there has been a long-term decline in the rate of traffic-related deaths, over 90% since 1925 as shown in Fig. 170-1.[7] This is primarily due to advances in the safety of vehicles and roads, and improvements in driver behavior[10] which have mitigated the negative

*Disclaimer: The findings and conclusions in this chapter are those of the authors and do not necessarily represent the official position of the Centers for Disease Control and Prevention.

TABLE 170-1 LEADING CAUSES OF DEATH IN THE UNITED STATES, 2018

	Age Groups									
Rank	**<1**	**1–4**	**5–9**	**10–14**	**15–24**	**25–34**	**35–44**	**45–54**	**55–64**	**65+**
1	Congenital anomalies	Other unintentional injury	Malignant neoplasms	Suicide	**Unintentional motor vehicle**	Other unintentional injury	Other unintentional injury	Malignant neoplasms	Malignant neoplasms	Heart disease
	4,473	864	393	596	**6,434**	17,552	17,448	37,301	113,947	526,509
2	Short gestation	Congenital anomalies	**Unintentional motor vehicle**	Malignant neoplasms	Suicide	Suicide	Malignant neoplasms	Heart disease	Heart disease	Malignant neoplasms
	3,679	384	**368**	450	6,211	8,020	10,640	32,220	81,042	431,102
3	Maternal pregnancy complications	**Unintentional motor vehicle**	Other unintentional injury	**Unintentional motor vehicle**	Other unintentional injury	**Unintentional motor vehicle**	Heart disease	Other unintentional injury	Chronic lower respiratory disease	Chronic lower respiratory disease
	1,358	**362**	366	**397**	5,610	**7,062**	10,532	17,534	18,804	135,560
4	SIDS	Homicide	Congenital anomalies	Other unintentional injury	Homicide	Homicide	Suicide	Suicide	Other unintentional injury	Cerebrovascular
	1,334	353	201	295	4,607	5,234	7,521	8,345	17,847	127,244
5	Other unintentional injury	Malignant neoplasms	Homicide	Congenital anomalies	Malignant neoplasms	Malignant neoplasms	**Unintentional motor vehicle**	Liver disease	Diabetes mellitus	Alzheimer's disease
	1,087	326	121	172	1,371	3,684	**5,219**	8,157	14,941	120,658
6	Placenta cord membranes	Influenza and pneumonia	influenza and pneumonia	Homicide	Heart disease	Heart disease	Homicide	Diabetes mellitus	Liver disease	Diabetes mellitus
	724	122	71	168	905	3,561	3,304	6,414	13,945	60,182
7	Bacterial sepsis	Heart disease	Chronic lower respiratory disease	Heart disease	Congenital anomalies	Liver disease	Liver disease	**Unintentional motor vehicle**	Cerebrovascular	Other unintentional injury
	579	115	68	101	354	1,008	3,108	**5,522**	12,789	49,102
8	Circulatory system disease	Perinatal period	Heart disease	Chronic lower respiratory disease	Diabetes mellitus	Diabetes mellitus	Diabetes mellitus	Cerebrovascular	Suicide	Influenza and pneumonia
	428	62	68	64	246	837	2,282	5,128	8,540	48,888
9	Respiratory distress	Septicemia	Cerebrovascular	Cerebrovascular	Influenza and pneumonia	Cerebrovascular	Cerebrovascular	Chronic lower respiratory disease	Septicemia	Nephritis
	390	54	34	54	200	567	1,704	3,807	5,956	42,232
10	Neonatal hemorrhage	Chronic lower respiratory disease	Septicemia	Influenza and pneumonia	Chronic lower respiratory disease	HIV	Influenza and pneumonia	Septicemia	Influenza and pneumonia	Parkinson's disease
	375	50	34	51	165	482	956	2,380	5,858	32,988

Source: CDC WISQARS, available at: https://www.cdc.gov/injury/wisqars/.

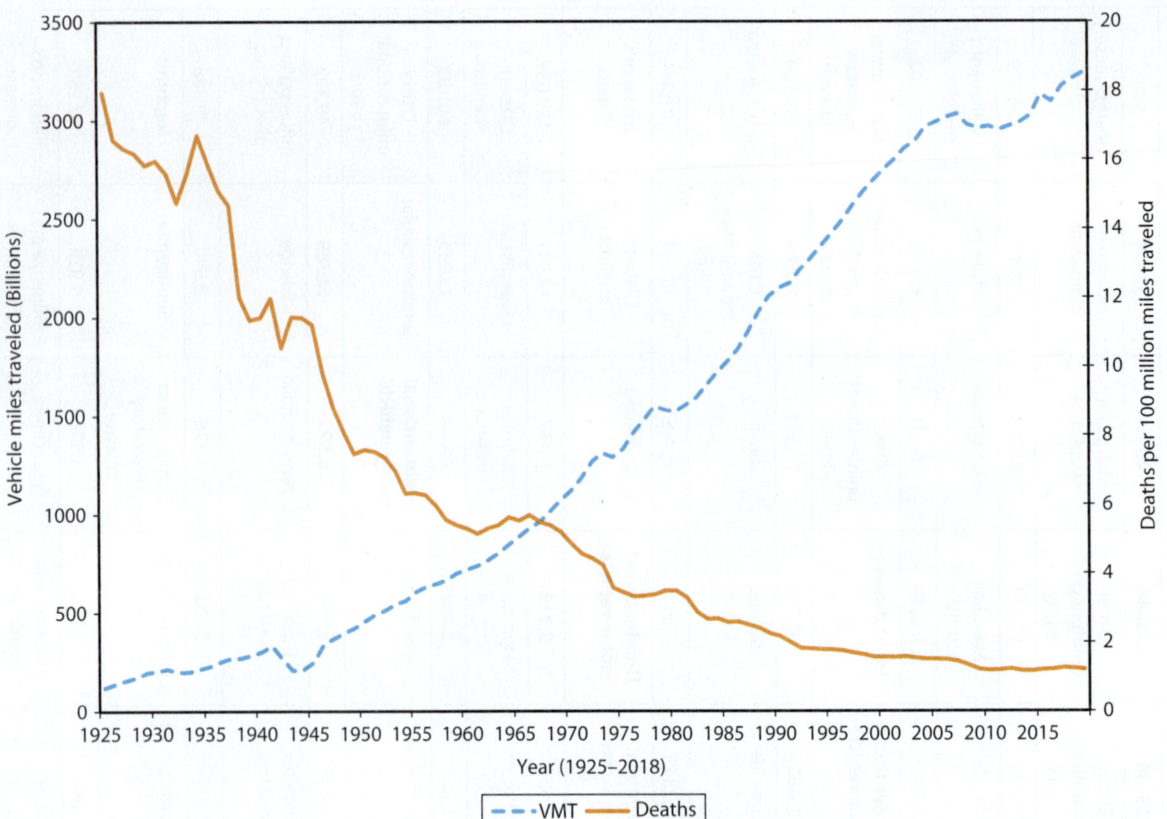

FIGURE 170-1. Annual vehicle miles traveled (VMT) and motor vehicle-related deaths, United States, 1925–2018. (*Source:* National Safety Council, Injury Facts, 2018 Data.)

effects of increased motorization. In spite of these declines, traffic crashes remain a leading cause of death among all age groups in the United States,[11] Table 170-1.

Traffic-related injuries have only recently been recognized as a fundamental part of public health practice. This chapter describes the current traffic safety context and the epidemiology of traffic-related deaths and injury highlighting the situation in the United States, but including what is known globally when information is available. It also reviews what is known about effective prevention strategies, with an emphasis on strategies that are most applicable to public health and medicine.

Definitions

Exposure to the road environment brings with it injury risks for all road users: drivers, passengers, motorcyclists, pedestrians, and cyclists. For the purposes of this chapter, drivers and passengers will refer to drivers and passengers of passenger cars, light/pickup trucks, vans and sport utility vehicles; motorcyclists refers to operators and passengers of motorcycles; pedestrians are persons traveling on foot; and cyclists are those traveling on nonmotorized, generally two-wheeled, vehicles.

Other important concepts include **risk factor**, that is, a factor that can make a crash or injury more likely to occur (e.g., speeding), and **protective factor**, which can make a crash or injury less likely to occur (e.g., wearing a seat belt).

Health Burden

Mortality—Global

As previously mentioned, at least 1.35 million people die each year in road traffic crashes worldwide. The most recent global data indicate that in 2016, the global road traffic death rate was 18.2 per 100,000 population.[1] For comparison, the United States had a road traffic death rate of 10.3 per 100,000 population during the same time period.[1,3]

Common across countries is the higher death rate among males, with young males especially at risk. A Global Burden of Disease Study revealed that in 2010, the number of road traffic deaths among males 15–49 years of age was 35 times higher than the number of road traffic deaths among females in the same age group.[12] This heightened risk of death comes at a time of vital economic productivity. The death of a family breadwinner can have serious financial consequences regardless of country of residence.

LMICs, defined by the World Bank as those countries with a gross national income (GNI) per capita of $1005 (in U.S. dollars) or less for low-income, and between $1006 and $12,235 GNI for middle-income, have the highest death rates—more than double those seen in the world's high-income countries (Fig. 170-2).[1,13] In addition, the situation does not seem to be improving. Out of the 104 countries that have seen more than a 2% increase in the number of road traffic deaths since 2013, 87 (84%) are LMICs. Moreover, no low-income country saw a reduction in the number of road traffic deaths between 2013 and 2016.[1]

Differences in the risk of crash death have at their core differences in country income status. Income status influences several factors related to the risk of death on the road. For example, income status influences the number and distribution of motorized versus nonmotorized (pedestrians and cyclists) road users, and the number and distribution of two-wheeled versus four-wheeled vehicle operators. Nonmotorized and two-wheeled road users are typically at increased risk of death in a crash. Income status also affects the level of available medical care and the infrastructure (or lack of infrastructure) to get the injured to care. In the latest global survey, the proportion of injured people who die before reaching a hospital in LMICs is over twice that in high-income countries.[1]

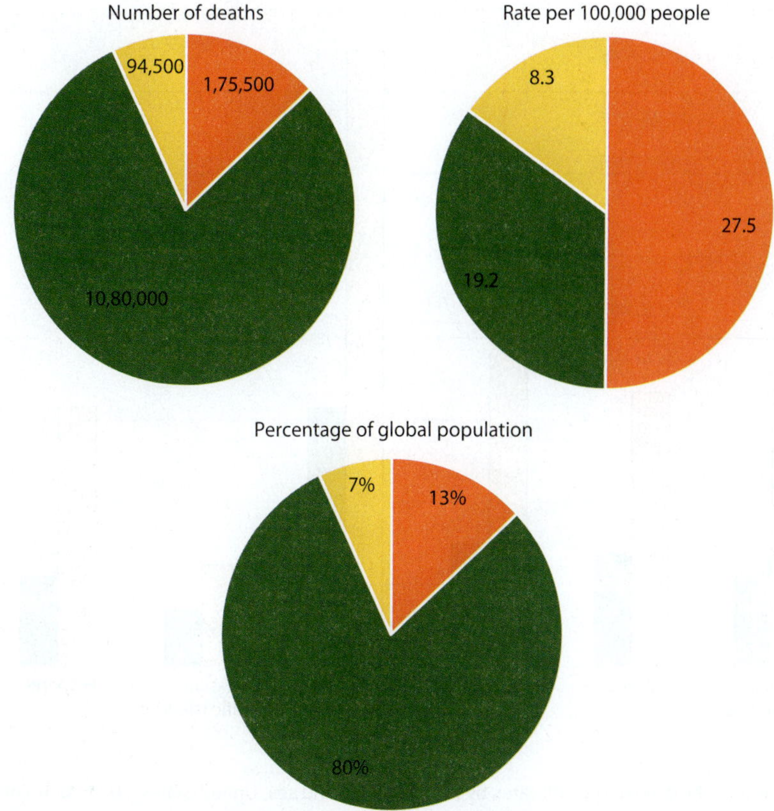

FIGURE 170-2. Estimated global road traffic injury-related deaths by country income status (2016). (*Source:* Global Status Report on Road Safety 2018, available at: https://www.who.int/violence_injury_prevention/road_safety_status/2018/en/.)

The World Health Organization (WHO) African Region continues to have the highest regional rate of road traffic deaths, with a death rate of 26.6 per 100,000 population. Notably, all but one of the 44 African region countries that provided road traffic death data in 2016 are classified as LMICs. On the other hand, the European region has the lowest road traffic death rate, and is also the region with the highest percentage of countries classified as high-income. At 9.3 per 100,000 population, the European death rate is about half of the world rate.[1]

LMICs often face challenges accurately documenting the size of their road traffic injury problem. This can result in the underrecognition of crashes as a public health problem, and hamper efforts to garner support to address the issue. In response, many LMICs have made a concerted effort to improve data collection to better estimate the burden of road traffic injury. Nevertheless, data remain subpar in many countries, and estimates of road traffic injury deaths greatly exceed the number of deaths captured in data systems. For example, the National Transport and Safety Authority of Kenya reported a total of 2965 road traffic deaths in Kenya in 2016; however, the WHO estimates that the number of road traffic deaths was over 4.5 times greater than what was recorded in the country's data systems for the same period.[1]

Mortality—United States

Traffic crashes result in about 37,000 deaths in the United States each year.[4,11] The risk of death varies by many factors including sex, age, race/ethnicity, type of road user and location (e.g., state, urban/rural setting). There is a significant risk difference in mortality by sex. Males have death rates at least twice that of females overall; for vehicle occupants, motorcyclists, pedestrians, and cyclists; and for all age groups after the age of licensure. The difference is especially high for motorcyclists (death rate 11 times higher among males) and cyclists (six times higher among males).[11]

Death rates also vary widely by age, with the lowest rates among children too young to drive (ages 0–14 years), and the highest rates among those ages 15–24 years and 80 years and older.[11] Children killed in traffic crashes can be vehicle occupants (74% of children killed in crashes), pedestrians (19% of children killed in crashes), or bicyclists (5% of children killed in crashes).[14] They are especially vulnerable when riding as passengers of drinking drivers; 54% of children killed in crashes with an alcohol-impaired driver were passengers of the alcohol-impaired driver.[14]

The population age 65 years and older increased 32% over a 10-year period (2009–2018), and during that time the number of older driver fatalities increased; older male driver fatalities increased by 36% and older female driver fatalities increased by 17%.[15] Older adults are more likely to be restrained and less likely to be involved in alcohol-involved crashes.[15] Moreover, their contributions to crash morbidity and mortality is generally a result of injuries to self rather than to others.[16]

By race/ethnicity, American Indian and Alaska Native populations have the highest death rates while Asian and Pacific Islander populations have the lowest; African American, white (non-Hispanic), and Hispanic populations (of all races) have similar death rates[11] (Fig. 170-3). However, when adjusting for time on the road, or vehicle miles traveled, vehicle occupants who are African American and Hispanic have higher death rates than whites.[17] For all racial/ethnic groups, males have higher death rates than females; American Indian and Alaska Native males have higher deaths rates than all other groups.[11]

Morbidity—Global

For every person who dies in a road traffic crash globally, there are at least 20 more individuals who are injured.[1,2,18] These nonfatal injuries can greatly affect an individual's quality of life and in many cases can cause long-term or permanent disability. Unfortunately, accurate

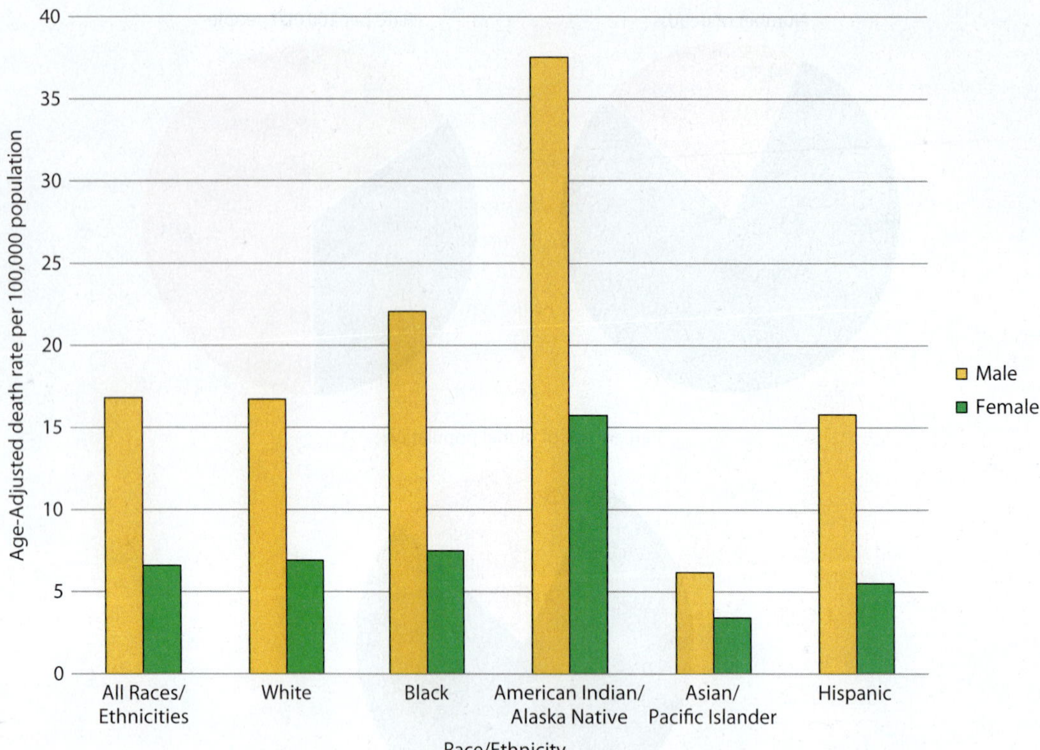

FIGURE 170-3. Age-adjusted motor vehicle-related death rates by race/ethnicity and sex, United States, 2018. All unintentional motor vehicle-related deaths are included in these rates. Rates are per 100,000 population and are standardized to the 2000 U.S. population. Data for White, Black, American Indian/Alaska Native, and Asian/Pacific Islander only include non-Hispanic ethnicity. Data for Hispanic ethnicity include all races. (*Source:* CDC WISQARS, available at: https://www.cdc.gov/injury/wisqars/.)

global data capturing the number and burden of nonfatal road traffic injuries is limited, especially in LMICs. In the most recent global survey only 29 of 175 countries provided estimates of the proportion of road crash victims left with permanent disabilities.[1]

In many countries, there are two separate systems of data collection that provide information related to road traffic crashes and any resulting deaths and injuries, the transportation system and the health or medical system. In general, the data collected by these two systems are not integrated. In the transportation system, police are responsible for responding to road traffic crashes and officially collecting road traffic injury data while collecting other information about the incident, for instance, location, type of road, weather conditions, or suspicion of drunk driving. However, police often do not have specialized training in the collection of data for public health purposes or the accurate assessment of injury severity. In addition, some traffic crashes and resulting injuries are never reported to the police and are therefore not captured in the data system.[1]

Information about road traffic injury is also collected in the health sector, most commonly at hospitals. Although this can provide information on the most severe injuries, it does not capture the full burden of nonfatal injuries. Moreover, since the objective of medical care is the health and survival of the patient, important public health risk and protective factor data such as whether the patient was using a seat belt or helmet, alcohol/drug use, type of road user (driver, bicyclist, pedestrian), seating position in vehicle, and other important information is not typically collected. Unfortunately, many hospitals have weak data collection systems and have no way of sharing or linking their data outside of the hospital.[1]

Despite the difficulty in quantifying the amount of road traffic injuries, there are gross disparities in injury outcomes between high-income countries and LMICs. This is primarily due to the level of care received immediately after a crash, as well as the level of care received in health facilities. If trauma care systems for severely injured road traffic victims in LMICs could be brought up to the levels of high-income countries, it is estimated that a half million lives could be saved every year.[2]

Morbidity—United States

Traffic crashes result in more than 3 million nonfatal injuries treated in hospital emergency departments each year in the United States.[11] Similar to deaths, the risk of nonfatal motor vehicle injury varies by many factors, including sex and age. Males have higher motor vehicle crash injury rates overall and by road user type (motorcyclists, pedestrians, etc.) than females. The exception is in the case of motor vehicle occupants, where the injury rate among females is 1.3 times higher than that among males.[11]

The patterns of injury rates by age group are similar to the patterns seen in death rates per age group. The lowest rates are among children 0–14 years of age, and the highest rates are among those 20–29 years of age, with about 2000 injuries per 100,000 population. For individuals 55 years of age and older, the injury rate drops below 1000 and continually declines as individuals advance in age.[11] Part of this decline can be explained by a reduction in exposure for older age groups, they are on the road fewer miles than younger groups. Because racial/ethnic information is often unknown or inaccurate for injured individuals, it is not customary to calculate national rates by racial/ethnic group since those rates could be unstable or misleading.[19]

Economic Burden

Globally, an estimated 3–5% of GDP is lost because of road traffic deaths and injuries.[2,20,21] A 2017 World Bank report demonstrated that reducing the number of road traffic deaths and injuries, especially in developing countries, can substantially increase income growth and generate significant benefits to societies.[22]

Although the economic burden is greatest in developing countries, motor vehicle crashes cause a significant economic burden in the United States as well. A study of the economic and societal impact of motor vehicle crashes in the United States in 2010 determined that the economic costs of crashes totaled $242 billion, which was 1.6% of the GDP for that year. This cost estimate included lost productivity, medical costs, legal/court costs, emergency service costs (EMS), insurance administration costs, congestion costs, property damage, and workplace losses. The total value of societal harm, which includes quality of life valuations, was $836 billion.[23]

RISK AND PROTECTIVE FACTORS

Global

Many road safety strategies can be implemented regardless of country income status or the distribution of vehicles or road users. There are five priority strategies that the WHO and partners across the globe are promoting to reduce the burden of road crashes.[2] These strategies represent evidence-based best practice that focus on behavior and can make large impacts on road safety:

- Setting and enforcing 0.05 g/dL blood alcohol concentration (BAC) limits; also lower BAC limits for young and novice drivers;
- Setting and enforcing national speed limits with urban maximum limits lower than 50 km/h (equivalent to 31 mph); and local authority to reduce limits;
- Comprehensive seat belt legislation that is enforced and covers all occupants and all seating positions;
- Comprehensive CSS legislation that is enforced and based on age, height, or weight, and applies an age restriction for sitting in the front seat; and
- Comprehensive helmet legislation for motorcycle riders that is enforced, covers all motorcyclists, includes a helmet standard and requires helmets to be fastened.

There is much room for improvement. In an analysis of 175 countries covering 98% of the world's population, 45 countries met best practice for drunk driving legislation; 46 countries met best practice for speed limit legislation; 105 countries met best practice for seat belt legislation; 33 countries met best practice for CSS legislation; and 49 countries met best practice for motorcycle helmet legislation.[1]

United States

Major Risk Factors

Alcohol-impaired driving and speeding have been consistent risk factors for crashes over many decades in the United States. Moreover, these two risk factors often occur concurrently. When a crash involving alcohol-impaired driving occurs, speeding is often a contributing factor, and vice versa. To illustrate, in 2018, 37% of all speeding drivers involved in fatal crashes were alcohol-impaired (BAC $\geq$ 0.08 g/dL), compared to 16% of nonspeeding drivers involved in fatal crashes.[24] Historically, speeding and alcohol-impairment are two of the most important contributors to crash risk; therefore, these factors are an essential part of any road safety strategy. The following section describes common risk factors for crashes that have significant effects on road safety and public health.

Alcohol

In 2018, 29% of all traffic deaths[5,10,11] involved an alcohol-impaired driver (i.e., a driver with a BAC of $\geq$ 0.08 g/dL, a level illegal in every U.S. state).[5,25] Each year millions of adults in the United States admit to an estimated 121 million episodes of alcohol-impaired driving,[26] yet only a small proportion, 1.02 million, are arrested for this offense.[27] Furthermore, 85% of drinking and driving episodes are reported by binge drinkers, and the 4.5% of the adult population who reported binge drinking at least four times per month accounted for 55% of all alcohol-impaired driving episodes.[26] Progress has stalled in this area; while the number of traffic deaths involving an alcohol-impaired driver has declined with the overall decline in all traffic deaths, the proportion of traffic deaths that involve an alcohol-impaired driver has remained relatively constant. The proportion of motor vehicle traffic deaths involving at least one alcohol-impaired driver has hovered around 30% since the late 1990s.[5]

Speed

Speed affects both the likelihood of a crash and the severity of a crash. Crashes at higher speeds are more severe given the greater change in velocity at impact; therefore, the risk of injury is higher.[28,29] For vulnerable road users such as pedestrians and cyclists, this is especially problematic. The European Transport Safety Council estimates that 30–50% of drivers in 30 highly motorized European countries violate speed limits.[29] Speeding is also prevalent in the United States. A 2018 study of self-reported speeding behaviors indicated that almost half (49%) of surveyed drivers admitted to driving 15 miles per hour above the speed limit on freeways in the previous 30 days, and 40% admitted to driving 10 miles per hour above the speed limit on a residential (neighborhood) street.[30] These results are worrisome, even more so because the same drivers considered it at least moderately dangerous to perform these very same behaviors (82% for driving 15 miles per hour over the limit on freeways, and 88% for driving 10 miles per hour over the limit on residential streets).[30]

In 2018, in the United States, 26% of traffic fatalities (9378 fatalities) were among persons killed in crashes where at least one driver was speeding.[24] These speeding-related fatalities are not equally distributed across driver groups; young male drivers aged 15–20 years are most likely to be involved in fatal speeding crashes. In 2018, 30% of young male drivers involved in fatal crashes were speeding.[24] Additionally, motorcyclists are more likely than other road users to be speeding when involved in fatal crashes; almost one-third (31%) of motorcyclists involved in fatal crashes in 2018 were speeding, more than drivers of any other vehicle type.[24] While this situation is problematic from a public health perspective, it also means that the opportunity for prevention is considerable.

Young Drivers

Young drivers have higher crash involvement rates per 100,000 licensed drivers than any other age group; this holds true for fatal crashes, injury crashes, and property-damage-only crashes.[5,31] Novice teen drivers have especially high death rates given their lack of experience driving and risk-taking behaviors. Young drivers are overrepresented in both police-reported and fatal crashes; they represent 5.4% of all licensed drivers in the United States, but 12% of drivers in police-reported crashes and 8.3% of drivers in fatal crashes.[31] Although too young to legally purchase alcohol, 19% of young drivers in fatal crashes have alcohol in their system.[31]

An issue related to teen driver safety is driver education that results in early licensure. Early licensure can lead to increased exposure of inexperienced drivers and to more crashes. School-based driver education training can often lead to earlier licensure, which in turn can lead to increased exposure.[32] Studies by Levy, Vernick et al., and Roberts and Kwan[32–34] have consistently indicated that young drivers who take driver education tend to get their licenses earlier than young drivers who do not. Any potential safety benefit from the driver training could be offset by the increase in exposure of teens to unsupervised driving.[32–34] A more recent trend, that could reduce the added risk from early licensure, is for fewer teens to get their driver's licenses; in 2009, 31% of 16-year olds were licensed drivers compared to 26% in 2018.[35,36]

Rural Location

States vary in the number and rate of traffic crash deaths, the use of seat belts, the incidence of self-reported drinking and driving, the coverage of level one trauma-care centers, and many other factors related to the risk of a crash and the risk of death or injury given a crash has occurred (Fig. 170-4). One of the main reasons for these differences is geography, more specifically, the level of rurality.

A long-standing safety disparity has existed between urban versus rural locations; about one in five (19%) people live in rural

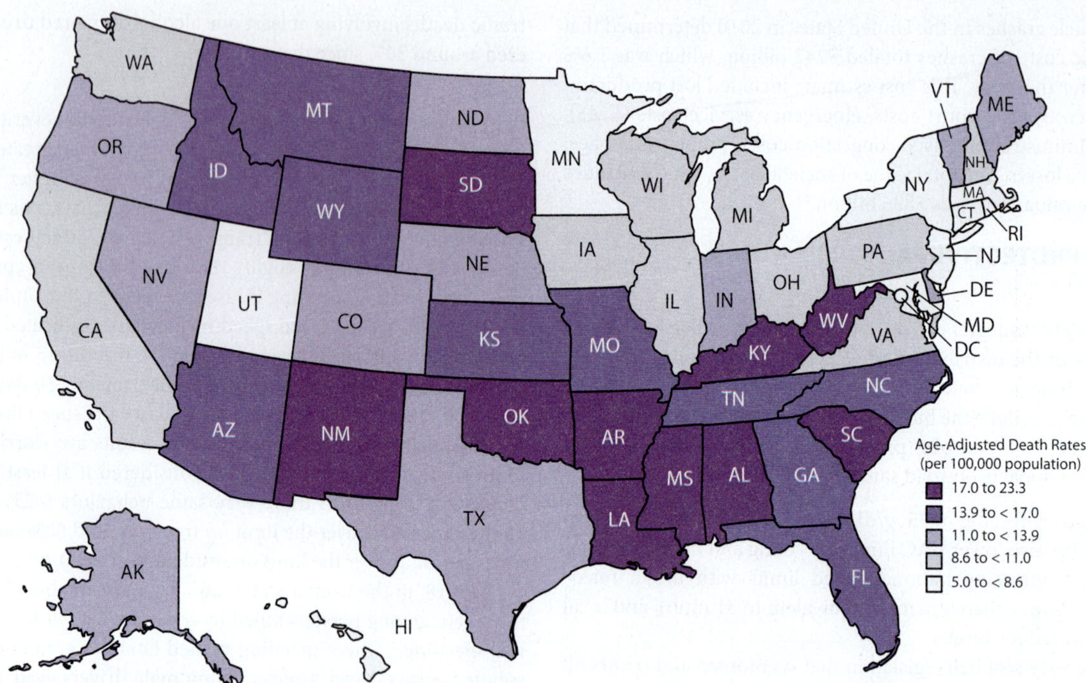

FIGURE 170-4. Age-adjusted motor vehicle-related death rates by U.S. state, 2018. All unintentional motor vehicle-related deaths are included in these rates. Rates are per 100,000 population and are standardized to the 2000 U.S. population. Map created using mapchart.net. (*Source:* CDC WISQARS, available at: https://www.cdc.gov/injury/wisqars/.)

areas, yet nearly half of all crash fatalities occur in rural areas.[37] The crash death rate in rural areas is about two times greater than the rate in urban areas.[37] An analysis using a more precise, six-level gradient of urban/rural designation, found even greater differences; the most rural counties had driver/passenger crash death rates that were three to ten times higher than those in the most urban counties.[38] This disparity can be at least partly explained by lower seat belt use in rural locations, the higher incidence of rollover crashes (a particularly deadly type of crash when not using a seat belt), and time to medical care.[37,38]

There are indications that the disparity might be declining. A 2016 comparison found that the proportion of speeding-related fatalities was similar between urban and rural areas, and that the proportion of alcohol-related fatalities decreased 23% in rural areas and increased 23% in urban areas over a 10-year period.[37] In addition, exposure is declining in rural areas, between 2000 and 2016 the amount driven increased 33% in urban areas and decreased 12% in rural areas.[39]

Vulnerable Road Users

Simply put, vulnerable road users are those not protected by the "shell'" of a vehicle such as motorcyclists, pedestrians, and cyclists. While motor vehicle occupants (drivers and passengers) represent the majority of crash deaths (67%), motorcyclists represent 14%, pedestrians 16%, cyclists 2%, and others 1%.[5] However, these unadjusted statistics do not account for exposure to the road environment. For example, motorcyclists represent 14% of all crash deaths, but only 3% of all registered vehicles and less than 1% of all vehicle miles traveled.[40] Adjusting for miles traveled, in 2017, motorcyclist fatalities occurred nearly 27 times more frequently than those in passenger cars.[40]

Alcohol is also prevalent in fatal crashes among motorcyclists: The percent of motorcyclists involved in fatal crashes who had a BAC of ≥ 0.08 g/dL (27%) was higher than the percent of passenger car drivers (21%); light truck drivers (20%); and large truck drivers (3%).[40] Among cyclists killed in crashes, 20% had a BAC of 0.08 g/dL or higher.[41] Among pedestrians killed in crashes, 33% had a BAC of 0.08 g/dL or higher.[42]

The number of fatalities in each of these groups has changed to varying degrees over the last 10 years; motorcyclist deaths have decreased 3%,[40] cyclist deaths have increased 37%,[41] and pedestrian deaths have increased 53%.[42] The increase in cyclist and pedestrian deaths is particularly disturbing given the renewed focus on active travel (i.e., bicycling and walking) as a way to increase physical activity for a variety of health benefits. In particular, more than 6000 pedestrians were killed representing 17% of all road fatalities in 2018[42]; this was the largest proportion of road fatalities in decades.[43]

Major Protective Factors

Once a crash occurs, protective factors are important to decrease the likelihood of an injury or decrease the severity of injury. For vehicle occupants, restraints such as seat belts, CSSs and booster seats provide this protection. For users of motorcycles and bicycles, helmets provide protection from head injury.

Restraints

Occupant restraints, including lap and shoulder belts, CSSs and booster seats, are among the most effective injury prevention interventions available. Seat belts provide the greatest protection available to drivers and other occupants. Seat belts reduce the risk of death and serious injury in a crash by about half.[44,45] Despite this substantial reduction in risk, the United States has the third lowest use of front seat belts among 19 high-income countries.[3]

When used correctly, CSS reduce the risk of death by 71% among infants and 54% among toddlers.[46] An estimated 325 children under 5 years of age were saved in 2017 by CSS.[47] Booster seats are 45% more effective than adult seat belts alone in reducing injury among age- and size-appropriate children.[48]

Helmets

Motorcycle helmets are estimated to be 42% effective in preventing fatal injury to motorcyclists and 69% effective in reducing head injury.[49] Helmet use is especially important given the high risk of fatal injury to motorcyclists in a crash.[40,50] Helmets saved an estimated 1872 motorcyclists' lives in 2017, and another 749 more could have been saved if all motorcyclists had worn helmets that year.[40,47]

Bicyclists are considered vehicle operators and as such are required to ride in the same direction as traffic and to obey the same rules of the road as other drivers.[41] Bicycle helmets are effective in preventing head injury, brain injury, facial injury, and death[51–53]; however, only about half of children ages 5–14 years always wear their helmets when riding.[54]

Evidence-based Strategies

Alcohol

Zero tolerance laws. These laws make it illegal for persons under age 21 to drive after any drinking, but the threshold is usually set at 0.02 g/dL BAC because of the possibility for slight imprecision in breathalyzer testing. These laws have been associated with declines in alcohol-related deaths[55–57]; Voas, Tippetts, and Fell found declines from 19% to 24% in underage drinking drivers in fatal crashes.[58] All states have passed zero tolerance laws for young drivers.

Minimum legal drinking age laws. Age 21 minimum legal drinking age (MLDA) laws are effective in reducing alcohol-related crashes and injuries.[56,59] This type of law is especially important given the high crash and death rates of young drivers.[58,60–62] At the same blood alcohol level, crash risk is higher for young drivers than older drivers.[63] NHTSA estimates 538 lives saved in 2017 due to MLDA laws in all states.[47] Lowering the state MLDA so that younger people can legally purchase alcohol has been associated with an increase in alcohol-impaired crashes by a median of 10%.[56]

Sobriety checkpoints. Alcohol roadside checkpoints, whether randomly or selectively implemented, can be an effective law enforcement intervention. Sobriety checkpoints have been shown to decrease fatal and nonfatal alcohol-involved injury crashes by a median of 9%.[64] Sobriety checkpoints are generally paired with media efforts to publicize the effort, which helps to increase the perceived risk of arrest.

Lower BAC. BAC laws make it illegal to operate a motor vehicle at or above a specified BAC. Originally set at 0.10 or 0.15, the maximum limits of these laws have been lowered over time; 0.08 g/dL BAC laws have been found effective in reducing alcohol-impaired driving.[55,56,61] As of 2004, all states have passed 0.08 g/dL BAC laws that place the legal limit for driving after drinking (for adults above the minimum legal drinking age) below 0.08 g/dL. One state, Utah, has since passed a 0.05 BAC g/dL limit, which went into effect at the end of 2018.[57,65] The United States lags behind many other countries that have reduced their legal BAC limit for drivers to under 0.05 g/dL.[1,2]

Ignition interlocks. These devices prevent a drinking driver from starting the vehicle by requiring the driver to provide a breath sample before starting the vehicle. If the breath sample exceeds a specified BAC, the ignition is locked and the vehicle will not start. State-administered ignition interlock programs can range from strictly judicial (i.e., judges decide on the interlock requirements), administrative (e.g., operated through the department of motor vehicles), or a hybrid of the two. Reports that have combined data from multiple studies estimate that interlocks account for 65% reductions in driving while impaired (DWI) recidivism, a beneficial effect that is usually limited to the period of installment.[66–68] An innovative study in Florida paired ignition interlocks with treatment for alcohol use disorder. The interlock plus treatment group experienced 32% lower recidivism than the nontreatment group. This level of effectiveness translated into an estimated 41 fewer rearrests and 13 fewer crashes.[69] Because drivers with a prior DWI violation are seven times more likely to have a subsequent violation than drivers without a history of DWI,[70] ignition interlocks could be considered for all convicted DWI offenders, including first-time and repeat offenders.

Server intervention training programs and dram shop liability. These programs are designed for servers at commercial establishments that serve alcohol to be consumed on site (such as bars and restaurants, also known as "dram shops").[57,71] Servers are trained to prevent patron intoxication and alcohol-impaired driving by offering food with drinks, delaying service to rapid drinkers, and refusing service to intoxicated patrons. Evidence for effectiveness of these training programs comes from studies of establishments that volunteered to participate in training servers; therefore, management support was well established, and server training was intensive, high-quality, and face-to-face (not video training); questions remain about whether server training is effective as a stand-alone intervention.[56] There is stronger evidence for dram shop liability, which holds the owner(s) or server(s) at the location that provided the last alcoholic drink to a patron responsible for harms inflicted by that patron on others. Dram shop liability has been shown to be effective in reducing alcohol-related crash fatalities.[71]

Alcohol screening and brief intervention. Screening for excessive alcohol use and subsequent brief intervention has been found effective in emergency departments,[72] trauma centers,[73] and primary-care settings.[74] The outcome measures of interest vary across studies, but have included reduced alcohol intake, reduced excessive drinking, reduced injury frequency and other outcomes.[72–74] A study by Fleming et al. found that two 15-minute sessions with a physician followed by two 5-minute telephone calls from an office nurse resulted in sustained effects over a 48-month period. The treatment group had significant reductions in 7-day alcohol use, number of binge drinking episodes, and frequency of excessive drinking compared to controls. In addition, the treatment group had fewer days of hospitalization and fewer emergency department visits. The largest cost savings were due to fewer motor vehicle-related events.[74] These results indicate that a modest investment in time and resources can have a clinically important effect that is maintained over years.

Alcohol pricing strategies. Alcohol pricing strategies can be implemented at the state and federal levels, and are beverage-specific (i.e., they differ for beer, wine, and spirits). Studies have shown that increasing alcohol taxes and higher alcohol prices raise revenue and reduce excessive drinking and alcohol-related harms (such as fewer deaths from liver cirrhosis and all-cause mortality), as well as reduce alcohol-impaired driving and motor vehicle crash fatalities.[57,75–77] Some studies have also shown effects for reducing outcomes of violence, sexually transmitted diseases, and alcohol dependence.[78] Despite the strong evidence showing that increased alcohol taxes reduce a wide variety of alcohol-related harms, the revenue from these taxes does not cover alcohol-related costs to society and have declined in inflation-adjusted terms (at both the federal and state levels).[57,74,78,79]

Speed

Speeding is a difficult issue to address, but two interventions have been shown to work, speed limits and automated enforcement.[80] Speed limits are effective *when enforced and obeyed*, however, many drivers admit to speeding under a range of circumstances, so their effectiveness is reduced in practice.[30,80] Automated enforcement (using speed and red light cameras) is one way to supplement conventional enforcement, which requires law enforcement officers to stop drivers and issue citations. Automated speed enforcement has been shown to reduce speeds and speeding violations.[81] Reviews of the effectiveness of speed cameras have found decreases in both crashes and injuries in the United States and around the world.[51,82,83]

Another form of automated enforcement is red light cameras. As of January 2018, 422 communities in the United States have red light camera programs.[84] A recent study[85] looked at the effectiveness of red light cameras in two ways: they measured the effect of turning the cameras on, and also the effect of turning off existing red light cameras. The investigators found that the cameras were effective in preventing crash deaths; fatal crashes were reduced when cameras were turned on, and higher when turned off. In a survey of U.S. drivers, most (93%) considered it unacceptable for a driver to drive through a light that had already turned red when they could have stopped safely, yet, more than one in three (36%) admitted to doing this in the past 30 days.[30]

Young Drivers

Graduated drivers licensing (GDL) systems address the high risks faced by new drivers by requiring an apprenticeship of planned and supervised practice (learners permit stage), followed by a provisional license that places temporary restrictions on unsupervised driving.[86] Two commonly imposed restrictions are limits on nighttime driving and passenger limits for the number of teen passengers allowed to ride with the new driver. These restrictions are lifted (full licensure) as new drivers gain experience and teenage drivers mature. Although the specific requirements for advancing through the three stages of GDL vary across jurisdictions, they provide a protective environment while new drivers become more experienced. GDL has proven effective in reducing new driver crash risk, and the stronger the system the stronger the effect.[87–91] The most comprehensive GDL systems were associated with a 38% reduction in fatal crashes among 16-year-old drivers.[92] All states have some form of GDL system, but the strength of the system varies greatly by state.[93]

Although not definitive, there are studies of the positive safety effect of parental monitoring (i.e., parents spending practice time with their teens and creating parent-teen driver agreements) on young driver safety. Results have varied from indicating no effect to modest effects on risky driving behaviors.[80] However, parents are in a strong position to delay licensure and to restrict driving under higher risk conditions such as night-time driving and driving with teenage passengers [94,95] whether these restrictions are part of their states' GDL system or not. Research has shown that teens whose parents set and maintain strict limits are less likely to engage in risky driving behaviors, have traffic violations, or to crash during the first year of licensure.[95] *Parents are the Key to Safe Teen Driving* is a campaign from the Centers for Disease Control and Prevention that provides materials for parents, pediatricians, and community groups to help keep teen drivers safe on the road (https://www.cdc.gov/parentsarethekey/).

Restraints

Seat belts. The National Occupant Protection Use Survey (NOPUS) conducted in 2019 found seat belt use to be 91% nationwide.[96] Although seat belt use at the national level is high, about 27.5 million people still do not buckle up.[97] The small percentage of drivers and passengers who do not always buckle up represent a large proportion of crash deaths, between 44% and 61%, depending on level of rurality.[38] In addition, seat belt use continues to be much lower in the rear seating positions, at only 81%.[96]

To date, 49 states, the District of Columbia (DC), Puerto Rico, and all U.S. territories have adult seat belt use laws in place. Primary enforcement laws allow a law enforcement officer to stop a motorist based on a seat belt violation alone, while secondary enforcement laws require another reason to stop a motorist other than a seat belt infraction. Both primary and secondary enforcement laws are effective in increasing belt use and reducing fatal and nonfatal injury, with primary enforcement laws showing the greatest effectiveness.[98–101] Evidence suggests that primary laws covering all seating positions might be particularly effective.[102] State primary enforcement laws became operative from 1984 through 2015; however, as of January 2018, 16 states do not have primary enforcement seat belt laws for front or rear seating positions.[103] Enhanced enforcement programs of seat belt laws, through more officers on patrol, or by increasing the number of citations issued, are also effective in reducing fatal and nonfatal injuries, and increasing belt use.[98]

Child safety seats. All states require children to be restrained, although the specifics of coverage vary.[103] CSS laws require children to be restrained in federally approved safety seats appropriate for the child's age, height, and weight. CSS laws decrease fatal and nonfatal injury, and increase CSS use. CSS education programs combined with distribution of CSS have been found to decrease fatal and nonfatal injury, increase CSS use, and increase possession of CSSs.[103,104] Community-wide information plus enhanced enforcement campaigns have also been found to increase CSS use.[103,104] Finally, incentive plus education programs (including rewards for either parents or children for correctly using CSS) have been shown to increase CSS use.[104,105]

Booster seats. Booster seats are designed to raise a child so that the vehicle lap and shoulder belts fit properly. The American Academy of Pediatrics recommends that all children use a booster seat until they reach 4 feet, 9 inches in height, which usually occurs between 8 and 12 years of age.[106] A systematic review of the impact of various legislative, educational, and promotional interventions among children aged 4–8 years found that interventions that combined education with distribution of booster seats or incentives such as discounted coupons had the greatest positive impact.[107,108] Moreover, booster seat legislation has been shown to increase booster seat use, reduce injury, and save costs.[109–112]

Rear seating position. The number of children sitting in the front seat is declining. By 2008, 95% of infants, 98% of toddlers, and 88% of children 4–7 years of age rode in the rear seating position.[106] Although the catalyst for moving children to the rear seat was the danger from passenger-side air bags, rear seating position is still the safest place for children whether or not there is a passenger-side air bag present.[113–115] Studies have found that children in the rear row(s) of the vehicle are 40–70% less likely to sustain injury than those in the front, depending on the specific characteristics of each study.[106–116]

Motorcycle and Bicycle Helmets

Motorcycle helmet use laws are effective in increasing helmet use among riders. In states with mandatory or universal (covers riders of all ages) helmet use laws, 76% of motorcyclists wear them—without a law, use is 40%.[117] In states that repealed universal helmet laws, helmet use declined (a median of 39 percentage points) and deaths increased (a median of 42 percentage points).[117] In 2018, 19 states plus the DC required helmet use by all operators and passengers, 28 states required some motorcyclists to wear helmets, and 3 states had no helmet use law.[118] An estimated 54% of motorcyclists wore helmets in 2010, compared with 71% in 2019.[119]

No state law requires adults to wear bicycle helmets; however, 21 states have laws in place that require young riders to wear bicycle helmets.[120] Interventions designed to increase bicycle helmet use generally target children and adolescents, as does legislation requiring helmet use. Legislation with supporting helmet promotional activities has successfully increased observed helmet use and reduced injury and death in the United States and abroad. Higher increases in helmet use tend to be among groups with the lowest prelaw use rates; several studies have reported helmet use rates doubling or tripling after legislation is enacted.[18,121–123] Community-based interventions that included free helmets and an educational component had the strongest evidence of effectiveness, along with school-based interventions and those that subsidized helmets.[124]

EMERGING ISSUES

Older Adults

The age distribution of the U.S. population is changing. Beginning in 2011, 10,000 people in the United States reach the age of 65 every day and this trend will hold for 20 years (http://pewresearch.org/databank/dailynumber/?NumberID=1150). This aging of the Baby Boomer generation has important implications for our nation in a variety of ways, including our ability to meet the mobility needs of an increasing older adult population. People reaching age 65 today will, on average, live another 19 years.[125]

Some emerging changes that will have direct effects on mobility and transportation needs are apparent now. For example, in 1998, 18% of people aged 65–74 participated in the civilian labor force; in 2018, this proportion had risen to 27% and by 2028, it is estimated to reach 33%.[126] More participation in the labor force could result in more exposure to the traffic environment among older adults.

Older adults frequently choose to age in place; one consequence of this is the proportion of older adults living alone, 28% or 14.3 million older people in 2017.[125] This differs between men, 21% living alone, and women, 34% living alone.[125] People age 65+ are less likely to change their residence than any other age group; between 2016 and 2017 just 4% moved versus 11% for those younger than 65.[125] Living alone can make driving critical for meeting everyday needs. For those older adults who are not able to drive safely due to physical and/or cognitive impairments, few mobility options might exist in their neighborhood. However, ride-hailing services such as Uber or Lyft could help older adults maintain their mobility, if these services were able to meet the needs of this special population. In a survey of residents in seven major U.S. cities, 4% of those aged 65 and older had used a ride-hailing service versus 36% of those aged 18–29.[127]

Older drivers, age 65 years and older, represent a fast growing segment of the driving population. In just 10 years' time, from 2009 to 2018, the number of older licensed drivers grew 37% to more than 45 million, nearly 20% of the driving population in the country.[35,36] The proportion of the population who are licensed drivers has also increased in this age group; for example, in 2009, 58% of persons aged 85 and older were licensed drivers, in 2018, this had increased to 62%.[35,36]

Per mile traveled, fatal crash rates increase notably starting at age 70–74 years and are highest among drivers 85 years of age and older.[128] This is largely due to an increased susceptibility to injury and medical complications among older drivers rather than an increase in crash involvement.[5,128] However, age-related declines in vision and cognitive functioning, as well as physical changes, might affect some older adults' driving abilities. The American Medical Association has collaborated with the National Highway Traffic Safety Administration to create resources for physicians to assess and counsel their patients on their ability to drive safely.[129]

Autonomous Vehicles

Autonomous vehicles, what many people think of as "self-driving cars," have the potential for many societal benefits, including a significant decline in the number of road traffic crashes, deaths, and injuries. The potential for significant declines stems from the estimate that some component of human error is involved in 94% of all car crashes,[130] and if this human behavioral component can be eliminated from driving, the potential for a reduction in car crashes will follow. Although self-driving cars will not be a large part of the vehicle fleet for many years, there are vehicle safety features available now that impart some level of automation and gains in safety. For example, forward collision warning systems warn the driver of an imminent collision, and the driver must act to avoid the collision; forward collision warning systems with automatic emergency braking engage when a collision is imminent without the need for driver action. Data from 22 states were analyzed to explore the effectiveness of these features for crash reduction.[131] Results indicated that forward collision warning plus automatic emergency braking reduced police-reported rear-end crashes by 50%. Moreover, the authors estimated 400,000 injuries in such crashes could have been prevented if all vehicles were equipped with these features during the study period.[131]

This example supports the view that the difference between self-driving vehicles and vehicles requiring drivers is actually a continuum that has many possibilities. For example, the Society of Automotive Engineers defines six levels of possible automation ranging from zero to fully automated:

- Zero automation—driver performs all driving tasks;
- Driver assistance—driver controls vehicle but some driving assist features might be present in the vehicle design such as adaptive cruise control and lane assist;
- Partial automation—driver must remain engaged with the driving task at all times, but vehicle has some automatic functions like acceleration and steering;
- Conditional automation—driver is necessary but not required to monitor the environment, driver must be ready to take control of the vehicle at all times;
- High automation—driver might have the option to control the vehicle, but the vehicle is capable of performing all driving functions under certain conditions such as urban roads with low speeds; and
- Full automation—driver might have the option to control the vehicle, but the vehicle is capable of performing all driving functions under all conditions.[132]

Autonomous vehicles hold promise for safety improvements, but also generate new challenges that will need to be addressed in order to maximize public health impact (e.g., crash liability, data privacy, regulations, security).[133]

Drug-Impaired Driving

Drugs other than alcohol are involved in about 16% of motor vehicle crashes.[134,135] Marijuana-impaired driving has become an issue of increasing concern, especially with the recent expansion of state marijuana legislation (both medical and recreational) within many states.[135] All states have laws prohibiting driving while *impaired* by alcohol and other drugs, including marijuana, and marijuana remains an illegal Schedule I drug at the federal level.[136] At the same time, as of June 2019, 33 states and the DC have legalized marijuana use in some manner, and 11 states and DC have legalized marijuana for recreational use (http://www.governing.com/gov-data/state-marijuana-laws-map-medical-recreational.html).

The effects of alcohol on driving performance are well understood. Alcohol metabolizes at a relatively steady rate and can be measured by the concentration of alcohol in the blood (BAC). In addition, level of impairment corresponds reasonably well with BAC; therefore, BAC can be used to measure impairment.[136] In contrast, the primary psychoactive substance in marijuana is delta-9-tetrahydrocannabinal (THC). It is fat-soluble and stores in fatty tissues in the body. THC can be released back into the blood long after ingestion and long after the psychoactive effects can be felt; therefore, blood levels of THC are not a good measure of impairment.[136] However, like alcohol, marijuana impairs an individual's ability to drive safely, including slowing reaction time and reducing coordination.[137] Despite the negative effects of marijuana use on driving performance, there are currently no known effective strategies to address this issue.

Driving under the influence of opioids is another issue of increasing concern in the field of injury prevention, especially because the United States is in the midst of an opioid overdose epidemic. More than 47,000 Americans died from opioid-involved overdose in 2017.[138] Studies exploring the effects of opioid use on driving ability and motor vehicle crash risk are limited, including the effects of prescription opioid use for managing pain or treating substance use disorder, as well as prescription opioid misuse or illicit opioid use. A 2013 Canadian case-control study found that among drivers who were prescribed opioids, those prescribed opioids in a dosage > 20 morphine milligram equivalents per day had increased odds (between 21% and 42% higher, depending on dose) of road trauma resulting in an emergency department visit compared to those prescribed lower dosages.[139] A 2017 self-report study of medical and nonmedical prescription opioid use and crash history found that medical use of prescription opioids was associated with a 62% increase in odds for a motor vehicle collision.[140] Given available evidence, the *CDC Guideline for Prescribing Opioids for Chronic Pain* recommends that clinicians discuss with patients the effects that opioids might have on ability to safely operate a vehicle, particularly when opioids are initiated, when dosages are increased, or when other central nervous system depressants, such as benzodiazepines or alcohol, are used concurrently.[141]

Distracted Driving

Distracted driving, defined as any activity that diverts a driver's attention from safety-critical driving tasks,[142] is a significant source of injury and mortality in road crashes.[143–145] Distracted driving can impair a driver's performance in multiple ways, including increasing reaction time when critical events arise, impairing the ability to maintain lane position, and reducing overall awareness of the driving environment.[146,147]

Cell phone use is an important in-vehicle distraction associated with a substantial number of distraction-related fatal crashes. Research has shown that drivers using cell phones are two to nine times more likely to be involved in a car crash.[143,148–150] Texting while driving could be especially risky because it involves three types of driver distraction: visual (eyes off the road), physical (hands off the steering wheel), and cognitive (mind not on the driving task).[142,151]

Research by the American Automobile Association (AAA) Foundation found that 81% of drivers view texting and emailing very serious threats to safety, yet 40% of drivers admitted to having read a text or email message, and 31% admitted to typing or sending a text message or email while driving in the past 30 days.[30] The prevalence of texting while driving is similarly high among adolescents, with 39% of student drivers admitting to texting while driving at least once in the past 30 days in the school administered 2017 Youth Risk Behavior Survey.[152]

Cell phone legislation varies by state and by locality, with some states or localities banning hand-held devices for all drivers, some banning use among certain populations (such as young drivers, novice drivers, or bus drivers), some banning use in certain situations (such as while driving in school zones or work zones) and some banning texting while driving but allowing for other uses of hand-held devices. As of June, 2020, 25 states and the DC had legislation prohibiting talking on a hand-held cell phone while driving for all drivers.[153] For young and/or novice drivers, the use of cell phones while driving was restricted in 38 states and DC.[153] Texting while driving is banned for all drivers in 48 states and the DC.[153]

Although most people agree that using a cell phone while driving is unsafe, the effectiveness of legislation to address this problem has yielded inconsistent results at this time,[30,153] especially because enforcing these laws can be challenging.[153] Technological approaches, for example, automatic disabling of cell phones while the vehicle is moving, might hold promise.

Vision Zero and the Path Forward

In response to the increasing global threat of road traffic injury deaths, and to accelerate action to reduce this burden, the United Nations General Assembly adopted Resolution 64/255, which established the Decade of Action for Road Safety (2011–20).[1,2,154] The Global Plan for the Decade of Action provides a roadmap and an overall framework to achieve a substantial reduction in road traffic injury deaths. The plan includes the following five primary categories of activities, along with accompanying indicators to measure progress in each of these areas: (1) building road safety management capacity; (2) improving road safety and mobility; (3) developing safer vehicles; (4) enhancing the behavior of road users; and (5) improving postcrash response.[154] Although some countries have made progress in strengthening road safety laws, making vehicles and roads safer, and/or improving postcrash care, the number of deaths and serious injuries on the world's roads is far too high.[1]

United Nations Member States also recognized that road traffic injuries present a formidable obstacle to development efforts. To that end, when the Sustainable Development Goals were adopted in 2015 as part of the 2030 Agenda for Sustainable Development, Member States included two specific targets committed to road traffic injury prevention and safe mobility. Target 3.6 aims to halve the number of global road traffic deaths and injuries by 2020. Some modest progress has been made in reducing road traffic deaths, however this target has not been met. Although the number of estimated deaths increased from 1.25 million in 2013 to 1.35 million in 2016,[1,2] the road traffic death rates have begun to stabilize.[1] Target 11.2 calls for safe, affordable, accessible, and sustainable transport systems to be available to all by 2030.[155] This can be achieved by improving road safety and by expanding public transportation, with a special emphasis on the needs of vulnerable members of society such as women, children, persons with disabilities, and older adults.[155]

While these goals and targets are challenging, Sweden's Vision Zero initiative points the way forward.[156] Sweden's Vision Zero starts with the ultimate target of no deaths or serious injuries on their roads. Their approach, termed the Safe Systems Approach, acknowledges that human error is inevitable, and that vehicles and the environment must be designed and built to accommodate these mistakes. In addition, improving driver behavior and enforcement to complement infrastructure and vehicle enhancements are included. A Safe Systems approach was implemented by Parliament in 1997 and has led to more than a 50% reduction in road traffic deaths.[156]

To complement Vision Zero and the Decade of Action, as well as to address the concerning number of preventable traffic deaths in the United States, the National Safety Council joined with partners such as the U.S. Department of Transportation and the National Highway Traffic Safety Administration to form the Road to Zero Coalition.[157] Announced in October of 2016, the coalition has set a goal of eliminating traffic deaths on U.S. roads by 2050. To achieve that vision, the coalition has brought together a diverse array of stakeholders and organizations to work together to develop a coordinated strategy focused on a Safe Systems approach similar to that pioneered by Sweden.[157]

CONCLUSIONS

Improvements in road safety at the global level require the use of a variety of effective strategies that match the particular problems in each country. There are problems such as speed and alcohol-impaired driving that are universal concerns, and others that are more specific to countries with a higher proportion of vulnerable road users, such as the lack of motorcycle helmet use. However, all countries can benefit from the considerable momentum created by the Decade of Action for Road Safety and the more recent Sustainable Development Goals. These efforts have brought the international road safety community, including the United States, together to acknowledge the problem of road traffic crashes, document burden, implement prevention strategies and track progress.

Despite the great success in reducing motor vehicle-related death rates in the United States in the past 50 years, motor vehicle crashes remain a leading cause of death. Future challenges in road safety include making progress in areas that have been long-standing problems, such as safety belt use and alcohol-impaired driving, and new issues such as the increasing number of older drivers, changes in technology, impaired driving from drugs such as marijuana and opioids, and an increasing number of in-vehicle distractions, including cellular phones.

References

1. World Health Organization (WHO). Global Status Report on Road Safety 2018. https://www.who.int/violence_injury_prevention/road_safety_status/2018/en/. Accessed June 20, 2020.
2. World Health Organization (WHO). Global Status Report on Road Safety 2015. https://www.who.int/violence_injury_prevention/road_safety_status/2015/en/. Accessed July 20, 2020.
3. Sauber-Schatz EK, Ederer DJ, Dellinger AM, Baldwin GT. Vital signs: Motor vehicle injury prevention—United States and 19 comparison countries. *MMWR Morb Mortal Wkly Rep.* 2016;65(26):672–7.

4. National Highway Traffic Safety Administration (NHTSA). 2018 Fatal Motor Vehicle Crashes: Overview. Traffic Safety Facts Research Note. Report No. DOT HS 812 826. https://crashstats.nhtsa.dot.gov/Api/Public/ViewPublication/812826. Published October 2019. Accessed July 20, 2020.
5. National Highway Traffic Safety Administration (NHTSA). Traffic Safety Facts Annual Report Tables. (Online). https://cdan.nhtsa.gov/tsftables/tsfar.htm#. Accessed July 20, 2020.
6. US Department of State, Foreign Service Institute. So You're an American? A Guide to Answering Difficult Questions Abroad. (Online). https://www.state.gov/so-youre-an-american-a-guide-to-answering-difficult-questions-abroad/. Accessed July 20, 2020.
7. National Safety Council (NSC). Motor vehicle. *Injury Facts, 2018 Edition.* Itasca, IL: NSC Press; 2018.
8. U.S. Census Bureau. Table B08201: Household Size by Vehicles Available. 2013–2017 American Community Survey 5-Year Estimates. (Online). https://factfinder.census.gov/faces/nav/jsf/pages/searchresults.xhtml?refresh=t&keepList=f. Accessed July 25, 2019.
9. US Department of Transportation, Federal Highway Administration, Office of Highway Policy Information. Highway Statistics 2016. (Online). https://www.fhwa.dot.gov/policyinformation/statistics/2016/. Released September 2017. Accessed July 20, 2020.
10. Dellinger AM, Sleet DA, Jones BH. Drivers, wheels and roads: Motor vehicle safety in the 20th century. In: Ward J, Warren C, eds. *Silent Victories: Public Health Triumphs of the 20th Century.* Oxford, UK: Oxford University Press; 2007.
11. Centers for Disease Control and Prevention (CDC), National Center for Injury Prevention and Control. Web-based Injury Statistics Query and Reporting System (WISQARS). (Online). https://www.cdc.gov/injury/wisqars/index.html. Accessed July 20, 2020.
12. Lozano R, Naghavi M, Foreman K, et al. Global and regional mortality from 235 causes of death for 20 age groups in 1990 and 2010: A systematic analysis for the Global Burden of Disease Study 2010. *Lancet.* 2012;380(9859):2095–128.
13. The World Bank. The DATA Blog. New Country Classifications. (Online). https://blogs.worldbank.org/opendata/new-country-classifications. Accessed July 20, 2020.
14. National Highway Traffic Safety Administration (NHTSA). Children: 2017 data. Traffic Safety Facts. Report No. DOT HS 812 719. https://crashstats.nhtsa.dot.gov/Api/Public/Publication/812719. Published May 2019. Accessed July 20, 2020.
15. National Highway Traffic Safety Administration (NHTSA). Older Population: 2018 data. Traffic Safety Facts. Report No. DOT HS 812 928. https://crashstats.nhtsa.dot.gov/Api/Public/Publication/812928. Published April 2020. Accessed July 20, 2020.
16. Dellinger AM, Kresnow M, White DD, Sehgal M. Risk to self versus risk to others: How do older drivers compare to others on the road? *Am J Prev Med.* 2004;26(3):217–21.
17. Braver ER. Race, Hispanic origin, and socioeconomic status in relation to motor vehicle occupant death rates and risk factors among adults. *Accid Anal Prev.* 2003;35(3):295–309.
18. World Health Organization (WHO). In: Peden M, Scurfield R, Sleet D, et al., eds. *World Report on Road Traffic Injury Prevention.* Geneva, World Health Organization; 2004. http://www.who.int/violence_injury_prevention/publications/road_traffic/world_report/en/. Published 2004. Accessed July 20, 2020.
19. Zhang Y, Lin G. Disparity surveillance of nonfatal motor vehicle crash injuries. *Traffic Inj Prev.* 2013;14(7):697–702.
20. Dahdah S, McMahon K. The true cost of road crashes: Valuing life and the cost of a serious injury. International Road Assessment Programme (iRAP) and World Bank Global Road Safety Facility. https://pdfs.semanticscholar.org/9fd8/4da172d099b96b7ce515f892b11a2f39bd1b.pdf. Released 2008. Accessed April 13, 2018.
21. Jacobs G, Aeron-Thomas A, Astrop A. Estimating global road fatalities. Transportation Research Laboratory (TRL), Report No. 445. 2000. https://trl.co.uk/reports/TRL445. Published 2000. Accessed July 20, 2020.
22. World Bank. The High Toll of Traffic Injuries: Unacceptable and Preventable. https://openknowledge.worldbank.org/handle/10986/29129. Published December 2017. Accessed July 20, 2020.
23. Blincoe LJ, Miller TR, Zaloshnja E, Lawrence BA. National Highway Traffic Safety Administration (NHTSA). The Economic and Societal Impact of Motor Vehicle Crashes, 2010 (Revised). Report No. DOT HS 812 013. https://crashstats.nhtsa.dot.gov/Api/Public/ViewPublication/812013. Published May 2015 (revised). Accessed July 20, 2020.
24. National Highway Traffic Safety Administration (NHTSA). Speeding: 2018 Data. Traffic Safety Facts. Report No. DOT HS 812 932. https://crashstats.nhtsa.dot.gov/Api/Public/ViewPublication/812932. Published April 2020. Accessed July 20, 2020.
25. National Highway Traffic Safety Administration (NHTSA). Alcohol-Impaired Driving: 2018 Data. Traffic Safety Facts. Report No. DOT HS 812 864. https://crashstats.nhtsa.dot.gov/Api/Public/ViewPublication/812864. Published December 2019. Accessed July 20, 2020.
26. Jewett A, Shults RA, Banerjee T, Bergen G. Alcohol-impaired driving among adults—United States, 2012. *MMWR Morb Mortal Wkly Rep.* 2015;64(30):814–7.
27. US Department of Justice, Federal Bureau of Investigation, Criminal Justice Information Services Division. 2016 Crime in the United States: Uniform Crime Reports. Table 18—Estimated Number of Arrests (United States, 2016). (Online). https://ucr.fbi.gov/crime-in-the-u.s/2016/crime-in-the-u.s.-2016/tables/table-18. Accessed July 20, 2020.
28. National Transportation Safety Board (NTSB). Reducing Speeding-Related Crashes Involving Passenger Vehicles. Safety Study NTSB/SS-17/01. https://www.ntsb.gov/safety/safety-studies/Pages/SS1701.aspx. Adopted July 25, 2017. Accessed July 20, 2020.
29. Elvik R. Speed limits, enforcement, and health consequences. *Ann Rev Public Health.* 2012;33:225–38.
30. AAA Foundation for Traffic Safety. 2018 Traffic Safety Culture Index. https://aaafoundation.org/2018-traffic-safety-culture-index/. Published June 2019. Accessed July 20, 2020.
31. National Highway Traffic Safety Administration (NHTSA). Young Drivers: 2017 Data. Traffic Safety Facts. Report No. DOT HS 812 753. https://crashstats.nhtsa.dot.gov/Api/Public/ViewPublication/812753.pdf. Published May 2019. Accessed July 20, 2020.
32. Levy DT. Youth and traffic safety: The effects of driving age, experience, and education. *Accid Anal Prev.* 1990;22(4):327–34.
33. Vernick JS, Li G, Ogaitis S, MacKenzie EJ, Baker SP, Gielen AC. Effects of high school driver education on motor vehicle crashes, violations, and licensure. *Am J Prev Med.* 1999;16(1):40–6.
34. Roberts IG, Kwan I. School-based driver education for the prevention of traffic crashes. *Cochrane Database Syst Rev.* 2001;(3):CD003201.
35. Federal Highway Administration, Department of Transportation (US). *Highway Statistics 2009.* Washington, DC: FHWA. (Online). https://www.fhwa.dot.gov/policyinformation/statistics/2009/dl20.cfm. Accessed July 20, 2020.
36. Federal Highway Administration, Department of Transportation (US). *Highway Statistics 2018.* Washington, DC: FHWA. (Online). https://www.fhwa.dot.gov/policyinformation/statistics/2018/dl20.cfm. Accessed July 20, 2020.
37. National Highway Traffic Safety Administration (NHTSA). Traffic Safety Facts Rural/Urban comparison of traffic fatalities. Washington, DC: US Department of Transportation. https://crashstats.nhtsa.dot.gov/Api/Public/Publication/812957. Accessed July 20, 2020.
38. Beck LF, Downs J, Stevens MR, Sauber-Schatz EK. Rural and urban differences in passenger-vehicle-occupant deaths and seat belt use among adults—United States, 2014. *MMWR Surveill Summ.* 2017;66(17):1–13.
39. Sivak M, Schoettle B. Recent diverging trends in the amount of urban and rural driving in the United States. 2017 Report No. SWT-2017-11. Ann Arbor, Michigan: University of Michigan Sustainable Worldwide Transportation.
40. National Highway Traffic Safety Administration (NHTSA). Traffic Safety Facts, Motorcycles. 2019 Report No. DOT HS 812-785. Washington, DC: US Department of Transportation. https://crashstats.nhtsa.dot.gov/Api/Public/Publication/812785. Accessed July 20, 2020.
41. National Highway Traffic Safety Administration (NHTSA). Traffic Safety Facts, Bicyclists and Other Cyclists. 2020 Report No. DOT HS 812-884. Washington, DC: US Department of Transportation. https://crashstats.nhtsa.dot.gov/Api/Public/ViewPublication/812884. Accessed July 20, 2020.
42. National Highway Traffic Safety Administration (NHTSA). Traffic Safety Facts, Pedestrians. 2020 Report No. DOT HS 812-850. Washington, DC: US Department of Transportation. https://crashstats.nhtsa.dot.gov/Api/Public/ViewPublication/812850. Accessed July 20, 2020.
43. Retting R. *Pedestrian Traffic Fatalities by State: 2017 Preliminary Data.* Washington, DC: Governors Highway Safety Association; 2018.
44. Kahane CJ. Fatality reduction by safety belts for front-seat occupants of cars and light trucks: Updated and expanded estimates based on 1986-99 FARS data. 2000 Report No. DOT HS 809 199. Washington, DC: National Highway Traffic Safety Administration (NHTSA), US Department of Transportation. https://crashstats.nhtsa.dot.gov/Api/Public/ViewPublication/809199. Accessed July 20, 2020.

45. National Highway Traffic Safety Administration (NHTSA). Traffic Safety Facts, Research Note, Seat Belt Use in 2017—Overall Results. 2017 Report No. DOT HS 812-465. Washington, DC: US Department of Transportation. https://crashstats.nhtsa.dot.gov/Api/Public/ViewPublication/812465. Accessed July 20, 2020.
46. National Highway Traffic Safety Administration (NHTSA). Traffic Safety Facts, Children. 2017 Report No. DOT HS 812 383. Washington, DC: US Department of Transportation. https://crashstats.nhtsa.dot.gov/Api/Public/Publication/812383. Accessed July 20, 2020.
47. National Highway Traffic Safety Administration (NHTSA). Traffic Safety Facts Lives Saved in 2017 by Restraint Use and Minimum Drinking Age Laws. 2017 Report No. DOT HS 812 683. Washington, DC: US Department of Transportation. https://crashstats.nhtsa.dot.gov/Api/Public/Publication/812683. Accessed July 20, 2020.
48. Durbin DR, Elliott MR, Winston FK. Belt-positioning booster seats and reduction in risk of injury among children in vehicle crashes. *JAMA.* 2003;289(21):2835–40.
49. Liu B, Ivers R, Norton R, Boufous S, Blows S, Lo SK. Helmets for preventing injury in motorcycle riders. *Cochrane Database Syst Rev.* 2008;(1):CD004333.
50. National Highway Traffic Safety Administration (NHTSA). Traffic Safety Facts. Motorcycles 2017 Data. 2019 Report No. DOT HS 812 785. Washington, DC: US Department of Transportation. https://crashstats.nhtsa.dot.gov/Api/Public/ViewPublication/812785. Accessed July 20, 2020.
51. Elvik R, Vaa T, eds. *The Handbook of Road Safety Measures.* 2nd ed. UK: Elsevier Ltd; 2009.
52. Thompson DC, Rivara FP, Thompson R. Helmets for preventing head and facial injuries in bicyclists. *Cochrane Database Syst Rev.* 2000;1999(2):CD001855.
53. Attewell RG, Glase K, McFadden M. Bicycle helmet efficacy: A meta-analysis. *Accid Anal Prev.* 2001;33:345–52.
54. Dellinger AM, Kresnow M. Bicycle helmet use among children in the United States: The effects of legislation, personal and household factors. *J Safety Res.* 2010;41:375–80.
55. Hingson R, Heeren T, Winter M. Effects of recent 0.08% legal blood alcohol limits on fatal crash involvement. *Inj Prev.* 2000;6:109–14.
56. Shults RA, Elder RW, Sleet DA, et al. Reviews of evidence regarding interventions to reduce alcohol-impaired driving. *Am J Prev Med.* 2001;21(4S):66–88.
57. National Academies of Sciences, Engineering, and Medicine. *Getting to Zero Alcohol-Impaired Driving Fatalities: A Comprehensive Approach to a Persistent Problem.* Washington, DC: The National Academies Press; 2018. https://www.nap.edu/catalog/24951/getting-to-zero-alcohol-impaired-driving-fatalities-a-comprehensive-approach. Accessed July 20, 2020.
58. Voas RB, Tippetts AS, Fell JC. Assessing the effectiveness of minimum legal drinking age and zero tolerance laws in the United States. *Accid Anal Prev.* 2003;35:579–87.
59. McCartt AT, Hellinga LA, Kirley BB. The effects of minimum legal drinking age 21 laws on alcohol-related driving in the United States. *J Safety Res.* 2010;41:173–81.
60. Zwerling C, Jones MP. Evaluation of the effectiveness of low blood alcohol concentration laws for younger drivers. *Am J Prev Med.*1999; 16(1S):76–80.
61. Wagenaar AC, O'Malley PM, LaFond C. Lowered legal blood alcohol limits for young drivers: Effects on drinking, driving, and driving-after-drinking behaviors in 30 states. *Am J Public Health.* 2001;91:801–4.
62. Wagenaar AC, Toomey TL. Effect of minimum drinking age laws: Review and analyses of the literature from 1960 to 2000. *J Stud Alcohol.* 2002;(Suppl 14):206–25.
63. Zador PL, Krawchuk SA, Voas RB. Alcohol-related relative risk of driver fatalities and driver involvement in fatal crashes in relation to driver age and gender: An update using 1996 data. *J Stud Alcohol.* 2000;61:387–95.
64. Bergen G, Pitan A, Qu S, et al. Publicized sobriety checkpoint programs: A community guide systematic review. *Am J Prev Med.* 2014;46(5):529–39.
65. National Highway Traffic Safety Administration (NHTSA). State Alcohol-Impaired-Driving Estimates: 2018 data. Traffic Safety Facts. Report No. DOT HS 812 917. https://crashstats.nhtsa.dot.gov/Api/Public/ViewPublication/812917. Accessed July 20, 2020.
66. Marques PR. The alcohol ignition interlock and other technologies for the prediction and control of impaired drivers. In: Verster JC, Pandi-Perumal SR, Ramaekers JG, de Gier JJ, eds. *Drugs, Driving and Traffic Safety.* Switzerland: Birkhauser Verlag; 2009, pp. 457–76.
67. Willis C, Lybrand S, Bellamy N. Alcohol ignition interlock programmes for reducing drink driving recidivism. *Cochrane Database Syst Rev.* 2004 Oct 18;2004(4):CD004168.
68. Elder RW, Voas R, Beirness D, Shults RA, Sleet DA, Nichols JL, Compton R. Task Force on Community Preventive Services. Effectiveness of ignition interlocks for preventing alcohol-impaired driving and alcohol-related crashes. *Am J Prev Med.* 2011;40(3):362–76.
69. Voas RB, Tippetts AS, Bergen G, Grosz M, Marques P. Mandating treatment based on interlock performance: Evidence for effectiveness. *Alcohol Clin Exp Res.* 2016;40(9):1953–60.
70. Rauch WJ, Zador PL, Ahlin EM, Howard JM, Frissell KC, Duncan GD. Risk of alcohol-impaired driving recidivism among first time offenders and multiple offenders. *Am J Public Health.* 2010;100:919–24.
71. Rammohan V, Hahn RA, Elder R, et al. Effects of dram shop liability and enhanced overservice law enforcement initiatives on excessive alcohol consumption and related harms: Two Community Guide systematic reviews. *Am J Prev Med.* 2011;41(3):334–43.
72. Nilsen P, Baird J, Mello MJ et al. A systematic review of emergency care brief alcohol interventions for injury patients. *J Subst Abuse Treat.* 2008;35:184–201.
73. Schermer CR, Moyers TB, Miller WR, Bloomfield LA. Trauma center brief interventions for alcohol disorders decrease subsequent driving under the influence arrests. *J Trauma.* 2006;60:29–34.
74. Fleming MF, Mundt MP, French MT, Manwell LB, Stauffacher EA, Barry KL. Brief physician advice for problem drinkers: Long-term efficacy and benefit-cost analysis. *Alcohol Clin Exp Res.* 2002:26(1):36–43.
75. Elder RW, Lawrence B, Ferguson A, et al. Task Force on Community Preventive Services. The effectiveness of tax policy interventions for reducing excessive alcohol consumption and related harms. *Am J Prev Med* 2010;38(2):217–29.
76. Wagenaar AC, Tobler AL, Komro KA. Effects of alcohol tax and price policies on morbidity and mortality: A systematic review. *Am J Public Health.* 2010;100(11):2270–8.
77. Wagenaar AC, Livingston MD, Staras SS. Effects of a 2009 Illinois alcohol tax increase on fatal motor vehicle crashes. *Am J Public Health.* 2015;105(9):1880–5.
78. Naimi TS. Blanchette JG, Xuan Z. Chaloupka FJ. Erosion of state alcohol excise taxes in the United States. *J Stud Alcohol.* 2018;79:43–8.
79. Sacks JJ, Gonzales KR, Bouchery EE, Tomedi LE, Brewer RD. 2010 National and state costs of excessive alcohol consumption. *Am J Prev Med.* 2015;49(5):e73–9.
80. Richard CM, Magee K, Bacon-Abdelmoteleb P, Brown JL. *Countermeasures That Work: A Highway Safety Countermeasure Guide for State Highway Safety Offices.* Report No. DOT HS 812 478. 9th ed. Washington, DC: US Department of Transportation, National Highway Traffic Safety Administration (NHTSA); April 2018. https://www.nhtsa.gov/sites/nhtsa.dot.gov/files/documents/812478_countermeasures-that-work-a-highway-safety-countermeasures-guide-9thedition-2017v2_0.pdf. Accessed July 20, 2020.
81. Retting RA. Two decades of photo enforcement in the United States: A brief summary of experience and lessons learned. *ITE J.* 2010;80(11):20–9.
82. Pilkington P, Kinra S. Effectiveness of speed cameras in preventing road traffic collisions and related casualties: Systematic review. *BMJ.* 2005;330:331–4.
83. Decina LE, Thomas L, Srinivasan R, Staplin L. *Automated Enforcement: A Compendium of Worldwide Evaluations of Results.* Report No. DOT HS 810 763. Washington, DC: US Department of Transportation; 2010. https://www.bing.com/search?q=dot%20hs%20810%20763&qs=n&form=QBRE&sp=-1&pq=dot%20hs%20810%20763&sc=0-14&sk=&cvid=AF2DAE8D729E49E6A165F8897958C45A. Accessed July 20, 2020.
84. Insurance Institute of Highway Safety (IIHS). *Red Light Running.* Arlington, VA: Insurance Institute for Highway Safety, Highway Loss Data Institute; 2018. (Online). https://www.iihs.org/topics/red-light-running. Accessed July 20, 2020.
85. Hu W, Cicchino JB. Effects of turning on and off red light cameras on fatal crashes in large US cities. *J Safety Res.* 2017;61:141–8.
86. Williams AF, Ferguson SA. Rationale for graduated licensing and the risks it should address. *Inj Prev.* 2002;8(Suppl II):ii9–16.
87. Shope JT, Molnar LJ. Graduated driver licensing in the United States: Evaluation results from the early programs. *J Safety Res.* 2003;34:63–9.
88. Simpson HM. The evolution and effectiveness of graduated licensing. *J Safety Res.* 2003;34:25–34.
89. Begg D, Stephenson S. Graduated driver licensing: The New Zealand experience. *J Safety Res.* 2003;34(1):99–105.
90. Hartling L, Wiebe N, Russell K, Petruk J, Spinola C, Klassen TP. Graduated driver licensing for reducing motor vehicle crashes among young drivers. *Cochrane Database Syst Rev.* 2004;(2):CD003300.

91. Pressley JC, Benedictor CB, Trieu L, et al. Motor vehicle injury, mortality, and hospital charges by strength of graduated driver licensing laws in 36 states. *J Trauma*. 2009;67(1):S43–53.

92. Baker SP, Chen L-H, Li G. *Nationwide Review of Graduated Driver Licensing*. Washington, DC: AAA Foundation for Traffic Safety; 2007.

93. Insurance Institute for Highway Safety (IIHS). *Teenagers. Graduated Licensing*. Arlington, VA: Insurance Institute for Highway Safety, Highway Loss Data Institute; 2020. (Online). https://www.iihs.org/topics/teenagers#graduated-licensing. Accessed July 20, 2020.

94. Simons-Morton B, Quimet MC, Catalano RF. Parenting and the young driver problem. *Am J Prev Med*. 2008;35(3S):S294–303.

95. Simons-Morton B, Quimet MC. Parent involvement in novice teen driving: A review of the literature. *Inj Prev*. 2006;12(Suppl. I):i30–7.

96. National Highway Traffic Safety Administration (NHTSA). Seat Belt Use in 2019—Use Rates in States and Territories, A Brief Statistical Summary. Report No. DOT HS 812 947. Washington, DC: US Department of Transportation; 2020.

97. National Highway Traffic Safety Administration (NHTSA). Seat Belts: Overview. (Online). https://www.nhtsa.gov/risky-driving/seat-belts. Accessed July 20, 2020.

98. Dinh-Zarr TB, Sleet DA, Shults RA, et al. Reviews of evidence regarding interventions to increase the use of safety belts. *Am J Prev Med*. 2001;21(4S):48–65.

99. Beck LF, West BA. Vital signs: Nonfatal motor vehicle occupant injuries (2009) and seat belt use among adults—United States. *MMWR Morb Mortal Wkly Rep*. 2011;59(51):1681–6.

100. Beck LF, Shults RA. Seat belt use in states with primary and secondary use laws—United States, 2006. *J Safety Res*. 2009;40:469–72.

101. Lee LK, Monuteaux MC, Burghardt LC, et al. Motor vehicle crash fatalities in states with primary versus secondary seat belt laws: A time-series analysis. *Ann Inter Med*. 2015;163(3):184–90.

102. Bhat G, Beck L, Bergen G, Kresnow M-J. Predictors of rear seat belt use among US adults, 2012. *J Safety Res*. 2015;53:103–6.

103. Insurance Institute for Highway Safety (IIHS). *Safety Belts and Child Safety Seats*. Arlington, VA: Insurance Institute for Highway Safety, Highway Loss Data Institute; 2018. (Online). http://www.iihs.org/iihs/topics/laws/safetybeltuse. Accessed July 20, 2020.

104. Zaza S, Sleet DA, Thompson RS, Sosin DM, Bolen JC, the Task Force on Community Preventive Services. Reviews of evidence regarding interventions to increase use of child safety seats. *Am J Prev Med*. 2001;21(4S):31–47.

105. Grossman DC, Garcia CC. Effectiveness of health promotion programs to increase motor vehicle occupant restraint use among young children. *Am J Prev Med*. 1999;16(1S):12–22.

106. Durbin DR, Hoffman BD, AAP Council on Injury, Violence, and Poison Prevention. Child passenger safety. *Pediatrics*. 2018;142(5):e20182460.

107. Ehiri JE, Ejere HO, Hazen AE, Emusu D, King B, Osberg SJ. Interventions to increase children's booster seat use: A review. *Am J Prev Med*. 2006;31(2):185–92.

108. Yellman MA, Rodriguez MA, Colunga MI, et al. Evaluation of give kids a boost: A school-based program to increase booster seat use among urban children in economically-disadvantaged areas. *Traffic Inj Prev*. 2018;19(4):378–84.

109. Sun K, Bauer MJ, Hardman S. Effects of upgraded child restraint law designed to increase booster seat use in New York. *Pediatrics*. 2010;126(3):484–9.

110. Pressley JC, Trieu L, Barlow B, Kendig T. Motor vehicle occupant injury and related hospital expenditures in children aged 3 years to 8 years covered versus uncovered by booster seat legislation. *J Trauma Acute Care Surg*. 2009;67(1):S20–9.

111. Eichelberger AH, Chouinard AO, Jermakian JS. Effects of booster seat laws on injury risk among children in crashes. *Traffic Inj Prev* 2012;13(6):631–9.

112. Mannix R, Fleegler E, Meehan WP, et al. Booster seat laws and fatalities in children 4 to 7 years of age. *Pediatrics*. 2012;130(6):996–1002.

113. Berg MD, Cook L, Corneli HM, Vernon DD, Dean JM. Effect of seating position and restraint use on injuries to children in motor vehicle crashes. *Pediatrics*. 2000;105(4 Pt 1):831–5.

114. Durbin DR, Kallan M, Elliott M, Cornejo RA, Arbogast KB, Winston FK. Risk of injury to restrained children from passenger air bags. *Traffic Inj Prev*. 2003;4:58–63.

115. Durbin DR, Elliott M, Arbogast KB, Anderko RL, Winston FK. The effect of seating position on risk of injury for children in side impact collisions. *Pediatrics*. 2005;115(3):e305–9.

116. Arbogast KB, Kallan MJ, Durbin DR. Front versus rear seat injury risk for child passengers: Evaluation of newer model year vehicles. *Traffic Inj Prev*. 2009;10:297–301.

117. Peng Y, Vaidya N, Finnie R, et al. Universal motorcycle helmet laws to reduce injuries: A community guide systematic review. *Am J Prev Med*. 2017;52(6):820–32.

118. Insurance Institute of Highway Safety (IIHS), Highway Loss Data Institute. Motorcycles. 2020. (Online). https://www.iihs.org/topics/motorcycles. Accessed July 20, 2020.

119. National Highway Traffic Safety Administration (NHTSA). Traffic Safety Facts. Motorcycle Helmet Use in 2019—Overall Results. Report No. DOT HS 812 936. Report No. DOT HS 812 936. Washington, DC: US Department of Transportation; 2020 https://crashstats.nhtsa.dot.gov/Api/Public/Publication/812936. Accessed July 20, 2020.

120. Insurance Institute of Highway Safety (IIHS), Highway Loss Data Institute. Pedestrians and Bicyclists. 2020. (Online). http://www.iihs.org/iihs/topics/laws/bicycle-laws?topicName=pedestrians-and-bicyclists. Accessed July 20, 2020.

121. Lee BH, Schofer JL, Koppelman FS. Bicycle safety helmet legislation and bicycle-related non-fatal injuries in California. *Accid Anal Prev*. 2005;37:93–102.

122. Wesson DE, Stephens D, Lam K, Parsons D, Spence L, Parkin PC. Trends in pediatric and adult bicycling deaths before and after passage of a bicycle helmet law. *Pediatrics*. 2008;122(3):605–10.

123. Towner E, Dowswell T, Burkes M, Dickinson H, Towner J, Hayes M. *Bicycle Helmets: Review of Effectiveness (No. 30)*. London, UK; Department for Transport; 2002.

124. Royal ST, Kendrick D. Coleman T. Non-legislative interventions for the promotion of cycle helmet wearing by children (Review). *Cochrane Database Syst Rev*. 2005;(2):CD003985.

125. Administration on Aging, Administration for Community Living. A profile of older Americans: 2018. US Department of Health and Human Services. (Online). https://www.acl.gov/sites/default/files/Aging%20and%20Disability%20in%20America/2018OlderAmericansProfile.pdf. Accessed July 20, 2020.

126. Bureau of Labor Statistics. Employment projections. US Department of Labor. Civilian labor force participation rate, by age, sex, race, and ethnicity. Table 3.3. (Online). https://www.bls.gov/emp/tables/civilian-labor-force-participation-rate.htm. Accessed July 20, 2020.

127. Clewlow RR, Mishra GS. *Disruptive Transportation: The Adoption, Utilization, and Impacts of Ride-hailing in the United States*. Research Report UCD-ITS-RR-17-07. Davis, CA: University of California Davis Institute of Transportation Studies; 2017.

128. Insurance Institute for Highway Safety (IIHS). Fatality Facts 2018, Older People. Arlington, VA: IIHS; 2018. (Online). http://www.iihs.org/iihs/topics/t/older-drivers/fatalityfacts/older-people/2016. Accessed July 20, 2020.

129. Carr DB, Schwartzberg JG, Manning L, Sempek J, Physician's Guide to Assessing and Counseling Older Drivers, 2nd ed, Washington, DC: NHTSA. 2010. https://www.nhtsa.gov/staticfiles/nti/older_drivers/pdf/811298.pdf. Accessed July 20, 2020.

130. National Highway Traffic Safety Administration (NHTSA). Critical reasons for crashes investigated in the National Motor Vehicle Crash Causation Survey. Report No. DOT HS 812 115. Washington, DC: US Department of Transportation; 2015.

131. Cicchino J. Effectiveness of forward collision warning and autonomous emergency braking systems in reducing front-to-rear crash rates. *Accid Anal Prev*. 2017;99:142–52.

132. National Highway Traffic Safety Administration (NHTSA). *Automated Driving Systems: A Vision for Safety*. Report No. DOT HS 812 442. Washington, DC: US Department of Transportation; 2017.

133. Insurance Institute for Highway Safety (IIHS). *Self-driving Vehicle could Struggle to Eliminate Most Crashes*. Arlington, VA: IIHS; 2020. (Online). https://www.iihs.org/news/detail/self-driving-vehicles-could-struggle-to-eliminate-most-crashes. Accessed July 20, 2020.

134. Centers for Disease Control and Prevention (CDC). Impaired driving: Get the facts. (Online). https://www.cdc.gov/motorvehiclesafety/impaired_driving/impaired-drv_factsheet.html. Accessed July 20, 2020.

135. Compton RP, Berning A. *Drug and Alcohol Crash Risk*. Traffic Safety Facts Research Note. DOT HS 812 117. Washington, DC: National Highway Traffic Safety Administration; 2015, February. https://www.nhtsa.gov/staticfiles/nti/pdf/812117-Drug_and_Alcohol_Crash_Risk.pdf. Accessed July 20, 2020.

136. National Highway Traffic Safety Administration (NHTSA). Marijuana-Impaired Driving. A Report to Congress. Report No. DOT HS

812-440. Washington, DC: US Department of Transportation; 2017. https://www.nhtsa.gov/sites/nhtsa.dot.gov/files/documents/812440-marijuana-impaired-driving-report-to-congress.pdf. Accessed July 20, 2020.

137. Centers for Disease Control and Prevention (CDC). What you need to know about marijuana use and driving. (Online). https://www.cdc.gov/marijuana/pdf/marijuana-driving-508.pdf. Accessed July 20, 2020.

138. Wilson N, Kariisa M, Seth P, Smith H, Davis NL. Drug and opioid-involved overdose deaths—United States, 2017–2018. *MMWR Morb Mortal Wkly Rep*. 2020;69(11):290–7.

139. Gomes T, Redelmeier DA, Juurlink DN, Dhalla IA, Camacho X, Mamdani MM. Opioid dose and risk of road trauma in Canada: A population-based study. *JAMA Intern Med*. 2013;173(3):196–201.

140. Wickens CM, Mann RE, Ialomiteanu AR, et al. The impact of medical and non-medical prescription opioid use on motor vehicle collision risk. *Transp Res Part F Traffic Psychol Behav*. 2017;47:155–62.

141. Dowell D, Haegerich TM, Chou R. CDC guideline for prescribing opioids for chronic pain—United States, 2016. *MMWR Recomm Rep*. 2016;65:1–49.

142. Regan MA, Lee JD, Young K. *Driver Distraction: Theory, Effects, and Mitigation*. Boca Raton, FL: CRC Press; 2008.

143. Klauer SG, Guo F, Simons-Morton BG, et al. Distracted driving and risk of road crashes among novice and experienced drivers. *N Engl J Med*. 2014;370:54–9.

144. Redelmeier DA, Tibshirani RJ. Association between cellular-telephone calls and motor vehicle collisions. *N Engl J Med*. 1997;336:453–8.

145. Wilson FA, Stimpson JP. Trends in fatalities from distracted driving in the United States, 1999 to 2008. *Am J Public Health*. 2010;100:2213–9.

146. Harbluk JL, Noy YI, Trbovich PL, et al. An on-road assessment of cognitive distraction: Impacts on drivers' visual behavior and braking performance. *Accid Anal Prev*. 2007;39:372–9.

147. Shen S, Neyens DM. Assessing drivers' response during automated driver support system failures with non-driving tasks. *J Safety Res*. 2017;61:149–55.

148. McCartt AT, Hellinga LA, Braitman KA. Cell phones and driving: Review of research. *Traffic Inj Prev*. 2006;7:89–106.

149. McEvoy SP, Stevenson MR, McCartt AT, et al. Role of mobile phones in motor vehicle crashes resulting in hospital attendance: A case-crossover study. *BMJ*. 2005;331:428.

150. Coben JH, Zhu M. Keeping an eye on distracted driving. *JAMA*. 2013;309:877–8.

151. Caird JK, Johnston KA, Willness CR, et al. A meta-analysis of the effects of texting on driving. *Accid Anal Prev*. 2014;71:311–8.

152. Kann L, McManus T, Harris WA, et al. Youth Risk Behavior Surveillance—United States, 2017. *MMWR Surveill Summ*. 2018;67(No. SS 8):12.

153. Insurance Institute for Highway Safety (IIHS). *Distracted Driving*. Arlington, VA: Insurance Institute for Highway Safety, Highway Loss Data Institute; 2019. (Online). https://www.iihs.org/topics/distracted-driving. Accessed July 20, 2020.

154. World Health Organization. *Global Plan for the Decade of Action for Road Safety 2011–2020*. Geneva, Switzerland: World Health Organization; 2011. (Online). http://www.who.int/roadsafety/decade_of_action/plan/plan_english.pdf?ua=1. Accessed July 20, 2020.

155. United Nations. Sustainable Development Goads: 17 goals to transform our world. United Nations, New York, USA. 2015. (Online). https://www.un.org/sustainabledevelopment/sustainable-development-goals/. Accessed July 20, 2020.

156. Vision Zero Network. (Online). https://visionzeronetwork.org/about/what-is-vision-zero/. Accessed July 20, 2020.

157. National Safety Council. Road to Zero (Online). https://www.nsc.org/road-safety/get-involved/road-to-zero. Accessed July 20, 2020.

CHAPTER

171

Fall Burden and Prevention Across the Lifespan*

Robin Lee • Briana Moreland

INTRODUCTION

While definitions vary, researchers typically define a fall as the occasion in which an individual loses their balance causing them to hit the ground or other object at a lower level.[1] Falls occur at home, the workplace, school, or in recreational settings. They can occur while walking on a flat surface, ascending or descending from a staircase, or when standing on an object such as a ladder or step stool. Falls can also occur from substantial height, such as falling from a window or roof top. The location and the circumstances of falls vary by age group.

Unintentional falls are the leading cause of nonfatal injuries seen in emergency departments in the United States among all age groups except 10- to 24-year olds where they are the second leading cause.[2] In the past 15 years, the rate of fatal falls remained relatively constant among individuals less than 65 years old (Fig. 171-1). In contrast, the fatal fall rate among older adults, persons 65 and older, has increased considerably (Fig. 171-1).[2]

Given the high and increasing burden among older adults, more research has been conducted and reported on the circumstances and prevention of falls among persons 65 and older. Therefore, this chapter focuses primarily on older adults, yet also touches upon what is known about falls among infants, children, and adults younger than 65. This includes an overview of the predominant risk factors and circumstances associated with falls, the health and economic burden, and effective strategies for preventing falls for all age groups. We also spotlight global trends in falls.

INFANTS, CHILDREN, AND ADULTS UNDER 65

Incidence and Mortality

In 2017, falls accounted for 24% (5,620,191 fall injuries) of all unintentional injuries among infants, children, and adults less than 65 years of age.[2] The occurrence of nonfatal fall injuries resulting in emergency department (ED) visits or hospitalizations has a "U"-shaped curve representing a large number of injuries among infants and toddlers 1–2 years of age followed by a decrease until age 65 when nonfatal fall injury rates rise again (Fig. 171-2). Deaths from falls among individuals under 65 are relatively infrequent, occurring at a rate of 1.9 per 100,000 individuals.[2]

Risk Factors and Circumstances

The predominant risk factors for fall injuries among infants, children, and adults under 65 are extrinsic factors. Extrinsic risk factors originate outside the body and include hazards that are located in or around the home (e.g., stairs), workplace (ladders, scaffolding), or recreational areas (e.g., jungle gym, playscape).[3–5]

Infants and Children

In infants and toddlers, fall injuries are more likely to occur in the home than in other locations such as daycare facilities.[5–7] Infants and toddlers fall from furniture including baby changing tables, couches, and high chairs.[8] As children begin to walk around the age of one, they also become more likely to fall down stairs.[4] Falls from stairs are often associated with not using a barrier such as a baby gate to block access to stairs or the improper installation of a baby gate.[9] The use of infant walkers also poses a risk for stair-related falls.[10] Falls from beds account for 30% of traumatic brain injuries (TBIs) associated with a consumer product in infants and toddlers.[8] Specifically, bunk beds are associated with a large number of falls, most often among children 2–6 years old.[11]

Aside from furniture and stairs, falls from windows and balconies account for fall-related injuries in infants and toddlers.[5] Annually, more than 5000 children in the United States are treated for falls that occur by falling from a window.[12] Falls from windows are more common in children 1–2 years of age than any other age group.[12] The majority of these falls are from second story windows.

For children 5–9 years old, playground injuries are common.[13,14] Climbers (monkey bars or jungle gyms), swings, and slides specifically pose a risk.[13] Falls from treehouses have also been studied in this age group. In the United States, there are an estimated 2700 ED visits from treehouse-related falls each year.[15] Although there were no significant gender differences among falls from playground equipment, boys were more likely than girls to sustain an injury from a treehouse-related fall.[14,15] Less is reported on the circumstances related to falls in youth between 10 and 17 years old. However, some studies suggest sports and recreational injuries are associated with falls in this age group.[4,16]

Adults Under 65 Years Old

In adults 18–49 years old, the most common mechanism for falls is slipping or tripping.[17] The proportion of indoor falls compared to outdoor falls increases with age. Across all adults under 65, women had a higher proportion of indoor falls.[18] Alcohol use is also associated with falls in this age group.[17]

Falls account for 21.6% of all occupational injuries.[3] Occupation-related falls are associated with transportation, movers, food preparation, and construction work. Younger construction workers (less than 40 years old) make up 65% of fall injuries at construction sites and falls account for 42% of construction fatalities in the United States.[19,20] Construction-related deaths are often due to falls from elevated work surfaces, such as rooftops or ladders.[19,20]

*The findings and conclusions in this chapter are those of the authors and do not necessarily represent the official position of the Centers for Disease Control and Prevention.

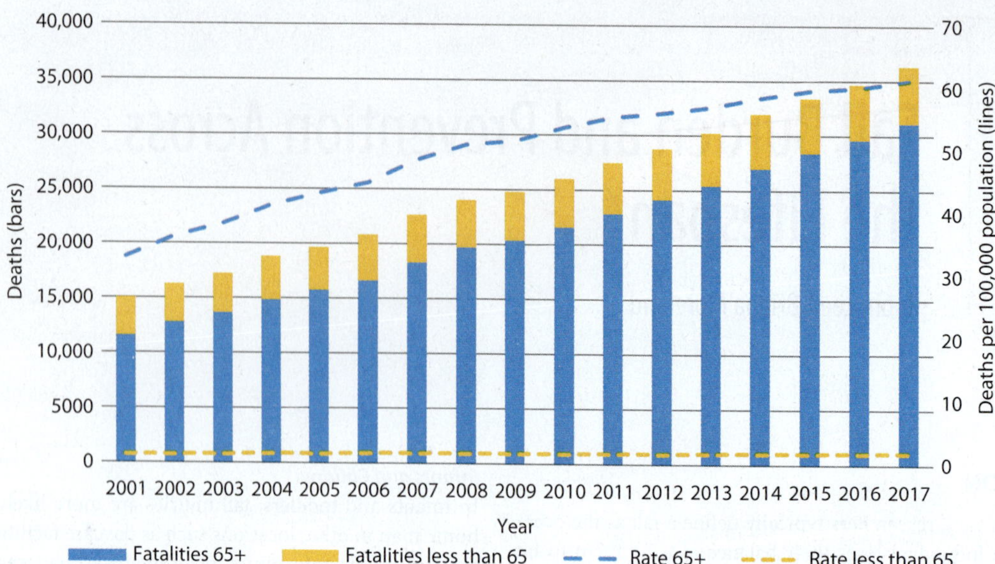

FIGURE 171-1. Fall deaths and death rates by age group and year, United States, 2001–2017. (*Source:* Data from Centers for Disease Control and Prevention: Web-based Injury Statistics Query and Reporting System (WISQARS). https://www.cdc.gov/injury/wisqars/index.html.)

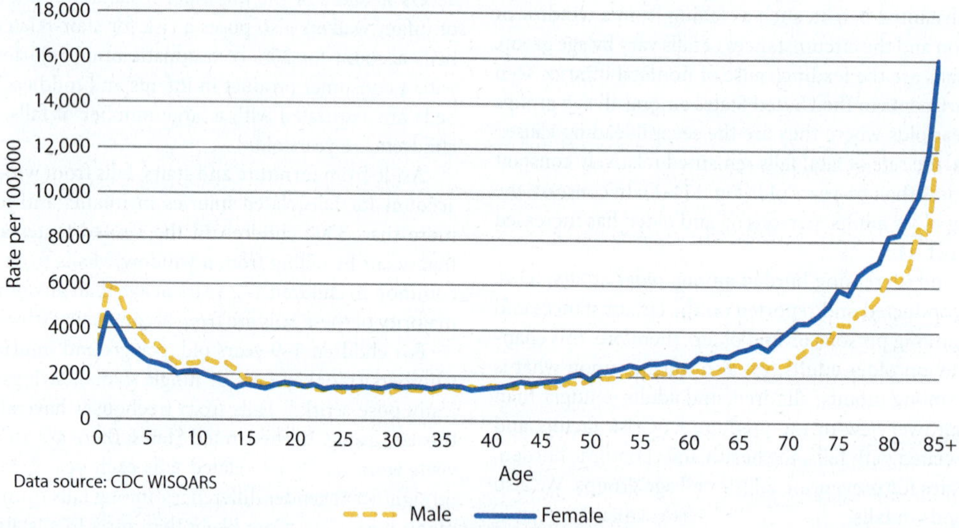

FIGURE 171-2. Rate of emergency department visits and hospitalizations for fall injuries by age and sex, United States, 2017. (*Source:* Data from Centers for Disease Control and Prevention: Web-based Injury Statistics Query and Reporting System (WISQARS). https://www.cdc.gov/injury/wisqars/index.html.)

HEALTH AND ECONOMIC BURDEN

While not all falls result in an injury, as many as one in five can cause minor to severe health complications in older adults.[21] Among individuals less than 65 years old, the prominent injuries are TBIs, upper extremity fractures, and contusions and abrasions.

Falls are the leading cause of TBI across all age groups.[22] Among infants and toddlers less than 5 years old, fall-related TBIs account for 72% of TBIs.[22] Falls from beds and falls down stair cases were the most common mechanisms of fall-related TBIs in infants and toddlers.[8,23] Infants and toddlers who fell from a height of more than three stories or landed on a hard surface were more likely to sustain a fracture or a TBI.[12]

Upper extremity fractures among children are more common in 3- to 8-year olds than other age groups and lower extremity injuries are more common in 13- to 16-year olds.[4] Twenty-eight percent of fall-related injuries from bunkbeds resulted in a fracture.[11] Upper extremity fractures are the most commonly reported injury associated with playground falls and falls from treehouses.[13,15] Playground surfaces have changed over time to protect against injuries.[24] However, these materials are not protective against extremity fractures.[24]

Contusions and abrasions are common among construction-related falls, followed by sprains/strains. The areas of the body most often injured are the trunk and extremities.[25] Ten percent of fall-related construction injuries seen in EDs required hospitalization.[25]

In 2010, the average lifetime cost of a nonfatal fall requiring hospitalization was approximately $154,000 per individual when including both medical expenses and lifetime loss of work.[2] The average cost per individual seen and discharged from the ED was $6800.[2]

Effective Interventions

There are few evidence-based interventions for preventing falls among individuals under 65. Interventions described in the literature tend to focus on reducing falls among infants and toddlers and construction-related falls (Table 171-1). Reduction in infant walker use is one example. The American Academy of Pediatrics recommended a ban on mobile infant walkers in 2001 due to their risk of injury and no clear benefit to their use.[26] Research has shown that providing education about the dangers of infant walkers was effective in reducing the number of parents who use infant walkers.[10] However, warning labels have not shown a reduction in injuries from infant walkers.[26] Educational interventions have also been effective for increasing baby gate use. However,

TABLE 171-1 COMMON INTERVENTION STRATEGIES USED TO PREVENT FALLS*

Intervention	Target Population	Clinical Support
Restricting the use of infant walkers	Parents and caregivers of infants	• The American Academy of Pediatrics recommended a ban on mobile infant walkers due to their risk of injury.
Use of stair gates	Parents and caregivers of toddlers	• Although the evidence is limited, some educational interventions have increased the use of stair gates.
Window guards laws	Parents of infants/ children	• Although the evidence is limited, some communities with laws requiring window guards have reported a reduction in hospital admissions for falls from windows.
Occupational fall prevention policies and guidance	Working adults	• The National Institute for Occupational Safety and Health provides information on preventing falls in the workplace, with specific guidance on preventing falls from ladders.
Strength, gait, and balance programs	Community-dwelling older adults	• The U.S. Preventive Services Task Force conducted a pooled analysis of 18 trials and found a 13% reduction in fall risk. • The American and British Geriatrics Society Guideline gave a grade A recommendation to exercise programs that target strength, gait, and balance.
Home modification led by an occupational therapist	Community-dwelling older adults	• The American and British Geriatrics Society Guideline gave a grade A recommendation for home environment assessment and intervention for older persons who have fallen or who have risk factors for falling, and for mitigation of identified home hazards, with evaluation and intervention to promote safe behavior.
Medication management	Older adults	• The American and British Geriatrics Society Guideline gave a B recommendation for recommending withdrawal or minimization of psychoactive medications.
Cataract surgery	Older women	• The American and British Geriatrics Society Guideline gave a B grade recommendation for expedited first eye cataract surgery among older women in whom cataract surgery is indicated.
Review of foot health and footwear	Older adults	• Although the evidence is not strong enough for an American and British Geriatrics Society Guideline recommendation, footwear does affect balance, gait, and posture. Therefore, wearing shoes with a low heel height and shoes with slip resistant soles is logical.
Hospital falls prevention policies	Hospitalized persons of any age	• Agency for Healthcare Research and Quality has a toolkit to assist in the implementation of best practices for fall prevention in hospitals.

*The CDC STEADI initiative, for older adults, has tools and resources to help with conducting many of these interventions (www.cdc.gov/STEADI).

there is little research to suggest that these interventions work to reduce the number of falls in children under four.[10] In some cities in the United States, window guards were made mandatory.[7,27] In New York City, window guard laws require window guards be installed in all apartments housing children under the age of 10. Since this law took effect, there has been a 96% reduction in hospital admissions for falls from windows.[7] To reduce occupational falls, the National Institute for Occupational Safety and Health provides information on preventing falls in the workplace, with specific guidance on preventing falls from ladders.[28]

OLDER ADULTS

Incidence and Mortality

Approximately one in four older adults report falling each year.[29] This constitutes approximately 30 million falls annually. There are about 3 million fall injuries that result in an ED visit or hospitalizations each year, resulting in a crude rate of over 5800 fall injuries per 100,000 older adults.[2] By 2030, there will be an estimated 49 million falls, 12 million fall-related injuries, and 59,000 fall deaths among older adults annually.[29,30] This increase is likely due to many factors, including but not limited to the aging population as well as increased survival after the onset of common diseases such as heart disease, cancer, and stroke.[31] Among older adults, fall rates continue to increase as people age. Twenty-seven percent of 65- to 74-year olds reported a fall in the past year.[29] The percent increases to 30% for adults 75–84 years of age and more than 37% for persons 85 and older. [29]

Older women are more likely to report a fall in the past year (30%) than men (27%). In addition, women are more likely to report a fall-related injury (12.6% of women compared to 8.3% for men).[29] Fall rates differ by race and ethnicity. American Indian and Alaskan Natives are more likely to report a fall in the past year (34%) compared to Caucasians (30%), persons of Hispanic origin (26%), African Americans (23%), and Asian or Pacific Islanders (20%).[29]

As well as being the leading cause of nonfatal injuries among older adults, falls are also the leading cause of fatal injuries among older adults. In 2017, there were more than 31,000 fatal falls.[2] This translates into roughly 85 deaths per day because of falls. Fall deaths among older adults have steadily increased over the past decade (Fig. 171-3). Between 2001 and 2017, the crude death rate increased more than 86% from 32.9 to 61.3 per 100,000 older adults.[2] In 2017, the age-specific death rate for adults 65–74 years old was 16.0 per 100,000, 62.7 among adults 75–84, and 266.2 among adults 85 and older.[2] The annual percent increase in fall death rates is highest among the oldest age groups.[32]

While more females die because of a fall, the rate is higher for men (Fig. 171-3). This is due to the gender imbalance in the older age groups; older women (27 million) outnumber older men (21 million).[29] Women are more likely to sustain severe injuries, such as a hip fractures than men.[33]

Fatal fall rates also differ by race/ethnicity. In the United States, White non-Hispanic older adults have the highest age-adjusted fall death rate per 100,000 population (68.7) followed by American Indian/Alaskan Natives (47.0), Asian/Pacific Islanders (36.7), and Black non-Hispanic Americans (27.1).[30]

Risk Factors and Circumstances

Epidemiological studies report numerous fall risk factors for older adults age 65 and older.[34–36]

Intrinsic Risk Factors

Intrinsic risk factors refer to an attribute or characteristic of an individual that increases their likelihood of falling. These risk factors include a person's age or gender, as well as, whether they have fallen in the past, poor gait and balance from vestibular disorders, fear of falling, impaired vision, dizziness, and foot and ankle disorders.[35–41]

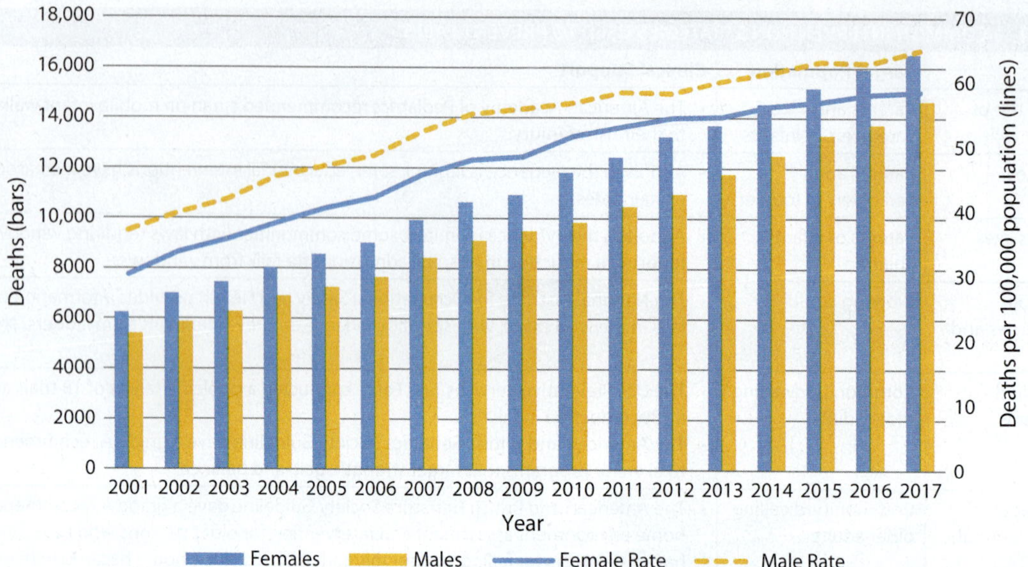

FIGURE 171-3. Falls deaths for older Americans (65 and older) by year and sex, United States, 2001–2017. (*Source:* Data from Centers for Disease Control and Prevention: Web-based Injury Statistics Query and Reporting System (WISQARS). https://www.cdc.gov/injury/wisqars/index.html.)

Extrinsic Risk Factors

Extrinsic risk factors, those that originate outside the body, include hazards around the home (e.g., throw rugs; stairs; wrinkled, torn or uneven flooring; poor lighting; trailing cords; misuse of walking aids or devices) or outside the home (uneven sidewalks, curbs, streets, lighting, cords, or garden hose).[4,35,36]

Medications and Vision

Other important factors include the use of certain medications.[42,43] Specifically, psychoactive medications that directly affect cognition and brain function are associated with side effects that may increase fall risk, such as orthostatic hypotension, confusion, lethargy, and vision changes.[42] These include sedative hypnotics, opioids, antidepressants, antipsychotics, and antiepileptics. While these medications can have valuable health benefits, they can also cause adverse drug events. For example, the use of opioids, dopaminergic agents, anxiolytics, antidepressants, and sedatives/hypnotics have been associated with an increased risk of hip fractures among adults 75 and older.[44] Similarly, antidepressants and opioids can cause orthostatic hypotension that in turn causes dizziness and may increase fall risk.[42,45,46] Psychoactive polypharmacy, or the use of multiple psychoactive medications (medications which act on the central nervous system or cross the blood brain barrier), further increases fall risk due to the synergistic effect some medications have on cognition and physical function.[42,45] Certain chronic conditions like stroke, arthritis, diabetes, dementia, depression, and Parkinson's disease are associated with an increased risk of falls.[35] Falls are also associated with vision impairment and the use of inappropriate eyewear.[47,48]

In older adults, fall risk increases with each risk factor present. In an early study of community-dwelling older adults, Tinetti et al. found that the likelihood of falling increases linearly with the number of fall risk factors present.[49] The annual risk of falling when one risk factor is present is 19%. Risk increases to 32% when two risk factors are present, 60% with three risk factors, and 78% with four or more fall risk factors.[49]

While falls can occur in any location, more than half of falls occur in the home.[50,51] The circumstances surrounding falls suggest that more falls (35.3%) occur while walking or standing on the same level compared to falls that occurred on stairs (6.5%), or from furniture (4.4%).[52] The latter includes falls that might occur while transferring from a bed to a chair or a fall that occurs while standing on a step stool or ladder. While more falls occur in the home, nursing home residents, and hospitalized older adults have higher rates of falls than community dwelling older adults.[53] Half of nursing home residents fall annually, and residents with certain conditions (e.g., dementia) have even higher fall incidence, ranging as high as 80% annually.[54]

The fall rate is higher among nursing home residents than among community-dwelling older adults.[55,56] The increased incidence rate is likely a result of increased frailty among the residents, cognitive impairment, and the greater likelihood that nursing home residents had a previous fall or fall injury. Subsequent falls often result in more severe injury or death. The national incidence of hip fractures among nursing home residents is 3.1 per 100 person-years.[56] Among U.S. nursing homes, there is considerable variability in hip fracture rates. Resident characteristics (e.g., frailty, comorbidity) and staff characteristics (e.g., clinical expertise and care management) might explain the difference in nursing home hip fracture rates. New data suggest that hip fracture incidence may also be associated with a resident's use of psychoactive medications, a risk factor for falls.[56]

The fall rate in U.S. hospitals is estimated to be 3.5 falls per 1000 person days and 0.91 injurious falls per 1000 person days.[57] Within hospitals, fall rates differ by the type of hospital unit, with higher rates in medical units compared to surgical units. While these rates include falls among all ages, falls occur more often among older adult patients.[58] The high frequency of falls in hospitals has been associated with gait and balance problems, cognitive impairment, urinary incontinence, fall history, and the use of specific medications (e.g., sedative/hypnotics).[59]

Health and Economic Burden

Hip fractures and TBIs are among the most severe nonfatal fall injuries affecting older adults. Eight out of ten TBIs in older adults are caused by a fall.[22] Between 2006 and 2014, TBIs caused by a fall climbed steadily.[22] ED visits for fall-related TBIs more than doubled, reaching more than 394,000 visits. Hospitalizations for fall-related TBIs increased by 50%, resulting in more than 91,000 stays. While hip fracture rates had decreased between 2002 and 2012, more recent data suggest hip fractures are no longer on the decline. Between 2013 and 2015, hip fracture rates increased.[60] In adults 65 and older, falls cause approximately 95% of hip fractures.[61,62] Hip fractures often result in long-term disability and loss of independence.[63] The mortality rate for hip fracture ranges from 14% to 36% within 1 year of surgery.[64]

Falls can also result in social consequences. Studies show that up to 39% of older adults who fall develop a fear of falling.[65] Fear of falling can cause older adults to further limit their daily activities, leading to increased muscle weakness, a risk factor for falls.[66]

The average cost of a fall-related hospitalization is $30,000.[67] In 2015, the estimated medical costs attributable to both fatal and nonfatal falls was approximately $50 billion.[68] Seventy-five percent ($38 billion) is paid by public health insurance programs (Medicare and Medicaid). Overall, medical spending for fatal falls was estimated to be $754 million.[68] These statistics will only worsen as America's baby boomer population (born between 1946 and 1964) continues to turn 65 years of age. By 2030, one in five Americans will be at least 65 years of age, and without preventive efforts, the CDC estimates there may be 49 million falls and 12 million fall-related injuries among older adults annually.[29,69] The high incidence of falls, long-term health effects, and costs of falls will severely impact the U.S. healthcare system.

Effective Interventions

Among older adults, there are many effective fall prevention interventions (Table 171-1).[70–72] There are interventions that focus on one specific risk factor and those that address multiple modifiable risk factors.[73,74] Multifactorial interventions that include exercise along with other intervention strategies (e.g., vision improvement, removal of home hazards) tend to be the most effective at reducing injurious falls.[75] Implementation of these interventions, at the population level, are estimated to have the potential to prevent thousands of falls and avert millions in healthcare costs.[76]

Physical Activity

Exercises that target strength, gait, and balance, have been found to reduce falls or how many times people fall. The effect of exercise on falls differs by duration, intensity, type, time for follow-up, and other factors.[73,77–81] The U.S. Preventive Services Task Force (Task Force) reviewed 18 trials involving exercise or physical therapy and found a 13% reduction in the risk of falling in a pooled analysis.[80] A review of 59 systematic reviews found exercise consistently effective for community residents, but not for those in care facilities.[79] Exercise was found effective as a single intervention and as part of a multifactorial strategy. The American Geriatrics Society and British Geriatrics Society Clinical Practice Guideline for Prevention of Falls in Older Persons (AGS/BGS Guideline) gave the highest grade A recommendation to exercise programs that target strength, gait, and balance (i.e., a strong recommendation that physicians provide the intervention to eligible patients) and that exercise be included as a component of multifactorial interventions.[77] There are a variety of community-based exercise programs that providers can refer their patients to; two have also been shown to have a positive return on investment. These include Stepping On and Tai Chi.[82–84]

Home Modifications

Hazards in the home are common and can be reduced by conducting home modifications. Home modifications led by an occupational therapist have been shown to reduce both the fall rate and number of fallers.[73,77,79,85,86] The trial reported by Cumming et al. showed a 36% reduction in the proportion of people falling, although only among those with a history of falls.[85] The AGS/BGS Guideline gives a grade A recommendation (a strong recommendation that physicians provide the intervention to eligible patients) for home environment assessment and intervention for older persons who have fallen or who have risk factors for falling, and for mitigation of identified home hazards, with evaluation and intervention to promote safe behavior.[77]

Changes in Medication

Both a Cochrane systematic review and the review for the updated AGS/BGS Guidelines found that withdrawal of certain medications, especially psychoactive medications, was an effective strategy as a single intervention or as a component of a multifactorial intervention.[73,77] The updated AGS/BGS Guideline recommends withdrawal or minimization of psychoactive medications with a B grade (i.e., recommendation that clinicians provide this intervention to eligible patients). Beyond the AGS/BGS Guideline, medications that cause dizziness, sedation, confusion, blurred vision, or orthostatic hypotension represent a modifiable risk factor for falls. Stopping these medications when possible, switching to safer alternatives, or reducing medications to their lowest effective dose may help prevent falls (www.cdc.gov/steadi).

Improve Vision

Harwood et al. found that first eye cataract surgery reduced fall rate and fracture risk among older women.[87] While additional research is needed to determine whether men would also benefit from cataract surgery, The AGS/BGS Guideline currently recommends expedited first eye cataract surgery with a B grade (clinicians provide this intervention to eligible patients) for older women in whom cataract surgery is indicated.[77]

Proper Footwear

Foot problems and footwear have been identified as risk factors for falls, but there are few studies that document the effectiveness of addressing these issues as a fall prevention strategy.[73,77,88,89] Spink et al. showed a 36% reduction in the fall rate when measured as the number of falls per person but did not show a difference in the proportion of fallers between the intervention and control groups.[89] Although the evidence is not strong enough for an AGS/BGS Guideline recommendation, footwear does affect balance, gait, and posture. Therefore, wearing shoes with a low heel height and shoes with slip resistant soles is logical.[90]

Fall Prevention in Hospitals and Nursing Homes

Fall prevention interventions in nursing homes are similar to those for community-dwelling older adults and have been effective at reducing falls by 33%.[91] Recurrent falls were reduced by 21%.[91] In hospital settings, a systematic review found certain multifactorial interventions could reduce falls by up to 30%, but pooled risk reduction was not statistically significant.[92] The use of bed alarms and wearable movement sensors have been developed but the evidence for their ability to prevent falls in hospitals is inconsistent.[93] Successful hospital interventions included standardized assessments to identify risk factors, such as delirium, and the development of patient specific care plans to reduce the identified risk. Patient and provider education, alert signs, and medication review were important components.[92,94]

The Agency for Healthcare Research and Quality has a toolkit to assist in the implementation of best practices for fall prevention in hospitals.[95] The Centers for Medicare and Medicaid Services has designated falls occurring during hospitalization as preventable; therefore, any additional cost of care or increased length of stay because of an in-hospital fracture or brain injury is the hospital's responsibility. Professional organizations, such as the American Academy of Nursing, recommend against the use of physical restraints with older hospitalized patients.[96] The use of restraints can increase the risk of injurious falls.[97] There is limited evidence on the effectiveness of multifactorial fall prevention interventions in hospital settings.[98]

While fall prevention can occur in many settings, healthcare providers are uniquely equipped to offer individualized clinical fall risk assessment and treatment to their older patients. Such strategies are also in line with clinical recommendations made by the AGS/BGS. The AGS/BGS guidelines on fall prevention recommend providers assess older patients fall risk annually.[77] The CDC's STEADI (Stopping Elderly Accidents Death and Injuries) initiative offers resources and tools to help members of the healthcare team (e.g., physicians, nurses, pharmacists, physical therapists) integrate the AGS/BGS guidelines into their clinical practice (www.cdc.gov/STEADI). Providers such as those at the Oregon Health and Science University (OHSU) and the United Health Services in New York have successfully implemented STEADI.[99–101]

Real-world Examples

In New York, a clinical champion from United Health Services (UHS) pilot tested STEADI and then rolled it out to 17 primary-care clinics. The champion worked with each clinic to improve integration success and address concerns. Before implementing STEADI, physicians at United Health Services did not regularly speak to their older patients about falls, whereas 79% of older patients were screened 12 months after implementation.[101] In 2018, Johnston et al. reported that at-risk older adults who were screened and received a treatment plan to reduce fall risk were less likely to have a fall-related hospitalization than those at-risk who were screened but not treated. This evaluation demonstrated STEADI can be implemented in primary-care settings and has potential to reduce fall-related hospitalizations among older adults.[102]

At OHSU, STEADI was integrated first within their internal medicine and geriatrics clinics and later into family medicine practice.[99] Integration included outlining roles and responsibilities for each healthcare team member (physicians, nurses, medical assistants, and even front desk staff). They also created electronic health record-based (EHR) clinical decision support tools for fall risk assessment, including structured note templates, data-entry tables for scored measures, and all-in-one order sets that resembled EHR tools frequently used by clinic staff. Within 6 months postimplementation, providers were able to screen 64% of eligible patients and intervene to reduce risk in 85% of community-dwelling older adults with gait impairment, 97% with orthostatic hypotension, 82% with vision impairment, 90% with inadequate vitamin D intake, 75% with foot issues, and 22% taking high-risk medications.[100] Conducting clinical fall prevention can be challenging. At UHS, challenges included the need to retrain staff on a regular basis and the need to provide ongoing performance monitoring and feedback to each site. Results indicated that during the first 12 months of implementation, 79% of patients aged 65 and older were screened, but during the second 12-month period, providers only screened 49% of patients. Instituting regular training and performance monitoring led to 12 of 14 practices improving screening rates in year three.[101]

STEADI implementation at UHS and OHSU were used to inform the development of the CDC Coordinated Care Plan to Prevent Older Adult Falls.[103] The Plan offers practical suggestions to incorporate and evaluate fall prevention in primary-care settings. Although the Plan was developed for primary care, STEADI-based programs can be implemented in different healthcare settings, and steps described in the plan can be adapted accordingly. The Plan is complimented by the CDC STEADI: Evaluation Guide for Older Adult Clinical Fall Prevention Programs.[104] The Evaluation Guide is adapted from CDC's Framework for Program Evaluation in Public Health, and describes key steps to measure and report on the success of implementing a STEADI-based clinical fall prevention program. Evaluating the implementation and use of STEADI-based programs can help providers and organizations increase the quality of care provided to their older patients, and demonstrate program-related successes and areas for improvement.

GLOBAL TRENDS IN FALLS BURDEN

Although the majority of this chapter explores falls in the United States, falls are a major concern in all countries. In 2012, the World Health Organization reported that falls ranked 21st among the leading causes of death worldwide. By 2030, falls are predicted to rise to the 17th leading cause of death.[105] Falls are the second leading cause of unintentional injury death worldwide, surpassed only by road traffic injuries.[106] Annually there are an estimated 650,000 fall-related deaths reported among all ages and more than 80% of these deaths occur in low- and middle-income countries.[106] As in the United States, fall deaths rates are higher among children 1–4 years old and among individuals 65 and older. One percent of all deaths in children 1–4 years old are caused by falls.[107] Male deaths from falls exceeded female deaths in all age groups. In addition to fall deaths, annually, there are approximately 172 million falls resulting in short-term or long-term disability in all age groups.[108]

Falls are the most frequent mechanism of injury in Ethiopia, Peru, Vietnam, and India.[109] In Turkey, Tanzania, Australia, Switzerland, and Ghana toddlers and infants are more likely to sustain an injury from a fall than older children.[110–114] Falls from furniture, stairs, balconies, and windows are the most common mechanism of falls among children.[110,113,115,116] The majority of falls among young children occur at home, although in Pakistan this was only true for girls.[117–119]

Falls in older children are also common.[120–122] In children in sixth to tenth grade, falls account for 14.6% of all injuries in Southeast Asian countries and 11.4% of injuries in Caribbean countries.[121,122] Falls account for 58.6% of unintentional injuries in children under 12 in Columbia, Bangladesh, Egypt, and Pakistan.[123] Most falls in these countries occur at home among boys 5 years of age and older.[123] Falls from trees are common in the Solomon Islands, Burkina-Faso, Iran, and Fiji mostly in males between 10 and 15 years old.[124–128] The majority of cases are from farm work or fruit picking except in Iran where most falls from trees are due to leisure activities.[124–128] In India and Brazil, falls have occurred from unprotected roof tops where children play.[129,130]

Falls from playground equipment are a common mechanism of injury in Singapore, Australia, and Greece, especially in children between 5 and 9 years old.[112,131–133] Sports-related falls are a frequently reported mechanism in adolescents.[111,117,134]

Research on falls in adults under 65 years of age in LMICs is limited. In Mozambique, falls from a height, not including trees, are the most reported mechanism in men and falls from the same level or from vehicles are the most reported in women.[135] Head injuries are the most common type of injury from falls seen in a Maputo province hospital.[135] In Andhra Pradesh, India, between 2007 and 2008, 10% of study participants (adults 30 and over) reported a nonfatal fall in the past year.[136] Upper and lower limbs were the most frequently injured body part and sprains/strains were the most reported injury. Among women, injuries occurred most often in the home, while men were most frequently injured on the farm.[136]

Alcohol use, medication use, falls from ladders, and occupational injuries are common risk factors for falls in 18- to 64-year olds in high-income countries.[137–145] Workers in construction, farming, and recreational professions are most likely to fall.[142–145] In the United Kingdom and Canada, falls in adults are a common cause of TBIs.[146,147]

As in the United States, globally falls account for most (90%) fractures in older adults.[148] Fall injuries in older people can result in reduced independence, early death and development of a fear of falling; mortality following a hip fracture is around 20% in the following year.[149–151]

Falls among older adults in LMICs was often based on self-report and varied from 10% to 54% annually.[152] Across six LMICs (India, China, Mexico, Ghana, Russian Federation, and South Africa) prevalence of fall-related injuries in the past year was 4% among persons 50 and older.[153] Environmental hazards may differ in LMIC countries, resulting in more falls from factors relating to street and house design, transport, and rural locations.[136,152,154–156] In addition, osteoporotic fractures may differ across settings due to variations in diet and in load-bearing work or exercise.[157]

CONCLUSION

Across the globe and across the lifespan, falls can severely affect health. In the United States, there are more than 8.5 million fall-related injuries per year.[2] This is especially concerning for children under 5 years of age and older adults who experience the greatest burden of falls in the United States and worldwide. Additional research is needed to evaluate effective interventions for children under 5 years old. For older adults, there are many effective interventions, yet fall rates continue to rise. This is alarming given the aging of the American baby boomer population. By the year 2030, 18% of the U.S. population will be age 65 or older.[158] If fall rates continue to increase, in the United States we can anticipate 49 million falls and 12 million injuries at an estimated annual cost of $100 billion.[29,159] The increase in the rate of falls in older adults suggests an urgent need to support fall-prevention efforts. In the United States, more than 90% of older adults see a medical provider at least once a year.[160] This gives providers the opportunity to screen patients for fall risk, assess their modifiable risk factors, and develop individualized care plans to reduce fall risk. Patients should be encouraged to select intervention strategies tailored to their specific fall risk factors and their health goals. Addressing an older adult's multiple risk factors has shown to reduce the rate of falls by up to 24%.[73]

References

1. Hauer K, Lamb SE, Jorstad EC, et al. Systematic review of definitions and methods of measuring falls in randomised controlled fall prevention trials. *Age Ageing.* 2006;35(1):5–10.
2. Centers for Disease Control and Prevention. Web-based Injury Statistics Query and Reporting System (WISQARS). https://www.cdc.gov/injury/wisqars/. 2019.
3. Yeoh HT, Lockhart TE, Wu X. Non-fatal occupational falls on the same level. *Ergonomics.* 2013;56(2):153–65.
4. Wang D, Zhao W, Wheeler K, Yang G, Xiang H. Unintentional fall injuries among US children: A study based on the National Emergency Department Sample. *Int J Inj Contr Saf Promot.* 2013;20(1):27–35.
5. Khambalia A, Joshi P, Brussoni M, et al. Risk factors for unintentional injuries due to falls in children aged 0–6 years: A systematic review. *Inj Prev.* 2006;12(6):378–81.
6. Powell EC, Tanz RR. Adjusting our view of injury risk: The burden of nonfatal injuries in infancy. *Pediatrics.* 2002;110(4):792–6.
7. Gielen AC, McDonald EM, Shields W. Unintentional home injuries across the life span: Problems and solutions. *Annu Rev Public Health.* 2015;36:231–53.
8. Kamboj A, Chounthirath T, Xiang H, Smith GA. Traumatic brain injuries associated with consumer products at home among US children younger than 5 years of age. *Clin Pediatr.* 2017;56(6):545–54.
9. Cheng Y-W, Fletcher EN, Roberts KJ, McKenzie LB. Baby gate-related injuries among children in the United States, 1990–2010. *Acad Pediatr.* 2014;14(3):256–61.
10. Kendrick D, Coupland C, Mason-Jones AJ, et al. Home safety education and provision of safety equipment for injury prevention. *Cochrane Database Syst Rev.* 2007;(1):CD005014.
11. Mack KA, Gilchrist J, Ballesteros MF. Bunk bed-related injuries sustained by young children treated in emergency departments in the United States, 2001–2004, National Electronic Injury Surveillance System—All Injury Program. *Inj Prev.* 2007;13(2):137–40.
12. Harris VA, Rochette LM, Smith GA. Pediatric injuries attributable to falls from windows in the United States in 1990–2008. *Pediatrics.* 2011;128(3):455–62.
13. Vollman D, Witsaman R, Comstock RD, Smith GA. Epidemiology of playground equipment-related injuries to children in the United States, 1996–2005. *Clin Pediatr.* 2009;48(1):66–71.
14. Phelan KJ, Khoury J, Kalkwarf HJ, Lanphear BP. Trends and patterns of playground injuries in United States children and adolescents. *Ambul Pediatr.* 2001;1(4):227–33.
15. Randazzo C, Stolz U, Hodges NL, McKenzie LB. Pediatric tree house-related injuries treated in emergency departments in the United States: 1990–2006. *Acad Emerg Med.* 2009;16(3):235–42.
16. Nathanson BH, Ribeiro K, Henneman PL. An analysis of US Emergency Department visits from falls from skiing, snowboarding, skateboarding, roller-skating, and using nonmotorized scooters. *Clin Pediatr.* 2016;55(8):738–44.
17. Chen CM, Yoon Y-H. Usual alcohol consumption and risks for nonfatal fall injuries in the United States: Results from the 2004–2013 National Health Interview Survey. *Subst Use Misuse.* 2017;52(9):1120–32.
18. Timsina LR, Willetts JL, Brennan MJ, et al. Circumstances of fall-related injuries by age and gender among community-dwelling adults in the United States. *PLoS One.* 2017;12(5):e0176561.
19. Nadhim EA, Hon C, Xia B, Stewart I, Fang D. Falls from height in the construction industry: A critical review of the scientific literature. *Int J Environ Res Public Health.* 2016;13(7):638.
20. Dong XS, Largay JA, Choi SD, et al. Fatal falls and PFAS use in the construction industry: Findings from the NIOSH FACE reports. *Accid Anal Prev.* 2017;102(Supplement C):136–43.
21. Schwenk M, Lauenroth A, Stock C, et al. Definitions and methods of measuring and reporting on injurious falls in randomised controlled fall prevention trials: A systematic review. *BMC Med Res Methodol.* 2012;12:50.
22. Peterson AB, Xu L, Daugherty J, Breiding MJ. Surveillance Report of Traumatic Brain Injury-related Emergency Department Visits, Hospitalizations, and Deaths—United States, 2014. Centers for Disease Control and Prevention. U.S. Department of Health and Human Services. https://www.cdc.gov/traumaticbraininjury/pdf/TBI-Surveillance-Report-508.pdf. 2019.
23. Zielinski AE, Rochette LM, Smith GA. Stair-related injuries to young children treated in US emergency departments, 1999–2008. *Pediatrics.* 2012;129(4):721–7.
24. Norton C, Nixon J, Sibert J. Playground injuries to children. *Arch Dis Child.* 2004;89(2):103–8.
25. Shishlov KS, Schoenfisch AL, Myers DJ, Lipscomb HJ. Non-fatal construction industry fall-related injuries treated in US emergency departments, 1998–2005. *Am J Ind Med.* 2011;54(2):128–35.
26. American Academy of Pediatrics. Committee on Injury and Poison Prevention. Injuries associated with infant walkers. *Pediatrics.* 2001;108(3):790–2.
27. Pressley JC, Barlow B. Child and adolescent injury as a result of falls from buildings and structures. *Inj Prev.* 2005;11(5):267–73.
28. National Institute for Occupational Safety and Health (NIOSH). Falls in the Workplace. https://www.cdc.gov/niosh/topics/falls/. 2019.
29. Bergen G, Stevens MR, Burns ER. Falls and fall injuries among adults aged >/=65 years—United States, 2014. *MMWR Morb Mortal Wkly Rep.* 2016;65(37):993–8.
30. Burns E, Kakara R. Deaths from aalls among persons aged >/=65 years—United States, 2007–2016. *MMWR Morb Mortal Wkly Rep.* 2018;67(18):509–14.
31. Paulozzi LJ, Ballesteros MF, Stevens JA. Recent trends in mortality from unintentional injury in the United States. *J Safety Res.* 2006;37(3):277–83.
32. Hartholt KA, Lee R, Burns ER, van Beeck EF. Mortality from falls among US adults aged 75 years or older, 2000–2016. *JAMA.* 2019;321(21):2131–.
33. Wolinsky FD, Fitzgerald JF, Stump TE. The effect of hip fracture on mortality, hospitalization, and functional status: A prospective study. *Am J Public Health.* 1997;87(3):398–403.
34. Masud T, Morris RO. Epidemiology of falls. *Age Ageing.* 2001;30 Suppl 4:3–7.
35. Ambrose AF, Paul G, Hausdorff JM. Risk factors for falls among older adults: A review of the literature. *Maturitas.* 2013;75(1):51–61.
36. Rubenstein LZ. Falls in older people: Epidemiology, risk factors and strategies for prevention. *Age Ageing.* 2006;35 Suppl 2:ii37–41.
37. Lord SR. Visual risk factors for falls in older people. *Age Ageing.* 2006;35 Suppl 2:ii42–5.
38. Muir SW, Berg K, Chesworth B, Klar N, Speechley M. Quantifying the magnitude of risk for balance impairment on falls in community-dwelling older adults: A systematic review and meta-analysis. *J Clin Epidemiol.* 2010;63(4):389–406.
39. Verghese J, Ambrose AF, Lipton RB, Wang C. Neurological gait abnormalities and risk of falls in older adults. *J Neurol.* 2010;257(3):392–8.
40. Agrawal Y, Carey JP, Della Santina CC, Schubert MC, Minor LB. Disorders of balance and vestibular function in US adults: Data from the National Health and Nutrition Examination Survey, 2001–2004. *Arch Intern Med.* 2009;169(10):938–44.
41. Moreland JD, Richardson JA, Goldsmith CH, Clase CM. Muscle weakness and falls in older adults: A systematic review and meta-analysis. *J Am Geriatr Soc.* 2004;52(7):1121–9.
42. Woolcott JC, Richardson KJ, Wiens MO, et al. Meta-analysis of the impact of 9 medication classes on falls in elderly persons. *Arch Intern Med.* 2009;169(21):1952–60.
43. American Geriatrics Society. 2015 Updated beers criteria for potentially inappropriate medication use in older adults. *J Am Geriatr Soc.* 2015;63(11):2227–46.
44. Thorell K, Ranstad K, Midlov P, Borgquist L, Halling A. Is use of fall risk-increasing drugs in an elderly population associated with an increased risk of hip fracture, after adjustment for multimorbidity level: A cohort study. *BMC Geriatr.* 2014;14:131.
45. Hartikainen S, Lonnroos E, Louhivuori K. Medication as a risk factor for falls: Critical systematic review. *J Gerontol A Biol Sci Med Sci.* 2007;62(10):1172–81.
46. Leipzig RM, Cumming RG, Tinetti ME. Drugs and falls in older people: A systematic review and meta-analysis: I. Psychotropic drugs. *J Am Geriatr Soc.* 1999;47(1):30–9.

47. Lord SR, Dayhew J, Howland A. Multifocal glasses impair edge-contrast sensitivity and depth perception and increase the risk of falls in older people. *J Am Geriatr Soc.* 2002;50(11):1760–6.
48. Reed-Jones RJ, Solis GR, Lawson KA, et al. Vision and falls: A multidisciplinary review of the contributions of visual impairment to falls among older adults. *Maturitas.* 2013;75(1):22–8.
49. Tinetti ME, Speechley M, Ginter SF. Risk factors for falls among elderly persons living in the community. *N Engl J Med.* 1988;319(26):1701–7.
50. Deprey SM, Biedrzycki L, Klenz K. Identifying characteristics and outcomes that are associated with fall-related fatalities: Multi-year retrospective summary of fall deaths in older adults from 2005–2012. *Inj Epidemiol.* 2017;4(1):21.
51. Mack KA, Rudd RA, Mickalide AD, Ballesteros MF. Fatal unintentional injuries in the home in the U.S., 2000–2008. *Am J Prev Med.* 2013;44(3):239–46.
52. Stevens JA, Rudd RA. Circumstances and contributing causes of fall deaths among persons aged 65 and older: United States, 2010. *J Am Geriatr Soc.* 2014;62(3):470–5.
53. Rubenstein LZ, Josephson KR, Robbins AS. Falls in the nursing home. *Ann Intern Med.* 1994;121(6):442–51.
54. Shaw FE. Prevention of falls in older people with dementia. *J Neural Transm (Vienna).* 2007;114(10):1259–64.
55. Sugarman JR, Connell FA, Hansen A, et al. Hip fracture incidence in nursing home residents and community-dwelling older people, Washington State, 1993–1995. *J Am Geriatr Soc.* 2002;50(10):1638–43.
56. Zullo AR, Zhang T, Banerjee G, et al. Facility and state variation in hip fracture in U.S. nursing home residents. *J Am Geriatr Soc.* 2018;66(3):539–45.
57. Bouldin EL, Andresen EM, Dunton NE, et al. Falls among adult patients hospitalized in the United States: Prevalence and trends. *J Patient Saf.* 2013;9(1):13–7.
58. Hitcho EB, Krauss MJ, Birge S, et al. Characteristics and circumstances of falls in a hospital setting: A prospective analysis. *J Gen Intern Med.* 2004;19(7):732–9.
59. Oliver D, Daly F, Martin FC, McMurdo ME. Risk factors and risk assessment tools for falls in hospital in-patients: A systematic review. *Age Ageing.* 2004;33(2):122–30.
60. Michael Lewiecki E, Wright NC, Curtis JR, et al. Hip fracture trends in the United States, 2002 to 2015. *Osteoporos Int.* 2018;29(3):717–22.
61. Hayes WC, Myers ER, Morris JN, et al. Impact near the hip dominates fracture risk in elderly nursing home residents who fall. *Calcif Tissue Int.* 1993;52(3):192–8.
62. Parkkari J, Kannus P, Palvanen M, et al. Majority of hip fractures occur as a result of a fall and impact on the greater trochanter of the femur: A prospective controlled hip fracture study with 206 consecutive patients. *Calcif Tissue Int.* 1999;65(3):183–7.
63. Dyer SM, Crotty M, Fairhall N, et al. A critical review of the long-term disability outcomes following hip fracture. *BMC Geriatr.* 2016;16:158.
64. Mundi S, Chaudhry H, Bhandari M. Systematic review on the inclusion of patients with cognitive impairment in hip fracture trials: a missed opportunity? *Can J Surg.* 2014;57(4):E141–5.
65. Scheffer AC, Schuurmans MJ, van Dijk N, van der Hooft T, de Rooij SE. Fear of falling: Measurement strategy, prevalence, risk factors and consequences among older persons. *Age Ageing.* 2008;37(1):19–24.
66. Visschedijk J, Achterberg W, Van Balen R, Hertogh C. Fear of falling after hip fracture: A systematic review of measurement instruments, prevalence, interventions, and related factors. *J Am Geriatr Soc.* 2010;58(9):1739–48.
67. Burns ER, Stevens JA, Lee R. The direct costs of fatal and non-fatal falls among older adults—United States. *J Safety Res.* 2016;58:99–103.
68. Florence C, Bergen G, Atherly A, Burns E, Stevens J, Drake C. Medical costs of fatal and non-fatal falls in older adults. *J Am Geriatr Soc.* 2018;66(4):693–8.
69. Colby SL, Ortman J. Projections of the Size and Composition of the U.S. Population: 2014 to 2060. https://www.census.gov/content/dam/Census/library/publications/2015/demo/p25-1143.pdf. 2015.
70. Gillespie LD, Robertson MC, Gillespie WJ, et al. Interventions for preventing falls in older people living in the community. *Cochrane Database Syst Rev.* 2009;(2):CD007146.
71. Stevens JA, Burns ER. *A CDC Compendium of Effective Fall Interventions: What Works for Community-Dwelling Older Adults.* Atlanta, GA: Centers for Disease Control and Prevention (CDC); 2015. https://www.cdc.gov/homeandrecreationalsafety/falls/compendium.html.
72. Dellinger A. Older adult falls: Effective approaches to prevention. *Curr Trauma Rep.* 2017;3(2):118–23.
73. Gillespie LD, Robertson MC, Gillespie WJ, et al. Interventions for preventing falls in older people living in the community. *Cochrane Database Syst Rev.* 2012;(9):CD007146.
74. Stubbs B, Brefka S, Denkinger MD. What works to prevent falls in community-dwelling older adults? Umbrella review of meta-analyses of randomized controlled trials. *Phys Ther.* 2015;95(8):1095–110.
75. Tricco AC, Thomas SM, Veroniki AA, et al. Comparisons of interventions for preventing falls in older adults: A systematic review and meta-analysis. *JAMA.* 2017;318(17):1687–99.
76. Stevens JA, Lee R. The potential to reduce falls and avert costs by clinically managing fall risk. *Am J Prev Med.* 2018;55(3):290–7.
77. AGS/BGS. Summary of the Updated American Geriatrics Society/British Geriatrics Society clinical practice guideline for prevention of falls in older persons. *J Am Geriatr Soc.* 2011;59(1):148–57.
78. Thomas S, Mackintosh S, Halbert J. Does the 'Otago exercise programme' reduce mortality and falls in older adults?: A systematic review and meta-analysis. *Age Ageing.* 2010;39(6):681–7.
79. Rimland JM, Abraha I, Dell'Aquila G, et al. Effectiveness of non-pharmacological interventions to prevent falls in older people: A systematic overview. The SENATOR Project ONTOP Series. *PLoS One.* 2016;11(8):e0161579.
80. Michael YL, Whitlock EP, Lin JS, et al. Primary care-relevant interventions to prevent falling in older adults: A systematic evidence review for the U.S. Preventive Services Task Force. *Ann Intern Med.* 2010;153(12):815–25.
81. Barnett A, Smith B, Lord SR, Williams M, Baumand A. Community-based group exercise improves balance and reduces falls in at-risk older people: A randomised controlled trial. *Age Ageing.* 2003;32(4):407–14.
82. Carande-Kulis V, Stevens JA, Florence CS, Beattie BL, Arias I. A cost-benefit analysis of three older adult fall prevention interventions. *J Safety Res.* 2015;52:65–70.
83. Clemson L, Cumming RG, Kendig H, et al. The effectiveness of a community-based program for reducing the incidence of falls in the elderly: A randomized trial. *J Am Geriatr Soc.* 2004;52(9):1487–94.
84. Li F, Harmer P, Fisher KJ, et al. Tai Chi and fall reductions in older adults: A randomized controlled trial. *J Gerontol A Biol Sci Med Sci.* 2005;60(2):187–94.
85. Cumming RG, Thomas M, Szonyi G, et al. Home visits by an occupational therapist for assessment and modification of environmental hazards: A randomized trial of falls prevention. *J Am Geriatr Soc.* 1999;47(12):1397–402.
86. Voigt-Radloff S, Ruf G, Vogel A, van Nes F, Hull M. Occupational therapy for elderly. Evidence mapping of randomised controlled trials from 2004–2012. *Z Gerontol Geriatr.* 2015;48(1):52–72.
87. Harwood RH, Foss AJ, Osborn F, et al. Falls and health status in elderly women following first eye cataract surgery: A randomised controlled trial. *Br J Ophthalmol.* 2005;89(1):53–9.
88. Karlsson MK, Vonschewelov T, Karlsson C, Coster M, Rosengen BE. Prevention of falls in the elderly: A review. *Scand J Public Health.* 2013;41(5):442–54.
89. Spink MJ, Menz HB, Fotoohabadi MR, et al. Effectiveness of a multifaceted podiatry intervention to prevent falls in community dwelling older people with disabling foot pain: Randomised controlled trial. *BMJ.* 2011;342:d3411.
90. Menant JC, Steele JR, Menz HB, Munro BJ, Lord SR. Optimizing footwear for older people at risk of falls. *J Rehabil Res Dev.* 2008;45(8):1167–81.
91. Vlaeyen E, Coussement J, Leysens G, et al. Characteristics and effectiveness of fall prevention programs in nursing homes: A systematic review and meta-analysis of randomized controlled trials. *J Am Geriatr Soc.* 2015;63(2):211–21.
92. Hempel S, Newberry S, Wang Z, et al. Hospital fall prevention: A systematic review of implementation, components, adherence, and effectiveness. *J Am Geriatr Soc.* 2013;61(4):483–94.
93. Kosse NM, Brands K, Bauer JM, Hortobagyi T, Lamoth CJ. Sensor technologies aiming at fall prevention in institutionalized old adults: A synthesis of current knowledge. *Int J Med Inform.* 2013;82(9):743–52.
94. Miake-Lye IM, Hempel S, Ganz DA, Shekelle PG. Inpatient fall prevention programs as a patient safety strategy: A systematic review. *Ann Intern Med.* 2013;158(5 Pt 2):390–6.
95. AHRQ. Preventing falls in hospitals. A toolkit for improving quality of care. 2013. http://www.ahrq.gov/sites/default/files/publications/files/fallpxtoolkit.pdf. Accessed February 14, 2019.
96. American Academy of Nursing. Don't use physical restraints with an older hospitalized patient. http://www.aannet.org/initiatives/choosing-wisely/physical-restraints. 2018.

97. Rubenstein LZ, Josephson KR. The epidemiology of falls and syncope. *Clin Geriatr Med.* 2002;18(2):141–58.
98. Stern C, Jayasekara R. Interventions to reduce the incidence of falls in older adult patients in acute-care hospitals: A systematic review. *Int J Evid Based Healthc.* 2009;7(4):243–9.
99. Casey CM, Parker EM, Winkler G, et al. Lessons learned from implementing CDC's STEADI falls prevention algorithm in primary care. *Gerontologist.* 2017;57(4):787–96.
100. Eckstrom E, Parker EM, Lambert GH, et al. Implementing STEADI in academic primary care to address older adult fall risk. *Innov Aging.* 2017;1(2):igx028.
101. Stevens J, Smith M, Parker E, Jiang L, Floyd F. Implementing a clinically based fall prevention program. *Am J Lifestyle Med.* 2020;14(1):71–7.
102. Johnston YA, Bergen G, Bauer M, et al. Implementation of the stopping elderly accidents, deaths, and injuries initiative in primary care: An outcome evaluation. *Gerontologist.* 2019;59(6):1182–91.
103. Eckstrom E, Parker E, Shakya I, Lee R. *Coordinated Care Plan to Prevent Older Adult Falls.* Atlanta, GA: Centers for Disease Control and Prevention; 2019. https://www.cdc.gov/steadi/pdf/Steadi-Coordinated-Care-Final-4_24_19.pdf.
104. Bergin G, Shakya I. *CDC STEADI: Evaluation Guide for Older Adult Clinical Fall Prevention Programs.* Atlanta, GA: Centers for Disease Control and Prevention; 2019. https://www.cdc.gov/steadi/pdf/Steadi-Evaluation-Guide_Final_4_30_19.pdf.
105. World Health Organization. Injuries and violence the facts. http://www.who.int/violence_injury_prevention/media/news/2015/Injury_violence_facts_2014/en/. 2014.
106. WHO. Falls fact sheet. http://www.who.int/mediacentre/factsheets/fs344/en/. 2018.
107. Lozano R, Naghavi M, Foreman K, et al. Global and regional mortality from 235 causes of death for 20 age groups in 1990 and 2010: A systematic analysis for the Global Burden of Disease Study 2010. *Lancet.* 2012;380(9859):2095–128.
108. GBD. Global, regional, and national incidence, prevalence, and years lived with disability for 354 diseases and injuries for 195 countries and territories, 1990–2017: A systematic analysis for the Global Burden of Disease Study 2017. *Lancet.* 2018;392:1789–858.
109. Howe LD, Huttly SRA, Abramsky T. Risk factors for injuries in young children in four developing countries: The Young Lives Study. *Trop Med Int Health.* 2006;11(10):1557–66.
110. Bulut M, Koksal O, Korkmaz A, Turan M, Ozguc H. Childhood falls: Characteristics, outcome, and comparison of the Injury Severity Score and New Injury Severity Score. *Emerg Med J.* 2006;23(7):540–5.
111. Kamala B, Wilson ML, Hasselberg M. Pattern of childhood falls in a low-income setting: A cross-sectional study in Dar es Salaam. *Int J Inj Contr Saf Promot.* 2011;18(4):305–11.
112. Moorin RE, Hendrie D. The epidemiology and cost of falls requiring hospitalisation in children in Western Australia: A study using linked administrative data. *Accid Anal Prev.* 2008;40(1):216–22.
113. Mayer L, Meuli M, Lips U, Frey B. The silent epidemic of falls from buildings: Analysis of risk factors. *Pediatr Surg Int.* 2006;22(9):743–8.
114. Gyedu A, Nakua EK, Otupiri E, et al. Incidence, characteristics and risk factors for household and neighbourhood injury among young children in semiurban Ghana: A population-based household survey. *Inj Prev.* 2015;21(e1):e71–9.
115. Samuel N, Jacob R, Eilon Y, Mashiach T, Shavit I. Falls in young children with minor head injury: A prospective analysis of injury mechanisms. *Brain Inj.* 2015;29(7–8):946–50.
116. Pickett W, Streight S, Simpson K, Brison RJ. Injuries experienced by infant children: A population-based epidemiological analysis. *Pediatrics.* 2003;111(4):e365–70.
117. Cartaxo CKA, Nunes MdS, Raposo OFF, Fakhouri R, Hora EC. Fall-related traumas in urgent care centers. *Clinics.* 2012;67(10):1133–8.
118. Chaveepojnkamjorn W, Pichainarong N, Pooltawee S. Unintentional injuries among children aged 1–4 years at home. *Southeast Asian J Trop Med Public Health.* 2002;33(3):642–6.
119. Bhatti JA, Farooq U, Majeed M, et al. Fall-related injuries in a low-income setting: Results from a pilot injury surveillance system in Rawalpindi, Pakistan. *J Epidemiol Glob Health.* 2015;5(3):283–90.
120. Pant P, Towner E, Ellis M, et al. Epidemiology of unintentional child injuries in the Makwanpur District of Nepal: A household survey. *Int J Environ Res Public Health.* 2015;12(12):14967.
121. Peltzer K, Pengpid S. Injury and social correlates among in-school adolescents in four Southeast Asian countries. *Int J Environ Res Public Health.* 2012;9(8):2851–62.
122. Peltzer K, Pengpid S. Unintentional injury and social correlates among in-school adolescents in seven Caribbean countries. *Mediterr J Soc Sci.* 2014;5(20):2321.
123. Hyder AA, Sugerman D, Ameratunga S, Callaghan JA. Falls among children in the developing world: A gap in child health burden estimations? *Acta Pædiatr.* 2007;96(10):1394–8.
124. Rehan R, Jones PD, Abdeen H, Rowas H, Dhaliwal J. The dangers to children from coconut tree trauma, in KiraKira, Solomon Islands: A retrospective clinical audit. *Arch Public Health.* 2016;74(1):14.
125. Mulford J, Oberli H, Tovosia S. Coconut palm-related injuries in the pacific islands. *ANZ J Surg.* 2001;71(1):32–4.
126. Dakouré PW, Diallo M, Traoré A-CV, et al. Trauma related to falls from trees treated in a specialized trauma centre in Burkina-Faso—One hundred and six cases treated in one year. *Int Orthop.* 2015;39(12):2451–6.
127. Gupta A, Reeves B. Fijian seasonal scourge of mango tree falls. *ANZ J Surg.* 2009;79(12):898–900.
128. Zargar M, Khaji A, Karbakhsh M. Injuries caused by falls from trees in Tehran, Islamic Republic of Iran. *East Mediterr Health J.* 2005;11(1–2):235–9.
129. Bartlett SN. The problem of children's injuries in low-income countries: A review. *Health Policy Plan.* 2002;17(1):1–13.
130. Rudelli BA, Silva MVAd, Akkari M, Santili C. Accidents due to falls from roof slabs. *Sao Paulo Med J.* 2013;131(3):153–7.
131. Petridou E, Sibert J, Dedoukou X, Skalkidis I, Trichopoulos D. Injuries in public and private playgrounds: The relative contribution of structural, equipment and human factors. *Acta Paediatr.* 2002;91(6):691–7.
132. Möller H, Falster K, Ivers R, et al. Closing the aboriginal child injury gap: Targets for injury prevention. *Aust N Z J Public Health.* 2017;41(1):8–14.
133. Leung KWP, Mahadev A. The cost of sustaining playground related extremity fractures in Singapore. *Injury.* 2011;42(4):352–5.
134. Keays G, Dumas A. Longboard and skateboard injuries. *Injury.* 2014;45(8):1215–9.
135. Taibo CL, Moon TD, Joaquim OA, et al. Analysis of trauma admission data at an urban hospital in Maputo, Mozambique. *Int J Emerg Med.* 2016;9(1):6.
136. Dandona R, Kumar GA, Ivers R, et al. Characteristics of non-fatal fall injuries in rural India. *Inj Prev.* 2010;16(3):166–71.
137. Thornley S, Kool B, Marshall RJ, Ameratunga S. Alcohol intake, marijuana use, and sleep deprivation on the risk of falls occurring at home among young and middle-aged adults: A case-crossover study. *N Z Med J.* 2014;127(1406):32.
138. Kool B, Ameratunga S, Robinson E, Crengle S, Jackson R. The contribution of alcohol to falls at home among working-aged adults. *Alcohol.* 2008;42(5):383–8.
139. Kool B, Ameratunga S, Jackson R. The role of alcohol in unintentional falls among young and middle-aged adults: A systematic review of epidemiological studies. *Inj Prev.* 2009;15(5):341–7.
140. Kool B, Ameratunga S, Robinson E. Association between prescription medications and falls at home among young and middle-aged adults. *Inj Prev.* 2012;18(3):200–3.
141. Vallmuur K, Eley R, Watson A. Falls from ladders in Australia: Comparing occupational and non-occupational injuries across age groups. *Aust N Z J Public Health.* 2016;40(6):559–63.
142. Mangharam J, Moorin R, Straker L. A comparison of the burden and resultant risk associated with occupational falls from a height and on the same level in Australia. *Ergonomics.* 2016;59(12):1646–60.
143. Mattila TE, Kaustell KO, Rautiainen RH, et al. Slip, trip and fall injuries in potato, sugar beet and open field vegetable production in Finland. *Ergonomics.* 2008;51(12):1944–59.
144. Bentley T, Tappin D, Moore D, et al. Investigating slips, trips and falls in the New Zealand dairy farming sector. *Ergonomics.* 2005;48(8):1008–19.
145. Son HM, Kim SH, Shin SD, et al. Occupational fall injuries presenting to the emergency department. *Emerg Med Australas.* 2014;26(2):188–93.
146. Wei W, Liu M, Fergenbaum J, Comper P, Colantonio A. Work-related mild–moderate traumatic brain injuries due to falls. *Brain Inj.* 2010;24(11):1358–63.
147. Friedland D, Brunton I, Potts J. Falls and traumatic brain injury in adults under the age of sixty. *J Community Health.* 2014;39(1):148–50.
148. Court-Brown CM, McQueen MM. Global forum: Fractures in the elderly. *J Bone Joint Surg Am.* 2016;98(9):e36.
149. Haines TP, Hill AM, Hill KD, et al. Cost effectiveness of patient education for the prevention of falls in hospital: Economic evaluation from a randomized controlled trial. *BMC Med.* 2013;11:135.
150. Panula J, Pihlajamaki H, Mattila VM, et al. Mortality and cause of death in hip fracture patients aged 65 or older: A population-based study. *BMC Musculoskelet Disord.* 2011;12:105.

151. Vellas BJ, Wayne SJ, Romero LJ, Baumgartner RN, Garry PJ. Fear of falling and restriction of mobility in elderly fallers. *Age Ageing.* 1997;26(3):189–93.
152. Kalula SZ, Scott V, Dowd A, Brodrick K. Falls and fall prevention programmes in developing countries: Environmental scan for the adaptation of the Canadian Falls prevention curriculum for developing countries. *J Safety Res.* 2011;42(6):461–72.
153. Stewart Williams J, Kowal P, Hestekin H, et al. Prevalence, risk factors and disability associated with fall-related injury in older adults in low- and middle-incomecountries: Results from the WHO Study on global AGEing and adult health (SAGE). *BMC Med.* 2015;13:147.
154. Jagnoor J, Keay L, Jaswal N, Kaur M, Ivers R. A qualitative study on the perceptions of preventing falls as a health priority among older people in Northern India. *Inj Prev.* 2014;20(1):29–34.
155. Jitapunkul S, Yuktananandana P, Parkpian V. Risk factors of hip fracture among Thai female patients. *J Med Assoc Thai.* 2001;84(11):1576–81.
156. Ranaweera AD, Fonseka P, PattiyaArachchi A, Siribaddana SH. Incidence and risk factors of falls among the elderly in the District of Colombo. *Ceylon Med J.* 2013;58(3):100–6.
157. Lau EM, Suriwongpaisal P, Lee JK, et al. Risk factors for hip fracture in Asian men and women: The Asian osteoporosis study. *J Bone Miner Res.* 2001;16(3):572–80.
158. Pew Research Center: Baby Boomers Approach 65—Glumly. http://www.pewsocialtrends.org/2010/12/20/baby-boomers-approach-65-glumly/. 2010.
159. Houry D, Florence C, Baldwin G, Stevens J, McClure R. The CDC Injury Center's response to the growing public health problem of falls among older adults. *Am J Lifestyle Med.* 2016;10(1):74–7.
160. O'Hara B, Caswell K. Health Status, Health Insurance, and Medical Services Utilization: 2010. Current Population Reports. www.census.gov/prod/2012pubs/p70-133.pdf. 2013.

CHAPTER

172 Fire and Burns

Karin A. Mack • Michael F. Ballesteros • Shane Diekman • Leila Cuttle*

BACKGROUND

This chapter covers damage to a body resulting from acute exposure to thermal energy—that is burns and scalds, but also smoke inhalation. Further, this review focuses on unintentional fire and burn injuries. Intentional burn injuries (self-inflicted or homicidal) happen worldwide,[1,2] but are especially concerning in certain regions in the world, particularly among young women.[1,3] The prevention of intentional burn injuries are more appropriately covered by interventions related to violence and self-directed harm.

Exposure to fires, flames, and hot items can lead to serious health outcomes, including painful long-lasting scars, impaired lung function, and loss of life. Generally, the most serious injuries among these result from fires (e.g., home fires, cooking fires), but they can result from numerous sources, including hot liquids or surfaces, fireworks, or blast explosions.[1,4–6] Most burn injuries in the home are caused by a hot liquid (scalds), a hot solid (contact burns), or a flame (flame burns).[7] Thermal burns to the skin can occur from contact with a hot object, liquid, or surface such as irons, heaters, microwaved liquids, metal playground slides exposed to the sun, electrical outlets, or open flames. Contact with hot liquids such as grease, heated food, leaking hot water bottles, or steam, through spills or immersion, causes scald burns. Inhalation burns caused by breathing in the products of combustion during a fire, are a key concern in structure fires.[8] This harmful smoke may contain chemicals or poisons such as carbon monoxide. Inhaling harmful smoke can cause the lungs and airways to become irritated, swollen, and blocked.[9] A damaged airway and lungs prevent oxygen from getting into the blood stream (asphyxiation) and respiratory failure may develop.

Preventing unintentional fire and burn injuries covers a broad landscape from preventing the precipitating event (e.g., preventing a fire from starting or preventing skin contact with a hot liquid) to preventing an injury even if the event has occurred (e.g., creating lifesaving egress from a fire). Advances in both of these areas have significantly reduced fire and burn injury rates,[10] and yet the United States fire death rate is at least double that of some other industrialized countries such as Australia, Spain, and Germany.[11] Major concerns for fire morbidity and mortality worldwide include structure fires, but regional concerns exist as well (e.g., wildfires in the United States; cook stove-related injuries in some developing countries). The authors of this chapter reviewed the nature and burden of residential fire and burns in the United States, risk and protective factors, and interventions to prevent fires and injuries. They also examined the burden and prevention of wildfires in the United States. Finally, as examples of fire concerns outside the United States, the authors considered the fire burden and prevention measures in three other countries (China, India, and Australia).

NATURE AND BURDEN OF THE PROBLEM

Home fires are a major public health concern that result in substantial morbidity and mortality. In 2017, 499,000 structure fires were reported to local fire departments in the United States, 72% (n = 357,000) of which occurred in homes.[12] The actual number of fires is much greater as fire departments attend to only 3.4% of fires.[13]

In 2017, fires and burns caused 3398 U.S. deaths[14] and was the seventh most common cause of unintentional injury death in the United States. Among these, 2432 persons died in a residential fire.[14] The overall age-adjusted fire and burn death rate has decreased from 1.41 deaths per 100,000 in 1999 to 0.94 in 2017, a 33% reduction.[14] There were more than 355,000 U.S. emergency department visits for a fire or burn injury (age-adjusted rate = 112.14 per 100,000) where the patient was treated and released in 2017.[14] This number decreased from 497,000 (174.31 per 100,000) in 2001. Additionally, there were another 35,500 visits where the patient was hospitalized or transferred (10.88 per 100,000) in 2017, which was a substantial increase from the 18,200 visits in 2001 (6.42 per 100,000).[14]

Fire risk also varies by region within the United States. The Southeast region contains nearly half of the total U.S. rural population and has historically had the highest fire death rates (see Fig. 172-1).[14] States with the highest fire death rates generally tended to have larger percentages of people living in poverty, people living in rural areas, current smokers, and adults with lower education.[15]

Consequences

After the initial healing and recovery, burn victims also face long-term health challenges such as scarring, restriction in range of motion (if the injury was over a joint), and potential reconstructive surgery.[16] Many burn patients will also experience changes in sensation, including paresthesia and chronic pain.[17,18] Long-term psychological outcomes may include depression and posttraumatic stress disorder.[19,20] Furthermore, physical rehabilitation may improve function and to prevent secondary complications.[21]

Economic Burden

The economic costs of fire and burn injuries can also be substantial. The total cost of fire in 2014 was \$328.5 billion or roughly 1.9% of the U.S. gross domestic product.[22] Property damage represented only \$13.2 billion of this total. Additional costs included net fire insurance (\$23.6 billion), career fire departments operating costs (\$41.9 billion), new building costs for fire protection (\$57.4 billion), and the monetary value of donated time from volunteer firefighters (\$46.9 billion). Fire and burn *injuries* that occurred in 2017 cost \$6.9 billion in direct medical (\$1.4 billion) and work loss costs (\$5.5 billion).[14]

*The findings and conclusions in this chapter are those of the authors and do not necessarily represent the official position of the Centers for Disease Control and Prevention.

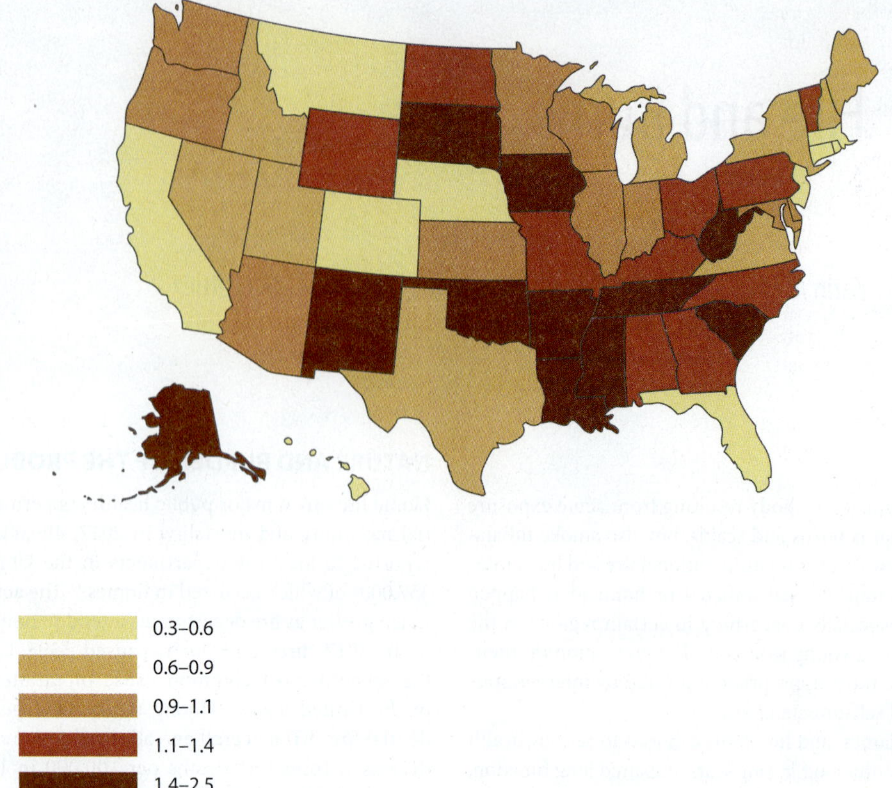

FIGURE 172-1 . Fire/flame deaths per 100,000 population (age adjusted), 2017, United States. (*Source:* Centers for Disease Control and Prevention. Web-based Injury Statistics Query and Reporting System (WISQARS). 2019; www.cdc.gov/ncipc/wisqars. Accessed January 2018.)

This includes $3.3 billion for deaths, $2.2 billion for nonfatal ED visits, and $1.4 billion for hospitalizations.

RISK AND PROTECTIVE FACTORS

According to Turner, Johnson, Weightman, et al. (2017) a robust literature exists to describe risk factors for injury and death from residential fires. Many of these are related to individual limitations that prevent quick escape from a fire (e.g., mobility limitations, hearing impairment, young age, older age, being under the influence of a substance such as alcohol).[4,23,24] Other individual risk factors related to a fire event occurring include the presence of a smoker in the home or a child playing with the ignition source. Populations with higher fire death rates often face multiple health disparities (including persons living in poverty and those with lower levels of education or income).[15,25] Black and American Indian/Eskimo/Aleut individuals face a higher risk of fire death and injury compared to white or Asian individuals.[26,27]

Risk factors related to the home environment and whether a fire event occurs or is amplified include the absence of a smoke alarm, the presence of flammable materials, blocked egress, fewer exits, building code violations, use of candles, lack of a telephone, older homes, mobile homes manufactured prior to 1976, lack of appliance maintenance, and crowded conditions.[4,7,24,28,29] Location can also play a role such as living in the Southeastern United States or living in a rural area, as both are associated with a higher fire death rate.[30]

Protective factors include having a fire escape plan that has been practiced, working smoke alarms placed in appropriate locations, the presence of a residential sprinkler system, properly installed and maintained heating equipment, and being a nonsmoker.[10] Quick fire department response times can also protect against fire-related deaths. In addition, organizations such as the International Code Council (ICC; https://codes.iccsafe.org/content/IFC2018) and the National Fire Protection Association (NFPA; https://www.nfpa.org/Codes-and-Standards) develop, publish, and revise standards and model codes that inform construction and building occupancy to safeguard public health and safety. These codes address and regulate fire-resistance construction, fire protection systems, means of egress, and smoke control. Local governments are responsible for selecting, adopting, and enforcing building codes, and they sometimes rely on these published documents as a resource to set legal requirements.

INTERVENTIONS/BEST AVAILABLE EVIDENCE

Smoke Alarms

Working smoke alarms are effective, reliable, and inexpensive devices that provide early warning during home fires. Results from a 2010 telephone survey showed that 96% of all homes have at least one smoke alarm.[31] Working smoke alarms reduce the risk of dying in home fires[32]; however, the death rate was higher in fires in which smoke alarms were present, but failed to operate, than in homes that had no smoke alarms at all. Compared to homes with no smoke alarms or automatic extinguishing systems (sprinklers), the death rate was 42% lower when smoke alarms were present, and 90% lower when hardwired smoke alarms and sprinklers were present.[32] During 2011–15, almost three of every five home fire deaths resulted from fires where there were no working smoke alarms, including 40% of deaths that resulted from fires with no smoke alarms at all and 17% from fires in which smoke alarms were present, but failed to operate.[4] In reported home fires in which the smoke alarms were present, but did not operate, almost half (46%) of the smoke alarms had missing or disconnected batteries. Nuisance activations (e.g., activations from cooking or low battery warning chirp) were the leading reason for disconnected smoke alarms.[33]

Smoke alarms can be single-station (battery powered) units or hardwired into the home's electrical system. Interconnected smoke alarms are more likely to operate and alert occupants to a fire.[13] Therefore, smoke alarms should be interconnected so that if one sounds, they all do. Whereas most interconnected smoke alarms are hardwired, wireless technology can interconnect single-station battery-powered smoke alarms.[32]

Most home smoke alarms use ionization or photoelectric sensor technology to detect a fire: photoelectric alarms respond faster to smoldering fires and ionization alarms respond faster to flaming fires. Combination alarms that include both technologies in a single device are available and may offer the best protection.[33]

Extended-life, lithium batteries have been promoted in recent years to address the issue of battery replacement. These batteries are typically advertised as lasting 10 years, which coincides with recommendations to replace the entire smoke alarm unit regardless of battery type or power source. Batteries that are not lithium should be replaced annually and the entire unit should be replaced every 10 years.[34] Current NFPA recommendations for smoke alarm placement and number are based on sleeping location and home design: one alarm should be located on each level of the home (including the basement) and one inside and outside of each sleeping area. Larger homes may require additional smoke alarms to provide a minimum level of protection.[34]

Installing, maintaining, and testing smoke alarms according to the manufacturer's instructions are important to ensure they are working properly. The presence of a working smoke alarms at all times is important for protecting occupants in the event of a home fire. Although smoke alarms provide early warning of a fire, they do not stop the danger posed by a growing fire. Occupants must therefore develop and practice an escape plan (https://www.nfpa.org/Public-Education/Staying-safe/Preparedness/Escape-planning).

Lighter/Cigarette Changes

The NFPA reports on yearly estimates related to reported fires involving "play" as a contributing factor.[35] Between 2007 and 2011, among home structure fires involving play, over half (52%) were started with cigarette lighters, compared to 18% by matches and 5% by candles. Forty-three percent of home structure fires involving play were started by a child under the age of 6 years. Older children were more likely to start outside fires, with two out of five (38%) of all outside or unclassified fires started by a child between the ages of 10 and 12 years.

The NFPA recommends that individuals exclusively purchase and use child-resistant lighters. When not in use, matches and lighters should be stored in a locked cabinet, high out of the reach of children.[34] In 1994, Consumer Product Safety Commission (CPSC) introduced a safety standard for cigarette lighters requiring that disposable or novelty lighters have a child-resistant mechanism that makes them difficult for children younger than 5 years to operate. Lighter manufacturers are required to test their products using panels of children between 42 and 51 months of age, 85% of which must not be able to operate them within a defined time limit.[36] The same study showed a 58% reduction in lighter fires started by children younger than 5 years after the introduction of the CPSC standard. Study estimates also showed that the child-resistant standard prevented 3300 fires, 100 deaths, 660 injuries, and $52.5 million in property losses in 1998.

Fire-safe Cigarettes

Fire-safe cigarettes (FSCs) are designed to be less likely than previous cigarettes to ignite household materials such as furniture and mattresses and to self-extinguish when they are not being smoked.[37,38] FSCs typically include two or three thin bands of less-porous paper that act as "speed bumps"—if a FSC is left unattended, the burning tobacco will reach one of these speed bumps and self-extinguish.[37,39] In June 2004, New York was the first U.S. state to pass legislation for the use of FSCs and Canada became the first country to adopt requirements for FSCs the following year. By 2011, all 50 states and the District of Columbia had passed legislation and began implementing FSC laws.[37,40] Folz and Shults (2017) analyzed 2005–12 pooled cross-sectional time series or pooled data for all states (except for New York) to determine whether or not states' FSC laws impacted annual smoking-related home fire fatalities, injuries, and incidents. Their analysis determined that the FSC legislation adopted by the states, when compared to the preimplementation period, was associated with a significant and substantial reduction in the rates of both smoking-related fire deaths and fire incidents started by tobacco products. The analysis also indicated a modest, but statistically nonsignificant impact of the FSC laws on smoking-related injuries. Other work by Bonander, Jakobsson, and Nilson (2018) has suggested that there is a need for stronger evidence of the effects of FSCs on ignition risk and cited inconsistent evidence of the impact of state laws regarding FSCs.

Conversely, while FSCs may be contributing to fire reductions, new concern has risen over the potential for fires and burns from electronic cigarettes.[42–45] Injuries have occurred while the devices were being held in pockets[43,46–48] or while being used.[45] Between 2009 and 2016, researchers examined 195 separate e-cigarette fire and explosion incidents in the United States, and described 133 acute injuries.[49]

Arc Fault Circuit Interrupters

Every time an electrical switch is flipped, an arc of electricity crosses a circuit. Unintentional arc faults occur when the electricity crosses through loose connections or damaged wires.[50] These arc faults can cause sparks and high temperatures that can result in fire by igniting nearby combustibles. Most home fires due electrical failure are due to arc faults.[50] Conventional circuit breakers operate in response to overloads or short circuits, not the erratic current flow associated with unintentional arcing. Arc fault circuit interrupters (AFCIs) continuously monitor and detect these arcs and disconnect electrical power before a fire starts. The 2017 edition of the *National Electrical Code* required the installation of AFCIs in all new residential construction excluding bathrooms, garages, and outside areas. In addition to new construction, AFCI protection is now required in areas where electrical outlets are replaced.[51] These AFCIs should only be installed by a licensed, qualified electrician.

Home Fire Sprinklers

Home fire sprinkler systems are designed to automatically control or extinguish fires allowing occupant(s) time to escape. Sprinkler systems can react to fires as quickly as 35 seconds. A 2017 NFPA report derived estimates using 2010–14 data to characterize the United States experience with fire sprinkler systems.[52] During this time, sprinklers were present in 10% of reported U.S. fires. Sprinklers operated 92% of the time in fires considered large enough to activate them. In those fires, they effectively controlled the fire 96% of the time. The civilian death rate of 1.4 per 1000 reported fires was more than 80% lower in homes with sprinklers than in homes with no automatic extinguishing systems (7.5 per 1000 reported fires).[52]

Wet pipe sprinklers have sprinkler heads directly attached to pipes containing water, and are the most common type of fire sprinkler.[53] One of the major arguments offered against installing sprinkler systems has been the cost, but recent studies have shown it is much lower than expected and can be made lower still by innovative methods. One study of the cost of adding sprinklers to 51 different houses in 17 U.S. cities and 1 Canadian city showed that the average cost to the home builder was $1.35 per sprinklered square foot.[54] This was lower than the $1.61 per sprinklered square foot mean cost found in a similar 2008 study.[55] The authors suggested that the reduction in costs during the 5-year period was likely due to "increased adoption of sprinkler ordinances, improved installation methods, standardized practices, and increased contractor competition...." Both studies (2008 and 2013) showed that higher costs were associated with greater use of copper piping, lack of a municipal water supply, higher permit fees, and local requirements for sprinklers in additional areas such as garages and attics. Numerous demonstration projects have been conducted to reduce installation costs, simplify installation, and to investigate infrastructure and code alternatives and incentives for installing these systems.[56]

WILDFIRES IN THE UNITED STATES

Wildfires are common in the United States. The record for the number of acres burned was set in 2015 when 68,151 fires burned 10.1 million acres.[57] More fires occurred in 2017 (71,499), but slightly fewer acres burned (10 million). However, 2017 was an especially challenging year for California because historic fires damaged or destroyed more than 32,000 homes and 4300 businesses across the state.[58] The combined destruction of four of the wildfires (Tubbs, Atlas, Nuns, and Redwood Valley) represented the costliest wildfire event on record.[59]

Wildfires destroy property, but they also pose a significant public health threat and contribute to premature mortality, increased need for healthcare, lost productivity, lower quality of life, and compromised drinking water quality.[60] Adverse health outcomes occur near the burn area, but also extend well beyond that due to smoke dispersion. The adverse health outcomes from exposure to the particulate matter of wildfires can include respiratory morbidity (respiratory tract irritation, asthma exacerbation, bronchitis, and decreased lung function) as well as contribute to cardiovascular/cerebrovascular events and all-cause mortality.[61–63] Children and older adults may be especially susceptible to these adverse health outcomes.[62]

Researchers have developed an online tool that can identify at-risk populations for wildfire smoke hazards. This has been incorporated into the Center for Disease Control and Prevention's (CDC) National Environmental Public Health Tracking Network (http://ephtracking.cdc.gov).[61] The purpose of the tool is to strengthen existing situational awareness and expedite response and recovery efforts during wildfire episodes.

INTERNATIONAL EXAMPLES

There has been a decrease of burn incidence, severity, and mortality worldwide in recent years.[64,65] The burden and source of these injuries, however, varies by country. Structure fires are cause for concern in every country, but the source of the fire can vary widely—consider electrical wiring failure as a source versus open fire cooking. In many low- and middle-income countries (LMICs), cookstoves are a primary source of cooking and heating, and as such are a major source of fires, burns, and air-quality issues.[66] Cookstoves may represent the single most important modifiable risk factor for burn injuries in LMICs because they are amenable to multiple technological and behavioral modifications.[66] While considered a clean fuel, the use of liquefied petroleum gas has also contributed to the fire and burn problem in LMICs because of cylinder leaks.[67–69] Interventions to reduce exposure to fires and flames seem intuitively correct, but have largely not yet been formally tested for effectiveness in reducing burn injuries.

Individuals at risk for fire and burn injury can also vary widely by country. For example, gender differences between high-income countries and low-income countries for fire deaths can be polar opposites.[65] In the United States, the 2017 fire/burn death rate was higher for males (1.26; crude rate) than for females (0.83).[14] However, the death rate for females is higher than for males in countries where cooking is done primarily by women with an open flame.[70,71]

International Burn Registry

Tertiary hospitals specializing in burn care often collect information about their admitted patients. This information allows those hospitals to track morbidity, disability, cost, and use of resources; inform and evaluate prevention strategies, programs, and policies; and to generate reports for research. Burn registries, which collect defined datasets from these types of hospitals, can provide global surveillance information about this topic. Burn centers located in large metropolitan areas and in higher income countries typically collect data about hospitalized patients. This results in underestimates of burns in LMICs because of the paucity of such specialty centers in many developing nations. In 2014, researchers piloted a Global Burn Registry (GBR) form and online data entry systems[71] to standardize and validate formats that would enable assembling national data into centralized burn registries. Based on the findings from the GBR pilot, the World Health Organization (WHO) now maintains a Global Burn Registry (http://www.who.int/violence_injury_prevention/burns/gbr/en/). The GBR moves burn injury data collection from a range of fragmented approaches to an improved, standardized, and global system for this important public health problem. Conceivably, the GBR should enable cross-country comparisons, including burn injuries related to combustion of household fuels used for cooking (e.g., cookstoves), heating, and lighting.

China

Mortality from fire and burns has decreased gradually in the past several decades in China[72–74] and studies show significant progress in burn care and treatment.[75] Reportedly, 9000–12,000 fire/burn-related deaths occur per year, with overall death rates ranging from 0.74 to 0.89 per 100,000.[74,76] Burns are more common among males, young children (less than 5 years) and young adults (20–30 years), with scalds and flames being the common cause of hospitalizations.[72,75,77] Fire-related deaths exhibit a seasonal pattern with a higher occurrence in the early Spring.[73]

Emerging concerns in China include those associated with liquefied petroleum gas and wildfires. A recent study showed an exponential increase in liquefied petroleum gas burns between 2011 and 2015, with most (83%) occurring at home.[67] Forest fires are also a concern, with recent events causing many firefighter fatalities.[78]

India

The death rate from unintentional fire in India was 3 per 100,000 in 2005.[79] Findings from Sanghavi, Bhalla, and Das (2009) uncovered more than 163,000 fire-related deaths in 2001 in India, which was 2% of all deaths in the country. Other reports show that 7 million burn incidents occur annually.[81] According to recent studies of burn cases in India, most victims are female[79,82] and adolescents/young adults (ages 12–26 years).[82] The high proportion of fire-related deaths among young adult women in India has been concerning[79] and has been attributed to unsafe cooking practices and traditional clothing that easily ignites, as well as to intentional fires from self-immolation and domestic violence.[80,82,83]

India has begun a national program to prevent burn injuries (http://dghs.gov.in/content/1357_3_ National ProgrammePrevention-Management.aspx) which includes prevention, burn injury patient management, and rehabilitation programs for burn victims.[81,84] More than 50 medical colleges and 17 district hospitals have been approved to establish burn units.

Australia

Most fatal burns are caused by exposure to smoke, fire, and flames, predominantly due to residential fires. Ten-year data (2007–16) from the Australian Bureau of Statistics shows that the average number of deaths due to exposure to smoke fire and flames (ICD-10-AM codes X00-09) or contact with heat and hot substances (X10-19) has been decreasing.[85] An average of 87 people per year lost their lives due to fire or burns during this period. The mortality rate from burns has remained low, reported as 0.62/100,000 in the state of Victoria.[86] The rate is higher among males and increases with age, such that the rate is 2.71/100,000 for adults aged 80+ years.[86]

Hospital admissions for burn injury are increasing at each burn center; however due to inconsistencies in data collection between time periods, determining overall Australian temporal trends is difficult.[87,86] Males and children under the age of 4 years are overrepresented[88] and the single leading cause of hospital admission is scalds from hot drinks and food.[86] Young children and the elderly are more commonly burned by contact with hot water, whereas young people aged 15–24 years and adults are more commonly affected by ignition of highly flammable material and flame burns. Most burns (84%) are less than 10% total body surface area (TBSA), with only 3% of total hospitalized burns being > 20% TBSA.[87]

As most burns occur in the home, Australian burn prevention initiatives have focused on improvements to building codes and legislation. To prevent hot water scalds, all newly installed water heaters are required by Australian building codes and standards to ensure that water temperature does not exceed 50°C or 45°C for child-care facilities, schools, clinics/hospitals, and nursing homes.[89] Data show that the rate of hospital admissions for hot tap water scalds has decreased, particularly for children under the age of 4 years after these regulations were introduced into the state of New South Wales in 1999.[90] To prevent deaths from house fires, each Australian state and territory adopted the National Construction Code (NCC; https://www.abcb.gov.au/Connect/Categories/National-Construction-Code) in 2011, which required the mandatory installation of smoke alarms. Australian Standard 3786 also regulates manufacturing standards for smoke alarms.[91] However, legal requirements still vary across states for houses built prior to the NCC. Rental homes fall under other code requirements.

Gaps exist in population-level data related to residential fire deaths, smoke alarm use in houses from different fire service jurisdictions, water temperature-valve installations in residential properties, and in burn injury rates (hospitalized and otherwise), which makes it difficult to assess the effectiveness of these interventions. Most recently, Australian burn prevention campaigns have used smartphone apps and social media strategies to reach broad audiences. Education regarding burn prevention and burn first aid treatment can be targeted to discrete populations via social media and changes in public knowledge can be assessed using the smartphone technology platform.[92]

RESOURCES

Fire-*prevention* strategies aim to prevent a fire from occurring, for example, by making materials harder to ignite or by changing the environment so that a heat source is prevented from combining with fuel to start a fire.[93] Fire *protection* strategies apply after ignition occurs and play an important role in reducing injuries and deaths.[93] For example, home escape planning and fire drills help ensure that if a fire occurs, everyone present will know how to get out quickly and safely. Many fire-prevention and protection strategies can help reduce residential fire injuries and death [see especially World Health Organization (2011)]. The following section provides information and resources related to implementing prevention and protection strategies, and about the Federal Emergency Management Agency's (FEMA) innovative grant programs.

General Fire Safety Tips and Prevention Programs

Several U.S. organizations provide home fire prevention and safety tips, and materials for community education programs. They include the American Red Cross (https://www.redcross.org/get-help/how-to-prepare-for-emergencies/types-of-emergencies/fire.html), the U.S. Fire Administration (https://www.usfa.fema.gov/prevention/outreach/education_programs.html), the NFPA (https://www.nfpa.org/Public-Education/Resources/Education-Programs), the National Safety Council (https://www.nsc.org/home-safety/safety-topics/emergency-preparedness/fire), Safe Kids Worldwide (https://www.safekids.org/fire), and the U.S. Consumer Product Safety Commission (https://www.cpsc.gov/safety-education/safety-guides/home/fire/). Local fire departments often use these materials to develop and deliver prevention programs that are administered at schools and community centers and events.

Smoke Alarms

Reviews that rate the evidence for certain fire injury prevention interventions consider smoke alarms effective [see World Health Organization (2011), Warda, and Ballesteros (2007)]. Smoke alarms (a fire protection strategy) provide early warning of a developing fire, which can allow for additional escape time, but homes need to have operational and properly placed alarms. Information about lessons learned from smoke alarm giveaway and installation programs have been presented in the research literature.[95–104] Guidance also exists for program implementation. Both the NFPA and the FEMA have webpages devoted to smoke alarm installation and outreach (https://www.nfpa.org/Public-Education/By-topic/Smoke-alarms/Installing-and-maintaining-smoke-alarms; https://www.usfa.fema.gov/prevention/outreach/smoke_alarms.html). The NFPA has a guide for planning and implementing a successful smoke alarm installation program (https://www.nfpa.org/-/media/Files/Public-Education/By-topic/Smoke-alarms/Smoke-Alarm-Installation-Guide.pdf) and a free desk reference of the most current smoke alarm prevention education messages.[34] The National Fire Safety Council (https://nfsc.org/materials) offers fire safety educational materials. Implementation resources are also available for targeted/certain groups such as the FEMA/CDC toolkit that was designed to run a comprehensive fire safety program for older adults (https://www.usfa.fema.gov/prevention/outreach/fire_safe_seniors.html).[105]

Working carbon monoxide (CO) detectors are also important. Carbon monoxide is an odorless, colorless gas which can cause sudden illness and death and is produced any time a fossil fuel is burned. Resources for preventing CO poisoning are available from CDC (https://www.cdc.gov/co/default.htm) and a prevention toolkit is also offered to help keep communities safe (https://www.nphic.org/toolkits/carbon-monoxide).

Residential Sprinklers

One strategy listed by Warda, and Ballesteros (2007), that had insufficient evidence at the time was the use of residential sprinklers; however, they can be a life-saving technology. Diffusion of this technology has begun and efforts to require sprinklers in new home construction are underway. The NFPA's Fire Sprinkler Initiative (https://www.nfpa.org/Public-Education/Campaigns/Fire-Sprinkler-Initiative) helps stakeholders navigate the code process to establish fire sprinkler requirements for new homes in their communities. The initiative offers resources and on-the-ground support to promote the life-saving impact of home fire sprinklers.

Wildfires

As more people move into areas that are prone to wildfires, special consideration should be taken to prepare a home and landscaping to reduce the risk of injury. The Johns Hopkins Bloomberg School of Public Health held a symposium where speakers discussed health and safety concerns for homeowners in fire-prone areas and ways to mitigate risks.[106] CDC has resources on protection from a wildfire, safe evacuation during a wildfire, and how to stay healthy when returning home after a wildfire (https://www.cdc.gov/disasters/wildfires/ and https://www.cdc.gov/air/wildfire-smoke/default.htm). The U.S. Environmental Protection Agency (EPA) has developed an infographic about how to reduce exposure to wildfire smoke, select the correct respirator mask, and how to properly wear the mask to protect your health (https://www.epa.gov/air-research/how-order-infographic-card-reduce-health-risks-areas-wildfire-smoke) and a guide for public health professionals to help prepare for smoke events (https://www3.epa.gov/airnow/wildfire_may2016.pdf). In addition, EPA is conducting a citizen science study using a mobile application to evaluate health effects from wildland fires and to test whether health risks can be communicated effectively through resources and engagement from the app. *Smoke Sense* is a mobile app available in the Google Play Store and the Apple App Store. Finally, local health

BOX 172.1 Make a Wildfire planruled

- Know your **wildfire risk** (http://www.nps.gov/fire/wildland-fire/learning-center/fire-in-depth/understanding-fire-danger.cfm).
- Familiarize yourself with local emergency plans. Know where to go and how to get there should you need to evacuate.
- Make a wildfire emergency plan including an evacuation plan and a communication plan.
- Many communities have text or email alerting systems for emergency notifications. To find out what alerts are available in your area, search the Internet with your town, city, or county name and the word "alerts."
- Build or restock your emergency preparedness kit, including a flashlight, batteries, cash, and first-aid supplies.
- Stay tuned to your phone alerts, TV, or radio, for weather updates, emergency instructions or evacuation orders.

Source: https://www.ready.gov/wildfires.

departments, responders, and the general public can find assistance with preparing and responding to wildfire events at (http://nacchopreparedness.org/wildfire-health-and-safety-information-resources).

Firefighter Safety and Advanced Fire Safety Practices

FEMA's Assistance to Firefighters Grant (AFG) program and the Fire and Prevention Safety (FP&S) Grants program provide funding and support for projects that enhance the safety of firefighters and the public from fire and related hazards. The main focus of the FP&S grants is to reduce injury and to prevent death in high-risk populations. In 2005, Congress reauthorized funding for FP&S and expanded the eligible uses of funds to include Firefighter Safety Research and Development. More about this program, including success stories, can be found at https://www.fema.gov/fire-prevention-safety-grants.

Data Visualization Tools

Two notable tools are available to examine the fire problem in the United States. An NFPA tool (https://data.nfpa.org/dataportal/index.html) captures national fire incidents, incident causalities and provides a *Remembering When*™ Map. It allows users to explore and compare two national data sets on a dynamic platform that maps historical data on fires using NFPA's custom geolocation of information from the U.S. Fire Administration's National Fire Incident Reporting System. CDC's Web-based Injury Statistics Query and Reporting System (WISQARS) Fatal Injury Data Visualization (https://wisqars-viz.cdc.gov:8006/) can be used to query death data over time (2001–17), create state maps, and look at the distribution of injury-related deaths by demographics such as sex and age. CDC's Environmental Public Health Tracking Network (https://ephtracking.cdc.gov/) is a dynamic, web-based data system that individuals can use to track environmental and health factors over time. For example, an individual can get 48-hour forecasts for smoke in areas down to the census travel level.

CONCLUSIONS

Despite substantial reductions in fire-related deaths in the United States overall, one civilian fire death occurred every 2.5 hours in 2017[12] Cooking was the leading cause of home fires and home fire injuries, while smoking was the leading cause in home fire deaths.[5] Many people are aware of lifesaving and fire-prevention interventions; however, they are not fully used across the population. For example, the United States has yet to achieve full saturation of working smoke alarms in homes.

Although authors discussed the public health burden of fire injury across populations, this chapter did not cover all fire- and burn-related conditions. For example, it does not cover vehicle fires which account for 8% of fire-related deaths in the United States.[107] Authors also did not review changes in post event treatment, which can reduce the impact of thermal injuries including increased survival and improved functional recovery. Burn trauma treatment advancements include novel graft options and innovations in wound closure and imaging.[108]

Technology improvements can certainly prevent fires and save lives. These range from simple modifications to more complex system modifications. For example, some appliances now have automatic shutoffs to prevent fires. Portable electric heaters employ automatic shutoffs if tipped over, and coffee makers and irons have timers that will shut the equipment off after a period of time if not actively in use. Complex home system modifications have great potential, but are not yet fully developed for widespread application. Nevertheless, systems such as continuous home monitoring through smart technology could detect risks, deploy shutoffs, notify residents and the fire department, and activate suppression systems.[10]

References

1. Peck MD. Epidemiology of burns throughout the World. Part II: Intentional burns in adults. *Burns.* 2012;38(5):630–7.
2. Reiland A, Hovater M, McGwin G Jr, Rue LW 3rd, Cross JM. The epidemiology of intentional burns. *J Burn Care Res.* 2006;27(3):276–80.
3. Gupta S, Mahmood U, Gurung S, et al. Intentional burns—A form of gender based violence in Nepal. *Burns.* 2016;42(3):713.
4. Ahrens M. *Home Structure Fires.* Quincy, MA: National Fire Protection Association; 2018. https://www.nfpa.org/-/media/Files/News-and-Research/Fire-statistics-and-reports/Building-and-life-safety/oshomes.pdf.
5. National Fire Protection Association. *An Overview of the U.S. Fire Problem.* 2017. https://www.nfpa.org/-/media/Files/News-and-Research/Fire-statistics/Fact-sheets/FireLossFacts.pdf.
6. Aherns M. *Fireworks.* Quincy, MA: National Fire Protection Association; 2016. https://www.nfpa.org/-/media/Files/News-and-Research/Fire-statistics-and-reports/US-Fire-Problem/Fire-causes/osfireworks.ashx?la=en.
7. World Health Organization. *Burn Prevention Success Stories Lessons Learned.* Geneva, Switzerland; 2011. http://apps.who.int/iris/bitstream/10665/97938/1/9789241501187_eng.pdf.
8. National Fire Protection Association. Reporter's Guide: The consequences of fire. https://www.nfpa.org/News-and-Research/Publications-and-media/Press-Room/Reporters-Guide-to-Fire-and-NFPA/Consequences-of-fire. Accessed June, 2019.
9. Dries DJ, Endorf FW. Inhalation injury: Epidemiology, pathology, treatment strategies. *Scand J Trauma Resusc Emerg Med.* 2013;21:31.
10. Gielen AC, Frattaroli S, Pollack KM, Peek-Asa C, Yang JG. How the science of injury prevention contributes to advancing home fire safety in the USA: Successes and opportunities. *Inj Prev.* 2018;24(Suppl 1):i7–13.
11. U.S. Department of Homeland Security, U.S. Fire Administration. *Fire Death Rate Trends: an International Perspective.* Emmitsburg, MD: National Fire Data Center; 2011. https://www.usfa.fema.gov/downloads/pdf/statistics/v12i8.pdf.
12. Evarts B. *Fire Loss in the United States During 2017.* Quincy, MA: National Fire Protection Association; 2018. https://www.nfpa.org/-/media/Files/News-and-Research/Fire-statistics-and-reports/US-Fire-Problem/osFireLoss.pdf.
13. Greene MA, Andres C. *2004–2005 National Sample Survey of Unreported Residential Fires.* Washington, DC: U.S. Commission Product Safety Commission; 2009. https://www.cpsc.gov/s3fs-public/UnreportedResidentialFires.pdf.
14. Centers for Disease Control and Prevention. Web-based Injury Statistics Query and Reporting System (WISQARS). 2019. www.cdc.gov/ncipc/wisqars. Accessed January, 2018.
15. Ahrens M. *U.S. Fire Death Rates by State.* Quincy, MA: National Fire Protection Association; 2018. https://www.nfpa.org/-/media/Files/News-and-Research/Fire-statistics-and-reports/US-Fire-Problem/osstate.pdf.
16. Falder S, Browne A, Edgar D, et al. Core outcomes for adult burn survivors: A clinical overview. *Burns.* 2009;35(5):618–41.
17. Malenfant A, Forget R, Papillon J, Amsel R, Frigon JY, Choinière M. Prevalence and characteristics of chronic sensory problems in burn patients. *Pain.* 1996;67(2–3):493–500.
18. Dauber A, Osgood PF, Breslau AJ, Vernon HL, Carr DB. Chronic persistent pain after severe burns: A survey of 358 burn survivors. *Pain Med.* 2002;3(1):6–17.

19. Thombs BD, Haines JM, Bresnick MG, Magyar-Russell G, Fauerbach JA, Spence RJ. Depression in burn reconstruction patients: Symptom prevalence and association with body image dissatisfaction and physical function. *Gen Hosp Psychiatry*. 2007;29(1):14–20.
20. Baur KM, Hardy PE, Van Dorsten B. Posttraumatic stress disorder in burn populations: A critical review of the literature. *J Burn Care Rehabil.* 1998;19(3):230–40.
21. Sliwa JA, Heinemann A, Semik P. Inpatient rehabilitation following burn injury: Patient demographics and functional outcomes. *Arch Phys Med Rehabil.* 2005;86(10):1920–3.
22. Zhuang J, Payyappalli V, Behrendt A, Lukasiewicz K. *Total Cost of Fire in the United States*. Quincy, MA: National Fire Protection Association; 2017. https://www.nfpa.org/-/media/Files/News-and-Research/Fire-statistics-and-reports/US-Fire-Problem/RFTotalCost.pdf.
23. Turner S, Johnson R, Weightman A, et al. Risk factors associated with unintentional house fire incidents, injuries and deaths in high-income countries: A systematic review. *Inj Prev*. 2017;23(2):131–7.
24. Xiong L, Bruck D, Ball M. Preventing accidental residential fires: The role of human involvement in non-injury house fires. *Fire Mater*. 2017;41:3–16.
25. Ahrens M. *Characteristics of Home Fire Victims*. Quincy, MA: National Fire Protection Association; 2014.
26. Bishai D, Lee S. Heightened risk of fire deaths among older African Americans and native Americans. *Public Health Rep*. 2010;125(3):406–13.
27. Flynn J. *Characteristics of Home Fire Victims*. Quincy, MA: National Fire Protection Association; 2010. http://tkolb.net/FireReports/HomeFireVictims2010.pdf.
28. Shai D. Income, housing, and fire injuries: A census tract analysis. *Public Health Rep*. 2006;121(2):149–54.
29. National Fire Protection Association. Fire safety in manufactured homes. https://www.nfpa.org/Public-Education/By-topic/Safety-in-the-home/Escape-planning/Fire-safety-in-manufactured-homes. Accessed March, 2018.
30. National Fire Protection Association. *Demographic and Other Characteristics Related to Fire Deaths or Injuries*. 2010. https://www.nfpa.org/-/media/Files/News-and-Research/Fire-statistics/Victim-Patterns/ossocfactors.ashx?la=en.
31. Harris Poll National Quorum. *Smoke Alarms*. Quincy, MA: National Fire Protection Association; 2010.
32. Ahrens M. *Smoke Alarms in U.S. Home Fires*. Quincy, MA: National Fire Protection Association; 2019. https://www.nfpa.org/-/media/Files/News-and-Research/Fire-statistics-and-reports/Detection-and-signaling/ossmokealarms.pdf.
33. Ahrens M. *Smoke Alarms in U.S. Home Fires*. Quincy, MA: National Fire Protection Association; 2014.
34. National Fire Protection Association. *NFPA Educational Messages Desk Reference*. 2017.
35. Campbell R. *Playing with Fire*. Quincy, MA: National Fire Protection Association; 2014. https://www.nfpa.org/-/media/Files/News-and-Research/Fire-statistics-and-reports/US-Fire-Problem/Fire-causes/oschildplay.ashx?la=en.
36. Smith LE, Greene MA, Singh HA. Study of the effectiveness of the US safety standard for child resistant cigarette lighters. *Inj Prev*. 2002;8(3):192–6.
37. Folz DH, Shults C. The impact of state fire safe cigarette policies on fire fatalities, injuries, and incidents. *J Emerg Manag*. 2017;15(6):379–89.
38. Butry DT, Thomas DS. Cigarette fires involving upholstered furniture in residences: The role that smokers, smoker behavior, and fire standard compliant cigarettes play. *Fire Technol*. 2017;53(3):1123–46.
39. Hall J. *The Smoking-Material Fire Problem*. Quincy, MA: National Fire Protection Association; 2012.
40. Coalition for Fire-Safe Cigarettes. https://www.nfpa.org/public-education/by-topic/top-causes-of-fire/smoking/coalition-for-fire-safe-cigarettes.
41. Bonander C, Jakobsson N, Nilson F. Are fire safe cigarettes actually fire safe? Evidence from changes in US state laws. *Inj Prev*. 2018;24(3):193–8.
42. Ramirez JI, Ridgway CA, Lee JG, et al. The unrecognized epidemic of electronic cigarette burns. *J Burn Care Res*. 2017;38(4):220–4.
43. Simpson LJ, Lye G. Burns injuries from e-cigarettes kept in pockets. *BMJ*. 2019;364:l554.
44. Hassan S, Anwar MU, Muthayya P, Jivan S. Burn injuries from exploding electronic cigarette batteries: An emerging public health hazard. *J Plast Reconstr Aesthet Surg*. 2016;69(12):1716–8.
45. Kumetz EA, Hurst ND, Cudnik RJ, Rudinsky SL. Electronic cigarette explosion injuries. *Am J Emerg Med*. 2016;34(11):2252.e2251–3.
46. Treitl D, Solomon R, Davare DL, Sanchez R, Kiffin C. Full and partial thickness burns from spontaneous combustion of e-cigarette lithium-ion batteries with review of literature. *J Emerg Med*. 2017;53(1):121–5.
47. Maraqa T, Mohamed MAT, Salib M, Morris S, Mercer L, Sachwani-Daswani GR. Too hot for your pocket! Burns from e-cigarette lithium battery explosions: A case series. *J Burn Care Res*. 2018;39(6):1043–7.
48. Hickey S, Goverman J, Friedstat J, Sheridan R, Schulz J. Thermal injuries from exploding electronic cigarettes. *Burns*. 2018;44(5):1294–1301.
49. McKenna L. *Electronic Cigarette Fires and Explosions in the United States 2009–2016*. U.S. Fire Administration; 2017. https://www.usfa.fema.gov/downloads/pdf/publications/electronic_cigarettes.pdf.
50. Campbell R. *Home Electrical Fires*. Quincy, MA: National Fire Protection Association; 2019.
51. National Fire Protection Association. *NFPA 70-2017 Edition: National Electrical Code (NEC)*. https://www.nfpa.org/codes-and-standards/all-codes-and-standards/list-of-codes-and-standards/detail?code=70.
52. Ahrens M. *US Experience with Sprinklers*. Quincy, MA: National Fire Protection Association; 2017. https://www.nfpa.org/-/media/Files/News-and-Research/Fire-statistics-and-reports/Suppression/ossprinklers.pdf.
53. Butry DT. Comparing the performance of residential fire sprinklers with other life-safety technologies. *Accid Anal Prev*. 2012;48:480–94.
54. Newport Partners. *Home Fire Sprinkler Cost Assessment*. Quincy, MA: Fire Protection Research Foundation; 2013. https://www.nfpa.org/-/media/Files/News-and-Research/Fire-statistics-and-reports/Suppression/HomeFireSprinklerCostAssessment2013.ashx?la=en.
55. Newport Partners. *Home Fire Sprinkler Cost Assessment*. Quincy, MA: Fire Protection Research Foundation; 2008.
56. National Fire Protection Association. Sprinkler performance and benefits research. https://www.nfpa.org/Public-Education/Staying-safe/Safety-equipment/Home-fire-sprinklers/Fire-Sprinkler-Initiative/Benefits-of-home-fire-sprinklers/Sprinkler-performance-and-benefits-research. Accessed July 22, 2019.
57. National Interagency Coordination Center. *Wildland Fire Summary and Statistics Annual Report*. 2017. https://www.predictiveservices.nifc.gov/intelligence/2017_statssumm/annual_report_2017.pdf.
58. California Department of Insurance. California statewide wildfire insurance claims nearly $12 billion [press release]. 2018.
59. National Oceanic and Atmospheric Administration. Billion-dollar weather and climate disasters: Table of events. https://www.ncdc.noaa.gov/billions/events/US/2017. Accessed March, 2019.
60. Cascio WE. Wildland fire smoke and human health. *Sci Total Environ*. 2018;624:586–95.
61. Vaidyanathan A, Yip F, Garbe P. Developing an online tool for identifying at-risk populations to wildfire smoke hazards. *Sci Total Environ*. 2018;619–20:376–83.
62. Reid CE, Brauer M, Johnston FH, Jerrett M, Balmes JR, Elliott CT. Critical review of health impacts of wildfire smoke exposure. *Environ Health Perspect*. 2016;124(9):1334–43.
63. Wettstein ZS, Hoshiko S, Fahimi J, Harrison RJ, Cascio WE, Rappold AG. Cardiovascular and Cerebrovascular Emergency Department visits associated with wildfire smoke exposure in California in 2015. *J Am Heart Assoc*. 2018;7(8):e007492.
64. Smolle C, Cambiaso-Daniel J, Forbes AA, et al. Recent trends in burn epidemiology worldwide: A systematic review. *Burns*. 2017;43(2):249–57.
65. Peck MD. Epidemiology of burns throughout the world. Part I: Distribution and risk factors. *Burns*. 2011;37(7):1087–100.
66. Diekman ST, Pope D, Falk H, et al. WHO indoor air quality guidelines: Household fuel combustion. *Review 10: Burns and Poisoning*. Geneva: WHO; 2014.
67. Jin R, Wu P, Ho JK, Wang X, Han C. Five-year epidemiology of liquefied petroleum gas-related burns. *Burns*. 2018;44(1):210–7.
68. Tarim MA. Evaluation of burn injuries related to liquefied petroleum gas. *J Burn Care Res*. 2014;35(3):e159–63.
69. Paliwal G, Agrawal K, Srivastava RK, Sharma S. Domestic liquefied petroleum gas: Are we using a kitchen bomb? *Burns*. 2014;40(6):1219–24.
70. World Health Organization. Facts about injuries: Burns. 2018. http://www.who.int/mediacentre/factsheets/fs365/en/.
71. Peck MD, Falk H, Meddings D, Sugerman D, Mehta S, Sage M. The design and evaluation of a system for improved surveillance and prevention programmes in resource-limited settings using a hospital-based burn injury questionnaire. *Inj Prev*. 2016;22(Suppl 1):i56–62.
72. Cheng W, Wang S, Shen C, Zhao D, Li D, Shang Y. Epidemiology of hospitalized burn patients in China: A systematic review. *Burns Open*. 2018;2(1):8–16.

73. Lu S, Li G, Mei P, Zhang H. Suppressive effects of fire prevention campaign in China: A time series analysis. *Saf Sci.* 2016;86:69–77.
74. Zhou M, Wang H, Zhu J, et al. Cause-specific mortality for 240 causes in China during 1990–2013: A systematic subnational analysis for the Global Burden of Disease Study 2013. *Lancet.* 2016;387(10015):251–72.
75. Fan X, Ma B, Zeng D, et al. Burns in a major burns center in East China from 2005 to 2014: Incidence and outcome. *Burns.* 2017;43(7):1586–95.
76. Wang SY, Li YH, Chi GB, et al. Injury-related fatalities in China: An under-recognised public-health problem. *Lancet.* 2008;372(9651):1765–73.
77. Li H, Wang S, Tan J, Zhou J, Wu J, Luo G. Epidemiology of pediatric burns in southwest China from 2011 to 2015. *Burns.* 2017;43(6):1306–17.
78. Myers S. 30 Die fighting forest fire in China. New York Times. April 1, 2019.
79. Jagnoor J, Suraweera W, Keay L, Ivers RQ, Thakur J, Jha P. Unintentional injury mortality in India, 2005: Nationally representative mortality survey of 1.1 million homes. *BMC Public Health.* 2012;12(1):487.
80. Sanghavi P, Bhalla K, Das V. Fire-related deaths in India in 2001: A retrospective analysis of data. *Lancet.* 2009;373(9671):1282–8.
81. Gupta JL, Makhija LK, Bajaj SP. National programme for prevention of burn injuries. *Indian J Plast Surg.* 2010;43(Suppl):S6–10.
82. Bhansali C, Gandhi G, Sahastrabudhe P, Panse N. Epidemiological study of burn injuries and its mortality risk factors in a tertiary care hospital. *Indian J Burns.* 2017;25(1):62–6.
83. Bhate-Deosthali P, Lingam L. Gendered pattern of burn injuries in India: A neglected health issue. *Reprod Health Matters.* 2016;24(47):96–103.
84. Sachan D. India launches major programme to treat burn injuries. *BMJ.* 2014;348:g1658.
85. Australian Bureau of Statistics. 3303.0 Causes of death, Australia, 2016. 2017.
86. Wasiak J, Spinks A, Ashby K, Clapperton A, Cleland H, Gabbe B. The epidemiology of burn injuries in an Australian setting, 2000–2006. *Burns.* 2009;35(8):1124–32.
87. Tracy L, McInnes J, Gong J, Gabbe B, Thomas T. *Burns Registry of Australia and New Zealand—Annual Report.* Monash University Department of Epidemiology and Preventative Medicine; 2017. https://www.branz.org/__data/assets/pdf_file/0005/1411349/BRANZ-8th-Annual-Report-Jul-16-Jun-17_0.pdf.
88. Australian Institute of Health and Welfare, Pointer S, Tovell A. *Hospitalised Burn Injuries, Australia, 2013–2014.* Canberra: Australian Institute of Health and Welfare; 2016. https://www.aihw.gov.au/getmedia/aa910281-ad80-4963-808e-c41bc7191039/20432.pdf.aspx?inline=true.
89. Australian/ New Zealand Standard. *3500.4:2003 Plumbing and drainage. Part 4: Heated water services.* 2003.
90. Harvey LA, Poulos RG, Finch CF, Olivier J, Harvey JG. Hospitalised hot tap water scald patients following the introduction of regulations in NSW, Australia: Who have we missed? *Burns.* 2010;36(6):912–9.
91. Legal and Constitutional Affairs References Committee, Commonwealth of Australia. *Use of Smoke Alarms to Prevent Smoke and Fire Related Deaths.* Canberra: Department of the Senate, Parliament House; 2016. https://www.aph.gov.au/Parliamentary_Business/Committees/Senate/Legal_and_Constitutional_Affairs/Fire_safety/~/media/Committees/legcon_ctte/Fire_safety/report.pdf.
92. Burgess JD, Watt KA, Kimble RM, Cameron CM. Knowledge of childhood burn risks and burn first aid: Cool Runnings. *Inj Prev.* 2019;25:301–6.
93. Diekman S, Ballesteros MF, Ahrens M. Home fires in America: Progress and opportunities. *Am J Lifestyle Med.* 2012;6(2):141–51.
94. Warda L, Ballesteros M. Interventions to prevent residential fire injury In: Doll B, Mercy, Sleet, eds. *Handbook of Injury and Violence Prevention.* New York: Springer; 2007, pp. 97–115.
95. Omaki EC, Frattaroli S, Shields WC, et al. Pilot study of a novel partnership for installing smoke alarms. *Matern Child Health J.* 2018;22(7):1025–32.
96. Omaki E, Shields WC, Frattaroli S, McDonald E, Jones V, Gielen A. Six-month follow-up of lithium-battery smoke alarms and self-reported reasons for disabling. *Inj Prev.* 2017;23(1):67–9.
97. Gielen AC, Perry EC, Shields WC, McDonald E, Frattaroli S, Jones V. Changes in smoke alarm coverage following two fire department home visiting programs: What predicts success? *Inj Epidemiol.* 2014;1(1):30.
98. Diamond-Smith N, Bishai D, Perry E, Shields W, Gielen A. Economic evaluation of smoke alarm distribution methods in Baltimore, Maryland. *Inj Prev.* 2014;20(4):251–7.
99. Istre GR, McCoy MA, Moore BJ, et al. Preventing deaths and injuries from house fires: An outcome evaluation of a community-based smoke alarm installation programme. *Inj Prev.* 2014;20(2):97–102.
100. Yellman MA, Peterson C, McCoy MA, et al. Preventing deaths and injuries from house fires: A cost-benefit analysis of a community-based smoke alarm installation programme. *Inj Prev.* 2018;24(1):12–8.
101. Jackson M, Wilson J, Akoto J, Dixon S, Jacobs DE, Ballesteros MF. Evaluation of fire-safety programs that use 10-year smoke alarms. *J Community Health.* 2010;35(5):543–8.
102. Liu Y, Mack KA, Diekman ST. Smoke alarm giveaway and installation programs: An economic evaluation. *Am J Prev Med.* 2012;43(4):385–91.
103. Arai L, Roen K, Roberts H, Popay J. It might work in Oklahoma but will it work in Oakhampton? Context and implementation in the effectiveness literature on domestic smoke detectors. *Inj Prev.* 2005;11(3):148–51.
104. Warda L, Tenenbein M, Moffatt ME. House fire injury prevention update. Part II. A review of the effectiveness of preventive interventions. *Inj Prev.* 1999;5(3):217–25.
105. Diekman S, Huitric M, Netterville L. The development of the residential fire HELP tool kit: A resource to protect homebound older adults. *J Public Health Manag Pract.* 2010;16(5):S61–7.
106. Johns Hopkins Center for Injury Research & Policy. 2019 *Daniel J. Raskin Memorial Symposium Wildfires and Public Health,* Baltimore, Maryland. 2019.
107. National Fire Protection Association. *Fact Sheet: Research.* 2017. https://www.nfpa.org/-/media/Files/News-and-Research/Fire-statistics/Fact-sheets/FireLossFacts.pdf.
108. Rowan MP, Cancio LC, Elster EA, et al. Burn wound healing and treatment: Review and advancements. *Crit Care.* 2015;19:243.

CHAPTER

173

The Epidemiology and Prevention of Drowning

Linda Quan • Julie Gilchrist

INTRODUCTION

Drowning is a leading cause of death among children and young adults in every region of the world; an estimated 372,000 people die from drowning each year.[1] Worldwide, it is the major cause of death among children 1–4 years and the second major cause of unintentional injury deaths among those 10–29 years.[2] This serious public health problem disproportionately affects those in low- and middle-income countries (LMIC) where 90% of global drowning deaths occur. However, it remains a concern even in the high-income countries (HIC) like the United States (US). In the US, drowning kills more children 1–4 years of age than anything else except birth defects.[3] In 2016, almost 5000 Americans lost their lives to drowning of all intents, even more if one includes those related to boating, motor vehicle crashes, flooding, and other natural disasters.[4] Unintentional drowning rates have been decreasing (Fig. 173-1)[5] but the rate of decrease has slowed in the past two decades. Although studies have revealed some effective interventions, continued drowning research, and development and implementation of prevention programs remain largely neglected. In this chapter, drowning is defined and the epidemiology, risk factors, and prevention are discussed. Two frameworks are presented for considering prevention interventions and implementation strategies.

Drowning has been defined as "the process of experiencing respiratory impairment from submersion/immersion in liquid."[6] Outcomes depend on when in the process one intervenes to reestablish effective ventilation and how damaged the organs may be due to the effects of hypoxia (lack of oxygen at the tissue level). Victims can recover without morbidity, be left with a variety of lasting consequences as severe as a persistent vegetative state, or die.

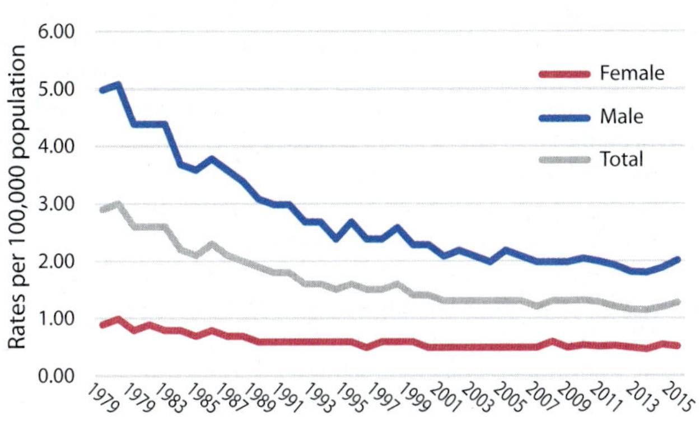

FIGURE 173-1. Fatal unintentional drowning—United States, 1999–2016.

The Burden of Drowning

Drowning is an injury mechanism which can occur from different intents (homicide, suicide, unintentional, or undetermined), although unintentional intent predominates (Fig. 173-2).[5] Each year in the US, there are about 4300 emergency department (ED) visits for unintentional drowning and an additional 3300 hospitalizations and 3500 deaths.[4] Studies suggest that about half of emergency department visits for drowning result in hospitalization or transfer for further care, compared with about 6% of ED visits for all unintentional injuries.[7,8] For most other injury mechanisms, each more serious level of disposition (ED visits, hospitalizations, deaths) vastly outnumbers the next, creating a pyramid that describes the burden of injury.[9] However, the drowning "pyramid" is more like a column; in 2013, there were 3701 unintentional drowning deaths, 3115 victims hospitalized and 2664 treated and released from emergency departments.[5,10] This demonstrates that a greater proportion of drowning injuries, compared with other mechanisms, is severe, resulting in hospitalization or death.

The long-term mortality rate, up to 20 years postdrowning event, among those discharged from the hospital was 23% (16/70) (95% CI: 13–34%) and higher among those with severe neurologic sequelae at hospital discharge.[11] Importantly, survivors with severe neurologic sequelae do not improve significantly over time. They require an estimated $100,000 per year of medical and other care. The annual cost of medical care associated with injuries and deaths from drowning is almost 200 million US dollars. Additionally, the associated productivity losses reach more than 8 billion dollars.[4]

The Pathophysiology of Submersion Injuries

Drowning as an injury mechanism is so lethal because it causes global anoxia, lack of oxygen in every body organ. When the victim's airway is submerged in water, breathing and the replenishment of oxygen in the blood are impaired either by laryngospasm or aspiration of the fluid. Aspirated fluid washes out surfactant in the pulmonary alveoli which collapse limiting ventilation. When the victim's airway stays submerged, asphyxia (the lack of breathing) leads to anoxia.

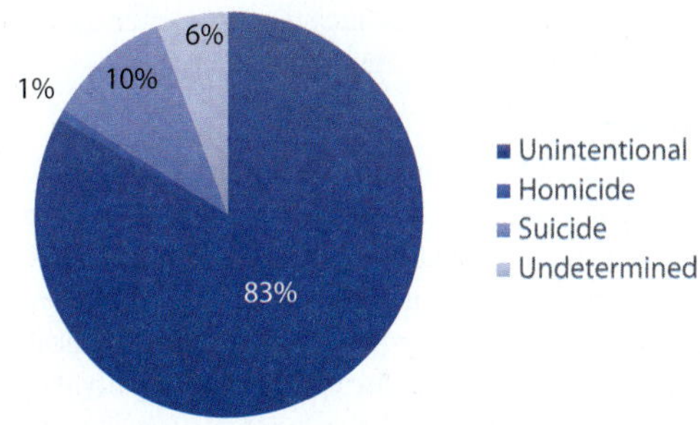

FIGURE 173-2. Fatal drowning by intent—United States, 2012–2016.

The key organs respond immediately to the anoxic insult. Within minutes, lack of oxygen to the brain leads to loss of consciousness and respiratory arrest (cessation of breathing). Within another few minutes, the hypoxic myocardium develops nonperfusing rhythms which manifest as cardiac arrest.[12] If, at this point, the drowning process is interrupted and ventilation and oxygenation are restored, cardiac and respiratory activity may return. However, the victim may develop multiorgan failure as other injured organs (e.g., gastrointestinal, coagulation, lung, and renal) display the effects of anoxia at a slower pace.

Among those victims resuscitated from cardiac and respiratory arrest (no breathing or heart beat), most die of brain death within 12–24 hours after the drowning incident. In a recent US cardiac arrest registry, the case fatality rate (died prior to hospital admission) after drowning-related cardiac arrest was 83% (1021/1236) (95% CI: 80–85%) for all victims, and 47% (192/407) (95% CI: 42–52%) for those who had had an attempted resuscitation.[11] Approximately 5–7% survive with severe neurologic sequelae: hypoxic encephalopathy with no self-help skills, communication or mobility. About 10% (range 0.8–47%) of victims of cardiac arrest survive with seemingly favorable neurologic outcomes at hospital discharge.[13–16] However, long term and more thorough neurologic evaluations than those conducted at hospital discharge show that many survivors deemed normal at discharge have some neurologic sequelae.[17,18] In one study of patients admitted to the ICU of a children's hospital, 49% died, 19% survived with severe sequelae dependent in care, communication and mobility, and 26% left the hospital with no identified functional disability.[19]

The progression of the physiologic response of anoxic injury to organs can be stopped if the drowning process is interrupted. Proven strategies to limit the anoxic injury include early rescue and early resuscitation; CPR at the scene by a bystander prior to arrival of EMS has been associated with a greater likelihood of favorable survival.[15] The victim who is cyanotic, unresponsive and not breathing can often be revived by a bystander and resume breathing spontaneously and become responsive. Some of these victims may develop respiratory distress within the next few hours due to the effects of hypoxia on the lungs, but this can resolve.

The earlier the restoration of oxygenation, the lower the likelihood of death or survival with brain injury. Submersion duration is the most robust predictor of outcome.[20] Victims with short submersion durations, < 5–6 minutes, have very high rates of favorable outcome, survival with no or mild neurologic sequelae. Those with submersion durations of 10–11 minutes have lower likelihoods of favorable outcome while those submerged greater than 15–25 minutes rarely have favorable outcomes. Meta-analyses find that neither young age nor submersion in cold or very cold water have consistently shown a protective effect despite beliefs that young children tolerate hypoxia better than adults and that cold water induced hypothermia saves brain cells.[21]

Of the clinical findings, coma on arrival to hospital or a history of cardiac arrest postdrowning predicts death for the majority of hospitalized drowning victims.[22] Additionally, various physiologic scores that reflect brain and cardiac function are predictive. Unfortunately, later interventions in the process such as advanced in-hospital medical care are not associated with improved outcomes.[23]

Data Limitations

Valid drowning data are limited by the availability of data and variability in its quality. In many countries, fatal and nonfatal injury data are collected through the death registration and healthcare systems. In LMIC countries, many drowning victims who die at the scene or are cared for at home and subsequently die without medical care may not be included in statistics. Intensive efforts to identify these victims in several Asian countries with verbal autopsy surveys at the community level showed that drowning surpassed motor vehicle crashes as the leading cause of child death.[24] Even in the US, drowning-related deaths that occur long after the initial event may not be identified as drownings. Thus, existing surveillance data, the basis for public health priorities and programs, may underestimate the drowning problem.

In addition, drowning deaths in certain circumstances either are not included or cannot be included in reported drowning statistics. By international standards, drownings related to boating, motor vehicle crashes and other forms of transportation are reported as transportation-related deaths and excluded from the drowning statistics.[25] Drownings due to motor vehicle crashes into bodies of water are not coded in a way that they can be captured and included in drowning statistics. Similarly, drowning deaths during floods and other natural disasters are reported as such and the codes for natural disasters do not include one specific to drowning.[25] The intent is to ensure that drownings in different countries are reported similarly to aid in comparisons and research; however, it reduces the reportable burden of drowning.

There may be misclassifications in the intent behind a drowning. In the US, 1% of drownings are classified as homicide; some homicides by drowning may be missed. However, Child Death Review efforts and other medical examiner processes improve the likelihood of identifying homicide by drowning. One review of hospitalized or autopsied children with submersion injuries found that 8% of all submersions and 26% of bathtub submersions were judged to be intentional injuries. These victims were young (mean age of 2.1 years). They also commonly had objective physical signs of abuse and incompatibilities between the physical findings or the child's developmental stage and the history of the incident.[26] In the US, 10% of drownings are classified as suicide. However, suicide as a designation of intent may be influenced by the victim's age, sex, and country leading to classification as unintentional or undetermined.[27] See chapters on homicide and suicide for more details on the epidemiology and prevention of violence.

Medical records and death certificates often lack details on known risk and protective factors such as the victim's activities, swimming ability, the body of water, weather conditions, health conditions, use of life jackets, type and functionality of fences or barriers, supervision type and quality (e.g., impaired), presence of lifeguards, alcohol use, and whether CPR was performed by a bystander.[3] These measures could be used to explore drowning risks and to guide the development and effectiveness of targeted prevention programs.

In HIC where water exposure is more likely to be recreational, lack of exposure data is a major limitation in epidemiologic studies of drowning. Without information on exposure to aquatic activities in different settings (e.g., swimming pools, natural water environments), researchers can only provide population-based rates and cannot accurately determine those groups at highest risk. Exposure to recreational water settings likely varies substantially by age, sex, level of swimming skill, race/ethnicity, and other factors.[3]

Above all, good data should drive development, evaluation, and implementation of drowning prevention programs. Yet detailed drowning surveillance is conducted in only a few states, such as Texas. Drowning data collected needs to be expanded to include more than the usual demographic and basic descriptors; this includes data relevant to natural water settings, supervision, rescue responses and prevention opportunities.[28] There have been efforts to expand the information collected on drowning incidents. Child Death Review aims to bring together the circumstances of drowning, as well as other causes of child death, to identify places to intervene.[29] In Washington State, the data needs of each of the multiple agencies (police, EMS, coroners/medical examiners, boating) involved with a drowning were sought, put into one document, and shared to minimize duplication of data collection efforts.[30]

RISK FACTORS FOR UNINTENTIONAL DROWNING

Risks for drowning vary by intrinsic victim characteristics (sex, age, race/ethnicity, health conditions), knowledge and behavior (risk taking, alcohol use, swim skill), and the environment (setting). These identified risk factors are often interrelated.

Victim-related Risk Factors

Sex

As with most injuries, males outnumber females in fatal drowning in all studies. In the US, the overall ratio of 3.1 increases to 8:1 amongst 15- to 24-year olds and in 2012–16 was highest among those 15–19 at 9:1. This may be due to different supervision styles for male children, increased water exposure, riskier activities or increased alcohol use among males. Males have a lower perception of risk and a higher perception of their own swim competency.[31,32]

Age

In almost all countries, children have the highest risks for drowning. In LMICs, drowning is the most common cause of injury death by far making the drowning burden among children a leading public health problem. In Bangladesh, a country with one of the highest reported pediatric drowning rates, fatal drownings represented 42% of deaths in one cohort of children under 5 years.[33] In the US, fatal drowning rates are highest among those 1–4 with a secondary peak from 15 to 24 years. These two age groups share similar lethal combinations of developmentally based behaviors including exploration of their environment, lack of judgment, inattention to hazards and avoidance of supervision. US school age children, 5–14 years have the lowest fatal drowning rates.[8] Fatal drowning rates have increased among Americans > 65 years of age likely due to increases in health conditions contributing to the risk of drowning.[34]

Characteristics and setting of the drowning event vary by age group.[35,36] In the US, those at the extremes of age drown in bathtubs; infants less than 1 year drown because of lack of supervision while those 80+ years likely have acute cardiovascular or other health events leading to drowning. Children 1–5 years commonly drown in private residential swimming pools during a lapse in supervision. The contribution of drowning in natural waters such as lakes, rivers, and ponds increases with age.[36] The exception in the US is minority urban school age children who commonly drown in apartment or public pools.[37]

Race/Ethnicity

As with so many injury mechanisms, race and ethnicity are identified risk factors for fatal drowning. Race or ethnicity may be a proxy for differences in exposure and experiences. In the US, white toddlers and preschoolers have the highest drowning rates compared to other race/ethnicities and other age groups. However, from school age through adulthood, Native Americans, blacks, and Hispanics have disproportionately higher drowning rates compared to whites.[3] The higher risks among racial and ethnic minorities have been noted in other HIC. In Canada, Australia, and New Zealand, indigenous/aboriginal peoples have higher drowning rates than whites.[38] Additionally, racial and ethnic minorities have increased drowning rates in these countries and the Netherlands.[39]

Race and ethnic disparities may relate to socioeconomic factors. In the state of Georgia, US, white children 1–4 years of age, representing the majority of drowning fatalities, drowned in private residential pools in high-income communities while black children 5–14 years from low-income and low education level neighborhoods drowned in public swimming pools.[40] Cost of lessons and pool entrance, as well as reduced access to swimming pools in poor neighborhoods where minority groups may live, are barriers to learning to swim and attending pools. Among families surveyed in nine major US cities, increased household income was associated with higher percentages of family members who could swim and who encouraged swimming.[41] Among Alaskan native populations, high drowning rates may be related to their exposure to occupational fishing or subsistence activities and water transportation as well as increased use of alcohol.[42]

However, socioeconomic status alone does not explain all of the increased drowning risk among many racial and ethnic minorities. In the Netherlands, ethnic minorities were more likely to drown than native Dutch RR 2.51 (95% CI 1.84, 3.41) even after adjusting for age, sex, income, and urbanization.[39] Among black males, swimming pool drowning risk remained higher even after controlling for income.[37] Among urban youth, black children report lower swimming ability even after controlling for income.[43] Underlying reasons are complex, likely including cultural, historical, and environmental influences.

For some groups, recreational water sports are not part of their culture. The parents of urban black children in the US report more fear of drowning and less likelihood of swim lessons.[41,43,44] The history of exclusion from public swimming pools and lessons among blacks may explain these fears and avoidance of swimming activities. Avoidance as a drowning prevention strategy fails once someone encounters the water either willingly or unwillingly; they are then left without the skills to survive. Immigrant Vietnamese-Americans reported not having engaged in aquatic recreation in Vietnam.[45] In New Zealand, 43% of new immigrants surveyed had never participated in recreational aquatics prior to moving to New Zealand yet 72% of them did presently.[46] Thus, cultural behaviors affect exposure to, familiarity with and skills around water.

Lack of familiarity with local waters may put groups at risk. Several countries have reported higher drowning rates among foreigners and travelers compared to local populations.[47] International tourists in Australia had higher drowning rates in surf than native Australians.[48] They reported less knowledge about rip currents and less ability to manage them compared to native beachgoers.[49] The most revealing reports come from China which document that citizens who have migrated within China have higher fatal and nonfatal drowning rates than the local population.[50] These findings suggest that unfamiliarity with water-related activities and the waters themselves contribute to risk; race and ethnicity may only help identify those who are more likely to be unfamiliar.

Comorbidities

Certain diseases, health conditions and their associated medications can increase the risk of drowning. Anything causing loss of consciousness can be catastrophic if it occurs in water. Conditions of concern are those that result in a sudden drop in blood pressure or blood sugar, seizure, arrhythmia, heart attack or stroke. Chronic disease incidence varies with the age group studied. Not surprisingly, those 65 years and older had more pre-existing conditions.[51] Of these, neuropsychiatric conditions, dementia and depression, were more commonly linked to drowning among those 65 and older compared to the general population.

Pre-existing conditions can also affect drowning risk among children. The most common high risk condition among children in HIC is epilepsy. In an 11-year study of fatal drownings among Australian children less than 14 years of age, epilepsy was the only significantly increased medical risk, present in 35.8% of their cohort.[52] Drowning among those with epilepsy commonly occurs in bathtubs when unattended as well as in swimming pools.[53] In most studies, victims have had poorly controlled seizures that cause drowning either because they fall into water or are in the water, often a bathtub, during their seizure. In fact, the most common cause of injury death to those with epilepsy is drowning. Prevention of drowning is a well-known issue for those managing patients with epilepsy. Best practice recommendations include showering instead of using bathtubs, swimming where there is a lifeguard, controlling the epilepsy and avoiding swimming until seizure free for a period of time. However, effectiveness of these recommendations has not been evaluated.[54] It has been suggested that chronic medical conditions among children may increase drowning risk in one of three ways: (a) increase the likelihood of seeking hazardous settings, (b) increase drowning risk when in the water, or (c) decrease the likelihood of successful rescue.[52]

Children with Autism Spectrum Disorder have increased drowning risk because these children tend to wander.[55] Other developmental disorders have not been evaluated for drowning risk.

An intriguing and silent comorbidity is the Long-QT syndrome. This rare autosomal dominant syndrome is due to various genetic mutations and can result in sudden cardiac death triggered by swimming. These mutations allow prolongation of the QT interval in the cardiac cycle that leads to development of torsades or ventricular fibrillation, lethal cardiac arrhythmias. Some are specifically triggered by immersion but also can be triggered by anxiety, fear, or exercise. Case reports and small series of victims with usually unexplained drowning scenarios describe finding these gene mutations.[56] Screening all drowning victims has been of low yield because of the low incidence of this mutation.[57] Interestingly, over 200 pharmaceuticals in common use prolong the QT interval. However, their role in increasing drowning risk has not been evaluated.[58]

Behavioral Risk Factors

Risk taking is a commonly identified cause of drowning, especially among teens and young adult males. Risk taking around water is a developmental age-related behavior, documented in surveys as well as in brain imaging studies among adolescents and young adults, especially males. Whether surveyed in the US, New Zealand, or China, males report greater risk taking behavior than females along with greater estimation of skills and lower estimation of risks or less safety knowledge.[31,32,59] Similarly, observational studies showed that male teenagers were more likely to enter restricted drowning risk zones at Yosemite falls.[60,61]

Alcohol use is a common behavior that increases risk of drowning. Alcohol is a neurologic agent affecting risk taking, judgment, coordination and balance, and a depressant affecting the response to drowning. It also has cardiotoxic potential to evoke arrhythmias. Blood alcohol content (BAC) levels were positive in 30–70% of adults and 20–30% of teenage drowning fatalities.[62] Although alcohol intake is a common component of recreational water activities like boating, pool parties and going to the beach, its contributory role was defined in a case control study of drowning deaths.[63] This study showed increased likelihood of boat-related drowning death at all BAC > 0. Furthermore, risk increased with increasing blood alcohol levels, with a 10 times risk for BAC > 100 mg. Routine blood alcohol testing on drowning victims older than 10 years has been recommended.[62] Drug or alcohol intoxications may appear on the death certificate if, in the judgment of the coroner or medical examiner, they contributed to the death or the circumstances leading to death. However, in some states, these data may be considered confidential patient information. The contribution of other drugs has not been evaluated; forensic evaluations commonly include only toxicology screens that evaluate for drugs of abuse.

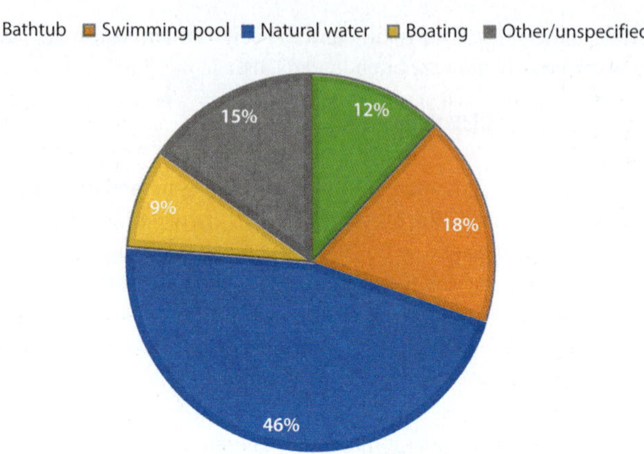

FIGURE 173-3. Fatal unintentional drowning by setting—United States, 2012–2016.

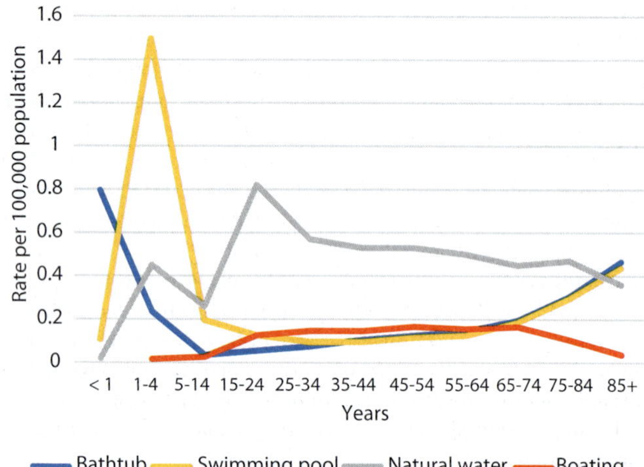

FIGURE 173-4. Fatal unintentional drowning rate by setting and age group—United States, 2007–2016.

Environmental Risks: Drowning Settings

Drowning characteristics and risk factors vary by the environmental setting (Fig. 173-3).[5] When including boating-related drowning, more than half of all unintentional drowning occurs in natural water settings. Almost one fifth occur in swimming pools. The risk by setting also varies by age group (Fig. 173-4).[5]

Bathtubs

Bathtubs are one of the two unique drowning settings that are commonly built and used in HIC (swimming pools being the other). Most fatal bathtub drownings involve the extremes of age, young children and older adults. Inadequate supervision is the key risk factor among the young who are left unsupervised in the bathtub containing water.[35,64] Often, the drowned child is the youngest of a large family, left alone or with another child < 5 years. In a survey conducted in an urban emergency department, 13% of parents reported leaving young children unsupervised an average of 15 minutes, ranging from a few minutes to as long as 1 hour; 16% left the child with an older sibling. Parents have reported that they thought they would hear noise if the child had difficulty.[65] Child neglect is often identified through Child Death Review. Drowning related to child abuse is most likely to be recognized among bathtub drownings. Recognizing homicide can be difficult; studies suggest looking for an inconsistent history of the drowning scenario and not, necessarily, the presence of physical signs of abuse.[26]

Bathtub drowning rates decrease as children reach school age. Outside of early childhood, those who drown in bathtubs usually have a comorbidity (e.g., seizures, arrhythmias, cardiovascular disease). Most older children, adolescents and young adults who drown in bathtubs have a history of seizures. Bathtub drowning rates rise again among those > 65 years of age. A study in Japan documented bathtub drowning rates among the elderly that are the highest reported, 10 times those of older Americans.[66] The Japanese have the oldest population in the world and bathing in hot tubs is a cultural activity that increases exposure. Health conditions that can cause loss of consciousness such as hypotension, hypoglycemia, heart attack, seizure or stroke may be survivable on land but fatal if occurring in water. Many older adult drowning victims may have had a heart attack while in the bathtub which can be indistinguishable at autopsy from drowning. Correct classification of the cause of death poses a challenge in this age group.

Swimming Pools

Swimming pools are generally considered safer sites for recreational swimming because they lack many of the hazards of natural water settings. Pools have known depths, relatively short distances, and lack currents, obstacles and waves that pose risks to swimmers.[3] However, swimming pools pose a major risk to those under 5 years of age.[3,67] The number of residential swimming pools in the US result in US children 1–59 months of age having the highest fatal drowning rates among the HIC.[1] Additionally, among older children, there are significant racial and ethnic disparities among swimming pool drowning deaths possibly complicated by lack of basic swim skills among many in the black community.[3,37] One study examining swimming pool-related drownings among those 5–24 years found that risks were highest among black males even after controlling for income.[37]

The rates of swimming pool drownings vary by age as well. The highest drowning rates occur among toddler and preschool children who drown in swimming pools. These occur most commonly in residential backyard pools at their own home or the home of a caretaker.[67,68] This age group is particularly at risk since they may not have yet acquired the judgment and skills to survive. There are two common scenarios: young children escape the house or yard during a lapse in supervision and enter the pool when not expected to be swimming. These children often are in play clothes rather than swim suits. In this case, barriers like door locks, door alarms and isolation pool fencing can delay water entry until supervision is re-established. In the second scenario, the victims intended to be in the water but drown due to a lapse in supervision/lifeguarding and a lack of survival swim skills and/or a complicating health condition.

Among school age children and young adults, settings of swimming pool drowning vary by race and ethnicity.[37] This may be related to the extent to which children without skills have increased exposure to pools. In one examination of US swimming pool drowning data among those 5–24 years, 51% of black victims drowned in public pools, 55% of white victims drowned in residential pools, and 35% of Hispanic victims drowned in community (e.g., apartment) pools.[37]

Finally, among all ages, males predominate in fatal swimming pool drownings, representing 70%.[7,8,37,69]

Natural Water

In the US and globally, natural water is where most people of school age and older drown. Natural water includes fresh water (lakes, rivers, ponds) and oceans. Fatal and nonfatal drownings most commonly occur in freshwater rivers, lakes, and ponds.[8,47,70–72] Not surprisingly, natural water drowning rates are higher in rural areas. Case fatality rates are highest (70%) in recreational natural water drownings compared to those in swimming pools or bathtubs. Longer emergency response times may contribute to the higher case fatality rates.[73]

Natural water drowning primarily involves those > 5 years of age.[7,36] This is true even in arid states, inland states, and states with high preschooler drowning rates in pools. Male to female ratios are highest in natural water drownings where males represent 90% of drownings.[69] In the US, natural water drowning overwhelmingly involves recreational activities such as boating, swimming, wading or diving. Studies document alcohol use by 30–70% of victims who died.[35,62] In a 10-year Australian study, fatal drownings in rivers involved mostly adults swimming, but also children falling into the water, and nonaquatic transport (such as vehicles).[70]

Risk factors for drowning include warmer weather. Drowning is a seasonal injury, most common in the summer months. Not surprisingly, drowning is more likely during hot days. In Ontario, Canada, between 1999 and 2009, risk for fatal drowning outdoors increased 69% when ambient temperatures were > 30C (>86F; OR = 1.69, CI 1.23–2.25) but not for indoor drownings.[74] Thus, with greater exposure to natural waters with increasing environmental temperatures, drownings may increase.

Boating

In the US, boating-related drownings represent about 9% of all unintentional drownings.[69] Even though boating deaths in the US are usually recreational, a boat-related drowning is coded and reported as a transportation-related death and may be excluded from state or national drowning reports. Boat-related fatal drownings are described annually by the US Coast Guard (USCG).[75] In 2016, fatal drowning accounted for 80% (n = 509) of 701 boat-related accidental deaths. Drowning deaths primarily involved small boats, < 21 feet in length, most of which were motorboats; 83% of victims were not wearing a life jacket. However, drowning involving kayaks and canoes is increasing, probably due to their low cost and increasing popularity. While alcohol remains a leading contributory factor, its role is underestimated since boat operators' alcohol data is not always obtained nor made available. Victims' swimming ability and life jacket use also are often not reported. In Canada, among 2678 recreational and daily living boating drowning deaths occurring between 1991 and 2010, victims with average swimming ability had almost two times the odds of wearing a life jacket compared to nonswimmers and weak swimmers combined (95% 1.06–3.40).[76,77] This suggests that those with some water experience were more prepared.

In LMIC, boat use is often for transportation. Transportation involving ferries or other large ships commonly claim hundreds of lives in one sinking. Vessels' maintenance, safety procedures, and lifesaving equipment are factors. The United Nations Refugee Agency (UNHCR) reported that 5096 migrants drowned while being transported in overcrowded and illegal watercraft in the Mediterranean alone in 2017 and 3119 in 2017.[78] Moreover, drownings in unofficial transport in small boats, rafts or other watercraft are often not recorded.

Other Transportation

Motor vehicle-related drownings occur when vehicles drive or crash into bodies of water. This can occur intentionally or unintentionally. Since these are coded as transportation-related deaths, they are not routinely included in drowning surveillance data.

Other Settings

Nonrecreational settings that pose drowning risk include waters used for domestic chores. In the 1990s, the toddler-drowning rate in five gallon buckets was 0.367 per 100,000 two-year olds in the US.[79] In rural US and Canada, irrigation ditches remain a major drowning hazard for children. Other large water collecting containers in the residential setting account for many drownings of young children in LMIC. Residential ponds for drinking water, washing and fish propagation that are within meters of the house, pose threats to children in LMIC who fall in them while playing, bathing or performing chores such as obtaining water, fish, or washing.[71] Older children walking to school or in the course of other daily activities, cross over bodies of water into which they can fall or are in unsafe water transport. Moreover, many live in houses on water or in houseboats.[80]

Occupational Settings

Occupational drowning is most commonly associated with the commercial fishing industry. Commercial fishing is consistently one of the most dangerous occupations in the US, with a rate of 86 fatalities per 100,000 workers reported during 2016, 24 times higher than the average workplace fatality rate of 3.6 per 100,000.[81] In this industry, 86% of fatalities are due to drowning.[82] These most commonly occur due to vessel disasters and falls overboard. The use of personal flotation devices (life jackets) reduces these risks. CDC's National Institute of Occupational Safety and Health (NIOSH) has conducted research to determine how to increase use of life jackets and some manufactures have incorporated the findings.[83] NIOSH also maintains the Commercial Fishing Incident Database, which allows examination of injury and fatality data to monitor trends and identify preventive strategies. Occupational injuries are discussed elsewhere in this book.

Flooding and Natural Disasters

Drowning is often the most common cause of death during hurricanes and other natural disasters that involve flooding.[84–87] These drownings often occur at home or when driving a motor vehicle through flooded roads.

DROWNING PREVENTION STRATEGIES

Primary, Secondary, and Tertiary Prevention

The strategies to prevent any public health problem can be categorized as primary, secondary, or tertiary. For injury mechanisms, primary prevention is preventing exposure to the harmful condition, secondary prevention is reducing the risk of harm should the condition be encountered and tertiary is acting to reduce the consequences and improve outcomes from injuries due to encountering the condition.[88] Although the drowning process is swift, several very different and unique opportunities to intervene occur in its short timeline. The drowning chain of survival provides an approach to drowning prevention strategies based on this timeline.[89] We present strategies to prevent drowning based on these categorizations: Primary—prevent exposure to the water; secondary—keep swimmers/bathers/boaters safe while in, on or around the water; and tertiary—improve the outcomes of a drowning event.

No single intervention will prevent all drowning. Implementing layers of protection provides multiple opportunities to prevent negative outcomes. Hyder first described four major drowning prevention interventions: barriers, lifeguards, swimming lessons, and lifejackets.[90] These plus supervision are the five evidence-based interventions placed into the Circle of Drowning Prevention developed by the American Red Cross.[91] The prevention recommendations of the World Health Organization (WHO) added developing safe places, managing flooding, and improving boating and shipping.[80]

Each of these proven and some promising interventions are discussed presenting:

- Data on effectiveness of the intervention;
- Existing policies and/or legislation;
- Example of successful programs;
- Challenges and limitations; and
- What's needed.

Primary Prevention—Prevent Access to Water

Barriers

Barriers are the key prevention strategy among the very young (before they are able to open an appropriately latched gate or door). Pool fencing is the most researched drowning prevention intervention. A systematic review of pool fencing through the Cochrane Collaboration presented evidence from case control studies demonstrating that pool fencing is effective in preventing child drowning. The odds ratio for fatal or nonfatal drowning risk in a fenced compared to unfenced pool was 0.27 (95% CI: 0.16–0.47). Four sided or isolation pool fencing (which prevents access to the pool directly from the house) is more effective in preventing drowning compared to perimeter or three-sided fencing (in which the house forms the fourth side allowing unsupervised access to the pool). The odds ratio of drowning risk with four-sided as compared with three-sided fencing was 0.17 (95% CI 0.07–0.44). Since most young children access the pool directly from the house, isolation fencing combined with a functional self-closing and self-latching gate is the most effective barrier.[92]

Other barriers such as door locks (special latches placed out of a child's reach to restrict egress) and motorized, weight-bearing pool safety covers might delay a child's unintended entry into the water. However, neither has been rigorously evaluated. Additional products have been developed to alert caregivers to potential pool access. Door alarms are intended to signal unexpected exit from the home and pool alarms are intended to signal unexpected water entry. However, effectiveness has not been established for these adjunctive devices.

Barriers remain the obvious, effective solution for drowning prevention for many nonpool waters too. They are likely effective for ponds, irrigation ditches, even some natural waterways. Barriers can keep children from falling into water by which they play or walk or vehicles from accidentally driving into rivers along roads. In Bangladesh, the Anchal program provided cribs for children < 18 months along with organized, supervised day care (creches) for children 1–4 years. The program also included home visits to identify and reduce access to home hazards. The increased supervision and home improvements (barriers) resulted in an 82% decrease in pediatric drowning mortality compared to a retrospective matched cohort.[93] This program was cost effective.

The US Consumer Product Safety Commission has developed residential pool barrier guidelines.[94] While these are guidelines and not part of federal nor state law, they have been adapted by some jurisdictions for inclusion in building codes and other regulations. The state of Florida enacted a residential pool safety act which requires that, to pass final inspection, all new pools include at least one of five options to improve safety: a barrier around the pool, a pool safety cover, door, and window alarms on any that provide access to the pool, self-closing and latching devices with release at least 54 inches from the ground on all doors leading to the pool, or a swimming pool alarm to sound with unexpected water entrance.[95] However, in a national telephone survey between 2001 and 2003, inadequate fencing was associated with higher income, owning the home and having a detached house. This study estimated more than 488,000 homes had children under 5 years with access to an inadequately fenced swimming pool.[96] Innovative programs to increase residential pool fencing are needed.

There are many challenges and limitations to implementing and enforcing barrier policies. In the US, fencing laws are most often addressed through local ordinances or building codes. These are rarely at the state level making widespread passage and implementation very difficult. Moreover, laws most often apply to new pools, leaving existing pools unprotected. Requirements are usually enforced upon final inspection of a newly constructed pool and continued enforcement is difficult. Finally, although isolation fencing is most protective for small children, opposition to fencing requirements makes passing, maintaining, and enforcing barrier requirements difficult. Pool owners, as well as some within the industry, often resist new requirements or work to overturn existing ones. Often interventions considered less than ideal (door locks and alarms as opposed to isolation fencing) are put into place as a compromise to ensure that all pools can have some measure of protection.[97]

As with pool fencing, challenges to constructing other barriers include cost, political will, and esthetics. However, it is possible. For instance, the US National Park Service erected fences in the untamed wilderness of Yosemite National Park, in risk zones where almost half the visitor drowning deaths have occurred. Despite these fences, visitors, primarily males, still entered these restricted risk zones.[61]

A barrier is to limit access to areas at risk; this can be achieved legislatively, without physical structures. Some communities prohibit swimming in high-risk natural waters, such as waterways or rivers, sometimes seasonally. In the city of Seattle, a law prohibiting swimming in its busy Ship Canal prevented further drowning deaths in this waterway.

Secondary Prevention—Reduce Risks While In, On, or Around the Water

Life Jackets

Life Jackets for Boating Life jacket use remains the most effective drowning prevention strategy in boating by keeping boaters safer should they end up in the water. In national and state studies of boating fatalities, life jacket wear decreases fatalities by 50%.[22,98,99]

In the US, a national law requires only that each boater has a USCG approved lifejacket that fits and is in the boat. Additionally, national law requires all children less than 13 years actually wear a

USCG approved life jacket in a boat while underway. The boating law applies only to certain vessels. It does not apply to inflatable rafts, inflated tires, or flotation toys such as inflated mattresses or tubes. Nationally, observed voluntary life jacket wear is highest among those kayaking or sailing, and lowest among those in small motorboats (<19 feet) and those fishing. Legislation at the state or local level may require that life jackets actually be worn. All 50 states require USCG approved life jackets be worn on personal watercraft and by those being towed or skiing behind a boat. Some states require boaters to wear lifejackets in specific bodies of water, water conditions, or times of the year.

Successful programs that increased use among children involved educational efforts prior to mandated use. Following a county-wide awareness campaign promoting life jacket use, when surveyed, parents reported increased ownership (11%; 95% CI 3–17%) and use (OR = 1.6; 95% CI 1.1–2.5) of child life jackets in WA State; greater use was significantly associated with owning a life jacket, poor swimming ability of the child, parental confidence in fitting a life jacket and parent recall of the campaign.[100]

The most successful educational effort without mandate occurred within the sailing community. Among those observed in various boat types over 12 years, only those in sailboats increased life jacket use with no change in laws, from 13.6% to 31.1%. This remarkable change may be related to the US Sailing Organization's efforts.[101]

Life jacket use is highest in children; rates increased from 80% to 92% in nationwide observations conducted between 1999 and 2015.[102] During this period, most states had passed laws mandating their use by children aged < 6 to < 12 years, depending on the state; in 2017, 45 states had mandates in place.[103,30]

The best evidence demonstrating the effectiveness of mandating life jacket wear comes from Victoria, Australia, where recreational boating drowning deaths fell 50% when life jacket wear became compulsory.[99] Three years after the US Army Corps of Engineers mandated life jacket use among boaters in certain locales in Mississippi, boaters' life jacket wear rates increased from 13.7% at baseline to 68.1% while wear rates at control sites were unchanged.[104,105]

Among mandated groups in WA State, observed life jacket wear rates have been 90–95%, although they dropped to 80% in 2015.[106] Most encouraging, although not mandated, life jacket wear among adolescents increased from 24% to 37.2% nationally between 1999 and 2010 and was 50% in WA State in 2010.[101,106] This suggests that adolescents familiarized and trained to use life jackets as required in childhood may continue to use them. Importantly, use by an adult in a boat markedly increased likelihood that a child wore a life jacket (RR 20.0, 95% CI 7.1, 55.8), a modeling phenomenon seen in other injury prevention interventions such as seat belt use.[106]

The biggest challenge is the need to develop new strategies to influence life jacket use. Despite 20 years of the USCG's continuous educational efforts aimed at boaters, overall wear rates in the US remained unchanged among adults between 1999 and 2014, from 9% to 11.1% over a 13-year period.[105] In fact, national life jacket wear rates actually decreased to 3.9% among those in all powerboats, the largest group of boaters. Moreover, a regional educational campaign to increase life jacket use in California led to negligible increases in use among adults (from 8.5% at baseline to 10.5% three years postintervention) compared to regions with no campaign.

Communication without culturally appropriate risk perspectives can limit a program's effectiveness. Canada's program failed to increase life jacket use among its northern Aboriginal peoples when delivered by "water experts" instead of elders.[107] This highlighted the need to use trusted, respected, and community-based authorities to deliver risk communication. In contrast, appropriate risk communication through the US Sailing organization's efforts may have led to the higher wear rates subsequently observed among adult sailors.

Risk perspectives need to be addressed. In focus groups, northwest American boaters reported that they were aware of the drowning prevention role of life jackets, but that they believed their drowning risk was lower in good weather and because they were experienced, disliked the discomfort and limitation wearing a life jacket and that they would only wear a life jacket if required to do so.[108,109] In a recent study of canoers, the boating group with the highest risk of drowning, those newest to canoeing were least likely to recognize risk and to use a life jacket.[110] Thus, the message needs to clarify misinformation held by boaters, old and new. Safe boating education may be effective just not widely implemented; in 2016, of the 351 boaters who fatally drowned and whose boating educational status was known, 77% had not had boating safety education.[75] In 2017, 48 states required some segment of the boating population to take a state approved course.[103] However, these courses have not been thoroughly evaluated.

What is needed is standardization of life jacket requirements to decrease confusion based on location/jurisdiction or water craft. Policy makers should consider the benefits of mandating wear of USCG approved life jackets among all ages or at least children under 18 years, and expanding requirements to include other vessels such as paddle craft (e.g., canoes, kayaks, standup paddleboards). Additionally, more comfortable and appealing life jackets need to be developed. A focused marketing approach needs to address each low-user/high-risk boating group such as fishermen, power boaters, teens, and older age groups. Lessons could be learned from the research involving life jacket use among commercial fishermen.[82,111]

Finally, to improve compliance, boating safety education needs to be provided in conjunction with any legislation. It should also be promoted among those outside of the "boating community," the more casual users, especially those using paddle craft. Boating safety education should be evaluated to ensure it is meeting the educational and cultural needs of different boaters. Better evaluation of mandatory boating education safety education for recreational boaters might encourage more widespread passage and enforcement of education requirements.

Life Jackets Use When In or Near Water Wearing life jackets around swimming pools or other water settings provides an added layer of protection for children who might fall into the water. Life jacket use can also protect inexperienced or nonswimmers who plan to be in the water.

While the concept of life jacket use for swimming is not mainstream, the concept of flotation assistance is. In recent observation studies of people in the water at designated natural water swim sites, 25% of all ages were using or playing with something that assists flotation.[21] Life jackets were worn by 50% of those less than 6 years of age but rarely after that age. Natural water swimmers use various foam or air-filled toys and products to provide flotation assistance but are not designed to keep swimmers safe.

Policy around life jacket use outside of boating varies. Surveyed in 2016, most responding International Life Saving organizations reported allowing life jacket use in the "shallow end" at their facilities, as did national organizations in the US.[112] Additionally, the American Red Cross teaches life jacket use in its swim programs. Following the refusal of a summer camp to allow a child's request to use a life jacket and his subsequent drowning, Massachusetts passed "Christian's law" that ensures that camps allow and provide life jackets to nonswimmers or at-risk swimmers or those requesting them.[113]

Inconsistent and shifting policies regarding life jacket use around swimming pools is a challenge. Swimming pool operators have only recently allowed life jacket use in their pools; previously, there has been concern that life jacket use precluded learning how to swim. The lack of consistent policy toward use of life jackets in controlled water environments may undermine their use in riskier water environments where most drownings occur.

Accepted and routine use of life jackets needs to expand beyond boating to include most water activities, including swimming. The observed popularity of toys that provide flotation assistance presents an opportunity to create and market safer, dependable, approved, and acceptable flotation.

Swimming Lessons/Water Competency

Several studies demonstrate that swim instruction confers some drowning protection. Swim lessons were associated with safer behaviors and some swim skills in preschoolers.[114] A history of swim lessons was associated with lower fatal drowning rates in case-controlled studies of US children and of Chinese children ages less than 5 years.[115,116] The converse has been shown, that lack of swim skill contributes to drowning risk. However, what aspects of these swim lessons conferred protection was not clear from these studies.

While in-water training is ideal, some water safety knowledge transfer can be achieved among children taught in a classroom setting; in a randomized controlled trial in the US, a 6-week integrated in-school injury prevention curriculum that included water safety resulted in increased knowledge about water-related injury and drowning.[117] However, the effectiveness of knowledge transfer has rarely been evaluated; in China, migrant children had lower risk of nonfatal drowning if they had water safety knowledge, knew it was dangerous to swim alone and if a parent accompanied them to school.[50]

Learning to swim has been the longstanding sine qua non of drowning prevention. The best evidence for the effectiveness of swim skills comes from recent large studies conducted with children in Bangladesh. Extensive scientific examination of the risks for drowning and the effect of increased swim skill in Bangladesh suggests that acquisition of swim skills reduces drowning risk dramatically among those receiving lessons [RR of 0.072 (CI: 0.017–0.307, $p < 0.0001$)].[93] Importantly, a follow-up survey reported that children who had learned to swim showed no greater risk taking or water exposure compared to those who learned naturally.[118]

What constitutes basic swim skills was defined operationally by the swim community as those skills needed to be able to swim in "the deep end." Based on a survey of multiple international, national, and local organizations' practices, a definition for minimal water competency was proposed. It consisted of five skills: entering with submersion, floating or treading, propulsion for 25 yards/meters, turning 360 degrees and exiting.[119] Many organizations require greater swimming distances, up to 200 meters. However, swim skills learned in one setting, such as a pool, may not adequately protect a swimmer in another water environment, such as when in surf or following a fall out of a boat.[120,121] Experiential training has become recognized as key to expanding skills. Thus, swimming lessons have begun to be taught in the sea or in simulated waves and while wearing clothing. However, even strong swimmers can drown.

Physical swimming skills alone do not protect against drowning; broader water safety knowledge is needed. This is why a young child who can perform all the swim competencies well is still not "water safe" and why no one can be "water-proofed." Any drowning event is a confluence of water safety knowledge, physical skill, and environmental conditions. This has recently led to developing the concept of water competency as a holistic approach incorporating basic swim skills plus water safety knowledge, safe attitudes, appropriate behaviors, and other skills such as safe rescue and CPR; 15 competencies have been proposed[122] (Table 173-1A, 1B). These competencies guide what each person needs to achieve and demonstrate they have achieved prior to going near, in, or on water.

Existing policy on swimming competency resides within organizations providing swimming lessons. Once a mainstay of graduation from school, taking swimming lessons or passing a swim test is now rarely required. In Washington State, of 78 randomly surveyed public schools, none required swimming for graduation. Reasons cited

TABLE 173-1A THE 15 WATER COMPETENCIES

Knowledge/Attitudes/Behaviors	Skills
Knowledge of local hazards	Safe entry • Entry into water • Surface and level off
Coping with risks • Recognize and avoid risk • Judgment of risk and action	Breath control—integrated and effective breathing
Assessment of personal competencies	Stationary surface competencies • Float front and back • Tread water
Water safety attitudes and values	Water orientation • Roll from front to back, back to front • Turn, L and R, on front and back
Use of personal flotation device	Swimming skills • Swim on front • Swim on back
	Underwater competencies • Surface dive • Swim underwater
	Safe exit
	Clothed water competencies
	Open water competencies
	Recognition of and assistance to a drowning victim • Rescue • CPR

TABLE 173-1B 15 WATER COMPETENCIES BASED ON NEEDED CHANGE IN KNOWLEDGE OR PHYSICAL SKILL

Knowledge	Physical Skills
Knowledge of local hazards	Safe entry • Entry into water • Surface and level off
Coping with risks • Recognize and avoid risk • Judgment of risk and action	Breath control—integrated and effective breathing
Assessment of personal competencies	Stationary surface competencies • Float front and back • Tread water
Water safety attitudes and values	Water orientation • Roll from front to back, and back to front • Turn, left and right, on front and back
How to fit and use personal flotation device	Swimming skills • Swim on front • Swim on back
	Underwater competencies • Surface dive • Swim underwater
	Safe exit Clothed water competencies Open water competencies Recognition of and assistance to a drowning victim (Rescue)

included lack of funding, time, and access to pools. Several swim programs in Vietnam solved this by bringing large portable pools to schools. One county in Florida buses children to local pools for 10 days of 30 minutes in water training during the school day (reference Swim Central http://www.broward.org/Parks/ProgramsClasses/Pages/SwimCentral.aspx). In Canada, the Swim to Survive program aims to provide swim lessons to children in third grade.[123] In the Netherlands, passing a swim test remains a national requirement.

Successful programs are rarely able to show decreased drowning mortality. In a remarkable drowning prevention effort in Bangladesh, the Swimsafe program provided swimming lessons and water safety instruction including rescue to 79,421 children ages 6–12 years.[93] The relative risk for fatal drowning was 0.072 ($p < 0.0001$) compared with an untrained matched cohort. This program was cost effective. In HIC, programs are unlikely to be able to demonstrate statistically significant decreases in fatal drownings because of their lower baseline drowning rates.

Challenges to acquiring water competency start with the continuing focus on swim skills, not safe judgment and behaviors, and use of the pool environment rather than natural water environments. Furthermore, how to screen for the minimum set of water competency swim skills remains a challenge. In one US study, being able to meet minimal water competency swim skills as judged by lifeguards (e.g., able to swim in the deep end) was positively correlated with self- or parental reports that the child had "good" swim skills (as a opposed to poor or none) or was "comfortable in deep water."[124]

Real barriers are the time and cost of water competency. The number of swim lessons needed to achieve minimal swim skills requires a large commitment of time and money.[125] In the American Red Cross swim program, this is usually achieved after 20 lessons or more (in ARC Level 5 classes) and in Bangladesh's SwimSafe program, 17 lessons. In Australia, the Swim and Survive program addresses swim skills and water safety in three progressive age-based programs starting at 6 months and running through 14 years.[125]

Supervision

Data evaluating the effectiveness of supervision is sparse because it has been poorly defined. Supervision as an injury prevention strategy has been conceptualized as including three dimensions: attention, proximity, and continuity.[126] The level of each dimension required to ensure the ability to intervene appropriately varies depending on the risks in the environment and the abilities of those near or in the water. Supervision as a drowning prevention measure is critical when children or others are playing near or are in the water. However, observational studies of New Zealand parents at beaches showed 29% and 46% failed to adequately supervise children < 5 years and 5–9 years, respectively; instead they were engaged in sunbathing, talking with others, or using cellphones.[127,128] Lapses in supervision over time are normal and expected; for instance, lifeguards generally have a rotation schedule with breaks to ensure attention does not wane. The level of supervision necessary to prevent drowning is not possible on a continuous, long-term basis which is why barriers are necessary and effective when children are not intended to be in the water. Poor supervision is more easily recognized than good supervision.

The components of adequate supervision around the water have been delineated over time but remain poorly documented and evaluated. The description of adequate supervision for drowning prevention most often applies primarily to young children who are nonswimmers and includes that the supervising adult should be within arm's reach of the child (close proximity).[126] The American Red Cross describes the qualities of an appropriate supervisor as being an adult or person trained in rescue, undistracted, not using alcohol or recreational drugs, and aware of how to call for help. In China, fatal drowning risk was higher among children supervised by grandparents, presumably who were either incapable or limited in their ability to watch or respond to the child near the water.[116] As seen with other interventions that induce false security, parents of children in swim lessons reported lower likelihood of supervising them.[129]

Successful programs that improved supervision addressed the risk that swim lessons incur. Parents of children in swim lessons must learn that supervision is still needed despite the child's swimming ability. Parents in programs that specifically sought to educate them of their continued role in protecting children in swim lessons reported improved supervisory behaviors.[130,131]

Additionally, many parents cannot recognize the swimmer in distress. Drowning occurs quickly and quietly and potentially in full view of supervisors who are unfamiliar with and cannot identify the process of drowning. Adequate supervision includes not only the ability to identify a drowning person, but also the knowledge of how to conduct a safe rescue and the ability to do so. Finally, a supervising person should be able to initiate CPR and call for emergency medical service.

An educational approach to relaying the responsibilities and characteristics required of someone who supervises children, adolescents or others in or around water is needed. To develop a program to provide the knowledge and skills to be an appropriate supervisor, research is needed to determine how to effectively convey what qualities of supervision (attentiveness, proximity, continuity) are needed in different situations/settings, and how to identify the drowning process. A critical mass of laypersons trained in rescue is needed to ensure someone with skills is present when needed. Finally, cultural barriers exist regarding skills to prevent drowning; information on how to identify and overcome these barriers is needed.

Lifeguards

Evaluation of lifeguards' role in risk reduction is poor; United States Lifesaving Association (USLA) reports that the risk of fatal drowning on surf beaches is 1 per 18 million beach visits and that three quarters of drowning deaths at surf beaches guarded by USLA lifeguards occurred afterhours when lifeguards were not on duty.[132] Similarly, a review of lifeguard records at waterparks reported one death per 15.9 million visits.[133] Ecologic case studies of drowning incidents before and after initiation or discontinuation of lifeguard services suggest lifesaving benefits.[132,134] While it is well known that lifeguards are trained to rescue drowning victims, what they do to decrease fatal and nonfatal drowning risk has been poorly described and evaluated. In a recent evaluation of surf beach lifeguard activities, prevention interventions represented 54.8% while rescues represented 1.9% of their interactions with beachgoers.[135]

In a US study of drowning deaths in lifeguarded pools, most occurred in municipal pools (38%), community organizations' pools (15%), or school pools (14%) and fatal events were twice as likely to be identified by a nonlifeguard than a lifeguard.[136] Drownings occur in lifeguarded swimming areas because surveillance requires constant scanning of an area affected by multiple factors including as light, water and surface conditions as well as responding to high rates of risk taking behaviors by swimmers and occasional distractions.[137]

In the US, pool lifeguard training and certification are standardized, but operations and monitoring are highly variable. Unlike emergency medical services and fire departments, few state, county, or municipal laws govern lifeguard services. To address this variability, the Model Aquatic Health Code (MAHC), includes recommended standards for pool lifeguard staffing based on best practices and evidence regarding zones and rotation procedures.[138] For example, the MAHC recommends that pool lifeguards be limited to a maximum 60 minutes of surveillance followed by a 10-minute break. The MAHC outlines the need for management to maintain staffing plans, record keeping, and regular pool inspections and includes forms to do so.[138] The MAHC does not address open water lifeguarding. Training and policy related to open water lifeguarding are based at the agency level and as such are variable.

Successful ways to improve lifeguarding have primarily focused on evaluating and improving performance of specific tasks such as recognition of the swimmer in distress, swim efficiency in reaching the swimmer, and CPR.[139–141] In one study, a single mid-summer brief intervention with lifeguards directly increased lifeguard surveillance and indirectly decreased swimmer risk taking.[142] Researchers suggest that, similar to other industries, frequent role-playing can improve lifeguard performance and, to decrease lifeguard surveillance fatigue, organizations can limit surveillance time with breaks and have a manager onsite.[143]

In Australia, New Zealand, and the United Kingdom, open water lifeguarding is regulated, its activities are compiled and evaluated. In Australia, this includes annual surveillance data of rescues and drownings with trend, G.I.S., and critical incident analysis, which inform drowning prevention strategies.[144] Australia has subsequently noted a decrease in coastal drownings.

The biggest challenge is the reduced number of public recreational sites with lifeguards over the past decades due to funding shortages. Lifeguard recruitment has become more difficult, especially where racial diversity is needed. The lack of systematic, reliable, and timely data collection systems is a challenge to documentation and evaluation of lifeguard services. Useful data are either not collected, not evaluated, or surveillance systems are incomplete. Existing data collection efforts are hampered by lack of real-time systems and reporting bias, which threaten the reliability and validity of reports and conclusions derived from such methods.[135,145]

Evaluation of the cost-effectiveness of lifeguard services in the US is needed. In the United Kingdom and Australia, studies of the cost-effectiveness of their lifeguarding services on coastal beaches identified the benefit they provided the communities.[146,147] Similar examination in the US might provide the justification for some communities to commit to lifeguard staffing at public sites and support learn-to-swim and junior lifeguard programs in the community. Development of lifeguard data systems similar to that of EMS might improve staffing, effectiveness and community support for lifeguarding. Increased training of lifeguards, of diverse backgrounds, especially in high-risk areas and populations could increase involvement of minority groups in water activities. For example, the American Red Cross has included lifeguard training in its Centennial Swim program conducted in 100 high-risk cities and regions.[148]

Other

Alcohol use is a known risk factor for drowning. There is indirect evidence that reductions in alcohol use around water might be related to reductions in drowning deaths.[23] All 50 states have Boating Under the Influence (BUI) laws restricting alcohol use by the boat operator but the details and penalties vary widely (https://www.boat-ed.com/bui-laws.html). There has generally been support for BUI laws given the documented effectiveness in the reduction of motor vehicle crashes, deaths, and injuries following Driving Under the Influence laws. However, research suggests that, unlike with motor vehicles where the operator's sobriety is key, the passengers on a boat are also at risk of drowning if they drink. In one study, 46% of boating-related fatalities occurred when the boat was docked, drifting, or anchored, meaning that the operator's sobriety was not a contributing factor.[31] A major challenge to support for alcohol control policies and programs is the current culture of alcohol use during water recreation. The role of alcohol control policies in drowning prevention has not been well examined. Finally, a culture change is needed regarding the acceptability of alcohol use in the recreational water setting.

Signage is a common intervention to promote water safety, including signage to designate safe swim areas, use of life jackets and hazards. However, no studies have evaluated its efficacy in drowning prevention.

Tertiary Prevention of Drowning—Improve Outcomes

Rescue

The chain of survival for drowning has similarities but important differences from the cardiac chain of survival. Recognition of the swimmer in distress, reaching the victim, and safely bringing the victim to land are unique to the drowning chain of survival. These involve unfamiliar skills and equipment. Furthermore, these need to be used as quickly as possible so that resuscitation, treatment, and reversal of anoxia, can begin as quickly as possible.[89]

While the focus has been to provide the drowning victim CPR, the critical but ignored step in the chain of survival for drowning has been rescue. Recognition of drowning is difficult; it is a learned skill. The timeline from distress to submersion and sinking is less than a minute or two. In the early stage, the victim loses forward momentum in the horizontal plane in the water and goes vertical.[149] Panic and air hunger make the breathing effort all-consuming, leaving no air for yelling; instead of waving for help, the victim uses his arms underwater to try to lift his upturned face and airway above the water. Furthermore, ultimate aspiration of fluid silences the victim. By the time the person in distress begins to submerge, a few bobs up and down, if at all, are swiftly followed by sinking. Commonly, tragedies result when the untrained witness thinks the victim is "fooling around" when they see the underwater arm flapping or the body bobbing. Teaching recognition of the person in distress is a key concept in the chain of survival of the drowning victim, just as recognition of the collapsed victim as a possible cardiac arrest is for the cardiac chain of survival.[89,149]

Compared to intervening on a collapsed cardiac victim, people are more willing to respond to a drowning victim. In New Zealand, 47% of festival go-ers said they would jump in to rescue a person. In Bangladesh, children 6–14 years reported commonly performing a rescue in ponds and ditches within 10 m of the bank.[150] Once a distressed swimmer is recognized, throwing the victim a floating object to grab can help safely bring the victim to land.

However, skills to perform a safe rescue need to be learned because a rescue attempt can lead to the would-be rescuer's death. A layperson attempting an in-water rescue of a drowning victim can be overwhelmed by the struggling victim, his own panic or fatigue, or the environmental conditions (e.g., waves, cold water). Rescuers who die may represent as many as 10% of fatal drownings.[50,151] In this not uncommon tragedy, the would-be rescuer is often the victim's father, is not wearing a life jacket, and ultimately drowns while the initial victim often survives.[151,152]

The common best practice, "reach or throw, don't go" requires practice. Even throwing a lifeline from the shore to someone in the water takes practice.[153] Further study is needed to define which technological interventions, such as throw rings, ropes or rescue tubes, are most effective and more easily and safely mastered. Additionally, other more common, inexpensive, and widely available home-made alternatives need to be identified.

Increasing rescue capacity among families, supervisors, and the public is needed. Just as CPR in the 1970s extended beyond professionals to citizens, safe rescue needs to be a more widely disseminated skill. Parents and those who supervise children are likely to be around, intervene, and conduct a rescue; they need to be taught safe rescue along with CPR.[151] Surfers are also a likely group for rescue training since they are water experienced, spend a lot of time in water, and 63% reported having saved a life.[154] In large surveys in Bangladesh, both female and male 6- to 14-year olds reported having safely and successfully rescued younger children while doing house chores or bathing in natural water.[150] Thus, older children represent a group who are willing and able to conduct safe rescues in some settings as well as perform CPR.

CPR

Rescue and CPR need to be taught together since early CPR improves favorable survival for drowning. Waiting for EMS to arrive and provide CPR represents a tremendous prolongation of anoxia even among urban rapid response. Drownings in natural waters commonly occur far from EMS. Delays of 9–10 minutes from the first call to arrival of EMS are associated with poor outcomes.[73] Bystander CPR prior to EMS arrival was associated with improved outcomes among drowning victims (adjusted OR 3.02, 95% CI 1.85–4.92).[15] Wide dissemination of rescue with CPR training programs to adults as well as middle school and high school children is needed to build capacity to safely respond to a drowning victim.

Additional interventions have not been helpful in reducing consequences of a drowning event. Early defibrillation has a minimal role in drowning since a shockable rhythm occurs in only 5–7% of cardiac arrests following drowning. In fact, use of an automatic external defibrillator was associated with a lower likelihood of favorable outcome. Between 1975 and 1995, advanced medical care was not associated with improved outcomes for drowning victims.[23] More recently, in a randomized controlled multicenter trial, the longest and most studied medical intervention, therapeutic hypothermia, did not improve outcome of drowned children.[155] Over the past decade, extra corporeal membrane oxygenation, which oxygenates the blood outside the body thus bypassing injured lungs, resulted in survival of some very hypothermic victims, although most treated victims died.[156,157] These highly invasive, very expensive, resource intensive, advanced life support interventions have not been evaluated with randomized or case controlled studies. Only basic life support interventions at the scene have been demonstrated to improve outcomes.

IMPLEMENTATION OF DROWNING PREVENTION STRATEGIES: FUTURE DIRECTIONS

The Three Pillars of Injury Prevention

A second framework to consider for drowning prevention includes how interventions can be implemented through the three pillars of injury prevention: education, engineering the environment, and legislation. Of these, education is the most commonly embraced approach. Drowning prevention education globally has focused on children, especially in classroom settings where they are an accessible, captured audience. The goal is for children to gain safety knowledge and behaviors that they will use when in, at or near water. However, these programs need evaluation and long-term follow-up. Strategies to change adult behaviors regarding alcohol and lifejacket use need to be pursued.

Educational messages should be standardized so that they are reinforced and become familiar. An international task force, representing 18 countries, sought to develop global messages for prevention of natural (or open) water drowning.[158] Members prioritized and developed 16 concise statements to provide message clarity and to improve message retention. Additionally, these prioritized messages may provide a focus for drowning prevention programs and an agenda for future research in the area.

Engineering and technology can be used to improve swimmer safety. Lifejackets and safe flotation devices remain technologies that are still underdeveloped, underpromoted, and underutilized. Redesigning beaches to eliminate hazards can make natural waters safer. The introduction of drones as adjuncts to lifeguarding can potentially enhance surveillance and more quickly deliver flotation to rescue swimmers in distress.

Legislation and policy represent the third pillar for implementation. Not surprisingly, legislation is most common for the built environment of swimming pools; these are most often at the local and state level. To address the confusing range of codes and rules for pools, the MAHC covers the design, construction, operation, and maintenance of swimming pools, spas, hot tubs, and other public disinfected aquatic facilities.[138] The MAHC is a model for preventive legislation and includes a process for periodic updates and changes. However, while it evaluates emergency department visits for waterborne illnesses or pool chemical exposures, it does not evaluate rescues, drownings, or deaths as outcome measures. Moreover, it only applies to pools.[138] In contrast, very little drowning prevention legislation and oversight apply to natural water.

To address the problem of hazardous natural water recreational swim sites, Australia developed the concept of managing risks at natural water sites.[159] These efforts include assessing of physical hazards in the area and water, including drop off, bottom irregularity, current, bacteria, chemicals, and dangerous aquatic creatures and mitigating risks by providing lifeguards, rescue equipment, and/or life jacket loaner boards. The US Army Corps of Engineers used many of these interventions to reduce drowning risks at its lake shores.[160] Washington State developed a list of potential criteria to define designated swim areas in natural water sites and rate them.[161] These criteria were used by some communities to develop or enhance existing local swim sites. States that have regulations for designated swim sites have lower fatal natural water drowning rates; however, this strategy has not been fully evaluated.

The tragedy of drowning deaths can be very powerful drivers of drowning prevention legislation. Following the drowning death of a young child who was not allowed to use his lifejacket at a summer camp, Christian's law in Massachusetts was passed, requiring camps to have lifejackets that children could use. The revised law requires municipal and recreational programs and camps to determine the swimming ability of each minor at the beginning of its swimming program at marine or freshwater beaches.[113] Following the death of children in suction drains in pools and spas, the Virginia Graham Baker Act was passed. This national law requires replacement of unsafe drains in semipublic and public pools and spas; it also supports pool safety educational activities by the Consumer Product Safety Commission.[162] Many parents become strong advocates, leading, guiding, and supporting drowning prevention in many ways.

Toward Comprehensive Programs

Very few multifaceted community drowning prevention programs have been evaluated.[163] The Bangladesh Anchal and Swimsafe programs were implemented on a large scale in multiple communities that included before and after mortality assessments. An Iranian multi agency collaboration involved a quasiexperimental design with a control and an intervention region along the Caspian Sea.[164] The interventions included education of the public and healthcare providers about drowning risks and the need for supervision of children, identification, and removal of hazards in the beach environment with some fencing of reservoirs, and markedly increasing the number of lifeguards along the recreational beaches. Three years after the intervention, the fatal drowning rates decreased significantly in the intervention region and proved cost effective regarding the increase in lifeguard services. Rates did not change significantly in the control region. This program incorporated many of the interventions and approaches recommended by the World Health Organization.

The World Health Organization developed an implementation guide for drowning prevention that included: (1) providing safe places for children, (2) installing barriers, (3) providing swimming lessons for school age children, (4) managing flood risks, (5) teaching safe rescue, and resuscitation, and (6) developing safe boating and shipping.[80] It recommends increasing public awareness, promoting collaboration, establishing national water safety (drowning prevention) plans, and research to identify effective drowning prevention strategies. Countries including Australia, Ireland, New Zealand, Scotland, the United Kingdom, Sri Lanka, and Canada have put

TABLE 173-2 SUMMARY OF PROVEN AND PROMISING INTERVENTION STRATEGIES

Strategy	Summary
Barriers	Four-sided isolation fencing is the most effective fencing configuration. Laws requiring four-sided fencing decrease deaths, especially if enforced. Other adjunctive barriers like door locks and weight bearing pool covers have not been evaluated.
Life jacket use	Life jackets are effective in reducing drowning risks but only if they are worn. Laws requiring they be worn decrease drowning deaths.
Lifeguarding	Lifeguards provide supervision and routinely intervene to reduce risky behaviors. Additionally, they are trained to recognize distressed swimmers, and perform rescues and resuscitation.
CPR	Bystander CPR has been proven to improve outcomes because it can halt the drowning process more quickly than waiting for emergency medical response. Lifeguards also can provide timely CPR.
Supervision	When young children are not supposed to be in the water, supervision cannot be expected to be constant enough to ensure children are protected from the water. When swimmers are supposed to be in the water, supervision can be effective if it is attentive, continuous and close enough to allow intervention. Supervisors must be able to recognize and respond to a swimmer in distress.
Alcohol use reduction	Alcohol is a known risk factor for drowning as it affects balance, judgment, coordination, risk taking, and response to drowning. Reduction of alcohol use is a promising intervention.
Entrapment prevention	Federal requirements now effectively prevent suction entrapments in compliant swimming pools and hot tubs.
Environmental changes	Designated swim areas and reduction in lake front slope gradients can prevent unexpected submersion.

forth national water safety plans while other nations' plans are in the works. Above all, good data should drive development, evaluation, and implementation of drowning prevention programs.

Summary

Since drowning is a very severe injury, occurring quickly and generally not reversed by current medical treatments, prevention is critical in reducing the burden of drowning. Implementation of proven prevention strategies is needed (Table 173-2).

There are concerns that drowning prevention interventions used in HIC may not be relevant in LMIC based on social, cultural, and behavioral factors.[33] For instance, socioeconomic resources limit safety infrastructure, widespread ownership of lifejackets and decreases in water risks in domestic settings. However, the basic drowning prevention interventions remain the same though applied in a different manner, considerate of cultural and social differences. The Bangladesh experience showed that the HIC-based swimming program could be modified for the LMIC setting and be effective there. Moreover, the program provided interventions for HIC's consideration; the Bangladesh intervention demonstrated that children can be taught to perform safe rescue and the Vietnam program showed the usefulness of portable swimming pools as training venues. What is clear is that drowning risks and settings are local and prevention efforts would likely improve with a community-based collaborative approach. Yet they need to be part of a larger effort and plan, with the support, resources, and dissemination abilities that a national commitment can provide.

Drowning prevention is not simple; progress will require multiple actions, focused on the risk factors and appropriate to the specific target group and setting. As a major public health challenge, drowning is preventable provided people have appropriate knowledge, skills, attitudes, and behaviors. Environments also can be altered and technologies leveraged to reduce risks. Drowning is a serious public health threat that has been neglected relative to other public health conditions. The exciting increase in global efforts and collaboration will rapidly disseminate efforts that can be adapted to each region's cultural, economic, and geographic specifics. However, drowning prevention research and programs should receive support commensurate with the burden and preventability.

References

1. World Health Organization. *Global Report on Drowning: Preventing a Leading Killer*. Geneva: World Health Organization; 2014.
2. Patton GC. Global patterns of mortality in young people: A systematic analysis of population health data. *Lancet.* 2009;374:881–92.
3. Gilchrist J, Parker EM. Racial and ethnic disparities in fatal unintentional drowning among persons less than 30 years of age—United States, 1999–2010. *J Safety Res.* 2014;50:139–42.
4. Centers for Disease Control and Prevention. Web-based Injury Statistics Query and Reporting System. http://www.cdc.gov/ncipc/wisqars. Accessed January, 2010.
5. Centers for Disease Control and Prevention (CDC). Injury Prevention and Control: WISQARS (Web-based Injury Statistics Query and Reporting System). http://www.cdc.gov/ncipc/wisqars/. Updated 2018. Accessed February 18, 2018.
6. Idris AH, Berg RA, Bierens J, et al. Recommended guidelines for uniform reporting of data from drowning: The "Utstein style." *Resuscitation.* 2003;59(1):45–57.
7. Gilchrist J, Gotsch K, Ryan G. Nonfatal and fatal drownings in recreational water settings—United States, 2001–2002 (Reprinted from MMWR, vol 53, pg 447-452, 2004). *JAMA.* 2004;53(2):164–6.
8. Laosee O, Gilchrist J, Rudd R. Drowning—United States, 2005–2009. *MMWR Morb Mortal Wkly Rep.* 2012;61(19):344.
9. Wadman MC, Muelleman RL, Coto JA, Kellermann AL. The pyramid of injury: Using ecodes to accurately describe the burden of injury. *Ann Emerg Med.* 2003;42(4):468–78.
10. Healthcare Cost and Utilization Project. https://hcupnet.ahrq.gov/. 2014.
11. Reynolds JC, Michiels EA, Nasiri M, Reeves MJ, Quan L. Observed long-term mortality after 18,000 person-years among survivors in a large regional drowning registry. *Resuscitation.* 2017;110:18–25.
12. Bierens JJ, Lunetta P, Tipton M, Warner DS. Physiology of drowning: A review. *Physiology.* 2016;31(2):147–66.
13. Nitta M. Out-of-hospital cardiac arrest due to drowning among children and adults form the Utstein Osaka Project. *Resuscitation.* 2013;84(11):1568–73.
14. Vahatalo RP, Lunetta P, Olkkola KT, Suominen PK. Drowning in children: Utstein style reporting and outcome. *Acta Anesthesiol Scand.* 2014;58:604–10.
15. Tobin JM, Ramos WD, Pu Y, Wernicki PG, Quan L, Rossano JW. Bystander CPR is associated with improved neurologically favourable survival in cardiac arrest following drowning. *Resuscitation.* 2017;115:39–43.
16. Youn C, Choi SP, Yim ea. Out-of-hospital cardiac arrest due to drowning: An Utstein Style report of 10 years of experience from St. Mary's Hospital. *Resuscitation.* 2009;80:778 –83.
17. Suominen PK, Vahatalo R. Neurologic long term outcome after drowning in children. *Scand J Trauma Resusc Emerg Med.* 2012;20:55.
18. Suominen PK, Sutinen N, Valle S, Olkkola KT, Lonnqvist T. Neurocognitive long term follow-up study on drowned children. *Resuscitation.* 2014;85(8):1059–64.
19. Spack L, Gedeit R, Splaingard M, et al. Failure of aggressive therapy to alter outcome in pediatric near-drowning. *Pediatr Emerg Care.* 1997;13(2):98–102.
20. Quan L, Bierens JJ, Lis R, Rowhani-Rahbar A, Morley P, Perkins GD. Predicting outcome of drowning at the scene: A systematic review and meta-analyses. *Resuscitation.* 2016;104:63–7.

21. Quan L, Mangione T, Bennett E, Chow W. Use of life jackets and other types of flotation for in-water recreation in designated swim areas in Washington State. *Inj Prev*. 2018;24(2):123–8.
22. Cummings P, Mueller BA, Quan L. Association between wearing a personal floatation device and death by drowning among recreational boaters: A matched cohort analysis of United States Coast Guard data. *Inj Prev*. 2011;17(3):156–9.
23. Cummings P, Quan L. Trends in unintentional drowning: The role of alcohol and medical care. *JAMA*. 1999;281(23):2198–202.
24. Linnan M, Lanh EV, Cuong PV. Child mortality and injury in Asia: Survey results and evidence. Innocenti Working Papers 2007–06, Special Series on Child Injury No. 33, 2007.
25. World Health Organization. *ICD-10 International Classification of Diseases and Related Health Problems*. Vol 2. 10th ed. Malta: World Health Organization; 2010. http://www.who.int/classifications/icd/ICD10Volume2_en_2010.pdf. Accessed February 15, 2018.
26. Gillenwater JM, Quan L, Feldman KW. Inflicted submersion in childhood. *Arch Pediatr Adolesc Med*. 1996;150(3):298–303.
27. Haw C, Hawton K. Suicide and self-harm by drowning: A review of the literature. *Arch Suicide Res*. 2016;20(2):95–112.
28. Quan L, Pilkey D, Gomez A, Bennett E. Analysis of paediatric drowning deaths in Washington State using the child death review (CDR) for surveillance: What CDR does and does not tell us about lethal drowning injury. *Inj Prev*. 2011;17(Suppl 1):28–33.
29. National Center for Fatality Review and Prevention. Child Death Review Case Reporting System Case Report Version 4.1. https://www.ncfrp.org/wp-content/uploads/NCRPCD-Docs/CDRPrintCase_v4-1.pdf. Updated 2016. Accessed February 18, 2018.
30. Washington State Open Water Drowning Reporting Tool. http://www.seattlechildrens.org/pdf/washington-state-open-water-drowning-reporting-tool.pdf. 2016.
31. Howland J, Hingson R, Mangione TW, Bell N, Bak S. Why are most drowning victims men? Sex differences in aquatic skills and behaviors. *Am J Public Health*. 1996;86(1):93–6.
32. McCool J, Moran K, Ameratunga S, Robinson E. New Zealand beachgoers' swimming behaviours, swimming abilities and perception of drowning risk. *Int J Aquat Res Educ*. 2008;2(1):7–15.
33. Hyder AA, Alonge O, He S, et al. Saving of children's lives from drowning project in Bangladesh. *Am J Prev Med*. 2014;47(6):842–5.
34. Hu G, Mamady K. Impact of changes in specificity of data recording on cause-specific injury mortality in the United States, 1999–2010. *BMJ Public Health*. 2014;14:1010.
35. Quan L, Cummings P. Characteristics of drowning by different age groups. *Inj Prev*. 2003;9(2):163–8.
36. Xu JQ. Unintentional drowning deaths in the United States, 1999–2010. *NCHS Data Brief*. 2014;149:1–8.
37. Saluja G, Brenner RA, Trumble AC, Smith GS, Schroeder T, Cox C. Swimming pool drownings among US residents aged 5–24 years: Understanding racial/ethnic disparities. *Am J Public Health*. 2006;96(4):728–33.
38. Golob MI, Giles AR, Rich KM. Enhancing the relevance and effectiveness of water safety education for ethnic and racial minorities. *Int J Aquat Res Educ*. 2013;7(1):5.
39. Stirbu I, Kunst AE, Bos V, van Beeck EF. Injury mortality among ethnic minority groups in the Netherlands. *J Epidemiol Community Health*. 2006;60(3):249–55.
40. Dai D, Zhang Y, Lynch CA, Miller T, Shakir M. Childhood drowning in Georgia: A geographic information system analysis. *Appl Geogr*. 2013;37:11–22.
41. Irwin CC, Irwin RL, Ryan TD, Drayer J. Urban minority youth swimming (in)ability in the United States and associated demographic characteristics: Toward a drowning prevention plan. *Inj Prev*. 2009;15(4):234–9.
42. Strayer HD, Lucas DL, Hull-Jilly DC, Lincoln JM. Drowning in Alaska: Progress and persistent problems. *Int J Circumpolar Health*. 2010;69(3):253–64.
43. Irwin R, Drayer J, Irwin C, Ryan T, Southall R. *Constraints Impacting Minority Swimming Participation*. Memphis: University of Memphis; 2008.
44. Irwin CC, Irwin RL, Ryan TD, Drayer J. The legacy of fear: Is fear impacting fatal and non-fatal drowning of African American children? *J Black Stud*. 2011;42(4):561–76.
45. Quan L, Crispin B, Bennett E, Gomez A. Beliefs and practices to prevent drowning among Vietnamese-American adolescents and parents. *Inj Prev*. 2006;12(6):427–9.
46. Moran K, Willcox S. Water safety practices and perceptions of 'new' New Zealanders. *Int J Aquat Res Educ*. 2013;7(2):136–46.
47. Peden AE, Franklin RC, Leggat PA. International travelers and unintentional fatal drowning in Australia—A 10 year review 2002–12. *J Travel Med*. 2016;23(2):tav031.
48. Morgan D, Ozanne-Smith J, Triggs T. Descriptive epidemiology of drowning deaths in a surf beach swimmer and surfer population. *Inj Prev*. 2008;14(1):62–5.
49. Hatfield J, Williamson A, Brander R, Sherker S, Hayen A, Dunn N. Development and evaluation of campaigns to reduce rip current-related beach drowning in Australia. *Inj Prev*. 2012;18(Suppl 1):A135.
50. Zhu Y, Xu G, Li H, Huang Y, Ding K, Chen J. Epidemiology and risk factors for nonfatal drowning in the migrant children. *Southeast Asian J Trop Med Public Health*. 2015;46(6):1112–23.
51. Mahony AJ, Peden E, Franklin RC, Pearn JH, Scarr J. Fatal, unintentional drowning in older people: An assessment of the role of preexisting medical conditions. *Healthy Aging Res*. 2017;6(1):e7.
52. Franklin RC, Pearn JH, Peden AE. Drowning fatalities in childhood: The role of pre-existing medical conditions. *Arch Dis Child*. 2017;102(10):888–93.
53. Diekema DS, Quan L, Holt VL. Epilepsy as a risk factor for submersion injury in children. *Pediatrics*. 1993;91(3):612–6.
54. Appleton RE. Seizures, safety and submersion: Sense and sensibility. *Arch Dis Child*. 2017;102(10):883–4.
55. Mouridsen SE. Mortality and factors associated with death in autism spectrum disorders: A review. *Am J Autism*. 2013;1:17–25.
56. Splawski I, Shen J, Timothy KW, et al. Spectrum of mutations in long-QT syndrome genes. KVLQT1, HERG, SCN5A, KCNE1, and KCNE2. *Circulation*. 2000;102(10):1178–85.
57. Tzimas I, Bajanowski T, Poetsch M. The role of hereditary KCNQ1 mutations in water-related death. *Int J Legal Med*. 2016;130(2):361–3.
58. Pajunen T, Vuori E, Vincenzi FF, Lillsunde P, Smith G, Lunetta P. Unintentional drowning: Role of medicinal drugs and alcohol. *BMC Public Health*. 2017;17(1):388.
59. Shen J, Pang S, Schwebel DC. Cognitive and behavioral risk factors for unintentional drowning among rural Chinese children. *Int J Behav Med*. 2016;23(2):243–50.
60. Girasek DC, Marschall JS, Pope D. Understanding hikers who approached a hazardous river in Yosemite National Park. *Inj Prev*. 2016;22(2):110–6.
61. Girasek DC, Marschall JS, Pope D. Patterns of behaviour that pose potential drowning risk to hikers at Yosemite National Park. *J Travel Med*. 2016;23(1):1–7.
62. Driscoll TR, Harrison JA, Steenkamp M. Review of the role of alcohol in drowning associated with recreational aquatic activity. *Inj Prev*. 2004;10(2):107–13.
63. Smith GS, Keyl PM, Hadley JA, et al. Drinking and recreational boating fatalities: A population-based case-control study. *JAMA*. 2001;286(23):2974–80.
64. Peden AE, Franklin RC, Queiroga AC. Epidemiology, risk factors and strategies for the prevention of global unintentional fatal drowning in people aged 50 years and older: A systematic review. *Inj Prev*. 2018;24(3):240–7.
65. Simon HK, Tamura T, Colton K. Reported level of supervision of young children while in the bathtub. *Ambul Pediatr*. 2003;3(2):106–8.
66. Satoh F, Osawa M, Hasegawa I, Seto Y, Tsuboi A. "Dead in hot bathtub" phenomenon: Accidental drowning or natural disease? *Am J Forensic Med Pathol*. 2013;34(2):164–8.
67. Yang T. Pool or Spa Submersion: Estimated Injuries and Reported Fatalities, 2014 Report. https://www.cpsc.gov/s3fs-public/pdfs/2014H005.pdf. 2014.
68. Worldwide SK. Dangerous Waters Research. https://www.safekids.org/research-report/dangerous-waters-research-report. Updated 2016.
69. U.S. Department of Health and Human Services. CDC Wonder. CDC WONDER Web site. https://wonder.cdc.gov/. Updated 2018. Accessed February, 2018.
70. Peden AE, Franklin RC, Leggat PA. Fatal river drowning: The identification of research gaps through a systematic literature review. *Inj Prev*. 2016;22(3):202–9.
71. Peden MM, McGee K. The epidemiology of drowning worldwide. *Inj Control Saf Promot*. 2003;10(4):195–9.
72. Brenner RA, Trumble AC, Smith GS, Kessler EP, Overpeck MD. Where children drown, United States, 1995. *Pediatrics*. 2001;108(1):85–9.

73. Claesson A, Svensson L, Silfverstolpe J, Herlitz J. Characteristics and outcome among patients suffering out-of-hospital cardiac arrest due to drowning. *Resuscitation.* 2008;76(3):381–7.
74. Fralick M, Denny CJ, Redelmeier DA. Drowning and the influence of hot weather. *PLoS One.* 2013;8(8):e71689.
75. U.S. Department of Homeland Security, United States Coast Guard. 2016 Recreational Boating Statistics. https://www.uscgboating.org/library/accident-statistics/Recreational-Boating-Statistics-2016.pdf. 2017.
76. Barss P, Olsen K, Hamilton J, Dalke S. Non-wearing of floatation devices and swimming ability of boating immersion victims in Canada. *Inj Prev.* 2016;22(Suppl 2):a296.
77. Barss P, Olsen K, Hamilton J, Dalke S. Twenty years of PFD non-wearing and wearing among child and youth boating immersion victims in Canada. *International Life Saving Federation: World Conference on Drowning Prevention*, Penang, Malaysia, 2015, p. 141.
78. UNHCR. Mediterranean Statistics Dead and missing. http://data2.unhcr.org/en/situations/mediterranean. Updated 2018. Accessed February 15, 2018.
79. Mann NC, Weller SC, Rauchschwalbe R. Bucket-related drownings in the United States, 1984 through 1990. *Pediatrics.* 1992;89(6):1068–71.
80. World Health Organization. *Preventing Drowning: An Implementation Guide.* Geneva: World Health Organization; 2017.
81. Department of Labor, Bureau of Labor Statistics. National Census of fatal occupational injuries in 2016. USDL-17-1667. https://www.bls.gov/news.release/pdf/cfoi.pdf. 2017.
82. Lincoln JM, Lucas DL. Occupational fatalities in the United States commercial fishing industry, 2000–2009. *J Agromed.* 2010;15(4):343–50.
83. National Institute for Occupational Safety and Health. PFD manufacturer adopts NIOSH research into product development process. https://www.cdc.gov/niosh/docs/2015-119/pdfs/2015-119.pdf. 2014.
84. Centers for Disease Control and Prevention (CDC). Morbidity and mortality associated with Hurricane Floyd—North Carolina, September–October 1999. *MMWR Morb Mortal Wkly Rep.* 2000;49(17):369–72.
85. Zane DF, Bayleyegn TM, Hellsten J, et al. Tracking deaths related to Hurricane Ike, Texas, 2008. *Disaster Med Public Health Prep.* 2011;5(1):23–8.
86. Brunkard J, Namulanda G, Ratard R. Hurricane Katrina Deaths, Louisiana, 2005. *Disaster Med Public Health Prep.* 2008;2(4):215–23.
87. Centers for Disease Control and Prevention (CDC). Deaths associated with Hurricane Sandy—October–November 2012. *MMWR Morb Mortal Wkly Rep.* 2013;62(20):393–7.
88. Pless IB, Hagel BE. Injury prevention: A glossary of terms. *J Epidemiol Community Health.* 2005;59(3):182–5.
89. Szpilman D, Webber J, Quan L. Creating a drowning chain of survival. *Resuscitation.* 2014;85(9):1149–52.
90. Hyder AA, Borse NN, Blum L, Khan R, El Arifeen S, Baqui AH. Childhood drowning in low- and middle-income countries: Urgent need for intervention trials. *J Paediatr Child Health.* 2008;44(4):221–7.
91. Ramos WD, Beale A, Chambers P, et al. Primary and secondary drowning interventions: The American Red Cross Circle of Drowning Prevention and Chain of Drowning Survival. *Int J Aquat Res Educ.* 2015;9:89–101.
92. Thompson DC, Rivara FP. Pool fencing for preventing drowning in children. *Cochrane Database Syst Rev.* 1998;2000(2):CD001047.
93. Rahman F, Bose S, Linnan M, et al. Cost-effectiveness of an injury and drowning prevention program in Bangladesh. *Pediatrics.* 2012;130(6):e1621–8.
94. Consumer Product Safety Commission. Safety Barrier Guidelines for Residential Pools. https://www.cpsc.gov/s3fs-public/362%20Safety%20Barrier%20Guidelines%20for%20Pools.pdf. 2012
95. Florida. Florida Statutes: Chapter 515 Residential swimming pool safety act. http://www.leg.state.fl.us/statutes/index.cfm?App_mode=Display_Statute&URL=0500-0599/0515/0515.html. 2017.
96. Gilchrist J, Mack K. Prevalence of pools and adequate pool fencing in the United States, 2001–2003. *Int J Aquat Res Educ.* 2008;2(1):3.
97. Scott I. Prevention of drowning in home pools. In: Bierens JJLM, ed. *Handbook on Drowning Prevention, Rescue and Treatment.* Berlin Heidelberg, Germany: Springer-Verlag; 2006, p. 105. 10.1007/3-540-29656-5.
98. Stempski S, Schiff M, Bennett E, Quan L. A case-control study of boat-related injuries and fatalities in Washington State. *Inj Prev.* 2014;20(4):232–7.
99. Bugeja L, Cassell E, Brodie L, Walter S. Effectiveness of the 2005 compulsory personal flotation device (PFD) wearing regulations in reducing drowning deaths among recreational boaters in Victoria, Australia. *Inj Prev.* 2014;20:387–92.
100. Bennett E, Cummings P, Quan L, Lewis FM. Evaluation of a drowning prevention campaign in King County, Washington. *Inj Prev.* 1999;5(2):109–13.
101. Mangione TW, Chow W, Nguyen J. Trends in life jacket wear among recreational boaters: A dozen years (1999–2010) of US observational data. *J Public Health Policy.* 2012;33:59–74.
102. Mangione TW, Imre M, Chow W, et al. 2015 Life Jacket Wear Rate Observation Study. JSI Research & Training Institute, Inc. https://uscgboating.org/library/national-live-jacket-wear-study/2015-life-jacket-wear-rate-observation-study-report.pdf. 2016.
103. National Association of State Boating Legislators. State boating laws. www.nasbla.org Web site. https://www.nasbla.org/home. Accessed February 15, 2018.
104. US Army Corps of Engineers. Life Jacket Policy Study. 2012.
105. Mangione T, Chow W. Changing life jacket wearing behavior: An evaluation of two approaches. *J Public Health Policy.* 2014;35(2):204–18.
106. Chung C, Quan L, Bennett E, Kernic MA, Ebel BE. Informing policy on open water drowning prevention: An observational survey of life jacket use in Washington State. *Inj Prev.* 2014;20(4):238–43.
107. Giles AR, Castleden H, Baker AC. "We listen to our Elders. You live longer that way": Examining aquatic risk communication and water safety practices in Canada's North. *Health Place.* 2010;16(1):1–9.
108. Quistberg DA, Bennett E, Quan L, Ebel BE. Low life jacket use among adult recreational boaters: A qualitative study of risk perception and behavior factors. *Accid Anal Prev.* 2014;62:276–84.
109. Quistberg DA, Quan L, Ebel BE, Bennett EE, Mueller BA. Barriers to life jacket use among adult recreational boaters. *Inj Prev.* 2014;20(4):244–50.
110. Franklin RC, Leggat PA. The epidemiology of injury in canoeing, kayaking and rafting. *Med Sport Sci.* 2012;58:98–111.
111. Lucas D, Lincoln J, Somervell P, Teske T. Worker satisfaction with personal flotation devices (PFDs) in the fishing industry: Evaluations in actual use. *Appl Ergon.* 2012;43(4):747–52.
112. Seattle Children's Hospital. Open water drowning prevention policy strategy: Life Jackets. https://www.seattlechildrens.org/pdf/life-jackets.pdf. 2016.
113. Public Health Council. 105 CMR 432.00: Minimum Requirements for Personal Flotation Devices for Minor Children at Municipal and Recreational Programs and Camps. [Christian's law]. https://www.mass.gov/files/documents/2017/09/11/105cmr432.pdf. 2016.
114. Asher KN, Rivara FP, Felix D, Vance L, Dunne R. Water safety training as a potential means of reducing risk of young children's drowning. *Inj Prev.* 1995;1(4):228–33.
115. Brenner RA, Taneja GS, Haynie DL, et al. Association between swimming lessons and drowning in childhood: A case-control study. *Arch Pediatr Adolesc Med.* 2009;163(3):203–10.
116. Yang L, Nong Q, Li C, Feng QM, Lo SK. Risk factors for childhood drowning in rural regions of a developing country: A case-control study. *Inj Prev.* 2007;13:178–82.
117. Gresham LS, Zirkle DL, Tolchin S, Jones C, Maroufi A, Miranda J. Partnering for injury prevention: Evaluation of a curriculum-based intervention program among elementary school children. *J Pediatr Nurs.* 2001;16(2):79–87.
118. Mecrow TS, Linnan M, Rahman A, et al. Does teaching children to swim increase exposure to water or risk-taking when in the water? Emerging evidence from Bangladesh. *Inj Prev.* 2015;21(3):185–8.
119. Quan L, Ramos WD, Harvey C, et al. Toward defining water competency: An American Red Cross definition. *Int J Aquat Res Educ.* 2015;9:12–23.
120. Quieroga AC, Blitvich J, McElroy KD, Moran K, Fernandes RJ, Soares S. Can You Swim? Project: Evaluation of perceived and real water safety skills of children and adolescents aged 5-16 years old. *World Drowning Prevention Conference*, Book of Abstracts, #364, 2013, p. 109. http://www.ilsf.org/sites/ilsf.org/files/filefield/wcdp_abstracts_web.pdf#overlay-context=drowning-prevention/conference/2013.
121. Kjendlie PL, Pedersen T, Thoresen T, Setlo T, Moran K, Stallman R. Can you swim in waves? Children's swimming, floating, and entry skills in calm and simulated unsteady water conditions. *Int J Aquat Res Educ.* 2013;7(4):301–13.
122. Stallman RK, Moran K, Quan L, Langendorfer S. From swimming skill to water competence: Towards a more inclusive drowning prevention future. *Int J Aquat Res Educ.* 2017;10(2):3.
123. Lifesaving Society Canada. Swim to Survive. http://www.lifesaving.mb.ca/files/SwimToSurvive.pdf.

124. Mercado MC, Quan L, Bennett E, et al. Can you really swim? Validation of self and parental reports of swim skill with an inwater swim test among children attending community pools in Washington state. *Inj Prev*. 2016;22(4):253–60.

125. Royal Life Saving. Swim and Survive. http://www.swimandsurvive.com.au/content_common/pg-swim-and-survive.seo. Accessed February 15, 2018.

126. Saluja G, Brenner R, Morrongiello BA, Haynie D, Rivera M, Cheng TL. The role of supervision in child injury risk: Definition, conceptual and measurement issues. *Inj Control Saf Promot*. 2004;1:17–22.

127. Moran K. Parent/caregiver perceptions and practice of child water safety at the beach. *Int J Inj Contr Saf Promot*. 2009;16(4):215–21.

128. Moran K. Watching parents, watching kids: Water safety supervision of young children at the beach. *Int J Aquat Res Educ*. 2010;4:269–77.

129. Morrongiello BA, Sandomierski M, Spence JR. Changes over swim lessons in parents' perceptions of children's supervision needs in drowning risk situations: "His swimming has improved so now he can keep himself safe." *Health Psychol*. 2014;33(7):608–15.

130. Moran K, Stanley T. Toddler drowning prevention: Teaching parents about water safety in conjunction with their child's in-water lessons. *Int J Inj Contr Saf Promot*. 2006;13(4):254–6.

131. Morrongiello BA, Sandomierski M, Schwebel DC, Hagel B. Are parents just treading water? The impact of participation in swim lessons on parents' judgments of children's drowning risk, swimming ability, and supervision needs. *Accid Anal Prev*. 2013;50:1169–75.

132. United States Lifesaving Association. American Lifeguard Rescue and Drowning Statistics for Beaches. http://www.usla.org/?page=STATISTICS.

133. Hunsucker JL, Davison SJ. Analysis of rescue and drowning history from a lifeguarded waterpark environment. *Int J Inj Contr Saf Promot*. 2011;18(4):277–84.

134. Branche CM, Stewart S. *Lifeguard Effectiveness: A Report of the Working Group*. Atlanta: Centers for Disease Control and Prevention, National Center for Injury Prevention and Control; 2001.

135. Koon W, Rowhani-Rahbar A, Quan L. The ocean lifeguard drowning prevention paradigm: How and where do lifeguards intervene in the drowning process? *Inj Prev*. 2018;24(4):296–9.

136. Pelletier AR, Gilchrist J. Fatalities in swimming pools with lifeguards: USA, 2000–2008. *Inj Prev*. 2011;17(4):250–3.

137. Schwebel DC, Simpson J, Lindsay S. Ecology of drowning risk at a public swimming pool. *J Safety Res*. 2007;38(3):367–72. doi: https://doi.org/10.1016/j.jsr.2007.01.010.

138. Centers for Disease Control and Prevention (CDC). Model Aquatic Code (MAHC): An all-inclusive model public swimming pool and spa code. https://www.cdc.gov/mahc/index.html. Updated 2016. Accessed February 15, 2018.

139. Barcala-Furelos R, Szpilman D, Palacios-Aguilar J, et al. Assessing the efficacy of rescue equipment in lifeguard resuscitation efforts for drowning. *Am J Emerg Med*. 2016;34(3):480–5.

140. Barcala-Furelos R, Abelairas-Gomez C, Romo-Perez V, Palacios-Aguilar J. Effect of physical fatigue on the quality CPR: A water rescue study of lifeguards: Physical fatigue and quality CPR in a water rescue. *Am J Emerg Med*. 2013;31(3):473–7.

141. Adelborg K, Dalgas C, Grove EL, Jørgensen C, Al-Mashhadi RH, Løfgren B. Mouth-to-mouth ventilation is superior to mouth-to-pocket mask and bag-valve-mask ventilation during lifeguard CPR: A randomized study. *Resuscitation*. 2011;82(5):618–22.

142. Schwebel DC, Lindsay S, Simpson J. Brief report: A brief intervention to improve lifeguard surveillance at a public swimming pool. *J Pediatr Psychol*. 2007;32(7):862–8.

143. Schwebel DC, Jones HN, Holder E, Marciani F. Lifeguards: A forgotten aspect of drowning prevention. *J Inj Violence Res*. 2010;2(1):1–3.

144. Surf Life Saving Australia. Australian National Coastal Safety Report. https://issuu.com/surflifesavingaustralia/docs/ncsr-2017_lr_3298b910d49b62/59. Published December 11, 2017. Accessed February 15, 2018.

145. Williamson A. Feasibility study of a water safety data collection for beaches. *J Sci Med Sport*. 2006;9(3):243–8.

146. Logan A, Oxford Economics, MORI I. The economic and social benefits of lifeguard provision—RNLI. RNLI Research Project ID 13-1, 2013.

147. Myers M. What is the economic contribution of Surf Lifesaving. https://sls.com.au/surf-life-savings-economic-contribution-community-valued-36-billion/. Updated 2011. Accessed February 20, 2018.

148. American Red Cross. A Century of Aquatics: Making the Water Safe for Everyone. https://www.redcross.org/take-a-class/swimming/centennial. Updated 2017. Accessed February 17, 2018.

149. Pia F. Observations on the drowning of non-swimmers. *J Phys Educ*. 1974;71(6):164–7.

150. Mecrow TS, Rahman A, Linnan M, et al. Children reporting rescuing other children drowning in rural Bangladesh: A descriptive study. *Inj Prev*. 2015;21(e1):e51–5.

151. Franklin RC, Pearn JH. Drowning for love: The aquatic victim-instead-of-rescuer syndrome: drowning fatalities involving those attempting to rescue a child. *J Paediatr Child Health*. 2011;47(1–2):44–7.

152. Turgut A, Turgut T. A study on rescuer drowning and multiple drowning incidents. *J Safety Res*. 2012;43(2):129–32.

153. Pearn JH, Franklin RC. "Flinging the Squaler" lifeline rescues for drowning prevention. *Int J Aquat Res Educ*. 2009;3(3):315–21.

154. Attard A, Brander RW, Shaw WS. Rescues conducted by surfers on Australian beaches. *Accid Anal Prev*. 2015;82:70–8.

155. Moler FW, Hutchison JS, Nadkarni VM, et al. Targeted temperature management after pediatric cardiac arrest due to drowning: Outcomes and complications. *Pediatr Crit Care Med*. 2016;17(8):712.

156. Weuster M, Haneya A, Panholzer B, et al. The use of extracorporeal membrane oxygenation systems in severe accidental hypothermia after drowning: A centre experience. *ASAIO J*. 2016;62(2):157–62.

157. Burke CR, Chan T, Brogan TV, et al. Extracorporeal life support for victims of drowning. *Resuscitation*. 2016;104:19–23.

158. Quan L, Bennett E, Moran K, Bierens J. Use of a consensus-based process to develop international guidelines to decrease recreational open water drowning deaths. *J Health Promot Educ*. 2012;50(3):135–44.

159. NHMRC. *Guidelines for Managing Risks in Recreational Water*. Canberra: Australian Government; 2008. https://www.nhmrc.gov.au/_files_nhmrc/publications/attachments/eh38.pdf.

160. Gilchrist J, Branche C. Lifeguard effectiveness. In: Tipton M, Wooler A, eds. *The Science of Beach Lifeguarding*. Cleveland, OH: CRC Press; 2016, p. 29.

161. Washington State DOH. Washington State Designated Swim Area Guidelines. DOH 333-211. https://www.doh.wa.gov/Portals/1/Documents/Pubs/333-211.pdf. 2015.

162. Consumer Product Safety Commission. Virginia Graeme Baker Law. https://www.poolsafely.gov/wp-content/uploads/2016/04/pssa.pdf. 2012.

163. Wallis BA, Watt K, Franklin RC, Taylor M, Nixon J, Kimble RM. Interventions associated with drowning prevention in children and adolescents: Systematic literature review. *Inj Prev*. 2015;21:195–204.

164. Davoudi-Kiakalayeh A, Mohammadi R, Yousefzade-Chabok S, Jansson B. Evaluation of a community-based drowning prevention programme in northern Islamic Republic of Iran. *East Mediterr Health J*. 2013;19(7):629–37.

CHAPTER

174 Poisoning Prevention*

Tamara M. Haegerich • Erin Parker • Pierre-Olivier Cote • Debra Houry

BACKGROUND/INTRODUCTION

Over the past 15 years, poisoning death rates have increased in the United States from a rate of 9.19 per 100,000 in 2002, to 23.13 per 100,000, or 75,354 poisoning deaths in 2017. Increases in drug poisonings have contributed significantly to the increase in poisonings overall. This chapter provides a broad overview of the nature and burden of fatal and nonfatal poisonings and in addition to drug poisonings includes nondrug poisonings such as ingestion or exposure to household substances. Poisonings related to environmental factors such as lead, pesticides, and carbon monoxide are included within morbidity and mortality statistics, but are more closely associated with environmental health topics and risk factors and prevention strategies will not be discussed further in this chapter. The primary focus is on poisoning in the United States; however, some sections highlight where data from other countries are important to understanding effectiveness of interventions and the public health problem in a global perspective. The majority of poisonings are unintentional and preventable. Intentional poisonings are covered briefly in this chapter, specifically demographics, type of poisonings, and poisoning-specific prevention strategies, but for more information the reader is referred to Holland et al., in this textbook. Outlined in Chapter 175: The Epidemiology and Prevention of Self-Directed Violence are risk and protective factors separated by age group, in particular children compared to adolescents and adults. For example, parental characteristics such as younger maternal age, less supervision, single parent status, and a greater number of children in the household have been associated with increased risk for unintentional poisoning in children. Interventions specific to removing household risks, including safe storage of medications and household cleaning supplies, as well as parental education and training can reduce these poisonings. In comparison, unintentional poisonings in adults are largely due to drug overdoses. Interventions for drug overdoses, in particular opioid overdoses, include safe prescribing to prevent people from opioid use disorder, using lowest effective dosages of medication, minimizing drug interactions, and increasing access to naloxone. More recently, interventions have been focused on addressing the problem of illicit opioids, such as heroin and illicitly manufactured fentanyl. By focusing on intent, age group, and type of substance involved in the poisoning, implementing evidence-based interventions for poisonings can decrease burden.

NATURE AND BURDEN OF THE PROBLEM

Definitions

Definitions of poisoning have varied depending on perspective, analysis intent, and data source considered.[1] Consensus recommendations for national and state poisoning surveillance have defined poisoning as "an exposure to any extrinsic substance by ingestion, inhalation, injection, or absorption through the skin or mucous membranes that results in at least one related adverse clinical effect." Excluded from this definition are bites and stings without envenomation, infections, and exposure to radiation sources external to the body.[2] A subset of poisoning involving drugs is of particular interest given the public health burden, and is often referred to as "overdose." A drug is defined as "any chemical compound that is chiefly used by or administered to humans or animals as an aid in the diagnosis, treatment, or prevention of disease or injury, for the relief of pain or suffering, to control or improve any physiologic or pathologic condition, or for the feeling it causes." This includes illicit drugs, prescription drugs, over-the-counter drugs, supplements, etc. but excludes alcohol, tobacco, and solvents used for other purposes.[2] Drug overdose can be unintentional or intentional, and includes being given the wrong drug, taking a drug in error, or taking a drug inadvertently.[3] The definition of poisoning using the International Classification of Diseases for surveillance purposes is presented in Table 174-1.

Health Burden

Mortality

Information about poisoning mortality comes from national Vital Statistics data. In 2017, there were 75,354 poisoning deaths in the United States, at an age-adjusted rate of 23.19 per 100,000. Poisoning rates were twice as high among men (31.29) compared to women (15.15). Asian/Pacific Islanders had notably lower poisoning age-adjusted rates (4.00) than Whites (25.66), Blacks (20.66), and American Indian/Alaskan Natives (20.85). The majority of poisonings were unintentional (86.0%) (see Table 174-2). Unintentional poisoning was the leading cause of injury death in the United States in 2017. Burden varied across different age groups, with the highest rates concentrated among those aged 25–59 years.[8]

Determining manner of death—that is, whether a poisoning death is intentional or unintentional—can be challenging, particularly for drug-overdose death. There is wide variability across states in how manner of death is determined. Factors driving this variability include multidisciplinary differences in or lack of training, ambiguity of scene evidence, overlapping risk factors, fear of litigation, variations in burden of proof needed for certification, variations in toxicology and autopsy training and practice, variations in resources, and differences in social and cultural contexts.[9] Further, regardless of intent, estimating the prevalence of poisoning associated with specific drugs is a challenge because states differ greatly in toxicology testing practices. For example, in 2014, 19% of drug-overdose deaths did not include information on the death certificate about the specific types of drug involved in the death.[10] In one study, variation across states in

*The findings and conclusions in this chapter are those of the authors and do not necessarily represent the official position of the Centers for Disease Control and Prevention.

TABLE 174-1 INTERNATIONAL CLASSIFICATION OF DISEASES CODES FOR POISONING

Poisoning Codes	Unintentional	Self-inflicted	Assault	Undetermined	Other
ICD-9-CM ++ (morbidity)	E850-E869	E950-E952	E962, E979.7	E980-E982	E972, E997.2
ICD-10 (mortality)	X40-X49	X60-X69	X85-X90, *U01.6-.7*	Y10-Y19	Y35.2

Note: Items in *italics* are used when assessing terrorism. http://c.ymcdn.com/sites/www.cste.org/resource/resmgr/Injury/ISW7.pdf. Use of specific codes is recommended for surveillance of drug overdose, and can be found elsewhere.[3,4]
++ Final ICD-10-CM guidance is forthcoming. Guidance on transitioning from ICD-9-CM to ICD-10CM for analysis and reporting of nonfatal injuries (including poisonings) by mechanism and intent is available from the Safe States Alliance.[5] A framework has been proposed for presenting injury data using ICD-10-CM external cause of injury codes and diagnosis codes[6,7]; final guidance with recommendations for analyzing drug and opioid overdose specifically may differ from originally proposed framework and is forthcoming in 2019.

TABLE 174-2 POISONING DEATH RATES (CRUDE) PER 100,000 BY AGE, UNITED STATES, 2017

Age Group	All Cases Count	All Cases Rate	Unintentional Count	Unintentional Rate	Intentional[a] Count	Intentional[a] Rate	Undermined Count	Undetermined Rate
0–4	92	0.46	38	0.19	21	0.11	33	0.17
5–9	**	**	**	**	**	**	**	**
10–14	82	0.39	39	0.19	40	0.19	**	**
15–19	915	4.33	687	3.25	175	0.83	53	0.25
20–24	4,872	22.03	4,343	19.64	302	1.37	227	1.03
25–29	8,571	36.67	7,781	33.29	393	1.68	397	1.7
30–34	9,628	43.82	8,697	39.58	441	2.01	490	2.23
35–39	9,326	43.92	8,368	39.41	510	2.4	448	2.11
40–44	7,618	38.78	6,664	33.92	610	3.11	344	1.75
45–49	8,476	40.41	7,257	34.6	808	3.85	411	1.96
50–54	8,742	40.85	7,450	34.81	816	3.81	476	2.22
55–59	8,008	36.39	6,731	30.58	812	3.69	465	2.11
60–64	4,774	23.88	3,850	19.26	657	3.29	267	1.34
65–69	2,275	13.51	1,709	10.15	437	2.6	129	0.77
70–74	878	6.83	532	4.14	290	2.26	56	0.44
75–79	436	4.99	250	2.86	158	1.81	28	0.32
80–84	261	4.38	156	2.62	94	1.58	**	**
85+	374	5.78	224	3.46	136	2.1	**	**
Total	75,354	23.13	64,795	19.89	6,705[a]	2.06	3,854	1.18

WISQARS, available at https://www.cdc.gov/injury/wisqars/fatal.html.
ICD-10 Codes: X40-X49, X60-X69, X85-X90, Y10-Y19, Y35.2, *U01(.6,.7)
** = Rates are unstable, < 20 deaths.
[a]Suicides account for approximately 98% of intentional poisoning deaths.

the percentage of drug-overdose deaths with the drugs specified on the death certificate ranged from 30% to 95%.[11] As an additional concern, continued emergence of novel substances (aka "designer drugs" and fentanyl analogs) has posed challenges for toxicology testing and laboratory detection.[12] Although prescription and illicit drugs remain the predominant substances involved in intentional poisonings, other nonpharmacological substances are sometimes involved in these poisonings. A study analyzing nonpharmacological poisoning suicides between 2000 and 2012 in San Diego County, CA found that carbon monoxide ($n = 103$), helium ($n = 65$), and ethylene glycol ($n = 12$) were the primary poisoning mechanisms in about 85% of cases but other substances were involved in the remaining deaths.[13] This chapter focuses primarily on substances associated with a high morbidity and mortality burden, with the recognition that a variety of other substances are involved in unintentional and intentional poisonings.

Over 93% of all poisoning deaths were due to drug overdose in 2017. Drug-overdose death rates more than tripled from 1999 (6.1 per 100,000) to 2017 (21.7 per 100,000), with the rate increasing from 1999 to 2006 by 10% per year on average; from 2006 to 2014 the rate increased by 3% per year, and from 2014 to 2017 the rate increased by 16% per year.[3] See Table 174-3 for a display of the most common drugs in overdose deaths, and how drugs involved have changed over time (with the most recent data from 2016). Among the 70,237 people who died of drug overdose in 2017, 67.8% of deaths involved an opioid, including natural and semisynthetic opioids and methadone (commonly referred to as "prescription" opioids), synthetic opioids other than methadone, and heroin.[14] Other drugs commonly involved in drug overdose were cocaine (involved in 19.8% of deaths) and psychostimulants (14.7%); nearly three fourths of cocaine-involved deaths and half of psychostimulant-involved deaths also involved opioids.[15] The burden of opioid-related overdose is greatest for men, non-Hispanic whites, and those aged 25–54. Death rates vary significantly across states, with those living in the northeastern and southern regions of the United States affected the greatest. From 2016 to 2017, counties in large central, large fringe, and medium metro areas as well as micropolitan areas experienced the largest absolute increases in deaths involving opioids. Death rates are highest for synthetic opioids other than methadone (9.0) and prescription opioids (5.2); the most dramatic increases in mortality have been seen for synthetic opioids

TABLE 174-3 MOST COMMON DRUGS INVOLVED IN DRUG OVERDOSE DEATHS, 2010–16

Rank	2010	2011	2012	2013	2014	2015	2016
1	Oxycodone	Oxycodone	Heroin	Heroin	Heroin	Heroin	Fentanyl
2	Methadone	Cocaine	Oxycodone	Cocaine	Cocaine	Fentanyl	Heroin
3	Cocaine	Heroin	Cocaine	Oxycodone	Oxycodone	Cocaine	Cocaine
4	Alprazolam	Methadone	Methadone	Morphine	Alprazolam	Oxycodone	MET
5	Heroin	Alprazolam	Alprazolam	Alprazolam	Fentanyl	MET	Alprazolam
6	Morphine	Morphine	Morphine	Methadone	Morphine	Alprazolam	Oxycodone
7	Hydrocodone	Hydrocodone	Hydrocodone	MET	MET	Morphine	Morphine
8	Fentanyl	MET	MET	Hydrocodone	Methadone	Methadone	Methadone
9	Diazepam	Diazepam	Fentanyl	Fentanyl	Hydrocodone	Hydrocodone	Hydrocodone
10	MET	Fentanyl	Diazepam	Diazepam	Diazepam	Diphenhydramine	Diazepam

Notes: MET—Methamphetamine. Deaths are classified using the International Classification of Diseases, Tenth Revision. Drug overdose deaths are identified using underlying cause-of-death codes X40-X44, X60-X64, X85, and Y10-Y14.
Sources: CDC/NCHS, National Vital Statistics System Mortality File.[18] Hedegaard H, Bastian BA, Trinidad JP, Warner M. Drugs most frequently involved in drug overdose deaths: United States, 2011–16. National Vital Statistics Reports 2018;67(9):1–14.[19]

TABLE 174-4 PRIMARY SOURCES OF POISONING DATA IN THE UNITED STATES

Resource	Underlying Data Source	Description	Sample/Population	Poisoning Variables	Website
WISQARS (Web-based Injury Statistics Query and Reporting System) Fatal Injury Data	National Vital Statistics System (NVSS) from CDC's National Center for Health Statistics	Presents mortality data in five report formats: fatal injury, leading causes of death, years of potential life lost, fatal injury mapping, and costs of injury reports.	Death certificates and census data at the national level (since 1981).	Intent of injury, mechanism of injury, body region, nature of injury, geographic location, and sex, race/ethnicity, and age of the injured person.	https://www.cdc.gov/injury/wisqars/fatal.html
WISQARS Nonfatal Injury Data	U.S. Consumer Product Safety Commission's National Electronic Injury Surveillance System—All Injury Program (NEISS-AIP)	Presents nonfatal injury data from emergency department (ED) visits in two reports: nonfatal injury and leading causes of nonfatal injury reports.	National probability sample of hospitals in the United States and its territories (since 2000).	Cause (mechanism) of injury, intent of injury, disposition (where injured person went after release from ED), and year, sex, and race/ethnicity of the injured person.	https://www.cdc.gov/injury/wisqars/nonfatal.html
WONDER (Wide-ranging Online Data for Epidemiological Research) Underlying Cause of Death database	WONDER. Compressed Mortality, Multiple Cause of Death, and Infant Deaths databases also available.	Unlike WISQARS, WONDER offers county-level information, data prior to 1981, and specification of user-defined causes of death codes.	Mortality and population counts for all U.S. counties based on death certificates for U.S. residents.	Cause of death, injury intent and mechanism, place of residence (region, state, or county), urbanization, age, race/ethnicity, gender, and year.	https://wonder.cdc.gov/
Healthcare Cost and Utilization Project (HCUP) databases	Healthcare Cost and Utilization Project, sponsored by the Agency for Healthcare Research and Quality (AHRQ).	Data on healthcare utilization, access, charges, quality, and outcomes. Files available for SAS, SPSS, and Stata.	Varies by database. Both nationwide and state-level data.	Varies by database.	https://www.hcup-us.ahrq.gov/databases.jsp
National Poison Data System (NPDS) Annual Reports	American Association of Poison Control Centers (AAPC) member poison centers	Data on over 62 million poison exposure case records and consumer product data going back to 1983. Annual Reports are freely available.	Poisoning cases from 55 poison control centers (as of 2017) uploaded into electronic health record collection systems in near real-time.	Medical outcome, intent/reason of poisoning, route of exposure, exposure site and duration, substance quantity, caller location, and age and sex.	http://www.aapcc.org/annual-reports/

other than methadone (a 45.2% increase in rate from 2016 to 2017). This dramatic increase in mortality in 1 year has been attributed to the increasing availability of illicitly-manufactured fentanyl, which is commonly sold as or mixed with heroin.[14] Drug-poisoning death rates have also been found to be significantly correlated with prescription opioid sales.[16] Opioid-involved drug overdose has contributed significantly to the first decline in life expectancy in the United States since 1993, contributing an estimated loss of 0.21 years to the change in life expectancy from 2000 to 2015.[17]

Morbidity

Information about poisoning morbidity comes from emergency department, hospitalization, and poison control center data (see Table 174-4). Using data from the U.S. Consumer Product Safety Commission National Electronic Injury Surveillance System—All

TABLE 174-5 POISONING NONFATAL INJURY ESTIMATED COUNTS AND RATES (AGE-ADJUSTED) PER 100,000, UNITED STATES, 2017

Age Group	All Cases Count (95% CI)	All Cases Rate	Unintentional Count (95% CI)	Unintentional Rate	Intentional[a] Count	Intentional[a] Rate
0–4	41,053 (32,588–49,518)	205.89	40,952 (32,486–49,419)	205.39	**	**
5–9	7,832 (5,679–9,985)	38.57	7,800 (5,649–9,951)	38.42	**	**
10–14	30,716 (20,835–40,597)	147.83	14,197 (9,668–18,726)	68.33	16,519 (9,984–23,054)	79.50
15–19	139,495 (106,400–172,590)	660.12	91,501 (65,819–117,183)	433.00	47,994 (37,358–58,630)	227.12
20–24	188,783 (151,784–225,782)	853.50	155,110 (119,965–190,255)	701.26	33,673 (27,005–40,341)	152.24
25–29	228,752 (174,468–283,037)	978.81	200,915 (148,166–253,663)	859.70	27,838 (22,933–32,742)	119.12
30–34	224,839 (167,937–281,742)	1,023.29	200,904 (145,422–256,386)	914.35	23,935 (19,314–28,556)	108.93
35–39	191,966 (142,370–241,562)	904.14	171,160 (121,098–221,222)	806.14	20,806 (15,908–25,704)	97.99
40–44	169,535 (119,738–219,333)	863.06	150,107 (100,612–199,602)	764.16	19,429 (16,363–22,495)	98.91
45–49	173,413 (124,547–222,279)	826.81	152,670 (105,651–199,689)	727.91	20,743 (16,026–25,460)	98.90
50–54	203,827 (141,383–266,272)	952.41	184,774 (123,033–246,515)	863.39	19,053 (14,742–23,364)	89.03
55–59	164,361 (118,753–209,970)	746.83	148,621 (103,864–193,378)	675.31	15,740 (11,857–19,624)	71.52
60–64	106,074 (79,844–132,305)	530.70	96,668 (70,771–122,565)	483.64	9,406 (7,086–11,726)	47.06
65–69	57,321 (42,924–71,717)	340.46	52,430 (38,359–66,501)	311.41	4,891 (3,106–6,675)	29.05
70–74	38,350 (28,084–48,615)	298.51	36,447 (26,769–46,125)	283.70	1,903 (945–2,861)	14.81
75–79	20,910 (12,451–29,370)	239.21	19,151 (11,035–27,268)	219.09	1,759 (797–2,721)	20.12
80–84	17,126 (10,993–23,259)	287.09	16,035 (10,303–21,768)	268.81	**	**
85+	14,485 (8,845–20,126)	223.93	13,785 (8,324–19,246)	213.10	**	**
Total (age-adj. rate)	2,020,800 (1,568,353–2,473,247)	624.07	1,755,044 (1,314,343–2,195,744)	539.76	265,756[a] (218,521–312,991)	84.31

**Injury estimate is unstable because of small sample size.
[a]Self-harm accounts for approximately 98% of intentional nonfatal poisoning injuries.

Injury Program (NEISS-AIP), in 2017, there were an estimated 2,020,800 nonfatal poisonings seen in emergency departments in the United States, at an age-adjusted rate of 624.07 per 100,000 (see Table 174-5). Similar to mortality, the burden was higher among men (766.64 per 100,000) than women (484.59). The majority of nonfatal poisonings were unintentional (86.8%). Burden varied across different age groups, with the highest rates concentrated among those aged 15–59 years; among children under the age of 15, those under the age of 5 had the highest burden. There are some important differences in morbidity burden based on intent, however. For example, while the overall burden of poisoning is higher among men, in 2017, women had higher age-adjusted rates of self-harm poisoning (108.83) than men (57.70).[8]

Overdoses involving opioids pose a high burden for emergency department poisoning visits. Using data from the Healthcare Cost and Utilization Project (HCUP), in 2014 the rate of opioid-related emergency department (ED) visits was estimated at 177.7 per 100,000 population, reflecting an almost 100% increase since 2005 (an 8.0% average annual growth rate). The rate of opioid-related inpatient stays was estimated at 224.6 per 100,000, reflecting a 64.1% increase during this same time period (a 5.7% average annual growth rate). Significant variation was seen across states, with a tenfold variation in burden.[20] Although inpatient stays and ED visits increased for both sexes 2005–14, the greatest increase in rates was seen for women.[21] There is a significant delay in availability of data through the HCUP system. However, syndromic surveillance methods are beginning to allow faster detection of opioid overdose trends and outbreaks. For example, in early 2018, estimates from rapidly available emergency department medical claims and syndromic surveillance data were reported from 52 areas in 45 states, showing that the rate of ED visits for opioid overdoses went up 30% from July 2016 through September 2017. The rate of overdoses seen in emergency departments increased for men and women, people ages 25 and over, and in most states, with greatest increases seen in the Midwestern region.[22] While promising, the use of syndromic surveillance data for poisoning surveillance is relatively new and subject to a number of limitations, including variation in participation of hospitals over time and variation in coding and data quality across hospitals.[22]

One might expect that poisoning morbidity may differ among children as compared to adults. Of note, analysis of NEISS-AIP data illustrated that among children less than 5 years of age, the majority of poisonings seen in emergency departments involved drugs, such as analgesics (pain relievers) and supplements (60%); much less common were poisonings involving cleaning products, drugs and ointments, and personal-care products.[23] Over 80% of medication overdoses among children $<$ 18 years of age seen in emergency departments have been reported to be as a result of unsupervised ingestion, with only 14% as a result of medication errors and misuse.[24]

Rates of poisoning estimated with emergency department data correlate positively with frequency of poison control center calls.[25] Poison control data offer a more nuanced understanding of the types of substances involved in poisonings and rates of exposure, particularly for exposures where individuals do not seek healthcare. In 2017, the National Poison Data System (NPDS) reported an estimated 640 exposures per 100,000 population, with the most common route of exposure through ingestion (83.4% of all cases).[26] The majority of cases did not involve a visit to a healthcare facility (65.5%). The top five substances most frequently involved in human exposures included analgesics (11.1%), household cleaning substances (7.4%), cosmetics/personal care products (6.8%), sedatives/hypnotics/antipsychotics

(5.7%), and antidepressants (5.0%). Exposures were similar among adults and children, with the exception of children being exposed more frequently to foreign bodies/toys/miscellaneous and topical preparations, rather than sedatives and antidepressants.

Among young children, cleaning substances of particular concern include laundry detergent pods that began distribution in the United States in 2010. In 2012, using NPDS data, there were an estimated 17,230 children younger than 6 years of age who were exposed to laundry detergent pods, with 4.4% hospitalized and 7.5% experiencing a moderate or major medical outcome including symptoms such as vomiting, choking, ocular irritation, lethargy, and in a small number of cases, coma, and seizures.[27] In just a one-month period in 2012, poison centers reported over 1000 laundry detergent exposures to the NPDS, of which 48% involved laundry detergent pods.[28]

Similar to trends in morbidity and mortality involving opioid analgesics among adults, from 2000 to 2010 poison control data revealed a 33% increase in pharmaceutical-related exposures in children younger than 6 years, with the top exposure category including analgesics; in this same time period, there was a 2.8% decline in the number of nonpharmaceutical-related exposures. This trend also included a 53% increase in serious medical outcomes among young children, a category that ranges from moderate effects (i.e., more pronounced, more prolonged, or more systematic than minor effects, but not requiring specific intervention) to death.[29] A more recent study of national poison system data examining prescription opioid exposures among children and adolescents illustrated that the number and rate of exposures increased from 2000 to 2009, but then started to decline through 2015, except for buprenorphine exposures which increased from 2014 to 2015.[30] The declines in exposures are consistent with declines in opioid prescribing overall during this period.[31] Given the focus on increasing medication-assisted treatment for opioid use disorder among adults and adolescents to help address the opioid overdose epidemic, there is an increasing concern about adverse effects among those with a buprenorphine prescription, in addition to unintentional exposure to young children. In Utah, from 2002 to 2011, 462 exposures were reported to the Utah Poison Control Center, 54.1% were among adults aged >20 years, and 38.7% were among children <5 years, a significant increase, particularly among young children; however, exposures were relatively low compared to the rate with which it was prescribed.[32]

A substance of particular concern related to intentional poisoning, relative to unintentional poisoning, is acetaminophen. An analysis of acetaminophen toxicity-related emergency department visits from 2006 to 2010 illustrated 411,811 observed visits (a rate of 27 per 100,000). Intentional self-harm was indicated in 58.4% of the visits, with percentages of visits significantly higher among those 12–20 years of age, and among women. Depression was the most common comorbidity noted.[33] Among cases of unintentional poisoning involving acetaminophen, liver failure, or renal dysfunction are the most notable toxicity outcomes, particularly among young patients exposed to high doses and adults aged 65 years and older with chronic exposure.[34]

Economic Burden

Poisonings account for 2.6% of medical and work loss costs associated with nonfatal injury[35]; however, drug poisonings account for the highest percentage of costs among fatal injuries, estimated at 26%.[36] The annual economic burden of prescription opioid overdose, abuse, and dependence was estimated at more than $78.5 billion per year in 2013, with more than a third of this amount attributable to healthcare, including treatment costs for opioid use disorder.[37] More recently, the total cost of the opioid crisis, including costs associated with the use and misuse of prescription and illicit opioids, and calculated through methods estimating the value of a statistical life, was estimated at over $500 billion.[38] There are also significant costs associated with acetaminophen overdose. In 2014, the estimated economic burden of acetaminophen-toxicity-related emergency department visits was over $1 billion per year, with nearly 60% of costs associated with intentional self-harm.[33]

International Perspective

Compared to other high-income countries, the burden of unintentional poisoning is higher in the United States, with stark differences seen more clearly in recent years. Examining available data for comparison, from 2000 to 2014, Mack and colleagues[39] documented a dramatic increase in unintentional poisoning mortality rates in the United States, an increase of 189.4% from 4.5 per 100,000 to 13.1 per 100,000. In comparison, in 2012, unintentional poisoning mortality rates in Canada (4.8) and Australia (4.1) were much lower, with no increase in Australia seen since 2000, and a small increase observed in Canada during this time period.[40] A detailed investigation of the cause for such differences was not conducted; however, differences could be due to variations in societal-level risk factors across countries. For example, in the United States, rapid increases in opioid prescribing paralleled rapid increases in prescription opioid-involved mortality.[41]

RISK AND PROTECTIVE FACTORS

Different mechanisms are at play that increase risk for poisoning or protect individuals from poisoning across childhood, adolescence, and adulthood. Among children, exposure is primarily unintentional; in turn, the most influential factors include supervision and proper storage and disposal of substances that can be toxic. Among adolescents and adults, while poisoning from the substance is commonly unintentional, initial exposure to the substance is often intentional (e.g., voluntary taking of a drug), signifying a different process at play.

Factors Associated with Unintentional Poisoning Among Children

Both demographic and contextual risk factors are notable for unintentional poisoning among children. Lower socioeconomic status, younger maternal age, single parent status, and a greater number of children in the household have been associated with increased risk for unintentional poisoning internationally—all perhaps related to and illustrating the importance of capacity for supervision.[42–45] Such risk factors related to supervision are most important for children under the age of 5, during the years in which the risk for morbidity and mortality among children is greatest.

Availability of toxic substances in easy reach is the greatest contextual risk factor for child poisoning. Analysis of the Researched Abuse, Diversion, and Addiction-Related (RADAR) Surveillance System Poison Center Program and Reckitt Benckiser Pharmaceuticals' pharmacovigilance system revealed that the most common causes of unintentional exposure among young children included the medication being stored in sight, accessed from a bag or purse, and not stored in the original packaging (e.g., placed in a cup).[46] A case-control study of poisoning cases aged 0–4 seen in healthcare facilities in England, found that compared to community controls, parents of cases were more likely to not store medicines locked or out of reach and more likely to not put medicines and household products away immediately after use.[47] Examining the processes at play, a study in Australia examined factors associated with unintentional poisoning among children ages 1–3, compared to children who were injured, sick, or otherwise healthy. The authors discovered that in addition to medication being stored in more accessible locations, risk for unintentional poisoning increased with greater levels of maternal distress and less maternal supervision during risk-taking activities.[48] Such findings illustrate the importance of parenting capacity and skill to supervise young children and ensure proper storage of hazards.

The opioid overdose epidemic and corresponding increase in opioid availability may have spillover effects on children. Analysis of data from poison control centers participating in the RADAR system found 9179 exposures to a prescription opioid among children 6 and under between 2003 and 2006, and that 92% of these exposures occurred in the home.[49] The number of exposures in a zip code was correlated with the number of opioid analgesic prescriptions dispensed by retail pharmacies.[49] Some prescription drug forms may be protective of accidental exposure. The analysis of RADAR and Reckitt Benckiser Pharmaceuticals' pharmacovigilance system found that for children 28 days to less than 6 years the child exposure rate per unique recipients of a dispensed drug (URDD) was greater for buprenorphine tablets (rate ratio 3.5) and buprenorphine-naloxone tablets (rate ratio 8.8) than for buprenorphine-naloxone film.[46] The reason for this could not be determined from the data; however, the authors note that the film form is generally dispensed in a single-dose child resistant packaging, while tablets are generally dispensed in bottles with 30-day supplies.

Factors Associated with Poisoning Among Adolescents and Adults

Factors associated with poisoning among adults and adolescents vary significantly according to intent; that is, whether the poisoning is unintentional or self-inflicted (suicide or self-harm). Risk factors for suicide and self-harm are covered in detail in another chapter within this text (see Holland et al.).

Among those aged 15–65 in the United States, 95% of unintentional poisoning deaths involved drugs.[8] Both individual and contextual risk factors contribute to risk of unintentional drug poisoning among adolescents and adults. Individual risk factors include demographic characteristics, substance use and substance use disorders, and comorbid health conditions. Contextual risk factors include prescribing-related characteristics, geographic location, and limited access to treatment and prevention services.

Demographic Characteristics

While not modifiable, certain demographic characteristics are associated with a higher risk of a fatal drug poisoning. The likelihood of experiencing a drug-poisoning death in the United States is greatest in the 25–34, 35–44, and 45–54 age groups. Overall drug-poisoning death rates are higher for men than women.[3] This difference is driven by unintentional drug-poisoning deaths; the age-adjusted rate of drug-poisoning suicides for females exceeds the rate for males.[8] The highest age-adjusted rates of unintentional drug-poisoning deaths as of 2017 are among non-Hispanic White and American Indian/Alaska Native populations, followed by non-Hispanic black, and Hispanic populations; the unintentional drug-poisoning death rate among the Asian/Pacific Islander population are substantially lower.[8] Non-Hispanic Whites and American Indian/Alaska Natives also have the highest rates of intentional drug overdose deaths, with much lower rates among Black, Hispanic, and Asian/Pacific Islander populations.[8]

Substance Use and Substance Use Disorders

Having a substance use disorder is a key risk factor for drug poisoning.[50–53] About two-thirds of drug overdose deaths in 2016 involved an opioid, highlighting the importance of opioid use and opioid use disorders as risk factors for drug overdose.[3] Use of illicit opioids, such as heroin, and misuse of prescription opioids are both associated with overdose risk. Misuse includes use in any way not directed by a doctor, including in greater amounts, more often, or longer than told, or use of a prescription that is not one's own.[54] A case control study in Utah found that among those that reported using a prescription opioid in the prior year, those that obtained prescription opioids from nonprescription sources were about five times more likely to die of an overdose, while those that used more than prescribed were more than 16 times more likely to die of an overdose than those not reporting such behaviors.[55] Injection drug use has also been associated with an increased risk for nonfatal overdose.[56] In one surveillance study of persons who injected drugs across three U.S. cities in 2012, on average 45% of respondents indicated a lifetime history of nonfatal overdose.[57] Prior experience of a nonfatal overdose is associated with subsequent overdose risk among injection drug users.[58]

The United States has experienced a recent increase in heroin use, which has contributed to an increasing rate of fatal poisonings involving heroin.[59] The rate of past-year heroin use in the United States increased 62.5% from 2002–04 to 2011–13, with a parallel increase in those reporting past-year heroin abuse or dependence.[59] There is some evidence that heroin use began to stabilize from 2014 to 2016.[54] Among people who use heroin, multiple substance use and co-occurring substance use disorders are common, with 96% of those who use heroin in the past-year reporting use of more than one substance in the last year, 45% meeting the diagnostic criteria for opioid pain reliever abuse or dependence, more than 35% reporting alcohol use consistent with an abuse or disorder diagnosis, and about 25% reporting cocaine or marijuana use consistent with abuse or dependence.[56] The presence of multiple substances, including alcohol, is common in drug-poisoning deaths.[60–62]

Other Comorbid Health Conditions

Among those taking prescription opioids, a number of health conditions are associated with an increased risk of drug poisoning. Factors that increase the risk of a drug poisoning in this group include chronic pain,[55] depression,[50,63] and other psychiatric illness.[51,52] While mental health disorders and substance use disorders are risk factors for both unintentional and intentional drug poisoning, the prevalence of mental health risk factors tends to be higher among intentional poisonings, while the prevalence of substance use problems is higher among unintentional poisonings.[64]

Opioid Prescribing-Related Risk Factors

Approximately 35% of opioid overdose deaths involve prescription opioids,[14] and a number of factors have been associated with an increased risk of overdose among those receiving opioid prescriptions.[65] There is strong evidence of a dose-response relationship between opioid prescription dose and risk of a drug poisoning.[50–53,66–70] Increased risk of drug poisoning is found above prescribed doses of 50 morphine milligram equivalents (MMEs) per day, and some studies show increased risk with as little as 20–50 MME per day.[50,52] Use of extended release/long-acting opioids has also been shown to increase overdose risk.[53,71] Other prescribing-related characteristics associated with increased risk of opioid poisoning include number of prescribers,[69,72] number of prescriptions,[66] overlapping prescriptions[50]; and number of pharmacies used by the patient.[50,51,69,72]

Polypharmacy, or the simultaneous use of multiple prescription drugs, increases the risk of drug poisoning, particularly among patients taking prescription opioids. Specific drug classes that have been associated with increased risk of drug poisoning include benzodiazepines and other sedative/hypnotics[50,51,53,63,65] and antidepressants.[53,63] However, although having depression increases the risk of overdose, antidepressant use may be protective against poisoning among those with depression.[63]

Geographic Risk Factors

There is substantial variation in drug-poisoning death rates between states, with about a sevenfold difference between the states with the highest and lowest drug-poisoning death rate in 2017.[3] States with the highest rates of drug-poisoning deaths in 2017 were West Virginia, Ohio, and the District of Columbia, while states with the lowest rates were Nebraska, North Dakota, and South Dakota.[3] One of the drivers of variation in drug-poisoning death rates between states is differences in availability of both prescription and illicit opioids. With prescription opioids, there is a relationship between prescription opioid sales in a geographic area and prescription opioid-involved deaths.[41] For illicit drugs, of particular concern is a recent influx of illicitly manufactured fentanyl, an opioid with up to 100 times the potency of morphine. A CDC report on drug poisoning in ten states in the second half of 2016 found fentanyl in more than half of opioid poisoning deaths in those states.[74] Some states, including New Hampshire, reported fentanyl involvement in nearly 90% of opioid deaths. When mixed with heroin without the user's knowledge, fentanyl users may not be aware they are being exposed to this highly potent drug, increasing the already inherent riskiness of heroin use in settings experiencing an influx of illicitly manufactured fentanyl. DEA drug seizures show variation in the illicit drug supply across the United States.[75] For example, in the West, a higher proportion of seizures are methamphetamine. This regional variation is reflected in differences in substances involved in drug poisonings.[76]

Once considered an urban problem, drug poisoning has increased substantially in rural areas in the early part of the twenty-first century, and is now a problem across the rural/urban continuum.[77] In 2015, unintentional drug-poisoning death rates in the United States were slightly higher in nonmetro areas than in metro areas; this is a reversal from 1999, when unintentional drug-poisoning death rates were higher in metro areas than in nonmetro areas.[39] However, the absolute burden on metro areas is greater than on nonmetro areas, with more than six times as many deaths in metro than nonmetro areas in the United States in 2015. Rates of suicide drug-poisoning deaths were similar in nonmetro and metro areas in 2015, with nonmetro areas experiencing larger rate increases since 1999.[39]

Other Contextual Factors

Contextual factors that limit access to prevention and treatment services can increase risk of drug poisoning in a community, in particular. Such factors may include limited access to and reimbursement for alternative treatments for pain, limited access to harm reduction approaches such as comprehensive syringe services programs, limited availability of medication-assisted treatment (MAT) programs to treat opioid use disorder, and limited access to naloxone to reverse opioid overdoses. For example, in the United States it has been demonstrated that there are significant gaps between treatment need and capacity to provide MAT for opioid use disorder.[78] Individuals released from incarceration are at extremely high risk for overdose upon release,[79] likely due to the contextual factors of enforced abstinence and discontinuation of drug treatment services. In a survey of organizations reporting distribution of naloxone to laypersons, over 26,000 reversals were reported from 1999 to 2014 among 109 organizations collecting reversal data, illustrating the powerful life-saving potential of naloxone availability.[80] Interventions to address contextual risk factors will be discussed in more detail the next section on Interventions/Best Available Evidence (Fig. 174-1).

INTERVENTIONS/BEST AVAILABLE EVIDENCE

Given that risk and protective factors influencing poisoning vary across intent, population, and contexts, tailored intervention strategies are key. Table 174-6 summarizes intervention strategies by target population (child, adolescent, adult) and stage of prevention (primary, secondary, tertiary). Next, we discuss the context for the development of these intervention strategies and what is known about their effectiveness in impacting poisoning outcomes and risk factors.

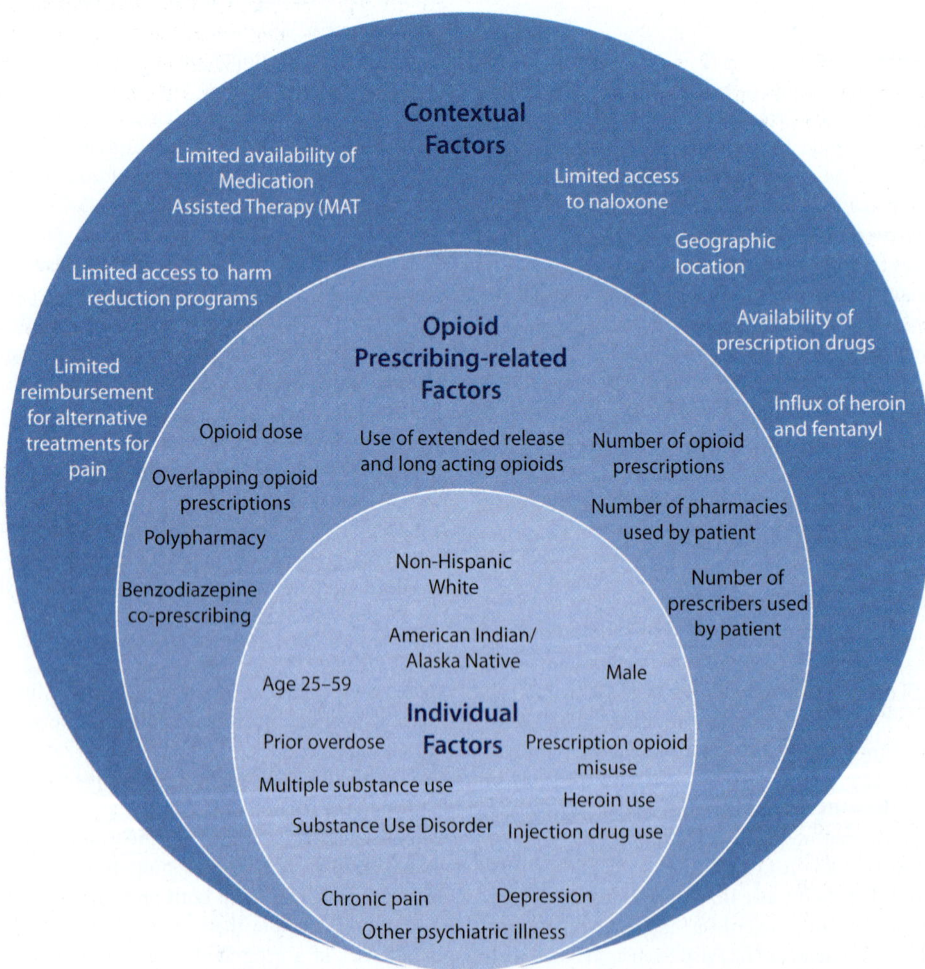

FIGURE 174-1. Risk factors for unintentional poisoning among adolescents and adults.

TABLE 174-6 INTERVENTION STRATEGIES FOR THE PREVENTION OF POISONING

Intervention	Target Population	Stage of Prevention
Product packaging	Child	Primary
	Adolescent/Adult	
Home safety interventions	Child	Primary
Education on safe storage and disposal	Child	Primary
Prescription drug monitoring programs	Adolescent/Adult	Primary
Drug formulary management	Adolescent/Adult	Primary
Opioid prescribing guidelines	Adolescent/Adult	Primary
Communication Campaigns	Adolescent/Adult	Primary
Pill mill legislation	Adolescent/Adult	Primary
Family/school-based development programs	Child/Adolescent	Primary
Overdose education and naloxone distribution	Adolescent/Adult	Secondary
Safe injection facilities	Adolescent/Adult	Secondary
Drug supply testing in the community	Adolescent/Adult	Secondary
Medication-assisted treatment/behavioral therapy	Adolescent/Adult	Tertiary
Linkage to treatment (e.g., hospital, law enforcement)	Adolescent/Adult	Tertiary

Prevention of Unintentional Poisoning Among Children

The prevention of unintentional poisoning among children has been an important public health objective in the United States for several decades. The nation's first poison control center was established in Chicago in 1953 and focused on preventing unintentional poisoning in children that occurred in the home.[81] Today, Poison Control Centers operate in all 50 states, D.C., and all U.S. territories, managing over 2.7 million cases in 2016. Staffed by physicians, nurses, pharmacists, and toxicology specialists, these centers provide poisoning information and advice by phone.[82] During the 1960s, child-resistant containers were developed and widely tested. Following the development of effective child-resistant containers, the Poison Prevention Packaging Act was enacted in 1970 to mandate their use. More recently, buprenorphine packaging has been the target of prevention efforts. Poisoning prevention efforts have focused on different interventions over the years and even recommendations for basic first-aid measures following ingestion have seen changes. The safe storage and disposal of medicine and poisonous substances however, have been important components of poisoning prevention interventions throughout this period. Educating children on the dangers of medicine and common household supplies has also played a large role in the prevention of unintentional poisonings among children. Moving forward, poisoning prevention strategies will continue to evolve along with evidence-based prevention interventions and safety recommendations.

After the rapid increase in the availability of household chemicals after World War II, the Food and Drug Administration (FDA) partnered with the American Medical Association (AMA) to advocate for policies that would mandate the appropriate labeling of dangerous toxic substances. This led to the Hazardous Substances Labeling Act, which was enacted in 1960.[81] In 1966, the Child Protection Act was passed to give the FDA greater authority in banning hazardous products and substances used by children.[83] During that year, the FDA began looking at child-resistant packaging as a new approach for preventing unintentional poisoning among children.[81] A 1967 randomized control trial compared a newly designed plastic container with a child-resistant top to the snap-top container that was already in use in most pharmacies at the time. The new design, which required two coordinated maneuvers (depression of the cap and a counterclockwise turn), proved to be far superior to the existing container, especially in preventing access to children under the age of 5.[84] The introduction of child-resistant containers for prescription medications dispensed at Madigan General Hospital and McChord Air Force Base in 1967 led to a decrease in the overall poisoning rate from 15.8 to 8.2 poisonings per 10,000 pediatric outpatient visits.[85] The following year, there was a 70% decrease in poisonings related to tablets and capsules dispensed in the new child-resistant containers.[85] Both studies showed that child-resistant containers could be a cost-effective strategy to prevent poisonings from prescription medications.

With the success of new child-resistant prescription medication containers, Congress passed the Poison Prevention Packaging Act (PPPA) in 1970. The PPPA, which was administered by the U.S. Consumer Product Safety Commission (CPSC), required prescription drugs, aspirin, acetaminophen, and hazardous household products to be packaged in containers that were both child-resistant and adult-friendly.[81] The effectiveness of child-resistant packaging and the Poison Prevention Packaging Act in reducing unintentional child poisonings have been well documented.[86–88] Since most regulations became effective in 1973, Walton evaluated the effect of the legislation on child poisonings between 1973 and 1978 and found that the rate of ingestion of substances covered by the regulations declined from 5.7 to 3.4 per 1000 children in only 6 years.[86] A quarter of a century after the passage of the PPPA, Rodgers evaluated the impact of the legislation on prescription drug-related mortality in children under the age of 5.[87] Child-resistant packaging was estimated to have reduced the oral prescription drug-related mortality rate of children under the age of 5 by 1.40 per million over the previous two decades.[87] Before the PPPA, aspirin alone accounted for an average of 120 fatal poisonings of children under the age of 5 each year between 1958 and 1963.[88] The PPPA included regulations on aspirin packaging that focused on children under the age of 5 that became effective in 1972. Rodgers estimated that child-resistant aspirin packaging reduced related mortality by 34% and prevented 90 deaths between 1973 and 1990.[88]

In 1997, the FDA issued a final rule, requiring label warning statements and unit-dose packaging for iron supplements meeting certain criteria (the unit-dose packaging requirement was ultimately withdrawn in 2003 following a court challenge).[89] An evaluation of this packaging requirement found a significant decrease in the average number of iron ingestion calls to poison control centers for children less than 6 years of age, as well as the number of deaths.[90] More recently, efforts to improve the safety of buprenorphine prescriptions by compartmentalizing packaging into individual doses has been evaluated by Budnitz et al.[91] Previous to 2010, buprenorphine/naloxone was only available in multidose child-resistant bottles but between 2013 and 2015, 86.9% of buprenorphine prescriptions were dispensed as either unit-dose packaged tablets or film strips. Adjusting for prescribing frequency, ED visits for the unintentional ingestion by children decreased by 65.3% between 2013 and 2015.[91] Flow restrictors on liquid medicine bottles have also been shown to be effective at reducing the amount of liquid young children can remove from open medicine bottles[92] and could therefore be used alongside child-resistant packaging as a comprehensive approach to safer packaging. Restricting packaging size has proven effective in decreasing intentional overdoses in England and Wales[93] and efforts to use similar restrictions to prevent the unintentional poisoning of children show similar promise.

Over the years, recommendations for basic first aid after the ingestion of poisonous substances have changed significantly. For many years, the American Academy of Pediatrics (AAP) recommended that parents keep a 1-oz bottle of syrup of ipecac in the home that could be used to induce vomiting after poisoning if deemed appropriate by a poison control center or physician.[94] In 2003, the AAP's Committee on Injury and Poison Prevention declared that syrup of ipecac should no longer be used as a routine poison treatment intervention in the home.[94] Since then, syrup of ipecac has greatly decreased in popularity and is no longer sold in most retail stores and pharmacies. Similarly, activated charcoal, which is used by healthcare providers to induce vomiting after poisoning, is not recommended for in-home use.[94] According to the AAP, consulting with the local poison control center should be the first step taken by the caregiver of a child that has ingested poison. Having the phone number to the local poison control center readily available is therefore recommended by the AAP.[94] According to a 2012 Cochrane Database Review, home safety interventions significantly increase the odds that poison control numbers are accessible in a home (OR 3.30, 95% CI 1.70–6.39).[95] Although such interventions have resulted in making numbers more accessible, studies evaluating their effect on injury reduction are lacking.

Educating parents about the dangers of prescription medications and other poisonous substances in the home and about effective safety interventions is an important element of current poisoning prevention efforts. Many prevention strategies focus on comprehensive home interventions and a Cochrane Database Review evaluated the effectiveness of several such interventions in educating parents about safety practices.[95] Home interventions evaluated included a wide array of approaches such as hazard identification during home visits, parent education interventions, safe storage of medicine and cleaning supplies, and the provision of safety equipment for the home. Based on 45 studies that reported poisoning-related outcomes, home safety interventions, defined as interventions that focus on home safety education or the provision of tools supporting poison-prevention practices, increased having easy access to poison control center numbers (OR 3.30, 95% CI 1.70–6.39).[95] Home safety interventions also increased the safe storage of medicines (OR 1.53, 95% CI 1.27–1.84) and cleaning products (OR 1.55, 95% CI 1.22–1.96) out of the reach of children. Three studies included in the meta-analysis evaluated the effectiveness of home safety interventions in educating parents about the safe storage of plants and keeping toxic plants out of the home but evidence was lacking (OR 1.18, 95% CI 0.40–3.48). Although home safety interventions were shown to be effective at increasing safety practices, their effect on preventing injuries was only evaluated in four studies and the reduction in the poisoning incidence observed was not significant (IRR 0.93, 95% CI 0.65–1.32), though notably studies were small and likely underpowered.[95]

Although interventions that focus on the safe storage and proper disposal of medicine and other poisonous household products have been popular for the last several decades in the United States, more attention needs to be placed on education that targets populations of various socioeconomic groups and educational backgrounds. For example, Crosslin et al. noted that Hispanic parents with a high school education or less were at least three times more likely to improperly store household cleaners compared to Hispanic parents with a college degree.[96] Additionally, the risk for improper storage increased by 44% with each additional child in the household.[96] According to Patel et al., substances perceived less likely to be harmful by parents were also the least likely to be stored safely, including dishwasher tablets (68%), toilet cleaner (71%), bleach (74%), oven cleaner (78%), oral contraceptives (80%), and essential oils (81%).[97] Safe storage interventions such as installing child-resistant latches on medicine cabinets or keeping cleaning supplies locked can help diminish the accessibility of potentially poisonous substances within the home. The proper disposal of unused or expired substances and medications reduces overall availability and is therefore just as important. The Up and Away educational campaign, developed in collaboration with the CDC, the CHPA Educational Foundation, and a range of partners provides specific action steps for parents and caregivers to safety store medicines and be prepared in case of emergency (see http://www.upandaway.org/#resources). State-level disposal campaigns and drug take-back events have been popular interventions in the midst of this current opioid overdose epidemic but rigorous evaluations of such interventions, that focus on health outcomes, are lacking.[98] Although the effect of such campaigns on poisoning rates remains unclear, many studies have evaluated their impact on the disposal rates of unused or expired medicine. For example, exposure to a drug take-back and disposal campaign was a significant predictor of disposing unused medicine at a collection site (OR = 2.14) which was promoted through the campaign.[99] Overall, safe storage and disposal interventions show promise in reducing the availability and accessibility of dangerous substances within the home but their impact on preventing poisonings remains unclear.

Home safety interventions often focus on parent education but educating children about the dangers of prescription medicines and poisonous household substances is an important complement. Children need to be able to recognize poisoning dangers around the household and understand the importance of getting help from an adult if poisoning occurs. According to a study by Rodgers et al. analyzing U.S. hospital emergency department data, imitative behavior may contribute to 20% of poisonings involving children under the age of 5 and 30% of poisonings involving children aged 20–59 months.[100] Based on the study results, Rodgers et al. argue that parents should never ingest medicines in front of their children.[100] Although imitative behavior may not place children at a greater poisoning risk from the ingestion of household cleaners, parental behavior may impact the child's attitude toward medicines such as prescription opioids. The proper storage of both medicine and other poisonous household products and the disposal of unused or expired substances may therefore also provide a second benefit in teaching children that such substances are dangerous and should be treated accordingly. Unfortunately, poisoning prevention education interventions targeting children have not been rigorously evaluated and therefore their impact on poisoning rates is unknown. The prevention of unintentional poisonings in children requires a multifaceted approach, and more research is needed to rigorously evaluate many interventions that could prove effective by themselves or as a component of a comprehensive prevention strategy.

Prevention of Unintentional Poisoning Among Adolescents and Adults

Most contemporary evaluations of poisoning prevention strategies for adolescents and adults have focused on the prevention of opioid overdose to address the exploding epidemic in the United States, given the predominance of the burden among poisoning deaths.[98,101] Approaches include primary prevention strategies that aim to prevent opioid misuse and overdose before it occurs among the general population, secondary prevention strategies aimed at addressing overdose in high-risk individuals, and tertiary prevention strategies aimed at long-term treatment.

Given that opioid prescribing is a key risk factor for overdose from both prescription and illicit opioids, one primary prevention approach has been to focus on improving the safety of opioid prescribing. For example, legislatures have established state-level prescription drug monitoring programs in 49 states and require pharmacies to submit information on controlled substance prescriptions, including opioids, to a central database managed by entities such as a state health department or board of pharmacy. States have passed legislation to regulate pain clinics that limit the ownership, prescribing, and dispensing of opioids in clinics, with registration and inspection requirements. State Medicaid programs, Medicare, and private insurers have implemented formulary management strategies, such as patient review and restriction programs that limit patients to using one provider and pharmacy, or require prior authorization for or impose quantity limits on specific medications.[102] States, local governments, and health systems, as well as the U.S. Centers for Disease Control and Prevention,[103] have developed guidelines for prescribing opioids, with recommendations about dose limits, formulations, initiation and titration of dose, and risk management strategies (e.g., urine drug testing). Finally, communication campaigns have been developed to increase community awareness of the risks of prescription opioids. Although the quality of evidence for many of these prevention strategies is moderate, there are some promising data to suggest that they can reduce morbidity and mortality.[98]

For example, states that have combined mandated use of prescription drug monitoring programs and pain clinic regulation have evidenced a decrease in the amount of opioids prescribed by 8%, and a decline in prescription opioid overdose death rates of 12%; with higher decreases in states implementing such policies than in comparison states.[104] After an academic detailing campaign accompanying issuance of an opioid prescribing guideline in New York City, there were significant improvements in provider knowledge and decreases in high-dose prescribing in intervention areas, accompanied by significant decreases in opioid overdose mortality.[61,105] In the Pennsylvania Medicaid program, plans that implemented prior authorization policies for opioids for pain management evidenced lower rates of opioid use disorder and overdose among enrollees compared to plans with no prior authorization.[106] Opioid prescribing, including indicators of high-risk prescribing was found to significantly decrease at a greater rate after the publication of the CDC Guideline for Prescribing Opioids for Chronic Pain.[107] And in Utah, implementation of the *Use Only As Directed* statewide media campaign was associated with a 14% one-year reduction in unintentional opioid-related drug-overdose deaths.[108] A newly developed CDC campaign, *Rx Awareness*, aims to increase awareness that prescription opioids can be addictive and dangerous, and decrease the number of people who misuse opioids. The campaign was piloted in four states in 2017, and is currently expanding in additional states with the support of an implementation and evaluation toolkit that could allow for the production of evaluation data to assess impact. In the pilot evaluation, more than 65% of respondents in implementation areas reported hearing a radio ad, seeing the campaign online or in digital media, or saw campaign billboards. Over 70% reported that the campaign was meaningful and believable, and that the message was effective. During the pilot, display ads, testimonial videos, and bumper videos gained over 141 million impressions, 5.47 million interactions, and over 360,000 click throughs, with a rate higher than standard government benchmarks.[109]

For the primary prevention of opioid misuse in adolescence, a key risk factor for overdose later in early- to mid-adulthood, middle schools have implemented curricula that promote social skills and youth competencies to prevent opioid misuse, with some success. For example, compared to middle school youth not participating in a program, youth participating in the Iowa Strengthening Families Program for Parents and Youth 10-14 (SFP 10-14); SFP 10-14 plus Life Skills training; SFP 10-14 plus Project Alert; or SFP 10-14 plus All Stars showed significant reductions in prescription opioid misuse and lifetime prescription drug misuse.[110] These programs generally modify family and school environments and build youth competencies to reduce risk factors for substance misuse.

A key secondary prevention strategy for opioid overdose is naloxone distribution. Naloxone is an opioid antagonist, a drug that can reverse an overdose when it occurs. Naloxone can be accompanied by overdose education and distributed through community-based programs, carried by law enforcement, made available in pharmacies, prescribed by a provider (e.g., when high dosages of opioids are prescribed to manage pain or when medication-assisted treatment for opioid use disorder is prescribed), or distributed to patients, families, and friends after a person overdoses and is treated in the emergency department. Evaluations have illustrated that community-based naloxone distribution results in naloxone administrations in the community as well as reductions in overdose death in high-implementation areas, without an apparent increase in risk behavior.[111] Further, Coffin and colleagues demonstrated that co-prescribing naloxone to patients receiving long-term opioid therapy for pain in primary-care safety-net clinics can reduce opioid-related emergency department visits.[112] And, an innovative approach in Rhode Island from the Overdose Prevention and Rescue Coalition pairs distribution of naloxone kits with referral to treatment for opioid use disorder and recovery coaches for patients who are treated in the emergency department for overdose. Although promising, rigorous evaluation data illustrating impact on overdose death at the community level are not yet available.[113] Moreover, naloxone prescribing remains underutilized, with only one naloxone prescription is dispensed for every 69 high-dose opioid prescriptions.[114]

Internationally, safe injection facilities (SIFs) are a harm reduction approach taken by several locations, including Canada, Australia, and Europe. Such facilities are not sanctioned by federal law in the United States; however, some localities are considering authorizing safe injection facilities in their jurisdictions. One such example is the city of Philadelphia, which recently announced its intent to open the first legalized facility in America,[115] and there have been reports of other unsanctioned facilities.[116]

Safe injection facilities are locations where individuals can inject drugs in the presence of healthcare professionals, with the provision of sterile syringes, referral to health services including treatment for substance use disorder, and response to overdose should it occur (e.g., naloxone administration, EMS services). An evaluation of a safe injection facility in Vancouver Canada illustrated a 35% reduction in the fatal overdose rate after the opening of the facility, compared to a decrease of 9% during the same period in the remainder of the city.[117]

An innovative harm reduction approach that is being tried in some U.S. localities to address the increasing concern about potent illicitly manufactured fentanyl in the drug supply is drug product testing. In three cities in the Northeast United States, public health workers tested samples of drugs provided by users to identify the presence and concentration of fentanyl and fentanyl analogues. A pilot study revealed that users were concerned about fentanyl and interested in testing drugs to help protect them from overdose, indicating that test results could help change their behavior (e.g., not use the drugs or use with others who have naloxone).[118]

Finally, tertiary prevention for opioid overdose includes treating opioid use disorder with medications in combination with behavioral therapies. Medication-assisted treatment (MAT) for opioid use disorder includes methadone (an opioid agonist that activates opioid receptors), buprenorphine (a partial opioid agonist that activates receptors with diminished response), and naltrexone (an opioid antagonist that blocks opioid receptors and interferes with reward). Methadone is available through outpatient treatment programs that include daily visits for medication administration, buprenorphine is available through certified physicians, and naltrexone can be prescribed by any provider who is licensed to prescribe medications, but has challenging initiation with patients and is most likely to be effective with highly motivated individuals.[119] Discontinuation of MAT is high, and relapse is higher with naltrexone[120]; however once successfully initiated, effectiveness of naltrexone and buprenorphine may be similar.[121] Patients treated with buprenorphine or methadone maintenance therapy are retained in treatment longer and misuse opioids less often compared to patients not receiving medication treatment.[122] Retention in treatment is associated with decreases in overdose mortality.[123] Initiating buprenorphine treatment in the emergency department with referral to primary care can increase engagement in treatment and reduce opioid use for those at highest risk for overdose compared to brief intervention and referral.[124] Initiation of naltrexone prior to prison release, a point at which overdose risk is extremely high, can result in greater abstinence use and retention in treatment compared to initiation after release, although more research is needed to determine effects on overdose.[125]

The changing nature of the opioid overdose epidemic with a shift to burden of overdose from illicit substances, including heroin and illicitly manufactured fentanyl,[10,126] and an increase in overdoses involving cocaine or methamphetamine in addition to opioids,[15] has raised the importance of collaboration between public health and law enforcement to address the epidemic. Evaluations of such strategies are limited. Promising approaches include an addiction treatment referral program led by the Gloucester Massachusetts police department which accommodated 75% of participants who sought a referral[127] and a training on opioid overdose prevention and naloxone administration for law enforcement officers with a referral to treatment component that resulted in about 20% of patients seeking treatment after an overdose.[128] More rigorous evaluations of law enforcement and public health collaboration interventions are needed to determine their effectiveness in improving access to MAT and long-term health outcomes.

Prevention of Intentional Poisoning

Similar to risk factors for intentional poisoning, the preventive interventions available for addressing self-directed violence, including intentional drug overdose, are multifaceted. A detailed review of effective suicide prevention strategies is presented elsewhere in this text and can be consulted (see Holland et al.). In addition, the CDC had released a technical package to help states and communities make decisions about suicide prevention strategies that are based on the best available evidence.[129] However, a few specific strategies are noteworthy for discussion related to poisoning prevention.

Because chronic pain is a risk factor for suicide, and opioid prescribing increases access to a lethal means for overdose, the Veterans' Health Administration has developed a Stratification Tool for Opioid Mitigation to assist with identifying and monitoring patients prescribed opioids for chronic pain to prevent suicide-related events. This tool allows for decision support through the electronic health record for providers to identify patients who are at risk. Risk factors include variables such as previous overdose or suicide-related event, substance use disorder diagnosis, detoxification, inpatient mental health treatment, and previous emergency department visit for injury. With information about such risk factors at their fingertips, providers can then address risk with targeted interventions, such as referral to behavioral health treatment.[130] Although further evaluation of impact on patient outcomes is needed, there is reason to believe this approach is promising. Other studies indicate that following evidence-based guidelines on opioid prescribing and risk mitigation strategies can reduce suicide risk among patients receiving opioids long term for pain management.[131] Note, however, that such strategies might prevent suicide more broadly, and not just through intentional poisoning.

Internationally, evaluations have investigated the effectiveness of medication packaging legislation on suicide by paracetamol (acetaminophen) poisoning. Restricted pack sizes are thought to increase the difficulty of intentionally overdosing on drugs given that intentional overdoses are often impulsive, with individuals relying on drugs available in the home.[132,133] An interrupted time series evaluation in England and Wales of packaging legislation found a decrease in level and trend in intentional overdose deaths involving paracetamol.[93] More broadly, there is some evidence that restricting access to specific medications overall could reduce suicide by any means. For example, in Denmark, regulatory restrictions on the prescribing of barbiturates was found to be associated with a decrease in the number of suicides overall and suicides by self-poisoning with barbiturates; it was estimated that a 10% increase in sales was associated with a 1% increase in overall suicide rate. This was during a time when suicides from multiple methods were decreasing; however, suicides from other means declined to a lesser degree.[134]

CONCLUSIONS

Over the past 15 years, poisonings have increased significantly in the United States, in large part due to the opioid overdose epidemic. The cost to society through medical costs, work loss costs, and impact on families is tremendous. As outlined in this chapter, strategies such as safer prescribing and utilizing prescription drug monitoring programs can impact opioid overdoses in adults and focusing on safe storage of medications and other household chemicals can reduce poisonings in children. By focusing on interventions specific to etiology of the poisonings, many of these exposures can be reduced. As new substances continue to be manufactured, there is a need for more timely data and better toxicology testing so that poison centers, hospitals, and health departments are aware of emerging threats. Finally, what works theoretically or in one setting needs to be evaluated directly in other contexts while addressing barriers to implementation.

References

1. Committee on Poison Prevention and Control. *Forging a Poison Prevention and Control System*. Washington, DC: National Academies Press; 2004. https://www.ncbi.nlm.nih.gov/books/NBK215795/pdf/Bookshelf_NBK215795.pdf
2. Injury Surveillance Workgroup 7. *Consensus Recommendations for National and State Poisoning Surveillance*. Atlanta, GA: The Safe States Alliance; 2012. http://c.ymcdn.com/sites/www.cste.org/resource/resmgr/Injury/ISW7.pdf. Accessed October 25, 2017.
3. Hedegaard H, Miniño AM, Warner M. *Drug Overdose Deaths in the United States, 1999–2017. NCHS Data Brief, No 329*. Hyattsville, MD: National Center for Health Statistics; 2018.
4. Centers for Disease Control and Prevention. *Annual Surveillance Report of Drug-Related Risks and Outcomes—United States, 2017. Surveillance Special Report 1*. Atlanta, GA: Centers for Disease Control and Prevention, US Department of Health and Human Services; 2017. https://www.cdc.gov/drugoverdose/pdf/pubs/2017-cdc-drug-surveillance-report.pdf. Accessed October 25, 2017.
5. Injury Surveillance Workgroup 9. *The Transition from ICD-9-CM to ICD-10-CM: Guidance for Analysis and Reporting of Injuries by Mechanism and Intent*. Atlanta, GA: The Safe States Alliance; 2016. http://c.ymcdn.com/sites/www.safestates.org/resource/resmgr/isw9/ISW9_FINAL_Report.pdf. Accessed February 2, 2018.
6. Annest J, Hedegaard H, Chen L, Warner M, Small E. Proposed Framework for Presenting Injury Data Using ICD-10-CM External Cause of Injury Codes. Atlanta, GA: National Center for Injury Prevention and Control, National Center for Health Statistics, Centers for Disease Control and Prevention; 2014. https://www.cdc.gov/injury/wisqars/pdf/icd-10-cm_external_cause_injury_codes-a.pdf.
7. Hedegaard H, Johnson RL, Warner M, Chen L, Annest JL. Proposed framework for presenting injury data using the International Classification of Diseases, Tenth Revision, Clinical Modification (ICD-10-CM) Diagnosis Codes. *Natl Health Stat Rep*. 2016;89:1–19.
8. Centers for Disease Control and Prevention. Web-based Injury Statistics Query and Reporting System. 2019. https://www.cdc.gov/injury/wisqars/index.html. Accessed May, 2019.
9. Stone DM, Holland KM, Bartholow B, et al. Deciphering suicide and other manners of death associated with drug intoxication: A Centers for Disease Prevention and Control consultation meeting summary. *Am J Public Health*. 2017;107:1233–9.
10. Rudd RA, Aleshire N, Zibell JE, Gladden RM. Increases in drug and opioid-involved overdose deaths—United States, 2010–2015. *MMWR Morb Mortal Wkly Rep*. 2016;65:1378–82.
11. Sabel J, Poel A, Tuazon E, et al. *Recommendations and Lessons Learned from Improved Reporting of Drug Overdose Deaths on Death Certificates*. Atlanta, GA: Council of State and Territorial Epidemiologists; 2016. http://c.ymcdn.com/sites/www.cste.org/resource/resmgr/PDFs/PDFs2/4_25_2016_FINAL-Drug_Overdos.pdf.
12. Liu L, Wheeler SE, Venkataramanan R, et al. Newly emerging drugs of abuse and their detection methods: An ACLPS critical review. *Am J Clin Pathol*. 2018;149:105–16.

13. Cantrell L, Lucas J. Suicide by non-pharmaceutical poisons in San Diego County. *Clin Toxicol.* 2014;52(3):171–5.
14. Scholl L, Seth P, Kariisa M, Wilson N, Baldwin G. Drug and opioid-involved overdose deaths—United States, 2013–2017. *MMWR Morb Mortal Wkly Rep.* 2019;67:1419–27.
15. Kariisa M, Scholl L, Wilson N, Seth P, Hoots B. Drug overdose deaths involving cocaine and psychostimulants with abuse potential—United States, 2003–2017. *MMWR Morb Mortal Wkly Rep.* 2019;68:388-395.
16. Paulozzi LJ, Ryan GW. Opioid analgesics and rates of fatal drug poisoning in the United States. *Am J Prev Med.* 2006;31:506–11.
17. Dowell D, Arias E, Kochanek K, Anderson R, Guy GP, Losby J, Baldwin G. Contribution of opioid-involved overdose to change in life expectancy, United States, 2000–2015. *JAMA.* 2017;318:1065–7.
18. National Center for Health Statistics. Provisional counts of drug overdose deaths, as of 8/6/2017. Centers for Disease Control and Prevention. https://www.cdc.gov/nchs/data/health_policy/monthly-drug-overdose-death-estimates.pdf. Accessed October 25, 2017.
19. Hedegaard H, Bastian BA, Trinidad JP, Warner M. Drugs most frequently involved in drug overdose deaths: United States, 2011–2016. *Natl Vital Stat Rep.* 2018;67(9):1–14.
20. Weiss AJ, Elixhauser A, Barrett ML, Steiner CA, Bailey MK, O'Malley L. *Opioid-Related Inpatient Stays and Emergency Department Visits by State, 2009–2014. HCUP Statistical Brief #219.* Rockville, MD: Agency for Healthcare Research and Quality; December 2016. http://www.hcup-us.ahrq.gov/reports/statbriefs/sb219-Opioid-Hospital-Stays-ED-Visits-by-State.pdf.
21. Weiss AJ, Bailey MK, O'Malley L, Barrett ML, Elixhauser A, Steiner CA. *Patient Characteristics of Opioid-Related Inpatient Stays and Emergency Department Visits Nationally and by State, 2014. HCUP Statistical Brief #224.* Rockville, MD: Agency for Healthcare Research and Quality; June 2017. www.hcup-us.ahrq.gov/reports/statbriefs/sb224-Patient-Characteristics-Opioid-Hospital-Stays-ED-Visits-by-State.pdf.
22. Vivolo-Kantor A, Seth P, Gladden M, et al. Vital signs: Trends in emergency department visits for suspected opioid overdoses—United States, July 2016–September 2017. *MMWR Morb Mortal Wkly Rep.* 2018;67:1–8.
23. Franklin RL, Rodgers GB. Unintentional child poisonings treated in United States hospital emergency departments: National estimates of incident cases, population-based poisoning rates, and product involvement. *Pediatrics.* 2008;122(6):1244–51.
24. Schillie SF, Shehab N, Thomas KE, Budnitz DS. Medication overdoses leading to emergency department visits among children. *Am J Prev Med.* 2009;37(3):181–7.
25. Albertson TE, Tharratt RS, Marquardt K, Alsop J, Ninomiya JK, Foulke GE. Poisoning hospitalization correlates with poison center call frequency. *J Med Toxicol.* 2008;4:151–6.
26. Gummin DD, Mowry JB, Spyker DA, Brooks DE, Osterthaler KM, Banner W. 2017 Annual Report of the American Association of Poison Control Centers' National Poison Data System (NPDS): 35th Annual Report. *Clin Toxicol (Phila).* 2018:1–203.
27. Valdez AL, Casavant MJ, Spiller HA, Chounthirath T, Xiang H, Smith GA. Pediatric exposure to laundry detergent pods. Pediatrics. 2014;134:1127-35.
28. Centers for Disease Control and Prevention. Health hazards associated with laundry detergent pods—United States, May–June 2012. *MMWR Morb Mortal Wkly Rep.* 2012a;61:825–9.
29. Spiller HA, Beuhler MC, Ryan ML, Borys DJ, Alequas A, Bosse GM. Evaluation of changes in poisoning in young children: 2000 to 2010. *Pediatr Emerg Care.* 2013;29(5):635–40.
30. Allen JD, Casavant MJ, Spiller HA, Chounthirath T, Hodges NL, Smith GA. Prescription opioid exposures among children and adolescents in the United States: 2000–2015. *Pediatrics.* 2017;139:e20163382.
31. Guy GP, Zhang K, Bohm MK, et al. Vital signs: Changes in opioid prescribing in the United States, 2006–2015. *MMWR Morb Mortal Wkly Rep.* 2017;66:697–704.
32. Centers for Disease Control and Prevention. Buprenorphine prescribing practices and exposures reported to a poison center—Utah, 2002–2011. *MMWR Morb Mortal Wkly Rep.* 2012b;61:997–1001.
33. Altyar A, Kordi L, Skrepnek G. Clinical and economic characteristics of emergency department visits due to acetaminophen toxicity in the USA. *BMJ Open.* 2015;5:e007368.
34. Blieden M, Paramore LC, Shah D, Ben-Joseph R. A perspective on the epidemiology of acetaminophen exposure and toxicity in the United States. *Expert Rev Clin Pharmacol.* 2014;7:341–8.
35. Florence C, Simon T, Haegerich T, Luo F, Zhou C. Estimated lifetime medical and work-loss costs of fatal injuries—United States, 2013. *MMWR Morb Mortal Wkly Rep.* 2015;64(38):1074–7.
36. Florence C, Haegerich T, Simon T, Zhou C, Luo F. Estimated lifetime medical and work-loss costs of emergency department-treated nonfatal injuries—United States, 2013. *MMWR Morb Mortal Wkly Rep.* 2015;64(38):1078–82.
37. Florence CS, Zhou C, Luo F, Xu L. The economic burden of prescription opioid overdose, abuse, and dependence in the United States, 2013. *Med Care.* 2016;54(10):901–6.
38. White House Council of Economic Advisors. The underestimated cost of the opioid crisis. Executive Office of the President of the United States. 2017. https://www.whitehouse.gov/sites/whitehouse.gov/files/images/The%20Underestimated%20Cost%20of%20the%20Opioid%20Crisis.pdf.
39. Mack KA, Jones CM, Ballesteros MF. Illicit drug use, illicit drug use disorders, and drug overdose deaths in metropolitan and nonmetropolitan areas—United States. *Am J Transplant.* 2017;17(12):3241–52.
40. Mack KA, Clapperton AJ, Macpherson A, et al. Trends in the leading causes of injury mortality, Australia, Canada, and the United States, 2000–2014. *Can J Public Health.* 2017;108:e185–91.
41. Centers for Disease Control and Prevention. Vital signs: Overdoses of prescription opioid pain relievers—United States, 1999–2008. *MMWR Morb Mortal Wkly Rep.* 2011;60(43):1487–92.
42. Beautrais AL, Fergusson DM, Shannon FT. Accidental poisoning in the first three years of life. *Aust Paediatr J.* 1981;17:104–9.
43. Groom L, Kendrick D, Coupland C, Patel B, Hippisley-Cox J. Inequalities in hospital admission rates for unintentional poisoning in young children. *Inj Prev.* 2006;12:166–70.
44. Hjern A, Ringbäck-Weitoft G, Andersson R. Socio-demographic risk factors for home-type injuries in Swedish infants and toddlers. *Acta Paediatr.* 2001;90:61–8.
45. Tyrrell EG, Orton E, Tata LJ, Kendrick D. Children at risk of medicinal and non-medicinal poisoning: A population-based case-control study in general practice. *Br J Gen Pract.* 2012;62(605):e827–33.
46. Lavonas EJ, Banner W, Bradt P, et al. Root causes, clinical effects, and outcomes of unintentional exposures to buprenorphine by young children. *J Pediatr.* 2013;163:1377–83.
47. Kendrick D, Majsak-Newman G, Benford P, et al. Poison prevention practices and medically attended poisoning in young children: Multicentre case-control study. *Inj Prev.* 2017;23(2):93–101.
48. Schmertmann M, Williamson A, Black D, Wilson L. Risk factors for unintentional poisoning in children aged 1–3 years in NSW Australia: A case-control study. *BMC Pediatr.* 2013;13:88.
49. Bailey JE, Campagna E, Dart RC. The underrecognized toll of prescription opioid abuse on young children. *Ann Emerg Med.* 2009;53(4):419–24.
50. Yang Z, Wilsey B, Bohm M, et al. Defining risk of prescription opioid overdose: Pharmacy shopping and overlapping prescriptions among long-term opioid users in Medicaid. *J Pain.* 2015;16:445–53.
51. Dilokthornsakul P, Moore G, Campbell JD, et al. Risk factors of prescription opioid overdose among Colorado Medicaid beneficiaries. *J Pain.* 2016;17(4):436–43.
52. Bohnert AS, Valenstein M, Bair MJ, et al. Association between opioid prescribing patterns and opioid overdose-related deaths. *JAMA.* 2011;305(13):1315–21.
53. Zedler B, Xie L, Wang L, et al. Risk factors for serious prescription opioid-related toxicity or overdose among Veterans Health Administration patients. *Pain Med.* 2014;15(11):1911–29.
54. Substance Abuse and Mental Health Services Administration. *Key Substance Use and Mental Health Indicators in the United States: Results from the 2016 National Survey on Drug Use and Health (HHS Publication No. SMA 17-5044, NSDUH Series H-52).* Rockville, MD: Center for Behavioral Health Statistics and Quality, Substance Abuse and Mental Health Services Administration; 2017. https://www.samhsa.gov/data/.
55. Lanier WA, Johnson EM, Rolfs RT, Friedrichs MD, Grey TC. Risk factors for prescription opioid-related death, Utah, 2008–2009. *Pain Med.* 2012;13(12):1580–9.
56. Mateu-Gelabert P, Guarino H, Frank D, et al. Factors associated with nonfatal overdose among young opioid users: Heroin and benzodiazepine use, prescription opioid and heroin injection and HCV status. *Drug Alcohol Depend.* 2017;171:e131.
57. Robinson W, Kazbour C, Tanner N, et al. Brief report: Nonfatal overdose events among persons who inject drugs: Findings from seven national HIV behavioral surveillance cities 2009 and 2012. *J Acquir Immune Defic Syndr.* 2017;75:S341–5.
58. Coffin PO, Tracy M, Bucciarelli A, Ompad D, Vlahov D, Galea S. Identifying injection drug users at risk of nonfatal overdose. *Acad Emerg Med.* 2007 Jul 1;14(7):616–23.

59. Jones CM, Logan J, Gladden RM, Bohm MK. Vital signs: Demographic and substance use trends among heroin users—United States, 2002–2013. *MMWR Morb Mortal Wkly Rep*. 2015;64(26):719–25.
60. Piercefield E, Archer P, Kemp P, Mallonee S. Increase in unintentional medication overdose deaths: Oklahoma, 1994–2006. *Am J Prev Med*. 2010;39(4):357–63.
61. Paone D, Tuazon E, Kattan J, et al. Decrease in rate of opioid analgesic overdose deaths—Staten Island, New York City, 2011–2013. *MMWR Morb Mortal Wkly Rep*. 2015;64:491–4.
62. Daniulaityte R, Juhascik MP, Strayer KE, et al. Overdose deaths related to fentanyl and its analogs—Ohio, January–February 2017. *MMWR Morb Mortal Wkly Rep*. 2017;66(34):904.
63. Turner BJ, Liang Y. Drug overdose in a retrospective cohort with non-cancer pain treated with opioids, antidepressants, and/or sedative-hypnotics: Interactions with mental health disorders. *J Gen Intern Med*. 2015;30:1081–96.
64. Hempstead K. Manner of death and circumstances in fatal poisonings: Evidence from New Jersey. *Inj Prev*. 2006;12(suppl 2):ii44–8.
65. Park TW, Lin LA, Hosanagar A, Kogowski A, Paige K, Bohnert AS. Understanding risk factors for opioid overdose in clinical populations to inform treatment and policy. *J Addict Med*. 2016;10(6):369–81.
66. Paulozzi LJ, Kilbourne EM, Shah NG, et al. A history of being prescribed controlled substances and risk of drug overdose death. *Pain Med*. 2012;13(1):87–95.
67. Dunn KM, Saunders KW, Rutter CM, et al. Opioid prescriptions for chronic pain and overdose: A cohort study. *Ann Intern Med*. 2010;152(2):85–92.
68. Gomes T, Mamdani MM, Dhalla IA, Paterson JM, Juurlink DN. Opioid dose and drug-related mortality in patients with nonmalignant pain. *Arch Intern Med*. 2011;171(7):686–91.
69. Baumblatt JAG, Wiedeman C, Dunn JR, Schaffner W, Paulozzi LJ, Jones TF. High-risk use by patients prescribed opioids for pain and its role in overdose deaths. *JAMA Intern Med*. 2014;174(5):796–801.
70. Liang Y, Turner BJ. Assessing risk for drug overdose in a national cohort: Role for both daily and total opioid dose? *J Pain*. 2015;16:318–25.
71. Miller M, Barber CW, Leatherman S, et al. Prescription opioid duration of action and the risk of unintentional overdose among patients receiving opioid therapy. *JAMA Intern Med*. 2015;175:608–15.
72. Peirce GL, Smith MJ, Abate MA, Halverson J. Doctor and pharmacy shopping for controlled substances. *Med Care*. 2012;50(6):494–500.
73. Park TW, Saitz R, Ganoczy D, Ilgen MA, Bohnert AS. Benzodiazepine prescribing patterns and deaths from drug overdose among US veterans receiving opioid analgesics: Case-cohort study. *BMJ*. 2015;350:h2698.
74. O'Donnell JK, Halpin J, Mattson CL, Goldberger BA, Gladden RM. Deaths involving fentanyl, fentanyl analogs, and U-47700-10 states, July–December 2016. *MMWR Morb Mortal Wkly Rep*. 2017;66(43):1197–202.
75. Drug Enforcement Administration (DEA), Diversion Control Division. *National Forensic Laboratory Information System: NFLIS-Drug Midyear Report 2018*. Springfield, VA: US Department of Justice, Drug Enforcement Administration; 2019.
76. Gladden RM, O'Donnell J, Mattson CL, Seth P. Changes in opioid-involved overdose deaths by opioid type and presence of benzodiazepines, cocaine, and methamphetamine—25 States, July–December 2017 to January–June 2018. *MMWR Morb Mortal Wkly Rep*. 2019;68:737–44.
77. Paulozzi LJ, Xi Y. Recent changes in drug poisoning mortality in the United States by urban-rural status and by drug type. *Pharmacoepidemiol Drug Saf*. 2008;17(10):997–1005.
78. Jones CM, Campopiano M, Baldwin G, McCance-Katz E. National and state treatment need and capacity for opioid agonist medication-assisted treatment. *Am J Public Health*. 2015;105:e55–63.
79. Binswanger IA, Blatchford PJ, Mueller SR, Stern MF. Mortality after prison release: Opioid overdose and other causes of death, risk factors, and time trends from 1999 to 2009. *Ann Intern Med*. 2013;159:592–600.
80. Wheeler E, Jones TS, Gilbert MK, Davidson PJ. Opioid overdose prevention programs providing naloxone to laypersons—United States, 2014. *MMWR Morb Mortal Wkly Rep*. 2015;64:631–5.
81. United States Consumer Product Safety Commission. Poison prevention packaging: A guide for healthcare professionals. https://www.cpsc.gov/s3fs-public/384.pdf. Revised 2005. Accessed January 3, 2018.
82. American Association of Poison Control Centers (AAPCC). Poison Control Centers. https://www.aapcc.org/. Accessed May 3, 2019.
83. United States Food and Drug Administration. This week in FDA history—Nov. 3, 1966. https://www.fda.gov/AboutFDA/WhatWeDo/History/ThisWeek/ucm117876.htm. Updated 2009. Accessed January 3, 2018.
84. Stracener CE, Scherz RG, Crone RI. Results of testing a child-resistant medicine container. *Pediatrics*. 1967;40(2):286–8.
85. Scherz RB, Latham GH, Stracener CE. Child resistant containers can prevent poisoning. *Pediatrics*. 1969;43(1):84–7.
86. Walton WW. An evaluation of the poison prevention packaging act. *Pediatrics*. 1982;69(3):363–70.
87. Rodgers GB. The safety effects of child-resistant packaging for oral prescription drugs. Two decades of experience. *JAMA*. 1996;275(21):1661–5.
88. Rodgers GB. The effectiveness of child-resistant packaging for aspirin. *Arch Pediatr Adolesc Med*. 2002;156(9):929–33.
89. United States Food and Drug Administration. Guidance for Industry: Iron-Containing Supplements and Drugs: Label Warning Statements: Small Entity Compliance Guide. 2003. https://www.fda.gov/regulatory-information/search-fda-guidance-documents/guidance-industry-iron-containing-supplements-and-drugs-label-warning-statements-small-entity. Accessed October 18, 2019.
90. Tenenbein M. Unit-dose packaging of iron supplements and reduction of iron poisoning in young children. *Arch Pediatr Adolesc Med*. 2005;159:557–60.
91. Budnitz DS, Lovegrove MC, Sapiano MR, Kegler MJ, Geller AI, Hampp C. Notes from the field: Pediatric emergency department visits for buprenorphine/naloxone ingestion—United States, 2008–2015. *MMWR Morb Mortal Wkly Rep*. 2016;65:1148–9.
92. Lovegrove MC, Hon S, Geller RJ, et al. Efficacy of flow restrictors in limiting access of liquid medications by young children. *J Pediatr*. 2013;163(4):1134–9.
93. Hawton K, Bergen H, Simkin S, et al. Long term effect of reduced pack sizes of paracetamol on poisoning deaths and liver transplant activity in England and Wales: Interrupted time series analyses. *BMJ*. 2013;346:f403.
94. Committee on Injury, Violence, and Poison Prevention. Poison treatment in the home. *Pediatrics*. 2003;112(5):1182–5.
95. Kendrick D, Young B, Mason-Jones AJ, et al. Home safety education and provision of safety equipment for injury prevention. *Cochrane Database Syst Rev*. 2012;(9):CD005014.
96. Crosslin KL, Tsai R, Romo CV, Tsai A. Acculturation in Hispanics and childhood poisoning: Are medicines and household cleaners stored properly? *Accid Anal Prev*. 2011;43:1010–4.
97. Patel B, Groom L, Prasad V, Kendrick D. Parental poison prevention practices and their relationship with perceived toxicity: Cross-sectional study. *Inj Prev*. 2008;14(6):389–95.
98. Haegerich TM, Jones CM, Cote PO, Robinson A, Ross L. Evidence for state, community and systems-level prevention strategies to address the opioid crisis. *Drug Alcohol Depend*. 2019;204:107563.
99. Yanovitzky I. The American medicine chest challenge: Evaluation of a drug take-back and disposal campaign. *J Stud Alcohol Drugs*. 2016;77(4):549–55.
100. Rodgers GB, Franklin RL, Midgett JD. Unintentional paediatric ingestion poisonings and the role of imitative behaviour. *Inj Prev*. 2012;18(2):103–8.
101. Haegerich TM, Paulozzi LJ, Manns BJ, Jones CM. What we know, and don't know, about the impact of state policy and sytems-level interventions on prescription drug overdose. *Drug Alcohol Depend*. 2014;145:34–47.
102. Prescription Drug Monitoring Program Training and Technical Assistance Center (PDMP TTAC). PDMP Maps and Tables. https://www.pdmpassist.org/content/pdmp-maps-and-tables. Accessed July 22, 2019.
103. Dowell D, Haegerich TM, Chou R. CDC guideline for prescribing opioids for chronic pain—United States, 2016. *MMWR Morb Mortal Wkly Rep*. 2016;65:1–49.
104. Dowell D, Zhang K, Noonan RK, Hockenberry JM. Mandatory provider review and pain clinic laws reduce the amounts of opioids prescribed and overdose death rates. *Health Aff (Millwood)*. 2016;35:1876–83.
105. Kattan JA, Tuazon E, Paone D, et al. Public health detailing—A successful strategy to promote judicious opioid analgesic prescribing. *Am J Public Health*. 2016;106:1430–8.
106. Cochran G, Gordon AJ, Gellad WF, et al. Medicaid prior authorization and opioid medication abuse and overdose. *Am J Manag Care*. 2017;23:e164–71.
107. Bohnert SB, Guy GP, Losby JL. Opioid prescribing in the United States before and after the Centers for Disease Control and Prevention's 2016 opioid guideline. *Ann Intern Med*. 2018;169:367–75.
108. Johnson EM, Porucznik CA, Anderson JW, Rolfs RT. State-level strategies for reducing prescription drug overdose deaths: Utah's prescription safety program. *Pain Med*. 2011;12:S66–72.

109. Centers for Disease Control and Prevention. Rx Awareness. https://www.cdc.gov/rxawareness/pdf/Overview-Rx-Awareness-Resources.pdf.

110. Spoth R, Trudeau L, Shin C, et al. Longitudinal effects of universal preventive intervention on prescription drug misuse: Three randomized controlled trials with late adolescents and young adults. *Am J Public Health*. 2013;103:665–72.

111. Walley AY, Xuan Z, Hackman HH, et al. Opioid overdose rates and implementation of overdose education and nasal naloxone distribution in Massachusetts: Interrupted time series analysis. *BMJ*. 2013;346:f174.

112. Coffin PO, Behar E, Rowe C, et al. Nonrandomized intervention study of naloxone coprescription for primary care patients receiving long-term opioid therapy for pain. *Ann Intern Med*. 2016;165:245–52.

113. Samuels E. Emergency department naloxone distribution: A Rhode Island department of health, recovery community, and emergency department partnership to reduce opioid overdose deaths. *R I Med J*. 2014;97:38–9.

114. Guy GPJr., Haegerich TM, Evans ME, Losby JL, Young R, Jones CM. Vital signs: Pharmacy-based naloxone dispensing—United States, 2012–2018. *MMWR Morb Mortal Wkly Rep*. 2019;68:679–86.

115. Ducharme J. The country's first safe injection facility may soon open in Philadelphia: Here's what you need to know. February 6, 2018. http://time.com/5128626/safe-injection-facilities-us-philadelphia/.

116. Davidson PJ, Lopez AM, Kral AH. Using drugs in un/safe spaces: Impact of perceived illegality on an underground supervised injecting facility in the United States. *Int J Drug Policy*. 2018;53:37–44.

117. Marshall BDL, Milloy J, Wood E, Montaner J, Kerr T. Reduction in overdose mortality after the opening of North America's first medically supervised safer injecting facility: A retrospective population-based study. *Lancet*. 2011;9775:23–9.

118. Johns Hopkins Bloomberg School of Public Health, Bloomberg American Health Initiative. Fentanyl overdose reduction checking analysis study (FORECAST), 2018. http://americanhealth.jhu.edu/assets/pdfs/FORECAST__Summary_Report.pdf.

119. Volkow ND, Frieden TR, Hyse P, Cha SS. Medication-assisted therapies—Tackling the opioid overdose epidemic. *N Engl J Med*. 2014;370:2063–6.

120. Morgan JR, Schackman BR, Leff JA, Linas BP, Walley AY. Injectable naltrexone, oral naltrexone, and buprenorphine utilization and discontinuation among individuals treated for opioid use disorder in a United States commercially insured population. *J Subst Abuse Treat*. 2018;85:90–6.

121. Lee JD, Nunes EV, Novo P, et al. Comparative effectiveness of extended-release naltrexone versus buprenorphine-naloxone for opioid relapse prevention (X:BOT): A multicenter, open-label, randomized controlled trial. *Lancet*. 2018;391:309–18.

122. Connock M, Juarez-Garcia A, Jowett S, et al. Methadone and buprenorphine for the management of opioid dependence: A systematic review and economic evaluation. *Health Technol Assess*. 2007;11:9.

123. Sordo L, Barrio G, Bravo MJ, et al. Mortality risk during and after opioid substitution treatment: systematic review and meta-analysis of cohort studies. *BMJ*. 2017;357:j1550.

124. D'Onofrio GD, Chawarski MC, O'Connor PG, et al. Emergency department-initiated buprenorphine with opioid dependence with continuation in primary care: Outcomes during and after intervention. *J Gen Intern Med*. 2017;32:660–6.

125. Friedmann PD, Wilson D, Hoskinson R, Poshkus M, Clarke JG. Initiation of extended release naltrexone (XR-NTX) for opioid use disorder prior to release from prison. *J Subst Abuse Treat*. 2018;85:45–8.

126. Rudd RA, Paulozzi LJ, Bauer MJ, et al. Increases in heroin overdose deaths—28 States, 2010 to 2012. *MMWR Morb Mortal Wkly Rep*. 2014;63(39):849.

127. Schiff DM, Drainoni ML, Weinstein ZM, Chan L, Bair-Merritt M, Rosenbloom D. A police-led addiction treatment referral program in Gloucester, MA: Implementation and participants' experiences. *J Subst Abuse Treat*. 2017;82:41–7.

128. Dahlem CHG, King L, Anderson G, Marr A, Waddell JE, Scalera M. Beyond rescue: Implementation and evaluation of revised naloxone training for law enforcement officers. *Public Health Nurse*. 2017;34(6):516–21.

129. Stone DM, Holland KM, Bartholow B, Crosby AE, Davis S, Wilkins N. *Preventing Suicide: A Technical Package of Policies, Programs, and Practices*. Atlanta, GA: National Center for Injury Prevention and Control, Centers for Disease Control and Prevention; 2017. https://www.cdc.gov/violenceprevention/pdf/suicideTechnicalPackage.pdf. Accessed October 18, 2019.

130. Oliva EM, Bowe T, Tavakoli S, et al. Development and applications of the Veterans Health Administration's Stratification Tool for Opioid Risk Mitigation (STORM) to improve opioid safety and prevent overdose and suicide. *Psychol Serv*. 2014;14:34–49.

131. Brennan PL, Del Re AC, Henderson PT, Trafton JA. Healthcare system-wide implementation of opioid-safety guideline recommendations: The case of urine drug screening and opioid-patient suicide- and overdose-related events in the Veterans Health Administration. *Transl Behav Med*. 2016;6:605–12.

132. Hawton K, Ware C, Mistry H, et al. Paracetamol self-poisoning. Characteristics, prevention and harm reduction. *Br J Psychiatry*. 1996;168(1):43–8.

133. Hawton K, Ware C, Mistry H, et al. Why patients choose paracetamol for self poisoning and their knowledge of its dangers. *BMJ*. 1995;310(6973):164.

134. Nordentoft M, Qin P, Helweg-Larsen K, Juel K. Restrictions in means for suicide: An effective tool in preventing suicide: The Danish experience. *Suicide Life Threat Behav*. 2007;37:688--97.

CHAPTER 175

The Epidemiology and Prevention of Self-directed Violence

Kristin M. Holland • Alex E. Crosby

Suicide is a significant public health problem affecting countries worldwide. Globally, approximately 800,000 suicides occur every year, making it the 17th leading cause of death in the world. In 2016, the international annual age-adjusted suicide rate was 11.2 per 100,000 population.[1] In the United States, suicide resulted in over 48,000 deaths in 2018, and it has been one of the top ten leading causes of death for the country since 2008.[2] While suicide rates have been declining globally, rates in the United States have been rising since the late 1990s (Fig. 175-1).[3–5] In fact, the overall decrease in Americans' average life expectancy in 2015–17 has been attributed in part to increasing suicide rates, which rose by 33% from 1999 to 2017,[2,6,7] underlining the public health significance of the growing problem.

Unfortunately, suicide is simply the tip of the iceberg contributing to the public health problem encompassing all self-directed violence (SDV). Indeed, many more people attempt suicide than die by suicide every year, and even more contemplate suicide than attempt it. In fact, for every one suicide in the United States, there are an estimated 29 suicide attempts, and 248 people who seriously consider suicide.[2,8] Ultimately, every year, over 1.4 million American adults attempt suicide, and almost 12 million seriously consider suicide.[8,9] Because suicidal ideation and suicide attempts in particular are strong predictors of suicide, suicide prevention efforts must take into account the full spectrum of suicidal thoughts and behavior to be effective.

Research indicates that suicide is not just a mental health problem, but that it is generally the influenced by risk factors at the individual, relationship, community, and societal levels.[10] Problems such as substance use, intimate partner and other relationship problems, exposure to adverse childhood experiences, financial problems, job problems, and physical health issues also serve as risk factors for suicide.[10–12] Given all of these risk factors, a comprehensive public health approach is needed that prevents suicide risk in the first place through upstream prevention, that identifies and supports people at increased risk of suicide, prevents reattempts, and assists people who are survivors of suicide loss. The purpose of this chapter is to describe the nature and burden of the problem of suicide, identify risk and protective factors, and highlight evidence-based prevention strategies.

DEMOGRAPHIC PATTERNS IN SUICIDE RISK

Suicide is but one behavior encompassed by a broad range of SDV, which includes fatal and nonfatal suicidal behavior. Suicidal ideation—that is, thoughts about or plans for suicide—is also associated with SDV and included in the spectrum of SDV. The Centers for Disease Control and Prevention (CDC) defines suicide as death caused by self-directed injurious behavior where the decedent's intent is to die as a result of the behavior. A suicide attempt is defined as a nonfatal, self-directed, potentially injurious behavior where the victim intends to die as a result of the behavior. However, it is important to note that not all suicide attempts result in an injury. In fact, most suicide attempts do not even result in an injury serious enough to require medical attention.[8,13] The act of thinking about, considering, or planning suicide is referred to as suicidal ideation.[14]

The burden associated with suicide varies by many factors, including sex, age, race, and geography. For example, in 2016, males experienced higher rates of suicide globally (15.6 per 100,000) than did females (7.0 per 100,000).[1] However, suicide rates by sex vary with respect to countries' economic status. For instance, in wealthier countries, males die by suicide approximately three times more often than females; whereas, in poorer countries, males account for only about 1.5 times as many suicide deaths as females. Further, while almost 80% of suicides occur in developing countries, suicide remains a major public health problem in developed countries, including the United States, often ranking among the leading causes of death.[12]

Just as they do globally, rates of suicide and suicidal behavior vary by age, sex, geographic location, and occupation in the United States. For instance, while suicide is the tenth leading cause of death overall in the United States, it was the second leading cause of death among individuals aged 10–34 years in 2018. Although suicide was the second leading cause of death among youth and young adults, working aged adults—those aged 25–64 years—contribute the greatest burden to the problem of suicide, with this group making up a total of 32,426 (67.0%) of the 48,344 suicides that occurred in the United States in 2018 (Fig. 175-2). More males than females die by suicide in the United States, where males make up about three-quarters of suicides every year. Middle-aged men (i.e., 35–64 years), in particular, have seen a 39.5% increase in suicide rates from 1999 to 2018 and experience a rate more than twice that of the national average (30.0 vs. 12.0 per 100,000 population).[2] Research suggests this rise in suicide rates among middle-aged men could be related to the economic recession impacting the United States in the late 2000s, as well as a rise in intentional drug poisoning that may coincide with increased availability of prescription opioids since the late 1990s.[15–18] Further, although rates have increased dramatically for men in the middle years, males aged 85+ experience the highest rates of suicide annually (47.2 per 100,000 population in 2018). On the other hand, among females, suicide rates are highest between the ages of 45 and 49.[2] Table 175-1 highlights these and other demographic groups at risk of suicide and self-harm.[2,19]

Research has also demonstrated that certain racial and ethnic groups in the United States experience higher suicide rates than others. For instance, from 2001 to 2015, suicide rates were consistently highest among American Indian/Alaska Natives (AIAN).[5] Additionally, a recent analysis of trends in male and female suicide rates by race/ethnicity from 1999 through 2017 indicated that for males, age-adjusted suicide rates increased 71% among non-Hispanic

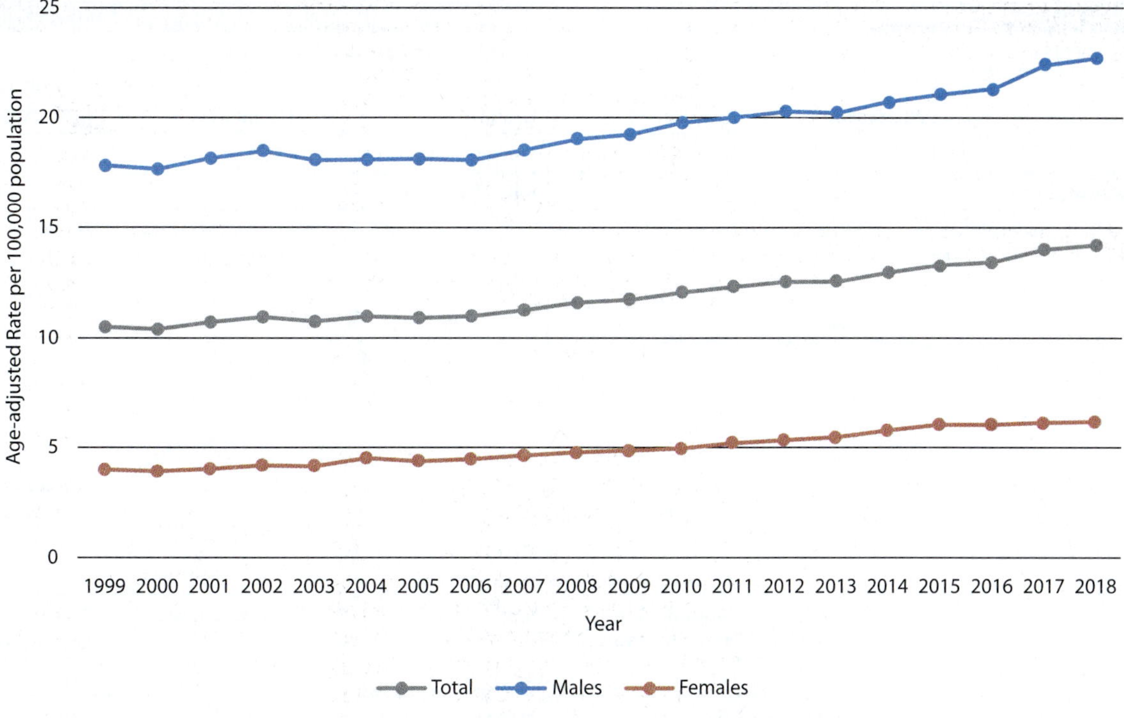

FIGURE 175-1. Suicide rates by year and by sex, United States, 1999–2018. (*Source:* CDC, National Center for Health Statistics (NCHS), National Vital Statistics System, produced by National Center for Injury Prevention and Control (NCIPC), Web-based Injury Statistics Query and Reporting System [WISQARS].)

	Age Groups										
Rank	<1	1-4	5-9	10-14	15-24	25-34	35-44	45-54	55-64	65+	All Ages
1	Congenital Anomalies 4,473	Unintentional Injury 1,226	Unintentional Injury 734	Unintentional Injury 692	Unintentional Injury 12,044	Unintentional Injury 24,614	Unintentional Injury 22,667	Malignant Neoplasms 37,301	Malignant Neoplasms 113,947	Heart Disease 526,509	Heart Disease 655,381
2	Short Gestation 3,679	Congenital Anomalies 384	Malignant Neoplasms 393	Suicide 596	Suicide 6,211	Suicide 8,020	Malignant Neoplasms 10,640	Heart Disease 32,220	Heart Disease 81,042	Malignant Neoplasms 431,102	Malignant Neoplasms 599,274
3	Maternal Pregnancy Comp. 1,358	Homicide 353	Congenital Anomalies 201	Malignant Neoplasms 450	Homicide 4,607	Homicide 5,234	Heart Disease 10,532	Unintentional Injury 23,056	Unintentional Injury 23,693	Chronic Low. Respiratory Disease 135,560	Unintentional Injury 167,127
4	SIDS 1,334	Malignant Neoplasms 326	Homicide 121	Congenital Anomalies 172	Malignant Neoplasms 1,371	Malignant Neoplasms 3,684	Suicide 7,521	Suicide 8,345	Chronic Low. Respiratory Disease 18,804	Cerebro-vascular 127,244	Chronic Low. Respiratory Disease 159,486
5	Unintentional Injury 1,168	Influenza & Pneumonia 122	Influenza & Pneumonia 71	Homicide 168	Heart Disease 905	Heart Disease 3,561	Homicide 3,304	Liver Disease 8,157	Diabetes Mellitus 14,941	Alzheimer's Disease 120,658	Cerebro-vascular 147,810
6	Placenta Cord Membranes 724	Heart Disease 115	Chronic Low. Respiratory Disease 68	Heart Disease 101	Congenital Anomalies 354	Liver Disease 1,008	Liver Disease 3,108	Diabetes Mellitus 6,414	Liver Disease 13,945	Diabetes Mellitus 60,182	Alzheimer's Disease 122,019
7	Bacterial Sepsis 579	Perinatal Period 62	Heart Disease 68	Chronic Low. Respiratory Disease 64	Diabetes Mellitus 246	Diabetes Mellitus 837	Diabetes Mellitus 2,282	Cerabro-vascular 5,128	Cerabro-vascular 12,789	Unintentional Injury 57,213	Diabetes Mellitus 84,946
8	Circulatory System Disease 428	Septicemia 54	Cerabro-vascular 34	Cerabro-vascular 54	Influenza & Pneumonia 200	Cerabro-vascular 567	Cerabro-vascular 1,704	Chronic Low. Respiratory Disease 3,807	Suicide 8,540	Influenza & Pneumonia 48,888	Influenza & Pneumonia 59,120
9	Respiratory Distress 390	Chronic Low. Respiratory Disease 60	Septicemia 34	Influenza & Pneumonia 51	Chronic Low. Respiratory Disease 165	HIV 482	Influenza & Pneumonia 956	Septicemia 2,380	Septicemia 5,956	Nephritis 42,232	Nephritis 51,386
10	Neonatal Hemorrhage 375	Cerebro-vascular 43	Benign Neoplasms 19	Benign Neoplasms 30	Complicated Pregnancy 151	Influenza & Pneumonia 457	Septicemia 829	Influenza & Pneumonia 2,339	Influenza & Pneumonia 5,858	Parkinson's Disease 32,988	Suicide 48,344

FIGURE 175-2. Top ten leading causes of death in the United States by age group, 2018. (*Source:* CDC, National Center for Health Statistics (NCHS), National Vital Statistics System, produced by National Center for Injury Prevention and Control (NCIPC), Web-based Injury Statistics Query and Reporting System [WISQARS].)

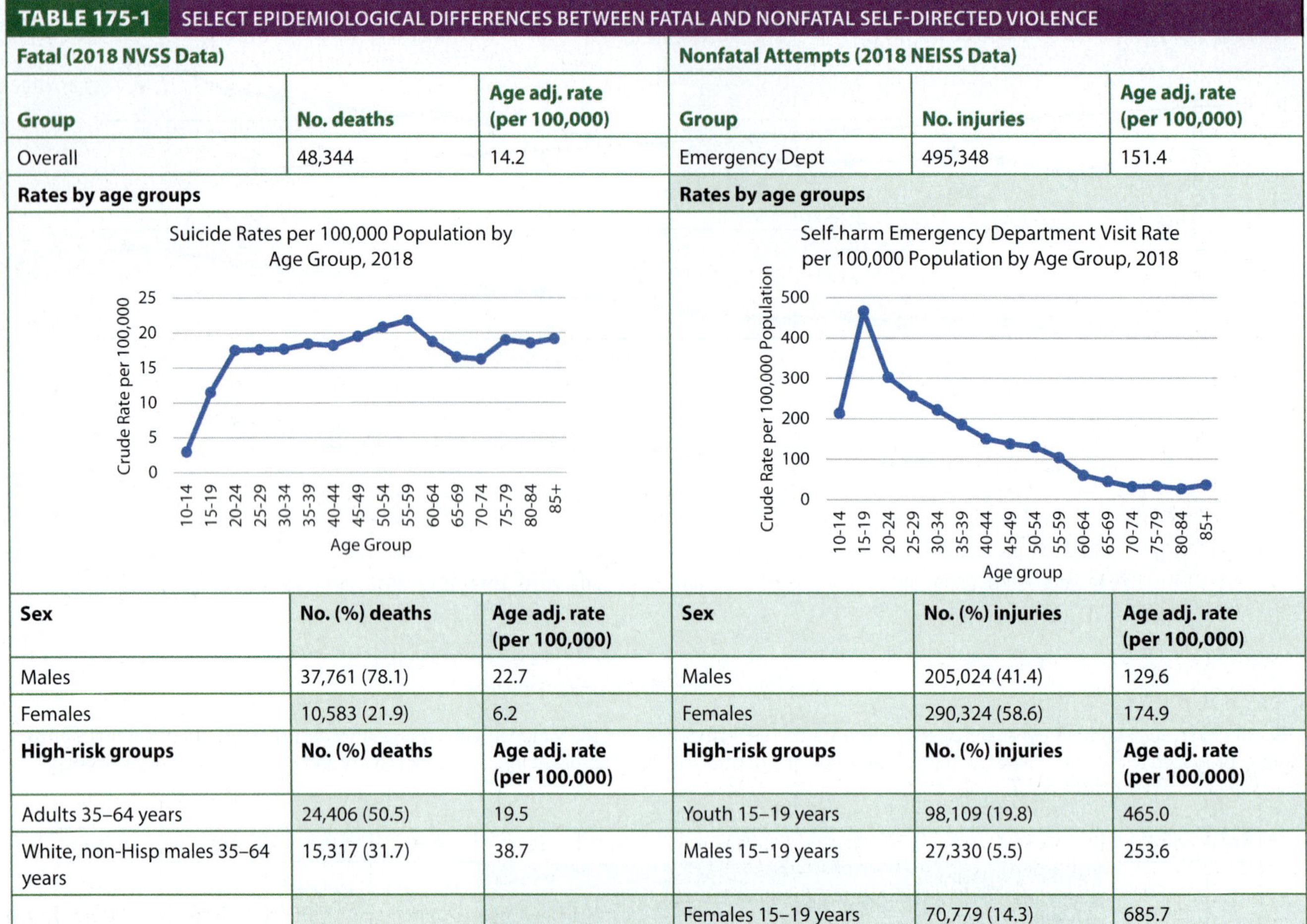

TABLE 175-1 SELECT EPIDEMIOLOGICAL DIFFERENCES BETWEEN FATAL AND NONFATAL SELF-DIRECTED VIOLENCE

Fatal (2018 NVSS Data)			Nonfatal Attempts (2018 NEISS Data)		
Group	**No. deaths**	**Age adj. rate (per 100,000)**	**Group**	**No. injuries**	**Age adj. rate (per 100,000)**
Overall	48,344	14.2	Emergency Dept	495,348	151.4
Rates by age groups			**Rates by age groups**		
Suicide Rates per 100,000 Population by Age Group, 2018			Self-harm Emergency Department Visit Rate per 100,000 Population by Age Group, 2018		
Sex	**No. (%) deaths**	**Age adj. rate (per 100,000)**	**Sex**	**No. (%) injuries**	**Age adj. rate (per 100,000)**
Males	37,761 (78.1)	22.7	Males	205,024 (41.4)	129.6
Females	10,583 (21.9)	6.2	Females	290,324 (58.6)	174.9
High-risk groups	**No. (%) deaths**	**Age adj. rate (per 100,000)**	**High-risk groups**	**No. (%) injuries**	**Age adj. rate (per 100,000)**
Adults 35–64 years	24,406 (50.5)	19.5	Youth 15–19 years	98,109 (19.8)	465.0
White, non-Hisp males 35–64 years	15,317 (31.7)	38.7	Males 15–19 years	27,330 (5.5)	253.6
			Females 15–19 years	70,779 (14.3)	685.7

AIAN and 39.6% among non-Hispanic white males. The suicide rate for 15- to 24- and 25- to 44-year old males were highest for non-Hispanic AIAN males in 2017 (53.7 and 58.1, respectively); in fact, the suicide rate among this group was over three times the 2017 national average of 14.0 per 100,000 population. During the same time period, suicide rates for females increased for all racial and ethnic groups, except non-Hispanic Asian or Pacific Islanders (API). The greatest increases among females were observed among non-Hispanic AIAN females (89%) and non-Hispanic white females (60%). The highest suicide rate among females was experienced by 45–64-year-old non-Hispanic white females (12.6 per 100,000).[20]

Much research has described the geographic variation in suicide rates in the United States. For instance, there are differences in suicide rates by region, where the Rocky Mountain states tend to have the highest age-adjusted rate.[21] In addition, suicide rates are higher in rural compared to urban areas. One study found that suicide rates increased from 1999 to 2015 in the United States across all levels of urbanization—that is, in rural and urban areas.[22] However, the gap in suicide rates between more rural and more urban areas widened over time, with rates in more rural areas beginning to increase at a more rapid pace in 2007–08 around the time of the economic downturn, which disproportionately impacted rural areas and also involved longer recovery times in these areas.[22,23]

With respect to occupation, Peterson and colleagues examined occupational data included in the National Violent Death Reporting System (NVDRS) data from 32 states in 2016 and found that persons in five industry groups experienced suicide rates significantly higher than the national average: (1) males working in mining, quarrying, and oil and gas extraction, (2) males working construction, (3) males working other services (e.g., automotive repair), (4) males working agriculture, forestry, fishing, and hunting, and (5) males and females working in transportation and warehousing. Among males, the five occupations with the highest suicide rates included fishing and hunting workers (119.9 per 100,000), musicians, singers, and related workers (96.5), artists and related workers (93.5), structural iron and steel workers (79.0), and millwrights (78.7). Among females, the highest suicide rates were experienced by those working as artists and related workers (45.5), laborers and freight, stock, and material movers (20.9), personal-care aides (12.1), and retail salespersons (11.5). Factors that may put individuals who work in industries with the highest suicide rates at increased risk for suicide may include stressful work environments, social isolation related to the job, access to lethal means on the job, and socioeconomic inequalities such as lower income and education level, as well as less access to healthcare.[24]

Additionally, much work has been done to assess suicide risk among Veterans. In 2017, after adjusting for age and sex differences, the suicide rate among Veterans was 1.5 times higher than for civilian adults. Further, Veterans accounted for 13.5% of all adult suicide deaths in the United States in 2017, but only made up 7.9% of the adult population, demonstrating the disparity in suicide deaths.[25] Further, as did the general population, Veterans experienced an increase in suicide rates over time; from 2005 to 2017, there was a 6.1% increase among Veteran suicides.

SUICIDE MEANS

The most prevalent means of suicide also differ globally and within the United States. For instance, globally, suffocation, pesticide ingestion, and carbon monoxide poisoning are common methods of suicide.[26–29] One systematic review of global data from 1990 to 2007 suggested that pesticide ingestion may contribute to as many as 30% of suicides globally; this method is most commonly used in low- and middle-income countries.[12,29] In the United States, the most prevalent means of suicide are firearms (50.5%), suffocation (including hanging; 28.6%), and poisoning (12.9%).[2] One recent study demonstrated that both the percentage of suicides involving firearms and poisoning decreased from 1999 through 2014, but the percentage of suicides involving suffocation increased during that time.[4] However, in light of the opioid crisis in the United States, it is important to note that while poisoning-related suicides have shown a decline in recent years, suicides where poisoning specifically by opioids was listed as a contributing cause of death experienced a statistically significant increase from 0.3 per 100,000 in 1999 to 0.7 per 100,000 in 2009 and remained steady from 2009 through 2014.[30] This increase may be related to the simultaneous increase in unintentional poisoning deaths, which have been increasing in the United States since around 1999.[31]

DEMOGRAPHIC PATTERNS IN NONFATAL SELF-DIRECTED VIOLENCE AND SUICIDAL IDEATION RISK

The most prevalent means involved in suicide attempts differs from those used in suicides. The National Electronic Injury Surveillance System, All Injury Program (NEISS-AIP) maintained by the U.S. Consumer Product Safety Commission houses data on all first-time visits for nonfatal injuries treated in 66 U.S. emergency departments through stratified probability sampling, which allows for the generation of national prevalence estimates for nonfatal injuries. NEISS data on SDV indicates that in 2018, there were almost half a million medically serious incidents of nonfatal SDV, with an age-adjusted rate of 158.2 per 100,000 population. Like suicide, rates of nonfatal SDV vary by age group, with adolescents and young adults aged 15–24 experiencing the highest rates (465.0 per 100,000 among 15–19 year olds and 301.1 among 20–24 year olds). Whereas males contribute the greatest burden to suicide rates, females contribute the greatest burden to nonfatal self-harm rates (females: 174.9 per 100,000 vs. 129.6 per 100,000 rate for males). For instance, while the overall rate of nonfatal self-harm among 15–19 year olds is 465.0 per 100,000, the rate among females in the same age range is 685.7 per 100,000 (Table 175-1). Further, the prevalence of means used in nonfatal SDV differs from means used in suicides, primarily because the means used in nonfatal events are less lethal. For instance, according to NEISS, the most prevalent means for nonfatal SDV in 2018 was poisoning (including drug overdose), which contributed to over 240,000 emergency department visits for nonfatal SDV at an age-adjusted rate of 73.9 per 100,000. The second most common means of nonfatal SDV was injury by a sharp object, contributing to over 135,000 ED visits (41.3 per 100,000). The prevalence of firearm and suffocation-involved nonfatal SDV is too low to estimate because of instability due to the small sample size, likely because of the highly lethal nature of these mechanisms.[2] Table 175-1 demonstrates some key epidemiological differences between suicide and nonfatal SDV based on 2018 NVSS and NEISS data.[2,19]

Finally, similar to suicide, recent studies have demonstrated increases in nonfatal SDV over time. An analysis of data from the nationally representative National Epidemiologic Survey on Alcohol and Related Conditions indicated that the percentage of U.S. adults who made a recent suicide attempt significantly increased from 0.62% (221 adults out of 34,629) in 2004–05 to 0.79% (305 of 34,712) in 2012–13. Olfson, Blanco, Wall et al. (2017) found that while the percentage of all adults who attempted suicide from 2004–05 to 2012–13 increased, several groups in particular, including younger adults with lower educational attainment and adults with anxiety disorders, personality disorders, and depressive disorders, as well as those with a history of violence, were disproportionately impacted by the increases.[32] Another study examining NEISS data from 2000 through 2015 demonstrated that among youth, rates of medically serious nonfatal SDV remained relatively stable through 2008, but thereafter increased 5.7% per year, ultimately reaching 303.7 per 100,000 population in 2015. As the trends for males during this time

TABLE 175-2 SUICIDE PREVENTION STRATEGIES AND APPROACHES BASED ON THE BEST AVAILABLE EVIDENCE

Strategy	Approach
Strengthen economic supports	• Strengthen household financial security • Housing stabilization policies
Strengthen access and delivery of suicide care	• Coverage of mental health conditions in health insurance plans • Reduce provider shortages in underserved areas • Safer suicide care through systems change
Create protective environments	• Reduce access to lethal means among persons at risk of suicide • Organizational policies and culture • Community-based policies to reduce excessive alcohol use
Promote connectedness	• Peer norm programs • Community engagement activities
Teach coping and problem-solving skills	• Social-emotional learning programs • Parenting skill and family relationship programs
Identify and support people at risk	• Gatekeeper training • Crisis intervention • Treatment for people at risk of suicide • Treatment to prevent re-attempts
Lessen harms and prevent future risk	• Postvention • Safe reporting and messaging about suicide

period remained relatively stable, the overall increases were driven by increases in SDV among females, who experienced an overall increase of 8.4% per year from 2009 to 2015. Further driving the increasing rates among girls were, specifically, the rates among 10- to 14-year-old females, who saw an increase in SDV rates of 18.8% per year from 2009 to 2015. This study also identified an increase in the rate at which poisoning was used in nonfatal SDV, particularly after 2007.[33]

Research suggests that more than 50% of people who engage in suicidal behavior never seek medical treatment.[8] The National Survey on Drug Use and Health indicates that in 2019, over 1.4 million U.S. adults attempted suicide, only a portion of whom sought medical attention following their attempt. Further, 3.5 million adults made a suicide plan and 12.0 million seriously thought about suicide, and these numbers have risen annually.[34] Finally, 2019 Youth Risk Behavior Survey data indicate that 18.8% of 9th- to 12th-grade students in the United States. Seriously considered attempting suicide, 15.7% made a plan about how they would attempt suicide, 8.9% attempted suicide at least once, and 2.5% of made a medically serious suicide attempt.[35]

THE SOCIAL AND ECONOMIC TOLL OF SUICIDE

The social and economic impacts of suicide and nonfatal suicide attempts are profound, and the consequences are far-reaching. One researcher suggested that for every one suicide in the United States, six individuals are personally impacted,[36] but this has long been considered a conservative estimate. One study suggests the impact of suicide is much broader, estimating that approximately 7% of adults knew someone who died by suicide in the 12 months prior to the survey and that for each suicide, over 400 adults were exposed or reported knowing about the death.[37] Another study found that almost 50% of Americans knew at least one person in their lifetime who died by suicide.[38] Importantly, the social impact having known someone who died by or attempted suicide is extensive. For instance, survivors of suicide loss (i.e., individuals who have lost a loved one to suicide) may experience feelings of depression, anger, guilt, and resentment experienced by friends and family of suicide victims or attempt survivors.[39–42] Further, suicide attempts that do not result in death can be associated with considerable physical and financial costs. Nonfatal suicide attempts can result in minor to debilitating injuries sustained during the attempt and can be accompanied by costly medical bills, lost productivity, and other expenses. The economic toll associated with suicide and nonfatal suicide attempts is great. One study suggested that lifetime medical and work lost expenses alone associated with suicide resulted in costs of an estimated $50.8 billion in 2013.[43] A more complex calculation, which takes into account nonfatal suicide attempts and the likelihood that suicide is underreported, as well as healthcare expenditures per capita, gross domestic product per capita, and variation in per capita healthcare expenditures and income, suggested that the cost of nonfatal suicide attempts and deaths was approximately $93.5 billion in 2013.[44]

RISK FACTORS FOR SUICIDE

Suicide and suicidal behavior are complex problems influenced by a number of biological, psychological, and social risk factors at multiple levels of the social ecology (i.e., the individual, relationship, community, and societal levels).[45,46] Examples of risk factors at the individual level of the social ecology include mental health problems, substance use, history of suicide attempts, physical illness, pain, and socioeconomic status. At the relationship level, family problems (e.g., adverse childhood experiences), family history of suicide, relationship problems with peers (e.g., bullying), intimate partner problems, and social isolation have all been shown to be associated with suicide. Examples of risk factors at the community level include inadequate access to mental health treatment and social services. Finally, at the societal level, easy access to lethal means and stigma associated with mental health problems and help-seeking behaviors are factors that increase risk for suicide.[11]

Given that risk for suicide varies by age, it follows that the types of risk factors vary by age as well. For instance, the factors that increase adolescents' risk for suicide are not necessarily the same ones that older adults experience that put them at increased risk for suicide. During youth and adolescence, risk factors include family problems, particularly problems with parents, easy access to lethal means, exposure to the suicide or death of a friend or loved one, poor problem solving and coping skills, and the potential onset of depression and other mental health problems during the teenage years.[47] Further, some youth experience school-related problems, such as bullying and troubled peer relationships, which may be exacerbated by school-age and biological changes experienced during this time period (e.g., a move from elementary to middle or middle to high school and the onset of puberty).[48–51]

Risk factors for suicide among young adults overlap with those experienced by youth and adolescents to an extent. Mental health problems (particularly depression), access to lethal means, exposure to others' suicidal behavior, and troubled relationships are still very much risk factors. Additionally, a feeling of being discouraged by life and alcohol and substance use may become more prominent risk factors during this time period.[52,53]

In addition to the common risk factors experienced by other age groups, including mental illness, history of suicidal behavior, and intimate partner problems, middle adulthood may present unique life situations uncommon to younger age groups. For instance, challenges during this time period may include changes in marital and family relationships (e.g., intimate partner problems and divorce, children leaving the home), employment changes, caring for a dependent parent, and changes in one's own physical health. While more risk factor research has been conducted among younger age groups than middle-aged adults, some factors known to increase suicide risk among this age group include depression, lack of connectedness, legal problems, intimate partner problems and other relationship problems, and job and financial problems.[54,55]

Additionally, older adults, who contribute the highest rate of suicide in the United States, often experience a number of challenges during this phase of life, potentially including managing chronic health conditions, changes in social roles and networks, and overall physical functioning. These changes may also impact mental health of older adults. Thus, older adults may experience physical health problems, loss of loved ones and lack of social connectedness, and mental illness, particularly depression, as risk factors for suicide. Additionally, a greater intent to die and access to lethal means also put older adults at risk for suicide.[56] Stigma associated with mental health problems and seeking access to mental healthcare may also prevent middle-aged and older adults from effectively addressing factors that increase their risk for suicide.[57,58]

Although all of the factors described herein can increase the risk of suicide, it is important to note that the majority of individuals who are depressed, attempt suicide, or experience the other risk factors highlighted here, do *not* die by suicide.[59] Indeed, while suicide attempts are the strongest predictor of suicide, only between 5% and 10% of people who have attempted suicide will go on to die by suicide.

PROTECTIVE FACTORS

While there is much research on factors that put certain individuals and groups at risk for suicide, less research exists on factors that protect against suicide. Protective factors are those that serve to reduce suicide risk or serve as a buffer against risk factors.[11] Protective factors may be biopsychosocial, environmental, or sociocultural in nature. For example, biopsychosocial protective factors include effective coping and problem-solving skills and genetic history.[60] Environmental factors include policies, services, and systems that serve to reduce risk for suicide. For instance, increased availability of high quality and continuous physical and mental healthcare can serve as protective factors for suicide.[61,62] Additionally, research has suggested that environmental factors reducing access to lethal means through practices related to safe storage of firearms, development of barriers or nets in places where suicides by falls are common, and blister packaging of medications can reduce suicide.[63–65] Finally, social factors may include moral or cultural objections to suicide; strong and supportive relationships with partners, friends, and family; and connectedness to school, community, and other social institutions. In fact, connectedness was highlighted as the CDC's strategic direction for suicide prevention in 2009 and remains critical to its current strategy along with other key national strategies, including the National Strategy for Suicide Prevention.[66,67]

Prevention Strategies

In 2017, the Injury Center's Division of Violence Prevention released "Preventing Suicide: A Technical Package of Policy, Programs, and Practices." This resource describes a collection of strategies and approaches based on the best available evidence that have been shown to reduce and prevent suicide and suicidal behaviors. The package was developed to assist communities and states in focusing their suicide prevention efforts on those strategies that have the greatest potential for preventing suicide among their population(s) of interest. Each strategy highlighted in the technical package is accompanied by multiple approaches that can be used to advance the strategy through specific policy, programs, or practices. While strategies and approaches can be implemented in isolation, a comprehensive approach to suicide prevention whereby multiple strategies and approaches are implemented to achieve synergistic effects in reducing suicide at the community level may be best suited to prevent suicide at the population level.[67]

Table 175-2 lists the seven strategies and their corresponding approaches contained in the technical package beginning with those strategies that have the best ability to impact suicide at the population level and ending with strategies more likely to impact individual-level risk factors for suicide. These strategies are: (1) strengthen economic supports; (2) strengthen access to and delivery of suicide care; (3) create protective environments; (4) promote connectedness; (5) teach coping and problem-solving skills; (6) identify and support people at risk; and (7) lessen harm and prevent future risk.

Strengthen Economic Supports

The first strategy focuses on strengthening economic supports—a strategy likely to have broad impacts at the societal level. This strategy recognizes that suicides increase during economic downturns and that financial strain due to unemployment, housing concerns, and other unanticipated financial stress are associated with suicide.[15,68,69] Two approaches to strengthen economic supports and buffer risk of suicide include strengthening household financial security and housing stabilization policies. Research related to strengthening economic supports has demonstrated that policies such as increased unemployment benefits and increased state social spending have been associated with offset or decreased rates of suicide at the state level.[70,71] The second approach focuses on housing and aims to keep people in their homes and provide affordable housing options, especially during times of financial insecurity. Examples of such programs include the National Neighborhood Stabilization Program.[72]

Strengthen Access and Delivery of Suicide Care

The second strategy highlighted in the technical package focuses on strengthening access to and delivery of suicide/mental healthcare. While most people with mental disorders do not attempt or die by suicide, we know that mental health problems are a risk factor for suicide and, according to survey data, we know that a minority of people in the United States with mental health disorders receive mental health treatment. [59,73] Lack of access to such treatment and stigma is one of the factors related to this underutilization. Coverage of mental health conditions (i.e., mental health parity) is an approach that helps ensure that mental health services, such as copays, inpatient and outpatient services, prescription drugs, and hospitalizations, are covered by health insurance policies at the same level as physical health concerns. And indeed, evidence indicates that states had increased utilization of mental health services after implementation of state mental health parity laws.[74] Further, research has shown that mental health parity laws are associated with a reduction in suicide rates.[62,75]

It is also important to ensure that individuals across the country have access to care—particularly in rural areas that experience provider shortages and suffer from increased suicide rates. One approach that may help to ensure that individuals in rural areas have access to quality mental healthcare is through provision of telemental health services, which can be delivered remotely.[76]

Finally improving health systems through systems change ensures consistent, coordinated, and timely follow-up with patients at increased risk of suicide and focuses on effectiveness, safety, patient centeredness, efficiency, and equity. Such programs like Perfect Depression Care, the precursor to Zero Suicide, have been found to be associated with reductions in suicide.[61,77]

Create Protective Environments

Ensuring that people are protected in the environments in which they live, work, and play is one way to prevent suicide. Promoting safety in these areas can involve reducing access to lethal means among those at risk for suicide. For instance, storing firearms unloaded and in a locked place or secured with a safety device has been shown to be protective against suicide attempts among adolescents.[78] Safely securing and storing firearms and medication can also put time between one's suicidal thoughts and access to lethal means, which is important given that researchers have long demonstrated that many suicidal thoughts are fleeting and may be resolved with time.[65,79,80] Further, some countries where suicide by intentional ingestion of pesticides is a common means of suicide have implemented policies to reduce access to pesticides and thereby reduced suicide rates. For instance, in Sri Lanka, national policies related to the import and sales of toxic pesticides commonly used in suicides were implemented in the mid-1990; the suicide rate decreased dramatically thereafter (over 34%) from 47 per 100,000 in 1995 to 30.9 per 100,000 in 2005.[81,82] A number of countries (e.g., Jordan, Bangladesh, Korea, Taiwan) have implemented similar policies reducing access to lethal pesticides, and most saw decreases in suicide rates afterward.[83] Further, promoting positive organizational policies and culture in workplaces (e.g., by promoting help-seeking, providing counseling through employee assistance programs), and implementing community-based policies to reduce excessive alcohol use, a risk factor for suicide (e.g., creating zones to limit alcohol outlet density and implementing alcohol taxes) can also help to prevent suicide.[84–87]

Promote Connectedness

Connectedness has long been recognized as factor that can protect against suicide. Promoting connectedness is the primary strategic direction of suicide prevention at CDC, particularly because social connections can be promoted at each level of the social ecology. For instance, people can be connected to friends and family and the relationship level, to neighborhoods, churches, and schools at the community level, and through cultural groups at the societal level. Approaches that can advance connectedness include peer norms programs and community engagement activities, which can enhance connectedness at the community level.[67] Sources of Strength is a school-based program that has evidence of effectiveness in normalizing protective factors through peer norms, ensuring that people at risk of suicide seek help and reach out and communicate with adults in the community, and promoting connectedness between peers.[88] Additionally, evaluations of programs like a vacant lot greening initiative have shown that engaging community members in shared work to clean and beautify city lots can resulted in decreased stress levels, decreased depressive symptoms, and increased physical activity.[89,90]

Teach Coping and Problem-solving Skills

Life skills are crucial to protecting against suicide and suicidal behaviors. Life skills that can help protect against suicide include coping and problem-solving skills, conflict resolution, emotion regulation, and critical thinking. Some suicide prevention programs that focus on enhancing coping and problem-solving skills include social-emotional learning programs, such as the Good Behavior Game, and parenting skill and family relationship programs, such as Strengthening Families 10–14. These programs have been shown to reduce a number of negative outcomes, including depression, anxiety, conduct problems, and substance use.[91–93] Thus, programs like these are beneficial for those who may or may not be at increased risk for suicide, as they help to ensure that individuals have the skills necessary to successfully navigate stressful problems and cope with trauma and adversity using healthy strategies.

Identifying and Supporting People at Risk

Identifying and supporting people at increased risk of suicide is imperative to preventing suicide. People at risk of suicide can be identified and supported through a number of approaches, such as gatekeeper training and crisis intervention which involve training community members to identify and effectively respond to people at risk of suicide and to connect people in crisis with appropriate services.[94,95] It is important to note that identifying people at risk is only the first step in preventing suicide; these individuals also need to be referred to and be able to engage in evidence-based treatment strategies, such as Dialectical Behavioral Therapy or Collaborative Assessment and Management of Suicidality.[96–98] Further, engaging in therapies that are collaborative between the patient and provider and involve ongoing follow-up care may be most effective at preventing suicide.[96,97] Importantly, participating in many treatment strategies can be costly and often requires health insurance coverage. Thus, ensuring access to quality mental healthcare is a strategy that closely overlaps with supporting people at risk of suicide and is necessary in order to ensure that people at risk can obtain the help they need.

Lessen Harms and Prevent Future Risk

Finally, the risk of suicide is known to be increased among individuals mourning the loss of a friend or family member to suicide.[11] Mitigating the risk that people bereaved by suicide experience is critical to preventing future risk. This can be done at both an individual level and more broadly at the societal level. At the individual level, postvention services such as bereavement support groups and counseling for survivors of suicide (i.e., those who have survived the loss of a loved one to suicide) have been shown to reduce feelings of guilt, depression, and complicated grief associated with having a loved one die by suicide.[99] At the societal level, safe reporting and messaging about suicide is of utmost importance, as there is a contagion factor associated with the manner in which suicides are reported.[100] Reporting on the facts about suicide, if necessary, can be done in a safe way to mitigate the risk of contagion. For instance, avoiding reports that glamorize suicide and highlight details regarding means and precipitating factors, and providing information for a suicide prevention hotline as well as accompanying reports of suicide with reports of people who have overcome odds and mastered crisis situations can help to reduce rates in suicide at the societal level.[100]

IMPLEMENTATION CONSIDERATIONS

Suicide is a preventable public health problem; however, preventing it will require a comprehensive approach that engages multiple sectors and addresses risk and protection across the social ecology. Research has demonstrated that there is no single cause for suicide; thus, it is unlikely that any one prevention strategy alone can prevent suicide. While strategies that have the potential to make an impact at the population level (e.g., policies impacting unemployment benefits, insurance coverage, and access to lethal means) are imperative to suicide prevention, so too are the prevention approaches that target individuals at increased risk (e.g., individual therapy to prevent reattempts and postvention efforts). Thus, a comprehensive approach to suicide prevention involves recognizing that prevention, supported by multisectoral partnerships and informed by data and science, occurs across the ecological levels. Comprehensive suicide prevention also involves understanding the link between suicide and other health outcomes so that prevention efforts can be maximized. For instance, recognizing the associations and shared root causes between suicide and other forms of violence and negative health experiences (e.g., sexual and intimate partner violence and adverse childhood experiences) can help to ensure that programs with a widespread impact that prevent multiple forms of violence are implemented. Coordinating and integrating such violence prevention efforts can help to move the focus of suicide prevention "upstream"—that is, ensure that suicide prevention efforts are implemented early in life before exposure to risk occurs.[101] While comprehensive suicide prevention efforts should adopt evidence-based prevention strategies that have been shown to reduce suicide and/or other related outcomes, there is still a need for documentation of the manner in which such approaches are integrated, as well as outcome and cost evaluation of comprehensive suicide prevention approaches as a whole. Rigorous evaluation of comprehensive suicide prevention efforts can provide the field with valuable information related to risk reduction, the number of lives saved by these efforts, and the cost effectiveness of such efforts.

Finally, effective suicide prevention involves enhancing all community members' understanding that everyone has a role to play in suicide prevention—individuals, families, schools, faith-based organizations, and businesses can all help prevent suicide. Everyone can learn the signs and symptoms of suicidal behavior and safely store firearms and medications if someone in their home is thinking of suicide; schools can implement evidence-based programs that build coping and problem-solving skills, which can continue to serve youth into adulthood; clergy members, physicians, and other community leaders can serve as gatekeepers who can help to identify people at risk of suicide and refer them to appropriate services; and employers can implement programs and policies that provide support to employees in need and create a positive culture that encourages help-seeking behavior. Further, local, state, and federal governments can work to strengthen policies that may impact suicide at the broader societal level. The public health sector can serve to guide data collection efforts to continually monitor the problem of suicide, help identify effective prevention strategies through research and evaluation, and disseminate information about what works to key stakeholders. Other sectors that play a critical role in suicide prevention efforts include social and mental health services, justice, housing, and community organizations that serve youth, and the media to name a few.[67] In order to ensure that evidence-based prevention strategies are adopted and effectively implemented, the involvement of multiple sectors is essential.

CONCLUSION

Suicide and suicidal behavior takes an enormous toll on our society. These tragedies are societal issues that warrant a public health response and have implications for public health practice. Although suicide rates have been increasing for more than a decade in the United States, it is important to note that suicide is preventable. Suicide is more than a mental health concern so framing suicide as a public health problem is one of the first steps in reducing and preventing suicide. Taking a public health approach to suicide prevention will require that ongoing surveillance be conducted to track and monitor the problem over time and to provide a continuous feedback loop that can inform prevention and intervention efforts. Also from a public health perspective, developing and evaluating prevention strategies that target populations, as opposed to individuals, is needed. Most importantly, recognizing that suicide is a public health problem calls for acknowledging the fact that everyone has a role to play in suicide prevention—individuals, schools, businesses, the private sector, and government. These individuals and groups can work together to implement comprehensive prevention strategies that impact all layers of the social ecology in an effort to have the greatest potential to impact suicide rates at the population level.

References

1. Naghavi M. Global, regional, and national burden of suicide mortality 1990 to 2016: Systematic analysis for the Global Burden of Disease Study 2016. *BMJ*. 2019;364:l94.
2. CDC. Web-based Injury Statistics Query and Reporting System (WISQARS) [online]. 2019. www.cdc.gov/injury/wisqars/index.html.
3. Case A, Deaton A. Mortality and morbidity in the 21st century. *Brookings Pap Econ Act*. 2017;2017:397–476.
4. Curtin S, Warnger M, Hedegaard H. Increase in suicide in the United States, 1999–2014. *NCHS Data Brief*. 2016;(241):1–8.
5. Ivey-Stephenson AZ. Suicide trends among and within urbanization levels by sex, race/ethnicity, age group, and mechanism of death—United States, 2001–2015. *MMWR Surveill Summ*. 2017;66(18):1–16.
6. Woolf SH, Aron L. Failing health of the United States. *BMJ*. 2018;360:k496.
7. Murphy SL, Xu JQ, Kochanek KD, Arias E. Mortality in the United States, 2017. *NCHS Data Brief*. 2018;(328):1–8.
8. Ahrnsbrak R, Bose J, Hedden S, Lipari R, Park-Lee E. *Key Substance Use and Mental Health Indicators in the United States: Results from the 2016 National Survey on Drug Use and Health*. Rockville, MD: Center for Behavioral Health Statistics and Quality, Substance Abuse and Mental Health Services Administration; 2017.
9. David-Ferdon C. CDC grand rounds: Preventing suicide through a comprehensive public health approach. *MMWR Morb Mortal Wkly Rep*. 2016;65(34);894–7.

10. Stone D, Simon T, Fowler K, et al. Vital signs: Trends in state suicide rates—United States, 1999–2016 and circumstances contributing to suicide—27 states, 2015. *MMWR Morb Mortal Wkly Rep*. 2018;67(22):617.
11. U.S. Department of Health and Human Services (HHS) Office of the Surgeon General, National Action Alliance for Suicide Prevention. *2012 National Strategy for Suicide Prevention: Goals and Objectives for Action*. Washington, DC: HHS; 2012.
12. World Health Organization. *Suicide Prevention: A Global Imperative*. Geneva, Switzerland: World Health Organization; 2014, p. 92.
13. Kann L, McManus T, Harris WA, et al. Youth Risk Behavior Surveillance—United States, 2015. *MMWR Surveill Summ*. 2016;65(SS-6):1–174.
14. Crosby A, Ortega L, Melanson C. *Self-directed Violence Surveillance: Uniform Definitions and Recommended Data Elements*. Atlanta, GA: Centers for Disease Control and Prevention; National Center for Injury Prevention and Control; 2011.
15. Luo F, Florence CS, Quispe-Agnoli M, Ouyang L, Crosby AE. Impact of business cycles on US suicide rates, 1928–2007. *Am J Public Health*. 2011;101(6):1139–46.
16. Reeves A, Stuckler D, McKee M, Gunnell D, Chang S-S, Basu S. Increase in state suicide rates in the USA during economic recession. *Lancet*. 2012;380(9856):1813–4.
17. Rockett IRH, Regier MD, Kapusta ND, et al. Leading causes of unintentional and intentional injury mortality: United States, 2000–2009. *Am J Public Health*. 2012;102(11):e84–92.
18. Sullivan E, Annest JL, Luo F, Simon T, Dahlberg L. Suicide among adults aged 35–64 years—United States, 1999–2010. *Morb Mortal Wkly Rep*. 2013;62(17);321–5.
19. Centers for Disease Prevention and Control. *Underlying Cause of Death 1999–2016 on CDC WONDER Online Database*, released December, 2018. Atlanta, GA: National Center for Health Statistics; 2019.
20. Curtin SC, Hedegaard H. Suicide rates for females and males by race and ethnicity: United States, 1999 and 2017. *NCHS Health E-Stat*. 2019.
21. Phillips JA. Factors associated with temporal and spatial patterns in suicide rates across US states, 1976–2000. *Demography*. 2013;50(2):591–614.
22. Kegler S, Stone D, Holland K. Trends in suicide by level of urbanization—United States, 1999–2015. *Morb Mortal Wkly Rep*. 2017;66(10):270.
23. Hertz T, Kusmin L, Marré A, Parker T. Rural employment in recession and recovery. *Amber Waves*. 2014.
24. Peterson C, Sussell A, Li J, Schumacher P, Yeoman K, Stone D. Suicide rates by industry and occupation—National Violent Death Reporting System, 32 States, 2016. *MMWR Morb Mortal Wkly Rep*. 2020;69(3):57–62.
25. U.S. Department of Veterans Affairs. 2019 National Veteran Suicide Prevention Annual Report. Office of Mental Health and Suicide Prevention, 2019.
26. Bertolote JM, Fleischmann A, Butchart A, Besbelli N. Suicide, suicide attempts and pesticides: A major hidden public health problem. *Bull World Health Organ*. 2006;84(4):260.
27. Chen Y-Y, Bennewith O, Hawton K, et al. Suicide by burning barbecue charcoal in England. *J Public Health*. 2012;35(2):223–7.
28. Gunnell D, Eddleston M. Suicide by intentional ingestion of pesticides: A continuing tragedy in developing countries. *Int J Epidemiol*. 2003;32(6):902–9.
29. Gunnell D, Eddleston M, Phillips MR, Konradsen F. The global distribution of fatal pesticide self-poisoning: Systematic review. *BMC Public Health*. 2007;7(1):357.
30. Brennan Braden J, Edlund M, Sullivan M. Suicide deaths with opioid poisoning in the United States: 1999–2014. *Am J Public Health*. 2017;107(3):421–6.
31. Chen LH, Hedegaard H, Warner M. Drug-poisoning deaths involving opioid analgesics: United States, 1999–2011. *NCHS Data Brief*. 2014(166):1–8.
32. Olfson M, Blanco C, Wall M, et al. National trends in suicide attempts among adults in the United States. *JAMA Psychiatry*. 2017;74(11):1095–103.
33. Mercado MC, Holland K, Leemis RW, Stone DM, Wang J. Trends in emergency department visits for nonfatal self-inflicted injuries among youth aged 10 to 24 years in the United States, 2001–2015. *JAMA*. 2017;318(19):1931–3.
34. Substance Abuse and Mental Health Services Administration. *Key Substance Use and Mental Health Indicators in the United States: Results from the 2019 National Survey on Drug Use and Health*. Rockville, MD: Center for Behavioral Health Statistics and Quality, Substance Abuse and Mental Health Services Administration; 2020.
35. Ivey-Stephenson A, Demissie Z, Crosby A, et al. Suicidal ideation and behaviors among high school students—Youth risk behavior survey, United States, 2019. *MMWR Morb Mortal Wkly Rep*. 2020;69(1):47.
36. Shneidman ES, American Association of Suicidology. *On the Nature of Suicide*. San Francisco: Jossey-Bass; 1969, p. 146.
37. Crosby AE, Sacks JJ. Exposure to suicide: Incidence and association with suicidal ideation and behavior: United States, 1994. *Suicide Life Threat Behav*. 2002;32(3):321–8.
38. Cerel J, Maple M, van de Venne J, Moore M, Flaherty C, Brown M. Exposure to suicide in the community: Prevalence and correlates in one US state. *Public Health Rep*. 2016;131(1):100–7.
39. Cerel J, McIntosh JL, Neimeyer RA, Maple M, Marshall D. The continuum of "survivorship": Definitional issues in the aftermath of suicide. *Suicide Life Threat Behav*. 2014;44(6):591–600.
40. Chapman AL, Dixon-Gordon KL. Emotional antecedents and consequences of deliberate self-harm and suicide attempts. *Suicide Life Threat Behav*. 2007;37(5):543–52.
41. Mitchell AM, Kim Y, Prigerson HG, Mortimer-Stephens M. Complicated grief in survivors of suicide. *Crisis*. 2004;25(1):12–8.
42. Sudak H, Maxim K, Carpenter M. Suicide and stigma: A review of the literature and personal reflections. *Acad Psychiatry*. 2008;32(2):136–42.
43. Florence C, Simon T, Haegerich T, Luo F, Zhou C. Estimated lifetime medical and work-loss costs of fatal injuries—United States, 2013. *MMWR Morb Mortal Wkly Rep*. 2015;64(38):1074–7.
44. Shepard DS, Gurewich D, Lwin AK, Reed GA, Silverman MM. Suicide and suicidal attempts in the United States: costs and policy implications. *Suicide Life Threat Behav*. 2016;46(3):352–62.
45. Bunney W, Kleinman A, Pellmar T, Goldsmith S. *Reducing Suicide: A National Imperative*. Washington, DC: National Academies Press; 2002.
46. Dahlberg LL, Krug EG. Violence—A global public health problem. In: Krug E, Dahlberg LL, Mercy JA, Zwi AB, Lozano R, eds. *World Report on Violence and Health*. Geneva, Switzerland: World Health Organization; 2002, pp. 1–56.
47. Gould MS, Greenberg TED, Velting DM, Shaffer D. Youth suicide risk and preventive interventions: A review of the past 10 years. *J Am Acad Child Adolesc Psychiatry*. 2003;42(4):386–405.
48. Bolger N, Downey G, Walker E, Steininger P. The onset of suicidal ideation in childhood and adolescence. *J Youth Adolesc*. 1989;18(2):175–90.
49. Robinson NS, Garber J, Hilsman R. Cognitions and stress: Direct and moderating effects on depressive versus externalizing symptoms during the junior high school transition. *J Abnorm Psychol*. 1995;104(3):453.
50. Windle M, Spear LP, Fuligni AJ, et al. Transitions into underage and problem drinking: Developmental processes and mechanisms between 10 and 15 years of age. *Pediatrics*. 2008;121(Suppl 4):S273–89.
51. Holland KM, Vivolo-Kantor AM, Logan JE, Leemis RW. Antecedents of suicide among youth aged 11–15: A multistate mixed methods analysis. *J Youth Adolesc*. 2017;46(7):1598–610.
52. Gutierrez P, Rodriguez P, Garcia P. Suicide risk factors for young adults: Testing a model across ethnicities. *Death Stud*. 2001;25(4):319–40.
53. Silenzio V, Pena J, Duberstein P, Cerel J, Knox K. Sexual orientation and risk factors for suicidal ideation and suicide attempts among adolescents and young adults. *Am J Public Health*. 2007;97(11):2017–9.
54. Lachman ME. Development in midlife. *Annu Rev Psychol*. 2004;55:305–31.
55. Schiff L, Holland K, Stone D, et al. Acute and chronic risk preceding suicidal crises among middle-aged men without known mental health and/or substance abuse problems. *Crisis*. 2015;36(5):304–15.
56. Conwell Y, Duberstein P, Caine E. Risk factors for suicide in later life. *Biol Psychiatry*. 2002;52(3):193–204.
57. Corrigan P. How stigma interferes with mental health care. *Am Psychol*. 2004;59(7):614.
58. Sareen J, Jagdeo A, Cox BJ, et al. Perceived barriers to mental health service utilization in the United States, Ontario, and the Netherlands. *Psychiatr Serv*. 2007;58(3):357–64.
59. Owens D, Horrocks J, House A. Fatal and non-fatal repetition of self-harm. Systematic review. *Br J Psychiatry*. 2002;181:193–9.
60. Becker-Weidman EG, Jacobs RH, Reinecke MA, Silva SG, March JS. Social problem-solving among adolescents treated for depression. *Behav Res Ther*. 2010;48(1):11–8.
61. Coffey CE, Coffey MJ, Ahmedani BK. An update on perfect depression care. *Psychiatr Serv*. 2013;64(4):396.
62. Lang M. The impact of mental health insurance laws on state suicide rates. *Health Econ*. 2013;22(1):73–88.

63. Cox GR, Owens C, Robinson J, et al. Interventions to reduce suicides at suicide hotspots: A systematic review. *BMC Public Health*. 2013;13(1):214.
64. Hawton K. United Kingdom legislation on pack sizes of analgesics: Background, rationale, and effects on suicide and deliberate self-harm. *Suicide Life Threat Behav*. 2002;32(3):223–9.
65. Runyan CW, Becker A, Brandspigel S, Barber C, Trudeau A, Novins D. Lethal means counseling for parents of youth seeking emergency care for suicidality. *West J Emerg Med*. 2016;17(1):8.
66. Centers for Disease Control and Prevention. Strategic direction for suicide prevention: Promoting individual, family, and community connectedeness to prevent suicidal behavior. 2009. www.cdc.gov/violenceprevention/pdf/Suicide_Strategic_Direction_Full_Version-a.pdf.
67. Stone DM, Holland KM, Bartholow BN, Crosby AE, Jack SPD, Wilkins N. *Preventing Suicide: A Technical Package of Policies, Programs, and Practices*. Atlanta, GA: National Center for Injury Prevention and Control, Centers for Disease Control and Prevention; 2017.
68. Fowler KA, Gladden RM, Vagi KJ, Barnes J, Frazier L. Increase in suicides associated with home eviction and foreclosure during the US housing crisis: Findings from 16 national violent death reporting system states, 2005–2010. *Am J Public Health*. 2015;105(2):311–6.
69. Classen TJ, Dunn RA. The effect of job loss and unemployment duration on suicide risk in the United States: A new look using mass-layoffs and unemployment duration. *Health Econ*. 2012;21(3):338–50.
70. Cylus J, Glymour MM, Avendano M. Do generous unemployment benefit programs reduce suicide rates? A state fixed-effect analysis covering 1968–2008. *Am J Epidemiol*. 2014;180(1):45–52.
71. Flavin P, Radcliff B. Public policies and suicide rates in the American states. *Soc Indic Res*. 2009;90(2):195–209.
72. Development USDoHaU. Neighborhood Stabilization Program. 2017.
73. Wang PS, Demler O, Kessler RC. Adequacy of treatment for serious mental illness in the United States. *Am J Public Health*. 2002;92(1):92–8.
74. Cunningham PJ. Beyond parity: Primary care physicians' perspectives on access to mental health care. *Health Aff (Millwood)*. 2009;28(3):w490–501.
75. Harris KM, Carpenter C, Bao Y. The effects of state parity laws on the use of mental health care. *Med Care*. 2006;44(6):499–505.
76. Hailey D, Roine R, Ohinmaa A. The effectiveness of telemental health applications: A review. *Can J Psychiatry*. 2008;53(11):769–78.
77. Coffey MJ, Coffey CE, Ahmedani BK. Suicide in a health maintenance organization population. *JAMA Psychiatry*. 2015;72(3):294–6.
78. Grossman DC, Mueller BA, Riedy C, et al. Gun storage practices and risk of youth suicide and unintentional firearm injuries. *JAMA*. 2005;293(6):707–14.
79. Deisenhammer EA, Ing CM, Strauss R, Kemmler G, Hinterhuber H, Weiss EM. The duration of the suicidal process: How much time is left for intervention between consideration and accomplishment of a suicide attempt? *J Clin Psychiatry*. 2009;70(1):19–24.
80. Simon OR, Swann AC, Powell KE, Potter LB, Kresnow MJ, O'Carroll PW. Characteristics of impulsive suicide attempts and attempters. *Suicide Life Threat Behav*. 2001;32(1 Suppl):49–59.
81. Gunnell D, Fernando R, Hewagama M, Priyangika W, Konradsen F, Eddleston M. The impact of pesticide regulations on suicide in Sri Lanka. *Int J Epidemiol*. 2007;36(6):1235–42.
82. World Health Organization. *Suicide Mortality Rate: Data Tables*. Geneva, Switzerland: World Health Organization Statistics; 2017.
83. Gunnell D, Knipe D, Chang S-S, et al. Prevention of suicide with regulations aimed at restricting access to highly hazardous pesticides: A systematic review of the international evidence. *Lancet Glob Health*. 2017;5(10):e1026–37.
84. Gruenewald PJ, Remer L. Changes in outlet densities affect violence rates. *Alcohol Clin Exp Res*. 2006;30(7):1184–93.
85. Knox KL, Litts DA, Talcott GW, Feig JC, Caine ED. Risk of suicide and related adverse outcomes after exposure to a suicide prevention programme in the US Air Force: Cohort study. *BMJ*. 2003;327(7428):1376.
86. Lipton R, Gruenewald P. The spatial dynamics of violence and alcohol outlets. *J Stud Alcohol*. 2002;63(2):187–95.
87. Rush BR, Gliksman L, Brook R. Alcohol availability, alcohol consumption and alcohol-related damage. I. The distribution of consumption model. *J Stud Alcohol*. 1986;47(1):1–10.
88. Wyman PA, Brown CH, LoMurray M, et al. An outcome evaluation of the sources of strength suicide prevention program delivered by adolescent peer leaders in high schools. *Am J Public Health*. 2010;100(9):1653–61.
89. Branas CC, Cheney RA, MacDonald JM, Tam VW, Jackson TD, Ten Have TR. A difference-in-differences analysis of health, safety, and greening vacant urban space. *Am J Epidemiol*. 2011;174(11):1296–306.
90. Branas CC, Kondo MC, Murphy SM, South EC, Polsky D, MacDonald JM. Urban blight remediation as a cost-beneficial solution to firearm violence. *Am J Public Health*. 2016;106(12):2158–64.
91. Kellam SG, Brown CH, Poduska JM, et al. Effects of a universal classroom behavior management program in first and second grades on young adult behavioral, psychiatric, and social outcomes. *Drug Alcohol Depend*. 2008;95(Suppl 1):S5–28.
92. Petras H, Kellam SG, Brown CH, Muthen BO, Ialongo NS, Poduska JM. Developmental epidemiological courses leading to antisocial personality disorder and violent and criminal behavior: Effects by young adulthood of a universal preventive intervention in first- and second-grade classrooms. *Drug Alcohol Depend*. 2008;95(Suppl 1):S45–59.
93. Spoth RL, Guyll M, Day SX. Universal family-focused interventions in alcohol-use disorder prevention: Cost-effectiveness and cost-benefit analyses of two interventions. *J Stud Alcohol*. 2002;63(2):219–28.
94. Gould MS, Cross W, Pisani AR, Munfakh JL, Kleinman M. Impact of applied suicide intervention skills training on the National Suicide Prevention Lifeline. *Suicide Life Threat Behav*. 2013;43(6):676–91.
95. Gould MS, Kalafat J, Harrismunfakh JL, Kleinman M. An evaluation of crisis hotline outcomes. Part 2: Suicidal callers. *Suicide Life Threat Behav*. 2007;37(3):338–52.
96. Comtois KA, Jobes DA, O'Connor SS, et al. Collaborative assessment and management of suicidality (CAMS): Feasibility trial for next-day appointment services. *Depress Anxiety*. 2011;28(11):963–72.
97. Jobes DA. The collaborative assessment and management of suicidality (CAMS): An evolving evidence-based clinical approach to suicidal risk. *Suicide Life Threat Behav*. 2012;42(6):640–53.
98. Linehan MM, Comtois KA, Murray AM, et al. Two-year randomized controlled trial and follow-up of dialectical behavior therapy vs therapy by experts for suicidal behaviors and borderline personality disorder. *Arch Gen Psychiatry*. 2006;63(7):757–66.
99. Szumilas M, Kutcher S. Post-suicide intervention programs: A systematic review. *Can J Public Health*. 2011;102(1):18–29.
100. Bohanna I, Wang X. Media guidelines for the responsible reporting of suicide: A review of effectiveness. *Crisis*. 2012;33(4):190–8.
101. Wilkins N, Tsao B, Hertz M, Davis R, Klevens J. *Connecting the Dots: An Overview of the Links Among Multiple Forms of Violence*. Atlanta, GA: National Center for Injury Prevention and Control, Centers for Disease Control and Prevention. Oakland, CA: Prevention Institute; 2014.

CHAPTER

176

Child Abuse and Neglect

Katie A. Ports • Beverly L. Fortson

BACKGROUND

Child abuse and neglect (CAN) is a serious public health problem that affects millions of children around the world.[1,2] While some populations are more vulnerable to CAN, exposure affects everyone—all races, genders, socioeconomic statuses, and geographic boundaries. Exposure to CAN has far-reaching impacts beyond a single time-period, person, or generation. CAN is often associated with short-term health consequences, such as broken bones, bruises, and mental health issues [e.g., posttraumatic stress disorder (PTSD), anxiety and depressive symptoms]. However, the science of brain development, childhood adversity, and toxic stress demonstrate strong associations between CAN and longer-term health consequences, including changes in the physiological development of the nervous, endocrine, and immune systems, physical and mental health problems, engagement in risky health behaviors, limited life opportunities, and premature death.[3–9] Addressing and treating exposure to CAN is important, but the goal in preventing CAN is clear—to stop this violence from happening in the first place. In this chapter, we define and describe CAN from a public health perspective, including both the magnitude and the health and social burden of CAN, as well as risk and protective factors for exposure. We will also provide evidence-based strategies for the prevention of CAN and prevention implementation considerations.

NATURE AND BURDEN OF THE PROBLEM

Definitions

Consistent definitions for CAN are important for two main reasons. First, monitoring the problem of CAN relies on a stable definition to track trends over time. Second, a clear definition helps us understand the scope of the problem and allows for comparisons of the issue across international, national, state, and local jurisdictions. CAN is defined as any act or series of acts of commission or omission by a parent, caregiver, or another person in a custodial role that result in harm, potential for harm, or threat of harm to a person under 18 years of age.[10] CAN, also referred to as child maltreatment, includes four common types: physical abuse, sexual abuse, emotional abuse, and neglect. Brief definitions for each type of CAN developed by the Centers for Disease Control and Prevention (CDC) are presented in Table 176-1.[10] These definitions align with the World Health Organization's (WHO) definitions and support Article 19 of the United Nations Convention on the Rights of a Child, which serve to protect children from violence, exploitation, and abuse while in the care of parents and other caregivers.[11–13]

A caregiver is defined as a person who at the time of the maltreatment is in a permanent (primary caregiver) or temporary (substitute caregiver) role.[10] In a custodial role, the person is responsible for care and control of the child and for the child's overall health and welfare.

TABLE 176-1 BRIEF DEFINITIONS OF CHILD ABUSE AND NEGLECT DEVELOPED BY THE CENTERS FOR DISEASE CONTROL AND PREVENTION

Type of Child Abuse/Neglect	Definition
Acts of Commission (Child abuse)	
Physical	Intentional use of force against a child that results in, or has the potential to result in, physical injury.
Psychological	Intentional caregiver behavior that conveys to a child that he/she is worthless, flawed, unloved, unwanted, endangered, or valued only in meeting another's need.
Sexual	Any completed or attempted sexual act, sexual contact with, or exploitation (i.e., noncontact sexual interaction) of a child by a caregiver.
Acts of Omission (Child neglect)	
Failure to provide	Failure by a caregiver to meet a child's basic physical, emotional, medical/dental, or educational needs, or combination thereof.
Failure to supervise	Failure by caregiver to ensure a child's safety within and outside the home given the child's emotional and developmental needs.

A primary caregiver lives with the child at least part of the time and can include, but is not limited to, a relative or biological, adoptive, step-, or foster parent(s); a legal guardian(s); or their intimate partner.[10] A substitute caregiver may or may not live with the child and can include coaches, clergy, teachers, relatives, babysitters, residential facility staff, or others who are not the child's primary caregiver(s).

Additional events that negatively impact children's ability to thrive, and that are related to CAN, include child sexual exploitation,[14] child trafficking,[15] other adverse childhood experiences (ACEs),[5,16,17] child marriage,[18] corporal punishment,[12,19] and child poverty.[20] These areas are highlighted in Table 176-2. Additional surveillance and research efforts are needed to better understand the magnitude and epidemiology of these surreptitious problems that also affect the health and well-being of children around the world.

Magnitude of the Problem

Nonfatal abuse and neglect. One billion children, which is roughly half of all children around the world, have experienced violence in the past year.[1] Global, lifetime estimates for exposure to specific types of abuse and neglect suggest that approximately 36% of children are emotionally abused,[21] 23% are physically abused,[22] 18% of girls and

TABLE 176-2 ADDITIONAL TYPES OF MALTREATMENT IN CHILDHOOD

Other Maltreatment Types	
Child sexual exploitation	Sexual exploitation of a child is the sexual abuse of children and youth through the exchange of sex or sexual acts for drugs, food, shelter, protection, other basics of life, and/or money. Sexual exploitation also includes involving children and youth in pornographic performances or materials and the solicitation of children for sexual purposes.[14]
Child trafficking	The United Nations defines human trafficking as the recruitment, transportation, transfer, harboring, or receipt of persons by improper means (e.g., by force, abduction, fraud, or coercion) for an improper purpose. Child trafficking involves any person under 18 years of age. Trafficking can include forced labor, commercial sexual exploitation, illegal adoption, and recruitment and use of children in armed conflict.[15]
Adverse Childhood Experiences (ACEs)	Adverse Childhood Experiences, or ACEs, are indicators of traumatic experiences that occur during the first 18 years of life, and, in the absence of protective factors, can affect optimal development. ACEs generally include child abuse and neglect and household challenges (i.e., witnessing intimate partner violence, parental separation or divorce, mental illness in the household, substance abuse in the household, or parental incarceration).[5] Contemporary ACE studies have included additional items, such as loss of a loved one, bullying, peer and community violence, discrimination and poverty.[16,17] ACEs have been linked to over 40 different adverse adult health outcomes to date, including opioid misuse, sexual violence, suicide, high school noncompletion, cancer, and premature mortality.
Child marriage	Child marriage is a formal marriage or informal union before age 18 years, and can occur among boys and girls, although girls are disproportionately affected. A social norm in communities and countries where it is prevalent, child marriage is widespread and can lead to a lifetime of disadvantage and deprivation.[18] The marriage of girls under age 18 is rooted in gender discrimination, and encourages premature and continuous child bearing among girls and gives preference to boys' education and life opportunities.[18] Child marriage is also a strategy for economic survival as families marry off their daughters at an early age to reduce their economic burden.[18]
Corporal punishment	Corporal punishment includes actions taken by a parent or caregiver that are intended to cause a child physical pain or emotional distress as a way to correct and/or act as a deterrent for child misbehavior.[12,19] Corporal punishment of children, including hitting, punching, kicking, or beating, is socially and legally accepted in many countries. It can be a significant problem in schools and other institutions, including penal systems for young offenders.[12,19] Decades of research on corporal punishment highlight its negative effects for children.[12,19] In the short term, it kills thousands of children each year and injures and handicaps many more. In the longer term, it may lead to mental health problems, violent behavior, and other problems in childhood and later life.[19,64]
Child poverty	Many children around the world live in poverty whereby they lack the means necessary to meet basic personal needs, including food, clothing, and shelter. Poverty is an important determinant of health and well-being. Children who grow up in poverty are at increased risk of remaining in poverty for the rest of their lives.[20] Children living in poverty are at increased risk of experiencing early adversity, including child abuse and neglect.[20]

8% of boys are sexually abused,[23] and 16% of children are neglected.[24] The prevalence of different forms of CAN, however, are not consistent across societies[1,21–25] and vary widely by the method of data collection. For example, girls in armed conflict and refugee settings are particularly vulnerable to sexual violence, exploitation and abuse by combatants, security forces, members of their communities, and aid workers.[26]

National surveys of children's exposure to violence, conducted around the world, reveal that rates vary by country, and many countries have much higher rates of childhood physical, sexual and emotional abuse than the global rates. For instance, findings from the Violence against Children Surveys conducted in Kenya, the Republic of Tanzania, Swaziland, and Zimbabwe indicate that about one in three girls experienced sexual abuse during their childhood.[27–30] For boys, the reported prevalence of childhood sexual abuse ranged from 9% in Zimbabwe to 18% in Kenya.[27–30] Between 53% and 76% of children in Kenya, the Republic of Tanzania, and Zimbabwe reported exposure to physical abuse, with somewhat higher rates of childhood physical abuse experienced by boys than girls.[28–30] And in Swaziland, the reported prevalence of childhood physical abuse of girls was much lower at 22%.[27] The reported prevalence of emotional abuse during childhood for the four countries was between 24% and 38%, with similar rates indicated by both boys and girls.[27–30]

In the United States (US), approximately 676,000 children (9.1 per 1000) were victims of CAN in 2016 according to official reports by Child Protective Services (CPS).[31] However, official CPS reports underestimate the true occurrence of these exposures, because only a fraction of children experiencing CAN come to the attention of child and family protection agencies or other social services. Indeed, estimates from self-reported data indicate that more than one in seven children in the US have experienced one or more forms of CAN in the past year, and one in four experienced CAN in their lifetime.[32] Furthermore, many children are at risk for experiencing multiple types of violence, or polyvictimization. Data from the Kaiser Permanente-CDC ACE Study found that 87% of respondents who reported experiencing one type of early adversity reported experiencing at least one additional type of adverse event.[33] In addition, researchers using data from a national, longitudinal probability sample in the US demonstrated that approximately 22% of children in the sample experienced four or more different kinds of victimizations in the past year.[34,35]

CAN is more prevalent in some groups, because of the structural and social conditions that influence how children and families interact with their environments. For example, US data from official reports show higher rates of victimization among girls compared to boys (9.5 vs. 8.7 per 1000, respectively) with the highest rate of victimization among children under 1 year (24.8 per 1000 children).[31] However, exposure rates are more complex than official reports might suggest; rates of CAN vary by the type of exposure as well as sociodemographic characteristics. For example, physical abuse rates tends to peak in early childhood and sexual abuse rates peak in adolescence. In general, however, younger children are more likely to experience fatal abuse and neglect[31] and 14- to 17-year-olds are more likely to experience nonfatal abuse and neglect.[32] Official reports also demonstrate higher victimization rates among some racial and ethnic categories; however, these differences are generally attributed to various community and societal factors, including differences in reporting and investigation among racial/ethnic groups as well as poverty.[31] Indeed, children living in families with a low socioeconomic status (SES) in the United States have rates of CAN that are five times higher than those of children living in families with a higher SES.[36] Furthermore, Maker and colleagues note that studies on physical abuse among Latino, Asian, and Middle Eastern families commonly use low SES, shelter, or clinical samples, highlighting the narrow focus on certain populations, which greatly restricts the generalizability of the results.[37] While it is generally accepted that poverty, unemployment, single-parent households, and other factors put children and families at increased risk for abuse and neglect, more rigorous research that can fully account for potential confounding variables are needed to fully examine and understand the associations among race, ethnicity, class, and CAN.[36] These and other risk factors of CAN will be discussed further in the next section.

Fatal abuse and neglect. The most tragic consequence of CAN is child fatalities. In 2016, approximately 1750 children in the United States died from abuse and neglect across the country—a rate of 2.36 deaths per 100,000 children.[31] Globally, in 2015, there were approximately 70,000 deaths from intentional injuries among children under 15 years of age.[38] These numbers underestimate the true extent of the problem, as a significant proportion of deaths due to CAN may be incorrectly attributed to falls, burns, drowning, or other unintentional injury causes. Furthermore, child deaths are not routinely investigated, and postmortem examinations often are not carried out. As such, it is difficult to establish the precise number of fatalities resulting from CAN.[39–41]

Data considerations. Although recent national surveys in several low- and middle-income countries have highlighted the prevalence of CAN on a more global level, data from many countries is still lacking and estimates often vary widely based on the country and the method of data collection. This results in uncertainty about the precise magnitude of the issue. Data regarding the prevalence of CAN come from a variety of sources, including official reports, case reports, population-based surveys, and national surveillance systems. Each of these sources differ in regards to their strengths, limitations, and ultimately, their usefulness in describing the magnitude of the problem. Of the available data, problems with data quality, cultural variations in parenting and related social norms, and varied definitions as to what constitutes CAN among the multiple sectors, limit the utility and reliability of the data.

Typically, CAN victimization rates are based on reports from a single source, which can yield varied estimates depending on the data source utilized. For example, exposure to CAN is not always reported to officials, and even when it is, cases may not be investigated. As such, studies relying on data from official sources underestimate the true magnitude of the problem. In addition, data from official sources can distort descriptions of the individuals at greatest risk and characteristics of the problem. Given this, data from official sources are often discordant from self-report data.[42] Self-report surveys can provide a better estimate of the true magnitude of CAN, but they too can be problematic. Sampling biases and problems with memory contribute to issues with the reliability of data. Irrespective of data source, definitions, and measures, the true magnitude of CAN is likely underestimated, and thus, reliance on multiple indicators and sources in the assessment and surveillance of CAN may lead to better estimates.

Health Burden

The millions of children who survive exposure to violence can go on to experience both immediate and long-term health consequences. The consequences of CAN are profound and may endure long after the maltreatment occurs. Adverse consequences can appear in childhood, adolescence, adulthood, and even in future generations.[9] In the absence of protective factors (e.g., supportive adult relationships, social connectedness, stable housing),[43] CAN may impact multiple aspects of an individual's development (e.g., physical, psychological, social, and behavioral; see Fig. 176-1).[44]

Physical health consequences. CAN is often associated with immediate physical injuries and health outcomes, which may include bruises, burns, broken bones, and sexually transmitted infections. Infants and young children (aged 0–4 years) are particularly

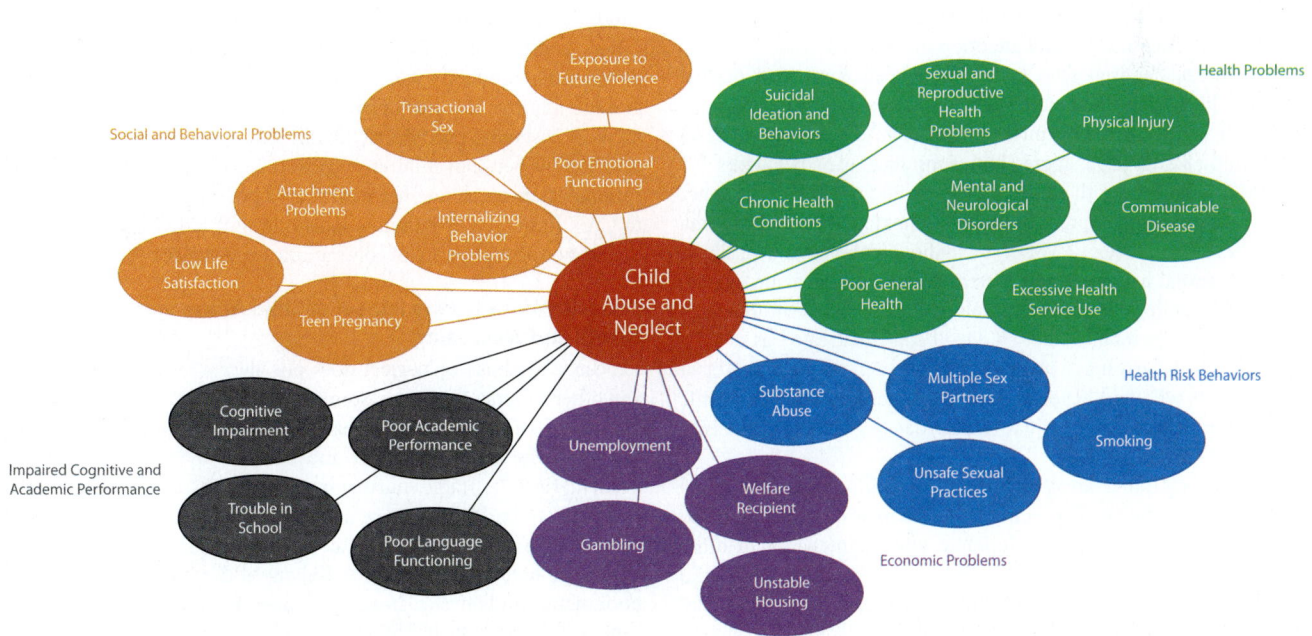

FIGURE 176-1. Common consequences of child abuse and neglect.

vulnerable to the immediate physical consequences caused by abuse. For example, when children under 5 years of age experience abuse they are at highest risk of experiencing head trauma that can lead to death or severe nonfatal consequences (e.g., blindness, cerebral palsy, cognitive impairments).[45]

Beyond immediate physical injuries, exposure to CAN also predicts longer-term health problems.[46] For example, the Adverse Childhood Experiences (ACE) study has repeatedly demonstrated a strong relationship between exposure to abuse, neglect, and other household challenges during childhood and several of the leading causes of death in adulthood in the United States (e.g., ischemic heart disease, cancer, chronic lung disease, and liver disease).[5] The findings of this large-scale study also indicate that the impact of these adverse experiences on adult health status is cumulative, such that as exposure to early adversity increases (e.g., exposure to multiple forms of abuse and neglect), the greater the likelihood of negative health outcomes.[5]

Exposure to CAN may result in toxic stress responses that can impede a child's development by producing changes at molecular, cellular, and behavioral levels: at the molecular level, changes in gene expression are possible[47]; at the cellular level, changes in brain connectivity and immune function are possible,[9] and at the behavioral level, changes in the type of coping strategies adopted are possible.[48] While many coping strategies are healthy and help reduce acute stress, some (e.g., smoking cigarettes, drinking alcohol, using substances, engaging in risky sexual behavior) present additional risks to health and well-being. As such, exposure to CAN and other early adversity can increase risk of later chronic and infectious health conditions through changes in physiological mechanisms, as well as increased engagement in risky health behaviors, ultimately resulting in premature death.[8,49]

Pscyhosocial and behavioral consequences. Children who experience CAN are more likely than their peers to experience difficulties with learning and school performance,[50,51] which persist even after controlling for potential individual and familial confounders (e.g., maternal drug and alcohol use, prematurity and low birth weight, and maternal anxiety and depression).[52] Similarly, children exposed to family violence (physical and/or sexual abuse, witnessing domestic violence) are more likely to exhibit poorer executive functioning, including impairments with cognitive processes such as working memory, inhibition, auditory attention, and processing speed, relative to their peers.[53] Studies have also found robust connections between exposure to CAN and attention disorders.[54,55]

In general, children who have experienced abuse and neglect are more likely than their nonmaltreated peers to experience mental health issues, including internalizing (e.g., depression, anxiety) and externalizing (e.g., aggression, substance use) behaviors.[56–58] Specifically, children with a history of abuse and neglect are at higher risk for experiencing depressive disorders, anxiety disorders, trauma and stress disorders (e.g., PTSD), suicidality, alcohol and drug abuse, high-risk sexual behaviors and increased bullying behavior, aggression, and juvenile delinquency compared to their peers without such histories.[12,59–64] In longitudinal studies, being maltreated as a child increased risk of arrest as a juvenile by 59%,[65] and as many as 80% of young adults who had histories of maltreatment met the diagnostic criteria for at least one psychiatric disorder (e.g., major depressive disorder, PTSD) at age 21.[66]

CAN affects other areas of life that are influential for optimal health and well-being. For example, CAN may have severe negative consequences on the development and maintenance of other close relationships throughout the life course.[67,68] The parent–child relationship is influential in how children develop other close relationships, and exposure to CAN may result in a disorganized attachment style that interferes with the formation of stable, affectionate relationships that are essential to health and well-being.[68] Children exposed to maltreatment are also at increased risk of exposure to other types of violence later in life[69–72] and for engaging in violent and criminal behavior themselves, including maltreatment of their own children.[73–77]

Many of the negative developmental consequences experienced by victims of CAN have neurobiological explanations, at least, in part. Abuse and neglect can interfere with optimal brain growth and development resulting in improper functioning of important regions of the brain, which, in turn, have consequences for development.[78,79] Brain development is dependent upon activity and experience. As an individual interacts with their environment, brain synapses and pathways are formed and strengthened; more interaction results in stronger pathways. Brain development is also cumulative; it is built in a series of sequential steps—interactions result in the formation of synapses, which lead to circuits that lead to pathways, which ultimately lead to consciousness and behavior. When children are continually exposed to threats, their brain remains on high alert and their stress response system is continuously activated creating a new pattern of behaviors that are "hard-wired." For example, the stress of chronic abuse may cause a "hyperarousal" response in certain areas of the brain, which may result in hyperactivity and sleep disturbances.[80,81] This stress may also strengthen the pathway among neurons that are involved in the fear response, and as a result, the brain may become predisposed to experience the world as hostile, which, in turn, may lead to anxious and aggressive behaviors.[82] In this example, the child becomes accustomed to living and dealing with toxic stress and develops a toxic stress response whereby the child may have difficulty discriminating between events that require immediate attention and those that do not. This toxic stress response can interfere with life-long learning, emotional self-regulation, social interactions, and other important developmental milestones.

Economic consequences. Some countries and regions have used their available data to estimate the economic consequences of CAN. Combined, these estimates highlight the substantial financial toll of CAN. For example, in the East Asia and Pacific region, it is estimated that the economic costs of CAN, which considers the costs of only a few known health consequences, were equivalent to between 1.4% and 2.5% of the region's annual GDP.[83] According to data from the United States, the total lifetime economic burden associated with new or incident cases of CAN occurring in 2008 was $124 billion.[84] This latter estimate was based on costs associated with healthcare in both childhood and adulthood, child welfare, criminal justice, special education, and loss of productivity. The estimated average lifetime cost per victim of nonfatal CAN is $210,012 in 2010 dollars. The estimated average lifetime cost per death from CAN is $1,272,900, including medical costs and productivity losses. Other studies have noted the associations between children's exposure to violence and limited educational attainment, unemployment, and poverty.[3,4] In sum, exposure to CAN limits the economic opportunities of individuals, as well as the economic prosperity of communities and society.

Considerations for the Impact of Child Abuse and Neglect on Health and Well-being

Exposure to abuse or neglect does not always result in toxic stress and other adverse outcomes. Some research indicates that nearly one quarter of children who are maltreated have no long-term symptoms.[85] If the stressor is brief and buffered by protective factors, particularly safe, stable, nurturing relationships and environments, children can build confidence and resilience. However, if abuse and neglect is chronic, severe, or excessive, a toxic stress response may trigger biological and behavioral changes that are risk factors for poor mental and physical health outcomes in the short-term and over time. Characteristics of children's exposure to abuse or neglect can also influence the risk of adverse outcomes. Characteristics that contribute to the heterogeneity in both short- and long-term outcomes can result from multiple, interacting factors, including the child's stage of development or age when the abuse occurred, the relationship of the perpetrator to the child, the length of time over which the abuse happened, severity of abuse, and other factors in the child's environment.[59,86–91]

RISK AND PROTECTIVE FACTORS

Researchers studying CAN have identified factors in multiple areas of children's lives that either increase their risk of experiencing abuse and neglect and related problems (i.e., risk factors) or that prevent abuse and neglect and support healthy development and behavior (i.e., protective factors). Exposure to CAN is rooted in a number of social, economic, and cultural factors that impact individuals, relationships and families, communities, and societies. The WHO and CDC have utilized the social ecological model[91,92] to depict factors at the individual, relationship, community, and societal levels that contribute to experiences of CAN. Risk and protective factors are not static and change over time. A factor that increases risk of abuse or neglect at one life stage may or may not put the same child at risk at a later stage in development.[93] Although risk and protective factors can occur at any level of the social ecology, most research has focused on individual- and relationship-level factors. However, evidence has expanded understanding of the important contributions that the community and broader sociopolitical environment play in exposure to CAN.[94,95]

Risk Factors

Risk of CAN perpetration and victimization is influenced by a number of individual, family, and environmental factors, all of which interact to increase or decrease risk over time and within specific contexts. Risk factors may differ depending on the type of CAN being studied; however, most of the risk factors associated with early adversity are dual risk factors in that they often put children and families at risk for multiple types of adversity and violence exposures.

Although children are not responsible for the harm inflicted upon them, some individual child characteristics have repeatedly been found to increase risk of being a victim of CAN; these characteristics include special needs that may increase caregiver burden (e.g., developmental and intellectual disabilities, mental health issues, and chronic physical illnesses).[91]

Risk factors for perpetration of CAN include parental or caregiver characteristics such as a lack of understanding of child development and parenting skills; history of CAN; substance abuse and/or mental health issues; young parental age; low education; single parenthood; large number of dependent children; low income; and nonbiological, transient caregivers in the home (e.g., mother's male partner).[91] Other risk factors for perpetration include limited social connections and support; other forms of family violence in the home (e.g., intimate partner violence); poor parent–child relationships; family disorganization; parenting stress; community violence; and concentrated neighborhood disadvantage (e.g., high poverty and residential instability, high unemployment rates).[91,96–98] Although risk factors provide information about who is most at risk for being a perpetrator of CAN, these factors are not direct causes and cannot predict who will be a perpetrator.

Protective Factors

Protective factors also exist at various levels of the social ecology but have been studied less extensively than risk factors, despite being equally important. For example, supportive family environments and social networks characterized by warmth, trust, and support can break the cycle of abuse and neglect across generations[74,76,77,99,100] and consistently emerge as protective factors.[91,101] Strong perceived social support, a good relationship between at least one parental figure and a child, and having a familial SES above the poverty level have also been continually associated with lower risk for CAN perpetration.[67,102] Other factors such as parental employment, adequate housing, and access to healthcare and social services may also reduce CAN perpetration risk.[103] Household financial security can reduce CAN by improving parents' ability to satisfy their children's basic needs (e.g., food, shelter, medical care), provide quality childcare, and improve parental mental health. As such, evidence suggests that economic supports to families, including child support payments,[104] tax credits,[105] paid leave,[106] nutrition assistance programs,[107] and subsidized childcare,[94] can reduce the risk of CAN perpetration. Access to quality care and education early in life through Child Parent Centers and/or Early Head Start[108,109] and enhancing positive parenting skills[110,111] can also be protective of abuse and neglect. In addition, research supports that safe, stable, nurturing relationships between parents and other adults may help prevent CAN, especially among parents who experienced abuse during their own childhood.[100] Unfortunately, no single factor tells the entire story about how and why CAN occurs; however, when positive experiences outweigh negative experiences, a child's likelihood of positive outcomes will be greater.

Interconnections between different forms of violence. Multiple forms of violence—CAN, youth violence, intimate partner violence, sexual violence, elder abuse, and self-directed violence (i.e., suicide)—are strongly connected to each other, often sharing risk and protective factors[112] that accumulate throughout childhood and carry into adulthood. In particular, exposure to violence in childhood increases risk for later violent experiences, which can have a cumulative and compounding impact on health and well-being across one's lifespan and future generations. Given the linkages across different forms of violence starting with exposure in childhood, the need for comprehensive prevention programs that address risk and protective factors across the social ecology and that start early in life is clear.

INTERVENTIONS/BEST AVAILABLE EVIDENCE

Comprehensive approaches to CAN prevention that address risk factors and promote protective factors at all levels of the social ecology are critical. To date, the bulk of violence prevention research has focused on addressing individual- and relational-level risk factors, whereas strategies that work at the community- or societal-level with the potential for broader public health impact with minimal individual effort have been studied less extensively.[103,113] While there is a need to continually expand the evidence base, particularly for community- and societal-level strategies to prevent CAN, it is also imperative to utilize the current and best available evidence for prevention. The *Essentials for Childhood* framework proposes four goal areas that communities can consider when implementing comprehensive approaches to prevent CAN.[138] The four goal areas can guide implementation and strengthen the impact of prevention approaches, and while each individual goal is important, implementation of activities in each of the four goal areas are more likely to build the comprehensive foundation of safe, stable, nurturing relationships and environments for all children and families. Goals 1 and 2 focus on building commitment for the prevention of CAN and using available data to educate communities about the importance of prevention and estimate the value of any prevention efforts. Goals 3 and 4 focus on the use of policies, programs, and norms change activities with the best available evidence to prevent CAN. CDC's Division of Violence Prevention developed a technical package to prevent CAN focused on goals 3 and 4 of the *Essentials for Childhood* framework. Technical packages also have been developed to assist communities in taking advantage of the best available evidence to prevent other forms of interpersonal, as well as self-directed, violence.[103,114–117] The strategies included in these technical packages focus on different levels of the social ecology, but all are intended to work together and reinforce each other to prevent violence against children.[92,103] The technical packages also are designed to help focus prevention efforts on

TABLE 176-3 STRATEGIES FOR PREVENTING CHILD ABUSE AND NEGLECT IN THE UNITED STATES

Strategy	Approach	Description
Strategy 1: Strengthen economic supports for families	Strengthening household financial security	Allows parents to satisfy their children's basic needs (e.g., food, shelter, medical care) and provide childcare appropriate to the child's age and level of development.
	Family-friendly work policies	Allows parents to improve the balance between work and family.
Strategy 2: Change social norms to support parents and positive parenting	Public engagement and education campaigns	Uses communication strategies (e.g., framing and messaging or social marketing), communication channels (e.g., mass or social media) and community-based efforts (e.g., town hall meetings, neighborhood screenings and discussions) to support parents.
	Legislative approaches to reduce corporal punishment	Establishes norms around safe, more effective discipline strategies.
Strategy 3: Provide quality care and education early in life	Preschool enrichment with family engagement	Ensures the provision of high-quality early education and care to economically disadvantaged children; also ensures support and educational opportunities for parents.
	Improved quality of child care through licensing and accreditation	Ensures that the quality of children's daily experiences are positive and supportive.
Strategy 4: Enhance parenting skills to promote healthy child development	Early childhood home visitation	Uses a home setting to provide information, caregiver support, and training about child health, development, and care to families.
	Parenting skill and family relationship approaches	Provides parents and caregivers with support and teaches behavior management and positive parenting skills.
Strategy 5: Intervene to lessen harms and prevent future risk	Enhanced primary care	Allows for the identification and treatment of problems (e.g., parental depression, intimate partner violence, substance abuse) that serve as risk factors for child abuse and neglect.
	Behavioral parent training programs	Allows parents to learn specific skills to build a safe, stable, nurturing relationship with their children.
	Treatment to lessen harms of abuse and neglect exposure	Mitigates the health consequences of abuse and neglect exposure and decreases the likelihood of intergenerational transmission of abuse.
	Treatment to prevent problem behavior and later involvement in violence	Provides support and treatment for youth in their social networks as a means to address current problems and prevent future violence.

Source: Adapted from the Centers for Disease Control and Prevention's *Preventing Child Abuse and Neglect: A Technical Package for Policy, Norm, and Programmatic Activities.*

specific strategies that have demonstrated effectiveness in preventing the varied forms of violence and include the specific ways in which strategies can be advanced, which are referred to as "approaches."[118] The evidence associated with each approach also is included, thereby clearly outlining those strategies and approaches with the best available evidence for preventing violence.

Child Abuse and Neglect Technical Package

Five strategies have been identified for preventing CAN in the US (see Table 176-3).[103] To maximize impact, these strategies are intended to be part of a comprehensive CAN prevention portfolio. Moreover, the implementation of each of the strategies requires collaboration of multiple sectors (e.g., public health, social services, justice, and government), as no one entity has the capacity or expertise to implement each of the strategies.[103]

Strategy 1: Strengthen economic supports for families. As noted previously, the socioeconomic conditions in which families live and raise children can influence health and life opportunities and impact how parents interact with their children.[3,119] Thus, one strategy for preventing CAN is to strengthen economic supports for families, which includes strengthening household financial security and supporting family-friendly work policies. These supports and policies ensure that parents are able to satisfy their children's basic needs (e.g., through the use of tax credits and child support passed on to the custodial parent), provide child care that is safe and developmentally appropriate for the child (e.g., through subsidized child care) and provide opportunities to balance work and family life (e.g., through paid leave and livable wages).[94,104,107,120–126] Research has demonstrated that abusive head trauma, a form of child abuse, decreases when certain policies, including tax credits and paid leave, are provided to families.[105,106] Moreover, many families have all adults working. Both work and family suffer when there is not enough flexibility and resources to meet parental responsibilities at work and at home. Family-friendly policies in the workplace, such as paid family leave, can make a big difference in parents' ability to raise their children to succeed. For example, state and/or organizational policies that include paid leave for 6 weeks after the birth of a child for all new parents may result in fewer instances of new parents worrying about losing their jobs or returning to work sooner because they cannot afford to stay home or provide for their families without working and being paid. Ultimately, this can reduce parental stress, allowing parents to focus on the health and well-being of their child. Thus, other risk and protective factors (e.g., parental depression and stress) are positively impacted when strategies are implemented to strengthen economic supports for families.[127–133] Family-friendly workplace policies also benefit employers in the form of increased productivity, improved employee retention and lower absenteeism—they also give employers a competitive advantage in recruiting and retaining skilled employees.[134]

Strategy 2: Change social norms to support parents and positive parenting. A second strategy that aims to prevent CAN focuses on changing how we think and talk about CAN and how we can best support parents and positive parenting. In the United States, there is a common belief that what happens in families stays in families (i.e., the family bubble) and others outside of the family are not to interfere.[135,136] In reality, however, the responsibility of preventing CAN is a shared responsibility of all adults in that child's life, as all children thrive when others around them also thrive.[137–139] Public engagement and education campaigns have demonstrated success in changing norms, reframing how we think and talk about CAN, and who is responsible for preventing it.[138,140,141] This includes how we think and talk about issues such as corporal punishment or harsh physical discipline of children. Approximately 60–70% of parents in the United States think, "it is sometimes necessary to discipline a child with a good hard spanking."[142] These beliefs persist although, as noted previously, there are decades of research that demonstrate its harmful effects.[19,64] At present, 53 countries have bans on corporal punishment; however, it is still permissible in much of American culture.[143] In the United States, 19 states still allow physical discipline in schools and it is still widely used in the home.[144] The use of corporal punishment remains high because many parents lack positive parenting skills, they believe it works, and alternative (i.e., positive parenting) skills are not acceptable among many racial/ethnic groups.[145,146] It is important, however, that adults not accept or allow indifference to violence toward children but instead support positive parenting and acceptability of help-seeking for when parents struggle. Behavioral parent training programs may be helpful for parents in addressing challenging child behaviors (see Strategy 4 in Table 176-3). Changing social norms may assist in addressing misperceptions about parenting and the fact that the ultimate responsibility of any child resides with all adults in that child's life, not just those who have some biological relation to the child.[139,147] Legislative approaches to reduce corporal punishment have been used in other countries, and over time have resulted in changes in norms about the acceptability of corporal punishment.[148]

Strategy 3: Provide quality care and education early in life. The third strategy for preventing CAN focuses on opportunities to ensure optimal learning environments for young children through quality care and education.[103] Children growing up in high-risk environments characterized by poverty and violence have a reduced chance of graduating from high school and tend to earn lower wages as adults, among other negative outcomes.[149–151] Heckman and Masterov argue that investments in young children from disadvantaged environments is logical from a productivity perspective.[152] Specifically, they note that interventions that can mitigate the effects of adverse environments can have a high economic return.[152] For example, preschool enrichment with family engagement provides a supportive early learning environment wherein there is an opportunity to reverse some of the harm of disadvantage, as these programs can enhance parenting practices and attitudes as well as family involvement in children's education.[109] Research on Child Parent Centers in Chicago and Early Head Start have documented relationships between participation in the programs and high school completion, lower rates of juvenile and violent arrest, lower rates of grade retention and special education services, and decreases in rates of child abuse.[108,153–155] Quality child care also is important for healthy child development, with stronger positive effects observed when children are from more at-risk backgrounds.[156–158] Moreover, quality child care is associated with positive social and cognitive development in children, which contributes to better academic achievement and less parental stress and conflict.[159]

Strategy 4: Enhance parenting skills to promote healthy child development. Much of the evidence in CAN prevention has focused on behavior change as a way to prevent the occurrence or re-occurrence of abusive behavior. The fourth strategy for preventing CAN focuses on enhancing parenting skills to promote healthy child development.[103] Early childhood home visitation (e.g., Nurse Family Partnership, Family Connects) and parenting skill and family relationship approaches (e.g., Adults and Children Together against Violence: Parents Raising Safe Kids, Incredible Years, SafeCare) aim to protect children from violence and its long-term consequences and build safe, stable, nurturing relationships and environments for children and families by influencing familial child-rearing practices.[160–162] These programs have been associated with positive outcomes for youth and families, including reductions in CAN perpetration, reductions in risk factors for CAN (e.g., child behavior problems), and improvements in parenting-related behaviors (e.g., nurturing behaviors, child behavior management).[110,111,163–166]

Strategy 5: Intervene to lessen harms and prevent future risk. Approximately 50–90% of children who experience CAN do not receive any intervention or treatment, irrespective of whether the case comes to the attention of child welfare agencies,[167] thereby highlighting the importance of the fifth strategy identified in the CAN technical package, which is to intervene to lessen harms and prevent future risk. As noted previously, the effects of CAN are far-reaching and may affect both physical and mental health, as well as biological systems and structures.[48] To mitigate these negative health effects, a number of approaches can be used depending on the level of risk and whether abuse has happened or not. Some approaches may be targeted toward high-risk populations to prevent CAN (e.g., enhanced primary care with the Safe Environments for Every Kid program), whereas families where abuse has already occurred may benefit from behavioral parent training using programs such as Parent–Child Interaction Therapy, SafeCare, or the Incredible Years.[168–175] Collectively, these programs are associated with fewer reports to child protective services, fewer occurrences of physical assaults, and decreased maternal psychological aggression, among other positive outcomes.[170,171] Moreover, several of these programs have demonstrated efficacy in preventing the reoccurrence for abuse in families with confirmed cases of CAN, while also reducing risk factors of CAN in high-risk families (e.g., those who use harsh/punitive parenting practices).[168,169,174,176,177]

Exposure to CAN may increase risk of future exposure to violence, as both a victim and perpetrator, thereby highlighting the necessity of treatment.[178–180] Trauma-Focused Cognitive Behavioral Therapy is one evidence-based approach that targets emotional and behavioral symptoms resulting from CAN exposure. The treatment is associated with reductions in PTSD, depression, and behavior problems.[181] Other programs, including Children with Problematic Sexual Behavior Cognitive-Behavioral Treatment Program: School-age Program and Multisystemic Therapy, have been used to address behavioral issues (e.g., reoffending, inappropriate parent-child interactions and parenting behaviors) and psychological symptoms for the youth and caregiver.[182–185]

Inspire Technical Package

As noted previously, roughly half of all children around the world experienced violence in the past year.[1] While the aforementioned strategies are based on the best available evidence for preventing CAN, they are based primarily on research conducted in the US context; however, strategies and approaches that work in the US may not be scalable or applicable in an international context, such as in low- and middle-income countries. The WHO partnered with technical experts from a number of global agencies, as well as other partners, to identify seven strategies for preventing violence against children globally.[92] The INSPIRE technical package focuses on strategies to prevent all forms of violence against children, not just CAN. Like its US counterpart, the strategies are most effective when implemented as part of a comprehensive prevention plan that includes multiple sectors working together to fulfill a common goal, which is to prevent and respond to violence against children. Each of the seven strategies is represented by the INSPIRE acronym.[92] Broadly, the strategies focus on the importance of changes in laws, norms and values, and environments to prevent violence against children. In addition, the strategies reflect the importance of positive parenting, economic security and stability, access to quality response and intervention services, and gender-equitable education and school environments.[92]

IMPLEMENTATION CONSIDERATIONS

In efforts to prevent CAN and assure that all children reach their full potential, it is important to understand the factors that may influence implementation and dissemination of prevention strategies. The feasibility of successfully implementing CAN prevention strategies will vary according to the selected strategy and the context in which it will be implemented. The specific strategies that are implemented, when the strategies are implemented, and in what order the strategies are implemented should depend on what is already happening in the community, as well as the unique needs of the selected community. One of the first steps in this process is to build commitment for the prevention of CAN. Other implementation considerations, including the use of data to select and evaluate strategies, are included below.

Ensure sufficient awareness and support. A challenge that is often noted when communities are implementing comprehensive strategies for prevention, particularly at the societal and community levels, is the lack of commitment to do something about the issue.[113] To best prevent CAN, communities will need the support of government and civil society, and all must adopt a unifying vision. While it takes time to get everyone to support and adopt a unifying vision, communities can begin to garner support for preventing CAN by presenting the issue in a way that others understand and value and that goes beyond just noting that CAN is a problem or bad for children. The more other entities (e.g., businesses, media) "buy in" to the issue and vision, the greater the likelihood that communities can move from commitment to action.[139] For example, as noted previously, the prevention of CAN may have positive benefits for businesses, including increased productivity, retention of talented employees, and lower absenteeism.[134] This information may be useful when engaging businesses to adopt and champion initiatives that have a high return on investment and prevent CAN.

Use data to select and evaluate strategies. Data can be particularly powerful when highlighting social issues such as abuse and neglect. Data allows communities to identify population needs, gaps in services, high-risk groups, and protective factors to name a few. Data also helps communities understand the size and nature of the problem, how to best direct prevention resources, and monitor the impact of prevention strategies; thus, communities may want to ensure partnerships include those who can assist in gathering and synthesizing data. Once partnerships are established, communities will need to examine what data already exists in the community and identify steps that can be taken to fill critical gaps in data. Most communities have existing systems that include vital statistics, as well as health, criminal justice, child protection and welfare, educational, and basic demographic (e.g., number of children living in poverty, number of parents unemployed) data.[139] Data from other community or national level surveys or surveillance systems also may be available and customizable to the community. Partnerships may be used to develop new data systems and fill critical data gaps. For example, questions could be added to existing surveys such as the Youth Risk Behavior Survey. Once data has been collected, it can be used to support activities that are part of a comprehensive prevention portfolio.[139]

Support beneficial social and economic policies. An important first step in ensuring that policies support children and families is to identify and assess (within the community) which policies have the potential to positively impact the lives of children and families and make individuals' default decisions healthy ones. Consideration of how policies are implemented (e.g., the coverage, cost, and eligibility requirements) at the appropriate community level is critical in understanding potential impacts of a policy on children and families. Moreover, awareness among stakeholders, including policy makers, employers, and the public, about the relationship between family-friendly policies and decreased risk for multiple forms of violence, may be helpful in encouraging buy-in and support for policies that positively impact children and families. Public health and other research fields are in a unique position to provide decision-makers and community leaders with information on the benefits of evidence-based strategies and rigorous evaluation to ensure that any activities being implemented, including policies, are providing optimal benefits and worth any investments being made.[138] For example, health impact assessments and paid leave analyses (e.g., cost-benefit analysis of worker retention and productivity) may be helpful in understanding potential gains and barriers to the provision of family-friendly work supports at the national and local level.

Invest in staff/implementer education and retention. Staff turnover is a major concern in many of the agencies and service systems working to prevent and treat CAN. Training for many of the programs included in the CAN technical package require a training time commitment of 40 hours or more, as well as practice and ongoing supervision by individuals trained in the model. Previous research has noted reduced staff turnover when evidence-based programs are implemented with fidelity monitoring (i.e., ongoing supervision and consultation).[186] This may include opportunities to identify and share best practices and create feedback loops for communication. Thus, staff education, training, and on-going learning are important considerations in the implementation of any activities aimed at preventing CAN.

Consider transportability and cost. Strategies at the outer levels of the social ecology will likely have greater population impact in preventing CAN, than programs focused on individuals or families, when they can be successfully implemented.[103] It is more difficult for individual or family level prevention and intervention programs to have population impact, relative to policy and norms change strategies, because of the substantial cost of scaling them up to reach a sufficient number of individual and families to change conditions at a population level. Moreover, many programs developed for preventing CAN or the re-occurrence of CAN are not easily transportable into systems where families can benefit and often require extensive efforts to build the capacity of governments and other organizations and systems serving families.[187] Finally, the costs associated with implementation of programs to prevent CAN are often a barrier to implementation. Start-up costs for the programs often include the costs of materials, as well as training of staff. Agencies with high staff turnover may have to provide training several times a year to ensure staff are trained appropriately in implementing services. To this end, it will also likely be helpful to consider the type and number of policies or programs that are introduced at any one time.

Build partnerships. The technical packages discussed previously for preventing CAN and violence against children are based on the best available evidence.[92,103] For some of the strategies identified, public health agencies are well positioned to bring leadership and resources to implementation efforts; however, for other strategies, leadership, and commitment from other sectors such as business/labor, government, social services, healthcare, education, and justice are critical to implementation.[92,103] Moreover, the sectors that are in the best position to enact and lead implementation of the various strategies and approaches will likely depend on whether implementation is occurring in the US or globally. In most cases, implementation is best when multiple sectors partner in implementation efforts. For example, although public health will not be directly responsible for changes in policy, public health agencies may provide government leaders with data that can provide support for or against certain policy-level changes. In general, any implementation of laws and policies will require commitment and/or support of governments to enact changes at the local, state, or federal/country levels. Organizational policy changes (when occurring without a broader governmental mandate) will require the engagement of business and labor. Public health agencies are poised to lead norms change activities focused on supporting parents and positive parenting, whereas commitment and/or support of the government is necessary for legislative approaches to reduce corporal punishment and to improve the quality of child care through licensing and accreditation.[103]

Other considerations. In the implementation of programs to enhance parenting skills or interventions to lessen harms and prevent future risk, parents and/or children attend face-to-face sessions, whether in the home or clinic/therapeutic setting, with highly skilled professionals from various sectors (e.g., nurses, mental health providers). Moreover, the populations of focus often vary depending on the program being implemented. Implementation of these programs should also be mindful of context, as well as culture and history. Depending on the programs being implemented, the programming may be delivered to those deemed most "at risk" or those who have already experienced abuse or neglect, which will ultimately have implications for the cost and burden of implementation. Like other activities that are part of a comprehensive child abuse prevention portfolio, program implementation will likely require interaction among multiple sectors (e.g., public health, healthcare, social services, justice), each of whom plays a role in enhancing parenting skills and lessening harms and preventing future risk.[92,103]

CONCLUSIONS

CAN is a serious public health issue with far-reaching consequences. While CAN is a significant public health problem, it is also a preventable one. The policies, social norms, and programmatic strategies and approaches highlighted in this chapter are intended to help guide the creation of neighborhoods and communities where every child has safe, stable, nurturing relationships and environments, and ultimately, a world where every child can thrive. Together we can assure that all children reach their full health and life potential.

References

1. Hillis S, Mercy J, Amobi A, Kress H. Global prevalence of past-year violence against children: A systematic review and minimum estimates. *Pediatrics*. 2016;137(3):e20154079.
2. Pinheiro PS. *World Report on Violence against Children*. Geneva: United Nations; 2006.
3. Metzler M, Merrick MT, Klevens J, Ports KA, Ford DC. Adverse childhood experiences and life opportunities: Shifting the narrative. *Children and Youth Services Review*. 2017;72:141–9.
4. Font SA, Maguire-Jack, K. Pathways from childhood abuse and other adversities to adult health risks: The role of adult socioeconomic conditions. *Child Abuse Negl*. 2016;51:390–9.
5. Felitti VJ, Anda RF, Nordenberg D, et al. Relationship of childhood abuse and household dysfunction to many of the leading causes of death in adults. The Adverse Childhood Experiences (ACE) Study. *Am J Prev Med*. 1998;14(4):245–58.
6. Gilbert LK, Breiding MJ, Merrick MT, et al. Childhood adversity and adult chronic disease: An update from ten states and the District of Columbia, 2010. *Am J Prev Med*. 2015;48(3):345–9.
7. Merrick MT, Ports KA, Ford DC, Afifi TO, Gershoff ET, Grogan-Kaylor A. Unpacking the impact of adverse childhood experiences on adult mental health. *Child Abuse Negl*. 2017;69:10–9.
8. Brown DW, Anda RF, Tiemeier H, et al. Adverse childhood experiences and the risk of premature mortality. *Am J Prev Med*. 2009;37(5):389–96.
9. Shonkoff JP. Capitalizing on advances in science to reduce the health consequences of early childhood adversity. *JAMA Pediatr*. 2016;170(10):1003–7.
10. Leeb RT, Pailozzi L, Melanson C, Simon T, Arias I. *Child Maltreatment Surveillance: Uniform Definitions for Public Health and Recommended Data Elements*. Atlanta, GA: Centers for Disease Control and Prevention, National Center for Injury Prevention and Control; 2008. https://www.cdc.gov/violenceprevention/pdf/cm_surveillance-a.pdf.
11. World Health Organization. *Global Status Report on Violence Prevention 2014*. Geneva, Switzerland: World Health Organization; 2014. http://www.who.int/violence_injury_prevention/violence/status_report/2014/en/.
12. Runyan D, Wattam C, Ikeda R, Hassan F, Ramiro L. Child abuse and neglect by parents and other caregivers. In: Krug EG, Dahlberg LL, Mercy JA, Zwi AB, Lozano R, eds. *World Report on Violence and Health*. Geneva: World Health Organization; 2002, pp. 59–85.
13. United Nations Children's Fund. A summary of the United Nations convention on the rights of the child. https://www.unicef.org/crc/files/Rights_overview.pdf.
14. Institute of Medicine and National Research Council. *Confronting Commercial Sexual Exploitation and Sex Trafficking of Minors in the United States*. Washington, DC: The National Academies Press; 2013.
15. United Nations. Protocol to prevent, suppress, and punish trafficking in persons, especially women and children. Geneva; 2000. http://www.unodc.org/unodc/en/treaties/CTOC/index.html.
16. Finkelhor D, Shattuck A, Turner H, Hamby S. A revised inventory of Adverse Childhood Experiences. *Child Abuse Negl*. 2015;48:13–21.
17. Cronholm PF, Forke CM, Wade R, et al. Adverse childhood experiences: Expanding the concept of adversity. *Am J Prev Med*. 2015;49(3):354–61.
18. United Nations Children's Fund. *The State of the World's Children 2009*. New York: United Nations Children's Fund; 2008.
19. Gershoff ET, Grogan-Kaylor A. Spanking and child outcomes: Old controversies and new meta-analyses. *J Fam Psychol*. 2016;30(4):453–69.
20. Pascoe JM, Wood DL, Duffee JH, et al. Mediators and adverse effects of child poverty in the United States. *Pediatrics*. 2016;137(4):e20160340.
21. Stoltenborgh M, Bakersmans-Kranenburg MJ, Alink LRA, van Ijzendoorn MH. The universality of childhood emotional abuse: A meta-analysis of worldwide prevalence. *J Aggression, Maltreatment Trauma*. 2012;21(8):300–20.
22. Stoltenborgh M, Bakermans-Kranenburg MJ, van Ijzendoorn MH, Alink LRA. Cultural-geographical differences in the occurrence of child physical abuse? A meta-analysis of global prevalence. *Int J Psychol*. 2013;48(2):81–94.
23. Stoltenborgh M, van Ijzendoorn MH, Euser EM, Bakermans-Kranenburg MJ. A global perspective on child sexual abuse: Meta-analysis of prevalence around the world. *Child Maltreat*. 2011;16(2):79–101.
24. Stoltenborgh M, Bakermans-Kranenburg MJ, van Ijzendoorn MH. The neglect of child neglect: A meta-analytic review of the prevalence of neglect. *Soc Psychiatry Psychiatr Epidemiol*. 2013;48(3):345–55.
25. Klevens J, Ports KA, Austin C, Ludlow IJ, Hurd J. A cross-national exploration of societal-level factors associated with child physical abuse and neglect. *Glob Public Health*. 2018;13(10):1495–1506.
26. World Health Organization: Child Maltreatment Fact Sheet 2016. http://www.who.int/mediacentre/factsheets/fs150/en/.
27. Reza A, Breiding MJ, Gulaid J, et al. Sexual violence and its health consequences for female children in Swaziland: A cluster survey study. *Lancet*. 2009;373(9679):1966–72.
28. United Nations Children's Fund, Centers for Disease Control and Prevention, Muhimbili University of Health and Allied Sciences. *Violence against Children in Tanzania: Findings from a National Survey 2009*. Dar es Salaam: United Nations Children's Fund; 2011. https://www.unicef.org/media/files/VIOLENCE_AGAINST_CHILDREN_IN_TANZANIA_REPORT.pdf.
29. United Nations Children's Fund Kenya Country Office, Division of Violence Prevention, National Center for Injury Prevention and Control, Centers for Disease Control and Prevention, the Kenya National Bureau of Statistics. *Violence against Children in Kenya: Findings from a 2010 National Survey*. Nairobi, Kenya: United Nations Children's Fund; 2012. https://www.unicef.org/esaro/VAC_in_Kenya.pdf.
30. Zimbabwe National Statistics Agency, United Nations Children's Fund, Collaborating Centre for Operational Research and Evaluation. *National Baseline Survey on Life Experiences of Adolescents in Zimbabwe 2011*. Harare: Zimbabwe National Statistics Agency; 2013. https://www.unicef.org/zimbabwe/UNICEF_NBSLEA-Report-23-10-13.pdf.
31. U.S. Department of Health & Human Services, Administration for Children and Families, Administration on Children, Youth and Families, Children's Bureau. *Child Maltreatment 2016*. 2018. https://www.acf.hhs.gov/cb/resource/child-maltreatment-2016.
32. Finkelhor D, Turner HA, Shattuck A, Hamby SL. Prevalence of childhood exposure to violence, crime, and abuse: Results from the National Survey of Children's Exposure to Violence. *JAMA Pediatr*. 2015;169(8):746–54.
33. Dong M, Giles WH, Felitti VJ, et al. Insights into causal pathways for ischemic heart disease: Adverse childhood experiences study. *Circulation*. 2004;110(13):1761–6.
34. Finkelhor D, Ormrod RK, Turner HA. Polyvictimization and trauma in a national longitudinal cohort. *Dev Psychopathol*. 2007;19(1):149–66.
35. Turner HA, Shattuck A, Finkelhor D, Hamby S. Polyvictimization and youth violence exposure across contexts. *J Adolesc Health*. 2016;58(2):208–14.
36. Sedlak AJ, Mettenburg J, Basena M, et al. *Fourth National Incidence Study of Child Abuse and Neglect (NIS-4): Report to Congress, Executive Summary*. Washington, DC: U.S. Department of Health and Human Services, Administration for Children and Families; 2010.

37. Maker AH, Shah PV, Agha Z. Child physical abuse: Prevalence, characteristics, predictors, and beliefs about parent-child violence in South Asian, Middle Eastern, East Asian, and Latina women in the United States. *J Interpers Violence*. 2005;20(11):1406–28.
38. World Health Organization. *Global Health Estimates 2015: Deaths by Cause, Age, Sex, Country and Region, 2000–2015. Geneva: Health Statistics and Information Systems*. Geneva: World Health Organization; 2016. http://www.who.int/healthinfo/global_burden_disease/en/.
39. Herman-Giddens ME, Brown G, Verbiest S, et al. Underascertainment of child abuse mortality in the United States. *JAMA*. 1999;282(5):463–7.
40. Meadow R. Unnatural sudden infant death. *Arch Dis Child*. 1999;80(1):7–14.
41. Adinkrah M. Maternal infanticides in Fiji. *Child Abuse Negl*. 2000;24(12):1543–55.
42. Pinto RJ, Maia AC. A comparison study between official records and self-reports of childhood adversity. *Child Abuse Review*. 2012;22:354–66.
43. Turner HA, Merrick MT, Finkelhor D, Hamby S, Shattuck A, Henly M. *The Prevalence of Safe, Stable, Nurturing Relationships among Children and Adolescents. Juvenile Justice Bulletin*. Washington, DC: Office of Juvenile Justice and Delinquency Prevention. 2017. https://www.ojjdp.gov/pubs/249197.pdf.
44. World Health Organization. *Violence Info: Child Maltreatment*. Geneva, Switzerland: World Health Organization; 2016. http://apps.who.int/violence-info/child-maltreatment/.
45. Parks SE, Annest JL, Hill HA, Karch DL. *Pediatric Abusive Head Trauma: Recommended Definitions for Public Health Surveillance and Research*. Atlanta, GA: Centers for Disease Control and Prevention; 2012. https://www.cdc.gov/violenceprevention/pdf/pedheadtrauma-a.pdf.
46. Thompson MP, Arias I, Basile K, Desai S. The association between childhood physical and sexual victimization and health problems in adulthood in a nationally representative sample of women. *J Interpers Violence*. 2002;17:1115–29.
47. Brockie TN, Heinzelmann M, Gill J. A framework to examine the role of epigenetics in health disparities among Native Americans. *Nurs Res Pract*. 2013;2013:410395.
48. Shonkoff JP, Garner AS, Committee on Psychosocial Aspects of Child and Family Health, et al. The lifelong effects of early childhood adversity and toxic stress. *Pediatrics*. 2012;129(1):e232–46.
49. Division of Violence Prevention, Centers for Disease Control and Prevention. Adverse Childhood Experiences: ACE Pyramid. Atlanta, GA: CDC; 2016. https://www.cdc.gov/violenceprevention/acestudy/about.html.
50. Kerr MA, Black MM, Krishnakumar A. Failure-to-thrive, maltreatment and the behavior and development of 6-year-old children from low-income, urban families: A cumulative risk model. *Child Abuse Negl*. 2000;24(5):587–98.
51. Perez CM, Widom CS. Childhood victimization and long-term intellectual and academic outcomes. *Child Abuse Negl*. 1994;18(8):617–33.
52. Mills R, Alati R, O'Callaghan M, et al. Child abuse and neglect and cognitive function at 14 years of age: Findings from a birth cohort. *Pediatrics*. 2011;127(1):4–10.
53. DePrince AP, Weinzierl KM, Combs MD. Executive function performance and trauma exposure in a community sample of children. *Child Abuse Negl*. 2009;33(6):353–61.
54. Heneghan A, Stein RE, Hurlburt MS, et al. Mental health problems in teens investigated by U.S. child welfare agencies. *J Adolesc Health*. 2013;52(5):634–40.
55. Briscoe-Smith AM, Hinshaw SP. Linkages between child abuse and attention-deficit/hyperactivity disorder in girls: Behavioral and social correlates. *Child Abuse Negl*. 2006;30(11):1239–55.
56. Bolger KE, Patterson CJ. Pathways from child maltreatment to internalizing problems: Perceptions of control as mediators and moderators. *Dev Psychopathol*. 2001;13(4):913–40.
57. Johnson RM, Kotch JB, Catellier DJ, et al. Adverse behavioral and emotional outcomes from child abuse and witnessed violence. *Child Maltreat*. 2002;7(3):179–86.
58. Rogosch FA, Cicchetti D, Aber JL. The role of child maltreatment in early deviations in cognitive and affective processing abilities and later peer relationship problems. *Development and Psychopathology*. 1995;7:591–609.
59. Briere J, Jordan CE. Childhood maltreatment, intervening variables, and adult psychological difficulties in women: An overview. *Trauma Violence Abuse*. 2009;10(4):375–88.
60. Kaplow JB, Widom CS. Age of onset of child maltreatment predicts long-term mental health outcomes. *J Abnorm Psychol*. 2007;116:176–87.
61. Lo CC, Cheng TC. The impact of childhood maltreatment on young adults' substance abuse. *Am J Drug Alcohol Abuse*. 2007;33(1):139–46.
62. MacMillan HL, Fleming JE, Streiner DL, et al. Childhood abuse and lifetime psychopathology in a community sample. *Am J Psychiatry*. 2001;158(11):1878–83.
63. Hankin B. Childhood maltreatment and psychopathology: Prospective tests of attachment, cognitive vulnerability, and stress as mediating processes. *Cognit Ther Res*. 2005;29:645–71.
64. Afifi TO, Ford D, Gershoff ET, et al. Spanking and adult mental health impairment: The case for the designation of spanking as an adverse childhood experience. *Child Abuse Negl*. 2017;71:24–31.
65. Widom CS, Maxfield MG. *An Update on the "Cycle of Violence."* Washington, DC: US Dept of Justice; 2001. Publication NCJ 184894.
66. Silverman AB, Reinherz HZ, Giaconia RM. The long-term sequelae of child and adolescent abuse: A longitudinal community study. *Child Abuse Negl*. 1996;20(8):709–23.
67. Muller RT, Goebel-Fabbri AE, Diamond T, Dinklage D. Social support and the relationship between family and community violence exposure and psychopathology among high risk adolescents. *Child Abuse Negl*. 2000;24(4):449–64.
68. Kobak R, Madsen S. *Disruptions in Attachment Bonds: Implications for Theory, Research, and Clinical Intervention. Handbook of Attachment: Theory, Research, and Clinical Applications*, 2nd ed. New York: Guilford Press; 2008.
69. Holt S, Buckley H, Whelan S. The impact of exposure to domestic violence on children and young people: A review of the literature. *Child Abuse and Negl*. 2008;32:197–810.
70. Renner LM, Slack KS. Intimate partner violence and child maltreatment: Understanding intra- and intergenerational connections. *Child Abuse Negl*. 2006;30(6):599–617.
71. Ports KA, Ford DC, Merrick MT. Adverse childhood experiences and sexual victimization in adulthood. *Child Abuse Negl*. 2016;51:313–22.
72. Barnes JE, Noll JG, Putnam FW, Trickett PK. Sexual and physical revictimization among victims of severe childhood sexual abuse. *Child Abuse Negl*. 2009;33:412–20.
73. Berlin LJ, Appleyard K, Dodge KA. Intergenerational continuity in child maltreatment: Mediating mechanisms and implications for prevention. *Child Dev*. 2011;82(1):162–76.
74. Conger RD, Schofield TJ, Neppl TK, Merrick MT. Disrupting intergenerational continuity in harsh and abusive parenting: The importance of a nurturing relationship with a romantic partner. *J Adolesc Health*. 2013;53(4 Suppl):S11–7.
75. Herrenkohl TI, Klika JB, Brown EC, Herrenkohl RC, Leeb RT. Tests of the mitigating effects of caring and supportive relationships in the study of abusive disciplining over two generations. *J Adolesc Health*. 2013;53(4 Suppl):S18–24.
76. Jaffee SR, Bowes L, Ouellet-Morin I, et al. Safe, stable, nurturing relationships break the intergenerational cycle of abuse: A prospective nationally representative cohort of children in the United Kingdom. *J Adolesc Health*. 2013;53(4 Suppl):S4–10.
77. Thornberry TP, Henry KL, Smith CA, Ireland TO, Greenman SJ, Lee RD. Breaking the cycle of maltreatment: The role of safe, stable, and nurturing relationships. *J Adolesc Health*. 2013;53(4 Suppl):S25–31.
78. Office of the Surgeon General, National Center for Injury Prevention and Control, National Institutes of Health, Center for Mental health Services. *Youth Violence: A Report of the Surgeon General*. Rockville, MD: Office of the Surgeon General; 2001. https://www.ncbi.nlm.nih.gov/pubmed/20669522.
79. Watts-English T, Fortson BL, Gibler N, Hooper SR, De Bellis MD. The psychobiology of maltreatment in childhood. *Social Issues*. 2006;62(4):717–36.
80. Dallam SJ. The long-term medical consequences of childhood maltreatment. In: Franey K, Geffner R, Falconer R, eds. *The Cost of Child Maltreatment: Who Pays? We All Do*. San Diego, CA: Family Violence & Sexual Assault Institute; 2001.
81. Perry BD. The neurodevelopmental impact of violence in childhood. In: Schetky D, Benedek EP, eds. *Textbook of Child and Adolescent Forensic Psychiatry*. Washington, DC: American Psychiatric Press, Inc.; 2001, pp. 221–38.
82. Perry BD, Pollard R, Blakely T, Baker W, Vigilante D. Childhood trauma, the neurobiology of adaptation and "use-dependent" development of the brain: How "states" become "traits." *Infant Ment Health J*. 1995;16:271–91.
83. Fang X, Fry DA, Brown DS, et al. The burden of child maltreatment in the East Asia and Pacific region. *Child Abuse Negl*. 2015;42:146–62.

84. Fang X, Brown DS, Florence CS, Mercy JA. The economic burden of child maltreatment in the United States and implications for prevention. *Child Abuse Negl.* 2012;36(2):156–65.
85. McGloin J, Widom CS. Resilience among abused and neglected children grown up. *Dev Psychopathol.* 2001;13:1021–38.
86. Briere JN, Elliott DM. Immediate and long-term impacts of child sexual abuse. *Future Child.* 1994;4(2):54–69.
87. Bulik CM, Prescott CA, Kendler KS. Features of childhood sexual abuse and the development of psychiatric and substance use disorders. *Br J Psychiatry.* 2001;179:444–9.
88. Collishaw S, Pickles A, Messer J, Rutter M, Shearer C, Maughan B. Resilience to adult psychopathology following childhood maltreatment: Evidence from a community sample. *Child Abuse Negl.* 2007;31(3):211–29.
89. Keiley MK, Howe TR, Dodge KA, Bates JE, Petti GS. The timing of child physical maltreatment: A cross-domain growth analysis of impact on adolescent externalizing and internalizing problems. *Dev Psychopathol.* 2001;13(4):891–912.
90. Manly JT, Kim JE, Rogosch FA, Cicchetti D. Dimensions of child maltreatment and children's adjustment: Contributions of developmental timing and subtype. *Dev Psychopathol.* 2001;13(4):759–82.
91. Centers for Disease Control and Prevention. *Child Maltreatment: Risk and Protective Factors.* Atlanta, GA: CDC; 2017. www.cdc.gov/ViolencePrevention/childmaltreatment/riskprotectivefactors.html.
92. World Health Organization. *INSPIRE: Seven Strategies for Ending Violence against Children.* Geneva, Switzerland: World Health Organization; 2016. http://apps.who.int/iris/bitstream/10665/207717/1/9789241565356-eng.pdf?ua=1.
93. Cicchetti D, Toth SL. Child maltreatment. *Annu Rev Clin Psychol.* 2005;1:409–38.
94. Klein S. The availability of neighborhood early care and education resources and the maltreatment of young children. *Child Maltreat.* 2011;16(4):300–11.
95. Coulton CJ, Crampton DS, Irwin M, Spilsbury JC, Korbin JE. How neighborhoods influence child maltreatment: A review of the literature and alternative pathways. *Child Abuse Negl.* 2007;31:1117–42.
96. Jent JM, Merrick MT. Child neglect. In: Gellman M, Rick TJ, eds. *Encyclopedia of Behavioral Medicine.* New York: Springer Science and Business Media; 2013.
97. Merrick MT, Jent JM. Child abuse. In: Gellman M, Rick TJ, eds. *Encyclopedia of Behavioral Medicine.* New York: Springer Science and Business Media; 2013.
98. Stith SM, Liu T, Davies LC, et al. Risk factors in child maltreatment: A meta-analytic review of the literature. *Aggress Violent Behav.* 2009;14:13–29.
99. Merrick MT, Leeb RT, Lee RD. Examining the role of safe, stable, and nurturing relationships in the intergenerational continuity of child maltreatment—Introduction to the special issue. *J Adolesc Health.* 2013;53(4 Suppl):S1–3.
100. Schofield TJ, Lee RD, Merrick MT. Safe, stable, nurturing relationships as a moderator of intergenerational continuity of child maltreatment: A meta-analysis. *J Adolesc Health.* 2013;53(4 Suppl):S32–8.
101. Development Services Group, Inc. *Protective Factors for Populations Served by the Administration on Children, Youth, and Families: A Literature Review and Theoretical Framework.* Bethesda, MD: Administration on Children, Youth, and Families; 2013. https://ncfy.acf.hhs.gov/library/2013/protective-factors-populations-served-administration-children-youth-and-families.
102. Freisthler B, Bruce E, Needell B. Understanding the geospatial relationship of neighborhood characteristics and rates of maltreatment for black, hispanic, and white children. *Soc Work.* 2007;52(1):7–16.
103. Fortson BL, Klevens J, Merrick MT, Gilbert LK, Alexander SP. Preventing child abuse and neglect: A technical package for policy, norm, and programmatic activities. Atlanta, GA: National Center for Injury Prevention and Control, Centers for Disease Control and Prevention; 2016. https://www.cdc.gov/violenceprevention/pdf/can-prevention-technical-package.pdf.
104. Cancian M, Yang M, Slack KS. The effect of additional child support income on the risk of child maltreatment. *Soc Serv Rev.* 2013;87(3):417–37.
105. Klevens J, Schmidt B, Luo F, Xu L, Ports KA, Lee RD. Effect of the earned income tax credit on hospital admissions for pediatric abusive head trauma, 1995–2013. *Public Health Rep.* 2017;132(4):505–11.
106. Klevens J, Luo F, Xu L, Peterson C, Latzman NE. Paid family leave's effect on hospital admissions for pediatric abusive head trauma. *Inj Prev.* 2016;22(6):442–5.
107. Lee BJ, Mackey-Bilaver L. Effects of WIC and food stamp program participation on child outcomes. *Youth Serv Rev.* 2007;29:501–17.
108. Green BL, Ayoub C, Bartlett JD, et al. The effect of Early Head Start on child welfare system involvement: A first look at longitudinal child maltreatment outcomes. *Child Youth Serv Rev.* 2014;42:127–35.
109. Reynolds AJ, Robertson DL. School-based early intervention and later child maltreatment in the Chicago Longitudinal Study. *Child Dev.* 2003;74(1):3–26.
110. Olds DL, Eckenrode J, Henderson CR, et al. Long-term effects of home visitation on maternal life course and child abuse and neglect: Fifteen-year follow-up of a randomized trial. *J Am Med Assoc.* 1997;278(8):637–43.
111. Portwood SG, Lambert RG, Abrams LP, Nelson EB. An evaluation of the Adults and Children Together (ACT) Against Violence Parents Raising Safe Kids program. *J Prim Prev.* 2011;32(3–4):147–60.
112. Wilkins N, Tsao B, Hertz M, Davis R, Klevens J. *Connecting the Dots: An Overview of the Links Among Multiple Forms of Violence.* Atlanta, GA: National Center for Injury Prevention and Control, Centers for Disease Control and Prevention; Oakland, CA: Prevention Institute; 2014. https://www.cdc.gov/violenceprevention/pdf/connecting_the_dots-a.pdf.
113. Frieden TR. A framework for public health action: The health impact pyramid. *Am J Public Health.* 2010;100(4):590–5.
114. Basile KC, DeGue, S, Jones, K, et al. *STOP SV: A Technical Package to Prevent Sexual Violence.* Atlanta, GA: National Center for Injury Prevention and Control, Centers for Disease Control and Prevention; 2016. https://www.cdc.gov/violenceprevention/pdf/sv-prevention-technical-package.pdf.
115. David-Ferdon C, Vivolo-Kantor AM, Dahlberg LL, Marshall KJ, Rainford N, Hall JE. *A Comprehensive Technical Package for the Prevention of Youth Violence and Associated Risk Behaviors.* Atlanta, GA: National Center for Injury Prevention and Control, Centers for Disease Control and Prevention; 2016. https://www.cdc.gov/violenceprevention/pdf/yv-technicalpackage.pdf.
116. Niolon PH, Kearns M, Dills J, et al. *Preventing Intimate Partner Violence Across the Lifespan: A Technical Package of Programs, Policies, and Practices.* Atlanta, GA: National Center for Injury Prevention and Control, Centers for Disease Control and Prevention; 2017. https://www.cdc.gov/violenceprevention/pdf/ipv-technicalpackages.pdf.
117. Stone DM, Holland KM, Bartholow B, Crosby AE, Davis S, Wilkins N. *Preventing Suicide: A Technical Package of Policies, Programs, and Practices.* Atlanta, GA: National Center for Injury Prevention and Control, Centers for Disease Control and Prevention; 2017. https://www.cdc.gov/violenceprevention/pdf/suicidetechnicalpackage.pdf.
118. Frieden TR. Six components necessary for effective public health program implementation. *Am J Public Health.* 2014;104(1):17–22.
119. Doepke M, Zilibotti F. Parenting with style: Altruism and paternalism in intergenerational preference transmission. *Econometrica.* 2017;85(5):1331–71.
120. Chatterji P, Markowitz, S. Does the length of maternity leave affect maternal health? *South Econ J.* 2005;72(1):16–41.
121. Forget E. The town with no poverty: The health effects of a Canadian guaranteed annual income field experiment. *Can Public Policy.* 2011;37:283–305.
122. Gibson-Davis C, Foster EM. A cautionary tale: Using propensity scores to estimate the effect of Food Stamps on food insecurity. *Soc Serv Rev.* 2006;80:93–126.
123. Klevens J, Barnett SB, Florence C, Moore D. Exploring policies for the reduction of child physical abuse and neglect. *Child Abuse Negl.* 2015;40:1–11.
124. Pressman S. Policies to reduce child poverty: Child allowances versus tax exemptions for children. *J Econ Issues.* 2011;45:323–32.
125. Schnitzer PG, Ewigman BG. Child deaths resulting from inflicted injuries: Household risk factors and perpetrator characteristics. *Pediatrics.* 2005;116(5):e687–93.
126. Tiehen L, Jolliffe D, Gunderson C. *Alleviating Poverty in the United States: The Critical Role of SNAP Benefits.* Washington, DC: U.S. Department of Agriculture, Economic Research Service; 2012.
127. Aumann K, Galinsky E. *The State of Health in the American Workforce: Does having an Effective Workplace Matter?* New York: Families and Work Institute: 2009. http://familiesandwork.org/downloads/StateofHealthinAmericanWorkforce.pdf.
128. Morrissey TW, Warner ME. Why early care and education deserves as much attention, or more, than prekindergarten alone. *Appl Dev Sci.* 2007;11(2):47–70.

129. Milligan K, Stabile M. Do child tax benefits affect the well-being of children? Evidence from Canadian child benefit expansions. *Am Econ J Econ Policy*. 2011;3:175–205.

130. Cancian M, Meyer DR. Testing the economic independence hypothesis: The effect of an exogenous increase in child support on subsequent marriage and cohabitation. *Demography.* 2014;51(3):857–80.

131. Gordon RA, Usdansky ML, Wang X, Guzman A. Child care and mothers' mental health: Is high-quality care associated with fewer depressive symptoms? *Fam Relat.* 2011;60:446–60.

132. Ludwig J, Duncan G, Gennetian LA, et al. Neighborhood effects on the long term well-being of low-income adults. *Science.* 2012;337(3101):1505–10.

133. Sanbonmatsu L, Marvakov J, Potter NA, et al. The long term effects of moving to opportunity on adult health and economic self-sufficiency. *Cityscape.* 2012;14:109–35.

134. Centers for Disease Control and Prevention. *VetoViolence. Making the Case: Engaging Businesses.* 2018. https://vetoviolence.cdc.gov/apps/child-abuse-neglect-biz/.

135. Aubrun A, Grady J. Two Cognitive Obstacles to Preventing Child Abuse: The "Other-Mind" Mistake and the "Family Bubble." Washington, DC: FrameWorks Institute; 2003. http://frameworksinstitute.org/toolkits/canp/resources/pdf/TwoCognitiveObstacles.pdf.

136. O'Neil M. The family bubble, achievement gap, and development as competition: Media frames on youth. *New Dir Youth Dev.* 2009;124:39–49.

137. Carrell SE, Hoekstra ML. Externalities in the classroom: How children exposed to domestic violence affect everyone's kids. *Am Econ J Appl Econ.* 2010;2(1):211–28.

138. Kendall-Taylor N, Simon A, Volmert A. Taking Responsibility for Solutions: Using Values to Reframe Child Maltreatment in the United Kingdom. Washington, DC: FrameWorks Institute [online]; 2014. https://frameworksinstitute.org/assets/files/ECD/nspcc_values.pdf.

139. Centers for Disease Control and Prevention. *Essentials for Childhood: Steps to Create Safe, Stable, Nurturing Relationships and Environments.* Atlanta, GA: National Center for Injury Prevention and Control; 2014. https://www.cdc.gov/violenceprevention/pdf/essentials_for_childhood_framework.pdf.

140. Henley N, Donovan RJ, Morehead H. Appealing to positive motivations and emotions in social marketing: Example of a positive parenting campaign. *Soc Mar Q.* 1998;Summer:49–53.

141. Stannard S, Hall, S, Young J. Social marketing as a tool to stop child abuse. *Soc Mar Q.* 1998;Summer:64–8.

142. ChildTrends. Attitudes Toward Spanking: Indicators of Child and Youth Well-being. Bethesda, MD: ChildTrends; 2015. https://www.childtrends.org/wp-content/uploads/2015/11/51_Attitudes_Toward_Spanking.pdf.

143. Global Initiative to End All Corporal Punishment of Children. London, UK. 2018. www.endcorporalpunishment.org.

144. Gershoff ET, Font SA. Corporal punishment in U.S. public schools: Prevalence, disparities in use, and status in state and federal policy. *Soc Policy Rep.* 2016;30:1.

145. Knox M. On hitting children: A review of corporal punishment in the United States. *J Pediatr Health Care.* 2010;24(2):103–7.

146. Patton S. *Spare the Fids: Why Whupping Children won't Save Black America.* Boston: Beacon Press; 2017.

147. Daro D, Dodge KA. Creating community responsibility for child protection: Possibilities and challenges. *Future Child.* 2009;19(2):67–93.

148. Bussman K, Erthal C, Schroth A. Effects of banning corporal punishment in Europe. In: Durrant JE, Smith AB, eds. *A Five Nation Comparison: Global Pathways to Abolishing Physical Punishment.* New York: Routledge; 2011, pp. 229–322.

149. Leventhal T, Brooks-Gunn J. The neighborhoods they live in: The effects of neighborhood residence on child and adolescent outcomes. *Psychol Bull.* 2000;126(2):309–37.

150. Wodtke GT, Harding DJ, Elwert F. Neighborhood effects in temporal perspective: The impact of long-term exposure to concentrated disadvantage on high school graduation. *Am Sociol Rev.* 2011;76:713–36.

151. Galster G, Marcotte DE, Mandell M., et al. The influence of neighborhood poverty during childhood on fertility, education, and earnings outcomes. *Housing Studies.* 2007;2(5):723–51.

152. Heckman JJ, Masterov DV. The productivity argument for investing in young children. *Appl Econ Perspect Policy.* 2007;29(3):446–93.

153. Reynolds AJ, Temple JA, Ou SR, et al. Effects of a school-based, early childhood intervention on adult health and well-being: A 19-year follow-up of low-income families. *Arch Pediatr Adolesc Med.* 2007;161(8):730–9.

154. Reynolds AJ, Temple JA, Robertson DL, Mann EA. Long-term effects of an early childhood intervention on educational achievement and juvenile arrest: A 15-year follow-up of low-income children in public schools. *JAMA.* 2001;285(18):2339–46.

155. Love JM, Kisker EE, Ross C, et al. The effectiveness of early head start for 3-year-old children and their parents: Lessons for policy and programs. *Dev Psychol.* 2005;41(6):885–901.

156. Peisner-Feinberg ES, Burchinal MR, Clifford RM, et al. The relation of preschool child-care quality to children's cognitive and social developmental trajectories through second grade. *Child Dev.* 2001;72(5):1534–53.

157. Pluess M, Belsky J. Differential susceptibility to rearing experience: The case of childcare. *J Child Psychol Psychiatry.* 2009;50(4):396–404.

158. Watamura SE, Phillips DA, Morrissey TW, McCartney K, Bub K. Double jeopardy: Poorer social-emotional outcomes for children in the NICHD SECCYD experiencing home and child-care environments that confer risk. *Child Dev.* 2011;82(1):48–65.

159. Mersky JP, Topitzes, JD, Reynolds SW. Maltreatment prevention through early childhood intervention: A confirmatory evaluation of the Chicago child-parent center preschool program. *Child Youth Serv Rev.* 2011;33:1454-63.

160. Kaminski JW, Valle LA, Filene JH, Boyle CL. A meta-analytic review of components associated with parent training program effectiveness. *J Abnorm Child Psychol.* 2008;36(4):567–89.

161. Lundahl B, Risser HJ, Lovejoy MC. A meta-analysis of parent training: Moderators and follow-up effects. *Clin Psychol Rev.* 2006;26(1):86–104.

162. Taylor TK, Biglan A. Behavioral family interventions for improving child-rearing: A review of the literature for clinicians and policy makers. *Clin Child Fam Psychol Rev.* 1998;1(1):41–60.

163. Carta JJ, Lefever JB, Bigelow K, Borkowski J, Warren SF. Randomized trial of a cellular phone-enhanced home visitation parenting intervention. *Pediatrics.* 2013;132 Suppl 2:S167–73.

164. Dodge KA, Goodman WB, Murphy RA, O'Donnell K, Sato J, Guptill S. Implementation and randomized controlled trial evaluation of universal postnatal nurse home visiting. *Am J Public Health.* 2014;104 Suppl 1:S136–43.

165. Knox MS, Burkhart K, Hunter KE. ACT against Violence Parents Raising Safe Kids program: Effects on maltreatment-related parenting behaviors and beliefs. *J Fam Issues.* 2011;32:55–74.

166. Webster-Stratton C, Reid MJ, Hammond M. Preventing conduct problems, promoting social competence: A parent and teacher training partnership in head start. *J Clin Child Psychol.* 2001;30(3):283–302.

167. Leeb RT, Lewis T, Zolotor AJ. A review of physical and mental health consequences of child abuse and neglect and implications for practice. *Am J Lifestyle Med.* 2011;5:454–68.

168. Chaffin M, Funderburk B, Bard D, Valle LA, Gurwitch R. A combined motivation and parent-child interaction therapy package reduces child welfare recidivism in a randomized dismantling field trial. *J Consult Clin Psychol.* 2011;79(1):84–95.

169. Chaffin M, Silovsky JF, Funderburk B, et al. Parent-child interaction therapy with physically abusive parents: Efficacy for reducing future abuse reports. *J Consult Clin Psychol.* 2004;72(3):500–10.

170. Dubowitz H, Feigelman S, Lane W, Kim J. Pediatric primary care to help prevent child maltreatment: The Safe Environment for Every Kid (SEEK) Model. *Pediatrics.* 2009;123(3):858–64.

171. Dubowitz H, Lane WG, Semiatin JN, Magder LS. The SEEK model of pediatric primary care: Can child maltreatment be prevented in a low-risk population? *Acad Pediatr.* 2012;12(4):259–68.

172. Gershater-Molko RM, Lutzker JR, Wesch D. Using recidivism data to evaluate project safecare: Teaching bonding, safety, and health care skills to parents. *Child Maltreat.* 2002;7(3):277–85.

173. Linares LO, Montalto D, Li M, Oza SV. A promising parent intervention in foster care. *J Consult Clin Psychol.* 2006;74:32–41.

174. Silovsky JF, Bard D, Chaffin M, Hecht D, Burris L, Owora A, Lutzker J. Prevention of child maltreatment in high-risk rural families: A randomized clinical trial with child welfare outcomes. *Child Youth Serv Rev.* 2011;33:1435–44.

175. Webster-Stratton C, Reid M. Adapting the incredible years: An evidence-based parenting programme for families involved in the child welfare system. *J Child Serv.* 2010;5(1):25–42.

176. Hurlburt MS, Nguyen K, Reid J, Webster-Stratton C, Zhang J. Efficacy of the incredible years group parent program with families in head start who self-reported a history of child maltreatment. *Child Abuse Negl.* 2013;37(8):531–43.

177. Letarte MJ, Normandeau S, Allard J. Effectiveness of a parent training program "Incredible Years" in a child protection service. *Child Abuse Negl.* 2010;34(4):253–61.

178. Milaniak I, Widom CS. Does child abuse and neglect increase risk for perpetration of violence inside and outside the home? *Psychol Violence.* 2015;5(3):246–55.

179. Oshima KMM, Jonson-Reid M, Seay KD. The influence of childhood sexual abuse on adolescent outcomes: The roles of gender, poverty, and revictimization. *J Child Sex Abuse.* 2014;23:367–86.

180. Widom CS, Wilson HW. Intergenerational transmission of violence. In: Lindert J, Levav I, eds. *Violence and Mental Health.* New York: Springer; 2015, pp. 27–45.

181. Cary CE, McMillen, JC. The data behind the dissemination: A systematic review of trauma-focused cognitive behavioral therapy for use with children and youth. *Child Youth Serv Rev.* 2012;34:748–57.

182. Brunk M, Henggeler SW, Whelan JP. Comparison of multisystemic therapy and parent training in the brief treatment of child abuse and neglect. *J Consult Clin Psychol.* 1987;55(2):171–8.

183. Carpentier MY, Silovsky JF, Chaffin M. Randomized trial of treatment for children with sexual behavior problems: Ten-year follow-up. *J Consult Clin Psychol.* 2006;74(3):482–8.

184. Swenson CC, Schaeffer CM, Henggeler SW, Faldowski R, Mayhew AM. Multisystemic Therapy for child abuse and neglect: A randomized effectiveness trial. *J Fam Psychol.* 2010;24(4):497–507.

185. Schaeffer CM, Swenson CC, Tuerk EH, Henggeler SW. Comprehensive treatment for co-occurring child maltreatment and parental substance abuse: Outcomes from a 24-month pilot study of the MST-Building Stronger Families program. *Child Abuse Negl.* 2013;37(8):596–607.

186. Aarons GA, Sommerfeld D, Hecht D, Silovsky J, Chaffin M. The impact of evidence-based practice implementation and fidelity monitoring on staff turnover: Evidence for a protective effect. *J Consult Clin Psychol.* 2009;77(2):270–80.

187. Wilson R, Fortson BL. Treatment of parent-child violence. In: Sturmey P, ed. *The Wiley Handbook of Violence and Aggression.* Hoboken, NJ: John Wiley and Sons; 2017.

CHAPTER

177 Prevention of Youth Violence*

Jeffrey H. Herbst • Khiya J. Marshall • Bradford Bartholow • Jennifer L. Matjasko

INTRODUCTION

Youth violence is a significant public health problem worldwide. This form of violence involves youth and young adults between the ages of 10 and 24 years who either intentionally use physical force or power to threaten or harm others or are victims of violence perpetrated by other youth.[1,2] The consequences of youth violence include homicides, injuries requiring medical attention, psychological trauma, poor development and deprivation, and impact peers, families, schools, and entire communities.[3,4] Exposure to youth violence has been associated with the development of health-risk behaviors such as alcohol and drug use, smoking and unsafe sexual practices; and associated with many adult forms of violent behavior including perpetration of child maltreatment, sexual violence, intimate partner violence, and self-harming behaviors through shared risk and protective factors.[5]

Public health efforts demonstrate youth violence is preventable. A public health approach to youth violence prevention involves a systematic understanding of the magnitude of the problem, identifying important risk and protective factors, developing and testing strategies to address risk and promote protective factors, and widely disseminating effective strategies.[2,6] To effectively prevent youth violence, it is important to address risk and protective factors at multiple levels of the social ecology including the individual, relational, community, and societal levels. Youth violence primary prevention strategies may be directed to age groups early in the developmental lifespan when aggression and other violent behaviors commonly emerge and intensify and continue through adolescence and young adulthood.[7]

This chapter begins with an overview of the nature and burden of youth violence. Next, the social ecological model is used to describe the research on risk and protective factors for youth violence within a developmental framework.[2] Next, programs, policies, and practices with the best available evidence for preventing youth violence are discussed. Finally, considerations are explored to enhance the implementation of evidence-based youth violence prevention programs, policies, and practices, and ultimately produce the greatest public health impact. While most studies cited in this chapter are from the United States (US), evidence from international studies are presented when available.

NATURE AND BURDEN OF THE PROBLEM

Definitions

Youth violence involves the use of physical force or power, threatened or actual, by a person 10–24 years old, against another person that either results in or has a high likelihood of resulting in injury, death, psychological harm, maldevelopment, or deprivation.[4] This form of violence encompasses an array of harmful behaviors that begins in childhood and continues into young adulthood. Youth violence can take many forms including peer-to-peer violence that occurs in communities, school-based violence, bullying, and youth involved in gang violence. Some behaviors, such as bullying, cyberbullying, slapping, and hitting, can have significant consequences but do not always result in serious injury or death.[3] Conversely, physically violent behaviors, such as fighting and assaults with or without a weapon, can lead to serious injury and even death. Youth violence commonly takes place outside the home, in the streets, or in institutional settings such as schools.[3]

School violence is a type of youth violence that occurs on school property, on the way to or from school or school-sponsored events, or during a school-sponsored event. School violence typically involves peer-on-peer violence, but may involve adults including teachers and school staff. While school-associated violent deaths are generally rare, schools do report cases of nonfatal violent victimizations among students aged 12–18 years of age, and school-associated student homicides represent approximately 1% of homicides that occur among school-aged youths.[8]

Bullying is a specific type of youth violence that involves threats to other young people's well-being. The US Centers for Disease Control and Prevention (CDC) defines bullying as "any unwanted aggressive behavior(s) by another youth or group of youths, who are not siblings or current dating partners, involving an observed or perceived power imbalance. These behaviors are repeated multiple times or are highly likely to be repeated."[9] Bullying commonly occurs in person or by use of technological devices. Bullying behaviors include aggression that can be physical (hitting, tripping), verbal (name calling, teasing), or social (spreading rumors, leaving out of group). Electronic bullying (or *cyberbullying*) involves aggressive acts directed at other youths via technological devices (e.g., email, chat rooms, instant messaging, websites, text messages, or social media platforms). Regardless of method, bullying and cyberbullying can inflict significant distress on targeted youth, and often results in harmful physical, psychological, social, or educational consequences.[10]

Youth gang violence involves violence and criminal behavior by young people affiliated with gangs.[11] Youth join gangs for a variety of reasons, including money, sense of support and belonging, peer status, perceived sense of protection, enjoyment, respect, or to demonstrate an outlaw mentality.[11,12] The most common ages for youth to join a gang is 13–15 years. Youth are at high risk for joining a gang if they engage in delinquent behaviors, are aggressive or violent,

*Disclaimer: The findings and conclusions in this chapter are those of the authors and do not necessarily represent the views of the Centers for Disease Control and Prevention.

experience multiple adverse childhood experiences, have problems at school, associate with other gang-involved youth, or live in communities where they feel unsafe and where many youth get in trouble.[11,13] Research suggests that youth in gangs are more likely to abuse drugs, engage in high-risk sexual behaviors, experience long-term health and social consequences and are likely to die due to gang-related homicide.[14,15] While gang members are typically boys, girls join gangs in large numbers, contrary to stereotypes, and many affiliate with gangs through their male dating or sex partners due to many of the reasons stated above.[12] ***Magnitude of Youth Violence*** Worldwide, an estimated 200,000 homicides (43% of all homicides) occur each year among youth and young adults aged 10–29 years. Homicide rates among youth vary dramatically between and across jurisdictions within countries. Globally, 83% of youth homicide victims are males, and, in all countries, males constitute the majority of perpetrators. For every young person killed by violence, many more sustain injuries that require hospital treatment.[4]

Physical fighting and bullying are common among youth. Nearly 40% of young people reported in 2015 that they were in a physical fight during the past year.[16] A study of 40 developing countries showed that an average of 42% of boys and 37% of girls reported exposure to bullying. Youth homicide and nonfatal violence not only contribute greatly to the global burden of premature death, injury, and disability, but also have a serious, often lifelong, impact on a person's psychological and social functioning.

While youth violence is a global problem, the US youth homicide rate is seven times higher than the rate in other high-income countries.[17] Youth violence is a leading cause of fatal and nonfatal injuries in the US. Homicide was the third leading cause of death among youth aged 10–24 years (Web-based Injury Statistics Query and Reporting System).[18] In terms of age groups, homicide was the fourth leading cause of death among youth aged 10–14 years, and the third leading cause of death among young persons aged 15–24 years.[18] Among all youth homicide victims, 87% were killed with a firearm.[18] Each day 1374 young people between the ages of 10 and 24 are treated in emergency departments for nonfatal physical assault-related injuries, a number more than 115 times higher than the number killed.[18] An analysis of nonfatal assault injuries reported in US emergency departments from 2001 to 2015 among young persons aged 10–24 years found higher rates among males (vs. females) and young adults aged 20–24 years (vs. 10–14 and 15–19 years).[19] In addition, rates of nonfatal assaults declined for all groups from 2011 to 2015, with the lowest rate reported in 2015 (753.2 per 100,000 population).[19]

In the US, males aged 10–24 experience a disproportionate burden of fatal injuries resulting from violence. In 2016, 86% of the homicide deaths were male while 14% were female. Overall, crude rates of homicide per 100,000 population were substantially higher among males than females, especially in the 15–19 and 20–24 age groups. Also among these age groups, deaths were stable from 1999 to 2006, declined from 2006 to 2014, and increased from 2014 to 2016. Figure 177-1 presents crude homicide rates by race and ethnicity from 2009 to 2016. Black youth experienced much higher rates of homicide than the other groups across the entire timespan, with marked increases from 2014 to 2016.

Racial and ethnic minority youth in the US experience a disproportionate burden of youth violence. Among 10- to 24-year olds in 2016, homicide was the leading cause of death for non-Hispanic black youth; the second leading cause of death for Hispanics; the third leading cause of death American Indians and Alaska Natives; and fourth leading cause of death among Asian/Pacific Islanders and non-Hispanic whites.[18] Homicide rates reported in 2016 among non-Hispanic, black males (60.5 per 100,000) were five times higher than those of Hispanic males (11.88 per 100,000) and 19 times higher than those of non-Hispanic, white males (3.2 per 100,000).[18] Examination of data from the National Survey on Drug Use and Health, a population-based study of youths aged 12–17, reported a 29% decrease in prevalence of youth fighting and violence among all racial and ethnic groups from 2002 to 2014.[20] However, year-by-year point estimates for these behaviors were consistently highest among non-Hispanic black youths, followed by Hispanics and then non-Hispanic whites.

The CDC's Youth Risk Behavior Surveillance System (YRBS) monitors health-risk behaviors that contribute to the leading causes of death, disability, and social problems among youth and young adults.[21] YRBS provides representative student-reported estimates of different forms of youth violence and is conducted every 2 years. In 2015, nearly a quarter (22.6%) of youth reported being in a physical fight in the 12 months preceding the survey; 16.2% reported carrying a weapon (i.e., gun, knife, or club) on one or more days in the 30 days preceding the survey; and 5.3% reported carrying a gun on one or more days in the 30 days preceding the survey.[22] Data from 2015 also revealed that lesbian, gay, and bisexual (LGB) students, relative to their heterosexual counterparts, reported higher rates of physical fights (28% vs. 22%), physical dating violence (18% vs. 8%), and cyberbullying (28% vs. 14%).[23] An examination of trends in YRBS data over time showed that overall rates of physical fighting and weapon carrying decreased from 2009 to 2015; other forms of violence behavior remained stable.[24]

Biennial YRBS data from 2009 to 2015 are presented in Table 177-1 for male and female students.[22,25–27] Data reported in 2015 are compared to prior years. In 2015, fewer females reported physical fights (compared to 2009 and 2011), being in a physical fight on school property (compared to 2011), and not attending school because of safety concerns (compared to 2013). However, females reported greater bullying on school property in 2013 and 2015 than in 2011. For males, several violence-related behaviors were lower in 2015 than in 2009 and 2011. Compared to the earlier years, fewer males reported in 2015 they carried a weapon on school property, were threatened or injured with a weapon on school property, were in a physical fight, and were in a physical fight on school property. Fewer males reported being bullied on school property in 2015 than in 2009. It should be noted that the latest YRBS data collected in 2015 occurred before the upticks in youth violence rates suggested by homicide data from vital statistics.

Health and Economic Burden of Youth Violence

The health and economic consequences of youth violence are substantial. Nonfatal youth violence often results in medical care to treat cuts, lacerations, bruises, broken bones, and gunshot wounds. Some injuries, like gunshot wounds, can lead to disabilities and mental health treatment. As youth can be exposed to violence as a perpetrator, a victim, or a witness of behavior committed by others, the impact of these exposures produce lasting psychological and physical harm on youth, their families, schools, and communities. These exposures also increase the likelihood of future violence victimization and perpetration. Individual-level consequences of youth violence may include academic difficulties and not attending school due to fear or feeling unsafe,[28,29] engaging in risky behaviors,[30] depression and social isolation,[10,31] and self-injury including suicide.[32,33] Relational- and familial-level consequences may include poor peer relationships[34–38] and low levels of attachment to parents or caregivers.[39] Community and societal consequences may include increased medical and justice costs, decreased property values in neighborhoods, and disruption of services.[40]

A WHO review of the international literature reports considerable consequences of youth violence on health, social, and behavioral problems, as well as academic performance.[16] The association of youth violence with health-related problems includes an over twofold increased likelihood of mental and neurological disorders (including suicidal ideation and behavior, depressive symptoms and somatic symptoms), increased likelihood of poor general health, and

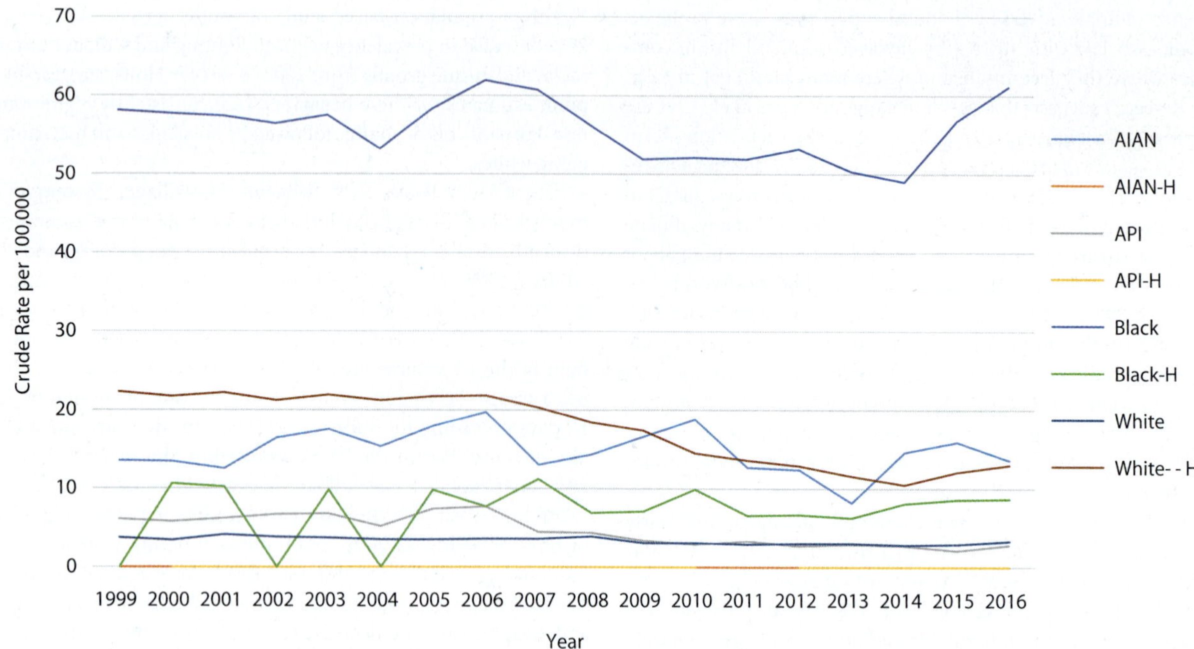

FIGURE 177-1. Violence-related injury deaths (crude rates per 100,000 population) by race and ethnicity among youth aged 10–24 Years, United States, 1999–2016. (*Source:* Centers for Disease Control and Prevention, National Center for Injury Prevention and Control. Web-based Injury Statistics Query and Reporting System (WISQARS). Available online: www.cdc.gov/injury/wisqars [accessed on 29 March 2019].

increased likelihood of health-risk behaviors including drug use. In addition, exposure to youth violence was associated with an increase in externalizing behavior problems, subsequent violence perpetration, and violent victimization.

The economic burden of youth violence extends well beyond physical consequences and constitutes a major burden on health systems. For example, in the US homicides and nonfatal physical assault-related injuries among youth result in an estimated $18.6 billion (US dollars) annually in combined medical and lost productivity costs alone.[18] This estimate is a fraction of the true economic consequences of youth violence because it does not include criminal justice system costs, such as arrests, prosecutions, incarcerations, and re-entry, or the costs associated with addressing the psychological and social consequences for victims, perpetrators, and their families.

Cost estimates also do not factor in medical costs due to longer-term consequences (e.g., mental health or impact on infectious or chronic diseases), only immediate costs of treating injuries are included in these estimates. Moreover, estimates do not include the costs incurred by communities to address victims' needs (e.g., property damage, lost wages) that result from youth violence and crime or the substantial economic impacts on communities' healthcare system, property values, and social services systems. The costs of responding to youth violence significantly limits the resources states, communities, and countries possess to address other needs and goals.

RISK AND PROTECTIVE FACTORS

To prevent the health and social consequences of youth violence, stopping perpetration is essential. A focus on protecting victims will not address the root causes of violence. Research on risk and protective factors for violence perpetration among youth often frames those factors within the social ecological model. There is a complex interplay of different characteristics and conditions that cause youth violence, and risk and protective factors are situated at the individual, relational, community, and societal levels. In addition, risk and protective factors for youth violence can be examined from a developmental perspective. Various developmental trajectories of youth violence identify risk factors extending back into early childhood.[41,42] Regardless of pathway, it is important to keep in mind that the presence of risk is not deterministic; no single risk factor leads to youth violence and the presence of risk does not mean a particular youth will perpetrate violence.

Individual-level Risk and Protective Factors

Risk factors for various forms of youth violence include individual characteristics along with traumatic experiences. The individual characteristics that are consistently associated with youth violence include impulsiveness, substance use, antisocial or aggressive beliefs and attitudes, low achievement, weak connection to school, history of child abuse and neglect, exposure to violence in the home and community, depression, anxiety, chronic stress, and trauma. A lack of personal connection to prosocial individuals and institutions is also a risk factor for violence among youth. Developmental research shows that individuals who engage in violent behavior during adolescence are more likely to be male, demonstrate aggressive behavior in childhood, and display impulsivity and inattentiveness throughout the lifespan.[16,43]

Individual-level protective factors buffer youth from perpetrating violence. They also include a mix of individual characteristics, skills, and experiences. They include school achievement, high educational aspirations, positive peer relationships, social skills, problem-solving and planning skills, and religiosity.[34,36–38] Fostering opportunities for youth to achieve emotional and behavioral autonomy, resolving identity issues, and acquiring education and other experiences needed to make a successful transition to adulthood provide opportunities to protect youth from becoming involved with violence.

Relational- and Familial-level Risk and Protective Factors

Risk factors for youth violence at the relationship and familial levels involve an array of parenting/caregiver characteristics as well as peer relationships.[34–38] Family risk factors include lack of parental supervision, parenting styles characterized by harsh, inconsistent, or uninvolved parenting, as well as family dysfunction, and family instability. Parental characteristics include low parental education and income,

TABLE 177-1 PERCENTAGE (AND 95% CONFIDENCE INTERVAL) OF HIGH SCHOOL STUDENTS WHO REPORTED WEAPON CARRYING AND VIOLENCE-RELATED BEHAVIORS, YOUTH RISK BEHAVIOR SURVEILLANCE (YRBS) SURVEY, 2009–15

	Years			
	2009	**2011**	**2013**	**2015**
Female				
Carried a weapon[a]	7.1 (6.3–7.9)	6.8 (6.1–7.7)	7.9 (6.8–9.1)	7.5 (6.1–9.3)
Carried a gun[a]	1.7 (1.3–2.3)	1.4 (1.1–1.8)	1.6 (1.2–2.2)	1.6 (1.2–2.0)
Carried a weapon on school property[a]	2.9 (2.5–3.4)	2.3 (2.0–2.8)	3.0 (2.2–3.9)	2.0 (1.5–2.7)
Threatened or injured with a weapon on school property[b]	5.5 (4.8–6.3)	5.2 (4.5–6.0)	6.1 (5.3–7.0)	4.6 (3.9–5.5)
In a physical fight[b]	22.9 (21.4–24.4)	24.4 (22.6–26.3)	19.2 (17.8–20.7)	16.5 (14.5–18.7)
Injured in a physical fight[b]	2.2 (1.8–2.8)	2.6 (2.2–3.0)	2.4 (1.9–2.9)	1.8 (1.4–2.3)
In a physical fight on school property[b]	6.7 (5.9–7.6)	7.8 (7.0–8.7)	5.6 (4.9–6.5)	5.0 (4.1–6.0)
Bullied on school property[c]	21.2 (19.6–22.7)	18.2 (16.6–20.1)	23.7 (22.3–25.2)	24.8 (22.8–26.9)
Did not go to school because of safety concerns[a]	5.3 (4.6–6.1)	6.0 (5.0–7.3)	8.7 (7.4–10.2)	6.0 (5.1–7.1)
Electronically bullied[c,d]	NA	22.1 (20.9–23.3)	21.0 (19.2–22.9)	21.7 (20.1–23.4)
Male				
Carried a weapon[a]	27.1 (24.3–30.2)	25.9 (23.8–28.2)	28.1 (25.6–30.9)	24.3 (21.9–27.0)
Carried a gun[a]	9.8 (8.3–11.7)	8.6 (7.6–9.7)	9.4 (8.1–11.0)	8.7 (7.3–10.3)
Carried a weapon on school property[a]	8.0 (7.1–9.2)	8.2 (7.1–9.5)	7.6 (6.3–9.1)	5.9 (5.0–6.9)
Threatened or injured with a weapon on school property[b]	9.6 (8.5–10.8)	9.5 (8.7–10.3)	7.7 (6.7–8.9)	7.0 (6.1–8.1)
In a physical fight[b]	39.3 (36.9–41.7)	40.7 (39.2–42.2)	30.2 (28.0–32.4)	28.4 (26.3–30.5)
Injured in a physical fight[b]	5.1 (4.4–6.0)	5.1 (4.6–5.8)	3.8 (3.3–4.4)	3.7 (3.1–4.5)
In a physical fight on school property[b]	15.1 (13.1–17.3)	16.0 (14.9–17.2)	10.7 (9.6–11.8)	10.3 (8.8–12.0)
Bullied on school property[c]	18.7 (17.4–20.1)	18.2 (16.6–20.1)	15.6 (14.2–17.0)	15.8 (14.5–17.2)
Did not go to school because of safety concerns[a]	4.6 (3.8–5.6)	5.8 (5.0–6.9)	5.4 (4.4–6.7)	5.0 (4.2–5.9)
Electronically bullied[c,d]	NA	10.8 (9.6–12.0)	8.5 (7.7–9.5)	9.7 (8.4–11.1)

Note: NA = not asked in survey. YRBS data drawn from CDC MMWRs.[22,25–27]
[a]On at least 1 day during the 30 days before the survey.
[b]One or more times during the 12 months before the survey.
[c]During the 12 months before the survey.
[d]Includes being bullied through e-mail, chat rooms, instant messaging, Web sites, or texting.

parental substance abuse, and deviant behavior. Peer relationships are also important risk factors for youth violence and include involvement with delinquent peers, gang involvement, as well as peer conflict and rejection. Developmental research shows that family, parental, and peer factors come together to predict violent behavior during adolescence.[42,43] Those youth tend to have parents who offer little supervision and guidance, which likely provide opportunities to engage in violence. Violent peers might also provide a context in which violence is accepted and encouraged.[43]

Protective factors include connectedness to parents and prosocial adults and peers. The quality of the parent-adolescent relationship is important in buffering youth from violence. Those youth who have warm relationships with their parents and have the ability to discuss problems with them are less likely to engage in violent behavior. The activities that youth engage in also matter. Youth who have frequent shared activities with their parents and are involved in prosocial activities with peers (e.g., extracurricular activities) report less involvement with violence.[36–38,44]

Community- and Societal-level Risk and Protective Factors

Risk factors at the community and societal levels involve important contextual conditions that provide the conditions or opportunities for youth to engage in violence. These include neighborhood conditions associated with poverty and blight (e.g., residential instability, crowded housing, a high alcohol outlet density, poor economic growth or stability, unemployment, concentrated poverty, neighborhood violence and crime, lack of positive relationships among residents, and positive norms around community drug use and crime).[45,46] Societal-level conditions include policies and other social conditions that might contribute to individuals' sense that there are limited opportunities for success. This may result in individuals turning to violence to gain feelings of power and status. These societal-level risk factors include economic and limited opportunities to secure safe and affordable housing.[47,48]

Protective factors include the physical conditions and social processes at the neighborhood level that promote health and safety. Neighborhoods with safe greenspaces and parks are associated with lower community violence. Communities with thriving businesses are also associated with lower rates of crime and violence.[49,50] Neighborhood social processes that encourage collective efficacy, or the extent to which residents monitor and look out for each other, also buffer youth from becoming involved with violence.[45]

BEST AVAILABLE EVIDENCE

The field of youth violence prevention is well developed due to decades of research. Research shows that the prevention of youth violence requires a crosscutting approach from every level of the social ecological model.[2] Prevention must also address the social determinants of violence, such as income inequality, rapid demographic and social change, and low levels of social protection.[51] Further, youth should be provided ample opportunity to meet the developmental needs of adolescence and young adulthood.[52] To implement such a crosscutting approach, specific strategies are necessary to prevent youth violence.

CDC released several technical packages to prevent various forms of violence.[53] The technical packages highlight strategies and approaches with evidence to support effective public health program implementation.[54] The technical packages serve as a resource to guide and inform decision-making in communities, and can be used across sectors to address and reduce multiple forms of violence.

The technical package, *A Comprehensive Technical Package for the Prevention of Youth Violence and Associated Risk Behaviors*,[56] represents a core set of strategies and approaches based on the best available evidence in youth violence prevention.[54] *Strategies* provide the direction or actions to achieve the goal of preventing youth violence, and *approaches* describe the specific ways to advance each strategy. Evidence for each approach includes programs, practices, or policies that have been evaluated for impact on youth violence outcomes or associated risk and protective factors. The six strategies in the youth violence technical package include:

1. ***Promote family environments that support healthy development;***
2. ***Provide quality education early in life;***
3. ***Strengthen youth's skills;***
4. ***Connect youth to caring adults and activities;***
5. ***Create protective community environments; and***
6. ***Intervene to lessen harms and prevent future risk.***

These six strategies, along with corresponding approaches and specific programs, practices, or policies, are listed in Table 177-2. Strategies and approaches included in the technical package represent different levels of the social ecology, with prevention focused on impacting individual behaviors, relationships, and communities that influence risk and protective factors for youth violence.[55] Table 177-2 is not intended to be an exhaustive list of effective strategies for preventing youth violence, but merely highlights example programs with evidence of reducing violence. Several comprehensive registries or compendia of evidence-based and evidence-informed youth violence prevention programs are available online.[56–60] As the youth violence prevention field continues to expand, additional approaches, programs, and polices to address community and societal influences of youth violence will be added to the technical package.

Promote Family Environments that Support Healthy Development

Promotion of family environments that support both parents and their children may prevent youth violence. The family is essential for the development of a child's behavioral, physical, emotional, and social health, which can have lasting effects throughout life.[61,62] Two approaches with evidence of helping families create and maintain the healthy development of their children include *early childhood home visitation programs* and *parenting skill and family relationship programs*. Early childhood home visitation programs provide information, caregiver support, training about child development, and help with accessing services. *Nurse Family Partnership® (NFP)* is one type of home visitation program that has successfully reduced childhood behavior problems (arrests, convictions, and probation violations) as well as parental coping problems.[63,64] *Incredible Years®* and *Coping Power* are examples of parenting skill and family relationship programs. These programs assist caregivers with support by providing communication, problem solving, monitoring, and behavior management skills training. *Incredible Years®* focuses on youth up to 12 years old and their families. The program has shown decreases with disruptive behaviors at home and school and increases in prosocial behaviors.[65] *Coping Power* focuses on older youth aged 10–17, which is a critical time in an adolescence's life and can lead to an increase in risk behaviors. Evidence suggests that *Coping Power* decreases aggressive acts and delinquency, substance use, and parent's lack of support.[66–68]

Provide Quality Education Early in Life

Providing children with quality education at a young age not only helps the child with their socioemotional and cognitive development but also allows the child to have positive long-term impacts on academic success and health, including lower rates of violence and problem behaviors.[69,70] Provision of a safe, stable, nurturing relationships, and environment improve when children receive quality education early in life.

Preschool enrichment with family engagement is one approach to providing quality education early in life. This approach helps set the foundation for a child's development, including academic, social, and behavioral components. Many of these programs help support

TABLE 177-2 EVIDENCE-BASED STRATEGIES, APPROACHES AND PROGRAMS TO PREVENT YOUTH VIOLENCE BASED ON CDC'S YOUTH VIOLENCE TECHNICAL PACKAGE[55]

Strategy	Approach	Program, Practice, or Policy
Promote family environments that support healthy development	Early childhood home visitation	Nurse–Family Partnership®[a,b,c,d,e,f,g]
	Parenting skill and family relationship programs	The Incredible Years®[a,b,c,d,e,f,g]
		Parent Management Training—Oregon Model™[c]
		Strengthening Families 10–14[a,b,c,d,e,f]
		Coping Power[b,d,e,f]
		Familias Unidas™[b,c,d,e,f]
Provide quality education early in life	Preschool enrichment with family engagement	Child-Parent Centers[d,e,g]
		Early Head Start[b,g]
Strengthen youth's skills	Universal school-based programs	Good Behavior Game[a,b,c,d,e,f]
		Promoting Alternative THinking Strategies (PATHS)®[b,c,d,e,f,g]
		LifeSkills® Training[a,b,c,d,e,f,g]
		Steps to Respect®: A Bullying Prevention Program[b,c,d,e,f]
Connect youth to caring adults and activities	Mentoring programs[$]	Big Brothers Big Sisters of America[b,c,d,e,f,g]
	After-school programs	Los Angeles' Better Educated Students for Tomorrow (LA's BEST)[g]
		After School Matters
Create protective community environments	Modify the physical and social environment	Business improvement districts[b,d,g]
		Crime Prevention through Environmental Design (CPTED)[b,g]
	Reduce exposure to community-level risks	Tax credits (Earned Income Tax Credit, Child Tax Credit, Low Income Housing Tax Credit)[g]
		Alcohol policies (outlet density pricing)[b,g]
	Street outreach and community norm change	Cure Violence (formerly Chicago CeaseFire)[b,d,e]
		Safe Streets
Intervene to lessen harms and prevent future risk	Treatment to lessen harms of violence exposure	Trauma-focused Cognitive Behavioral Therapy (TF-CBT)®[b,c,d,e]
		Cognitive Behavioral Intervention for Trauma in Schools (CBITS)[c,d,e,f]

TABLE 177-2 EVIDENCE-BASED STRATEGIES, APPROACHES AND PROGRAMS TO PREVENT YOUTH VIOLENCE BASED ON CDC'S YOUTH VIOLENCE TECHNICAL PACKAGE[55] *(Continued)*

Strategy	Approach	Program, Practice, or Policy
	Treatment to prevent problem behavior and future violence	Functional Family Therapy[a,b,c,d,e,f,g]
		Multidimensional Treatment Foster Care (now called Treatment Foster Care Oregon)[a,b,d,e,f]
		Multisystemic Therapy®[a,b,c,d,e,f,g]
	Hospital-community partnerships	SafERteens[e]
		Caught in the Crossfire

[a]Programs and policies with demonstrated economic benefits that exceed implementation costs (see David-Ferdon et al., page 37).[55]
[b]Included in CDC's *STRYVE Selector Tool*: https://vetoviolence.cdc.gov/apps/stryve/strategyselector; no categories describing program effectiveness.[56]
[c]Included in SAMHSA's *National Registry of Evidence-based Programs and Practices*: https://www.samhsa.gov/nrepp; no categories describing program effectiveness.[58]
[d]Included in National Institute of Justice's *Crime Solutions*: http://www.crimesolutions.gov; categories include effective, promising, no effects.[59]
[e]Included in Office of Juvenile Justice and Delinquency Prevention's Model Program Guide: https://www.ojjdp.gov/mpg; categories include effective, promising, no effects[57]
[f]Included in University of Colorado Boulder's *Blueprints*: http://www.blueprintsprograms.com/; categories include model plus, model, promising.[60]
[g]Included in World Health Organization's *Preventing Youth Violence: An Overview of the Evidence*: http://www.who.int/violence_injury_prevention/violence/youth/youth_violence/en/.[4]

economically disadvantaged families and they include parental involvement to help the child succeed in school. These programs occur across the developmental spectrum and may extend into early or middle childhood. *Child Parent Centers (CPCs)* and *Early Head Start (EHS)* are two programs with extensive evidence. Evidence demonstrates reductions in arrest rates, aggressive behavior, physical or sexual abuse encounters, substance use, and grade retention as well as increases high school completion, 4-year college attendance, and full-time employment for children participating in these programs.[69–74]

Strengthen Youth's Skills

Research demonstrates that strengthening youth's skills prevents both youth violence perpetration and victimization. Communication, problem solving, and empathy are important skills needed to prevent youth violence.[75] *Universal school-based programs* (sometimes also referred to as social-emotional learning approaches) work to enhance interpersonal and emotional skills as well as provide education and skills necessary to change behaviors.[75,76] These programs are available to all youth regardless of current or prior behavioral problems. Evidence shows that from prekindergarten through high school, *universal school-based programs* decreased violent behavior within diverse school environments (i.e., race/ethnicity, socioeconomic status, and crime rates).[76] Two school-based programs, *Life Skills® Training* and *Steps to Respect*, showed significant reductions in youth violence. Youth that participated in *Life Skills® Training* showed decreases in delinquency, fighting, substance abuse, smoking, and HIV risk behaviors compared to youth not participating in the program.[77] *Steps to Respect* participants experienced decreases in bullying and victimization and increases in positive bystander behavior compared to youth not participating in the program.[78,79]

Connect Youth to Caring Adults and Activities

Parents and caring adults (i.e., teachers, coaches, extended family members, neighbors, community volunteers) play a critical role in creating positive environments that help youth decide not to engage in risk behaviors such as substance use, risky sexual behaviors, and violence.[80] Two approaches include *mentoring programs* and *after-school programs*. Mentoring programs allow youth to build positive relationships with adults that will help with their skill development, academic achievement, and have an opportunity for personal growth.[81,82] *Big Brothers Big Sisters of America* is one mentoring program that showed a delay in substance use and engaging in a physical fight over an 18-month period.[83]

In addition to mentoring programs, after-school programs allow youth to improve their social and academic skills during a critical time of the day (3:00–6:00 pm) when violence increases among youth.[84] Youth are able to complete obtain assistance with their schoolwork and are able to participate in community activities. *Los Angeles' Better Educated Students for Tomorrow (LA's Best)* is one after-school program that has shown improvements in academic achievement and reductions in youth arrest rates.[85]

Create Protective Community Environments

Protective community environments include areas where the community gathers and interacts (e.g., schools, parks, and business districts) to reduce risk behaviors and increase protective factors for youth violence.[55] According to the technical package, three community-level approaches have promise for improving settings associated with youth violence victimization and perpetration: *modifying the physical and social environment*, *reduce exposure to community-level risks*, and *street outreach and community norm change*. Modifying physical and social environments can prevent violence by establishing and maintaining community connectedness and social interaction. *Crime Prevention Through Environmental Design (CPTED)* is a type of environmental design activity that provides updates to the visual structure with adequate maintenance to encourage social interactions and the improved use of spaces (e.g., updating green spaces).[86] *CPTED* has been able to reduce robberies, gun assaults, youth homicide, violent crime, and disorderly conduct.[87–92]

Reducing exposure to community-level risks can reduce risks such as poverty, housing instability, and alcohol-density outlets by creating and imposing laws. For example, the *Low-Income Housing Tax Credit (LIHTC)* helps communities develop urban communities with safe and affordable rental housing.[93] *LIHTC* not only reduced poverty in these communities, but also reduced crime and aggravated assault.[93,94]

Street outreach and community norm change programs help prevent violence by engaging youth with community supports and help mediate conflicts.[95] *Cure Violence* (formerly known as *Ceasefire*) is a type of street outreach program that resulted in reductions in assaults and shootings, as well as aggravated battery in half of the communities that implemented the program.[96]

Intervene to Lessen Harms and Prevent Future Risk

Programs that lessen harms and trauma experienced by youth can help prevent future violence. Three approaches that address risk and prevent the continuation or escalation of violence include: *treatment to lessen the harms of violence exposures*, *treatment to prevent problem behavior and further involvement in violence*, and *hospital-community partnerships*. Therapeutic treatment can help lessen the harms of violence exposures. *Trauma-Focused Cognitive Behavioral Therapy® (TF-CBT)* is one example of therapeutic treatment that reduces depression, PTSD symptoms, and helps to improve parenting skills.[97,98] Treating youth that have been involved in violence, crime, and delinquency is critical to the prevention of future violence. *Multisystemic Therapy® (MST)* is a type of program that has demonstrated benefits for youth and their families. *MST* has shown reductions in violent felony arrests, child abuse, substance use, and improved parental practices.[99–101]

Hospital-community partnerships connect acute treatment of violence-related injuries and community assistance to prevent future health-risk behaviors. *SafERteens* is one hospital-based program that uses motivational interviewing for youth with a history of alcohol use and problem violent behaviors.[102] *SafERteens* has been shown to reduce both victimization and perpetration of peer violence[102] and decrease dating violence victimization and alcohol use.[103,104] *ProjectSYNC* is an adaptation of *SafERteens* for youth without a history of violence or alcohol use. The program decreased violence perpetration and increased self-efficacy to avoid a fight.[105]

International Evidence

In 2015, the WHO published *Preventing Youth Violence: An Overview of the Evidence*[4] to describe the evidence of 21 prevention programs, practices, and polices (programs highlighted in Table 177-2, see footnote). Many of the programs identified by WHO are based on US studies and categorized into the following four areas:

1. Parenting and early childhood development (*Nurse-Family Partnership®* and *The Incredible Years®*);
2. School-based academic and social skills development (*Promoting Alternative THinking Strategies®, LifeSkills® Training, and Los Angeles' Better Educated Students for Tomorrow*);
3. Young people at higher risk of or already involved in violence (*Big Brothers Big Sisters of America; Functional Family Therapy*; and *Multisystemic Therapy®*); and
4. Community and societal level (*Business Improvement Districts, Crime Prevention through Environmental Design*, tax credits, and alcohol policies).

Additional strategies include the *Olweus Bullying Prevention Program*[106,107] for elementary and middle school youth shown to reduce self-reported bullying and victimization, and financial grants and housing vouchers. In another example, the United Kingdom's *Cardiff Model* for the prevention of violence involved data sharing between hospital emergency departments and police to identify community-based violence hotspots. The identification of hotspots combined with an effort to identify the drivers and context of violence in these hotspots led to interventions resulting in reduced rates of violence-related injuries treated in hospitals and violence-related injuries reported to the police.[108]

IMPLEMENTATION CONSIDERATIONS

Research suggests that each of the six strategies listed in the CDC's youth violence technical package has evidence for preventing youth violence, and/or associated risk and protective factors. The implementation of a single strategy or approach will be beneficial but may not produce maximum impact on preventing youth violence. Instead, comprehensive prevention involves the implementation of multiple evidence-based strategies and approaches, across several levels of the social ecology, in a variety of settings and in collaboration with various sectors to produce long-term and widespread effects on youth violence outcomes.[109] Implementation of a comprehensive approach to youth violence prevention must consider several challenges. These challenges include few empirically supported approaches at the community and societal levels, determination of the best approaches to implement and evaluate prevention at scale, focus on conditions that perpetuate inequities in violence among youth, and involvement of multisectoral coalitions to enhance impact.

The current evidence base for youth violence prevention contains few empirically supported approaches at the outer levels of the social ecology (i.e., community and societal levels).[110] Although several approaches listed in Table 177-2 aim to modify the physical and social environments, reduce exposure to community-levels risks, and involve street outreach to change community norms, additional community-level approaches are needed to complement the robust evidence base of individual- and relationship-level prevention strategies. Community-level risk factors that could be addressed by youth violence prevention approaches include reducing the density of risky venues in neighborhoods and communities, altering social norms favorable of violence, and stabilizing neighborhoods experiencing mobility of residents and social disorganization. Feasible and sustainable approaches may include policies that seek to improve the conditions of neighborhoods and communities. For example, an urban blight remediation program involving the restoration of abandoned buildings significantly and sustainably reduced firearm violence by 39% in one community.[90] Policies, in conjunction with other approaches, can be evaluated for potential impact on youth violence outcomes in different communities and settings.

Another important consideration involves understanding how to implement and evaluate multiple youth violence prevention programs at scale to enhance reach and impact. This involves developing and testing ways to adapt programs that encourage community-wide uptake of evidence-based youth violence prevention strategies. Potential adaptations may include re-structuring the timing of the sessions (e.g., condensing six weekly 1-hour sessions into two 3-hour weekend sessions), training community members to facilitate programs, and identifying and delivering key components of programs.[111] There are also data-driven strategic prevention models (otherwise known as prevention operating systems) that show promise, including Communities That Care (CTC)[112] and PROmoting School-community-university Partnerships to Encourage Resiliency (PROSPER).[113] The CTC system uses community data to identify multifaceted interventions to prevent violence. Results from a community randomized trial demonstrated significant reductions in delinquent behaviors (e.g., stealing, damaging property, carrying a handgun, being arrested), violent acts, and substance use up to 8 years after implementation of CTC.[112] Results of an evaluation of the PROSPER partnership delivery system showed that 1–5 years after implementation, intervention participants compared to controls exhibited fewer conduct problems (e.g., truancy, stealing, physical fighting, damaging property, and carrying a concealed weapon).[113]

Evidence from the CDC's National Centers of Excellence in Youth Violence Prevention (or Youth Violence Prevention Centers; YVPCs) demonstrates both successes and challenges to implementing and evaluating comprehensive evidence-based approaches for youth violence prevention.[114] Since 2000, the YVPCs established academic-community partnerships to gather data for understanding the magnitude and nature of youth violence in communities, to understand key youth violence risk and protective factors, and to develop and test youth violence prevention interventions. Since their inception, the YVPCs demonstrated success in reducing youth violence in targeted communities while also generating a body of generalizable science to inform prevention activities in other communities.[114–116]

Myriad implementation challenges were reported by the YVPC researchers. One challenge involves the identification, systematic collection and analysis of community-level youth violence outcome, and indicator data to assess the impact of prevention interventions.[117] The YVPCs employ a range of creative sources for data on youth violence within the communities they have worked with including data on fatal outcomes (e.g., violent deaths including homicides, death certificates, uniform crime reports) and nonfatal outcomes (e.g., crime incidents, school discipline incidents, juvenile justice services, emergency department data, ambulance pick-ups, and YRBS school-based risk behaviors). Another implementation challenge involves developing community-informed processes for the selection of a comprehensive set of evidence-based prevention programs.[118] Key considerations the YVPCs and their community partners use include community capacity, infrastructure, and readiness for program implementation, the roles of researchers and community stakeholders in program selection and sustainability, use of data to inform program decision-making, and determination of program reach, resources, and dosage. Another challenge relates to the evaluation of comprehensive youth violence prevention programs. YVPCs use study designs to effectively measure impact (e.g., interrupted time series and multiple baseline designs as opposed to randomized controlled trials).[119] A final implementation challenge reported by the YVPCs pertains to engaging and partnering with community stakeholders to achieve and sustain participation in evidence-based programs.[120] The YVPCs are finding that building trust is the foundation of a strong partnership with community stakeholders. In many of the high-risk communities where rates of youth violence are highest, there is unfortunately a history of mistrust, especially of science. The YVPCs found building trust requires investment of time in partnership development; transparency about level of community involvement and acknowledging and respecting different agendas among partners; critical importance of tactful and direct communication when voicing concerns and attending to feedback from all partners; and indicating commitment by building upon the strengths and assets within a community.[120]

Prior research demonstrates that a focus on the conditions that perpetuate inequities in violence among youth can inform ways to reduce risk and increase resilience among youth and their communities. Globally, low-income communities and communities of color often accumulate an overwhelming number of risk factors for violence, and many of these same communities lack resources to protect against violence.[4] Young people who reside in neighborhoods and communities that experience social inequities also often experience persistent or chronic traumatic stress and violence that may perpetuate health inequities and other adverse health conditions.[51,121] It is important to address the daily circumstances (e.g., quality education early in life, quality housing and transportation, and adequate working conditions) and the structural dynamics of resources and power to help prevent youth violence.[51,122] Implementation of violence prevention strategies can help reduce health inequities and other related outcomes among youth.[122] This will require a comprehensive approach that includes informing policy, bringing together networks to achieve broader goals, providing knowledge to community members and providers, increasing individual knowledge and skills, and modifying organizational norms and practices.[123]

Another important consideration for implementation relates to the involvement of multisectoral coalitions to address youth violence. Communities can raise awareness of youth violence as a public health problem with their leaders, local or state health departments (or ministries of health) and other decision makers[4] by collaborating with the following sectors: education, healthcare, justice, social services, business, housing, and the media.[55] Nongovernmental organizations, such as faith-based organizations, youth-serving organizations and foundations, can also contribute to youth violence prevention activities within communities. By raising awareness and developing collaborations with disparate sectors, communities can marshal resources to address the context and underlying risk factors contributing to youth violence.[124]

CONCLUSION

Youth violence is a significant public health problem that is preventable. Risk and protective factors for youth violence have been identified, and numerous evidence-based prevention strategies are available for implementation. While most prevention strategies to reduce youth violence focus on individuals and relationships with peers and families, evidence is emerging that multifaceted, comprehensive youth violence prevention strategies at all levels of the social ecology are needed to produce the population-level impact.[55,114] In addition, efforts to prevent other forms of violence, including child abuse and neglect, dating violence and sexual violence, may also impact youth violence through shared risk and protective factors.[5] The prevention strategies and approaches reviewed in this chapter inform a public health approach to violence prevention and health promotion, lesson harms, and prevent future violence among youth.[6] Additional research is needed to identify additional prevention strategies at the outer levels of the social ecology, examine the efforts of multiple sectors to prevent youth violence and its consequences, and determine the most efficient and effective ways to implement comprehensive youth violence prevention strategies that result in the greatest public health impact.

References

1. David-Ferdon C, Simon, TR. *Preventing Youth Violence: Opportunities for Action*. Atlanta, GA: Centers for Disease Control and Prevention; 2014:1–54.
2. Dahlberg LL, Krug EG. Violence: A global public health problem. In: Krug EG, Dahlberg LL, Mercy JA, Zwi AB, Lozano R, eds. *World Report on Violence and Health*. Geneva, Switzerland: World Health Organization; 2002:1–56.
3. Centers for Disease Control and Prevention. *Youth Violence*. Atlanta, GA: National Center for Injury Control and Prevention, Division of Violence Prevention; 2017. https://www.cdc.gov/violenceprevention/youthviolence/index.html. Accessed December 4, 2017.
4. World Health Organization. *Preventing Youth Violence: An Overview of the Evidence*. Geneva, Switzerland: World Health Organization; 2015:1–96.
5. Wilkins N, Tsao B, Hertz M, Davis R, Klevens J. *Connecting the Dots: An Overview of the Links Among Multiple Forms of Violence*. Atlanta, GA: National Center for Injury Prevention and Control, Centers for Disease Control and Prevention; 2014:1–16.
6. Sood AB, Berkowitz SJ. Prevention of youth violence: A public health approach. *Child Adolesc Psychiatr Clin N Am*. 2016;25:243–56.
7. Heinze JE, Stoddard SA, Aiyer SM, Eisman AB, Zimmerman MA. Exposure to violence during adolescence as a predictor of perceived stress trajectories in emerging adulthood. *J Appl Dev Psychol*. 2017;49:31–8.
8. Centers for Disease Control and Prevention. School-associated student homicides—United States, 1992–2006. *MMWR Morb Mortal Wkly Rep*. 2008;57(2):33–6.
9. Gladden RM, Vivolo-Kantor AM, Hamburger ME, Lumpkin CD. *Bullying Surveillance Among Youths: Uniform Definitions for Public Health and Recommended Data Elements, Version 1.0*. Atlanta, GA: National Center for Injury Prevention and Control, Centers for Disease Control and Prevention and US Department of Education; 2014:1–116.
10. Arseneault L, Walsh E, Trzesniewski K, Newcombe R, Caspi A, Moffitt TE. Bullying victimization uniquely contributes to adjustment problems in young children: A nationally representative cohort study. *Pediatrics*. 2006;118(1):130–8.
11. Howell JC. *Gang Prevention: An Overview of Research and Programs*. Washington, DC: Office of Juvenile Justice and Delinquency Prevention, Office of Justice Programs, US Department of Justice; 2010:1–24. https://www.ncjrs.gov/pdffiles1/ojjdp/231116.pdf. Accessed December 11, 2017.
12. Centers for Disease Control and Prevention. *Prevent Gang Membership*. Atlanta, GA: Division of Violence Prevention, NCIPC, CDC; 2017. https://www.cdc.gov/violenceprevention/youthviolence/preventgang-membership/index.html. Accessed December 11, 2017.
13. Ross L, Arsenault S. Problem analysis in community violence assessment: Revealing early childhood trauma as a driver of youth and gang violence. *Int J Offender Ther Comp Criminol*. 2018;62(9):2726–41.
14. Kittle J. A literature review on gang violence. *J Trauma Nurs*. 2017;24(4):270–9.
15. Quinn K, Pacella ML, Dickson-Gomez J, Nydegger LA. Childhood adversity and the continued exposure to trauma and violence among adolescent gang members. *Am J Community Psychol*. 2017;59(1–2):36–49.
16. World Health Organization. *Violence Info: Youth Violence*. Geneva, Switzerland: World Health Organization; 2017. http://apps.who.int/violence-info/youth-violence/. Accessed January 5, 2018.
17. Grinshteyn E, Hemenway D. Violent death rates: The US compared with other high-income OECD countries, 2010. *Am J Med*. 2016;129:266–73.

18. Centers for Disease Control and Prevention. *Web-based Injury Statistics Query and Reporting System (WISQARS)*. Atlanta, GA: Centers for Disease Control and Prevention; 2018. http://www.cdc.gov/injury/wisqars/.
19. David-Ferdon CF, Haileyesus T, Liu Y, Simon TR, Kresnow MJ. Nonfatal assaults among persons aged 10–24 years—United States, 2001–2015. *MMWR Morb Mortal Wkly Rep*. 2018;67(5):141–5.
20. Salas-Wright CP, Nelson EJ, Vaughn MG, Reingle Gonzalez JM, Cordova D. Trends in fighting and violence among adolescents in the United States, 2002–2014. *Am J Public Health*. 2017;107(6):977–82.
21. Centers for Disease Control and Prevention. *Youth Risk Behavior Surveillance System (YRBSS)*. Atlanta, GA: Division of Adolescent and School Health, National Center for HIV/AIDS, Viral Hepatitis, STD and TB Prevention, Centers for Disease Control and Prevention; 2016. https://www.cdc.gov/healthyyouth/data/yrbs/index.htm. Accessed February 14, 2018.
22. Kann L, McManus T, Harris WA, et al. Youth risk behavior surveillance—United States, 2015. *MMWR Surveill Summ*. 2016;65(6)1–174.
23. Kann L, Olsen EO, McManus T, et al. Sexual identity, sex of sexual contacts, and health-related behaviors among students in grades 9–12—United States and selected sites, 2015. *MMWR Surveill Summ*. 2016;65(9):1–202.
24. Centers for Disease Control and Prevention. Trends in the prevalence of behaviors that contribute to violence national YRBS: 1991–2015. Atlanta, GA: Centers for Disease Control and Prevention; 2017. https://www.cdc.gov/healthyyouth/data/yrbs/pdf/trends/2015_us_violence_trend_yrbs.pdf. Accessed December 18, 2017.
25. Eaton DK, Kann L, Kinchen S, et al. Youth risk behavior surveillance—United States, 2009. *MMWR Surveill Summ*. 2010;59(5):1–142.
26. Eaton DK, Kann L, Kinchen S, et al. Youth risk behavior surveillance—United States, 2011. *MMWR Surveill Summ*. 2012;61(4):1–162.
27. Kann L, Kinchen S, Shanklin S, et al. Youth risk behavior surveillance—United States, 2013. *MMWR Surveill Summ*. 2014;63(4):1–168.
28. McGill TM, Self-Brown SR, Lai BS, et al. Effects of exposure to community violence and family violence on school functioning problems among urban youth: The potential mediating role of posttraumatic stress symptoms. *Front Public Health*. 2014;2(8):1–8. doi: 10.3389/fpubh.2014.00008.
29. Telleen S, Kim YOR, Stewart-Nava H, Pesce RC, Maher S. Implementing comprehensive safe school plans: Effective school and community mental health collaborations to reduce youth violence. *Handbook of School Violence and School Safety: From Research to Practice*. Mahwah, NJ: Lawrence Erlbaum Associates Publishers; US; 2006:567–86.
30. Okumu M, Mengo C, Ombayo B, Small E. Bullying and HIV risk among high school teenagers: The mediating role of teen dating violence. *J Sch Health*. 2017;87(10):743–50.
31. Benedict FT, Vivier PM, Gjelsvik A. Mental health and bullying in the United States among children aged 6 to 17 years. *J Interpers Violence*. 2015;30(5):782–95.
32. Alavi N, Reshetukha T, Prost E, et al. Relationship between bullying and suicidal behaviour in youth presenting to the emergency department. *J Can Acad Child Adolesc Psychiatry*. 2017;26(2):70–7.
33. Farrell C, Zimmerman GM. Violent lives: Pathways linking exposure to violence to suicidal behavior in a national sample. *Arch Suicide Res*. 2019;23(1):100–21. doi:10.1080/13811118.2017.1404517.
34. Department of Health and Human Services. *Youth Violence: A Report of the Surgeon General [online]*. Washington, DC: Department of Health and Human Services; 2001. www.surgeongeneral.gov/library/youthviolence/toc.html.
35. Lipsey MW, Derzon JH. Predictors of violent and serious delinquency in adolescence and early adulthood: A synthesis of longitudinal research. In: Loeber R, Farrington DP, eds. *Serious and Violent Juvenile Offenders: Risk Factors and Successful Interventions*. Thousand Oaks, CA: Sage Publications; 1998:86–105.
36. Resnick MD, Ireland M, Borowsky I. Youth violence perpetration: What protects? What predicts? Findings from the National Longitudinal Study of Adolescent Health. *J Adolesc Health*. 2004;35(424):e1–10.
37. Dubow E, Huesmann L, Boxer P, Smith C. Childhood and adolescent risk and protective factors for violence in adulthood. *J Crim Justice*. 2016;45:26–31.
38. Lösel F, Farrington DP. Direct protective and buffering protective factors in the development of youth violence. *Am J Prev Med*. 2012;43(2):S8–23.
39. Elsaesser C, Gorman-Smith D, Henry D, Schoeny M. The longitudinal relation between community violence exposure and academic engagement during adolescence: Exploring families' protective role. *J Interpers Violence*. 2020;35(17–18):3264–85.
40. Welsh BC, Loeber R, Stevens BR, et al. Costs of juvenile crime in urban areas: A longitudinal perspective. *Youth Violence Juv Justice*. 2008;6(1):3–27.
41. Kratzer L, Hodgins S. A typology of offenders: A test of Moffitt's theory among males and females from childhood to age 30. *Crim Behav Ment Health*. 1999;9:57–73.
42. Moffitt TE, Caspi A, Harrington H, Milne BJ. Males on the life-course-persistent and adolescence-limited antisocial pathways: Follow-up at age 26 years. *Dev Psychopathol*. 2002;14:179–207.
43. Moffitt TE. Adolescence-limited and life-course-persistent offending: A complementary pair of developmental theories. In: Thornberry T, ed. *Advances in Criminological Theory: Developmental Theories of Crime and Delinquency*. London: Transaction Press; 1997:11–54.
44. Farb AF, Matjasko JL. Recent advances in research on extracurricular activities and adolescent development. *Dev Rev*. 2012;32:1–48.
45. Morenoff JD, Sampson RJ, Raudenbush SWL. Neighborhood inequality, collective efficacy, and the spatial dynamics of violence. *Criminol*. 2001;39:517–60.
46. Resko SM, Walton MA, Bingham CR, et al. Alcohol availability and violence among inner-city adolescents: A multi-level analysis of the role of alcohol outlet density. *Am J Community Psychol*. 2010;3:253–62.
47. Pickett KE, Wilkinson RG. Income inequality and health: A causal review. *Soc Sci Med*. 2015;128:316–26.
48. Applied Research Center. *Racial Profiling and Punishment in U.S. Public Schools: How Zero Tolerance Policies and High Stakes Testing Subvert Academic Excellence and Racial Equality*. Oakland, CA: Applied Research Center; 2001.
49. MacDonald J, Golinelli D, Stokes RJ, Bluthenthal R. The effect of business improvement districts on the incidence of violent crimes. *Inj Prev*. 2010;16:327–32.
50. Heinze JE, Reischl TM, Bai M, et al. A comprehensive prevention approach to reducing assault offenses and assault injuries among youth. *Prev Sci*. 2016;17(2):167–76.
51. Commission on Social Determinants of Health. *A Conceptual Framework for Action on the Social Determinants of Health*. Geneva, Switzerland: World Health Organization; 2007.
52. Matjasko JL, Bacon S. Evidence for global violence prevention during adolescence and emerging adulthood. *Evidence for Violence Prevention Across the Lifespan and Around the World: Workshop Summary*. Washington, DC: The National Academies Press; 2013:II-8–14.
53. Centers for Disease Control and Prevention. *Technical Packages for Violence Prevention: Using Evidence-Based Strategies in Your Violence Prevention Efforts*. Atlanta, GA: Centers for Disease Control and Prevention; 2017. https://www.cdc.gov/violenceprevention/pub/technical-packages.html. Accessed January 31, 2018.
54. Frieden TR. Six components necessary for effective public health program implementation. *Am J Public Health*. 2014;104(1):17–22.
55. David-Ferdon C, Vivolo-Kantor AM, Dahlberg LL, Marshall KJ, Rainford N, Hall JE. *A Comprehensive Technical Package for the Prevention of Youth Violence and Associated Risk Behaviors*. Atlanta, GA: National Center for Injury Prevention and Control, Centers for Disease Control and Prevention; 2016.
56. Centers for Disease Control and Prevention. *STRYVE Online*. Atlanta, GA: Centers for Disease Control and Prevention; 2017. https://vetoviolence.cdc.gov/apps/stryve/. Accessed January 31, 2018.
57. Office of Juvenile Justice and Delinquency Prevention. *OJJDP Model Programs Guide*. Washington, DC: Office of Justice Programs, US Department of Justice; 2018. https://www.ojjdp.gov/mpg. Accessed January 31, 2018.
58. Substance Abuse and Mental Health Services Administration. *National Registry of Evidence-based Programs and Practices (NREPP)*. Rockville, MD: Substance Abuse and Mental Health Services Administration; 2018. https://www.samhsa.gov/nrepp. Accessed January 31, 2018.
59. National Institute of Justice. *Evidence-based Programs and Practices—What Works in Criminal Justice—CrimeSolutions.gov*. Washington, DC: Office of Justice Programs, National Institue of Justice; 2018. https://www.crimesolutions.gov/default.aspx. Accessed January 31, 2018.
60. Center for the Study and Prevention of Violence. *Blueprints for Healthy Youth Development*. Boulder, CO: University of Colorado Boulder, Institute of Behavioral Science; 2018. http://www.blueprintsprograms.com/. Accessed January 31, 2018.
61. DeVore ER, Ginsburg KR. The protective effects of good parenting on adolescents. *Curr Opin Pediatr*. 2005;17(4):460–5.
62. National Scientific Council on the Developing Child. *Young Children Develop in an Environment of Relationships. Working Paper No. 1*. Boston,

MA: Center on the Developing Child at Harvard University; 2004. http://developingchild.harvard.edu/wp-content/uploads/2004/04/Young-Children-Develop-in-an-Environment-of-Relationships.pdf.

63. Olds D, Henderson CR Jr, Cole R, et al. Long-term effects of nurse home visitation on children's criminal and antisocial behavior: 15-Year follow-up of a randomized controlled trial. *JAMA*. 1998;280(14):1238–44.
64. Olds DL, Henderson CR Jr, Kitzman H. Does prenatal and infancy nurse home visitation have enduring effects on qualities of parental caregiving and child health at 25 to 50 months of life? *Pediatrics*. 1994;93(1):89–98.
65. Menting AT, Orobio de Castro B, Matthys W. Effectiveness of the incredible years parent training to modify disruptive and prosocial child behavior: A meta-analytic review. *Clin Psychol Rev*. 2013;33(8):901–13.
66. Lochman JE, Wells KC. Effectiveness of the coping power program and of classroom intervention with aggressive children: Outcomes at a 1-year follow-up. *Behav Ther*. 2003;34(4):493–515.
67. Lochman JE, Wells KC. The coping power program for preadolescent aggressive boys and their parents: Outcome effects at the 1-year follow-up. *J Consult Clin Psychol*. 2004;72(4):571–8.
68. Lochman JE, Wells KC, Qu L, Chen L. Three year follow-up of coping power intervention effects: Evidence of neighborhood moderation? *Prev Sci*. 2013;14(4):364–76.
69. Braveman P, Gottlieb L. The social determinants of health: It's time to consider the causes of the causes. *Public Health Rep*. 2014;129 (Suppl 2):19–31.
70. Manning M, Homel R, Smith C. A meta-analysis of the effects of early developmental prevention programs in at-risk populations on non-health outcomes in adolescence. *Child Youth Serv Rev*. 2010;32(4):506–19.
71. Green BL, Ayoub C, Bartlett JD, et al. The effect of early head start on child welfare system involvement: A first look at longitudinal child maltreatment outcomes. *Child Youth Serv Rev*. 2014;42:127–35.
72. Love JM, Kisker EE, Ross C, et al. The effectiveness of early head start for 3-year-old children and their parents: Lessons for policy and programs. *Dev Psychol*. 2005;41(6):885–901.
73. Reynolds AJ, Temple JA, Ou SR, et al. Effects of a school-based, early childhood intervention on adult health and well-being: A 19-year follow-up of low-income families. *Arch Pediatr Adolesc Med*. 2007;161(8):730–9.
74. Reynolds AJ, Temple JA, White BA, Ou SR, Robertson DL. Age 26 cost-benefit analysis of the child-parent center early education program. *Child Dev*. 2011;82(1):379–404.
75. Durlak JA, Weissberg RP, Dymnicki AB, Taylor RD, Schellinger KB. The impact of enhancing students' social and emotional learning: A meta-analysis of school-based universal interventions. *Child Dev*. 2011;82(1):405–32.
76. Hahn R, Fuqua-Whitley D, Wethington H, et al. Effectiveness of universal school-based programs to prevent violent and aggressive behavior: A systematic review. *Am J Prev Med*. 2007;33(2 Suppl):S114–29.
77. Botvin GJ, Griffin KW, Nichols TD. Preventing youth violence and delinquency through a universal school-based prevention approach. *Prev Sci*. 2006;7(4):403–8.
78. Frey KHM, Edstrom L, Snell JL. Observed reductions in school bullying, nonbullying aggression, and destructive bystander behavior: A longitudinal evaluation. *J Educ Psychol*. 2009;101(2):466–81.
79. Brown EC, Low S, Smith BH, Haggerty KP. Outcomes from a school-randomized control trial of steps to respect. *School Psych Rev*. 2011;40(3):423–43.
80. DuBois DL, Portillo N, Rhodes JE, Silverthorn N, Valentine JC. How effective are mentoring programs for youth? A systematic assessment of the evidence. *Psychol Sci Public Interest*. 2011;12(2):57–91.
81. Tolan PH, Henry DB, Schoeny MS, Lovegrove P, Nichols E. Mentoring programs to affect delinquency and associated outcomes of youth at-risk: A comprehensive meta-analytic review. *J Exp Criminol*. 2014;10(2):179–206.
82. DuBois DL, Karcher MJ, eds. *Handbook of Youth Mentoring*. 2nd ed. Thousand Oaks, CA: Sage Publications; 2014.
83. Grossman J, Tierney JP. Does mentoring work? An impact study of the big brothers big sisters program. *Eval Rev*. 1998;22(3):403–26.
84. Sickmund M, Puzzanchera C, eds. *Juvenile Offenders and Victims: 2014 National Report*. Pittsburgh, PA: National Center for Juvenile Justice; 2014. http://www.ojjdp.gov/ojstatbb/nr2014/.
85. Goldschmidt P, Huang D, Chinen M. *The Long-Term Effects of After-School Programming on Educational Adjustment and Juvenile Crime: A Study of the LA's BEST After-School Program*. Los Angeles, CA: National Center for Research on Evaluation, Standards, and Student Testing and University of California Los Angeles; 2007. http://www.chapinhall.org/research/brief/after-school-programs-and-academic-impact.
86. Crowe TD. *Crime Prevention Through Environmental Design: Applications of Architectural Design and Space Management Concepts*. Boston, MA: Butterworth-Heinemann; 2000.
87. Casteel C, Peek-Asa C. Effectiveness of crime prevention through environmental design (CPTED) in reducing robberies. *Am J Prev Med*. 2000;18(4 Suppl):99–115.
88. Bogar S, Beyer KM. Green space, violence, and crime: A systematic review. *Trauma Violence Abuse*. 2016;17(2):160–71.
89. Branas CC, Cheney RA, MacDonald JM, Tam VW, Jackson TD, Ten Have TR. A difference-in-differences analysis of health, safety, and greening vacant urban space. *Am J Epidemiol*. 2011;174(11):1296–306.
90. Branas CC, Kondo MC, Murphy SM, South EC, Polsky D, MacDonald JM. Urban blight remediation as a cost-beneficial solution to firearm violence. *Am J Public Health*. 2016;106(12):2158–64.
91. Culyba AJ, Jacoby SF, Richmond TS, Fein JA, Hohl BC, Branas CC. Modifiable neighborhood features associated with adolescent homicide. *JAMA Pediatr*. 2016;170(5):473–80.
92. Donnelly P, Kimble CE. Community organizing, environmental change, and neighborhood crime. *Crime Delinquency*. 1997;43(4):493–511.
93. Ellen IG, O'Regan KM, Voicu I. Siting, spillovers, and segregation: A reexamination of the Low Income Housing Tax Credit Program. In: Glaeser EL, Quigley JM, eds. *Housing Markets and the Economy: Risk, Regulation, and Policy*. Cambridge, MA: Lincoln Institute of Land Policy; 2009, pp. 233–67.
94. Freedman M, Owens EG. Low-income housing development and crime. *J Urban Econ*. 2011;70(2):115–31.
95. Butts JA, Roman CG, Bostwick L, Porter JR. Cure violence: A public health model to reduce gun violence. *Annu Rev Public Health*. 2015;36:39–53.
96. Skogan WG, Hartnett SM, Bump N, Dubois J. *Evaluation of Cease-Fire-Chicago*. Evanston, IL: Northwestern University; 2008. http://www.skogan.org/files/Evaluation_of_CeaseFire-Chicago_Main_Report.03-2009.pdf.
97. Cary CE, McMillen JC. The data behind the dissemination: A systematic review of trauma-focused cognitive behavioral therapy for use with children and youth. *Child Youth Serv Rev*. 2012;34(4):748–57.
98. de Arellano MA, Lyman DR, Jobe-Shields L, et al. Trauma-focused cognitive-behavioral therapy for children and adolescents: Assessing the evidence. *Psychiatr Serv*. 2014;65(5):591–602.
99. Sawyer AM, Borduin CM. Effects of multisystemic therapy through midlife: A 21.9-year follow-up to a randomized clinical trial with serious and violent juvenile offenders. *J Consul Clin Psychol*. 2011;79(5):643–52.
100. Wagner DV, Borduin CM, Sawyer AM, Dopp AR. Long-term prevention of criminality in siblings of serious and violent juvenile offenders: A 25-year follow-up to a randomized clinical trial of multisystemic therapy. *J Consul Clin Psychol*. 2014;82(3):492–9.
101. Multisystemic Therapy Services. *Multisystemic Therapy (MST) Research at a Glance: Published MST Outcome, Implementation, and Benchmarking Studies*. Mount Pleasant, SC: Multisystemic Therapy Services; 2016. http://mstservices.com/files/outcomestudies.pdf.
102. Cunningham RM, Chermack ST, Zimmerman MA, et al. Brief motivational interviewing intervention for peer violence and alcohol use in teens: One-year follow-up. *Pediatrics*. 2012;129(6):1083–90.
103. Cunningham RM, Whiteside LK, Chermack ST, et al. Dating violence: Outcomes following a brief motivational interviewing intervention among at-risk adolescents in an urban emergency department. *Acad Emerg Med*. 2013;20(6):562–9.
104. Walton MA, Chermack ST, Shope JT, et al. Effects of a brief intervention for reducing violence and alcohol misuse among adolescents: A randomized controlled trial. *JAMA*. 2010;304(5):527–35.
105. Carter PM, Walton MA, Zimmerman MA, Chermack ST, Roche JS, Cunningham RM. Efficacy of a universal brief intervention for violence among Urban Emergency Department Youth. *Acad Emerg Med*. 2016;23(9):1061–70.
106. Olweus D. A useful evaluation design, and effects of the Olweus Bullying Prevention Program. *Psychol Crime Law*. 2005;11(4):389–402.
107. Olweus D. Bullying among school children: Intervention and prevention. In: Peters RD, McMahon RJ, Quinsey VL, eds. *Aggression and Violence Throughout the Life Span*. Newbury Park, CA: Sage Publications; 1992:100–25.
108. Florence C, Shepherd J, Brennan I, Simon T. Effectiveness of anonymised information sharing and use in health service, police, and local government partnership for preventing violence related injury: Experimental study and time series analysis. *BMJ*. 2011;342:d3313.

109. Centers for Disease Control and Prevention. *Preventing Multiple Forms of Violence: A Strategic Vision for Connecting the Dots.* Atlanta, GA: Division of Violence Prevention, National Center for Injury Prevention and Control, Centers for Disease Control and Prevention; 2016. https://www.cdc.gov/violenceprevention/overview/strategicvision.html. Accessed March 18, 2018.
110. Fagan AA, Catalano RF. What works in youth violence prevention: A review of the literature. *Res Social Work Practice.* 2013;23(2):141–56.
111. Perkinson L, Freire K, Stocking M. *Using Essential Elements to Select, Adapt and Evaluate Violence Prevention Approaches.* Atlanta, GA: Division of Violence Prevention, National Center for Injury Prevention and Control, Centers for Disease Control and Prevention; 2017. https://www.cdc.gov/violenceprevention/pdf/adaptationguidance.pdf. Accessed March 18, 2018.
112. Hawkins JD, Oesterle S, Brown EC, Abbott RD, Catalano R. Youth problem behaviors 8 ears after implementing the communities that care prevention system: A community-randomized trial. *JAMA Pediatr.* 2014;168(2):122–9.
113. Spoth RL, Trudeau LS, Redmond CR, et al. PROSPER partnership delivery system: Effects on adolescent conduct problem behavior outcomes through 6.5 years past baseline. *J Adolesc.* 2015;45:44–55.
114. Matjasko JL, Massetti GM, Bacon S. Implementing and evaluating comprehensive evidence-based approaches to prevent youth violence: Partnering to create communities where youth are safe from violence. *J Primary Prev.* 2016;37(2):109–19.
115. Holland KM, Vivolo-Kantor AM, Dela Cruz J, Massetti GM, Mahendra R. A qualitative evaluation of the 2005–2011 National Academic Centers of Excellence in Youth Violence Prevention Program. *Eval Program Plann.* 2015;53:80–90.
116. Vivolo AM, Matjasko JL, Massetti GM. Mobilizing communities and building capacity for youth violence prevention: The National Academic Centers of Excellence for Youth Violence Prevention. *Am J Community Psychol.* 2011;48(1–2):141–5.
117. Masho SW, Schoeny ME, Webster D, Sigel E. Outcomes, data and indicators of violence at the community level. *J Primary Prev.* 2016;37:121–39.
118. Kingston B, Bacallao M, Smokowski P, Sullivan T, Sutherland K. Constructing "packages" of evidence-based programs to prevent youth violence: Processes and illustrative examples from the CDC's Youth Violence Prevention Centers. *J Primary Prev.* 2016;37:141–63.
119. Farrell AD, Henry D, Bradshaw C, Reischl T. Designs for evaluating the community-level impact of comprehensive prevention programs: Examples from the CDC Centers of Excellence in Youth Violence Prevention. *J Primary Prev.* 2016;37:165–88.
120. Morrel-Samuels S, Bacallao M, Brown S, Bower M, Zimmerman M. Community engagement in youth violence prevention: Crafting methods to context. *J Primary Prev.* 2016;37:189–207.
121. Matjasko JL, Barnett SB, Mercy JA. Maceroeconomic factors and inequities in youth violence: The cyclical relationship between community conditions, family factors, and youth violence. In: Rosenfeld R, Edberg M, Fang X, Florence CS, eds. *Economics and Youth Violence: Crime, Disadvantage, and Community.* New York: New York University Press; 2013.
122. Cohen L, Davis D, Realini A. Communities are not all created equal: Strategies to prevent violence affecting youth in the United States. *J Public Health Policy.* 2016;37(S1):S81–94.
123. Cohen L, Erlenborn J. *Cultivating Peace in Salinas: A Framework for Violence Prevention.* Oakland, CA: Prevention Institute; 2001. http://preventioninstitute.org/publications/cultivating-peace-in-salinas-a-framework-for-violence-prevention. Accessed March 28, 2018.
124. Kim BE, Gilman AB, Hawkins JD. School- and community-based preventive interventions during adolescence: Preventing delinquency through science-guided collective action. In: Morizot J, Kazemian L, eds. *The Development of Criminal and Antisocial Behavior.* Switzerland: Springer International Publishing; 2015:447–60.

CHAPTER

178 Intimate Partner Violence Prevention*

Megan C. Kearns • Ashley Schappell D'Inverno • Jenny Dills • Phyllis Holditch Niolon

Intimate partner violence (IPV) represents a significant and preventable public health issue. Also known as domestic violence, IPV describes physical violence, sexual violence, stalking, and/or psychological aggression by a current or former intimate partner (who may or may not be cohabiting).[1] Importantly, IPV occurs across the lifespan and can affect individuals, including adolescents who have just started dating or having intimate relationships. IPV in adolescence is often referred to as teen dating violence (TDV). The purpose of this chapter is to outline the nature and burden of IPV across the lifespan (including TDV), discuss current data on risk and protective factors for IPV, and describe best available evidence for preventing violence in intimate relationships.

NATURE AND BURDEN OF THE PROBLEM

Definitions

Intimate partners can include current or former spouses, boyfriends or girlfriends, dating partners or sexual partners. Although not all of the following relationship characteristics may be present, an intimate partner is generally defined as a close personal relationship that may involve emotional connectedness, regular contact, ongoing physical and/or sexual contact, identity as a couple, and familiarity about each other's lives.[1] IPV can occur in heterosexual or same-sex couples and does not require sexual intimacy. Broadly, IPV encompasses multiple forms of partner violence, several methods or tactics to perpetrate IPV, and can vary in frequency and severity, including both single episodes of IPV as well as chronic and severe episodes occurring over a longer period of time.[1]

In order to facilitate consistency of IPV surveillance across organizations, the Centers for Disease Control and Prevention (CDC) consulted a panel of IPV subject matter experts and developed a document that provides uniform definitions and recommended data elements for IPV.[1] Table 178-1 outlines definitions for IPV and other related terms that are used when reporting the prevalence of IPV. Additionally, while the definitions included in Table 178-1 refer to IPV in adulthood, they may also be used when describing TDV.

Health Burden Across Demographic Characteristics

IPV is a serious public health problem with long-lasting impacts on physical and mental health. IPV can begin in adolescence and affects millions of American men and women across the lifespan. A few key findings about IPV from the CDC's National Intimate Partner and Sexual Violence Survey (NISVS)[2] are highlighted below:

- Over one in three women (36.4%) and about one in three men (33.6%) in the United States have experienced contact sexual violence, physical violence, and/or stalking by an intimate partner in their lifetime.
- About one in four women (25.1%) and one in ten men (10.9%) in the United States reported an impact as a result of experiencing IPV during their lifetime.
- Over one in five women (21.4%) and one in seven men (14.9%) in the United States experienced severe physical violence in their lifetime from an intimate partner.
- Approximately 18.3% of U.S. women and 8.2% of U.S. men experienced some form of contact sexual violence by an intimate partner during their lifetime.
- An estimated 10.4% of U.S. women and 2.2% of U.S. men have experienced stalking in their lifetime by an intimate partner.
- Over one-third of women (36.4%) and men (34.2%) in the United States report that they have experienced psychological aggression by an intimate partner in their lifetime.

In addition, romantic relationships often emerge during adolescence,[3] and as romantic relationships begin to develop, some teens experience dating violence. National U.S. estimates show that 7.1% of female victims and 3.7% of male victims of IPV report first experiencing partner violence (i.e., rape, physical violence, and/or stalking) before the age of 18.[4] Data from the 2017 Youth Risk Behavior Survey, which surveys a nationally representative sample of U.S. high school students, indicate that among students who dated in the year prior to the survey, 8.0% had experienced physical dating violence (9.1% of female students and 6.5% of male students), and 6.9% had experienced sexual dating violence (10.7% of female students and 2.8% of male students).[5] The prevalence of TDV highlights the importance of adolescence as a critical period for teens to learn healthy relationship behaviors and skills. Preventing TDV has implications for disrupting the trajectory of IPV, as youth experiencing TDV are at a higher risk of IPV later in life.[6,7]

Importantly, IPV occurs across the globe, with some countries experiencing higher rates of IPV than others. The World Health Organization's (WHO) Multicountry Study on Women's Health and Domestic Violence against Women collected data from ten countries and over 24,000 women in diverse cultural settings, including both rural and urban populations. The countries included were Bangladesh, Brazil, Ethiopia, Japan, Namibia, Peru, Samoa, Serbia and Montenegro, Thailand, and the United Republic of Tanzania. Lifetime physical violence by an intimate partner ranged from 13% in Japan to 61% in Peru; lifetime sexual violence by an intimate partner ranged from 6% in Japan to 59% in Ethiopia.[8] With the exception of rural Bangladesh, Ethiopia, and urban Thailand, sexual violence was

*The findings and conclusions in this chapter are those of the authors and do not necessarily represent the official position of the Centers for Disease Control and Prevention.

TABLE 178-1 DEFINITIONS OF INTIMATE PARTNER VIOLENCE AND RELATED TERMS

Term	Definition
Intimate partner violence[a]	Physical violence, sexual violence, stalking, and/or psychological aggression by a current or former intimate partner who may or may not be cohabiting. An intimate partner may include a spouse, boyfriend/girlfriend (may be of the same or opposite sex), dating partner, or ongoing sexual partners.
Physical violence[a]	The intentional use of physical force that may cause harm, injury, disability, or death. This includes behaviors such as hitting, punching, pushing, shoving, choking, throwing, grabbing, biting, slapping, use of a weapon, or using restraints or one's body against another person.
Severe physical violence[a]	A subset of physical violence, severe physical violence includes being kicked, hit with a fist or something hard, hurt by pulling hair, slammed against something, tried to hurt by choking or suffocating, beaten, choked, burned on purpose, or having a knife or gun used against the victim.
Sexual violence[a]	A committed or attempted sexual act by another person in which the victim does not provide consent or is unable to consent or refuse the sexual act. Acts of sexual violence include, but are not limited to: intentional unwanted sexual touching; forced or alcohol/drug facilitated penetration; forced or alcohol/drug facilitated instances where the victim was made to penetrate someone else (may include the perpetrator); unwanted noncontact acts of a sexual nature; unwanted penetration whereby the victim is pressured in a nonphysical manner.
Rape[b]	A form of sexual violence, rape is completed or attempted unwanted vaginal, oral, or anal penetration through the use of physical force or threats to harm a victim or through the use of alcohol/drugs in which the victim is incapacitated, unconscious, or not aware enough to provide consent.
Penetration[a]	Physical insertion of the penis into the vulva, to any degree; physical insertion of a hand, finger, or other object into the anus or genital opening of another individual; physical contact between the mouth and penis, vulva, or anus.
Made to penetrate[a]	A committed or attempted act where the victim is made to sexually penetrate someone else (may include the perpetrator) without the victim's consent due to force or threat of physical harm (e.g., assaulting the victim, pinning down the victim's arms, use of a weapon, or using one's body to prevent moving or escaping), or use of alcohol/drugs in which the victim is incapacitated, unconscious, or not aware enough to provide consent.
Noncontact unwanted sexual violence[b]	Unwanted sexual experiences that do not involve touching or penetration. Examples include flashing, masturbating in front of the victim, making the victim look at or participate in sexual media, or verbally sexually harassing the victim.
Contact sexual violence[b]	A combined measure that includes rape, being made to penetrate someone else, sexual coercion, and/or unwanted sexual contact.
Stalking[a]	Multiple harassing or threatening tactics by the same perpetrator or a single tactic multiple times by the same perpetrator that makes the victim very fearful or makes them believe that they or someone close to them would be harmed or killed as a result of the perpetrator's behavior. Examples include, but are not limited to: unwanted phone calls, text messages, emails, or messages; watching or following from a distance; showing up in places when the victim does not want to see the person; damaging the victim's property; making threats to physically harm the victim.
Psychological aggression[a]	The use of verbal or nonverbal communication with the intent to harm the victim emotionally or mentally and/or exert control over the victim. These acts may be covert and manipulative including, but not limited to: expressive aggression such as name-calling, humiliating, or degrading a victim; coercive control of a victim's whereabouts and communications; threats of physical or sexual violence through words, gestures, or weapons; control of reproductive or sexual health (e.g., birth control or abortions); exploitation of a victim or perpetrator's vulnerability such as immigration status, disability, or sexual orientation; gaslighting or playing mind games with the intent to make the victim doubt their own memory, perception, and sanity.

[a]Definitions were obtained from the CDC's Intimate Partner Violence Surveillance Uniform Definitions and Recommended Data Elements document;[1] more detailed definitions of these terms, and others, can be found in this document, which can be located at https://stacks.cdc.gov/view/cdc/31292.
[b]Definitions were meant to be consistent with the way in which these terms were defined in CDC's National Intimate Partner and Sexual Violence Survey (NISVS), 2015 Data Brief—Updated Release[2] (the NISVS 2015 Data Brief can be located at https://stacks.cdc.gov/view/cdc/60893).

less common than physical violence. Additionally, the study found that among women who experienced IPV, many reported experiencing severe violence (i.e., being hit with a fist, kicked, dragged, threatened with a weapon, or having a weapon used against them at some point). More recently, a systematic review conducted by the WHO used additional analyses of the Multicountry Study, as well as data from 155 other studies, to examine the prevalence of IPV in 81 countries.[9] The results indicate that worldwide, 30% of women aged 15 and above have experienced physical and/or sexual violence by an intimate partner in their lifetime, with large variation by geographic region.[9] The variation in prevalence of IPV for different regions and countries suggests the importance of societal and cultural norms in influencing rates of IPV.

It is important to note that some populations, particularly racial and sexual minorities, as well as those with disabilities, are disproportionately affected by IPV. Racial and ethnic minorities report large disparities. Figure 178-1 illustrates differences in prevalence estimates by race/ethnicity among men and women in the United States, with multiracial men and women reporting the highest prevalence estimates of IPV and Asian and Pacific Islander men and women reporting the lowest prevalence estimates of IPV.[4] Other minorities, such as sexual minorities and those with disabilities, are also disproportionately affected by IPV. A 2010 NISVS special report[10] found that 44% of lesbian women, 61% of bisexual women, and 35% of heterosexual women in the U.S. experienced rape, physical violence, and/or stalking by an intimate partner in their lifetime. The report also found that 26% of gay men, 37% of bisexual men, and 29% of heterosexual men in the United States experienced rape, physical violence, and/or stalking by an intimate partner in their lifetime. In addition, higher rates of IPV victimization have been documented among individuals with mental and physical disabilities,[11,12] with some research indicating that women with physical, mental, or

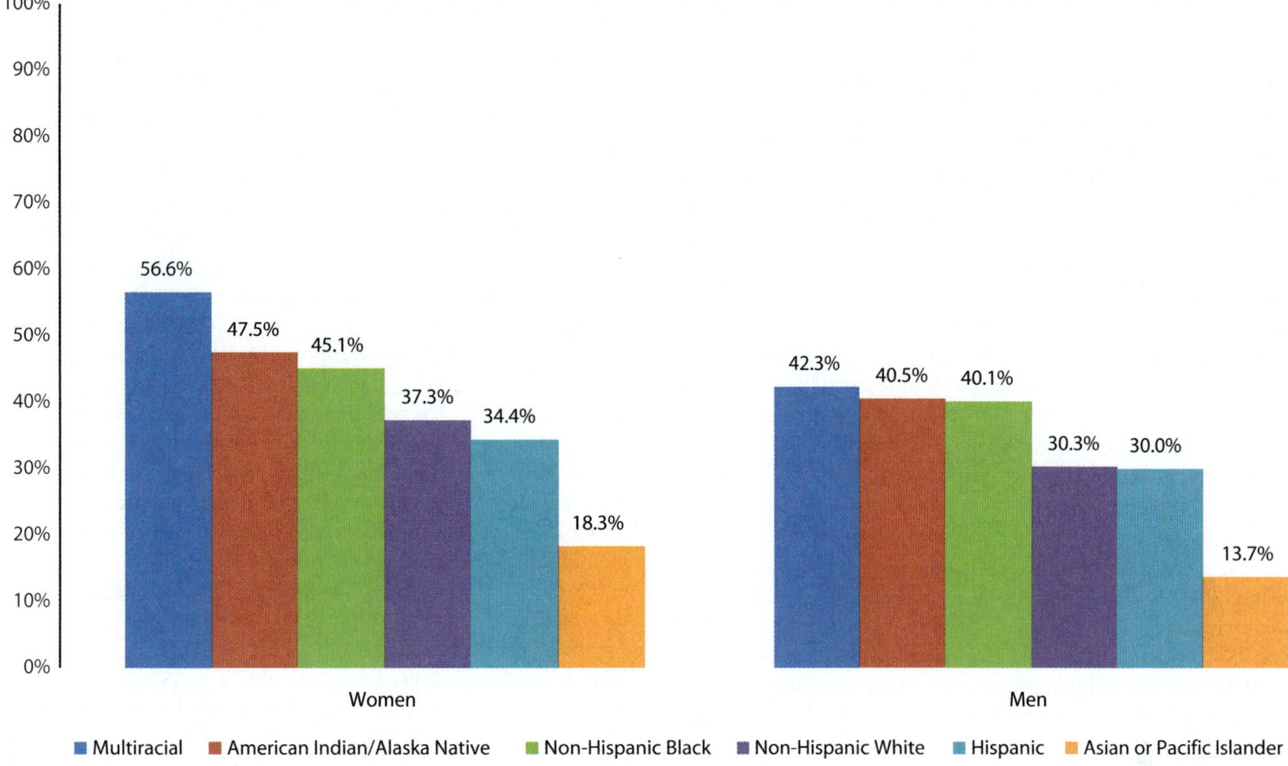

FIGURE 178-1. Prevalence of IPV by Race/Ethnicity, U.S. Women and Men (NISVS 2010–12). (*Source:* Prevalence estimates reported in Smith SG, Chen J, Basile KC, et al. The National Intimate Partner and Sexual Violence Survey (NISVS): 2010–2012 State Report. Atlanta, GA: National Center for Injury Prevention and Control, Centers for Disease Control and Prevention; 2017.)[4]

emotional disabilities experience approximately twice the rate of IPV as those without these disabilities.[13]

Furthermore, the consequences and impact of IPV victimization are not shared equally across all groups. While the data clearly demonstrate that men are victims of IPV, it does not suggest that victimization, or its impact, is equal for men and women. Female victims are more likely than male victims to experience multiple forms of IPV.[14] In addition, 25.1% of women and 10.9% of men experienced a form of IPV in their lifetime and at least one measured negative impact (e.g., fear, concern for safety, being injured, missing school or work, needing services).[2] Over 20% of women (20.5%) and 5.3% of men reported being concerned for their safety.[15] Furthermore, the most recent report of IPV fatalities indicates that female homicide victims in the United States are nearly six times as likely to be killed by an intimate partner than male homicide victims in the United States (41.5% versus 7.1%).[16] Generally, one out of five murder victims in the United States (16.3%) were killed by an intimate partner from 1980 to 2008.[16]

Health and Social Consequences of Intimate Partner Violence

The impact of IPV on health is vast and includes multiple negative effects on physical health, mental health, social services, and economic, educational, and criminal justice systems. IPV puts a strain on medical and mental health resources and lowers the quality of life for victims and their loved ones. Victims of IPV suffer both direct and indirect effects, in the short term and long term, even after the abuse has ended.[17–19] A large, cross-sectional public health survey with over 70,000 respondents in 18 U.S. states/territories reported that persons who report experiencing IPV during their lifetimes have a significantly greater likelihood of reporting adverse chronic health conditions and risk behaviors.[20] Although this study was cross-sectional and could not establish causality, basic scientific research indicates that chronic psychological stress caused by IPV, including length of time spent in an abusive relationship, is associated with shortened telomeric DNA length, which is a marker of biological age and predictor of early morbidity and mortality.[21] Consistent with this research, other studies have also established that IPV can lead to chronic health problems such as fainting, seizures, gastrointestinal disorders, hypertension, colds and influenza, asthma, chest pain, and other chronic pain symptoms, such as headaches, back pain, and joint diseases.[20,22–32] Abused women are more likely to have gynecological problems including sexually transmitted diseases, invasive cervical cancer, fibroids, vaginal bleeding, pelvic pain, painful intercourse, and urinary tract infections.[22,23,25,26,29,33–37] Victims of IPV are also more likely to experience PTSD, depression, anxiety, insomnia, and suicidal tendencies.[38–43] Similar findings on the mental health consequences of IPV have been documented in international research conducted in developing countries, such as Nicaragua and Pakistan.[44,45] Furthermore, women who are victims of IPV report engaging in a higher number of risky health behaviors including smoking, drinking, drugs, unprotected sex, and more sexual partners than nonvictims.[20,25,30,32,38,42,46–50]

In addition, IPV has been associated with multiple harms related to maternal and child health outcomes. Seeking medical care is particularly important during pregnancy, yet pregnant IPV victims are more likely to delay prenatal care[51,52] and experience increased risk for health problems, which may lead to harm or death of the fetus and/or mother.[53,54] IPV during pregnancy is associated with increased risk of miscarriages, premature labor, fetal distress, sexually transmitted diseases, mental health symptoms, as well as destructive and risky health behaviors such as substance use.[22,55–63] A commonly reported infant outcome of IPV during pregnancy is low birth weight, which is associated with infant death, particularly in developing countries. A meta-analysis of studies conducted in North American and European countries showed a small, but significant relationship between IPV during pregnancy and low birth weight.[64] Children may also be injured during episodes of IPV if they try to intervene or are being held by the victim. Nearly half of children injured during an IPV episode are less than 2 years old.[65]

In sum, the consequences of IPV are serious and substantial. IPV results in nearly 2.0 million injuries each year, causing victims to lose approximately 8.0 million days of paid work and 5.6 million days of household productivity.[66] The economic magnitude of IPV should not be understated, with an estimated lifetime economic burden of nearly $3.6 trillion (2014 USD) in the United States, including costs related to medical care, lost productivity among victims and perpetrators, criminal justice activities, and other costs such as victim property loss or damage.[67] These significant and wide-ranging consequences to individuals, families, and society as a whole further illustrate the public health burden IPV represents and highlights the importance of identifying risk and protective factors associated with IPV, as well as enhancing prevention efforts.

Risk and Protective Factors for IPV

In order to address IPV across the lifespan and develop effective prevention strategies, the public health approach to violence emphasizes identifying and understanding risk and protective factors associated with IPV perpetration and victimization. In this section, we focus on describing risk and protective factors established from longitudinal research, but also include information on cross-sectional studies when appropriate. Importantly, we describe factors associated with both perpetration and victimization, as many studies on this topic include both outcomes. Where possible, we have specified when evidence for a risk or protective factor is relevant to both perpetration and victimization. However, some studies examined the couple as a unit and measured reports of perpetration and victimization from both partners. In these cases, it was not always possible to attribute the findings to reports of victimization or perpetration (or both). Additionally, we present the risk and protective factors according to the levels of the social ecological model,[68,69] which takes into account the interconnected relationships between risk and protective factors at the individual, relationship, community, and societal levels. Understanding and preventing violence requires recognition of the way each of these levels interact with one another, since individuals have relationships (friends, family, peers, etc.), are a part of communities (schools, faith communities, neighborhoods, etc.), and exist in a broader society (with laws, norms, media, global influence). The interplay among these factors plays an important role in determining who is at risk and who may be protected from perpetrating violence against an intimate partner. It is worth noting that there is a dearth of research examining protective factors at the various levels of the social ecological model, but we present the limited evidence that exists.

Risk and protective factors for IPV at the individual-level are the most widely researched. As previously mentioned, several demographic and developmental factors are associated with increased risk of IPV perpetration and/or victimization. Low income and low verbal IQ increase risk of perpetrating IPV,[70,71] while older age is a protective against violence between intimate partners.[72–74] Racial/ethnic minority groups are also at increased risk of experiencing IPV, as evidence suggests that African American and Hispanic couples are more likely to report IPV compared to White couples;[75,76] however, the effects of race/ethnicity may be mediated by other factors such as age, marital status, and income.[77] The research on acculturation has been mixed, but there is some evidence that Hispanics born in the United States are at a higher risk for IPV perpetration than foreign-born individuals.[78,79] Stress stemming from finances, parenting, acculturation, and other life events are risk factors for IPV perpetration and victimization.[80–86] Adverse childhood experiences, specifically witnessing IPV in parents and childhood abuse and neglect, are important predictors of IPV perpetration and victimization later in life, and they are also related to other IPV risk factors, such as behavioral problems and substance use.[87–92] While it is difficult to tease apart the distinct effect that each of these factors has on IPV, research indicates that certain individual demographic and childhood historical factors increase risk for IPV perpetration and victimization.

Mental and behavioral health have been extensively researched as risk factors for IPV. Antisocial behavior and conduct problems in adolescence consistently predict IPV perpetration later in life.[87,93–96] Research on internalizing factors such as self-esteem, depression, and suicide is less clear.[97] Cross-sectional studies have found some evidence for an association between low self-esteem and risk for IPV perpetration,[98–100] but a significant relationship between self-esteem and IPV perpetration has not been detected in studies using a longitudinal design.[96,101] The research examining the link between depression and IPV perpetration shows there may be some relationship, but the findings are not robust once other variables are accounted for in the analyses;[72,95,96,99,102] similarly, the research on suicide as a risk factor for IPV perpetration and victimization is mixed, but one longitudinal study found that suicide attempts in adolescence are a predictor of IPV perpetration in young adulthood.[103–105] Substance use has been associated with increased risk of IPV perpetration and victimization. Alcohol use, cannabis, hallucinogens, and nicotine, which are often used in combination, are predictors of IPV perpetration;[73,106,107] the relationship between alcohol consumption and IPV victimization has also been examined and found to be significant.[108,109] Finally, individual attitudes and beliefs are related to IPV perpetration; examples include hostility toward women and attitudes accepting or justifying IPV.[93,110–112] For example, White and colleagues[112] found that among males, hostility toward women predicted physical and verbal aggression toward intimate partners. Moreover, other studies suggest that males that endorse more gender-equitable attitudes are less likely to be perpetrators of IPV.[113–115]

Less research has examined relationship-level risk and protective factors for IPV. Within an intimate relationship, frequent disagreements, conflict, or relationship discord is associated with IPV perpetration and victimization.[109,116–120] Jealousy, possessiveness, and a tendency to experience negative emotions (e.g., anxiety, anger) in a relationship are also related to IPV perpetration.[104,121,122] Relationship status is a robust predictor of IPV, with single, divorced, and separated marital statuses at high-risk of IPV victimization, as well as cohabitating couples;[75,77,123–126] being married is protective against women experiencing IPV.[74] Beyond the intimate partner relationship, relationships with other individuals and the quality of these relationships may offer protective benefits or put the person at risk for IPV. For instance, association with antisocial and aggressive peers is a predictor of perpetrating dating violence,[96,127–130] while higher friendship quality is associated with lower levels of dating violence.[88] Research examining social support and IPV perpetration is mixed, although the bulk of the evidence suggests that certain types of social support (e.g., tangible help, support from neighbors) are protective against IPV perpetration and victimization.[85,131] For teens, close social bonds with parents, school, and the neighborhood is generally protective against TDV perpetration and victimization (with some exceptions for boys).[101,128,132–134] Conversely, aversive family communication and relationships, hostility in parents' marital relationships, and engaging in peer violence are risk factors for TDV perpetration at the relationship-level.[135–138]

A dearth of evidence exists at the outer levels of the social ecology (i.e., the community and societal levels). Community factors include the characteristics of settings, such as schools, workplaces, and neighborhoods, that are associated with being victims or perpetrators of violence; societal factors include broad factors that help create a climate in which violence is encouraged or prohibited, including social and cultural norms, and policies that perpetuate inequalities between different groups of people.[139] Recently researchers have started to focus on the outer levels and investigate how these factors can influence IPV, particularly how community- and society-level factors can protect individuals from experiencing IPV. For example, research suggests that higher densities of alcohol outlets, or the number of locations where alcohol can be purchased (calculated per area or per population), are associated with higher rates of IPV.[140] Using data aggregated at the neighborhood level, one longitudinal study found that higher levels of collective efficacy in a neighborhood, which is comprised of factors like community cohesiveness, mutual trust, and willingness to intervene for the common good, was associated with reduced individual risk of IPV victimization for men, but not women.[141] In a similar vein, a cross-sectional study with an adolescent sample found that low collective efficacy and social control, and high neighborhood disorder aggregated at the neighborhood level predicted TDV perpetration.[142] Some characteristics of the school context may place teens at risk for dating violence. For example, attending an economically disadvantaged school is a predictor of TDV victimization for males and it moderates the relationship between family disadvantage and TDV victimization in females, such that girls with disadvantaged families are more likely to report TDV victimization if they attend a more advantaged school as measured at the school-level.[143] Additionally, poverty is a key risk factor for IPV as rates of IPV in the lowest-income households are nearly 15 times greater than in the highest income households.[144]

At the societal-level, gender inequality has been associated with greater risk of IPV and/or sexual violence against women by men.[145–148] Depriving women of social and economic status creates power inequities in relationships, families, work, and communities.[145,146,149] For example, in a study that examined women's status in 44 countries, results indicated that gender bias in ownership property rights and societal norms accepting violence (aggregated at the country level) predicted prevalence of partner violence.[150] Thus, altering traditional hegemonic gender norms to improve attitudes and beliefs about women as equals may be beneficial to preventing IPV.

Many of the aforementioned risk and protective factors for TDV and IPV have also been identified for other forms of violence (e.g., child maltreatment, sexual violence, youth violence, bullying, suicide, and elder maltreatment). For example, substance use and mental health problems are risk factors for youth violence and suicide, in addition to TDV and IPV.[151] Additionally, individuals who experience violence are more likely to experience other forms of violence and perpetrate violence toward others.[151] This is illustrated by research that shows children who experience abuse and neglect, which have been identified as adverse childhood experiences, are more likely to experience IPV later in life.[97] Nonetheless, if the overlapping root causes of violence are properly addressed, it is possible to prevent multiple, connected forms of violence through prevention programs, policies, and strategies.

BEST AVAILABLE EVIDENCE TO PREVENT INTIMATE PARTNER VIOLENCE

Although public health research aimed at better identifying and monitoring the problem of IPV is still ongoing, evidence is also accumulating on the best ways to effectively prevent IPV before it starts, which is considered primary prevention. Because IPV is such a complex social problem, successful primary prevention efforts will likely require a comprehensive approach. To this effect, a growing body of research points to strategies that have evidence of effectiveness.

A technical package is a collection of strategies and approaches with evidence to support effective public health program implementation.[152] Technical packages are meant to help communities and prevention practitioners understand the best available evidence on what works to prevent different forms of violence, and prioritize what they will implement in order to achieve significant and synergistic impact. In 2017, CDC released the technical package, *Preventing Intimate Partner Violence Across the Lifespan: A Technical Package of Programs, Policies, and Practices*, which outlines six evidence-based strategies for IPV.[153] A strategy is the preventive direction or actions to achieve the goal of preventing IPV, and the approaches are the specific ways to advance each strategy. Strategies described in this technical package included:

1. Teach Safe and Healthy Relationship Skills;
2. Engage Influential Adults and Peers;
3. Disrupt the Developmental Pathways Toward Partner Violence;
4. Create Protective Environments;
5. Strengthen Economic Supports for Families; and
6. Support Survivors to Increase Safety and Lessen Harms.

These strategies represent the current best available evidence for addressing IPV and include approaches with a focus on primary prevention of IPV across the lifespan, as well as approaches that can lessen the immediate and long-term harms of partner violence. The research on the most effective ways to prevent IPV is less prolific than for some other areas of violence, such as youth violence.[153,154] For some strategies, there is a dearth of evidence demonstrating the impact on IPV directly, but in this case, the package presents evidence of approaches within that strategy impacting proven risk and protective factors for IPV. The following sections describe each strategy and its relevant approaches. In addition, Table 178-2 includes a summary of these strategies and describes specific programs, policies, or practices relevant to each approach, as outlined in *Preventing Intimate Partner Violence Across the Lifespan: A Technical Package of Programs, Policies, and Practices*.[153] Although this is not intended to be an exhaustive list of effective strategies for preventing IPV, this table highlights some example programs and details relevant research evidence supporting each approach for its impact on violence outcomes or risk or protective factors for IPV.

Teach Safe and Healthy Relationship Skills

Evidence suggests that teaching healthy relationship skills, such as conflict resolution and communication skills, can reduce risk for perpetration and victimization of IPV.[122,138,155] *Social-emotional learning programs for youth* represent one approach for teaching safe and healthy relationship skills. Many of these programs involve multisession classroom curricula implemented in school-based settings and focus on developing and practicing skills related to positive communication, anger management, conflict resolution, and respect. In addition to evidence suggesting that these programs are effective at reducing dating violence perpetration and victimization, this approach has also been linked to reductions in associated risk factors such as aggression, weapon carrying, and sexual violence.[156]

For adults who are already in a relationship, but who are not experiencing IPV, *healthy relationship programs for couples* represents another evidence-based approach for teaching safe and healthy relationship skills. Although couples-based programs are not recommended for relationships where severe violence and fear is already occurring,[157] there is evidence that providing these programs to nonviolent couples can be an effective approach for preventing future IPV.[153]

Engage Influential Adults and Peers

Another effective strategy for preventing IPV involves programs that engage influential adults and peers who are able to promote positive, healthy relationship behaviors among adolescents and young adults. Utilizing trusted peers and adults to change social norms about the acceptability of violence and gender equity can decrease tolerance for IPV.[158] As a result, these social contexts can encourage positive bystander behaviors that interrupt violence from occurring and discourage potential perpetrators from engaging in IPV.[158]

For example, a growing body of evidence supports the *bystander empowerment and education approach*. This approach engages a wide

TABLE 178-2 BEST AVAILABLE EVIDENCE FOR STRATEGIES AND APPROACHES TO PREVENT IPV

Strategy	Approach	Example Program, Practice or Policy	IPV Outcomes	Risk and Protective Factors for IPV
Teach safe and healthy relationship skills	Social-emotional learning programs for youth	*The Fourth R: Strategies for Healthy Teen Relationships*	Decrease in TDV perpetration for boys only[183]	
	Healthy relationship programs for couples	*Premarital Relationship Enhancement Program (PREP)*	Decrease in physical IPV perpetration and victimization[184]	Increase in positive communication skills and decrease in negative communication skills[184]
Engage influential adults and peers	Bystander empowerment and education	*Green Dot*	Decrease in IPV perpetration and victimization, sexual violence, sexual harassment, and stalking[185]	
	Men and boys as allies in prevention	*Coaching Boys into Men*	Decrease in TDV perpetration[186]	Decrease in negative bystander behavior[186]
	Family-based programs	*Families for Safe Dates*	Decrease in report of physical TDV victimization[161]	Decrease in acceptance of dating abuse and negative communication with teens, increase in parental/caregiver efficacy in resolving teen relationship conflicts[161]
Disrupt the developmental pathways toward partner violence	Early childhood home visitation	*Nurse Family Partnership*	Decrease in IPV exposure for nurse-visited women[187]	Decrease in child abuse and neglect, parental substance use, use of welfare, and criminal behavior[188,189] Decrease in child behavioral problems, arrests, convictions, probation violations, and substance use[190–192]
	Preschool enrichment with family engagement	*Early Head Start*		Increase in parent-child engagement, fewer child welfare encounters, fewer reports of substantiated physical or sexual abuse[193]
	Parenting skill and family relationship programs	*Parent Management Training Oregon*		Decrease in coercive and harsh parenting, increase in positive parenting practices and adaptive family functioning[194,195] Decrease in child behavior problems, youth aggression, deviant peer associations, substance use, and arrest rates[165,196]
	Treatment for at-risk children, youth, and families	*Multidimensional Treatment Foster Care*		Decrease in child behavioral problems, adolescent violent crimes, incarceration, and substance use[166,167]
Create protective environments	Improve school climate and safety	*Shifting Boundaries* building-level component	Decrease in sexual violence victimization in dating relationships[197]	Decrease in sexual violence perpetration by peers and sexual harassment perpetration[197]
	Improve organizational policies and workplace climate	*IPV and the Workplace Training*		Increase in tangible help and social support in the workplace (e.g., providing information to employees on resources and state law protections for work leave for IPV survivors)[198]
	Modify the physical and social environments of neighborhoods	*Alcohol-related policies (e.g., outlet density)*		Decrease in excessive alcohol use at the community-level[140]
Strengthen economic supports for families	Strengthen household financial security	*Microfinance programs*	Decrease in physical and sexual IPV[199,200]	Increase in female empowerment[200]
	Strengthen work-family supports	*Paid-leave policies*	Decrease in physical and emotional IPV[201]	Decrease in depressive symptoms after birth of child[202]
Support survivors to increase safety and lessen harms	Victim-centered services	*Domestic Violence Advocacy Services*	Decrease in IPV victimization[203,a]	
	Housing programs	*Domestic Violence Housing First*	N/A[b]	N/A[b]
	First responder and civil legal protections	*Lethality Assessment Programs* *Protection Orders*	Decrease in severity and frequency of physical and emotional IPV[204] Decrease in IPV victimization[205,206]	Increase in help-seeking behavior (e.g., applying for and receiving a protective order, removing or hiding a partner's weapons, and seeking medical care)[204]

TABLE 178-2 BEST AVAILABLE EVIDENCE FOR STRATEGIES AND APPROACHES TO PREVENT IPV *(Continued)*

Strategy	Approach	Example Program, Practice or Policy	IPV Outcomes	Risk and Protective Factors for IPV
	Patient-centered approaches	*Education with tailored intervention for specific risk such as reproductive coercion*	Decrease in IPV victimization[207]	
	Treatment and support for survivors of IPV, including TDV	*Cognitive Behavioral Therapy (CBT)*	Decrease in IPV victimization[177,a]	Decrease in PTSD and depression symptoms[177]

Note: This table provides an overview of strategies and approaches identified in CDC's Preventing Intimate Partner Violence Across the Lifespan: A Technical Package of Programs, Policies, and Practices.[153] It includes example programs, practices, and policies for each approach and relevant research-based outcomes for each example provided. This is not an exhaustive list of evidence-based approaches for each of the described strategies and approaches for preventing IPV. For more information, see CDC's Preventing Intimate Partner Violence Across the Lifespan: A Technical Package of Programs, Policies, and Practices.[153]

[a]This approach decreases risk for IPV victimization, but is also intended to mitigate consequences of IPV among survivors and their families.

[b]This example program is aimed at mitigating consequences of exposure to IPV (e.g., PTSD, depression).

range of community members as bystanders (e.g., informal helpers, popular opinion leaders, or larger social groups) with programs that offer training in specific strategies for how to intervene to prevent violence or situations that condone IPV.[159,160] Other approaches specifically target *men and boys as allies in prevention*, frequently delivered in peer groups like athletic teams or fraternities. These programs often include bystander training, but also promote social norms that are protective against risk for IPV perpetration. The final approach under this strategy is *family-based programs*, which engage parents or caretakers to improve awareness and knowledge about TDV, parental attitudes about the acceptability of violence, communication skills, and skills for assisting their teens with conflict resolution. Programs have been successful in reducing risk factors, such as acceptance of IPV, as well as reductions in rates of TDV victimization.[161]

Disrupt the Developmental Pathways toward IPV

An accumulating body of evidence from longitudinal research suggests that many risk factors for IPV perpetration emerge in childhood and early adolescence, including exposure to child abuse and neglect, family conflict, negative parenting behaviors, involvement with deviant peers, and antisocial behavior.[97,138] Thus, an important strategy for prevention of IPV is one that focuses on disrupting these developmental pathways through approaches that focus on early childhood development and offer parenting skills and other types of supports to parents and children at risk. For example, *early childhood home visitation programs* represent one approach for engaging with families in order to provide education, training, and support to caregivers and families. There are several different models for home visitation programs, but many are delivered by nurses, professionals, or paraprofessionals, and provide support to first time mothers during pregnancy and after the birth of a child in order to improve maternal and child health outcomes.[162]

Programs that focus on *preschool enrichment with family engagement* also have potential to disrupt the developmental pathways toward IPV. *Early Head Start* and *Child Parent Centers* represent two examples of programs that provide high-quality early education to economically disadvantaged families, with research suggesting long-term benefits to school achievement and high school completion, as well as reduced rates of youth involvement in crime and violence.[163] Other approaches that can reduce risk for IPV include *parenting skill and family relationship programs*, which offer support to parents and caregivers in developing positive parenting skills.[164] These programs are associated with decreases in child behavior problems and reductions in youth violence, association with deviant peers, and rates of arrest.[165]

Finally, *treatment for at-risk children, youth, and families* also offers an approach for decreasing risk factors for IPV by providing interventions for youth who are already experiencing conduct problems or report exposure to child abuse and neglect. These interventions are designed to lessen harms associated with these experiences and have demonstrated effectiveness at reducing risk for violent crime, behavioral problems, substance use, and subsequent arrests.[166–168]

Create Protective Environments

Another critical strategy for advancing a public health approach to preventing IPV is developing approaches that work to create protective environments. Implementing prevention approaches that more broadly target schools, workplaces, and neighborhoods has potential to have wide-reaching effects through improved awareness and disclosure of IPV, increased resources for IPV survivors, and social norms change that decreases tolerance for IPV and promotes bystander intervention.[169]

One approach for creating protective environments is to focus on school settings as an opportunity to *improve school climate and safety*. These types of approaches can promote respectful boundaries and reduce tolerance for violence, as well as increase student awareness about TDV and feelings of safety. For adults, the workplace represents an important context and opportunity for IPV prevention, through approaches that *improve organizational policies and workplace climate*. Similar to school-based approaches, these efforts can reduce tolerance for violence among employees in the workplace and promote protective factors, such as providing tangible aid and social support to individuals at risk for IPV. Finally, *modifying the physical and social environment of neighborhoods* is another important approach that involves changing, enacting, or enforcing laws and regulations that can address neighborhood risk factors (e.g., reducing alcohol outlet density), as well as approaches that can strengthen a community's ties and promote willingness to monitor and respond to problem behavior.[153] Together, these community-level approaches aimed at creating protective environments represent an important element of a public health approach to preventing IPV.

Strengthen Economic Supports for Families

Research suggests that strengthening economic supports for families and improving financial stability has the potential to impact multiple socioeconomic factors associated with risk for IPV, such as poverty, financial stress, and unemployment.[97,153] Furthermore, improving education, employment, and income opportunities for women in particular may also be critical to prevention, as studies suggest that gender inequality also increases risk for IPV.[147,170,171]

Efforts to *strengthen household financial security* represent one approach for improving economic factors associated with IPV risk, including supports like income supplements, tax credits, and child-care subsidies. Household financial security can also be enhanced through programs that promote employment or income-generating opportunities. Similarly, approaches that aim to *strengthen work-family supports*, such as paid leave policies, represent another opportunity to improve economic supports to families. Access to these types of work supports can be beneficial in multiple ways for reducing risk for IPV, including reducing financial stress, mitigating the impact of work interruptions on future earning potential, and promoting gender equality.[172]

Support Survivors to Increase Safety and Lessen Harms

As described previously, IPV can have long-lasting negative health outcomes on survivors and their children. In addition to identifying strategies for primary prevention, it is also essential to develop secondary prevention approaches that can support IPV survivors and their children in an effort to increase safety, decrease subsequent IPV experiences, and try to mitigate the negative consequences of IPV for survivors and their children. In the immediate aftermath of violence, *victim-centered services*, which includes crisis intervention, counseling, safe shelter, and medical and legal advocacy, are often the first resources needed by a survivor. Another important resource for supporting survivors involves *housing programs* that assist survivors and their children in quickly finding a safe place to reside following the occurrence of IPV. Programs that support permanent, stable, affordable housing allows survivors to focus on other needs, without fear of homelessness, instability, or future violence from their abuser.[173]

Another approach that can increase safety for survivors involves *first responder and civil legal protections*, which represents an area where public health can form partnerships with other sectors. Tools like lethality assessment programs, protection orders, and supervised visitation and exchange can be utilized by law enforcement, courts, and social services to decrease risk for subsequent IPV.[153] In addition to these approaches, existing federal laws limit access to firearms for individuals who have restraining orders or who have been convicted of a misdemeanor or felony crime of domestic violence. Policies that reduce abusers' access to lethal means have been shown to significantly decrease risk for IPV homicides.[174]

The healthcare sector offers another important opportunity for supporting survivors of IPV, as well as an opportunity to provide universal prevention education that is focused on healthy relationships. *Patient-centered approaches*, such as brief interventions delivered in a primary-care setting, can improve physical and mental health, increase safety behaviors, and reduce risk for experiencing future IPV.[175,176] Finally, *treatment and support for survivors of intimate partner violence, including teen dating violence,* are associated with improved psychological health and long-term positive impacts for survivors.[177] Trauma-informed interventions delivered by licensed mental health providers that consider the complex ways that trauma can influence a survivor's well-being are particularly important.[178] Importantly, evidence suggests that individuals who receive these treatments also report decreased risk for subsequent experiences of IPV victimization.[177]

IMPLEMENTATION CONSIDERATIONS

While research findings indicate that each of these six strategies has evidence for preventing IPV and/or associated risk and protective factors, effect sizes differ from program to program with wide variation in the types of approaches, outcomes, and overall impact on IPV. More research and evidence is needed to support communities in identifying interventions that can fit best with community needs and can have the greatest impact in preventing IPV within different settings and with diverse populations. However, given the significant costs and consequences associated with IPV, immediate action steps are needed based on the best available evidence. Effective public health efforts will require implementing multiple strategies, in an array of settings, to a variety of audiences, in order to achieve a significant decrease in rates of IPV. Comprehensive prevention strategies are critical to having broad and sustained impact on IPV.[179,180] Using a comprehensive strategy would mean that communities are implementing multiple evidence-based approaches that focus on the modifiable risk and protective factors at each level of the social ecology. Existing evidence for IPV prevention strategies and approaches is largely at the individual and relationship level. However, the violence prevention field is beginning to recognize the importance of identifying more outer level (community and societal) and comprehensive approaches in order to reach a greater number of individuals and achieve broader population impact. For example, a recent randomized controlled trial of the Dating Matters comprehensive model for TDV prevention demonstrated significant program effects on TDV perpetration and victimization outcomes among youth in high-risk urban areas relative to the standard of care.[179] This research highlights the potential for comprehensive approaches to enhance IPV prevention efforts. Moreover, approaches implemented at the community- or societal-level can require less individual effort,[181] which is particularly important given that many of the individual-level programs can be resource intensive (e.g., many hours of instructor time, time away from the core curriculum instruction, salary and benefits of outside trainers, and space and materials). Comprehensive prevention of IPV also means prevention efforts are implemented in coordination with victim advocacy and response efforts. Survivors of IPV will be in the audience, in the classroom, and in the community during prevention programs and ensuring that resources and support are in place for them is key.

Another important consideration for implementation relates to the high degree of overlap between IPV and other forms of violence, such as child abuse and neglect, sexual violence, youth violence, and suicide.[153] Given this overlap and the role of shared risk and protective factors that may be influencing rates of violence,[151] communities may benefit from selecting and implementing approaches with cross-cutting prevention effects. This creates opportunities to form nontraditional partnerships and streamline prevention efforts to benefit community health outcomes in multiple ways. In order to accomplish this, multiple sectors are also necessary for prevention—public health can provide leadership and support prevention efforts, but other sectors are needed to implement, support, and reinforce the strategies and approaches listed in this chapter.[153] Forming partnerships across sectors creates opportunities to better support survivors of IPV and reinforce prevention efforts that address the extensive and diverse populations and settings where IPV can occur.

CONCLUSION

IPV across the lifespan represents a significant burden on the health of our society, both in terms of the prevalence of IPV and its far-reaching consequences for survivors, their children, their families, and communities. Once seen as a private issue between husbands and wives,[182] we now recognize IPV as an important public health issue that should be documented, examined, and prevented utilizing a scientific approach that can lead to widespread dissemination and implementation of effective prevention strategies. Although further research is still needed in order to fully understand how to best prevent IPV and its negative consequences, communities can act now to implement strategies based on the best available evidence to work to prevent IPV and stop its negative consequences from affecting society as a whole.[153] Implementing strategies that prevent IPV through reduction of risk factors and promotion of protective factors may also prevent other forms of violence that share these risk and protective factors and will bring us closer to having safer, healthier, and violence-free communities where all people can thrive.

References

1. Breiding MJ, Basile KC, Smith SG, Black MC, Mahendra RR. *Intimate Partner Violence Surveillance: Uniform Definitions and Recommended Data Elements, Version 2.0.* Atlanta, GA: National Center for Injury Prevention and Control, Centers for Disease Control and Prevention; 2015.
2. Smith SG, Zhang X, Basile KC, et al. *The National Intimate Partner and Sexual Violence Survey (NISVS): 2015 Data Brief—Updated Release.* Atlanta, GA: National Center for Injury Prevention and Control, Centers for Disease Control and Prevention; 2018.
3. Connolly J, Furman W, Konarski R. The role of peers in the emergence of heterosexual romantic relationships in adolescence. *Child Dev.* 2000;71(5):1395–408.
4. Smith SG, Chen J, Basile KC, et al. *The National Intimate Partner and Sexual Violence Survey (NISVS): 2010-2012 State Report.* Atlanta, GA: National Center for Injury Prevention and Control, Centers for Disease Control and Prevention; 2017.
5. Kann L, McManus T, Harris WA, et al. Youth risk behavior surveillance—United States, 2017. *MMWR Surveill Summ.* 2018;67(SS-8):1–114.
6. Exner-Cortens D, Eckenrode J, Rothman E. Longitudinal associations between teen dating violence victimization and adverse health outcomes. *Pediatrics.* 2013;131(1):71–8.
7. Smith PH, White JW, Holland, LJ. A longitudinal perspective on dating violence among adolescent and college-age women. *Am J Public Health.* 2003;93(7):1104–9.
8. Garcia-Moreno C, Jansen H, Ellsberg M, Heise L, Watts C. *WHO Multi-Country Study on Women's Health and Domestic Violence Against Women: Initial Results on Prevalence, Health Outcomes, and Women's Responses.* Geneva, Switzerland: World Health Organization; 2005.
9. World Health Organization. *Global and Regional Estimates of Violence Against Women: Prevalence and Health Effects of Intimate Partner Violence and Non-partner Sexual Violence.* Geneva: World Health Organization; 2013.
10. Walters ML, Chen J, Breiding MJ. *The National Intimate Partner and Sexual Violence Survey (NISVS): 2010 Findings on Victimization by Sexual Orientation.* Atlanta, GA: National Center for Injury Prevention and Control, Centers for Disease Control and Prevention; 2013.
11. Breiding MJ, Armour BS. The association between disability and intimate partner violence in the United States. *Ann Epidemiol.* 2015;25(6):455–7.
12. Hahn JW, McCormick MC, Silverman JG, Robinson EB, Koenen KC. Examining the impact of disability status on intimate partner violence victimization in a population sample. *J Interpers Violence.* 2014;29(17):3063–85.
13. Smith DL. Disability, gender and intimate partner violence: Relationships from the behavioral risk factor surveillance system. *Sex Disabil.* 2008;26(1):15–28.
14. Black MC, Basile KC, Breiding MJ, et al. *The National Intimate Partner and Sexual Violence Survey (NISVS): 2010 Summary Report.* Atlanta, GA: National Center for Injury Prevention and Control, Centers for Disease Control and Prevention; 2011.
15. D'Inverno AS, Smith SG, Zhang X, Chen J. *The Impact of Intimate Partner Violence: A 2015 NISVS Research-in- Brief.* Atlanta, GA: National Center for Injury Prevention and Control, Centers for Disease Control and Prevention; 2019.
16. Cooper A, Smith EL. *Homicide Trends in the United States, 1980–2008.* Washington, DC: Bureau of Justice Statistics; 2011.
17. Campbell JC. Health consequences of intimate partner violence. *Lancet.* 2002;359(9314):1331–6.
18. Campbell JC, Lewandowski LA. Mental and physical health effects of intimate partner violence on women and children. *Psychiatr Clin North Am.* 1997;20(2):353–74.
19. Mouton CP, Rovi S, Furniss K, Lasser NL. The associations between health and domestic violence in older women: Results of a pilot study. *J Womens Health Gend Based Med.* 1999;10(9):861–6.
20. Breiding MJ, Black MC, Ryan GW. Chronic disease and health risk behaviors associated with intimate partner violence—18 U.S. states/territories, 2005. *Ann Epidemiol.* 2008;18(7):538–44.
21. Humphreys J, Epel ES, Cooper BA, Lin J, Blackburn EH, Lee KA. Telomere shortening in formerly abused and never abused women. *Biol Res Nurs.* 2012;14(2):115–23.
22. Black MC. Intimate partner violence and adverse health consequences: Implications for clinicians. *Am J Lifestyle Med.* 2011;5(5):428–39.
23. Campbell J, Jones AS, Dienemann J, et al. Intimate partner violence and physical health consequences. *Arch Internal Med.* 2002;162(10):1157–63.
24. Cascardi M, Langhinrichsen J, Vivian D. Marital aggression: Impact, injury and health correlates of husbands and wives. *Arch Intern Med.* 1992;152:357–63.
25. Coker AL, Smith PH, Bethea L, King MR, McKeown RE. Physical health consequences of physical and psychological intimate partner violence. *Arch Fam Med.* 2000;9(5):451–7.
26. Kramer A, Lorenzon D, Mueller G. Prevalence of intimate partner violence and health implications for women using emergency departments and primary care clinics. *Womens Health Issues.* 2004;14:19–29.
27. Leserman J, Drossman DA. Relationship of abuse history to functional gastrointestinal disorders and symptoms. *Trauma Violence Abuse.* 2007;8:331–43.
28. Leserman J, Li D, Drossman DA, Hu YJB. Selected symptoms associated with sexual and physical abuse among female patients with gastrointestinal disorders: The impact on subsequent health care visits. *Psychol Med.* 1998;28:417–25.
29. Letourneau EJ, Holmes M, Chasedunn-Roark J. Gynecologic health consequences to victims of interpersonal violence. *Womens Health Issues.* 1999;9(2):115–20.
30. Plichta SB. Violence and abuse: Implications for women's health. In: Falik MF, Collins KS, eds. *Women's Health: Results from the Commonwealth Fund Survey.* Baltimore: MD: Johns Hopkins University Press; 1996, pp. 237–70.
31. Tollestrup K, Sklar D, Frost FJ, et al. Health indicators and intimate partner violence among women who are members of a managed care organization. *Prev Med.* 1999;29(5):431–40.
32. Weinbaum Z, Stratton TL, Chavez G, Motylewski-Link C, Barrera N, Courtney JG. Female victims of intimate partner physical domestic violence (IPP-DV), California 1998. *Am J Prev Med.* 2001;21(4):313–9.
33. Coker AL, Sanderson M, Fadden MK, Pirisi L. Intimate partner violence and cervical neoplasia. *J Womens Health Gend Based Med.* 2000;10(9):861–6.
34. Eby KK, Campbell JC, Sullivan CM, Davidson WS. Health effects of experiences of sexual violence for women with abusive partners. *Health Care Women Int.* 1995;16(6):563–76.
35. Plichta SB, Abraham C. Violence and gynecologic health in women <50 years old. *Am J Obstet Gynecol.* 1996;174:903–7.
36. Schei B. Physically abusive spouse: A risk factor for pelvic inflammatory disease? *Scand J Prim Health Care.* 1991;9(1):41–5.
37. Schei B, Bakketeig LS. Gynaecological impact of sexual and physical abuse by spouse: A study of a random sample of Norwegian women. *Br J Obstet Gynaecol.* 1989;96(12):1379–83.
38. Coker AL, Davis KE, Arias I, et al. Physical and mental health effects of intimate partner violence for men and women. *Am J Prev Med.* 2002;23(4):260–8.
39. Golding JM. Intimate partner violence as a risk factor for mental disorders: A meta-analysis. *J Fam Viol* 1999;14(2):99–132.
40. Ratner PA. The incidence of wife abuse and mental health status in abused wives in Edmonton, Alberta. *Can J Public Health.* 1993;84(4):246–9.
41. Silva C, McFarlane J, Soeken K, Parker B, Reel S. Symptoms of post-traumatic stress disorder in abused women in a primary care setting. *J Womens Health.* 1997;6(5):543–52.
42. Silverman JG, Raj A, Mucci L, Hathaway J. Dating violence against adolescent girls and associated substance use, unhealthy weight control, sexual risk behavior, pregnancy, and suicidality. *JAMA.* 2001;286(5):572–9.
43. Warshaw C, Brashler P, Gil J. Mental health consequences of intimate partner violence. In: Mitchell C, Anglin D, eds. *Intimate Partner Violence, A Health-Based Perspective.* Oxford: Oxford University Press; 2009, pp. 147–72.
44. Ellsberg M, Caldera T, Herrera A, Winkvist A, Kullgren G. Domestic violence and emotional distress among Nicaraguan women: Results from a population-based study. *Am Psychol.* 1999;54(1):30–6.
45. Fikree FF, Bhatt LI. Domestic violence and health of Pakistani women. *Internat J Gynaecol Obstet.* 1999;65:195–201.
46. Champion JD, Shain RN, Piper J, Perdue ST. Sexual abuse and sexual risk behaviors of minority women with sexually transmitted diseases. *West J Nurs Res.* 2001;23(3):241–54.
47. Hathaway JE, Mucci LA, Silverman JG, Brooks DR, Mathews R, Pavlos CA. Health status and health care use of Massachusetts women reporting partner abuse. *Am J Prev Med.* 2000;19(4):302–7.
48. Lemon SC, Verhoek-Oftedahl W, Donnelly EF. Preventive healthcare use, smoking, and alcohol use among Rhode Island women experiencing intimate partner violence. *J Womens Health Gend Based Med.* 2002;11(6):555–62.

49. Rickert VI, Wiemann CM, Harrykissoon SD, Berenson AB, Kolb E. The relationship among demographics, reproductive characteristics, and intimate partner violence. *Am J Obstet Gynecol.* 2002;187(4):1002–7.
50. Roberts TA, Auinger P, Klein JD. Intimate partner abuse and the reproductive health of sexually active female adolescents. *J Adolesc Health.* 2005;36(5):380–5.
51. Goodwin MM, Gazmararian JA, Johnson CH, Gilbert BC, Saltzman, LE. Pregnancy intendedness and physical abuse around the time of pregnancy: Findings from the Pregnancy Risk Assessment Monitoring System, 1996–1997. PRAMS Working Group. *Matern Child Health J.* 2000;4(2):85–92.
52. Taggart L, Mattson S. Delay in prenatal care as a result of battering in pregnancy: Cross-cultural implications. *Health Care Women Int.* 1996;17(1):25–34.
53. Parsons LH, Harper MA. Violent maternal deaths in North Carolina. *Obstet Gynecol.* 1999;94(6):990–3.
54. Pearlman MD, Tintinalli JE, Lorenz RP. Blunt trauma during pregnancy. *N Engl J Med.* 1990;323(23):1609–13.
55. Amaro H, Fried L, Cabral H, et al. Violence during pregnancy and substance use. *Am J Public Health.* 1990;80(5):575–9.
56. Bailey BA. Partner violence during pregnancy: Prevalence, effects, screening, and management. *Int J Womens Health.* 2010;2:183–97.
57. Cokkinides VE, Coker AL, Sanderson M, Addy C, Bethea L. Physical violence during pregnancy: Maternal complications and birth outcomes. *Obstet Gynecol.* 1999;93(5 Pt. 1):661–6.
58. Jejeebhoy SJ. Associations between wife-beating and fetal and infant death: Impressions from a survey in rural India. *Stud Fam Plann.* 1998;29(3):300–8.
59. Maman S, Campbell JC, Sweat M, Gielen AC. The intersection of HIV and violence: Directions for future research and interventions. *Soc Sci Med.* 2000;50(4):459–78.
60. Martin SL, Kilgallen B, Tsui AO, et al. Sexual behaviors and reproductive health outcomes: Associations with wife abuse in India. *JAMA.* 1999;282(20):1967–72.
61. McFarlane JM. Pregnancy following partner rape: What we know and what we need to know. *Trauma Violence Abuse.* 2007;8(2):127–34.
62. Rosales Ortiz J, Loaiza E, Primante D, Barberena A, Blandon Sequeira L, Ellsberg M. *Encuesta Nicaraguense de Demografia y Salud, 1998 [SPA] [1998 Nicaraguan Demographic and Health Survey].* Managua, Nicaragua: Instituto Nacional de Estadisticas y Censos; 1999.
63. Sarkar NN. The impact of intimate partner violence on women's reproductive health and pregnancy outcome. *J Obstet Gynaecol.* 2008;28(3):266–71.
64. Murphy CC, Schei B, Myhr TL, Du Mont J. Abuse: A risk factor for low birth weight? A systematic review and meta-analysis. *CMAJ.* 2001;164(11):1567–72.
65. Christian CW, Scribano P, Seidl T, Pinto-Martin JA. Pediatric injury resulting from family violence. *Pediatrics.* 1997;99(2):E8.
66. Centers for Disease Control and Prevention, National Center for Injury Prevention and Control. *Costs of Intimate Partner Violence Against Women in the United States.* Atlanta, GA: Centers for Disease Control and Prevention; 2003.
67. Peterson C, Kearns MC, McIntosh WL, et al. Lifetime economic burden of intimate partner violence among United States adults. *Am J Prev Med.* 2018;55(4):433–44.
68. Bronfenbrenner U. Contexts of child rearing: Problems and prospects. *Am Psychol.* 1979;34(10):844–50.
69. Centers for Disease Control and Prevention. *Sexual Violence Prevention: Beginning the Dialogue.* Atlanta, GA: Centers for Disease Control and Prevention; 2004.
70. Cunradi CB, Caetano R, Schafer J. Socioeconomic predictors of intimate partner violence among White, Black, and Hispanic couples in the United States. *J Fam Violence.* 2002;17(4):377–89.
71. Lussier P, Farrington DP, Moffitt TE. Is the antisocial child father of the abusive man? A 40-year prospective longitudinal study on the developmental antecedents of intimate partner violence. *Criminology.* 2009;47(3):741–80.
72. Kim HK, Laurent HK, Capaldi DM, Feingold A. Men's aggression toward women: A 10-year panel study. *J Marriage Fam.* 2008; 70(5):1169–87.
73. Rodriguez E, Lasch KE, Chandra P, Lee J. Family violence, employment status, welfare benefits, and alcohol drinking in the United States: What is the relation? *J Epidemiol Community Health.* 2001;55(3):172–8.
74. Yakubovich AR, Stöckl H, Murray J, Melendez-Torres GJ, Steinert JI, Glavin CEY, Humphreys DK. Risk and protective factors for intimate partner violence against women: Systematic review and meta-analyses of prospective-longitudinal studies. *Am J Public Health.* 2018;108:e1–11.
75. Caetano R, Field CA, Ramisetty-Mikler S, McGrath C. The 5-year course of intimate partner violence among White, Black, and Hispanic couples in the United States. *J Interpers Violence.* 2005;20(9):1039–57.
76. Huang CC, Son E, Wang LR. Prevalence and factors of domestic violence among unmarried mothers with a young child. *Fam Soc.* 2010;91(2):171–7.
77. Vest JR, Catlin TK, Chen JJ, Brownson RC. Multistate analysis of factors associated with intimate partner violence. *Am J Prev Med.* 2002;22(3):156–64.
78. Jasinski JL. The role of acculturation in wife assault. *Hisp J Behav Sci.* 1998;20(2):175–91.
79. Kantor GK, Jasinski JL, Aldarondo E. Sociocultural status and incidence of marital violence in Hispanic families. *Violence and Vict.* 1994;9(3):207–22.
80. Caetano R, Ramisetty-Mikler S, Vaeth PAC, Harris TR. Acculturation stress, drinking, and intimate partner violence among Hispanic couples in the U.S. *J Interpers Violence.* 2007;22(11):1431–47.
81. Jasinski JL, Asdigian NL, Kantor GK. Ethnic adaptations to occupational strain. *J Interpers Violence.* 1997;12(6):814–31.
82. Jasinski JL, Kantor GK. Pregnancy, stress and wife assault: Ethnic differences in prevalence, severity, and onset in a national sample. *Violence Vict.* 2001;16(3):219–32.
83. Neff JA, Holamon B, Schluter TD. Spousal violence among Anglos, Blacks, and Mexican Americans: The role of demographic variables, psychosocial predictors, and alcohol consumption. *J Fam Violence.* 1995;10(1):1–21.
84. Probst JC, Wang J-Y, Martin AB, Moore CG, Paul BM, Samuels ME. Potentially violent disagreements and parenting stress among American Indian/Alaska native families: Analysis across seven states. *Matern Child Health J.* 2008;12(Suppl1):S91–102.
85. Smith Slep AMS, Foran HM, Heyman RE, Snarr JD. Unique risk and protective factors for partner aggression in a large scale Air Force survey. *J Community Health.* 2010;35(4):375–83.
86. Schwab-Reese LM, Peek-Asa C, Parker E. Associations of financial stressors and physical intimate partner violence perpetration. *Inj Epidemiol.* 2016;3(1):6.
87. Ehrensaft MK, Cohen P, Brown J, Smailes E, Chen HN, Johnson JG. Intergenerational transmission of partner violence: A 20-year prospective study. *J Consult Clin Psychol.* 2003;71(4):741–53.
88. Linder JR, Collins WA. Parent and peer predictors of physical aggression and conflict management in romantic relationships in early adulthood. *J Fam Psychol.* 2005;19(2):252–62.
89. Renner LM, Slack KS. Intimate partner violence and child maltreatment: Understanding intra- and intergenerational connections. *Child Abuse Negl.* 2006;30(6):599–617.
90. Roberts AL, Gilman SE, Fitzmaurice G, Decker MR, Koenen KC. Witness of intimate partner violence in childhood and perpetration of intimate partner violence in adulthood. *Epidemiology.* 2010;21(6):809–18.
91. Swinford SP, DeMaris A, Cernkovich SA, Giordano PC. Harsh physical discipline in childhood and violence in later romantic involvements: The mediating role of problem behaviors. *J Marriage Fam.* 2000;62(2):508–19.
92. White HR, Widom CS. Intimate partner violence among abused and neglected children in young adulthood: The mediating effects of early aggression, antisocial personality, hostility and alcohol problems. *Aggress Behav.* 2003;29(4):332–45.
93. Capaldi DM, Dishion TJ, Stoolmiller M, Yoerger K. Aggression toward female partners by at-risk young men: The contribution of male adolescent friendships. *Dev Psychol.* 2001;37(1):61–73.
94. Huesmann LR, Dubow EF, Boxer P. Continuity of aggression from childhood to early adulthood as a predictor of life outcomes: Implications for the adolescent-limited and life-course-persistent models. *Aggress Behav.* 2009;35(2):136–49.
95. Kim HK, Capaldi DM. The association of antisocial behavior and depressive symptoms between partners and risk for aggression in romantic relationships. *J Fam Psychol.* 2004;18(1):82–96.
96. Smith CA, Greenman SJ, Thornberry TP, Henry KL, Ireland TO. Adolescent risk for intimate partner violence perpetration. *Prev Sci.* 2015;16(6): 862–72.
97. Capaldi DM, Knoble NB, Shortt JW, Kim HK. A systematic review of risk factors for intimate partner violence. *Partner Abuse.* 2012;3(2):231–80.

98. Ellison CG, Anderson KL. Religious involvement and domestic violence among US couples. *J Sci Study Relig*. 2001;40(2):269–86.
99. Capaldi DM, Crosby L. Observed and reported psychological and physical aggression in young, at-risk couples. *Soc Dev*. 1997;6(2):184–206.
100. Diaz-Aguado MJ, Martinez R. Types of adolescent male dating violence against women, self-esteem, and justification of dominance and aggression. *J Interpers Violence*. 2015 Sep;30(15):2636–58.
101. Cleveland HH, Herrera VM, Stuewig J. Abusive males and abused females in adolescent relationships: Risk factor similarity and dissimilarity and the role of relationship seriousness. *J Interpers Violence*. 2003;18(6):325–39.
102. Spencer C, Mallory AB, Cafferky BM, Kimmes JG, Beck AR, Stith SM. Mental health factors and intimate partner violence perpetration and victimization: A meta-analysis. *Psychol Violence*. 2019;9(1):1–17.
103. Howard DE, Wang MQ, Yan F. Psychological factors associated with reports of physical dating violence among U.S. adolescent females. *Adolescence*. 2007;42(166):311–24.
104. Kerr DCR, Capaldi DM. Young men's intimate partner violence and relationship functioning: Longterm outcomes associated with suicide attempt and aggression in adolescence. *Psychol Med*. 2011;41(4):759–69.
105. Seedat S, Stein MB, Forde DR. Association between physical partner violence, posttraumatic stress, childhood trauma, and suicide attempts in a community sample of women. *Violence Vict*. 2005;20(1):87–98.
106. Feingold A, Kerr DCR, Capaldi DM. Associations of substance use problems with intimate partner violence for at-risk men in long-term relationships. *J Fam Psychol*. 2008;22(3):429–38.
107. Okuda M, Olfson M, Wang S, Rubio JM, Xu Y, Blanco C. Correlates of intimate partner violence perpetration: Results from a National Epidemiologic Survey. *J Trauma Stress*. 2015;28(1):49–56.
108. Schluter PJ, Abbott MW, Bellringer ME. Problem gambling related to intimate partner violence: Findings from the Pacific Islands families study. *Int Gambl Stud*. 2008;8(1):49–61.
109. Spencer CM, Stith SM, Cafferky B. Risk markers for physical intimate partner violence victimization: A meta-analysis. *Aggress Violent Behav*. 2019;44:8–17.
110. Fite JE, Bates JE, Holtzworth-Munroe A, Dodge KA, Nay SY, Pettit GS. Social information processing mediates the intergenerational transmission of aggressiveness in romantic relationships. *J Fam Psychol*. 2008;22(3):367–76.
111. Connolly J, Nocentini A, Menesini E, Pepler D, Craig W, Williams TS. Adolescent dating aggression in Canada and Italy: A cross-national comparison. *Int J Behav Dev*. 2010;34(2):98–105.
112. White JW, Merrill LL, Koss MP. Predictors of premilitary courtship violence in a Navy recruit sample. *J Interpers Violence*. 2001;16(9):910–27.
113. Das M, Ghosh S, Verma R, O'Connor B, Fewer S, Catrina Virata M, Miller E. Gender attitudes and violence among urban adolescent boys in India. *Int J Adolesc Youth*. 2014;19(1):99–112.
114. McCauley HL, Tancredi DJ, Silverman JG, et al. Gender equitable attitudes, bystander behavior, and recent abuse perpetration against heterosexual dating partners of male high school athletes. *Am J Public Health*. 2013;103(10):1882–7.
115. Santana MC, Raj A, Decker MR, La Marche A, Silverman JG. Masculine gender roles associated with increased sexual risk and intimate partner violence perpetration among young adult men. *J Urban Health*. 2006;83(4):575–85.
116. Aldarondo E, Sugarman DB. Risk marker analysis of the cessation and persistence of wife assault. *J Consult Clin Psychol*. 1996;64(5):1010–9.
117. Bookwala J, Sobin J, Zdaniuk B. Gender and aggression in marital relationships: A life-span perspective. *Sex Roles*. 2005;52(11–12):797–806.
118. DeMaris A, Benson ML, Fox GL, Hill T, Van Wyk J. Distal and proximal factors in domestic violence: A test of an integrated model. *J Marriage Fam*. 2003;65(3):652–67.
119. O'Leary KD, Tintle N, Bromet E. Risk factors for physical violence against partners in the US. *Psychol Violence*. 2014;4(1):65–77.
120. Shortt JW, Capaldi DM, Kim HK, Tiberio SS. The interplay between interpersonal stress and psychological intimate partner violence over time for young at-risk couples. *J Youth Adolescence*. 2013;42(4):619–32.
121. Brownridge DA. Understanding women's heightened risk of violence in common-law unions: Revisiting the selection and relationship hypotheses. *Violence against Women*. 2004;10(6):626–51.
122. Moffitt TE, Krueger RF, Caspi A, Fagan J. Partner abuse and general crime: How are they the same? How are they different? *Criminology*. 2000;38(1):199–232.
123. Cui M, Durtschi JA, Donnellan MB, Lorenz FO, Conger RD. Intergenerational transmission of relationship aggression: A prospective longitudinal study. *J Fam Psychol*. 2010;24(6):688–97.
124. Herrera VM, Wiersma JD, Cleveland HH. The influence of individual and partner characteristics on the perpetration of intimate partner violence in young adult relationships. *J Youth Adolesc*. 2008;37(3):284–96.
125. Hyman L, Forte T, Mont JD, Romans S, Cohen MM. The association between length of stay in Canada and intimate partner violence among immigrant women. *Am J Public Health*. 2006;96(4):654–9.
126. Slashinski MJ, Coker AL, Davis KE. Physical aggression, forced sex, and stalking victimization by a dating partner: An analysis of the National Violence Against Women Survey. *Violence Vict*. 2003;18(6):595–617.
127. Arriaga XB, Foshee VA. Adolescent dating violence: Do adolescents follow in their friends', or their parents', footsteps? *J Interpers Violence*. 2004;19(2):162–84.
128. Foshee VA, Reyes HLM, Ennett ST, et al. Risk and protective factors distinguishing profiles of adolescent peer and dating violence perpetration. *J Adolesc Health*. 2011;48(4):344–50.
129. Schnurr MP, Lohman BJ. How much does school matter? An examination of adolescent dating violence perpetration. *J Youth Adolesc*. 2008;37(3):266–83.
130. Williams JR, Ghandour RM, Kub JE. Female perpetration of violence in heterosexual intimate relationships: Adolescence through adulthood. *Trauma Violence Abuse*. 2008;9(4):227–49.
131. Lanier C, Maume MO. Intimate partner violence and social isolation across the rural/urban divide. *Violence Against Women*. 2009;15(11):1311–30.
132. Banyard VL, Modecki KL. Interpersonal violence in adolescence—Ecological correlates of self-reported perpetration. *J Interpers Violence*. 2006;21(10):1314–32.
133. Maas CD, Fleming CB, Herrenkohl TI, Catalano RF. Childhood predictors of teen dating violence victimization. *Violence Vict*. 2010;25(2):131–49.
134. Espelage DL, Leemis RW, Niolon PH, Kearns M, Basile KC, Davis JP. Teen dating violence perpetration: Protective factor trajectories from middle to high school among adolescents. *J Res Adolesc*. 2020;30(1):170–88. doi: 10.1111/jora.12510
135. Stocker CM, Richmond MK. Longitudinal associations between hostility in adolescents' family relationships and friendships and hostility in their romantic relationships. *J Fam Psychol*. 2007;21(3):490–7.
136. Foshee VA, Reyes HL, Ennett ST. Examination of sex and race differences in longitudinal predictors of the initiation of adolescent dating violence perpetration. *J Aggress Maltreat Trauma*. 2010;19(5):492–516.
137. Ozer E, Tschann J, Pasch L, Flores E. Violence perpetration across peer and partner relationships: Co-occurrence and longitudinal patterns among adolescents. *J Adolesc Health*. 2004;34(1):64–71.
138. Vagi KJ, Rothamn E, Latzman NE, Tharp AT, Hall DM, Breiding MJ. Beyond correlates: A review of risk and protective factors for adolescent dating violence perpetration. *J Youth Adolesc*. 2013;42(4):633–49.
139. Dahlberg LL, Krug EG. Violence-a global public health problem. In: Krug E, Dahlberg LL, Mercy JA, Zwi AB, Lozano R, eds. *World Report on Violence and Health*. Geneva, Switzerland: World Health Organization; 2002, pp. 1–56.
140. Kearns MC, Reidy DE, Valle LA. The role of alcohol policies in preventing intimate partner violence: A review of the literature. *J Stud Alcohol Drugs*. 2015;76(1):21–30.
141. Jain S, Buka SL, Subramanian SV, Molnar BE. Neighborhood predictors of dating violence victimization and perpetration in young adulthood: A multilevel study. *Am J Public Health*. 2010;100(9):1737–44.
142. Rothman EF, Johnson RM, Young R, Weinberg J, Azrael D, Molnar BE. Neighborhood-level factors associated with physical dating violence perpetration: Results of a representative survey conducted in Boston, MA. *J Urban Health*. 2011;88(2):201–13.
143. Spriggs AL, Halpern CT, Herring AH, Schoenbach VJ. Family and school socioeconomic disadvantage: Interactive influences on adolescent dating violence victimization. *Soc Sci Med*. 2009;68(11):1956–65.
144. McKinsey Global Institute. *The Power of Parity: Advancing Women's Equality in the United States*. New York: McKinsey & Company; 2016.
145. Baron L, Straus MA. *Four Theories of Rape in American Society: A State-Level Analysis*. New Haven: Yale University Press; 1989.
146. World Health Organization. *Social Determinants of Sexual and Reproductive Health: Informing Future Research and Programme Implementation*. Geneva, Switzerland: WHO; 2010.
147. Gressard LA, Swahn MH, Tharp AT. A first look at gender inequality as a societal risk factor for dating violence. *Am J Prev Med*. 2015;49(3):448–57.
148. Willie TC, Kershaw TS. An ecological analysis of gender inequality and intimate partner violence in the United States. *Prev Med*. 2019;118:257–63.
149. Jewkes R, Sen P, Garcia-Moreno C. Sexual violence. In: Krug E, Dahlberg L, Mercy J, Zwi A, Lozano R, eds. *World Report on Violence*

and Health. Geneva, Switzerland: World Health Organization; 2002, pp. 147–81.

150. Heise LL, Kotsadam A. Cross-national and multilevel correlates of partner violence: An analysis of data from population-based surveys. *Lancet Glob Health*. 2015;3(6):e332–40.
151. Wilkins N, Tsao B, Hertz M, Davis R, Klevens, J. *Connecting the Dots: An Overview of the Links Among Multiple Forms of Violence*. Atlanta, GA: National Center for Injury Prevention and Control, Centers for Disease Control and Prevention; 2014.
152. Frieden TR. Six components necessary for effective public health program implementation. *Am J Public Health*. 2014;104(1):17–22.
153. Niolon PH, Kearns MC, Dills J, et al. *Preventing Intimate Partner Violence Across the Lifespan: A Technical Package of Programs, Policies and Practices*. Atlanta, GA: National Center for Injury Prevention and Control, Centers for Disease Control and Prevention; 2017.
154. David-Ferdon C, Vivolo-Kantor AM, Dahlberg LL, Marshall KJ, Rainford N, Hall JE. *A Comprehensive Technical Package for the Prevention of Youth Violence and Associated Risk Behaviors*. Atlanta, GA: National Center for Injury Prevention and Control, Centers for Disease Control and Prevention; 2016.
155. Feldman CM, Ridley CA. The role of conflict-based communication responses and outcomes in male domestic violence toward female partners. *J Soc Pers Relat*. 2000;17(4–5):552–73.
156. Foshee VA, Reyes LM, Agnew-Brune CB, et al. The effects of the evidence-based Safe Dates dating abuse prevention program on other youth violence outcomes. *Prev Sci*. 2014;15(6):907–16.
157. McCollum EE, Stith SM. Couples treatment for interpersonal violence: A review of outcome research literature and current clinical practices. *Violence Vict*. 2008;23(2):187–201.
158. Banyard VL. *Toward the Next Generation of Bystander Prevention of Sexual and Relationship Violence: Action Coils to Engage Communities*. New York: Springer; 2015.
159. Banyard VL, Moynihan MM, Plante EG. Sexual violence prevention through bystander education: An experimental evaluation. *J Community Psychol*. 2007;35(4):463–81.
160. Coker AL, Fisher BS, Bush HM, et al. Evaluation of the Green Dot bystander intervention to reduce interpersonal violence among college students across three campuses. *Violence Against Women*. 2015;21(12):1507–27.
161. Foshee VA, Reyes HLM, Ennett ST, Cance JD, Bauman KE, Bowling JM. Assessing the effects of Families for Safe Dates, a family-based teen dating abuse prevention program. *J Adolesc Health*. 2012;51(4):349–56.
162. Avellar S, Paulsell D, Sama-Miller E, Del Grosso P, Akers L, Kleinman R. *Home Visiting Evidence of Effectiveness Review: Executive Summary*. Washington, DC: Office of Planning, Research and Evaluation, Administration for Children and Families, U.S. Department of Health and Human Services; 2016. http://homvee.acf.hhs.gov/. February, 2018.
163. Reynolds AJ, Temple JA, Robertson DL, Mann EA. Long-term effects of an early childhood intervention on educational achievement and juvenile arrest: A 15-year follow-up of low-income children in public schools. *JAMA*. 2001;285(18):2339–46.
164. Piquero AR, Jennings WG, Diamond B, et al. A meta-analysis update on the effects of early family/parent training programs on antisocial behavior and delinquency. *J Exp Criminol*. 2016;12(2):229–48.
165. Forgatch MS, Patterson GR, DeGarmo DS, Beldavs Z. Testing the Oregon delinquency model with 9-year follow-up of the Oregon Divorce Study. *Dev Psychopathol*. 2009;21(5):637–60.
166. Task Force on Community Preventive Services. Recommendations to reduce violence through early childhood home visitation, therapeutic foster care, and firearm laws. *Am J Prev Med*. 2005;28(251):6–10.
167. Fisher PA, Gilliam KS. Multidimensional treatment foster care: An alternative to residential treatment for high risk children and adolescents. *Interv Psicosoc*. 2012;21(2):195–203.
168. Sawyer AM, Borduin CM. Effects of multisystemic therapy through midlife: A 21.9-year follow-up to a randomized clinical trial with serious and violent juvenile offenders. *J Consult Clin Psychol*. 2011;79(5):643–52.
169. Browning CR. The span of collective efficacy: Extending social disorganization theory to partner violence. *J Marriage Fam*. 2002;64(4):833–50.
170. World Health Organization/London School of Hygiene and Tropical Medicine. *Preventing Intimate Partner and Sexual Violence Against Women: Taking Action and Generating Evidence*. Geneva: World Health Organization; 2010.
171. Vyas S, Watts C. How does economic empowerment affect women's risk of intimate partner violence in low- and middle-income countries? A systematic review of published evidence. *J Int Dev*. 2009;21(5):577–602.
172. D'Inverno A, Reidy DE, Kearns MC. Paid parental leave policies: Can they reduce intimate partner violence? *Prev Med*. 2018;114:18–23.
173. Mbilinyi L. *The Washington State Domestic Violence Housing First Program: Cohort 2 Agencies Final Evaluation Report*. Washington State Coalition Against Domestic Violence. 2015. https://wscadv.org/resources/the-washington-state-domestic-violence-housing-first-program-cohort-2-agencies-final-evaluation-report-september-2011-september-2014/. February, 2018.
174. Zeoli AM, Webster DW. Effects of domestic violence policies, alcohol taxes and police staffing levels on intimate partner homicide in large US cities. *Inj Prev*. 2010;16(2):90–5.
175. Nelson HD, Bougatsos C, Blazina I. Screening women for intimate partner violence: A systematic review to update the U.S. Preventive Services Task Force Recommendation. *Ann Intern Med*. 2012;156(11):796–808.
176. Bair-Merritt MH, Lewis-O'Connor A, Goel S, et al. Primary care-based interventions for intimate partner violence: A systematic review. *Am J Prev Med*. 2014;46(2):188–94.
177. Iverson KM, Gradus JL, Resick PA, Suvak MK, Smith KF, Monson CM. Cognitive-behavioral therapy for PTSD and depression symptoms reduces risk for future intimate partner violence among interpersonal trauma survivors. *J Consult Clin Psychol*. 2011;79(2):193–202.
178. Elliott DE, Bjelajac P, Fallot RD, Markoff LS, Reed BG. Trauma-informed or trauma-denied: Principles and implementation of trauma-informed services for women. *J Community Psychol*. 2005;33(4):461–77.
179. Niolon PN, Vivolo-Kantor AM, Tracy AJ, et al. An RCT of dating matters: Effects on teen dating violence and relationship behaviors. *Am J Prev Med*. 2019;57(1):13–23.
180. David-Ferdon C, Simon TR. *Preventing Youth Violence: Opportunities for Action*. Atlanta, GA: National Center for Injury Prevention and Control, CDC; 2014.
181. Frieden TR. A framework for public health action: The health impact pyramid. *Am J Public Health*. 2010;100(4):590–5.
182. Fagan J. *The Criminalization of Domestic Violence: Promises and Limits*. Washington, DC: US Department of Justice, Office of Justice Programs, National Institute of Justice; 1996.
183. Wolfe DA, Crooks C, Jaffe P, et al. A school-based program to prevent adolescent dating violence: A cluster randomized trial. *Arch Pediatr Adolesc Med*. 2009;163(8):692–9.
184. Markman HJ, Renick MJ, Floyd FJ, Stanley SM, Clements M. Preventing marital distress through communication and conflict management training: A 4-and 5-year follow-up. *J Consult Clin Psychol*. 1993:61(1):70.
185. Coker AL, Bush HM, Cook-Craig PG, et al. RCT testing bystander effectiveness to reduce violence. *Am J Prev Med*. 2017;52(5):566–78.
186. Miller E, Tancredi DJ, McCauley HL, et al. One-year follow-up of a coach-delivered dating violence prevention program: A cluster randomized controlled trial. *Am J Prev Med*. 2013;45(1):108–12.
187. Olds DL, Robinson J, Pettitt L, et al. Effects of home visits by paraprofessionals and by nurses: Age 4 follow-up results of a randomized trial. *Pediatrics*. 2004;114(6):1560–8.
188. Olds DL, Eckenrode J, Henderson CR, et al. Long-term effects of home visitation on maternal life course and child abuse and neglect: Fifteen-year follow-up of a randomized trial. *JAMA*. 1997;278(8):637–43.
189. Olds DL, Kitzman H, Hanks C, et al. Effects of nurse home visiting on maternal and child functioning: Age-9 follow-up of a randomized trial. *Pediatrics*. 2007;120:e832–45.
190. Olds DL, Henderson CR, Kitzman H. Does prenatal and infancy nurse home visitation have enduring effects on qualities of parental caregiving and child health at 25 to 50 months of life? *Pediatrics*. 1994;93(1):89–98.
191. Olds DL, Henderson CR, Cole R, et al. Long-term effects of Nurse Home Visitation on children's criminal and antisocial behavior: 15-Year follow-up of a randomized controlled trial. *JAMA*. 1998;280(14):1238–44.
192. Eckenrode J, Campa M, Luckey DW, et al. Long-term effects of prenatal and infancy nurse home visitation on the life course of youths: 19-Year follow-up of a randomized trial. *Arch Pediatr Adolesc Med*. 2010;164(1):9–15.
193. Green BL, Ayoub C, Bartlett JD, et al. The effect of Early Head Start on child welfare system involvement: A first look at longitudinal child maltreatment outcomes. *Child Youth Serv Rev*. 2014;42:127–35.
194. Kjøbli J, Ogden T. A randomized effectiveness trial of brief parent training in primary care settings. *Prev Sci*. 2012;13(6):616–26.
195. Patterson GR, Forgatch MS, DeGarmo DS. Cascading effects following intervention. *Dev Psychopathol*. 2010;22(4):949–70.
196. Martinez C, Eddy M. Effects of culturally adapted Parent Management Training on Latino youth behavioral health outcomes. *J Consult Clin Psychol*. 2005;73(4):841–51.

197. Taylor BG, Stein ND, Mumford EA, Woods D. Shifting boundaries: An experimental evaluation of a dating violence prevention program in middle schools. *Prev Sci.* 2013;14(1):64–76.

198. Glass N, Hanson GC, Laharnar N, Anger WK, Perrin N. Interactive training improves workplace climate, knowledge, and support towards domestic violence. *Am J Ind Med.* 2016;59(7):538–48.

199. Pronyk PM, Hargreaves JR, Kim JC, et al. Effect of a structural intervention for the prevention of intimate-partner violence and HIV in rural South Africa: A cluster randomised trial. *Lancet.* 2006;368:1973–83.

200. Kim JC, Watts CH, Hargreaves JR, et al. Understanding the impact of a microfinance-based intervention on women's empowerment and the reduction of intimate partner violence in South Africa. *Am J Public Health.* 2007;97(10):1794–802.

201. Gartland D, Hemphill SA, Hegarty K, Brown SJ. Intimate partner violence during pregnancy and the first year postpartum in an Australian pregnancy cohort study. *Matern Child Health J.* 2011;15(5):570–8.

202. Chatterji P, Markowitz S. Does the length of maternity leave affect maternal health? *South Econ J.* 2005;72(1):16–41.

203. Sullivan CM. *Domestic Violence Shelter Services: A Review of the Empirical Evidence.* Harrisburg, PA: National Resource Center on Domestic Violence; October 2012. http://www.dvevidenceproject.org. February, 2018.

204. Messing JT, Campbell J, Wilson JS, Brown S, Patchell B, Shall C. *Police Departments' Use of the Lethality Assessment Program: A Quasi-Experimental Evaluation.* Washington, DC: US Department of Justice (document # 247456); 2014.

205. Benitez CT, McNiel DE, Binder RL. Do protection orders protect? *J Am Acad Psychiatry Law.* 2010;38(3):376–85.

206. Holt VL, Kernic MA, Lumley T, Wolf ME, Rivara FP. Civil protection orders and risk of subsequent police-reported violence. *JAMA.* 2002;288(5):589–94.

207. Miller E, Decker MR, McCauley HL, et al. A family planning clinic partner violence intervention to reduce risk associated with reproductive coercion. *Contraception.* 2011;83(3):274–80.

CHAPTER 179

Sexual Violence*

Tracy N. Hipp • Sarah DeGue

Sexual violence is a major public health problem that exacts a toll on the health and well-being of millions of individuals, communities, and broader society. Decades of research have improved our understanding of the nature and scope of the problem, including disparities in the burden of sexual violence across populations. Researchers have also documented the substantial short- and long-term effects of sexual violence on survivors and estimated the economic burden to society that results. In recent years, the field has made strides by identifying evidence-based approaches for primary prevention of sexual violence at each level of the social ecology. Perhaps most importantly, the field has begun to move toward a focus on shared risk and protective factors for co-occurring and interconnected forms of violence, a new strategic direction for violence prevention aimed at maximizing the impact of prevention efforts and resources. This chapter reviews what we know about the nature and burden of sexual violence—and how we can prevent it.

UNDERSTANDING SEXUAL VIOLENCE AND ITS CONSEQUENCES

Sexual violence, as defined by the Centers for Disease Control and Prevention (CDC), includes any sexual act committed or attempted by another person without the victim's freely given consent or against someone unable to consent or refuse.[1] This definition encompasses a range of unwanted sexual behaviors, including sexual penetration of a victim or being made to sexually penetrate someone else resulting from the use of physical force, alcohol/drug intoxication, or nonphysical pressure (i.e., sexual coercion). Sexual violence also includes intentional sexual touching or noncontact acts of a sexual nature that are unwanted and without victim consent.[1] Sexual violence can occur at any age (e.g., against children or adults), anywhere (e.g., at home, work, school, or in public), and by any type of perpetrator (e.g., friend, spouse or intimate partner, relative, coworker, acquaintance, or stranger). As such, it overlaps substantially with other domains of violence research. For example, sexual violence against children is frequently considered in the context of research on childhood abuse and neglect (see Chapter 176: Child Abuse and Neglect), while sexual violence within the context of an intimate relationship is often addressed in research on intimate partner violence (see Chapter 178: Intimate Partner Violence Prevention). Although a majority of sexual violence involves a male perpetrator and a female victim, sexual violence can also occur between people of the same sex and can involve a woman perpetrating sexual violence.[2–4]

The term sexual violence—used most often in social science and public health research and practice—captures a broad range of sexually violating behaviors that may or may not meet the legal standards for criminal behavior in every state or jurisdiction.[5] In contrast, the terms rape and sexual assault originate in legal definitions of criminal sexual behavior, capturing more defined subsets of unwanted sexual acts that vary by jurisdiction. Rape typically refers—in a legal context—to nonconsensual sexual penetration that results from the use or threat of physical force, while sexual assault can include other forms of nonconsensual or forced sexual acts and contact (e.g., fondling). This chapter will generally use the term sexual violence to refer to any behaviors falling within the CDC definition. Table 179-1[1,3] provides key terms and definitions to guide the reader throughout this chapter.

Measuring Sexual Violence

Despite calls for the use of uniform definitions and measurement,[1] sexual violence research often uses definitions and survey instruments that vary in the types of sexual violence assessed, the wording used to assess those forms of sexual violence, and the reference periods during which the violence occurred. As a result, the field has yielded varying prevalence estimates. Studies that measure attempted or completed rape will yield smaller estimates than studies that measure sexual violence—a broader construct that includes more behaviors. Understanding which forms of sexual violence are included in sexual violence research and how those forms of sexual violence were defined and measured is important. For example, research suggests that asking respondents whether they have "ever been raped" can produce artificially low estimates of the true number of rape victims. Many people who have experienced unwanted or forced sex—even experiences meeting the legal definition of rape—have not labeled those experiences as "rape" themselves.[6,7] Thus, asking whether this term applies to them relies on their own understanding of their experience and definitions of rape, something which can shift over time. Instead, researchers ask *behaviorally specific* questions in which they embed the definition of the behavior within the survey question. For example, a behaviorally specific item assessing rape victimization might ask: "Have you ever had vaginal, oral, or anal sex when you didn't want to because someone threatened or used some degree of physical force (twisting your arm, holding you down, etc.) to make you?" The practice of behaviorally specific wording became standard in the field after the development of the Sexual Experiences Survey (SES) in the mid-1980s.[8] The SES has been revised and updated

*The findings and conclusions in this chapter are those of the authors and do not necessarily represent the official position of the Centers for Disease Control and Prevention.

TABLE 179-1 OPERATIONAL DEFINITIONS FOR DIFFERENT FORMS OF SEXUAL VIOLENCE MEASURED BY THE NATIONAL INTIMATE PARTNER AND SEXUAL VIOLENCE SURVEY (NISVS)

Term	Definition
Sexual violence	A sexual act that is committed or attempted by another person without freely given consent of the victim or against someone who is unable to consent or refuse. It includes: forced or alcohol-/drug-facilitated penetration of a victim; forced or alcohol-/drug-facilitated incidents in which the victim was made to penetrate a perpetrator or someone else; nonphysically pressured unwanted penetration; intentional sexual touching; or noncontact acts of a sexual nature. Sexual violence can also occur when a perpetrator forces or coerces a victim to engage in sexual acts with a third party.
Contact sexual violence	A combined measure of sexual violence that includes rape, being made to penetrate someone else, sexual coercion, and/or unwanted sexual contact.
Rape	Any completed or attempted unwanted vaginal, oral, or anal penetration involving physical force or threats to physically harm and includes times when the victim was unable to give consent due to incapacitation resulting from drugs or alcohol. Rape is further separated into three types: completed forced penetration, attempted forced penetration, and completed alcohol- or drug-facilitated penetration.
Made to penetrate	Being made to penetrate another person due to force, threat of harm, or when unable to consent due to the effects of drugs or alcohol. This definition also includes being forced to receive oral sex.
Sexual coercion	Unwanted penetration that occurred due to nonphysical pressure, such as using one's authority to pressure the victim, threatening to lie or spread rumors about the victim, or wearing someone down by repeatedly verbally pressuring someone for sex.
Unwanted sexual contact	Sexual touching that does not involve penetration, such as groping or fondling.
Noncontact sexual violence	Unwanted sexual experiences that do not involve touching or penetration, such as someone exposing themselves or flashing their sexual body parts, masturbating in front of the victim, forcing a victim to expose their own body parts, making a victim participate in or view sexually explicit photographs or movies, or harassing the victim (in a public place) in a way that made the victim feel unsafe.

Source: From Smith SG, Zhang X, Basile KC, et al. *The National Intimate Partner and Sexual Violence Survey (NISVS): 2015 Data Brief—Updated Release.* Atlanta, GA: National Center for Injury Prevention and Control, Centers for Disease Control and Prevention; 2018.

over time to assess both victimization and perpetration, and is still the most widely used measure of self-reported sexual violence for research purposes. The latest version of this instrument uses gender-neutral wording in order to capture female perpetration and male victimization,[9] an important advancement in the field.

Research instruments may ask whether or how frequently a behavior occurred during a prespecified timeframe. This *reference period* is important for violence researchers to consider. Some surveys ask about sexual violence experienced across the survivor's lifetime (e.g., "Have you *ever* experienced…") while others ask about victimization since the age of 14 or 18 years old to differentiate child sexual abuse from victimization in adolescence or adulthood. In other cases, asking about victimization or perpetration during the prior calendar year, or since the start of a school year, may be most useful. There are a number of reasons that researchers may choose different reference periods. Researchers may want to establish the incidence or the prevalence of the problem. Assessing *incidence*, or new cases (or incidents) that occur within a specific timeframe, enables researchers to track trends in violence over time, assessing whether rates of sexual violence are increasing, decreasing, or remaining stable. Establishing what proportion of individuals within a population have ever experienced sexual violence provides the *lifetime prevalence* of the problem and allows researchers, public health experts, service providers, policy-makers, and others to better understand the *burden* of the problem. *Period prevalence* can also be assessed within a specific timeframe, such as the last 12 months, to understand the proportion of the population affected by violence during that period. When assessed repeatedly, prevalence estimates also allow for the identification of trends in victimization over time and changes in the total burden. Asking about victimization or perpetration during a shorter, more recent time period (e.g., in the last 6 months) may be useful for assessing reductions in sexual violence following an intervention. The important thing to remember is that estimates using different reference periods cannot be directly compared. In this chapter we rely primarily on lifetime prevalence data—the proportion of individuals surveyed that have experienced sexual violence at any point during their lives—in order to highlight disparities in the burden of sexual violence across populations.

Sexual Violence Victimization around the World

In 2013, the World Health Organization (WHO) published the first global systematic review—based on data from 79 countries and 2 territories—estimating the prevalence of two forms of violence against women: intimate partner violence (IPV; including physical and sexual violence by a partner) and nonpartner sexual violence.[10] Worldwide, approximately 30% of all ever-partnered women reported IPV, while about 7% of all women reported nonpartner sexual violence. Estimates for partner-perpetrated sexual violence, specifically, were not available. While rates of IPV tended to be highest in low- and middle-income regions, nonpartner sexual violence was highest in the WHO-defined high-income regions (13%; e.g., United States of America, Australia, Canada, and a number of European countries), as well as in African nations (12%) and the Americas (11%). The South-East Asian region reported high rates of IPV (37%) but the lowest rates of nonpartner sexual violence (5%). WHO estimated that, on average, almost 36% of women worldwide have experienced one or both of these forms of violence.[10]

Global prevalence rates for childhood sexual abuse, specifically, are limited. A seven-country national household survey of 13- to 24-year olds conducted by CDC in partnership with the United Nations International Children's Emergency Fund (UNICEF) and local governments sought to establish the prevalence of sexual violence against children in Cambodia, Haiti, Kenya, Malawi, Swaziland, Tanzania, and Zimbabwe.[11] The survey measured lifetime sexual violence experienced before 18 years of age. Cambodia reported the lowest prevalence of sexual violence among girls (4.4%) and boys (5.6%) while Swaziland reported the highest rates among girls (37.6%). Rates among boys were not assessed in Swaziland.

Sexual Violence Victimization in the US

The CDC's National Intimate Partner and Sexual Violence Survey (NISVS) provides the most comprehensive national- and state-level data on the prevalence of sexual violence in the United States (www.cdc.gov/violenceprevention/datasources/nisvs). Since 2010, this telephone survey has tracked the 12 month and lifetime prevalence of sexual violence, intimate partner violence, and stalking victimization in the United States on an ongoing basis. The most recent figures from NISVS, using data collected in 2015, indicate that approximately two in five women and one in four men in the United States have experienced contact sexual violence (e.g., rape, coerced sex, unwanted touching) in their lifetime, while one in five women and 2.6% of men have experienced attempted or completed rape at some point in life.[12] State-level prevalence estimates of lifetime contact sexual violence from 2010 to 2012, the most recent data years available, ranged from 29.5% (Louisiana) to 47.5% (Oregon) among women and 10.4% (Utah) to 29.3% (Washington, DC) among men.

Rates of sexual violence vary by demographic characteristics of the victim. Historically marginalized groups experience a disproportionate burden of the problem. In the sections that follow, we provide prevalence rates for individuals within a number of demographic categories, as well as prevalence rates among college students.

Race/Ethnicity

As shown in Fig. 179-1,[3] individuals who are multiracial and American Indian and Alaskan Native (AIAN) tend to report the highest rates of lifetime sexual violence victimization while both men and women identifying as Asian or Pacific Islander reported the lowest rates. Disparities in sexual violence victimization by race or ethnicity may reflect, in part, the impacts of systemic disadvantage. Factors such as limited educational and employment opportunities and high poverty rates, which disproportionately impact AIAN populations and other racial and ethnic minority groups, may increase risk for sexual violence victimization by acting as a barrier to escaping violent families or relationships.[13] Some have also hypothesized that certain racial or ethnic groups, such as Asian American women, may be less likely to report sexual violence, even in anonymous surveys, due to cultural beliefs about privacy in intimate and family matters.[14]

Sexual Orientation and Gender Identity

Bisexual women report higher rates of sexual violence victimization than other women or men.[4] Nationally representative data from a 2010 survey suggests that 46% of all bisexual women experienced rape and 75% experienced other forms of sexual violence in their lifetimes.[4] In contrast, lesbian and heterosexual women reported substantially lower rates of rape (13% and 17%) and sexual violence other than rape (46% and 43%), respectively. Both gay (40%) and bisexual (47%) men reported more sexual violence other than rape than heterosexual men (21%). Rates of rape for gay and bisexual men could not be calculated in this national survey due to small sample sizes; less than 1% of heterosexual men reported having experienced rape.[4]

The 2015 U.S. Transgender Survey, an anonymous online survey of 27,715 transgender American adults, determined that almost half (47%) of transgender people experience sexual violence at some point in their lifetime.[15] An earlier study of transgender and gender-nonconforming individuals found that 10% of individuals experienced a bias-motivated sexual assault—that is, sexual violence *due to* their transgender or gender-nonconforming status.[16] Male-to-female transgender individuals had the highest rates of bias-motivated sexual violence victimization with more than one in four reporting victimization (26%).[16]

Research on sexual violence among sexual and gender minorities is a relatively new area of study, and as such, theory to explain why certain subpopulations (e.g., bisexual women, transgender individuals) experience the highest burden of sexual violence is lacking. Negative stereotypes about bisexuals, such as the belief that bisexuals are promiscuous and nonmonogamous,[17] and cultural norms that eroticize sexual relationships among women[18] may influence perpetrators' motivations and behavior. Stigma enacted on multiple levels, such as discriminatory housing and employment laws,[19] which can contribute to higher rates of poverty and homelessness[20] and interpersonal stigma enacted by family members, dating partners, and the public, all likely contribute to higher rates of sexual violence toward transgender individuals.[21] Relatedly, high rates of homelessness among lesbian, gay, bisexual, transsexual, or queer (LGBTQ) youth due to experiences of family rejection and violence[21,22] may predict higher levels of economic insecurity throughout their lives which can increase their risk for sexual violence victimization.[23] Compounding these issues, minority stress[24] or the additive stress of prejudice and stigma experienced by LGBTQ individuals, may lead to maladaptive coping processes such as alcohol and drug use, which further increases vulnerability to sexual violence.[25–27]

Income

Data from the 2010 NISVS indicate that both women and men who reported high levels of housing and food insecurity in the 12 months preceding the survey were more likely to report experiencing sexual violence during that same timeframe than individuals reporting low levels of economic insecurity.[23] Federal data from the National Crime Victimization Survey indicate that lower income women (i.e., household income < \$25,000 per year) report approximately twice the rate of rape and sexual violence than women in higher income brackets.[28] Theories examining the relationship between income and sexual violence suggest that women living in poverty may be at an increased risk for victimization due to having insufficient financial means to avoid or escape violent relationships, to leave unsafe workplaces, or to choose alternatives to unsafe commuting options.[29] However, women of greater financial means—particularly when their economic status meets or exceeds that of men's—may actually face an increased risk of sexual violence, particularly at the hands of intimate partners.[5,30] More research is needed to understand the reasons for this differential risk among women. And given a dearth of research in this area, much remains to be learned about the relationship between men's socioeconomic status and risk for sexual violence.

Disability Status

Women with conditions or disabilities that impact sensory, physical, or cognitive functioning face more than twice the risk of sexual

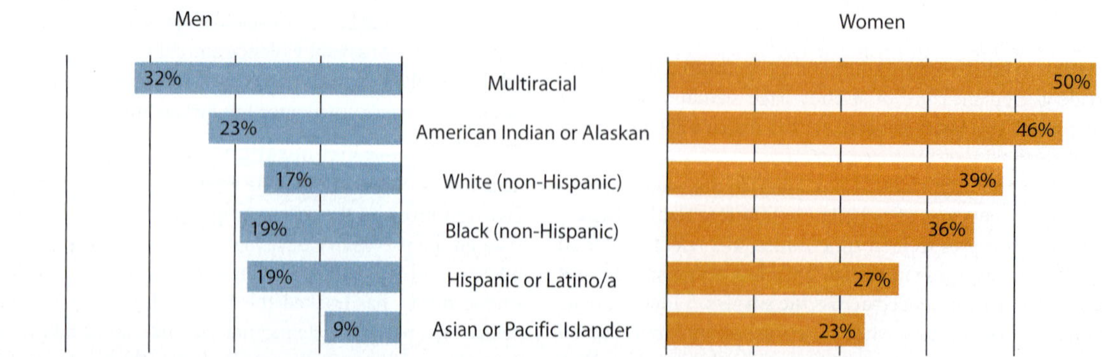

FIGURE 179-1. Weighted lifetime prevalence of contact sexual violence by race and sex, NISVS 2010–12. (*Source:* From Smith SG, Chen J, Basile KC, et al. *The National Intimate Partner and Sexual Violence Survey (NISVS): 2010–2012 State Report*. Atlanta, GA: National Center for Injury Prevention and Control, Centers for Disease Control and Prevention; 2017.)

violence compared to women without a disability,[31] with some estimates suggesting that this risk may be up to four times higher.[32,33] People with disabilities may be vulnerable to abuse by caregivers or others who perceive them as unable or less likely to resist or report their victimization.[33] Those living with multiple disabilities[34] and more severe disabilities[32] are most at risk. Individuals with cognitive disabilities experience more violent victimization, including sexual violence, than those living with other types of disabilities, and one in five survivors with cognitive disabilities say that their assault was bias-motivated.[34] Even as young as high school, girls with physical disabilities are more likely to be raped than girls without a disability.[35] Less is known about the experiences of men living with disabilities who have survived sexual violence, but one nationally representative survey demonstrated that men with a disability were more likely to report experiencing sexual violence in the past 12 months than men without a disability.[36] Sexual violence is an underreported crime across all communities. Some scholars suggest that survivors with disabilities may be even less likely to report sexual violence than the general population, and less likely to seek out supportive services after an assault has occurred.[37]

College Students

High rates of sexual violence on college campuses have been described for decades[38] but recent national efforts to address the problem have elevated the issue further in the public consciousness.[39] Prevalence estimates of sexual violence on college campuses vary widely across studies.[40] The most recent data available come from a random sample of undergraduate students drawn from two different college campuses in 2016. This study found that approximately 22% of students reported sexual violence victimization—defined as nonconsensual sexual touching or attempted/completed penetration—since beginning college, including 28% of women, 12.5% of men, and 38% of gender-nonconforming students.[41] Among college women, the most common forms of sexual violence are unwanted sexual contact—which includes unwanted kissing or touching (but excludes intercourse)[40]—and alcohol- or drug-facilitated rape involving a victim who was incapacitated and unable to consent or refuse.[40,41] Research suggests that the transition into college can mark a period of elevated risk for sexual violence victimization and perpetration, potentially due to the increased availability and excessive use of alcohol during this period.[42] However, while high rates of sexual violence have been well-documented among college students, research also suggests that 18- to 24-year-old *non*students may actually experience even higher rates.[43]

Age

Sexual violence often begins early in the lifespan. A 2015 survey found that among all U.S. women who experienced a completed or attempted rape, more than 80% were under the age of 25 at the time of their first victimization; about 43% were under 18; approximately 30% were between 11 and 17 years old; and almost 13% were age 10 or younger.[12] An alarming 35% of women raped as a child or adolescent reported experiencing rape again as an adult—a pattern often described as *sexual revictimization*.[2] While less is known about the age at which men are first raped, 26% of men with a history of rape were first victimized by age 10.[12] Among men who reported being made to sexually penetrate someone else—a form of sexual violence assessed in CDC's NISVS—71% were younger than 25 years old and 21% were younger than 18.[44] Given the early onset of sexual violence, prevention efforts must begin early and continue across the lifespan in order to protect against the negative health and social outcomes of victimization.

Addressing Disparities through the Social Determinants of Health

Disparities in rates of sexual violence experienced across groups based on gender, age, race and ethnicity, sexual orientation and gender identity, ability, and region are not inevitable—they are driven by inequitable access to economic and social resources.[45–47] Inequitable distribution of resources also influences how survivors fare in the aftermath of experiencing sexual violence.[48,49] Addressing these disparities and improving the health and welfare of survivors means focusing on the social determinants of health.

Social determinants of health are the circumstances in which we live, influenced by our positioning in complex social hierarchies.[50] For example, in most countries, women are afforded an inequitable share of social power compared to men.[51] Within the same country, two women who experience gender inequality may also experience stigma and discrimination differently based upon systems of racism, classism, or heteronormativity (viewing heterosexuality as the only normal or natural way of being; www.merriam-webster.com/dictionary/heternormative). Their positioning within the social hierarchy likely influences their access to vital resources such as education and employment—this social positioning also differentially influences their vulnerability to sexual violence. In order to prevent sexual violence, public health partnerships with other sectors (e.g., education, criminal justice, business) are important in order to address the root causes of social inequalities: policies and cultural values that promote gender inequality and other inequitable social stratifications.

One example of how health inequity impacts rates of violence, including sexual violence, comes from work on structural stigma with sexual and gender minorities. Today, LGBTQ individuals have fewer protections under the law compared to heterosexual and cisgender individuals (those whose gender identity conforms to their sex assigned at birth) in terms of family and relationship protections; nondiscrimination laws (e.g., for employment, housing, public accommodations, and in schools); medical decision-making; and protections against bias-motivated assault (e.g., hate crimes).[52–54] Such inequities can negatively impact the health and well-being of sexual and gender minorities. For example, research suggests that LGB students living in areas with protective school climates (e.g., Gay-Straight Alliances, safe spaces, nondiscrimination policies) and social environments (e.g., higher proportion of same-sex couples) reported fewer past-year suicidal thoughts than students with less protective climates.[55,56] Other work points to the potential harms of structural stigma, defined as social norms, environmental conditions, and institutional laws and policies that limit resources, opportunities, and well-being, on transgender people by generating chronic stress with direct effects on physical and mental health.[21] Preventing sexual violence and promoting health equity among marginalized populations that experience a disproportionate burden of sexual violence necessitates greater research attention to these social and structural stigmas that impact health and increase vulnerability to violence victimization.[46]

Health Consequences of Sexual Violence Victimization

Sexual violence victimization is associated with a host of negative short- and long-term health effects.[2,10] Sexual violence may result in injury due to the assault itself or may result in maladaptive coping behaviors (e.g., smoking, alcohol or drug use) that are the root causes of other health problems.[3] Some long-term health problems may also be due to the cumulative effects of the body's biological response to chronic stress brought on by surviving sexual violence.[57] Women with a victimization history (sexual violence, stalking, and intimate partner violence) are more likely to report asthma, irritable bowel syndrome, diabetes, high blood pressure, frequent headaches, chronic pain, difficulty sleeping, and limitations to their activity compared to women never victimized.[2] Survivors of violence are also more likely to rate their overall physical health and mental health as poor compared to women with no victimization history.[2] Men report some of the same concerns as women, including a higher prevalence of frequent headaches, chronic pain, difficulty sleeping, and activity limitations—and they subjectively rate their physical and mental health as being poorer than men without a victimization history.[2] A number of short- and long-term mental health problems are also commonly reported among survivors. Depression, anxiety, posttraumatic stress disorder, eating disorders, and suicidal behavior are reported at higher rates among women with a history of sexual violence victimization.[58-61] The severity of these mental health outcomes may be determined in part by the severity of the assault, the age at which victimization occurred, or the level of support a survivor received from friends, family members, and partners after assault.[59,61] Integrated and trauma-informed care for survivors may lessen some of these negative impacts.[62]

The Costs of Rape

Sexual violence, including childhood sexual abuse, has economic consequences that extend well beyond the victim to impact the larger economy. When considering the costs of short- and long-term medical care for victims, criminal justice system activities, and lost work productivity for victims and incarcerated perpetrators, researchers have estimated that the lifetime cost of rape is $122,461 per victim, or an estimated $3.1 trillion over the lives of the 25 million men and women who have been raped in the U.S. population.[63] This total economic burden includes $1.6 trillion in lost work productivity, $1.2 trillion in medical costs, $234 billion in criminal justice activities, and $36 billion in other expenses, of which about one-third is paid by government sources.[61] The economic burden of childhood sexual abuse is estimated to be $9.3 billion.[64] With such steep costs to individuals and the economy, policymakers and others can expect that investing in the prevention of sexual violence, including childhood sexual abuse, will actually conserve health and economic resources—in addition to saving lives.

Risk Factors for Victimization

Research has identified factors associated with a disproportionate risk for experiencing sexual violence victimization. These factors do not cause or explain sexual violence on their own, and their identification does not—and should not—suggest that survivors of sexual violence are responsible in any way for their own assault. Instead, these factors may be useful for identifying situations or circumstances in which individuals may be more vulnerable to perpetrators and, thus, where intervention may be possible or needed. Some research on risk factors for victimization has focused on identity characteristics—nonmodifiable characteristics of individuals. While women and girls, younger individuals, sexual and gender minorities, and women of color may experience a disproportionate burden of sexual violence, these do not constitute modifiable risk factors for intervention or prevention programs; therefore, these factors are discussed earlier in the chapter related to the nature and burden of sexual violence.

The World Health Organization identified several modifiable risk factors for victimization based on global sexual violence research including: consumption of alcohol and drugs, having numerous sexual partners, involvement in sex work, and poverty. To date, the strongest and most consistent risk factor for sexual violence victimization is a previous history of sexual violence victimization.[30] A number of theories have been proposed to explain why sexual revictimization occurs,[65,66] with substantial evidence suggesting that survivors use unhealthy coping strategies (e.g., sex, alcohol, and drug use) to avoid or numb the pain of their early abuse, but these behaviors create more opportunities for future victimization.[67,68] Effective prevention strategies for sexual violence victimization tend to primarily address the proximal, contextual risk factors that can increase the risk for experiencing sexual violence in the moment.[69] While these strategies (e.g., self-defense, consent communication) may reduce victimization risk for those individuals using them and are an important piece of the prevention puzzle, they do not address the underlying risk level of potential perpetrators. Thus, in order to reduce the overall risk for sexual violence, research and strategies that consider modifiable risk factors for perpetration may have the greatest potential for achieving population-level reductions in sexual violence.

TABLE 179-2 RISK FACTORS FOR SEXUAL VIOLENCE PERPETRATION ORGANIZED BY LEVEL OF THE SOCIAL ECOLOGY

Individual factors	Alcohol and drug use
	Delinquency
	Empathic deficits
	General aggressiveness and acceptance of violence
	Early sexual initiation
	Coercive sexual fantasies
	Preference for impersonal sex and sexual risk-taking
	Exposure to sexually explicit media
	Hostility toward women
	Adherence to traditional gender role norms
	Hypermasculinity
	Suicidal behavior
	Prior sexual victimization or perpetration
Relationship factors	Family environment characterized by physical violence and conflict
	Childhood history of physical, sexual, or emotional abuse
	Emotionally unsupportive family environment
	Poor parent–child relationships, particularly with fathers
	Association with sexually aggressive, hypermasculine, and delinquent peers
	Involvement in a violent or abusive intimate relationship
Community factors	Poverty
	Lack of employment opportunities
	Lack of institutional support from police and judicial system
	General tolerance of sexual violence within the community
	Weak community sanctions against sexual violence perpetrators
Societal factors	Societal norms that support sexual violence
	Societal norms that support male superiority and sexual entitlement
	Societal norms that maintain women's inferiority and sexual submission
	Weak laws and policies related to sexual violence and gender equity
	High levels of crime and other forms of violence

Source: From Centers for Disease Control and Prevention, National Center for Injury Prevention and Control, Division of Violence Prevention. Risk and Protective Factors. 2019. Retrieved from https://www.cdc.gov/violenceprevention/sexualviolence/riskprotectivefactors.html.

Risk Factors for Perpetration

In order to prevent sexual violence from happening, researchers have sought to better understand the thoughts, attitudes, and behaviors of perpetrators, as well as characteristics of their relationships and environments that increase their risk for perpetration. Researchers have identified a range of risk factors across the social ecology—characteristics of the individual, their relationships, their community, and society-at-large—that contribute to higher rates of sexual violence perpetration (Table 179-2[70]). None of these risk factors, in isolation, *cause* sexual violence perpetration. Rather, a confluence of multiple risk factors across an individual's lifetime can create a psychological, behavioral, social, and physical environment that makes perpetration more likely than not.[70] Proximal circumstances—stress, alcohol or drug use, peer influence, perceived opportunity and risk—can trigger this underlying risk for perpetration in the moment. Understanding how these proximal risk factors interact with other factors to contribute to the risk of perpetration informs the design of interventions to prevent sexual violence.

Most research identifying risk factors for sexual violence perpetration focuses on individual or relationship-level factors.[70] Some of these factors focus on the role of sex in people's lives, such as becoming sexually active at a young age, having casual attitudes toward sex, being exposed to sexually explicit media, and having a greater number of sex partners. Other individual-level risk factors include the ways people think about gender, such as rigid beliefs about how men and women should act and whether there should be consequences for violating traditional gender role norms. General acceptance of violence and difficulty negotiating social relationships may also influence risk for sexual violence perpetration, as does having a history of sexual violence victimization or perpetration.

A number of empirically supported factors associated with family, peer, and intimate partner relationships may also place individuals at an increased risk for perpetrating sexual violence.[70] Childhood maltreatment, particularly childhood emotional and physical abuse, are associated with an increased risk for sexual violence perpetration in adolescence and adulthood. Exposure to family conflict and parental violence, as well as poor parent-child relationship quality, may also impact perpetration risk. Similar risk factors exist within the context of intimate partner relationships. How individuals handle conflict within their relationships, the extent to which individuals use controlling behaviors, and the use of physical or emotional abuse may indicate risk of perpetrating sexual violence toward an intimate partner. Research also demonstrates that one's peer group impacts risk of perpetration—having friends with attitudes and beliefs that condone sexual violence or friends who perpetrate sexual violence is associated with one's risk of sexual violence perpetration. These harmful ideologies and behaviors may be more common among certain all-male peer groups, such as fraternities and some sports teams, when hypermasculine beliefs and gender norms are reinforced by the peer group culture.[71]

A number of community- and societal-level risk factors for sexual violence have been hypothesized[30]—but few of these have been tested and validated.[70] Some of these factors include community-level poverty and norms supporting male superiority and entitlement to sex. Laws, policies, and social norms that support the use of violence as a legitimate means to achieve one's goals have also been hypothesized as risk factors at the societal level.[70] A major next step in the field of sexual violence prevention involves identifying and addressing risk factors at the community and society level. A focus on change at these outer levels of the social ecology is essential to achieving population-level reductions in the prevalence of sexual violence.[72,73]

Child Sexual Abuse Perpetration

Child sexual abuse perpetrators often display a unique pattern of risk behaviors and characteristics that set them apart from the general risk population described above. There are many myths surrounding child sexual abuse that are helpful to debunk.[74] First, child sexual abuse by a stranger accounts for fewer than one in ten cases known to law enforcement. Instead, the vast majority of abuse reported to law enforcement is perpetrated by a family member (59%) or an acquaintance (34%).[75] Second, while it is common for the general public to think of child sex offenders as "sick"—and they do have higher rates of mental illness than the general population—the vast majority (75%) are not seriously mentally ill.[76] Third, only about half of child sex offenders have a sexual preference disorder—clinically diagnosed as *pedophiles* (those sexually attracted to prepubescent minors) or *hebephiles* (those sexually attracted to pubescent minors).[77] The remainder may perpetrate childhood sexual abuse for a number of reasons. Many have psychosocial deficits (e.g., poor social skills and impulse control) which make establishing healthy relationships with appropriate-aged partners difficult.[77] Many are young people themselves; more than one-third of childhood sexual abuse perpetrators are adolescents or other children, and one-in-eight are under the age of 12 themselves.[74,78,79] Widespread endorsement of these myths, coupled with deep concerns raised by the public and policymakers in response to high-profile sexual abuse cases, has resulted in public policies, such as sex offender registration and residency restrictions, that some have criticized as controversial, lacking evidence, or potentially increasing risk of recidivism.[80,81]

Adolescents who perpetrate sexual violence against other adolescents (e.g., peer sexual violence) tend to display risk characteristics and behaviors similar to adult perpetrators of rape, while youth who offend against children under 12 display offense patterns (e.g., "grooming" behaviors) more like that of adults who perpetrate childhood sexual abuse. Like adult perpetrators, adolescent perpetrators may have histories of childhood adversity, including child abuse and neglect, and may struggle with social skills, but the abuse they perpetrate is typically less severe and more infrequent (in terms of duration and number of incidents) than adults.[82] These youth are more likely to perpetrate as a crime of opportunity (e.g., while babysitting) and are more likely to desist or stop perpetrating sexual abuse on their own, particularly as they age out of adolescence.[82] There are important differences in the likelihood of reoffending between different types of perpetrators, but most sex offenders known to law enforcement —both adolescents and adults—will not re-offend once they are identified.[83,84]

Although most survivors of childhood sexual abuse never go on to perpetrate sexual violence, many perpetrators were abused themselves as children. This tendency of perpetrators to have a history of childhood victimization has been described as the "victim-to-abuser cycle."[85] Some theories attempting to explain why this happens suggests that early sexual abuse may impact the way the child thinks about the abuser, the abuse, and sex more generally—leading the child to develop hypersexual behavior, identify with the perpetrator, and ultimately become an abuser themselves.[85] Other suggested risk factors for the perpetration of sexual violence toward children, particularly among those with a "sexual preference disorder," include differences in the structure or functioning of the brain, potentially caused by prenatal hormone exposure, early traumatic experience (e.g., sexual abuse), head trauma in early life, or lower IQ.[77,85] Nevertheless, childhood sexual abuse victimization has not been identified as a key, causal factor for perpetration. Research suggests that childhood neglect is actually a stronger predictor of later sexual abuse perpetration than is sexual abuse victimization.[86]

Perpetrators of childhood sexual abuse are difficult to study. Research participants must be willing to admit to behavior that is not only illegal but also highly stigmatized by society. Most of the existing research on perpetration of childhood sexual abuse comes from clinical or incarcerated populations, which may bias the findings.[85]

Perpetrators who go undetected by the criminal justice system may differ in important ways (e.g., cognitive functioning, type of offense) from those incarcerated or remanded into treatment. Programs for the primary prevention of childhood sexual abuse are incredibly limited—the most common approach to responding to child sexual abuse perpetration involves medical, psychiatric, and legal intervention.[77,82]

Theories of Rape and Sexual Aggression

Early theories attempting to explain why rape occurs arose from evolutionary, social learning, and feminist perspectives.[87] *Evolutionary theory*, also referred to as sociobiological theory, emphasized the role that genes may have played in the perpetration of rape as the species evolved. Evolutionary theory suggests that natural selection would have favored males who reproduced with as many different females as possible, including through rape or forced copulation tactics. *Social learning theory* emphasizes the role of imitation and modeling in the development of behavior. This theory suggests that sexual aggression may be learned from family and peers, culture, and mass media wherein a perpetrator imitates depictions of violence toward women. This theory posits that perpetrators may learn to associate sex with violence and ultimately become desensitized to the suffering of victims. *Feminist theories* highlight the role of power and control—conceptualizing rape as the consequence of women's lower political and economic status compared to men. Feminist theory suggests that a feedback process occurs whereby women restrict their behavior and activities in order to minimize the threat of rape, but these self-imposed restrictions reinforce the political, occupational, and economic inequality that men then use to perpetrate rape.[87]

As is commonly the case in social science research, the field has progressed to recognize that the problem of sexual violence is multifaceted and cannot be attributed to one specific cause or theory. As a result, the most promising advances in the study of sexual violence have taken into account multiple interacting factors, drawn from different schools of thought, in order to predict risk for sexual violence perpetration. The most prominent of these contemporary theories is the Confluence Model of Sexual Aggression.[88,89] The Confluence Model, which includes elements of earlier social learning and feminist theories of rape, attempts to predict risk for perpetration by considering the degree to which potential perpetrators possess certain risk characteristics, endorse certain attitudes, and display specific behaviors. Specifically, this model demonstrates how each of these components interact to potentially increase or decrease risk for violent behavior. This model highlights the central roles that hostile masculinity (an orientation that distrusts and denigrates women) and impersonal sex (an orientation focused on sex with multiple partners outside of the context of a caring or committed relationship) play in the development of sexual aggression, potentially exacerbated by early experiences of violence and abuse (e.g., childhood abuse and neglect). The Confluence Model has been shown to successfully predict risk for sexual violence perpetration over a 10-year period.[89] It has provided such a useful framework for understanding the various influences that may cause perpetrators to be violent generally, and sexually aggressive toward women specifically, that it has served as the foundational theory for a number of subsequent research endeavors attempting to further understand risk for sexual violence.[88,90–93] Such insights have been key to identifying points of intervention for the prevention of sexual violence.

PREVENTING SEXUAL VIOLENCE

Sexual violence is prevalent, often starts early, and is associated with multiple negative health outcomes for victims, as well as an increased risk for future victimization. As such, it comes at a high cost to society and creates an enormous public health burden. Fortunately, sexual violence <u>can</u> be prevented. Effective prevention strategies are grounded in an evidence-based understanding of the problem, including its nature and scope, and modifiable risk and protective factors. Once effective approaches are identified, widespread implementation is critical to ensure the greatest potential for impact on rates of sexual violence at the population-level. Identifying and disseminating the most cost-effective approaches to preventing sexual violence—before it starts—is a critical role for the field of public health.

Comprehensive Prevention

Sexual violence is a multifaceted problem—and, as such, requires a multifaceted solution. As discussed in the previous section and as illustrated in Table 179-2,[30,70] there are many risk factors for sexual violence perpetration, and these factors interact with one another across the lifespan to influence perpetration risk. To be effective at reducing the overall rates of sexual violence, prevention approaches cannot focus only on one or two risk factors or operate at only one level of the social ecology. Nor can we anticipate that a brief, one-time prevention program will be able to counteract the multiple influencers at play across an individual's lifetime. Unfortunately, most prevention efforts to date have been brief interventions—often less than 1 hour long—focused on awareness-raising and changing individual attitudes or knowledge about sexual violence.[70,94] Not surprisingly, these efforts have been largely unsuccessful.[94] Prevention efforts will likely only be effective if they are comprehensive—addressing numerous risk factors at each level of the social ecology, using consistent messaging across contexts and across the lifespan.[72,73]

Evidence-based Prevention Strategies

Based on more than four decades of research, theory, and practice to understand the problem, the CDC developed *STOP SV: A Technical Package to Prevent Sexual Violence*[95] in order to guide the field of sexual violence prevention toward evidence-based strategies. A *technical package* is a compilation of a core set of public health strategies intended to achieve and sustain substantial reductions in a specific risk factor or health outcome. STOP SV outlines five key strategies, based on the best available research evidence, for the prevention of sexual violence. Within each broader strategy, specific approaches (i.e., the ways to achieve the strategy) are highlighted with example programs, policies, and practices, as promising means for achieving a reduction in sexual violence. The technical package focuses on violence over the lifespan with approaches addressing risk at each level of the social ecology. The strategies and approaches are intended to be synergistic—they work together to create safer workplaces, schools, neighborhoods, relationships, and families. Table 179-3[95] summarizes the strategies and approaches outlined in STOP SV.

The first strategy focuses on **promoting social norms that protect against violence**. Group-level beliefs and expectations about violence—for example, seeing violence as normal or being indifferent to the problem of sexual violence—allows the problem to continue unabated. Strategies aimed at changing these norms reinforce the idea that sexual violence is unacceptable. Approaches that engage individuals as active bystanders to stand up and speak out against violence-supportive beliefs and behaviors may change social norms and perceptions of peer support for violence. Mobilizing men and boys as allies in sexual violence prevention is another approach that can foster healthy, positive norms about masculinity and violence, changing social norms and individual risk for perpetration.

The second strategy involves **teaching skills to prevent sexual violence.** Social-emotional skills (e.g., conflict management, empathy), healthy relationship skills, skills to promote healthy sexuality, and empowerment-based training help to prevent both sexual violence perpetration and victimization. Many of these skill-based approaches are designed to improve communication and problem-solving in relationships, leading to more respectful and caring relationships free of violence. Comprehensive sex education programs that focus on sexual communication, respect, and consent not only reduce the risk

TABLE 179-3 STRATEGIES AND APPROACHES TO PREVENT SEXUAL VIOLENCE FROM THE CDC'S STOP SV TECHNICAL PACKAGE

	Strategy	Approach
S	Promote *social norms* that protect against violence	Bystander approaches
		Mobilizing men and boys as allies
T	*Teach* skills to prevent sexual violence	Social-emotional learning
		Teaching healthy, safe dating, and intimate relationship skills to adolescents
		Promoting healthy sexuality
		Empowerment-based training
O	Provide *opportunities* to empower and support girls and women	Strengthening economic supports for women and families
		Strengthening leadership and opportunities for girls
P	Create *protective* environments	Improving safety and monitoring in schools
		Establishing and consistently applying workplace policies
		Addressing community-level risks through
		environmental approaches
SV	*Support victims/* survivors to lesson harms	Victim-centered services
		Treatment for victims of SV
		Treatment for at-risk children and families to prevent problem behavior including sex offending

Source: From Basile KC, DeGue S, Jones K, et al. *STOP SV: A Technical Package to Prevent Sexual Violence.* Atlanta, GA: National Center for Injury Prevention and Control, Centers for Disease Control and Prevention; 2016.

of sexual violence but may also reduce risk for sexually transmitted infections and unintended pregnancy. Empowerment-based training builds women's ability to assess risk for violence in their relationships and the situations they encounter and reduces barriers to action that could reduce exposure to sexual violence.

The third strategy focuses on **empowering girls and women.** Gender inequality in education, employment, and income increases women and girls' risk of experiencing sexual violence.[47,96] Policies and programs that address gender inequality, such as those that improve economic security and access to education and employment, can mitigate this risk.[97–100] One approach that strengthens economic supports for women and their families involves closing the gender wage gap and providing paid family and medical leave. For example, in the United States, women earn approximately 80 cents on the dollar compared to men.[101] The Lillie Ledbetter Fair Pay Act, enacted in 2009, promotes equal pay for equal work, providing legal recourse to those who experience wage discrimination based on their sex, race, national origin, age, religion, or disability.[102] Additionally, programs that build girls' leadership skills can also improve their educational and occupational opportunities for many years to come, assisting in the prevention of sexual violence across their lifetimes. Including women and other historically marginalized communities in positions of upper management may further reduce unfair wage discrimination[103] and improve health equity, including reductions in violence.

The fourth strategy involves **creating protective environments**. Changing characteristics of schools, neighborhoods, cities, organizations, and institutions to promote positive behavior and inhibit harmful behavior is a powerful way to prevent sexual violence at the community level. Improving safety and monitoring in schools can prevent sexual violence by altering areas of the school where students feel unsafe and by promoting a school culture where harassment and violence are not tolerated. In the workplace, proactive sexual harassment policies that are consistently enforced can create a workplace culture where all individuals understand and follow standards of behavior that prohibit bullying and harassment. Environmental approaches that alter neighborhoods or communities, such as those that reduce alcohol outlet density or increase the price of alcohol, may prevent sexual violence by deterring excessive alcohol use, a known risk factor for sexual violence perpetration.

Finally, **supporting survivors to lessen harms** not only reduces the likelihood of experiencing long-term consequences of violence, but it may also prevent future sexual violence perpetration and victimization. In addition to a host of negative physical and mental health outcomes, experiencing violence early in life is also associated with a number of negative behaviors in adolescence and adulthood, including sexual violence perpetration. Victim-centered services and treatment for survivors of sexual violence can help ameliorate the health effects of victimization, while treatment for children and families at-risk for behavioral problems, including sexual offending, can reduce those children's risk for future perpetration. Victim-centered services, such as those offered at rape crisis centers, provide resources and victim advocacy in a safe and supportive environment. Survivors who have utilized these services report more positive experiences with medical and legal systems. Trauma-focused Cognitive Behavioral Therapy is an evidenced-based approach that effectively treats psychological problems resulting from traumatic experiences, such as rape. There are also evidence-based therapeutic approaches focused on children who have experienced violence and who may be at risk of perpetrating sexual violence in the future. These programs may help deter risk of future perpetration by focusing on skills, belief systems, and attitudes conducive to violence and by promoting healthy and age-appropriate relationships and behaviors.

Connecting the Dots: Opportunities for Preventing Multiple Forms of Violence

Violence takes many forms, and many forms of violence co-occur or overlap. For example, different forms of childhood abuse (e.g., physical, sexual, and emotional) tend to co-occur,[104,105] and the more forms of childhood abuse experienced, the greater the likelihood of experiencing violence in adulthood.[106] Among girls, specifically, those who have experienced childhood sexual abuse are more likely to experience later intimate partner violence and sexual revictimization.[107] Among adolescents, those who have experienced rape are disproportionately likely to contemplate suicide.[108] And young people who perpetrate bullying are more likely to also perpetrate homophobic name-calling, sexual harassment, and sexual violence later in their adolescence.[109,110] These forms of violence often share the same root causes. Selecting violence prevention approaches that focus on shared risk factors across these various forms of violence is the most efficient way to prevent violence, including sexual violence.[111]

Shared risk and protective factors for multiple forms of violence exist at each level of the social ecology.[111] The CDC has begun work to break down the disciplinary silos that have historically limited researchers' ability to identify these shared risk and protective factors. We can achieve greater public health impact by encouraging intervention programs to broaden their curriculum to focus on factors for multiple forms of violence. Table 179-4[111] provides information to begin identifying some of these shared factors to inform more comprehensive prevention approaches.[111] From this table we can see that, at the societal level, norms about violence and gender roles are not only risky for sexual violence, but may also increase risk for child maltreatment, teen dating violence, intimate partner violence, and youth violence. At the relational level, poor parent-child relationships have been associated with almost every form of violence. At the individual level, substance use and lack of problem-solving skills have been associated with every form of violence, including sexual

TABLE 179-4 SHARED RISK FACTORS ACROSS MULTIPLE FORMS OF VIOLENCE

		Child Maltreatment	Teen Dating Violence	Intimate Partner Violence	Sexual Violence	Youth Violence	Bullying	Suicide	Elder Maltreatment
Societal	Cultural norms that support aggression toward others	X	X	X	X	X			X
	Media violence				X	X	X	X	
	Societal income inequality	X		X		X	X		
	Weak health, educational, economic, and social policies/laws	X		X	X			X	
	Harmful norms around masculinity and femininity	X	X	X	X	X	X		
Community	Neighborhood poverty	X		X	X	X		X	
	High alcohol outlet density	X		X		X		X	
	Community violence	X			X	X	X		
	Diminished economic opportunities/high unemployment rates	X		X	X	X		X	
	Poor neighborhood support and cohesion	X	X	X		X		X	
Relationship	Social isolation/Lack of social support	X	X	X			X	X	X
	Poor parent-child relationships	X	X	X	X	X	X	X	
	Family conflict	X	X	X	X	X	X		
	Economic stress	X		X		X		X	X
	Associating with delinquent peers		X	X	X	X	X		
	Gang involvement		X	X	X	X			
Individual	Low educational achievement	X	X	X		X	X	X	
	Lack of nonviolent social problem-solving skills	X	X	X	X	X	X	X	X
	Poor behavioral control/Impulsiveness	X	X	X	X	X		X	
	History of violent victimization	X	X	X	X	X	X	X	X
	Witnessing violence	X	X	X	X	X	X	X	
	Psychological/Mental health problems	X	X	X		X		X	X
	Substance use	X	X	X	X	X	X	X	X

Source: From Wilkins N, Tsao B, Hertz M, Davis R, Klevens J. Connecting the Dots: *An Overview of the Links Among Multiple Forms of Violence.* Atlanta, GA: National Center for Injury Prevention and Control, Centers for Disease Control and Prevention; Oakland, CA: Prevention Institute; 2014.

violence. Prevention strategies that focus on some of these factors should have broad impact on preventing all of these interconnected forms of violence, including sexual violence.

Applying some of the evidence-based strategies described in the STOP SV Technical Package as part of a comprehensive prevention plan that addresses risk at multiple levels of the social ecology increases the likelihood of achieving reductions in sexual violence rates at the population level. However, these strategies are not one-size-fits-all. Every community is unique and prevention efforts should address the specific needs and characteristics of their contexts and populations in order to achieve the greatest possible effects. Evidence-based interventions may need to be adapted to increase the relevance of programming, to encourage participation in programs, to create or maintain relationships with participants, or due to resource constraints. In other cases, new and innovative interventions may better suit the needs of a community. Such approaches are most likely to succeed when they are grounded in theory, knowledge about sexual violence, best practices for effective prevention, and when they are evaluated.[112] The challenges of adapting effective programs to new contexts and settings, or the need for innovative approaches, is particularly salient when considering the implementation of primary prevention activities in international settings and special contexts (e.g., in times of war or natural disasters).

Sexual Violence Prevention around the World and in Special Contexts

Sexual violence in other parts of the world may take different forms with unique risk and protective factors that are not typically addressed by domestic prevention efforts. For example, rape as an act of war or sexual violence in the context of extreme poverty or social disruption may necessitate strategies and approaches that differ from those discussed here. Further, sexual violence in times of natural disaster, whether domestic or abroad, also warrants special consideration. These unique needs and concerns have led to the development and implementation of prevention strategies that address the complex challenges posed by sexual violence in these contexts. Three examples highlight the range of approaches applied around the world to address sexual violence.

Laws and policies are an essential part of preventing sexual violence both domestically and abroad. During war and armed conflict, rape and sexual violence abound.[113] Rape as a tool of war is used to intimidate, destabilize, and eradicate the enemy, particularly during ethnic conflicts when rape is strategically used as a means of genocide.[113–115] It was not until 2002 that The International Criminal Court (ICC) began investigating and prosecuting genocide, war crimes, and crimes against humanity, which include the systematic rape of civilians.[116] The ICC secured the first conviction of rape as an act of war in 2016 against Jean-Pierre Bemba, the former vice-president of the Democratic Republic of the Congo and commander-in-chief of the Movement for the Liberation of Congo. This landmark ruling affirms that military commanders, whether or not personally engaged in the perpetration of rape, can be held accountable for campaigns of sexualized violence occurring under their command.[117] Today 11 cases are under investigation by the ICC[116] and coordinated efforts to train health professionals and human rights workers to document human rights abuses continue with the goal of enabling future prosecutions and ending the widespread practice of rape as a weapon of war.[118]

In underresourced areas, microfinance programs provide small loans that allow women to develop income-generating projects or businesses. These programs can prevent sexual violence by increasing women's economic and social power. Such programs frequently include skill-building and norm-changing components. For example, South Africa's Intervention with Microfinance for AIDS and Gender Equity (IMAGE) program works with rural women living in extreme poverty. The program not only alleviates poverty for these women by providing small loans and financial training, but changes social norms by engaging men and boys as allies, ultimately leading to a reduction in both sexual and physical violence within the home.[99,100,119]

Times of emergency such as natural disasters can create contexts more vulnerable to sexual violence, such as when safe housing, transportation, friends and family, law enforcement, and healthcare resources become unavailable. Further, disasters typically have the most detrimental effect on those already vulnerable to violence, such as individuals living in poverty, people of color, and those living with a disability.[120] In the wake of Hurricane Katrina, the National Sexual Violence Resource Center and the Louisiana Foundation Against Sexual Assault developed guidelines to reduce the risk of sexual violence during times of natural disaster, specifically in evacuation shelters.[121] Some of these guidelines include having private spaces for changing clothes and attending to personal hygiene, ensuring evacuees are aware of safe places with constant security presence, and closing any shelter areas that cannot be made safe. Local law enforcement agencies may be unable to take reports of sexual violence if they are focused on other disaster relief efforts. Therefore, these guidelines also recommend coordination with neighboring districts and states to take such reports on behalf of the local jurisdiction.[121]

Other resources exist to guide in the prevention of violence toward children in international contexts.[98] Although not specific to childhood sexual abuse, the CDC's INSPIRE Technical Package outlines a number of evidence-based strategies and approaches that can be taken to prevent violence, including sexual violence, against children. More can be found on this topic in Chapter 176: Child Abuse and Neglect.

CONCLUSIONS

Sexual violence is a major public health problem with long-lasting impacts on survivors and society as a whole. Yet our understanding of the nature and burden of sexual violence internationally is incomplete—researchers, federal governments, and international organizations define and measure sexual violence differently, which makes collating and comparing reports challenging. Nevertheless, knowledge of the nature and scope of sexual violence has grown exponentially over the past five decades. We know that it is a costly and multifaceted problem, that risk and protective factors exist at each level of the social ecology, and that strategies and approaches to preventing sexual violence need to be comprehensive—multilevel prevention approaches addressing multiple risk and protective factors. We also know that the burden of this problem is not distributed equally—individuals, particularly women, who are low income, multiracial or American Indian/Alaskan Native, bisexual, transgender, or living with a disability are more likely to be victimized than their higher income, white, heterosexual, cisgender, nondisabled counterparts. Addressing health disparities among these diverse populations and preventing sexual violence more broadly requires promoting health equity and coordination across disciplines—working with experts in other domains of violence prevention as well as working together with communities engaged in social justice action aimed at promoting overall health and wellbeing of historically marginalized communities. By connecting the dots between fields and promoting health equity for all, we should achieve substantial gains in the movement to end sexual violence. Sexual violence is preventable. The field is evolving to identify and address shared risk and protective factors for sexual violence along with other forms of violence, in order to maximize public health impact and promote the health and wellbeing of everyone, everywhere, across the lifespan.

References

1. Basile KC, Smith SG, Breiding MJ, Black MC, Mahendra R. *Sexual Violence Surveillance: Uniform Definitions and Recommended Data Elements.* Atlanta, GA: National Center for Injury Prevention and Control, Centers for Disease Control and Prevention; 2014, pp. 1–136. https://www.cdc.gov/violenceprevention/pdf/sv_surveillance_definitionsl-2009-a.pdf.
2. Black MC, Basile KC, Breiding MJ, et al. *The National Intimate Partner and Sexual Violence Survey (NISVS): 2010 Summary Report.* Atlanta, GA: National Center for Injury Prevention and Control, Centers for Disease Control and Prevention; 2011, pp. 1–124. https://www.cdc.gov/violenceprevention/pdf/nisvs_report2010-a.pdf.
3. Smith SG, Basile KC, Gilbert LK, et al. *National Intimate Partner and Sexual Violence Survey (NISVS): 2010–2012 State Report.* Atlanta, GA: National Center for Injury Prevention and Control, Centers for Disease Control and Prevention; 2017, pp. 1–272. https://www.cdc.gov/violenceprevention/pdf/NISVS-StateReportBook.pdf.
4. Walters ML, Chen J, Breiding MJ. *The National Intimate Partner and Sexual Violence Survey: 2010 Findings on Victimization by Sexual Orientation.* Atlanta, GA: National Center for Injury Prevention and

Control, Centers for Disease Control and Prevention; 2013, pp.1–48. https://www.cdc.gov/violenceprevention/pdf/nisvs_sofindings.pdf.

5. Hipp TN, Cook SL. Rape and sexual assault on campus, in diverse populations, and in the spotlight, In: Renzetti CM, Edleson JL, Bergen RK, eds. *Sourcebook on Violence Against Women*. Los Angeles, CA: SAGE Publications; 2017.
6. Cook SL, Gidycz CA, Koss MP, Murphy M. Emerging issues in the measurement of rape victimization. *Violence Against Women.* 2011;17(2):201–18.
7. Fisher BS. The effects of survey question wording on rape estimates: Evidence from a quasi-experimental design. *Violence Against Women.* 2009;15:133–47.
8. Koss MP, Gidycz CA. Sexual experiences survey: Reliability and validity. *J Consult Clin Psychol.* 1985;53(3):422–3.
9. Koss MP, Abbey A, Campbell R, et al. Revising the SES: A collaborative process to improve assessment of sexual aggression and victimization. *Psychol Women Q.* 2007;31(4):357–70.
10. World Health Organization. *Global and Regional Estimates of Violence Against Women: Prevalence and Health Effects of Intimate Partner Violence and Non-partner Sexual Violence.* Geneva, Switzerland: World Health Organization; 2013. http://apps.who.int/iris/bitstream/10665/85239/1/9789241564625_eng.pdf.
11. Sumner SA, Mercy A, Saul J, et al. Prevalence of sexual violence against children and use of social services-seven countries, 2007-2013. *MMWR Surveill Summ.* 2015;64(21):565–9.
12. Smith SG, Zhang X, Basile KC, et al. *The National Intimate Partner and Sexual Violence Survey (NISVS): 2015 Data Brief—Updated Release.* Atlanta, GA: National Center for Injury Prevention and Control, Centers for Disease Control and Prevention; 2018, pp. 1–32.
13. Bachman R, Zaykowski H, Lanier C, Poteyeva M, Kallmyer R. Estimating the magnitude of rape and sexual assault against American Indian and Alaska Native (AIAN) women. *Aust N Z J Criminol.* 2010;43(2):199–222.
14. White JW, Yuan NP, Cook SL, Abbey A. Ethnic minority women's experiences with intimate partner violence: Using community-based participatory research to ask the right questions. *Sex Roles.* 2013;69(3–4):226–36.
15. James SE, Herman JL, Rankin S, Keisling M, Mottet L, Anafi M. *The Report of the United States Transgender Survey.* Washington, DC: National Center for Transgender Equality; 2016, pp. 1-302. https://www.transequality.org/sites/default/files/docs/USTS-Full-Report-FINAL.PDF.
16. Grant JM, Mottet LA, Tanis J, Harrison J, Herman JL, Keisling M. *Injustice at Every Turn: A Report of the National Transgender Discrimination Survey.* Washington, DC: National Center for Transgender Equality and National Gay and Lesbian Task Force; 2011, pp. 1–228. https://www.transequality.org/sites/default/files/docs/resources/NTDS_Report.pdf.
17. Yost MR, Thomas GD. Gender and binegitivity: Men's and women's attitudes toward male and female bisexuals. *Arch Sex Behav.* 2011;41:691–702.
18. Hequembourg AL, Brallier SA. An exploration of sexual minority stress across the lines of gender and sexual identity. *J Homosex.* 2009;56:273–98.
19. Movement Advancement Project. "Equality Maps: State Non-Discrimination Laws." http://www.lgbtmap.org/equality-maps/non_discrimination_laws. Accessed February 8, 2019.
20. Crissman HP, Berger MB, Graham LF, Dalton VK. Transgender demographics: A household probability sample of US adults, 2014. *Am J Public Health.* 2017;107(2):213–5.
21. White Hughto JMW, Reisner SL, Pachankis JE. Transgender stigma and health: A critical review of stigma determinants, mechanisms, and interventions. *Soc Sci Med.* 2015;147:222–31.
22. Morton M, Dworsky A, Matjasko J, Curry D, Schlueter R, Farrell A. Prevalence and correlates of youth homelessness in the United States. *J Adolesc Health.* 2018;62(1):14–21.
23. Breiding MJ, Basile KC, Klevens J, Smith SG. Economic insecurity and intimate partner and sexual violence victimization. *Am J Prev Med.* 2017;53(4):457–64.
24. Meyer IH. Prejudice, social stress, and mental health in lesbian, gay, and bisexual populations: Conceptual issues and research evidence. *Psychol Sex Orientat Gend Divers.* 2013;1:3–26.
25. Bandermann KM, Szymanski DM. Exploring coping mediators between heterosexist oppression and posttraumatic stress symptoms among lesbian, gay, and bisexual persons. *Psychol Sex Orientat Gend Divers.* 2014;1:213–24.
26. Gold SD, Dickstein BD, Marx BP, Lexington JM. Psychological outcomes among lesbian sexual assault survivors: An examination of the roles of internalized homophobia and experiential avoidance. *Psychol Women Q.* 2009;33:54–66.
27. Lehavot K, Simoni JM. The impact of minority stress on mental health and substance use among sexual minority women. *J Consult Clin Psychol.* 2011;79:159–70.
28. Planty M, Langton, L, Krebs, C, Berzofsky, M, Smiley-McDonald, H. *Female Victims of Sexual Violence, 1994–2010.* Washington, DC: Bureau of Justice Statistics; 2016. https://www.bjs.gov/content/pub/pdf/fvsv9410.pdf.
29. Martin K, Vieraitis LM, Britto S. Gender equality and women's absolute status: A test of the feminist models of rape. *Violence Against Women.* 2006;12(4):321–39.
30. Jewkes R, Sen P, Garcia-Moreno C. Sexual violence. In: Krug EG, Dahlberg LL, Mercy JA, Zwi AB, Lozano R, eds. *World Report on Violence and Health.* Geneva, Switzerland: World Health Organization; 2002.
31. Rand M, Harrell E *National Crime Victimization Survey: Crime Against People with Disabilities, 2007.* Washington, DC: Bureau of Justice Statistics; 2009. https://www.bjs.gov/content/pub/pdf/capd07.pdf.
32. Casteel C, Martin SL, Smith JB, Gurka KK, Kupper LL. National study of physical and sexual assault among women with disabilities. *Inj Prev.* 2008;14(2):87–90.
33. Martin SL, Ray N, Sotres-Alvarez D, et al. Physical and sexual assault of women with disabilities. *Violence Against Women.* 2006;12(9):823–37.
34. Harrell E. *Crime Against Persons with Disabilities, 2009–2015—Statistical Tables.* Washington, DC: Bureau of Justice Statistics; 2017. https://www.bjs.gov/content/pub/pdf/capd0915st.pdf.
35. Alriksson-Schmidt AI, Armour BS, Thibadeau JK. Are adolescent girls with a physical disability at increased risk for sexual violence? *J Sch Health.* 2010;80(7):361–7.
36. Basile KC, Breiding MJ, Smith SG. Disability and risk of recent sexual violence in the United States. *Am J Public Health.* 2016;106(5):928–33.
37. Anderson ML, Kobek Pezzarossi CM. Is it abuse? Deaf female undergraduates' labeling of partner violence. *J Deaf Stud Deaf Educ.* 2011;17(2):273–86.
38. Koss M, Gidycz CA, Wisniewski N. The scope of rape: Incidence and prevalence of sexual aggression and victimization in a national sample of higher education students. *J Consult Clin Psychol.* 1987;55(2):162–70.
39. White House Task Force to Protect Students from Sexual Assault. The second report of the White House Task Force to Protect Students from Sexual Assault. 2017. http://www.changingourcampus.org/resources/not-alone/Second-Report-VAW-Event-TF-Report.PDF.
40. Fedina L, Holmes JL, Backes BL. Campus sexual assault: A systematic review of prevalence research from 2000 to 2015. *Trauma Violence Abuse.* 2018;19(1):76–93.
41. Mellins CA, Walsh K, Sarvet AL, et al. Sexual assault incidents among college undergraduates: Prevalence and factors associated with risk. *PLoS One.* 2017;12(11):e0186471.
42. Krebs CP, Lindquist CH, Warner TD, Fisher BS, Martin SL. College women's experiences with physically forced, alcohol-or other drug-enabled, and drug-facilitated sexual assault before and since entering college. *J Am Coll Health.* 2009;57(6):639–49.
43. Sinozich S, Langton L. *Rape and Sexual Assault Victimization among College-Age Females, 1995–2013.* Washington, DC: Bureau of Justice Statistics; 2014. https://www.bjs.gov/content/pub/pdf/rsavcaf9513.pdf.
44. Breiding MJ, Smith S, Basile K, Walters M, Chen J, Merrick M. Violence, stalking, and intimate partner violence victimization-National intimate partner and sexual violence survey, United States, 2011. *MMWR Surveill Summ.* 2014;63(SS08):1–18.
45. National Academies of Sciences, Engineering, and Medicine. *Communities in Action: Pathways to Health Equity.* Washington, DC: The National Academies Press; 2017.
46. Hatzenbuehler ML, Phelan JC, Link BG. Stigma as a fundamental cause of population health inequalities. *Am J Public Health.* 2013;103(5):813–21.
47. Malarcher S, World Health Organization, Department of Reproductive Health and Research. *Social Determinants of Sexual and Reproductive Health: Informing Future Research and Programme Implementation.* Geneva, Switzerland: World Health Organization; 2010, pp. 1–157. http://www.ncdsv.org/images/WHO_SocialDeterminantsSexualHealth_2010.pdf.
48. Bryant-Davis T, Ullman S, Tsong Y, Tillman S, Smith K. Struggling to survive: Sexual assault, poverty, and mental health outcomes of African American women. *Am J Orthopsychiatry.* 2010;80(1):61–70.
49. Campbell R, Dworkin E, Cabral G. An ecological model of the impact of sexual assault on women's mental health. *Trauma Violence Abuse.* 2009;10(3):225–46.
50. Solar O, Irwin A. *A Conceptual Framework for Action on the Social Determinants of Health. Social Determinants of Health Discussion Paper 2 (Policy and Practice).* Geneva, Switzerland: World

Health Organization; 2010, pp. 1–79. http://www.who.int/sdhconference/resources/ConceptualframeworkforactiononSDH_eng.pdf.

51. World Health Organization. Gender: Definitions. http://www.euro.who.int/en/health-topics/health-determinants/gender/gender-definitions.
52. Redcay A, McMahon S, Hollinger V, Mabry-Kourt HL, Cook TB. Policy recommendations to improve the quality of life for LGBT older adults. *J Hum Rights Soc Work.* 2019;4(4):267–74.
53. Williams Institute. *Same-Sex Parenting in the US.* Los Angeles, CA: The Williams Institute; 2018. https://williamsinstitute.law.ucla.edu/uncategorized/same-sex-parenting-in-the-u-s/.
54. Williams Institute. *LGBT People in the US not Protected by State Nondiscrimination Statutes.* Los Angeles, CA: The Williams Institute; 2019. https://williamsinstitute.law.ucla.edu/wp-content/uploads/Equality-Act-April-2019.pdf.
55. Hatzenbuehler ML. The social environment and suicide attempts in lesbian, gay, and bisexual youth. *Pediatrics.* 2011;127(5):896–903.
56. Hatzenbuehler ML. Structural stigma and the health of lesbian, gay, and bisexual populations. *Curr Dir Psychol Sci.* 2014;23(2):127–32.
57. Sutherland CA, Bybee DI, Sullivan CM. Beyond bruises and broken bones: The joint effects of stress and injuries on battered women's health. *Am J Community Psychol.* 2002;30(5):609–36.
58. Chen LP, Murad MH, Paras ML, et al. Sexual abuse and lifetime diagnosis of psychiatric disorders: Systematic review and meta-analysis. *Mayo Clin Proc.* 2010;85(7):618–29.
59. Goodman LA, Koss MP, Russo NF. Violence against women: Physical and mental health effects. Part I: Research findings. *Appl Prev Psychol.* 1993;2(2):79–89.
60. Tomasula JL, Anderson LM, Littleton HL, Riley-Tillman TC. The association between sexual assault and suicidal activity in a national sample. *Sch Psychol Q.* 2012;27(2):109–19.
61. Yuan NP, Koss MP, Stone M. *The Psychological Consequences of Sexual Trauma.* Harrisburg, PA: VAWnet, a project of the National Resource Center on Domestic Violence; 2006, pp. 1–11. https://vawnet.org/sites/default/files/materials/files/2016-09/AR_PsychConsequences.pdf.
62. World Health Organization. *Responding to Intimate Partner Violence and Sexual Violence Against Women: WHO Clinical and Policy Guidelines.* Geneva, Switzerland: World Health Organization; 2013, pp. 1–56. https://apps.who.int/iris/bitstream/handle/10665/85240/9789241548595_eng.pdf.;jsessionid=649D0DC2C7C9E67B959CA0D65D789E53?sequence=1.
63. Peterson C, DeGue S, Florence C, Lokey CN. Lifetime economic burden of rape among US adults. *Am J Prev Med.* 2017;52(6):691–701.
64. Letourneau E, Brown D, Fang X, Hassan A, Mercy J. The economic burden of child sexual abuse in the United States. *Child Abuse Negl.* 2018;79:413–22.
65. Breitenbecher KH. Sexual revictimization among women: A review of the literature focusing on empirical investigations. *Aggress Violent Behav.* 2001;6(4):415–32.
66. Messman-Moore TL, Long PJ. The role of child sexual abuse sequelae in the sexual revictimization of women: An empirical review and theoretical reformulation. *Clin Psychol Rev.* 2003;23(4):537–71.
67. Messman-Moore TL, Long PJ. Alcohol and substance use disorders as predictors of child to adult sexual revictimization in a sample of community women. *Violence Vict.* 2002;17(3):319–40.
68. Polusny MA, Follette VM. Long-term correlates of child sexual abuse: Theory and review of the empirical literature. *Appl Prev Psychol.* 1995;4(3):143–66.
69. Senn CY, Eliasziw M, Barata PC, et al. Efficacy of a sexual assault resistance program for university women. *N Engl J Med.* 2015;372(24):2326–35.
70. Tharp AT, DeGue S, Valle LA, Brookmeyer KA, Massetti GM, Matjasko JL. A systematic qualitative review of risk and protective factors for sexual violence perpetration. *Trauma Violence Abuse.* 2013;14(2):133–67.
71. Sønderlund AL, O'Brien K, Kremer P, et al. The association between sports participation, alcohol use and aggression and violence: A systematic review. *J Sci Med Sport.* 2014;17(1):2–7.
72. DeGue S, Holt MK, Massetti GM, Matjasko JL, Tharp AT, Valle LA. Looking ahead toward community-level strategies to prevent sexual violence. *J Womens Health.* 2012;21(1):1–3.
73. DeGue S, Hipp TN, Herbst JH. Community-level approaches to prevent sexual violence. In: Jeglic EL, Calkins C, eds. *Sexual Violence: Evidence Based Policy and Prevention.* Switzerland AG: Springer International Publishing; 2016, pp. 161–79.
74. Jeglic E, Calkins C. *Protecting Your Child from Sexual Abuse.* New York: Skyhorse Publishing; 2018, pp. 1–176.
75. Snyder HN. *Sexual Assault of Young Children as Reported to Law Enforcement: Victim, Incident, and Offender Characteristics: A NIBRS Statistical Report.* Washington, DC: U.S. Department of Justice; 2000. https://files.eric.ed.gov/fulltext/ED446834.pdf.
76. Marshall WL. The sexual offender: Monster, victim, or everyman? *Sex Abuse.* 1996;8(4):317–35.
77. Tenbergen G, Wittfoth M, Frieling H, et al. The neurobiology and psychology of pedophilia: Recent advances and challenges. *Front Hum Neurosci.* 2015;9(344):1–20.
78. Finkelhor D, Ormrod R, Chaffin M. *Juveniles who Commit Sex Offenses against Minors. Juvenile Justice Bulletin.* Washington, DC: Office of Juvenile Justice and Delinquency Prevention; 2009, pp. 1–12. www.ojp.usdoj.gov/ojjdp.
79. Finkelhor D, Vanderminden J, Turner H, Shattuck A, Hamby S. Youth exposure to violence prevention programs in a national sample. *Child Abuse Negl.* 2014;38(4):677–86.
80. Savage J, Windsor C. Sex offender residence restrictions and sex crimes against children: A comprehensive review. *Aggress Violent Behav.* 2018;43:13–25.
81. Lussier P, Mathesius J. Trojan horse policies: Sexual predators, sorn laws and the American experience. *Psychol Crime Law.* 2018;25(2):133–56.
82. Letourneau DJ, Schaeffer CM, Bradshaw CP, Feder KA. Preventing the onset of child sexual abuse by targeting young adolescents with universal prevention programming. *Child Maltreat.* 2017;22(2):100–11.
83. Richards K. Misperceptions about child sex offenders. *Trends Issues Crime Criml Justice.* 2011;(429):1–7.
84. Schmucker M, Lösel F. The effects of sexual offender treatment on recidivism: An international meta-analysis of sound quality evaluations. *J Exp Criminol.* 2015;11(4):597–630.
85. Hall RCW, Hall RCW. A profile of pedophilia: Definition, characteristics of offenders, recidivism, treatment outcomes, and forensic issues. *Mayo Clin Proc.* 2007;82(4):457–71.
86. Widom CS, Massey C. A prospective examination of whether childhood sexual abuse predicts subsequent sexual offending. *JAMA Pediatr.* 2015;169(1):e143357.
87. Ellis L. *Theories of Rape: Inquiries Into The Causes of Sexual Aggression.* New York: Taylor & Francis; 1989.
88. Malamuth N, Sockloskie R, Koss M, Tanaka J. Characteristics of aggressors against women: Testing a model using a national sample of college students. *J Consult Clin Psychol.* 1991;59:670–82.
89. Malamuth N, Linz D, Heavey C, Barnes G, Acker M. Using the confluence model of sexual aggression to predict men's conflict with women: A ten year follow-up study. *J Pers Soc Psychol.* 1995;69:353–69.
90. Abbey A, Jacques-Tiura AJ, LeBreton JM. Risk factors for sexual aggression in young men: An expansion of the Confluence Model. *Aggress Behav.* 2011;37(5):450–64.
91. Nguyen D, Parkhill MR. Integrating attachment and depression in the Confluence Model of Sexual Assault Perpetration. *Violence Against Women.* 2014;20(8):994–1011.
92. Testa M, Cleveland MJ. Does alcohol contribute to college men's sexual assault perpetration? Between and within-person effects over five semesters. *J Stud Alcohol Drugs.* 2017;78(1):5–13.
93. Troche SJ, Yorck Herzberg P. On the role of dominance and nurturance in the Confluence Model: A person-centered approach to the prediction of sexual aggression. *Aggress Behav.* 2017;43(3):251–62.
94. DeGue S, Valle LA, Holt MK, Massetti GM, Matjasko JL, Tharp AT. A systematic review of primary prevention strategies for sexual violence perpetration. *Aggress Violent Behav.* 2014;19(4):346–62.
95. Basile KC, DeGue S, Jones K, et al. *STOP SV: A Technical Package to Prevent Sexual Violence.* Atlanta, GA: National Center for Injury Prevention and Control, Centers for Disease Control and Prevention; 2016, pp. 1–48. https://www.cdc.gov/violenceprevention/pdf/sv-prevention-technical-package.pdf.
96. Baron L, Straus MA. *Four Theories of Rape in American Society: A State-Level Analysis.* New Haven, CT: Yale University Press; 1989.
97. World Health Organization/London School of Hygiene and Tropical Medicine. *Preventing Intimate Partner and Sexual Violence against Women: Taking Action and Generating Evidence.* Geneva: World Health Organization; 2010, pp. 1–102.
98 World Health Organization. *INSPIRE Handbook: Action for Implementing the Seven Strategies* for Ending Violence against Children. Geneva: World Health Organization; 2018, p. 301. License; CC-BY-NC-SA 3.0 IGO.
99. Kim JC, Watts CH, Hargreaves JR, et al. Understanding the impact of a microfinance-based intervention on women's empowerment and

the reduction if intimate partner violence in South Africa. *Am J Public Health.* 2007;97(10):1794–802.

100. Pronyk PM, Hargreaves JR, Kim JC et al. Effect of a structural intervention for the prevention of intimate-partner violence and HIV in rural South Africa: A cluster randomized trial. *Lancet.* 2006;368:1973–83.
101. American Association of University Women. *The Simple Truth about the Gender Pay Gap.* Washington, DC: American Association of University Women; 2017, pp. 1–36. https://www.aauw.org/aauw_check/pdf_download/show_pdf.php?file=The-Simple-Truth.
102. Sorock CE. Closing the gap legislatively: Consequences of the Lilly Ledbetter Fair Pay Act. *Chi-Kent L Rev.* 2010;85:1199.
103. Cohen PN, Huffman ML. Working for the woman? Female managers and the gender wage gap. *Am Sociol Rev.* 2007;72(5):681–704.
104. Cloitre M, Stolbach BC, Herman JL, et al. A developmental approach to complex PTSD: Childhood and adult cumulative trauma as predictors of symptom complexity. *J Trauma Stress.* 2009;22(5):399–408.
105. Messman-Moore TL, Walsh KL, DiLillo D. Emotion dysregulation and risky sexual behavior in revictimization. *Child Abuse Negl.* 2010;34(12):967–76.
106. Chiu GR, Lutfey KE, Litman HJ, Link CL, Hall SA, McKinlay JB. Prevalence and overlap of childhood and adult physical, sexual, and emotional abuse: A descriptive analysis of results from the Boston Area Community Health (BACH) survey. *Violence Vict.* 2013;28(3):381–402.
107. Trickett PK, Noll JG, Putnam FW. The impact of sexual abuse on female development: Lessons from a multigenerational, longitudinal research study. *Dev Psychopathol.* 2011;23(2):453–76.
108. Basile KC, Black MC, Simon TR, Arias I, Brener ND, Saltzman LE. The association between self-reported lifetime history of forced sexual intercourse and recent health-risk behaviors: Findings from the 2003 National Youth Risk Behavior Survey. *J Adolesc Health.* 2006;39(5):752.e1–7.
109. Espelage DL, Basile KC, Hamburger ME. Bullying perpetration and subsequent sexual violence perpetration among middle school students. *J Adolesc Health.* 2012;50(1):60–5.
110. Espelage DL, Basile KC, Lemis RW, Hipp TN, Davis JP. Longitudinal examination of the bullying-sexual violence pathway across early to late adolescence: Implicating homophobic name-calling. *J Youth Adolesc.* 2018;47(9):1880–93.
111. Wilkins N, Tsao B, Hertz MF, Davis R, Klevens J. *Connecting the Dots: An Overview of the Links among Multiple Forms of Violence.* Atlanta, GA: National Center for Injury Prevention and Control, Centers for Disease Control and Prevention; Oakland, CA: Prevention Institute; 2014, pp. 1–16. https://www.cdc.gov/violenceprevention/pdf/connecting_the_dots-a.pdf.
112. Nation M, Crusto C, Wandersman A, et al. What works in prevention: Principles of effective prevention programs. *Am Psychol.* 2003;58(6–7):449–56.
113. De Brouwer A. *Supranational Criminal Prosecution of Sexual Violence: The ICC and the Practice of the ICTY and the ICTR.* Antwerpen-Oxford: Intersentia; 2005.
114. The PLoS Medicine Editors. Rape in war is common, devastating, and too often ignored. *PLoS Med.* 2009;6(1):e1000021.
115. Russell-Brown S. Rape as an act of genocide. *Berkeley J Int L.* 2003;21(2):350–74.
116. International Criminal Court. About. The Hague, Netherlands. 2018. https://www.icc-cpi.int/about.
117. United Nations. UN News: UN welcomes ICC's first conviction for rape as war crime. 2016. https://news.un.org/en/story/2016/03/525132-un-welcomes-iccs-first-conviction-rape-war-crime.
118. GOV.UK. Preventing Sexual Violence Initiative. London. https://www.gov.uk/government/organisations/preventing-sexual-violence-initiative.
119. World Health Organization. *Violence Prevention: The Evidence: Promoting Gender Equality to Prevent Violence Against Women.* Geneva, Switzerland: World Health Organization; 2009. http://www.who.int/violence_injury_prevention/violence/gender.pdf.
120. National Sexual Violence Resource Center. *Sexual Violence in Disasters: Fact Sheet.* Enola, PA: National Sexual Violence Resource Center; 2009. http://www.nsvrc.org/sites/default/files/Factsheet_sv-in-disasters.pdf.
121. Klein A. *Sexual Violence in Disasters: A Planning Guide for Prevention and Response.* Enola, PA: National Sexual Violence Resource Center; 2008. http://www.nsvrc.org/sites/default/files/Publications_NSVRC_Guides_Sexual-Violence-in-Disasters_A-planning-guide-for-prevention-and-response.pdf.

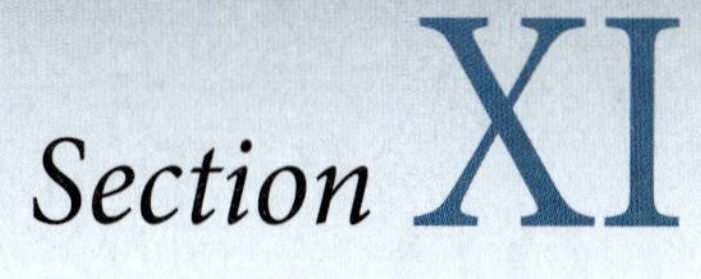

Section XI

Section Editor
Karen Peterson

Nutrition and Physical Activity

CHAPTER 180

The Principles of Nutritional Sciences: Nutrients, Nutrition Recommendations, and Dietary Guidelines

Olivia S. Anderson • Robin L. García • Yue Wu

INTRODUCTION TO NUTRIENTS

Food consists of nutrients, some of which are essential for the body to function on a daily basis. Digestion of food starts in our mouths, and food continues to break down as it travels from the mouth through the esophagus, stomach, and small intestine by a combination of mechanical forces and chemical reactions. Enzymes that are produced within the saliva, stomach, pancreas, liver, and small intestine target-specific chemical bonds holding complex nutrient structures together. Ultimately, those complex structures are broken down to simple nutrients that transporters along the stomach, small intestine, and large intestine can absorb into the body.

There are six main classes of nutrients existing in our dietary sources. They are categorized as (1) carbohydrates, (2) lipids, (3) proteins, (4) water, (5) vitamins, and (6) minerals. Carbohydrates, lipids proteins, and water are all considered macronutrients while vitamins and minerals are micronutrients (see following sections for more detail). Food also contains other bioactive substances that may not be essential for the human body to function but over the past decades have been found to have beneficial effects on human health. Such substances include phytochemicals, pre- or probiotics, and polyphenols. For example, phytochemicals contained in plant-based food products have been found to have protective effects on chronic disease such as hypertension, cancer and heart disease.[1-3] This chapter will focus on the six main classes of nutrients by describing the different subclasses within each nutrient, defining their roles in the body, and relating their role to key health outcomes or development towards disease states.

MACRONUTRIENTS

Macronutrients encompass the nutrient classes of carbohydrates, lipids, proteins, and water. These nutrients are energy yielding, with the exception of water, and are needed in relatively large amounts (thus "macro-"). Macronutrients are essential for cells to function because of the energy they provide. The energy that macronutrients yield is measured in kilocalories, a unit representing the amount of heat required to raise the temperature of 1 kilogram of water by 1°C. Kilocalorie is commonly presented as Calorie on food labels and other dietary resources (note the capital "C" represents "kilo-" while a lowercase "c" technically represents 1/1000 of a kilocalorie). Although water is not energy yielding it is also categorized as a macronutrient because it is needed in larger amounts on a daily basis and is essential for the body to function. The recommended amount of macronutrients required for normal body functioning are typically expressed in grams or kilograms per day. The amount of energy one requires from macronutrients depends on factors such as age, gender, weight, level of physical activity, and height. All of these things can this can vary even in people within the same life stage. A dietary guideline called the Acceptable Macronutrient Distribution Range provides a range of percent of Calories that one should get from each macronutrient per day. The recommendations include obtaining 45–65% of Calories from carbohydrates, 20–35% of Calories from fat, and 10–35% of Calories from protein. By meeting this recommended combination of macronutrients, there is evidence that one will likely be taking in adequate micronutrient levels and reduce their risk to chronic disease.[4]

CARBOHYDRATES

Basic Definition and Dietary Sources

Carbohydrates are organic compounds containing hydrogen, carbon, and oxygen molecules. Carbohydrates contain 4 Calories per gram. There are some forms of carbohydrates that are readily digested and absorbed while other forms of carbohydrates, also referred to as fibers, are resistant to digestive enzymes and rather remain in the digestive tract and play a role in digestive health or other health outcomes. The carbohydrates that can be broken down in the digestive tract are readily available and preferred as an energy source for the majority of cell types within the human body. In the Westernized diet, carbohydrates make up an estimated 52% of Calories consumed on a daily basis.[5] In regard to fiber intake, an adult eats about 16 g per day, yet the recommended intake is 25 g per day for females and 38 g per day in males.[6] Carbohydrates are found in a variety of food products including breads, pasta, beans, vegetables, fruits, milk, yogurt, and juices.

Carbohydrate Structure

Carbohydrate is commonly abbreviated as CHO, giving us insight into its basic structural components. Carbohydrates are made of *carbon* chains with *hydrogen* and *oxygen* groups having the standard molecular formula of $C_n(H_20)_n$. The carbohydrate structure contains two types of functional groups—(1) hydroxyl (-OH) and (2) carbonyl. A carbonyl group contains a carbon double bonded to oxygen. There are two types of carbonyl groups that a carbohydrate can contain—either an aldehyde or a ketone. The structure of an aldehyde carbohydrate includes a carbon double bonded to oxygen at the end of the carbon chain, while for a ketone, the double bond is in the middle of the carbon chain.

Classes of Carbohydrates

Carbohydrates fall into one of three classes: (1) monosaccharides, (2) oligosaccharides, or (3) polysaccharides. Of the three classes, monosaccharides have the simplest structure and are made up of a single sugar unit. Monosaccharides exist in the structural form available for absorption within the digestive tract. The two other classes are made up of monosaccharide unit chains. Glycosidic bonds link monosaccharides to form oligo- and polysaccharides. The glycosidic bond is named after the direction (alpha- or beta-) of the hydroxyl group attached to the anomeric carbon, the anomeric carbon number and the carbon number of the subsequent monosaccharide linking the units together. To form oligo- or polysaccharides through glycosidic bonding, the monosaccharides undergo condensation to eliminate a water group. Alternatively, the oligo- or polysaccharides can be broken down to their respective monosaccharide units through hydrolysis, or the addition of a water molecule. Hydrolysis is the key reaction that occurs during digestion that will break apart oligo- and polysaccharides contained in food into monosaccharide units that are readily available for absorption in the small intestine.

First Class of Carbohydrates: Monosaccharides The first and simplest class is monosaccharides, often referred to as simple sugars. Monosaccharides include glucose, fructose, and galactose. They are found in food sources such as honey, fruits, and corn syrup. Typically, carbohydrates are not in this simple form in food sources but rather as di- or polysaccharides (see following sections), but during digestion humans break down these larger carbohydrates to simple sugars. Once in the form of glucose, fructose, or galactose, these simple sugars are capable of absorption at the small intestine via sugar transporters. Before discussing the larger carbohydrate classes, it is important to understand the glycosidic bond that links monosaccharides.

Second Class of Carbohydrates: Oligosaccharides The next class of carbohydrates is oligosaccharides. They contain two to ten monosaccharides units with each unit linked by a glycosidic bond. Disaccharides are two monosaccharides linked by glycosidic bonds and are the most common type of oligosaccharides present in dietary sources. The three major disaccharides in dietary source are maltose, lactose, and sucrose. Maltose consists of two glucose units linked by a glycosidic bond. Sucrose consists of a glucose linked to fructose. Lactose contains a glucose linked to a galactose. Lactose is the main carbohydrate existing in dairy products and often associated with "lactose intolerance," the overarching symptom of lactase e nonpersistence that can develop in humans over the course of their lifetime and as early as in childhood.

Lactase Nonpersistence Lactose intolerance is a common term used to describe the overarching symptom of the condition of lactase nonpersistence. This condition results from a deficiency of the digestive enzyme lactase. In mammals, the lactase gene is highly active during the lactation period when the sole dietary intake is from the mother's lactose-containing breast milk. Following the introduction to other food products, in other words, exposure to foods containing carbohydrates other than lactose, the production of lactase rapidly declines, as there is a lesser need for its activity. Humans are unique as mammals because the domestication of milk-producing animals allows individuals access to milk and milk-products throughout one's life. As such, humans continue to take in these types of food products beyond the lactation period, and thus, have a lifetime exposure to lactose.[7]

Over time humans developed a genetic polymorphism in the lactase gene resulting in sufficient production of lactase throughout adulthood when there is continuous exposure to lactose-containing foods. Because milk-producing agriculture is a recent event in regard to evolution, this polymorphism is thought to arise from a high-frequency haplotype due to the benefit of ingesting lactose in cultures that raise milk-producing animals.[7,8] Individuals lacking this polymorphism will have a decline in lactase resulting in symptoms that indicate someone is intolerant to lactose as early as in the toddler lifestage. Symptoms include bloating, cramping, and diarrhea because lactose will not be properly digested for absorption and instead will travel to the large intestine where it can absorb water. Of note, it has also been evidenced that individuals who are lactase persistent but do not expose themselves to milk-containing products will have a steady decline of lactase production overtime and may also exhibit symptoms of lactose intolerance when reintroducing milk products.[9]

Third Class of Carbohydrate: Polysaccharides Polysaccharides contain 11 or more and up to 10,000,000 monosaccharide units. The monosaccharide units of the polysaccharide can be the same (homopolysaccharide) or have varying monosaccharide units (heteropolysaccharide). Another characteristic of polysaccharides are the degree of branching. Some are linear and contain zero branching units while others have varying degrees of branching. The branching units are significant for storage capacity, which will be discussed in more detail in the following subsections covering specific polysaccharides. There are three polysaccharides to discuss that have relevant implications in human nutrition—starch, glycogen, and cellulose. Common among these three polysaccharides is that they are all homopolysaccharides containing only glucose units.

Starch Starch is the most abundant polysaccharide found in plants (e.g., tubers, seeds, roots). Starch is found in two forms, amylose and amylopectin. Amylose is linear, unbranched, and made of glucose connected by alpha 1,4 glycosidic bonds. Amylopectin is moderately branched and a homopolymer of glucose linked by alpha 1,4 bonds on the linear chains but by alpha 1,6 bonds at the branching points (Fig. 180-1). The typical lengths of a linear chain between branching points is 20–25 glucose units. In uncooked starch food sources, the linear structure of amylose allows it to be tightly packed. This creates a structure that is not as readily digestible as the branched less packed structure of amylopectin. In contrast, the processing and heating of amylose-containing foods (i.e., cooking) can loosen hydrogen bonds within the structure making it more accessible for digestion.

Glycogen Glycogen is a highly branched, homopolymer of glucose. Glycogen is abundant in skeletal muscle and liver tissue of mammals. The glucose units are linked by alpha 1,4 bonds on the linear chains but by alpha 1,6 bonds at the branching points (just like amylopectin). The typical lengths of a linear chain between branching points is 10–14 glucose units. More branching allows for a higher degree of accessibility for metabolic enzymes, thus glycogen is a ready source of energy for humans (and other mammals).

Fibers The structural components of a fiber are similar to that of a digestible carbohydrate except that the glycosidic bonds are resistant to enzymatic breakdown and forgo absorption in the gastrointestinal (GI) tract. There are many types of fibers we consume in food such as cellulose, resistant starch, bran, pectin, and inulin. Fibers are found in plants, specifically within the cellular walls. Common dietary sources of fiber include fruits, vegetables, grains, and legumes. Fibers can also be synthetically added to food sources such as cereals, yogurt, juices, and even artificial sweeteners. Fibers have an array of functions, characteristics, and physiological effects.

Characteristics (and Physiological Effects) *Solubility* As the name of this characteristic suggests, fibers that are water-soluble will dissolve in water whereas fibers that are water-insoluble will not. The solubility of a fiber results in unique physiological effects. Fibers with a higher water-solubility form a more gel-like substance as it moves through the tract. They also tend to have a high viscosity, ability to adsorb, and are typically fermentable (see other characteristics sections below for more detail). Alternatively, insoluble fibers will stay intact as they travel through the digestive tract. Upon reaching the colon insoluble fiber will add to the bulk of fecal matter decreasing its transit time through the large intestine. This property of insoluble fibers helps to relieve constipation.[10,11]

Fermentable Whether a fiber is fermentable depends on whether the bacteria in our large intestine can ferment it (i.e., metabolize it). Byproducts of fermentation include short-chained fatty acids (acetate, propionate, and butyrate), carbon dioxide, and hydrogen. The short-chained fatty acids (SCFA) that are produced through the fermentation process are either used as an energy source by colon cells or to support bacterial growth.

Other Characteristics Water-soluble fibers are typically viscous. The viscosity turns the material more gel-like and slows the movement of food through the digestive tract. Viscous fibers delay gastric emptying leaving chyme in the stomach for a longer period of time and

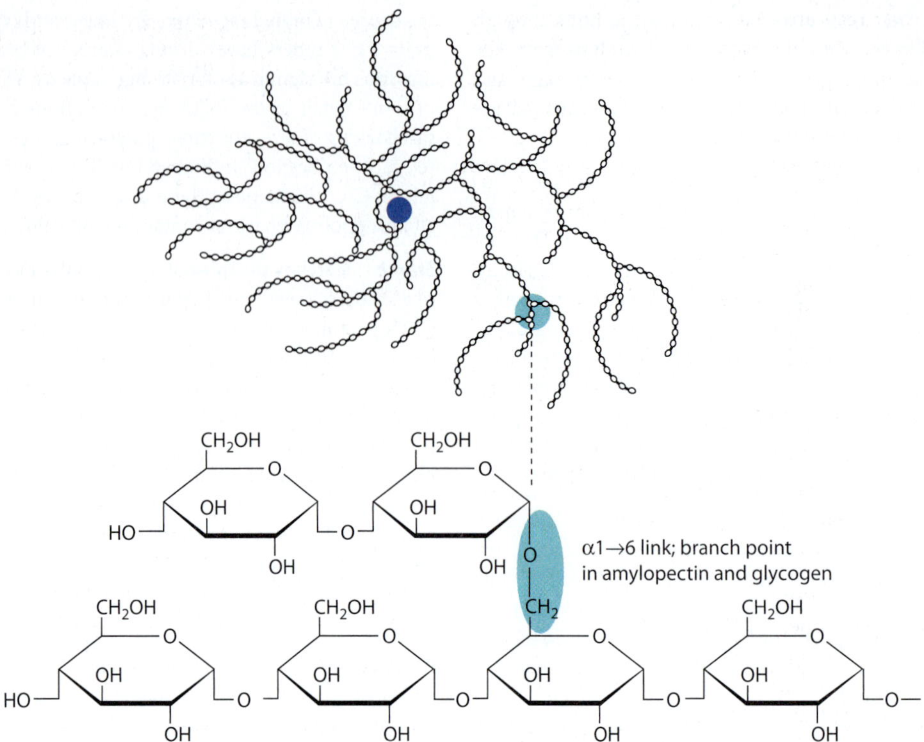

FIGURE 180-1. The structure of starch and glycogen. Amylose is a linear polymer of glucose residues linked α1→4, which coils into a helix. Amylopectin and glycogen consist of short chains of glucose residues linked α1→4 with branch points formed by α1→6 glycoside bonds. The glycogen molecule is a sphere ~21 nm in diameter that can be seen in electron micrographs. It has a molecular mass of ~10^7 Da and consists of polysaccharide chains, each containing about 13 glucose residues. The chains are either branched or unbranched and are arranged in 12 concentric layers. The branched chains (each has two branches) are found in the inner layers and the unbranched chains in the outermost layer. The blue dot at the center of the glycogen molecule is glycogenin, the primer molecule for glycogen synthesis. (*Source*: Used with Permission from Rodwell VW, Bender DA, Botham KM, Kennelly PJ, Weil P. Harper's Illustrated Biochemistry, 31e; 2018. Available at: https://accessmedicine.mhmedical.com/content.aspx?bookid=2386§ionid=187832287&-jumpsectionid=187832333 Accessed: March 05, 2020.)

increasing the time of feeling full.[12] The slower gastric emptying can play a role in the rate of glucose absorption at the small intestine which aides in the well-controlled flux of glucose levels into circulation following food intake. In addition to sequestering carbohydrates, viscous fibers can also sequester proteins and lipids inhibiting their exposure to digestive enzymes. This can impede absorption of these macronutrients at the small intestine. Thus, fiber has been consistent as a staple food source to help with weight management and the control of blood sugar for type 1 and 2 diabetes.[13–15]

Some fibers have the ability to adsorb (i.e., to bind) to molecules and other nutrients. Relevant to human health, some fibers bind fatty acids, cholesterol, and bile acids within the digestive tract. Once bound the material travels to the large intestine and is added to the bulk of fecal matter to be excreted or bacteria in the large intestine can metabolize the bound molecules. Focusing on the potential of increased bile excretion via feces by fiber, the liver will need to synthesize more bile to keep up with lipid digestion and absorption. Part of the basic structure of bile includes cholesterol, thus low-density lipoprotein (LDL) cholesterol will be taken from circulation and incorporated into bile ultimately decreasing serum cholesterol.[16] Although, this is a well-proposed mechanism, evidence shows that high intake of fiber (equivalent to > 3 servings of oatmeal per day) on a regular basis is needed to result in significant decrease in LDL blood cholesterol. Fiber can also adsorb specific minerals like calcium and iron. This can have either a positive or negative consequence. If the fiber is highly fermentable with bound minerals, the breakdown of the fiber by gut bacteria releases the minerals and allow for additional mineral absorption at the large intestine. Instead, if the fiber is poorly fermented the minerals will remain intact with the fiber material and be incorporated into and lost through fecal matter.

Other Considerations of Carbohydrates

Unrefined Versus Refined Carbohydrates Although it is appropriate as a health professional to discuss carbohydrates in relation to their structures which will dictate their function in the body, often individuals broadly refer to carbohydrates as either refined or unrefined. Unrefined carbohydrates exist in whole food products, in other words, a food product that has undergone zero to minimal processing keeping its nutrients intact at the time of consumption. Examples of unrefined, whole food sources of carbohydrates are legumes, fresh fruits, fresh vegetables, and grains. The wheat grain is a great example of a carbohydrate that can be both unrefined and refined. The unrefined wheat grain contains layers including the bran, germ, and endosperm. The bran contains nutrients such as fiber and B vitamins. The germ contains polyunsaturated fatty acids, iron, zinc, magnesium, and vitamin E. The endosperm is rich in carbohydrates and contains protein. Thus, consumption of an unrefined wheat grain product provides an individual with a nutrient-rich food source with the potential to reap health benefits from these nutrients. The intake of unrefined grains has shown to be protective of the development of obesity, heart disease, hypertension, and type 2 diabetes.[17,18] If a wheat grain were to undergo a refinement process, the nutrient-rich layers of the bran and germ are removed. This provides a food product that has an increased shelf life and an altered the taste but lacks nutrients that are essential to the body. Over the past century there has been an increase in the consumption of refined grains and is associated with lower fiber intake and increased risk of chronic disease like type 2 diabetes.[19]

Added Sugars Added sugars are those that are intentionally added to food or beverages when they are being processed or prepared for the consumer. These sugars exclude naturally occurring sugars such as the sugar content existing in fruits and lactose-rich milk products. Over the past few decades there has been a rise in the consumption of added sugars in all life-stages, except during infancy, and has been closely associated with the rise in obesity and chronic disease in the United States especially in childhood and adolescence.[20–22] Added sugars pose a threat to human health because they add on Calories to a food product without adding on any nutrient value. It has been estimated that about 15% of total daily Calories in adults come from added sugars alone; this is 10% higher than the recommendation from the World Health Organization.[23,24] Added sugars will be listed in the food label under the ingredients section. Some examples of common added sugars include, but are not limited to: anhydrous dextrose, brown sugar, corn syrup, high-fructose corn syrup (HFCS), honey, invert sugar, malt syrup, maple syrup, molasses, nectars (e.g., peach nectar, pear nectar), and sugar.

Protein

Basic Definition and Dietary Sources

Proteins contain four Calories per gram. In the United States, protein deficiency is quite rare as sources of protein such as meat, eggs, grains, legumes, and dairy products are readily available. As such, protein is estimated to make up about 15% of the Calories consumed on a daily basis in the United States.[5]

Protein Structure

Protein molecules consist of amino acids linked together by peptide bonds. There are approximately 20 amino acids that are consistently found within dietary proteins (Table 180-1). Amino acids are molecules that are made of a central carbon attached to a hydrogen group, carboxyl group, amino group, and a side chain. The nitrogen present in the amino group differentiates its structural make-up from carbohydrates and lipids. The side chain is unique for each particular amino acid and is what differentiates each amino acid from one another. The make-up of the side-chain gives each amino acid specific properties, and thus, dictates the role of the protein.

The amino acids are linked together by the carboxyl group of one amino acid to the nitrogen of the amino group of another amino acid, otherwise known as a peptide bond. Proteins can be as small as two or three amino acids linked together (i.e., dipeptide or tripeptides, respectively) or more than three amino acids linked together (polypeptide). Dietary proteins are broken down to single amino acids, di- or tripeptides within the GI tract. Transporters at the small intestine are able to transfer these molecules from the GI tract to circulation. Once amino acids are present within the body they are available for protein synthesis. Polypeptides can stand-alone or form larger proteins with other polypeptides. The chemical properties of the amino acid side chains result in bending, folding, attraction, coiling, etc. of the polypeptide resulting in varying functional capabilities within the human body. The polypeptides that form take on the role of hormones, enzymes, and transporters and have structural properties within the body.

Essentiality

Of the 20 amino acids in Table 180-1, there are nine that are considered to be essential. Essential amino acids are required to be taken in through the diet because the body cannot biosynthesize them. Most proteins consist of at least some of each of the amino acids which means we cannot generate new proteins unless we have a dietary supply of the essential amino acids.[25] The remaining 11 are nonessential and are not required to be taken in through the diet although they are commonly contained within animal food sources.

Although there are 11 nonessential amino acids, there are instances when they do become essential to take in through the diet. When this occurs, the amino acid is called "conditionally essential." A clear example of a nonessential amino acid changing into a conditionally essential amino acid is in a condition referred to as phenylketonuria. This is a condition that results from a mutation on phenylalanine hydroxylase gene.[26] Tyrosine is normally a nonessential amino acid that can be made when phenylalanine is available (Table 180-1). This conversion is stimulated by the enzyme phenylalanine hydroxylase. When the mutation in the enzyme's gene is present, this conversion of phenylalanine to tyrosine is almost completely nonexistent resulting in tyrosine becoming conditionally essential. Other examples of conditionally essential amino acids are indicated in Table 180-1.

TABLE 180-1 THE ESSENTIAL AND NONESSENTIAL AMINO ACIDS[a]

Essential	Nonessential
Histidine	Alanine
Isoleucine	Arginine[b]
Leucine	Asparagine
Lysine	Aspartate
Methionine	Cysteine[b]
Phenylalanine	Glutamate
Threonine	Glutamine[b]
Tryptophan	Glycine[b]
Valine	Proline[b]
	Serine[b]
	Tyrosine[b]

[a]Essential amino acids are required to obtain through the diet because the body cannot biosynthesize them.
[b]Conditionally essential amino acids.

Protein Quality

As stated, the amount of protein taken in through the Westernized diet is likely enough to satisfy an individual's daily requirement. Needs are different dependent on life-stage, physical activity levels, and general size of a human. For example, infants and children need more protein per kilogram of body weight per day than adults due to the rapid tissue deposition occurring with normal growth and development (i.e., 1.5–0.95 g/kg body weight vs. 0.8 g/kg body weight, respectively).

Although the amount taken in is generally sufficient, the make-up of the protein, or quality of the protein, is something to consider, especially in a time when vegetarian and vegan diets are an option. A high-quality protein food source is one that contains all to most of the nine essential amino acids in proper proportions that once ingested, digested, and absorbed will adequately support protein synthesis. Animal sources are considered complete proteins. The types of proteins derived from animal muscles are myosin and actin. These form the contractile units of muscle and are the major component in both meat and in building muscle tissue. Since mammalian-derived meat and human skeletal muscle are similar in composition, these proteins contain high levels of all the essential amino acids needed for muscle growth. Whey and casein are also proteins that are animal-derived. Casein is abundant in milk products and makes up about 80% of all protein in cow's milk. Whey is derived from leftover materials after milk is coagulated for cheese. Whey proteins are isolated from the leftover material and are digested efficiently.[27] Although soy proteins are derived from plant sources, they contain adequate levels of amino acids and are considered to be a complete protein source.

On the other hand, incomplete proteins contain some essential amino acids; but not all, though two incomplete proteins can be put together to form a complete protein source. For example, wheat products contain all essential amino acids except they lack lysine.

Alternatively, legumes are low in methionine. To overcome these essential amino acid deficiencies, individuals on a vegetarian or vegan diet often practice combining a wheat- and legume-derived protein to form a complete protein source (e.g., rice and beans).

Celiac Disease

Celiac disease is an autoimmune reaction to gluten, a protein found in wheat, barley, semolina, farro, and rye. Celiac is prevalent worldwide with an estimated 1 in 100 people affected by this heritable disease. An individual carrying a HLA2 DQ2 or DQ8 allele is genetically predisposed and has a one in ten chance of developing Celiac in their lifetime.

Specifically, the disease is characterized by a response that occurs when the body is exposed to gliadin, a glycoprotein component of gluten. This triggers a T-cell mediated response resulting in the destruction of villi in the small intestine. Villi are essential for complete digestion and absorption of nutrients to occur. They house digestive enzymes that complete digestion as well as peptide and amino acid transporters that allow for absorption to circulation. With damaged villi resulting from the autoimmune response, nutrients are unable to be digested down to their absorbable forms and there is lack of surface area and transporters to allow of absorption even for completely digested nutrients. Unabsorbed nutrients then travel to the large intestine resulting in stomach discomfort and other related symptoms such as fatigue, bloating, and diarrhea. Long-term insufficient nutrient absorption deprives the body of essential nutrients and can result in unintentional weight loss, several types of anemia, osteoporosis, intestinal cancer, and, in children, failure to thrive.

Since this autoimmune response is triggered by exposure to gliadin, removing the gluten exposure through dietary sources, including medicine and foods manufactured in the same facilities as gluten-containing products, will eliminate the autoimmune response. Without this response occurring, the villi remain intact, functional, and can regenerate for those who have been exposed to gluten for any amount of time.

Lipids

Basic Definition and Dietary Sources

Lipids contain nine Calories per gram. Like carbohydrates and proteins, there are several different types of dietary fat with different functions and effects in regard to human health. Common types of dietary fat include triglycerides, saturated fatty acids, trans-fatty acids, monounsaturated fatty acids, polyunsaturated fatty acids, cholesterol, and phospholipids. Foods often associated with higher fat content include red meats, cooking oils, butter, nuts, avocado, and certain fish. The energy that is taken in from lipids in the Westernized diet is about 33% on a daily basis.[5] Of the percent of Calories coming from lipids about 11% of that is made up of saturated fatty acids which exceeds the recommendation of the 2015–20 *Dietary Guidelines for Americans* to consume less than 10% of Calories from saturated fatty acids.[28] Instead of focusing on reducing lipid intake in the diet, there is an emphasis on focusing on specific types of lipids taken in through the diet to support body functioning and health.

Lipid Structure

Triglycerides and Fatty Acids Triglycerides consist of a three-carbon chain (glycerol) with a fatty acid esterified to each carbon. Triglycerides are the most-widely consumed type of lipid within the diet. The make-up of fatty acids vary and will dictate the properties that they give food (e.g., whether a lipid-containing food is liquid at room temperature or solid). Triglycerides are digested down to free fatty acids within the GI tract. The fatty acids are then absorbed to circulation and, once absorbed, will have different functions and effects on the human body dependent on their chemical make-up. Each differs by the number of carbons atoms on its chain (i.e., short-, medium-, or long-chained), number or existence of double bonds (e.g., mono- or polyunsaturated), and the arrangement of double bonds (i.e., cis- versus trans- configuration). Fatty acids abundant in our dietary sources include saturated, trans, monounsaturated, and polyunsaturated, which will be discussed later in this chapter. The body can synthesize many fatty acids. Humans do lack an enzyme necessary to facilitate the double bond position in the omega-6 and -3 ends of the fatty acids making these types of fatty acids essential in terms of consumption within the diet.

Cholesterol Cholesterol is a lipid that is only found in animal food sources, thus oils or plant-based foods do not contain cholesterol. The liver has the ability to synthesize cholesterol so it is not considered to be essential to obtain through the diet. Cholesterol consists of a steroid nucleus. In dietary sources, cholesterol is either found as such or esterified to a fatty acid. Because of the steroid nucleus, cholesterol is key for the synthesis of many steroid hormones such as estrogen or testosterone.

Phospholipids Like triglycerides, phospholipids also consist of glycerol as its backbone but instead of three fatty acids attached to each carbon of the glycerol, there are only two. The third carbon consists of a phosphate group, thus the name, phospholipid. This structural make-up allows it to be amphipathic giving it the ability to act as an emulsifier allowing oils and water to mix giving a product a certain texture. In the human body phospholipids are integral parts of the cellular membrane and help regulate the substances that transport to and from a cell.

Lipid Properties and Their Significance on Select Health Outcomes

Saturated Fatty Acids These fatty acids are considered saturated because the carbons along the fatty acid chain are bound to four atoms and thus is saturated. Over the past decades, saturated fatty acid intake has been deemed as a major influencer for the rise in cardiovascular disease resulting in health practitioners recommending limited saturated fatty acid intake for those at risk or recovering from a cardiovascular event.[18] The results from a meta-analysis completed in 2010,[29] caused researchers to question this long-time theory and expand research to look at the entire make-up of macro- and micronutrients within one's diet in regard to the risk of cardiovascular disease.[30,31] Other patterns of the diet important to consider include high calcium intake, added or refined sugar intake, and high protein intake.

Trans Fatty Acids When carbons along the fatty acid chain contain a double bond, the hydrogens attached to each carbon of the double bond either exist in a cis or trans formation. Trans fatty acids differ than other fatty acids containing double bonds because the hydrogens attached to the carbons are in the trans orientation versus cis. In the trans orientation the hydrogens are on the opposite sides of the double bonds. This trans configuration gives the fatty acid a higher melting point, and when present in food, can keep food solid at room temperature (e.g., margarine) or lengthen shelf life (e.g., chips, crackers, granola bars). There are few trans fatty acids found in natural food products but the majority in the human diet come from synthetic trans fatty acids. Fatty acids undergo a process called hydrogenation where double bonds become saturated. Between the saturation of double bonds and the arrangement of hydrogens, this configuration makes it shaped like a saturated fatty acid with similar properties. Research has illustrated a positive association between trans fatty acid intake and circulating cholesterol levels and inflammation making this type of fat a risk for cardiovascular disease. Studies have shown that even just a few grams of trans fatty acid intake per day can result in as much of a 23% increased risk of cardiovascular disease.[32,33] Because of this heightened risk for cardiovascular events, the FDA has required that food labels present the amount of trans-fatty acids within a product.

Polyunsaturated—Omega-3 and Omega-6 Fatty Acids A focus on dietary consumption of omega-3 and -6 fatty acids has been suggested by health officials and government agencies over the years as evidence has brought to light their protective affects against heart disease, cancers, and their anti-inflammatory properties. Omega-3 derivatives, EPA and DHA, from animal sources such as fish and fish oil supplements, reduce risk of coronary heart disease by lowering circulating LDL and triglycerides without affecting high-density lipoprotein (HDL) levels, which reduces the buildup of plaque leading to atherosclerosis. Omega-3 intake has also been associated with a reduced risk of thrombosis and arrhythmias.[34] Low to moderate consumption of omega-6 fatty acids can stimulate inflammatory markers protective of coronary heart disease. The ratio of omega-6 to -3 intake has been evaluated over the years in terms of the resulting health outcomes. The typical Westernized diet results in a high omega-6 to -3 ratio (about 16:1).[35] A high intake of omega-6 saturates the inflammatory response and there has been evidence that it can lead to the oxidation of circulating LDL, leading to atherosclerosis. Therefore, the current recommendations are to take in a ratio of 5–10:1 to reap the optimal health benefits from omega -6 and -3 fatty acids and their derivatives.[36]

Monounsaturated Fatty Acids Monounsaturated fatty acids also have lowering effects of circulating LDL. There are certain regions in the world, like Mediterranean countries, with typical diets high in monounsaturated fat due to the high use of olive oils during the cooking and preparation process. Mediterranean populations have lower incidence of coronary heart disease in comparison to the United States. While intake of monounsaturated fats certainly plays a role in the mechanisms to reduce the risk of heart disease, it is likely not the only driver in Mediterranean diets as these diets are rich in fruits, vegetables, fatty fish, and nuts.

Cholesterol The steroid core of cholesterol is not used for energy but rather is an essential component of all cellular membranes, aiding in their fluidity, as well as a component of other compounds in the body like hormones and bile. Cholesterol is found in animal products and is commonly taken in through the diet. Although cholesterol is consumed through the diet, our body is fully capable of biosynthesizing cholesterol within the liver in times of need. On the other hand, if much cholesterol is consumed through the diet, the liver suppresses the internal synthesis of cholesterol. Hypercholesterolemia, high blood cholesterol, arises when there is a mutation in the low-density lipoprotein receptor gene. When this mutation is present, there is inhibition of a negative feedback loop during cholesterol biosynthesis resulting in accelerated synthesis of internal cholesterol and high blood levels. Over the years, associations between circulating cholesterol and cardiovascular events suggested restrictions of dietary cholesterol to be prudent, but more recent research has shown that dietary cholesterol plays an insignificant role in modulating blood cholesterol levels.[37] The evidence is strong enough that the 2015–20 *Dietary Guidelines for Americans* no longer recommend restricting dietary cholesterol.[38]

WATER

Basic Definition and Dietary Sources

Water is essential for the human body to function. So much so that humans can survive weeks without food intake but only a few days without water. Water is a polar molecule and serves as an ideal solvent within the body. It is the medium in which chemical reactions occur, nutrients and hormones are transported, body temperature is regulated, and serves to regulate acid-base balance. Dietary consumption of water occurs through beverages like water, juice, coffee, and tea as well as foods containing water. Foods with high content of water include fruits, vegetables, and soups.

Distribution and Key Functions

In a normal healthy adult, water makes up about 60% of the total body weight. In other words, there is about 40 L of water in the body at any given time. About 66.7% (25 L) of that water is contained in intracellular environments, and the remaining 15 L is in extracellular compartments like plasma and interstitial fluid (i.e., surrounding cells). Each tissue type across the body has varying levels of water; for example, blood is about 90% water, muscle is about 75% water, bone is about 25% water, and adipose tissue is about 10% water.

Because water is the most abundant constituent of the human body, it plays an important role in maintaining cellular homeostasis, and thus, daily functioning. Water has many roles in metabolism, pH balance, and as a solvent (i.e., medium in which substances dissolve). Water holds heat so it affects body temperature. As part of the interstitial fluid, it provides a passageway for nutrients and other substances throughout the body. Water provides protection as a lubricant, rids toxicants via urine or foreign objects (e.g., tears), and provides buoyancy (e.g., to cushion walking).

Loss and Intake

The amount of water in the human body is not stored, yet the amount remains constant over time. Water is lost from our body (about 2500 mL per day) on a daily basis by obvious routes such as urine, feces, and sweat. Other routes of water loss include exhalation and skin diffusion. Because humans are constantly overturning water, individuals must obtain water by ingesting it. Dietary consumption of water occurs through beverages as well as water contained in food. Minimal amounts of water are also obtained from byproducts of metabolism (<10% of water "intake").

Water Regulation ***Glomerular Filtration*** The filtering and excretion functions of the kidney help maintain fluid balance. The filtering process begins in the Bowman's capsule, which encapsulates a series of capillaries called the glomerulus. The glomerulus receives blood (water, ions, amino acids, glucose, etc.) and filters it. Larger molecules like red blood cells return to circulation via the efferent arteriole. The filtered blood, called glomerular filtrate, crosses the wall of Bowman's capsule and continues to the tubules along the nephron unit. The tubules have variable permeability along their length making them more pervious (or porous) to specific to certain solutes and water.

The formation of urine in the kidney rids the body of waste, potential toxins, and excess water and solutes. Urine is synthesized following reabsorption along the kidney. During reabsorption certain filtrates will reenter the blood stream, such as water and electrolytes, to ensure intra- and extracellular homeostasis. Of the glomerular filtrate that enters the kidney, only about 1% of it is actually incorporated into urine and excreted on a daily basis.

Osmolality Osmotic pressure plays a significant role in the intra- and extracellular distribution of water. Cellular membranes may be impermeable to solutes but not to water, thus, it will move from a high water concentration (low solute concentration) compartment to where there is a low water concentration. This gradient creates equilibrium of "water to solute."

Vasopressin Vasopressin is a hormone produced in the hypothalamus and released to the kidney by the pituitary gland. Its main function is to retain water levels in the body. Vasopressin is released in response to an increase of extracellular osmolality (low water volume) and increased sodium concentration in circulation. Upon reaching the kidney, vasopressin binds to V2 receptors on the basolateral end of the kidney tubules that trigger an increase of permeability to water by recruiting transport proteins called Aquaporin w and Aquaporin 3/4 to the apical and basolateral membranes of the kidney tubules, respectively. Aquaporins are selective water channels allowing for water reabsorption back to the bloodstream from the kidney.

MICRONUTRIENTS

Micronutrients are vitamins and minerals that, compared to macronutrients, are needed in smaller amounts by the body. Micronutrients are essential to human health and are used to maintain various systems in the body, including the brain, muscles, blood circulation, and the immune system. Although essential, humans are unable to produce micronutrients and therefore are required to intake them through dietary consumption.[39]

Vitamins

Basic Definition

Vitamins are mostly derived from the diet, although may also be partially generated by the body.[39] However, since vitamins or their precursors must be obtained through the diet, all vitamins are considered essential. These organic compounds are needed to prevent disease and used in enzymatic reactions. Thirteen known vitamins exist today—the water-soluble vitamins B complex (B1, B2, B3, B6, B12, folic acid, biotin, pantothenic acid) and C, and the fat-soluble vitamins A, D, E, and K.

Water-soluble Vitamins

The body handles the water-soluble vitamins differently than that of the fat-soluble vitamins. Water-soluble vitamins are absorbed into the portal blood after digestion and are transported via proteins throughout the body by binding to enzymes. They are excreted through the urine when levels are in excess of what is needed by the body.

B-Complex Vitamins The B-complex vitamins consist of B1 (thiamin), B2 (riboflavin), B3 (niacin), pantothenic acid (B5), biotin (B7), B6 (pyridoxine), folate (B9), and B12 (cobalamin). Each of these has different structures and functions in maintaining health.

Thiamin Basic Definition and Dietary Sources Vitamin B1, also known as thiamin, was the first B vitamin to be identified. The structure of thiamin is a pyrimidine ring (2,5-dimethy-6-aminopyrimidine) joined to a thiazolium ring (4-methyl-5-hydroxy ethyl thiazole) by a methylene bridge. Among multiple functions, thiamin is required by transketolase, an enzyme essential for the pentose shunt that supplies NADP for synthetic pathways.[40]

Thiamin is naturally found in many foods, including meats (especially pork), legumes, sunflower seeds, vegetables, and whole grains and has been added to enriched grain products.[41] Processing and heating foods will reduce the thiamin content. Foods containing antithiamin factors, such as thiaminases in raw fish, can cleave and destroy thiamin. Polyhydroxyphenols can also inactivate thiamin through oxyreductive processes, and are found in coffee, tea, betel nuts, blueberries, black currents, brussels sprouts, and red cabbage.[42]

Most dietary thiamin is in phosphylated forms, freed by intestinal phosphatases prior to absorption in the jejunum. Thiamin is stored in the liver, but in small amounts, and is needed in a continuous supply from the diet.

Key Functions About 80% of the thiamin in the body exists as thiamin pyrophosphate (TPP, also known as thiamin diphosphate),[36] which is the main metabolically active form of thiamin. TPP has many roles in energy metabolism. First, it is a cofactor for reactions that cleave alpha-ketoacids and decarboxylation of pyruvate to form acetyl CoA. This then goes onto the pyruvate pathway to oxidize glucose. TPP also is a cofactor in decarboxylation of alpha-ketoglutarate dehydrogenase, used in the citric acid cycle (also known as TCA cycle or Krebs cycle),[40] a cascade of chemical reactions that releases stored energy from carbohydrates, proteins, and fats, into adenosine triphosphate (ATP) and carbon dioxide.

Deficiency Thiamin deficiency can be caused by low dietary intakes, low absorption or high excretion rates due to alcoholism, dialysis, chronic diarrhea, and long-term use of high doses of diuretics. Although rare, thiamin deficiency can be caused by genetic mutations. Early symptoms of thiamin deficiency include weight loss and anorexia, confusion, short-term memory loss, muscle weakness, and cardiovascular symptoms.[43] Beriberi is the most common effect of a thiamin deficiency, which is characterized by peripheral neuropathy, wasting, and impaired sensory motor and reflex functions. Rarely does it result in congestive heart failure, edema in lower limbs, and death. Wernicke-Korsakoff syndrome more commonly occurs concurrently with thiamin deficiency, and is more common in people with chronic alcoholism, severe gastric disorders, drug use disorders, or AIDS. Most patients experience two phases, the first being acute, life-threatening Wernicke's encephalopathy, characterized by peripheral neuropathy. Those who survive this stage develop Korsakoff's psychosis, which is due to chronic thiamin deficiency and characterized by severe short-term memory loss, disorientation, and confabulation.[44]

Riboflavin Basic Definition and Dietary Sources Riboflavin, also known as vitamin B2, is a yellow, fluorescent compound, necessary for redox reactions.[45] Its structure, 7,8-dimethyl-10-ribityl-isoalloxaine, lends itself to be essential for two major coenzymes, flavin mononucleotide (FMN) and flavin adenine dinucleotide (FAD). Both of these coenzymes are critical in energy production and electron transport, cell function and development, and metabolism of fats and drugs. Riboflavin is key to the 2-electron acceptor/donor and 1-electron acceptor/donor complexes in the electron transport chain (complexes I-IV and coenzyme Q10).[46]

The majority of dietary riboflavin is in the form of FMN or FAD. Foods rich in riboflavin include eggs, organ meat, lean meats, dairy products, and green vegetables, as well as fortified cereals and grains.[46,47]

Key Functions Riboflavin, as the form of FMN and FAD, are distributed widely to body tissues. It is involved in the metabolism of macronutrients and the production of some other B complex vitamins, which make it an essential vitamin in growth and development. Riboflavin also serves as an antioxidant because its role in the regeneration of glutathione, a free radical scavenger.[48]

Deficiency Riboflavin deficiency is characterized by a sore throat, hyperemia, and edema of the pharyngeal and oral mucous membranes, cheilosis, angular stomatitis, glossitis, seborrheic dermatitis, and normochromic normocytic anemia.[45] People with riboflavin deficiency often present with other nutrient deficiencies as well.

Niacin Basic Definition and Dietary Sources Niacin (vitamin B3) encompasses several forms, including nicotinic acid (NA), nicotinamide (nicotinic acid amide, NM), nicotinic acid (pyridine-3-carboxylic acid), and the biologically active derivatives of nicotinamide.[49] Niacin is initially incorporated into nicotinamide adenine dinucleotide (NAD), which can be phosphorylated to form nicotinamide adenine dinucleotide phosphate (NADP) for more than 400 enzymatic activities. The redox potential of NAD and NADP is used in energy production, the Krebs cycle, glycolysis, ethanol oxidation, and other reactions.[50]

Food sources of niacin include animal products, including milk, eggs, fish, lean meats, poultry; legumes, rice; and enriched grains. The amino acid, tryptophan, is a precursor of nicotinamide and the conversion requires two major steps: metabolic conversion of tryptophan to α-amino-β-carboxymuconate-ε-semialdehyde (ACMS), then metabolic conversion of ACMS to nicotinamide. However, the conversion of tryptophan into nicotinamide is effected at low efficiency. The concept of niacin equivalents (NEs) is estimated as total food NE $=$ mg niacin $+1/60$ mg tryptophan.[50]

Key Functions All tissues in the body are able to convert absorbed niacin into its main metabolically active form. As one of the water-soluble vitamins, urinary excretion, not a blood sample, is the most sensitive and reliable measure of niacin status. Niacin, in the form of nicotinic acid, is used pharmacologically to reduce serum LDL cholesterol and increase serum HDL cholesterol. In patients with dyslipidemia, niacin intake has shown to correct the HDL:LDL cholesterol ratio and improve markers for atherosclerosis.[51] High doses of NA leads to the "niacin flush," characterized by an intense itching or burning sensation on the skin.[49]

Deficiency Niacin deficiency results in pellagra. The classic manifestation of pellagra is a pigmented rash the develops in areas exposed to sunlight; digestive conditions such as vomiting, constipation, diarrhea; a bright red tongue; and neurological symptoms such as depression, apathy, headache, fatigue, and loss of memory. Pellagra is common when corn is the dietary staple because corn is low in tryptophan and digestible niacin. It usually requires alkaline food to release the niacin from niacytin, so the human body can digest and absorb appropriately.[52] Pellagra has largely disappeared in developed countries thanks to niacin-enriched cereals and refined grain products. Individuals with chronic alcoholism or tryptophan pathway disruptions may develop secondary pellagra.[45]

Vitamin B6 Basic Definition and Dietary Sources Vitamin B6 is the generic name for a group of six compounds with vitamin B6 activity: pyridoxal (PL), pyridoxine (PN), pyridoxamine (PM), and their respective 5'-phosphates, pyridoxal 5' phosphate (PLP), pyridoxine 5' phosphate (PNP), and pyridoxamin 5' phosphate (PMP). PLP and PMP are coenzymes for more than 100 enzymatic reactions, including amino acid metabolism, heme biosynthesis, transsulfration, and methyl group transfer. PLP is also involved with the metabolism of one-carbon units, carbohydrates, and lipids. Vitamin B6 is found in a variety of foods, including fish, organ meats, potatoes and other starchy vegetables, and noncitrus fruits. The majority of vitamin B6 in the United States comes from fortified foods, potatoes, and noncitrus fruits.

Key Functions The human body absorbs vitamin B6 in the jejunum through passive diffusion. Vitamin B6 is essential in cognitive development through biosynthesis of neurotransmitters, including serotonin, dopamine, epinephrine, norepinephrine, and gamma-aminobutyric acid (GABA). Vitamin B6 also plays an important role in gluconeogenesis, glycogenolysis, as well as biosynthesis of sphingolipids and ceramide. Additionally, vitamin B6 serves as a coenzyme in the synthesis of hemoglobin and humoral, cell-mediated immune responses. Some current evidence also suggests that vitamin B6 might decrease the risks of cardiovascular disease and cancer as well as alleviate premenstrual syndrome and "morning sickness" in pregnancy.

Deficiency Deficiency of vitamin B6 is uncommon, but inadequate B6 status is usually associated with inadequacies of other B vitamins. Deficiency is associated with microcytic anemia, electroenecephalographic abnormalities, dermatitis with cheilosis and glossitis, depression and confusion, and weakened immune function. Mild deficiency patients may not have symptoms or signs for months or years.

Folate Basic Definition and Dietary Sources Folate is found in the forms folate and folic acid. Folic acid consists of a p-aminobenzoic molecule linked to a pteridine ring and one molecule of glutamic acid. Folate is a coenzyme or cosubstrate in single-carbon transfers in the synthesis of nucleic acids, metabolism of amino acids, and purine synthesis. Folic acid is the fully oxidized monoglutamate form of the folate that is used in fortified foods and dietary supplements.

Folate is found naturally in vegetables (especially dark green leafy vegetables), fruits and fruit juices, nuts, beans, peas, dairy products, poultry and meat, eggs, seafood, and grains. The highest levels of folate are found in spinach, liver, yeast, asparagus, and brussels sprouts. Fortified bread, flour, cornmeal, pasta, rice, and cereals are also good sources of folic acid. Dietary folate equivalents (DFEs) adjust for bioavailability of food folate versus folic acid, and 1 ug DFE = 0.6 ug of folic acid from fortified foods or supplement with meals = 1 ug of food folate = 0.5 ug of supplement on empty stomach.[53]

Key Functions Folate is essential in making red and white blood cells in the bone marrow, converting carbohydrates into energy, and producing DNA and RNA. Folate-dependent one-carbon metabolism is also required for *de novo* synthesis of purine nucleotides, thymidylate (dTMP), and methylation of homocysteine into methionine.

Deficiency Deficiency of folate exists with other nutrient deficiencies in poor diets, alcoholism, and malabsorptive disorders. Folate deficiencies are characterized by megaloblastic anemia; soreness and shallow ulcerations in the tongue and oral mucosa; and changes in skin and hair pigmentation. Women with low intakes of folate are at higher risk for giving birth to infants with neural tube defects.[54]

Cobalamin Basic Definition and Dietary Sources Cobalamin, also known as vitamin B12, consists of a cobalt atom coordinated by four nitrogens from four pyrrole rings (or tetrapyrrole) collectively. Methylcobalamin and 5-deoxyadenosylcobalamin are the active forms of vitamin B12. Food sources of vitamin B12 include animal products, such as fish, meat, poultry, eggs, milk and milk products, and fortified grains. Vegetarians and vegans need to eat supplemented B12 or nutritional yeast to ensure adequate intake. As B12 is bound to protein in food, hydrochloric acid and gastric protease in the stomach are needed to release B12. Fortified foods and supplements are in the free form and thus do not require this step. B12 is then bound to intrinsic factor for absorption from the small intestine.

Key Functions B12 is essential for red blood cell formation, neurological function, and DNA synthesis. Vitamin B12 is a cofactor for methionine synthase, which is used to catalyze homocysteine to methionineto form S-adenosylmethionine. Vitamin B12 is also critical for converting L-methylmalonyl-coenzyme A (CoA) to succinyl-CoA needed for hemoglobin synthesis.

Deficiency Pernicious anemia, an autoimmune disease, affects the gastric mucosa and leads to failure of production of intrinsic factor, which is necessary for absorption of vitamin B12. This results in B12 deficiency, megaloblastic anemia, and neurological disorders. Other symptoms of deficiency include difficulty maintaining balance, depression, confusion, dementia, poor memory, and soreness of mouth or tongue. In infants with deficiency, failure to thrive, movement disorders, developmental delays, and megaloblastic anemia can be present.[55]

Vitamin C Basic Definition and Dietary Sources Also known as ascorbic acid, vitamin C is required for collagen and neurotransmitter synthesis, protein metabolism, and wound healing.[56] Vitamin C cannot be made within the body, and therefore dietary intake is essential. Fruits and vegetables are the best sources, with high concentrations of vitamin C in citrus fruits, tomatoes, red and green peppers, strawberries, kiwi, and broccoli. Many foods are also fortified with vitamin C, such as breakfast cereals and grains. Ascorbic acid may be reduced through prolonged storage and can be destroyed by heat.[57]

The bioavailability of vitamin C is dependent on intestinal absorption and renal excretion. When ascorbic acid levels are high, the kidney will filter it out for excretion. When serum vitamin C levels are low, small intestinal absorption increases and renal tubule reabsorption of ascorbic acid increases.[56]

Key Functions Vitamin C is a co-factor in many enzymes used for biosynthesis of collagen, carnitine, and neurotransmitters.[56] Two enzymes involved with procollagen biosynthesis require vitamin C for formation and secretion of stable collagen helixes. Without vitamin C, the collagen structures weaken and lead to tooth loss, joint pain, bone and connective tissues disorders, and poor wound healing. The biosynthesis of carnitine is essential for transporting long-chain fatty acids; without vitamin C, the body may feel fatigued and lethargic. Vitamin C is also essential in converting dopamine to norepinephrine. Mood changes, depression, and hypochondria can occur with vitamin C deficiency.[58]

Vitamin C is also an essential antioxidant. As defined by the Panel on Dietary Antioxidants and Related Compounds of the Food and Nutrition Board, "a dietary antioxidant is a substance in foods that significantly decreases adverse effects of reactive oxygen species, reactive nitrogen species, or both on normal physiological function in humans."[59] Vitamin C has low one-electron reduction potential and is stable in the ascorbyl radical form when ascorbate reacts with reactive oxygen or nitrogen species. Vitamin C is therefore a free radical scavenger and helps to protect cells against reactive oxygen molecules. Furthermore, vitamin C is a co-antioxidant with vitamin E, as it can help regenerate α-tocopherol.[58]

Deficiency Scurvy results from acute vitamin C deficiency, with signs appearing within one month of low or no vitamin C intake. Symptoms include fatigue, lethargy, inflammation of gums, weakened connective tissues, petechiae, joint pain, poor wound healing, hyperkeratosis, and corkscrew hairs.[60] Vitamin C deficiency is rare in developed countries; however those with limited food variety and supply can still develop scurvy. Smokers need 35 mg more vitamin C per day due to their increased oxidative stress decreasing vitamin C levels.[57,61]

Disease Prevention Vitamin C's function as an antioxidant has led to research into vitamin C's role in cancer prevention. Vitamin C can limit the formation of carcinogens, and case-control studies have found an inverse association between dietary vitamin C intake and lung, breast, colon, rectum, stomach, oral cavity, larynx, pharynx, and esophageal cancers.[58] However, prospective cohort studies on dietary vitamin C intake and clinical trials of supplemental vitamin C intake show mixed to no results on cancer prevention.

The common cold is often attributed to requiring high levels of vitamin C intake. In the general population, evidence shows vitamin C levels of 200 mg/day or more do not reduce the risk of developing the common cold; however, in populations with extreme exercise or cold environments, higher doses may be helpful.[62]

Fat-soluble Vitamins

In contrast to the water-soluble vitamins previously described, the fat-soluble vitamins are absorbed and transported with lipids throughout the body. Their absorption in the digestive tract requires bile salts and transport by chylomicrons,[42] where they are then stored in lipids until they are utilized by the body.

Vitamin A ***Basic Definition and Dietary Sources*** Vitamin A is a group of retinoids, including retinol, retinal, and retinyl esters. Vitamin A exists in two forms in the diet: preformed vitamin A (retinol and retinyl ester) and provitamin A carotenoids (beta-carotene, alpha-carotene, and beta-cryptoxanthin). The body converts both forms into retinal and retinoic acid to become active and function. Vitamin A contains a beta-ionone ring, a conjugated polyene side chain and a terminal functional group. All-*trans*-retinol is the parent molecule that can be esterified with long chain fatty acids into retinyl esters. Retinol is also sequentially oxidized in the body to retinal then to retinoic acid; different forms of retinoic acid modulate the function of retinol in the body.

Vitamin A needs can be met with preformed vitamin A or provitamin A. Preformed vitamin A is found in animal sources, such as dairy products, fish, meat, and organ meats such as liver. Provitamin A can be found in plants, fungi, and bacteria. Foods are often enriched with retinyl ester or beta-carotene, such as fortified milk and breakfast cereals.

Key Functions Vitamin A is required for many key functions in the body. Most notable is the use of retinal in the transduction of light in the eye for vision. Retinoic acid is necessary for differentiation of the cornea and conjunctival membranes to prevent xerophthalamia and essential for rod and cone cells in the retina. The retinal in the rods are photoisomerized when light is absorbed to trigger the signaling of neurons. The photoisomerized retinal is then released and through a series of steps is added to the storage pool of retinyl esters for another photo cycle.

Vitamin A is also essential in epithelial cells to regulate genes for structural proteins such as keratin, enzymes such as alcohol dehydrogenase, extracellular matrix proteins and retinol binding proteins. Retinoic acid is also necessary in the embryonic development of the hindbrain, limbs, heart, eyes, and ears. Retinoids are needed for immune function through cell differentiation, antiviral and antitumor activity, phagocytic activity, and production of cytokines during inflammation.

Deficiency Although rare in the United States, vitamin A deficiency is common in many developing countries due to limited access to preformed vitamin A from animal sources and beta-carotene foods. During infancy, childhood, pregnancy, and lactation, vitamin A requirements increase, and therefore deficiency is mostly found in these populations. Other groups at risk for vitamin A deficiency include premature infants and patients with cystic fibrosis.

Most common symptoms of vitamin A deficiency include xerophthalmia, which includes night blindness or inability to see in low light, and Bitot's spots. Vitamin A deficiency is often seen with low iron status, which can lead to anemia.

Vitamin D ***Basic Definition and Dietary Sources*** Vitamin D is unique in that it can be synthesized endogenously or through dietary intake. Vitamin D has two major forms, vitamin D_2 (ergocalciferol), which is added to foods, and vitamin D_3 (cholecalciferol), synthesized in the skin and consumed from animal-based foods. Both forms of vitamin D are considered inactive until converted into calcitriol [1,25-dihydroxyvitamin D, or 1,25(OH)2D3] through two enzymatic reactions. The precursor to calcitriol, 25-hydroxyvitamin D (25(OH) D), is the major circulating form of vitamin D and binds to vitamin D binding protein throughout the body.

Since endogenous vitamin D synthesis varies due to location and sun exposure, most people require dietary vitamin D to maintain adequate vitamin D stores. Dietary sources include food and supplements. Natural sources high in vitamin D include fatty fish, fish liver oil, and egg yolks. In the United States and Canada, milk and infant formula are also fortified with vitamin D.

Vitamin D is absorbed with other dietary fats in the small intestine, and its absorption is dependent on fat in the lumen. Bile acids assist in the formation of chylomicrons in the intestines, which packages lipids and vitamin D for transport across the intestinal lining. Adipose and skeletal tissues then take up vitamin D during chylomicron hydrolysis, with the remaining vitamin D taken up by the liver.

Key Functions Vitamin D, in its biologically active form, 25(OH)D, formed in the liver, is required for bone mineralization through its mechanisms associated with calcium homeostasis. Calcitriol elevates ionized calcium levels through stimulating intestinal calcium absorption in the intestine when calcium levels are low. Furthermore, calcitriol mobilizes calcium from bone stimulating the formation and activation of osteoclasts. Calictriol also works with parathyroid hormone (PTH) to stimulate the renal distal tubule reabsorption of calcium for retention. These three actions increase serum calcium levels, which in turn decreases PTH secretion, closing the feedback loop. Calcitriol also suppresses the parathyroid gene expression to decrease PTH when calcium levels are high through the vitamin D receptor (VDR).[63]

Vitamin D also plays a role in phosphorous homeostasis. Phosphate deficiency stimulates production of calcitriol, which then stimulates phosphate absorption in the small intestine and induces the secretion of FGF23 by osteocytes to reabsorb phosphate in the kidney.

Deficiency Low vitamin D levels can be associated with inadequate dietary intake or insufficient sun exposure. Vitamin D is synthesized in the skin to contribute to serum 25(OH)D levels, but seasonal effects, latitude, and skin pigmentation can all impact 7-dehydrocholesterol's role in producing 25(OH)D.

Vitamin D deficiency can result in low bone mineralization, and can lead to rickets and osteomalacia (see "Calcium" below).

Vitamin E ***Basic Definition and Dietary Sources*** Vitamin E structures consist of a chromanol ring and a saturated tocopherol or unsaturated tocotrienol side chain. Natural vitamin E comes in eight forms (alpha-, beta-, gamma- and delta-tocopherol, and alpha-, beta-, gamma- and delta-tocotrienol). The term "vitamin E" refers to these eight forms, yet alpha-tocopherol is the only form of vitamin E that is required for humans, and the only form used to determine the DRI for vitamin E. Alpha-tocopherol is high in foods such as nuts, seeds, and plant-based oils, and is also available in green leafy vegetables and fortified grains and cereals.

Since vitamin E is fat soluble, it is absorbed through the intestine via chylomicrons and is taken up by the liver via the hepatic alpha-tocopherol transfer protein. Vitamin E is then metabolized into other forms for its antioxidant properties. All forms of vitamin E are absorbed and incorporated into chylomicrons, and no one form appears to be preferentially absorbed from the intestine. However, the liver preferentially releases alpha-tocopherol into plasma, regulated by alpha-tocopherol transfer protein (alpha-TTP).

Key Functions As previously stated, vitamin E acts as a key antioxidant in the body. Vitamin E scavenges for reactive oxygen species and stops their production as fat undergoes oxidation. Vitamin E breaks chains to prevent propagation of free-radical reactions and protects polyunsaturated fatty acids (PUFAs) from reacting with peroxyl radicals by binding to the reactive species. The resulting tocopheroxyl radical can be reduced by other antioxidants to tocopherol, react with another tocopheroxyl radical to form nonreactive products, undergo further oxidation to tocopheryl quinone, or act as a prooxidant and oxidize other lipids.

Furthermore, alpha-tocopherol is involved in immune function, cell signaling, and gene expression. It inhibits protein kinase C activity to inhibit cell proliferation and differentiation. It also decreases adhesion of blood cell components to the endothelium and increases production of phospholipases to inhibit platelet aggregation and increase vasodilation.

Deficiency Vitamin E deficiency is rare in humans, but is accompanied by symptoms of peripheral neuropathy, spinocerebellar ataxia, skeletal myopathy, and pigmented retinopathy.[64] Neurologic symptoms could progress in children who have deficiency within their first 10 years of life.

Disease Prevention Vitamin E is found to inhibit low-density lipoprotein (LDL) oxidation,[65] smooth muscle proliferation,[66] plasma generation of thrombin to reduce platelet aggregation, as well as induces synthesis of prostacyclin for vasodilation.[59] Although several observational studies have shown inverse associations between vitamin E intake and risk of heart disease,[67,68] randomized clinical trials have not found associations between supplementation of vitamin E and prevention of coronary heart disease.[69–71]

The antioxidant nature of vitamin E has led to the hypothesis proposing that vitamin E protects against the damaging effects of free radicals leading to cancers. However, trials have not shown such an association for breast,[72,73] lung,[72] or prostate cancers,[74,75] but have shown a slight inverse association between risk of colon[76] and esophageal cancers[77] with vitamin E supplementation.

Vitamin K ***Basic Definition and Dietary Sources*** Vitamin K is a group of compounds with the 2-methyl-1,4-napthoquinone structure, which is primarily present as phylloquinone (K_1) or menaquinones (K_2) in the diet.[78]

Phylloquinone is present in green leafy vegetables, such as spinach and collards. Darker leaves have higher concentrations. Other plant sources include soybean, canola, cottonseed, and olive oils. Menaquinones are found in modest amounts in animal-based products, such as dairy products like milk, butter, and cheeses, and fermented foods, such as the Japanese soy-product *natto*.[78] The bacteria in the human digestive tract also produce menaquinones.

Key Functions As a fat soluble vitamin, vitamin K is incorporated into micelles once ingested for absorption from the small intestine, which is then delivered to chylomicrons and transported to the liver for repackaging into very low-density lipoproteins before being transported to the liver, brain, heart, pancreas, and bone. Due to its nature, only small amounts of vitamin K circulate in the blood; it is quickly metabolized and excreted via urine and feces.[79]

Vitamin K functions as a coenzyme for vitamin K-dependent carboxylase, which is required for synthesis of proteins needed for blood clotting and bone metabolism. Prothrombin is a protein that is involved with blood clotting, and in vitamin K deficiency; prothrombin time increases and can lead to hemorrhagic events. Vitamin K-dependent proteins include matrix Gla-protein and osteocalcin. Matrix Gla-protein is used in vascular smooth muscle, bone, and cartilage while osteocalcin is needed for bone mineralization.[80]

Vitamin D and calcium intake throughout the lifespan is important for bone mass and to reduce the risk of osteoporosis, a condition characterized by porous and fragile bones. Vitamin K's role in the prevention of osteoporosis is less well-known, but studies have shown that supplementation of vitamin K can improve bone mineral density and reduce fractures by inducing osteocalcin synthesis.[81–86]

Deficiency Vitamin K deficiency can occur in the first few weeks of life due to low placental transfer, low clotting factor levels, and low vitamin K content in breast milk. Deficiency is rare in adults and can be attributed to malabsorption or medications that interfere with vitamin K metabolism. Patients on anticoagulants, such as Warfarin (Coumadin), should maintain a consistent vitamin K intake to avoid increased prothrombin time.[79]

In vitamin K deficiency, prothrombin time increases due to the decrease in prothrombin activity. This leads to bleeding and, in severe cases, hemorrhaging. As vitamin K is necessary for bone mineralization, reduction in mineralization and osteoporosis can also occur.[81]

Minerals

Minerals can be divided into major and trace minerals, depending on their essential quantity within the body. Major minerals are required in amounts greater than 100 mg per day, where as adults need trace minerals in less than 100 mg per day.[42] Minerals are obtained via the diet and are used in maintaining electrolyte balance, enzymatic reactions, and ensuring normal functioning throughout the body.

Calcium

Basic Definition and Dietary Sources Calcium is known to build strong bones and teeth, but the mineral's functions encompass more than just bone health. Calcium in the body is fundamental to shape proteins for catalytic and mechanical functions, regulates body processes, and acts as a signal transmitter for cells. The calcium ion (Ca^{2+}) is unique for its ability to fit into the folds of peptide chains to allow for triggering the shaping for protein function.

Dairy sources provide more than 70% of the calcium in the diet within the United States.[87] Milk and milk products, canned fish with bones, greens such as broccoli, kale, and mustard greens, as well as legumes, are considered great natural sources of calcium. Food items that have been fortified with calcium, including fortified tofu, soy milk, orange juice, and enriched grain products also contribute to a large portion of the calcium intake in the United States. For example, some ethnic groups receive most of their calcium from calcium-fortified corn tortillas with lime and dried beans.

Calcium intake can be impacted by its bioavailability. Inhibitors of calcium absorption include oxalic acid, which is high in spinach, rhubarb, sweet potatoes, and dried beans. Phytic acid also is an inhibitor of calcium absorption, which is the storage form of phosphorous in beans, and can be found in wheat bran and dried beans.

Distribution and Key Functions Calcium performs key functions in the body: calcium acts as an intracellular messenger, cofactor for enzymes and proteins, and maintains the structure of bones and teeth.

As a signal transmitter, calcium can bind to both extracellular and intracellular proteins. When a stimulus occurs, the cell releases a store of calcium and, depending on the action necessary, is released from the cell or to enter the cell. Calcium is critical for the mediation of vascular contraction, vasodilation, muscle function, nerve transmission, and hormonal secretion.

Calcium also maintains bone and teeth structure and function. About 50–70% of bone is mineral, most of which is calcium hydroxyapatite. Calcium is required for both bone formation and remodeling and is deposited into the organic matrix of the skeletal for rigidity, strength, and elasticity.

Deficiency Rickets and osteomalacia develop when calcium levels are low. In young children and infants, rickets is the end-stage condition when bones and cartilage fail to mature and lead to irreversible changes in the skeletal structure. Children with rickets present with symptoms of stunted growth and bowing of the extremities. Osteomalacia is seen in adults and children and is the defective mineralization of bone and softening of bone. Bone pain, muscle weakness, and impaired bone mineralization are key symptoms, and results in the undermineralization of bone.

Osteoporosis is associated with aging and reduced bone mass and bone quality. Low bone mineral density increases bone fragility, and in turn, increases the risk of fractures. Menopause can initiate osteoporosis through increased bone remodeling in women, and men experience comparable bone loss 5–10 years later than women.[63]

Sodium

Basic Definition and Dietary Sources Sodium (Na+) is one of the major minerals and an essential electrolyte that plays an important role in a host of normal metabolic functions. The major source of sodium is sodium chloride, commonly known as table salt. Protein foods generally contain more naturally existing sodium than vegetables, fruits, or grains.[88] High sodium content can be found in most convenience and fast-food products, as addition of table salts, flavored salts, preservatives, etc.

The 2015–20 *Dietary Guidelines for Americans* recommend consuming less than 2300 mg of sodium per day as part of a healthy eating pattern, though collected statistics present that the vast majority of adults in America eat an average of more than 3400 mg sodium each day. Healthy kidneys are usually able to excrete excess sodium intake, but persistent excessive sodium intake has been found to be associated with elevated risks of hypertension and osteoporosis.

Distribution and Key Functions Approximately 35–40% of the total body sodium is in the skeleton, and the normal sodium concentration in serum is 136–145 mEq/L. Secretions such as bile and pancreatic juice also contain substantial amounts of sodium.[88] Sodium is a cation of extracellular fluid and is needed for proper fluid balance, maintenance of acid-base balance, nerve transmission, and muscle contraction. The Na/K ATPase pump is an active transport system that requires sodium, potassium, and energy for proper function, and works to keep sodium extracellular through exchange with potassium. Exportation of sodium from the cell is the driving force for facilitated transporters that import glucose, amino acids, and other nutrients into the cells.

Regulation of Sodium Balance Changes in either intracellular or extracellular sodium concentrations can have a major effect on bodily functions. Sodium balance involves the function of the kidneys, the renin-angiotensin-aldosterone system, the sympathetic nervous system, circulating catecholamines, certain hormone concentrations, and blood pressure. The syndrome of inappropriate antidiuretic hormone secretion (SIADH) is one of the medical situations caused by disrupted sodium and fluid regulations.[88]

Potassium

Basic Definition and Dietary Sources Potassium (K+) is the major cation of intracellular fluid and is present in all body tissues.

Potassium can be found in a wide variety of plant and animal foods and beverages. Fresh fruits, vegetables, meat, and dairy products are all good sources of potassium. Insufficient potassium intake has been associated with hypertension and cardiac arrhythmia.

Distribution and Key Functions The total amount of potassium in the average adult body is about 45 mmol/kg body weight, and most potassium resides intracellularly. The potassium concentration difference between intracellular and extracellular fluids forms a transmembrane electrochemical gradient that is maintained via the sodium-potassium (Na+/K+) ATPase transporter. Therefore, sodium and potassium together, play an essential role in maintaining a normal water balance, osmotic equilibrium, acid-base balance, nerve transmission, and muscle contraction. In addition, potassium promotes cellular growth, and an adequate supply is essential when muscle is being formed.

Phosphorus

Basic Definition and Dietary Sources Phosphorus is an essential mineral that is required in cell function, acid-base balance, as well as energy and bone metabolism. Approximately 85% of phosphorus in adult is present in the skeleton and teeth as calcium phosphate crystals. Almost 50% of phosphorus that is present in serum exists as free ions (H2PO4- and H2PO42-), and the remainder is bound to protein or other compounds.[88] Phosphorus can be found in almost all protein sources, mainly in the form of phosphates and phosphate esters, such as meat, fish, poultry, eggs, milk, nuts, legumes, and grains. Phosphorus in seeds and unleavened breads is in the form of phytic acid. It can also be found in processed foods and soda soft drinks

Distribution and Key Functions Approximately 700 g of phosphorus exists in adult tissues. Of this amount, 85% is stored in bones and teeth, and the other 15% is distributed in the blood and soft tissues. In the form of phosphates, phosphorus is an essential component of DNA, RNA, ATP, and cAMP. In the form of phospholipids, phosphorus is a component of every cell membrane in the body. Phosphorus also plays key roles in gene transcription regulation, enzyme activation, energy production, and extracellular fluid pH maintenance.

Deficiency Phosphorus deficiency is very rare because first, its hemostasis is efficiently and effectively regulated by the kidneys, bones, and intestines, as well as hormones such as estrogen and adrenaline; and secondly, it is so widely available from both natural sources and processed foods. However, phosphate deficiency could develop in individuals who take phosphate binders for renal disease, use phosphate-binding antacids long term, or have poor intake in general. Severe phosphate depletion could lead to neural, muscular, skeletal, hematologic, and renal dysfunction and damage.[88]

Magnesium

Basic Definition and Dietary Sources Magnesium (Mg^{2+}) is the second-most abundant intracellular cation after potassium in the human body. The adult human body, on average, contains approximately 20–28 of magnesium.[88] The unique chemical structure and properties of magnesium allow it to position H_2O in a manner that promotes catalytic activity. It is also able to induce a conformational rearrangement that exposes catalytic sites and provides stability as the phosphate backbone is hydrolyzed.

Magnesium is fairly ubiquitous in whole, unrefined foods. Major food sources include nuts and seeds, legumes, leafy vegetables, seafood, chocolate, and artichokes.

Distribution and Key Functions An abundance of total magnesium is found in bones (60–65%) and in muscle (26%) with most of the remainder in soft tissues and body fluids. Less than 1% of total magnesium is in blood serum, making it difficult to assess magnesium status. Magnesium homeostasis is tightly controlled by the kidneys, which typically excrete about 120 mg magnesium in the urine per day.

Key functions of magnesium are threefold. First, magnesium is a required cofactor for over 300 enzymes that are involved in the metabolism of food, synthesis of fatty acids and proteins, phosphorylation of glucose, as well as the formation of cyclic adenosine monophosphate (cAMP). In these metabolic pathways, magnesium usually acts as a stabilizer to neutralize the (-) charge of ATP and regulate ATP-dependent enzyme reactions. Secondly, magnesium plays an important role in regulating calcium flux from intracellular organelles as well as extracellular calcium flux into a cell. Healthy function of vascular and other smooth cells requires a balanced ratio of calcium and magnesium in the blood.[88] Lastly, animal studies and human observational studies have found that magnesium has an effect on maintenance of healthy learning and memory functions.

Deficiency Serum magnesium concentration is commonly stable, under well-adjusted absorption, excretion, and transmembranous cation flux systems. Although very rare, severe magnesium deficiency symptoms such as tremors, muscle spasms, anorexia, nausea, vomiting, and personality changes have been observed in patients with diabetes, chronic renal failure, nephrolithiasis, osteoporosis, aplastic osteopathy, and heart and vascular diseases.[88] Moderate depletion of magnesium is prevalent in older populations in Western nations due to low intake of magnesium-rich foods, increased loss of electrolytes, or certain chronic diseases.

Sulfur

Basic Definition and Dietary Sources Sulfur is one of the most abundant mineral elements found in the human body, and it exists as a constituent of cystine, cysteine, and methionine amino acids. Methionine and cysteine provide nearly 100% of the sulfur in the human diet.[88] Sulfur functions almost entirely as a component of organic molecules in cells and extracellular compartments.[88] The unique tertiary structure of proteins indicate sulfur results from many biochemical reactions and structural modifications, which is essential for the activity of insulin, certain enzymes, proteins, and cellular reactions. Sulfur can be obtained almost exclusively from protein-rich food items including meats, poultry, fish, eggs, milk, legumes, and nuts. A very small proportion of sulfur exits in the form of inorganic sulfates in food items such as garlic, onion, and broccoli. Maintaining adequate dietary sulfur intake is necessary because methionine, an essential amino acid, cannot be synthesized by the human body, and therefore, has to be supplied through diet.[89]

Distribution and Key Functions The body contains approximately 140 grams of sulfur, and it is mostly distributed in proteins. Since sulfur is contained in so many amino acids, and plays a role in the synthesis of a very large number of key metabolic intermediates, sulfur has many key health functions. Sulfur can be considered as an antioxidant because glutathione (a tripeptide-containing cysteine) serves as a donor for the reduction of hydrogen peroxide and organic peroxides.[88] Taurine, another sulfur-containing amino acid made by liver cells, helps to regulate lipid metabolism. Studies have found that taurine supplementation is linked to a significant decrease in total hepatic lipid content and slightly increased bile flow and secretion of bile salts.[90] Sulfur is also part of the molecule known as S-adenosylmethionine, which serves as a cosubstrate in methyl group transfer, trans-sulfuration, and aminopropylation.

Trace Elements

Trace elements are minerals present in living tissues in small amounts; some of them are considered to be nutritionally essential, and the remainder are nonessential. Trace elements function primarily as catalysts in enzyme systems and include iron, zinc, copper, iodine, manganese, cobalt, fluoride, and selenium. In this section, we will concentrate our discussion on the first four trace minerals since the deficiency and/or toxicity of these four elements are relatively more common and have significant and close associations with the development of chronic diseases as well as other health dysfunctions.

Iron

Basic Definition and Dietary Sources

Iron is a mineral essential to catalytic reactions in the body. Two oxidative states of iron exist, the ferrous form (Fe^{2+}) and the ferric form (Fe^{3+}). These two states allow for redox reactions to occur, with ferrous iron oxidizing to ferric iron. In the body, iron can exist in one of three forms: bound to protein as heme, such as in hemoglobin or myoglobin; as heme enzymes; or as nonheme compounds such as in storage. Ferritin is the storage form of iron and consists of 24 protein units surrounding a ferric core. Ferritin releases iron when blood levels are low. Transferrin functions as a transport mechanism by binding to iron and can limit its toxic effects when levels of iron are high.

Iron can take two forms in food, heme and nonheme iron. Heme iron is derived from hemoglobin or myoglobin and is found in animal products, mostly red meats, fish, and poultry. In contrast, nonheme iron is found in plant foods, along with enriched and fortified foods. Nonheme iron is less bioavailable than heme iron, with only 2–20% of nonheme iron assimilated into the body compared to 15–35% of heme iron. Iron absorption is facilitated by ascorbate and citrate, while inhibited by phytates, polyphenols, and calcium.

Distribution and Key Functions

About 66% of the body's iron is found as hemoglobin, 15% bound to myoglobin in the muscle for oxygen, and 25% in the storage form.[91] Iron homeostasis is tightly regulated as its use in the body is diverse. As iron is not actively excreted from the body, absorption through the gastrointestinal system regulates iron balance. Through a feedback loop, iron is transferred across the intestines during iron deficiency and is then transported to cells or bone marrow by transferrin. When iron levels are high, the divalent metal transporter 1 in the intestines decreases transport of iron.[92]

In addition to transferrin, hepcidin is a hepatic peptide hormone that assists with iron homeostasis. Hepcidin binds to ferroportin in the intestines, macrophages, and placenta. Ferroportin is a transport protein of iron, and when bound to hepcidin, is degraded and leads to lower iron transport into plasma. This decrease in iron levels leads to lower saturation of transferrin and a feedback loop to decrease hepcidin production by the liver.[92]

Iron is essential for metabolic processes, including oxygen transport, electron transport, cell differentiation, and DNA and RNA synthesis. Iron is a key component of many enzymes for electron transport and DNA synthesis, and is used in oxidases, catalases, peroxidases, cytochromes, ribonucleotide reductases, aconitases, and nitric oxide synthases.[93]

Iron Deficiency and Anemia

Iron deficiency is prevalent in 39% of children less than 5 years of age, 48% of 5–14 year olds, and 52% of women in developing countries. Deficiency can be categorized in terms of severity and can present with or without anemia. Mild iron deficiency results in increased oxygen delivery due to lower hemoglobin and myoglobin status and redistribution of blood flow that results in enhanced cardiac output. Severe iron deficiency can result in acidosis and affects cognitive development and immune function.[42,92] Iron deficiency can be caused by low iron absorption, blood loss, increased iron requirements due to pregnancy or menstruation, and poor dietary intake.

Anemia occurs when the count of red blood cells is low or the amount of hemoglobin is below normal. Hemoglobin delivers oxygen from the lungs to other cells and when hemoglobin or red blood cells are not functioning at full capacity, fatigue, shortness of breath, and increased heart rate can occur. The most common cause of anemia is iron deficiency, which can result from poor dietary intake.

Zinc

Basic Definition and Dietary Sources

Zinc is an intracellular ion, required for catalytic activity in more than 300 different enzymes. Though zinc is abundant in the cytosol, almost all of it is bound to proteins that form "zinc fingers." Good food sources of zinc include red meats, poultry, shellfish, cereals, milk, and milk products. Zinc intestinal absorption does not appear to be influenced by total body zinc levels, but phytates readily bind to zinc and inhibit its absorption.

Distribution and Key Functions

The human body has approximately 2–3 g of zinc, with the highest concentrations stored in the liver, pancreas, kidneys, bone, and muscles.[88] Zinc homeostasis is maintained largely through pancreatic secretions regulated by zinc transporters. Metallothionein is the most abundant, nonenzymatic, zinc-containing protein and serves as an intracellular reservoir that donates zinc ions to other proteins.

Zinc has structural, catalytic, and regulatory functions in the cell, including gene expression, cell signaling, and cell proliferation and differentiation. It plays essential structural roles as components of many enzymes that are involved in either synthesis or degradation of carbohydrates, lipids, proteins, and nucleic acids. In addition, zinc stabilizes RNA and DNA structure, and is required for the activity of RNA polymerases. It also protects against age-related macular degenerative disease, and is able to stimulate bone formation.

Deficiency

Zinc deficiency is very rare in Western nations because of the abundance of fortified breads, cereals, and refined grains. However, zinc deficiency is one of the ten major factors contributing to disease in developing countries.[94] The clinical signs of zinc deficiency include short stature, hypogonadism, mild anemia, and low plasma zinc levels. Additional symptoms are delayed sexual maturation, poor wound healing, impaired taste acuity, immune dysfunction, alopecia, and dermatitis-like lesions.

Copper

Basic Definition and Dietary Sources

Copper is another essential trace mineral that serves as a normal constituent of blood. Copper has two oxidative statuses: cuprous (Cu^{+}) and cupric (Cu^{2+}), with cupric the most common biological form of copper. The redox capability of copper is utilized in numerous enzymatic reactions.

Most copper in the diet is bound to proteins, and good food sources of copper include shellfish, nut/seeds, cocoa powder, legumes, the germ component of grains, and organ meats. Some studies have shown that high ascorbic acid intake, high zinc intake, and therapeutic doses of iron may lead to a poorer copper status.

Distribution and Key Functions

Copper does not exist as a free ion in the body. Approximately 90% of the copper in serum is incorporated into ceruloplasmin, a copper-containing protein. The remaining 10% is bound loosely to albumin, transcuprein (a plasma protein that binds copper), other proteins, free amino acids, and histidine.[88] Copper is transported bound to albumin, and it is the temporary reservoir for copper. The liver provides long-term storage for copper where it binds to metallothionein.

Copper is a cofactor for a number of enzymes (metallo or cuproenuzymes) involved in electron transfer reactions, which is the primary role of copper. Some examples include reactions that are responsible for metabolism of catecholamines, development of connective tissues (copper-dependent lysol oxidase), iron oxidation, synthesis of norepinephrine and melanin, as well as electron transport.

Deficiency and Toxicity

Copper deficiency is characterized by anemia, neutropenia, skeletal demineralization, subperiosteal hemorrhages, hair and skin depigmentation, and defective elastin formation. Failure of erythropoiesis because of copper deficiency may lead to death. Copper deficiency is extremely rare among healthy humans consuming a balanced diet. However, premature infants and infants who were poorly nourished are likely to have copper deficiency. Two genetic disorders, known as Menkes' syndrome and Wilson's disease, could result in an abnormal distribution of copper among organs and within cells. Menke's syndrome is an X-linked recessive defect that affects the gene-encoding ATP7A. Menke's syndrome leads to generalized copper deficiency and marked cerebral degeneration, and is fatal by about three years of age. Wilson's disease, in contrast, is an autosomal recessive gene disorder that affects the gene encoding ATP7B. Wilson's disease leads to accumulated copper toxicity because the body is unable to excrete copper in bile or export copper from neuronal tissue. The onset of Wilson's disease is variable but usually presents with liver dysfunction by 30 years of age, accompanied with neuropsychiatric symptoms. Wilson's disease is usually treated by limiting copper in the diet and administering chelating agents and high doses of zinc.

Iodine

Basic Definition and Dietary Sources

Iodine is a trace mineral of crucial importance to health and well-being and diet is the sole source. Iodine is required at all stages of life, with fetal life and early childhood being the most critical phases for its availability. Good food sources of iodine are seafood (fish, shellfish, and seaweed), iodized salt, meats, and eggs. Vegetables and grains also contain iodine, but their content level depends on exposure to iodine through rain, glaciation, and soil.

Distribution and Key Functions

Dietary iodine is primarily needed for the synthesis of thyroid hormones, which are involved in numerous metabolic and developmental processes. Iodine is stored in the thyroid gland, and is used in synthesis of triiodothyronine (T3) and thyroxine (T4).[88] Three types of deiodinases regulate plasma and intracellular iodine levels, and thyroid hormone actions.

Deficiency and Toxicity

Iodine deficiency in the developed Western nations has practically been eliminated with the use of iodized salt. Yet, people living in many mountainous areas or developing countries of the world may still have low intake because of the low iodine content in the soil or high consumption of goitrogens (substances that disrupt the production of thyroid hormones by interfering with iodine uptake). Very low iodine intake is associated with the development of endemic goiter. Iodine deficiency during gestation and early postnatal growth can result in mental deficiency, deaf-mutism, and shortened stature.

Acute excessive intake of iodine results in the Wolff-Chaikoff effect, characterized by short-term, high intracellular iodine levels and decreased organification. Chronic excessive intake of iodine can disturb the thyroid gland's regulatory mechanisms and lead to hypothyroidism.

DIETARY REFERENCE INTAKE

Dietary reference intakes (DRIs), developed and published by the National Academy of Medicine (formerly the Institute of Medicine or IOM), are reference values that provide quantitative estimates of macro- and micronutrient intake, serving as a guide for good nutrition among healthy populations and provide the scientific basis for the development of dietary guidelines in the United States and Canada. DRI is an umbrella term that includes at least four nutrient-based reference values: Recommended Dietary Allowance (RDA), Estimated Average Requirement (EAR), Adequate Intake (AI), and Tolerable Upper Intake Level (UL). These recommendations include over 40 nutrients taken in through diet for ten different age groups across the life course, in addition to significant life-stages in females including pregnancy (taking into consideration different needs for each trimester) and lactation (addressing different needs for the age of the infant or child). The RDA is the average daily dietary intake level that is sufficient to meet the nutrient requirements of 9–98% of healthy individuals in a particular life stage and gender group. The EAR is the daily intake value that is estimated to meet half of the healthy individuals (median usual intake value) by life stage and gender group. The AI is based on experimentally derived intake levels or approximations of observed mean nutrient intake by a group or groups of healthy people. The UL is the highest level of daily nutrient intake that is unlikely to pose risks of adverse health effects in almost all individuals in the specified life-stage group.[95]

There are four overarching steps of the DRI development: (1) Indicator review and selection; (2) Intake-response assessment and specification of reference values; (3) Intake assessment; and (4) Discussion of implications and special concerns. The "indicator" that initiates the entire process refers to clinical endpoints, surrogate endpoints, biomarkers, or risk factors for a chronic disease. Selecting an appropriate indicator for a given nutrient and DRI usually starts with a review and interpretation of published literature by the DRI committee. After the selection of indicators, the intake-response relationships is determined, which includes responses of nutrient adequacy, excess, or relationship to a chronic disease outcome. Then, these values are compared to current levels of intake and implications of the determined reference values, and special concerns will be thoroughly discussed. Afterward, adjustments for special groups are conducted and risk assessments surrounding the DRIs will be included before publication.

Nutrient assessment for DRI review and update is based on annual nutrient nominations. Then, DRI committees are jointly prioritizing nutrients for government-funded review and subsequent commissioning of an expert review to re-establish reference values. The most recent DRI activity update is the DRI for sodium and potassium in the 2019 report.[96]

DIETARY GUIDELINES FOR AMERICANS

The history of USDA nutrition guides includes over 100 years of American nutrition advice. Both the *Dietary Goals* and the *Dietary Guidelines for Americans* have been updated over time, to reflect evolving scientific evidence, changed historical focus on nutrient adequacy, and new public health marketing techniques. There have been many versions of USDA food guides. For example, the influential MyPyramid food guide was introduced along with the *Dietary Guidelines for Americans* in 2005. It continued the "pyramid concept," which was first introduced in the 1992 Food Guide with a more simplified illustration. This version also added the concept of physical activity. The most recent USDA food guides, the MyPlate, was introduced along with an update of USDA food patterns for the 2010 *Dietary Guidelines for Americans*. It used a general plate shape and different colors on the plate to help grab consumers' attention and emphasize the importance of portion size.

The *Dietary Guidelines for Americans* have been developed jointly by the U.S. Department of Health and Human Services (HHS) and the U.S. Department of Agriculture (USDA) since 1980. Starting in 1985, the Dietary Guidelines Advisory Committee was established. A Federal advisory committee of nine nutrition scientists selected from outside the Federal Government was convened to review and make recommendations to HHS and USDA about the first edition of the Dietary Guidelines. New Advisory Committees are established every 5 years for each revision of the dietary guidelines. HHS and USDA collaborate during a three-stage process: review the science, develop the dietary guidelines, and implement the dietary guidelines. In the first stage, an external Dietary Guidelines Advisory Committee (Advisory Committee) is appointed. The advisory committee used four state-of-the-art approaches to review and analyze the available evidence, summarizing all of the evidence in a comprehensive scientific report. In the second stage, the scientific report is translated into more consumer-friendly language to create the actual dietary guidelines used by HHS and USDA. The most recent 2015–20 Dietary Guidelines is built around five Guidelines and Key Recommendations that provide detail on the elements of healthy eating patterns. In the third and final stage, the Federal Government implements the recommendations in the Dietary Guidelines. Federal programs apply the Dietary Guidelines to meet the needs of Americans and specific population groups through food, nutrition, and health policies and programs and in nutrition education materials for the public.

Nutrient recommendations in the United States have obviously evolved substantially over the past 100 plus years. They were first established with a focus solely on recommendations for macronutrients because knowledge about micronutrients was widely lacking. They also initially focused more on preventing infectious disease like polio or tuberculosis, leading causes of illness and death at that time. Because of medical advances including the use of vaccines, antibiotics and improvements in public health, the recommendations have now shifted to focus on chronic diseases like obesity and heart disease. Currently, the overarching goals of the recommendations are to prevent over- or undernutrition, ensure normal development and health status and to support pregnancy and lactation when nutritional needs are altered.

References

1. Pagliaro B, Santolamazza C, Simonelli F, Rubattu S. Phytochemical compounds and protection from cardiovascular diseases: A state of the art. *Biomed Res Int*. 2015;2015:918069.
2. Rodriguez-Casado A. The health potential of fruits and vegetables phytochemicals: Notable examples. *Crit Rev Food Sci Nutr*. 2016;56(7):1097–107.
3. Ruiz RB, Hernández PS. Cancer chemoprevention by dietary phytochemicals: Epidemiological evidence. *Maturitas*. 2016;94:13–9.
4. Institute of Medicine. *Dietary Reference Intakes for Energy, Carbohydrate, Fiber, Fat, Fatty Acids, Cholesterol, Protein, and Amino Acids*. Washington, DC: National Academies Press; 2005.
5. Wright JD, Wang CY, Kennedy-Stephenson J, Ervin RB. *Dietary Intake of Ten Key Nutrients for Public Health, United States: 1999–2000: Advance Data from Vital and Health Statistics*. Report No. 334. Hyattsville, MD: National Center for Health Statistics; 2003.
6. Hoy MK, Goldman JD. Fiber intake of the U.S. population: What we eat in America, NHANES 2009–2010. Food Surveys Research Group Dietary Data Brief No. 12. September 2014.
7. Itan Y, Powell A, Beaumont MA, Burger J, Thomas MG. The origins of lactase persistence in Europe. In: Tanaka MM, ed. *PLoS Comput Biol*. 2009;5(8):e1000491.
8. Harvey CB, Hollox EJ, Poulter M, et al. Lactase haplotype frequencies in Caucasians: association with the lactase persistence/non-persistence polymorphism. *Ann Hum Genet*. 1998;62(3):215–23.
9. Gerbault P, Liebert A, Itan Y, et al. Evolution of lactase persistence: An example of human niche construction. *Philos Trans R Soc B Biol Sci*. 2011;366(1566):863–77.
10. Kenny KA, Skelly JM. Dietary fiber for constipation in older adults: A systematic review. *Clin Eff Nurs*. 2001;5(3):120–8.
11. Dukas L, Willett WC, Giovannucci EL. Association between physical activity, fiber intake, and other lifestyle variables and constipation in a study of women. *Am J Gastroenterol*. 2003;98(8):1790.
12. Willis HJ, Eldridge AL, Beiseigel J, Thomas W, Slavin JL. Greater satiety response with resistant starch and corn bran in human subjects. *Nutr Res*. 2009;29(2):100–5.
13. Hjorth MF, Bray GA, Zohar Y, et al. Pretreatment fasting glucose and insulin as determinants of weight loss on diets varying in macronutrients and dietary fibers: The POUNDS LOST Study. *Nutrients*. 2019;11(3):586.
14. Howarth NC, Saltzman E, Roberts SB. Dietary fiber and weight regulation. *Nutr Rev*. 2001;59(5):129–9.
15. Chandalia M, Garg A, Lutjohann D, von Bergmann K, Grundy SM, Brinkley LJ. Beneficial effects of high dietary fiber intake in patients with type 2 diabetes mellitus. *N Engl J Med*. 2000;342(19):1392–8.

16. Brown L, Rosner B, Willett WW, Sacks FM. Cholesterol-lowering effects of dietary fiber: A meta-analysis. *Am J Clin Nutr*. 1999;69(1):30–42.
17. Liu S, Willett WC, Manson JE, Hu FB, Rosner B, Colditz G. Relation between changes in intakes of dietary fiber and grain products and changes in weight and development of obesity among middle-aged women. *Am J Clin Nutr*. 2003;78(5):920–7.
18. Fung TT, Rimm EB, Spiegelman D, et al. Association between dietary patterns and plasma biomarkers of obesity and cardiovascular disease risk. *Am J Clin Nutr*. 2001;73(1):61–7.
19. Gross LS, Li L, Ford ES, Liu S. Increased consumption of refined carbohydrates and the epidemic of type 2 diabetes in the United States: An ecologic assessment. *Am J Clin Nutr*. 2004;79(5):774–9.
20. Marriott BP, Olsho L, Hadden L, Connor P. Intake of added sugars and selected nutrients in the United States, National Health and Nutrition Examination Survey (NHANES) 2003–2006. *Crit Rev Food Sci Nutr*. 2010;50(3):228–58.
21. Shonkoff ET, Dunton GF, Chou C-P, Leventhal AM, Bluthenthal R, Pentz MA. Direct and indirect effects of parent stress on child obesity risk and added sugar intake in a sample of Southern California adolescents. *Public Health Nutr*. 2017;20(18):3285–94.
22. Vos MB, Kaar JL, Welsh JA, et al. Added sugars and cardiovascular disease risk in children: A scientific statement from the American Heart Association. *Circulation*. 2017;135(19):e1017–34.
23. Nishida C, Uauy R, Kumanyika S, Shetty P. The joint WHO/FAO expert consultation on diet, nutrition and the prevention of chronic diseases: Process, product and policy implications. *Public Health Nutr*. 2004;7(1a):245–50.
24. Yang Q, Zhang Z, Gregg EW, Flanders WD, Merritt R, Hu FB. Added sugar intake and cardiovascular diseases mortality among US adults. *JAMA Intern Med*. 2014;174(4):516–24.
25. Bowes JH, Kenten RH. The amino-acid composition and titration curve of collagen. *Biochem J*. 1948;43(3):358.
26. Blau N, van Spronsen FJ, Levy HL. Phenylketonuria. *Lancet*. 2010; 376(9750):1417–27.
27. Luhovyy BL, Akhavan T, Anderson GH. Whey proteins in the regulation of food intake and satiety. *J Am Coll Nutr*. 2007;26(6):704S–12S.
28. Dietary Guidelines Advisory Committee. *Scientific Report of the 2015 Dietary Guidelines Advisory Committee: Advisory Report to the Secretary of Health and Human Services and the Secretary of Agriculture*. Washington, DC: U.S. Department of Agriculture, Agricultural Research Service; 2015.
29. Siri-Tarino PW, Sun Q, Hu FB, Krauss RM. Meta-analysis of prospective cohort studies evaluating the association of saturated fat with cardiovascular disease. *Am J Clin Nutr*. 2010;91(3):535–46.
30. Hoenselaar R. Saturated fat and cardiovascular disease: The discrepancy between the scientific literature and dietary advice. *Nutrition*. 2012;28(2):118–23.
31. Astrup A, Dyerberg J, Elwood P, et al. The role of reducing intakes of saturated fat in the prevention of cardiovascular disease: Where does the evidence stand in 2010? *Am J Clin Nutr*. 2011;93(4):684–8.
32. Mozaffarian D, Katan MB, Ascherio A, Stampfer MJ, Willett WC. Trans fatty acids and cardiovascular disease. *N Engl J Med*. 2006;354(15):1601–13.
33. Willett WC, Stampfer MJ, Manson JE, et al. Intake of trans fatty acids and risk of coronary heart disease among women. *Lancet*. 1993;341(8845): 581–5.
34. Kris-Etherton PM, Harris WS, Appel LJ. Fish consumption, fish oil, omega-3 fatty acids, and cardiovascular disease. *Circulation*. 2002;106(21): 2747–57.
35. Simopoulos AP. Omega-6/Omega-3 essential fatty acid ratio and chronic diseases. *Food Rev Int*. 2004;20(1):77–90.
36. Harris WS, Mozaffarian D, Rimm E, et al. Omega-6 fatty acids and risk for cardiovascular disease. *Circulation*. 2009;119(6):902–7.
37. Fernandez ML, Calle M. Revisiting dietary cholesterol recommendations: Does the evidence support a limit of 300 mg/d? *Curr Atheroscler Rep*. 2010;12(6):377–83.
38. DeSalvo KB, Olson R, Casavale KO. Dietary guidelines for Americans. *JAMA*. 2016;315(5):457–8.
39. Kramer K, Badhman J, Christian P, Rah JH. *Micronutrients, Macro Impact: The Story of Vitamins and a Hungry World*. Basel, Switzerland: Sight and Life Press; 2011. https://issuu.com/sight_and_life/docs/micronutriens_macro_impact. Accessed July 22, 2018.
40. Lonsdale D. Thiamin(e): The spark of life. In: Stanger O, ed. *Water Soluble Vitamins: Clinical Research and Future Applications*. Dordrecht, Netherlands: Springer; 2012.
41. Frank LL. Thiamin in clinical practice. *J Parenter Enter Nutr*. 2015;39(5): 503–20.
42. Gropper SS, Smith JL. *Advanced Nutrition and Human Metabolism*. 6th ed. Belmont, CA: Wadsworth; 2013.
43. Institute of Medicine (US) Standing Committee on the Scientific Evaluation of Dietary Reference Intakes and its Panel on Folate, Other B Vitamins, and Choline. Thiamine. In: *Dietary Reference Intakes for Thiamine, Riboflavin, Niacin, Vitamin B6, Folate, Vitamin B12, Pantothenic Acid, Biotin, and Choline*. Washington, DC: National Academies Press; 1998.
44. Office of Dietary Supplements, National Institutes of Health. Thiamin: Fact Sheet for Health Professionals. https://ods.od.nih.gov/factsheets/Thiamin-HealthProfessional. Accessed July 22, 2018.
45. Institute of Medicine (US) Standing Committee on the Scientific Evaluation of Dietary Reference Intakes and its Panel on Folate, Other B Vitamins, and Choline. Riboflavin. In: *Dietary Reference Intakes for Thiamine, Riboflavin, Niacin, Vitamin B6, Folate, Vitamin B12, Pantothenic Acid, Biotin, and Choline*. Washington, DC: National Academies Press; 1998.
46. Pinto JT, Zempleni J. Riboflavin. *Adv Nutr*. 2016;7(5):973–5.
47. Powers HJ. Riboflavin (vitamin B-2) and health. *Am J Clin Nutr*. 2003;77(6):1352–60.
48. Peechakara BV, Gupta M. *Vitamin B2 (riboflavin)*. InStatPearls [Internet]. Treasure Island, FL: StatPearls Publishing. October 1, 2019.
49. MacKay D, Hathcock J, Guarneri E. Niacin: Chemical forms, bioavailability, and health effects. *Nutr Rev*. 2012;70(6):357–66.
50. Meyer-Ficca M, Kirkland JB. Niacin. *Adv Nutr*. 2016;7(3):556–8.
51. Goldie C, Taylor AJ, Nguyen P, McCoy C, Zhao X-Q, Preiss D. Niacin therapy and the risk of new-onset diabetes: A meta-analysis of randomised controlled trials. *Heart*. 2016;102(3):198–203.
52. Carpenter KJ. The relationship of pellagra to corn and the low availability of niacin in cereals. In: *Nutritional Adequacy, Nutrient Availability and Needs. Basel*. Switzerland: Springer; 1983, pp. 197–222.
53. Institute of Medicine (US) Standing Committee on the Scientific Evaluation of Dietary Reference Intakes and its Panel on Folate, Other B Vitamins, and Choline. Folate. In: *Dietary Reference Intakes for Thiamine, Riboflavin, Niacin, Vitamin B6, Folate, Vitamin B12, Pantothenic Acid, Biotin, and Choline*. Washington, DC: National Academies Press; 1998.
54. Ryan-Harshman M, Aldoori W. Folic acid and prevention of neural tube defects. *Can Fam Physician*. 2008;54(1):36–8.
55. Office of Dietary Supplements, National Institutes of Health. Vitamin B12: Fact Sheet for Health Professionals. https://ods.od.nih.gov/factsheets/VitaminB12-HealthProfessional. Accessed July 22, 2018.
56. Li Y, Schellhorn HE. New developments and novel therapeutic perspectives for vitamin C. *J Nutr*. 2007;137(10):2171–84.
57. U.S. Department of Agriculture, Agricultural Research Service. USDA National Nutrient Database for Standard Reference, Release 24. Nutrient Data Laboratory Home Page. https://www.ars.usda.gov/northeast-area/beltsville-md-bhnrc/beltsville-human-nutrition-research-center/nutrient-data-laboratory. Accessed July 1, 2018.
58. Carr AC, Frei B. Toward a new recommended dietary allowance for vitamin C based on antioxidant and health effects in humans. *Am J Clin Nutr*. 1999;69(6):1086–107.
59. Panel on Dietary Antioxidants and Related Compounds. *Dietary Reference Intakes for Vitamin C, Vitamin E, Selenium, and Carotenoids*. Washington, DC: National Academies Press; 2000.
60. Office of Dietary Supplements, National Institutes of Health. Vitamin C: Fact Sheet for Health Professionals. https://ods.od.nih.gov/factsheets/VitaminC-HealthProfessional. Accessed July 1, 2018.
61. Jacob RA, Sotoudeh G. Vitamin C function and status in chronic disease. *Nutr Clin Care*. 2002;5(2):66–74.
62. Hemilä H, Chalker E, Douglas B, Treacy B. Vitamin C for preventing and treating the common cold. In: Hemilä H, ed. *Cochrane Database of Systematic Reviews*. Chichester, UK: John Wiley & Sons, Ltd; 2007, p. CD000980.
63. Institute of Medicine (US) Committee to Review Dietary Reference Intakes for Vitamin D and Calcium. *Dietary Reference Intakes for Calcium and Vitamin D*. Washington, DC: National Academies Press (US); 2011.
64. Sokol RJ, Butler-Simon N, Conner C, et al. Multicenter trial of d-alpha-tocopheryl polyethylene glycol 1000 succinate for treatment of vitamin E deficiency in children with chronic cholestasis. *Gastroenterology*. 1993;104(6):1727–35.
65. Epstein FH, Steinberg D, Parthasarathy S, Carew TE, Khoo JC, Witztum JL. Beyond cholesterol. *N Engl J Med*. 1989;320(14):915–24.

66. Azzi A, Boscoboinik D, Marilley D, Ozer NK, Stäuble B, Tasinato A. Vitamin E: A sensor and an information transducer of the cell oxidation state. *Am J Clin Nutr.* 1995;62(6):1337S–46S.
67. Stampfer MJ, Hennekens CH, Manson JE, Colditz GA, Rosner B, Willett WC. Vitamin E consumption and the risk of coronary disease in women. *N Engl J Med.* 1993;328(20):1444–9.
68. Knekt P, Reunanen A, Järvinen R, Seppänen R, Heliövaara M, Aromaa A. Antioxidant vitamin intake and coronary mortality in a longitudinal population study. *Am J Epidemiol.* 1994;139(12):1180–9.
69. Saremi A, Arora R. Vitamin E and cardiovascular disease. *Am J Ther.* 2010;17(3):e56–65.
70. Traber MG. Heart disease and single-vitamin supplementation. *Am J Clin Nutr.* 2007;85(1):293S–9S.
71. Sesso HD, Buring JE, Christen WG, et al. Vitamins E and C in the prevention of cardiovascular disease in men. *JAMA.* 2008;300(18):2123.
72. Lonn E, Bosch J, Yusuf S, et al. Effects of long-term vitamin E supplementation on cardiovascular events and cancer. *JAMA.* 2005;293(11):1338.
73. Lee IM, Cook NR, Gaziano JM, et al. Vitamin E in the primary prevention of cardiovascular disease and cancer. *JAMA.* 2005;294(1):56.
74. Wang L, Sesso HD, Glynn RJ, et al. Vitamin E and C supplementation and risk of cancer in men: posttrial follow-up in the Physicians' Health Study II randomized trial. *Am J Clin Nutr.* 2014;100(3):915–23.
75. Lippman SM, Klein EA, Goodman PJ, et al. Effect of selenium and vitamin E on risk of prostate cancer and other cancers. *JAMA.* 2009;301(1):39.
76. Luo H, Fang Y-J, Lu M-S, et al. Dietary and serum vitamins A and E and colorectal cancer risk in Chinese population. *Eur J Cancer Prev.* 2019;28(4):268–77.
77. Cui L, Li L, Tian Y, Xu F, Qiao T. Association between dietary vitamin E intake and esophageal cancer risk: An updated meta-analysis. *Nutrients.* 2018;10(7):801.
78. Booth SL. Vitamin K: Food composition and dietary intakes. *Food Nutr Res.* 2012;56(1):5505.
79. Shearer MJ, Newman P. Metabolism and cell biology of vitamin K. *Thromb Haemost.* 2008;100(4):530–47.
80. Institute of Medicine (US) Panel on Micronutrients. *Dietary Reference Intakes for Vitamin A, Vitamin K, Arsenic, Boron, Chromium, Copper, Iodine, Iron, Manganese, Molybdenum, Nickel, Silicon, Vanadium, and Zinc.* Washington, DC: National Academies Press; 2001.
81. Jagannath VA, Fedorowicz Z, Thaker V, Chang AB. Vitamin K supplementation for cystic fibrosis. In: Jagannath VA, ed. *Cochrane Database of Systematic Reviews.* Vol. 1. Chichester, UK: John Wiley & Sons, Ltd; 2015, p. CD008482.
82. Yaegashi Y, Onoda T, Tanno K, Kuribayashi T, Sakata K, Orimo H. Association of hip fracture incidence and intake of calcium, magnesium, vitamin D, and vitamin K. *Eur J Epidemiol.* 2008;23(3):219–25.
83. Feskanich D, Weber P, Willett WC, Rockett H, Booth SL, Colditz GA. Vitamin K intake and hip fractures in women: A prospective study. *Am J Clin Nutr.* 1999;69(1):74–9.
84. Booth SL, Broe KE, Gagnon DR, et al. Vitamin K intake and bone mineral density in women and men. *Am J Clin Nutr.* 2003;77(2):512–6.
85. Cockayne S, Adamson J, Lanham-New S, Shearer MJ, Gilbody S, Torgerson DJ. Vitamin K and the prevention of fractures. *Arch Intern Med.* 2006;166(12):1256.
86. Knapen MHJ, Drummen NE, Smit E, Vermeer C, Theuwissen E. Three-year low-dose menaquinone-7 supplementation helps decrease bone loss in healthy postmenopausal women. *Osteoporos Int.* 2013;24(9):2499–507.
87. U.S. Department of Health and Human Services and U.S. Department of Agriculture. *2015–2020 Dietary Guidelines for Americans.* 8th ed. Washington, DC: U.S. Department of Health and Human Services; 2015. http://health.gov/our-work/food-nutrition/2015-2020-dietary-guidelines/guidelines. Accessed June 20, 2018.
88. Mahan LK, Escott-Stump S, Raymond JL, eds. *Krause's Food and the Nutrition Care Process.* St. Louis, MO: Elsevier; 2012.
89. Nimni ME, Han B, Cordoba F. Are we getting enough sulfur in our diet? *Nutr Metab.* 2007;4:24.
90. Ibrahim WH, Bailey N, Sunvold GD, Bruckner GG. Effects of carnitine and taurine on fatty acid metabolism and lipid accumulation in the liver of cats during weight gain and weight loss. *Am J Vet Res.* 2003;64(10):1265–77.
91. Trumbo P, Yates AA, Schlicker S, Poos M. Dietary reference intakes. *J Am Diet Assoc.* 2001;101(3):294–301.
92. Abbaspour N, Hurrell R, Kelishadi R. Review on iron and its importance for human health. *J Res Med Sci.* 2014;19(2):164–74.
93. Lieu PT, Heiskala M, Peterson PA, Yang Y. The roles of iron in health and disease. *Mol Aspects Med.* 2001;22(1–2):1–87.
94. Shrimpton R, Marinho H. The effects of zinc supplementation on zinc, retinol and carotene levels in lactating Amazonian women. *WNJ.* 2018;9(1):4–21.
95. Institute of Medicine (US) Standing Committee on the Scientific Evaluation of Dietary Reference Intakes and its Panel on Folate, Other B Vitamins, and Choline. Choline. In: *Dietary Reference Intakes for Thiamine, Riboflavin, Niacin, Vitamin B6, Folate, Vitamin B12, Pantothenic Acid, Biotin, and Choline.* Washington, DC: National Academies Press; 1998.
96. Committee to Review the Dietary Reference Intakes for Sodium and Potassium. *Dietary Reference Intakes for Sodium and Potassium.* Washington, DC: National Academies Press (US); 2019.

CHAPTER

181 Obesity Prevention and Control: A Public Health Perspective*

Deborah A. Galuska • Latetia V. Moore

INTRODUCTION

Obesity is common, affecting over 93 million adults and nearly 4 million children[1]; costs the U.S. healthcare system billions of dollars[2,3]; and puts both children and adults at risk for multiple health consequences including type 2 diabetes and coronary heart disease.[4,5] With the high prevalence of obesity, associated consequences, and forecasted increases,[6] preventing individuals from developing obesity and treating those who have it is the focus of many health initiatives across the country. Because obesity is a population-wide problem, this chapter examines the problem of obesity through a public health lens. Specifically, it focuses on the epidemiology of obesity including how it is defined, who is most affected, the health and economic effects of obesity; the modifiable risk factors for obesity; and strategies for prevention and treatment.

MEASUREMENT

Although obesity is most simply defined as excess body fat, methods to assess obesity vary. Body mass index (BMI) is most often used as a screening tool to identify obesity in clinical and research settings and in public health surveillance to track obesity among populations over time. BMI is a person's weight in kilograms divided by their height in meters squared. A BMI at or above 30.0 kg/m^2 in adults aged 20 years and older is defined as obesity by various expert bodies including the World Health Organization, the National Institutes of Health, and the Centers for Disease Control and Prevention.[5,7–9] Because children are still growing, BMI for children and adolescents must be interpreted relative to their peers of the same sex and age. A BMI at or greater than the 95th percentile in children and adolescents aged 2–19 years is classified as obesity.[10] In infants and children under 2 years of age, there is not a defined cutoff for obesity. Although no evidence-based guidelines for treating obesity in infancy exist, early recognition of a tendency toward obesity might appropriately trigger interventions to slow weight gain.[11] As such, in the United States, World Health Organization growth charts are used to monitor high weight for length.[11,12]

Although not the focus of this chapter, the classification overweight is also commonly used to characterize weight status, particularly in concert with obesity. Overweight is defined as a BMI of 25.0–29.9 kg/m^2 among adults and a BMI-for-age between the 85th percentile and <95th percentile among children and adolescents aged 2–19 years.[9,10]

Obesity can also be further categorized by levels of severity. Adults with a BMI 35.0–39.9 kg/m^2 and those with a BMI at or above 40.0 kg/m^2 are classified as having class II and class III obesity, respectively.[7] Some debate exists on how to classify severe obesity in children and adolescents.[13,14] To facilitate tracking changes in BMI status over time and interpretation of high-BMI values, some expert bodies suggest severe obesity in children and adolescents $\geq$ 2 years of age be defined as a BMI $\geq$ 120% of the 95th percentile based on age and sex or an absolute BMI $\geq$ 35 kg/m^2, whichever is lower.[13]

Although BMI is often used for clinical assessment, public health surveillance, and research, it does have limitations. BMI can overestimate body fat in those who weigh more because of a high-muscle mass and underestimate body fat in certain populations.[15–18] In addition, surveillance and research studies that depend on self-reported instead of measured weight and height can over- or underestimate obesity. Adults tend to underreport weight and overreport height, which may underestimate BMI; conversely, proxy reports of younger children's height by parents tend to be lower than measured heights, which may overestimate BMI.[19,20] Standard BMI cutoffs of $\geq$ 30 kg/m^2 also may not be the most appropriate measurement tool in determining obesity in all racial ethnic groups. For example, Rahman et al. concluded that current BMI cutoff values did not identify about half of non-Hispanic white and Hispanic reproductive-aged women as having obesity who had a percent body fat of greater than 35%; the standard BMI cutoff also did not identify 25% of non-Hispanic black women as having obesity.[21] Other direct measures of body fat may also be associated with health-risk factors when BMI is not. For example, in a convenience sample of over 100 non-Hispanic black women, percent body fat was significantly associated with systolic and diastolic blood pressure but BMI was not.[18] A World Health Organization report also found that the proportion of Asian people with a high risk of type 2 diabetes and cardiovascular disease is substantial at BMIs lower than the standard cut-off point for obesity.[17] Among children, evidence also exists that at equivalent levels of BMI-for-age, black children have less body fatness than white children, and Asian girls have slightly higher levels of body fat than white girls.[22]

Alternatives to BMI are direct measures of body fat including skinfold thickness measurements, bioelectrical impedance, densitometry (underwater weighing), and dual energy x-ray absorptiometry. Each of these direct measures may provide more accurate individual assessments of levels of body fat relative to BMI but may be difficult to perform correctly or be impractical or expensive, especially for large-scale research study or surveillance. Furthermore, obesity defined by BMI is correlated with more direct measures of body fat, higher all-cause mortality, and other obesity-related biologic factors such as blood pressure and plasma lipid levels.[15,23–27] For example, BMI was as strongly associated with levels of lipids and lipoproteins as was percent body fat calculated from Slaughter skinfold

*Disclaimer: The findings and conclusions in this chapter are those of the authors and do not necessarily represent the official position of the Centers for Disease Control and Prevention.

thickness and dual energy x-ray absorptiometry among 8- to 19-year olds who participated in the (U.S.) National Health and Nutrition Examination Survey from 1999 to 2004.[15] In this same study, systolic blood pressure was more strongly associated with BMI than the other measures.[15]

CONSEQUENCES

The effects of obesity are already apparent in childhood. Research shows that during their childhood years, children with obesity are more likely to experience psychological or psychiatric problems including low self-esteem and behavioral problems, high-blood pressure, dyslipidemia, abnormalities in left ventricular mass and/or function, abnormalities in endothelial function, hyperinsulinemia and/or insulin resistance, and asthma than children who do not have obesity.[4] Girls are often at greater risk than boys of psychological morbidity and risk increases with age.[4,28]

Evidence on the longer-term consequences of childhood obesity is sparse but suggest that childhood obesity is associated with poorer health outcomes later in life.[4] First, evidence indicates that obesity in children and adolescents persists into later years.[4,29] In one study, children at the 50th percentile of BMI at 5 years of age had a 6% probability of developing obesity at 14 years of age compared to 47% among those at the 95th percentile.[29] The probability of developing obesity between 5 and 14 years of age varied by sex, race/ethnicity, and income.[29] For example, 16.8% of non-Hispanic black and 14.3% of Hispanic children developed obesity between these ages compared to 10.1% of non-Hispanic white children. Second, a few studies have shown that obesity in youth is associated with adult mortality. One cohort study found that being overweight (BMI of >25 kg/m^2) at 18 years of age was associated with significantly increased mortality within 20 and 32 years of follow up compared to having a BMI 19.0–19.9 kg/m^2.[30] In another study, participants who reported having obesity at 21 years of age experienced mortality rates that were 64% higher than normal weight participants regardless of race, sex, and obesity status in later life.[31] Finally, among those with obesity, children and adolescents with more severe obesity may suffer from poorer immediate and long-term health outcomes and an increased likelihood of having obesity and associated chronic diseases as adults.[13]

In adulthood, obesity is associated with a variety of health conditions. Adults who have obesity, compared to those with a normal or healthy weight, are at increased risk for all-cause mortality, developing risk factors such as hypertension and dyslipidemia, and various chronic conditions including type 2 diabetes, coronary heart disease, stroke, gallbladder disease, and osteoarthritis.[5,7] Adults with obesity also have a higher risk of sleep apnea and breathing problems, low quality of life, mental illnesses including clinical depression and anxiety, body pain, and difficulty with physical functioning.[7,9,32–34] Overweight ($25.0 \leq$ BMI < 30.0 kg/m^2) and obesity combined are associated with at least 13 different types of cancer (adenocarcinoma of the esophagus; cancers of the breast in postmenopausal women, colon and rectum, endometrium, gallbladder, gastric cardia, kidney, liver, ovary, pancreas, and thyroid; meningioma; and multiple myeloma).[35] These cancers made up 40% of all cancers diagnosed in 2014 and have increased over time.[36] Severe obesity in adults as in children is associated with even poorer health outcomes.[37,38]

ECONOMIC COSTS

A substantial and rising percentage of healthcare costs are associated with obesity across the United States.[39] Estimates for how much obesity costs the United States in medical-care range significantly. For example, one study estimated obesity costs at approximately 147 billion in U.S. dollars (2008 dollars) with medical spending for someone with obesity 1429 dollars higher (42% higher) per year compared to those of normal weight.[2] Another study estimated higher costs of about 315.8 billion dollars per year or 3508 dollars higher for someone with obesity (2010 dollars).[40] Studies have also estimated that obesity-related costs have increased 14.3–29% over 10–15 years in adults and that costs differ across states.[3,40,41] One study estimated obesity-related costs were lowest in Wyoming [203 million dollars per year (2009 dollars)] and highest in California (15.2 billion dollars per year).[3] A quarter to half of these state-level costs of obesity are estimated to be financed by federal and state government programs (i.e., Medicare and Medicaid).[3]

Higher medical expenditures for obesity among adults and children have been attributed to increased costs of office-based visits, outpatient hospital care, in-patient care, and prescription drugs. For example, compared with normal and underweight children, children with obesity had 100–200 dollars' higher outpatient visit expenditures and prescription drug expenditures and slightly higher emergency room costs over a 2-year period.[42] Childhood obesity was associated with 14.1 billion dollars in additional prescription drug, emergency room, and outpatient visit costs annually.[42]

Higher grades of obesity are associated with higher medical costs. For example, one study estimates healthcare costs rise rapidly for individuals with severe obesity (BMI ≥ 35) but not for those with class I obesity.[40] Another study indicated that per capita healthcare expenditures for adults with severe obesity were 81% greater than normal-weight adults and 47% greater than adults with class I obesity.[43] Aggregate U.S. healthcare expenditures associated with excess body weight among adults with severe obesity have been estimated at more than 11 billion dollars in 2000.[43] The estimated savings in annual medical-care costs from a 5% reduction in weight is 2137 dollars for those with class III obesity, 528 dollars for those with class II obesity, and 69 dollars for those with class I obesity.[40]

DEMOGRAPHIC PATTERNS

Obesity varies in the United States by race/ethnicity, age, education, income, and area of the country.[44] Among adults in 2015–16, obesity was 24% higher in Hispanic and non-Hispanic black adults than non-Hispanic white adults and 36% more prevalent than in non-Hispanic Asian adults (Fig. 181-1).[1] Representative data for other racial/ethnic groups comes from studies using self-reported weights and heights. In one study, obesity was 33% higher in American Indians/Alaska Natives and 76% higher in Native Hawaiian/other Pacific Islanders compared to whites.[45] Obesity does not vary by sex for non-Hispanic whites but for other racial ethnic groups obesity is about 20–50% higher among women than men. Obesity is also 20% higher among middle-aged adults than younger adults. Obesity decreases with increasing income in women, but not among men, and is lower among college graduates than among persons with less education for both non-Hispanic whites, non-Hispanic black women, and Hispanic women.[46]

In addition to the above variation, obesity also varies by area of the United States. Although all states had more than 20% of adults with obesity based on self-reported data in 2017, obesity was higher in the South (32.4%), and Midwest (32.3%) than the Northeast (27.7%) and West (26.1%).[47] Obesity ranged from 23.9% in Hawaii to 38.1% in West Virginia (Fig. 181-2) and was almost 20% higher among adults in nonmetropolitan counties than among those in metropolitan counties.[47,48]

Obesity patterns in children and adolescents by race/ethnicity are similar to those in adults. In 2015–16, obesity was higher among non-Hispanic black (22.0%) and Hispanic (25.8%) youth than non-Hispanic white (14.1%) and Asian (11.0%) youth.[1] Among very young (2–4 years), low-income children, obesity prevalence was highest among American Indians/Alaska Natives and Hispanics.[49] Also similar to adults, obesity among children and adolescents varies by age, income, education, and area of the country. Obesity increases with age; 13.9% of preschool-aged children (2–5 years) had obesity in 2015–16 versus 18.4% of 6–11 year olds and 20.6% of 12- to 19-year

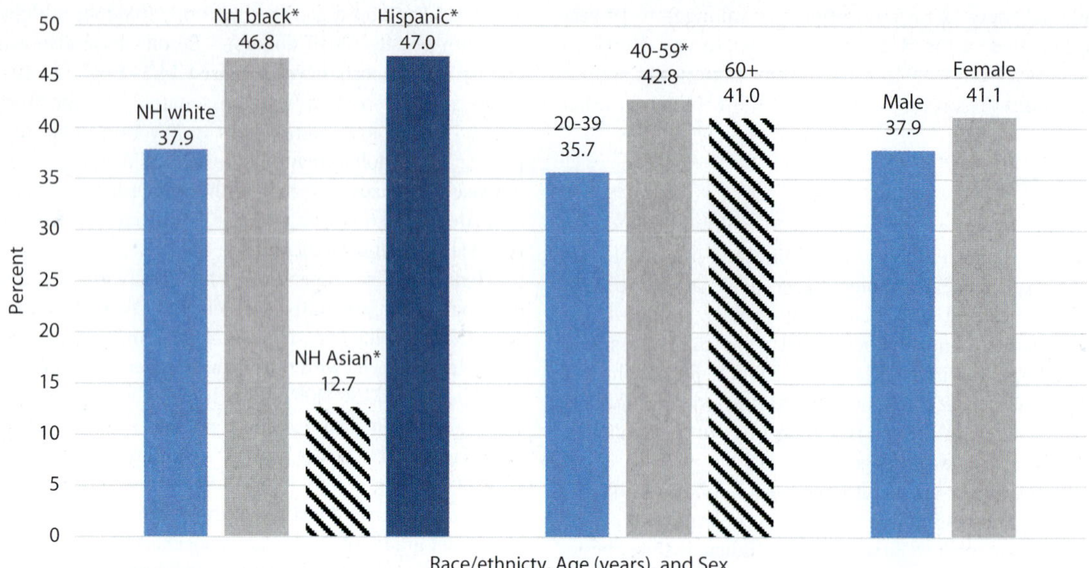

FIGURE 181-1. Prevalence of obesity among adults 20 and over by race/ethnicity, age, and sex, United States. (*Source:* National Health and Nutrition Examination Survey, 2015–2016.)

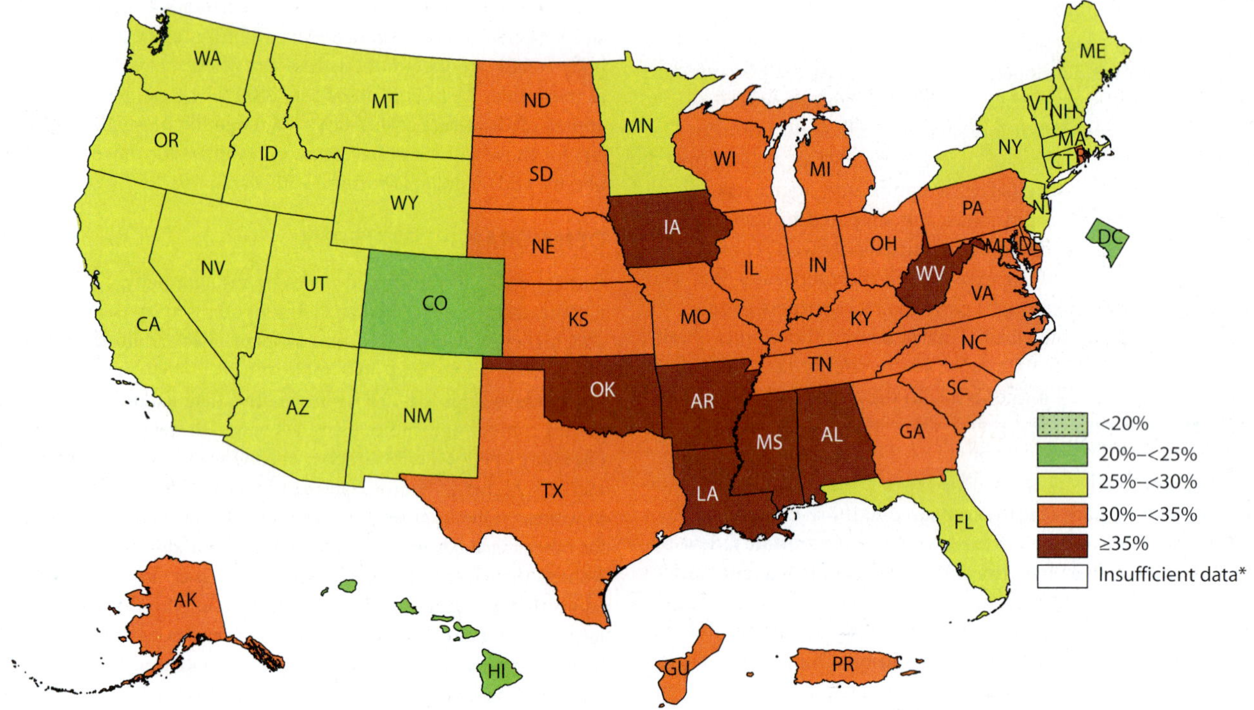

FIGURE 181-2. Prevalence of self-reported obesity among U.S. adults by state and territory. (*Source:* Division of Nutrition, Physical Activity, and Obesity, National Center for Chronic Disease Prevention and Health Promotion, Centers for Disease Control and Prevention. Adult Obesity Prevalence Maps. https://www.cdc.gov/obesity/data/prevalence-maps.html.)

olds.[1] Childhood obesity was lower in higher-income groups and among those with higher level of education of the head of household.[46,50] State by state data are not available for all age groups, but among very young low-income children obesity prevalence ranged from 8.2% in Utah to 20% in Virginia.[49]

TRENDS OVER TIME

The prevalence of obesity was fairly consistent among adults over 20 years of age from 1960 through 1980, but has increased since 1976–80.[51] Obesity increased from 14.5% in 1976–80 to 22.5% in 1988–94.[51] Increases have continued from 30.5% in 1999–2000 to 39.8% in 2015–16 (Fig. 181-3).[52,53] However, increases are not consistently evident across all sociodemographic groups over time.[52,53] For example, obesity has increased significantly during past decade among women but not men, and among adults older than 40 years of age but not among those who are younger.[53]

Among youth, there have been similar increases in obesity over time but the prevalence plateaued between 2007–08 and 2015–16.[53] Modest declines in obesity prevalence from 2010 to 2014 were observed overall and in all five racial/ethnic groups among 2- to 4-year-old, low-income children based on data from 56 WIC state agencies, the District of Columbia, and U.S. territories.[49] Statistically significant declines were observed in 34 of the 56 WIC agencies.

MODIFIABLE RISK FACTORS FOR OBESITY

Because obesity is common, costly, and associated with many serious health outcomes, understanding how to prevent obesity has the potential to significantly impact the economic and physical health of

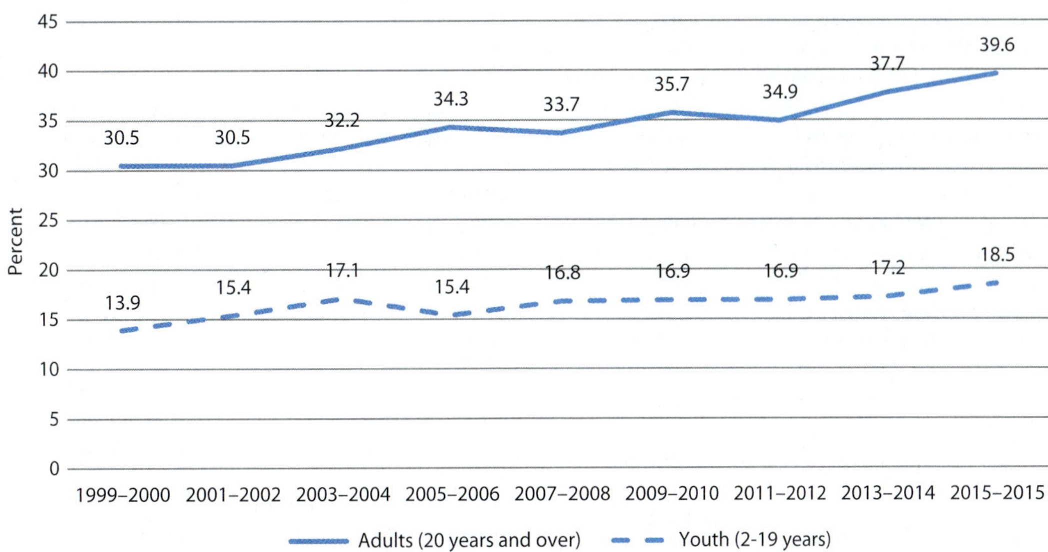

FIGURE 181-3. Trends in obesity prevalence among adults aged 20 and over (age adjusted) and youth aged 2–19 years. (*Source:* United States, National Health and Nutrition Examination Survey, 1999–2000 through 2015–2016.)

the country. The first step to successful prevention is identifying the modifiable risk factors for obesity.

A primary mechanism for excessive weight gain and obesity is the gap between energy intake and energy expenditure, that is, energy imbalance. Positive energy gaps lead to weight gain and negative energy gaps to weight loss. Relatively small changes in this gap are hypothesized to have contributed to the increase in obesity in the United States. One model estimated that an average positive energy gap of about 7 kcal/per day contributed to the increase in adult obesity in the United States between the 1980s and early 2000s.[54] However, because the population became heavier and energy needs are higher at increased weights, it is hypothesized that to move the population back to average weights in the 1980s, a population-wide positive energy gap of about 200 kcal/day would be need to be addressed.[54]

Although the concept of energy imbalance is theoretically simple, weight gain is influenced by an incredibly complex group of factors including individual behaviors related to energy consumption and expenditure, individual, environmental, and societal factors that influence these behaviors, and individual physiological mechanisms that affect energy metabolism.[55,56] A review of all these topics is beyond the scope of the chapter. Therefore, the next section will focus on individual-level risk factors that have the potential to be decreased through public health strategies.

Prenatal Exposures and Early-life Exposures

The risk for obesity starts early. Maternal-risk factors during pregnancy most consistently and positively linked with childhood weight status include maternal weight at the start of pregnancy,[57] gestational diabetes,[57] excessive weight gain during pregnancy,[57–59] and tobacco use during pregnancy.[57,60] The mechanisms that explain the relationships between these maternal risk factors and the child's weight are still unclear but at least three hypotheses have been proposed.[61] The first hypothesis is that children of women with any of these four risk factors experience different intrauterine exposures either through diet, chemical exposures from diet or tobacco smoke, or metabolic exposures (e.g., inflammation, high insulin levels) than other children. These exposures may cause permanent epigenetic changes in the offspring that predispose them to adverse weight outcomes.[61,62] The second potential explanation is that the mother and child share common genes; women who have a genetic propensity to gain weight may have children with the same propensity.[61] The final potential explanation is that the mother and child share a common environment once the child is born. For example, if a woman has less healthy dietary habits during pregnancy these may persist after pregnancy and affect the dietary habits of the child.[61]

Early dietary exposures and patterns during infancy may also affect later diet and weight status. Some studies report associations between adverse childhood weight outcomes with formula feeding (vs. breastfeeding),[57,63] early introduction of solid foods,[64] or high protein intake.[65] However, the evidence is inconsistent and whether links are causal is unclear. Infancy is also thought to be a time that dietary preferences for certain flavors such as sweet and salty start to be established and may affect later dietary patterns.[66]

Diet

Although early dietary exposures may affect later obesity risk as explained above, diet through the life course in general is also an important risk factor for weight gain and obesity and can contribute in multiple ways. The primary mechanism is contributing to energy imbalance through excessive energy (calorie) intake. Calories are obtained from four dietary sources: carbohydrates, proteins, fats, and alcohol. In general, the energy density of fats (9 kcal/g) and alcohol (7 kcal/g) are approximately twice that of carbohydrates (4 kcal/g) and proteins (4 kcal/g).[67] Calorie needs vary by age, sex, and activity level. For example, estimated calorie needs for subgroups in the population range from about 1000 calories for a sedentary toddler to 3000 calories for an active teen-aged boy.[68]

A number of aspects of diet can contribute to excess energy consumption and weight gain. First, the physical characteristics of foods may contribute to caloric consumption. For example, foods higher in fiber and/or water content, such as fruits and vegetables and whole grains, are thought to be more satiating and thus are less likely to be overconsumed. Studies have found some evidence of an inverse relationship between consumption of fruits and vegetables and whole grains with weight outcomes.[69] Second, the form of the foods also appears to matter. For example, the energy consumed from liquid foods as compared to semisolid or solid foods tends to be less compensated for in later food encounters, potentially leading to overconsumption of total calories in the day.[70] As such, while a person who consumes a large amount of calories from food early in the day may reduce their calorie intake later in the day, this may not be as true for calories from liquids. This is one explanation for the consistent positive relationship between sugar-sweetened beverage consumption and higher weight status.[69,71,72] Third, the palatability or the sensory properties of foods also affect consumption. People tend to choose more highly palatable foods (e.g., foods higher in sugar or fat content) when they are available. This effect may occur even when a person is not hungry.[73] Because these foods tend to also be higher in calories, overconsumption of them can contribute to excess calorie intake. Fourth, where foods and meals are consumed may also affect weight status. For example, more frequent consumption of meals away from home has been associated with increased caloric consumption[74] and increased weight.[75]

Finally, an emerging way that diet might affect obesity is through its potential impact on the gut microbiome. Those with obesity appear to have a different gut microbiome than those without.[76] Although the reasons are not yet entirely understood, the gut microbiome may impact obesity by more effectively harvesting energy from foods or by influencing metabolic and immunological pathways associated with obesity.[76] Diet appears to interact with the microbiome to affect obesity by either changing the composition of the microbiome or by causing the production of microbiotic products that influence metabolic pathways.[77]

Although managing one's weight is an important consideration in planning a healthy diet, a person's diet also needs to provide the nutrients needed for growth and function and to address the nutritional risk factors for other chronic diseases and conditions. As such, current Dietary Guidelines for Americans recommend consuming a healthy dietary pattern within an individual's calorie needs.[68] This includes diets higher in fruits and vegetables and whole grains, moderate in lean proteins and low-fat dairy products and lower in saturated fat, added sugar and sodium.[68] This dietary pattern has been associated with favorable weight-related outcomes.[78]

Physical Activity

Another factor that contributes to weight gain is energy expenditure that is not commensurate with energy intake; this also contributes to an energy imbalance or a positive energy gap. Components of energy expenditure include basal and resting metabolic rate, thermic effect of eating, and physical activity.[79,80] However, individuals have the most control over physical activity and changing it is the focus of population strategies for weight control.

Lower levels of physical activity are related to larger increases in weight status and adiposity measures in children and adults[81] and the incidence of obesity in adults.[81] However, the amount of physical activity needed to prevent unhealthy weight gain varies by person, as it is affected by dietary intake as discussed above, the type of physical activity, and characteristics of the person. Energy expenditure during physical activity is a function of both the volume and intensity of the activity.[82] For example, a 120-pound adult expends approximately 120 calories during a brisk 30-minute walk; that same person expends about 190 calories if they jogged during that 30 minutes. Energy expended during physical activity also varies by body size and fitness level.[81,82] A person who is less fit or weighs more will in general expend more energy engaging in the same activity compared to their counterparts. For example, compared to the 120-pound adult above, a 220-pound adult would expend about 215 calories briskly walking and 350 jogging over the same time period.

Currently about 150–250 minutes of moderate to vigorous physical activity per week are recommended for adults to prevent weight gain.[83] Although weight specific recommendations for children do not exist, current health recommendations for 60 minutes per day of physical activity for children 6 and older are a reasonable starting goal.[84]

In addition to affecting weight directly though activity specific energy expenditure, physical activity may also assert its effect by improving appetite control[85] or by increasing muscle mass and thus basal metabolic rate.[86]

Sedentary Behaviors

Sedentary behaviors are defined as behaviors done while either sitting or reclining that have low-energy expenditure and include activities such as television watching, computer use or other screen viewing.[81] They have been hypothesized to contribute to weight status because of their low-energy expenditure or because they are correlated with other behaviors that might be occurring simultaneously such as increased snacking or exposure to advertising of less healthy foods.[87]

In contrast to the dose–response relationship between physical activity and weight, the relationship between sedentary behaviors and weight is less clear. Recent reviews for both children and adults have found limited or inconsistent evidence of a positive relationship between time spent in sedentary behaviors and higher weight status[81,87–89]; for children, the relationship may be more consistent for television viewing.[81]

Sleep

Shorter duration of sleep is associated with increased risk of obesity[90,91] or weight gain[90,92]; this relationship appears more consistent in children and younger adults than in older adults.[92,93] Several plausible mechanisms have been proposed to explain the association. These include the association of sleep with behavioral factors (e.g., increased time awake increases opportunities for additional calorie consumption); with alterations to hormones that affect appetite control or basal metabolic rate such as leptin, ghrelin or TSH; or with cognitive factors such as mood or impulse control that could affect eating behaviors.[90,91]

Some research also suggests that the relationship between sleep duration and weight gain may be u-shaped and that those who sleep long periods of time may also have a higher risk for obesity.[92] However, this relationship is less consistently reported and it is unclear if longer bouts of sleep cause obesity or if obesity results in problems that cause individuals to sleep longer.

Chemical Exposures

An emerging area of research is the role a group of chemicals called endocrine disruptors have on obesity. When exposure to these chemicals occurs during sensitive developmental periods in early life, they are thought to permanently alter the susceptibility to obesity.[62,94] Hypothesized mechanisms that link exposure of these exogenous chemicals to weight or weight gain include[1]: altering adipogenesis, the development of the size, number, or storage capacity of fat cells, or[2] altering neuroendocrine pathways that control appetite and other aspects of eating behaviors.[62,94] At least 20 chemicals have been hypothesized to have obesogenic properties with mixed levels of evidence. Examples include dichlorodiphenyldiclorethylene and cigarette smoke.[62,95]

WEIGHT LOSS

Given the high existing prevalence of obesity, understanding who is trying to lose weight, what benefits they might expect, and the most effective strategies individuals can use is also important for identifying public-health strategies to control obesity.

Trying to lose weight is a common behavior for adults and adolescents. In 2013–16, nearly half (49.1%) of adults were trying to lose weight.[96] Similarly, in 2017, 47.1% of adolescents were trying to lose weight.[97] For both groups, weight loss attempts were more common in females than males.

Weight loss can have short-term and long-term health impacts. Intentional weight loss positively affects metabolic risk factors for chronic diseases. For example, in adults, positive changes in blood pressure, lipid profiles, and blood glucose are observed with even small amounts of weight loss—in the range of 5–10% of baseline.[5] Similar associations are found for children; one meta-analysis found a significant association between weight loss and improvements in systolic blood pressure, triglycerides, and high-density lipoproteins.[98] Weight loss is also associated with improvements in functional status. For example, those with osteoarthritis experience reduced pain and improved quality of life after losing weight.[99]

Whether weight loss results in reduced chronic disease risk is less clear and may depend on whether or not the weight loss is intentional

have the potential to impact a large number of adults and adolescents and have a positive impact on both the employer and employee. Numerous expert bodies, including the Community Preventive Services Task Force[149] and the IOM,[56] recommend intervening in the worksite to prevent or control obesity.

Federal and state governments can impact the health of workers by setting laws or other policies that affect the availability and usage of worksite health programs, employee benefits, or active transportation to and from work. For example, in 2013, approximately half of states had laws related to worksite health programs that included policy elements for weight management ($n = 26$); physical activity ($n = 24$), and nutrition ($n = 21$). Examples of policy elements authorized or funded in these laws include grants and funding provided to worksites to implement programs, tax credits for worksite expenditures on health programs and certification programs to ensure worksites offer quality programs.[150]

At the facility level, interventions can be implemented with the sole focus of weight management or as part of a larger worksite wellness program designed to affect multiple health outcomes. Strategies can include implementing individually focused programs or changing worksite environments or policies to make a healthy diet and physical activity easier.[56,151] Based on systematic reviews, the evidence that worksite interventions can improve weight status or BMI ranges from limited to strong.[149,152] Similar to the evidence in schools, intensity of the intervention appears to matter. Multicomponent (those addressing both diet and physical activity) and multilevel (those that target the needs of the individual at work as well as change their surrounding work environment to be more for supportive diet and/or physical activity) tend to be more effective.[149,152]

One example of a facility-level intervention that resulted in weight loss was the adaption of the Diabetes Prevention Program (DPP) intervention in a university worksite in Ohio. The intervention group, workers with prediabetes, were randomly assigned to receive a 16-week intervention that addressed losing weight, increasing physical activity, and reducing fat consumption. The group received written materials, participated in weekly group meetings, and set individual goals. The control group received written materials only. The intervention group had significantly more weight loss, a 5.5% reduction in comparison to a 0.4% reduction in the control group.[153]

An example of a policy that can be incorporated into worksite wellness programs is nutrition standards for foods served or sold at the worksite. The *Food Service Guidelines for Federal Facilities* provides federal worksite best practices to increase healthy and safe food options that can be incorporated into food-services contracts.[154] However, these guidelines can be used by other worksites to improve their own food environments.

Healthcare Setting

Approximately 85% of adults and 92% of youth under 18 years of age had contact with a healthcare provider in the past year.[155] This provides opportunities for healthcare providers to address weight and weight-related behaviors.

Within a medical-care setting, healthcare providers can address obesity by following recommended standards of care.[56] Multiple clinical groups recommend regular assessment of weight, height, and BMI for patients of all ages.[14,156,157] Using these assessments to specifically screen for obesity is recommended for both adults and children 6 years and older. The U.S. Preventive Clinical Services Task Force recommends that patients be screened for obesity using BMI for adults or body mass percentile for children. If obesity is present, patients should receive intensive multicomponent behavioral interventions.[105,106] For adults, intensive interventions last 1–2 years with 12 or more sessions during the first year,[105] whereas for children, they include 25 hours or more of contact time over a 6-month period.[106] Multicomponent interventions include diet, physical activity, and teaching behavioral modification strategies for the patient and their families.

The interventions for referral can be located within the healthcare setting or in the community. One example of an intensive intervention for childhood obesity available in the community setting is Mind, Exercise, Nutrition, Do It (MEND).[158] This program is a family centered intervention, focusing on education, skill building, and motivation related to diet, physical activity, and sedentary behavior. The randomized control trial that tested MEND found that eighteen 2-hour sessions across 2–3 months led to significant reductions in measures of adiposity and BMI at the end of 12 months. This program has been scaled up and is delivered by the YMCA across the country to school-aged children aged 7–13. For adults, the previously described Diabetes Prevention Program, which now has certified programs throughout the country, illustrates an example of a community-level program where those with prediabetes (who often also have obesity) can be referred.

In addition to clinical guidelines that establish a standard of care, other system-level policies and supports can facilitate the actions of healthcare providers. One example is the Healthcare Effectiveness Data and Information Set (HEDIS).[159] These standard measures allow healthcare plans to document performance and progress on important dimensions of care and service. Assessment of adult BMI is one of the measures. Another recommended system-level strategy in the healthcare setting is ensuring coverage of, access to, and incentives for obesity prevention and treatment services in the public and private sector.[56]

Communities

In addition to the role specific community settings have in helping people prevent and manage their weight, the community at large also has a role. Outside of their homes, schools, and worksites, people interact with their community to buy foods at retail venues, travel between places, and participate in community programs, all offering opportunities to affect diet and physical activity. As such, expert groups have recommended that local governments, businesses, and nonprofit groups all have a role to play in their community's health both individually and in collaboration with other settings.[56,130,160]

Two types of community-level interventions exist. The first focuses on simultaneously implementing interventions across multiple settings in a community with a goal of improving population-level weight status. These interventions are relatively rare and have been primarily tested in children. The most successful programs have included the school setting as one of the targets for the intervention.[135] A case study of four communities that reported childhood obesity declines in the early 2000s identified other potential elements for success in these multifaceted interventions including having a local champion, cross-sector partnerships, and the layering of diet and physical activity strategies at the individual, community, state, and federal level.[161]

An example of this type of intervention was Shape Up Somerville, whose goal was to prevent weight gain in young children in a small Massachusetts community.[162,163] This intervention simultaneously targeted homes, schools, and community settings and included interventions to educate parents and children as well as policy and environmental interventions to improve foods offered in schools and community restaurants and to increase opportunities for physical activity in the school and community. The project found a small but significant decline in BMI z-score for children in the intervention community compared to the control communities over 2 years[162,163] and some evidence that the intervention also reduced the BMI of the parents of the children.[164]

The second type of community intervention aims to change an obesity-related behavior, such as physical activity or diet, through an intervention targeting a specific community policy or practice. For example, the Community Preventive Services Task Force (CPSTF) has recommended several strategies communities can implement based on evidence that they improve physical activity levels. One group of strategies improves the built environment in the community to support physical activity. One recommended built environment strategy is improving access to places for physical activity (e.g., parks or community recreation centers) combined with informational outreach (e.g., training on how to use equipment a setting). Another recommended strategy to improve the built environment for physical activity is to use interventions that combine improvements in transportation systems (e.g., pedestrian and cyclist friendly street design) and improvements in land use and environmental design (e.g., mixed use land development).[165,166] Another group of recommended strategies from the Community Guide target individuals in the communities. Two recommended strategies are providing social support programs or providing individually adapted behavior change programs.[165] Social support programs bring people together to support each other in being active; an example is a weekly free walking program at the community recreation center. Individually adapted behavior change programs are designed to meet the unique needs of certain types of individuals such as those with arthritis who may need to learn about types of physical activities that do not cause more pain.

Another example of a community-level strategy designed to change a specific behavior is one attempting to change diet by increasing the relative cost of less healthy foods. For example, in Berkeley, California, a policy intervention that increased the excise tax of sugar-sweetened beverages resulted in a decrease in sugar sweetened beverage consumption and an increase in water consumption in low-income adults when compared to similar communities during the same time period.[167] In addition to pricing strategies, other community-level strategies related to diet include providing healthy food retail (e.g., supermarkets, farmers markets) in underserved communities and establishing nutrition standards for foods served in government venues.[56,130,160]

CONCLUSION

In summary, this chapter demonstrates that the problem of obesity is common, costly, and serious. However, the problem can be addressed through public-health strategies that are evidence-based and that target individuals as well as the places they live, learn, and work.

References

1. Hales CM, Carroll MD, Fryar CD, Ogden CL. Prevalence of obesity among adults and youth: United States, 2015–2016. *NCHS Data Brief.* 2017(288):1–8.
2. Finkelstein EA, Trogdon JG, Cohen JW, Dietz W. Annual medical spending attributable to obesity: Payer-and service-specific estimates. *Health Aff (Millwood).* 2009;28(5):822–31.
3. Trogdon JG, Finkelstein EA, Feagan C, Feagan CW, Cohen J, Cohen JW. State- and payer-specific estimates of annual medical expenditures attributable to obesity. *Obesity.* 2012;20(1):214–20.
4. Reilly JJ, Methven E, McDowell ZC, et al. Health consequences of obesity. *Arch Dis Child.* 2003;88(9):748–52.
5. National Institutes of Health, National Heart, Lung, and Blood Institute. *Managing Overweight and Obesity in Adults: Systematic Evidence Review from the Obesity Expert Panel, 2013.* Rockville, MD: Agency for Healthcare Research and Quality; 2013, pp. 1-501. https://www.nhlbi.nih.gov/health-topics/managing-overweight-obesity-in-adults. Accessed May 7, 2019.
6. Finkelstein EA, Khavjou OA, Thompson H, et al. Obesity and severe obesity forecasts through 2030. *Am J Prev Med.* 2012;42(6):563–70.
7. National Institutes of Health, National Heart, Lung, and Blood Institute. *Clinical Guidelines on the Identification, Evaluation, and Treatment of Overweight and Obesity in Adults.* Bethesda, MD: National Heart, Lung, and Blood Institute; 1998. https://www.nhlbi.nih.gov/files/docs/guidelines/ob_gdlns.pdf. Accessed August 8, 2018.
8. World Health Organization. Obesity: Preventing and managing the global epidemic. *World Health Organ Tech Rep Ser.* Report of a WHO Consultation. WHO Technical Report Series 894. 2000, pp. i–xii, 1–253. http://whqlibdoc.who.int/trs/WHO_TRS_894.pdf. Accessed August 8, 2018
9. Division of Nutrition, Physical Activity, and Obesity, National Center for Chronic Disease Prevention and Health Promotion, Centers for Disease Control and Prevention. Defining adult overweight and obesity. https://www.cdc.gov/obesity/adult/defining.html. Accessed August 8, 2018.
10. Division of Nutrition, Physical Activity, and Obesity, National Center for Chronic Disease Prevention and Health Promotion, Centers for Disease Control and Prevention. Defining childhood obesity. https://www.cdc.gov/obesity/childhood/defining.html. Accessed August 8, 2018.
11. Grummer-Strawn LM, Reinold C, Krebs NF. Use of World Health Organization and CDC Growth Charts for children aged 0–59 months in the United States. *MMWR Morb Mortal Wkly Rep.* 2010;59(RR09):1.
12. World Health Organization. Child growth standards. https://www.who.int/childgrowth/en/. Accessed May 1, 2019.
13. Kelly AS, Barlow SE, Rao G, et al. Severe obesity in children and adolescents: Identification, associated health risks, and treatment approaches: A scientific statement from the American Heart Association. *Circulation.* 2013(128):1689–712.
14. Barlow SE. Expert committee recommendations regarding the prevention, assessment, and treatment of child and adolescent overweight and obesity: Summary report. *Pediatrics.* 2007;120(Suppl 4):S164–92.
15. Freedman DS, Ogden CL, Kit BK. Interrelationships between BMI, skinfold thicknesses, percent body fat, and cardiovascular disease risk factors among U.S. children and adolescents. *BMC Pediatr.* 2015;15:188.
16. Garrow JS, Webster J. Quetelet's index (W/H2) as a measure of fatness. *Int J Obes.* 1985;9(2):147–53.
17. WHO Expert Consultation. Appropriate body-mass index for Asian populations and its implications for policy and intervention strategies. *Lancet.* 2004;363(9412):157–63.
18. Clark AE, Taylor JY, Wu CY, Smith JA. Alternative methods for measuring obesity in African American women. *Yale Jl of Biol and Med.* 2013;86(1):29–39.
19. Gorber SC, Tremblay M, Moher D, Gorber B. A comparison of direct vs. self-report measures for assessing height, weight and body mass index: a systematic review. *Obes Rev.* 2007;8(4):307–26.
20. Weden MM, Brownell PB, Rendall MS, Lau C, Fernandes M, Nazarov Z. Parent-reported height and weight as sources of bias in survey estimates of childhood obesity. *Am J Epidemiol.* 2013;178(3):461–73.
21. Rahman M, Berenson AB. Accuracy of current body mass index obesity classification for white, black and Hispanic reproductive-age women. *Obstet Gynecol.* 2010;115(5):982–8.
22. Freedman DS, Wang J, Thornton JC, et al. Racial/ethnic differences in body fatness among children and adolescents. *Obes.* 2008;16(5):1105–11.
23. Flegal KM, Kit BK, Orpana H, Graubard BI. Association of all-cause mortality with overweight and obesity using standard body mass index categories: A systematic review and meta-analysis. *JAMA.* 2013;309(1): 71–82.
24. Flegal KM, Graubard BI. Estimates of excess deaths associated with body mass index and other anthropometric variables. *Am J Clin Nutr.* 2009;89(4):1213–9.
25. Sun Q, Van Dam RM, Spiegelman D, Heymsfield SB, Hu FB. Comparison of dual-energy x-ray absorptiometric and anthropometric measures of adiposity in relation to adiposity-related biologic factors. *Am J Epidemiol.* 2010;172(12):1442–54.
26. Hetherington-Rauth M, Bea JW, Lee VR, et al. Comparison of direct measures of adiposity with indirect measures for assessing cardiometabolic risk factors in preadolescent girls. *Nutr J.* 2017;16:15.
27. Alves Junior CA, Mocellin MC, Andrade Goncalves EC, Silva DA, Trindade EB. Anthropometric indicators as body fat discriminators in children and adolescents: A systematic review and meta-analysis. *Adv Nutr.* 2017;8(5):718–27.
28. Latzer Y, Stein D. A review of the psychological and familial perspectives of childhood obesity. *J Eating Disorders.* 2013;1:7–7.
29. Cunningham SA, Kramer MR, Narayan KMV. Incidence of childhood obesity in the United States. *NEJM.* 2014;370(5):403–11.
30. Hoffmans MD, Kromhout DF, De Lezenne CC. The impact of body mass index of 78,612 18-year old Dutch men on 32-year mortality from all causes. *J Clinl Epidemiol.* 1988;41(8):749–56.
31. Hirko KA, Kantor ED, Cohen SS, Blot WJ, Stampfer MJ, Signorello LB. Body mass index in young adulthood, obesity trajectory, and premature mortality. *Am J Epidemiol.* 2015;182(5):441–50.
32. Kasen S, Cohen P, Chen H, Must A. Obesity and psychopathology in women: A three decade prospective study. *Int J Obes.* 2008;32(3): 558–66.
33. Roberts RE, Deleger S, Strawbridge WJ, Kaplan GA. Prospective association between obesity and depression: Evidence from the Alameda County Study. *Int J Obes Relat Metab Disord.* 2003;27(4):514–21.

34. Luppino FS, De Wit LM, Bouvy PF, et al. Overweight, obesity, and depression: A systematic review and meta-analysis of longitudinal studies. *Arch Gen Psychiatry*. 2010;67(3):220–9.

35. Lauby-Secretan B, Scoccianti C, Loomis D, Grosse Y, Bianchini F, Straif K. Body fatness and cancer—Viewpoint of the IARC Working Group. *NEJM*. 2016;375(8):794–8.

36. Steele CB, Thomas CC, Henley SJ, et al. Vital signs: Trends in incidence of cancers associated with overweight and obesity—United States, 2005–2014. *MMWR Morb Mortal Wkly Rep*. 2017;66(39):1052–8.

37. Pi-Sunyer X. The medical risks of obesity. *Postgrad Med*. 2009;121(6):21–33.

38. Nyberg ST, Batty GD, Pentti J, et al. Obesity and loss of disease-free years owing to major non-communicable diseases: A multicohort study. *Lancet Public Health*. 2018;3(10):e90–7.

39. Tremmel M, Gerdtham UG, Nilsson PM, Saha S. Economic burden of obesity: A systematic literature review. *Int J Environ Res Public Health*. 2017;14(4):435.

40. Cawley J, Meyerhoefer CF, Biener AF, Hammer MF, Wintfeld N. Savings in medical expenditures associated with reductions in body mass index among US adults with obesity, by diabetes status. *Pharmacoeconomics*. 2015;33(7):707–22.

41. Biener A, Cawley J, Meyerhoefer C. The impact of obesity on medical care costs and labor market outcomes in the US. *Clin Chem*. 2018;64(1):108–17.

42. Trasande L, Chatterjee S. The impact of obesity on health service utilization and costs in childhood. *Obes*. 2009;17(9):1749–54.

43. Arterburn DE, Maciejewski Ml, Tsevat J. Impact of morbid obesity on medical expenditures in adults. *Int J Obes*. 2005;29(3):334–9.

44. Wang Y, Beydoun MA. The obesity epidemic in the United States—Gender, age, socioeconomic, racial/ethnic, and geographic characteristics: A systematic review and meta-regression analysis. *Epidemiol Rev*. 2007;29(1):6–28.

45. Blackwell DL, Villarroel MA; US Department of Health and Human Services, Centers for Disease Control and Prevention, National Center for Health Statistics. Summary Health Statistics: National Health Interview Survey, 2016: Table A-15a. Age-adjusted percent distribution (with standard errors) of body mass index among adults aged 18 and over, by selected characteristics: United States, 2016. https://ftp.cdc.gov/pub/Health_Statistics/NCHS/NHIS/SHS/2016_SHS_Table_A-15.pdf. Accessed June 15, 2018.

46. Ogden CL, Fakhouri TH, Carroll MD, et al. Prevalence of obesity among adults, by household income and education—United States, 2011–2014. *MMWR Morb Mortal Wkly Rep*. 2017;66(50):1369.

47. Division of Nutrition, Physical Activity, and Obesity, National Center for Chronic Disease Prevention and Health Promotion, Centers for Disease Control and Prevention. Adult Obesity Prevalence Maps. https://www.cdc.gov/obesity/data/prevalence-maps.html. Accessed June, 7, 2018.

48. Lundeen E, Park S, Pan L, O'Toole T, Matthews K, Blanck H. Obesity prevalence among adults living in metropolitan and nonmetropolitan counties—United States, 2016. *MMWR Morb Mortal Wkly Rep*. 2018;67:653–8.

49. Pan L, Freedman DS, Sharma AJ, et al. Trends in obesity among participants aged 2–4 years in the special supplemental nutrition program for women, infants, and children—United States, 2000–2014. *MMWR Morb Mortal Wkly Rep*. 2016;65(45):1256–60.

50. Ogden CL, Fryar CD, Hales CM, Carroll MD, Aoki YA, Freedman DS. Differences in obesity prevalence by demographics and ubanization in US children and adolescents. *JAMA*. 2018;319(23):2410–8.

51. Flegal KM, Carroll MD, Kuczmarski RJ, Johnson CL. Overweight and obesity in the United States: Prevalence and trends, 1960–1994. *Int J Obes Relat Metab Disord*. 1998;22(1):39–47.

52. Flegal KM, Kruszon-Moran D, Carroll MD, Fryar CD, Ogden CL. Trends in obesity among adults in the United States, 2005 to 2014. *JAMA*. 2016;315(21):2284–91.

53. Hales CM, Fryar CD, Carroll MD, Freedman DS, Ogden CL. Trends in obesity and severe obesity prevalence in US youth and adults by sex and age, 2007–2008 to 2015–2016. *JAMA*. 2018;319(16):1723–5.

54. Hall KD, Sacks G, Chandramohan D, et al. Quantification of the effect of energy imbalance on bodyweight. *Lancet*. 2011;378(9793):826–37.

55. US Department of Health and Human Services. *The Surgeon General's Vision for a Healthy and Fit Nation*. Rockville, MD: U.S. Department of Health and Human Services, Office of the Surgeon General; 2010, pp. 1–21. https://www.ncbi.nlm.nih.gov/books/NBK44660/. Accessed January 4, 2019.

56. Institute of Medicine, Committee on Accelerating Progress in Obesity Prevention, Food and Nutrition Board. In: Glickman D, Parker L, Sim LJ, Cook HDV, Miller EA, eds. *Accelerating Progress in Obesity Prevention: Solving the Weight of the Nation*. Washington, DC: National Academies Press (US); 2012. http://nationalacademies.org/hmd/Reports/2012/Accelerating-Progress-in-Obesity-Prevention.aspx. Accessed January 4, 2019.

57. Woo Baidal JA, Locks LM, Cheng ER, Blake-Lamb TL, Perkins ME, Taveras EM. Risk factors for childhood obesity in the first 1,000 days: A systematic review. *Am J Prev Med*. 2016;50(6):761–79.

58. Lau EY, Liu J, Archer E, McDonald SM, Liu J. Maternal weight gain in pregnancy and risk of obesity among offspring: A systematic review. *J Obes*. 2014;2014:524939.

59. Mamun AA, Mannan M, Doi SA. Gestational weight gain in relation to offspring obesity over the life course: A systematic review and bias-adjusted meta-analysis. *Obes Rev*. 2014;15(4):338–47.

60. Ino T. Maternal smoking during pregnancy and offspring obesity: Meta-analysis. *Pediatr Int*. 2010;52(1):94–9.

61. Gaillard R. Maternal obesity during pregnancy and cardiovascular development and disease in the offspring. *Eur J Epidemiol*. 2015;30(11):1141–52.

62. Heindel JJ, Newbold R, Schug TT. Endocrine disruptors and obesity. *Nat Rev Endocrinol*. 2015;11(11):653–61.

63. Victora CG, Bahl R, Barros AJ, et al. Breastfeeding in the 21st century: Epidemiology, mechanisms, and lifelong effect. *Lancet*. 2016;387(10017):475–90.

64. Pearce J, Taylor MA, Langley-Evans SC. Timing of the introduction of complementary feeding and risk of childhood obesity: A systematic review. *In J Obes*. 2013;37(10):1295–306.

65. Pearce J, Langley-Evans SC. The types of food introduced during complementary feeding and risk of childhood obesity: A systematic review. *Int J Obes*. 2013;37(4):477–85.

66. Beauchamp GK, Mennella JA. Early flavor learning and its impact on later feeding behavior. *J Pediatr Gastroenterol Nutr*. 2009;48(Suppl 1): S25–30.

67. National Research Council (US) Committee on Diet and Health. *Diet and Health: Implications for Reducing Chronic Disease Risk*. Washington, DC: National Academies Press (US); 1989.

68. U.S. Department of Agriculture and U.S Department of Health and Human Services. *2015-2020 Dietary Guidelines for Americans*. 8th ed. Washington, DC: US Department of Agriculture and US Department of Health and Human Services; 2015, pp. 1–144. https://health.gov/dietaryguidelines/2015/guidelines/. Accessed January 4, 2019.

69. Fardet A, Boirie Y. Associations between food and beverage groups and major diet-related chronic diseases: An exhaustive review of pooled/meta-analyses and systematic reviews. *Nutr Rev*. 2014;72(12):741–62.

70. Almiron-Roig E, Palla L, Guest K, et al. Factors that determine energy compensation: A systematic review of preload studies. *Nutr Rev*. 2013;71(7):458–73.

71. Malik VS, Pan A, Willett WC, Hu FB. Sugar-sweetened beverages and weight gain in children and adults: A systematic review and meta-analysis. *Am J Clin Nutr*. 2013;98(4):1084–102.

72. Malik VS, Hu FB. Fructose and cardiometabolic health: What the evidence from sugar-sweetened beverages tells us. *J Amer Coll Cardiol*. 2015;66(14):1615–24.

73. Johnson F, Wardle J. Variety, palatability, and obesity. *Adv Nutr*. 2014;5(6):851–9.

74. Nguyen BT, Powell LM. The impact of restaurant consumption among US adults: Effects on energy and nutrient intakes. *Public Health Nutr*. 2014;17(11):2445–52.

75. Bezerra IN, Curioni C, Sichieri R. Association between eating out of home and body weight. *Nutr Rev*. 2012;70(2):65–79.

76. Sanmiguel C, Gupta A, Mayer EA. Gut microbiome and obesity: A plausible explanation for obesity. *Curr Obes Rep*. 2015;4(2):250–61.

77. Chen J, He X, Huang J. Diet effects in gut microbiome and obesity. *J Food Sci*. 2014;79(4):R442–51.

78. Dietary Guidelines Advisory Committee. *Scientific Report of the 2015 Dietary Guidelines Advisory Committee*. Washington, DC: US Department of Agriculture and US Department of Health and Human Services; 2015, pp. 1–436. https://health.gov/dietaryguidelines/2015-scientific-report/. Accessed January 4, 2019.

79. Bouchard CE, Shephard RJ, Stephens TE. *Physical Activity, Fitness, and Health: International Proceedings and Consensus Statement*. Champaign, IL, England: Human Kinetics Publishers; 1994.

80. US Department of Health Human Services. *Physical Activity and Health: A Report of the Surgeon General*. Atlanta, GA: U.S. Department of Health and Human Services, Centers for Disease Control and Prevention,

National Center for Chronic Disease Prevention and Health Promotion; 1996, pp. 1–300. http://www.cdc.gov/nccdphp/sgr/pdf/execsumm.pdf. Accessed January 4, 2019.

81. US Department of Health and Human Services, Physical Activity Guidelines Advisory Committee. *2018 Physical Activity Guidelines Advisory Committee Scientific Report.* Washington, DC: US Department of Health and Human Services; 2018. https://health.gov/paguidelines/second-edition/report/. Accessed January 4, 2019.

82. Ainsworth BE, Haskell WL, Herrmann SD, et al. 2011 Compendium of physical activities: A second update of codes and MET values. *Med Sci Sports Exer.* 2011;43(8):1575–81.

83. Donnelly JE, Blair SN, Jakicic JM, Manore MM, Rankin JW, Smith BK. American College of Sports Medicine Position Stand. Appropriate physical activity intervention strategies for weight loss and prevention of weight regain for adults. *Med Sci Sports Exerc.* 2009;41(2):459–71.

84. US Department of Health and Human Services. *Physical Activity Guidelines for Americans, 2nd edition.* Washington, DC: U.S. Department of Health and Human Services; 2018, pp. 1–118. https://health.gov/paguidelines/second-edition/. Accessed January 4, 2019.

85. Blundell JE, Gibbons C, Caudwell P, Finlayson G, Hopkins M. Appetite control and energy balance: Impact of exercise. *Obes Rev.* 2015;16(Suppl 1): 67–76.

86. Speakman JR, Selman C. Physical activity and resting metabolic rate. *Proc Nutr Soc.* 2003;62(3):621–34.

87. Biddle SJH, Pearson N, Salmon J. Sedentary behaviors and adiposity in young people: Causality and conceptual model. *Exerc Sport Sci Rev.* 2018;46(1):18–25.

88. Campbell SDI, Brosnan BJ, Chu AKY, et al. Sedentary behavior and body weight and composition in adults: A systematic review and meta-analysis of prospective studies. *Sports Med.* 2018;48(3):585–95.

89. Cliff DP, Hesketh KD, Vella SA, et al. Objectively measured sedentary behaviour and health and development in children and adolescents: Systematic review and meta-analysis. *Obes Rev.* 2016;17(4):330–44.

90. Miller MA, Kruisbrink M, Wallace J, Ji C, Cappuccio FP. Sleep duration and incidence of obesity in infants, children, and adolescents: A systematic review and meta-analysis of prospective studies. *Sleep.* 2018;41(4).

91. Ruan H, Xun P, Cai W, He K, Tang Q. Habitual sleep duration and risk of childhood obesity: Systematic review and dose-response meta-analysis of prospective cohort studies. *Sci Rep.* 2015;5:16160.

92. Magee L, Hale L. Longitudinal associations between sleep duration and subsequent weight gain: A systematic review. *Sleep Med Rev.* 2012;16(3):231–41.

93. Patel SR, Hu FB. Short sleep duration and weight gain: A systematic review. *Obes.* 2008;16(3):643–53.

94. Janesick AS, Blumberg B. Obesogens: An emerging threat to public health. *Am J Obstet Gynecol.* 2016;214(5):559–65.

95. Tang-Peronard JL, Andersen HR, Jensen TK, Heitmann BL. Endocrine-disrupting chemicals and obesity development in humans: A review. *Obes Rev.* 2011;12(8):622–36.

96. Martin CB, Herrick KA, Sarafrazi N, Ogden CL. Attempts to lose weight among adults in the United States, 2013–2016. *NCHS Data Brief.* 2018;(313):1–8. https://www.cdc.gov/nchs/products/databriefs/db313.htm. Accessed January 4, 2019.

97. Kann L, McManus T, Harris WA, et al. Youth risk behavior surveillance—United States, 2017. *MMWR Surveill Summ.* 2018;67(8):1–114.

98. Rajjo T, Almasri J, Al Nofal A, et al. The association of weight loss and cardiometabolic outcomes in obese children: Systematic review and meta-regression. *J Clin Endocrinol Metab.* 2017;102(3):758–62.

99. Bliddal H, Leeds AR, Christensen R. Osteoarthritis, obesity and weight loss: Evidence, hypotheses and horizons—A scoping review. *Obes Rev.* 2014;15(7):578–86.

100. Knowler WC, Barrett-Connor E, Fowler SE, et al. Reduction in the incidence of type 2 diabetes with lifestyle intervention or metformin. *N Engl J Med.* 2002;346(6):393–403.

101. Birks S, Peeters A, Backholer K, O'Brien P, Brown W. A systematic review of the impact of weight loss on cancer incidence and mortality. *Obes Rev.* 2012;13(10):868–91.

102. Ma C, Avenell A, Bolland M, et al. Effects of weight loss interventions for adults who are obese on mortality, cardiovascular disease, and cancer: Systematic review and meta-analysis. *BMJ.* 2017;359:j4849.

103. Pack QR, Rodriguez-Escudero JP, Thomas RJ, et al. The prognostic importance of weight loss in coronary artery disease: A systematic review and meta-analysis. *Mayo Clin Proc.* 2014;89(10):1368–77.

104. Wing RR, Bolin P, Brancati FL, et al. Cardiovascular effects of intensive lifestyle intervention in type 2 diabetes. *N Engl J Med.* 2013;369(2):145–54.

105. U.S. Preventive Services Task Force. Behavioral weight loss interventions to prevent obesity-related morbidiy and mortality in adults: U.S. Preventive Services Task Force Recommendation statement. *JAMA.* 2018:320(11):1163–71.

106. Grossman DC, Bibbins-Domingo K, Curry SJ, et al. Screening for obesity in children and adolescents: US Preventive Services Task Force Recommendation Statement. *JAMA.* 2017;317(23):2417–26.

107. Gow ML, Ho M, Burrows TL, et al. Impact of dietary macronutrient distribution on BMI and cardiometabolic outcomes in overweight and obese children and adolescents: A systematic review. *Nutr Rev.* 2014;72(7):453–70.

108. Johns DJ, Hartmann-Boyce J, Jebb SA, Aveyard P. Diet or exercise interventions vs combined behavioral weight management programs: A systematic review and meta-analysis of direct comparisons. *J Acad Nutr Diet.* 2014;114(10):1557–68.

109. Ho M, Garnett SP, Baur LA, et al. Impact of dietary and exercise interventions on weight change and metabolic outcomes in obese children and adolescents: A systematic review and meta-analysis of randomized trials. *JAMA Pediatr.* 2013;167(8):759–68.

110. Swift DL, Johannsen NM, Lavie CJ, Earnest CP, Church TS. The role of exercise and physical activity in weight loss and maintenance. *Prog Cardiovasc Dis.* 2014;56(4):441–7.

111. Shaw K, Gennat H, O'Rourke P, Del Mar C. Exercise for overweight or obesity. *Cochrane Database Syst Rev.* 2006;(4):Cd003817.

112. Physical Activity Guidelines Scientific Committee. *Physical Activity Guidelines Advisory Committee Report, 2008.* Washington, DC: US Department of Health and Human Services; 2008, pp. 1–76. https://health.gov/paguidelines/2008/report/. Accessed January 4, 2019.

113. Kelley GA, Kelley KS, Pate RR. Effects of exercise on BMI z-score in overweight and obese children and adolescents: A systematic review with meta-analysis. *BMC Pediatr.* 2014;14:225.

114. Apovian CM, Aronne LJ, Bessesen DH, et al. Pharmacological management of obesity: An Endocrine Society clinical practice guideline. *J Clinl Endocrin Meta.* 2015;100(2):342–62.

115. Greig SL, Keating GM. Naltrexone ER/Bupropion ER: A review in obesity management. *Drugs.* 2015;75(11):1269–80.

116. Nuffer WA, Trujillo JM. Liraglutide: A new option for the treatment of obesity. *Pharmacotherapy.* 2015;35(10):926–34.

117. Yanovski SZ, Yanovski JA. Long-term drug treatment for obesity: A systematic and clinical review. *JAMA.* 2014;311(1):74–86.

118. Khera R, Murad MH, Chandar AK, et al. Association of pharmacological treatments for obesity with weight loss and adverse events: A systematic review and meta-analysis. *JAMA.* 2016;315(22):2424–34.

119. Shoar S, Mahmoudzadeh H, Naderan M, et al. Long-term outcome of bariatric surgery in morbidly obese adolescents: A systematic review and meta-analysis of 950 patients with a minimum of 3 years follow-up. *Obes Surg.* 2017;27(12):3110–7.

120. Kwok CS, Pradhan A, Khan MA, et al. Bariatric surgery and its impact on cardiovascular disease and mortality: A systematic review and meta-analysis. *Int J Cardiol.* 2014;173(1):20–8.

121. Chang SH, Stoll CR, Song J, Varela JE, Eagon CJ, Colditz GA. The effectiveness and risks of bariatric surgery: An updated systematic review and meta-analysis, 2003–2012. *JAMA Surg.* 2014;149(3):275–87.

122. Pratt JS, Lenders CM, Dionne EA, et al. Best practice updates for pediatric/adolescent weight loss surgery. *Obes.* 2009;17(5):901–10.

123. Frieden TR. A framework for public health action: The health impact pyramid. *Am J Public Health.* 2010;100(4):590–5.

124. Halliday JA, Palma CL, Mellor D, Green J, Renzaho AM. The relationship between family functioning and child and adolescent overweight and obesity: A systematic review. *Int J Obes.* 2014;38(4):480–93.

125. O'Connor EA, Evans CV, Burda BU, Walsh ES, Eder M, Lozano P. Screening for obesity and intervention for weight management in children and adolescents: Evidence report and systematic review for the US Preventive Services Task Force. *JAMA.* 2017;317(23):2427–44.

126. Sung-Chan P, Sung YW, Zhao X, Brownson RC. Family-based models for childhood-obesity intervention: A systematic review of randomized controlled trials. *Obes Rev.* 2013;14(4):265–78.

127. Showell NN, Fawole O, Segal J, et al. A systematic review of home-based childhood obesity prevention studies. *Pediatrics.* 2013;132(1):e193–200.

128. Haines J, McDonald J, O'Brien A, et al. Healthy habits, happy homes: Randomized trial to improve household routines for obesity prevention among preschool-aged children. *JAMA Pediatr.* 2013;167(11):1072–9.

129. U.S. Department of Education, National Center for Education Statistics. Early Childhood Program Participation Survey of the National Household Education Surveys Program (ECPP-NHES:2005). https://

nces.ed.gov/programs/digest/d09/tables/dt09_044.asp. Accessed August 22, 2018.

130. Khan LK, Sobush K, Keener D, et al. Recommended community strategies and measurements to prevent obesity in the United States. *MMWR Recomm Rep*. 2009;58(RR-7):1–26.

131. United States Department of Agriculture. Child and Adult Care Food Program (CACFP): Child care centers. https://www.fns.usda.gov/cacfp/child-day-care-centers. Accessed July 30, 2018.

132. National Resource Center for Health and Safety in Child Care and Early Education Healthy Weight. http://nrckids.org/HealthyWeight. Accessed July 29, 2018.

133. Centers for Disease Control and Prevention. The spectrum of opportunities framework for state-level obesity prevention efforts targeting the early care and education setting. https://www.cdc.gov/obesity/strategies/early-care-education/pdf/TheSpectrumofOpportunitiesFramework_May2018_508.pdf. Accessed January 4, 2019.

134. Sisson SB, Krampe M, Anundson K, Castle S. Obesity prevention and obesogenic behavior interventions in child care: A systematic review. *Prev Med*. 2016;87:57–69.

135. Wang Y, Cai L, Wu Y, et al. What childhood obesity prevention programmes work? A systematic review and meta-analysis. *Obes Rev*. 2015;16(7):547–65.

136. Zhou YE, Emerson JS, Levine RS, Kihlberg CJ, Hull PC. Childhood obesity prevention interventions in childcare settings: Systematic review of randomized and nonrandomized controlled trials. *Am J Health Prom*. 2014;28(4):e92–103.

137. Ward DS, Welker E, Choate A, et al. Strength of obesity prevention interventions in early care and education settings: A systematic review. *Prev Med*. 2017;95(Suppl):S37–52.

138. Alkon A, Crowley AA, Neelon SE, et al. Nutrition and physical activity randomized control trial in child care centers improves knowledge, policies, and children's body mass index. *BMC Public Health*. 2014;14:215.

139. Centers for Disease Control and Prevention. School health guidelines to promote healthy eating and physical activity. *MMWR Recomm Rep*. 2011;60(RR-5):1–76.

140. United States Department of Agriculture, Food and Nutrition Service. Team nutrition: Local school wellness policy. https://www.fns.usda.gov/tn/local-school-wellness-policy. Accessed July 30, 2018.

141. United States Department of Agriculture, Food and Nutrition Service. National School Lunch Program. https://www.fns.usda.gov/nslp/national-school-lunch-program-nslp. Accessed July 30, 2018.

142. Shape America—Society of Health and Physical Educators. Shape of the nation: Status of physical education in the USA. https://www.shapeamerica.org/advocacy/son/2016/upload/Shape-of-the-Nation-2016_web.pdf. Accessed July 30, 2018.

143. Langford R, Bonell CP, Jones HE, et al. The WHO Health Promoting School framework for improving the health and well-being of students and their academic achievement. *Cochrane Database System Rev*. 2014;(4):Cd008958.

144. Waters E, De Silva-Sanigorski A, Hall BJ, et al. Interventions for preventing obesity in children. *Cochrane Database System Rev*. 2011;(12):Cd001871.

145. Coleman KJ, Tiller CL, Sanchez J, et al. Prevention of the epidemic increase in child risk of overweight in low-income schools: The El Paso coordinated approach to child health. *Arch Pediatr Adoles Med*. 2005;159(3):217–24.

146. Hoelscher DM, Springer AE, Ranjit N, et al. Reductions in child obesity among disadvantaged school children with community involvement: The Travis County CATCH Trial. *Obes*. 2010;18(Suppl 1):S36–44.

147. U.S. Department of Labor, Bureau of Labor Statistics. Labor force statistics from the Current Population Survey. https://www.bls.gov/cps/cpsaat08.pdf. Accessed July 29, 2018.

148. Yarborough CM 3rd, Brethauer S, Burton WN, et al. Obesity in the workplace: Impact, outcomes, and recommendations. *J Occup Environ Med*. 2018;60(1):97–107.

149. Anderson LM, Quinn TA, Glanz K, et al. The effectiveness of worksite nutrition and physical activity interventions for controlling employee overweight and obesity: A systematic review. *Am J Prev Med*. 2009;37(4):340–57.

150. Vanderveur J, Gilchrist S, Matson-Koffman D. An overview of state policies supporting worksite health promotion programs. *Am J Health Prom*. 2017;31(3):232–42.

151. Harvard T.H. Chan—School of Public Health. Worksite obesity prevention recommendations: Complete list. https://www.hsph.harvard.edu/obesity-prevention-source/obesity-prevention/worksites/worksites-obesity-prevention-recommendations-complete-list. Accessed July 29, 2018.

152. Gudzune K, Hutfless S, Maruthur N, Wilson R, Segal J. Strategies to prevent weight gain in workplace and college settings: A systematic review. *Prev Med*. 2013;57(4):268–77.

153. Weinhold KR, Miller CK, Marrero DG, Nagaraja HN, Focht BC, Gascon GM. A randomized controlled trial translating the Diabetes Prevention Program to a university worksite, Ohio, 2012–2014. *Prev Chronic Dis*. 2015;12:e2.

154. U.S. Department of Health and Human Services. Food service guidelines federal workgroup food service guidelines for federal facilities. https://www.cdc.gov/obesity/downloads/guidelines_for_federal_concessions_and_vending_operations.pdf. Accessed January 4, 2019.

155. National Center for Health Statistics. Ambulatory care use and physician office visits. https://www.cdc.gov/nchs/fastats/physician-visits.htm. Accessed July 30, 2018.

156. Daniels SR, Hassink SG. The role of the pediatrician in primary prevention of obesity. *Pediatrics*. 2015;136(1):e275–92.

157. Jensen MD, Ryan DH, Apovian CM, et al. *2013 AHA*/ACC/TOS guideline for the management of overweight and obesity in adults: A report of the American College of Cardiology/American Heart Association Task Force on Practice Guidelines and The Obesity Society. *Circulation*. 2014;129(25 Suppl 2):S102–38.

158. Sacher PM, Kolotourou M, Chadwick PM, et al. Randomized controlled trial of the MEND program: A family-based community intervention for childhood obesity. *Obes*. 2010;18(Suppl 1):S62–8.

159. National Committee for Quality Assurance. HEDIS and performance measurement. http://www.ncqa.org/hedis-quality-measurement. Accessed July 30, 2018.

160. Institute of Medicine, National Research Council, Committee on Childhood Obesity Prevention Actions for Local Governments. In: Parker L, Burns AC, Sanchez E, eds. *Local Government Actions to Prevent Childhood Obesity*. Washington, DC: National Academies Press (US); 2009. https://www.nap.edu/catalog/12674/local-government-actions-to-prevent-childhood-obesity. Accessed January 4, 2019.

161. Ottley PG, Dawkins-Lyn N, Harris C, et al. Childhood obesity declines project: An exploratory study of strategies identified in communities reporting declines. *Child Obes*. 2018;14(S1):S12–21.

162. Economos CD, Hyatt RR, Goldberg JP, et al. A community intervention reduces BMI z-score in children: Shape Up Somerville first year results. *Obes*. 2007;15(5):1325–36.

163. Economos CD, Hyatt RR, Must A, et al. Shape Up Somerville two-year results: A community-based environmental change intervention sustains weight reduction in children. *Prev Med*. 2013;57(4):322–7.

164. Coffield E, Nihiser AJ, Sherry B, Economos CD. Shape Up Somerville: Change in parent body mass indexes during a child-targeted, community-based environmental change intervention. *Am J Public Health*. 2015;105(2):e83–9.

165. Task Force on Community Preventive Services. Increasing physical activity. A report on recommendations of the Task Force on Community Preventive Services. *MMWR Recomm Rep*. 2001;50(RR-18):1–14.

166. Community Preventive Services Task. *Physical Activity: Built Environment Approaches Combining Transportation System Interventions with Land Use and Environmental Design*. Atlanta, GA: Community Preventive Services Task; 2016. https://www.thecommunityguide.org/findings/physical-activity-built-environment-approaches. Accessed July 30, 2018.

167. Falbe J, Thompson HR, Becker CM, Rojas N, Mcculloch CE, Madsen KA. Impact of the Berkeley excise tax on sugar-sweetened beverage consumption. *Am J Public Health*. 2016;106(10):1865–71.

CHAPTER

182

Nutritional Epidemiology

James R. Hebert

INTRODUCTION

Eating food is something that most people do every day of their lives. Indeed, to go for too long without food will lead to disability, disease and, ultimately, death. Therefore, it should not be surprising that cultures throughout history have sought to understand the role of dietary exposures (i.e., the foods we eat) in determining health and well-being. Interest in understanding the role of diet in health extends back millennia in the Greek, Ayurvedic, and Chinese traditional medicine systems[1–5]; that is, long before scientific medicine, as we know it, came to the West. It is interesting to note that in the modern (post-Medieval) Western tradition the first clinical trial, conducted by Lind in the middle of the eighteenth century,[6] focused on a dietary factor (i.e., ascorbic acid-rich limes for the prevention and treatment of scurvy among sailors on long journeys). That work preceded by a century that of John Snow,[7] who showed that cholera was spread by contaminated water (and even that is a nutritional exposure of sorts!) and is widely credited to be the father of modern epidemiology.

Careful observations regarding the role of diet in health have been recorded throughout human history and have become part of cultural traditions all over the world including in: East Asia (e.g., Chinese Traditional Medicine); South Asia (e.g., Ayurvedic and Siddha Medicine); West Asia/Middle East (e.g., Persian Medicine); Africa (e.g., Herbalism); the Americas (Herbalism and Culinary Traditions); and Europe (e.g., Greek Medicine).[1–5] These traditions incorporate the concept of balance, with the specific understanding that manifestation of imbalance, including a clinical diagnosis of a disease, can be rectified through changes in lifestyle behaviors. All of these traditions credit dietary factors with playing an essential role in restoring equilibrium to the body. While specific, culture-bound explanations may differ from the kind of evidence that we associate with modern medical science, the conclusions are strikingly similar. For example, specific foods that are recommended in the Asian tradition include ginger, garlic, onion, cloves, cardamom, nutmeg, and pepper[8,9]; all of which we now know can reduce chronic systemic inflammation.[10–13]

Many dietary traditions began as part of larger systems of religious and spiritual thought, philosophy, and practice.[14,15] While it might be unusual to encounter a patient who understands the concept of balance and the role of nutrition in restoring biological systems to a state of homeostasis, and rarer still to find someone who understands the philosophical underpinnings in these traditions, most people understand the importance of a healthy diet in maintaining or restoring good health. So, it is not surprising that patients often present with strong feelings about diet. These may include a desire or intention to reverse or slow the progression of some specific condition or disease, and evidence has existed for several decades that heart disease, type 2 diabetes, and even prostate cancer may be reversible.[16–21] All of these findings are consistent with the ability of nutrition to modulate metabolic inflammation.[22]

THE NATURE OF EVIDENCE FOR THE ROLE OF DIET IN HEALTH

As through most of history, in the modern era there is legitimate concern regarding competing claims as to the role of specific dietary factors in maintaining and restoring health. So, it is important to understand how we come to make inferences about the role of diet in health. A common complaint that we hear from the general public is that the evidence regarding the effect of a particular nutrient, food, or way of eating on health outcomes is constantly changing. Some of the frustration, no doubt reflected in patients' opinions, appears to be well warranted.[23,24] However, we need to put this into perspective. A useful way to do this is to consider the Criteria for Judging Causality, developed by Bradford Hill[25] in the early 1950s. This schema is based on Hill's work with Sir Richard Doll on the role of smoking in lung cancer.[26] It was later popularized in the 1964 Surgeon General Report on Smoking and Health.[27] This way of thinking, which employs the hierarchy of criteria shown in Box 182-1, provides a very useful framework for keeping a perspective on evidence in relation to assessing causality. Plausibility, which is often a concern of basic scientists and is inherent in the didactic method of medical education, is accorded less weight because it is the evidence, not simply a plausible story, that matters most when we need to decide whether or not something works.

This framework assigns the greatest weight to relationships that are stronger. It is no accident, therefore, that tobacco was deemed to be a cause of cancer, even in the absence of experimental evidence, because of the very strong risk estimates observed in the studies by Doll and Hill in the United Kingdom[26] and Wynder and Graham in the United States.[28] While there had only been a handful of studies on the subject of tobacco smoke in relation to lung cancer before the 1964 Surgeon General's report was published, virtually all of the studies that had been conducted produced very strong risk estimates that were consistent with the hypothesis that smoking causes lung cancer

BOX 182-1 Criteria for Judging Causality

1. Strength
2. Consistency
3. Specificity
4. Temporality
5. Dose-response
6. Plausibility
7. Coherence
8. Experiment
9. Analogy

Based on Hill, 1953[25]; later popularized in the 1964 Surgeon General's Report on Smoking and Health,[27] in which only the first six were listed.[b]The only *sine qua non* on the list; a cause must precede its effect in time.Refers to the story of how it works.

(and a variety of other chronic diseases). Contrast this with the situation regarding the effects of dietary factors. While the risk estimates are not so large, there are over a million references linking different aspects of diet to a wide variety of health outcomes. Far from being equivocal on most relationships, the evidence is remarkably consistent across a variety of study designs in humans.[29,30]

Other criteria on the list also are important to consider. Specificity was deemed by Hill to be important because there are things about how human beings organize their lives that underlie, and are universally associated with, other important factors that may determine health. For example, we now know that socioeconomic status is associated with numerous health outcomes, as discussed in detail in Chapter 29: The Social Determinants of Health. So, anticipating this, Hill was careful not to conflate association with causality which, after all, was the point of developing the schema in the first place. Still, a legitimate question would be: How does socioeconomic status affect health? While people who are more affluent (and are often more well educated) might eat a better diet, they also are well positioned to do other things that may improve their health. Michael Marmot, also a collaborator on the Whitehall study, has produced fascinating work on the role of social status, itself, in producing positive health outcomes. [31,32] While this is interesting and important to understand as a clinician, it is also essential to keep in mind that diet is a ubiquitous set of exposures that is related to a wide variety of health outcomes and is important even after controlling for social status and economic wealth.[33,34] So, part of what people buy with their higher social and economic status is often, but hardly always, healthier food.

Dietary factors that affect inflammation, which is a substrate for many disease-related mechanisms, will exert an effect on a wide variety of outcomes. However, the consistency of results as we point out in a recent narrative review of hundreds of articles on the Dietary Inflammatory Index (DII®) takes precedence over the fact that there tend to be few single dietary exposures that are strongly associated with a single outcome.[35] This is not too surprising given that for the vast majority of the chronic diseases responsible for most morbidity and mortality in places like the United States, we are not talking about a single infectious disease agent that causes a single disease. Even in the world of established infectious disease agents, it is interesting and important to note that Epstein-Barr virus can, depending on the nutritional status of the host, produce a wide range of outcomes from none at all to mononucleosis or even Burkitt's lymphoma.[36,37]

Temporality should be considered in light of the kinds of studies that provide us with information on diet-health outcome relationships. Although we discuss this later in the chapter, it is important to mention here that the vast majority of evidence linking dietary factors to health outcomes is from observational, not experimental, studies.[29] Clearly, this is analogous to the situation Hill and colleagues faced when considering the role of tobacco in lung cancer, where there never was (or ever will be) a randomized controlled trial (RCT) to establish the association between tobacco and cancer (or any other health outcome). Some of the observational; that is, prospective cohort, studies have a longitudinal component in that diet and other risk factors are measured prior to the time when cohort members would be diagnosed with a disease. Case-control studies, on the other hand, typically measure diet after a health condition has been diagnosed. This leaves these studies particularly vulnerable to information bias, for example, individuals modifying their recall of typical diet in the past based on their current health status, which includes the clinical diagnosis of the disease under study. Regarding dose response, it is important to note that while some dietary factors exert their effects in a dose-response manner, many do not. For example, the recommended dietary reference intakes (DRIs), described in Chapter 180: The Principles of Nutritional Sciences: Nutrients, Nutrition Recommendations, and Dietary Guidelines, are set to prevent nutrient deficiencies and these clearly relate to threshold effects—not linear dose effects.[38]

DIETARY EXPOSURES—EVERYONE EATS!

Unlike many of the exposures that we study in epidemiology, diet is unique in that one cannot go for very long without eating. So, diet is a set of ubiquitous, if widely varying, exposures. For many years, the exposures of interest in nutritional epidemiology were specific nutrients. With notable failures in the single-agent approach to assessing diet-health outcome relationships including trials of β-carotene and α-tocopherol to prevent lung cancer[39,40] and selenium and α-tocopherol to prevent prostate cancer,[41] over the past quarter century there has been a move toward focusing on overall patterns of intake. These can be: (1) deduced from data within a particular study or population (e.g., from principal components analysis or other regression techniques)[42,43]; (2) defined according to a particular cuisine (e.g., the Mediterranean diet)[44,45]; (3) determined by a set of dietary recommendations such as the Alternative Healthy Eating Index [46,47]; or (4) generated on the basis of primary research results, either from laboratory analyses (e.g., the glycemic index[48]) or in the published literature (e.g., the DII®[10]). This "whole dietary pattern" approach produces results that are imminently useful to conscientious clinicians who wish to encourage their patients to eat healthier diets.

HOW WE MEASURE THE EFFECT OF DIET

Study Designs

The evidence on which dietary recommendations are based comes from a wide variety of sources. These represent a potentially bewildering range of designs from ecological, cross-sectional, observational, and experimental studies of humans to laboratory animal and cell culture experimental. While RCTs are considered the "purest" source of evidence, they represent only a tiny fraction of the > 1 million references on diet and health in the National Library of Medicine database.[29] Also, there are a host of problems with using RCTs to test diet-related hypotheses.[30] These include: (1) the need to focus narrowly (diet is a wide-ranging set of exposures that are related to other things like stress and sleep); (2) subjects are volunteers probably different in important ways from the general population; (3) unlike a single-agent trial, blinding of dietary interventions is not possible; (4) perceived asymmetry of treatment in relation to need (e.g., for primary prevention, there may be little perceived need to participate at all, while in a secondary prevention trial subjects may want the intervention no matter random assignment to the control condition); (5) temporal relationships between dietary exposures and health outcomes (i.e., it takes an impractically long time to reach most disease endpoints); (6) the strict adherence to the intervention protocol, despite potential clinical counterindications (e.g., to lower or increase dose to improve outcome for a particular patient); and (7) the need to maintain methodological rigor including measuring diet carefully, frequently and at the right time to understand effects on metabolism and disease processes.

Clearly, RCTs are not the only way to get relevant answers to important questions about diet and health. Virtually none of the evidence regarding associations of tobacco use and health came from RCTs and the few studies that have been designed to test the hypothesis that individual micronutrients would prevent lung cancer have failed.[39,40,49,50] So, too, is this the case with prostate cancer.[51] Indeed, there are few examples of single-agent trials actually preventing or reversing disease. By contrast, that those trials that have worked to reverse chronic diseases involve whole dietary approaches that often also include other aspects of life, including stress reduction and physical activity.[16–21]

Although the sheer number of articles is biased toward observational epidemiologic studies, there is a hierarchy of types of studies that contribute evidence regarding specific diet-health relationships. This is reflected in developing the DII®[10] in which weights were assigned in this order (i.e., from highest to lowest): experiments in humans; prospective studies in humans; case-control studies in humans; cross-sectional studies in humans; laboratory animal experiments; and cell culture experiments.

Measurement Methods

Both the general public and scientists unfamiliar with the methods and philosophy of nutritional epidemiology may see results from observational studies as unreliable and confusing.[24,52–61] Over the years, there have been many reasoned responses to this so-called complaint literature, including ours.[62–71] We were able to address these concerns because we had become very familiar with sources of bias, mainly due to social approval (the desire to seek approval in a situation perceived to be a test) or social desirability (the defensive tendency to portray oneself more in keeping with perceived positive social norms) in measuring dietary intake among free living people.[72–77]

There is a large, well-established literature on methods used to measure dietary intake and examine the effect of diet on a variety of health outcomes.[29] Common methods to assess individual's diet in clinical and public health settings include structured questionnaires; that is, those with a limited food list in response categories for frequency of consumption and, usually, typical portion size consumed. The instrument most often used in these settings is the food frequency questionnaire (FFQ). Other methods include: (1) dietary recalls, usually focused on a 24-hour period or a calendar day,[78,79] but sometimes focusing on a longer period of time[80]; (2) food diaries or records, which are often used in clinical studies[81] or for counseling patients with eating disorders[82,83]; (3) short screeners[84]; and, more recently, (4) remote food photography.[85] Because these instruments rely heavily on self-report of foods consumed they may be subject to inaccuracy (e.g., from incomplete recall), imprecision (e.g., by estimating portion size incorrectly), or biases in recall (e.g., intentional or unintentional errors).

Methods such as dietary recalls or food diaries tend to be both time consuming and expensive. However, their use may be warranted in smaller-scale or more intensive studies. In most validation studies of self-reported diet, repeat 24-hour recall interviews are used as the comparator.[86,87] It is well known that individuals' dietary intake varies from day-to-day, thus data from a single administration will have extraneous variation that makes it harder to discern the "signal" of the dietary effect from the "noise" of day-to-day. Therefore, in most studies it is necessary to measure at least several days of intake, usually a minimum of three randomly selected days over a 2- to 3-week period.

Because structured questionnaires such as the FFQ are relatively inexpensive, both in terms of actual monetary cost and logistical complexity, most epidemiologic studies use these methods to assess dietary intake. Although results are fairly consistent across different populations using different versions of FFQs to answer the same research question,[35] as noted above, significant self-report biases encountered in their use have been documented within North American populations.[72–77] Because the social approval and social desirability that most reliably bias the results are sensitive to cultural norms of behavior and definitions of what foods are considered good and bad, it is conceivable that different patterns of bias might be evident in other parts of the world or in racial and ethnic subgroups. However, we have found that in the U.S. education supplants the effects of race or ethnicity; that is, highly educated women, irrespective of race, tend to underreport calorie-dense foods according to social desirability.[75]

Other methods that can be used in clinical practice include the National Cancer Institute's Fruit and Vegetable[84,88] and Percent Fat[73,89] screeners and mobile phone-based apps. These alternative methods of assessment may be useful for clinical decision-making and screening. However, they will not provide data of sufficient quality to serve as research-competent measurement devices.

WHAT KIND OF RECOMMENDATIONS CAN WE MAKE BASED ON EXISTING EVIDENCE?

There are over a million references on diet and health and the results are overwhelmingly consistent in support of diet as an important determinant of overall health. In this section, we will focus on: (1) specific nutrition-related mechanisms and conditions that are of practical interest and high importance to primary care and preventive medicine physicians, (2) characteristics of healthy diets, and (3) making recommendations fit individual's motivation and readiness to change.

Health Outcomes range from biological markers that are well known to be associated with risk of numerous diseases to actual physical and mental health outcomes.

Inflammatory and Immune Response. It is known that an acute inflammatory response is necessary for mounting a competent immune response. Acute inflammatory responses are time-limited and require negative feedback signaling between proinflammatory cytokines that turn on the response and anti-inflammatory cytokines that signal it to cease.[90,91] In contrast to acute inflammation, chronic systematic inflammation results when negative feedback does not occur, or is incomplete or inefficient.[90,92] The chronic phase is characterized by specified cellular immune response along with specific humoral responses.[93,94] In addition to diet's role in regulating acute inflammatory responses, it also has been implicated in regulating chronic inflammation.[95,96] Ironically, chronic systemic inflammation is a state of hypervigilance during which mounting a competent inflammatory response is virtually impossible. Thus, people who are in a state of chronic systemic inflammation are more likely to suffer from infections and high rates of chronic disease. For example, natural killer cell activity, an important first-line defense against cancer,[97] is diminished by calorie-dense diets with high levels of saturated fat and ω-6 polyunsaturated fats.[98,99]

Lipid Markers. It has been known for over a half-century that serum lipid concentrations predict cardiovascular disease outcomes. In the 1950s and 1960s, Ancel Keys in Minnesota[100,101] and Mark Hegsted at Harvard[102] showed in carefully conducted feeding studies that changes in the composition of dietary fatty acids could, on average, predict serum lipid changes. We confirmed this among free-living adults of both sexes when we validated the 7-day dietary recall; that is, showing that after controlling for social approval and social desirability bias we could predict actual serum LDL and total cholesterol changes within 10% and 15%, respectively, using the Keys and Hegsted predictive equations.[80]

Infections. Because of the unique nutritional needs of children and the imperative to deal with enteric and other infections, to which children are especially vulnerable, much of the initial focus of the field of immunology was on children and childhood nutrition.[103,104] It is now firmly established that infections occur more readily and are more severe in individuals with nutritional deficiencies or, in more affluent societies, among people consuming excessive amounts of calorie-dense, nutrient-sparse foods.[103,105] Over the past decade, obesity has emerged as a risk factor for complications from influenza virus infection and duration of influenza A viral shedding in adults, due to its effects on immune function and inflammation.[106–109]

Type 2 Diabetes Mellitus (T2DM). Type 2 diabetes mellitus (T2DM) produces a variety of debilitating and potentially deadly direct effects, such as peripheral vascular disease,[110–113] renal disease,[114–116] and retinopathy.[117–121] T2DM also underlies a variety of other lethal and destructive chronic diseases, including heart disease,[122–124] other cardiovascular diseases,[124–126] and a variety of cancers.[127–132] T2DM rates have risen dramatically with the epidemic of obesity.[133,134] This has occurred at alarming rates in middle-aged people (i.e., between 50 and 64 years of age).[135,136] This age group represents a window in time that is amenable to behavioral modifications for control and prevention of T2DM; that is, before the disease has progressed to cause irreversible damage. While obesity (high weight for height) is positively associated with adiposity (fat mass) in human populations, it is adiposity (primarily central adiposity),[137–146] and its strong association with inflammation, that increases disease risk.[147–153] T2DM and prediabetes are strongly proinflammatory conditions that are associated with poor dietary quality (i.e., calorie-dense, nutrient-sparse) diets. In addition to overall energy balance, specific dietary factors have been implicated in T2DM.[46]

Cancer. The observation that inflammation is related to cancer was first made in the Western tradition by Virchow in the nineteenth century.[154] Diet is related to cancer via a number of mechanisms, many associated with inflammation (e.g., nitrative and oxidative DNA damage). Although there clearly is variability with respect to different anatomic sites; in general, a nutrient-dense, calorie-sparse diet tends to lower overall risk of cancer. The cancer with the strongest connection to inflammation through its precursor condition, inflammatory bowel disease, is colorectal cancer.[155–164] Because tobacco also is a strongly proinflammatory agent it would be expected that if diet could exert a powerful enough effect it would be observable in tobacco-related cancers. Indeed, virtually all of the cancers of the upper aerodigestive tract, including laryngeal cancer,[165–167] nasopharyngeal cancer,[167–169] and esophageal cancer[167,169–174] are strongly influenced by diet-associated inflammation. Other tobacco-related cancers, including lung,[175–177] bladder,[178,179] and kidney[180–182] cancers, are similarly associated as are other cancers of the digestive tract, including pancreatic cancer,[167,183–185] liver cancer,[186,187] and gastric cancer.[188,189]

Of the hormone-sensitive cancers, prostate[167,190–199] and ovarian cancer [200–202] are more strongly related to diet (and dietary inflammation in particular) than breast cancer, for which there are some positive results,[203–207] but also some studies that have observed no relationship.[208–210] There also seems to be a relationship with non-Hodgkin Lymphoma,[211] but not with Hodgkin Lymphoma.[212]

Logically, one might conclude that having a strongly proinflammatory condition such as T2DM would place individuals at higher risk of cancer. Indeed, this is what has been observed with respect to colorectal cancer,[127] and the effects appear to be more strongly expressed in African-Americans, who are both more likely to be diagnosed with colorectal cancer and to have more virulent disease and poorer survival once diagnosed.[213–216]

Cardiovascular Diseases (CVD). CVDs encompass diseases of the heart and vascular system. Based on work completed before Stamler's description of the epidemiology of coronary heart disease (CHD) in 1979,[217] it became clear that the relationship of diet with CHD was confounded by physical activity. Once it became clear that the more physically active individuals also required greater caloric intake, it became possible to discern the role of specific dietary factors in CHD. This follows, by several decades, careful metabolic ward studies showing that saturated fatty acids increased serum cholesterol levels in middle-aged men.[100,102,218] At that time, it was thought that serum cholesterol was the most important factor in CHD and other CVDs. With the work of Paul Ridker in the 1990s,[219,220] it became clear that C-reactive protein (CRP) and, by logical extension, other factors affecting chronic systemic inflammation also were important in causing CVDs. Over the years, these observations have been confirmed in a wide variety of studies.[221–230] Specific effects include increased histamine release by damaged mast cells, increased foam cell production, and direct effects on vascular structure and function.[230,231] Many of the same foods that have been shown to be protective for other health outcomes also affect CVDs, including fruits and vegetables[123,232–234] and higher polyunsaturated dietary fats consumed as part of a healthful dietary pattern.

Depression, Anxiety, and Cognitive Decline. Concerns about the upsurge in depression and anxiety across the population and cognitive decline associated with age and premature aging in certain groups (e.g., increased allostatic load and weathering in people experiencing discrimination-related stress[235–241]), has prompted great interest in the role of diet in preventing or retarding these processes. There is strong and consistent evidence linking diet with depression [91,242–250] and anxiety.[251–253]

As the population ages, there is concern with cognitive decline. There is now good evidence that a proinflammatory diet is associated with earlier and more rapid onset of cognitive decline.[254–260] This also is consistent with a literature showing both that diet-related inflammation is associated shorter telomeres[261–264] and with a more rapid shortening of telomere length over time.[261]

Musculoskeletal Issues. Important sequelae of the upsurge in unhealthy eating patterns (e.g., fast food consumption), sedentariness, and obesity include musculoskeletal problems.[265] With the aging of the population and concern about unhealthy aging, this represents a serious problem in clinical medicine and public health. Because inflammation is so strongly associated with musculoskeletal complaints, it stands to reason that diet, as an important modulator of inflammation, would be an important part of the solution. There is a larger literature showing the benefit of a healthy, anti-inflammatory diet on these outcomes. Studies range from RCTs of Mediterranean diet in the elderly[266] to a variety of observational studies across the lifespan.[265,267–277]

Characteristics of Healthy Diets

With the constant barrage of new findings in the study of the role of diet in health, it is easy to lose sight of some simple truths. First, most new results consider a set of relationships about which much is known, across numerous studies.[29] Second, there is neither a single bad diet nor a single good diet. What is known as the Mediterranean diet, for example, with its focus on fruits, vegetables, nuts, sea fish, and whole grains, appears to improve a variety of health outcomes including metabolic syndrome and type 2 diabetes,[278–280] cancer,[167,281] heart disease,[282] and cognitive decline.[283] Despite that we might wish to think of "the Mediterranean Diet" as a single thing, there are 21 countries that have coastlines on the Mediterranean Sea and many of these have more than one culinary tradition. In addition, there is an increase in obesity and inflammation-related conditions in many Mediterranean countries, especially among the young.[284] Also, there are many other healthy diets from around the world that are not at all Mediterranean; for example, South Asian [285,286] and East Asian.[287,288]

In work with the dietary inflammatory index we have defined characteristics of proinflammatory diets as per Table 182-1. Selecting and eating foods that meet the characteristics in the right-hand column the table will result in reduced risk of all of the health conditions listed above and will inevitably lead to better control of body weight.

In examining studies on single nutrient approaches to intervening on diet, two important implications emerge for clinical practice. First, that vitamin and mineral supplementation, while well advised in certain situations, is not generally a good strategy for improving overall health. Second, the whole dietary pattern approach implies the

TABLE 182-1 CHARACTERISTICS OF PROINFLAMMATORY AND ANTI-INFLAMMATORY FOODS

Proinflammatory Foods Are Generally:	Anti-inflammatory Foods Are Generally:
White or colorless	Colorful; the darker the better
Not flavorful (though they may have a strong taste, e.g., sweet)	Flavorful and aromatic
Calorie dense	Calorie sparse (i.e., low energy/weight)
Nutrition sparse	Nutrient dense (i.e., contain lots of micronutrients and phytochemicals)

existence of final common pathways involving nutrition. Inflammation represents the largest platform for a variety of these mechanisms ranging from insulin resistance to nitrative and oxidative DNA damage, foam cell formation, immune response, and oxidation.

Thinking Holistically about Diet in the Context of Healthy Lifestyle and Motivation and Readiness to Change

People purchase, prepare, and eat foods in contexts that represent a complex mix of social, personal, health-related, religious/spiritual, and economic factors. Clearly, diet does not happen in isolation; it is related to social and cultural contexts, physical activity, stress, the built and natural environments, and chronobiological factors, including sleep and how people organize their lives including timing of both diet and physical activity.

Clinicians and public health professionals have to deal with the reality of making dietary recommendations against which there may be concerns about practicality and cost. As shown in Table 182-1, healthful foods reflected in anti-inflammatory diets and other dietary indices such as the Healthy Eating Index, that measures compliance with the U.S. Dietary Guidelines (described in Chapter 180: The Principles of Nutritional Sciences: Nutrients, Nutrition Recommendations, and Dietary Guidelines), tend to be colorful, flavorful, nutrient dense, and are naturally appealing if prepared correctly. If we are going to make inroads into how people think about diet, we are going to need to consider concepts related to cost per unit nutritional value versus cost per unit calorie. The DII represents a way to think about the quality of diet using a summary score that, in turn, relates to a set of biological processes that have implications for risk of chronic diseases. Clinicians on the frontline will be in an excellent position to move the population in the direction of nutritional balance and overall well-being.

Clearly, thinking about lifestyle and life experiences as a whole is critically important. Highly processed fast foods have been a feature of the American food landscape now since the 1950s; that is, for over two generations. Consequently, children are battling obesity and other chronic health conditions much earlier in life in the face of advertising by food companies and peer-pressure to eat calorically dense, nutrient-sparse foods. So, there is an important educational component that must be addressed. And it is not simply didactic. We need to change the experience of healthy food. At the other end of the age spectrum, older people tend to require fewer calories. So, achieving nutritional adequacy may be very difficult when overall dietary intake is very low. Energy flux, or the amount of energy that moves through a biological system,[289–292] would naturally favor active children who have high caloric requirements because of the need to grow and to obtain sufficient calories to support physical activity. Opportunities for increasing children's physical activity in school setting are described in Chapter 184: Strategies to Address Physical Activity in Schools. By increasing physical activity not only do individuals experience the salubrious effects of movement and flexibility, but doing so also allows one to have much more latitude in selection of nutritious foods.[290,291,293] The frail elderly are particularly high risk because the core requirements are so very low. Of course, this applies to very sedentary children as well. Likewise, when individuals are under stress or have disturbed sleep they may be less likely to want to participate in physical activity, to prepare foods at all, or to eat in a relaxed way. Sleep duration, quality, and timing have been positively related to healthy dietary patterns, including fruit and vegetable intake, as well as plasma concentrations of long chain fatty acids (DHA and archacidonic acid) among adolescents and young adults.[294–296]

It also is important to consider the individuals' motivations which is often not discerned in clinical encounters. Feelings and beliefs about the inherent properties of food may affect people's perception of what they eat. Given that the same part of the brain that processes the chemical senses of taste, flavor and smell; that is the limbic lobe,[297–300] also is the region responsible for emotion and instinctual behavior.[301–303] This has significant implications for identifying ways to tap into the emotional basis and motivation for dietary change. In addition, psychological traits such as acquiescence or the tendency to engage in active coping, that may predispose individuals to do particularly well, or poorly, in identifying the need to make changes in their diet and in implementing and sustaining change.[72]

Future Directions

We will need to continue to get better in pinpointing the role of dietary exposures in determining health outcomes. This should include use of innovative means, such as the DII, to assess dietary "exposures" that are known to be related via inflammation to major chronic health conditions. We can also be more clever in how we use our understanding of basic psychology to assist with the processes of behavior change, by involving not only patients but also clinicians in the design of RCTs and other study designs to evaluate nutrition interventions.[304,305] After all, who is better situated to help design trials and enroll participants than the people on the frontline of patient care? This way of looking at things would broaden our perspective with respect to personalizing medicine and nutrition. This will, no doubt, require partnerships that acknowledge that many clinicians think the diet is important and build opportunities to incorporate training in nutrition into medical and public health school curricula. In the meantime, we know much about the role of diet and health and can make recommendations to patients based on solid scientific evidence that is regularly reviewed and updated by professional groups, government agencies, and expert panels.[233,234,306–308]

References

1. Sigerist HE. *A History of Medicine: Primitive and Archaic Medicine*. Vol. I. Oxford: Oxford Univerity Press; 1951.
2. Sigerist HE. *A History of Medicine: Early Greek, Hindu, and Persian Medicine*. Vol. I. Oxford: Oxford Univerity Press; 1961.
3. Critchley JA, Zhang Y, Suthisisang CC, Chan TY, Tomlinson B. Alternative therapies and medical science: Designing clinical trials of alternative/complementary medicines—Is evidence-based traditional Chinese medicine attainable? *J Clin Pharmacol*. 2000;40(5):462–7.
4. Samuels N. Chronotherapy in traditional Chinese medicine. *Am J Chin Med*. 2000;28(3–4):419–23.
5. Kiefer D, Pitluk J, Klunk K. An overview of CAM: Components and clinical uses. *Nutr Clin Pract*. 2009;24(5):549–59.
6. Lind J. *Treatise on the Scurvey*. Edinburgh: Sands, Murray, and Cochran; 1753.
7. Snow J. *On the Mode of Communication of Cholera*. 2nd ed. London: John Churchill; 1860.
8. Sengupta A, Ghosh S, Bhattacharjee S, Das S. Indian food ingredients and cancer prevention: An experimental evaluation of anticarcinogenic effects of garlic in rat colon. *Asian Pac J Cancer Prev*. 2004;5(2):126–32.
9. Ferrucci LM, Daniel CR, Kapur K, et al. Measurement of spices and seasonings in India: Opportunities for cancer epidemiology and prevention. *Asian Pac J Cancer Prev*. 2010;11(6):1621–9.
10. Shivappa N, Steck SE, Hurley TG, Hussey JR, Hebert JR. Designing and developing a literature-derived population-based dietary inflammatory index. *Public Health Nutr*. 2014;17(6):1689–96.
11. Azimi P, Ghiasvand R, Feizi A, Hariri M, Abbasi B. Effects of cinnamon, cardamom, saffron, and ginger consumption on markers of glycemic control, lipid profile, oxidative stress, and inflammation in type 2 diabetes patients. *Rev Diabet Stud*. 2014;11(3–4):258–66.
12. Li F, Yang XW, Krausz KW, et al. Modulation of colon cancer by nutmeg. *J Proteome Res*. 2015;14(4):1937–46.
13. Han SS, Keum YS, Seo HJ, Chun KS, Lee SS, Surh YJ. Capsaicin suppresses phorbol ester-induced activation of NF-kappaB/Rel and AP-1 transcription factors in mouse epidermis. *Cancer Lett*. 2001;164(2):119–26.
14. Henderson VP, Clemow L, Massion AO, Hurley TG, Druker S, Hebert JR. The effects of mindfulness-based stress reduction on psychosocial outcomes and quality of life in early-stage breast cancer patients: A randomized trial. *Breast Cancer Res Treat*. 2012;131(1):99–109.
15. Fardet A, Rock E. Toward a new philosophy of preventive nutrition: From a reductionist to a holistic paradigm to improve nutritional recommendations. *Adv Nutr*. 2014;5(4):430–46.

16. Ornish D, Brown SE, Scherwitz LW, et al. Can lifestyle changes reverse coronary heart disease? The Lifestyle Heart Trial. *Lancet.* 1990;336:129–33.
17. Ornish D, Weidner G, Fair WR, et al. Intensive lifestyle changes may affect the progression of prostate cancer. *J Urol.* 2005;174(3):1065–9.
18. Steven S, Lim EL, Taylor R. Population response to information on reversibility of type 2 diabetes. *Diabet Med.* 2013;30(4):e135–8.
19. DeFronzo RA, Ferrannini E, Groop L, et al. Type 2 diabetes mellitus. *Nat Rev Dis Prim.* 2015;1:15019.
20. Hebert JR, Hurley TG, Harmon BE, Heiney S, Hebert CJ, Steck SE. A diet, physical activity, and stress reduction intervention in men with rising prostate-specific antigen after treatment for prostate cancer. *Cancer Epidemiol.* 2012;36 (2):e128–36.
21. Saxe GA, Hebert JR, Carmody JF, et al. Can diet, in conjunction with stress reduction, affect the rate of increase in prostate specific antigen after biochemical recurrence of prostate cancer? *J Urol.* 2001;166:2202–7.
22. Kirwan AM, Lenighan YM, O'Reilly ME, McGillicuddy FC, Roche HM. Nutritional modulation of metabolic inflammation. *Biochem Soc Trans.* 2017;45(4):979–85.
23. Fraser GE. A search for truth in dietary epidemiology. *Am J Clin Nutr.* 2003;78(3 Suppl):521S–5S.
24. Taubes G. What if it's all been a big fat lie? *New York Times Magazine.* 2002:22–7.
25. Hill AB. Observation and experiment. *N Engl J Med.* 1953;248:3–9.
26. Doll R, Hill AB. Smoking and carcinoma of the lung. *BMJ.* 1950;2:739–48.
27. U.S. Department of Health Education and Welfare. *Smoking and Health: Report of the Advisory Committee to the Surgeon General of the Public Health Services.* Washington, DC: U.S. Department of Health Education and Welfare; 1964, P.H.S. Publ. No. 1103, .
28. Wynder EL, Graham EA. Tobacco smoking as a possible etiologic factor in bronchiogenic carcinoma: A study of six hundred and eighty-four proved cases. *Cancer.* 1950;143:329–36.
29. Hebert JR, Hurley TG, Steck SE, et al. Considering the value of dietary assessment data in informing nutrition-related health policy. *Adv Nutr.* 2014;5(4):447–55.
30. Hebert JR, Frongillo EA, Adams SA, et al. Perspective: Randomized controlled trials are not a panacea for diet-related research. *Adv Nutr.* 2016;7(3):423–32.
31. Marmot MG. Status syndrome: A challenge to medicine. *Cancer.* 2006;295(11):1304–7.
32. Marmot M, Friel S. Global health equity: Evidence for action on the social determinants of health. *J Epidemiol Comm Health.* 2008;62(12):1095–7.
33. Marmot MG, Syme SL. Acculturation and coronary heart disease in Japanese-Americans. *Am J Epidemiol.* 1976;104(3):225–47.
34. Marmot M, Shipley M, Hemingway H, Head J, Brunner E. Biological and behavioural explanations of social inequalities in coronary heart disease: The Whitehall II study. *Diabetologia.* 2008;51(11):1980–8.
35. Phillips CM, Chen LW, Heude B, et al. Dietary inflammatory index and non-communicable disease risk: A narrative review. *Nutrients.* 2019;11(8):pii:E1873.
36. Brady G, MacArthur GJ, Farrell PJ. Epstein–Barr virus and Burkitt lymphoma. *J Clin Pathol.* 2007;60(12):1397–402.
37. Dunmire SK, Hogquist KA, Balfour HH. Infectious mononucleosis. *Curr Top Microbiol Immunol.* 2015;390:211–40.
38. Kumanyika S, Oria MP. *Guiding Principles for Developing Dietary Reference Intakes Based on Chronic Disease.* Washington, DC: National Academies of Sciences, Engineering, and Medicine; 2017.
39. The Alpha Tocopherol Beta Carotene Cancer Prevention Group. The effect of vitamin E and beta carotene on the incidence of lung cancer and other cancers in male smokers. *N Engl J Med.* 1994;330(15):1029–35.
40. Omenn GS, Goodman G, Thornquist M, et al. The beta-carotene and retinol efficacy trial (CARET) for chemoprevention of lung cancer in high risk populations: Smokers and asbestos-exposed workers. *Cancer Res.* 1994;54:2038S–43S.
41. Sharma AK, Amin S. Post SELECT: Selenium on trial. *Future Med Chem.* 2013;5(2):163–74.
42. Arthur AE, Peterson KE, Shen J, et al. Diet and proinflammatory cytokine levels in head and neck squamous cell carcinoma. *Cancer.* 2014;120(17):2704–12.
43. Hunt MK, Hebert JR, Sorensen G, et al. Measuring changes in eating pattern messages in worksite participating in a Cancer Prevent program. *J Nutr Educ.* 1993;25:236–44.
44. Estruch R, Ros E, Salas-Salvado J, et al. Primary prevention of cardiovascular disease with a Mediterranean diet. *N Engl J Med.* 2013;368(14):1279–90.
45. Hodge AM, Bassett JK, Dugue PA, et al. Dietary inflammatory index or Mediterranean diet score as risk factors for total and cardiovascular mortality. *Nutr Metab Cardiovasc Dis.* 2018;28(5):461–9.
46. Qiao Y, Tinker L, Olendzki BC, et al. Racial/ethnic disparities in association between dietary quality and incident diabetes in postmenopausal women in the United States: The Women's Health Initiative 1993–2005. *Ethn Health.* 2013;19(3):328–47.
47. Shivappa N, Hebert JR, Kivimaki M, Akbaraly T. Alternative Healthy Eating Index 2010, Dietary Inflammatory Index and risk of mortality: Results from the Whitehall II cohort study and meta-analysis of previous Dietary Inflammatory Index and mortality studies. *Br J Nutr.* 2017;118(3):210–21.
48. Blasetti A, Franchini S, Comegna L, Prezioso G, Chiarelli F. Role of nutrition in preventing insulin resistance in children. *J Pediatr Endocrinol Metab.* 2016;29(3):247–57.
49. Albanes D, Heinonen OP, Huttunen JK, et al. Effects of alpha-tocopherol and beta-carotene supplements on cancer incidence in the Alpha-Tocopherol Beta-Carotene Cancer Prevention Study. *Am J Clin Nutr.* 1995;62(6 Suppl):1427S–30S.
50. Omenn GS, Goodman GE, Thornquist MD, et al. Risk factors for lung cancer and for intervention effects in CARET, the Beta-Carotene and Retinol Efficacy Trial. *J Natl Cancer Inst.* 1996;88(21):1550–9.
51. Lippman SM, Goodman PJ, Klein EA, et al. Designing the Selenium and Vitamin E Cancer Prevention Trial (SELECT). *J Natl Cancer Inst.* 2005;97(2):94–102.
52. Taubes G. Epidemiology faces its limits. *Science.* 1995;269:164–9.
53. Taubes G. The (political) science of salt. *Science.* 1998;281(5379):898–901.
54. Taubes G. The soft science of dietary fat. *Science.* 2001;291:2536–45.
55. Taubes G. Nutrition. The epidemic that wasn't? *Science.* 2001;291(5513):2540.
56. Taubes G. Nutrition. What if Americans ate less saturated fat? *Science.* 2001;291(5513):2538.
57. Feinstein AR. Scientific standards in epidemiologic studies of the menace of daily life. *Science.* 1988;242:1257–63.
58. Ioannidis JP. Implausible results in human nutrition research. *BMJ.* 2013;347:f6698.
59. Archer E, Blair SN. Implausible data, false memories, and the status quo in dietary assessment. *Adv Nutr.* 2015;6:229–30.
60. Archer E. The NHANES dietary data are physiologically implausible and inadmissible as scientific evidence. *Am J Clin Nutr.* 2017;106(3):951–2.
61. Archer E. The use of implausible data without caveats is misleading. *Am J Clin Nutr.* 2017;106(3):949–50.
62. Savitz D, Greenland S, Stolley P, Kelsey J. Scientific standards of criticism: A reaction to "scientific standards in epidemiologic studies of the menace of daily life," by A. R. Feinstein. *Epidemiol.* 1990;1:78–83.
63. Gori GB. Epidemiology faces its limits. [letter]. *Science.* 1995;269:1328.
64. Miller RW. Epidemiology faces its limits. [letter]. *Science.* 1995;269:1327.
65. Rapp J. Epidemiology faces its limits. [letter]. *Science.* 1995;269:1327.
66. Saah AJ. Epidemiology faces its limits. [letter]. *Science.* 1995;269:1327.
67. Trichopoulos D. Epidemiology faces its limits. [letter]. *Science.* 1995;269:1326.
68. Willett W, Greenland S, MacMahom B, et al. Epidemiology faces its limits. [letter]. *Science.* 1995;269:1325–6.
69. Greenland S. Induction versus Popper: Substance versus semantics. *Int J Epidemiol.* 1998;27(4):543–8.
70. Hebert JR, Hurley TG, Steck SE, et al. Reply to E Archer and SN Blair: Implausible data, false memories, and the status quo in dietary assessment. *Adv Nutr.* 2015;6(2):230–3.
71. Satija A, Yu E, Willett WC, Hu FB. Understanding nutritional epidemiology and its role in policy. *Adv Nutr.* 2015;6(1):5–18.
72. Hebert JR. Social desirability trait: Biaser or driver of self-reported dietary intake? *J Acad Nutr Diet.* 2016;116(12):1895–8.
73. Hebert JR, Hurley TG, Peterson KE, et al. Social desirability trait influences on self-reported dietary measures among diverse participants in a multicenter multiple risk factor trial. *J Nutr.* 2008;138(1):226S–34S.
74. Hebert JR, Ebbeling CB, Matthews CE, et al. Systematic errors in middle-aged women's estimates of energy intake: Comparing three self-report measures to total energy expenditure from doubly labeled water. *Ann Epidemiol.* 2002;12:577–86.
75. Hebert JR, Peterson KE, Hurley TG, et al. The effect of social desirability trait on self-reported dietary measures among multi-ethnic female health center employees. *Ann Epidemiol.* 2001;11(6):417–27.
76. Hebert JR, Ma Y, Clemow L, et al. Gender differences in social desirability and social approval bias in dietary self report. *Am J Epidemiol.* 1997;146:1046–55.

77. Hebert JR, Clemow L, Pbert L, Ockene IS, Ockene JK. Social desirability bias in dietary self-report may compromise the validity of dietary intake measures. *Int J Epidemiol.* 1995;24:389–98.
78. Ma Y, Olendzki BC, Pagoto SL, et al. Number of 24-hour diet recalls needed to estimate energy intake. *Ann Epidemiol.* 2009;19(8):553–9.
79. Hebert JR, Hurley TG, Cavicchia P, et al. Response to Dr. Arab et al. on "Number of 24-hour diet recalls needed to estimate energy intake." *Ann Epidemiol.* 2010;20(1):87–8.
80. Hebert JR, Ockene IS, Hurley TG, Luippold R, Well AD, Harmatz MG. Development and testing of a seven-day dietary recall. *J Clin Epidemiol.* 1997;50:925–37.
81. Kim Y, Chen J, Wirth MD, Shivappa N, Hebert JR. Lower Dietary Inflammatory Index scores are associated with lower Glycemic Index scores among college students. *Nutrients.* 2018;10(2):E182.
82. Taren DL, Tobar M, Hill A, et al. The association of energy intake bias with psychological scores of women. *Eur J Clin Nutr.* 1999;53(7):570–8.
83. Shah N, Passi V, Bryson S, Agras WS. Patterns of eating and abstinence in women treated for bulimia nervosa. *Int J Eating Disord.* 2005;38(4):330–4.
84. Peterson KE, Hebert JR, Hurley TG, et al. Accuracy and precision of two short screeners to assess change in fruit and vegetable consumption among diverse populations participating in health promotion intervention trials. *J Nutr.* 2008;138(1):218S–25S.
85. Stumbo PJ. New technology in dietary assessment: A review of digital methods in improving food record accuracy. *Proc Nutr Soc.* 2013;72(1):70–6.
86. Hebert JR, Ockene IS, Botelho L, Luippold R, Merriam P, Saperia G. Development and validation of a seven-day diet recall. Paper presented at: American Public Health Association 120th Annual Meeting. 1992; Washington, DC.
87. Hebert JR, Gupta PC, Bhonsle RB, Sinor PN, Mehta H, Mehta FS. Development and testing of a quantitative food frequency questionnaire for use in Gujarat, India. *Public Health Nutr.* 1999;2(1):39–50.
88. Greene GW, Resnicow K, Thompson FE, et al. Correspondence of the NCI Fruit and Vegetable Screener to repeat 24-H recalls and serum carotenoids in behavioral intervention trials. *J Nutr.* 2008;138(1):200S–4S.
89. Williams GC, Hurley TG, Thompson FE, et al. Performance of a short percentage energy from fat tool in measuring change in dietary intervention studies. *J Nutr.* 2008;138(1):212S–7S.
90. Elenkov IJ, Iezzoni DG, Daly A, Harris AG, Chrousos GP. Cytokine dysregulation, inflammation and well-being. *Neuroimmunomodulation.* 2005;12(5):255–69.
91. Kiecolt-Glaser JK, Derry HM, Fagundes CP. Inflammation: Depression fans the flames and feasts on the heat. *Am J Psychiatry.* 2015;172(11):1075–91.
92. Mathe E, Nguyen GH, Funamizu N, et al. Inflammation regulates microRNA expression in cooperation with p53 and nitric oxide. *Int J Cancer.* 2012;131(3):760–5.
93. Larsen JM. The immune response to Prevotella bacteria in chronic inflammatory disease. *Immunology.* 2017;151(4):363–74.
94. Kagnoff MF. Immunology of the intestinal tract. *Gastroenterology.* 1993;105(5):1275–80.
95. Saita E, Kondo K, Momiyama Y. Anti-inflammatory diet for atherosclerosis and coronary artery disease: Antioxidant foods. *Clin Med Insights Cardiol.* 2014;8(S3):61–5.
96. Ramallal R, Toledo E, Martinez JA, et al. Inflammatory potential of diet, weight gain, and incidence of overweight/obesity: the SUN cohort. *Obesity.* 2017;25(6):997–1005.
97. Whiteside TL, Herberman RB. The role of natural killer cells in immune surveillance of cancer. *Curr Opin Immunol.* 1995;7(5):704–10.
98. Hebert JR, Barone J, Reddy MM, Backlund JYC. Natural killer cell activity in a longitudinal dietary fat intervention trial. *Clin Immunol Immunopathol.* 1990;54:103–16.
99. Hebert JR, Miller DR, Barone J, Richie JJ, Reddy M. Erythrocyte membrane fatty acids and natural killer cell activity in a longitudinal intervention trial. *Immun Infect Dis.* 1991;1:341–8.
100. Keys A, Anderson JT, Grande F. Prediction of serum-cholesterol response of man to changes in fats in the diet. *Lancet.* 1957;7003:959–66.
101. Keys A, Anderson JT, Grande F. Serum cholesterol response to changes in the diet-IV. Particular fatty acids in the diet. *Metabolism.* 1965;14:776–87.
102. Hegsted DM, McGandy RB, Myers ML, Stare FJ. Quantitative effects of dietary fat on serum cholesterol in man. *Am J Clin Nutr.* 1965;17:281–95.
103. Jones KD, Thitiri J, Ngari M, Berkley JA. Childhood malnutrition: Toward an understanding of infections, inflammation, and antimicrobials. *Food Nutr Bull.* 2014;35(2 Suppl):S64–70.
104. Hebert JR. Growth monitoring: The "G" in GOBI FFF. In: Cash R, Keusch GT, Lamstein J, eds. *Child Health and Survival: The UNICEF GOBI FFF Program.* London: Croom Helm; 1987, pp. 11–20.
105. Lopez AD, Mathers CD, Ezzati M, Jamison DT, Murray CJL. Global and regional burden of disease and risk factors, 2001: Systematic analysis of population health data. [see comment]. *Lancet.* 2006;367(9524):1747–57.
106. Van Kerkhove MD, Vandemaele KA, Shinde V, et al. Risk factors for severe outcomes following 2009 influenza A (H1N1) infection: A global pooled analysis. *PLoS Med.* 2011;8(7):e1001053.
107. Maier HE, Lopez R, Sanchez N, et al. Obesity increases the duration of influenza A virus shedding in adults. *J Infect Dis.* 2018;218(9):1378–82.
108. Mancuso P. Obesity and respiratory infections: Does excess adiposity weigh down host defense? *Pulm Pharmacol Ther.* 2013;26(4):412–9.
109. Milner JJ, Beck MA. The impact of obesity on the immune response to infection. *Proc Nutr Soc.* 2012;71(2):298–306.
110. Thorud JC, Plemmons B, Buckley CJ, Shibuya N, Jupiter DC. Mortality after nontraumatic major amputation among patients with diabetes and peripheral vascular disease: A systematic review. *J Foot Ankle Surg.* 2016;55(3):591–9.
111. Jagadapillai R, Rane MJ, Lin X, et al. Diabetic microvascular disease and pulmonary fibrosis: The contribution of platelets and systemic inflammation. *Int J Molec Sci.* 2016;17(11):08.
112. Dryden M, Baguneid M, Eckmann C, et al. Pathophysiology and burden of infection in patients with diabetes mellitus and peripheral vascular disease: Focus on skin and soft-tissue infections. *Clin Microbiol Infect.* 2015;21 Suppl 2:S27–32.
113. Bowling FL, Rashid ST, Boulton AJ. Preventing and treating foot complications associated with diabetes mellitus. *Nat Rev Endocrinol.* 2015;11(10):606–16.
114. Tesch GH. Diabetic nephropathy—Is this an immune disorder? *Clin Sci (Colch).* 2017;131(16):2183–99.
115. Pichler R, Afkarian M, Dieter BP, Tuttle KR. Immunity and inflammation in diabetic kidney disease: Translating mechanisms to biomarkers and treatment targets. *Am J Physiol Renal Physiol.* 2017;312(4):F716–31.
116. Shen Y, Cai R, Sun J, et al. Diabetes mellitus as a risk factor for incident chronic kidney disease and end-stage renal disease in women compared with men: A systematic review and meta-analysis. *Endocrine.* 2017;55(1):66–76.
117. Zerbini G, Maestroni S, Turco V, Secchi A. The eye as a window to the microvascular complications of diabetes. *Dev Ophthalmol.* 2017;60:6–15.
118. Liew G, Wong VW, Ho IV. Mini review: Changes in the incidence of and progression to proliferative and sight-threatening diabetic retinopathy over the last 30 years. *Ophthalmic Epidemiol.* 2017;24(2):73–80.
119. Roy S, Kern TS, Song B, Stuebe C. Mechanistic insights into pathological changes in the diabetic retina: Implications for targeting diabetic retinopathy. *Am J Pathol.* 2017;187(1):9–19.
120. Guzman DC, Olguin HJ, Garcia EH, Peraza AV, de la Cruz DZ, Soto MP. Mechanisms involved in the development of diabetic retinopathy induced by oxidative stress. *Redox Rep.* 2017;22(1):10–6.
121. Li C, Miao X, Li F, et al. Oxidative stress-related mechanisms and antioxidant therapy in diabetic retinopathy. *Oxid Med Cell Longev.* 2017;2017:9702820.
122. Gopalan C. Rising incidence of obesity, coronary heart disease and diabetes in the Indian urban middle class. Possible role of genetic and environmental factors. *World Rev Nutr Diet.* 2001;90:127–43.
123. Micha R, Shulkin ML, Penalvo JL, et al. Etiologic effects and optimal intakes of foods and nutrients for risk of cardiovascular diseases and diabetes: Systematic reviews and meta-analyses from the Nutrition and Chronic Diseases Expert Group (NutriCoDE). *PLoS One.* 2017;12(4):e0175149.
124. Leong DP, Joseph PG, McKee M, et al. Reducing the global burden of cardiovascular disease, part 2: Prevention and treatment of cardiovascular disease. *Circ Res.* 2017;121(6):695–710.
125. Thornburg KL. The programming of cardiovascular disease. *J Dev Orig Health Dis.* 2015;6(5):366–76.
126. Volkova N, McClellan W, Soucie JM, Schoolwerth A. Racial disparities in the prevalence of cardiovascular disease among incident end-stage renal disease patients. *Nephrol Dial Transplant.* 2006;21(8):2202–9.
127. Cavicchia PP, Adams SA, Steck SE, et al. Racial disparities in colorectal cancer incidence by type 2 diabetes mellitus status. *Cancer Causes Control.* 2012;24(2):277–85.
128. La Vecchia C, Giordano SH, Hortobagyi GN, Chabner B. Overweight, obesity, diabetes, and risk of breast cancer: Interlocking pieces of the puzzle. *Oncologist.* 2011;16(6):726–9.

129. Gouveri E, Papanas N, Maltezos E. The female breast and diabetes. *Breast.* 2011;20(3):205–11.
130. He J, Stram DO, Kolonel LN, Henderson BE, Le Marchand L, Haiman CA. The association of diabetes with colorectal cancer risk: The Multiethnic Cohort. *Br J Cancer.* 2010;103(1):120–6.
131. Flood A, Strayer L, Schairer C, Schatzkin A. Diabetes and risk of incident colorectal cancer in a prospective cohort of women. *Cancer Causes Control.* 2010;21(8):1277–84.
132. Vinikoor LC, Long MD, Keku TO, Martin CF, Galanko JA, Sandler RS. The association between diabetes, insulin use, and colorectal cancer among Whites and African Americans. *Cancer Epidemiol Biomarkers Prev.* 2009;18(4):1239–42.
133. Singh PN, Arthur KN, Orlich MJ, et al. Global epidemiology of obesity, vegetarian dietary patterns, and noncommunicable disease in Asian Indians. *Am J Clin Nutr.* 2014;100 Suppl 1:359S–64S.
134. Hebert JR, Allison DB, Archer E, Lavie CJ, Blair SN. Scientific decision making, policy decisions, and the obesity pandemic. *Mayo Clin Proc.* 2013;88(6):593–604.
135. Hales CM, Carroll MD, Fryar CD, Ogden CL. Prevalence of obesity among adults and youth: United States, 2015–2016. *NCHS Data Brief.* 2017;(288):1–8.
136. Hedley AA, Ogden CL, Johnson CL, Carroll MD, Curtin LR, Flegal KM. Prevalence of overweight and obesity among US children, adolescents, and adults, 1999–2002. *Cancer.* 2004;291(23):2847–50.
137. Mueller WH, Reid RM. A multivariate analysis of fatness and relative fat patterning. *Am J Phys Anthropol.* 1979;50(2):199–208.
138. Kissebah AH, Vydelingum N, Murray R, et al. Relation of body fat distribution to metabolic complications of obesity. *J Clin Endocrinol Metab.* 1982;54(2):254–60.
139. Gray DS, Fujioka K, Colletti PM, et al. Magnetic-resonance imaging used for determining fat distribution in obesity and diabetes. *Am J Clin Nutr.* 1991;54(4):623–7.
140. Dulloo AG, Jacquet J. An adipose-specific control of thermogenesis in body weight regulation. *Int J Obes Relat Metab Disord.* 2001;25 Suppl 5:S22–9.
141. Krekoukia M, Nassis GP, Psarra G, Skenderi K, Chrousos GP, Sidossis LS. Elevated total and central adiposity and low physical activity are associated with insulin resistance in children. *Metabolism.* 2007;56(2):206–13.
142. Hermsdorff HH, Zulet MA, Puchau B, Martinez JA. Central adiposity rather than total adiposity measurements are specifically involved in the inflammatory status from healthy young adults. *Inflammation.* 2011;34(3):161–70.
143. Lumeng CN, Saltiel AR. Inflammatory links between obesity and metabolic disease. *J Clin Invest.* 2011;121(6):2111–7.
144. Muller MJ, Lagerpusch M, Enderle J, Schautz B, Heller M, Bosy-Westphal A. Beyond the body mass index: Tracking body composition in the pathogenesis of obesity and the metabolic syndrome. *Obes Rev.* 2012;13 Suppl 2:6–13.
145. Yerrakalva D, Mullis R, Mant J. The associations of "fatness," "fitness," and physical activity with all-cause mortality in older adults: A systematic review. *Obesity (Silver Spring, Md).* 2015;23(10):1944–56.
146. Martin-Calvo N, Moreno-Galarraga L, Martinez-Gonzalez MA. Association between body mass index, waist-to-height ratio and adiposity in children: A systematic review and meta-analysis. *Nutrients.* 2016;8(8):20.
147. Sen S, Rifas-Shiman SL, Shivappa N, et al. Associations of prenatal and early life dietary inflammatory potential with childhood adiposity and cardiometabolic risk in Project Viva. *Pediatr Obes.* 2018;13(5):292–300.
148. Connaughton RM, McMorrow AM, McGillicuddy FC, Lithander FE, Roche HM. Impact of anti-inflammatory nutrients on obesity-associated metabolic-inflammation from childhood through to adulthood. *Proc Nutr Soc.* 2016;75(2):115–24.
149. Bag-Ozbek A, Giles JT. Inflammation, adiposity, and atherogenic dyslipidemia in rheumatoid arthritis: Is there a paradoxical relationship? *Curr Allergy Asthma Rep.* 2015;15(2):497.
150. Tsatsoulis A, Mantzaris MD, Bellou S, Andrikoula M. Insulin resistance: An adaptive mechanism becomes maladaptive in the current environment—An evolutionary perspective. *Metabolism.* 2013;62(5):622–33.
151. Guffey CR, Fan D, Singh UP, Murphy EA. Linking obesity to colorectal cancer: Recent insights into plausible biological mechanisms. *Curr Opin Clin Nutr Metab Care.* 2013;16(5):595–600.
152. Yehuda-Shnaidman E, Schwartz B. Mechanisms linking obesity, inflammation and altered metabolism to colon carcinogenesis. *Obes Rev.* 2012;13(12):1083–95.
153. Ouchi N, Parker JL, Lugus JJ, Walsh K. Adipokines in inflammation and metabolic disease. *Nature Rev Immunol.* 2011;11(2):85–97.
154. Balkwill F, Mantovani A. Inflammation and cancer: Back to Virchow? [see comment]. *Lancet.* 2001;357(9255):539–45.
155. Shivappa N, Prizment AE, Blair CK, Jacobs DR Jr, Steck SE, Hebert JR. Dietary Inflammatory Index (DII) and risk of colorectal cancer in Iowa Women's Health Study. *Cancer Epidemiol Biomarkers Prev.* 2014;23(11):2383–92.
156. Shivappa N, Zucchetto A, Montella M, et al. Inflammatory potential of diet and risk of colorectal cancer: A case-control study from Italy. *Br J Nutr.* 2015;114(1):152–8.
157. Tabung FK, Steck SE, Ma Y, et al. The association between dietary inflammatory index and risk of colorectal cancer among postmenopausal women: results from the Women's Health Initiative. *Cancer Causes Control.* 2015;26(3):399–408.
158. Wirth MD, Shivappa N, Steck SE, Hurley TG, Hebert JR. The dietary inflammatory index is associated with colorectal cancer in the National Institutes of Health-American Association of Retired Persons Diet and Health Study. *Br J Nutr.* 2015;113(11):1819–27.
159. Zamora-Ros R, Shivappa N, Steck SE, et al. Dietary inflammatory index and inflammatory gene interactions in relation to colorectal cancer risk in the Bellvitge colorectal cancer case-control study. *Genes Nutr.* 2015;10(1):447.
160. Harmon BE, Wirth MD, Boushey CJ, et al. The Dietary Inflammatory Index is associated with colorectal cancer risk in the Multiethnic Cohort. *J Nutr.* 2017;147(3):430–8.
161. Niclis C, Pou SA, Shivappa N, Hebert JR, Steck SE, Diaz MDP. Proinflammatory dietary intake is associated with increased risk of colorectal cancer: Results of a case-control study in Argentina using a multilevel modeling approach. *Nutr Cancer.* 2017;70(1):61–8.
162. Sharma I, Zhu Y, Woodrow JR, et al. Inflammatory diet and risk for colorectal cancer: A population-based case-control study in Newfoundland, Canada. *Nutrition.* 2017;42:69–74.
163. Shivappa N, Godos J, Hebert JR, et al. Dietary inflammatory index and colorectal cancer risk: A meta-analysis. *Nutrients.* 2017;9(9):E1043.
164. Shivappa N, Hebert JR, Steck SE, et al. Dietary Inflammatory Index and odds of colorectal cancer in a case-control study from Jordan. *Appl Physiol Nutr Metab.* 2017;42(7):744–9.
165. Shivappa N, Hebert JR, Rosato V, Serraino D, La Vecchia C. Inflammatory potential of diet and risk of laryngeal cancer in a case-control study from Italy. *Cancer Causes Control.* 2016;27(8):1027–34.
166. Mazul AL, Shivappa N, Hebert JR, et al. Proinflammatory diet is associated with increased risk of squamous cell head and neck cancer. *Int J Cancer.* 2018;143(7):1604–10.
167. Accardi G, Shivappa N, Di Maso M, et al. Dietary Inflammatory Index and cancer risk in the elderly: A pooled-analysis of Italian case-control studies. *Nutrition.* 2019;63-64:205–10.
168. Shivappa N, Hebert JR, Zucchetto A, et al. Increased risk of nasopharyngeal carcinoma with increasing levels of diet-associated inflammation in an Italian case-control study. *Nutr Cancer.* 2016;68(7):1123–30.
169. Abe M, Shivappa N, Ito H, et al. Dietary Inflammatory Index and risk of upper aerodigestive tract cancer in Japanese adults. *Oncotarget.* 2018;9(35):24028–40.
170. Shivappa N, Hebert JR, Rashidkhani B. Dietary Inflammatory Index and risk of esophageal squamous cell cancer in a case-control study from Iran. *Nutr Cancer.* 2015;67(8):1253–9.
171. Shivappa N, Zucchetto A, Serraino D, Rossi M, La Vecchia C, Hebert JR. Dietary Inflammatory Index and risk of esophageal squamous cell cancer in a case-control study from Italy. *Cancer Causes Control.* 2015;26(10):1439–47.
172. Lu Y, Shivappa N, Lin Y, Lagergren J, Hebert JR. Diet-related inflammation and oesophageal cancer by histological type: A nationwide case-control study in Sweden. *Eur J Nutr.* 2016;55(4):1683–94.
173. Shivappa N, Hebert JR, Anderson LA, et al. Dietary inflammatory index and risk of reflux oesophagitis, Barrett's oesophagus and oesophageal adenocarcinoma: A population-based case-control study. *Br J Nutr.* 2017;117(9):1323–31.
174. Tang L, Shivappa N, Hebert JR, Lee AH, Xu F, Binns CW. Dietary Inflammatory Index and risk of oesophageal cancer in Xinjiang Uyghur Autonomous Region, China. *Br J Nutr.* 2018;119(9):1068–75.
175. Maisonneuve P, Shivappa N, Hebert JR, et al. Dietary Inflammatory Index and risk of lung cancer and other respiratory conditions among heavy smokers in the COSMOS screening study. *Eur J Nutr.* 2015;55(3):1069–79.
176. Hodge AM, Bassett JK, Shivappa N, et al. Dietary Inflammatory Index, Mediterranean diet score, and lung cancer: A prospective study. *Cancer Causes Control.* 2016;27(7):907–17.

177. Shivappa N, Wang R, Hebert JR, Jin A, Koh WP, Yuan JM. Association between inflammatory potential of diet and risk of lung cancer among smokers in a prospective study in Singapore. *Eur J Nutr.* 2018;58(7):2755–66.

178. Shivappa N, Hebert JR, Rosato V, et al. Dietary Inflammatory Index and risk of bladder cancer in a large Italian case-control study. *Urology.* 2017;100:84–9.

179. Shivappa N, Hebert JR, Mirsafa F, Rashidkhani B. Increased inflammatory potential of diet is associated with increased risk of bladder cancer in an Iranian case-control study. *Nutr Cancer.* 2019;71(7):1086–93.

180. Shivappa N, Blair CK, Prizment AE, Jacobs DRJr, Hebert JR. Dietary Inflammatory Index and risk of renal cancer in the Iowa Women's Health Study. *Eur J Nutr.* 2017;57(3):1207–13.

181. Shivappa N, Hebert JR, Rosato V, et al. Dietary Inflammatory Index and renal cell carcinoma risk in an Italian case-control study. *Nutr Cancer.* 2017;69(6):833–9.

182. Bondonno NP, Blekkenhorst LC, Bird AL, et al. Dietary Inflammatory Index and the aging kidney in older women: A 10-year prospective cohort study. *Eur J Nutr.* 2020;59(7):3201–11.

183. Shivappa N, Bosetti C, Zucchetto A, Serraino D, La Vecchia C, Hebert JR. Dietary inflammatory index and risk of pancreatic cancer in an Italian case-control study. *Br J Nutr.* 2015;113(2):292–8.

184. Antwi SO, Oberg AL, Shivappa N, et al. Pancreatic cancer: Associations of inflammatory potential of diet, cigarette smoking, and long-standing diabetes. *Carcinogenesis.* 2016;37(5):481–90.

185. Antwi SO, Bamlet WR, Pedersen KS, et al. Pancreatic cancer risk is modulated by inflammatory potential of diet and ABO genotype: A consortia-based evaluation and replication study. *Carcinogenesis.* 2018;39(8):1056–67.

186. Shivappa N, Hebert JR, Polesel J, et al. Inflammatory potential of diet and risk for hepatocellular cancer in a case-control study from Italy. *Br J Nutr.* 2016;115(2):324–31.

187. Wang XY, Fang AP, Chen PY, et al. High dietary inflammatory index scores are associated with an elevated risk of hepatocellular carcinoma in a case-control study. *Food Funct.* 2018;9(11):5832–42.

188. Shivappa N, Hebert JR, Ferraroni M, La Vecchia C, Rossi M. Association between dietary inflammatory index and gastric cancer risk in an Italian case-control study. *Nutr Cancer.* 2016;68(8):1262–8.

189. Vahid F, Shivappa N, Faghfoori Z, et al. Validation of a Dietary Inflammatory Index (DII) and association with risk of gastric cancer: A case-control study. *Asian Pac J Cancer Prev.* 2018;19(6):1471–7.

190. Graffouillere L, Deschasaux M, Mariotti F, et al. The dietary inflammatory index is associated with prostate cancer risk in French middle-aged adults in a prospective study. *J Nutr.* 2016;146(4):785–91.

191. Hoang DV, Shivappa N, Pham NM, Hebert JR, Binns CW, Lee AH. Dietary Inflammatory Index is associated with increased risk for prostate cancer among Vietnamese men. *Nutrition.* 2019;62:140–5.

192. McMahon DM, Burch JB, Hebert JR, et al. Diet-related inflammation and risk of prostate cancer in the California Men's Health Study. *Ann Epidemiol.* 2019;29:30–8.

193. Shivappa N, Bosetti C, Zucchetto A, et al. Association between Dietary Inflammatory Index and prostate cancer among Italian men. *Br J Nutr.* 2014;113:278–83.

194. Shivappa N, Jackson MD, Bennett F, Hebert JR. Increased Dietary Inflammatory Index (DII) is associated with increased risk of prostate cancer in Jamaican men. *Nutr Cancer.* 2015;67(6):941–8.

195. Shivappa N, Hebert JR, Askari F, Kardoust Parizi M, Rashidkhani B. Increased inflammatory potential of diet is associated with increased risk of prostate cancer in Iranian men. *Int J Vitam Nutr Res.* 2017;86(3–4):161–8.

196. Shivappa N, Miao Q, Walker M, Hebert JR, Aronson KJ. Association between a dietary inflammatory index and prostate cancer risk in Ontario, Canada. *Nutr Cancer.* 2017;69(6):825–32.

197. Shivappa N, Niclis C, Coquet JB, Román MD, Hébert JR, Diaz MDP. Increased inflammatory potential of diet is associated with increased odds of prostate cancer in Argentinian men. *Cancer Causes Control.* 2018;29(9):803–13.

198. Vazquez-Salas RA, Shivappa N, Galvan-Portillo M, Lopez-Carrillo L, Hebert JR, Torres-Sanchez L. Dietary Inflammatory Index and prostate cancer risk in a case-control study in Mexico. *Br J Nutr.* 2016;116(11):1945–53.

199. Vidal AC, Oyekunle T, Howard LE, et al. Dietary Inflammatory Index (DII) and risk of prostate cancer in a case-control study among Black and White US Veteran men. *Prostate Cancer Prostatic Dis.* 2019;(22)4:580–7.

200. Shivappa N, Hebert JR, Rosato V, et al. Dietary Inflammatory Index and ovarian cancer risk in a large Italian case-control study. *Cancer Causes Control.* 2016;27(7):897–906.

201. Nagle CM, Ibiebele T, Shivappa N, et al. The association between the inflammatory potential of diet and risk of developing, and survival following, a diagnosis of ovarian cancer. *Eur J Nutr.* 2019;58(4):1747–56.

202. Shivappa N, Hebert JR, Paddock LE, Rodriguez-Rodriguez L, Olson SH, Bandera EV. Dietary Inflammatory Index and ovarian cancer risk in a New Jersey case-control study. *Nutrition.* 2018;46:78–82.

203. Shivappa N, Sandin S, Lof M, Hebert JR, Adami HO, Weiderpass E. Prospective study of dietary inflammatory index and risk of breast cancer in Swedish women. *Br J Cancer.* 2015;113(7):1099–103.

204. Huang WQ, Mo XF, Ye YB, et al. A higher dietary inflammatory index score is associated with a higher risk of breast cancer among Chinese women: A case-control study. *Br J Nutr.* 2017;117(10):1358–67.

205. Shivappa N, Blair CK, Prizment AE, Jacobs DR, Hebert JR. Prospective study of the Dietary Inflammatory Index and risk of breast cancer in postmenopausal women. *Mol Nutr Food Res.* 2017;61(5).

206. Shivappa N, Hebert JR, Rosato V, Montella M, Serraino D, La Vecchia C. Association between the Dietary Inflammatory Index and breast cancer in a large Italian case-control study. *Mol Nutr Food Res.* 2017;61(3).

207. Jalali S, Shivappa N, Hebert JR, Heidari Z, Hekmatdoost A, Rashidkhani B. Dietary Inflammatory Index and odds of breast cancer in a case-control study from Iran. *Nutr Cancer.* 2018;70(7):1034–42.

208. Ge I, Rudolph A, Shivappa N, Flesch-Janys D, Hebert JR, Chang-Claude J. Dietary inflammation potential and postmenopausal breast cancer risk in a German case-control study. *Breast.* 2015;24(4):491–6.

209. Gardeazabal I, Ruiz-Canela M, Sanchez-Bayona R, et al. Dietary Inflammatory Index and incidence of breast cancer in the SUN project. *Clin Nutr.* 2019;38(5):2259–68.

210. Obon-Santacana M, Romaguera D, Gracia-Lavedan E, et al. Dietary Inflammatory Index, dietary non-enzymatic antioxidant capacity, and colorectal and breast cancer risk (MCC-Spain Study). *Nutrients.* 2019;11(6):E1406.

211. Shivappa N, Hebert JR, Taborelli M, et al. Dietary Inflammatory Index and non-Hodgkin lymphoma risk in an Italian case-control study. *Cancer Causes Control.* 2017;28(7):791–9.

212. Shivappa N, Hebert JR, Taborelli M, et al. Association between Dietary Inflammatory Index and Hodgkin's lymphoma in an Italian case-control study. *Nutrition.* 2018;53:43–8.

213. Laryea JA, Siegel E, Klimberg S. Racial disparity in colorectal cancer: The role of equal treatment. *Dis Colon Rectum.* 2014;57(3):295–302.

214. Siegel R, Desantis C, Jemal A. Colorectal cancer statistics, 2014. *CA Cancer J Clin.* 2014;64(2):104–17.

215. Tammana VS, Laiyemo AO. Colorectal cancer disparities: Issues, controversies and solutions. *World J Gastroenterol.* 2014;20(4):869–76.

216. Xirasagar S, Li Y-T, Hurley TG, et al. Colorectal cancer prevention by an optimized colonoscopy protocol in routine practice. *Int J Cancer.* 2015;136(6):E731–42.

217. Stamler J. Population studies. In: Levy RRB, Dennis B, Ernst N. eds. *Nutrition, Lipids, and Coronary Heart Disease.* New York: Raven Press; 1979, pp. 25–88.

218. McGandy R, Hegsted D. Quantitative effects of dietary fat and cholesterol on serum cholesterol in man. In: Vergroesen AJ, ed. *The Role of Fats in Human Nutrition.* New York: Academic Press; 1975, pp. 212–30.

219. Ridker PM, Glynn RJ, Hennekens CH. C-reactive protein adds to the predictive value of total and HDL cholesterol in determining risk of first myocardial infarction. *Circulation.* 1998;97(20):2007–11.

220. Albert MA, Ridker PM. The role of C-reactive protein in cardiovascular disease risk. *Curr Cardiol Rep.* 1999;1(2):99–104.

221. Yu H, Rifai N. High-sensitivity C-reactive protein and atherosclerosis: From theory to therapy. *Clinical Biochemistry.* 2000;33(8):601–10.

222. Blake GJ, Ridker PM. C-reactive protein and other inflammatory risk markers in acute coronary syndromes. *J Am Coll Cardiol.* 2003;41(4 Suppl S):37S–42S.

223. Calabro P, Golia E, Yeh ET. CRP and the risk of atherosclerotic events. *Semin Immunopathol.* 2009;31(1):79–94.

224. Ramallal R, Toledo E, Martinez-Gonzalez MA, et al. Dietary Inflammatory Index and incidence of cardiovascular disease in the SUN Cohort. *PLoS One.* 2015;10(9):e0135221.

225. Neufcourt L, Assmann KE, Fezeu LK, et al. Prospective association between the Dietary Inflammatory Index and cardiovascular diseases in the SUpplementation en VItamines et Mineraux AntioXydants (SU.VI.MAX) Cohort. *J Am Heart Assoc.* 2016;5(3):e002735.

226. Ruiz-Canela M, Bes-Rastrollo M, Martinez-Gonzalez MA. The role of Dietary Inflammatory Index in cardiovascular disease, metabolic syndrome, and mortality. *Int J Mol Sco.* 2016;17(8):E1265.

227. Wirth MD, Shivappa N, Hurley TG, Hebert JR. Association between previously diagnosed circulatory conditions and a dietary inflammatory index. *Nutr Res.* 2016;36(3):227–33.

228. Boden S, Wennberg M, Van Guelpen B, et al. Dietary Inflammatory Index and risk of first myocardial infarction; a prospective population-based study. *Nutr J.* 2017;16(1):21.

229. Mazidi M, Shivappa N, Wirth MD, et al. Dietary Inflammatory Index and cardiometabolic risk in US adults. *Atherosclerosis.* 2018;276:23–7.

230. Shivappa N, Godos J, Hebert JR, et al. Dietary Inflammatory Index and cardiovascular risk and mortality: A meta-analysis. *Nutrients.* 2018;10(2):E200.

231. Messner B, Bernhard D. Smoking and cardiovascular disease: Mechanisms of endothelial dysfunction and early atherogenesis. *Arterioscler Thromb Vasc Biol.* 2014;34(3):509–15.

232. Sjogren P, Becker W, Warensjo E, et al. Mediterranean and carbohydrate-restricted diets and mortality among elderly men: A cohort study in Sweden. *Am J Clin Nutr.* 2010;92(4):967–74.

233. Wang DD, Li Y, Chiuve SE, et al. Association of specific dietary fats with total and cause-specific mortality. *JAMA Intern Med.* 2016;176(8):1134–45.

234. Sacks FM, Lichtenstein AH, Wu JHY, et al. Dietary fats and cardiovascular disease: A Presidential Advisory from the American Heart Association. *Circulation.* 2017;136(3):e1–23.

235. Geronimus AT. The weathering hypothesis and the health of African-American women and infants: Evidence and speculations. *Ethn Dis.* 1992;2(3):207–21.

236. Seeman TE, Singer BH, Rowe JW, Horwitz RI, McEwen BS. Price of adaptation-allostatic load and its health consequences. *Arch of Int Med.* 1997;157:2259–68.

237. Seeman TE, McEwen BS, Rowe JW, Singer BH. Allostatic load as a marker of cumulative biological risk: MacArthur studies of successful aging. *Proc Natl Acad Sci U S A.* 2001;98(8):4770–5.

238. Stevens-Simon C. The weathering hypothesis. *Am J Public Health.* 2002;92(4):507–8.

239. McEwen BS. Sleep deprivation as a neurobiologic and physiologic stressor: Allostasis and allostatic load. *Metabolism.* 2006;55(10 Suppl 2):S20–3.

240. Lekan D. Sojourner syndrome and health disparities in African American women. *Adv Nursing Sci.* 2009;32(4):307–21.

241. Simons RL, Lei MK, Beach SR, et al. Economic hardship and biological weathering: The epigenetics of aging in a U.S. sample of black women. *Soc Sci Med.* 2016;150:192–200.

242. Krauchi K, Wirz-Justice A, Graw P. The relationship of affective state to dietary preference: Winter depression and light therapy as a model. *J Affect Disorders.* 1990;20:43–53.

243. Luciano M, Mottus R, Starr JM, et al. Depressive symptoms and diet: Their effects on prospective inflammation levels in the elderly. *Brain Behav Immun.* 2012;26(5):717–20.

244. Sanchez-Villegas A, Ruiz-Canela M, de la Fuente-Arrillaga C, et al. Dietary Inflammatory Index, cardiometabolic conditions and depression in the Seguimiento Universidad de Navarra cohort study. *Br J Nutr.* 2015;114(9):1471–9.

245. Akbaraly T, Kerlau C, Wyart M, et al. Dietary Inflammatory Index and recurrence of depressive symptoms: Results from the Whitehall II Study. *Clin Psychol Sci.* 2016;4(6):1125–34.

246. Shivappa N, Schoenaker DAJM, Hebert JR, Mishra GD. Association between inflammatory potential of diet and risk of depression in middle-aged women: The Australian Longitudinal Study on Women's Health. *Br J Nutr.* 2016;116(6):1077–86.

247. Adjibade M, Andreeva VA, Lemogne C, et al. The inflammatory potential of the diet is associated with depressive symptoms in different subgroups of the general population. *J Nutr.* 2017;147(5):879–87.

248. Wirth MD, Shivappa N, Burch JB, Hurley TG, Hebert JR. The Dietary Inflammatory Index, shift work, and depression: Results from NHANES. *Health Psychol.* 2017;36(8):760–9.

249. Molendijk M, Molero P, Ortuno Sanchez-Pedreno F, Van der Does W, Angel Martinez-Gonzalez M. Diet quality and depression risk: A systematic review and dose-response meta-analysis of prospective studies. *J Affect Disord.* 2018;226:346–54.

250. Shivappa N, Hebert JR, Veronese N, et al. The relationship between the Dietary Inflammatory Index (DII®) and incident depressive symptoms: A longitudinal cohort study. *J Affect Disord.* 2018;235:39–44.

251. Goode AD, Winkler EAH, Reeves MM, Eakin EG. Relationship between intervention dose and outcomes in living well with diabetes: A randomized trial of a telephone-delivered lifestyle-based weight loss intervention. *Am J Health Promot.* 2014;30(2):120–9.

252. Phillips CM, Shivappa N, Hebert JR, Perry IJ. Dietary Inflammatory Index and mental health: A cross-sectional analysis of the relationship with depressive symptoms, anxiety and well-being in adults. *Clin Nutr.* 2017;37(5):1485–91.

253. Shivappa N, Hebert JR, Rashidkhani B. Association between inflammatory potential of diet and stress levels in adolescent women in Iran. *Archi Iran Med.* 2017;20(2):108–12.

254. Panickar KS, Jewell DE. The beneficial role of anti-inflammatory dietary ingredients in attenuating markers of chronic low-grade inflammation in aging. *Horm.* 2015;23(2):59–70.

255. Williams RJ, Mohanakumar KP, Beart PM. Neuro-nutraceuticals: The path to brain health via nourishment is not so distant. *Neurochem Int.* 2015;89:1–6.

256. Hayden KM, Beavers DP, Steck SE, et al. The association between an inflammatory diet and global cognitive function and incident dementia in older women: The Women's Health Initiative Memory Study. *Alzheimers Dement.* 2017;13(11):1187–96.

257. Kesse-Guyot E, Assmann KE, Andreeva VA, et al. Long-term association between the dietary inflammatory index and cognitive functioning: Findings from the SU.VI.MAX study. *Eur J Nutr.* 2017;56(4):1647–55.

258. Assmann KE, Adjibade M, Shivappa N, et al. The inflammatory potential of the diet at midlife is associated with later healthy aging in French adults. *J Nutr.* 2018;148(3):437–44.

259. Frith E, Shivappa N, Mann JR, Hebert JR, Wirth MD, Loprinzi PD. Dietary Inflammatory Index and memory function: Population-based national sample of elderly Americans. *Br J Nutr.* 2018;119(5):552–8.

260. Shin D, Kwon SC, Kim MH, et al. Inflammatory potential of diet is associated with cognitive function in an older adult Korean population. *Nutrition.* 2018;55–6:56–62.

261. Garcia-Calzon S, Zalba G, Ruiz-Canela M, et al. Dietary Inflammatory Index and telomere length in subjects with a high cardiovascular disease risk from the PREDIMED-NAVARRA study: Cross-sectional and longitudinal analyses over 5 y. *Am J Clin Nutr.* 2015;102(4):897–904.

262. Shivappa N, Wirth MD, Hurley TG, Hebert JR. Association between the Dietary Inflammatory Index (DII) and telomere length and C-reactive protein from the National Health and Nutrition Examination Survey—1999–2002. *Mol Nutr Food Res.* 2017;61(4).

263. De Meyer T, Bekaert S, De Buyzere ML, et al. Leukocyte telomere length and diet in the apparently healthy, middle-aged Asklepios population. *Sci Rep.* 2018;8(1):6540.

264. Meinila J, Perala MM, Kautiainen H, et al. Healthy diets and telomere length and attrition during a 10-year follow-up. *Eur J Clin Nutr.* 2019;73(10):1352–60.

265. Vincent HK, Adams MC, Vincent KR, Hurley RW. Musculoskeletal pain, fear avoidance behaviors, and functional decline in obesity: Potential interventions to manage pain and maintain function. *Reg Anesth Pain Med.* 2013;38(6):481–91.

266. Hardman RJ, Kennedy G, Macpherson H, Scholey AB, Pipingas A. A randomised controlled trial investigating the effects of Mediterranean diet and aerobic exercise on cognition in cognitively healthy older people living independently within aged care facilities: The Lifestyle Intervention in Independent Living Aged Care (LIILAC) study protocol [ACTRN12614001133628]. *Nutr J.* 2015;14:53.

267. Chopra A. Ayurvedic medicine and arthritis. *Rheum Dis Clin North Am.* 2000;26(1):133–44.

268. Seaman DR. The diet-induced proinflammatory state: A cause of chronic pain and other degenerative diseases? *J Manip Physiol Ther.* 2002;25(3):168–79.

269. Adam O, Beringer C, Kless T, et al. Anti-inflammatory effects of a low arachidonic acid diet and fish oil in patients with rheumatoid arthritis. *Rheumatol Int.* 2003;23(1):27–36.

270. Smith SM, Sumar B, Dixon KA. Musculoskeletal pain in overweight and obese children. *Int J Obes.* 2014;38(1):11–5.

271. Shivappa N, Hebert JR, Karamati M, Shariati-Bafghi SE, Rashidkhani B. Increased inflammatory potential of diet is associated with bone mineral density among postmenopausal women in Iran. *Eur J Nutr.* 2016;55(2):561–8.

272. Duchesne E, Dufresne SS, Dumont NA. Impact of inflammation and anti-inflammatory modalities on skeletal muscle healing: from fundamental research to the clinic. *Phys Ther.* 2017;97(8):807–17.

273. Mazidi M, Shivappa N, Wirth MD, Hebert JR, Vatanparast H, Kengne AP. The association between dietary inflammatory properties and bone mineral density and risk of fracture in US adults. *Eur J Clin Nutr.* 2017;71(11):1273–7.
274. Orchard T, Yildiz V, Steck SE, et al. Dietary Inflammatory Index, bone mineral density and risk of fracture in postmenopausal women: Results from the Women's Health Initiative. *J Bone Miner Res.* 2017;32(5):1136–46.
275. Shivappa N, Stubbs B, Hebert JR, et al. The relationship between the Dietary Inflammatory Index and incident frailty: A longitudinal cohort study. *J Am Med Dir Assoc.* 2018;19(1):77–82.
276. Veronese N, Shivappa N, Stubbs B, et al. The relationship between the dietary inflammatory index and prevalence of radiographic symptomatic osteoarthritis: Data from the Osteoarthritis Initiative. *Eur J Nutr.* 2017;58(1):253–60.
277. Veronese N, Stubbs B, Koyanagi A, et al. Pro-inflammatory dietary pattern is associated with fractures in women: An eight-year longitudinal cohort study. *Osteoporos Int.* 2018;29(1):143–51.
278. Viscogliosi G, Cipriani E, Liguori ML, et al. Mediterranean dietary pattern adherence: Associations with prediabetes, metabolic syndrome, and related microinflammation. *Metab Syndr Relat Disord.* 2013;11(3):210–16.
279. Echeverria G, McGee EE, Urquiaga I, et al. Inverse associations between a locally validated mediterranean diet index, overweight/obesity, and metabolic syndrome in Chilean adults. *Nutrients.* 2017;9(8):862.
280. Giugliano D, Ceriello A, Esposito K. The effects of diet on inflammation: Emphasis on the metabolic syndrome. *J Am Coll Cardiol.* 2006;48(4):677–85.
281. Boden S, Myte R, Wennberg M, et al. The inflammatory potential of diet in determining cancer risk: A prospective investigation of two dietary pattern scores. *PLoS One.* 2019;14(4):e0214551.
282. Puddu PE, Shivappa N, Menotti A, et al. Energy-adjusted Dietary Inflammatory Index scores predict long-term cardiovascular disease mortality and other causes of death in an ecological analysis of the Seven Countries Study. *Eur J Prev Cardiol.* 2020. [Epub ahead of print].
283. Caracciolo B, Xu W, Collins S, Fratiglioni L. Cognitive decline, dietary factors and gut-brain interactions. *Mech Ageing Dev.* 2014;136–7:59–69.
284. Bawaked RA, Schroder H, Ribas-Barba L, et al. Association of diet quality with dietary inflammatory potential in youth. *Food Nutr Res.* 2017;61(1):1328961.
285. Gupta PC, Hebert JR, Bhonsle RB, Sinor PN, Mehta H, Mehta FS. Dietary factors in oral leukoplakia and submucous fibrosis in a population-based case-control study in Gujarat, India. *Oral Dis.* 1998;4:200–6.
286. Gupta PC, Hebert JR, Bhonsle RB, Murti PR, Mehta H, Mehta FS. Influence of dietary factors on oral precancerous lesions in a population-based case-control study in Kerala, India. *Cancer.* 1999;85(9):1885–93.
287. Nakamura M, Tajima S, Yoshiike N. Nutrient intake in Japanese adults—From The National Nutrition Survey, 1995–99. *J Nutr Sci Vitaminol (Tokyo).* 2002;48(5):433–41.
288. Kimura Y, Nanri A, Matsushita Y, Sasaki S, Mizoue T. Eating behavior in relation to prevalence of overweight among Japanese men. *Asia Pac J Clin Nutr.* 2011;20(1):29–34.
289. Swinburn BA, Sacks G, Lo SK, et al. Estimating the changes in energy flux that characterize the rise in obesity prevalence. *Am J Clin Nutr.* 2009;89(6):1723–8.
290. Paris HL, Foright RM, Werth KA, et al. Increasing energy flux to decrease the biological drive toward weight regain after weight loss: A proof-of-concept pilot study. *Clin Nutr ESPEN.* 2016;11:e12–20.
291. Hume DJ, Yokum S, Stice E. Low energy intake plus low energy expenditure (low energy flux), not energy surfeit, predicts future body fat gain. *Am J Clin Nutr.* 2016;103(6):1389–96.
292. Rarick KR, Pikosky MA, Grediagin A, et al. Energy flux, more so than energy balance, protein intake, or fitness level, influences insulin-like growth factor-I system responses during 7 days of increased physical activity. *J Appl Physiol.* 2007;103(5):1613–21.
293. Manore MM, Larson-Meyer DE, Lindsay AR, Hongu N, Houtkooper L. Dynamic energy balance: An integrated framework for discussing diet and physical activity in obesity prevention—Is it more than eating less and exercising more? *Nutrients.* 2017;9(8):19.
294. Jansen EC, Conroy DA, Burgess HJ, et al. Plasma DHA is related to sleep timing and duration in a cohort of Mexican adolescents. *J Nutr.* 2020;150(3):592–8.
295. Jansen EC, Peterson KE, Lumeng JC, et al. Associations between sleep and dietary patterns among low-income children attending preschool. *J Acad Nutr Diet.* 2019;119(7):1176–87.
296. Jansen EC, She R, Rukstalis MM, Alexander GL. Sleep duration and quality in relation to fruit and vegetable intake of US young adults: A secondary analysis. *Int J Behav Med.* 2020. [Epub ahead of print].
297. Castillo M. The complicated equation of smell, flavor, and taste. *AJNR Am J Neuroradiol.* 2014;35(7):1243–5.
298. Sclafani A. Gut-brain nutrient signaling. Appetition vs. satiation. *Appetite.* 2013;71:454–8.
299. Ruijschop RM, Boelrijk AE, de Ru JA, de Graaf C, Westerterp-Plantenga MS. Effects of retro-nasal aroma release on satiation. *Br J Nutr.* 2008;99(5):1140–8.
300. Dalenberg JR, Weitkamp L, Renken RJ, Nanetti L, Ter Horst GJ. Flavor pleasantness processing in the ventral emotion network. *PLoS One.* 2017;12(2):e0170310.
301. Rolls ET. Functions of the orbitofrontal and pregenual cingulate cortex in taste, olfaction, appetite and emotion. *Acta Physiol Hung.* 2008;95(2):131–64.
302. Rolls ET. Taste, olfactory, and food texture processing in the brain, and the control of food intake. *Physiol Behav.* 2005;85(1):45–56.
303. Rolls ET. Convergence of sensory systems in the orbitofrontal cortex in primates and brain design for emotion. *Anat Rec A Discov Mol Cell Evol Biol.* 2004;281(1):1212–25.
304. Haynes SC, Rudov L, Nauman E, Hendryx L, Angove RSM, Carton T. Engaging stakeholders to develop a patient-centered research agenda: Lessons learned from the Research Action for Health Network (REACHnet). *Med Care.* 2018;56 Suppl 10 Suppl 1:S27–32.
305. Sheridan S, Schrandt S, Forsythe L, Advisory Panel on Patient Engagement, Hilliard TS, Paez KA. The PCORI Engagement Rubric: Promising practices for partnering in research. *Ann Fam Med.* 2017;15(2):165–70.
306. Nutrition Evidence Systematic Review. Systematic reviews for the 2020 Dietary Guidelines Advisory Committee. https://nesr.usda.gov/2020-dietary-guidelines-advisory-committee-systematic-reviews. Accessed March 5, 2020.
307. The Academy of Nutrition and Dietetics Evidence Analysis Library. https://www.cdrnet.org/evidence. Accessed March 5, 2020.
308. Community Preventive Services Task Force (CPSTF). The Community Guide—Nutrition. https://www.thecommunityguide.org/topic/nutrition. Accessed March 5, 2020.

CHAPTER

183 Physical Activity Epidemiology in Health and Disease

Robin P. Shook • Michael D. Wirth • Steven N. Blair

INTRODUCTION

Ancient philosophers and medical scientists, English Lords, and United States Presidents have noted the health benefits of living an active life for thousands of years. Attempts to quantify the role of physical activity and health using scientific methods have been much more recent, beginning in earnest during the mid-twentieth century with a series of foundational epidemiological studies.[1,2] In the decades since, cohort epidemiological studies have demonstrated clear and consistent benefits of physical activity on a broad range of health outcomes and mortality using a variety of different techniques to quantify activity. National and global surveillance systems provide population-level physical activity prevalence data, which is used to guide public health recommendations for optimal health. To understand how epidemiology informs our understanding the role of lifestyle and physiology in preventive medicine and disease treatment, it is important to define the different aspects physical activity and fitness.

Defining Physical Activity and Physical Fitness

Physical activity is defined as any bodily movement produced by skeletal muscles that results an increase in metabolic rate over a period of time.[3] This concept is intentionally broad in scope, and there are numerous domains of physical activity including leisure-time physical activity (which include exercise and sport), work-based physical activity, household physical activity, and transportation physical activity (Fig. 183-1 for average energy expenditure by each domain for a representative U.S. sample of adults). Structured **exercise** is one component of leisure-time physical activity and is defined as an activity that is performed repeatedly over an extended period of time (bout) with the specific external intention of improvement in fitness, physical performance, or health.[3] **Sport** is another form of leisure-time physical activity, and is generally defined as a competitive activity under the context of rules (though some parts of the world consider all exercise as sport).[3] **Work, household, and transport physical activity** refer to bodily movement that occurs while performing task related to the relevant domain (lifting boxes, caring for a child, biking to work, etc.). **Fitness** refers the ability to perform work, and can be either health- or performance-related. **Performance** aspects of fitness can include muscular power, speed, endurance, agility, etc. **Health-related fitness** can refer to muscular, motor, metabolic, and cardiorespiratory components.

PROGRESSION OF PHYSICAL ACTIVITY EPIDEMIOLOGY: HISTORICAL OVERVIEW

Epidemiologists have been exploring the association between physical activity and health for over six decades using a variety of techniques. Before the establishment of a national surveillance system related to physical activity, Morris et al. creatively compared London transportation workers by classifying them by the occupational tasks in a landmark 1953 study. Double-decker bus conductors, who spent the majority of their day walking through the aisle and climbing the bus steps to collect fares and supervising passenger loading/unloading, experienced lower rates of cardiovascular disease compared to the sedentary bus drivers, who spent the majority of their day seated (Table 183-1).[1,4] Similar analysis of occupational physical activity and health was subsequently conducted among civil servants (postmen, telegraph officers, telephonists, and supervisors)[1] and San Francisco longshoremen (handling cargo vs. less active jobs).[5] In an effort to identify the role of leisure-time physical activity on health in 1966, Paffenbarger et al. asked college alumni from Harvard University and the University of Pennsylvania to subjectively report their participation in sports using a questionnaire. Those engaging in ≥ 10 hours/week of exercise were less likely to die from coronary heart disease compared to their sedentary peers after 40 years of follow-up (Fig. 183-2, 8.9% vs. 17.4%).[2] Importantly, by using a questionnaire that included detailed questions about duration and intensity of exercise, Paffenbarger was able quantify for the first time the dose-dependent relationship between amount of physical activity performed and health outcomes (Fig. 183-3).[6]

Attempting to further quantify this association, Blair et al. in 1989 objectively measured cardiorespiratory fitness (CRF) using a

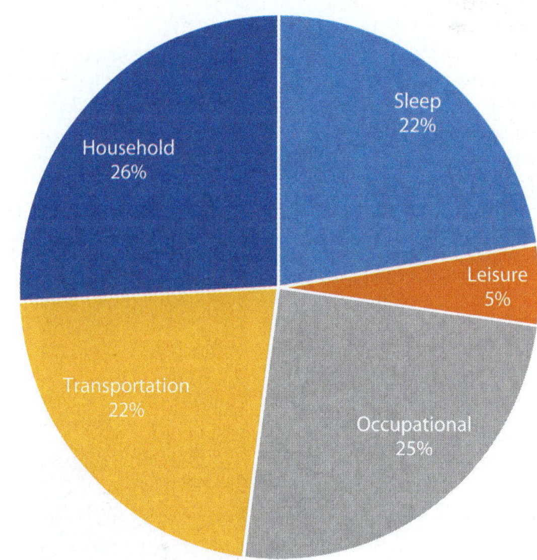

FIGURE 183-1. Energy expenditure by activity domain estimated from the National Human Activity Patterns Survey. (*Source:* Adapted from Dong L, Block G, Mandel S. Activities contributing to total energy expenditure in the United States: Results from the NHAPS Study. *Int J Behav Nutr Phys Act.* 2004;1(1):4.)

maximal treadmill exercise test in 13,344 adults and found a 58% higher relative risk for unfit men and 94% relative risk for unfit women compared to their fit counterparts after 110,482 person years of follow-up (Table 183-2).[7] Further advancements in 1995 involved multiple assessments of CRF separated by years, which controlled for confounders associated with one-time assessments, and found those who improved from unfit to fit had a reduction in mortality risk of 44% compared to those who were unfit at both assessments.[8]

Physical activity epidemiology has continued to progress and offer insights into the role of an active lifestyle on human health. Researchers have described temporal declines in occupational,[9] household,[10] and transportation-related[11] physical activity over several decades, corresponding with increases in population-level obesity rates. Monitoring devices such as pedometers[12] and accelerometers[13] have been included in variety of surveillance systems and have added to the large body of evidence describing the protective effects of physical activity and human health. More recently, data from smartphones equipped with accelerometers have provided worldwide data from nearly a million users across hundreds of countries.[14]

ASSESSING PHYSICAL ACTIVITY

An ever-growing array of physical activity assessment tools exist, and the user should select a method based on the cost, participant burden, sample size, collection time frame, type of information required (e.g., steps, counts, energy expenditure), data management,

TABLE 183-1 RATES OF CARDIOVASCULAR-RELATED DEATH AMONG ACTIVE BUS CONDUCTORS VS. SEDENTARY BUS DRIVERS

	Age-standardized Rates per 1000/year	
	"Sudden Death" in First Clinical Episode	Deaths Later, within First 3 Months of First Episode
Men ages 35–64		
Conductors	0.5	0.3
Drivers	1.1	0.5
Men ages 35–59		
Postmen	0.4	0.3
Telephonists	0.8	0.6

Source: Morris JN, Heady JA, Raffle PA, Roberts CG, Parks JW. Coronary heart-disease and physical activity of work. *Lancet.* 1953;265(6795):1053–7.

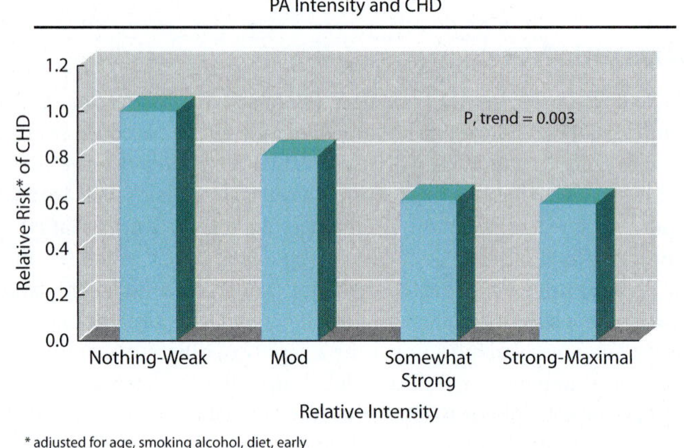

FIGURE 183-3. (*Source:* Lee IM, Paffenbarger RS Jr. Associations of light, moderate, and vigorous intensity physical activity with longevity: The Harvard Alumni Health Study. *Am J Epidemiol.* 2000;151(3):293–9.)

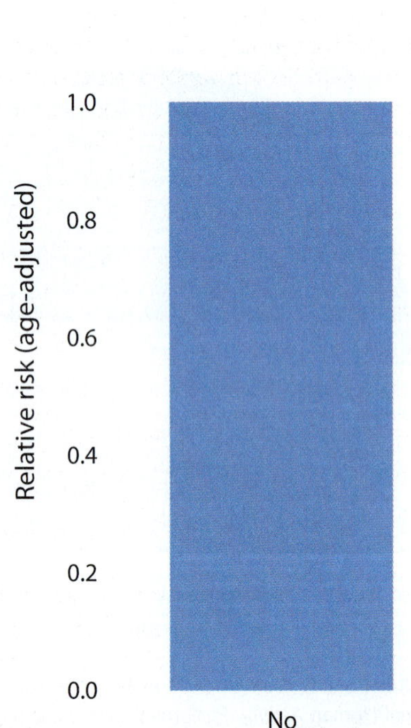

FIGURE 183-2. Participation in varisity athletics. (*Source:* Paffenbarger RS Jr, Wolf PA, Notkin J, Thorne MC. Chronic disease in former college students. I. Early precursors of fatal coronary heart disease. *Am J Epidemiol.* 1966;83(2):314–28.)

TABLE 183-2 AGE-ADJUSTED ALL-CAUSE DEATH RATES PER 10,000 PERSON-YEARS OF FOLLOW-UP (1970–85) BY PHYSICAL FITNESS GROUPS IN MEN AND WOMEN IN THE AEROBICS CENTER LONGITUDINAL STUDY

Fitness Group	Person-Years of Follow-up	No. of Deaths	Age-Adjusted Rates per 10 000 Person-Years	Relative Risk	95% Confidence Limits
Men					
1 (low)	14 515	75	64.0	3.44*	2.05, 5.77
2	16 898	40	25.5	1.37	0.76, 2.50
3	17 287	47	27.1	1.46	0.81, 2.63
4	18 792	43	21.7	1.17	0.63, 2.17
5 (high)	17 557	35	18.6	1.00	. . .
Women					
1 (low)	4916	18	39.5	4.65†	2.22, 9.75
2	5329	11	20.5	2.42	1.09, 5.37
3	5053	6	12.2	1.43	0.60, 3.44
4	5522	4	6.5	0.76	0.27, 2.11
5 (high)	4613	4	8.5	1.00	. . .

*Test for linear trend, slope = −4.5; 95% confidence limits, −7.1, −1.9.
†Test for linear trend, slope = −5.5; 95% confidence limits, −9.2, −1.9.

Source: Data from Blair SN, Kohl HW 3rd, Paffenbarger RS Jr, Clark DG, Cooper KH, Gibbons LW. Physical fitness and all-cause mortality. A prospective study of healthy men and women. *JAMA*. 1989;262(17):2395–401.

and measurement error.[15,16] The following section provides a brief overview of physical activity assessment tools. Additional information can be found in recent reviews by McClung,[17] Ainsworth et al.,[18] Slyvia et al.,[19] Welk et al.,[20] and the Physical Activity Resource Center for Public Health (http://www.parcph.org/). Physical activity assessment techniques are summarized in Table 183-3.

Self-report Assessment Tools

Self-report physical activity measures include traditional written logs or diaries and questionnaires. Questionnaires have been used to identify the dimensions and domains of physical activity behaviors from either written responses or interviews.[21] The strengths of self-report assessments are their simplicity, low-cost, and ease of administration, as well as strong correlation to vigorous-intensity physical activity.[22–24] However, these assessments are limited by issues with recall, difficulty in measuring compliance, and dose-response outcomes in research.[18]

Device-based Assessment Tools

Physical activity can also be assessed using a wide range of mechanical or electrical devices that are worn on the body. Pedometers (small, step-counting devices) may utilized be at a population level with great validity,[25] reliability,[26] and affordability.[27] For these same reasons, pedometers are often recommended for use in "real-world" settings to promote physical activity, and public health guidelines for the accumulation of physical activity have been translated into terms of steps per day.[26,28,29]

Accelerometers measure physical activity volume and intensity by recording movement in multiple geometric axis (e.g., anteroposterior, mediolateral, vertical). They can be worn on the wrist or hip, with the hip location providing better accuracy but the wrist providing better participant compliance.[30–32] Accelerometers allow users to collect large amounts of data, estimation of intensity level, and avoid potential participant recall bias. Limitations include a greater cost compared to devices such as pedometers, the inability to provide contextual information (e.g., leisure vs. occupational activity), and need for specific training in data analysis.

Consumer Devices

Consumer wearable devices from companies such as Fitbit, Jawbone, Garmin, and Apple designed to measure physical activity are generally affordable, easy to use, and popular (an estimated 45 million were sold in 2017),[33] but have varying levels of validity and reliability.[34–36] New devices and algorithm updates are released frequently, making longitudinal comparisons challenging. Additionally, modern smartphones often include onboard accelerometers within their hardware, and many applications ("apps") collect continuous data from their owners throughout the day. For example, a 2017 manuscript reported physical activity data on 717,527 individuals from 111 countries, consisting of 68 million days of minute-by-minute step recordings.[14] This information was combined with user-entered age, sex, and body weight, and overlayed with location data, providing insights on physical activity throughout the world.

Cardiorespiratory Fitness

As described earlier, cardiorespiratory fitness (CRF) is an excellent predictor of a variety of health outcomes as it represents multiple physiological systems (cardiovascular, pulmonary, musculoskeletal, etc.). CRF is determined by a combination of intrinsic factors (e.g., heredity) and recent (e.g., past 3–6 months) physical activity level; as a result, it has become a desirable outcome for many surveillance systems. A meta-analysis involving both objectively measured CRF and subjectively reported physical activity found consistently lower rates of risk reduction for all-cause mortality among studies utilizing self-reported physical activity compared to objectively measured CRF.[37] One study involving 6213 men which included both variables measured simultaneously among the same cohort found a poor correlation between the two methods ($r = 0.09$), though high levels of each were associated with reductions in mortality (high CRF: HR = 0.28, $p < 0.0001$; high physical activity: HR = 0.38, $p < 0.001$).[38] Despite the superiority of using objective methods, maximal exercise testing requires participants to exercise to volitional fatigue and may require medical supervision,[39] making implementation in large cohort studies typically unfeasible. Conversely, self-report

TABLE 183-3 SUMMARY OF PHYSICAL ACTIVITY ASSESSMENT TOOLS IN THE FIELD

Type	Method/Tool	Appropriate Applications (e.g., Population, Timeline, etc.)	Outcome Measure	Attributes	Limitations	Validity	Research Gaps	References
Reported (subjective)	Questionnaires	Large populations; epidemiologic and surveillance	Different dimensions of PA, including EE estimates	Rank order based on activity levels; ease of administration; low cost; multiple validated questionnaires for different populations; assesses the domain in which PA occurred; ability to assess previous PA levels	Reliance on self-report; potential for recall bias; difficulty establishing a dose–response relationship	Validity correlations range from 0.14 to 0.36, with the exception of the Seven-Day Physical Activity Recall, which had validity correlations of 0.53 with accelerometers	Combining questionnaires with objective PA measures in order to identify the specific domain (occupation, leisure, lifestyle, transport, household) in which PA occurred	21–24
	Diaries/logs	Detailed hour-by-hour assessment of PA	EE estimate based on the Compendium of Physical Activities	Time, intensity rating, and type of PA; information can then be scored and EE estimated	Reliance on self-report	Correlations range from 0.2 to 0.3 against accelerometers	Being used in conjunction with ecological momentary assessment	63, 64
Device-based (objective)	Consumer wearables (Fitbit, Jawbone, Apple)	Large population; behavior change within individuals	EE	Popular; ease of collection and data upload (wireless); large amounts of data collected	Not a valid measure of TEE; underestimates free-living EE; overestimates PAEE; algorithms change with updates; not designed for research; cost to obtain data	Correlation between consumer activity monitors and accelerometers for sleep count and step count, $r > 0.8$; for TDEE, $r = 0.74–0.81$; and MVPA, $r = 0.52–0.91$	More accuracy research is needed	65–69
	Accelerometers	Large populations	Minutes of physical activity, intensity	Commonly used in research settings and by NHANES; ability to collect large amounts of data	Expense; inability to provide contextual information; data collection protocols (e.g., hip vs. wrist placement, waking-hour vs. 24-hour registration period) and data analysis approaches (e.g., nonwear-time definition, valid day criteria, cut-points for intensity classification) vary, making it very difficult to compare across studies using accelerometry	Correlations between daily PAEE and activity counts for the hip-worn ActiGraph range from $r = 0.77–0.90$; compared to wearable cameras measuring PA, hip-worn accelerometers had 89.4% accuracy and wrist-worn accelerometers had 84.6% accuracy	Lack of consensus regarding data processing	30–32, 70–75
	GPS	Large populations; outdoors	Distance and speed	Ideal use outdoors (free-living walking and running) or field testing	Underestimates EE for field activities; not a standalone measure for EE; not appropriate for indoor activities; issues with battery life	Compared to accelerometers, GPS underestimates EE by 42–50%	Stronger association with EE measure (accelerometer use)	76–82

TABLE 183-3 SUMMARY OF PHYSICAL ACTIVITY ASSESSMENT TOOLS IN THE FIELD *(CONTINUED)*

Type	Method/Tool	Appropriate Applications (e.g., Population, Timeline, etc.)	Outcome Measure	Attributes	Limitations	Validity	Research Gaps	References
	HR	Supervised exercise	HR, activity intensity	Direct measure, high-validity to clinical measures	Uncomfortable when worn for long periods of time; not a valid estimate of EE at rest; must have a HR-O_2 consumption curve for each person to measure their intensity; TDEE is hard to predict because daily HR is not linear	During PA, EE error rates are $< 3\%$ compared to whole-room calorimetry; however, when doing light or sedentary activity, they have poor predictive power in terms of EE	Improved estimates of TEE	83–86
	Multisensor	Populations with a wide range of activities	Minutes of PA, EE	Multiple mechanical and physiological sensors improve estimates	Cost, availability	Sensewear: EE and activity ICC of 0.81–0.85 compared to DLW; IDEEA: EE within $98.9\% \pm 9.0\%$ compared to indirect calorimetry	Improved estimates of individual-level estimates	87–94
	ActivPAL	Large populations	Sedentary time, steps/day	Can be worn 24 hours/day	Relatively small body of literature compared to other accelerometers	Correlations range from 0.78 to 0.99 against direct observation	Validation for EE	95–99
	Pedometers	Large populations	Steps/day	Affordable; best used to assess walking; steps/day is well understood by the lay population; newer versions store data	Inaccurate at slow speeds; interindividual variability-based difference; in some models, must manually record steps; readings vary according to anatomical location (e.g., hip or ankle)	Varies by model	Estimations of EE and exercise intensity	100–106

Abbreviations: EE = energy expenditure; ICC = intraclass correlation coefficient; NHANES = National Health and Nutrition Examination Survey; PA = physical activity; PAEE = physical activity energy expenditure; TDEE = total daily energy expenditure; TEE = total energy expenditure. (*Source:* McClung H, Ptomey L, Shook RP, et al. Dietary intake and physical activity assessment: Current tools, techniques, and technologies for use in adult populations. *Am J Prev Med*. 2018;55(4):e93–104.)

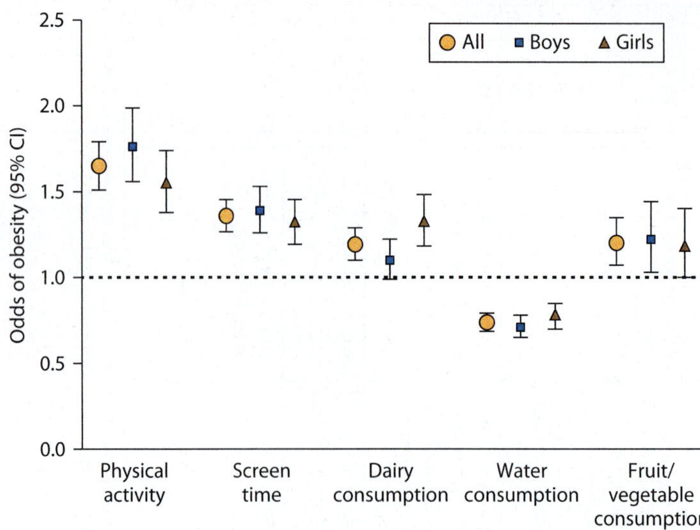

FIGURE 183-4. Odds of obesity if not meeting recommendations for specific lifestyle behaviors, adjusted for race/ethnicity, insurance type, year of visit, and other lifestyle behavior responses. (*Source:* Reproduced with Permission from Shook RP, Halpin K, Carlson JA, et al. Adherence with multiple national healthy lifestyle recommendations in a large pediatric center electronic health record and reduced risk of obesity. *Mayo Clin Proc.* 2018;93(9):1247-1255.)

questionnaires, which are limited by recall bias and misreporting,[40] have been typically utilized in large population-based studies.

The Fitness Registry and the Importance of Exercise National Database (FRIEND) was created in 2013 to provide national standards CRF values across a variety of populations.[38,41–44] Currently, the database include values from ten different clinical research centers involving nearly 8000 individuals ranging in age from 20 to 79 years. One of the primary goals of FRIEND is to serve as a tracking device for CRF levels in the U.S. population, complementing present physical activity surveillance systems, which lack robustness.[44]

Assessments in the Electronic Health Record

With increasing widespread adoption of electronic health record (EHR), opportunities are emerging for improved surveillance of health outcomes, such as childhood obesity and cardiovascular disease outcomes, at the local and population level.[45–48] The global initiative Exercise is Medicine (http://www.exerciseismedicine.org/) encourages primary-care physicians and other healthcare providers to include physical activity when designing treatment plans, and includes the tracking of physical activity as a "vital sign," just as a provider would track a patient's heart rate, body weight, and blood pressure. There is growing momentum in healthcare systems to track exercise levels in EHRs[49–51] due to the clear role of physical activity and cardiorespiratory fitness in improving health[7,52–56] and in preventing/treating obesity.[9,10,57–59] The assessment of physical activity level as vital sign in EHR using a brief (<30 seconds) question (e.g., "Please describe your level of physical activity in minutes per day and days per week") has generally resulted in good concurrent validity and strong correlations with longer, more detailed physical activity questionnaires,[60] in addition to clear discriminant validity to identify chronic diseases associated with low levels of physical activity.[61] In Kansas City, Missouri, researchers and clinicians at Children's Mercy Hospital have embedded five simple questions related to physical activity and eating behavior, and compared response to national recommendations for each lifestyle factor.[62] Among 24,255 patients aged 2–18 years old, prevalence of meeting recommendations for lifestyle behaviors was highest for physical activity (84%), followed by screen time (61%), consumption of water (51%), dairy (27%), and fruit/vegetables (10%). When merged with clinic-measured body weight, they observed that insufficient physical activity was the strongest predictor of obesity (OR 1.65, 95% CI 1.51–1.79), followed by excess screen time (OR 1.36, 95% CI 1.27–1.45; Fig. 183-4). Those youths who met 0 or 1 lifestyle recommendation were 1.45 (95% CI 1.06, 1.99) to 1.71 (95% CI 1.22, 2.41) times more likely to have obesity than those meeting all five recommendations.

NATIONAL SURVEILLANCE SYSTEMS

National surveillance systems are the backbone for the valid and reliable assessment of physical activity in all segments of the U.S. population.[107,108] There are multiple governmental surveys currently performing surveillance activities across a variety of populations and domains (Table 183-4),[107,109] including the American Community Survey (active transportation), American Time Use Survey (active transportation, leisure time, household, occupational), Behavioral Risk Factor Surveillance System (nonoccupational), National Household Transportation Survey (active transportation), National Health and Nutrition Examination Survey (NHANES; active transportation, leisure time, work, accelerometry), and the National Health Interview Survey (active transportation, leisure); the Youth Risk Behavior Surveillance System (YRBSS; physical activity specifically among middle and high school students). Assessment of physical activity is conducted via self-reported questionnaire, interviewer-assessed questions, or device-based measures (accelerometry), depending on the surveillance system. Additionally, health assessments are completed either by self-reporter in-person, which allows for associations with physical activity.

Surveillance of physical activity over the past several decades has led to the development, implementation, and evaluation of programs at the local, national, and global levels.[110] Surveillance systems will continue to incorporate standardized objective measures such as accelerometers and CRF into their assessments. There are increasingly new opportunities to include emerging technologies and innovative data sources, such as smartphone apps[14] and consumer devices[14,67,111] to assess physical activity at both a national and global scale with a relatively low cost. Additionally, comprehensive surveillance should also include indicators for macro-level determinants of physical activity, such as governmental support, national policy, local zoning codes, and infrastructure for physical activity.[110,112–114]

TABLE 183-4 CURRENT U.S. GOVERNMENT SURVEILLANCE SYSTEMS THAT COLLECT PHYSICAL ACTIVITY BEHAVIOR AMONG U.S. ADULTS

Survey (website)	Collection Method (\mode)	Physical Activity Domains	Survey Years	Measure
American Community Survey (http://www.census.gov/acs/)	Survey questions (on-line/mail/in person)	Active transportation	2008–2012	Usual mode of transportation to work last week
ATUS (http://www.bls.gov/tus/)	One day activity diary (telephone)	Active transportation	2003–2013	Minutes of specific activity for 24 h
		Leisure time	2003–2013	
		Household	2003–2013	
		Occupational	2003–2013	
Behavioral Risk Factor Surveillance System (http://www.cdc.gov/brfss/)	Survey questions (Telephone)	Nonoccupational	2011–2014[a]	Minutes of top two physical activities in past week or past month
NHTS (http://nhts.ornl.gov/)	One day travel diary survey question (telephone)	Active transportation	1969–2009	Participants logged all trips on 1 d, including mode of travel and purpose; mode of transportation to work used for most of the distance in the past week
NHANES (http://www.cdc.gov/nchs/nhanes.htm)	Survey questions (in person)	Active transportation	2007–2014	Minutes of walking and bicycling for transportation in typical week
		Leisure time	2007–2014	Minutes of vigorous- and moderate-intensity leisure-time activity in typical week
		Work (paid/unpaid)	2007–2014	Minutes of vigorous- and moderate-intensity work activity in typical week
NHIS: Cancer Supplement (http://www.cdc.gov/nchs/nhis.htm)	Survey questions (in person)	Active transportation	2005, 2010	Minutes of transportation walking in past 7 d
NHIS: Sample Adult Survey (http://www.cdc.gov/nchs/nhis.htm)	Survey questions (in person)	Leisure time	1997–2014	Minutes of vigorous- and light- to moderate-intensity activity in respondent selected recall period

[a]Inactivity surveyed every year, all physical activity surveyed in odd years.

Source: Reproduced with Permission Fulton JE, Carlson SA, Ainsworth BE, et al. Strategic priorities for physical activity surveillance in the United States. *Med Sci Sports Exerc.* 2016;48(10):2057-2069.

References

1. Morris JN, Heady JA, Raffle PA, Roberts CG, Parks JW. Coronary heart-disease and physical activity of work. *Lancet.* 1953;265(6795):1053–7.
2. Paffenbarger RS Jr, Wolf PA, Notkin J, Thorne MC. Chronic disease in former college students. I. Early precursors of fatal coronary heart disease. *Am J Epidemiol.* 1966;83(2):314–28.
3. Bouchard C, Blair SN, Haskell WL, Haskell W. *Physical activity and health.* Champaign, IL: Human Kinetics; 2007.
4. Morris JN, Heady JA, Raffle PA, Roberts CG, Parks JW. Coronary heart-disease and physical activity of work. *Lancet.* 1953;262(6795):1053–7.
5. Paffenbarger RS Jr, Laughlin ME, Gima AS, Black RA. Work activity of longshoremen as related to death from coronary heart disease and stroke. *N Engl J Med.* 1970;282(20):1109–14.
6. Lee IM, Paffenbarger RS Jr. Associations of light, moderate, and vigorous intensity physical activity with longevity: The Harvard Alumni Health Study. *Am J Epidemiol.* 2000;151(3):293–9.
7. Blair SN, Kohl HW 3rd, Paffenbarger RS Jr, Clark DG, Cooper KH, Gibbons LW. Physical fitness and all-cause mortality. A prospective study of healthy men and women. *JAMA.* 1989;262(17):2395–401.
8. Blair SN, Kohl HW 3rd, Barlow CE, Paffenbarger RS Jr, Gibbons LW, Macera CA. Changes in physical fitness and all-cause mortality: A prospective study of healthy and unhealthy men. *JAMA.* 1995;273(14):1093–8.
9. Church TS, Thomas DM, Tudor-Locke C, et al. Trends over 5 decades in U.S. occupation-related physical activity and their associations with obesity. *PLoS One.* 2011;6(5):e19657.
10. Archer E, Shook RP, Thomas DM, et al. 45-year trends in women's use of time and household management energy expenditure. *PLoS One.* 2013;8(2):e56620.
11. McDonald NC. Active transportation to school: Trends among US schoolchildren, 1969–2001. *Am J Prev Med.* 2007;32(6):509–16.
12. Dwyer T, Pezic A, Sun C, et al. Objectively measured daily steps and subsequent long term all-cause mortality: The Tasped Prospective Cohort Study. *PLoS One.* 2015;10(11):e0141274.
13. Troiano RP, Berrigan D, Dodd KW, Masse LC, Tilert T, McDowell M. Physical activity in the United States measured by accelerometer. *Med Sci Sports Exerc.* 2008;40(1):181–8.
14. Althoff T, Sosic R, Hicks JL, King AC, Delp SL, Leskovec J. Large-scale physical activity data reveal worldwide activity inequality. *Nature.* 2017;547(7663):336–9.
15. Schutz Y, Weinsier RL, Hunter GR. Assessment of free-living physical activity in humans: An overview of currently available and proposed new measures. *Obes Res.* 2001;9(6):368–79.
16. Hills AP, Mokhtar N, Byrne NM. Assessment of physical activity and energy expenditure: An overview of objective measures. *Front Nutr.* 2014;1:5.
17. McClung H, Ptomey L, Shook RP, et al. Dietary intake and physical activity assessment: Current tools, techniques, and technologies for use in adult populations. *Am J Prev Med.* 2018;55(4):e93–104.
18. Ainsworth B, Cahalin L, Buman M, Ross R. The current state of physical activity assessment tools. *Prog Cardiovasc Dis.* 2015;57(4):387–95.
19. Sylvia LG, Bernstein EE, Hubbard JL, Keating L, Anderson EJ. A practical guide to measuring physical activity. *J Acad Nutr Diet.* 2014;114(2):199–208.
20. Welk GJ, Morrow J, Saint-Maurice P. *Measures Registry User Guide: Individual Physical Activity.* Washington, DC: National Collaborative on Childhood Obesity Research; 2017, pp. 1–72. http://nccor.org/

tools-mruserguides/wp-content/uploads/2017/NCCOR_MR_User_Guide_Individual_PA-FINAL.pdf.

21. Strath SJ, Kaminsky LA, Ainsworth BE, et al. Guide to the assessment of physical activity: Clinical and research applications. *Circulation.* 2013;128(20):2259–79.
22. Jacobs DR Jr, Ainsworth BE, Hartman TJ, Leon AS. A simultaneous evaluation of 10 commonly used physical activity questionnaires. *Med Science Sports Exerc.* 1993;25(1):81–91.
23. Ainsworth BE, Richardson MT, Jacobs DR, Leon AS, Sternfeld B. Accuracy of recall of occupational physical activity by questionnaire. *J Clin Epidemiol.* 1999;52(3):219–27.
24. Strath SJ, Bassett DR, Swartz AM. Comparison of the college alumnus questionnaire physical activity index with objective monitoring. *Ann Epidemiol.* 2004;14(6):409–15.
25. Tudor-Locke C, Williams JE, Reis JP, Pluto D. Utility of pedometers for assessing physical activity: Construct validity. *Sports Med.* 2004;34(5):281–91.
26. Tudor-Locke C, Burkett L, Reis JP, Ainsworth BE, Macera CA, Wilson DK. How many days of pedometer monitoring predict weekly physical activity in adults? *Prev Med.* 2005;40(3):293–8.
27. Welk GJ, Differding JA, Thompson RW, Blair SN, Dziura J, Hart P. The utility of the Digi-walker step counter to assess daily physical activity patterns. *Med Sci Sports Exerc.* 2000;32(9 Suppl):S481–8.
28. Tudor-Locke C, Craig CL, Aoyagi Y, et al. How many steps/day are enough? For older adults and special populations. *Int J Behav Nutr Phys Act.* 2011;8:80.
29. Department of Health and Human Services. *2008 Physical Activity Guidelines for Americans.* Washington, DC: Department of Health and Human Services; 2008.
30. Tudor-Locke C, Barreira TV, Schuna JM Jr. Comparison of step outputs for waist and wrist accelerometer attachment sites. *Med Sci Sports Exerc.* 2015;47(4):839–42.
31. Ellis K, Kerr J, Godbole S, Lanckriet G, Wing D, Marshall S. A random forest classifier for the prediction of energy expenditure and type of physical activity from wrist and hip accelerometers. *Physiol Meas.* 2014;35(11):2191–203.
32. Ellis K, Kerr J, Godbole S, Staudenmayer J, Lanckriet G. Hip and wrist accelerometer algorithms for free-living behavior classification. *Med Sci Sports Exerc.* 2016;48(5):933–40.
33. Alger K. Wearable technology is revolutionizing fitness. 2014. https://www.raconteur.net/technology/wearables-are-the-perfect-fit.
34. El-Amrawy F, Nounou MI. Are currently available wearable devices for activity tracking and heart rate monitoring accurate, precise, and medically beneficial? *Healthc Inform Res.* 2015;21(4):315–20.
35. Lee J-M, Kim Y, Welk GJ. Validity of consumer-based physical activity monitors. *Med Sci Sports Exerc.* 2014;46(9):1840–48.
36. Murakami H, Kawakami R, Nakae S, et al. Accuracy of wearable devices for estimating total energy expenditure: Comparison with metabolic chamber and doubly labeled water method. *JAMA Intern Med.* 2016;176(5):702–3.
37. Lollgen H, Bockenhoff A, Knapp G. Physical activity and all-cause mortality: An updated meta-analysis with different intensity categories. *Int J Sports Med.* 2009;30(3):213–24.
38. Myers J, Kaykha A, George S, et al. Fitness versus physical activity patterns in predicting mortality in men. *Am J Med.* 2004;117(12):912–8.
39. ACSM. Physical fitness testing and interpretation. In: American College of Sports Medicine, ed. *ACSM's Guidelines for Exercise Testing and Prescription.* 8th ed. Baltimore, MD: Lipencott, Williams, and Williams; 2009.
40. Sallis JF, Saelens BE. Assessment of physical activity by self-report: Status, limitations, and future directions. *Res Q Exerc Sport.* 2000;71(2 Suppl):S1–14.
41. Myers J, Kaminsky LA, Lima R, Christle JW, Ashley E, Arena R. A reference equation for normal standards for VO2 max: Analysis from the Fitness Registry and the Importance of Exercise National Database (FRIEND Registry). *Prog Cardiovasc Dis.* 2017;60(1):21–9.
42. Kaminsky LA, Imboden MT, Arena R, Myers J. Reference standards for cardiorespiratory fitness measured with cardiopulmonary exercise testing using cycle ergometry: Data from the Fitness Registry and the Importance of Exercise National Database (FRIEND) registry. *Mayo Clin Proc.* 2017;92(2):228–33.
43. Kaminsky LA, Arena R, Myers J. Reference standards for cardiorespiratory fitness measured with cardiopulmonary exercise testing: Data from the Fitness Registry and the Importance of Exercise National Database. *Mayo Clin Proc.* 2015;90(11):1515–23.
44. Kaminsky LA, Arena R, Beckie TM, et al. The importance of cardiorespiratory fitness in the United States: The need for a national registry: A policy statement from the American Heart Association. *Circulation.* 2013;127(5):652–62.
45. Hawkins SS, Gillman MW, Rifas-Shiman SL, Kleinman KP, Mariotti M, Taveras EM. The Linked CENTURY Study: Linking three decades of clinical and public health data to examine disparities in childhood obesity. *BMC Pediatr.* 2016;16:32.
46. Kranz AM, Browner DK, McDermid L, Coleman TR, Wooten WJ. Using electronic health record data for healthy weight surveillance in children, San Diego, California, 2014. *Prev Chronic Dis.* 2016;13:E34.
47. Tomayko EJ, Weinert BA, Godfrey L, Adams AK, Hanrahan LP. Using electronic health records to examine disease risk in small populations: Obesity among American Indian children, Wisconsin, 2007–2012. *Prev Chronic Dis.* 2016;13:E29.
48. Funk LM, Shan Y, Voils CI, Kloke J, Hanrahan LP. Electronic health record data versus the National Health and Nutrition Examination Survey (NHANES): A comparison of overweight and obesity rates. *Med Care.* 2017;55(6):598–605.
49. Grant R, Schmittdiel J, Neugebauer R, Uratsu C, Sternfeld B. Exercise as a vital sign: A quasi-experimental analysis of a health system intervention to collect patient-reported exercise levels. *J Gen Intern Med.* 2014;29(2):341–8.
50. Joy E. Time for a new 'vital sign': Providers should monitor patients' physical activity in battle against obesity. *Mod Healthc.* 2013;43(13):29.
51. Sallis R, Franklin B, Joy L, Ross R, Sabgir D, Stone J. Strategies for promoting physical activity in clinical practice. *Prog Cardiovasc Dis.* 2015;57(4):375–86.
52. Arem H, Moore SC, Patel A, et al. Leisure time physical activity and mortality: A detailed pooled analysis of the dose-response relationship. *JAMA Intern Med.* 2015;175(6):959–67.
53. Blair S. Physical inactivity: The biggest public health problem of the 21st century. *Brit J Sport Med.* 2009;43(1):1–2.
54. Diabetes Prevention Program Research Group, Knowler WC, Fowler SE, et al. 10-year follow-up of diabetes incidence and weight loss in the Diabetes Prevention Program Outcomes Study. *Lancet.* 2009;374(9702):1677–86.
55. Castro-Pinero J, Perez-Bey A, Segura-Jimenez V, et al. Cardiorespiratory fitness cutoff points for early detection of present and future cardiovascular risk in children: A 2-year follow-up study. *Mayo Clin Proc.* 2017;92(12):1753–62.
56. Lavie CJ, Kokkinos P, Ortega FB. Survival of the fittest—Promoting fitness throughout the life span. *Mayo Clin Proc.* 2017;92(12):1743–5.
57. Donnelly JE, Honas JJ, Smith BK, et al. Aerobic exercise alone results in clinically significant weight loss for men and women: Midwest Exercise Trial 2. *Obesity.* 2013;21(3):E219–28.
58. Bouchard C, Tremblay A, Despres JP, et al. The response to exercise with constant energy intake in identical twins. *Obes Res.* 1994;2(5):400–10.
59. Shook RP. Obesity and energy balance: What is the role of physical activity? *Expert Rev Endocrinol Metab.* 2016;11(6):511–20.
60. Ball TJ, Joy EA, Gren LH, Shaw JM. Concurrent validity of a self-reported physical activity "vital sign" questionnaire with adult primary care patients. *Prev Chronic Dis.* 2016;13:E16.
61. Coleman K, Ngor E, Reynolds K, et al. Initial validation of an exercise "vital sign" in electronic medical records. *Med Sci Sports Exerc.* 2012;44(11):2071–6.
62. Shook RP, Halpin K, Carlson JA, et al. Adherence with multiple national healthy lifestyle recommendations in a large pediatric center electronic health record and reduced risk of obesity. *Mayo Clin Proc.* 2018;93(9):1247–55.
63. Ainsworth BE, Haskell WL, Herrmann SD, et al. 2011 Compendium of physical activities: A second update of codes and MET values. *Med Sci Sports Exerc.* 2011;43(8):1575–81.
64. Macfarlane DJ, Lee CC, Ho EY, Chan K-L, Chan D. Convergent validity of six methods to assess physical activity in daily life. *J Appl Physiol.* 2006;101(5):1328–34.
65. Morabito V. Wearable technologies. In: Morabito V, ed. *The Future of Digital Business Innovation: Trends and Practices.* Switzerland: Springer International Publishing; 2016.
66. Case MA, Burwick HA, Volpp KG, Patel MS. Accuracy of smartphone applications and wearable devices for tracking physical activity data. *JAMA.* 2015;313(6):625–6.

67. Nelson MB, Kaminsky LA, Dickin DC, Montoye A. Validity of consumer-based physical activity monitors for specific activity types. *Med Sci Sports Exerc*. 2016;48(8):1619–28.

68. Ferguson T, Rowlands AV, Olds T, Maher C. The validity of consumer-level, activity monitors in healthy adults worn in free-living conditions: A cross-sectional study. *Int J Behav Nutr Phy*. 2015;12(1):42.

69. Murakami H, Kawakami R, Nakae S, et al. Accuracy of wearable devices for estimating total energy expenditure: Comparison with metabolic chamber and doubly labeled water method. *JAMA Intern Med*. 2016;176(5):702–3.

70. Zhang S, Rowlands AV, Murray P, Hurst TL. Physical activity classification using the GENEA wrist-worn accelerometer. *Med Sci Sports Exerc*. 2012;44(4):742–8.

71. Migueles JH, Cadenas-Sanchez C, Ekelund U, et al. Accelerometer data collection and processing criteria to assess physical activity and other outcomes: A systematic review and practical considerations. *Sports Med*. 2017;47(9):1821–45.

72. Troiano RP, McClain JJ, Brychta RJ, Chen KY. Evolution of accelerometer methods for physical activity research. *Brit J Sport Med*. 2014;48(13):1019–23.

73. Liu S, Gao RX, Freedson PS. Computational methods for estimating energy expenditure in human physical activities. *Med Sci Sports Exerc*. 2012;44(11):2138–46.

74. Staudenmayer J, He S, Hickey A, Sasaki J, Freedson P. Methods to estimate aspects of physical activity and sedentary behavior from high-frequency wrist accelerometer measurements. *J Appl Physiol*. 2015;119(4):396–403.

75. Hildebrand M, Van Hees VT, Hansen BH, Ekelund U. Age group comparability of raw accelerometer output from wrist- and hip-worn monitors. *Med Sci Sports Exerc*. 2014;46(9):1816–24.

76. Terrier P, Schutz Y. How useful is satellite positioning system (GPS) to track gait parameters? A review. *J Neuroeng Rehabil*. 2005;2(1):28.

77. Witte T, Wilson A. Accuracy of WAAS-enabled GPS for the determination of position and speed over ground. *J Biomech*. 2005;38(8):1717–22.

78. Wieters KM, Kim J-H, Lee C. Assessment of wearable global positioning system units for physical activity research. *J Phys Act Health*. 2012;9(7):913–23.

79. Stopher P, FitzGerald C, Zhang J. Advances in GPS technology for measuring travel. Paper presented at: *22nd ARRB Conference: Research into Practice*; October 29–November 2, 2006; Canberra, Australia.

80. Stopher P, FitzGerald C, Zhang J. Search for a global positioning system device to measure person travel. *Transport Res C-Emer*. 2008;16(3):350–69.

81. Hongu N, Orr BJ, Roe DJ, Reed RG, Going SB. Global positioning system watches for estimating energy expenditure. *J Strength Cond Res*. 2013;27(11):3216–20.

82. Rodriguez DA, Brown AL, Troped PJ. Portable global positioning units to complement accelerometry-based physical activity monitors. *Med Sci Sports Exerc*. 2005;37(11):S572.

83. Church TS, Blair SN, Cocreham S, et al. Effects of aerobic and resistance training on hemoglobin A1c levels in patients with type 2 diabetes: A randomized controlled trial. *JAMA*. 2010;304(20):2253–62.

84. Church TS, Earnest CP, Skinner JS, Blair SN. Effects of different doses of physical activity on cardiorespiratory fitness among sedentary, overweight or obese postmenopausal women with elevated blood pressure: A randomized controlled trial. *JAMA*. 2007;297(19):2081–91.

85. Freedson PS, Miller K. Objective monitoring of physical activity using motion sensors and heart rate. *Res Q Exer Sport*. 2000;71(Suppl 2):21–9.

86. Dong L, Block G, Mandel S. Activities contributing to total energy expenditure in the United States: Results from the NHAPS Study. *Int J Behav Nutr Phys Act*. 2004;1(1):4.

87. Herrmann SD, Barreira TV, Kang M, Ainsworth BE. Impact of accelerometer wear time on physical activity data: A NHANES semisimulation data approach. *Brit J Sport Med*. 2014;48(3):278–82.

88. Jakicic JM, Marcus M, Gallagher K, et al. Evaluation of the SenseWear Pro Armband™ to assess energy expenditure during exercise. *Med Sci Sports Exerc*. 2004;36(5):897–904.

89. Johannsen DL, Calabro MA, Stewart J, Franke W, Rood JC, Welk GJ. Accuracy of armband monitors for measuring daily energy expenditure in healthy adults. *Med Sci Sports Exerc*. 2010;42(11):2134–40.

90. St-Onge M, Mignault D, Allison DB, Rabasa-Lhoret R. Evaluation of a portable device to measure daily energy expenditure in free-living adults. *Am J Clin Nutr*. 2007;85(3):742–9.

91. Welk GJ, McClain JJ, Eisenmann JC, Wickel EE. Field validation of the MTI Actigraph and BodyMedia armband monitor using the IDEEA monitor. *Obesity*. 2007;15(4):918–28.

92. Correa JB, Apolzan JW, Shepard DN, Heil DP, Rood JC, Martin CK. Evaluation of the ability of three physical activity monitors to predict weight change and estimate energy expenditure. *Appl Physiol Nutr Metab*. 2016;41(7):758–66.

93. Zhang K, Pi-Sunyer FX, Boozer CN. Improving energy expenditure estimation for physical activity. *Med Sci Sports Exerc*. 2004;36(5):883–9.

94. Zhang K, Werner P, Sun M, Pi-Sunyer FX, Boozer CN. Measurement of human daily physical activity. *Obes Res*. 2003;11(1):33–40.

95. Kozey-Keadle S, Libertine A, Lyden K, Staudenmayer J, Freedson PS. Validation of wearable monitors for assessing sedentary behavior. *Med Sci Sports Exerc*. 2011;43(8):1561–7.

96. Bassett DR Jr, John D, Conger SA, Rider BC, Passmore RM, Clark JM. Detection of lying down, sitting, standing, and stepping using two activPAL monitors. *Med Sci Sports Exerc*. 2014;46(10):2025–9.

97. Dowd KP, Harrington DM, Donnelly AE. Criterion and concurrent validity of the activPAL professional physical activity monitor in adolescent females. *PLoS One*. 2012;7(10):e47633.

98. Lyden K, Keadle SK, Staudenmayer J, Freedson PS. The activPALTM accurately classifies activity intensity categories in healthy adults. *Med Sci Sports Exerc*. 2017;49(5):1022–8.

99. Edwardson CL, Winkler EAH, Bodicoat DH, et al. Considerations when using the activPAL monitor in field-based research with adult populations. *J Sport Health Sci*. 2017;6(2):162–78.

100. Normand MP. Increasing physical activity through self-monitoring, goal setting, and feedback. *Behav Intervent*. 2008;23(4):227–36.

101. Berlin JE, Storti KL, Brach JS. Using activity monitors to measure physical activity in free-living conditions. *Phys Ther*. 2006;86(8):1137–45.

102. Crouter SE, Schneider PL, Karabulut M, Bassett DR. Validity of ten electronic pedometers for measuring steps, distance, and kcals. *Med Sci Sports Exerc*. 2003;35(8):1455–60.

103. Abel MG, Peritore N, Shapiro R, Mullineaux DR, Rodriguez K, Hannon JC. A comprehensive evaluation of motion sensor step-counting error. *Appl Physiol Nutr Metab*. 2011;36(1):166–70.

104. Le Masurier GC, Lee SM, Tudor-Locke C. Motion sensor accuracy under controlled and free-living conditions. *Med Sci Sports Exerc*. 2004;36(5):905–10.

105. Crouter SE, Schneider PL, Bassett DR Jr. Spring-levered versus piezo-electric pedometer accuracy in overweight and obese adults. *Med Sci Sports Exerc*. 2005;37(10):1673–9.

106. Bassey E, Dallosso H, Fentem P, Irving J, Patrick J. Validation of a simple mechanical accelerometer (pedometer) for the estimation of walking activity. *Eur J Appl Physiol Occup Physiol*. 1987;56(3):323–30.

107. Fulton JE, Carlson SA, Ainsworth BE, et al. Strategic priorities for physical activity surveillance in the United States. *Med Sci Sports Exerc*. 2016;48(10):2057–69.

108. Pate RR, Berrigan D, Buchner D. *Actions to Improve Physical Activity Surveillance in the United States*. Washington, DC: National Academy of Sciences; 2018.

109. Katzmarzyk PT, Lee I-M, Martin CK, Blair SN. Epidemiology of physical activity and exercise training in the United States. *Prog Cardiovasc Dis*. 2017;60(1):3–10.

110. Ding D. Surveillance of global physical activity: Progress, evidence, and future directions. *Lancet Glob Health*. 2018;6(10):e1046–7.

111. Evenson KR, Wen F, Furberg RD. Assessing validity of the Fitbit indicators for U.S. public health surveillance. *Am J Prev Med*. 2017;53(6):931–2.

112. Chriqui JF, Nicholson LM, Thrun E, Leider J, Slater SJ. More active living-oriented county and municipal zoning is associated with increased adult leisure time physical activity—United States, 2011. *Environ Behav*. 2016;48(1):111–30.

113. Strauss WJ, Nagaraja J, Landgraf AJ, et al. The longitudinal relationship between community programmes and policies to prevent childhood obesity and BMI in children: The Healthy Communities Study. *Pediatr Obes*. 2018;13(S1):82–92.

114. Breda J, Jakovljevic J, Rathmes G, et al. Promoting health-enhancing physical activity in Europe: Current state of surveillance, policy development and implementation. *Health Policy*. 2018;122(5):519–27.

CHAPTER

184 Strategies to Address Physical Activity in Schools

Jennifer Sacheck • Sarah Amin

INTRODUCTION

Children spend over half of their waking hours in school for a major portion of the year. Schools are increasingly in the spotlight for not only enhancing children's learning and well-being, but are also a critical point of engagement for promoting children's physical health. In the context of the national obesity epidemic, schools have further been complimented or criticized for both dietary and physical activity influences,[1] as discussed in Chapters 181 and 185. A major focus within the context of the obesity epidemic has been school food—the National School Lunch Program, competitive foods, removing vending and sodas, and school breakfast, but increasingly physical education and physical activity programming are a major focus.[2,3] In a concerted effort to address the many different personal and environmental factors that holistically shape the integral link between student health and educational attainment, the Centers for Disease Control and Prevention (CDC) in collaboration with the Association for Supervision and Curriculum Development (ASCD) developed the "Whole School, Whole Community, Whole Child" (WSCC) model. Under this framework, the Comprehensive School Physical Activity Program (CSPAP) is one of eight central components that are addressed for health promotion and disease prevention and underlies many of the school-based physical activity approaches described in this chapter.[1]

Over the past decade, there has been a greater focus on children's physical activity and movement within the school setting given the contribution of physical activity to energy balance, but also in part due to the decline in physical education offerings throughout the elementary, middle, and high school years given tighter budgets. Beyond obesity prevention, efforts to address physical activity in schools have gained momentum in recent years given mounting evidence surrounding the impact of these behaviors on student behavior, attention-to-task, cognitive health, and academic achievement.[4] Importantly, there is also renewed attention on increasing children's fitness levels in terms of military preparedness. Historically, physical education and school-based fitness testing were aligned with the goals of having a healthy military. A 2018 report from the Council for a Strong America, "Unhealthy and Unprepared," estimated that an alarming 71% of individuals between the ages of 17–24 do not qualify for military service and obesity prevents 31% of youth from serving if they choose to, which has major implications for recruitment and the future of our armed services.[5,6]

Given the breadth of potential benefits of enhancing school-time physical activity, the National Academy of Sciences (formerly the Institute of Medicine) recommends that elementary school children and middle/high school children engage in 30 minutes and 45 minutes of school-time moderate-to-vigorous physical activity (MVPA) per day, respectively.[7] Contextually, children should be accruing approximately half of the current U.S. Physical Activity Guidelines recommendation of 60 minutes of MVPA per day in school.[8] Objective national and international data using accelerometry indicate that anywhere from less than 50% to 3–5% of children (depending on the cut-points used for analysis—see following section) are reaching the recommended 60 minutes of daily MVPA,[9,10] and even fewer are meeting the school-time recommendation.[11] Racial/ethnic and socioeconomic status disparities in physical activity and childhood obesity rates underscore the need for concerted efforts to target children disproportionately at risk for low activity levels.[11–13] Further, there are striking gender and age-related differences in these behaviors. Not only do studies demonstrate that elementary-aged girls on average accrue 18 minutes less of MVPA compared to boys on a daily basis,[11] but there is also a decline in physical activity from childhood to adolescence with this trend more pronounced in girls.[14–16]

In response to this public health issue, the 2013 Institute of Medicine (IOM) report, "Educating the Student Body: Taking Physical Activity and Physical Education to School," recommended that schools adopt a "whole school" approach to physical activity and physical education in schools. To accomplish this, the committee advised that key stakeholders, teachers, parents, and administrators be leveraged and physical activity-promoting strategies be adopted across multiple school environments (unique examples beyond traditional recess and physical education are presented in Table 184-1). Other approaches that have been suggested for increasing physical activity during the school day include: recess/playground strategies, classroom-based physical activity, active transport, before/after school physical activity clubs or intramural sports, and the built environment.[17,18] This chapter will take a deeper dive into each of these domains for improving physical activity among children, with a specific focus on intervention studies and key behavioral and health outcomes.

SCHOOL PHYSICAL ACTIVITY INTERVENTION TARGET OUTCOMES

A large portion school-based physical activity intervention studies have focused on increasing physical activity, including total activity, MVPA, and decreasing sedentary time. These studies have included objectively measured physical activity as measured by accelerometry, pedometry (step counts), and heart rate. Accelerometry is still considered the gold standard for objectively measured physical activity utilizing either waist-worn (most common) or wrist-worn accelerometers.[19] The accelerometers measure movement in three planes and capture varying epoch lengths, which include counts.[20] Counts represent movement and utilizing validated cut-points that equate to a certain amount of time at different activity intensities (sedentary, light, moderate, and vigorous). Many other studies have utilized parent/teacher report and child self-report (typically from children in the third grade or higher) of select activities such as different sports

TABLE 184-1 SCHOOL ENVIRONMENT STRATEGIES FOR PROMOTING PHYSICAL ACTIVITY FROM THE COMMUNITY TO CLASSROOM

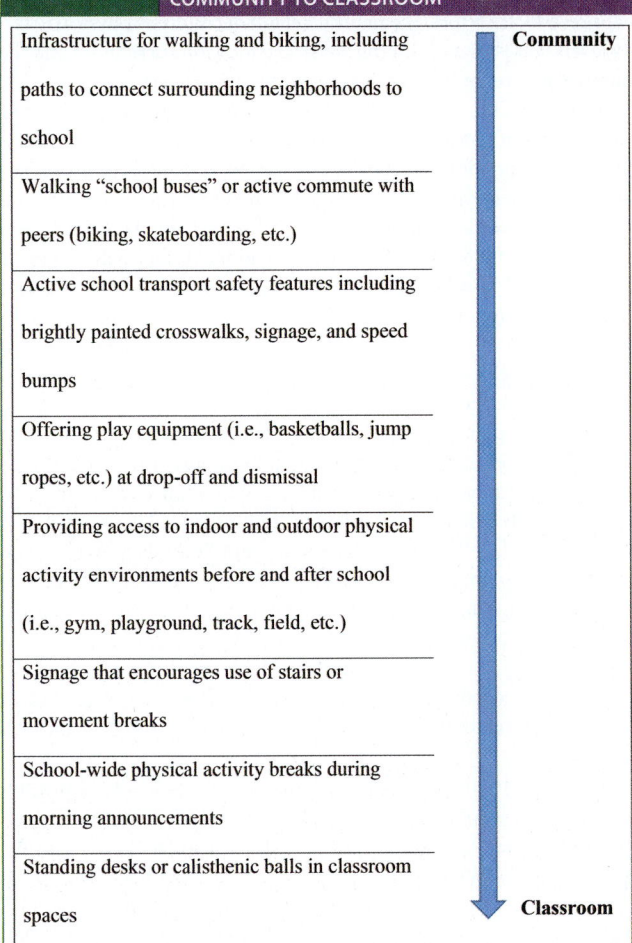

Strategy	
Infrastructure for walking and biking, including paths to connect surrounding neighborhoods to school	Community
Walking "school buses" or active commute with peers (biking, skateboarding, etc.)	↓
Active school transport safety features including brightly painted crosswalks, signage, and speed bumps	↓
Offering play equipment (i.e., basketballs, jump ropes, etc.) at drop-off and dismissal	↓
Providing access to indoor and outdoor physical activity environments before and after school (i.e., gym, playground, track, field, etc.)	↓
Signage that encourages use of stairs or movement breaks	↓
School-wide physical activity breaks during morning announcements	↓
Standing desks or calisthenic balls in classroom spaces	Classroom

and/or time spent in different movements or movement intensities. Studies have also included validated visual assessments (i.e., System for Observing Fitness Instruction Time, SOFIT) of children's movement and activity levels (often during a structured time such as during physical education class or recess).[21,22]

In addition, fitness as an outcome measure has been the focus of numerous studies, especially given the link between physical activity and physical fitness levels. In 1956, the President's Council on Youth Fitness was formed, and in 1958, the first Youth Fitness Test was published and used as a national survey.[23] The test included the shuttle run, 50-yd dash, 500-yd run-walk, pull-ups (boys), modified pull-ups (girls), softball throw, long jump, and sit-ups. In 1966, the Presidential Physical Fitness Awards Program was launched to commend students who performed at or above the 85th percentile for all seven tests, with the goal to measure fitness with an eye toward skills and military performance.

Today, school-based fitness testing is linked more directly to health outcomes—cardiovascular and respiratory health, metabolic health and obesity, mental and cognitive health, and musculoskeletal health.[24] The components of fitness linked to these outcomes include: body composition, cardiorespiratory endurance, musculoskeletal fitness, and flexibility. The two most common national fitness batteries include Fitnessgram and the President's Council on Fitness, Sports, and Nutrition (PCFSN). The Fitnessgram includes the following tests: Progressive Aerobic Cardiovascular Endurance Test (PACER) or mile run/walk (cardio respiratory endurance), skinfold measurement (body composition), curl-up (strength and endurance), trunk lift (strength and flexibility), push-ups (strength and endurance), sit and reach (flexibility).[25] The PCFSN measures shuttle run (speed and agility), curl-ups (strength and endurance), endurance run/walk (cardiorespiratory endurance), pull-up (strength and endurance), and sit and reach (flexibility).[23]

Routine assessment of fitness in schools is not mandated nationally and is not currently part of national surveillance, although some states are conducting annual assessments (e.g., Texas and California). Often, researchers will need to conduct fitness assessments themselves or with the assistance of a physical educator. Many studies utilizing fitness as an outcome have focused on cardiovascular fitness (as commonly assessed by the shuttle run or PACER test and the 1 mile run) given that cardiorespiratory fitness is associated with physical activity engagement and often tightly linked with health outcomes.[26] The importance of the different dimensions of fitness and its close association with physical activity makes it a natural target for interventions.

In addition to the physical activity and fitness outcomes, there are the health-related outcomes such as changes in weight status or BMI, adiposity, cardiometabolic risk factors (including lipids and blood pressure), and cognitive health that are often examined as a result of school-based interventions. Given the sensitivity and need for privacy for doing more invasive measures within the school environment, body composition assessments typically include BMI and less frequently measures of skinfolds, waist circumference, and body composition by bioelectrical impedance. Studies have been successful in doing phlebotomy in the school setting, however, it is understandably challenging. Blood biomarkers typically include cardiometabolic risk factors and inflammatory markers.[27]

There are clear challenges of performing interventions within the school environment. Given the growth of the evidence in terms of the positive impact of physical activity and physical fitness on cognitive health among children, investigators have shifted some of the focus from long-term health impacts (i.e., chronic disease prevention) to more proximal outcomes (i.e., acute changes in academic performance). This offers a win-win scenario for researchers to promote physical activity interventions with the potential benefit of student academic achievement, which is the overriding priority of the school. Furthermore, popular culture and school administrators have picked up on some of the fundamental findings from researchers such as the work of Ratey [28] and are beginning to see the potential benefits of incorporating more physical activity within the school day without risking a decline in student achievement.

Typical measures of student academic success include examination of school attendance records and standardized test scores, with the major limitation of the latter measure is that children begin testing in third grade. These tests are typically conducted annually and include scores in the mathematics and English language arts (ELA) subject areas which have been positively associated with physical activity,[29] thus can be considered an indicator of academic achievement. Studies surrounding academic achievement have extended beyond physical activity as a predictor with recent studies suggesting a positive school physical activity environment may enhance the academic success of students, particularly for underserved students. In low-income schools, a supportive physical activity environment was associated with Math standardized test score achievement (OR $= 5.40$, 95% CI $= 2.52–11.54$ $p < 0.001$).[30] Cognitive performance uses tests such as the digit span forward and backward subtests of the Wechsler Intelligence Scales for Children,[31] which have been validated in young children and takes 5–7 minutes to administer with little equipment required.[31] This standardized test measures short-term memory and attention, while the Stroop Color Word test measures disinhibition, both of which have been linked to physical activity.[32] Others include the Eriksen Flanker task, which assesses conflict monitoring and represents one facet of cognitive control whereby an individual needs to respond to stimuli that is "flanked" by irrelevant stimuli.[33] Attention-to-task is an observational measure of attentiveness that may be more cumbersome for researchers. Teacher-reported or parent-report of student behavior is also used but is less objective.[34]

In conjunction with academic outcomes, other measures of effects of physical activity interventions in schools have included psychosocial outcomes such as child perception of physical activity self-efficacy/confidence, motivation, and fun. Noteworthy is that the construct of physical literacy is being revitalized in recent research. To increase physical activity in childhood and over the life course, organizations such as the Society of Health and Physical Educators (SHAPE) America and the Aspen Institute have made physical literacy a centerpiece of their recommendations for physical education and other youth physical activity programs.[7–9] Physical literacy incorporates: (1) *physical competence*—the ability of an individual to develop movement skills and patterns, along with a variety of movement intensities and durations; and (2) *confidence and motivation*—enthusiasm for, enjoyment of, and self-assurance in adopting physical activity as an integral part of life.[11]

Physical competence can be measured by instruments such as the PLAYfun tool. PLAYfun is an observational assessment that has undergone reliability and validity evaluation in the laboratory for motor competence and includes five domains: running, locomotion, balance, and lower/upper body object control. Physical literacy confidence and motivation are assessed by self-report with validated questionnaires such as the Harter Self-Perception Profile[35] and the Canadian Assessment of Physical Literacy (CAPL).[36]

Physical literacy has become a centerpiece of national recommendations for physical education and other school-based programs that aim to increase physical activity. These are based on a large body of theoretical and empirical evidence demonstrating that competence, confidence, and motivation are independently associated with children's physical activity in both the short and long terms.[12,13] In fact, research historically has focused only on the individual constructs of physical literacy rather than on the relationship between constructs fundamental to physical literacy. While the core constructs of physical literacy have been found to independently predict children's physical activity in the near term,[14–18] little empirical research has assessed the synergistic effect. Better understanding of whether and how those constructs influence each other has important implications for intervention design. Due to the newness of the concept, longitudinal studies establishing a link between programs designed to develop physical literacy and their efficacy to increase physical activity have yet to appear. Moreover, since competence, motivation, and confidence are disproportionately low among girls and overweight/obese children,[19,20] programs that effectively and simultaneously enhance these domains of physical literacy may have particular benefit for increasing physical activity among priority groups.[14,21–25]

SCHOOL-DAY DOMAINS FOR INCORPORATION OF PHYSICAL ACTIVITY

This section will highlight the segments of the school-day that provide opportunities to incorporate physical activity and that have served as prime target of school-based interventions. Different approaches for increasing active time in these segments are discussed including: physical education, recess, active classroom breaks and below and after-school activities, along with a summary of the evidence base surrounding a variety of health and academic outcomes linked to these strategies. Examples of specific physical activity interventions and best practices surrounding their implementation are also highlighted.

Physical Education

Physical education (PE) is a curricular subject that, by definition, aims to empower students with the necessary "knowledge, skills, abilities, and confidence, to be physically active throughout their lifetime" while also promoting daily physical activity for all students.[37] Historically, the overriding assumption has been that incorporation of physical activity during school-time occurs during PE (and perhaps recess); therefore, the natural default of children's physical activity levels falls primarily on the physical education curriculum and the implementation of this curriculum by the PE teacher.

Providing PE to support both children's *physical literacy* and engagement in physical activity has been a hot-button issue for physical activity and for public health practitioners and policymakers. The importance of improving these policies and practices surrounding PE has been pressed by organizations including SHAPE America as well as the IOM.[18,38,39] SHAPE America is a national leader behind efforts to address PE in schools and provides the necessary programs and resources to support physical educators.[38] Central to its mission *is the push to recognize PE as a core academic subject that allows for 150 minutes and 225 minutes per week for elementary and middle/high school students, respectively.*[39]

Despite legislative and advocacy efforts, no federal law currently mandates the number of days and minutes of PE each week.[18] Without federal backing, schools may lack the time and resources to implement PE policies. This is largely an unintended consequence of the "No Child Left Behind Elementary and Secondary Act," which prioritized student academic achievement and accountability in core subjects, including reading and mathematics.[17,37] However, in 2015 this act was reauthorized with the name "Every Student Success Act," and now acknowledges that health and PE are key components of a well-rounded education.[17] Though this was a promising shift at the federal level, there is wide latitude in implementing PE-focused policies.

For PE in particular, state- and district-level policies are integral to mobilizing school-level efforts since these set the stage for PE standards including time requirements, teacher qualifications, and professional development.[37] In fact, it has been shown that the odds of elementary schools providing the recommended 150 min/week of PE increased if they were located in states or school districts that had such a law or policy.[40] Current estimates suggest that only 3.7% of schools required daily PE for the entire school year[41] and that PE sessions may only provide 10–20 minutes of daily MVPA.[7]

Schools can choose from a variety of evidence-based PE curricula and programs that have been developed and disseminated nationally across elementary, middle, and high schools. For elementary-aged children, programs include Sports, Play, and Active Recreation for Kids (SPARK) and the Coordinated Approach to Child Health, formerly the Child and Adolescent Trial for Cardiovascular Health (CATCH).[37,42–44] CATCH, an NIH-funded research study (National Heart, Lung, and Blood Institute) conducted by researchers at The University of Texas Health Science Center at Houston, represents the largest school-based health promotion study in the United States. CATCH is based on the CDC WSCC model and thus aims to promote healthy student behaviors around physical activity, diet, and tobacco use through addressing a variety of environmental influences both in and out of school.[43] The central goal of CATCH PE is to promote increased MVPA during class time to align with the National Association for Sport & Physical Exercise (NASPE) goal of having at least 50% of PE emphasizing activities that encourage student activity to a moderate-to-vigorous level. To achieve this, the PE programs guide teachers throughout the school year using age-appropriate lesson plans that include nonelimination activities that motivate and engage all students.[43]

SPARK, dating back to the 1980s, is an NIH-funded research study (National Heart, Lung, and Blood Institute, NHLBI) conducted by researchers at San Diego State University that addresses both PE and school-based physical activity. While the original research-based curriculum focused on elementary school PE, additional research has led to the development of programs for early childhood, middle school

PE (grades 6–8), afterschool (ages 5–14), high school PE, and classroom activity and recess.[44,45] To best promote changes to the school environment and student behavior, SPARK provides a curriculum, teacher training (onsite), technical assistance, and content-matched equipment.[44] Both CATCH and SPARK have been associated with increases in MVPA, and SPARK has also been related to improvements in fitness, sports skills, and academic achievement.[42,45–47]

Evidence-based programs for middle school and high school students include the Middle School Physical Activity and Nutrition intervention (M-SPAN).[48] This intervention was implemented during the late-1990s by researchers at San Diego State University and informed by a large randomized trial of 24 middle schools and approximately 25,000 students. M-SPAN broadly focused on utilizing environmental, policy, and social marketing strategies to increase physical activity and reduce fat intake with PE representing an important aspect of the intervention. The 2-year PE component of M-SPAN comprises: (1) PE teacher professional development (five 3-hour sessions) with an emphasis on equipping teachers to enhance existing instructional strategies to increase MVPA versus providing a specific curriculum, and (2) on-site consultations that emphasized motivational feedback and technical assistance. Physical activity was assessed using direct observation through the SOFIT (see *Target Outcomes* section above) and findings indicate that the M-SPAN increased MVPA by 18% with a greater increase for boys compared to girls.[48]

Given the marked gender disparities in physical activity that worsen as youth transition from elementary to middle and high school, programs including the Trial of Activity for Adolescent Girls (TAAG) and Lifetime Education for Activity Program (LEAP) aim to close the gender gap in these behaviors for middle and high school girls, respectively.[37] TAAG was a multicenter group randomized trial funded by the NHLBI that used a socioecological approach that included PE, health education with activity challenges, partnerships among TAAG investigators, schools, and community partners, as well as promotional activities.[49] The impact of the program on the physical activity of participating adolescent girls was modest, amounting to approximately 1.6 minutes of MVPA per day.[50]

Physical education continues to be the centerpiece by which children in schools are exposed to physical activity and movement skills. Renewed awareness of the importance of movement during the school day, along with budget cuts that constrain many schools from offering PE on a daily basis has made the delivery of "quality physical education" a priority. Teacher training, innovative curricula, and creative engagement with diverse children to embrace movement for health and sport is bringing more attention to research in improving the PE experience for schools and providing data on the importance of offering PE at least once weekly for children of all ages.

Recess Strategies

The second prime target for incorporation of school-time physical activity is recess. Recess is defined as "the noncurricular time allocated by schools between classes for youth to engage in leisure activities."[51] NASPE, SHAPE America, and the CDC among other national organizations recommend that all elementary school children have at least 20 minutes of recess each day.[52] Research suggests that recess can help children achieve anywhere from 5% to 40% of the 60 minute daily physical activity recommendation.[51] Similar to PE, schools may be pressed to reduce the frequency and duration of recess sessions in favor of classroom instruction time. Allocation of recess declines across the elementary and middle school years as well. Data show that approximately two-thirds of schools meet the recommendation of 20 minutes of recess per week for elementary school children.[53]

In an effort to guide schools' adoption of positive practices surrounding recess, the CDC and SHAPE America issued a report, "Strategies for Recess in Schools," in 2017.[52] Examples of key national guidance for recess include strong recommendations against replacing PE with recess. Both school-based opportunities are needed to help children meet school-time physical activity recommendations. Schools should provide children with a sufficient and safe environment for recess with ample equipment and supplies and be supported by staff who have ongoing professional training. Timing of recess is important; it is recommended that recess take place before the lunch period. Finally, the report emphasized that disciplinary actions should not impact the provision of recess time.[52]

Several systematic reviews point to successful strategies and factors that positively impact youth physical activity behaviors during recess.[54–56] Ridgers et al. used a socioecological lens and found positive relationships between physical activity and access to school facilities that support activity during recess, unfixed equipment (e.g., balls, skipping ropes), and perceived encouragement from friends, family, and schools.[54] The importance of the playground environment and design has been corroborated in a separate review of recess interventions which found that playground markings plus physical structures, specifically were associated with increased physical activity of children during recess in the short to medium term.[55] Clearly, a supportive built environment, sufficient resources, and positive social support play an important role in supporting children's physical activity behaviors during recess. Notably, many of these strategies including playground markings and games equipment are cost-effective and may be more feasible for schools to readily implement.[51] Structured recess programs, like Playworks, aim to enhance youth safety, engagement, and empowerment through on-site staffing, consultative support, professional development, and resources that can be implemented on the playground. This evidence-based program has been supporting schools for over 20 years and a randomized control trial by Stanford University found that Playworks participants engaged in high levels of physical activity and that this program supported improvements in important student outcomes like perceptions of safety and bullying.[57] Overall, higher quality intervention research surrounding recess-focused physical activity interventions is needed.[56]

Recess offers the opportunity for children to re-charge and be active. Promotion of movement during this time is encouraged independent of the space allocated for this break (i.e., indoors if the weather is not conducive to outdoor time). Innovative strategies to engage all children, with special consideration of age, sex, culture, different fitness levels, and even seasonality, are encouraged. Timing of recess is also important so that the movement time offers the children a break from other more sedentary academic periods.

Classroom-based Physical Activity

In-class physical activity breaks represent an important and emerging opportunity for integrating additional minutes of active time into the classroom in order to help achieve policy recommendations for school-time physical activity. This approach is marked by "physical activity carried out during regular classroom time, and can occur either inside or outside the classroom (i.e., hallway, playground) and is distinct from school recess/lunch break times."[58] Although using instruction time for physical activity may seem counterintuitive to school administrators and teachers who are impacted by competing academic demands, a 2017 meta-analysis by Watson et al. indicated that in-class physical activity breaks improved on-task and reduced off-task classroom behavior. Classroom-based physical activity also supported improvements on academic achievement when a progress-monitoring tool was used.[58]

There are different ways that physical activity can be implemented in the classroom environment as evidenced by the variety of intervention studies that have evaluated these approaches. *Active breaks* consist of brief bouts of physical activity that provide children with a break from an academic lesson. *Curriculum-focused active breaks* on the other hand reinforce previous lesson content from specific subject areas into the bout of physical activity often in shorter bursts (GoNoodle,[59] CHALK/Just Move [60]). *Physically active lessons* utilize physical activity to teach lessons in key learning areas other than physical education and are typically designed to deliver 10–15 minutes of physical activity [examples include Energizers,[61] Take 10,[62] Physical Activity Across the Curriculum,[63,64] Texas Initiatives for Children's Activity and Nutrition (I-CAN!)[65]]. These classroom-based physical activity approaches vary not only in characteristics such as intensity and duration, but also in terms of the physical activity type (i.e., yoga vs. jumping jacks).[66] Although classroom-based physical activity does not necessarily need to be carried out in the classroom, studies that used this setting often required minimal equipment or set-up needs.[58]

Studies surrounding the implementation and effectiveness provide insight into potential factors that may foster the success of classroom-based physical activity outside of a controlled intervention study. Interviews and process evaluation with teachers regarding implementing classroom physical activity breaks suggest that key barriers include time, adequate infrastructure,[67] space constraints,[68] and fear that breaks will take away from instruction time.[34,69,70] When adopting this physical activity promoting strategy, it is important to consider: developing a district plan that is tailored to specific needs, identifying a district-level coordinator to organize teacher trainings, offering support groups, engaging parents, community members and school staff, and providing accompanying resources such as materials such as instruction books or videos.[69,71] One study found that incorporating a social media campaign into teacher training and facilitator support boosted teachers' self-efficacy to lead activity breaks.[69] With adequate training, boosting of teacher confidence, and demonstrating to teachers that classroom physical activity may be beneficial to student behavior and attention, consistent and long-term physical activity across the school day may be more fully realized.[34]

Two evidence-based programs that promote physical activity in the classroom and have been widely implemented across the United States include Take10 and GoNoodle. Take10 which uniquely was designed by teachers, promotes academic instruction within 10-minute bouts of classroom-based physical activity and includes more than 40 different types of activities per grade level.[72] A summary of Take10 points to its impact on health-related outcomes including increased physical activity and decreased BMI z-scores as well as academic improvements in reading, math, spelling, and composite scores and reduced off-task behavior.[73] GoNoodle distinguishes itself from Take10 as a web-based application that features a variety of 1- to 20-minute activity videos that can be played on a projector or monitor. Classrooms can access a YouTube channel that contains additional activities and classrooms can also add their own videos to this forum.[59] This online feature of GoNoodle enhances its potential to be adopted by teachers in variety of classroom settings since it does not require physical materials to implement.

Active classroom breaks remain a major opportunity for which many classrooms can continue to incorporate physical activity. Important factors to consider are the relative buy-in and physical activity self-efficacy of the teachers, school administrators' support for these approaches, and encouraging curricula incorporate movement breaks with changes over time so that students continue to be engaged. This type of programming has the potential to reach all children regardless of fitness status, sex, or race/ethnicity. Age-appropriate movements clearly need to be considered as children get older. Finally, ownership of some of this programming by the schoolchildren themselves (i.e., the students leading the classroom breaks) can enhance their engagement.

Active School Transport

In 2016, 17% of U.S. children walked to school—a number that has substantially declined since the 1960s. Reasons for this decline include factors such as school distance, traffic-related dangers, and weather.[74,75] Active school transport (AST) represents a noncurricular re-emerging opportunity for fitting more minutes of physical activity into the day without compromising instruction time. These nonmotorized opportunities for commuting to school can include but are not limited to walking, biking, and skateboarding.[76] Active transport to school represents an important milestone for children's independent mobility, which corresponds with a number of psychosocial and cognitive benefits—including a sense of identity, responsibility, self-esteem, and social skills.[77] As far as impact on physical health outcomes, evidence suggests that AST supports increases in physical activity and that cycling to and from school is associated with improved cardiovascular fitness.[78]

There are a variety of factors associated with active school transport including socioeconomic status, access to a car, child age (increasing likelihood for older children), facets of the built environment, safety, urbanicity, and school distance from home.[79–84] Although distance from home to school has been found to be the biggest predictor of active school transport,[79,82] concern of safety surrounding active school transport and other forms of independent mobility is significant and widely held by both parents/caregivers and children. While children value independence, their concerns surrounding strangers, traffic, bullying, and getting lost are shared with parents/caregivers.[75,77,85–87] Further, many of the concerns around active transport may be exacerbated or unique to underserved communities.[83,84] For example, in low-income neighborhoods, parents who perceive their neighborhood as unpleasant for activity are less likely to have children engage in active school transport.[79,87] In low-income communities, efforts to improve the neighborhood environment in terms of safety and aesthetics are needed to address parental concerns.

The National Center for Safe Routes to School aims to help communities to implement active school transport with safety being the organization's central priority. To meet this goal, it utilizes evidence-based research and translates this to actionable resources including education, professional development, and community technical support.[88] One key initiative of the National Center launched in 2015 is "Vision Zero," which aims to eliminate traffic fatalities and serious injuries. Other advocacy efforts spearheaded by the National Center for Safe Routes to School include "Walk to School Day" in October and "Bike to School Day" in May, which aim to build awareness and enthusiasm around active school transportation.[88]

Key strategies that can support active school transport include "walking school buses" (a parent and/or staff member has a walking route and pick up kids who walk on the way so that they may walk as a group), brightly painted crosswalks so that they are more visible to pedestrians and motorists, flashing walking signs at the crosswalks, speed bumps in high foot-traffic areas, and more paths on school grounds that can connect the schools directly to more neighborhoods.[76,89,90] As far as the effectiveness of active school transport interventions, a recent systematic review found that while these strategies can increase rates of active commuting there is little evidence to suggest improvements in physical fitness. Further, more rigorous research is needed in this area.[91]

Before/After School Physical Activity

Before or after-school physical activity provides children with opportunities to be active outside the constraints of school hours and classroom time, but is linked to the school day to enable potential broad reach of programming. Included within this space are *before/after school programming* (also referred to as *out-of-school time programs*) or *physical activity clubs* that provide a less specialized and flexible approach to physical activity. This is in contrast to *intramural/interscholastic sports*, which involve tailored instruction and a focus on specific athletic skills and performance.[92–95]

Before/after-school physical activity programs take the form of an extracurricular or enrichment programs that are open to all children with physical activity often representing one of various activities offered to students whereas *physical activity clubs* hone in on physical activity engagement, exclusively.[93,96] Given that nearly half (43%) of youth participate in some form of afterschool program,[97] these have immense potential to positively influence activity behaviors.

These are typically supervised by a teacher, school/community staff member, or volunteers either at the school or separate location in the surrounding community.[92] A review of reviews highlights that this research area is still relatively new and that there is modest evidence to support that these programs increase physical activity levels and impact body composition.[92]

Promising examples of *physical activity clubs* include walking or running clubs that consist of "running laps" or games that involve running.[19,60] Evidence suggests that running "game day" sessions can help children reach the nationally recommended intensity of 50% MVPA for afterschool activities.[19] Evidence-based programs that have national scope include *Build Our Kids Success (BOKS)*, a before/after school 12-week functional fitness curriculum with each session lasting roughly 45 minutes across 3 days each week. Each session focuses on a specific functional fitness skill (i.e., squat, plank) and is typically divided into six segments: drop-off and free play, warm up, running-related activity, a featured skill of the week, end of class game, and a cool down/stretching.[98] A recent study surrounding the impact of this programming suggests that *BOKS* yields improvements in BMI-z score and student engagement.[99] Other evidence-based afterschool physical activity programs include the nationally recognized *Girls on the Run (GOTR)*, a 10-week program for both elementary and middle school girls that culminates with a 5K running event. What distinguishes this program is that it not only addresses PA behaviors but also has an over-arching goal of preparing girls for "a lifetime of self-respect and healthy living" with lessons promoting positive emotional, social, mental, and physical development.[100] This represents a crucial component of *GOTR* since research suggests that physical activity competence, motivation, and confidence tend to be lower in girls compared to boys.[16,101] Findings suggest that *GOTR* produces beneficial changes in self-esteem, body-size satisfaction, physical activity commitment, and physical activity frequency.[102]

Incorporating physical activity programming before and/or after school offers the potential for broad reach for all children, extending beyond youth sport programs that can be more intimidating and selective. Inclusiveness and convenience for families is a huge draw for families and children given that children are in an environment where they feel comfortable among their peers and often teachers already employed by the schools. Often, these programs do not require supplemental funding by families and are funded by school districts and grants. Thinking creatively about different opportunities for children with different demographic characteristics while also keeping things "new" will keep students with diverse interests engaged.

Intramural Sports

Intramural/interscholastic sports are anchored to the school or a school/community partnership in contrast with extramural or club sports, thus boosting their potential to reach all children irrespective of factors such as socioeconomic barriers.[93,95] Promoting school adoption of *intramural/interscholastic sports* is recommended by the IOM with a heightened focus on inclusion of low-income and racial/ethnic minority children who typically have lower levels of physical activity.[7,95] However, these opportunities are fundamentally important for all children. Findings from a 2017 Aspen Institute report demonstrate that although household income is a major factor in sports engagement, there continues to be a steady decline in sports participation across all youth, with the majority of children dropping out of organized sports by age 11.[103] This trend is further marked by increasing concern about the extent to which organized sports get children moving at recommended levels.[104–106] Although a systematic review supports that sport participants are more physically active than nonparticipants,[106] the actual quantity of active time for participants is questionable.[104,105] One study surrounding sports practices (i.e., soccer and baseball/softball) indicated that only 24% of children 7–14 years met the 60-minute physical activity guideline, with even bleaker results with increasing age and sex.[104] Activity levels are also low during athletic competition, with evidence that children spent on average 49% of a 50-minute soccer match in sedentary time.[105] Nonetheless, the benefits of sports participation may transcend physical benefits and correspond with important social and psychological benefits for youth, including perceived athletic competence [107] due to factors such as inspiring coaches and a motivational climate.[108,109]

There is clearly room for improvement for youth sports—the Aspen Institute 2017 Project Play Summit gave stakeholders a "C" grade for getting youth active through sports.[103] Investing in intramural and interscholastic sports opportunities should be a priority for schools to not only reach more children, but also to improve the quality and quantity of physical activity options offered. With this in mind, the National Afterschool Association has adopted standards that align with the United States Department of Health and Human Services 2018 Physical Activity Guidelines and provides key guidance regarding program content and quality, staff training, social support, program support, and environmental support.[94]

CONSIDERATION OF OPPORTUNITIES AND BARRIERS

Presenting opportunities to be physically active is key for the success of children's school-time engagement. The physical activity environment is a term that encompasses these opportunities, policies, physical environment of schools that promotes physical activity—all are domains that have been discussed above.

Other items to be considered within the school environment that may or may not be captured by survey instruments include the overall institutional energy around the promotion of physical activity. The term "champion" often is used to characterize that one key individual who spearheads new programming and initiatives. This can be a principal, physical education teacher, wellness staff, nurse, and/or parent. Having a champion and even more than one has been linked to a more positive environment and engagement in programming. Role models are also important. The champion may or may not serve as a positive role model, but engagement of a critical number of teachers and staff in healthy behaviors has also been linked with the success of implementation of programming.[29,65] Similarly, these factors, if they are not in place, can make it extremely difficult to shift the culture of a school and empower teachers and staff. Although the research is continuing to accumulate on the benefits of physical activity for children throughout the school day, many schools are still hesitant to allocate more time to physical activity.

Barriers to students' physical activity can also include the simple lack of infrastructure (no permanent gym or outdoor play space) and warrant extra creativity, but innovative solutions are emerging especially around engaging children in movement in the classroom and changing the classroom environment so that movement throughout the day is a natural default. The urbanicity of the school and surrounding safety also is important to consider, especially in terms active transport and before and after school programming.

One also needs to consider the reach of the programming. *First, is it feasible?* For example, a school wants to incorporate more physical education, but the funding for PE teachers is lacking or a policy is not in place to support this goal. Or, a principal may want all teachers to engage their students in active classroom breaks, but the support for this initiative from teachers may be low. Research studies designed as randomized controlled trials have also attempted to deliver programming, but schools may have difficulty implementing or the program is not the right fit for the school population. The FLEX Study randomized two school-based programs to lower-income schools, active classroom breaks (CHALK/Just Move), and a running/walking club (100 Mile Club) and noted barriers to implementation even with strong initial program support.[34,70]

Does the program/initiative have broad reach? Does it enable students to comfortably be involved regardless of age, sex, socioeconomic status, or race/ethnicity/cultural background? For instance, does a child need to have sneakers to participate? Or can the activities be performed if a child is wearing a skirt or dress? Similar to the issue of feasibility, children may or may not engage in programming, making it difficult to measure true impact, especially in a randomized trial. Some programming may have major impacts on student physical activity and associated outcomes, but the reach is not broad. This may be the case for a before school program, for example, that limits class size and accessibility to only those who can get to school early.

Finally, it *is important to consider sustainability and scalability.* Having programming and infrastructure that is financially viable and interesting to the students and the school is critical for long-term success. The evolution of stakeholders, the environment, policies, and programs occurs over time, but programming needs to be maintained as a priority if the goal is to meet the current school-time physical activity guidelines—that have been recommended in terms of impact on both short- and long-term health.

References

1. Lewallen TC, Hunt H, Potts-Datema W, Zaza S, Giles W. The whole school, whole community, whole child model: A new approach for improving educational attainment and healthy development for students. *J Sch Health*. 2015;85(11):729–39.
2. Council on Sports Medicine and Fitness, Council on School Health. Active healthy living: Prevention of childhood obesity through increased physical activity. *Pediatrics*. 2006;117(5):1834–42.
3. Poitras VJ, Gray CE, Borghese MM, et al. Systematic review of the relationships between objectively measured physical activity and health indicators in school-aged children and youth. *Appl Physiol Nutr Metab*. 2016;41(6 Suppl 3):S197–239.
4. Donnelly JE, Lambourne K. Classroom-based physical activity, cognition, and academic achievement. *Prev Med*. 2011;52(Suppl 1):S36–42.
5. Gagnon M, Stephens MB. Obesity and national defense: Will America be too heavy to fight? *Mil Med*. 2015;180(4):464–7.
6. Maxey H, Bishop-Josef S, Goodman B. *Unhealthy and Unprepared*. Washington, DC: Council for a Strong America; 2018.
7. Institute of Medicine. *Education the Student Body: Taking Physical Activity and Physical Education to School*. Washington, DC: The National Academies Press; 2013.
8. U.S. Department of Health and Human Services. *Physical Activity Guidelines for Americans*. Washington, DC: U.S. Department of Health and Human Services; 2018.
9. Troiano RP, Berrigan D, Dodd KW, Masse LC, Tilert T, McDowell M. Physical activity in the United States measured by accelerometer. *Med Sci Sports Exerc*. 2008;40(1):181–8.
10. Cooper AR, Goodman A, Page AS, et al. Objectively measured physical activity and sedentary time in youth: The International Children's Accelerometry Database (ICAD). *Int J Behav Nutr Phys Act*. 2015;12:113.
11. Hubbard K, Economos CD, Bakun P, et al. Disparities in moderate-to-vigorous physical activity among girls and overweight and obese schoolchildren during school- and out-of-school time. *Int J Behav Nutr Phys Act*. 2016;13:39.
12. Kwon S, Mason M, Welch S. Physical activity of fifth to sixth graders during school hours according to school race/ethnicity: Suburban Cook County, Illinois. *J Sch Health*. 2015;85:382–7.
13. Singh GK, Siahpush M, Kogan MD. Rising social inequalities in US childhood obesity, 2003–2007. *Ann Epidemiol*. 2010;20(1):40–52.
14. Pate RR, Freedson PS, Sallis JF, et al. Compliance with physical activity guidelines: Prevalence in a population of children and youth. *Ann Epidemiol*. 2002;12(5):303–8.
15. Sherar LB, Esliger DW, Baxter-Jones AD, Tremblay MS. Age and gender differences in youth physical activity: Does physical maturity matter? *Med Sci Sports Exerc*. 2007;39(5):830–5.
16. Ziviani J, Macdonald D, Ward H, Jenkins D, Rodger S. Physical activity of young children: A two-year follow-up. *Phys Occup Ther Pediatr*. 2008;28(1):25–39.
17. Cooper KH, Greenberg JD, Castelli DM, Barton M, Martin SB, Morrow JR. Implementing policies to enhance physical education and physical activity in schools. *Res Q Exerc Sport*. 2016;87(2):133–40.
18. Institute of Medicine. *Educating the Student Body: Taking Physical Activity and Physical Education to School*. Washington, DC: The National Academies Press; 2013.
19. Puyau MR, Adolph AL, Vohra FA, Butte NF. Validation and calibration of physical activity monitors in children. *Obesity*. 2002;10(3):150–7.
20. Cain KL, Salis JF, Conway TL, Van Dyck D, Calhoon L. Using accelerometers in youth physical activity studies: A review of methods. *J Phys Act Health*. 2013;10(3):437–50.
21. Pope RP, Coleman KJ, Gonzalez EC, Barron F, Heath EM. Validity of a revised system for observing fitness instruction time (SOFIT). *Pediatr Exerc Sci*. 2002;14(2):135–46.
22. Rowe PJ, Schuldheisz JM, vanderMars H. Validation of SOFIT for measuring physical activity of first- to eighth-grade students. *Pediatr Exerc Sci*. 1997;9(2):136–49.
23. President's Council on Sports Fitness & Nutrition. Presidential Youth Fitness Program 2019. https://www.pyfp.org/about-us. Accessed August 5, 2019.
24. Janssen I, LeBlanc AG. Systematic review of the health benefits of physical activity and fitness in school-aged children and youth. *Int J Behav Nutr Phys Act*. 2010;7:40.
25. Plowman SA, Meredith MD, eds. *Fitnessgram/Activitygram Reference Guide*. Dallas, TX: The Cooper Institute; 2013.
26. Pillsbury L, Oria M, Pate R. *Fitness Measures and Health Outcomes in Youth*. Washington, DC: National Academies Press; 2013.
27. Ekelund U, Luan J, Sherar LB, et al. Moderate to vigorous physical activity and sedentary time and cardiometabolic risk factors in children and adolescents. *JAMA*. 2012;307(7):704–12.
28. Ratey JJ. *Spark: The Revolutionary New Science of Exercise and the Brain*. New York: Little, Brown and Company; 2008.
29. Sibley BA, Etnier JL. The relationship between physical activity and cognition in children: A meta-analysis. *Pediatr Exerc Sci*. 2003;15(3):243–56.
30. Amin SA, Wright CM, Boulos R, et al. The physical activity environment and academic achievement in Massachusetts schoolchildren. *J Sch Health*. 2017;87(12):932–40.
31. Wechsler D. Wechsler intelligence scale for children-revised. 1974.
32. Taylor AF, Kuo FE. Children with attention deficits concentrate better after walk in the park. *J Atten Disord*. 2009;12(5):402–9.
33. Drollette ES, Pontifex MB, Raine LB, et al. Effects of the FITKids physical activity randomized controlled trial on conflict monitoring in youth. *Psychophysiology*. 2018;55(3).
34. Sacheck JM, Wright CM. What do teachers see? Perceptions of school-time physical activity programs on student behavior. *J Sport Health Sci*. 2020;9(1):50–2.
35. Harter S. The perceived competence scale for children. *Child Dev*. 1982;53(1):87–97.
36. Healthy Active Living and Obesity Research Group. Canadian Assessment of Physical Literacy. 2019. https://www.capl-ecsfp.ca. Accessed August 7, 2019.
37. Sallis JF, McKenzie TL, Beets MW, Beighle A, Erwin H, Lee S. Physical education's role in public health: Steps forward and backward over 20 years and HOPE for the future. *Res Q Exerc Sport*. 2012;83(2):125–35.
38. SHAPE America. About SHAPE America. 2018. https://www.shapeamerica.org/about/default.aspx. Accessed June 4, 2018.
39. National Association for Sport and Physical Education. *Moving into the Future: National Standards for Physical Education*. Reston, VA: McGraw-Hill; 2004.
40. Slater SJ, Nicholson L, Chriqui J, Turner L, Chaloupka F. The impact of state laws and district policies on physical education and recess practices in a nationally representative sample of us public elementary schools. *Arch Pediatr Adolesc Med*. 2012;166(4):311–6.
41. Centers for Disease Control and Prevention. *School Health Policies and Practices Study (SHPPS): Physical Education and Physical Activity*. Atlanta, GA: U.S. Department of Health and Human Services; 2014.
42. Webber LS, Osganian SK, Feldman HA, et al. Cardiovascular risk factors among children after a 212-year intervention—The CATCH study. *Prev Med*. 1996;25(4):432–41.
43. CATCH Global Foundation. CATCH: How Does CATCH Work? 2019. https://catchinfo.org/about/. Accessed July 24, 2019.
44. What is SPARK? 2019. https://sparkpe.org/what-is-spark/. Accessed July 24, 2019.
45. Sallis JF, McKenzie TL, Alcaraz JE, Kolody B, Faucette N, Hovel, MF. The effects of a 2-year physical education program (SPARK) on physical activity and fitness in elementary school students. *Am J Public Health*. 1997;87(8):1328–34.
46. McKenzie TL, Sallis JF, Rosengard P. Beyond the stucco tower: Design, development, and dissemination of the SPARK physical education programs. *Quest*. 2009;61(1):114–27.

47. McKenzie TL, Nader PR, Strikmiller PK, et al. School physical education: Effect of the Child and Adolescent Trial for Cardiovascular Health. *Prev Med.* 1996;25(4):423–31.
48. McKenzie TL, Sallis JF, Prochaska JJ, Conway TL, Marshall SJ, Rosengard P. Evaluation of a two-year middle-school physical education intervention: M-SPAN. *Med Sci Sports Exerc.* 2004;36(8):1382–8.
49. Stevens J, Murray DM, Catellier DJ, et al. Design of the Trial of Activity in Adolescent Girls (TAAG). *Contemp Clin Trials.* 2005 Apr;26(2):223–33.
50. Webber LS, Catellier DJ, Lytle LA, et al. Promoting physical activity in middle school girls: Trial of Activity for Adolescent Girls. *Am J Prev Med.* 2008 Mar;34(3):173–84.
51. Ridgers ND, Stratton G, Fairclough SJ. Physical activity levels of children during school playtime. *Sports Med.* 2006;36(4):359–71.
52. Centers for Disease Control and Prevention and SHAPE America. *Strategies for Recess in Schools.* Atlanta, GA: U.S. Department of Health and Human Services; 2017.
53. Turner L, Chaloupka FJ, Chriqui JF, Sandoval A. *School Policies and Practices to Improve Health and Obesity: National Elementary School Survey Results: School Years 2006–2007 and 2007–2008.* Chicago, IL: Bridging the Gap Program, Health Policy Center, Institute for Health Research and Policy, University of Illinois at Chicago; 2010.
54. Ridgers ND, Salmon J, Parrish AM, Stanley RM, Okely AD. Physical activity during school recess: A systematic review. *Am J Prev Med.* 2012;43(3):320–8.
55. Escalante Y, García-Hermoso A, Backx K, Saavedra JM. Playground designs to increase physical activity levels during school recess: A systematic review. *Health Educ Behav.* 2014;41(2):138–44.
56. Parrish AM, Okely AD, Stanley RM, Ridgers ND. The effect of school recess interventions on physical activity. *Sports Med.* 2013;43(4):287–99.
57. Fortson J, James-Burdumy S, Bleeker M, et al. *Impact and Implementation Findings from an Experimental Experimental Evaluation of Playworks: Effects on School Climate, Academic Learning, Student Social Skills and Behavior.* Princeton, NJ: Mathematica Policy Research; 2013.
58. Watson A, Timperio A, Brown H, Best K, Hesketh KD. Effect of classroom-based physical activity interventions on academic and physical activity outcomes: A systematic review and meta-analysis. *Int J Behav Nutr Phys Act.* 2017;14(1):114.
59. GoNoodle. About GoNoodle. 2018. https://www.gonoodle.com. Accessed July 11, 2018.
60. Wright CM, Duquesnay PJ, Anzman-Frasca S, et al. Study protocol: The Fueling Learning through Exercise (FLEX) study—A randomized controlled trial of the impact of school-based physical activity programs on children's physical activity, cognitive function, and academic achievement. *BMC Public Health.* 2016;16(1):1078.
61. Mahar MT, Murphy SK, Rowe DA, Golden J, Shields AT, Raedeke TD. Effects of a classroom-based program on physical activity and on-task behavior. *Med Sci Sports Exerc.* 2006;38(12):2086–94.
62. Kibbe DL, Hackett J, Hurley M, et al. Ten years of TAKE 10!(®): Integrating physical activity with academic concepts in elementary school classrooms. *Prev Med.* 2011;52(Suppl 1):S43–50.
63. Donnelly JE, Greene JL, Gibson CA, et al. Physical Activity Across the Curriculum (PAAC): A randomized controlled trial to promote physical activity and diminish overweight and obesity in elementary school children. *Prev Med.* 2009;49(4):336–41.
64. Donnelly JE, Greene JL, Gibson CA, et al. Physical Activity and Academic Achievement Across the Curriculum (A + PAAC): Rationale and design of a 3-year, cluster-randomized trial. *BMC Public Health.* 2013;13:307.
65. Bartholomew JB, Jowers EM. Physically active academic lessons in elementary children. *Prev Med.* 2011;52(Supp):S51–4.
66. Schmidt M, Benzing V, Kamer M. Classroom-based physical activity breaks and children's attention: Cognitive engagement works! *Front Psychol.* 2016;7:1474.
67. Dinkel D, Schaffer C, Snyder K, Lee JM. They just need to move: Teachers' perception of classroom physical activity breaks. *Teach Teach Educ.* 2017;63:186–95.
68. Goh TL, Hannon JC, Webster CA, Podlog L. Classroom teachers' experiences implementing a movement integration program: Barriers, facilitators, and continuance. *Teach Teach Educ.* 2017;66:88–95.
69. Delk J, Springer AE, Kelder SH, Grayless M. Promoting teacher adoption of physical activity breaks in the classroom: Findings of the Central Texas CATCH Middle School Project. *J Sch Health.* 2014;84(11):722–30.
70. Wright CM, Chomitz VR, Duquesnay PJ, Amin SA, Economos CD, Sacheck JM. The FLEX study school-based physical activity programs—Measurement and evaluation of implementation. *BMC Public Health.* 2019;19(1):73.
71. Carlson JA, Engelberg JK, Cain KL, et al. Implementing classroom physical activity breaks: Associations with student physical activity and classroom behavior. *Prev Med.* 2015;81:67–72.
72. TAKE10. About TAKE10. 2018. http://take10.net/about-take10/. Accessed July 11, 2018.
73. Kibbe DL, Hackett J, Hurley M, et al. Ten Years of TAKE 10!®: Integrating physical activity with academic concepts in elementary school classrooms. *Prev Med.* 2011;52:S43–50.
74. Pullen-Seufert NLS, Marchetti L, Heiny S, Lusk Dudley K. National Center for Safe Routes to School. 2019. http://www.saferoutesinfo.org. Accessed August 6, 2019.
75. Weir LA, Etelson D, Brand DA. Parents' perceptions of neighborhood safety and children's physical activity. *Prev Med.* 2006;43(3):212–7.
76. Faulkner GEJ, Buliung RN, Flora PK, Fusco C. Active school transport, physical activity levels and body weight of children and youth: A systematic review. *Prev Med.* 2009;48(1):3–8.
77. Crawford SB, Bennetts SK, Hackworth NJ, et al. Worries, 'weirdos,' neighborhoods and knowing people: A qualitative study with children and parents regarding children's independent mobility. *Health Place.* 2017;45:131–9.
78. Larouche R, Saunders TJ, Faulkner G, Colley R, Tremblay M. Associations between active school transport and physical activity, body composition, and cardiovascular fitness: A systematic review of 68 studies. *J Phys Act Health.* 2014;11(1):206–27.
79. DeWeese RS, Yedidia MJ, Tulloch DL, Ohri-Vachaspati P. Neighborhood perceptions and active school commuting in low-income cities. *Am J Prev Med.* 2013;45(4):393–400.
80. Timperio A, Ball K, Salmon J, et al. Personal, family, social, and environmental correlates of active commuting to school. *Am J Prev Med.* 2006;30(1):45–51.
81. Rodriguez A, Vogt CA. Demographic, environmental, access, and attitude factors that influence walking to school by elementary school-aged children. *J Sch Health.* 2009;79(6):255–61.
82. Panter JR, Jones AP, Van Sluijs EM, Griffin SJ. Neighborhood, route, and school environments and children's active commuting. *Am J Prev Med.* 2010;38(3):268–78.
83. McDonald NC, Brown AL, Marchetti LM, Pedroso MS. U.S. school travel, 2009: An assessment of trends. *Am J Prev Med.* 2011;41(2):146–51.
84. Babey SH, Hastert TA, Huang W, Brown ER. Sociodemographic, family, and environmental factors associated with active commuting to school among US adolescents. *J Public Health Policy.* 2009;30(Suppl 1):S203–20.
85. Veitch J, Bagley S, Ball K, Salmon J. Where do children usually play? A qualitative study of parents' perceptions of influences on children's active free-play. *Health Place.* 2006;12(4):383–93.
86. O'Connor J, Brown A. A qualitative study of 'fear' as a regulator of children's independent physical activity in the suburbs. *Health Place.* 2013;24:157–64.
87. Veitch J, Carver A, Salmon J, et al. What predicts children's active transport and independent mobility in disadvantaged neighborhoods? *Health Place.* 2017;44:103–9.
88. National Center for Safe Routes to School. Safe Routes. 2018. http://www.saferoutesinfo.org/. Accessed June 25, 2018.
89. Carver A, Veitch J, Sahlqvist S, Crawford D, Hume C. Active transport, independent mobility and territorial range among children residing in disadvantaged areas. *J Transp Health.* 2014;1(4):267–73.
90. Larouche R, Mammen G, Rowe DA, Faulkner G. Effectiveness of active school transport interventions: A systematic review and update. *BMC Public Health.* 2018;18(1):206.
91. Jones RA, Blackburn NE, Woods C, Byrne M, van Nassau F, Tully M. Interventions promoting active transport to school in children: A systematic review and meta-analysis. *Prev Med.* 2019;123:232–41.
92. Demetriou Y, Gillison F, McKenzie TL. After-school physical activity interventions on child and adolescent physical activity and health: A review of reviews. *Adv Phys Educ.* 2017;7(2):191–215.
93. Centers for Disease Control and Prevention. *Physical Activity Before and After School.* Atlanta, GA: U.S. Department of Health and Human Services; 2018.
94. National AfterSchool Association. *Healthy Eating and Physical Activity in Out-of-School Time.* Oakton, VA: National AfterSchool Association; 2011.
95. Bocarro JN, Kanters MA, Edwards MB, Casper JM, McKenzie TL. Prioritizing school intramural and interscholastic programs based on observed physical activity. *Am J Health Promot.* 2014;28(3_suppl):S65–71.
96. Kahan D, McKenzie TL. Physical activity and psychological correlates during an after-school running club. *Am J Health Educ.* 2018;49(2):113–23.

97. Branscum P, Sharma M, Wang, LL, Wilson BR, Rojas-Guyler L. A true challenge for any superhero: An evaluation of a comic book obesity prevention program. *Fam Community Health*. 2013;36(1):63–76.

98. BOKS. What is BOKS. 2018. https://www.bokskids.org/program/. Accessed July 11, 2018.

99. Whooten RC, Perkins ME, Gerber MW, Taveras EM. Effects of before-school physical activity on obesity prevention and wellness. *Am J Prev Med*. 2018;54(4):510–8.

100. Girls on the Run. What We Do. 2018. https://www.girlsontherun.org/What-We-Do. Accessed July 11, 2018.

101. Tergerson JL, King KA. Do perceived cues, benefits, and barriers to physical activity differ between male and female adolescents? *J Sch Health*. 2002;72(9):374–80.

102. Debate RD, Pettee Gabriel K, Zwald M, Huberty J, Zhang Y. Changes in psychosocial factors and physical activity frequency among third- to eighth-grade girls who participated in a developmentally focused youth sport program: A preliminary study. *J Sch Health*. 2009;79(10):474–84.

103. The Aspen Institute Sport & Society Program. *State of Play 2017: Trends and Developments*. Washington, DC: The Aspen Institute; 2017.

104. Leek D, Carlson JA, Cain KL, et al. Physical activity during youth sports practices. *Arch Pediatr Adolesc Med*. 2011;165(4):294–9.

105. Sacheck JM, Nelson T, Ficker L, Kafka T, Kuder J, Economos CD. Physical activity during soccer and its contribution to physical activity recommendations in normal weight and overweight children. *Pediatr Exerc Sci*. 2011;23(2):281–92.

106. Nelson TF, Stovitz SD, Thomas M, LaVoi NM, Bauer KW, Neumark-Sztainer D. Do youth sports prevent pediatric obesity? A systematic review and commentary. *Curr Sports Med Rep*. 2011;10(6):360–70.

107. Eime RM, Young JA, Harvey JT, Charity MJ, Payne WR. A systematic review of the psychological and social benefits of participation in sport for children and adolescents: Informing development of a conceptual model of health through sport. *Int J Behav Nutr Phys Act*. 2013;10(1):98.

108. Gould D, Flett R, Lauer L. The relationship between psychosocial developmental and the sports climate experienced by underserved youth. *Psychol Sport Exerc*. 2012;13(1):80–7.

109. Anderson-Butcher D, Riley A, Amorose A, Iachini A, Wade-Mdivanian R. Maximizing youth experiences in community sport settings: The design and impact of the LiFE Sports Camp. *J Sport Manage*. 2014;28(2):236–49.

CHAPTER

185

Food and Physical Activity Environments: Influences on Diet and Physical Activity

Brisa N. Sánchez • Maria Acosta • Robin L. García • Amihan F. Crisostomo • Emma V. Sanchez-Vaznaugh

INTRODUCTION

Diet and physical activity are shaped by multiple and complex pathways, including individual-level factors, social and cultural norms, as well as the environment. In turn, as is well documented, diet and physical activity influence myriad clinical outcomes including obesity—the result of an imbalance caused by physical inactivity and poor nutrition—and its association with health, morbidity, and mortality. In 2017, most of the leading causes of death in the United States, including heart disease, cancers, chronic lower respiratory diseases, cerebrovascular diseases, diabetes, kidney disease, and hypertension[1] can be linked to obesity. The trends in leading chronic diseases and associated causes of death in the United States are also seen globally.

There is an impetus among the scientific, medical, and policy communities to devote attention to how characteristics of the environment influence diet and physical activity. This growing concern is, in part, driven by the need to complement individual-level treatments or programs addressing diet and physical activity with policies and environmental interventions that support healthy choices and behaviors for entire populations.[2–12] Independent of individual-level factors well known to be associated with health (e.g., income), growing evidence indicates that the environment (including its social and physical dimensions) may influence a person's ability to be physically active [13–17] and to consume nutritious and/or nonhealthful foods.[18–20] In particular, community-level resources and characteristics of the built environment may influence diet and physical activity through a variety of pathways, and may interact with individual factors (Fig. 185-1). The built environment refers to the physical, human-made space within which humans live, work, and recreate on a day-to-day basis. It includes all of the physical aspects of a person's life, such as the residential and school/work neighborhood environments, infrastructure that supports those places, and physical space. Studies have noted that specific aspects of the built environment are associated with a plethora of biological factors for which diet and physical activity serve as pathways, including glucose levels[21] and obesity,[22,23] cholesterol levels, triglycerides,[24,25] and increased risk for chronic diseases, including cancer, diabetes,[26,27] and cardiovascular disease.[28,29]

It is increasingly clear that environmental factors play a role in diet and physical activity above and beyond other individual-level characteristics. Crucially, the work of the medical and public health communities, along with other sectors, to alleviate the burden of chronic disease can leverage research on the health effects of the built environment. In addition to providing high-quality medical care within the clinic walls, healthcare providers may seek to broaden the lens to include built environments as part of assessments of patients' risks, exposures, and vulnerabilities to health outcomes, and in devising treatment strategies, incorporate the built environment.

This chapter is organized as follows: First, we highlight how the medical community has engaged with built environment research along with implications for current and future clinical practice as well as research. Second, we provide an overview of the lexicon and research methods that have been used to examine the influence of food and physical activity environments outside of homes and work/school on diet and physical activity. Subsequently, we summarize

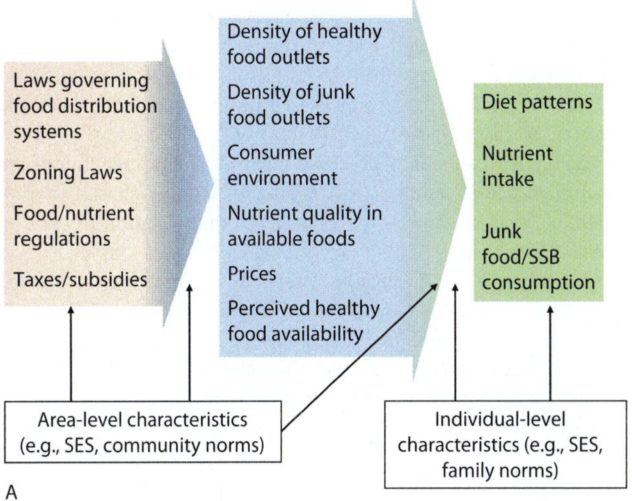

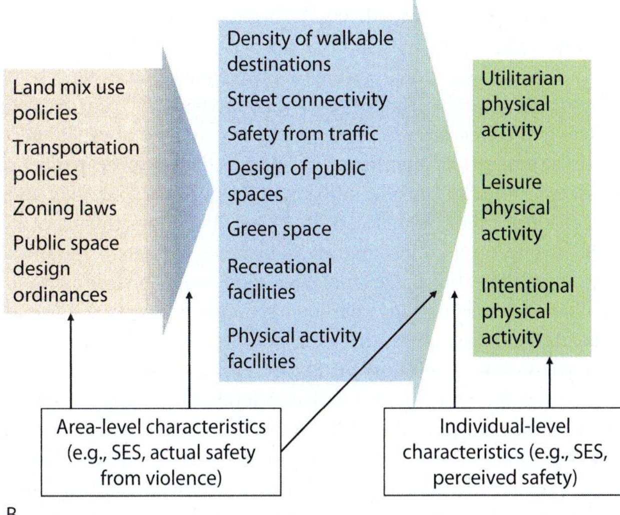

FIGURE 185-1. Conceptual frameworks describing how policies and broader community factors influence specific features of the (A) food and (B) physical activity environment, and, in concert with individual- and other community-level characteristics, influence diet and physical activity.

research findings in this area, separately for the food and physical environment and, within these for adults and children. Next, we discuss the role of said environmental attributes on social disparities in health along dimensions of race/ethnicity, socioeconomic advantage, and sex. We end with a discussion of future directions for research in this area along with ways in which clinicians may engage to conduct related research or support the development of policy and population-level interventions.

GEOMEDICINE AND IMPLICATIONS FOR CLINICAL PRACTICE AND RESEARCH

The field of geomedicine emerged as a result of increased awareness within the medical community about the ways in which environments shape health outcomes[30,31] and the importance to conduct empirical research on this topic for preventive medicine. In recent years, the National Academy of Medicine (NAM), formerly the Institute of Medicine (IOM), recommended the standardization and routine collection of patients' neighborhood physical and social factors, and their systematic linkage to electronic health records (EHRs).[32,33] In addition, the proposed "All of Us" research program, initially known as the "precision medicine cohort,"[34–36] will attempt to characterize the environments in which all study participants live.[37,38] The primary objectives of generating this linked information are: to study how healthcare outcomes, including adherence to treatment,[39] vary by contextual or environmental factors,[32,33] and to capitalize on the rich clinical, objectively-measured information available in the medical records to shape clinical practice. The emergence of so-called "precision medicine" and "precision environments" thus underscore the importance of capturing environmental factors relevant to each individual patient or person and using that information in crafting treatment strategies.

Of particular importance for clinicians is that research findings about the links between environment and health, along with the use of data about environmental factors tied to the patients and embedded in EHR, can impact (enhance) their ability to manage individual patients' disease.[40] Emerging research indicates that it is plausible to strengthen the impact of clinical interventions on patients' health outcomes through a better understanding of the environmental circumstances of specific patients.[41,42] Improved understanding of research findings on the built environment plus the linkage of individuals' EHRs to databases of community resources[42] can enhance clinical interventions and their effectiveness. For example, clinical recommendations for individual patients can be developed in ways that incorporate additional features of the patient's circumstances.[43–45] As a simple example, taking into account patients' proximity to parks when counseling them about physical activity can help tailor the intervention to recommend in-home exercises when parks are far away. Similarly, considering proximity to famers markets and/or routes from their home/work to stores with fresh produce could result in improved counseling and adherence to dietary modifications. Available knowledge and data about built environments of individual patients provides unique opportunities to expand overall medical effectiveness.[43]

Beyond clinical settings, healthcare professionals can also help support the development of population-level policies and built environment interventions. Population policy interventions hold strong potential to shape health behaviors because they typically apply to entire populations and improve health outcomes for all.[2–12] Thus, they are fundamental complements for disease prevention and management. However, the effective design of comprehensive built environment interventions and policies hinges upon our nuanced understanding of the combinations of environmental features that impact health behaviors of patients with varying clinical profiles. That is, developing successful population-level policies requires understanding the views of all stakeholders in the health arena and other sectors, from the needs of communities, to how people's health or disease profiles manifest, and how clinicians address those in the delivery of healthcare. Physicians may extend their impact beyond healthcare settings by engaging in the development of built environment policy. For example, physicians may lead efforts within their communities or lend their expertise on clinical outcomes to others' efforts, such as supporting policies to regulate sugar-sweetened beverages.

In parallel to research about physical activity and diet moving from individual to neighborhood/environmental factors, health disparities research has advanced from describing to understanding and developing ways to reduce or eliminate disparities and to identifying how differences in environmental exposures across population subgroups may impact disparities in health and health behaviors.[46–49] This knowledge can inform how individual- and population-wide interventions can be designed to reduce disparities or to mitigate any detrimental intervention effects on disparities.[50,51] For clinicians, this may entail understanding the degree to which differential access to environments that promote health effects of physical activity and diet in their patients of color. Additionally, it may involve developing treatment strategies to better support patients, for example, in disease management, medication adherence, or reduction of risks. Clinicians have predominantly focused on improving healthcare disparities, for instance, through the establishment of cultural competency training and enhancing patient-physician communications.[52] However, understanding the larger contextual circumstances that facilitate or impede patients' behavioral options/decisions, and incorporating that knowledge into clinical practice may expand clinician's "toolboxes" to further support patients.

While the link between clinical outcomes and built environments may appear far and fuzzy, mounting empirical evidence, as reviewed in the next sections, suggests its growing significance, both for population-level strategies and for tailoring of clinical, individual-level treatments.

RESEARCH OVERVIEW

Over the past several decades, neighborhood environments research has grown exponentially. Along with the volume of research, scientists have developed definitions and measures of the built environment, which has resulted in an entire taxonomy and language to describe environmental "exposures." Though initially broad area-level features of neighborhoods were used, this rapidly expanding body of research has increased its focus on more granular, specific features of "the food environment" and the "physical activity environment" (described in more detail below), and has used advanced methods to more precisely measure diet and physical activity. Within both of these broad topics, the research conducted to date includes both adults and children. Additionally, in some but not all instances, scientific inquiry has evaluated the influence of these environments on social disparities in health, defined based on race/ethnicity, income, education, and sex.

Measurement Tools and Methods

Geographic information systems (GIS) are undoubtedly an important methodological tool that propelled research forward on built environments and health.[53–55] GIS permits mapping and cross-referencing locations of individuals to geographic areas (e.g., census tracts) and/or point locations (e.g., grocery stores). The widespread availability of GIS has made it increasingly possible to link large health-related databases, including cohort studies and EHRs, with databases that characterize the built environment and community resources,[56–61] enabling scholarly research in this area. Databases that included rich measures of individual-level measures of diet and physical activity can be readily linked to participants' community resources, for example, supermarkets and gyms, provided person/patient-level addresses (or other area-unit such as ZIP code) for each person, enabling rich hypotheses testing and advancing empirical work.

In addition to GIS, several quantitative technologies and qualitative tools have been used to empirically study the health effects of neighborhood environments, as discussed in more detail in the chapter "Connecting Neighborhoods and Health" in this book. For example, emerging technologies now make it possible to track individuals' activity spaces over time[62–67] through the use of global positioning systems (GPS) and synchronously measure the locations of study subjects (e.g., closeness to a park or gym) and their levels of physical activity using accelerometers.[68,69] While these rich data sources require novel methods to capitalize on emerging "big data" to study environmental influences on behaviors, health, and disease, such data sources will continue to advance high-quality research in this area. Presently, this area is also capitalizing on the availability of EHRs to build cross-sectional and longitudinal cohorts from EHR data that have been geocoded to link it to patient's neighborhoods or places.[44,70] Several other quantitative tools include systematic field observations (where observers conduct visual audits of places, in person or virtually, to collect specific data elements such as presence of fast food or sidewalk quality[71]); social media and internet data[72]; and self-reported questionnaires about the environment.[73]

Although qualitative tools (e.g., go-along interviews,[74] ethnography [75,76]) cannot be readily processed and linked with large databases, they contribute critically important information about the underlying causal mechanisms that link environmental features to health behaviors. As an example, go-along interviews inform researchers on how built environment features, like sidewalk quality, influence the interviewee's decision to participate in walking for either transport or exercise and/or if instead other factors are at play.[77] When participants see, in real time, the walking infrastructures while they are interviewed, that closely connects the interviewee to the actual context under investigation. Thus, this experiential type of qualitative research provides potentially more accurate information. For instance, it could reveal that a particular route is discouraged given the neighborhood reputation despite excellent sidewalks. Ethnography, which involves direct, open-ended (vs. structured) observation of participants during their daily lives, provides a deeper level of understanding as to why participants do what they do in the specific places and contexts in which their life develops. This can be particularly important when researchers and study participants are from distinct backgrounds, including social class and community environment characteristics. Qualitative methods can also be used to test hypotheses.[78,79] Therefore, these methods can play a critically important role: aiding the researcher to generate and test hypotheses about the environment. Further, these methods also help develop approaches to measure features of the environment that matter the most to the study population and can be subsequently used to empirically test hypothesis in the quantitative context.

Research Designs

As is in many other health areas, built environment-health inquiry begun with cross-sectional studies, but existing cohort studies have now compiled a wealth of environmental data that can be linked to each participant in a time varying fashion.[19,80–82] Longitudinal cohort studies improved the rigor of prior research studies and provided more robust evidence supporting causal inferences about environmental effects on health and disease, given that changes in outcomes can be related to changes in the environment. Importantly, a growing body of research uses study designs that can quantify the effects of "natural experiments" (such as the effects on physical activity associated with the opening of a new rapid transit station[83,84]), or how actual, randomized relocation of study participants to new neighborhoods influenced obesity status and other outcomes.[85] In addition to the strength of study designs, a critical component in evaluating the quality of built environment research is a deeper understanding about the causal mechanisms that can give rise to the associations of interest.

Mechanisms

Community design can provide varying levels of support to improve, leave unchanged or erode healthy lifestyles for the entire population in that community. Having ready access to safe green spaces can make it easy for people to engage in recreational physical activity. Additionally, environments that feature a variety of produce markets and other food stores offering nutritious foods can facilitate healthy diets. The premise behind these notions is that easy accessibility and availability of resources can support individuals to make "health-promoting" decisions, or those that would exert healthier effects on their bodies. Proximity and availability have been the most widely tested mechanisms in the food and physical activity environments, likely due to the more prevalent availability of data to measure these mechanisms.[86] Undoubtedly, the mere presence of a produce market will not necessarily entice a person with low economic resources to make purchases if the market is unaffordable or perceived as such. Likewise, availability of sidewalks in one's neighborhood will not necessarily support walking if the neighborhood is unsafe due to the threat of physical violence, or is only feasible to use during the day because streetlights are unavailable at night. That is, the mechanisms may be more complex, involving the interaction of person-level characteristics or preferences and the available infrastructure or resources, and not equally applicable to all persons across all places. Conceptualizing a mechanism before testing hypotheses is critical to enable more rigorous inferences. Technological advancements have enabled researchers to pose and answer more complex research questions involving single or multiple mechanisms hypothesized to shape health and disease.

Reverse Causation/Residential Self-selection Bias

Residential self-selection bias arises due to the sorting of individuals into neighborhoods according to preferences that are often correlated with health outcomes and has long been discussed as a threat to causal inferences in this field.[87–94] For example, people who prefer walking for transportation will be more likely to choose to live in pedestrian-friendly environments and as a result (continue to) have higher physical activity levels. Similarly, people who like shopping for fresh produce at farmers markets may consider their proximity when making choices about where to live and support their (already established) fruit- and vegetable-rich diet. Thus, residential selection bias may give rise to "significant associations" that are due to "reverse causation." However, recent studies have examined empirically the extent to which residential self-selection may be present in diet and physical activity studies.[87–94] In conducting research in this area, investigators distinguish between aspirational preferences, defined as those that are not constrained due to cost or other competing interests, compared to actual residential decisions that consider realized opportunity costs. Importantly, findings by Li et al. suggest that residential self-selection biases are likely stronger for populations that have more economic resources[95] and have not endured structural exclusionary housing policies (e.g., redlining). Moreover, studies that adjust for residential self-selection effects, or employ robust longitudinal designs or natural experiments, have improved the rigor of the studies in this field and lend credence to the existing findings about built environment influences on health outcomes.

THE FOOD ENVIRONMENT

Nutrient-rich diets, especially those with plentiful fruits and vegetables high in antioxidants or fish rich in omega fatty acids, as well as meals or snacks low in sugar, fat, and salt have been consistently associated with multiple positive health outcomes (see Chapter 180: The Principles of Nutritional Sciences: Nutrients, Nutrition Recommendations, and Dietary Guidelines). Conversely, high caloric density food, including snacks with high content of trans fatty acids and sugary beverages, have been associated with ill health and disease.[96–100] Naturally, these relationships apply to both children and adults, although examining the food environment effects on children's nutrition is even more important because it can potentially impact life long patterns of nutrition-related behaviors and health. Current evidence shows that, at least among several population subgroups, food environments affect diet.

What Is the Food Environment?

The food environment can be defined as the collective physical, economic, policy and sociocultural surroundings, opportunities, and conditions that influence a person's food choices and nutritional status.[101] Food systems and the policies that govern them ultimately determine the types of food and food quality available to consumers.[102] Unhealthy food, snacks, and beverages (e.g., high in harmful types of fats,[103] salt, and sugar) tend to be pervasive in the food supply.[104,105] In turn, these items are distributed to individuals through food outlets in/near residential, workplace, and school environments and other supply systems. While metrics to characterize the food policy environments, including globalization of the food environment, have been developed,[106,107] the vast majority of research linking food environments to individual-level diet has focused on two more proximal types of environments: the community food environment, which describes the distribution of food outlets within a community's physical space; and the consumer food environment, which entails what consumers encounter while inside local food outlets.[108] Some key terms that have been used to characterize community food environments in popular media and research include "food desert" and "food swamp." The former is commonly used to describe food environments that "lack affordable fruits, vegetables, whole grains, lowfat milk, and other foods that make up a full and healthy diet."[109] Food deserts are often found in rural, minority, and low-income communities that lack large supermarkets and, instead, have a preponderance of convenience stores. Food swamp refers to the overwhelming availability of junk food outlets.[110–112] However, as compared to broad categorizations like food swamp or desert, the majority of research has devoted attention to more granular measures of the environment.

Measuring the Food Environment

The food environment is typically (but not always) measured in three different domains: (1) physical food environment, (2) social food environment, and (3) the person-centered food environment. The domains address the availability and access of foods (physical environment); the social support and role modeling from peers, family, neighbors, and society to make food choices (social environment); and, finally, an individual's own relationship with, attitudes, and preferences for food (person-centered environment).[113] Within these domains, the food environment encompasses five dimensions: (i) availability, (ii) accessibility, (iii) affordability, (iv) acceptability, and (v) accommodation (Table 185-1). In this review, we address the physical environment domain.

TABLE 185-1 DIMENSIONS OF THE FOOD ENVIRONMENT

Dimension	Definition, How Dimension Is Operationalized in Research, and/or Example
Availability	• Adequate supply of healthy food[108] • GIS-based methods for store presence, density of stores per mile or per population within an area • Perceived higher availability of healthy foods is associated with consuming a healthier diet[114,231]; GIS metrics have results mixed[108]
Accessibility	• Proximity to food outlets and the ease of getting to these establishments • Includes physical distance, geographic boundaries, and transportation[232] • Inconsistent results on accessibility and diet outcomes
Affordability	• Individual's perceptions of affordability; price of food and beverages as well as perceptions of worth relative to cost • Ways to measure: Index of food prices, perceptions of affordability, store audits
Acceptability	• Attitudes about one's local food environment and whether the supply meets personal standards
Accommodation	• Ability of local food sources to accept and adapt to local residents' needs and preferences

Influence of Food Environments on Adults' Diet

Residential Food Environment

Most studies linking the food environment with eating behaviors and health indicators such as obesity have examined exposures within neighborhoods of residence. The Multi-Ethnic Study of Atherosclerosis (MESA) study, for example, investigated food environments in relation to healthy diets. Participants with no supermarkets near their home were 25–46% less likely to report having a healthy diet, described by a "fats and processed meats" dietary pattern and the Alternative Healthy Eating Index (AHEI).[114] Several other U.S.-based cohorts have also observed associations between the community food environment and adult diet and obesity.[115,116] In a Canadian study, food destination density, measured by the density, diversity, and presence of specific food destination types around a 400-meter radius of a participant, was positively associated with the Canadian Healthy Eating Index.[117] Meta-analysis and systematic reviews of observational studies have documented links between food environment factors and downstream clinical outcomes including body mass index (BMI), blood pressure, and metabolic syndrome.[118,119]

Intervention studies add rigor to observational studies, enhancing causal inferences. A systematic review assessing effects of retail food environment interventions reported at least one positive effect on dietary outcomes (which included price or purchasing, dietary intake, dietary quality, or other health measures) in 67% of the 86 articles reviewed.[120] The systematic review of policies and natural or quasiexperiments by Mayne et al. found improvements in diet following bans/restrictions on unhealthy foods, mandates offering healthier foods, and altering purchase/payment rules on foods purchased using low-income food vouchers.[4] While the Mayne et al. study did not find significant effects following the introduction of new supermarkets into communities, studies conducted after the review identified improvements in population diet following opening of supermarkets, including systematic reviews,[121–123] although the exact mechanism remained unclear.[122] The evidence from observational, longitudinal, and natural experiments supports an association between food environment and diet. Most of these studies have focused primarily on where people live and do not take into account the environments surrounding workplaces.[124]

Food Environment Near Workplaces

There is increasing recognition that dietary behaviors are likely to be influenced by exposures in nonresidential environments as well. U.S. adults spend a large proportion of their time at work and likely procure food at or near work environments. While research has examined food environment exposures *inside* workplaces, here we describe research related to food environments *surrounding* or near workplaces to help provide a more comprehensive understanding of how neighborhoods and place affect health beyond the residential neighborhoods described above.

To date, few studies have considered food environments near workplaces. A literature review revealed that less than 5% of neighborhood environment studies consider the characteristics of the neighborhoods near workplaces.[124] This relatively small body of research has examined its impact on healthy food choices, dietary intake, BMI, and obesity. A cross-sectional study conducted in Cambridgeshire in the United Kingdom (UK) described the food environments that a sample of working adults were exposed to at home, work, and along their commute routes between home and work. Food environments were composed of a mix of retail food outlets including supermarkets, restaurants, and fast food options, which could either promote or discourage healthy eating habits. Overall, the study found that participants were exposed to food environments near work and along the commute in addition to exposure to food environments near their home, although food environments near work and along the commute route differed from the residential food environment. For instance, among participants with the highest exposure to takeaway food outlets, workplaces accounted for most of the exposure.[125] In a subsequent study among a similar cross-section of working adults in Cambridgeshire, UK, Borgoine et al. found that exposure to takeaway food outlets was positively associated with consumption of takeaway food, and that exposure to fast food outlets near the workplace of UK adults yielded stronger associations with fast food consumption than exposure near home or along commuting routes.[126] The total exposure to takeaway food outlets in home, work, and commuting environments was significantly associated with increased BMI and with greater odds of obesity.[126] Similarly, in another cross-sectional study, Watts et al. observed that among young adults in the Minneapolis/St. Paul metropolitan area, working within a 5-minute walk of a fast food outlet was associated with increased likelihood of consuming fast food more than 3 days a week.[127] Conversely, a 2013 cross-sectional study using data from women in Australia, found that having access to healthy foods near the workplace was associated with consumption of healthier foods. Having supermarkets within walking distance (0.8 km) from the workplace, for example, was positively associated with greater vegetable and fruit intake.[128]

Child-specific Evidence of the Food Environment Influences

Residential Food Environment

Many studies have linked residential neighborhood food environments to children's health outcomes, including eating patterns, with several longitudinal studies observing positive associations between the built environment and overweight and obesity status and trajectory. The Cohort Study of Young Girls' Nutrition, Environment and Transitions (CYGENT) found that living in California neighborhoods with high availability of convenience stores was associated with overweight and obesity after three years. Conversely, availability of produce vendors/farmer's markets was associated with a lower risk of overweight and obesity.[129] The Early Childhood Longitudinal Study—Kindergarten Cohort (ECLS-K) also found a protective association of supermarket density and obesity in girls, but found no associations between neighborhood food environments and risk of obesity in boys after 3 years.[7] The Neighborhood Impact on Kids study found that children who lived in high physical activity/high nutritional environment neighborhoods were less likely to have overweight or obesity after 2 years compared with other neighborhoods.[130]

A systematic review of local food environments and obesity, looking specifically at availability of food (both distance to food outlets and density of types of food outlets), found mixed evidence among children, although the studies included were generally low quality as they were mostly cross-sectional. About half of the 14 studies looking at the association between convenience store availability and obesity found at least one positive association. Most associations with fast food availability and obesity in children were null; however for low-income children, 12 of 19 associations tested demonstrated positive relationships between fast food availability and obesity.[8]

The Food Environment Within Neighborhoods Surrounding Schools

The food environment near schools,[131,132] particularly the availability of fast food restaurants and convenience stores, may be uniquely important because children spend a large proportion of their waking time in or around schools.[133,134] The availability of junk food outlets near schools can influence diet directly through purchases, or indirectly through exposure to advertisements and thus subsequent purchases elsewhere. Indeed, food outlet availability near schools has been associated with purchases and consumption of unhealthy foods.[135] Additionally, multiple, though not all,[136–142] studies, including a systematic review,[143] have found that the density and/or proximity of food retailers to schools was positively associated with obesity.[144–150]

The food environment near schools could act synergistically with other interventions within communities, schools, homes, and clinics to influence health outcomes. That is, community, clinical, behavioral, and policy interventions to improve child health may be strengthened or undermined by the food environment near schools and homes. For example, policy interventions that ban or restrict students' access to high calorie food and drinks on campus can be undermined easily in a school neighborhood with high access to those same foods and beverages. Knowledge about these environments and their potential influence on child health can strengthen strategies for interventions, including in clinical settings. Importantly, as further described in the penultimate section within this chapter, junk food outlets (e.g., fast food restaurants) tend to be more prominent near schools attended by more socioeconomically deprived populations or located in economically disadvantaged neighborhoods,[151] highlighting the importance of these patterns to research and practice related to social disparities in health.

PHYSICAL ACTIVITY ENVIRONMENT

The benefits of physical activity are widely known and extend to many aspects of health. Regular physical activity can help with weight control and reduction, lowering the risk of cardiovascular disease, type 2 diabetes, and metabolic syndrome, reducing risk of some cancers, strengthening bones and muscles to slow loss of bone density, and improving mental health and mood.[152] There is a continuum in the ways in which activity is conceptualized, measured, and assessed for its effects on health: from no-activity or sedentariness such as sitting or television watching, to vigorous physical activity that induces sweating. Many levels of this continuum have been associated with health outcomes.[153] Sedentariness itself is associated with poor health outcomes, thus any activity is better than no activity.[154] The National Academies of Sciences recommended that physical activity be routinely recorded as part of a set of social and behavioral indicators in EHRs.[33]

Physical activity also benefits a wide range of outcomes among children, including health and mental health.[153] Studies have shown that compared to more fit and active children, those who are not active have lower high-density lipoprotein (HDL) levels. Aerobic exercise training can be related to reducing both systolic and diastolic blood pressure, especially in youth with high blood pressure. As metabolic syndrome becomes more prevalent in children, more studies are showing that physical activity is inversely related to metabolic syndrome and positively associated with cardiorespiratory fitness in a dose-response pattern. Bone mineral density, especially important in growing children, also benefits from as little as 10 minutes of physical activity. Depression also improves in children with moderate physical activity.[155]

Measured subjectively through surveys and/or objectively using accelerometers and other similar monitors, physical activity can be categorized into two domains: (1) recreational physical activity for exercise and/or fitness and (2) utilitarian physical activity as a means of active transport. Recreational physical activity measures often include intentional exercise. Each of these domains, and thus total physical activity, can be impacted by features of the physical activity environment, including overall access to green spaces, recreational facilities, walkability, crime, and safety.

What Is the Physical Activity Environment?

The physical activity environment includes spaces or space configurations that either inhibit or encourage those accessing them to be physically active.[156] Examining the contexts and domains of the physical activity environment is important when attempting to understand the environmental influence on physical activity.[157] The dimensions of the physical activity environment encompass both the built and natural environments. The built environment dimension includes the buildings, spaces, and objects created or modified by people, and is shaped by land-use and transportation policies. For example, road and pedestrian infrastructure, traffic, public transport, street connectivity, and residential density [158] are all attributes of the built environment. The natural environment includes parks, trails, and other green spaces. The effects of both of these dimensions on physical activity can be modified by climate and weather, other neighborhood-level factors including social norms and safety,[6] as well as person-level characteristics including perceptions and psychosocial factors.[159,160]

Measuring the Physical Activity Environment

Measurement of the physical activity environment has a long history with several metrics used in research.[156] As with the food environment, measures of physical activity environments may include proximity to (the nearest entrance to) a park or other address-based locations such as gyms or community centers. As mentioned above, GIS analysis has been widely used to quantify characteristics of the built and natural environment hypothesized to influence levels of physical activity (Table 185-2). However, the physical activity environment has also included area-level measures, such as the density of intersections near one's residence—with a higher density of intersections typically meaning smaller streets and thus more walkable areas, and area-level density of walking destinations. Given the high intercorrelation among many of these indices, composite measures, such as the WalkScore™, have also been used in research.[161–163]

Most recently, GPS have enabled more precise measurement of the actual paths taken by individuals from one place to another. Coupling GPS with accelerometers to measure physical activity facilitates ascertainment of where and when physical activity occurs and the quality of physical activity (whether it is moderate or vigorous). Although this new frontier in measurement methods is not without limitations, it opens the door to answering richer questions about the ways in which individuals interact in the physical environments.

The domains of physical activity, recreational and utilitarian, are often studied separately. In research studies, these classifications are paired with a physical activity environment metric that is more plausibly related to the specific dimension (e.g., green space and recreational activity vs. street connectivity and utilitarian physical activity).

TABLE 185-2 DEFINITIONS OF COMMONLY USED BUILT ENVIRONMENT ATTRIBUTES

Domain	Attribute	Definition
Macroscale: layout of communities	Walkability	• How the physical environment favors walking • Combination of mixed land use, moderate-to-high residential density, street connectivity • Traversable (move without impediments), compact to provide short distances between destinations, safe areas for walking, physically enticing[233]
	Street connectivity	• How well streets are connected to each other, density of intersections, directness of connections[234] • High connectivity characterized by short links to streets and fewer cul de sacs and dead ends
	Residential density/ urbanization	• Size and density of neighborhood one lives in • High urbanization/density may lead to critical mass, which can lead to safety concerns
	Access to/ availability of stores, services, and destinations	• Distance and ease to reach a certain place
Microscale: design of setting and affects experience	Infrastructure and street design	• Presence and quality of bicycle and pedestrian infrastructure, bus stop shelters and signage, and other transportation systems[235,236]
	Design of public spaces	• Quality of spaces and characteristics that are or are not conducive to activity
Social: people in the environment and behaviors	Safety (includes general, traffic-related, crime-related)	• Perceived safety influences physical activity behavior • Indicators of social disorder (graffiti, litter) diminish physical activity

Adult-specific Evidence About Physical Activity Environments

Residential Environments

High-quality physical environments can promote greater quantities of recreational physical activity in adults. Specifically, in a review of recreational walking and cycling, physical environments with higher ratings of traffic-related safety were associated with walking and cycling.[164,165] A study among French adults found that residents of communities with available, high-quality green/open spaces, accessible services, and fewer nuisances such as traffic had higher likelihood of recreational walking within their neighborhood.[166] Moreover, Nehme et al. support the idea that recreational walking may be more influenced by environmental factors that support a safe, enjoyable, and social experience, but not necessarily environmental features that are prioritized for transportation walking.[165]

Active transport has a positive relationship with access to shops, services (such as recreational facilities), and work.[167] A more walkable environment leads to higher odds of walking or cycling for transportation.[164,167] Urbanization has been associated with cycling for transportation as it increases infrastructure of both bicycle lanes and sidewalks, which contrasts with the evidence found for street connectivity and physical activity in children.[157] Hilliness is negatively associated with walking and cycling for transportation[164] whereas greenery and public/open space has been linked to higher levels of total walking, with walking for transport also associated with proximity to public transit.[164,167]

In a meta-analysis of studies relating neighborhood environments to cardiovascular disease, higher levels of physical activity and walking were associated with safe walkways and recreational facilities. Neighborhoods with higher indices of street connectivity, residential density, recreational facilities and availability of traffic devices had improved walkability and lower incidence of cardiovascular disease.[118] Furthermore, living in a walkable neighborhood is associated with lower prevalence of high BMI, diabetes, and metabolic syndrome risk.[118]

Systematic reviews of natural experiments support a link between physical activity environments and physical activity.[168] Kärmeniemi et al. found that accessibility to and creation of new infrastructure for walking, cycling, and public transportation was related to higher total and utilitarian physical activity, and that existing evidence supports a link between perceived aesthetics and safety as determinants of physical activity.[168] Similarly, in their systematic review, Smith et al. found that making improvements to neighborhoods' walkability including active transport infrastructure and improving the quality of parks and playgrounds can have a positive impact on activity in children and adults.[84] However, they noted variations across levels of socioeconomic advantage were observed in some studies (see below). In summary, there is strong evidence that residential physical activity environments influence levels and types of physical activity.

Physical Activity Environments Near the Workplace

Multiple studies have investigated the impact of physical environments within worksites and wellness interventions on sedentary behavior, productivity, and physical activity[169–172] while few investigations have linked various elements of the built environment surrounding workplaces to increased physical activity. Researchers maintain that the influence of workplace neighborhoods is potentially important because adults spend about half of their waking hours at/near workplaces. A cross-sectional study of 2015 employed adults residing in four Missouri metropolitan areas found that sidewalks and walkable access to transit were significantly associated with physical activity around workplaces.[173] Bike facilities around workplaces and the presence of interesting things to look at in the surrounding neighborhood were also significantly associated with physical activity.[173] Similarly, in a cross-sectional study of 148 adults in Massachusetts, Troped et al. reported significant associations with both the home and workplace built environments and measures of physical activity occurring near the home and workplace. Using accelerometer and GPS devices, researchers found that within 1 kilometer of work, population and housing unit density were associated with moderate-to-vigorous physical activity (MVPA) occurring within areas around work locations.[174] In another study, Hoener et al. examined the association of workplace neighborhood characteristics with health-related outcomes, specifically, cardiorespiratory fitness (CRF) and BMI. In the cross-sectional study of 4734 adults aged 20–88 years old residing in 12 Texas counties, higher street connectivity, the number of exercise facilities, and neighborhood vegetation around the workplace were positively yet weakly associated with higher levels of CRF.[175]

Other studies have similarly shown that the physical environment around the workplace, such as neighborhood vegetation, can influence engagement in physical activity. Adams et al. associated commuter walking with the presence of convenient routes to work and well-maintained pavements for walking in the workplace neighborhood.[176] In a 2009 study among 117 adults, self-reported workplace neighborhood factors were not associated with overall physical activity; however, built environment features like sidewalks and crosswalks were correlated with taking at least one walking trip from the workplace in the past month.[177] And, in a cross-sectional study among employed adults in Australia, physical activity during the work day was influenced by unsupportive physical environments surrounding the workplace, such as lack of safety in the outside environment.[172]

Watts et al. described the workplace environments of young adults and examined the associations with diet, physical activity, and BMI in a cross-sectional study of 1538 employed young adult participants in Project EAT (Eating and Activity among Teens and Young Adults). They found that reporting that it is easy to be active at work was associated with significantly greater likelihood of engaging in more than 2.5 hours per week of MVPA and participating in transportation-related activity, and a lower prevalence of obesity. Additionally, living within a 30-minute walk of work was significantly related to participating in transportation-related activity while distance to a fitness facility and perceiving that coworkers think physical activity is important were unrelated to PA or BMI.[127]

Child-Specific Evidence About Physical Activity Environments

Residential Environments

The infrastructure and street design of neighborhoods can encourage or limit children's physical activity. Youth who live on a side street, cul-de-sac, dead end, or one-way street are more physically active compared to those who live on main streets.[178] Mixed-use areas, which include both commercial and residential spaces, are less likely to be used for physical activity among children. Instead, most activity outside of school occurs in residential or green spaces.[179] Urban versus rural environments also play a role in physical activity. Children who live in urban areas are more likely to play in parks and streets compared to rural children who are more active in farms and grasslands.[179] In addition to the infrastructure of the residential environment, children who have friends that live in the same neighborhood or within walking distance are more likely to be physically active.[180] Moreover, children who have greater access to recreational facilities within one's neighborhood have higher likelihood of engaging in physical activity than those who have less access.[180]

Safety is an important factor to consider when surveying the physical activity of children. As described above, there is perceived overall safety, traffic safety, and crime-related safety that come into play. Parents are concerned over their children's use of outside spaces to be active, both for leisure time activities and for walking or bicycling as transportation.[179] In addition to crime-related safety, traffic, and pedestrian[157] safety is an attribute of active transport. For example, sidewalks are positively associated and intersection density is negatively associated with parental concern of children walking and biking.[179]

Active Transport—Near Homes and Schools

Active transport among children is increasingly used as a strategy to improve health. In particular, for children and youth, scientific inquiry has often examined transportation to and from school.[181,182] Walking, biking, and/or skating to school, now commonly referred to as active school transport (AST), has received increased attention as a strategy to promote and enhance levels of physical activity and to prevent obesity among children.[153,183,184] Children and youth who engage in AST are generally more likely to be physically active than their peers who do not use AST.[153,184–190] A systematic review and meta-analysis of studies with more rigorous designs (e.g., controlled quantitative designs, such as randomized controlled trials, cluster RCTs, and quasiexperimental studies) concluded that active travel interventions were effective in increasing physical activity among children in elementary schools.[182] Nevertheless, other built environment factors can facilitate or hinder active transport among children and youth, thus interfering with the ability of children to practice physical activity. A review which included a mix of study designs (cross-sectional and longitudinal) found consistent evidence to suggest a positive association between street connectivity (measured as street intersection density) and physical activity measures including overall physical activity, moderate to vigorous physical activity, active transport, walking, and sedentary behaviors among children.[191] Additionally, features of the built environment including traffic safety, crime-related safety, street connectivity, and physical barriers have been identified as parental concerns in relation to active transport to school[192] among children and youth. However, the contribution of AST to health and health promoting behaviors may be more complex. AST may be associated with obesity and related behaviors. For example, AST has been positively associated with junk food purchases and higher BMIz scores[193] as well as fast food intake among some adolescents. This is plausible due to the surrounding food environment on the route to school.

Recreation Facilities, Parks, and Green Space

Green areas, including parks, are environmental resources humans can use to promote health and prevent disease. Park availability/accessibility and health among children is positively associated[180] which contrasts evidence on the association between green space and activity in adults.[194] Gender also plays a role in children's activity patterns.[195] A study found physical activity among boys is more influenced by the availability of park facilities whereas physical activity among girls is more affected by social aspects of the environment (e.g., the presence of other children).[179,196]

Compared with younger children, youth have greater independence and mobility and are more likely to use public spaces. Access to recreational and sports facilities is positively associated with physical activity in youth.[197] Furthermore, features that are well maintained, such as creeks, ponds, and trees, are related to greater visitation and use of green spaces.[198] In contrast, as expected, empirical work has found that if an area is unclean or vandalized, youth are less likely to use these areas due to the perceived safety issues.[198]

INEQUALITIES IN FOOD AND PHYSICAL ACTIVITY ENVIRONMENTS

Why should clinicians heed inequalities in food and physical activity environments? There are plenty of reasons. Most importantly, the racial/ethnic and socioeconomic disparities in diet, physical activity, and obesity, together with demographic shifts in the U.S. population, will substantially impact the healthcare system, including challenges in healthcare costs, management of chronic illnesses in the presence of obesity, adherence to treatments, and quality of care. Moreover, the Center for Medicare and Medicaid Services recently sponsored a special issue on health services research focused on disparities, which included community environments as important components of clinical care. Similarly, in a recent position paper,[199] the American College of Physicians offered recommendations on how to better integrate social determinants of health to address health equity. This reflects increasing efforts to improve understanding of disparities and their causes among healthcare providers, along with the need for additional efforts by the medical community to improve health equity.[200,201]

It is unsurprising that preventing obesity and eliminating health disparities are two significant goals of major health importance in the twenty-first century.[202] As detailed in Chapter 30: Race and Ethnic Health Disparities of this book, Latino, African American, and low-income children and adults are typically less likely to consume healthy diets, less likely to meet physical activity guidelines, and more likely to be overweight/obese than other racial/ethnic groups and higher income groups. While Asians tend to have lower body weight, they have greater risk for ill health at lower levels of body weight than other racial/ethnic populations.[203] The significance of all of these patterns and trends is amplified by demographic shifts in the U.S. population. Children under 15 years of age are the most racially/ethnically diverse section of U.S. society; half of all children in this age group are of racial/ethnic minority backgrounds.[204] Therefore, it is especially important that stakeholders across multiple sectors, including healthcare providers, work together to minimize the potentially negative effects of these trends on the overall health of the nation. Understanding the causes behind health disparities[205] and understanding disparities in comorbidities (and thus cumulative risks) can help shift paradigms toward an expanded view of health and related disparities and to accelerate progress.[206]

Inequities in environments remain significant barriers to achieving major public health goals. To that end, we underscore the need to consider disease vulnerabilities within the patient's historical, sociopolitical, and economic contexts.[207] Healthy People 2020 contextualizes health disparities by defining a health disparity as "a particular type of health difference that is closely linked with economic, social, or environmental disadvantage." Health disparities adversely affect groups of people who have systematically experienced greater social or economic obstacles to health based on their racial or ethnic group, religion, socioeconomic status, gender, age, or mental health; cognitive, sensory, or physical disability; sexual orientation or gender identity; geographic location; or other characteristics historically linked to discrimination or exclusion.[208]

Places in the United States have been shaped by historical segregation.[209,210] In turn, this has given rise to place-level differences in the environments in which people live, work, play, and attend school. While individual-level factors are likely to be implicated in the well-documented and persistent social disparities, they do not fully explain health disparities.[211–213] Furthermore, it is important to understand that the high correlation between individual-level socioeconomic advantage (i.e., income) and the socioeconomic advantage of the places[214] where people live, work, or go to school resulted from historical macrolevel social and political processes that have sorted different people into distinct places and neighborhoods.

In relation specifically to diet and physical activity environments, the segregation of neighborhoods and schools by race/ethnicity or social class has resulted in unequal distribution of health-promoting and health-damaging food and physical activity environments. For example, socioeconomically affluent compared to disadvantaged neighborhoods tend to have greater availability and density of healthy foods.[215–217] Conversely, there is greater concentration of unhealthy food within socioeconomically disadvantaged than advantaged neighborhoods. Neighborhoods with higher concentrations of Latino or African Americans are less likely to have health-promoting resources such as accessible recreational facilities, clean parks, and trails. Thus, differences in the distribution of environmental factors driving physical activity and diet are related to health disparities. Although both adults and children are affected by unequal distribution of environmental factors, we provide illustrative examples about children.

Evidence from cross-sectional data suggests that children from socioeconomically disadvantaged and racial/ethnic minority backgrounds are more likely to be exposed to unhealthy food outlets near their residential neighborhoods as well as near the schools to which they attend. Multiple descriptive studies have examined the distribution of fast food restaurants near schools by neighborhood socioeconomic advantage, race/ethnicity, and urbanicity levels using mostly cross-sectional data. Schools located in socioeconomically disadvantaged neighborhoods tended to be surrounded by greater concentrations of fast food restaurants compared with those located in affluent neighborhoods [131,132,218–221] though there are exceptions to this pattern.[222] Most, but not all, studies[132] observed greater fast food restaurant concentrations near schools attended by majority Latino and African American students relative to schools attended by majority White students.[146,150,223,224] Previous research has also observed greater fast food restaurant densities near schools in urban versus nonurban areas.[132] More recently, studies using data from New Zealand and California found that fast food restaurant concentrations increased over time in socioeconomically deprived neighborhoods compared with less deprived neighborhoods[225] and particularly if those schools where the majority of students were of Black and Latino backgrounds.[151]

Linking inequalities in the built environment near homes and schools to health outcomes requires explicit analyses of these associations by dimensions of social inequalities in health, such as race/ethnicity, socioeconomic status, and gender. This area of research is more challenging because it requires greater disaggregation of the data by these dimensions as well as sufficient sample sizes for each specific sociodemographic subgroup. A systematic review of the literature assessing evidence on the associations between fast food availability near schools and body weight found only 14 studies that investigated associations either by race/ethnicity, gender, or socioeconomic disadvantage. They found that fast food availability was linked with obesity mostly among Latino children, although the evidence varied across racial/ethnic groups.[84]

Many, though not all, studies have also found that children from socioeconomically disadvantaged and racial/ethnic minority backgrounds face many obstacles to physical activity opportunities because they are more likely to live in neighborhoods with limited opportunities for active living. Importantly, although children from disadvantaged and racial minority backgrounds are more likely to use active school transport than their White counterparts,[226-228] other research has observed that children who use active transport to or from school purchase unhealthy foods on their way to schools and are more likely to report fast food intake, with stronger AST-fast food intake associations among Latino children.[229]

The food and physical activity environments may, independently and in combination, promote or undermine health outcomes for all individuals. However, given the unequal distribution of the quality and quantity of health-promoting resources in environments of low income and minority populations, the interactions between environmental features are especially salient in the context of reducing social disparities in health. This requires greater understanding and awareness among healthcare providers about environmental effects and to use that information judiciously to tailor clinical care. For example, although active transport generally has beneficial effects on physical activity, this particular strategy may not work well for all patients. Greater active transport among children and adults who live in poor environments may translate into greater exposure to health-damaging resources (e.g., more fast food stores) unless environmental interventions increase health-promoting resources in those neighborhoods.

Clinical interventions that broaden the scope to incorporate the built environment have the potential to significantly improve patient-related outcomes, enhance clinical effectiveness, reduce health disparities, and advance population health. In particular, the reduction of disparities in obesity—a major risk factor for several chronic diseases—could have a major impact on health and healthcare costs, improve minority health overall and reduce racial/ethnic differences in morbidity, quality of life, and life expectancy.

CONCLUSIONS

Mounting evidence increasingly supports causal links between food and physical activity environments and realized diet and physical activity among adults and children, though the evidence is stronger for some population subgroups and/or specific exposure-outcome pairs. This evidence invites the medical, public health and policymaking communities to move to the next frontiers of research and implementation of policies/interventions to support physical activity and healthy diets, thus preventing human disease and improving population health.

For those in clinical practice, several frontiers lie ahead. One is to fully implement the National Academies of Science recommendations to include patients' home/work/school neighborhood information into EHRs.[32,33] This effort, if done systematically and with rigor, will enable clinicians to tailor interventions in ways analogous to how genetic data are used to inform treatment strategies. This will help advance population health and has the potential to contribute to reduction of disparities and enhance overall clinical effectiveness through improved patient outcomes. Second, clinicians can reach out beyond the clinic walls to develop and/or support policies or interventions in the community overall as well as areas near schools and work centers. For example, in light of strong evidence for population interventions and diet,[4] clinicians can lend their support to bans and restrictions on unhealthy foods and mandates to offer healthier foods. Third, clinicians can collaborate with other researchers in conducting empirical work that utilizes EHR data linked to environments, including research on social disparities in health and potential approaches to mitigate them. Clinical records provide unique opportunities for longitudinal designs to address questions that lie at the intersection of healthcare and community environments: Is medical care more cost effective in middle-income neighborhoods? How can healthcare resources be more targeted to better serve underresourced communities such as those with the worst food and/or physical activity environments? These and several other recommendations have been drafted in recent years to address important policy and causal inference questions in this area.[125,126,176,177,230]

Frontiers in medical training include institutionalizing the implementation of recommendations by the American College of Physicians, specifically that "Healthcare professionals should be knowledgeable about screening and identifying social determinants of health and approaches to treating patients whose health is affected by social determinants."[199] All medical schools can make steps to institutionalize this recommendation by establishing neighborhood and environmental determinants of health as part of the medical curriculum and training of the next generation of physicians.

Poor or good health is not just a result of individual choices, but also a consequence of environmental attributes of the neighborhoods where people live, work, and attend school. Current and future empirical research on physical and food environments, along with further engagement of the medical community in environmental determinants of health, hold immense potential to impact future environmental and policy interventions for obesity and to fundamentally shape the practice of preventive medicine in years to come.

References

1. Kochanek KD, Murphy SL, Xu J, Arias E. *Deaths: Final Data for 2017.* National Vital Statistics Reports; Vol. 68, No. 9. Hyattsville, MD: U.S. Department of Health and Human Services; 2019.
2. Brownson RC, Baker EA, Housemann RA, Brennan LK, Bacak SJ. Environmental and policy determinants of physical activity in the United States. *Am J Public Health.* 2001;91(12):1995–2003.
3. Exworthy M, Peckham S. Access, choice and travel: Implications for health policy. *Soc Policy Admin.* 2006;40(3):267–87.
4. Mayne SL, Auchincloss AH, Michael YL. Impact of policy and built environment changes on obesity-related outcomes: A systematic review of naturally occurring experiments. *Obes Rev.* 2015;16(5):362–75.
5. National Complete Streets Coalition. *The Best Complete Streets Policies of 2013.* Washington, DC: Smart Growth America; 2013. https://smartgrowthamerica.org/resources/best-complete-streets-policies-of-2013.
6. Sallis JF. Measuring physical activity environments: A brief history. *Am J Prev Med.* 2009;36(4 Suppl):S86–92.
7. Chen HJ, Wang Y. Changes in the neighborhood food store environment and children's body mass index at peripuberty in the United States. *J Adolesc Health.* 2016;58(1):111–8.
8. Cobb LK, Appel LJ, Franco M, Jones-Smith JC, Nur A, Anderson CA. The relationship of the local food environment with obesity: A systematic review of methods, study quality, and results. *Obesity.* 2015;23(7):1331–44.
9. Henriksen L. The retail environment for tobacco: A barometer of progress towards the endgame. *Tob Control.* 2015;24(e1):e1–2.
10. Sanders-Jackson A, Parikh NM, Schleicher NC, Fortmann SP, Henriksen L. Convenience store visits by US adolescents: Rationale for healthier retail environments. *Health Place.* 2015;34:63–6.
11. Belay B, Dietz WH. Obesity prevention and control: From clinical tools to public health strategies. *Acad Pediatr.* 2009;9(5):291–2.
12. Jeffery RW. Public health strategies for obesity treatment and prevention. *Am J Health Behav.* 2001;25(3):252–9.
13. Humpel N, Owen N, Leslie E. Environmental factors associated with adults' participation in physical activity: A review. *Am J Prev Med.* 2002;22(3):188–99.
14. Cunningham GO, Michael YL. Concepts guiding the study of the impact of the built environment on physical activity for older adults: A review of the literature. *Am J Health Promot.* 2004;18(6):435–43.
15. Bauman AE, Bull FC. *Environmental Correlates of Physical Activity and Walking in Adults and Children: A Review of Reviews.* London: National Institute of Health and Clinical Excellence; 2007.
16. Diez Roux AV, Evenson KR, McGinn AP, et al. Availability of recreational resources and physical activity in adults. *Am J Public Health.* 2007;97(3):493–9.
17. Saelens BE, Handy SL. Built environment correlates of walking: A review. *Med Sci Sports Exerc.* 2008;40(7 Suppl):S550–66.
18. Rahmanian E, Gasevic D, Vukmirovich I, Lear SA. The association between the built environment and dietary intake—A systematic review. *Asia Pac J Clin Nutr.* 2014;23(2):83–96.
19. Boone-Heinonen J, Gordon-Larsen P, Kiefe CI, Shikany JM, Lewis CE, Popkin BM. Fast food restaurants and food stores: Longitudinal associations with diet in young to middle-aged adults: The CARDIA study. *Arch Intern Med.* 2011;171(13):1162–70.

20. Jeffery RW, Baxter J, McGuire M, Linde J. Are fast food restaurants an environmental risk factor for obesity? *Int J Behav Nutr Phys Act.* 2006;3:2.

21. Auchincloss AH, Diez Roux AV, Brown DG, Erdmann CA, Bertoni AG. Neighborhood resources for physical activity and healthy foods and their association with insulin resistance. *Epidemiology.* 2008;19(1):146–57.

22. Ding D, Gebel K. Built environment, physical activity, and obesity: What have we learned from reviewing the literature? *Health Place.* 2012;18(1):100–5.

23. Feng J, Glass TA, Curriero FC, Stewart WF, Schwartz BS. The built environment and obesity: A systematic review of the epidemiologic evidence. *Health Place.* 2010;16(2):175–90.

24. Bisciglia A, Pasceri V, Irini D, Varveri A, Speciale G. Risk factors for ischemic heart disease. *Rev Recent Clin Trials.* 2019;14(2):86–94.

25. Scordo K, Pickett KA. Triglycerides: Do they matter? *Am J Nurs.* 2017;117(1):24–31.

26. Diez Roux AV, Jacobs DR, Kiefe CI. Neighborhood characteristics and components of the insulin resistance syndrome in young adults: The coronary artery risk development in young adults (CARDIA) study. *Diabetes Care.* 2002; 25(11):1976–82.

27. Auchincloss AH, Diez Roux AV, Mujahid MS, Shen M, Bertoni AG, Carnethon MR. Neighborhood resources for physical activity and healthy foods and incidence of type 2 diabetes mellitus: The Multi-Ethnic Study of Atherosclerosis. *Arch Intern Med.* 2009;169(18):1698–704.

28. Mujahid MS, Diez Roux AV, Cooper R, Shea S, Ni H. Neighborhood walkability and healthy foods are related to hypertension in a multiethnic sample. *Am J Epidemiol.* 2006;163:S253.

29. Diez Roux AV. Residential environments and cardiovascular risk. *J Urban Health.* 2003;80(4):569–89.

30. Beck AF, Simmons JM, Huang B, Kahn RS. Geomedicine: Area-based socioeconomic measures for assessing risk of hospital reutilization among children admitted for asthma. *Am J Public Health.* 2012;102(12):2308–14.

31. Jusatz HJ. Current state of medical geography and geomedicine. *Internist.* 1980;21(8):410–16.

32. Institute of Medicine. *Capturing Social and Behavioral Domains and Measures in Electronic Health Records: Phase 1.* Washington, DC: The National Academies Press; 2014.

33. Institute of Medicine. *Capturing Social and Behavioral Domains and Measures in Electronic Health Records: Phase 2.* Washington, DC: The National Academies Press; 2014.

34. Ashley EA. The precision medicine initiative: A new national effort. *JAMA.* 2015;313(21):2119–20.

35. Collins FS, Varmus H. A new initiative on precision medicine. *N Engl J Med.* 2015;372(9):793–5.

36. National Institutes of Health. All of Us Research Program. https://allofus.nih.gov. Accessed March 12, 2020.

37. National Instituted of Health. Request for Information: NIH Precision Medicine Cohort (NOT-OD-15-096). http://grants.nih.gov/grants/guide/notice-files/NOT-OD-15-096.html. 2015.

38. Hills AP, Farpour-Lambert NJ, Byrne NM. Precision medicine and healthy living: The importance of the built environment. *Prog Cardiovasc Dis.* 2019;62(1):34–8.

39. Feathers A, Aycinena AC, Lovasi GS, et al. Food environments are relevant to recruitment and adherence in dietary modification trials. *Nutr Res.* 2015;35(6):480–8.

40. Wilkie S, Townshend T, Thompson E, Ling J. Restructuring the built environment to change adult health behaviors: A scoping review integrated with behavior change frameworks. *Cities Health.* 2018;2(2):198–211.

41. Soril LJ, Leggett LE, Lorenzetti DL, et al. Effective use of the built environment to manage behavioural and psychological symptoms of dementia: A systematic review. *PLoS One.* 2014;9(12):e115425.

42. Goddu AP, Roberson TS, Raffel KE, Chin MH, Peek ME. Food Rx: A community-university partnership to prescribe healthy eating on the South Side of Chicago. *J Prev Interv Community.* 2015;43(2):148–62.

43. Bazemore AW, Cottrell EK, Gold R, et al. "Community vital signs": Incorporating geocoded social determinants into electronic records to promote patient and population health. *J Am Med Inform Assoc.* 2016;23(2):407–12.

44. Schinasi LH, Auchincloss AH, Forrest CB, Diez Roux AV. Using electronic health record data for environmental and place based population health research: A systematic review. *Ann Epidemiol.* 2018;28(7):493–502.

45. Tamariz L, Medina H, Suarez M, Seo D, Palacio A. Linking census data with electronic medical records for clinical research: A systematic review. *JESM.* 2018;43(1–2):105–18.

46. Powell LA, Chaloupka FJ, Bao Y. The availability of fast-food and full-service restaurants in the United States: Associations with neighborhood characteristics. *Am J Prev Med.* 2007;33(4):S240–5.

47. Dai D. Black residential segregation, disparities in spatial access to health care facilities, and late-stage breast cancer diagnosis in metropolitan Detroit. *Health Place.* 2010;16(5):1038–52.

48. Casagrande SS, Whitt-Glover MC, Lancaster KJ, Odoms-Young AM, Gary TL. Built environment and health behaviors among African Americans: A systematic review. *Am J Prev Med.* 2009;36(2):174–81.

49. Moore LV, Diez Roux AV. Associations of neighborhood characteristics with the location and type of food stores. *Am J Public Health.* 2006;96(2):325–31.

50. Brown AF, Ma GX, Miranda J, et al. Structural interventions to reduce and eliminate health disparities. *Am J Public Health.* 2019;109(S1):S72–8.

51. McGill R, Anwar E, Orton L, et al. Are interventions to promote healthy eating equally effective for all? Systematic review of socioeconomic inequalities in impact. *BMC Public Health.* 2015;15(1):457.

52. Torres-Ruiz M, Robinson-Ector K, Attinson D, Trotter J, Anise A, Clauser S. A portfolio analysis of culturally tailored trials to address health and healthcare disparities. *Int J Environ Res Public Health.* 2018;15(9):E1859.

53. Moore DA, Carpenter TE. Spatial analytical methods and geographic information systems: Use in health research and epidemiology. *Epidemiol Rev.* 1999;21(2):143–61.

54. Rushton G. Public health, GIS, and spatial analytic tools. *Annu Rev Public Health.* 2003;24(1):43–56.

55. Thornton LE, Pearce JR, Kavanagh AM. Using Geographic Information Systems (GIS) to assess the role of the built environment in influencing obesity: A glossary. *Int J Behav Nutr Phys Act.* 2011;8(1):71.

56. Fleischhacker SE, Evenson KR, Sharkey J, Pitts SB, Rodriguez DA. Validity of secondary retail food outlet data: A systematic review. *Am J Prev Med.* 2013;45(4):462–73.

57. Kelly CM, Wilson JS, Baker EA, Miller DK, Schootman M. Using Google Street View to audit the built environment: Inter-rater reliability results. *Ann Behav Med.* 2013;45(Suppl 1):S108–12.

58. Silva V, Grande AJ, Rech CR, Peccin MS. Geoprocessing via Google Maps for assessing obesogenic built environments related to physical activity and chronic noncommunicable diseases: Validity and reliability. *J Healthc Eng.* 2015;6(1):41–54.

59. Walls D. *National Establishment Time-series (NETS) Database: 2008 Database Description.* Oakland, CA: Walls & Associates; 2009.

60. InfoUSA. InfoUSA Business Listing Description. https://www.infousa.com/product/business-lists. 2015.

61. Company N. Retail Site Database, The Ultimate Source in Retail Site Database—The Ultimate Source, a.s.o.N.C. Trade Dimensions. 2008.

62. Crawford TW, Jilcott Pitts SB, McGuirt JT, Keyserling TC, Ammerman AS. Conceptualizing and comparing neighborhood and activity space measures for food environment research. *Health Place.* 2014;30:215–25.

63. Drewnowski A, Buszkiewicz J, Aggarwal A, Rose C, Gupta S, Bradshaw A. Obesity and the built environment: A reappraisal. *Obesity.* 2020;28(1):22–30.

64. Hirsch JA, Winters M, Clarke P, McKay H. Generating GPS activity spaces that shed light upon the mobility habits of older adults: A descriptive analysis. *Int J Health Geogr.* 2014;13(1):51.

65. Kestens Y, Lebel A, Chaix B, et al. Association between activity space exposure to food establishments and individual risk of overweight. *PLoS One.* 2012;7(8):e41418.

66. Mitchell JT, Schick RS, Hallyburton M, et al. Combined ecological momentary assessment and global positioning system tracking to assess smoking behavior: A proof of concept study. *J Dual Diagn.* 2014;10(1):19–29.

67. Widener MJ, Minaker LM, Reid JL, Patterson Z, Ahmadi TK, Hammond D. Activity space-based measures of the food environment and their relationships to food purchasing behaviours for young urban adults in Canada. *Public Health Nutr.* 2018;21(11):2103–116.

68. Irwin ML, Lowry D, Neuhouser ML, et al. Transdisciplinary Research in Energetics and Cancer early career investigator training program: First year results. *Transl Behav Med.* 2020. [Epub ahead of print].

69. James P, Jankowska M, Marx C, et al. "Spatial energetics": Integrating data from GPS, accelerometry, and GIS to address obesity and inactivity. *Am J Prev Med.* 2016;51(5):792–800.

70. Mayne SL, Pellissier BF, Kershaw KN. Neighborhood physical disorder and adverse pregnancy outcomes among women in Chicago: A cross-sectional analysis of electronic health record data. *J Urban Health.* 2019;96(6):823–34.

71. Lafontaine SJ, Sawada M, Kristjansson E. A direct observation method for auditing large urban centers using stratified sampling, mobile GIS technology and virtual environments. *Int J Health Geogr.* 2017;16(1):6.
72. Leypunskiy E, Kiciman E, Shah M, et al. Geographically resolved rhythms in twitter use reveal social pressures on daily activity patterns. *Curr Biol.* 2018;28(23):3763–75.
73. Mujahid MS, Diez Roux AV, Morenoff JD, Raghunathan T. Assessing the measurement properties of neighborhood scales: From psychometrics to ecometrics. *Am J Epidemiol.* 2007;165(8):858–67.
74. Zandieh R, Flacke J, Martinez J, Jones P, van Maarseveen M. Do inequalities in neighborhood walkability drive disparities in older adults' outdoor walking? *Int J Environ Res Public Health.* 2017;14(7):E740.
75. McKernan C, Montemurro G, Chahal H, Veugelers PJ, Gleddie D, Storey KE. Translation of school-learned health behaviours into the home: Student insights through photovoice. *Can J Public Health.* 2019;110(6):821–30.
76. Visser SS, Hutter I, Haisma H. Building a framework for theory-based ethnographies for studying intergenerational family food practices. *Appetite.* 2016;97:49–57.
77. Adams EJ, Sherar LB. Community perceptions of the implementation and impact of an intervention to improve the neighbourhood physical environment to promote walking for transport: A qualitative study. *BMC Public Health.* 2018;18(1):714.
78. Krieger N. Epidemiology and the web of causation: Has anyone seen the spider? *Soc Sci Med.* 1994;39(7):887–903.
79. Krieger N, Davey Smith G. The tale wagged by the DAG: Broadening the scope of causal inference and explanation for epidemiology. *Int J Epidemiol.* 2016;45(6):1787–808.
80. Richardson AS, Meyer KA, Howard AG, et al. Neighborhood socioeconomic status and food environment: A 20-year longitudinal latent class analysis among CARDIA participants. *Health Place.* 2014;30:145–53.
81. Hirsch JA, Moore KA, Clarke PJ, et al. Changes in the built environment and changes in the amount of walking over time: Longitudinal results from the multi-ethnic study of atherosclerosis. *Am J Epidemiol.* 2014;180(8):799–809.
82. Hirsch JA, Diez Roux AV, Moore KA, Evenson KR, Rodriguez DA. Change in walking and body mass index following residential relocation: The multi-ethnic study of atherosclerosis. *Am J Public Health.* 2014;104(3):E49–56.
83. Hirsch JA, DeVries DN, Brauer M, Frank LD, Winters M. Impact of new rapid transit on physical activity: A meta-analysis. *Prev Med Rep.* 2018;10:184–90.
84. Smith M, Hosking J, Woodward A, et al. Systematic literature review of built environment effects on physical activity and active transport—An update and new findings on health equity. *Int J Behav Nutr Phys Act.* 2017;14(1):158.
85. Ludwig J, Sanbonmatsu L, Gennetian L, et al. Neighborhoods, obesity, and diabetes—A randomized social experiment. *N Engl J Med.* 2011;365(16):1509–19.
86. Papas MA, Alberg AJ, Ewing R, Helzlsouer KJ, Gary TL, Klassen AC. The built environment and obesity. *Epidemiol Rev.* 2007;29(1):129–43.
87. Boone-Heinonen J, Gordon-Larsen P, Guilkey DK, Jacobs DRJr, Popkin BM. Environment and physical activity dynamics: The role of residential self-selection. *Psychol Sport Exerc.* 2011;12(1):54–60.
88. Boone-Heinonen J, Guilkey DK, Evenson KR, Gordon-Larsen P. Residential self-selection bias in the estimation of built environment effects on physical activity between adolescence and young adulthood. *Int J Behav Nutr Phys Act.* 2010;7(1):70.
89. Cao X, Mokhtarian PL, Handy SL. Examining the impacts of residential self-selection on travel behaviour: A focus on empirical findings. *Transp.* 2009;29(3):359–95.
90. Frank LD, Saelens BE, Powell KE, Chapman JE. Stepping towards causation: Do built environments or neighborhood and travel preferences explain physical activity, driving, and obesity? *Soc Sci Med.* 2007;65(9):1898–914.
91. Heinen E, van Wee B, Panter J, Mackett R, Ogilvie D. Residential self-selection in quasi-experimental and natural experimental studies: An extended conceptualization of the relationship between the built environment and travel behavior. *J Transp Land Use.* 2018;11(1):939–59.
92. Howell NA, Farber S, Widener MJ, Allen J, Booth GL. Association between residential self-selection and non-residential built environment exposures. *Health Place.* 2018;54:149–54.
93. Rummo PE, Guilkey DK, Ng SW, et al. Understanding bias in relationships between the food environment and diet quality: The Coronary Artery Risk Development in Young Adults (CARDIA) study. *J Epidemiol Community Health.* 2017;71(12):1185–90.
94. Rummo PE, Guilkey DK, Shikany JM, Reis JP, Grodon-Larsen P. How do individual-level sociodemographics and neighbourhood-level characteristics influence residential location behaviour in the context of the food and built environment? Findings from 25 years of follow-up in the CARDIA Study. *J Epidemiol Community Health.* 2017;71(3):26–8.
95. Li J, Auchuncloss AH, Roriguez DA, Moore KA, Diez Roux AV, Sánchez BN. Determinants of residential preferences related to built and social environments and concordance between neighborhood characteristics and preferences. *J Urban Health.* 2020;97(1):62–77.
96. Hu FB, Malik VS. Sugar-sweetened beverages and risk of obesity and type 2 diabetes: Epidemiologic evidence. *Physiol Behav.* 2010;100(1):47–54.
97. Malik VS, Schulze MB, Hu FB. Intake of sugar-sweetened beverages and weight gain: A systematic review. *Am J Clin Nutr.* 2006;84(2):274–88.
98. Moreno LA, Rodriguez G. Dietary risk factors for development of childhood obesity. *Curr Opin Clin Nutr Metab Care.* 2007;10(3):336–41.
99. Rosenheck R. Fast food consumption and increased caloric intake: A systematic review of a trajectory towards weight gain and obesity risk. *Obes Rev.* 2008;9(6):535–47.
100. Islam MA, Amin MN, Siddiqui SA, Hossain MP, Sultana F, Kabir MR. Trans fatty acids and lipid profile: A serious risk factor to cardiovascular disease, cancer and diabetes. *Diabetes Metab Syndr.* 2019;13(2):1643–7.
101. Swinburn B, Sacks G, Vandevijvere S, et al. INFORMAS (International Network for Food and Obesity/non-communicable diseases Research, Monitoring and Action Support): Overview and key principles. *Obes Rev.* 2013;14(Suppl 1):1–12.
102. Stuckler D, Nestle M. Big food, food systems, and global health. *PLoS Med.* 2012;9(6):e1001242.
103. Raper NR, Marston RM. Levels and sources of fat in the US food supply. *Prog Clin Biol Res.* 1986;222:127–52.
104. Basu S, Lewis K. Reducing added sugars in the food supply through a cap-and-trade approach. *Am J Public Health.* 2014;104(12):2432–8.
105. Basu S, Yoffe P, Hills N, Lustig RH. The relationship of sugar to population-level diabetes prevalence: An econometric analysis of repeated cross-sectional data. *PLoS One.* 2013;8(2):e57873.
106. Popkin BM, Reardon T. Obesity and the food system transformation in Latin America. *Obes Rev.* 2018;19(8):1028–64.
107. Rincón-Gallardo Patiño S, Rajamohan S, Meaney K, et al. Development of a responsible policy index to improve statutory and self-regulatory policies that protect children's diet and health in the America's region. *Int J Environ Res Public Health.* 2020;17(2):E495.
108. Caspi CE, Sorensen G, Subramanian SV, Kawachi I. The local food environment and diet: A systematic review. *Health Place.* 2012;18(5):1172–87.
109. Centers for Disease Control and Prevention. A Look Inside Food Deserts. https://www.cdc.gov/features/fooddeserts. Published September 24, 2012.
110. Cooksey-Stowers K, Schwartz MB, Brownell KD. Food swamps predict obesity rates better than food deserts in the United States. *Int J Environ Res Public Health.* 2017;14(11):E1366.
111. Phillips AZ, Rodriguez HP. Adults with diabetes residing in "food swamps" have higher hospitalization rates. *Health Serv Res.* 2019;54(Suppl 1):217–25.
112. Luan H, Law J, Quick M. Identifying food deserts and swamps based on relative healthy food access: A spatio-temporal Bayesian approach. *Int J Health Geogr.* 2015;14(1):37.
113. Lytle L, Myers A. *Measures Registry User Guide: Food Environment.* Washington, DC: National Collaborative on Childhood Obesity Research. Published January 2017. http://nccor.org/tools-mruserguides/wp-content/uploads/2017/NCCOR_MR_User_Guide_Food_Environment-FINAL.pdf.
114. Moore LV, Diez Roux AV, Nettleton JA, Jacobs DR Jr. Associations of the local food environment with diet quality—A comparison of assessments based on surveys and geographic information systems: The multi-ethnic study of atherosclerosis. *Am J Epidemiol.* 2008;167(8):917–24.
115. Hickson DA, Diez Rouz AV, Smith AE, et al. Associations of fast food restaurant availability with dietary intake and weight among African Americans in the Jackson Heart Study, 2000–2004. *Am J Public Health.* 2011;101(S1):S301–9.
116. Richardson AS, Meyer KA, Howard AG, et al. Multiple pathways from the neighborhood food environment to increased body mass index through dietary behaviors: A structural equation-based analysis in the CARDIA study. *Health Place.* 2015;36:74–87.
117. McInerney M, Csizmadi I, Friedenreich CM, et al. Associations between the neighbourhood food environment, neighbourhood socioeconomic status, and diet quality: An observational study. *BMC Public Health.* 2016;16:984.

118. Malambo P, Kengne AP, De Villiers A, Lambert EV, Puoane T. Built environment, selected risk factors and major cardiovascular disease outcomes: A systematic review. *PLoS One*. 2016;11(11):e0166846.

119. Holsten JE. Obesity and the community food environment: A systematic review. *Public Health Nutr*. 2009;12(3):397–405.

120. Mah CL, Luongo G, Hasdell R, Taylor NGA, Lo BK. A systematic review of the effect of retail food environment interventions on diet and health with a focus on the enabling role of public policies. *Curr Nutr Rep*. 2019;8(4):411–28.

121. Hollis-Hansen K, Vermont L, Zafron ML, Seidman J, Leone L. The introduction of new food retail opportunities in lower-income communities and the impact on fruit and vegetable intake: A systematic review. *Transl Behav Med*. 2019;9(5):837–46.

122. Dubowitz T, Ghosh-Dastidar M, Cohen DA, et al. Diet and perceptions change with supermarket introduction in a food desert, but not because of supermarket use. *Health Aff (Millwood)*. 2015;34(11):1858–68.

123. Rogus S, Athens J, Cantor J, Elbel B. Measuring micro-level effects of a new supermarket: Do residents within 0.5 mile have improved dietary behaviors? *J Acad Nutr Diet*. 2018;118(6):1037–46.

124. Moore K, Diez Roux AV, Auchincloss A, et al. Home and work neighbourhood environments in relation to body mass index: The Multi-Ethnic Study of Atherosclerosis (MESA). *J Epidemiol Community Health*. 2013;67(10):846–53.

125. Burgoine T, Monsivais P. Characterising food environment exposure at home, at work, and along commuting journeys using data on adults in the UK. *Int J Behav Nutr Phys Act*. 2013;10(1):85.

126. Burgoine T, Forouhi NG, Griffin SJ, Wareham NJ, Monsivais P. Associations between exposure to takeaway food outlets, takeaway food consumption, and body weight in Cambridgeshire, UK: Population based, cross sectional study. *BMJ*. 2014;348:g1464.

127. Watts AW, Laska MN, Larson NI, Neumark-Sztainer DR. Millennials at work: Workplace environments of young adults and associations with weight-related health. *J Epidemiol Community Health*. 2016;70(1):65–71.

128. Thornton LE, Lamb KE, Ball K. Employment status, residential and workplace food environments: Associations with women's eating behaviours. *Health Place*. 2013;24:80–9.

129. Leung CW, Laraia BA, Kelly M, et al. The influence of neighborhood food stores on change in young girls' body mass index. *Am J Prev Med*. 2011;41(1):43–51.

130. Saelens BE, Glanz K, Frank LD, et al. Two-year changes in child weight status, diet, and activity by neighborhood nutrition and physical activity environment. *Obesity*. 2018;26(8):1338–46.

131. Simon PA, Kwan D, Angelescu A, Shih M, Fielding JE. Proximity of fast food restaurants to schools: Do neighborhood income and type of school matter? *Prev Med*. 2008;47(3):284–8.

132. Zenk S, Powell L. US secondary schools and food outlets. *Health Place*. 2008;14(2):336–46.

133. Dale D, Corbin CB, Dale KS. Restricting opportunities to be active during school time: Do children compensate by increasing physical activity levels after school? *Res Q Exerc Sport*. 2000;71(3):240–8.

134. Hofferth S, Sandberg J. How American children spend their time. *J Marriage Fam*. 2001;63(2):295–308.

135. Borradaile KE, Sherman S, Vander Veur SS, et al. Snacking in children: The role of urban corner stores. *Pediatrics*. 2009;124(5): 1293–8.

136. Buck C, Börnhorst C, Pohlabein H, et al. Clustering of unhealthy food around German schools and its influence on dietary behavior in school children: A pilot study. *Int J Behav Nutr Phys Act*. 2013;10:65.

137. Harris DE, Blum JW, Bamptom M, et al. Location of food stores near schools does not predict the weight status of Maine high school students. *J Nutr Educ Behav*. 2011;43(4):274–8.

138. Heroux M, Iannotti RJ, Currie D, Pickett W, Janssen I. The food retail environment in school neighborhoods and its relation to lunchtime eating behaviors in youth from three countries. *Health Place*. 2012;18(6):1240–7.

139. Sturm R, Datar A. Body mass index in elementary school children, metropolitan area food prices and food outlet density. *Public Health*. 2005;119(12): 1059–68.

140. Powell LM, Han E, Chaloupka FJ. Economic contextual factors, food consumption, and obesity among U.S. adolescents. *J Nutr*. 2010;140(6): 1175–80.

141. An R, Sturm R. School and residential neighborhood food environment and diet among California youth. *Am J Prev Med*. 2012;42(2):129–35.

142. Rossen LM, Curriero FC, Cooley-Strickland M, Pollack KM. Food availability en route to school and anthropometric change in urban children. *J Urban Health*. 2013;90(4):653–66.

143. Williams J, Scarborough P, Matthews A, et al. A systematic review of the influence of the retail food environment around schools on obesity-related outcomes. *Obes Rev*. 2014;15(5):359–74.

144. Davis B, Carpenter C. Proximity of fast-food restaurants to schools and adolescent obesity. *Am J Public Health*. 2009;99(3):505–10.

145. Gilliland JA, Rangel CY, Healy MA, et al. Linking childhood obesity to the built environment: A multi-level analysis of home and school neighbourhood factors associated with body mass index. *Can J Public Health*. 2012;103(9 Suppl 3):eS15–21.

146. Howard PH, Fitzpatrick M, Fulfrost B. Proximity of food retailers to schools and rates of overweight ninth grade students: An ecological study in California. *BMC Public Health*. 2011;11:68.

147. Li M, Dibley MJ, Yan H. School environment factors were associated with BMI among adolescents in Xi'an City, China. *BMC Public Health*. 2011;11:792.

148. Park S, Choi BY, Wang Y, Colantuoni E, Gittelsohn J. School and neighborhood nutrition environment and their association with students' nutrition behaviors and weight status in Seoul, South Korea. *J Adolesc Health*. 2013;53(5):655–62.

149. Powell LM, Auld MC, Chaloupka FJ, O'Malley PM, Johnston LD. Associations between access to food stores and adolescent body mass index. *Am J Prev Med*. 2007;33;S301–7.

150. Sánchez BN, Sanchez-Vaznaugh EV, Uscilka A, Baek J, Zhang L. Differential associations between the food environment near schools and childhood overweight across race/ethnicity, gender, and grade. *Am J Epidemiol*. 2012;175(12):1284–93.

151. Sanchez-Vaznaugh EV, Weverka A, Matsuzaki M, Sánchez BN. Changes in fast food outlet availability near schools: Unequal patterns by income, race/ethnicity, and urbanicity. *Am J Prev Med*. 2019;57(3):338–45.

152. Division of Nutrition, Physical Activity, and Obesity, National Center for Chronic Disease Prevention and Health Promotion. Physical activity and health: The benefits of physical activity. https://www.cdc.gov/physicalactivity/basics/pa-health/index.htm. Updated February 25, 2020.

153. Kohl HW3rd, Cook HD, eds. *Educating the Student Body: Taking Physical Activity and Physical Education to School*. Washington DC: National Academies Press; 2013.

154. Vallance JK, Gardiner PA, Lynch BM, et al. Evaluating the evidence on sitting, smoking, and health: Is sitting really the new smoking? *Am J Public Health*. 2018;108(11):1478–82.

155. Janssen I, Leblanc AG. Systematic review of the health benefits of physical activity and fitness in school-aged children and youth. *Int J Behav Nutr Phys Act*. 2010;7:40.

156. Sallis JF. Measuring physical activity environments: A brief history. *Am J Prev Med*. 2009;36(4 Suppl):S86–92.

157. Ding D, Sallis JF, Kerr J, Lee S, Rosenberg DE. Neighborhood environment and physical activity among youth a review. *Am J Prev Med*. 2011;41(4):442–55.

158. McGrath LJ, Hopkins WG, Hinckson EA. Associations of objectively measured built-environment attributes with youth moderate-vigorous physical activity: A systematic review and meta-analysis. *Sports Med*. 2015;45(6):841–65.

159. Wang X, Conway TL, Cain KL, et al. Interactions of psychosocial factors with built environments in explaining adolescents' active transportation. *Prev Med*. 2017;100:76–83.

160. Thornton CM, Kerr J, Conway TL, et al. Physical activity in older adults: An ecological approach. *Ann Behav Med*. 2017;51(2):159–69.

161. Carr LJ, Dunsiger SL, Marcus BH. Walk score™ as a global estimate of neighborhood walkability. *Am J Prev Med*. 2010;39(5):460–3.

162. Forjuoh SN, Ory MG, Won J, Towne SD Jr, Wang S, Lee C. Determinants of walking among middle-aged and older overweight and obese adults: Sociodemographic, health, and built environmental factors. *J Obes*. 2017;2017:9565430

163. Hirsch JA, Winters M, Clarke PJ, Ste-Marie N, McKay HA. The influence of walkability on broader mobility for Canadian middle aged and older adults: An examination of Walk Score™ and the Mobility Over Varied Environments Scale (MOVES). *Prev Med*. 2017;95 Suppl:S60–7.

164. Van Holle V, Deforche B, Van Cauwenberg J, et al. Relationship between the physical environment and different domains of physical activity in European adults: A systematic review. *BMC Public Health*. 2012;12:807.

165. Nehme EK, Oluyomi AO, Calise TV, Kohl HW 3rd. Environmental correlates of recreational walking in the neighborhood. *Am J Health Promot*. 2016;30(3):139–48.

166. Chaix B, Simon C, Charreire H, et al. The environmental correlates of overall and neighborhood based recreational walking (a cross-sectional analysis of the RECORD Study). *Int J Behav Nutr Phys Act*. 2014;11(1):20.

167. Barnett DW, Barnett A, Nathan A, Van Cauwenberg, Cerin E, Council on Environment and Physical Activity (CEPA)—Other Adults Working Group. Built environmental correlates of older adults' total physical activity and walking: A systematic review and meta-analysis. *Int J Behav Nutr Phys Act.* 2017;14(1):103.
168. Kärmeniemi M, Lankila T, Ikäheimo T, Koivumaa-Honkanen H, Korpelainen R. The built environment as a determinant of physical activity: A systematic review of longitudinal studies and natural experiments. *Ann Behav Med.* 2018;52(3):239–51.
169. Candido C, Thomas L, Haddad S, Zhang F, Mackey M, Ye W. Designing activity-based workspaces: Satisfaction, productivity and physical activity. *Building Res Inf.* 2019;47(3):275–89.
170. Bergman F, Wahlström V, Stomby A, et al. Treadmill workstations in office workers who are overweight or obese: A randomised controlled trial. *Lancet Public Health.* 2018;3(11):e523–35.
171. Lin YP, McCullagh MC, Kao TS, Larson JL. An integrative review: Work environment factors associated with physical activity among white-collar workers. *West J Nurs Res.* 2014;36(2):262–83.
172. Bennie J, Salmon J, Crawford D. How do workplace environments influence physical activity? A qualitative study of employee's perceptions of influences on physical activity within the workplace. *J Sci Med Sport.* 2010;12:e95.
173. Adlakha D, Hipp AJ, Marx C, et al. Home and workplace built environment supports for physical activity. *Am J Prev Med.* 2015;48(1):104–7.
174. Troped PJ, Wilson JS, Matthews CE, Cromley EK, Melly SJ. The built environment and location-based physical activity. *Am J Prev Med.* 2010;38(4):429–38.
175. Hoehner CM, Allen P, Barlow CE, Marx CM, Brownson RC, Schootman M. Understanding the independent and joint associations of the home and workplace built environments on cardiorespiratory fitness and body mass index. *Am J Epidemiol.* 2013;178(7):1094–105.
176. Adams EJ, Bull FC, Foster CE. Are perceptions of the environment in the workplace 'neighbourhood' associated with commuter walking? *J Transp Health.* 2016;3(4):479–84.
177. Schwartz MA, Aytur SA, Evenson KR, Rodríguez DA. Are perceptions about worksite neighborhoods and policies associated with walking? *Am J Health Promot.* 2009;24(2):146–51.
178. Kaczynski AT, Besenyi GM, Child S, et al. Relationship of objective street quality attributes with youth physical activity: Findings from the Healthy Communities Study. *Pediatr Obes.* 2018;13(Suppl 1):7–13.
179. Masoumi HE. Associations of built environment and children's physical activity: A narrative review. *Rev Environ Health.* 2017;32(4):315–31.
180. Oliveira A, Moreira C, Abreu S, Mota J, Santos R. Environmental determinants of physical activity in children: A systematic review. *Arch Exerc Health Dis.* 2014;4(2):254–61.
181. Smith M, Amann R, Cavadino A, et al. Children's transport built environments: A mixed methods study of associations between perceived and objective measures and relationships with parent licence for independent mobility in Auckland, New Zealand. *Int J Environ Res Public Health.* 2019;16(8):E1361.
182. Jones RA, Blackburn NE, Woods C, Byrne M, van Nassau F, Tully MA. Interventions promoting active transport to school in children: A systematic review and meta-analysis. *Prev Med.* 2019;123:232–41.
183. National Center for Safe Routes to School. Safe Routes to School and Health: Understanding the Physical Activity Benefits of Walking and Bicycling to School. http://www.saferoutesinfo.org/sites/default/files/resources/SRTS%20and%20health_final.pdf
184. Faulkner GE, Buliung RN, Flora PK, Fusco C. Active school transport, physical activity levels and body weight of children and youth: A systematic review. *Prev Med.* 2009;48(1):3–8.
185. Cooper AR, Page AS, Foster LJ, Qahwaji D. Commuting to school: Are children who walk more physically active? *Am J Prev Med.* 2003;25(4):273–76.
186. Mendoza JA, Watson K, Baranowski T, Nicklas TA, Uscanga DK, Hanfling MJ. The walking school bus and children's physical activity: A pilot cluster randomized controlled trial. *Pediatrics.* 2011;128(3):e537–44.
187. Cooper AR, Andersen LB, Wedderkopp N, Page AS, Froberg K. Physical activity levels of children who walk, cycle, or are driven to school. *Am J Prev Med.* 2005;29(3):179–84.
188. Active Living Research. *Walking and Biking to School, Physical Activity, and Health Outcomes.* San Diego, CA: Active Living Research, a National Program of the Robert Wood Johnson Foundation. Published May 2009. https://activelivingresearch.org/sites/activelivingresearch.org/files/ALR_Brief_ActiveTransport_0.pdf.
189. Denstel KD, Broyles ST, Larouche R, et al. Active school transport and weekday physical activity in 9-11-year-old children from 12 countries. *Int J Obes Suppl.* 2015;5(Suppl 2):S100–6.
190. Larouche R, Saunders TJ, Faulkner G, Colley R, Tremblay M. Associations between active school transport and physical activity, body composition, and cardiovascular fitness: A systematic review of 68 studies. *J Phys Act Health.* 2014;11(1):206–27.
191. Jia P, Zou Y, Wu Z, et al. Street connectivity, physical activity, and childhood obesity: A systematic review and meta-analysis. *Obes Rev.* 2019. Online ahead of print.
192. Aranda-Balboa MJ, Huertas-Delgado FJ, Herrador-Colmenero M, Cardon G, Chillón P. Parental barriers to active transport to school: A systematic review. *Int J Public Health.* 2020;65(1):87–98.
193. Madsen KA, Gosliner W, Woodward-Lopez G, Crawford PB. Physical activity opportunities associated with fitness and weight status among adolescents in low-income communities. *Arch Pediatr Adolesc Med.* 2009;163(11):1014–21.
194. Evenson KR, Jones SA, Holliday KM, Cohen DA, McKenzie TL. Park characteristics, use, and physical activity: A review of studies using SOPARC (System for Observing Play and Recreation in Communities). *Prev Med.* 2016;86:153–66.
195. Floyd MF, Bocarro JN, Smith WR, et al. Park-based physical activity among children and adolescents. *Am J Prev Med.* 2011;41(3):258–65.
196. Bocarro JN, Floyd MF, Smith WR, et al. Social and environmental factors related to boys' and girls' park-based physical activity. *Prev Chronic Dis.* 2015;12:E97.
197. Davison KK, Lawson CT. Do attributes in the physical environment influence children's physical activity? A review of the literature. *Int J Behav Nutr Phys Act.* 2006;3(1):19.
198. Van Hecke L, Ghekiere A, Veitch J, et al. Public open space characteristics influencing adolescents' use and physical activity: A systematic literature review of qualitative and quantitative studies. *Health Place.* 2018;51:158–73.
199. Daniel H, Bornstein SS, Kane GC, Health and Public Policy Committee of the American College of Physicians. Addressing social determinants to improve patient care and promote health equity: An American College of Physicians position paper. *Ann Intern Med.* 2018;168(8):577–8.
200. Dulin A, Risica PM, Mello J, et al. Examining neighborhood and interpersonal norms and social support on fruit and vegetable intake in low-income communities. *BMC Public Health.* 2018;18(1):455.
201. James CV. Putting patients first: Today's disparities research leading to health equity tomorrow. *Health Serv Res.* 2019;54(Suppl 1):203–5.
202. Office of Disease Prevention and Health Promotion. *Healthy People 2020, About Health People.* Washington, DC: U.S. Department of Health and Human Services. Updated March 13, 2020. https://www.healthypeople.gov/2020/About-Healthy-People.
203. Palaniappan LP, Wong EC, Shin JJ, Fortmann SP, Lauderdale DS. Asian Americans have greater prevalence of metabolic syndrome despite lower body mass index. *Int J Obes.* 2011;35(3):393–400.
204. Frey W. *Less than Half of Children under 15 are White, Census Shows.* Washington DC: Brookings Institution. Published June 24, 2019. https://www.brookings.edu/research/less-than-half-of-us-children-under-15-are-white-census-shows.
205. Woolf SH, Braveman P. Where health disparities begin: The role of social and economic determinants—And why current policies may make matters worse. *Health Aff (Millwood).* 2011;30(10):1852–9.
206. Hicken M, Gragg R, Hu H. How cumulative risks warrant a shift in our approach to racial health disparities: The case of lead, stress, and hypertension. *Health Aff (Millwood).* 2011;30(10):1895–901.
207. Kumanyika S, Taylor WC, Grier SA, et al. Community energy balance: A framework for contextualizing cultural influences on high risk of obesity in ethnic minority populations. *Prev Med.* 2012;55(5):371–81.
208. The Secretary's Advisory Committee on National Health Promotion and Disease Prevention Objectives for 2020. Phase I Report: Recommendations for the Framework and Format of Healthy People 2020. Section IV: Advisory Committee Findings and Recommendations. https://www.healthypeople.gov/sites/default/files/PhaseI_0.pdf. Published October 28, 2008.
209. Massey DS. Segregation and stratification: A biosocial perspective. *Du Bois Rev.* 2004;1(1):7–25.
210. Williams DR, Collins C. Racial residential segregation: A fundamental cause of racial disparities in health. *Public Health Rep.* 2001;116(5):404–16.
211. Finkelstein EA, Khavjou OA, Mobley LR, Haney DM, Will JC. Racial/ethnic disparities in coronary heart disease risk factors among WISEWOMAN enrollees. *J Womens Health.* 2004;13(5):503–18.
212. Gorman BK, Sivaganesan A. The role of social support and integration for understanding socioeconomic disparities in self-rated health and hypertension. *Soc Sci Med.* 2007;65(5):958–75.

213. Kramer H, Han C, Post W, et al. Racial/ethnic differences in hypertension and hypertension treatment and control in the multi-ethnic study of atherosclerosis (MESA). *Am J Hypertens.* 2004;17(10):963–70.
214. Mode NA, Evans MK, Zonderman AB. Race, neighborhood economic status, income inequality and mortality. *PLoS One.* 2016;11(5):e0154535.
215. Dubowitz T, Heron M, Bird CE, et al. Neighborhood socioeconomic status and fruit and vegetable intake among whites, blacks, and Mexican Americans in the United States. *Am J Clin Nutr.* 2008;87(6):1883–91.
216. Sallis JF, Saelens BE, Frank LD, et al. Neighborhood built environment and income: Examining multiple health outcomes. *Soc Sci Med.* 2009;68(7):1285–93.
217. Smoyer-Tomic KE, Spence JC, Raine KD, et al. The association between neighborhood socioeconomic status and exposure to supermarkets and fast food outlets. *Health Place.* 2008;14(4):740–54.
218. Kestens Y, Daniel M. Social inequalities in food exposure around schools in an urban area. *Am J Prev Med.* 2010;39(1):33–40.
219. Neckerman K, Bader MD, Richards CA, et al. Disparities in the food environments of New York City public schools. *Am J Prev Med.* 2010;39(3):195–202.
220. Powell LM, Chaloupka FJ, Bao Y. The availability of fast-food and full-service restaurants in the United States: Associations with neighborhood characteristics. *Am J Prev Med.* 2007;33(4 Suppl):S240–5.
221. Coffee NT, Kennedy HP, Niyonsenga T. Fast-food exposure around schools in urban Adelaide. *Public Health Nutr.* 2016;19(17):3095–105.
222. Austin SB, Melly SJ, Sanchez BN, Patel A, Buka S, Gortmaker SL. Clustering of fast food restaurants around schools: A novel application of spatial statistics to the study of food environments. *Am J Public Health.* 2005;95(9):1575–81.
223. Kwate N, Loh J. Separate and unequal: The influence of neighborhood and school characteristics on spatial proximity between fast food and schools. *Prev Med.* 2010;51(2):153–6.
224. Sturm R. Disparities in the food environment surrounding US middle and high schools. *Public Health.* 2008;122(7):681–90.
225. Day PL, Pearce JR, Pearson AL. A temporal analysis of the spatial clustering of food outlets around schools in Christchurch, New Zealand, 1966 to 2006. *Public Health Nutr.* 2015;18(1):135–42.
226. Babey SH, Hastert TA, Huang W, Brown ER. Sociodemographic, family, and environmental factors associated with active commuting to school among US adolescents. *J Public Health Policy.* 2009;30(Suppl 1):S203–20.
227. Martin SL, Lee SM, Lowry R. National prevalence and correlates of walking and bicycling to school. *Am J Prev Med.* 2007;33(2):98–105.
228. McDonald NC. Critical factors for active transportation to school among low-income and minority students: Evidence from the 2001 National Household Travel Survey. *Am J Prev Med.* 2008;34(4):341–4.
229. Sanchez-Vaznaugh EV, Bécares L, Sallis JF, Sánchez BN. Active school transport and fast food intake: Are there racial and ethnic differences? *Prev Med.* 2016;91:281–6.
230. Lucan SC. Concerning limitations of food-environment research: A narrative review and commentary framed around obesity and diet-related diseases in youth. *J Acad Nutr Diet.* 2015;115(2):205–12.
231. Inglis V, Ball K, Crawford D. Socioeconomic variations in women's diets: What is the role of perceptions of the local food environment? *J Epidemiol Community Health.* 2008;62(3):191–7.
232. Aggarwal A, Cook AJ, Jiao J, et al. Access to supermarkets and fruit and vegetable consumption. *Am J Public Health.* 2014;104(5):917–23.
233. Forsyth A. What is a walkable place? The walkability debate in urban design. *Urban Des Int.* 2015;20(4):274–92.
234. Mecredy G, Pickett W, Janssen W. Street connectivity is negatively associated with physical activity in Canadian youth. *Int J Environ Res Public Health.* 2011;8(8):3333–50.
235. U.S. Department of Transportation. Connectivity: Relationship to public health. https://www.transportation.gov/mission/health/connectivity. Updated August 24, 2015.
236. Carlson J, Dean K, Sallis JF. *Measures Registry User Guide: Physical Activity Environment.* Washington DC: National Collaborative on Childhood Obesity Research. Published January 2017. http://nccor.org/tools-mrusergudes/wp-content/uploads/2017/NCCOR_MR_User_Guide_Physical_Activity-FINAL.pdf.

CHAPTER

186

Nutrition and Global Food Systems

Eileen Kennedy

INTRODUCTION

In 2016, the United Nations declared a worldwide Decade of Action on Nutrition.[1] The focus of this decade is the elimination of malnutrition in all its forms, including undernutrition, micronutrient deficiencies, and overnutrition. This is a sharp departure from the historical emphasis of the United Nations agencies on the undernutrition component of the nutrition continuum. A key element of the global strategy to address malnutrition in all its forms is a food systems approach. Indeed, food systems are identified as one of six actions to promote healthy diets.[1] This chapter has a twofold purpose: (1) summarize our knowledge of typologies of food systems and pathways of impact on diet quality and nutritional status and (2) analyze policies and programs that can enhance the diet quality and nutrition impacts of food systems.

WHAT IS A FOOD SYSTEM?

A food system includes all the elements from production to consumption that influence the ability to access a healthy diet.[2] In colloquial terms, a food system is farm to table, or farm to fork, or in some cases, farm to flush. The renewed emphasis on a food systems approach to improving nutritional status globally is largely driven by the overweight and obesity crisis.

There have been a variety of publications that have focused on the diet and nutrition effects of food systems[3,4] in all regions and all countries. These reports have attempted, in part, to develop typologies of food systems that exist globally. There is a general consensus that food systems range from the more traditional, rural food systems to the modern, industrialized type. In the traditional food system, food is mainly produced by smallholder farmers in the immediate area, and most of the foods that are available are local and seasonal.[3] For the modernized food system, a wide variety of foods are available year-round, produced from many farms, from small farms to those that are industrial in size. Production is global and therefore foods are available at any time in a modernized food system.

Each type of food system is associated with differential effects on diet and nutrition. Rural food systems are found in most developing countries, which have high rates of stunting, underweight, micronutrient deficiencies, but, until recently, low levels of overweight, obesity, and noncommunicable diseases (NCDs).[3] In contrast, modern, industrialized systems, such as in the United States (U.S.), have low levels of short stature, underweight, and micronutrient deficits yet high levels of overweight, obesity, and NCDs.[3] The most recent evidence, however, indicates that overweight and obesity are now increasing in all regions, even in the poorest countries of the world.[5]

Embedded in food systems are food value chains and food environments, both of which are critical to understanding the impact on diet quality and nutrition. A food value chain includes all the activities and actors that take crops and livestock from production to consumption.[2] The value chain includes several steps linking agriculture to the consumer including production, storage, distribution, processing, packaging, and sale.[2] Food value chains vary by commodity; for example, the critical issues for improving nutrition for a dairy value chain can be quite different than those influencing a vegetables value chain. This will be discussed further in the section below.

The food environment is the physical, economic, political, and sociocultural context in which consumers interact with the food system to obtain their food.[2] In essence, the food environment is the context in which a household or individual accesses their food. For the rural food system, the food environment might be limited to consumption from own, on-farm production and purchases from a near-by local market, whereas the modern system can include foods produced globally, with a reliance on formal markets and purchases from supermarkets. Figure 186-1 illustrates a conceptual framework for a food system.

There are numerous points in the food system where actions can either enhance or detract from the effects of policies and programs on dietary quality and nutrition. The starting point in understanding effects of food systems on diet and nutrition is the agricultural production side of the framework. Whether in the U.S. or globally, the agriculture sector is critical in providing access to both the quantity and quality of food needed for a healthful diet. Additionally, trade can be an important component of agriculture and the influence of trade on commodity availability varies tremendously across countries. In the U.S., for example, a large share of fruit is imported. For other countries, exports are a significant part of the overall economy and, thus, the revenues derived can be an important part of improving national level food security. The monies obtained from exports, however, are affected by global shocks. Liberia illustrates the impact of exports on the economy.[6] Positive economic growth was being achieved until 2016, when the country's main foreign exchange earning commodities, rubber and iron ore, were affected dramatically by the fall in world prices. This price shock reversed the country's economic growth leading to a fall in GDP from 8.7% to 0.7%.[6]

AGRICULTURE, DIET QUALITY, AND NUTRITION

Agriculture has a critical role to play in ensuring food security, diet quality, and improving nutritional status.

The framework in Fig. 186-1 provides a road map to "unpackage" the significance of individual steps in the pathway from agriculture, to diet, to nutrition. Historically, the primary goal of agriculture was to ensure adequate national food supplies. The advances in biotechnology in the late 1970s and beyond were focused on increasing worldwide food supplies, with an emphasis on grains—rice, maize, and wheat. An underlying assumption was that increases in commodities would increase overall caloric consumption which, in turn, would translate into improved diets. This was not entirely true.

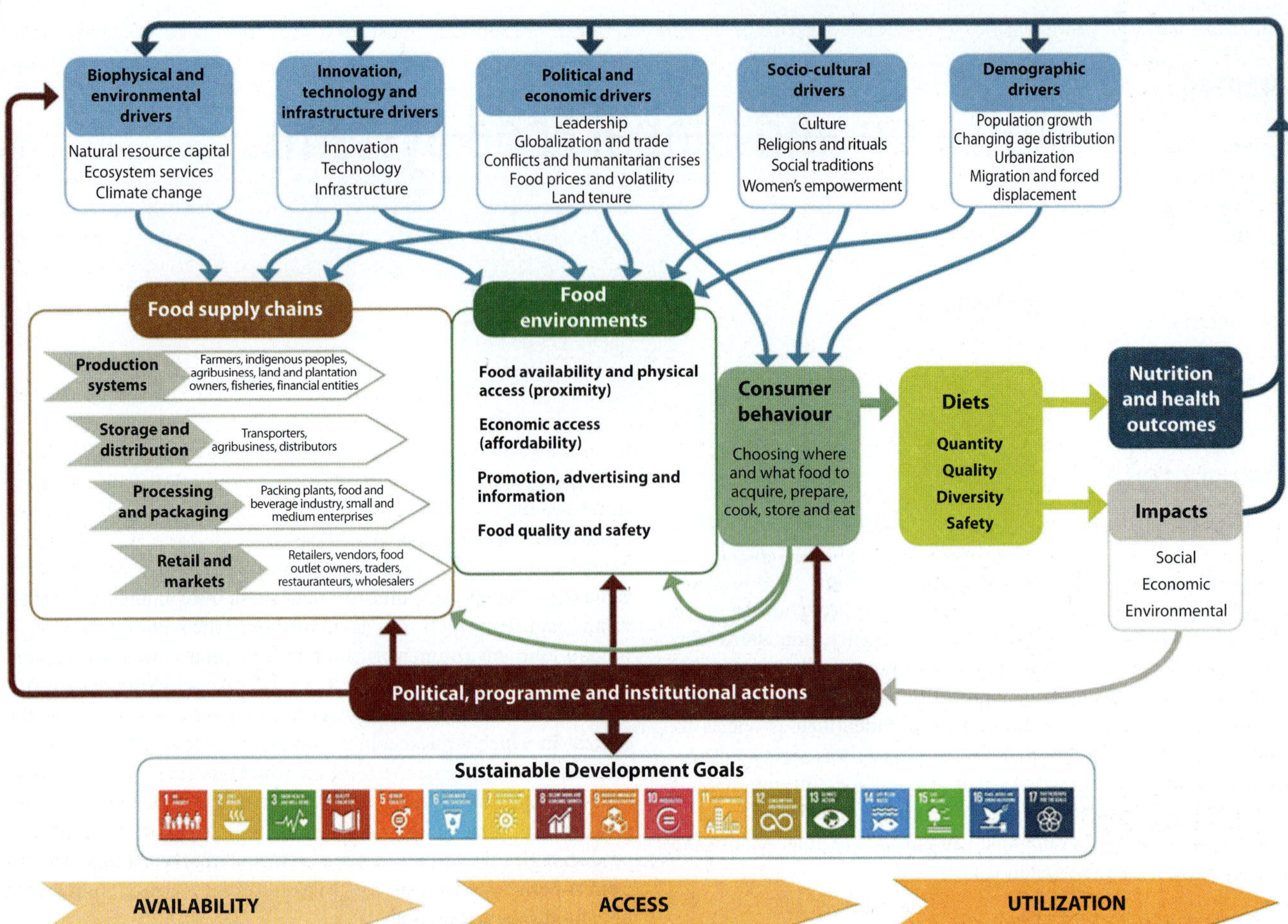

FIGURE 186-1. Food systems and their drivers influence our dietary choices and health outcomes. (*Source:* Reproduced with Permission from High Level Panel of Experts on Food Security and Nutrition (HLPE). HLPE Report #12: Nutrition and Food Systems. Rome: Committee on World Food Security, Food and Agriculture Organization of the United Nations. 2017. http://www.fao.org/3/a-i7846e.pdf.)

The Green Revolution, a term used to describe the advances associated with the use of improved technologies, resulted in increased food supplies globally, and on average, improvement in calories available.[7] Dramatic results were most apparent in Asia where investments in manmade irrigation contributed to the success of the improved technologies. The Green Revolution is not without controversy, including the emphasis placed on the quantity not the quality of food, and in some countries, also led to a depletion of natural resources.[7] As a result, the United Nations Decade of Action on Nutrition[1] is now stressing improvement in both quantity and the quality of food produced in a sustainable manner.[1]

Prior research on the links between agricultural production and diet quality and nutrition has shown only weak or nonsignificant results.[8] Some of this ambiguity was related to the assumptions underlying the concept of agriculture-nutrition linkages. The links between the agriculture sector, diet quality, and nutrition are more complex than originally conceptualized. Typically, policy officials in developing countries expect the beneficial effects of agriculture on nutrition to operate through three main pathways at the farm level: (1) increased crop/livestock production improves household diet quality by increasing own consumption of nutrient dense foods; (2) increased marketing of crops/livestock improves income which, in turn, improves diet quality; and (3) enhanced female-controlled income leads to greater expenditures on food and other health-promoting activities. The impacts on dietary quality and nutrition can vary depending on the agricultural pathway pursued.

In the U.S. and other developed countries, the link between agriculture and diet relates most often to ensuring the availability of food (geographic access) and proving access to food, which involves providing food to consumers at a reasonable price point.

PRODUCTION DIVERSITY AND DIET QUALITY

Is diet diversity good or bad? The answer to this question depends heavily on how diet diversity is defined. In developing countries, diet diversity is often considered a proxy measure for diet quality.[9] This is related to the fact that in low- and middle-income countries, an increase in the number of foods consumed is associated with better diet quality, including increases in the micronutrient content of the diet. Diet diversity is typically measured as either the number of unique foods consumed or the number of food groups eaten in a given period. The impacts of dietary diversity in U.S. and other developed countries are less straightforward. In one study, where diet diversity was defined as increases in fruit and vegetable consumption, individuals were less likely to be overweight or obese.[10] However, in this same study, diversity in consumption of snack foods, which were primarily high-energy density but low-nutrient content foods, increased the likelihood of being overweight or obese.[10]

The results on crop production diversity and dietary diversity are also mixed. A four-country study including Indonesia, Kenya, Ethiopia, and Malawi reported that production diversity at the farm level was associated with diet diversity in some, but not all, cases.[11] Another more recent study in Ethiopia posed the question, "What is the relative extent to which household dietary diversity is explained by production diversity?"[12] Maybe surprisingly, the relationship between total production diversity and diet diversity was small and nonsignificant.[12] In this same study, the production of specific food crops, not total production diversity, was associated with diet diversity. Specifically, households that produced pulses, eggs, fruits, and dairy were more likely to consume these products and thus, enhanced the nutrient density of the diet. This finding indicates that policies and programs that promote the cultivation of specific crops may be more effective in improving diet quality in low-income countries than simply an increase in overall agricultural production.

The effect of agricultural production strategies is modified by the degree of market integration. The case of dairy illustrates this phenomenon. Data from 93 woredas (villages) in Ethiopia reveal that cow ownership is strongly associated with an increased frequency of milk and dairy consumption among children; these effects, however, are two to three times higher in nonmarket villages.[13] These significant effects disappear in market villages, indicating that milk can now be sold, rather than simply consumed. In another study in rural Ethiopia, cow ownership had a large and positive effect on dairy consumption and linear growth of preschool-aged children.[14] Here again, however, in villages where there were large functioning markets, cow ownership had no impact on linear growth. Milk and dairy may be unique products since they are perishable and therefore must either be sold or consumed. If milk cannot be sold in the market, it will need to be consumed at the household level. Thus, the availability and structure of existing markets influences the household's decisions on whether to sell or consume a particular product. A study by Stifel and Minten in Ethiopia reinforces the larger literature; households in more remote areas in Ethiopia have significantly less agricultural production (likely due to less access to inputs) and market 50% less of their agricultural surplus.[15] The net effect is that more remote households in this East African setting are significantly more likely to be food insecure.

The implications of these findings are that understanding the impact of specific production strategies on diet has important implications for the policies and program implemented by governments to improve diet quality.

COMMERCIALIZATION OF AGRICULTURE

It is common for agricultural policy to encourage commercialization of agriculture with the dual goal of meeting the growing demand for national food supplies, in part spurred by urbanization, while also increasing household income and, in turn, improving household dietary quality.[16]

Households have to decide whether to consume their own farm production or market these commodities (cash crops). The effects of commercialization of agriculture on diet and nutrition, however, have been controversial. The early studies of cash cropping on diet and nutrition in Asia, Africa, and Latin America settings provided mixed results. A meta-analysis of a multicountry study in sub-Saharan Africa, Asia, and Latin America, however, found that household incomes, diet quality, and nutritional status of preschool-aged children were better, on average, than in noncash cropping households.[16] The major positive effects of cash cropping occurred because of increases in household income, which led to improvements in household food intake and food consumption by preschool children. The effect of cash cropping on preschool nutritional status, however, was more muted.

Data from Ethiopia found that agriculture income, as a proxy for agricultural commercialization (almost all cash income comes from crop and livestock sales), was significantly and positively associated with diet diversity.[12] This effect was independent of obvious confounders such as wealth and nonagricultural income. Households in the highest agricultural income quartile were 2.5 times more likely to have consumed vegetables, 2.1 times more likely to have consumed dairy, and 1.9 times more likely to have consumed oils and fats compared to those in the lowest quartile of income.[12] Cash cropping households, in general, have more diverse diets than subsistence farmers.[16] In addition, households with greater levels of commercialization that were headed by women had an even higher level of diet diversity; thus, there is a multiplicative effect of cash crop income and female-controlled income on diet quality.[12]

The decision for households either to sell or consume agricultural production must consider local context. In many countries rural, smallholder households are small, have limited access to markets, credit, and the inputs that are needed to effectively commercialize commodities. This finding transcends any particular regions or individual country.

GENDER, DIET QUALITY, AND NUTRITION

A large amount of literature documents that female-controlled income is related to better diet quality and improved child nutritional status when compared to male-controlled income.[17,18] Mental accounting, or the practice of treating different sources of income as not fully fungible, has emerged to explain this pattern.[19] Income and assets controlled by women tend to be used differently than male-controlled income. Women are the "gatekeepers" for home production activities—food, healthcare, and care of children. Research from Kenya and Malawi show that children from female-headed households, at lower levels of income, had higher energy intake and better nutritional status than children from male-headed households.[20] In addition, in Ethiopia, research indicates that female asset ownership was associated with a significantly higher probability of consumption of roots, vegetables, oils/fats, sugar/honey, and meat.[12] In addition, at a national level in Ethiopia, female-controlled income was also associated with greater household diet diversity. Finally, above and beyond female-controlled income, evidence documents that women's involvement in decision-making is positively and significantly related to better-quality household diets.[12]

The positive effects of women-controlled income are not limited to sub-Saharan African countries but have also been observed in Asia and Latin America.[18]

FOOD VALUE CHAINS FOR IMPROVED DIET AND NUTRITION

There are a number of ways the food supply chain can be enhanced to increase the positive effects on diet and nutrition. At the production end, strategies to reduce contamination with aflatoxin, promote use of extension services, and use of improved seed varieties are just some of the examples for maximizing nutrition entering the supply chain.[2] Similarly, at the consumer side, incorporating nutrition communications at the point of consumer purchases, targeting vulnerable groups through specific programs such as school feeding, and improving the variety of low cost, nutritious foods at point of purchase are just a few examples.[2] What is clear is that there are potentialities at each link in the supply chain to improve the impact on nutrition. The range of options for maximizing nutrition entering the food chain must be context specific. For example, the use of biofortification—enhancing the nutrient content of a food by incorporating naturally occurring traits—has demonstrated significant effects on intake of beta-carotene in households.[21] Biofortification would likely be less beneficial in a modern food system that has a wide variety of foods, including fortified products that address the nutrient needs of consumers, readily available. Similarly, the degree of contamination and spoilage of crops differs in rural versus modern food systems and therefore the types of investment in minimizing food losses will vary. Data from the Food and Agriculture Organization (FAO) indicate that about one-third of world food supplies are lost through waste in developed countries; this mainly occurs immediately postharvest through improper storage and handling.[22,23] In developed countries, the major portion of food waste occurs after purchase through spoilage and waste.[22,23]

FOOD ENVIRONMENTS, DIET, AND NUTRITION

The food environment is where production and consumption decisions interact to reach the consumer. A key issue is availability of a variety of nutrient-dense foods. Nutrient density is typically measured by computing the ratio of nutrients to calories consumed; a nutrient-dense food has a lot of nutrients for the number of calories consumed. Fruits, vegetables, and whole grains are nutrient dense. A nutrient-poor food has few nutrients per the number of calories consumed and these foods tend to be more expensive.[24]

There is concern that the proliferation of food deserts and food swamps, particularly in urban areas, compromise the ability of households to purchase a healthful diet. Food deserts are areas where proximity to outlets that provide a variety of healthy foods is limited. Food swamps are localities where there is an abundance of retail facilities selling foods of minimal nutritional value. Both food deserts and food swamps challenge the ability of households to acquire a healthy diet.

A number of cities in the U.S. have implemented policies to increase the availability of healthier foods. For example, in New York City, vendor licenses were given to Green Carts that sell fresh fruits and vegetables, at a reasonable cost, in low-income neighborhoods.[25] Evaluation results indicate that this approach is reaching at-risk areas and having some positive impact on increasing fruit and vegetable consumption.

Access to nutritious foods entails physical proximity as well as economic access—affordability. Policies that increase the incomes of vulnerable households increase access to healthy foods. Programs such as the U.S. Supplemental Nutrition Assistance Program (SNAP) provide increased purchasing power for food. Studies have documented that SNAP households purchase more nutritious foods when compared to eligible, nonparticipating households,[26] and further research corroborates the findings that the increased purchasing power provided by SNAP benefits results in improved diet quality.[27] In addition, a program to increase fruit and vegetable purchases by SNAP households provides added value of so-called "Green Stamps," and evaluation data indicate that this program has resulted in increased purchases of fruits and vegetables.[28]

Another example of success in improving diet quality is the Special Supplemental Nutrition Program for Women, Infants, and Children (WIC) program in the U.S. National evaluation results indicate that participation in WIC by preschool-aged children increased the consumption of calcium, vitamins A and C, and iron when compared to nonparticipating children.[29]

Several factors need to be considered in optimizing changes in a food system for improving diet quality and nutrition. First, the points of interventions to improve diet and nutrition vary by type of food system. Second, actions that target availability, affordability, marketing, and food safety also vary by food system. Therefore, the points for policy interventions need to be modified to address the context of the dominant food system. In addition, it is likely that there is no "silver bullet"—that is, it is unlikely that any single approach, by itself, will be sufficient to significantly improve the food environment.

CONSUMER BEHAVIOR AND FOOD SYSTEMS

Figure 186-1 highlights the critical role of consumer food choice behaviors in determining the ultimate effect on dietary choices and quality. Enhancing consumers' information and knowledge about healthy eating is one strategy to positively affect consumer behavior. Indeed, a number of approaches have been used to influence consumer demand for healthier food choices. These include nutrition education, mass media campaigns, and social/behavior change interventions. There are some elements across each of these strategies that are effective[30] including focus on a specific behavior, understanding the dose of exposure necessary for the desired change, and the ability to respond to the information provided. Food labeling and marketing can also affect a person's food choices. The role of food advertising has been controversial. If advertising influences a person to buy less nutritious foods, there will be a net, negative nutrition effect. Food advertising to children is particularly problematic and has led many countries to implement mandatory or voluntary guidelines to limit advertising to children. Policies to strengthen regulations for advertising and marketing can be a powerful tool to increase the positive nutrition impacts of food systems.

FOOD SYSTEMS AND SUSTAINABLE DIETS

The United Nations sustainable development goals[31] emphasize that a healthy diet is a sustainable diet. As defined by the FAO,

> Sustainable diets are those with low-environmental impacts which contribute to food and nutrition security, and to healthy life for present and future generations. Sustainable diets are protective and respectful of biodiversity and ecosystems, culturally acceptable, accessible, economically fair and affordable, nutritionally adequate, safe and healthy, while optimizing natural and human resources.[32]

Diets need to be environmentally as well as nutritionally sustainable. This has implications for appropriateness of food systems. Sustainable diets have a low-carbon footprint and, as such, put pressure to reduce the consumption of animal sourced foods in developed countries. A report on sustainable agriculture and the level of livestock production needed to meet an increasing demand for animal-sourced foods (ASF) highlighted the significant impacts on the environment—both positive and negative—of livestock production.[33] On the one hand, ASF have a significant positive effect on reducing stunting in preschool aged children and improving micronutrient intakes.[33] ASFs, however, have an enormous carbon footprint, which left unchecked, can lead to negative effects on the environment. This example illustrates that there can be trade-offs between environmental and nutritional goals which can complicate the policy making process.

The agriculture production practices of food systems put enormous pressure on natural resources. Evolving food systems are required to address the underlying drivers of food systems (Fig. 186-1) to contribute more effectively to sustainable diets.

POLICIES FOR EVOLVING FOOD SYSTEMS

Agricultural sector initiatives offer enormous potential for improving diet quality and household-level food security. The research summarized in this chapter highlights the nuances involved in analyzing agriculture-diet diversity linkages. The apparent modest or weak evidence from many prior studies linking agriculture to diet quality may be related, in part, to the tendency to treat agricultural production strategies as entailing homogeneous approaches. Information presented in this chapter disaggregated agriculture and examined production diversity, individual food group production, commercialization, and gender-controlled income as separate entities that may, independently, influence diet quality.

Some policy and programmatic recommendations emerged from the evidence in this chapter that suggest possible interventions to enhance the impacts on diet quality. Policies to increase the commercialization of agriculture can have powerful effect on increasing diet diversity globally. In order to expand the opportunities for smallholder farmers to participate in cash cropping, governments should invest in infrastructure to provide better linkages to the market economy.

Many of the poorest agricultural households worldwide have limited access to inputs into commercial agriculture including into the adoption of improved seed varieties. The provision of inputs and/or credit can increase the access to important inputs.

Data in this chapter suggest that on-farm production of specific, nutrient-dense crops have more of an effect on improving diet quality than simply emphasizing overall increased production. Agricultural strategies should focus on cultivation of individual crops as one strategy for enhancing diet quality.

Women and men's incomes are often used differently, suggesting that examining the effects of total household income on diet and nutrition may miss important household dynamics. An assessment of different sources of gender specific control of income may more effectively identify points of entry for improvement of diet diversity. Agricultural programs that educate and empower women to have greater control over assets and other decision-making will likely see improved dietary diversity independent of commercialization efforts.

Agricultural programs are typically targeted at the level of the agro-ecosystem, not the individual or household. The most vulnerable households may not be reached through geographical targeting. Given this, additional strategies for generating program demand such as outreach around farmer demonstrations and extension activities should be employed to expand the participant base of nutrition sensitive approaches.

Interventions should facilitate increased access to a healthier food environment, by considering how to improve market access, decrease the real cost of, and increase the convenience of healthy, nutritious food. Nutrition education must focus on informing healthy food purchasing decisions.

This chapter highlights the fact that linkages between agriculture and nutrition are more complex than originally conceptualized in the 1970s and 1980s. Governments and donors should use this newer information to maximize the effects on policies and programs on diet quality and nutrition.

References

1. United Nations. Decade of action on nutrition. 2016. https://www.un.org/nutrition.
2. High Level Panel of Experts on Food Security and Nutrition (HLPE). *HLPE Report #12: Nutrition and Food Systems*. Rome: Committee on World Food Security, Food and Agriculture Organization of the United Nations; 2017. http://www.fao.org/3/a-i7846e.pdf.
3. International Food Policy Research Institute. *Global Nutrition Report 2015: Actions and Accountability to Advance Nutrition and Sustainable Development*. Washington, DC: IFPRI; 2015. https://www.ifpri.org/publication/global-nutrition-report-2015.
4. Global Panel on Agriculture and Food Systems on Nutrition. *Foresight Report on Foods Systems and Diets*. London: Foresight; 2016.
5. Popkin B, Corvalan C, Grummer-Strawn L. Dynamics of the double burden of malnutrition and the changing nutrition reality. *Lancet*. 2020;395(10217);65–74.
6. World Food Programme. Zero hunger strategic review: Republic of Liberia. 2017. https://docs.wfp.org/api/documents/WFP-0000040056/download.
7. Pingali P. Green revolution: Impacts, limits, and the path ahead. *Proc Natl Acad Sci U S A*. 2012;109(31):12302–8.
8. Webb P, Kennedy E. Impacts of agriculture on nutrition: Nature of the evidence and research gaps. *Food Nutr Bull*. 2014;35(1):126–32.
9. Arimond M, Ruel MT. Diet diversity is associated with child nutritional status: Evidence form 11 demographic and health surveys. *J Nutr*. 2004;134(10):2579–85.
10. Kennedy E. Dietary diversity, diet quality, and body weight regulation. *Nutr Rev*. 2004;62(2):S78–81.
11. Carletto G, Ruel MT, Winters P, Zezza A. Farm-level pathways to improved nutritional status: Introduction to the special issue. *J Dev Stud*. 2015;51(8):945–57.
12. Kennedy E, Kershaw M, Coates J. Food systems: Pathways for improved diets and nutrition. *Curr Dev Nutr*. 2018;2(9):nzy027.
13. Sibhatu KT, Krishna VV, Qaim M. Production diversity and dietary diversity in smallholder farm households. *Proc Natl Acad Sci U S A*. 2015;112(34): 10657–62.
14. Hoddinott J, Headey D, Dereje M. Cows, missing milk markets, and nutrition in rural Ethiopia. *J Dev Stud*. 2015;51(8):958–75.
15. Stifel D, Minten B. *Market Access, Welfare, and Nutrition: Evidence from Ethiopia*. Washington, DC: International Food Policy Research Institute; 2016. https://www.ifpri.org/publication/synopsis-market-access-welfare-and-nutrition-evidence-ethiopia.
16. Von Braun J, Kennedy E. *Agricultural Commercialization, Economic Development and Nutrition*. Baltimore: Johns Hopkins University Press; 1986.
17. Engle P. Influences of mothers' and fathers' income on children's nutritional status in Guatemala. *Soc Sci Med*. 1993;37(11):1303–12.
18. Food and Agriculture Organization of the United Nations. Strengthening sector policies for better food security and nutrition results, Report #6: Gender Equality. 2017. http://www.fao.org/3/i7218en/I7218EN.pdf.
19. Villa KM, Barrett CB, Just DR. Whose fast and whose feast? Intrahousehold asymmetries in dietary diversity response among East African pastoralists. *Am J Agr Econ*. 2011;93(4):1062–81.
20. Kennedy E, Peters P. Household food security and child nutrition: The interaction of income and gender of household head. *World Dev*. 1992;20(8): 1077–85.
21. Bouis HE, Saltzman A. Improving nutrition through biofortificaiton: A review of evidence from Harvest Plus, 2003 through 2016. *Glob Food Sec*. 2017;12:49–58.
22. Willett W, Rockström J, Loken B, et al. Food in the Anthropocene: The EAT–Lancet Commission on healthy diets from sustainable food systems. *Lancet*. 2019;393(10170):447–92.
23. Gustavsson J, Cederberg C, Sonesson U, van Otterdijk R, Meybeck A. *Global Food Losses and Food Waste*. Rome: Food and Agriculture Organization of the United Nations; 2011. http://www.fao.org/3/a-i2697e.pdf.
24. Drewnowski A, Fulgoni V. Nutrient profiling of foods: Creating a nutrient-rich food index. *Nutr Rev*. 2008;66(1):23–39.
25. Down S, Fanzo J. Managing value chains for improved nutrition. In: Eggersdorfer M, et al., eds. *Good Nutrition: Perspectives for the 21st Century*. Basel: Kraeger Publications; 2016, pp. 45–59.
26. Nguyen BT, Shuval K, Bertmann F, Yaroch AL. The Supplemental Nutrition Assistance Program, food insecurity, dietary quality, and obesity among U.S. adults. *Am J Public Health*. 2015;105(7):1453–9.
27. Kennedy E, Guthrie JF. Nutrition assistance programs: Cause or solution to obesity. *Curr Obes Rep*. 2016;5(2):176–83.
28. Olsho LE, Klerman JA, Wilde PE, Bartlett S. Financial incentives increase fruit and vegetable intake among Supplemental Nutrition Assistance Program participants: A randomized controlled trial of the USDA Healthy Incentives Pilot. *Am J Clin Nutr*. 2016;104(2):423–35.
29. Rush D, Leighton J, Sloan NL, et al. The National WIC evaluation: Evaluation of the Special Supplemental Food Program for women, infants and children. VI. Study of infants and children. *Am J Clin Nutr*. 1988;48(2 Suppl):484–511.
30. Contento IR. Nutrition education: Linking research, theory, and practice. *Asia Pac J Clin Nutr*. 2008;17(Suppl 1):176–9.
31. United Nations. *The Sustainable Development Goals Report*. New York: United Nations Publications; 2016. https://www.unodc.org/documents/commissions/CND_CCPCJ_joint/2030Agenda/The_Sustainable_Development_Goals_Report_2016.pdf.
32. Burlingame B. Sustainable diets: Nutrition's role in the sustainability negotiations. 2016. http://www.unscn.org/files/Annual_Sessions/UNSCN_Meetings_2013/burlingame_scn_sustainable_diets_MoM.pdf.
33. High Level Panel of Experts on Food Security and Nutrition (HLPE). *HLPE Report #10: Sustainable Agricultural Development for Food Security and Nutrition: What Roles for Livestock?* Rome: Committee on World Food Security, Food and Agriculture Organization of the United Nations; 2016. http://www.fao.org/3/a-i5795e.pdf.

Index

F

G

I

O

P

S

V

X

Y